Principles and Practice
of
Medical Intensive Care

PRINCIPLES & PRACTICE OF
MEDICAL INTENSIVE CARE

Richard W. Carlson, M.D., Ph.D.
Professor and Chairman
Department of Medicine
University of Illinois College of Medicine—Peoria
Peoria, Illinois

formerly

Professor and Division Chief
Pulmonary (1983–1990) and
Critical Care Medicine (1983–1992)
Wayne State University
School of Medicine/Detroit Medical Center
Chief of Medicine
Detroit Receiving Hospital
Detroit, Michigan

Michael A. Geheb, M.D.
Professor of Medicine
Associate Dean for Clinical Affairs
School of Medicine
State University of New York at Stony Brook
Attending Physician, University Hospital
Stony Brook, New York

formerly

Associate Professor of Medicine
Vice-Chairman, Department of Internal Medicine
Wayne State University
School of Medicine/Detroit Medical Center
Attending Physician, Harper Hospital
Detroit Receiving Hospital
Detroit, Michigan

W.B. SAUNDERS COMPANY
Harcourt Brace Jovanovich, Inc.
Philadelphia   London   Toronto   Montreal   Sydney   Tokyo

W.B. SAUNDERS COMPANY
Harcourt Brace Jovanovich, Inc.

The Curtis Center
Independence Square West
Philadelphia, Pennsylvania 19106

Library of Congress Cataloging-in-Publication Data

Principles and practice of medical intensive care / [edited by]
Richard W. Carlson, Michael A. Geheb.

    p.   cm.

ISBN 0–7216–3396–X

1. Critical care medicine.   I. Carlson, Richard W.
    II. Geheb, Michael A.

[DNLM: 1. Critical Care.   2. Emergencies.   WB 105 P9575]

RC86.7.P743   1993

616′.028—dc20

DNLM/DLC   91–45005

PRINCIPLES AND PRACTICE OF MEDICAL INTENSIVE CARE   ISBN 0–7216–3396–X

Last digit is the print number: 9   8   7   6   5   4   3   2   1

CONTRIBUTORS

Steven M. Albelda, M.D.

Assistant Professor of Medicine, University of Pennsylvania School of Medicine; Faculty, Medical Staff, Hospital of the University of Pennsylvania, Philadelphia, Pennsylvania
Life-Threatening Pulmonary Hemorrhage

David W. Allen, M.D.

Chief Medical Resident, The Johns Hopkins University School of Medicine, Baltimore, Maryland
Pneumonia

Judith C. Andersen, M.D.

Associate Professor of Internal Medicine, Wayne State University School of Medicine; Medical Director, Apheresis Unit, Harper Hospital, and Staff Physician, Harper Hospital, Detroit Receiving Hospital, and Hutzel Hospital–Detroit Medical Center, Detroit, Michigan
Hematology/Oncology: Introduction; Clinical Apheresis

Derek C. Angus, M.B., Ch.B., M.R.C.P.(U.K.)

Investigator, International Resuscitation Research Center, University of Pittsburgh Medical Center, Pittsburgh, Pennsylvania
Modern Medical Response to Disasters

Eugenio Armendariz, M.D.

Assistant Professor of Medicine, Wayne State University School of Medicine; Assistant Director, Intensive Care Unit, Hutzel Hospital, Detroit, Michigan
Hemodynamic Monitoring

Mark E. Astiz, M.D.

Associate Professor of Medicine, New York Medical College; Associate Chairman, Department of Medicine, and Program Director, Critical Care Medicine, St. Vincent's Hospital and Medical Center, New York, New York
Circulatory Shock

Frank A. Baciewicz, Jr., M.D.

Associate Professor of Surgery, Division of Cardiothoracic Surgery, Wayne State University School of Medicine; Chief, Thoracic Surgery, Grace Hospital, Director, Cardiopulmonary Transplantation, and Cardiothoracic Surgeon, Harper Hospital, Detroit, Michigan
Cardiac Assist Devices and Transplantation

Ann Sullivan Baker, M.D.

Associate Professor of Medicine, Harvard Medical School; Director, Infectious Diseases, Massachusetts Eye and Ear Infirmary, and Physician, Infectious Disease Unit, Massachusetts General Hospital, Boston, Massachusetts
Upper Respiratory Tract Infections

Robert A. Balk, M.D.

Associate Professor of Medicine, Rush Medical College; Director, Medical Intensive Care Unit, and Medical Director, Respiratory Therapy, Rush–Presbyterian–St. Luke's Medical Center, Chicago, Illinois
The Septic Syndrome and Septic Shock; Pathophysiology of Sepsis

Jeffrey D. Band, M.D.

Associate Clinical Professor of Medicine, Wayne State University School of Medicine, Detroit; Corporate Epidemiologist and Director, Division of Infectious Diseases and International Medicine, William Beaumont Hospital, Royal Oak, Michigan
Control and Prevention of Infection

Joseph Bander, M.D., F.C.C.M.

Associate Professor of Medicine, Wayne State University School of Medicine; Director, Medical Intensive Care Unit, and Chief, Section of Critical Care Medicine, Harper Hospital, Detroit, Michigan
Long-Term Airway Management

Joseph A. Barbera, M.D.

Assistant Professor of Medicine, Albert Einstein College of Medicine; Bronx Municipal Hospital Center, Bronx, New York
Modern Medical Response to Disasters

Jamie S. Barkin, M.D.

Professor of Medicine, University of Miami School of Medicine, Miami; Chief, Division of Gastroenterology, Mt. Sinai Medical Center, Miami Beach, Florida
Pancreatitis

Steven L. Beck, M.D.

Professor and Chairman, Department of Medicine, East Tennessee State University, James H. Quillen College of Medicine, Johnson City, Tennessee
Pneumonia

Michael F. Beers, M.D.

Research Associate, Institute for Environmental Medicine, University of Pennsylvania School of Medicine; Attending Physician, Medical Intensive Care Unit, Hospital of the University of Pennsylvania, Philadelphia, Pennsylvania
Oxygen Toxicity

Carolyn Bekes, M.D., F.A.C.P., F.C.C.M.

Associate Professor of Clinical Medicine and Anesthesia, University of Medicine and Dentistry of New Jersey, Robert Wood Johnson Medical School at Camden; Director, Intensive Care Unit, Chief, Section of Critical Care Medicine, and Director of Clinical Outcomes, Cooper Hospital/University Medical Center, Camden, New Jersey
Standards

**Michael A. Belfort, M.D., M.B., B.Ch., D.A.(S.A.),
D.Mid.C.O.G.(S.A.), M.R.C.O.G., F.R.C.S.(C.)**

Clinical Instructor, Division of Maternal Fetal Medicine, Department of Obstetrics and Gynecology, Baylor College of Medicine; Clinical Instructor, Ben Taub Hospital and St. Luke's Episcopal Hospital, Houston, Texas
Obstetrics and Gynecology in the Intensive Care Unit

Richard C. Berchou, M.D.

Assistant Professor of Medicine and of Pharmacy, Wayne State University School of Medicine; Staff, Sinai Hospital, Lafayette Clinic, and Detroit Psychiatric Institute, Detroit, Michigan
Hyperpyretic-Rigidity Syndrome (Neuroleptic Malignant Syndrome)

Henry J. Binder, M.D.

Professor of Medicine, Yale University School of Medicine; Director, General Clinical Research Center, Yale—New Haven Medical Center, New Haven, Connecticut
Pathophysiology of Acute Diarrhea in the Intensive Care Unit

Andres T. Blei, M.D.

Associate Professor of Medicine, Northwestern University School of Medicine; Attending Physician, Northwestern Memorial Hospital, and Staff Physician, Lakeside Veterans Administration Medical Center, Chicago, Illinois
Pathophysiology and Therapy of Hepatic Encephalopathy

Roger C. Bone, M.D.

Dean, Rush Medical College, Vice President, Medical Affairs, The Ralph C. Brown, M.D., Professor of Medicine; Chief, Section of Pulmonary Medicine, Rush–Presbyterian–St. Luke's Medical Center, Chicago, Illinois
The Septic Syndrome and Septic Shock

Frank V. M. Booth, B.M., B.Ch., M.A., M.Sc.

Associate Professor of Surgery and Anesthesia, School of Medicine and BioMedical Sciences, State University of New York at Buffalo; Chief, Division of Surgical Critical Care, Director, Surgical Intensive Care Units, and Director, Nutrition Support Service, Buffalo General Hospital, Buffalo, New York
Computers in Critical Care Units

Michael J. Borucki, M.D.

Assistant Professor of Medicine, University of Texas Medical Branch, Galveston, Texas
Fulminant Viral Infections

Roderick J. Boyes, M.D., F.R.C.P.(C.), F.A.C.E.P.

Assistant Professor of Medicine, Wayne State University School of Medicine; Associate Director, Medical Intensive Care Unit, Harper Hospital, Detroit, Michigan
Selected Nonvascular Procedures

Eugene M. Bozynski, M.D.

Professor of Medicine, University of North Carolina at Chapel Hill School of Medicine; Attending Physician, University of North Carolina Hospital, Chapel Hill, North Carolina
Lower Gastrointestinal Tract Hemorrhage

Robert W. Bradsher, M.D.

Professor of Medicine, and Director, Division of Infectious Diseases, University of Arkansas for Medical Sciences; Attending Physician, University Hospital of Arkansas and John L. McClellan Veterans Administration Hospital, Little Rock, Arkansas
Fungal Infections

Sidney S. Braman, M.D.

Professor of Medicine, Brown University School of Medicine; Director, Division of Pulmonary and Critical Care Medicine, Rhode Island Hospital, Providence, Rhode Island
Transporting Critically Ill Patients

Lawrence J. Brandt, M.D.

Professor of Medicine, Albert Einstein College of Medicine; Director, Division of Gastroenterology at the Moses Division of Montefiore Medical Center and North Central Bronx Hospital, Bronx, New York
Acute Mesenteric Ischemia

John C. M. Brust, M.D.

Professor of Clinical Neurology, Columbia University College of Physicians and Surgeons; Director, Department of Neurology, Harlem Hospital Center, New York, New York
Alcoholism

Phillip J. Burke, M.D.

Professor of Oncology and Medicine, The Johns Hopkins University School of Medicine; Director, Adult Leukemia Program, and Director, Clinical Laboratories, The Johns Hopkins Hospital, Baltimore, Maryland
Bone Marrow Disorders Associated with Excessive Production

Alfred E. Buxton, M.D.

Associate Professor of Medicine, University of Pennsylvania School of Medicine; Director, Clinical Electrophysiology Laboratory, Hospital of the University of Pennsylvania, Philadelphia, Pennsylvania
Disorders of Cardiac Rhythm and Conduction in the Medical Intensive Care Unit

Mark A. Camp, B.S., M.D.

Instructor of Medicine, University of Oklahoma Health Sciences Center; Staff Physician, University of Oklahoma Teaching Hospitals, Oklahoma City, Oklahoma
Pulmonary Edema: Lung Water Balance in Relation to Physiologic Monitoring and Clinical Outcome in the Critically Ill

Ellis S. Caplan, M.D.

Associate Professor of Medicine, University of Maryland School of Medicine; Chief, Infectious Diseases, Maryland Institute for Emergency Medical Services Systems, University of Maryland, Baltimore, Maryland
Infections in the Multitrauma Patient

Richard W. Carlson, M.D., Ph.D.

Professor and Chairman, Department of Medicine, University of Illinois College of Medicine; Academic Chairman, St. Francis Medical Center and Methodist Medical Center of Illinois, Peoria, Illinois
Artificial Intelligence and Expert Systems in Critical Care Medicine; Cold Exposure Injuries; Electrical and Lightning Injuries; Anaphylaxis; Injuries by Venomous and Poisonous Animals

Donald B. Chalfin, M.D., M.S.

Assistant Professor of Medicine, State University of New York Health Sciences Center at Stony Brook, Stony Brook; Director, Surgical Intensive Care Unit, Winthrop-University Hospital, Mineola, New York
Severity Scoring in Intensive Care Units

Pranatharthi Chandrasekar

Associate Professor of Medicine, Division of Infectious Diseases, Wayne State University School of Medicine; Staff Physician, Division of Infectious Diseases, Department of Internal Medicine, Harper Hospital, Detroit, Michigan
Infections in Cancer Patients

Vivian L. Clark, M.D.

Clinical Instructor, University of Michigan School of Medicine, Ann Arbor; Senior Staff Physician, Henry Ford Hospital, Detroit; Consulting Staff, St. Mary Hospital, Livonia, Michigan
Vascular Procedures

Steven E. Come, M.D.

Associate Professor of Medicine, Harvard Medical School; Director, Hematology-Oncology Units, Beth Israel Hospital, and Assistant Physician, Dana–Farber Cancer Institute, Boston, Massachusetts
Complications of Therapy of Neoplastic Disease: An Overview

David B. Cotton, M.D., F.A.C.O.G.

Professor, Chairman, and Chief, Department of Obstetrics and Gynecology, Wayne State University School of Medicine; Chief, Obstetrics and Gynecology, Detroit Medical Center Affiliated Hospitals, Detroit, Michigan
Obstetrics and Gynecology in the Intensive Care Unit

Lawrence R. Crane, M.D.

Associate Professor of Medicine, Division of Infectious Diseases, Wayne State University School of Medicine; Staff Physician, Harper Hospital, Detroit, Michigan
Human Immunodeficiency Virus Infection and the Acquired Immunodeficiency Syndrome

Simon Cronin, Pharm.D.

Associate Professor, Department of Pharmacy Practice, College of Pharmacy, Southeastern University of the Health Sciences, North Miami Beach, Florida
Pharmacologic Agents and Poisoning: Pharmacokinetics in Critically Ill Patients

J. Randall Curtis, M.D.

Clinical Scholar, Robert Wood Johnson Clinical Scholars Program, and Acting Instructor of Medicine, University of Washington, Seattle, Washington
Acute Respiratory Failure in Chronic Obstructive Pulmonary Disease

William C. Darrah, M.B., B.Ch., M.R.C.P., F.F.A.R.C.S.

Senior Resident, Critical Care and Trauma Center, Victoria Hospital, London, Ontario, Canada
Multiple Organ System Failure in Sepsis

F. D. Daschner, M.D.

Professor and Chief, Department of Hospital Epidemiology, University Hospital Freiburg, Freiburg, Germany
Infections Associated with Intravascular Devices

Tusar K. Desai

Assistant Professor of Medicine, Division of Gastroenterology, Wayne State University School of Medicine; Staff Physician, Harper Hospital, Detroit, Michigan
Clinical Disorders of Calcium and Magnesium Metabolism in Critically Ill Patients

Fernando G. Diaz, M.D., Ph.D.

Professor and Chairman, Department of Neurosurgery Wayne State University School of Medicine; Neurosurgeon in Chief, Detroit Medical Center, Detroit, Michigan
Critical Care Management of Traumatic Brain Injury and Spinal Cord Injury

Lawrence M. Diebel, M.D.

Assistant Professor, Wayne State University School of Medicine, Detroit, Michigan
Emergency Vascular Surgery in Patients in the Intensive Care Unit

Gary A. Dildy, M.D.

Assistant Professor of Obstetrics/Gynecology, University of Utah School of Medicine, Salt Lake City; Director of the Perinatal Center, Utah Valley Regional Medical Center, Provo, Utah
Obstetrics and Gynecology in the Intensive Care Unit

Andrew C. Dixon, M.D.

Fellow, Sections of Pulmonary and Critical Care Medicine, Rush–Presbyterian–St. Luke's Medical Center, Chicago, Illinois
Cardiovascular Dysfunction in Septic Shock

Scott Dulchavsky, M.D.

Assistant Professor of Surgery, Wayne State University School of Medicine; Director, Surgical Intensive Care Units, Harper Hospital, Staff Physician, Trauma Team, Detroit Receiving Hospital, Attending Staff, Detroit Receiving, Harper, Hutzel, and Grace Hospitals, and Consulting Staff, Rehabilitation Institute of Michigan, Detroit, Michigan
The Acute Abdomen

Michael P. Earnest, M.D.

Professor of Neurology and Preventive Medicine, University of Colorado School of Medicine; Director of Neurology, Denver General Hospital, Denver, Colorado
Brain Damage from Cardiac Arrest: Pathophysiology, Intensive Care Unit Management, and Outcome, Including Brain Death

H. Tristram Engelhardt, Jr., Ph.D., M.D.

Professor of Medicine, Baylor College of Medicine, Professor of Philosophy, Rice University, and Adjunct Research Fellow, The Institute of Religion; Member of the Center for Ethics, Medicine, and Public Issues, Houston, Texas
Ethical Decision Making in Critical Care

Gordon A. Ewy, M.D.

Director, University Heart Center, Professor and Chief, Section of Cardiology, University of Arizona College of Medicine; Director of Diagnostic Cardiology, University Medical Center, Tucson, Arizona
Cardiopulmonary Resuscitation: Current Status and New Horizons

Thomas J. Fahey III, M.D.

Administrative Chief Resident, Department of Surgery, The New York Hospital–Cornell Medical Center, New York, New York
Cytokines, Tumor Necrosis Factor, and Other Mediators of Sepsis

Stephen L. Farrow, M.D.

Assistant Professor, Endocrinology Division, Wayne State University School of Medicine, Detroit; Staff Physician, Harper and Detroit Receiving Hospitals, and Veterans Administration Medical Center, Allen Park, Michigan
Catecholamines and Pressor Agents

I. Alan Fein, M.D.

Chief, Division of Surgical Critical Care, Associate Professor of Surgery, and Assistant Professor of Medicine, Albany Medical College of Union University; Director, Surgical Intensive Care Unit, and Attending Physician, Albany Medical Center Hospital, Albany, New York
Organization of Critical Care Units

Sandra L. Fein, R.N., M.A.

Consulting Community Psychologist, Albany, New York
Organization of Critical Care Units

Robert Fekety, M.D., F.A.C.P.

Professor of Internal Medicine and Chief, Division of Infectious Diseases, Department of Internal Medicine, University of Michigan, School of Medicine; Chief, Adult Infectious Diseases Service, University of Michigan Hospitals, Ann Arbor, Michigan
Gastroenteric Infections

George M. Feldman, M.D.

Associate Professor of Medicine and of Physiology, Medical College of Virginia; Chief, Renal Section, McGuire Veterans Affairs Medical Center, Richmond, Virginia
Acid-Base Homeostasis

Pedro C. Fernandez, M.D.

Professor of Medicine, The Medical College of Pennsylvania, and Adjunct Associate Professor of Medicine, University of Pennsylvania School of Medicine; Director, Dialysis Unit, Veterans Affairs Medical Center, Philadelphia, Pennsylvania
Dialysis and Hemoperfusion: Principles of Dialysis Therapy

Victor A. Ferrari, M.D.

Instructor in Medicine, University of Pennsylvania School of Medicine; Staff Echocardiographer, Cardiovascular Division, Hospital of the University of Pennsylvania, Philadelphia, Pennsylvania
Mechnical Respiratory Failure

James E. Fish, M.D.

Professor of Medicine, Jefferson Medical College, Thomas Jefferson University; Director Pulmonary Medicine and Critical Care, Thomas Jefferson University Hospital, Philadelphia, Pennsylvania
Acute Severe Asthma

Aron B. Fisher, M.D.

Professor of Physiology and of Environmental Medicine, and Director, Institute for Environmental Medicine, Hospital of the University of Pennsylvania, Philadelphia, Pennsylvania
Oxygen Toxicity

Rosemarie L. Fisher, M.D.

Professor of Medicine, Yale University School of Medicine; Director, Residency Training Programs, Internal Medicine and Attending Physician, Yale–New Haven Hospital, and Consultant, West Haven Veterans Administration Medical Center, New Haven, Connecticut
Upper Gastrointestinal Tract Hemorrhage

U. Frank, M.D.

Fellow, Division of Infectious Diseases, San Francisco General Hospital, San Francisco, California
Infections Associated with Intravascular Devices

Bruce Friedman, M.D., F.C.C.P.

Assistant Professor of Medicine and Anesthesia and Co-Director, Critical Care Fellowship Program, University of Medicine and Dentistry of New Jersey, Robert Wood Johnson Medical School at Camden; Administrative Director, Nutrition Support Services, and Attending Physician, Intensive Care Unit, Cooper Hospital/University Medical Center, Camden, New Jersey
Standards

William J. Fulkerson, Jr., M.D.

Associate Professor of Medicine, Duke University School of Medicine; Director, Critical Care Medicine, Duke University Medical Center, Durham, North Carolina
Hemodynamic Effects of Mechanical Ventilation

Carol V. Garner, M.D.

Assistant Professor of Surgery and Medicine, Brown University; Assistant Director of Medical Intensive Care Unit, Miriam Hospital, Providence, Rhode Island
Upper Respiratory Tract Infections

Michael A. Geheb, M.D.

Professor of Medicine, and Associate Dean for Clinical Affairs, State University of New York at Stony Brook Health Sciences Center; Senior Attending Physician, University Hospital, Stony Brook, New York
Clinical Disorders of Calcium and Magnesium Metabolism in Critically Ill Patients; Drug Dosing Adjustments in Renal Failure; Heat Injuries; Pharmacologic Agents and Poisoning: Pharmacokinetics in Critically Ill Patients

Jeffrey A. Gelfand, M.D.

Professor and Vice-Chairman, Department of Medicine, Tufts University School of Medicine; Associate Physician-in-Chief, New England Medical Center, Boston, Massachusetts
Burns

W. Lance George, M.D.

Professor of Medicine, University of California, Los Angeles, School of Medicine; Chief, Infectious Diseases Division, and Director, Clinical Microbiology Laboratory, West Los Angeles Veterans Administration Medical Center, Los Angeles, California
Life-Threatening Skin and Soft Tissue Infections

Joanne E. Getsy, M.D.

Assistant Professor of Medicine, University of Pennsylvania School of Medicine; Medical Director, Penn Center for Sleep Disorders, University of Pennsylvania Medical Center, Philadelphia, Pennsylvania
Central Respiratory Failure, Including Sleep Disorders

Marla J. Gold, M.D.

Clinical Assistant Professor of Medicine, Medical College of Pennsylvania; Assistant Health Commissioner for Infectious Disease Control, Philadelphia, Department of Public Health, Philadelphia, Pennsylvania
Endocarditis

Stanley Goldfarb, M.D.

Associate Professor of Medicine, Hospital of the University of Pennsylvania, Philadelphia, Pennsylvania
Phosphorus Homeostasis

Francisco Gonzalez-Scarano, M.D.

Associate Professor of Neurology and of Microbiology, University of Pennsylvania School of Medicine; Attending Physician, Hospital of the University of Pennsylvania, Philadelphia, Pennsylvania
Viral Encephalitis

James J. Gordon, M.D.

Assistant Professor of Medicine, Michigan State University School of Medicine; Director of Infectious Diseases, McLaren Regional Medical Center, Flint, Michigan
Gram-Positive Bacterial Sepsis

Jonathan E. Gottlieb, M.D.

Associate Professor of Medicine, Jefferson Medical College, Thomas Jefferson University; Director, Medical/Respiratory Intensive Care Unit, Thomas Jefferson University Hospital, Philadelphia, Pennsylvania
Acute Severe Asthma

Steven A. Gould, M.D.

Professor of Surgery, University of Illinois at Chicago; Chief of Service, Department of Surgery, Humana Hospital–Michael Reese, Chicago, Illinois
Artificial Blood

Bradford Grassmick, M.D.

Associate Director, Cardiac Surgical Unit, Providence Hospital, Southfield, Michigan
Long-Term Airway Management

Barry A. Gray, M.D., Ph.D.

Professor of Medicine, University of Oklahoma College of Medicine; Director, Medical Intensive Care Unit, Department of Veterans Affairs Medical Center, and Staff Physician, University of Oklahoma Teaching Hospitals, Oklahoma City, Oklahoma
Physiology of Gas Exchange; Pulmonary Edema: Lung Water Balance in Relation to Physiologic Monitoring and Clinical Outcome in the Critically Ill

Michael A. Grippi, M.D.

Assistant Professor and Vice-Chairman, Clinical Affairs, Department of Medicine, Pulmonary and Critical Care Division, Hospital of the University of Pennsylvania, Philadelphia, Pennsylvania
Mechanical Properties of the Respiratory System; Adjunct Methods of Respiratory Therapy

Jeffrey S. Groeger, M.D.

Associate Professor of Medicine, Cornell University Medical College; Medical Director, Special Care Unit, and Associate Attending Physician, Memorial Sloan–Kettering Cancer Center, New York, New York
Severity Scoring in Intensive Care Units

Guillermo Gutierrez, M.D.

Associate Professor and Director, Division of Pulmonary and Critical Care Medicine, The University of Texas Health Science Center; Chief of Service, Pulmonary Medicine, Hermann Hospital and Lyndon B. Johnson Hospital, Houston, Texas
Abnormalities of Oxygen Delivery and Uptake in Sepsis

Steven D. Ham, D.O.

Assistant Professor of Neurosurgery, Wayne State University School of Medicine; Vice-Chief of Neurosurgery, Detroit Receiving Hospital, and Attending Physician, Children's Hospital of Michigan, Harper Hospital, and William Beaumont Hospital, Detroit, Michigan
Clinical Neurophysiology in the Intensive Care Unit

Stephen B. Hanauer, M.D.

Associate Professor of Medicine, University of Chicago Pritzker School of Medicine; University of Chicago Medical Center, Chicago, Illinois
Inflammatory Bowel Disease

John H. Hansen-Flaschen, M.D.

Associate Professor of Medicine and Director, Pulmonary and Critical Care Division, University of Pennsylvania School of Medicine, Philadelphia, Pennsylvania
Adult Respiratory Distress Syndrome: Clinical Features

Marilyn T. Haupt, M.D.

Associate Professor of Medicine and Chief, Division of Critical Care Medicine, Wayne State University School of Medicine; Chief, Section of Critical Care Medicine, Detroit Receiving Hospital, Detroit, Michigan
Anaphylaxis

Bassam N. Helou, M.D.

Intensivist, Community Hospital, Indianapolis, Indiana
Electrical and Lightning Injuries

Timothy L. Hooper, M.D., F.R.C.S.

Consultant for Cardiothoracic Surgery, Wythenshowe Hospital, Manchester, United Kingdom
Cardiac Assist Devices and Transplantation

Leonard D. Hudson, M.D.

Professor of Medicine and Head, Division of Pulmonary and Critical Care Medicine, University of Washington School of Medicine; Medical Director, Medical Intensive Care Unit, and Attending Physician, Harborview Medical Center, and Attending Physician, University of Washington Medical Center, Seattle, Washington
Acute Respiratory Failure in Chronic Obstructive Pulmonary Disease

H. David Humes, M.D.

Professor of Internal Medicine, University of Michigan Medical Center; Chief of Medicine, Veterans Administration Medical Center, Ann Arbor, Michigan
Acute Renal Failure

Jodie L. Hurwitz, M.D.

Assistant Professor of Medicine, University of Pennsylvania School of Medicine; Assistant Professor of Medicine/Cardiology, Hospital of the University of Pennsylvania, Philadelphia, Pennsylvania
Disorders of Cardiac Rhythm and Conduction in the Medical Intensive Care Unit

Robert C. Hyzy, M.D.

Clinical Assistant Professor, University of Michigan School of Medicine, Ann Arbor; Senior Staff Physician and Director, Medical Intensive Care Units, Henry Ford Hospital, Detroit, Michigan
Mechanical Ventilation and Weaning

Thomas J. Iberti, M.D.

Late Associate Professor of Surgery, Anesthesiology, and Medicine, Mount Sinai Medical Center; Director, Critical Care Division, and Director, Surgical Intensive Care Unit, Mount Sinai Medical Center, New York, New York
Preoperative Care

Kim L. Isaacs, M.D., Ph.D.

Assistant Professor of Medicine, University of North Carolina at Chapel Hill; Attending Physician, University of North Carolina Hospitals, Chapel Hill, North Carolina
Lower Gastrointestinal Tract Hemorrhage

Matthew A. Ivanovich, M.D.

Pulmonary Fellow, Rush–Presbyterian–St. Luke's Medical Center, Chicago; Associate Attending Physician, Sherman Hospital and St. Joseph's Hospital, Elgin, and Good Shepherd Hospital, Barrington, Illinois
Pathophysiology of Sepsis

T. M. Jiva, M.D.

Clinical Instructor and Fellow in Pulmonary and Critical Care Medicine, University of Rochester School of Medicine and Dentistry, Rochester, New York
Cold Exposure Injuries

Richard K. Kasama, M.D.

Assistant Professor of Medicine, University of Medicine and Dentistry of New Jersey, Stratford; Staff Nephrologist, Kennedy Memorial Hospital, Stratford, New Jersey
Dialysis and Hemoperfusion: Principles of Dialysis Therapy

Brian S. Kaufman, M.D.

Assistant Professor of Anesthesiology and Medicine, and Director, Section of Critical Care Medicine, New York University Medical Center; Medical Director, Respiratory Therapy, Tisch University Hospital, New York, New York
Fluid Resuscitation

Mark A. Kelley, M.D.

Professor of Medicine and Vice-Dean for Clinical Affairs, University of Pennsylvania School of Medicine, Philadelphia, Pennsylvania
Pulmonary Embolism in the Critically Ill Patient

Karl B. Kern, M.D.

Associate Professor of Medicine, University of Arizona College of Medicine; Associate Director, Cardiac Catheterization Laboratory, University Medical Center, Tucson, Arizona
Cardiopulmonary Resuscitation: Current Status and New Horizons

Thomas S. Kickler, M.D.

Associate Professor of Laboratory Medicine and of Internal Medicine (Hematology), The Johns Hopkins University School of Medicine; Associate Director of the Blood Bank and Transfusion Service, Johns Hopkins Hospital, Baltimore, Maryland
Blood Banking and Transfusion Principles in Critical Care

Gary T. Kinasewitz, M.D.

Professor of Medicine and of Physiology and Biophysics, University of Oklahoma College of Medicine; Chief, Pulmonary Disease and Critical Care, University of Oklahoma Health Sciences Center, and Director, Intensive Care Unit, Oklahoma Memorial Hospital, Oklahoma City, Oklahoma
Physiology of Gas Exchange; Pleural Disease

Lisa L. Kirkland, M.D.

Associate Director, Intensive Care Units, and Active Staff, Department of Critical Care Medicine, St. John's Mercy Medical Center, St. Louis, Missouri
Arterial Pressure Monitoring

Lewis R. Kline, M.D.

Associate Professor of Medicine, University of Pennsylvania School of Medicine, Philadelphia; Director, Center

for Sleep Disorders, West Penn Hospital, Pittsburgh, Pennsylvania
Mechanical Respiratory Failure

Robert A. Kloner, M.D., Ph.D.

Professor of Medicine, Section of Cardiology, University of Southern California School of Medicine; Director of Research, Heart Institute, Hospital of the Good Samaritan, Los Angeles, California
Metabolic and Toxic Effects on the Cardiovascular System

Sidney M. Kobrin, M.D.

Assistant Professor of Medicine, University of Pennsylvania School of Medicine; Director, In-Patient Dialysis Unit, Hospital of the University of Pennsylvania, Philadelphia, Pennsylvania
Phosphorus Homeostasis; Dialysis and Hemoperfusion: Intermittent Renal Replacement Therapy in Treating the Critically Ill Patient with Acute Renal Failure; Hemoperfusion and the Treatment of Poisoning

Dennis L. Kolson, M.D., Ph.D.

Assistant Professor of Neurology, University of Pennsylvania School of Medicine; Attending Physician in Neurology, Hospital of the University of Pennsylvania, Philadelphia, Pennsylvania
Viral Encephalitis

Jacob Korula, M.D., F.R.C.P.C.

Associate Professor of Clinical Medicine, University of Southern California School of Medicine, Los Angeles; Attending Physician, Liver Unit, Rancho Los Amigos Medical Center, Downey, California
Portal Hypertension and Variceal Hemorrhage

Oksana M. Korzeniowski, M.D.

Associate Professor of Medicine, Division of Infectious Diseases, Medical College Hospitals, Philadelphia, Pennsylvania
Endocarditis

D. Charles Kowalewski, Jr., D.O.

Critical Care Fellow, Wayne State University School of Medicine, Detroit, Michigan
Artificial Intelligence and Expert Systems in Critical Care Medicine

Robert A. Kreisberg, M.D.

Professor of Medicine, University of Alabama at Birmingham School of Medicine, Birmingham, Alabama
Diabetic Ketoacidosis and Hypoglycemia

Willane S. Krell, M.D.

Assistant Professor of Medicine, Wayne State University School of Medicine; Director, Pulmonary Diagnostics, Harper Hospital, Detroit, Michigan
Bronchoscopic Procedures in Critically Ill Patients

James A. Kruse, M.D., F.C.C.M.

Associate Professor of Medicine, Division of Critical Care Medicine, Wayne State University School of Medicine; Director, Medical Intensive Care Unit, and Director, Pulmonary Care Unit, Detroit Receiving Hospital, Detroit Michigan
Selected Nonvascular Procedures; Vascular Procedures; Blood Gas Analysis and Related Techniques; Hemodynamic Monitoring; Lactic Acidosis; Pharmacologic Agents and Poisoning: Methanol, Ethylene Glycol, and Related Intoxications

Vladimir Kvetan, M.D., F.C.C.M.

Associate Professor of Anesthesiology and of Critical Care Medicine, and Director, Critical Care Medicine Fellowship Programs, Albert Einstein College of Medicine; Director, Critical Care Medicine, Montefiore Medical Center, Bronx, New York
Modern Medical Response to Disasters

Jeffrey V. Kyff, D.O., F.A.O.C.A., F.C.C.P.

Assistant Clinical Professor of Anesthesiology, Michigan State University College of Osteopathic Medicine, East Lansing; Senior Staff Anesthesiologist, Director, Anesthesia Critical Care Services, Director, Post Anesthesia Care Unit, and Co-Director, Cardiothoracic Intensive Care Unit, Henry Ford Hospital, Detroit, Michigan
Airway Management and Endotracheal Intubation

Paul N. Lanken, M.D.

Associate Professor of Medicine, University of Pennsylvania School of Medicine; Medical Director, Medical Intensive Care Unit, Hospital of the University of Pennsylvania, Philadelphia, Pennsylvania
Respiratory Failure: An Overview; Adult Respiratory Distress Syndrome: Clinical Management

Steven J. Lavine, M.D.

Associate Professor of Internal Medicine, Wayne State University School of Medicine; Director, Noninvasive Laboratory, Harper Hospital, Detroit Receiving Hospital, and University Health Center, Detroit, Michigan
Right-Sided Heart and Pericardial Disease; Noninvasive Techniques

Carl V. Leier, M.D.

James W. Overstreet Professor of Medicine and Pharmacology; Ohio State University School of Medicine; Director, Division of Cardiology, and Attending Physician, The Ohio State University Hospitals, Columbus, Ohio
Left-Sided Heart Failure

Donald P. Levine, M.D.

Associate Professor of Medicine, Wayne State University School of Medicine; Chief, Section of Infectious Diseases, Detroit Receiving Hospital, Detroit, Michigan
Infections in Intravenous Drug Abusers

Steven R. Levine, M.D.

Clinical Associate Professor of Neurology, University of Michigan Medical School, Ann Arbor; Director, Clinical Stroke Service and Acute Stroke Unit, Center for Stroke Research, Department of Neurology, Henry Ford Hospital and Health Science Center, Detroit, Michigan
Cerebrovascular Disease

Matthew E. Levison, M.D.

Professor of Medicine, Medical College of Pennsylvania; Chief, Division of Infectious Diseases, Medical College Hospitals, Philadelphia, Pennsylvania
Selection of Antimicrobial Agents: Pharmacokinetic and Pharmacodynamic Principles

Richard P. Lewis, M.D.

Professor of Internal Medicine, Ohio State University College of Medicine; Attending Physician, The Ohio State University Hospitals, Columbus, Ohio
Left-Sided Heart Failure

Peter A. LeWitt, M.D.

Professor of Neurology, Wayne State University School of Medicine; Director, Clinical Neuroscience Program, Sinai Hospital, Detroit, Michigan
Hyperpyretic-Rigidity Syndrome (Neuroleptic Malignant Syndrome)

Robert P. Lisak, M.D.

Professor and Chairman, Department of Neurology, and Professor of Immunology/Microbiology, Wayne State University School of Medicine; Neurologist-in-Chief, Detroit Medical Center, Chief of Neurology, Harper Hospital, Attending Neurologist, Detroit Receiving Hospital, and Consultant, Rehabilitation Institute of Michigan, Detroit, Michigan
Neuromuscular Diseases

Warren E. Lockette, M.D.

Assistant Professor of Medicine, Division of Endocrinology and Hypertension Research, and Associate Professor of Physiology and of Neurosurgery, Wayne State University School of Medicine, Detroit; Staff Physician, Veterans Administration Medical Center, Allen Park, Michigan
Catecholamines and Pressor Agents; Hypertensive Urgencies and Emergencies

Jacob Loke, M.D.

Clinical Professor of Medicine, Yale University School of Medicine; Attending Physician, Yale–New Haven Hospital, New Haven, Connecticut
Acute Smoke Inhalation

Daniel Luba, M.D.

Postdoctoral Fellow in Medicine (Gastroenterology), Stanford University Medical Center, Stanford, California
Hepatic Emergencies

John M. Luce, M.D.

Associate Professor of Medicine and of Anesthesia, University of California, San Francisco, School of Medicine; Associate Director, Medical–Surgical Intensive Care Unit, San Francisco General Hospital, San Francisco, California
Pulmonary Consequences of Trauma

Rebecca E. Martin, M.D.

Assistant Professor of Medicine, University of Arkansas for Medical Sciences; Attending Physician, University Hospital of Arkansas and John L. McClellan Veterans Administration Hospital, Little Rock, Arkansas
Fungal Infections

Martin Mayers, M.D.

Assistant Professor of Ophthalmology, Albert Einstein College of Medicine; Director, Cornea Service, Montefiore Medical Center, Bronx Municipal Hospital Center, and WHAECOM, and Consultant, Cornea and External Eye Diseases, Lawrence Hospital, Bronx, New York
Ophthalmic Infections

Kathleen A. McCarroll, M.D.

Assistant Professor of Radiology, Wayne State University School of Medicine; Vice-Chief, Department of Radiology, Detroit Receiving Hospital, Detroit, Michigan
Imaging the Chest

Prabodh M. Mehta, M.D.

Assistant Professor of Medicine, Section of Cardiology, East Carolina University School of Medicine; Medical Director, Cardiac Catheterization Laboratory, Pitt County Memorial Hospital, Greenville, Consulting Staff, Onslow Memorial Hospital, Jacksonville, Beaufort County Hospital, Washington, Roanoke-Chowan Hospital, Ahoskie, Washington County Hospital, Lenoir Memorial Hospital, Kinston, and Wayne Memorial Hospital, Goldsboro, North Carolina
Metabolic and Toxic Effects on the Cardiovascular System

Karen A. Mello, M.D.

Instructor in Medicine, Tufts University School of Medicine, Boston; Chairperson, Infection Control, Lawrence General Hospital, Lawrence, Massachusetts
Burns

Stephen A. Mette, M.D.

Clinical Assistant Professor of Medicine, University of Pennsylvania School of Medicine; Director, Medical Intensive Care Unit, The Graduate Hospital, Philadelphia, Pennsylvania
Life-Threatening Pulmonary Hemorrhage

Michael M. Millenson, M.D.

Instructor in Medicine, Harvard Medical School; Associate Physician, Department of Medicine, Division of Hematology/Oncology, Beth Israel Hospital, Boston, Massachusetts
Complications of Therapy of Neoplastic Disease: An Overview

Michael H. Miller, M.D.

Professor and Head, Division of Infectious Diseases Albany Medical College; Attending Physician, Albany Medical Center, Albany, New York
Ophthalmic Infections

Richard P. Millman, M.D.

Associate Professor of Medicine, Brown University School of Medicine; Director, Pulmonary Function Laboratory and Sleep Disorders Center, Rhode Island Hospital, Providence, Rhode Island
Transporting Critically Ill Patients

Barry A. Mizock, M.D.

Associate Professor of Medicine, University of Health Sciences/The Chicago Medical School, North Chicago; Associate Director, Medical Intensive Care Unit, Department of Medicine, Cook County Hospital, Chicago, Illinois
Introduction: History and Destiny of Critical Care Medicine

Gerald S. Moss, M.D.

Professor of Surgery and Dean, University of Illinois College of Medicine at Chicago, University of Illinois Hospital and Humana/Michael Reese Hospital, Chicago, Illinois
Artificial Blood

Joseph A. Moylan, M.D.

Professor of Surgery, Duke University School of Medicine and Duke University Medical Center, Durham, North Carolina
Burn Injury

David M. F. Murphy, M.D.

Chairman, Department of Pulmonary Medicine, Deborah Heart and Lung Center, Browns Mills, New Jersey
Respiratory Failure in Cardiac Disease

Charles Natanson, M.D.

Senior Investigator, National Institutes of Health, Bethesda; Associate Professor of Anesthesia, University of Maryland, Baltimore, Maryland, and Assistant Professor of Medicine, George Washington University, Washington, D.C.
Treatment of Sepsis and Septic Shock: Standard and Experimental Therapies

Loren D. Nelson, M.D.

Associate Professor of Surgery and of Anesthesiology, and Director, Surgical Critical Care, Vanderbilt University School of Medicine, Nashville, Tennessee
Care of the Trauma Patient

Ronald Lee Nichols, M.D.

Henderson Professor of Surgery, Tulane University School of Medicine, New Orleans, Louisiana
Abdominal Infections

John M. Oropello, M.D.

Assistant Professor of Surgery and of Medicine, and Director, Critical Care Fellowship, and Director, Neurosurgical Intensive Care Unit, Mount Sinai Medical Center, New York, New York
Preoperative Care

Gregory R. Owens, M.D.

Associate Professor of Medicine, Division of Pulmonary Medicine, University of Pittsburgh School of Medicine, Pittsburgh, Pennsylvania
Aspiration

Allan I. Pack, M.D., Ph.D.

Associate Professor of Medicine, Pulmonary and Critical Care Division, University of Pennsylvania School of Medicine; Director, Center for Sleep and Respiratory Neurobiology, University of Pennsylvania Medical Center, Philadelphia, Pennsylvania
Central Respiratory Failure, Including Sleep Disorders

Harold I. Palevsky, M.D.

Associate Professor of Medicine, Pulmonary and Critical Care Division, University of Pennsylvania School of Medicine; Medical Director, Lung Transplant Program, and Medical Director, Respiratory Care Services, Hospital of the University of Pennsylvania, Philadelphia, Pennsylvania
Pulmonary Hypertension and Right-Sided Heart Failure

Paul M. Palevsky, M.D.

Assistant Professor of Medicine, Renal-Electrolyte Division, University of Pittsburgh School of Medicine; Chief, Hemodialysis, Department of Veterans Affairs Medical Center, and Staff Physician, Presbyterian University Hospital and Montefiore University Hospital, Pittsburgh, Pennsylvania
Water and Tonicity Homeostasis

Charles J. Parker, M.D.

Associate Professor of Medicine, University of Utah School of Medicine; Chief, Hematology Subsection, Veterans Administration Medical Center, Salt Lake City, Utah
Acute Hemolytic Disorders

Joseph E. Parrillo, M.D.

James B. Herrick Professor of Medicine, Rush Medical College; Chief, Section of Cardiology and Section of Critical Care Medicine, and Medical Director, Rush Heart Institute, Chicago, Illinois
Cardiovascular Dysfunction in Septic Shock

David A. Paulus, M.S., M.D.

Associate Professor of Anesthesiology and of Mechanical Engineering, University of Florida College of Medicine; Attending Physician, Shands Hospital at the University of Florida and the Veterans Administration Medical Center, Gainesville, Florida
Noninvasive Monitoring of Oxygen and Carbon Dioxide

Paul E. Pepe, M.D., F.A.C.P., F.C.C.M., F.C.C.P., F.A.C.E.P.

Associate Professor of Medicine, Surgery, and Pediatrics, Baylor College of Medicine and the Ben Taub General Hospital Emergency Trauma Center; Director, City of Houston Emergency Medical Services, Houston, Texas
Emergency Medical Service Systems and Prehospital Management of Patients Requiring Critical Care

Michael P. Peppers, Pharm.D.

Pharmacology Instructor, Central Methodist College of School of Nursing, Flat River; Clinical Coordinator, Department of Pharmacy, Mineral Area Regional Medical Center, Farmington, Missouri
Drug Dosing Adjustments in Renal Failure; Pharmacologic Agents and Poisoning: Pharmacokinetics in Critically Ill Patients; Pharmacologic Poisoning

Patti L. Peterson, M.D.

Associate Professor of Neurology, Wayne State University School of Medicine; Chief of Neurology, Detroit Receiving Hospital and University Health Center, Detroit, Michigan
Clinical Neurophysiology in the Intensive Care Unit; Disorders of Consciousness

Claude A. Piantadosi, M.D.

Associate Professor of Medicine, Duke University School of Medicine; Director, F. G. Hall Hyperbaric Center, Duke University Medical Center, and Attending Physician, Durham Veterans Administration Medical Center, Durham, North Carolina
Hemodynamic Effects of Mechanical Ventilation

Richard J. Pisani, M.D.

Assistant Professor of Thoracic Disease and Critical Care Medicine, Mayo Medical School; Consultant, St. Mary's Hospital and Rochester Methodist Hospital, Rochester, Minnesota
Acute Drug-Induced Lung Injury

Philip A. Pizzo, M.D.

Professor of Pediatrics, Uniformed Services University of the Health Sciences; Chief, Pediatric Branch, and Head, Section of Infectious Diseases, National Cancer Institute, Bethesda, Maryland
Infections in Granulocytopenic Patients

Richard B. Pollard, M.D.

Professor of Internal Medicine and of Microbiology, University of Texas Medical Branch, Galveston, Texas
Fulminant Viral Infections

Elizabeth Poplin, M.D.

Assistant Professor of Medicine, Wayne State University School of Medicine; Attending Physician, Harper Hospital, Detroit, Michigan
Acute Effects of Neoplastic Disease

John Popovich, Jr., M.D.

Clinical Associate Professor of Medicine, University of Michigan Medical School, Ann Arbor; Division Head, Pulmonary and Critical Care Medicine, Henry Ford Hospital, Detroit, Michigan
Mechanical Ventilation and Weaning

Laurel C. Preheim, M.D.

Professor of Medicine and of Medical Microbiology, and Chief, Infectious Diseases Section, Creighton University School of Medicine; University of Nebraska Medical Center and Omaha Veterans Affairs Medical Center, Omaha, Nebraska
Tuberculosis and Other Mycobacterial Infections

Kristen Price, M.D.

Assistant Professor of Medicine, Division of Pulmonary and Critical Care Medicine, The University of Texas Health Science Center; Assistant Professor of Medicine, Pulmonary Medicine, Lyndon B. Johnson Hospital, Houston, Texas
Abnormalities of Oxygen Delivery and Uptake in Sepsis

Donald S. Prough, M.D.

Professor and Chairman, Department of Anesthesiology, The University of Texas Medical Branch at Galveston, Galveston, Texas
Neurologic Monitoring

Eric C. Rackow, M.D.

Professor and Vice-Chairman, Department of Medicine, New York Medical College, Valhalla; Chairman, Department of Medicine, St. Vincent's Hospital and Medical Center, New York, New York
Circulatory Shock

Thomas A. Raffin, M.D.

Associate Professor of Medicine, Chief, Division of Pulmonary and Critical Care Medicine, and Co-Director, Stanford University Center for Biomedical Ethics; Medical Director, Department of Respiratory Therapy, Stanford University Hospital, Stanford, California
Ethical and Legal Aspects of Forgoing Life-Sustaining Treatments

Dean Railey, M.D.

Attending Physician, Florida Medical Center, Miami Beach, Florida
Pancreatitis

Nabih M. Ramadan, M.D.

Director, Cerebrovascular Disease Laboratory, Department of Neurology, Henry Ford Hospital and Health Science Center; Staff Neurologist, Henry Ford Hospital, Detroit, Michigan
Cerebrovascular Disease

Sushma Reddy, M.D.

Assistant Professor of Medicine, Division of Endocrinology, Wayne State University School of Medicine; Staff Physician, Harper Hospital and Detroit Receiving Hospital, Detroit, Michigan
Disorders of the Adrenal Cortex

Herbert Y. Reynolds, M.D.

Professor and Chairman, Department of Medicine, The Milton S. Hershey Medical Center, The Pennsylvania State University, Hershey, Pennsylvania
Lung Defense

Elizabeth B. D. Ripley, M.D.

Clinical Instructor of Medicine, Medical College of Virginia; Staff Nephrologist, Hospitals of the Medical College of Virginia, Richmond, Virginia
Acid-Base Homeostasis

John L. Rombeau, M.D.

Associate Professor of Surgery, University of Pennsylvania School of Medicine; Attending Physician, Hospital of the University of Pennsylvania, Philadelphia, Pennsylvania
Indications for and Administration of Enteral and Parenteral Nutrition in Critically Ill Patients

Edward C. Rosenow III, M.D.

Chair, Division of Thoracic Diseases, and Arthur M. and Gladys D. Gray Professor of Medicine, Mayo Medical School, Mayo Clinic, Rochester, Minnesota
Acute Drug-Induced Lung Injury

Robert H. Rubin, M.D.

Associate Professor of Medicine, Harvard Medical School; Chief, Transplantation Infectious Disease, and Director, Clinical Investigation Program, Massachusetts General Hospital, Boston, Massachusetts
Infections in the Organ Transplant Recipient

Edmund J. Rutherford, M.D.

Assistant Professor of Surgery, Vanderbilt University, Medical Center, Nashville, Tennessee
Care of the Trauma Patient

David R. Rutledge, Pharm.D.

Associate Professor, University of Florida, College of Pharmacy; Consultant, Shands Hospital, Gainesville, Florida
Drug Dosing Adjustments in Renal Failure; Pharmacologic Agents and Poisoning: Pharmacokinetics in Critically Ill Patients

Linea L. Rydstedt, M.D.

Assistant Clinical Professor of Internal Medicine, Wayne State University School of Medicine; Medical Director, Harper Hospital Weight Management Program, and Staff Physician, Harper Hospital and Detroit Receiving Hospital, Detroit, and Veterans Administration Medical Center, Allen Park, Michigan
Hypertensive Urgencies and Emergencies

Dennis R. Schaberg, M.D.

Professor of Internal Medicine, University of Michigan College of Medicine; Associate Chairman, Graduate Medical Education, University of Michigan Medical Center, Ann Arbor, Michigan
Gram-Positive Bacterial Sepsis

W. Michael Scheld, M.D.

Professor of Internal Medicine and of Neurosurgery, University of Virginia School of Medicine; Associate Chair for Residency Programs, Department of Internal Medicine, University of Virginia Health Sciences Center, Charlottesville, Virginia
Bacterial Meningitis

Rick J. Schiebinger, M.D.

Associate Professor of Surgery, Wayne State University School of Medicine, Detroit; Staff Physician, Veterans Administration Medical Center, Allen Park, Harper Hospital, and Detroit Receiving Hospital, Detroit, Michigan
Disorders of the Adrenal Cortex

Paula C. Schuman, M.D.

Assistant Professor of Medicine, Division of Infectious Diseases, Wayne State University School of Medicine; Staff Physician, Harper Hospital, Detroit, Michigan
Human Immunodeficiency Virus Infection and the Acquired Immunodeficiency Syndrome

Richard J. Schwab, M.D.

Assistant Professor of Medicine, Pulmonary and Critical Care Division, Center for Sleep and Respiratory Neurobiology, University of Pennsylvania School of Medicine; Hospital of the University of Pennsylvania, Philadelphia, Pennsylvania
Central Respiratory Failure, Including Sleep Disorders

Harold M. Schwartz, M.D.

Senior Fellow, Section of Digestive Diseases, Yale University School of Medicine; Clinical Fellow, Department of Internal Medicine, Yale–New Haven Hospital, New Haven, Connecticut
Esophageal Emergencies

W. Eric Scott, M.D., F.C.C.M., F.A.C.P.

Associate Professor of Anesthesiology, University of Medicine and Dentistry of New Jersey, Robert Wood Johnson Medical School at Camden; Chief, Department of Anesthesia, Director, Intermediate Intensive Care Unit, and Attending Intensivist, Division of Pulmonary and Critical Care Medicine/Department of Medicine, Cooper Hospital/University Medical Center, Camden, New Jersey
Standards

Hansa L. Sehgal, B.S., M.T.

Supervisor and Research Associate, Department of Surgical Research, Humana/Michael Reese Hospital, Chicago, Illinois
Artificial Blood

Lakshman R. Sehgal, Ph.D.

Assistant Professor of Surgery, University of Chicago School of Medicine; Director, Surgical Research, Department of Surgery, Humana/Michael Reese Hospital, Chicago, Illinois
Artificial Blood

Lyle L. Sensenbrenner, M.D.

Lecturer in Pharmacology and in Hematology, Wayne State University School of Medicine; Associate Director for Hematology, Harper Hospital, Professor of Pediatrics, Children's Hospital, Attending Physician in Hematology, Hutzel Hospital, Detroit, Michigan
Hematology/Oncology: Introduction; Bone Marrow Failure and Transplantation

Fuad Shihab, M.D.

Fellow, Division of Nephrology, University of Pennsylvania School of Medicine, Philadelphia, Pennsylvania
Dialysis and Hemoperfusion: Intermittent Renal Replacement Therapy in Treating the Critically Ill Patient with Acute Renal Failure; Hemoperfusion and the Treatment of Poisoning

William J. Sibbald, M.D.

Clinical Professor of Medicine, University of Western Ontario; Coordinator, Critical Care Trauma Center, Victoria Hospital Corporation, London, Ontario, Canada
Multiple Organ System Failure in Sepsis

Frederick R. Sidell, M.D.

Director, Medical Management Chemical Casualties Course, The Chemical Casualty Care Office, U.S. Army Medical Research Institute of Chemical Defense, Aberdeen Proving Ground, Maryland
Chemical Exposure

Alan M. Siegal, M.D.

Professor of Medicine, Divisions of Gerontology and Endocrinology and Metabolism, University of Alabama at Birmingham School of Medicine; Attending Physician, University of Alabama at Birmingham Hospitals and Clinics and Birmingham Veterans Administration Medical Center, Birmingham, Alabama
Diabetic Ketoacidosis and Hypoglycemia

Jerome H. Siegel, M.D., F.A.C.P., F.A.C.G.

Associate Clinical Professor of Medicine, Mt. Sinai School of Medicine of City University of New York; Chief, Endoscopy, Beth Israel Medical Center, North Division, New York, New York
Endoscopic Management of Biliary Emergencies

Miles H. Sigler, M.D., F.A.C.P.

Clinical Professor of Medicine, Thomas Jefferson University Medical College; Chief, Division of Nephrology, Lankenau Hospital, and Research Associate, Lankenau Medical Research Center, Philadelphia, Pennsylvania
Dialysis and Hemoperfusion: Continuous Renal Replacement Therapy in Treating the Critically Ill Patient with Acute Renal Failure

Dale H. Sillix, M.D.

Assistant Professor of Medicine and Transplant Nephrologist, Wayne State University School of Medicine; Staff Physician, Harper Hospital, Detroit, Michigan
Complications of Renal Transplantation

Jack D. Sobel, M.D.

Professor of Medicine and Chief, Division of Infectious Diseases, Wayne State University School of Medicine; Chief, Division of Infectious Diseases, Detroit Medical Center, Detroit, Michigan
Candida Infections

Michael A. Solomon, M.D.

Senior Critical Care Fellow, National Institutes of Health, Bethesda, Maryland
Treatment of Sepsis and Septic Shock: Standard and Experimental Therapies

James R. Sowers, M.D.

Professor of Medicine and Director, Division of Endocrinology and Hypertension, and Professor of Physiology, Wayne State University School of Medicine; Staff Physician, Harper Hospital and Detroit Receiving Hospital, Detroit, and Veterans Administration Medical Center, Allen Park, Michigan
Catecholamines and Pressor Agents; Hypertensive Urgencies and Emergencies

Michael R. Sperling, M.D.

Associate Professor of Neurology, University of Pennsylvania School of Medicine; Director, Electroencephalography Laboratory, Graduate Hospital, and Chief, Medical/Surgical Program, Comprehensive Epilepsy Center, Graduate Hospital, Philadelphia, Pennsylvania
Seizures and Status Epilepticus

A. Robert Spitzer, M.D.

Assistant Professor of Neurology and Adjunct Assistant Professor of Electrical and Computer Engineering, Wayne State University School of Medicine; Director, Electromyography Laboratory, Harper Hospital, and Vice-Chief, Department of Neurology, Detroit Receiving Hospital, Detroit, Michigan
Clinical Neurophysiology in the Intensive Care Unit

Charles L. Sprung, M.D., J.D.

Professor of Medicine, The Hebrew University of Jerusalem School of Medicine; Director, Intensive Care Unit, Hadassah Hebrew University Medical Center, Jerusalem, Israel
The Future of Ethical Issues in Critical Care Medicine

Steven M. Steinberg, M.D.

Assistant Professor of Surgery, Tulane University School of Medicine, New Orleans, Louisiana
Abdominal Infections

Larry W. Stephenson, M.D.

Professor and Chief, Cardiothoracic Surgery, Wayne State University School of Medicine; Chief, Cardiothoracic Surgery, Harper Hospital, Detroit, Michigan
Cardiac Assist Devices and Transplantation

Martin A. Strosberg, M.P.H., Ph.D.

Associate Professor of Management and Director, Health Administration Program, Graduate Management Institute, Union College, Schenectady, New York
Organization of Critical Care Units

Uma Sundaram, M.D.

Assistant Professor of Medicine, Yale University School of Medicine; Attending Physician, Yale–New Haven Medical Center and West Haven Veterans Administration Medical Center, New Haven, Connecticut
Pathophysiology of Acute Diarrhea in the Intensive Care Unit

Harold M. Szerlip, M.D.

Associate Professor of Medicine, Tulane University School of Medicine; Chief, Tulane Medical Service, Charity Hospital, New Orleans, Louisiana
Sodium and Volume Homeostasis

Brendan P. Teehan, M.D., F.A.C.P.

Clinical Professor of Medicine, Thomas Jefferson University Medical College; Director of Dialysis Program, Lankenau Hospital, and Research Associate, Lankenau Medical Research Center, Philadelphia, Pennsylvania
Dialysis and Hemoperfusion: Continuous Renal Replacement Therapy in Treating the Critically Ill Patient with Acute Renal Failure

Stephen R. Thom, M.D., Ph.D.

Assistant Professor of Medicine, University of Pennsylvania School of Medicine; Chief, Hyperbaric Medicine, Institute for Environmental Medicine, Philadelphia, Pennsylvania
Barotrauma, Decompression Sickness, and Air Embolism

Gregory Tino, M.D.

Fellow, Pulmonary and Critical Care Division, Department of Medicine, Hospital of the University of Pennsylvania, Philadelphia, Pennsylvania
Adjunct Methods of Respiratory Therapy

Kevin J. Tracey, M.D.

Chief, Department of Neurosurgery, North Shore University Hospital–Cornell Medical Center, Manhasset, New York
Cytokines, Tumor Necrosis Factor, and Other Mediators of Sepsis

Morris Traube, M.D.

Associate Professor of Medicine, Yale University School of Medicine; Attending Physician and Director, Gastrointestinal Procedure Center, Yale–New Haven Hospital, New Haven, Connecticut
Esophageal Emergencies

Allan R. Tunkel, M.D., Ph.D.

Assistant Professor of Medicine and Assistant Program Director, Medical Residency Training Program, Medical College of Pennyslvania, Philadelphia, Pennsylvania
Bacterial Meningitis

John S. Urbanetti, M.D., F.R.C.P.(C.)

Clinical Assistant Professor of Medicine, Yale University School of Medicine, New Haven; Senior Staff, Lawrence Memorial Hospital, New London, Connecticut
Chemical Exposure

Luis R. Urbina, M.D.

Fellow in Pulmonary and Critical Care Medicine, Wayne State University School of Medicine, Detroit, Michigan
Blood Gas Analysis and Related Techniques

Annamalai Veerappan, M.D.

Assistant Attending Physician, Washington Hospital, Fremont, and Valley Health Care Hospital, Pleasanton and Livermore, California
Endoscopic Management of Biliary Emergencies

Christopher Veremakis, M.D.

Assistant Clinical Professor and Director, Critical Care Fellowship, St. Louis University School of Medicine; Chairman, Department of Critical Care Medicine, St. John Mercy Medical Center, St. Louis, Missouri
Arterial Pressure Monitoring

Thomas J. Walsh, M.D.

Senior Investigator, Section of Infectious Diseases Pediatric Branch, National Cancer Institute, Bethesda, Maryland
Infections in Granulocytopenic Patients

Alexander J. Walt, M.D., Ch.B., M.S.(Minn.), F.R.C.S.(Eng.), F.R.C.S.(C.), F.A.C.S.

Distinguished Professor of Surgery, Wayne State University School of Medicine; Attending Physician in Surgery, Harper Hospital, and Senior Attending Physician in Surgery, Detroit Receiving Hospital, Detroit, Michigan
The Acute Abdomen

John W. Warren, M.D.

Professor of Medicine, University of Maryland School of Medicine; Head, Division of Infectious Diseases, Department of Medicine, University of Maryland Medical Center, Baltimore, Maryland
Nosocomial Urinary Tract Infections

John A. Washington, M.D.

Chairman, Department of Microbiology, The Cleveland Clinic Foundation, Cleveland, Ohio
Diagnostic Methods and the Laboratory in Intensive Care Unit Patients

Alan G. Wasserstein, M.D.

Associate Professor of Medicine, University of Pennsylvania School of Medicine; Director, Dialysis Programs and Stone Evaluation Center, Hospital of the University of Pennsylvania, Philadelphia, Pennsylvania
Renal Insufficiency

Max Harry Weil, M.D., Ph.D.

Distinguished University Professor, University of Health Sciences/The Chicago Medical School, North Chicago, Illinois, and Professor of Medicine, University of Southern California; President, Institute of Critical Care Medicine, Palm Springs, California
Introduction: History and Destiny of Critical Care Medicine; Circulatory Shock

Lawrence S. Weisberg, M.D.

Assistant Professor of Medicine, University of Medicine and Dentistry of New Jersey, Robert Wood Johnson Medical School at Camden; Medical Director of Dialysis, Cooper Hospital/University Medical Center, Camden, New Jersey
Potassium Homeostasis

Donna I. Whittle, M.D.

Attending Physician, Infectious Diseases, Mercy Hospital, Pittsburgh, Pennsylvania
Infections in the Multitrauma Patient

Laurel Wiegand, M.D.

Assistant Professor of Medicine, Pulmonary Critical Care Division, Pennsylvania State University College of Medicine, Hershey, Pennsylvania
Lung Defense

Robert F. Wilson, M.D.

Professor of Surgery, Wayne State University School of Medicine; Chief of Surgery, Director, Trauma Services, and Director, Surgical Intensive Care Units, Detroit Receiving Hospital, Detroit, Michigan
Emergency Vascular Surgery in Patients in the Intensive Care Unit

Richard G. Wood, D.O.

Clinical Instructor in Medicine, University of Oklahoma Health Sciences Center, Oklahoma City; Director, Cardiopulmonary, Edmond Regional Hospital, Edmond, Oklahoma
Pleural Disease

Antoinette Wozniak, M.D.

Assistant Professor of Medicine, Wayne State University School of Medicine, Detroit; Staff Oncologist, Veterans Administration Hospital, Allen Park, Michigan
Acute Effects of Neoplastic Disease

Joshua Wynne, M.D.

Professor of Medicine and Chief, Division of Cardiology, Wayne State University School of Medicine; Chief, Section of Cardiology, Harper Hospital, Detroit, Michigan
Acute Myocardial Ischemia

Ernest L. Yoder, M.D., F.A.C.P.

Assistant Professor of Medicine and Director of Curriculum Development, Wayne State University School of Medicine; Vice-Chief, Department of Medicine and Director, Critical Care, Grace Hospital, Detroit, Michigan
Heat Injuries; Cold Exposure Injuries

Rowen K. Zetterman, M.D.

Professor of Internal Medicine, University of Nebraska Medical Center, and Clinical Professor of Internal Medicine, Creighton University School of Medicine; University of Nebraska Hospital and Omaha Department of Veterans Affairs Medical Center, Omaha, Nebraska
Liver Transplantation

Irene Zielinski, R.N.

Staff Nurse, Pheresis Department, Harper Hospital, Detroit, Michigan
Clinical Apheresis

Foreword

How does one know when a new field of medicine has crystallized out of the saturated solution of modern medicine? The appearance of a major new textbook such as this is surely one indication. But in the case of critical care medicine, the signs of independent existence are much stronger still. In a remarkably short time, this field has evolved from a few self-styled intensivists working in critical care units in a handful of quaternary hospitals to a full-fledged—some would say overblown—discipline with specialty societies replete with continuing medical education courses, accreditation mechanisms for training programs, and specialty boards offering fancy certificates. How did all this happen? More important, why did all this happen?

Perhaps only an "outsider" can fully appreciate the explosive emergence of the field of critical care medicine over a scant few years—an emergence that, given the brief time involved, is still occurring even as we bask in the accomplishments represented in the pages of this impressive text. No one can seriously question any longer the need for physicians with special training and a heavily skewed, if not an exclusive, dedication to the care of critically ill patients. Only by such highly focused attention can one optimize the delivery of the most sophisticated, technologically intensive care that modern medicine has to offer. The dilettante intensivist may play a useful supporting role but cannot be expected to have the extraordinary knowledge and special skills required to bring a contemporary standard of care to the management of the desperately ill patients who now populate critical care units.

Despite the overwhelming rationale for the emergence of critical care medicine, many nettlesome questions remain, and several more years will be required before we know the answers. Is critical care *a* field or *many* fields? Is critical care a natural, seamless extension of a mother discipline or does it have sharply defined borders? Should there be a final common pathway for the training of critical care specialists regardless of their primary discipline or should such training be tailored to a sharply delimited scope of practice? In other words, should critical care training be generic or boutique? Who should have primary responsibility for the care of patients in the critical care unit? Is it the role of the intensivist to be a sometime consultant or to be the primary physician for all critically ill patients? Who should decide how many resources to allocate to the unit or to a given patient? What portion of the modern hospital should be given over to expansion of critical care units? Does every hospital need one or more such units? Does every such unit need one or more certified intensivists? Does every patient in the unit need one or more certified intensivists?

The fact that this text has been prepared for the critical care internist—the *medical* intensivist—serves to acknowledge that some of these questions have yielded provisional answers in keeping with the current political landscape, a landscape still subject to potential upheaval. In "prehistoric" times, that is, a decade or so ago, it was not at all clear that internal medicine would develop its own, separate subspeciality dealing with internal medicine–based critical care. Indeed, many struggled long and hard to establish the principle that critical care was *not* discipline specific. These ardent supporters of an integrated critical care specialty argued that the public interest would best be served by a broadly trained physician who could man (or woman) the ramparts of a general-purpose critical care unit besieged by an onslaught of very ill people, all of whom required expert intensive care according to the same set of precepts and standards. In pursuit of this unifying principle, valiant efforts were made to establish a single set of training requirements and a single set of certifying standards for all intensivists, whether they came from internal medicine, surgery, anesthesia, or pediatrics. This noble undertaking was, however, doomed to run aground on the shoals of parochialism. Those in anesthesia insisted that 1 year of specialized training was adequate for their purposes, given the nature of basic training in that discipline; all the others remained convinced that a minimum of 2 years was required. Surgery was never quite comfortable that postoperative care would be incorporated into a common curriculum, and pediatrics had its problems with the idiosyncratic needs of neonates. So, the four primary disciplines went their separate ways, each formulating its own set of special requirements for accrediting subspecialty training programs in critical care medicine and each constructing its own examination for certifying individual diplomates. Although some visionaries remain optimistic that integration will ultimately prevail, it will not be easy to put Humpty Dumpty back together again, even for those accustomed to resuscitating train wrecks!

Even after its sister disciplines parted company, internal medicine was faced with a fractious house of its own. Pulmonologists were hard to convince that critical care meant something more than pulmonary medicine writ serious. Endless dialogue, thoughtful compromise, and some gentle arm twisting ultimately succeeded in crafting the boundary conditions and in identifying the unique domain of this newest of internal medicine's subspecialties. Special requirements for training programs in internal medicine–based critical care were drawn up to ensure that the norm for this demanding field included broad-based training in a densely academic setting, under the tutelage of a well-seasoned, diversified faculty utilizing a carefully thought-out curriculum. Adherence to these high standards has limited the number of institutions that have been accredited to offer critical care training, and this limitation has created its own political fallout.

Witnessing critical care medicine differentiate itself from its ancestors and from its contemporaries has been fascinating, and the future should be equally enthralling. Despite the intrigues surrounding these sideshow events, however, it is comforting to know that the main attraction—taking care of the critically ill patient—has not been ignored. If proof were needed that critical care medicine knows full well what the main attraction is, this ambitious textbook provides us with unequivocal evidence.

JORDAN J. COHEN, M.D.
Dean, School of Medicine
State University of New York
at Stony Brook

PREFACE

The genesis of PRINCIPLES AND PRACTICE OF MEDICAL INTENSIVE CARE was based on our observation that the role of the internist practicing intensive care is increasingly central to the provision of comprehensive critical care services in major hospitals throughout the United States. Within that context, we view critical care medicine as the final common path of general internal medicine for the care of acutely ill patients with organ failure. The field of general internal medicine may be characterized by a spectrum of activities that include the historic models of ambulatory care and general inpatient care, as well as the newer practices of critical and geriatric care. The field of critical care has been created as a result of the development of complex treatment and support modalities and the need for dedicated, highly trained personnel to provide care on a round-the-clock basis in a unique technical environment. Shared responsibility and interdisciplinary cooperation are essential for delivery of high-quality intensive care services. In contrast, the development of geriatrics has been driven by the marked increase in life span of our population. Both of these newer specialties represent medical success stories that require specific commitments to a unique base of clinical knowledge and expertise.

The specific knowledge base required of the practitioner of critical care is both detailed and broad in scope. We recognize the enormous contributions of many subspecialties of internal medicine to the curriculum of the internist-intensivist. In particular, a substantial portion of critical care is acute pulmonary medicine. However, cardiovascular, renal, fluid and electrolyte, and infectious complications account for significant proportions of the intensivist's practice. We also recognize the increasing number and variety of disorders, especially neurologic, related to other organ systems that are commonly encountered by the intensivist. In fact, the typical patient in an intensive care unit suffers from simultaneous or consecutive failure of multiple organ systems. Detailed knowledge and skills that cross traditional specialties of medicine as well as other disciplines are therefore required of the successful intensivist. In turn, the practice of critical care requires an integration of a broad range of clinical data and therapeutic plans that often involve consultants drawn from multiple specialties to achieve a unified approach to diagnosis and treatment. This integration requires skill and tact and the recognition that the role of the intensivist is to serve as the custodian but not the owner of patients in his or her charge. The rights and prerogatives of the various primary and consulting physicians must be respected; however, it is the intensive care unit team that provides a safety net for continuous delivery of emergent, often lifesaving, interventions.

Although PRINCIPLES AND PRACTICE OF MEDICAL INTENSIVE CARE is aimed at the internist who wishes to acquire the knowledge and skills for intensive care, we recognize that critical care is a multidisciplinary and interdisciplinary enterprise. Respect for the roles of other health care professionals has been a key to the emergence of the discipline during the past two decades.

We are particularly thankful that we were given the opportunity to develop and apply these principles as we participated in the development of critical care services at Wayne State University and the Detroit Medical Center in the past decade. Simultaneous with our experience in Detroit, interest in the field of critical care medicine by internists has grown to an exceptional level as gauged by any number of parameters, including the dramatic demand to attain certification in critical care through the American Board of Internal Medicine. After only three examination cycles (1987, 1989, and 1991), approximately 3000 internists have attained certification of added qualification in critical care medicine. This number far exceeds the number of certificates issued by anesthesia and surgery, the other boards offering a certifying process for adult critical care. It would appear that the role of the internist in providing critical care services will continue to thrive and expand, with many exciting clinical and academic challenges.

The goal of PRINCIPLES AND PRACTICE OF MEDICAL INTENSIVE CARE is to provide the internist-intensivist with a precise, up-to-date, and well-organized text in intensive care. Our book is meant to be useful at the bedside and as a reference. The intent is to present a text that is comprehensive and covers a broad range of topics, and one that can serve as a core curriculum for medical-based fellowships in critical care.

Special emphasis has been placed on the pathophysiology of disease processes and their presentation in the critically ill patient. In addition, current management is stressed. To that end, we encourage your feedback to improve and make more usable further editions of this text.

We would like to thank several colleagues who encouraged the production of this text, including Dr. Max Harry Weil, whose seminal influence in the development of this field is a matter of record. As the mentor and trainer of many of the leaders in critical care medicine, he is regarded by many as a distinguished "father" of this new endeavor.

We are particularly grateful to our section editors and contributors. No project of this size can be carried out by two editors alone. A truly distinguished group of individuals, each of whom has made significant contributions to the field of critical care medicine, became our partners. A terrific group of section editors helped marshal this effort, and an enthusiastic group of contributors responded. To all of them we give special thanks.

We also acknowledge the vision, skill, and encouragement of the many talented individuals at W. B. Saunders Company who have made this project possible, especially Mr. Richard Zorab and Mr. Leslie E. Hoeltzel, who have been of invaluable help in proceeding with this large task.

We would like to thank especially Ms. Camilla Longley, who worked tirelessly on this project. Her efforts in cajoling contributors and in retrieving, retyping, and collating manuscripts have given her a special role in this text. Special thanks also go to Drs. Hugh Greville and James Kruse, who were always available to help answer questions and provide valuable input.

RICHARD W. CARLSON, M.D., Ph.D.
MICHAEL A. GEHEB, M.D.

ACKNOWLEDGMENTS

Thanks are due to individuals who recognized the need and who provided the encouragement for the development of critical care services at Wayne State University and the Detroit Medical Center. They include Vainutis K. Vaitkevicius, Professor and Chairman, Department of Internal Medicine, 1982–1988, and Robert E. Mack, Professor of Medicine, Associate Dean for Academic Affairs, and Senior Vice President for Medical Affairs at the Detroit Medical Center. A personal tribute from one of us (M.A.G.) is given to Liborio Tranchida, Professor and Chairman, Department of Internal Medicine, 1988–present.

CONTENTS

Introduction: History and Destiny of Critical Care Medicine 1

Barry A. Mizock and Max Harry Weil

SECTION ONE
Sequential and Organizational Aspects of Intensive Care 9

Section Editors, Richard W. Carlson and Michael A. Geheb

CHAPTER 1
Emergency Medical Service Systems and Prehospital Management of Patients Requiring Critical Care 9

Paul E. Pepe

CHAPTER 2
Modern Medical Response to Disasters 25

Derek C. Angus, Joseph A. Barbera, and Vladimir Kvetan

CHAPTER 3
Chemical Exposure 48

John S. Urbanetti and Frederick R. Sidell

CHAPTER 4
Transporting Critically Ill Patients 54

Richard P. Millman and Sidney S. Braman

CHAPTER 5
Organization of Critical Care Units 57

I. Alan Fein, Martin A. Strosberg, and Sandra L. Fein

CHAPTER 6
Standards 67

Carolyn Bekes, W. Eric Scott, and Bruce Friedman

CHAPTER 7
Severity Scoring in Intensive Care Units 77

Donald B. Chalfin and Jeffrey S. Groeger

CHAPTER 8
Computers in Critical Care Units 88

Frank V. M. Booth

CHAPTER 9
Artificial Intelligence and Expert Systems in Critical Care Medicine 95

D. Charles Kowalewski, Jr., and Richard W. Carlson

SECTION TWO
Resuscitation and Monitoring 109

Section Editor, James A. Kruse

CHAPTER 10
Airway Management and Endotracheal Intubation 109

Jeffrey V. Kyff

CHAPTER 11
Cardiopulmonary Resuscitation: Current Status and New Horizons 118

Karl B. Kern and Gordon A. Ewy

CHAPTER 12
Fluid Resuscitation 129

Brian S. Kaufman

CHAPTER 13
Artificial Blood 151

Steven A. Gould, Lakshman R. Sehgal, Hansa L. Sehgal, and Gerald S. Moss

CHAPTER 14
Selected Nonvascular Procedures 160

Roderick J. Boyes and James A. Kruse

CHAPTER 15
Vascular Procedures 177

Vivian L. Clark and James A. Kruse

CHAPTER 16
Bronchoscopic Procedures in Critically Ill Patients 192

Willane S. Krell

CHAPTER 17
Noninvasive Monitoring of Oxygen and Carbon Dioxide ... 203

David A. Paulus

CHAPTER 18
Neurologic Monitoring 221
 Donald S. Prough

CHAPTER 19
Blood Gas Analysis and Related Techniques 235
 Luis R. Urbina and James A. Kruse

CHAPTER 20
Arterial Pressure Monitoring 251
 Lisa L. Kirkland and Christopher Veremakis

CHAPTER 21
Imaging the Chest 257
 Kathleen A. McCarroll

SECTION THREE
The Septic Syndrome 295
 Section Editor, Robert A. Balk

CHAPTER 22
The Septic Syndrome and Septic Shock 295
 Robert A. Balk and Roger C. Bone

CHAPTER 23
Pathophysiology of Sepsis 301
 Matthew A. Ivanovich and Robert A. Balk

CHAPTER 24
**Cytokines, Tumor Necrosis Factor, and
Other Mediators of Sepsis** 311
 Thomas J. Fahey III and Kevin J. Tracey

CHAPTER 25
Cardiovascular Dysfunction in Septic Shock 323
 Andrew C. Dixon and Joseph E. Parrillo

CHAPTER 26
Multiple Organ System Failure in Sepsis 340
 William J. Sibbald and William C. Darrah

CHAPTER 27
Abnormalities of Oxygen Delivery and Uptake in Sepsis .. 352
 Guillermo Gutierrez and Kristen Price

CHAPTER 28
**Treatment of Sepsis and Septic Shock: Standard and
Experimental Therapies** 365
 Michael A. Solomon and Charles Natanson

SECTION FOUR
Infectious Diseases 381
 Section Editor, Jack D. Sobel

CHAPTER 29
Control and Prevention of Infection 381
 Jeffrey D. Band

CHAPTER 30
Fulminant Viral Infections 391
 Michael J. Borucki and Richard B. Pollard

CHAPTER 31
Gram-Positive Bacterial Sepsis 408
 James J. Gordon and Dennis R. Schaberg

CHAPTER 32
Tuberculosis and Other Mycobacterial Infections 422
 Laurel C. Preheim

CHAPTER 33
***Candida* Infections** 434
 Jack D. Sobel

CHAPTER 34
Fungal Infections 444
 Rebecca E. Martin and Robert W. Bradsher

CHAPTER 35
Life-Threatening Skin and Soft Tissue Infections 448
 W. Lance George

CHAPTER 36
Bacterial Meningitis 454
 Allan R. Tunkel and W. Michael Scheld

CHAPTER 37
Ophthalmic Infections 466
 Martin Mayers and Michael H. Miller

CHAPTER 38
Upper Respiratory Tract Infections 474
 Carol V. Garner and Ann Sullivan Baker

CHAPTER 39
Pneumonia 480
 Steven L. Berk and David W. Allen

CHAPTER 40
Endocarditis 491
 Marla J. Gold and Oksana M. Korzeniowski

CHAPTER 41
Gastroenteric Infections 500
 Robert Fekety

CHAPTER 42
Abdominal Infections 513
 Steven M. Steinberg and Ronald Lee Nichols

CHAPTER 43
Burns 521

Karen A. Mello and Jeffrey A. Gelfand

CHAPTER 44
Nosocomial Urinary Tract Infections 527

John W. Warren

CHAPTER 45
Infections in Granulocytopenic Patients 532

Thomas J. Walsh and Philip A. Pizzo

CHAPTER 46
Infections in Cancer Patients 545

Pranatharthi Chandrasekar

CHAPTER 47
Infections in the Multitrauma Patient 556

Donna I. Whittle and Ellis S. Caplan

CHAPTER 48
Infections in Intravenous Drug Abusers 566

Donald P. Levine

CHAPTER 49
Infections in the Organ Transplant Recipient 579

Robert H. Rubin

CHAPTER 50
**Human Immunodeficiency Virus Infection and the
Acquired Immunodeficiency Syndrome** 589

Lawrence R. Crane and Paula C. Schuman

CHAPTER 51
Infections Associated with Intravascular Devices 601

U. Frank and F. D. Daschner

CHAPTER 52
**Diagnostic Methods and the Laboratory in
Intensive Care Unit Patients** 608

John A. Washington

CHAPTER 53
**Selection of Antimicrobial Agents: Pharmacokinetic and
Pharmacodynamic Principles** 614

Matthew E. Levison

**SECTION FIVE
The Nervous System** 621

Section Editor, Robert P. Lisak

CHAPTER 54
Clinical Neurophysiology in the Intensive Care Unit 621

A. Robert Spitzer, Patti L. Peterson, and Steven D. Ham

CHAPTER 55
Disorders of Consciousness 631

Patti L. Peterson

CHAPTER 56
**Brain Damage from Cardiac Arrest: Pathophysiology,
Intensive Care Unit Management, and Outcome,
Including Brain Death** 639

Michael P. Earnest

CHAPTER 57
Cerebrovascular Disease 648

Steven R. Levine and Nabih M. Ramadan

CHAPTER 58
Seizures and Status Epilepticus 663

Michael R. Sperling

CHAPTER 59
Neuromuscular Diseases 672

Robert P. Lisak

CHAPTER 60
Viral Encephalitis 687

Dennis L. Kolson and Francisco Gonzalez-Scarano

CHAPTER 61
**Hyperpyretic-Rigidity Syndrome (Neuroleptic Malignant
Syndrome)** 698

Peter A. LeWitt and Richard C. Berchou

CHAPTER 62
Alcoholism 706

John C. M. Brust

CHAPTER 63
**Critical Care Management of Traumatic Brain Injury and
Spinal Cord Injury** 714

Fernando G. Diaz

**SECTION SIX
The Pulmonary System** 719

Section Editor, Mark A. Kelley

CHAPTER 64
Mechanical Properties of the Respiratory System 719

Michael A. Grippi

CHAPTER 65
Physiology of Gas Exchange 732

Gary T. Kinasewitz and Barry A. Gray

CHAPTER 66
Lung Defense 748

Laurel Wiegand and Herbert Y. Reynolds

CHAPTER 67
Respiratory Failure: An Overview 754
  Paul N. Lanken

CHAPTER 68
Mechanical Respiratory Failure 763
  Lewis R. Kline and Victor A. Ferrari

CHAPTER 69
Central Respiratory Failure, Including Sleep Disorders 773
  Richard J. Schwab, Joanne E. Getsy, and Allan I. Pack

CHAPTER 70
Respiratory Failure in Cardiac Disease 786
  David M. F. Murphy

CHAPTER 71
Acute Respiratory Failure in Chronic Obstructive Pulmonary Disease 793
  J. Randall Curtis and Leonard D. Hudson

CHAPTER 72
Acute Severe Asthma 805
  Jonathan E. Gottlieb and James E. Fish

CHAPTER 73
Adult Respiratory Distress Syndrome 816

Clinical Features 816
  John H. Hansen-Flaschen

Clinical Management 826
  Paul N. Lanken

CHAPTER 74
Pulmonary Hypertension and Right-Sided Heart Failure ... 838
  Harold I. Palevsky

CHAPTER 75
Pulmonary Embolism in the Critically Ill Patient 849
  Mark A. Kelley

CHAPTER 76
Pleural Disease 860
  Richard G. Wood and Gary T. Kinasewitz

CHAPTER 77
Aspiration 872
  Gregory R. Owens

CHAPTER 78
Life-Threatening Pulmonary Hemorrhage 876
  Stephen A. Mette and Steven M. Albelda

CHAPTER 79
Acute Smoke Inhalation 883
  Jacob Loke

CHAPTER 80
Pulmonary Consequences of Trauma 887
  John M. Luce

CHAPTER 81
Acute Drug-Induced Lung Injury 896
  Edward C. Rosenow III and Richard J. Pisani

CHAPTER 82
Barotrauma, Decompression Sickness, and Air Embolism 902
  Stephen R. Thom

CHAPTER 83
Pulmonary Edema: Lung Water Balance in Relation to Physiologic Monitoring and Clinical Outcome in the Critically Ill 911
  Mark A. Camp and Barry A. Gray

CHAPTER 84
Mechanical Ventilation and Weaning 924
  Robert C. Hyzy and John Popovich, Jr.

CHAPTER 85
Hemodynamic Effects of Mechanical Ventilation 944
  William J. Fulkerson, Jr., and Claude A. Piantadosi

CHAPTER 86
Oxygen Toxicity 949
  Michael F. Beers and Aron B. Fisher

CHAPTER 87
Adjunct Methods of Respiratory Therapy 957
  Gregory Tino and Michael A. Grippi

CHAPTER 88
Long-Term Airway Management 967
  Bradford K. Grassmick and Joseph Bander

SECTION SEVEN
The Cardiovascular System 978
  Section Editor, Joshua Wynne

CHAPTER 89
Circulatory Shock 978
  Mark E. Astiz, Eric C. Rackow, and Max Harry Weil

CHAPTER 90
Acute Myocardial Ischemia 989
  Joshua Wynne

CHAPTER 91
Left-Sided Heart Failure 1015
  Richard P. Lewis and Carl V. Leier

CHAPTER 92
Right-Sided Heart and Pericardial Disease 1025
Steven J. Lavine

CHAPTER 93
**Metabolic and Toxic Effects on the Cardiovascular
System** 1038
Prabodh M. Mehta and Robert A. Kloner

CHAPTER 94
**Disorders of Cardiac Rhythm and Conduction in the
Medical Intensive Care Unit** 1049
Alfred E. Buxton and Jodie L. Hurwitz

CHAPTER 95
Hemodynamic Monitoring 1079
James A. Kruse and Eugenio Armendariz

CHAPTER 96
Noninvasive Techniques 1103
Steven J. Lavine

CHAPTER 97
Cardiac Assist Devices and Transplantation 1120
Frank A. Baciewicz, Jr., Timothy L. Hooper, and
Larry W. Stephenson

CHAPTER 98
**Emergency Vascular Surgery in Patients in the
Intensive Care Unit** 1133
Robert F. Wilson and Lawrence M. Diebel

**SECTION EIGHT
The Renal System and Metabolic Function** 1155
Section Editor, Malcolm Cox

CHAPTER 99
Sodium and Volume Homeostasis 1155
Harold M. Szerlip

CHAPTER 100
Water and Tonicity Homeostasis 1168
Paul M. Palevsky

CHAPTER 101
Potassium Homeostasis 1179
Lawrence S. Weisberg

CHAPTER 102
**Clinical Disorders of Calcium and Magnesium
Metabolism in Critically Ill Patients** 1196
Michael A. Geheb and Tusar K. Desai

CHAPTER 103
Phosphorus Homeostasis 1212
Sidney M. Kobrin and Stanley Goldfarb

CHAPTER 104
Acid-Base Homeostasis 1219
George M. Feldman and Elizabeth B. D. Ripley

CHAPTER 105
Lactic Acidosis 1231
James A. Kruse

CHAPTER 106
Diabetic Ketoacidosis and Hypoglycemia 1245
Robert A. Kreisberg and Alan M. Siegal

CHAPTER 107
Acute Renal Failure 1256
H. David Humes

CHAPTER 108
Renal Insufficiency 1267
Alan G. Wasserstein

CHAPTER 109
Dialysis and Hemoperfusion 1275

Principles of Dialysis Therapy 1275
Richard K. Kasama and Pedro C. Fernandez

**Intermittent Renal Replacement Therapy in Treating the
Critically Ill Patient with Acute Renal Failure** 1280
Fuad Shihab and Sidney Kobrin

**Continuous Renal Replacement Therapy in Treating the
Critically Ill Patient with Acute Renal Failure** 1287
Miles H. Sigler and Brendan P. Teehan

Hemoperfusion and the Treatment of Poisoning 1291
Fuad Shihab and Sidney Kobrin

CHAPTER 110
Complications of Renal Transplantation 1293
Dale H. Sillix

CHAPTER 111
Drug Dosing Adjustments in Renal Failure 1304
David R. Rutledge, Michael A. Geheb, and
Michael P. Peppers

CHAPTER 112
Disorders of the Adrenal Cortex 1310
Sushma Reddy and Rick J. Schiebinger

CHAPTER 113
Catecholamines and Pressor Agents 1318
Stephen L. Farrow, Warren E. Lockette, and
James R. Sowers

CHAPTER 114
Hypertensive Urgencies and Emergencies 1327

Linea L. Rydstedt, Warren E. Lockette, and
James R. Sowers

SECTION NINE
Hematology/Oncology 1335

Section Editors, Lyle L. Sensenbrenner and Judith C. Andersen

CHAPTER 115
Hematology/Oncology: Introduction 1335

Judith C. Andersen and Lyle L. Sensenbrenner

CHAPTER 116
Bone Marrow Failure and Transplantation 1339

Lyle L. Sensenbrenner

CHAPTER 117
Bone Marrow Disorders Associated with
Excessive Production 1359

Philip J. Burke

CHAPTER 118
Acute Hemolytic Disorders 1370

Charles J. Parker

CHAPTER 119
Blood Banking and Transfusion Principles in
Critical Care 1387

Thomas S. Kickler

CHAPTER 120
Acute Effects of Neoplastic Disease 1393

Elizabeth Poplin and Antoinette Wozniak

CHAPTER 121
Complications of Therapy of Neoplastic Disease:
An Overview 1403

Michael M. Millenson and Steven E. Come

CHAPTER 122
Clinical Apheresis 1419

Irene Zielinski and Judith C. Andersen

SECTION TEN
The Gastrointestinal System 1432

Section Editor, Rosemarie L. Fisher

CHAPTER 123
Esophageal Emergencies 1432

Harold M. Schwartz and Morris Traube

CHAPTER 124
Upper Gastrointestinal Tract Hemorrhage 1439

Rosemarie L. Fisher

CHAPTER 125
Portal Hypertension and Variceal Hemorrhage 1445

Jacob Korula

CHAPTER 126
Lower Gastrointestinal Tract Hemorrhage 1457

Kim L. Isaacs and Eugene M. Bozymski

CHAPTER 127
Pathophysiology of Acute Diarrhea in the
Intensive Care Unit 1464

Uma Sundaram and Henry J. Binder

CHAPTER 128
Inflammatory Bowel Disease 1470

Stephen B. Hanauer

CHAPTER 129
The Acute Abdomen 1474

Alexander J. Walt and Scott Dulchavsky

CHAPTER 130
Acute Mesenteric Ischemia 1485

Lawrence J. Brandt

CHAPTER 131
Endoscopic Management of Biliary Emergencies 1490

Jerome H. Siegel and Annamalai Veerappan

CHAPTER 132
Pancreatitis 1499

Dean Railey and Jamie S. Barkin

CHAPTER 133
Hepatic Emergencies 1506

Gabriel Garcia and Daniel Luba

CHAPTER 134
Liver Transplantation 1514

Rowen K. Zetterman

CHAPTER 135
Pathophysiology and Therapy of Hepatic
Encephalopathy 1519

Andres T. Blei

SECTION ELEVEN
Nutrition 1528

Section Editor, John L. Rombeau

CHAPTER 136
Indications for and Administration of Enteral and
Parenteral Nutrition in Critically III Patients 1528

John L. Rombeau

SECTION TWELVE
Special Topics 1552
Section Editors, Richard W. Carlson and Michael A. Geheb

CHAPTER 137
Preoperative Care 1552
John M. Oropello and Thomas J. Iberti

CHAPTER 138
Care of the Trauma Patient 1574
Edmund J. Rutherford and Loren D. Nelson

CHAPTER 139
Obstetrics and Gynecology in the Intensive Care Unit ... 1593
Michael A. Belfort, Gary A. Dildy, and David B. Cotton

CHAPTER 140
Burn Injury 1616
Joseph A. Moylan

CHAPTER 141
Heat Injuries 1626
Ernest L. Yoder and Michael A. Geheb

CHAPTER 142
Cold Exposure Injuries 1633
T. M. Jiva, Ernest L. Yoder, and Richard W. Carlson

CHAPTER 143
Electrical and Lightning Injuries 1645
Bassam N. Helou and Richard W. Carlson

CHAPTER 144
Anaphylaxis 1650
Marilyn T. Haupt and Richard W. Carlson

CHAPTER 145
Injuries by Venomous and Poisonous Animals 1660
Richard W. Carlson

CHAPTER 146
Pharmacologic Agents and Poisoning 1686

Pharmacokinetics in Critically Ill Patients 1686
David R. Rutledge, Michael A. Geheb, Simon Cronin, and Michael P. Peppers

Pharmacologic Poisoning 1702
Michael P. Peppers

Methanol, Ethylene Glycol, and Related Intoxications 1714
James A. Kruse

SECTION THIRTEEN
Ethics 1724
Section Editor, Charles L. Sprung

CHAPTER 147
Ethical Decision Making In Critical Care 1724
H. Tristram Engelhardt, Jr.

CHAPTER 148
Ethical and Legal Aspects of Forgoing Life-Sustaining Treatments 1731
Thomas A. Raffin

CHAPTER 149
The Future of Ethical Issues in Critical Care Medicine ... 1740
Charles L. Sprung

INDEX 1745

Introduction: History and Destiny of Critical Care Medicine

Barry A. Mizock
Max Harry Weil

HISTORY OF CRITICAL CARE MEDICINE

Critical care medicine evolved as a distinct specialty because of a combination of events. The first was that patients whose lives were immediately threatened after traumatic injuries or surgical operations or during the course of a severe illness were sequestered in a hospital area, which facilitated closer observation. Second, striking medical and nursing advances made available lifesaving diagnostic and therapeutic interventions, including antibiotics, defibrillation and resuscitation, external cardiac pacing, endotracheal intubation, mechanical ventilation, neuromuscular blockade, and anticoagulation. Cardiac catheterization, open heart surgery, peritoneal dialysis and hemodialysis, and organ transplantation became realities. The more radically invasive procedures were contingent on uniquely skillful intraoperative and postoperative care. These techniques were of themselves of moment, such as to make it possible to intervene immediately for life preservation, provided that they were available and exercised within the time pressure of an acute event. Third, the special training and, especially, the unique skills and temperament of physicians and nurses who provide such acute care were a scarce resource, and the intensive care unit (ICU) provided an efficient pool of talents to secure their availability. Finally, the life-support environment, including the bedside, with its monitors, and physical space for life-support devices such as ventilators, cardiac assist devices, hemodialysis machines, and infusion pumps, together with the ready availability of special supplies and drugs, called for a physically specialized unit.

Evolution of the Intensive Care Unit

The modern ICU had as its predecessor the postoperative recovery room, stemming from the era of Florence Nightingale. In the 1860s, she brought to the public's attention the importance of establishing a separate area within the hospital in which postoperative patients could be closely monitored during their recovery after surgical operations. In 1923, W. E. Dandy helped to establish the first American ICU for postoperative recovery of neurosurgical patients. The creation of surgical units was in part spurred on by catastrophic events with mass casualties, especially the Cocoanut Grove fire in Boston in 1942. Because of the need to care efficiently for a very large number of burn casualties, a special unit was created at the Massachusetts General Hospital. Postoperative recovery units were also established at the Mayo Clinic and at the Strong Memorial Hospital in 1942, at New York Hospital in 1944, and at the Ochsner Clinic in 1947. The first postoperative cardiac unit was established in 1951 in Boston by Dwight Harken, a founder of heart surgery at the Harvard Medical School and Peter Bent Brigham Hospital. For practical purposes, these were anesthesia recovery units that provided primarily monitoring for patients in the hours after a surgical procedure. The current ICUs, for postoperative care for intervals exceeding 24 hours, were to evolve some 15 years later. The modern surgical ICU with a capacity for prolonged monitoring was a development of the 1960s.

Historically, ICUs were organized to serve specific purposes. We have already mentioned postoperative monitoring and the postanesthesia recovery unit. Subsequently, medical units that would improve airway management and provide for mechanical ventilation, the current respiratory care units, evolved. This was followed by units for cardiac rhythm monitoring, which were the predecessors of the modern coronary care units.

The earliest respiratory care units were also developed in response to a crisis, the poliomyelitis epidemic, in an effort to treat acute ventilatory failure more efficiently. During the late 1940s, respiratory support for poliomyelitis victims was limited to negative pressure ventilation, using tank ventilators, or manual bagging of patients by armies of volunteers after endotracheal intubation or tracheostomy. In Los Angeles (between 1948 and 1949) and Scandinavia (in 1949 and 1952), such lifesaving sustenance of patients with bulbar poliomyelitis was recognized. In 1952 the newly developed Engström positive pressure ventilator was shown to be an effective life-support device for patients with paralytic poliomyelitis, with improved survival compared with that with negative pressure ventilation. Other technologic developments would facilitate management of the airway and prolonged mechanical ventilation. Respiratory care with mechanical ventilation was subsequently extended to the care of patients with respiratory failure of other causes. Specialized respiratory care units were subsequently established in Toronto, Canada; Southampton, England; Baltimore, Maryland; and Uppsala, Sweden.

The introduction of hemodynamic monitoring and management was spurred by the shock and trauma units. The first shock unit was established at the University of Southern California in 1959 by Weil and Shubin. It was initially a clinical research unit with a focus on improving understanding of the pathophysiology and therapy of shock by study of patients. Patients who presented with circulatory shock caused by myocardial infarction, drug overdose, sepsis, and hypovolemia were initially investigated. Invasive techniques of hemodynamic monitoring were evolved, together with respiratory and metabolic measurements. Measurements of central venous pressure, arterial pressure, blood lactate concentration, and arterial blood gases became routine for diagnosis and assessment of the severity of shock states, and concepts of titrated fluid and drug therapy guided by these measurements were developed. The first bedside computer system was also developed in this unit to facilitate monitoring, data acquisition, trend plotting, and automation of procedures. Special devices for computer-controlled measurements of cardiac output, urine flow, and respiratory frequency and pumps for automated infusion of fluids were developed. A "stat" laboratory was installed adjacent to the ICUs. This laboratory demonstrated the value of automated testing, supported by a computer system, for measurements of blood and urine.

The concept of coronary care was sparked to a large extent by Claude Beck's observations that the sudden deaths that followed even minor myocardial injury with no major structural changes were due to ventricular fibrillation. This could be reversed by electrical cardioversion and potentially prevented by pharmacologic interventions. Because many of these fatalities occurred before hospital transfer, and especially within the first 1 to 2 hours after myocardial infarction, a parallel system of mobile coronary care units was evolved to facilitate monitoring and resuscitation during the vulnerable period before admission to the coronary care unit. This mobile resuscitation system was deemed a major advance because of the capability to resuscitate approximately one third of patients who had out-of-hospital cardiac arrest after myocardial infarction. Ventricular arrhythmias, especially

1

ventricular fibrillation, were the major cause of mortality after myocardial infarction, and immediate defibrillation by electrical countershock was remarkably effective.

The first cardiac care units were established in the early 1960s in Kansas City by Day, in Philadelphia by Meltzer, and in Toronto by Brown. These units were intended to monitor and treat potentially fatal arrhythmias after myocardial infarction. After hospital admission, the coronary care unit provided continuous electrocardiographic monitoring with preparation for immediate electrical and pharmacologic interventions by which otherwise fatal ventricular arrhythmias were prevented or reversed.

The intermediate coronary care unit was proposed as part of progressive coronary care in which cardiac patients could be transferred to an area where noninvasive monitoring could be extended for periods of a week or more. Routine monitoring of patients beyond the fifth hospital day in a specially equipped and staffed area separate from the cardiac care unit was implemented in 1971 by the late William Grace. The step-down concept itself had been implemented as early as 1968 for noninvasive monitoring of noncardiac patients after discharge from the ICU, in part with aid of telemetric monitors. Accordingly, the intermediate care unit now served as a bidirectional resource for intensive care—as a step-up area for patients requiring more intensive monitoring or nursing care than could be provided on the general wards as well as a step-down unit from the highest level of intensity of care. The intermediate care unit thereby decreases demand for scarce ICU beds and improves critical care availability.

Neonatal ICUs had their origins in premature nurseries that were organized in France during the late 19th century. The first premature nurseries in the United States were established in Chicago at the Lying-In Hospital in 1900. Modern neonatal care was fostered not only by electrical and mechanical cardiac and respiratory advances of monitoring and management but also by advances in microchemistry techniques developed in Scandinavia during the 1950s. These techniques made it possible to monitor arterial blood gases and electrolytes in low-birth-weight infants. Neonatal care in the United States was subsequently regionalized, with a system of referral centers for high-risk infants. Remarkable improvement in survival was observed in populations served by this system. However, other pediatric ICUs were opened only after the evolution of adult units in the late 1960s.

We currently recognize four systems by which critical care services are organized within the hospital: (1) by traditional specialty service (e.g., medical ICU, surgical ICU); (2) by organ system (e.g., gastrointestinal unit, respiratory care unit); (3) by clinical syndrome (e.g., shock unit, trauma unit, burn unit, stroke unit); and (4) by defined population of patients (e.g., neonatal unit, pediatric unit, obstetric unit).

Critical Care Nursing

Florence Nightingale was influential in proposing a new role for the nurse in the hospital setting. Rather than offering only comfort and body care, the nurse should be a professionally trained and qualified expert who would best assume an active role. Accordingly, Nightingale identified a primary role for the nurse in data gathering and analysis and in the initiation and monitoring of therapy to complement and even control the quality of care of patients. As detailed earlier, her initial focus was on the postoperative setting. Yet, as late as 1953, patients were still transferred from the operating room directly to private rooms or to wards that had more than 30 beds. Their postanesthesia care was typically entrusted to a private duty nurse after the surgical procedure was completed. The private duty nurse

therefore was the sole resource of what is now termed postanesthesia recovery and postoperative care, and the patient was managed in a conventional, nonspecialized medical-surgical bed. Both the training and in-service updating of these nurses were highly variable. Because private duty practice was often independent of the mainstream of the hospital nursing services, these nurses had little opportunity for systematic in-service training and updating.

With the emergence of postoperative units, a new generation of hospital-employed or contracted nurse specialists was born. Their training and practices provided unique competence beyond that of general medical-surgical nursing practitioners. They learned how to operate high-technology devices such as defibrillators and ventilators and became well versed in the indications for and appropriate use of lifesaving drugs. These critical care nurse specialists proved to be the major asset for operation of special care units. Their presence was also of paramount importance in the vast majority of medical centers during the two decades that preceded the availability and full-time dedication of critical care physician specialists. Unfortunately, rapid expansion of the number of intensive care beds was impeded by the limited availability of well-trained and dedicated critical care nurses. The extraordinary demand for their services therefore prompted expansion of training and recruitment programs. Beds were often "closed" because of the shortage of qualified critical care nurses, and in the United States many nurse specialists were recruited from abroad (especially from England, Scandinavia, and the Philippine Islands). Nevertheless, the demand is still not met. Rapid turnover because of irregularity of work hours, extraordinary demands, psychologic stresses in life-and-death settings, and options for financially more rewarding employment perpetuates this shortage. Increases in pay, in part initiated by private nurse registries, have provided some, but incomplete, relief.

The professional critical care nurses in the United States are formally organized as the American Association of Critical Care Nurses, which was established in 1969. The association subsequently developed professional standards and formal examinations for certification of critical care nurse specialists, whom it designated as CCRN (critical care registered nurses). In 1980 the essential role of the nurse specialists was further recognized when they were accepted to full membership in the Society of Critical Care Medicine on a parallel with physician intensivists.

Advances in Monitoring

Critical care monitoring evolved from intraoperative and postoperative monitoring, especially that related to cardiac surgery. Technology for continuous monitoring was also related to that developed for the crewed space efforts during the 1960s. Yet current methods of invasive hemodynamic monitoring had their origin more than 250 years ago. Arterial blood pressure was first measured directly by Hales in 1733 by inserting a brass tube into the carotid artery of a horse. This "cannula" was connected to a glass tube that extended to a height of 9 feet! Internal jugular cannulation was first performed by Bernard in 1844. Ludwig introduced the kymograph for recording arterial waveforms in 1847. Marey in 1881 utilized a pressure transducer made of a rigid tube leading to a metal cage in which a rubber membrane served as the transducing element. Forssmann, in 1929, catheterized his own right atrium under fluoroscopic guidance, for which he was essentially discharged from his hospital post, only to receive a Nobel Prize many years later. The first percutaneous cannulation of the subclavian vein was performed by Aubaniac in 1952. Methods for measuring central venous pressures were developed starting in the

1940s and were clinically applied in the 1950s, especially for patients undergoing thoracotomy. Hughes and Magovern observed that right atrial pressure was a useful indicator of the effective circulating blood volume in the clinical setting.

The flow-directed pulmonary arterial catheter, which has been the most striking innovation in hemodynamic monitoring, was introduced into clinical practice by Swan and Ganz in the early 1970s. This allowed not only intracardiac pressure measurements outside the catheterization laboratory but also routine sampling of mixed venous blood. It made practical use of the Fick equation to estimate cardiac output from the oxygen content of arterial and mixed venous blood and the oxygen consumption, the standard method employed in conjunction with diagnostic cardiac catheterization since the mid-1940s. It also provided the option of measuring cardiac output by the thermodilution technique, which was initially described by Fegler in 1954.

The early method for measuring the oxygenation of blood, and specifically the oxygen content for calculation of oxygen saturation, was a formidable gasometric method of Van Slyke. In 1945 Riley described a method for the direct determination of oxygen and carbon dioxide tensions in blood using a somewhat less cumbersome but still demanding bubble technique. Advances in blood gas analyses followed the development of glass electrodes for blood pH measurements in the 1950s, Severinghaus' PCO_2 electrode in 1958, and the Clark PO_2 electrode in 1956. The availability of routine blood gas measurements by increasingly automated, rapid, and accurate electrode methods revolutionized respiratory management.

Advances in Resuscitation

The history of modern cardiopulmonary resuscitation is rooted in early techniques of open chest cardiac massage described by Schiff in 1874. Its current application is attributed to Claude Beck, who spoke of "hearts too young to die" in the late 1940s. The first successful open chest defibrillation was performed by Beck in 1947. In 1956 Zoll successfully reversed ventricular fibrillation on 11 occasions in four patients with externally applied alternating-current countershocks, and this was followed by external direct-current defibrillation based on work by Peleska and Lown in the mid-1950s. Transthoracic needle puncture of the heart, first performed by Pike in 1908, was subsequently used widely to administer cardiotonic drugs directly into the left ventricle but was abandoned when central venous catheters came into routine use. Hyman, in 1932, pioneered electrical pacing of the heart with transthoracic needles, which were advanced into the right atrium. Epicardial electrodes were implanted during heart surgery for postoperative use in 1957, and Furman and Schwedel made a major contribution to cardiology, and subsequently to emergency and critical care practice, when they introduced the transvenous route for insertion of ventricular pacemakers in 1958. The era of closed chest cardiac massage followed a landmark report by Kouwenhoven and colleagues in 1960. The National Research Council, in collaboration with the American Heart Association, first published the consensus of experts as recommendations for cardiopulmonary resuscitation in 1966. These were directed to the training of medical and allied health workers and stressed airway management and external chest compression. Protocols for advanced life support were subsequently developed during the National Conference on Cardiopulmonary Resuscitation in 1973. Safar and colleagues more recently introduced the concept of brain resuscitation, that is, cardiopulmonary cerebral resuscitation.

The issue of brain death, particularly global cerebral ischemia after initially successful cardiac resuscitation, was brought up by Mollaret and Goulon in 1959. It provoked both professional and legal dilemmas. An ad hoc committee of the Harvard Medical School agreed on clinical criteria of brain death in 1968. This prompted revision of the legal definition of death by each of the state legislatures and abandonment of absence of the heartbeat as the sole criterion of death.

The Shock Unit at the University of Southern California pioneered protocols for fluid resuscitation guided by invasive hemodynamic monitoring for patients with circulatory shock. The first trauma units in the United States were established in the early 1960s at Cook County Hospital by Shoemaker and at the University of Maryland Hospital in Baltimore by Cowley. Remarkable improvements in the survival of trauma victims were ushered in by establishment of paramedic-staffed emergency medical systems and trauma centers staffed by well-trained surgical specialists and anesthesiologists who were, in fact, specialized surgical intensivists.

Advances in Organ Support

The earliest organ support devices were developed to sustain the airway and support ventilation. The endotracheal tube, devised by Pugh in 1754, was intended for resuscitation of neonates. It was an air pipe constructed from coiled wire and covered with soft leather and was inserted into the trachea through the mouth without direct visualization. The first endotracheal tube that included an inflatable cuff was designed in 1871 by the famed surgeon Trendelenburg. This was a major advance because the cuff prevented aspiration and strikingly reduced the incidence of postoperative pneumonia.

The earliest tank ventilator was developed during the 1920s by Drinker and manufactured by the Emerson Company of Boston. It had its largest application for life support of poliomyelitis victims. The next major advances in mechanical ventilation were the positive pressure valve and the subsequent work by Barach with the introduction of continuous positive pressure breathing. This technique used a pressure source of gas and the patient's exhalation against a specific resistance. Ibsen first used a positive pressure ventilator for clinical management of patients during the poliomyelitis epidemic in Scandinavia in 1952 as an alternative to negative pressure ventilators. This greatly facilitated access to the patient for nursing care. Nevertheless, tank ventilators remained the standard of care in the United States until about 1960. Initially, pressure-controlled valves were hazardous or the intermittent positive pressure devices delivered unpredictable volumes with changes in airway resistance. Mörch is credited with the development in 1955 of the first volume-controlled ventilator using a piston, but it had the disadvantage that there was no means of override by or coordination with the patient. The Engström constant-volume ventilator, introduced in the late 1950s, largely resolved the problem of coordinating the demands of the patient and the output of the ventilator. Positive end-expiratory pressure was subsequently introduced as an option for improving alveolar oxygen exchange. It was brought forth for wide clinical application in 1969 by Ashbaugh and Petty, who pioneered the recognition of adult respiratory distress syndrome and provided impressive guidelines for its management.

One of the most striking advances was in the management of acute renal failure. Hemodialysis was invented by Kolff in 1938 and introduced in the United States in 1947. Its application was greatly simplified and expedited with development of routines for both arterial and venous catherization and the ready availability of systems for both arterio-venous and venovenous dialysis. Lifesaving reversal of renal failure was further secured by the subsequent introduction of peritoneal dialysis.

Blood banking, begun by Fantus at Cook County Hospital in Chicago in 1937, was perhaps the single important life-support development that allowed rapid advances in highly invasive surgical procedures and in the resuscitation of trauma victims, both civilian and military. It opened the door to the development of radical cancer surgery and cardiac surgery.

In 1953 Gibbon succeeded, after a professional lifetime of dedication, in developing extracorporeal circulation, the heart-lung machine, which in turn started the era of open heart operations. The intra-aortic balloon counterpulsation catheter became available for more protracted circulatory support in 1962.

Multidisciplinary Approach to Management of the Critically Ill Patient

The early postoperative recovery rooms and ICUs were largely the domain of anesthesiologists and surgeons. It was the special skills of the anesthesiologists in airway management, ventilatory support, and pharmacologic support of the circulation that allowed them to extend their professional care to the immediate postoperative setting. The involvement of internists was primarily by way of the early cardiac care (and shock) units. Yet, it was soon apparent to those who provided acute care that a commonality of knowledge, skills, technology, and support services was involved. This prompted a multidisciplinary approach to both the medical and surgical management by doctors and nurses who were to provide full-time services in acute care units. The concept of multidisciplinary intensive care together with emergency care was developed and implemented first in 1958 by Safar at Baltimore City Hospital and subsequently by his group of anesthesiologists at the University of Pittsburgh. The first center that specifically included internal medicine, surgery, anesthesia, obstetrics-gynecology, and neurosurgery with a multidisciplinary team of dedicated intensivists was established at the University of Southern California by Weil and Shubin in 1967. This approach is not yet universally accepted, although it is apparent that the alternative of care by multiple subspecialists who focused on one specific organ or organ system ("organ protectionism") often failed to provide comprehensive and predictable lifesaving care in the absence of a responsible and qualified intensivist.

Essential for this multidisciplinary approach was the presence 24 hours a day of a physician trained in diagnosis and management of life-threatening diseases. In major medical centers, the model that evolved was that of a team headed by a physician, anesthesiologist, pediatrician, or surgeon who assumed responsibility for the overall clinical management of the patient; coordinated and implemented the recommendations made by consultants; directed the team with support for the essential role of nurses, therapists, and technicians; and served as a continuing source of information and advocate for the patient and the family. In teaching hospitals, this physician also served as an educator for house staff, nursing staff, therapists, and technicians. This physician's duties further included an administrative role, especially that of priority assignments of beds when there was competing need. His or her continuing presence not only facilitated clinical and operational decision making but also improved staff morale and retention and especially the quality of care of patients.

Yet the initial efforts to establish multidisciplinary units were often constrained by a perceived conflict with the traditional autonomy of the attending physician and the conventional independent authority of the consulting physician.

Parallel developments in emergency medicine were instrumental in bringing national focus on the critically ill and injured. Indeed, this served as a stimulus for the Highway Safety Act of 1966, which provided for improvements in ambulance services and provision for life-support training for ambulance personnel, and the subsequent evolution of the paramedic-staffed emergency medical systems in the United States. The early emergency rooms were previously staffed by primary care physicians. Emergency medicine itself evolved into a recognized and certifiable specialty with formal residency training programs in the late 1970s.

With the recognition that the practice of critical care medicine would require a substantial number of specially trained physicians, fellowship training programs in critical care medicine were begun at the University of Southern California in 1961 and at the University of Pittsburgh in 1963.

In 1968, a group of physicians assembled in Los Angeles at the invitation of Max Harry Weil and Herbert Shubin and with the close collaboration of Peter Safar, William Shoemaker, and William Grace. Some 20 physicians, surgeons, anesthesiologists, and pediatricians became the founders of the Society of Critical Care Medicine in 1970. Their initial focus was on education and organization. Critical Care Medicine began as the journal of the society in 1973. Soon thereafter, discussions with the subspecialty organizations were initiated to identify relationships between the practice of critical care medicine and the conventional acute subspecialty disciplines. Ake Grenvik of Pittsburgh formally approached the American Board of Medical Specialities as the representative of the Society of Critical Care Medicine with the proposal that formal board certification be accorded to critical care medicine. There was initial support for a multidisciplinary career-structured intensivist, but the specialty boards were not in accord on the content, duration, and operation of training programs and the requirements for multidisciplinary certification. This ultimately led four of the major specialty boards, namely the American Boards of Medicine, Surgery, Pediatrics, and Anesthesia, to elect separate subspecialty or specialized competence certification under each of their separate auspices.

Growth of Critical Care Medicine

There is increasing demand for critical care. In 1960, there were organized ICUs in less than 10% of American hospitals of more than 200 beds. In 1981, more than 95% of all American hospitals had ICUs. The overall number of ICU beds has increased annually by approximately 4%. A consensus development conference held at the National Institutes of Health in 1973 defined critical care medicine as "a multidisciplinary and multiprofessional medical-nursing field concerned with patients who have sustained or are at risk of sustaining acutely life-threatening single- or multiple-organ failure because of disease or injury."

CRITICAL CARE MEDICINE: FUTURE TRENDS

The role of the intensivist has gradually expanded beyond conventional bedside care in the ICU. There have been changes in the economic milieu, the emergence of complex ethical and legal issues related to the indications for critical care, and developments in both evaluation and care of patients who are at high risk before surgery, after traumatic injuries, or for other reasons and who may be hospitalized outside the ICU.

The Cost-Benefit Issues of Critical Care

One of the key issues that has both ethical and economic implications is whether there is objective evidence that the benefits of critical care outweigh their emotional stress on patients, invasiveness, and high economic costs. It is difficult because of both ethical and strategic restraints to conduct randomized trials by which benefits and both biologic and economic detriments would be better exposed. However, there is consensus that survival alone is not likely to be the sole criterion. Critical care may be appropriate because of its beneficial effect on subsequent function and lifestyle of the patient and the efficiency of hospital care. Even more, the responsibility perceived by both society and physicians is to provide life-threatened patients with critical care for both professional and humanistic reasons, even at the twilight of life.

These considerations notwithstanding, there is evidence for improved outcome when critically ill patients are managed in competent ICU settings, especially when physicians who are trained in critical care medicine are in attendance. Especially in teaching hospitals, care of the most critically ill patients, particularly at times other than the usual workday, was traditionally delegated to the most junior house staff. This has been referred to as the inverse hierarchy principle. These trends have been substantially reversed. Brown and collaborators reported that ICU mortality was reduced by 52% when responsibility for management of patients was maintained on a full-time, in-house basis by a qualified intensivist. Such observations and especially increases in survival of critically ill patients have been supported by other observers. There are also economic considerations in that the length of ICU stay may be abbreviated when care is directed by a critical care specialist. This may be explained, at least in part, by earlier diagnosis and intervention and prompt recognition of failure of response to a specific therapeutic intervention.

Nevertheless, both government and industry with the involvement of third-party payers are cognizant of seemingly escalating costs for critical care. The cost of delivering care in an ICU is approximately 3.8 times greater than that of general medical-surgical care. Furthermore, the costs of hospitalization in an ICU are consumed disproportionately by the patients who have the least likelihood of survival at the terminus of life. The critical care provider is therefore challenged to reduce the high cost of procedure-oriented care that is currently rendered without rigorous test of clinical benefit. Moreover, the implementation of diagnosis-related groups in which reimbursement is primarily related to diagnosis rather than the services rendered has made critical care services a special target for cost savings. This focus on cost containment in critical care has brought forth the concept of more selective care for patients who do not have high likelihood of benefit. Yet, the capability for predicting outcome is, as yet, primitive when it is applied to individual patients. The intensivist therefore is in the uncomfortable role of the gatekeeper. More recently, this had engendered some emotional debates on the subject of "rationing." The profession has responded by increasing utilization of intermediate care beds and hospices. It is also recognized that quality-of-life issues are appropriately addressed when critical care services are offered to the individual patient and his or her family. Patients and their surrogates increasingly reject prolongation of life unless it is meaningful. The issues become more complex when either or both the patient and the family regard benefits of critical care independently of the advice of physicians or nurses. Nevertheless, the obligation of the intensivist is to present the options objectively, including those that apply to the terminally ill or functionally deprived, and abide by the decisions that reflect the wishes of the patient or his or her surrogate. Demand for ICU beds may therefore be reduced with full ethical and medical justification when patients choose to forgo ICU treatment. Greater availability of hospice care would be likely to decrease the demand for ICU beds and provide for the terminally ill, who so often choose to "die with dignity."

Access to Medical Technology—Health Care: A Right or a Luxury?

The rapid evolution of complex and expensive life-support technology has created stressful ethical and economic dilemmas. Are patients to be kept alive by this technology for protracted periods, and who will pay for the costs of this care? Court decisions, in contrast to those of the government and industry, generally reject cost-benefit concepts. The current epidemic of acquired immunodeficiency syndrome has created an especially urgent call for resolution of such dilemmas. Comparable dilemmas involve organ transplantation, especially who is an appropriate candidate, who will provide the organs, and who will be responsible for the extraordinarily high costs of initial and continuing care.

The resolution of such questions will in part come from intensive research through which the natural history and outcomes of critical illnesses are better understood and quantitated. Potential improvement in utilization and efficiency of critical care services may be forthcoming from the developing technology itself. Perhaps the most likely and historically most potent option is that of preventive medicine, by which the causes of degenerative diseases are addressed and treated and requirements for critical care services are decreased. Yet, this may not suffice because increases in life expectancy, in part related to the survival of critically ill patients of itself, increase the demand. Even though the patients are progressively older and may be less diseased at younger ages, we are likely to struggle to keep up with the demands of a rapidly enlarging geriatric population.

We therefore respect the skills of modern intensivists not only because of the clinical acumen and medical expertise that they bring to the bedside but also because of their important human, ethical, and leadership roles in the delivery of critical care services. We quote Leigh Thompson from his chapter in the book The ICU—A Cost Benefit Analysis: "Critical care physicians must be leaders in defining realistic resources, employing them with maximum efficiency, and educating all their peers and their patients to the benefits and risks of critical care."

Bibliography

Ad Hoc Committee of the Harvard Medical School: A definition of irreversible coma: Report of the Ad Hoc Committee of the Harvard Medical School to examine the definition of brain death. JAMA 205:337, 1968.

American Hospital Association: Hospital Statistics—1981. Chicago, American Hospital Association, 1982.

Ashbaugh DG, Petty TL, Bigelow DB, et al: Continuous positive-pressure breathing (CPPB) in adult respiratory distress syndrome. J Thorac Cardiovasc Surg 57:31, 1969.

Aubaniac R: L'injection intraveineuse sousclaviculaire: avantage et technique. Presse Med 60:1456, 1952.

Avery EE, Mörch ET, Benson D: Critically crushed chest: A new method of treatment with continuous mechanical hyperventilation to produce alkalotic apnea and internal pneumatic stabilization. J Thorac Surg 32:291, 1956.

Ayers SM: Introduction: Critical care medicine. In: Ayers SM, Schlichtig R, Sterling MJ (eds): Care of the Critically Ill. Chicago, Year Book Medical Publishers, p xvii, 1988.

Barach AL, Martin J, Eckman M: Positive pressure respiration and its application to the treatment of acute pulmonary edema. Ann Intern Med 12:754, 1938.

Basson MD: Choosing among candidates for scarce medical resources. J Med Philos 4:313, 1979.

Bayer R, Callahan D, Fletcher J, et al: The care of the terminally ill: Morality and economics. N Engl J Med 309, 1490, 1983.

Beck CS, Leighninger DS: Death after a clean bill of health. JAMA 174:133, 1960.

Beck CS, Pritchard H, Feil SH: Ventricular fibrillation of long duration abolished by electric shock. JAMA 135:985, 1947.

Beck CS, Weckesser EC, Barry FM: Fatal heart attack and successful defibrillation. JAMA 161:434, 1956.

Bernard C: Leçons sur la Chaleur Animale. Paris, Ballière, p 42, 1876.

Birnbaum JL: Cost-containment in critical care. Crit Care Med 14:1068, 1986.

Blackhall LJ, Cobb J, Moskowitz MA: Discussions regarding aggressive care with critically ill patients. J Gen Intern Med 4:399, 1989.

Bone RC: Let's represent the interest of our patients. Chest 91:317, 1987.

Bone RC: Outcomes in critical care medicine. JAMA 260:3487, 1988.

Bower AG, Bennett VR, Dillon JR: Investigation on the care and treatment of poliomyelitis patients. Ann West Med Surg 4:561, 687, 1950.

Brown JJ, Sullivan G: Effect on ICU mortality of a full-time critical care specialist. Chest 96:127, 1989.

Brown KWG, MacMillan RL, Forbath N: Coronary unit: An intensive care centre for acute myocardial infarction. Lancet 2:349, 1963.

Bryan-Brown CW: Pathway to the present: A personal view of critical care. In: Civetta JA, Taylor RW, Kirby RR (eds): Critical Care. Philadelphia, JB Lippincott, p 1641, 1988.

Cady LD Jr, Whitston CW, Weil MH: Optimizing the use of critical care beds. Hospitals 46:58, 1972.

Civetta JM: Setting objectives: Perspectives for care. In: Civetta JA, Taylor RW, Kirby RR (eds): Critical Care. Philadelphia, JB Lippincott, p 5, 1988.

Clark LC: Monitor and control of blood and tissue oxygen tensions. Trans Am Soc Artif Intern Organs 2:41, 1956.

Claus KE, Bailey JT: Living with Stress and Promoting Well-Being: A Handbook for Nurses. St Louis, CV Mosby, 1980.

Consensus conference: Critical care medicine. JAMA 250:798, 1983.

Cullen DJ: Reassessing critical care: Illness, outcome and cost. Crit Care Med 17:S172, 1989.

Danis M, Gerrity MS, Southerland LI, et al: A comparison of patient, family and physician assessments of the value of medical intensive care. Crit Care Med 16:594, 1988.

Day HW: An intensive coronary care area. Dis Chest 44:423, 1963.

Drinker P, Shaw LA: Apparatus for prolonged administration of artificial respiration: Design for adults and children. J Clin Invest 7:229, 1929.

Engelhardt HT, Rie MA: Intensive care units, scarce resources, and conflicting principles of justice. JAMA 255:1159, 1986.

Engström CG: Treatment of severe cases of respiratory paralysis by the Engström Universal Respirator. Br Med J 2:666, 1954.

Fairly HB: The Toronto General Hospital Respirator Unit. Anaesthesia 16:267, 1961.

Fantus B: Therapy of Cook County Hospital; blood preservation. JAMA 109:128, 1937.

Fegler G: Measurement of cardiac output in anaesthetized animals by a thermodilution method. Q J Exp Physiol 39:153, 1954.

Fick A; Hoff HE, Scott HJ, trans: Über die Messung des Blutquantums in den Herzventrikeln. 1870. N Engl J Med 239:122, 1948.

Field BE, Devich LE, Carlson RW: Impact of a comprehensive supportive care team on management of hopelessly ill patients with multiple organ failure. Chest 96:353, 1989.

Forssmann W: Die Sondierung des rechten Herzens. Klin Wochenschr 8:2085, 1929.

Franklin CM, Rackow EC, Mamdani B, et al: Decreases in mortality on a large urban medical service by facilitating access to critical care. Arch Intern Med 148:1403, 1988.

Frumin MJ, Bergman NA, Holaday DA, et al: Alveolar-arterial O_2 differences during artificial respiration in man. J Appl Physiol 14:694, 1959.

Gibbon JH: Application of a mechanical heart and lung apparatus to cardiac surgery. Minn Med 37:171, 1954.

Gotsman MS, Schrire V: Acute myocardial infarction—an ideal concept of progressive coronary care. S Afr Med J 42:829, 1968.

Grace WJ, Keyloun V: The natural history of patients with acute myocardial infarction. In: Grace WJ, Keyloun V (eds): The Coronary Care Unit. New York, Appleton-Century-Crofts, p 2, 1970.

Grace WJ, Yarvote PM: Acute myocardial infarction: The course of the illness following discharge from the coronary care unit. Chest 59:15, 1971.

Harvey AM: Neurosurgical genius—Walter Edward Dandy. Johns Hopkins Med J 135:358, 1974.

Hilberman M: The evolution of intensive care units. Crit Care Med 3:159, 1975.

Hill DW, Dolan AM: The measurement of blood pressure. In: Hill DW, Dolan AM (eds): Intensive Care Instrumentation. London, Academic Press, p 1, 1982.

Holmdahl MH: The respiratory care unit. Anesthesiology 23:559, 1962.

Hughes RE, Magovern GJ: The relationship between right atrial pressure and blood volume. Arch Surg 79:238, 1959.

Hyman AS: Resuscitation of the stopped heart by intra-cardiac therapy. Arch Intern Med 50:283, 1932.

Ibsen B: The anesthetist's viewpoint on the treatment of respiratory complications in poliomyelitis during the epidemic in Copenhagen in 1952. Proc R Soc Med 47:72, 1954.

Jennett B: The way ahead for acute hospital services: Delay cure or deny rescue? Lancet 2:1235, 1976.

Jennett B: Inappropriate use of intensive care. Br Med J 289:1709, 1984.

Jude JR, Kouwenhoven WB, Knickerbocker GC: External cardiac resuscitation. Monogr Surg Sci 1:59, 1964.

Kalb PE, Miller DH: Utilization strategies for intensive care units. JAMA 261:2389, 1989.

Kelley MA: Critical care medicine—a new specialty? N Engl J Med 318:1613, 1988.

King EG: Accreditation without certification: Critical care training in Canada. Crit Care Med 15:978, 1987.

King EG, Sibbald WJ: The territorial imperative. Chest 93:1121, 1988.

Klaus MH, Kennell JH: Mothers separated from their newborn infants. Pediatr Clin North Am 17:1015, 1970.

Klem SA, Pollack MM, Getson PR: Cost, resource utilization and severity of illness in intensive care. J Pediatr 116:231, 1990.

Knaus WA: Rationing, justice and the American physician. JAMA 255:1176, 1986.

Knaus WA, Draper EA, Wagner DP: The use of intensive care: New research initiatives and their implications for national health policy. Milbank Mem Fund Q 61:561, 1983.

Koch EB, Reiser SJ: Critical care: historical development and ethical considerations. In: Fein IA, Strosberg MA (eds): Managing the Critical Care Unit. Rockville, MD, Aspen Publishers, p 3, 1987.

Kolff WJ: New Ways of Treating Uraemia. London, Churchill Livingstone, 1947.

Kouwenhoven WB, Jude JR, Knickerbocker GC: Closed chest cardiac massage. JAMA 173:1064, 1960.

Landis EM, Hortenstine JC: Functional significance of venous blood pressure. Physiol Rev 30:1, 1950.

Langrehr D, Miranda DR, West KJ: The benefits of intensive care. In: Miranda DR, Langrehr D (eds): The ICU—A Cost-Benefit Analysis. Amsterdam, Elsevier, p 127, 1986.

Lassen HCA: Preliminary report on the 1952 epidemic of poliomyelitis in Copenhagen. Lancet 1:37:1953.

Li TCM, Phillips MC, Shaw L, et al: On-site physician staffing in a community hospital intensive care unit. JAMA 252:2023, 1984.

Lown B, Neuman J, Amarasingham R, et al: Comparison of alternating current with direct current electroshock across the closed chest. Am J Cardiol 10:233, 1962.

Luce JM, Dalen JE, Soffer A: Critical care medicine is here to stay. Chest 90:309, 1986.

Ludwig C: Beitrage zur Kenntniss des Einflusses der Respirations Bewegungen auf den Blutlauf im Aortensysteme. Muller's Arch Anat, p 240, 1847.

Mason RL: Preoperative and Postoperative Care. Philadelphia, WB Saunders, p 108, 1937.

Massachusetts General Hospital: Management of the Cocoanut Grove Burns at the Massachusetts General Hospital. Philadelphia, JB Lippincott, 1943.

McKay JE: Historical review of emergency medical services, EMT roles and EMT utilization in emergency departments. J Emerg Med 11:27, 1985.

Meltzer LE, Kitchell JB: The incidence of arrhythmias associated with acute myocardial infarction. Prog Cardiovasc Dis 9:50, 1966.

Mollaret P, Goulon M: Le coma dépasse. Rev Neurol 101;3, 1959.

Mörch ET: History of mechanical ventilation. In: Kirby RR, Smith RA, Desautels DA (eds): Mechanical Ventilation. New York, Churchill Livingstone, p 1, 1985.

Mouloupoulos SD, Topaz S, Kolff WJ: Diastolic balloon pumping (with carbon dioxide) in the aorta: Mechanical assistance to the failing circulation. Am Heart J 63:669, 1962.

Nightingale F: Notes on Hospitals. 3rd ed. London, Longman & Green, p 89, 1863.

Ochsner AJ: Recovery rooms contribute to better patient care. Hospitals 24:50, 1950.

Olsen GN: Certification in critical care medicine: Why? Ann Intern Med 106:914, 1987.

Paneth N, Kiely JL, Wallenstein S, et al: Newborn intensive care and neonatal mortality in low-birth-weight infants: A population study. N Engl J Med 307:149, 1982.

Pantridge JF: Mobile coronary care. Chest 58:229, 1970.

Pantridge JF, Geddes JS: Cardiac arrest after myocardial infarction. Lancet 1:807, 1966.

Pantridge JF, Geddes JS: A mobile intensive-care unit in the management of myocardial infarction. Lancet 2:271, 1967.

Pearce DJ: Experiences in a small respiratory unit of a general hospital. Anaesthesia 16:308, 1961.

Peleska B: Transthoracic and direct defibrillation. Rozhl Chir 36:731, 1957.

Pike FJ, Guthrie CC, Steward GN: Studies in resuscitation. J Exp Med 10:371, 1908.

Relman AS: Intensive-care units: Who needs them? N Engl J Med 302:965, 1980.

Rettig R: End-Stage Renal Disease and the "Cost" of Medical Technology. Santa Monica, CA, Rand Corporation, October 1977. Rand Paper Series.

Reynolds HN, Haupt MT, Thill-Baharozian MC, et al: Impact of critical care physician staffing on patients with septic shock in a university hospital medical intensive care unit. JAMA 260:3446, 1988.

Riley RL, Proemmel DD, Frank RE: Direct method for determination of oxygen and carbon dioxide tensions in blood. J Biol Chem 161:621, 1945.

Safar P: The critical care medicine continuum from scene to outcome. In: Parillo JE, Ayres SM (eds): Major Issues in Critical Care Medicine. Baltimore, Williams & Wilkins, p 71, 1984.

Safar P (ed): Advances in Cardiopulmonary Resuscitation: Proceedings of the Wolf Creek Conference. New York, Springer-Verlag, 1975.

Safar P, DeKornfeld TJ, Person JM: The intensive care unit. Anaesthesia 16:275, 1961.

Schecter DC: Background of clinical cardiac electrostimulation. VII. Modern era of artificial cardiac pacemakers. NY State J Med 72:1166, 1972.

Schragg MA, Albertson TE: Moral, ethical and legal dilemmas in the intensive care unit. Crit Care Med 12:62, 1984.

Severinghaus JW: Recent developments in blood O_2 and CO_2 electrodes. In: Woolmer RF (ed): pH and Blood Gas Measurements. London, Churchill, p 126, 1959.

Shubin H, Weil MH: Bacterial shock: A serious complication in urological practice. JAMA 185:850, 1963.

Swan HCJ, Ganz W, Forrester JS, et al: Catheterization of the heart in man with use of a flow directed balloon-tipped catheter. N Engl J Med 283:447, 1970.

Thompson MH, Khot AS: Impact of neonatal intensive care. Arch Dis Child 60:213, 1985.

Thompson WL: Critical care tomorrow: Economics and challenges. Crit Care Med 10:561, 1982.

Thompson WL: The future of critical care in the United States of America. In: Miranda DR, Langrehr D (eds): The ICU—A Cost-Benefit Analysis. Amsterdam, Elsevier, p 199, 1986.

Trendelenburg F: Beiträge zu den Operationen an den Luftwegen. Tamponade der Trachea. Arch Klin Chir 12:121, 1871.

Wagner DP, Wineland TD, Knaus WA: The hidden costs of treating severely ill patients: Charges and resource consumption in an intensive care unit. Health Care Finance Rev 5:81, 1983.

Weil MH: Current concepts on the management of shock. Circulation 16:1097, 1957.

Weil MH, Rackow EC: Critical care medicine: Caveat emptor. Arch Intern Med 143:1391, 1983.

Weil MH, Shubin H: Critical care medicine. I. the "VIP" approach to the bedside management of shock. JAMA 207:337, 1969.

Weil MH, Shubin H: Centers for the critically ill. Symposium on care of the critically ill. Mod Med 39:86, 1971.

Weil MH, Shubin H, Biddle M: Shock caused by gram negative microorganisms: Analysis of 169 cases. Ann Intern Med 60:384, 1964.

Weil MH, Shubin H, Rand W: Experience with a digital computer for study and improved management of the critically ill. JAMA 198:1011, 1966.

Weil MH, Shubin H, Faber DA, et al: A new approach to critical care units. Hospitals 45:65, 1971.

Weil MH, Michaels S, Puri VK, et al: The stat laboratory. Am J Clin Pathol 76:34, 1981.

Weil MH, Shoemaker WC, Rackow EC: Competent and continuing care of the critically ill. Crit Care Med 16:298, 1988.

Weil MH, Von Planta M, Rackow EC: Critical care medicine: Introduction and historical perspective. In: Shoemaker WC, Ayres S, Grenvik A, et al (eds): Textbook of Critical Care. Philadelphia, WB Saunders, p 1, 1989.

White GMJ: Evolution of endotracheal and endobronchial intubation. Br J Anaesth 32:235, 1960.

Wiklund PE: Intensive care units: Design, location, staffing, ancillary areas, equipment. Anesthesiology 31:122, 1969.

Williams RL, Chen P: Identifying the sources of the recent decline in perinatal mortality rates in California. N Engl J Med 306:207, 1982.

Williamson J: Geriatric medicine: Whose specialty? Ann Intern Med 91:774, 1979.

Wright MP: pH measurement with the glass electrode. In: Woolmer RF (ed): pH and Blood Gas Measurements. London, Churchill, p 250, 1959.

Zoll PM, Linenthal AJ, Gibson W, et al: Termination of ventricular fibrillation in man by externally applied countershock. N Engl J Med 254:727, 1956.

SECTION ONE

Sequential and Organizational Aspects of Intensive Care

Section Editors

Richard W. Carlson and Michael A. Geheb

Emergency Medical Service Systems and Prehospital Management of Patients Requiring Critical Care

Paul E. Pepe

The entity of emergency medical service (EMS), as a formal profession, is only two decades old; yet it is now demanded as a public service and almost taken for granted in the United States.[1] However, few members of the medical community (let alone the public at large) know the difference between various levels of prehospital care providers. This lack of knowledge becomes relevant because in many cases, by law, members of the medical community are explicitly accountable for determining (and guaranteeing) the level of care provided by both individuals and groups of EMS personnel.[2, 3] Specifically, critical care practitioners not only receive but also send patients by ground ambulance, yet few practitioners have a working knowledge of the actual capabilities and government regulations involved in the operation of the various medical transport vehicles. Furthermore, the prehospital setting is rapidly becoming *the* key venue for resuscitation research as well as early critical care interventions, including those for cardiac arrest, serious trauma, myocardial infarction, and respiratory insufficiency. This chapter reviews (1) the scope of EMS as a *system of care*, (2) the basic training levels for various EMS personnel, and (3) the management strategies for two key critical care functions of EMS, trauma and cardiopulmonary resuscitation (CPR).

SYSTEM COMPONENTS
Emergency Medical Service System: The Chain of Survival Concept

Most people who die prematurely in our communities do so as a result of unheralded cardiac arrest caused by sudden primary ventricular fibrillation (VF).[4–6] It is the first symptom in as many as 25% of those with coronary artery disease.[4] Without intervention, VF is lethal within a few minutes. Similarly, provision for the earliest possible definitive care for many types of critical injury (the number one killer of Americans under the age of 45) has been shown to be pivotal to survival. As a result, intensive care of the critically ill or injured must begin in the prehospital setting. Therefore, both lifesaving trauma care and successful management of most cardiac arrests require a strong "chain of survival." This chain includes (1) a well-known universal access to the EMS system (e.g., 911 phone call in the United States, 120 in China, 03 in Russia, and 119 in Japan); (2) bystanders (average citizens) with a fundamental knowledge of proper first aid, hazard recognition, and basic CPR; (3) a well-integrated first-responder program (e.g., fire department, police, or other professionals who can arrive within 3 to 4 minutes to provide immediate basic life support [BLS] and even automated external defibrillation); (4) a rapid response and transport service, whose components are preferably capable of delivering advanced life support (ALS); and (5) specialized receiving facilities capable of immediately managing victims of acute injury and myocardial reperfusion in their emergency centers, operating rooms, intensive care units, and, later, rehabilitation units.[5, 7–9] Each link of the chain must be intact and strong enough to ensure the best possible outcome. Therefore, the chain requires a highly integrated, well-scrutinized continuum of care intensely overseen by physician directors of that care.[2, 7] Physician supervisors must therefore be completely familiar with both the in-hospital and prehospital environments. In the prehospital setting, multiple factors must be overcome. These include difficult extrications of victims, lifting and evacuation, weather, hostile crowds, hazardous conditions, and limited resources, which change the priorities and ability not only to deliver optimal care but also to recognize and monitor for potential complications of acute illness and injury. In critical care cases, management of patients must be modified and tailored to the environment in which it is delivered.

Training Levels of Emergency Medical Service Personnel

Despite the critical nature of prehospital care, few physicians (let alone the average citizen) understand either the differences between an emergency medical technician (EMT), paramedic, and first responder (FR) or the purpose and need for each of these types of personnel.

For the majority of injuries to which EMS systems respond, the use of physicians as primary prehospital care providers is not only impractical but also unnecessary in most settings in North America. Most injury cases initially seen by EMS personnel do not require advanced, invasive skills such as endotracheal intubation (ETI) or intravenous infusions. Careful and expeditious extrication, skeletal splinting or immobilization, low-flow oxygen administration, and evacuation are often the only skills required. Nevertheless, for approximately 10% of trauma cases, especially those involving severe head injuries or penetrating truncal injuries with unstable vital signs, more advanced judgment, skills, and monitoring may be required.[7] Correspondingly, two major categories of EMS personnel have evolved that are recognized and granted certifications by most state governments.[10] The first of these training certification levels is the basic emergency medical technician (EMT-B). The other is the paramedic (also known as EMT-P). Although the training requirements for both of these levels may vary, not only from state to state but also according to local requirements, most states set forth comparable minimum basic requirements while encouraging further training and higher standards within local systems. Such standards are usually determined by the local accountable medical director (or sometimes a local EMS medical advisory committee).[2] For such purposes, the U.S. Department of Transportation has developed minimal standards and objectives for EMT-B. There is also a national registry that grants a nationally recognized certification for reciprocity purposes. Generally, a basic EMT course has been 120 hours in length and involves approximately 80 hours of didactic instruction and "skill laboratories" with an additional 40 hours of "clinical" work that includes measuring vital signs and history taking in an environment of caring for patients. After passing written and skills tests, these persons are certified as being capable of handling the first tier of prehospital trauma care, primarily involving basic extrication, immobilization, and evacuation. With such skills, they can also manage many other minor medical emergencies.

Spectrum of Paramedic Training

Requirements for paramedic (EMT-P) certification are much more variable and range from less than 500 hours to over 3000 hours, depending on the locale. For example, some programs are just over 400 hours in length. They may involve hospital, community college, or allied health school educators. The curriculum usually commits 300 or so hours to job-specific didactic training in medical-legal issues, pharmacology, communications, basics of shock, and other key clinical overviews (e.g., pediatrics, obstetrics and gynecology, respiratory and cardiovascular systems). Another 200 hours of clinical training may involve ambulance "ride-alongs" and observation in various settings (e.g., emergency departments, delivery rooms). Because of resource restrictions, ETI and defibrillation may be taught only in a simulated setting, and

some states still may grant certification before paramedic performance in the actual clinical setting. In contrast, other systems require paramedic students to have more extensive training before certification. For example, it may involve a minimum of several years of basic EMT experience followed by thousands of hours of advanced training and probationary status. These courses often include training by "streetwise" physicians both in the classroom and in the "field." In essence, in such systems, EMS training is a type of apprenticeship or internship in the actual setting of caring for patients. Hundreds of hours are dedicated to this aspect of training, and paramedic students must directly demonstrate relative expertise in the prehospital management of critically ill or injured patients before the supervising physicians authorize their certification to function independently without direct on-scene supervision.

Therefore, the term paramedic generally indicates a person who has been trained in ETI, peripheral intravenous catheter placement, defibrillation, drug administration, and other emergency ALS skills. However, the term encompasses a variety of individuals with a vast spectrum of training that varies with local requirements.

Although the EMT-B may also have some training in special skills, such as defibrillation (EMT-D) or placement of intravenous lines or intubation (EMT-I), the two basic categories of EMT and paramedic are, for the most part, used to delineate those trained in BLS and ALS techniques, respectively. Some states have now allowed nurses to "challenge" parts of the paramedic requirements by testing in lieu of certain training requirements. Nevertheless, the states still require formal EMS certification (EMT or paramedic) to function in the out-of-hospital setting, including responses to emergency scenes and interhospital transport.

Key Element of First-Responder Crews

The term *first responder* is becoming a part of everyday jargon for sophisticated EMS systems. There are FR training courses and certifications. However, the term remains generic because of variations in configurations, philosophy, and deployment strategies among EMS systems. In general, FR refers to a nearby, nontransporting response team sent by dispatchers in addition to ambulance (EMS transport unit) personnel. The FR is usually the local neighborhood fire truck (e.g., engine company) or police unit. On occasion it may be a BLS ambulance (EMT-B crew) or a specialized rescue vehicle. In other cases, the FR may be a volunteer responding in a private vehicle. Most FR units are staffed with at least one EMT-B trained in CPR and bag-valve-mask ventilation. However, the FR may consist of minimally trained personnel (basic CPR and oxygen providers). In some locales, FR units may be staffed with paramedics carrying ALS equipment such as defibrillators, intravenous fluids, and endotracheal tubes. Therefore, depending on the system, the FR unit, when used (some places still do not use FR crews), may have personnel of various training levels, who may, on occasion, also accompany the patient to the hospital.

The FR units are key to early CPR and automated defibrillation programs. As a result, the goal is to have them arrive as soon as possible, and it is hoped within 3 to 4 minutes after the call for help. They also can play a vital role in trauma care in scene logistics, hemorrhage control, extrication and rescue, basic airway and spinal immobilization techniques, and expediting "packaging" and lifting of patients, particularly when multiple patients are involved. Typically, fire department engine companies may also wash down leaking fuel and help to identify and suppress hazards. In cases of cardiac arrest, basic FR crews not only arrive earlier but also act as part of the "arrest team," performing basic CPR, ventilation, and record keeping so that ALS personnel can concentrate and expedite the advanced techniques and procedures.[11]

Direct On-Line Medical Control

Because of the high demand for ALS services in urban areas, most cities and suburban areas have paramedic services or at least a tiered system of paramedic and basic EMT services. Whereas some cities have all paid-professional paramedic services (private and/or public sector), nonurban areas often have little or no paramedic service. In this instance, care is provided primarily by volunteer EMT services. Regardless of the staffing composition, EMTs and paramedics generally report to a base hospital or "base station" (often there is more than one in larger cities) for on-line physician direction, advice, or back-up.[12] In prehospital trauma management, the base station is also contacted by radio (or occasionally telephone) to inform the receiving facility about the incoming injury victim(s) to better prepare trauma center or hospital teams, particularly for more serious cases. The base station may not be contacted in less serious cases or in other circumstances, where the other receiving facilities may be contacted directly. For the most part, EMS base stations are centralized and placed in a regional trauma center that will receive most of the critical injury cases. Being prewarned of the patient's probable injuries, mental status, and approximate vital signs, trauma center teams are better prepared to continue the vital continuum of trauma care as soon as the patient arrives. Specialized EMS courses for medical directors have been created for those providing these base station services. In fact, in some states, completion of these courses is required by law for physicians wishing to serve in such capacities.

Supervision of Emergency Medical Service Care

Prehospital care of patients sets the stage and tone for all subsequent care. As a result, meticulous prehospital management results in improved emergency care in hospital. Recognizing this, many states have enacted laws to ensure that EMS systems are supervised closely by physician medical directors.[2, 3] In the past, medical direction has frequently lacked the important component of intense, direct field supervision to ensure such standards. Today, progressive EMS systems make full-time physician involvement a priority. Municipalities, particularly large cities, have begun to hire full-time (or full-time equivalent) physician directors for EMS systems. In addition, many academic centers provide residents and fellows with dedicated EMS experience to enhance prehospital care training and research and to facilitate better role modeling for EMS supervision.[13] It is well recognized that, despite their medical degrees, physicians unfamiliar with the prehospital setting may complicate care of patients in the field.[2, 14]

Deployment Strategies

In addition to understanding the unique aspects of prehospital care of patients and management priorities, physician managers who are thoroughly familiar with both prehospital and hospital phases of care should be involved in EMS system design. For example, experience has shown that simply training more paramedics and buying more ambulances to improve ALS response time is not necessarily the correct approach to improving the delivery of prehospital medical care.[5, 15] Instead, in some settings, it may be better to maintain strategic placement of a relatively few, but busy,

ALS specialists who can be more closely supervised by physician directors.[16] In such systems, by virtue of a dispatch priority triage system, most EMS responses are managed and carried out by well-trained, properly supervised, but basic-level EMTs.[16-18] As a result, the manipulative skills and knowledge base of ALS providers (paramedics) are continually focused on cases requiring their expertise (which account for only 10 to 15% of EMS responses). For example, with respect to trauma care, call history data demonstrate that in most urban EMS systems, unless the dispatcher has evidence of confirmed serious injuries, a pin-in (persons trapped), confirmed unconsciousness, a roll-over, or a completely demolished vehicle, supervised basic EMTs can be dispatched with confidence to most motor vehicle collisions (unless a pedestrian, bicyclist, or motorcyclist is involved).[18] In most locales, basic EMTs can readily manage nearly 90% of all motor vehicle collisions as well as more than 95% of other (unspecified) injury and assault cases. Such injuries alone account for more than a third of all emergency medical dispatches.[19] Without the need for an ALS response in such situations, ALS personnel can be kept more available for major incidents by using a so-called ALS-BLS tiered or dual-response dispatch triage system.[5, 15, 16, 18] As a result, a smaller cadre of highly skilled ALS personnel still achieve a better response time (when needed) because they are not preoccupied with the large number of (time-consuming) basic calls. Furthermore, with the automated defibrillation capabilities and rapid access of FRs, concerns regarding the critical element of time to defibrillation, traditionally provided by paramedics, are further diminished.[5, 20] Again, such principles of management are not intuitive and require sophisticated, knowledgeable medical direction, management, and scrutiny to be effective.

STRATEGIES FOR CARE OF TRAUMA PATIENTS
Overview of Trauma Care

Trauma is often treated as a generic disease in prehospital management schemes. However, like cancer, trauma is not generic, but rather a group of different processes whose management depends on the mechanism, staging, and anatomic extent of involvement.

Most injury patients seen by EMS personnel require only meticulous BLS techniques such as neck and back immobilization or splinting of extremity fractures.[7, 19] Most of these procedures are simply precautionary, as subsequent emergency department evaluations fortunately show no evidence of unstable spinal (or other) fractures in the great majority of cases. Nevertheless, the absence of such abnormalities is usually difficult to determine clinically, particularly in the field, where patients may be intoxicated, upset, embarrassed, scared, or even denying symptoms so that they can avoid the "hassle" or even cost of emergency department evaluation. Therefore, reassurance, methodic skeletal immobilization, and expeditious transportation of the patient to an appropriate facility are the most common and basic features of good prehospital injury care. Even though a very small percentage of these patients are later found to have radiographic abnormalities, the volume of these patients who have some risk for spinal injuries is extremely high. In turn, the number of patients truly spared by early spinal immobilization still rivals the number truly spared by advanced trauma life-support techniques. Thus, the injured patient presenting in critical condition is not the only concern of rescue personnel, and "scoop and run" rapid evacuation is not always the appropriate priority.[7]

Need for Trauma Centers

Certain injury patients clearly need to be transported as soon as possible to a trauma center so that immediate definitive care can be provided for conditions such as progressive internal hemorrhage or intracranial hematoma.[7, 21, 22] It is the ability to delineate such patients that allows one to determine the proper management strategy. As a rule, the key to management of trauma patients is to prioritize the sparing of red blood cells. If bleeding from an extremity can be stopped by direct pressure, rapid transport is no longer a high priority. Conversely, if bleeding (or potential bleeding) is uncontrollable or cannot be ruled out (e.g., penetration of the abdomen), rapid evacuation to a trauma center is the overall priority. At the trauma center, experienced trauma surgeons are standing by and ready, not only to ensure the staving of hemorrhage but also, in extreme cases, to replace critical losses of blood. Likewise, if a motor vehicle collision victim has altered mental status and cannot clearly tell you that his chest, abdomen, and pelvis do not bother him, you must presume that internal bleeding is occurring. Alternatively, the cooperative, alert woman with a bump on her forehead who has no chest, abdominal, or pelvic pain or tenderness but does have cervical spine tenderness deserves more meticulous, careful extrication. The need to evacuate her is of less priority, assuming the mechanism of injury is minor and no other worrisome symptoms exist. Similarly, the cool, clammy, and pale young man with an accidental radial artery laceration needs direct control of the bleeding site, but intravenous catheter placement and initiation of rapid fluid infusion are not unreasonable before evacuation, assuming hemorrhage has not been too extreme. In essence, the critical tenets of prehospital care are (1) to spare red blood cells (either at the scene, if possible, or by evacuation to definitive surgical intervention); (2) to saturate the red blood cells with oxygen; and (3) to circulate the oxygenated red blood cells to vital organs while ensuring spinal immobilization. Therefore, step 1 is to ask, "Is the patient still bleeding or possibly bleeding?" (that is, "Is rapid evacuation a priority?"). The next step is to ask, "Is the patient able to generate adequate lung inflations bilaterally?" (while providing supplemental oxygen), and to ensure that there is adequate blood pressure (while ensuring spinal immobilization and evaluating the patient for any neurologic disability as needed). In the best of all worlds, these would be accomplished simultaneously, and obviously these are only generic principles of initial management.

Prehospital Triage Decisions

Real-life triage decisions made by EMS personnel (i.e., where to transport patients) often have been influenced or motivated by political, proprietary, or even personal interests. Various "objective" triage scoring systems have been developed that take into account cardinal vital signs and neurologic status, but such trauma schemas usually lack specificity and sometimes sensitivity. A stable-looking, wide-awake patient with a gunshot wound to the buttocks is a classic example of a patient whose condition can suddenly turn critical because of an occult internal iliac artery injury. Therefore, any decision to transport or refer to a facility that can offer immediate definitive care should not be based solely on a trauma score; the mechanism of injury is also a critical consideration. Many victims of blunt injury with slight sternal or retrosternal pain or tenderness may be at high risk for myocardial contusion, pericardial tamponade, and other significant complications, although they give an initial clinical impression that they are doing well. They should be monitored and treated as are patients with possible myocardial ischemia and should be transported rapidly to a trauma center. Likewise, victims of rapid deceleration accidents—falls over 6 ft or car accidents at speeds over 20 mph—deserve close evaluation and concern, especially for occult aortic and abdominal injury, even when they appear to be stable. Patients with punctures near the sternum are obviously of concern despite initial appearances. Subsequent development of cardiac tamponade is not uncommon. Such patients therefore deserve careful monitoring and rapid intervention if necessary.

Occasionally, because of embarrassment, anxiety, avoidance, stoicism, or intoxication (endogenous or exogenous), patients report that they are doing fine at the scene, but continued observation may still be important. Patients with the "lucky save syndrome"—that is, those who have walked away unscathed from a catastrophic event or a demolished vehicle in which others died—are of major concern. Despite their intact appearance and lack of complaints, such patients with histories or mechanisms of injury suggestive of high risk for occult internal injury should also be transported to a trauma center. For such patients, "overtriage" is considered acceptable. This also emphasizes the importance of emergency department physicians listening carefully to the EMT's description of the scene and of prehospital care providers meticulously gathering this information.

With these concepts in mind, recognized algorithms have been established to assist EMS personnel in their triage decisions regarding direct transport to a trauma center (Fig. 1–1).[23] As it usually turns out, the experience and intuition of a well-trained, well-supervised EMT or paramedic are the best triage tools. Nevertheless, the consensus scheme developed by the American College of Surgeons Committee on Trauma (see Fig. 1–1) is an excellent training guideline that can work well, particularly in urban areas where EMS personnel are busy and therefore well versed in recognizing patients at high risk for delayed or occult problems. A narrative summary of this American College of Surgeons flow sheet is shown in Table 1–1.

The basic objective of a trauma center is to provide a readily available, experienced staff of surgeons and other support personnel who routinely deal with major injuries and can immediately render rapid hemorrhage control, particularly in cases of intrathoracic, abdominal, or intracranial injury. The major correlates with survival in moribund injury victims are the prehospital provision of patent airway, preferably by endotracheal tube placement, coupled with rapid evacuation to a major trauma center for immediate thoracotomy or surgical intervention.[24] If the total prehospital interval (from injury to trauma center arrival) exceeds 20 minutes, it is unheard of for a victim of injury-related cardiopulmonary arrest to survive, even if intubated, unless there is an improvement soon after initial ETI. Therefore, if an injured patient has already lapsed into asystolic cardiopulmonary arrest and the trip to the trauma center will take more than 15 minutes, it is probably reasonable to avoid further danger to others by not racing all the way to that center, particularly if the patient has blunt injuries. Similarly, if an airway is completely obstructed, EMS personnel should try to go to the nearest facility capable of opening the airway, especially if transport time to the trauma center is over 10 to 15 minutes. There are other situations in which direct transport to the trauma center may be unnecessary; for example, isolated, external bleeding in an extremity can often be easily controlled, in which case immediate transport to the trauma center may not be necessary. In addition, unless there is significant external bleeding, patients with isolated critical head injuries (definitely isolated to the head alone) may be initially resuscitated with ETI and drug therapy outside the trauma center. However, this may be only to provide a potential candidate for organ donation.

In general, when these triage guidelines are used in urban areas, approximately one half of all injury patients are transported to trauma centers and the other half go to other

TRIAGE DECISION SCHEME

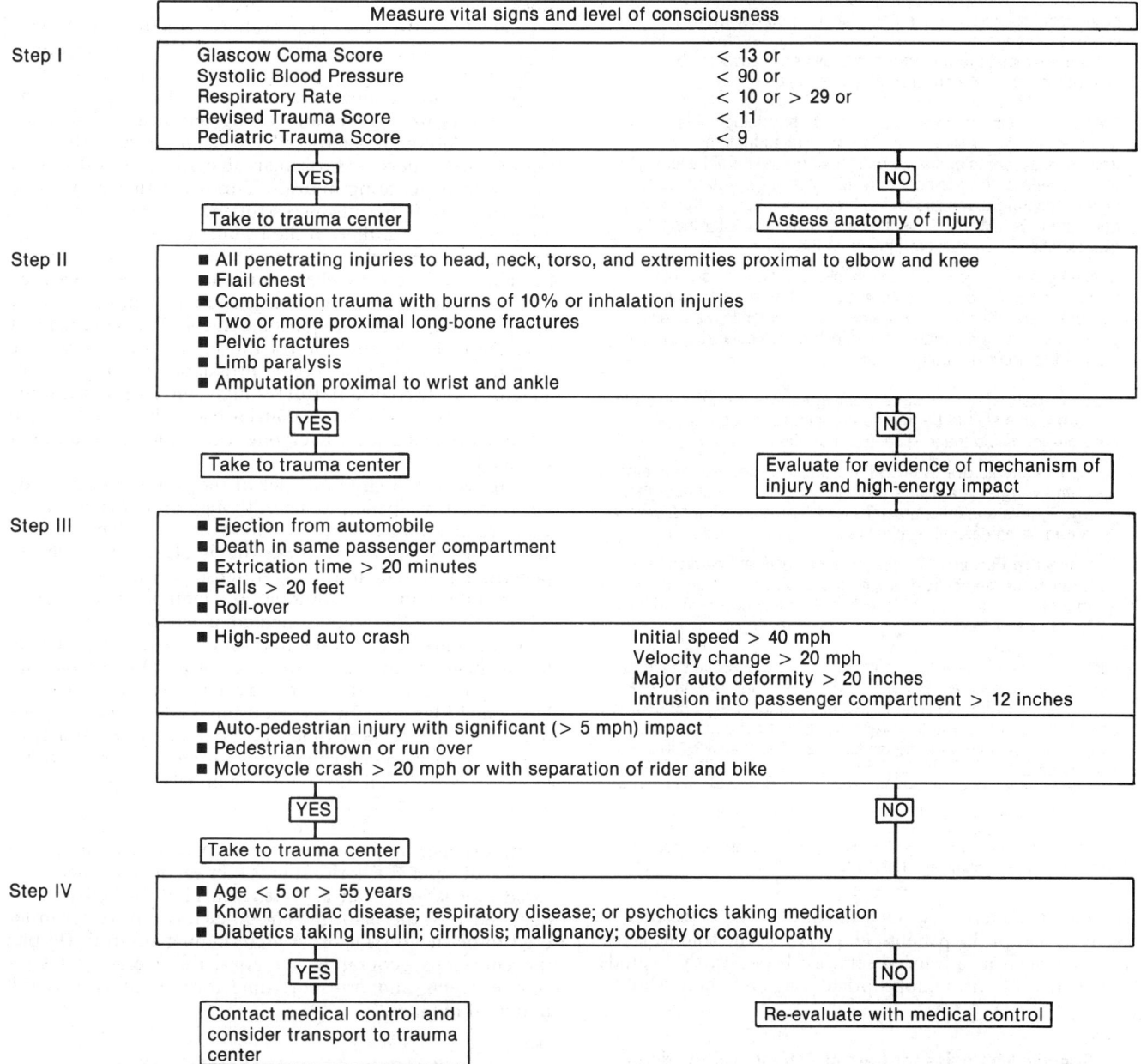

Figure 1–1. Triage decision algorithm. The American College of Surgeons Committee on Trauma criteria for direct transport of patients to a trauma center. (From Field categorization of trauma patients (field triage). In: Task Force of the Committee on Trauma of the American College of Surgeons Staff, Gere M [ed]: Resources for Optimal Care of the Injured Patient. Rev. ed. Chicago, American College of Surgeons, 1990, p 15.)

TABLE 1-1

NOTES TO FIGURE 1-1

Step I   Physiologic status thresholds are values of the Glasgow Coma Score, blood pressure, and respiratory rate from which further deviations from normal are associated with less than a 90 percent probability of survival. Used in this manner, prehospital values can be included in the admission trauma score and the quality assessment process.

A variety of physiologic severity scores have been used for prehospital triage and have been found to be accurate. The scores contained in the triage guidelines, however, are believed to be the simplest to perform, and provide an accurate basis for field triage based on physiologic abnormality.

Step II   Even in the presence of normal physiology, it is important to evaluate the likely presence of injuries that should be treated in a trauma center. A patient who has normal vital signs at the scene of the accident may still have a serious or lethal injury. Accurate diagnosis of life-threatening injury at the accident scene is unlikely. Thus, it is essential to look for indications that significant forces were applied to the body.

Evidence of damage to the automobile can be a helpful guideline to the change in velocity (ΔV), A ΔV of 20 mph will produce an ISS of greater than 15 in 90 percent of automobile crash occupants. ΔV can be estimated if one inch of vehicular deformity is equated to approximate one mph of ΔV.

Step III   Certain other factors that might lower the threshold at which patients should be treated in trauma centers must be considered in field triage. These incude the following:

A. Age   Patients over age 55 have an increased risk of death from even moderately severe injuries. Patients younger than age 5 have certain characteristics that may merit treatment in a trauma center with special resources for children.

B. Co-morbid Factors   The presence of significant cardiac, respiratory, or metabolic diseases are additional factors that may merit the triage of patients with moderately severe head injury to trauma centers.

Step IV   It is the general intention of these triage guidelines to select patients with an ISS of greater than 15 for trauma center care. Patients with this level of ISS have at least a 10 percent risk of dying from a single severe or multiple serious injuries. When there is doubt, the patient is often best evaluated in a trauma center.

From Field categorization of trauma patients (field triage). In: Task Force of the Committee on Trauma of the American College of Surgeons Staff, Gere M (ed): Resources for Optimal Care of the Injured Patient. Rev. ed. Chicago, American College of Surgeons. 1990, p 15.

community emergency departments.[19, 23] In retrospect, as many as half of the patients who arrive at the trauma center may not need its advanced services; however, these guidelines generally ensure appropriate triage for those who do.

Specific Strategies for Care of Patients with Various Types of Trauma

Most injury victims can be categorized into three main groups: (1) those with penetrating injuries, (2) those with blunt trauma, and (3) those with thermal and toxic injuries (burns, inhalation injuries). These groups should be subcategorized further into those with potential or known truncal injuries and those with clearly isolated head injuries or those with clearly isolated extremity injuries. In explosions, blasts, and bombings, however, all three of these categories may be involved and therefore all of the following strategies may need to be integrated.

Penetrating Injuries

It should be presumed that there is active substantial internal bleeding in patients with penetrating truncal injuries, particularly those with missile-type penetrations, despite a favorable-appearing clinical status on initial encounter. Again, this implies the need for rapid evacuation, preferably to facilities that can provide immediate thoracotomy, laparotomy, or both. As patients fare much better with their own blood than with massive transfusions, the earliest possible hemostasis is of primary concern.

Control of the airway in the prehospital setting, preferably by ETI, is one intervention that also correlates with improved outcome.[7, 24–27] In a Seattle study of 131 patients with prehospital cardiopulmonary arrest associated with trauma, the 31 survivors were generally "young, intubated, and penetrated."[24] Although almost all (90%) of those with blunt injuries died, there was a remarkable 70% survival rate in those with penetrating injuries. This dramatic survival rate correlated not only with successful endotracheal tube placement but also with time to the trauma center. The average response, scene, and transport time in this study was about 21 minutes. These excellent survival rates were achieved most likely because penetrations, especially knifings, usually involve a single lesion requiring control of hemorrhage. It is easier to locate and control the injury proximal to the wound (as opposed to an occult intra-abdominal injury after a motor vehicle collision). Interestingly, the 10% in this study who did survive with blunt injuries had only a single-organ intramediastinal injury. Everyone with multiple-organ injuries died.

In retrospect, a large number of the "saves" in this study involved cardiac penetrations. Although an injury to such a vital organ would be expected to lead to cardiopulmonary arrest, the potential for lifesaving is also quite high. In penetrating wounds to the heart, tense pericardial tamponade is quite common.[28] Although the tamponade may cause a faster demise, the state of hemodynamic compromise and shock of tamponade is easier to reverse than that of extensive hemorrhage (exsanguination). Thus, ironically, such an apparently lethal wound may be easier to treat if it is treated in a timely fashion. In the Houston EMS system, despite much longer transport times, approximately two thirds of patients with isolated penetrating cardiac injuries who are hypotensive (or even moribund) on initial field presentation are salvaged (over 75% of stab wounds and 40% of gunshot wounds in one study when antishock garments were not used), despite the presence of tense pericardial tamponade in 75% of cases.[28] Prioritization of airway management and rapid evacuation to an aggressive surgical facility (well acquainted with the management of such cases) were considered to be the key factors in determining survival. Despite the enormous geographic territory, the average total response, scene, and transport time for trauma care is still under 30 minutes.

Key Role of Endotracheal Intubation

In essence, in view of the studies just discussed, the classic "golden hour" of trauma could more appropriately be condensed to the "platinum half-hour" for serious blunt trauma and the "superconductor quarter-hour" for penetrating truncal injuries. In neither study, however, did the administration of intravenous fluids appear to provide any advantage. On the other hand, early ETI made a difference, probably because those who are apneic or in deep shock (and therefore not capable of spontaneous generation of adequate lung inflation) have deflated lungs.[25] Therefore, there is rapid development of profound intrapulmonary shunting (critical hypoxemia with substantial hemoglobin desaturation).[25] As a result, whatever red blood cells still are being circulated are delivering little oxygen. Particularly with basic CPR, the lung becomes extremely noncompliant and difficult to reinflate except by direct control of the intrathoracic airway through ETI. It is speculated that ETI, by supporting adequate oxygenation of the remaining circulating red blood cells, "buys" the moribund injury victim the few extra minutes needed to survive before definitive surgery. In a study of prehospital cardiopulmonary arrest after trauma, ETI significantly extended the average CPR time tolerated by survivors more than 5 minutes.[29] Without ETI, it is rare for any trauma victim to survive much more than 5 minutes of an apneic or pulseless state, even with basic CPR. Therefore, in the absence of such an airway and rapid access to a definitive care facility, moribund patients with penetrations are often considered to be "expectant" (probably will die).

Other Shock Interventions

In the case of penetrating wounds, other modalities such as the pneumatic antishock garment or military antishock trousers do not appear to offer any significant advantage, at least in the urban paramedic–trauma center system.[28, 30–32] The pneumatic antishock garment generally raises blood pressure by a peripheral resistance effect but does not appear to have a tamponade effect on bleeding (as previously thought) in certain abdominal injuries.[30, 33] Currently, intravenous volume infusions are recommended by most practitioners, especially in the case of hypoperfusing patients. However, intravenous volume infusions should be started only while en route, unless transport is unavoidably delayed and an intravenous catheter and infusion can be initiated readily. In this case cannulation is obviously acceptable as long as transport is not impeded just for the catheter placement. Fluids are classically infused under pressure through large-bore intravenous cannulas.

Evolving Directions in Early Hemorrhagic Shock Management

Although there has been a widely accepted belief that volume infusion can be beneficial en route to definitive hemostasis, this particular intervention is now coming under closer scrutiny and study.[34, 35] Continuous infusion of fluids without blood or hemostasis for extended periods may be harmful, particularly after more than several liters of volume infusion. In addition to the dilution of clotting factors or mechanical disruption of any forming clot, fluid overload may become a complication. More important, it has also been postulated by some that increasing blood pressure (or at least hydraulic flow) with fluids may serve only to accelerate hemorrhage if hemostasis has not yet been achieved. Therefore, the timing of fluid infusion is now being questioned. Experimental work has clearly reaffirmed the importance of fluids *after hemostasis*. For example, hypertonic (7.5%) saline in dextran has been found to be extremely effective in animals whose severe hemorrhage has been controlled.[36] However, there is concern about raising intravascular pressure before control of hemorrhage. A 250-mL infusion of hypertonic saline in dextran can be delivered in just a few minutes and has hemodynamic effects comparable to those of 4 L of isotonic fluids.[36, 37] This may therefore accelerate uncontrolled hemorrhage. Both experimental data and preliminary clinical findings confirming this hypothesis under certain circumstances (i.e., penetrating vascular injury) have prompted large prospective clinical trials evaluating early versus delayed fluid infusion in patients

with uncontrolled hemorrhage secondary to penetrating truncal injuries. These studies may better define the role and timing of volume infusion. The most important survival factors may simply be the type of penetrating injury and time to eventual definitive care.[38]

The benefits of both basic CPR chest compressions and advanced cardiac life-support drug protocols in pulseless trauma patients are debatable, particularly because it is likely that the pulseless patient has either massive brain injury, extreme hypovolemia or exsanguination pericardial tamponade, or unrecognized tension pneumothorax. In all of these situations, basic CPR is theoretically worthless. However, in the Seattle study of injury patients with cardiopulmonary arrest, basic CPR was an integral part of the care, along with aggressive, expeditious ETI and intravenous fluid resuscitation. It is reasonable to rationalize that when personnel are limited and priorities must be chosen, evacuation and ETI probably should not be delayed solely to perform basic CPR. Epinephrine and other catecholamines have been contraindicated in classic hemorrhagic shock when the patient is already vasoconstricted. However, the use of even high doses of epinephrine may have value in the moribund patient who has now developed vascular collapse. But even if the use of epinephrine and even bicarbonate were to be of some benefit, their use should not delay definitive hemostasis and transfusion. Therefore, under certain circumstances, there may be a theoretic place for basic and advanced CPR in trauma care, but the value of these interventions still needs to be proved explicitly.

Spinal Injury After Penetrating Wounds

The incidence of spinal fracture with penetrating injury is higher than is generally recognized, particularly with gunshot wounds to the neck. In a Los Angeles County study of 110 gunshot penetrations of the neck, the incidence of cervical fracture was 22% with neurologic interruption in 8%.[7, 39] Although spinal stabilization (cervical, thoracic, and lumbar) has not been clearly proved to alter outcome in this setting, medical logic mandates it be done as needed (until documented otherwise) in patients who have been shot in the head, neck, shoulders, upper chest, flank, abdomen, buttocks, and upper thighs. This may simply involve a long back board for patients with wounds below the chest and the addition of cervical spine immobilization as well for gunshots that enter above the mid-chest. For wounds near the neck, airways must be closely observed in case there is an evolving occult hematoma deep in the throat. In critical cases, simple manual immobilization may have to suffice in order to expedite evacuation, and further "packaging" is accomplished subsequently en route. Such techniques are described in detail in the following.

Open Penetrating Chest Wounds

Sucking chest wounds (open pneumothorax) and tension pneumothorax can be insidiously lethal but also are usually easy to reverse. They simply require quick recognition and action. When chest wounds larger than the tracheal diameter (3 to 4 cm) are present, air is inspired preferentially into the thoracic cavity through this path of least resistance during the inspiratory cycle (when intrathoracic pressure becomes negative). As a result, air does not readily enter the airways and inflate the lungs. Respiratory arrest ensues. Although positive pressure lung inflations should help to control this problem, simple manual sealing often solves the problem if the patient is still attempting to breathe. A sterile petroleum gauze is a preferred method, especially when accompanied by a sealed thoracostomy or one-way flutter valve to release any air remaining in the pleural space. Alternatively, one end of the gauze should be left untaped to allow outward release of air, anticipating that tension pneumothorax may ensue.

Tension Pneumothorax

Tension pneumothorax generally occurs when there is a rent in the visceral pleura. This tear may form a flap that closes on expiration but opens outward during inspiration, allowing air to flow one way into the pleural space. Air builds up under pressure in the thorax and the great vessels, heart, trachea, and lungs are all compressed and shifted to the contralateral side, collapsing the lung, impairing venous return, and compromising cardiac output. This situation is relatively uncommon. However, when present, it results in immediate respiratory and hemodynamic failure. Insertion of a small catheter or a one-way flutter valve relieves the tension, and although a sealed thoracostomy tube is eventually preferable to aid in full inflation of the lung, the critical nature of the problem mandates speedy relief in the field using a needle or catheter before tube placement. Chest tubes are also best left to in-hospital placement under most circumstances. Immediate decompression is best accomplished by placement of the needle into the thoracic cavity in the mid-clavicular line at the second or third intercostal space and over the superior aspect of the rib.

Tension pneumothorax coexists within a category of injuries associated with chest trauma and shock. It must be differentiated from massive hemothorax, pericardial tamponade, massive air leak, diaphragmatic rupture, and air embolism. Although hemodynamic compromise is the basic problem with tension pneumothorax (not necessarily hypoxemia or hypoventilation), hypotension is not always present. Occasionally patients may have systemic systolic blood pressures of 120 to 140 mm Hg, particularly when antishock trousers or vigorous fluid replacement is used. When the pneumothorax is discovered and relieved, the blood pressure suddenly rises even higher and the pulse rate falls. Nevertheless, the blind placement of flutter valves is probably unnecessary if asymmetric breath sounds are the only abnormal findings. If there is no evidence of significant tension (such as tympanic hemithorax or subcutaneous emphysema with decreased blood pressure or increased neck veins), an airway and high oxygen flow may suffice in the prehospital setting. Close monitoring of those with chest trauma is required, especially if the patient is intubated and receiving positive pressure breaths.

Blunt Injury

Prehospital management of blunt trauma presents a complex challenge. Certain field interventions, if performed efficiently, can be of value in patients with multiple blunt injuries, especially if severe head injury is involved. For example, the outcome of patients with severe head injury may be significantly improved by early prehospital ETI. However, the need for field procedures (ETI, spinal immobilization, and splinting techniques) must be carefully balanced with the need for rapid evacuation, because internal bleeding (e.g., liver, spleen, mesentery hemorrhage) always must be suspected, particularly if the abdomen and chest evaluation is rendered difficult or impossible by an altered mental status or age and language barriers.

Antishock Garments and Fluid Infusion in Blunt Injuries

The question of possible acceleration of internal hemorrhage by prehemostasis volume infusion is more complicated in the case of blunt trauma. Intravascular fluid infusion needs for blunt injuries are also affected by multiple factors including edema formation, cerebral perfusion, and anatomic considerations. Therefore, it is generally accepted that intravenous volume replacement should be initiated in patients who are hypoperfusing (or even at risk for hypovolemia), such as those with major fractures who bleed into and have edema formation in the soft tissue. Those with crushed limbs or muscles may also benefit in case of subsequent rhabdomyolosis and potential kidney failure. However, intravenous fluid replacement should not delay transport for more than a few minutes in blunt trauma, and this intervention preferably should be carried out en route if cannulation would delay evacuation, especially in the urban setting. The efficacy of the pneumatic antishock garment in blunt trauma has not been confirmed in controlled scientific studies.[31] Such studies, particularly in cases of pelvic fractures and/or long transports, would provide long overdue insight into this issue.

Basic Cardiopulmonary Resuscitation for Blunt Injuries

Basic CPR in a blunt injury case is generally considered to be futile. However, one must first consider the presence of a underlying reversible medical condition. For example, a motor vehicle collision may have been caused by a sudden run of sustained ventricular tachycardia (VT) with some minimal circulatory perfusion. This may then evolve into (pulseless) VF just before arrival of rescuers. Aggressive therapy for the medical condition is still warranted. Even an asystolic patient may be the victim of a sudden hypoxic event (seizure or choking) that is potentially reversible. Therefore, even with blunt trauma, such considerations must still be made before resuscitation of the injury patient is deferred.

Spinal Immobilization

After blunt injury, immobilization of the cervical spine should be performed liberally in the prehospital arena even when symptoms (e.g., neck pain) are absent. Most victims are anxious, extremely reticent to go to the emergency center, or "feeling no pain," either because of endogenous or exogenous substances, at the time of evaluation. Subsequent re-evaluation may be done in the emergency department, but unless the patient is completely alert, cooperative, and painless without any mechanism or other distracting sensory input (e.g., femur fracture), he or she should receive immediate meticulous prehospital spinal precautions. Rigid cervical collars provide some restriction to range of motion when applied properly, but further immobilization must still be achieved with some type of form-fitting packaging around the head and neck that is firmly secured to a long back board, scoop stretcher, vacuum body splint, or similar device. If the neck is immobilized in a standing or sitting patient, a second pair of hands should support the weight of the head against gravity and maintain an in-line neutral position until the horizontal position is secured. If the patient complains of pain induced while gently moving the head into the midline, "neutral" position, the rule is to "splint it where it lies," again always maintaining good manual control of the neck's position. Thoracic spine injuries receive some intrinsic stabilization from the thoracic cage, but those at risk still deserve attention, particularly if found in the upright position, in which gravity may have a deleterious effect. When packaged on the spine board, all parts of the body (pelvis, chest, head, and neck) should be secured in line to prevent angulated sliding of the torso against a fixed head and neck. In certain critical cases, meticulous spinal immobilization may have to be modified to expedite evacuation or airway management. Manual stabilization and alignment of the spine (at the least, the cervical spine) may have to substitute for meticulous packaging when immediate life-threatening hazards, airway compromise, or deterioration of vital signs alters the immediate priorities.

Consideration of Underlying Conditions

It must be remembered that reversible underlying medical problems may accompany or may even have been the cause of a subsequent accident or injury. Hypoglycemia should be a consideration in those with altered mental status even when other causes seem more likely (e.g., head injury, ethanol). Certain reagent strips, although quantitatively inaccurate on occasion, are reliable in detecting hypoglycemia.[40, 41]

Management of Serious Blunt Head Injury

Almost 40% of patients with serious blunt head injuries (Glasgow Coma Scale score less than 8) have a mass lesion (e.g., subdural or epidural hematoma) that may be amenable to surgical intervention if accomplished within 1 to 2 hours (and maximally 4 hours). About 75% of head-injured patients who "talked and died" proved to have intracranial hematomas.[21] The sooner these patients reach a center with a computed tomography scanner, in-house technicians, scan interpreters, and neurosurgical support, the better they fare. In the meantime, however, early respiratory support is critical.[7, 25] In cases of serious head injury, early ETI may alter the outcome.[25] With the sole exception of eventual neurosurgical control of epidural and subdural bleeding, ensuring oxygen delivery to the brain by (1) ETI (which facilitates adequate lung inflation and 100% oxygen) and (2) maintenance of an adequate blood pressure is more important than any other current potential therapeutic interventions.

Therapeutic Hyperventilation in Perspective

Although medical care providers are classically taught to "hyperventilate" the patient, this concept is often poorly understood. Lowering arterial carbon dioxide tensions can lead to vasoconstriction of cerebral vessels and subsequent decreased intracranial pressure by virtue of diminished cerebral blood volume, but this reflex may not function when mechanical or hypoxic brain damage is already severe enough to distort local reflexes or when there is severe hypotension or hypoxemia.[42, 43] Therefore, ensuring adequate oxygen transport to the brain (sparing red blood cells, providing adequate lung inflation with 100% oxygen, and supporting blood pressure) becomes the medical care provider's priority, even before attempts at therapeutic hyperventilation (i.e., the purposeful lowering of the blood carbon dioxide tension).[25]

Ensuring Adequate Lung Inflation

Appreciation of these concepts provides the most compelling rationale for aggressive ETI in patients with severe head injury (and other critically injured patients). Hypoxemia is extremely common in these patients. Although accompanying lung contusion or aspiration of gastric contents is often a contributing factor, the mechanism more often than not is inadequate lung inflation.[25] Therefore, ETI, which can help guarantee delivery of a selected tidal volume, is of considerable help. By ensuring adequate lung inflation (tidal volume of 10 to 15 mL/kg), ETI helps to prevent or reverse even critical hypoxemia, especially when 100% oxygen (an inspired fraction of oxygen of 1.00) is administered. As long as blood pressure is maintained, attempts to lower the arterial carbon dioxide are then justified. The typical self-inflating resuscitation bag used by prehospital care providers has a volume of 1500 to 1600 mL. Therefore, an adequate squeeze of the bag should provide close to 1000 to 1200 mL when the patient is intubated. This would be appropriate for the average 70- to 80-kg adult. Providers should be familiar with the volume of the resuscitation bags that they use and the approximate tidal volume delivered with each squeeze. Shallow breaths should be avoided, except in assisting the patient who is breathing spontaneously. Even then, a minimal number of large inflations (10 to 15 mL/kg) is often recommended (four or five per minute) to guarantee maintenance of adequate lung inflation whether or not therapeutic hyperventilation is indicated. Although pulse oximetry and electrocardiography (ECG) are becoming valuable monitoring adjuncts in such circumstances, it is rare for patients to become significantly desaturated if these empirical guidelines are used. Therefore, even positive end-expiratory pressure (PEEP) valves are unnecessary in the first phases of care. On the other hand, if hypovolemia is not a concern, low levels of PEEP (5 to 10 cm H_2O) are unlikely to be harmful and may support oxygenation enough to lower the fractional inspired oxygen if long transport is anticipated. Pulse oximeters may be useful for guiding therapy under such circumstances.

Specific Approaches to Therapeutic Hyperventilation

Lowering of the arterial carbon dioxide tension to 24 to 30 mm Hg generally is accepted as standard therapy in the neurosurgical community.[42, 43] Lower tensions are to be avoided because of certain inferential data. For example, cerebral oxygen extraction has been shown to become markedly increased below tensions of 20 mm Hg. This is interpreted as the consequence of inadequate blood flow to certain regions of the brain because of excessive vasoconstriction. Although this observation and its presumed consequences have not been elucidated completely, most patients still seem to fare just as well when they are moderately or mildly hypocapnic. However, without blood gas analyzers, the arterial carbon dioxide tension is difficult to determine in the field. Empirical experience has demonstrated that most patients who are ventilated with a tidal volume of about 15 mL/kg reach a desired arterial carbon dioxide range when they receive about 16 to 18 breaths per minute (or about one breath every 3 to 4 seconds), assuming an endotracheal tube is in place. Although this approach may be inadequate for a specific patient, it is successful for the great majority with severe head injury until an arterial blood gas analysis becomes available to better titrate the respiratory rate.

Problems in Effecting Prehospital Intubation

Although ETI may be indicated or desirable, several factors (e.g., clenched teeth) can preclude its ready performance, particularly with patients with head injuries. The performance of ETI in head-injured patients often has been discouraged because of concern about manipulating a possible cervical spine injury or aggravating increased intracranial pressure. All of these issues have been addressed in great detail elsewhere.[25] Briefly, there are multiple strategies that one can use to obviate these difficulties. In the case of possible cervical spine injuries, a modified procedure that simply emphasizes stabilization of the neck in a neutral position by gentle in-line manual control (not active countertraction), using a second pair of hands, usually overcomes these concerns. The high incidence of serious hypoxemia would appear to outweigh the 5 to 10% chance of cervical spine fracture in the patient with serious head injury.[25] Therefore, when proper technique is used, apprehension about the risk of inducing paraplegia by endotracheal placement in a patient with serious head injury should not stand in the way of ensuring airway control and proper ventilatory technique. During the past two decades in the cities of Seattle and Houston, using extremely liberal indications for ETI by paramedics, we have not found a single incident in which ETI exacerbated or induced cervical spine injury. However, it must be strongly emphasized that proper training and meticulous quality control by physician supervisors are key elements that must be present.[2, 25]

Nasotracheal Versus Orotracheal Intubation

The use of the nasotracheal tube, generally attempted in those who are spontaneously breathing but biting down, has been suggested but never proved to be a superior technique.[25] Although uncommon, significant complications such as gagging, retropharyngeal perforation, laryngospasm, and severe bleeding can occur and may be difficult to control in the prehospital setting. The patient with severe head injury also may have facial fractures that further complicate the ability to pass the tube blindly. Most important, the main rationale in such cases has been to diminish manipulation of the cervical spine, yet the noxious stimulus may induce head jerking in the semicomatose patient. Although nasotracheal intubation is extremely useful, it is recommended generally as an alternative to direct orotracheal placement and it requires just as much spinal precaution.[25]

Other Airway Interventions

Aside from nasotracheal intubation, there are several other options for the patient with clenched teeth. One is to use a muscle relaxant (e.g., succinylcholine); another is to use a "jaw screw" that wedges the mouth open. Use of the jaw screw is somewhat limited in edentulous patients and worrisome in those with loose or fractured teeth, and it is therefore generally discouraged. The usual arguments against the use of succinylcholine are that some spontaneous ventilation is much better than the risk of potential intubation failure and that the muscle relaxant obscures the neurologic examination. However, even with use by paramedics, such as in the Seattle EMS system over the past 15 years, there has been quite a favorable experience. Authorized by direct on-line permission from base station physicians, the use of succinylcholine has not only offered an extremely useful adjunct (without incurring further complications) but also, because the action of succinylcholine is short-lived, has not significantly complicated neurosurgical evaluations. However, the use of succinylcholine should be strongly discouraged in any system in which a supervising physician's meticulous control and accountability are not key features.[2]

Likewise, cricothyrotomies, jet ventilation, and tracheotomies are all plausible airway procedures in similar appropriate circumstances.[2]

Other Adjuncts to Blunt Head Injury Management

Because maintenance of cerebral perfusion is critical, maintenance of systemic blood pressure is also a key component of care. It is usually difficult to exclude other injuries (especially internal injuries) in patients with blunt head trauma, except in unusual circumstances. Therefore, rapid transport is a priority if internal (truncal) bleeding cannot be excluded. Nevertheless, most patients with isolated serious head injury are generally not hypotensive but, in fact, hypertensive. Therefore, rapid fluid infusions are not necessarily indicated. Infusions of dextrose-in-water solutions are avoided because of the presumed exacerbation of brain swelling from the "free water." Therefore, intravenous lines are usually established with isotonic solutions and kept at a minimal flow rate. Conversely, if the patient has risk for hypotension (or becomes hypotensive), it would probably be a result of neurogenic vascular collapse or occult internal bleeding, and isotonic fluid infusions should be initiated. It is possible that hypertonic saline solutions currently under study may offer some advantages under the right circumstances.[36, 37] Judicious prehospital use of furosemide, mannitol, lidocaine, and other pharmacologic agents is best left to local practice with input from the neurosurgeons who will care for these patients. Experience with prehospital use of these agents has revealed no problems in well-controlled systems.

Isolated Extremity and Head Injuries

A relative exception to the immediate transport rule is the management of most patients with isolated extremity or isolated head injuries. Bleeding usually can be controlled in extremity injuries distal to mid-thigh or mid–upper arm. Even with major femur fractures, where significant bleeding and edema formation can occur into the thigh tissues, the bleeding is still somewhat self-limited. If this is the only injury, the worry of further hemorrhage is not as pressing, and intravenous isotonic fluid infusions can be started to restore or prevent any compromise of perfusion and shock from intravascular volume losses. As mentioned before, careful splinting is a tenet of good prehospital care in cases in which rapid evacuation is not indicated. For alert and oriented patients who can tell you that they have no chest, abdominal, or pelvic pain or tenderness (and considering the mechanism of injury), the chance of internal hemorrhage is relatively low and splinting before transport is desirable. For example, expeditious traction splinting of a closed midshaft femur fracture not only relieves pain but also can diminish further morbidity.

Major Burns

Adult patients suffering major burns (e.g., 25% partial, 10% full thickness), having lost integument protection, are at great risk for fluid and body heat loss. This is of major significance in a disaster situation in which multiple burn patients may be exposed to the elements. Therefore, certain field interventions (followed by transport to a burn center) are a standard approach, including liberal intravenous fluid administration en route. Likewise, meticulous sterile technique, dry sterile covering of serious burns, and insulation against the enhanced heat loss are recommended in the immediate prehospital phase of management of major burns. If possible, early ETI and 100% oxygen should be considered for airway swelling or for altered mental status (carbon monoxide poisoning). If ETI is precluded by factors such as a strong gag reflex, 100% oxygen should still be provided by masks with oxygen reservoir bags and suction readily available, as nausea and vomiting are common with carbon monoxide poisoning and other inhalation injuries. In alert and oriented burn patients, pain relief is reasonable at times. Small incremental doses of morphine sulfate or self-administered nitrous oxide–oxygen mixtures can be given safely, assuming that no blunt trauma or blast was involved. Rapid, "uncontrolled" transport usually is not as much a priority, except in the case of those suspected of having internal (truncal) injuries or those deeply obtunded, which is often presumed to be from carbon monoxide poisoning but also may represent associated head injury.

STRATEGIES FOR CARE OF PATIENTS WITH CARDIOPULMONARY ARREST

Overview of Out-of-Hospital Cardiac Arrest

Only about 1% of all EMS incidents involve cardiopulmonary arrest secondary to nontraumatic causes and, in most EMS systems, less than 50% of these present as VF. Nevertheless, most people who die in our communities do so as the result of unheralded VF. Therefore, resuscitation and survival rates of patients with out-of-hospital cardiac arrest have become the yardsticks of EMS system success. The pages that follow provide strategies for achieving such successes.

Sudden Death and Cardiac Arrest in Perspective

Although "sudden death syndrome" is the number one killer in the American population (nearly 400,000 deaths a year in the United States alone), it is now known that, under certain circumstances, nearly one half of these patients are salvageable and many have an underlying problem that is amenable to subsequent therapy (i.e., isolated ischemic coronary artery disease).[4, 5] Interestingly, the average age of VF victims is about 60 years. Therefore VF is not really a disease of the elderly. Because cardiac arrest is often reported as the first symptom for 25% of those with coronary artery disease, it is not surprising that out-of-hospital VF is frequently observed in 40- and 50-year-old men. Some U.S. studies find that 20% of males with coronary artery disease experience their first symptom by the age of 50. Therefore, sudden death resulting from VF is clearly a major if not the major health issue of our time, not only because of the sheer numbers (more than a 0.3 million Americans annually) but also because of what we now know about the reversibility of VF. In addition to sudden death, many other out-of-hospital deaths occur because of reversible cardiac or respiratory arrests that have resulted from a multitude of etiologies, including chronic heart diseases, chronic lung diseases, seizure, asthma, toxic overdose, drowning, and electrocution. Many of these arrests are also reversible with proper EMS interventions.

Out-of-Hospital Versus In-Hospital Cardiac Arrests

Many critical care practitioners manage in-hospital arrests that are generally associated with end-stage diseases, and therefore they often lack enthusiasm about resuscitation attempts, particularly in the elderly.[6, 44] This attitude is not surprising if cardiac arrest is seen as a single or generic disease process. But if the various pathways leading to this common-appearing clinical condition are better understood, appropriate enthusiasm for resuscitation can be better directed, especially in the case of out-of-hospital arrests.[5, 6, 45]

We have now learned that only one half of the patients resuscitated after out-of-hospital cardiac arrest associated with VF or VT have sustained any evidence of permanent heart damage (i.e., no evidence of infarction by ECG or enzymes).[5, 46] As Claude Beck (who performed the first successful human defibrillation in 1947) pointed out, in the majority of cases, "the heart's too good to die." Indeed, studies have demonstrated a very high salvage rate for patients whose VF- or VT-associated cardiac arrest was witnessed by a paramedic who could immediately provide defibrillation and other ALS interventions (Fig. 1–2).[5, 47]

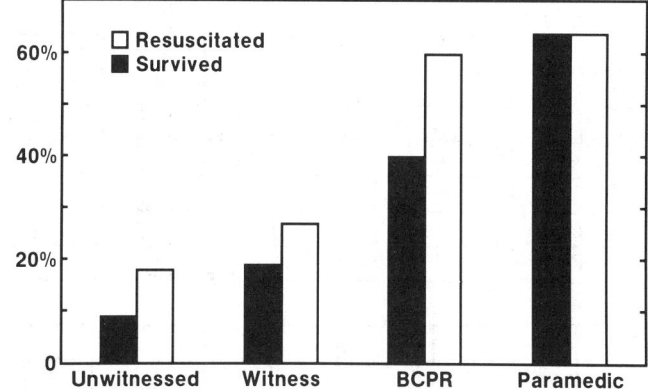

Figure 1–2. Effect of witnessing persons on the outcome of sudden death associated with out-of-hospital VF or VT. If no one hears or sees the collapse (Unwitnessed), chances for long-term survival (successful hospital discharge) are only 1 in 10. Even without performing CPR, a bystander witnessing the event (Witness) more than doubles the chances of long-term survival (successful hospital discharge). If that witness performs bystander CPR (BCPR), the survival rate is again doubled (to about 40%). If an ALS provider (Paramedic) witnesses the event (monitored arrest), the great majority (nearly two thirds) survive. The chances of resuscitation of the cardiovascular system (resuscitation of spontaneous circulation) are nearly the same with BCPR as with ALS providers, indicating a key physiologic contribution of BCPR.

Approximately two thirds (or more) of these patients can be resuscitated and successfully discharged from the hospital neurologically intact (and quite functional). Therefore, although VF, a sudden, unexpected chaotic twitching of the heart muscle resulting in immediate loss of all cardiac output, is obviously lethal, it is also quite treatable. Interestingly, the few who do not survive are simply not even resuscitated. On closer analysis, those who did not survive generally had hypotension when they presented to paramedics, whereas most of the survivors had good vital signs before their sudden cardiac arrest.[47] This implies that in the smaller group who did not survive the VF or VT was probably secondary to evolving cardiogenic shock and severe myocardial dysfunction, whereas the VF was more of an ischemia-produced primary "electrical" problem in the much larger group of survivors.

Dynamics of Cardiac Arrest

VF or VT rhythms are the initiating event in 70 to 80% of primary cardiac arrests in the out-of-hospital setting, but only a percentage of these patients are found to have VF or VT by the time rescuers arrive. Cardiac arrest is often seen as a rather static process. However, in VF the immediate loss of organized heartbeat caused by the sudden, chaotic, short-circuiting of the heart's electrical system leads to immediate loss of coronary artery perfusion. Therefore, the sources of the metabolic nutrients needed to produce the high-energy phosphates (e.g., ATP) used to fuel the heart's various functions, including pacemaker activity, conduction of electrical impulses, and myocardial contractility, are suddenly shut off. Depending on the individual, the degree of previous underlying cardiac disease, and external factors such as the timing (or absence) of basic CPR, the VF activity consumes all remaining energy sources. As minutes pass, the VF is less vigorous and its ECG appearance becomes less coarse. Eventually, the VF becomes more and more fine until the complete depletion of energy supplies leaves the heart at a standstill (Fig. 1–3).

With a very rapid response of FR crews with monitoring

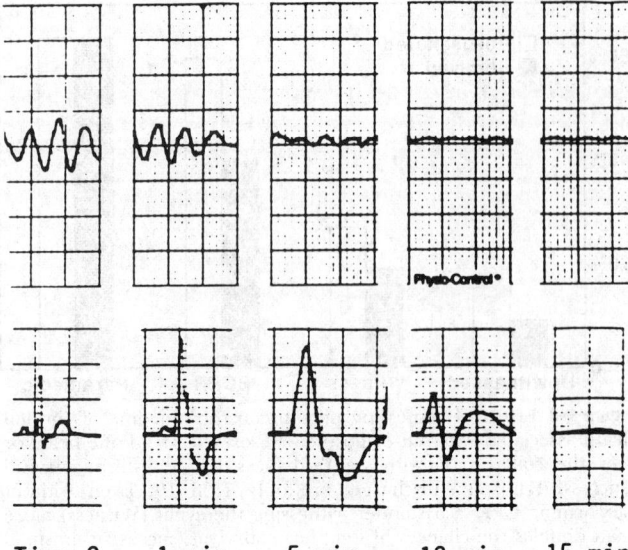

Time 0   1 min   5 min   10 min   15 min

Figure 1–3. Sample (compressed) time course of the VF waveform (*upper panels*) demonstrating a deterioration of coarse to fine fibrillation over 15 minutes. The lower panels show samples of the concomitant conversion rhythms one might expect as time elapses.

equipment, high rates of VF or VT are found on presentation (over 50%). However, in most prehospital care systems, VF or VT is the presenting rhythm in 40% or less of cases. Asystole or agonal rhythms therefore reflect long "downtimes" and depletion of the energy sources necessary to resume spontaneous circulation and predict a poor prognosis. Even in the best of EMS systems, prognosis for long-term survival of patients with unmonitored primary cardiac arrest presenting with asystole on ECG is rarely greater than 1 to 2%.[48] This is why most "last-ditch" attempts to resuscitate with artificial pacemakers are futile, despite "capture." In fact, the survival rate for asystole generally is zero in most places. Those who do survive usually are patients who had an easily reversible underlying cause of arrest, such as transient hypoxemia or transient loss of blood pressure. Nonetheless, despite low survival "rates," initial resuscitation efforts are strongly encouraged in view of the overall significant contribution of such efforts toward total potential survivorship in a given community.[49]

Effect of Bystander Cardiopulmonary Resuscitation

Compared with long-term survival rates of patients with paramedic-witnessed arrests, those of patients who are given bystander-initiated CPR are somewhat lower but still remarkably good (see Fig. 1–2). The lower survival rates probably reflect a delay or inadequacy of bystander CPR to protect the brain against irreversible ischemic damage for extended periods of time, as when ALS care is delayed or when a single rescuer must leave temporarily to call for help. Most studies indicate that when bystander CPR is performed, it is usually initiated within the first 4 minutes. As a result, on the average, 40% of the patients who received bystander CPR from someone who witnessed the VF- or VT-associated arrest are successfully discharged from the hospital (see Fig. 1–2).[5, 6, 18] This is a remarkable rate of reversibility for this unpredicted, rapidly fatal clinical entity that occurs out in the community. On the average, bystander CPR at least doubles the survival rates for VF- or VT-associated arrests.[5]

Relative Contribution of Bystander Cardiopulmonary Resuscitation

One essential aspect of the training of the lay public in basic CPR techniques is instructing them in the when and how of accessing the EMS system quickly (calling 911, or some equivalent). Another important aspect of public CPR training is that the earlier BLS is given, the better the results. Studies show that very early bystander CPR is associated with an initial rhythm of coarse VF and a more organized conversion rhythm (e.g., sinus tachycardia) after initial countershocks.[50] The patient is also more apt to be making respiratory efforts or have some observable motor function when ALS arrives. More recently, it has been recognized that if the bystander CPR is begun within seconds (and continued), it is apt to "buy the patient more time" (e.g., survival despite the passage of more than 10 to 15 minutes before ALS arrives). On the other hand, if bystander CPR is not initiated until 3 minutes after collapse, it may also buy some time but it may be of value for only 2 or 3 more minutes. Therefore, early bystander CPR may have a more pronounced physiologic effect if it is provided almost immediately (the earlier the better). Nevertheless, these observations should not prevent the lone bystander-rescuer from first calling for professional help. With two bystanders, one should call for help while the other immediately begins BLS.

Other Factors Associated with Resuscitation Success

Studies of successful outcomes in out-of-hospital VF (long-term survival rates > 20%) are usually conducted in EMS systems in which there are (1) a minimum of two paramedics per ALS unit and (2) simultaneous dispatch of an accompanying neighborhood FR fire truck crew who assist with the basic CPR, ventilation, and drug set-ups. In addition, community CPR training is usually a major feature.[5, 50] In the city of Seattle, where for years the survival rate for VF has exceeded 25%, bystander CPR occurs in nearly 40% of cases.[5, 50] The addition of automated defibrillators on FR fire trucks now has further increased the chances of survival to over 30% (Fig. 1–4). Not only is there earlier delivery of

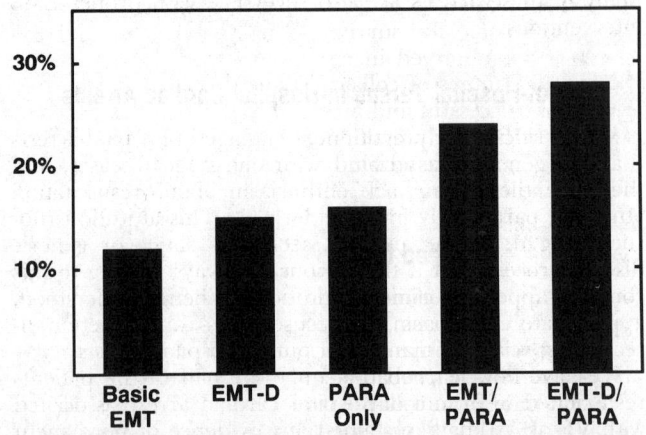

Figure 1–4. Comparison of average survival (successful hospital discharge) rates after out-of-hospital cardiac arrest associated with VF for various types of EMS system configurations: basic emergency medical technicians (Basic EMT) only, EMTs who can defibrillate (EMT-D), paramedics (PARA) only, "tiered" EMT and paramedic (EMT/PARA) services, and tiered systems in which EMTs also defibrillate (EMT-D/PARA). (Adapted from Eisenberg MS, Horwood BT, Cummins RO, et al: Cardiac arrest and resuscitation: A tale of 29 cities. Ann Emerg Med 19:179, 1990.)

countershocks, but also there is an increase in the number of patients presenting with VF or VT (because of earlier arrival). Thus a higher percentage of a larger number of patients is saved. Often, patients receiving FR defibrillation have pulses long before the other ALS modalities and care are available. A large percentage of patients refibrillate (about 60%), but obviously there is still a significant number who do not. It has now been shown that lives can be saved in systems with BLS providers who also have a defibrillator, even without the immediate provision of other ALS modalities such as ETI and intravenous lidocaine.[5] Although paramedic services have an additional effect, the earliest possible initiation of bystander CPR and defibrillation are clearly the key lifesaving factors in cardiac arrest management.

Contribution of Advanced Life-Support Interventions

There is significant inferential evidence to support the value of both ETI and postresuscitative intravenous lidocaine administration, namely that higher survival rates are found in systems using them than in those without these modalities.[4, 5, 25] Similarly, experimental data indicate that outcomes are improved by epinephrine administration; however, the absolute clinical value of epinephrine (and other such drugs) only now are being proved in a rigorous scientific fashion.[6, 51] Experimental evidence suggests that the doses of drugs currently used for resuscitation may actually be ineffectual in a large percentage of cardiac arrest cases. The recommended dose of epinephrine in adults during cardiac arrest has been 0.5 to 1.0 mg (about 0.01 mg/kg) every 5 minutes. However, studies in canines and swine have now demonstrated that there is no significant improvement in aortic diastolic pressure (AODP), myocardial oxygen delivery, or myocardial blood flow at this dosage after extended periods (e.g., 10 minutes) of circulatory arrest.[52] Because of the progressive loss of vascular tone and/or adrenergic uncoupling, epinephrine dosage appears to increase with time. Human studies have now been performed that demonstrate a significant increase in AODP after prolonged arrest (over 0.5 hour) when higher doses of epinephrine (5 to 15 mg) are administered.[53] In those studies, the higher doses were also associated with unexpected resuscitation but unfortunately not an increase in long-term survival. Nevertheless, in multicenter trials, flushed intravenous epinephrine doses of approximately 15 to 20 mg significantly improved neurologic outcome for survivors, and a trend for improved survival was observed in the subgroup of patients treated within 10 minutes of collapse.[54] Such single large doses are not often successful and are more likely to be successful in cases in which early bystander CPR was performed or the time to epinephrine administration was less than 10 minutes after collapse.[6, 55]

Need for Further Research

Despite the experimental data and preliminary results in humans, a consensus regarding doses of epinephrine required to effect human resuscitation is still evolving. Dosage requirements are probably determined by multiple factors (weight, time from collapse, bystander CPR, individual variability). It is less likely that those with a monitored arrest who are treated immediately will need any epinephrine (let alone the higher doses discussed earlier). Also, as discussed earlier, bystander CPR may have a profound physiologic effect if administered within seconds. It is speculated that the immediate provision of some basic circulation delays the decline in peripheral vascular tone enough to maintain AODP. With delays in bystander CPR, vascular tone deteriorates and the initial AODP with CPR is much lower. Thus

CPR is less effective, creating a vicious cycle. Because the timing of CPR may alter the rate at which vascular receptors lose their tone, it may also affect their sensitivity to administered epinephrine. Both relative weight (lean body versus actual) and individual variation may also play significant roles in determining the relative need for and dose of epinephrine. Therefore, further scientific investigations must be conducted not only to examine the dosing required for efficacy but also to rule out undesirable complications.

Atropine and Lidocaine Administration

In view of the previous discussion, the efficacy and proper dosing of other ALS drugs such as atropine and lidocaine during CPR conditions (circulatory arrest) may also need to be re-examined. For example, the common understanding that 2 mg of atropine is the total vagolytic dose may be true in a human adult with normal circulation. On the other hand, this dose may not be as effective after 10 to 15 minutes of profound vascular collapse and minimal circulatory blood flow. In fact, there is now concern that lidocaine administration before restoration of spontaneous circulation may be detrimental.[56] However, after restoration of spontaneous circulation, immediate loading of up to 3 mg/kg of lidocaine (followed by a drip of 2 to 4 mg/min) is still strongly advised.[4]

Advanced Cardiac Life Support in Perspective

Despite the experimental and theoretic data, most current drug therapy may be simply "icing on the cake" with respect to the contributions of very early bystander CPR and early defibrillation. Perhaps in the future, drugs that restore energy supplies or mechanical devices that immediately restore more than adequate myocardial blood flow will be found to be more efficacious. Until then, the initial approach to VF is to provide (1) the earliest possible defibrillation; (2) airway protection and adequate lung inflation (usually with an endotracheal tube) along with 100% oxygen; (3) basic CPR techniques and, if needed, enhancement of the basic CPR effect by epinephrine (or other alpha$_2$-vasopressors); and (4) appropriate administration of stabilizing antiarrhythmic agents after restoration of spontaneous circulation. With this background, the following sections review the latest rationales and accepted clinical approaches to management of out-of-hospital cardiac arrest.

PRACTICAL APPROACH TO MANAGEMENT OF OUT-OF-HOSPITAL CARDIAC ARREST
Aggressive Restoration of Circulation

The key to successful resuscitation of the cardiac arrest patient is maintaining an organized, prioritized approach that will effectively accomplish the appropriate interventions as rapidly as possible. Although the pathophysiologies and outcomes of individual cardiopulmonary arrests may vary, an approach to management still can be simplified. In essence, the approach to all cases is to rapidly restore brisk coronary artery perfusion with oxygenated blood. In all cases, the primary mechanisms used to achieve this goal are to (1) adequately inflate the lungs bilaterally (tidal volume of 15 mL/kg) with 100% oxygen (which should always allow nearly full oxygen saturation of red blood cells), (2) circulate the oxygenated red blood cells with basic CPR (chest compressions), and (3) enhance the basic CPR with potent vasopressors (epinephrine, norepinephrine) as needed (pulselessness, persistent hypotension).

For the electrical short-circuiting syndromes (i.e., VF and VT), one must first clear a pathway for organized electrical

TABLE 1–2

GENERAL APPROACH TO NONTRAUMATIC CARDIAC ARREST MANAGEMENT

I. Clear out ventricular fibrillation or ventricular tachycardia (VF/VT), while considering spinal injury, and follow these "ABCs":
  A. Adequate lung inflation bilaterally with O_2 (check endotracheal tube centimeter mark, stomach sounds, bite block).
  B. Blood pressure or chest compressions adequate? (Check compression depth, and rate 80–100/min.)
  C. Catheter(s): drips and patency? (Use large bore if possible.)
  D. Drugs = "LEAP ABC." Consider each one and go back again.
    L. Lidocaine: always in VF/VT (except with wide, slow QRS on electrocardiogram not "driven" by P wave). Remember to load (3 mg/kg).
    E. Epinephrine: pulseless despite good O_2 and CPR or pulseless and definite long interval of time after arrest.
    A. Atropine: (1) hypotensive and (2) rate 60 or less (or AV block).
    P. Pressors (e.g., levarterenol or dopamine): pulses present but hypotensive (or epinephrine wearing off). Set up ahead of time in anticipation of need.
    A. Altered mental status considerations (e.g., glucose test strip, naloxone).
    B. Bicarbonate: no significant response to initial rounds of therapy.
    C. Chemical imbalances (e.g., M^{2+}, Ca^{2+}, K^+).
  E. ECG functions ("GAMES") and pacemaker trial:
    Gain?
    Attached leads?
    Mode (paddles versus chest leads)
    ECG vector (check several leads)
    Strip (document with a hard copy)
  F. Further history and physical examination (e.g., medications, recent symptoms or injury, auto-PEEP).
II. Rapidly repeat foregoing steps over and over.

impulses (defibrillation) and then help to maintain electrical stability with antiarrhythmic agents (e.g., lidocaine). But these are the simple "book end" additions to the basic strategies of proper lung inflation, chest compressions, and enhancement of the basic CPR effect with vasopressors. If additional drugs such as atropine and sodium bicarbonate are used, their use must be considered supplemental to the basic strategies for restoring strong perfusion of the coronaries. To be more specific, when one defibrillates a victim of unmonitored VF and finds wide QRS complexes on the postconversion ECG with a rate of 40/min, a common reaction is to administer atropine because of the bradycardia. Although this drug may actually be helpful in some patients, in the prolonged pulseless state the bradycardia is most likely to be secondary to an oxygen-starved conduction system that first needs to be reperfused with a supernormal oxygen supply. With the minimal coronary blood flow, successful drug actions during CPR conditions probably result from indirect stimulation of the heart through restoration of adequate AODP. Therefore, considering the use of atropine would be more of a secondary thought after the priorities of basic CPR, ETI, oxygen, and epinephrine.

A summary approach, listed in Table 1–2, represents an A-B-C-D-E-F mnemonic that can be applied almost universally to nontraumatic cardiac arrest management in which other reversible factors such as hypovolemia, tension pneumothorax, and pericardial tamponade processes have at least been considered and tentatively ruled out. The following sections elaborate on each of the aspects of this practical approach.

Clearing Ventricular Fibrillation

Spontaneous circulation does not occur until the VF is therapeutically removed. Therefore, the priority in VF- or VT-associated circulatory arrest is to clear out the ventricular arrhythmia with defibrillatory countershocks in order to allow a clear path for spontaneous, organized, cardiac electrical impulses. It can be argued that defibrillation may not occur until there is blood oxygenation by ETI or reversal of acidosis with sodium bicarbonate. However, it is more likely that very early defibrillation will allow the heart to beat spontaneously again, even obviating the need for these other ALS procedures. Therefore, in VF- or VT-associated arrest, the patient should first receive successive countershocks until the VF or VT clears, at least for the first three or four shocks.

Energy Levels for Countershocks

There is some evidence that cardiac arrest "stuns" the myocardium and that the conduction system is also more apt to be stunned by higher energies, at least transiently. Although a few VF patients can be successfully defibrillated with only 100 J (or less) of defibrillatory energy, more than 90% of out-of-hospital patients can be cleared of VF using three shocks (or less) at 200 J.[57] Therefore, this seems to be the most efficient lower energy level. Nevertheless, a small percentage of patients may have a larger than usual mass of fibrillating myocardium.[4] Some experts believe that these patients should receive higher energies if the first one or two shocks fail to convert the VF, reasoning that the sooner the defibrillation occurs the better the result. Thus, in adults, the current American Heart Association Advanced Cardiac Life Support (ACLS) algorithm calls for 200 J for the first shock, 200 (or 300) J for the second, and up to 360 J for the third if necessary. This wording leaves leverage for clinical judgment, let alone different points of view.[4]

Although most adults have about the same heart size (regardless of body weight), a child's heart size and mass of fibrillating myocardium are obviously smaller. It is recommended as a rough guideline that children receive a starting "dose" of 2 J/kg. However, the correct level of defibrillation energy has not yet been clearly established for the pediatric population.[4, 5]

Adequate Lung Inflation Bilaterally with Oxygen

The "A" in cardiac arrest management stands for adequate lung inflation bilaterally (with oxygen). Because experimental data support the effectiveness of epinephrine in augmenting the effects of basic CPR, intravenous epinephrine infusion is often considered to be the next recommended action in a pulseless patient (with or without VF).[4] However, in most settings, at least two ALS providers are available and ETI can (and should) be performed simultaneously. In the most advanced EMS systems, defibrillation is managed by the FR crew's automated defibrillator while paramedics intubate and infuse epinephrine (as indicated), thus expediting the patient's care.[11]

ETI is important not only in terms of airway protection from aspiration of gastric contents but also because it is the definitive way to restore the adequate lung inflation required to reverse the critical hypoxemia that usually occurs when gas exchange units collapse after cardiopulmonary arrest.[25] Because lung compliance falls dramatically with both apnea and chest compressions, it may be difficult to reinflate the lung with a bag-valve-mask system alone. The use of ETI guarantees the 10 to 15 mL/kg that is probably needed to reverse the intrapulmonary shunt resulting from CPR-associated collapse of gas exchange units. If the patient receives ETI, properly placed and accompanied by the delivery of a tidal volume of 10 to 15 mL/kg and 100% oxygen given during a 1.5 to 2.0-second period per breath, PaO_2 levels leading to significant red blood cell (hemoglobin) desaturation are rarely seen regardless of the etiology and severity of any accompanying lung disease.

Blood Pressure

The "B" in this mnemonic approach is not the well-known "breathing" of BLS but rather blood pressure. After red blood cell saturation with oxygen, the next end point is to restore a strong AODP and briskly perfuse the coronaries with those oxygenated cells. There is current speculation that a transient 15- to 20-minute period of relative hypertension may actually be therapeutic immediately after restoration of spontaneous circulation. In fact, if the systolic blood pressure is less than 110 to 120 mm Hg, the coronary artery perfusion pressure (AODP) may not be adequate.[58] Despite the fact that pulses have returned, if the blood pressure remains less than 90 to 100 mm Hg (e.g., absence of radial pulse or strong femoral pulses), this still may not be enough to adequately restore the oxygen debt to the stunned myocardium, let alone supply the steady-state circulation required to support coronary perfusion. It is not unreasonable in some cases to sustain chest compressions to augment spontaneous circulation while pressors are being initiated.

Catheters

The "C" is for catheters, as in intravenous catheter. Although endotracheal administration of drugs (such as epinephrine) can be attempted when intravenous access is not available, this is probably a poor route in the absence of adequate circulation. Lidocaine and atropine are not even absorbed well in a patient with normal circulation. Therefore, one should establish intravenous access (or eventually several accesses) as soon as possible with a catheter of as large a bore as feasible (e.g., No. 14 or 16 French). This is best accomplished at either antecubital, forearm, or external jugular sites (not central intravenous access initially). As drugs are administered during CPR conditions, they should be subsequently flushed in vigorously. In an antecubital site, the intravenous solution can be squeezed in under pressure with the arm elevated well above heart level for 15 to 20 seconds. This flush is probably very adequate, especially if positive pressure breathing and chest compressions are transiently withheld during the last 5 seconds of the flush. This helps to overcome any obstruction to flow from the associated increases in intrathoracic pressure. In the case of external jugular or direct central venous access, a shorter flush (with immediate CPR and ventilation interruption) is acceptable. Multiple cannulations are eventually preferred, as long as the initial therapeutic interventions are not delayed. This is encouraged so that there are multiple sites, not only for various interventions (e.g., lidocaine drip or norepinephrine drip) but also in anticipation of intravenous site infiltration or accidental dislodging. Because there have been concerns regarding poor neurologic outcomes in those found to have hyperglycemia after resuscitation, it may be preferable to use normal saline solutions for flushes and intravenous access.[59]

Drugs

The "D" is for drugs. It should be remembered that even those who regain their pulse after a period of cardiac arrest are at great risk for refibrillation or further deterioration if the perfusion of the coronaries is not adequate to restore sorely needed nutrients for functional cardiac requirements. Therefore, in hypotensive postresuscitative patients, the aggressive use of pressor agents is generally recommended for transient augmentation of AODP sufficient to establish a stabilized and adequate spontaneous circulation (e.g., systolic systemic arterial blood pressure greater than 100 or 110 mm Hg for 10 to 15 minutes). It may take several minutes or even hours of continued pressor support before this stabilization will occur.

In cases of ventricular dysrhythmias, lidocaine administration is strongly recommended, particularly when pressors are being used. A minimal initial dose of 1 mg/kg is recommended,[4] to achieve a reasonably "suppressive" level. In successful EMS systems, a full 100-mg intravenous push has been routinely given to most adults, followed by another dose within minutes if VF persists and often 50 to 100 mg more within another few minutes if it still remains. However, as stated before, there is growing concern that lidocaine should be withheld until restoration of spontaneous circulation has been established. After an adequate spontaneous circulation is achieved, the patient is loaded with 3 mg/kg (if not already done) and a maintenance drip of 2 mg/min (initially) is also provided. This is often increased to 3 or 4 mg/min if ventricular ectopy persists. Bretylium is now considered a second-line drug in VF because of its potential hypotensive effects and, with our current approach, is rarely needed.

Sodium bicarbonate administration is generally not recommended early in the arrest. Many practitioners now believe that the correction of blood pH is largely "cosmetic" and does not alter outcome. Others even believe it to be harmful. Although a lower blood pH usually correlates with a bad outcome, this may simply mean that the degree of metabolic acidosis is just a marker for the patient's intolerance of the cardiac arrest state. For example, sprinters and seizure patients often experience a substantially lower blood pH without adverse effect. Thus, this agent is usually not given until after the first or second round of therapy has failed. Restoration of spontaneous circulation generally suggests that sodium bicarbonate should be deferred, although this concept is now being reassessed. Clinical trials to examine which subset of patients are benefited (or even harmed) by supplemental bicarbonate are being considered.

Electrocardiographic Functions

The "E" is for ECG functions. It is important to interpret the ECG properly. Asystole is not a flat line on the ECG. It is a clinical state evidenced by no pulse, apnea, and no detectable electrical activity in the heart. Therefore one must be sure of the detection apparatus. The ECG monitor gain position should be adjusted properly to establish standard amplitude calibration. If gain adjustment is desired, notation of the increased or decreased gain should accompany the ECG interpretations. Standard coarse VF may resemble torsades de pointes (atypical polymorphic VT) if the gain is too high or a normal sinus rhythm may be mistaken for asystole if the gain is too low, particularly in some patients, such as those with chronic obstructive pulmonary disease, who have electrical "insulation."

Detachment of an ECG lead is a key problem in patients receiving continuous chest compressions and multiple body jolts (during countershocks), not to mention the relatively chaotic emergency situation that predisposes to accidental detachment.

One of the mistakes occasionally made by prehospital care providers is failure to recognize that they did not switch from the "quick-look" paddle mode to the "lead" mode when they placed the standard ECG leads. Thus absent electrical activity on the monitor can be misleading. Clearly, the best safeguard is always to check for pulses and/or apical heartbeat (no matter what shows up on the monitor). In addition, constant reassessment is wise, and in cases of flat line or possible atypical VF waveforms one should consider looking at both modes and various ECG vectors before drawing final conclusions.

Further History and Physical Examination

The "F" is for further history and physical examination. Although often there is little time to obtain much history, one should still try to gain background information that might be useful in guiding further therapy. A history of hypoglycemic medications might indicate the need for glucose administration. However, there is some current thinking that hyperglycemia may exacerbate neurologic injury after cardiac arrest.[59] Therefore, measurement of blood glucose by a reagent strip (e.g., Chemstrip) is recommended. A history of tricyclic antidepressant use might steer one away from the use of antiarrhythmics that might widen the QT interval, or a history of furosemide and digoxin use in a patient with coarse VF or recurrent VT might make one consider hypomagnesemia and/or hypokalemia and treat accordingly. Medications such as beta-blockers (e.g., propranolol) or vasodilators (nitroglycerin, hydralazine, or other afterload reducers) may explain refractory bradycardia or hypotension. Nitroglycerin pads on the chest wall should be removed and wiped clean during resuscitations. A patient with a prolonged expiratory phase (e.g., chronic obstructive pulmonary disease or asthma patient) may appear to be in electromechanical dissociation when pulses have been diminished by an "auto-PEEP effect."[60] This occurs in patients who are unable to expel an entire tidal volume rapidly before delivery of the next positive pressure breath, resulting in inadvertent PEEP. In such cases there is a severely diminished venous return because of persistently high intrathoracic pressures. This can be detected by a transient (10-second) cessation of breathing, which allows complete expulsion of gas and may then allow return of palpable pulses. Treatment directed at bronchospasm, slowing of respiratory rates, and even fluid challenges may be of value here. In all cases, other reversible causes of shock (e.g., tension pneumothorax, cardiac tamponade, and hypovolemia) should be considered (and continually reconsidered).

Future Directions

Some of the future directions of management standards for cardiac arrest have been suggested earlier in this discussion. Whether or not these hypotheses are eventually validated, the key to successful management is the fastest possible restoration of adequate spontaneous circulation.[61] We have learned that the earlier the intervention, the better the results. At present, the earliest possible basic CPR and the earliest possible defibrillation (and probably aggressive use of epinephrine and ETI) are the keys to achieving better survival rates. Lidocaine probably also plays a significant role in preventing the recurrence of VF, particularly when adequate perfusion has been restored. In the future, other modalities, such as modified emergency cardiopulmonary bypass, may replace our present priorities and methodologies.[62] For now, we will probably see automated FR defibrillation becoming universal.[63] Specifically, the automated defibrillator will evolve as a routine part of BLS. FR crews will become the fundamental defibrillation specialists throughout a resuscitation, allowing paramedics to go directly to intu-

bation and intravenous access and thus expediting the efforts.

References

1. Pepe PE: The past, present, and future of emergency medical services. Prehosp Disaster Med 4(1):47, 1989.
2. Pepe PE, Bonnin MJ, Mattox KL: Regulating the scope of EMS. Prehosp Disaster Med 5(1):59, 1990.
3. Stewart RD: Medical direction in emergency medical services: The role of the physician. Emerg Med Clin North Am 5:119, 1987.
4. Emergency Cardiac Care Committee, American Heart Association: Standards and guidelines for cardiopulmonary resuscitation and emergency cardiac care. JAMA 255:2841, 1986.
5. Cummins RO, Ornato JP, Thies WH, et al: State-of-the-art review—Improving survival from sudden cardiac arrest: The "chain of survival" concept. A statement for health professionals from the Advanced Cardiac Life Support Subcommittee and the Emergency Cardiac Care Committee, American Heart Association. Circulation 83:1832, 1991.
6. Pepe PE: Advanced cardiac life support: State of the art. In: Vincent JL (ed): Emergency and Intensive Care. Berlin, Springer-Verlag, p 565, 1990.
7. Pepe PE, Copass MK: Prehospital care. In: Moore EE (ed): Early Care of the Injured Patient. 4th ed. Toronto, BC Decker, p 34, 1990.
8. Hartmann J: A system approach to intravenous thrombolysis in acute myocardial infarction in community hospitals: The influence of paramedics. Clin Cardiol 11:812, 1988.
9. American College of Emergency Physicians Committee on Emergency Medical Services: Guidelines for the Use of Thrombolytic Agents in the Prehospital Setting. Dallas, American College of Emergency Physicians Distribution Center, September 1990.
10. Pepe PE, Almaguer DR: Emergency medical services personnel and ground transport vehicles. Probl Crit Care 4:470, 1990.
11. Hoekstra JW, Banks J, Martin D, et al: The effect of EMT-defibrillation on time to the therapeutic interventions during cardiac arrest. Ann Emerg Med 20:446, 1991.
12. Braun O, Callaham ML: Direct medical control. In: Kuehl AE (ed): National Association of EMS Physicians. EMS Medical Directors' Handbook. St Louis, CV Mosby, p 175, 1989.
13. Stewart RD, Paris PM, Heller M: Design of a resident in-field experience for an emergency medicine residency curriculum. Ann Emerg Med 16:175, 1987.
14. American College of Emergency Physicians Position Statement: Control of advanced life support at the scene of medical emergencies. Ann Emerg Med 13:547, 1984.
15. Pepe PE, Bonnin MJ, Almaguer DR, et al: The effect of tiered system implementation on sudden death survival rates. Prehosp Disaster Med 4(1):71, 1989.
16. McManus WF, Tresch DD, Darin JC: An effective prehospital emergency system. J Trauma 17:304, 1977.
17. Clawson JJ: Emergency medical dispatching. In Roush WR, Aranosian RD, Blair TMH, et al (eds): Principles of EMS Systems: A Comprehensive Text for Physicians. Dallas, American College of Emergency Physicians. p 119, 1989.
18. Curka PA, Pepe PE, Ginger VF, et al: Computer-aided EMS priority dispatch: Ability of a computerized triage system to safely spare paramedics from responses not requiring advanced life support. Ann Emerg Med 20:446, 1991.
19. Pepe PE, Mattox KL, Fischer RP, et al: Geographic patterns of urban trauma according to mechanism and severity of injury. J Trauma 30:1125, 1990.
20. Pepe PE, Kelly JE, Ivy MV, et al: Resource utilization and impact of using fire apparatus for a fully-integrated EMS first-responder program. Ann Emerg Med 20:488, 1991.
21. Stone JL, Lowe RJ, Jonasson O, et al: Acute subdural hematoma: Direct admission to a trauma center yields improved results. J Trauma 26:445, 1986.
22. Bowers SA, Marshall LP: Outcome in 200 consecutive cases of severe head injury treated in San Diego county: A prospective analysis. Neurosurgery 6:237, 1980.
23. American College of Surgeons Committee on Trauma: Hospital and Prehospital Resources for Optimal Care of the Injured Patient and Appendices A–J. Chicago, American College of Surgeons, 1987.
24. Copass MK, Oreskovich MR, Bladergroen MR, et al: Prehospital cardiopulmonary resuscitation of the critically injured patient. Am J Surg 148:20, 1984.
25. Pepe PE, Copass MK, Joyce TH: Prehospital endotracheal intubation—Rationale for training emergency medical personnel. Ann Emerg Med 14:1085, 1985.
26. Gildenberg PL, Makela M: The effect of early intubation and ventilation on outcome following head trauma. In Dacey RG, Winn HR, Rimmell RW, et al (eds): Trauma of the Central Nervous System. New York, Raven Press, p 79, 1985.
27. Miller JD, Butterworth JF, Gudeman SK, et al: Further experience in the management of severe head injury. J Neurosurg 54:289, 1981.

28. Pepe PE, Wyatt CH, Bickell WH, et al: Use of MAST in penetrating cardiac injuries. Chest 89(suppl):452, 1986.
29. Durham LA, Richardson RJ, Wall MJ, et al: Emergency center thoracotomy: Impact of prehospital resuscitation. J Trauma 32:775, 1992.
30. Bickell WH, Pepe PE, Bailey ML, et al: Randomized trial of pneumatic antishock garments in the prehospital management of penetrating abdominal injuries. Ann Emerg Med 16:653, 1987.
31. Pepe PE, Bass RR, Mattox KL: Clinical trials of the pneumatic antishock garment in the urban prehospital setting. Ann Emerg Med 15:1407, 1986.
32. Mattox KL, Bickell WH, Pepe PE, et al: Prospective MAST study in 911 patients. J Trauma 29:1104, 1989.
33. McSwain NE: Pneumatic anti-shock garment: State of the art. Ann Emerg Med 17:506, 1988.
34. Bickell WH, Shaftan GW, Mattox KL: Intravenous fluid administration and uncontrolled hemorrhage (editorial). J Trauma 29:409, 1989.
35. Martin RR, Bickell WH, Mattox KL, et al: Prospective evaluation of preoperative volume resuscitation in hypotensive patients with penetrating truncal injuries—Preliminary report. J Trauma 33:354, 1992.
36. Maningas PA, Mattox KL, Pepe PE, et al: Hypertonic saline-dextran solutions for the prehospital management of traumatic hypotension. Am J Surg 157:528, 1989.
37. Mattox KL, Maningas PA, Moore EE, et al: Prehospital hypertonic saline/dextran infusion for post-traumatic hypotension—The U.S.A. multi-center trial. Ann Surg 213:482, 1991.
38. Pepe PE, Wyatt CH, Bickell WH, et al: The relationship between total prehospital time and outcome in hypotensive patients with penetrating trauma. Ann Emerg Med 16:293, 1987.
39. Ordog GJ, Ablvin D, Wasserberger J, et al: 110 bullet wounds to the neck. J Trauma 25:238, 1985.
40. Pepe PE, Ginger VF, Ritter A: Prehospital detection of hypoglycemia. Prehosp Disaster Med 5(3):313, 1990.
41. Lavery RF, Allegra JR, Cody RP, et al: A prospective evaluation of glucose reagent test strips in the prehospital setting. Am J Emerg Med 9:304, 1991.
42. Jones PW: Hyperventilation in the management of cerebral oedema. Intensive Crit Care Dig 1:17, 1982.
43. McGillicuddy JE: Cerebral protection: Pathophysiology and treatment of increased intracranial pressure. Chest 87:85, 1985.
44. Taffett G, Teasdale TA, Luchi RJ: In-hospital cardiopulmonary resuscitation. JAMA 260:2069, 1988.
45. Bonnin MJ, Pepe PE, Clark PS: Survival prognosis for the elderly after out-of-hospital cardiac arrest. Ann Emerg Med 18:469, 1989.
46. Myerburg RJ, Conde CA, Sung RJ, et al: Clinical, electrophysiologic and hemodynamic profile of patients resuscitated from prehospital cardiac arrest. Am J Med 68:568, 1980.
47. Pepe PE, Bonnin MJ, Clark PS: Clinical predictors of survival in paramedic-witnessed cardiac arrest. Prehosp Disaster Med 4(1):71, 1989.
48. Weaver WD, Cobb LA, Hallstrom AP, et al: Considerations for improving survival from out-of-hospital cardiac arrest. Ann Emerg Med 15:1181, 1986.
49. Pepe PE, Levine RL, Fromm RE, et al: Cardiac arrest presenting with rhythms other than ventricular fibrillation: Contribution of resuscitation efforts toward total survivorship. Crit Care Med. In press.
50. Weaver WD, Cobb LA, Dennis D, et al: Amplitude of ventricular fibrillation wave form and outcome after cardiac arrest. Ann Intern Med 102:53, 1985.
51. Ornato JP: High-dose epinephrine during resuscitation: A word of caution (editorial). JAMA 265:1160, 1991.
52. Brown CG, Weman HA, Davis EA, et al: The effects of graded doses of epinephrine on regional myocardial blood flow during cardiopulmonary resuscitation in swine. Circulation 75:491, 1987.
53. Gonzalez ER, Ornato JP, Garnett AR, et al: Dose-dependent vasopressor response to epinephrine during CPR in humans. Ann Emerg Med 18:920, 1989.
54. Brown CG, Martin DR, Pepe PE, et al: Standard versus high-dose epinephrine in out-of-hospital cardiac arrest—A controlled clinical trial. N Engl J Med 327:1051, 1992.
55. Brown CG, Werman HA: Adrenergic agonists during cardiopulmonary resuscitation. Resuscitation 19:1, 1990.
56. Wesley RC, Resh W, Zimmerman D: Reconsiderations of the routine and preferential use of lidocaine in the emergent treatment of ventricular arrhythmias. Crit Care Med 19:1439, 1991.
57. Weaver WD, Cobb LA, Copass MK, et al: Ventricular defibrillation: A comparative trial using 175-J and 320-J shocks. N Engl J Med 307:1101, 1982.
58. Spivey WH, Abramson NS, Safar P, et al: Correlation of blood pressure with mortality and neurologic recovery in comatose postresuscitation patients. Ann Emerg Med 20:453, 1991.
59. Nielsen MM, Barsan WG, Dimlich RVW: Effect of IV glucose on survival and neurologic outcome after cardiac arrest. Ann Emerg Med 20:454, 1991.
60. Pepe PE, Marini JJ: Occult positive end-expiratory pressure in mechanically-ventilated patients with airflow obstruction. Am Rev Respir Dis 126:166, 1982.
61. Bonnin MJ, Pepe PE, Clark PS: Key role of prehospital resuscitation in survival from out-of-hospital cardiac arrest. Ann Emerg Med 19:466, 1990.
62. Tisherman S, Grenvik A, Safar P: Cardiopulmonary-cerebral resuscitation: Advanced and prolonged life support with emergency cardiopulmonary bypass. Acta Anaesthesiol Scand 34(suppl 94):63, 1990.
63. Kerber RE: Early Defibrillation. Position statement of the American Heart Association Emergency Cardiac Care Committee. Circulation 83:2233, 1991.

CHAPTER 2

Modern Medical Response to Disasters

Derek C. Angus
Joseph A. Barbera
Vladimir Kvetan

Disaster is defined as "an occurrence causing widespread destruction and distress."[1] Whether natural or of human origin, a disaster can strike unpredictably and produce a large number of injuries and fatalities, which can easily overwhelm local medical capabilities. Furthermore, disasters manifest in many different fashions, resulting in a large volume of specific syndromes (e.g., toxic gas exposure in Bhopal and radiation injury in Chernobyl), which severely strain national medical specialized resources. Proper analysis of hazards likely to lead to a catastrophe may reduce or even prevent a disaster. In addition, prior training of professional personnel and the lay public for rapid response to an emergency should logically reduce morbidity and mortality.

The critical care physician in the United States traditionally functions in the relatively isolated environment of the intensive care unit (ICU), where resources are focused on resuscitation and life support of the individual patient. Disasters, especially those occurring in remote areas or scenarios in which the medical infrastructure has been overwhelmed, may not lend themselves to this type of focused, individual care. The critical care physician, therefore, must adapt his or her skills to respond appropriately to the ensuing chaos. This involves the use of triage, an algorithmic approach to decision making, and the institution of standardized care. To function effectively in a disaster situation, the critical care physician must also have a basic understanding of the common disaster syndromes and an awareness of his or her expected role in the medical response to disaster.

This chapter reviews the terminology and the evolution of the modern medical response to common disaster types and resulting medical syndromes, in addition to current local, state, and national policies for disaster response in the United States.

TERMINOLOGY AND HISTORY

The Armenian earthquake of 1988 caused widespread destruction and distress, rendering hundreds of thousands homeless and killing 25,000 people.[2] Likewise, earthquakes in other regions of the world (for example, the Mexico City earthquake in 1985 and the 1980 earthquake in Italy) fit this description of widespread destruction and distress.[3-5] The Union Carbide chemical plant explosion in Bhopal in 1984 did not cause an undue amount of destruction of property but did claim many lives and caused great distress.[6] Similarly, the radiation leak at Chernobyl, a nuclear disaster, claimed many lives without widespread destruction.[7]

There are, however, examples of great loss of life that are more difficult to classify. The droughts of Ethiopia have caused massive loss of life during the past 20 years, yet opinions are split in defining such events as disasters. In contrast, the Loma Prieta earthquake of 1989 caused the death of only 63 people, yet it was generally considered a disaster.[8] Aircraft accidents are also often considered disasters, even though they too have considerably less death and injury than earthquakes.[9] The explosion of Pan American flight 103 over Lockerbie, Scotland, in 1988, captured massive media attention yet claimed only a fraction of the deaths that occurred later that year in Armenia.[10]

Without minimizing the tragedy of these incidents, health care professionals concerned with the analysis of the medical response to disasters must decide on a common nomenclature and classification. Without such a system, there is no means by which to share and contrast different experiences scientifically.[11] Emergency management, which encompasses the overall approach to disaster management at a systems level, is rapidly evolving into a sophisticated specialty. For medical systems to develop effective disaster response capability, they must be closely integrated into this management system. Consideration of emergency management nomenclature is, therefore, of value.

Hazards are events with potential to cause catastrophic damage. These may be naturally occurring phenomena such as earthquakes, hurricanes, fires, and droughts. They may also be human-made, such as war with its accompanying injuries and destruction. *Disasters* are hazards that have an impact on human lives, causing adverse physical, psychologic, social, economic, or even political effects.[12, 13] The scope of this impact exceeds the affected community's ability to manage the resultant damage. For example, a tornado that strikes an area distant from a population base is a hazard; a tornado striking an urban area quickly becomes a disaster. *Medical disasters* constitute a disaster subset in which physical and/or psychologic injuries exceed the medical response capabilities of the communities affected. Many medical disasters include a component of property disaster and disrupt essential services (including local emergency medical systems).

An early and practical delineation of medical disasters came from Peter Safar, who suggested dividing disasters into three types.[14] The first is an event that, regardless of its size, is containable by the local emergency medical service (EMS). This is termed a multicasualty incident (MCI). The second is an event that overwhelms local response capability and is termed a mass disaster (sometimes called a mass casualty incident).[15] The third type is termed an endemic disaster (e.g., the recurrent famines of Ethiopia).

Medical disasters may also be classified by the speed of impact and the requisite response phase. For example, earthquakes and tornadoes are of sudden onset and necessitate an effective rapid response, whereas famines are more characteristically slow-onset disasters. Birnbaum suggested further classifying MCIs and mass disasters by type and scope.[11] The type reflects the incident's cause (a train wreck, an earthquake, and a flood, for example), whereas the scope defines the extent of the event in terms of fatalities, injuries, and required response.

From an operational perspective, an event becomes an MCI when its impact exceeds the routine response capability of the local systems and significant local adjustments have to occur. This is often called a level I response. A level II

response develops when this enhanced local response is overwhelmed and neighboring or regional resources are activated for assistance. A level III response involves state, interstate, and federal resources in the rescue and recovery process.[16] Depending on the human impact and the degree of deviation from normal response capability, mass disasters may require a level II or level III response.

Factors other than overwhelming numbers of casualties may generate a disaster situation. For example, disruption of rapid transport systems to the hospital may prevent the timely delivery of necessary services. A moderately increased number of patients in a narrow diagnostic category may overwhelm specific critical care services (e.g., pulmonary care, renal dialysis, burn care, and confined-space medical care to entrapped persons).[17] With the onset of a medical disaster, operational priorities change from the provision of optimal care to each patient to the provision of the best care possible to the greatest number of patients.

For many years, the only organized medical involvement in disasters was the public health response. This tended to focus on long-term support for mass disasters and for endemic disasters. Since the formation of the Club of Mainz in 1968 (later the World Association for Emergency and Disaster Medicine), physicians concerned with organizing a more effective approach to handle these situations have generated interest in an area called disaster resuscitation (or reanimatology). This field is concerned primarily with the logistics of applying the principles of emergency medicine to the much larger scales of mass disasters.[18] Meanwhile, considerable experience was being gained in military medicine from the application of resuscitation techniques in combat situations. The Vietnam War demonstrated that effective medical care practiced outside the traditional hospital setting (using field medics, rapid transport, and field hospitals) could dramatically reduce morbidity and mortality.[19-21] The subsequent development of EMS systems throughout the United States, the development of the fields of emergency medicine and critical care, and the dissemination of first aid concepts throughout society provided the foundation for the delivery of immediate and effective prehospital and emergency medical care to disaster victims. Sophisticated medical response to disasters in the forms of mobile critical care teams (Armenian earthquake in 1988; pipeline explosion in Ufa, Commonwealth of Independent States, in 1989), renal dialysis teams (Armenian earthquake in 1988; Ufa pipeline explosion in 1989), orthopedic and trauma teams (Armenia), burn teams (Ufa), disaster medical assistance teams (Hurricane Hugo in St. Croix, Virgin Islands, 1989), and emergency medical teams (Armenia; Philippine earthquake, 1990) further expanded the evolving field of disaster medicine[22-26] (Collins AJ, personal communication, 1990).

In 1989, the Society of Critical Care Medicine developed a Task Force on Disasters to provide a didactic and clinical forum for intensive care specialists interested in the delivery of services in disasters, adverse environments, and armed conflict. The task force has a clinical response capability; its members have worked on civilian and military disaster response teams.[22] The need for a high-quality multidisciplinary critical care response was noted during one of the largest potential human-made disasters: Operation Desert Storm in the Persian Gulf. At the request of the U.S. Office of Army Surgeon General, the task force recruited 42 large multidisciplinary teams from 22 states to augment military medical resources at U.S. military hospitals in Germany.[27]

Through the World Association for Emergency and Disaster Medicine and other forums, such as the Society of Critical Care Medicine, medical personnel share their experiences and exchange research ideas from their primary

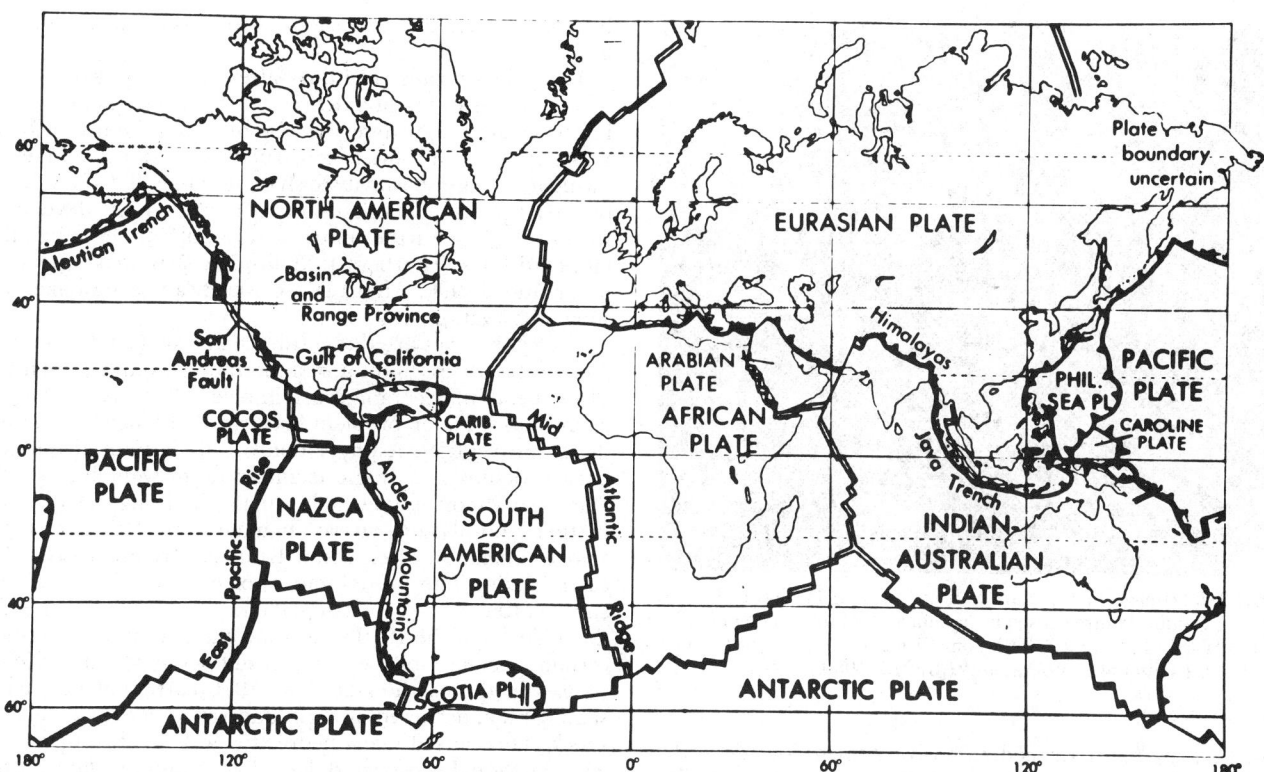

Figure 2–1. U.S. Geological Survey map depicting the major tectonic plates of the world. Most earthquakes occur in the areas of plate boundaries. (From Tilling RI: Volcanoes. Washington, DC, US Government Printing Office. US Department of the Interior, Division of Geological Survey, general interest publication.)

specialties with those who have responded to disasters.[18] These are also media in which clinicians interact with experts in public health and epidemiology in an effort to more clearly define the prehospital and disaster setting as an area of investigation.

DISASTER TYPES

The scale of a disaster is dependent not only on the size but also the site and timing of the event. For example, the 1989 Loma Prieta, California, earthquake caused the loss of 63 lives and $6 billion of damage. However, if an earthquake of the same size had occurred farther north on the Hayward, California, fault line, it would have been centered on the cities of Oakland, Fremont, and Berkeley, California. The

TABLE 2–1			
TEN MOST LETHAL EARTHQUAKES IN THE TWENTIETH CENTURY			
Year	Place	Deaths	Richter Magnitude Scale
1908	Italy	75,000	7.5
1915	Italy	29,000	7.0
1920	China	180,000	8.6
1923	Japan	43,000	8.3
1927	China	200,000	8.3
1932	China	70,000	7.6
1935	India	30,000	7.5
1939	Chile	30,000	8.3
1970	Peru	66,000	7.8
1976	China	242,000	8.0

Courtesy of Abrams J, Department of Civil Engineering, University of Pittsburgh.

predicted damage would then have been 1500 to 4500 deaths and more than $70 billion damage.[28, 29]

Therefore, it is important to understand and predict the impact of such disasters to identify high-risk areas and plan effectively. The first step in planning is to understand the effects of the different natural and human-made phenomena that may occur. Some common disaster types are reviewed, with a focus on earthquakes because they are the most overwhelming natural disasters.[30, 31] Other disaster types can be reviewed elsewhere.[16, 31–33]

Earthquakes

An earthquake is the oscillatory movement of the earth's surface, resulting from the underlying movements of tectonic plates, that follows a release of energy in the earth's crust.[32] The vast majority of the world's earthquakes occur around the Pacific rim at the edge of the Pacific plate (Fig. 2–1). The most well-known section of this plate is in California, the San Andreas fault. More than 1 million earthquake deaths and serious injuries have occurred worldwide during the past 20 years.[34] Table 2–1 lists the 10 most severe earthquakes of the 20th century.

In addition to the primary movement of the earth's crust, secondary effects also occur including tsunamis, landslides, fire, and flooding. Tsunamis are tidal waves generated by the sudden movement of ocean beds (earthquakes occurring on the sea floor) and can be up to 50 ft in height and travel at up to 600 mph. When they hit coastal regions, the effect can be devastating. The 1964 earthquake in Alaska was complicated by tsunamis, which caused severe damage as far south as Crescent City, California, and some waves raced across the entire Pacific Ocean to the coasts of Japan.[32] Landslides are caused by the liquefaction of weak soils by the vibration from the earthquake. The Marina district in

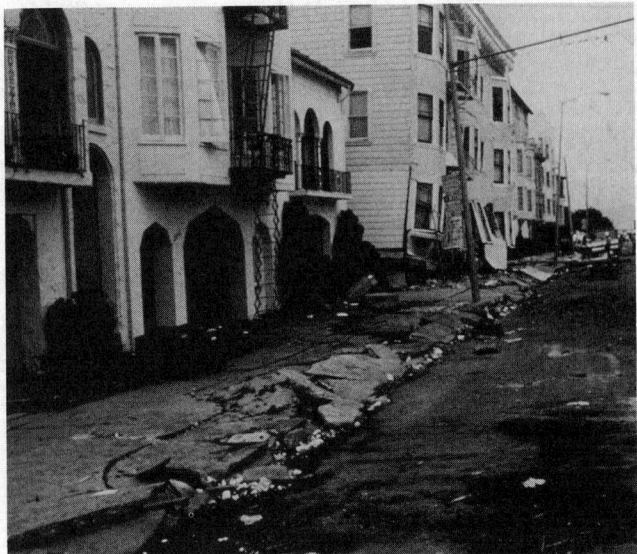

Figure 2–2. Damage in the Marina district of San Francisco demonstrating ground failure caused by liquefaction of underlying landfill. (From Ward PL, Page RA: The Loma Prieta earthquake of October 17, 1989. Earthquakes Volcanoes 21[6]:215, 1989.)

San Francisco experienced extensive damage owing to the complete liquefaction of the landfill on which it was built[35] (Fig. 2–2). The principal destruction from the 1906 earthquake in San Francisco was due to subsequent fire. Flooding, resulting from changes in the levels of artesian wells or destruction of dams, is also a major source of destruction after an earthquake.[36]

The size of an earthquake is determined by the Richter magnitude scale, which is a logarithmic scale measuring the amplitude of the reverberations that an earthquake produces.[37] An earthquake of magnitude 7 is 100 times more powerful than one measuring 5. Because the Richter scale does not measure damage caused, a subjective scale (the modified Mercalli Intensity Scale) was developed (Table 2–2). This scale is based on the degree of structural damage caused by an earthquake at particular sites. As such, the modified Mercalli Intensity Scale for the Marina area of San Francisco in the Loma Prieta earthquake was higher than that of neighboring districts, which were built on solid

bedrock and experienced significantly less damage[36] (see Fig. 2–2).

The primary cause of injury after an earthquake is structural collapse and falling debris.[16, 31, 36, 38] Consequently, building types are major determinants of injury. Non-reinforced masonry and mud-brick construction are most dangerous owing to its high sensitivity to shaking forces. This is reflected by the large casualty tolls after earthquakes in the developing world.[2, 16, 31, 39–41] Further injury can result from flooding, fire, and landslides[42] (Barbera J, Philippine earthquake, personal observation, 1990; Angus DC, Costa Rican earthquake, personal observation, 1991).

Typical injuries are due to direct trauma (Table 2–3) and include fractures, blunt and penetrating wounds, open and closed head injuries, and crush injuries.[2, 31, 39, 41] Airway injury represents a major problem because of the need for immediate intervention. Asphyxiation of mildly injured but concussed victims is a tragic example of preventable death.[14] Dust generation is inevitable during building collapse and further complicates airway management.[43, 44] Burns and smoke inhalation often result from the frequent fires after earthquakes. The most famous example of fire injury occurred after the 1906 earthquake in San Francisco, in which the majority of the 1900 deaths were due to fire. In addition, certain peculiar injuries may result from specific circumstances in the earthquake. The 1976 earthquake in Tangshan, China, occurred at night and was preceded by a small shock. This caused many people to awake and sit up in bed. The earthquake occurred less than a minute later, while many people sat upright, and the ensuing building collapse caused a large number of spinal injuries. The thousands of paraplegic patients continue to present a significant financial and logistical burden to the region today.[45]

Volcanoes

A volcano is a hill or mountain built around a vent that connects with reservoirs of molten rock below the earth's surface.[46] Buoyancy and gas pressure can cause the molten rock to be driven up through these vents, breaking through weaknesses in the surface of the volcano. Molten rock can pour over the edge of the volcano as nonexplosive, slow-moving lava flows or there can be the violent explosion of lava fragments propelled into the air with hot gases (Figs. 2–3 and 2–4). These fragments may fall back onto the volcano and slip down the mountain as ash flows. The finer

	TABLE 2–2				
	MODIFIED MERCALLI INTENSITY SCALE				
		Amount of Structural Damage			
Scale	Human Impression	*Poor Construction*	*Good Construction*	*Specially Designed*	General
I	Not felt	Nil	Nil	Nil	
II	Felt by few on upper floors	Nil	Nil	Nil	
III	Felt by some indoors like truck passing	Nil	Nil	Nil	
IV	Felt by many indoors	Nil	Nil	Nil	Cars rocked
V	Felt by nearly all	Nil	Nil	Nil	Windows broken
VI	Felt by all, many frightened	Slight	Slight	Slight	Heavy furniture moved
VII		Considerable	Moderate	Slight	Heavy furniture overturned
VIII		Great	Considerable	Slight	
IX		Great	Great	Considerable	
X		Destroyed	Destroyed	Some destroyed	
XI		Destroyed	Destroyed	Many destroyed	Bridges destroyed
XII		Total destruction	Total destruction	Total destruction	Objects thrown in the air

Adapted from US Geological Survey: The Severity of an Earthquake. Washington, DC, US Government Printing Office, 1990. US Department of the Interior, Division of Geological Survey, general interest publication 0-273-494 QL3.

TABLE 2–3
INJURIES IN EARTHQUAKES BY NUMBER (PERCENTAGE)

Type of Injury	Saidi (1963)*	De Goyet (1979)	Gueri (1979)	Ortiz (1986)	Noji (1989)
Fracture (clavicle)		18 (11.5)			
Fracture (skull, face)				16 (1.0)	130 (2.7)
Fracture (cervical and dorsal vertebrae)	10 (9.0)			37 (2.3)	388 (8.0)
Fracture (upper extremity)	49 (44.1)	5 (3.2)		80 (4.9)	265 (5.5)
Fracture (lower extremity)		10 (6.4)		189 (11.7)	584 (12.1)
Fracture (pelvis)	7 (6.3)	4 (2.6)			
Brain concussion					417 (8.6)
Other internal head trauma					173 (3.6)
Open head, facial wounds					320 (6.6)
Traumatic amputation, arms					197 (4.1)
Open wounds, legs					102 (2.1)
Traumatic amputation, legs					170 (3.5)
Vascular injuries					5 (0.1)
Elective amputation, arms					13 (0.3)
Elective amputation, legs					59 (1.2)
Dislocations				12 (0.7)	61 (1.3)
Sprains and tears				139 (8.6)	
Intracranial injury without fracture				95 (5.9)	
Internal injury to chest, abdomen, or pelvis				4 (0.3)	70 (1.5)
Wound of the head, neck, and trunk	19 (17.1)		80 (35.8)	219 (13.5)	
Wound, upper extremity			11 (4.9)	122 (7.5)	
Wound, lower extremity			87 (39.0)	217 (13.4)	
Superficial injury or minor contusion	26 (23.4)			415 (25.6)	1203 (24.9)
Bruises				7 (0.4)	
Injury to nerves and spinal column			10 (4.5)	7 (0.4)	30 (0.6)
Complications of unspecified injury				16 (1.0)	
Crush syndrome					533 (11.0)
Burns					56 (1.2)
Frostbite					4 (0.8)
Nonearthquake related injuries					52 (1.1)
Others		120 (76.4)	35 (15.7)	48 (3.0)	
TOTAL	111 (100)	157 (100)	223 (100)	1623 (100)	4832 (100)

*References as given in original publication.
Adapted from Pollander GS, Rund DA: Analysis of medical needs in disasters caused by earthquake: The need for a uniform injury reporting scheme. Disasters 13:365, 1989, in Noji E: Natural disasters in disaster management. Crit Care Clin 7:271, 1991.

ash particles can be carried in the atmosphere and spread as clouds of hot ash. The heat generated from these flows of gas, ash, and molten rock can melt snowcaps and liquefy soils, causing landslides, fast-moving mud flows (lahars), and floods.[47] The most lethal consequences are pyroclastic flows (Fig. 2–5), because of their speed. These are flows of lava fragments and ash that accelerate down the side of a volcano at speeds of hundreds of miles per hour and can spread for several miles.[16, 31, 48]

Injury patterns depend on the characteristics of the eruption. One recurring feature, however, is the high proportion of lethal injuries.[49] Contrary to popular belief, lava flows are not the main danger, because they are easily avoided.[16] The major causes of death and injury are lahars, ashfalls, and

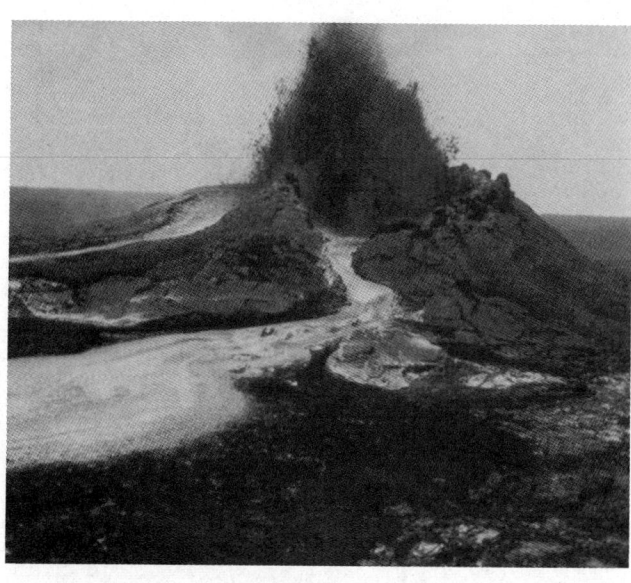

Figure 2–3. 1983 eruption of Pu'u'O'o demonstrating both slow lava flow and violent ash and gas eruption. (From Heliker C: Volcanic and Seismic Hazards on the Island of Hawaii. Washington, DC, US Government Printing Office, 1990. US Department of the Interior, Division of Geological Survey, general interest publication 259-799.)

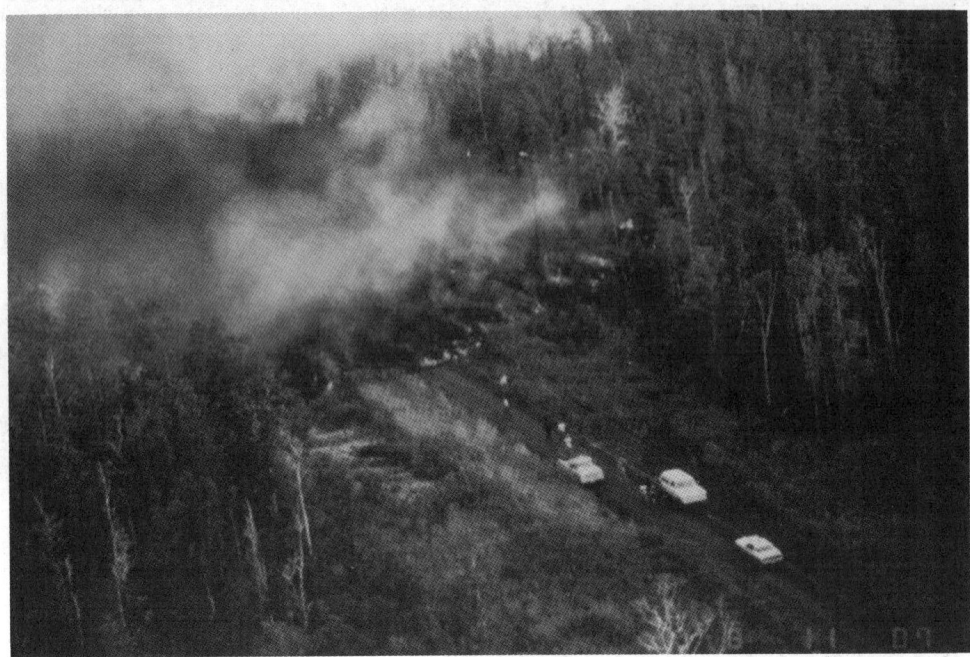

Figure 2–4. Slow-moving lava after 1983 eruption of the Pu'u'O'o volcano, Hawaii. (From Heliker C: Volcanic and Seismic Hazards on the Island of Hawaii. Washington, DC, US Government Printing Office, 1990. US Department of the Interior, Division of Geological Survey, general interest publication 259-799.)

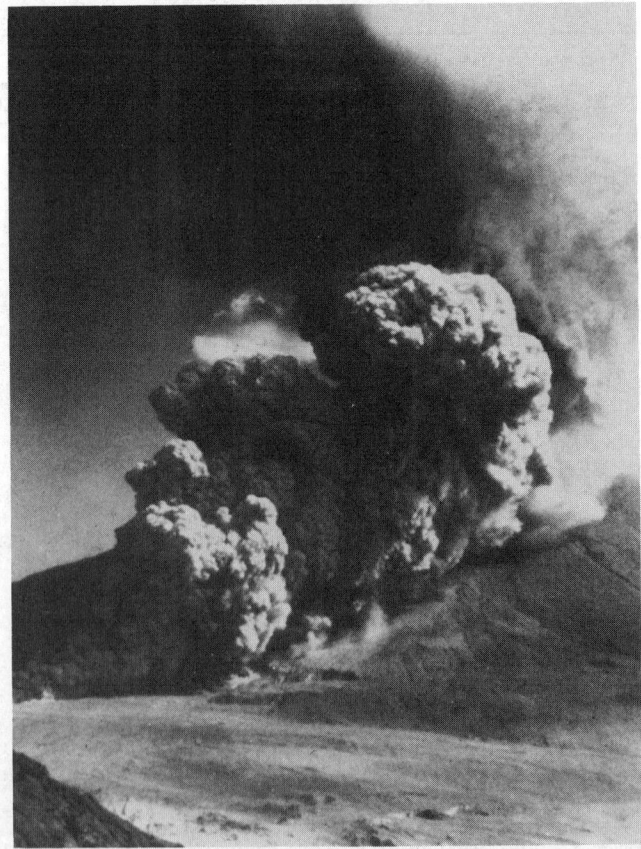

Figure 2–5. Pyroclastic flow after eruption of Mount St. Helens on August 7, 1980. (From Crandell DR, Nichols DR: Volcanic hazards at Mount Shasta, California. Washington, DC, US Government Printing Office, 1989. US Department of the Interior, Division of Geological Survey, publication 0-235-707.)

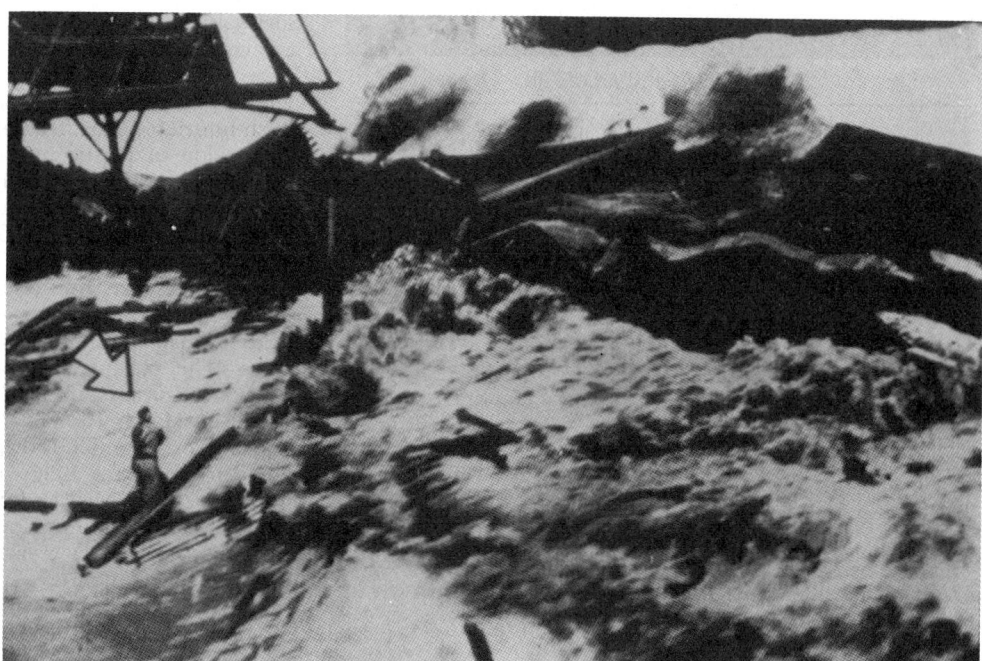

Figure 2–6. A giant wave engulfs the Hilo pier during the 1946 tsunami. The arrow points to a man who was swept away seconds later. (From Heliker C: Volcanic and Seismic Hazards on the Island of Hawaii. Washington, DC, US Government Printing Office, 1990. US Department of the Interior, Division of Geological Survey, general interest publication 259-799.)

pyroclastic flows. The relatively small eruption of snow-capped Nevada del Ruiz in Columbia in 1986 caused considerable lahars owing to melting of the icecap. Twenty-three thousand people died from engulfment in these lahars.[48, 49] The proportion of dead to injured was 5:1. The eruption of Mt. Vesuvius in AD 79 buried the towns of Pompeii and Herculaneum under falling ash in only a few hours. They were inundated so completely that their ruins were not discovered for 1700 years. A striking example of a pyroclastic flow was the 1902 eruption of Mt. Pelee in Martinique in which one surge left only a handful of people alive of the 28,000 inhabitants of St. Pierre.[16, 49] In those who survive volcanic eruptions, the most common injuries are burns and inhalation injuries. Death is usually by incineration, asphyxiation, or drowning.

Cyclones

Cyclones are large rotating weather systems that form seasonally over tropical oceans.[16] They consist of a calm inner portion of low pressure known as the eye, surrounded by a wall of rain and high-velocity winds. The wind circles fastest at the inner edge of the eye and can travel up to 150 mph. They are called hurricanes in the Caribbean Sea and western Atlantic Ocean and typhoons in the western Pacific Ocean and South China Sea.[31] The most devastating hurricane in the United States hit Galveston, Texas, in 1900 and killed 6000 people. This remains the most catastrophic disaster in North American history.[36]

The major cause of death and destruction is storm surges.[50–52] These are caused by a rise in sea level in response to the profound barometric depression at the center of the cyclone. Consequently, up to 90% of fatalities are from drowning.[53] The Bangladesh cyclones of 1970 and 1991 caused 300,000 and 100,000 deaths, respectively.[54] Other early causes of injury include trauma from building collapse and floating debris.[55] A common injury during the Bangladesh cyclone in 1970 was severe abrasion of skin in persons attempting to cling to trees in fast-moving water.[54] Late morbidity is due to postdisaster cleanup accidents (including electrocution), starvation and dehydration, outbreaks of communicable diseases, and wound contamination.[56]

Tornadoes

A tornado is a funnel-shaped cloud extending toward the ground from the base of a thundercloud. The funnel is composed of high-velocity winds encircling a low-pressure hollow cavity.[57] Circular wind speeds can exceed 300 mph and are strong enough to propel objects as heavy as automobiles.[16] Tornadoes occur worldwide but are particularly common and severe in the Midwest and South of the United States. Although there are hundreds every year in the United States, most occur over remotely populated regions and only 3% cause casualties.[57] Of the 14,600 tornadoes recorded from 1952 to 1973, only 497 caused fatalities and 26 alone caused more than 50% of the deaths.[58]

In the past 50 years, 9000 people have died in tornadoes.[59] The most common causes of death were craniocerebral trauma and crush injuries to the trunk.[60] Other causes of injury and death include fractures, spinal cord injuries, lacerations, and contusions.[61]

Floods

Floods can be divided into three types: flash floods (caused by heavy rains or dam failures), coastal floods (including storm surges and tsunamis), and river floods[62] (Fig. 2–6). Together, they are the most common type of disaster and account for about half of all disaster-related deaths.[34, 63] The most lethal flood in recorded history was the 1887 flood of the Hwang Ho (Yellow River) in China, killing 900,000 and leaving 2 million people homeless.[31] The worst flood in the United States was the flash flood in Johnstown, Pennsylvania, in 1889, which killed 2200 people.[52]

The primary cause of death is drowning.[64] Other causes are principally related to trauma from floating debris and hypothermia.[65] Of those who survive, few (less than 2%) require extensive medical intervention.[54, 63] Later complications include public health concerns such as contamination of water supplies, overcrowded conditions of refugee shelters, and outbreaks of communicable diseases.[66] Wound infection is common because of contamination.[67] A notable concern is the displacement of wildlife. In 1973, Ussher reported numerous snake bites including six deaths after a

TABLE 2–4

DISASTERS OF HUMAN ORIGIN

Event	Type of Injuries
Building collapse	Mechanical trauma, crush injuries
Airplane crash	Mechanical trauma, thermal burns, inhalation injuries
Train/bus wreck	Mechanical trauma
Nuclear power plant accident	Radiation injuries (irradiation, external contamination, incorporation)
Hazardous materials accident	Chemical burns, inhalation injuries, systemic toxicity
Terrorist activities	Depending on event: gunshot wounds, blast injuries, shrapnel/penetrating injuries

Adapted from Leonard RB, Teitelman U: Manmade disasters in disaster management. Crit Care Clin 7:293, 1991.

flood in the Philippines. The snakes were cobras driven to higher ground near towns and villages.[67]

Human-Made Disasters

Table 2–4 lists important causes of disasters of human origin and their likely injury patterns. Transport accidents, structural collapses, and acts of war and terrorism produce many injuries similar to those seen after natural disasters and in urban EMS systems. Other types, such as release of chemicals or radioactive materials, may produce syndromes rarely seen by a practicing intensivist.[33]

Transport Accidents

Motor Vehicle Accidents. Although motor vehicle accidents cause many deaths per year, single incidents rarely constitute a medical disaster. When there are large numbers of casualties, a complicating factor (such as the spillage of chemicals from trucks) is often present. In 1982, more than 1000 deaths occurred after an accident involving a petroleum tanker in the Salang Tunnel in Afghanistan. The majority of deaths were caused by inhalation of carbon monoxide released from the combustion of petroleum.[68] However, the usual injury pattern is of multiple trauma and fractures.

Rail Transport. Rail transport is considered one of the safest modes of transportation with an estimated 0.05 deaths per million hours of travel.[69] However, disasters do occur. More than 800 people perished in June 1981 when a train crashed into the Bagmati River in India.[70] There are aspects of particular importance with rail crashes. First, access is often difficult. For example, trains may crash in narrow cuttings or in tunnels, resulting in delayed rescue. Second, there are often hazardous materials on board. Unlike the case with road transport, a train may be carrying several different chemicals in different cars. During a train crash, these chemicals may mix, releasing new and unexpected toxic chemicals, further hampering the rescue response.[71]

Injury patterns depend on the circumstances of the crash. The most common injuries are multiple trauma and fractures. However, burns and chemical injuries can be common, depending on the cargo and secondary effects of the crash. Furthermore, exposure, hypothermia, and drowning are obviously likely if the train crashes into water.

Air Transport. There are approximately 60 fatal airline crashes per year worldwide and more than half are nonsurvivable.[69] In general, most crashes occur at an airport.[72]

Survival is more likely if the aircraft has a wide rather than a narrow body and if the crash occurs at an airport.[69, 73] Moreover, if there are survivors, they are usually outnumbered by the dead. Injury patterns are multiple trauma and crush injuries, burns, fractures, and asphyxiation caused by combustion of plastic products lining the cabin. Of those who survive, one third will have long-term disability.[69]

The most important feature of aircraft disaster management is airport planning. Guidelines are published by the International Civil Aviation Organization, and implementation of all aspects of these guidelines is mandatory if an effective response is to be achieved.[74]

Sea Transport. Shipwrecks have caused disasters for centuries. The collapse of the Titanic is one of the most infamous disasters in modern times. More recently, the sinking in March 1987 of the Herald of Free Enterprise, a British cross-channel ferry, less than 5 minutes after its departure from the Belgian port of Zeebrugge caused just less than 200 deaths. Unfortunately, despite vast improvements in ship design during the past 100 years, shipwrecks continue to occur for a variety of reasons, including storm damage, collision, fire, explosions, chemical leakage, and war.[75] The main causes of death and injury are due to immersion (leading to drowning, hypothermia, and oil contamination), starvation, dehydration, and exposure.

Hazardous Materials Spills

Hazardous materials spills are more unusual, producing diverse injury patterns, such as chemical burns, toxic inhalations, and systemic injuries. Furthermore, although the risk of such spills is rising with the ever-increasing volume of chemical production (more than 60,000 chemicals and radioactive isotopes are produced in the United States) and transport, accidents are relatively rare. Consequently, medical and EMS reponders have little experience dealing with such disasters.

A hazardous material is defined in the United States as "a substance or material which has been determined by the Secretary of Transportation to be capable of posing an unreasonable risk to health, safety, and property when transported in commerce."[76] A detailed review of hazardous materials is available[33] (see also Chapter 3).

Terrorism

The most common terrorist act is detonating an explosive device among a large group of people. An analysis of 220 bombings shows that, although 89.5% of persons requiring surgery have bone and soft tissue injury, head injury results in 71.4% of immediate and 52% of late deaths. Pulmonary blast injury, the most common thoracic trauma syndrome, accounts for 11% of the mortality.[77] The lessons learned have resulted in the development of focused medical response capabilities, such as the U.S. Air Force FAST teams (flying ambulance surgical trauma teams) organized after the 1983 bombing of the Marine barracks in Beirut.

MEDICAL SYNDROMES IN DISASTERS

The clinical management of individual casualties after an MCI or mass disaster is often compromised by insufficient personnel or inadequate equipment and supplies. It is the responsibility of the medical personnel to be knowledgeable in the optimal management of the injuries likely to be sustained and to adapt that management as effectively as possible to the specific disaster situation.

Common disaster injury patterns are listed in Table 2–5. The major early consequences are hypovolemic shock, loss

TABLE 2–5

COMMON INJURY PATTERNS IN DISASTERS

Disaster	Injury Type										
	Trauma	Crush	Head Injury	Spinal Injury	Fracture	Laceration	Burns	Hypothermia	Inhalation	Drowning	Late Complications*
Natural											
Earthquake	x	x	x	x	x	x	x	x	x		x
Volcano	x						x		x		
Cyclone	x									x	x
Tornado	x	x	x	x	x						
Flood								x		x	x
Human-Made											
Motor vehicle accident	x	x	x	x	x	x					
Rail accident	x	x	x	x	x	x	x				
Aircraft accident	x	x	x	x	x	x	x		x		
Sea accident								x	x	x	x
Hazardous material spill							x		x		
Terrorism	x	x	x	x	x	x					

*Includes starvation, dehydration, wound infection, and communicable disease.

of consciousness, airway compromise, hypoxia, and ventilatory failure. Later problems include renal failure (often secondary to crush syndrome), wound infection, sepsis, and multiple organ system failure.[2, 78] In addition, public health problems such as contaminated water supplies, overcrowding, and lack of shelter can further hamper management of initial injuries. We discuss crush syndrome and the management of certain other conditions that occur frequently after a disaster.

Crush Syndrome

Crush syndrome is the systemic manifestation of extensive muscle damage sustained by patients trapped under debris. These consequences most significantly affect cardiac, renal, and metabolic functions and often cause deterioration and even sudden death shortly after extrication of seemingly stable persons. Survivors who are not treated early in their rescue course frequently experience acute renal failure secondary to crush injury.[23]

Crush syndrome was extensively described in patients injured during the London bombings of 1940 and 1941 and has been commonly observed in victims trapped in the rubble of structures that collapse because of earthquakes, terrorist bombings, and spontaneous structural failure.[79] Severe crush syndrome is unusual outside these scenarios. The primary bodily insult is prolonged compression of a large skeletal muscle bed, most often the thigh or the calf, leading to rhabdomyolysis.[80]

Clinical Manifestations

Local Effects. Muscle damage results from ischemia (interruption of the arterial supply caused by either direct compression of the artery proximal to the muscle or a diminished arteriocompartmental pressure gradient), and direct compression on the muscle bed.[81, 82] Skeletal muscles in the forearm and the lower leg are encased in compartments surrounded by inelastic fascial sheaths. In health, the intracompartmental pressures are low, with an arteriocompartmental pressure gradient that allows normal blood flow.

With compression of a muscle, intracompartmental pressures rise dramatically, inhibiting intracompartmental tissue perfusion and leading to ischemic injury, cell dysfunction, and early cell death.[83–85]

This entity is called the compartmental syndrome and is usually seen in patients with a pure arterial ischemic insult, as in patients with peripheral vascular disease and acute arterial obstruction. For surgical purposes, it can be defined as an intracompartmental pressure in excess of 40 mm Hg, lasting longer than 8 hours.[83, 86, 87] In compartmental syndrome secondary to crush injury, intracompartmental pressures of up to 240 mm Hg may be generated. This results in muscle cell injury with resultant cell swelling and capillary leak after 60 minutes of compression. Reperfusion of severely damaged muscle leads to further swelling of both the intracellular and extracellular spaces, causing severe myoedema and progressive intracompartmental tissue injury.

Systemic Effects. Because of the tamponade effect of overlying debris, the compressed limb may be isolated from the central circulation of the patient until rescue occurs. On rescue, the patient may appear deceptively stable, until the patient is extricated from the debris. At that time, reperfusion of and venous washout from the affected limb occurs and multiple pathologic processes commence, leading to the systemic manifestations of the crush syndrome. Without immediate intervention, these patients may experience rapid deterioration and death.[84]

The most immediate threat is hypovolemia (Table 2–6). Massive accumulation of fluid in the injured muscle tissue (myoedema) may cause hemoconcentration and severe

TABLE 2–6

CAUSES OF HYPOVOLEMIA IN CRUSH SYNDROME

Third spacing
Distant hemorrhage
Dehydration
Vasodilation
Inadequate resuscitation

shock. Several other mechanisms may magnify this hypovolemic effect. The patient may have bled significantly from other injuries. Trapped persons rarely have access to fluids before rescue and may be significantly dehydrated in the absence of overt hemorrhage. Lactic acid and other products of cell damage may cause failure of autoregulation of the vasculature. In this setting, fluid resuscitation may be inadequate owing to delayed intravenous (IV) access and the failure of the medical team to assess appropriately the amount of blood or fluid deficits.

An elevation in serum potassium levels and sudden acidemia can lead to severe dysrhythmias and cardiac arrest shortly after extrication.[88] Hyperkalemia with its attendant cardiovascular effects can occur rapidly and necessitates immediate therapy[89] (Barbera JA, unpublished series, 1990).

Renal Effects. Surviving patients are at high risk for the development of acute renal failure because of volume depletion and myoglobinuria.[90] Early intervention is imperative to prevent oliguric renal failure. This is particularly important in the mass disaster setting, where the technologic support for prompt dialysis may be destroyed or overwhelmed.[24]

Diagnosis

Because early treatment is essential in the management of patients with crush injury, the diagnosis is ideally made before extrication of the patient. Unfortunately, the signs and symptoms can be subtle, especially before limb extrication and early in the postextrication course.

While entombed, the patient may be hemodynamically stable. Severe muscle injury may occur with little damage to overlying skin, making initial assessment misleading. Myoedema is not clinically apparent until release and reperfusion of the limb. If a limb has been compressed for a significant period, it may become insensate and the patient may deny pain, until release from entrapment. The injury itself may present with muscle dysfunction and overlying skin anesthesia, mimicking a spinal cord lesion. The compressed anatomic component may not be accessible for examination. Normal distal pulses and skin color may be present, despite proximal crush injury from direct compression. After the patient's release, the patient may indicate severe pain without having obvious external signs of trauma.

After the patient's release from entrapment, myoglobin in the urine is confirmed with urinalysis strips. Often, the urine is dark reddish brown because of myoglobin. The hospital laboratory can differentiate myoglobinuria from hemoglobinuria.

Early biochemical indicators include hyperkalemia out of proportion to the rise in creatinine, hyperphosphatemia, and elevated creatine kinase level. In the absence of significant bleeding, an elevated hematocrit can indicate hemoconcentration. Hypocalcemia is also common.

Management

The first trial of specific therapy for crush syndrome in humans was reported in 1984 by Ron and coworkers, who treated seven young men trapped in a collapsed building after a terrorist bomb attack in Lebanon in 1982.[91] The protocol consisted of high-volume, isotonic fluid resuscitation (with lactated Ringer's solution) begun before or immediately after extrication. High-volume crystalloid administration was continued in the ICU. This was augmented by mannitol to attain a forced diuresis of greater than 300 mL/h of urine. Sodium bicarbonate and acetazolamide were administered to alkalize the urine to a pH of 6.5 or greater. These objectives were reached quickly and maintained until visible myoglobinuria and rising serum potassium levels resolved.

All seven patients in this study had clinical and biochemical evidence of severe crush injury, but none developed renal failure. In contrast, another patient from the same incident was misdiagnosed as having a spinal cord injury. An aggressive fluid replacement and alkalization protocol was not used and acute renal failure occurred, necessitating 3 weeks of dialysis.

After the Armenian earthquake of 1988, a delay of 24 to 48 hours occurred before treatment of many patients with crush syndrome was initiated and at least 600 patients required hemodialysis.[78] Although no prospective, randomized studies exist to support the effectiveness of these protocols, experience suggests that institution of high-volume fluid therapy and bicarbonate administration early in the management of these patients may provide renal protective effects. Hypocalcemia is common and its management is reviewed elsewhere.[13, 84, 92] Patients who survive, even those who require dialysis, have a relatively good prognosis.

Another life-threatening risk is infection, particularly that arising from the injured muscle. In the past, fasciotomy was often performed early to decrease intracompartmental pressure when compartmental syndrome was suspected. The procedure was associated with a high risk of infection when the necrotic muscle tissue was exposed. With the advent of direct manometry, the arteriocompartmental gradient is now easily calculated and the indications for fasciotomy are better defined. In a review of their patient series, Better and Stein concluded that fasciotomy should be done only when there is interruption of arterial blood flow (loss of distal pulses) from high intracompartmental pressures.[84] They concluded that the risk of infection from exposure of necrotic tissue did not justify the use of surgery in traumatic rhabdomyolysis and that the skin should be considered a natural dressing for the underlying muscle.[93] Although all of the 1982 subjects had demonstrable rhabdomyolysis, none sustained compartmental syndrome or required a fasciotomy; still the controversy about fasciotomy continues. It is clear that manometry plays a useful role in monitoring the intracompartmental perfusion pressures, however, and that further study using this measurement is needed.

Experience has shown that, with meticulous medical and surgical care, extremities sustaining severe crush injury may survive with relatively good functional recovery.[93] Scrupulous wound care is essential and IV antibiotic therapy should be administered promptly for suspected infection. It appears that the use of military antishock trousers should be avoided, as should air splints and compressive dressings.[94, 95] Injured extremities are best stabilized by splinting in neutral position using methods that minimize the application of pressure to the tissues. The extremity should be kept at heart level, because raising it may critically decrease perfusion pressure and lowering it may increase dependent edema.[80]

Some authors have recommended the use of tourniquets in the prehospital management of crush injury to avoid systemic sequelae.[96] Both venous and arterial tourniquets, however, can have deleterious effects. Venous obstruction increases the formation of myoedema, and both types of tourniquets worsen muscle ischemia. The systemic risks of reperfusion are not lessened by tourniquet application but simply delayed, perhaps to be dealt with later by an overwhelmed emergency department. With the increased risk of limb loss and little obvious benefit over fluid resuscitation and electrolyte control, tourniquet application should be reserved for life-threatening situations with inadequate treatment options.

Experience with the large numbers of crush injuries in the Armenian earthquake resulted in the development of a

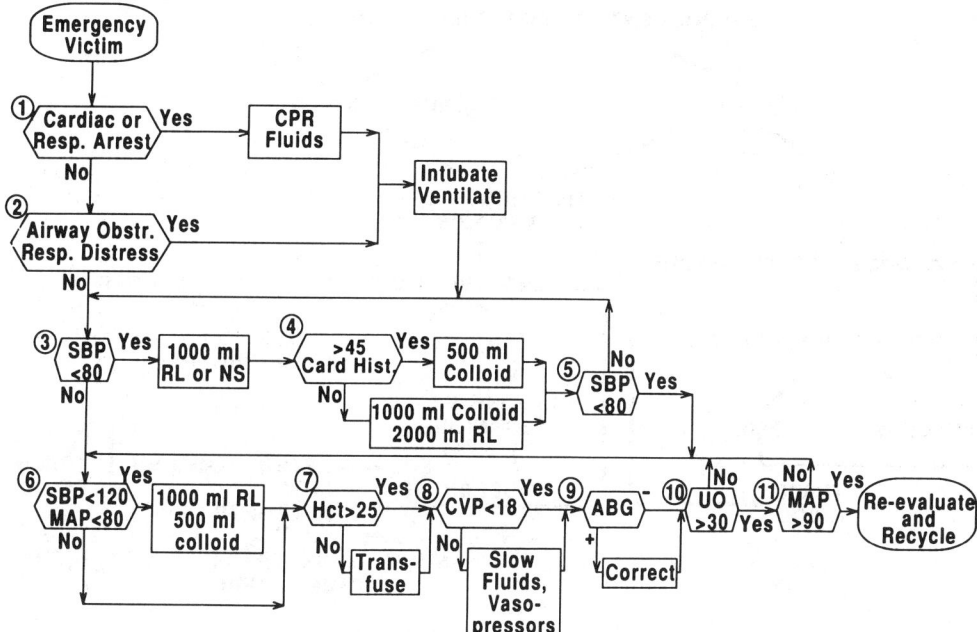

Figure 2–7. Emergency disaster algorithm. (From Shoemaker W, Kvetan V, Fyodorov V, et al: Clinical algorithm for initial fluid resuscitation in disasters. Crit Care Clin 7:363, 1991.)

specialized U.S. disaster dialysis team. The indication for the deployment of the team is the occurrence of a large number of trapped victims, at a remote site, with limited access to adequate fluid resuscitation. Because the weight of fluid requirements make peritoneal dialysis impractical for transport, other techniques are usually considered.[24] Continuous arteriovenous hemofiltration and continuous arteriovenous hemodialysis present hemorrhagic problems aggravated by the use of heparin and immobilization. The most efficient technique appears to be intermittent hemodialysis through venovenous access via dual-lumen femoral or subclavian catheters, if adequate water treatment and technical support can be guaranteed.

Circulatory and Respiratory Compromise

Circulatory support of individuals in a mass disaster situation requires an organized approach to fluid resuscitation. After the development of a successful clinical algorithm for emergency resuscitation,[95] a modified algorithm to use for disaster victims was proposed,[97] with the following requirements: (1) initial resuscitation should be started in the field or in an emergency receiving area that has the capability to deliver fluid therapy and (2) fluid therapy should continue if hematocrit monitoring, central venous pressure catheter insertion, and blood gas analysis are possible (Fig. 2–7, Appendix 2–1). The algorithm may need to be modified for specific circumstances such as burns or crush injury. Management of patients with trauma can be improved by pulmonary arterial catheter–guided physiologic support.[98] Although this is rapidly accomplished in a modern hospital, there are no data available on the use of advanced hemodynamic monitoring at remote disaster sites.

Airway Injury

Airway compromise is common in disasters. Building collapse generates large, dense clouds of suspended dust particles, with concrete, brick, and adobe structures causing the most severe consequences.[99, 100] Survivors, who must be reached and extricated, endure repeated airway insults from resuspension of dust particles during the rescue activities. Therefore, the patient must be provided with airway pro-

tection as soon as possible. Protection may vary from a wet cloth or simple dust mask to a non-rebreathing oxygen mask or a self-contained breathing apparatus. Victims exposed to heavy volcanic ash may asphyxiate from airway plugs formed by the airborne ash and mucus.[101] Burn and hazardous material inhalation may cause further airway insult by inducing upper airway edema and adult respiratory distress syndrome.[102]

Management of these conditions involves preventing further insult and administering humidified oxygen. If respiratory embarrassment is significant, early intubation may be required. Positive pressure ventilation, humidified oxygen, and positive end-expiratory pressure should be available if necessary to maintain adequate ventilation and oxygenation. Portable pulse oximetry, portable ventilators and suction apparatus, and other technologic advances make sophisticated prehospital airway evaluation and management feasible.

The field of trauma anesthesia is rapidly evolving into a structured subspecialty with advanced approaches to the difficult airway (see ref 103, p 191) (Fig. 2–8). This approach must be available to critical care specialists involved in the early management of disaster victims.[104–107]

Blunt Trauma

After extrication, the patient with blunt trauma should be transferred as rapidly as possible to the designated definitive care center. Control of internal hemorrhage is not possible in the prehospital environment and the only interventions likely to make a difference before transfer are endotracheal intubation and immobilization. Although prehospital fluid administration is of value for a trapped person, delaying transit to establish IV access in cases of blunt trauma is controversial.

The argument against attempting IV access in the field is that it delays transport to a trauma center where definitive therapy can be delivered. Thus, precious minutes of the "golden hour" are wasted.[108, 109] Lewis suggested that the average volume of fluid that paramedics can infuse is between 1 and 2 L. Using a computer model, he calculated that, for field times of less that 30 minutes or for any victim

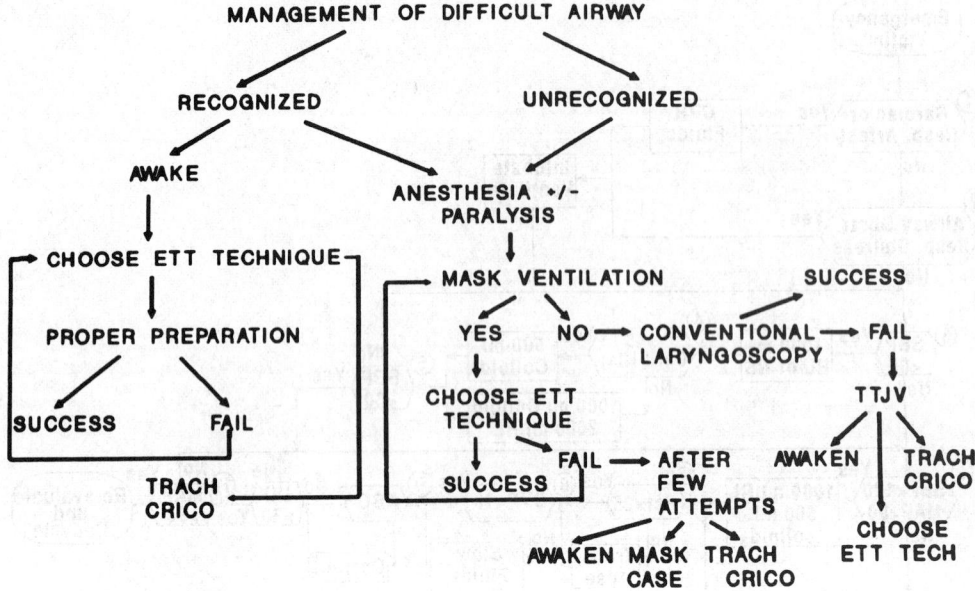

Figure 2–8. Preliminary ASA Airway Task Force Algorithm. (Excerpted from Benumof JL: Management of the difficult or impossible airway. Annual Refresher Course Lectures, American Society of Anesthesiologists, Las Vegas, 1990, p 163. A copy of the full text can be obtained from ASA, 520 N. Northwest Highway, Park Ridge, Illinois 60068-2573.)

with bleeding in excess of 100 mL/min, this volume is inadequate to sustain life.[110, 111]

The argument for prehospital IV administration of fluid assumes that the earlier studies are misrepresentative of experiences elsewhere in the country. Specifically, many centers report shorter downtimes and highlight differences in the training and capability of paramedics in different areas. Rottman pointed out that infusion rates through standard IV tubing are slow and that the use of wide-bore tubing, 14-gauge catheters, and pneumatic pressure bags can raise the infusion rate to 370 mL/min or more, providing significant fluid resuscitation capability.[112]

There is merit to both arguments. The lesson for the medical triage officer in the field is that he or she must know the resources available. We suggest that airway control and stabilization be achieved in the field. With regard to IV access, if there are a large number of patients, few prehospital staff, and well-staffed local hospitals, we recommend rapid transport, with IV access being attempted in transit. Conversely, if local hospital resources are overwhelmed, with only prolonged transport to the nearest care center available, and good support is present at the disaster site, establishment of IV access and fluid administration in the field should be attempted.[112]

Hypothermia

If rescue of trapped individuals is delayed, large numbers of patients can experience hypothermia. For example, in Armenia, many persons who survived the earthquake were rendered homeless in freezing winter conditions.[113] Consideration of hypothermia in the trapped person can be particularly important: even before extrication, wet clothing should be removed and the patient should be protected with heat-reflective, waterproof blankets if possible. IV fluids should be prewarmed, if necessary by placing IV fluid bags inside the shirts of rescue personnel, and drug doses adjusted as necessary.

Other Medical Considerations

Patients with penetrating truncal injuries should be transported to a definitive care center with the objects left in place. Awareness of the possibility of tension pneumothorax

and the ability to treat it with needle decompression are essential in the field. Formal tube thoracostomy should probably be delayed until arrival at the definitive care center. In the management of burns, attention should be focused on aggressive fluid replacement and suspicion should be high for smoke inhalation. Head injury is common and often fatal in mass disasters. Management is no different from that of head injuries sustained in the day-to-day environment: attention to airway control is crucial.

DISASTER PREPAREDNESS

Responses to disasters vary by type, size and location of disaster, and the available resources. One of the most em-

---

TABLE 2–7

COMMON WAYS IN WHICH DISASTER IS FIRST DISCOVERED

Lay Public (Bystanders)
Many multicasualty incidents are witnessed only by the lay public. Therefore, the disaster manager must be able to receive immediately any warning communicated through a 911 call or direct contact of the emergency services (if telephone lines are damaged). For example, if fire, police, or ambulance are contacted by 911 or directly, they must be responsible for immediately notifying the manager, often by radio in the event of busy or damaged telephone lines.

Seismic Recording Laboratories
The manager must have direct contact at all times with these stations for warning of any significant seismic activity in case it causes damage or catastrophe.

Chemical, Nuclear, and Other Industrial Plants
Ideally, local disaster planning should include direct links between the disaster manager and any large installation capable of causing a human-made hazard. This facilitates early warning and evacuation.

Coast Guard, Weather Stations, Emergency Services (Police, Fire, EMS)
Warnings of hurricanes, typhoons, tornadoes, tsunamis, and other natural hazards must obviously be communicated early to the disaster manager.

Other Disaster Managers
Good communication with disaster managers in surrounding communities and with state disaster managers is clearly imperative not only for advance warning of an impending catastrophe but also for recruiting help.

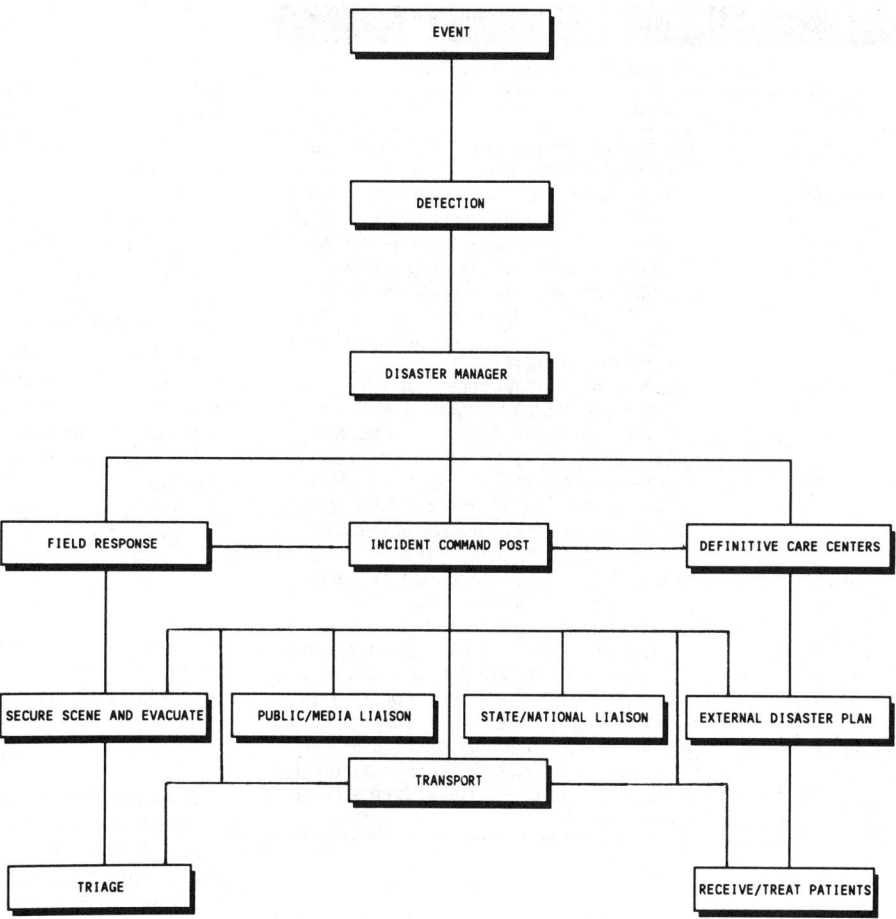

Figure 2–9. Simplified disaster response plan.

phatic conclusions of the official Soviet investigation of the Armenian earthquake of 1988 was that the response was significantly handicapped by a lack of any disaster planning and the lack of qualified disaster management personnel[114] (Kvetan V, Armenian earthquake, unpublished findings, 1989). Figure 2–9 outlines the principal features of a U.S. disaster plan.

Local Disaster Planning

The first rule in disaster response is to preplan. Although differences in jurisdictions, resources, and catastrophes necessitate different systems, the following principles hold true.

In planning a disaster response, the initial step is to conduct a careful survey of the plan's jurisdiction to identify all potential sites (e.g., industry, nuclear reactors, highways and hazardous materials allowed on them, airports, prisons, and schools) and types of hazardous events. A response network must then be designed and a disaster manager designated. His or her function is to command and coordinate this network during response activation. The disaster manager may be the local fire chief, the local EMS supervisor, or most likely, a local government official. The next step is to ensure that the disaster manager will receive early, accurate information to activate the disaster response plan. This necessitates that he or she be directly linked to various information sources that function under a variety of situations (Table 2–7).

Each governmental and nongovernmental organization that could be needed in a local disaster response must develop a disaster plan. If the disaster manager determines that a disaster is evolving, she or he activates the disaster response plan and immediately contacts the responsible managers of the relevant emergency services (Table 2–8), who initiate their organizations' plans.

The individual plans must be carefully coordinated, particularly the command and communication aspects, within the overall community disaster response plan. Mock disaster responses, or drills, must be run periodically to assess the plan's effectiveness and to identify problem areas. The drills

TABLE 2–8
COMMON DISASTER RESPONSE ENTITIES AND THEIR FUNCTIONS

Ambulance/Paramedic Service
To provide basic life support, advanced life support, and medical transport
Law Enforcement
To ensure crowd control, maintenance of communication routes, and crime surveillance
Fire and Rescue Services
To ensure building safety, fire control, and extrication of victims
Utility Services
To provide damage reports of gas lines, water systems, and electrical systems and to repair or discontinue gas and electric supply as necessary
Hospitals and Medical Support Services
To receive and treat victims
Other Specialty Services Relevant to Certain Geographic Areas
Coast Guard, hazardous materials agencies, and so on
Neighboring Resources
To implement mutual aid agreements between neighboring locales, which greatly facilitate effective disaster response

TABLE 2-9

INCIDENT COMMAND SYSTEM STRUCTURE

Section	Function
Command	Organizes and manages the overall structure of the response.
Operations	Performs the actual response work in the incident. This would include medical teams if the response requires medical care for victims. (Medical care for incident command system responders is provided under the logistics section, although the same medical personnel may provide both services.)
Planning	Gathers relevant information and prepares possible response strategies as the incident progresses. This group includes technical specialists with expertise required for the specific incident. It often includes a medical specialist if the response involves casualties or medical risk to response personnel.
Logistics	Includes both a service branch (responsible for communications, medical care, food and drink for incident command system personnel) and a support branch (responsible for providing and servicing equipment, for obtaining supplies, and for arranging necessary facilities).
Finance	Provides financial management, authorizes expenditures, arranges contracts, and maintains records and documentation of the incident.

must test functional areas that most often fail in a real disaster response.

Incident Command System

To facilitate a response that involves the interaction of many agencies, the disaster response plan should be organized using the incident command system.[115] This is an organizational structure originally developed to coordinate response to large wilderness fires in the western United States. It was designed to be adaptable to any emergency response and originated as a means to overcome problems arising in a response involving multiple organizations. Nonstandard terminology for command, for organizational divisions, for equipment, and for other details has consistently made interaction between organizations difficult during disaster responses. The incident command system specifies a common terminology and a common command structure with five functional sections (Table 2-9).

Development of a disaster plan under the incident command system includes the establishment of an incident command post with central communication. This is predetermined in the plan so that all concerned parties know the location of the central headquarters. It may be at the scene of the event, an example being the Sioux City airliner crash.[116] There, the city was warned of an incoming, handicapped jet and established the command post at the airport. In other situations such as in an earthquake-prone region where massive building collapse may occur, the plan could include a list of alternative sites, dependent on what remains intact. Planning and establishing an effective communication system are also essential. The system must be independent of the telephone system (which may be incapacitated by the hazard).

Emergency Service Response

Once each emergency service (e.g., law enforcement, fire suppression, and EMS) is activated, its response is prescribed by its individual disaster plan. In addition to its operational response, other key actions must be taken, including assessing availability of personnel, equipment, and support services.

The disaster plan for emergency services must involve, for instance, a prior determination of how many crews are needed to maintain coverage of the unaffected areas, how many crews can be relied on from neighboring regions, and how off-duty crews can be contacted.

In addition, deployment of personnel to assess the families and homes of emergency workers and help alleviate the personal fears of these workers can be of significant value. Emergency personnel may be required to work for prolonged periods without knowing the fate of their families. Removing this unknown was seen as a major contribution to the ability of emergency teams to effectively function during the Loma Prieta disaster.[8]

Medical Response

Although each medical disaster response is unique, they all have distinct phases that must be addressed in planning and managing the response (Table 2-10).

Initial Field Response

Disaster Scene Considerations. Many aspects of the disaster scene affect the response personnel. For example, after an earthquake, workers may be confronted by many injured, dead, and dying persons with panic behavior among the survivors. There may be severe property damage with the loss of all utility services, including telephones, electrical power, and natural gas sources, and aftershocks of the earthquake may be completely unpredictable and severe.[22, 23] The potential for hazardous materials release from a variety of sites must be considered. Explosive hazards from disruption of natural gas lines, sewers, and other sources are possible. The stress of dealing with a critical incident may affect the responders' ability to perform and may have long-term psychologic implications.[117, 118]

Multiple disaster scene considerations directly affect the function of a medical unit. These include the potential devastation of the local emergency medical and hospital-based medical systems, as occurred in Soviet Armenia.[3] Destruction of transportation infrastructures necessary for prompt evacuation may also occur.

Bystander Response. Within this disarray, there may be casualties with injuries that require immediate intervention. Reviews of many catastrophic disasters repeatedly note that the first available help in a disaster area is the local population.[45, 119, 120] They rescue the majority of lightly trapped survivors soon after the event occurs. A crucial development in the field of disaster research was the recognition that the

TABLE 2-10

PHASES OF MEDICAL RESPONSE IN DISASTER OR MULTICASUALTY INCIDENTS

1. Initial field response
2. Field medical support and extrication/rescue of victims (if indicated)
3. Establishment of a triage system and casualty collection site
4. Transport of injured to appropriate definitive care centers
5. Organization of definitive care centers

ability to save lives in a mass disaster is dependent on the ability of the lay public to perform life-supporting first aid.[2] Techniques of value include airway protection, control of hemorrhage, and attention to spinal injuries during positioning and transport.[2, 121, 122] Disaster preparedness should include a program to train the lay public in life-supporting first aid.[123, 124] In regions prone to collapsed structure disasters (earthquakes), disaster preparedness should also include teaching basic extrication skills to the public.[14, 123, 125]

Organized Disaster Response Resources. The first organized response personnel to reach the scene are usually police, fire, or EMS crews. The senior individual present from the lead agency for the disaster assumes on-scene command, makes a brief assessment, and communicates the information to the command center. A determination is then made that routine response resources are inadequate and the disaster response plan is activated.

A primary role of the first trained responders to arrive, including medical personnel, is to consider scene safety. Because the underlying principle of disaster response is to save the maximal number of lives, the first rule in an unstable environment is to protect the uninjured, the mildly injured, and the rescuers.[15] This includes evacuation of civilians from the scene. The perimeter of the scene must also be secured to effect crowd control.

Unless adequately trained and equipped, rescue workers should not enter into any potentially dangerous, unstable situation until the environment has been stabilized.[15] Stabilization includes the shoring up of structures at risk of further collapse. Other safety procedures include disconnecting utility lines, extinguishing fires, and containing leaking chemicals or gasoline from transport wrecks, holding tanks, and pipelines.[43] This intervention is usually done by trained personnel to avoid injury to the rescuers. After the scene is stabilized, the rescue and medical teams may enter.

Back-up for the initial EMS responders in an emergency could be provided by extra paramedics, EMS physicians, or physicians from local hospitals trained in field resuscitation. The value of physicians who have not had previous experience in disaster management is not clear (Barbera J, Philippine earthquake, personal observation, 1990; McDermott R, Philippine earthquake, personal communication, August 1990).[2] The potential value of well-equipped and trained intensivists, emergency physicians, and trauma anesthesiologists in the field is currently being explored.[126]

Establishment of Triage System

Triage was first used by Napoleon's chief medical officer Baron Dominique Jean Larrey, who separated soldiers on the basis of the perceived severity of their injury and then performed surgery on the most seriously injured.[127] Modern triage still uses the technique of dividing patients by severity of illness but differs from Larrey's initial concept in that the emphasis is not necessarily on the management of the most severely injured but rather on those who are likely to survive.[15, 128]

In assessing the extent of damage, the disaster manager must assess whether to set up a triage site at the scene. In general, a disaster that involves a significant number of casualties may overload the capacity to evacuate all victims to definitive care centers immediately. Furthermore, the unorganized departure of a fleet of ambulances with untriaged injured individuals to the nearest hospital could be catastrophic. It is crucial to consider the potential of the hospitals in performing triage. Pooling of victims in one transport vehicle bound for one destination increases the efficiency of the response. The triage officer should not be involved in patient transport or individual patient care but

should be devoted to quick patient assessment and the subsequent priority for staging and dispatch of patients. This officer should be identified in the disaster plan and is often a senior experienced physician.

After extrication and provision of basic life support, patients are brought to the initial triage area from the scene of injury. At this point, the triage officer assesses the patient and categorizes her or him according to the triage system selected in the disaster response plan. Triage personnel should limit any patient treatment to basic airway maintenance and bleeding control. The principal patient categories are as follows:

Category 1 patients require immediate intervention to save life. These patients are usually in shock, frequently are bleeding extensively, may have an impaired level of consciousness, and often have a compromised airway. In addition, they often have closed chest or abdominal wounds, major fractures, or extensive second- and third-degree burns.

Category 2 patients require second-priority intervention to avoid significant deterioration and possible death. Although significantly ill, these patients are well enough to withstand stabilization at the triage site before transfer. The airway is usually uncompromised, and they are usually conscious. Burns are less than 10% third degree or less than 30% second degree, and blood loss is less than 1 L.

Category 3 patients can wait for delayed intervention without undue compromise. These patients have only minor injury for which no initial medical treatment is necessary.

Category 4 patients are either dead on arrival at the triage site or have sustained injuries thought to be incompatible with life. For example, patients with more than 60% third-degree burns, those who are unconscious after severe head injury with their brain exposed, and those who have cardiorespiratory arrest with injuries that preclude feasible cardiorespiratory resuscitation fall into this category.[129]

After categorization, the patient may be tagged at the triage center according to a casualty triage code[128, 130] (e.g., color-coded tag or Mettag). Category 1 patients receive the maximal deployment of personnel and equipment (including transport). Category 2 patients also receive close observation to determine outcome. Category 3 patients are less intensively observed and may even be used to help in the emergency response if needed. Category 4 patients should be treated with respect; preserving identifying information and forensic evidence is vitally important.

A separate transport officer, often an EMS supervisor, should be designated at the casualty collection site. Her or his job is to match patients according to triage class with available transport and to coordinate ground and air evacuation. In determining the definitive care centers for individual patients, the transport officer should communicate with the disaster manager. The disaster management personnel should have knowledge of the nearby hospitals' capabilities at the time of the disaster and their designations as trauma centers, burn centers, pediatric capabilities, ICU facilities, and so on.

Transport of Injured to Appropriate Care Centers

Transport of victims after a major disaster is rarely ideal. There is often delay: roads may be blocked; helicopter flight may be impaired by dust clouds; and the demand may grossly outstrip the supply. However, in the management of the individual patient, the same goals apply as in day-to-day EMS transport. The principles are to move patients expeditiously from the scene to definitive care while preventing deterioration. An estimate of the level of medical support required during transit should be made before departure.

Guidelines for the transport of the critically ill, regardless of who accompanies the patient, include the following:

1. Monitor mental status, vital signs, electrocardiographic findings, and pulse oximetry if possible.
2. Attempt only simple procedures en route, such as establishing peripheral IV access.
3. Proceed to the planned destination as expeditiously as possible (and at as low an altitude as possible during air transport).
4. Consider detour to a nearer hospital only if monitoring reveals a significant deterioration.
5. Stabilize the patient as much as possible if transport is prolonged or delayed.[131]

The ambulance personnel transferring the patient should have basic life-support training and, if possible, advanced life-support capacity.

Organization of Definitive Care Centers

Hospital Response. Hospitals are required by the Joint Commission on Accreditation of Healthcare Organizations to have both internal disaster plans (for mishaps within the hospital) and external disaster plans (for events outside the hospital).[132] These must be periodically updated and exercised through semiannual drills. Although most hospital disaster plans have not been tested in a mass disaster, disaster drills have highlighted certain logistic issues that should be considered.

The reception point for the arrival of casualties should be larger than the average emergency department. The hospital entrance is often a good choice, especially if it is close to the elevator (if operable), emergency department, and operating suites. This area should be considered more as a staging area (or secondary triage center) than a treatment area.

The hospital should receive prior warning of incoming casualties, should be able to inform the disaster manager of its potential to receive casualties—both by number and by severity—and should then activate its external disaster plan. This would involve a prearranged notification and deployment of in-house staff for staffing the triage/reception area; commencing evacuation of stable patients from the ICUs and step-down unit areas; staffing the emergency department, which is usually designated as the immediate treatment area for category 1 patients; and staffing the operating room and recovery room for category 1 patients requiring surgery (e.g., Presbyterian-University Hospital disaster plan, University of Pittsburgh). In addition, off-duty staff would be called in from home as needed.

In developing the external disaster plan, guidelines include preparing for realistic types of disasters from the hospital's area. Hospitals near chemical plants, for example, should be prepared for hazardous materials spills and carry stocks of appropriate antidotes and treatments. The most common external disasters that hospitals anticipate are those that generate a heavy trauma toll, such as transportation mishaps. These are usually large MCIs.[15] Realistic preparation for a major disaster (with thousands of injuries, crippled local response, concomitant involvement of the hospital in the catastrophe, and impaired transport and communication) is rarely adequately accomplished.[15]

Critical Care and Emergency Medical Response. In a disaster response, any beds that can be created in the ICU are of importance. Because this is frequently implausible, most disaster plans utilize the emergency department as an ICU. It must be provided with an adequate cadre of physicians, equipment, and support personnel to allow full advanced trauma life-support and prolonged life-support procedures. This capability should be attained by the formation of teams that stabilize patients until transfer to the operating room or other appropriate disposition.

A coordinator should be designated in the emergency department. Her or his function is to triage the patients using laboratory blood test results and radiologic procedures on a priority basis similar to that used for field triage of patients.[129]

The ICU response is characterized by the recruitment of all available staff to provide critical care both in the existing ICU and makeshift ICUs elsewhere in the hospital. An integrated plan with trauma, emergency medical, and critical care physicians is imperative for a smoothly functioning response. Scheduling of staff should involve designated rotations to decrease stress and avoid fatigue in a prolonged disaster response. Finally, disaster planning should include critical incident stress debriefing teams composed of similar support personnel and mental health professionals. This debriefing is considered highly important for the effective function and recuperation of those involved in the response.

State Response

All thorough local (municipal and county) disaster response plans incorporate a mechanism for accessing additional resources if a disaster exceeds the local response capability. If a determination is made by the local disaster manager that an incident requires outside resources, the mechanism is activated.

The most common level of outside aid is accessed typically by activating pre-existing mutual aid agreements with neighboring jurisdictions. Additional resources (e.g., fire suppression and police support) may quickly become available through this avenue. In addition, EMS systems are often grouped by county with supervision by regional EMS councils (mandated by federal law), which coordinate many regional issues. This coordination may include a system for a regional EMS response to disasters.

The disaster manager may subsequently appeal to the next level of aid, asking the state government for disaster assistance. States are mandated to have an emergency management capability. Commonly, the responsibility is through a state emergency management agency or emergency services sector. The make-up and capabilities of these entities vary markedly among the 50 states. Some, such as California's Office for Emergency Services, are organized operational and educational entities. They have grouped the state's counties into regions to provide an intermediate response level to the local and full state responses.

Each state's medical disaster response is typically coordinated by the state's emergency management agency and the state's department of health. Historically, the primary organized medical response to disasters has consisted of triage performed by EMS responders and then transport of victims to appropriate facilities.

National Response

In the event of a truly catastrophic occurrence, the state's governor may appeal to the President of the United States to declare the affected area a disaster. A presidential disaster declaration allows activation of considerable federal resources.

The federal resources are catalogued, coordinated, and mobilized through a detailed and complex Federal Response Plan. Within the plan, federal agencies, the Department of Defense, the American Red Cross, and other resources are organized to provide a multitude of emergency support functions (ESF) (Table 2–11).

The primary federal agency in charge of emergency

TABLE 2–11

EMERGENCY SUPPORT FUNCTIONS

1. Transportation
2. Communications
3. Public works and engineering
4. Firefighting
5. Information and planning
6. Mass care
7. Resource support
8. Health and medical services
9. Urban search and rescue
10. Hazardous materials
11. Food
12. Energy

support function 8 (health and medical services) is the U.S. Public Health Service, and both its own medical personnel and military medical units can be accessed and deployed in addition to the civilian response (Table 2–12).

National Disaster Medical System

Within emergency support function 8, the organization given the task of providing the majority of the prehospital medical care, patient evacuation, and definitive medical care is the National Disaster Medical System (NDMS). It consists of elements from the Department of Health and Human Services, Department of Veterans Affairs, Department of Defense, and Federal Emergency Management Agency.

The predecessor of NDMS, the Civilian-Military Contingency Hospital System, was conceived in the early 1980s as a back-up to the military medical system for casualties of a non-nuclear military conflict. This system evolved into NDMS as an organized national mutual aid system to be activated in the event of an overwhelming disaster.[133] The system's concept is to provide medical care resources at the disaster site, air evacuation for patients unable to be cared for by local resources, and a commitment of hospital beds nationwide to be made available for these evacuated patients. The participating hospitals are organized into NDMS regions centered around receiving airports. NDMS' air evacuation systems utilize military and civilian aircraft. Patients are to be transported by air from casualty collection sites in the disaster area to the designated airports, where they would be retriaged and distributed to the participating hospitals in the region.

The NDMS plan also incorporates entities known as disaster medical assistance teams (DMATs) to staff the casualty collection points and the receiving airport's reception areas. The original DMAT concept was based on the military model with a specified personnel composition (Table 2–13). A command and support unit was also devised and, when combined with three DMATs, was designated as the clearing-staging unit.

The original NDMS concept was to provide medical care at receiving areas near disaster sites and to continue the care through the evacuation stage until definitive care could be delivered at fixed medical facilities that were recruited through the system. This original NDMS/DMAT concept, however, was noted to have several major deficiencies in adequately covering the many areas of medical need arising from a truly major disaster. It was also difficult to develop adequate numbers of equipped and trained DMATs because little financial support was available.

The original DMAT concept has since been developed into highly organized DMAT units that can set up field hospital units and provide hospital care in the prehospital environment. There are currently 36 of these in the United States, many believed to be operational on the basis of successful response drills (Gray E, Office of Emergency Preparedness, U.S. Public Health Service, personal communication, 1991). Two DMAT units successfully deployed and provided care in St. Croix after Hurricane Hugo's devastation of the island in September 1988.[26]

In addition to these DMATs, the concept of specialized DMATs is evolving. The NDMS National Medical Response Steering Committee includes organized provision of critical care services within this scope. Advance teams (evaluation and resuscitation) evaluate the need on site within a few hours in preparation for deployment of a DMAT or clearing-staging unit augmented by specialized teams. The categories of specialization, each having operational groups identified, are listed in Table 2–14. The concept of a rapidly deployed resuscitation/critical care group by rotary wing aircraft was recommended by Safar for insertion within NDMS some years ago.[14] This had not been implemented until 1988 when a critical care team was airlifted to Armenia in the early phase of the earthquake response. Because of the success of this experience, the critical care specialized team consists of a multidisciplinary group of 11 specialists able to staff an 11-bed ICU facility. The modular units can be used for critical care transport and limited field operating room capability and are supported by a diagnostic unit. This team may also extend its function into difficult triage decisions,

TABLE 2–12

HEALTH AND MEDICAL SERVICES:* SCOPE OF CARE

1. Assessment of health/medical needs
2. Health surveillance
3. Medical care personnel
4. Health/medical equipment and supplies
5. Patient evacuation
6. In-hospital care
7. Food/drug/medical device safety
8. Worker health/safety
9. Radiation health issues
10. Chemical (hazardous materials)
11. Biologic health issues
12. Mental health
13. Public health information
14. Disease vector control
15. Water safety/wastewater and solid waste disposal
16. Victim identification/mortuary services

*Emergency support function 8.

TABLE 2–13

DISASTER MEDICAL ASSISTANCE TEAM

Number	Minimal Qualification
2	Medical officers
1	Supervising nurse clinician
2	Staff nurses (registered nurses)
4	Licensed practical or vocational nurses, registered nurses, or paramedics
2	Surgical technicians
1	Laboratory technician
1	Pharmacy technician
3	Emergency medical technicians
2	Medical records clerks
1	Pharmacy clerk
1	Supply clerk
9	Ward attendants-litterbearers
29	TOTAL

TABLE 2–14

SPECIALIZED DISASTER MEDICAL ASSISTANCE TEAMS

Advance team
Trauma team
Pediatric team
Burn team
Hazardous materials team
Dialysis team
ICU team
Mortuary team
Critical incident debriefing team

critical care transport, and consultation to other groups in the field.

Bringing all of the medical entities into NDMS provides multiple benefits. It markedly improves the federal government's ability to expeditiously respond to realistic disaster problems, and it provides local medical teams logistic support at the disaster site. The NDMS also provides licensure and liability for medical teams to cross state lines.

Military Response

The U.S. military maintains a large medical establishment with some 100,000 personnel. The capabilities are considerable, varying from small rapid-response teams to 1000-bed ship hospitals and large medical centers. A number of these assets have been used in disaster relief operations, and collaboration between civilian and military disaster medical organizations has begun. In a national disaster situation, military medical resources can be accessed after a state has requested assistance from the Federal Emergency Management Agency and presidential approval for declaration of a disaster has been received. Some of the specialized resources of military medicine are ideally configured for disaster response. The U.S. Air Force developed a number of FAST teams after the 1983 bombing of U.S. Marine barracks in Beirut. Four of these teams are deployed in Europe. The teams consist of 20 individuals who can be en route within 2 hours, are self-sufficient for up to 48 hours, and have capabilities for providing advanced trauma life support and post-traumatic surgical care for up to 50 casualties. An example of deployment occurred during the crash in Ethiopia of an aircraft carrying Congressman Leland of Texas. The U.S. Army maintains similar FAST teams (forward Army surgical teams). In addition to major trauma surgical capabilities, the Army teams have enhanced critical care capabilities, which include hemodynamic monitoring and mechanical ventilation. The U.S. Navy supports 10 mobile medical augmentation teams with similar capabilities. In addition, the naval preventive/environmental medical teams are available for disease control, most recently utilized during the deployment of a U.S. Marine task force in the aftermath of hurricanes and floods in Bangladesh in 1991. The U.S. military also has a number of mobile hospital facilities ranging from the Air Force Air Transportable Hospital, which is a self-sufficient 50-bed hospital, to naval hospital ships, which have up to 1000 beds and 80 ICU beds with full diagnostic capabilities.

The formal response to a request of a foreign government for assistance is coordinated by the Office of Foreign Disaster Assistance within the Agency for International Development under the State Department. This organization has sponsored medical groups specializing in search and rescue. In addition, resources of the armed services may be requested and contracted by the State Department from the Department of Defense.

SPECIAL CONSIDERATIONS
Care of Trapped Persons

Disasters involving structural collapse present unique and extreme obstacles to rescue personnel. Earthquakes, flash floods, tornadoes, hurricanes, explosions, and other hazards may leave in their aftermath a large number of trapped survivors. Although bystanders may extricate the lightly entangled victims, many patients may be deeply entombed. Because of concomitant multiple medical emergencies, survival of trapped persons falls off dramatically after the first 24 hours.[2, 118] The ability of advanced search and rescue teams to rapidly respond is crucial to reducing morbidity among these patients. The urban search and rescue team system has been developed to achieve this goal. A sophisticated medical unit is an essential component of these teams.

The components of urban search and rescue teams are listed in Table 2–15. The management group interacts with the overall disaster management structure (incident command staff) and provides logistic support. Communications are vital in this environment and portable radios are carried by most team members. The technical support unit provides expertise in hazardous materials, structural engineering, and technical search capabilities (e.g., sensitive listening devices and fiberoptic telescopes). The search unit includes specially trained canines and their handlers. The rescue personnel are equipped and trained to penetrate dense debris rapidly to reach trapped individuals. The medical unit is composed of experienced emergency physicians and paramedics trained to provide medical care in this environment.[44] Protective clothing, hard hats, atmospheric monitoring devices (for oxygen, carbon monoxide, and methane), and eye, airway, and hearing protection are necessary. The entire team must be self-sufficient in its equipment and supplies.[134]

These teams are designed to be activated and to respond within hours of the disaster onset. Trapped persons that they reach have survived the golden hour of trauma management but may yet have severe and progressive medical problems requiring nonoperative intervention.[14, 135] The process of extricating these patients may cause a precipitous decline in their medical stability, particularly if crush syndrome, unstable long bone and pelvic fractures, severe hypothermia, spinal fractures, dust inhalation, or tamponaded vascular injuries are present. Medical evaluation and management should, therefore, begin at the time these patients are reached.

Evaluation of a patient within a confined space can be difficult and tax the clinical acumen of the strongest diagnostician. A brief goal-directed physical examination that follows the usual approach of advanced cardiac life support, advanced trauma life support, and other resuscitation guides is required[33, 136–141] (see ref 103, p 130).

Critical Care Transport

In addition to the guidelines regarding transport during evacuation from a disaster site, specific aspects of critical care transport depend on the mode of transport, the patient's medical condition, and the medical equipment available.

TABLE 2–15

COMPONENTS OF URBAN SEARCH AND RESCUE TEAM

Management and logistics group	Search unit
Communications unit	Rescue unit
Technical support unit	Medical unit

TABLE 2–16

CHARACTERISTICS OF AERIAL CRITICAL CARE TRANSPORT

Subject to sudden three-dimensional forces
Subject to gravitational and centrifugal forces
Gas space expansion/contraction coincident with alterations in altitude
Subject to rapid and extreme temperature changes
Increased and varied visual, auditory, and olfactory stimuli
Increased vibration
Limited cabin space with secondary difficulties in patient care (cabin room, floor space)
Limitations in amount of electrical power (especially during engine shutdown) and in the type of electrical equipment that can be used (e.g., interface with avionics equipment)
Diminished levels of ambient P_{O_2} in cabin (dependent on cabin pressurization)
Limitations in payload and thus in weight and bulk of passengers and supplies
Access doors may be small, have steps, or be high above the ground, making it difficult to move patients into and out of the aircraft

From Grande CM: Critical care transport: A trauma perspective. An overview of trauma anesthesia and critical care. Crit Care Clin 6:165, 1990.

Air Transport

Air transport can be via fixed or rotary wing aircraft. With both, it is important to appreciate that there are certain features of flight that may adversely affect the critically ill patient (Table 2–16). For example, in the patient with a head injury, unwanted rises in intracranial pressure may be caused by intracranial venous pooling resulting from the accelerative and decelerative forces during takeoff and landing.[142]

The extent to which altitude affects cabin pressure and oxygen content is demonstrated in Figures 2–10 and 2–11. It can be seen that a height of 8000 ft will correlate with an arterial P_{O_2} of 55 mm Hg, with normal ventilation. This is clinical hypoxia and, although it may be tolerated by healthy individuals, it is clearly dangerous in the critically ill patient.[143] Furthermore, cabin pressurization is not usually available in helicopters and is able to produce an atmospheric pressure that is only equivalent of 8000 ft in most fixed wing aircraft. To avoid or reverse arterial hypoxia, transport should be at as low an altitude as possible and the physician should expect to provide the patient with supplemental oxygenation as necessary, including intubation and mechanical ventilation.[142]

Both fixed and rotary wing aircraft have a role in medical transport but both have advantages and disadvantages. Helicopters (rotary wing) are capable of vertical takeoff, and therefore, the horizontal accelerative and decelerative forces are avoided. In addition, they are capable of being rapidly deployed and do not require an airfield for landing. However, disadvantages include short flight range (300 to 500 mi), small passenger/patient load capabilities, vibration and noise (uncomfortable for the patient and difficult for auscultation and examination), limits imposed by weather conditions, and lack of pressurization capability.[144] Although the fixed wing aircraft is not as hampered by these restrictions, it necessitates both an airfield and more preflight planning.[143]

Ground Transport

Ground ambulances have the advantages of immediate deployment, high mobility, and lower cost. However, they are obviously much slower than aircraft, they still cause more noise and vibration than the hospital and can produce significant horizontal forces, especially on deceleration.[144]

Medical Considerations

Certain medical conditions and equipment present particular problems during transport. They are most important in long, high-altitude flights.

Hemorrhagic Shock. The effects of altitude hypoxia are exacerbated in the patient with a low serum hemoglobin level. An acute drop to a hemoglobin concentration of 10 g/dL at sea level is equivalent to an altitude hypoxia effect of 6000 ft (see Fig. 2–11). The patient with trauma with uncontrolled hemorrhage or partially corrected bleeding is therefore particularly sensitive to hypoxia. Attempts should be made to stabilize and transfuse the patient before flight if prolonged transport is anticipated.[143]

Thoracoabdominal Trauma. The major concern with air transport in patients with thoracic trauma is the development of a tension pneumothorax. With falling atmospheric pressure, intrathoracic air spaces enlarge.[145] A previously missed small pneumothorax or an improperly decompressed pneumothorax could become life threatening in flight. It is, therefore, often prudent to insert thoracostomy tubes prophylactically before transport. Drainage should be via a Heimlich valve attached to the distal end of the tube unless water-sealed suction is available aboard the aircraft.[131] Throughout the flight, the physician should be prepared to manage the possibility of the new development of a pneumothorax.

In the management of abdominal trauma during flight, the main concerns are aspiration, intra-abdominal gas expansion, and ongoing hemorrhage. The insertion of a nasogastric tube is essential.[142] This relieves gas build-up and secondary pressure changes and reduces the risk of aspiration.

Fever. Fever raises the basal metabolic rate and consequently increases oxygen consumption. Supplemental oxygen by mask may be inadequate at high altitude to meet oxygen demand and the patient may require intubation and ventilation.

Eye and Maxillofacial Injuries. The retina is extremely oxygen sensitive and avoidance of hypoxia is essential to prevent further exacerbation of retinal injuries. Open eye injuries are also susceptible to pressure changes, and orbital contents can extrude from the globe if care is not paid to reducing the effects of pressurization changes.[143]

Facial fractures may be accompanied by sinus damage with subcutaneous emphysema. The swelling may cause pain and local ischemia. Most important, if swelling is severe, it may spread around the jaw and neck and cause soft tissue airway obstruction. Any suspicion of this should prompt immediate airway control by intubation. Prophylactic intubation should be performed if the physician is in doubt. Interhospital transfer of patients with wired jaws can also be dangerous for similar reasons. It is clearly essential that the physician be equipped with wire cutters if transporting this type of patient.[142]

Spinal Injuries. The patient should be fully stabilized at the scene using a back board and cervical collar with sandbags or equivalent device. Additional precautions for flight include insertion of a nasogastric tube in cases of paralytic ileus (which may be exacerbated by intraviscous gas expansion) and a urinary catheter to relieve a neurogenic bladder.[142]

Interfacility transport may involve moving a patient in free-weight traction. This is undesirable in most ground and air ambulances. Therefore, the traction frame should be replaced (for example, by a cervical traction frame that

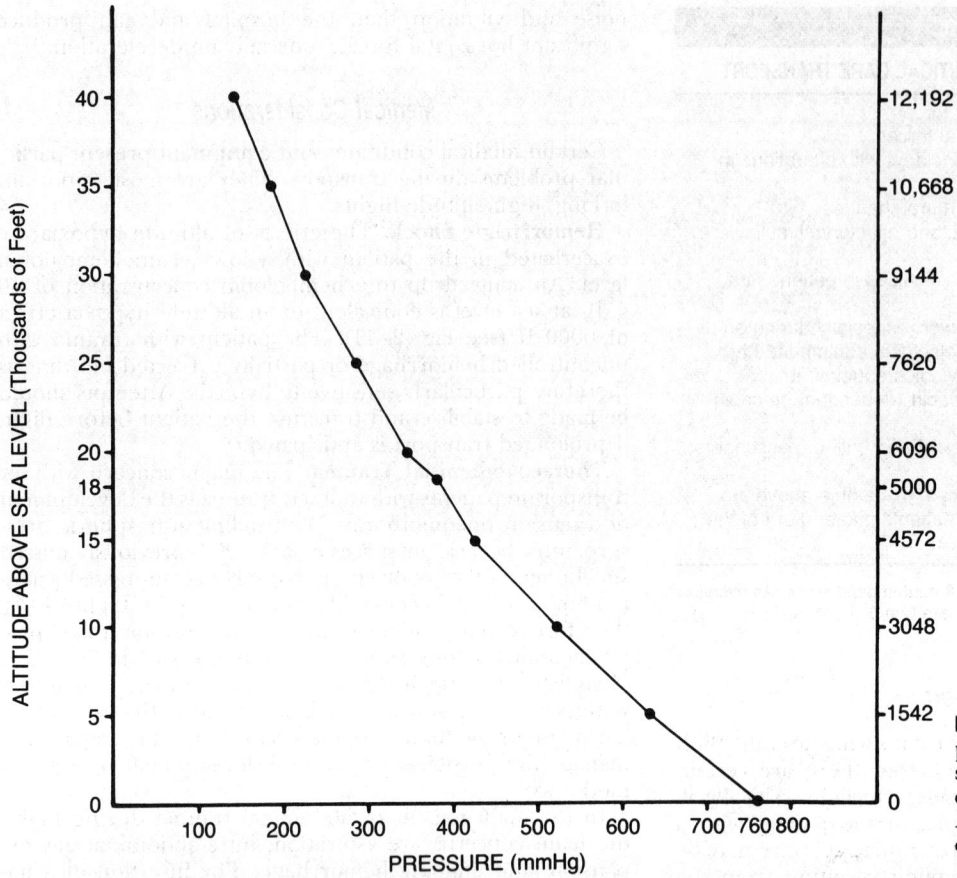

Figure 2–10. Relation of atmospheric pressure and altitude (shown in two scales). (From Grande CM: Critical care transport: A trauma perspective. An overview of trauma anesthesia and critical care. Crit Care Clin 6:165, 1990.)

substitutes a spring system for free weights and attaches to the head of the stretcher). Other devices, such as a halo vest, are free of traction and, therefore, comparatively easy to manage.[142]

Head Injuries. Patients with head injuries present perhaps the most challenging transport problems. They are particularly sensitive to pressure-volume changes, hypoxia, and gravitational and centrifugal forces. The aim of the physician is to maintain a normal intracranial pressure, ensure airway control, and provide adequate oxygenation and ventilation.

Flights should be pressurized and at low altitude. Careful management of the intra-arterial and central IV catheters is of crucial importance, because an intracranial arterial gas embolus can be devastating with depressurization causing gas expansion and compression of surrounding ischemic tissue. Likewise, intracranial venous pooling can markedly increase intracranial pressure, causing a precipitous drop in cerebral perfusion during takeoff, landing, and banking turns. The physician must alert the pilot to his or her needs and the patient should be transported in a head-raised,

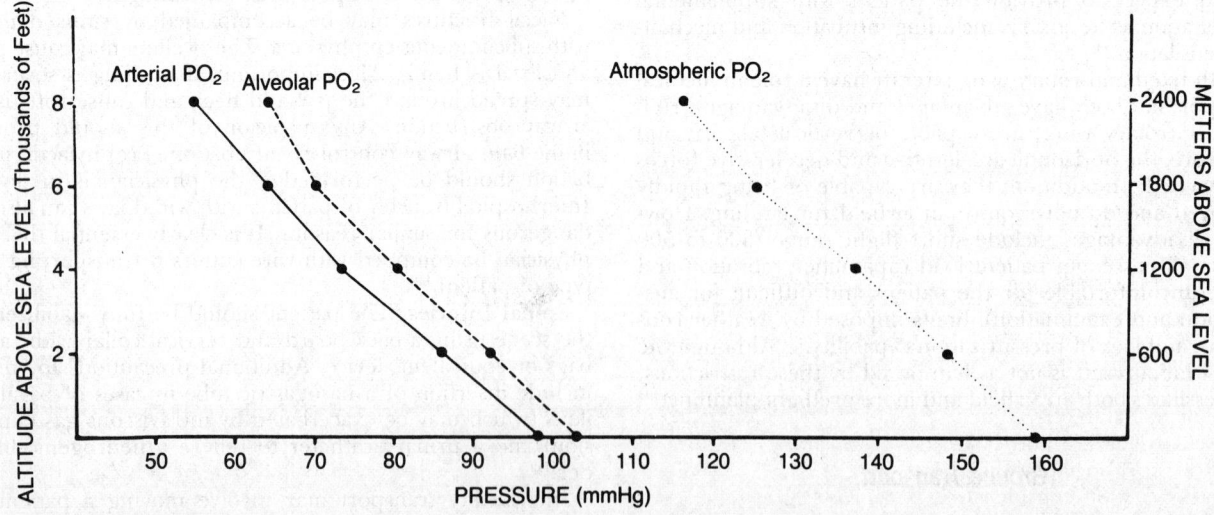

Figure 2–11. The diminishing relationship of atmospheric, alveolar, and arterial oxygen partial pressure with each other and with altitude (shown in two scales). (From Grande CM: Critical care transport: A trauma perspective. An overview of trauma anesthesia and critical care. Crit Care Clin 6:165, 1990.)

TABLE 2–17

MEDICAL EQUIPMENT THAT CONTAINS GAS AND REQUIRES SPECIAL ATTENTION IN CRITICAL CARE AIR TRANSPORT

Orthopedic air splints
Pneumatic antishock garments (military antishock trousers)
Intravenous fluid reservoirs containing air
Blood pressure cuffs
Balloon cuffs (endotracheal tubes, esophageal obturator airway, Foley's catheters)
Medication, fluid, and suction bottles

From Grande CM: Critical care transport: A trauma perspective. An overview of trauma anesthesia and critical care. Crit Care Clin 6:165, 1990.

cross-cabin position if possible. Careful observation is imperative and the physician should request a drop in altitude or emergency landing if he or she believes that the patient's condition is deteriorating owing to the effects of transport.[142, 143, 146]

Orthopedic Injuries. In stabilizing fractures before flight, pneumatic splints should not be used because they expand at high altitudes and threaten limb viability.[142] Plaster casts, if recently applied, can also cause underlying ischemia, and the physician should be able to monitor the limb and split the cast if necessary. Traction should be with springs rather than free weights as with spinal injuries. Pelvic fractures may be managed with military antishock trousers, but the physician should be aware of changing gas pressures and release air as required during flight.

Burns. The major concerns of transporting patients with complicated burns are airway management and fluid status. There are considerable fluid losses with large burns and appropriate replacement is difficult.[147] Inadequate fluid volume exacerbates altitude hypoxia as discussed earlier, whereas over-resuscitation may cause tissue swelling. This is particularly dangerous in the patient with facial and neck burns who may develop airway obstruction. Such patients, therefore, may benefit from prophylactic intubation, especially if a long transport (during which extensive fluid shifts may occur) is anticipated.[133] Patients with burns may also have experienced inhalation injury requiring intubation and positive end-expiratory pressure to ensure adequate oxygenation at high altitude.[148]

Medical Conditions. Various medical conditions may exacerbate the management of the patient with trauma during transport. For example, in the patient with pre-existing heart disease, venous pooling during accelerative and decelerative forces may cause a critical drop in end-diastolic filling, leading to coronary insufficiency and profound cardiac compromise.[142, 144] Patients with chronic obstructive pulmonary disease are also at risk, and prophylactic intubation and mechanical ventilation may be indicated.[142]

Medical Equipment

The physician must ensure that electrical power for essential equipment will be supplied during all phases of the transport. There must also be accessibility to an emergency battery pack. Equipment must be compatible with regard to size, weight, and ability to operate with the battery supply. It should be suitable, compact, and multifunctional (e.g., multilead monitor), and if electromagnetically sensitive, it should be appropriately shielded.

Another major consideration is the effect of changing ambient pressure. Table 2–17 lists equipment affected by altitude. Adjustments may be necessary to maintain steady flow rates during IV fluid administration as the air in the bag and drip chamber expands; pressure bags exert a changing effect on rate of administration. Blood pressure cuffs should be forcibly expelled of air and be left vented. They should not remain on the patient's limb between readings. Air in endotracheal tube and Foley's catheter cuffs should be replaced fully or in part with saline to avoid cuff expansion, with ensuing tissue compression, ischemia, and necrosis. Mechanical ventilators that are pneumatically driven do not work properly unless a compressed gas source is available. Flowmeters are calibrated at 1 atm and become inaccurate at higher altitudes.

Finally, the physician should check all vital supplies and equipment. For example, he or she must check that oxygen cylinders do indeed contain oxygen. This is especially important in foreign disaster settings where regulations and color coding of gas cylinders vary.[142]

SUMMARY

In Europe, critical care medicine has long been recognized as an integral part of emergency care, the provision of which begins in the field and is continued through to the ICU. Although modern critical care in the United States owes much of its early development to the experiences of military medicine during the Korean and Vietnam Wars, development has been more insulated and confined to the ICU.

It is necessary for the critical care physician to explore his or her role outside the ICU, to gain an understanding of critical care in the field, and to prepare for a more effective response to future disasters.

References

1. American Heritage Dictionary, 2nd College Edition. New York, Houghton Mifflin, p 401, 1982.
2. Klain M, Ricci E, Safar P, et al: Disaster reanimatology potentials: A structured interview study in Armenia I. Methodology and preliminary results. Prehosp Disaster Med 4(2):135, 1989.
3. Romo CR: The Mexico City earthquake—An international disaster. An overview. Prehosp Disaster Med 2(1):4, 1986.
4. Safar P, Kirimli N, Agnes A, et al: Anecdotes on resuscitation potentials following the earthquake of 1980 in Italy (abstract). In: Proceedings of the Fourth World Congress on Emergency and Disaster Medicine, Brighton, United Kingdom, June 1985.
5. De Bruycker M, Greco D, Lechat MF: The 1980 earthquake in Southern Italy: Morbidity and mortality. Int J Epidemiol 14:113, 1985.
6. Hines K: Chemical accidents. In: Baskett P, Weller R (eds): Medicine for Disasters. Littleton, MA, PSG Publishing, p 376, 1988.
7. Chernobyl, USSR (editorial). Lancet 1:1321, 1986.
8. Comfort L: Reconnaisance report: The Loma Prieta earthquake, October 17, 1989. Communication and co-ordination in emergency response and recovery. Submitted to the Earthquake Engineering Research Institution and National Science Foundation.
9. Fahey M: The challenge of survival. J World Assoc Emerg Disaster Med 1(2):101, 1985.
10. Pan Am 103. Presentation from International Trauma, Anesthesia and Critical Care Society, Baltimore, May 1991.
11. Birnbaum M: Disaster medicine: Fact or fiction? Prehosp Disaster Med 4(2):107, 1989.
12. Petroni JJ: Systems affecting the disaster rescue and EMS response. Presented at EMS Today, San Diego, CA, March 8, 1989.
13. Meroney WH, et al: The acute calcification of traumatized muscle, with particular reference to acute post-traumatic renal insufficiency. J Clin Invest 36:825, 1957.
14. Safar P: Resuscitation potentials in mass disasters. J World Assoc Emerg Disaster Med 2(1):34, 1986.
15. Pepe P, Stewart RD, Copass MK: Ten golden rules for urban multicasualty incident management. Prehosp Disaster Med 4(2):131, 1989.
16. Mahoney LE, Lasek RW, Paris PM: Natural disaster management. In: Auerbach PS, Geehr EC (eds): Management of Wilderness and Environmental Emergencies. St Louis, CV Mosby, p 453, 1989.
17. Bissell R, Young K, Abbott L, et al: Management of the Medical

Response to Mass Casualties in a Catastrophic Disaster. A Planning Guidance Document. US Public Health Service. In press.

18. Safar P: Introduction to "Disaster Resuscitology." J World Assoc Emerg Disaster Med 1(suppl I):11, 1985.

19. Elseman B: Combat casualty management in Vietnam. J Trauma 7:53, 1967.

20. Heaton LD: Army medical services activities in Vietnam. Milit Med 131:646, 1966.

21. Peel S: Army aeromedical evacuation procedures in Vietnam: Implications for rural America. JAMA 4:99, 1968.

22. Pesola G, Bayshtok V, Kvetan V: American critical care team at a foreign disaster site: The Armenian experience. Crit Care Med 17:582, 1989.

23. Collins AJ: Kidney dialysis treatment for victims of the Armenian earthquake. N Engl J Med 320:1291, 1989.

24. Collins AJ, Burnstein S: Renal failure in disasters. Crit Care Clin 7:421, 1991.

25. Barbera J: Report of Special Medical Response Team response to earthquake in Baguio City, Philippines. Office of Foreign Disaster Assistance, 1990.

26. Roth PB, Vogel A, Key G, et al: The St Croix disaster and the National Disaster Medical System. Ann Emerg Med 20:391, 1991.

27. Kvetan V: Operation Desert Storm: Task force on disasters and critical care. Crit Care Med 19:854, 1991.

28. An Assessment of the Consequences and Preparations for a Catastrophic California Earthquake: Findings and Action Taken. Report of an Ad Hoc committee for the National Security Council, Federal Emergency Management Agency, M and R-2, January 1981.

29. San Francisco: Earthquake Planning Scenario for a Magnitude 7.5 Earthquake in the Hayward Fault in the San Francisco Bay Area. California Department of Conservation, Division of Mines and Geology, 1987. Special publication 78.

30. Wackerle JF: Disaster planning and response. N Engl J Med 324:815, 1991.

31. Noji EK: Natural disasters in disaster management. Crit Care Clin 7:271, 1991.

32. Pakiser LC: Earthquakes. Washington, DC, US Government Printing Office, 1990. US Department of the Interior, Division of Geological Survey, publication 0-273-042 QL3.

33. Leonard RB, Teitelman U: Manmade disasters in disaster management. Crit Care Clin 7:293, 1991.

34. Office of US Foreign Disaster Assistance: Disaster History: Significant Data on Major Disasters Worldwide, 1900–Present. Washington, DC, Agency for International Development, p 1, 1990.

35. Ward PL, Page RA: The Loma Prieta earthquake of October 17, 1989. Earthquakes & Volcanoes 21(6):215, 1989.

36. American Association for World Health: Should disaster strike—Be prepared. World Health Day Bull April 7, 1991.

37. US Geological Survey: The Severity of an Earthquake. Washington, DC, US Government Printing Office, 1990. US Department of the Interior, Division of Geological Survey, general interest publication 0-273-494 QL3.

38. Glass RI, Urrutia JJ, Sibony S, et al: Earthquake injuries related to housing in a Guatemalan village. Science 197:638, 1977.

39. Saidi F: The 1962 earthquake in Iran. N Engl J Med 268:929, 1963.

40. De Ville de Goyet C, Del Cid E, Romero E, et al: Earthquake in Guatemala: Epidemiologic evaluation of the relief effort. Bull Pan Am Health Organ 10:95, 1976.

41. Berberian M: Tabas-e-Golshan (Iran) catastrophic earthquake of 16 September, 1978; a preliminary field report. Disasters 2:207, 1979.

42. Philippines earthquake. Earthquake Eng September:3, 1990.

43. Barbera JA, Cadoux CG: Search, rescue, and evacuation. In disaster management. Crit Care Clin 7:321, 1991.

44. Kunkle RF: Medical care of entrapped patients in confined spaces. International Workshop on Earthquake Injury. Epidemiology for mitigation and response. In: Johns Hopkins University Proceedings, July 10–12, 1989, p 338.

45. Sheng CY: Medical support in the Tangshan earthquake: A review of the management of mass casualties and certain major injuries. J Trauma 27:1130, 1987.

46. Tilling RI: Volcanoes. Washington, DC, US Government Printing Office. US Department of the Interior, Division of Geological Survey, general interest publication.

47. Heliker C: Volcanic and Seismic Hazards on the Island of Hawaii. Washington, DC, US Government Printing Office, 1990. US Department of the Interior, Division of Geological Survey, general interest publication 259-799.

48. Baxter PJ: Volcanoes. In: Gregg MB (ed): The Public Health Consequences of Disasters. Atlanta, Centers for Disease Control, p 25, 1989.

49. Sigurdsson H, Carey S: Volcanic disasters in Latin America and the 13 November 1985 eruption of Nevada del Ruiz volcano in Colombia. Disasters 10:205, 1986.

50. French JG: Hurricanes. In: Gregg MB (ed): The Public Health Consequences of Disasters. Atlanta, Centers for Disease Control, p 33, 1989.

51. Orlowskii J: Floods, hurricanes and tsunamis. In: Baskett P, Weller R (eds): Medicine for Disasters. Littleton, MA, PSG Publishing, p 291, 1988.

52. Frazier K: The Violent Face of Nature: Severe Phenomena and Natural Disasters. New York, William Morrow, 1979.

53. Gueri M, Perez LJ: Medical aspects of the "El Ruiz" avalanche disaster, Colombia. Disasters 10:150, 1986.

54. Sommer A, Mosley WH: East Bengal cyclone of November, 1970. Lancet 1:1029, 1972.

55. Centers for Disease Control: Medical examiner/coroner reports of deaths associated with Hurricane Hugo—South Carolina. MMWR 38:754, 1989.

56. Centers for Disease Control: Update: Work related electrocutions associated with Hurricane Hugo. MMWR 38:718, 1989.

57. Sanderson LN: Tornadoes. In: Gregg MB (ed): The Public Health Consequences of Disasters. Atlanta, Centers for Disease Control, p 39, 1989.

58. Galway G: Relationship of tornado death to severe weather watch areas. Mon Weather Rev 103:737, 1975.

59. Glass RI, Craven RB, Bregman DG, et al: Injuries from the Witchita Falls tornado: Implications for prevention. Science 207:734, 1980.

60. Bakst HJ, Berg RL, Foster FD, et al: The Worchester County Tornado: Medical Study of the Disaster. Washington, DC, National Research Council, Committee on Disaster Studies, p 1, 1954.

61. Mandelbaum I, Nahrwold D, Boyer DW: Management of tornado casualties. J Trauma 6:353, 1966.

62. French JG, Holt KW: Floods. In: Gregg MB (ed): The Public Health Consequences of Disaster. Atlanta, Centers for Disease Control, 1989.

63. Seaman J: Epidemiology of natural disasters. Contrib Epidemiol Biostatistics 5:1, 1984.

64. French J, Ing R, Von Allmen S, et al: Mortality from flash flood: A review of national weather reports, 1969–1981. Public Health Rep 98:584, 1983.

65. Beinin L: Medical Consequences of Natural Disasters. New York, Springer-Verlag, p 1, 1985.

66. Pan American Health Organization: Assessing Needs in the Health Sector after Floods and Hurricanes. Washington, DC, Pan American Health Organization, p 1, 1987. Technical paper 11.

67. Ussher JH: Philippine flood disaster. J R Nav Med Serv 59:81, 1973.

68. Fisher J: Road traffic accidents. In: Baskett P, Weller R (eds): Medicine for Disasters. Littleton, MA, PSG Publishing, p 318, 1988.

69. Fahey M: Airport and aircraft accidents. In: Baskett P, Weller R (eds): Medicine for Disasters. Littleton, MA, PSG Publishing, p 354, 1988.

70. Robertson B: Railway accidents. In: Baskett P, Weller R (eds): Medicine for Disasters. Littleton, MA, PSG Publishing, p 340, 1988.

71. Guzzardi L: Toxic products of combustion. Top Emerg Med 7:45, 1985.

72. Auffret R: Airport disasters. In: Proceedings of the 7th World Congress on Emergency and Disaster Medicine, Montreal. In press.

73. Bergot GP: Medical equipment for disaster at airports. J World Assoc Emerg Disaster Med 1(2):124, 1985.

74. Airport Emergency Planning—Part 7. 1980 International Civil Aviation Organization document 9137-AN/898.

75. Golden F: Shipwreck and exposure. In: Baskett P, Weller R (eds): Medicine for Disasters. Littleton, MA, PSG Publishing, p 363, 1988.

76. Code of Federal Regulations 49, Parts 100 to 177 (Transportation). Washington, DC, Office of the Federal Register, National Archives and Records Service, part 171.8, October 1, 1981.

77. Frykberg ER, Tepas JJ: Terrorist bombings. Ann Surg 208:569, 1988.

78. Safar P, Pretto E, Bircher N: Disaster resuscitation including management of severe trauma. In: Baskett P, Weller R (eds): Medicine for Disasters. Littleton, MA, PSG Publishing, p 36, 1988.

79. Bywaters EGL, Beall D: Crush injuries with impairment of renal function. Br Med J 1:427, 1941.

80. Kitka MJ, Meyer JP, Bishard RA, et al: Crush syndrome due to limb compression. Arch Surg 122:1078, 1987.

81. Better OS, Abassi Z, Rubinstein I, et al: The mechanism of muscle injury in the crush syndrome: Ischemic versus pressure-stretch myopathy (editorial). Miner Electrolyte Metab 16:181, 1990.

82. Odeh M: The role of reperfusion-induced injury in the pathogenesis of the crush syndrome. N Engl J Med 324:1417, 1991.

83. Owen CA, Mubarak SJ, Hargens AR, et al: Intramuscular pressures with limb compression: Clarification of the pathogenesis of the drug-induced muscle-compartment syndrome. N Engl J Med 300:1169, 1979.

84. Better OS, Stein JH: Early management of shock and prophylaxis of acute renal failure in traumatic rhabdomyolysis. N Engl J Med 322:825, 1990.

85. Odeh M: The role of reperfusion-induced injury in the pathogenesis of crush syndrome. N Engl J Med 324:1417, 1991.

86. Matsen FA III: Compartmental syndrome: A unified concept. Clin Orthop 113:8, 1975.

87. Whitesides TE, Haney TC, Morimoto K: Tissue pressure measurements as a determinant for the need of fasciotomy. Clin Orthop 113:43, 1975.

88. Allister C: Cardiac arrest after crush injury (case report). Br Med J 287:531, 1983.

89. Braunwald E, Isselbacher KJ, Petersdorf RG, et al (eds): Harrison's Principles of Internal Medicine. 11th ed. New York, McGraw-Hill, p 208, 880, 1987.

90. Zagar RA: Studies of mechanisms and protective maneuvers in myoglobinuric acute renal injury. Lab Invest 60:619, 1989.

91. Ron D, et al: Prevention of acute renal failure in traumatic rhabdomyolysis. Arch Intern Med 144:277, 1984.

92. Serum calcium derangements in rhabdomyolysis (editorial). N Engl J Med 305:161, 1981.

93. Reis ND, Michaelson M, et al: Crush injury to the lower limbs. Treatment of the local injury. J Bone Joint Surg [Am] 68:414, 1986.

94. Christensen KS: Pneumatic antishock garments (PASG): Do they precipitate lower-extremity compartment syndromes? J Trauma 26:1102, 1986.

95. Godbout B, Burchard KW, Slotman GJ, et al: Crush syndrome with death following pneumatic antishock garment application. J Trauma 24:1052, 1984.

96. Aprosio PN: Le syndrome d'ensevelissement. Med Catastrophes 38:11, 1986.

97. Hopkins JA, Shoemaker WC, Chang PC, et al: Results of clinical trial on the use of an emergency resuscitation algorithm. Crit Care Med 11:621, 1983.

98. Shoemaker W, Kvetan V, Fyodorov V, et al: Clinical algorithm for initial fluid resuscitation in disasters. Crit Care Clin 7:363, 1991.

99. Shoemaker WC, Kram HB, Appel PL, et al: The efficacy of central venous and pulmonary artery catheters and therapy based upon them in reducing mortality and morbidity. Arch Surg 125:1332, 1990.

100. Hingston RA, Hingston L: Respiratory injuries in earthquakes in Latin America in the 1970's: a personal experience in Peru (1970), Nicaragua (1972–3), and Guatemala (1976). Disaster Med 1:425, 1983.

101. Yong C, et al (eds): The Great Tangshan Earthquake of 1976: An Anatomy of a Disaster. New York, Pergamon Press, p 58, 1988.

102. Eisele JW, O'Halloran R, Reay D, et al: Death during the May 18, 1980 eruption of Mount St. Helens. N Engl J Med 305:931, 1981.

103. Borak J, Callan M, Abbott W: Hazardous Materials Exposure: Emergency Response and Patient Care. Englewood Cliffs, NJ, Brady, p 191, 1991.

104. Benumof JL: Management of the Difficult or Impossible Airway. Las Vegas, NV, American Society of Anesthesiologists, p 163, 1990.

105. Kingsley CP: Anesthesia care under austere conditions. Crit Care Rep 2:71, 1990.

106. Baskett PJF: The trauma anesthesia/critical care specialist in the field. Crit Care Clin 6:13, 1990.

107. Grande C, Baskett PJF, Donchin Y, et al: Trauma anesthesia for disasters: Anything, anytime, anywhere. Crit Care Clin 7:339, 1991.

108. Donchin Y, Wiener M, Grande C, et al: Military medicine: Trauma anesthesia and critical care on the battlefield. Crit Care Clin 6:185, 1990.

109. McSwain GR, Garrison WB, Artz CP: Evaluation of resuscitation from cardiopulmonary arrest by paramedics. Ann Emerg Med 9:341, 1980.

110. Lewis FR: Prehospital intravenous fluid therapy: Physiologic computer modeling. J Trauma 26:804, 1986.

111. Lewis FR: Ineffective treatment and delayed transport. Prehosp Disaster Med 4(2):129, 1989.

112. Rottman S: Prehospital fluid administration in trauma. Prehosp Disaster Med 4(2):127, 1989.

113. Bishop M, Shoemaker W, Jackson G, et al: Evaluation of a blunt and penetrating trauma algorithm for truncal injury. Crit Care Clin 7:383, 1991.

114. Aznaurian AV, Haroutunian GM, Atabekian AL, et al: Medical aspects of the consequences of earthquake in Armenia. In: Proceedings of the International Symposium on Medical Aspects of Earthquake Consequences in Armenia, 1990, p 9.

115. The skywalk collapse: A personal response (editorial). Ann Emerg Med 12:651, 1983.

116. Irwin RI: The incident command system (ICS). In: Auf der Heide E (ed): Disaster Response: Principles of Preparation and Coordination. St Louis, CV Mosby, p 133, 1989.

117. Kerns DE, Anderson PB: Emergency medical services response to a major aircraft incident: Sioux City, Iowa. Prehosp Disaster Med 5(2):159, 1990.

118. Sanner PH, Wolcott BW: Stress reactions among participants in mass casualty simulations. Ann Emerg Med 7:426, 1983.

119. Gunn SW: Medical management in international relief. UN Disaster Relief Organ News September/October:8, 22, 1987.

120. Noji EK, Kelen GD, Armenian HK, et al: The 1988 earthquake in Soviet Armenia: A case study. Ann Emerg Med 19:891, 1990.

121. Cowley RA: The resuscitation and stabilization of major multiple trauma patients in a trauma center environment. Clin Med 83:14, 1976.

122. Abrams T: The feasibility of prehospital medical response teams for foreign disaster assistance. Prehosp Disaster Med 5(3):241, 1990.

123. Borden FW: A Government and Community Approach to Disaster Response in Los Angeles. Disaster Preparedness Division, Los Angeles City Fire Department, Los Angeles, October 1990.

124. Angus D, Pretto E, Abrams J, et al: Life supporting first aid training of the lay public for disaster preparedness (abstract). Prehosp Disaster Med 6(2):257, 1991.

125. Abrams J, Pretto E, Angus D, et al: Basic extrication training of the lay public for disaster preparedness. Prehosp Disaster Med 6(2):257, 1991.

126. Vayer JS, Ten Eyck RP, Cowan ML: New concepts in triage. Ann Emerg Med 15:927, 1986.

127. Winslow GR: Triage and Justice. Los Angeles, University of California Press, 1982.

128. Champion HR, Sacco WJ: Triage of trauma victims. In: Trunkey DD, Lewis FR (eds): Current Treatment of Trauma—2. Philadelphia, BC Decker, 1986.

129. Champion HR, Moreau MM, Gainer PS: Assessment and triage. In:

Baskett P, Weller R (eds): Medicine for Disasters. Littleton, MA, PSG Publishing, p 19, 1988.

130. Auf der Heide E (ed): Disaster Response: Principles of Preparation and Coordination. St Louis, CV Mosby, 1989.

131. Lachenmyer J: Physiological aspects of transport. Int Anesthesiol Clin 25:15, 1987.

132. Joint Commission on Accreditation of Healthcare Organizations: Accreditation Manual for Hospitals, 1991. Standard PL.1-7. Chicago, Joint Commission On Accreditation of Healthcare Organizations, p 201, 1990.

133. Mahone LE, Reutershan TP: Catastrophic disasters and the design of disaster medical care systems. Ann Emerg Med 16:1085, 1987.

134. Urban Search and Rescue Response System: A Component of the Federal Response Plan Under Emergency Support Function 9. Washington, DC, US Government Printing Office, 1991. Federal Emergency Management Agency. Publication 523-835/40339.

135. Cowley RA: The resuscitation and stabilization of major multiple trauma patients in a trauma center environment. Clin Med 93:14, 1976.

136. Textbook of Advanced Cardiac Life Support. Dallas, American Heart Association, 1987.

137. Advanced Trauma Life Support Instructor's Manual. Chicago, American College of Surgeons Committee on Trauma, 1988.

138. Bender EM, Moore EE, Kashuk JL, et al: Conservative management of sand aspiration: A case report. Milit Med 149:98, 1984.

139. Mateer JR, Thompson BM, Aphramian C, et al: Rapid fluid resuscitation with central venous catheters. Ann Emerg Med 12:149, 1983.

140. Kunkle RF: Delivery of medical care in confined spaces. In: Proceedings of the Structural Collapse Rescue Technologies Workshop, Los Alamos National Laboratories, October 3, 1989. IAO-90-384.

141. Castillo CJ: Philippine earthquake: International disaster with an international response. Fire Eng 143(12):20–27, 1990.

142. Grande CM: Critical care transport: A trauma perspective. An overview of trauma anesthesia and critical care. Crit Care Clin 6(1):165, 1990.

143. McNeil EL: Airborne Care of the Ill and Injured. New York, Springer-Verlag, 1983.

144. Gilman JI: Carrier and vendor selection. Int Anesthesiol Clin 24:117, 1987.

145. Dhenin G: Aviation Medicine: Physiology and Human Factors. London, Tri-Med, 1978.

146. Pearl RG, Mihm FG, Rosenthal MH: Care of the adult patient during transport. Int Anesthesiol Clin 25:43, 1987.

147. American College of Surgeons Committee on Trauma (Collicott PE, et al): Advanced Trauma Life Support Course for Physicians. Chicago, American College of Surgeons, 1984.

148. Wong L, Grande CM, Muenster AM: Burns and associated non-thermal trauma: An analysis of management, outcome and relation to the Injury Severity Score. J Burn Care Rehabil 6:10, 1989.

Appendix 2–1

Clinical Algorithm for Initial Fluid Resuscitation of Disaster Victims

Step 1. If cardiac or respiratory arrest occurs, begin cardiopulmonary resuscitation, start fluids, intubate, and ventilate. If not, proceed to step 2.

Step 2. If upper airway obstruction or respiratory distress is present, clear nasopharynx, intubate, and ventilate. If not, proceed to step 3.

Step 3. If systolic blood pressure < 80 mm Hg, start 1 L of Ringer's lactate or normal (physiologic) saline. If not, proceed to step 6.

Step 4. If the patient is older than 45 years of age or has a history of cardiac problems, give 500 mL of a colloid solution: 5% albumin, 5% plasma protein solution, or hydroxyethyl starch. If not, give a second liter of Ringer's lactate (or physiologic saline) and 500 mL of colloids.

Step 5. If systolic blood pressure has increased to >80 mm Hg, proceed to step 6; if not, repeat through step 6; if not, steps 3 through 5. If after repeating two or three times without systolic blood pressure response, consider immediate surgical exploration for occult bleeding.

Step 6. If systolic blood pressure < 120 mm Hg or mean arterial pressure < 80 mm Hg, give 1 L of Ringer's lactate and 500 mL of a colloid.

Step 7. If hematocrit < 25%, transfuse with whole blood or packed red blood cells until hematocrit of at least 25% is reached.

Step 8. Place central venous pressure catheter; if central venous pressure > 18, slow or stop fluids, give vasopressors (dopamine, norepinephrine) to maintain mean arterial pressure of >80 mm Hg.

Step 9. Obtain arterial blood gas analysis, if available, and correct acidosis, hypoxemia, and so on.

Step 10. Place Foley's catheter and measure hourly urine output. If <30 mL/h, recycle for additional fluids.

Step 11. If mean arterial pressure not restored, repeat steps 6 to 11. If mean arterial pressure is restored, continue maintenance fluids, re-evaluate clinically, and recycle if there is subsequent deterioration.

Adapted from Shoemaker WC, Kvetan V, Fyodorov V, et al: Clinical algorithm for initial fluid resuscitation in disasters. Crit Care Clin 7:363, 1991.

CHAPTER 3

Chemical Exposure

John S. Urbanetti
Frederick R. Sidell

OVERVIEW OF CHEMICAL EXPOSURE

In April 1915 at Ypres, Belgium, modern gas warfare[1] began when the Germans released chlorine gas on the front lines, creating havoc and casualties in the opposing French and British forces. On July 12, 1917, the Germans first used mustard gas, which caused more than 20,000 casualties over the ensuing weeks. Because of the topical effects of that substance, gas masks alone were inadequate protection, and by the end of the war 1,300,000 chemical casualties were recorded among all combatants. During World War II the Germans developed and produced two nerve agents (Tabun and Sarin) in substantial quantities. Since World War II many examples of chemical use in combat have been recorded, most recently in the Iran-Iraq conflict.[2] United Nations investigation teams have identified both mustard gas and nerve agents as having been used in that conflict. The "success" of such use makes future use of similar substances highly likely. The Persian Gulf military conflict in 1991 raised the consciousness of the medical community about toxic chemical exposures.

Toxic Chemical Agents

There is a threat that chemical casualties may develop in settings outside a military or combat scenario. Industrialized nations manufacture, transport, and use large quantities of particularly toxic substances, and there are occasional acci-

dental releases of these substances. It is not possible here to discuss all the chemical warfare agents that are produced. The commonly available chemical agents are discussed, and these include riot control agents, choking agents, cyanide, nerve agents, vesicant agents, and incapacitating compounds.

Riot control agents[3] have been in regular use since the French police's first use of ethyl bromoacetate against rioters in 1910 to 1914. Since World War I these compounds have continued in regular use with some periodic notoriety (e.g., U.S. use in Vietnam and Londonderry use in 1969).[4, 5] Riot control agents[6, 7] include chloroacetophenone (CN), dibenzoxazepine (CR), o-chlorobenzylidenemalononitrile (CS). Characteristics shared by these agents are their rapid onset of effect (seconds to minutes), brief duration of effect (15 to 30 minutes after exposure terminates), high safety ratio (ratio of lethal dose and effective dose), and effects caused by sensory irritation.

Phosgene (carbonyl chloride) was produced by John Davy in 1812 from CO, Cl, and sunlight (hence phos-gene). The Germans first used phosgene as a chemical warfare agent during World War I. Phosgene produces severe irritation of the respiratory system and was classed as a choking agent during World War I. It is a colorless gas that may hydrolyze slightly in moist air to produce a white cloud. A vapor density greater than air causes phosgene to hug the ground and flow into trenches. An odor of newly mown hay is just detectable at concentration levels that have a mild degree of toxicity.

Hydrogen cyanide was discovered by Scheele in 1782, when he made it by heating sulfuric acid with Prussian blue (hence the name prussic acid). Cyanide is a colorless gas or liquid with a peach kernel or bitter almond odor. The odor is just barely detectable by trained observers at slightly less than toxic levels. Because of the additional fact of very rapid onset of toxic effect, hydrogen cyanide is regarded as having poor warning properties. As a gas hydrogen cyanide is lighter than air. Because of its volatility and low density, cyanide is a nonpersistent substance. Therefore, shortly after the gas is used the area can be occupied by personnel.

Nerve agents were first developed in a search for better insecticides. Organophosphate (OP) compounds were studied by a German industrial research team headed by Gerhard Schrader, resulting in the discovery of a particularly potent OP chemical, Tabun, in 1936. By the end of the war two additional highly potent OP compounds had been developed.

Sulfur mustard, a vesicant agent, was first synthesized in the mid-1800s. It was investigated by the Germans as a possible chemical warfare agent and introduced on the battlefield at Ypres in 1917. Despite its relatively late deployment, sulfur mustard came to be the principal chemical agent during World War I and was responsible for the greatest number of chemical casualties during that conflict.

Sulfur mustard is a slightly yellow and/or brown oily substance (depending on the manufacturing process) that may contain up to 30% of impurities. An odor of garlic or mustard is characteristic. The odor is not reliably identified. Because olfactory adaptation may occur over time, odor does not serve as an adequate warning. Nitrogen mustard is also considered as a chemical warfare vesicant agent and has similar chemical effects. However, it should not be considered identical to sulfur mustard, as it appears to have more severe systemic and central nervous system effects.

Incapacitating compounds are agents that create a disability in the combatant without causing physical damage. During the 1950s the U.S. military studied a variety of substances. These included tranquilizers, cannabinols, indoles (including lysergic acid diethylamide), and anticholinergics.[8] The glycolate anticholinergics were primarily studied, and of these 3-quinuclidinyl benzilate (BZ) was identified for further study. However, it has been found that these compounds produce unpredictable behavior. They are not stockpiled as U.S. chemical agents. The possibility of terrorist use and similarity in effect to atropine, however, prompt this review. Atropine, which is currently used as a specific nerve agent antidote, might be misused by the soldier. Consequently, the soldier might suffer medical effects similar to those of BZ intoxication.

BZ is a solid and is disseminated as a fine powder or by aerosol for inhalational exposures. By the inhalational route, 6 to 8 μg/kg may produce some drowsiness within 15 to 30 minutes. Lower doses may produce effects up to 4 hours later. Dermal and topical exposures may produce effects 4 to 24 hours after the exposure. The duration of the effect averages 5 days and may last as long as 7 to 10 days.

GENERAL MANAGEMENT IN CHEMICAL EXPOSURES[9]

Protective Equipment

Protective masks are available and are of the filtration type or are self-contained respiratory units. The masks with charcoal-based filter elements provide filtration of all known military chemical agents in both vapor and aerosol form. These filters also effectively remove particulate material, including smoke, dusts, and aerosolized bacterial particles. Ammonia and carbon monoxide are inadequately filtered by charcoal-based masks, and self-contained breathing units must be used. Cyanide and vaporized acids such as hydrogen sulfide and hydrogen fluoride rapidly degrade charcoal-based filter capabilities, reducing their effective life by 50% or more. Dermal protective equipment includes protective suits and protective wraps for casualties. The U.S. military suits and wraps consist of carbon-impregnated fabrics that protect individuals from all known military chemical agents for up to 6 hours—a time similar to the effective period of mask filters.

Triage in Chemical Warfare

Chemical warfare exposure is likely to result in mass casualties in which an arriving population of patients may overwhelm the medically available personnel and/or the equipment pool. Consequently, triage is used to evaluate and classify casualties for purposes of treatment and evacuation. Triage is intended (1) to provide immediate treatment, (2) to delay treatment for casualties with less than life-threatening injuries, (3) to set aside at least temporarily casualties requiring care beyond current medical or equipment capability, and (4) to conserve medical resources by not treating casualties expected to die.

Such an approach to care of patients at first seems foreign to both the medical training and practice of the U.S. physician. However, wartime experience has repetitively reinforced the need to develop a confident and smoothly functional triage system utilizing officers who are experts in such matters.

Decontamination of Chemical Exposures

Decontamination may be "spot" decontamination, in which decontaminating solutions (such as 5% bleach) are used both to remove and to degrade chemical agents. Specialized decontamination kits are available that contain chemicals specifically designed for the removal of particular known agents. An integral part of the training of personnel in decontamination includes instruction in removal of contaminated clothing.

Laboratory Precautions

Patients with chemical exposure who enter a medical facility present additional difficulties for laboratory personnel. Questions of contaminations with bodily fluids are typically raised. However, a properly decontaminated patient presents a minimal exposure risk for laboratory personnel. Blood, urine, blister fluid, feces, and other bodily secretions contain nontoxic amounts of chemical agents and thus do not present a significant threat of chemical contamination. Surface contamination with most chemical agents is easily removed by the previously mentioned decontamination process. Material not removed from the surface has been fixed to deeper layers of skin or combined with various tissues or blood in a wound site in such a way as to be relatively nontoxic to subsequent care providers.

GENERAL CONCEPTS OF EMERGENCY SUPPORT OF CHEMICAL INJURIES

Protect Yourself

The medical care provider must be alert to the possibility that a chemical casualty is contaminated with the substance in question. Unless certain that decontamination has been accomplished, the initial investigating medical care provider must be wearing protective clothing and a functional gas mask.

Immediate Chemical Therapy

Certain chemical exposures create medical illness that may be lethal if allowed to progress even for a matter of minutes. Recognition of these types of chemical exposures is therefore critically important.

Cyanide Exposures. The rapidity with which cyanide inhibits intracellular oxygen utilization and hence has a lethal effect is well known. Vapor exposures are so rapidly lethal that counteracting chemical therapy may be of no particular lifesaving benefit unless applied within seconds to minutes of an observed exposure. Ingested cyanide has a more delayed onset of effect and prolonged action. Therapy is with the standard antidote kit (described later).

Nerve Agent. Exposure to OP (by inhalation or by a transdermal route) creates a rapidly progressive respiratory failure that requires immediate chemical therapy. Routine support techniques of airway protection, endotracheal intubation, and mechanical ventilation do not salvage a nerve agent casualty unless a specific antidote (atropine) is provided concurrently.

Airway Support

Airway support in a chemical environment may be necessary for (1) vesicants causing laryngeal edema or laryngospasm, (2) vesicants causing severe facial edema, and (3) nerve agents causing acute respiratory failure by central apnea, muscle weakness, and airway compromise (bronchospasm and secretions). Clinical indications for airway support include hoarseness and stridor. Intubation, if required, should be accomplished under direct vision by the most experienced individual available. Rapidly progressive laryngospasm may occur if endotracheal tube placement is not possible, and cricothyrotomy may be urgently required.

Symptoms of dyspnea and/or chest tightness may be an early indication of alveolar capillary leak and impending pulmonary edema in the absence of radiologic chest abnormalities. Application of a continuous positive airway pressure mask may be appropriate in this setting. Individuals with heightened airway sensitivity (irritable airways disease) may have asthma triggered by virtually any inhalational exposure. Standard therapeutic interventions for bronchospasm should be considered in this setting. Adrenergic agents, theophylline, and ultimately corticosteroids may be indicated, depending on the severity of disease. Resistant ventricular tachyarrhythmias may be seen if atropine is employed in a setting of arterial hypoxemia.

In the most severe form of respiratory failure, there is diffuse alveolar capillary membrane damage leading to the adult respiratory distress syndrome. Ventilatory support should be instituted early, particularly when ventilation and perfusion abnormalities may severely compromise oxygen exchange and the resulting hypoxia may compromise other organ functions.

Other Medical Support

Cardiovascular System. Circulatory failure occurring as a result of chemical agent exposure is of such serious consequence that the likelihood of recovery of such an individual is low unless immediate medical support at the level of the intensive care unit is available and can be provided without compromising the care available to others who are less severely injured.[10]

Central Nervous System. Various central nervous system effects may be seen after chemical exposures. Seizure activity may be a primary effect of nerve agent or cyanide exposure. Seizures with other chemical exposures should be further investigated.

Immunosuppression. Vesicant exposures may result in substantial systemic absorption of sulfur mustard with a resulting blood cell line suppression. Neutropenia may occur and can be sufficiently severe to render the patient immunosuppressed. A progressive neutropenia may begin at 3 days with a nadir several days later. The resulting syndromes most often seen in the critical care setting are septic shock and pneumonia.

Burns. Vesicant burns are not associated with the same fluid balance difficulties as thermal burns of similar size. The difficulties associated with vesicant burns are those of mechanical compromise of the affected part. There is no active vesicant in the burn and blister fluid.

Nosocomial Infection. Inhalational trauma to the respiratory system compromises the normal protective mechanisms of mucociliary function of the lung. Secondary bacterial infections are commonly seen. The major source of the organisms may be another colonized and/or infected patient whose bacterial organisms are spread (generally on the hands of medical personnel) to the compromised patient. There is no evidence that prophylactic antibiotic treatment is beneficial.

MEDICAL MANAGEMENT OF SPECIFIC TOXIC AGENTS
Riot Agents

CN was first synthesized in the 1800s and used in World War I. It is a solid or powder that is generally disseminated by burning munitions. This produces a blue and white cloud with an odor of orange blossoms. Until the 1950s this substance was a standard riot control agent used by the U.S. military and various law enforcement groups. Although it has been replaced by CS, it is still sold for self-protection as Mace. CN is a more potent skin irritant[11] than CS and a more potent skin sensitizer as well, with a high likelihood of causing allergic dermatitis. Ocular effects are seen with sprays; corneal epithelial edema is noted but remits quickly. Eye injury may also occur with close range use of riot guns, generally as a result of a blast effect or a mechanical effect of cartridge particles. Pulmonary pathology includes pneumonitis with diffuse pseudomembrane development. It appears more severe than the pathology associated with CS.[12]

CR was first synthesized in 1962. It is a solid that is generally dispersed in a solution. It has an irritating odor and is persistent. Studies have shown a transient elevation of blood pressure with a "drench" of the skin.[3] CR typically is used as a solution and erythema is noted 1 to 2 hours after exposure. There is no vesication or skin sensitization,[11] and the effects on airways or lung parenchyma are minimal.

CS was synthesized in 1928 (by Corson and Stoughton, hence CS). Because of its effectiveness, CS replaced CN for both military and law enforcement use. CS is a white solid that is dispersed by spraying a solution or burning munitions. The clinical effect of this substance is to produce eye burning, blepharospasm, lacrimation, oropharyngeal burning, and chest burning. CS is a primary skin irritant that can produce an allergic contact dermatitis. Higher doses of CS, especially with abraded skin, increased temperature, and increased humidity, produce an intense erythema with subsequent edema and vesication.[13]

When the casualty is removed from contamination most effects remit within 20 to 30 minutes. The recommended mixture for skin decontamination is composed of 6% sodium bicarbonate, 1% benzalkonium chloride, and 3% sodium carbonate.

Exposed individuals should be evaluated for respiratory distress. There is a potential for exacerbation of subclinical bronchospasm. Severe respiratory effects may not appear for 12 hours. Hospitalization is indicated if respiratory complaints increase and are associated with hypoxemia. As in any dry chemical ocular injury, the eyes should be flushed thoroughly and the use of topical anesthetics should be minimal. Severe skin erythema and inflammation may be treated with topical corticosteroids with wet dressings for oozing lesions.

Phosgene

In an aqueous environment phosgene hydrolyzes, producing both HCl and a carbonyl group (C=O). Both chemical species are reactive and toxic. At low-dose exposure, the phosgene reaches the peripheral airways before the development of a substantial cough caused by free HCl irritation of the trachea. In the smaller airways, the free HCl is well buffered. The carbonyl group, however, interacts with the alveolar capillary membrane and increases its permeability. Consequently, there is capillary leak into the pulmonary interstitium and the alveoli as well. Clinically evident pulmonary edema ensues. At higher-dose exposure, the free HCl interacts with the more central airways, producing intense inflammatory change. In higher concentrations, early laryngospasm with death may occur. Alveolar capillary membrane leak occurs relatively slowly. It is stabilized to some extent by normal lymphatic drainage system function. The clinical effect of this prolonged pathophysiologic process is such that early symptoms of interstitial edema (such as chest tightness and dyspnea) may precede clear signs of increased lung water. Physical examination and laboratory tests (e.g., arterial blood gas assays and chest radiograph) may be normal up to 4 hours after exposure. Despite such apparent clinical stability, the exposure may still produce a lethal outcome.[14, 15]

With the onset of pulmonary edema an adult respiratory

distress syndrome–like picture is produced. Therapy[16] is directed toward the obvious abnormal physiology, that is, pulmonary edema. Stabilization of the patient is undertaken until spontaneous resolution of the alveolar capillary membrane leak occurs. The increase in interstitial lung water and alveolar edema interferes with gas exchange and decreases intravascular volume. The early application of positive end-expiratory pressure or positive pressure ventilation stabilizes gas exchange. If positive end-expiratory pressure is applied after substantial intravascular volume loss has occurred, hypotension may appear. Systemic hypoxia and acidosis may subsequently occur. The risk of multiple organ system failure with hypotension dictates the need to be aggressive and expeditious with volume replacement. Pressors are utilized only pending appropriate volume loading. Individuals with chronic bronchitic secretions have an increase in quantity of secretions, although there is little difficulty with clearance unless bronchospasm supervenes. Individuals with underlying bronchospastic airways disease often demonstrate increased bronchospasm as a result of a phosgene exposure. Therapy of the bronchospasm should be similar to that applied to an asthmatic with an acute inflammatory exacerbation. Bronchodilators should be used aggressively and corticosteroids may be needed if bronchodilators fail. Infectious complications are commonly noted 3 to 4 days after toxic inhalational exposure. Careful attention must be paid to anticipating these infections in a setting of what is generally considered a nosocomial problem. Surveillance sputum cultures and chest radiographs may help identify an infectious complication early. The use of prophylactic antibiotics is of no apparent benefit.

Phosgene-exposed individuals recover from the acute process within 2 to 4 days. Superinfections may require long-term antibiotic therapy. Persistent, indolent postexposure infections may lead to varying degrees of interstitial fibrosis.[17] In the absence of infection an exposed lung generally recovers well.

Cyanide

Cyanide produces a histotoxic hypoxia by inhibiting the final step of mitochondrial oxidative phosphorylation. Thus, cellular death is due to inhibition of intracellular respiration. Tissues that are highly metabolically active (i.e., the central nervous system and heart) are most sensitive to the effects of cyanide.

The clinical effects of cyanide[18] include immediate and intense stimulation of the respiratory system with hyperpnea and uncontrollable hyperventilation. There is subsequent severe respiratory depression with respiratory center failure ultimately leading to death.

Artificial respiration was suggested in 1840 as a specific therapy.[19] Chen and coworkers[20] later proposed the use of an antidotal combination of amyl nitrite, sodium nitrite, and sodium thiosulfate. This therapeutic approach takes advantage of cyanide's affinity for porphyrin pigments by making the hemoglobin in erythrocytes more available. In developing the technique of methemoglobin production for cyanide binding, it has been observed that methemoglobin levels above 30% of the total hemoglobin are dangerous. An additional observation that amyl nitrite improved both respiratory and cardiac effects in dogs before substantial methemoglobin was formed suggested that the vasodilating effect of amyl nitrite may be an important therapeutic process.[21] However, the exceptional rapidity with which cyanide poisons an individual makes therapeutic intervention generally impractical. With the exception of cyanide-exposed individuals who are directly observed in their exposure by individuals immediately prepared to treat them, even intravenous therapy is unlikely to be of significant benefit.

Specific therapy for inhalational cyanide exposure includes the giving of amyl nitrite (one or two pearls are crushed and inspired). If amyl nitrite is not available, sodium nitrite is given as 30 mg/mL intravenously to a total of 300 mg for a 70-kg individual and the individual is observed for hypotension. (Note that the combination of amyl nitrite and sodium nitrite may produce excessive methemoglobin levels.) Sodium thiosulfate is given intravenously at 250 mg/mL in a 50-mL volume (12.5 g) in a 70-kg individual to provide an adequate thiol pool and supply sulfur necessary for hepatic rhodanese to catalyze the production of thiocyanate (SCN^-), which can be excreted by the kidney. Casualties are subsequently observed for signs of hypoxic damage of critical organs.

Nerve Agents

The primary recognized effect of OP agents is inhibition of the enzyme acetylcholinesterase.[22, 23] In a manner similar to inhibition by carbamates (e.g., pyridostigmine, physostigmine), OP agents bind by their organic phosphorus atoms to the site in acetylcholinesterase normally occupied by acetylcholine, ultimately inhibiting the normal metabolism of acetylcholine and resulting in its accumulation.[24] This initially hyperstimulates the end organs and ultimately inhibits them. The time course of these effects varies with route of exposure. Inhalational exposure results in effects within seconds to minutes. Percutaneous (liquid) exposure may lead to effects up to 18 hours after contamination; once these effects become evident, however, the rapidity of progression is equivalent to that with inhalational exposure. Duration of effect depends on dose and the use of therapeutic interventions.

Initial effects of low-dose vapor exposure include miosis with complaints of dim vision. Complaints of copious rhinorrhea are noted, and complaints of dyspnea are frequent, although there is often no confirming clinical sign. The classic triad of miosis, rhinorrhea, and slight respiratory impairment is the clinical finding in individuals exposed to small amounts of nerve agent vapor. More intense exposures lead to increased oropharyngeal secretions with increased lower respiratory tract symptoms of both copious secretions and bronchospasm. Hypoxia may be present. More severe exposures may result in sudden loss of consciousness and subsequent convulsions with cessation of respiration. Respiratory failure with subsequent death[25] may occur if immediate medical intervention is not available. Muscle twitching is prominent and progresses to a flaccid paralysis.[26]

Liquid exposure produces initial local effects of sweating and muscle fasciculation with subsequent progression to systemic effects that include respiratory distress and major muscular effects, similar to those of vapor exposure. Small droplets of liquid on the skin may have onset of effect up to 18 hours after skin contact, depending on the site of contact, temperature, and other variables. Systemic effects may begin up to 3 hours after decontamination of the skin because of delayed penetration through the dermis.[27]

Rapid aggressive antidotal therapy is vitally important in the care of OP-exposed individuals. With knowledgeable application of appropriate medical therapy,[28–32] most exposed individuals can recover. The therapy consists of termination of exposure, maintenance of a patent airway and/or ventilatory support, blockade of accumulated acetylcholine, regeneration of cholinesterase, and treatment of complications. Because the clinical effects of liquid exposures may be delayed up to 18 hours, decontamination should always be undertaken even in the absence of symptoms.

Ventilatory embarrassment attributable to secretion excess and bronchospasm responds to atropine.[33] The appropriate dose of atropine is titrated by the parameters of bronchospasm and/or secretions. Up to 20 mg may be needed for severe nerve agent exposure. Hypoxia may increase the sensitivity of the myocardium for ventricular arrhythmias induced by atropine.

The OP-acetylcholinesterase bond in some nerve agent exposures may be disrupted by the use of an oxime,[34, 35] pralidoxime chloride. The Mark 1 nerve agent antidote kit consists of an Atropen (containing 2 mg of atropine) and a ComboPen (containing 600 mg of pralidoxime). These autoinjectors allow rapid intramuscular injection of the antidote. Pralidoxime in a dose of up to 1.8 g is given intramuscularly initially with an additional 1.0 g given every hour either intramuscularly or intravenously. This therapy is titrated by its effect on muscle twitching. Because some nerve agents become irreversibly bound ("aged") to acetylcholinesterase, failure to reduce muscle twitching with an oxime would mitigate against further use.

Seizure activity may follow a nerve agent exposure and hypoxia should be considered as a possible trigger. Diazepam[36] is utilized specifically for seizure control. The U.S. military has autoinjectors containing 10 mg of diazepam for this purpose. Most patients have substantial clearance of symptoms within 7 to 10 days. Some long-term central nervous system effects,[37] including difficulty in concentrating, restlessness, and other cognitive changes, require careful neurologic examination before the patient is cleared to return to duty.

Vesicant Agents

Mustard is an alkylating agent. In the presence of water, the mustard side chains each attach to the guanine nitrogen in a DNA strand. The DNA strand then cross-links and becomes damaged, and cell death ensues. Cell lines that have the most active DNA turnover (e.g., hematopoietic and gastrointestinal tract cells) are most affected by mustard.[38] Mustard is poorly metabolized by the human body. In addition, sensitization may occur so that with repeated exposures the toxic effect increases geometrically.

Mustard fixes to exposed tissues within 2 minutes. Decontamination within this time eliminates its topical effects. Decontamination after 2 minutes is of value in protecting others and minimizing further systemic absorption of the agent but does not prevent blistering.

Mustard[39, 40] is toxic to the ocular, dermal, and respiratory systems[41] of individuals exposed to the vapor. Intense vapor or liquid exposure may have systemic effects as well. Hematopoietic effects of mustard exposure include leukocytopenia, which may be severe enough to lead to lethal pneumonitis and/or sepsis at 7 to 10 days after the exposure.

Intense exposures produce injury to the airways as well, forming an inflammatory and necrotic debris and a "pseudomembrane" that may peel from the wall and block more peripheral airways. An inflammatory and necrotic bronchitis is almost universally complicated by bacterial superinfection. With inflammation of more peripheral airways and parenchyma, diffuse pulmonary infiltrates are seen radiologically. These may be confused with bacterial pneumonitis.

Mild symptoms of cough or sore throat need no therapy. Bacterial superinfection should be treated specifically when an organism has been identified. Impending laryngospasm requires careful endotracheal tube placement. Oxygen therapy and continuous positive airway pressure may be necessary. Exposures of this intensity are associated with up to 80% mortality.[42]

Bronchospasm may occur in 15% of an exposed population. Many of these casualties have had no prior episode of significant bronchospasm. Routine bronchodilator therapy is given and corticosteroids may be needed if the bronchospasm is severe.

Most eye lesions are mild. With vapor exposure there is a latent period with onset commencing at 4 to 12 hours; 75% of the ocular lesions recover spontaneously, although photophobia may last for 2 to 6 weeks. During the recovery phase there may be severe blepharospasm. More intense exposures lead to earlier symptoms with added corneal changes. There may be permanent eye changes of corneal opacity and alteration and perforation of anterior chamber. Liquid mustard exposure of the eyes, if not decontaminated within 2 minutes, produces a severely debilitated "blind eye." Sterile petrolatum jelly on the eyelids helps prevent lid adhesions, and mydriatics may help reduce the painful ciliary muscle spasm.

An amount of vesicant as small as 10 μg on the skin can produce a blister if not decontaminated within 2 minutes. An effective decontamination solution is 5% (household) bleach diluted 1:10 (to 0.5%). With vapor exposures, erythema appears and acts much like a sunburn. The erythema appears 2 to 48 hours after the exposure and may progress (depending on the intensity of exposure) to blisters in 2 to 12 hours after it appears. These blisters are not the equivalent of those in thermal burns. The erythema may respond to calamine lotion. Topical corticosteroids may be useful for severe itching. Generally, blisters in noncritical areas should be left alone. Larger blisters or those in critical areas (e.g., intertriginous) respond to drainage and débridement. Blister fluid is not a vesicant. Vesicant burns are generally second-degree burns. Although there is some fluid loss, it does not approach that of thermal burns.

Intense exposures are associated with early nausea and vomiting. This may be partly a cholinergic effect and partly a reaction to swallowed mustard. Atropine and/or antiemetics may be effective. Autopsies of individuals who died after acute mustard exposure have shown duodenal ulceration and necrosis and desquamation of epithelium in the small intestine.

Intense systemic exposures suppress the hematopoietic system with effects on all cell lines. White blood cell suppression is the most significant effect and may be severe enough to lead to sepsis and death. Leukopenia begins to appear at 3 to 5 days with a nadir at 7 to 9 days. At this time, gastrointestinal sterilization may be of value. The use of parenteral thiols (e.g., sodium thiosulfate) may be of value as sulfur scavengers within the first 20 minutes after a sulfur mustard exposure.

Incapacitating Agents

Anticholinergic agents act primarily to block the effects of acetylcholine at muscarinic sites in the body.[43] The peripheral effects include decreased sweating, which is a potentially serious effect in a warm or hot environment. There is a decrease in oral and gastrointestinal secretions. Mydriasis occurs with an onset that may be delayed for 1 to 2 hours, and paralyzed accommodation may be seen up to weeks after exposure. Gastrointestinal tone and bladder tone are decreased and can lead to ileus and urinary retention. The cardiac rhythm abnormalities vary with the agent. BZ may produce an early bradycardia, and atropine may cause a tachycardia. The central nervous system effects are more complex, with all anticholinergic agents producing generally similar effects although the effective dose varies. The level of consciousness depends on the dose and is associated with mood changes from euphoria to apprehension. Disturbances of perception and judgment occur, with both illusions and hallucinations. Memory defects (especially short-term) are noted. Disorientation is often seen, especially in relation to both time and place. Behavior is variable and may fluctuate from quiet confusion to restlessness, suspicion, and agitation.

Generally, medical therapy is not critically urgent. These patients most often require management and should be constantly supervised or placed in a protected environment, as an acutely psychotic patient would be. Two additional special problems are sweat gland inhibition leading to an increase in temperature and acute bladder distention.

Specific antidotal therapy is available in the form of carbamates. Of the carbamates, only physostigmine is both peripherally and centrally active; it presumably acts to produce an excess of acetylcholine to overcome a cholinergic receptor blockade. Carbamates are relatively ineffective during the induction phase. With onset of stupor, physostigmine effectively treats the mental confusion. However, therapy must be repeated frequently, about every 40 to 60 minutes. Furthermore, specific therapy does not alter the time course of illness.[44] Specific physostigmine therapy[45] for BZ (or other anticholinergic intoxication) should be given promptly to patients with hallucinations and delirium with signs of flushing, dry mouth, mydriasis, tachycardia, and hyperthermia. Intramuscular administration of physostigmine (3 to 4 mg) is preferred because there have been reports of sudden death[46] resulting from intravenous use. Oral maintenance can be given in the form of 2 to 5 mg of physostigmine salicylate every 1 to 2 hours.

References

1. Urbanetti J: Battlefield chemical inhalation injury. In: Loke J (ed): Pathophysiology and Treatment of Inhalational Injuries. New York, Marcel Dekker, p 281, 1988.
2. Hu H, Cook-Deegan R, Shukri A: The use of chemical weapons. Conducting an investigation using survey epidemiology. JAMA 262:640, 1989.
3. Ballantyne B: Riot control agents. In: Scott RB, Fraser J (eds): Medical Annual. Bristol, Wright, p 7, 1977.
4. Himsworth H: Report of the Enquiry into the Medical and Toxicological Aspects of CS (Orthochlorobenzylidene Malonitrile). Part I. Enquiry into the Medical Situation Following the Use of CS in Londonderry on 13th and 14th of August, 1969. London, Her Majesty's Stationery Office, p 1, 1971. Command 4775.
5. Himsworth H: Report of the Enquiry into the Medical and Toxicological Aspects of CS. (Orthochlorobenzylidene Malonitrile). Part II. Enquiry into Toxicological Aspects of CS and Its Use for Civil Purposes. London, Her Majesty's Stationery Office, p 1, 1971. Command 4775.
6. Bestwick FW: Chemical agents used in riot control and warfare. Hum Toxicol 2:247, 1983.
7. Hu H, Fine J, Epstein P, et al: Tear gas—harassing agent or toxic chemical weapon? JAMA 262:660, 1989.
8. Sidell FR: Use of Physostigmine by the Intravenous, Intramuscular, and Oral Routes in the Therapy of Anticholinergic Drug Intoxication. Aberdeen Proving Ground, MD, Headquarters, Edgewood Arsenal, 1976. Biomedical Laboratory publication EB-Tr-76012.
9. Departments of the Army, Navy, and Air Force: Treatment of Chemical Agent Casualties and Conventional Military Chemical Injuries. Washington, DC, US Government Printing Office, 1990. Army FM 8-285; Navy Navmed P5041; Air Force AFM 160-11.
10. Hassler CR, Moutvic RR, Hamlin RL: Studies of the action of chemical agents on the heart. In: Proceedings of the Sixth Medical Chemical Defense Bioscience Review. Aberdeen Proving Ground, MD, US Army Medical Research Institute of Chemical Defense, 1986. Publication AD B121516.
11. Holland P, White RG: The cutaneous reactions produced by o-chlorobenzylidene malononitrile and 1-chloroacetophenone when applied directly to the skin of human subjects. Br J Dermatol 86:150, 1972.
12. Chapman AJ, White C: Death resulting from lacrimatory agents. J Forensic Sci 23:527, 1978.
13. Weigand DA: Cutaneous reaction to the riot control agent CS. Milit Med 134:437, 1969.
14. Bruner HD, Coman DR: The pathologic anatomy of phosgene poisoning in relation to the pathologic physiology. In: Fasciculus on Chemical Warfare Medicine, Volume II, Respiratory Tract. Washington, DC,

Committee on Treatment of Gas Casualties, Division of Medical Services of the National Research Council, p 234, 1945.
15. Clay JR, Rossing RG: Histopathology of exposure to phosgene. Arch Pathol 78:544, 1964.
16. Diller WF: Medical phosgene problems and their possible solution. J Occup Med 20:189, 1978.
17. Cucinell SA: Review of the toxicity of long-term phosgene exposure. Arch Environ Health 28:272, 1974.
18. Hall AH, Rumack BH: Clinical toxicology of cyanide. Ann Emerg Med 15:1067, 1986.
19. Blake J: Observations and experiments on the mode in which various poisonous agents act on the animal body. Edinburgh Med Surg J 53:35, 1840.
20. Chen KK, Rose CL, Clowes GHA: Amylnitrite and cyanide poisoning. JAMA 100:1920, 1933.
21. Way JL, Leung P, Sylvester DM, et al: Methemoglobin formation in the treatment of acute cyanide intoxication. In: Ballantyne B, Marrs TC (eds): Clinical and Experimental Toxicology of Cyanide. Bristol, Wright, p 402, 1987.
22. Anzueto A, Berdine GG, Moore GT, et al: Pathophysiology of soman intoxication in primates. Toxicol Appl Pharmacol 86:56, 1986.
23. Holmstedt B: Pharmacology of organophosphorus cholinesterase inhibitors. Pharmacol Rev 11:567, 1959.
24. Craig AB, Woodson GS: Observations on the effects of accidental exposure to nerve gas. I. Clinical observations and cholinesterase depression. Am J Med Sci 238:49, 1959.
25. DeCandole CA, Douglas WW, Lovatt-Evans C, et al: The failure of respiration and death by anticholinesterase poisoning. Br J Pharmacol Chemother 8:466, 1953.
26. Rickett DL, Glenn JF, Beers ET: Central respiratory effects versus neuromuscular actions of nerve agents. Neurotoxicology 7:225, 1986.
27. Craig FN, Cummings EG, Sim VM: Environmental temperature and the precutaneous absorption of a cholinesterase inhibitor, VX. J Invest Dermatol 68:357, 1977.
28. DeJong RH: Drug Therapy of Nerve Agent Poisoning. Edgewood, MD, US Army Medical Research and Development Command, p 1, 1985. ICD Technical Report 85-01.
29. Dunn MA, Sidell FR: Progress in medical defense against nerve agents. JAMA 262:649, 1989.
30. Keeler JR: Interactions between nerve agent pretreatment and drugs commonly used in combat anesthesia. Milit Med 155:527, 1990.
31. Rickett DL, Glenn JF, Houston WE: Medical defense against nerve agents: New directions. Milit Med 152:35, 1987.
32. Sidell FR: Soman and sarin: Clinical manifestations and treatment of accidental poisoning by organophosphates. Clin Toxicol 7:1, 1974.
33. Davies DP, Green AC, Willey GL: Hydroxyiminomethyl-N-methyl-pyridinium methane sulfonate and atropine in the treatment of severe organophosphate poisoning. Br J Pharmacol 14:5, 1958.
34. Childs AF, Davies DR, Green AL, et al: The reactivation by oximes and hydroxamic acids of cholinesterase inhibited by organophosphorus compounds. Br J Pharmacol 10:462, 1955.
35. Grob D, Johns RJ: Use of oximes in the treatment of intoxication by anticholinesterase compounds in normal subjects. Am J Med 24:497, 1958.
36. Blick DW, Murphy MR, Fanton JW, et al: Incapacitation and performance recovery after high-dose soman: Effects of diazepam. In: Proceedings of the 1989 Medical Defense Bioscience Review. Aberdeen Proving Ground, MD, US Army Medical Research Institute of Chemical Defense, 1989. Publication AD B139550.
37. Duffy FH, Gurchfiel JL, Bartels PH, et al: Long-term effects of an organophosphate upon the human electroencephalogram. Toxicol Appl Pharmacol 47:161, 1979.
38. Fox M, Scott D: The genetic toxicology of nitrogen and sulfur mustard. Mutat Res 75:131, 1980.
39. Balali-Mood M, Navaeian A: Clinical and paraclinical findings in 233 patients with sulfur mustard poisoning. In: Proceedings of the Second World Congress on New Compounds in Biological and Chemical Warfare, Ghent, Belgium, 1986, p 464.
40. Beebe GW: Lung cancer in World War I veterans: Possible relation to mustard-gas injury and 1918 influenza epidemic. US Natl Cancer Inst J 25:1231, 1960.
41. Winternitz MC: Anatomical changes in the respiratory tract initiated by irritating gases. Milit Surg 44:476, 1919.
42. Willems JL: Clinical management of mustard gas casualties. Ann Med Milit Belg 3:S1, 1989.
43. Ketchum JS, Sidell FR, Crowell EB Jr, et al: Atropine, scopolamine, and ditran: Comparative pharmacology and antagonists in man. Psychopharmacologia 28:121, 1973.
44. Rumack BH: Anticholinergic poisoning: Treatment with physostigmine. Pediatrics 52:449, 1973.
45. Daunderer M: Physostigmine salicylate as an antidote. Int J Clin Pharmacol Ther Toxicol 18:523, 1980.
46. Lipka LJ, Lathers CM: Psychoactive agents, seizure production, and sudden death in epilepsy. J Clin Pharmacol 27:169, 1987.

CHAPTER 4

Transporting Critically Ill Patients

Richard P. Millman
Sidney S. Braman

The second half of the 20th century has provided extraordinary technologic advances in medical therapeutics and treatment. High cost and limited availability have caused many of these services to be concentrated in tertiary referral centers. Situations, therefore, frequently arise in which patients must be transferred to these centers. The transfer may be made when specific diagnostic tests (such as pulmonary angiography) or treatment modalities (such as hemodialysis) are not available in the referring hospital. In addition, many critically ill patients are transported to allow treatment by more specialized physicians.

Even within hospitals, patients must be transported to highly specialized testing and treatment areas. Although transport by stretcher or wheelchair causes minimal risk and discomfort for the majority of patients, transport of critically ill patients can be potentially hazardous. This chapter reviews the common problems of both interhospital and intrahospital transport of critically ill patients and suggests guidelines for minimizing these risks.

INTERHOSPITAL TRANSPORT

An early study by Waddell and coworkers[1] demonstrated a high incidence of complications in critically ill patients transferred by ambulance from peripheral hospitals to a central intensive therapy unit. Of 46 patients, 6 became hypertensive during transport, 6 became hypotensive, 1 had a seizure, and 13 had an increase in arterial P_{CO_2}. Areas of inadequacy in care of patients before or during transfer may have contributed to these complications. These include poor communications between the transferring and receiving hospitals, inadequate cardiac and respiratory monitoring, inadequate airway protection and oxygenation, and lack of intravenous access.[2] Adequate stabilization before transfer, the use of a trained team to transfer the patient, and aggressive monitoring and treatment of patients during transport can prevent the development of dangerous complications.[1, 3–5]

Physiologic Aspects of Transport

Environmental conditions can adversely influence interhospital transport (Table 4–1). Ground transport of critically ill patients can be hindered by excessive noise and vibration. The high noise levels make auscultation with a stethoscope impossible and air leaks around an endotracheal tube undetectable. Vibration can make it difficult to perform procedures such as changing intravenous lines and can cause electrical artifacts on monitoring equipment.

Besides vibration and noise, air transportation presents a host of additional problems for the patient and the transport team. These effects have been extensively reviewed[6] and are discussed here in detail. Many of these effects are related to altitude. Typically, patients and team members are exposed to a cabin pressure equivalent to an altitude of 8000 ft when

flying in pressurized airplanes. Helicopters are unpressurized, and when it is necessary for a helicopter to exceed an altitude of 8000 ft during flight the clinical effects are further accentuated.

One problem encountered at increased altitude is a decrease in ambient oxygen concentration. Whereas the alveolar P_{O_2} is 110 mm Hg at sea level (assuming a water pressure of 47 mm Hg and a P_{CO_2} of 40 mm Hg), it is only 69 mm Hg at 8000 ft because of a fall in barometric pressure to 565 mm Hg. Thus borderline patients may experience significant compromise as the plane ascends. The team members may also be affected, with a reduced ability to perform physical work and an impaired ability to perform skilled tasks.

Disturbances can also result from differences between ambient pressure and the pressure of gases within body cavities, tissues, and fluid. At a cabin pressure equivalent to an altitude of 8000 ft there is an approximately 30% increase in the volume of air within a closed or semiclosed cavity. This increase in volume causes an increase in pressure. As the plane descends the reverse occurs; the volume of air contracts and pressure within these cavities falls.

One example of this effect is in the tympanic cavity. With descent, the gas in the tympanic cavity contracts and the air pressure within the cavity is reduced relative to ambient pressure. Yawning or swallowing normally equalizes the pressure during descent. A depressed mental state or an upper respiratory tract infection with blockage of the eustachian tubes may prevent equalization of these pressures. As a result, the tympanic membrane may retract, causing pain, and there is even a potential for membrane rupture.

Small pneumothoraces can expand as the plane ascends, and these should be treated before flight with chest tube drainage. Trapped intestinal gas, caused by an ileus or volvulus, can expand further during flight, thus compromising bowel circulation. Intestinal gas expansion can also exert marked pressure on recent surgical anastomoses and compromise ventilation by upward pressure on the diaphragm. Thus nasogastric or rectal tubes may be necessary to allow gas elimination. Patients being transported to hyperbaric chambers for treatment of an air embolism must be transported in specialized planes with cabins pressurized at sea level.

This air expansion can also affect equipment. During ascent and descent, pressure changes can induce changes in the flow rate of fluids, so intravenous lines should be controlled by volume regulation rather than rate. Glass bottles for intravenous fluids should not be used because of the danger of breakage. During ascent the cuffs on endotracheal tubes may expand enough to cause mucosal damage, and with descent there may be enough contraction to cause a cuff leak. Because of the gas expansion with ascent, it is

TABLE 4–1
ADVERSE ENVIRONMENTAL INFLUENCES DURING INTERHOSPITAL TRANSPORT
Ground transportation
Noise
Vibration
Air transportation
Noise
Vibration
Reduced ambient oxygen concentration
Dysbarisms
Hemodynamic changes with acceleration
Reduced humidity

better to fill Foley's catheter balloons with water rather than air.

There are also potential gravitational effects during take-off. These are acceleration effects from the front to the back of the plane. If the patient is in the supine position with the head toward the front of the plane, there is a transient increase in venous return during acceleration. This may adversely affect patients in congestive heart failure or with increased intracranial pressure.

Significant falls in ambient humidity in the plane can also occur because moisture and air are supplied to the cabin from the surrounding atmosphere. The content of moisture drops as the plane ascends because the surrounding air is quite cold. This theoretically may affect patients with obstructive airways disease who have difficulty mobilizing secretions.

Special Considerations in Cardiac Patients

With the advent of aggressive interventional thrombolytic therapy in the early hours of an acute myocardial infarction, more patients are being transferred to tertiary centers for therapy. This means that many have chest pain, hypotension, or arrhythmias before the transport.[7] Despite this, these patients can be successfully transported to the tertiary centers without ill effects.[7, 8] Part of the success is dependent on the skill of the team, the level of monitoring, and the capability of giving intravenous antiarrhythmics, pressors, and nitroglycerin as needed during transport. There is also evidence that intravenous thrombolytic therapy with tissue plasminogen activator or streptokinase can be given safely before transporting the patient. In fact, there was a higher incidence of more complete infarct vessel patency in patients treated with these agents before transport than in an untreated control group.[9]

It is sometimes necessary to transfer cardiac patients who have an intra-aortic balloon pump. Indications for inserting the device include an evolving myocardial infarction, postinfarction angina, unstable angina, and cardiogenic shock. LoCicero and coworkers[10] reported the transfer of 50 patients with an intra-aortic balloon pump to a tertiary center for open heart surgery; all 50 were successfully transported without significant complications. It is important to remember, however, that the balloon also expands and contracts as the plane ascends and then descends. Balloon pressure has to be closely monitored and intermittently purged, that is, equilibrated with ambient air.[11]

Special Considerations in the Transport of the Pregnant Woman

Safe transport of the pregnant woman is dependent on an understanding of the physiologic changes of pregnancy.[12] Supine hypotension caused by compression of the vena cava by a gravid uterus may impair preload sufficiently to reduce stroke volume by 30%. This is problematic in a patient with preeclampsia or other conditions with reduced intravascular volume. In fact, there have been several reports of cardiopulmonary arrest related to supine hypotension in pregnancy. Even if there is no evidence of maternal compromise, one must be aware that aortocaval compression could lead to a decrease in uterine blood flow because the uterine vasculature constricts during periods of relative hypotension. In addition, interruption of inferior vena caval blood flow has the potential to produce placental separation.

The supine position can also cause respiratory compromise because the gravid uterus displaces the diaphragm and compresses the lung parenchyma. Hypoxemia may result, and this can be extremely hazardous to the fetus because of differences in oxygen affinity between maternal and fetal hemoglobin; small changes in maternal P_{O_2} may lead to large changes in fetal P_{O_2}.

These complications can be prevented by adequate volume replacement, oxygen, and displacement of the pregnant uterus by placing a wedge or pillow under the right hip.

Monitoring Techniques

The sophistication of monitoring depends on the severity of the clinical condition. Routine monitoring includes direct observation, electrocardiography, and blood pressure monitoring. Because of the low complication rate in most patients, there should be a low threshold for insertion of arterial catheters.[3] This is essential in patients who are hypertensive because of administration of intravenous nitroprusside or who are being treated with vasopressors because of hypotension. Furthermore, noninvasive blood pressure monitoring may be difficult because of the noise. In hemodynamically unstable patients a pulmonary arterial catheter may be necessary. Useful respiratory monitoring techniques include pulse oximetry, end-tidal carbon dioxide measurements, and assessment of airway pressure.

INTRAHOSPITAL TRANSPORT

Removing the seriously ill patient from the intensive care unit for even short periods subjects the patient to many potential hazards in the unprotected environment of hospital hallways, elevators, and waiting areas. It is mandatory that a decision to transport the patient from the intensive care unit for testing or therapy be made after carefully weighing the anticipated benefits against the potential risks.

Indications for Transport

The most common indication for intrahospital transport of critically ill patients is computed tomographic (CT) scanning.[13, 14] In most instances, CT scanning is used to evaluate the chest, abdomen, or head as a possible focus of infection or source of bleeding. In general, CT scanning of the critically ill patient is more useful than conventional roentgenography for localizing lesions and defining their extent in relationship to surrounding structures. For example, CT scanning of the chest can be helpful in showing pneumothorax, loculated pleural fluid, pericardial fluid, and tracheoesophageal fistulas when these abnormalities are not apparent on the chest roentgenogram. A series of 87 CT scans of the thorax performed on 50 major trauma patients detected 15 cases of empyema, 4 cases of lung abscesses, and 2 cases of bronchiectasis that developed as a complication of adult respiratory distress syndrome.[15] Golding and colleagues[16] evaluated the impact of CT scanning on clinical outcome in critically ill patients. In 15 of 20 patients studied, the chest CT scans were judged useful because they led to a change in strategy (5 patients) or supported the working diagnosis (10 patients). The authors stressed the need to ask precisely formulated clinical questions before subjecting the patient to intrahospital transport. Other sites to which critically ill patients are often transported include the operating room, radiation therapy department, angiography suite, and diagnostic imaging department for radionuclide scanning and ultrasonography.

Complications of Transport

Although several prospective studies of intrahospital transport have shown that mortality is quite low, mishaps such as interruption of monitoring or therapy and hemodynamic and respiratory instability are quite common. Furthermore, deaths have been reported and therefore careful planning and adequate support personnel are essential. Potential complications of transport are listed in Table 4–2.

In 1970 Taylor and coworkers[17] showed that 84% of 50 high-risk cardiac patients developed a new arrhythmia during intrahospital transport. In 44% of these cases, the arrhythmias (frequent or multifocal ventricular premature contractions, ventricular tachycardia, severe bradycardia, atrial fibrillation with a rapid ventricular response, and complete heart block) were severe enough to require treatment. Several years later Waddell[18] reported on the outcome of a 5-month study of medical and surgical intensive care unit patients who were observed during routine movement within the hospital. During this period there were seven episodes of major cardiorespiratory collapse or death as a result of transport. Because baseline readings showed that most of the patients were stable, it was thought that these untoward effects were due directly to transport of the patients. Specific observations were renewed bleeding of a fractured pelvis, acute airway obstruction, movement-induced arrhythmias, and compression of the heart and great vessels by intrathoracic bleeding in patients with major chest trauma.

Moving critically ill patients to and from the operating room, particularly during the first few hours after surgery, is also fraught with hazards. The immediate postoperative period is often marked by cardiovascular changes. For example, significant increases in systolic blood pressure and heart rate have been reported after general and vascular surgery. This can be related to acute emergence from inhalation anesthesia or rewarming after induced hypothermia. Sudden increases in blood pressure during transport may be quite severe and require emergency treatment with intravenous nitroprusside. Hypotension during postoperative transport is another potential complication. However, with appropriate hemodynamic monitoring, transport of the postoperative patient within the hospital is safe and is associated with extremely low mortality and morbidity.[18, 19]

The critically ill patient who requires continuous mechanical ventilatory support is at a particularly high risk for

TABLE 4–2
COMPLICATIONS OF INTRAHOSPITAL TRANSPORT
Interruption of monitoring or therapy
Power failure or disconnection of monitors
Infiltration of venous line
Disconnection of arterial and venous lines
Interruption of medication schedule
Uncontrolled fluid management
Hemodynamic complications
Arrhythmias
Hypertension
Hypotension
Myocardial ischemia
Heart failure
Respiratory complications
Hypoxemia
Hypoventilation or hyperventilation
Occult positive end-expiratory pressure
Barotrauma
Extubation
Intubation of right main bronchus
Mucus plugging
Aspiration

complications during transport. Because inadequate ventilation may result in severe hypoxemia or sudden change in the patient's acid-base status, life-threatening complications may arise. Our experience in a prospective study of ventilator-dependent patients requiring procedures outside the intensive care unit showed that clinically significant respiratory and hemodynamic changes occurred in the majority of patients when mechanical ventilatory support was replaced by manual ventilation.[13] These changes occurred despite the presence of a registered nurse, a physician, and a registered respiratory therapist who ventilated the patient with a resuscitation bag. Four of these patients developed hypoventilation with a mean change in Pco_2 of 15 mm Hg. Ten other patients showed hyperventilation with resulting alkalosis. The drop in Pco_2 ranged up to 22 mm Hg with an

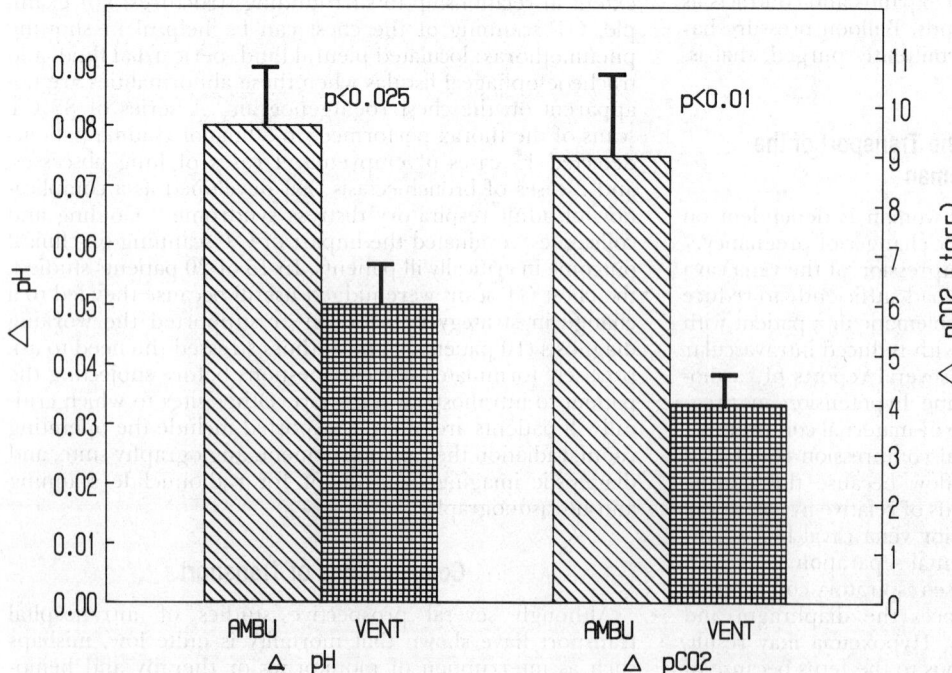

Figure 4–1. Comparison of mean changes in pH and Pco_2 in critically ill patients receiving ventilatory support through a manual resuscitation bag (ambu) or portable ventiltor (vent) during intrahospital transport. (Reproduced, with permission, from Braman SS, Dunn SM, Amico CA, et al, Complications of intrahospital transport in critically ill patients. Ann Intern Med 1987;107:469–473.)

TABLE 4–3

SIGNS OF CLINICAL DETERIORATION

System	Signs
General	Agitation, diaphoresis
Cardiac	Tachycardia, bradycardia, arrhythmia, hypotension
Central nervous system	Somnolence, coma, twitching, seizures
Respiratory	Cyanosis, tachypnea, apnea, suprasternal and intercostal retraction, use of accessory muscles, detection of paradoxical motion of ribs and abdomen

increase in pH as high as 0.18. Five patients became hypotensive, with the drop in systolic blood pressure ranging from 40 to 60 mm Hg, and two patients developed new cardiac arrhythmias of bradycardia and ventricular irritability.

A second group of critically ill patients were transported using a portable ventilator rather than manual ventilation. Although a few complications still occurred, including mechanical failure of the ventilator, the mean changes in pH and Pco_2 were significantly less than in the manually ventilated group (Fig. 4–1). No patient died in either group as a result of the transport, but the severe systemic hypotension and cardiac arrhythmias were potentially life threatening. These complications were directly related to the alterations in acid-base status.

This study underscores the potential hazards of intrahospital transport even in the presence of a skilled health care team. Adequate oxygenation can be easily and uniformly achieved. However, hyperventilation and hypoventilation are more difficult to prevent. Ideally, the arterial blood gas derangements can be minimized by using a portable ventilator. Although we and other centers[20] prefer this modality, other intensivists have had reasonable success transporting patients with manual ventilation aided by a tidal volume meter at the exhalation valve.[21]

Monitoring Techniques

As with interhospital monitoring, the sophistication of monitoring depends on the severity of the clinical condition. Close observation of the patient for signs of clinical deterioration (Table 4–3) is an essential first step. Because respiratory and hemodynamic complications are quite frequent in these patients, special attention should be given to monitoring the heart and lung. These include frequent blood pressure measurements and a continuous electrocardiographic tracing. Because portable ventilators have been shown to provide stable arterial blood gas values during transport,[13, 20] respiratory monitoring may be optional. Pulse oximetry or measurements of end-tidal Pco_2 to ensure the adequacy of oxygenation and ventilation during transport may be useful in conjunction with manual ventilation.

References

1. Waddell G, Scott PDR, Lees NW, et al: Effects of ambulance transport in critically ill patients. Br Med J 1:386, 1975.
2. Olson CM, Jastremski MS, Vilogi JP, et al: Stabilization of patients prior to interhospital transfer. Am J Emerg Med 5:33, 1986.
3. Bion JF, Edlin SA, Ramsay G, et al: Validation of a prognostic score in critically ill patients undergoing transport. Br Med J [Clin Res] 291:432, 1985.
4. Ehrenwerth J, Sorbo S, Hackel A: Transport of critically ill adults. Crit Care Med 14:543, 1986.
5. Pearl RG, Mihm FG, Rosenthal MH: Care of the adult patient during transport. Int Anesthesiol Clin 25:43, 1987.
6. Lachenmyer J: Physiological aspects of transport. Int Anesthesiol Clin 25:15, 1987.
7. Gore JM, Corrao JM, Goldberg RJ, et al: Feasibility and safety of emergency interhospital transport of patients during early hours of acute myocardial infarction. Arch Intern Med 149:353, 1989.
8. Kaplan L, Walsh D, Burney RE: Emergency aeromedical transport of patients with acute myocardial infarction. Ann Emerg Med 16:55, 1987.
9. Topol EJ, Fung AY, Kline E, et al: Safety of helicopter transport and out-of-hospital intravenous fibrinolytic therapy in patients with evolving myocardial infarction. Cathet Cardiovasc Diagn 12:151, 1986.
10. LoCicero J III, Hartz RS, Sanders JH Jr, et al: Interhospital transport of patients with ongoing intraaortic balloon pumping. Am J Cardiol 56:59, 1985.
11. Mertlich G, Quaal SJ: Air transport of the patient requiring intra-aortic balloon pumping. Crit Care Nurs Clin N Am 1:443, 1989.
12. Katz VL, Hansen AR: Complications in the emergency transport of pregnant women. South Med J 83:7, 1990.
13. Braman SS, Dunn SM, Amico CA, et al: Complications of intrahospital transport in critically ill patients. Ann Intern Med 107:469, 1987.
14. Smith I, Fleming S, Cernaianu A: Mishaps during transport from the intensive care unit. Crit Care Med 18:278, 1990.
15. Mirvis SE, Tobin KD, Kostrubiak I, et al: Thoracic CT in detecting occult disease in critically ill patients. AJR 148:685, 1987.
16. Golding RP, Knape P, Strack RJM, et al: Computed tomography as an adjunct to chest x-rays of intensive care unit patients. Crit Care Med 16:211, 1988.
17. Taylor JO, Landers CF, Chulay JD, et al: Monitoring high-risk cardiac patients during transportation in hospital. Lancet 2:1205, 1970.
18. Waddell G: Movement of critically ill patients within hospital. Br Med J 2:417, 1975.
19. Insel J, Weissman C, Kemper M, et al: Cardiovascular changes during transport of critically ill and postoperative patients. Crit Care Med 14:539, 1986.
20. Hurst JM, Davis K Jr, Branson RD, et al: Comparison of blood gases during transport using two methods of ventilatory support. J Trauma 29:1637, 1989.
21. Gervais HW, Eberle B, Konietzke D, et al: Comparison of blood gases of ventilated patients during transport. Crit Care Med 15:761, 1987.

CHAPTER 5

Organization of Critical Care Units

I. Alan Fein
Martin A. Strosberg
Sandra L. Fein

The philosopher Alfred North Whitehead wrote that organized education should ideally progress through three stages: romance, in which the student develops a fascination and interest in the subject of study; discipline, in which the student acquires the skills and methods to study and analyze the subject properly; and finally fruition, whereby the concepts and methods are used to understand the subject fully and perhaps improve it by their application.[1] Critical care medicine and its practitioners seem to be moving through similar stages. As the Introduction details, critical care units (CCUs) have evolved from the rudimentary recovery rooms of Florence Nightingale's day to the sophisticated monitoring and interventionist units of today. In examining this evolutionary process, one might argue that these units have grown simply in response to logistic, financial, and personnel demands, or simply for the convenience of busy nurses or physicians. Although this unstructured development may have been acceptable in Whitehead's romance phase, it is increasingly apparent that critical care medicine has now entered the era of discipline and that the demands of economics are already insisting on fruition. As the costs of critical care exceed 1% of the U.S. gross national product, as the population ages and becomes increasingly knowledgeable, and as resources decline and demand increases, the pressure for cost-effective health care delivery is paramount. The time has come for the management of CCUs to be assessed, evaluated, and demystified.

The progressive decline in available resources for the care of the critically ill in the face of an increasing demand for these services is a compelling reason for implementing a rational hospital-wide approach to the management of all CCUs. Specific goals should include the following:

1. An efficient intersection of scheduling, admissions, and discharge systems should be worked out by the emergency department, postanesthesia care units, operating rooms, critical care and step-down units, and the general hospital floors to facilitate interhospital and intrahospital transfer of patients.

2. Formal written procedures should be established to guide resource allocation decisions, and the elucidation of the decision-making process, to minimize, if not eliminate, the inevitable conflicts over "last bed" admissions and discharges.

3. The manager or managers responsible for the CCU must find ways to build teams and to change the attitude and behavior of independent physicians who still regard the hospital as the physician's domain, so that they can accommodate to the new collaborative practice–oriented CCU staff.[2]

Social scientists have studied organizational structures, processes, and functions for some time. The corporate community has certainly recognized the relationships between organizational structure and outcome (e.g., profits). The medical community has also begun to recognize the importance of understanding organization and management, partly in response to changing economic realities and partly as a result of a heightened demand for quality assurance.[3] CCUs are, in fact, structured organizations; there is increasing evidence that the nature of these structures may directly affect patient outcome and cost. Knaus and colleagues, in a study of 13 CCUs, suggested that there was a positive relationship between the degree of organizational coordination in those units and the severity of illness-adjusted outcomes of patients.[4]

There is also a rapidly growing body of medical literature exploring the application of industrial management and quality assurance technology to the medical arena.[5–7] Industrial quality improvement systems developed during the past 60 years by Deming,[8] Shewhart,[9] Juran,[10] and others have had a profound influence on organizational structures, process, and outcomes. If and how these techniques can be applied to the critical care environment remains to be determined but will certainly be the subject of extensive investigation as the pressure for cost-effectiveness and quality improvement intensifies.

A seminal editorial by Teres briefly discussed the growing need for physicians to become more knowledgeable and actively involved in the administration of CCUs, an area heretofore left almost entirely to nurses.[11] The nursing profession has in the past assumed, one might argue by default, the burden of organization, management, and administration of CCUs. Despite the lack of medical input, or

perhaps because of it, there is a remarkably sound nursing organizational structure to be found in most units, even given their wide diversity. Consider one set of criteria for assessing organizational structures developed by the Aston Group on Industrial Administration Research (University of Aston-in-Birmingham, United Kingdom):

- Specialization of functions and roles
- Standardization of procedures
- Formalization of documentation
- Centralization of authority
- Configuration of role structure[12]

In spite of the great diversity of special care units, most nursing organizational structures are generally stable and similar when judged by these criteria. Professional nursing organizations such as the American Association of Critical Care Nurses and accrediting agencies such as the Joint Commission on Accreditation of Healthcare Organizations (JCAHO) have been active in promoting and examining administrative and managerial concerns.

During the nursing shortage of the 1970s and 1980s, there was an increased interest in improving the work environment as an aid to staff retention. For example, there have been numerous studies assessing burnout in health care professionals, its causes, and strategies for prevention and management.[13–15] It is generally accepted that organizational structure can influence employee satisfaction and consequently turnover and retention. However, one might argue that there has been little improvement in the overall work environment of CCUs for a number of reasons. First, most of the strategies for the management of burnout and stress have been directed at individual rather than organizational changes. Second, organizational inertia is notorious. According to the organizational theorist Richard Hall, "there are limits to the variation possible in organizational characteristics—given the constraints of size, the technology employed, the market conditions, and other environmental factors. Organizations cannot change simply to be more pleasant places in which to work."[16] Finally, physicians, an obviously key component of both the health care process and the CCU work environment, have only recently become actively involved in the management and administration of CCUs and have been viewed by some as a threat to the established order. One might suggest that the environment will not improve until physicians are successfully integrated into the organizational structure.

The 1983 National Institutes of Health Consensus Conference on Critical Care Medicine concluded that "the organizational structure [of CCUs] should promote and require that nurses and physicians work together as colleagues at all levels—especially the medical director and the nursing director."[17] Indeed, the concept of nurse-physician collaboration in critical care has been strongly supported by the Society of Critical Care Medicine and the American Association of Critical Care Nurses,[18] the Joint Commission on Accreditation of Hospitals,[19] and the National Commission on Nursing.[20] The literature is replete with studies examining the nurse-physician relationship,[21,22] and there is general agreement that collaborative practice is both desirable and necessary for optimal functioning of the unit.

In fact, nursing has achieved a high degree of collaborative practice at the grassroots level: coordination, communication, and cooperation is extensive among nurses, ancillary service personnel, and physicians at the bedside. Yet for all of the discussion, there is little evidence of widespread collaborative practice on an either formal or informal basis at the managerial level; much of the problem-solving process involving nurses and physicians has been described as competitive.[21, 23, 24]As physicians become as involved in unit management as they have been in patient management, the need to formally integrate them into the organizational structure will only grow; integration, in turn, will be accomplished only if collaboration replaces competition between the professions.

TEAM MANAGEMENT

Teres and colleagues have long advocated a team or triad approach to the management and organization of CCUs.[25] This approach requires the collaboration of dedicated physicians, nurses, and administrators, each with specified roles and responsibilities. As mentioned earlier, the role of nurses, whether director, head nurse, supervisor, coordinator, or staff nurse, has traditionally been well defined. The role of hospital administration in the CCU has been less well defined, and the role of the physician in unit management has also been unclear.

The nurse, the administrator, and the physician director should work together as equal members of a team, each with their respective roles, skills, and responsibilities. Nurses have traditionally been the permanent staff of the unit, unlike physicians and administrators who were part-time, or transient, members of the staff. As such, nurses have had a clear interest in the management of the CCU. The key to the active, interested participation of administrative personnel and physicians is in creating roles that provide them with a vested interest in the functioning of the unit.

Nursing Director

The role of the nurse director has been well established over time. This position has assumed administrative responsibility not only for the education and management of the nursing staff but also for virtually all activities in the CCU. With that responsibility has come authority. Although in many cases the responsibility and consequently the authority may have been reluctantly assumed, nurses have proved eminently capable and now guard their advances in the administrative heirarchy carefully.

True collaborative practice suggests that responsibility, accountability, and authority must be shared by both physician and nurse managers; sharing the latter is difficult for all involved. Joint management can be achieved only when the involved parties are all committed to this concept and have developed a high level of communication and trust. This requires frequent meetings of the managerial team on a regular basis, open and honest communications, and concerted efforts at team building.[26]

Administrative Liaison

A designated hospital administrator who also functions as part of the unit management team would benefit by assuring her or his supervisor (e.g., the hospital's chief executive officer) that the most expensive segment of the hospital was indeed operated at peak efficiency. This person would be involved in fiscal affairs, budget preparation, purchasing, financial planning, and personnel management, such as staffing patterns and strategies for recruitment and retention of staff. Rather than functioning in an adversarial or watchdog manner, an actively participating administrator can be useful as an informed, educated ally, functioning as a resource person and liaison with the chief executive officer and other administrative personnel. This individual would facilitate the interaction of the unit not only with the hospital administration but also with the external environment, including federal, state, and other regulatory agencies such as JCAHO. Finally, an administrator committed to working with the critical care team can be invaluable in creating and maintaining a positive image of the unit.

When there is a gap between administrators and the caregivers, the CCU can easily be viewed as a drain on hospital personnel and finances. The unit should be seen as a valuable resource that facilitates the activities of the rest of the institution. The administrator and the unit medical director should understand the mission and direction of the hospital and ensure that the role of the CCU is appropriate and well understood. Properly managed units can be viewed as revenue centers in that they make possible the admission of remunerative, high-risk patients (e.g., for elective vascular surgery). Maintaining the "through-put" of short-term patients may well balance the long-term occupants of the CCU financially, while providing the community with an irreplaceable service.

Medical Director

The role of the medical director is the most difficult to define, yet it is central to the organization of the CCU. In sharp contrast to the generally well-defined roles of critical care nursing directors, the medical directors of many CCUs find that they may be writing their own job descriptions. Hospital administrations may instinctively know that they need a medical director for their units but may not know exactly what to do with one or what to expect of one. Given the variety of hospitals with CCUs, from urban to rural, large to small, and teaching and nonteaching, and the variety of political situations, each institution must carefully define the role of the director given its own particular needs. Surprisingly, although institutional needs and situations are diverse, the functions of a medical director are often remarkably uniform. A singular purpose of this chapter is to provide a generic framework for exploring the essential roles most medical directors must fulfill, regardless of their particular environment.

A key function of a medical director is to foster the development of a collaborative practice, within the particular constraints of the institution. As alluded to earlier, although collaborative practice is an eminently desirable goal, it is often equally elusive to achieve. This is not surprising in a complex organization with multiple constituencies of greatly differing backgrounds and expectations. Medical directors would be well served by familiarizing themselves not only with the nursing literature on collaborative practice (see earlier) but also with the industrial management literature on team building.[27, 28] Indeed, even some of the popular management literature, such as Peters' Thriving on Chaos[29] may be appropriate reading for the new or veteran manager of a CCU.

Regardless of the type of hospital in which a CCU resides, some common management tools, devices, and tenets should be implemented by a medical director:

Review and update the formal unit policies, especially as pertaining to the role, expectations, responsibilities, authority, jurisdiction, and reporting relationships of both the nursing and medical directors.

Review, update, and clarify the role and responsibilities of the critical care services committee.

Establish regular meetings with the management of the unit, both physicians and nurses. Weekly sessions are generally appropriate.

Establish regular meetings with the nursing staff. This should be an open-ended opportunity for the staff to express their concerns and be heard by the unit management, again both physicians and nurses; the managers should create a listening environment of trust in which the staff can freely discuss problems without fear of reprisal and with assurances that the sessions will result in both action and feedback.

Establish regular multidisciplinary educational sessions.

Establish multidisciplinary (e.g., physician and nurse) committees to address issues of common interest, including quality assurance, risk management, and morbidity and mortality evaluation; these foster a sense of togetherness and trust and also address JCAHO requirements.

ORGANIZATIONAL MODELS OF CRITICAL CARE UNITS

Medical directors may be full-time or part-time staff, salaried or contractual employees, and members of a faculty practice plan or volunteer physicians. Full-time salaried medical directors were rare in the past; however, given the demands of the position and regulatory agencies such as JCAHO, this is becoming commonplace for large and moderate-sized institutions. Many hospitals are finding that it is cost- and quality-effective for both the institution and the medical community to hire or contract with a group of intensivists to manage the CCUs in a manner comparable to the management of many emergency departments.

Similarly, CCUs may be open, semiopen, or closed units (Table 5–1). Open units are those in which admission of patients is relatively uncontrolled and management of patients is at the discretion of each private attending physician. The medical director may or may not be consulted on all patients, and his or her primary functions may be largely administrative, including overseeing general care, quality assurance, risk management, education of staff, involvement in ethical and legal affairs, purchasing of equipment, and policy making and/or policy enforcing, to name but a few. The advantage of this structure is that it invites, in fact necessitates, the active participation of the medical community at large in all aspects of care. An adept physician director can begin to implement a collaborative practice by instituting protocols involving nursing in the decision-making process. The disadvantage is that, given the vagaries of human nature, some physicians invariably are less than cooperative. The director of an open unit may have difficulty controlling the flow of patients; ensuring the availability of beds for elective and emergent cases may be difficult if there are no mechanisms to prevent inappropriate admissions or ensure timely discharge of recovering patients. Furthermore, although the director may be responsible for quality assurance, this may prove problematic if there is no direct involvement in patient care.

Semiopen units are those in which the director and/or designees screen all admissions to the unit and may or may not take a more active role in direct patient care. Given the decline in the number of beds and the increasing demand for them, this role of gatekeeper is becoming more necessary and commonplace. This requires a 24-hour presence and, consequently, the services of more than one individual. The gatekeeping role is examined in detail later. Some hospitals have found that contracting with a group of intensivists to serve this function works well on several levels. If the intensivists are indeed independent, decision making regarding admissions can theoretically be made on the basis of medical need rather than political expediency. Although this may upset some traditional power structures, it best serves both the institution and the patients. Although many medical communities may initially resent the intrusion of a group of new specialists, many private practitioners soon come to appreciate their efforts.

Critical care is perhaps the most labor intensive of all specialties, requiring long hours at the bedside and frequent and repeated visits for proper care. This is problematic for even highly dedicated private practitioners, most of whom spend long hours in their offices, clinics, or operating rooms: caring for the critically ill is simply not cost-effective or an efficient use of time when patients are spread over several hospitals, clinics, or offices. The intensivist who, by his or her actions, proves not to be a threat to the private physician is often greatly appreciated for the assistance he or she

	TABLE 5–1		
	ORGANIZATIONAL MODELS OF CRITICAL CARE UNITS		
Parameter	**Open Unit**	**Semiopen Unit**	**Closed Unit**
Admissions	Can be approved by any qualified physician	Must be approved by medical director (or designee)	Must be approved by medical director (or designee)
Patient care	Any qualified physician	Any qualified medical director	By intensivists (on medical director's service)
Conflict resolution	By medical director	By medical director	By medical director
Advantages	Invites active participation of medical staff Medical director may be a full-time or dedicated volunteer physician	Improved control of patient flow and bed availability Improved accountability for quality assurance, risk management, and cost containment Staff participation a plus Facilitates collaborative practice	Absolute control and accountability for beds and patient flow, quality assurance, risk management, and cost containment Easiest situation to create collaborative practice
Disadvantages	Patient through-put and bed availability may be difficult to maintain Accountability for quality assurance, risk management, and cost containment may be difficult May be difficult to implement collaborative practice	Requires 24 h/d availability of medical director (or designee)	Requires 24 h/d availability of medical director (or designee) May alienate medical staff if not properly managed

renders in the unit. This requires not only medical skills but also political and communicative interpersonal skills of a reasonably high order to be successful.

The closed unit is one in which patients are transferred to the service of the intensivist for direct patient care at the time of admission to the unit. This requires the services of several full-time intensivists who may be employees of the hospital, members of a faculty plan, or a part of a group that contracts their services to the hospital. Administratively, this is the simplest structure: both accountability and responsibility for quality patient care, as well as risk management, cost containment, and appropriate resource utilization, rest with the same individuals. Open structures may develop a schism between accountability and responsibility in that those charged with ensuring cost-effective quality care are not the ones providing direct patient care. The effectiveness of a director certainly depends on a multiplicity of diverse factors, including interpersonal skills, rapport with the administration and the medical community, and support of department heads, to name but a few. Drawbacks to closed units stem largely from the possibility of alienating the private practice community. Not only can this generate ill will in the medical community at large if not managed properly, but also patients and staff can be deprived of the valuable input of many knowledgeable physicians, both primary practitioners and specialists. Referrals and admissions may also decline if the closed unit is perceived as elitist. An astute medical director needs to devote a significant amount of effort to education and public relations with all segments of the service and client populations.

MANAGERIAL ROLES FOR CRITICAL CARE UNIT MEDICAL DIRECTORS

Consider the position of the CCU medical director in relation to the nursing chain of command. The positions in the nursing hierarchy have been formalized with written position descriptions, task objectives, performance measures, and performance assessment criteria. Managerial responsibilities such as objective setting, budgeting, staffing, and performance monitoring are usually well delineated. There is hierarchic accountability starting with the bedside nurse and rising through the head nurse to the nursing director. In contrast, the position description of the medical director and his or her place in the organizational chart is often unclear. Nurses frequently distinguish between working medical directors and "paper" medical directors. Paper directors may report to or chair JCAHO-mandated committees and be officially accountable to the organized medical staff but take little part in the day-to-day running of the unit. Working directors take an active part in CCU operations, including quality assurance, education, policy development and enforcement, and triage.[30]

The distinction between working and paper directors does not necessarily parallel part-time and full-time status. A survey of nursing supervisors and their perception of the nighttime availability of medical directors or their designates to make triage decisions and resolve conflict showed a surprising number of units with full-time directors without availability as perceived by the nurses.[31] On the other hand, from the perspective of the nurses, a medical director of a small, low-intensity case-mix unit who maintains good rapport with the nurses may need to work only several hours a week to be effective.

How should the role of the medical director be characterized? How should the range of activities and responsibilities that should make up the medical director's position be described? In contrast to critical care nurse management, there is scant information on working medical directors.

There is no comprehensive information on training of critical care specialists, establishment of credentials, patterns of reimbursement, and types of patients treated, nor is information available regarding the types and numbers of special care units.

In the absence of hard data, is there any way to describe the decision-making roles of the working CCU medical director? Fortunately, management and organizational theories, both descriptive and prescriptive, provide frameworks and concepts for understanding the conditions, constraints, and challenges faced.

Management of Critical Care Units

The danger lies in the tendency to teach the principles of administration as though they were scientific laws, when they are really little more than administrative expedients found to work well in certain circumstances but never tested in any systematic way.[32]
Joan Woodward

All organizations face the dual challenge of dividing work up into tasks and then coordinating the tasks to accomplish the overall objectives of the organization (i.e., differentiation and integration).[33] The concept of illness trajectory, introduced by sociologist Anselm Strauss and colleagues, is particularly useful in illustrating the coordination challenges posed by critically ill patients. The illness trajectory encompasses "not only the physiological unfolding of a patient's disease but the total organization of work done over that course plus the impact on those involved with the work and its organization" (see ref 34, p 8). According to Strauss (see ref 34, pp 26–27),

> . . . under conditions of contemporary hospital practice, it is not always a simple matter to say who is in charge of managing the trajectory. In routine cases, the principal physician is primarily responsible for visualizing the trajectory: for ordering, evaluating, and acting on diagnostic tests: for utilizing the ward's organizational machinery. When the course of illness becomes problematic, however, when things get out of hand, when other physiological systems go awry, when other chronic illnesses impinge on the primary one—and even begin to take priority—then the trajectory management begins to get shared with other medical specialists. And . . . these specialists may disagree or their orders may conflict, so that problems of coordination can play havoc with house staff and, not incidentally, also with patient care. Lack of coordination amounts to a blurring of the division of labor, with untoward consequences then flowing from unclear or disagreed upon conceptions of responsibility. On the other hand, the specialists may work well together, sharing in the shaping of the trajectory. It is important to understand that with complex trajectories, this shaping, which involves a complicated division of labor, may be parcelled out, not only among several specialists, including a psychiatrist, but also involve the efforts of kin. Patients themselves may enter this process at key option points, entering as intensely interested parties or being invited in by the physicians, who may even press them to make certain decisions when the options are very risky, or their potential psychological or physiological impact is great.

From this description it should be abundantly clear that it is more appropriate to talk about managing the illness trajectory than managing the illness. Critical care specialists, to the extent that they are uniquely qualified to understand the complex interactions of multiple organ system failure, claim that they are in the best position to manage the erratic trajectories common to the critically ill. But unlike emergency medical specialists, they seldom have full control of the patients in the unit.

Three managerial roles are suggested for CCU medical directors (Table 5–2). The first role involves coordinating the care of the patient (i.e., illness trajectory management).

TABLE 5–2
MANAGERIAL FUNCTIONS OF CRITICAL CARE UNIT MEDICAL DIRECTORS

Role	Focus
1. Manager of illness trajectory	Individual patient
2. Allocator of scarce resources/gatekeeper to beds	Unit and patient
3. Strategy maker	Hospital, unit, and patient

The focus of illness trajectory management is the individual patient and the quality of care he or she receives. The second role involves the allocation of resources and, in particular, gatekeeping. These functions necessitate a broader perspective and a longer time frame than is typically applied to the individual patient. The focus is the entire unit. The third role calls for the CCU director to participate in strategy making: determining the basic tasks of the CCU vis-à-vis the rest of the hospital, the types of services delivered, the design of the appropriate structure for carrying out those tasks. All three roles, but in particular the third, require collaboration with a variety of professionals and administrators.

Management of Illness Trajectories

Because of JCAHO requirements, most medical directors are involved, at least minimally, in monitoring the quality of care (e.g., retrospective review of mortalities and readmissions) and establishment of credentials (who is qualified to do what procedures). A well-known cybernetic model of management responsibility conceptualizes the manager as monitor[35] (Fig. 5–1). The CCU medical director measures the outcomes (e.g., deaths, readmissions, and complications) and compares them with expectations (what is versus what should be). Expectations or performance standards can be formally generated and codified by internal committees of the hospital or by external accrediting bodies and professional societies. They can also come from implicit standards that have been developed during medical training and socialization. When performance does not meet expectations, the medical director may take corrective action in the form of education or sanctions.

Alternatively, it is necessary to periodically review and reassess existing expectations and performance standards to

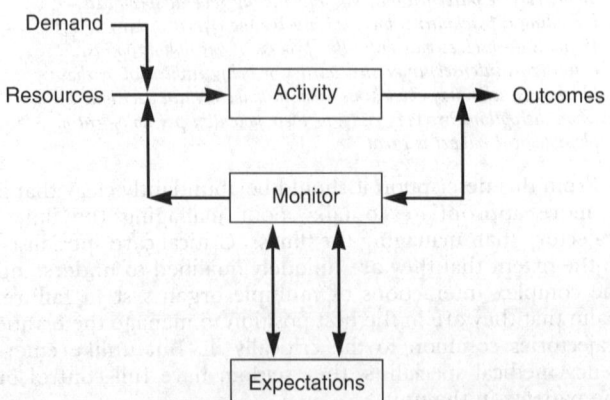

Figure 5–1. Cybernetic model for hospitals. (From Griffith JR: The Well-Managed Community Hospital. Ann Arbor, Health Administration Press, p 63, 1987.)

ensure appropriateness. Some directors may choose to become the primary manager of the illness trajectory, not only for their own patients but also for selected other or all patients entering the unit. Although these situations are often politically difficult, these actions may occasionally be necessary for patient safety. In the absence of a structured closed unit, when and how a director assumes direct patient care is both situation and personality dependent.

Resource Allocation and Gatekeeping

There are many parallels between managing the patient needing critical care (i.e., managing the trajectory of the critically ill patient) and managing the CCU. Trajectory management can be used as a metaphor for CCU management. Just as the physiologic functions of critically ill patients may fluctuate dramatically and unpredictably and an array of drugs, hardware, and personnel must be deployed to balance the patient's unstable condition, so too the workload, case mix, and available staff may fluctuate greatly and unpredictably. It is management's objective to develop strategies to cope with and reduce the impact of uncertainties and fluctuations as much as possible.[36] The goal is to create and maintain a degree of order in a dynamic environment where uncertainty is the norm.

Strategies that may help CCU managers cope with the uncertainties confronting them daily might include the following:

Surround CCU with intermediate care units and step-down units to help smooth the flow of patients into and out of the unit.

Maintain redundant capacity in the recovery room, the emergency room, and other units to temporarily absorb unmet demand.

Schedule elective surgery for times of off-peak demand.

Use downtime or troughs in demand for training periods.

Disguise troughs in demand to protect against budget and staff cutbacks (i.e., keep personnel busy all of the time to ensure that there will be enough resources for times of peak demand).

Dilute case mix with patients with less severe illnesses to fill beds, preserve slack time, and temporarily slow admissions.

Show leniency in supervision of rules during downtime as a way of creating obligations for subordinates to respond energetically to an emergency.

These strategies are based on propositions set forth in organization theory literature and codified by Thompson.[36] In their general applications, they are certainly not unique to hospital settings. Their effective application is situation dependent and requires the skills of a politically aware and adept management team. Ultimately, however, as with any organization, when demand overwhelms capacity, the CCU must ration services, by diluting the level of care provided, by prematurely discharging patients, or by restricting access. In the words of the late organizational theorist JD Thompson (see ref 36, p 23),

Rationing is an unhappy solution, for its use signifies that the technology is not operating at its maximum. Yet some system of priorities for the allocation of capacity under adverse conditions is essential if a technology is to be instrumentally effective—if action is to be other than random.

Increasingly, CCUs are faced with difficult admission and discharge decisions, especially in light of the nursing shortage. Both the JCAHO and the Society for Critical Care Medicine define a gatekeeping role for the medical director:

It is the responsibility of the ICU [CCU] director (or designee) to

decide if the patient meets eligibility requirements for ICU. In case of conflict regarding admission or discharge criteria, the ICU director (designee) will decide which patient should be given priority. A procedure to implement this policy should be specified for each ICU. A mechanism should also exist to review retrospectively cases wherein the attending physician disagrees with the decision of the ICU director (designee). Whenever possible, objective measures of illness and prognosis should be considered when reaching decisions to continue, limit, or terminate ICU support.[37]

It should be pointed out that gatekeeping is greatly simplified in those CCUs that are dedicated solely to serve the needs of physicians of a particular service, e.g., cardiothoracic surgery. Single-specialty units reduce the diversity of patients, promote scheduling and the certainty of bed availability, and eliminate the climate of competition endemic in a multiple-specialty unit. However, for a variety of reasons, both political and economic, multiple-specialty units are the norm in most hospitals.

When there are available beds in the CCU, gatekeeping remains in the background as an important managerial function. It is only when demand exceeds supply that gatekeeping becomes problematic. When beds are filled, a specific protocol must be in place and activated to deal with admissions and discharges effectively. This can be accomplished only when an appropriate individual (preferably the unit's medical director or designee) has been vested with both the responsibility and the authority to take the necessary action. This individual must also be fully accountable for those decisions. There are probably as many approaches to gatekeeping as there are CCUs.

Decisions to admit and discharge patients are complex: when all beds are filled, the only way to admit a patient is to discharge a patient. The competing claims of patients already in the unit must be weighed against those waiting to be admitted. Not only are patient-centered physiologic variables considered but also organizational variables such as staffing levels, capacity of the next best alternative unit, and the demand from the operating room, emergency department, and other hospitals. A full-time intensivist describes a typical mode of decision making when the beds are completely filled:

> You come down to the floor to look at the patient. You look at the number of tubes and what is being secreted. You see how many nurses you've got on the floor. You know whether Betsy's pregnant and whether Tony is not coming in that night and you decide whether you can handle the patient.

Admission and discharge decisions are collaborative, made jointly by the physician and the nurse, each supplying a vital piece of information (e.g., medical and nursing diagnoses, resource requirements, and staffing availability on the floors and in the CCU). Although all CCUs have written admission and discharge policies, they are of little use at the bedside. Subjective global assessments are far more relevant.

There are other factors to consider, including the patient's and the family's understanding of the prognosis and their options, legal ramifications, ethical considerations, and family psychodynamics. Dealing with patients and their families is time consuming and demands extraordinary patience and sensitivity yet is worth the effort. Developing and maintaining a solid rapport with families are essential, especially if patients are unconscious or otherwise unable to make their own decisions. Hospital-wide, or preferably state-wide, policies regarding patient health care proxies, living wills, and do-not-resuscitate decision making are essential in minimizing conflict. New York State has passed legislative guidelines on these issues; although the full impact of these regulations has yet to be fully assessed, they have raised the level of discussion and awareness in both lay and medical communities.[38]

Keeping the key constituents of the CCU satisfied is a Sisyphean task. It is virtually inevitable that there will be parties with valid yet conflicting and/or competitive interests placing constant demands on the CCU. For example, a tertiary care hospital that serves as a regional trauma center would place a high priority on receiving emergent trauma patients. These patients can easily overwhelm the resources of most CCUs, limiting the bed availability for high-risk elective surgical patients. This can result in an unbalanced surgical CCU population, possibly compromising the education of house staff and also having a serious impact on finances as treatment of trauma is significantly underreimbursed.

Complicating the situation may be whatever regulatory or contractual agreements the hospital may have entered into with federal, state, or local regulatory agencies for special status or funding. The unit director must be well informed as to the hospital's overall mission, direction, and standing within the external medical, social, and economic environment if he or she is to adequately represent and protect both patients and the CCU. The immediate demands on the CCU medical director would be

Maintaining bed availability for emergency cases commensurate with the institution's accepted commitment to the community

Maintaining the operating room schedule

Keeping the stress levels of CCU nurses at a tolerable level

Preventing a backlog in the emergency department

Just as the role of the medical director in the management of illness trajectories can be described as ranging from minor to major, one can also characterize the role of the medical director in gatekeeping. Here the concepts of centralization and decentralization are germane. Centralization and decentralization should not be considered in terms of absolutes but as degrees as indicated by the following description of steps in the decision-making process:

1. Information—what can be done
2. Advice—what should be done
3. Choice—what is intended to be done
4. Authorization—what is authorized to be done
5. Execution—what is in fact done[39]

Decision making is most centralized when one decision maker unilaterally controls all the steps. For example, she or he collects information on the potential admission; analyzes that information in connection with information about the patients currently in the unit and other candidates for admission; makes the choice to admit, not admit, or discharge; needs no authorization; and executes the decision.[33] To the extent that some of these steps are shared with or controlled by others, decision making is decentralized. For example, frequently, the CCU director must depend on others for steps 1 and 2. Thus, the collection of information and the interpretation of that information (which is perhaps selectively filtered and reported) sets the premises (what should be done) for the actual choice. Compare this with a process in which the decision maker has the willingness and the ability to go physically to the emergency department, recovery room, or patient care floors to observe and make independent judgments.

Decentralization is obviously required when the complexity of information is so great that it would overload any single person. In such a fluid environment, an adhocracy may be appropriate. Adopted from Alvin Toffler's Future Shock,[40] the term *adhocracy* describes a structure that is designed for innovation and the solution of unique problems. Information processing, innovating, and problem solving necessitate a collaborative effort. Relationships among these cooperating persons are informal and nonhierarchic. Coordination is achieved through interaction rather than through command and control. For example, Singer and associates reported that attending physicians, when faced with a substantial reduction in CCU beds, spontaneously and naturally adjusted their individual admission and discharge decisions to achieve a more efficient use of a smaller number of beds.[41] No central direction or explicit administrative rules were required. There was coordination through "mutual adjustment."[41]

In the absence of a central decision maker such as a working medical director, decision making necessarily remains decentralized and adhocratic. When there are no bed or resource shortages, this may be preferred. What structure should be adopted when there are resource constraints? Given the uncertainty of the physiologic variables and the unpredictability of demand, and given the array of parties who legitimately must participate in the management of illness trajectories and the many aspects of admission, discharge, and treatment, is the decentralized adhocratic approach the best approach? It depends. Physicians may have an interest in maintaining a weak medical directorship because it maximizes their access to the CCU and its technologies. When decision making is diffused, so is accountability. Furthermore, adhocracy tends to be conflict ridden because many individuals have input. Because of the informality of adhocracy, hierarchic channels are often not available to resolve conflict.

Strategy Making

The question of what kind of organizational structure the CCU should have is subsumed under strategy making. Conceptually, strategy making calls for the CCU medical director to go beyond the role of illness trajectory manager and gatekeeper to participate in the formation of hospital-wide strategy. Logically, the question of what are the goals of the CCU and how do they relate to the overall mission of the hospital should be answered before determining an organizational structure (Table 5–3).

The types of services that are produced in the CCU are related to the type of institution, such as functioning as a tertiary center or community hospital; serving low-income or middle- and upper-income populations; and emphasizing trauma care or elective surgery. Analytic tools can help strategy makers make these choices: marketing studies, reimbursement analysis, capital budgeting, area-wide and institutional planning, and so on. Unfortunately, the process is seldom as linear or logical as it appears in management textbooks.

Strategy making is a complex interactive process. Organization design entails more than producing organizational charts or formulating position descriptions, procedures, and policies. Consider the concept of centralization. To the extent that it restricts the freedom of other physicians, and given the fragmented nature of hospital authority and the necessity of multiple-specialty participation in illness trajectory management, centralization is likely to be conflict ridden. Centralization is not decided by a hospital policy board; rather, it is a process, sometimes subtle, always political.

The organized medical staff and its standing committees, a standard fixture in the governance system of American hospitals, play a role in the process. An important aspect of this role is symbolic. There is legitimacy to committee policies because due process, representation, voting, appeals mechanisms, written rules, and official minutes have been painstakingly built into the policy-making process to reassure organization members of its accountability and its legitimacy.

However, the public and official nature of the committee deliberations limits its effectiveness in resolving conflict through the formal issuance of written policies. Implicit in the policies is a structure of economic relationships built on admitting and operating privileges. To even acknowledge the existence of these economic relationships, let alone to engage the committee policy-making process seriously and publicly is to invite controversy. There are other, more subtle, and less controversial ways of adjusting differences. The concept of *negotiated order* is appropriate.

According to Strauss and colleagues, a negotiated order is a set of understandings, agreements, and informal contracts, among various professionals and nonprofessionals.[42] In contrast to written rules backed by formal sanction (the traditional notion of hierarchy), unwritten understandings, sometimes implicit and arrived at through negotiation and renegotiation, govern relationships in the hospital.

As an example of the negotiated order, consider the variety of tactics that can be used in controlling not only the admission of patients to the unit but also the influence of outside physicians. Written admission policies might include the following proviso:

> The surgical intensive care unit will serve surgical patients who require preoperative insertion of invasive monitoring devices for preoperative monitoring. These admissions are subject to space availability and can be cancelled if a critically ill patient must be admitted.

This policy does not give the CCU director or designee control over admissions or control over who can perform what procedures. The ability to make beds available does give de facto control as the following hypothetic conversation shows:

Surgeon: Do you have any beds available?

CCU physician: I don't know, I'll see. By the way, if I do, do you want me to put in the lines?

One issue is, of course, who is going to place the preoperative monitoring catheters: the intensivists or other credentialled specialists, such as the cardiologists or pulmonologists. Subtle pressure is placed on the surgeon to tip the balance in favor of the CCU physicians. Furthermore, CCU physicians can legitimately argue that if they are being asked to provide the beds, they should be able to influence patient care.

Carried to its logical conclusion, centralization leads to a closed unit with a central decision maker controlling not only entry and exit but also the treatment of the patients within the unit. In a busy CCU, centralizing or coordinating decision making requires the reduction in the uncertainty

TABLE 5–3	
STRATEGY MAKING	
Activities	**Tools**
• Elaborating tasks and mission of hospital CCU	• Area-wide and institutional planning
• Delineating types of services to be delivered and markets to be served	• Marketing
	• Reimbursement analysis
• Designing organizational structure to achieve objectives	• Capital budgeting
	• Strategic planning

posed by a number of independent variables external to the immediate boundaries of the CCU. For example, we expect that a central decision maker would have the option to participate in preoperative screening of surgical candidates to determine their suitability for critical care, mandate ambulance diversion when beds are at full capacity, and cancel elective surgery. At the extreme end of the continuum, there is the emergence of what Mintzberg describes as the "simple structure" with a single, well-informed, decision maker, typical of the small, flexible, nonbureaucratic, albeit autocratic, entrepreneurial firm.[33]

The extent to which the centralized, simple structure is characteristic of CCUs is not known. The presence of a full-time working medical director is probably a necessary but not sufficient condition. Given the formality of the nursing chain of command and its separate professional identity, the working medical director is at best only half of the two-manager matrix. Furthermore, in busy CCUs, admission, discharge, and triage decision making may involve additional physicians (designees or associate directors) to share the 24-hour responsibility. Nevertheless, in a centralized mode, even a solitary medical director can have a significant impact on CCU organizational functioning.

Expectation Setting

Assuming that the anarchy of the open unit with weak managerial leadership is avoided, must one be forced to accept the personal fiefdom of the CCU medical director? How can one design an organization-wide accountability system that transcends the personal control system of the medical director? This issue revolves around the central question of how to recognize a well-managed, high-performance, cost-effective CCU. Third-party payers, quality assurance groups, and government in general are interested in this issue. Unfortunately, there is little to tell them about the efficiency of treatments, who can benefit most by the treatments, and the cost-effectiveness of the treatments. To answer the questions, the expectations and performance standards (see Fig. 5–1) for each managerial function must be better defined: illness trajectory management, resource allocation and gatekeeping, and strategy making. This is not to say that there are not expectations of each function, but they are not explicitly defined and formally recognized so that managers can be systematically held accountable for the achievement of expectations. As an example, consider the gatekeeping role. Although the decision of who gets the CCU bed is obviously important and triage is a central preoccupation in many units, gatekeeping has not been conceptualized as an administrative task with defined performance standards. How do we recognize a good triage decision?

Criteria for triage decisions vary among hospitals, among units within the same hospital, and by personnel within each unit. There has been little research on what criteria triage decision makers use. With regard to the discharge of patients, readmission information is sometimes collected, but it is not clear how it is used to evaluate unit performance. Similarly, little is known about denied or delayed admissions originating from within the hospital or from outside the hospital, and hospitals almost never examine the implicit or explicit criteria used in decision making to see if there is consistent application among patients with similar conditions.[43]

Thus, decision makers struggle to meet the minimal acceptable achievement levels for a set of expectations generated by its many internal and external constituencies: patients, families, physicians, nurses, attorneys, administrators, personnel from other units and hospitals, quality assurance

committees, state regulators, and house staff, among others. The demands of these constituencies are not treated as goals to be maximized but rather as constraints to be satisfied. For example, a CCU medical director might typically face the following performance expectations:

Allow every salvageable patient fair access to the CCU.
Minimize legal risk of foregoing nonbeneficial treatment.
Keep risk management activities from being triggered.
Satisfy formal institutional policies.
Calm angry private physicians who want their patients in the unit or do not want them discharged.
Keep nurses from walking out.
Keep the operating room on schedule and the emergency department open.
Keep readmission rates at an acceptable level.
Satisfy demands of powerful medical interests (e.g., do not cancel elective surgery even in the face of frequent emergency or trauma admissions).

In the face of resource cutbacks or if the CCU is continually operating at full capacity, the solution is to find a constituent to whom a lower level of performance would be acceptable. The search is an exercise in political rationality and individual survival; it is also invariably frustrating and often futile. Obviously, what is needed are well-supported and recognized performance expectations about access to CCU beds. All other constituency demands must be met in light of the primary expectation. Along with public recognition and support comes public accountability.

CONCLUSIONS

Both medical and nurse directors of CCUs must have a clear vision and perspective of their short-term and long-term goals as a first step to survival in such a complex environment. Organizational theory provides some useful insights for the practitioner. In describing the rational contingency model, Hall says that "organizations are viewed as attempting to attain goals and deal with their environment, with the realization that there is not one best way to do so (see ref 16, p 312).

As with any organization, there are barriers to the CCU's achieving optimal effectiveness. The CCU may have multiple and conflicting goals that constrain the decision-making process. The unit also has multiple internal and external constituencies placing often contradictory and conflicting demands on the unit and its management team. The unit also faces multiple environmental constraints, both internal and external. Whether these restrictions, such as protocols for quality assurance and cost containment, are self-imposed or arise from external sources (e.g., government agencies and JCAHO), they are often in conflict with one another and must be acknowledged. Actions designed to satisfy one constraint may directly oppose the meeting of another constraint. The larger and more complex the organization is, the greater the range and variety of environmental constraints to be met.

Improving the efficacy of any organization can be difficult. The first problem is defining what constitutes an effective unit, and some researchers have urged that effectiveness be used in a relative as opposed to an absolute sense.[44–46] As Hall says (ref 16, p 264), organizations may be considered to be

more or less effective in regard to the variety of goals which they pursue; the variety of resources which they attempt to acquire; the variety of constituents inside and outside of the organization, whether or not they are part of the decision-making process; and the variety of time frames by which effectiveness is judged. The idea of variety . . . is key . . . since it suggests that an organization can be effective in some aspects of its operations and less so in others.

Medical and nursing directors of CCUs should assess the role of their units within the context of the mission of their hospital and how it pertains to the community at large. A thorough understanding of the internal and external environments, the unit's multiple constituencies and their respective goals and time frames, and the existing negotiated order of the institution as a whole is vital if the management team is to be successful. This necessitates sophisticated interpersonal, communicative, and political skills if the unit directors are to build the multidisciplinary coalitions necessary for them to function properly.

Locally, CCU directors need to engage in networking and the development of cooperative multiple-hospital systems for the regionalization of health care delivery, especially as it pertains to the critically ill patient. The Society of Critical Care Medicine has already published guidelines for the categorization of CCUs.

On a national level, performance standards for quality assurance and cost-effective medical care will have to be developed for serious progress to be made in the continuing evolution of CCUs. Berwick has discussed the need for information gathering and analysis required to meet the exigencies of health care in the 1990s:

[We] must pursue at least four intellectual agendas: the study of efficacy (knowing what works), the study of appropriateness (using what works), the study of the execution of care (doing well what works), and the study of the purposes of care (the values that underlie action). The responsibility for the financing and conduct of the research agendas varies with the level of aggregation of data and the effort needed for each topic. All four topics must be pursued effectively if health care quality is to be successfully defined, measured, and protected.[6]

These agendas were posited for the health care industry at large but are especially appropriate for critical care. As one of the most visible and arguably the most expensive segments of health care, it will undoubtedly be most carefully scrutinized in the near future. Because critical care is one of the newest and most politically complex specialties, little information is available about its structure, process, function, and outcomes. Nurse and physician managers would do well to pool their resources and act collaboratively in pursuing these agendas.

References

1. Whitehead AN: The Aims of Education. New York, Macmillan, 1929.
2. Strosberg MA, Fein IA: Policy and management issues in rationing care for the critically ill. Hosp Admin Curr 31:1, 1987.
3. Griner PF: The relationship between managerial and clinical decision making in the hospital. Med Decis Making 8:151, 1988.
4. Knaus WA, Draper EA, Wagner DP, Zimmerman JE: An evaluation of outcome from intensive care in major medical centers. Ann Intern Med 104:410, 1986.
5. Berwick DM: Toward an applied technology for quality measurement in health care. Med Decis Making 8:253, 1988.
6. Abramowitz KS: The Future of Health Care Delivery in America. New York, Sanford C Bernstein, 1988.
7. Berwick DM: Health services research and quality of care—assignments for the 1990s. Med Care 27:763, 1989.
8. Deming WE: Out of the Crisis. Cambridge, MA, Massachusetts Institute of Technology, Center for Advanced Engineering Study, 1986.
9. Shewhart WA: Economic Control of Quality of Manufactured Product. New York, D Van Nostrand, 1931.
10. Juran JM: Managerial Breakthrough. New York, McGraw-Hill, 1964.
11. Teres D: Enter: The era of management. Crit Care Med 13:137, 1985.
12. Pugh DS, Hickson DJ: Writers on Organizations. Newbury Park, CA, Sage Publications, 1989.
13. Fein SL: Burnout in nursing: Prevention and management. In: Fein IA, Strosberg MA (eds): Managing the Critical Care Unit. Rockville, MD, Aspen Publishers, p 96, 1987.
14. Maslach C: Burnout—The Cost of Caring. Englewood Cliffs, NJ, Prentice-Hall, 1982.
15. Muldary TW: Burnout and Health Professionals: Manifestations and Management. Garden Grove, CA, Capistrano Press, 1983.
16. Hall RH: Organizations: Structures, Processes, and Outcomes. 4th ed. Englewood Cliffs, NJ, Prentice-Hall, 1987.
17. Consensus Development Conference: Critical care medicine. JAMA, 250:798, 1983.
18. American Association of Critical Care Nurses and Society of Critical Care Medicine: The organization of human resources in critical care units. Focus Crit Care 10:43, 1983.
19. Joint Commission on Accreditation of Hospitals: Accreditation Manual for Hospitals. Chicago, Joint Commission on Accreditation of Hospitals, 1982.
20. Initial Report and Preliminary Findings. Chicago, National Commission on Nursing, 1981.
21. Alt-White AC, Charns M, Strayer R: Personal, organizational and managerial factors related to nurse physician collaboration. Nurs Adm Q 8:8, 1983.
22. Prescott PA, Bowen SA: Physician-nurse relationships. Ann Intern Med 103:127, 1985.
23. Gill S, Gill M, Spence S: Five roadblocks to effective partnership in a competitive health care environment. Hosp Health Serv Admin 33:4, 1988.
24. Pluckhan M: Professional territoriality: A problem affecting the delivery of health care. Nurs Forum 11:300, 1972.
25. Teres D, Chandler RE, Riddle MM: Critical care unit administration: The management team approach. In: Fein IA, Strosberg MA (eds): Managing the Critical Care Unit. Rockville, MD, Aspen Publishers, p 32, 1987.
26. Kuhn R: Nurse and physician collaboration: How to strengthen the team. Heart Lung 14:18, 1985.
27. Dyer WG: Team Building: Issues and Alternatives. Reading, MA, Addison-Wesley, 1977.
28. Shonk JH: Working in Teams. New York, Shonk and Associates, 1980.
29. Peters T: Thriving on Chaos. New York, Alfred A Knopf, 1987.
30. Adler DC: Hospital management of critical care. In: Parrillo JE, Ayres SN (eds): Major Issues in Critical Care Medicine. Baltimore, Williams & Wilkins, 1984.
31. Strosberg MA, Teres D, Fein IA, et al: Nursing perception of the availability of the intensive care unit medical director for triage and conflict resolution. Heart Lung 19:452, 1990.
32. Woodward J: Industrial Organization: Theory and Practice. 2nd ed. London, Oxford University Press, 1981.
33. Mintzberg H: The Structuring of Organizations. Englewood Cliffs, NJ, Prentice-Hall, 1979.
34. Strauss A, Fagerhaugh S, Suczek B, et al: Social Organization of Medical Work. Chicago, University of Chicago Press, 1985.
35. Griffith JR: The Well-Managed Community Hospital. Ann Arbor, MI, Health Administration Press, 1987.
36. Thompson JD: Organizations in Action. New York, McGraw-Hill, 1967.
37. Society of Critical Care Medicine Task Force on Guidelines: Recommendations for intensive care unit admission and discharge criteria. Crit Care Med 16:807, 1988.
38. Baker R, Dersch V, Fein IA, et al: Ethical implications of New York State's DNR law. Crit Care Med 18:52, 1990.
39. Paterson TT: Management Theory. London, Business Publications, p 150, 1969.
40. Toffler A: Future Shock. New York, Bantam Books, 1970.
41. Singer DE, Carr PL, Mulley AG, Thibault GE: Rationing intensive care: Physician responses to a resource shortage. N Engl J Med 309:1150, 1981.
42. Strauss A, Schatzman L, Ehrlich D, et al: The hospital and its negotiated order. In: Friedson E (ed): The Hospital in Modern Society. New York, Free Press of Glencoe, p 147, 1963.
43. Strosberg MA: Intensive care units in the triage mode: An organizational perspective. Hosp Health Serv Admin 36:95, 1991.
44. Hannan MT, Freeman JH: Obstacles to comparative studies. In: Goodman PS, Pennings JM (eds): New Perspectives on Organizational Effectiveness. San Francisco, Jossey-Bass, 1977.
45. Kahn RL: Organizational effectiveness: An overview. In: Goodman PS, Pennings JM (eds): New Perspectives on Organizational Effectiveness. San Francisco, Jossey-Bass, 1977.
46. Campbell JP: On the nature of organizational effectiveness. In: Goodman PS, Pennings JM (eds): New Perspectives on Organizational Effectiveness. San Francisco, Jossey-Bass, 1977.

CHAPTER 6

Standards

Carolyn Bekes
W. Eric Scott
Bruce Friedman

TERMINOLOGY

Any attempt to discuss the creation and utilization of standards in the practice of medicine immediately leads to the problem of definition. Eddy, in one of a series of articles on practice policies, discussed terminology.[1] He indicated that the term *standard*, in this context, refers to a recommendation that is intended to be inflexible, whereas *guidelines* are intended to be more flexible, and *options* are so flexible that they provide no guidance. In this chapter, we use the term standard in a more generic sense to encompass a spectrum of meaning that ranges from rigid standards to options. We acknowledge, however, that each policy must specify into which category its recommendations fall (see later).

GENERAL CONSIDERATIONS

Multiple factors are responsible for the increasing formulation and use of standards in many fields of medical practice. These relate not only to the complexity and hazards of the area of practice, but also to its cost and the perceived cost/benefit ratio. With this in mind, it is easy to understand that the practice of critical care medicine is, and will continue to be, subject to the formulation of standards. Not only is it an extremely costly area of care delivery, but it is one in which questions of cost/benefit ratio are immediately apparent. Critical care medicine has multidisciplinary origins, and its practitioners have variable training backgrounds and are working in a highly technical setting with tremendous potential for iatrogenic complications. Theories, therapies, and technology at the cutting edge have often been implemented before being established by rigorous scientific process and need to be evaluated under controlled conditions if needless expenditure and morbidity are to be avoided.

These factors call not only for the application of scientifically derived guidelines to the practice of critical care medicine, but also for the development of standards pertaining to the environment in which it takes place as well as to the qualifications, knowledge, and skills of its practitioners.

Thus, it is important for the intensivist to have some knowledge of the historical background of standards and the present forces shaping their development and application in the practice arena. The methods of standard formulation as well as the criticisms thereof should also be appreciated by the practitioner to enable informed, reasoned evaluation of proposed standards.

HISTORICAL BACKGROUND

Any group of individuals joining cooperatively to achieve common goals need to agree on rules of behavior. Thus, social interaction breeds standards. Indeed, in all societies that have attained any measure of order or organization, there is an obligation placed on all members to deal with each other in a reasonable manner. Furthermore, should damage or injury be caused to an individual because of the unreasonable behavior of another, the former may be entitled to compensation by the latter. The practical application of this concept requires, of course, definitions of what constitutes reasonable and unreasonable behaviors, and thus standards for behavior must be developed by that society.

Standards may evolve gradually through a process of general consensus, but as the societal structure increases in complexity, they are undoubtedly modified, molded, and formalized by more discrete groups of individuals representing the power structure and religiophilosophic beliefs of that society. It may be important to note that the goals of these groups may not always be apparent to the society utilizing the standards, even when the standards have been generally accepted.

Judicial Standards of Medical Practice

Present ideas about professional malpractice stem from an extension of the principle of reasonable behavior between individuals to the behavior of members of the society who provide services to others. Here, also, there is a requirement to determine reasonable standards of behavior. This has been one of a number of important forces driving the formulation of standards of medical practice by the judicial system.

The judicial system determines standards of practice by relying on expert testimony rendered during the conduct of malpractice cases. Standards so derived therefore tend to apply more to individuals in specific situations than to groups of people or categories of patients. Because of the nature of the process, the standards that have been established have been largely based on expressions of personal opinion by practitioners whom the court has accepted as experts in a particular field under review. Alternatively, standards have been derived from medical texts that the court has accepted as learned treatises.[2]

This approach to the construction of standards illustrates a method still much in use in medicine today, that is, the utilization of the opinion of the experienced practitioner generally considered by his or her peers to be an expert in the field. Publications and presentations at meetings by such individuals, unless rebutted or countered by others, often lead to the development of standards for given situations. In court proceedings, a balance of viewpoints is sought by allowing both the plaintiff and the defendant to introduce expert testimony regarding the standard of practice in the matter under litigation. On the basis of this evidence, the judge or the judge and jury decide on the standard and whether it has been met.

Measures of medical practice may be promulgated by different bodies with different goals in mind. Standards generated primarily to reduce cost may not be suitable for court proceedings, because the betterment of patient welfare is not the sole concern of such standards.[2] Historically, the determination of standards by courts has been based almost entirely on the individual patient's needs and welfare. The cost to society has generally not been weighed against the benefit to the patient. Whether courts will continue to ignore costs in considering medical standards remains to be seen. This is important because, as discussed later, the judicial process is one of the most important mechanisms in mandating the application of standards formulated by the medical profession and others.

Standards Originating with Physicians

If standards are viewed as a directive regarding how best to achieve a defined goal in a specific situation, the writing of standards is hardly a new phenomenon in medicine. Textbooks, publications, and proclamations from innumerable medical and specialty societies have outlined ideal diagnostic and therapeutic schemes for countless medical problems for as long as the practice of medicine has been viewed as a profession. However, during the past 10 to 15 years, many medical organizations and groups have become increasingly interested in both formulating and disseminating many more practice standards in almost every field. This interest has been stimulated by a number of factors.

The explosion in medical knowledge and technology presents individual practitioners with a serious problem. It has become increasingly difficult to remain current both cognitively and procedurally. A partial solution to this problem might be provided by the generation and wide dissemination of standards or practice policies.[3] Physicians often appear to prefer to receive this type of information in a concise format with specific directives.[4] By utilizing standards, the practitioner would not have to review every publication on each situation encountered in the practice of medicine; he or she could simply refer to the appropriate practice policy. In this way, it might be possible to improve the quality of care. Viewed in this light, the dissemination of standards may also offer the benefit of providing continuing medical education in a condensed and easy to digest format. However, with the rapidly burgeoning publication of standards in recent years, a number of issues have been raised regarding their method of formulation in relation to their validity.[5-7] There has been an increasing interest in the processes used to examine the underlying data bases and draw conclusions, as well as the steps taken to ensure clarification and agreement on the desired goals to be attained by applying the standard.

Although the publication and promulgation of standards of medical practice is as old as the profession, the process has been variable and usually informal. Only in recent years have attempts been made to survey much wider data bases to formulate standards. Accordingly, many groups and medical organizations have organized and sponsored opportunities for respected and expert practitioners to discuss issues together and then to generate recommendations reached by consensus. These groups have included the American Medical Association, the American College of Physicians, the National Institutes of Health (NIH), the Centers for Disease Control, and universities, medical schools, and specialty societies.

Joint Commission for the Accreditation of Healthcare Organizations

The Joint Commission for the Accreditation of Healthcare Organizations (JCAHO) plays a key and ever-increasing role in the setting of standards for medical care. In fact, the setting of standards is one of its most important activities, and most hospitals voluntarily endeavor to meet these standards.

The process used by the JCAHO to define standards has been described in depth elsewhere.[8] Although quite complex and cumbersome, this procedure allows for change when advances in the knowledge base or in practice techniques occur. A three-phase standards development process has evolved, which is designed to elicit significant input from the field, ensure a scientific basis for the standards, and explore the difficulties that institutions will encounter in their efforts to implement the new or revised standards (Figs. 6–1 and 6–2). After new standards are adopted or old standards revised or deleted, each change in recommendations has been well studied and its implications for health care organizations are well understood. A built-in feedback loop ensures constant reappraisal.

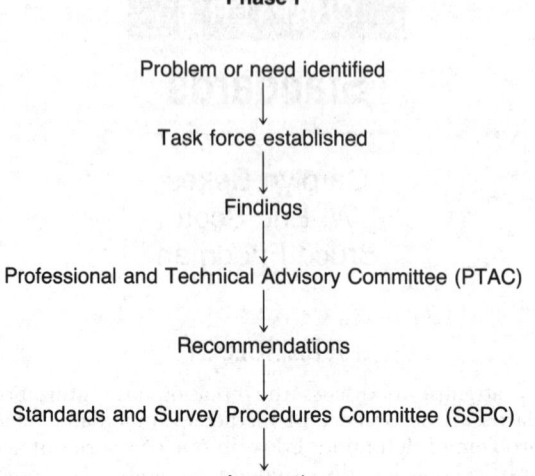

Figure 6–1. First phase of the standards development process.

To understand standards development by the JCAHO, it is important to have some insight into the Agenda for Change program, which was instituted in 1987.[8] Most previous standards emphasizing compliance with elements of care delivery focused on structure and process. With the Agenda for Change, the JCAHO encouraged organizations, through their quality assurance process, to examine indicators of performance and outcome. If an institution focuses on outcome, and then takes action to improve it, a higher quality of care should be achieved. This allows the JCAHO to be less prescriptive in its standards, merely mandating the review process. As a result, the JCAHO standards focus on continuous comprehensive monitoring, evaluating activities, and developing opportunities to improve care. Standards

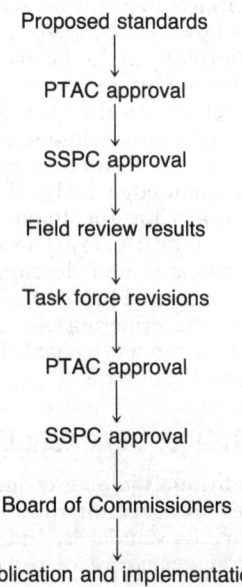

Figure 6–2. Second phase of the standards development process.

TABLE 6-1
QUALITY ASSURANCE PROCESS

Step No.	Action
1	Assign responsibility
2	Delineate scope of care
3	Identify important aspects of care
4	Identify indicators
5	Establish thresholds for evaluation
6	Collect and organize data
7	Evaluate care
8	Take actions to solve identified problems
9	Assess actions and document improvement
10	Communicate relevant information to the organization-wide quality assurance program

also stress the importance of documenting these activities and reporting the results through designated channels.

The process that the JCAHO recommends that hospitals adopt in constructing a quality assurance program consists of 10 steps[9] (Table 6–1). The JCAHO examines each plan to ensure compliance with each of the 10 steps. An example of such a 10-step plan, which has been implemented in a multidisciplinary intensive care unit (ICU), can be seen in Table 6–2.

Standards Derived by Payers and Regulatory Agencies

Many nonphysician groups are becoming involved in the development of standards with the goal of containing costs.[4] The Healthcare Financing Administration,[10] Physician Payment Review Commission,[11] and the Agency for Health Care Policy and Research have all emphasized standards of care.[12] In fact, the U.S. General Accounting Office suggested in 1988 that a federal entity be developed to define practice standards and monitor quality assurance programs, incorporating them into the quality assurance program for Medicare.[13] The Professional Standard Review Organization system has already engaged in the development of standards; perhaps because of inadequate resources, the results to date have been disappointing.[14]

Because of a worsening economic situation and the need to control health care costs, governmental agencies, third-party payers, businesses and corporations, and purveyors of managed health care are all exceedingly interested in promoting outcome studies on which to base reimbursement decisions. Examples of these efforts are the work of Blue Cross and Blue Shield in its Medical Necessity Project[15] and the U.S. Preventive Services Task Force.[16]

A measure of governmental concern with these issues is the rapidly increasing funding of research projects relating to technology assessment and outcome research, which should lead to increased standard and policy formulation. In 1988, federal funding of patient outcome research totaled approximately $1.9 million. In 1989, this rose to $5.5 million, and for 1990, it is somewhat in excess of $30 million.[12] The creation by the federal government of such agencies as the Agency for Health Care Policy and Research (to replace the now defunct National Center for Healthcare Technology) and the federal allocation of almost $600 million to be spent on outcome research and the appropriateness of some aspects of medical care (Omnibus Budget Reconciliation Act, 1989) are further indications of the intense governmental interest in determining whether the money spent on health care is being efficiently expended and whether the expenditure can be reduced or limited.

PROCESS OF DEVELOPING STANDARDS

Many factors are driving the development of standards of care. It seems inevitable that this will continue; physicians should at least participate in, if not lead, the process. There are, however, many issues that must be addressed if it is to proceed in a logical or systematic fashion. First comes the question of who sponsors and funds these efforts. Thereafter, it is necessary to define goals and to select the technique or techniques to be utilized for the formulation of standards. After development of the policy, a policy statement must be written and the policy must be introduced to the community. Each of these steps is examined later.

Sponsoring and Funding

It is unlikely that the private sector can afford the necessary funding; public funds will undoubtedly be needed.[5] This is appropriate, because practice policies benefit the population as a whole. However, if the development of standards is sponsored by the federal government, it is unlikely that many practitioners would cooperate, and the results might not be credible to many practitioners. Accordingly, it has been proposed that a sponsoring organization be identified that is prestigious enough to attract cooperation, possesses political independence from the government and organized medicine (so standards will be accepted), and has the internal management expertise to oversee the project.[5]

Membership on a team or a panel developing standards probably varies depending on the topic to be addressed.[5] Certainly, any group considering medical practice standards should include practitioners representing academic and private practice medicine from varying geographic locations, modes of practice, and if indicated, differing specialities. Nurses and others should be included if they have any major role in the delivery of the care; consumer (patient) input is appropriate mainly to ensure that defined goals truly reflect patients' preferences.

After the sponsoring organization is identified, the next important task is identification of outcome goals.

Identifying Goals
Cost Limitation

As discussed earlier, many governmental agencies and health care providers have been active in the formation and promulgation of standards of care. On initial examination, this would appear to be an excellent trend, whereby various aspects of medical practice are evaluated; the basis of the results, practice policies and standards can be generated and widely disseminated, leading to an ongoing educational process for practitioners. The problem lies in the need for assurance that the goals of standards so formulated are indeed those of the practitioner and the patient. Although federal agencies responsible for health care finance are clearly concerned with the quality of care, they are also greatly concerned with its cost, and the thrust of practice standards developed by those agencies undoubtedly is not just to ensure quality but also to limit and contain costs.

In the past, physicians tended to address only the individual patient's condition and to present to the patient the prevailing medical opinion regarding the options pertaining to that particular situation without addressing issues of societal resources or their distribution. Regardless of whether this is right or wrong, it may require a considerable readjustment on the part of most physicians to be guided by policies whose goals stress significant reductions in health care expenditures. A further difficulty for physicians facing

---

TABLE 6–2

EXAMPLE OF INTENSIVE CARE UNIT QUALITY ASSURANCE PLAN

Step 1
The ICU director is responsible for proposing a quality assurance plan to the critical care committee and reporting to the critical care committee on a monthly basis.

Step 2
The chairperson of the critical care committee is responsible for reporting to the executive committee and to the quality assurance committee.

Scope of Care
The ICU ordinarily accepts any patient age 17 y or older with a presently or potentially life-threatening medical or surgical condition, excluding acute myocardial infarction, postcraniotomy or neurosurgical patients, or post-trauma patients, who would usually go to a specialized unit. See ICU policy book for full admission criteria.

Step 3
Important Aspects of Care
1. Avoidance of nosocomial infection
2. Education and support of family
3. Close monitoring of fluid balance
4. Removal of life support performed consistent with hospital policy
5. Avoidance of complications of life-support therapy
6. Transfer patient out of unit when patient meets discharge criteria
7. Coordination of care by primary attending physician
8. Interhospital transport accomplished safely

Steps 4 and 5

Indicators	Criteria	Threshold	Responsible Person	Months
1. Avoidance of nosocomial infection and identification of significant cases for individual review (aspect 1)	Infection rate: 15%	Review if >15%	Infection control coordinator and unit director	All
2. Antibiotic coverage narrowed when possible (aspect 1)	Antibiotic regimen based on cultures *and* clinical picture	All cases of documented bacteremia studied	Infectious disease physician	All
3. Education and support of family (aspect 2)	Family receives informational booklet	90%	ICU nurse manager	All
4. ICU house staff assess fluid balance (aspect 3)	Assessment mentioned in progress note	95%	ICU fellow	All
5. Withdrawal of life support consistent with hospital policy (aspect 4)	Progress notes written by physician, which specify that nurse and family have participated in discussion. Specific orders written or countersigned immediately by attending level physician	All reviewed	Utilization review nurse	All
6. Daily progress noted by primary attending physician (aspect 7)	Progress note by attending physician	95%	ICU director	All
7. Ventilated patient evaluated for ventilation weaning on an ongoing basis (aspect 5)	Vital capacity and negative inspiratory force measured daily in appropriate patients	75%	Respiratory therapy coordinator	All
8. Interhospital transport accomplished in a safe fashion (aspect 8)	Patients have appropriate medical/nursing observation and monitoring during transport to ICU	All cases examined	ICU nurse manager and ICU Director	All

Volume Indicators	Threshold	Responsible Person
9. Incident reports	All reviewed	ICU nurse manager and ICU director
10. Nursing documentation	95%	ICU nurse manager
11. Number of inappropriate utilizations	All reviewed	Utilization review nurse
12. Number of readmissions within 7 d (aspect 6)	All reviewed	Member of quality assurance committee responsible
13. Predicted/actual mortality; do in June and December	Actual must be within 15% of predicted	Hospital administrator

TABLE 6–2

EXAMPLE OF INTENSIVE CARE UNIT QUALITY ASSURANCE PLAN *Continued*

Other
14. Morbidity and mortality conference
15. Referrals from other quality assurance activities

Step 6
Data are collected monthly and reported in tabular form to the critical care committee.

Step 7
The critical care committee evaluates any cases that indicate problems with care.

Step 8
When problems are identified, the chairperson of the critical care committee communicates with the appropriate department by memorandum or directly with the individuals involved.

Step 9
Action taken is evaluated at the next meeting of the critical care committee and documented in the minutes.

Step 10
Minutes of the critical care committee are forwarded to the executive committee of the medical staff and the quality assurance committee.

Approved	_____		_____
	Chairperson, Critical Care Committee		Director, Intensive Care Unit
Date	_____	Date	_____
Approved	_____		_____
	Director of Nursing, Critical Care Medicine		Nurse Manager, Intensive Care Unit
Date	_____	Date	_____

such policies is the assumption that the primary motivation of the physician is to be a contributor to the delivery of health care services to the public. In fact, physicians practice medicine for widely diverse reasons. Although many physicians are motivated by compassion and a desire to serve, other practitioners are primarily driven by scientific curiosity, the need to discover, or the need to create. This diversity in motivation leads to a variety of professional goals such that many practitioners may have difficulty accepting practice policies wherein the primary goal may be to contain the service costs rather than to encourage the search for and discovery of new technologies and knowledge. Although policy-directed practice may be inevitable in the current economic climate, it may nevertheless be unfortunate because advances in medicine probably stem more from the contributions of curiosity-driven practitioners than from those of individuals concerned with the organization and delivery of services to a society with limited resources. Clearly, however, at this time, the limitation of available resources makes the promulgation of standards in medicine that have cost containment as a goal inevitable.

Education of Physicians and Improvement in Care of Patients

Other reasons for the development of standards may be more easily accepted. Physicians recognize that most decisions are complicated and cannot be based on the expertise of only one practitioner. With the explosion of medical knowledge and its documentation in the literature, it has become difficult, if not impossible, for each physician to review all of the available scientific data, examine it critically, and select the best treatment plan. Therefore, one of the processes in the development of standards should be a critical and exhaustive review of the literature, pooling the lessons of research and clinical judgment, to identify the treatment option or options most likely to achieve the desired outcome. If this results in the publication and appropriate

introduction and dissemination of a succinctly written guide to treatment, based on sound data, not only may patient care be improved but also a contribution will have been made to physician education. Furthermore, the utilization of standards as an objective basis for establishing credentials for physicians, particularly in discipline such as critical care medicine, may make another indirect contribution to improving patient care.

Another goal of standard formulation, often neglected in the past, must be the identification of the results desired by the individual patient or group of patients whose care is being considered; these may not necessarily correspond to the goals of the health care practitioner or the funding agencies. This is particularly important in critical care medicine in which issues of quality of life versus longevity often assume great importance. In these cases, the standard of care should often concern itself more with ensuring the thorough and complete presentation of relevant information (both treatment and nontreatment options) to patients and/ or the family so that they can make an informed choice, rather than make assumptions regarding the desired outcome.

Establishing Data Base

Different techniques have been used by the various groups involved in the formulation of standards to facilitate the personal interactions necessary to reach worthwhile consensus. The Delphi Process, the Nominal Group, the consensus conferences organized by the NIH, and the consensus conferences organized by Glaser are some of the better known examples and are well described elsewhere;[17] they constitute a rather traditional approach to the generation of standards. The basic concept in all of these approaches has been to arrive at a standard by reaching agreement among experts in the field.

Two examples of this ongoing standard-setting consensus process are examined in detail. The NIH Consensus Development Program, administered by the NIH Office of Medical Applications of Research, involves scientists, medical practitioners, and informed lay people in the public evaluation of scientific information about biomedical technologies. Meeting for 2.5 days, these panels review scientific evidence then meet in executive session to seek consensus on key questions posed in advance. The findings of the panel are thereafter presented as a consensus statement, which is widely disseminated both in the medical literature and directly to practicing physicians, other health care professionals, and the research community.

This process has been criticized.[18] It offers the potential to translate a large unit of evidence into concise policy, brings together conflicting viewpoints, draws public attention to important issues, obtains input of practitioners, and increases exposure of all parties to research evidence. Nonetheless, there may be too much focus on compromise, final recommendations may be ambiguous, proceedings may be dominated by a vocal few, there probably is too little time for considered conclusions, and there is poor or nonexistent impact on clinical practice.[18] The compression of writing a policy, hearing reaction to it, and rewriting the policy in just 1 day may not allow for a well-thought-out approach.

Although not ideal, the NIH consensus process can have an impact and result in a change in practice. In 1983, such a conference addressed issues related to the practice of critical care. Specifically, essential capabilities of an ICU, personnel training, organization of ICU personnel, and directions for critical care research were addressed.[19]

Canada modified this process somewhat for their National Consensus Statement on Cesarian Delivery sponsored by the Society of Obstetricians and Gynaecologists, which was developed and published in 1986. Although it was similar to the NIH process in many ways, there are a few significant differences.[20] A needs assessment phase was introduced, which analyzed in detail where clinical practice and research diverged. The panel, drawn from a wide spectrum of interests, including involved professional organizations, was extensively prepared for the conference by project staff who reviewed the literature, sending it to the panel in advance for review.

At the 2.5-day conference of the Canadian group, public input was sought. Although an interim statement was prepared at the conclusion of the conference, a final statement was not released until several months of reconsideration and review were undertaken. Thus, much emphasis was placed on consideration of evidence during policy development.

The consensus conference format probably provides the best compromise to meet the needs of policy development when compared with the other processes described to date. It synthesizes and reinforces research findings, serves an educational role, provides a forum for the resolution of conflict among various researchers and clinicians, and focuses on problems needing attention.

These traditional approaches are popular because (1) it is possible to involve many in the development of practice policies, (2) the logistics are not complicated, and (3) the costs may be relatively low. However, these traditional methods have many drawbacks, including (1) the standard may simply reflect current practice, which may or may not be based on scientific evidence; (2) there is an intrinsic assumption that subjective decision making (without explicit evaluation of evidence) is effective; and (3) the assumption that desired outcomes are known intuitively leads to the failure to examine critically the goals to be achieved. These traditional approaches have been employed by both the American Association of Critical Care Nurses (AACN) and the Society of Critical Care Medicine (SCCM) when formulating their standards and guidelines (see discussion later).

During the past 10 years, other approaches have been suggested. Several of these are well described by Eddy in a series of articles in the Journal of the American Medical Association.[1, 6, 7, 21–23] In addition to the traditional subjective approaches, he defines the evidence-based, outcomes-based, and preference-based approaches.[6] The evidence-based approach requires an explicit examination of all available data, both clinical and research, before the development of any practice policy. The outcomes-based approach adds an objective assessment of outcome data, and the preference-based approach requires, in addition, that the patient's desires for results be a part of the decision-making process.

The closest to ideal is probably the preference-based approach, which combines the advantages of the first two (explicit examination of the evidence and an estimation of the outcomes of alternative practices) with an explicit assessment of patients' preferences for outcomes. A move toward these techniques, all of which attempt to use data explicitly to shape practice policies, is probably appropriate because the traditional consensual methods of policy formation have as their aim a summary of accepted and usual practices, not changes in approach.[5] Because these newer approaches require explicit examination of the scientific literature, outcomes, and patient preferences, they can be logistically complicated and expensive; thus, funding and sponsorship issues (discussed earlier) must be resolved.

Categorizing Policy

It is important to determine if the policy will be in the form of standards, guidelines, or options (see earlier). The development of these policies is difficult because, by definition, the recommendations are for groups of patients rather than individuals and recommendations that affect many patients magnify uncertainties.[1] Therefore, when outcomes are unclear or variable, it is important to allow the practitioner flexibility. Standards, designed to be rigid, should be utilized only when there is unanimous agreement on a specific approach to a specific problem, which is supported by outcome data and widespread patient agreement on desired result. Policy should usually be presented as guidelines, which should be followed most of the time but can be tailored for individual patient needs; these require majority, but not unanimous, support. When a problem is so controversial that none of several approaches is clearly superior, policy should be presented as options, which are neutral and allow the practitioners a great deal of choice.

Writing Policy Statements

The policy statement, if accepted and applied correctly, should improve outcomes for patients and should present the policy in a manner that ensures its acceptance; elements of such a statement have been described.[22] If the given statement conflicts with other policies, this should be explained and reconciled, and the policy or recommended approach should be compared with other possible interventions.[23]

It is also important that any expected developments, which might require future modification or urgent needs for research, be explicitly mentioned, as should suggested dates for review of the policy. Authors of the policy should be identified. The degree of complexity and detail of the document depend on the subject under review.[22]

Introducing Standards

Development of a policy statement is not the end of the process. If a policy is to be implemented and accepted, close attention must be given to the method used to introduce it to the medical community. It is clear that, although physicians might be aware of new practice policies, objective behavior may not be significantly modified, despite stated agreement with the policy. Possible reasons for noncompliance include perceived threats of malpractice, inadequate technical skills, socioeconomic disincentives, and pressure from patients.[24]

For the process to be effective, the policy statement must be well constructed, reflective of a consensus, issued by an organization with scientific and professional credibility, and written in clear and unambiguous language.[5, 22] Physicians must be provided with convincing evidence, both research and clinical. Ideally, subsequent educational efforts should be narrowly focused on the area of practice needing improvement, conducted by a respected physician who speaks directly with the physicians to be affected by the policy, and followed by reinforcement at the state and local levels.[3, 5]

FUTURE STANDARDS

In any field of human endeavor, a standard ideally represents a consensus opinion on the most effective and efficient approach to a specific problem. The potential benefit of a standard increases directly with both the complexity of a problem and the size of the population utilizing it.

For the process to achieve maximal success, the technique for constructing standards and for ensuring their adoption must be both scientific and carefully planned. The definition of goals, though of paramount and obvious importance, does not always receive the attention it is due.[6]

Standards being formulated today that are designed to influence the practice of medicine and the operation of health care services seek to achieve at least two goals: (1) improvement in health care and individual patient satisfaction and (2) cost control of health care expenditures. Although these two goals are not necessarily mutually exclusive, the final form of a standard attempting to meet them both must be a compromise between standards addressing each exclusively.

It is thus clear that future standard writing must involve two processes, which for the sake of clarity may be considered separately. The first is a strictly medical assessment of the benefit/risk ratio of a given therapeutic pathway in terms of health goals as defined by the informed patient with whom all alternatives have been discussed. This should be a completely objective process based on the scientific medical evidence, the only subjective aspect being the individual patient's preferences.

The second process in arriving at the standard is much less scientific and objective. It is a value judgment, which must determine what financial cost is justified for the purchase of a defined medical benefit applied to groups of patients within the population as a whole.

How are these standards to be arrived at, who will write them, and what part should be played by the medical profession? Although nurses began the process of writing standards in the field of critical care, physicians have become increasingly active, particularly through the SCCM, accepting responsibility for the definition of standards for several discrete areas of practice (see discussion later).

In the past, as noted, standards for medical practice were largely generated by physicians, but their mandatory application has resulted from the ongoing conduct of malpractice cases in the courts. It is only more recently that legislative activity, through restrictions on reimbursement to and billing by physicians, has started to have a significant impact on medical practice.

To a significant extent, the courts continue to play a part in forming mandatory medical standards. It remains to be seen whether, under the influence of governmental concern for cost containment, court decisions about necessary standards of care will start to address the question of the cost of such care and weigh them against the medical benefits. It may well be that these court decisions will act as a compromising process in the development of standards addressing both medical benefits and cost containment.

It is of vital importance that physicians remain active and continue as a major force in medical standards formulation, so that there is no question about issues of medical benefit. The primary responsibility of physicians in societal decision-making mechanisms (e.g., the judicial system and the legislature) for arriving at reasonable and fair conclusions regarding health care standards should be to provide scientific evidence regarding therapeutic risk/benefit ratios and patient preferences. To the greatest extent possible, the data should be firmly based on scientifically obtained evidence; only when this is lacking or incomplete should guidelines be based solely on consensus opinions. Physicians may also have input and should attempt to influence decision making with regard to the value judgments of society regarding the resources to be allocated to health care endeavors and the financial value of a given health care benefit. In this regard, they are functioning more as members of society than as trained professionals with a pertinent area of expertise. It is rather in the area of pure medicine that physicians have a duty to provide the firm data base without which no rational medical standard can be formulated.

STANDARDS IN CRITICAL CARE MEDICINE

Perhaps in no area of patient care practice is there a greater need for practice policies and standards than in critical care medicine. This need arises not only from the peculiar aspects of the medical practice of critical care medicine but also from the enormous costs associated with this field of medicine.

Critical care medicine is a label, lacking precise definition, that is used to denote a variety of practices. Similarly, critical care practitioners are not a homogeneous group and include a wide range of traditional specialists, as well as critical care specialists.

This conglomeration of practices and practitioners is a reflection of the multiple organ system dysfunction experienced by the critically ill patient. However, the multidisciplinary nature of critical care medicine creates special problems with respect to the coordination of activities of various caregivers who must focus their efforts on a single patient. Although this problem is not new or unique to critical care, it is particularly salient in critical care. Additionally, the demands frequently made by the acutely ill patient for multiple, complex support technologies can be met only in a strictly controlled and constantly evolving environment wherein a variety of ancillary and support technologists must be able to ply their expertise. In no other field is a smooth interface among physicians, nurses, technicians, and ancillary staff more essential to the welfare of and satisfactory outcome for patients.[25]

It follows that each caregiver must know and accept his or her role, his or her areas of expertise and limitations, and the goals to be achieved at the various stages of the therapeutic plan. Thus, care of patients in this setting is invariably a complex operation involving many people with diverse skills and a large data base. Furthermore, because of the interventional nature of critical care, there is great potential for iatrogenic complications relating to ill-conceived or inexpertly applied care.

All of these characteristics of critical care medicine incontestably demand that its practice be governed and guided by

---

TABLE 6–3

CRITERIA FOR ADMISSION AND DISCHARGE

Priority 1 Patients
Critically ill, unstable, requiring intensive treatment and intervention. No limits are placed on therapy.

Priority 2 Patients
Not critically ill on admission, but require intensive monitoring. No limits are placed on therapy.

Priority 3 Patients
Critically ill, unstable, but underlying disease, state of health, or acute illness reduces likelihood of recovery and benefit from ICU care.

Priority 4 Patients
Patients not meeting routine admission criteria:
1. Brain-dead patients (can admit for organ donation).
2. Patients competently refusing life support.
3. Patients with nontraumatic coma with permanent vegetative state.
Admitted only under unusual circumstances by discretion of ICU director.

Discharge Criteria
1. Patients for whom intensive treatment is no longer necessary.
2. Patients of advanced age with three or more organ failures, who are unresponsive to initial therapy for more than 72 h.
3. Patients with limits on care (comfort care).
4. Patients with end-stage diseases who fail to respond to ICU therapy and for whom no potential therapy exists to alter prognosis.
5. Patients needing low-risk monitoring (e.g., carotid endarterectomy, aortofemoral bypass, transsphenoidal hypophysectomy, uncomplicated diabetic ketoacidosis, self-inflicted drug overdose, concussion, or mild congestive heart failure, who may benefit from intermediate care facility if available.

Adapted from Society of Critical Care Medicine Task Force on Guidelines: Recommendations for intensive care unit admission and discharge criteria, Crit Care Med, 16, 8, 807–808, © by Williams & Wilkins, 1988.

policies and standards. These should be soundly conceived to achieve agreed-on goals. This need was recognized by the American Hospital Association's Committee on Medical Education in 1975 when it called for the establishment of qualifications for those practicing critical care at all levels.[26]

It cannot be overemphasized that standards and policies developed for the care of patients in ICUs must be scientifically constructed on a foundation of carefully gathered evidence, which has widespread and justified acceptance. The costs of critical care are, in relation to those of many other fields of medicine, large indeed. This fact serves as a further stimulus for the creation of standards in an attempt to control such costs; it also makes it imperative to ensure that standards to improve patient outcome are based on strong evidence. Implementation of such standards may be extremely costly and can be justified only if demonstrable advances are being made toward agreed-on goals. Accordingly, standards should be written only when an extremely strong evidentiary base exists, although it may be permissible to publish guidelines or indicate practice options with lesser weights of evidence.[20]

Development of Standards by Critical Care Organizations

With these considerations in mind, two of the major organizations in critical care practice, SCCM and AACN, embarked almost simultaneously on the task of developing standards in critical care medicine. The initiatives that they have taken provide a foundation on which the process of further standard development may rest.

SCCM, established in 1970, represents physicians, nurses, and other critical care personnel throughout the world. The group mandated as early as 1978 that a standard of practice must be developed for the critical care practitioner and that this was a primary mission of the SCCM.

The practical expression of this commitment to quality care was the creation of the SCCM Task Force on Guidelines in 1985. The charge to this group was to evaluate current practice and thereafter to develop a consensus on the best possible methods for the delivery of quality critical care. Members of this group included physicians, nurses, technicians, and other health care professionals. Through their efforts, standards were initially generated for two distinct areas of critical care medicine: the critical care body of knowledge (curriculum)[27] and standards for fellowship directors.[28] Since then, guidelines have been proposed for ICU design,[29] ICU admission and discharge criteria,[30] services and personnel,[31] categorization of services,[32] and guidelines for the care of the mechanically ventilated patient in acute respiratory failure.[33] Some of these recommendations are outlined on Tables 6–3 to 6–6. All are based on the recommendation that the care of the critically ill patient be directed by a physician who, on the basis of training, experience, and availability, has been granted privileges by the hospital medical staff to care for patients with life-threatening complex problems. In addition, these guidelines recommend ratios of properly trained nursing and support personnel that are based on measures of acuity. Finally, they recommend the availability of certain equipment and support services that are deemed essential to provide safe care to critically ill patients, while recognizing that many hospitals exceed these suggested minimal requirements. After approval by the Council of the SCCM (which represents the general membership), these recommendations were published for distribution to critical care practitioners.[27–33]

In addition to serving as educational tools, the SCCM recommendations form the basis for updating and evaluating the practice of critical care medicine both within the

---

TABLE 6–4

GUIDELINES FOR CATEGORIZATION OF SERVICES FOR CRITICALLY ILL PATIENTS

1. ICUs appropriately concentrate critically ill patients in specified areas of the hospital.
2. ICUs have equipment, supplies, and personnel with special training and expertise to care for the critically ill.
3. Nurses in ICU are specially trained, based on AACN standards, to care for the critically ill.
4. Physicians trained and tested in the field of critical care medicine must be involved in the management of critically ill patients and be available on 24-h basis.
5. ICU design should be coordinated by critical care specialist–led multidisciplinary team and conform to known standards.
6. Definitions of levels of care and system of regional categorization are developed to triage patients based on needed resources. In this way, critical care system is cost-effective and maintains logical use of limited resources.
7. Providers of critical care have quality assurance and administrative duties to assure parties financing medical care that the unit management is cost-effective and delivers high-quality care.
8. Critical care medicine should provide ongoing educational and research activities.

Adapted from Society of Critical Care Medicine Task Force on Guidelines: Guidelines for the categorization of services for the critically ill patient, Crit Care Med, 19, 2, 279–285, © by Williams & Wilkins, 1991.

TABLE 6-5

RECOMMENDATIONS FOR SERVICES AND PERSONNEL SPECIFIC TO CRITICAL CARE DELIVERY

1. Care for severely ill and/or potentially severely ill patients
2. Specially trained nurses
3. Appropriate and expedient support services
4. Qualified physician as director
5. Technical services, consultants of all relevant medical subspecialties, and qualified ancillary personnel
6. Equipment and trained personnel for intrahospital and interhospital transport of severely ill patients
7. Cardiopulmonary resuscitation and advanced cardiac life support, necessary equipment, and pharmaceutical agents
8. Airway management, including endotracheal intubation and ventilation
9. Oxygen delivery systems and qualified respiratory therapists or registered nurses to provide oxygen therapy
10. Emergency and other temporary cardiac pacing
11. Continuous electrocardiographic monitoring
12. Rapid comprehensive specified laboratory services
13. Nutritional support services
14. Titrated therapeutic interventions with infusion pumps
15. All aspects of hemodynamic monitoring (e.g., pulmonary arterial catheter, central venous pressure monitoring, arterial line, intracranial pressure monitoring, capnography, pulse oximetry, temperature measurement, and cardiac output monitoring)
16. Access to specialized technology (e.g., computed tomography, magnetic resonance imaging, cardiac catheterization, bronchoscopy, fluoroscopy, extracorporeal membrane oxygenator, assistive devices, intra-aortic balloon pump, hyperbaric chambers, and computerized data management)
17. Continuing education for all critical care personnel
18. Quality assurance and control as well as policies and procedures specific to each facility
19. Ongoing educational and research activities in critical care medicine

Adapted from Society of Critical Care Medicine Task Force on Guidelines: Recommendations for services and personnel for delivery of care in a critical care setting, Crit Care Med, 16, 8, 809–811, © by Williams & Wilkins, 1988.

specialty and by other specialty groups and monitoring agencies. The SCCM standards may not reflect true national standards, because all specialties and boards were not represented when they were developed, and they were mostly formulated using traditional consensus methods and not always based on strong evidence. The SCCM recommendations indicate directions and provide a solid basis for formulating future guidelines.

In parallel with the efforts of the SCCM, the AACN developed standards for the nursing care of the critically ill[34] (Table 6–7). The formulation of these standards has been the goal of the AACN since 1969, and eventually they were generated by a designated standards task force, in collaboration with the American Nurses' Association, between 1975 and 1980.

The similarities between the AACN and SCCM recommendations are remarkable and reflect the commonality of goals arrived at independently. Through their parallel efforts, the two groups have formed a foundation for the development of national critical care standards. These documents and their implementation must spearhead the setting of true standards in the field of critical care, which may eventually gain acceptance by the entire health care community.

Such standards, however, to be credible and to serve their purpose, must adhere strictly to the constructional and developmental principles discussed earlier. Failure to do this

will inevitably result in increasing criticism of critical care medicine on grounds of cost, or risk a serious decline in quality of care resulting from inadequate financial support.

For standards to have a greater impact on the practice of critical care medicine, it will probably also be necessary to

TABLE 6-6

RECOMMENDATIONS FOR STANDARDS OF CARE FOR PATIENTS WITH ACUTE RESPIRATORY FAILURE RECEIVING MECHANICAL VENTILATORY SUPPORT

Available Personnel
Physician, 24 h/d in-house personnel, nurses, respiratory therapists, ancillary support staff

Available Monitoring
Cardiac, oxygen saturation, end-tidal carbon dioxide, hemodynamic apparatus, core temperature

Available Support Services
1. Radiographic services 24 h/d
2. Laboratory services 24 h/d, with special laboratory results available at least once per day and routine laboratory tests available within 1 h on an acute basis
3. Respiratory services

Available Equipment
1. Multifaceted mechanical ventilators
2. Resuscitation equipment accessible at bedside
3. Endotracheal tubes and equipment for intubation, including suction

General Management
1. Initial laboratory evaluation
2. Hourly vital signs
3. Complete, continuous monitoring of the hemodynamically unstable patient
4. Measurements of the following at least q 4 h: fractional inspired oxygen, minute volume, tidal volume, positive airway pressure, temperature of inspired gas, alarm checks, oxygen saturation
5. Input and output measurements q 8 h
6. Capabilities to institute:
   a. Analysis of blood gases
   b. Respiratory measurements
   c. Nutritional support services
   d. Continuous intravenous access
   e. Endotracheal tube cuff pressure measurements
   f. Patient weights
7. Preventive measures, such as prophylaxis of deep venous thrombosis, stress ulcer coverage, and avoidance of nosocomial infection
8. Available diagnostic and therapeutic modalities: cardiac pacing, special beds, temperature control devices, thoracentesis, tube thoracostomy, tracheostomy, anticoagulation, dialysis

Ventilator Management
1. Management of the airway: secure airway and endotracheal tube, prevent self-extubation, appropriate sedation, secretion control
2. Ventilatory support:
   a. Maintain oxygen saturation greater than 90%, except in congenital cyanotic heart disease and advanced chronic obstructive pulmonary disease
   b. Avoid fractional inspired oxygen greater than 50% to reduce oxygen toxicity
   c. Ensure adequate oxygen delivery and measurements as needed
   d. Provide appropriate sedation, minimize arterial blood gas draws
3. Remove ventilatory support in a timely manner by objective measures of pulmonary mechanics, clinical observation, and resolution of the problem necessitating ventilation

Adapted from Committee on Guidelines of the Society of Critical Care Medicine: Recommendations for standards of care for patients with acute respiratory failure receiving mechanical ventilatory support, Crit Care Med, 19, 2, 275–278, © by Williams & Wilkins, 1991.

TABLE 6-7
STANDARDS FOR NURSING CARE OF CRITICALLY ILL

1. The ICU shall be designed to ensure safe and supportive environments for critically ill patients and for personnel who care for them.
2. The ICU shall be constructed, equipped, and operated in a manner that protects patients, visitors, and personnel from hazards, including fire.
3. The ICU shall have essential equipment and supplies immediately available at all times.
4. The ICU shall have a comprehensive infection control program.
5. The ICU shall be managed in a manner that ensures the delivery of safe and effective care to the critically ill.
6. The ICU shall have appropriately qualified staff to provide care on a 24-h basis.
7. The critical care nurse shall be competent and current in critical care nursing.
8. The critical care nurses' performance appraisal shall be based on the roles and responsibilities identified in the job description.
9. The ICU shall have a well-defined, organized written program to evaluate care of the critically ill.
10. Critical care nursing practice shall include both the conduct and the utilization of clinical research.
11. The critical care nurse shall ensure delivery of safe nursing care to patients, being cognizant of the various causes of action for which the nurse may be liable.

Adapted from Structure standards. In: Sanford S, Disch J (eds): Standards for Nursing Care of the Critically Ill. Aliso Viejo, CA, American Association of Critical Care Nurses, p 16, 1989.

follow their development and publication with organized educational opportunities, such as national or regional symposia wherein practitioners become familiar with the recommendations and explore their implications in daily practice. In this way, it may be possible to achieve the dual goals of encouraging qualified practitioners to deliver a high quality of care while practicing in a fiscally responsible manner.

In the future, standards will need to address several areas of concern. Although some documents examined certain administrative issues,[27-33] many related topics remain unresolved, such as the role of the critical care specialist in relation to the primary attending physician and other consultants, as well as requirements for obtaining privileges to do procedures. These issues are extremely controversial and not well studied; thus, agreement will not be easy. Other subjects that will undoubtedly be approached by those developing standards include the management of certain disease states and the application of life-support technology. These topics are also controversial and not well studied to date. However, most practitioners would probably welcome guidelines addressing such matters as the maintenance of central venous catheters, for instance.

Individual ICU directors, thus, are faced with an ever-expanding number of standards that have been developed externally and must grapple with the issue of local application. It might be appropriate for each hospital to convene a group of critical care physicians, critical care nurses, respiratory therapists, and administrators to examine standards collaboratively and recommend how those standards should be applied in a particular ICU. This group might also begin to develop standards to meet local needs (perhaps identified through the quality assurance process) if no national standard exists. In this manner, local units participate in establishing practical standards.

On the national level, SCCM, AACN, and other concerned

organizations should continue to develop standards designed to ensure the delivery of high-quality critical care to appropriate patients in an efficient and ethical fashion. An important area of endeavor must be to secure a credible and meaningful working relationship with the various governmental health care and financing regulatory agencies. Standards developed cooperatively in this manner have the best chance of maintaining a proper balance among cost containment, quality of care, and the achievement of consumer goals. Much could be done, for example, to shape and influence the development of regionalization in the delivery of critical care as well as related educational and research activities.

In all of these endeavors, however, one should never lose sight of the basic goal of humane and efficient care of patients. Only in this way can we ensure that the patient does not get lost in the maelstrom of our technology and that care be provided in a manner that minimizes pain and discomfort and preserves the dignity of the patient.

References

1. Eddy DM: Designing a practice policy—Standards, guidelines and options. JAMA 263:3077, 1990.
2. Hirshfeld EB: Practice parameters and the malpractice liability of physicians. JAMA 263:1556, 1990.
3. Kosecoff J, Kanouse DE, Rogers WH, et al: Effects of the National Institutes of Health Consensus Development Program on physician practice. JAMA 258:2708, 1987.
4. Kanouse DE, Winkler JD, Kosecoff J, et al: Changing Medical Practice Through Technology Assessment: An Evaluation of the NIH Consensus Development Program. Ann Arbor, MI, Health Administration Press, 1989.
5. Chassin MR: Standards of care in medicine. Inquiry 25:437, 1988.
6. Eddy DM: Practice policies: Where do they come from? JAMA 263:1265, 1990.
7. Eddy DM: The challenge. JAMA 263:287, 1990.
8. Joint Commission for the Accreditation of Healthcare Organizations: Committed to quality: An introduction to the Joint Commission. Chapter 3, 1989.
9. Joint Commission for the Accreditation of Healthcare Organizations: Examples of Monitoring and Evaluation in Special Care Units. Chicago, Joint Commission for the Accreditation of Healthcare Organizations, 1988.
10. Roper W, Winkenwerder W, Hackbarth GM, et al: Effectiveness in health care: An initiative to evaluate and improve medical practice. N Engl J Med 319:1197, 1988.
11. Lee PR, Ginsburg PB, Leroy LB, et al: The Physician Payment Review Commission Report to Congress. JAMA 261:2383, 1989.
12. Epstein AM: Sounding board—The outcomes movement—Will it get us where we want to go? N Engl J Med 233:266, 1990.
13. General Accounting Office: Report to the Chairman, Subcommittee on Health, Committee on Ways and Means, House of Representatives: Medicare: Improving Quality of Care Assessment and Assurance. Publication GAO-PEMD-88-10. Washington, DC, US Government Printing Office, p 17, May 1988.
14. Brook, RH: Practice guidelines and practicing medicine. Are they compatible? JAMA 262:3027, 1989.
15. Goodman C (ed): Medical Technology Assessment Directory. A Pilot Reference to Organizations, Assessment, and Information Resources. Washington, DC, National Academy Press, p 27, 1988.
16. US Preventive Services Task Force: Guide to Clinical Preventive Services: An Assessment of the Effectiveness of 169 Interventions. Baltimore, Williams & Wilkins, 1989.
17. Fink A, Kosecoff J, Chassin M, et al: Consensus methods: Characteristics and guidelines for use. Am J Public Health 74:979, 1984.
18. Lomas J: The consensus process and evidence dissemination. Can Med Assoc J 134:1340, 1986.
19. Office of Medical Application of Research, National Institutes of Health: Critical care medicine. JAMA 250:798, 1983.
20. Lomas J, Anderson G, Enken M, et al: The role of evidence in the consensus process. JAMA 259:3001, 1988.
21. Eddy DM: Practice policies—What are they? JAMA 263:877, 1990.
22. Eddy DM: Guidelines for policy statements: The explicit approach. JAMA 263:2239, 1990.
23. Eddy DM: Resolving conflicts in practice policies. JAMA 264:389, 1990.
24. Lomas J, Anderson GM, Domnick-Pierre K, et al: Do practice guidelines guide practice? N Engl J Med 321:1306, 1989.
25. Knaus WA, Draper EA, Wagner DP, et al: An evaluation of outcome from intensive care in major medical centers. Ann Intern Med 104:410, 1986.

26. Robinson DJ: Legal aspects of critical care medicine: An evolving standard of care. In: Textbook of Critical Care. 2nd ed. Shoemaker WC, Ayres SM, Grenvik A, et al (eds): Philadelphia, WB Saunders, p 1474, 1989.
27. Society of Critical Care Medicine Task Force on Guidelines: Recommendations for program content for fellowship training in critical care medicine. Crit Care Med 15:971, 1987.
28. Society of Critical Care Medicine Task Force on Guidelines: Recommendations for the qualifications of a director of a fellowship training program in critical care medicine. Crit Care Med 15:977, 1987.
29. Society of Critical Care Medicine Task Force on Guidelines: Recommendations for critical care unit design. Crit Care Med 16:796, 1988.
30. Society of Critical Care Medicine Task Force on Guidelines: Recommendations for intensive care unit admission and discharge criteria. Crit Care Med 16:807, 1988.
31. Society of Critical Care Medicine Task Force on Guidelines: Recommendations for services and personnel for delivery of care in a critical care setting. Crit Care Med 16:809, 1988.
32. Society of Critical Care Medicine Task Force on Guidelines: Guidelines for the categorization of services for the critically ill patient. Crit Care Med 19:279, 1991.
33. Society of Critical Care Medicine Task Force on Guidelines: Guidelines for standards of care for patients with acute respiratory failure on mechanical ventilatory support. Crit Care Med 19:275, 1991.
34. American Association of Critical Care Nurses Standards Committee: Standards for Nursing Care of the Critically Ill. Reston, VA, Reston Publishing, p 1, 1981.

CHAPTER 7

Severity Scoring in Intensive Care Units

Donald B. Chalfin
Jeffrey S. Groeger

Intensive care physicians and practitioners continually face the task of predicting outcomes and identifying patients who may benefit from intensive care and ultimately survive hospitalization. Since the inception of intensive care units (ICUs), technologic advances in intensive care medicine have radically altered the scope of medical care to the point where prolongation of life represents the rule rather than the exception.[1] Patients and their families often seek prognostic estimates to help them make difficult decisions and cope with the physical and emotional stresses of life-threatening illness and prolonged ICU stays.

As ICUs have proliferated, the services they provide have come under careful scrutiny, especially in view of heightened concerns about growing financial and economic inequities in the health care sector. ICUs account for only 5 to 7% of all hospital beds in the United States, yet they consume between 15 and 20% of all hospital budgets, a level amounting to nearly 1% of the nation's gross national product.[2-9] Related issues focus on concerns about the effectiveness and ultimate benefit of intensive care. Some patients admitted to an ICU may receive lifesaving care that results in a return to good health, whereas ICU admission and the subsequent aggressive intervention may only prolong suffering and delay the inevitable demise of others.[10]

Limited resources and curtailed reimbursement, coupled with growing questions about the efficacy of ICU care, have dictated the need for sound, objective measures of the outcome of patient care. Implicitly and even subconsciously,

physicians in all specialties make routine prognostic assessments of patients and incorporate these intuitive predictions into clinical regimens. All too often these assessments are highly uncertain and lead to great variability in decisions concerning ICU admission and intensity of treatment.[11] Factors such as bed availability, patient age, and even personal bias and physician zeal also influence ICU admission and clinical practice.[11-16]

Because of these concerns about the growing scarcity of resources and the inherent uncertainties of qualitative clinical assessment, several quantitative indices, specific for the intensive care patient, have been developed to provide the ICU practitioner with an objective and reliable measure of severity of illness and probability of survival. The purpose of this chapter is to review the theory and application of these scoring systems, particularly as they pertain to critically ill and injured patients.

PROGNOSTIC INDICES OUTSIDE THE INTENSIVE CARE UNIT

Quantitative assessment and clinical prognostication have been increasingly incorporated into intensive care. However, scoring systems and indices have had wide use in other related clinical settings, with various levels of use and acceptance. These measures reflect the desire of physicians to comfortably group patients into clinical categories that have universal meanings with respect to therapeutic response and eventual outcome. To state that one patient is "critical" and another is "unstable" provides no reproducible clinical information, for such subjective terms may lead to many different interpretations. Furthermore, the provision of a subjective ordinal rating, such as a statement that a patient's angina "is a 9 on a scale of 1 to 10" or that an illness is a "3+ or 4+" does little to reduce these intuitive differences.[17, 18]

Some of the more familiar empirical scoring indices were developed for cardiovascular patients. In 1967, Killip and Kimball described a method of classifying patients with acute myocardial infarctions based on a simple and easily reproducible clinical classification in which estimated mortality correlated closely with each class[19] (Table 7–1). Forrester

TABLE 7–1

KILLIP'S CLASSIFICATION OF PATIENTS WITH ACUTE MYOCARDIAL INFARCTION

Class	Definition	Patients With Acute Myocardial Infarction Admitted to ICU in This Category (%)	Approximate Mortality (%)*
I	Absence of rales over the lung fields and absence of S₃	30–40	8
II	Rales over 50% or less of the lung fields or the presence of an S₃	30–50	30
III	Rales over more than 50% of the lung fields (frequently pulmonary edema)	5–10	44
IV	Shock	10	80–100

*Estimated mortality in the 1960s. Mortality still rises with increased class, although the values in each class are lower today than in the 1960s.

Adapted from Killip T, Kimball JT: Treatment of myocardial infarction in a coronary care unit: A two-year experience with 250 patients. Am J Cardiol 20:457, 1967.

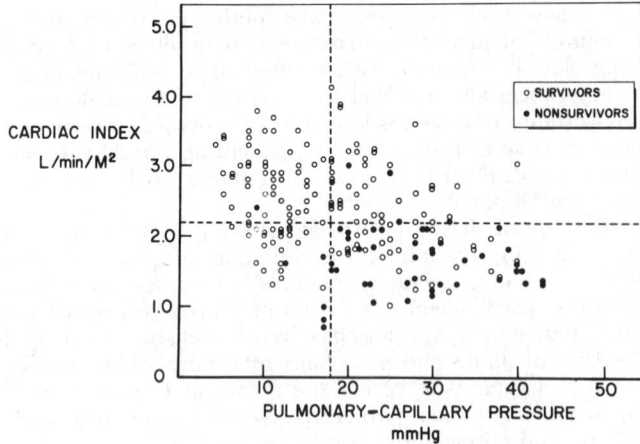

Figure 7–1. Relation between pulmonary capillary pressure and cardiac index in 200 patients at the time of admission to Cedars-Sinai Medical Center Myocardial Infarction Research Unit. The dotted lines are placed at the levels of 18 mm Hg for pulmonary capillary pressure and 2.2 L/min/m² for cardiac index. There is a wide degree of variability in left ventricular performance in patients with acute myocardial infarction, and mortality rate increases as cardiac performance deteriorates. (From Forrester JS, Diamond G, Chatterjee K, et al: Medical therapy of acute myocardial infarction by application of hemodynamic subsets. Reprinted, by permission of the New England Journal of Medicine, 295;1361, 1976.)

and coworkers also developed a highly objective and reproducible measure of outcome assessment for patients with acute myocardial infarction based on hemodynamic variables (cardiac index and pulmonary capillary wedge pressure) obtained via pulmonary arterial catheter.[20, 21] This index (Fig. 7–1) has been useful as an adjunctive guide to assist physicians in the selection of appropriate clinical strategies. As in the Killip classification, patient outcome in the Forrester schema is inversely related to increasing class, with a progressively worsening prognosis for each successive class.

Related to these indices are the objective measures that assess cardiovascular functional disability: the New York Heart Association Functional Classification, the Canadian Cardiovascular Society Functional Classification, and the Specific Activity Scale[22–25] (Table 7–2). Like the Killip and Forrester systems, these methods are easily reproducible and provide the clinician with meaningful measures of patient performance and therapeutic response. A physician may base therapy on the flux in a patient's objective functional status and clinical information. Evaluation (and communi-

TABLE 7–2

A COMPARISON OF THREE METHODS OF ASSESSING CARDIOVASCULAR DISABILITY

Class	New York Heart Association Functional Classification	Canadian Cardiovascular Society Functional Classification	Specific Activity Scale
I	Patients with cardiac disease but without resulting limitations of physical activity. Ordinary physical activity does not cause undue fatigue, palpitation, dyspnea, or anginal pain.	Ordinary physical activity, such as walking and climbing stairs, does not cause angina. Angina with strenuous or rapid or prolonged exertion at work or recreation.	Patients can perform to completion any activity requiring ≥7 metabolic equivalents, e.g., can carry 24 lb up eight steps; carry objects that weigh 80 lb; do outdoor work (shovel snow, spade soil); do recreational activities (skiing, basketball, squash, handball, jog/walk 5 mph).
II	Patients with cardiac disease resulting in slight limitation of physical activity. They are comfortable at rest. Ordinary physical activity results in fatigue, palpitation, dyspnea, or anginal pain.	Slight limitation of ordinary activity. Walking or climbing stairs rapidly, walking uphill, walking or stair climbing after meals, in cold, in wind, or when under emotional stress, or only during the few hours after awakening. Walking more than two blocks on the level and climbing more than one flight of ordinary stairs at a normal pace and in normal conditions.	Patients can perform to completion any activity requiring ≥5 metabolic equivalents but cannot and do not perform to completion activities requiring ≥7 metabolic equivalents, e.g., have sexual intercourse without stopping, garden, rake, weed, roller skate, dance fox trot, walk at 4 mph on level ground.
III	Patients with cardiac disease resulting in marked limitation of physical activity. They are comfortable at rest. Less than ordinary physical activity causes fatigue, palpitation, dyspnea, or anginal pain.	Marked limitation of ordinary physical activity. Walking one to two blocks on the level and climbing more than one flight in normal conditions.	Patients can perform to completion any activity requiring ≥2 metabolic equivalents but cannot and do not perform to completion any activities requiring ≥5 metabolic equivalents, e.g., shower without stopping, strip and make bed, clean windows, walk 2.5 mph, bowl, play golf, dress without stopping.
IV	Patients with cardiac disease resulting in inability to carry on any physical activity without discomfort. Symptoms of cardiac insufficiency or of the anginal syndrome may be present even at rest. If any physical activity is undertaken, discomfort is increased.	Inability to carry on any physical activity without discomfort—anginal syndrome *may be* present at rest.	Patients cannot or do not perform to completion activities requiring ≥2 metabolic equivalents. *Cannot* carry out activities listed above (Specific Activity Scale, class III).

From Goldman L, Hashimoto B, Cook EF, et al: Comparative reproducibility and validity of systems for assessing cardiovascular functional class: Advantages of a new specific activity scale. Circulation 64:1227–1234, 1981, by permission of the American Heart Association, Inc.

cation) is more meaningful when it can be stated that a patient improved from a New York Heart Association class III to a class II, as opposed to a vague report that a patient "got better."

The clinical and pathologic staging of malignant disease is analogous to scoring indices, as it conveys a distinct and uniform meaning with respect to time-dependent prognosis and specific therapeutic alternatives. Similarly, systems for the classification of hepatic and pancreatic disease have also gained wide clinical acceptance. Child and Turcotte described a system for determining outcome and prognosis based on hepatic functional reserve for patients with liver failure requiring surgical shunts. This system, referred to as the Child-Turcott Classification or Child's Criteria, stratifies patients into three different categories based on five simple laboratory and clinical criteria: serum bilirubin level, serum albumin level, presence of ascites, neurologic impairment, and nutritional status[26] (Table 7–3). Scales designed to aid in the determination of severity of illness and guide therapeutic decisions have also been developed and subsequently disseminated for patients with acute pancreatitis. For example, Ranson and colleagues defined a scale of 11 objective criteria obtained either at presentation or during the first 48 hours,[27–29] and Imrie and coworkers derived a closely related measure based on patient age and eight other laboratory parameters[30] (Table 7–4).

The identification of preoperative factors predictive of surgical risk has also been widely studied and reduced to objective indices. Anesthesiologists often use a simple yet comprehensive scoring system to assess the risk for perioperative morbidity.[31–33] This system, referred to as the American Society of Anesthesia Physical Status Classification, is based on the routine preoperative history and physical examination and classifies patients into one of five distinct classes: the first class represents patients with no significant systemic disease and the fifth category represents the most seriously ill patients who are not expected to survive, even with surgery (Table 7–5). Although the American Society of Anesthesia system is capable of meaningfully assessing the risk of noncardiac perioperative complications, it often fails to identify and predict cardiac morbidity for noncardiac surgery.[33] To this end, Goldman and coworkers developed a quantitative tool capable of assessing cardiac risk. They prospectively studied 1001 consecutive patients over the age of 40.[34–36] Using multivariate discriminate analysis, they identified nine independent variables that correlated with the subsequent development of life-threatening cardiac complications (Table 7–6). From these variables, a numeric scale was derived to classify patients into four distinct groups for the ultimate purpose of stratifying patients according to their probability of developing morbid or mortal cardiac

events. This Multifactorial Cardiac Risk Index ranges from 0 to 53; the risk of serious cardiac complication rises with increased score and for each successive class. Class I patients (5 points or less) have a 0.7% chance of morbidity and a 0.2% mortality rate. For class II patients (6 to 12 points), the risk for complication rises to 5% and the risk of death increases 10-fold to 2%. Class III patients (13 to 25 points) have the same risk of death as the class II group, but the probability of serious cardiac complication more than doubles to 11%. For class IV patients (26 points or more), the complication rate exceeds 25% and the mortality rate rises dramatically to 56%.

Goldman's index has remained useful because of its statistical validity and clinical applicability.[16, 36] The index is easy to apply and is based on the routine clinical assessment and examination that physicians perform for all patients with cardiac disease. Likewise, the Glasgow Coma Scale (GCS), an index with perhaps the greatest familiarity and acceptance, has attained broad use because of its underlying ease and implicit relationship to clinical practice. The GCS, used for grading the severity of neurologic impairment, provides

---

TABLE 7–4

MULTIPLE CRITERIA FOR THE PREDICTION OF SEVERE ACUTE PANCREATITIS*

Ranson et al†	Imrie et al‡
On admission	**During the first 48 h**
Age > 55 y	Arterial Po_2 < 60 torr
Blood dextrose > 11 mmol/L	Serum albumin < 32 g/L
White blood cell count > 16 × 10⁹/L	Serum calcium < 2.0 mmol/L
SGOT > 120 IU/L	White blood cell count > 15 × 10⁹/L
LDH > 350 IU/L	SGOT > 100 IU/L
During the first 48 h	LDH > 600 IU/L
Fall in hemocrit > 10%	Blood dextrose > 10 mmol/L
Serum calcium < 2.0 mmol/L	Plasma urea > 16 mmol/L
Base deficit > 4.0 mmol/L	Age > 55 y
Blood urea increase > 1.0 mmol/L	
Fluid sequestration > 61	
Arterial Po_2 < 60 torr	

Severe disease is indicated by the presence of three or more factors in each case.

*SGOT = serum glutamic-oxaloacetic transaminase; LDH = lactate dehydrogenase.

†Ranson JHC, Rifkind KM, Turner JW: Prognostic signs and nonoperative peritoneal lavage in acute pancreatitis. Surg Gynecol Obstet 143:209, 1976.

‡Imrie CW, Benjamin IS, Ferguson JC, et al: A single-center double-blind trial of Trasylol therapy in primary acute pancreatitis. Br J Surg 65:337, 1978.

From McMahon MJ, Playforth MJ, Pickford IR: A comparative study of methods for the prediction of severity of attacks of acute pancreatitis. Br J Surg 67:22, 1980, by permission of the publishers Butterworth-Heinemann Ltd.

TABLE 7–3

CRITERIA FOR CHILD-TURCOTTE CLASSIFICATION

Parameter	Group A	Group B	Group C
Serum bilirubin (mg %)	<2.0	2.0–3.0	>3.0
Serum albumin (g %)	>3.5	3.0–3.5	<3.0
Ascites	None	Easily controlled	Poorly controlled
Neurologic disorder	None	Minimal	Advanced "coma"
Nutrition	Excellent	Good	Poor, "wasting"

From Child CG, Turcotte JG: Surgery and portal hypertension. In: Child CG (ed): The Liver and Portal Hypertension. Philadelphia, WB Saunders, p 50, 1964.

TABLE 7–5

AMERICAN SOCIETY OF ANESTHESIA PHYSICAL STATUS CLASSIFICATION

Class	Description
1	Normal
2	Mild systemic disease
3	Systemic disease that limits activity but does not incapacitate
4	Incapacitating, life-threatening disease
5	Not expected to survive with or without operation

TABLE 7-6

COMPUTATION OF MULTIFACTORIAL INDEX SCORE TO ESTIMATE CARDIAC RISK IN NONCARDIAC SURGERY

Factor	Points
S₃ gallop or jugular venous distention on preoperative physical examination	11
Transmural or subendocardial myocardial infarction in the previous 6 mo	10
Premature ventricular beats, more than 5/min documented at any time	7
Rhythm other than sinus or presence of premature atrial contractions on last preoperative electrocardiogram	7
Age over 70 y	5
Emergency operation	4
Intrathoracic, intraperitoneal, or aortic site of surgery	3
Evidence for important valvular aortic stenosis*	3
Poor general medical condition†	3

*Findings of a cardiologist's examination, noninvasive testing, or cardiac catheterization.

†As evidenced by electrolyte abnormalities (potassium < 3.0 mEq/L; HCO₃ < 20 mEq/L), renal insufficiency (blood urea nitrogen > 50 mg/dL; creatinine > 3.0 mg/dL), abnormal blood gases (Po₂ < 60 mm Hg; Pco₂ > 50 mm Hg), abnormal liver status (elevated aspartate transaminase or signs at physical examination of chronic liver disease), or any condition that has caused the patient to be chronically bedridden.

Adapted, with permission, from Goldman L, Cardiac risks and complications of noncardiac surgery. Ann Intern Med 1983; 98:504–513.

a relatively objective measure of brain injury and greatly eliminates interobserver, subjective assessment of coma.[37–39] As Kirby stated, coma is usually defined by an inability to open one's eyes, speak, or follow simple commands, and the GCS scores patients on the basis of their ability to perform these functions[40] (Table 7–7). The GCS ranges from 3 to 15, and severe neurologic impairment is usually present with a score of 8 or less. Patients with a GCS score of 7 or less usually require mechanical ventilation, and patients with a GCS score of 3 or those without any spontaneous motor response, verbal response, or eye opening have poor ultimate prognoses.

OUTCOME ASSESSMENT AND SCORING IN THE INTENSIVE CARE UNIT

Reasons for Scoring in the Intensive Care Unit

The GCS, the Multifactorial Cardiac Risk Index, and other related clinical scoring systems represent attempts by physicians to provide accurate estimates of patient outcome and reduce subjective implications to well-delineated, objective, numeric measures.[17] As the range and complexity of clinical practice in the ICU grew, it became apparent that appropriate standards and a common language to express prognostic information were needed.[18, 41–46] The many questions and issues raised by the rapid and continuing expansion and scope of ICU care accelerated this need. The need for more objective measures of severity was also prompted by concerns about identifying which patients truly benefit from intensive care and which ones do not.[47] Closely related to these issues are concerns about the economics and cost-effectiveness of intensive care and the implicit and often difficult questions related to the marginal effectiveness and diminishing returns of services provided to critical, often moribund patients.[8, 47–49] Profound accomplishments often coexist in proximity to wanton waste in the ICU, and efforts are rarely made to distinguish between these extremes.[50] As Detsky and others have shown, patients who consume the most resources in ICUs are often those with the lowest chances for survi-

val.[49, 51–53] These concerns, as Sax and Charlson stated, were strong enough to lead a National Institutes of Health consensus panel to recommend delineated restriction of ICU beds for patients with no meaningful or probable chance of recovery.[54, 55]

These economic concerns are joined by demands for universal measures of comparison and for uniform, unambiguous methods of communicating both obvious and subtle similarities and differences. The increase in clinical alternatives and improved diagnostic and therapeutic options dictate the need for standardized measures of comparison. The variable interhospital scope of ICU services and the variable range of patients served greatly limit the usual crude comparisons based on simple statistics such as mortality rate, length of stay, and morbid incidence. Statistically valid indices provide physicans and researchers with precise ways to describe the patients they treat and serve. Changes in outcome and response that may or may not occur can be documented, and difficult scientific and clinical questions may thus be answered quantitatively. Other issues concerning ICU performance and quality assurance can also be addressed. Prognostic scoring and probabilistic models allow verifiable standards of care and models of performance to be established.[42, 56]

Outcome Determinants in the Intensive Care Unit

Prognostic models such as the Killip and Forrester classifications, which were developed for specific specialties or disease processes, differ from the broader ICU models of prediction in that their applications are confined to relatively specific groups of patients or diseases. Intensive care medicine differs from most other specialties in that the scope of practice is not limited to any one organ system or age group. The intensivist must have a keen understanding of pathophysiologic processes for a wide spectrum of diseases and patients and must possess an intimate knowledge of the different approaches to patient management used by all clinical specialties. At a more fundamental level, the ICU practitioner must understand the basic factors that determine patient outcome and that consequently must be incorporated into any predictive or prognostic instrument. Furthermore, intensivists must recognize and explicitly stipulate the intentions, implications, and goals of these predictive models and tasks.

Knaus has noted that outcome is influenced by the di-

TABLE 7-7

GLASGOW COMA SCALE

Sign	Finding	Value
Eye opening	Spontaneous	4
	To voice	3
	To pain	2
	None	1
Verbal response (arousal with voice or noxious stimulus)	Oriented	5
	Confused	4
	Inappropriate speech	3
	Incomprehensible speech	2
	None	1
Motor response (response to command or noxious stimulus)	Obeys command	6
	Localizes pain	5
	Withdraws from pain	4
	Flexion (decorticate posturing)	3
	Extension (decerebrate posturing)	2
	None	1

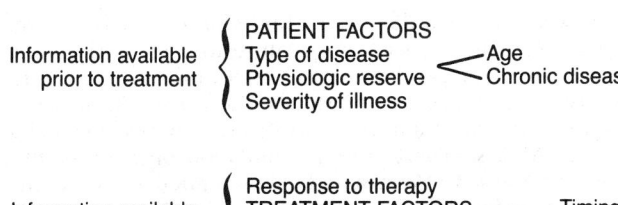

Information available
prior to treatment { PATIENT FACTORS
Type of disease —— Age
Physiologic reserve —— Chronic disease
Severity of illness

Information available
after treatment { Response to therapy
TREATMENT FACTORS —— Timing
Type of therapy available —— Process
Use of application of therapy

Figure 7–2. Determinants of outcome from an acute illness. (From Knaus WA: The science of prediction and its implications for the clinician today. Theor Surg 3:93, 1988.)

chotomous effects of both patient factors and treatment factors.[57] Patient factors include the type of disease, underlying physiologic reserve (which is closely related to age and chronic disease), and the severity or acuity of illness. Treatment factors consist primarily of the specific type of therapy provided, along with its timing and the method of administration (Fig. 7–2). The importance of these latter, interrelated treatment factors can be illustrated by some of the newer thrombolytic agents for acute myocardial infarctions. These agents may be efficacious in restoring coronary artery patency and reducing myocardial damage when used in the appropriate patient population during the first few hours after the acute event. However, they also have diminished efficacy in certain cardiac conditions and are associated with significant side effects and clinical contraindications.[58–60]

Specific diagnostic entities are obviously associated with outcome. However, a practitioner must recognize the limitations and restrictions of narrow diagnostic labels and groups.[61] As Figure 7–2 shows, diagnosis is only one of several factors that influence ultimate response. In the multidisciplinary nature of intensive care and acute critical illness, diagnosis may be a small and perhaps even minor determinant of inevitable outcome. Critically ill patients are often afflicted by several simultaneous processes and suffer from multiple organ system failure. Thus, no single disease entity will encompass the total "nature" of their illness, and therefore patients should not and perhaps cannot be grouped into any single diagnostic category. To accurately reflect the scope of critical illness, ICU scoring systems should therefore attempt to incorporate the many interrelated and often subtle factors that ultimately determine therapeutic response and clinical outcome.

SPECIFIC INDICES IN THE INTENSIVE CARE UNIT

The earliest studies on outcome assessment in the ICU were performed simultaneously with the development of the cardiac indices of Killip and Kimball, Forrester, and Norris.[19–21, 62] Yet, as Farmer noted, these first attempts were primarily retrospective and generally descriptive.[63] As awareness of the need for appropriate assessment grew, statistical and mathematic models were increasingly adopted by researchers in this area. Descriptions and rationales of the major and most familiar ICU scoring systems are presented here.

Therapeutic Intervention Scoring System

In 1974, Cullen and coworkers devised the Therapeutic Intervention Scoring System (TISS) based on their experience with the ICU population at the Massachusetts General Hospital.[64] The basic premise of this early index was that severity of illness can be determined and quantified by the amount and level of specific therapeutic interventions. According to Cullen and Nemeskal, "regardless of the diagnosis

TABLE 7–8
EXAMPLES FROM THE THERAPEUTIC INTERVENTION SCORING SYSTEM 1983 UPDATE

4 points
   Pulmonary arterial catheter
   Intra-aortic balloon pump
   Controlled mechanical ventilation (with or without positive end-expiratory pressure)
   Vasoactive drug therapy (more than one drug)
3 points
   Chest tubes
   Continuous positive airway pressure
   Intermittent mandatory or assisted ventilation
   Arterial catheter
2 points
   Central venous pressure
   Two peripheral intravenous catheters
   Spontaneous ventilation via endotracheal tube or tracheostomy (T piece or tracheostomy mask)
   Multiple dressing changes
1 point
   Electrocardiographic monitoring
   One peripheral intravenous catheter
   Routine dressing changes
   Urinary catheter

From AR Keene, DJ Cullen: Therapeutic Intervention Scoring System: Update 1983, Crit Care Med, 11, 1, 1–3, © by Williams & Wilkins, 1983.

causing critical illness, the physiologic derangements requiring therapeutic support result from the severity of the illness."[65]

Determination of a specific TISS score involves daily assessment of all therapeutic interventions for a given ICU patient during the previous 24 hours of care. Briefly, each therapeutic measure or procedure is assigned an integer value between 1 and 4, and the "points" for all of the interventions are totaled to yield a single score or measure (Table 7–8). As intuition and the basic premise of TISS dictate, a worsening condition should result in a higher TISS value, secondary to more aggressive management. Conversely, clinical improvement should lead to less intervention and a lower total score. TISS was subsequently updated and revised in the early 1980s to reflect the changing patterns and technologic innovations of ICU care.[66]

TISS essentially stratifies patients into four major classes (Table 7–9), of which the class II, III, and IV patients generally require ICU care.[65, 66] Class I patients do not usually require admission to an ICU. As Table 7–9 shows, the other three classes require progressively closer monitoring and more aggressive interventions. Knaus has suggested that the therapeutic interventions of TISS be divided into four major groups that closely match Cullens's classifications: standard care, technology-intensive ICU monitoring, personnel-intensive ICU monitoring, and active therapy.[49, 67] As expected from the basic premise of TISS, higher scores and

TABLE 7–9
THERAPEUTIC INTERVENTION SCORING SYSTEM: PATIENT CLASSES

Class	Description
I	Routine postanesthesia care and standard floor care
II	Close observation and monitoring
III	Extensive nursing care
IV	Extensive physician and nursing care

Adapted from Cullen DJ, Nemeskal AR: Therapeutic intervention scoring system (TISS). Probl Crit Care 3:545, 1989.

classes have been correlated with increased in-hospital mortality.[49, 66, 67]

Several administrative, management, and clinical uses have been suggested for TISS. Aside from its use as a measure of patient acuity, TISS has been applied to the following situations: (1) utilization review or determination of the appropriate allocation of ICU facilities; (2) cost and economic analysis of ICU care; (3) clinical stratification according to severity of illness; and (4) determination of appropriate nurse/patient ratios.[64, 66] With respect to the latter, Keene and Cullen have suggested that a class IV patient may require the services of one or more intensive care nurses to provide a satisfactory level of care, whereas four class I patients may be looked after, in most cases, by a single nurse.[66]

As the first quantitative measure of ICU services, TISS received great attention and is still applied to multiple ICU situations. However, it also has limitations. The basic premise of TISS—that the amount and level of therapeutic interventions patients receive are directly related to the underlying pathologic processes and physiologic derangements—is certainly subject to question. Also, TISS provides only information concerning therapy and does not specifically measure physiologic derangements and alterations.[49, 66] Even if the underlying premise of TISS is accepted, one must recognize that the relationship between therapy provided and patient illness may represent an indirect association.

In addition to clinical severity, factors that determine which services are provided to patients range from access and availability to individual physician preferences and specialty bias. Interinstitutional variations may also influence the type and level of care. For example, tertiary care facilities and university medical centers would be expected to provide a broader and perhaps more aggressive range of services than voluntary community hospitals. TISS requires periodic revision to reflect the dynamic nature of ICU care, and it must at least be tailored to specific institutional and physician practices. Furthermore, the collection and interpretation of TISS data require substantial, labor-intensive effort, as well as proficiency in data analysis and interpretation. Cullen and colleagues suggested that data collection be performed by trained personnel, preferably intensive care nurses, who are familiar with ICU care.[64, 66] This endeavor represents a significant commitment and undertaking.

Acute Physiology and Chronic Health Evaluation

In 1981, Knaus and colleagues published the first version of the Acute Physiology and Chronic Health Evaluation (APACHE) prognostic scoring system.[68] Like TISS, APACHE was designed in response to the need for standardized and uniform information capable of classifying ICU patients. However, APACHE differs from TISS in that it is based primarily on data reflecting a patient's physiologic status and underlying reserve. The basic premise and hypothesis of APACHE are that, as Knaus stated, "outcome from an acute illness is in part related to the degree of disturbances in the body's major physiologic organ systems and that the risk imposed by these physiologic abnormalities could be estimated on the basis of deviations from normal physiology and on past experience treating acutely ill patients."[69]

The original APACHE system consisted of two parts: a physiology score (termed the Acute Physiology Score [APS]) and an assessment of preadmission health status (or Chronic Health Evaluation [CHE]). The APS was derived from 34 distinct physiologic measurements that included such parameters as vital signs, hematocrit, serum electrolytes, urine output, liver function tests, and the GCS. These measurements were obtained during the first 32 hours of ICU care. Patients were assigned a score from 0 to 4 for each of the 34 parameters, depending on the level of derangement. In the case of multiple tests or values, the worst-case scenario was used for evaluation. All scores were summed to yield a singular APS, similar to the accumulation of TISS points. As Knaus and coworkers stated: "The higher the score, the sicker the patient."[68]

The chronic health evaluation or the preadmission health status was determined by a careful review of the patient's medical history, including such factors as functional status, the presence of comorbid conditions (e.g., diabetes mellitus or chronic renal insufficiency), and the extent of a patient's medical attention and care during the 3 to 6 months before admission. As a result of this review, patients were placed into one of four different categories, labeled A to D. Class A represented an individual with no functional limitation or no prior medical history, and class D represented either a patient with severe restriction secondary to underlying poor health or a bedridden or institutionalized individual. Thus, the original APACHE score consisted of two parts that reflected both acute illness and baseline status. Patients received a numeric score to indicate the acute physiologic processes and a letter designation to account for pre-ICU condition.[70]

The specific parameters for the APACHE score were developed by two of the original authors and five other intensive care practitioners. The APACHE system was subsequently validated over an 8-month period using a data base derived from 582 consecutive ICU admissions at the George Washington University Hospital and 223 consecutive ICU admissions at a neighboring community hospital. The APS correlated with both in-hospital mortality and the number of therapeutic interventions as measured by TISS. Each additional APS point, for example, raised the probability of an in-hospital death by approximately 2% in both the community and the tertiary care setting. A strong relationship was also noted between chronic health status and short-term survival. In view of these results, authors suggested that APACHE could be used for collective assessments and comparisons of ICU patients in such situations as utilization review, evaluation of therapeutic efficacy, and case mix controls.[70]

Simplified Acute Physiology Score

APACHE was significantly limited, perhaps more than TISS, by the need for significant data collection by individuals acutely familiar with the important issues of intensive care management. The APS required the collection of 34 parameters during the first 32 hours of ICU care, many of which were recorded several times or even continuously during this period. In addition, because certain parameters were not measured for all patients or were not even routinely collected, no points would accrue and thus these measures would be implicitly recorded as normal.[70, 71]

In response to these limitations, LeGall and colleagues in the early 1980s described a Simplified Acute Physiology Score (SAPS) to facilitate outcome comparison among similar groups of ICU patients.[70, 72] Instead of a 34-parameter physiology score plus another measure of preadmission health, SAPS employed a single, 14-variable scale consisting of 13 easily collected parameters plus patient age (Table 7–10). Data for SAPS are collected during the first 24 hours of ICU admission and, as with APACHE, are assigned on a scale of 0 to 4 (the grade for age, however, is doubled) to reflect acute physiologic derangement. Scoring with SAPS involves far less time and results in fewer data omissions.[70]

SAPS was initially validated with 679 successive patients

TABLE 7–10

SIMPLIFIED ACUTE PHYSIOLOGY SCORE VARIABLES

Age (years)
Heart rate (beats/min)
Systolic blood pressure (mm Hg)
Body temperature (°C)
Spontaneous respiratory rate (breaths/min)
or
Ventilation or continuous positive airway pressure (yes/no)
Urine output (L/24 h)
Blood urea nitrogen level (mmol/L)
Hematocrit (%)
White blood cell count (10^3/mm³)
Serum glucose level (mmol/L)
Serum potassium level (mEq/L)
Serum HCO_3 (mEq/L)
Glasgow Coma Scale score (3–15)

From JR LeGall, P Loirat, A Alperovitch, et al: A simplified acute physiology score for ICU patients, Crit Care Med, 12, 11, 975–977, © by Williams & Wilkins, 1984.

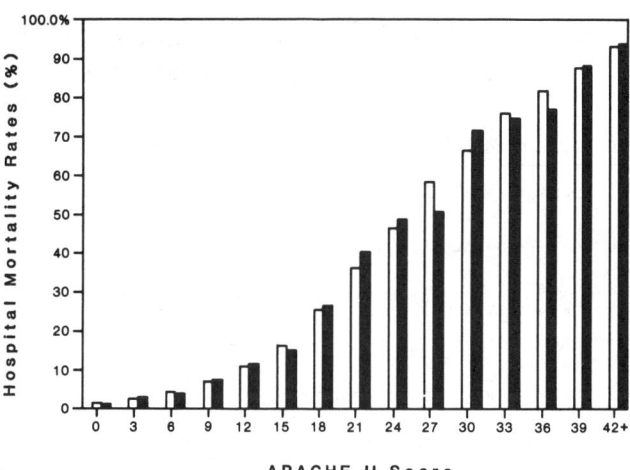

Figure 7–3. APACHE II scores and hospital mortality rates. (Reproduced, with permission, from Knaus WA, Draper EA, Wagner DP, et al, An evaluation of outcome from intensive care in major medical centers. Ann Intern Med 1986; 104:410–418.)

admitted to eight different ICUs throughout France. Analysis of receiver operating characteristic curves for both SAPS and the APS of APACHE demonstrated similar predictive ability.[72] Based on a French multicenter study of 38 ICUs (3687 patients), researchers noted a close correlation among SAPS score, severity of illness, and in-hospital mortality. The correlation was particularly evident when patients were divided into three categories: medical, surgical-elective, and surgical-emergent[73] (Table 7–11). SAPS has been used as a measure of severity and for group comparisons in French and other European hospitals.

THE APACHE II

Knaus and colleagues subsequently updated and simplified APACHE with the introduction of APACHE II in 1985.[74] APACHE II is based on the same premise as its predecessor, but it requires only 12 variables for the APS, instead of the 34 variables used to determine the APS for the original APACHE. In addition, the APS total is combined with points for age and chronic health to yield a single APACHE II score that may be more inclusively reflective of both pre-morbid state and acute critical illness.[74] Table 7–12 shows the format and mechanism of APACHE II.

Whereas the initial APACHE system was validated with only 805 patients admitted to two hospitals, APACHE II was subsequently tested on 5030 patients treated in 13 different tertiary medical centers in the United States.[75] Total

TABLE 7–11

CONVERTING SIMPLIFIED ACUTE PHYSIOLOGY SCORE TO PROBABILITY OF HOSPITAL MORTALITY

SAPS	Medical Probability of Mortality (%)	Surgical (Unscheduled) Probability of Mortality (%)	Surgical (Scheduled) Probability of Mortality (%)
0–4	1.8	6.8	0.0
5–9	7.9	8.3	0.9
10–14	14.5	16.8	3.1
15–19	34.9	38.1	13.3
20–24	50.3	61.0	13.0
25–29	76.1	88.9	66.7
30+	82.4	77.8	–

From LeGall JR, Loirat P, Alperovitch A: The Simplified Acute Physiology Score (SAPS): Probl Crit Care 3:581, 1989.

APACHE II scores correlated significantly with hospital mortality; however, closer and direct correlations were observed when patients were classified into distinct medical or surgical diagnostic categories (Fig. 7–3). For each of these diagnostic categories, a group estimate of the probability of mortality may be obtained by logistic regression.[76] APACHE II has also compared favorably with other severity scores and methods.[42, 76, 77] It is important to note, however, that certain diagnoses or classes of patients cannot be classified under the APACHE II system. These include those admitted to ICUs for management of burns or after coronary artery bypass surgery; such patients were not included in the initial data analysis.[74, 75]

More than any other system and perhaps because of its broad visibility, APACHE II brought the "science" of prediction into the clinical and investigational mainstream of intensive care. In addition to its use in administration, planning, quality assurance, and resource allocation, APACHE II has been utilized in clinical trials to randomize patients and to evaluate the therapeutic efficacy of new clinical measures. For example, in investigations on the use of monoclonal antibodies in the treatment of sepsis, APACHE II scores were used to evaluate the level of acuity and make comparisons with studies of similar agents.[78, 79] APACHE II has also demonstrated that differences in outcome among hospitals may be related to issues of organization and communication between physicians and nurses.[75] APACHE II has also been incorporated into health care financing administration for use in severity adjustment[76, 80, 81] and has further been applied to international comparisons of ICUs.[82, 83]

THE APACHE III

The APACHE system was updated in a large prospective multicenter study.[84, 85, 85a] Stated goals of the APACHE III study include improved accuracy of the scoring system; development of a predictive instrument to estimate hospital mortality for individual patients on a scientific basis; and evaluation of process of care indicators, including delayed ICU admission, complications and iatrogenesis, and unmonitored or untreated abnormal parameters.[84, 85, 85a]

The APACHE III study prospectively evaluated 17,440 medical and surgical ICU admissions at 40 U.S. hospitals between May 1988 and November 1989. The likelihood of survival to hospital discharge was determined from data that reflected acute physiologic abnormalities, patient age, co-

TABLE 7–12

THE APACHE II SEVERITY OF DISEASE CLASSIFICATION SYSTEM

Physiologic Variable	High Abnormal Range				Low Abnormal Range				
	+4	+3	+2	+1	0	+1	+2	+3	+4
Temperature, rectal (°C)	≥41	39–40.9		38.5–38.9	36–38.4	34–35.9	32–33.9	30–31.9	≤29.9
Mean arterial pressure, mm Hg	≥180	130–159	110–129		70–109		50–69		≤49
Heart rate (ventricular response)	≥180	140–179	110–139		70–109		55–69	40–54	≤39
Respiratory rate (nonventilated or ventilated)	≥50	35–49		25–34	12–24	10–11	6–9		≤5
Oxygenation P_{AO_2} – Pa_{O_2} or Pa_{O_2} (mm Hg) a. F_{IO_2} ≥ 0.5 record P_{AO_2} – Pa_{O_2}	≥500	350–499	200—349		<200				
b. F_{IO_2} < 0.5 record only Pa_{O_2}					Po_2>70	Po_2 61–70		Po_2 55–60	Po_2<55
Arterial pH	≥7.7	7.6–7.69		7.5–7.59	7.33–7.49		7.25–7.32	·7.15–7.24	<7.15
Serum sodium (mmol/L)	≥180	160–179	155–159	150–154	130–149		120–129	111–119	<110
Serum potassium (mmol/L)	≥7	6–6.9		5.5–5.9	3.5–5.4	3–3.4	2.5–2.9		<2.5
Serum creatinine (mg/100 mL) (double point score for acute renal failure)	≥3.5	2–3.4	1.5–1.9		0.6–1.4		<0.6		
Hematocrit (%)	≥60		50–59.9	46–49.9	30–45.9		20–29.9		<20
White blood cell count (total/mm³) (in 1000s)	≥40		20–39.9	15–19.9	3–14.9		1–2.9		<1
Glasgow Coma Score (GCS): Score = 15 minus actual GCS									
A Total APS: Sum of the 12 individual variable points Serum HCO_3 (venous, mmol/L) (Not preferred; use if no arterial blood gases)	≥52	41–51.9		32–40.9	22–31.9		18–21.9	15–17.9	<15

B **Age points:**
Assign points to age as follows:

Age (y)	Points
≤44	0
45–54	2
55–64	3
65–74	5
≥75	6

C **Chronic health points**
If the patient has a history of severe organ system insufficiency or is immunocompromised, assign points as follows:
a. for nonoperative or emergency postoperative patients—5 points
  or
b. for elective postoperative patients—2 points

APACHE II SCORE
Sum of A + B + C
A APS points _____
B Age points _____
C Chronic health points _____
Total APACHE II _____

Definitions
Organ insufficiency or immunocompromised state must have been evident prior to this hospital admission and conform to the following criteria:

Liver: Biopsy-proven cirrhosis and documented portal hypertension; episodes of past upper gastrointestinal bleeding attributed to portal hypertension; or prior episodes of hepatic failure/encephalopathy/coma.

Cardiovascular: New York Heart Association class IV.

Respiratory: chronic restrictive, obstructive, or vascular disease resulting in severe exercise restriction, i.e., unable to climb stairs or perform household duties; or documented chronic hypoxia, hypercapnia, secondary polycythemia, severe pulmonary hypertension (>40 mm Hg), or respirator dependency.

Renal: Receiving chronic dialysis.

Immunocompromised: The patient has received therapy that suppresses resistance to infection, e.g., immunosuppression, chemotherapy, radiation, long-term or recent high-dose steroids, or has a disease that is sufficiently advanced to suppress resistance to infection, e.g., leukemia, lymphoma, AIDS.

From WA Knaus, EA Draper, DP Wagner, et al, APACHE II: A severity of disease classification system, Crit Care Med, 13, 10, 818–829, © by Williams & Wilkins, 1985.

morbid status, pre-existing functional abilities and limitations, medical and surgical diagnoses, and location of the patient immediately before ICU admission. Two prognostic options were developed from this study: (1) a numeric APACHE III score (range of 0 to 299, mean of 50) for risk stratification of patient groups and (2) a predictive equation to provide a quantitative, objective, and reproducible estimate of individual mortality on admission to the ICU and for each day thereafter.[85a] The results of the APACHE III study show some promise for the expanded use of scoring systems in ICU quality assurance and clinical research, and they may even assist clinicians in the decision-making process for individual patients. Future reports on the implications, validation, and potential uses of APACHE III are eagerly awaited.

Mortality Prediction Models

The original APACHE, APACHE II, and SAPS are similar in that a unique numeric score is assigned to patients with certain physiologic derangements based on measurable parameters and variables. The total score is associated with a particular outcome and prognosis based on comparison with clinical experience (SAPS) or by the statistical conversion of a numeric score to a probability estimate (APACHE II). Higher mortality and greater severity correlate with higher SAPS and APACHE II scores, thereby justifying the use of these indices in patient prognostication and outcome prediction. In spite of the strong statistical evidence for these associations, it must be noted that the variables and their weights in each of the indices were selected by expert consensus a priori, based on the clinical judgment of intensive care physicians.[17]

Lemeshow and coworkers approached the issue of outcome prediction and assessment in a different way, using multiple logistic regression to select the variables and their appropriate weights. Their system, initially termed the Mortality Prediction Model but more recently changed to the Mortality Probability Model (MPM), is based on a large data base containing 377 possible variables. Multiple logistic regression is applied to objectively determine which of these variables best correlates with patient outcome and what weights should be assigned. Unlike APACHE II and SAPS, MPM yields a direct probability of death instead of a numeric score for each patient.[17, 86]

Data for the development of MPM were derived from 755 consecutive admissions to the general medical-surgical ICU at Baystate Medical Center in Springfield, Massachusetts, during a 7-month period in 1983. As with APACHE II, cardiac, coronary artery bypass surgery, and burn patients were excluded from the analysis. However, unlike APACHE II and SAPS in which data were only collected during the first 24 hours of ICU admission, data for MPM were collected at five different points during hospitalization: at the time of ICU admission and at 24 hours, 48 hours, ICU discharge, and hospital discharge. From these data, an MPM was developed, based on seven variables determined from multiple logistic regression, for use at the time of ICU admission; another MPM was developed for patients remaining in the ICU at 24 hours[86] (Table 7–13). A subsequent analysis of 2783 patients, using the same approach and similar multiple logistic regression techniques, led to the derivation of separate MPMs for admission, at 24 hours, and at 48 hours, and an MPM that reflects probability over time.[87] MPM compares favorably with other scoring systems based on a study of 1997 patients,[88, 89] and its performance has also been validated for use in a diverse case mix of patients by a multi-institutional study.[90]

The information required by MPM is relatively simple to collect, and unlike APACHE II and SAPS, the variables analyzed are predominantly dichotomous and independent of treatment.[86–89] MPM, at least in the most recent derivations, incorporates serial observations and measurements and may therefore be more sensitive to the dynamic nature of critical illness, thereby providing a mechanism for the refinement of probability over time.[87] Because a direct probability estimate is provided by MPM, patients need not be placed into a single medical or surgical diagnostic category.[91] This latter feature is important and may be a significant advantage of MPM. Patients in ICUs frequently suffer from multiple processes and multiple organ system dysfunction and thus cannot be easily classified into a single diagnostic category.

PEDIATRIC AND SURGICAL SCORING SYSTEMS AND INDICES

Scoring indices have also been developed for surgical and pediatric intensive care patients. Yeh and colleagues devel-

TABLE 7–13

VARIABLES AND RESPONSE CATEGORIES OF ADMISSION AND 24-HOUR MORTALITY PROBABILITY MODELS

Variable	Response
Admission MPM	
Level of consciousness (coma/deep stupor)	Yes, no
Type of admission	Elective, emergency
CPR before ICU admission	Yes, no
Cancer part of present problem	Yes, no
History of chronic renal failure	Yes, no
Probable infection	Yes, no
Age	Age (y)
Previous ICU admission within 6 mo	Yes, no
Heart rate at ICU admission	Beats/min
Surgical service at ICU admission	Yes, no
Systolic blood pressure at admission	Number of mm Hg
Systolic blood pressure, squared	mm Hg^2
Constant	
24-Hour MPM	
Coma/deep stupor at 24 h	Yes, no
Cancer part of present problem	Yes, no
Emergency admission	Yes, no
Prothrombin time > 3 s above laboratory standard during first 24 h	Yes, no
Probable shock during first 24 h	Yes, no
Urine output < 150 mL in any 8 h during first 24 h	Yes, no
Infection confirmed at 24 h	Yes, no
Po$_2$ < 60 torr in first 24 h	Yes, no
Fio$_2$ > 0.50 in first 24 h	Yes, no
Creatinine > 2.0 mg/dL in first 24 h	Yes, no
Age	Age (y)
Hours of mechanical ventilation	Hours
Number of "lines" at 24 h	Number
Surgical service at 24 h	Yes, no
Constant	

Adapted from Teres D, Lemeshow S, Harris D, et al: Mortality prediction models (MPM) for ICU patients. Probl Crit Care 3:587, 1989.

oped the Physiologic Stability Index for critically ill pediatric patients. This index, a physiology-based classification system similar to APACHE, was validated by comparison with observed hospital mortality and with the TISS clinical classifications.[64, 65, 92] This physiologic index was later modified by Pollack and colleagues into a simpler measure with fewer variables: the Pediatric Risk of Mortality, or PRISM.[93]

For surgical and trauma patients, Kirkpatrick and Youmans developed the Trauma Index, based on information about the injured region, the type of injury, and the presence and degree of cardiovascular, respiratory, and neurologic dysfunction.[94] Champion and colleagues developed the Triage Score and the Trauma Score on the basis of variables derived from the initial physical examination.[95] Other indices include the Hannover Intensive Score for mortality prediction in the surgical ICU,[96] and the CRAMS (circulation, respiration, abdomen, motor, and speech) Scale developed for field triage.[97]

LIMITATIONS OF SCORING SYSTEMS

The development and use of ICU prognostic indices represent the desire among intensive care practitioners to quantitively assess the severity of illness of the patients they treat and thereby provide reasonable and reliable prognostic estimates. Scoring systems have been used for multiple purposes, including evaluation of therapeutic efficacy of new treatments, quality assurance, and interhospital comparisons of morbidity and mortality. Despite their limitations, scoring systems have increased the awareness among ICU practitioners of the need to objectify severity of illness and efficacy of ICU care. However, it is important to recognize the current limitations of these systems as well.

Most authors and experts suggest that scoring should not be applied to individual patients and individual management issues. Although the more established scoring models have achieved a relatively high degree of collective accuracy, the systems are most appropriately applied to groups or populations. Individual patients may fall outside the predicted outcome based on a given score or range. Nevertheless, scoring may be helpful when discussing prognosis with patients and families.

Concerns have been raised about scoring system performance and whether clinical scoring is able to predict mortality more accurately than bedside clinical assessment. Kruse and colleagues addressed this issue in a comparison of the predictive accuracy of APACHE II and that of intensive care physicians and nurses. In this analysis of 366 medical ICU patients, clinical judgment was as predictive as APACHE II scores.[98] McClish and Powell arrived at a similar conclusion in their investigation of 523 medical ICU patients.[99] They further made the important yet subtle distinction between discrimination (or resolution) and calibration. Discrimination refers to the ability to distinguish among different outcomes and therefore provide an appropriate decision criterion, whereas calibration (or reliability) is the ability to accurately assign a specific numeric probability.[99] Their data showed that physicians exhibited better discrimination than APACHE II, which perhaps demonstrates an innate clinical ability to distinguish those who will eventually die from those who will eventually survive. APACHE II demonstrated better calibration, but this difference changed in favor of the physicians at the lowest and highest probability values.[99]

In addition to the issues related to individual patient decisions and the incremental utility of scoring systems, it is important to note that the generalized scoring instruments cannot currently be applied to certain patient populations. Cardiac and coronary bypass patients, for example, were not included in either the testing or the validation populations for either APACHE II or MPM. Smith and coworkers also showed the inability of APACHE II to predict the probability of death for patients with acquired immunodeficiency syndrome who require ICU care. In their study, APACHE II significantly underestimated mortality, especially among the subgroup with *Pneumocystis carinii* pneumonia who required mechanical ventilation.[100]

Other confounding and important factors that influence mortality are not measurable with current scoring indices. Escarce and Kelley have suggested an independent association between patient origin (i.e., emergency room versus the general medical or surgical ward) and hospital mortality for intensive care patients.[101] Rapoport and colleagues further noted a relationship between mortality and the timing of the initiation of ICU care relative to hospital admission.[102] In this study predicted (by MPM) mortality and observed mortality both rose as the interval between hospital and ICU admission increased. They also showed a higher observed and predicted mortality for patients transferred from other institutions. Further research must be devoted to these and other issues, as source and timing of admissions are among the factors that may be subject to modification.

It is also important to distinguish between probability and prediction. Prediction is usually measured in a binary, dichotomous fashion (i.e., survival or death, positive or negative); probability is expressed as a number between 0 and 1, and it refers to the chance of occurrence for any particular and possible event. Confusion and misconceptions develop when probability measures are interpreted as dichotomous predictions. To use an example described by Lemeshow and coworkers, if a patient is given a 0.46 probability of survival (by MPM), a significant chance exists for either survival or death. If this probability estimate were reduced to a dichotomous prediction in which the cutoff for survival is 50%, patients with a value of 50% or greater would be predicted to die, whereas patients with a value of 49% or less would be predicted to survive. Thus, the patient with a 46% probability of mortality would be grouped with a patient having a 5% probability. The two patients are clearly different in terms of survival probability; however, dichotomous predictions with sharp cutoffs fail to make this distinction.[103]

The incorporation of measures that evaluate clinical change over time will also improve the utility and effectiveness of scoring systems. Whereas APACHE II and SAPS measure data during the initial 24 hours of ICU care, a stated aim of the APACHE III study is the provision of outcome estimates on a continuous basis. MPM addresses the dynamic nature of critical illness with the use of multiple models for different points in time. Chang and colleagues also used trend analysis and daily APACHE II scores instead of single measurements on admission to demonstrate improved predictive ability.[104–106] Future efforts should therefore be devoted to the measurement of clinical change and therapeutic response.

TRENDS AND FUTURE USES

The results of the APACHE III study may herald new applications and uses for ICU scoring. As Bastos and colleagues stated, the goals of this project are the development of a dynamic predictive index as an aid to physicians for individual patient decisions.[85] Aside from the current limitations of scoring systems that generally preclude application to individual clinical cases, a fear remains that such measures may excessively guide diagnostic and therapeutic choice and subsequently alter one's clinical threshold.[107] Although one multicenter study seems to show only slight evidence of such alteration in clinical behavior,[108] further study will be needed. Despite advances in the methodology of prognostication, scoring is at best adjunctive and should not replace sound clinical judgment.

Scoring systems will most likely continue to develop to the point at which the techniques and applications of scoring and prediction will help ICU practitioners better manage their resources and evaluate the quality of the care that they provide.

References

1. Schwartz S, Cullen DJ: How many intensive care beds does your hospital need? Crit Care Med 9:625, 1981.
2. Bekes C, Fleming S, Scott WE: Reimbursement for intensive care services under diagnosis-related groups. Crit Care Med 6:478, 1988.
3. Chalfin DB: Diagnosis-related groups (DRGs) and intensive care. Intensive Care World 7:198, 1990.
4. Spivack D: The high cost of acute health care: A review of escalating costs and limitations of such exposure. Am Rev Respir Dis 136:1007, 1987.
5. Sloan FA, Morrissey MA, Valvona J: Medicare prospective payment and the use of medical technologies in hospitals. Med Care 26:837, 1988.
6. Butler PW, Bone RC, Field T: Technology under Medicare diagnosis-related groups prospective payment. Implications for medical intensive care. Chest 87:229, 1985.
7. Ahmed M, Fergus L, Stothard P, et al: Impact of diagnosis-related groups' prospective payment. Chest 93:176, 1988.
8. Douglas PS, Roses RL, Butler PW, et al: DRG payment for long-term ventilator patients. Chest 91:413, 1987.
9. Jacobs P, Noseworthy TW: National estimates of intensive utilization and costs: Canada and the United States. Crit Care Med 18:1282, 1990.
10. Raffin TA: Intensive care unit survival of patients with systemic illness. Am Rev Respir Dis 140:S28, 1989.

11. McClish DK, Powell SH: How well can physicians estimate mortality in a medical intensive care unit? Med Decis Making 9:125, 1989.
12. Chalfin DB, Carlon GC: Age and utilization of intensive care unit resources of critically ill cancer patients. Crit Care Med 18:694, 1985.
13. Strauss MJ, LoGerfo JP, Yeltatzie JA, et al: Rationing intensive care unit services. JAMA 255:1143, 1986.
14. McLean RF, McIntosh JD, Kung GY, et al: Outcome of respiratory intensive care for the elderly. Crit Care Med 13:625, 1985.
15. Poses RM, Bekes C, Copare FJ, et al: The answer to "What are my chances, Doctor?" depends upon whom is asked: Prognostic disagreement and inaccuracy for critically ill patients. Crit Care Med 17:827, 1989.
16. Zimmerman JE, Knaus WA: Outcome prediction in adult intensive care. In: Shoemaker WC, Ayres S, Grenvik A, et al (eds): Textbook of Critical Care. Philadelphia, WB Saunders, p 1477, 1989.
17. Kiefe C: Statistical methods used by prognostic indices. Probl Crit Care 3:514, 1989.
18. Charlson ME, Sax FL, MacKenzie R, et al: Morbidity during hospitalization: Can we predict it? J Chronic Dis 40:705, 1987.
19. Killip T, Kimball JT: Treatment of myocardial infarction in a coronary care unit: A two-year experience with 250 patients. Am J Cardiol 20:457, 1967.
20. Forrester JS, Diamost G, Chatterjee K, et al: Medical therapy of acute myocardial infarction by application of hemodynamic subsets (first of two parts). N Engl J Med 295:1356, 1976.
21. Forrester JS, Diamost G, Chatterjee K, et al: Medical therapy of acute myocardial infarction by application of hemodynamic subsets (second of two parts). N Engl J Med 295:1404, 1976.
22. Goldman L, Hashimoto B, Cook EF, et al: Comparative reproducibility and validity of systems for assessing cardiovascular function class: Advantages of a new specific activity scale. Circulation 64:1227, 1981.
23. The Criteria Committee of the New York Heart Association: Diseases of the Heart and Blood Vessels: Nomenclature and Criteria for Diagnosis. 6th ed. Boston: Little, Brown, 1964.
24. Campeau L: Grading of angina pectoris. Circulation 64:522, 1975.
25. Goldman L, Hashimoto B, Cook EF, et al: Comparative reproducibility and validity of systems for assessing cardiovascular functional class: Advantages of a new specific activity scale. Circulation 64:1227, 1981.
26. Child CG, Turcotte JG: Surgery and portal hypertension. In: Child CG (ed): The Liver and Portal Hypertension. Philadelphia, WB Saunders, p 50, 1964.
27. McMahon MJ, Playforth MJ, Pickford IR: A comparative study of methods for the prediction of severity of attacks of acute pancreatitis. Br J Surg 67:22, 1980.
28. Ranson JHC, Rifkind KM, Roses DF, et al: Prognostic signs and the role of operative management in acute pancreatitis. Surg Gynecol Obstet 139:69, 1974.
29. Ranson JHC, Pasternak BS: Statistical methods for quantifying the severity of clinical acute pancreatitis. J Surg Res 22:79, 1977.
30. Imrie CW, Blumgart LH: Acute pancreatitis: A prospective study of some factors in mortality. Bull Soc Int Chir 34:601, 1975.
31. New classification of physical status (editorial). Anesthesiology 24:111, 1963.
32. Dripps RD, Lamont A, Eckenhoff JE: The role of anesthesia in surgical mortality. JAMA 178:261, 1961.
33. Vacanti CJ, van Houten RJ, Hill RC: A statistical analysis of the relationship of physical status to postoperative mortality in 68,388 cases. Anesth Analg 49:564, 1970.
34. Goldman L, Caldera DL, Nussbaum SR, et al: Multifactorial index of cardiac risk in noncardiac surgical procedures. N Engl J Med 297:845, 1977.
35. Goldman L, Caldera DL, Southwick FS, et al: Cardiac risk factors and complications in non-cardiac surgery. Medicine 37:357, 1978.
36. Goldman L: Cardiac risks and complications of noncardiac surgery. Ann Intern Med 95:504, 1983.
37. Teasdale G, Jennett B: Assessment of coma and impaired consciousness: A practical scale. Lancet 2:81, 1974.
38. Jennett B: Assessment of the severity of brain injury. J Neurol Neurosurg Psychiatry 39:647, 1976.
39. Dean JM, Kaufman ND: Prognostic indicators in pediatric near drowning: The Glasgow Coma Scale. Crit Care Med 9:536, 1981.
40. Kirby RR: Monitoring of neurologic function. In: Civetta JM, Taylor RW, Kirby RR (eds): Critical Care. Philadelphia, JB Lippincott, p 351, 1988.
41. Charlson ME, Sax FL, MacKenzie CR, et al: Assessing illness severity: Does clinical judgement work? J Chronic Dis 39:439, 1986.
42. Seneff M, Knaus WA: APACHE, a prognostic system. Probl Crit Care 3:563, 1989.
43. Civetta JM: The clinical limitations of ICU scoring. Probl Crit Care 3:681, 1989.
44. Knaus WA, Wagner DP, Draper EA: The value of measuring severity of disease in clinical research on acutely ill patients. J Chronic Dis 37:455, 1984.
45. Wagner DP, Knaus WA, Draper EA, et al: Identification of low-risk monitor patients within a medical-surgical intensive care unit. Med Care 21:425, 1983.
46. Wagner DP, Draper EA, Campos RA, et al: Initial international use of APACHE. Med Decis Making 3:297, 1984.

47. Cullen DJ: Results and costs of intensive care. Anesthesiology 47:203, 1977.
48. Spicack D: The high cost of acute health care: A review of escalating costs and limitations of such exposure in intensive care units. Am Rev Respir Dis 136:1007, 1987.
49. Cullen DJ, Keene R, Waternaux C, et al: Results, charges, and benefits of intensive care for critically ill patients: Update 1983. Crit Care Med 12:102, 1984.
50. Carlon C: Just say no. Crit Care Med 17:106, 1989.
51. Detsky AS, Stickler SC, Mulley AG, et al: Prognosis, survival, and the expenditure of hospital resources for patients in an intensive care unit. N Engl J Med 305:667, 1981.
52. Thibault GE, Mulley AG, Barnett GO, et al: Medical intensive care: Indications, interventions, and outcomes. N Engl J Med 302:938, 1980.
53. Bloom BS, Peterson OL: End results, cost and productivity of coronary care units. N Engl J Med 288:72, 1973.
54. Sax FL, Charlson ME: Utilization of critical care units: A prospective study of physician triage and patient outcome. Arch Intern Med 147:929, 1987.
55. NIH Consensus Development Conference on Critical Care Medicine. Crit Care Med 11:466, 1983.
56. Civetta JM: Prediction and definition of outcome in a cost-sensitive era. In: Civetta JM, Taylor RW, Kirby RR (eds): Critical Care. Philadelphia, JB Lippincott, p 1677, 1988.
57. Knaus WA: The science of prediction and its implication for the clinician today. Theor Surg 3:93, 1988.
58. TIMI Study Group: Comparison of invasive and conservative strategies after treatment with intravenous tissue plasminogen activator in acute myocardial infarction: Results of the Thrombolysis in Myocardial Infarction (TIMI) Phase II Trial. N Engl J Med 19:129, 1989.
59. TIMI Study Group: Immediate versus delayed catheterization and angioplasty following thrombolytic therapy for acute myocardial infarction: TIMI IIA results. JAMA 260:2849, 1988.
60. Wall TC, Phillips HR 3rd, Stack RS, et al: Results of high dose intravenous urokinase for acute myocardial infarction. Am J Cardiol 65:124, 1990.
61. Gonella JS, Hornbrook MC, Louis DZ: Staging of disease. A case-mix measurement. JAMA 251:637, 1984.
62. Norris RM, Brandt PWT, Caughey DE, et al: A new coronary prognostic index. Lancet 1:294, 1969.
63. Farmer JC: Intensive care: How do we measure outcome? Problems Crit Care 3:511, 1989.
64. Cullen DJ, Civetta JM, Briggs BA, et al: Therapeutic intervention scoring system: A method for quantitative comparison of patient care. Crit Care Med 2:57, 1974.
65. Cullen DJ, Nemeskal AR: Therapeutic intervention scoring system (TISS). Probl Crit Care 3:545, 1989.
66. Keene AR, Cullen DJ: Therapeutic intervention scoring system: Update 1983. Crit Care Med 11:1, 1983.
67. Knaus WA, Wagner DP, Draper EA, et al: The range of intensive care services today. JAMA 246:2711, 1981.
68. Knaus WA, Zimmerman JE, Wagner DP, et al: APACHE—Acute physiology and chronic health evaluation: A physiology-based classification system. Crit Care Med 9:591, 1981.
69. Knaus WA: Prognosis with mechanical ventilation: The influence of disease, severity of disease, age, and chronic health status on survival from an acute illness. Am Rev Respir Dis 1989; 140:S8, 1989.
70. LeGall JR, Loirat P, Alperovitch A: Simplified acute physiology score for intensive care patients. Lancet 2:741, 1983.
71. LeGall JR, Loirat P, Nicholas F, et al: Utilization d'un indice de gravité dans huit services de réanimation multidisciplinaires. Nouv Presse Med 12:1757, 1983.
72. LeGall JR, Loirat P, Alperovitch A, et al: A simplified acute physiology for ICU patients. Crit Care Med 12:975, 1984.
73. French Multicenter Group of ICU Research: Factors related to outcome in intensive care: French multicenter study. Crit Care Med 17:305, 1989.
74. Knaus WA, Draper EA, Wagner DP, et al: APACHE II: A severity of disease classification system. Crit Care Med 13:818, 1985.
75. Knaus WA, Draper EA, Wagner DP, et al: An evaluation of outcome from intensive care in major medical centers. Ann Intern Med 104:410, 1986.
76. Lemeshow S, Teres D, Avrunin JS, et al: A comparison of methods to predict mortality of intensive care patients. Crit Care Med 15:715, 1987.
77. Silverstein ME: Predictive instruments and clinical judgement in critical care. JAMA 260:1758, 1988.
78. Zeigler EJ, Fischer CJ, Sprung CL, et al: Treatment of gram-negative bacteremia and septic shock with HA-1A human monoclonal antibody against endotoxin. N Engl J Med 324:429, 1991.
79. Greenman RL, Schein RMH, Martin MA, et al: A controlled clinical trial of E5 murine monoclonal IgM antibody to endotoxin in the treatment of gram-negative sepsis. JAMA 266:1097, 1991.
80. Coulton CJ, McClish D, Doremus HG, et al: Implications of DRG payments for medical intensive care. Med Care 23:977, 1985.
81. Daly J, Jenck S, Draper D, et al: Predicting hospital-associated mortality for Medicare patients with stroke, pneumonia, acute myocardial infarction, and congestive heart failure. JAMA 260:3617, 1988.

82. Zimmerman JE, Knaus WA, Judson JA, et al: Patient selection for intensive care: A comparison of New Zealand and United States hospitals. Crit Care Med 16:318, 1988.

83. Rauss A, Knaus WA, Patois E, et al: Prognosis for recovery from multiple organ system failure: The accuracy of objective estimates of chances for survival. Med Decis Making 10:155, 1990.

84. Wagner D, Draper E, Knaus W: Development of APACHE III. In: Zimmerman JE (ed): APACHE III Study Design: Analytic Plan for Evaluation of Severity and Outcome. Crit Care Med 17:S199, 1989.

85. Bastos PG, Knaus WA: APACHE III study: A summary. Intensive Care World 8:35, 1991.

85a. Knaus WA, Wagner DP, Draper EA, et al: The APACHE III prognostic system. Risk prediction of hospital mortality for critically ill hospitalized adults. Chest 100:1619, 1991.

86. Lemeshow S, Teres D, Pastides H, et al: A method for predicting survival and mortality of ICU patients using objectively derived weights. Crit Care Med 13:519, 1985.

87. Lemeshow S, Teres D, Avrunin JS, et al: Refining intensive care unit outcome prediction by using changing probabilities of mortality. Crit Care Med 16:470, 1988.

88. Lemeshow S, Avrunin JS, Teres D: A comparison of models to predict mortality of intensive care unit patients (abstract). Crit Care Med 14:356, 1986.

89. Lemeshow S, Teres D, Avrunin JS, et al: A comparison of methods to predict mortality of intensive care unit patients. Crit Care Med 15:715, 1987.

90. Teres D, Lemeshow S, Avrunin JS, et al: Multicenter validation of mortality prediction model (abstract). Crit Care Med 16:412, 1988.

91. Teres D, Lemeshow S, Harris D, et al: Mortality prediction models (MPM) for ICU patients. Probl Crit Care 4:585, 1989.

92. Yeh TS, Pollack MM, Holbrook PR, et al: Validation of a physiologic stability index for use in critically ill infants and children. Pediatr Res 1984; 18:445, 1984.

93. Pollack MM, Ruttiman UE, Getson PR. The pediatric risk of mortality (PRISM) score. Crit Care Med 16:1110, 1988.

94. Kirkpatrick JR, Youmans RL. Trauma index: An aid in the evaluation of injury victims. J Trauma 11:711, 1971.

95. Champion HR, Sacco WJ, Carnazzo AJ, et al: Trauma score. Crit Care Med 9:672, 1981.

96. Lehmkul P, Ludwig M, Pichlmayr I: The use of scoring systems as a prognostic parameter after surgery and trauma. In: Schlag G, Redl H (eds): First Vienna Shock Forum, Part B, Monitoring and Treatment of Shock. New York, Alan R Liss, p 17, 1987.

97. Gormican SP: CRAMS scale: Field triage of trauma victims. Ann Emerg Med 11:132, 1982.

98. Kruse JA, Thill-Baharozian MC, Carlson RW: Comparison of clinical assessment with APACHE II for predicting mortality risk in patients admitted to a medical intensive care unit. JAMA 260:1739, 1988.

99. McClish DK, Powell SH: How well can physicians estimate mortality in a medical intensive care unit? Med Decis Making 9:125, 1989.

100. Smith RL, Levine SM, Lewis ML: Prognosis of patients with AIDS requiring intensive care. Chest 96:857, 1989.

101. Escarce JJ, Kelley MA: Admission source to the medical intensive care unit predicts hospital death independent of APACHE II score. JAMA 264:2389, 1990.

102. Rapoport J, Teres D, Lemeshow S, et al: Timing of intensive care unit admission in relation to ICU outcome. Crit Care Med 18:1231, 1990.

103. Lemeshow S, Teres D, Klar J: Use of a probability model for predicting ICU outcome. Update Intensive Care Emerg Med 14:574, 1991.

104. Chang RWS, Jacobs S, Lee B, et al: Predicting deaths among intensive care unit patients. Crit Care Med 16:34, 1988.

105. Chang RS: Individual outcome prediction models for intensive care units. Lancet 2:143, 1989.

106. Chang RWS, Jacobs S, Lee B: Predicting outcome among intensive care unit patients using computerized trend analysis of daily APACHE II scores corrected for organ system failure. Intensive Care Med 14:558, 1988.

107. Hickman DH: Do severity of disease classification tools change patient care? Med Decis Making 10:155, 1990.

108. Knaus WA, Rauss A, Alperovitch A, et al: Do objective chances for survival influence decisions to withhold or withdraw treatment? Med Decis Making 10:163, 1990.

CHAPTER 8

Computers in Critical Care Units

Frank V. M. Booth

No medical textbook contains a section on the use of the telephone in critical care. This is not because critical care units (CCUs) could function without telephones, but because they are so fundamental to communication in a CCU that their presence and use are taken for granted. The telephone is intuitively easy to use and is extraordinarily reliable, and although the inner workings may be extremely complex, this complexity is not apparent to the user. In computer terms, the telephone is a "transparent" device. Anyone using an institution's switchboard to transfer a call or "camp on" a busy number is actually using a computer to do these things.

Similarly, modern ventilators in many CCUs employ sophisticated computers that process a stream of information "on the fly," allowing complex patterns of ventilation to be administered. It is not externally obvious, however, that a computer is what makes this possible. When computers have reached a level of sophistication such that they are no longer "visible" as distinct entities in CCUs, chapters such as this one will no longer be necessary in critical care textbooks.

This chapter will describe areas of critical care practice and unit management in which the application of computer technology may improve the quality of care, enhance communication, or simply improve management. The software developed for many other industries is immediately adaptable to the critical care setting provided the potential user understands the processes of the critical care milieu. This chapter is therefore intended to serve as an introduction to computer systems in the critical care environment and to help the critical care practitioner better understand the commercial systems utilized in critical care. Practical examples of the development and implementation of computer-assisted CCU activities are described. The areas to be discussed include

- Clinical information handling in the CCU
- Computer-assisted decision making in critical care
- Medical informatics
- Staff communication within a CCU
- Computer-assisted quality assurance
- Inventory, budget, and other financial control systems

CLINICAL INFORMATION SYSTEMS

Care of the critically ill patient involves an enormous amount of data. Much of this information undergoes repeated manual transcription. The goals of computerization in this area of critical care include eliminating all handwriting, maximizing the use of keyboard entry, and eliminating duplication of data entry.

Acquisition and Management of Information

An information system is only as good as the input it receives. For a system to be useful to the clinician, it must enhance that activity without imposing any additional burdens on the user. Many optimistic schemes for computerization have foundered because the system designers underestimated the process of data entry. This resulted either in excessive amounts of additional time being spent to enter data or in the entering of inaccurate or incomplete information. When this occurs, the problem lies with software design and not with the user.

The data entry problem is still not understood by all vendors. The author had the experience of serving on a committee that was taken to an institution by a vendor for demonstration of a CCU data management system the vendor had installed. Although the clinical information system had made it possible to produce an impressive array of computer graphics describing the state of a patient, *not a single element of the previous manual data entry or written record had been eliminated.* The normal clerical overhead conventionally estimated to take up to 30% of the CCU nurse's time had in fact *increased* to nearly 40% for very little tangible gain.

Ironically, almost all information about a critically ill patient in the CCU is in electronic form at some stage. The demographic information is in the hospital billing system, and all the laboratory values are measured by instruments using a current or voltage. Most of the vital signs are continuously monitored by instruments that transform these vital signs into electronic signals.[1] Critical care record keeping has traditionally consisted of converting these signals to marks on a piece of paper. It matters not whether this transcription is done with a quill pen or laser printer. Once the information has been put on paper, it is no longer readily accessible for data analysis.

In designing a computerized system for clinical data management, it is important to avoid this "paper" trap. Although printed output will often be important for archival purposes, the final resting place of information for data management purposes should always be in a computer-accessible form (i.e., a data base).

User Interfaces

The term *user interface* encompasses many elements of the transaction between the workers in a CCU and the computers handling the information. The words *user friendly* are frequently but not always appropriately applied. To be truly user friendly, an interface should incorporate physical devices to communicate with the computer that are convenient and comfortable for the user. Examples of input devices include a keyboard, a mouse, a trackball, a light pen, a touch-sensitive screen, a digital pad, and a bar code reader. These devices must be designed and situated according to the physical circumstances of the users. It makes little sense, for example, to use touch-screen technology with the screen mounted next to the CCU monitor where a short nurse cannot reach all of the screen.[2] Finally, the way in which

TABLE 8–1
NEGOTIABLE ITEMS FOR DATA TRANSFER UNDER PROPOSED INSTITUTE OF ELECTRICAL AND ELECTRONICS ENGINEERS STANDARDS FOR THE MEDICAL INFORMATION BUS
What kind of device is this?
Is the transferred information discrete or continuous?
What is the name of these data?
What is their value?
Is this value read only, write only, or read and write?
What are the dimensions of this value?
How often is it coming or going?
Is this value a mean value (if so, over what time frame)?

TABLE 8–2
SYSTEMS TO WHICH A CCU SYSTEM MIGHT BE REQUIRED TO RELATE TO OBTAIN A COMPLETE CCU CHART
Hospital medical information system
Blood gas laboratory
Laboratory system
Pharmacy system
Radiology reporting system
Medical records word-processing system for operating room records
Central supply inventory system

a device interacts with the software is also crucially important.

Interfaces to Critical Care Unit Equipment

Some manufacturers have recognized the need to communicate information gathered by patient-monitoring devices to an information system or to another computer. Unfortunately, there is currently no standard method of communication between devices from different manufacturers. The lack of a communication standard is analogous to the difficulties faced by manufacturers of other high-technology products, such as high-definition television or digital audio tape, but the communication protocol problems with patient-monitoring devices are much more severe because the intended receiver is another machine. Table 8–1 provides a list of items that must be negotiated in any communication protocol for medical devices. A draft engineering standard has been proposed to address these concerns, but consumer demand will ultimately determine the degree of industrial compliance with this voluntary standard.

A common but misleading practice among vendors of critical care monitoring equipment involves devices sold with an RS232 port. The clinician with limited experience with personal computers will recall that the serial communications port of many personal computers also uses the RS232 standard. It may then be imagined that all that is necessary for the device to communicate with the computer is two plugs and a cable, but this is not so! The RS232 standard addresses very few of the questions raised in Table 8–1. Sales representatives are often unaware of this problem.

As a general rule *the bulk of the programming work for communication between a device and a computer (or information system) must be done by the computer and not by the device.* Because there are many different systems and many users who have no systems at all, the manufacturers have naturally taken the line of greatest economy and least resistance by including only the most rudimentary communication capabilities or none at all.

Interfaces to Other Computer Systems

Similar to the problem of communication among individual machines within a CCU computer system, there are often complex problems involved in exchanging information between a CCU system and other computer systems. A partial list of systems with which a CCU computer might be required to communicate is provided in Table 8–2.

The concept of communicating through a single "gateway" is gaining favor in commercial data base applications.* In

---

*The gateway concept will be familiar to users of commercial data bases such as COMPUSERVE or PRODIGY. The user connects his or her computer to a large computer, usually by modem or telephone. This large computer then offers a menu of other services, many of which actually run on completely different computers far removed from the machine to which the user was originally connected. To the user, however, this is a transparent process that gives no indication of where the transaction is actually taking place. The more user-transparent this process is, the easier it is likely to be for the consumer.

practice, however, many institutions have acquired their computer equipment in a piecemeal fashion. A general principle of information management is that two systems having elements of information in common can be made to share that information. However, unless systems have been designed to interface with one another, the process of accomplishing this communication is often time-consuming and expensive.

When contemplating the purchase of computer information systems, the ability of the system to communicate with existing equipment is a prime consideration. This is almost as important a consideration as the functionality of the system and is an area in which the purchaser should be extremely skeptical of vendor promises. The most reliable test of the ability to interface any two systems is a demonstration that the vendor has previously accomplished a working interface between the two systems contemplated. Vendor claims to this effect should be verified. The process of implementing the interface was probably more difficult and time-consuming than either party anticipated. However, the key question relates to the degree of functionality achieved. If this is high, discussions with the potential vendor can proceed with confidence.

Design Philosophy Behind Clinical Information Systems

The first electronic device to appear in the CCU was the oscilloscope in the form of a cardiograph. For many years, the predominance of monitoring in critical care was reflected in the way in which information systems were constructed. The same companies that manufactured monitors also made information systems. The focus of the information system was sometimes intentionally narrow (e.g., software for the management of arrhythmia detection and analysis). At other times, the focus was broader.[3, 4]

In the 1980s, the great debates in clinical information management systems centered on hardware architecture, that is, the physical design and relationship between the output seen by the user at the bedside or nursing station and the bedside monitoring devices. The objective of such systems was reproduction of the flow sheet without human intervention. The debates about architecture often focused on whether one central computer should support many terminals or if many interdependent and interchangeable computers were more advantageous. Both views had merit. However, little attention was paid to the fundamental nature of the critical care process. The result was the generation of a number of systems that with varying degrees of success, automated the vital signs segment of clinical record keeping. In some implementations, a modicum of artificial intelligence was also added, but this was usually confined to simple exception reporting or rudimentary trend analysis.

Although this design philosophy offered the possibility of improved documentation of critical care activities and events, the results were disappointing. The majority of critical care functions—nursing care, pharmacotherapeutics, laboratory investigations, ventilator support, physical therapy, and the like—did not easily fit into a monitoring system. Thus, the clinical information systems of the 1980s consisted mainly of machines to process vital signs, with add-on interfaces (of variable quality) for other aspects of the medical record.[5]

Despite these intrinsic limitations, there were a few successful implementations of critical care computerization, notably at the Latter Day Saints facilities in Salt Lake City, the Cedars-Sinai Medical Center in Los Angeles, and the Michael Reese Hospital in Chicago. At these centers, it became quickly apparent that a team of dedicated software engineers and computer-orientated clinicians were the sine

qua non for success. Despite their success, these systems were neither transparent nor "robust" (i.e., capable of operating in variable environments).

Motivated in part by the seminal thinking of Gardner and Brimm,[3, 6] software engineers started to analyze the nature of the critical care process more carefully, and they concluded that it is the patient as a whole that drives critical care. Thus, the core activity of a clinical information system is not the recording of vital signs but the management and documentation of tasks within a given period. This seemingly revolutionary concept arose from a better understanding of the medical setting.

The engineers realized that, short of medical catastrophes, nothing happens in a CCU without orders. These orders may originate with physicians, nurses (the nursing care plan), or protocol for a given situation. These orders define what is done for a patient. When orders are made central to information management, other functions flow naturally and logically. The gathering of vital signs takes its place with the administration of medications, the ordering of laboratory tests, and the updating of problem lists and care plans. From a nursing point of view, the rational ordering and listing of tasks, with timed prompts where appropriate, can relieve an extraordinary clerical burden. Documentation and detailing of tasks accomplished become simply an acknowledgement to the system that the task list was completed. Thus, the system is largely self-documenting. Anything that has been overlooked remains on the system as a reminder to the next nurse.

This philosophy represents a tremendous advance in software design for the critical care setting. Software based on the new philosophy is now being implemented in a number of settings, including Harbor View Hospital in Seattle and Shriners' Burn Institute in Galveston.

PRESENTATION OF INFORMATION

The traditional method of organizing the large quantity of data associated with care of the critically ill has been the familiar CCU flow sheet based on an extended list of vital signs and supplemented by other information such as fluid balance, ventilatory support, inotropic drugs, and limited laboratory results. A well-designed flow sheet is efficient when used by experienced critical care staff.

One of the challenges software designers have faced is to create an electronic tool that can match or exceed the efficiency and simplicity of the flow sheet. Until recently, the physical limitations of display terminals have not allowed more than one fifth of the information on a typical flow sheet to be presented on a single screen. This has been a major handicap for the clinician attempting to use such a system. Much of the information processing that occurs when a patient's situation is reviewed is associative. The need to switch back and forth between screens of data seriously interferes with the associative thought process. Fortunately, resolution of display devices continues to improve, and screen displays increasingly resemble a traditional flow sheet. However, the electronic version has the added advantage that it cannot easily be lost or applied to the wrong patient. Furthermore, in a network environment, many different people at various locations may examine the flow sheet simultaneously.

The availability of clinical information in a form that can be manipulated for the purposes of data analysis has enabled workers to obtain answers about the nature of critical care by making queries that were previously not practical. Examples include questions relating to the quality of care, morbidity, severity of illness, and prognostication.[7] Computer systems have proved useful in the quest for a better understanding of the pathophysiology of the critically ill and in optimizing care.

ASSISTED DECISION MAKING

Computers do not get tired. They are capable of processing millions of possible associations in a short space of time and, given sufficient storage, can retain the data in memory for as long as necessary. The science of artificial intelligence has already been applied to a number of diagnostic modalities, such as the likelihood of myocardial infarction,[8] the diagnosis of abdominal pain, and others.[9] The situation in medicine is analogous to computer chess programs. A good program performs at the level of an expert but cannot yet defeat a grand master. There are, however, other important functions that the user should demand of critical care computerized information systems, as follows.

Intelligent or Adaptive Alarms. For example, a creatinine value of 1.2 mg/dL may not be abnormal, but if the last two values were 0.6, a change of this magnitude should be flagged for further inspection.[10, 11]

Associated Prompts. If a certain condition is noted, the system should prompt considerations for work-up of potentially associated conditions.[12] For example, respiratory alkalosis and hypoxemia should alert the clinician to the possible diagnoses of pulmonary embolism, pneumonia, sepsis, or adult respiratory distress syndrome.

Drug and Allergy Interaction Monitoring. Although intellectually trivial, this modality is still surprisingly lacking in many CCUs, perhaps because the burden of data entry seems out of proportion to the length of stay of the average critical care patient. As more automated pharmacy systems become available, the CCU director should require this functionality to be made part of the pharmacy system (the preferable method) or that a stand-alone program be made available to providers in the unit.

MEDICAL INFORMATICS

The field of medical informatics is now the subject of a number of specialized journals. As in other areas of technologically driven medicine, there has been an explosion of information and activity in this field in the past decade.

Local Information Systems

The development of highly condensed storage media such as CD ROM* has made it possible for the entire contents of Index Medicus to be stored on fewer than a dozen disks. With the addition of "juke box" technology, the user can search the entire body of medical knowledge with incredible ease and speed. Menu-driven software allows the inexperienced user to do productive work almost immediately. The relatively low cost (a few thousand dollars a year) of subscribing to such services has meant that a rapidly growing number of medium- and small-sized institutions have this capability on-site. Access to such dial-up services as After Dark or BRS (Bibliographic Retrieval Service) or the National Library of Medicine may soon become a rare activity. With the addition of personal computer (PC) communications technology, this capability can now be brought directly to the CCU.

Expertise in accessing information systems, although in-

*This term means read only memory and refers to a disk that is physically identical with the familiar compact audio disk but that contains computer-readable information instead of music. The capacity of such disks is quite remarkable. Early floppy disks held an amount of information equivalent to approximately twice the length of this chapter, or 140 kilobytes. A typical CD ROM holds 650 megabytes, or 4000 times as much information.

cluded in few medical school curricula, is becoming a necessary qualification for practice in a fast-moving area such as critical care. Fortunately, the required techniques are easy to learn and are becoming more user friendly.

The dramatic improvements in ease of access to medical information may soon have an impact in the area of liability exposure. A CCU that does not provide sophisticated searching capabilities to its practitioners may soon be an undesirable place in which to work from a malpractice point of view.

Remote Information Management Systems

Institutions without the resources to offer facilities such as on-site access to Index Medicus may still access these resources with the simplest computer, suitable communications software, and a modem. Software such as Paperchase or Grateful Med have greatly simplified access to these data bases and thus save valuable connect time and money. Once a new user has gained some confidence in accessing such systems, there is almost no limit to the medical information that can be accessed. There are even data bases (or computerized lists) of the medical data bases maintained by commercial dial-up services such as GENIE, COMPUSERVE, and the SOURCE. Through services such as BRS, the user can access over 500 discrete medical services.

COMPUTER-ASSISTED QUALITY ASSURANCE

Although the science of industrial quality assurance may be said to have been developed in America by Wald,[13] it traveled around the world before becoming a hot topic in the American health care field.[14] Of all the contributions made to nursing and health care made by Florence Nightingale, the most important was undoubtedly the systematic application of statistical information to the process of quality assurance. Indeed, from a public health point of view, she may be said to have invented the process.[15] Quality assurance in the health care field still lacks a precise and generally agreed-upon set of principles, but after almost a decade of wild swings in the expectations of individual Joint Commission on Accreditation of Healthcare Organizations (JCAHO) inspectors, there appears to be an increasing degree of stability and unanimity in the procedures expected of health care providers by the JCAHO in the the area of quality assurance or *quality improvement* (the officially preferred term).

The JCAHO emphasizes 10 steps in the quality assurance process:

1. Assign responsibility.
2. Delineate the scope of care or service.
3. Identify important aspects of care or service. A properly constructed data base of activity in the CCU allows the prompt identification of those events or procedures that are likely targets for quality assurance efforts. (This may be accomplished by using the check list method described later in this chapter.)
4. Identify indicators. Although the identification of indicators in a particular critical care situation may follow published guidelines,[16] the locally generated data base allows the unit manager or director to assess compliance with such standards.
5. Establish thresholds for these indicators that will trigger a more detailed evaluation of the care rendered. Clearly, this can be accomplished only if the results of care are routinely collected into a data base.
6. Monitor the important aspects of care by collecting and organizing the data for each indicator. (Two specific

examples, one relating to adverse experiences at a low threshold and the other to certain aspects of patient support, will be described later.)

7. Evaluate care when thresholds are reached to identify problems or opportunities for improvement in care.

8. Take action to resolve identified problems.

9. Assess the actions and document improvement.

10. Communicate the relevant information. This last step is often taken for granted or accomplished by such relatively archaic and undocumented methods as the bulletin board or the communications book. A more reliable and verifiable computerized method will be described later.

Indices, Scoring Systems, and Politicians

The twin pressures of cost containment and liability exposure have greatly accelerated efforts toward establishing normative standards of care. The clinician is well aware of the difficulty of applying universal standards to various groups of patients or to a particular hospital in which the characteristics of the patients may not match those of the index population. The early development of diagnosis-related groups (DRGs) is perhaps the most notorious example of this tendency.[17] Critical care is awash with indices: Acute Physiology and Chronic Health Evaluation (APACHE) II, Simplified Acute Physiology Score (SAPS), APACHE III, Mortality Probability Model (MPM), a variety of trauma scores, and others. When carefully applied within the limits conceived by the original index designers, with care taken to assure true population comparability and homogeneity, many of these indices are powerful tools for comparing patient populations in different centers. The use of a scoring index that predicts an outcome or a relative risk of death or morbidity is particularly attractive to hospital administrators and politicians.[18] For a given clinical entity such as open heart surgery, if sufficient data are collected for each patient, it is possible to construct relative risk ratios for many different cardiac surgical procedures. Furthermore, it is possible to weight these risk ratios according to patient-related factors such as age, previous history, left ventricular function, and so on.

When sample size is sufficient, it is possible to compare the performance of different hospitals or even different surgeons by seeking deviations from the expected odds ratios that lie outside the confidence levels of the estimates—the so-called Z coefficient.* By using this process, the state of New York now publishes tables of the performance of cardiac surgical centers throughout the state. To the outside observer, this may seem a fair practice. However, aside from two centers whose relative risk ratio was more than two standard deviations from predicted levels, all of the centers were statistically indistinguishable. Nevertheless, the health department readily published a ranking list.[19]

A second hazard to which institutions may be exposed by the use of scoring systems results from the inclusion of inappropriate patient groups. Although this problem may be expected to diminish as scoring schemes become more sophisticated, it is by no means a dead issue. The costs of assembling data bases that allow more valid models to be constructed have created substantial hardships for the developers of such systems. This has resulted in what may be a unique blend of science and commercialism as developers race to be the first to sell their particular predictive model to health care providers, third-party payers, and legislative authorities.

---

*This general principle has also been used in trauma research, pediatric trauma, and other fields as well. The details are unimportant; the opportunity for abuse and the pitfalls are almost identical.

The best defense for an institution or a CCU is to have as clear a picture as possible of the nature of the patient population and the activity in that unit. If an outside regulatory body, such as a state agency, is using a particular model, it is essential that the hospital administrator collect the same data and examine it prospectively. This will provide maximal opportunity to spot trends, to isolate and correct sources of difficulty, and to practice true quality improvement. It is likely that accrediting agencies will increasingly emphasize data-driven quality assurance techniques.[20]

Information

The ultimate objective of a quality assurance program is changing behavior to eliminate practices that do not meet the desired standard. The leadership at the Buffalo (New York) General Hospital's Surgical Intensive Care Unit (SICU) developed and implemented methods of prospective record keeping that have allowed the identification of problem areas, and several changes have resulted in practice to avoid or reduce these problems. The working assumptions for the design of the SICU quality assurance program included

- Precise information is needed about bedside events.
- Such information is most reliably gathered prospectively.
- Information gathering must be integrated into daily activity but must not be an undue burden on the CCU staff.
- In a technologically oriented environment, constant attention to "readiness," in a military sense, is necessary. Equipment must work when needed; when broken, it must be promptly and reliably repaired.
- Effective communication with all staff in a unit is essential for the implementation of quality assurance policies.

A critical care quality assurance form was developed that contained demographic information about the patient—supplied by imprinting the hospital plate—and the date and time of admission. The remainder of the form consisted of a list of items relating to events that were to be tracked. The form was available for any professional caregiver to mark at any time during the patient's stay in the SICU. Considerable time was spent orienting the nursing staff to the objectives of the new procedure, and a regular review of the previous day's sheets was conducted by the head nurse and the attending physician. Information from the completed forms was then keyed into a PC by a clinical secretary using software designed for this purpose.

Accumulation of the data in a computer file format greatly simplified presentation and analysis of the data. Summaries of events and unscheduled repairs were made available monthly. Review of this data became part of the routine monthly agenda of the nurse-physician liaison committee, whose primary purpose is quality assurance at the implementation level.

This process of data accumulation has ensured that current data are available for review by the group of individuals who have the greatest influence on the actual care given in the CCU. It has allowed trends to be spotted and the subjective impressions of trends (e.g., "We're having a rash of unintended extubations!") to be confirmed or refuted. Problems have thus been promptly identified, and isolated incidents have been placed in perspective.

The use of a data base for analyzing equipment problems has meant that a variety of reports are easily generated. Information is typically sorted by an internal classification scheme. For example, all failures of intravenous pumps may be grouped together. The institutional property tag number is one of the items entered on the original form, making it easy to identify equipment that fails repeatedly. Inappropriate practices that contributed to equipment failure are identified and corrected.

Communication

A variety of actions might be recommended as a result of the review session. Correspondence or counseling may be initiated with an individual who appears to be a repeated source of deviation from standard practice. Attendance at a subsequent quality assurance meeting might be requested for a representative of a support service not normally attending the meetings to discuss a specific issue arising out of the monthly reports or other specific incidents.

It is possible to detect patterns of behavior in a number of areas (see the following examples). The availability of statistical evidence helps to modify the behavior in a rational manner.

EXAMPLE 1

In an SICU designed and staffed to accommodate only a certain number of overnight patients, it is important to post overnight stays in advance to allow the best allocation of resources. We found that there was a significant problem with elderly, high-risk patients who were undergoing surgery without appropriate overnight space in the CCU booked for them in advance. We thus selected inappropriate posting as a review category, which made it possible to produce lists of patients and to identify physicians who were posting inappropriately. In 1 month, we found that 60% of inappropriately posted patients originated from one surgical office. When this information was made available to the physicians in that office, the group communicated needs for CCU care in advance.

EXAMPLE 2

A study of patients revealed a group flagged as "hypoxic." Within this group we identified a major subgroup in which the hypoxemia was associated with transport from the operating room to the SICU without the use of tank oxygen. Most of these patients were young. Individuals who were associated with this practice were identified. When the data were discussed with them, compliance was improved for the routine use of supplemental oxygen for transfers of patients from the operating room to the SICU.

Unfortunately, denial is a major factor in the behavior of many well-intentioned practitioners. All physicians have complications, and almost all physicians occasionally do something less than appropriate. These complications and inappropriate behaviors, however, are soon forgotten. The province of quality assurance reviewers is to detect significant departures from normal patterns. We believe that the methods described here have improved our ability to detect such departures and have provided evidence to help modify this behavior.

A discussion of computer-assisted, quality assurance data gathering would be incomplete without mention of the achievements realized in a few centers with comprehensive clinical information systems. Shabot and coworkers[21] at Cedars-Sinai Medical Center and Carlon and colleagues at Memorial Sloan-Kettering Hospital have developed methods of extracting an analogue of the APACHE score directly from their clinical information system without operator intervention. The cost of such state-of-the-art methods of data collection is likely to limit applicability for some time.

STAFF COMMUNICATIONS WITHIN A CRITICAL CARE UNIT

The CCU is a complex environment with a rapidly changing melange of patients, personnel, policies, and procedures. In a well-run unit, there is a continual process of reevaluation, both of individual and group practice. Much of this activity can be broadly classified as quality assurance—the goal is to eliminate errors and improve care. Quality assurance activities can take many forms. Patients may be followed prospectively by using a broad range of clinical physiologic and administrative monitors. Outcomes may be monitored, and equipment breakdown and repairs may be vigorously tracked to ensure unit readiness. Regular chart review for completeness and decision content (from both physician and nursing standpoints) can also be an integral part of this process. An ad hoc committee may be convened to conduct an inquiry when a major incident occurs. All of these activities lead to a constant flow of information affecting those who work in the CCU. In addition, an upward channel of communication is also needed for managers and directors to know what issues are important to the staff.

At the Buffalo General Hospital SICU, the need to document the dissemination of information such as new policies and to satisfy accrediting agencies led to the development of MEMOS, an electronic mail system for staff members within the local area network in the SICU. Although the system could have run on an individual PC,[22] a network was used because of the physical configuration of the CCU. The system has been used by nurse managers for more than 3 years to keep staff members up to date. Features include

- Easy file maintenance
- Individual password access
- A defined group of system operators with access to all system functions
- Limited access for all other users
- As many as 40 definable subgroups for the purposes of mail distribution
- Easy identification of those delinquent in reading their mail
- Hard copy with a distribution list for all memorandums added to the system
- A browse feature to allow rereading of old memorandums
- A feedback channel

The system was designed to meet the following objectives:

1. The system must be able to be operated without outside help by the unit managers responsible for policies and communications.
2. The staff members in the unit must be able to use the system without extensive orientation.
3. The system should create a permanent record of communications.
4. The system must allow unit managers to identify staff members who are lax in keeping up with the flow of information.
5. A method of responding to staff turnover by updating files in an efficient manner is essential.

One of the senior nurses in the unit, without any previous computing experience, functioned as the unit's system manager, performing maintenance, supervision, communication, and documentation functions as required.

The system allows definition of subgroups of individuals to whom mail may be sent selectively. Thus users can avoid reading irrelevant material. A memorandum may be appended to the incoming mail for all users in the selected profiles, and a permanent copy is printed, which is dated, time stamped, and identified with the name of the operator. At the top of the memorandum is the list of staff members to whom it was sent. This paper is filed as part of the permanent quality assurance record to document the completeness of communications.

On request, the system prints a list of staff members with more than a given number of unread memorandums. This list may be posted on a bulletin board. We have rarely found it necessary to resort to this technique to ensure that individuals are using the system properly.

Results

There has been a dramatic improvement in the quality of communication within the unit. In a snapshot study of a routine communication 1 week after it was issued from the nursing office, the SICU was compared with another CCU to test nursing awareness of the information. This other unit uses conventional methods of communication—bulletin board, communications book, and staff meetings. There was a dramatic difference in nurse awareness of the content of the memorandums between the two units.

It has been claimed that CCUs function most efficiently when communication among workers is effective.[23] Although only a small body of evidence specific to CCUs has been adduced to support this view,[24] it is a well-recognized management principle.

The shift schedule in many nursing units is such that a staff member may not be scheduled to work for a week or more, during which much can happen. The system described here offers that individual an easy way to stay current and provides the supervisor with a method of determining whether staff members are indeed keeping themselves informed. This same system requires minimal equipment (an IBM PC clone with 256K memory, two floppy disks, and a simple printer), obtainable at a minimal cost. The equipment will also be available for many other tasks within the CCU.

INVENTORY AND EQUIPMENT MANAGEMENT
Consumable Item Inventory Control

As institutions seek to cut costs by reducing the size of consumable item inventories, the quality of record keeping and inventory tracking, particularly for high-cost, low-volume items, becomes more important. Although some hospital-wide inventory control systems are fully integrated into the hospital's medical information system, this function is still lacking in most special care units. Alternatively, many CCUs order needed items directly from an outside supplier. In these circumstances, the application of even a rudimentary inventory control system, preferably with an automated form of data entry such as bar coding, can pay for itself in 6 months or less.

Preventive and Emergency Maintenance

A typical CCU contains a complex array of equipment subject to heavy physical demands in environments that are often hostile to reliable performance. The ubiquitous presence of human secretions and concentrated intravenous fluids, as well as the normal hazards of heat, dust, and physical abuse, makes the CCU a difficult place in which to keep equipment functional.

One important yardstick of quality in a CCU, as in a military unit, is its degree of preparedness (i.e., how much of the theoretically available resources can actually be mobilized at any given time). There is a strong correlation between preparedness and staff morale. In managing the equipment for a CCU, there are several important objectives:

- As much of the equipment as possible must work at any given time.
- When equipment is broken, it must be repaired promptly.
- Equipment that is inadequately repaired or that requires repeated repair must be easily identified and documented so the causes can be addressed.
- The preventive maintenance program must make information accessible to unit managers.
- The staff members in the unit must feel they have a stake in the process of maintaining readiness.

A data base system was developed at the Buffalo General Hospital to address these objectives. Organizing repair activities into a data base made it possible to

- Provide prompt feedback to the individual reporting the problem.
- Detect problem patterns and attack their root causes.
- Demonstrate to hospital management that it would be more cost-effective to replace older equipment than to continue to repair it.

The heart of the scheme was the FIX-ME ticket, a three-part, carbonless form. Anyone discovering a malfunction completed six items on the top half of the form. The top copy was attached to the offending equipment, which was then taken out of service. The other two copies were given to the charge nurse, who was required to communicate with the department responsible for correcting the problem. The second copy became the preliminary work order, and the third copy was used to update the repairs data base. Entering details of all the repairs generated required less than an hour of clerical time weekly.

A simple data form using a commercially available forms-generation/data base program was used. The software selected was Versaform (Applied Software Technology, 170 Knowles Drive, Los Gatos, CA 95030). It will run on an IBM PC or compatible with a minimum of 512K memory and two floppy disk drives with a printer. The precise choice of software is relatively unimportant compared with the organization of management information into an accessible format.

This system allowed all repaired items to be tracked by their hospital property number, a unique serial number attached to every item of equipment when it first enters the hospital. The date of the next scheduled safety check or preventative maintenance was also entered into the data base at the time of an unscheduled repair. It has proved useful for the unit managers to have this information available from an independent source.

The strength of the system lies in the use of the reports. The following examples demonstrate some of the capabilities provided by repair documentation.

EXAMPLE 1

A print-out of unscheduled repairs month by month showed that more than 40 intravenous pumps per month had been sent out for repair in 3 consecutive months. When the manufacturer was confronted with this information in the form of a print-out, only a short time elapsed before company executives arrived to examine the problem. Two weeks later, company engineers were stationed in the hospital around the clock for a period of 7 days to troubleshoot problems. The net effect of this activity included the following:

- Better in-service programs on management of the pumps were provided by the department of nursing education to the actual nurse users.
- A number of practices likely to degrade the performance of the pumps were identified and steps taken to eliminate them.
- The medical electronics department was brought up-to-date on the latest maintenance procedures.

- The monthly pump failure rate declined to single figures.

EXAMPLE 2

Many of the electrocardiogram machines in the unit had been manufactured at a time when minimal ground current leakage standards were much less stringent than they are today. As a result, whenever electrocardiograms were obtained with exposed pacer wires, a battery-operated portable machine was used. This machine was continually being sent out for repair. In a short time, six successive repairs were documented. When the print-out of the chronologic sequence of repairs was attached to a request for emergency funding for the purchase of a new machine, the request was immediately granted. Before the institution of this recording scheme, requests for replacement of the equipment in the course of annual capital budgets had been denied for several years.

The data base showing equipment failure and unscheduled repairs provided powerful information for the unit managers. It ensured that both the hospital administration and outside vendors paid attention to the needs of the unit. It allowed for focused investigation of problems that in some cases led to changes in practice. The prompt and regular feedback of this information to the staff in the unit served to raise morale and reinforce the best practices in the use of complex equipment. Such a data base is simple to operate, requires little in the way of complex equipment, and is a highly cost-effective component of the overall quality assurance effort.

SUMMARY

The applications for computers in the critical care setting are widespread and diverse. A knowledge of the possibilities, a healthy skepticism when dealing with vendors, and a willingness to explore and seek help from other users are the prerequisites to the successful harnessing of this technology for use in the CCU.

References

1. Booth FVM: Patient monitoring in the intensive care unit (editorial). Crit Care Med 11:57, 1983.
2. Bradshaw KE, Sittig DF, Gardner RM, et al: Computer-based data entry for nurses in the ICU. MD Comput 6:274, 1989.
3. Gardner RM: Computerized management of intensive care patients. MD Comput 3:36, 1986.
4. Glaeser DH, Thomas LJ: Computer monitoring in patient care. Annu Rev Biophys Bioeng 4:449, 1975.
5. Milholland K: Patient data management systems (PDMS): Computer technology for critical care nurses. Comput Nurs 6:237, 1988.
6. Brimm JE: Computers in critical care. Crit Care Nurs Q 9:53, 1987.
7. Leyerle BJ, LoBue M, Shabot MM: Integrated databases for data management beyond the bedside. Int J Clin Monit Comput 7:83, 1990.
8. Goldman L, Cook EF, Brand DA, et al: A computer protocol to predict myocardial infarction in emergency department patients with chest pain. N Engl J Med 318:797, 1988.
9. De Dombal FT: Computer-aided decision support in acute abdominal pain, with special reference to the EC concerted action. Int J Biomed Comput 26:183, 1990.
10. Shabot MM, LoBue M, Leyerle BJ: Decision support ALERTS for clinical laboratory and blood gas data. Int J Clin Monit Comput 7:27, 1990.
11. Tate KE, Gardner RM, Weaver LK: A computerized laboratory alerting system. MD Comput 7:296, 1990.
12. Weed LL, Zimny NJ: The problem-oriented system, problem-knowledge coupling, and clinical decision making. Phys Ther 69:565, 1989.
13. Wald A: Sequential Analysis. New York, John Wiley & Sons, 1947.
14. Berwick DM: Health services research and quality of care: Assignments for the 1990s. Med Care 27:763, 1989.
15. Nutting MA, Dock LL: A History of Nursing. New York, GP Putnam & Sons, p 147, 1907.
16. Meisenheimer CG (ed): Quality Assurance: A Complete Guide to Effective Programs. Rockville, MD, Aspen Publishers, 1985.
17. Thompson J: Diagnosis-related groups and quality assurance. Top Health Care Financing 8:43, 1982.
18. Iezzoni LI: Using severity information for quality assessment: A review of three cases by five severity measures. QRB 15:376, 1989.
19. Hannan EL, Kilburn H Jr, O'Donnell JF: Adult open heart surgery in New York State: An analysis of risk factors and hospital mortality rates. JAMA 264:2768, 1990.
20. Patterson CH: Quality assurance, control, and monitoring: The future role of information technology from the Joint Commission's perspective. Comput Nurs 8:105, 1990.
21. Shabot MM, LoBue M, Leyerle BJ: Automatic extraction of intensity intervention scores from a computerized surgical ICU flowsheet. Am J Surg 154:72, 1987.
22. Booth FVM: Effective staff communications in a large ICU. Int J Clin Monit Comput 6:81, 1989.
23. Knaus WA: Organizational structure affects patient survival. Hospitals 61(13):62, 1987.
24. Knaus WA, Draper EA, Wagner DP, et al: An evaluation of outcome from intensive care units in major medical centers. Ann Intern Med 104:410, 1986.

CHAPTER 9

Artificial Intelligence and Expert Systems in Critical Care Medicine

D. Charles Kowalewski, Jr.
Richard W. Carlson

Computers and computer-related technology are increasingly evident in the critical care unit (CCU), where they excel in information retrieval, data storage, and patient monitoring. The computer systems used in the CCU are relatively passive; they function without much interaction from health care professionals. The various commercial computer systems that perform these operations are discussed elsewhere in this text.

Many clinicians believe the computer can and should play a more active role in the CCU. Exploiting the power and memory that newer computers possess, dedicated researchers have developed computer programs to simulate intelligence or cognition. Fagan loosely defined *intelligence* as the ability to solve complex problems accurately and dependably using the same incomplete or circumstantial information available to humans.[1] However, computers are not human, and their cognitive programming is *artificial*. "Intelligent" programs are unique in that they consider incomplete or incorrect data as well as valid, correct data and still develop useful conclusions. Other computer programs generally lack such a robust feature. Standard computer programs may perform calculations, data storage, or telecommunications quickly and accurately, but these programs often fail when offered information that is inconsistent with their task or when unexpected results are obtained.

As computers pervade the workplace, the development of artificially intelligent software directed toward solving medical programs is increasingly important. Intensivists are often regarded as the most technologically literate of the medical staff; they will therefore be called on to assess the need and standards for artificially intelligent programs in the CCU.

This chapter reviews the principles and applications of artificial intelligence (AI) in critical care medicine. Artificial intelligence in medicine (AIM) is a subset of a much larger field of computer science called medical informatics in which researchers investigate the diverse role of the computer in medicine.[2]

In addition to developing intelligent programs, AI researchers often examine the *reasoning* mechanisms that humans use to interpret different types of data when applying similar methods to computer programs. The study of these mechanisms often leads to novel concepts in learning how humans reason. In fact, AI research is a strong contributor to studies in cognitive science.

AI researchers look for areas of science in which methods of cognition are well defined, so that they might study computer applications that mimic intelligence. Modern medicine is a useful platform for the study of AI because it contains a wide variety of data sources that physicians utilize in structured ways. Critical care medicine is particularly useful because most information has already been encoded into a logical, predefined format. For example, advanced cardiac life support[3] and advanced trauma life support[4] protocols organize the complicated and sometimes confusing mass of data generated during emergencies into differential diagnoses and treatment algorithms. Structured methods such as these developed by medical science present enticing insights into the mechanisms of human decision making. Because medicine is based on a variety of diagnostic mechanisms, it can be used as a model for creating diverse clinical decision algorithms.

Table 9–1 lists a few of the applications currently under study for use in the CCU.

BAYESIAN DIAGNOSIS AND TREATMENT

AI applications are best known for their contribution to the development of differential diagnoses and treatment algorithms. This is because most physicians are taught a bayesian approach to diagnosis. That is, a list of differential diagnoses is prepared that applies to the patient's signs and symptoms, and the physician then attempts to prove or disprove members of that list in order of decreasing likelihood. This series of functions (retrieving data, quantifying probabilities, and sorting) is well suited to computer programming algorithms. One of the earliest models of medical expert systems was the Internist-1 medical diagnosis program developed at the University of Pittsburgh.[5] The program uses a highly stratified decision algorithm and numerous rules as the user provides information about patient findings. At each step, the program offers a differential

diagnosis or questions the user until a differential diagnosis can be made. During his or her progress through the algorithm, the user can check the working differential diagnosis or the logic the program is using to develop its differential. A personal computer–based extension of Internist-1, QMR (Quick Medical Reference), has also been introduced.[6]

In programs such as these, the machine functions as a surrogate consultant, bringing an expert's encoded knowledge to the user. This is useful when a human consultant may not be available. The programs' knowledge is not limited to values and clinical knowledge, but integrates to some degree the nuances and inferences that an expert develops over time. Although a program may be limited in that it is without human senses, it provides a wealth of knowledge and specialized insight not commonly available to the user. Optimally, the program educates the user about the problem and explains the reasoning by which it develops a conclusion. Limitations of hardware and concepts in AI require that the system focus on a particular problem in medicine. AI programs that provide the focal services of a specialist are termed *expert systems*.

THE EXPERT SYSTEM

To better explain the workings of an expert system, the rule-based expert system and some of its variations are briefly described here. Thomas L. Lincoln described an expert system as an active reference source that combines three components: a knowledge base, a reasoning engine, and a user interface (Table 9–2).

The knowledge base is a specially constructed data base that contains the weights, caveats, and accumulated expertise of its particular domain. The knowledge base may be intelligent (Fig. 9–1). It may be capable of learning from past experiences or sufficiently intuitive to seek out information when its own stores seem inadequate to the task at hand. However, the depth and breadth of medical knowledge may be too great to capture in a knowledge base, even when the knowledge base is constrained to a focused topic. Conversely, hardware limitations of more portable personal computers may prohibit the creation of a knowledge base with adequate intuitive capabilities, thereby limiting the expert system's portability or command of the specific topic.

Basic research in AI explores methods to efficiently store and apply information as knowledge, as well as how to exchange that knowledge with the outside world. The challenge is to store information so that it will be usable, affordable, and sufficiently expansive during use by other programs while operating within the constraints of the hardware used for the project. The precision, accuracy, quantity, volatility, and format of information all affect the recording of information.[7]

Often, information does not need to be stored literally; rather, the *essence* of the data must be recorded. Therefore, the problem in AI research may not be how to develop a workable system, but how to encode the essentials and nuances of the expert's knowledge.[8] An example of this symbolic (non-numeric) data storage would be to record that a patient has tachycardia rather than recording the actual heart rate. Tachycardia can be defined. Therefore, changing the definition for each patient in question can dynamically alter the qualities of the knowledge base. Creating symbolic forms of data such as this permits versatility in data storage. Knowledge comes in a variety of types, and this necessitates the development of different methods to store knowledge.

Combining the knowledge base with the user interface to emulate intelligence is the job of the reasoning engine. The reasoning engine (also called a logic or inference engine)

TABLE 9–1

APPLICATIONS FOR ARTIFICIAL INTELLIGENCE PROGRAMS IN THE CRITICAL CARE UNIT

Bayesian diagnosis and treatment algorithms
Closed-loop ventilator management
Waveform recognition
   Cardiac arrhythmias
   Arterial pressure monitoring
   Pulmonary arterial catheters and hemodynamics
   Intracranial pressures
   Epileptiform activity
Review and editing medical orders
Administration of CCU facilities
Education of intensivists in training
Formalization of treatment and test protocols
Evaluation of severity of illness and prognosis

TABLE 9–2

SIMPLIFIED STRUCTURE OF AN EXPERT SYSTEM

Knowledge Base	User Interface
Statistics	Typed input and output
Remote experience	Pointing devices
Temporal events	Handwriting recognition
Intuition	Voice recognition
Inferences	Nonhuman interfaces
Reasoning Engine	
If-then reasoning	
Fuzzy reasoning	
Causal modeling	
Blackboard architecture	
Distributed parallel processes	

IF:	1. The infection that requires therapy is meningitis, and
	2. The patient has evidence of a serious skin or soft tissue infection, and
	3. Organisms were not seen on the stain of the culture, and
	4. The type of infection is bacterial
THEN:	There is evidence that the organism (other than those seen on cultures or smears) that might be causing the infection is staphylococcus-coag-pos (0.75) or streptococcus (0.5).

Figure 9–2. Sample rule from MYCIN demonstrating the if-then structure. In this example, four conditions must be met for the premise to be considered true. (From Shortliffe EH, Fagan LM: Expert systems research: Modeling the medical decision making process. In: Gravenstein JS, Newbower RS, Ream AK, et al [eds]: An Integrated Approach to Monitoring. Stoneham, MA, Butterworth, p 183, 1983.)

applies and associates information in the knowledge base. Reasoning is made to be as versatile and intelligent as possible, so that one engine may be applied to several knowledge bases for multiple purposes. Some designs of engine types that have been studied are listed in Table 9–2. Keeping the medical knowledge base separate from the mechanism that applies the information makes both the knowledge base and the reasoning engine easier to manage.

Depending on the type and use of the expert system, both the input and the output of the system may incorporate automated data devices such as a CCU monitor; manually transferred data such as paper or speech; or internally created data such as the results of deductions or tests that can be further utilized in calculations or deductions. Although the development and testing of expert systems occupy the bulk of current applied AI research, the study of components of the expert system (data storage, reasoning engines, and user interfaces) constitutes the bench research aspects of AI.

MYCIN is an expert system developed by Shortliffe at Stanford University.[9] MYCIN combines information with rules to suggest diagnoses and treatments of bacteremia and meningitis (Fig. 9–2). The user inputs patient data, and the program responds with optimal antibiotic therapy. MYCIN uses an if-then architecture to operate its reasoning engine.

The *if* clause contains a test, and the *then* clause contains actions to perform. Most persons are comfortable with the if-then concept. If-then designs were among the first AI applications in medicine. A wide variety of well-known systems utilize this approach. If-then models have other advantages that are listed in Table 9–3.

One complaint about if-then reasoning engines is that some rules are too rigid or literal. However, this need not be the case. By assigning an arbitrary weight to a rule, the significance of a rule may be quantified. For example, checking for a life-threatening condition might carry greater weight than checking for a chronic illness. The reasoning engine could be directed to invoke a rule to establish the presence (or absence) of a critical disorder despite evidence that may be more convincing for a less serious condition.

Often, the program is empowered to modify its own rules, effectively rewriting its reasoning engine as different patient conditions are identified. The computer may also be permitted to carry its then clause onward, linking rules together sequentially to form a chain of inferences. In some cases, the inferences are later stored in the knowledge base for application to similar problems.

Probability assignments may be made to data in the knowledge base or to data in the patient records to indicate the dependability of the data. Such flexibility in rule making provides for highly versatile decision algorithms that are robust. The application of these weights to decision making has been termed *fuzzy reasoning*.

MYCIN is a program that uses inexact or fuzzy reasoning.[10] MYCIN establishes a "certainty factor" by calculating the difference between measures of belief and measures of disbelief. These measures weigh the attached datum by applying values to the terms *definite, probable, unlikely,* and so forth. The probability that a datum is true is scored by a numeric weight from -1 (absolutely false) to 1 (absolutely true). As the certainty factor of one diagnosis in the differential becomes large, that diagnosis and related treatment are identified as the most likely to be correct. This technique of scoring competing hypotheses is common to many expert systems where conditions are uncertain or different conclusions compete for greatest likelihood.

Some disadvantages of an if-then model are shown in Table 9–4. Most of these are related to limitations of the current hardware in computer systems. However, as hardware advances in scope and capability, many of these limitations will likely be overcome. AI concepts are also advancing to circumvent hardware and conceptual hurdles. An example is provided by one particular problem found with the MYCIN project. Clancy and coworkers discovered that

Question:	How many fellows graduated from Critical Care Medicine at General Hospital this year?
Data base:	Zero.
Knowledge base:	There is no critical care fellowship at General Hospital.

Figure 9–1. An intelligent data base.

TABLE 9–3

ADVANTAGES OF RULE-BASED MODELS

The knowledge base is relatively easy to maintain.
The reasoning engine may be modified without affecting the medical subject matter. One reasoning engine may be used for several knowledge bases in different applications.
The application of the entire system can be easily checked for logic.
Rule-based systems are more easily conceptualized and may be more acceptable than other systems.

TABLE 9–4
LIMITATIONS OF RULE-BASED MODELS
The knowledge base may become exceedingly large as the problem becomes more general (or more complicated).
Data must be defined by norms or ranges. Nondiscrete patterns may be difficult to encode.
Rules must be segregated from the data to which they apply. The distinction between rules and data may become clouded.
Rules designed for medical decision making are often insufficient to provide in-depth education to users.[63]
Time-dependent data are difficult to model in a set of rules.[64]
"Mesa effect": The system may fail unexpectedly and completely (like falling off a mesa) when data or results are encountered that substantially differ from expectations.

```
.. 1640..
** SUGGEST CONSIDER PLACING PATIENT ON T PIECE IF
** PAO2 > 70 on FIO2 < = .4        (measure of blood gas status)
** PATIENT AWAKE AND TRIGGERING VENTILATOR
** ECG IS STABLE


.. 1650....1700....1710....1720....1730....1740....1750....
.. 1800..
** HYPERVENTILATION
** PATIENT HYPERVENTILATING
** SUGGEST REDUCING EFFECTIVE ALVEOLAR VENTILATION
** TO REDUCE ALVEOLAR VENTILATION, REDUCE
   TIDAL VOLUME
** REDUCE RESPIRATION RATE, OR
** INCREASE DISTAL DEAD SPACE TUBING VOLUME


.. 1800..
** SYSTEM ASSUMES PATIENT STARTING T PIECE


.. 1813....1815....1817..
** HYPOVENTILATION
```

Figure 9–3. Sample output from VM. Note the time of day markers and the suggestions for correcting ventilatory abnormalities. (From Fagan LM, Kunz JC, Feigenbaum EA, et al: Extensions to the rule-based formalism for a monitoring task. In: Buchanan BG, Shortliffe EH [eds]: Rule-Based Systems: The MYCIN Experiments of the Standard Heuristic Programming Project. Reading, MA, Addison-Wesley, p 397, 1984.)

although the if-then architecture of MYCIN facilitates the review of decision logic, the if-then clauses do not readily adapt to educational purposes. Clancy demonstrated that programs such as MYCIN can be modified to be used as educational devices.[11] Other programs have explored diagnostic as well as therapeutic algorithms for the acutely ill.[12]

Another program, Nutritional Advisor, provides advice on nutritional assessment and support of critically ill patients. The system mimics the decisions of a gastroenterologist and is typical of expert systems in that it addresses a narrow problem area to attain the level of accuracy of a clinical expert.[13] Like MYCIN, the program accepts patient data as input and infers rules to critique the nutritional support provided to a patient. Suggestions may be given on an ongoing basis. In addition to formulating total parenteral nutrition, the program suggests appropriate parameters and criteria for initiating weaning from this type of nutrition.

VENTILATOR MANAGEMENT

The need for an autonomous mechanism to control ventilators has been voiced for several years. Several expert systems for ventilator management have been specifically designed for use in the CCU. The overall requirement of the software is to control a ventilator capable of autonomously monitoring, adjusting, and ultimately weaning the patient from the ventilator. The large amount of patient information readily available to potential ventilator management programs makes this an attractive area to AI researchers. These measurements are easily available and usually remain within well-contained ranges, and the respiratory information closely estimates the actual patient state. The ability to adequately quantify the patient state without human intervention enables AI researchers to more confidently develop autonomous expert systems to serve in critical roles, such as direct control of the ventilator. Systems that can operate without physician interaction are called *closed-loop* systems. Although there are no true, commercial closed-loop systems in existence at the time of this writing, several highly successful expert systems come close to achieving autonomous operation. Each program described here differs in structure and function, but all attempt to optimize the patient's physiologic status and wean the patient from the ventilator.

Strongly influenced by MYCIN's reasoning engine, Fagan and colleagues undertook an ambitious project to interpret on-line quantitative data for the purpose of managing postsurgical, ventilator-dependent patients (Figs. 9–3 and 9–4).[14–16] The system, VM (Ventilator Manager), monitors patients' physiologic status, maintains patient-specific goals, and recommends adjustments of the ventilator based on these goals. In addition, VM monitors patient parameters,

detecting and alarming adverse events and providing suggestions for corrective action. This program differs from MYCIN in that it collects data over time, interpreting both the patient's changing disease process and previous responses to therapeutic adjustments. Another system, VentPlan,[17, 18] evaluates arterial blood gas values and ventilator parameters and suggests alterations to ventilator settings (Fig. 9–5). Using a graphic approach for display, the program produces mathematic predictions of the resulting changes in pulmonary physiology and ventilator settings.

```
STATUS RULE: STABLE-HEMODYNAMICS
DEFINITION: Defines stable hemodynamics based on blood
   pressures and heart rates.
APPLIES to patients on VOLUME, CMV, ASSIST, T PIECE
COMMENT: Look at mean arterial pressure for changes in
   pressure and systolic blood pressure for maximal pressures.


IF:
   HEART RATE is ACCEPTABLE
   PULSE RATE does NOT CHANGE by 20 beats/min in 15 min
   MEAN ARTERIAL PRESSURE is ACCEPTABLE
   MEAN ARTERIAL PRESSURE does NOT CHANGE by
      15 torr in 15 min
   SYSTOLIC BLOOD PRESSURE is ACCEPTABLE


THEN:
   The HEMODYNAMICS are STABLE
```

Figure 9–4. An example of the if-then relationships in VM. There is strong similarity between this system and MYCIN. Note that "acceptable" varies with the clinical context, and the rule may apply to the type of ventilatory assistance for which VM has been given knowledge. (From Shortliffe EH, Fagan LM: Expert systems research: Modeling the medical decision making process. In: Gravenstein JS, Newbower RS, Ream AK, et al [eds]: An Integrated Approach to Monitoring. Stoneham, MA, Butterworth, p 183, 1983.)

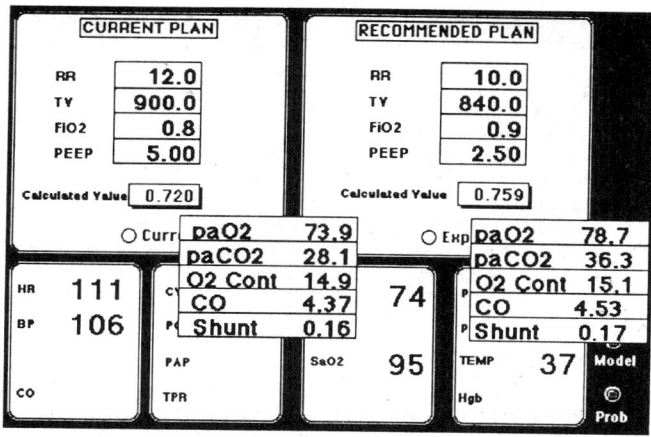

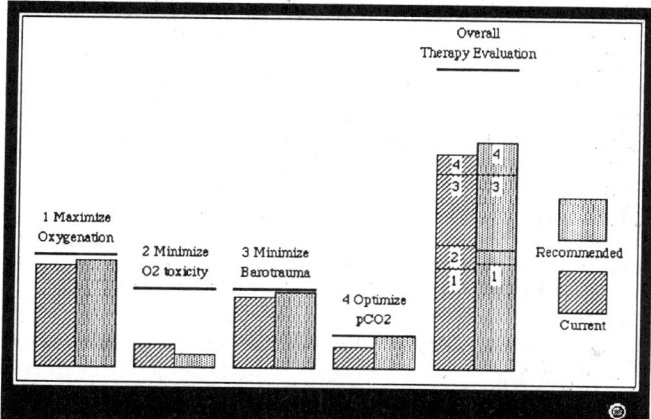

Figure 9–5. Sample output from VentPlan. The left upper box displays the current ventilator setting; the right upper box displays settings recommended by VentPlan. Mathematic calculations from the data are superimposed on the settings boxes. Note also the real-time data acquisition of vital signs and hemodynamics. (From Farr BR, Fagan LM: Decision-theoretic evaluation of therapy plans. Symp Comput Appl Med Care 13:188, 1989. © 1989 IEEE.)

Much like a human consultant, VM applies the underlying physiology and pathophysiology to documented interactions to determine which patient findings agree with the defined physiology.[19]

VentPlan incorporates a "belief network" of information with a mathematic model of pulmonary physiology (Fig. 9–6).[20] The two components are combined with a "plan evaluator" to generate and critique treatment plans for various physiologic states. A "control algorithm" manages communications between the user, as well as automated data inputs. For example, VentPlan mathematically assesses arterial blood gas values for a patient, then transmits its impression to the belief network. The belief network compares the new data to its patient data base and checks to see if it must modify its understanding of the current pulmonary physiology for the patient under consideration. If the system detects a change or violation of pulmonary rules, the belief network notifies the plan evaluator to reassess the current ventilator settings and to make further recommendations as necessary.

Use of a belief network is called *causal modeling*.[21] Causal modeling may optimally be used in systems that are dynamic, time varying, or homeostatic.[22]

Sittig and coworkers developed the COMPAS patient management system.[23, 24] This expert system uses data in ways much like VM, but COMPAS is designed to study the

patient with adult respiratory distress syndrome. Accessing the integrated hospital information system HELP gives COMPAS vast amounts of information about the patient without requiring health professionals to repeatedly input patient data.

COMPAS uses an interesting approach called *blackboard architecture* (Fig. 9–7). According to Sittig, this model is analogous to a group of experts from different fields who are able to communicate only by leaving messages one at a time on a "blackboard." All the information pertaining to the problem, in this case ventilator management, is available on the blackboard, and each expert writes an opinion and solution. Someone monitors the interactions between experts and decides which participant should be allowed to offer the next piece of advice. The accumulation of multiple solutions from multiple experts results in more complete solutions. In this analogy, the HELP system contains the information and COMPAS utilizes a reasoning engine as the moderator of the blackboard discussion.

Although each of the programs just mentioned discusses diagnosis and treatment plans for patients undergoing ventilation, none of these programs directly communicates with the ventilator in the closed-loop style discussed earlier. Kusivar, a system developed by Rudowski and colleagues, was developed to assess the feasibility of a closed-loop ventilator management system.[25, 26] The system accommodates long-term goals and monitors patient status for both unexpected changes and changes in response to therapy (Fig. 9–8). It has the potential to assess pulmonary status, critique current treatment plans, recommend new treatment plans, and modify ventilator settings directly. Only the first three functions are currently active. This expert system is being modified to operate on desktop-style personal com-

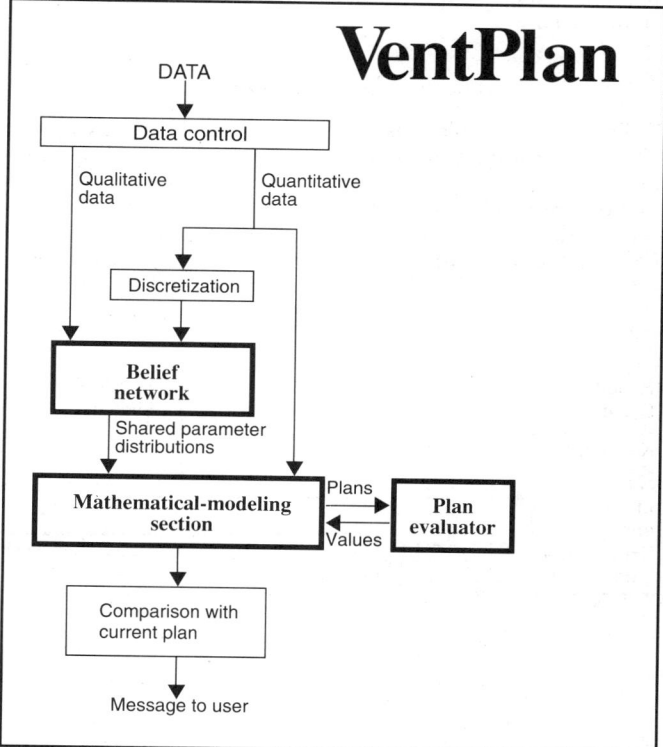

Figure 9–6. Diagram of the VentPlan control algorithm. (From Rutledge G, Thomsen G, Beinlich I, et al: Combining qualitative and quantitative computation in a ventilator therapy planner. Symp Comput Appl Med Care 13:315, 1989. © 1989 IEEE.)

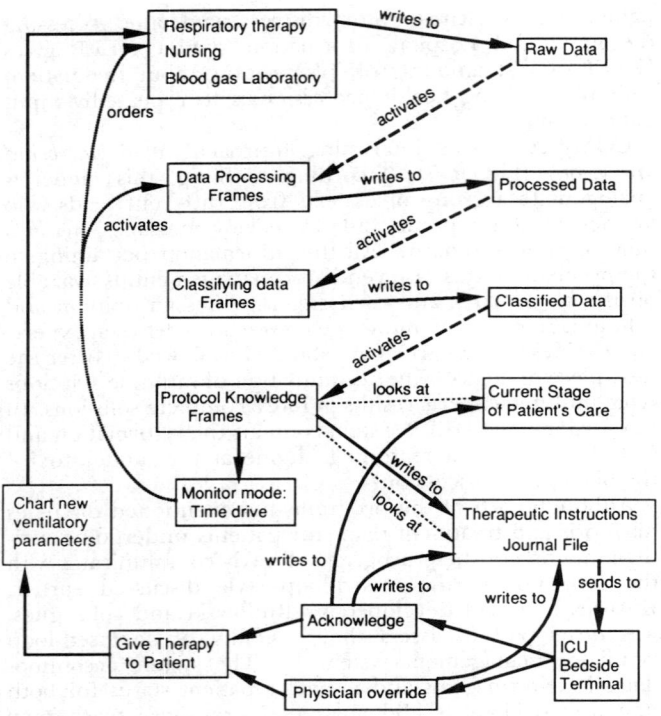

Figure 9–7. The blackboard control architecture is displayed in this schematic diagram of COMPAS, an expert ventilator management system. (From Sittig DF, Pace NL, Gardner RM, et al: Implementation of a computerized patient advice system using the HELP clinical information system. Comput Biomed Res 22:474, 1989.)

puters, so that it may be taken to the patient's bedside for clinical trials.

WAVEFORM RECOGNITION

The most conspicuous of all computer functions in the CCU is the waveform monitor. Computers record the various waveforms and optionally store or redisplay the information on remote terminals. Frequently, the patient monitor is also utilized as a data input and retrieval device. Data may be retained for later use or interpreted immediately and discarded. Regardless of how the waveform gets into the

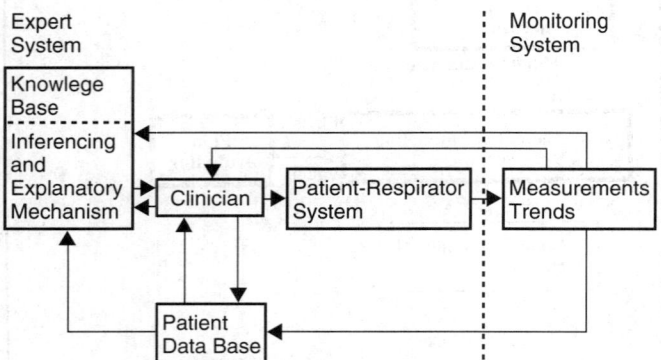

Figure 9–8. Schematic of data communication in the Kusivar system. (From Rudowski R, Frostell C, Gill H: A knowledge-based support system for mechanical ventilation of the lungs. The KUSIVAR concept and prototype. Comput Methods Programs Biomed 30:59, 1989.)

TABLE 9–5
STAGES OF INTERPRETING A WAVEFORM
Identify the waveform and its source. Visually scan an appropriate amount of the waveform. Conceptually isolate all noise and artifacts. Identify important and repetitive features. Classify (diagnose) the waveform. Determine the significance of the diagnosis. Include other medical information if needed. Develop a treatment plan.

computer, data in any format is not knowledge until it is utilized in a meaningful way. Stated another way, a device may be considered intelligent when it can use data as knowledge. Devices that record and redisplay physiologic waveforms are not intelligent. However, a device that recognizes normal and pathologic changes, suggests diagnoses or treatments, and functions as a useful surrogate consultant is intelligent.

The interpretation of waveforms is taken for granted by humans (Table 9–5). Without realizing it, health professionals accomplish most of the tasks required to interpret waveforms within 6 to 12 seconds. During this process, the clinician refers to his or her vast knowledge of waveform appearances and interpretations and applies rules of interpretation to the particular waveform under scrutiny. If this interpretation results in significant conclusions, the clinician may elect to institute or alter therapy.

Computer systems to interpret electrocardiographic (ECG) rhythms were under development long before the phrase *artificial intelligence* was coined. Originally, ECG waveforms were simply recorded and redisplayed to monitors at a remote nursing station. As computer processors eventually became fast enough for real-time observations, the task of continuous observation of the monitors was turned over to the computer. Many of the ECG monitoring programs are sophisticated, and they have been extensively reviewed in the literature.[27–30]

However, significant problems exist with many of the current arrhythmia monitors. For example, monitors with near-perfect sensitivity to detect life-threatening arrhythmias frequently generate false-positive alarms. Health professionals quickly "tune out" the alarms of these wolf-criers. Unfortunately, disregarding an alarm may have catastrophic results. The challenge is to develop a waveform monitor that distinguishes between true and artifactual arrhythmias, so that true arrhythmias are always alarmed and false arrhythmias are never alarmed. Signals that are not part of the ECG may frequently be the cause of the false alarms; these signals may be generically termed *noise* (Table 9–6). Mathematic attempts to remove noise have been met with varying degrees of success. At this time, no monitors claim both 100% sensitivity and 100% specificity.

The management of noise in cardiac arrhythmia monitors remains a concern for researchers.[31] Baseline wander and line noise do not look like the ECG signal, but if they are loud enough, they can mask it. This type of noise is relatively

TABLE 9–6
COMMON CLASSES OF NOISE
Baseline wander Line interference (50 or 60 Hz) Movement artifact Muscle contraction

easy to eliminate because it is regular, consistent, and distinctly different from the ECG signal. Mathematic methods of filtering out this type of noise have been described and are used commercially. More cumbersome are noise artifacts from muscle and patient motion, because they may closely approximate the amplitude and frequency of the QRS complex.

Analog signals are continuous variations of voltage or current displayed as an unbroken curve on an oscilloscope screen. Digital signals are not continuous; rather, they are "dots" of numbers placed so closely together that they merge to appear as a continuous curve on a graph. Figures 9–9 and 9–10 demonstrate differences in representing analog and digital signals. Current methods to extract noise from the ECG signal (and other physiologic recording systems) consist of analog and digital noise filters. Other techniques involve creating a set of templates to match and extract the QRS signal from the noise.

Digital filtering techniques are numeric algorithms performed on a series of numbers that represent a signal. They have superseded analog filters in many cases. A physiologic signal, once digitized into a computer, may be reviewed or filtered in many ways. In fact, digital filters for the types of noise just mentioned have been derived. However, these techniques are statistical or mathematic algorithms and may not be considered AI by AI purists. Figure 9–11 demonstrates four different types of filters for ECG analysis.

False alarms may also originate from unexpected signals. Occasionally, a normal rhythm with a bizarre appearance convinces the monitor that the patient has an arrhythmia. This also causes frequent, irritating false alarms. To solve this problem, some arrythmia-monitoring programs study the signal for a short period before actual arrhythmia processing. During that time, templates are created that the monitor uses for comparison to future waveforms. When templates are used in this capacity, AI researchers are challenged to create template-matching algorithms sufficiently robust to differentiate all divergent patterns while clustering all similar ones.

Another AI approach may be to acknowledge the presence of noise, identify it, and then exclude it from the decision-making process. AI programs that perform this function are being studied; one technique is described later in this chapter.

Electroencephalographic monitoring is a fertile field for AI to study waveform analysis, control of noise, and clinical interpretation. A discussion of such monitoring may be found in Chapter 54.

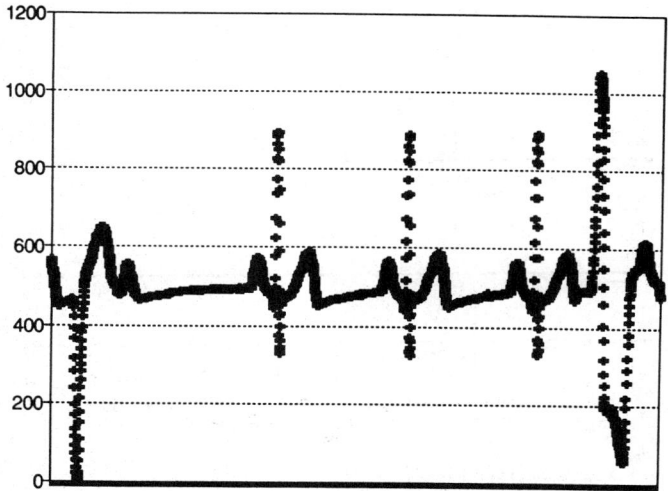

Figure 9–10. The same ECG signal as that shown in Figure 9–9 as represented here by the computer. By sampling the voltage of the signal at 500 Hz, a number is generated that represents the signal amplitude. When sampling is done quickly, the signal appears as an analog and mathematic algorithms may be performed on the series of numbers.

ORDER MANAGEMENT

An order management system can identify difficulties with order entry. This type of monitor may increase the efficiency of order placement, identify potential misuse or abuse of orders, and assist physicians in locating appropriate orders with greater ease than the paper audit systems currently in use by hospitals. AI has already been incorporated into the placement of orders at many medical centers. Typically, these are centers with physicians in training. Order management expert systems have access to patient information and a series of rules to determine if orders are appropriate and safe. Potentially hazardous orders are flagged and referred to physicians or quality assurance personnel for review.[32] Examples of such ordering controls include checking for potential idiosyncratic laboratory errors (e.g., prothrombin time may be decreased because of concurrent use of diuretics) or alerting health care personnel of treatments lacking appropriate indication (e.g., a bolus of potassium that has been ordered may not be required because the patient's most recent serum potassium level was normal).

These expert systems provide additional medical gains in that they may reduce the number of inappropriate treatments or tests, thereby conserving limited financial resources.

EDUCATION

Expert systems have also been used effectively in education. A Critical Care and Hemodynamic Monitoring Training System, which consists of a personal computer, software, and a replica of a human torso, is used to teach future intensivists how to manage a patient requiring hemodynamic monitoring (Fig. 9–12).[33] The intensivist in training may insert and pass a pulmonary arterial catheter into the torso, interpret pressure waveforms generated on a computer monitor, and work through various patient scenarios. Obviously, this type of training offers substantial advantages over current clinical training techniques, as the physician may learn and practice potentially dangerous maneuvers without risk or injury to a real patient.

Hundreds of other clinical simulators exist for personal

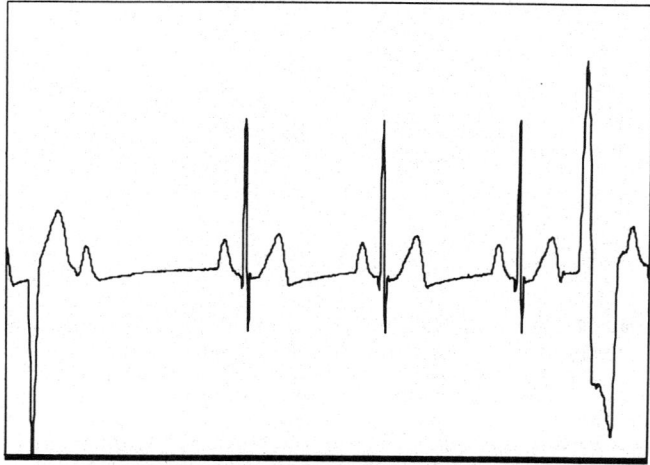

Figure 9–9. A computer-generated analog ECG signal.

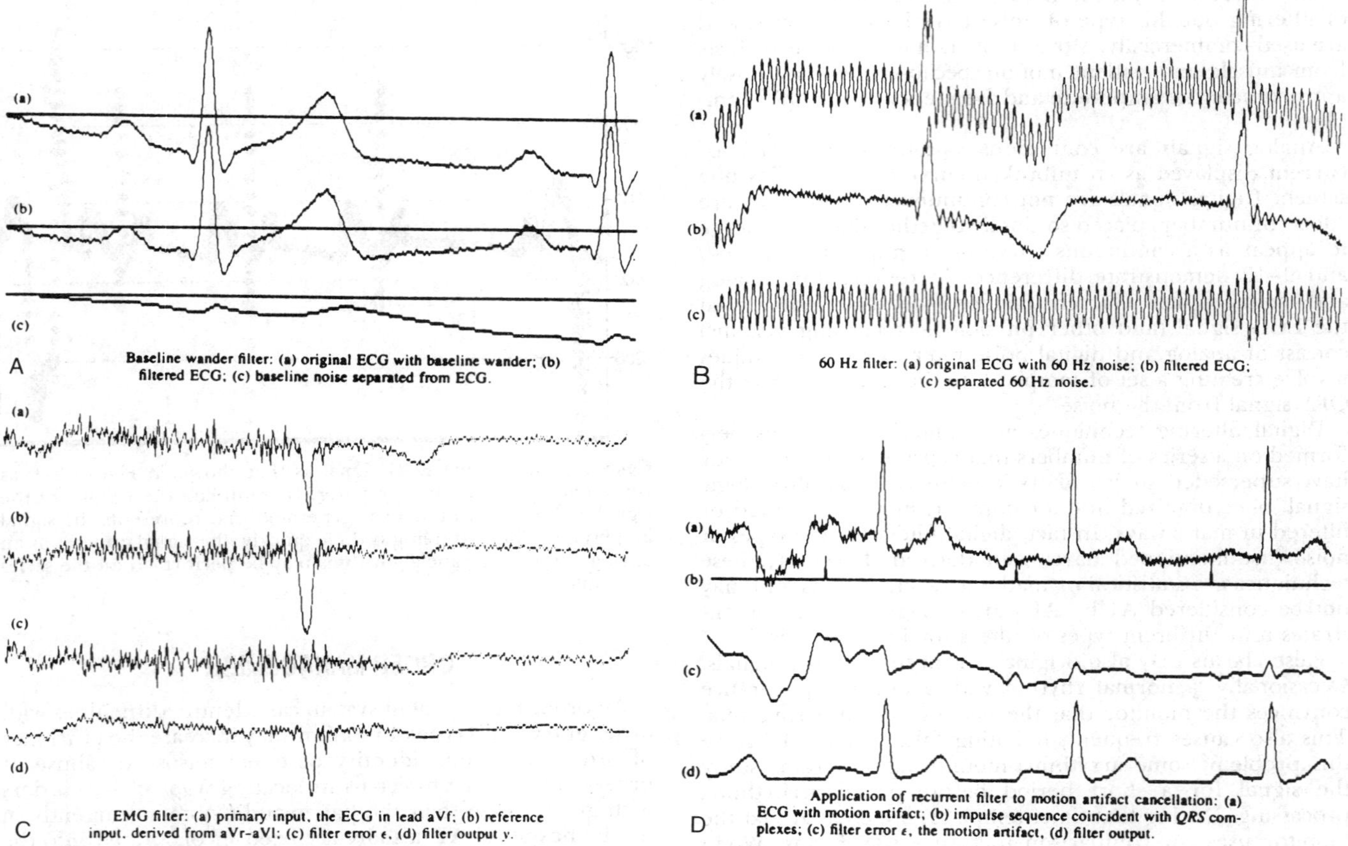

A
Baseline wander filter: (a) original ECG with baseline wander; (b) filtered ECG; (c) baseline noise separated from ECG.
B
60 Hz filter: (a) original ECG with 60 Hz noise; (b) filtered ECG; (c) separated 60 Hz noise.
C
EMG filter: (a) primary input, the ECG in lead aVf; (b) reference input, derived from aVr-aVl; (c) filter error ε, (d) filter output y.
D
Application of recurrent filter to motion artifact cancellation: (a) ECG with motion artifact; (b) impulse sequence coincident with *QRS* complexes; (c) filter error ε, the motion artifact, (d) filter output.

Figure 9–11. Four examples of noisy ECG recordings and the results of digital filters that are applied to them. *A.* Baseline wander. *B.* Line noise. *C.* Electromyogram noise. *D.* Motion artifact.

computers. Anbar and coworkers have developed a neonatal ventilator simulation program similar to some of the ventilator programs described earlier.[34] Using this simulator, a neonatologist may simulate 5 days of ventilator management in less than 1 hour. Analogous to the previously described hemodynamic monitoring training system, the program allows physicians to gain necessary experience rapidly while avoiding risk to real patients.

ADMINISTRATIVE ROLES

Intensivists are frequently called on to determine intensity of service, appropriateness of continued care, and similar qualitative and ethical issues that involve the critically and terminally ill. The highly social and emotional issues and the sometimes overwhelming body of medical information involved in making these decisions have prompted develop-

Dynacath Critical Care & Hemodynamic Monitoring Training System

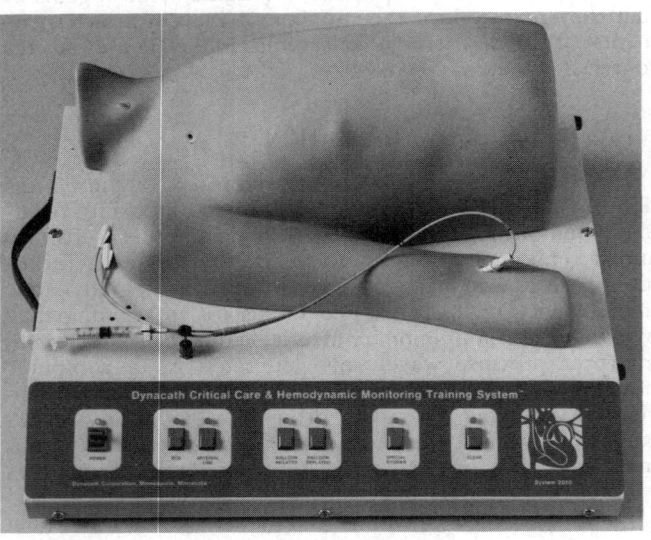

Figure 9–12. The Critical Care and Hemodynamic Monitoring Training System. A pulmonary arterial (PA) catheter may be inserted and advanced into wedge position. Insertion technique, balloon use, wedge time, and pulmonary arterial waveforms are generated or monitored by computer. Various patient conditions and technical obstacles may be simulated on the device. (From Saliterman SS: A computerized simulator for critical-care training: A new technology for medical education. Mayo Clin Proc 65:968, 1990.)

TABLE 9–7

OTHER MEDICAL EXPERT SYSTEMS*†

System	Function
MEDAS	Diagnostic expert system designed to handle patient with multiple disorders. Integrates the expert system with patient and medical data bases. Designed for operation on IBM PC, Apple Macintosh, and Digital Equipment Corporation VAX systems.
ARTEMIS	Records and tracks the long-term follow-up of hypertensive patients. Suggests tests and treatment plans.
ESPRE	Evaluates the indications and best use of platelet transfusions.
TA	Evaluates and suggests appropriate transfusion orders.
DESCL	Discriminates colonic adenoma and adenocarcinoma from normal tissue with 98% success.
DIABETEX	Collects outpatient blood glucose data from type I diabetics and suggests treatment plans.
SESAM-DIABETE	Provides for the education and tracking of outpatient type I diabetics.
IMEX	Tool to assist physicians in the diagnosis and treatment of malaria. Includes consideration of costs and ease of use (of treatment plan).
TraumAID	Expert system to guide the diagnosis and treatment of trauma.
ANEMIA	Evaluates the differential diagnosis of anemia and suggests appropriate tests.

*See refs 65–75.

†MEDAS = Medical Emergency Decision Assistance System; ESPRE = Expert System for Platelet Request Evaluation; TA = Transfusion Advisor; DESCL = Diagnostic Expert System for Colonic Lesions; IMEX = Integrated Malaria Expert System; TraumAid = Trauma Aid.

ment of a computer model that predicts mortality of patients in the CCU.[35] One program that has been developed is based on the presence, severity, and duration of organ failure using the Acute Physiology and Chronic Health Evaluation (APACHE) II score.[36] Based on this index and other calculations, the program predicts patient outcome on a daily basis. In the study, the results of the predictions were kept from experienced CCU teams, who made their own predictions of patient mortality. Presumably, predicting no chance of survival would result in a decision to withdraw treatment. In the test phase of this program, clinicians had a relatively high false-positive rate of predicting death, whereas the computer had no false-positive predictions. Chang and co-workers suggested that physicians are often loath to withdraw treatment, perhaps because of this fact. The researchers also found that deaths predicted by the computer varied widely from deaths predicted by the CCU team, suggesting that the decision-making process of the doctors and nurses differed widely from that of the computer. They emphasized that computer predictions should not be used as the sole source of information for clinical decisions but indicated that a decision to withdraw treatment should include referral to an artificially intelligent, emotionally detached computer program such as the one they described.

Other administrative roles for AI computers include managing bed occupancy, nursing schedules, and quality assurance goals.[37]

Table 9–7 describes a variety of other medical expert systems. Although these programs are not directly related to critical care medicine, their significant contributions to the AI in medicine field deserve merit. A program was presented that provides assistance to general practitioners in managing chronic heart failure.[38] This expert system does not attempt to make a diagnosis but accurately assesses current treatment plans and suggests alternative therapy for heart failure.

NEURAL NETWORKS

Models exist that do not incorporate an if-then design at all, thereby avoiding some of the inherent complications. An AI technique that may prove more successful than current statistical methods is called *neural networking*. In a relatively new field of AI, *artificial neural networks* (ANNs) have been developed that utilize pattern recognition as their logic and data storage mechanism.[39, 40] These algorithms are termed neural networks because of their greatly simplified mathematic similarity to functioning neurons and their ganglions (Fig. 9–13). Like a ganglion, multiple data inputs (x_i) are combined by a simple algebraic function, Σ (a linear equation or a sigmoidal function, for example). A qualifying weight (w_i) is attached to each input datum, the value of which depends on the importance of that datum to the final pattern recognition. The result of all the functions and their weights is an output (f_o) that is sent to yet another function, which also accepts many other inputs. Each function with its inputs and outputs is called a *neurode*. By clustering large numbers of neurodes together (Fig. 9–14), complex and intricate patterns of information may be processed and stored.

ANNs associate input patterns to output patterns based on pattern associations previously "taught" to them. The input pattern may be any group of data, such as a liver chemistry panel, a digitized image or waveform, or even

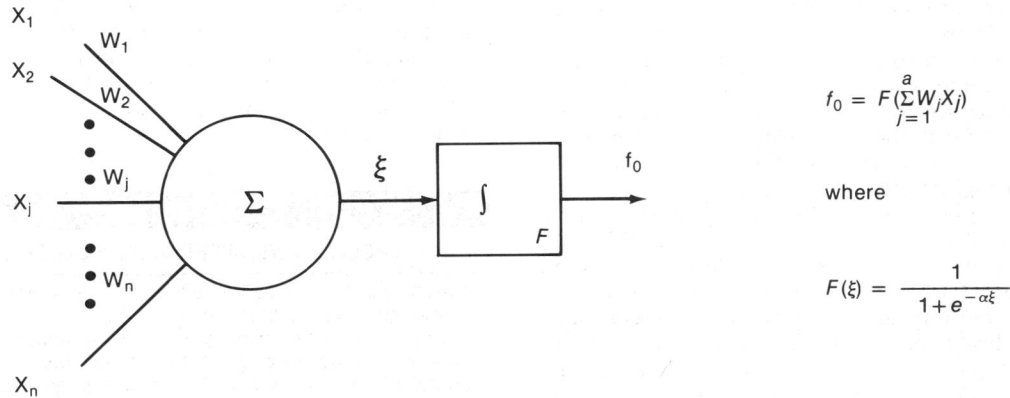

$$f_0 = F(\sum_{j=1}^{a} W_j X_j)$$

where

$$F(\xi) = \frac{1}{1+e^{-\alpha\xi}}$$

Figure 9–13. Schematic diagram of a single artificial neural network neurode.

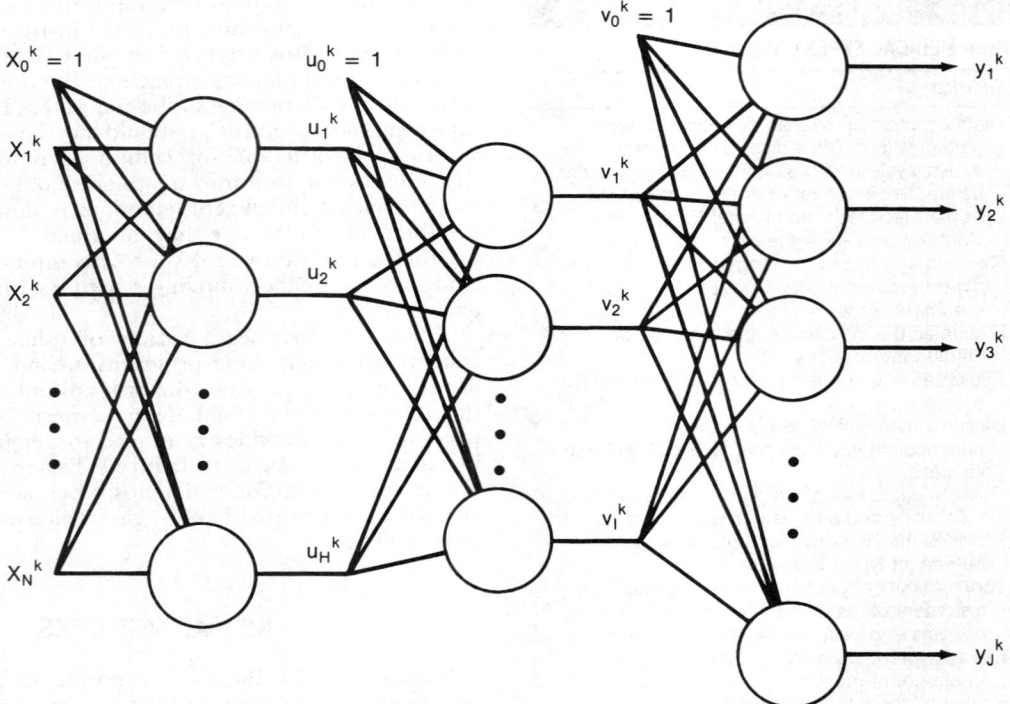

Figure 9–14. A typical ANN structure. Many neurodes connected together form a network that distributes the information, patterns, or knowledge across all of the ANN. Output from the X layer is sent to the U layer, output from the U layer connects to the V layer, and so forth. The number of layers, number of neurodes in each layer, and pattern of connections are all variables. During training, the squared sum of the error between the outputs (U) and the desired result are calculated. If significant error results, the variables and weight of the inner layers are modified until the error is tolerable.

sound. The output pattern may similarly be an encoded diagnosis, an image, or a digitized recording of speech.

ANNs must be taught patterns that they will be asked to recall. Teaching is accomplished by one of several methods. The two most common methods are *supervised learning* and *unsupervised learning*. In supervised learning, the ANN is given input data and the desired output pattern for each input pattern. An example of supervised learning is an ANN trained to recognize patterns created by the chest radiograph. After being "shown" digitized images of the chest radiograph and an output pattern that identifies the cardiac silhouette, the ANN might be able to identify cardiac silhouettes on future x-ray films.

Unsupervised learning consists of mapping the input pattern directly to the output pattern. The ANN is not given a desired output pattern by the user-trainer. Such training would teach an ANN to identify and remember a variety of patterns. An ANN using unsupervised learning might be presented several sets of different waveforms. The goal of this ANN is to create a network of inputs, outputs, and weights that capture the essence of the waveform patterns. Training is successful if the ANN can fill in and create a complete, defined output pattern of the waveform when presented with a slightly different or incomplete pattern.

A practical example of an ANN currently under study is the interpretation of the electromyogram.[41, 42] Traditionally, neurologists have attempted to identify electromyographic waveforms as they flash across the oscilloscope. Based on the neurologist's training, ability to read an oscilloscope, and awareness of applicable patient findings, a diagnosis is made. Waveforms from the electromyogram are infrequently recorded for reappraisal, yet they last less than a second, precluding any opportunity for careful study of the wave-

form morphology, frequency characteristics, or response to stimuli (Table 9–8).

ECGs are similar in scope to electromyograms, and the ANN treats them in the same manner. Our work, shown in Figures 9–15 and 9–16, demonstrates a signal and output from an ANN that has used unsupervised learning to discriminate normal QRS complexes in an ECG signal from premature ventricular complexes. Later, a different ANN will attempt to identify the rhythm that the QRS complexes represent. This ANN would likely be trained from a predefined set of arrhythmias using supervised learning.

Because an ANN does not use discrete rule sets, problems of the if-then model can be avoided. Large sets of data can be stored, provided the patterns are relatively similar in nature. Rules defining an association between data and diagnosis are not utilized; therefore, the ANN can encode knowledge that is not yet completely defined. This is quite useful in medicine, because relationships between signs and symptoms do not necessarily correlate with diagnoses in a clearly defined manner. Use of an ANN requires only that it be exposed to a pattern and an associated conclusion during training.

TABLE 9–8

PROBLEMS INTERPRETING PHYSIOLOGIC SIGNALS

Waveforms may not be predefined or of a common, expected type, such as electromyograms.
Waveforms may not follow a trend for individual electrical bursts.
Waveforms may not be predictably repetitious.
Waveforms may be superimposed on one another.
Criteria to identify the waveforms are difficult to specify.

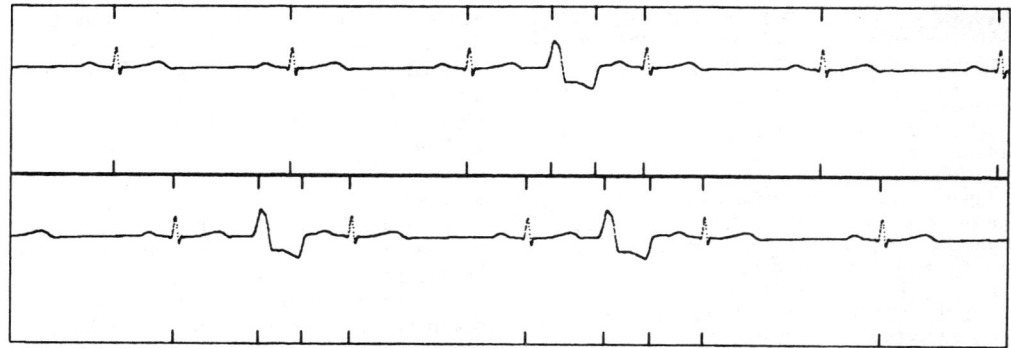

Figure 9–15. The raw signal used to generate Figure 9–16. Note that the larger premature ventricular complexes are counted twice. This is a function of the waveform detection algorithm and not of the ANN itself.

If no previously defined weights define the current waveform during training, a new set of weights is declared that identifies the new sample pattern, as well as all previous samples. Determination of weights that simultaneously describe all input patterns is performed by methods of probability and trial and error. Therefore, training may be a long and tedious task. However, once the ANN has discovered the numeric pattern of weight that describes all the waveforms in the training set, mapping and classification of other waveforms occur quite rapidly. Future test waveforms are classified as a member of the most similar set of previously recognized waveforms. If sufficient examples were used during training and the ANN was designed for the type of patterns in question, future test waveforms are categorized according to their correct classes. The resulting output pattern for each test waveform is the pattern that

had been assigned to similar patterns during training. Because all training has occurred before the ANN is presented with the test waveform, identification of the test waveform is quite rapid. This fact permits the use of ANNs in real-time applications.

ANNs are remarkably robust in the face of unexpected input. After training, any pattern can be associated with the training conclusion it most closely resembles. Patterns dissimilar from the training set of patterns (so-called unexpected input) may slow the ANN from making a comparison, but the ANN will not fail completely.

ANNs are not without inherent problems, some of which are discussed in Table 9–9. For instance, training patterns must not vary widely, or the ANN may not be able to assign weights that discretely describe the patterns. For example, the input vectors of numbers for the QRS patterns of the

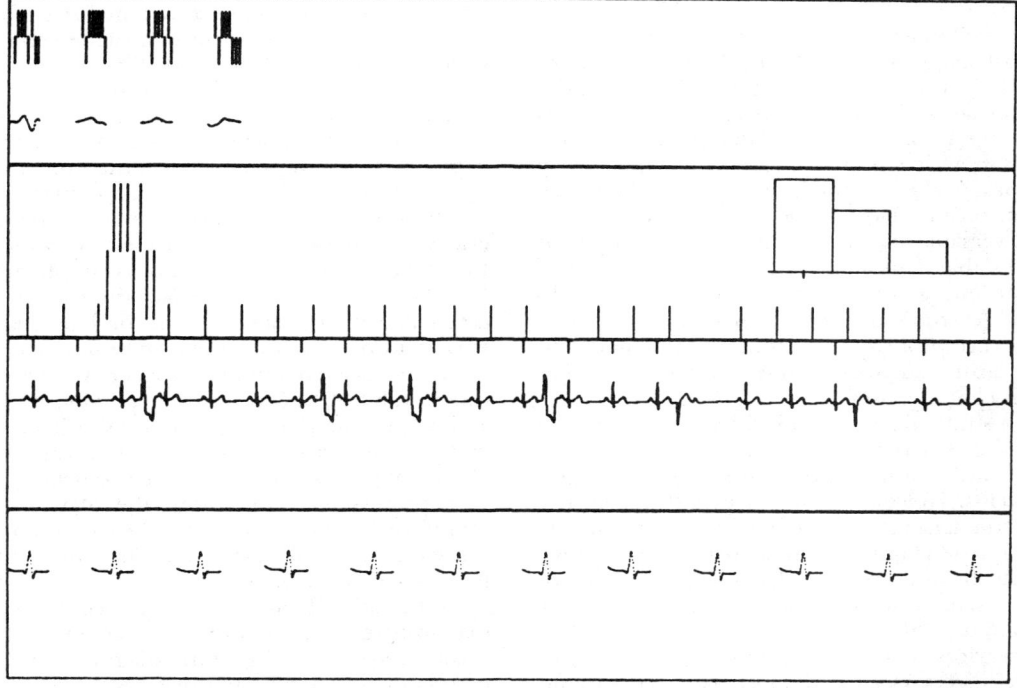

Figure 9–16. Screen output of an ECG rhythm that was used to train an ANN. The fine bars at the top left represent the "essence" of the QRS morphologies as identified by the ANN. The histogram at the top right displays the relative occurrence of the classes and marks this class as the most common (the largest bar). The second row describes the first classified complex and shows its relative position of occurrence in time. The third row displays the signal and marks the complexes the ANN found. The bottom row is an enlarged view of the first 12 complexes placed in this class. Because the premature ventricular complex duration is much longer than that of a normal QRS complex, the ANN identified both phases of the electrical waveform; therefore, there are four identified patterns instead of three. A different ANN will recognize the temporal association of the two premature ventricular complex sections and splice them into one complex.

TABLE 9–9
DIFFICULTIES USING ARTIFICIAL NEURAL NETWORK
ANNs are exquisitely sensitive to the precision and variability of the training patterns. Widely varying patterns will invalidate the resulting ANN associations.
ANNs are trained by example; they are dependent on accurate teaching data. Supervised training algorithms require that the output pattern be well described. Unfortunately, medical data are not always well defined or understood. Therefore, finding adequate patterns for training may be difficult.
The ANN's logic is: "It is this way because it *looks* this way." Therefore, the logic of the ANN is difficult to evaluate.
Training of a network involves trial and error and therefore is slow and tedious. There are currently no methods to pretrain the ANN to expedite learning.
ANNs may require large amounts of computer memory or specialized computer processors to operate, which limits their availability.

ECG must start and end within predefined ranges in relationship to the beginning of the QRS complex. If one QRS pattern begins at the start of the list of numbers, another at the middle of the list, and yet another at the end, the ANN will have difficulty determining similarities or differences among QRS complexes of future patterns. Also, an ANN cannot be trained on an unlimited number of patterns without adjusting the size of the network. A small network that is overtrained may be ambiguous when attempting to discriminate new input patterns. Neural networking remains a new field despite a long theoretic past. Concepts and applications of ANNs continue to be the focus of active research.

THE FUTURE: PITFALLS AND PROMISES

Despite the contributions that AI has already made to medicine, the vast majority of medical AI applications are under study in the controlled laboratory. Placing an expert system in the clinical setting and especially in the CCU is both expensive and labor intensive. Attempting to implement an expert system in the critical care environment may also be dangerous if the system has not been rigorously tested. Definition of an adequate medical knowledge base, establishment of versatile and robust rules, and development of user interfaces that appeal to health professionals in a variety of clinical settings represent an immense undertaking. Provided the AI community can offer solutions to these demands, health care professionals require testing and validation of an application, as well as convincing evidence that the application is clinically useful.

Mechanisms to study, develop, and distribute expert systems are expensive. Current AI techniques often require large, state-of-the-art computer processors and their requisite support systems. However, once an expert system has been developed, the large support structures are not necessary. The expert system must be miniaturized to be sufficiently portable to fit into existing CCU computer systems, personal computers, or implantable integrated circuits. Many existing CCU computers were neither designed nor installed to provide the services that AI programs require. Accordingly, some CCU directors and administrators have found that they must purchase new computer systems to support an expert system. Unless the expert system generates revenue to recoup these expenses, CCUs may not be able to afford the capital expense.

Many forms of medical knowledge currently defy concise or comprehensive means of storage. Furthermore, many mysteries remain in medicine. Some medical practices are the subject of ongoing debate or controversy; other practices and beliefs are rapidly evolving. This constant flux of medical knowledge and application necessitates frequent updating of knowledge bases, modifications of the research engine, and novel approaches to interface the expert system with the user. These hurdles present both financial and logical challenges to AI research.

Obstructions to the introduction of AI to medicine also exist at the user's level. Health care professionals may not be receptive to machine-assisted medical decision making. Many clinicians find it difficult to trust a computer-generated diagnosis or treatment plan, even when their own knowledge may be limited for the field in question. Furthermore, use of the computer often requires familiarity with the computer's interactive devices, such as the keyboard, touch-sensitive screen, and mouse. If use of these unfamiliar devices is infrequent, users may find that the learning curve outweighs the benefits of using the expert system. Unfortunately, efforts to design AI clinical applications have outpaced the development of intelligent user interfaces.[43] However, several approaches currently under development show great promise. For example, many physicians find the computer unsuitable for use because it is difficult to enter day-to-day information such as progress notes. To confront this problem, AI researchers are exploring handwriting and speech recognition. Notebook-sized entry tablets are commercially available to permit handwritten notes to be entered into the computer. In addition, dictation devices can recognize the physician's speech pattern for almost any type of transcription.[44–46] For the majority of physicians who remain committed to writing or dictating onto a paper medical record, these new developments in record keeping may substantially ease the burden of interfacing with the computer.

Validation of an expert system is not a simple process. Validation represents another factor that may delay the introduction of the expert system for clinical use. Fieschi pointed out that acceptance is dependent on numerous factors of varying importance that are unique to the user and the planned use of the system.[47] For example, one system might be judged on its ability, accuracy, or cost to reach the same conclusion as a human expert. Another expert system may be judged on the similarity of its internal operations and logic with a human expert.[48–51]

Setting the level of acceptance is a topic that often generates considerable debate. In many cases, a system that functions within a 5% tolerance is simply not good enough for clinical use. Engineers accustomed to the tolerances acceptable in mechanical, civil, or biomedical engineering may be unprepared for the degree of perfection demanded by the medical community (Spitzer AR, personal communication, July 1991). One example previously discussed is CCU arrhythmia monitoring. Absolute sensitivity for life-threatening arrhythmias is necessary; however, even a low false-alarm rate on such systems may quickly condition health care professionals to ignore the alarms. A system may therefore be considered imperfect or even impractical because it occasionally alarms insignificant events, even though it alarms all significant ones.

On the other hand, the level of acceptance for a bayesian diagnostic expert system may hinge on its ability to provide a comprehensive differential diagnosis. The user may tolerate substantial false-positive results in the hope that all possible diagnoses will be considered. In this case, acceptability is defined by the comprehensiveness of the expert system's differential diagnosis. Accordingly, a user would demand that an expert system be absolutely certain before dismissing meningococcal meningitis as a potential diagnosis in a child with neck stiffness. This system would be imperfect

---

TABLE 9–10

ADVANTAGES OF A MECHANICAL EXPERT ASSISTANT

Does not become fatigued.

Remains consistent and accurate provided appropriate data are available to the program.

Is emotionally detached from both the patient and the staff.

Is portable; therefore, is more readily available in areas where human specialists are sparse.

May be more immediately available because the device is usually ready and waiting.

The standard of care for a given problem is defined.

Epidemiologic trends or changes may be retrospectively studied more easily through continuous accumulation of patient data.

Costs may be contained by increasing test or treatment efficiency or by preventing redundant or superfluous tests or treatments.

Provides education for health care professionals.

---

if it *did not* alarm all serious events, regardless of their likelihood.

As public scrutiny increases, medicolegal considerations may affect the specifications and validation of expert systems. Medicolegal issues include establishing standards for clinical testing of the expert system, defining and certifying qualified users, and establishing a trail of responsibility and liability for the use of these systems.[52-56] Some expert systems, such as ANNs, defy a conventional assessment of logic. This leads to complicated issues in expert system verification.[57] The solutions to these complex questions will be determined by knowledge experts (e.g., AI researchers), medical consultants, lawyers, and the courts, as expert systems are introduced into the marketplace.

Despite the potential drawbacks, many critical care practitioners anxiously await the benefits of AI research and implementation (Table 9–10). Some medical centers have already been successful in applying expert systems to clinical medicine and have demonstrated that AI can function in the CCU by acting as an expert assistant, providing information and competent reasoning in various areas of clinical decision making.[58-61] Gardner and Shabot suggested that physician-oriented support services, demonstration of the utility of the system, and a nonthreatening presentation of the application are keys to successful implementation.[58] Other methods to circumvent physician skepticism and reward participation have also been discussed.[62]

Acknowledgment. The authors thank Robert Spitzer, M.D., assistant professor of neurology at Wayne State University and director of the Electromyography Laboratory, for his assistance in preparing this chapter.

References

1. Rennels GD, Miller PL: Artificial intelligence research in anesthesia and critical care. J Clin Monit 4:274, 1988.
2. Lincoln TL: Medical informatics: The substantive discipline behind health care computer systems. Int J Biomed Comput 26:73, 1990.
3. Montgomery WH, Donegan J, McIntyre K: Standards and guidelines for cardiopulmonary resuscitation (CPR) and emergency cardiac care (ECC). JAMA 255:2905, 1986. Published erratum in: JAMA 256:1727, 1986.
4. Advanced Trauma Life Support Student Manual. Chicago, American College of Surgeons, 1988.
5. Miller RA, Pople HE, Myers JD: INTERNIST-1, an experimental computer-based diagnostic consultant for general internal medicine. N Engl J Med 307:468, 1982.
6. Bankowitz RA, McNeil MA, Challinor SM, et al: A computer-assisted medical diagnostic consultation service. Ann Intern Med 110:824, 1989.
7. Washington R, Hayes-Roth B: Input data management in real-time AI systems. In: Proceedings of the Eleventh International Joint Conference on AI, 1989, Volume 1, p 250.
8. Shortliffe EH: Computer programs to support clinical decision making. JAMA 258:61, 1987.
9. Buchanan B, Shortliffe EH (eds): Rule-Based Systems: The MYCIN Experiments of the Standard Heuristic Programming Project. Reading, MA, Addison-Wesley, 1984.
10. Pis P, Mesiar R: Fuzzy model of inexact reasoning in medicine. Comp Method Prog Biomed 30:1, 1989.
11. Clancey, WJ: NEOMYCIN: Reconfiguring a rule-based expert system for application to teaching. In: Proceedings of the Ninth International Joint Conference on AI, 1981, Volume 1, p 829.
12. Ben-Bassat M, Carlson RW, Puri VK, et al: A hierarchical modular design for treatment protocols. Methods Inf Med, 19:93, 1980.
13. Fraser RB, Turney SZ: An expert system for the nutritional management of the critically ill. Comput Methods Programs Biomed 33:175, 1990.
14. Fagan LM, Shortliffe EH, Buchanan BG: Computer-based medical decision making: From MYCIN to VM. Automedica 3:97, 1980.
15. Shortliffe EH, Fagan LM: Expert systems research: Modeling the medical decision making process. In: Gravenstein JS, Newbower RS, Ream AK, et al (eds): An Integrated Approach to Monitoring. Woburn, MA, Butterworth, p 183, 1983.
16. Fagan LM, Kunz JC, Feigenbaum EA, et al: Extensions to the rule-based formalism for a monitoring task. In: Buchanan BG, Shortliffe EH (eds): Rule-Based Systems: The MYCIN Experiments of the Standard Heuristic Programming Project. Reading, MA, Addison-Wesley, p 387, 1984.
17. Rutledge G, Thomsen G, Beinlich I, et al: Combining qualitative computation in a ventilator therapy planner. Symp Comput Appl Med Care 13:315, 1989.
18. Thomsen G, Shiener L: SIMV: An application of mathematical modeling in ventilator management. Symp Comput Appl Med Care 13:320, 1989.
19. Farr BR, Fagan LM: Decision-theoretic evaluation of therapy plans. Symp Comput Appl Med Care 13:188, 1989.
20. Rutledge GW, Anderson SK, Polaschek JX, et al: A belief network model for interpretation of ICU data. Symp Comput Appl Med Care 14:785, 1990.
21. Rennels GD, Miller PL: Artificial intelligence in anesthesia and critical care. J Clin Monit 4:274, 1988.
22. Widman LE: Expert system reasoning about dynamic systems by semi-quantitative simulation. Comput Methods Programs Biomed 29:95, 1989.
23. Sittig DF: Computerized management of patient care in a complex, controlled clinical trial in the intensive care unit. Symp Comput Appl Med Care 11:225, 1987.
24. Sittig DF, Pace NL, Gardner RM, et al: Implementation of a computerized patient advice system using the HELP clinical information system. Comput Biomed Res 22:474, 1989.
25. Rudowski R, Frostell C, Gill H: A knowledge-based support system for mechanical ventilation of the lungs: The KUSIVAR concept and prototype. Comput Methods Programs Biomed 30:59, 1989.
26. Rudowski R, Skreta L, Baehrendtz S, et al: Lung function analysis and optimization during artificial ventilation: A personal computer-based system. Comput Methods Programs Biomed 31:33, 1990.
27. Bessette F, Nguyen L: Automated electrocardiographic analysis: The state of the art. Med Inf 14:43, 1989.
28. Van Bemmel JH, Kors JA, Willems JL, et al: Evolution and evaluation of ECG interpretation systems: An illustration of the validation of decision support systems. Symp Comput Appl Med Care 13:547, 1990.
29. Larsen JL, Jenkins JM: Computerized arrhythmia monitoring. J Cardiovasc Nurs 2:58, 1987.
30. Mirvis DM, Berson AS, Goldberger AL, et al: Instrumentation and practice standards for electrocardiographic monitoring in special care units. Circulation 79:464, 1989.
31. Thakor NV, Zhu Y: Applications of adaptive filtering to ECG analysis: Noise cancellation and arrythmia detection. IEEE Trans Biomed Eng 38:785, 1991.
32. Pryor TA, Dupont R, Clay J: A MLM based order entry system: The use of knowledge in a traditional HIS application. Symp Comput Appl Med Care 14:579, 1990.
33. Saliterman SS: A computerized simulator for critical-care training: New technology for medical education. Mayo Clin Proc 65:968, 1990.
34. Anbar RD, Anbar M: Computerized dynamic simulation of clinical management. A ventilation simulation program. NY State J Med 86:73, 1986.
35. Chang RW, Lee B, Jacobs S, et al: Accuracy of decisions to withdraw therapy in critically ill patients: Clinical judgement versus a computer model. Crit Care Med 17:1091, 1989.
36. Knaus WA, Draper EA, Wagner DP, et al: APACHE II: A severity of disease classification system. Crit Care Med 13:818, 1985.
37. Marks RJ, Morgan C, Duce G: Computerized administration in an intensive care unit: Experience with a personal computer system. Ann R Coll Surg Engl 71:397, 1989.
38. Perlini S, Piepoli M, Marti G, et al: Treatment of chronic heart failure: An expert system advisor for general practitioners. Acta Cardiol 14:365, 1990.
39. McClelland JL, Rumelhart DE, Hinton GE: The Appeal of Parallel Distributed Processing. In: Feldman JA, Hayes PJ, Rumelhart DE (eds): Parallel Distributed Processing, Volume I, Foundations. Cambridge, MA, MIT Press, p 3, 1988.
40. James PO: A Study on the Use of Neural Networks to Determine

Relationships Between Data. Long Beach, CA, California State University; 1990. Master's thesis.

41. Wasser DJ: Application of an Artificial Neural Network to Learning-Based Pattern Recognition and Control. Chapel Hill, NC, The University of North Carolina at Chapel Hill, 1990. Thesis.

42. Spitzer AR, Hassoun M, Wang C, et al: Signal decomposition and diagnostic classification of the electromyogram using a novel neural network technique. Symp Comput Appl Med Care 14:552, 1990.

43. Coiera E: Incorporating User and Dialogue Models into the Interface Design of an Intelligent Patient Monitor. HP Laboratories Technical Report HPL-91-42, 1991.

44. Shortliffe EH: Developing trends in clinical computing. Ann Acad Med Singapore 20:277, 1991.

45. Bergeron B, Locke S: Speech recognition as a user interface. MD Comput 7:329, 1990.

46. Landau JA, Norwich KH, Evans SJ: Automatic speech recognition: Can it improve the machine interface in medical expert systems? Int J Biomed Comput 24:111, 1989.

47. Fieschi M: Towards validation of expert systems as medical decision aids. Int J Biomed Comput 26:93, 1990.

48. McDonald CJ: Standards for the electronic transfer of clinical data: Progress, promises and the conductor's wand. Symp Comput Appl Med Care 14:9, 1990.

49. Detmer DE: The Institute of Medicine patient record study and its implications for health data standards. Symp Comput Appl Med Care 14:15, 1990.

50. Greenes, RA: Promoting productivity by propagating the practice of "plug-compatible" programming. Symp Comput Appl Med Care 14:22, 1990.

51. Clayton PD, Hripcsak G, Pryor TA: Emerging standards for medical logic. Symp Comput Appl Med Care 14:27, 1990.

52. Cannataci JA: Liability for medical expert systems: An introduction to the legal implications. Med Inf 14:226, 1989.

53. Wyatt J, Spiegelhalter D: Evaluating medical expert systems: What to test and how? Med Inf 15:205, 1990.

54. Miller RA, Schaffner KF, Meisel A: Ethical and legal issues related to the use of computer programs in clinical medicine. Ann Intern Med 102:529, 1985.

55. Dowie J: The evaluation of decision aids: The role of the decision owner. Med Inf 15:219, 1990.

56. Miller PL, Sittig DF: The evaluation of clinical decision support systems: What is necessary versus what is interesting. Med Inf 15:185, 1990.

57. Hart A, Wyatt J: Evaluating black-boxes as medical decision aids: Issues arising from a study of neural networks. Med Inf 15:229, 1990.

58. Gardner RM, Shabot MM: Computerized ICU data management: Pitfalls and promises. Int J Clin Monit Comput 7:99, 1990.

59. Sivak ED, Gochberg JS, Fronek R, et al: Lessons to be learned from the design, development, and implementation of a computerized patient care management system for the intensive care unit. Symp Comput Appl Med Care 11:614, 1987.

60. Lundsgaarde HP, Gardner RM, Menlove RL: Using attitudinal questionnaires to achieve benefits optimization. Symp Comput Appl Med Care 13:703, 1989.

61. Avila LS, Shabot MM: Keys to the successful implementation of an ICU patient data management system. Int J Clin Monit Comput 5:15, 1988.

62. Zibrak JD, Roberts MS, Nelick-Cohen LN, et al: Creating an environment conducive to physician participation in a hospital information system. Symp Comput Appl Med Care 14:779, 1990.

63. Clancey WJ: Transfer of Rule-Based Expertise Through a Tutorial Dialogue. Stanford, CA, Memo STAN-CS-79-769. In: Dept of Computer Science, Stanford University, September 1979.

64. Fagan LM, Shortliffe EH, Buchanan BG: Computer-based medical decision making: From MYCIN to VM. Automedica 3:97, 1980.

65. Trace D, Evens M, Naeymi-Rad F, et al: Medical information management: The MEDAS approach. Symp Comput Appl Med Care 14:635, 1990.

66. Georgakis DC, Trace DA, Naeymi-Rad F, et al: A statistical evaluation of the diagnostic performance of MEDAS—The Medical Emergency Decision Assistance System. Symp Comput Appl Med Care 14:815, 1990.

67. Degoulet P, Chatellier G, Devries C, et al: Computer-assisted techniques for evaluation and treatment of hypertensive patients. Am J Hypertens 3:156, 1990.

68. Connely DP, Sielaff BH, Scott EP: ESPRE-expert system for platelet request evaluation. Am J Clin Pathol 94(4 suppl 1):S19, 1990.

69. Spackman KA, Beck JR: A knowledge-based system for transfusion advice. Am J Clin Pathol 94(4 suppl 1):S25, 1990.

70. Graham AR, Paplanus SH, Bartels P: A diagnostic expert system for colonic lesions. Am J Clin Pathol 94(4 suppl 1):S15, 1990.

71. Zahlmann G, Franczykova M, Hening G, et al: DIABETEX—a decision support system for therapy of type I diabetic patients. Comput Methods Programs Biomed 32:297, 1990.

72. Levy M, Ferrand P, Chirat V: SESAM-DIABETE, an expert system for insulin-requiring diabetic education. Comput Biomed Res 22:442, 1989.

73. Suan OL: Computer-aided diagnosis and treatment of malaria: The IMEX system. Comput Biol Med 20:361, 1990.

74. Clarke JR, Cebula D, Webber BA: A computerized decision aid for trauma. J Trauma 28:1250, 1988.

75. Lanzola G, Stefanelli M, Barosi G, et al: NEOANEMIA: A knowledge-based system emulating diagnostic reasoning. Comput Biomed Res 23:560, 1990.

SECTION TWO

Resuscitation and Monitoring

Section Editor

James A. Kruse

CHAPTER 10

Airway Management and Endotracheal Intubation

Jeffrey V. Kyff

Airway management and endotracheal intubation are essential skills for physicians working in intensive care units or with critically ill patients in other settings. They are, however, skills that require effort both to learn and to maintain. One does not become an expert at airway management by virtue of having a medical degree and having read this chapter or other materials. Ideally, physician trainees working in the intensive care setting should rotate through the anesthesiology department to gain a solid base of experience in airway management. In addition, a working relationship with the personnel in the anesthesiology department helps ensure both good care of patients and the resources to help maintain skills. In many institutions the anesthesiology department is routinely called for airway management. When a relationship already exists between departments, asking the anesthesiologist to stand by, if the situation permits, while trainees do the intubation will not cause bruised egos or other problems. Elective intubations occur only in the operating suite, so all discussions in this chapter are in the context of urgent or emergent airway management. The material in this chapter also gives some insight into the times when only a skilled practitioner should attempt to manage the airway.

RECOGNIZING THE DIFFICULT INTUBATION

The failed intubation or difficult airway results in approximately 600 deaths per year worldwide.[1] In addition, it is the most common cause of litigation related to anesthesia mishaps, representing 31% of all claims. Of these, 74% are related to inadequate ventilation, difficult intubation, and esophageal intubation.[2] It is important to remember that

these figures are based on cases involving anesthesiologists, experts in airway management. Figures would be expected to be much higher in cases handled by those less skilled.

Many potentially difficult airways, such as those associated with skeletal deformity or facial trauma, are readily apparent at first glance. Patients with short necks, obesity, protruding incisors, limited opening of the mouth, limited neck extension, or high arched palates are usually more difficult to intubate.[3] Of particular concern, however, are patients who have none of these characteristics but are, in fact, difficult to intubate. Measurements of various anatomic parameters have been described in an effort to predict the difficulty of tracheal intubation in otherwise normal-appearing individuals.[3–12] However, there is little agreement on most of these parameters. Many of the measurements are too complex to be carried out in everyday practice and certainly not in an urgent situation. One of the most accepted parameters involves the atlanto-occipital gap.[13–16] Lateral neck radiographs taken with the neck in neutral position demonstrating minimal or no atlanto-occipital gap are predictive of limited neck extension and thus difficulty in endotracheal intubation.

The most accepted clinical scoring system is that described by Mallampati and colleagues.[7] Their conclusions have been supported and later modified by others.[17] In this system there are four classes of airways based on the structures observed during visual inspection of the oral pharynx. Patients are examined in the sitting position, neck neutral, with the tongue maximally protruded. The larynx of patients in classes 1 and 2 is easily visualized and intubation should follow accordingly (Table 10–1). Difficulty with endotracheal intubation should be anticipated in patients in categories 3 and 4. The interdental gap (distance between upper and lower front teeth on jaw opening) is commonly assessed and should be equal to or greater than two finger widths (approximately 4.6 cm).[10–12] It is also important to assess mandibular subluxation, that is, the maximal forward protrusion of the lower incisors in relation to the upper incisors. Free movement of the temporomandibular joint in this plane significantly increases the ability to visualize the trachea during laryngoscopy.[18] A chin-to-larynx (thyromental) distance of less than three finger widths may also indicate a difficult intubation. This assessment is made by noting the number of finger widths that can be placed between the top of the thyroid cartilage and the mandible with the head fully

TABLE 10–1

MALLAMPATI AIRWAY CLASSIFICATION SYSTEM

Class	Anatomy Visualized During Oral Inspection*
1	Soft palate, fauces, uvular pillars
2	Soft palate, uvula
3	Soft palate, uvular base
4	No soft palate

*Visualization of the larynx and related structures during intubation is most likely to be inadequate in class 3 and class 4 patients.[7]

extended. In the end, no single parameter accurately determines the difficulty of intubation; however, these signs should at least alert you that more experienced help may be necessary.

In general, no more than two attempts should be made to intubate the trachea of a normal-appearing patient. If the second attempt is unsuccessful, continue to ventilate the patient with 100% oxygen until more experienced help becomes available.[19] Further attempts at intubation place the patient at increased risk and make subsequent attempts more difficult. Even experienced anesthesiologists set limits on the number of intubation attempts before calling for help or selecting other means of airway management, such as returning to spontaneous ventilation or advancing to cricothyrotomy.[11, 19]

AIRWAY MANAGEMENT

More important than the ability to intubate the trachea is the ability to manage the airway, that is, to ventilate as well as oxygenate the patient and to know when intervention is and is not necessary. Initial assessment of the patient must include both the history and physical examination, even if only of a cursory nature. This chapter does not provide an extensive review of the various causes of respiratory insufficiency and failure. Some criteria to look for are a respiratory rate of 40 breaths/min or more, use of accessory respiratory muscles (as in a patient who is using the arms for support to fix the rib cage), retraction of the tissue just above the suprasternal notch during inspiration, and inability or refusal to lie flat. This may be accompanied by tachycardia of 120 to 170 beats/min. In addition, the following laboratory values are significant: arterial blood gases demonstrating respiratory acidosis with a pH less than 7.35, a $PaCO_2$ value greater than 50 torr, and a PaO_2 value less than 50 torr. Patients with a decreased level of consciousness and loss of the gag reflex are unable to protect their airway from aspiration and therefore warrant intubation. With the exception of some patients in this last category, all patients requiring endotracheal intubation should be given mechanical ventilation. Conversely, patients who require mechanical ventilation for any reason also require endotracheal intubation.

Ventilating patients by bag and mask is a skill that requires practice and experience to maintain. It is, in fact, a more important skill than intubation. The initial step is to establish an open airway. This can be accomplished by several methods. The method most frequently used is the head tilt maneuver. The airway is opened by placing the fingers of one hand under the mandible and lifting up and backward, extending the patient's neck. The same result is achieved (sometimes more effectively) by using the index fingers of both hands to lift the mandible from the angles of the jaw while standing behind the patient, in what is known as the jaw lift. This method has the obvious disadvantage of requiring the use of both hands. An oral airway also may be

inserted, but care must be taken to ensure that the proper size is selected and that correct positioning is achieved. This point is critical. The size should be measured by holding the oral airway against the cheek of the patient; an airway of the proper size reaches from the corner of the patient's mouth to the tragus of the ear. The tongue must be pushed anteriorly against the lower jaw with a tongue blade and the oral airway inserted behind it. A properly inserted oral airway sits flush against the lips. If it does not, it is likely that the airway has forced the tongue posteriorly (instead of anteriorly), occluding the oropharynx and preventing full insertion. In this case the oral airway must be removed and reinserted.

Ventilation is carried out using either a bag-valve mask device or, increasingly in many hospitals, a mouth-to-mask device. The most important aspect of ventilation, however, is the establishment of a patent airway as described earlier. The mask is then placed over the bridge of the nose; the patient's jaw is rocked up and backward by the third, fourth, and fifth fingers of the left hand (regardless of whether the operator is left or right handed) to meet the flanges of the mask; and a seal of tissue to rubber is made. It is not as important to press down firmly on the mask as it is to lift the jaw and establish an open air passage. The often-described "death-like grip on mask and jaw" usually results in air leakage because of uneven pressure. In addition, excessive pressure under the mandible can damage the facial nerve and certainly tires the operator after only a short time. If the operator's fingers blanch white from pressure, too much pressure is being applied. A good mask and a well-established airway obviate the need for excessive pressure to seal the mask. With edentulous patients, who lack the underlying tissue support usually provided by teeth, it is often necessary to have a second person lift upward on the right cheek to create a seal.

Care should be taken not to generate excessive airway pressure when ventilating patients by bag and mask. Airway pressures exceeding 24 mm Hg are likely to overcome the resistance of the gastroesophageal sphincter and fill the patient's stomach with gases.[20, 21] This usually causes patients to regurgitate not only the insufflated air but also the gastric contents. Aspiration of this material into the lungs is of serious consequence and, depending on the pH, volume, and particulate nature of the material, may result in significant morbidity and mortality.[21] When ventilation is effective, the chest rises with each squeeze of the ventilating bag, the pulse rate of the patient (and the person managing the airway) may decrease or increase depending on whether tachycardia or bradycardia was initially present, and signs of cyanosis disappear. Interestingly, patients who are hypercapnic are often both tachycardic and hypertensive because of release of endogenous catecholamines. As carbon dioxide is removed by effective ventilation, the catecholamine-provoking stimulus is removed and both heart rate and blood pressure decrease, sometimes to hypotensive levels. The response of heart rate is variable: initially hypoxemia may cause tachycardia, but ultimately hypoxemia results in bradycardia and cardiac arrest. A rule of thumb is that if you see bradycardia and you think of atropine, think of oxygen first!

When a patent airway has been established and the patient is adequately ventilated (except for the risk of aspiration), you may take as much time as you need to intubate the trachea. It is important first to assemble the necessary equipment and personnel and then to stabilize and position the patient for the planned procedure. When the patient is stable, consideration should be given to sedating the patient. Paralyzing patients with muscle relaxants for endotracheal intubation in settings outside the operating suite should be done rarely. When muscle relaxants have been administered, only one option remains: the patient must be ventilated. When patients are breathing spontaneously, even if not entirely adequately, there is a margin of safety not present when muscle relaxants are used. When spontaneous ventilation has stopped, because of use of muscle relaxants or excessive sedation, it is up to the person managing the airway to ventilate the patient and intubate the trachea, neither of which is ever a certainty even in skilled hands. Therefore, it is strongly recommended that only persons who are highly skilled in airway management and regularly use those skills be permitted to use muscle relaxants. In almost all cases a small dose of a benzodiazepine, titrated slowly, can provide patients with amnesia for the procedure without producing apnea or adverse hemodynamic response. When a benzodiazepine reversal agent becomes available in the United States, higher doses of these drugs may be given more routinely. When additional sedation and relaxation are required, narcotics (e.g., morphine or meperidine) are good because their effects can be reversed with naloxone. Many patients are sufficiently obtunded that sedation or relaxation is not necessary. Semiconscious patients who are reluctant to open their mouths to permit laryngoscopy can usually be induced to do so by stimulating their gag reflex with a tongue depressor or by gently pinching shut both nostrils. In the end, it is better for a patient to remember being intubated than to die because of loss of a patent, ventilatable airway.

ORAL INTUBATION

Indications for oral endotracheal intubation include respiratory insufficiency, respiratory failure, and need to protect the airway because of either a decrease in the level of consciousness or the potential for later airway compromise resulting from progressive edema or sepsis. In urgent or emergent situations the most expedient method of securing the patient's airway is oral endotracheal intubation. For patients who are likely to remain intubated over a long period, nasal intubation has the advantages of improved comfort of the patient and a more stable and easily secured endotracheal tube. There has been concern about ulceration of nasal tissue and a reported propensity for maxillary sinus infections.[22–24] In any event, when the patient has been stabilized and is no longer in imminent danger, the endotracheal tube may be changed to a nasal tube electively. The first step in any procedure is to obtain all the necessary equipment, well in advance of any emergent situation. Therefore, it is essential to have an emergency airway kit available, either separate from the unit crash cart or as a part of it. This kit should be checked regularly for completeness and functionality (Table 10–2). Commonly overlooked is the brightness of the laryngoscope light bulb. The light should be bright white; any dullness or yellow color is a sign that the batteries must be replaced. The endoscopist should make all decisions concerning the airway, including the degree and type of sedation, if any is to be given. In the ideal situation, a pulse oximeter is used so that intubation can be attempted when the patient is maximally oxygenated. It also serves to warn the endoscopist when to abort the intubation attempt and return to bag-mask ventilation. The pulse oximeter also provides useful information about oxygenation of the patient when the endotracheal tube is in place.[25]

Ventilation is most easily provided with the patient's head flat on the surface of the bed. This allows maximal extension of the head and ease of ventilation. When intubation is attempted the head should be placed in the classic sniffing position, with the occiput on a pillow 10 cm high and the head extended maximally (Fig. 10–1). The laryngoscope

TABLE 10–2
BASIC AIRWAY MANAGEMENT EQUIPMENT (ADULT AND PEDIATRIC)*
Bag-valve mask ventilation device with oxygen source attachment
Assorted pediatric and adult masks, sizes 0 through 6
Oral airways, sizes 1 through 6, two each
Geudel's nasal airways, sizes 3.5 through 8.5, two each
Endotracheal tubes, 3.5 through 9 mm, two each (whole sizes only above 5.5 mm)
Laryngoscope handles, two
Miller's laryngoscope blades, sizes 1 to 3
MacIntosh's laryngoscope blades, sizes 3 and 4
Syringes, 10 mL, two
Endotracheal tube stylets, infant and adult, two each
Magill's forceps
Tape and skin preparation solution
Tongue blades
Tube-changing stylet

*All equipment must be regularly inspected for completeness and tested for function. This is particularly important for the laryngoscope handles and blades, which must have working batteries and bright lamps.

blade is placed in the oral pharynx, just to the right of midline, being careful to avoid trauma to the lips, teeth, and gums. There are two basic types of laryngoscope blades, straight and curved. The curved (e.g., MacIntosh's) blade is intended to be inserted into the vallecula (the area just cephalad to the epiglottis) and used indirectly to elevate the epiglottis; the straight (e.g., Miller's) blade is inserted beyond the epiglottis and drawn back until the vocal cords appear (Fig. 10–2). It is important that the endoscopist not obstruct the view of the landmarks with the endotracheal tube. This is especially true when using the straight blade. The inexperienced tend to use this instrument as a guide for the tube. When this happens the landmarks are obscured and the endoscopist unintentionally moves the blade, resulting in a failed intubation. In either case, once the blade is inserted, the tongue is swept slightly to the left and lift is applied to the laryngoscope in the direction of the laryngoscope handle points (approximately 45° from the horizon). Using the laryngoscope to pry results in damage to the teeth or gums and does not aid in visualization of the vocal cords. Important points to remember include keeping the elbow of the left arm tucked in close to the side. This allows you to use the muscles of the anterior chest and shoulder to help lift the mandible of the patient. The more the left elbow is abducted, the more the burden of lifting falls to the muscles of the left forearm alone. This makes prying more likely to occur. The endoscopist may obtain additional lifting support rotating his or her body slightly to the right and supporting the left elbow against the body. Finally, the laryngoscope should be held as low on the handle as possible. The higher up the handle is gripped, the more difficult it becomes to avoid prying. Gentle, yet firm, pressure applied by an assistant to the cricoid cartilage (Sellick's maneuver) may bring an anterior larynx into view. It also may close off the esophagus and protect against passive regurgitation and aspiration. Cricoid pressure is always applied with patients who are considered to have a full stomach. This means any patient who has had anything by mouth during the 6 hours before the procedure, and anyone with intra-abdominal pathology.

Occasionally, with patients who have an anterior larynx, it is necessary to use an endotracheal tube changer (also known as an endotracheal tube introducer). This is a long (45 to 60 cm), narrow, and stiff yet flexible piece of plastic

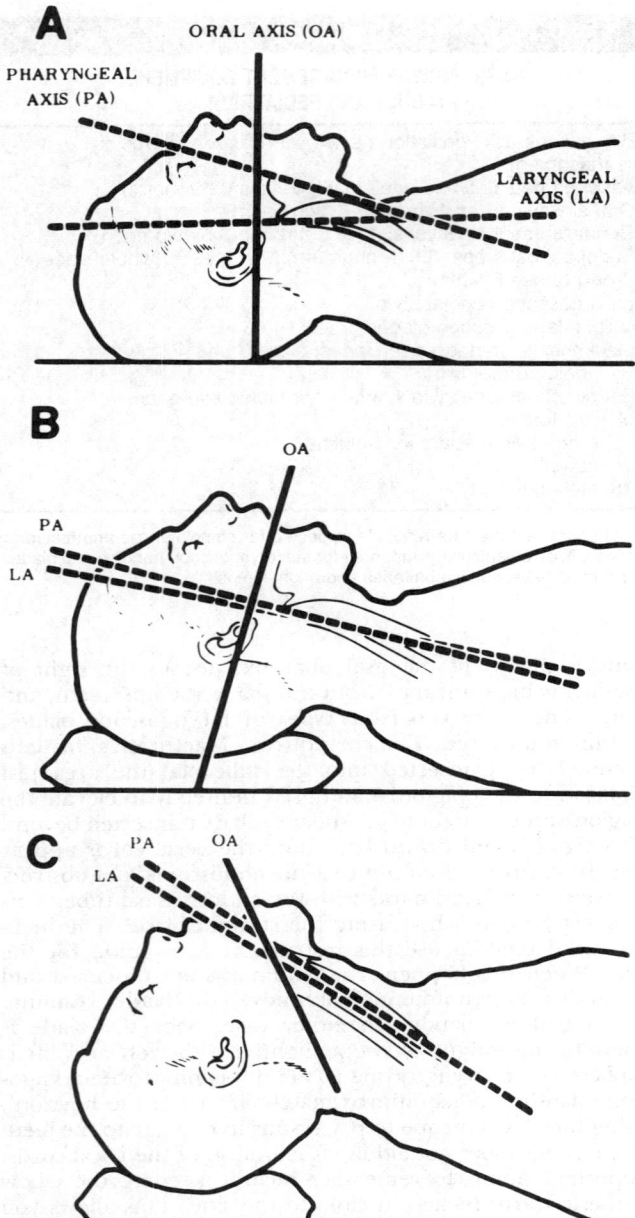

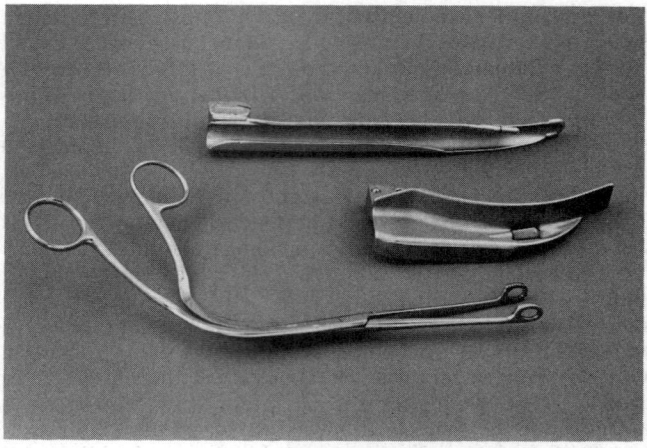

Figure 10–2. From top to bottom are the Miller (straight) laryngoscope blade, the MacIntosh (curved) laryngoscope blade, and the Magill forceps.

the changer and into the larynx. The tube changer is then removed, the cuff inflated, the patient ventilated, and the tube secured. Because this technique is not guaranteed, you must also be prepared to perform laryngoscopy.

As with any procedure, it is most important to have the patient positioned appropriately. In addition, the endoscopist should work in a comfortable position. It may be necessary to raise the height of the bed to a level that permits ease of access to the patient without requiring excessive bending. Also, it is important for those coming in contact with the airway and its secretions to be protected by both goggles and gloves.

Insertion of the endotracheal tube usually takes place when the vocal cords can be seen and the tube advanced under direct visualization (Fig. 10–4). Occasionally, only the arytenoid cartilages or the tip of the epiglottis can be seen. In this situation the tube may be advanced under the epiglottis and into the trachea by feel alone. This maneuver is sometimes aided by slight twisting or rotation of the tube as it reaches and passes the cords. However, in this situation, tube placement must be assessed with great care because intubation was not done under direct visualization.

Once the endotracheal tube has been inserted, the chest

Figure 10–1. Schematic diagram demonstrating head position for endotracheal intubation. *A.* Successful direct laryngoscopy requires alignment of the oral, pharyngeal, and laryngeal axes. *B.* Elevation of the head about 10 cm with pads under the occiput while the shoulders remain on the table aligns the laryngeal and pharyngeal axes. *C.* Subsequent head extension at the atlanto-occipital joint creates the shortest and most nearly straight line from the incisor teeth to glottic opening. (From Stoelting RK: Endotracheal intubation. In: Miller RD [ed]: Anesthesia. 2nd ed. Churchill Livingstone, New York, p 525, 1986.)

with a slight curve at the tip (Fig. 10–3). This may be passed into the trachea when it is not possible to pass an endotracheal tube. When it is in place, an endotracheal tube may be passed over it into the trachea. It can also be used, when necessary, to change an endotracheal tube in patients who are already intubated. When the patient has been well oxygenated, the tube changer is advanced down the endotracheal tube and the tube removed over the changer. The new endotracheal tube is then quickly advanced back over

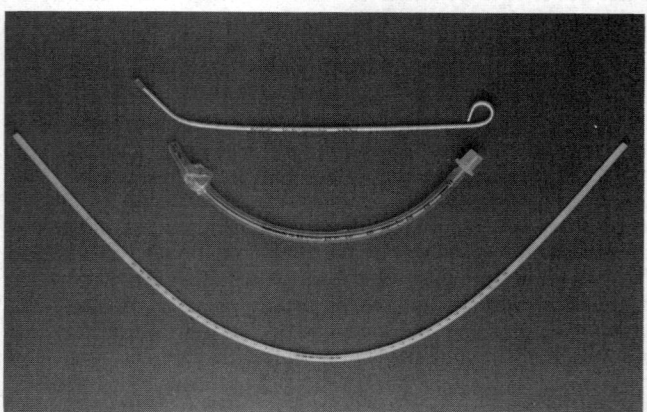

Figure 10–3. Photograph showing the usual shape and length of the endotracheal tube stylet *(top)* in relation to an adult endotracheal tube *(middle)* and an endotracheal tube changer, also called an intubating stylet *(bottom)*. Note the classic "hockey stick" deformity of the endotracheal tube stylet.

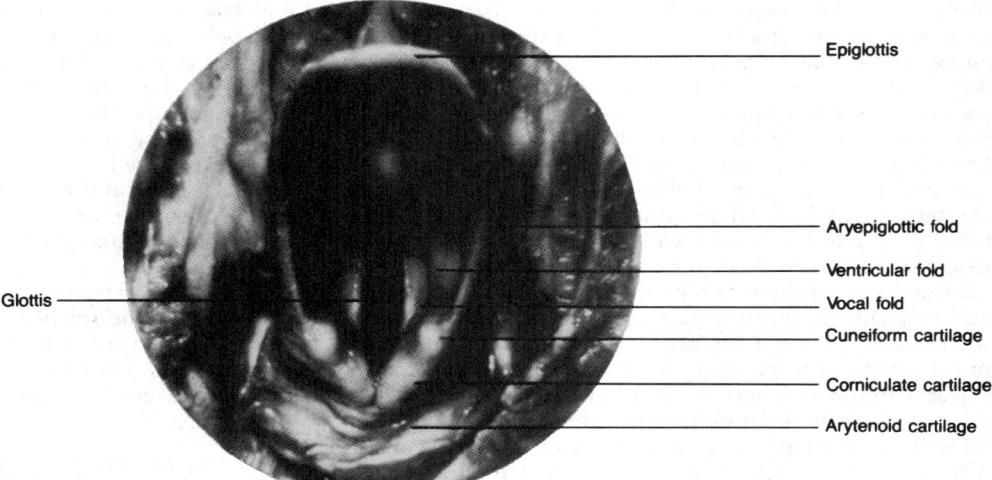

Figure 10–4. Anatomic specimen of adult human larynx. The perspective is similar to that seen during laryngoscopy. (From Stehling LC: Management of the airway. In: Barash PG, Cullen BF, Stoelting RK [eds]: Clinical Anesthesia. Philadelphia, JB Lippincott, p 544, 1990.)

Glottis

Epiglottis

Aryepiglottic fold

Ventricular fold

Vocal fold

Cuneiform cartilage

Corniculate cartilage

Arytenoid cartilage

should be inspected visually to determine that it is rising symmetrically and the inside of the tube should be inspected to ensure that it lightly mists with each breath. If monitored, significant end-tidal carbon dioxide levels can be detected within seconds and arterial saturation should rise and stabilize one half to several minutes later. When esophageal intubation has been done, the chest does not rise and harsh bubbling sounds can be auscultated over the stomach. Abdominal girth may increase and a belching sound may arise from the patient's mouth.[26, 27] The endotracheal tube may still mist, but end-tidal carbon dioxide and arterial saturation levels do not rise.[27–29] Initially a stethoscope should be placed over the fundus of the stomach to determine that oxygen is not being forced into the stomach via an esophageal intubation. Next, the stethoscope should be placed over the lungs laterally to determine that ventilation is occurring and equal in all fields. It is also essential to determine that the endotracheal tube is not located in either the right (most often, because of its more directly caudad path) or left mainstem bronchus. Visualization and direct palpation of the endotracheal tube passing anterior to the arytenoid cartilages are the only sure clinical signs of successful endotracheal intubation.[11, 30] The final confirmation of successful intubation is by laboratory test.[31] One test is to determine that a significant quantity of carbon dioxide is returned with each exhalation. This can be done by portable capnography, now available at some institutions, or by the use of a disposable in-line device that changes color when a threshold level of carbon dioxide is detected.[26, 28, 32] Obviously, significant quantities of carbon dioxide are detected only when tracheal intubation has taken place. Arterial blood gas levels can also be confirmatory, but there is a significant delay before results are available.

In the proverbial 70-kg patient, the endotracheal tube should be secured with the 20-cm mark at the lip. The usual distance from the carina to the vocal cords is approximately 6 to 8 cm and another 13 to 17 cm from the vocal cords to the front incisor.[33] Position of the endotracheal tube must be verified by clinical observation and chest roentgenogram. The endotracheal tube should be secured to the skin over the maxilla because this is a nonmovable body part. To secure the endotracheal tube to the skin over the mandible invites its untoward removal. The skin underlying the tape should be clean and dry and may be prepared with any of the commercially available substances that cause the tape to adhere more firmly. The endotracheal tube should never be secured to anything other than the patient. Endotracheal tubes should not be secured to the tapes securing things such as nasogastric tubes, because an incoherent patient could grasp one tube and, with one effort, remove both. There are as many ways to secure endotracheal tubes as there are people doing it, but these basic concepts should be adhered to. Another method of securing endotracheal tubes is tying them in place. This technique is particularly useful in patients with beards or facial wound dressings. Cloth "twill" or, for patients with facial wounds such as burns, intravenous tubing may be cut and used for this purpose. Intravenous tubing has the advantage of not absorbing liquids such as blood, pus, or secretions, and it can be prepared with povidone-iodine (Betadine) or other substances. The tie can be brought around the patient's neck and over both ears. Care must be taken not to let the tie slide down from the ears, as the tube would then have less support and there would be a greater likelihood of vascular compromise. It is of paramount importance that the tie not be secured so tightly that it obstructs either carotid or external jugular venous drainage. The result would be either to obstruct the supply of oxygen to the brain or to obstruct venous drainage, resulting in cerebral edema. The tie is first secured to the tube, making sure that it is snug without compromising the lumen of the tube. The two ends of the tie are brought together and secured with a knot.

When the tube is in place and secured, the patient should be well sedated so that he or she tolerates mechanical ventilation and does not self-extubate. An unfortunately common problem with mechanically ventilated patients in the intensive care unit has been inadequate sedation and the creation of airway emergencies by unplanned extubation. Long-acting narcotics such as morphine make excellent sedatives and may be combined with long-acting benzodiazepines. The advantage of using narcotics is that they may be reversed with naloxone, and even without reversal ventilation is seldom totally blocked. If untoward extubation occurs, the patient is probably self-ventilating to some degree. Not all patients can be ventilated, intubated, or reintubated, and the presence of spontaneous respirations, no matter how feeble, provides some measure of safety.

NASAL INTUBATION

Nasal intubation is seldom the method of choice for initial emergent intubation because it requires skills in addition to those needed for oral intubation. It has several advantages as well as potential risks. Oral tubes may be changed electively to nasal tubes when the benefits of a nasal endotracheal tube outweigh the risk of a change. The advantages of nasal endotracheal tubes include increased stability, improved access for providing oral care, and increased comfort of the patient. The disadvantages include the potential for sinus infection because of obstruction by the endotracheal tube, trauma to the nasal mucosa with epistaxis, and passage of the endotracheal tube submucosally or into the brain through an undetected or unsuspected basilar skull fracture.[23, 25, 34] There is always a risk that reintubation may be unsuccessful. Therefore, contraindications include a pre-existing sinus infection or a predilection for sinus infections, and suspicion or documentation of a basilar skull fracture, when there is a need for urgent control and management of the airway or when difficulty in intubation is anticipated.

Nasal intubation may be done either blindly or under direct visualization. In either case, the patient should first be well oxygenated and ventilated. Paint the nasal mucosa with either 4% cocaine, using cotton-tipped applicators, to a total dose of not more than 4.6 mg/kg, or a combination of 4% lidocaine with 0.25 to 0.50% phenylephrine. This serves to anesthetize and shrink the nasal mucosa, which enables passage of the endotracheal tube and reduces the chance of precipitating a nosebleed. If epistaxis occurs, often the best course of action is to continue to insert the tube or to leave it in place, allowing the tube to plug the bleeding. In normal situations, using information gained by painting the nasal mucosa with the cotton-tipped applicators, an assessment would be made concerning which nasal passage is more patent. The chosen nasal passage can be dilated by using progressively larger Guedel nasal airways from 6 through 8.5 mm. These airways can also be used as an aid in ventilating the patient. Because of the left-facing bevel on the end of the endotracheal tube, the right nasal passage is generally preferred. Only endotracheal tubes of 8 mm or smaller should be used. The tube should be lubricated with a water-soluble lubricant or lidocaine jelly. Insertion occurs along the floor of the nares and is directed straight back toward the occiput with firm steady pressure. Resistance is met and yields under gentle steady pressure. As the tube passes down into the oral pharynx, breath sounds become louder if the patient is breathing spontaneously.

If the blind nasal technique is used, it is essential for the person performing the intubation to keep an ear directly next to the opening of the endotracheal tube. Subtle changes in ventilation are heard as the tube nears the glottis. If all goes well, the tube enters the trachea. This is evidenced by fogging of the tube with the patient's ventilation, by the person doing the intubation feeling the patient's breath, and frequently by induction of a cough. If the tube does not enter the trachea, these signs are not present and the patient is able to speak when questioned. When the tube is in the trachea, phonation is not possible because the vocal cords cannot approximate and air does not flow against them. If the tube is advanced into the esophagus, breath sounds at the endotracheal tube cease. The endotracheal tube must be withdrawn until breath sounds are again at their best. At this point you must experiment with alternately flexing or extending the patient's neck and advancing the tube again while listening for optimal breath sounds. If after this experimentation the tube has not entered the trachea, direct visualization is necessary. Even though intubation may not be accomplished, the patient can usually be ventilated with the endotracheal tube in the posterior pharynx. To do so, seal the lips and the opposite nares with the fingers of the left hand and squeeze the ventilating bag with the right hand or have an assistant perform this task.

The direct visualization technique is the same even when blind nasal intubation has already been attempted. The endotracheal tube is inserted into the posterior pharynx. At this point an oxygen source or ventilating bag may be attached to the endotracheal tube to provide supplemental oxygen to the patient. When the patient is well oxygenated a laryngoscope blade is inserted into the mouth and the vocal cords are visualized. Then the tip of the endotracheal tube is visualized or advanced into the oral pharynx until it can be grasped using a Magill forceps (see Fig. 10–2). The tube is then directed toward the tracheal opening with the Magill forceps and advanced from above by an assistant. Care must be taken not to rupture the cuff of the endotracheal tube by grasping it with the forceps. Once the tube is inserted into the trachea, the cuff is inflated and the tube secured in the usual fashion. As always, the chest is then auscultated to ensure equality of the breath sounds bilaterally, and a chest roentgenogram is obtained to confirm proper placement.

RETROGRADE TECHNIQUE OF INTUBATION

When other techniques of endotracheal intubation fail and the patient can be ventilated or is breathing spontaneously, it may still be possible to intubate via the retrograde technique. At this stage it is probably too late to consider fiberoptic endoscopy as the pharynx of most patients contains a significant amount of blood and other secretions, which makes use of the endoscope difficult if not impossible. In general, fiberoptic endoscopy should be considered early in a difficult intubation, but a skilled endoscopist may wish to make an attempt. The retrograde technique involves insertion of a large-bore needle, bevel facing cephalad, straight down through the cricothyroid membrane. Aspiration of air from the catheter signals entry into the trachea. Either a guide wire or a long venous catheter is passed in a cephalad direction through the vocal cords. The catheter is grasped in the mouth with a Magill forceps and threaded from bottom up through an endotracheal tube. The endotracheal tube is next passed into the trachea using the catheter as a guide. When the tip of the endotracheal tube has just passed the vocal cords, the guidewire or catheter is withdrawn and the endotracheal tube inserted to an appropriate depth. The advantage of using a catheter is that air may be injected into it, and the catheter tip may be located in a blood- and secretion-filled posterior pharynx by noting bubbles. Many variations of this technique have been described.[35–43]

TRANSTRACHEAL VENTILATION

Transtracheal ventilation is an emergency lifesaving procedure undertaken when ventilation by mouth to mouth or bag and mask is inadequate and tracheal intubation has not been successful. This is accomplished by inserting the largest-bore intravenous catheter available through the cricothyroid membrane in a caudad direction (Figs. 10–5 and 10–6). Constant suction is applied to the syringe and catheter during insertion. Free aspiration of air signals entrance into the trachea.[43–47] The needle is removed and a 3-mL syringe, without plunger, is attached to the hub of the catheter. Next a 7-mm endotracheal tube connector (the part of the tube that attaches to the ventilator or ventilating bag) is inserted into the syringe barrel and a ventilating bag is connected. This system allows oxygenation, but ventilation (removal of carbon dioxide) may not be adequate and a more definitive method of airway control must be established as soon as possible.[45]

CRICOTHYROTOMY

Cricothyrotomy is performed only when control of a patient's airway is emergently required and other methods

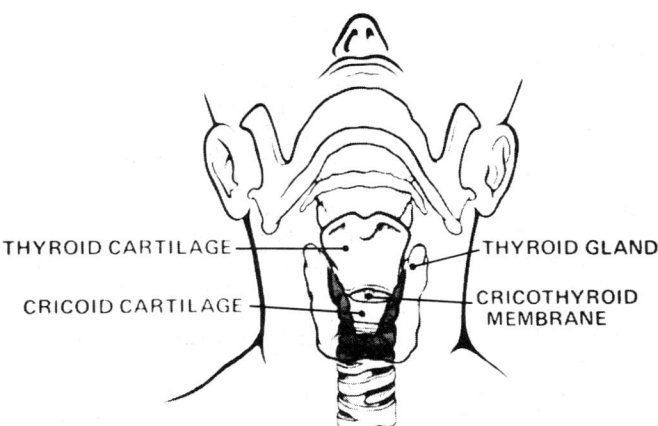

Figure 10–5. Laryngeal anatomy. (From Adjuncts for airway control, ventilation, and supplemental oxygen. In: Textbook of Advanced Cardiac Life Support. 2nd ed. Dallas, American Heart Association, p 33, 1987. Reproduced with permission. © Textbook of Advanced Cardiac Life Support, 1987. Copyright American Heart Association.)

have been unsuccessful. The cricothyroid membrane is located and prepared with povidone-iodine solution, if available. A scalpel blade is then inserted completely through the membrane and withdrawn (a stab wound), leaving an incision the size of the blade used (Fig. 10–7). Next, the handle of the scalpel is inserted through the incision and rotated 90° to increase the width of the incision by blunt dissection. Finally, a well-lubricated, size 6 endotracheal tube is gently inserted with steady, constant pressure into the trachea and ventilation is begun. The entire procedure should require approximately 60 seconds. Formal tracheostomy, or fiberoptic intubation, can be carried out in a more controlled fashion, if desired, once the patient has been stabilized. Formal tracheostomy should rarely or never be done emer-

gently (but should be done urgently). In general, it cannot be done rapidly enough to save a life or prevent serious brain damage.

COMPLICATIONS

Complications of airway management and endotracheal intubation may include damage to the teeth and soft tissue of the oral pharynx.[48–51] In general, if the laryngoscope is properly placed and forces are applied in the correct planes, no damage is done. Despite all precautions, adequate training, and experience, mishaps do occur. Undetected esophageal intubation, failed intubation, and inability to ventilate remain significant problems in airway management, but with today's technology (end-tidal carbon dioxide detectors and pulse oximeters) they are readily detectable.[26–32] They remain, however, the most serious, dreaded, and common of airway-related complications.

Next to airway obstruction, aspiration of gastric contents is the most feared complication of airway management. Depending on the nature of the aspirate (pH less than 2.5, volume greater than 0.5 mL/kg, and particulate content), the mortality resulting from aspiration is reported to average 30%.[50–52] Patients at increased risk include those with de-

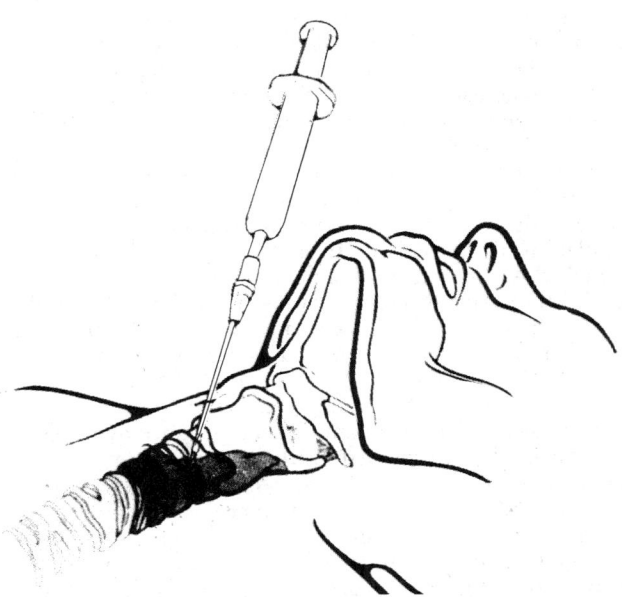

Figure 10–6. Method of catheter insertion for transtracheal ventilation. Note caudad direction of insertion to avoid injury to the vocal cords. (From Adjuncts for airway control, ventilation, and supplemental oxygen. In: Textbook of Advanced Cardiac Life Support. 2nd ed. Dallas, American Heart Association, p 34, 1987. Reproduced with permission. © Textbook of Advanced Cardiac Life Support, 1987. Copyright American Heart Association.)

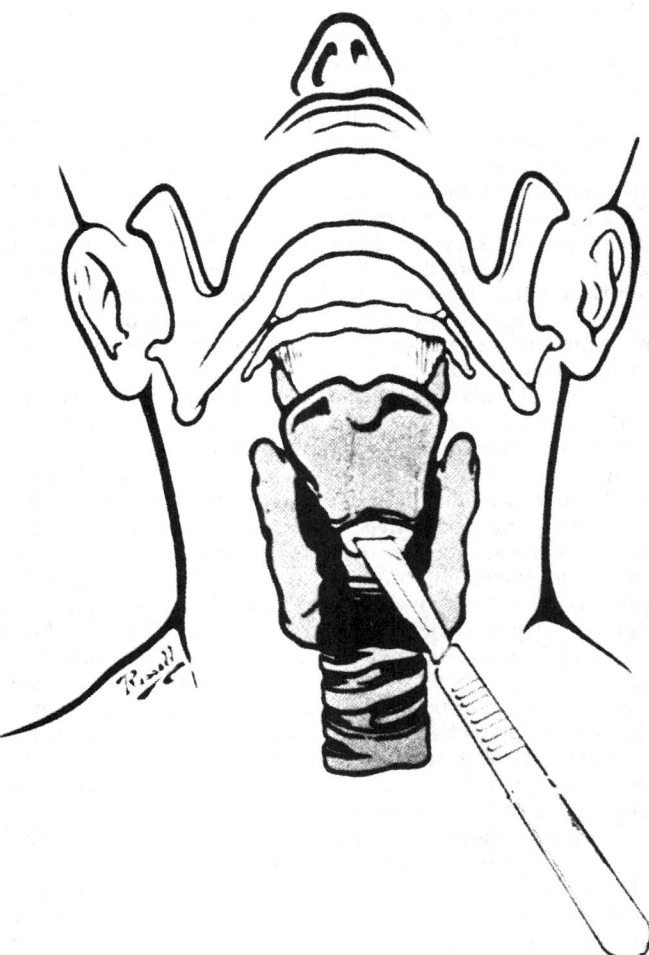

Figure 10–7. Scalpel insertion for cricothyrotomy. (From Adjuncts for airway control, ventilation, and supplemental oxygen. In: Textbook of Advanced Cardiac Life Support. 2nd ed. Dallas, American Heart Association, p 35, 1987. Reproduced with permission. © Textbook of Advanced Cardiac Life Support, 1987. Copyright American Heart Association.)

creased levels of consciousness, intra-abdominal pathology, ingestion of food or liquids within the previous 6 hours, delayed gastric emptying (diabetics, patients under stress or in pain), and low gastric pH. Of the two variables gastric pH and volume, low pH has been shown to be more detrimental to pulmonary function in animal models.[53, 54] Treatment is generally supportive and may include oxygen, mechanical ventilation, positive end-expiratory pressure, and fluids. Steroids are potentially harmful, and antibiotics should be given only if infection is present or suspected.[55, 57]

Submucosal dissection occurs most frequently when nasogastric tubes are inserted but may also occur with nasotracheal intubation. Detection is by palpation of the posterior oral pharynx. Suspicion of this diagnosis should be raised when undue resistance is met with insertion or when a tube (nasogastric or nasotracheal) has been inserted far enough to be visible in the oral pharynx but is not visible.[34]

Mucosal ischemia can result from prolonged intubation. The optimal time to perform a tracheostomy is a topic of extensive debate and is covered in Chapter 88. Within hours of intubation, tracheal cilia are inactivated in the area around the endotracheal tube cuff. Frank ischemia can develop when cuff pressures are increased above the tracheal capillary pressure of approximately 28 mm Hg. As a rule, endotracheal tube cuff pressures should be monitored every 8 hours and maintained below 25 mm Hg.[58, 59] Conflicts arise when the pressures required to ventilate patients exceed the cuff pressures. This dilemma is particularly likely to occur in patients with very high airway pressures. The choice must always be in favor of providing adequate ventilation. In these situations a lower cuff pressure accompanied by a minimal gas leak may be preferable to inducing mucosal ischemia if ventilation and oxygenation are not too adversely effected. Complications such as mucosal ulceration, tracheitis, and ultimately tracheal stenosis must be dealt with later, if the patient survives. Mucosal ulcerations and tracheitis generally heal on their own if the patient is adequately nourished and the source of the irritation is removed.[17, 60–63] Tracheal stenosis can be a long-term problem requiring multiple corrective surgical procedures and potentially permanent tracheostomy.

Laryngeal, submucosal, and facial edema can be serious and potentially lethal problems in airway management. The edema is most frequently the result of either trauma or fluid resuscitation. Trauma may be direct, in the form of injury resulting from inhalation of heat or chemicals or surgical injury (e.g., head and neck surgery), or caused by missiles, motor vehicles, or other objects. In addition, upper airway edema is extremely common after extensive surgery. In patients who have been in the head-down position (e.g., during surgery done in the prone or the Trendelenburg position) or who have received a significant fluid load (e.g., for surgery or burn resuscitation), intubation (and even tracheostomy) can be impossible. It is, therefore, imperative that such patients have their endotracheal tubes well secured and that adequate sedation (or even paralysis in rare situations) be provided. Every precaution must be taken to prevent an unintentional extubation.

Vocal cord paralysis is an infrequent but potentially lethal occurrence after intubation and is most commonly a complication of direct trauma during surgery near the recurrent laryngeal nerve.[64, 65] The result is usually relaxation of one or both vocal cords, which assume varying degrees of adduction. This results in a narrowed airway, stridor, and respiratory embarrassment. Treatment may range from observation to reintubation or tracheostomy.

Arytenoid cartilage displacement is a rare complication of endotracheal intubation and probably represents direct trauma to the vocal cords. The most likely presenting symptom is a weak voice with a recent history of laryngeal instrumentation. On laryngoscopy the affected cord is displaced laterally or posteriolaterally and held in abduction. Treatment is by surgical reduction.[66]

Hoarseness occurs in 3% of postsurgical patients and is usually benign, disappearing within a few days of extubation without any therapy other than vocal rest.[67] Sore throat occurs in 40% of patients after extubation. Patients should be reassured and even warned of this possible effect of intubation. Treatment consists of reassurance, use of warm or hot liquids when the larynx is again competent, and use of throat lozenges as needed. It is important to remember that the normal protective mechanisms of the larynx may not be entirely intact immediately after extubation.[68] Normal laryngeal function may not return for hours to days after extubation.

Tooth avulsions should be referred to an oral surgeon or dentist as soon as possible.[48] The treatment is to reinsert the tooth into its socket gently and slowly and hold steady pressure on it for 15 minutes. The sooner this is done, the more likely it is that the tooth will heal; even a delay of a few hours significantly reduces the chance of the tooth's being successfully reimplanted. If the tooth cannot be reinserted, because of the patient's level of consciousness or for other reasons, it should be kept in a solution of normal saline. Chipped teeth need not be treated immediately but should be referred to a dentist. Oral prostheses are more fragile than original equipment, and those that can be removed should be before instrumentation takes place. Those that cannot be removed should be located by questioning the patient beforehand and avoiding contact with them whenever possible. If a tooth or dental prosthesis is missing and is not found, a chest roentgenogram should be taken to make certain that it has not been aspirated into the lungs, which would require bronchoscopic retrieval.

Laryngospasm occurs most commonly in patients emerging from anesthesia but also may occur in other settings. It is a reflex contraction of the laryngeal muscles that results in total obstruction of the airway. It is recognized by cessation of ventilation, a rocking-boat motion of the patient's chest and abdomen during attempts to inhale against a closed glottis. On occasion these efforts have resulted in pulmonary edema because of creation of highly negative airway pressures behind a closed glottis.[69] Laryngospasm is treated by holding 10 to 20 cm H_2O constant pressure (not repeated attempts at ventilation against the closed glottis) for up to 60 seconds. Usually the laryngospasm breaks, permitting ventilation of the patient. If ventilation is still not possible, a small dose of succinylcholine (10 mg in a 70-kg patient) administered intravenously causes sufficient muscle relaxation to allow ventilation. Ventilation by bag and mask must then continue until the patient is again able to support spontaneous ventilatory efforts.

Other physiologic alterations that occur during intubation include release of catecholamines that produce hypertension, tachycardia, and increased cardiac output, none of which are beneficial for the patient with coronary artery disease.[70, 71] Intraocular pressure is increased, resulting in increased likelihood of eye loss in a patient with an open eye injury. Patients with increased intracranial pressure are at risk for further increases in intracranial pressure and brain herniation. When dealing with compounding factors in airway management such as these, experienced, highly skilled individuals should be called on to assist with airway management.

A foundation for the concepts presented here may be found in a text by Whitten.[72]

References

1. Utting JE: Pitfalls in anaesthetic practice. Br J Anaesth 59:877, 1987.
2. Caplan R, Todd D: Respiratory mishaps: Principal anesthetic of risk and implications for anesthetic care. Anesthesiology 67:A469, 1987.
3. Mathew M, Hanna L, Aldrete J: Pre-operative indices to anticipate difficult tracheal intubation. Anesth Analg 68:S187, 1989.
4. Bellhouse C, Dore C: Predicting difficult intubation. Br J Anaesth 62:469, 1989.
5. Bellhouse C, Dore C: Criteria for estimating likelihood of difficulty of endotracheal intubation with the MacIntosh laryngoscope. Anaesth Intensive Care 16:329, 1988.
6. Charters P, Fahy L, Horton W: Airways re-visited. Br J Anaesth 62:6, 1989.
7. Mallampati S, Gatt S, Gugino L, et al: A clinical sign to predict difficult tracheal intubation: A prospective study. Can Anaesth Soc J 32:429, 1985.
8. Samsoon G, Young J: Difficult tracheal intubation: A retrospective study. Anaesthesia 42:487, 1987.
9. White A, Kander P: Anatomical factors in difficult direct laryngoscopy. Br J Anaesth 47:468, 1975.
10. Cass N, James N, Lines V: Difficult direct laryngoscopy complicating intubation for anaesthesia. Br Med J 1:488, 1956.
11. King TA, Adams AP: Failed tracheal intubation. Br J Anaesth 65:400, 1990.
12. Zuck D: Factors in difficult direct laryngoscopy. Br J Anaesth 48:395, 1976.
13. Nichol H, Zuck D: Difficult laryngoscopy—the "anterior" larynx and the atlanto-occipital gap. Br J Anaesth 55:141, 1983.
14. Zuck D: Difficult tracheal intubation. Anaesthesia 40:1016, 1985.
15. Wilson M, Spiegelhalter D, Robertson J, et al: Predicting difficult intubation. Br J Anaesth 61:211, 1988.
16. Westhorpe R: The position of the larynx in children and its relationship to the ease of intubation. Anaesth Intensive Care 15:384, 1987.
17. Bishop MJ, Weymuller EA Jr, Fink BR: Laryngeal effects of prolonged intubation. Anesth Analg 63:335, 1984.
18. Block C, Brechner VL: Unusual problems in airway management. II. The influence of the temporomandibular joint, the mandible and associated structures on endotracheal intubation. Anesth Analg 50:114, 1971.
19. Turnstall M: Failed intubation drill. Anaesthesia 31:850, 1976.
20. Ruben H, Knudsen E, Carugati G: Gastric inflation in relation to airway pressure. Acta Anaesthesiol Scand 5:107, 1961.
21. Wycoff CC: Aspiration during induction of anesthesia. Anesth Analg 38:5, 1959.
22. Berry FA, Blankenbaker WL, Ball CG: A comparison of bacteremia occurring with nasotracheal and orotracheal intubation. Anesth Analg 52:873, 1973.
23. Dubick MN, Wright BD: Comparison of laryngeal pathology following long-term oral and nasal endotracheal intubations. Anesth Analg 57:663, 1978.
24. Arens JF, LeJeune FE, Webre DR: Maxillary sinusitis, a complication of nasotracheal intubation. Anesthesiology 40:415, 1974.
25. Warden J: Accidental intubation of the oesophagus and preoxygenation. Anaesth Intensive Care 8:377, 1980.
26. Birmingham P, Cheney F, Ward R: Esophageal intubation: A review of detection techniques. Anesth Analg 65:6, 1986.
27. Linko K, Paloheimo M, Tammisto T: Capnography for detection of accidental oesophageal intubation. Acta Anaesthesiol Scand 27:199, 1983.
28. Murry I, Modell J: Early detection of endotracheal tube accidents by monitoring carbon dioxide concentration in respiratory gas. Anesthesiology 59:344, 1983.
29. Guggenberger H, Lenz G, Federle R: Early detection of inadvertent oesophageal intubation: Pulse oximetry vs. capnography. Acta Anaesthesiol Scand 33:112, 1989.
30. Charters P, Wilkinson K: Tactile orotracheal placement test. A bimanual tactile examination of the positioned orotracheal tube to confirm laryngeal placement. Anaesthesia 42:801, 1987.
31. Ionescu T: Signs of endotracheal intubation. Anaesthesia 36:422, 1981.
32. O'Flaherty D, Adams A: The end-tidal carbon dioxide detector. Anaesthesia 45:653, 1990.
33. Gammage GW: Airway management. In: Civetta JM, Taylor RW, Kirby RR (eds): Critical Care Medicine. Philadelphia, JB Lippincott, p 197, 1988.
34. Seebacher J, Nozik D, Mathieu A: Inadvertent intracranial introduction of a nasogastric tube, a complication of severe maxillofacial trauma. Anesthesiology 42:100, 1975.
35. Bourke D, Levesque PR: Modification of retrograde guide for endotracheal intubation. Anesth Analg 53:1013, 1974.
36. Barriot P, Riou B: Retrograde technique for tracheal intubation in trauma patients. Crit Care Med 16:712, 1988.
37. Powell WF, Ozdil T: A translaryngeal guide for tracheal intubation. Anesth Analg 46:231, 1967.
38. Dhara S: Guided blind endotracheal intubation. Anaesthesia 35:81, 1980.
39. deLisser E, Muravchick S: Emergency transtracheal ventilation. Anesthesiology 55:606, 1981.
40. Akinyemi O: Complications of guided blind endotracheal intubation. Anaesthesia 34:590, 1979.
41. Barriot P, Riou B: Retrograde technique for tracheal intubation with trauma patients. Crit Care Med 16:712, 1988.
42. Abou-Madi M, Trop D: Pulling versus guiding: A modification of retrograde guided intubation. Can J Anaesth 36:336, 1989.
43. Aye L: Percutaneous transtracheal ventilation. Anesth Analg 62:619, 1983.
44. Benumof JL, Scheller MS: Jet ventilation and difficult airway. Anesthesiology 71:769, 1989.
45. Gildar JS: A simple system for transtracheal ventilation. Anesthesiology 58:106, 1983.
46. Patel R: Systems for transtracheal ventilation. Anesthesiology 59:165, 1983.
47. Scuderi P, McLesky C, Comer P: Emergency percutaneous transtracheal ventilation during anesthesia using readily available equipment. Anesth Analg 61:867, 1982.
48. Lind GL, Spiegel EH, Munson ES: Treatment of traumatic tooth avulsion. Anesth Analg 61:469, 1982.
49. Blanc VF, Tremblay NAG: The complications of tracheal intubation: A new classification with a review of the literature. Anesth Analg 53:202, 1974.
50. Zwillich CW, Pierson DJ, Creagh CE, et al: Complications of assisted ventilation. Am J Med 57:161, 1974.
51. Stauffer JL, Olson DE, Petty TL: Complications and consequences of endotracheal intubation and tracheotomy. Am J Med 70:65, 1981.
52. Mendleson CL: The aspiration of stomach contents into the lungs during obstetric anesthesia. Am J Obstet Gynecol 52:191, 1946.
53. Kennedy TP, Johnson KJ, Kunkel RG, et al: Acute acid aspiration lung injury in the rat. Anesth Analg 69:87, 1989.
54. James CF, Modell JH, Gibbs CP, et al: Pulmonary aspiration—effects of volume and pH in the rat. Anesth Analg 65:665, 1984.
55. Downs JB, Chapman RL, Modell JH, et al: An evaluation of steroid therapy in aspiration pneumonitis. Anesthesiology 40:129, 1974.
56. Wynne JW, Reynolds JC, Hood CL, et al: Steroid therapy for pneumonitis induced in rabbits by aspiration of foodstuff. Anesthesiology 51:11, 1979.
57. Modell JH, Boysen PG: Pulmonary aspiration of stomach contents. In: Shoemaker WC, Ayers S, Grenvik A, et al (eds): Textbook of Critical Care. 2nd ed. Philadelphia, WB Saunders, p 565, 1989.
58. Lindholm CE, Grenvik A: Tracheal tube and cuff problems. Int Anesthesiol Clin 20:103, 1982.
59. Bernhard WN, Cottrell JE, Sivakumaran C, et al: Adjustment of intracuff pressure to prevent aspiration. Anesthesiology 50:363, 1979.
60. Bishop MJ, Weymuller EA, Fink BR: Laryngeal effects of prolonged intubation. Anesth Analg 63:335, 1984.
61. Klainer AS, Turndorf H, Wu W, et al: Surface alterations due do endotracheal intubation. Am J Med 58:674, 1975.
62. Jackson C: Contact ulcer granuloma and other laryngeal complications of endotracheal anesthesia. Anesthesiology 14:425, 1953.
63. Snow JC, Harano M, Balogh K: Postintubation granuloma of the larynx. Anesth Analg 45:425, 1966.
64. Holley HS, Gildea JE: Vocal cord paralysis after tracheal intubation. JAMA 215:281, 1980.
65. Hahn FW, Martin JT, Lillie JC: Vocal-cord paralysis with endotracheal intubation. Arch Otolaryngol Head Neck Surg 92:226, 1970.
66. Prasertwanitch Y, Schwarz JJH, Vandam LD: Arytenoid cartilage dislocation following prolonged endotracheal intubation. Anesthesiology 41:516, 1974.
67. Jaffe BF: Postoperative hoarseness. Am J Surg 123:432, 1972.
68. Burgess GE, Cooper JR, Marino RJ, et al: Laryngeal competence after tracheal extubation. Anesthesiology 51:73, 1979.
69. Kyff JV, Finch JS: Hemoptysis following anesthesia and surgery. Respir Care 32:117, 1987.
70. Stoelting RK: Circulatory changes during direct larygoscopy and tracheal intubation. Anesthesiology 47:381, 1977.
71. Cole WL, Stoelting VK: Blood gases during intubation following two types of oxygenation. Anesth Analg 50:68, 1971.
72. Whitten CE: Anyone Can Intubate. San Diego, CA, Medical Arts Press, 1989.

CHAPTER 11

Cardiopulmonary Resuscitation: Current Status and New Horizons

Karl B. Kern
Gordon A. Ewy

More than 0.5 million individuals will suffer cardiac arrest this year in the United States alone.[1] With current cardiopulmonary resuscitation (CPR) techniques, fewer than 20% of these people will survive in the long term. CPR is intended to restore circulation after respiratory or circulatory arrest. It must be emphasized, however, that the use of external chest compression and assisted ventilation is merely a temporizing therapy.

VENTRICULAR FIBRILLATION AND DEFIBRILLATION

Seventy percent of cardiac arrests are secondary to ventricular fibrillation. Ventricular fibrillation almost invariably requires defibrillation for definitive therapy. Patients with ventricular fibrillation have a good chance of survival provided that basic and advanced life support is provided in a timely manner.

Fifty to seventy percent of the annual deaths from coronary artery disease occur suddenly and are the result of ventricular fibrillation.[2, 3] Fortunately, primary ventricular fibrillation is usually responsive to immediate defibrillation.[4] Patients who have experienced witnessed, exertion-related cardiac arrest in established cardiac rehabilitation units have been reported to respond uniformly to prompt defibrillation.[5] Similarly, nearly 40% of patients who are promptly treated for out-of-hospital cardiac arrest with CPR and early defibrillation survive in the long term.[6, 7] Because the rapidity with which defibrillation is delivered is a major determinant in survival from cardiac arrest secondary to ventricular fibrillation, early administration of such therapy is assuming increasing importance.[8–10]

Increasing the speed of delivery of defibrillation can be accomplished by innovative programs such as training emergency medical technicians to perform defibrillation.[11, 12] Automatic external defibrillators can also be applied by emergency medical technicians and by others with a minimum of training. Placement of automatic external defibrillators at locations where large numbers of individuals gather, such as football stadiums or large office buildings, may be an important step in improving survival in unexpected cardiac arrest.[13]

Implantation of automatic internal cardioverter defibrillators in patients who are at high risk of sudden arrhythmic death has resulted in markedly improved survival in the subgroup of patients with recurrent ventricular tachycardia or ventricular fibrillation.[14, 15] Figure 11–1 shows the improved survival rate of patients at high risk of sudden death who have implanted automatic internal cardioverter defibrillators.

The amount of energy desirable for direct-current external defibrillation is controversial.[16] It is clear that a defibril-

lation threshold exists and that shocks of inadequate strength do not defibrillate.[17–23] Yet excessively strong defibrillation shocks are known to produce dysrhythmias and myocardial damage.[19] Observations of human adults indicate that body weight is not a major determinant of the energy levels necessary for defibrillation.[23–26] It is now generally agreed that, although there is a relationship between body size and the energy needed for defibrillation (infants and small children require less energy than large adults) over the range of weights in most people, size does not appear to be a clinically important variable.[27] Two clinical studies have suggested that an initial shock energy of no more than 200 J should be used. In a prospective out-of-hospital study, Weaver and associates compared the effects of low- and high-energy shocks in 249 patients with ventricular fibrillation.[28] "Low-energy" shocks (two 175-J shocks and, if ineffective, an additional 320-J shock) were compared on alternate days with "high-energy" shocks (three 320-J shocks). Defibrillation rates were virtually identical with either shock energy, as was the proportion of patients resuscitated and subsequently discharged from the hospital. Kerber and associates conducted a prospective in-hospital study of 183 patients who received direct-current shocks for ventricular fibrillation.[29] Patients received initial shocks of either 200 J or 300 to 400 J. This study also showed no difference in the first-shock or cumulative success rates of shocks at these two energy levels. Neither study showed any benefit from initial shocks above 200 J. Moreover, using a lower energy may be safer. Weaver and associates found a higher incidence of atrioventricular block in patients receiving 320-J shocks than in those receiving the lower-energy shocks; it was particularly evident in patients who received several shocks at the higher energy level.[28]

The appropriate energy level for the second shock is still somewhat controversial. The advanced cardiac life-support guidelines suggested that the initial shock and the second shock should be of similar energies.[30] This recommendation was based on two lines of evidence. First, defibrillation appears to be a probability function; that is, at any given energy there is a specific probability that defibrillation can be achieved.[31] Therefore if the first shock fails, it is possible that a second shock of the same energy will succeed. Second, the rationale for a second shock of the same energy is that

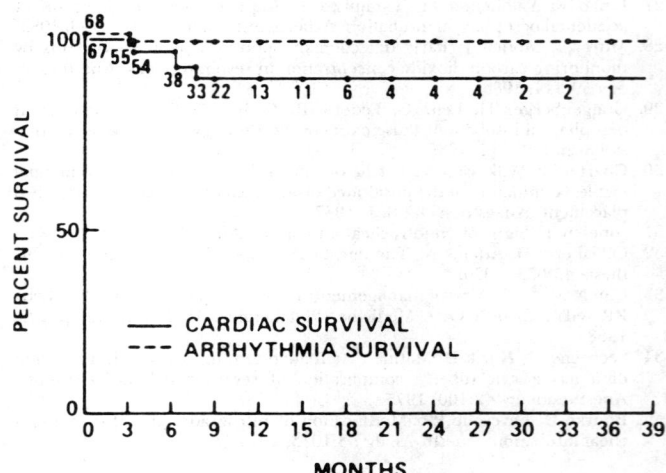

Figure 11–1. Excellent survival curves (Kaplan-Meier) for patients with the implantable cardioverter/defibrillator. Historical controls typically show an approximately 50% mortality rate by 24 months. (From Echt DS, Armstrong K, Schmidt P, et al: Clinical experience, complications, and survival in 70 patients with the automatic implantable cardioverter/defibrillator. Circulation 71:289, 96, 1985.)

transthoracic impedance decreases with repeated shocks.[32, 33] Such a decrease results in greater current flow for any given energy, and this increase in current flow should improve the chance of achieving defibrillation with a second shock of the same energy. However, Kerber and associates have shown that, although the transthoracic impedance in humans does fall with repeated shocks, the change is modest.[34] They concluded that a greater and more predictable increase in current flow occurs if the shock energy is raised. The present recommendation for the strength of the second shock remains 200 to 300 J.[30] Should the first two shocks fail to defibrillate, a third shock of not more than 360 J should be delivered immediately. This sequence was incorporated in the 1986 guidelines for advanced cardiac life support.[30]

Because the success of defibrillation is significantly decreased by a delay of even a few minutes, the present guidelines suggest three immediate and consecutive shocks when needed.[30, 35] For recurrent ventricular fibrillation, it may not be necessary to increase the defibrillation energy on successive shocks. If ventricular fibrillation is recurrent, it is reasonable to use the same energy level that was previously effective. If ventricular fibrillation recurs frequently, it may in fact be desirable to reduce the energy of subsequent defibrillatory shocks. This approach has the theoretic advantage of minimizing electrical injury to the heart. Appropriate external chest compression and assisted ventilation should be performed until a defibrillator is available and between shocks while the defibrillator capacitor is charging, except with automatic or semiautomatic external defibrillators. These devices require a period of time for diagnosis and capacitor charging. During this time, external chest compression interferes with the diagnostic process and delays or aborts discharge. Therefore a period of up to 1.5 minutes is, by consensus, acceptable for diagnosing and delivering three shocks by automatic or semiautomatic external defibrillators *without* chest compression.[36]

Defibrillation is accomplished by passing through the heart an electric current of sufficient energy to depolarize a critical mass of the myocardium. Although the operator selects the energy (in joules), it is the current flow (in amperes) that is responsible for defibrillation. Current flow is determined by the shock strength and the transthoracic resistance (impedance). Many of the factors determining transthoracic impedance to direct-current defibrillator discharge are known. They include the energy level,[37] electrode size,[38–41] interface between the skin and the electrode,[40, 42, 43] number of previous shocks and time interval between them,[32, 33] phase of ventilation,[44] distance between electrodes,[34] and paddle electrode pressure.[34] Human transthoracic impedance to cardioversion or defibrillator shock ranges between 14 and 143 Ω.[45] If the impedance is high, low-energy shocks fail to defibrillate.[46] Factors affecting transthoracic impedance are less important for high-energy defibrillations. However, if all three defibrillation attempts fail, one should evaluate not only electrode position but also factors that may contribute to a high transthoracic impedance or resistance to defibrillation. These factors include pneumothorax, inadequate electrode–chest wall interface, inadequate electrode position or skin contact, excessive distance between electrodes, and inadequate electrode pressure.

Our current understanding is that defibrillation depends on an adequate current traversing the myocardium; hence paddle electrode placement is critical. The electrodes should be placed in a position that maximizes current flow through the ventricular myocardium. There are two accepted locations for paddle placement. The standard placement is with one electrode with its edge just to the right of the upper sternum and below the clavicle and the other paddle to the left of the nipple with the center of the electrode in the

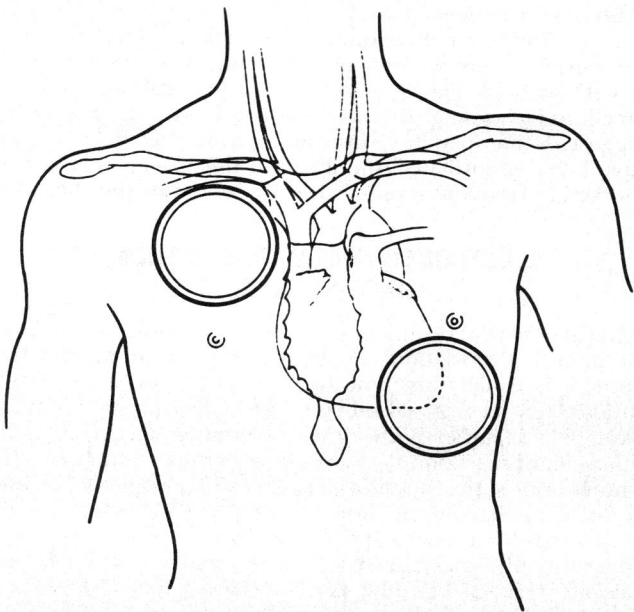

Figure 11–2. Correct paddle placement for the anterior-apical approach. Note that the anterior paddle is on the right side of the upper sternum. (From Tilkian AG: Cardiovascular Procedures—Diagnostic Techniques and Therapeutic Procedures. St Louis, CV Mosby, p 281, 1986.)

midaxillary line (Fig. 11–2). An alternative approach is to place one paddle anteriorly over the left or right precordium and the other posteriorly behind the heart (Fig. 11–3). The paddle should be applied to the chest wall with firm pressure (about 25 lb).

Paddle electrode size is another factor that alters transthoracic resistance to defibrillation discharge.[16] However, paddle size seems to be less important for successful defibrillation than is correct placement.

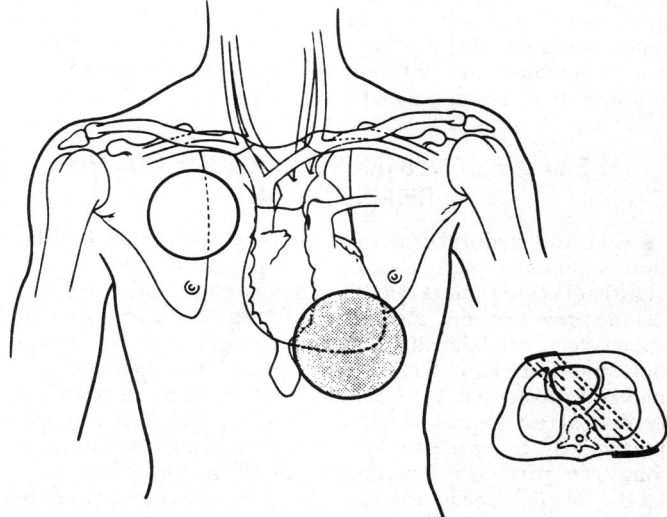

Figure 11–3. Optional paddle position for the anteroposterior approach to cardioversion or defibrillation. Again note that the posterior paddle is placed to the right of the spine. (From Tilkian AG: Cardiovascular Procedures—Diagnostic Techniques and Therapeutic Procedures. St Louis, CV Mosby, p 282, 1986.)

On occasion, external cardioversion or defibrillation is necessary in patients with permanent pacemakers. The external defibrillation electrodes should not be placed too near the subcutaneous pacemaker generator (not closer than 5 inches), as defibrillation shocks may cause pacemaker malfunction by raising the pacing threshold.[47] It has been suggested that patients with permanent pacemakers who have been defibrillated should have the pacing thresholds checked at frequent intervals for 6 weeks after the shock.[47]

ELECTROMECHANICAL DISSOCIATION AND ASYSTOLE

Cardiac arrest resulting from either asystole or electromechanical dissociation usually has a poor prognosis. Indeed, it is usually an indication of a large ischemic insult and is often seen as an end result of cardiac arrest that may have begun earlier with either ventricular tachycardia or ventricular fibrillation that was not responsive to therapy. In a number of series, attempts at successful treatment of these arrhythmias have been shown to be poor, if not uniformly unsuccessful. In a series of 143 cardiac arrests seen at the University of Arizona over a 1-year period, 61 (43%) of the patients were successfully resuscitated. Asystole and electromechanical dissociation were almost uniformly associated with nonsurvival. Only 1 of 33 patients with electromechanical dissociation survived. No patient with asystole survived.[48]

Because of their integral role in myocardial excitation-contraction coupling, calcium ions have been postulated to be useful during profound cardiovascular collapse when accompanied by electromechanical dissociation, and they restore electrical rhythm in some instances of electrical standstill. However, there are few experimental data to support this postulate,[49] and intravenous injections in the quantities usually given result in potentially dangerously high serum calcium levels in the patient.[50, 51] When 5 mg of 10% calcium chloride was administered as an intravenous bolus to victims of cardiac arrest, serum calcium levels were found to vary from 12.9 to 18.2 mg/dL.[51] The mean serum calcium level was 15.3 mg/dL at 5 minutes and 11.2 mg/dL at 10 minutes. Calcium has the potential of being particularly dangerous in patients receiving digitalis. Finally, no evidence exists that calcium improves the outcomes of patients suffering electromechanical dissociation or asystole.[52–54] Accordingly, the revised American Heart Association standards and guidelines deleted the previous recommendations for using calcium chloride in the treatment algorithms for electromechanical dissociation and asystole.

THE VALUE OF BYSTANDER CARDIOPULMONARY RESUSCITATION

Successful defibrillation of patients in ventricular fibrillation depends on many factors, including the duration of the ventricular fibrillation and the environment and condition of the myocardium. As mentioned earlier, the speed at which electrical defibrillation is provided is crucial for a good outcome. Data from Seattle indicate that early defibrillation makes a substantial difference in the long-term outcomes of cardiac arrest victims. Early initiation of basic life support, particularly by witnesses or bystanders, can also improve long-term survival if it is followed by electrical defibrillation. In the Seattle experience, in which definitive therapy (defibrillation) was provided within 8 minutes of collapse and basic life support (CPR) was begun within 4 minutes of collapse, 43% of the patients survived. If basic CPR was not performed before the arrival of paramedics and defibrillation, only 7% survived. If both therapies were delayed, with no

TABLE 11–1

CARDIAC ARREST: TIME TO INITIATION OF THERAPY AND SUBSEQUENT SURVIVAL

Time at Which CPR Given (min)	Survival (%) with Defibrillation at		
	<8 min	8–16 min	>16 min
<4	43	19	10
4–8	27	19	6
>8	—	7	0

Data from Eisenberg MS, Bergner L, Hallstrom A: Cardiac resuscitation in the community: Importance of rapid provision and implications for program planning. JAMA 241:1905, 1979.

CPR within 10 minutes after collapse and no attempt at defibrillation within 16 minutes after collapse, no patients survived (Table 11–1).[7]

Other studies from major cities showing the clear benefit of the use of early or bystander CPR include those from Oslo, Birmingham, and Pittsburgh.[55–57] Only the Milwaukee study has failed to show such a benefit.[58–61]

The benefits of bystander CPR seem to extend beyond simple myocardial survival and into neurologic outcomes. Thompson and coworkers have reported that more patients receiving bystander CPR regained consciousness and they regained it earlier than patients who did not receive this form of treatment. Patients who received early basic life support CPR had fewer neurologic deficits, and fewer patients needed extended-care placement on discharge.[62] Copley and colleagues also demonstrated the benefit of early CPR in terms of significantly less residual central nervous system impairment on hospital discharge.[56] In an experimental model at the University of Arizona, we have shown improved neurologic outcomes with the use of early CPR.[63] Twenty-two mongrel dogs were subjected to 5 minutes of electrically induced ventricular fibrillation. In 11 dogs, closed chest massage and ventilation with room air were begun immediately and were continued for 5 minutes. The other 11 dogs received no chest compression or assisted ventilation for 5 minutes. At 5 minutes defibrillation was attempted and advanced cardiac life-support protocols were followed until the animals were resuscitated or died. No statistical difference in resuscitability or 24-hour survival between the two groups was demonstrated. Eight of 11 early-CPR animals were resuscitated and survived 24 hours; 6 of 11 no-early-CPR dogs were resuscitated, and 5 lived for 24 hours. There was a significant difference in neurologic deficit and in the ease of resuscitation. Early-CPR dogs had no neurologic deficit, whereas no-early-CPR dogs had a neurologic deficit of 41% ($P < .01$).

MECHANISM OF BLOOD PRESSURE DURING CARDIOPULMONARY RESUSCITATION

One of the continuing questions concerning CPR is the rate at which external chest compression should be applied. In 1977, Taylor and coworkers suggested that over a range of 40 to 80 compressions per minute the duration of chest compression was more important than the rate of chest compression.[64] A duty cycle of 50% (with 50% chest compression and 50% relaxation) at 60 compressions per minute was thought to be optimal.[64] However, work from Duke University indicated that a higher chest compression rate produces better blood flow during closed chest CPR.[65, 66] Some of these data were available at the time of the 1985 national conference on CPR.[2] Consequently, this information

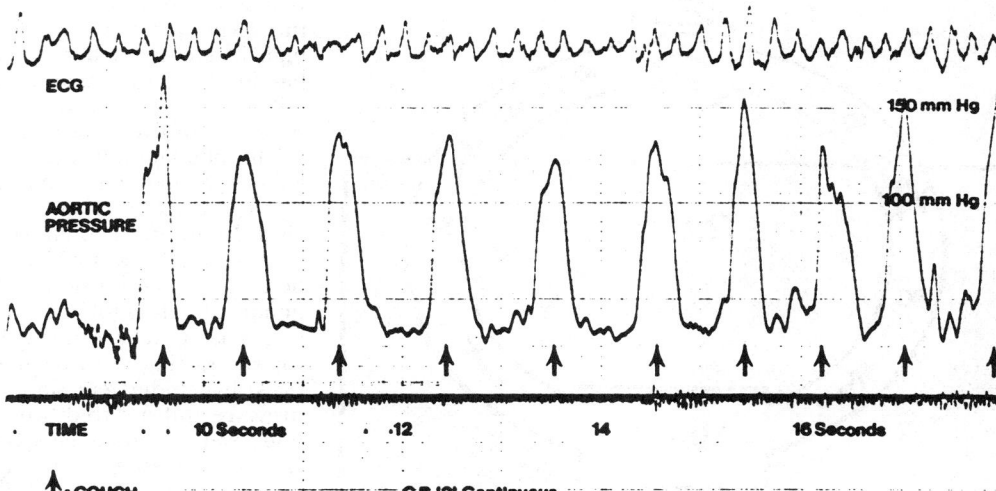

Figure 11–4. Hemodynamic results of cough CPR. (From Ewy GA, Bressler R: Cardiovascular Drugs and the Management of Heart Disease. New York, Raven Press, p 364, 1982.)

played a role in the recommendation of a chest compression rate of 80 to 100 compressions per minute.[2]

Physiologists and physicians alike have assumed that external chest compression created temporary circulation by compressing the heart in much the same manner as open chest internal cardiac massage. It was assumed that during sternal compression there was cardiac compression and that blood moved from the left ventricle into the aorta as closure of the mitral valve prevented retrograde blood flow. This widely held concept was challenged during the late 1970s by Weisfeldt and associates.[67–71] These investigators from Johns Hopkins University thought that this concept was inconsistent with a number of observations. They noted that when sternal compression was performed in a patient with a flail chest no arterial blood pressure was recorded until the remainder of the chest was bound to prevent paradoxical expansion.[67, 69] Their second clinical observation was that patients with chronic obstructive pulmonary disease, a marked increase in anteroposterior chest diameter, and a relatively small heart could be resuscitated by sternal compression.[67, 69] The third observation was that during conventional CPR the compression cycle that followed ventilation often resulted in increased blood pressure and carotid blood flow.[67, 69] Weisfeldt's group extended these observations by maintaining airway pressure with a bag-mask device and noted that this technique increased radial artery pressure during external chest compression.[67] These findings suggested that forward blood flow was related to an increase in intrathoracic pressure. This theory was supported by the studies of Criley and associates on "cough CPR."[72, 73]

Cough CPR is accomplished by having the patient with recent-onset asystole or ventricular fibrillation cough forcefully about every second.[72, 73] The obvious disadvantage of this technique is that it must be initiated before the patient loses consciousness. Forceful cough results in an abrupt increase in intrathoracic pressures, which can result in striking aortic systolic pressures (Fig. 11–4). By employing cough CPR in the cardiac catheterization laboratory, Criley and associates have had patients sustain consciousness for up to 40 seconds after the onset of ventricular fibrillation.[72, 73] Cough CPR has several advantages. It enables laboratory personnel to turn their full attention to preparing for and using the defibrillator rather than performing cardiac massage; it can be performed by a patient in any position and on any surface, including the lateral position of the angiographic cradle; it avoids the hazards of fracture; and ventilation also occurs spontaneously.[72, 73] The potential for using

cough CPR in areas other than the cardiac catheterization laboratory has failed to meet initial expectations. Cough has been used not only for resuscitation but also for termination of ventricular tachycardia.[74]

Another important observation was the rediscovery that the pressures in the aorta and right atrium were often similar during external sternal compression. This observation had been reported by Weale and Rothwell-Jackson in 1962 but had received little attention.[75] Weisfeldt and associates found that during chest compression not only were the central venous and aortic pressures similar, but also the pressures in all cardiac chambers and the intrapleural pressure were nearly equal. In the fluid-filled system of the heart and great vessels there must be a pressure gradient across a resistance for the production of flow. When the heart is pumping normally, there is a large pressure gradient between the aorta and the right atrium and central veins. The lack of a gradient during external chest compression suggested that the heart was not functioning as a pump, but rather the entire thorax was the "pump."[67, 69]

In contrast to the similar pressures found inside the thorax, Weisfeldt and associates found a significant pressure difference between the extrathoracic carotid artery and the jugular veins. This pressure gradient was thought to be responsible for producing cerebral blood flow. The reason for the pressure difference between the intrathoracic and extrathoracic veins was initially not clear.[69] At the same time, Criley and coworkers demonstrated that the jugular venous valves were operative during coughing.[76] This observation led to a renewed appreciation of the internal jugular valves that were well described by early anatomists.[77] Figure 11–5 illustrates how the thorax, in conjunction with these jugular venous valves, produces pressure gradients such that the thorax acts as the pump.

Further support for the theory that increasing intrathoracic pressure was the driving force for the forward blood flow during external chest compression came from echocardiographic studies during cardiopulmonary resuscitation.[78, 79] Two different two-dimensional echocardiographic studies during cardiopulmonary resuscitation in humans showed that the mitral valve did not close and that the left ventricular internal diameter was constant.[78, 79] These findings supported the observation that in some patients increased intrathoracic pressure and not cardiac compression accounted for the forward blood flow during external chest compression.

Cardiac compression does occur in some humans.[67] In a few of the patients studied by the Johns Hopkins group,

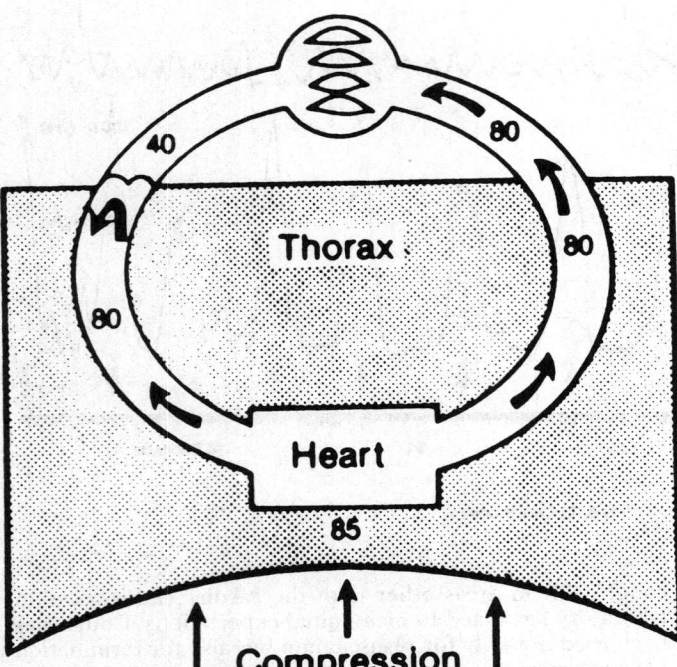

Figure 11-5. Schematic representation of the thoracic pump mechanism for blood flow production during CPR. A gradient across the central nervous system capillary bed is produced by the presence of venous valves in the internal jugular system. (From Ewy GA, Bressler R: Cardiovascular Drugs and the Management of Heart Disease. New York, Raven Press, p 358, 1982.)

simultaneous central venous pressures were lower than arterial pressures during external chest compression, indicating cardiac compression.[67] It is of interest that in patients in whom cardiac compression is present the arterial pressure generated is generally higher than that found in patients without cardiac compression (Fitzgerald KR, Babbs CF, Frissors HA, personal communication).

If in most patients blood flow during external chest compression depends on increased intrathoracic pressure, the question that logically follows is whether alternative techniques to conventional CPR could enhance blood flow during external chest compression. Accordingly, the group from Johns Hopkins explored two basic strategies: simultaneous chest compression and ventilation and abdominal binding.[69] Although increased intrathoracic pressure could be obtained by clamping the endotracheal tube during chest compression, the initial increase in pressure and flow dissipated rapidly, undoubtedly because venous return is inhibited by the continuous high intrathoracic pressure.[67] The Johns Hopkins group then reported that maintaining inflated lungs during external chest compression resulted in significant increases in arterial pressure and carotid flow over those observed with conventional CPR.[69] These results have been confirmed by other investigators using simultaneous high-pressure ventilation and chest compression in large[80] but not small[80, 81] dogs. In small dogs, true cardiac compression evidently occurs with relatively good blood pressure and flow, and the addition of simultaneous high-pressure ventilation does not appear to improve these hemodynamics.[82] In large animals, in which cardiac compression plays a small role, the addition of simultaneous ventilation improves peripheral circulation.[81]

The second approach to augmenting blood flow during CPR was abdominal binding. Redding was the first to show that abdominal binding during CPR improves survival as well as hemodynamics.[82] However, further investigation of this technique was interrupted by studies that reported a high incidence of liver laceration secondary to abdominal binding.[83] Studies that applied abdominal binding using military antishock trousers during CPR also revealed a high incidence of liver laceration and exsanguination.[84]

The ultimate utility of simultaneous high-pressure ventilation or abdominal binding would be determined by whether these interventions resulted in an increase in survival. In an effort to answer this question, an experimental form of CPR that involved high-pressure (60 torr) ventilation, chest compression with a broad flat surface, and abdominal binding (60 torr) was compared with standard CPR in our laboratory. Standard or experimental CPR was performed during ventricular fibrillation.[85] Five of the six animals that underwent standard CPR had a return of blood pressure and survived, whereas none of the six animals that underwent simultaneous high-pressure ventilation, diffuse chest compression, and abdominal pressure had a return of blood pressure after defibrillation and none could be resuscitated despite intensive efforts.[85] A clinical trial of simultaneous compression-ventilation CPR was also performed. A total of 994 patients were enrolled in a field trial in which ambulance crews were randomly assigned to use simultaneous compression-ventilation CPR or conventional CPR procedures in the prehospital setting. Survival to hospital admission and to discharge was greater in the conventional CPR group than in the experimental group ($P < .01$). In a subset of adult patients whose causes of arrest were nontraumatic, survivor rates still favored the conventional CPR group, with 34% of 337 versus 23% of 365 surviving ($P < .001$). It was concluded that survival in the simultaneous compression-ventilation CPR group was lower, probably reflecting a deleterious effect of the experimental technique of resuscitation.[86] The results of these studies showed that simultaneous chest compression and ventilation did not improve survival, and this technique is therefore not recommended.

In contrast to the "thoracic pump" mechanism of blood flow during CPR, Rankin and associates were convinced from their clinical experience that higher chest compression rates were more effective and that cardiac compression was the mechanism of blood flow during CPR. Maier, Rankin, and associates from Duke University studied the effects of varying the manual compression rate, force, and duration in large, chronically instrumented dogs.[65, 66] They reported that the relative contributions of the thoracic pump and direct cardiac compression mechanisms to blood flow varied with the method of CPR being performed.[65, 66] Direct cardiac compression seemed to be more significant during high-impulse (increased-frequency) CPR, and the thoracic pump mechanism was predominant during low-momentum compression techniques. Echocardiographic studies by Deshmukh and associates[87, 88] in anesthetized minipigs demonstrated cardiac valve motion and a change in left ventricular dimensions during the early phases of closed chest CPR, adding further support for direct cardiac compression as the mechanism of blood flow during CPR. Transesophageal echocardiography in an experimental cardiac arrest model[89] and in clinical cardiac arrest[90] has also shown left ventricular compression and competent mitral valve function.

As in the case of most disagreements, there is probably truth on both sides. It is our conclusion that the mechanism of blood flow during CPR can be cardiac and vascular compression or thoracic pump or a combination of both. Open chest cardiac massage and high-impulse, closed chest compression in small subjects produce blood flow predominantly by cardiac and vascular compression. Cough and vest forms of CPR produce little thoracic compression but pro-

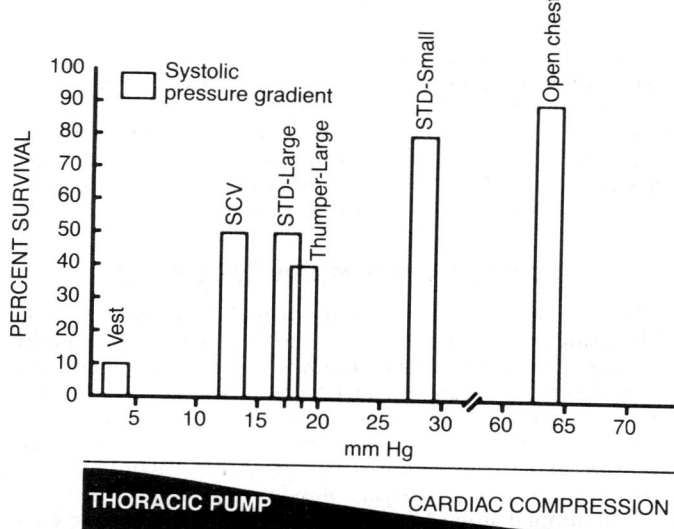

Figure 11–6. Relationship among the systolic or peak pressure gradient between cardiac chambers, mechanism of blood flow during CPR, and 24-hour survival after cardiac arrest. (From Raessler KL, Kern KB, Sanders AB, et al: Aortic and right atrial systolic pressures during cardiopulmonary resuscitation: A potential indicator of the mechanism of blood flow. Am Heart J 115:1021, 1988.)

duce large fluctuations in intrathoracic pressure and hence produce blood flow via the thoracic pump mechanism.

Our conclusion is based on the following observations. In patients with sinus rhythm and subjects in cardiac arrest who are undergoing open chest cardiac compression, there is a large difference between the aortic and right atrial systolic pressures. In contrast, there appears to be little or no difference in systolic pressure between the aorta and the right atrium in subjects in whom blood moves by the thoracic pump mechanism during CPR. Because of this observation, we evaluated the absolute difference between aortic and right atrial systolic pressure (which we call the systolic pressure gradient) in 63 adult mongrel dogs undergoing five types of CPR.[91] After 3 minutes of "downtime" during which no CPR was performed, the animals were ventilated and one of five methods of CPR was initiated. Systolic pressure gradients were measured after 1, 7, and 17 minutes of CPR. The systolic pressure gradient was greatest during open chest cardiac massage (true cardiac compression), intermediate with external mechanical (thumper) and standard CPR, and lowest with CPR performed with a combined thoracic and abdominal vest apparatus (predominantly thoracic pump).[91] The findings are shown in Figure 11–6. It was also noted that 24-hour survival was greatest in the groups treated with cardiac compression and least in those treated with the thoracic pump mechanism.[91] The latter observation is of interest in light of the report by Deshmukh and associates concerning a two-dimensional echocardiographic study of eight minipigs.[87, 88] The aortic and mitral valves demonstrated appropriate systolic and diastolic behavior for the first 5 minutes of CPR in all animals. In the three minipigs that were successfully resuscitated, this valve competence continued for 12 minutes.[87, 88]

We concluded that the mechanism of blood flow during CPR varies according to the technique employed; cardiac and vascular compression is greatest with the open chest technique and high-impulse CPR and lowest with vest CPR. The mechanism also varies with the duration of CPR. Cardiac compression predominates as the mechanism early in CPR, and the thoracic pump mechanism seems to predom-

inate later. The initial human studies performed during CPR at Johns Hopkins and during echocardiography[69, 78, 79] were in fact performed late in the resuscitation effort. Therefore, by the time these measurements were made, the thoracic pump mechanism was predominant. The third determinant of blood flow during closed chest CPR is the anatomic makeup of the subject. Patients with narrow anteroposterior chest diameters and large hearts have more cardiac compression than do emphysematous patients with large anteroposterior chest diameters and small hearts. In summary, the mechanism of blood flow during closed chest CPR depends on the anatomy and pathology of the patient, the duration of CPR, and the technique used. We continue to recommend a compression rate of at least 100 per minute with a 50% compression/50% relaxation ratio.

IMPORTANCE OF MYOCARDIAL PERFUSION PRESSURE

Myocardial perfusion pressure during CPR is defined as the aortic diastolic pressure minus the right atrial diastolic pressure. This pressure gradient correlates well with myocardial blood flow produced in experimental models of CPR.[92–94] Both myocardial perfusion pressure and myocardial blood flow correlate with resuscitation success. Myocardial perfusion pressure has also been correlated not only with initial resuscitation but also with 24-hour survival after CPR.[95]

Myocardial perfusion pressure has been measured in several clinical human series. Because of the requirement of invasive catheterization with catheters placed in the aorta and the right atrium, this hemodynamic parameter is not easy to obtain in the clinical setting. There have been reports of more than 150 patients who have had this gradient measured during CPR.[96–104]

Unfortunately, so much time is required to insert the catheters that when insertion is complete many subjects are well beyond the usual time period when resuscitation success can be expected. What is needed is a simple, rapid, and preferably noninvasive measure of the effectiveness of CPR. Such a measure could then be applied early in the resuscitation effort.

The monitoring of end-tidal carbon dioxide during CPR is one such possibility. This is a noninvasive technique whereby the partial pressure of carbon dioxide is measured from the endotracheal tube at the end of expiration during the performance of CPR. Laboratory studies have shown excellent correlations between end-tidal carbon dioxide and cardiac output, coronary perfusion pressure, and resuscitation success.[105–109]

The utility of monitoring end-tidal carbon dioxide in humans has also been investigated.[110–113] Garnett and coworkers, studying 28 patients undergoing CPR after out-of-hospital cardiac arrest, found that immediately on successful restoration of effective circulation, end-tidal carbon dioxide levels rapidly increased.[111] Falk and coworkers, from the University of Chicago, similarly showed that end-tidal carbon dioxide levels fell rapidly with cardiac arrest and rose on restoration of effective circulation.[112] To determine whether end-tidal carbon dioxide monitoring during CPR could be used as a prognostic indicator of resuscitation and survival in patients, we performed a prospective study of 34 hospitalized patients suffering 35 cardiac arrests.[113] All adult patients seen at our hospital over the period of a year were eligible for the study. Patients were excluded from this trial if they had traumatic cardiac arrest. We equipped the standard cardiac arrest cart with an infrared capnometer. The sensor was placed at the external end of the endotracheal tube when the patient was intubated. End-tidal carbon

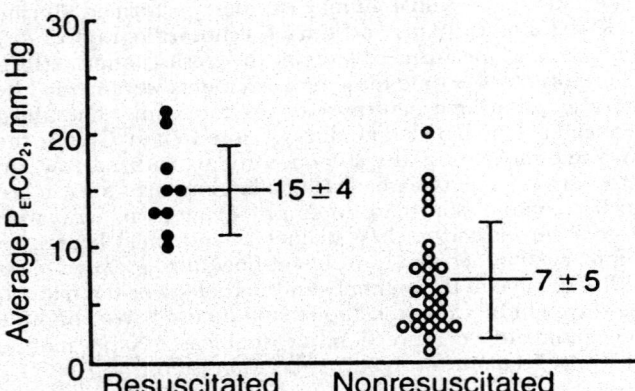

Figure 11–7. Average end-tidal partial pressures of carbon dioxide during CPR in 34 inpatients suffering cardiac arrest. The patients who were eventually resuscitated had a significantly higher mean average end-tidal carbon dioxide level. No patient with an end-tidal carbon dioxide level of less than 10 torr (10 mm Hg) during CPR was resuscitated. (From Sanders AB, Kern KB, Otto CW, et al: End-tidal carbon dioxide monitoring during cardiopulmonary resuscitation. JAMA 262:1347, 1989. Copyright 1989, American Medical Association.)

dioxide values were measured for each patient and categorized as initial, maximal, minimal, final, and average. Carbon dioxide values obtained within the first 5 minutes after bicarbonate administration were excluded from analysis. The 9 patients who were successfully resuscitated from cardiac arrest had significantly greater expired end-tidal carbon dioxide values than the 26 patients who could not be resuscitated. This held for all values, including average, initial, final, maximal, and minimal values. No patient with an end-tidal carbon dioxide pressure of less than 10 torr was resuscitated (Fig. 11–7). This identified a subgroup of patients who, with continued unchanged efforts of CPR, will expire. Although the numbers were small, end-tidal carbon dioxide values were also able to differentiate between patients who were resuscitated but subsequently died and those who survived to leave the hospital. These findings suggest that end-tidal carbon dioxide levels can be used as a prognostic guide during the performance of CPR. More important, monitoring end-tidal carbon dioxide during CPR can be a noninvasive method for determining the quality of CPR and thereby telling whether alterations in resuscitative technique or adjunctive therapy are necessary. Such a prognostic indicator may allow a more rational approach to the treatment of individual patients with cardiac arrest.

FUTURE DIRECTIONS IN ADJUNCTIVE THERAPY

Appropriate drug therapy can increase the effectiveness of CPR. The objectives of drug therapy during CPR are to augment arterial blood pressure and thereby blood flow, to improve the metabolic milieu associated with cardiac arrest, and to stabilize the cardiac rhythm.

An important aspect of advanced cardiac life support is the establishment of intravenous access for drug administration.[21] However, because of effective alternative routes, administration of critically important drugs should not be delayed for placement of an intravenous line. When peripheral injection sites are used, large volumes of flushing solution should be used to ensure more rapid and complete delivery of the drug into the central circulation. Caution is appropriate in avoiding distal veins in the hands, wrists, and feet because of the marked diminution of peripheral blood flow during CPR.[114] Intracardiac injections are feasible but

are not routinely performed because of potential complications.

The endotracheal tube provides an alternative route for drug administration in cardiac emergencies.[115–119] Epinephrine given endotracheally is rapidly absorbed, with peak blood concentrations occurring within 15 seconds. Drugs that have been shown to be well absorbed via the endotracheal route include atropine, lidocaine,[120] propranolol,[121] naloxone, and diazepam (for status epilepticus).[122]

Drugs for Cardiopulmonary Resuscitation

No drug has proved as useful during CPR as epinephrine. The primary benefit of epinephrine during CPR is its ability to cause alpha-adrenergic receptor stimulation, producing vasoconstriction. Through such vasoconstriction, particularly of the peripheral vasculature, central aortic diastolic and coronary perfusion pressures rise. Increasing the aortic diastolic and coronary perfusion pressures during CPR results in improved myocardial blood flow and survival.[92, 93]

The optimal alpha-adrenergic agonist for use during CPR is unknown. Theoretically, pure alpha-agonists may have several advantages. Pure alpha-agonists stimulate myocardial oxygen consumption less than agonists with beta-adrenergic properties.[123, 124] To date, no pure alpha-adrenergic agonist has yet been shown to be superior to epinephrine in restoring spontaneous circulation or in terms of neurologic benefit after treatment of cardiac arrest.[125, 126]

The optimal dosing regimen for adrenergic agonists during CPR remains elusive. The American Heart Association standards and guidelines state that 0.5 to 1.0 mg of epinephrine should be given every 5 minutes during the performance of CPR.[114] Work by Brown and coworkers has shown that this dose, which extrapolates to approximately 0.02 mg/kg, has little effect on hemodynamics or blood flow during resuscitation efforts.[127, 128] However, a dose of 0.2 mg/kg is quite effective in raising aortic pressure, coronary perfusion pressure, and regional myocardial and cerebral blood flow during CPR. Several anecdotal reports and one clinical series have appeared that both advocate and denounce high-dose epinephrine therapy in the treatment of cardiac arrest.[129–132]

Two drugs, sodium bicarbonate and calcium chloride, are often used in excess during CPR. Investigation has shown that sodium bicarbonate given alone during CPR does not promote return of cardiac contractility.[133] In fact, accurate correction of metabolic acidosis is often not feasible until cardiac resuscitation had been successful and improved tissue perfusion has mobilized the acid metabolites sequestered in the tissues. Administration of bicarbonate has not potentiated the effect of suboptimal doses of epinephrine, whereas epinephrine was found to be effective in raising perfusion pressures even in the presence of severe metabolic acidosis.[133]

The benefit of calcium in improving the outcome of cardiac arrest has been even harder to verify. Without question, calcium can be a lifesaving drug in some patients with cardiac arrest, particularly those with hyperkalemia. However, no evidence exists that calcium is effective in asystole or electromechanical dissociation. The most recent guidelines state, "Thus, except when hyperkalemia, hypocalcemia (e.g., after multiple blood transfusions), or calcium channel blockade toxicity is present, calcium should not be employed."[2]

Lidocaine and bretylium have been used in cardiac arrest treatment protocols for several years. Lidocaine increases the ventricular fibrillation threshold and reverses the fall in this threshold associated with myocardial ischemia. Bretylium also increases the ventricular fibrillation threshold, especially during acute ischemia. A number of clinical trials have compared lidocaine and bretylium during cardiac arrest. Harrison reported no difference in the rate of successful defibrillation in a nonrandomized, retrospective study.[134] Haynes and associates performed a randomized, controlled trial of bretylium and lidocaine therapy in out-of-hospital ventricular fibrillation.[135] No difference in either successful defibrillation or resuscitation was seen among the 146 study patients.

Noting the hemodynamic advantages of lidocaine (less hypotension), the American Heart Association standards and guidelines recommended that lidocaine be used as the drug of first choice for the treatment of ventricular arrhythmias associated with cardiac arrest, including ventricular fibrillation.

Atropine is often used during bradycardiac-asystolic cardiac arrest. Its utility in hemodynamically compromising sinus bradycardia and atrioventricular nodal block is well established. Atropine's effectiveness in infranodal block or asystole is much less certain. Several clinical trials have failed to show a significant effect of atropine's use in successfully treating asystolic cardiac arrest.[136, 137] The key to success in all forms of cardiac arrest is early restoration of adequate myocardial and cerebral blood flow. Current schemes for treatment of asystolic-bradycardiac arrests emphasize the use of epinephrine both for peripheral vasoconstriction (raising perfusion pressures to the myocardium and cerebrum) and for its chronotropic effect.

Alternative Compression Techniques

In an attempt to improve on the current success rate with standard CPR, a number of alternative methods have been suggested. After the discovery of cough CPR circulatory support, efforts were made to produce chest compression techniques that would optimize intrathoracic pressure changes.

The first technique employed was that of simultaneous compression and ventilation CPR, which was developed through the efforts of Criley in Los Angeles and Weisfeldt in Baltimore. Experimental evidence was found for increased carotid blood flow with this "new" form of CPR.[68–70] This was interpreted as indicating a distinct advantage of this form of chest compression. However, further work in animals and people has shown that increased carotid flow does not equate with improved survival.[85, 86, 138]

Other adjunctive forms of chest compression include vest CPR. In animal models, vest CPR has been shown to improve 24-hour survival[139, 140] (Table 11–2); however, in other experimental studies such encouraging results could not be confirmed.[138] In a clinical trial measuring hemodynamics during CPR in humans, Swenson and colleagues found no particular benefit of pneumatic vest CPR, with or without simultaneous ventilation and abdominal binding, compared with standard manual forms of CPR.[101]

Two other alternative forms of CPR, interposed abdominal compression CPR and rapid manual CPR, have been examined. Interposed abdominal compression has not been shown to be superior to standard conventional chest compression in experimental models,[141] but it continues to find some clinical interest.[142] Rapid manual CPR (in which manual chest compressions are performed at 100 to 120/min in lieu of the standard 60 to 80) has been shown in experimental models to improve both myocardial perfusion and 24-hour survival[143] (Fig. 11–8). Further investigations of all of these alternative compression techniques continue.

Invasive Cardiopulmonary Resuscitation

Approximately three decades ago open chest cardiac massage was replaced with closed chest compression and external

TABLE 11–2

SUMMARY OF FINDINGS ON SURVIVAL AND TRAUMA WITH MANUAL AND VEST CARDIOPULMONARY RESUSCITATION*

CPR	Survival		Severe Trauma†	
	Yes	No	Yes	No
Vest	7	0	0	7
CF manual	1	6‖	2	5
HF manual	3	4§	4	3§
CF + HF manual	4	10‖	6	8¶

*Values are numbers of dogs. CF = conventional force; HF = high force; CF + HF = combined conventional force and high force.
†Severe trauma consisted of liver laceration with hemoperitoneum or flail chest.
§$P < .04$ vs. vest.
‖$P < .003$ vs. vest.
¶$P = .055$ vs. vest.
From Halperin HR, Guerci AD, Chandra N, et al: Vest inflation without simultaneous ventilation during cardiac arrest in dogs: Improved survival from prolonged cardiopulmonary resuscitation. Circulation 74:1407, 1986.

defibrillation as the principal treatment for cardiac arrest. The current American Heart Association standards and guidelines for advanced cardiac life support recognize that direct cardiac massage often provides better hemodynamics than closed chest compression.

Several investigators have shown improvements in cardiac output with open chest techniques compared with closed chest compression. Weiser and associates found that open chest CPR produced three times the cardiac output achieved with closed chest CPR.[144] In one of the few human clinical trials, Del Guercio and coworkers found that open chest cardiac massage doubled the cardiac index achieved with closed chest resuscitation.[145] Others have likewise shown direct hemodynamic benefits from the use of internal cardiac massage, including significant rises in aortic mean pressure, aortic diastolic pressures, cerebral perfusion pressure, and coronary perfusion pressure.[146] More important, open chest cardiac massage has been shown experimentally to improve not only hemodynamics but also resuscitation success.[147]

If open chest cardiac massage can produce superior hemodynamics, cardiac output, cerebral perfusion, myocardial perfusion, and myocardial blood flow with resulting improvement in resuscitation success, when should such a technique be employed? Specifically, when should open chest cardiac massage be entertained as an alternative to a failed closed chest compression effort? Before open chest compression is used, "ineffective closed chest compression" must be defined. Once closed chest compression has been determined to be ineffective or to have failed, when should open chest cardiac massage be started? If efforts at closed resuscitation persist too long, it is predictable that open chest massage will also fail. To address these questions we performed a series of experiments in our laboratory to determine whether the time to initiation of open chest massage after closed chest compression influenced resuscitation success.[148]

We found that open chest massage improves hemodynamics when it is instituted as late as 30 minutes after the institution of closed chest compressions, but it improves initial resuscitation success only when applied early, that is, within 15 to 20 minutes of the onset of cardiac arrest and ineffective closed chest compressions. Improving perfusion pressures after a lengthy period of poor blood flow may be ineffective in reversing the myocardial damage resulting from prolonged global ischemia. Open chest cardiac massage can be strikingly effective in improving resuscitation if efforts at ineffective closed chest compression are not continued for lengthy periods.

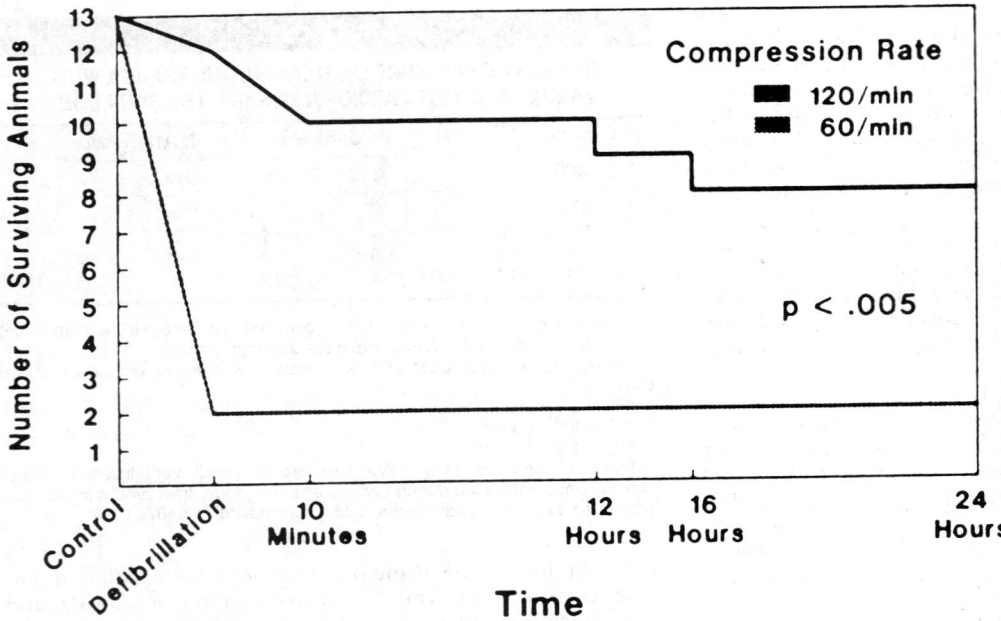

Figure 11–8. Improved 24-hour survival with rapid manual (120 compressions per minute) CPR. (From Feneley MP, Maier GW, Kern KB, et al: Influence of compression rate on initial success of resuscitation and 24 hour survival after prolonged manual cardiopulmonary resuscitation in dogs. Circulation 77:240, 1988.)

In spite of some enthusiasm for open chest cardiac massage, some precautions must be emphasized. In one of the few clinical trials of open chest massage, results similar to those of our experimental work have been found.[149] Open chest CPR is not successful if it is instituted after 30 minutes of cardiac arrest and closed chest compression efforts. Before embracing this invasive form of therapy, additional information is needed concerning the role of open chest massage after various downtimes of untreated arrest. Examining this question, we have found that open chest cardiac massage, when instituted after 20 minutes of untreated ventricular fibrillation, is capable of improving hemodynamics to a degree similar to that seen with open chest resuscitation efforts after ineffective closed chest compression. After 20 minutes of untreated ventricular fibrillation, initial resuscitation results are significantly better with open chest techniques than with closed chest efforts, but morbidity is high and results in a high 24-hour mortality. If long-term survival is to be improved, the maximal period of untreated cardiac arrest that can be successfully treated by open chest cardiac massage appears to be 10 to 15 minutes.

Finally, the last remaining key appears to be a technique that can realistically assess the time of total cardiac arrest (including downtime) or that can assess the prognosis with ongoing resuscitation efforts. Increasing evidence indicates that monitoring end-tidal expired carbon dioxide levels during cardiopulmonary resuscitation may be able to provide this important information. We are hopeful that routine monitoring of expired end-tidal carbon dioxide during cardiac arrest therapy will enable us to better identify the subgroup of patients who are doomed to die with standard closed chest procedures. If the technology is confirmed, this should enable the identification of a subpopulation of cardiac arrest victims who do not respond to current standard therapy and who are good candidates for more aggressive invasive procedures.

RESUSCITATION RESULTS

Numerous studies have been performed to assess the overall outcome of CPR in community programs. Perhaps the most meaningful data come from the Seattle area.

Eisenberg and associates have shown a direct relationship among the response time, the time to initiation of CPR, and the time to definitive care and outcome results. The sooner CPR is begun and the sooner defibrillation is attempted, the higher the survival rate in cardiac arrest.[7] Weaver and colleagues, also of Seattle, have shown that early defibrillation improves not only survival but also neurologic recovery.[150]

Survival after CPR in the hospital has also been carefully examined. Bedell and colleagues have shown that the results of inpatient cardiac arrest treatment are directly related to the time needed for such resuscitation efforts.[151] In their study in Boston, they found that the mortality was 66% in patients whose cardiac arrests lasted fewer than 15 minutes. Patients whose arrests lasted from 15 to 30 minutes had a 95% mortality rate. Patients whose arrests lasted more than 30 minutes had 100% mortality.

Several studies have examined whether the elderly are reasonable candidates for CPR therapy. Tresch and colleagues reported on 214 consecutive cardiac arrest patients who were divided into two age groups, those older than 70 and those younger than 70.[152] The hospital course of the patients was then reviewed retrospectively. They concluded that resuscitation of elderly patients in whom out-of-hospital cardiac arrest occurs is reasonable and appropriate. They found that hospital deaths were more common in the elderly, 71% versus 53%, but that the length of hospitalization and stay in intensive care units was not significantly different for the two age groups. The neurologic outcomes were also similar, in terms of both residual neurologic impairment and neurologic deaths. They concluded that, although elderly patients are more likely than younger patients to die during hospitalization after out-of-hospital cardiac arrest, the hospital stay for the elderly is not longer and the neurologic impairment is not greater than for a similar cohort of younger victims of cardiac arrest. In contrast, Murphy and colleagues from Boston reported on 500 consecutive patients over the age of 70 who had received CPR.[153] They found that though initial resuscitation was 22%, only 4% survived to be discharged from the hospital. The poorest outcomes were those of patients with unwitnessed arrest or terminal arrhythmias, such as asystole or electromechanical disassociations. They concluded that CPR in elderly patients is rarely effective, particularly for those with out-of-hospital, unwitnessed, or associated asystolic or electromechanical disassociation cardiac arrest. It is apparent that this issue is not yet completely resolved, but certainly at the present time it seems unreasonable to deny an elderly patient the chance of possible resuscitation by withholding such therapy.

CONCLUSIONS

Sudden cardiac death and the need for CPR remain prominent problems. Advances have been made over the past several decades. The advent of early defibrillation has had the most profound effect on long-term outcome. In spite of the continued controversy about the mechanism of blood flow generation during CPR, it is now apparent that myocardial perfusion pressure is of paramount importance for success. A noninvasive measure of the perfusion pressure gradient appears to be obtained by monitoring end-tidal carbon dioxide production during the performance of CPR. It is hoped that future studies will validate the usefulness of this parameter, not only for prognostication but also for alteration of ongoing resuscitation efforts to the benefit of the individual patient.

References

1. 1988 Heart Facts. Dallas, American Heart Association, 1988.
2. Standards and guidelines for cardiopulmonary resuscitation and emergency cardiac care. JAMA 255:2908, 1986.
3. Julian DG: Toward preventing coronary death from ventricular fibrillation. Circulation 54:370, 1976.
4. Eisenberg MS, Copass MK, Hallstrom, AP et al: Treatment of out-of-hospital cardiac arrests with rapid defibrillation by emergency medical technicians. N Engl J Med 302:1379, 1980.
5. Hossack KF, Hartwig R: Cardiac arrest associated with supervised cardiac rehabilitation. J Cardiac Rehabil 2:402, 1982.
6. Cobb LA, Hallstrom AP: Community based cardiopulmonary resuscitation: What have we learned? Ann NY Acad Sci 382:330, 1982.
7. Eisenberg MS, Bergner L, Hallstrom AP: Cardiac resuscitation in the community: Importance of rapid provision and implications for program planning. JAMA 241:1905, 1979.
8. Stults KR, Brown DD, Schug VL, et al: Pre-hospital defibrillation performed by emergency medical technicians in rural communities. N Engl J Med 310:219, 1984.
9. Rozkovec A, Crossley J, Walesby R, et al: Safety and effectiveness of a portable external automatic defibrillator-pacemaker. Clin Cardiol 6:527, 1983.
10. Weaver WD, Copass MK, Cobb LA, et al: A new, compact, automatic external defibrillator designed for layperson use (abstract). J Am Coll Cardiol 5:457, 1985.
11. Eisenberg MS, Cummins RO: Defibrillation performed by the emergency medical technician. Circulation 74(suppl IV):9, 1986.
12. Stults KR, Brown DD: Special considerations for defibrillation performed by emergency medical technicians in small communities. Circulation 74(suppl IV):13, 1986.
13. Weaver WD, Sutherland K, Wirkus MI, et al: Emergency medical care requirements for large public assemblies and a new strategy for managing cardiac arrest in this setting. Ann Emerg Med 18:155, 1989.
14. Mirowski M, Reid PR, Mower MM, et al: Termination of malignant ventricular arrhythmias with an implanted automatic defibrillator in human beings. N Engl J Med 303:322, 1980.
15. Echt DS, Armstrong K, Schmidt P, et al: Clinical experience, complications, and survival in 70 patients with the automatic implantable cardioverter/defibrillator. Circulation 71:289, 1985.
16. Ewy GA, Tacker WA, Jr: Transchest electrical ventricular defibrillation. Am Heart J 91:403, 1976.
17. Garrey WE: The nature of fibrillatory contractions of the heart and its relation to tissue mass and form. Am J Physiol 33:397, 1914.
18. Zipes DP, Fisher J, King RM, et al: Termination of ventricular fibrillation in dogs by depolarizing a critical amount of myocardium. Am J Cardiol 36:37, 1975.
19. Geddes LA, Tacker WA, Rosborough JP, et al: Electrical dose for ventricular defibrillation of large and small animals using precordial electrodes. J Clin Invest 53:310, 1974.
20. Gutgesell HP, Tacker WA, Geddes LA, et al: Energy dose for defibrillation in children. Pediatrics 58:898, 1976.
21. Dahl CF, Ewy GA, Warner ED, et al: Myocardial necrosis from direct current countershock. Circulation 50:956, 1974.
22. Warner ED, Dahl CF, Ewy GA: Myocardial injury from transthoracic defibrillator countershock. Arch Pathol 99:55, 1975.
23. Pantridge JR, Adgey AAJ, Webb SW, et al: Electrical requirements for ventricular defibrillation. Br Med J 2:313, 1975.
24. Adgey AA: Electrical energy requirements for ventricular defibrillation. Br Heart J 40:1197, 1978.
25. Crampton JA, Crampton RS, Sipes JN, et al: Energy levels and patient weight in ventricular defibrillation. JAMA 242:1380, 1984.
26. Gascho JA, Crampton RS, Cherwek ML, et al: Determinants of ventricular defibrillation in adults. Circulation 60:231, 1979.
27. Lown B, Crampton RS, DeSilva RA, et al: The energy for ventricular fibrillation—Too little or too much? N Engl J Med 298:1252, 1978.
28. Weaver WD, Cobb LA, Copass MK, et al: Ventricular defibrillation—A comparative trial using 175 J and 320 J shocks. N Engl J Med 307:1101, 1982.
29. Kerber RE, Jensen SR, Gascho JA, et al: Determinants of defibrillation: Prospective analysis of 183 patients. Am J Cardiol 52:739, 1985.
30. Standards and guidelines for cardiopulmonary resuscitation (CPR) and emergency cardiac care (ECC). JAMA 244:453, 1980.
31. Tacker WA, Geddes LA: Electrical Defibrillation. Boca Raton, FL, CRC Press, p 141, 1980.
32. Geddes LA, Tacker WA, Cabler DP, et al: Decrease in transthoracic resistance during successive ventricular defibrillation trials. Med Instrum 9:179, 1975.
33. Dahl CF, Ewy GA, Thomas ED: Transthoracic impedance to direct current discharge: Effect of repeated countershocks. Med Instrum 10:151, 1976.
34. Kerber RE, Grayzel J, Hoyt R, et al: Transthoracic resistance of human defibrillation: Influence of body weight, chest size, serial shocks, paddle size and paddle contact pressure. Circulation 63:676, 1981.
35. Yakaitis RW, Ewy GA, Otto CW, et al: Influence of time and therapy on ventricular defibrillation in dogs. Crit Care Med 8:157, 1980.
36. Ewy GA: Electrical therapy for cardiovascular emergencies. Circulation 74(suppl IV):111, 1986.
37. Ewy GA, Ewy MD, Nuttall AJ, et al: Canine transthoracic resistance. J Appl Physiol 32:91, 1972.
38. Thomas ED, Ewy GA, Dahl CF: Effectiveness of direct current defibrillation: Role of paddle electrode size. Am Heart J 93:463, 1977.
39. Patel AS, Galysh FT: Experimental studies to design safe external pediatric paddles for DC defibrillation. IEEE Trans Biomed Eng 19:228, 1972.
40. Connell PN, Ewy GA, Dahl CF, et al: Transthoracic impedance to defibrillation discharge: Effect of electrode size and electrode chest wall interface. J Electrocardiol 6:313, 1973.
41. Ewy GA, Horan WJ: Effectiveness of direct current defibrillations II. Role of paddle electrode size. Am Heart J 93:674, 1977.
42. Ewy GA, Horan WJ: Disposable defibrillator electrodes. Heart Lung 6:127, 1977.
43. Ewy GA, Taren D: Comparison of paddle electrode pastes used for defibrillation. Heart Lung 6:847, 1977.
44. Ewy GA, Hellman DA, McClung S, et al: Influence of ventilation phase on transthoracic impedance and defibrillation effectiveness. Crit Care Med 3:164, 1980.
45. Ewy GA, Ewy MK, Silverman J: Determinants of human transthoracic resistance to direct current discharge. Circulation 46(suppl II):150, 1972.
46. Kerber RE, Kouba C, Martins J, et al: Advanced prediction of transthoracic impedance in human defibrillation and cardioversion: Importance of impedance in determining the success of low energy shocks. Circulation 70:303, 1984.
47. Levine PA, Barold SS, Fletcher RD, et al: Adverse acute and chronic effects of electrical defibrillation and cardioversion on implanted unipolar cardiac pacing systems. J Am Coll Cardiol 1:1413, 1983.
48. Sanders AB, Kern KB, Otto CW, et al: End-tidal carbon dioxide monitoring during cardiopulmonary resuscitation—A prognostic indicator for survival. JAMA 262:1347, 1989.
49. White BC, Petinga TJ, Hoehner PJ, et al: Incidence, etiology and outcome of pulseless idioventricular rhythm treated with dexamethasone during advanced CPR. JACEP 8:188, 1979.
50. Carlon GC, Howland WS, Kahn RC, et al: Calcium chloride administration in normocalcemic critically ill patients. Crit Care Med 8:209, 1980.
51. Dembo DH: Calcium in advanced life support. Crit Care Med 9:358, 1981.
52. Stueven HA, Thompson BM, Aprahamian C, et al: Use of calcium in prehospital cardiac arrest. Ann Emerg Med 12:136, 1983.
53. Stueven HA, Thompson BM, Aprahamian C, et al: Calcium chloride: Reassessment of use in asystole. Ann Emerg Med 13:820, 1984.
54. Harrison EE, Amey BD: Use of calcium in electromechanical dissociation. Ann Emerg Med 13:844, 1984.
55. Lund I, Skulberg A: Cardiopulmonary resuscitation by lay people. Lancet 2:702, 1976.
56. Copley DP, Mantle JA, Rodgers WJ, et al: Improved outcome for prehospital cardiopulmonary collapse with resuscitation by bystanders. Circulation 56:901, 1977.
57. Roth R, Steward RD, Rogers K, et al: Out-of-hospital cardiac arrest: Factors associated with survival. Ann Emerg Med 13:237, 1984.
58. Kowalski R, Thompson BM, Horwitz L, et al: Bystander CPR in prehospital coarse ventricular fibrillation. Ann Emerg Med 13:1016, 1984.

59. Pionkowski RS, Thompson BM, Gruchow HW, et al: Resuscitation time in ventricular fibrillation—A prognostic indication. Ann Emerg Med 12:733, 1983.

60. Stueven HA, Troiano P, Thompson B, et al: Bystander/first responder CPR: Ten-year experience in a paramedic system (abstract). Ann Emerg Med 14:510, 1985.

61. Thompson BM, Stueven HA, Mateer JR, et al: Comparison of clinical CPR studies done in Milwaukee and elsewhere in the United States. Ann Emerg Med 14:750, 1985.

62. Thompson RG, Hallstrom AP, Cobb LA: Bystander initiated cardiopulmonary resuscitation in the management of ventricular fibrillation. Ann Intern Med 90:737, 1979.

63. Sanders AB, Kern KB, Bragg S, et al: Neurologic benefits from the use of early cardiopulmonary resuscitation. Ann Emerg Med 16:142, 1987.

64. Taylor Gj, Tucker WM, Green HL, et al: Importance of prolonged compression duration during cardiopulmonary resuscitation in man. N Engl J Med 296:1515, 1977.

65. Maier GW, Tyson GS, Olsen CO, et al: The physiology of external cardiac massage. High impulse cardiopulmonary resuscitation. Circulation 70:86, 1984.

66. Maier GW, Tyson GS, Olsen CO, et al: Optimal techniques of external cardiac massage. Surg Forum 33:282, 1982.

67. Weisfeldt MI, Chandra N, Tsitlik JE, et al: New attempts to improve blood flow during CPR. In: Schluger J, Lyon AF (eds): CPR and Emergency Cardiac Care: Looking to the Future. New York, EM Books, p 29, 1980.

68. Chandra N, Rudikoff MT, Tsitlik J, et al: Augmentation of carotid flow during cardiopulmonary resuscitation (CPR) in the dog by simultaneous compression and ventilation with high airway pressure. Am J Cardiol 43:422, 1979.

69. Rudikoff MT, Maughan WL, Effron M, et al: Mechanism of blood flow during cardiopulmonary resuscitation. Circulation 61:345, 1980.

70. Chandra N, Rudikoff MT, Weisfeldt ML: Simultaneous chest compression and ventilation at high airway pressure during cardiopulmonary resuscitation. Lancet 1:175, 1980.

71. Chandra N, Snyder LD, Weisfeldt ML: Abdominal binding during cardiopulmonary resuscitation in man. JAMA 246:351, 1981.

72. Criley JM, Blaufuss AH, Kissel GL: Cough-induced cardiac compression. JAMA 236:1246, 1976.

73. Criley JM: Cough CPR. In: Schluger J, Lyon AF (eds): CPR and Emergency Cardiac Care: Looking to the Future. New York, EM Books, p 47, 1980.

74. Wei JY, Greene HL, Weisfeldt ML: Cough facilitated conversion of ventricular tachycardia. Am J Cardiol 45:174, 1980.

75. Weale FE, Rothwell-Jackson RL: The efficiency of cardiac massage. Lancet 1:1990, 1962.

76. Niemann JT, Garner D, Rosborough JP, et al: The mechanism of blood flow in closed chest cardiopulmonary resuscitation (abstract). Circulation 59(suppl II):74, 1979.

77. Weathersby HT: The valves of the axillary, subclavian, and internal jugular vein (abstract). Anat Rec 124:379, 1956.

78. Werner JA, Greene JL, Janko C, et al: Visualization of cardiac valve motion in man during external chest compression using two-dimensional echocardiography: Implications regarding the mechanism of blood flow. Circulation 63:1417, 1981.

79. Rich S, Wix HL, Shapiro E: Two dimensional echocardiography resuscitation in man. Am J Cardiol 47:398, 1981.

80. Babbs CF, Tacker WA, Paris RJ, et al: Cardiopulmonary resuscitation with simultaneous compression and ventilation at high airway pressure in four animal models. In: Abstracts of the Fourth Purdue Conference on Cardiac Defibrillation and Cardiopulmonary Resuscitation, Purdue University, September 15–17, 1981, p 5.

81. Redding JS, Haynes RR, Thomas JD: "Old" and "new" CPR manually performed in dogs. Crit Care Med 9:386, 1981.

82. Redding JS: Abdominal compressions in cardiopulmonary resuscitation. Anesth Analg 50:668, 1971.

83. Harris LC Jr, Kirimli B, Safar P: Augmentation of artificial circulation during cardiopulmonary resuscitation. Anesthesiology 28:730, 1967.

84. Alifimoff JK, Barnett WM, Safar P, et al: Comparisons of standard cardiopulmonary resuscitation, new CPR, abdominal restraint–Augmented CPR and open-chested CPR. In: Abstracts of the Fourth Purdue Conference on Cardiac Defibrillation and Cardiopulmonary Resuscitation, Purdue University, September 15–17, 1981, p 2.

85. Sanders A, Ewy GA, Alferness C, et al: Failure of one method of simultaneous chest compression, ventilation, and abdominal binding during cardiopulmonary resuscitation. Crit Care Med 10:509, 1982.

86. Krischer JP, Fine EG, Weisfeldt ML, et al: Comparison of prehospital conventional and simultaneous compression-ventilation cardiopulmonary resuscitation. Crit Care Med 17:1263, 1989.

87. Deshmukh HG, Weil MH, Gudipati CV, et al: Blood flow during CPR is maintained by direct cardiac compression (abstract). Clin Res 34:88A, 1986.

88. Deshmukh HG, Weil MH, Rackow EC, et al: Echocardiographic observation during cardiopulmonary resuscitation: A preliminary report. Crit Care Med 13:904, 1985.

89. Feneley MP, Maier GW, Jaynor JW, et al: Sequence of mitral valve motion and transmitral blood flow during manual cardiopulmonary resuscitation in dogs. Circulation 76:363, 1987.

90. Higano ST, Oh JK, Ewy GA, et al: The mechanisms of blood flow during closed chest cardiac massage in humans: Transesophageal echocardiographic observations. Mayo Clin Proc 65:1432, 1990.

91. Raessler KL, Kern KB, Sanders AB, et al: Aortic and right atrial systolic pressures as an indicator of the mechanism of blood flow during CPR. Am Heart J 115:1021, 1988.

92. Ralston SH, Voorhees WD, Babbs CF: Intra-pulmonary epinephrine during prolonged cardiopulmonary resuscitation: Improved regional flow and resuscitation in dogs. Ann Emerg Med 13:79, 1984.

93. Michael JR, Guerci AD, Koehler RC, et al: Mechanisms by which epinephrine augments cerebral and myocardial perfusion during cardiopulmonary resuscitation in dogs. Circulation 69:822, 1984.

94. Kern KB, Lancaster LD, Goldman S, et al: The effect of coronary artery lesions on the relationship between coronary artery perfusion pressure and myocardial blood flow during cardiopulmonary resuscitation in pigs. Am Heart J 120:324, 1990.

95. Kern KB, Ewy GA, Voorhees WD, et al: Myocardial perfusion pressure: A predictor of 24-hour survival during prolonged cardiac arrest in dogs. Resuscitation 16:241, 1988.

96. Sanders AB, Ogle M, Ewy GA: Coronary perfusion pressure during cardiopulmonary resuscitation. Am J Emerg Med 3:11, 1985.

97. McDonald JL: Effect of interposed abdominal compression during CPR on central arterial and venous pressures. Am J Emerg Med 3:156, 1985.

98. Howard MA, Labadie LL, Martin GB, et al: Aortic and right atrial pressures during standard and simultaneous compression and ventilation CPR in human beings. Ann Emerg Med 15:125, 1986.

99. Howard MA, Labadie LL, Martin GB, et al: Improvement in coronary perfusion pressures after open-chest cardiac massage in humans: Preliminary report (abstract). Ann Emerg Med 15:664, 1986.

100. Howard M, Carrubba C, Foss F, et al: Interposed abdominal compression-CPR: Its effects on coronary perfusion in human subjects. Ann Emerg Med 16:253, 1987.

101. Swenson RD, Weaver WD, Niskanen RA, et al: Hemodynamics in humans during conventional and experimental use of cardiopulmonary resuscitation. Circulation 78:630, 1988.

102. Paradis NA, Martin GB, Goetting MG, et al: Simultaneous aortic, jugular bulb and right atrial pressures during cardiopulmonary resuscitation in humans: Insights into mechanisms. Circulation 80:361, 1989.

103. Paradis NA, Martin GB, Rivers EP, et al: High-dose epinephrine and coronary perfusion pressure during cardiac arrest in human beings (abstract). Ann Emerg Med 18:478, 1989.

104. Paradis NA, Martin GB, Rivers EP, et al: Coronary perfusion pressure and the return of spontaneous circulation in human cardiopulmonary resuscitation. JAMA 263:1106, 1990.

105. Weil MH, Bisera J, Trevino RR, et al: Cardiac output and end-tidal carbon dioxide. Crit Care Med 13:907, 1985.

106. Sanders AB, Atlas M, Ewy GA, et al: Expired P_{CO_2} as an index of coronary perfusion pressure. Am J Emerg Med 3:147, 1985.

107. Sanders AB, Ewy GA, Bragg S, et al: Expired P_{CO_2} as a prognostic indicator of successful resuscitation from cardiac arrest. Ann Emerg Med 14:948, 1985.

108. Gudipati CV, Weil MH, Bisera J, et al: Expired carbon dioxide: A noninvasive monitor of cardiopulmonary resuscitation. Circulation 77:234, 1988.

109. Kern KB, Sanders AB, Voorhees WD, et al: Changes in expired end-tidal carbon dioxide during cardiopulmonary resuscitation in dogs: A prognostic guide for resuscitation efforts. J Am Coll Cardiol 13:1184, 1989.

110. Kalenda Z: The capnogram as a guide to the efficacy of cardiac massage. Resuscitation 6:259, 1978.

111. Garnett AR, Ornato JP, Gonzales ER, et al: End-tidal carbon dioxide monitoring during cardiopulmonary resuscitation. JAMA 257:512, 1987.

112. Falk JL, Rackow EC, Weil MH: End-tidal carbon dioxide concentration during cardiopulmonary resuscitation. N Engl J Med 318:607, 1988.

113. Sanders AB, Kern KB, Otto CW, et al: End-tidal carbon dioxide monitoring during cardiopulmonary resuscitation. JAMA 262:1347, 1989.

114. Standards and guidelines for cardiopulmonary resuscitation (CPR) and emergency cardiac care (ECC). JAMA 255:2905, 1986.

115. Redding JS, Asuncion JS, Pearson JW: Effective routes of drug administration during cardiac arrest. Anesth Analg 46:253, 1967.

116. Roberts JR, Greenberg MI, Knaub MA, et al: Blood levels following intravenous and endotracheal epinephrine administration. JACEP 8:53, 1979.

117. Roberts JR, Greenberg MI, Baskin SI, et al: Endotracheal epinephrine in cardiorespiratory collapse. JACEP 8:515, 1979.

118. Greenberg MI, Roberts JR, Baskin SI, et al: Endotracheal naloxone reversal of morphine-induced respiratory depression in rabbits. Ann Emerg Med 9:289, 1980.

119. Greenberg MI, Roberts JR, Krusz JC, et al: Endotracheal epinephrine in a canine anaphylactic shock model. JACEP 8:500, 1979.

120. Ward JT: Endotracheal drug therapy. Am J Emerg Med 1:71, 1983.

121. Scott B, Martin GF, Matchett J, et al: Canine cardiovascular responses to endotracheally and intravenously administered atropine, isoproterenol, and propranolol. Ann Emerg Med 16:1, 1987.

122. Barsan WG, Ward JT, Otten EJ: Blood levels of diazepam after endotracheal administration in dogs. Ann Emerg Med 11:242, 1982.

123. Ditchey RV: High dose epinephrine does not improve the balance between myocardial oxygen supply and demand during cardiopulmonary resuscitation in dogs. J Am Coll Cardiol 3:596, 1984.

124. Linder KH, Ahnefeld FW, Schurmann W, et al: Effects of epinephrine and norepinephrine on myocardial oxygen delivery and consumption during cardiopulmonary resuscitation. Chest 97:1458, 1990.

125. Brillman JC, Sanders AB, Otto CW, et al: Outcome of resuscitation from fibrillatory arrest using epinephrine and phenylephrine in dogs. Crit Care Med 13:912, 1985.

126. Brown CG, Katz SE, Werman HA, et al: The effect of epinephrine versus methoxamine on regional myocardial blood flow and defibrillation rates following a prolonged cardiorespiratory arrest in a swine model. Am J Emerg Med 5:362, 1987.

127. Brown CG, Werman HA, Davis EA, et al: Comparative effect of graded doses of epinephrine on regional brain blood flow during CPR in a swine model. Ann Emerg Med 15:1138, 1986.

128. Brown CG, Taylor RB, Werman HA, et al: Effect of standard doses of epinephrine on myocardial oxygen delivery and utilization during cardiopulmonary resuscitation. Crit Care Med 16:536, 1988.

129. Marwick TH, Siskind V, Case C, et al: Adverse effect of early high-dose adrenaline on outcome of ventricular fibrillation. Lancet 1:66, 1988.

130. Koscove EM, Paradis NA: Successful resuscitation from cardiac arrest using high-dose epinephrine therapy. JAMA 259:3031, 1988.

131. Goetting MG, Paradis NA: High dose epinephrine in refractory pediatric cardiac arrest. Crit Care Med 17:1258, 1989.

132. Gonzalez ER, Ornato JP, Garnett AR, et al: Dose-dependent vasopressor response to epinephrine during CPR in human beings. Ann Emerg Med 18:920, 1989.

133. Bishop RL, Weisfeldt ML: Sodium bicarbonate administration during cardiac arrest. JAMA 235:506, 1976.

134. Harrison EE: Lidocaine in prehospital countershock refractory ventricular fibrillation. Ann Emerg Med 10:420, 1981.

135. Haynes RE, Chinn TL, Copass MK, et al: Comparison of bretylium tosylate and lidocaine in management of out of hospital ventricular fibrillation: A randomized clinical trial. Am J Cardiol 48:353, 1981.

136. Myerburg RJ, Estes D, Zaman L, et al: Outcome of resuscitation from bradyarrhythmic or asystolic prehospital cardiac arrest. J Am Coll Cardiol 4:1118, 1984.

137. Stueven HA, Tonsfeldt DJ, Thompson BM, et al: Atropine in asystole: Human studies. Ann Emerg Med 13:815, 1984.

138. Kern KB, Carter AB, Showen RL, et al: Comparison of mechanical techniques of cardiopulmonary resuscitation: Survival and neurologic outcome in dogs. Am J Emerg Med 5:190, 1987.

139. Niemann JT, Rosborough JP, Niskanen RA, et al: Mechanical "cough" cardiopulmonary resuscitation during cardiac arrest in dogs. Am J Cardiol 55:194, 1985.

140. Halperin HR, Guerci AD, Chandra N, et al: Vest inflation without simultaneous ventilation during cardiac arrest in dogs: Improved survival from prolonged cardiopulmonary resuscitation. Circulation 74:1407, 1986.

141. Kern KB, Carter AB, Showen RL, et al: Twenty-four hour survival in a canine model comparing three methods of manual cardiopulmonary resuscitation. J Am Coll Cardiol 7:859, 1986.

142. Sack JB, Kesselbrenner M, Bregman D: Interposed abdominal couterpulsation (IAC) during human CPR: Initial clinical study (abstract). Circulation 82(suppl III):III-484, 1990.

143. Feneley MP, Maier GW, Kern KB, et al: Influence of compression rate on initial success of resuscitation and 24-hour survival after prolonged manual cardiopulmonary resuscitation in dogs. Circulation 77:240, 1988.

144. Weiser FM, Adler LN, Kuhn LA: Hemodynamic effects of closed and open chest cardiac resuscitation in normal dogs and those with acute myocardial infarction. Am J Cardiol 10:555, 1962.

145. Del Guercio LRM, Feins NR, Cohn JD, et al: Comparison of blood flow during external and internal cardiac massage in man. Circulation 31(suppl I):171, 1965.

146. Byrne D, Pass HI, Neely WA, et al: External versus internal cardiac massage in normal and chronically ischemic dogs. Am Surg 46:657, 1980.

147. Kern KB, Sanders AB, Badylak SF, et al: Long-term survival with open chest cardiac massage after ineffective closed chest compression in a canine preparation. Circulation 75:498, 1987.

148. Sanders AB, Kern KB, Atlas M, et al: Importance of the duration of inadequate coronary perfusion pressure on resuscitation from cardiac arrest. J Am Coll Cardiol 6:113, 1986.

149. Geehr EC, Lewis FR, Auerbach PS: Failure of open heart massage to improve survival after pre-hospital non-traumatic cardiac arrest. N Engl J Med 314:1189, 1986.

150. Weaver WD, Copass MK, Bufi D, et al: Improved neurologic recovery and survival after early defibrillation. Circulation 69:943, 1984.

151. Bedell SE, Delbanco TL, Cook EF, et al: Survival after cardiopulmonary resuscitation in the hospital. N Engl J Med 309:569, 1983.

152. Tresch DD, Thakur RK, Hoffman RG, et al: Should the elderly be resuscitated following out-of-hospital cardiac arrest? Am J Med 86:145, 1989.

153. Murphy DJ, Murray AM, Robinson BE, et al: Outcomes of cardiopulmonary resuscitation in the elderly. Ann Intern Med 111:199, 1989.

CHAPTER 12

Fluid Resuscitation

Brian S. Kaufman

Plasma volume deficits are frequently present in critically ill patients. Untreated, these deficits can contribute to the pathophysiologic derangements that characterize disorders such as hemorrhage, sepsis, pancreatitis, anaphylaxis, and diabetic ketoacidosis. When hypovolemia is severe, tissue oxygenation becomes impaired and the clinical and metabolic features of circulatory shock appear. The need for prompt restoration of adequate plasma volume under such circumstances is well recognized.[1, 2] Few issues in critical care medicine have prompted as much diversity of opinion as the ongoing debate regarding the most appropriate asanguineous fluid to accomplish this goal.[3–5]

This chapter attempts not to end the colloid versus crystalloid controversy but rather to provide the reader with a framework for understanding the issues involved.

FLUID DISTRIBUTION

The total body water content of humans is approximately 60% of body weight and is contained within distinct fluid compartments. Harrison and coworkers calculated that two thirds of total body water is located in the intracellular and one third in the extracellular compartment.[6] The extracellular compartment can be further subdivided into interstitial and intravascular compartments. Usually 75% of the extracellular water is located within the interstitium and 25% is in the vasculature. There are marked differences in electrolyte content between intracellular and extracellular fluids; potassium is predominantly intracellular, and sodium and chloride are the major extracellular ions.[7] An energy-consuming Na^+-K^+ pump is required to maintain this concentration gradient. Distribution of water between the intracellular and extracellular compartments is determined by osmosis.

Cell membranes are normally relatively impermeable to ions but permeable to water. A decrease in extracellular sodium concentration and osmolarity, for example, after infusion of 5% dextrose in water, is followed by diffusion of water into the cells until the osmotic pressure between the two compartments equalizes. Conversely, an increase in extracellular sodium concentration and osmolarity, for instance, after infusion of hypertonic saline, is followed by movement of water from the intracellular to the extracellular compartment. Infusion of an isotonic electrolyte solution does not alter the osmolarity of the extracellular compartment and therefore does not lead to shifts of water into or out of the intracellular compartment.

Water movement between the two components of the extravascular space is determined primarily by differences in protein concentration. Colloid osmotic pressure (COP) is the net osmotic pressure across the capillary membrane resulting from the impermeability of the endothelium to plasma proteins. Because physical confinement of protein molecules produces an osmotic imbalance, water moves from the interstitial space into the blood stream. Crystalloid molecules cannot establish a pressure gradient because they move freely across the capillary membrane (Fig. 12–1).

Protein molecules are negatively charged and attract a

BODY COMPARTMENT FLUID DISTRIBUTION

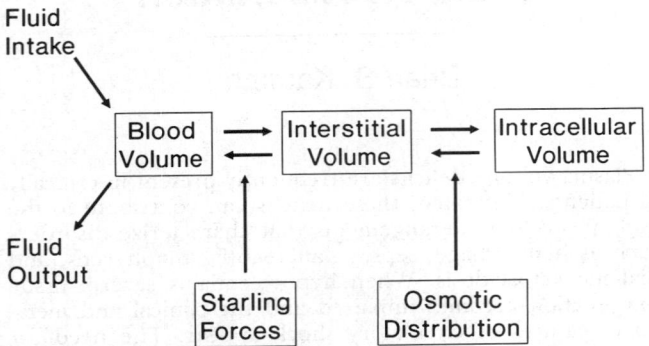

Figure 12–1. Body fluid compartments and the forces that influence fluid distribution between the compartments.

small number of positive ions, preventing them from diffusing across the endothelium. These retained ions produce an additional osmotic pressure (called the Donnan equilibrium effect). Sixty percent of normal COP is produced by protein molecules (75% by albumin and most of the remainder by globulins and fibrinogen). The other 40% is produced by the electrostatically held cations. However, if the plasma protein concentration rises, the influence of the Donnan equilibrium effect on COP increases disproportionately. There is therefore a curvilinear relationship between total protein concentration and COP (Fig. 12–2).

Landis and Pappenheimer derived an empirical equation by which COP may be calculated from measurement of the total plasma protein (TP).[8]

$$COP = 2.1TP + 0.16TP^2 + 0.009TP^3$$

Weil and colleagues demonstrated a low correlation between calculated and measured plasma COP in normal subjects; an even poorer correlation has been noted in critically ill patients.[9, 10] These findings can be explained by alteration of the albumin/globulin ratio in patients, which affects the number of cations associated with the negatively charged proteins.

COP is measured by placing a protein solution on one side of a semipermeable membrane and a protein-free solution on the other side. Fluid moves through the membrane until a pressure is generated that prevents further osmosis. This pressure is defined as the COP.[10] Plasma COP in normal ambulatory subjects is approximately 25 mm Hg; in supine individuals, 22 mm Hg; and in a critical care unit population, 18 to 20 mm Hg.[11–13]

Infusion of an iso-oncotic solution in isotonic saline, such as 5% albumin, expands the intravascular space without producing an acute shift of water from other compartments. Administration of a hyperoncotic solution, such as 25% albumin, expands blood volume to a greater extent than the volume infused by shifting water and electrolytes from the interstitium. Water does not, however, diffuse from the intracellular space if extracellular osmolarity remains unchanged.

In 1896 Starling first defined the forces that influence the bulk movement of water between the vascular and interstitial compartments.[14] In 1948 Pappenheimer and Soto-Rivera derived a mathematic expression for these forces that is referred to as the Starling equation of transcapillary exchange:[15]

$$Q_f = K_f [(P_c - P_i) - \sigma(\pi_c - \pi_i)]$$

where Q_f = total fluid flow across the capillary membrane
K_f = fluid filtration coefficient
P_c = capillary hydrostatic pressure
P_i = interstitial hydrostatic pressure
σ = osmotic reflection coefficient
π_c = capillary oncotic pressure
π_i = interstitial oncotic pressure

The four pressures in this equation are called the Starling forces. The net driving pressure favoring filtration is $P_c - P_i$. The hydrostatic pressure within the capillary is the major force driving fluid into the interstitium and is essentially unopposed by the interstitial hydrostatic pressure. This is usually slightly negative and approaches zero or becomes slightly positive only when substantial amounts of edema accumulate.[16, 17] The plasma COP is thus the only force acting to retain fluid within the intravascular space. The interstitial COP works in the opposite direction; the net effect of these opposing forces is described by $\pi_c - \pi_i$.

K_f, the filtration coefficient, has two components: L_p, the hydraulic conductivity, which describes how rapidly fluid can pass through the microvascular exchange barrier (capillary membrane, interstitial gel, and terminal lymphatics), and S, the capillary surface area available for filtration.[18–20] If either component of K_f increases, for example, because of damage to the endothelial membrane or precapillary vascular dilatation in response to increased cardiac output (CO), the rate and amount of fluid filtered increase independently of changes in the Starling forces.[21]

The reflection coefficient σ defines the capacity of the membrane to prevent translocation of proteins. If $\sigma = 1$, the membrane is totally impermeable and proteins are able to exert their full oncotic force; if it is 0, the membrane permits the substance to pass without impedance.[21] σ is different for different capillary membranes throughout the body. It is approximately 0.9 for systemic capillaries and 0.7 for pulmonary vessels.[22] The net effect of the Starling forces

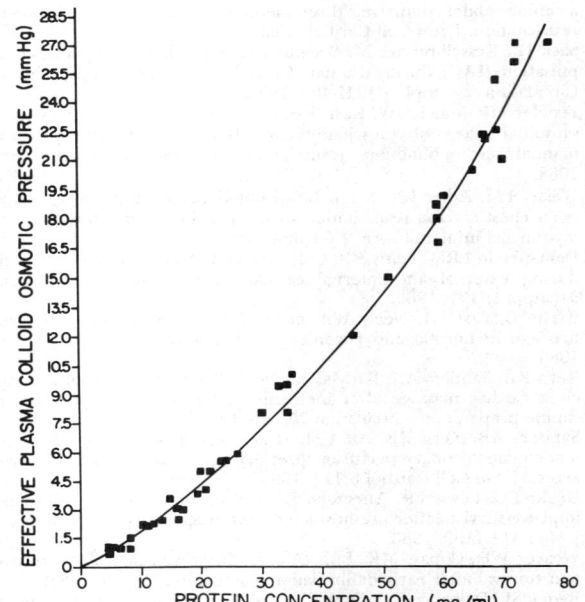

Figure 12–2. Plot of plasma colloid osmotic pressure and plasma total protein concentration. The plasma colloid osmotic pressure was directly measured using an oncometer. (From Prather JW, Gaar KA Jr, Guyton AC: Direct continuous recording of plasma colloid osmotic pressure of whole blood. J Appl Physiol 24:602, 1968.)

TABLE 12–1

IONIC COMPOSITION OF CRYSTALLOIDS

Fluid	Na$^+$ (mEq/L)	Cl$^-$ (mEq/L)	K$^+$ (mEq/L)	Ca^{2+} (mEq/L)	Lactate (mEq/L)	COP (mm Hg)	Osmolarity (mOsm/L)	pH
Ringer's lactate	130	109	4	3	28	0	273	5.1
Normal saline	154	154	0	0	0	0	308	6.0

across the capillaries is to produce fluid movement from the intravascular to the interstitial space. Because accumulation of interstitial fluid in the lung is much more threatening to survival of the patient than peripheral edema formation, there has been great interest in evaluating the safety factors that decrease the risk of development of clinically significant pulmonary edema.[23–25]

Modest increases in pulmonary capillary hydrostatic pressure, or decreases in plasma oncotic pressure, do not result in pulmonary edema because the lung has mechanisms for resisting accumulation of interstitial fluid. The pulmonary interstitial hydrostatic pressure (P_i) is normally slightly negative.[24, 26, 27] When fluid first begins to accumulate in the interstitium, the pressure rapidly increases (compliance is low). This hydrostatic pressure increase opposes any further fluid entry (by decreasing the hydrostatic pressure gradient, $P_c - P_i$).[23] However, as interstitial fluid pressure rises above atmospheric, resistance to fluid transport through the interstitium decreases markedly; further increases in fluid volume then cause only minimal increases in interstial hydrostatic pressure.[26, 28] This may reflect a change in the resistance of the interstitial gel to bulk fluid flow as the gel becomes hydrated.[25, 29] The P_i appears to level off between 1 and 5 mm Hg in severe pulmonary edema.[30]

A second compensatory mechanism is a decrease in the interstitial oncotic pressure resulting from accumulation of protein-poor fluid in the interstitium.[18] The pulmonary interstitial oncotic pressure is normally approximately 75% of the plasma level; the oncotic gradient across the pulmonary capillary membrane ($\pi_c - \pi_i$) is only 4 to 6 mm Hg. If serum COP decreases, the interstitial oncotic pressure decreases proportionally as fluid enters the interstitial space and thereby helps limit the change in the oncotic gradient.[24, 31, 32] π_i decreases not only because of simple dilution but also because a greater proportion of the interstitial water becomes available for protein distribution, and increased amounts of protein are removed from the interstitium by the pulmonary lymphatics.[18]

Proteins are normally excluded from a large portion of the interstitial fluid volume because the density of the matrix is high in certain areas and large protein molecules like albumin cannot fit. However, as the degree of hydration increases, the fibers in the interstitial gel are pulled apart, allowing protein to enter previously unavailable space.[18] This effect helps lower π_i, widens the transcapillary oncotic gradient ($\pi_c - \pi_i$), and thereby opposes further pulmonary edema formation.

Lymphatic drainage is the third and probably most important safety factor. Experimental studies have demonstrated that the lymph flow rate can increase by a factor of about 10 when interstitial fluid volume or pressure increases.

CRYSTALLOID SOLUTIONS

Normal Saline and Ringer's Lactate

Crystalloid solutions are sodium-containing solutions devoid of protein or other macromolecules. Normal saline (NS) and Ringer's lactate (RL) are the two crystalloids most frequently utilized for fluid resuscitation. The volume-expanding effects of these fluids are identical.[33] Both are freely permeable across the vascular membrane and therefore distribute evenly throughout the extracellular space. In normal individuals approximately 25% of the infused volume remains within the blood vessels when equilibrium is achieved, which usually takes 20 to 30 minutes. Studies of critically ill patients have demonstrated that less than 20% of infused crystalloid may remain in the circulation 1 to 2 hours after infusion.[34, 35] The ionic characteristics of these two fluids are compared in Table 12–1. There have been several theoretic concerns regarding the use of these fluids for resuscitation of patients in circulatory shock:

1. Does the 28 mEq/L of lactate in RL exacerbate lactic acidosis?
2. Does the use of RL complicate interpretation of the blood lactate level as a marker of the degree of tissue hypoxia?
3. Does the use of large amounts of unbuffered NS result in hyperchloremic acidosis, which could exacerbate preexisting metabolic acidosis?
4. Is the blood pH decreased because of the acidotic pH of most commercial solutions of RL and NS?

Lowery and associates compared the use of RL to that of NS in patients with traumatic shock.[36] Fluids and blood were infused until the clinical signs of shock resolved. There was no evidence that RL infusion exacerbated lactic acidosis, and acid-base balance was similar in both groups. Patients resuscitated with NS had significantly higher serum chloride levels, but these were never high enough to be of concern and were not associated with dilutional acidosis.[36]

Although commercial preparations of both RL and NS have acid pH values, the solutions are unbuffered; therefore only minimal neutralization is needed to restore the blood pH to 7.4 after administration of these solutions. The sodium lactate in RL is not an acid and is metabolized in the liver to bicarbonate, producing a mild alkalizing effect.[37]

Crystalloid solutions are nontoxic and do not produce anaphylactoid reactions. Interstitial edema is a necessary consequence of volume resuscitation with crystalloids and should not be interpreted as evidence of intravascular overload. Whether there are any clinical consequences of the edema and whether excessive administration of crystalloid solutions predisposes the patient to development of pulmonary edema are discussed subsequently.

Hypertonic Saline

Sodium is largely confined to the extracellular compartment. Infusion of hypertonic saline solutions expands the extracellular space by a volume greater than that of the fluid infused, because water is extracted from the intracellular compartment. The hemodynamic effects of hypertonic saline infusion cannot be entirely explained by extracellular volume expansion, because the increase in plasma volume is transient and of far shorter duration than the improvement in cardiovascular function.[38] These solutions produce a positive inotropic effect and lower systemic and pulmonary vascular resistance by producing precapillary dilation.[39, 40] A vagally mediated reflex venoconstriction, triggered by the arrival of hypertonic solutions within the pulmonary vasculature, also plays a significant role in the therapeutic response.[40–42] Hypertonic crystalloid solutions have been used to resuscitate patients with severe burns since the 1970s. The benefits of these preparations in burn patients include decreased wound and peripheral edema as a result of a smaller positive fluid balance during the resuscitative phase of treatment. Conventional treatment with isotonic crystalloids is usually associated with appreciable sodium and water retention; weight gains of as much as 10% of baseline body weight often occur by the time clinically adequate resuscitation is achieved.[43] Monafo and associates administered hypertonic saline solution with a sodium level of 300 mEq/L to 106 severely burned patients.[43] Resuscitation was accomplished with 20 to 25% less fluid than is called for by the Parkland protocol. A "striking" decrease in the severity of wound edema was reported.

Jelenko and colleagues compared the effects of a hypertonic albumin-containing fluid (240 mEq sodium, 12.5 g albumin) with those of RL and hypertonic saline solution in patients with severe burns.[44] The patients in the albumin group were resuscitated more quickly, developed less peripheral edema, and had significantly fewer respiratory complications than those receiving the other solutions.

In the 1980s there was renewed interest in the use of hypertonic sodium chloride for the treatment of hypovolemic shock.[45] Superior immediate hemodynamic improvement and improved survival were documented with the use of hypertonic solutions compared to isotonic crystalloids in several animal models of hemorrhagic shock.[45] In 1980 De Felippe and associates reported the use of a hypertonic saline solution for resuscitation.[46] In this uncontrolled trial, 12 patients in "hypovolemic shock refractory to other fluids and dopamine" were given 100 to 400 mL of 7.5% sodium chloride solution. Shock was promptly reversed in 11 of the 12 patients.

Resuscitation of trauma patients may require large volumes of isotonic crystalloids. This need creates problems in the prehospital setting, because percutaneous insertion of large-bore catheters into the constricted veins of severely hypovolemic patients is difficult. The amount of fluid that can be infused during stabilization of the patient and transport to the hospital is therefore limited. Hypertonic saline solutions would seem to be an attractive choice in this situation.[47]

Intraoperative use of 3% sodium chloride (maximal infusion of 12 mL/kg) was compared with that of RL in severely injured patients.[47] Maintenance of blood pressure and urine output were the end points of treatment. Patients resuscitated with RL received significantly larger fluid volumes (24 ± 9 L) than the 3% sodium chloride group (15 ± 12 L). Significant deterioration in pulmonary gas exchange was seen in patients receiving RL but not in the 3% sodium chloride group.

Similar beneficial effects of hypertonic saline infusion have been described in patients undergoing aortic reconstruction.[48, 49]

Hyperosmolarity, hypernatremia, hyperchloremic acidosis, and hypokalemia may all result from use of hypertonic crystalloid solutions. Severe cerebral dehydration may result in disorientation, confusion, and seizures. If a patient has unsuspected hyponatremia, the rapid increase in serum sodium level may produce central pontine myelinolysis.[50] In the patient with limited cardiac reserve, pulmonary edema may develop.

Another potentially dangerous effect of hypertonic crystalloid resuscitation of uncontrolled traumatic hemorrhage has been described.[51] When a blood vessel is lacerated in a traumatic injury, bleeding continues until the blood pressure drops to so low a level that the pressure gradient across the laceration approaches zero. Active vasoconstriction aids this process. The physiologic effects of hypertonic solutions include increased blood pressure and vasodilation. Both of these effects increase vascular wall tension and could draw lacerated edges of vessels apart and produce renewed blood loss from vessels that had previously stopped bleeding. In a rat model of uncontrolled hemorrhagic shock, infusion of hypertonic saline resulted in increased intra-abdominal bleeding, hypotension, and early mortality.[51]

Despite these theoretic objections, untoward effects were not reported in any of the clinical studies just described. However, the infusions of hypertonic fluid were generally discontinued when the serum sodium concentration exceeded 160 mOsm/L or when serum osmolarity exceeded 350 mOsm/L. The dangers of uncontrolled or poorly monitored infusion of hypertonic solutions are obvious.[52] Although it appears that certain patients might benefit from resuscitation with hypertonic crystalloids or hypertonic crystalloid-colloid mixtures, the optimal osmolarity, the amount and rate of fluid infusion, and the acceptable upper limits of serum sodium concentration and osmolarity need to be more carefully defined before these preparations are accepted for first-line management.

COLLOID SOLUTIONS

Albumin

Albumin is the major protein produced by the liver, constituting up to 50% of its normal synthetic output.[53] Albumin is a highly flexible molecule with a molecular weight between 66,000 and 69,000, depending on the technique used for measurement.[54] The molecule contains 584 amino acids, is extremely water soluble, and has a negative charge of 19 at a pH of 7.4. Albumin makes up about 50% of the plasma protein content and produces two thirds to three fourths of the plasma COP.[55]

Albumin is synthesized in the liver at a rate of 130 to 200 mg/kg/d.[53] It is released into the hepatic sinusoids and thus enters the systemic circulation. The half-life of albumin in the plasma is about 16 hours; 10% leaves the vascular space within 2 hours and 75% by 2 days.[53] From the plasma, albumin passes to its main extravascular storage sites, the interstitial spaces of the skin, muscles, and viscera. These regions contain 60% of the total exchangeable albumin pool.[56] Some of this is tissue bound and therefore is unavailable to the circulation. Unbound albumin can return to the blood stream via lymphatic drainage. The half-life of albumin in the body is 20 days. Approximately 8% of the total exchangeable albumin is degraded daily.[57] The site (or sites) of albumin degradation is uncertain.

The average plasma level of serum albumin is 4.0 g/dL with a range of 3.5 to 5.0 g/dL.[53] Albumin synthesis is regulated primarily by colloid osmoreceptors in the interstitial space near the hepatic sites of synthesis and is not controlled by the serum albumin concentration itself except through its contribution to the COP.[58] If a non–albumin-containing colloid is infused, albumin synthesis decreases.[34, 54] Albumin synthesis is also decreased in malnourished patients, primarily because of inadequate amino acid supply to the liver.

When acute loss of albumin occurs from the intravascular space, as in severe blood loss, the extravascular exchangeable albumin can be rapidly mobilized into the plasma. If the patient begins with normal albumin stores, any decrease in the serum albumin level is transient. The ensuing extravascular deficit is corrected more slowly by an increased rate of albumin synthesis.[59] If the patient is chronically ill and has been in a prolonged catabolic state, a different response is seen: the serum albumin level is initially maintained by a gradual transfer of extravascular albumin to the circulation and begins to drop only when the extravascular stores are markedly depleted. An acute albumin loss in the presence of chronic depletion is associated with a rapid, profound, and prolonged drop in the circulating albumin level.[59]

Human serum albumin is available for intravenous infusion as either a 5% or a 25% solution. The 5% solution contains 50 g of albumin per liter of isotonic saline, producing a COP of 20 mm Hg; the 25% solution contains 12.5 g of albumin in 50 mL of isotonic saline and results in a COP of approximately 100 mm Hg.

Albumin infusions are effective in restoring blood volume and hemodynamic stability after intravascular volume depletion. Clinical indications for infusion of albumin or other colloids are controversial, however, as discussed later. A 500-mL infusion of 5% albumin expands the intravascular volume 450 to 500 mL.[35] After 2 hours and under conditions of normal capillary permeability, 90% remains within the intravascular space.[60] Eventually the administered albumin is distributed throughout the extracellular space.[60]

The 25% solution of albumin is often referred to as "salt-poor" albumin. This terminology is misleading because the sodium content of all albumin preparations is 145 mEq/L. In the 1940s albumin solutions were stabilized with salt-rich solution containing sodium at 300 mEq/L. These preparations are no longer available.[60] After infusion of 100 mL of 25% albumin, the plasma volume continues to increase over the next 30 to 60 minutes to achieve a final blood volume expansion of 450 mL.[34] Redistribution of 350 mL of interstitial fluid to the intravascular space is necessary for this to occur. In patients with extracellular or total body water depletion, equilibration is slow and incomplete.[61] Therefore, in acute hypovolemia, 5% albumin should be given rather than the hyperoncotic form. The 25% albumin solution is usually used in patients with concomitant hypovolemia and elevated extracellular fluid volume.

The duration of vascular retention and the hemodynamic effects of infused albumin solutions vary greatly depending on the patient's disease state. Although this variability may result from "leakage" into the interstitium, it may also reflect preferential binding of albumin in the skin and wound (e.g., after operative procedures) or increased catabolism.

Significant complications of albumin infusion are unusual if iatrogenic fluid overload is avoided by appropriate use of hemodynamic monitoring. The incidence of albumin-induced anaphylaxis is 0.11%.[62] There is no risk of hepatitis with albumin because the solution is heated to 60°C for 10 hours during processing.[60] There is also no known risk of transmission of acquired immunodeficiency syndrome. Two studies have shown that infusion of large volumes of albumin may lower the serum ionized calcium concentration, producing a negative inotropic effect; however, these results are controversial because the patients had significant fluid overload.[63, 64] The same group of investigators reported that traumatically injured patients resuscitated with albumin required larger amounts of transfused blood and plasma than patients resuscitated with crystalloid infusions.[65, 66] However, studies of both animal models and patients have demonstrated dilutional effects of albumin infusion on coagulation factors that did not differ from those seen in subjects resuscitated with crystalloids.[67, 68]

Albumin has several unique effects that differentiate it from other colloids as well as from crystalloids.[69] Albumin can bind reversibly with both anions and cations. This characteristic allows albumin to regulate the extracellular

concentration of various substances such as iron, lipids, and bilirubin.[69] It has been suggested that these properties may eventually become the major reason for choosing albumin as a resuscitative fluid. Albumin, for example, has the ability to act as a free radical scavenger and may limit lipid peroxidation.[70–73] Fluid resuscitation is often utilized in pathologic states resulting from tissue damage caused by free radicals and lipid peroxidation, and albumin infusion might be efficacious in limiting this damage. Albumin is also able to bind to toxic substances generated in inflammatory disease states.

Albumin may also play a role in the maintenance of normal microvascular permeability to protein molecules. Endothelial cells contain pores through which proteins may leave the vascular space. Albumin may help regulate the permeability of these pores, which may be increased in the presence of hypoalbuminemia. The intravascular albumin level necessary to maintain normal microvascular permeability is unknown, but work by Demling and associates demonstrates that reducing the blood albumin concentration increases capillary leakage and restoration of the albumin level restores permeability toward normal.[19, 20]

Plasma Protein Fraction

Plasma protein fraction (PPF) is a pasteurized plasma product that is utilized for fluid resuscitation infrequently because of its side effects.[74, 75] It is available as a 5% solution. The protein content of PPF is 83% albumin, the remainder consisting of alpha and beta globulins.[60] Prekallikrein activators (Hageman's factor fragments) are frequently present in PPF but are rarely found in albumin solutions.[74, 75] Hypotension and circulatory collapse can follow infusion of PPF, the former developing within 2 minutes of the initiation of infusion in the majority of patients.[75] A correlation exists between levels of prekallikrien activators in various lots of PPF and the incidence and severity of reactions. Animal studies indicate that generation of bradykinin plays a major role in producing hypotension during PPF infusion.[75]

PPF is still manufactured, primarily because it is easier to produce than albumin solutions (requiring one less fractionation step) and because a higher protein yield is obtained.[74]

Dextrans

Dextrans were introduced into clinical medicine in the late 1940s to meet the wartime demand for a safe and easily stored plasma substitute.[76] The dextrans are mixtures of glucose polymers of various sizes and molecular weights produced by the bacterium *Leuconostoc mesenteroides* when grown on a sucrose medium. The molecular weight of the polymer mixture may vary from a few thousand to several million. Dextrans of different molecular weights can be produced by acid hydrolysis of the parent macromolecules. The two dextran preparations most often used clinically are dextran 70 (Macrodex) and dextran 40 (Rheomacrodex).

The molecular weight of polydisperse macromolecules such as dextran can be presented as the number average molecular weight, the arithmetic mean molecular weight of all the molecules, or as the weight average molecular weight, the sum of the number of molecules at each number average molecular weight times that weight divided by the total weight of all the molecules.

Dextran 70 has a weight average molecular weight of 70,000, with 90% of the molecules falling between 25,000 and 125,000.[76] It is available as a 6% solution in normal saline. Dextran 40 has a weight average molecular weight of 40,000, with 90% of the molecules falling between 10,000 and 80,000. It is available as a 10% solution in either normal saline or 5% dextrose. Infusion of either dextran 70 or dextran 40 results in plasma volume expansion. The duration and degree of this effect are influenced by the total amount infused, the rate of infusion, the molecular weight distribution, and the rate of clearance from the plasma.[76] The smallest dextran molecules are rapidly filtered by the kidneys and produce mild diuresis or pass through the endothelium to the interstitial space and eventually return to the blood stream via the lymphatics. Larger dextran molecules are stored briefly in hepatocytes, renal tubular cells, and reticuloendothelial cells without producing any known toxicity and are eventually metabolized to carbon dioxide and water.

The larger average molecular weight of dextran 70 results in slower excretion of this product than of dextran 40. Infusion of dextran 70 therefore results in a greater and more prolonged volume effect. Unless a transient effect is desired, dextran 70 is preferable for plasma volume expansion.[76]

Seventy percent of an infused volume of dextran 70 is retained within the plasma after 3 hours, and 30% remains after 24 hours.[57] Lamke and Liljedahl evaluated plasma volume changes after infusion of 1 L of dextran 70 in postoperative patients.[35] Dextran 70 produced an average plasma volume increase of 790 mL, which was comparable to the effect of infusion of the same amount of 6% hetastarch and was clearly superior to the volume effects of 5% albumin. Both 6% dextran 70 and 6% hetastarch solutions are hyperoncotic compared with 5% albumin, and this difference most likely explains their superior plasma volume–expanding effects.[35]

A 10% dextran 40 solution is an even more potent volume expander than dextran 70 because of the greater oncotic pressure of dextran 40. However, because it is cleared much more quickly by the kidneys, the effect is short-lived.[77] In patients with normal renal function, approximately 60% of infused dextran 40 is excreted in the urine after 6 hours.[78] In healthy patients who received 500 mL of 10% dextran 40 during 1 hour, maximal plasma volume expansion (1 to 1.5 times the volume infused) occurred at the end of infusion and the effect persisted for only 1.5 hours.[77, 79]

A similar volume effect of dextran 40 was observed in patients with circulatory shock. However, greater hemodynamic and oxygen transport improvement was observed in critically ill patients than in healthy volunteers.[79, 80] Matsuda and Shoemaker postulated that this increased effect in critically ill patients was caused not only by plasma volume expansion but also by an improvement in microcirculatory blood flow distribution.[79, 80] Dextran 40 and, to a much smaller extent, dextran 70 decrease blood viscosity and thereby may promote peripheral blood flow and tissue oxygenation. Several factors may contribute to the rheologic effects of dextran, including (1) coating of endothelial surfaces, resulting in decreased interaction between the endothelium and the cellular elements of the blood; (2) hemodilution; (3) decreased red blood cell aggregation and rigidity; and (4) decreased platelet adhesiveness and aggregation.[76] Under normal conditions blood has nearly perfect rheologic properties; thus dextran 40 infusion does not improve peripheral flow properties. In patients with circulatory shock, however, red blood cell sludging may contribute to the hypoxic tissue insult; under these circumstances, dextran 40 infusion may improve blood rheology.[76, 79, 81, 82]

Several potentially life-threatening toxic effects may complicate dextran administration, including acute renal failure, anaphylaxis, and bleeding diathesis.[76] Dextran 40 has been associated with the development of acute renal failure, although it is difficult to determine whether the underlying illness or the infusion itself is the etiologic factor.[83, 84] Signif-

icant amounts of dextran 40 are rapidly filtered by the kidneys and enter the renal tubules. A highly viscous urine results, and, as tubular reabsorption of water continues, the dextran may precipitate, causing irreversible plugging of the renal tubules and acute renal failure.[83] Renal damage may be more likely when renal dysfunction or pre-existing dehydration is present. It is therefore recommended that use of dextran 40 should be avoided in patients with incipient or established renal failure.[84] Dextran 70 is rarely associated with the development of acute renal failure, probably because much fewer molecules are filtered by the glomeruli.[85]

Anaphylaxis after dextran infusion most likely involves a reaction between immunoglobulin G or immunoglobulin M antibodies and dextran. Natural antibodies to dextran exist in the general population and probably result from exposure to the substance in food products, from dextran-producing bacteria in the gastrointestinal tract, or from exposure to bacteria possessing antigens that cross-react with dextran. Severe reactions occur predominantly in patients with high antidextran antibody titers, although other factors are necessary for a severe anaphylactoid reaction to occur.[86, 87]

The incidence of anaphylactoid reactions after dextran administration was reported to be 0.032% by Ring and Messmer, with dextran 40 producing many fewer reactions than dextran 60 or 75.[62] Severe reactions occurred in only 0.008% of patients in this series. In a prospective study of patients undergoing major surgery, Paull found a much higher incidence of dextran-induced anaphylactoid reactions (0.26%), with life-threatening anaphylaxis after 0.12% of dextran infusions.[88] In all cases, the reaction appeared within a maximum of 5 minutes after the commencement of the infusion.[88] The highest incidence of dextran-induced anaphylactoid reactions was reported by Thompson, who reviewed observations in 10 studies involving 2462 patients given dextran and noted that 5.3% of the patients experienced a reaction.[57]

The incidence of dextran-induced anaphylactoid reactions can be reduced by administrating a solution of monovalent hapten dextran before the infusion.[89, 90] This preparation has an average molecular weight of 1000 and is called dextran 1 (Promit). Dextran 1 occupies one binding site of the antidextran antibody and prevents the formation of immune complexes. Twenty milliliters of a 15% solution of dextran 1 should be given 2 minutes before starting dextran 40 or 70.[90] This significantly reduces the incidence of severe anaphylaxis but may not influence the number of mild reactions, which probably have a different pathophysiologic mechanism.[87]

Dextran 40 and dextran 70 both produce a dose-related hemostatic defect. Its cause is multifactorial but is primarily related to a reduction in platelet adhesion and aggregation mediated through factor VIIIR:ag activity.[91] Primary hemostasis is affected; clinically the picture mimics that in von Willebrand's disease. Dextran also lowers levels of all the clotting factors by hemodilution, coats blood vessel walls and cellular elements, and impairs the elasticity and tensile strength of fibrin clots.[92–96] Dextran 70 impairs coagulation more significantly than does dextran 40, but both products affect coagulation more profoundly than does hetastarch.[95]

To minimize the risk of bleeding, the volume of dextran infused should be limited to no more than 20 mL/kg/d or 1.5 g/kg/d.[92] Bleeding may occur more readily in patients with pre-existing coagulation abnormalities such as thrombocytopenia; patients with renal failure are especially at risk because of uremic platelet dysfunction combined with a prolonged intravascular dextran half-life.[94]

HYDROXYETHYL STARCH (HETASTARCH)

Hetastarch is a generic term used to describe a broad class of starch molecules having various molecular weights and degrees of hydroxyethylation. For clinical use hetastarch consists of a 6% solution of hydroxyethyl starch ranging in molecular weight from 10,000 to more than 1 million in an isotonic saline solution.[97] The number average molecular weight of hetastarch is approximately 71,000, which is similar to that of human serum albumin. The solution has an osmolarity of 310 mOsm/L, an oncotic pressure of 30 mm Hg, and a pH of 5.5.[97]

Hetastarch is produced by chemical modification of amylopectin, a highly branched polymer of glucose. Amylopectin itself is quickly hydrolyzed in blood by amylase. Hydroxyethylation of the molecule with ethylene oxide results in a product that is resistant to amylase activity. There is a direct relationship between the degree of hydroxyethylation and the resistance of the molecule to enzymatic degradation.

The pharmacokinetics of hetastarch are complex because of the heterogeneity of molecular weights and hydroxyethylation of the substance in solution. Molecules with a molecular weight of less than 50,000 are rapidly excreted in the urine or distributed in body tissues. Larger molecules may also enter body tissues (at a lower rate), may be taken up by the reticuloendothelial cells, or are degraded in the blood stream by amylases and then excreted in urine and bile. In normal patients, 46% of a 500-mL infusion of hetastarch is excreted in the urine within 2 days and 64% within 8 days.[98] The disappearance curve of hetastarch from the plasma is complex, with three exponential components representing fractions with slow, intermediate, and rapid elimination.[99] Because the biologic half-life of hetastarch changes as a function of time, it is necessary to define the time period being studied.[97] Metcalf and associates found that 30% of infused hetastarch was excreted with a half-life of 67 hours, 17.1% was eliminated more rapidly with a half-life of 8.5 hours, and 18% was excreted with a half-life of only 2 hours.[99] Tissues with relatively high macrophage activity, such as liver and spleen, take up a small percentage of the infused hetastarch and retain it for an extended period. The presence of hetastarch molecules within the reticuloendothelial cells does not appear to depress their function or increase mortality in animal models of sepsis.[100] Hetastarch molecules are also stored transiently in renal tubular epithelial cells and can produce morphologic changes. However, renal tubular function is not altered.[101]

Because renal excretion is the major route of hetastarch elimination, the elimination half-life and duration of plasma volume expansion would be expected to be prolonged in patients with significant renal impairment. However, clinical data suggest that patients with moderate reductions in glomerular filtration rate can eliminate hetastarch in a nearly normal fashion.[102] Studies of patients with severe renal failure are not available.

Hetastarch has been consistently demonstrated to be an effective plasma volume expander in both normal volunteers and hypovolemic patients.[99, 103] Most of the studies that have measured changes in plasma volume have demonstrated that intravascular volume increases are in excess of the quantity of hetastarch infused.[103] The patient's hemodynamic status may improve for more than 24 hours after the infusion. Metcalf and associates found that 24 hours after administration of 1000 mL of hetastarch, plasma volume averaged 285 mL above baseline.[99] The duration of volume expansion is directly related to intravascular persistence of the larger hetastarch molecules. Clinical studies that have directly compared the effects of hetastarch and of 5% albumin demonstrate that the former is an equivalent or superior volume expander, probably as a result of the higher COP of 6% hetastarch.[35, 104, 105]

For plasma volume expansion, the dosage of hetastarch must be titrated on an individual basis. Although most hypovolemic patients respond to 500 to 1000 mL, patients with ongoing blood loss or septic shock may require much larger amounts to restore hemodynamic stability. For example, Shatney and colleagues infused an average of 3600 mL of hetastarch to resuscitate patients with multisystem trauma and shock, and Rackow and associates required an average of 4568 mL of hetastarch to resuscitate patients in hypovolemic and septic shock.[106, 107] Despite the large amount of hetastarch administered in these studies within 24 hours, adverse effects on renal, hepatic, or pulmonary function were either not detected or no worse than those seen with other resuscitative fluids.

The effects of hetastarch infusion on blood coagulation have been extensively studied.[68, 108–112] Strauss reviewed these effects and concluded that moderate infusions, defined as those not exceeding 1500 mL or 20 mL/kg during a 24-hour period, have transient and clinically insignificant effects on coagulation.[108] Clinical data on the effects of massive infusion of hetastarch are limited. In the study by Rackow and coworkers, which compared 6% hetastarch to 5% albumin and normal saline, changes in prothrombin time, partial thromboplastin time, and platelet count were seen in all three groups and were thought to reflect only hemodilution.[68, 107] There were no significant differences in coagulation among the three groups, and increased clinical bleeding was not evident. In the study by Shatney and colleagues of traumatically injured patients with hemorrhagic shock, hetastarch-resuscitated patients did not exhibit any increased incidence of local bleeding or systemic coagulopathy compared with injured patients resuscitated with PPF.[106]

Nonetheless, animal studies have demonstrated that hetastarch adversely affects blood coagulation in a dose-dependent fashion.[108, 113] The mechanisms responsible for the clotting abnormalities have not been clearly established by these studies. Possibilities include hemodilution, poorly formed fibrin clots, prolongation of bleeding time secondary to abnormalities of platelet number and function, and prolongation of partial thromboplastin time resulting from adverse effects on factor VIII.[108, 111, 113]

Although the available clinical studies do not demonstrate a significantly increased risk of bleeding after hetastarch infusion, one should be cautious when considering the use of doses greater than 20 mL/kg during a 24-hour period. Both clinical and laboratory evidence of coagulopathy should be anticipated.

Anaphylactoid reactions to hetastarch infusion occur infrequently. Only 14 reactions were reported in 16,405 infusions, an incidence of 0.085%.[62] Only one of these reactions was considered life threatening.

Serum amylase levels often are elevated after hetastarch infusion.[114, 115] After administration of 500 mL of hetastarch in healthy volunteers, the amylase level peaked at an average of 290% of baseline.[114] The amylase increase appears to result from binding of hetastarch to amylase, which impairs the normal urinary amylase excretion. This hyperamylasemia may obscure the diagnosis of pancreatitis. There is no evidence that hetastarch affects the pancreas. If pancreatitis is suspected, serum lipase measurements should be used to help confirm the diagnosis for at least 3 to 5 days after the last hetastarch infusion.[114]

Low-Molecular-Weight Hydroxyethyl Starch (Pentastarch)

Pentastarch is an analogue of hetastarch with a lower weight average molecular weight, a lower number average molecular weight, and fewer hydroxyethyl groups added per molecule (lower molar substitution ratio). These structural characteristics explain the much shorter duration of plasma volume expansion with this solution compared with hetastarch. More than 90% of a single infusion of pentastarch is cleared from the blood stream within 24 hours, and it is undetectable in the blood after 96 hours.[116] Pentastarch expands the plasma volume approximately 1.5 times the volume infused; its effect lasts less than 12 hours. The greater volume effect of pentastarch compared with 5% albumin or 6% hetastarch probably results from its higher COP of 40 mm Hg.[117]

Because of its lower molar substitution ratio, pentastarch is more rapidly and completely degraded by circulating amylase than is hetastarch. The low-molecular-weight fraction can penetrate the endothelium and enter the interstitial space or can be directly excreted in the urine. Larger molecules are enzymatically degraded in the liver and then excreted in urine and stool.[118] The largest molecules are phagocytized by the reticuloendothelial system.

A 10% solution of pentastarch in NS (Pentaspan) has been approved in the United States for leukapheresis.[119] The shorter persistence of pentastarch in the circulation permits more frequent granulocyte donation. Because pentastarch is a potent plasma volume expander with minimal toxicity, including fewer effects on coagulation than hetastarch in granulocte donors, there has been interest in this fluid for volume resuscitation of the critically ill.[120] Pentastarch has been investigated in a number of clinical settings, including burn resuscitation, septic shock, and postoperative hypovolemia.[118, 121, 122] These studies demonstrated that the hemodynamic effects of pentastarch were equal or superior to those of equal volumes of 5% albumin. Effects on coagulation were similar with both fluids and were dilutional in nature. Pentastarch, however, is an investigational agent in the United States.

High-Molecular-Weight Hydroxyethyl Starch

Hetastarch has a wide spectrum of molecular sizes, and fractions of the solution with a higher average molecular weight and a narrower molecular mass distribution can be separated out with appropriate filters.[123] Animal studies have evaluated different fractions of high-molecular-weight hetastarch to see if capillary endothelial leaks could be sealed by infusion of hetastarch molecules of appropriate size and shape.[123, 124] Zikria and associates demonstrated significantly decreased leakage of albumin across capillaries in areas of scald injury when a fraction of hetastarch with a molecular weight between 100,000 and 300,000 (Fm fraction) was infused, compared with two other hetastarch fractions, RL, or 5% albumin solution.[123] The authors thought that the Fm fraction produced biophysical sealing of capillary leaks. In a subsequent study the same group used a rat limb ischemia-reperfusion injury and demonstrated that animals receiving the Fm fraction of hetastarch had significantly lower ischemic tissue water content and necrosis.[124]

Webb and associates evaluated the effects of a different hydroxyethyl starch derivative, produced by diafiltration of pentastarch, in a porcine model of sepsis secondary to induction of fecal peritonitis.[125] After fecal peritonitis was produced, animals were resuscitated with either 6% hetastarch or diafiltered pentastarch (6% Pentafraction), a hydroxyethyl starch product that is devoid of both small and extremely large molecules. The number average molecular weight of this experimental product is 120,000, compared with 71,000 for hetastarch. Fluid infusion rates were adjusted to maintain the plasma volumes at baseline levels (as estimated by measurements of hematocrit). Despite the greater oncotic pressure of the 6% hetastarch solution, a significantly greater volume of this fluid was needed to maintain the hematocrit at baseline levels. Because urine

output and hemodynamic variables were similar in both groups, the authors postulated that a larger amount of the hetastarch than of diafiltered pentastarch solution leaked into the interstitial spaces and the peritoneal cavity. Evaluation of lung tissue by electron microscopy demonstrated a greater alveolar capillary barrier thickness in the hetastarch group, consistent with increased pulmonary interstitial edema.

The potential clinical implications of these studies are enormous, as capillary leak plays a significant role in a diverse group of disorders including shock, myocardial ischemia, and adult respiratory distress syndrome (ARDS).

GELATINS

In Europe, collagen derivatives are extensively used for fluid resuscitation. These modified gelatins were developed by the Swiss Red Cross for use in mass civilian and military disasters.[126] Several of these substances are commercially available. Modified fluid gelatin (Plasmagel) and urea-bridged gelatin (Haemaccel) are cattle bone gelatin derivatives. Modified fluid gelatin is produced by controlled heating and chemical hydrolysis of the raw material followed by coupling of the resulting gelatin polymers into larger complexes by reacting them with succinic anhydride. Urea-bridged gelatin is produced by thermal degradation of the raw material, producing small polypeptides that are cross-linked by urea bridges to form larger polymers. Both of these modified gelatin products have molecular weights of approximately 35,000.

Urea-bridged gelatin is available as a 3.5% solution in NS, and modified fluid gelatin is a 4% solution in NS. Both solutions have been shown to be effective plasma volume expanders in critically ill patients.[126, 127] In normovolemic volunteers, modified fluid gelatin provides volume expansion with an intravascular concentration half-life of 2.5 hours.[127] Their low molecular weights lead to rapid renal elimination of a large percentage of the infused gelatin. In anuric patients, however, repeated infusion does not lead to significant accumulation, suggesting that extrarenal elimination is possible.

The most significant side effects of modified gelatins are anaphylactoid reactions, which occurred after urea-bridged gelatin infusion in 0.146% of patients in Ring and Messmer's series, with severe reactions occurring in 0.048%.[62, 86] Rapid infusion of this colloid is usually associated with histamine release, probably secondary to a direct effect on mast cells and basophils.[128] Although antihistamines can prevent these reactions in volunteers, effective prophylaxis has not been demonstrated under clinical conditions.[128] The incidence of severe allergic reactions to modified fluid gelatin is less than that associated with urea-bridged gelatin.[62] True anaphylactic reactions may also occasionally develop secondary to gelatin–antigelatin antibody immune complex–induced mediator activation.[86]

Neither gelatin product is associated with renal failure or coagulopathy, even when several liters are infused within 24 hours. The physicochemical properties of colloids are compared in Table 12–2.

CIRCULATORY SHOCK

Circulatory shock is a clinical syndrome of acute perfusion failure with inadequate tissue oxygen delivery (DO_2) resulting in decreased tissue oxygen consumption (VO_2), anaerobic metabolism, and lactic acidosis.[129] Weil and Henning classified shock into four categories: hypovolemic, cardiogenic, distributive, and obstructive.[129] Reduction of plasma volume is the primary abnormality in hypovolemic shock, but abso-

TABLE 12–2

PHYSIOCHEMICAL PROPERTIES OF SEVERAL COLLOIDS

Fluid	Weight Average Molecular Weight	Number Average Molecular Weight	COP (mm Hg)	Osmolarity (mOsm/L)	pH
5% albumin	69,000	69,000	20	290	6.6
10% dextran 40	40,000	25,000	68*	320	6.7
6% dextran 70	70,000	39,000	70*	320	6.3
6% hetastarch	450,000	71,000	70*	310	5.5

*Represents maximal COP. This decreases rapidly as smaller molecules leave the intravascular space.

lute or relative plasma volume deficits frequently contribute to the disturbances of tissue oxygenation in the other three types of circulatory shock. Decreased plasma volume produces a decrease in left ventricular end-diastolic volume and stroke volume. Although sympathetic nervous system activation can initially maintain CO by inducing tachycardia and arterial pressure by producing vasoconstriction, at some point compensatory limits are reached and CO and systemic blood pressure may suddenly fall.

There is clear agreement that the major goal of treatment of circulatory shock associated with hypovolemia is rapid restoration of blood volume and tissue oxygenation.[107, 129] The use of asanguineous fluids for initial resuscitation produces better restoration of capillary blood flow than does immediate transfusion. Moderate hemodilution, for example, to a hemoglobin level of 10 to 12 g/dL, is well tolerated by most patients and does not lower $\dot{D}o_2$ if intravascular volume is maintained.[130]

The hemodynamic response to fluid infusion is influenced by the choice of fluid, vascular tone, and cardiac compliance. Several studies have directly compared the plasma volume–expanding and hemodynamic effects of colloids and crystalloids. In these studies a preselected volume of fluid was infused rather than a volume adjusted on the basis of physiologic response. Lamke and Liljedahl compared plasma volume responses to 1-L infusions of 6% dextran 70, 6% hetastarch, 5% albumin, 3.5% urea-bridged gelatin, and NS in stable postoperative patients.[35] Significant increases in plasma volume occurred with all colloids but not with NS. The greatest increases in plasma volume were with dextran 70 (790 mL) and 6% hetastarch (710 mL) (Fig. 12–3).

Lazrove and associates evaluated responses to infusion of 500 mL of 5% albumin and 6% hetastarch during 1 hour in

acutely ill postoperative patients using a prospective, randomized crossover design.[104] Both solutions produced significant increases in plasma volume, CO, $\dot{D}o_2$, and $\dot{V}o_2$. Plasma volume expansion persisted for 1.5 hours with albumin and at least 3 hours with hetastarch. Similar hemodynamic effects of 5% albumin and 6% hetastarch were reported in a series of critically ill patients studied by Puri and coworkers.[131]

Shoemaker compared the relative effectiveness of a 1-hour infusion of 500 mL of whole blood, 5% albumin, 6% dextran 70, and 10% dextran 40 and 1000 mL of RL in critically ill patients.[1] Blood and colloid infusion produced significant increases in blood volume, CO, stroke volume, left ventricular stroke work index, central venous pressure (CVP), and pulmonary arterial wedge pressure (PAWP), but insignificant improvements occurred after crystalloid infusion even though twice the volume was infused (Fig. 12–4). In a subsequent study by the same group involving critically ill patients with ARDS, 100 mL of 25% albumin was compared with 1000 mL of RL.[34] Plasma volume increased an average of 465 mL with the albumin but only 194 mL with RL. Significant increases in $\dot{D}o_2$ and $\dot{V}o_2$ were seen only in the albumin group. The more potent volume-expanding properties of colloids compared to crystalloids may permit more rapid restoration of hemodynamic stability in hypotensive critically ill patients.[132, 133]

Changes in vascular and cardiac compliance in the shock patient make it difficult to rely on any single hemodynamic measurement to define adequate resuscitation. Isolated measurements of CVP or PAWP do not correlate well with direct measurements of blood volume.[134] CVP may decrease

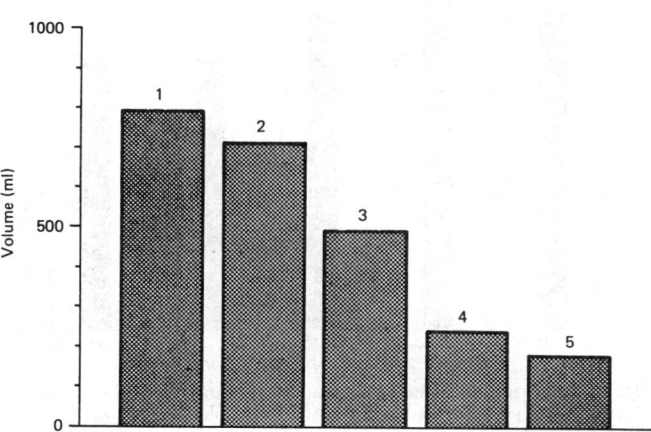

Figure 12–3. Plasma volume expansion after infusion of 1 L of (1) dextran 70, (2) 6% hetastarch, (3) 5% albumin, (4) modified fluid gelatin, and (5) NS in postoperative patients. (From Lamke LO, Liljedahl SO: Plasma volume changes after infusion of various plasma expanders. Resuscitation 5:93–100, 1976.)

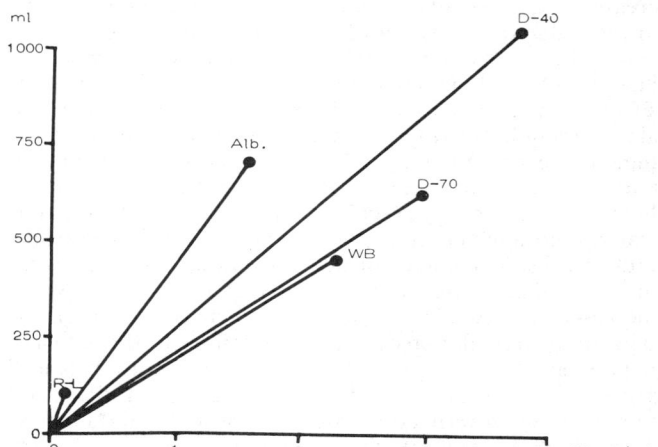

Figure 12–4. Maximal changes in blood volume (mL) versus change in cardiac output (L/min) after infusion of 500 mL of whole blood or colloids and 1000 mL of RL in critically ill patients. (From WC Shoemaker, Comparison of the relative effectiveness of whole blood transfusions and various types of fluid therapy in resuscitation, Crit Care Med, 4, 71–78, © by Williams & Wilkins, 1976.)

TABLE 12–3

GUIDELINES FOR FLUID CHALLENGE UTILIZING PULMONARY ARTERIAL DIASTOLIC OR PULMONARY ARTERIAL WEDGE PRESSURE MONITORING: 7/3 RULE FOR FLUID CHALLENGE

Steps: Observe PAWP/PADP	PAWP/PADP*	Fluid Infusion Rate
For 10 min before challenge	<12	200 mL × 10 min
	<16	100 mL × 10 min
	≥16	50 mL × 10 min
During 10-min infusion	Change >7	Stop
Immediately after 10-min infusion	Change ≤3	Continue infusion without interruption
After 10-min wait	Change >3, ≤7	Wait 10 min
	Change >3	Stop
	Change ≤3	Repeat fluid challenge

*PAWP = pulmonary arterial wedge pressure (mm Hg); PADP = pulmonary arterial diastolic pressure (mm Hg).
Adapted from Weil MH, Henning RJ: New concepts in the diagnosis and fluid treatment of circulatory shock. Anesth Analg 58:124, 1979.

during fluid infusion if blood volume expansion results in decreased autonomic nervous system–induced arteriolar and venous vasoconstriction.[135] Changes in left ventricular compliance during fluid resuscitation may also limit the usefulness of PAWP as a measure of left ventricular end-diastolic volume (preload).[136]

Nonetheless, for clinical purposes the hemodynamic response to fluid resuscitation should be assessed using the fluid challenge technique originally described by Weil and Henning (Table 12–3).[129] When this is combined with sequential measurements of CO and measurement of variables that help assess adequacy of tissue oxygenation (lactate, $\dot{D}o_2$, $\dot{V}o_2$, mixed venous oxygen saturation), the risks of under- and over-resuscitation are minimized.[137]

The basic disagreement that initiated the colloid versus crystalloid controversy was a conceptual one. Crystalloid advocates believe that an extracellular fluid deficit plays a primary role in the pathophysiology of hypovolemic shock and therefore repletion of this deficit is essential for optimal survival of patients. Colloid proponents believe that decreased blood volume and reduced oxygen transport are the critical pathophysiologic factors; therefore, rapid and complete repletion of the intravascular compartment is critical for resuscitation.

In a series of experimental and clinical studies initiated in the early 1960s, Shires and associates demonstrated that severe hemorrhagic shock was associated with a large decrease in extracellular volume, caused predominantly by intracellular translocation of interstitial fluid in addition to external losses or shift to the intravascular space (transcapillary refill).[138–140] In their studies, using a canine hemorrhagic shock model, animals resuscitated with shed whole blood alone or whole blood plus 10 mL/kg plasma had significantly higher mortality than animals resuscitated with whole blood and 50 mL/kg RL[138] (Fig. 12–5). In a baboon model of hemorrhagic shock, microelectrodes were used to monitor transmembrane potential gradients across individual skeletal muscle cells. Sustained cell depolarization, a 49% decrease in extracellular water, a 6% increase in intracellular water, increased intracellular sodium, and decreased intracellular potassium were all noted, suggesting failure of the ATPase-dependent Na⁺-K⁺ pump.[139] Resuscitation with balanced salt solution produced a return of the potential difference to normal along with a decrease in intracellular and increase in extracellular volume. Similar alterations in water distribution were described in patients with circulatory shock and in patients undergoing major operative procedures.[141, 142] These changes also resolved with infusion of balanced salt solutions.

There is, however, substantial controversy regarding the methods used by Shires and colleagues to measure extracel-

lular fluid volume.[1, 143] Several groups using different techniques and models have found either that the decrease of extracellular volume in hemorrhagic shock was minimal and could be accounted for by the plasma volume loss or that the volume was actually increased.[143–145] Similar controversy exists regarding changes in extracellular volume after major surgery, with no significant alteration measurable in patients after cholecystectomy and increases seen in patients after cardiac surgery.[143]

Despite this controversy, there is considerable evidence from experimental models of severe hemorrhagic shock and from clinical studies of traumatic shock that subjects can be successfully resuscitated with the use of balanced salt solutions and blood (whole blood or packed red blood cells) without the need for administration of colloidal solutions.[2, 146–148] Lowe and associates studied 141 patients with traumatic abdominal injuries requiring laparotomy.[146] Patients were resuscitated randomly with either RL or 4% albumin together with washed red blood cells for the entire emergency room and intraoperative period. Only crystalloids were used postoperatively. Clinical criteria were used as the end points for resuscitation (systemic blood pressure, pulse, and urine output). Both groups of patients were successfully resusci-

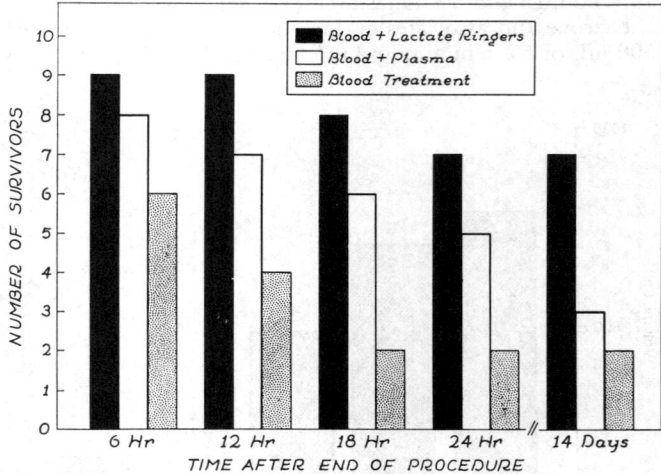

Figure 12–5. Survival after resuscitation of dogs from hemorrhagic shock. Each group consisted of 10 dogs, bled into shock by the Wiggers method. The RL group received fluid equivalent to 5% of body weight followed by return of shed blood. The plasma group received 10 mL/kg of donor plasma plus shed blood. The blood group received shed blood alone. (From Shires T, Coln D, Carrico J, et al: Fluid therapy in hemorrhagic shock. Arch Surg 88:688–693, 1964. Copyright 1964, American Medical Association.)

tated; overall mortality was low (4.3%) and there was no difference between the two groups in the need for postoperative ventilatory support. Because most of the patients in this study were not in shock on admission, the results might not be applicable to patients in severe hemorrhagic shock. Moss and coworkers repeated the study in a group of patients with traumatic shock (systolic arterial pressure 80 mm Hg or need for five or more red blood cell transfusions before surgery) with similar results.[147] Pulmonary edema did not complicate use of colloid or crystalloid in either of these studies. One interesting aspect of these two studies was that similar volumes of colloid and crystalloid were required for resuscitation. This surprising finding may be explained by the use of clinical rather than physiologic end points for fluid resuscitation. Whether the successful outcome with crystalloid resuscitation in these studies is related to replacement of an interstitial fluid deficit or to the limited amount of the infused solution that remains in the circulation has not been ascertained.

The current recommendations of the American College of Surgeons for initial resuscitation of patients with traumatic injury (hemorrhagic shock) include rapid infusion of up to 2 L of RL until hemodynamic stability is restored. Packed red blood cells are then infused if the patient remains unstable. The use of two to four large-bore intravenous lines can compensate for the much more limited volume expansion produced by crystalloids. Complications of fluid infusion with this approach are minimal.[147]

Much more controversial is the choice of fluid in patients with massive bleeding that is difficult to control or in patients who are chronically ill before their acute problem. The potential complications of infusion of large volumes of crystalloid in these settings are discussed later.

SEPTIC SHOCK

Intravascular pooling resulting from an increase in venous capacitance occurs in experimental models of endotoxic shock.[149–151] Decreases in right atrial pressure despite normal blood volume have been documented in patients with septic shock, suggesting that a similar phenomenon may occur in humans.[152]

A close relationship has been demonstrated between plasma volume and CO in patients with septic shock.[153] Hypovolemia is frequently present in patients with severe sepsis and may contribute to the development of hypotension and septic shock. Several factors may contribute to an absolute intravascular volume deficit, including pre-existing illness, decreased fluid intake, increased insensible loss as a consequence of fever, third spacing into the peritoneal cavity in patients with peritonitis, vomiting, diarrhea, and a generalized increase in capillary permeability with resulting interstitial fluid accumulation.

Absolute or relative intravascular volume deficits are associated with inadequate CO and tissue perfusion. Most studies of hemodynamics early in septic shock in humans used baseline measurements made after significant volume resuscitation was accomplished. Rackow and associates evaluated 18 septic shock patients in whom baseline measurements were made before any significant fluid infusion.[154] They found that both the mean PAWP and mean cardiac index were in the low-normal range. Only after the patients underwent fluid resuscitation did the more typical high-CO state become evident. Similar observations have been made in animal experiments.[155]

Repleting intravascular volume by fluid infusion is the most important initial step in resuscitation; this increases venous return, improves CO, and enhances nutrient flow to tissues. Blood volume expansion corrects hypotension and oliguria in almost 50% of septic shock patients.[156]

Improvement of $\dot{D}O_2$ is an important goal in treatment of septic shock. When resuscitation with colloids or crystalloids increases $\dot{D}O_2$, $\dot{V}O_2$ increases and lactic acidosis decreases.[157–160] In severely septic patients without elevated blood lactate levels, fluid-induced increases in $\dot{D}O_2$ are not associated with increases in $\dot{V}O_2$, suggesting that the blood lactate level can predict whether attempts to improve $\dot{D}O_2$ with fluid infusion or other interventions will be effective in increasing $\dot{V}O_2$.[159] Unfortunately, $\dot{D}O_2$ does not predictably increase during fluid resuscitation of septic shock patients. Thirty percent of the patients in the study by Haupt and associates had decreases in $\dot{D}O_2$ secondary to hemodilution, which outweighed the effects of increased CO produced by the fluid infusion.[159] Hemodynamic monitoring with a pulmonary arterial catheter permits calculation of $\dot{D}O_2$ and early detection of this potentially unfavorable response to fluid loading.

Various goals of resuscitation have been proposed, including restoration of normal systemic blood pressure, urine output, or lactate level.[161] Shoemaker and colleagues have suggested that the most important therapeutic goal in critically ill postoperative patients is induction of a hyperdynamic circulation with preset end points for $\dot{D}O_2$ and $\dot{V}O_2$.[162] The authors were able to reach these goals 68% of the time with fluid resuscitation alone.[163]

The potential benefits of improved tissue oxygenation produced by fluid resuscitation must be weighed against the risks of deterioration in pulmonary function. Hemodynamic monitoring with a pulmonary arterial catheter permits rapid fluid infusion while minimizing the possibility of inadvertent circulatory overload. Monitoring of the CVP alone may provide misleading data regarding the ability of the left ventricle to handle a fluid load.[164–166] The CVP may be elevated in septic shock because of acute right ventricular failure at the same time as left-sided preload is decreased.[164, 166] A poor correlation has been reported between the direction and magnitude of changes in CVP and those of the PAWP in septic shock patients.[165]

During fluid resuscitation, the patient's cardiac function curve should be assessed and an "optimal" wedge pressure should be determined at which the CO is either adequate to achieve oxygen transport end points or is maximized, before other therapeutic interventions are considered. In a series of patients in septic shock who underwent fluid resuscitation, Packman and Rackow found that the CO peaked at a PAWP of 12 mm Hg, which is considerably lower than the value (18 mm Hg) usually considered optimal for patients with cardiogenic shock secondary to acute myocardial infarction[165] (Fig. 12–6). The difference may result from a decrease in left ventricular compliance after myocardial infarction.

Whether colloids or crystalloids are preferable for fluid resuscitation of patients with septic syndrome or septic shock remains controversial. Colloid infusion helps maintain the plasma COP, which should aid intravascular fluid retention. However, when microvascular permeability is increased, an oncotic gradient between the intravascular and extravascular compartments may be difficult to maintain.

Crystalloid proponents suggest that infused colloid extravasates into the interstitium of the lung, increasing the interstitial oncotic pressure and producing further extravascular fluid accumulation.[167] Sturm and associates measured extravascular lung water (EVLW) in a sheep septic shock model. Animals resuscitated with Plasmanate had significantly greater amounts of EVLW and a greater degree of pulmonary dysfunction than animals resuscitated with RL solution. The use of a human protein solution in this study complicates interpretation of the data and may explain the

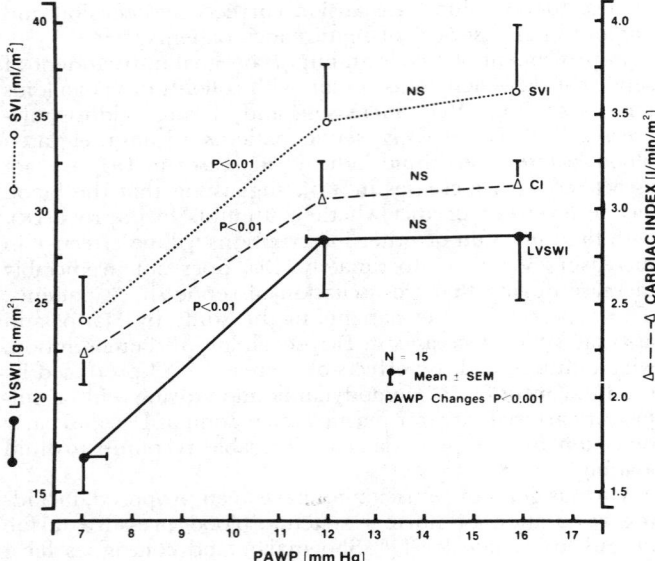

Figure 12–6. Changes in stroke volume index (SVI), left ventricular stroke work index (LVSWI), and cardiac index (CI) as PAWP is increased during fluid resuscitation of patients in septic shock. Note the plateau that occurred at a mean PAWP of 12 mm Hg. (From MI Packman, EC Rackow, Optimum left heart filling pressure during fluid resuscitation of patients with hypovolemic and septic shock, Crit Care Med, 11, 165–169, © by Williams & Wilkins, 1983.)

surprising finding that approximately equal volumes of crystalloid and colloid were required to achieve the same hemodynamic end point.[167, 168]

Crystalloid supporters suggest that decreases in COP during fluid resuscitation do not influence pulmonary water distribution as long as excessive increases in pulmonary capillary pressure do not occur. In an experimental sepsis model, lowering the COP by plasmapheresis while a normal pulmonary capillary hydrostatic pressure was maintained did not exacerbate the pre-existing pulmonary dysfunction.[169]

Colloid advocates believe that there is little clinical evidence that vascular membrane integrity is lost completely in septic shock.[170] Even when sepsis injures the capillary membrane, the basement membrane and interstitial matrix play important roles in preventing fluid movement.[19, 20] Experimental studies provide evidence that early in the course of sepsis, systemic and pulmonary microvascular integrity is intact and a colloid oncotic gradient can be maintained.[171] Altered permeability of the microcirculation may develop as a result of tissue hypoperfusion and ischemia when resuscitation is not initiated promptly. Colloids may permit more rapid resuscitation with significantly smaller infusion volumes and achieve the same hemodynamic end points.[107, 161, 170] Colloid resuscitation in septic shock may be associated with a lower risk of postresuscitation pulmonary edema than crystalloid infusion.[107] Hypoalbuminemia develops in most patients in septic shock; crystalloid resuscitation may exacerbate the fall in the level of this protein and contribute to an increased risk of pulmonary edema formation.[172]

The primary goal of resuscitation of the patient in septic shock is to reverse tissue hypoperfusion and restore hemodynamic stability. Fluid infusion is essential for this purpose; however, some degree of respiratory dysfunction may have to be accepted as an expected and usually manageable side effect.

CARDIOGENIC SHOCK

When cardiogenic shock develops as a complication of acute myocardial infarction, the left ventricular end-diastolic pressure is not necessarily increased above normal. In the classic paper by Forrester and associates in which the four hemodynamic subsets of acute myocardial infarction were described, approximately 15% of the patients had marked decreases in cardiac index (less than 2.2 L/min/m²) with a pulmonary capillary wedge pressure of 18 mm Hg or less (subset III).[173] Most of the patients in this subset have a low stroke volume and compensatory tachycardia. Recognition of patients in this group is important because clinical and metabolic features of hypoperfusion may improve with judicious use of plasma volume expansion.[173–175]

Edwards and colleagues described the clinical features and course of 18 patients with cardiogenic shock secondary to acute myocardial infarction whose initial PAWP was less than 18 mm Hg.[175] All 18 patients had a right atrial pressure that exceeded the PAWP, and 14 of the 18 had electrocardiographic evidence of an inferior wall myocardial infarction. It is likely, therefore, that most of these patients had sustained a right ventricular infarction. The importance of volume resuscitation in this setting was demonstrated by the complete reversal of signs of perfusion failure with volume expansion alone in 7 of the 18 patients.

Hypovolemia may also complicate the management of acute cardiogenic pulmonary edema. A sudden increase in left ventricular end-diastolic pressure (often induced by ischemia) increases the pulmonary capillary wedge pressure and leads to transudation of hypo-oncotic fluid from the intravascular space into the interstitium of the lung and alveoli. Although intravascular volume may occasionally decrease to a level at which perfusion failure and hypotension occur, more commonly these manifestations of shock develop after the pulmonary edema is treated with pharmacologic agents such as morphine and furosemide, which acutely increase venous capacitance.[176, 177] Hemodynamic measurements at this point reveal a low pulmonary capillary wedge pressure associated with a low CO. Despite the presence of clinical signs of pulmonary congestion such as rales and despite pulmonary edema on the chest x-ray film, volume repletion guided by monitoring of pulmonary capillary wedge pressure is a logical and effective therapeutic maneuver.[178] Whether colloids or crystalloids are preferable in this situation has not been evaluated.

ANAPHYLACTIC SHOCK

Anaphylactic syndromes range in severity from mild to fatal. Anaphylactic shock is the most common life-threatening expression of anaphylaxis.[179] It results from vasodilation, peripheral pooling of blood, and increased systemic microvascular permeability. Pulmonary edema is seen on occasion and is caused by altered pulmonary microvascular permeability.[180] If pulmonary edema occurs, the plasma volume deficit is exacerbated. This deficit develops acutely and may be severe. Up to 50% of the plasma volume may leak into the interstitium, with most of the loss occurring within 15 minutes.[179, 181]

The essential components of treatment are sympathomimetics and fluid resuscitation. Because there are no prospective clinical trials comparing colloid to crystalloid in anaphylactic shock, the choice of fluid must be based on experimental studies and anecdotal clinical experience. Anaphylaxis is difficult to study because of its explosive onset, unpredictable severity, and rapid response to treatment. Clinical experience suggests that colloids or crystalloids can be used successfully in mild cases; in severe anaphylaxis, colloids may be more effective in restoring plasma volume and decreasing resuscitation time.[179] When pulmonary edema is present, the increase in pulmonary hydrostatic pressure resulting from fluid infusion may not produce further gas exchange abnormalities as the permeability alteration appears to be a short-lived phenomenon.[180]

FLUID RESUSCITATION IN CONDITIONS ASSOCIATED WITH INCREASED MICROVASCULAR PERMEABILITY

Adult Respiratory Distress Syndrome

An increase in microvascular permeability to both water and macromolecules is characteristic of several clinical conditions, including the septic syndrome, ARDS, burns, anaphylaxis, and certain poisonings. The duration of the permeability alteration may be brief as in anaphylaxis, or it may last for days as in ARDS.[182] Because redistribution of water from the intravascular to the interstitial space is associated with mediator-induced vasodilation, absolute or relative hypovolemia may develop. If it is not treated, it may progress to hypovolemic shock with critical decreases in blood pressure and oxygen transport.

Plasma volume expansion usually reverses hypotension and increases $\dot{D}o_2$ and $\dot{V}o_2$ in hypovolemic shock.[157] These effects not only are important for immediate survival of the patient but also may be major factors in preventing, or decreasing the severity of, later complications of shock including ARDS.[133, 183, 184]

Indications for and choice of resuscitation fluids for patients with established ARDS remain extremely controversial.[185] Under conditions of increased microvascular permeability to water and plasma proteins, the pulmonary microvascular hydrostatic pressure becomes the major determinant of the rate of fluid movement from the intravascular to the interstitial space. The influence of plasma COP on fluid movement decreases as microvascular permeability increases, because the normal oncotic gradient cannot develop. The threshold pressure at which edema formation begins is decreased when permeability is altered, and fluid flux in response to a given pressure gradient is increased.

Animal studies of ARDS have demonstrated that reduction of PAWP is associated with decreased pulmonary edema formation.[186] Sibbald and associates demonstrated a positive association among PAWP, fluid flux, and accumulation of EVLW in patients with ARDS.[187, 188] Simmons and colleagues prospectively evaluated fluid balance in 113 patients with ARDS.[189] Surviving patients lost weight, whereas nonsurvivors gained weight. In addition, survivors had a significantly smaller positive fluid balance than nonsurvivors. However, a cause-and-effect relationship between positive fluid balance and poor outcome was not demonstrated.

Although therapeutic maneuvers (diuresis, fluid restriction) that decrease PAWP might decrease EVLW in ARDS, the decrease in left ventricular end-diastolic volume may also produce decreases in CO and $\dot{D}o_2$. Patients with isolated ARDS may tolerate modest decreases in $\dot{D}o_2$ without developing evidence of tissue hypoperfusion, but this may not be true in critically ill patients with multiple organ system failure. In these patients, attempts are often made to increase $\dot{D}o_2$ with fluids to achieve a hyperdynamic circulation.[162, 163] Increased EVLW is an expected consequence of this approach.

Prospective comparisons of these two markedly different approaches to fluid management of patients with ARDS are, unfortunately, not available. A study by Eisenberg and associates, however, begins to address this issue.[190] In their protocol, hypotensive patients were randomized to two groups. The first group was managed by using routine hemodynamic measurements (PAWP) to guide the use of fluid and/or catecholamines for treatment of hypotension. Therapeutic decisions in the second group were determined by measurements of EVLW. When EVLW was normal, hypotension was treated with volume infusion, regardless of PAWP. When EVLW was increased, fluid infusion was restricted and hypotension was treated with catecholamines, whatever the PAWP. Diuresis was then initiated in patients with increased EVLW when hemodynamic stability was restored. Although overall survival was not improved in the protocol group, there was a significantly better survival rate in patients with elevated EVLW and PAWP less than 18 mm Hg managed by fluid restriction and catecholamine infusion. The results of this study suggest that outcome might be improved by restricting excessive intravascular volume expansion in patients with ARDS.

Until more clinical studies of this difficult issue are available, my approach is to attempt to correct relative or absolute plasma volume deficits with fluid infusion if there is either clinical (decreased urine output, hypotension) or metabolic (increased lactate, $\dot{V}o_2$ dependent on $\dot{D}o_2$) evidence of tissue hypoperfusion. I try to prevent excessive fluid administration by using sequential measurements of CO while PAWP is increased with a fluid challenge.[129]

The choice of colloid or crystalloid in patients with ARDS requiring fluid resuscitation is influenced by their effectiveness in improving peripheral perfusion and by their effects on lung water accumulation. If microvascular membranes are freely permeable to protein and other macromolecules, then the plasma volume–expanding effects of colloids and crystalloids should be similar. However, microvascular leakage is not an all-or-none phenomenon, and an oncotic gradient can be maintained to some extent. Therefore, the degree of retention of a colloid infusion within the intravascular space is influenced by the oncotic properties of the fluid and the functional integrity of the endothelium.

Several animal models have been utilized to study the effects of colloid and crystalloid resuscitation in conditions of altered pulmonary microvascular permeability.[191–193] Unfortunately, in many of these experiments the pulmonary vascular pressures were maintained at low values, which would tend to minimize differences in pulmonary effects of the two types of fluids.[191–193] For example, Pearl and associates used an oleic acid infusion to alter pulmonary microvascular permeability in a canine model.[193] Twenty-four hours later, 25% of the blood volume was removed and the animals were resuscitated with NS, 5% albumin, or 6% hetastarch until CO was within 90% of baseline. Although the authors reported that there was no significant difference in EVLW among the three groups during or 24 hours after resuscitation, it is important to recognize that the mean PAWP was always less than 4 mm Hg in all the groups.

In a similar canine model, Jing and coworkers[191] investigated whether increasing COP with infusion of 25% albumin could decrease EVLW. Attempts were made to "keep the PAWP stable" in animals receiving the albumin solution as well as in a control group receiving RL. EVLW was similar in both groups, providing evidence that colloid infusion does not exacerbate pulmonary dysfunction by leakage into the pulmonary interstitium.

Experimental models that combine altered pulmonary microvascular permeability and a shock state in which fluid is infused to achieve a maximal CO at elevated microvascular hydrostatic pressures are of greater clinical relevance. Finch and associates used a canine model of oleic acid infusion followed by blood removal to induce hemorrhagic shock.[185] After 2 hours of hypotension the shed blood was reinfused, followed by 500 mL of RL, 5% albumin, 6% dextran, or 6%

hetastarch. RL was then infused in all four groups to achieve "optimal hemodynamic performance" (PAWP 12 to 15 mm Hg). EVLW was markedly greater in the RL group than in the 5% albumin and 6% hetastarch groups. In a model of microthromboembolism that leads to moderate increases in pulmonary vascular permeability to fluid and proteins, Schaeffer and colleagues tested the effects of colloids and crystalloids on lung edema under conditions of increased microvascular hydrostatic pressure.[194, 195] They found no differences in lung water among the various fluid groups.

Results of clinical studies comparing colloid and crystalloid resuscitation in patients with ARDS are consistent with the findings in animal models. Appel and colleagues demonstrated that colloids were much more potent plasma volume expanders than twice the volume of crystalloids early in the course of ARDS.[183] In addition, there was no evidence that administration of colloids had a deleterious effect on intrapulmonary shunt or lung function. However, when either colloid or crystalloid was infused within the last 48 hours of life in nonsurviving patients, minimal improvement in hemodynamic and oxygen transport parameters was seen. Hauser and associates compared infusion of 100 mL of 25% albumin with administration of 1000 mL of RL in a prospective randomized crossover study of patients in ARDS.[34] The RL infusion did not increase PAWP significantly, expanded the plasma volume only an average of 194 mL at the completion of infusion (with a rapid decrease subsequently), and did not produce significant increases in blood pressure, CO, $\dot{D}o_2$, or $\dot{V}o_2$. In contrast, 25% albumin produced an average increase in plasma volume of 465 mL, associated with significant increases in blood pressure, CO, $\dot{D}o_2$, and $\dot{V}o_2$. Intrapulmonary shunt did not increase with either fluid.

Metildi and associates compared RL to 5% albumin resuscitation in surgical patients with ARDS. They also concluded that colloid administration did not adversely affect pulmonary function.[196] Most experimental and clinical studies of fluid resuscitation in early ARDS demonstrate that colloid infusion does not adversely affect pulmonary function when compared with crystalloids. Colloids might be more effective than two or more times their volume of crystalloid infusion in increasing $\dot{D}o_2$. Neither colloids nor crystalloids appear to be effective plasma volume expanders in the preterminal phase of ARDS.

NEUROLOGIC INJURY

Little information is available on the effects of colloid or crystalloid administration on cerebral edema formation in normal subjects or in patients with brain injury and decreased intracranial compliance.[197] Hyposmolar solutions, such as 5% dextrose, increase brain water content and intracranial pressure (ICP). Concern exists as to whether resuscitation with hypo-oncotic saline solutions has similar effects on the brain.[197]

Zornow and associates evaluated the acute cerebral effects of changes in plasma osmolarity and plasma COP in normal rabbits with an intact blood-brain barrier.[198] In one group COP was decreased without a change in plasma osmolarity, whereas in a second group a hyposmolar condition was produced without change in the COP. Cerebral edema (as estimated by changes in brain specific gravity) developed only in the hyposmolar group, suggesting that changes in COP do not influence intracranial water distribution in the absence of brain injury (Fig. 12–7).

The unique structural characteristics of the cerebral capillaries (the blood-brain barrier) limit the influence of changes in COP on cerebral water distribution. The intercellular pores of peripheral capillaries are approximately 65

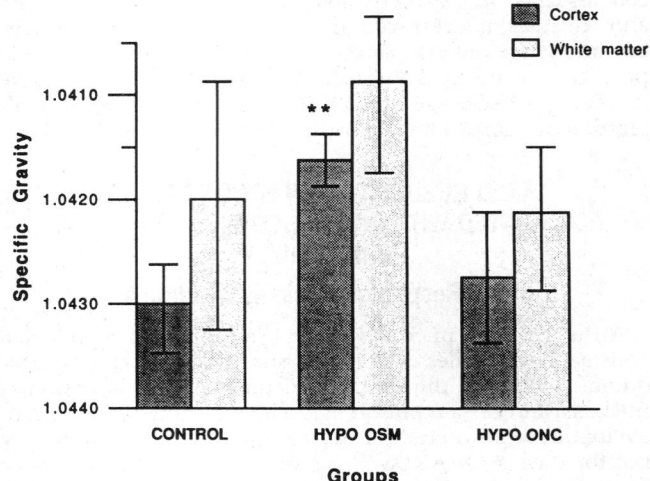

Figure 12–7. Acute cerebral effects of changes in plasma osmolality and oncotic pressure in normal rabbits. The lower the specific gravity, the greater the brain water content. **$P < .01$ vs. other groups. (From Zornow MH, Todd MM, Moore SS: The acute cerebral effects of changes in plasma osmolality and oncotic pressure. Anesthesiology 67:936, 1987.)

Å in diameter. Ionic solutes like sodium and chloride are able to migrate freely between the interstitium and the intravascular space and therefore have no influence on water distribution.[198] High-molecular-weight compounds like albumin and hetastarch are retained in the intravascular space and produce an oncotic gradient that tends to retain water in the capillaries. Because of the small pore size (8 Å) of cerebral capillaries, changes in serum electrolyte content (osmolarity) have significant effects on water movement. An osmotic gradient of 1 mOsm/L produces a hydrostatic gradient of 19.3 mm Hg. Because there are so few protein molecules compared with the number of inorganic ions, their effect is minimal.[199] A 10 mm Hg decrease in COP during crystalloid resuscitation has the same effect on cerebral water distribution as a decrease in serum osmolarity of only 0.5 mOsm/L. Clearly the influence of changes in osmolarity on cerebral water distribution dwarfs the effects of alteration of COP.

If the blood-brain barrier is damaged by traumatic injury, the capillaries become permeable to both proteins and electrolytes; neither osmotic nor oncotic gradients can be established in the region of injury.[197] Under these circumstances, the capillary hydrostatic pressure determines the rate at which edema forms. Several investigators have evaluated the effects of fluid resuscitation in experimental hemorrhagic shock on ICP and cerebral edema in animals with intact blood-brain barriers.[200-202] Although different models were used in these experiments, fluid resuscitation with hypertonic crystalloid solutions was consistently associated with a lower ICP than fluid resuscitation with RL, NS, or 10% dextran 40.[200, 201] Resuscitation with 6% hetastarch was associated with significantly lower ICP than resuscitation with RL.[202]

The results obtained in these studies are not unexpected, because hypertonic saline would be expected to shift water from the intracellular to the extracellular space. RL is a hyposmolar solution and 6% hetastarch is iso-osmolar, and the different effects of these solutions on ICP can be explained by the differences in their osmolarity.

The lower ICP after resuscitation with hypertonic crystalloid solutions is potentially advantageous for restoration of cerebral blood flow and $\dot{D}o_2$. However, Prough and associates found decreased cerebral blood flow and $\dot{D}O_2$ in animals resuscitated from hemorrhagic shock with 7.5% saline or RL, despite significantly lower ICPs in the 7.5% saline group.[203]

Ducey and associates used somatosensory evoked potentials to evaluate the effects of fluid resuscitation in hemorrhagic shock on neurologic function.[204] Swine were given 7.5% saline in 6% dextran 70, 6% hetastarch, or NS. Despite a significantly lower ICP in the hypertonic saline group, cerebral perfusion pressure was significantly greater in the 6% hetastarch group than in the other two groups. Neurologic function was also better in the hetastarch group, suggesting that restoration of cerebral perfusion pressure with fluid resuscitation is a more important goal than any isolated effect on ICP. The vasodilatory effect of hypertonic saline may have resulted in a lower mean arterial pressure than was produced by hetastarch.

Patients with severe traumatic injury often require resuscitation with large volumes of intravenous fluid to restore hemodynamic stability. When a significant head injury is also present, concern exists as to whether the choice of fluid for resuscitation can contribute to the development of cerebral edema.

Gunnar and associates compared the effects of fluid resuscitation with NS, 10% dextran 40, and 3% saline in a dog model of hemorrhagic shock combined with a space-occupying cerebral lesion.[205] The animals resuscitated with NS and 10% dextran 40 had four- to sevenfold ICP elevations, whereas the animals resuscitated with hypertonic saline maintained a normal ICP.

Wisner and colleagues compared 6.5% saline to RL for resuscitation from hemorrhagic shock in rats with a unilateral percussive injury to the brain.[206] Brain water was significantly reduced in areas of uninjured brain in animals resuscitated with the hypertonic saline, but the hypertonic saline had no effect on the degree of water accumulation in areas of injured brain where the blood-brain barrier was damaged.

COMPLICATIONS OF FLUID RESUSCITATION
Pulmonary Edema

Patients who develop pulmonary edema during or after resuscitation from circulatory shock have a significantly higher mortality rate than those who do not develop this complication.[3] One of the most controversial aspects of the colloid versus crystalloid controversy is whether the choice of fluid used for resuscitation of the critically ill influences the incidence and severity of pulmonary edema. This has been a difficult question to answer, as problems exist with both experimental and clinical studies. The use of an animal model has several major advantages, including access to tissues for direct measurement of water content and the ability to control several of the potential variables. However, there are many major disadvantages, including species differences in the response to hemorrhagic shock; different study designs with different severities and duration of shock, making comparisons difficult; and the use of animals without the concurrent diseases, which may have a major impact on the way humans respond to shock and fluid resuscitation. It has also been suggested that subconscious bias by experienced animal researchers can lead to selection of animals more likely to survive regardless of the experimental protocol.[3]

Problems abound with clinical studies as well, including the use of fixed fluid volumes independent of clinical response and variability in severity of shock, resuscitation times, and end points of resuscitation.

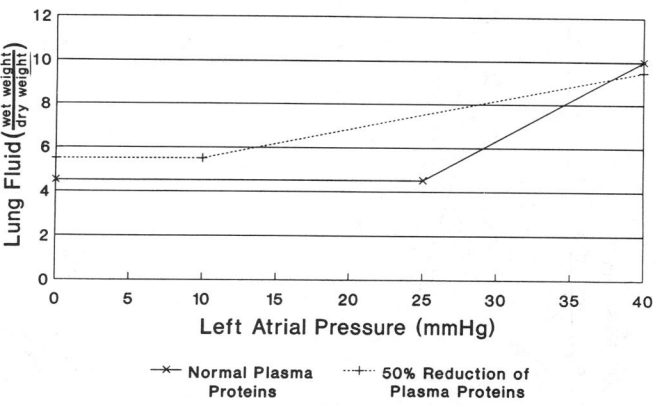

Figure 12–8. The "critical" left atrial pressure at which lung water begins to accumulate was approximately 25 mm Hg when plasma protein levels were normal and decreased to 11 mm Hg when the plasma protein level was reduced 50% by plasmapheresis. (Modified from Guyton AC, Lindsey AW: Effect of elevated left atrial pressure and decreased plasma protein concentration on the development of pulmonary edema. Circ Res 7:649–657, 1959. Reproduced with permission. Copyright 1959 American Heart Association.)

A problem common to both experimental and clinical studies is the method used to determine the degree of lung damage. There is no consensus about the most appropriate way to assess fluid-induced pulmonary dysfunction. Measurements of intrapulmonary shunt fraction, alveolar-arterial oxygen gradient, static pulmonary compliance, PaO_2, need for mechanical ventilation, and EVLW have all been utilized, as have sequential chest x-ray films.[207, 208] All of these have their limitations. Sibbald and associates found no correlation between measurement of EVLW and calculated intrapulmonary shunt fraction in patients with pulmonary edema, and Brigham and colleagues found a similar lack of correlation between EVLW and the alveolar-arterial oxygen gradient in patients with ARDS.[209, 210] EVLW may be statistically increased with no clinically significant effect on gas exchange, and the difficulty of assessing the presence and quantity of lung water with portable chest x-ray films limits their usefulness for research. With these limitations in mind, I review some of the more important work in this area.

Guyton and Lindsey studied the effects of increasing left atrial pressure by use of an aortic clamp and decreasing plasma COP by plasmapheresis on the dynamics of fluid exchange in a canine model.[211] They found a critical value for left atrial pressure of 25 mm Hg, above which transudation of fluid into the lungs would begin. After the plasma protein concentration was reduced approximately 50%, the critical pressure was reduced to 11 mm Hg (Fig. 12–8). The results of this study suggested that the decrease in COP produced a direct and equal decrease in the critical pulmonary capillary pressure and that the changes in pulmonary microvascular fluid flux could be explained completely by the balance between the intravascular Starling forces. These findings produced interest in using the COP-PAWP gradient to predict the risk of pulmonary edema in patients.[212–214]

Rackow and colleagues also used a canine model to evaluate the effects of fluid resuscitation on lung water accumulation in animals made hypoproteinemic by plasmapheresis.[215] After completion of plasmapheresis to obtain a plasma COP less than 40% of baseline, animals were resuscitated with NS, 5% albumin, or 6% hetastarch until the PAWP was increased to 10 mm Hg above the postplasmapheresis baseline (final PAWP 15 to 17 mm Hg). The PAWP was maintained at this level by fluid infusion for the next 5 hours. In addition to gross evidence of systemic edema in the crystalloid group, EVLW was significantly increased and

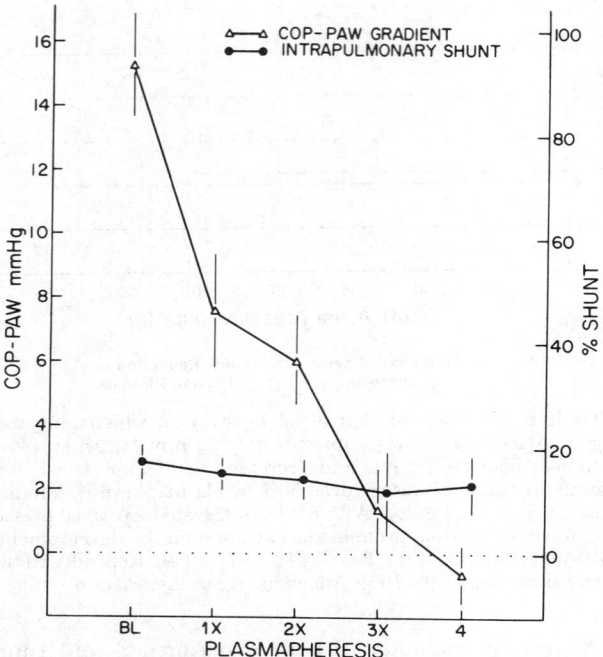

Figure 12-9. Effect of decreased COP-PAWP gradient on intrapulmonary shunt in healthy baboons. (From Zarins CK, Rice CL, Peters RM, et al: Lymph and pulmonary response to isobaric reduction in plasma oncotic pressure in baboons. Circ Res 43:925, 1978.)

oxygenation was significantly decreased. Similar results were reported by McKeen and coworkers for a sheep model of hemorrhagic shock.[216] In this study, blood was removed to produce hypotension and then either NS or autologous plasma was infused to restore systolic blood pressure to baseline. Shed blood was not administered. Lung lymph flow and EVLW were significantly greater in the saline-resuscitated animals. The pulmonary microvascular hydrostatic pressure was 50% above baseline after saline resuscitation but only 20% above baseline after plasma infusion. Both of these studies combine a hypo-oncotic state with elevation of pulmonary capillary hydrostatic pressure by fluid administration.

In contrast, Zarins and associates evaluated the effects of an isolated reduction in plasma COP on lung fluid dynamics.[217] In baboons, plasma COP was reduced 76% by plasmapheresis while baseline PAWP (4 to 6 mm Hg) was maintained by infusion of RL. Although the plasma COP decreased below the PAWP (a negative COP-PAWP gradient), there was no significant change in pulmonary function, as assessed by measurement of intrapulmonary shunt or airway pressures (Fig. 12-9). There was, however, a sevenfold increase in lung lymph flow with a decrease in the protein content of the lymph. On postmortem examination, there was no gross or microscopic evidence of pulmonary edema, although marked peripheral edema and ascites were present. Similar findings were reported by Holcroft and Trunkey in a baboon model of hemorrhagic shock.[218] In this study, hemorrhagic shock was produced by blood removal and animals were then resuscitated with return of shed blood and RL to return the PAWP to preshock values (5 ± 2 mm Hg). Despite infusion of large volumes of RL and significant decreases in the blood albumin level, EVLW remained within normal limits.

On the basis of these experimental results, it can be concluded that an isolated decrease in plasma COP in the presence of intact pulmonary safety factors may not result in pulmonary edema even when the COP-PAWP gradient is markedly decreased.

In general, clinical studies support the experimental findings. Da Luz and associates evaluated 26 patients with acute myocardial infarction, of whom 14 developed pulmonary edema.[213] Patients with pulmonary edema had higher PAWPs and lower plasma COPs than patients without pulmonary edema. The COP-PAWP gradient was decreased from the normal range of 9 to 17 mm Hg to an average of 1.2 mm Hg in patients with pulmonary edema but averaged 9.7 mm Hg in the patients without pulmonary edema. These authors found that the COP-PAWP gradient was a more sensitive index for predicting pulmonary edema than measurement of the PAWP alone. Other clinical studies have substantiated that when decreases in plasma COP are combined with elevated or high normal PAWP, pulmonary edema is a likely consequence.[107, 212, 214]

Rackow and colleagues evaluated the cardiopulmonary effects of colloids and crystalloids during resuscitation of patients in hypovolemic shock (many of whom were septic).[107] Patients were randomized to receive NS, 5% albumin, or 6% hetastarch, infused to achieve and maintain a PAWP of 15 mm Hg for 24 hours. It required two to four times as much crystalloid as colloid to reach and maintain this PAWP. The COP-PAWP gradient decreased to less than 4 mm Hg for the 24-hour postresuscitation period in the NS group but was only minimally decreased in the two colloid groups. Radiologic evidence of pulmonary edema developed in 75% of the NS group compared to only 22% in each of the colloid groups.

Several other studies, however, have questioned the importance of the COP-PAWP gradient as a prognostic indicator for development of pulmonary edema.[4, 219, 220] Sise and associates did not find a correlation between intrapulmonary shunt fraction and the lowest COP-PAWP gradient in critically ill surgical patients.[219] Rafferty and coworkers also did not find a significant relationship between the COP-PAWP gradient and pulmonary edema estimated by either chest roentgenogram or intrapulmonary shunt fraction in a series of 17 patients admitted postoperatively to a surgical critical care unit.[220]

Virgilio and coworkers compared the effects of RL and 5% albumin for fluid maintenance during and after aortic reconstructive surgery.[4] Hemodynamic and clinical end points were used to determine the quantity of fluid infused. Twice as much RL as 5% albumin was required on the operative day. The plasma COP decreased 40% and the COP-PAWP gradient decreased 80% compared with preoperative values in the RL group, but no significant changes occurred in the 5% albumin group. This decrease in COP-PAWP gradient was entirely secondary to a fall in the COP as the PAWP did not change from its preoperative value of 10 mm Hg. The postoperative intrapulmonary shunt fraction did not differ between the two groups, and there was no relationship between this value and the COP-PAWP gradient.

Similar results were reported by Shires and colleagues when comparing RL with Plasmanate for fluid maintenance during major vascular surgery.[221] Despite large decreases in COP and COP-PAWP gradient in the RL group, EVLW was not increased.

Based on the available clinical studies, the following conclusions can be made: (1) when the PAWP is above the normal range, pulmonary edema is more likely to occur if the plasma COP is decreased; (2) when the PAWP is normal, pulmonary edema is unlikely regardless of plasma COP, if the decrease in COP is acute and the patient was previously healthy and therefore has sufficient albumin stores to allow rapid restoration of plasma protein levels; (3) pulmonary

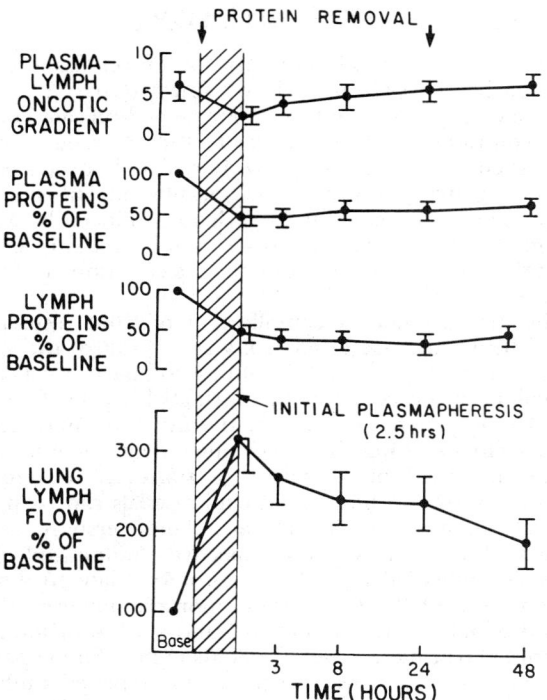

Figure 12–10. Effect of sustained decrease in plasma protein concentration produced by repeated plasmapheresis on lung lymph flow at 48 hours, despite re-establishment of a normal plasma-lymph oncotic gradient. (Adapted from Demling RH, Harms B, Kramer G, et al: Acute versus sustained hypoproteinemia and posttraumatic pulmonary edema. Surgery 92:79, 1982.)

edema may occur when the PAWP is normal, if plasma COP is decreased and the patient is chronically ill and therefore has depleted protein stores. These patients have sustained decreases in plasma and interstitial COP and more limited defenses against pulmonary edema formation.[212]

Experimental support for the last two conclusions is provided by Demling and associates.[19, 20] These investigators used an unanesthetized sheep model to evaluate the effects of acute and sustained decreases in plasma COP on pulmonary microvascular fluid flux. Acute decreases in plasma COP were produced by plasmapheresis, combined with infusion of RL to maintain CVP and CO. Sustained decreases in plasma COP were accomplished in a second group of sheep by intermittent plasmapheresis during a 24-hour period. In the acute study, lung lymph flow was significantly increased immediately after plasmapheresis when the plasma-lymph oncotic gradient was maximally decreased. However, despite re-establishment of a normal gradient after 8 hours, lung lymph flow remained elevated for an additional 8 hours before returning to baseline at 24 hours. When a sustained reduction in COP was induced by repeated plasmapheresis, pulmonary lymph flow remained significantly increased for 24 to 36 hours after the Starling forces returned to baseline (Fig. 12–10). Because lung lymph flow (as a measure of increased intravascular-to-interstitial fluid flux) remained elevated despite return of the Starling forces to baseline and microvascular permeability was not altered, as indicated by a low lymph protein content, the authors suggested that the decrease in interstitial oncotic pressure produced by hypoproteinemia altered the capillary filtration coefficient (K_f), augmenting the movement of water from the capillaries to the interstitium. These results may be due to an increase in the size of the endothelial pores resulting from decreased albumin binding or to increased interstitial

compliance caused by protein depletion and gel hydration. The relatively rapid return of the rate of lung lymph flow to normal after acute and nonsustained decreases in plasma COP demonstrates the effectiveness of mechanisms available to the lung to prevent pulmonary edema. These findings may help explain why clinical studies of acute plasma COP decreases, such as those in trauma patients, do not support the value of maintaining plasma COP for preventing pulmonary edema, whereas studies of chronically ill patients do. When a chronically hypoproteinemic patient requires fluid resuscitation, the full complement of pulmonary defenses against edema formation is no longer available and pulmonary edema is more likely.

Systemic Edema

Systemic edema is quite common in critically ill patients. Fluid resuscitation is one factor that contributes to edema. Organs that may become edematous include the intestines, heart, brain, skin, muscle, and fat. Until recently, the colloid versus crystalloid controversy revolved around issues of cost, efficacy (primarily evaluated by hemodynamic effects), and cardiopulmonary side effects. Although some groups were concerned about renal function, for the most part the adverse effects of fluid resuscitation on the systemic organs were not well studied because of the general belief that systemic edema was merely a cosmetic problem.[222, 223]

Some studies suggest that systemic edema may not be entirely benign.[224, 225] Because infusion of large volumes of crystalloid for resuscitation of the patient in shock is invariably associated with a much greater degree of systemic edema than administration of colloids, any influence of systemic edema on hospital cost, morbidity, or mortality may add fuel to the colloid versus crystalloid controversy.

The soft tissues (skin, fat, muscle) are the major sites of fluid retention during crystalloid resuscitation. In an experimental model that simulated the use of a massive volume of crystalloids for treatment of acute plasma loss, Pappova and coworkers demonstrated that 25% of the fluid was retained within fat tissue, 25% within muscle, and 37% within the skin.[226]

Heughan and associates investigated the potential significance of soft tissue edema by evaluating the effects of mild saline solution overload on soft tissue oxygenation.[225] After infusion of only 2.5 mL/kg, a dramatic and statistically significant decrease in tissue oxygen tension was detected in a rabbit model. Because arterial oxygen tension remained stable and changes in hematocrit were minimal, the most likely explanation for this observation was increases in intercapillary distances produced by tissue edema. After saline infusion of 10 mL/kg, it took 3.5 days for tissue oxygen tensions to return to baseline.

Critically ill patients may remain in positive water balance (with resultant soft tissue edema) for prolonged periods after traumatic or surgical injury and sepsis, even when cardiac and renal functions are normal.[227] Gump and associates documented delayed water excretion that persisted for 8 to 22 days in 6 of 20 patients resuscitated predominantly with crystalloid solutions.[227]

Soft tissue edema–induced increases in the oxygen diffusion distance to active cells have several potentially important clinical implications: (1) wound healing may be adversely affected as lower tissue oxygen tensions inhibit collagen formation and epithelialization of wounds;[228, 229] (2) tensile strength of sutured wounds may be decreased;[230] (3) leukocyte bactericidal activity may be decreased, which could increase the risk of wound infection;[231, 232] (4) anaerobic metabolism may persist despite restoration of oxygen transport to normal levels. Few clinical data have not demonstrated a causal relationship between edema and stasis ulceration, although they are commonly seen together.[233] Controlled experimental or clinical comparisons of the effects of colloid versus crystalloid resuscitation on soft tissue oxygen tensions, wound healing, and wound infection are unfortunately not available.

Crystalloid infusion produces peripheral edema by lowering the COP to a greater extent than it decreases the interstitial oncotic pressure, while the capillary hydrostatic pressure is increasing. This unbalancing of the Starling forces favors outward fluid flux. In addition, a change in K_f caused by the acute decrease in plasma and interstitial COP may play a much more significant role in development of soft tissue edema than its previously described effects on lung fluid flux.[19, 20]

Harms and colleagues evaluated the effects of acute decreases in COP on soft tissue edema formation in a sheep model.[19] Peak increase in lymph flow occurred 2.5 hours after plasmapheresis at a time when the oncotic gradient between the intravascular and interstitial spaces was maximal. Even though a normal gradient was re-established 24 hours after plasmapheresis, soft tissue lymph flow remained elevated for the remainder of the 72-hour study period. Significantly, when plasma was reinfused and plasma COP returned to normal, lymph flow returned rapidly to baseline even though the oncotic gradient did not change (as interstitial COP also increased).

The gastrointestinal system may also be adversely affected by hypoproteinemia. A correlation exists between hypoalbuminemia, gut edema, and intolerance of enteral nutrition.[224, 234] In a preliminary report, Brinson and associates found that 12 of 35 patients studied prospectively in a medical critical care unit had diarrhea.[234] The mean serum albumin concentration of the patients with diarrhea was only 1.90 ± 0.14 (SEM) g/dL, which was significantly lower than the mean level of 3.40 ± 0.12 (SEM) g/dL in patients without diarrhea. Cobb and associates reported that all patients with a serum albumin level of less than 3 g/dL could not tolerate full-strength tube feeding, whereas all patients with an albumin level above 4 g/dL tolerated enteral nutrition without difficulty.[235]

Severe decreases in serum albumin level and COP can produce intestinal wall edema with associated disruption of normal villous structure.[236, 237] Milder hypo-oncotic states can increase intestinal interstitial pressure enough to interfere with passive water absorption from the intraluminal space, producing diarrhea. The accumulation of fluid within the bowel can produce a reflex decrease in bowel motility and subsequent ileus.[238] Both the intestinal edema and decreased motility may improve after administration of albumin.[237] However, controlled clinical trials evaluating this issue are not available.

Experimental and clinical studies provide evidence that the presence of nutrients in the gastrointestinal tract has a trophic effect on mucosal integrity and that failure to provide or inability to tolerate enteral nutrition may be associated with bacterial translocation through the epithelial mucosa into mesenteric lymph nodes or a greater incidence of septic complications.[238, 239] Gut mucosal failure has been postulated to be the initiating event for development of the multiple organ system failure syndrome.[239, 240]

Clearly, more work needs to be done in this field. However, if crystalloid resuscitation is associated with decreased ability to tolerate enteral feeding and if this decreased ability is associated with increased risk of sepsis and multiple organ system failure, the clinical implications are significant and obvious.

OTHER COMPLICATIONS

Adverse effects of albumin infusion on renal and cardiac function have been reported by a few groups.[63, 222, 223, 241, 242] In most cases, these results have not been duplicated or have been contradicted by the work of other investigators.[107, 131] In particular, studies done by Lucas and associates that report negative inotropic effects of albumin infusion most likely reflect iatrogenic fluid overload produced by a study design that attempted to restore serum albumin levels to normal after adequate volume resuscitation had been achieved.[63, 222, 241]

The most significant complication of fluid resuscitation would be an increase in mortality as a result of the specific fluid administered. Clinical studies comparing colloids to crystalloids rarely comment on mortality because of the small number of patients in each study and the multiplicity of other factors that may influence outcome in the critically ill. Velanovich used meta-analysis (a statistical technique in which data from a number of clinical trials can be pooled) to evaluate mortality in clinical colloid versus crystalloid studies.[5] Data from eight prospective randomized clinical trials that included mortality rates were analyzed. Overall, there were a 12.3% difference in mortality favoring the use of crystalloids in trauma patients and a 7.8% difference in mortality favoring the use of colloids in nontrauma patients. Although one can easily criticize this type of study, the results support the concept that the best resuscitation fluid may vary with the clinical circumstance.

Another important consideration in fluid resuscitation is its cost. Natural and artificial colloids are considerably more expensive than crystalloids. At Tisch University Hospital in April 1991, costs were $0.65 to $0.85 per liter of crystalloid, $52 for 500 mL of 5% albumin, and $48 for 500 mL of 6% hetastarch. Because albumin is a human blood product, its supply and therefore its price are more variable than those of the other fluids. For example, the price projected for 500 mL of 5% albumin in September 1991 is $76 to $80. Although fluid cost is clearly greater when colloid resuscitation is utilized, it is uncertain whether the use of colloids adversely affects the overall expense of hospitalization. For example, resuscitation from shock may be more rapidly and completely accomplished with colloid infusion, and this may result in a decreased incidence of costly complications of shock such as ARDS.[133]

Resuscitation with crystalloids results in greater weight gain and increased systemic edema formation. If this, for example, results in a 24-hour prolongation of hospital stay or the need to use parenteral rather than enteral nutrition, any economic benefits of crystalloid use are lost.

CONCLUSIONS

Restoration of plasma volume, CO, and $\dot{D}o_2$ is of primary importance during resuscitation of patients with shock secondary to, or exacerbated by, hypovolemia. In many clinical circumstances the choice of fluid may be less important than the skill employed to ensure rapid and complete resuscitation. Appropriate use of invasive hemodynamic monitoring and fluid challenge helps the clinician optimize tissue perfusion while minimizing the risks of fluid overload.

It has been suggested that the type of fluid used for resuscitation may have a minimal influence on the patient's outcome and represent a tossup situation.[243] The failure of multiple experimental and clinical trials to indicate a clear winner may mean that there is no winner. I do not agree with that suggestion. I believe it is generalization of the conclusions of clinical trials with totally different populations of patients that has made the subject so controversial. For example, it seems clear that the young and previously healthy trauma patient can be resuscitated successfully with either type of fluid, and because no benefit has been demonstrated with the more expensive colloids, crystalloids would be preferable in this circumstance. However, adequate crystalloid resuscitation may be more difficult to accomplish in older, debilitated patients, particularly if attempts are made to achieve hyperdynamic end points that may be associated with improved morbidity and mortality.[34, 107, 162, 163]

As we enter the 1990s new issues have replaced the old in the colloid versus crystalloid controversy. Interest has shifted away from the lung to other organs. Hypertonic solutions with or without the addition of colloids are being evaluated. Hetastarch derivatives that may "seal" capillary leaks are being investigated. The controversy is likely to remain.

References

1. Shoemaker WC: Comparison of the relative effectiveness of whole blood transfusions and various types of fluid therapy in resuscitation. Crit Care Med 4:71, 1976.
2. Shires GT, Canizaro PC: Fluid resuscitation in the severely injured. Surg Clin North Am 53:1341, 1973.
3. Shoemaker WC, Hauser CJ: Critique of crystalloid versus colloid therapy in shock and shock lung. Crit Care Med 7:117, 1979.
4. Virgilio RW, Rice CL, Smith DE, et al: Crystalloid vs. colloid resuscitation: Is one better? Surgery 85:129, 1979.
5. Velanovich V: Crystalloid versus colloid fluid resuscitation: A meta-analysis of mortality. Surgery 105:65, 1989.
6. Harrison N, Darrow D, Yannet H: The total electrolyte content of animals and its probable relation to distribution of body water. J Biol Chem 113:515, 1936.
7. Gamble J, Ross G, Tisdall F: The metabolism of fixed base during fasting. J Biol Chem 57:633, 1923.
8. Landis EM, Pappenheimer JR: Exchanges of substances through capillary walls. In: Field J (ed): Handbook of Physiology, Section 2, Circulation, Volume 2. American Physiological Society, Washington, DC, p 961, 1963.
9. Weil MH, Henning RJ, Puri VK: Colloid oncotic pressure: Clinical significance. Crit Care Med 7:113, 1979.
10. Morissette MP: Colloid osmotic pressure: Its measurement and clinical value. Can Med Assoc J 116:897, 1977.
11. Weil MH, Morissette M, Michaels S, et al: Routine plasma colloid osmotic pressure measurements. Crit Care Med 2:229, 1974.
12. Weil MH, Michaels S, Puri VK, et al: The stat laboratory: Facilitating blood gas and biochemical measurements for the critically ill and injured. Am J Clin Pathol 76:34, 1981.
13. Rackow EC, Fein IA, Leppo J: Colloid osmotic pressure as a prognostic indicator of pulmonary edema and mortality in the critically ill. Chest 72:709, 1977.
14. Starling EH: On the absorption of fluids from the connective tissue spaces. J Physiol (Lond) 9:312, 1896.
15. Pappenheimer JR, Soto-Rivera A: Effective osmotic pressure of the plasma proteins and other quantities associated with the capillary circulation in the hind limbs of cats and dogs. Am J Physiol 152:471, 1948.
16. Meyer BJ, Meyer A, Guyton A: Interstitial fluid pressure. Clin Res 22:263, 1968.
17. Guyton AC, Granger HJ, Taylor AE: Interstitial fluid pressure. Physiol Rev 51:527, 1971.
18. Granger JH: Role of the interstitial matrix and lymphatic pump in regulation of transvascular fluid balance. Microvasc Res 18:207, 1979.
19. Harms BA, Kramer GC, Bodal BI, et al: Effect of hypoproteinemia on pulmonary and soft tissue edema formation. Crit Care Med 9:503, 1981.
20. Demling RH, Harms B, Kramer G, et al: Acute versus sustained hypoproteinemia and posttraumatic pulmonary edema. Surgery 92:79, 1982.
21. Peters RM, Hargens AR: Protein vs. electrolytes and all of the Starling forces. Arch Surg 116:1293, 1981.
22. Wittmers LE, Bartlett M, Johnson JA: Estimation of capillary permeability coefficient of inulin in various tissues of the rabbit. Microvasc Res 11:67, 1976.
23. Allen SJ, Drake RE, Williams JP, et al: Recent advances in pulmonary edema. Crit Care Med 15:963, 1987.
24. Civetta JM: A new look at the Starling equation. Crit Care Med 7:84, 1979.
25. Crandall ED, Staub NC, Goldberg HS, et al: Recent developments in pulmonary edema. Ann Intern Med 99:808, 1983.
26. Levine OR, Mellins RB, Senior RM, et al: The application of Starling's law of capillary exchange to the lungs. J Clin Invest 46:934, 1967.
27. Taylor AE, Parker JC, Kvietys PR, et al: The pulmonary interstitium in capillary exchange. Ann NY Acad Sci 384:146, 1982.
28. Goldberg HS: Pulmonary interstitial compliance and microvascular filtration coefficient. Am J Physiol 239:H189, 1980.
29. Granger HS, Dhar J, Chen HI: Structure and function of the interstitium. In: Sgouris JT, Rene A (eds): Proceedings of the Workshop in Albumin. Bethesda, National Institutes of Health, p 114, 1975.
30. Bhattacharya J, Gropper MA, Staub NC: Interstitial fluid pressure gradient measured by micropuncture in excised dog lung. J Appl Physiol 56:271, 1984.
31. Demling RH: Lung fluid and protein dynamics during hemorrhagic shock, resuscitation and recovery. Circ Shock 7:149, 1980.
32. Demling RH, Manohar M, Will JA, et al: The effect of plasma oncotic pressure on the pulmonary microcirculation after hemorrhagic shock. Surgery 86:323, 1979.
33. Cervera AL, Moss G: Dilutional re-expansion with crystalloid after massive hemorrhage: Saline versus balanced electrolyte solution for maintenance of normal blood volume and arterial pH. J Trauma 15:498, 1975.
34. Hauser CJ, Shoemaker WC, Turpin I, et al: Oxygen transport responses to colloids and crystalloids in critically ill surgical patients. Surg Gynecol Obstet 150:811, 1980.
35. Lamke LO, Liljedahl SO: Plasma volume changes after infusion of various plasma expanders. Resuscitation 5:93, 1976.
36. Lowery BD, Cloutier CT, Carey LC: Electrolyte solutions in resuscitation in human hemorrhagic shock. Surg Gynecol Obstet 133:273, 1971.
37. Canizaro PC, Prager MD, Shires GT: The infusion of Ringer's lactate solution during shock: Changes in lactate, excess lactate and pH. Am J Surg 122:494, 1971.
38. Velasco IT, Pontieri V, Rocha E, et al: Hyperosmotic NaCl and severe hemorrhagic shock. Am J Physiol 239:H664, 1980.
39. Wildenthal K, Mierzviak DS, Mitchell JH: Acute effects of increased serum osmolarity on left ventricular performance. Am J Physiol 216:898, 1969.
40. Gazitua S, Scott JB, Swindall B, et al: Resistance responses to local changes in plasma osmolality in three vascular beds. Am J Physiol 220:384, 1971.
41. Younes RN, Aun F, Tomida RM, et al: The role of lung innervation in the hemodynamic response to hypertonic sodium chloride solutions in hemorrhagic shock. Surgery 98:900, 1985.
42. Lopes OU, Pontieri V, Rocha E, et al: Hyperosmotic NaCl and severe hemorrhagic shock: Role of the innervated lung. Am J Physiol 241:H883, 1981.
43. Monafo WW, Chuntrasakul C, Ayvazian VH: Hypertonic sodium solutions in the treatment of burn shock. Am J Surg 126:778, 1973.
44. Jelenko C, Williams JB, Wheeler ML, et al: Studies in shock and resuscitation, 1: Use of a hypertonic, albumin-containing, fluid demand regimen (HALFD) in resuscitation. Crit Care Med 7:157, 1979.
45. Maningas PA, Bellamy RF: Hypertonic sodium chloride solutions for the prehospital management of traumatic hemorrhagic shock: A possible improvement in the standard of care? Ann Emerg Med 15:1411, 1986.
46. De Felippe J, Timoner J, Velasco IT, et al: Treatment of refractory hypovolemic shock by 7.5% sodium chloride injections. Lancet 2:1002, 1980.
47. Holcroft JW, Vassar MJ, Turner JE, et al: 3% NaCl and 7.5% NaCl/dextran 70 in the resuscitation of severely injured patients. Ann Surg 206:279, 1987.
48. Shackford SR, Fortlage DA, Peters RM, et al: Serum osmolar and electrolyte changes associated with large infusions of hypertonic sodium lactate for intravascular volume expansion of patients undergoing aortic reconstruction. Surg Gynecol Obstet 164:127, 1987.
49. Shackford SR, Sise MJ, Fridlund PH, et al: Hypertonic sodium lactate versus lactated Ringer's solution for intravenous fluid therapy in operations on the abdominal aorta. Surgery 94:41, 1983.
50. Vassar MJ, Perry CA, Holcroft JW: Analysis of potential risks associated with 7.5% sodium chloride resuscitation of traumatic shock. Arch Surg 125:1309, 1990.
51. Gross D, Landau EH, Klin B, et al: Treatment of uncontrolled hemorrhagic shock with hypertonic saline solution. Surg Gynecol Obstet 170:106, 1990.
52. Mattar JA: Hypertonic and hyperoncotic solutions in patients. Crit Care Med 17:297, 1989.
53. Rothschild MA, Oratz M, Schreiber SS: Albumin synthesis. N Engl J Med 286:748, 1972.
54. Tullis JL: Albumin: 1. Background and use. JAMA 237:355, 1977.
55. Lewis RT: Albumin: Role and discriminative use in surgery. Can J Surg 23:322, 1980.
56. Rothschild MA, Bauman A, Yalow RS, et al: Tissue distribution of I[131] labeled human serum albumin following intravenous administration. J Clin Invest 34:1354, 1955.
57. Thompson WL: Rational use of albumin and plasma substitutes. Johns Hopkins Med J 136:220, 1975.
58. Rothschild MA, Oratz M, Evans CD, et al: Role of hepatic interstitial albumin in regulating albumin synthesis. Am J Physiol 210:57, 1966.
59. Lundsgaard-Hansen P, Pappova E: Component therapy of surgical hemorrhage: Red cells, plasma substitutes and albumin. Ann Clin Res 13(suppl 33):26, 1981.

60. Rainey TG, English JF: Pharmacology of colloids and crystalloids. In: Chernow B (ed): The Pharmacologic Approach to the Critically Ill Patient. Baltimore, Williams & Wilkins, p 219, 1988.

61. Beecher HK: Preparation of battle casualties for surgery. Ann Surg 121:769, 1945.

62. Ring J, Messmer K: Incidence and severity of anaphylactoid reactions to colloid volume substitutes. Lancet 1:466, 1977.

63. Dahn MS, Lucas CE, Ledgerwood AM, et al: Negative inotropic effect of albumin resuscitation for shock. Surgery 86:235, 1979.

64. Kovalik SG, Ledgerwood AM, Lucas CE, et al: The cardiac effect of altered calcium homeostasis after albumin resuscitation. J Trauma 21:275, 1981.

65. Johnson SD, Lucas CE, Gerrick SJ, et al: Altered coagulation after albumin supplements for treatment of oligemic shock. Arch Surg 114:379, 1979.

66. Lucas CE, Ledgerwood AM, Mammen EF: Altered coagulation protein content after albumin resuscitation. Ann Surg 196:198, 1982.

67. Cogbill TH, Moore EE, Dunn EL, et al: Coagulation changes after albumin resuscitation. Crit Care Med 9:22, 1981.

68. Falk JL, Rackow EC, Fein IA, et al: The effect of hetastarch, albumin and saline resuscitation on coagulation in shock patients. Crit Care Med 11:219, 1983.

69. Emerson TE: Unique features of albumin: A brief review. Crit Care Med 17:690, 1989.

70. Holt ME, Ryall ME, Campbell AK: Albumin inhibits human polymorphonuclear leucocyte luminol-dependent chemiluminescence: Evidence for oxygen radical scavenging. Br J Exp Pathol 65:231, 1984.

71. Wasil M, Halliwell B, Hutchison DC, et al: The antioxidant action of human extracellular fluids. Biochem J 243:219, 1987.

72. Stocker R, Glazer AN, Ames BN: Antioxidant activity of albumin-bound bilirubin. Proc Natl Acad Sci USA 84:5918, 1987.

73. Pirisino R, Di Simplicio P, Ignesti G, et al: Sulfhydryl groups and peroxidase-like activity of albumin as scavenger of organic peroxides. Pharmacol Res Commun 20:545, 1988.

74. Colman RW: Paradoxical hypotension after volume expansion with plasma protein fraction. N Engl J Med 299:97, 1978.

75. Alving BM, Hojima Y, Pisano JJ, et al: Hypotension associated with prekallikrein activator (Hageman-factor fragments) in plasma protein fraction. N Engl J Med 299:66, 1978.

76. Atik M: The uses of dextran in surgery: A current evaluation. Surgery 65:548, 1969.

77. Gelin LE, Solvell L, Zederfeldt B: The plasma volume expanding effect of low viscous dextran and Macrodex. Acta Chir Scand 122:309, 1961.

78. Arturson G, Granath K, Thoren L, et al: The renal excretion of low molecular weight dextran. Acta Chir Scand 127:543, 1964.

79. Matsuda H, Shoemaker WC: Cardiorespiratory responses to dextran 40: Hemodynamic and oxygen transport changes in normal subjects and critically ill patients. Arch Surg 110:296, 1975.

80. Mohr PA, Monson DO, Owczarski C, et al: Sequential cardiorespiratory events during and after dextran-40 infusion in normal and shock patients. Circulation 39:379, 1969.

81. Gelin LE: Studies in anemia of injury. Acta Chir Scand S210:1, 1956.

82. Baker RJ, Shoemaker WC, Suzuki F, et al: Low molecular weight dextran therapy in surgical shock. Arch Surg 89:373, 1964.

83. Mailloux L, Swartz CD, Capizzi R, et al: Acute renal failure after administration of low-molecular-weight dextran. N Engl J Med 277:1113, 1967.

84. Matheson NA, Diomi P: Renal failure after the administration of dextran 40. Surg Gynecol Obstet 131:61, 1970.

85. Feest TG: Low molecular weight dextran: A continuing cause of acute renal failure. Br Med J 2:1300, 1976.

86. Isbister JP, Fisher MM: Adverse effects of plasma volume expanders. Anaesth Intensive Care 8:145, 1980.

87. Hedin H, Richter W: Pathomechanisms of dextran-induced anaphylactoid/anaphylactic reactions in man. Int Arch Allergy Appl Immunol 68:122, 1982.

88. Paull J: A prospective study of dextran-induced anaphylactoid reactions in 5745 patients. Anaesth Intensive Care 15:163, 1987.

89. Hedin H, Richter W, Ring J: Dextran-induced anaphylactoid reactions in man: Role of dextran reactive antibodies. Int Arch Allergy Appl Immunol 52:145, 1976.

90. Renck H, Ljungstrom KG, Hedin H, et al: Prevention of dextran-induced anaphylactic reactions by hapten inhibition. III. A Scandinavian multicenter study on the effect of 20 ml dextran 1, 15% administered before dextran 70 or dextran 40. Acta Chir Scand 149:355, 1983.

91. Alexander B, Odake K, Lawlor D, et al: Coagulation, hemostasis and plasma expanders: A quarter century enigma. Fed Proc 34:1429, 1975.

92. Atik M: Dextran 40 and dextran 70. Arch Surg 94:664, 1967.

93. Weiss HJ: The effect of clinical dextran on platelet aggregation, adhesion and ADP release in man: In vivo and in vitro studies. J Lab Clin Med 69:37, 1967.

94. Adelson E, Crosby WH, Roeder WH: Further studies of a hemostatic defect caused by intravenous dextran. J Lab Clin Med 45:441, 1955.

95. Karlson KE, Garzon AA, Shaftan GW, et al: Increased blood loss associated with administration of certain plasma expanders: Dextran 75, dextran 40 and hydroxyethyl starch. Surgery 62:670, 1967.

96. Muzaffar TZ, Stalker AL, Bryce WAJ, et al: Quantitative studies on fibrin formation and effects of dextran. Bibl Anat 12:340, 1973.

97. Hulse JD, Yacobi A: Hetastarch: An overview of the colloid and its metabolism. Drug Intell Clin Pharm 17:334, 1983.

98. Yacobi A, Stoll RG, Sum CY: Pharmacokinetics of hydroxyethyl starch in normal subjects. J Clin Pharmacol 22:206, 1982.

99. Metcalf W, Papadopoulos A, Tufaro R, et al: A clinical physiologic study of hydroxyethyl starch. Surg Gynecol Obstet 131:255, 1970.

100. Shatney CH, Chaudry IH: Hydroxyethyl starch administration does not depress reticuloendothelial function or increase mortality from sepsis. Circ Shock 13:21, 1984.

101. Thompson WL, Fukushima T, Rutherford RB, et al: Intravascular persistence, tissue storage and excretion of hydroxyethyl starch. Surg Gynecol Obstet 131:965, 1970.

102. Hulse JD, Gibson TP, Look Z, et al: Pharmacokinetics of hetastarch in patients with renal impairment. Clin Pharmacol Ther 33:254, 1983.

103. Gollub S, Schechter DC, Hirose T, et al: Use of hydroxyethyl starch solution in extensive surgical operations. Surg Gynecol Obstet 128:725, 1969.

104. Lazrove S, Waxman K, Shippy C, et al: Hemodynamic, blood volume and oxygen transport responses to albumin and hydroxyethyl starch infusions in critically ill postoperative patients. Crit Care Med 8:302, 1980.

105. Haupt MT, Rackow EC: Colloid osmotic pressure and fluid resuscitation with hetastarch, albumin and saline solutions. Crit Care Med 10:159, 1982.

106. Shatney CH, Deepika K, Militello PR, et al: Efficacy of hetastarch in the resuscitation of patients with multisystem trauma and shock. Arch Surg 118:806, 1983.

107. Rackow EC, Falk JL, Fein IA, et al: Fluid resuscitation in circulatory shock: A comparison of the cardiorespiratory effects of albumin, hetastarch and saline solutions in patients with hypovolemic and septic shock. Crit Care Med 11:839, 1983.

108. Strauss RG: Review of the effects of hydroxyethyl starch on the blood coagulation system. Transfusion 21:299, 1981.

109. Macintyre E, Mackie IJ, Tinker J, et al: The haemostatic effects of hydroxyethyl starch (HES) used as a volume expander. Intensive Care Med 11:300, 1985.

110. Gold MS, Russo J, Tissot M, et al: Comparison of hetastarch to albumin for perioperative bleeding in patients undergoing abdominal aortic aneurysm surgery: A prospective, randomized study. Ann Surg 211:482, 1990.

111. Stump DC, Strauss RG, Henriksen RA, et al: Effects of hydroxyethyl starch on blood coagulation, particularly factor VIII. Transfusion 25:349, 1985.

112. Gollub S, Schaefer C, Squitieri A: The bleeding tendency associated with plasma expanders. Surg Gynecol Obstet 124:1203, 1967.

113. Garzon AA, Cheng C, Lerner B, et al: Hydroxyethyl starch (HES) and bleeding: An experimental investigation of its effect on hemostasis. J Trauma 7:757, 1967.

114. Mishler JM, Borberg H, Emerson PM, et al: Hydroxyethyl starch: An agent for hypovolemic shock treatment. 1. Serum concentrations in normal volunteers following three consecutive daily infusions. J Surg Res 23:239, 1977.

115. Conduit D, Freeman K, Brodman R: Hyperamylasemia in cardiac surgical patients receiving hydroxyethyl starch. J Crit Care 2:26, 1987.

116. Mishler JM, Hester JP, Huestis DW, et al: Panel II: Dosage and scheduling regimens for erythrocyte-sedimenting macromolecules. J Clin Apheresis 1:130, 1983.

117. Kohler H, Zschiedrich H, Clasen R, et al: The effects of 500 ml 10% hydroxyethyl starch 200/0.5 and 10% dextran 40 on blood volume, colloid osmotic pressure and renal function in human volunteers. Anesthetist 31:61, 1982.

118. Rackow EC, Mecher C, Astiz ME, et al: Effects of pentastarch and albumin infusion on cardiorespiratory function and coagulation in patients with severe sepsis and systemic hypoperfusion. Crit Care Med 17:394, 1989.

119. Strauss RG, Hester JP, Vogler WR, et al: A multicenter trial to document the efficacy and safety of a rapidly excreted analog of hydroxyethyl starch for leukapheresis with a note on steroid stimulation of granulocyte donors. Transfusion 26:258, 1986.

120. Strauss RG, Stansfield C, Henriksen, et al: Pentastarch may cause fewer effects on coagulation than hetastarch. Transfusion 28:257, 1988.

121. Waxman K, Holness R, Tominaga G, et al: Hemodynamic and oxygen transport effects of pentastarch in burn resuscitation. Ann Surg 209:341, 1989.

122. London MJ, Ho JS, Triedman JK, et al: A randomized clinical trial of 10% pentastarch (low molecular weight hydroxyethyl starch) versus 5% albumin for plasma volume expansion after cardiac operations. J Thorac Cardiovasc Surg 97:785, 1989.

123. Zikria BA, King TC, Stanford J, et al: A biophysical approach to capillary permeability. Surgery 105:625, 1989.

124. Zikria BA, Subbarao C, Oz MC, et al: Macromolecules reduce abnormal microvascular permeability in rat limb ischemia-reperfusion injury. Crit Care Med 17:1306, 1989.

125. Webb AR, Tighe D, Moss RF, et al: Advantages of a narrow-range, medium molecular weight hydroxyethyl starch for volume maintenance in a porcine model of fecal peritonitis. Crit Care Med 19:409, 1991.

126. Edwards JD, Nightingale P, Wilkins RG, et al: Hemodynamic and

oxygen transport response to modified fluid gelatin in critically ill patients. Crit Care Med 17:996, 1989.

127. Mishler J: Synthetic plasma volume expanders—Their pharmacology, safety and clinical efficacy. Clin Haematol 13:75, 1984.

128. Lorenz W, Doenicke A, Messmer K, et al: Histamine release in human subjects by modified gelatin (Haemaccel) and dextran: An explanation for anaphylactoid reactions observed under clinical conditions. Br J Anaesth 48:151, 1976.

129. Weil MH, Henning RJ: New concepts in the diagnosis and fluid treatment of circulatory shock. Anesth Analg 58:124, 1979.

130. Messmer K: Hemodilution. Surg Clin North Am 55:659, 1975.

131. Puri VK, Howard M, Pidipaty BB, et al: Resuscitation in hypovolemia and shock: A prospective study of hydroxyethyl starch and albumin. Crit Care Med 11:518, 1983.

132. Shoemaker WC, Schluchter M, Hopkins JA, et al: Comparison of the relative effectiveness of colloids and crystalloids in emergency resuscitation. Am J Surg 142:73, 1981.

133. Modig J: Effectiveness of dextran 70 versus Ringer's acetate in traumatic shock and adult respiratory distress syndrome. Crit Care Med 14:454, 1986.

134. Shippy CR, Appel PL, Shoemaker WC: Reliability of clinical monitoring to assess blood volume in critically ill patients. Crit Care Med 12:107, 1984.

135. Baek SM, Makabali GG, Bryan-Brown CW, et al: Plasma expansion in surgical patients with high central venous pressure (CVP); the relationship of blood volume to hematocrit, CVP, pulmonary wedge pressure and cardiorespiratory changes. Surgery 78:304, 1975.

136. Calvin JE, Driedger AA, Sibbald WJ: The hemodynamic effect of rapid fluid infusion in critically ill patients. Surgery 90:61, 1981.

137. Shoemaker WC, Czer LS: Evaluation of the biologic importance of various hemodynamic and oxygen transport variables: Which variables should be monitored in postoperative shock? Crit Care Med 7:424, 1979.

138. Shires T, Coln D, Carrico J, et al: Fluid therapy in hemorrhagic shock. Arch Surg 88:688, 1964.

139. Shires GT, Cunningham JN, Baker CRF, et al: Alterations in cellular membrane function during hemorrhagic shock in primates. Ann Surg 176:288, 1972.

140. Carrico CJ, Canizaro PC, Shires GT: Fluid resuscitation following injury: Rationale for the use of balanced salt solutions. Crit Care Med 4:46, 1976.

141. Shires GT: The role of sodium containing solution in the treatment of oligemic shock. Surg Clin North Am 45:365, 1965.

142. Shires GT, Williams J, Brown F: Simultaneous measurement of plasma volume, extracellular fluid volume and red blood cell mass in man utilizing I^{131}, S^{35}, O$_4$, Cr^{51}. J Lab Clin Med 55:776, 1960.

143. Roth E, Lax LC, Malone JV: Ringer's lactate solution and extracellular fluid volume in the surgical patient: A critical analysis. Ann Surg 169:149, 1969.

144. Serkes KD, Lang S: Changes in extracellular fluid volume after hemorrhage and tourniquet trauma. Surg Forum 17:58, 1966.

145. Moore FD, Dagher FJ, Boyden CM, et al: Hemorrhage in normal man. 1. Distribution and dispersal of saline infusions following acute blood loss: Clinical kinetics of blood volume support. Ann Surg 163:485, 1966.

146. Lowe RJ, Moss GS, Jilek J, et al: Crystalloid versus colloid in the etiology of pulmonary failure after trauma—A randomized trial in man. Crit Care Med 7:107, 1979.

147. Moss GS, Lowe RJ, Jilek J, et al: Colloid or crystalloid in the resuscitation of hemorrhagic shock: A controlled clinical trial. Surgery 89:434, 1981.

148. Weaver DW, Ledgerwood AM, Lucas CE, et al: Pulmonary effects of albumin resuscitation for severe hypovolemic shock. Surgery 113:387, 1978.

149. MacLean LD, Weil MH: Hypotension in dogs produced by *Escherichia coli* endotoxin. Circ Res 4:546, 1956.

150. MacLean LD, Weil MH, Spink WW, et al: Canine intestinal and liver weight changes induced by *E. coli* endotoxin. Proc Soc Exp Biol Med 92:602, 1956.

151. Teule GJJ, Den Hollander W, Bronsveld W, et al: Effect of volume loading and dopamine on hemodynamics and red-cell redistribution in canine endotoxin shock. Circ Shock 10:41, 1983.

152. Loeb HS, Cruz A, Teng CY, et al: Haemodynamic studies in shock associated with infection. Br Heart J 29:883, 1967.

153. Nishijima H, Weil MH, Shubin H, et al: Hemodynamic and metabolic studies on shock associated with gram negative bacteremia. Medicine 52:287, 1973.

154. Rackow EC, Kaufman BS, Falk JL, et al: Hemodynamic response to fluid repletion in patients with septic shock: Evidence for early depression of cardiac performance. Circ Shock 22:11, 1987.

155. Carroll GC, Snyder JV: Hyperdynamic severe intravascular sepsis depends on fluid administration in cynomolgus monkey. Am J Physiol 243:131, 1982.

156. Sugarman HG, Diaco JF, Pollack TW, et al: Physiologic management of septicemic shock in man. Surg Forum 22:3, 1971.

157. Kaufman BS, Rackow EC, Falk JL: The relationship between oxygen delivery and consumption during fluid resuscitation of hypovolemic and septic shock. Chest 85:336, 1984.

158. Astiz, ME, Rackow EC, Falk JL, et al: Oxygen delivery and consumption in patients with hyperdynamic septic shock. Crit Care Med 15:26, 1987.

159. Haupt MT, Gilbert EM, Carlson RW: Fluid loading increases oxygen consumption in septic patients with lactic acidosis. Am Rev Respir Dis 131:912, 1985.

160. Gilbert EM, Haupt MT, Mandanas RY, et al: The effect of fluid loading, blood transfusion and catecholamine infusion on oxygen delivery and consumption in patients with sepsis. Am Rev Respir Dis 134:873, 1986.

161. Allardyce DB: Parenteral fluid therapy in septic shock: An evaluation of crystalloid and colloid. Am Surg 542, 1974.

162. Shoemaker WC, Appel PL, Kram HB: Prospective trial of supranormal values of survivors as therapeutic goals in high-risk surgical patients. Chest 94:1176, 1988.

163. Shoemaker WC, Kram HB, Appel PL, et al: The efficacy of central venous and pulmonary artery catheters and therapy based upon them in reducing mortality and morbidity. Arch Surg 125:1332, 1990.

164. Kimchi A, Ellrodt G, Berman DS, et al: Right ventricular performance in septic shock: A combined radionuclide and hemodynamic study. J Am Coll Cardiol 4:945, 1984.

165. Packman MI, Rackow EC: Optimum left heart filling pressure during fluid resuscitation of patients with hypovolemic and septic shock. Crit Care Med 11:165, 1983.

166. Krausz MM, Perel A, Eimerl D, et al: Cardiopulmonary effects of volume loading in patients with septic shock. Ann Surg 185:429, 1977.

167. Sturm JA, Carpenter MA, Lewis FR, et al: Water and protein movement in the sheep lung after septic shock: Effect of colloid versus crystalloid resuscitation. J Surg Res 26:233, 1979.

168. Nylander WA, Hammon JW, Roselli RJ, et al: Comparison of the effects of saline and homologous plasma infusion on lung fluid balance during endotoxemia in the unanesthetized sheep. Surgery 90:221, 1981.

169. Kohler JP, Rice CL, Zarins CK, et al: Does reduced colloid oncotic pressure increase pulmonary dysfunction in sepsis? Crit Care Med 9:90, 1981.

170. Hillman K: Colloid versus crystalloid fluid therapy in the critically ill. Intensive Crit Care Dig 5:7, 1986.

171. D'Orio V, Wahlen C, Rodriguez LM, et al: Effects of intravascular volume expansion on lung fluid balance in a canine model of septic shock. Crit Care Med 15:863, 1987.

172. Deysine M, Lieblich N, Aufses AH: Albumin changes during clinical septic shock. Surg Gynecol Obstet 137:475, 1973.

173. Forrester JS, Diamond G, Chatterjee K, et al: Medical therapy of acute myocardial infarction by application of hemodynamic subsets. N Engl J Med 295:1356, 1976.

174. Kaufman BS, Rackow EC, Falk JL: Response to fluid challenge in patients with acute myocardial infarction and hypovolemia. Clin Res 31:824A, 1983.

175. Edwards D, Whittaker S, Prior A: Cardiogenic shock without a critically raised left ventricular end diastolic pressure: Management and outcome in eighteen patients. Br Heart J 55:549, 1986.

176. Figueras J, Weil MH: Blood volume prior to and following treatment of acute cardiogenic pulmonary edema. Circulation 57:349, 1978.

177. Dikshit K, Vyden JK, Forrester JS, et al: Renal and extrarenal effects of furosemide in congestive heart failure after myocardial infarction. N Engl J Med 288:1087, 1973.

178. Figueras J, Weil MH: Hypovolemia and hypotension complicating management of acute cardiogenic pulmonary edema. Am J Cardiol 44:1349, 1979.

179. Fisher M: Anaphylaxis. Dis Mon 33:433, 1987.

180. Carlson RW, Schaffer RC, Puri VK, et al: Hypovolemia and permeability pulmonary edema associated with anaphylaxis. Crit Care Med 9:883, 1981.

181. Fisher MM: Clinical observations on the pathophysiology and treatment of anaphylactic cardiovascular collapse. Anaesth Intensive Care 14:17, 1986.

182. Sugerman HG, Tatum JL, Burke TS, et al: Gamma scintigraphic analysis of albumin flux in patients with acute respiratory distress syndrome. Surgery 95:674, 1984.

183. Appel PL, Shoemaker WC: Evaluation of fluid therapy in adult respiratory failure. Crit Care Med 9:862, 1981.

184. Shoemaker WC, Appel P, Czer LSC, et al: Pathogenesis of respiratory failure (ARDS) after hemorrhage and trauma. Crit Care Med 8:504, 1980.

185. Finch JS, Reid C, Bandy K, et al: Compared effects of selected colloids on extravascular lung water in dogs after oleic acid–induced lung injury and severe hemorrhage. Crit Care Med 11:267, 1983.

186. Prewitt RM, McCarthy J, Wood LDH: Treatment of acute low pressure pulmonary edema in dogs. J Clin Invest 67:409, 1981.

187. Sibbald WJ, Driedger AA, Moffat JD, et al: Pulmonary microvascular clearance of radiotracers in human cardiac and noncardiac pulmonary edema. J Appl Physiol 50:1337, 1981.

188. Sibbald WJ, Short AK, Warshawski FJ, et al: Thermal dye measurements of extravascular lung water in critically ill patients: Intravascular Starling forces and extravascular lung water in the adult respiratory distress syndrome. Chest 87:585, 1985.

189. Simmons RS, Berdine GG, Seidenfeld JJ, et al: Fluid balance and the adult respiratory distress syndrome. Am Rev Respir Des 135:924, 1987.

190. Eisenberg PR, Hansbrough JR, Anderson D, et al: A prospective study of lung water measurements during patient management in an intensive care unit. Am Rev Respir Dis 136:662, 1987.

191. Jing DL, Kohler JP, Rice CL, et al: Albumin therapy in permeability pulmonary edema. J Surg Res 33:482, 1982.

192. Peitzman AB, Shires T, Illner H, et al: Pulmonary acid injury: Effects of positive end-expiratory pressure and crystalloid vs colloid fluid resuscitation. Arch Surg 117:662, 1982.

193. Pearl RG, Halperin BD, Mihm FG, et al: Pulmonary effects of crystalloid and colloid resuscitation from hemorrhagic shock in the presence of oleic acid–induced pulmonary capillary injury in the dog. Anesthesiology 68:12, 1988.

194. Schaeffer RC Jr, Barnhart MI, Carlson RW: Pulmonary fibrin deposition and increased microvascular permeability to protein following fibrin microembolism in dogs: A structure-function relationship. Microvasc Res 33:327, 1987.

195. Schaeffer RC Jr, Reniewicz RA, Chilton SM, et al: Effects of colloid or crystalloid solutions on edemagenesis in normal and thrombomicroembolized lungs. Crit Care Med 15:1110, 1987.

196. Metildi LA, Shackford SR, Virgilio RW, et al: Crystalloid versus colloid in fluid resuscitation of patients with severe pulmonary insufficiency. Surg Gynecol Obstet 158:207, 1984.

197. Zornow MH, Scheller MS, Todd MM, et al: Acute cerebral effects of isotonic crystalloid and colloid solutions following cryogenic brain injury in the rabbit. Anesthesiology 69:180, 1988.

198. Zornow MH, Todd MM, Moore SS: The acute cerebral effects of changes in plasma osmolality and oncotic pressure. Anesthesiology 67:936, 1987.

199. Albright AL, Latchaw RE, Robinson AG: Intracranial and systemic effects of osmotic and oncotic therapy in experimental cerebral edema. J Neurosurg 60:481, 1984.

200. Prough DS, Johnson JC, Poole GV, et al: Effects on intracranial pressure of resuscitation from hemorrhagic shock with hypertonic saline versus lactated Ringer's solution. Crit Care Med 13:407, 1985.

201. Gunnar W, Merlotti GJ, Jonasson O, et al: Resuscitation from hemorrhagic shock: Alterations of the intracranial pressure after normal saline, 3% saline and dextran-40. Ann Surg 204:686, 1986.

202. Poole GV, Johnson JC, Prough DS, et al: Cerebral hemodynamics after hemorrhagic shock: Effects of the type of resuscitative fluid. Crit Care Med 14:629, 1986.

203. Prough DS, Johnson JC, Stump DA, et al: Effects of hypertonic saline versus lactated Ringer's solution on cerebral oxygen transport during resuscitation from hemorrhagic shock. J Neurosurg 64:627, 1986.

204. Ducey JP, Lamiell JM, Gueller GE: Cerebral electrophysiologic effects of resuscitation with hypertonic saline-dextran after hemorrhage. Crit Care Med 18:744, 1990.

205. Gunnar W, Jonasson O, Merlotti G, et al: Head injury and hemorrhagic shock: Studies of the blood-brain barrier and intracranial pressure after resuscitation with normal saline solution, 3% saline solution and dextran-40. Surgery 103:398, 1988.

206. Wisner DH, Schuster L, Quinn C: Hypertonic saline resuscitation of head injury: Effects on cerebral water content. J Trauma 30:75, 1990.

207. Baudendistel L, Shields J, Kaminski D: Comparison of double indicator thermodilution measurements of extravascular lung water (EVLW) with radiographic estimation of lung water in trauma patients. J Trauma 22:983, 1982.

208. Turner AF, Lav FYK, Jacobson G: A method for the estimation of pulmonary venous and arterial pressure from the routine chest roentgenogram. Am J Radiol 116:96, 1972.

209. Sibbald WJ, Warshawski FJ, Short AK, et al: Clinical studies of measuring extravascular lung water by the thermal dye technique in critically ill patients. Chest 5:725, 1983.

210. Brigham KL, Kariman K, Harris TR, et al: Correlation of oxygenation with vascular permeability–surface area but not with lung water in humans with acute respiratory failure and pulmonary edema. J Clin Invest 72:339, 1983.

211. Guyton AC, Lindsey AW: Effect of elevated left atrial pressure and decreased plasma protein concentration on the development of pulmonary edema. Circ Res 7:649, 1959.

212. Puri VK, Weil MH, Michaels S, et al: Pulmonary edema associated with reduction in plasma oncotic pressure. Surg Gynecol Obstet 151:344, 1980.

213. Da Luz PL, Shubin H, Weil MH, et al: Pulmonary edema related to changes in colloid osmotic and pulmonary artery wedge pressure in patients after myocardial infarction. Circulation 51:350, 1975.

214. Stein L, Beraud JJ, Morissette M, et al: Pulmonary edema during volume infusion. Circulation 52:483, 1975.

215. Rackow EC, Weil MH, MacNeil AR, et al: Effects of crystalloid and colloid fluids on extravascular lung water in hypoproteinemic dogs. J Appl Physiol 62:2421, 1987.

216. McKeen CR, Bowers RE, Harris TR, et al: Saline compared to plasma volume replacement after volume depletion in sheep: Lung fluid balance. J Crit Care 1:133, 1986.

217. Zarins CK, Rice CL, Peters RM, et al: Lymph and pulmonary response to isobaric reduction in plasma oncotic pressure in baboons. Circ Res 43:925, 1978.

218. Holcroft JW, Trunkey DD: Pulmonary extravasation of albumin during and after hemorrhagic shock in baboons. J Surg Res 18:91, 1975.

219. Sise MJ, Shackford SR, Peters RM, et al: Serum oncotic pressure and oncotic-hydrostatic pressure differences in critically ill patients. Anesth Analg 61:496, 1982.

220. Rafferty TD, Ljungquist R, Firestone L, et al: Plasma colloid oncotic pressure–pulmonary artery occlusion pressure gradient: A poor predictor of pulmonary edema in surgical intensive care unit patients. Arch Surg 118:841, 1983.

221. Shires GT, Peitzman A, Albert S, et al: Response of extravascular lung water to intraoperative fluids. Ann Surg 197:515, 1983.

222. Lucas CE, Weaver D, Higgins RF, et al: Effects of albumin versus non-albumin resuscitation on plasma volume and renal excretory function. J Trauma 18:564, 1978.

223. Siegel DC, Cochin A, Geocaris T, et al: Effects of saline and colloid resuscitation on renal function. Ann Surg 177:51, 1973.

224. Kaminski MV, Williams SD: Review of the rapid normalization of serum albumin with modified total parenteral nutrition solutions. Crit Care Med 18:327, 1990.

225. Heughan C, Niinikoski J, Hunt TK: Effect of excessive infusion of saline solution on tissue oxygen transport. Surg Gynecol Obstet 135:257, 1972.

226. Pappova E, Bachmeier W, Crevoisier JL, et al: Acute hypoproteinemic fluid overload: Its determinants, distribution and treatment with concentrated albumin and diuretics. Vox Sang 33:307, 1977.

227. Gump FE, Kinney JM, Iles M, et al: Duration and significance of large fluid loads administered for circulatory support. J Trauma 10:431, 1970.

228. Hunt TK, Pai MP: The effect of varying ambient oxygen tensions on wound metabolism and collagen synthesis. Surg Gynecol Obstet 135:561, 1972.

229. Pai MP, Hunt TK: Effects of varying oxygen tensions on the healing of open wounds. Surg Gynecol Obstet 135:756, 1972.

230. Lundsgaarden-Hansen P, Blauhaut B: The relationship of hypoxia and edema in the intestinal wall and skin to colloid osmotic pressure. Anaesthetist 37:112, 1988.

231. Hohn DC, Makay RD, Halliday B, et al: The effect of O_2 tension on microbicidal function of leukocytes in wounds and in vitro. Surg Forum 27:18, 1976.

232. Hunt TK, Linsey M, Sonne M, et al: Oxygen tension and wound infection. Surg Forum 23:47, 1972.

233. Myers MB, Rightor M, Cherry G: Relationship between edema and the healing rate of stasis ulcers of the leg. Am J Surg 124:666, 1972.

234. Brinson R, Guild R, Kolts B: Diarrhea and hypoalbuminemia in a medical intensive care unit. Gastroenterology 88:1336, 1985.

235. Cobb LM, Cartmill AM, Gilsdorf RB: Early post-operative nutritional support using the serosal tunnel jejunostomy. JPEN 8:397, 1981.

236. Granger DW, Udrich M, Parks DA, et al: Transcapillary exchange during intestinal fluid absorption. In: Sheppard AP, Granger DW (eds): Physiology of the Intestinal Circulation. New York, Raven Press, p 107, 1984.

237. Moss G: Malabsorption associated with extreme malnutrition: Importance of replacing plasma albumin. J Am Coll Nutr 1:89, 1982.

238. Barden RP, Thompson WD, Ravdin IS, et al: The influence of serum protein on the motility of the small intestine. Surg Gynecol Obstet 66:819, 1958.

239. Moore FA, Moore EE, Jones TN, et al: TEN versus TPN following major abdominal trauma—Reducing septic mortality. J Trauma 29:916, 1989.

240. Deitch EA, Winterton J, Berg R: The gut as a portal of entry for bacteremia. Ann Surg 205:681, 1987.

241. Lucas CE, Ledgerwood AM, Higgins RF, et al: Impaired pulmonary function after albumin resuscitation from shock. J Trauma 20:446, 1980.

242. Lucas CE, Ledgerwood AM, Higgins RF: Impaired salt and water excretion after albumin resuscitation for hypovolemic shock. Surgery 86:544, 1979.

243. Fisher MM: The crystalloid versus colloid controversy: Bias, logic and toss-up. Theor Surg 4:205, 1989.

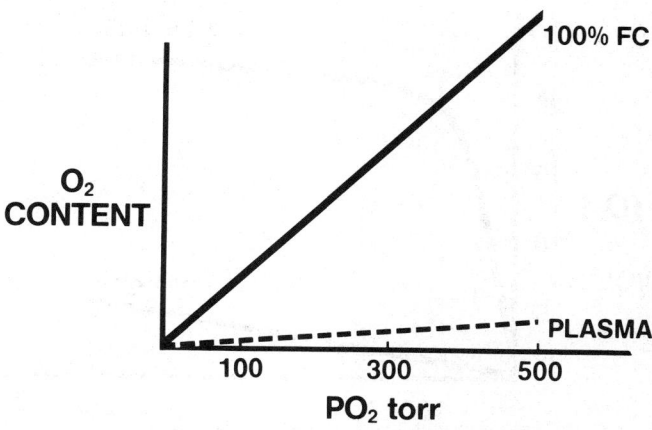

Figure 13–2. [O_2] curves for 100% FCs and plasma. (From Gould SA, Moss GS, Rosen AL, et al: Red cell substitutes. In: Civetta J, Taylor R, Kirby R [eds]: Critical Care. Philadelphia, JB Lippincott, p 1495, 1988.)

CHAPTER 13

Artificial Blood

Steven A. Gould
Lakshman R. Sehgal
Hansa L. Sehgal
Gerald S. Moss

The development of a safe and effective red blood cell (RBC) substitute for use in resuscitation is an exciting prospect. Such a product has been sought over the past century for several reasons. The most important functions of an RBC substitute are to transport oxygen and carbon dioxide effectively and to support circulatory dynamics. From a logistic point of view, a suitable product should be readily available, nontoxic, temperature stable, and universally compatible. In addition, it should have a long shelf life and satisfactory intravascular persistence, and it should be effective during room air breathing. Clinically, the risk/benefit ratio would be improved by the availability of such a product because serious transfusion hazards such as hepatitis and acquired immunodeficiency syndrome would not be a consideration. Fluorocarbon (FC) emulsions and hemoglobin solutions are the two products that have been most extensively evaluated.

PERFLUOROCHEMICAL EMULSIONS
Physiologic Considerations

The FCs are potential oxygen carriers because of their relatively high oxygen solubility compared with blood or plasma.[1] However, this high solubility exists only for pure FCs. Because they are not miscible with water (i.e., plasma), current FC products are prepared as an emulsion, which lowers their concentration. Their properties can best be understood by looking at several oxygen content ([O_2]) curves. The [O_2] curve for whole blood is actually the composite of the [O_2] curves for the RBC hemoglobin and the plasma (Fig. 13–1).[2] The majority of oxygen is chemically bound to the hemoglobin molecule, which becomes fully saturated at a P_{O_2} of 150 torr. Above this level, a further

increase in whole blood oxygen reflects the dissolved oxygen in the aqueous phase of plasma. Because this amount is only 0.3 mL/dL at the alveolar P_{O_2} of 100 torr, it is generally ignored when discussing [O_2].

The potential value of FCs as oxygen carriers is illustrated in Figure 13–2.[3] Pure FCs have a solubility coefficient that is approximately 10 to 20 times that of plasma. In a sense, they function as a "super water." Unfortunately, they cannot be administered in this form. A major development in FC research was the ability to make a stable emulsion using pluronic F-68 as the emulsifying agent. With this emulsion, the concentration of FC is lowered dramatically, as is the [O_2] (Fig. 13–3). The [O_2] depends on both the P_{O_2} and the volume concentration of FC (fluorocrit). For any given fluorocrit, the higher the P_{O_2}, the higher the concentration of dissolved oxygen. Similarly, for any given P_{O_2}, the higher the amount of FC, the higher the [O_2].

The commercially prepared FC emulsion is Fluosol-DA 20% (FL-DA 20%). This product has been evaluated extensively in animals and in humans in Japan and in several series in the United States. A comparison between whole blood with a hemoglobin content of 15 g/dL and FL-DA 20% is shown in Figure 13–4.[3] Although FL-DA 20% offers some value as an oxygen carrier, several limiting factors are present. First, the patient must breathe a high concentration

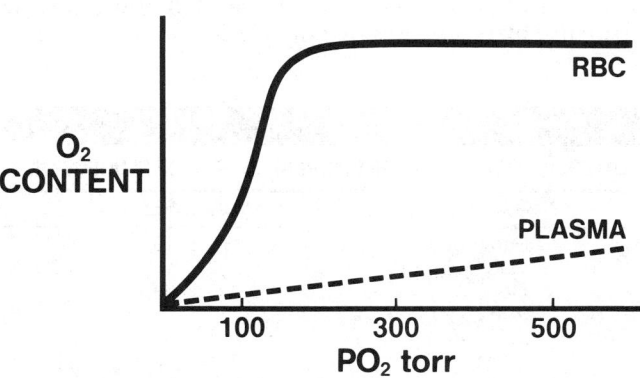

Figure 13–1. [O_2] curves for RBCs and plasma. (From Gould SA, Moss GS, Rosen AL, et al: Red cell substitutes. In: Civetta J, Taylor R, Kirby R [eds]: Critical Care. Philadelphia, JB Lippincott, p 1495, 1988.)

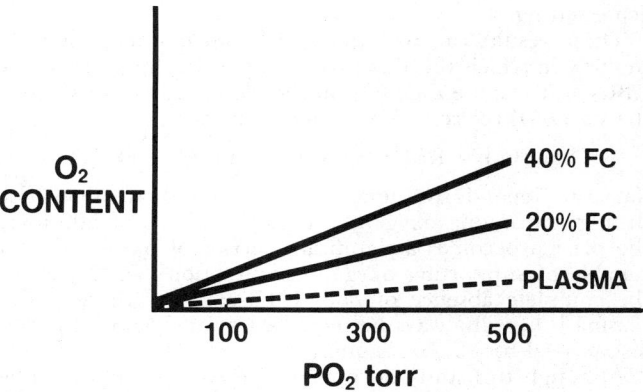

Figure 13–3. [O_2] curves for plasma and 20 and 40% FCs. (From Gould SA, Moss GS, Rosen AL, et al: Red cell substitutes. In: Civetta J, Taylor R, Kirby R [eds]: Critical Care. Philadelphia, JB Lippincott, p 1495, 1988.)

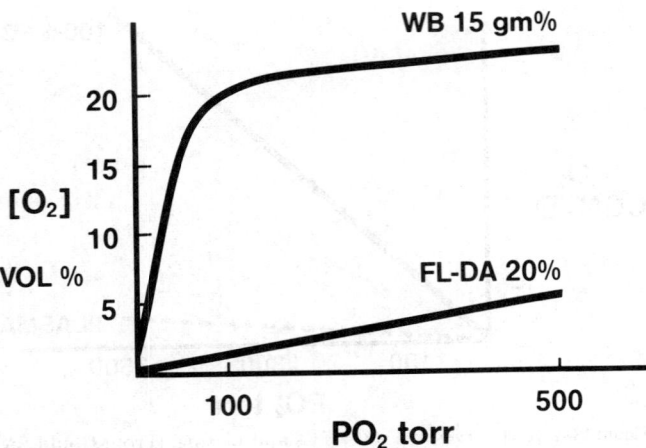

Figure 13–4. [O_2] curves for 15 g/dL hemoglobin in whole blood (WB) and for 20% FL-DA. (From Gould SA, Moss GS, Rosen AL, et al: Red cell substitutes. In: Civetta J, Taylor R, Kirby R [eds]: Critical Care. Philadelphia, JB Lippincott, p 1495, 1988.)

of inspired oxygen to maximize FL-DA [O_2]. Second, even at a PO_2 of 500 torr (fraction of inspired oxygen [FIO_2] = 1.0), with the maximal achievable fluorocrit, the [O_2] is still less than 5 mL/dL compared with the normal 20 mL/dL of whole blood. The infusion of FL-DA 20% thus adds little to the total [O_2] unless the hemoglobin content is considerably reduced from normal. Finally, the amount of FL-DA 20% that can be administered to any patient (40 mL/kg) limits the achievable fluorocrit, further decreasing the amount of oxygen that can be carried.

Laboratory Studies

Our initial concern was to answer the question: How good are FC emulsions as oxygen carriers? Because the principal requirement of any oxygen carrier is the ability to load and unload oxygen, these functions must be assessed accurately. We have shown that adult baboons can survive a total exchange transfusion to zero hematocrit with FL-DA, if they are ventilated with pure oxygen.[4] The animals maintain normal hemodynamic and oxygen transport functions in the virtual absence of RBCs. Although these data suggest that FL-DA is an effective oxygen carrier, we also demonstrated that control animals survive at zero hematocrit and an FIO_2 of 1.0 without FL-DA. This remarkable observation leads to the conclusion that FL-DA is not necessary, at least in this acute setting.

These results can be explained by an understanding of the way in which the FCs carry oxygen. In the presence of RBCs and FC, the total [O_2] in the blood can be considered the sum of three separate oxygen carriers:

$$Total\ [O_2] = RBC\ [O_2] + plasma\ [O_2] + FC\ [O_2]$$

Survival depends on total [O_2], but the body does not distinguish among oxygen carriers.[5] At a PO_2 of 500 torr, the plasma becomes a significant carrier of oxygen that is capable of supporting oxygen consumption ($\dot{V}O_2$), even in the complete absence of both RBC and FC. Because the plasma [O_2] will always be increased at an FIO_2 of 1.0, the actual need for FL-DA is unclear.

Although this study documents the efficacy of plasma as an oxygen carrier, we are concerned about the potential risk of pulmonary oxygen toxicity in the clinical setting. The safe level of supplemental oxygen is thought to be an FIO_2 less than 0.6. Although our data suggest that FL-DA is unnec-

essary at a FIO_2 of 1.0, we cannot assume the same is true at lower levels of supplemental oxygen.

Clinical Trials

The results of our animal study[4] led us to design a clinical trial.[6] We sought to distinguish between the contributions of the plasma [O_2] and FL-DA [O_2]. Further, we wanted to minimize the risk of toxicity associated with breathing 100% O_2. The objective, therefore, was to provide sufficient oxygen delivery with FL-DA at an FIO_2 less than 0.6. Unlike most clinical trials, the protocol for FL-DA was nonblinded and had a crossover design, with each patient serving as his or her own control for each oxygen carrier. This design allowed us to define the physiologic need for and evaluate the efficacy of FL-DA in acute anemia.

Physiologic criteria of need derived from our control studies in baboons included a hemoglobin concentration less than 3.5 g/dL, venous partial pressure of oxygen (PvO_2) less than 25 torr, and oxygen extraction ratio less than 50%. We evaluated 23 surgical patients with blood loss and religious objections to receiving blood transfusions. Of these 23, 15 moderately anemic patients with a mean hemoglobin concentration ($\pm$ SEM) of 7.2 $\pm$ 0.5 g/dL had no evidence of a physiologic need for increased arterial oxygen content and did not receive FL-DA. Eight severely anemic patients with a mean hemoglobin concentration of 3.0 $\pm$ 0.4 g/dL met one or more of our criteria and received FL-DA until the physiologic need disappeared or a maximal dose of 40 mL/kg of body weight was reached. All patients breathed supplemental oxygen. We observed no adverse reactions. The volume of FL-DA infused ranged from 2 to 10 U. Six of the eight patients received the maximal allowable dose; one patient survived after receiving only 2 U and another died before the total dosage had been infused.

The maximal FL-DA [O_2] ranged from 0.3 to 1.2 mL/dL, with a mean increment of 0.7 $\pm$ 0.1 mL/dL. The simultaneous level of arterial oxygen carried by the plasma was 1.3 $\pm$ 0.1 mL/dL, and the level of oxygen carried by the RBCs was 2.8 $\pm$ 0.6 mL/dL (Table 13–1).

Eighty-two percent of the plasma and FL-DA oxygen phases was unloaded. In contrast, only 19% was unloaded from the RBC phase (Table 13–2). The relative contribution to total $\dot{V}O_2$ for each of the three phases is also shown in Table 13–2. The plasma contributed 50%, whereas FL-DA contributed 28% and the RBCs only 22%.

The only statistically significant differences in hemodynamic and oxygen transport values before and after FL-DA were a minor reduction in heart rate and an increase in alveolar partial pressure of oxygen (PAO_2) (which followed an increased FIO_2 in one patient) (Table 13–3). Intravascular persistence of FL-DA was determined in five patients. The

TABLE 13–1

ARTERIAL OXYGEN CONTENT AT PEAK EFFECT OF FLUOSOL-DA

Measure	Mean ± SEM
PaO_2 (torr)	430 ± 19
Fluorocrit (%)	5 ± 1
FIO_2	1.0 ± 0.0
Arterial [O_2] (mL/dL)	
FL-DA phase	0.7 ± 0.1
Plasma phase	1.3 ± 0.1
RBCs	2.8 ± 0.6

From Gould SA, Moss GS, Rosen AL, et al: Red cell substitutes. In: Civetta J, Taylor R, Kirby R (eds): Critical Care. Philadelphia, JB Lippincott, p 1495, 1988.

TABLE 13–2

OXYGEN DYNAMICS OF THREE PHASES AT PEAK EFFECT OF FLUOSOL-DA (MEAN ± SEM)

Measure	Fluosol-DA	Plasma	Red Blood Cells
Arterial [O_2] (mL/dL)	0.7 ± 0.1	1.3 ± 0.1	2.8 ± 0.6
Venous [O_2] (mL/dL)	0.2 ± 0.1	0.2 ± 0.1	2.2 ± 0.4
Oxygen unloaded (%)	82 ± 5	82 ± 5	19 ± 5
Contribution to $\dot{V}O_2$ (%)	28 ± 5	50 ± 5	22 ± 7

From Gould SA, Moss GS, Rosen AL, et al: Red cell substitutes. In: Civetta J, Taylor R, Kirby R (eds): Critical Care. Philadelphia, JB Lippincott, p 1495, 1988.

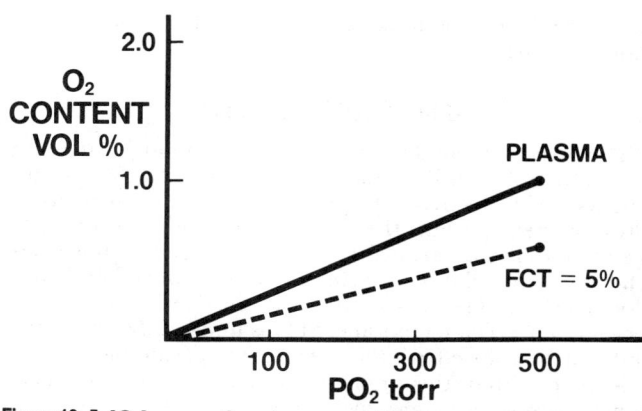

Figure 13–5. [O_2] curves for plasma and FL-DA at a fluorocrit of 5%. (From Gould SA, Moss GS, Rosen AL, et al: Red cell substitutes. In: Civetta J, Taylor R, Kirby R [eds]: Critical Care. Philadelphia, JB Lippincott, p 1495, 1988.)

mean half-life was 24.3 ± 4.3 hours, with a range of 12 to 37 hours.

Of the eight patients who received FL-DA, six died. The minimal hemoglobin level observed in these eight patients was 1.8 ± 0.4 g/dL. Fourteen of the 15 patients who did not receive FL-DA survived.

These data illustrate that FL-DA is a poor oxygen loader and that the fluorocrit that can be achieved clinically with the currently available product is only about 5%. A 5% concentration of FL-DA at a Po_2 of 430 torr carries 0.7 mL/dL of oxygen or approximately half the oxygen carried by plasma (1.3 mL/dL). This value is equivalent to an increase in hemoglobin content of only 0.5 g/dL. The relationship between FL-DA [O_2] at this fluorocrit and the amount carried by plasma holds regardless of the Po_2 because the [O_2] curves for both carriers are linear (Fig. 13–5). The potential benefit of FL-DA is that even this small amount of oxygen is additive to the amount carried by plasma. However, the observed increase in total [O_2] of 0.7 mL/dL was not clinically important, as evidenced by the absence of any discernible physiologic benefit after the FL-DA infusion.

In contrast, FL-DA unloads oxygen effectively. The difference between the arterial and venous FL-DA [O_2] is 0.5 mL/dL (see Table 13–2). Most of the oxygen carried by FL-DA is thus unloaded. However, the lack of any apparent physiologic benefit despite this efficient unloading again suggests that this contribution is inadequate.

The intravascular persistence of FL-DA is also insufficient, at least when RBCs cannot be used subsequently. The half-life of 24 hours and the maximal allowable dose of 40 mL/kg

TABLE 13–3

HEMODYNAMICS AND OXYGEN TRANSPORT BEFORE AND AFTER FLUOSOL-DA ADMINISTRATION (MEAN ± SEM)

Measure	Before Fluosol-DA	After Fluosol-DA*
Heart rate (beats/min)	117 ± 5	106 ± 4†
Mean arterial pressure (torr)	74 ± 6	78 ± 5
Cardiac index (L/min/m²)	4.5 ± 0.7	4.2 ± 0.7
Hemoglobin (g/dL)	3.0 ± 0.4	2.0 ± 0.4
Arterial [O_2] (mL/dL)	5.3 ± 0.5	4.8 ± 0.6
Oxygen delivery (mL/min/m²)	235 ± 27	197 ± 32
$\dot{V}O_2$ (mL/min/m²)	109 ± 13	88 ± 11
Pao_2 (torr)	356 ± 24	430 ± 19†
Pvo_2 (torr)	40.0 ± 3.9	78.2 ± 23.3
Oxygen extraction ratio (%)	46.0 ± 2.5	47.6 ± 3.8

*Data were obtained at peak arterial [O_2] after FL-DA.

†The difference between values before and after FL-DA is significant ($P < .05$).

From Gould SA, Moss GS, Rosen AL, et al: Red cell substitutes. In: Civetta J, Taylor R, Kirby R (eds): Critical Care. Philadelphia, JB Lippincott, p 1495, 1988.

led to a loss of FL-DA from the circulation before the patients were able to regenerate an adequate RBC mass to recover from their severe anemia. The mean hemoglobin level in the eight patients fell from an initial value of 3.0 g/dL to a low of 1.8 g/dL. This level usually is not compatible with survival. The combination of an insufficient increase in arterial [O_2] and an inadequate duration of FL-DA probably contributed to this unsatisfactory outcome. One of the two survivors eventually received RBCs against his wishes after the total FL-DA dose had been infused. An evaluation of FL-DA during short-term unavailability of RBCs might result in a better outcome.

In earlier reports representing a total of 200 patients, only 3 had a hemoglobin concentration less than 3 g/dL. Two of these three patients died. The less severely anemic patients receiving FL-DA had satisfactory outcomes. Fifteen of our 23 patients had no physiologic evidence of a need for increased arterial [O_2] despite their minimal hemoglobin level of 7.2 g/dL. Fourteen of these 15 moderately anemic patients survived without FL-DA. This good outcome raises some questions about the manner in which decisions about transfusions are made. The mortality rate is high among severely anemic patients who refuse RBCs, despite FL-DA therapy. Patients with less extreme blood loss who refuse RBCs do well, with or without FL-DA.

In conclusion, FL-DA is unnecessary when anemia is moderate and ineffective when it is severe. It is, therefore, an inadequate RBC substitute. New formulations of FCs that correct the observed shortcomings of FL-DA may be more effective by providing higher FC concentrations and longer intravascular persistence.[7, 8] In the near future, however, FCs are unlikely to be effective RBC substitutes.

HEMOGLOBIN SOLUTIONS

For many years, we have pursued the concept that a hemoglobin solution prepared from outdated blood could serve as a temporary substitute for RBCs.[9–11] This interest is based on several characteristics of the hemoglobin molecule. For example, 1 g of hemoglobin binds 1.39 mL of oxygen and is almost fully saturated with oxygen at ambient pressure. Few, if any, biologically acceptable substances have a greater oxygen-binding capacity. Oxygen is normally unloaded from hemoglobin in the capillaries at a Po_2 of approximately 40 torr, allowing oxygen molecules to diffuse from hemoglobin to the intracellular mitochondria without producing interstitial hypoxia. Despite these features, an acceptable hemoglobin solution has not yet been used in the clinical setting.

Unmodified Hemoglobin

The basic, unmodified hemoglobin solution is currently prepared from outdated blood, beginning with the washing and lysis of the RBCs with pyrogen-free water. A series of filtration steps permits the complete separation of the RBC membrane debris (stroma) from the hemoglobin molecules. The resultant solution is referred to as stroma-free hemoglobin (SFH) (Fig. 13–6). Because the RBC antigens are located on the cell membrane, SFH is universally compatible and can be infused without regard to specific blood type. The properties of this unmodified, tetrameric or "stripped" hemoglobin solution are given in Table 13–4.

Although SFH can be prepared with a hemoglobin concentration of 14 g/dL, this solution has a colloid osmotic pressure (COP) greater than 60 mm Hg, which renders it unacceptable for clinical use.[9] The hemoglobin concentration of 7 g/dL is iso-oncotic. The low P_{50} is due to the loss of the organic ligand, 2,3-diphosphoglycerate (2,3-DPG), during preparation. The $[O_2]$ curve of SFH (Fig. 13–7) is thus both anemic (hemoglobin content) and leftward shifted (P_{50}).

Despite these limitations, SFH supports life in primates in the absence of RBCs.[9] Animals survive a total exchange transfusion with SFH to zero hematocrit with maintenance of normal Vo_2, cardiac output, and arteriovenous oxygen content difference ($Cao_2 - Cvo_2$), although a decline from baseline values occurs in some of these measures. In addition, a considerable decrease occurs in the Pvo_2 from roughly 50 to 20 torr. The Pvo_2 is the partial pressure at which oxygen unloads from the hemoglobin molecule and is in equilibrium with the tissue Po_2. This decline indicates a marked increase in oxygen extraction and is the mechanism used to compensate for the fall in hemoglobin content and P_{50}. This low Pvo_2 is of some concern and led us to attempt to restore a more normal value.[12]

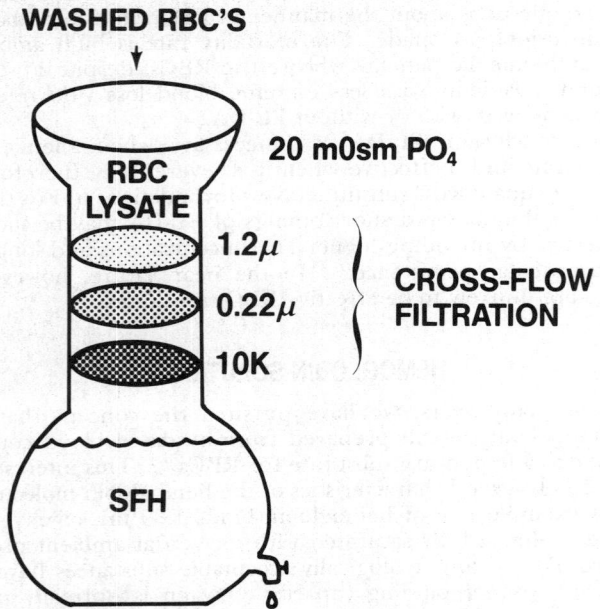

WASHED RBC'S

RBC LYSATE

20 mOsm PO$_4$

1.2µ

0.22µ

10K

CROSS-FLOW FILTRATION

SFH

Figure 13–6. Preparation of stroma-free hemoglobin (SFH). (From Gould SA, Moss GS, Rosen AL, et al: Red cell substitutes. In: Civetta J, Taylor R, Kirby R [eds]: Critical Care. Philadelphia, JB Lippincott, p 1495, 1988.)

TABLE 13–4

PROPERTIES AND PARAMETERS OF STROMA-FREE HEMOGLOBIN AND WHOLE BLOOD

Properties and Parameters	Stroma-Free Hemoglobin	Whole Blood
Hemoglobin content (g/dL)	6–8	12–14
Oxygen-carrying capacity (vol%)	8.0–11.0	16–19
Binding coefficient (mL O$_2$/g Hb)	1.30	1.30
P_{50} (torr) (Pco = 40 torr; pH = 7.40)	12–14	26–28
Methemoglobin (%)	<2	<1
Colloid osmotic pressure (torr)	18–25	18–25
Osmolarity (mOsm)	290–310	290–310
Total phospholipid (mg/dL)	0.4	
Viscosity (cp)	1.6 (8 g/dL)	3.2
Hill's coefficient	2.8	
Number average molecular weight	64,000	
Limulus amebocyte lysate assay (EU/mL)	<0.03	
Rabbit pyrogen test	Pass	
Bohr's coefficient	– 0.6	

From Moss GS, Sehgal LR, Gould SA, et al: Alternatives to transfusion therapy. Anesthesiol Clin North Am 8:569, 1990.

Pyridoxylated Hemoglobin

A leftward shift in the $[O_2]$ curve, with no change in Vo_2, cardiac output, or $Cao_2 - Cvo_2$, produces a decrease in the Pvo_2 (Fig. 13–8). Attempts to establish a normal P_{50} by the simple addition of 2,3-DPG to the hemoglobin solution were unsuccessful because the ligand disappears rapidly from the circulation after infusion. However, a modification of the hemoglobin molecule by the addition of pyridoxal phosphate results in a pyridoxylated hemoglobin (SFH-P) with a P_{50} of 20 to 22 torr, which is considerably higher than the P_{50} of unmodified SFH.[13, 14]

We evaluated SFH-P in eight baboons.[15] Four received SFH and four received SFH-P, with a hemoglobin content of 7 g/dL and zero hematocrit. The Pvo_2 levels were significantly higher at the end of the exchange in the animals receiving SFH-P. Although hemodynamic parameters were normal, a decline from the baseline values occurred in both groups.

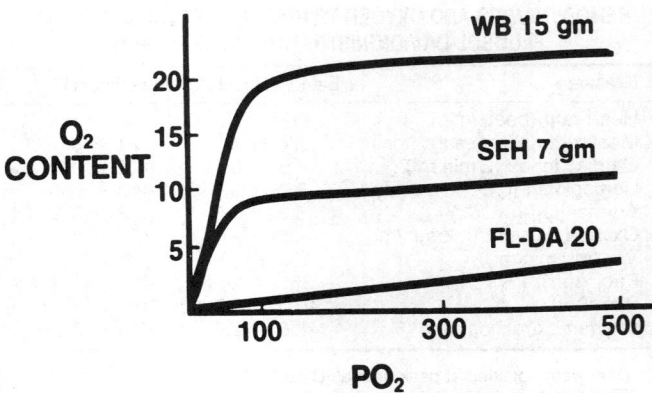

O_2 CONTENT

WB 15 gm

SFH 7 gm

FL-DA 20

100 300 500

PO$_2$

Figure 13–7. $[O_2]$ curves for 15 g/dL hemoglobin in whole blood (WB), 7 g/dL in SFH, and 20% FL-DA. (From Gould SA, Moss GS, Rosen AL, et al: Red cell substitutes. In: Civetta J, Taylor R, Kirby R [eds]: Critical Care. Philadelphia, JB Lippincott, p 1495, 1988.)

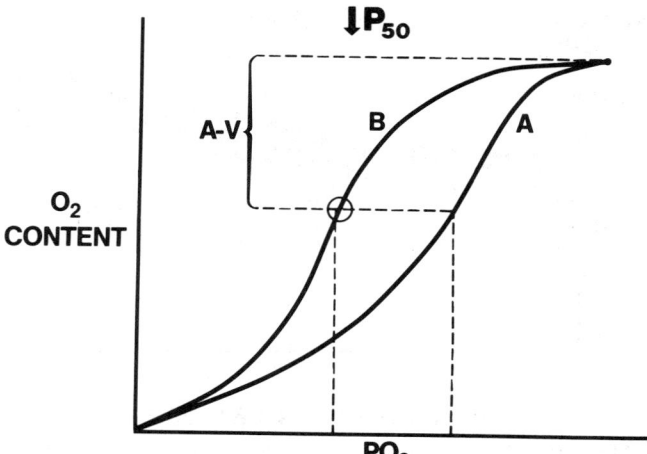

Figure 13–8. [O₂] curves showing how a leftward shift in P_{50} with a constant $CaO_2 - CvO_2$ leads to a lower PvO_2. Curve B is shifted to the left compared with curve A. (From Gould SA, Moss GS, Rosen AL, et al: Red cell substitutes. In: Civetta J, Taylor R, Kirby R [eds]: Critical Care. Philadelphia, JB Lippincott, p 1495, 1988.)

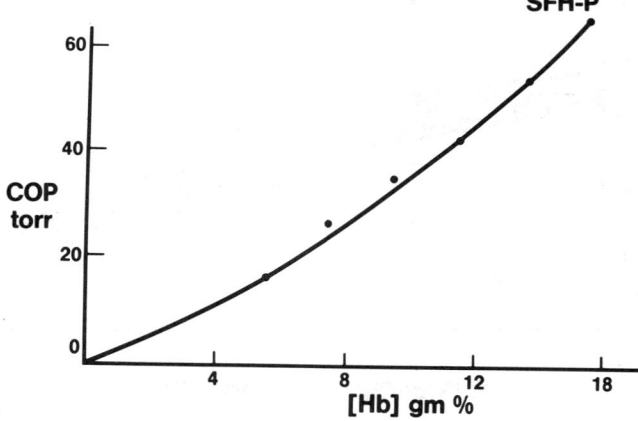

Figure 13–9. Relationship between COP and hemoglobin concentration for SFH-P. (From Moss GS, Sehgal LR, Gould SA, et al: Alternatives to transfusion therapy. Anesthesiol Clin North Am 8:569, 1990.)

These results illustrate three points. First, a rightward shift in the dissociation curve (P_{50}) results in an increased PvO_2 because all else remained constant. This observation is of physiologic importance because oxygen unloading can occur at a higher tissue PO_2. Second, although it was increased, the PvO_2 level in the animals treated with SFH-P was still substantially lower than the normal value of 40 to 50 torr found in control animals. Third, hemodynamic function still showed a reduction from the baseline values. It became apparent that a nonanemic hemoglobin solution was required.

Nonanemic Iso-oncotic Hemoglobin Solution

The advantages of a nonanemic hemoglobin solution are self-evident. Such a solution would have the same oxygen capacity as whole blood. In addition, according to our data, the infusion of a nonanemic solution should be associated with normal PvO_2 levels, even at zero hematocrit. The principal obstacle to normalization of hemoglobin concentration is the effect of an elevation in protein concentration on oncotic pressure.

The relationship between hemoglobin concentration and oncotic pressure is shown in Figure 13–9.[16] At hemoglobin concentrations of 7 g/dL, the oncotic pressure is similar to that of plasma (20 torr). In contrast, at hemoglobin levels of 15 g/dL, oncotic pressure increases by more than 300%. The infusion of such a solution would theoretically produce large shifts of fluid from the extravascular space into the intravascular space. These changes are likely to be exceedingly harmful.

One approach to producing a nonanemic hemoglobin solution with normal COP values is polymerization of the hemoglobin. The COP of any solution is proportional to the number of colloidal particles. If a 15 g/dL solution of hemoglobin could be polymerized, the result would be a reduction in COP, whereas no change would occur in hemoglobin concentration (Fig. 13–10).

This idea was tested in our laboratories.[17] Approximately 14 L of the hemoglobin solution thus obtained is pyridoxylated by modification of previously described techniques.[18, 19] Briefly, pyridoxal-5'-phosphate is added to the solution at a 4:1 molar ratio. The solution is transferred to a 20-L sealed

reservoir and deoxygenated with nitrogen (N_2) by using a gas exchanger. Deoxygenation of the solution is continued until the PO_2 is below 10 torr and the [O₂] is below 1 vol%.[17] Sodium borohydride is then added to the solution, and the reaction continues for 2 to 4 hours.

The goal of the polymerization is to normalize the oxygen capacity while maintaining the COP within normal limits (20 to 25 torr). Several parameters can be manipulated to obtain, in a reproducible manner, the polymerized solution of choice.[20] These are the hemoglobin concentration, the concentration of the polymerizing agent, the rate of addition of the latter, and the rate of mixing. Finally, the duration for which the above-mentioned parameters are controlled will in turn determine the reaction yield, molecular weight distribution of the polymeric species, oxygen affinity (P_{50}), and finally the viscosity of the solution.

The details of the polymerization have been previously described.[21] The polymerization is conducted to a physiologic end point with respect to COP. The reaction is thus monitored by the decrease in COP. Figure 13–11 shows the changes in COP monitored during the polymerization process conducted over a 3-hour period. As can be seen from the figure, the reproducibility of the process for five batches is acceptable.

The polymerization and evolution of the polymeric species are also followed by sodium dodecyl sulfate–polyacrylamide gel electrophoresis (SDS-PAGE). Figure 13–12 shows the formation of new polypeptide bands during the process.

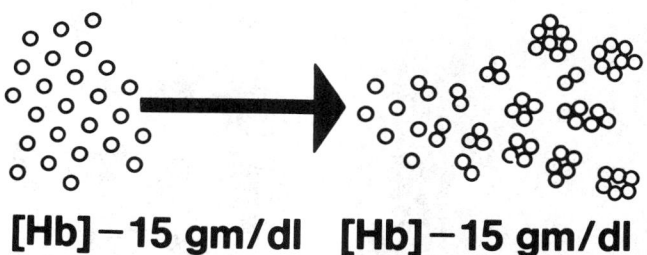

[Hb]–15 gm/dl   [Hb]–15 gm/dl
COP > 70 torr → COP = 25 torr

Figure 13–10. Polymerization. (From Moss GS, Sehgal LR, Gould SA, et al: Alternatives to transfusion therapy. Anesthesiol Clin North Am 8:569, 1990.)

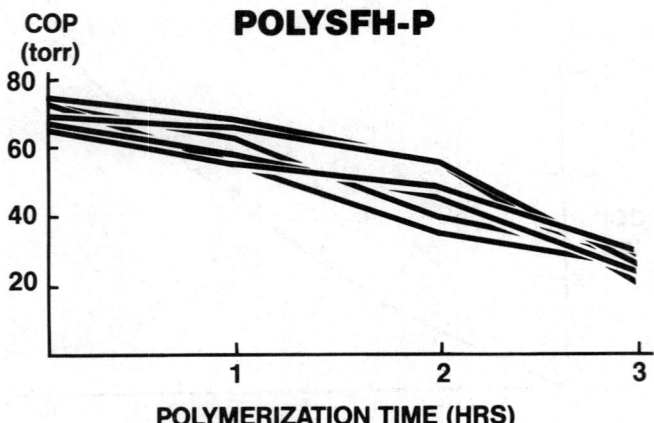

Figure 13–11. Decrease in COP measured during the course of polymerization for five different batches. (From Moss GS, Sehgal LR, Gould SA, et al: Alternatives to transfusion therapy. Anesthesiol Clin North Am 8:569, 1990.)

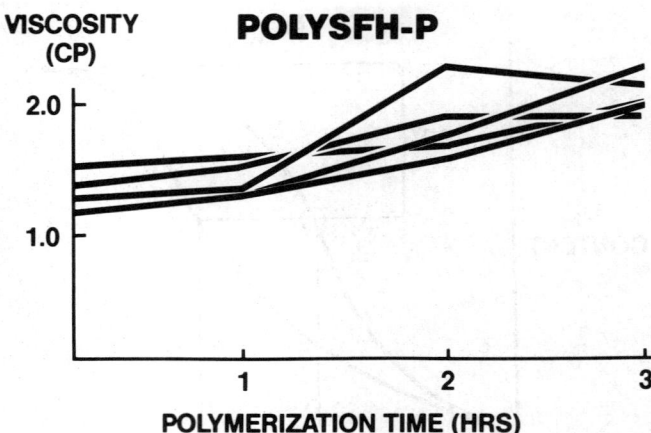

Figure 13–13. Changes in viscosity of five batches of hemoglobin solution during polymerization. (From Moss GS, Sehgal LR, Gould SA, et al: Alternatives to transfusion therapy. Anesthesiol Clin North Am 8:569, 1990.)

Typically, four to six bands are seen, ranging in molecular weights from 16,000 to 96,000. The first four bands (16,000 to 64,000 daltons) represent greater than 90% of all species.

With the formation of polymers, one would expect changes in the viscosity of the solution. Figure 13–13 shows the changes in viscosity observed for five different batches. The viscosity at the start of polymerization ranges from 1.0 to 1.5 cp and increases to reach a range of 1.9 to 2.1 cp at the end. This represents a relatively modest increase but is consistent with the absence of high-molecular-weight species in the solution, as demonstrated by SDS-PAGE.

The changes in P_{50} during the polymerization were followed and are shown in Figure 13–14. A modest increase in P_{50} was noted in all five batches shown. This increase reflects a decrease in buffering capacity of the solution with polymerization. It is consistent with the observation that a drop in pH is observed during the course of the polymerization. This is not surprising because it is some of the same amino groups that are involved in the buffering as well as the cross-linking.

The characteristics of the final product are listed in Table 13–5. The solution at 12 to 15 g/dL has a COP between 20 and 25 torr. The molecular weight based on SDS-PAGE and high-pressure liquid chromatography is between 16,000 and 96,000. The number average molecular weight calculated from the COP is 150,000. The weight average molecular weight obtained by ultracentrifugation is 120,000. The P_{50} of the solution under standard conditions (pH = 7.40, P_{CO_2} = 35 torr, temperature = 35°C) ranges from 18 to 22 torr. The viscosity of the solution (hemoglobin concentration = 8.0 g/dL) ranges from 1.9 to 2.2 cp. The phospholipid content is below the detection limits of the thin-layer chromatography technique used (<0.4 mg/dL).

We have followed the stability of the polymerized solution when stored at 4 to 8°C as a sterile, pyrogen-free product. The stability with respect to rate of conversion to methemoglobin is shown in Figure 13–15. The methemoglobin remains below 2% for a 150-day period.

The stability of the polymeric species was determined by monitoring the solution with high-pressure liquid chromatography, SDS-PAGE, and viscosity. No changes were observed for at least a 1-year period. Figure 13–16 shows the high-pressure liquid chromatography scans for three different batches at the time of manufacture and 150 days later.

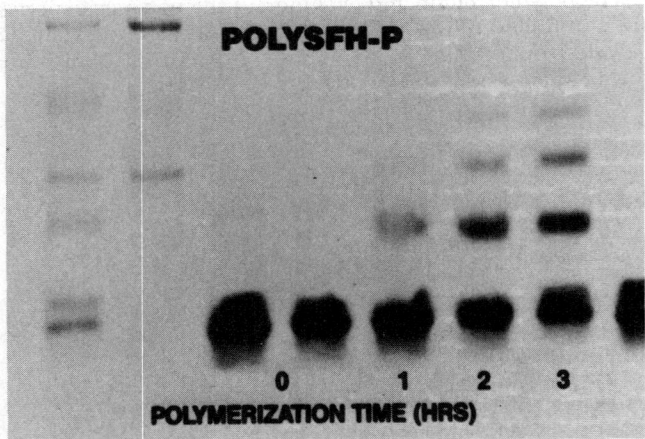

Figure 13–12. Evolution of new polypeptide bands over the course of the polymerization process, as monitored by SDS-PAGE. (From Moss GS, Sehgal LR, Gould SA, et al: Alternatives to transfusion therapy. Anesthesiol Clin North Am 8:569, 1990.)

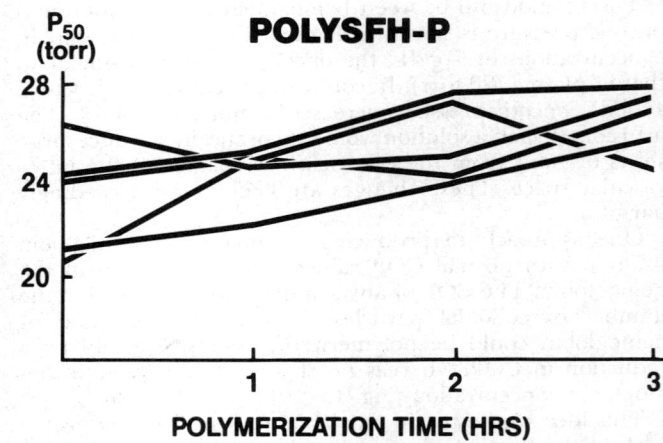

Figure 13–14. Alteration in P_{50} for five different batches of hemoglobin solution during polymerization. (From Moss GS, Sehgal LR, Gould SA, et al: Alternatives to transfusion therapy. Anesthesiol Clin North Am 8:569, 1990.)

TABLE 13–5

PROPERTIES OF POLYMERIZED PYRIDOXYLATED HEMOGLOBIN

Property	Parameter Range
Hemoglobin (g/dL)	12–14
Oxygen-carrying capacity (vol%)	16–19
Methemoglobin (%)	<5
Molecular weight range	64,000–400,000
Number average molecular weight	150,000
P_{50} (torr)	18–22
Binding coefficient (mL O_2/g Hb)	1.30
Hill's coefficient	1.5–2.0
Bohr's coefficient	−0.12 to −0.25
COP (torr)	20–25
Viscosity (cp)	1.9–2.2
Phospholipids (mg/dL)	<0.4
Limulus amebocyte lysate assay (EU/mL)	<0.625
Rabbit pyrogen test	Pass

From Moss GS, Sehgal LR, Gould SA, et al: Alternatives to transfusion therapy. Anesthesiol Clin North Am 8:569, 1990.

STABILITY OF POLYSFH-P

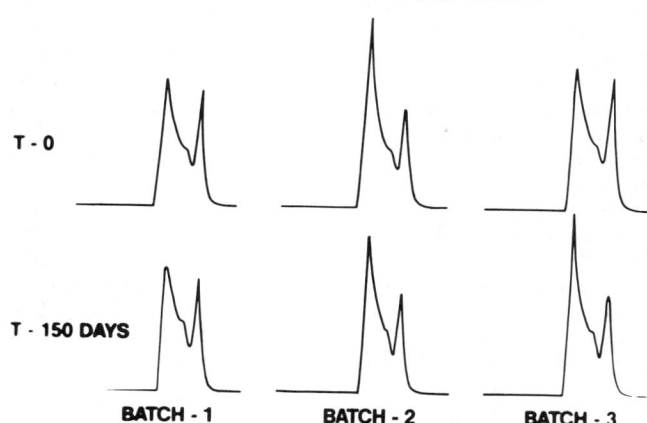

Figure 13–16. High-pressure liquid chromatography scans for three batches at the time of manufacture and 150 days later. No changes are noted. (From Moss GS, Sehgal LR, Gould SA, et al: Alternatives to transfusion therapy. Anesthesiol Clin North Am 8:569, 1990.)

No visible changes occurred. Finally, Figure 13–17 shows the changes in viscosity during a 150-day storage period. Once again, no change in viscosity was seen. Thus, the polymerized stroma-free hemoglobin (poly SFH-P), when stored at 4 to 8°C, appears to be quite stable.

Efficacy of Poly SFH-P

Seven adult baboons were anesthetized, paralyzed, intubated, and mechanically ventilated with room air. The respiratory rate and tidal volume were adjusted to maintain a $Paco_2$ between 35 and 45 torr before the start of the study and were not changed during the study. The animals were surgically prepared with arterial and central venous catheters for infusion, blood sampling, and monitoring. A thermal dilution balloon-tipped catheter was floated into the pulmonary artery. A Foley catheter was inserted into the urinary bladder. Standard hemodynamic monitoring was performed for electrocardiogram, arterial pressures, pulmonary capillary wedge pressure, and central venous pressure. Cardiac output was determined by the thermal dilution method.

The study was conducted with the use of ketamine anes-

thesia. After stabilization of the animals, a set of baseline measurements was obtained. An isovolemic exchange transfusion with the poly SFH-P was then performed. Whole blood was removed in 50-mL aliquots and was replaced with approximately equal volumes of the infusate. Additional volume adjustments were made as required to maintain the pulmonary capillary wedge pressure at baseline values. The exchange was stopped at hematocrits of 20, 10, and 5% to obtain additional sets of measurements. The exchange transfusion was then carried out to obtain a complete washout of the RBCs. A hematocrit of less than 1% was achieved.

These animals, at zero hematocrit, had a poly SFH-P concentration of approximately 10 g/dL. They were then exchange transfused with dextran 70 to a hemoglobin concentration of 1 g/dL. The data from the second half of the study were compared with a control group (n=6) that underwent an exchange transfusion with dextran 70 to a hemoglobin concentration of 1 g/dL.

Arterial and mixed venous blood gases were measured by standard electrodes (IL 813). Whole blood and plasma hemoglobin levels were determined on the IL 282 Co-

STABILITY OF POLYSFH-P

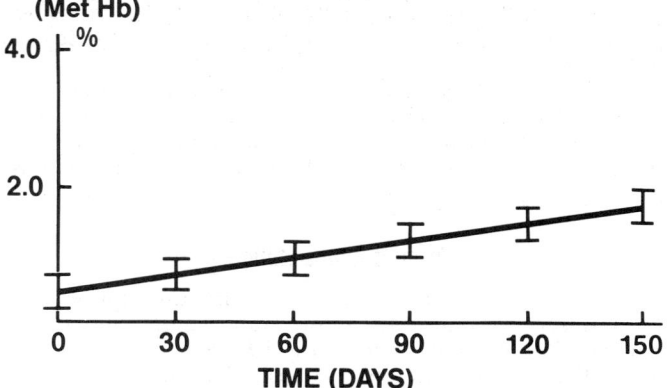

Figure 13–15. Changes in methemoglobin concentration on storage at 4 to 8°C, as a sterile, pyrogen-free solution. Each point represents the mean ± SEM. (From Moss GS, Sehgal LR, Gould SA, et al: Alternatives to transfusion therapy. Anesthesiol Clin North Am 8:569, 1990.)

STABILITY OF POLYSFH-P

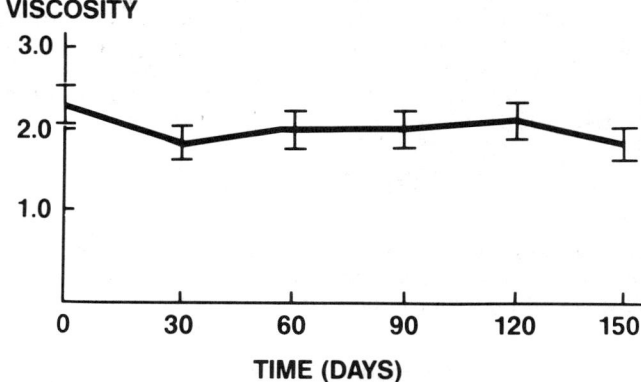

Figure 13–17. Changes in viscosity of five batches, observed during a 150-day period. Each point represents the mean ± SEM. No significant changes in viscosity are observed. (From Moss GS, Sehgal LR, Gould SA, et al: Alternatives to transfusion therapy. Anesthesiol Clin North Am 8:569, 1990.)

oximeter.[21] Oxygen carried by whole blood hemoglobin was measured by the IL 282 Co-oximeter. The physically dissolved oxygen in the aqueous phase was calculated from the PO_2 of the plasma separated by centrifugation. The poly SFH-P $[O_2]$ was measured by the IL 282 Co-oximeter. Hematocrits were determined by the microhematocrit method. P_{50} values of whole blood and plasma hemoglobin were determined with the hemoglobin oxygen dissociation curve analyzer (Hemo-O-Scan).[22]

The efficacy of the poly SFH-P was calculated as we have previously described.[23] At each hematocrit level, the arterial $[O_2]$ $([O_2]_a)$ was determined for each compartment by direct measurement or calculation. Total $\dot{V}O_2$ was calculated as the product of the cardiac output and $CaO_2 - CvO_2$. The contribution of poly SFH-P to oxygen delivery was calculated as the ratio of the poly SFH-P to total arterial $[O_2]$.[12]

$$\text{Poly SFH-P } O_2 \text{ delivery} = \frac{[O_2]_a, \text{ poly SFH-P}}{[O_2]_a, \text{ total}}$$

The contribution of poly SFH-P to $\dot{V}O_2$ was calculated as the ratio of poly SFH-P to total $CaO_2 - CvO_2$.

$$\text{Poly SFH-P } \dot{V}O_2 = \frac{\text{Poly SFH-P }(CaO_2 - CvO_2)}{\text{Total }(CaO_2 - CvO_2)}$$

All contributions were expressed as their percent values.

All animals receiving poly SFH-P survived the exchange transfusion, as did the previous animals receiving SFH-P.[15] The final hematocrit was $0.8 \pm 0.4\%$ (mean $\pm$ SEM). The difference in the initial bag P_{50} values of the two infusates was statistically significant ($P < .05$). However, the mean in vivo plasma P_{50} for the poly SFH-P was 17.0 ± 0.5 torr, which was not significantly different from the mean value of 17.6 ± 0.8 torr for the SFH-P. Both of these plasma P_{50} values are significantly below the mean baboon RBC P_{50} of 31.3 ± 0.8 torr. The poly SFH-P $[O_2]_a$ is significantly greater than the SFH-P value at all hematocrits ($P < .001$). At a hematocrit of 5%, the $[O_2]_a$ was 9.5 ± 0.2 vol% for poly SFH-P and 5.0 ± 0.4 vol% for SFH-P. The percent contributions of poly SFH-P to total oxygen delivery and total $\dot{V}O_2$ were compared with those of SFH-P. Poly SFH-P makes a significantly greater ($P < .02$) contribution to total oxygen delivery than SFH-P at all hematocrits. The contribution to total $\dot{V}O_2$ is greater by poly SFH-P at all hematocrits, with the difference significant ($P < .005$) at a hematocrit of 20%.

The in vivo P_{50} in the poly SFH-P animals undergoing the second exchange transfusion with dextran 70 ranged from 18 to 11 torr.[24] In contrast, the in vivo P_{50} of the control group ranged from 31.5 to 25.5 torr. The PvO_2 was significantly lower in the poly SFH-P group compared with the control group. Both groups of animals raised their cardiac output in an identical manner in response to their anemia. The critical oxygen delivery in the control group was 6.6 mL/min/kg of body weight compared with 5.7 mL/min/kg in the test group.

Safety of Poly SFH-P

So far, we have discussed the efficacy of hemoglobin solution with regard to oxygen dynamic properties. The next issue is safety. Our concern lies in two areas: nephrotoxicity and immunocompetence.

Nephrotoxicity

Nephrotoxicity was reported in early studies after infusion of the hemoglobin solution.[25] Further investigation suggested that the stroma was the toxic factor, probably on the basis of thrombosis of the small renal vasculature.[26] In 1967,

Rabiner and colleagues[27] reported that hemoglobin solution, relatively free of stroma, produced no deterioration in renal function after infusion into dogs. These findings were subsequently confirmed in monkeys, even in stressful circumstances of dehydration and shock.[28]

In 1977, Savitsky and colleagues[29] reported the results of a clinical safety trial in humans using SFH. Eight healthy male volunteers received a 250-mL infusion of SFH at a rate of 2 to 4 mL/min. The hemoglobin concentration of this solution was 6.4 g/dL. The P_{50} was not reported. Two control patients received similar infusions of 5% albumin.

The most striking finding of this study was a decline in creatinine clearance in the hemoglobin solution recipients from a baseline value of 148 to 73 mL/min 1 hour after infusion. This value returned to normal in the second hour after infusion. This alteration in kidney function was accompanied by a sharp decline in urine volume in these patients. In the albumin control patients, no changes were seen in urine volume or creatinine clearance. The authors stressed that this deterioration in kidney function was transient and not associated with permanent renal damage. Nevertheless, these results had a chilling effect on further clinical research.

As Savitsky and coworkers[29] pointed out, there are three possible explanations for the observed nephrotoxicity. The first is stromal toxicity. They did note a stroma lipid level of 1.6 mg/dL. Because this represents only 1% of the original level of phospholipid and the infusion of hemoglobin solution did not produce detectable disseminated intravascular coagulation in the recipients, stromal toxicity is an unlikely explanation.

A second possibility is the presence of a vasoactive substance in the hemoglobin solution that affects renal blood flow. This is supported by the observation that recipients developed transient bradycardia and mild hypertension during the infusion. We noted similar findings in our early hemoglobin solution studies in baboons. We therefore believe that prospective hemoglobin solutions should be tested for the presence of vasoactive substances by bioassay techniques before clinical testing.

A third possibility is that the changes in renal function were simply related to the filtration of free hemoglobin through the kidneys. Perhaps hemoglobin filtration in some way interferes with normal kidney function. Once the hemoglobinemia disappears, renal function returns to normal. This is an interesting argument, because the highest level of plasma hemoglobin in the human volunteers was only 57 mg/dL. In actual clinical practice, we expect plasma hemoglobin levels to rise to 6 to 8 g/dL, a 1000-fold increase over the levels seen in the clinical safety trials. It is likely that elevations of plasma hemoglobin of that magnitude would produce even greater changes in renal function, especially in a setting of hemorrhagic shock.

In this regard, polyhemoglobin has theoretic appeal. The large molecular size of a polymer should rule out renal excretion. The principal route of excretion is presumably the reticuloendothelial system. Thus, nephrotoxicity is less likely with a polymer than it is with the hemoglobin tetramer.

Immunocompetence

Our second concern is postinfusion immunosuppression. Because sepsis is one of the most serious complications that may develop in circumstances in which hemoglobin solution is used, it is important to establish that the infusion of hemoglobin solution does not impair the host defense mechanism.

The effect of hemoglobin solution on granulocyte function was studied by Hau and Simmons.[30] They showed that hemoglobin acted as an adjuvant in experimental peritonitis in rats by interfering with granulocyte phagocytosis and bacterial killing capability. However, the significance of this finding is not clear, because the hemoglobin acted as an adjuvant only when it was injected into the peritoneal cavity. It was not effective when it was injected intravenously or intramuscularly. In another report, Hoyt and colleagues[31] studied the ability of rats to withstand peritonitis after exposure to hemoglobin solution used as a volume expander in the treatment of hemorrhagic shock. They found no evidence that hemoglobin solution depressed host defense mechanisms.

Whether polyhemoglobin alters immunocompetence is unknown. It is known that the infusion of colloid particles produces blockage of the reticuloendothelial system and thereby enhances susceptibility to bacterial toxins.[32] Stein and Saba[33] have shown that the infusion of colloid particles not only blocks the reticuloendothelial system but also produces an acute depletion of plasma fibronectin levels. Thus, studies designed to investigate the effects of polyhemoglobin on immunocompetence would be necessary before clinical trials.

The solution passes the rabbit pyrogen test and from batch to batch has between 0.3125 and 0.625 EU/mL as determined by the limulus amebocyte lysate assay. In addition, the solution passes the U.S. Pharmacopeia safety and systemic toxicity tests and shows no pressor effects as measured by the U.S. Pharmacopeia pressor test.

In addition to these standard tests, baboons receiving poly SFH-P from 1 to 8 g/kg of body weight have been followed for a period of 3 to 6 months and have shown no alteration in renal function, blood chemistry, and coagulation profile.

On the basis of all the data on safety and efficacy, a further modification of the product was made, leading to the approval to initiate clinical trials on humans. Preliminary results from the trials confirm the preclinical data.[34]

SUMMARY AND CONCLUSION

Attempts to develop a hemoglobin-based RBC substitute have spanned many decades[34, 35] but have not yet resulted in a clinically useful product. The issues that have prevented clinical application have been primarily ones of safety and not efficacy.[23] Numerous animal studies have documented the efficacy of SFH.[3, 34] Although SFH was effective, there were limitations that were of concern. Oncotic considerations limit the concentration of infusate SFH to 6 to 8 g/dL, or half-normal. Owing to the loss of organic phosphate modulators of P_{50} such as 2,3-DPG, the P_{50} of SFH is typically between 12 to 14 torr, which again is half the normal value. Finally, the intravascular half-life of SFH is too short, ranging from 2 to 6 hours.[36]

Polymerization provides a means of correcting these limitations of SFH. The high oxygen affinity can be greatly diminished by covalent binding of pyridoxal-5'-phosphate to the NH_2 terminus of the beta-chains. COP exerted by a protein solution is proportional to the number of discrete colloid particles. By polymerization, the number of colloid particles is reduced, leading to a decrease in COP. Our data show that this can indeed be achieved in a reproducible fashion. The rate at which this diminution of COP is accomplished determines the yield of polymeric species, as well as their molecular weight distribution. We have demonstrated that the polymerization can be reproducibly controlled to result in a yield of 75 to 85% polymers, with a molecular weight distribution of 128,000 to 400,000. The number average and weight average molecular weights indicate that the large proportion of the polymers represent the cross-linking of two tetramers.

The data that reflect the interaction of oxygen with poly SFH-P indicate that the oxygen-carrying function of hemoglobin has not been significantly altered by the chemical modifications. The binding coefficient of oxygen is unchanged. As one would have anticipated, there is a loss of cooperativity (diminished Hill's coefficient) between the hemoglobin chains, suggesting structural restrictions in the polymeric species because of the cross-linking. A reduced alkaline Bohr's effect would be expected, and our data confirm that. Finally, some increase in oxygen affinity with polymerization would be expected. This is indeed the case, although the P_{50} of poly SFH-P is comparable to banked blood (18 to 22 torr).

A modified hemoglobin solution, to be clinically useful, would need to have a reasonable shelf life. Our data demonstrate that polymerized hemoglobin can be stored in the cold (4 to 8°C) for several months with minimal change in methemoglobin concentration. Furthermore, our HPLC and viscosity data clearly indicate that no significant alterations in the polymeric species occur during storage.

References

1. Biro GP, Blais P: Perfluorocarbon blood substitutes. Crit Rev Oncol Hematol 6:311, 1987.
2. Gould SA, Rosen AL, Sehgal LR, et al: Clinical experience with Fluosol-DA. In: Bolin RB, Geyer RP, Nemo GJ (eds): Advances in Blood Substitute Research. New York, Alan R Liss, p 331, 1983.
3. Gould SA, Sehgal LR, Rosen AL, et al: Red cell substitutes: An update. Ann Emerg Med 14:798, 1985.
4. Gould SA, Rosen AL, Sehgal LR, et al: How good are fluorocarbon emulsions as O_2 carriers? Surg Forum 32:299, 1981.
5. Gould SA, Rosen AL, Sehgal LR, et al: Red cell substitutes: Hemoglobin solution or fluorocarbon? J Trauma 22:736, 1982.
6. Gould SA, Rosen AL, Sehgal LR, et al: Fluosol-DA as a red cell substitute in acute anemia. N Engl J Med 315:1653, 1986.
7. Clark LC Jr, Clark EW, Moore RE, et al: Room temperature-stable biocompatible fluorocarbon emulsions. In: Bolin RB, Geyer RP, Nemo GJ (eds): Advances in Blood Substitute Research. New York, Alan R Liss, p 169, 1983.
8. Sloviter HA, Mukherji B: Prolonged retention in the circulation of emulsified lipid-coated perfluorochemicals. In: Bolin RB, Geyer RP, Nemo GJ (eds): Advances in Blood Substitute Research. New York, Alan R Liss, p 181, 1983.
9. Moss GS, DeWoskin R, Rosen AL, et al: Transport of oxygen and carbon dioxide by hemoglobin-saline solution in the red cell–free primate. Surg Gynecol Obstet 142:357, 1976.
10. Moss GS, Gould SA, Sehgal LR, et al: Hemoglobin solution. From tetramer to polymer. Surgery 95:249, 1984.
11. Gould SA, Sehgal LR, Rosen AL, et al: The development of polymerized pyridoxylated hemoglobin solution as a red cell substitute. Ann Emerg Med 15:1416, 1986.
12. Gould SA, Sehgal LR, Rosen AL, et al: Hemoglobin solution: Is a normal [Hb] or P_{50} more important? J Surg Res 33:189, 1982.
13. Benesch RE, Benesch R, Renthal RD, et al: Affinity labeling of the polyphosphate binding site of hemoglobin. Biochemistry 11:3576, 1972.
14. Greenburg AG, Hayashi R, Siefert I, et al: Intravascular persistence and oxygen delivery of pyridoxylated, stroma-free hemoglobin during gradations of hypotension. Surgery 86:13, 1979.
15. Gould SA, Rosen AL, Sehgal L, et al: The effect of altered hemoglobin-oxygen affinity on oxygen transport by hemoglobin solution. J Surg Res 28:246, 1980.
16. Sehgal LR, Rosen AL, Gould SA, et al: An appraisal of polymerized pyridoxylated hemoglobin as an acellular oxygen carrier. In: Bolin RB, Geyer RP (eds): Blood Substitutes. New York, Alan R Liss, p 19, 1983.
17. Sehgal LR, Rosen AL, Gould SA, et al: Preparation and in vitro characteristics of polymerized pyridoxylated hemoglobin. Transfusion 23:148, 1983.
18. Benesch RE, Benesch R, Renthal RD, et al: Affinity labeling of the polyphosphate binding site of hemoglobin. Biochemistry 11:3576, 1972.
19. Greenberg AG, Hayashi R, Siefert I, et al: Intravascular persistence and oxygen delivery of pyridoxylated, stroma-free hemoglobin during gradations of hypotension. Surgery 86:13, 1979.
20. Sehgal LR, Rosen AL, Gould SA, et al: Characteristics of polymerized pyridoxylated hemoglobin. Biomater Artif Cells Artif Organs 16:173, 1988.
21. Sehgal HL, Sehgal LR, Rosen AL, et al: Sensitivity of the IL 282 Co-oximeter to low hemoglobin concentration and high proportions of methemoglobin (letter). Clin Chem 26:362, 1980.
22. Sehgal HL, Sehgal LR, Rosen AL, et al: Performance of the oxygen-hemoglobin dissociation analyzer (Hem-O-Scan) compared with the IL 282 Co-oximeter (letter). Clin Chem 26:784, 1980.

23. Rosen AL, Gould SA, Sehgal LR, et al: Evaluation of efficacy of stroma-free hemoglobin solutions. In: Bolin RB, Geyer RP (eds): Blood Substitutes. New York, Alan R Liss, p 79, 1983.
24. Rosen AL, Gould SA, Sehgal LR, et al: Effect of hemoglobin solution on compensation to anemia in the red cell free primate. FASEB J 3:A686, 1989.
25. Hamilton PB, Hiller A, Van Slyke DD: Renal effects of hemoglobin infusions in dogs in hemorrhagic shock. J Exp Med 85:477, 1948.
26. Rabiner SF, Friedman LH: The role of intravascular hemolysis and the reticuloendothelial system in the production of a hypercoagulable state. Br J Haematol 14:105, 1968.
27. Rabiner SF, Helbert JR, Lopas H, et al: Evaluation of a stroma-free hemoglobin solution for use as a plasma expander. J Exp Med 126:1127, 1967.
28. Birndorf NI, Lopas H: Effects of red cell stroma-free hemoglobin solution on renal function in monkeys. J Appl Physiol 29:573, 1970.
29. Savitsky JP, Doczi J, Black J, et al: A clinical safety trial of stroma-free hemoglobin. Clin Pharmacol Ther 23:73, 1978.
30. Hau T, Simmons RL: Mechanisms of the adjuvant effect of hemoglobin in experimental peritonitis: III. The influence of hemoglobin on phagocytosis and intracellular killing by human granulocytes. Surgery 87:588, 1980.
31. Hoyt DB, Greenberg AG, Peskin CW, et al: Resuscitation with pyridoxylated stroma free hemoglobin: Tolerance to sepsis. J Trauma 21:938, 1981.
32. Litwin MD, Walter CW, Ejarque P, et al: Synergistic toxicity of gram-negative bacteria and free colloidal hemoglobin. Ann Surg 157:485, 1963.
33. Stein PM, Saba TM: Cardiovascular response to hemorrhage in the dog as modified by colloid induced opsonic deficiency and reticuloendothelial blockade. Fed Proc 38:1115, 1979.
34. Moss GS, Gould SA, Rosen AL, et al: Results of the first clinical trials with a polymerized hemoglobin solution. In: International Symposium on Red Cell Substitutes, Basel, Switzerland, University of Basel, March 18, 1989.
35. Mulder AG, Amberson WR, Steggerda FR, et al: Oxygen consumption with hemoglobin-ringer. J Cell Comp Physiol 5:383, 1934.
36. DeVenuto F, Friedman H, Neville JR, et al: Appraisal of hemoglobin solution as a blood substitute. Surg Gynecol Obstet 149:417, 1979.

CHAPTER 14

Selected Nonvascular Procedures

Roderick J. Boyes
James A. Kruse

THORACENTESIS

Thoracentesis is the temporary placement of a needle, cannula, or trocar in the pleural space for either diagnostic or therapeutic recovery of pleural fluid or air. The term is derived from the Greek words *thorakus* (chest) and *kentesis* (to pierce). It was described in the 18th century by Monro and Hewson, and Bowditch established the procedure in the 1830s.[1] Advances in the technique have been primarily due to the availability of improved instruments and the use of ultrasound imaging and computed tomography to direct cannula insertion.[2, 3] More recently, the role of thoracentesis has been expanded to include the placement of small-bore pleural catheters for pleurodesis, prolonged drainage of the pleural space, and relief of acute pneumothorax.[4-7]

Indications

Thoracentesis should be employed in the evaluation of any pleural effusion of unknown cause. It should also be used to alleviate respiratory distress caused by an expanding pleural effusion. Additional indications for thoracentesis include tension pneumothorax (before chest tube placement) and placement of a catheter for drainage of and sclerotherapy for persistent effusions secondary to malignancy. Thoracentesis is not done to verify the presence of pleural effusion; rather the presence of the effusion should be verified before performing the procedure. In most situations, this can be accomplished by physical examination and chest roentgenography. Decubitus chest radiographs should be taken to verify free fluid collections. Ultrasound imaging or computed tomography may be employed if there is any doubt about the presence of effusion.

Analysis of the pleural fluid obtained by thoracentesis is complementary to the clinical information obtained from the history, the physical examination, and other studies. Collins and Sahn reported on 129 prospective thoracenteses and found that in 18% the etiologic diagnosis could be based on the pleural fluid examination alone.[8] This contrasts with 56% of the cases in which the pleural fluid findings only supported the presumptive clinical diagnosis, and 26% of the procedures yielded no additive evidence for the diagnosis.

Contraindications

There are no absolute contraindications for thoracentesis, except lack of an indication. Most of the relative contraindications are associated with the increased incidence of complications when thoracentesis is performed in certain high-risk settings. These include patients with coagulopathy and/or thrombocytopenia, particularly with platelet counts of less than 50,000/mm³. When possible, pre-existing hemorrhagic diatheses should be corrected before attempting the procedure. Uncooperative patients may require sedation, careful monitoring, and restraints during the procedure. If patients are receiving mechanical ventilation with or without positive end-expiratory pressure, there should be careful consideration as to whether thoracentesis should be performed while they are undergoing positive pressure ventilation or deferred until they are able to ventilate spontaneously. No invasive procedure should be performed through a contaminated site, such as an area of cellulitis or herpes zoster. Other authors recommend that thoracentesis not be performed unless more than 10 mm of fluid is evident on the decubitus radiograph.[9, 10] Ultrasound imaging can be of considerable assistance in performing diagnostic thoracentesis in patients with small effusions that require evaluation.

Complications

Percutaneous needle drainage of the pleural space can result in both local and systemic complications (Table 14-1). Although uncommon, many of these complications, such as pneumothorax, re-expansion pulmonary edema, vasovagal reactions, and deep organ injury, are potentially life threatening and may necessitate specific treatment. Recognition of these complications is therefore paramount.

Pneumothorax occurs in 3 to 39% of patients undergoing thoracentesis.[10-12] The incidence may be as low as 5% if ultrasound imaging is employed.[11] Therefore, the use of ultrasound should be considered in high-risk patients, both to localize the pleural effusion and to estimate the depth of the fluid before thoracentesis. Vasovagal reactions typically manifest as lightheadedness or syncope associated with bradyarrhythmias or hypotension and usually respond promptly to intravenous atropine administration.[13] As with many percutaneous procedures, a knowledge of the under-

TABLE 14–1

COMPLICATIONS ASSOCIATED WITH THORACENTESIS

Pain[8, 11]
Dry tap[8, 11]
Cough[8]
Pleural fluid leakage[8]
Vasovagal reaction (bradycardia, hypotension)[9]
Intercostal artery bleeding[150]
Hematoma[11]
Pneumothorax[8, 11, 25]
Hemothorax[9]
Air embolism[16]
Infection (cellulitis, empyema)[151]
Needle track seeding with malignant cells[19]
Re-expansion pulmonary edema[152, 153]
Spleen or liver lacerations[154, 155]
Diaphragm injury[156]
Lung parenchyma laceration[8]
Catheter fragment sheared into thorax[18]
Hypoxemia[44]
Death[157]

lying anatomic features and the relationships to surface anatomic landmarks is fundamental to minimizing complications. Vital organs, such as the liver, the spleen, the heart, and the diaphragm, in proximity to the site of needle insertion, are at risk for puncture or laceration. The diaphragm is located more cephalad with the patient in the supine position than when the patient is upright. Thus, thoracentesis is not recommended below the eighth rib with the patient in the upright position and not below the sixth intercostal space in the supine patient. Strict adherence to aseptic technique minimizes the risk of bacterial contamination, which may result in empyema or soft tissue infection. Re-expansion pulmonary edema may occur and is often heralded by dyspnea or by marked, uncontrollable coughing.[14, 15]

Rare complications include air embolism,[16, 17] intercostal artery laceration, catheter shearing and lodgment within the thorax,[18] performance of the procedure on the wrong patient or the wrong side of the thorax,[8] and needle track seeding of malignancy.[19] Although inability to obtain fluid is not a true complication, it occurred in 12% of patients in one study.[8]

Procedure

Several techniques are in common use for accomplishing thoracentesis. The following description employs a modification of the Seldinger vascular technique,[20] which has the advantages of potentially allowing the use of a smaller-gauge needle, minimizing the time that the needle is in proximity to the lung. Substitution of a flexible catheter for a needle while drainage is performed increases patient comfort by allowing slight positional changes, while decreasing the risk of pneumothorax or lung laceration caused by movement of the patient or the drainage device. If the pleural fluid drainage ceases before the desired volume has been obtained, the position of the plastic catheter can be manipulated within the thorax, frequently resulting in further drainage. On the other hand, altering the position of a needle within the pleural space greatly increases the risk of inadvertent tissue penetration. For high-risk patients, including those receiving positive pressure ventilation, those with coagulopathies, patients who are too ill to be optimally positioned, and those with loculated fluid collections, ultrasound imaging should be used to evaluate the optimal site and depth of needle entry. If possible, the procedure should

be deferred in patients who are uncooperative. A similar risk-benefit analysis should be considered in patients receiving mechanical ventilation. In some cases, the procedure may be deferred until positive pressure ventilation is no longer required. If necessary, however, thoracentesis can be accomplished with relative safety in mechanically ventilated patients.[21]

1. If the procedure is done with the patient in the supine position, ultrasound imaging is used to locate the fluid and determine the optimal site of needle entry and depth. The patient should remain in this position until the thoracentesis is completed.

For patients who can tolerate it, the upright position is preferred and may carry a lesser risk of certain complications. While receiving support as required to maintain this position, the patient sits at the edge of the bed facing a bedside table, which has been raised to mid-chest level. The patient's folded arms rest comfortably on a pillow placed on the table, and the patient's head rests on the arms. This position should raise the scapulae above the sixth intercostal space posteriorly. Additional risk is likely entailed if an entry site below the eighth intercostal space is attempted, particularly without ultrasound guidance.

2. If necessary, an analgesic or sedative may be administered to the patient to limit discomfort or anxiety associated with the procedure.

3. The site of thoracentesis is percussed and one interspace below the superior level of dullness is selected posteriorly or posterolaterally. This is then marked with indelible ink or a small impression on the skin using a suitable instrument.

4. The area is thoroughly cleansed with an antiseptic solution, such as povidone-iodine, and allowed to dry. Hat, mask, sterile gown, and sterile gloves are donned by the physician, and sterile drapes are used to maintain an aseptic field.

5. A skin wheal is raised at the marked site by using a 25-gauge needle with 1% lidocaine with epinephrine. A 22-gauge needle is substituted, and further subcutaneous infiltration of anesthetic is then carried down to the rib inferior to the selected interspace. The periosteum is anesthetized and the needle is "walked up" the rib to its superior border. Because the intercostal neurovascular bundle lies at the inferior border of the rib, this area is avoided (Fig. 14–1). The needle is advanced just over the superior margin of the rib, down to the parietal pleura. The pleura may be anesthetized with a small amount of local anesthetic. Intentionally aspirating a small amount of pleural fluid into the anesthetic-containing syringe is helpful in confirming the presense of fluid at the chosen site. When fluid is aspirated, the depth of the needle is marked with the fingers or a small surgical clamp before its removal (see Fig. 14–1A); this depth measurement is then used to avoid overinsertion of the larger needle in the next step. After fluid is withdrawn into the syringe, however, there should be no further injection of local anesthetic as needle track seeding may occur if the effusion contains malignant cells.

6. After the infiltrating needle is removed, the insertion depth is noted and the clamp removed and placed at the same distance from the tip of a larger (18-gauge thin-walled) needle with attached syringe (see Fig. 14–1B). This needle is then directed along the same trajectory used earlier, inserting the needle just over the superior edge of the rib while applying continuous gentle aspiration. The clamp prevents overinsertion of the needle and mitigates the chance of puncturing the lung. After fluid is obtained, the syringe is carefully removed while the needle is stabilized, and a J-tipped guidewire is advanced through the needle and into the pleural space (see Fig. 14–1C). The hub of the

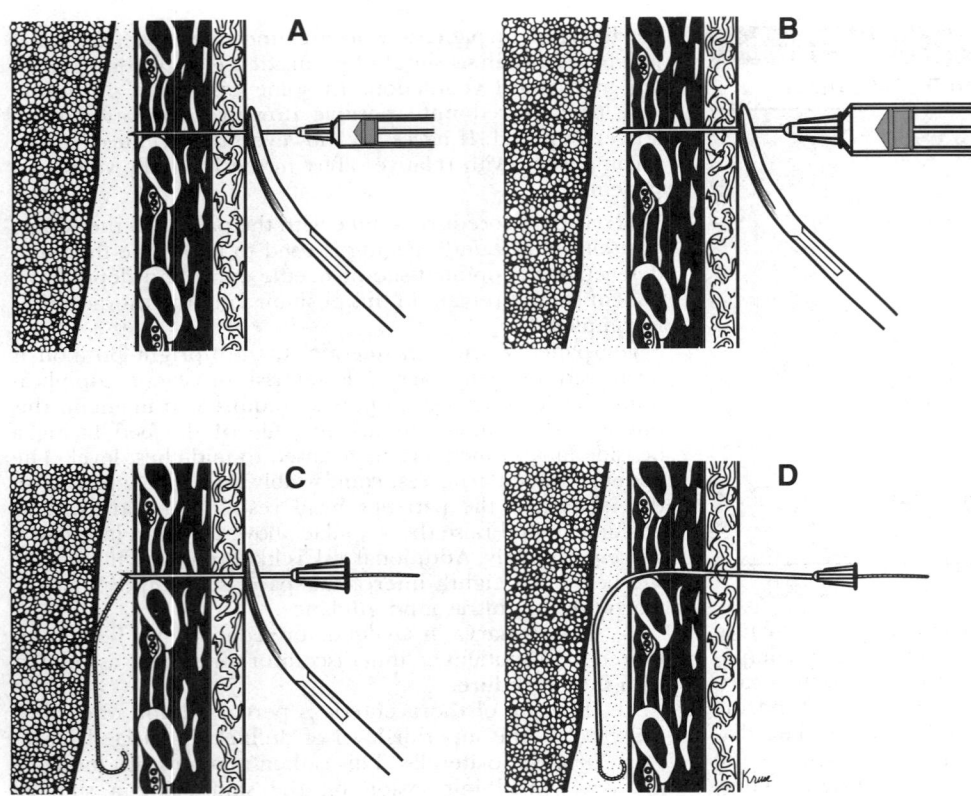

Figure 14–1. *A*. After infiltration of local anesthesia, the anesthetic syringe is advanced to the pleural space while aspiration is performed. At the point where pleural fluid is first aspirated, the depth of needle penetration is marked with a surgical clamp at the level of the skin. *B*. The clamp is repositioned on the Seldinger needle at the same level and advanced to the pleural space. Note the relationship between the needle and the intercostal neurovascular bundle. *C*. The J-tipped guidewire is inserted into the pleural space and the needle is removed. *D*. The thoracentesis catheter is advanced over the guidewire and the guidewire is removed.

needle should be open to the atmosphere only momentarily, otherwise air may be introduced into the pleural space, resulting in pneumothorax. After the guidewire has been successfully advanced well beyond the tip of the needle, the needle is withdrawn and an 18-gauge catheter is advanced over the guidewire (see Fig. 14–1*D*). Before the catheter makes contact with the skin, the operator should ensure that a portion of the guidewire visibly protrudes from the hub end of the catheter and is secured by the fingers. This ensures that the guidewire is not lost into the thorax as the catheter is inserted.

7. The guidewire is removed and the hub of the catheter immediately covered with the gloved finger. A syringe is quickly placed on the catheter to confirm free-flowing fluid.

8. Several options exist for effecting pleural fluid drainage. For diagnostic thoracentesis, a 50-mL syringe can be applied directly to the catheter and filled. For draining large volumes (e.g., during a therapeutic thoracentesis), repeatedly filling, disconnecting, emptying, and reconnecting the syringe not only become tiring but increase the likelihood that air will enter the pleural space. In this situation, other options are preferable.

For example, a sterile three-way stopcock with attached 50-mL syringe may be connected to the catheter hub, and a length of sterile tubing leading to a drainage container can be connected to the remaining stopcock port. The stopcock is first adjusted to allow aspiration of fluid from the thorax. After the syringe is full, the stopcock position is changed to allow the fluid to be expelled into the drainage container. Caution must be exercised to ensure that the stopcock is not inadvertently positioned such that the catheter is open to the atmosphere, resulting in air entry into the pleural space.

Sterile tubing can be used to connect a drainage bag or bottle directly to the catheter hub, and the effusion can be drained by gravity. However, unless a collapsed plastic bag is used as the collection chamber, or a water seal is employed,

there is a risk of inducing pneumothorax. Alternatively, a vacuum bottle may be attached directly to the catheter hub. Placing a stopcock between the catheter hub and the vacuum tubing allows the drainage to be easily controlled by turning the stopcock.

9. Regardless of the method employed, the quantity of fluid removed during large-volume diagnostic or therapeutic thoracentesis should be monitored to ensure that the desired volume is not exceeded. Re-expansion pulmonary edema more commonly occurs when more than 1 L of pleural fluid is removed at one time. If flow ceases before the desired amount of fluid has been obtained, the catheter tip may be occluded by contact with the visceral pleura. This can be corrected by releasing suction and gently repositioning the catheter slightly, and then resuming aspiration.

10. After the desired volume of drainage has been achieved, the catheter is removed while gentle suction is applied to avoid any air entrainment into the chest, a sterile bandage is placed over the puncture site, and the patient is repositioned for comfort.

11. A chest roentgenogram is routinely obtained after thoracentesis. Even if this radiograph shows no evidence of pneumothorax, one must be vigilant for the possible development of a subsequent, late pneumothorax. For the same reason, the patient should be closely monitored for signs or symptoms of pneumothorax during the initial 24 hours after thoracentesis, and a repeated chest x-ray film is obtained if there is any suspicion of delayed pneumothorax.

12. Pleural fluid specimens are sent for appropriate laboratory studies. Routine studies include complete and differential blood cell count, Gram's stain, microbiologic culture, and protein and glucose assays. Other studies may be indicated (e.g., smear and culture for acid-fast bacilli in suspected tuberculosis, amylase determination in pancreatitis, and cytologic cell block analysis if malignancy is suspected). Pleural fluid pH determination may be helpful in

evaluating parapneumonic effusions. To ensure accurate pleural fluid pH results, the specimen should be collected anaerobically in a heparinized syringe, any air bubbles immediately expelled, the syringe sealed, and the specimen assayed promptly.

Special Precautions for Ventilator-Dependent Patients in Supine Position

1. The patient should be given adequate sedation and/or analgesia, as necessary, before the procedure begins. The patient's arm on the side of the thoracentesis is abducted and secured either by an assistant or a soft restraint.

2. The fluid is localized with ultrasound imaging, and the effusion depth is noted. The preferred location is often the third or fourth intercostal space at or between the midaxillary and posterior axillary lines.

3. The rest of the procedure and precautions are similar to those for thoracentesis with the patient in the upright position, as detailed earlier.

4. After the procedure, the patient is carefully observed for possible development of pneumothorax. A chest roentgenogram should be obtained at the completion of the procedure and repeated the following day. Because of the increased risk of pneumothorax in patients receiving positive pressure ventilation, the patient should be monitored closely for respiratory and hemodynamic signs and symptoms suggestive of pneumothorax.

Draining Exudative Pleural Effusions

The technique described earlier to remove transudative effusions can be used to drain exudative and frankly purulent pleural effusions, except that a larger needle, guidewire, and catheter are necessary owing to the increased viscosity of the fluid. In a study by Reinhold and Ilescas, 15 patients with empyema were treated by percutaneous catheter drainage.[3] Twelve required no further surgical intervention; however, several required replacement of their catheters to improve drainage. This compares favorably with results with surgically placed tubes, which have a success rate of 35 to 80% in similar patients.[22]

Treatment of Simple Pneumothorax

Using needle aspiration or small-bore catheter aspiration to relieve simple pneumothorax was described by several authors.[5, 23, 24] This technique is suitable for small, uncomplicated pneumothoraces but should not be used as a substitute for conventional chest tube thoracostomy for patients who are receiving mechanical ventilation, patients with tension pneumothorax, or patients with significant hypoxemia. Several important points deserve mention:

1. The patient is supine, with the head of the bed elevated to 30°.

2. Needle entry is at the second or third intercostal space at the mid-clavicular line. After infiltration of the area with local anesthetic, the 22-gauge needle is advanced through the pleural membrane, with gentle aspiration to verify the presence of air, and the required depth is noted.

3. An 18-gauge needle attached to a 50-mL syringe is then advanced along the same trajectory and the pleural air collection is aspirated, or the Seldinger technique is used to place a flexible catheter for more complete aspiration with less risk of visceral pleura puncture.

A pigtail catheter may be employed in place of a conventional chest tube for continuous drainage of malignant effusions, for sclerotherapy,[6] or for initial drainage of empyema.[24, 25]

CLOSED CHEST TUBE THORACOSTOMY

Hippocrates was the first to describe a pleural drainage procedure,[26] and Playfair described a drainage tube with underwater seal in 1872.[27] Continuous drainage was introduced by Buelaw in 1875,[28] and Hewett was the first to describe the procedure in the English language literature when he used the procedure to drain an empyema in 1876.[29] Emergent placement of a thoracostomy tube was refined during the Korean War, and its use has since expanded to include traumatic and nontraumatic hemothorax, pneumothorax, chylothorax, malignant effusion, empyema, and a wide variety of infections in immunocompromised patients.[30, 31]

Urgent or emergent thoracostomy tube insertion is a common procedure in the intensive care unit. Patients receiving positive pressure ventilation, particularly those receiving high levels of positive end-expiratory pressure, are at increased risk of barotrauma, necessitating chest tube placement. Pneumothorax also occasionally occurs as a result of central venous catheterization via the subclavian vein and, rarely, via the internal jugular vein. Patients with severe lung diseases, such as necrotizing pneumonia and emphysema, are also at higher risk for barotrauma and spontaneous pneumothorax. In general, empyema and some parapneumonic effusions are optimally managed with continuous thoracostomy tube drainage. The intensivist should therefore be skilled in performing this procedure, as well as knowledgeable about its indications and complications.

The lungs are encased in a protective cage composed of the ribs and diaphragm. A neurovascular bundle consisting of intercostal vein, artery, and nerve lies at the inferior margin of each rib. Occasionally, a small vessel may lie on the superior margin of the ribs as well. The intercostal nerve supplies the parietal pleura and is involved in transmission of pleuritic pain sensation.[32] The lymphatic drainage of the parietal pleura is into the intercostal, substernal, and mediastinal lymphatic system. The lung has lymphatic drainage in the connective tissue adjacent to the pleura. Any injury to the lung or parietal pleura may cause fluid collections to accumulate between the visceral and parietal pleura for which a drainage procedure may be required.

Indications

Possible indications are listed in Table 14–2. Each listed indication may be handled in an alternative way. Hemorrhagic effusions have traditionally been considered an indication for chest tube placement. This was based on the belief that blood would not be reabsorbed and would serve as a culture medium for empyema or result in fibrous encasement of the pleura. It has been demonstrated that blood is generally reabsorbed from the pleural space, however, and hemorrhagic effusion per se is not necessarily an indication for tube thoracostomy.[33–35]

Contraindications

Bleeding diatheses increase the risk of hemorrhagic complications of chest tube placement. Therefore, strong consideration should be given to correcting coagulation abnormalities and severe thrombocytopenia before chest tube insertion. Similarly, if the patient is receiving heparin, administration of the drug should be discontinued before the procedure. Any patient with previous thoracic surgery or possible adhesions from previous surgery should have the

TABLE 14–2

INDICATIONS FOR CHEST TUBE INSERTION

1. Hemothorax
   a. Leakage from major vessel (e.g., aneurysm, arteriovenous malformation)[158]
   b. Iatrogenic injury during procedure, such as thoracentesis or central venous catheterization[159, 160]
   c. Trauma, blunt or penetrating[161, 162]
2. Pneumothorax
   a. Spontaneous (e.g., ruptured emphysematous bleb, asthma, necrotizing pneumonia)[163, 164]
   b. Iatrogenic (e.g., resulting from invasive procedure or positive pressure ventilation)[21, 165–167]
   c. Traumatic
   d. Surgical (e.g., after thoracotomy)
   e. Infectious (e.g., necrotizing pneumonia)
3. Empyema[32, 168]
   a. Sequela of lung infection
   b. Complication of procedure
   c. Direct spread from contiguous infection (e.g., from mediastinal source)
4. Pleurodesis[169, 170]
5. Chylothorax[159, 171]
6. Pleural effusion[172]
7. Thoracic trauma and hemodynamic instability
8. Prophylaxis
   a. Before surgery in patients with chest injuries
   b. When risk of barotrauma is high and personnel experienced with thoracostomy tube placement are not immediately available

procedure performed away from suspected sites of adhesions. Computed tomography may be helpful in delineating the optimal site in these situations. Patients with pleural malignancies require careful evaluation to avoid placement of the tube through a highly vascular area. All of these contraindications can be considered relative. For example, the potential benefits outweigh even these increased risks in the patient who is in extremis from a tension pneumothorax.

Complications

Serious technical complications associated with chest tube insertion are uncommon; in 447 patients with trauma, Millikan and colleagues demonstrated a 1% incidence.[36] With the elimination of the trocar as a placement technique, complications such as lung laceration and vascular injury are minimized. Following a protocol that includes digital probing of the track to feel for the lung and remove adhesions further minimizes the incidence of complications.[37] The routine use of prophylactic antibiotics is controversial. Decreased incidence of infection has been demonstrated in studies using prophylactic antibiotics in patients with trauma.[38, 39] Neugebauer and associates, on the other hand, reported an increase in infection rate with the use of prophylactic antibiotics in nontrauma patients.[40] For the trauma patient, prophylactic antibiotic use is not solely for covering the possibility of infection related to chest tube placement per se but also represents prophylaxis or therapy for possible bacterial contamination of chest or other injuries that may have been sustained.

As with thoracentesis, tube thoracostomy can produce re-expansion pulmonary edema.[41, 42] This usually occurs when there are marked pleural pressure shifts, typically to less than -20 cm H_2O, owing to pleural fluid drainage or relief of pneumothorax.[43] During drainage of pleural effusions, the risk of such pressure changes can be mitigated by clamping the chest tube when drainage exceeds 1000 mL

during several minutes, or if the patient has dyspnea or coughing. The onset of acute pulmonary edema may occur 1 to 2 hours after the procedure and is more likely if the lung has been collapsed for 72 hours or longer. Some patients may experience hypoxemia owing to worsened ventilation-perfusion mismatch through the re-expanded lung and may require supplemental oxygen. The need for oxygenation should therefore be monitored after chest tube insertion.[44]

Other complications include intercostal artery hemorrhage, subcutaneous tube placement, improper position of a chest tube with damage to intrathoracic structures, air leakage from a tube incompletely positioned in the chest, contusion or laceration of the lung parenchyma, diaphragm laceration, and subdiaphragmatic placement with or without injury to intra-abdominal organs (Table 14–3).

Procedure

The site of insertion and the technique used may vary depending on the reason for placement of the chest tube and the condition of the patient. The objective of adequately draining fluid or air, or providing access to the pleural space, should be accomplished by the tube thoracostomy. Careful placement is required to avoid discomfort to the patient and kinking of the tube and to ensure access to care of the tube by nursing personnel. With these considerations, the two most common sites chosen are the second intercostal space at the mid-clavicular line, and the fourth, the fifth, or the sixth intercostal space at the midaxillary line. Chest tube insertion at either site adequately relieves effusion or pneumothorax equivalently.[43, 45] Tube size is selected according to the viscosity of the fluid to be removed. Most simple pneumothoraces, as well as simple recurrent transudative effusions, are adequately drained using a No. 22 to 28 French tube. Fibrinous, exudative, hemorrhagic, and purulent effusions necessitate larger tubes (e.g., No. 32 to 42 French) to provide drainage without occluding. More than one tube may be required for large bronchopleural fistulas or for a loculated empyema.

The procedure for the lateral insertion site is described.

1. To obviate placing a chest tube in the wrong patient or the wrong hemithorax, it is important to examine each patient and review the chest radiograph before the procedure to verify the indication for placement and confirm on which side the tube is to be inserted. The chest x-ray film may show signs of adhesions or pleural thickening, which indicate that an alternative site should be considered.

TABLE 14–3

COMPLICATIONS OF CLOSED TUBE THORACOSTOMY

Intercostal bleeding[151]
Lung laceration[173–175]
Empyema[36, 176, 177]
Pulmonary edema[41, 153, 154, 178]
Lung entrapment[179]
Necrotizing fasciitis[180]
Arteriovenous fistula[181, 182]
Diaphragm paralysis[183, 184]
Diaphragm laceration[36]
Liver laceration[36]
Splenic injury[185]
Right atrial laceration[186]
Subcutaneous placement[36]
Abdominal placement[36]
Horner's syndrome[187–189]
Death[153, 190]

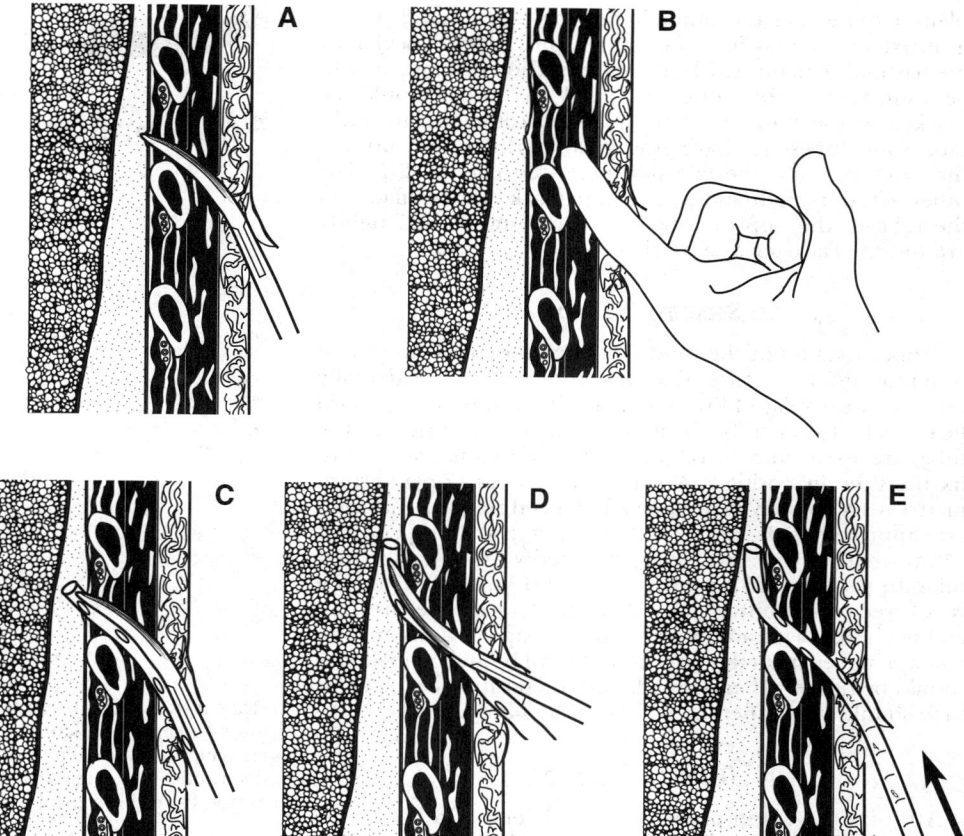

Figure 14–2. *A.* After a scalpel is used to make a skin incision, a surgical clamp is used for blunt dissection through the subcutaneous tissue, muscle, and pleura. Note that dissection begins one interspace inferior to the intended point of entry into the pleural space. *B.* Digital exploration of the track is performed to ensure that it reaches the pleural space and to ensure that the lung parenchyma is not fixed to the pleura. *C.* The thoracostomy tube is advanced into the pleural space with the surgical clamp. *D.* The clamp may be rotated to direct the tube to the desired position. *E.* The tube is then advanced into the chest until the last side hole is within the pleural space (further than shown here). Note graduated markings that denote distance from last drainage hole.

2. Adequate oxygenation and ventilation should be ensured before starting the procedure. If appropriate, sedation and systemic analgesia are provided.

3. The patient is placed in a 30° upright position with the arm on the side of insertion placed above the patient's head and secured by an attendant or an arm restraint. This allows the diaphragm to assume a lower position and provides easy access to the insertion site.

4. As noted earlier, the insertion site should be inspected for the presence of scars. The fifth or sixth intercostal space is identified by counting down from the second intercostal space, identified by the sternal angle of Louis. The diaphragm attaches at the tenth intercostal space laterally, but the dome of the diaphragm in the supine patient may extend to the fourth intercostal space.

5. The skin is cleansed with a suitable antiseptic, such as povidone-iodine solution, and allowed to dry. The operator must don surgical mask, hat, sterile gown, and sterile gloves, and a large sterile drape is used to provide a sterile field.

6. One uses a 25-gauge needle and syringe to raise a skin wheal with 1% lidocaine and epinephrine at both the fifth and sixth intercostal spaces. A 22-gauge needle is then used to infiltrate lidocaine into the subcutaneous tissue of the fifth and sixth intercostal spaces and the periosteum of the rib lying between the two interspaces over which the tube is to be inserted. The parietal pleura is anesthetized and aspiration for pleural air or fluid may be carried out to ensure proper position.

7. A skin incision, approximately 2 to 4 cm long, is made at the sixth intercostal space parallel to the ribs, and the subcutaneous tissue is spread and dissected using a Rochester-Pean clamp. A subcutaneous tunnel leading superiorly to the fifth intercostal space is made by blunt dissection. Thus, the chest tube enters the tunnel at the sixth intercostal space incision, but entry into the pleural space occurs at the level of the fifth intercostal space. This aids in securing the chest tube and reducing local fluid and air leakage.

8. After a sufficiently large track is made, the clamp is guided through the tunnel and up to the intercostal space where the tube is to be inserted. Continued blunt dissection though the intercostal muscles is accomplished by simultaneously spreading the jaws of the clamp as firm pressure is applied. It is necessary to concentrate the dissection at the superior margin of the inferior rib so that the vascular bundle at the lower aspect of the superior rib is avoided (Fig. 14–2A). When the tip of the clamp is at or nearly at the level of the pleural membrane, the index finger is positioned on the jaws of the clamp to provide guidance and a controlled force while the clamp is advanced through any remaining muscle fibers and while puncturing the pleura. This occasionally requires a reasonable amount of force.

9. After the tip of the clamp penetrates the pleura, a rush of air may be heard or fluid drainage observed. The clamp is then spread parallel to the ribs to open a space large enough to insert a finger into the thorax to verify the track and palpate for adhesions and ensure that the lung is not adherent to the chest wall (see Fig. 14–2B).

10. The tip of the tube is then grasped with the clamp and inserted through the hole in the pleura, either directly or by using the index finger as a guide. After it is inside the thoracic cavity, the clamp may be rotated to position the tube in the desired direction (see Fig. 14–2C and D). After this is accomplished, the clamp is released and removed, and the tube is advanced to the desired depth, ensuring that the last side hole of the tube is within the pleural space (see Fig. 14–2E).

11. The tube must be inserted to a sufficient depth to ensure that the last drainage hole is definitely inside the

pleural space. On the other hand, the tube should not be inserted so far that its tip impinges on central vascular or mediastinal structures. Ideally, the insertion distance should be estimated before insertion, and the tube should be marked at the position of the planned catheter-skin interface. Some tubes may have graduated markings that indicate the distance from the last side hole (see Fig. 14–2E). For tubes without graduations, a crimp mark can be made on the tube at the appropriate level, or a suture tied tightly around the catheter as a marker.

Securing the Tube

Proper fixation of the thoracostomy tube to the chest wall is important to ensure that the tube is not accidentally removed or displaced by patient activity or positioning. Two heavy (size 1-0 or 2-0) silk sutures, one on each side of the tube, are used both to provide skin approximation and to fix the tube in position. A simple skin suture or a vertical mattress suture may be employed. The edges of the incision are approximated and closed, leaving two long ends of suture that are then wrapped repeatedly around the chest tube (to provide additional security) and knotted. The tube is covered at the entry site with a sterile occlusive dressing and anchored with additional adhesive tape at a distance of about 8 inches from the insertion site. All tubing connections should be tightened and taped, and the position of the chest tube should be verified by a chest x-ray film.

Drainage Systems

After the tube is in place, the outside end of a chest tube cannot be allowed to remain exposed to the atmosphere. In spontaneously breathing patients, the pressure within the pleural space is normally negative with respect to atmospheric pressure, and this gradient would drive air into the tube, creating or worsening a pneumothorax. Although clamping the tube prevents this, it does not allow drainage of existing gas or fluid from the pleural space. The Heimlich valve (Fig. 14–3) is a simple instrument for preventing retrograde introduction of air into the pleural space while allowing free egress of gas or fluid from the tube.[46] This one-way rubber valve is often used in emergency situations in which a more complex drainage system is unavailable or would be unwieldy.

A water seal is more commonly used to provide the same function (Fig. 14–4). The water seal bottle is often connected to a vacuum source to facilitate removal of air from the

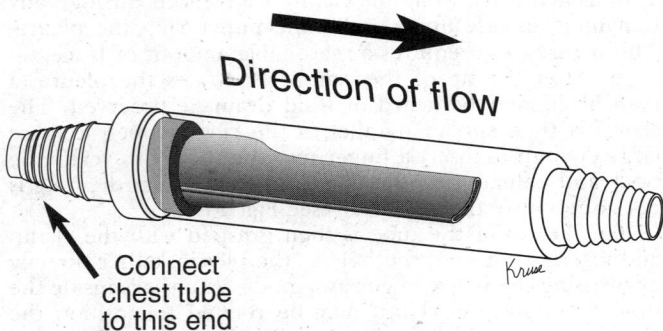

Figure 14–3. The Heimlich valve. When connected to a thoracostomy tube, this simple one-way valve allows decompression of a pneumothorax but prevents atmospheric air from entering the chest. This device is usually employed as a temporizing measure until a conventional water seal and drainage system can be applied. Note that connecting the valve backward can promote the development of a tension pneumothorax.

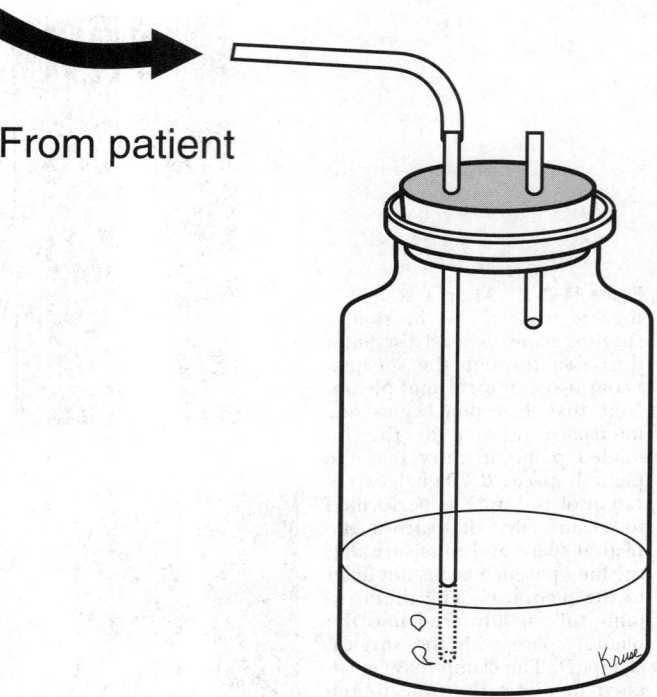

Figure 14–4. A single-bottle thoracostomy water seal. The water allows gas to escape the pleural space but prevents atmospheric air from entering the chest. The hydrostatic height of the water in the bottle determines the pressure that must be overcome before gas can escape from the pleural space.

pleural space. The height of the water seal, measured from the level of the submerged tube orifice to the surface of the water, represents the hydrostatic pressure that must be overcome before gas or fluid can escape from the chest. If the chest tube is connected directly to a water seal chamber, any pleural fluid that drains into the chamber increases the height of the water seal and eventually impedes drainage from the chest. This problem is obviated by using a two-bottle method, the first bottle acting as a simple trap for any pleural fluid drainage and the second bottle serving as the water seal.

Figure 14–5 depicts the more conventional three-bottle method. The chest tube is connected directly to a trap bottle for collecting any pleural fluid drainage, the second bottle is the water seal chamber, and the third bottle acts as a simple pressure-limiting device. The height of the fluid in the third bottle, measured vertically from the orifice of the submerged tubing to the surface of the water, represents the maximal negative pressure that can be applied to the system. For example, if this height is 25 cm, the maximal suction that can be applied to the chest tube is -25 cm H_2O. If the vacuum source exceeds this pressure, atmospheric air enters the center tube of this bottle, thus maintaining the system's pressure at -25 cm H_2O. Commercially available drainage systems are in common use in place of separate bottles. These devices incorporate the three-bottle method in an integral construction plastic unit and have the advantage of being preassembled and less cumbersome (Fig. 14–6).

Bubbling observed in the water seal chamber indicates that gas is exiting the pleural space or that there is a leak in the system somewhere between the chest tube insertion site and the water seal chamber. Briefly clamping the chest tube near the chest wall can aid in determining whether there is a leak in the system. If clamping the chest tube does not

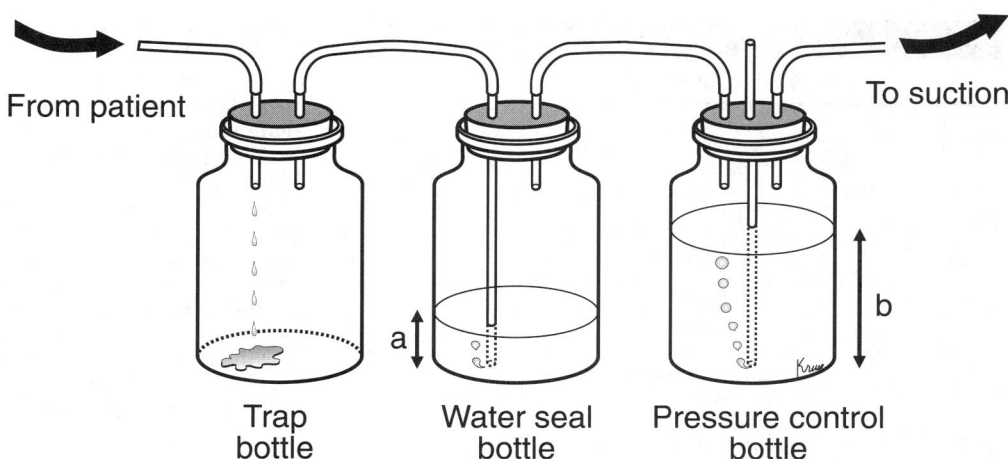

Figure 14–5. A three-bottle thoracostomy tube drainage system. The trap bottle collects pleural fluid drainage and prevents the drainage from raising the water seal level. The water seal acts as a one-way valve for gas flow. The height of level (a) determines the pressure that must be overcome for gas to escape the pleural space. The hydrostatic height in the pressure control bottle (b) determines the maximal suction that can be applied to the drainage system and thoracostomy tube.

halt bubbling at the water seal, atmospheric air is entering the tubing or tubing connections at some point between the clamp and the water seal. On the other hand, if bubbling ceases at the water seal after clamping, this indicates continued gas drainage from the pleural space or, alternatively, entry of atmospheric air into the chest tube at the incision site. The latter is particularly likely to occur if the last side hole of the chest tube is not completely within the thorax.

Bubbling at the water seal should not be confused with bubbling within the control chamber. Bubbles observed from the submerged tube of the control chamber indicate that the applied vacuum exceeds the hydrostatic pressure within this pressure control bottle. If suction is to be applied, it is desirable to adjust the applied vacuum so that bubbling is seen in the control chamber. This ensures that the negative pressure within the drainage system equals the hydrostatic height within the control chamber.

Chest Tube Removal

After the desired results have been accomplished, careful technique in chest tube removal may reduce the likelihood of pneumothorax. The patient should be positioned at 30° upright, with the arm secured over the head. The suture that is wrapped around the tube is cut using a scalpel or scissors and the suture is unwound from the tube. These free ends may be trimmed, and the suture and knot holding the incision in apposition can be left in place for a longer period if necessary. Thus, an advantage of the suturing technique described earlier is that the original sutures remain in place after the suture ends securing the tube have been cut. If a different knotting method necessitates removal of the entire suture, then depending on the size of the skin incision and the size of the tube, additional sutures may be required to approximate the wound edges and prevent air from entering the thorax. The chest tube should be removed while the patient expires or performs a mild Valsalva's maneuver; this increases intrathoracic pressure and minimizes the likelihood that air will enter the pleural space and induce pneumothorax. The incidence of pneumothorax after chest tube removal is about 4%, and it may be due to the original pathologic changes or induced during tube removal.[47–49] After the chest tube is removed, an occlusive dressing is immediately placed over the wound and held firmly in place for 3 to 5 minutes before placing any additional sutures, if required. If the tube was placed using the tunneling procedure described earlier, this limits the possibility of fluid leakage or entry of air into the chest. A regular occlusive sterile dressing is then placed and the wound is treated like any other surgical wound.

ABDOMINAL PARACENTESIS

Aspiration of peritoneal fluid was initially described by Saloman in 1906.[50] The original technique used a trocar through which a ureteral catheter was advanced. This technique was modified and used to control ascites in the 1940s.[51] With the advent of mercurial diuretics during the next decade, and subsequent refinements in dietary control and the use of loop diuretics, paracentesis was largely abandoned

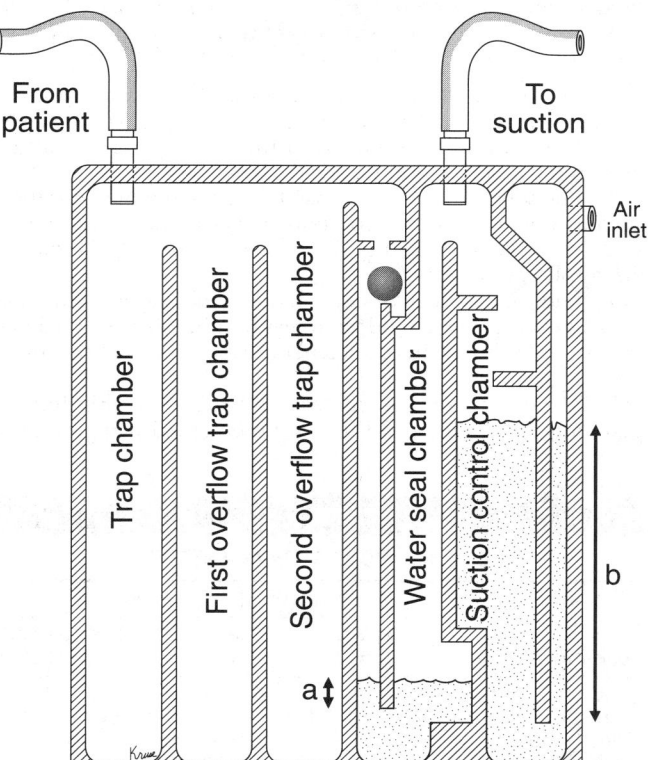

Figure 14–6. A modern integral thoracostomy tube drainage system. Note that there are three consecutive trap chambers. The water seal and control chambers function identically with those depicted in Figure 14–5. The height of level (a) determines the pressure that must be overcome for gas to escape from the pleural space. The hydrostatic height in the pressure control bottle (b) determines the maximal suction that can be applied to the drainage system and thoracostomy tube.

TABLE 14–4

DIFFERENTIAL DIAGNOSIS OF ASCITES

Peritonitis
  Fungal
  Tuberculous
  Bacterial
  Chemical
Pancreatic disease
Cardiac disease
  Congestive heart failure
  Constrictive pericarditis
  Tricuspid regurgitation
Malignancy
  Gastrointestinal
  Ovarian
  Breast
  Lymphoma
  Testicular
Hepatic disease
  Budd-Chiari syndrome
  Hepatic vein obstruction
  Hepatoma
  Cirrhosis
Vasculitis
Intestinal infarction
Urinary fistula
  Renal pelvis
  Ureter
  Bladder
Lymphatic obstruction
Thyroid disorder
  Myxedema
Hemoperitoneum
  Trauma
  Aneurysm

as a therapy for advanced ascites. Gines and colleagues elucidated the hemodynamic effects of large-volume paracentesis and demonstrated that this technique can be used with relative safety and may reduce the length of hospital stay without an increased incidence of complications.[52–54]

Indications

Paracentesis has become an invaluable procedure for the evaluation and/or therapeutic removal of ascitic fluid. The differential diagnosis of ascites is extensive (Table 14–4). Ascitic fluid analysis is essential in discriminating spontaneous bacterial peritonitis from other secondary causes of ascites. Paracentesis is therefore required for all patients with new-onset ascites and for those patients with ongoing ascites who experience clinical signs suggesting the possibility of peritonitis.[55, 56] This practice evolved from the understanding that there is a 10 to 25% incidence of spontaneous bacterial peritonitis in cirrhotic patients with ascites.[57–59]

In the past, therapeutic paracentesis was reserved for patients in respiratory distress or with excessive abdominal pressure from the ascites. Gines and colleagues demonstrated the safety and effectiveness of large-volume paracentesis (1 to 10 L) as a method of controlling ascites.[52–54] Large-volume paracentesis carries no more risks than do traditional methods to control ascites and may reduce the need for hospitalization.

Contraindications and Complications

Careful selection of patients to undergo paracentesis reduces the complications associated with this procedure. High-risk patients include those who are uncooperative and patients with severe coagulopathy, thrombocytopenia, or bowel obstruction. For patients with a significant hemorrhagic diathesis, efforts should be made to correct the coagulation disturbance before paracentesis, because local hemorrhage is one of the most frequent complications. Midline paracentesis may reduce the risk of abdominal wall bleeding. Bowel distention or obstruction increases the risk of inadvertent needle puncture of the bowel and resulting peritonitis. Moretz and Erickson showed in animal studies that bowel puncture in the absence of elevated intraluminal pressure is relatively innocuous, whereas puncture occurring in the face of increased pressures is likely to produce peritonitis.[60] Scars from prior abdominal surgery indicate the likely presence of underlying adhesions involving the bowel. Because adhesions increase the risk of puncture, these sites should be avoided. A summary of the complication rates from three studies is shown in Table 14–5.

Procedure

Paracentesis can be accomplished at a midline infraumbilical site or at either lower quadrant. The former site may be preferable because it should minimize the risk of abdominal wall hemorrhage; however, this potential advantage has not been conclusively demonstrated. The inferior epigastric arteries and large venous channels must be avoided if the lower quadrant approach is used. For patients with only small volumes of ascites or with questionable ascites, ultrasound imaging or computed tomography should be considered to confirm the presence of ascitic fluid as well as to localize the optimal site for paracentesis.[61] Preprocedure imaging may also be of value in defining the risk of bowel puncture for patients with distended loops of bowel or adhesions of bowel to the abdominal wall.

1. The bladder and the stomach should be decompressed using a urinary catheter and a nasogastric tube, respectively.
2. The patient is positioned in the supine or 30° head-up or semi-Fowler's position.
3. The selected area is cleansed using a suitable antiseptic, such as povidone-iodine solution. Surgical mask and hat, as well as sterile gown and gloves, are required. Sterile drapes are applied to the site.
4. The skin, subcutaneous tissue, and peritoneum are anesthetized using 1% lidocaine with epinephrine. To avoid intravascular injection of anesthetic, aspiration is always done before injection.
5. For diagnostic paracentesis, 50 mL of ascitic fluid is generally sufficient, and this can be obtained using either a

TABLE 14–5

COMPLICATIONS OF PARACENTESIS

Complications*	No. of Occurrences		
	Runyon[191] (n = 229)	Gines[52–54]† (n = 490)	Mallory[192] (n = 242)
Abdominal wall hematoma	4	3	4
Bloody tap	6	—	—
Peritonitis	—	2	2
Fluid leakage or abdominal wall edema	2	7	—

*Other cited complications included intraperitoneal embolization of catheter fragments, scrotal edema, cellulitis, mesenteric bleeding, and electrolyte imbalance. There were no reported deaths as a result of the procedure in any of the studies. Patient selection differed slightly in each study.

†Compilation of three studies.

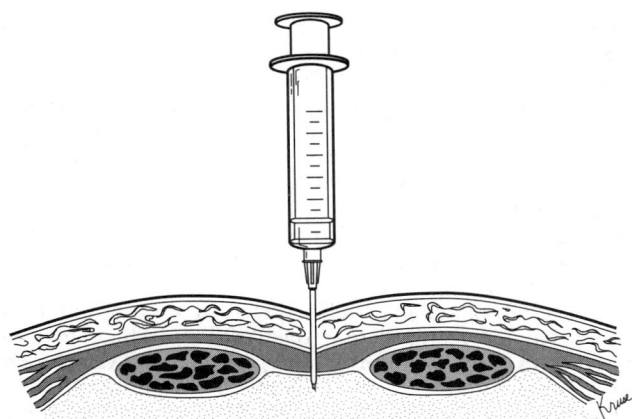

Figure 14–7. Cross-section of anterior abdomen at a level approximately 5 cm inferior to the umbilicus to illustrate the technique of abdominal paracentesis at the midline infraumbilical site. Either a 20-gauge needle or a 20-gauge catheter-over-needle device is carefully directed perpendicular to the skin through the previously anesthetized site until fluid is aspirated.

20-gauge needle or a 20-gauge catheter-over-needle device. In either case, a syringe should be attached to the hub and the needle slowly advanced through the previously anesthetized site and in a direction perpendicular to the skin until fluid is aspirated.

If a catheter-over-needle assembly is used, the assembly is advanced an additional 2 to 3 mm to ensure that the catheter is fully inside the peritoneum (Fig. 14–7). The needle is removed and a large syringe is attached to the plastic catheter.

6. Therapeutic paracentesis is similarly performed, with the exception that a larger needle (e.g., a 16-gauge or 18-gauge thin-walled needle) is employed and a J-tipped guidewire is threaded through the needle and into the peritoneum, after fluid has been aspirated. The needle is removed and a single-lumen catheter (e.g., 18 gauge) is then advanced over the guidewire into the peritoneal cavity and the desired volume of ascites is removed. Removal can be accomplished by using a sterile gravity drainage bag, a large-volume vacuum bottle, or a large syringe and three-way stopcock.

7. Pressure is applied to the site for at least 3 to 5 minutes after the catheter has been removed.

8. Ascitic fluid is sent to the laboratory for appropriate studies. For routine diagnostic paracentesis, this generally includes a Gram stain, total and differential blood cell counts, lactate dehydrogenase determination, total protein level, and glucose analysis. An aliquot should be immediately injected into aerobic and anaerobic blood culture bottles. Depending on the clinical situation, certain other tests may be desired (e.g., amylase determination, serologic studies, and smear and culture for acid-fast bacillus). If malignancy is specifically suspected, a large volume of fluid, at least 200 mL, should be obtained for cytologic analysis to increase the diagnostic yield.[62]

PERITONEAL LAVAGE

In 1954, Thompson and Brown used a spinal needle to perform abdominal paracentesis in the evaluation of 300 cases of abdominal trauma.[63] Root and associates, in 1965, reported the use of peritoneal lavage in 28 patients to evaluate for intraperitoneal injury.[64] The procedure correctly identified all 16 patients with significant intraperitoneal injury. In a subsequent review, Danto examined the sensitivity and specificity of lavage in 9588 cases, which included both blunt and penetrating abdominal trauma.[65] An abnormal lavage finding was 97% correct, resulting in only a 3% incidence of false-positive celiotomy results, whereas a normal lavage result was 99% correct.

Several methods have been described to identify lavage fluid as abnormal (i.e., indicative of likely intraperitoneal injury). Olsen and colleagues in 1972 based their judgment on the ability to read newsprint through the lavage tubing.[66] Significant hemoperitoneum was thought to be excluded if the newsprint could be read. It has since been common to employ the red blood cell count of the lavage fluid as a quantitative indicator of hemoperitoneum, with a red blood cell count of greater than 100,000/mm³ typically corresponding to an abnormal result using the newsprint technique. However, several investigators recommended that patients with red blood cell counts of less than 50,000/mm³ should still be admitted for observation, otherwise mesenteric or bowel injuries may occasionally be missed.[67–69]

Indications

Peritoneal lavage is primarily used to evaluate for significant intraperitoneal injury in cases of either blunt or penetrating trauma. The utility of peritoneal lavage in this evaluation derives from studies demonstrating that as many as 16% of patients without signs or symptoms of abdominal injury may have intraperitoneal injuries. This incidence rises to as high as 43% in patients with head trauma but no signs or symptoms of abdominal injury.[70] It has also been shown that a delay in diagnosis can result in increased mortality.[71–76]

Other indications for peritoneal catheterization include the need for peritoneal dialysis or intraperitoneal chemotherapy administration; the evaluation of certain nontraumatic intraperitoneal diseases, such as mesenteric ischemia and hemorrhagic pancreatitis; and large-volume paracentesis.[52, 54, 67, 77]

Contraindications

There are no absolute contraindications for peritoneal lavage, except when abdominal surgery is already indicated. Results obtained with peritoneal lavage have been shown to be reliable, even in the setting of coagulopathy.[77, 78] As is the case for paracentesis, certain patients are at increased risk for complications. These include patients with distended loops of bowel, uncooperative patients, and patients with abdominal scars or adhesions. Patients with retroperitoneal injuries or pelvic hematomas may have anterior abdominal wall hematomas, which may complicate the procedure. The supraumbilical approach may be preferable for these patients.

Complications

The incidence of complications has been correlated with both the inexperience of the operator and the failure to follow standard protocol.[65, 75] Danto compiled 9588 patients from 23 separate studies and found an overall complication rate of 1.4%.[65] Minor complications included abdominal wall or rectus sheath hematoma, incisional hernia, wound infection, mesenteric tears causing false-positive results, and mechanical difficulties with the catheter, such as kinking of the catheter or inadequate catheter drainage. Major complications have been associated with the use of the blind trocar procedure and include penetrations of bowel, bladder, stomach, and large vessels, including the abdominal aorta and iliac vessels.[72, 79–84] The complication rate has been substantially reduced since the advent of both the Lazarus-Nelson guidewire technique and the minilaparotomy technique. Bowel penetration is uncommon with these techniques, and even if it occurs, it is not usually associated with morbidity, provided that intraluminal pressure is not elevated.[85]

Procedure

Specialized kits for use with the guidewire technique are commonly available for performing peritoneal dialysis catheter placement and can also be employed for peritoneal lavage. An alternative procedure is the minilaparotomy. Both use a midline subumbilical approach through the linea alba, which is the most avascular area. Alternative sites are used in pregnancy, such as the upper midline, or when previous surgical scars are present, the left or right lower quadrant.

Guidewire Technique

1. The patient should be in the supine position. Nasogastric intubation and urinary bladder catheterization are required to decompress the stomach and the bladder, respectively.
2. Except as noted earlier, a midline site 3 to 6 cm below the umbilicus is generally preferred.
3. The area is prepared with a suitable antiseptic and draped in a sterile manner. The patient's hands should be at his or her side and restrained if necessary.
4. Gloves, gown, mask, and hat are required for the physician performing the procedure.
5. Local anesthesia is accomplished using 1% lidocaine with epinephrine to infiltrate the skin and subcutaneous tissue down to and including the peritoneum. To avoid intravascular injection of anesthetic, one should always aspirate before injecting. Care must be taken to ensure adequate local anesthesia; otherwise the procedure may not only be uncomfortable for the patient, but also pain results in muscle contraction and further difficulty in inserting the catheter.
6. A small skin incision is made using a No. 11 scalpel blade, and an 18-gauge thin-walled needle is inserted through the incision and into the peritoneal space. The operator will usually detect a palpable pop as the needle pierces the peritoneum. Alternatively, an 18-gauge needle may be directly inserted without an incision; however, after the guidewire is in place, an incision is still required to allow catheter advancement. A final option is to insert a catheter-over-needle device, as described earlier (see Fig. 14–7).
7. A flexible, J-tipped, metal guidewire is advanced through the needle or catheter and into the peritoneal cavity. Resistance likely indicates malposition of the cannula or failure to enter the peritoneal cavity. If this should occur, both the wire and the needle should be removed and the procedure reattempted. After the guidewire can be freely passed into the peritoneum, the cannula may be withdrawn over the guidewire.
8. A dilator may be used to facilitate subsequent placement of the catheter. The dilator is advanced over the guidewire and into the peritoneum and then removed. As with any Seldinger technique, one or the other end of the guidewire must remain visible and secured at all times to ensure that it is not inadvertently lost into the abdomen.
9. The lavage or dialysis catheter is then advanced over the guidewire and through the skin using a twisting motion. Because peritoneal fluid tends to accumulate first in the lower quadrants, an attempt should be made to direct the catheter to these locations during advancement. The guidewire is then removed.
10. The catheter is aspirated to see if any free blood is present. More than 10 mL indicates an abnormal lavage without the need for further evaluation.
11. If no blood returns, 15 mL/kg of sterile lactated Ringer's solution or normal (physiologic) saline solution is instilled into the peritoneum. An abnormal result is assumed if there is sudden appearance of fluid via an indwelling urinary catheter or nasogastric tube.
12. The patient is rolled first to one side then to the opposite side to ensure distribution of the fluid before allowing it to drain by gravity back into the intravenous fluid bag.
13. Poor drainage may be corrected by venting the intravenous bag or manipulating the catheter, which may be adherent to the omentum or the peritoneum. A representative sample is about 20% of the instilled volume.[85]
14. Catheters used for lavage should be allowed to remain in place until final evaluation of the fluid is completed. Repeated lavage may be required for cases in which analysis shows indeterminant results (e.g., 50,000 to 100,000 red blood cells per cubic millimeter[3]).[64, 69, 82, 86] A suture may be used to close the incision. Catheters to be used for peritoneal dialysis should be securely sutured in place and a sterile dressing affixed over the wound.

Minilaparotomy Technique

Steps 1 through 5 are the same as for the guidewire technique, except that a larger area of local anesthesia is required to allow for the larger skin incision.

6. The midline approach, 3 to 5 cm below the umbilicus, is preferred. A vertical incision, 4 to 8 cm long, is made through the skin into the subcutaneous tissue. A larger incision is necessary in the obese patient. Careful hemostasis is required.
7. Cautious blunt dissection is performed down to the preperitoneal fascia. Difficulties may occur when midline position has not been maintained and various layers at the rectus sheath are encountered. The fascia is grasped with sterile forceps or towel clips and elevated.
8. Under direct vision, the fascia is then opened 2 to 3 cm to allow visualization of the peritoneum,[86] and the catheter is then inserted.
9. A pursestring suture is placed around the catheter to prevent abdominal fluid leakage and, more important, to prevent any bleeding from the dissection from contaminating the lavage fluid.

Steps 10 through 15 are then performed as detailed earlier.

Lavage fluid should be submitted to the laboratory for full evaluation. Suggested tests include complete and differential cell counts, amylase determinations, Gram's stain and culture, and specific chemistry tests as indicated.[64, 69, 77, 84]

Peritoneal lavage is commonly used in the evaluation of trauma patients and for the temporary placement of peritoneal dialysis catheters. It is generally a safe procedure, provided the experienced operator follows guidelines cited earlier.

BALLOON TAMPONADE OF ESOPHAGEAL VARICES

In 1930, Westphal[87] used a Gottstein sound distended with water to accomplish tamponade of bleeding esophageal varices.[88] Twenty years later, the double-balloon Sengstaken-Blakemore tube was described.[89] Variations of this device include the Linton-Nachlas tube, a triple-lumen tube with a single gastric balloon,[90] and the Boyce modification of the Sengstaken-Blakemore tube,[91] in which a standard nasogastric tube is positioned just above the esophageal balloon and

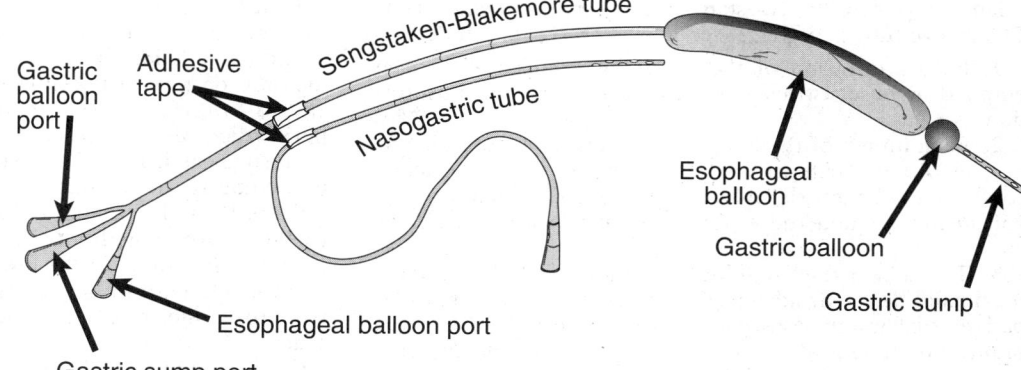

Figure 14–8. The Sengstaken-Blakemore tube. Note the standard nasogastric tube shown alongside the Sengstaken-Blakemore tube, and the adhesive tape markers used to ensure alignment of the two tubes during insertion.

used for suctioning (Fig. 14–8). Edlich and coworkers further modified the Sengstaken-Blakemore tube by including an integral lumen opening just above the esophageal balloon to provide the esophagus with a drainage port,[92] and this has come to be known as the Minnesota tube. A tube of advanced design is made of clear plastic and provides the ability to do diagnostic endoscopy through a central lumen; however, it does not allow for sclerotherapy.[93]

The use of these devices for bleeding esophageal varices has the potential for providing lifesaving hemostasis; however, acute mortality remains high. After successful tamponade, a more definitive therapeutic intervention may be considered because rebleeding occurs in as many as 35% of the cases within the first 24 hours after discontinuation of tamponade.[94, 95] Sclerotherapy, percutaneous transhepatic variceal embolization,[88, 96] emergent portal-systemic shunting,[96, 97] portal-azygous disconnection,[98] gastroesophageal staple gun transection,[99] thoracic variceal ligation,[100] and electrical[101] or laser obliteration[102] have all been described.

Indications

Criteria for placement of a Sengstaken-Blakemore tube have not been standardized. At some institutions,[103, 104] endoscopy is deemed a requirement before employing balloon tamponade to ensure that bleeding varices are indeed the cause of hemorrhage; however, other institutions may not have the capabilities of meeting that standard.

Contraindications

Contraindications include inability to control the airway, anatomic abnormalities that preclude the use of either the esophageal or the gastric balloon (e.g., Chagas' disease and previous esophageal surgery), lack of familiarity with the apparatus or the procedure, and lack of personnel trained in monitoring the patient intubated with this device. All patients undergoing this therapeutic modality should be monitored in an intensive care unit setting.[105] Cardiac monitoring, frequent pharyngeal suctioning, and the capability for rapid airway management are required. Attending personnel should be well versed in the care of patients with Sengstaken-Blakemore tubes, and policies should be in place to manage complications commonly associated with these devices. For example, scissors should be available at the bedside to cut the tube should it suddenly dislodge and occlude the airway.[106, 107]

Complications

Complications associated with the Sengstaken-Blakemore tube can be divided into major and minor. The reported

incidence of mortality directly related to the use of the Sengstaken-Blakemore or the Linton-Nachlas tube ranges from 8 to 22%.[108, 109] Bleeding from esophageal varices may itself carry a 50 to 80% mortality, and up to 90% of patients admitted for bleeding may die during that hospitalization.[88, 97, 109]

The most frequent major complication is pneumonitis resulting from aspirated esophageal secretions or gastric contents in an obtunded patient. Because this complication may be fatal,[110, 111] removal of gastric contents before tube insertion and prophylactic endotracheal intubation for obtunded patients have been suggested.[103, 108, 109, 110] Other potentially fatal complications include esophageal tear or rupture,[110, 111] tracheoesophageal fistula,[112] and esophageal necrosis.[105] The Sengstaken-Blakemore tube may become impacted,[113] and rarely surgical removal of the tube has been required if the lumina to the balloons become occluded.[114]

Airway obstruction may occur when the gastric balloon loses volume and the esophageal balloon pulls up into the upper airway.[107, 110, 115] Keeping scissors at the bedside to transect the tube quickly and allow decompression and rapid removal is advocated. Failure to control hemorrhage occurs in 10 to 50% of cases, with most series suggesting a 10 to 20% failure rate. Reasons for inadequate control include malposition of the balloon, low pressure in the esophageal balloon, and misdiagnosis (e.g., bleeding ulcer).[89, 105, 111] Rare complications include jejunal rupture when placed in the jejunal limb of a gastrojejunostomy[116] and innominate vein occlusion.[117]

Complications that are usually less serious include difficulty with insertion,[118] epistaxis,[111] hiccups,[103] chest pain, and pressure necrosis of the nares, the pharynx,[109] the esophagus, or the cardioesophageal junction.

Procedure

A number of clinical studies evaluated the utility of the Sengstaken-Blakemore tube in acutely controlling esophageal bleeding, and its efficacy varies from 50 to about 90%.[94, 119–122] Careful preparation and close monitoring are necessary to minimize complications. Before placement of the tube, all patients should have nasogastric lavage to clear blood from their stomach. Prophylactic intubation is recommended in the obtunded patient.

If a Minnesota tube is unavailable, the Boyce modification of the Sengstaken-Blakemore tube may be used to ensure esophageal drainage.[91] In this case, a standard nasogastric tube is held alongside the Sengstaken-Blakemore tube such that the distal end of the nasogastric tube is positioned just above the esophageal balloon. The proximal ends of both tubes are then marked with tape so that this positional relationship can be re-established after the Sengstaken-Blakemore tube is in place (see Fig. 14–8).

1. Before insertion of the tube, the stomach should be emptied by nasogastric suction to reduce the risk of aspiration.

2. Each lumen of the Sengstaken-Blakemore tube should be checked for patency and the integrity of the balloons confirmed. The gastric balloon is inspected by inflating with 250 mL of air and the esophageal balloon with 50 mL of air.

3. The tube is then well lubricated and, with the balloons maximally deflated, advanced through the nares while the patient sips water. Alternatively, the tube may be passed orally. The tube is always passed to at least the 50-cm mark to ensure placement within the stomach.

4. Tube position is checked by listening over the stomach while air is insufflated into the gastric aspiration lumen. After this verification, the gastric balloon is inflated with 250 mL of air. It is extremely important to ensure that the gastric balloon is never inflated while it is positioned within the esophagus. To this end, a more conservative approach is to inflate the gastric balloon initially with only 50 mL of air.[88] A chest roentgenogram is then done to visualize the radiolucent balloon and confirm an intragastric position. After this is confirmed, the gastric balloon is then fully inflated. Contrast media or other liquids should not be used to inflate either of the balloons, as this may result in inability to deflate the balloons, greatly complicating removal.

5. After the gastric balloon has been fully inflated, the tube is gently retracted to provide light pressure on the gastroesophageal junction. It is recommended that only gentle traction be applied and that the tube be taped to the nose[103] or to the faceguard of a football helmet.[88, 105, 110]

6. After the tube is secured, the gastric lumen is lavaged to confirm that bleeding has stopped. If hemorrhage is controlled with gastric balloon traction, inflation of the esophageal balloon is not necessary. The esophageal balloon is therefore inflated only if there is persistent bleeding.

7. If necessary, the esophageal balloon is inflated. Pressure within the esophageal balloon is monitored during inflation and maintained between 20 and 60 mm Hg. The lowest pressure that controls the hemorrhage should be used.

8. The esophageal balloon port (if used) and the gastric port are capped and double clamped to prevent air leakage, and the gastric aspiration lumen is connected to continuous suction. If a Minnesota tube is employed, the esophageal lumen is also connected to continuous suction. If a Sengstaken-Blakemore tube is used, a standard nasogastric tube must be inserted into the upper esophagus. Using the previously applied adhesive tape markers, the distal orifice is positioned just above the esophageal balloon and connected to continuous suction.

Oral and nasal secretions may reach 1500 mL/day; therefore, the application of continuous suction proximal to the esophageal balloon is imperative. During the first 24 hours, the balloons should remain inflated, although some have recommended transient deflation every 3 to 6 hours possibly to reduce the risk of mucosal pressure necrosis. Plans for adjunctive therapy should be made during this period. Sedation and the administration of narcotics for chest pain are frequently required and increase the risk of aspiration. Scissors should be immediately available at the bedside to cut all ports in case the tube becomes dislodged and threatens the airway.

PERICARDIOCENTESIS

Pericardiotomy was first performed by Romero in 1815.[123] Pericardiocentesis was first described in 1839 by Franz Schuh; he blindly aspirated pericardial fluid from a patient with malignant hemopericardium.[124] Since those first descriptions, opinion has been divided as to whether pericardiotomy or pericardiocentesis is the procedure of choice, and as to the preferred anatomic site for introducing the pericardiocentesis needle. At least six different sites have been suggested. In 1870, Dieulatoy used the fourth or fifth intercostal space just outside the area of cardiac dullness.[125] Baizeau,[126] in 1868, and Delorme and Mignon,[127] in 1896, used the fifth or sixth intercostal space just to the left of the sternum. Jaboulay (1899) used the left costophrenic angle, and Curschmann subsequently approached the pericardium from the posterior chest at the seventh or eighth intercostal space.[128] Of these indirect approaches, the subxiphoid, described by Marfan in 1911, is currently the most popular.[128] Owing to the relative ease and safety of subxiphoid pericardiotomy, several authors have recommended a surgical approach for all but the most emergent pericardial effusions.[129–131] The diagnostic yield is higher with an open procedure because it allows pericardial biopsy as well as fluid analysis.[131]

Indications

Analysis of pericardial fluid is often helpful in establishing the cause of pericardial effusion. The differential diagnosis of pericardial effusion is extensive (Table 14–6). Pericardiocentesis is also used therapeutically to relieve pericardial tamponade or to drain large or septic effusions. Although traumatic hemopericardium may be approached initially with pericardiocentesis, this should always be considered only a temporizing measure.[132–134] In a study of 459 patients with penetrating cardiac wounds, Sugg and associates found a 43% mortality when pericardiocentesis was used alone compared with 16% when early surgical intervention was performed.[135]

Contraindications

There are no absolute contraindications for pericardiocentesis to relieve cardiac tamponade. However, it is not always necessary to perform immediate pericardiocentesis on all patients with cardiac tamponade. Patients who are hemodynamically able to tolerate dialysis and have mild tamponade resulting from uremia may not require pericardiocentesis.[136] Similarly, patients with inflammatory causes of pericardial effusion with tamponade may, in selected cases, be treated with corticosteroids or other anti-inflammatory agents.[137] Relative contraindications for pericardiocentesis include coagulopathy or thrombocytopenia, an uncooperative patient, an inexperienced operator, and lack of proper monitoring and resuscitation equipment.

Complications

Using any of the locations or directions mentioned for pericardiocentesis puts several organs in the thorax and abdomen at risk. In the emergent situation of hemodynamic collapse caused by cardiac tamponade, a blind technique is used. For elective diagnostic pericardiocentesis, electrocardiographic guidance and/or echocardiographic guidance should be used.[137–141] Echocardiographic transducers have been fitted with a needle guide and used to accurately locate the effusion and guide pericardiocentesis.[140] Reported complications and their incidence are cited in Table 14–7. Complication rates are likely to be higher if the procedure is performed without monitoring.

TABLE 14–6

DIFFERENTIAL DIAGNOSIS OF PERICARDIAL EFFUSION

Cause*	% in Series		
	Markiewicz and Associates[143] (n = 215)	Krikorian and Hancock[193] (n = 120)	Guberman and Coworkers[194] (n = 56)
Neoplasia	21	16	32
Radiation	5.5	7.5	4
Idiopathic cause	26	13.5	14
Infection†	3.7	2.5	12.5
Uremia	9.8	5	9
Collagen-vascular disease‡	6.5	12	2
Anticoagulation	1	2	11
Aneurysmal leak	2	—	4
After open heart surgery	—	—	2
After myocardial infarction	8.4	—	—
Myxedema	—	—	4
Congestive heart failure	8.7	1.5	—
Trauma	—	9	—
Iatrogenic cause§	—	—	4.5
Other	7.4	30.5	—

*Other causes include the following:
  Sclerotherapy for esophageal varices[195]
  Drugs: hydralazine, minoxidil, phenytoin, procainamide, isoniazid, penicillin, daunorubicin, methysergide[196–198]
  Pancreatitis,[199] amyloidosis, Löffler's syndrome
  Scleroderma[200]
  Sarcoidosis[201]
  Cardiac transplantation[202]
  Chylopericardium[203]
  Iatrogenic injury during central venous catheter and pacemaker electrode insertion and myocardial biopsies[204]
†Tuberculous, bacterial, viral, and parasitic.
‡Lupus erythematosus, rheumatoid arthritis, and rheumatic fever.
§Related to diagnostic procedures.

Procedure

Only the most emergent pericardiocentesis should be performed outside an intensive care unit, cardiac catheterization laboratory, operating room, or similarly monitored setting. Except in the most extreme emergencies, echocardiography should be routinely performed before pericardiocentesis to identify or confirm the presence of effusion. Physical and electrocardiographic findings, such as pulsus paradoxus, elevated jugular venous pressure, faint heart sounds, and electrical alternans, are far less sensitive and specific for pericardial tamponade compared with the echocardiographic findings.[142] In one study of all patients with pericardial tamponade, 42% had the initial diagnosis made by echocardiography when they were referred for other reasons.[143] Although pericardiocentesis may alleviate the immediate crisis resulting from tamponade, it is generally necessary to consider more definitive, long-term therapy, such as a pericardial window procedure.

Several modern approaches have been recommended, including the left subxiphoid, the anterior intercostal, and the parasternal. For the subxiphoid approach, several different insertion trajectories have also been described. The recommended angle of insertion between the needle and the skin varies between 30 and 75°, and the recommended direction for aiming the needle has included the left

TABLE 14–7

COMPLICATIONS OF PERICARDIOCENTESIS

Parameter or Complication	% in Series				
	Kwasnik and Colleagues[136] (n = 34)	Krikorian and Hancock[193] (n = 123)	Wong and Colleagues[205] (n = 52)	Guberman and Associates[194] (n = 46)	Callahan and Coworkers[206] (n = 132)
Location of procedure*	Cath lab	Cath lab	Cath lab/echo lab	Echo lab	Echo lab
Success	100	86	69	87	98
Cardiac arrest	0	2	2†	2†	—
Ventricular puncture	2	2	9‡	6.5	2
Surgery required	2	39	—	26	29
Pneumothorax	1	—	—	—	—
Pneumoperitoneum	1	—	—	—	—
Induced hemopericardium	—	5	—	—	—
Death	0	5	1	1	0

*Cath lab = cardiac catheterization laboratory; Echo lab = echocardiography laboratory.
†One patient.
‡Five patients.

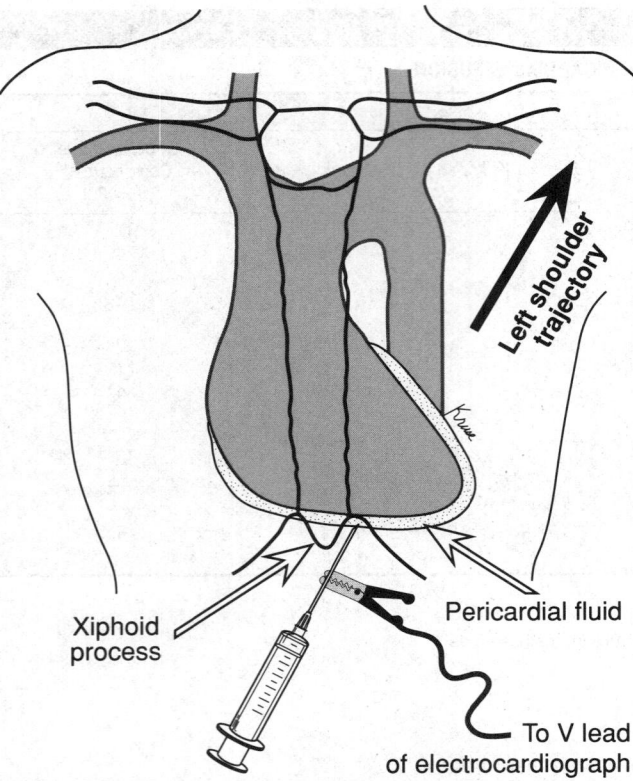

Figure 14–9. Pericardiocentesis from the left subxiphoid approach. The patient's left shoulder is used as a directive landmark. Note the alligator-style electrical connection that leads from the metal needle to the V lead of an electrocardiograph.

shoulder,[145, 146] the right shoulder,[145, 146] and a median approach.[147] The left subxiphoid approach may be preferred, unless dictated otherwise by echocardiographic findings, with an entry angle of about 45° and the left shoulder as a directive landmark. Most effusions lie on the diaphragmatic surface of the heart and to the left of the midline and thus lie directly in the path of the needle, minimizing the possibility of organ injury. Right-sided heart chamber puncture and hepatic puncture may be more likely if the needle is directed to the right shoulder. Coronary artery puncture is possible using the left shoulder as a landmark; however, the risk is small.

1. Continuous electrocardiographic monitoring is required during the procedure, and supplies and equipment for cardiac resuscitation must be on hand. A second electrocardiograph should be available if electrocardiographic guidance is to be used. The limb leads of this second electrocardiograph should be connected to the patient, and an alligator-type electrical connector fitted to the V lead for attachment to the paracentesis needle. Echocardiographic guidance during the procedure is ideal.

2. Adequate oxygenation and reliable intravenous access should be provided. Decompression of the stomach should be ensured via a nasogastric tube. Sedation or analgesia may be useful in some circumstances.

3. The patient is placed in the 30 to 45° upright position. The xiphoid process is palpated and the point of intended insertion selected: approximately 1 to 2 cm to the left of the xiphoid process, and 1 to 2 cm below the costal margin (Fig. 14–9). A skin impression can be made to mark the selected insertion point. The area is thoroughly cleansed with a

suitable antiseptic solution, such as povidone-iodine, and sterile drapes are positioned to surround the insertion point.

4. A 22-gauge needle is used to anesthetize the site with 1% lidocaine without epinephrine and the needle is advanced along the intended aspiration route at approximately a 45° angle to the skin and toward the left shoulder (see Fig. 14–9). As the needle is advanced, small amounts of additional anesthetic are injected after checking by aspiration for the position of the tip of the needle. Note that the pericardium can occasionally be reached with a 1.5-inch needle.

5. An 18-gauge spinal or similar needle attached to a 20-mL syringe is then inserted along the same trajectory. The V lead of the second electrocardiograph is connected to the shaft of the needle using the alligator clip. As the needle is advanced into the subcutaneous tissue, a surface electrocardiographic signal appears on the second monitor. If the needle makes contact with the myocardium, a characteristic high-amplitude epicardial injury pattern occurs, indicating that the needle should be immediately withdrawn. Continuous aspiration should be applied as the needle is advanced along the desired route. When the needle reaches the effusion (usually after inserting to a depth of 4 to 8 cm), the fluid may be directly aspirated, or a guidewire is inserted using the Seldinger technique and a catheter placed in the pericardial space for prolonged continuous drainage.[145, 148, 149]

If fluid is not aspirated after advancing at 45°, repeated attempts at 30 or 60° may prove successful; however, relocalization of the fluid by echocardiography should be considered first. In an emergency situation, if the fluid is suspected yet not aspirated by this technique, a second attempt may be made using the right shoulder as the directive landmark. Blind pericardiocentesis entails considerable risk and should be utilized only during a crisis situation.

References

1. Garrison FH: Introduction to the History of Medicine. 4th ed. Philadelphia, WB Saunders, p 632, 1929.
2. Merriam M, Cronan J, Dorfman G, et al: Radiographically guided percutaneous catheter drainage of pleural fluid collections. AJR 151:1113, 1988.
3. Reinhold C, Ilescas FF: Treatment of pleural effusions and pneumothorax with catheters placed percutaneously under imaging guidance. AJR 152:1189, 1989.
4. Wood PR, Tzakis A, Byers W, et al: A simplified technique for the treatment of simple pleural effusions. Surg Gynecol Obstet 164:283, 1987.
5. Hamilton AAD, Archer GJ: Treatment of pneumothorax by simple aspiration. Thorax 38:934, 1983.
6. Parker LA, Charnock GC, Delany DJ: Small bore catheter drainage and sclerotherapy for malignant pleural effusions. Cancer 64:1218, 1989.
7. Lorch DG, Gordon L, Wooten S, et al: Effect of patient positioning on distribution of tetracycline in the pleural space during pleurodesis. Chest 93:527, 1988.
8. Collins TR, Sahn SA: Thoracentesis. Clinical value, complications, technical problems and patient experience. Chest 91:817, 1987.
9. Bone RC: The techniques of diagnostic and therapeutic thoracentesis. J Crit Illness 5:371, 1990.
10. Hall WJ, Mayewski RJ: Position paper. Diagnostic thoracentesis and pleural biopsy in pleural effusions. Ann Intern Med 103:799, 1985.
11. Grogan DR, Irwin RS: Complications associated with thoracentesis. Arch Intern Med 150:873, 1990.
12. Seneff MA, Corwin RW: Complications associated with thoracentesis. Chest 90:97, 1986.
13. Lowell JR: Pleural Effusions: A Comprehensive Review. Baltimore, University Park Press, 1977.
14. Mahfood S, Hix WR: Reexpansion pulmonary edema. Ann Thorac Surg 45:340, 1988.
15. Wagaruddin M, Bernstein A: Reexpansion pulmonary edema. Thorax 30:54, 1975.
16. O'Quinn JR, Lahshminarayan S: Venous air embolism. Arch Intern Med 142:2173, 1982.
17. Diamond S, Koplitz S, Novich O: Cerebral air embolism as a complication of thoracentesis. Gen Practioner 30:87, 1964.

18. Sue DY, Lam K: Retention of catheter fragment after thoracentesis. Postgrad Med 72:101, 1982.
19. Agurlar-Torres FG, Schlueter DP, Perlman L, et al: Subcutaneous implantation of an adenocarcinoma following thoracentesis. Wis Med J 76:19, 1977.
20. Seldinger SI: Catheter replacement of the needle in percutaneous angiography: A new technique. Acta Radiol 39:368, 1953.
21. Godwin JE, Sahn SA: Thoracentesis: A safe procedure in mechanically ventilated patients. Ann Intern Med 113:800, 1990.
22. Lemmer JH, Bother MJ, Orringer MB: Modern management of adult thoracic empyema. J Thorac Cardiovasc Surg 90:849, 1985.
23. O'Rourke JP, Yee ES: Civilian spontaneous pneumothorax. Treatment options and long-term results. Chest 96:1302, 1989.
24. Fuhrman BP, Landrum BG, Ferrara TB, et al: Pleural drainage using modified pigtail catheters. Crit Care Med 14:575, 1986.
25. Henschke CI, Davis SD, Romano M, et al: The pathogenesis, radiologic evaluation and therapy of pleural effusions. Radiol Clin North Am 27:1241, 1989.
26. Hutchins RA: Hippocrates writings. In: Lust W (ed): Great Books of the Western World, Volume 29. Chicago, Encyclopaedia Britannica, p 142, 1952.
27. Hochberg LA: Thoracic Surgery Before the Twentieth Century. New York, Vantage Press, p 255, 1960.
28. Nissen R, Wilson RH: Pages in the History of Chest Surgery. Springfield, IL, Charles C Thomas, 1960.
29. Hewett FC: Thoracentesis: The plan of continuous aspiration. Br Med J 1:317, 1876.
30. Bartlett JG, Finegold SM: Anaerobic infections of the lung and pleural space. Am Rev Respir Dis 110:56, 1974.
31. Lawrence GH: Closed chest tube drainage for pleural space problems. Maj Probl Clin Surg 28:14, 1983.
32. Frumkin K: Tube Thoracostomy. Clinical Procedures in Emergency Medicine. Philadelphia, WB Saunders, p 99, 1985.
33. Courtice FC, Morris B: Effect of diaphragmatic movement on the absorption of protein and of red cells from the pleural cavity. Aust J Exp Biol Med Sci 31:227, 1953.
34. Wilson JL, Herrod CM, Searle GL, et al: The absorption of blood from the pleural space. Surgery 48:766, 1960.
35. Condon RE: Spontaneous resolution of experimental clotted hemothorax. Surg Gynecol Obstet 126:505, 1968.
36. Millikan JS, Moore EE, Steiner E, et al: Complications of tube thoracostomy for acute trauma. Am J Surg 140:738, 1980.
37. Vander Salm TJ: Chest tube insertion. In: Vander Salm TJ, Cutler BS, Wheeler HB (eds): Atlas of Bedside Procedures. 2nd ed. Boston, Little, Brown, p 259, 1988.
38. Grover FL, Richardson JD, Fewel JG, et al: Prophylactic antibiotics in the treatment of penetrating chest wounds. J Thorac Cardiovasc Surg 74:528, 1977.
39. Brunner RG, Vinsant GO, Alexander WF: The role of antibiotic therapy in the prevention of empyema in patients with an isolated chest injury (ISS 9-10): A prospective study. J Trauma 30:1148, 1990.
40. Neugebauer MK, Fosburg RG, Trummer MJ: Routine antibiotic therapy following pleural space intubation. J Thorac Cardiovasc Surg 61:882, 1971.
41. Childress ME, Moy G, Mottram M: Unilateral pulmonary edema resulting from treatment of spontaneous pneumothorax. Am Rev Respir Dis 104:119, 1971.
42. Sewell RW, Fewel JG, Grover FT, et al: Experimental evaluation of reexpansion pulmonary edema. Ann Thorac Surg 26:126, 1978.
43. Hegarty MM: A conservative approach to penetrating injuries of the chest. Injury 8:53, 1976.
44. Brandstetter RD, Cohen RP: Hypoxemia after thoracentesis. A predictable and treatable condition. JAMA 242:1060, 1979.
45. Duponselle EFC: The level of the intercostal drain and other determinant factors in the conservative approach to penetrating chest injuries. Cent Afr J Med 26:52, 1980.
46. Heimlich JH: Valve drainage of the pleural cavity. Dis Chest 52:282, 1968.
47. Graham JM, Mattox KL, Beall AC: Penetrating trauma of the lung. J Trauma 19:665, 1979.
48. Daly RC, Mucha P, Pairolero PC, et al: The risk of percutaneous chest tube thoracostomy for blunt trauma. Ann Emerg Med 14:865, 1985.
49. Sturm JT, Points BJ, Perry JF: Hemopneumothorax following blunt trauma of the thorax. Surg Gynecol Obstet 141:539, 1975.
50. Saloman H: Die diagnostische Punktion des Bauches. Berl Klin Wochenschr 43:45, 1906.
51. Reynolds T: Renaissance of paracentesis in the treatment of ascites. Adv Intern Med 35:365, 1990.
52. Gines P, Arroyo V, Quintero E, et al: Comparison of paracentesis and diuretics in the treatment of cirrhotics with tense ascites. Gastroenterology 93:234, 1987.
53. Gines P, Tito L, Arroyo E, et al: Randomized comparative study of therapeutic paracentesis with and without intravenous albumin in cirrhosis. Gastroenterology 94:1493, 1988.
54. Tito L, Gines P, Arroyo E, et al: Total paracentesis associated with intravenous albumin management of patients with cirrhosis and ascites. Gastroenterology 98:146, 1990.
55. Hoets JC, Runyon BA: Spontaneous bacterial peritonitis. Dis Mon 31:3, 1985.
56. Macrae F, St John DJ: Spontaneous bacterial peritonitis: Reversible cause of deterioration in patients with cirrhosis. Med J Aust 2:209, 1980.
57. Pinzello G, Simonette RG, Craxi A, et al: Spontaneous bacterial peritonitis: A prospective investigation in predominantly non-alcoholic cirrhotic patients. Hepatology 3:545, 1983.
58. Almdal TP, Shinhoj P: Spontaneous bacterial peritonitis in cirrhosis: Incidence, diagnosis and prognosis. Scand J Gastroenterol 22:295, 1987.
59. Attali P, Turner K, Pelletier G, et al: pH of ascitic fluid: Diagnostic and prognostic value in cirrhotic and noncirrhotic patients. Gastroenterology 90:1255, 1986.
60. Moretz WH, Erickson WB: Peritoneal tap as an aid in the diagnosis of acute abdominal disease. Am Surg 20:363, 1954.
61. Bard C, Lafortune M, Breton G, et al: Ascites: Ultrasound guidance or blind paracentesis. Can Med Assoc J 135:209, 1986.
62. Marshall JB: Finding the cause of ascites. The importance of accurate fluid analysis. Postgrad Med 83:189, 1988.
63. Thompson CT, Brown DR: Diagnostic paracentesis in the acute abdomen. Surgery 35:916, 1954.
64. Root HD, Hauser CW, McKinley CR, et al: Diagnostic peritoneal lavage. Surgery 57:633, 1965.
65. Danto LA: Paracentesis and diagnostic peritoneal lavage. In: Blaisdell FW, Trankey DO (eds): Trauma Management, Volume 1. New York, Thieme-Stratton, 1982.
66. Olsen WR, Redman HC, Hildreth DH: Quantitative peritoneal lavage in blunt abdominal trauma. Arch Surg 104:536, 1972.
67. Alyono D, Perry JF: Value of quantitative cell count and amylase activity of peritoneal lavage fluid. J Trauma 21:345, 1981.
68. Thal ER: Peritoneal lavage: State of the art. Ann Emerg Med 10:225, 1981.
69. Phillips TF, Bratman S, Cleveland S, et al: Perforating injuries of the small bowel from blunt abdominal trauma. Ann Emerg Med 12:75, 1983.
70. Wilson CB, Vidrine A, Rives JD: Unrecognized abdominal trauma in patients with head injuries. Ann Surg 162:608, 1965.
71. Keith LM, Zollinger RM, McCleery RS: Peritoneal fluid amylase determinations as an aid in diagnosis of acute pancreatitis. Arch Surg 61:930, 1950.
72. Williams RD, Zollinger RM: Diagnosis and prognostic factors in abdominal trauma. Am J Surg 97:575, 1959.
73. Perry JF: A five-year survey of 152 acute abdominal injuries. J Trauma 5:53, 1965.
74. Engrav LH, Benjamin CI, Strate RG, et al: Diagnostic peritoneal lavage in blunt abdominal trauma. J Trauma 15:854, 1975.
75. Bivins BA, Jona JZ, Berlin RP: Diagnostic peritoneal lavage in pediatric trauma. J Trauma 16:739, 1976.
76. Rothenberger DA, Quattlebaum MD, Zabel J, et al: Diagnostic peritoneal lavage for blunt trauma in pregnant women. Am J Obstet Gynecol 129:479, 1977.
77. Berry T, Flynn TC, Miller RW, et al: Diagnostic peritoneal lavage in trauma patients with coagulopathy. Ann Emerg Med 12:253, 1983.
78. Fischer RP, Beverlin BC, Engrav LH: Diagnostic peritoneal lavage fourteen years and 2,586 patients later. Am J Surg 136:701, 1978.
79. Brofen GJ, Liebler JB, Katz HM: A new method of abdominal paracentesis. Gastroenterology 21:426, 1952.
80. Veith FJ, Webber WB, Karl RC, et al: Peritoneal lavage in acute abdominal disease: Normal findings and evaluation in 100 patients. Ann Surg 166:290, 1967.
81. Krauz MM, Manny J, Ultsunomiya T, et al: Peritoneal lavage in blunt abdominal trauma. Surg Gynecol Obstet 152:327, 1981.
82. Moore JB, Moore EE, Markovchick VJ, et al: Diagnostic peritoneal lavage for abdominal trauma: Superiority of the open technique at the infraumbilical ring. J Trauma 21:570, 1981.
83. Myers RAM, Agarwal NN, Cowley RA: A safe, semi-open procedure for diagnostic peritoneal lavage. Surg Gynecol Obstet 153:739, 1981.
84. Parvin S, Smith DE: Effectiveness of peritoneal lavage in blunt abdominal trauma. Ann Surg 181:255, 1975.
85. Giacobine JW, Siler VE: Evaluation of diagnostic peritoneal lavage in blunt abdominal trauma. Ann Surg 165:70, 1967.
86. Perry JF Jr, Strate RG: Diagnostic peritoneal lavage in blunt abdominal trauma. Indication and results. Surgery 71:898, 1972.
87. Westphal K: Ueber eine Kompressionsbehandlung der Blutungen aus Oesophagusvarizen. Dtsch Med Wochenschr 56:1135, 1930.
88. Hanna SS, Warren WD, Galambos JJ, et al: Bleeding varices: Emergency management. Can Med Assoc J 124:29, 1981.
89. Sengstaken RW, Blakemore AH: Balloon tamponade for the control of hemorrhage from esophageal varices. Ann Surg 131:781, 1950.
90. Nachlas MM: A new triple lumen tube for the diagnosis and treatment of upper gastro-intestinal hemorrhage. N Engl J Med 252:720, 1955.
91. Boyce HW: Modification of the Sengstaken-Blakemore balloon tube. N Engl J Med 267:195, 1962.
92. Edlich RF, Lande AJ, Goodale RL, et al: Prevention of aspiration during esophagogastric tamponade and gastric cooling. Surgery 64:405, 1968.
93. Idezuki Y, Hagiwara M, Watanabe H: Endoscopic balloon tamponade for emergency control of bleeding esophageal varices using a new transparent tamponade tube. Trans Am Soc Artif Intern Organs 23:646, 1977.

94. Haddock G, Garden OJ, McKee RF, et al: Esophageal tamponade in the management of acute variceal hemorrhage. Dig Dis Sci 34:913, 1989.
95. Ramsburgh SR, Turcotte JG: Control of gastroesophageal variceal bleeding with balloon tamponade. In: Green RF, Turcotte J (eds): Upper Gastrointestinal Hemorrhage. New York, Grune & Stratton, p 286, 1980.
96. Nabseth DC, Johnson WC, Widrich WC, et al: Bleeding esophageal varices. Treatment by embolization and shunting. Jpn J Surg 11:8, 1981.
97. O'Donnell TF, Gembarowicz RM, Callow AD, et al: The economic impact of acute variceal bleeding: Cost effectiveness implications for medical and surgical therapy. Surgery 88:693, 1980.
98. Mafory WE, Sedgwick CE, Rossi RL: Nonshunting procedures in management of bleeding esophageal varices. Surg Clin North Am 60:281, 1980.
99. Sagar S, Harrison ID, Brearly R, et al: Emergency treatment of variceal hemorrhage. Br J Surg 66:824, 1979.
100. Schiff L, Schiff ER (eds): Diseases of the Liver. 5th ed. Philadelphia, JB Lippincott, p 894, 1982.
101. Taylor TV, Neilson JM: "Currents and clots"—An approach to the problem of acute variceal bleeding. Br J Surg 68:692, 1981.
102. Butler ML: Variceal hemorrhage: A review. Milit Med 145:766, 1980.
103. Pitcher JL: Safety and effectiveness of the modified Sengstaken-Blakemore tube: A prospective study. Gastroenterology 61:291, 1971.
104. Terblanche J: Treatment of esophageal varices by injection sclerotherapy. In: Maclean LD (ed): Advances in Surgery. Chicago, Year Book Medical Publishers, p 257, 1981.
105. Salam AA: Upper gastrointestinal bleeding: Differential diagnosis and management. In: Schwartz GR, Safar P, Stone JH, et al (eds): The Principles and Practice of Emergency Medicine. Philadelphia, WB Saunders, p 1036, 1986.
106. Zimmerman TA: Thinking critically about the Sengstaken-Blakemore tube. Crit Care Nurse 6:72, 1986.
107. Bennett HD, Baker L, Baker LA: Complications in the use of esophageal compression balloons. Arch Intern Med 90:196, 1952.
108. Conn HO, Simpson JA: Excessive mortality associated with balloon tamponade of bleeding varices. JAMA 202:137, 1967.
109. Chojkier M, Conn HO: Esophageal tamponade in the treatment of bleeding varices. Dig Dis Sci 25:267, 1980.
110. Bauer JJ, Kreel I, Kark HE: The use of the Sengstaken-Blakemore tube for immediate control of bleeding esophageal varices. Ann Surg 179:273, 1974.
111. Conn HO: Hazards attending the use of esophageal tamponade. N Engl J Med 259:701, 1958.
112. Akgun S, Lee DE, Weissman PS, et al: Hemoptysis and tracheoesophageal fistula in a patient with esophageal varices and Sengstaken-Blakemore tube. Am J Med 85:450, 1988.
113. Chawla Y, Singh R, Ramesh GN, et al: Impacted Sengstaken-Blakemore tube. Am J Gastroenterol 83:1438, 1988.
114. Bouchier IAD: Impact of Sengstaken-Blakemore tube. Gastroenterology 45:274, 1963.
115. Byrne WD, Washington DC, Samson PC, et al: Complications associated with the use of esophageal compression balloons. Am J Surg 104:250, 1962.
116. Goff JS, Thompson JS, Pratt CF, et al: Jejunal rupture caused by a Sengstaken-Blakemore tube. Gastroenterology 82:573, 1982.
117. Juffe A, Tellez G, Equaras MG, et al: Unusual complication of the Sengstaken-Blakemore tube. Gastroenterology 72:724, 1977.
118. Zamcheck N: Management of massive gastrointestinal hemorrhage on wards of Boston City Hospital. Arch Intern Med 96:78, 1955.
119. Teres J, Cecillia A, Bordas JM, et al: Esophageal tamponade for bleeding varices. Gastroenterology 75:566, 1978.
120. Feneyrou B, Hanana J, Daures JP, et al: Initial control of bleeding esophageal varices with the Sengstaken-Blakemore tube. Am J Surg 155:509, 1988.
121. Pones J, Teres J, Bosch J, et al: Efficacy of balloon tamponade in treatment of bleeding gastric and esophageal varices. Dig Dis Sci 33:454, 1988.
122. Moreto M, Zaballa M, Bernal A, et al: A randomized trial of tamponade or sclerotherapy as immediate treatment for bleeding esophageal varices. Surg Gynecol Obstet 167:331, 1988.
123. Husson HM, Merat FV: Extrait d'un mémoire de M. le docteur F. Romero, médecin de catalogue, sur l'hydrothorax et l'hydropéricarde; et du rapport qui en a été fait par MM. Huson et Mirat. Bull Fac Med Paris Soc 4:373, 1815.
124. Schuh F: Erfahrungen uber die Paracentese der Brust und des Herzbeutels. Med Jahrb Österr-Staates Wien [Neuste Folge 24] 33:388, 1841.
125. Dieulatoy G: A Treatise on the Pneumatic Aspiration of Morbid Fluids. London, Smith Elder, 1873.
126. Baizeau A: Mémoire sur la ponction du péricarde, envisagée au point de vue chirurgical. Gaz Hebd Med Paris 5:515, 562, 1868.
127. Delorme E, Mignon A: Sur la ponction et l'incision du péricarde. Rev Chir 15:797, 987, 1895; 16:56, 1896.
128. Marfan AB: Ponction du péricarde par l'épigastre. Ann Med Chir Inf 15:529, 1911.
129. Sutton GC, Tobin JR, Rox RT, et al: Study of the pericardium and ventricular myocardium. Exploratory mediastinotomy and biopsy in unexplained heart disease. JAMA 185:786, 1963.
130. Schwartz MJ, Nay HR, Fitzpatrick HF: Pericardial biopsy. Arch Intern Med 112:917, 1963.
131. Mills SA, Julian S, Holliday RH: Subxiphoid pericardial window for pericardial effusive disease. J Cardiovasc Surg 30:768, 1989.
132. Boyd T, Strieder J: Immediate surgery for traumatic heart disease. J Thorac Cardiovasc Surg 50:305, 1965.
133. Siemens R, Polk H, Gray L, et al: Indications for thoracotomy following penetrating thoracic injury. J Trauma 17:493, 1977.
134. Borja AR, Lansing A, Randell H: Immediate operative treatment for stab wounds of the heart. J Thorac Cardiovasc Surg 59:662, 1970.
135. Sugg WL, Rea WJ, Ecker RR, et al: Penetrating wounds of the heart: An analysis of 459 cases. J Thorac Cardiovasc Surg 56:531, 1968.
136. Kwasnik EM, Kostes JK, Lazarus JM, et al: Conservative management of uremic pericardial effusions. J Thorac Cardiovasc Surgery 76:629, 1978.
137. Tajik AJ: Echocardiography in pericardial effusion. Am J Med 63:29, 1977.
138. Clarke DP, Cosgrove DO: Real time ultrasound scanning in the planning and guidance of pericardiocentesis. Clin Radiol 38:119, 1987.
139. Pandian NG, Brockway B, Simonetti J, et al: Pericardiocentesis under two-dimensional echocardiographic guidance in loculated pericardial effusion. Ann Thorac Surg 45:99, 1988.
140. Hanaki Y, Kamiya H, Todoroki H, et al: New two-dimensional, echocardiographically directed pericardiocentesis in cardiac tamponade. Crit Care Med 18:750, 1990.
141. Kerber RE, Ridges JD, Harrison DC: Electrocardiographic indications of atrial puncture during pericardiocentesis. N Engl J Med 282:1142, 1979.
142. Singh S, Wann S, Klopfenstein HS, et al: Usefulness of right ventricular diastolic collapse in diagnosing cardiac tamponade and comparison to pulsus paradoxus. Am J Cardiol 57:652, 1986.
143. Markiewicz W, Borovik R, Ecker S: Cardiac tamponade in medical patients: Treatment and prognosis in the echocardiographic era. Am Heart J 111:1138, 1986.
144. Kotte JH, McGuire J: Pericardial paracentesis. Mod Concepts Cardiovasc Dis 20:102, 1951.
145. Patel AK, Kosolcharoen PK, Nallasivan M, et al: Catheter drainage of the pericardium: Practical method to maintain long-term patency. Chest 92:1018, 1987.
146. Treasure T, Cotter L: How to aspirate the pericardium. Br J Hosp Med 25:488, 1980.
147. Fowler NO: Recognition and management of pericardial disease and its complications. In: Hurst JW (ed): The Heart. 4th ed. New York, McGraw-Hill, 1978.
148. Shepherd FA, Morgan C, Evans WK, et al: Medical management of malignant pericardial effusion by tetracycline sclerosis. Am J Cardiol 60:1161, 1987.
149. Kaye W: Invasive therapeutic techniques: Emergency cardiac pacing, pericardiocentesis, intracardiac injections and emergency treatment of tension pneumothorax. Heart Lung 12:300, 1983.
150. Carney M, Ravin CE: Intercostal artery laceration during thoracentesis. Increased risk in elderly patients. Chest 75:520, 1979.
151. Emerson P: General investigation of pleural effusions. In: Emerson P: Thoracic Medicine. Woburn, MA, Butterworth, 1981.
152. Trapnell DH, Thurston JB: Unilateral pulmonary edema after pleural aspiration. Lancet 1:1367, 1970.
153. Ziskind MM, Weil H, George RA: Acute pulmonary edema following treatment of spontaneous pneumothorax with excessive negative intrapleural pressure. Am Rev Respir Dis 92:632, 1965.
154. Braveny I, Machka K: Delayed iatrogenic rupture of the spleen. Lancet 2:752, 1980.
155. Rauch RF, Korobkin M, Silverman PM, et al: CT detection of iatrogenic percutaneous splenic injury. J Comput Assist Tomogr 7:1018, 1983.
156. Heffner JE, Sahn SA: Abdominal hemorrhage after perforation of a diaphragmatic artery during thoracentesis. Arch Intern Med 141:1238, 1981.
157. Simpson K: Death from vagal inhibition. Lancet 1:558, 1949.
158. Williams KR, Burford TH: The management of chylothorax. Ann Surg 160:131, 1964.
159. Linos DA, Mucha P, van Heerden JA: Subclavian vein. A golden route. Mayo Clin Proc 55:315, 1980.
160. Mitchell SE, Clark RA: Complications of central venous catheterization. AJR 133:467, 1979.
161. Beall AC Jr, Crawford HW, DeBakey ME: Considerations in the management of acute traumatic hemothorax. J Thorac Cardiovasc Surg 52:351, 1966.
162. Oparah SS, Mandal AK: Operative management of penetrating wounds of the chest in civilian practice. Review of indications in 125 consecutive patients. J Thorac Cardiovasc Surg 46:331, 1963.
163. DeVries WC, Wolfe WG: The management of spontaneous pneumothorax and bullous emphysema. Surg Clin North Am 60:851, 1980.
164. Ruckley CV, McCormach RJ: The management of spontaneous pneumothorax. Thorax 21:139, 1966.
165. Zimmerman JE, Dunbar RS, Klingenmaier CH: Management of subcutaneous emphysema, pneumomediastinum and pneumothorax during respiratory therapy. Crit Care Med 3:69, 1975.
166. Zwillich DN, Pierson DJ, Creagh CE, et al: Complications of assisted

ventilation. A prospective study of 354 consecutive cases. Am J Med 57:161, 1974.

167. Bernard RW, Stahl WM: Subclavian vein catheterizations. A prospective study. Non-infecting complications. Ann Surg 173:184, 1971.

168. Light RW, Girard WM, Jenkinson SG, et al: Parapneumonic effusions. Am J Med 69:507, 1980.

169. Wallach HW: Intrapleural tetracycline for malignant pleural effusions. Chest 68:510, 1975.

170. Zalozink AJ, Oswald SG, Langon M: Intrapleural tetracycline in malignant pleural effusions. Cancer 51:752, 1983.

171. Kirsh MM, Sloan H: Blunt Chest Trauma. Boston, Little, Brown, p 49, 1977.

172. Sahn SA: Diagnosing and managing patients with parapneumonic effusions. J Respir Dis 1:13, 1980.

173. Moessinger AC, Driscoll JM, Wiggers HJ: High incidence of lung perforation by chest tube in neonatal pneumothorax. Pediatrics 92:635, 1978.

174. Fraser RS: Lung perforation complicating tube thoracostomy. Hum Pathol 19:518, 1988.

175. Hussain SA: Complication of inserting a chest tube. JAMA 238:1629, 1977.

176. Beall AC Jr, Bricker DL, Crawford WH, et al: Considerations in the management of penetrating thoracic trauma. J Trauma 8:408, 1968.

177. LeBlanc KA, Tucker WY: Empyema of the thorax. Surg Gynecol Obstet 158:66, 1984.

178. Murphy K, Tomlonovich MC: Unilateral pulmonary edema after drainage of a spontaneous pneumothorax: Case report and review of the world literature. J Emerg Med 1:29, 1983.

179. Stahly TL, Tench WD: Lung entrapment and infarction by chest tube suction. Radiology 122:307, 1977.

180. Pingleton SK, Jeter J: Necrotizing fasciitis as a complication of tube thoracostomy. Chest 83:925, 1983.

181. Cox PA, Keshishian JM, Blades BB: Traumatic arteriovenous fistula of the chest wall and lung. J Thorac Cardiovasc Surg 54:109, 1967.

182. Fein AB, Godwin JD, Moore AV, et al: Systemic artery to pulmonary vascular shunt: A complication of closed tube thoracostomy. AJR 140:917, 1983.

183. Palomeque A, Canadell D, Pastor X: Acute diaphragmatic paralysis after chest tube placement. Intensive Care Med 16:138, 1990.

184. Greene W, L'Hereny P, Hunt CE: Paralysis of the diaphragm. Am J Dis Child 129:1402, 1975.

185. Rauch RF, Korobkin M, Silverman PM, et al: CT detection of iatrogenic percutaneous splenic injury. J Comput Assist Tomogr 7:1018, 1983.

186. Meisel S, Ram Z, Priel I, et al: Another complication of thoracostomy—Perforation of the right atrium. Chest 98:772, 1990.

187. Bertino RE, Wesbey GE, Johnson RJ: Horner syndrome occurring as a complication of chest tube placement. Radiology 164:745, 1987.

188. Bourque PR, Paulus EM: Chest tube thoracostomy causing Horner's syndrome. Can J Surg 29:202, 1986.

189. Kahn SA, Brandt LJ: Iatrogenic Horner's syndrome: A complication of thoracostomy tube placement. N Engl J Med 312:245, 1985.

190. Lillen DA, Gobbel WG: Spontaneous Pneumothorax. London, Churchill Livingstone, p 209, 1968.

191. Runyon B: Paracentesis of ascitic fluid. Arch Intern Med 146:2259, 1986.

192. Mallory A: Complications of diagnostic paracentesis in patients with liver disease. JAMA 239:628, 1978.

193. Krikorian JG, Hancock EW: Pericardiocentesis. Am J Med 65:808, 1978.

194. Guberman BA, Fowler NO, Engel PJ, et al: Cardiac tamponade in medical patients. Circulation 64:633, 1981.

195. Knauer CM, Fogel MR: Pericarditis: Complication of esophageal sclerotherapy. Gastroenterology 93:287, 1987.

196. Krehlik JM, Hindson DA, Crowley JJ, et al: Minoxidil-associated pericarditis and fatal cardiac tamponade. West J Med 143:527, 1985.

197. Schoenwetter AH, Silber EN: Penicillin hypersensitivity, acute pericarditis and eosinophilia. JAMA 191:136, 1965.

198. Alarcon-Segovia D: Drug-induced lupus syndromes. Mayo Clin Proc 44:664, 1969.

199. Withrington R, Collins P: Cardiac tamponade in acute pancreatitis. Thorax 35:959, 1980.

200. Uhl GS, Kippes GM: Pericardial tamponade in systemic sclerosis. Br Heart J 42:345, 1979.

201. Verkleeren JL, Glover MV, Bloor C, et al: Cardiac tamponade secondary to sarcoidosis. Am Heart J 106:601, 1983.

202. Valantine HA, Hunt SA, Gibbons R, et al: Increasing pericardial effusion in cardiac transplant recipients. Circulation 79:603, 1989.

203. Rose DM, Colvin SB, Danilowicz D, et al: Cardiac tamponade secondary to chylopericardium following cardiac surgery: Case report and review of the literature. Ann Thorac Surg 34:333, 1982.

204. Bernstein V, Roten CE, Peretz DI: Permanent pacemakers: 8 year follow-up study. Incidence and management of congestive cardiac failure and perforations. Ann Intern Med 74:361, 1971.

205. Wong B, Murphy J, Chong CJ, et al: The risk of pericardiocentesis. Am J Cardiol 44:1110, 1979.

206. Callahan JA, Seward JB, Tajik AJ: Cardiac tamponade: Pericardiocentesis directed by two-dimensional echocardiography. Mayo Clin Proc 60:344, 1985.

CHAPTER 15

Vascular Procedures

Vivian L. Clark
James A. Kruse

The management of critically ill patients necessitates expertise in several vascular procedures used for both diagnostic and therapeutic purposes. This expertise encompasses competence in the technical aspects of the procedure as well as knowledge of the indications and potential complications of these procedures.[1] This chapter reviews the indications, techniques, and complications of vascular procedures commonly employed in the critical care setting. Although not discussed in this chapter, a high level of competence in the interpretation of measurements obtained from diagnostic vascular procedures is a prerequisite for the independent application of these skills.

GENERAL CONSIDERATIONS

At times, certain vascular procedures must be performed urgently and under less than ideal conditions, such as during cardiopulmonary resuscitation. In all other situations, however, strict attention to skin preparation and aseptic technique is of extreme importance in minimizing the risk of infectious complications. The intended site of catheterization should be cleansed thoroughly with a suitable antiseptic, such as a povidone-iodine solution, and carefully draped to expose the site and provide an ample sterile field. The exposed field should be kept as small as possible, although certain important proximate landmarks may remain visible (e.g., the clavicle and the suprasternal notch in subclavian catheterization). The sterile field should extend well beyond the perimeter of the site to provide a large area for placing instruments, catheters, and other supplies. Transducers, flush solutions, intravenous connections, and supplies should be ready and available before they are actually needed. The operator and any assistants should don sterile gowns and gloves and wear hats and masks as well as eye protection. Because infection is one of the most common complications of invasive vascular procedures, sterile technique should be followed as rigorously in the critical care unit as in the operating room or the cardiac catheterization laboratory.

Careful documentation of the catheterization procedure in the medical record is of utmost importance. This entry should include the date and time, a concise description of the procedure, the anatomic site employed, the indications, and any complications encountered. Except in emergency situations, informed consent should be obtained and documented. Hemodynamic measurements or other information obtained as a result of the procedure should also be recorded, along with an interpretation of these data and plans for intervention.

CENTRAL VENOUS CATHETERIZATION

One of the most frequently employed vascular procedures in the critical care unit is central venous catheterization.[1] The sites most commonly selected for central venous access include the internal jugular vein, the subclavian vein, and the femoral vein. There are several situations in which central venous access is desirable and may even be safer than peripheral catheterization.[2] These include fluid resuscitation for patients with circulatory shock and cardiopulmonary arrest,[2, 3] the administration of parenteral nutrition solutions, and access for acute hemodialysis. In addition, central venous catheterization allows measurement of central venous pressure and provides an access for the introduction of intracardiac catheters such as pulmonary arterial catheters and temporary pacing electrodes. Central venous catheterization may also be indicated in patients for whom peripheral access is not available (e.g., intravenous drug abusers).

Contraindications

There are relative but no absolute contraindications for central venous catheterization. Relative contraindications include extreme obesity and severe bleeding diatheses. If a bleeding diathesis is present, one may wish to avoid access sites where direct pressure cannot be applied to control bleeding. On the other hand, Goldfarb and Lebrec reported few bleeding complications with internal jugular cannulation in 1000 patients with abnormal clotting study results.[4] Catheters should not be placed at the site of active local infection or in veins contiguous to sites of previous vascular surgical procedures, nor on the same side as an arteriovenous fistula used for dialysis.

Procedure

Several different techniques are employed for the introduction of central venous catheters. The most commonly used, and the method that is described here in detail, is the Seldinger technique,[5] in which a needle is used to first insert a guidewire into the vessel, followed by advancement of a catheter over the guidewire (Fig. 15–1). Methods involving the insertion of a catheter through a needle have two major disadvantages. First, a large-bore needle is necessary and increases the risk of significant inadvertent tissue injury. In contrast, the Seldinger technique allows a smaller-bore needle to be used, because only a small-diameter guidewire is inserted through the needle rather than the catheter itself. Second, the catheter-through-needle approach presents a risk of shearing off a segment of the catheter if the latter is intentionally or inadvertently retracted back through the needle. In a modification of the Seldinger technique, a catheter-over-needle device, similar or identical to that commonly used for peripheral venous cannulation, is used in lieu of a thin-walled needle.

The first step in the insertion process is to select the catheterization site and prepare the area as outlined earlier. The choice of insertion site often depends on the experience of the operator. The subclavian and internal jugular sites are optimal in terms of patient comfort and catheter stability, but in certain situations, the femoral vessels may be most appropriate.[6, 7] Examples include the patient with a bleeding diathesis or the setting of cardiopulmonary resuscitation.[8] Although the femoral site is commonly thought to be associated with a higher incidence of infection, the risk of catheter-related sepsis at this site may actually be similar to that with the more conventional subclavian and internal jugular access sites.[9]

There are commercially available kits for venous catheterization, which may include an ampule of local anesthetic agent, needles, a guidewire, a catheter, and other supplies. The use of double- and triple-lumen catheters is increasing because these devices are particularly useful in critically ill patients requiring multiple incompatible intravenous medications. These devices also allow one to monitor central venous pressure and administer fluid or drug infusions simultaneously. If central venous access is necessary for

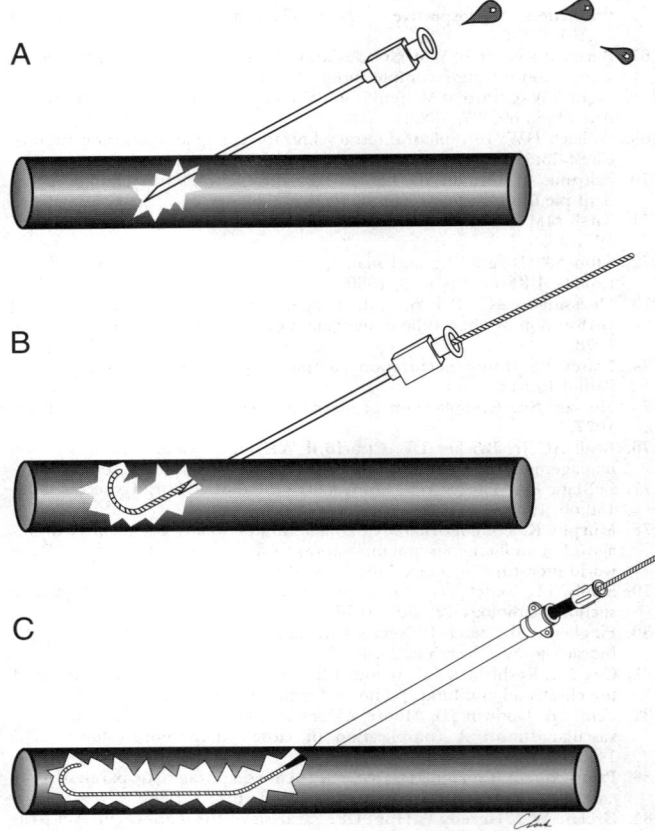

Figure 15–1. The Seldinger technique of vascular catheterization. *A.* The vessel is entered with thin-walled needle. *B.* A guidewire is advanced through the needle into the vessel. *C.* The catheter is advanced over the guidewire into the vessel.

insertion of a pulmonary arterial catheter or pacing electrode, a vascular introducer sheath is inserted over a tapered vein dilator.

The first step to cannulation of the femoral vein is to locate the femoral artery by palpation just below the inguinal ligament. The femoral vein lies just medial to the artery (Fig. 15–2). With a 25-gauge needle, 1% lidocaine without epinephrine is instilled intradermally and then subcutaneously to anesthetize the site. A small nick is made in the skin with a No. 11 scalpel blade to facilitate needle entry and subsequent catheter passage and to avoid the introduction of a plug of skin into the needle. Next, with the index and middle finger of one hand used to localize the position of the femoral artery, a thin-walled 18-gauge needle, attached to a syringe, is inserted with the bevel up and at approximately a 45° angle to the skin 1 cm medial to the artery (see Fig. 15–2). Constant gentle suction should be applied to the syringe as the needle is advanced. The sudden appearance of blood that is bright red or has pulsatile flow may signal inadvertent entry into the femoral artery. This can usually be confirmed by removing the syringe and noting pulsatile arterial flow from the needle. However, to minimize the risk of air embolism, the syringe should not be removed from the needle for more than 1 second. If pulsatile arterial flow is encountered, the needle should be withdrawn and pressure applied to the insertion site for several minutes to achieve hemostasis. Subsequent attempts to enter the vein should be made slightly medial to the initial entry site.

When venous blood is obtained, the needle should be held firmly in place and suction momentarily continued to ensure

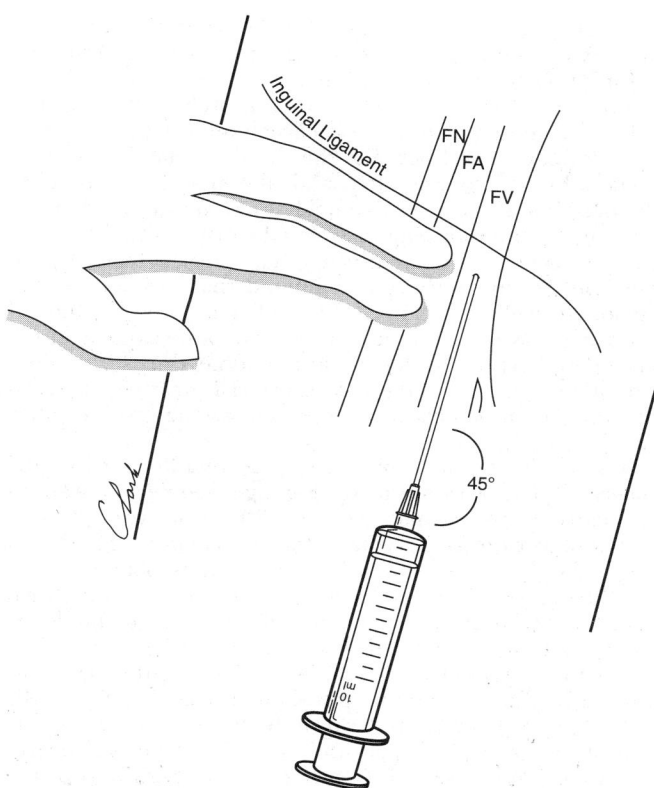

Figure 15-2. Femoral vein catheterization. The femoral artery is located just below the inguinal ligament, and the needle is inserted just medial to the artery at a 45° angle to the frontal plane while gentle suction is applied with a syringe, until free-flowing blood return is obtained. FN = femoral nerve; FA = femoral artery; FV = femoral vein.

free-flowing venous blood return. After satisfactory blood return is confirmed, the syringe is disconnected and a soft-tipped or J-tipped guidewire is immediately advanced through the needle and into the vein several centimeters beyond the tip of the needle. Another syringe design incorporates a small hole and one-way valve in the syringe plunger, which allows passage of a guidewire without disconnecting the syringe from the needle. There should be no resistance encountered while advancing the wire. If resistance is encountered, the wire should be withdrawn and blood return rechecked with a syringe. When blood return is confirmed, the wire may again be advanced. If resistance is still encountered, the wire is removed and the needle advanced or withdrawn slightly while aspirating to determine the position associated with optimal return. If after these manipulations the wire still cannot be advanced, the needle should be withdrawn and another attempt made after pressure is held briefly. Even seemingly slight resistance may be indicative of intimal or extravascular placement.

After the guidewire has been successfully advanced into the vessel and well beyond the tip of the needle, the needle should be immediately withdrawn and the wire then advanced to a point slightly beyond where the tip of the catheter is to be positioned. This is done to verify that there is no obstruction in the vessel and to ensure that the soft tip of the guidewire always remains beyond the tip of the advancing catheter, so that the catheter tracks the course of the guidewire and is less likely to injure the vessel intima. If not done previously, a No. 11 scalpel blade is used to make a nick in the skin wide enough to allow the catheter to pass

easily. To avoid possibly damaging the catheter, this should be done before the catheter is inserted into the skin.

The catheter is then advanced over the wire into the vessel. Advancement of the catheter is facilitated by grasping it close to the skin and using a slight twisting motion during insertion. Moderate resistance is sometimes encountered when advancing the catheter. A common source of excessive resistance is an inadequate skin nick. It is usually necessary to make this incision extend only just through the dermis because the subcutaneous tissue normally presents little additional resistance. However, it is important to ensure that the incision is sufficiently wide to allow catheter passage without stretching the incision. On the other hand, substantial subcutaneous scar tissue, such as might be encountered in sites of previous surgery or in intravenous drug abusers, may present considerable resistance and necessitate a deeper incision.

Occasionally, instead of tracking over the guidewire (Fig. 15-3*A* and *B*), the catheter may displace the proximal subcutaneous portion of the wire, creating a new and undesirable trajectory (see Fig. 15-3*C*). This usually is associated with a detectable increase in resistance during catheter advancement, but it may be difficult to distinguish from normally encountered resistance. A useful method for ensuring that the catheter is properly tracking the guidewire is to pause after the catheter has been advanced several

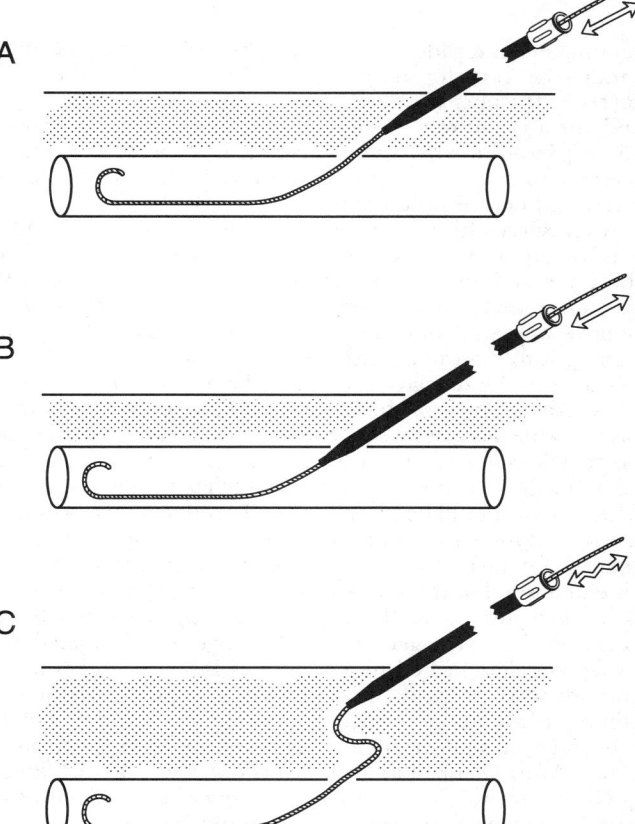

Figure 15-3. *A* and *B*. Catheter or dilator being advanced over the guidewire through subcutaneous tissue into the vessel. Proper tracking of the guidewire is shown. Gentle to-and-fro movement of the wire ensures correct tracking and facilitates catheter passage. *C*. Buckling of the guidewire in subcutaneous tissue creates a new and undesirable catheter trajectory. Increased resistance to both guidewire and catheter movement will be encountered in this situation.

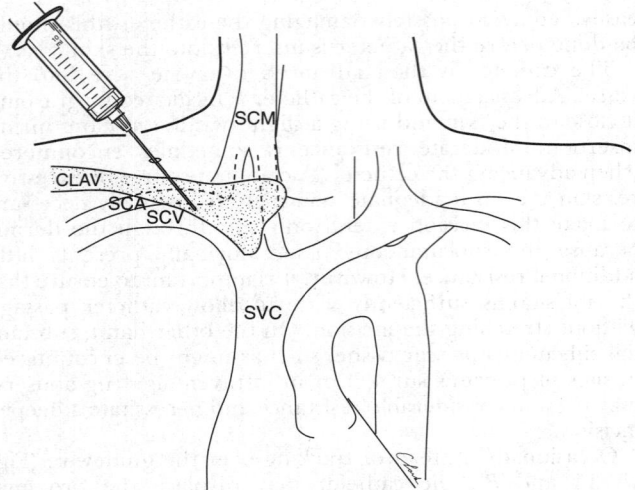

Figure 15–4. Supraclavicular subclavian vein catheterization. The needle is inserted just above the clavicle, approximately 3 cm lateral to the border of the sternocleidomastoid muscle, at a 0° or slightly negative angle to the frontal plane, and is advanced toward the opposite nipple while gentle suction is applied with a syringe, until free-flowing blood return is obtained. SCA = subclavian artery; SCV = subclavian vein; SCM = sternocleidomastoid muscle; CLAV = clavicle; SVC = superior vena cava.

centimeters and slide about 1 cm of the wire back and forth within the catheter (see Fig. 15–3B). If the catheter is correctly tracking the wire, there is essentially no resistance and the wire moves freely; substantial resistance (see Fig. 15–3C) indicates that the catheter is not correctly tracking the wire or some other problem is occurring that should be addressed before proceeding.

After successful advancement of the catheter, the guidewire is removed and a syringe is immediately connected to the catheter hub. A small amount of blood is aspirated to reconfirm that the catheter tip is within the vessel and to remove any air from the catheter dead space before connecting it to fluid-filled intravenous tubing.

Access to the subclavian vein may be obtained using either the supraclavicular or the infraclavicular approach. In either case a wide area above and below the clavicle should be prepared, as described earlier, and drapes placed so that the clavicle as well as the suprasternal notch area remain visible. The patient should be placed in the Trendelenburg position. This position increases the size of the vessels, optimizing the chances for successful cannulation and decreases the risk of air embolism. For the supraclavicular approach, 1% lidocaine is instilled just above the clavicle and approximately 3 cm lateral to the sternocleidomastoid muscle. A thin-walled 18-gauge needle attached to a syringe is inserted at this point and advanced toward the contralateral nipple while maintaining constant, gentle suction (Fig. 15–4). The needle should be at a 0° or slightly negative angle to the frontal plane. After venous blood return is obtained, the Seldinger guidewire technique is employed as described earlier. If the vessel is not entered, the needle should be withdrawn and reinserted at a slightly more positive angle. As with all other routes of percutaneous vascular cannulation, it is important to withdraw the needle to the level of the dermis before redirecting the angle of insertion. Adjusting the angle of insertion while the cutting edge of the needle is near the subclavian vein could result in laceration of the vein or artery. Some operators prefer to use a smaller-gauge needle

(e.g., 21-gauge needle) initially for localizing the vessel and identifying the appropriate angle and insertion trajectory before inserting the larger 18-gauge needle.

For the infraclavicular subclavian approach, the skin just below the mid-portion of the clavicle is anesthetized. Placing a small folded towel between the shoulder blades has traditionally been recommended, and although this may allow the needle and syringe to be held at a shallower angle from the skin, such positioning may actually distort the subclavian vein anatomy and decrease the chances of successful cannulation.[10] Some authors recommend that the point of insertion be at the junction of the medial and middle third of the clavicle, whereas other clinicians advocate starting at the junction between the lateral and middle thirds.[11-16] More lateral entry increases the risk of arterial puncture, and the position of the vessels is less constant as they course laterally.[17]

A skin nick is made just below the middle third of the clavicle, and the thin-walled 18-gauge needle is advanced toward the suprasternal notch at a 30° angle from the skin and kept as close as possible to the clavicle during insertion (Fig. 15–5). When venous blood return is obtained, one should proceed with the Seldinger technique as described earlier. If the vessel is not entered, the needle should be withdrawn and redirected either slightly above or slightly below the suprasternal notch. As with the supraclavicular approach, the operator may wish to use a smaller needle (e.g., 21-gauge needle) to localize the vessel and identify the appropriate angle and pathway of insertion before the 18-gauge needle is inserted. Gentle downward traction of the ipsilateral arm may be helpful if there is difficulty locating the vessel.

Another commonly used approach for central venous catheterization is via the internal jugular vein. The right side is preferred for this approach because there is a fairly straight path from the right internal jugular vein into the superior vena cava, thus minimizing the possibility of catheter malposition. In addition, the risk of pneumothorax, albeit low for this site, may be somewhat less on the right side owing to the more inferior pleural cupula on that side. For this approach, the lateral aspect of the neck and the

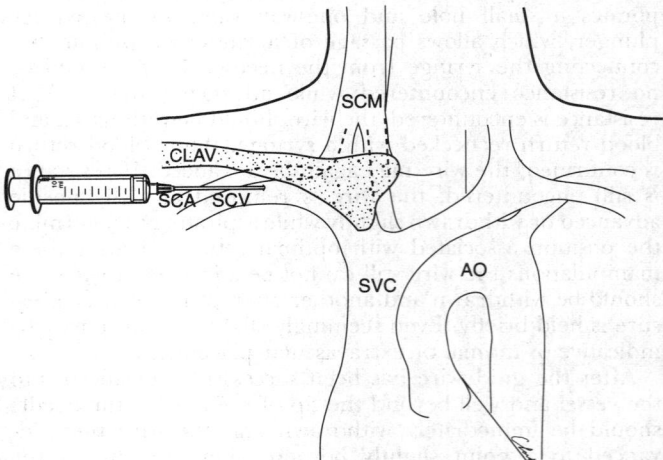

Figure 15–5. Infraclavicular subclavian vein catheterization. The needle is inserted just below the clavicle at its midpoint and is advanced toward the suprasternal notch while gentle suction is applied with a syringe, until free-flowing blood return is obtained. SCA = subclavian artery; SCV = subclavian vein; SVC = superior vena cava; AO = aorta; SCM = sternocleidomastoid muscle; CLAV = clavicle.

recommended because it may be associated with a higher risk of carotid puncture.

Central venous catheterization can be accomplished using the basilic vein, either percutaneously or via surgical cutdown, although this approach is rarely necessary. The percutaneous approach is done in a manner similar to the percutaneous femoral approach, except that a tourniquet is placed on the upper extremity to increase the size of the vein before catheterization. For an antecubital cutdown, local anesthetic is infiltrated just above the antecubital fossa, and a 2- to 3-cm transverse incision is made, extending medially from the point where the brachial artery is palpated. The subcutaneous tissue is dissected with a Kelly clamp until the vein is located. A silk tie may be used to ligate the vessel distal to the catheter insertion site, and another tie is placed loosely around the vein proximally to be used later in securing the catheter. A venotomy is made with a scalpel or eye scissors. After free blood flow is observed, a long catheter is advanced through the vein to the superior vena cava, a distance of 35 to 50 cm depending on the patient's size, and whether the right or left antecubital fossa is used. After the catheter tip is correctly positioned, the loose silk suture is tied around the vein to secure the catheter. The skin is closed with mattress sutures, and the catheter is anchored with a suture to the skin outside the incision. Care must be taken to avoid inadvertently nicking the catheter with the

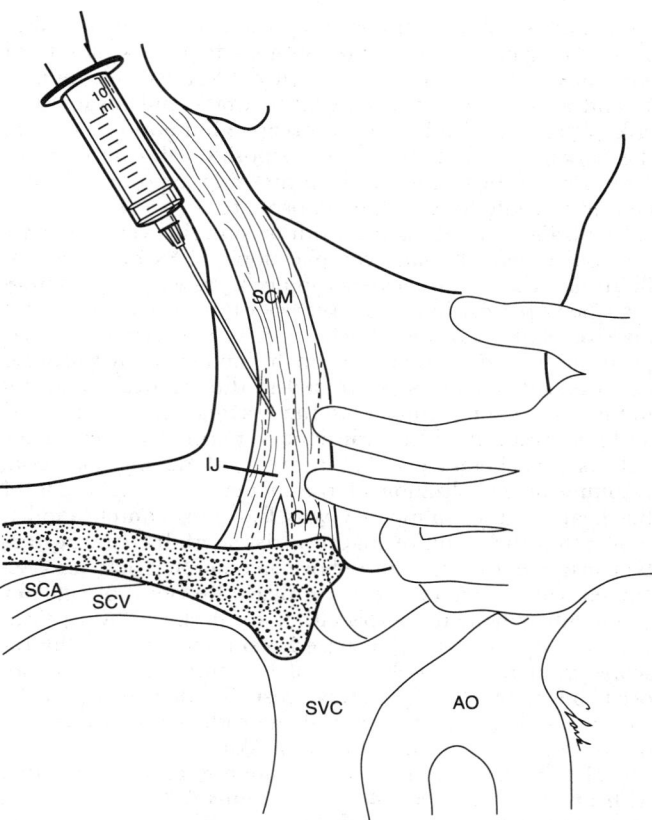

Figure 15–6. Posterior approach to internal jugular vein catheterization. The carotid artery is located with the nondominant hand. The needle is inserted along the lateral border of the sternocleidomastoid muscle approximately midway between the clavicle and the mastoid process and is advanced toward the suprasternal notch while gentle suction is applied with a syringe, until free-flowing blood return is obtained. SCA = subclavian artery; SCV = subclavian vein; SVC = superior vena cava; AO = aorta; CA = carotid artery; IJ = internal jugular vein; SCM = sternocleidomastoid muscle.

shoulder are prepared and draped so that the sternocleidomastoid muscle and the suprasternal notch are visible. The operator should stand at the head of the bed, with the patient in the Trendelenburg position. There are three commonly used approaches for internal jugular catheterization.

1. In the posterior approach, the needle with attached syringe is inserted behind the sternocleidomastoid muscle at the midpoint of the muscle between the clavicle and the mastoid process (Fig. 15–6). This is at approximately the level where the external jugular vein crosses the muscle, so care should be taken to avoid puncturing this more superficial vessel. The needle is advanced toward the suprasternal notch while gentle suction is applied with the syringe. When free-flowing venous blood return is confirmed, one should proceed with the Seldinger approach as described earlier.
2. In the middle approach, the needle is inserted at the apex of the triangle formed by the manubrial and clavicular heads of the sternocleidomastoid muscle and the clavicle (Fig. 15–7). The carotid artery is palpated with the nondominant hand and the needle is advanced lateral to it, aiming toward the ipsilateral nipple. When free-flowing venous blood return is confirmed, one should proceed with the Seldinger technique as described earlier.
3. An anterior approach has been described but is not

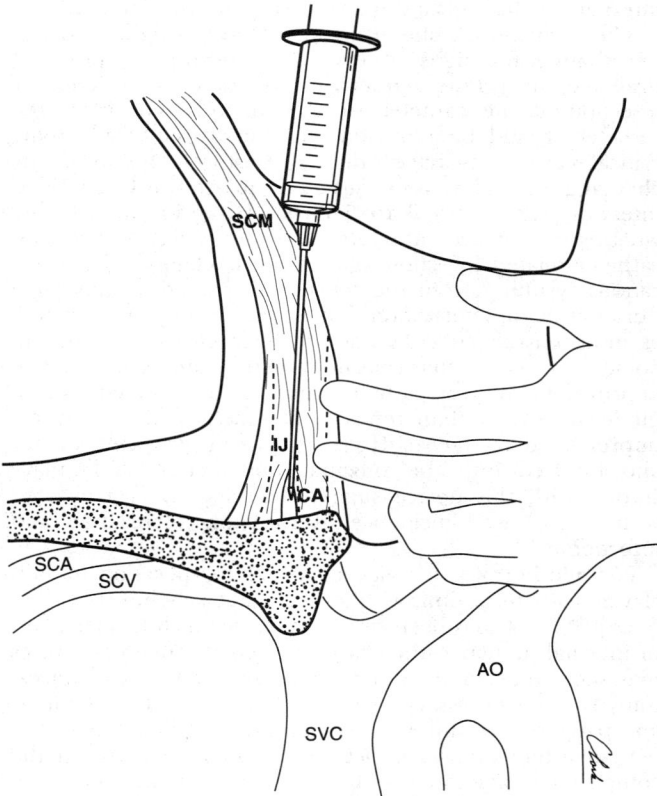

Figure 15–7. Middle approach to internal jugular vein catheterization. The carotid artery is located with the nondominant hand. The needle is inserted at the apex of the triangle formed by the clavicle and the manubrial and clavicular insertions of the sternocleidomastoid muscle and is advanced toward the ipsilateral nipple while gentle suction is applied with a syringe, until free-flowing blood return is obtained. SCA = subclavian artery; SCV = subclavian vein; SVC = superior vena cava; AO = aorta; CA = carotid artery; IJ = internal jugular vein; SCM = sternocleidomastoid muscle.

suture needle. Except for short catheters inserted via the femoral approach, the location of the catheter tip must be confirmed by a chest radiograph.

Meticulous catheter care after venous catheterization is important in preventing complications. Povidone-iodine ointment may be applied to the insertion site, and the site is always covered with a large sterile occlusive dressing affixed with tape. Intravenous tubing should be carefully secured to prevent traction on, or dislodgment of, the catheter. The dressing should be inspected frequently for signs of bleeding or drainage and changed daily or according to the institutional protocol.

Complications

The most common complications associated with central venous catheterization include infection, pneumothorax, and inadvertent arterial puncture.[18-28] The likelihood of a particular complication varies with the insertion site.[27-30] For example, pneumothorax is more common with subclavian catheterization, whereas arterial puncture probably occurs more often with the internal jugular approach.[26, 31]

Infectious complications of central venous catheterization include local cellulitis or abscess, septic phlebitis, bacteremia, and sepsis. The incidence of catheter-related infection has been reported to range from 0% to more than 25% and increases with the duration of catheterization.[18, 28, 32-43] Colonization of catheters may occur more frequently in the femoral site; however, the risk of infection is similar among internal jugular, subclavian, and femoral insertion sites.[27, 44]

The insertion site should be inspected during each dressing change for signs of erythema, induration, purulent drainage, or undue tenderness. If there is evidence of infection at the catheter site or unexplained fever, the catheter should be removed and the tip cultured. Some critical care units have adopted protocols for routinely changing central venous catheters at arbitrarily specified intervals (e.g., every 3 to 5 days). However, in deciding whether to replace catheters one must weigh the risk of catheter-related infection against the likelihood of complications resulting from the reinsertion procedure. An ideal duration of catheterization that minimizes infectious as well as insertion-related risks has not been clearly established. Some data suggest that routine catheter changes may not be appropriate or that catheters may be exchanged over a guidewire rather than replaced at a new site.[45-47] A silver-impregnated collagen cuff can be placed over the catheter and inserted into the subcutaneous tissues. Preliminary studies with this device suggest that its use is associated with a decreased incidence of catheter colonization and infection.[48, 49]

Pneumothorax is a well-recognized complication of subclavian catheterization, with an incidence ranging from 0 to 6%.[3, 18, 25, 26, 31] It has been reported but is much less frequent in internal jugular catheterization.[26] Small pneumothoraces may require no intervention; however, chest tube thoracostomy is often necessary, particularly in critically ill patients and patients receiving positive pressure ventilation.

Inadvertent arterial puncture accounts for many of the complications associated with internal jugular catheterization but is relatively uncommon during catheterization at other sites.[3, 26, 50] Despite its frequent occurrence, arterial puncture is rarely associated with significant bleeding, even in patients with coagulopathies.[4, 31]

There are also a number of less common but potentially serious complications. These include venous thrombosis, which may result in superior vena cava syndrome or pulmonary embolism,[51, 52] and air embolism, which can occur if the catheter hub is left exposed to the atmosphere.[21, 53, 54] Air

embolism, albeit uncommon, is a potentially fatal complication. Flanagan and colleagues showed that the quantity of air that can be entrained through a 14-gauge needle in 1 second may be sufficient to result in a fatal embolism.[55] The risk of this complication can be greatly minimized by placing the patient in the Trendelenburg position during catheter insertion and by compulsively minimizing exposure of catheter and needle hubs to the atmosphere.

Perforation of the right atrium or superior vena cava is a rare but potentially fatal complication.[56-60] Extravasation of fluids into the thoracic cavity can occur, as well as hemothorax, hemopericardium, or retroperitoneal bleeding with massive blood loss and shock.[18, 21, 57-60] The risk of cardiac perforation and tamponade can be mitigated by ensuring that the catheter tip is positioned in the vena cava and not in the right atrium. Injuries to the brachial plexus can occur and may result in either transient or permanent neurologic deficits.[18] Catheters can be sheared off during insertion, resulting in embolization of fragments to the right side of the heart or the pulmonary vessels.[51] This complication is most often the result of inappropriate withdrawal of catheters inserted through large-bore needles but has also occurred with catheters already in place. Retrieval of catheter fragments may be necessary either surgically or by a percutaneous approach using a snare in conjunction with fluoroscopic guidance. Embolization of the entire guidewire can occur but is avoidable by always ensuring that the tip of the wire is visible at the hub end of the catheter before the tip of the catheter is advanced into the skin.

Catheter malposition occurs frequently and is associated with an increased risk of complications.[23, 58, 61] In general, malpositioned catheters should be repositioned or removed. When reviewing a postcatheterization chest film, particular attention should be directed to ensuring that the catheter courses normally through the vasculature, ensuring that there is no pneumothorax, inspecting for evidence of intra-thoracic hematoma that could be related to the procedure, and ascertaining that the tip of the catheter does not extend into the right atrium.

ARTERIAL CATHETERIZATION

Arterial catheterization is frequently employed in critically ill patients. The most common arterial access sites are the radial, femoral, brachial, and axillary arteries.

Indications

There are two principal indications for arterial catheterization.

1. Continuous arterial pressure monitoring. This technique is commonly employed in the management of patients with hypotension or severe hypertension. It offers particular advantage in monitoring patients who require treatment with vasopressor agents, such as dopamine, or potent antihypertensive agents, such as sodium nitroprusside, that necessitate careful dosage titration to avoid precipitous changes in arterial pressure. In clinically stable patients, frequent measurement of blood pressure can be accomplished noninvasively with manual or automated blood pressure cuffs.

2. Frequent measurement of arterial blood gases. The most common situation is in patients with respiratory failure requiring mechanical ventilation, particularly when rapid changes in pulmonary status are expected and will likely require frequent modifications in ventilator settings. Frequent blood gas measurements may also be necessary in patients being weaned from mechanical ventilation.

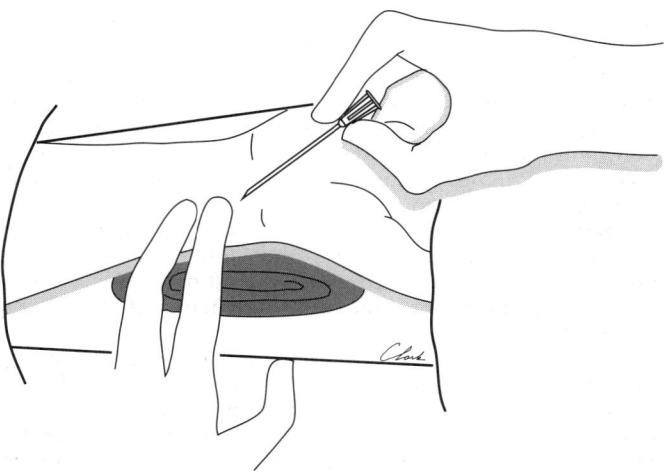

Figure 15–8. Radial arterial catheterization. The patient's hand is immobilized in a supinated position, and a small folded towel is placed under the wrist to maintain extension. The radial artery is located with the operator's nondominant hand, and the needle is advanced at a 30 to 45° angle until pulsatile blood return is obtained.

Contraindications

Relative contraindications for arterial catheterization include marked bleeding diatheses and severe peripheral vascular disease. Arterial puncture should be avoided in vessels with bruits or locally diminished pulsation suggesting the presence of significant atherosclerotic vascular disease. Catheterization should not be performed at sites of previous vascular surgery, through synthetic graft material, or in the vicinity of previous arterial thromboembolic events.

Procedure

A variety of catheters are available for arterial cannulation, including catheter-over-needle devices, which are used primarily for radial arterial insertion, and catheter-plus-guidewire devices. The first step in the insertion process is selection of an appropriate access site. The radial artery is frequently employed. Because of the dual circulation to the hand, the radial arterial approach has a low risk of serious vascular complications and is an optimal site in terms of patient comfort.[62] For patients with circulatory shock, the femoral artery may be more easily cannulated and yield more accurate measurements.[63] Before the radial artery is cannulated, the Allen test is performed to assess the adequacy of collateral circulation to the hand (see Chapter 19), although a favorable result does not ensure that collateral circulation is sufficient.[64–66] If femoral, axillary, or brachial arterial catheterization is planned, the adequacy of the peripheral circulation should be evaluated by examining the distal pulses and looking for other stigmata of arterial insufficiency.

For radial arterial catheter insertion, the hand should be supinated and immobilized. A small folded towel should be placed under the patient's wrist to maintain extension. After antisepsis and instillation of local anesthetic, the radial artery is located with the operator's nondominant hand and the needle is inserted parallel to the vessel at approximately a 30 to 45° angle and advanced slowly until blood return is obtained (Fig. 15–8). As with any arterial catheterization, a syringe should not be attached to the needle during radial arterial cannulation; it is unnecessary and may interfere with immediate recognition of arterial puncture. If the vessel is not entered, the needle is withdrawn, the site and/or the angle of insertion changed slightly, and insertion reattempted. To prevent laceration of the vessels, the direction of needle insertion should never be changed until the needle is completely or nearly completely withdrawn. After pulsatile blood return is obtained, the guidewire is advanced well beyond the tip of the needle and the needle is immediately withdrawn.

One should not attempt guidewire placement unless there is pulsatile blood flow from the needle hub. If blood flow is present but weakly pulsatile, it likely indicates either that the patient is hypotensive or that the needle is suboptimally positioned within the vessel. Slightly advancing the needle may result in more optimal positioning of the needle orifice within the central lumen of the vessel, resulting in increased blood flow and facilitating subsequent guidewire passage.

After successful guidewire insertion, a small nick is made in the skin with a No. 11 scalpel blade. After ensuring that the guidewire has been advanced sufficiently so that the tip of the wire lies farther upstream than the planned position of the catheter tip, the catheter is advanced over the wire. Pausing occasionally to check the guidewire for undue resistance (see Fig. 15–3) ensures that the catheter and the wire are not kinking within the subcutaneous space.

For radial arterial cannulation, a catheter-over-needle device may be used instead of the needle-and-guidewire method. Placement is similar to that in peripheral venous catheterization. After pulsatile blood return is observed, the catheter is advanced over the needle into the vessel and the needle then removed. Blood return from the catheter should be confirmed before connecting it to the transducer and flush device.

For brachial arterial cannulation, the forearm should be supinated and the arm immobilized on an arm board to prevent flexion at the elbow. After antiseptic preparation and local anesthesic instillation, the brachial artery is localized by palpation and entered just above the antecubital fossa. Femoral arterial catheterization is performed following the steps described for femoral venous catheterization.

After the arterial catheter is in place and pulsatile blood return confirmed, the catheter is connected to a transducer and continuous flush device using low-compliance tubing. A dressing is placed and the site is maintained as for central venous catheters. The involved extremity may be immobilized to prevent flexion at the catheter insertion site, which can result in spuriously low pressure readings. The extremity and the pulses distal to the insertion site should be checked regularly and if there is evidence of arterial insufficiency (e.g., diminished or absent pulses and coolness or mottling of the skin), the catheter should be removed to avert more serious complications.

Complications

The most common complication of arterial catheterization is infection, including local site infection or abscess, bacteremia, and overt sepsis. The risk of infection and sepsis is similar to that for venous catheters[67, 68] and increases with the duration of catheterization.[69] Arterial rupture resulting in hemorrhage or pseudoaneurysm formation has been reported as a rare consequence of catheter-related sepsis.[70] To minimize infectious complications, catheters should be removed as soon as the clinical situation warrants, and if infection is suspected, the catheter tip should be cultured using a semiquantitative technique.[71] Strict aseptic technique and meticulous catheter care reduce the risk of infectious complications.

Another common complication is bleeding, often a result of laceration of the vessel, which can range from a small localized hematoma to a major bleeding episode necessitating blood transfusions and open surgical repair. Bleeding complications are more common in patients with coagulopathies or in those receiving anticoagulants and are a particular threat in patients given thrombolytic agents. If possible, the administration of anticoagulants should be stopped or their effects reversed before insertion or removal of arterial catheters. Arterial puncture must be avoided in patients receiving thrombolytic agents, unless absolutely essential.

Local pulse deficits or ischemia may occur after arterial catheterization, generally as a result of thrombosis and/or embolization, vascular spasm, dissection, or rarely, cholesterol emboli. In most cases, significant sequelae are uncommon,[64, 72, 73] although surgical thrombectomy may be necessary,[74] and in rare instances, loss of digits or of the limb may occur.[65, 75] Persistent obstruction of the radial or ulnar artery has been documented by both angiography and Doppler ultrasonography; however, this rarely results in clinically significant ischemic complications.[64, 66, 72, 76–78] The risk of complications appears to be somewhat greater with the brachial approach than with either the radial or the femoral approach.[62, 79] Additional factors that increase the risk of vascular complications include the duration of catheterization, increased catheter diameter, concomitant use of vasopressor agents, and the presence of atherosclerosis, hypertension, and hypotension or low-flow states.[62, 64, 72]

Any evidence of limb ischemia mandates prompt removal of the catheter to minimize the risk of sequelae. Removal of the device often results in restoration of the pulse and alleviation of ischemia without the need for further intervention. Persistent clinical evidence of ischemia is generally an indication for exploration and thrombectomy.

Other potential complications of arterial catheterization include pseudoaneurysm and arteriovenous fistula formation, both of which generally necessitate surgical repair.[74, 80, 81] These types of complications are reported more commonly with diagnostic cardiac catheterization than with arterial cannulation for pressure monitoring, and this may be related to catheter size. Pseudoaneurysms and arteriovenous fistulas are most often noted after catheter removal and may not become apparent for several days after removal. The patient may complain of pain at the insertion site, and on examination, a pulsatile mass and bruit may be present. The presence of a pseudoaneurysm or a fistula can be confirmed by Doppler ultrasound imaging or by digital subtraction angiography.

TEMPORARY CARDIAC PACING

Temporary cardiac pacing can be accomplished either via a transvenous pacing catheter or through the use of a transcutaneous external pacemaker using precordial electrode patches. Clinical situations in which temporary pacing is used, either therapeutically or prophylactically, include (1) high-degree or complete atrioventricular block with significant symptoms or hemodynamic compromise, (2) severe symptomatic bradycardia, (3) new-onset bundle branch block in the setting of acute myocardial infarction,[82, 83] (4) overdrive pacing for control of supraventricular or ventricular tachycardia,[84–87] and (5) prophylactic use in patients with bifascicular or trifascicular blocks, or second degree atrioventricular block undergoing high-risk surgical procedures.[88]

Temporary transvenous pacing catheters generally range in size from No. 4 to 7 French. Smaller-diameter catheters are often equipped with a balloon at the tip to facilitate passage into the right ventricle.

Procedure

For pacing catheter insertion, central venous access is first accomplished using either the Seldinger or the catheter-over-needle technique. Pacing catheters are often introduced through venous introducer sheaths of compatible size, which should be equipped with a hemostasis valve to prevent bleeding and air embolism. Some sheaths also have a side arm connection, which allows for simultaneous central venous administration of fluids or drugs. The most common access sites are the subclavian, internal jugular, and femoral veins. Alternatively, an antecubital cutdown can be performed and the catheter introduced under direct vision into the basilic vein and advanced to the central venous circulation. However, the latter approach is least desirable, as there is a higher incidence of catheter dislodgment and pacemaker failure.[89, 90]

In emergencies, it may be necessary to advance pacing catheters blindly. Although this can often be accomplished when using the subclavian or jugular approach, blind positioning from the femoral or arm approach is technically more difficult. With this technique, the pacing catheter is advanced approximately 15 to 20 cm (from a jugular or subclavian site) and then connected to the pulse generator. The generator is set at a relatively high output current (e.g., 10 mA) and a rate exceeding the patient's intrinsic rate. The generator is switched on and the electrocardiographic monitor inspected for pacing spikes and ventricular capture as the electrode is advanced. If capture is observed, thresholds for sensing and capture should be checked, as described later, and if appropriate, the catheter is secured and its position checked radiographically. If capture is not observed, the catheter is advanced a few centimeters more. If capture is not apparent after a distance of approximately 30 cm is reached, it is likely that the catheter is curling in the atrium and should be withdrawn to the level of the introducer sheath and then readvanced. Use of a balloon-tipped electrode may facilitate successful catheter placement.

Under less urgent circumstances, the electrode catheter is advanced into the right ventricular apex using either electrocardiographic or fluoroscopic guidance. When using fluoroscopic control, the catheter is advanced to the right ventricular apex under direct vision. The electrocardiographic method uses the distal pacemaker catheter electrode to obtain an intracardiac electrogram, which guides insertion. The electrode is attached to one of the precordial leads of an electrocardiograph and a continuous recording is made as the catheter is slowly advanced toward the heart. Surface electrocardiographic leads are monitored simultaneously. If the catheter is balloon tipped, the balloon should be inflated at a distance of approximately 20 cm. When the catheter enters the right atrium, prominent P waves are evident (Fig. 15–9A). These P waves are upright if the catheter is advanced from the groin and inverted if the catheter is advanced from the neck or the arm. As the catheter enters the right ventricle, the P wave becomes smaller and the QRS complex more prominent (see Fig. 15–9B). ST elevation (injury current) or ventricular ectopy indicates that the catheter is in contact with the right ventricular endocardium (see Fig. 15–9C). After ST segment elevation is observed, the catheter need not be advanced farther. At this point, the catheter is attached to the pulse generator, and if pacing is confirmed, capture and sensitivity thresholds are evaluated.

To check capture threshold, the pacemaker generator should be set at a rate that exceeds the patient's intrinsic rate. First, one should confirm capture at a fairly high output current (e.g., 5 to 10 mA). If capture occurs consistently, the output is slowly reduced until the threshold for loss of capture is determined. Ideally, this should be at an output of 1 mA or less; higher thresholds indicate suboptimal positioning of the electrode. In practice, the current output of the generator is set to a level that is several milliamperes

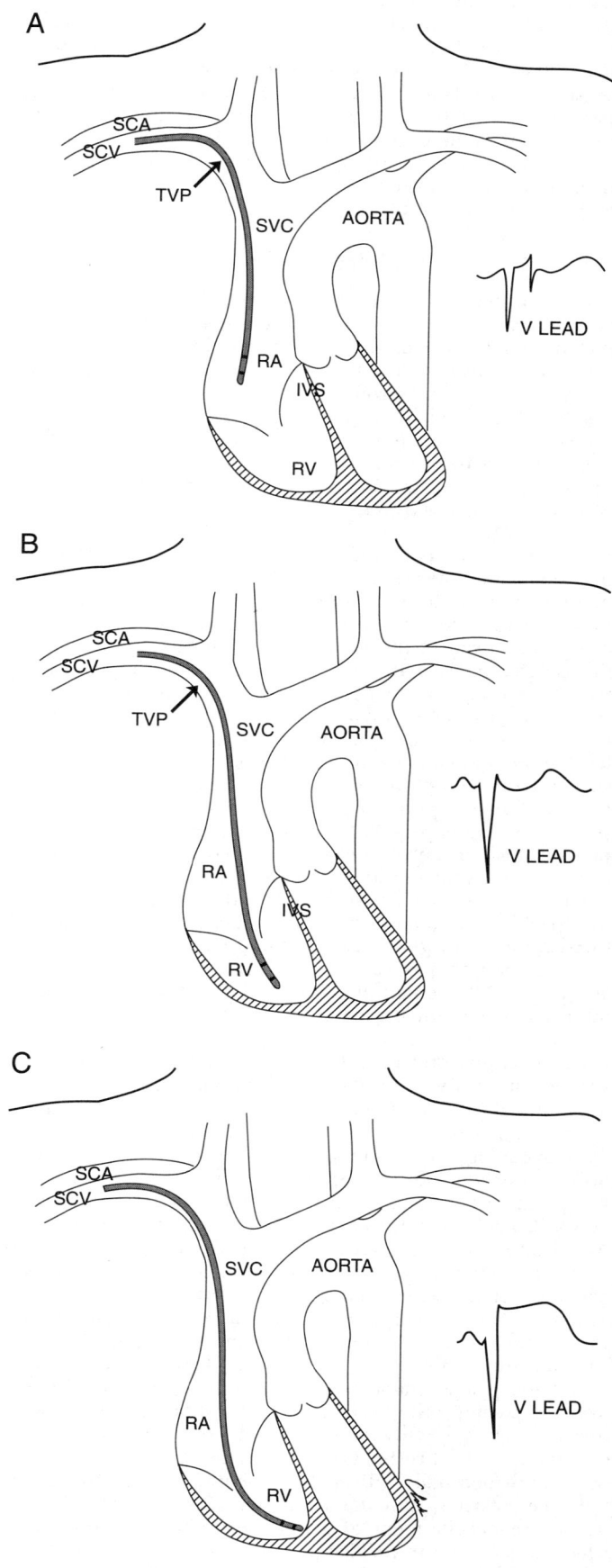

Figure 15–9. Insertion of a transvenous pacing catheter by using electrocardiographic guidance. The V lead of the electrocardiograph is attached to the distal pacing electrode by using a connecting wire with alligator clips. *A.* An intracardiac electrogram is shown with the electrode catheter's tip positioned high in the right atrium. Note the large inverted P wave and small QRS complex. *B.* An intracardiac electrogram with the catheter tip in the right ventricular cavity. Note the small upright P wave and large QRS complex with normal ST segment. *C.* An intracardiac electrogram with the electrode positioned in the right ventricular apex and in contact with the endocardium of the interventricular septum. Note the small upright P wave and large QRS complex with marked ST elevation (injury currrent). SCA = subclavian artery; SCV = subclavian vein; TVP = transvenous pacing catheter; SVC = superior vena cava; RA = right atrium; RV = right ventricle; IVS = interventricular septum.

higher than the determined threshold. The sensitivity threshold is of importance if the unit is being used in a demand mode. In demand mode, generator output is inhibited when a QRS complex is sensed. Generally, the lowest sensitivity threshold is selected. In the case of overdrive pacing for arrhythmia suppression, the sensitivity is set to the asynchronous position to allow pacing at a fixed rate. After appropriate pacing and sensing thresholds are confirmed, the pacemaker electrode position should be verified with a chest radiograph.

Complications

Complications of transvenous pacemaker insertion, aside from those associated with central venous catheterization, include perforation of the veins, the right ventricular free wall, or the interventricular septum; atrial or ventricular arrhythmias; venous thrombosis; and local or systemic infection.[88, 90, 91] After initial proper functioning, failure to capture or sense may occur. This may be due to movement of the electrode, fracture of the conductor leads, electrical failure of the generator or the battery, or perforation of the ventricle by the electrode.[89-95]

Right ventricular free wall perforation should be suspected when an audible pericardial rub appears after pacemaker insertion, when there is evidence of pacing of the diaphragm or intercostal muscles, or when the pacemaker tip extends to the cardiac apex or beyond on the chest radiograph. This complication can result in pericardial tamponade, although this is rare. Occasionally, a catheter perforates the interventricular septum and the tip enters the left ventricular cavity. A change in catheter tip position on the chest radiograph or a change in the morphology of the paced beats (from a left bundle branch pattern to a right bundle branch pattern) suggests this complication.[96] Such catheter migration may result in loss of capture or sensitivity but only rarely in more serious consequences. Withdrawal of the catheter by a centimeter or two usually brings it back into the right ventricular cavity. Pacing and sensing thresholds are then reconfirmed and catheter position again checked radiographically. If free wall perforation is suspected, the patient should be monitored closely for signs of cardiac tamponade.

Atrial arrhythmias can occur during catheter insertion and are usually benign and transient. Ventricular arrhythmias may occur during or after insertion. Ventricular arrhythmias occurring after pacemaker placement may represent excessive movement of the catheter tip within the ventricular cavity, and these arrhythmias are sometimes difficult to distinguish from those resulting from the patient's underlying cardiac disease. It may be helpful to compare the morphology of ectopic complexes recorded before pacemaker insertion with that of those observed after insertion. Ectopy arising from a pacing catheter should have a left bundle branch pattern and may closely resemble paced beats. Arrhythmias are sometimes abolished by repositioning the catheter. Failure to do so may lead to worsening arrhythmias and ventricular tachycardia or fibrillation.[89, 90, 94, 95]

Maintenance of temporary pacing catheters is the same as for central venous catheters. Pacing and sensing thresholds should be determined on a daily basis and adjustments made in catheter positioning as necessary. Applying a sterile sleeve over the pacing catheter during the insertion process allows the catheter to be advanced subsequently, if necessary, to obtain improved thresholds. Correct catheter position should be reconfirmed daily with a chest roentgenogram. In addition, daily cardiac auscultation is performed specifically to detect the development of a new pericardial friction rub, which could indicate cardiac perforation.[96] Electrode catheters should be removed as soon as the patient's clinical condition permits or after permanent pacemaker implantation.

PULMONARY ARTERIAL CATHETERIZATION

Pulmonary arterial catheterization has become increasingly common in the critical care unit setting during the past 20 years. Hemodynamic information derived from pulmonary arterial catheters can be valuable for both diagnosis and management of the critically ill patient. Specific hemodynamic syndromes are discussed in other chapters.

Indications

Indications for pulmonary arterial catheterization include the following:

1. The differential diagnosis and management of shock. Distinctive hemodynamic profiles characterize a number of shock syndromes.[97-99] The assessment of hemodynamic status on the basis of clinical evaluation alone may be unreliable and important changes in management can result from information derived from pulmonary arterial catheterization, particularly with regard to the administration of fluids or vasoactive agents.[99-101]

2. The identification and management of hemodynamic derangements associated with acute myocardial infarction. In this setting, pulmonary arterial catheterization has been shown to be a valuable clinical tool in differentiating low cardiac output caused by hypovolemia from pump failure. Pivotal management decisions can be based on the hemodynamic information obtained.[102-104] It is also useful in confirming the presence of significant right ventricular infarction, which can have important therapeutic implications in terms of fluid management.[105-107]

3. The identification of mechanical complications of acute myocardial infarction, such as ventricular septal defect and acute mitral valve dysfunction.[108] Hemodynamic information obtained is also of value in monitoring the effectiveness of therapy, such as afterload reduction or intra-aortic balloon counterpulsation.

4. The management of patients with adult respiratory distress syndrome. Pulmonary arterial catheterization is useful for monitoring the hemodynamic effects of positive end-expiratory pressure. Oxygen delivery can be quantitated from cardiac output and arterial blood gas results, and its assessment has been advocated as a means of identifying optimal levels of positive end-expiratory pressure.[109] In addition, measurement of pulmonary arterial occlusion pressure identifies patients with pulmonary edema caused by left ventricular failure versus those with noncardiogenic pulmonary edema.[110]

5. The management of patients with acute oliguria.[99] This is of particular value in assessing patients with left ventricular dysfunction or occult hypovolemia.

6. The assessment and titration of pharmacologic interventions in the management of acute and chronic heart failure.

7. The management of patients undergoing open heart surgery and of high-risk patients undergoing noncardiac surgery, such as abdominal aortic aneurysm repair.[111-113]

8. Preoperative assessment and management of patients with heart failure or significant left main coronary arterial stenosis.[114]

9. Evaluation for pericardial tamponade (see Chapters 92 and 95).

Contraindications

Pulmonary arterial catheterization entails central venous access and the same contraindications apply. Additional

TABLE 15–1

APPROXIMATE DISTANCES TO VENA CAVA AND CARDIAC CHAMBERS FROM DIFFERENT ACCESS SITES

Access Site	Distance (cm)*				
	SVC	RA	RV	PA	IVC
Right internal jugular vein	10–15	20–25	25–30	30–35	—
Left internal jugular vein	15–20	20–25	30–35	35–40	—
Right subclavian vein	10–15	20–25	25–30	30–35	—
Left subclavian vein	15–20	20–25	30–35	35–40	—
Right antecubital vein	35–40	40–45	45–50	50–55	—
Left antecubital vein	40–45	45–50	50–55	55–60	—
Right femoral vein	—	40–45	45–50	50–55	25–45
Left femoral vein	—	45–50	50–55	55–60	20–40

*SVC = superior vena cava; RA = right atrium; RV = right ventricle; PA = pulmonary artery; IVC = inferior vena cava.

relative contraindications include bacterial endocarditis involving the right side of the heart, thrombus within the chambers of the right side of the heart, prosthetic valves in the tricuspid or pulmonic positions, uncontrolled life-threatening cardiac arrhythmias, and cardiac conduction disturbances, such as bifascicular and trifascicular blocks. Pulmonary arterial catheters should also be avoided in general in patients with permanent transvenous pacemakers; if insertion is deemed necessary, they should be inserted using fluoroscopic guidance to avoid entangling the catheter with the pacing electrode.

Procedure

Pulmonary arterial catheters can be inserted percutaneously using vascular sheaths in the subclavian, the internal jugular, or the femoral vein; employing the Seldinger technique; or using a peripheral vein by means of an antecubital cutdown. The catheters are balloon tipped and designed to float into appropriate position without the use of fluoroscopic guidance. Occasionally, however, catheter positioning may be difficult and fluoroscopic guidance required, particularly in severe cases of pulmonary hypertension, dilated cardiomyopathy, or tricuspid insufficiency or when using the femoral approach. Catheters with a terminal S-shaped curvature are available to facilitate passage into the pulmonary artery from the femoral approach.

The first step in inserting the pulmonary arterial catheter is to obtain central venous access as described earlier. Standard No. 7, 7.5, and 8 French catheters are generally inserted through compatible No. 8 or 8.5 French vascular introducer sheaths. The sheath should be equipped with a diaphragm seal at the hub to prevent backflow of blood or entrainment of air into the circulation. If a vascular cutdown technique is employed, a sheath may be used, or alternatively, the catheter may be inserted directly into the peripheral vein. All infusion and pressure-monitoring ports should be flushed with heparinized saline and the integrity of the balloon checked before catheterization. The distal port is connected to a sterile stopcock for mixed venous blood sampling and to a pressure transducer using low-compliance tubing. After the electrical and pressure connections have been made, gently shaking the catheter and observing corresponding deflections on the monitor tracing confirm that it is ready to record pressures.

After the transducer has been properly leveled and calibrated (see Chapters 20 and 95), the catheter is advanced to about 20 cm (approximately 35 cm when using the antecubital approach), and the balloon inflated with air to its working volume (typically 1.5 mL). If a right-to-left shunt is suspected, carbon dioxide should be used for inflation, to prevent paradoxical air embolization into the systemic circulation in the event of balloon rupture. Fluid should never be injected into the balloon port, as this could prevent proper deflation of the balloon. The balloon should be inflated slowly enough to allow recognition of undue resistance to inflation. Resistance encountered during inflation may indicate that the balloon tip is still within the vascular sheath or has not yet reached the central circulation. In either case, the balloon is deflated, the catheter is advanced farther, and balloon inflation is cautiously reattempted.

The catheter should continue to be advanced until a right ventricular waveform is identified (see Chapter 95). At this point, the ventricular pressures should be documented and the insertion distance noted. The catheter is then farther advanced until a pulmonary arterial waveform is identified. The distance required to reach the pulmonary artery varies according to the insertion site (Table 15–1). If a pulmonary arterial waveform is not observed after advancing the catheter several centimeters farther, or if a right atrial waveform reappears, the catheter has probably coiled in the right ventricle. If coiling is suspected, the balloon is deflated and the catheter withdrawn to the right atrial position and readvanced after rotating it slightly. Fluoroscopic guidance may be necessary if the catheter cannot be advanced to the pulmonary artery after several attempts, but this is rarely necessary. Difficulty in reaching the pulmonary artery may be encountered in patients with severe heart failure, tricuspid insufficiency, or severe pulmonary hypertension.

When a pulmonary arterial waveform is identified, the catheter is advanced until a pulmonary arterial occlusion tracing is identified (see Chapter 95). The wedge pressure is generally within 4 to 5 mm Hg of the pulmonary arterial diastolic pressure, unless there is underlying pulmonary vascular disease. After an acceptable wedge waveform is obtained, the balloon is deflated and the pulmonary arterial waveform should return. If the occlusion waveform persists, the catheter is withdrawn slightly and the process is repeated until a wedge tracing is consistently seen with inflation of the balloon and an undamped pulmonary arterial tracing observed with deflation. To prevent balloon rupture, no more than the recommended volume of air should be used for balloon inflation. A greater likelihood of spontaneous wedging exists when the catheter wedges with a smaller than recommended volume of air. In the latter situation, there is also additional risk of pulmonary arterial rupture if the balloon is subsequently inflated with full volume. It is therefore best to position the catheter such that the full balloon inflation volume is required to achieve a wedge tracing.

Pulmonary arterial catheters are maintained similarly to central venous catheters. Generally, the proximal port is attached to a fluid infusion, which is maintained at a rate sufficient to keep the catheter open, although a three-way stopcock can be attached to the hub to allow connection to a pressure transducer for intermittent right atrial pressure measurement. Lumina should be flushed again with heparinized saline or dextrose solution before pressure is measured. A chest roentgenogram should be obtained on a daily basis while the catheter is in place, to monitor for possible complications or changes in catheter position. The application of a sterile sleeve over the distal portion of the catheter as it exits the introducer sheath allows for subsequent readjustment of catheter position.

Complications

A number of potential complications are associated with pulmonary arterial catheterization in addition to those related to central venous access. Atrial and ventricular arrhythmias or conduction disturbances are among the most common complications.[115-122] They are generally transient and resolve when the catheter is withdrawn, although life-threatening and fatal arrhythmias have been reported.[116] Arrhythmias are most likely to occur when the catheter tip is within the right ventricular outflow tract. Most arrhythmias occur during insertion, but they have been reported to develop hours to days after successful catheter placement and are sometimes related to looping of the catheter or tip displacement.[123] Catheter malposition also occurs frequently and may result in loss of ability to measure wedge pressure or persistent wedging.[118, 124]

Catheter-related infections and sepsis are common complications.[115, 118, 121, 125] Endocarditis has been reported in rare instances and should be considered in patients with bacteremia.[126]

Catheters may act as a nidus for intracardiac thrombus formation and can potentially lead to pulmonary emboli.[115, 127] Persistent wedging or sustained balloon inflation can result in pulmonary infarction or pulmonary arterial rupture.[118, 119, 127-129] Perforation of the right ventricle has also been reported.[119] Because these catheters have multiple connection hubs, care must be taken to avoid administering cardiac output injectate through the distal port or through the balloon lumen, which can result in pulmonary infarction or pulmonary arterial rupture.

Catheter knotting may occur if the catheter is allowed to coil in one of the cardiac chambers or in the vena cava. This can result from excessively advancing the catheter within the vena cava or one of the cardiac chambers, resulting in coiling.[130] Coiling can be avoided during catheter insertion by withdrawing the catheter if the pressure waveform fails to change (e.g., from right ventricular to pulmonary arterial) after the catheter has been advanced a reasonable distance (see Table 15-1). The catheter can also become tangled among the tricuspid valve chordae tendineae, which could potentially result in leaflet disruption and tricuspid insufficiency. Therefore, the catheter should never be withdrawn against resistance, which may be indicative of entanglement or knotting. A chest radiograph or fluoroscopic observation assists in determining the mechanism of the resistance.

INTRA-AORTIC BALLOON COUNTERPULSATION

Intra-aortic balloon counterpulsation is most often applied in the coronary care and cardiothoracic surgery unit settings and may be of value in supporting the circulation when standard pharmacotherapy fails. This device can potentially improve cardiac function by augmenting coronary perfusion pressure and by reducing afterload. Balloon inflation is synchronized with the patient's electrocardiogram or arterial pressure waveforms so that inflation is triggered in early

diastole, increasing coronary perfusion, and deflation occurs in late diastole, thereby decreasing afterload.

Indications

Indications for intra-aortic balloon insertion include the following:

1. Unstable angina that fails to respond to medical therapy. This is useful to treat patients awaiting revascularization and to stabilize patients before diagnostic cardiac catheterization.

2. Hemodynamic support and afterload reduction in patients with mechanical complications of acute myocardial infarction, including ventricular septal defect and severe mitral insufficiency from papillary muscle dysfunction.[131, 132]

3. Hemodynamic support of patients awaiting cardiac transplantation who are unresponsive to standard medical therapy.[133] Modest increases in cardiac output can be achieved with balloon counterpulsation, which may be sufficient to stabilize the critically ill patient with heart failure. Other types of circulatory support devices currently in use or under investigation may provide even greater increases in cardiac output.

4. Patients undergoing open heart surgery. Balloon counterpulsation is useful both preoperatively and postoperatively in patients who are at high risk, owing to either poor left ventricular function or left main coronary arterial disease.[134-136] In addition, intra-aortic balloon pumping is of value postoperatively when it is difficult to wean patients from cardiopulmonary bypass.[131, 137-139]

5. Support of patients with pump failure after acute myocardial infarction not due to a mechanical cause. This indication is somewhat controversial. Available data suggest that this intervention does not significantly improve survival in these patients, although some authors still advocate its use in this situation.[131, 133, 140, 141]

Contraindications

Absolute contraindications for intra-aortic balloon counterpulsation include aortic dissection and significant aortic insufficiency, because diastolic balloon inflation markedly increases regurgitation. Relative contraindications include abdominal aortic aneurysm, as well as severe peripheral vascular disease involving the lower extremity vessels. Because a large-bore introducer sheath (typically No. 10 to 12 French) is used for intra-aortic balloon insertion, this technique should be avoided in patients with severe, uncorrectable bleeding diatheses.

When intra-aortic balloon catheters were first introduced, insertion necessitated surgical exposure of the femoral artery and anastomosis of a Dacron graft through which the device was inserted. Thus, placement was performed only by surgeons skilled in vascular surgical techniques. In the late 1970s, catheters were developed for percutaneous insertion using the Seldinger technique.[142] A number of further advances occurred, including the development of long introducer sheaths and balloons with a central lumen to allow insertion over a guidewire, which further facilitated percutaneous balloon insertion and allowed pressure monitoring from the central aorta. Despite these advances, there is still the potential for significant vascular complications, so that insertion of these catheters should be performed only by physicians highly skilled in the Seldinger technique of arterial catheterization.

Procedure

Percutaneous insertion of intra-aortic balloon catheters is done through the femoral artery. Careful assessment of femoral and peripheral lower extremity pulses should be performed to determine which side should be used for insertion. In general, insertion should be avoided if femoral bruits or diminished peripheral pulses are present. The procedure is ideally carried out under fluoroscopic guidance, although successful insertion can be achieved at the bedside without fluoroscopy.

The groin should be cleansed with a povidone-iodine solution and draped to expose the femoral triangle. Ideally, the drapes should extend from the patient's neck to the foot of the bed, to provide a large sterile field. Access to the femoral artery should be obtained as described earlier for femoral arterial catheterization. A long J-tipped guidewire (e.g., 49 × 0.038 inch) is then advanced through the needle well into the abdominal aorta under fluoroscopic guidance. After the needle is removed, a small skin incision is made to facilitate the introduction of a No. 8 French vessel dilator to expand the arterial puncture site and subcutaneous tissues. The dilator is then removed and exchanged for the No. 10 or 12 French sheath-dilator assembly (depending on the size of balloon catheter used), which is advanced over the guidewire into the artery.

The balloon is prepared by applying negative pressure to the balloon lumen through a one-way valve using the large syringe supplied with the catheter. The balloon can then be removed from its protective tray. If fluoroscopic guidance is not used, the distance to the left subclavian artery should be estimated and noted using the balloon markings. The catheter should be moistened and, if a central lumen is present, flushed with sterile saline solution after removal of the inner stylet. The dilator is removed from the sheath, and the balloon is advanced over the guidewire until the tip is just distal to the origin of the left subclavian artery, using either fluoroscopic imaging or the markings on the catheter based on the previous estimate. The guidewire is then removed and the sheath partially withdrawn (6 inches for an 11-inch sheath and 10 inches for a 15-inch sheath). The balloon lumen is then connected to the balloon pump control console, and balloon pumping is initiated, usually by a technician trained in circulation technology. If the balloon catheter is placed without fluoroscopic guidance, radiographic verification that the entire balloon membrane has exited from the introducer sheath and ensurance of appropriate tip position is recommended before initiating counterpulsation (Fig. 15–10).

After balloon insertion, full anticoagulation with heparin should be initiated. The sheath and the balloon catheter are secured with several sutures and covered with a sterile occlusive dressing. The insertion site should be checked periodically for bleeding and the lower extremity observed for signs of arterial insufficiency. The catheter should be removed as soon as possible if evidence of limb ischemia is detected.

Complications

Intra-aortic balloon catheters are associated with a number of significant complications. The majority of these complications are vascular and involve arterial insufficiency and limb ischemia.[143–147] The risk of vascular complications is related to the duration of catheter placement.[144, 146] Other risk factors include older age, female sex, diabetes mellitus, and history of peripheral vascular disease.[131, 146] Limb ischemia may resolve spontaneously after catheter removal, although approximately one third of patients require surgical intervention and loss of limb has occurred on rare occasions.[144, 146, 148] Other infrequent complications include arterial or aortic dissection or perforation, bleeding and hematoma formation, infection, neuropathy, balloon rupture, and the

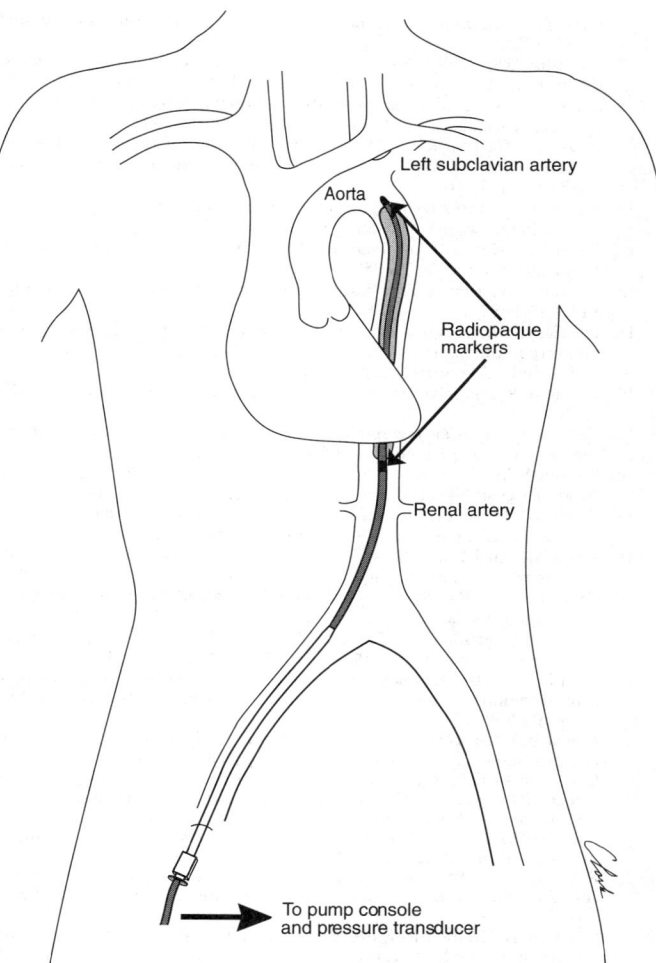

Figure 15–10. Proper positioning of the intra-aortic balloon catheter in the aorta. The tip lies just below the origin of the left subclavian artery. Radiopaque markers are located at each end of the balloon.

development of arterial pseudoaneurysms.[131, 143, 145, 147, 149, 150] Early recognition and treatment of complications may reduce the risk of long-term sequelae.[151]

CONCLUSION

Proficiency in a variety of vascular procedures is an integral part of overall competence in critical care medicine. Thorough knowledge of the technical aspects of these procedures, strict adherence to aseptic technique, and careful attention to detail allow the clinician to use invasive procedures to improve patient care with minimal risk of additional morbidity.

References

1. Kruse JA, Carlson RW: Training and practice patterns of Society of Critical Care Medicine internists. Crit Care Med 15:1065, 1987.
2. Giuffrida DJ, Bryan-Brown CW, Lumb PD, et al: Central vs peripheral venous catheters in critically ill patients. Chest 90:806, 1986.
3. Herbst CA: Indications, management, and complications of percutaneous subclavian catheters. Arch Surg 113:1421, 1978.
4. Goldfarb G, Lebrec D: Percutaneous cannulation of the internal jugular vein in patients with coagulopathies: An experience based on 1000 attempts. Anesthesiology 56:321, 1982.
5. Seldinger SI: Catheter replacement of the needle in percutaneous arteriography: A new technique. Acta Radiol 39:368, 1953.
6. Jastremski MS, Mathias HD, Randell PA: Femoral venous catheterization

during cardiopulmonary resuscitation: A critical appraisal. J Emerg Med 1:387, 1984.

7. Swanson RS, Uhlig PN, Gross PL: Emergency intravenous access through the femoral vein. Ann Emerg Med 13:244, 1984.

8. Standards and guidelines for cardiopulmonary resuscitation (CPR) and emergency cardiac care (ECC). JAMA 255:2905, 1986.

9. Kruse JA, Carlson RW: Infectious complications of femoral vs internal jugular and subclavian vein central venous catheterization. Crit Care Med 19:S84, 1991.

10. Joseph JM, Conces DJ, Augustyn GT: Patient positioning for subclavian vein catheterization. Arch Surg 122:1207, 1987.

11. Linos DA, Mucha P, van Heerden JA: Subclavian vein: A golden route. Mayo Clin Proc 55:315, 1980.

12. Pulliam CW, Reines HD: Subclavian vein catheterization. Am J Surg 149:416, 1985.

13. Eastridge CE, Hughes FA, Prather JR, et al: Use of central venous pressure in the management of circulatory failure: Review of indications and technic. Am J Surg 32:121, 1966.

14. Defalque RJ: Subclavian venipuncture: A review. Anesth Analg 47:677, 1968.

15. Tofield JJ: A safer technique of percutaneous catheterization of the subclavian vein. Surg Gynecol Obstet 128:1069, 1969.

16. Vander Salm TJ: Subclavian vein cannulation. In: Vander Salm TJ (ed): Atlas of Bedside Procedures. Boston, Little, Brown, p 25, 1979.

17. Borja AR, Hinshaw R: A safe way to perform infraclavicular subclavian vein catheterization. Surg Gynecol Obstet 560:673, 1970.

18. Ryan JA, Abel RM, Abbott WM, et al: Catheter complications in total parenteral nutrition. N Engl J Med 290:757, 1974.

19. Feliciano DV, Mattox KL, Graham JM, et al: Major complications of percutaneous subclavian vein catheters. Am J Surg 138:869, 1979.

20. Puri VK, Carlson RC, Bander JJ, et al: Complications of vascular catheterization in the critically ill. Crit Care Med 8:495, 1980.

21. Eisenhauer ED, Derveloy RJ, Hastings PR: Prospective evaluation of central venous pressure (CVP) catheters in a large city hospital. Ann Surg 196:560, 1982.

22. Pinilla JC, Ross DF, Martin T, et al: Study of the incidence of intravascular catheter infection and associated septicemia in critically ill patients. Crit Care Med 11:21, 1983.

23. Conces DJ, Holden RW: Aberrant locations and complications in initial placement of subclavian vein catheters. Arch Surg 119:293, 1984.

24. Lockwood AH: Percutaneous subclavian vein catheterization: Too much of a good thing? Arch Intern Med 144:1407, 1984.

25. Sitzmann JV, Townsend TR, Siler MC, et al: Septic and technical complications of central venous catheterization. Ann Surg 202:766, 1985.

26. Sznajder JI, Zveibil FR, Bitterman H, et al: Central vein catheterization: Failure and complication rates by three percutaneous approaches. Arch Intern Med 146:259, 1986.

27. Gil RT, Kruse JA, Thill-Baharozian, et al: Triple- vs single-lumen central venous catheters: A prospective study in a critically ill population. Arch Intern Med 149:1139, 1989.

28. Richet H, Hubert B, Nitemberg G, et al: Prospective multicenter study of vascular-catheter–related complications and risk factors for positive central-catheter cultures in intensive care unit patients. J Clin Microbiol 28:2520, 1990.

29. Kaiser CW, Koornick AR, Smith N, et al: Choice of route for central venous cannulation: Subclavian or internal jugular vein? A prospective randomized study. J Surg Oncol 17:345, 1981.

30. Dronen S, Thompson B, Nowak R, et al: Subclavian vein catheterization during cardiopulmonary resuscitation. JAMA 247:3227, 1982.

31. Seneff MG: Central venous catheterization: A comprehensive review. Part II. J Intensive Care Med 2:218, 1987.

32. Curry CR, Quie PG: Fungal septicemia in patients receiving total parenteral nutrition. N Engl J Med 285:1221, 1971.

33. Maki DG, Goldmann DA, Rhame FS: Infection control in intravenous therapy. Ann Intern Med 79:867, 1973.

34. Goldmann DA, Maki DG: Infection control in total parenteral nutrition. JAMA 223:1360, 1973.

35. Sanders RA, Sheldon GF: Septic complications of total parenteral nutrition: A five-year experience. Am J Surg 132:214, 1976.

36. Padberg FT, Ruggiero J, Blackburn GL, et al: Central venous catheterization for parenteral nutrition. Ann Surg 193:264, 1981.

37. Snydman DR, Murray SA, Kornfeld SJ, et al: Total parenteral nutrition–related infections. Am J Med 73:695, 1982.

38. Pinilla JC, Ross DF, Martin T, et al: Study of the incidence of intravascular catheter infection and associated septicemia in critically ill patients. Crit Care Med 11:21, 1983.

39. Collignon PJ, Munro R, Sorrell TC: Systemic sepsis and intravenous devices: A prospective study. Med J Aust 141:345, 1984.

40. Samsoondar W, Freeman JB, Coultish I, et al: Colonization of intravascular catheters in the intensive care unit. Am J Surg 149:730, 1985.

41. Sitzmann JV, Townsend TR, Siler MC, et al: Septic and technical complications of central venous catheterization: A prospective study of 200 consecutive patients. Ann Surg 202:766, 1985.

42. Pettigrew RA, Lang SDR, Haydock DA, et al: Catheter-related sepsis in patients on intravenous nutrition: A prospective study of quantitative catheter cultures and guidewire changes for suspected sepsis. Br J Surg 72:52, 1985.

43. Pemberton LB, Lyman B, Lander V, et al: Sepsis from triple-lumen versus single-lumen catheters during total parenteral nutrition in surgical or critically ill patients. Arch Surg 121:591, 1986.

44. Bozzetti F, Terno G, Camerini E, et al: Pathogenesis and predictability of central venous catheter sepsis. Surgery 91:393, 1982.

45. Eyer S, Brummitt C, Crossley K, et al: Catheter-related sepsis: Prospective randomized study of three methods of long term catheter maintenance. Crit Care Med 18:1073, 1990.

46. Newsome HH, Armstrong CW, Mayhall GC, et al: Mechanical complications from insertion of subclavian venous feeding catheters: Comparison of de novo percutaneous venipuncture to change of catheter over guidewire. JPEN 8:560, 1984.

47. Snyder RH, Archer FJ, Endy T, et al: Catheter infection: A comparison of two catheter maintenance techniques. Ann Surg 208:651, 1988.

48. Maki DG, Cobb L, Garman JK, et al: An attachable silver-impregnated cuff for prevention of infection with central venous catheters: A prospective randomized multicenter trial. Am J Med 85:307, 1988.

49. Flowers RH, Schwenzer KJ, Kopel RF, et al: Efficacy of an attachable subcutaneous cuff for the prevention of intravascular catheter-related infections. A randomized controlled trial. JAMA 261:878, 1989.

50. Johnson FE: Internal jugular catheterization: Prospective study. NY State J Med 78:2168, 1978.

51. Doering RB, Stemmer EA, Connolly JE: Complications of indwelling venous catheters: With particular reference to catheter embolus. Am J Surg 114:259, 1967.

52. Lynn KL, Maling TMJ: A major pulmonary embolus as a complication of femoral vein catheterization. Br J Radiol 50:667, 1977.

53. Ordway CB: Air embolus via CVP catheter without positive pressure. Ann Surg 179:479, 1974.

54. Peters JL, Armstrong R: Air embolism occurring as a complication of central venous catheterization. Ann Surg 18:375, 1978.

55. Flanagan JP, Gradisar IA, Gross RJ, et al: Air embolus—A lethal complication of subclavian venipuncture. N Engl J Med 281:488, 1969.

56. Brandt RL, Foley WJ, Fink GH, et al: Mechanism of perforation of the heart with production of hydropericardium by a venous catheter and its prevention. Am J Surg 119:311, 1970.

57. Mitchell SE, Clark RA: Complications of central venous catheterization. AJR 133:467, 1979.

58. Dunbar RD, Mitchell R, Lavine M: Aberrant locations of central venous catheters. Lancet 1:711, 1981.

59. Long R, Kassum D, Donen N, et al: Cardiac tamponade complicating central venous catheterization in total parenteral nutrition: A review. J Crit Care 2:39, 1987.

60. Chabanier A, Dany F, Brutus P, et al: Iatrogenic cardiac tamponade after central venous catheterization. J Clin Cardiol 11:91, 1988.

61. Johnston AOB, Clark RG: Malposition of central venous catheters. Lancet 2:1395, 1972.

62. Mortensen JD: Clinical sequelae from arterial needle puncture, cannulation, and incision. Circulation 35:1118, 1967.

63. Puri VK, Carlson RC, Bander JJ, et al: Complications of vascular catheterization in the critically ill. Crit Care Med 8:495, 1980.

64. Bedford RF, Wollman H: Complications of percutaneous radial-artery cannulation: An objective prospective study in man. Anesthesiology 38:228, 1973.

65. Mangano DT, Hickey RF: Ischemic injury following uncomplicated radial artery catheterization. Anesth Analg 58:55, 1979.

66. Slogoff S, Keats AS, Arlund C: On the safety of radial artery cannulation. Anesthesiology 59:42, 1983.

67. Band JD, Maki DG: Infections caused by arterial catheters used for hemodynamic monitoring. Am J Med 67:735, 1979.

68. Maki DG, McCormick RD, Uman SJ, et al: Septic endocarditis due to intra-arterial catheters for cancer chemotherapy. Cancer 44:1228, 1979.

69. Norwood SH, Cormier B, McMahon NG, et al: Prospective study of catheter-related infection during prolonged arterial catheterization. Crit Care Med 16:836, 1988.

70. Arnow PM, Costas CO: Delayed rupture of the radial artery caused by catheter-related sepsis. Rev Infect Dis 10:11035, 1988.

71. Maki DG, Weise CE, Sarafin HW: A semiquantitative culture method for identifying intravenous-catheter–related infection. N Engl J Med 296:1305, 1977.

72. Downs JB, Rackstein AD, Klein EF, et al: Hazards of radial-artery catheterization. Anesthesiology 38:283, 1973.

73. Moran KT, Halpin DP, Zide RS: Long-term brachial artery catheterization: Ischemic complications. J Vasc Surg 8:76, 1988.

74. Groome J, Vohra RJ, Cuschieri RJ, et al: Vascular injury after arterial catheterization. Postgrad Med J 65:86, 1989.

75. Baker RJ, Chunprapaph B, Nyhus LM: Severe ischemia of the hand following radial artery catheterization. Surgery 80:449, 1976.

76. Bjork L, Enghoff E, Grenvik A, et al: Local circulatory changes following brachial artery catheterization. Vasc Dis 2:283, 1965.

77. Gardner RM, Schwartz R, Wong HC, et al: Percutaneous indwelling radial-artery catheters for monitoring cardiovascular function: Prospective study of the risk of thrombosis and infection. N Engl J Med 290:1227, 1974.

78. Barnes RW, Foster EJ, Janssen GA, et al: Safety of brachial artery catheters as monitors in the intensive care unit: Prospective evaluation with the Doppler ultrasonic velocity detector. Anesthesiology 44:260, 1976.

79. Chiverton SG, Murie JA: Incidence and management of arterial injuries from left heart catheterization. J R Coll Physicians Lond 20:126, 1986.

80. Fleming R, Friedman S: Late sequelae after femoral artery catheterization. Am J Cardiol 53:1205, 1984.

81. Skillman JJ, Kim D, Baim DS: Vascular complications of percutaneous femoral cardiac interventions. Arch Surg 123:1207, 1988.

82. Hindman MC, Wagner GS, JaRo M, et al: The clinical significance of bundle branch block complicating acute myocardial infarction. 2. Indications for temporary and permanent pacemaker insertion. Circulation 58:689, 1978.

83. Lamas GA, Muller JE, Turi ZG, et al and the MILIS Study Group: A simplified method to predict occurrence of complete heart block during acute myocardial infarction. Am J Cardiol 64:1213, 1986.

84. Waldo AL, Wells JL, Cooper TB, et al: Temporary cardiac pacing: Applications and techniques in the treatment of cardiac arrhythmias. Prog Cardiovasc Dis 23:451, 1981.

85. Keren A, Tzivoni D, Gavish D, et al: Etiology, warning signs and therapy of torsade de pointes. Circulation 64:1167, 1981.

86. Bhandari AK, Scheinman M: The long QT syndrome. Mod Concepts Cardiovasc Dis 54:45, 1985.

87. Nguyen PH, Scheinman MM, Seger J: Polymorphous ventricular tachycardia: Clinical characterization, therapy, and the QT interval. Circulation 74:340, 1986.

88. Trancredi RG, McCallister BD, Mankin HT: Temporary transvenous catheter-electrode pacing of the heart. Circulation 36:598, 1967.

89. Hynes JK, Holmes DR, Harrison CE: Five year experience with temporary pacemakers in the coronary care unit. Mayo Clin Proc 58:122, 1982.

90. Austin JL, Preis LK, Cramton RS, et al: Analysis of pacemaker malfunction and complications of temporary pacing in the coronary care unit. Am J Cardiol 49:301, 1982.

91. Lumina FJ, Rios JC: Temporary transvenous pacemaker therapy: An analysis of complications. Chest 64:604, 1973.

92. Gordon AJ: Catheter pacing in complete heart block: Techniques and complications. JAMA 193:109, 1965.

93. Rosenberg AS, Grossman JI, Escher DJW, et al: Bedside transvenous cardiac pacing. Am Heart J 77:697, 1969.

94. Pandian NG, Kosowsky BD, Gurewich V: Transfemoral temporary pacing and deep vein thrombosis. Am Heart J 100:847, 1980.

95. Nolewajka AJ, Goddard MD, Brown TC: Temporary transvenous pacing and femoral vein thrombosis. Circulation 62:646, 1980.

96. Chung EK: Complications and malfunctions of artificial cardiac pacing. In: Chung EK (ed): Electrocardiography: Practical Applications with Vectorial Principles. 2nd ed. Philadelphia, JB Lippincott, p 513, 1980.

97. Cerra FB, Siegel JH, Border JR, et al: Correlations between metabolic and cardiopulmonary measurements in patients after trauma, general surgery, and sepsis. J Trauma 19:621, 1979.

98. Packman MI, Rackow EC: Optimum left heart filling pressures during fluid resuscitation of patients with hypovolemic and septic shock. Crit Care Med 11:165, 1983.

99. Connors AF, McCaffree DR, Gray BA: Evaluation of right heart catheterization in the critically ill patient without acute myocardial infarction. N Engl J Med 308:263, 1983.

100. Eisenberg PR, Jaffe AS, Schuster DP: Clinical evaluation compared to pulmonary artery catheterization in the hemodynamic assessment of critically ill patients. Crit Care Med 12:549, 1984.

101. Tuchschmidt J, Sharma OP: Impact of hemodynamic monitoring in a medical intensive care unit. Crit Care Med 15:840, 1987.

102. Forrester J, Diamond G, McHugh TJ, et al: Filling pressures in the right and left sides of the heart in acute myocardial infarction. N Engl J Med 285:190, 1971.

103. Forrester JS, Diamond G, Chatterjee K, et al: Medical therapy of acute myocardial infarction by application of hemodynamic subsets (part I). N Engl J Med 295:1365, 1976.

104. Gore JM, Goldberg RJ, Spodick DH, et al: A community-wide assessment of the use of pulmonary artery catheters in patients with acute myocardial infarction. Chest 92:721, 1987.

105. Cohn JN, Guiha NH, Broder MI, et al: Right ventricular infarction: Clinical and hemodynamic features. Am J Cardiol 33:209, 1974.

106. Lopez-Sendon J, Coma-Canella J, Gamallo C: Sensitivity and specificity of hemodynamic criteria in the diagnosis of acute right ventricular infarction. Circulation 64:515, 1981.

107. Lloyd EA, Gersh BJ, Kennelly BM: Hemodynamic spectrum of "dominant" right ventricular infarction in 19 patients. Am J Cardiol 48:1016, 1981.

108. Meister SG, Helphant RH: Rapid bedside differentiation of ruptured interventricular septum from acute mitral insufficiency. N Engl J Med 287:1024, 1987.

109. Suter PM, Fairley HB, Isenberg MD: Optimum end-expiratory pressure in patients with acute pulmonary failure. N Engl J Med 292:284, 1975.

110. Unger KM, Shibel EM, Moser KM: Detection of left ventricular failure in patients with adult respiratory distress syndrome. Chest 67:8, 1975.

111. Civetta JM, Gabel JC: Flow directed-pulmonary artery catheterization in surgical patients: Indications and modifications of technic. Ann Surg 176:753, 1972.

112. Sorensen MB, Bille-Brahe NE, Engell HC: Hemodynamic observations in relation to extensive surgical treatment of patients with increased operative risk. Acta Anaesthesiol Scand 22:287, 1978.

113. Rice CL, Hobleman CF, John DA, et al: Central venous pressure or pulmonary capillary wedge pressure as the determinant of fluid replacement in aortic surgery. Surgery 84:437, 1978.

114. Moore CH, Lombardo TR, Allums JA, et al: Left main coronary artery stenosis: Hemodynamic monitoring to reduce mortality. Ann Surg 26:445, 1978.

115. Elliot CG, Zimmerman GA, Clemmer TP: Complications of pulmonary artery catheterizations in the care of critically ill patients. Chest 76:647, 1979.

116. Sprung CL, Jacobs LJ, Caralis PV, et al: Ventricular arrhythmias during Swan-Ganz catheterization of the critically ill. Chest 79:413, 1981.

117. Sprung CL, Pozen RG, Rozanski JJ, et al: Advanced ventricular arrhythmias during bedside pulmonary artery catheterization. Am J Med 72:203, 1982.

118. Boyd KD, Thomas SJ, Gold J, et al: A prospective study of complications of pulmonary artery catheterization in 500 consecutive patients. Chest 84:245, 1983.

119. Shah KB, Rao LK, Laughlin S, et al: A review of pulmonary artery catheterization in 6,245 patients. Anesthesiology 61:271, 1984.

120. Iberti TJ, Benjamin E, Gruppi L, et al: Ventricular arrhythmias during pulmonary artery catheterization in the intensive care unit. Am J Med 78:451, 1985.

121. Damen J, Bolton D: A prospective analysis of 1400 pulmonary artery catheterizations in patients undergoing cardiac surgery. Acta Anaesthesiol Scand 30:386, 1986.

122. Sprung CL, Elser B, Schein RMH, et al: Risk of right bundle-branch block and complete heart block during pulmonary artery catheterization. Crit Care Med 17:1, 1989.

123. Voukydis PC, Cohen SI: Catheter-induced arrhythmias. Am Heart J 88:588, 1974.

124. Morris AH, Chapman RH, Gardner RM: Frequency of technical problems encountered in the measurement of pulmonary artery wedge pressure. Crit Care Med 12:164, 1984.

125. Hudson-Civetta JA, Civetta JM, Martinez OV: Risk and detection of pulmonary artery catheter–related infection in septic surgical patients. Crit Care Med 15:29, 1987.

126. Rowley KM, Clubb KS, Smith GJW, et al: Right-sided infective endocarditis as a consequence of flow-directed pulmonary-artery catheterization. N Engl J Med 311:1152, 1984.

127. Foote GA, Schabel SI, Hodges M: Pulmonary complications of the flow-directed balloon-tipped catheter. N Engl J Med 290:927, 1974.

128. Kelly TF, Morris GC, Crawford ES, et al: Perforation of the pulmonary artery with Swan-Ganz catheters: Diagnosis and surgical management. Ann Surg 193:686, 1981.

129. Cervenko FW, Shelley SE, Spence DG, et al: Massive endobronchial hemorrhage during cardiopulmonary bypass: Treatable complication of balloon-tipped catheter damage to the pulmonary artery. Ann Thorac Surg 35:326, 1983.

130. Lipp H, O'Donoghue K, Resnekov L: Intracardiac knotting of a flow-directed balloon catheter. N Engl J Med 284:220, 1971.

131. Goldberger M, Tabak SW, Shah PK: Clinical experience with intra-aortic balloon counterpulsation in 112 consecutive patients. Am Heart J 111:497, 1986.

132. Bolooki H: Emergency cardiac procedures in patients in cardiogenic shock due to complications of coronary artery disease. Circulation 79(suppl I):137, 1989.

133. Freed PS, Wasfie T, Zado B, et al: Intraaortic balloon pumping for prolonged circulatory support. Am J Cardiol 61:554, 1988.

134. Gunstensen J, Goldman BS, Scully HE, et al: Evolving indications for preoperative intraaortic balloon pump assistance. Ann Thorac Surg 22:535, 1976.

135. Feola M, Wiener L, Walinsky P, et al: Improved survival after coronary bypass surgery in patients with poor left ventricular function: Role of intraaortic balloon counterpulsation. Am J Cardiol 39:1021, 1977.

136. Cooper GN, Singh AK, Christian FC, et al: Preoperative intra-aortic balloon support in surgery for left main coronary stenosis. Ann Surg 185:242, 1977.

137. Lamberti JJ, Cohn LH, Lesch M, et al: Intra-aortic balloon counterpulsation; indications and long-term results in postoperative left ventricular power failure. Arch Surg 109:766, 1974.

138. Downing TP, Miller DC, Stinson EB, et al: Therapeutic efficacy of intraaortic balloon pump counterpulsation: Analysis with concurrent control subjects. Circulation 64(suppl II):108, 1981.

139. Di Lello F, Mullen DC, Flemma RJ, et al: Results of intraaortic balloon pumping after cardiac surgery: Experience with the Percor balloon catheter. Ann Thorac Surg 42:442, 1988.

140. Scheidt S, Wilner G, Meuller H, et al: Intra-aortic balloon counterpulsation in cardiogenic shock. Report of a cooperative clinical trial. N Engl J Med 299:979, 1973.

141. Willerson JT, Curry GC, Watson JT, et al: Intraaortic balloon counterpulsation in cardiogenic shock, medically refractory left ventricular failure and/or recurrent ventricular tachycardia. Am J Med 58:183, 1975.

142. Wolfson S, Karsh DL, Langou RA, et al: Modification of intraaortic balloon catheter to permit introduction by cardiac catheterization techniques. Am J Cardiol 41:733, 1978.

143. Harvey JC, Goldstein JE, McCabe JC, et al: Complications of percutaneous intraaortic balloon pumping. Circulation 64(suppl II):114, 1981.

144. Pelletier LC, Pomar JL, Bosch XB, et al: Complications of circulatory assistance with intra-aortic balloon pumping: A comparison of surgical and percutaneous techniques. J Heart Transplant 5:138, 1986.
145. Berg GA, Reece IJ, Davidson KG, et al: Recent clinical experience with percutaneous intra-aortic balloon pumping. Life Support Syst 4:249, 1986.
146. Alderman JD, Gabliani GI, McCabe CH, et al: Incidence and management of limb ischemia with percutaneous wire-guided intraaortic balloon catheters. J Am Coll Cardiol 9:524, 1987.
147. Curtis JJ, Boland M, Bliss D, et al: Intra-aortic balloon cardiac assist: Complication rates for the surgical and percutaneous techniques. Am Surg 54:142, 1988.
148. Goldberg MJ, Rubenfire M, Kantrowitz A, et al: Intraaortic balloon pump insertion: A randomized study comparing percutaneous and surgical techniques. J Am Coll Cardiol 9:515, 1987.
149. Biddle TL, Stewart S, Stuard ID: Dissection of the aorta complicating intraaortic balloon counterpulsation. Am Heart J 92:781, 1976.
150. Iverson LIG, Herfindahl G, Ecker RR, et al: Vascular complications of intraaortic balloon counterpulsation. Am J Surg 154:99, 1987.
151. Mills JL, Wiedeman JE, Robison JG, et al: Minimizing mortality and morbidity from iatrogenic arterial injuries: The need for early recognition and prompt repair. J Vasc Surg 4:22, 1986.

CHAPTER 16

Bronchoscopic Procedures in Critically Ill Patients

Willane S. Krell

Pulmonary complications are a frequent cause of morbidity and mortality in the intensive care unit patient population. The ability to make a specific diagnosis is complicated by the inherent instability of the patients, use of mechanical ventilation, and the wide variety of underlying illnesses in this nonhomogeneous population. The diagnostic considerations differ with the patient's underlying condition or disease process. For each case, from a postoperative patient with new chest x-ray findings to a patient with fever and cough after bone marrow transplantation, the physician must develop an appropriate differential diagnosis and have an understanding of the safety and the specificity of the available pulmonary diagnostic tools. Knowledge of the expected diagnostic yield of procedures versus the potential risks is especially important in caring for these compromised patients. Although the bronchoscope can be a valuable therapeutic and diagnostic tool in this population, there are some special concerns in performing bronchoscopy in critically ill patients. If appropriate judgment is used, the procedure is relatively safe[1, 2] and can provide significant information to the benefit of care of patients.

INDICATIONS FOR BRONCHOSCOPY IN THE INTENSIVE CARE SETTING

Therapeutic and diagnostic indications for bronchoscopy parallel those for the general medical population.[2, 3] The American Thoracic Society guidelines are a valuable reference regarding potential uses of the bronchoscope.[4]

Therapeutic Indications

Historically, the bronchoscope's primary use in the intensive care setting was as a therapeutic tool in airway management.[5, 6] When conventional maneuvers (e.g., endotracheal suctioning, postural drainage, and chest physiotherapy) failed to mobilize or clear secretions or to resolve atelectasis, bronchoscopic suctioning could achieve patency of the airways and improve gas exchange.[5-8] Direct visualization of the upper airway provides a means of achieving successful intubation in difficult cases, such as with cervicofacial trauma or known upper airway abnormalities.[1] Positioning of an endotracheal tube, particularly double-lumen tubes, can be ensured by direct visualization.

Other potential therapeutic uses of the bronchoscope include management of hemoptysis,[9, 10] removal of foreign bodies,[11, 12] and lung lavage.[13] In selected cases, therapeutic bronchoscopy may be beneficial in the management of lung abscess.[14]

Diagnostic Indications

In the critically ill, the general medical practice of proceeding from simple, noninvasive testing to more aggressive or invasive diagnostic measures is tempered by the fact that these patients are unstable and compromised either by poor cardiorespiratory function or immunodepression. The need for prompt and specific diagnosis requires that the physician review the expected yields of diagnostic procedures, potential risks of each procedure, and the urgency with which the diagnosis should be made.

Indications for diagnostic bronchoscopy include evaluation of lesions of unknown etiology on chest radiographs, hemoptysis, assessment of airway patency, evaluation of nonresolving chest radiographic lesions, and the acquisition of material for microbiologic cultures in suspected infections.

Evaluations of new or nonresolving chest radiographic lesions account for the bulk of diagnostic bronchoscopies performed in the intensive care setting.[1-3] Although up to 75% of new infiltrates in this population represent infectious processes,[15] the traditional clinical clues to infections such as tachycardia, fever, worsening oxygenation, and sputum production are difficult to interpret in severely compromised patients. Invasive procedures are often necessary when diagnosis is urgently needed and/or empirical therapy fails.

Assessment of the airway to determine extent of smoke or thermal inhalation injury, pathology related to endotracheal tubes, or damage related to aspiration, or to determine the source of hemoptysis, constitutes another major category of diagnostic uses of the bronchoscope. The relatively recent addition of accessory tools to the flexible bronchoscope, such as double-sheathed brushes, bronchoalveolar lavage (BAL), and Wang needles, has expanded the role of the bronchoscope for diagnosis of infections, malignancies, or inflammatory processes in the intensive care unit population.

CONTRAINDICATIONS

There are few absolute contraindications to bronchoscopy in the critically ill patient, although there is often an appreciable risk to performing bronchoscopy.[1-4] The physician must balance the relative risk of the procedure against the expected diagnostic yield. Absolute and relative risks are summarized in Table 16–1.

Refractory hypoxemia is an absolute contraindication to bronchoscopy.[4] If oxygenation cannot be maintained, the addition of the bronchoscope will further compromise the airway lumen and result in a further fall in arterial oxygen saturation (SaO_2).

TABLE 16-1

ABSOLUTE AND RELATIVE CONTRAINDICATIONS TO PERFORMANCE OF BRONCHOSCOPY IN THE CRITICALLY ILL PATIENT

Absolute
Refractory hypoxemia
Malignant arrhythmia
Unqualified bronchoscopist

Relative
Cardiovascular
  Recent myocardial infarction
  Unstable angina
  Pre-existent arrhythmias
Respiratory
  Severe hypoxemia
  Tracheal or major airway obstruction
  Asthma or severe obstructive airways process
  Hypercapnia
  Mechanical ventilation
  Lung abscess (spillage)
Risk of bleeding elevated
  Thrombocytopenia
  Uremia (functional platelet defect)
  Pulmonary hypertension
  Superior vena caval obstruction
  Bleeding diathesis, disseminated intravascular coagulation
General
  Lack of patient cooperation
  Debilitation
  Malnutrition
  Advanced age

Uncontrolled malignant arrhythmias obviously create circumstances in which the risk of inserting the bronchoscope cannot be justified. Passing the bronchoscope, particularly through the upper airway, risks further provocation because of stimulation of vagal afferents and irritant fibers within the airway.[16]

The third absolute contraindication to bronchoscopy is lack of skilled personnel to perform the procedure. Almost all critically ill patients are at higher risk for complications from bronchoscopy than the general medical population; thus, the procedure must be performed expediently and correctly to avoid undue risk to the patient. Although many institutions require a minimal number of 50 procedures under supervision to indicate that a physician is capable of performing bronchoscopy, a study by Dull indicated that true proficiency (as judged by diagnostic yield and complication rates) is achieved only after 100 or more supervised procedures.[17]

Relative contraindications to performing bronchoscopy exist for patients with unstable cardiovascular status, difficulty with oxygenation, bleeding diathesis, bronchospasm, or other airway obstruction. In addition, debilitation and malnutrition also contribute to increased risk.[1-4] The majority of patients in the intensive care setting manifest one or more of these high-risk conditions. As in other clinical situations, the possible benefits of bronchoscopy must be balanced against risk.

PHYSIOLOGIC CHANGES ASSOCIATED WITH BRONCHOSCOPY

It is important to understand which derangements of the cardiovascular and respiratory systems may be associated with bronchoscopy, as these known derangements relate directly to the major complications of the procedure. Risk modification demands that expected complications be con-sidered before beginning the procedure. Even in normal volunteers, bronchoscopy results in abnormalities in gas exchange. In the critically ill patient, the cardiorespiratory effects of bronchoscopy may adversely affect cardiac or pulmonary function, as the normal decrements in gas exchange are exaggerated and the underlying status is unstable.

The most consistent derangement noted during and after bronchoscopy is arterial hypoxemia. The average change in Pao_2 in healthy individuals is about 20 torr,[18-23] but Pao_2 may drop by as much as 30 to 60% in compromised individuals.[18, 23] The duration of the procedure also affects deoxygenation, with procedures exceeding 30 minutes resulting in greater decreases in Pao_2.[18] There is generally little change in $Paco_2$ during bronchoscopy. The decrease in Pao_2 may persist for several hours after completion of the procedure; thus, postprocedure monitoring is crucial.[20, 21, 24]

The mechanisms responsible for the drop in oxygenation are far from clear. Potential causes investigated include bronchospasm, airway occlusion by the bronchoscope, increased intrapulmonary shunting, and ventilation-perfusion mismatch. Increases in airway resistance and frank bronchospasm can occur, resulting in elevation of $Paco_2$,[18, 22] but this mechanism does not seem to be operative in most cases. Ventilation-perfusion mismatch, related either to increased intrapulmonary shunting in response to pulmonary reflexes or to direct effects of the bronchoscope, is an attractive mechanism to explain hypoxemia.[20, 25] Although scanning techniques to evaluate changes in ventilation or perfusion pre- and postbronchoscopy have not shown such changes,[26, 27] it may be that alterations in distribution of ventilation and perfusion are below the resolution level of these scanning methods.[26]

Cardiac derangements, primarily arrhythmias, are noted frequently.[28] Although generally of little clinical significance, even minor degrees of tachycardia or other "benign" arrhythmias can have important consequences in compromised patients. Mechanisms accounting for the arrhythmias may include the known decrease in oxygenation,[21, 28] but as arrhythmias are often noted during insertion of the bronchoscope or early in the procedure,[16] they are often most likely related to stimulation of vagal or irritant afferents in the airway. Patients with unstable angina or severe hypoxemia are at highest risk for complications.[16, 29]

PREPROCEDURE CONSIDERATIONS

Initial considerations before bronchoscopy obviously include ensuring that the procedure is indicated. Steps should be taken to minimize or correct abnormalities in high-risk patients, including control of arrhythmias, assurance of adequate oxygenation, and so forth.

Laboratory Evaluation

Important laboratory values to review before bronchoscopy are the platelet count and blood urea nitrogen level. If the platelet count is less than 20,000/mm³, the risk of bleeding during bronchoscopy is markedly elevated and either platelet transfusions should be given or another diagnostic procedure selected.[30] At platelet counts less than about 60,000/mm³, the risk of bleeding with bronchoscopic biopsies is high and the physician may opt not to use the forceps in such patients.[31] Blood urea nitrogen is evaluated because uremia produces a functional platelet defect that also increases the risk of bleeding.[32] Many physicians also routinely evaluate the coagulation system preprocedure via the partial thromboplastin time and prothrombin time.

These values may be of use if a bleeding disorder is suspected clinically.

Gastric Status

In awake, spontaneously breathing patients, liquid and solid intake is discontinued about 6 hours before bronchoscopy to allow for gastric emptying and to decrease the risk of aspiration during the procedure. In mechanically ventilated patients, gastric status must also be considered. The balloon of an endotracheal tube does not prevent aspiration, particularly when the tube is being moved and manipulated as during bronchoscopy. Stomach contents can be mechanically aspirated before bronchoscopy, or a dose of metoclopramide may be given to enhance gastric emptying and decrease the potential risk of aspiration.[33]

Premedications and Local Anesthetics

Premedications for the critically ill patient before bronchoscopy should not be given lightly. It is important to ensure that the patient is calm and cooperative to avoid trauma to the airways. Medications to decrease cough (to decrease the risk of barotrauma) are also often considered. On the other hand, complications related to sedatives and/or narcotics (such as hypotension and respiratory depression) are a large percentage of the total reported complications of bronchoscopy in any population, not just the critically ill.[1] Control of the effects of premedications is best achieved if small doses of narcotics or short-acting sedatives are given intravenously and only as necessary to ensure a quiet patient during the procedure.

Use of local anesthetics (e.g., lidocaine or cocaine) before and during the procedure should involve decisions similar to those for general premedications. The presence of an endotracheal or tracheostomy tube virtually eliminates upper airway irritation from bronchoscopy, but topical anesthetics for the lower airways should be used for any signs of cough or irritability of the airways.[5, 34]

Lidocaine, tetracaine, and cocaine are commonly used agents for topical anesthesia. These drugs are all absorbed systemically, but the blood levels achieved are difficult to predict. Neurologic and cardiac complications are the most commonly reported adverse effects of absorbed local anesthetics.[34, 35] The adult respiratory distress syndrome has been reported with local application of lidocaine.[36, 37]

To avoid toxicity with local anesthetics administered into the airway, a dose corresponding to a maximum of 400 mg of lidocaine is a safe guideline.[34] This admittedly conservative dose will result in acceptable blood levels even in compromised patients. Nonetheless, equipment for monitoring cardiac rhythm and capabilities for cardiopulmonary resuscitation should be close at hand.

PERFORMANCE OF BRONCHOSCOPY

Positioning of Patients

In the intensive care unit, it may be difficult to perform bronchoscopy from the "standard" position (patient supine, physician at the head of the bed). If possible, the headboard of the bed should be removed and the patient moved toward the head of the bed, moving aside any other obstacles such as ventilators, intravenous infusion pumps, and the like. If this arrangement cannot be achieved, the physician must be prepared to perform bronchoscopy from a position lateral or anterior to the patient. Although an experienced bronchoscopist will have little difficulty adapting to this altered perspective, trainees or less experienced physicians should

first attempt other approaches in more stable patients or in a bronchoscopic model before attempting them in the critically ill.

Roles of Ancillary Personnel

Ideally, both the patient's nurse and personnel skilled in assisting with bronchoscopy as well as ventilator management (such as a respiratory therapist) should be present before and during the bronchoscopy. The nurse can assist with positioning the patient, monitoring, and administering needed medications. The respiratory therapist ensures that ventilator settings allowing adequate oxygenation and ventilation are maintained during the procedure and assists with the bronchoscopy itself by making local anesthetic, brushes, suction containers, forceps, and the like available on command from the physician.[38] These personnel alert the physician to changes in vital signs and oxygenation and anticipate needs arising from the procedure (e.g., increase in the fraction of inspired oxygen or epinephrine for bleeding), enhancing the ability of the physician to complete the procedure safely and expediently.

Monitoring During Bronchoscopy

As hypoxemia is a known physiologic consequence of bronchoscopy, SaO_2 should be monitored throughout the procedure and for several hours afterward in critically ill patients.[18–24] This is most easily accomplished by ear or pulse oximetry. The probe for the oximeter may be placed on the ear lobe or a digit of the upper or lower extremity. Satisfactory readings of SaO_2 may be difficult to obtain in patients with poor peripheral vascular perfusion, so availability of various probes to deal with this problem is ideal. As the bronchoscopist directs primary attention to examination of the tracheobronchial tree, the respiratory therapist and/or nurse should periodically announce the saturation value and alert the physician if the SaO_2 falls by more than 4%. In intubated, mechanically ventilated patients, the inspired oxygen tension delivered via the ventilator is usually increased at the start of bronchoscopy to minimize falls in SaO_2.

Monitoring of the electrocardiogram during bronchoscopy is standard, as arrhythmias are not uncommon in the critically ill during bronchoscopy.[16, 21, 26, 28] Minimizing drops in SaO_2 is beneficial,[21, 26] but monitoring the electrocardiogram is routinely advised so that prompt recognition (and treatment if needed) of arrhythmias on insertion of the bronchoscope or during the procedure is possible.

Insertion Techniques

In the nonintubated patient, the two standard approaches to the lower airways are transnasal and transoral.[39] The transnasal approach (possibly using a soft latex nasal airway) has the advantage of virtually bypassing the gag reflex. This approach cannot be used in patients with nasal obstruction or with thrombocytopenia or functional platelet defects. The oral route (with a mouth guard to prevent the patient from biting the fiberoptic bundles) requires good upper airway anesthesia and provides good access to the airway.

In the intubated, mechanically ventilated patient, the means to ensure adequate ventilation during bronchoscopy must be planned before the procedure begins. Two major concerns are adequacy of the lumen of the artificial airway for both ventilation and the bronchoscope and continuation of mechanical ventilation during bronchoscopy.

The endotracheal tube must be fitted with an adaptor, usually a T piece, which allows simultaneous mechanical ventilation through one port and passage of the bronchoscope into the airway via another port.[5] Several such adaptors are commercially available.

The optimal diameter for the endotracheal or tracheostomy tube, which will permit adequate ventilation while the bronchoscope is in place, has been evaluated. Threefold increases in peak airway and ventilator pressures have been noted on insertion of the bronchoscope.[21] The smaller the tube, the higher the airway pressures generated. Expired tidal volume decreases and end-expiratory pressure increases.[21, 40]

Although an artificial airway of 7 mm could theoretically accommodate a 5-mm bronchoscope,[41] in practice most authorities recommend a tube diameter of at least 8 mm to avoid excessively high pressures and/or difficulties in maintaining ventilation.[5, 21, 41, 42] If too small a tube is in place, three methods may be used to overcome the problem: reintubation with a larger tube, ventilation during bronchoscopy with a hypodense gas mixture, or bypass of the endotracheal tube.

To perform fiberoptic reintubation, an endotracheal tube of the needed diameter is threaded onto the bronchoscope and held in place with the little finger. Once the existing endotracheal tube is visualized, its cuff is deflated and the bronchoscope is quickly passed below it and the vocal cords. The old tube is removed by an assistant as the new tube is placed, using the bronchoscope as a guide. In practice, this procedure is cumbersome and is not routinely recommended solely for the performance of bronchoscopy. If there is another reason to change the endotracheal tube, this method is a good means of minimizing the time the patient is without ventilatory support during tube changing for cuff leaks or other problems.

Theoretically, the high resistance created by the bronchoscope in a small tube can be decreased by ventilating the patient with a hypodense gas mixture such as 70% helium/30% oxygen.[43] As the density of helium is only 14% that of air, kinetic forces and turbulent flow are decreased, effectively lowering the resistance to airflow. This method has been used for bronchoscopy via endotracheal tubes ranging in size from 7.5 to 9 mm.[43]

If the patient is mechanically ventilated but does not require high levels of positive end-expiratory pressure, the bronchoscope may be passed to the side of the tube by temporarily deflating the cuff of the tube for passage, then reinflating as much as possible to restore the airway seal.[42, 44] By monitoring and adjusting tidal volume and pressures on the ventilator, adequate ventilation can be maintained.

Review of Basic Airway Anatomy

The physician performing bronchoscopy must know the normal anatomy of the upper airway and tracheobronchial tree and the common variants of that anatomy. In the critically ill or unstable patient, this is of great importance because the procedure must be done correctly and expediently to avoid compromising the patient's cardiopulmonary status unnecessarily. For the physician just learning to perform bronchoscopy, a text such as Stradling's Diagnostic Bronchoscopy[45] is a valuable adjunct to practicing the procedure.

In addition, the presence of an artificial airway requires the physician to recognize correct and incorrect tube placement (particularly one in the right mainstem bronchus). Lesions caused by the endotracheal tube, such as erosions or edema, should also be recognizable to the bronchoscopist. Once the trachea is entered, the character of the mucosa and any lesions or secretions should be noted. The carina should be visualized and any abnormalities of this structure noted. If a lesion is present radiographically, it is generally advisable to examine the normal side of the tracheobronchial tree first; otherwise, it is standard to begin with evaluation of the right side first.[39]

All 10 segments of the right lung's bronchial tree should be evaluated. The right upper lobe commonly has three segments: apical, anterior, and posterior. As one continues down the bronchus intermedius, the middle lobe and its two segments are identified: lateral and medial. The superior segment of the lower lobe (designated the apical segment in British terminology)[45] on the posterior wall of the bronchus intermedius should not be overlooked. The right lower lobe usually consists of four segments: a narrow orifice to the median basal segment, followed by linear series of orifices consisting of (from anterior to posterior) the anterior, lateral, and posterior segmental orifices. Common errors made by inexperienced bronchoscopists include missing the right upper lobe orifice and overlooking or misidentifying the superior segment of the lower lobe.

Although the left lung, by notation in anatomy texts, is said to have 8 bronchopulmonary segments, "bronchoscopic" anatomists designate 10 segments, similar to the right lung. As one enters the left side, the airway branches into upper and lower divisions. The upper division subdivides into upper lobe and lingular branches. The upper division subdivides into upper lobe and lingular branches. The upper lobe generally appears to have two segments: one smaller one known as the anterior segment and a larger orifice called the apicoposterior segment, equivalent to the apical and posterior segments on the right. The most common variant of left upper lobe anatomy is an appearance similar to the right side, with three distinct orifices. The lingula has two segments, called superior and inferior divisions. The left lower lobe is the most variable of the lung lobes. A distinct superior segment bronchus is seen. The most commonly reported lower lobe pattern is two large orifices that each divide into two sections. The two anterior orifices are the median basal and anterior segments, and the posterior orifices are the lateral and superior segments. One variant of the left lower lobe is to present as a mirror image of the right lower lobe.

Figure 16–1 depicts the anatomy of the tracheobronchial tree. Only the most common pattern of bronchial divisions is presented in this figure.

Complications

Rates for major complications with bronchoscopy range from less than 1 to 11%, depending on the population studied.[1, 5, 35, 46, 47] Hypoxemia occurs in varying degrees with bronchoscopy, but the incidence of related complications can be managed by monitoring SaO_2 during the procedure and using supplemental oxygen as required during and after the procedure.[18, 21, 24]

Cardiac complications, primarily arrhythmias, are recognized and managed by using the recommended electrocardiogram monitor before and during bronchoscopy. In a prospective study of 70 ambulatory patients, major cardiac arrhythmias occurred in about 11%.[28] Major arrhythmias were defined as those potentially causing hemodynamic compromise, such as sinus bradycardia, atrial fibrillation with rapid ventricular response, supraventricular tachycardia, premature ventricular contractions, and other ventricular arrhythmias. A retrospective study of more than 24,000 procedures noted a variety of potentially malignant arrhythmias, including one cardiac arrest resulting in death.[35] The overall incidence of cardiac complications in this series was low, which the authors ascribed to careful patient selection preprocedure and monitoring of the electrocardiogram during the procedure.

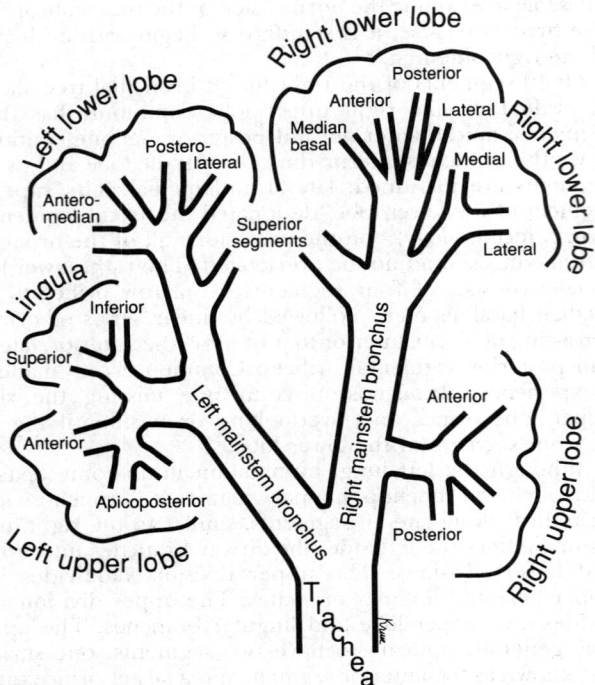

Figure 16–1. Anatomy of the tracheobronchial tree from the view of the bronchoscopist standing behind the head of a patient. Ten segments are identified on the right and the left.

The critically ill population cannot be directly compared with the ambulatory population, as the cardiopulmonary systems of the critically ill are often functioning at a marginal level.[21] Complication rates are generally higher, as would be predicted. In one study of a series of 309 patients in the intensive care unit, seven arrhythmias and three cardiopulmonary arrests occurred, one resulting in death.[5] Cardiac arrhythmias should be anticipated if patients have unstable angina or severe, pre-existing hypoxemia.[29] Careful monitoring of both the electrocardiogram and SaO_2, along with observation of the patient, should minimize cardiac complications.

Temperature above 101°F will develop in 10 to 20% of patients after bronchoscopy.[48, 49] The incidence of fever does not appear to be related to smoking history, underlying lung disease, oral or dental infection, concomitant disease process, use of antimicrobial agents, duration of the procedure, or special procedures performed as a part of the bronchoscopy. The only significant risk factor is age over 60 years.[48] Blood culture results are generally negative, although new pulmonary infiltrates may be noted on the chest radiograph.[48] Despite the low probability of bacteremia with bronchoscopy, attention must be given to proper cleaning of the bronchoscope by either glutaraldehyde solution or gas sterilization between procedures to avoid contamination by bacteria, fungi, mycobacteria, or viruses.[50-52]

Rates for other complications of bronchoscopy are relatively low.[35, 47] Complications may include severe bronchospasm, new pulmonary radiographic infiltrates with or without fever, dyspnea, epistaxis, sinusitis, or hysteria. As will be discussed later, any procedures performed as a part of the bronchoscopy carry their own level of risk over and above bronchoscopy alone.[35]

SPECIFIC PROCEDURES DURING THERAPEUTIC BRONCHOSCOPY

Therapeutic uses of the flexible bronchoscope in the intensive care setting are myriad. Use of the bronchoscope for intubation or replacement of endotracheal tubes has already been discussed. Other potential therapeutic uses include removal of mucous plugs or retained secretions, control of hemoptysis, and removal of selected foreign bodies.

Removal of Mucous Plugs and Excessive Secretions

Numerous studies have demonstrated improved oxygenation and ventilation and/or improvement in chest radiographic signs of atelectasis or collapse after bronchoscopic removal of mucous plugs or retained secretions.[5-7, 26, 53, 54] Despite the small diameter of the bronchoscopic suction channel, the flexible bronchoscope is remarkably effective at removing tenacious mucus.[7] When pooled secretions or mucous plugs are visually identified, moving the bronchoscope up and down in the area while intermittently actuating the suction control helps mobilize and remove mucus. Small quantities of saline injected repeatedly into the area of secretions facilitate bronchoscopic removal as well as potentially allow the patient to cough out remaining secretions after the procedure.[7]

Two cautions are necessary regarding this all-too-common procedure. First, despite the possibility of improved pulmonary function, the procedure carries the same risks and deserves the same precautions as any bronchoscopic procedure. Monitoring via electrocardiography and oximetry throughout the procedure is still required.[7] Second, bronchoscopy is not the first procedure to be used for removal of secretions. Encouragement of cough, postural drainage, and chest physiotherapy should generally be tried for at least 24 to 48 hours before resorting to bronchoscopy.[6, 7, 54]

Control of Hemoptysis

Massive amounts of blood are best handled by using a rigid bronchoscope to control bleeding. For active but submassive bleeding, the flexible bronchoscope may be useful. Acute bleeding can often be controlled with repeated saline lavage of the area.[55, 56] Application of dilute epinephrine solution (1:20,000) in 1-ml increments can also assist in achieving hemostasis.[55] Tamponade of the bleeding area can be accomplished by wedging the bronchoscope itself into the bleeding segment.[56] For larger airways, a Fogarty balloon catheter can be passed down alongside the bronchoscope and inflated under direct visualization in the bleeding segment, then left in place for up to 48 hours if needed.[9, 10]

Foreign Body Removal

Foreign body removal from the airways is generally performed by using a rigid bronchoscope, as the instrument's larger size accommodates large objects that may have entered the airway and any bleeding resulting from the foreign object can more easily be controlled. Several studies have demonstrated that, when undertaken cautiously, the flexible bronchoscope can be used for successful foreign body removal. A variety of small objects, such as pins, seeds, nuts, stray teeth, and small bones, have been successfully removed by using bronchoscopic forceps.[57] Up to 90% of commonly aspirated objects can be removed with the flexible bronchoscope, obviating the need for rigid bronchoscopy and general anesthesia.[12]

The general approach with the forceps is to visualize the object, then grasp it within the forceps. Care must be taken not to crush the foreign body or drive it further into the tracheobronchial tree. The forceps is left protruding from the bronchoscope while the entire instrument is removed from the patient's airway.

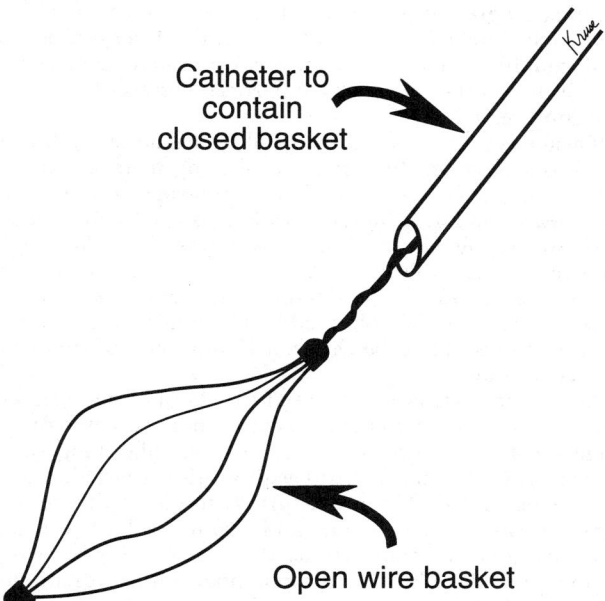

Figure 16–2. Wire basket for foreign body removal. The basket is passed down the bronchoscope's instrument channel in the closed position and then is opened as shown when in the vicinity of the object to be removed. Careful retraction at the proximal end tightens the basket around the foreign body, after which the bronchoscope with the basket protruding from the distal end is removed from the patient.

Two other methods for flexible foreign body removal have been successfully demonstrated. A deflated Fogarty's catheter can be passed distal to the foreign body under direct bronchoscopic visualization, then inflated and used to drag the object up and out of the airway.[58] A more elegant and practical method is to use a wire basket tool that can be passed into the area of the foreign body in a closed position, then carefully opened to encompass the object. The basket (Fig. 16–2) can enclose objects larger than the forceps can grasp and is less likely to crush the foreign body.[11]

DIAGNOSTIC BRONCHOSCOPY
Bronchial Washings

Simple bronchial aspirates are obtained by injecting small volumes of saline (2 to 20 mL) through the instrument channel of the bronchoscope, then aspirating material back to a trap chamber. When such specimens are used for microbiologic evaluation, considerable oropharyngeal contamination is present, with up to five different organisms cultured from a single bronchial aspirate.[59] Quantitative cultures for bacterial colony counts (with 10^5 to 10^6 colonies representing true infection and lesser counts representing contamination) can be performed;[60, 61] however, as other bronchoscopic procedures produce better specimens, this method is not generally preferred. Bronchial washings may be of more value for certain organisms such as mycobacteria, *Legionella, Pneumocystis,* and fungi.[60] Washings for cytology carry a low risk for complications, but the diagnostic yield is also generally low,[32, 62] on the order of 30%. If bronchoscopic biopsies cannot be performed because of potential complications, bronchial washings should be done.

Bronchial Brushings

Bronchial brushing by using an unsheathed or a single-sheathed brush is also subject to considerable contamination by upper airway flora, making identification of pathogenic organisms in the lower airways difficult. These types of brushings can be useful for making cytologic smears, but again the yield, even when combined with that of bronchial washings, is low. Unless there is a strong contraindication, biopsies are the preferred means of diagnosing malignancies, because of their much greater yield.[62, 63]

Protected brushes or double-sheathed brushes offer a theoretic means of obtaining uncontaminated lower respiratory tract samples.[64–70] This brush (Fig. 16–3) consists of two catheters shielding a sampling brush. The outer catheter is sealed with a wax or gelatin plug. After the brush is inserted through the instrument channel of the bronchoscope, the outer catheter with plug is visualized in the airway by the bronchoscopist. Extension of the inner catheter displaces the plug into the airway, where it dissolves or is coughed out. The brush is then extended from the inner catheter to obtain the specimen. In theory, the upper airway contaminants carried to the lower airways by the bronchoscope will touch only the outer catheter of the system, leaving the inner catheter and brush relatively sterile.

In practice, the brush does not remain absolutely contaminant free. Contamination has been demonstrated in studies comparing results from the brush to histologic specimens.[64] Quantitative culturing, with greater than 10^4 organisms representing true infections and fewer than 10^3 organisms indicating contamination, does increase the sensitivity and specificity of the protected brush for diagnosis of true lower respiratory tract infections.[71]

The reliability of the protected brush for obtaining specimens in intubated and mechanically ventilated patients has been specifically evaluated.[71–74] Overall sensitivity and specificity for bacteria in this population have been reported to be as high as 90% in some series;[66] most studies report yields in the range of 60 to 70%.[64, 65, 70, 71, 73]

The double-sheathed brush is unique among bronchoscopic procedures in that specimens suitable for recovery of anaerobic bacteria can be obtained.[64] If the brush is placed

Figure 16–3. Construction of the protected brush catheter and use in obtaining specimens. *(Left)* The structure of the brush includes inner and outer catheters shielding the specimen brush from contaminants. The outer catheter is sealed with a gelatin plug. *(Middle)* Extension of the inner catheter displaces the plug into the airway. *(Right)* The brush is extended from the inner catheter to obtain material for microbiologic studies.

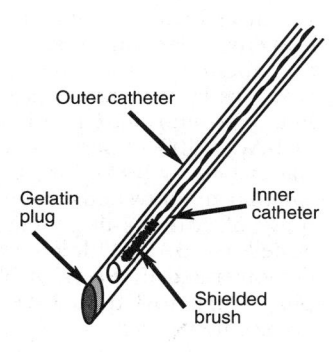
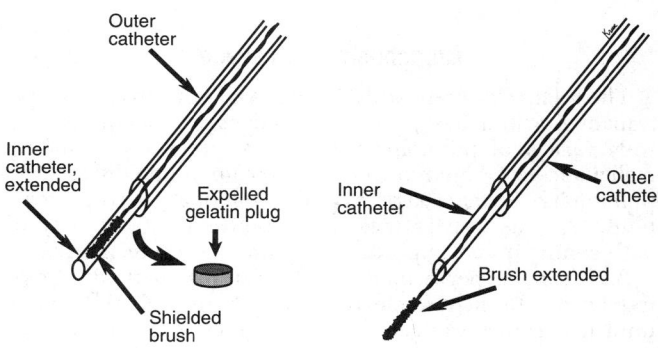

in sterile saline and transported to the laboratory within 30 minutes, anaerobic organisms can be recovered. The sensitivity for anaerobes is not high,[64, 66, 73] but use of the protected brush is the only common bronchoscopic procedure that provides acceptable anaerobic specimens.

Transbronchial Needle Aspiration

The use of needle aspiration to obtain cytologic specimens has a short but favorable history in bronchoscopy.[75–77] Yields positive for malignancy are reported as high as 77 to 90% for sampling of nodes from central bronchial locations.[75, 76] Reported yields for cytologic diagnosis of lung masses vary with the location of the lesion: yields are about 25% for central masses, whereas yields on the order of 65% are reported for more peripheral lesions (>2 mm from the carina).[77]

To use the transbronchial needle, a 22-gauge needle on a long, flexible catheter is passed down the instrument channel of the bronchoscope, with the needle retracted into the catheter to prevent damage to the bronchoscope. After the area of sampling is reached, the needle and catheter are extended from the bronchoscope. A guidewire inside the needle and catheter, used to stiffen and stabilize the system during puncture, is retracted inside the needle and the bronchoscopist punctures the bronchial wall. After the needle is imbedded, the guidewire is removed and a large syringe (20 to 50 mL) containing a few milliliters of sterile saline is attached to the proximal end of the catheter. While the bronchoscopist agitates the needle within the puncture site to loosen material, an assistant applies mild suction with the syringe to aspirate the loosened material. The procedure is illustrated in Figure 16–4. After sampling, the needle is retracted into the catheter and the needle and catheter are removed from the bronchoscope. The aspirate can be flushed into a sample container and sent for cytologic evaluation, or the material can be placed directly on slides to dry for cytologic examination.

If a larger needle is used, transbronchial sampling of cores of tissue for histologic examination can be performed with the same methodology.[75] Pneumothorax and hemoptysis are common complications associated with the use of this larger needle.[77]

Use of transbronchial aspiration or biopsy for culture has the potential to produce uncontaminated specimens for microbiologic studies, but obtaining specimens has been difficult in practice. Reported yields from aspirates taken from areas of suspected infections vary from quite low to as high as 73%.[70, 78] Transbronchial needle biopsies increase yields but often result in pneumothorax or bleeding.[78] In addition, up to 50% of specimens may contain organisms thought to be upper airway contaminants.[70] As the incidence of complications is high,[78] contaminants are frequent,[70] and similar yields can be obtained by other bronchoscopic procedures,[70] needle aspiration is not widely used for the diagnosis of infections.

Bronchoalveolar Lavage

The relatively recent addition of BAL to the bronchoscopic armamentarium has provided a means for diagnosis of a wide variety of pulmonary pathologic processes, including malignancies,[79–85] immune and inflammatory lung diseases,[86, 87] pulmonary hemorrhage,[88] and pulmonary drug reactions,[85, 89–92] as well as most importantly a wide variety of both common and opportunistic pulmonary infections.[93–111]

BAL can be performed by a variety of methods. Commonly, the bronchoscope is advanced through the airway until it becomes wedged in a subsegmental bronchus sub-

tending an area of parenchyma of interest. When the bronchoscope is firmly pressed into place, there should be minimal coughing, and the bronchoscopist may note a slight bluish hue to the mucosa as superficial vessels of the airway are compressed.

Lavage is accomplished by instilling sterile saline through the bronchoscope, then gently aspirating material back under low continuous suction. The total lavage volume should be at least 100 mL (generally instilled as five 20-mL aliquots, with suctioning between fluid additions).[112–116] Although a maximal lavage volume of 200 mL was once suggested,[113] more recent studies have demonstrated that larger volumes up to 300 mL are well tolerated.[114] The total returned volume on suctioning should be between 40 and 80% of the administered volume.

Several investigators proposed that lavage sampling need not involve bronchoscopy. So-called nonbronchoscopic lavage involves the use of a bronchoscope-like, long suction catheter wedged in an airway without direct visualization of the area sampled. The procedure as studied by these investigators was safe, economic, and produced high yields for some pathogens, notably *Pneumocystis carinii*.[117–119] Drawbacks to this procedure include the potential to miss a pathologic condition in the airway such as Kaposi's sarcoma or other endobronchial disease, as well as possibly overlooking other pathogens. More study is required before this technique should be generally used in the critically ill patient.

BAL is a relatively safe procedure, and the risk over bronchoscopy alone is increased very little. In normal volunteers, BAL caused a temporary fall in oxygenation, which was about 50% greater than that observed with bronchoscopy alone, and the oxygen desaturation persisted for up to 4 hours postprocedure.[25] In patients with underlying pulmonary disease, this decrease in oxygenation status is of a greater degree than in normal patients,[120] as would be expected given that effects of bronchoscopy alone are also magnified in the compromised patient.

Although the majority of more recent reports emphasize the usefulness of BAL for diagnosis of pulmonary infectious processes, particularly in patient with acquired immunodeficiency syndrome, BAL has also proved helpful in diagnosis of a number of noninfectious processes. As critically ill patients often present diagnostic dilemmas, knowledge of potential yields for these other processes is necessary to fully utilize the diagnostic capabilities of this technique.

BAL can be a useful tool for the diagnosis of pulmonary malignancies. Its utility has been specifically shown for acute myelomonocytic leukemia,[80] bronchioalveolar cell carcinoma,[81] and Hodgkin's[82] and non-Hodgkin's lymphoma.[83, 84] Diagnostic yield for malignancies with BAL alone is about 40%.[85] Despite this relatively low yield, morbidity with BAL is only slightly higher than that of bronchoscopy alone, and BAL can be performed in patients who are at high risk for complications from transbronchoscopic biopsies.

Cytologic examination of BAL fluid may provide evidence for drug toxicity, as has been shown for amiodarone,[89, 90] diphenylhydantoin (phenytoin),[91] and methotrexate.[92] There are questions as to the specificity of findings for drug reactions by cytopathic changes. Nonetheless, in a series of immunocompromised patients, the diagnosis was suggested by BAL in 40% of patients in whom pulmonary drug toxicity was eventually proved by other means.[85]

Other noninfectious diagnoses that may be present in the lungs of critically ill patients can be made or at least suggested by BAL. Pulmonary hemorrhage can be reliably demonstrated by Prussian blue staining of alveolar macrophages obtained from BAL fluid.[88] Scoring of the severity of bleeding based on the degree of staining may also be possible. In eosinophilic pneumonia, yields via BAL are

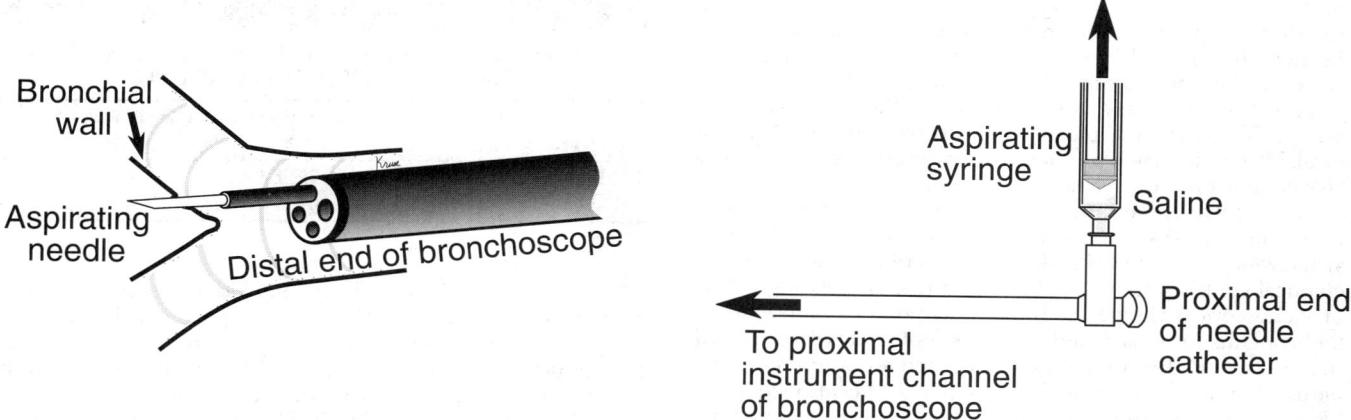

Figure 16–4. Transbronchial needle aspiration. *(Left)* The needle is imbedded through the bronchial mucosa via the distal end of the bronchoscope for sampling. The bronchoscopist agitates the needle in place to loosen material. *(Right)* A syringe applied to the proximal end of the catheter outside the bronchoscope is gently aspirated to obtain loosened material from the needle for samples.

comparable to those achieved by biopsy.[121] Pulmonary alveolar proteinosis can be diagnosed by finding the characteristic material in the lavaged fluid.[122] In some cases, flexible bronchoscopic lavage, using ventilation-perfusion mismatch scans to select areas for lavage, can also be used therapeutically in lieu of whole lung lavage.[123] Immunologic processes such as sarcoidosis or hypersensitivity pneumonitis may also be suggested diagnostically by examination of T cell populations in the lavage fluid.[86, 87]

BAL for diagnosis of infections in critically ill patients is attractive for two reasons. First, it may obviate the need for transbronchial biopsy or other more invasive procedures in this high-risk population. Second, a wide variety of special stains for many different organisms can be examined and reported within hours of the procedure, providing diagnostic information with a useful immediacy.

For patients with acquired immunodeficiency syndrome, BAL has proved safe and reliable in numerous studies for both infectious and noninfectious pulmonary involvement.[93–99] Yields of close to 100% for *Pneumocystis* have been demonstrated.[94, 100, 101] For other common pathogens seen with this syndrome, such as bacteria, cytomegalovirus, fungi, and mycobacteria, yields from BAL alone range from 60 to 85%.[93–96, 98, 102]

Diagnosis of pulmonary infections by BAL in patient populations other than those with acquired immunodeficiency syndrome produces less spectacular yields. Diagnosis of bacterial infections with reasonable yields by BAL is possible, provided quantitative cultures of the organisms obtained in lavage are performed.[103, 104] *Legionella* can also be detected in a majority of cases by fluorescent antibody staining, plus culture for the organism.[105] In immunocompromised patients (e.g., those with acute leukemia or after bone marrow transplantation), the diagnostic yield for opportunistic infections ranges from 15 to 66%, with somewhat higher reported yields if results of cultures of the fluid are included.[85, 106–111]

With respect to the rate of positive yields, the importance of the quality of the laboratory performing the stains and cultures of the lavage fluid cannot be overemphasized. It is worthwhile to ensure that the laboratory properly processes and centrifuges the lavage sample; performs special stain tests on the centrifuged fluid for bacteria, *Pneumocystis*, fungi, *Legionella*, mycobacteria, and viral inclusions in a reasonable time frame; and cultures all specimens properly[106] (Table 16–2). High-quality laboratories keep abreast of new developments such as enzyme-linked immunosorbent assay or newer culture systems for mycobacteria,[124, 125] DNA probes for hybridization studies (particularly for viruses),[126, 127] or other culture techniques[128] as they are developed to assist in expanding potential diagnostic yields from BAL.

Transbronchial and Endobronchial Biopsies

Endobronchial biopsies consist of tissue samples taken under direct visualization of lesions in airways. Generally, a large (alligator-type) forceps is used, as a larger cutting surface (often with a serrated edge) is more likely to produce adequate tissue samples from the tough bronchial walls.[129] Complications with endobronchial biopsies should be minimal if some simple precautions are observed. Lesions, such as the bluish endobronchial deposits of Kaposi's sarcoma, or highly vascular lesions, such as metastases from hypernephroma, adenomas, or carcinoid tumors, would not be biopsied in critically ill patients, as the risk of bleeding is high. In most cases, bleeding occurring postbiopsy can be controlled with saline rinses or topical application of a 1:20,000 epinephrine solution.

The bronchoscopic procedure with a high probability of producing useful diagnostic yields but also carrying a high probability of complications is the transbronchial lung bi-

TABLE 16–2
LABORATORY PROCEDURES FOR BRONCHOALVEOLAR LAVAGE SAMPLES
Filter particulate matter from specimens
Centrifuge sample
Perform special stains (30 min to 6 h)
Bacteria (Gram's stain)
Legionella (direct fluorescent antibodies or monoclonal antibodies)
Acid-fast bacilli (auramine-rhodamine)
Pneumocystis
Fungi (silver stain)
Cytologic preparation for viral inclusions
Setup cultures
Routine bacteria
Legionella
Mycobacteria
Fungus
Viral assays or shell cultures
Mycoplasma

opsy. Generally, a small cupped or ellipsoid forceps is used for these biopsies, as the smaller forceps can be passed the farthest distally and is most likely to grasp tissue containing alveoli rather than pieces of the bronchial wall.[129]

Transbronchoscopic lung biopsy in the intensive care setting has been a topic of controversy. On the basis of available studies, each physician must determine the patient's risk/benefit ratio on a case-by-case basis.

To perform these biopsies, the forceps is advanced carefully into the distal airways, beyond the range of direct visualization. In the critically ill, particularly those on mechanical ventilation or with increased risk of bleeding, many bronchoscopists wedge the bronchoscope in the subsegmental bronchus to be sampled. This allows for better control of hemostasis, as the bronchoscope is used to tamponade the biopsy segment. Continuous suction may be applied post-biopsy to appose the thin distal walls. Fluoroscopy may be used to visualize the site of biopsy, but as the logistics of fluoroscopy in the intensive care unit may be difficult and the safety of transbronchial lung biopsies without fluoroscopic guidance has been demonstrated,[130] radiographic assistance is not absolutely required.

Yields with transbronchial biopsies, particularly when combined with yields from brushings, washings, and lavage, are good in most populations of patients. Positive results are obtained in 32 to 84% of infectious processes, depending on the population studied.[32, 68, 93, 111, 131–136] For malignancies, yields of 50 to 70% positive results are reported.[79, 85] With other noninfectious, nonmalignant processes such as drug toxicity, the average positive yield is about 57%.[15, 62, 85, 88, 132, 133, 137] It has been shown that yields are not substantially improved if a second bronchoscopic procedure with repeat transbronchial biopsies is performed; therefore, if one procedure does not produce a result, there is little benefit in repeating the procedure.[138]

Unfortunately, despite improved diagnostic yields when transbronchial biopsies are performed during bronchoscopy, the physician must bear in mind that complication rates for biopsies are high in the critically ill patient population. The serious complications of biopsy are bleeding and pneumothorax.

The reported incidence of serious hemorrhage with biopsies ranges from 1.2 to 9% in a general population.[25, 31, 32] Pulmonary hypertension, thrombocytopenia, and functional platelet defects all predispose patients to increased risk of bleeding.[30] With platelet counts less than 60,000/mm³, serious bleeding occurs in 12% of cases.[127] Uremia, causing a functional platelet defect, has been associated with a 45% incidence of serious bleeding.[31] The risk of bleeding is also exceptionally high in immunocompromised patients with diffuse pulmonary infiltrates, occurring in about 29% of patients undergoing biopsy.[31, 32]

Pneumothorax may occur in up to 5% of patients undergoing transbronchial biopsy.[30, 32] Mechanical ventilation, especially with positive end-expiratory pressure, is a relative contraindication to biopsy. Serious bleeding may occur in up to 20% of cases, pneumothorax in up to 11%, and tension pneumothorax in 1.5%.[136, 139]

For each individual patient, the physician must balance the expected positive yield from transbronchial biopsy against the high risk of serious complications.[25, 30–32, 135, 136, 139]

In some cases, particularly if the course of the patient's illness is subacute or indolent, bronchoscopy without biopsy (using brushings and BAL) may be beneficial. In many cases, however, rapid progression of disease or poor patient status may make bronchoscopy less desirable than more invasive procedures such as open lung biopsy.[140] Despite general reluctance to subject a patient to open lung biopsy, it must be stressed that the complication rate for open lung biopsy

---

TABLE 16–3

POSITIVE YIELDS AND COMPLICATIONS FOR TRANSBRONCHIAL LUNG BIOPSY VERSUS OPEN LUNG BIOPSY

Procedure	Positive Diagnosis (%)	Complication Rate (%)
Transbronchial biopsy	32–84	11 (average)
Open lung biopsy	68–100	<3

is lower than that for transbronchial biopsy because superior control of bleeding and the pleural space is achieved with surgery.[15, 62, 132] In addition, the open procedure produces higher positive diagnostic yields.[62, 124, 140, 141] Rates of complications and rates of positive diagnostic yields for the two procedures are compared in Table 16–3. No intraoperative deaths have been reported. With open lung biopsy, incidences of bleeding, persistent pneumothorax, prolonged mechanical ventilation, or need for reoperation are reported to be 3 to 13%.[15, 62, 132, 142, 143]

The surgical approach may be guided by radiographic findings in some cases, but the standard procedure is generally a lingular biopsy with a small anterior thoracotomy.[143, 144] In diffuse lung disease, this approach produces excellent diagnostic yields.[144]

The presumption in selecting open lung biopsy for a critically ill patient is that more appropriate or effective therapy can be selected based on definitive results, with resulting improvement in survival.[143–148] There is no question that diagnostic yields from open lung biopsy are the highest of any pulmonary diagnostic approach, ranging from 68 to 100%.[15, 62, 132, 140, 142, 143, 149]

POSTPROCEDURE CONSIDERATIONS

Major concerns in the postbronchoscopy period are directed toward the patient's ventilatory and oxygenation status. Sedative medications given during the procedure may depress ventilatory drive and necessitate an increase in the amount of ventilatory support provided. Oxygen status should be monitored for several hours after the procedure, particularly if BAL or other procedures were part of the bronchoscopic procedure, as many patients will require an increase in supplemental oxygen.[20, 21, 24, 25, 120]

SUMMARY

Bronchoscopy can be an extremely useful diagnostic and therapeutic procedure in the critically ill patient population. Before undertaking the procedure, the physician should carefully assess the patient for any contraindications to bronchoscopy or biopsy. Expected diagnostic rates for suspected diagnostic yields should be carefully balanced against the risk of serious complications with bronchoscopy or its associated procedures. If an acceptable risk/benefit ratio is expected, careful monitoring of the patient during the procedure reduces morbidity.

The physician must decide whether specific diagnosis will be of benefit to the patient. Discouraging evidence has been provided by studies evaluating the benefits of making a specific diagnosis (by bronchoscopic or surgical means) on the ultimate outcome for patients.[133, 140, 145, 150–153] For bronchoscopy with transbronchial lung biopsy, although the overall diagnostic rate was 60%, no difference in survival was noted between the patients in whom a specific diagnosis was made and those in whom the nature of the pulmonary process remained unknown.[133] Similarly, in a series of patients who underwent open lung biopsy, although results of biopsy led to a therapeutic change for 70% of the patients, only 16.5% of patients benefited from this change in therapy.[140]

Many questions remain about the appropriate measures for critically ill patients with new-onset pulmonary disease. The importance of BAL for diagnosis of infections may be expanded in the future by use of newer microbiologic techniques. The development of DNA probes or monoclonal antibodies for rapid detection of a wide variety of viruses, *Legionella*, and so forth may increase the role of BAL in critically ill patients, particularly as more effective therapies are developed. Early reports provide evidence that earlier diagnosis and treatment may become possible.[154] The physician dealing with critically ill patients must follow developments in microbiologic diagnostic testing and pharmacology that may improve yields of bronchoscopy or other diagnostic procedures and provide possibilities for improved survival.

References

1. Sackner MA: Bronchofiberscopy. Am Rev Respir Dis 111:62, 1975.
2. Fulkerson WJ: Fiberoptic bronchoscopy. N Engl J Med 311:511, 1984.
3. Landa JF: Indications for bronchoscopy. Chest 73:686, 1978.
4. Sokolowski JW, Burgher LW, Jones FL, et al: Guidelines for fiberoptic bronchoscopy. Am Thorac Soc News 12:14, 1986.
5. Barrett CR: Flexible fiberoptic bronchoscopy in the critically ill patient. Chest 73:746, 1978.
6. Barrett CR, Vecchione JJ, Loomis Bell AL: Flexible fiberoptic bronchoscopy for airway management during acute respiratory failure. Am Rev Respir Dis 109:429, 1974.
7. Mahajan VK, Catron PW, Huber GL: The value of fiberoptic bronchoscopy in the management of pulmonary collapse. Chest 73:817, 1978.
8. Harada K, Mutsuda T, Saoyoma N, et al: Re-expansion of refractory atelectasis using a bronchofiberscope with a balloon cuff. Chest 84:725, 1983.
9. Swersky RB, Change JB, Wisoff BG, et al: Endobronchial balloon tamponade of hemoptysis in patients with cystic fibrosis. Ann Thorac Surg 27:262, 1979.
10. Saw EC, Gottlieb LS, Yokoyama T, et al: Flexible fiberoptic bronchoscopy and endobronchial tamponade in the management of massive hemoptysis. Chest 70:589, 1976.
11. McCullough P: Wire basket removal of a large endobronchial foreign body. Chest 87:270, 1985.
12. Cunanan OS: The flexible fiberoptic bronchoscope in foreign body removal: Experience in 300 cases. Chest 73:725, 1978.
13. Claypool WD, Rogers RM, Matuschak GM: Update on the clinical diagnosis, management and pathogenesis of pulmonary alveolar proteinosis (phospholipidosis). Chest 85:550, 1984.
14. Sosenko A, Glassroth J: Fiberoptic bronchoscopy in the evaluation of lung abscesses. Chest 87:489, 1985.
15. Fanta CH, Pennington JE: Fever and new lung infiltrates in the immunocompromised host. Clin Chest Med 2:19, 1981.
16. Katz AS, Michelson EL, Stawicki J, et al: Cardiac arrhythmias: Frequency during fiberoptic bronchoscopy and correlation with hypoxemia. Arch Intern Med 141:603, 1981.
17. Dull WL: Flexible fiberoptic bronchoscopy: An analysis of proficiency. Chest 77:65, 1980.
18. Albertini R, Harrell JH, Moser KM: Hypoxemia during fiberoptic bronchoscopy. Chest 65:117, 1974.
19. Salisbury BG, Metzger LF, Altose MD, et al: Effect of fiberoptic bronchoscopy on respiratory performance in patients with chronic obstructive pulmonary disease. Thorax 30:441, 1975.
20. Matsushima Y, Jones RL, King EG, et al: Alterations in pulmonary mechanics and gas exchange during routine fiberoptic bronchoscopy. Chest 86:184, 1984.
21. Lindholm CE, Ollman B, Snyder JV, et al: Cardiorespiratory effects of flexible fiberoptic bronchoscopy in critically ill patients. Chest 74:362, 1978.
22. Dubrawsky C, Awe RJ, and Jenkins DE: The effect of bronchofiberscopic examination on oxygenation status. Chest 67:137, 1975.
23. Ghows MB, Rosen MJ, Chuang MT, et al: Transcutaneous oxygen monitoring during fiberoptic bronchoscopy. Chest 89:543, 1986.
24. Albertini RE, Harrell JH, Moser KM: Management of arterial hypoxemia induced by fiberoptic bronchoscopy. Chest 67:134, 1975.
25. Burns DM, Shure D, Francoz R, et al: The physiologic consequences of saline lobar lavage in healthy adults. Am Rev Respir Dis 127:695, 1983.
26. Brach BB, Escano CG, Harrell JH, et al: Ventilation-perfusion alterations induced by fiberoptic bronchoscopy. Chest 69:335, 1976.
27. Phillips BA, Cooper KR, Fratkin MJ: Effect of bronchoscopy on localization of gallium citrate. Am Rev Respir Dis 127:342, 1983.
28. Schrader DL, Lakshminarayan S: The effect of fiberoptic bronchoscopy on cardiac rhythm. Chest 73:821, 1978.
29. Luck JC, Messender OH, Rubenstein MJ, et al: Arrhythmias from fiberoptic bronchoscopy. Chest 74:139, 1978.
30. Herf SM, Surratt PM, Arora NS: Deaths and complications associated with transbronchial lung biopsy. Am Rev Respir Dis 115:708, 1977.
31. Zavala DC: Pulmonary hemorrhage in fiberoptic transbronchoscopic biopsy. Chest 70:584, 1976.
32. Havson RR, Zavala DC, Rhodes RL, et al: Transbronchial biopsy via the flexible fiberoptic bronchoscope. Am Rev Respir Dis 114:67, 1976.
33. Givens CD, Lloyd JE: Bronchoscopy in patients with gastroparesis. Chest 88:482, 1985.
34. Perry LB: Topical anesthesia for bronchoscopy. Chest 73:691, 1978.
35. Credle WF, Smiddy JF, Elliot RC: Complications of fiberoptic bronchoscopy. Am Rev Respir Dis 109:67, 1974.
36. Woelke BJ, Tucker RA: ARDS after local lidocaine administration. Chest 83:933, 1983.
37. Howard JJ, Monsenifar Z, Simons SM: Adult respiratory distress syndrome following administration of lidocaine. Chest 81:644, 1982.
38. Coppolo DP, Brienza LT, Pratt DS, et al: A role for the respiratory therapist in flexible fiberoptic bronchoscopy. Respir Care 30:323, 1985.
39. Prakash UBS, Stubbs SE: Bronchoscopy: Indications and technique. Semin Respir Med 3:17, 1981.
40. Shinnick JP, Johnson RF, Oslick T: Bronchoscopy during mechanical ventilation using the fiberscope. Chest 65:613, 1974.
41. Grossman E, Jacobi AM: Minimal optimal endotracheal tube size for fiberoptic bronchoscopy. Anesth Analg 53:475, 1974.
42. Feldman NT, Sanders J: An alternative method for fiberoptic bronchoscopic examination of the intubated patient. Am Rev Respir Dis 11:562, 1975.
43. Pingleton SK, Bone RC, Ruth NC: Helium-oxygen mixtures during bronchoscopy. Crit Care Med 8:50, 1980.
44. Chung C: Fiberoptic bronchoscopy via the endotracheal tube. Chest 87:276, 1985.
45. Stradling P: Diagnostic Bronchoscopy: A Teaching Manual. New York, Churchill Livingstone, 1986.
46. Olopade CO, Prakash UBS: Bronchoscopy in the critical care unit. Mayo Clin Proc 64:1255, 1989.
47. Dreisin R, Albert RL, Talley PA, et al: Flexible fiberoptic bronchoscopy in the teaching hospital: Yield and complications. Chest 74:144, 1978.
48. Pereira W, Kounat D, Zacovino J: Fever and pneumonia following fiberoptic bronchoscopy. Am Rev Respir Dis 109:692, 1974.
49. Witte MC, Opal JM, Gilbert JG, et al: Incidence of fever and bacteremia following transbronchial needle aspiration. Chest 89:85, 1986.
50. Nelson KE, Larson P, Schraufragel DE, et al: Transmission of tuberculosis by flexible fiber bronchoscopes. Am Rev Respir Dis 126:99, 1983.
51. Dawson DJ, Armstrong JG, Blalock ZM: Mycobacterial cross-contamination of bronchoscopy specimens. Am Rev Respir Dis 126:1095, 1982.
52. Pappas SA, Schaaf DM, Costanza MB, et al: Contamination of flexible fiberoptic bronchoscopes. Am Rev Respir Dis 127:391, 1983.
53. Renz LE, Smiddy JF, Rauscher CR: Fiberoptic bronchoscopy during respiratory failure. Am Rev Respir Dis 103:904, 1971.
54. Wanner A, Landa J, Nelson RE. Bedside broncho-fiberscopy for atelectasis and lung abscess. JAMA 224:1284, 1973.
55. Conlan AA, Hurwitz SS: Management of massive hemoptysis with the rigid bronchoscope and cold saline lavage. Thorax 35:901, 1980.
56. Imgrund SP, Golberg SK, Waltenstein MD, et al: Clinical diagnosis of massive hemoptysis using the fiberoptic bronchoscope. Crit Care Med 13:438, 1985.
57. Zavala DC, Rhodes ML: Foreign body removal: A new role for the fiberoptic bronchoscope. Am Rev Respir Dis 109:691, 1974.
58. Banerjee A, Khanna SK, Haryanan PS: Use of Fogarty catheters for removal of tracheobronchial foreign bodies. Chest 85:452, 1984.
59. Bartlett JG, Alexander J, Mayhew J, et al: Should fiberoptic bronchoscopy aspirates be cultured? Am Rev Respir Dis 114:73, 1976.
60. Winterbauer RH, Hutchinson JF, Reinhardt GN, et al: The use of quantitative cultures and antibody coating of bacteria to diagnose bacterial pneumonia by fiberoptic bronchoscopy. Am Rev Respir Dis 128:98, 1983.
61. Jordan GW, Wong GA, Hoeprich PD: Bacteriology of the lower respiratory tract: Flexible fiberoptic bronchoscopy vs. transtracheal aspiration. J Infect Dis 134:428, 1976.
62. Wilson WR, Cockerill FR, Rosenow EC: Pulmonary disease in the immunocompromised host. Mayo Clin Proc 60:610, 1985.
63. Zisholtz BM, Eisenberg H: Lung cancer cell type as a determinant of bronchoscopy yield. Chest 84:428, 1983.
64. Bordelon JY Jr, Legrand P, Cewin WC, et al: The telescoping plugged catheter in suspected anaerobic infections: A controlled series. Am Rev Respir Dis 128:465, 1983.
65. Joshi JH, Wana KP, deJongh CA, et al: A comparative evaluation of two fiberoptic bronchoscopy catheters: The plugged telescoping catheter vs. the single sheathed nonplugged catheter. Am Rev Respir Dis 126:860, 1982.
66. Pollock HM, Hawkins EL, Bronner JR, et al: Diagnosis of bacterial pulmonary infections with quantitative protected catheter cultures obtained during bronchoscopy. J Clin Microbiol 17:255, 1983.
67. Teague RB, Wallace RJ, Awe RJ: The use of quantitative sterile brush

culture and gram stain analysis in the diagnosis of lower respiratory tract infection. Chest 79:157, 1981.

68. Wimberly NW, Bass JB, Boyd BW, et al: Use of a bronchoscopic protected catheter brush for the diagnosis of pulmonary infections. Chest 81:556, 1982.

69. Broughton WA, Bass JB, Kirkpatrick MB: The technique of protected brush catheter bronchoscopy. J Crit Illness 2:63, 1987.

70. Lorch DG, John JF Jr, Tomlinson JR, et al: Protected transbronchial needle aspiration and protected brush in the diagnosis of pneumonia. Am Rev Respir Dis 136:565, 1987.

71. Chastre J, Viau F, Brun P, et al: Prospective evaluation of the protected specimen brush for the diagnosis of pulmonary infections in ventilated patients. Am Rev Respir Dis 130:924, 1984.

72. Lambert RS, George RB: Diagnosing nosocomial pneumonias in mechanically ventilated patients. J Crit Illness 2:57, 1987.

73. Villers D, Derriennic M, Raffi F, et al: Reliability of the bronchoscopic protected brush catheter brush in intubated and ventilated patients. Chest 88:527, 1985.

74. Baughman RP, Thorpe JE, Staneck J, et al: Use of the protected specimen brush in patients with endotracheal or tracheostomy tubes. Chest 91:233, 1987.

75. Wang KP: Flexible transbronchial needle aspiration biopsy for histologic specimens. Chest 88:860, 1985.

76. Shure D, Fedullo PF: Transbronchial needle aspiration in the diagnosis of submucosal and peribronchial bronchogenic carcinoma. Chest 88:49, 1985.

77. Gay PC, Brutinel WM: Transbronchial needle aspiration in the practice of bronchoscopy. Mayo Clin Proc 64:158, 1989.

78. Shure D, Moser KM, Konopka R: Transbronchial needle aspiration in the diagnosis of pneumonia in a canine model. Am Rev Respir Dis 131:290, 1985.

79. Springmeyer SC, Hackman R, Carlson JJ, et al: Bronchiolo-alveolar cell carcinoma diagnosed by bronchoalveolar lavage. Chest 83:278, 1983.

80. Rossi GA, Repetto M, Ravazzoni C: Acute myelomonocytic leukemia: Demonstration of pulmonary involvement by bronchoalveolar lavage. Chest 87:259, 1985.

81. Fedullo AJ, Ettenson DB: Bronchoalveolar lavage in lymphangitic spread of adenocarcinoma to the lung. Chest 87:129, 1985.

82. Morales RM, Matthews JI: Diagnosis of parenchymal Hodgkin's disease using bronchoalveolar lavage. Chest 91:785, 1987.

83. Davis WB, Gadek JE. Detection of pulmonary lymphoma by bronchoalveolar lavage. Chest 91:787, 1987.

84. Pisani RJ, Witzig TE, Li C-Y, et al: Confirmation of lymphomatous pulmonary involvement by immunophenotypic and gene rearrangement analysis of bronchoalveolar lavage fluid. Mayo Clin Proc 65:651, 1990.

85. Stover DE, Zaman MB, Hajdi SI, et al: Bronchoalveolar lavage in the diagnosis of diffuse pulmonary infiltrates in the immunocompromised host. Ann Intern Med 101:1, 1984.

86. Hunninghake GW, Gadek JE, Kawanami O, et al: Inflammatory and immune processes in the human lung in health and disease: Evaluation by bronchoalveolar lavage. Am J Pathol 97:149, 1979.

87. Merrill WW, Reynolds HY: Bronchial lavage in inflammatory lung disease. Clin Chest Med 4:71, 1983.

88. Kahn FW, Jones JM, England DM: Diagnosis of pulmonary hemorrhage in the immunocompromised host. Am Rev Respir Dis 136:155, 1987.

89. Martin WJ, Osborn MJ, Douglas WW: Amiodarone pulmonary toxicity: Assessment by bronchoalveolar lavage. Chest 88:630, 1985.

90. Israel-Biet D, Venet A, Caubarrere I, et al: Bronchoalveolar lavage in amiodarone pneumonitis: Cellular abnormalities and their relevance to pathogenesis. Chest 91:214, 1987.

91. Chamberlain DW, Hyland RH, Rose DJ: Diphenylhydantoin induced lymphocytic interstitial pneumonia. Chest 90:458, 1986.

92. White DA, Rankin JA, Stover DE, et al: Methotrexate pneumonitis: Bronchoalveolar lavage finding suggest an immunologic disorder. Am Rev Respir Dis 139:18, 1989.

93. Broaddus C, Dake MD, Stulbarg MS, et al: Bronchoalveolar lavage and transbronchial biopsy for the diagnosis of pulmonary infections in the acquired immunodeficiency syndrome. Ann Intern Med 102:747, 1985.

94. Stover DE, White DA, Romano RA, et al: Diagnosis of pulmonary disease in AIDS: Role of bronchoscopy and BAL. Am Rev Respir Dis 130:659, 1984.

95. Hopewell PC, Luce JM: Pulmonary involvement in the acquired immunodeficiency syndrome. Chest 87:103, 1985.

96. Murray JF, Felton CP, Garay SM, et al: Pulmonary complications of the acquired immunodeficiency syndrome: Report of a National Heart Lung and Blood Institute workshop. N Engl J Med 310:1682, 1984.

97. White DA, Matthay RA: Noninfectious pulmonary complications of infection with human immunodeficiency virus. Am Rev Respir Dis 140:1763, 1989.

98. Murray JF, Mills J: Pulmonary infectious complications of human immunodeficiency virus infection (Part I). Am Rev Respir Dis 141:1356, 1990.

99. Murray JF, Mills J: Pulmonary infectious complications of human immunodeficiency virus infection (Part II). Am Rev Respir Dis 141:1582, 1990.

100. Golden JA, Hollander H, Stulbarg MS, et al: Bronchoalveolar lavage as the exclusive diagnostic modality for *Pneumocystis carinii* pneumonia: A prospective study among patients with the acquired immunodeficiency syndrome. Chest 90:18, 1986.

101. Ognibene FP, Shelhamer VG, Macher AM, et al: The diagnosis of *Pneumocystis carinii* pneumonia in patients with the acquired immunodeficiency syndrome using subsegmental bronchoalveolar lavage. Am Rev Respir Dis 129:929, 1984.

102. Polsky B, Gold JW, Whimbey E, et al: Bacterial pneumonia in patients with the acquired immunodeficiency syndrome. Ann Intern Med 104:38, 1986.

103. Kahn FW, Jones JM: Diagnosing bacterial respiratory infection by bronchoalveolar lavage. J Infect Dis 155:862, 1987.

104. Thorpe JE, Baughman RP, Frame PT, et al: Bronchoalveolar lavage for diagnosing acute bacterial pneumonia. J Infect Dis 155:855, 1987.

105. Kohorst WR, Schonfeld SA, Macklin JE, et al: Rapid diagnosis of Legionnaire's disease by bronchoalveolar lavage. Chest 84:186, 1983.

106. Martin WJ III, Smith TF, Sanderson DR, et al: Role of bronchoalveolar lavage in the assessment of opportunistic infections: Utility and complications. Mayo Clin Proc 62:549, 1987.

107. Saito H, Anaissie EJ, Morice RC, et al: Bronchoalveolar lavage in the diagnosis of pulmonary infiltrates in patients with acute leukemia. Chest 94:745, 1988.

108. Frankel LR, Smith DW, Lewiston NJ: Bronchoalveolar lavage for diagnosis of pneumonia in the immunocompromised child. Pediatrics 81:785, 1988.

109. Springmeyer SC, Hackman RC, Holle R, et al: Use of bronchoalveolar lavage to diagnose acute diffuse pneumonia in the immunocompromised host. J Infect Dis 154:604, 1986.

110. Krowka MJ, Rosenow EC, Hoagland HC: Pulmonary complications of bone marrow transplantation. Chest 87:237, 1985.

111. Cordonnier C, Bernaudin JF, Fleury J, et al: Diagnostic yield of BAL in pneumonitis occurring after allogenic bone marrow transplantation. Am Rev Respir Dis 132:1118, 1985.

112. Lam S, Leriche JC, Kijek K, et al: Effect of bronchial lavage volume on cellular and protein recovery. Chest 88:856, 1985.

113. Martin WJ III, Williams DE, Dines DE, et al: Interstitial lung disease: Assessment by bronchoalveolar lavage. Mayo Clin Proc 58:751, 1983.

114. Reynolds HY: Bronchoalveolar lavage: State of the art. Am Rev Respir Dis 135:250, 1987.

115. Pingleton SK, Harrison GF, Stechschulte DJ, et al: Effect of location, pH and temperature of instillate in BAL in normal volunteers. Am Rev Respir Dis 128:1035, 1983.

116. Crystal RG, Reynolds HY, Kalica AR. Bronchoalveolar lavage: The report of an international conference. Chest 90:122, 1986.

117. Mann JM, Altus CS, Webber CA, et al: Nonbronchoscopic lung lavage for diagnosis of opportunistic infection in AIDS. Chest 91:319, 1987.

118. Caughy G, Wong H, Gamsu G, et al: Nonbronchoscopic bronchoalveolar lavage for the diagnosis for *Pneumocystis carinii* pneumonia in the acquired immunodeficiency syndrome. Chest 88:659, 1985.

119. Piperno D, Baussorgues P, Bachmann P, et al: Diagnostic value of nonbronchoscopic bronchoalveolar lavage during mechanical ventilation. Chest 93:223, 1988.

120. Tilles DS, Goldenheim PD, Ginns LC, et al: Pulmonary function in normal subjects and patients with sarcoidosis after bronchoalveolar lavage. Chest 89:244, 1989.

121. Lieske TR, Sunderrajan EV, Passamonte PM: Bronchoalveolar lavage and technetium glucoheptonate imaging in chronic eosinophilic pneumonia. Chest 85:282, 1985.

122. Claypool WD, Rogers RM, Matuschak GM: Update on the clinical diagnosis, management and pathogenesis of pulmonary alveolar proteinosis (phospholipidosis). Chest 85:550, 1984.

123. Brach BB, Harrell JH, Moser KM: Alveolar proteinosis: Lobar lavage by fiberoptic bronchoscopic technique. Chest 69:224, 1979.

124. Daniel TM, Debane SM, van der Kuyp F: Enzyme-linked immunosorbent assay using Mycobacterium tuberculosis antigen and PPD for the serodiagnosis of tuberculosis. Chest 88:388, 1985.

125. Russell MD, Torrington KG, Tenholder MF: A ten-year experience with fiberoptic bronchoscopy for mycobacterial isolation: Impact of the BACTEC system. Am Rev Respir Dis 133:1069, 1986.

126. Tenover FC: DNA probes for infectious diseases. Clin Microbiol Newslett 7:105, 1985.

127. Hilbourne LH, Niebery RK, Cheng L, et al: Direct in situ hybridization for rapid detection of cytomegalovirus in bronchoalveolar lavage. Am J Clin Pathol 87:766, 1987.

128. Crawford SW, Bowden RA, Hackman RC, et al: Rapid detection of cytomegalovirus pulmonary infection by bronchoalveolar lavage and centrifugation culture. Ann Intern Med 108:180, 1988.

129. Smith LS, Seaquist M, Schillaci RF: Comparison of forceps used for transbronchial lung biopsy: Bigger may not be better. Chest 87:574, 1985.

130. Anders GT, Johnson JE, Bush BA, et al. Transbronchial biopsy without fluoroscopy: A seven-year perspective. Chest 94:557, 1988.

131. Feldman NT, Pennington JE, Ehrie MG: Transbronchial lung biopsy in the compromised host. JAMA 238:1377, 1977.

132. Masur H, Shelhamer J, Parillo JE: The management of pneumonia in immunocompromised patients. JAMA 253:1769, 1985.

133. Williams D, Yungbluth M, Adams G, et al: The role of fiberoptic bronchoscopy in the evaluation of immunocompromised hosts with diffuse pulmonary infiltrates. Am Rev Respir Dis 131:880, 1985.

134. Hedemark LL, Kronenbery RS, Rasp FL, et al: The value of bronchoscopy in establishing the etiology of pneumonia in renal transplant recipients. Am Rev Respir Dis 126:981, 1974.
135. Papin TA, Lynch JL, Weg JG: Transbronchial biopsy in the thrombocytopenic patient. Chest 88:549, 1985.
136. Papin TA, Grum GM, Weg JG: Transbronchial biopsy during mechanical ventilation. Chest 89:168, 1986.
137. Poletti V, Patelli M, Ferracini R, et al: Transbronchial lung biopsy in infiltrative lung disease. The importance of the pathologic approach. Sarcoidosis 5:43, 1988.
138. Che H: The diagnostic yield of repeat transbronchial lung biopsy. Chest 88:158, 1985.
139. Pincus PS, Kallenbach JM, Hurwitz MC, et al: Transbronchial biopsy during mechanical ventilation. Crit Care Med 15:1136, 1987.
140. McKenna RS Jr, Mountain CF, McMurtry MJ: Open lung biopsy in immunocompromised patients. Chest 86:671, 1984.
141. Chuang MT, Raskin J, Krellenstein DJ, et al: Bronchoscopy in diffuse lung disease: Evaluation by open lung biopsy in nondiagnostic transbronchial lung biopsy. Ann Otol Rhinol Laryngol 96:654, 1987.
142. Wilson WR, Cockerill FR: Pulmonary disease in the immunocompromised host. Mayo Clin Proc 70:610, 1985.
143. Matthay RA, Moritz ED: Invasive procedures for diagnosing pulmonary infection: A critical review. Clin Chest Med 2:3, 1981.
144. Wetstein L: Sensitivity and specificity of lingular segmental biopsies of the lung. Chest 90:383, 1986.
145. Robin ED, Burke CM: Lung biopsy in immunosuppressed patients. Chest 89:276, 1986.
146. Greenman RL, Goodall PT, King T: Lung biopsy in immunocompromised hosts. Am J Med 59:488, 1975.
147. Leight GS, Michalis LL: Open lung biopsy for the diagnosis of acute diffuse pulmonary infiltrates in the immunocompromised patient. Chest 73:477, 1978.
148. Toledo-Pereya LH, DeMeesterm TR, Churg A, et al: The benefits of open lung biopsy in patients with previous nondiagnostic transbronchial biopsy: A guide to appropriate therapy. Chest 77:647, 1980.
149. Early GL, Williams TE, Kilman JW: Open lung biopsy: Its effects on therapy in the pediatric patient. Chest 87:467, 1985.
150. Tenholder MF, Hooper RG: Pulmonary infiltrates in leukemia. Chest 78:468, 1980.
151. Rossiter SJ, Miller DC, Churg AM, et al: Open lung biopsy in the immunocompromised patient: Is it really beneficial? J Thorac Cardiovasc Surg 77:338, 1979.
152. Webster J, Clarke JC: A doctor's dilemma. Chest 78:417, 1980.
153. Puksa S, Hutcheon MA, Hyland RH: Usefulness of transbronchial biopsy in immunocompromised patients with pulmonary infiltrates. Thorax 38:146, 1983.
154. Emmanuel D, Peppard J, Stover D, et al: Rapid immunologic diagnosis of cytomegalovirus pneumonia by bronchoalveolar lavage using human and murine monoclonal antibodies. Ann Intern Med 104:476, 1986.

CHAPTER 17

Noninvasive Monitoring of Oxygen and Carbon Dioxide

David A. Paulus

Noninvasive gas monitoring has a long history. Just as invasive monitoring waited for suitable materials and technology, so noninvasive patient gas monitoring waited for computers, materials, technology, and ideas. Oxygen saturation and airway gas monitoring have become quite popular in intensive care units. This chapter considers the physiology of noninvasive gas monitoring, the problems it presents, and the avenues for solutions it provides. Measurement techniques and clinical applications (including the pitfalls) are discussed, and the technology behind the measurement techniques is briefly examined.

OXYGENATION

Kirchhoff and Bunsen[1] invented the stethoscope in 1860, and Stokes[2] observed in 1864 that oxygen was transported in blood by a colored substance. Hoppe-Seyler[3] recognized that absorption of green and blue light by blood was caused by hemoglobin and that absorption changed depending on the aeration of hemoglobin. Based on these observations, Mathes[4] built the first device that continuously measured saturation of hemoglobin with oxygen in arterial blood (SaO_2) in humans in 1935. However, calibration was a problem in this device, which measured the saturation by transilluminating tissue. During World War II, interest in a device that could measure SaO_2 accelerated when it was noted that pilots of nonpressurized aircraft became hypoxemic at high altitude. A servo system was built that varied the oxygen flow to a mask based on oximeter readings.[5] In the 1970s, Hewlett-Packard developed and marketed an ear oximeter that used eight wavelengths to determine SaO_2, but the instrument's bulk and expense severely limited its application. The first practical, noninvasive pulse oximeter was developed in the late 1970s and was marketed to pulmonary function laboratories.[6] A bit later, William New of Stanford found a market for pulse oximeters in the operating room and developed an oximeter that met the needs of both the operating room and the intensive care unit (New, personal communication, 1986). Today, pulse oximeters are found in many care units where hypoxemia is a concern.

PHYSIOLOGY AND PHYSICS OF PULSE OXIMETRY

Adult blood contains four species of hemoglobin: oxyhemoglobin (HbO_2), reduced hemoglobin (Hb), methemoglobin (MetHb), and carboxyhemoglobin (COHb). (In healthy persons, the latter two types are in small concentration.) Pulse oximetry is supposed to measure the proportion of hemoglobin that is oxygenated, but this presents a problem: Is oxygen saturation defined as the fraction of the sum of HbO_2 and Hb that is saturated with oxygen or as the fraction of total hemoglobin that is saturated with oxygen? Measuring saturation as the ratio of HbO_2 to total hemoglobin yields fractional hemoglobin saturation:

$$\text{Fractional } SaO_2 = \frac{HbO_2}{HbO_2 + Hb + COHb + MetHb} \times 100\%$$

The method of Van Slyke and Neill, on the other hand, defines oxygen capacity in terms of the volumetrically measured oxygen content and does not account for COHb or MetHb. This measure, which is the one reported by pulse oximetry, is now known as functional hemoglobin saturation:[7]

$$\text{Functional } SaO_2 = \frac{HbO_2}{HbO_2 + Hb} \times 100\%$$

The theoretic basis of pulse oximetry is the Beer-Lambert law.[6] The law states that the amount of light transmitted (I_{trans}) through a substance is a function of its concentration in a clear solution (C). To determine the concentration, one must know the intensity of the incident light (I_{in}), the path length (D), and the extinction coefficient (E) at the wavelength of the incident light. The extinction coefficient is a specific constant for a specific solute at a specific wavelength (Fig. 17–1). The equation for the Beer-Lambert law is

$$I_{trans} = I_{in}e^{-DC\epsilon}$$

Laboratory systems were developed in which a cuvette held the blood sample.[8] The path length was known, as were the frequency and intensity of the incident light. The transmitted light was measured and, because the extinction coef-

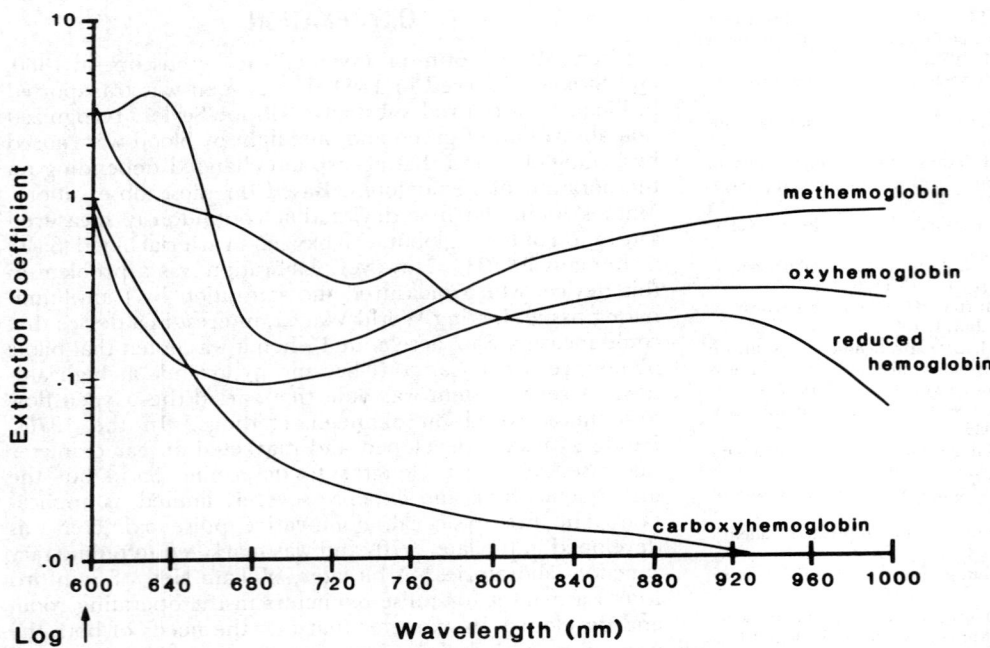

Figure 17-1. Transmitted light absorbance spectra of four hemoglobin species: Hb, HbO_2, COHb, and MetHb. (From Barker SJ, Tremper KK: Pulse oximetry: Applications and limitations. Reprinted with permission from International Anesthesiology Clinics, volume 25, p 155, 1987.)

ficients of each hemoglobin species were known, the equation for the Beer-Lambert law could be solved for the individual hemoglobin concentrations.

Unfortunately, light inside the body is scattered by skin surface and tissue and absorbed by tissues other than blood, and its optical characteristics are altered markedly by skin pigments. To counter these effects, early investigators tried to measure SaO_2 by compressing the tissue of interest so that they could initially transmit light through tissue that was free of blood. Nevertheless, the path length varied, making strict application of the Beer-Lambert law problematic.

Measurements of SaO_2 obtained by pulse oximetry (SpO_2) exploit the pulsatile nature of arterial blood. The light absorption of venous blood and other tissue can be eliminated because it is nearly constant, so the only variable is contributed by arterial blood. The absorption of incident light consists mostly of a continuous portion and a variable portion. The basic assumption underlying the design of the pulse oximeter is that the pulsatile portion of light absorption is contributed by arterial blood. The pulsatile flow of arterial blood rhythmically changes the path length and subsequently the absorption of incident light. The designers of the pulse oximeter recognized that to successfully measure arterial

saturation of tissue by applying the aspects of the Beer-Lambert equation, several conditions must exist: (1) The tissue must be reasonably transparent to the wavelengths of light that distinguish among the moieties of interest; (2) the absorption profile must be different among the specific species of interest; (3) the means of producing the wavelengths and detecting them must be readily available; and (4) the minimal number of wavelengths must equal the number of significant absorbers available.[6]

Red and near-infrared light satisfy the first criterion because tissue and pigments absorb blue, green, and yellow. Hemoglobin and HbO_2 are quite disparate in the range of 600 to 1000 nm, the range of red and infrared light. Fortunately, light-emitting diodes that produce light in the wavelengths of interest are readily available, as are detectors. The fourth criterion is problematic. Fortunately, the four hemoglobin moieties are the only significant absorbers found in normal blood for that wavelength segment (Fig. 17-2).

To develop a workable system, the pulsatile component of light absorption must be separated from the nonpulsatile component. The signal consists of two parts that we shall call the AC and the DC portions. To calculate SpO_2, the AC portion amplitude is divided by the DC amplitude at both

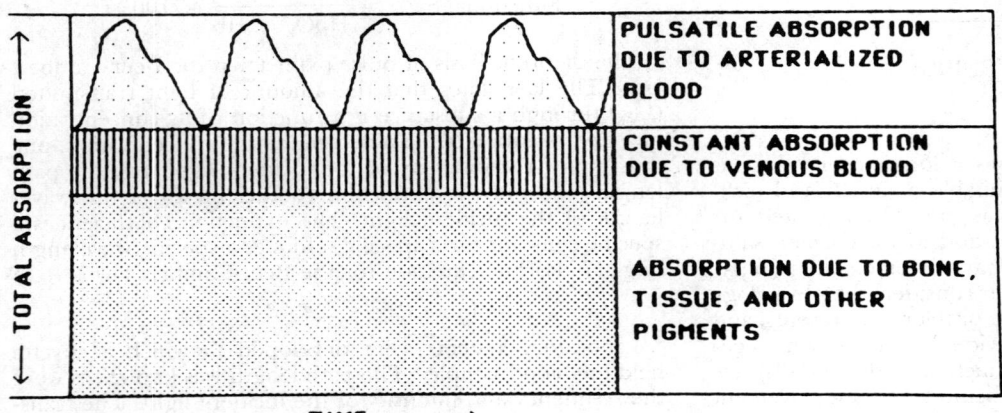

Figure 17-2. Contribution of tissue components to light absorption as a function of time. (From Alexander CM, Teller LE, Gross JB: Principles of pulse oximetry: Theoretical and practical considerations. Reprinted with permission from the International Anesthesia Research Society [Anesthesia and Analgesia, 1989, volume 68, pp 368-376].)

red (660 nm) and infrared (940 nm) wavelengths. The result is a scaled signal level for both the red and infrared wavelengths that eliminates the incident light intensity as a consideration. All variables have now been eliminated except the absorption related to arterial hemoglobin at the two wavelengths. The ratio of corrected red absorption to corrected infrared absorption can then be related to the SaO_2 (Fig. 17–3).

$$R = \frac{AC_{660}/DC_{660}}{AC_{940}/DC_{940}}$$

Figure 17–4 shows the relative plethysmographic signal amplitudes at both wavelengths.

The practical pulse oximeter uses these principles and applies them with due consideration of optics, signal-to-noise ratio, signal processing, human characteristics, data acquisition, and physiologic variabilities. The system measures the light levels three times in a cycle. First, the red light-emitting diode is illuminated, and the amount of light is measured by the detector. Next, the infrared light-emitting diode is illuminated and the light intensity is measured. Finally, the light-emitting diodes are both extinguished, and the ambient light level is ascertained. This final measurement allows the oximeter to compensate for ambient light levels. Sequencing the light timing rapidly as an integral multiple of the power line frequency allows the system to avoid the light flicker pulsations found with fluorescent lights (Fig. 17–5).

To report SpO_2 accurately, the AC/DC ratio is calculated many times per second. Then, through the use of some clever algorithms, the ratio is converted into an estimate of the SaO_2. This estimate has been shown to be accurate at saturation levels above 90%, even when the AC/DC ratio multiplied by 100 is as low as 0.2%. When the ratio diminishes further, the pulse oximeter indicates that the saturation measurement may be in error.

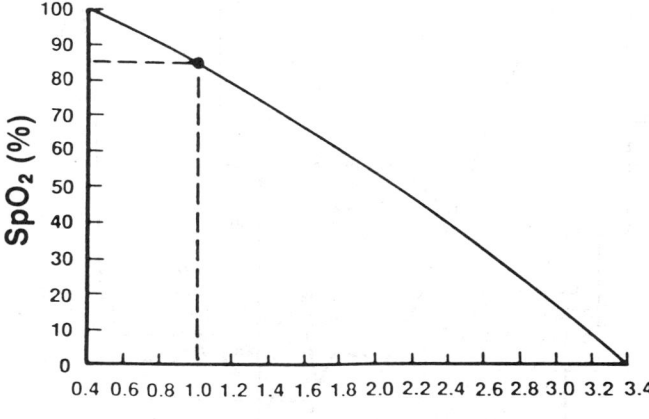

Figure 17–3. A typical pulse oximeter calibration curve. Note that the SaO_2 estimate is determined from the ratio (R) of the pulse-added red absorbance at 660 nm to pulse-added infrared absorbance at 940 nm. The ratios of red to infrared absorbances vary from approximately 0.4 at 100% saturation to 3.4 at 0% saturation. Note that the red-to-infrared absorbance is 1.0 at a saturation of approximately 85%. This curve can be approximately determined on a theoretic basis, but for accurate predictions of SpO_2, experimental data are required. (From Tremper KK, Barker SJ: Pulse oximetry. Anesthesiology 70:98, 1989.)

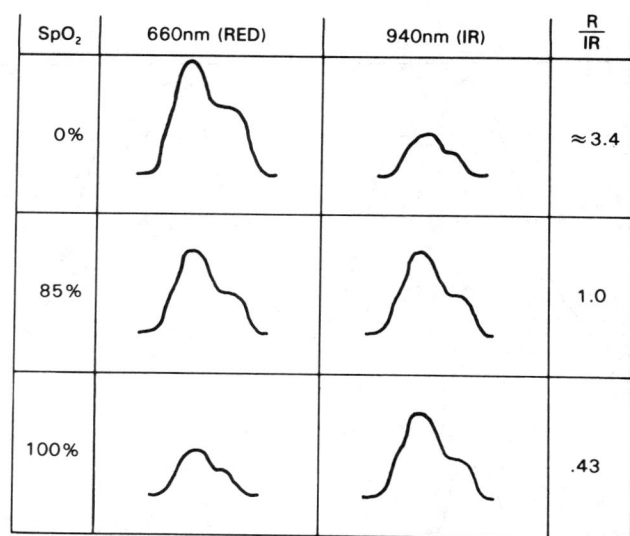

Figure 17–4. Relative plethysmographic signal amplitudes and SpO_2 values assuming the transmission intensities are equal. R = red; IR = infrared. (From Wukitsch MW, Petterson MT, Tobler DR, et al: Pulse oximetry: Analysis of theory, technology, and practice. Reprinted with permission from Journal of Clinical Monitoring, volume 4, pp 290–301, 1988.)

Clinical Application

The accuracy of pulse oximeters, confirmed by a number of studies, is remarkable. Generally, the manufacturers state the accuracy to be ±2% standard deviation (SD) for SpO_2 greater than 70% and ±3% SD for SpO_2 from 50 to 70%. This means that for values above 70%, 68% of the data can be expected to be within 2% of a line of identity and 95% of the data can be expected to be within 4%. Unfortunately, neither the bias nor the precision is indicated. The accuracy and responsiveness of the systems at lower levels are difficult to determine clinically.

Severinghaus and Sidi both investigated this accuracy question. In the study by Severinghaus and colleagues,[9] volunteers were subjected to severe and sudden desaturation to an SaO_2 of 40 to 70% (Fig. 17–6). A variety of pulse oximeters were used. The researchers found a lag time of about 15 seconds in the response of the ear probe after rapid desaturation and a much longer lag in the response of the finger probe (Fig. 17–7). The difference between the lag times of the two probes is probably a function of the difference in perfusion time constants. The inspired gas was suddenly oxygen enriched, but the lag time caused pulse oximeters to report a falling SpO_2 when SaO_2 was rising. The results among the different units cannot be exactly correlated because the averaging schemes vary among the units. Some pulse oximeters allow the operator to change the signal averaging time to "stabilize" the reading during disturbances.

Sidi and coworkers[10] investigated a steady-state desaturation condition in dogs. The hemoglobin of the dog has similar optical properties to human hemoglobin. The researchers found that the accuracy of pulse oximeter readings diminished at low saturations (Fig. 17–8).

Recognizing and Avoiding the Pitfalls of Pulse Oximetry

Perfusion to the measurement site must be sufficient to provide an adequate signal strength. If the patient is hypo-

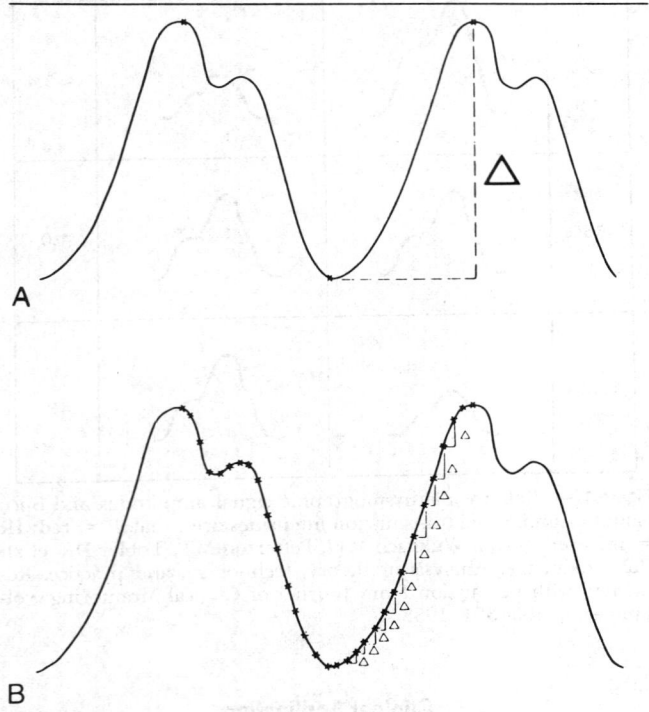

Figure 17–5. Changes in light intensity can be measured at the minimal and maximal points of the pulse wave or many times along the wave. X-X produces a change in the intensities (Δ) on both red and infrared wavelengths. *A* represents the change in light intensity from the minimal to the maximal point on the arterial pressure waveform from which saturation can be calculated once per heart beat. The multiple measurements depicted in *B* allow many sample points that can be subject to validation schemes, such as running weighted average. (From Wukitsch MW, Petterson MT, Tobler DR, et al: Pulse oximetry: Analysis of theory, technology, and practice. Reprinted with permission from Journal of Clinical Monitoring, volume 4, pp 290–301, 1988.)

Figure 17–6. The method of analysis of a step hypoxic test, showing the calculated saturation (Sco₂) from end-tidal Po₂ and Pco₂, and one pulse oximeter (Spo₂) response. The abrupt rise of a pulse oximeter recording was used to synchronize its trace with that of the calculated saturation value. The screen cursor was set to approximate mean values of the plateaus from 6 to 12 seconds before the end of each plateau. This setting accounts for blood transmission and sampling time and the one-breath lag between inspiration of an altered oxygen concentration and the recording of the Sco₂ from the subsequent end-tidal gases. The 9-second blood transmission time refers to the assumed lung-to-radial artery delay, not lung to finger or ear. (From Severinghaus JW, Naifeh KH, Koh SO: Errors in 14 pulse oximeters during profound hypoxia. Reprinted with permission from Journal of Clinical Monitoring, volume 5, pp 72–81, 1989.)

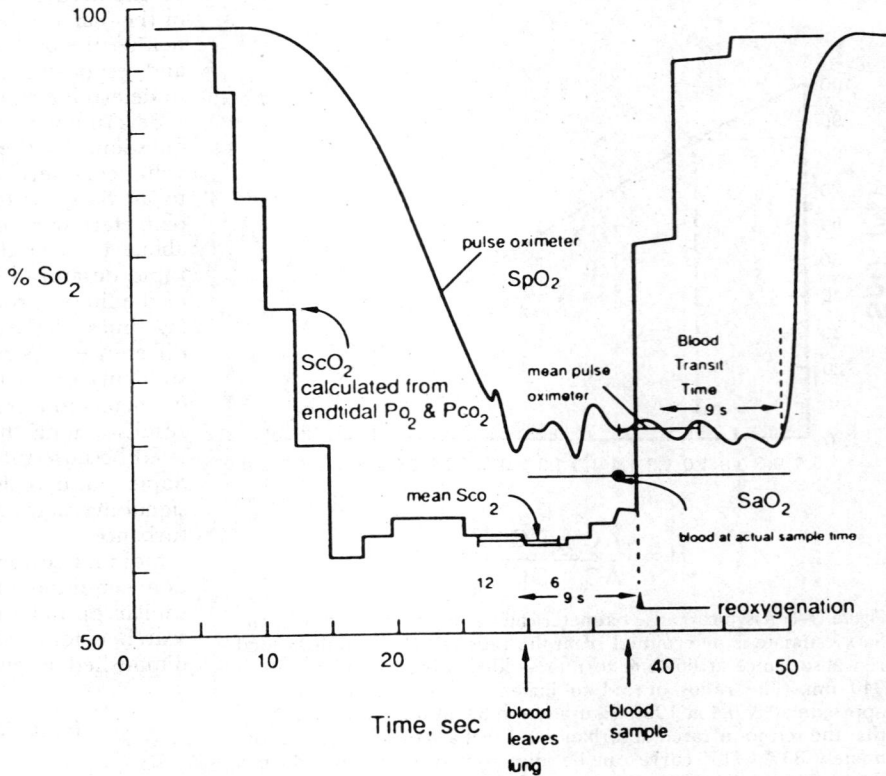

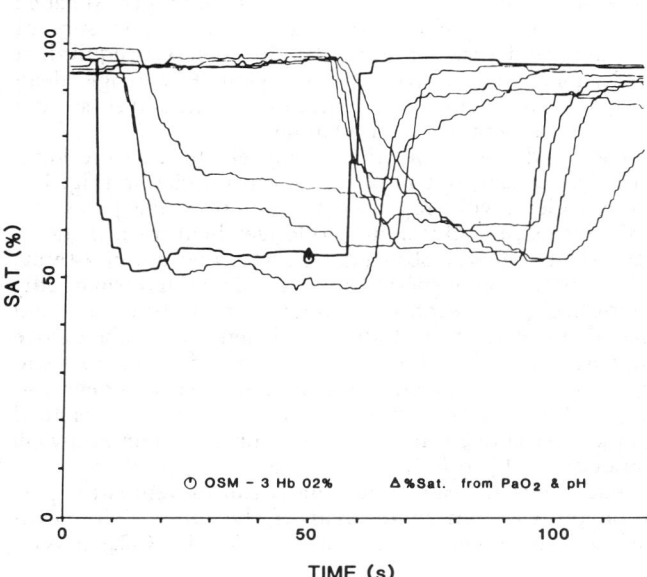

Figure 17–7. A typical step hypoxia test. The heavier line is calculated saturation, ScO_2. The symbols mark the measured blood HbO_2 percentage (O) and SaO_2 percentage calculated from pH and PO_2 (△). Simultaneous responses of three ear and four finger probes are shown. Finger response lag in this subject was about 50 seconds and ear lag was about 10 seconds. (From Severinghaus JW, Naifeh KH: Accuracy of response of six pulse oximeters to profound hypoxia. Anesthesiology 67:551, 1987.)

tensive or vasoconstricted because of hypothermia, drug therapy, or mechanical obstruction to flow, the AC portion of the signal may be insufficient. Correcting the cardiovascular problems or changing the measurement site may help. Local warming of the hand or foot can be helpful. Many of the instruments provide a signal indicative of pulse pressure.

Motion presents a different problem. Here, the instrument has difficulty distinguishing a cardiac-generated signal from an artifact created by motion. Mounting the probe securely to the site will help; however, mounting it too tightly can reduce perfusion and even cause local burns. Motion of the measurement site should always be minimized.

Because ambient light can be so bright as to overwhelm the sensor, it may be necessary to cover the probe with an opaque material such as foil. Frequently, moving the offending light source or covering the sensor with a towel will suffice.

In certain circumstances, hemoglobinopathies can be a problem. Barker and coworkers[11] artificially increased MetHb concentration in five dogs and found that pulse oximeters overestimate saturation in the presence of MetHb (Fig. 17–9). Fortunately, MetHb levels are usually less than 1%.

In an earlier study, Barker and Tremper[12] found that pulse oximeters tend to overestimate the SaO_2 by an amount roughly proportional to the percentage of COHb. For example, if the COHb is 10% and the SaO_2 is 80%, the SpO_2 will be 90%.

Vital dyes can affect pulse oximeter readings. Sidi and coworkers,[13] in a study with dogs, found that fluorescein did not affect pulse oximeter measurement, methylene blue decreased readings for about 30 minutes, and indocyanine green affected measurements for about 10 minutes.

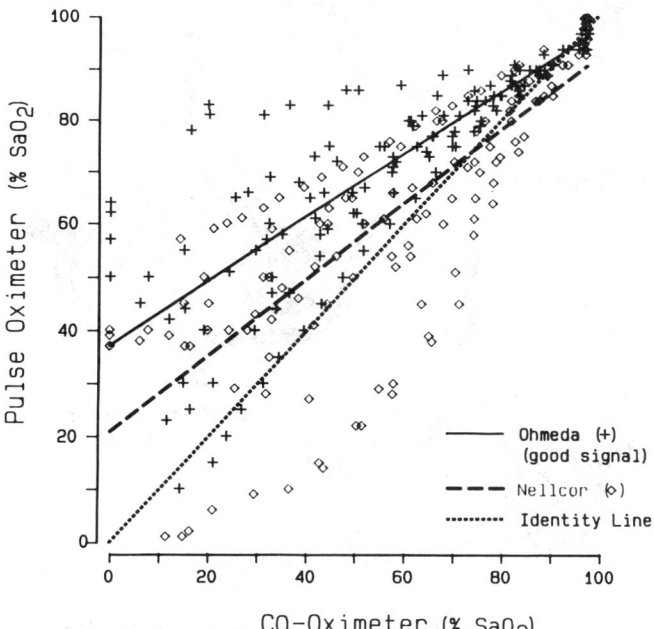

Figure 17–8. Linear regression analysis of the relationship between measurements of arterial hemoglobin oxygen saturation (SaO_2) obtained from an Ohmeda Biox 3700 pulse oximeter (+) and a Nellcor Model N-100 pulse oximeter (◇) as compared with corresponding values obtained with an IL 282 CO-Oximeter. Ohmeda versus CO-Oximeter regression line is represented by the dashes; Nellcor versus CO-Oximeter regression line is represented by the dots; the line of identity is solid. (From Sidi A, Rush W, Gravenstein N, et al: Pulse oximetry fails to accurately detect low levels of arterial hemoglobin oxygen saturation in dogs. Reprinted with permission from Journal of Clinical Monitoring, volume 3, pp 257–262, 1987.)

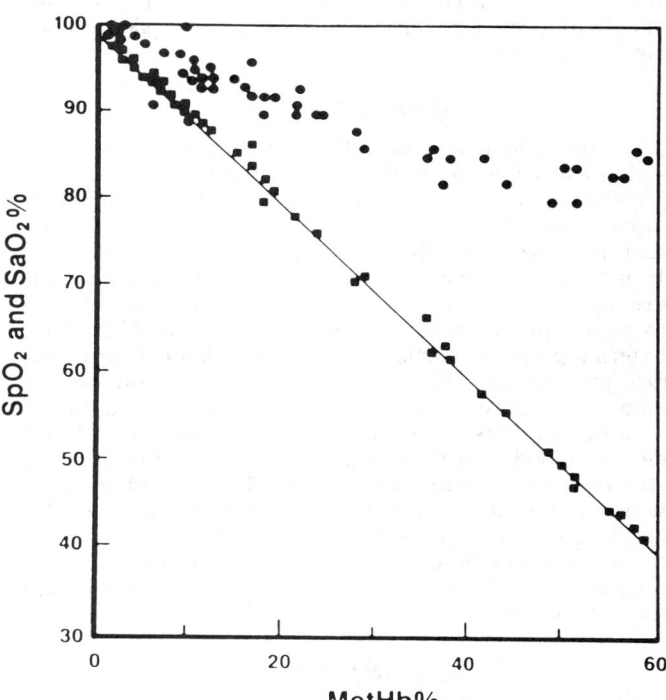

Figure 17–9. A plot of SpO_2 as reported by a Nellcor pulse oximeter (●) and SaO_2 as reported by an IL-282 (■) versus MetHb saturation (MetHb%) for FIO_2 = 1.0. The line represents SaO_2 = 100 – MetHb%. (From Barker SJ, Tremper KK: Effects of methemoglobinemia on pulse oximetry and mixed venous oximetry. Anesthesiology 70:112, 1989.)

Does Pulse Oximetry Help?

Proving effectiveness in monitoring has been problematic. A prospective study of 20,802 patients undergoing surgical procedures (excluding thoracic and neurologic operations) found that the presence or absence of pulse oximetry had no effect on the incidence of postoperative complications.[13a] However, pulse oximetry alerted anesthetists to the presence of hypoxemia and thus decreased the incidence of myocardial ischemia during anesthesia.[13b] Whether similar results occur in other areas of care remains to be seen.

Pulse oximetry has become a standard of practice in many medical jurisdictions. The American Society of Anesthesiologists has mandated its use for patients undergoing anesthesia. The Society of Critical Care Medicine designates capnography and the ability to measure transcutaneous P_{O_2} (P_{TCO_2}) as essential monitoring modalities for "the complicated, desperately ill patient."[13c] The Society of Critical Care Medicine also mandates that patients with acute respiratory failure who are receiving mechanical ventilatory support and whose cardiopulmonary status is unstable must have their circulation, oxygenation, and ventilation monitored continuously.[13d]

CAPNOGRAPHY

Capnography has been used for a number of years for specific clinical indications. In the operating room, for example, capnography helps clinicians detect air emboli and manage hyperventilation in patients undergoing neurosurgical operations. This latter application can be quite useful in the intensive care unit. More recently, however, capnography has found a routine place in the operating room, the emergency department, and a wide variety of intensive care units. Although capnography is probably just as important as pulse oximetry, clinical experience indicates that it is not as well understood as pulse oximetry and its applications are not as appreciated.

Physiologic Basis

For physiologic and pathologic reasons, pulmonary perfusion is usually not uniform to all alveoli. There are four physiologic causes of uneven or nonuniform pulmonary capillary blood flow.[14] First, blood flow is pulsatile. Hydrostatic pressure in the upright patient varies by approximately 15 mm Hg from the apex to the base of the lung. Even in the supine patient, hydrostatic pressure varies considerably from the uppermost to the most dependent part of the lung. External pressure, particularly from ventilators during positive pressure breathing, can exert great force on the pulmonary vasculature and thereby alter pulmonary resistence.

Pathologic reasons for nonuniform distribution of pulmonary blood flow include pulmonary emboli or thrombi, atherosclerotic disease, autoimmune disease, and compression of pulmonary vessels. Intraoperative "packing away" of the lung or the onset of a pneumothorax or hydrothorax can also contribute to pulmonary blood flow alterations, as can heart failure, shock, severe hypotension, and pulmonary arterial and venous shunts.

Ventilation

Just as pulmonary perfusion is nonuniform and at times not ideal, ventilation also varies, even across the lung fields of healthy persons. During both spontaneous breathing and mechanical ventilation, some ventilation is wasted. This wasted ventilation is termed *dead space*. If it is in the conducting airway (i.e., above the alveoli), it is called *anatomic dead space*. *Alveolar dead space* constitutes that amount of gas that enters alveoli but does not participate in gas exchange with the patient's blood with each breath. The sum of anatomic dead space and alveolar dead space is equivalent to physiologic dead space (Fig. 17–10). Physiologic dead space may be substantially increased during disease and certain intraoperative manipulations.

Like circulation, ventilation is uneven through the lung. Many factors can contribute to uneven ventilation (Fig. 17–11). In patients with emphysema, where pulmonary elasticity is diminished, the alveoli are no longer held open. Patients with regional airway obstruction, such as occurs in asthma, pulmonary cysts, or encroaching carcinoma, have markedly diminished gas flow rates. A combination of obstruction and changes in elasticity is found in patients with obstructive emphysema. If the alveoli cannot expand in response to airway pressure, a regional limitation to expansion develops. In patients with pneumonia, pleural effusion, interstitial disease, atelectasis, tumors, or even pneumothorax, alveoli cannot expand properly.

Ventilation-perfusion unevenness causes ventilation-perfusion mismatch in some areas of the lung. This means there is a difference in the carbon dioxide (CO_2) tension

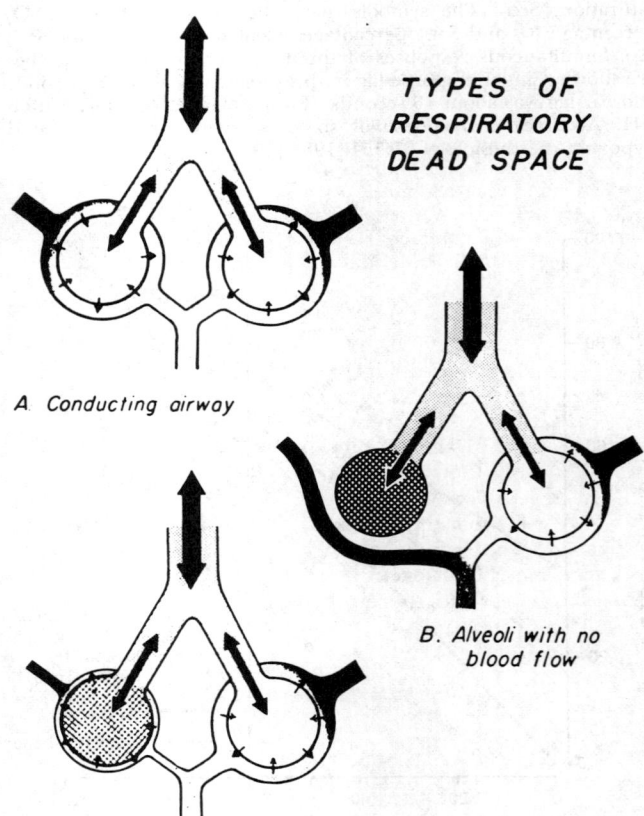

TYPES OF RESPIRATORY DEAD SPACE

A Conducting airway

B. Alveoli with no blood flow

C Ventilation in excess of blood flow

Figure 17–10. Circular parts of the structure represent the alveoli, where rapid gas exchange occurs. Arrows in the conducting airways signify the tidal volume entering and leaving the whole lung and its distribution to different regions. Width of the blood channel surrounding the alveoli indicates the volume of blood flow to each region: dark gray designates mixed venous blood entering and light gray indicates well-oxygenated blood leaving the pulmonary capillaries. Anatomic dead space is stippled. Physiologic dead space includes this and some (C) or all (B) of the gas volumes ventilating crosshatched areas. (From Forster RE II, DuBois AB, Briscoe WA, et al: The Lung: Physiologic Basis of Pulmonary Function Tests. 3rd ed. Chicago, Year Book Medical Publishers, p 38, 1986.)

CAUSES OF UNEVEN VENTILATION

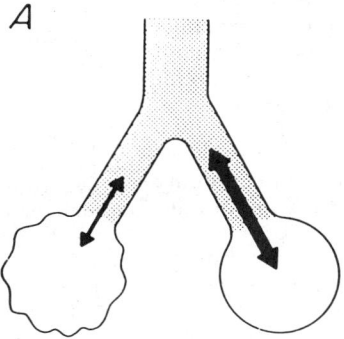

A

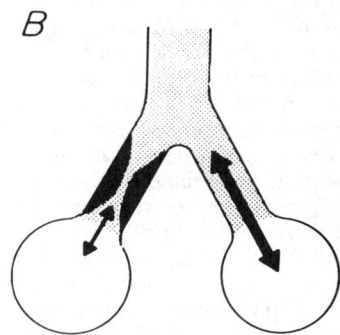

B

Regional changes in elasticity

Regional obstruction

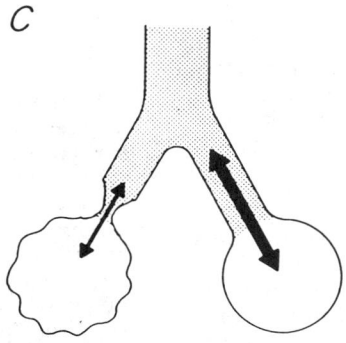

C

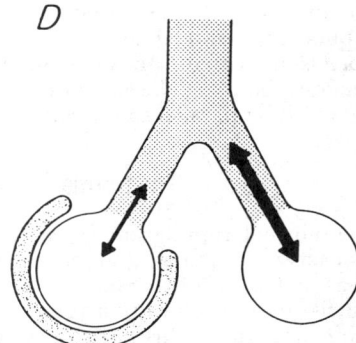

D

Regional dynamic compression

Regional limitation to expansion

Figure 17–11. Mechanisms responsible for nonuniform distribution of air ventilation. Circular areas represent the alveoli. The wavy lines in *A* and *C* designate alveoli that have lost their normal elastic recoil. The perialveolar band in *D* signifies alveoli that expand less than normally, although their elastic tissue is normal and there is no airway obstruction. Arrow size indicates the volume of gas ventilating each region. (From Forster RE II, DuBois AB, Briscoe WA, et al: The Lung: Physiologic Basis of Pulmonary Function Tests. 3rd ed. Chicago, Year Book Medical Publishers, p 50, 1986.)

between mixed end-capillary blood and mixed alveolar gas. For example, if there is an obstruction to gas flow into and out of alveolus A, then ventilation of alveolus B will exceed that of A (Fig. 17–12). If pulmonary blood flow is the same to both alveoli, the ratio of ventilation to blood flow will be altered. Mixed venous CO_2 will clearly be the same for both alveoli. We assume the end-pulmonary capillary blood PCO_2 is equal to that of alveolar gas for each alveolus. PCO_2, however, may be different in each alveolus because alveolus A is obstructed and therefore less ventilated than alveolus

B. For example, if alveolus B has a PCO_2 of 40 torr and alveolus A has a PCO_2 of 50 torr, the PCO_2 of the mixed blood from both A and B, assuming they are of the same blood volume, will be 45 torr.

Expired alveolar CO_2 concentration depends on the volume of each alveolus and the partial pressure of mixed venous CO_2. For example, if there are 3.0 L in alveolus B and 1.0 L in alveolus A, then the expired alveolar gas will have a PCO_2 of 42.5 torr. The difference between the alveolar and arterial concentrations of CO_2 is 45 − 42.5, or 2.5 torr.

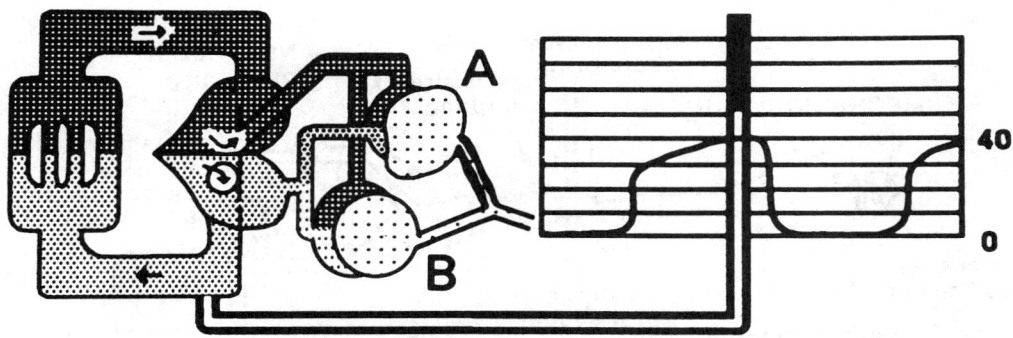

Figure 17–12. The partially obstructed airway. One bronchus (A) is partially obstructed as might be seen with asthma. The alveoli empty unevenly, and part of the lung is poorly ventilated but well perfused. An increased gradient of arterial to end-tidal PCO_2 results in a typical sloped plateau of the capnogram. As long as the plateau of the capnogram continues to rise, expiration continues; arterial values can therefore become significantly higher than end-tidal values of PCO_2. (From Gravenstein JS, Paulus DA, Hayes TJ: Capnography in Clinical Practice. Stoneham, MA, Butterworth, p 83, 1989.)

Monitoring Airway Carbon Dioxide

Airway CO_2 is monitored by the use of a capnograph. A capnograph is an instrument that indicates the presence and quantity of CO_2 in airway gases. A capnogram is a graphic plot of the concentration of CO_2 as a function of time. Although the digital representation of inspired and expired CO_2 is helpful, it can be misleading when compared with the values reported by the capnometer. For example, in the presence of uneven ventilation or respiratory effort, the portion designated by the capnogram to represent end-tidal CO_2 may not be truly end tidal. Therefore, it is important to analyze the capnogram when accuracy is desired.

Basically, there are two different types of capnographs. In one type, the sensor is mounted on the airway—either on a mask over the patient's face or on an endotracheal tube. An attractive feature of this type of capnograph is that measurements are not delayed by gas sampling, but the unit's bulk and weight may be objectionable. The other way to analyze gases in the airway is to place a small capillary tube at the location where gas is to be sampled. A small quantity of gas is removed continuously, delivered to the capnograph, and analyzed. The location of the analyzing port is important. In small infants, some clinicians even suggest obtaining the gas sample from the trachea from a second tube parallel to the endotracheal tube or within it.

The Normal Capnogram

A normal capnogram resembles the outline of a snake that has just swallowed an elephant, and it has four distinct phases (Fig. 17–13). Phase 1 is the tail of the snake and usually indicates 0 CO_2; it represents most of inspiration on the capnogram. This horizontal portion gives way to phase 2, which is the sharp ascent of the tail of the elephant. This phase corresponds with the appearance of CO_2 at the analyzer during exhalation. Phase 3 is the plateau, which is the back of the elephant proceeding toward its head. The plateau is usually relatively horizontal and represents a continuing part of exhalation during which most if not all of the gas at the sampling port is alveolar. Dead space gas has been replaced with CO_2-laden alveolar gas. Phase 4 occurs during inspiration and corresponds to the appearance of fresh gas and the washing out of CO_2 from the analyzer. The downstroke of phase 4 continues until the baseline is reached, where phase 1 begins again.

To demonstrate the four phases of the capnogram, a mechanical equivalent was configured (Fig. 17–14). Figure

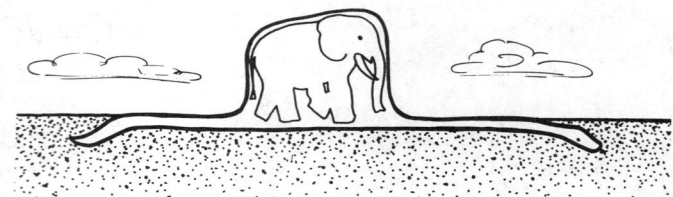

Figure 17–13. The "capnophant." The normal capnogram has the outline of an elephant swallowed by a snake hiding under sand. (From Gravenstein JS, Paulus DA, Hayes TJ: Capnography in Clinical Practice. Stoneham, MA, Butterworth, p 11, 1989.)

17–15 shows the relationship among the capnogram, pressure, flow, and tidal volume (V_T). Changing the rate of sampling flow can, in some instruments, alter the shape of the capnogram (Fig. 17–16).

The Abnormal Capnogram

Phase 1: Abnormal Baseline

If phase 1 of the capnogram is elevated, CO_2 is being inspired. This condition is not usual and not dangerous for the patient, but it may indicate a malfunction in some ventilating systems. If it is a "to-and-fro" ventilating system, then CO_2 may well be inspired. In a unidirectional ventilating system, however, only a malfunction or extremely shallow breaths (panting) can cause rebreathing of CO_2. If there is an extremely high respiratory rate, the frequency response of the system may be insufficient, and CO_2 is never cleared from the analyzer (Fig. 17–17).

Phase 2

The slope of phase 2 of the capnogram is important to consider. A slope that is not close to vertical but is more slanted instead may indicate that a sidestream analyzer has a prolonged sampling time. It may also indicate a partial occlusion of the sampling tube, which can happen frequently when there is moisture in the capillary tubing. The capnogram may also be slanted by prolonged exhalation, which indicates uneven or slow emptying of alveoli. The dead space is slowly cleared, which leads to slurring of the phase 2 portion of the curve. Biphasic capnograms secondary to kyphoscoliosis, secretions, endobronchial placement of an

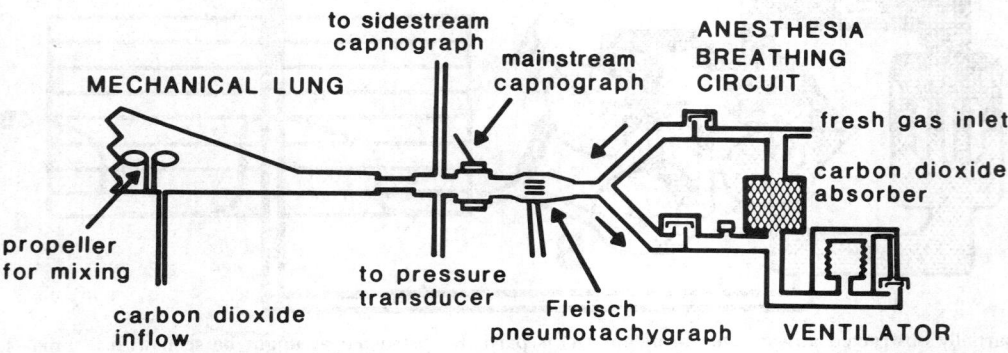

Figure 17–14. Equipment configuration to demonstrate the relationships between the capnogram and the pressure, flow, and volume of gas. CO_2, 300 mL/min, was infused into a mechanical lung in which a fan stirred the gas. The lung was connected to an anesthesia circle system with a ventilator, and both a mainstream and a sidestream capnograph were attached. (From Gravenstein JS, Paulus DA, Hayes TJ: Capnography in Clinical Practice. Stoneham, MA, Butterworth, p 13, 1989.)

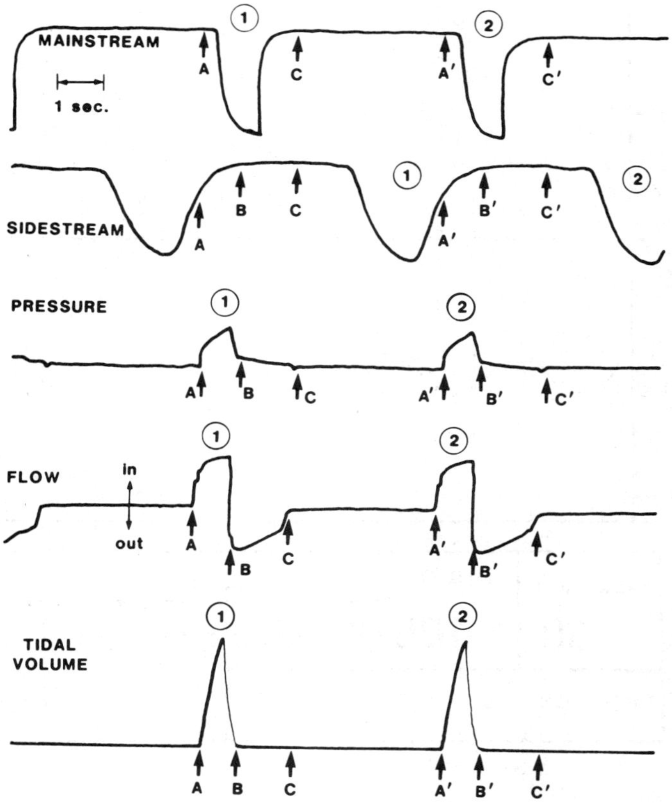

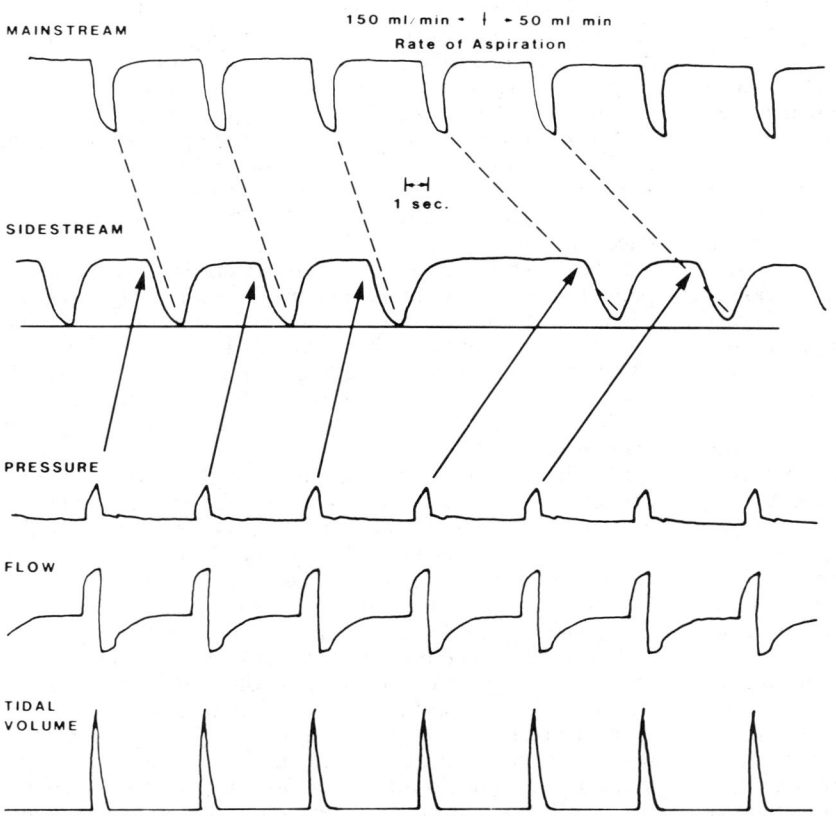

Figure 17–15. Capnograms and pressure, flow, and tidal volume. Data obtained experimentally (see Fig. 17–14) are from a Hewlett-Packard mainstream capnograph, a Datascope sidestream capnograph, a pressure transducer (upstroke = increased pressure), and a Fleisch pneumotachygraph for flow (upstroke = inspiration) and inspiratory tidal volume. The curves were recorded by a Grass polygraph, which records in a circular path. The arrows point to identical times but are not perfectly aligned because of the way traces are recorded. For breath 1, observe that pressure, flow, and volume are recorded nearly simultaneously at A; the capnogram of the mainstream analyzer responds in less than 0.5 second. B indicates the moment of flow reversal (from inspiration to expiration). At C, all flow ceases, but the mainstream capnogram registers CO_2 that remains under the sensor. Thus, capnographic evidence of CO_2 is indicated even though there is no gas flow. For breath 2 (A'), gas begins to flow again and the cycle repeats. The capnogram of the sidestream analyzer is almost one full breath out of phase. It shows deflections from previous expirations at A and A'. (From Gravenstein JS, Paulus DA, Hayes TJ: Capnography in Clinical Practice. Stoneham, MA, Butterworth, p 14, 1989.)

Figure 17–16. The effect of rate of sampling flow on sidestream analyzers. Sampling at a flow rate of 150 mL/min with an experimental model (see Figs. 17–14 and 17–15), a capnogram from a sidestream analyzer indicates almost identical data as the capnogram from the mainstream analyzer (the inspired values are slightly elevated on the sidestream capnogram). However, when the sampling rate is reduced to 50 mL/min, the sidestream capnograph does not have time to return to baseline before the next breath begins. Here it falsely reports CO_2 at 7 mm Hg during phase 4. With fast sampling, the respiratory pause and thus the plateau phase are long enough for the slower sidestream analyzer to reach its full response. Therefore, in the examples shown here, peak expired values of sidestream and mainstream capnograms are similar for the first three breaths. Slow sampling with a sidestream analyzer when respiratory rate is high can result in erroneous values during inspiration and expiration. (From Gravenstein JS, Paulus DA, Hayes TJ: Capnography in Clinical Practice. Stoneham, MA, Butterworth, p 15, 1989.)

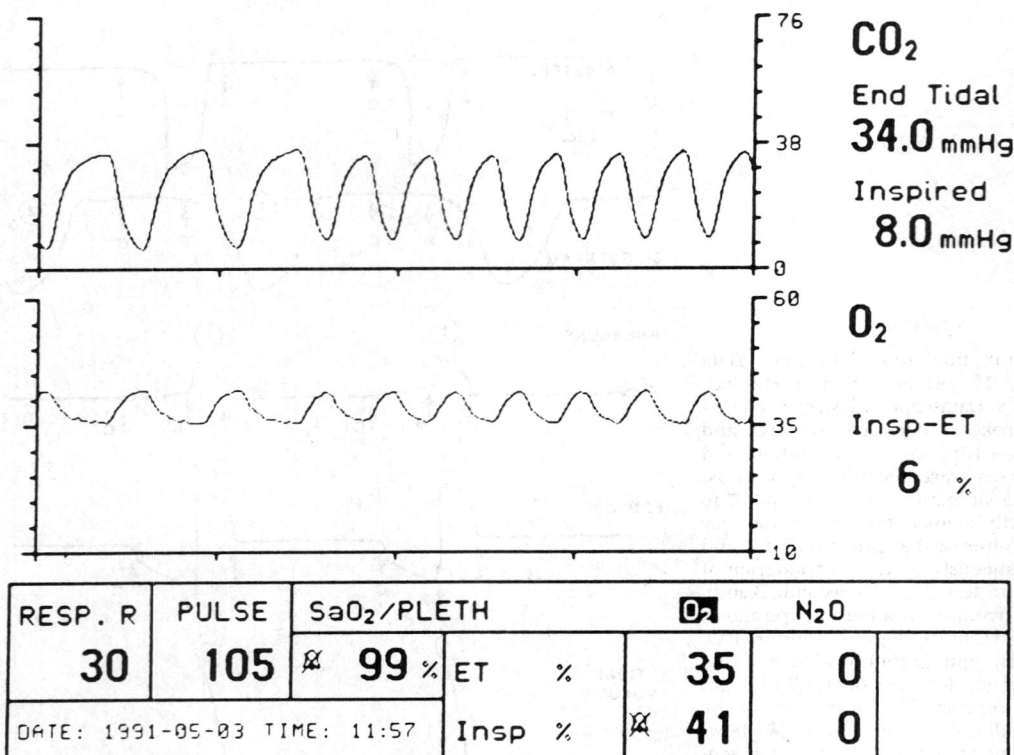

RESP. R	PULSE	SaO2/PLETH		O2	N2O
30	105	⌀ 99 %	ET %	35	0
DATE: 1991-05-03 TIME: 11:57		Insp %	⌀ 41	0

CO2
End Tidal
34.0 mmHg
Inspired
8.0 mmHg

O2
Insp-ET
6 %

Figure 17-17. A change in respiratory rate markedly alters the capnogram. Here, the patient's respiratory rate was voluntarily increased so that the gas at the analyzer was not cleared, which led to rebreathing. The indicated end-tidal CO_2 will decrease as well.

endotracheal tube, and altered mechanics after a single lung transplant have been seen (Fig. 17–18).

Phase 3: The Plateau

An elevated plateau (i.e., an end-tidal PCO2 [PETCO2] of greater than 44 torr) may indicate hypoventilation, increased production of CO_2, inhibition of nerve impulses to respiratory muscles, blockade of neuromuscular junction, weak respiratory muscle function, or obstructed airways, either intrinsic or extrinsic (Fig. 17–19).

There are also abnormally low plateaus. A plateau below 36 torr indicates that ventilation may be in excess of that needed to properly remove CO_2. Conversely, an increase in dead space may cause the capnogram to report low PETCO2 levels while arterial CO_2 levels are relatively high. In this case, ventilation of unperfused segments of lung causes gas free of CO_2 to mix with gas laden with CO_2, which results in a low PETCO2 tension.

Sometimes, the plateau associated with phase 3 is not smooth but is accentuated with bumps and dips. In Figure 17–20, a small breath appears as a dip in the plateau. The capnogram shows that the patient is making inspiratory effort during what is normally the expiratory phase. This perturbation could also be a hiccup or a disturbance in the capnogram brought on by clinical maneuvers. A breathlet may be the only evidence of a patient struggling to inhale oxygen.

A slanted plateau is most often associated with patients suffering from asthma or chronic obstructive lung disease. It indicates uneven or sequential emptying of both lungs. A leak around an endotracheal tube can allow other gas to dilute the exhaled gas carrying CO_2, and the plateau shown by the capnogram may be reduced proportional to the size of the leak.

Capnometers are also used during cardiac resuscitation. Schoonees[15] reported three cases in which capnography gave an early warning of ineffective cardiac massage or impending cardiovascular failure. Later, in a report of 13 episodes of cardiac arrest in 10 critically ill patients, Falk and coworkers[16] found that PETCO2 is a reliable indicator of the effectiveness of cardiopulmonary resuscitation. PETCO2 rises slightly during cardiopulmonary resuscitation and increases dramatically after successful resuscitation (Fig. 17–21).

During insertion of an automatic, implantable cardiac defibrillator, the device is tested by first inducing ventricular fibrillation. PETCO2 decreases rapidly after fibrillation and increases incrementally with defibrillation and return of adequate circulation (Fig. 17–22).

It has been suggested that inadvertent intubation of the patient's esophagus should not produce any CO_2. Actually, when a patient is ventilated by mask, some CO_2 may be entrained into the stomach. Carbonated beverages also cause CO_2 to be detected with esophageal intubation. However, if one "ventilates" a patient with an endotracheal tube located in the esophagus, the PETCO2 will drop substantially with every breath.[17, 18]

Slow inspiration or rebreathing of CO_2 is indicated by a capnogram in which phase 4 is slanted. An oscillatory pattern in phase 4 of the capnogram represents cardiogenic oscillations, which are small breathlets induced by pressure changes within the lung during the cardiac cycle (Fig. 17–23).

It is tempting to use capnography to estimate PaCO2. In anesthetized patients, several investigators have found a 1- to 5-torr difference between arterial and end-tidal CO_2.[19, 20] It was surmised that the gradient did not change significantly, so PETCO2 would be a good predictor of PaCO2, at least in patients undergoing anesthesia. This presumption was challenged in a study of 15 patients undergoing major surgery and was found to be in error. The difference between PaCO2 and PETCO2 reached 12 torr, and the patients were not critically ill.[21]

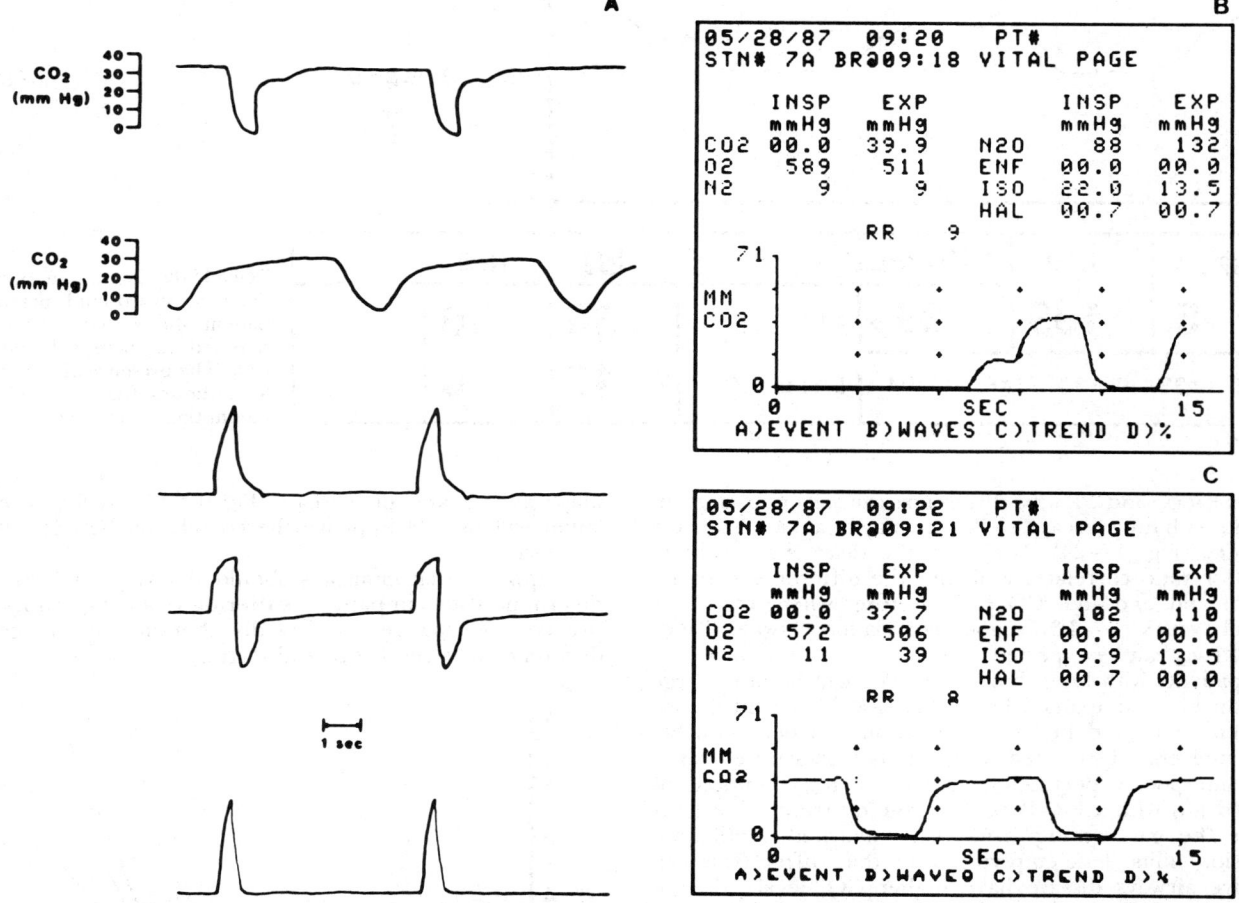

Figure 17–18. Capnogram showing uneven emptying of the lungs. A mechanical lung (see Fig. 17–15) with two bellows was connected to a trachea via two mainstem bronchi. *A*. Tracings *(from top to bottom)* are from a mainstream capnograph, a pressure transducer, and a pneumotachygraph (for flow and tidal volume). For one lung, compliance was set at 0.02 L/cm H_2O and bronchial resistance at 2.5 cm H_2O/L/s; the values for the other lung were set at 0.05 L/cm H_2O and 55 cm H_2O/L/s, respectively. During ventilation, the mainstream capnogram *(top tracing)* has a step increase in the plateau, which corresponds to one lung emptying before the other. The sidestream capnogram *(second tracing from top)* has a sloped plateau. The same type of capnogram was obtained from a patient under general anesthesia whose lungs emptied unevenly *(B)*. After the trachea was suctioned *(C)*, the capnogram returned to normal. Presumably, suctioning removed a mucous plug that had partially occluded one lung. (From Gravenstein JS, Paulus DA, Hayes TJ: Capnography in Clinical Practice. Stoneham, MA, Butterworth, p 22, 1989.)

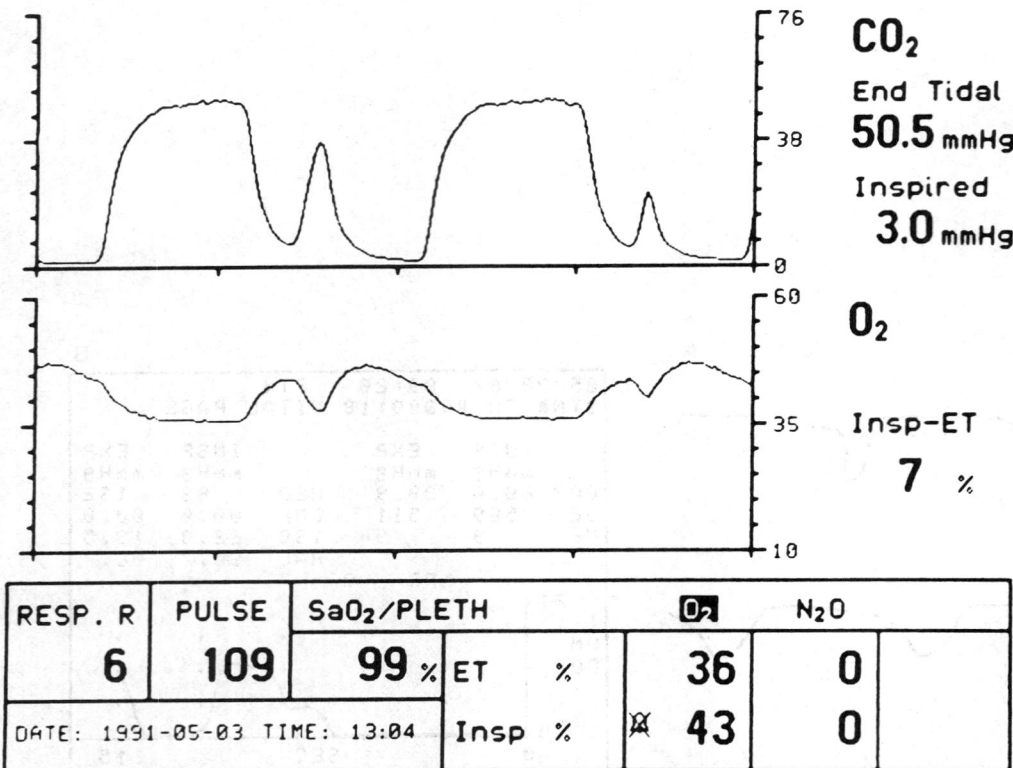

RESP. R	PULSE	SaO₂/PLETH			O₂	N₂O	
6	**109**	**99** %	ET	%	**36**	**0**	
DATE: 1991-05-03 TIME: 13:04			Insp	%	**43**	**0**	

Figure 17–19. Capnogram of a partially paralyzed and narcotized patient shows that hypoventilation led to increased end-tidal CO_2. The presence of the breathlet indicates that the patient is attempting to breathe.

The $PaCO_2$ and $PETCO_2$ difference can be quite large in patients with lung disease, so $PETCO_2$ may be a poor estimator of $PaCO_2$ (Fig. 17–24). However, the dead space volume (VDS)/VT ratio correlates well with the difference between arterial and end-tidal CO_2.[22] Therefore, when VDS/VT is normal ($VDS/VT \approx 2.3$), a good correlation between $PaCO_2$ and $PETCO_2$ can be expected.

In patients with lung disease, VDS/VT can be quite large and can be accompanied by an increase in the difference between $PaCO_2$ and $PETCO_2$. Ventilation and perfusion become unevenly distributed. Lung units that are well-ventilated but poorly perfused contribute a large amount of exhaled gas with a low PCO_2. Gas coming from these units dilutes the gas coming from better-matched ventilation-perfusion units. Late-emptying units that suffer from obstructive airways disease have higher CO_2 levels, do not contain as much volume, and may not empty completely before the next inhalation. The difference between $PaCO_2$ and $PETCO_2$ again widens. If $PETCO_2$ decreases, it may be associated with an equal decrease in $PaCO_2$. However, if the ventilation/perfusion ratio ($\dot{V}/\dot{Q}$) has worsened, the $PaCO_2$ may stay the same or increase (Fig. 17–25). A forced exhalation will usually improve the correlation between $PaCO_2$ and $PETCO_2$.

It appears that clinicians should not rely on $PETCO_2$ to determine $PaCO_2$ in patients suffering from respiratory failure because changes in $\dot{V}/\dot{Q}$ distribution can change the difference between $PaCO_2$ and $PETCO_2$.

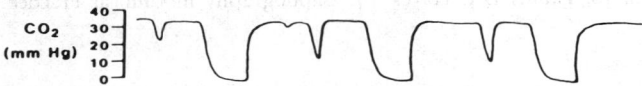

Figure 17–20. Capnogram showing a breathlet in the plateau (phase 3). This capnogram shows a patient making inspiratory efforts during mechanical ventilation, but the capnogram cannot reveal the circumstances of the inspiratory effort. Only examination of the patient and analysis of all clinical factors can guide the clinician in deciding to adjust the ventilator, administer drugs, or initiate other maneuvers. The patient's minute ventilation, level of anesthesia, degree of muscle relaxation, and metabolic state and the impact of external stimuli require consideration. (From Gravenstein JS, Paulus DA, Hayes TJ: Capnography in Clinical Practice. Stoneham, MA, Butterworth, p 19, 1989.)

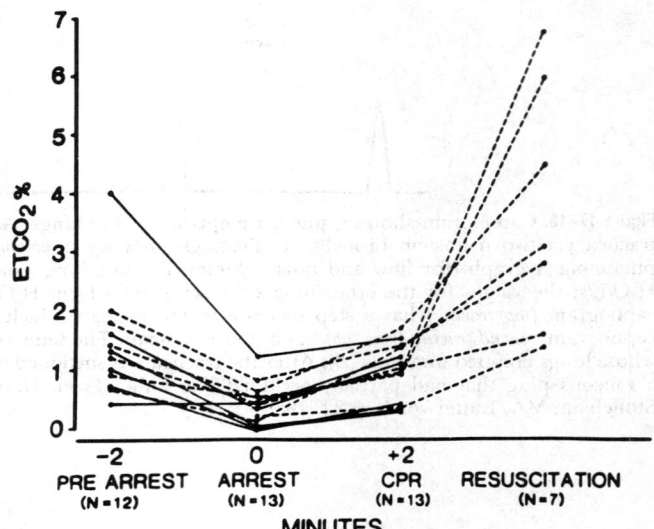

Figure 17–21. End-tidal CO_2 concentration before cardiac arrest, at the onset of cardiac arrest, 2 minutes after the start of cardiopulmonary resuscitation (CPR), and immediately after successful resuscitation. Solid lines represent nonresuscitated patients; broken lines represent resuscitated patients. (From Falk JL, Rackow EC, Weil MH: End-tidal carbon dioxide concentration during cardiopulmonary resuscitation. Reprinted by permission of the New England Journal of Medicine, 318; 607–611, 1988.)

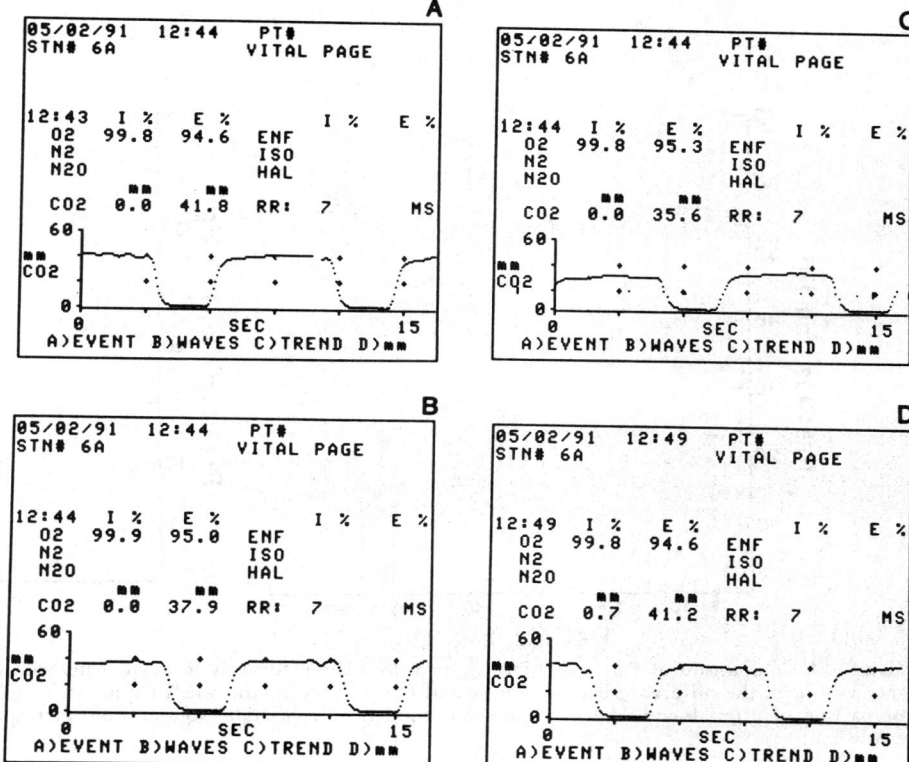

Figure 17–22. Capnogram after fibrillation of the heart. With each breath, end-tidal CO_2 falls until circulation is re-established with defibrillation.

AIRWAY OXYGEN MONITORING

Inspired oxygen monitoring has been essentially mandatory in ventilators for several years because clinicians have recognized the deleterious effects of both hyperoxia and hypoxemia. Inspired oxygen concentration can be regulated according to clinical needs. In addition, inspired oxygen monitoring can reduce the incidence of disasters caused by problems with oxygen supply.

Most hospitals have centralized oxygen supplies. Oxygen is delivered in liquid form and stored in large, insulated tanks; gaseous oxygen is stored in much smaller tanks as back-up and also for patient transport. The oxygen in gaseous form is piped throughout the hospital, and the pressure in the pipes is monitored continuously. Fittings are keyed through an index system so that only those expressly designed to handle the specific gas in question, in this case oxygen, can be used. Unfortunately, this system is not failsafe, and accidents have happened when pipes were crossed or the wrong gas was delivered to the hospital.

The only way to guard against such accidents is to monitor, as close to the airway as possible, the gas delivered to the patient and to monitor it specifically for oxygen. Several methods are used by oxygen analyzers. Most are standalone, single-function instruments that use either the polarographic or fuel cell method. The polarographic analyzer is based on the principle of the Clark electrode. Oxygen diffuses through a membrane covering a charged metal electrode and is reduced at the electrode. The current generated is a function of the amount of oxygen reaching the electrode, which is a function of the oxygen concentration being determined. The electrodes are changed about every 3 months and batteries may need changing just as often. Calibration is needed frequently. To avoid changing batteries, analyzers may be equipped with a reference metal in the electrode that creates a current. The reference metal obviates the need for a battery, but the analyzer still requires daily calibration and relatively frequent maintenance. Both these systems can work well but are additionally limited by a slow response time. They cannot respond quickly enough to measure both inspired and expired oxygen concentrations. Other technology is needed to accomplish this. The paramagnetic, Raman, hot zirconium wire, and mass spectrometry methods all allow inspired and expired measurements.[23, 24]

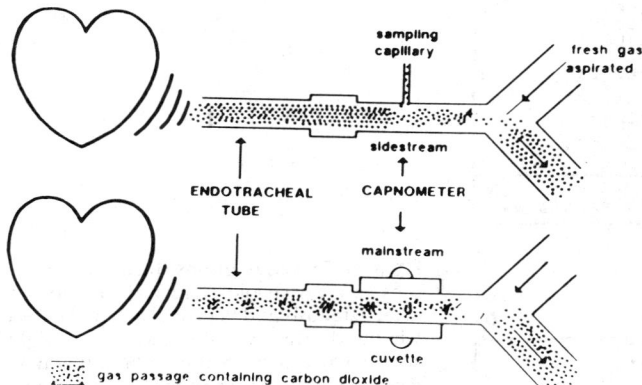

Figure 17–23. Causes of cardiogenic oscillations in the capnogram. Cardiogenic oscillations affect capnograms in different ways. A sidestream analyzer removes CO_2 from the sampling site and simultaneously pulls in fresh gas; the effect of the heartbeat on the gas column—here assumed to be filled with the homogeneous CO_2—registers on the capnogram because the CO_2 is mixed with fresh gas (*top*). With sidestream analyzers, this type of cardiogenic oscillation only occurs just before inspiration. Cardiogenic oscillation, however, can also be observed in the tracheal tube (and at the mouth) when cardiac activity propels gas from different segments of the lungs when they empty unevenly and have ventilation-to-perfusion abnormalities of varying degrees (*bottom*). This type of cardiogenic oscillation would be reflected on the capnogram from both sidestream and mainstream analyzers. (From Gravenstein JS, Paulus DA, Hayes TJ: Capnography in Clinical Practice. Stoneham, MA, Butterworth, p 29, 1989.)

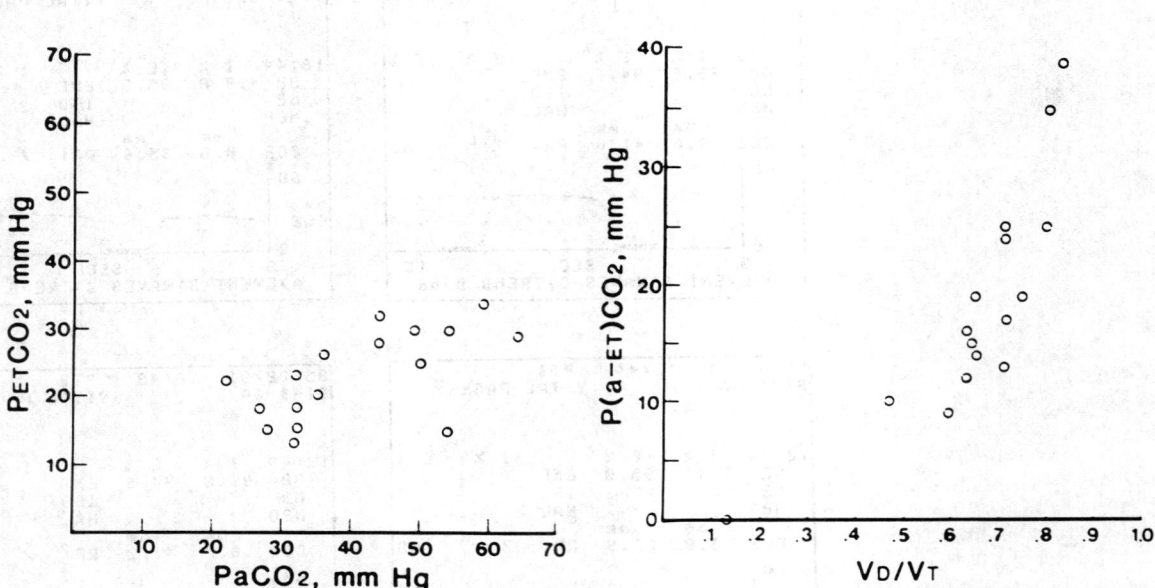

Figure 17–24. Comparison of $Paco_2$ and $Petco_2$ measured simultaneously in 17 patients with respiratory failure. $Petco_2$ does not predict $Paco_2$ well *(left)*; the difference between $Paco_2$ and $Petco_2$ predicts the Vds/Vt quite well *(right)*. (Modified from Yamanaka MK, Sue DY: Comparison of arterial–end-tidal Pco_2 difference and dead space/tidal volume ratio in respiratory failure. Chest 92:832–835, 1987, by permission.)

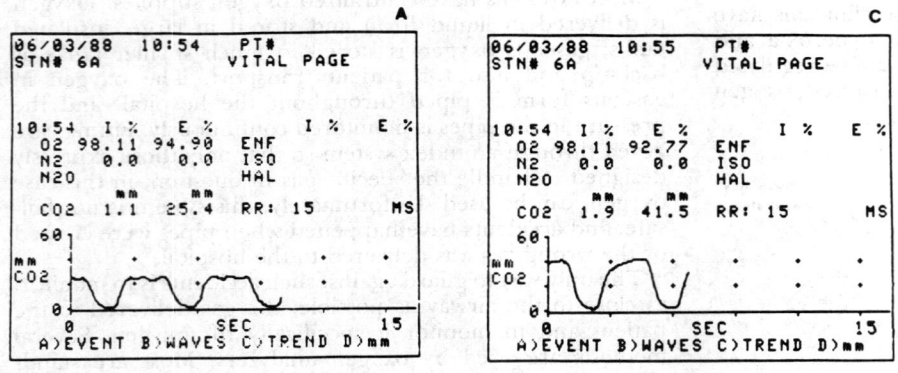

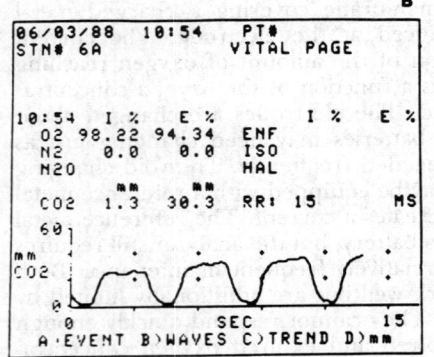

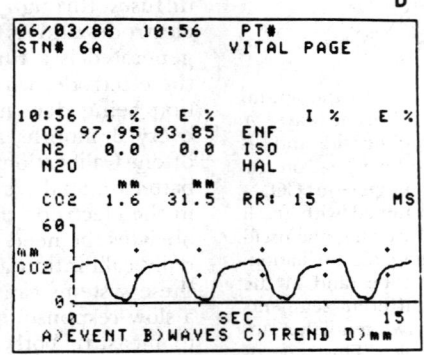

Figure 17–25. Capnograms during thoracotomy in a 2-year-old child with pulmonary artery stenosis and ventricular septal defect who underwent anastomosis of the right subclavian artery to the right pulmonary artery. *A.* Right lung compressed and subclavian and pulmonary artery clamped; $Paco_2$ is 58 mm Hg. *B.* Immediately after unclamping the vessels; $Paco_2$ rises immediately. *C.* One minute later. The lung is fully reinflated; dead space and shunt are reduced. *D.* Two minutes after unclamping. The $Paco_2$ is now 38 mm Hg. The arterial-to-alveolar Pco_2 gradient has dropped from 30 to 7 mm Hg. (From Gravenstein JS, Paulus DA, Hayes TJ: Capnography in Clinical Practice. Stoneham, MA, Butterworth, p 89, 1989.)

Clinical application of inspired and expired oxygen concentration measurement is rather recent. The inhaled oxygen fraction (FIO_2) of an endotracheally intubated patient is usually that of the delivered oxygen fraction unless air is entrained during inspiration or rebreathing is taking place. Factors that affect exhaled oxygen concentration (FEO_2) include oxygen consumption, oxygen delivery, and oxygen transport (cardiac output). The relationship is expressed by the equation

$$VO_2 = V(FIO_2 - FEO_2)$$

This equation is the numerator for the Fick equation. The Fick equation determines cardiac output by dividing oxygen consumption by the difference between arterial and mixed venous oxygen contents. Davies and colleagues[25] compared continuous Fick cardiac output to thermodilution. The thermodilution determinations were higher, particularly in low flow states, probably reflecting indicator loss as the cooled blood is warmed as it passes to the pulmonary artery.

In another application of inspired and expired oxygen concentration measurement, Linko and Paloheimo[26] anesthetized six pigs and subjected them to incrementally decreasing minute ventilation at inspired oxygen levels that varied from 0.2 to 1.0. They measured inspired and expired CO_2, oxygen, and N_2O and found that the difference between FIO_2 and $PETO_2$ was the most sensitive indicator of hypoventilation (Fig. 17–26). A breath-by-breath recording shows the rapid change in $PETO_2$ with a sudden decrease in ventilation (Fig. 17–27).

Oxygen uptake, if it can be measured, is a good indicator of a change in metabolic rate. For example, de las Alas and coworkers[27] found that oxygen consumption responded immediately and temperature lagged as an indicator in animals that were given 2,4-dinitrophenol to induce hyperthermia (Figs. 17–28 and 17–29).

Using end-tidal oxygen concentration, as an approximation of alveolar concentration, in combination with inspired concentration to find a value difference that can be monitored continuously may prove useful. In healthy persons, this difference is 4 to 5%, but the gap widens rapidly in response to hypoventilation or insufficient cardiac output. The increased difference is an indication that oxygenation at the cellular level is insufficient.

CUTANEOUS OXYGEN

Although the common name for the technique of measuring oxygen on the skin surface is *transcutaneous* measurement, the term *cutaneous* is probably more precise because the gases measured are those of the skin and its blood vessels.

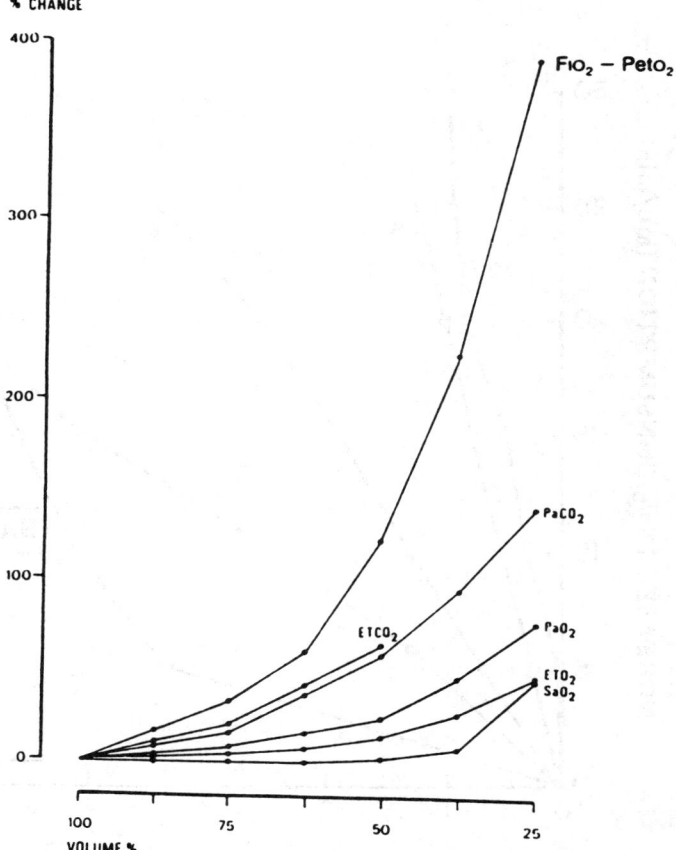

Figure 17–26. Percent change in the end-tidal gas concentrations, arterial blood gases, and SpO_2 (compared with the initial normoventilation values) during progressive hypoventilation. Each dot refers to a mean of seven determinations. (From L Linko, M Paloheimo, Inspiratory end-tidal oxygen content difference: A sensitive indicator of hypoventilation, Crit Care Med, volume 17, pp 345–348, © by Williams & Wilkins, 1989.)

In 1951, Baumberger and Goodfriend[28] demonstrated that a finger placed in a 45°C phosphate buffer would cause the PO_2 of the buffer to approach that of PaO_2 in 15 to 60 minutes. The secret to their success was heating the skin from 37°C, where the PO_2 on the surface would be close to 0. Twenty-two years after Baumberger and Goodfriend published their findings, Huch and colleagues[29] used the Clark polarographic electrode in combination with a heating

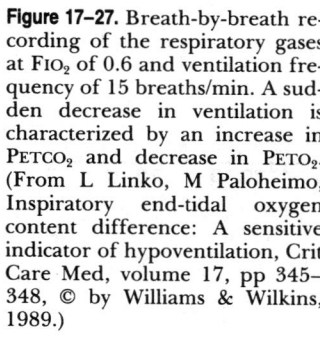

Figure 17–27. Breath-by-breath recording of the respiratory gases at FIO_2 of 0.6 and ventilation frequency of 15 breaths/min. A sudden decrease in ventilation is characterized by an increase in $PETCO_2$ and decrease in $PETO_2$. (From L Linko, M Paloheimo, Inspiratory end-tidal oxygen content difference: A sensitive indicator of hypoventilation, Crit Care Med, volume 17, pp 345–348, © by Williams & Wilkins, 1989.)

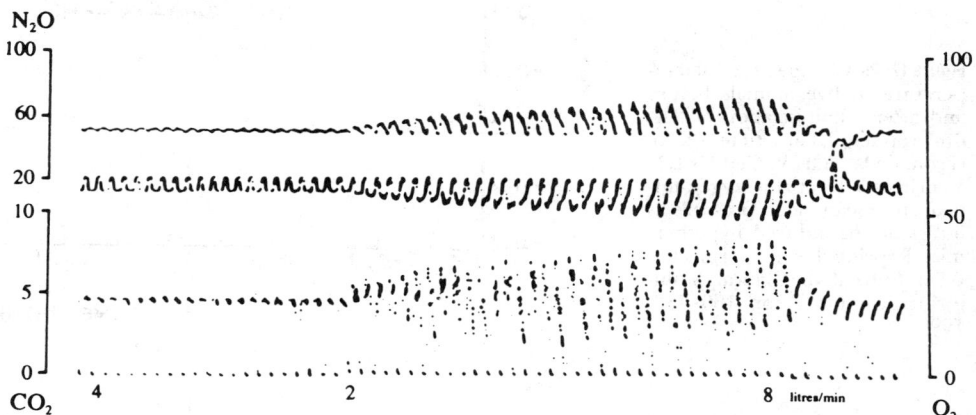

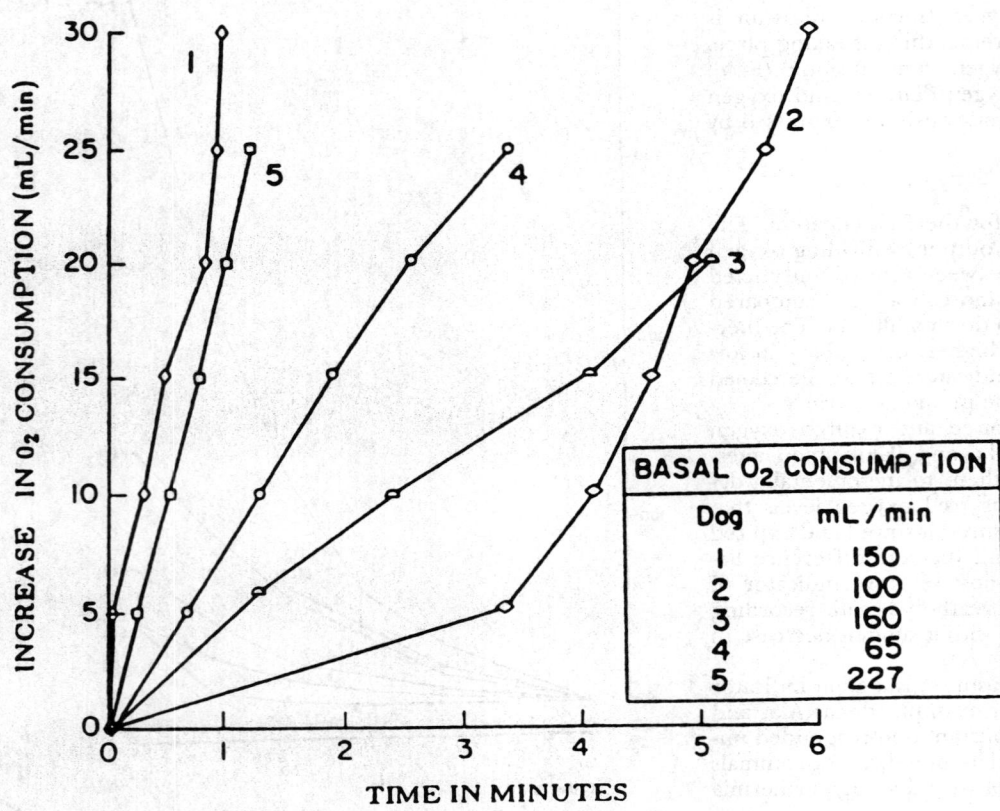

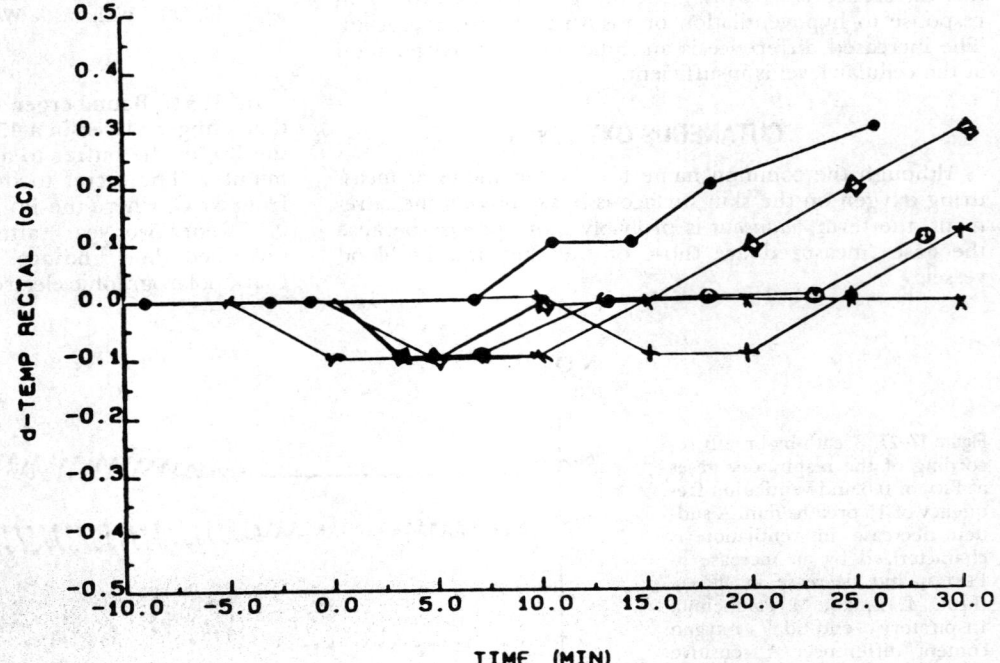

Figure 17–28. Increase in oxygen consumption in five animals after injection of 2,4-dinitrophenol at time zero. The inset shows the basal oxygen consumption before injecting 2,4-dinitrophenol. (From de las Alas V, Geddes LA, Voorhees WD, et al: Oxygen uptake and mean blood pressure as indicators of induced hypothermia. Reprinted with permission from Journal of Clinical Monitoring, volume 6, pp 186–188, 1990.)

Figure 17–29. Change in rectal temperature in five animals before and after administration of 2,4-dinitrophenol at time zero. (From de las Alas V, Geddes LA, Voorhees WD, et al: Oxygen uptake and mean blood pressure as indicators of induced hypothermia. Reprinted with permission from Journal of Clinical Monitoring, volume 6, pp 186–188, 1990.)

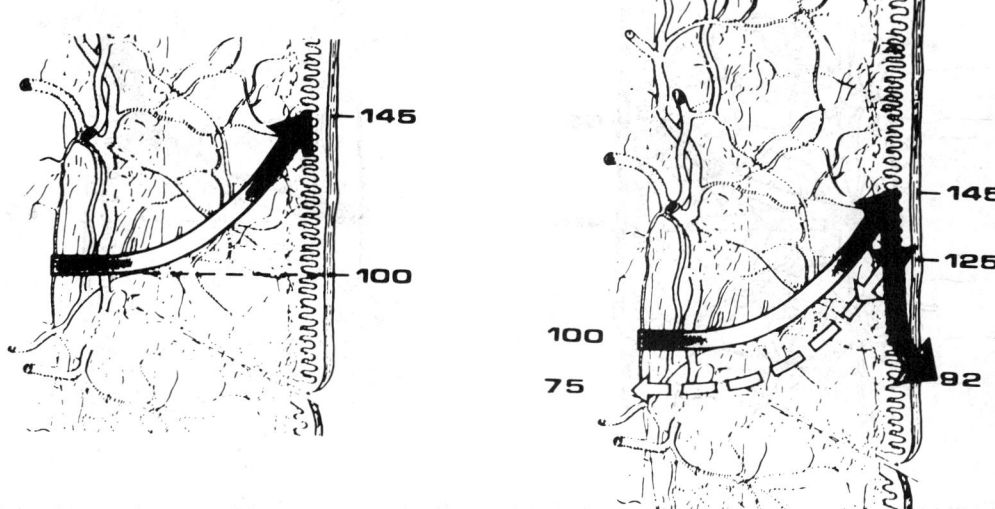

Figure 17–30. *(Left)* Blood PO_2 increases to about 145 mm Hg as it is heated by the overlying electrode. The distance from the capillary plexus at the arrow tip to the skin surface is only 0.3 mm. *(Right)* The blood PO_2 drops because of metabolic oxygen consumption and electrode oxygen consumption. The cooled venous blood drops to about 75 mm Hg before it mixes with other venous blood. (Modified from Baumbach P: Understanding Transcutaneous pO_2 and pCO_2 Measurements. Copenhagen, Denmark, Radiometer, p 10, 1986, by permission of Radiometer A/S, Copenhagen.)

element to measure cutaneous oxygen. They showed that the correlation between PaO_2 and $PTCO_2$ in infants was excellent ($r = .95$).

In a patient breathing room air at sea level, the arterial blood is initially approximately 100 torr. As the capillary blood approaches the stratum corneum, the increase in temperature caused by the overlying heated Clark electrode shifts the oxygen dissociation curve to the right, which gives the patient a higher PO_2 from the same total oxygen content (Fig. 17–30). The increase in blood PO_2 is approximately 6% per degree. However, oxygen diffuses out of the capillaries at the epidermal basement membrane to supply oxygen to the consuming tissue, and the partial pressure drops approximately 30 torr. The average mid-capillary PO_2 is about 125 torr. The oxygen then diffuses through the lipid-containing stratum corneum layer, the lipid liquefied by the heated electrode. The PO_2 decreases further as it supplies the metabolic needs of the cells. In addition, the electrode

itself consumes oxygen. In healthy persons, PO_2 typically decreases about 33 torr from the mid-capillary PO_2 of approximately 125 to 92 torr. The returning venous blood cools and reaches a PO_2 of about 75 torr.

The relationship between PaO_2 and $PTCO_2$ is therefore a function of three factors: (1) capillary temperature; (2) skin blood flow; and (3) metabolic and electrode oxygen consumption. Capillary temperature is perhaps the easiest to maintain because the overlying PO_2 electrode is heated to 42 to 45°C. The clinician can select the electrode temperature according to the manufacturer's directions. For neonates, a temperature setting of 44°C usually offers good correlation, whereas approximately 45°C is best for adults.

Because blood flow to the skin is a function of temperature, perfusion pressure, and drug effects, the correlation between PaO_2 and $PTCO_2$ can be adversely affected. For example, Tremper and Shoemaker[30] studied 106 adult patients and found that if cardiac index was above 2.2

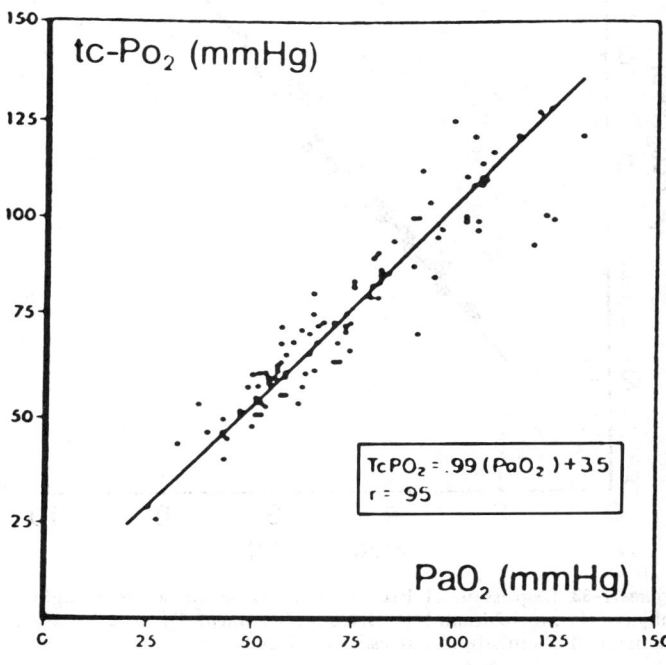

Figure 17–31. Relationship between $PTCO_2$ and PaO_2 in preterm infants with moderate to severe respiratory distress.

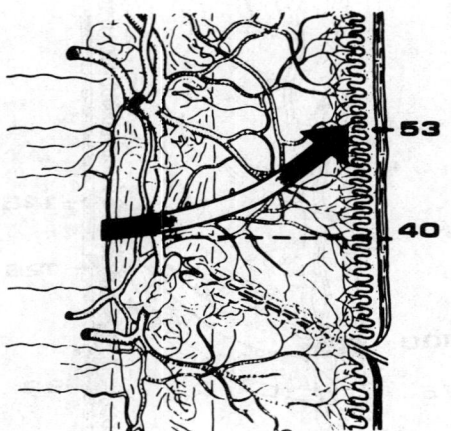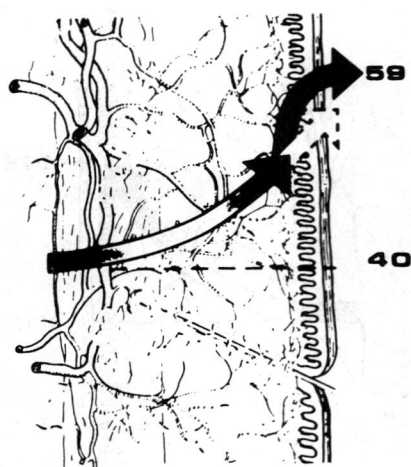

Figure 17–32. *(Left)* Increased temperature raises the blood Pco_2. *(Right)* Metabolic CO_2 production is the main contributor to increased blood Pco_2. Other factors contribute slightly to increased Pco_2. (Modified from Baumbach P: Understanding Transcutaneous pO_2 and pCO_2 Measurements. Copenhagen, Denmark, Radiometer, p 10, 1986, by permission of Radiometer A/S, Copenhagen.)

$L/min/m^2$, there was a correlation coefficient of 0.89. For patients with cardiac indices between 1.5 and 2.2 $L/min/m^2$, the correlation coefficient was 0.78. There was no correlation between cutaneous oxygen and arterial oxygen in patients with severe shock, but the cutaneous CO_2 ($Ptcco_2$) correlated well with the cardiac index. Typical of results with infants, a correlation coefficient of 0.95 was found in preterm infants with moderate or severe respiratory distress (Fig. 17–31).

It is the blood flow aspect that makes cutaneous oxygen measurements fortuitously convenient. Many clinicians believe that a sudden or gradual decrease in apparent oxygenation, as indicated by $Ptcco_2$ measurements, warns of patient difficulty. It may also be helpful in governing optimal ventilator setting, determining appropriate oxygen therapy, and obviating the need for repeated blood sampling.

The adequacy of vascular supply to a limb may also be indicated by $Ptco_2$ measurements. A low $Ptco_2$ may indicate peripheral vascular disease.[31] Similarly, skin flap viability assessment can be aided by cutaneous oxygen monitoring.[32] Cutaneous oxygen measurement is also used in hyperbaric chambers, where performing invasive blood gas analyses is sometimes difficult.[33]

CUTANEOUS CARBON DIOXIDE

A heated electrode is also used in the measurement of $Ptcco_2$. $Ptcco_2$ increases with temperature but only at a rate of 4.8% per degree (Fig. 17–32). Thus, if $Paco_2$ is 40 torr, it rises to approximately 53 torr when heated. In addition, Pco_2 rises across the epidermis because of the Pco_2 temperature coefficient in the interstitial fluid, and membrane cooling results in an additional 2 torr of pressure. The metabolic contribution of the epidermis raises Pco_2 an additional 4 torr.

Like $Ptco_2$ measurements, $Ptcco_2$ measurements are influenced by capillary blood temperature, metabolic activity, and blood flow. Perfusion has minimal effects on $Ptcco_2$ readings. However, metabolic influences and capillary blood temperature are problematic and must be compensated. Wimberley and coworkers[34] correct for capillary blood temperature by the formula

$$Ptcco_2\,(T) = Pco_2\,(37°C) \times 10^{0.021(T-37°C)}$$

The metabolic CO_2 contribution, which is thought to be about 4 torr, is then used with capillary blood temperature to correct the instrument reading.

Clinically, $Ptcco_2$ measurements have been shown to be quite accurate (Fig. 17–33). In one study,[35] $Paco_2$ was compared with $Ptcco_2$ in eight adults (seven patients and one normal subject). Forty simultaneous measurements of $Paco_2$ and $Ptcco_2$ were obtained from each subject, and $Ptcco_2$ was found to accurately reflect change in $Paco_2$. When $Paco_2$ changes rapidly, the cutaneous measurement will lag by a few minutes, and the measurement may be dampened as well.

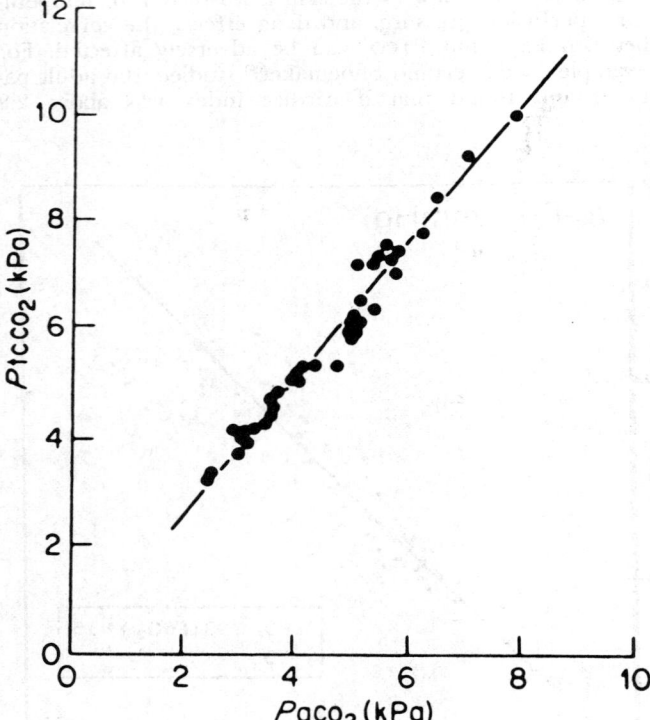

Figure 17–33. Regression of $Ptcco_2$ on $Paco_2$ at 40 points in eight subjects. (From Goldman MD, Gribbin HR, Martin RJ, et al: Transcutaneous Pco_2 in adults. Anaesthesia 37:944, 1982.)

References

1. Kirchhoff GR, Bunsen RWE: Chemiche Analyse Lurch Spectralbeobachtungen. Leipzig, Germany, Engelmann, 1860.
2. Stokes GG: On the reduction and oxygenation of the colouring matter of the blood. Dublin Philos Mag 28:391, 1864.
3. Hoppe-Seyler F: Uber die chemischen und optischen Eigenschafter des Blutfarbstoffs. Arch Pathol Anat Physiol 29:233, 1864.

4. Mathes K: Uber den Einfluss der Atmung auf die Sauerstoffsattigung des Arterienblutes. Arch Exp Pathol Pharmakol 176:683, 1934.

5. Severinghaus JW, Astrup PB: History of blood gas analysis, VI. Oximetry. J Clin Monit 2:270, 1986.

6. Wukitsch MW, Petterson MT, Tobler DR, et al: Pulse oximetry: An analysis of theory, technology and practice. J Clin Monit 4:290, 1988.

7. Tremper KK, Barker SJ: Pulse oximetry. Anesthesiology 70:98, 1989.

8. Nahas GG: A simplified lucite cuvette for the spectrophotometric measurement of hemoglobin and oxyhemoglobin. J Appl Physiol 13:147, 1958.

9. Severinghaus JW, Naifeh KH, Koh SO: Errors in 14 pulse oximeters during profound hypoxia. J Clin Monit 5:72, 1989.

10. Sidi A, Rush W, Gravenstein N, et al: Pulse oximetry fails to accurately detect low levels of arterial hemoglobin oxygen saturation in dogs. J Clin Monit 3:257, 1987.

11. Barker SJ, Tremper KK, Hyatt J: Effects of methemoglobinemia on pulse oximetry and mixed venous oximetry. Anesthesiology 70:112, 1989.

12. Barker SJ, Tremper KK: The effect of carbon monoxide inhalation on pulse oximetry and transcutaneous PO_2. Anesthesiology 66:677, 1987.

13. Sidi A, Paulus DA, Rush W, et al: Methylene blue and indocyanine green artifactually lower pulse oximetry readings of oxygen saturation: Studies in dogs. J Clin Monit 4:249, 1987.

13a. Moller JT, Pedersen T, Johannessen NW, et al: Pulse oximetry does reduce post-operative complications: A prospective study of 20,802 patients (abstract). Anesthesiology 75:A867, 1991.

13b. Moller JT, Pedersen T, Johannessen NW, et al: Pulse oximetry uncovers hypoxemia and decreases the incidence of evidence for myocardial ischemia during anesthesia: A prospective study of 20,802 patients (abstract). Anesthesiology 75:A1057, 1991.

13c. Task Force on Guidelines of the Society of Critical Care Medicine: Guidelines for Categorization of Services for the Critically Ill Patient. Anaheim, CA, Society of Critical Care Medicine, p 3, 1990.

13d. Task Force on Guidelines of the Society of Critical Care Medicine: Guidelines for Standards of Care for Patients with Acute Respiratory Failure on Mechanical Ventilatory Support. Anaheim, CA, Society of Critical Care Medicine, p 5, 1990.

14. Forster RE III, Dubois AB, Briscoe WA, et al: The Lung: Physiologic Basis of Pulmonary Function Tests. 3rd ed. Chicago, Year Book Medical Publishers, 1986.

15. Schoonees JA: Use of capnography to monitor pulmonary circulation during cardiac resuscitation. S Afr Med J 51:890, 1977.

16. Falk JL, Rackow EC, Weil MH: End-tidal carbon dioxide concentration during cardiopulmonary resuscitation. N Engl J Med 318:607, 1988.

17. Linko K, Paloheimo M, Tammisto T: Capnography for detection of accidental oesophageal intubation. Acta Anaesthesiol Scand 27:199, 1983.

18. Guggenberger H, Lenz G, Federle R: Early detection of inadvertent oesophageal intubation: Pulse oximetry vs. capnography. Acta Anaesthesiol Scand 33:112, 1989.

19. Nunn JF, Hill DW: Respiratory dead space and arterial to end-tidal CO_2 tension difference in anesthetized man. J Appl Physiol 15:383, 1960.

20. Whitesell R, Asiddleo C, Gollman D, et al: Relationship between arterial and peak expired carbon dioxide pressure during anesthesia and factors influencing the difference. Anesth Analg 60:508, 1981.

21. Raemer DB, Frannis D, Philip JH, et al: Variation in PCO_2 between arterial blood and peak expired gas during anesthesia. Anesth Analg 61:1065, 1983.

22. Yamanaka MK, Sue DY: Comparison of arterial–end-tidal PCO_2 difference and dead space/tidal volume ratio in respiratory failure. Chest 92:832, 1987.

23. Gravenstein JS, Paulus DA: Clinical Monitoring Practice. 2nd ed. Philadelphia, JB Lippincott, p 171, 1987.

24. Tremper KK, Barker SJ: Monitoring of oxygen. In: Lake CL (ed): Clinical Monitoring. Philadelphia, WB Saunders, p 283, 1990.

25. Davies GG, Jobson PJR, Glasgow BM, et al: Continuous Fick cardiac output compared to thermodilution cardiac output. Crit Care Med 14:881, 1986.

26. Linko K, Paloheimo M: Inspiratory end-tidal oxygen content difference: Sensitive indicator of hypoventilation. Crit Care Med 17:345, 1989.

27. de las Alas V, Geddes LA, Voorhees WD, et al: Oxygen uptake and mean blood pressure as indicators of induced hyperthermia. J Clin Monit 6:186, 1990.

28. Baumberger JP, Goodfriend RB: Determination of arterial oxygen tension in man by equilibration through intact skin. Fed Proc 10:10, 1951.

29. Huch R, Huch A, Lubbers DE: Transcutaneous measurement of blood PO_2 ($tcPO_2$): Method and application in perinatal medicine. J Perinat Med 1:183, 1973.

30. Tremper KK, Shoemaker WC: Transcutaneous oxygen monitoring of critically ill adults, with or without low flow shock. Crit Care Med 9:706, 1981.

31. Franzeck UK, Talke P, Bernstein EF, et al: Transcutaneous PO_2 measurements in health and peripheral arterial occlusive disease. Surgery 91:156, 1982.

32. Jensen HS, Alsbjörn BF: Variability in split-skin biopsies measured by a surface oxygen electrode. Scand J Clin Lab Invest 44:423, 1984.

33. Sheffield PJ, Workman WT: Cutaneous and Transcutaneous Blood Gas Monitoring. New York, Marcel Dekker, 1983.

34. Wimberley PD, Pedersen KG, Thode J, et al: Transcutaneous capillary PCO_2 and PO_2 measurements in healthy adults. Clin Chem 29:1471, 1983.

35. Goldman MD, Gribbin HR, Martin RJ, et al: Transcutaneous PCO_2 in adults. Anaesthesia 37:944, 1982.

CHAPTER 18

Neurologic Monitoring

Donald S. Prough

INTRODUCTION
New Technology Assessment

Many devices designed to monitor neurologic status are currently available or are under development. Some of these devices offer an unprecedented opportunity to recognize impending neurologic injury and, ideally, to reduce morbidity and mortality.

However, technologic developments must undergo intense scrutiny. Technology assessment in the 1990s has acquired a new, subjective dimension, which greatly complicates decisions regarding the application of existing equipment and newly available devices. Until recently, technology assessment emphasized safety and efficacy.[1] Today, however, technology assessment requires an even more demanding approach, incorporating traditional methods, such as the randomized clinical trial, but adding broader and more complex assessments of effectiveness, quality of life, patients' preferences, and costs and benefits.[1]

Fuchs and Garber have outlined three stages of technology assessment: assessment of technical characteristics; assessment of efficacy; and assessment of clinical, economic, and social end points.[1] The current status of brain monitoring devices is reviewed in these terms. Technical characteristics of each class of devices are discussed; the extent to which efficacy has been demonstrated is summarized; and the likely relationship between the device and the clinical, economic, and social end points is addressed.

Goals of Brain Monitoring

Monitoring devices cannot independently improve outcome. They can only contribute to decreased morbidity and mortality by providing physiologic data that can be integrated into a more effective therapeutic plan (Fig. 18–1). Neurologic monitoring falls into two distinct categories. The first category, which includes electroencephalography and evoked potential monitoring, defines a qualitative threshold beyond which additional morbidity becomes likely. The second category, which includes monitors of intracranial pressure, cerebral blood flow (CBF), and cerebral metabolism, provides quantitative physiologic information. Such devices can potentially define a threshold for intervention that provides a margin of safety between the level at which neurologic injury might occur and the level at which treatment can be implemented. For instance, pulse oximeters, which monitor a critical aspect of brain oxygenation, are widely applied in critically ill patients. The threshold of

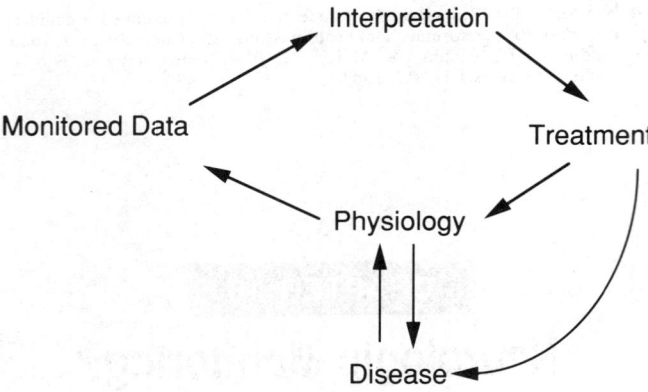

Figure 18–1. Monitored data are dynamically integrated into the management of critical neurologic illness. Acute neurologic disease produces alterations in physiology that are detected by monitors. The monitored data are then interpreted and, based on that interpretation, incorporated into a treatment plan. Treatment may alter the disease process or the physiologic expression of the disease process. In turn, monitored data change as a consequence of therapy.

hemoglobin (Hb) saturation below which tissue hypoxia becomes likely varies among individuals but is less than 75% (equivalent to $PaO_2 < 40$ mm Hg) in otherwise healthy persons. However, desaturation usually prompts intervention if Hb saturation declines below 90%.

Quantitative physiologic monitors may therefore be used to develop and test therapeutic goals that vary considerably from minimal threshold levels. For instance, Bland and colleagues have defined a threshold for systemic oxygen delivery (cardiac output × arterial oxygen content [CaO_2]) at 600 mL O_2/min/m², below which mortality and morbidity increase in high-risk surgical patients.[2, 3] Subsequently, by using that value as a threshold above which systemic oxygen delivery was maintained by hemodynamic support, they have demonstrated a decline in mortality and morbidity in comparison to those of patients managed without reference to the threshold.[4] That strategy provides a model for the definition of critical and interventional thresholds. Were the safety and efficacy of that approach validated, the third phase of technology assessment would remain: the assessment of more complex clinical, economic, and social end points.

Nevertheless, few data define thresholds for intervention that apply to brain monitoring. Few data even quantify the relationship between monitored variables and the risk of preventable neurologic injury. The development and utilization of brain monitoring devices therefore presuppose certain assumptions. First, reduced cerebral oxygen delivery ($CBF \times CaO_2$) is associated with avoidable neurologic morbidity in certain categories of critically ill patients. Second, the proportion of patients who develop avoidable injury is sufficiently large to justify extensive (and potentially expensive) application of brain monitoring devices. Third, thresholds for intervention can be defined on the basis of experimental and clinical evidence.

CEREBRAL ISCHEMIA

Cerebral ischemia, defined as inadequate oxygen delivery to the brain, can result from a critical reduction of any of the components of cerebral oxygen delivery, including CBF, Hb concentration, and arterial oxygen saturation. The brain constitutes only 2% of total body weight but receives 15% of cardiac output and accounts for 15 to 20% of total oxygen

consumption (Table 18–1). Certain regions of the brain, such as the cerebellum, the basal ganglia, the CA1 layer of the hippocampus, and the arterial boundary zones between major branches of the intracranial vessels, appear to be selectively vulnerable to ischemic injury.[5]

The severity of brain damage secondary to cerebral ischemia is proportional to the magnitude and duration of the insult. In monkeys, paralysis develops if regional CBF declines below about 23 mL/100 g/min.[6] Infarction of brain tissue, however, requires that CBF remain below 18 mL/100 g/min.[6] Therefore, prolonged paralysis is potentially reversible if the paralysis is associated with CBF values of 18 to 23 mL/100 g/min. The tolerable duration of more profound ischemia is inversely proportional to the severity of CBF reduction; CBF less than 10 mL/100 g/min for 2 hours results in infarction (Fig. 18–2).

TABLE 18–1

COMPARISON OF SYSTEMIC AND CEREBRAL OXYGENATION VARIABLES

Variable	Systemic	Cerebral
Blood flow (mL/100 g/min)	7.0	50
Oxygen consumption (mL/100 g/min)	0.3	3.4
Oxygen delivery (mL/100 g/min)	1.4	10
Arteriovenous oxygen content difference (mL O_2/100 mL)	5.0	7.0
Venous saturation (%)	75	65

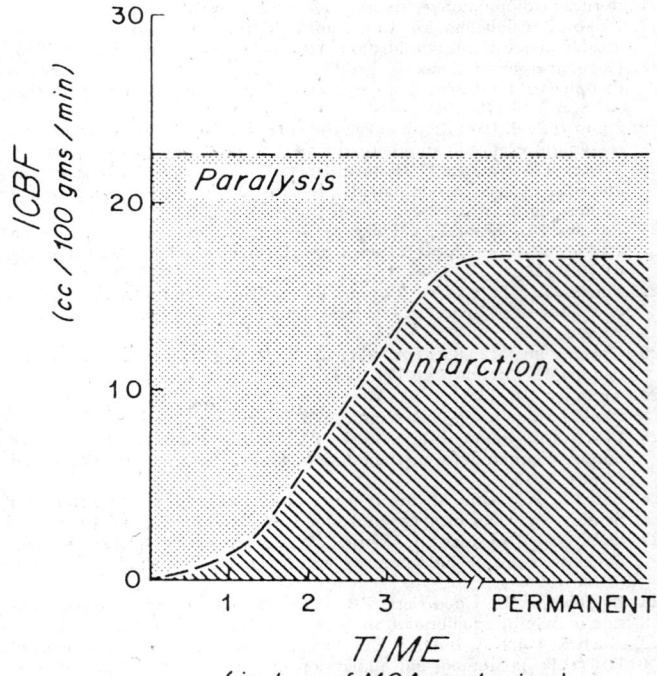

Figure 18–2. Schematic representation of ischemic thresholds in awake monkeys. The threshold for reversible paralysis occurs at a local cerebral blood flow (lCBF) of approximately 23 mL/100 g/min. Irreversible injury (infarction) is a function of the magnitude of blood flow reduction and the duration of that reduction. Relatively severe ischemia is potentially reversible if the duration is sufficiently short. (From Jones TH, Morawetz RB, Crowell RM, et al: Thresholds of focal cerebral ischemia in awake monkeys. J Neurosurg 54:773, 1981.)

TABLE 18–2

CHARACTERISTICS OF TYPES OF CEREBRAL ISCHEMIC INSULTS

Characteristics	Examples
Global, incomplete	Hypotension, hypoxemia, cardiopulmonary resuscitation
Global, complete	Cardiac arrest
Focal, incomplete	Stroke, subarachnoid hemorrhage with vasospasm

Cerebral ischemia is traditionally characterized as focal or global and complete or incomplete (Table 18–2). From a practical standpoint, a clinically useful brain monitor should detect focal cerebral ischemia. Most global cerebral insults, such as hypotension, hypoxemia, and cardiac arrest, are readily detected by systemic monitors. Therefore, brain-specific monitors can provide additional information primarily in situations, such as stroke, subarachnoid hemorrhage with vasospasm, and cerebral trauma, in which regional cerebral oxygenation may be impaired despite adequate systemic oxygenation and perfusion.

OVERVIEW OF BRAIN MONITORS

Brain monitors directly or indirectly assess cerebral perfusion, brain metabolism, or cerebral function (Table 18–3). Blood pressure monitoring and pulse oximetry provide important clues about the adequacy of global brain oxygenation. The normal brain autoregulates cerebral perfusion, that is, maintains stable CBF at perfusion pressures ranging from 50 to 150 mm Hg.[7, 8] Pulse oximetry monitors arterial oxygen saturation, a primary determinant of CaO_2 and therefore cerebral oxygen delivery. The brain normally increases CBF in response to decreasing CaO_2, whether the reduction is secondary to a decrease in Hb or in arterial oxygen saturation.[9–12] Consequently, brain-specific monitors are of greatest value in patients in whom global or regional CBF cannot increase in response to either decreasing oxygen supply or increasing metabolic requirements.

Cerebral ischemia may necessitate admission to an intensive care unit or may develop during the course of hospitalization. Nevertheless, the value of brain monitoring has been poorly defined in most critical neurologic and neurosurgical illnesses. Many clinicians assume that ischemic damage (such as that associated with stroke or cardiac arrest) is irreversible by the time patients are first seen by a physician. In addition, many brain monitors, such as those that record CBF, intracranial pressure (ICP), and computer-processed electroencephalograms (EEGs), require specially trained technicians. Therefore, no generally accepted protocols have been developed that establish clinically important thresholds for intervention, that define appropriate therapeutic interven-

tions, and that have been demonstrated to improve outcome. In the absence of such protocols, highly individualized approaches have arisen.

Operational Characteristics

Brain monitors can be classified in terms of the validity of the measurements performed and in terms of the ease with which monitored information can be incorporated in the clinical reasoning process (Tables 18–4 and 18–5). The design and utilization of monitoring devices necessitate trade-offs among various performance characteristics. For instance, a monitor that has high positive predictive value (i.e., that falls outside threshold values only when cerebral ischemia is unequivocally present) is unlikely to detect sensitively less profound ischemia. A monitor that is highly sensitive to changes in cerebral oxygenation frequently warns of small changes that are unlikely to produce brain injury. For example, pulse oximetry frequently demonstrates transient declines in arterial oxygen saturation that would result in no adverse sequelae were no action taken. Presumably, prompt correction of episodes of desaturation that would result in no harm in most patients prevents unexpected injury in an occasional patient.

Practical use of brain monitors requires definition of critical thresholds at which therapeutic interventions should be undertaken. Thresholds of CBF that correlate with various clinical outcomes, physiologic changes, and changes in monitored variables have been defined on the basis of animal experiments[6, 13–15] and to a lesser extent clinical data[16] (Table 18–6). If a monitor of brain function detects cerebral ischemia, the actual severity is not established. All that is known is that cerebral oxygenation in a region of brain that contributes to that function has fallen below a critical threshold. The shortfall could be slight or severe. Because more severe ischemia produces neurologic injury in less time, it is impossible to predict with certainty whether changes in function will be followed by cerebral infarction. In addition, if regional ischemia involves structures that do not participate in the monitored function, infarction could develop without warning. This predictable relationship no doubt explains the failure of monitors to detect cerebral ischemia in patients who subsequently develop clinical evidence of brain infarction as well as reports of profound changes in monitored variables that are followed by no apparent change in clinical condition. The complexity and heterogeneity of brain tissue virtually preclude development of a single, perfectly predictive brain monitor.

TABLE 18–3

CEREBRAL MONITORING DEVICES

Cerebral Perfusion	Cerebral Metabolism	Cerebral Function
Cerebral blood flow	Oxygen extraction	Evoked potentials
Cerebral blood flow velocity	Jugular bulb saturation	EEG Raw
Intracranial pressure	Near-infrared spectroscopy	Processed

TABLE 18–4

MONITOR CHARACTERISTICS

Accuracy	Incorporation into Clinical Reasoning
Bias	Sensitivity
Precision	Positive predictive value
	Specificity
	Negative predictive value
	Threshold definition
	Speed
	Utility in clinical reasoning
	Diagnosis
	Surveillance
	Prognosis
	Goal-directed therapy

From DS Prough: Brain monitoring. In: W Shoemaker, R Taylor (eds): Critical Care: State of the Art, Volume 12. Fullerton, CA, Society of Critical Care Medicine, p 164, © by Williams & Wilkins, 1991.

TABLE 18–5

BRAIN MONITOR CHARACTERISTICS: GLOSSARY

Term	Definition
Bias	Average difference (positive or negative) between monitored values and "gold standard" values
Precision	Standard deviation of the differences (bias) between the measurements
Sensitivity	Probability that the monitor will demonstrate cerebral ischemia when cerebral ischemia is present
Positive predictive value	Probability that cerebral ischemia is present when the monitor suggests cerebral ischemia
Specificity	Probability that the monitor will not demonstrate cerebral ischemia when cerebral ischemia is not present
Negative predictive value	Probability that cerebral ischemia is not present when the monitor reflects no cerebral ischemia
Threshold value	Value used to separate acceptable (i.e., no ischemia present) from unacceptable (i.e., ischemia present)
Speed	Time elapsed from the onset of ischemia until the monitor recognizes ischemia

From DS Prough: Brain monitoring. In: W Shoemaker, R Taylor (eds): Critical Care: State of the Art, Volume 12. Fullerton, CA, Society of Critical Care Medicine, p 164, © by Williams & Wilkins, 1991.

SPECIFIC BRAIN MONITORING MODALITIES

This section reviews techniques that provide direct or indirect data regarding CBF or cerebral perfusion pressure (CPP), techniques that estimate the adequacy of CBF to meet cerebral metabolic demand, and, more briefly, electrophysiologic techniques (somatosensory and brain stem evoked potentials).

Cerebral Blood Flow Monitoring

Xenon-133 Clearance (Table 18–7)

The first quantitative method for measuring human CBF was the Kety-Schmidt technique,[17, 18] in which global CBF was calculated from the difference between the arterial and jugular bulb saturation curves of an inhaled, inert gas. Shortly thereafter, techniques were developed that were based on the clearance from the brain of an intra-arterially injected radioisotope such as ^{133}Xe as detected by scintillation counters positioned over the scalp.[19, 20] Subsequently, mathematic techniques were devised to correct clearance curves for recirculation of ^{133}Xe, thereby permitting measurement of CBF after inhaled[21, 22] or intravenous administration of ^{133}Xe (Figs. 18–3 and 18–4).

CBF measurements have never become a routine part of management of critically ill patients, although considerable quantities of descriptive data have been generated, particularly for patients with severe head trauma. Human acute head injury sufficiently severe to produce coma (Glasgow Coma Scale score ≤ 8) is associated with decreased cerebral metabolic rate of oxygen consumption (CMRo$_2$), moderately decreased CBF, and highly variable autoregulation and carbon dioxide reactivity. The measurement of CBF, usually performed using ^{133}Xe clearance, is complicated by the fact that many clearance curves for head-injured patients do not have the normal biexponential shape.

The uninjured cerebral circulation is responsive to changes in metabolic demand, CPP, Paco$_2$ and Pao$_2$. Figure 18–5 depicts the normal "coupled" relationship in which CBF is dependent on CMRo$_2$. Metabolic demand varies directly with body temperature and with the level of brain activation, examples being increases in CMRo$_2$ produced by fever, seizures, or pain. Changes in CPP do not alter CBF over a range of pressures of approximately 50 to 130 mm Hg. Normally, Paco$_2$ powerfully regulates cerebrovascular resistance over a range of Paco$_2$ of 20 to 80 mm Hg. CBF is acutely halved if Paco$_2$ is halved and doubles if CBF doubles; therefore Paco$_2$ must be carefully monitored and controlled in head-injured patients.

In some patients with head injury, coupling is preserved, that is, both CMRo$_2$ and CBF are proportionately reduced, whereas in others uncoupling occurs, with CBF substantially in excess of CMRo$_2$[23] (Fig. 18–6). In the majority of comatose, head-injured patients, CBF is less than the normal value of 50 mL/100 g/min and CMRo$_2$ is well below the normal value of 3.5 mL/100 g/min.[24] Ninety percent of

TABLE 18–6

CLINICAL, PATHOPHYSIOLOGIC, AND MONITORING THRESHOLDS IN CEREBRAL ISCHEMIA

CBF (mL/100 g/min)	Clinical Effects	Pathophysiologic Changes	Monitored Changes
50	Normal		
23	Reversible paralysis		EEG slowing EP* change
20		Na$^+$-K$^+$ pump dysfunction	
18	Infarction		EEG flat
15			EP absent
10		K$^+$ efflux, Ca^{2+} influx	

*EP = evoked potential.
From DS Prough: Brain monitoring. In: W Shoemaker, R Taylor (eds): Critical Care: State of the Art, Volume 12. Fullerton, CA, Society of Critical Care Medicine, p 165, © by Williams & Wilkins, 1991.

TABLE 18–7

CHARACTERISTICS: CEREBRAL BLOOD FLOW MONITORING (XENON-133 CLEARANCE)

Characteristic	Grade*
Bias (vs. Kety-Schmidt)	±5%
Precision (vs. Kety-Schmidt)	±5%
Sensitivity	Good for 5% change
Positive predictive value	Good for CBF decrease
Specificity	Poor for ischemia; good for decreased CBF
Negative predictive value	Poor for ischemia
Threshold definition	CBF 24 mL/100 g/min (can be set at higher level)
Speed	Poor
Utility in clinical reasoning	
Diagnosis	Poor
Surveillance	Poor
Prognosis	Fair
Goal-directed therapy	Poor (untested)

*Subjective four-point scale: excellent, good, fair, poor.
From DS Prough: Brain monitoring. In: W Shoemaker, R Taylor (eds): Critical Care: State of the Art, Volume 12. Fullerton, CA, Society of Critical Care Medicine, p 173, © by Williams & Wilkins, 1991.

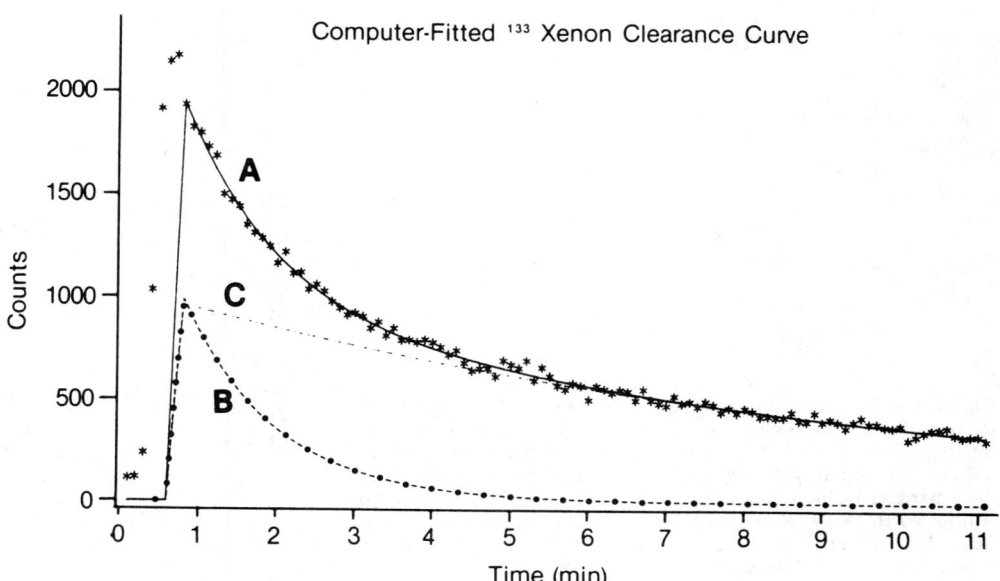

Figure 18–3. ^{133}Xe clearance curve after intra-arterial injection. After rapid bolus arrival in the cerebral circulation, clearance of the radioisotope usually is biexponential. The asterisks represent actual counted gamma emissions with the computer-fitted, computer-smoothed curve (A) superimposed. The rapidly clearing compartment (predominantly gray matter flow) is represented by curve B. The slowly clearing compartment is designated C. (From Prough DS, Michenfelder JD: Cerebral blood flow and metabolism: Implications for clinical monitoring. In: Cerra FB, Shoemaker WC [eds]: Critical Care: State of the Art, Volume 8. Fullerton, CA, Society of Critical Care Medicine, p 43, 1987.)

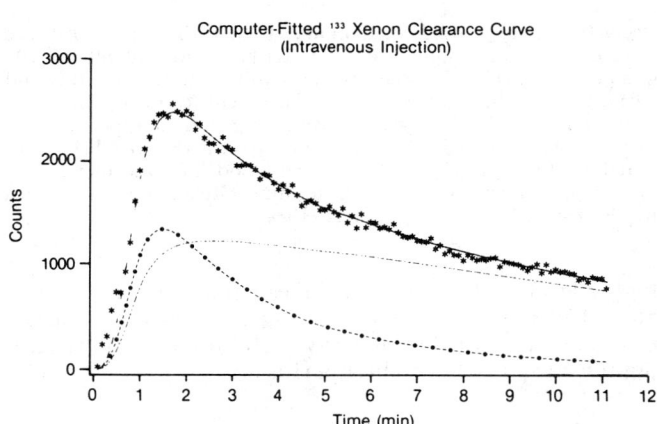

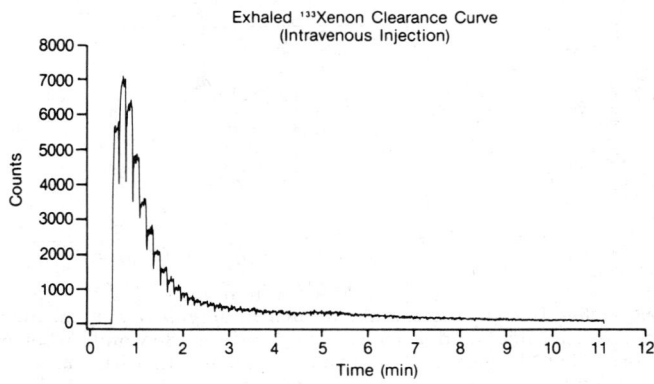

Figure 18–4. *(Top)* In contrast to the ^{133}Xe clearance curve generated by intra-arterial injection, an intravenous injection produces a later, broader peak in the gamma emission rate. Because larger doses are necessary for intravenous studies, recirculation of ^{133}Xe slows the clearance rate. *(Bottom)* Correction of the ^{133}Xe clearance curve for recirculation requires estimation of the decline in arterial ^{133}Xe clearance by counting the rate of gamma emissions in end-tidal exhaled gas. (From Prough DS, Michenfelder JD: Cerebral blood flow and metabolism: Implications for clinical monitoring. In: Cerra FB, Shoemaker WC [eds]: Critical Care: State of the Art, Volume 8. Fullerton, CA, Society of Critical Care Medicine, p 43, 1987.)

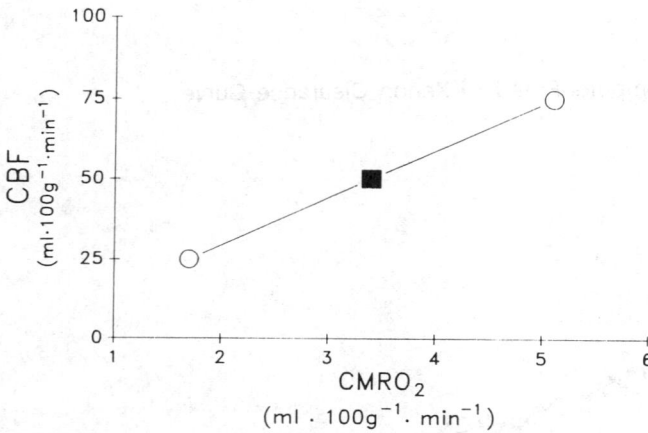

Figure 18–5. The normal relationship between $CMRO_2$ and CBF is characterized by closely coupled changes in both variables. Normally, CBF is 50 mL/100 g/min at a $CMRO_2$ of 3.4 mL/100 g/min in adults (filled square). As $CMRO_2$ increases or decreases, CBF changes in a parallel fashion (solid line). (Reprinted with permission from Butterworth JF IV, Prough DS: Head trauma. In: Rippe JR, Irwin RS, Alpert JS, et al [eds]: Intensive Care Medicine. 2nd ed. Boston, Little, Brown and Company, p 1463, 1991.)

patients less than 18 years old have cerebral hyperemia (CBF exceeding metabolic demand) at some point during intensive monitoring.[25] In contrast, many older patients have persistently subnormal CBF of 15 to 20 mL/100 g/min.[26]

CBF after head trauma may be pressure dependent at levels of CPP normally associated with unchanged CBF (Fig. 18–7). However, because both $CMRO_2$ and CBF tend to be low at baseline, CBF may not increase to normal levels, even at high levels of CPP. The status of autoregulation cannot be predicted on the basis of ICP, neurologic status, or baseline CBF.[24] Most patients with mass lesions have defective autoregulation; conversely, autoregulation remains intact in many patients without intracranial mass lesions.[24] In children, either abnormally high or abnormally low CBF is associated with impaired autoregulation.[27] In head-injured patients in whom autoregulation is intact, mannitol reduces ICP and does not change CBF; if autoregulation is defective, ICP changes little and CBF increases.[28]

The regional distribution of CBF is more variable in head-injured patients than in normal individuals.[29, 30] Nonsurviving patients and those who survive in a persistent vegetative state frequently have regional CBF values less than 20 mL/100 g/min, especially in the frontal and parietal lobes.[29] Low flow in arterial boundary regions in the frontoparietal cortex, often secondary to high ICP, contributes to poor neurologic outcome.[30] However, even in patients who ultimately progress to good recovery, CBF may be less than 20 mL/100 g/min in some brain regions.

In many patients, reduced CBF appears not to represent cerebral ischemia but rather to represent the expected coupling between low $CMRO_2$ and low CBF.[23] However, patients with low but coupled CBF may be vulnerable to excessive vasoconstriction during acute hyperventilation. Nearly 20% of patients develop a wide cerebral arteriovenous oxygen content difference during hyperventilation (Table 18–8), suggesting that hyperventilation therapy should be accompanied by an estimate of the adequacy of cerebral perfusion.[23] In some patients with severely reduced $CMRO_2$, acute hyperventilation actually increases $CMRO_2$.[31] Excessive regional vasoconstriction is a possible mechanism for the reported worsening of outcome in patients hyperventilated after head trauma compared with those maintained at a

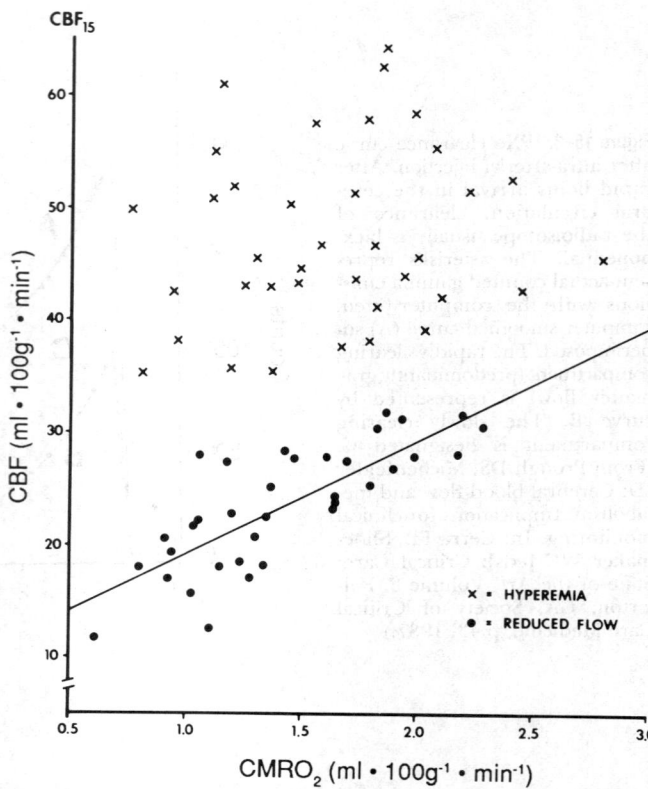

Figure 18–6. After closed head injury, both $CMRO_2$ and CBF are reduced. (Normal values are 3.4 mL/100 g/min and 50 mL/100 g/min, respectively.) In some patients (filled circles), $CMRO_2$ and CBF appear to be reduced to a similar extent (coupled). In others (represented by crosses), global CBF is higher than appears necessary to meet metabolic demand (uncoupled). (From Obrist WD, Langfitt TW, Jaggi JL, et al: Cerebral blood flow and metabolism in comatose patients with acute head injury. Relation to intracranial hypertension. J Neurosurg 61:241, 1984.)

higher level of $PaCO_2$.[32] If CBF measurements are unavailable, calculation of the cerebral oxygen extraction or lactate extraction may provide clinically useful information regarding the adequacy of cerebral perfusion.[33]

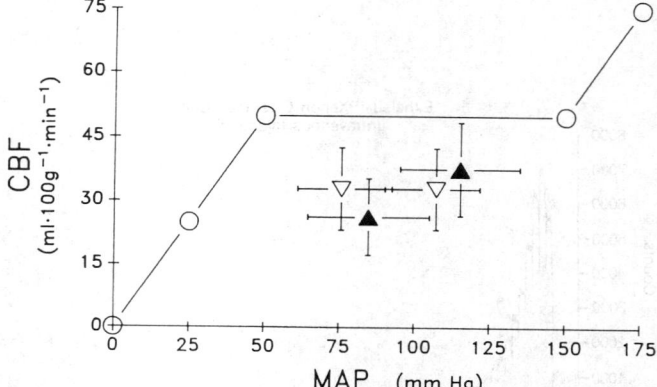

Figure 18–7. In comparison to the normal autoregulatory curve, after closed head injury, adult patients have reduced flow and, in some cases (filled triangles), impaired autoregulation. Other patients have reduced flow and preserved autoregulation (open triangles). (Data replotted from Muizelaar JP, Lutz HA III, Becker DP: Effect of mannitol on ICP and CBF and correlation with pressure autoregulation in severely head-injured patients. J Neurosurg 61:700, 1984.)

TABLE 18–8

CEREBRAL OXYGENATION IN 10 PATIENTS WITH GREATLY INCREASED CEREBRAL OXYGEN EXTRACTION*

Hemodynamic Variable	Hyperventilated Patients	Normal Value
$CMRo_2$ (mL/100 g/min)	1.9 ± 0.5	3.3 ± 0.4
CBF_{15} (mL/100 g/min)	18.6 ± 4.4	53.3 ± 6.8
$Cao_2 - Cvo_2$ (mL/100 mL)	10.5 ± 0.7	6.3 ± 1.2
Pvo_2 (mm Hg)	22.3 ± 1.8	37.5 ± 5.6

*Of 31 patients who were acutely hyperventilated ($Paco_2$ 18–26 mm Hg) after severe head injury, 10 demonstrated increased oxygen extraction. $CMRo_2$ = cerebral metabolic rate for oxygen consumption; CBF_{15} refers to the specific formula used to calculate CBF; $Cao_2 - Cvo_2$ = cerebral arteriovenous oxygen content difference; and Pvo_2 = jugular venous oxygen tension.
Modified from Obrist WD, Langfitt TW, Jaggi JL, et al: Cerebral blood flow and metabolism in comatose patients with acute head injury. Relation to intracranial hypertension. J Neurosurg 61:241, 1984.

CBF has also been investigated in patients who have suffered cardiac arrest because of the well-documented experimental phenomenon of postischemic hypoperfusion.[34, 35] Clinical data support the concept that some patients develop postischemic hypoperfusion after cardiac arrest,[36, 37] but $CMRo_2$ tends to be proportionately reduced.[36] Because of increased CBF and improved neurologic outcome in animals treated with the cerebral vasodilator nimodipine after complete cerebral ischemia,[38, 39] immediate postresuscitation administration of nimodipine was investigated in patients.[40] However, neurologic outcome was not improved.

[133]Xe clearance estimates of regional cortical CBF represent a powerful research technique. Nevertheless, despite the prognostic value of CBF measurements in patients who have suffered closed head injury,[133]Xe clearance has not been generally useful for primary diagnosis, surveillance, or goal-directed management. Among the obstacles to wider utilization are the cumbersome regulations governing the administration of radionuclides, the technically demanding nature of the measurements, and the sustained stable conditions (5 to 15 minutes) required to perform a single measurement.

Transcranial Doppler Flow Velocity (Table 18–9)

In most patients arterial flow velocity can be readily measured in intracranial vessels, especially the middle cerebral artery, using commercially available transcranial Doppler (TCD) equipment. TCD measurements initially appeared to offer useful diagnostic information in a variety of acute and chronic cerebrovascular problems. However, the diagnostic value of the technique has now been seriously questioned[41, 42] in "patients with brain tumors, familial and degenerative diseases of the cerebrum, brainstem, cerebellum, basal ganglia, and motor neurons, infectious and inflammatory conditions, psychiatric disorders, and epilepsy,"[42] although value appears to be established in noninvasively "detecting severe stenosis (>65%) in the major basal intracranial arteries; assessing patterns and extent of collateral circulation . . . ; evaluating and following vasoconstriction . . . , especially after subarachnoid hemorrhage (SAH); detecting arteriovenous malformations . . . ; and assessing patients with suspected brain death."[42]

TCD assesses blood flow velocity rather than blood flow per se. Velocity is a function not only of blood flow rate but also of vessel diameter. Therefore, when CBF declines as a consequence of cerebral vasospasm after SAH, flow velocity in the middle cerebral artery first increases[43–45] and then decreases as vasospasm resolves.[43] If the diameter of the middle cerebral artery remains constant, changes in velocity are proportional to changes in CBF measured using ^{133}Xe clearance; however, intersubject differences in flow velocity correlate poorly with intersubject differences in CBF measured using ^{133}Xe clearance (Fig. 18–8).[46]

TCD measurements of flow velocity in the middle cerebral artery have been extensively investigated in patients with progressive intracranial hypertension leading to brain death. Used in this manner, the TCD provides diagnostic and prognostic information because of characteristic changes in the systolic and diastolic components of the waveform (Fig. 18–9).[47, 48] As ICP increases, the flow during diastole decreases first; therefore, diastolic flow velocity declines. Severe intracranial hypertension results first in reversal of flow during diastole (negative flow velocity) and then in cessation of flow.[47, 48]

As a monitor for patients who are at risk for ischemic cerebral complications, TCD appears promising. Entirely noninvasive, TCD measurements can be repeated at frequent intervals or even applied continuously. Therefore, TCD could potentially be applied not only in a limited role as a diagnostic and prognostic tool but also as a surveillance monitor and as an essential component of goal-directed therapy. However, further work is necessary to define the situations in which the excellent capacity for rapid trend monitoring can be exploited. One possible approach is to combine intermittent ^{133}Xe clearance measurements with continuous TCD monitoring. In effect, ^{133}Xe clearance measurements could be used to "calibrate" the TCD, improving its quantitative value in individual patients.

Intracranial Pressure Monitoring (Table 18–10)

CPP is determined by the equation

$$CPP = MAP - ICP$$

where MAP is mean arterial pressure and ICP exceeds jugular venous pressure. Although CBF cannot be directly inferred from knowledge of MAP and ICP, severe increases in ICP reduce both CPP and CBF. In head-injured patients and children with Reye's syndrome, ICP monitoring is an

TABLE 18–9

CHARACTERISTICS: TRANSCRANIAL DOPPLER FLOW VELOCITY

Characteristic	Grade*
Bias	Not applicable
Precision	Not applicable
Sensitivity	Good for CBF change (relative), good for vasospasm in SAH
Positive predictive value	Good for CBF change; good for vasospasm in SAH
Specificity	Good for CBF change; good for vasospasm in SAH
Negative predictive value	Poor for ischemia; good for vasospasm in SAH
Threshold definition	Interpatient variation
Speed	Poor
Utility in clinical reasoning	
Diagnosis	Good
Surveillance	Fair in SAH
Prognosis	Fair in SAH
Goal-directed therapy	Untested

*Subjective four-point scale: excellent, good, fair, poor.
From DS Prough: Brain monitoring. In: W Shoemaker, R Taylor (eds): Critical Care: State of the Art, Volume 12. Fullerton, CA, Society of Critical Care Medicine, p 175, © by Williams & Wilkins, 1991.

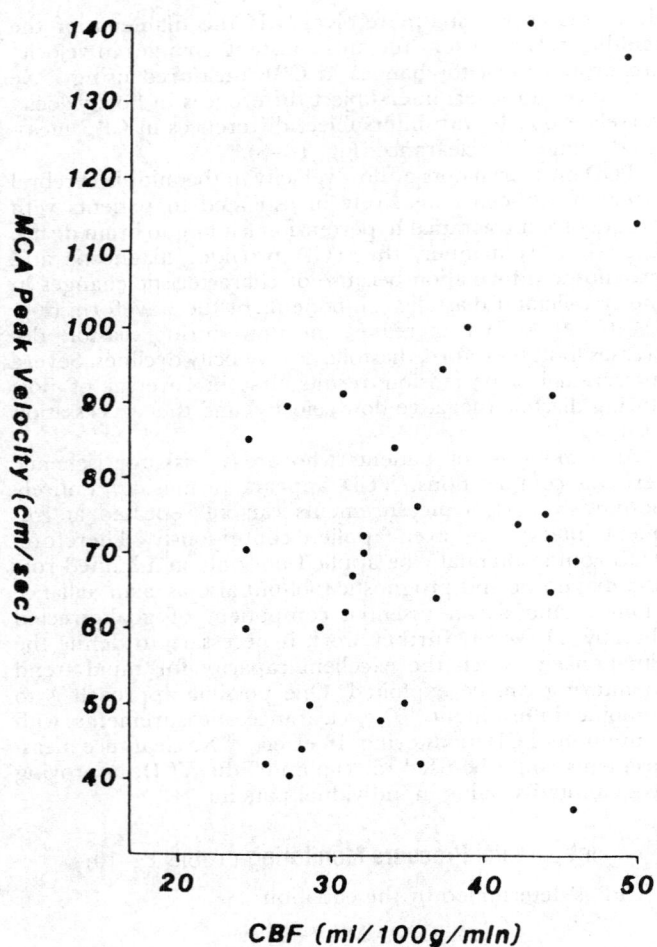

Figure 18–8. Relationship between CBF, measured using ^{133}Xe, and peak flow velocity in the middle cerebral artery (MCA), measured using the transcranial Doppler method. The intersubject correlation is poor ($r = .0424$). However, reactivity to changes in Pa_{CO_2} demonstrates that intrasubject changes in CBF, measured using ^{133}Xe, correlate better with changes in MCA peak velocity ($r = .489$). (From Bishop CCR, Powell S, Rutt D, et al: Transcranial Doppler measurement of middle cerebral artery blood flow velocity: A validation study. Stroke 17:913, 1986.)

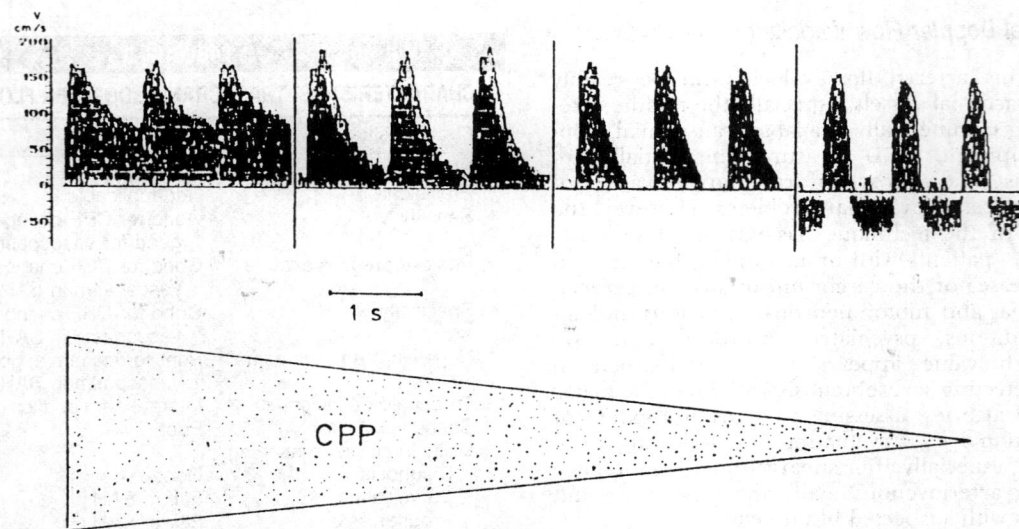

Figure 18–9. As CPP declines, the characteristic flow velocity (V), measured using transcranial Doppler of the middle cerebral artery, changes in a characteristic fashion. Systolic flow velocity is well maintained, but diastolic flow velocity gradually declines. Ultimately, as CPP approaches 0 mm Hg, flow in the middle cerebral artery becomes bidirectional. (From Hassler W, Steinmetz H, Galowski J: Transcranial Doppler ultrasonography in raised intracranial pressure and in intracranial circulatory arrest. J Neurosurg 68:745, 1988.)

TABLE 18–10

CHARACTERISTICS: INTRACRANIAL PRESSURE MONITORING

Characteristic	Grade*
Bias	Excellent
Precision	Excellent
Sensitivity	Good for ICP change; poor for CBF change or ischemia
Positive predictive value	Good for ICP change; poor for CBF change or ischemia
Specificity	Good for ICP change; poor for CBF change or ischemia
Negative predictive value	Good for ICP change; poor for CBF change or ischemia
Threshold definition	15–20 mm Hg or cerebral perfusion pressure < 50 mm Hg
Speed	Poor
Utility in clinical reasoning	
Diagnosis	Poor
Surveillance	Good (closed head trauma)
Prognosis	Good (closed head trauma)
Goal-directed therapy	Fair (closed head trauma; Reye's syndrome)

*Subjective four-point scale: excellent, good, fair, poor.
From DS Prough: Brain monitoring. In: W Shoemaker, R Taylor (eds): Critical Care: State of the Art, Volume 12. Fullerton, CA, Society of Critical Care Medicine, p 178, © by Williams & Wilkins, 1991.

accepted part of management.[49–56] In other clinical situations, including severe central nervous system infections, anoxic cerebral insults, SAH, and hepatic failure,[57–64] ICP monitoring has provided interesting descriptive information but has not been widely employed.

Lundberg and colleagues first proposed the concept that changes in therapy based on ICP monitoring could be used to improve the outcome of patients with closed head trauma,[51] based on the underlying assumption that intracranial hypertension, if untreated, may cause herniation or cerebral hypoperfusion. Head injury may increase intracranial volume and ICP through the mechanisms listed in Table 18–11. Most clinicians treat ICP if it exceeds a threshold of 20 mm Hg, a level that approximately one third of head-injured patients sometimes exceed.[52] Although ICP monitoring has been credited by some investigators with improving the prognosis in acute closed head injury,[49, 50, 53, 54] others question whether concurrent improvements in management, rather than ICP monitoring, explain the improvement.[65]

The equipment used for ICP monitoring has progressively evolved. The risk of infection associated with intraventricular cannulation slowed widespread application of ICP monitoring. The introduction of the subarachnoid screw facilitated effective, safe monitoring.[66] Despite occasional errors in measurement,[67, 68] most major centers now routinely provide ICP monitoring, especially for severely injured head trauma patients.[69] Many centers have begun to use fiberoptic catheters which are less susceptible to short-term malfunction than the previous generation of fluid-filled, subdural catheters.[70, 71]

Unlike the other modalities previously discussed, ICP monitoring has been used for surveillance and for goal-directed therapy. Particularly for head-injured patients and children who have Reye's syndrome, clinicians have applied systematic, although institutionally specific, protocols for avoidance of intracranial hypertension and for reduction of increased ICP when a threshold of 15 or 20 mm Hg is exceeded. In particular, decisions about diuretics, hyperventilation, positional changes, and additional diagnostic procedures may be determined by ICP information. The infor-

mation is considered necessary for patients who are being given neuromuscular blocking agents as part of the treatment to reduce ICP, because it is not possible to perform a comprehensive neurologic examination. If intracranial hypertension is refractory to conventional therapy, ICP monitoring is one of the alternative techniques used to titrate barbiturate coma,[72] although prophylactic barbiturate coma has failed to improve neurologic outcome after head injury.[73]

When ICP monitoring is used in other clinical situations, the rationale and strategies are similar. However, data defining the impact of ICP monitoring on outcome are more fragmentary and less convincing than those available for traumatized patients. Whenever ICP monitoring is employed, the potential complications, the most important of which is infection, must be considered.[74–76] Most clinicians agree that intraventricular catheters carry a greater risk of infection than subdural monitors.

Numerous authors have investigated ways to enhance the clinical value of ICP monitoring. The pressure-volume index (PVI) is calculated by removing or adding volume to cerebrospinal fluid through a ventricular cannula according to the equation

$$ \text{PVI} = \frac{V}{\log P_0/P_{m \text{ or } p}} $$

where V = volume withdrawn or injected
P_0 = pressure before withdrawing or injecting fluid
P_m = minimal pressure after fluid withdrawal
P_p = peak pressure after volume addition

A lower PVI, implying reduced brain compliance, is associated with the subsequent development of intracranial hypertension and with poorer neurologic outcome.[77] The critical value for PVI appears to be approximately 13 mL, below which level treatment is likely to be necessary either to reduce ventricular fluid pressure or to improve compliance.[78] If the PVI is less than 10 mL, reduction of ICP is nearly always required. Robertson and coworkers correlated the PVI with a computerized frequency analysis of the ICP waveform in 55 severely head-injured patients and determined that this continuous technique provided information

TABLE 18–11

CAUSES OF INTRACRANIAL HYPERTENSION AFTER HEAD TRAUMA

Cause	Mechanism
Mass lesions	Local expansion
Intracerebral hematoma	
Extra-axial hematoma	
Brain swelling	Vascular congestion, hyperemia
Brain edema	
Cytotoxic	Cellular swelling secondary to hypoxia or ischemia
Vasogenic	Breakdown of blood-brain barrier, interstitial accumulation of protein
Interstitial	Hydrocephalus
Secondary vasodilation	
Hypercarbia	Increased extracellular H^+ concentration
Hypoxia	Mechanism unclear; possibly increased local metabolite (adenosine?) concentration
Hypertension	Impaired autoregulation

Reprinted with permission from Butterworth JF IV, Prough DS: Head trauma. In: Rippe JR, Irwin RS, Alpert JS, et al (eds): Intensive Care Medicine. 2nd ed. Boston, Little, Brown and Company, p 1468, 1991.

that correlated highly with the PVI, provided earlier evidence of changes in intracranial compliance than ICP alone, and did not require manipulation of intracranial fluid volume.[79]

Brain Metabolic Monitoring

Jugular Venous Saturation (Table 18–12)

Measurements of oxygen in blood obtained from the jugular venous bulb provide information about the adequacy of CBF equivalent to that given by systemic "mixed venous" blood about the adequacy of cardiac output. CBF, $CMRo_2$, Cao_2, and jugular venous oxygen content ($Cjvo_2$) are related according to the following equation:

$$CMRo_2 = CBF(Cao_2 - Cjvo_2)$$

Rearranged, the equation becomes

$$Cjvo_2 = Cao_2 - \frac{CMRo_2}{CBF}$$

By inference, jugular venous oxygen saturation ($Sjvo_2$), a major determinant of $Cjvo_2$, represents a monitor of the adequacy of CBF. The jugular venous bulb was first used as a sampling site more than 60 years ago.[80] Today, retrograde cannulation of the jugular bulb is a low-risk, technically simple procedure.[81, 82] Continuous monitoring of $Sjvo_2$ is feasible using commercially available oximetry catheters. However, because of the configuration of the jugular bulb, continuous monitoring requires frequent repositioning and recalibration. In addition, mixed cerebral venous blood, like mixed systemic blood, is a global average of effluent from a variety of brain regions and may not reflect marked regional hypoperfusion. Therefore, abnormally low jugular venous saturation suggests the possibility of cerebral ischemia, but

TABLE 18–12	
CHARACTERISTICS: BRAIN METABOLIC MONITORING (JUGULAR VENOUS SATURATION)	
Characteristic	**Grade***
Bias	"Gold standard"
Precision	Gold standard
Sensitivity	Good for global desaturation; poor for regional change
Positive predictive value	Good for global desaturation; poor for regional change
Specificity	Good
Negative predictive value	Good
Threshold definition	Saturation < 50–60%
Speed	Fair (individual samples); good if continuously monitored
Utility in clinical reasoning	
Diagnosis	Poor
Surveillance	Poor unless continuously monitored
Prognosis	Untested
Goal-directed therapy	Untested

*Subjective four-point scale: excellent, good, fair, poor.
From DS Prough: Brain monitoring. In: W Shoemaker, R Taylor (eds): Critical Care: State of the Art, Volume 12. Fullerton, CA, Society of Critical Care Medicine, p 180, © by Williams & Wilkins, 1991.

normal or elevated jugular venous saturation, while reassuring, is not adequate evidence of satisfactory cerebral perfusion. Because of the limitations of the technique, insufficient data have been accumulated to allow firm conclusions about the utility of jugular bulb monitoring.

Robertson and coworkers reported extensive experience with monitoring of the cerebral arteriovenous oxygen content difference.[83] In a series of 100 patients, they accumulated evidence that measurements of the cerebral arteriovenous differences of lactate and oxygen content could be

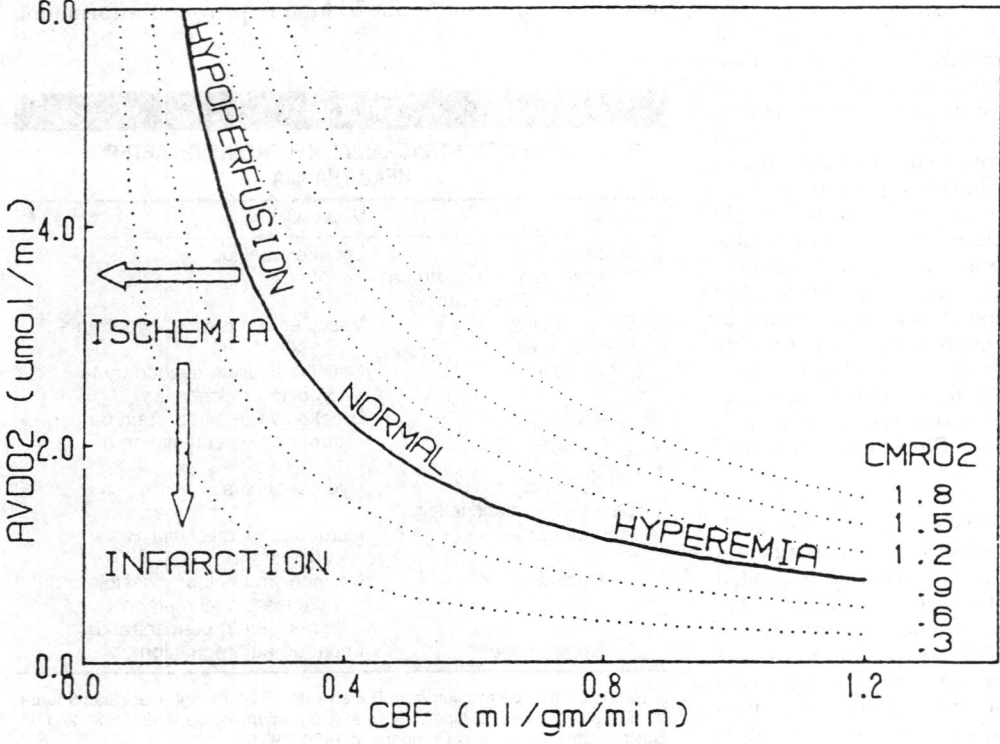

Figure 18–10. Conceptual model of the relationship between CBF and cerebral metabolism in comatose, head-injured patients. In nonischemic brain, the arteriovenous oxygen difference ($AVDo_2$) and CBF vary reciprocally as illustrated by the solid curve, representing a $CMRo_2$ averaging 0.9 μmol/g/min (note that this is substantially less than $CMRo_2$ in normal individuals of 1.5 μmol/g/min; 15 μmol/g/min = 3.4 mL O_2/100 g/min). In the presence of cerebral ischemia or infarction (*open arrows*), the arteriovenous oxygen difference and CBF have an unpredictable relationship. (From Robertson CS, Narayan RK, Gokaslan ZI, et al: Cerebral arteriovenous oxygen difference as an estimate of cerebral blood flow in comatose patients. J Neurosurg 70:222, 1989.)

used to predict CBF and to differentiate patients with patterns consistent with ischemia or infarction, normal CBF, cerebral hyperemia, and compensated hypoperfusion (Fig. 18–10).[83]

Near-Infrared Spectroscopy (Table 18–13)

Near-infrared spectroscopy may eventually offer the opportunity to assess the adequacy of brain oxygenation continuously, thereby facilitating either surveillance or goal-directed therapy. Near-infrared light penetrates the skull and, during transmission through or reflection from brain tissue, undergoes changes in wavelength that are proportional to the relative concentrations of oxygenated and deoxygenated Hb in the tissue beneath the field.[84]

The basic physical theories underlying near-infrared spectroscopy have been developed over the past 30 years. Extensive preclinical and clinical data demonstrate the sensitivity of the technique for the detection of qualitative changes in brain oxygenation[84–87] (Fig. 18–11). However, clinical application has been delayed because of uncertainties regarding quantification of the signal, especially differentiation of venous saturation from combined saturation in the pool of arterial, venous, and capillary blood between the light source and the detection system. More recent data suggest that quantification of the signal may be practical.[88–90] If subsequent clinical validation of one or more of the current approaches is satisfactory, a noninvasive, continuous monitor of cerebral circulatory adequacy will be possible. The availability of an inexpensive, simple-to-operate surveillance monitor as well as a monitor that could be used for goal-directed therapy provides an unprecedented opportunity to manage the cerebral circulation as comprehensively as the systemic circulation can now be managed. The challenge then will be to demonstrate that improved therapy based on enhanced monitoring improves outcome.

Evoked Potential Monitoring (Table 18–14)

Sensory evoked potentials (EPs), which include somatosensory evoked potentials (SSEPs), brain stem auditory evoked

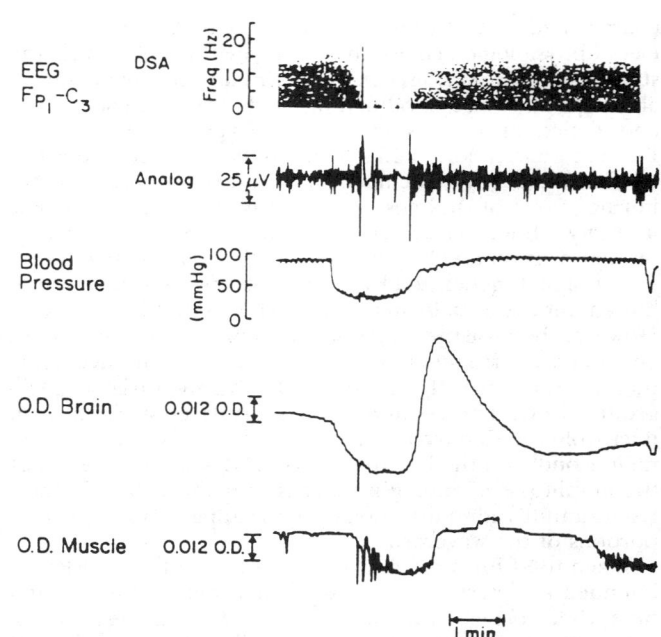

Figure 18–11. EEG (density spectral array display), analog EEG, blood pressure, and near-infrared spectroscopic estimation of Hb saturation in brain and muscle (O.D. = optical density) during an episode of ventricular fibrillation in a patient undergoing implantation of an automatic implantable defibrillator. With abrupt cessation of cerebral circulation, optical density in brain and muscle declined abruptly. After an interval of absent circulation, defibrillation resulted in restoration of perfusion. The postdefibrillation increase in optical density in brain may represent transient postischemic hyperemia. (From Smith DS, Levy W, Maris M, et al: Reperfusion hyperoxia in brain after circulatory arrest in humans. Anesthesiology 73:12, 1990.)

potentials (BAEPs), and visual evoked potentials, can be used as qualitative threshold monitors to detect severe neural ischemia. EPs are generated by integrated neural networks, including the initial sensory structure, the transmitting pathways, and cortical and subcortical stimulus-processing centers. As the response to a stimulus is transmitted centrally,

TABLE 18–13

CHARACTERISTICS: BRAIN METABOLIC MONITORING (NEAR-INFRARED SPECTROSCOPY)

Characteristic	Grade*
Bias	Not established (most devices qualitative)
Precision	Not established (most devices qualitative)
Sensitivity	Good for severe global desaturation
Positive predictive value	Not established
Specificity	Not established
Negative predictive value	Not established
Threshold definition	Probably similar to jugular saturation
Speed	Excellent
Utility in clinical reasoning	
Diagnosis	Untested
Surveillance	Should be excellent (continuous monitor)
Prognosis	Untested
Goal-directed therapy	Potentially valuable but untested

*Subjective four-point scale: excellent, good, fair, poor.
From DS Prough: Brain monitoring. In: W Shoemaker, R Taylor (eds): Critical Care: State of the Art, Volume 12. Fullerton, CA, Society of Critical Care Medicine, p 182, © by Williams & Wilkins, 1991.

TABLE 18–14

CHARACTERISTICS: EVOKED POTENTIAL MONITORING

Characteristic	Grade*
Bias	Not applicable
Precision	Not applicable
Sensitivity	High for ischemia
Positive predictive value	Good for ischemia
Specificity	High for ischemia
Negative predictive value	Good for ischemia
Threshold definition	Ischemia (CBF 15–23 mL/100 g/min)
Speed	Good
Utility in clinical reasoning	
Diagnosis	Good
Surveillance	Poor
Prognosis	Good
Goal-directed therapy	Poor

*Subjective four-point scale: excellent, good, fair, poor.
From DS Prough: Brain monitoring. In: W Shoemaker, R Taylor (eds): Critical Care: State of the Art, Volume 12. Fullerton, CA, Society of Critical Care Medicine, p 167, © by Williams & Wilkins, 1991.

characteristic waveforms are generated that correspond to electrophysiologic activity in structures through which the stimulus passes. EPs, especially BAEPs, are relatively robust, although they are modified by sedatives, narcotics, and anesthetics, as well as by trauma, hypoxia, or ischemia. Because obliteration of EPs occurs only under conditions of profound cerebral ischemia or mechanical trauma, EP monitoring is one of the most specific ways to assess neurologic integrity. However, EPs are insensitive to less severe deterioration of cerebral or spinal cord oxygen availability.

The signals generated by individual sensory stimuli are of low amplitude, usually lower than background EEG activity. However, because the responses are reproducible, the signals generated by frequent repetitive stimuli can be averaged, thereby removing the noise of the highly variable background EEG. The resulting signal, displayed as voltage (in microvolts or nanovolts) on the vertical axis and time (in milliseconds) on the horizontal axis, is described in terms of the amplitude of individual peaks and the delay (latency) from stimulus administration until the appearance of specific portions of the waveform.

When used for brain and spinal cord monitoring, EPs are intended to detect deterioration in neurologic function at a time when corrective action may still reverse changes. Thus, they have been most extensively utilized for monitoring during neurosurgical procedures[91, 92] and for diagnosis in such diseases as multiple sclerosis.[93, 94] However, neurologic deficits occur that have not been predicted by changes in EPs,[95] and apparently severe changes in EPs may not be followed by neurologic deficits. The former probably represent damage to tissue that has not been part of the conducting pathway for the monitored response; the latter presumably reflect either ischemia of insufficient duration to produce irreversible injury or ischemia of insufficient magnitude to produce cell death.

In critically ill patients, EP monitoring has been employed primarily as a diagnostic and prognostic aid in cases of head trauma[96–105] or spinal cord injury.[106–111] BAEPs correlate less well with clinical outcome after head injury than do cortical SSEPs,[96–99] the disappearance of which is a particularly ominous prognostic sign.[97] Multimodality EPs improve the prognostic accuracy of the clinical examination and measurement of ICP in head-injured patients.[98, 101, 103–105] After acute spinal cord injury, SSEPs differentiate complete from incomplete transection but do not accurately predict recovery of function.[106–110] Li and coworkers reported that a combination of quantitative SSEP assessment in the ulnar and posterior tibial regions, a motor index score, and a pinprick sensory score provided a strong prognostic battery in patients with cervical spinal cord injury.[111]

To a limited extent, EPs have been used to facilitate diagnosis and prognostication in ischemic and hypoxic brain injury. Central conduction time is prolonged by ischemia in primates[112] and in humans who have ischemic complications of SAH.[113] With impending brain death, cortical SSEPs disappear first; BAEPs disappear only when brain death is imminent.[114, 115] Persistence of the medullary components of the SSEP, at a time when the cortical components are no longer present, confirms brain death.[114] In children, absence of the cortical components of SSEPs with preserved brain stem function suggests the likelihood of a chronic vegetative state.[116]

SSEPs persist, although in altered form, during barbiturate administration; BAEPs are resistant to the effects of barbiturates.[117] Central conduction time, a measure of the time required to transmit the response to a stimulus from the periphery to the cortex, appears to be unaffected even by high levels of barbiturates.[118] Therefore, EPs assist in assessing neurologic status even in patients in barbiturate coma.

However, despite extensive development of hardware and software to support clinical EP monitoring, various factors have limited extensive use of these techniques. First, the equipment is expensive, although less costly devices have now been introduced. Second, highly trained technicians are essential for recording accurate data and for frequent observation of ongoing monitoring. Third, interpretation of changes requires considerable clinical sophistication in the art of pattern recognition. Perhaps most important, EP monitoring appears to have little value for either surveillance or goal-directed therapy in critically ill patients, in contrast to its possible value for intraoperative monitoring.

Electroencephalographic Monitoring (Table 18–15)

The cortical EEG, altered by mild cerebral ischemia and abolished by profound cerebral ischemia, is another qualitative monitor that indicates potentially damaging hypoperfusion. The sensitivity of EEG monitoring is similar to that of EP monitoring. Traditionally used to document brain death, the EEG is otherwise little used in critically ill patients. However, progressive development over the past decade of improved computer processing may improve the practicality of day-to-day monitoring of high-risk patients.

The unprocessed EEG is a complex waveform that consists of components of different frequencies and amplitudes. The spectrum of EEG frequencies is divided into delta (<4 Hz), theta (4 to 8 Hz), alpha (8 to 13 Hz), and beta (>13 Hz). Monitoring of the unprocessed EEG requires the presence of an expert technician or physician who can rapidly recognize changes in the pattern of the waveform. If the complex waveform is filtered and digitized, a computer-driven rapid Fourier analysis of the digitized data can determine the relative amplitude present in each frequency band. In the most commonly employed software programs, the data are then displayed as a compressed spectral array or density spectral array.[119] Computerized compression of the data permits frequent, repetitive assessment of the EEG with a minimum of specific training.

TABLE 18–15
CHARACTERISTICS: ELECTROENCEPHALOGRAPHIC MONITORING

Characteristic	Grade*
Bias	Not applicable
Precision	Not applicable
Sensitivity	Good for ischemia; sensitive to drug effects
Positive predictive value	Poor for ischemia
Specificity	Poor for ischemia
Negative predictive value	Fair for ischemia
Threshold definition	Ischemia (CBF 18–23 mL/100 g/min)
Speed	Good
Utility in clinical reasoning	
Diagnosis	Good
Surveillance	Fair
Prognosis	Fair
Goal-directed therapy	Poor

*Subjective four-point scale: excellent, good, fair, poor.
From DS Prough: Brain monitoring. In: W Shoemaker, R Taylor (eds): Critical Care: State of the Art, Volume 12. Fullerton, CA, Society of Critical Care Medicine, p 170, © by Williams & Wilkins, 1991.

Because of the sensitivity of the EEG to drug effects, either unprocessed or processed EEG monitoring can be used to assess sedation in critically ill patients. It can also be used to provide early evidence of seizure activity or cerebral ischemia.[120] However, despite considerable interest in the intraoperative use of computer-processed EEG monitoring,[120–132] particularly in patients undergoing carotid endarterectomy and cardiac surgery, few centers have extensively used EEG monitoring techniques in the intensive care unit.

Cant and Shaw monitored 51 patients using a compressed spectral array device[133] and reported that persistence or return of a peak of activity in the theta or alpha frequency bands within 10 days of the onset of coma was associated with a favorable recovery. In contrast, patients in whom such a peak was lost were likely to die or suffer residual neurologic damage. In patients comatose as a result of a mixture of traumatic and ischemic injuries, an alternating pattern of compressed spectral array activity was associated with a more favorable outcome.[134] Alpha coma, unconsciousness associated with an EEG pattern resembling normal wakefulness occurring after brain stem stroke or hypoxic or anoxic cerebral injury, suggests a poor prognosis for survival.[135] Serial EEGs have been used to improve prognostication in children with nontraumatic coma; the worst prognostic findings were low-amplitude activity or electrocerebral silence.[136]

As noted previously with regard to EP monitoring, extensive development and marketing of hardware and software suitable for EEG monitoring in critically ill patients have not appreciably increased utilization. Equipment is relatively expensive, depends for successful use on the ready availability of dedicated technicians if accurate data are to be obtained, and requires a modest level of sophistication for interpretation of changes. Also, like EP monitoring in critically ill patients, EEG monitoring appears to have little value either for surveillance or goal-directed therapy in critically ill patients, in contrast to its possible value for intraoperative monitoring.

SUMMARY

Various powerful techniques, all of which can be performed at the bedside of the critically ill patient, are available for assessing the cerebral circulation. The next step in the evolution of neurologic monitoring necessitates the development of physiologically and pharmacologically sound protocols for goal-directed therapy. These must then be carefully tested to determine whether they can reduce morbidity and mortality in patients with critical neurologic illness.

References

1. Fuchs VR, Garber AM: What is new about the new technology assessment? N Engl J Med 323:673, 1990.
2. Bland RD, Shoemaker WC, Abraham E, et al: Hemodynamic and oxygen transport patterns in surviving and nonsurviving patients. Crit Care Med 13:85, 1985.
3. Bland RD, Shoemaker WC: Probability of survival as a prognostic and severity illness score in critically ill surgical patients. Crit Care Med 13:91, 1985.
4. Shoemaker WC, Appel PL, Kram HB, et al: Prospective trial of supranormal values of survivors as therapeutic goals in high-risk surgical patients. Chest 94:1176, 1988.
5. Graham DI: The pathology of brain ischaemia and possibilities for therapeutic intervention. Br J Anaesth 57:3, 1985.
6. Jones TH, Morawetz RB, Crowell RM, et al: Thresholds of focal cerebral ischemia in awake monkeys. J Neurosurg 54:773, 1981.
7. Strandgaard S, Paulson OB: Cerebral autoregulation. Stroke 15:413, 1984.
8. Strandgaard S: Cerebral blood flow in hypertension. Acta Med Scand Suppl 678:11, 1983.
9. Tommasino C, Moore S, Todd MM: Cerebral effects of isovolemic hemodilution with crystalloid or colloid solutions. Crit Care Med 16:862, 1988.
10. Todd MM, Tommasino C, Moore S: Cerebral effects of isovolemic hemodilution with a hypertonic saline solution. J Neurosurg 63:944, 1985.
11. Phillis JW, Preston G, DeLong RE: Effects of anoxia on cerebral blood flow in the rat brain: Evidence for a role of adenosine in autoregulation. J Cereb Blood Flow Metab 4:586, 1984.
12. Hoffman WE, Albrecht RF, Miletich DJ: The role of adenosine in CBF increases during hypoxia in young vs. aged rats. Stroke 15:124, 1984.
13. Symon L: Flow thresholds in brain ischaemia and the effects of drugs. Br J Anaesth 57:34, 1985.
14. Holbach K-H, Wassmann HW, Hohelüchter KL: Reversibility of the chronic post-stroke state. Stroke 7:296, 1976.
15. Hossmann K-A, Olsson Y: Suppression and recovery of neuronal function in transient cerebral ischemia. Brain Res 22:313, 1970.
16. Sharbrough FW, Messick JM Jr, Sundt TM Jr: Correlation of continuous electrocephalograms with cerebral blood flow measurements during carotid endarterectomy. Stroke 4:674, 1973.
17. Kety SS, Schmidt CF: The determination of cerebral blood flow in man by the use of nitrous oxide in low concentrations. Am J Physiol 143:53, 1945.
18. Kety SS, Schmidt CF: The nitrous oxide method for the quantitative determination of cerebral blood flow in man: Theory, procedure and normal values. J Clin Invest 27:476, 1948.
19. Hoedt-Rasmussen K, Sveinsdottir E, Lassen NA: Regional cerebral blood flow in man determined by intra-arterial injection of radioactive inert gas. Circ Res 18:237, 1966.
20. Olesen J, Paulson OB, Lassen NA: Regional cerebral blood flow in man determined by the initial slope of the clearance of intra-arterially injected [133]Xe. Stroke 2:519, 1971.
21. Obrist WD, Thompson HK Jr, Wang HS, et al: Regional cerebral blood flow estimated by [133]xenon inhalation. Stroke 6:245, 1975.
22. Risberg J, Ali Z, Wilson EM, et al: Regional cerebral blood flow by [133]xenon inhalation. Stroke 6:142, 1975.
23. Obrist WD, Langfitt TW, Jaggi JL, et al: Cerebral blood flow and metabolism in comatose patients with acute head injury. Relationship to intracranial hypertension. J Neurosurg 61:241, 1984.
24. Bruce DA, Langfitt TW, Miller JD, et al: Regional cerebral blood flow, intracranial pressure, and brain metabolism in comatose patients. J Neurosurg 38:131, 1973.
25. Muizelaar JP, Marmarou A, DeSalles AA, et al: Cerebral blood flow and metabolism in severely head-injured children. Part 1: Relationship with GCS score, outcome, ICP, and PVI. J Neurosurg 71:63, 1989.
26. Cold GE, Jensen FT: Cerebral blood flow in the acute phase after head injury. Part 1: Correlation to age of the patients, clinical outcome and localization of the injured region. Acta Anaesthesiol Scand 24:245, 1980.
27. Muizelaar JP, Ward JD, Marmarou A, et al: Cerebral blood flow and metabolism in severely head-injured children. Part 2: Autoregulation. J Neurosurg 71:72, 1989.
28. Muizelaar JP, Lutz HA III, Becker DP: Effect of mannitol on ICP and CBF and correlation with pressure autoregulation in severely head-injured patients. J Neurosurg 61:700, 1984.
29. Overgaard J, Mosdal C, Tweed WA: Cerebral circulation after head injury. Part 3: Does reduced regional cerebral blood flow determine recovery of brain function after blunt head injury? J Neurosurg 55:63, 1981.
30. Overgaard J, Tweed WA: Cerebral circulation after head injury. Part 4: Functional anatomy and boundary-zone flow deprivation in the first week of traumatic coma. J Neurosurg 59:439, 1983.
31. Obrist WD, Clifton GL, Robertson CS, et al: Cerebral metabolic changes induced by hyperventilation in acute head injury. In: Meyer JS, Lechner H, Reivich M (eds): Cerebral Vascular Disease, Volume 6. New York, Elsevier Science Publishers, p 251, 1977.
32. Ward JD, Choi S, Marmarou A, et al: Effect of prophylactic hyperventilation on outcome in patients with severe head injury. In: Hoff JT, Betz AL (eds): Intracranial Pressure, Volume VII. New York, Springer-Verlag, p 630, 1989.
33. Robertson CS, Grossman RG, Goodman JC, et al: The predictive value of cerebral anaerobic metabolism with cerebral infarction after head injury. J Neurosurg 67:361, 1987.
34. Snyder JV, Nemoto EM, Carroll RG, et al: Global ischemia in dogs: Intracranial pressures, brain blood flow and metabolism. Stroke 6:21, 1975.
35. Steen PA, Michenfelder JD, Milde JH: Incomplete versus complete cerebral ischemia: Improved outcome with a minimal blood flow. Ann Neurol 6:389, 1979.
36. Beckstead JE, Tweed WA, Lee J, et al: Cerebral blood flow and metabolism in man following cardiac arrest. Stroke 9:569, 1978.
37. Cohan SL, Mun SK, Petite J, et al: Cerebral blood flow in humans following resuscitation from cardiac arrest. Stroke 20:761, 1989.
38. Steen PA, Newberg LA, Milde JH, et al: Nimodipine improves cerebral blood flow and neurologic recovery after complete cerebral ischemia in the dog. J Cereb Blood Flow Metab 3:38, 1983.
39. Steen PA, Gisvold SE, Milde JH, et al: Nimodipine improves outcome

when given after complete cerebral ischemia in primates. Anesthesiology 62:406, 1985.

40. Forsman M, Aarseth HP, Nordby HK, et al: Effects of nimodipine on cerebral blood flow and cerebrospinal fluid pressure after cardiac arrest: Correlation with neurologic outcome. Anesth Analg 68:436, 1989.
41. Caplan LR, Brass LM, DeWitt LD, et al: Transcranial Doppler ultrasound: Present status. Neurology 40:696, 1990.
42. American Academy of Neurology: Assessment: Transcranial Doppler. Neurology 40:680, 1990.
43. Seiler RW, Grolimund P, Aaslid R: Cerebral vasospasm evaluated by transcranial ultrasound correlated with clinical grade and CT-visualized subarachnoid hemorrhage. J Neurosurg 64:594, 1986.
44. Aaslid R, Huber P, Nornes H: Evaluation of cerebrovascular spasm with transcranial Doppler ultrasound. J Neurosurg 60:37, 1984.
45. Sekhar LN, Wechsler LR, Yonas H, et al: Value of transcranial Doppler examination in the diagnosis of cerebral vasospasm after subarachnoid hemorrhage. Neurosurgery 22:813, 1988.
46. Bishop CCR, Powell S, Rutt D, et al: Transcranial Doppler measurement of middle cerebral artery blood flow velocity: A validation study. Stroke 17:913, 1986.
47. Hassler W, Steinmetz H, Galowski J: Transcranial Doppler ultrasonography in raised intracranial pressure and in intracranial circulatory arrest. J Neurosurg 68:745, 1988.
48. Werner C, Kochs E, Rau M, et al: Transcranial Doppler sonography as a supplement in the detection of cerebral circulatory arrest. J Neurosurg Anesth 2:159, 1990.
49. Miller JD, Butterworth JF IV, Gudeman SK, et al: Further experience in the management of severe head injury. J Neurosurg 54:289, 1981.
50. Becker DP, Miller JD, Ward JD, et al: The outcome from severe head injury with early diagnosis and intensive management. J Neurosurg 47:491, 1977.
51. Lundberg N, Troupp H, Lorin H: Continuous recording of the ventricular-fluid pressure in patients with severe acute traumatic brain injury. J Neurosurg 22:581, 1965.
52. Miller JD, Becker DP, Ward JD, et al: Significance of intracranial hypertension in severe head injury. J Neurosurg 47:503, 1977.
53. Marshall LF, Smith RW, Shapiro HM: The outcome with aggressive treatment in severe head injuries. Part I: The significance of intracranial pressure monitoring. J Neurosurg 50:20, 1979.
54. Saul TG, Ducker TB: Effect of intracranial pressure monitoring and aggressive treatment on mortality in severe head injury. J Neurosurg 56:498, 1982.
55. Shaywitz BA, Leventhal JM, Kramer MS, et al: Prolonged continuous monitoring of intracranial pressure in severe Reye's syndrome. Pediatrics 59:595, 1977.
56. Shaywitz BA, Rothstein P, Venes JL: Monitoring and management of increased intracranial pressure in Reye syndrome: Results in 29 children. Pediatrics 66:198, 1980.
57. Mickell JJ, Reigel DH, Cook DR, et al: Intracranial pressure: Monitoring and normalization therapy in children. Pediatrics 59:606, 1977.
58. Tasker RC, Matthew DJ, Helms P, et al: Monitoring in non-traumatic coma. Part I: Invasive intracranial measurements. Arch Dis Child 63:888, 1988.
59. Barnett GH, Ropper AH, Romeo J: Intracranial pressure and outcome in adult encephalitis. J Neurosurg 68:585, 1988.
60. Hanid MA, Davies M, Mellon PJ, et al: Clinical monitoring of intracranial pressure in fulminant hepatic failure. Gut 21:866, 1980.
61. Bailes JE, Spetzler RF, Hadley MN, et al: Management morbidity and mortality of poor-grade aneurysm patients. J Neurosurg 72:559, 1990.
62. Sarnaik AP, Preston G, Lieh-Lai M, et al: Intracranial pressure and cerebral perfusion pressure in near-drowning. Crit Care Med 13:224, 1985.
63. Nussbaum E, Galant SP: Intracranial pressure monitoring as a guide to prognosis in the nearly drowned, severely comatose child. J Pediatr 102:215, 1983.
64. Griswold WR, Viney J, Mendoza SA, et al: Intracranial pressure monitoring in severe hypertensive encephalopathy. Crit Care Med 9:573, 1981.
65. Colohan AR, Alves WM, Gross CR, et al: Head injury mortality in two centers with different emergency medical services and intensive care. J Neurosurg 71:202, 1989.
66. Vries JK, Becker DP, Young HF: A subarachnoid screw for monitoring intracranial pressure. Technical note. J Neurosurg 39:416, 1973.
67. Miller JD, Bobo H, Kapp JP: Inaccurate pressure readings from subarachnoid bolts. Neurosurgery 19:253, 1986.
68. Allen R: Intracranial pressure: A review of clinical problems, measurement techniques and monitoring methods. J Med Eng Technol 10:299, 1986.
69. Ward JD: Intracranial pressure monitoring. In: Cerra FB, Shoemaker WC (eds): Critical Care: State of the Art. Fullerton, CA, Society of Critical Care Medicine, p 173, 1989.
70. Crutchfield JS, Narayan RK, Robertson CS, et al: Evaluation of a fiberoptic intracranial pressure monitor. J Neurosurg 72:482, 1990.
71. Chambers IR, Mendelow AD, Sinar EJ, et al: A clinical evaluation of the Camino subdural screw and ventricular monitoring kits. Neurosurgery 26:421, 1990.

72. Eisenberg HM, Frankowski RF, Contant CF, et al: High-dose barbiturate control of elevated intracranial pressure in patients with severe head injury. J Neurosurg 69:15, 1988.
73. Ward JD, Becker DP, Miller JD, et al: Failure of prophylactic barbiturate coma in the treatment of severe head injury. J Neurosurg 62:383, 1985.
74. Kanter RK, Weiner LB, Patti AM, et al: Infectious complications and duration of intracranial pressure monitoring. Crit Care Med 13:837, 1985.
75. Aucoin PJ, Kotilainen HR, Gantz NM, et al: Intracranial pressure monitors. Epidemiologic study of risk factors and infections. Am J Med 80:369, 1986.
76. Clark WC, Muhlbauer MS, Lowrey R, et al: Complications of intracranial pressure monitoring in trauma patients. Neurosurgery 25:20, 1989.
77. Maset AL, Marmarou A, Ward JD, et al: Pressure-volume index in head injury. J Neurosurg 67:832, 1987.
78. Tans JT, Poortvliet DC: Intracranial volume-pressure relationship in man. Part 2: Clinical significance of the pressure-volume index. J Neurosurg 59:810, 1983.
79. Robertson CS, Narayan RK, Contant CF, et al: Clinical experience with a continuous monitor of intracranial compliance. J Neurosurg 71:673, 1989.
80. Myerson A, Halloran RD, Hirsch HL: Technic for obtaining blood from the internal jugular vein and internal carotid artery. Arch Neurol Psychiatry 17:807, 1927.
81. Swedlow DB, Kettrick RG, Raphaely RC: Jugular venous bulb catheterization in children (abstract). Crit Care Med 9:287, 1981.
82. Goetting MG, Preston G: Jugular bulb catheterization: Experience with 123 patients. Crit Care Med 18:1220, 1990.
83. Robertson CS, Narayan RK, Gokaslan ZI, et al: Cerebral arteriovenous oxygen difference as an estimate of cerebral blood flow in comatose patients. J Neurosurg 70:222, 1989.
84. Jöbsis-VanderVliet FF, Fox E, Sugioka K: Monitoring of cerebral oxygenation and cytochrome aa_3 redox state. Int Anesthesiol Clin 25:209, 1987.
85. Proctor HJ, Cairns C, Fillipo D, et al: Brain metabolism during increased intracranial pressure as assessed by niroscopy. Surgery 96:273, 1984.
86. Brazy JE, Lewis DV, Mitnick MH: Noninvasive monitoring of cerebral oxygenation in preterm infants: Preliminary observations. Pediatrics 75:217, 1985.
87. Smith DS, Levy W, Maris M, et al: Reperfusion hyperoxia in brain after circulatory arrest in humans. Anesthesiology 73:12, 1990.
88. Ferrari M, Wilson DA, Hanley DF, et al: Noninvasive determination of hemoglobin saturation in dogs by derivative near-infrared spectroscopy. Am J Physiol 256:H1493, 1989.
89. Prough DS, Scuderi PE, Lewis G, et al: Initial clinical experience using in vivo optical spectroscopy to quantify brain oxygen saturation. Anesthesiology 73:A424, 1990.
90. McCormick PW, Stewart M, Goetting MG, et al: Regional cerebrovascular oxygen saturation measured by optical spectroscopy in humans. Stroke 22:596, 1991.
91. Grundy BL: Intraoperative monitoring of sensory-evoked potentials. Anesthesiology 58:72, 1983.
92. Grundy BL, Jannetta PJ, Procopio PT, et al: Intraoperative monitoring of brain-stem auditory evoked potentials. J Neurosurg 57:674, 1982.
93. Chiappa KH, Ropper AH: Evoked potentials in clinical medicine (first of two parts). N Engl J Med 306:1140, 1982.
94. Chiappa KH, Ropper AH: Evoked potentials in clinical medicine (second of two parts). N Engl J Med 306:1205, 1982.
95. Lesser RP, Raudzens P, Lüders H, et al: Postoperative neurological deficits may occur despite unchanged intraoperative somatosensory evoked potentials. Ann Neurol 19:22, 1986.
96. Seales DM, Rossiter VS, Weinstein ME: Brainstem auditory evoked responses in patients comatose as a result of blunt head trauma. J Trauma 19:347, 1979.
97. Ganes T, Lundar T: EEG and evoked potentials in comatose patients with severe brain damage. Electroencephalogr Clin Neurophysiol 69:6, 1988.
98. Greenberg RP, Newlon PG, Hyatt MS, et al: Prognostic implications of early multimodality evoked potentials in severely head-injured patients. J Neurosurg 55:227, 1981.
99. Hume AL, Cant BR: Central somatosensory conduction after head injury. Ann Neurol 10:411, 1981.
100. Cant BR, Hume AL, Judson JA, et al: The assessment of severe head injury by short-latency somatosensory and brain-stem auditory evoked potentials. Electroencephalogr Clin Neurophysiol 65:188, 1986.
101. Anderson DC, Bundlie S, Rockswold GL: Multimodality evoked potentials in closed head trauma. Arch Neurol 41:369, 1984.
102. Newlon PG, Greenberg RP, Hyatt MS, et al: The dynamics of neuronal dysfunction and recovery following severe head injury assessed with serial multimodality evoked potentials. J Neurosurg 57:168, 1982.
103. Greenberg RP, Mayer DJ, Becker DP, et al: Evaluation of brain function in severe human head trauma with multimodality evoked potentials. Part 1: Evoked brain-injury potentials, methods, and analysis. J Neurosurg 47:150, 1977.
104. Greenberg RP, Becker DP, Miller JD, et al: Evaluation of brain function in severe head trauma with multimodality evoked potentials. Part 2:

Localization of brain dysfunction and correlation with posttraumatic neurological conditions. J Neurosurg 47:163, 1977.

105. Narayan RK, Greenberg RP, Miller JD, et al: Improved confidence of outcome prediction in severe head injury. J Neurosurg 54:751, 1981.

106. Rowed DW, McLean JAG, Tator CH: Somatosensory evoked potentials in acute spinal cord injury: Prognostic value. Surg Neurol 9:203, 1976.

107. Powers SK, Bolger CA, Edwards MSB: Spinal cord pathways mediating somatosensory evoked potentials. J Neurosurg 57:472, 1982.

108. McGarry J, Friedgood DL, Woolsey R, et al: Somatosensory-evoked potentials in spinal cord injuries. Surg Neurol 22:341, 1984.

109. Dorfman LJ, Perkash I, Bosley TM, et al: Use of cerebral evoked potentials to evaluate spinal somatosensory function in patients with traumatic and surgical myelopathies. J Neurosurg 52:654, 1980.

110. Chabot R, York DH, Watts C, et al: Somatosensory evoked potentials evaluated in normal subjects and spinal cord–injured patients. J Neurosurg 63:544, 1985.

111. Li C, Houlden DA, Rowed DW: Somatosensory evoked potentials and neurological grades as predictors of outcome in acute spinal cord injury. J Neurosurg 72:600, 1990.

112. Hargadine JR, Branston NM, Symon L: Central conduction time in primate brain ischemia—A study in baboons. Stroke 11:637, 1980.

113. Symon L, Hargadine J, Zawirski M, et al: Central conduction time as an index of ischaemia in subarachnoid hemorrhage. J Neurol Sci 44:95, 1979.

114. Goldie WD, Chiappa KH, Young RR, et al: Brainstem auditory and short-latency somatosensory evoked responses in brain death. Neurology 31:248, 1981.

115. Garcia-Larrea L, Bertrand O, Artru F, et al: Brain-stem monitoring. II. Preterminal BAEP changes observed until brain death in deeply comatose patients. Electroencephalogr Clin Neurophysiol 68:446, 1987.

116. Frank LM, Furgiuele TL, Etheridge JE Jr: Prediction of chronic vegetative state in children using evoked potentials. Neurology 35:931, 1985.

117. de Weerd AW, Groeneveld C: The use of evoked potentials in the management of patients with severe cerebral trauma. Acta Neurol Scand 72:489, 1985.

118. Hume AL, Cant BR, Shaw NA: Central somatosensory conduction time in comatose patients. Ann Neurol 5:379, 1979.

119. Levy WJ, Shapiro HM, Maruchak G, et al: Automated EEG processing for intraoperative monitoring: A comparison of techniques. Anesthesiology 53:223, 1980.

120. Cant BR, Shaw NA: Electroencephalography and compressed spectral array in severe intracranial disease. Int Anesthesiol Clin 17:343, 1979.

121. Quasha AL, Tinker JH, Sharbrough FW: Hypothermia plus thiopental: Prolonged electroencephalographic suppression. Anesthesiology 55:636, 1981.

122. Rampil IJ, Holzer JA, Quest DO, et al: Prognostic value of computerized EEG analysis during carotid endarterectomy. Anesth Analg 62:186, 1983.

123. Rampil IJ, Matteo RS: Changes in EEG spectral edge frequency correlate with the hemodynamic response to laryngoscopy and intubation. Anesthesiology 67:139, 1987.

124. Smith NT, Dec-Silver H, Sanford TJ Jr, et al: EEGs during high-dose fentanyl-sufentanil-, or morphine-oxygen anesthesia. Anesth Analg 63:386, 1984.

125. Algotsson L, Messeter K, Rehncrona S, et al: Cerebral hemodynamic changes and electroencephalography during carotid endarterectomy. J Clin Anesth 2:143, 1990.

126. Silbert BS, Kluger R, Cronin KD, et al: The processed electroencephalogram may not detect neurologic ischemia during carotid endarterectomy. Anesthesiology 70:356, 1989.

127. Yamamura T, Fukuda M, Takeya H, et al: Fast oscillatory EEG activity induced by analgesic concentrations of nitrous oxide in man. Anesth Analg 60:283, 1981.

128. Sebel PS, Bovill JG, Wauquier A, et al: Effects of high-dose fentanyl anesthesia on the electroencephalogram. Anesthesiology 55:203, 1981.

129. Cucchiara RF, Sharbrough FW, Messick JM, et al: An electroencephalographic filter-processor as an indicator of cerebral ischemia during carotid endarterectomy. Anesthesiology 51:77, 1979.

130. Fleming RA, Smith NT: An inexpensive device for analyzing and monitoring the electroencephalogram. Anesthesiology 50:456, 1979.

131. Berger MS, Kincaid J, Ojemann GA, et al: Brain mapping techniques to maximize resection, safety, and seizure control in children with brain tumors. Neurosurgery 25:786, 1989.

132. Muizelaar JP: The use of electroencephalography and brain protection during operation for basilar aneurysms. Neurosurgery 25:899, 1989.

133. Cant BR, Shaw NA: Monitoring by compressed spectral array in prolonged coma. Neurology 34:35, 1984.

134. Karnaze DS, Marshall LF, Bickford RG: EEG monitoring of clinical coma: The compressed spectral array. Neurology 32:289, 1982.

135. Westmoreland BF, Klass DW, Sharbrough FW, et al: Alpha-coma. Electroencephalographic, clinical, pathologic, and etiologic correlations. Arch Neurol 32:713, 1975.

136. Tasker RC, Boyd S, Harden A, et al: Monitoring in non-traumatic coma. Part II. Electroencephalography. Arch Dis Child 63:895, 1988.

CHAPTER 19

Blood Gas Analysis and Related Techniques

Luis R. Urbina
James A. Kruse

It has been known for many years that dissolved gases are present in blood and that the acidity of blood varies over a relatively narrow range. Even though measurement of blood pH and gas partial pressures has been possible for decades, these techniques were initially restricted to the physiology laboratory for investigational purposes. It was not until the early 1950s, in the midst of the poliomyelitis epidemic in Denmark, that the analysis of blood pH was first used for clinical purposes.[1] Since then, many technical advances have occurred, and blood gas monitoring is now routinely employed in the clinical assessment of critically ill patients in intensive care units, emergency departments, and operating suites. Blood gas measurements are now among the most frequently performed laboratory tests in many hospitals.[2] This widespread use has become possible in part through the development of easy-to-use, accurate, and fully automated instruments that are able to analyze small-volume samples in as little as 1 minute.

This chapter covers the technical aspects of blood gas measurement, including sampling technique, potential sources of inaccuracy and how to avoid them, the assay methodology employed by modern analyzers, and the calculation of parameters derived from measured blood gas results.

OBTAINING THE SAMPLE

Blood gas analysis is generally performed on arterial blood obtained either by arterial puncture or from an indwelling arterial catheter and is used to assess gas exchange and systemic acid-base status. Assays are also performed on mixed venous blood, sampled through indwelling pulmonary arterial catheters, to assess systemic perfusion and oxygen utilization.

Selecting the Site. Several sites are available for sampling arterial blood. The most common include the radial, brachial, and femoral arteries. The radial artery offers a safe and easily accessible approach. It has the added advantage that there is normally good collateral circulation to the hand via the ulnar artery. In addition, it may be the site of choice for arterial puncture in patients with bleeding diatheses. The femoral artery is large and therefore easiest to localize by palpation and to cannulate. Both the femoral and brachial arteries, however, pose the problem of lack of significant collateral circulation should an occlusive complication occur. The proposed site should be free of signs of local infection or scars that may denote previous vascular surgery. Strict aseptic technique must be observed, and the procedure should be performed only by, or under direct supervision of, qualified experienced staff, which may include trained nurses[3, 4] and respiratory therapy personnel.[5] If frequent blood gas determinations are anticipated or if the critical condition of the patient warrants continuous arterial pressure monitoring, an indwelling arterial catheter may be indicated and may be preferable to frequent intermittent arterial punctures.

Assessing Collateral Artery Patency. Most authors recommend that the patency and adequacy of the collateral circulation be evaluated before radial artery cannulation, because 2% of normal adults have no palmar arch and 8% have inadequate collateral flow.[6] This can be assessed by the Allen test. As originally described,[7] this maneuver tests for the presence of arterial occlusion in vessels distal to the wrist. The examiner applies thumb pressure over the patient's radial artery to occlude blood flow while the patient forms a tight fist. After 1 minute the patient partially extends the fingers while the examiner continues to occlude the radial vessel and observes the patient's palm and fingers for color change. If the hand remains pale, the ulnar circulation is inadequate. If rubor develops, there is adequate collateral circulation from the ulnar artery. When the patient's fist is opened, it is important that the hand be in a neutral, relaxed position, as opposed to a fully extended position, which might impede the inflow of blood to the hand.[8]

In a modification of the Allen test,[9–11] the patient's fist is tightly clenched during digital occlusion of both the radial and ulnar vessels simultaneously. While the vessels are still occluded, the hand appears blanched after the fist is relaxed. The ulnar artery is then released. If the blanching resolves within 2 to 10 seconds, collateral circulation is adequate. The Allen test may be done in a more objective fashion by means of a Doppler ultrasound instrument applied to the palmar arch while compression maneuvers are done at the wrist arteries.[6] Digital pulse oximetry has been similarly used to assess collateral patency.[12]

Although the presence of a normal Allen test does not preclude the development of ischemic necrosis of the digits,[13] some practitioners consider the lack of adequate collateral circulation, as evidenced by the Allen test, a contraindication for puncture of the radial artery because a thrombotic complication could jeopardize perfusion to the hand,[8] leading to gangrene of the digits.[14] On the other hand, the low incidence of complications of radial artery puncture has prompted some authors to consider the Allen test optional rather than mandatory.[15, 16] It has been proposed that the words *positive* and *negative* not be used to report the outcome of this test, because the meaning of these terms may be reversed or misunderstood.[17, 18] Concise description of the test result avoids confusion. Although the result is usually reported qualitatively (e.g., as adequate or inadequate collateral circulation), a quantitative result is possible by reporting the time elapsed from release of compression to the appearance of palmar blushing.

Performing the Puncture. All of the necessary equipment and supplies should be at hand, including suitable antiseptic solution (e.g., povidone-iodine), sterile gauze, syringe, a small-gauge (20- to 25-gauge) needle with a short bevel, a cap for plugging the sample syringe, a container of ice slush for transporting the sample, an identification label for the sample, and a completed requisition form. Unless a preheparinized syringe is employed, a supply of heparin solution must also be available. Gloves should be worn when drawing and handling blood.[19, 20] If an indwelling arterial catheter is to be inserted, the operator should don cap and mask, sterile gloves, and gown, and a wide sterile field should be used to ensure rigorous aseptic technique. For the radial approach, a rolled towel placed under the wrist is helpful for optimal positioning (Fig. 19–1). Optionally, a small volume of local anesthetic may be injected at the site but this is usually unnecessary for puncture alone, particularly if an extremely small caliber needle (e.g., 25 gauge) is used.[21–23] Although concern has been expressed that the minor discomfort associated with arterial puncture might induce hyperventi-

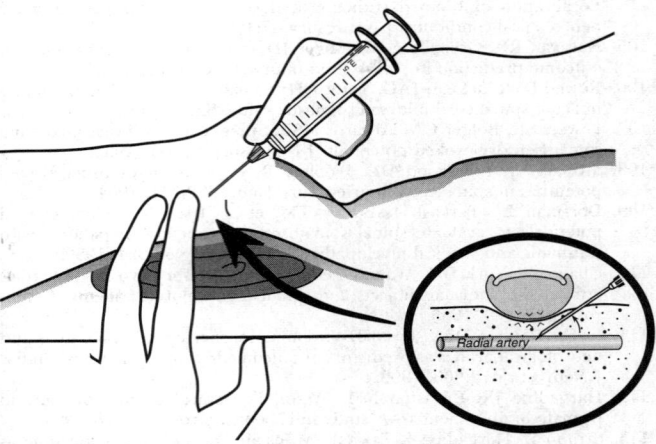

Figure 19–1. Technique of radial artery puncture. The artery is identified by palpation and the needle advanced at an approximately 45° angle with the bevel directed upward. Note that the artery is palpated immediately proximal to the point of needle entry and that the plunger of the syringe should not be used to aspirate the sample.

lation or breath holding and influence gas tensions,[24] it has been shown that blood gas results obtained after puncture without anesthetic do not differ from results obtained after instillation of local anesthetic or after drawing blood from an indwelling arterial catheter.[25, 26]

The artery to be punctured is identified by palpation and the needle advanced at an approximately 45° angle with the bevel directed upward. Unless sterile gloves are worn, the actual puncture site should not be touched; rather the artery is palpated immediately proximal to the point of needle entry. Some practitioners recommend quickly transfixing the artery and then slowly withdrawing the needle until its orifice is within the vessel lumen. This technique may occasionally be helpful for elderly patients with severe atherosclerotic disease who have hardened vessels that tend to roll away from the advancing needle. However, it is unnecessary for routine use and needlessly traumatizes the artery. It may also increase the possibility of entraining venous blood into the arterial sample.[27] Furthermore, the likelihood of touching the periosteum with the needle is greater if a deep puncture is performed, resulting in unnecessary pain for the patient. The plunger of the syringe should not be used to aspirate the sample. Allowing the blood to enter the syringe under the force of arterial pressure helps to ensure that the specimen is indeed arterial and avoids collapsing the artery or entraining air or creating foam in the sample. This is usually attainable with glass syringes that have been thoroughly lubricated with heparin and with most plastic syringes. It may not be possible, however, in severely hypotensive patients. It has been demonstrated in vitro that blood does not spontaneously flow into certain syringes when the driving pressure is less than about 70 mm Hg.[28] Spontaneous filling may not occur in normotensive patients when extremely small (25-gauge) needles are employed. After withdrawing the needle, firm pressure must be applied over the puncture site with a gauze pad for a minimum of 5 minutes.[11, 27, 29] The patient should not be asked to do this. Pressure must be held for a longer period if there is a bleeding diathesis or if hematoma formation is noted. Ideally, a second person should be available to provide pressure while the operator tends to the sample. Any air bubbles in the specimen syringe must be quickly expelled and the syringe capped to maintain a sealed, anaerobic sample. Air bubbles are particularly difficult to expel from plastic compared with glass syringes.[30] An identification label is attached to the sample syringe, which is then placed in the ice-slush mixture and immediately transported to the blood gas or "stat" laboratory.

Use of Heparin. Heparin is used to prevent the blood specimen from clotting during puncture, transport, and analysis. Preheparinized syringes are convenient and used routinely at some institutions. Alternatively, heparin solution (1000 U/mL) may be drawn into a sterile syringe immediately before performing the puncture. In this case, the syringe is rinsed with the heparin solution, which is then expelled through the needle. The heparin remaining in the dead space of the needle and syringe is generally sufficient to prevent coagulation.[31–33] The remaining heparin also displaces air that would otherwise remain in the dead space volume of the syringe and needle and result in an air bubble in the sample. Heparin further acts to wet the inside of the syringe and serve as a lubricant that facilitates spontaneous syringe filling. This wetting effect is particularly important when glass syringes are employed. Some practitioners use a scalp vein needle and tubing attached to the specimen syringe. This technique facilitates exchanging syringes when additional blood samples are desired for other laboratory tests. Although this is an acceptable procedure, the practitioner must ensure that the heparin is expelled from the syringe before the scalp vein assembly is attached. Otherwise the heparin from the syringe will be ejected into the scalp vein tubing and then return to the syringe during the puncture, resulting in dilution of the sample with excess heparin (see later).[24] Because there is no heparin in the scalp vein tubing, air enters the specimen syringe. Using the first syringe of blood for tests other than blood gases or immediately expelling the resulting air bubble prevents this from affecting the accuracy of the measurements.

Complications of Arterial Puncture and Cannulation. Various complications and sequelae have been reported in the literature, but most of these are, in fact, descriptions of complications related to arterial catheterization rather than simple puncture. Petty and coworkers found no complications in 475 punctures in 54 patients.[34] Fleming and Bowen[4] reported a 0.58% incidence of hematoma formation in 4342 arterial punctures. In a study by Mortensen in 1967,[35] which included 3193 arterial entries, the incidence of complications was 11.3% for percutaneous arterial puncture and was 17.7% when a catheter was inserted using the Seldinger technique. The brachial artery had the highest rate of complications from puncture. Risk factors identified by this study were wide pulse pressure resulting from aortic valve insufficiency (74% of patients with a pulse pressure of 75 mm Hg or more had complications), anticoagulation, hypertension, arteriosclerosis, and age less than 10 years. Among the major complications were local obstruction with distal ischemia, external hemorrhage, massive ecchymosis, arterial dissection, and false aneurysm formation. Minor complications included pain, ecchymosis, hematoma, arteriospasm, occlusion without symptoms of ischemia, and external hemorrhage.[35] Both partial and complete arterial thromboses have been reported as complications of arterial puncture and catheter insertion.[36, 37] The risk of developing radial artery occlusion after cannulation increases with increasing catheter diameter and smaller vessel diameter.[38] Wrist circumference correlates with vessel diameter and has been shown to predict the risk of radial artery occlusion.[39] These studies examined both cannulation and simple puncture of a variety of arteries, including the carotid, abdominal aorta, and subclavian arteries, and many were carried out for purposes of arteriography. Therefore, their findings may not be applicable to cases of simple puncture for arterial blood gas sampling. Although serious complications have been associated with

puncture-related ischemia, the incidence of such complications is exceedingly low considering the frequency of sampling for arterial blood gas analysis.[15, 16, 40]

Bleeding is a particular risk in the presence of coagulopathy, thrombocytopenia, or qualitative platelet disorders. Hemorrhagic complications can be minimized in these situations by using a 25-gauge needle and by applying prolonged direct pressure after the puncture or after removal of indwelling catheters. Care must be taken to apply pressure to the artery at the point where the needle or catheter actually penetrated the vessel wall and not at the skin puncture site. In obese patients and when the femoral site has been selected, the actual vessel wall defect may be located an inch or more proximal to the skin entry site. This is especially important when arterial catheters are removed because the relatively large defect remaining in the arterial wall can permit significant bleeding. Sandbags are by no means a good substitute for direct manual pressure. Excessive bleeding may occur and result in hematoma formation superficially or within the deep structures of the extremity. In one large series, hematoma formation was the most common complication, occurring with an incidence 0.58%.[4] Compartmental syndrome may occur but is rare.[16] Compression neuropathy has been observed as a complication of brachial artery puncture in anticoagulated patients.[41, 42] Peripheral neuropathy in anticoagulated patients has also been associated with femoral artery puncture. This complication should be diagnosed and treated as early as possible to minimize the likelihood of permanent sequelae.[43] Other complications of arterial cannulation are reviewed in Chapter 15.

PREANALYTICAL SOURCES OF ERROR

A common source of inaccuracy in blood gas determinations is incorrect specimen collection and handling.[44, 45] In one study such errors were suspected in up to 16% of arterial samples.[46] A number of specific factors have been identified that can cause spurious results. These factors should be considered when developing institutional protocols for routine collection and preanalytical handling of blood gas specimens.

Effects of Air Bubbles and Time Delays. Air bubbles entrapped in the sample syringe cause a time-dependent change in PO_2 and O_2 saturation. Because smaller bubbles have a larger surface area per unit volume, the effect may occur more rapidly if the entrapped air takes the form of froth.[47, 48] An air bubble as small as 0.5% of the blood sample volume is significant if there is a time delay before the sample is processed.[48, 49] Mixing and temperature cycling before analysis also augment the effect of air bubbles.[50] Temperature cycling occurs when the specimen is stored on ice and later injected into the blood gas analyzer, which then equilibrates the sample to 37°C. As the blood cools during the delay period, the solubility of dissolved gases increases. However, the solubility of O_2 increases more rapidly than that of nitrogen, resulting in a higher PO_2/PN_2 ratio. When the sample temperature is rapidly increased in the blood gas analyzer, the PO_2 of the liquid phase is spuriously increased because of this hysteresis effect.[48, 51]

Although a small air bubble (less than 5% of the sample volume) has no appreciable effect on blood gas results if the analysis is performed within 3 minutes, longer delay times can result in measurable errors. Exposure to a bubble with a volume of 10% of the sample volume leads to significant changes in both PCO_2 and PO_2 within 2 to 3 minutes.[47] The directional change in PO_2 caused by the presence of air bubbles depends on the initial PO_2 of the specimen. The air bubble contains room air with a PO_2 of approximately 150

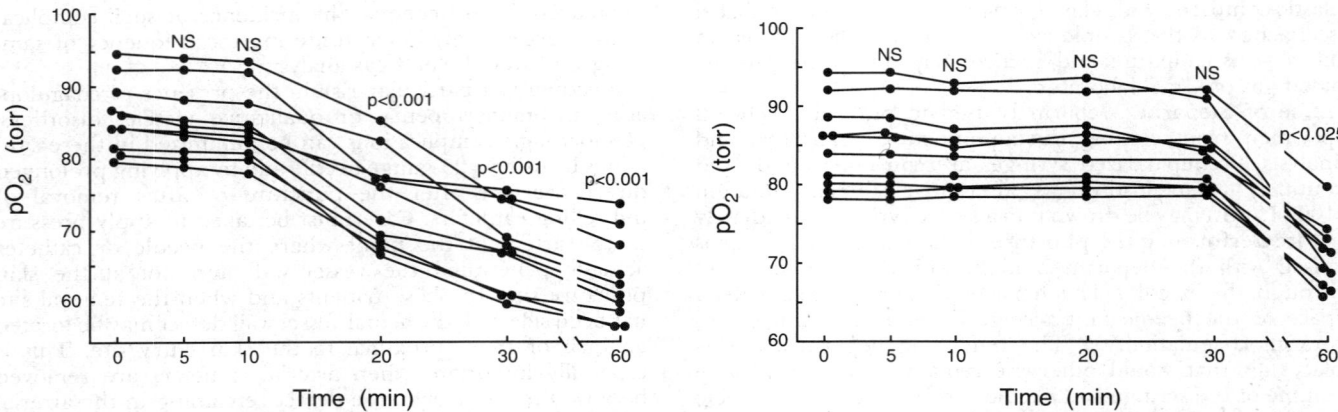

Figure 19–2. Change in blood Po_2 over time during storage in syringes at room temperature *(left)* and at 0°C *(right)*. (Modified from Biswas CK, Ramos JM, Agroyannis B, et al: Blood gas analysis: Effect of air bubbles in syringe and delay in estimation. Br Med J 284:923, 1982.)

torr. The specimen Po_2 and the air bubble Po_2 gradually equilibrate over time. Thus, a sample Po_2 that is initially higher than about 150 torr decreases as it equibrates with the air bubble Po_2. Hemoglobin saturation is not significantly affected because at a Po_2 of 150 torr or higher the oxyhemoglobin saturation (So_2) is for all practical purposes already maximal. On the other hand, if the sample Po_2 is below that of room air, air bubbles in the syringe spuriously increase the measured Po_2 and O_2 saturation.

Because of the sigmoid shape of the O_2-hemoglobin dissociation curve (see Fig. 142–4), O_2 saturation is affected to a greater extent when the sample Po_2 is below 60 torr. pH is less affected by air bubbles or froth.[47, 50]

If it can be absolutely ensured that the sample will be processed immediately after it is drawn, there is no need to place it in ice. This might occur, for example, in pulmonary function laboratories that have their own blood gas equipment on the premises or when portable point-of-care blood gas instruments are used at the patient's bedside or within the operating suite. Under most circumstances, however, the specimen must be sealed and placed in an ice bath. Partially or even completely burying the sample syringe in a container of cubed or crushed ice does not ensure rapid cooling of the specimen to 0°C. The ice should contain liquid water as well, to ensure equilibration of the bath to 0°C. Ice water provides greater surface contact area with the syringe to conduct heat away from the specimen and results in more rapid cooling. Properly iced samples may be stored for up to 30 minutes without significant change in Po_2 (Fig. 19–2). Pco_2 tends to change with storage time, but to a lesser extent than Po_2.[47] pH changes are of similarly small magnitude. When the sample is stored on ice, its pH typically changes by 0.01 to 0.05 pH units per hour.[44, 47, 52]

To avoid spurious results, air bubbles should be expelled from the sample syringe within 30 to 60 seconds of drawing the specimen and the syringe tightly capped. Samples containing obvious froth should be discarded.[47, 53] Analyzing the specimen within 10 minutes of collection obviates errors caused by time delay even if the specimen is maintained at room temperature.[29, 46, 47, 52, 54] For specimens stored on ice, this time delay can be safely extended to 30 minutes.

Effects of Heparin. An excessive volume of heparin remaining in the sample syringe may result in spurious blood gas results. Even if the heparin is fully expelled from the syringe, a certain amount remains in the needle and the tip of the syringe. This dead space volume varies with the size and brand of the syringe as well as the needle length and gauge. A typical 5-mL syringe with a 22-gauge needle has a dead space volume of approximately 0.2 mL.[55] The degree

of dilution of the sample also varies with the volume of blood aspirated. For example, if the dead space volume of a 5-mL syringe with needle is 0.2 mL, a 5-mL blood sample is diluted by 4%. If only 1 mL of blood is drawn into the same syringe, the dilution is 20%. A 20% dilution can result in a Pco_2 error of 20% or more,[31, 32, 56] and the drop in Pco_2 is proportional to the dilution of the sample. Although excessive heparin can decrease Pco_2 substantially, it has little effect on $Poo1_2$ and O_2 saturation and essentially no effect on pH (Fig. 19–3).[31, 32, 55–58] Even though most sodium heparin solutions are acidic, typically with a pH ranging from 5.0 to 7.0,[24, 59] the buffer capacity of whole blood maintains a constant pH even with substantial heparin dilution. Because pH is essentially unaffected by heparin while Pco_2 decreases, bicarbonate concentration, as calculated from pH and Pco_2 using the Henderson-Hasselbalch equation, likewise decreases. This may result in a discrepancy between the calculated bicarbonate or CO_2 content and the measured CO_2 content in simultaneously obtained nonheparinized blood.[55]

Heparin-induced errors are avoided by ensuring that all the anticoagulant is expelled except that remaining in the dead space of the syringe and needle and that at least 3 mL of blood is obtained.[11, 46, 55]

Indwelling Catheter Dead Space. Similar preanalytical dilution errors can occur when aspirating arterial or mixed venous blood from indwelling catheters.[60] To avoid a dilutional effect, sufficient fluid must be aspirated from the catheter and connecting tubing before obtaining the sample. Overestimating the discard volume, on the other hand, results in unnecessary blood loss and may increase transfusion requirements.[61] Judging discard volume by the color of the specimen is poor technique and can result in significant errors. Rules of thumb have been suggested, such as ensuring a discard volume equivalent to at least five times the total dead space volume. However, such recommendations are often overly conservative and increase blood wastage.[44, 62–64] Ideally, each institution or intensive care unit should have a standard configuration for catheters, stopcocks, and connection tubing; determine the total dead space of the setup; and establish a policy regarding discard and sample volumes.[62, 64] The dead space volume of arterial and pulmonary arterial catheter systems can be minimized by selecting the shortest practical connector tubing lengths.

Plastic Versus Glass Syringes. Glass syringes have traditionally been used for obtaining blood gas specimens. Cost considerations, disposability, and concern over breakage have led to increasing popularity of plastic syringes. Because certain plastics may absorb O_2 or allow a diffusion effect,

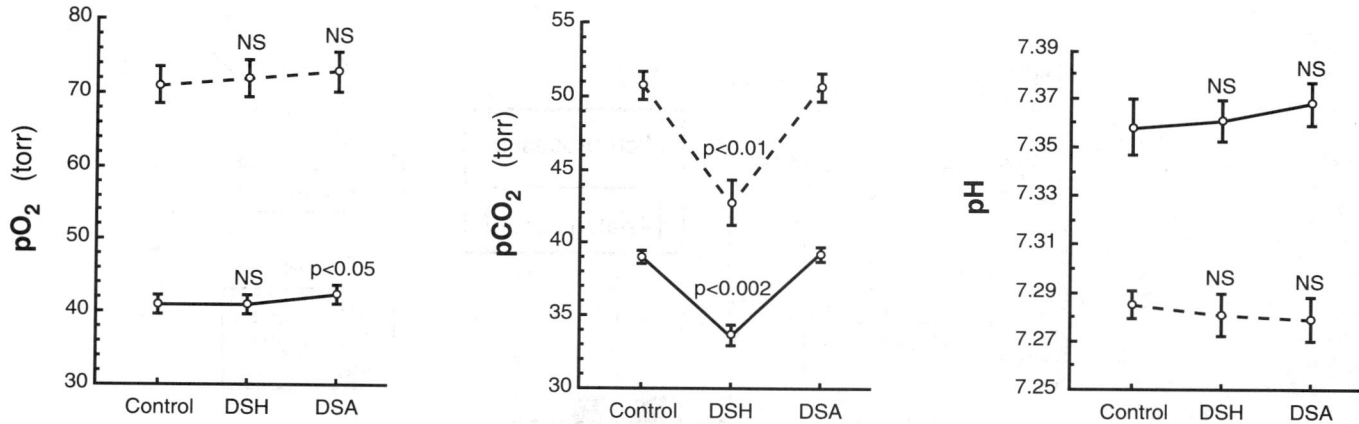

Figure 19–3. Effect of heparin-filled (DSH) versus air-filled dead space (DSA) in blood gas syringe on Po_2, Pco_2, and pH (mean ± SE). Samples were tonometered with 7% O_2, 7% CO_2 (——) and 12% O_2, 9% CO_2 (-----). (Modified from Fan LL, Dellinger KT, Mills AL, et al: Potential errors in neonatal blood gas measurements. J Pediatr 97:650, 1980.)

plastic syringes have been questioned as a source of preanalytical error.[53, 65, 66] At high levels of Po_2 (more than 400 torr) appreciable O_2 loss from the sample may occur, but this is of limited clinical relevance.[66] Most reports show that at lower levels of O_2 tension these differences are small or negligible and plastic syringes are generally held to be acceptable for clinical use.[29, 30, 53, 67] Polystyrene and polyethylene syringes pose more of a potential problem in this regard, but plastic syringes manufactured from polypropylene appear to be acceptable.[44, 68]

Other Preanalytical Factors. Increases in Pco_2 and decreases in pH and Po_2 observed during sample storage are in part due to ongoing metabolism by blood cells. In cases of severe leukocytosis, such as in leukemia, it is even more important to lower the temperature of the sample quickly because leukocytes remain metabolically active and rapidly decrease the Po_2 unless their metabolic rate is slowed. In extreme cases this artifactual hypoxemia may occur even in specimens that are rapidly cooled with ice.[69] Some laboratories have utilized fluoride salts to mitigate this effect, but this may not completely eliminate the metabolic effect and can itself cause spurious pH changes.[44]

Blood gas results may not reflect steady-state conditions if sampling is performed immediately after a change in fraction of inspired O_2 or ventilator settings that influence minute ventilation. A prolonged delay is not required, however, and intervals as short as 10 minutes have been demonstrated to yield equilibrium values.[70]

Halothane mimics O_2 in Po_2 electrodes.[71] This presents a clinical problem for blood gas determinations in patients anesthetized with this agent.[72] More disconcerting are reports that polarographic electrodes may be rendered inaccurate for prolonged periods after exposure to halothane-tainted blood,[73, 74] but not all studies have corroborated this carry-over effect.[75]

In the past it was common practice to place a bead or lead pellet in the syringe before obtaining the sample, to facilitate thorough mixing of the specimen just before performing the measurements. This is not recommended, however, because it increases the dead space volume and increases the likelihood of dilutional error caused by heparin.[76] Instead, the technician should roll the specimen syringe between the hands for 1 minute to ensure that the aliquot injected into the analyzer is representative of the specimen. This should be done with one hand over the other and the syringe parallel with the floor. This positioning is particularly important when glass syringes are used, because the plunger

may otherwise fall out, risking breakage, technician injury, and loss of the sample.[44]

It is of obvious importance that the specimen be properly labeled with the patient's name, bed number, and other required identifying information. The fraction of inspired O_2 must be recorded to interpret the O_2 tension and saturation results.

THE MODERN BLOOD GAS ANALYZER

Automated blood gas analyzers use specialized electrodes to measure simultaneously Pco_2 and Po_2 and blood pH. Required sample volumes typically range from 0.1 to 0.5 mL.[77] The blood specimen is either injected or aspirated through an inlet port of the instrument and into a sample chamber, where the assays take place (Fig. 19–4). The sample chamber houses four electrodes: one each for measuring Po_2, Pco_2, and pH and a reference electrode that works in conjunction with the pH electrode. The Po_2 and Pco_2 electrodes include integral Ag/AgCl half-cells, which constitute their reference electrodes and complete the electrical circuit. A thermostatically controlled heat exchanger equilibrates the chamber and the specimen to 37°C. The assays are then automatically performed, and the results are typically displayed on digital read-outs or a video monitor, along with printed hard copy. Many machines are equipped with a data interface that allows direct transfer of results to laboratory or hospital-wide data processing systems. After the assay, the sample chamber and associated connector tubing are automatically rinsed and the instrument is then ready for the next specimen. A complete assay cycle typically takes between 1 and 3 minutes with modern instruments.[77]

The pH Electrode. The term *pH* refers to the logarithmic transformation of the molar concentration or activity of hydrogen ions in a solution:

$$pH = -\log [H^+]$$

This nomenclature was first used by Sorensen[78] and allows convenient expression of the extremely small hydrogen ion concentrations typical of biologic systems. For example, the normal hydrogen ion concentration of blood is 0.00004 mmol/L, equivalent to pH 7.40. In 1906 Cremer discovered that an electrical voltage develops across a thin glass membrane separating solutions of different pH.[79] This voltage is linearly proportional to the difference in pH between the two solutions. Measurements based on quantitating a change in electrical potential or voltage are known as *potentiometric*

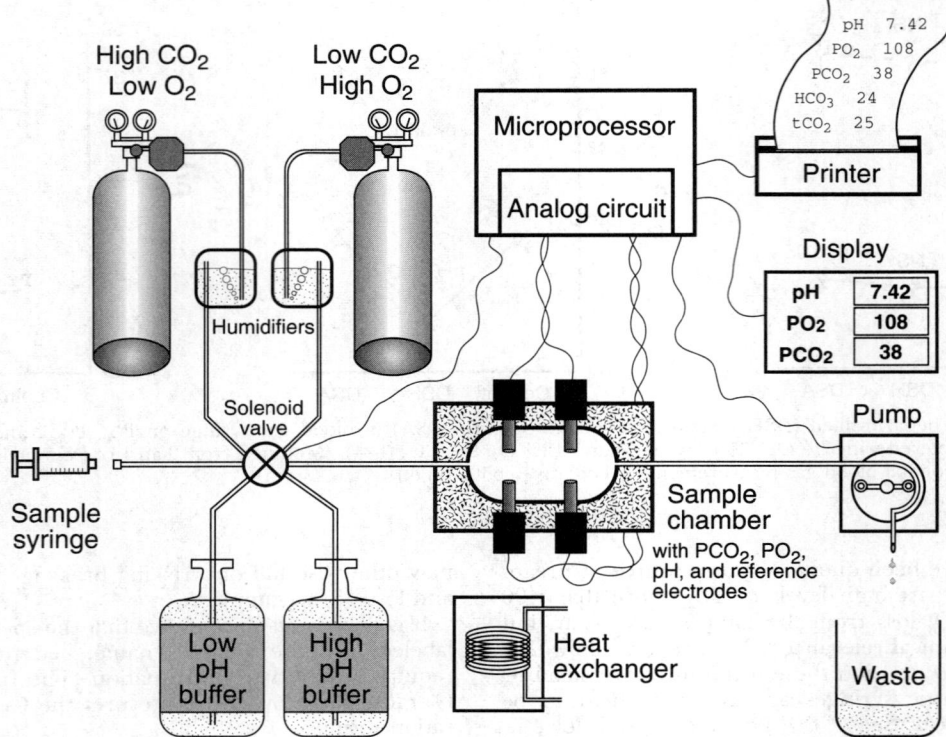

Figure 19–4. Simplified schematic representation of a modern blood gas analyzer. Under microprocessor control, either calibration solution or blood specimen is pumped into the temperature-equilibrated sample chamber, which contains the electrochemical electrodes (see text).

assays. Based on this principle, the glass pH electrode was developed in 1909 by Haber and Klemensiewicz and later used for analyzing blood pH.[80] The composition of the glass is important in determining which specific ions can induce an electrical potential across the glass. Quartz and Pyrex, for example, are essentially insensitive to pH gradients.[81] The ideal glass would be highly sensitive to hydrogen ions but show no response to gradients of other ionic species. Mac-Innes and Dole determined that a formula consisting of 72%

SiO_2, 22% Na_2O, and 6% CaO approaches this ideal, at least for pH levels below 9.[81, 82] This particular formula has been widely adopted for pH electrodes and is known as *Corning 015 pH glass.*

Blood pH is measured using a glass electrode in conjunction with a Hg/Hg_2Cl_2 (calomel) reference electrode (Fig. 19–5). The buffer solution inside the electrode is formulated to have a specific and constant pH. The electrical potential developed by the electrode varies as the sample pH deviates

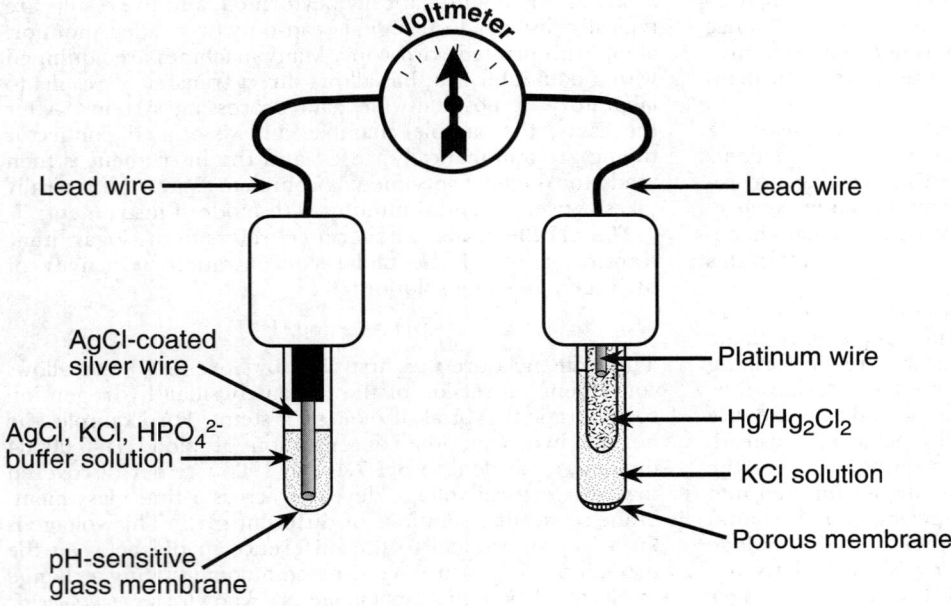

Figure 19–5. Schematic depiction of pH electrode (*left*) and reference electrode (*right*). pH electrode contains buffer solution of known pH. Voltage developed across the pH-sensitive glass membrane is proportional to the difference between this buffer pH and the sample pH.

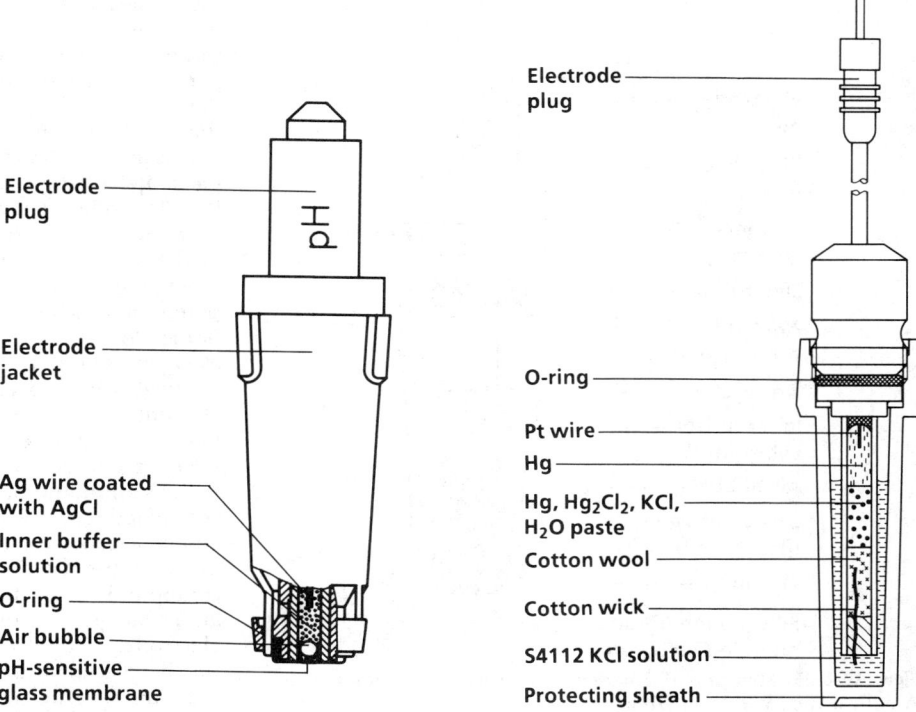

Figure 19–6. Construction of a modern pH electrode *(left)* and reference electrode *(right).* (© Radiometer America, Inc., Westlake, OH.)

from this reference pH, and the potential difference can be measured with a high-impedance voltmeter. The sample pH is then calculated using the Nernst equation, which relates the potential difference to pH:

$$pH_{sample} = pH_{reference} + \frac{V\mathscr{F}}{2.303TR}$$

where V = developed voltage (in volts)
T = temperature (in kelvins)
$\mathscr{F}$ = Faraday constant (96,496 coulombs)
R = molar gas constant (8.315 J/K/mol)[83]

Note from the equation that if the voltage is zero, the pH of the sample equals that of the reference solution. At 37°C, each millivolt developed by the electrode is equivalent to a pH difference of approximately 0.016 pH unit between the sample and the reference solution. The necessity of tightly regulating the temperature of the sample chamber is apparent from the inclusion of a temperature factor in the Nernst equation. Similarly, the pH of the reference buffer solution must be accurately known. Diagrammatic cross-sections of actual pH and reference electrodes are shown in Figure 19–6.

The P_{CO_2} Electrode. As with pH measurement, assay of blood P_{CO_2} is also performed potentiometrically. The P_{CO_2} electrode is, in fact, a slightly modified pH electrode (Fig. 19–7). An inner buffer solution is separated from an outer buffer solution by pH-sensitive glass covered with a porous cellulose, cellophane, or nylon spacer. An Ag/AgCl reference electrode is also positioned within the outer buffer solution to complete the electrical circuit. A plastic membrane made from Teflon, polyethylene, or silicone rubber separates the outer NaCl/NaHCO₃ buffer solution from the sample and acts as a barrier to charged and polar molecular species, permitting only uncharged particles to pass through to the pH-sensitive glass. Thus, dissolved CO_2 gas can diffuse through the outer layer of the electrode, but hydrogen ions cannot. CO_2 that passes through the outer membrane combines with water to form carbonic acid, which dissociates to form HCO_3^- and H^+. Hydrogen ions so generated in the outer buffer solution are responsible for inducing a potential difference across the glass membrane, exactly as in the glass pH electrode. At equilibrium the hydrogen ion concentra-

Figure 19–7. Principle of operation of the P_{CO_2} electrode. CO_2 gas dissolved in the sample diffuses through a layer of plastic that is impermeable to hydrogen ions. A nylon or cellophane spacer separates the CO_2-permeable membrane from the pH-sensitive glass electrode. CO_2 in this space combines chemically with water, forming bicarbonate and hydrogen ions. Hydrogen ion activity measured at pH electrode therefore reflects CO_2 tension, but not hydrogen ion activity, of the sample.

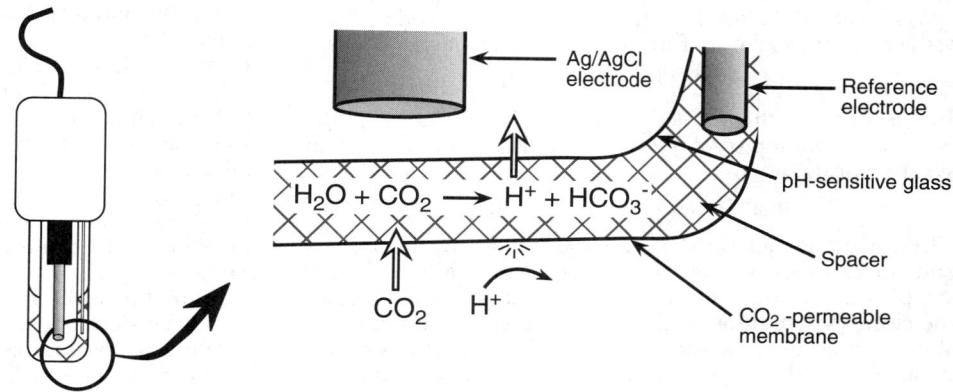

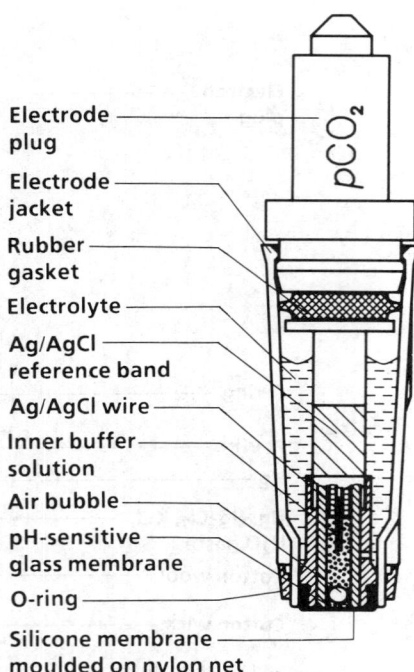

Electrode plug
Electrode jacket
Rubber gasket
Electrolyte
Ag/AgCl reference band
Ag/AgCl wire
Inner buffer solution
Air bubble
pH-sensitive glass membrane
O-ring
Silicone membrane moulded on nylon net

Figure 19–8. Construction of a modern P_{CO_2} electrode. (© Radiometer America, Inc., Westlake, OH.)

tion (pH) in the outer buffer solution is proportional to the P_{CO_2} or concentration of dissolved CO_2 gas in the sample. Thus, the P_{CO_2} electrode indirectly measures blood P_{CO_2} by monitoring the change in pH in the outer buffer solution caused by the selective diffusion of CO_2 from the sample across the Teflon membrane.[84] As with the pH electrode, precise temperature regulation is critically important to obtaining accurate results. In addition to affecting electrode function, changes in temperature also affect the solubility of CO_2 in the sample. Defects in the outer plastic membrane obviously introduce error in the measurement. A diagrammatic cross-section of an actual P_{CO_2} electrode is shown in Figure 19–8.

The P_{O_2} Electrode. Whereas the pH and P_{CO_2} electrodes are based on potentiometric measurements, the O_2 electrode is a *polarographic* device. Polarographic electrodes rely on the measurement of a generated electrical current; hence, this method is also classified as an *amperometric* determination. The Clark electrode, developed in the 1950s by Leland Clark,[85] consists of a platinum cathode and an Ag/AgCl anode, which are in electrical continuity by way of a potassium chloride and phosphate buffer solution (Fig. 19–9). The cathode is protected from protein contamination by a polypropylene membrane. When a constant polarizing voltage of 630 mV is applied across the two electrodes, O_2 is reduced at the cathode, forming hydroxide ions:

$$O_2 + 2H_2O + 4e^- \rightarrow 4OH^-$$

In response to the reduction of O_2, chloride ions in the electrolyte solution combine with silver at the anode to form silver chloride:

$$4Cl^- + 4Ag \rightarrow 4AgCl + 4e^-$$

Thus, electrons liberated at the anode flow to the cathode and an electrical current is generated. O_2 present in the sample diffuses through the plastic membrane and through the electrolyte solution to the cathode, creating this current. With increasing O_2 tension, a proportionately greater electrical current develops. Because O_2 is actually consumed at

the cathode, the P_{O_2} of the sample decreases as the reaction proceeds. To minimize this potential source of error, the cathode is constructed as a short section of extremely fine platinum wire, often only 20 to 25 μm in diameter, to limit the amount of O_2 consumed. However, this also attenuates the resulting current, and sensitive electronic circuitry is necessary to measure these weak currents, which are in the picoampere range. A diagrammatic cross-section of an actual P_{O_2} electrode is shown in Figure 19–10.

Other Ion-Selective Electrodes. Altering the composition of the glass electrode can result in glass that is sensitive to other ionic species besides hydrogen ions.[81] Alternatively, a potentiometric electrode can be covered with a plastic membrane doped with an appropriate ionophore to create an electrode selective to a particular ion.[86] These ion-selective electrodes have been designed for sensing many different elemental ions, including sodium, potassium, calcium, magnesium, lithium, chloride, bromide, and iodide.[81, 87–93] Ion-selective electrodes that assay more complex ionic species, such as ammonium, bicarbonate, thiocyanate, salicylate, and acetylcholine, have also been developed.[81, 86, 91] By coupling an ion-selective electrode with a biocatalytic reaction, sensors can be constructed for detecting ionic and nonionic organic compounds such as urea, glucose, CO_2, lactate, ammonia, amino acids, and even serum enzymes.[88, 94–97] Ion-selective electrodes can be made physically small enough that several can be placed in a single compact instrument designed to measure several analytes simultaneously in a single specimen.[86, 88, 98] Some of these electrodes are employed in currently available blood gas instruments for assaying sodium, potassium, calcium, and other ionic species commonly determined in the clinical laboratory, along with conventional blood gas and pH analysis.[86, 98] Some blood gas machines can also measure hematocrit using conductivity sensors.[86]

Quality Control. Before an assay is performed, the three conventional electrodes making up the basic clinical blood gas instrument must be calibrated. Calibration must be done frequently because electrical drift is an inherent problem with these electrodes. The calibration procedure consists of exposing the electrodes to solutions standardized with respect to pH, P_{O_2}, and P_{CO_2}. Two standard solutions, a high-pH and a low-pH buffer, each tonometered to specific P_{CO_2} and P_{O_2} values, are used to perform a two-point calibration of the electrodes. In modern blood gas machines the calibration is automated; the instrument performs a self-calibration at frequent and regular intervals under the control of a microprocessor (see Fig. 19–4). Under optimal conditions P_{O_2} and P_{CO_2} determinations are typically accurate to within ±0.5 torr and blood pH measurements accurate to within 0.005 pH unit. Accuracy may vary between different instrument models and over the range of the measured parameter. Reproducibility is typically within ±2% for P_{CO_2}, ±3% for P_{O_2}, and ±0.01 pH unit.[29] In practice, these specifications may not be attained. In one survey involving over 130 laboratories, 95% of the participants demonstrated errors of less than 4.5 torr for P_{CO_2}, 13 torr for P_{O_2}, and less than 0.05 pH unit.[99]

Automated blood gas machines are subject to electrical and mechanical failure. Accuracy and precision deteriorate over time as the electrodes become contaminated with residual material from within the measuring chamber, plastic tubing ages, membrane integrity alters, electrode output drifts, and other changes occur.[100] Limitations in accuracy are evidenced by interinstrument variability because of differences in design, construction, and calibration.[101, 102] To minimize the likelihood of error, quality assurance programs have been developed.[99] Some programs include processing of "blinded" test samples mailed periodically to participating laboratories. The California Thoracic Society Proficiency

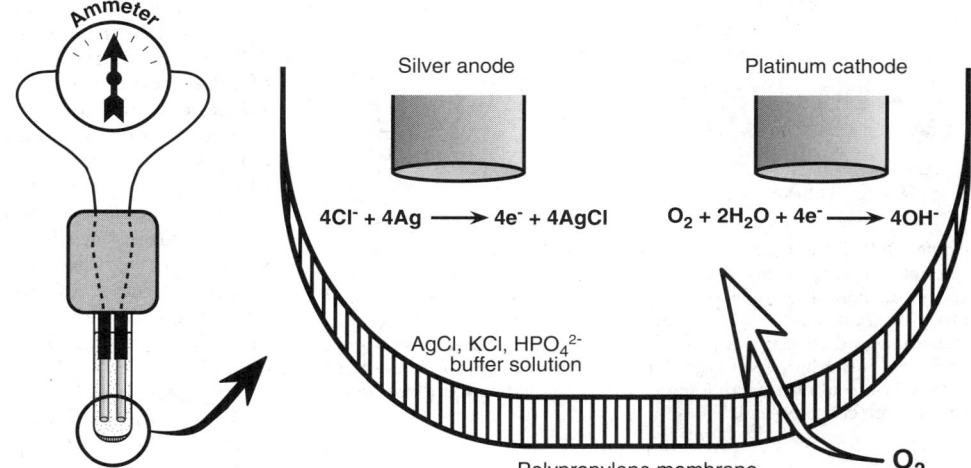

Figure 19–9. Principle of operation of the polarographic PO₂ electrode. Reduction of O₂ at the platinum cathode is accompanied by formation of silver chloride at the silver anode, resulting in an electrical current that is proportional to the quantity of O₂ present.

Testing Program demonstrated substantial variability in PO₂ measurements between laboratories but minimal differences when comparisons were limited to instruments of the same make and model.[103, 104]

Several types of proficiency testing control solutions are in current use. The "gold standard" test material is heparinized fresh blood that has been equilibrated with known PO₂ and PCO₂ values. Samples are prepared in a temperature-controlled precision instrument called a tonometer. Using blood has certain disadvantages, however. Ideally, only fresh blood should be used for quality controls. Blood easily forms bubbles or foam within tonometers, it is costly, it cannot be used for testing pH, mailing test samples poses problems, and blood presents an infectious risk to laboratory personnel.[99, 103] Preparing controls by tonometry also requires expensive equipment and a greater time commitment from blood gas laboratory personnel. The practicality of tonometrically preparing whole blood controls each shift in the blood gas laboratory for quality assurance purposes may be logistically problematic for smaller laboratories. For these reasons alternative test materials have been developed and are commercially available in glass ampules containing solutions with known pH and known PO₂ and PCO₂ values. These materials can be divided into three major categories: aqueous buffer solutions, hemoglobin-containing solutions, and fluorocarbon-containing emulsions. Aqueous and blood-containing solutions have the property of being sensitive to temperature changes; their PO₂ varies with the temperature of the ampule at the time it is opened.[105] When used, these ampules should therefore be warmed following the manufacturer's recommendations. The fluorocarbon-containing emulsions are not affected by temperature change. In addition, their O₂ affinity and O₂-buffering capacity closely mimic those of blood,[106] which results in improved reproducibility compared with aqueous controls.[107] Fluorocarbon emulsions may be preferable test materials for interinstitutional quality assurance surveys.[99]

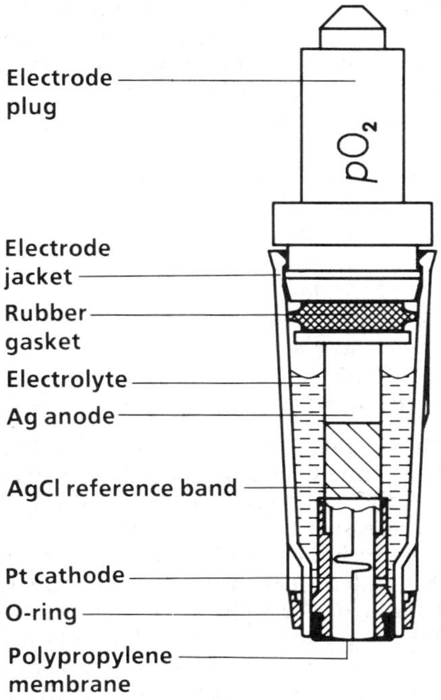

A quality assurance program should at a minimum include per shift analysis of control materials of known PO₂, PCO₂, and pH, as well as periodic (e.g., quarterly) proficiency testing with multiple blinded test samples.[99, 108, 109] Laboratories may be required to demonstrate testing results showing satisfactory proficiency to obtain and renew operating licenses.

CO-OXIMETRY

White light consists of a mixture of wavelengths of the electromagnetic radiation spectrum ranging from 400 to 800 nm. The wavelengths of light reflected, transmitted, and absorbed by a substance are physical characteristics of that substance, and color is the subjective perception of particular wavelengths of visible light. For example, if white light is directed through a translucent substance that absorbs blue and green wavelengths, that substance appears red. Hemoglobin, an iron-containing protein that has the ability to bind O₂, has different absorption characteristics, and therefore a different color, depending on the amount of O₂ bound to it (see Fig. 17–1). Fully oxygenated hemoglobin is bright red, deoxygenated hemoglobin dark red. SO₂ is the ratio of oxyhemoglobin to total hemoglobin and is measured in the clinical laboratory by spectrophotometric analysis using an instrument called the hemoximeter.

A blood specimen is introduced into an optically clear cuvette maintained at 37°C in the oximeter (Fig. 19–11) and the sample is hemolyzed to reduce light scattering. White light is focused through the sample and then through a prism or diffraction grating, which separates the wavelengths

Electrode plug

Electrode jacket

Rubber gasket

Electrolyte

Ag anode

AgCl reference band

Pt cathode

O-ring

Polypropylene membrane

Figure 19–10. Construction of a modern PO₂ electrode. (© Radiometer America, Inc., Westlake, OH.)

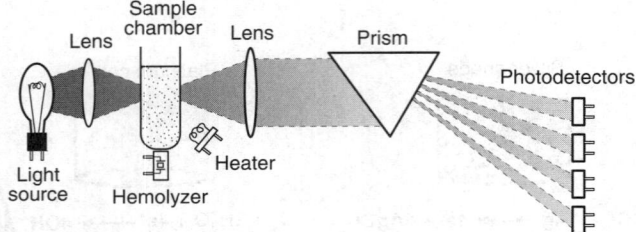

Figure 19–11. Schematic illustration of a CO-oximeter. A high-frequency vibrating piezoelectric crystal is used to hemolyze the blood specimen contained in the temperature-controlled, optically clear analysis chamber. A white light source is focused through the specimen and through a prism or diffraction grating, which separates wavelengths of transmitted light. Specific spectral bands are focused onto photosensitive semiconductors that convert light intensity into electrical signals.

of the transmitted light. Specific spectral bands are then focused onto photosensitive semiconductors that convert light intensity into electrical signals. According to the Lambert-Beer formula,[81, 87] optical density or absorbance (A) is related to the molar concentration of the absorbent as

$$ A = \frac{I_0}{I} \epsilon c l $$

where I_0 = intensity of the incident light
I = intensity of the transmitted light
ϵ = molar extinction coefficient
c = concentration
l = thickness of the sample

Thus, for a given wavelength of light, absorbance is directly proportional to the number of molecules of the substance under analysis.

Two wavelengths of light are usually used to determine SO_2. One wavelength may be used to measure oxyhemoglobin and another to determine either total or reduced hemoglobin. Simple hemoximeters do not measure other forms of hemoglobin, such as that bound to CO (carboxyhemoglobin). For example, if the instrument employs a wavelength of approximately 600 nm, carboxyhemoglobin is indistinguishable from oxyhemoglobin. Wavelengths such as these, at which two different substances show the same absorbance, are termed *isosbestic points*. Although carboxyhemoglobin normally accounts for a nearly negligible fraction of the total hemoglobin, it can be significantly increased in smokers and patients suffering from smoke inhalation. CO poisoning cannot be detected by oximeters that interpret the presence of carboxyhemoglobin as oxyhemoglobin. Carboxyhemoglobin saturation may be determined indirectly on such machines, however, by employing a deoxygenation reagent such as sodium dithionite. This substance reduces oxyhemoglobin without affecting carboxyhemoglobin or pre-existing reduced hemoglobin. When this deoxygenated blood specimen is then processed in the usual fashion, the reported oxyhemoglobin result actually represents carboxyhemoglobin saturation.

Hemoglobin can also exist in the form of methemoglobin and sulfhemoglobin. As with carboxyhemoglobin, levels of these forms are normally quite small but are significantly elevated in patients with methemoglobinemia or sulfhemoglobinemia. The CO-oximeter, a clinical instrument more sophisticated than the hemoximeter, measures oxyhemoglobin, reduced hemoglobin, carboxyhemoglobin, methemoglobin, and total hemoglobin. Although these instruments generally do not assay for sulfhemoglobin, significant elevations of this form are exceedingly rare. These machines operate on the same spectrophotometric principles but utilize multiple wavelengths and more complex mathematic processing.

Spectrophotometric techniques are subject to several types of measurement error. The presence of certain exogenous substances or abnormally high concentrations of certain endogenous blood constituents may result in spurious results if the substance shows an absorbance pattern similar to that of hemoglobin. This type of interference is highly dependent on the specific wavelengths employed. Elevated bilirubin concentrations in the range of 5 mg/dL, for example, may significantly affect oxyhemoglobin results obtained with certain instruments. Other machines that employ different wavelengths may be unaffected by even severe hyperbilirubinemia (>20 mg/dL). Intravenously administered methylene blue (used to treat methemoglobinemia) and indocyanine green (used as an indicator dye for cardiac output and lung water determinations) can result in spurious saturation results.[29] Differences in hemoglobin structure impart different absorption characteristics. Hence, with some instruments problems may be encountered if there are high levels of fetal hemoglobin or in the research setting when attempting to measure oxyhemoglobin saturation in nonhuman blood. Other instruments can be programmed to analyze accurately fetal hemoglobin and hemoglobins from certain animal species. Parenteral nutrition formulas containing lipids may also cause interference.[110]

DERIVED PARAMETERS

The incorporation of microprocessors in automated blood gas machines has facilitated routine calculations based on blood gas findings. Modern instruments report a number of calculated results in addition to the directly measured results. Certain of these derived parameters may be helpful to the clinician, but an understanding of their limitations is important to meaningful interpretation.

Saturation. As described previously, oxyhemoglobin saturation can be directly measured by spectrophotometric oximetry. The relationship between PO_2 and hemoglobin saturation is defined by the oxyhemoglobin dissociation curve (see Fig. 142–4). If PO_2 is measured by blood gas analysis, saturation may be estimated graphically by plotting PO_2 and determining the corresponding saturation. It may also be calculated using a mathematic equation that approximates this curve.[111–114] One polynomial function that closely approximates the curve is given by

$$ SO_2 = \frac{a_1 PO_2 + a_2 PO_2{}^2 + a_3 PO_2{}^3 + PO_2{}^4}{a_4 + a_5 PO_2 + a_6 PO_2{}^2 + a_7 PO_2{}^3 + PO_2{}^4} \times 100\% $$

where a_1 = −8532.2289
a_2 = 2121.4010
a_3 = −67.073989
a_4 = 935960.87
a_5 = −31346.258
a_6 = 2396.1674
a_7 = −67.104406[115]

Whereas the overall shape of the oxyhemoglobin dissociation curve is essentially constant, the horizontal position of the curve shifts in response to several physiologic factors.[116, 117] Increasing body temperature and PCO_2 shift the curve to the right; hypothermia (see Fig. 142–4) and hypocapnia result in a leftward shift. pH influences the position as well, shifting it to the right as pH decreases and to the left with increasing pH. Increasing 2,3-diphosphoglycerate concentration in the erythrocyte also displaces the curve rightward and facilitates O_2 unloading at the tissue level. These factors present a major shortcoming to estimating saturation by formula or nomogram. The effects of pH,

PCO_2, and temperature can be taken into account by using standard formulas to determine what the PO_2 would be under standard conditions, namely pH 7.40, PCO_2 40 torr, and temperature 37°C. Standard PO_2 can be calculated as[115, 118, 119]

$$stdPO_2 = mPO_2 \times 10^{[0.024(37 - T) + 0.4(pH - 7.40) + 0.06(\log 40 - \log PCO_2)]}$$

where $stdPO_2$ = standard PO_2
mPO_2 = measured PO_2
T = body temperature in degrees Celsius

Although this formula takes into account the effects of pH, PCO_2, and temperature, it does not correct for dissociation shifts caused by changes in 2,3-diphosphoglycerate concentration.

Assuming that P_{50} is known (see next section), the Hill equation provides an alternative method of calculating saturation from PO_2:[120]

$$SO_2 = \frac{PO_2{}^n}{PO_2{}^n + P_{50}{}^n}$$

where n is an empirical factor usually considered to be approximately 2.6.

An even stronger argument against the clinical use of calculated saturation values is illustrated by considering a patient poisoned with CO and receiving supplemental O_2. If the inspired O_2 concentration approaches 100%, arterial blood gas analysis may reveal a PO_2 of 600 torr, and calculated SO_2 would be essentially 100%. Both the measured PO_2 and the calculated saturation imply that the patient's blood is well oxygenated. Yet the actual SO_2 depends on the carboxyhemoglobin level. If the carboxyhemoglobin level were 40%, the arterial saturation could not be higher than 60%. O_2 content (CO_2), the volume of O_2 in milliliters carried by each deciliter of blood, can be calculated as

$$CO_2 = 1.39Hb \times SO_2 + 0.0031PO_2$$

where Hb is the hemoglobin concentration in grams per deciliter. Some blood gas analyzers with oximetry capabilities automatically calculate this parameter. The formula illustrates that CO_2 content is determined principally by the fraction of O_2 bound to hemoglobin, represented by the SO_2 term, and not the portion in physical solution in plasma, represented by the PO_2 term. The patient described is therefore profoundly hypoxemic, despite the high PO_2 and the spuriously high saturation. Measuring saturation using a CO-oximeter is the only reliable way to determine saturation under these circumstances. Similar errors can result if SO_2 is calculated in the presence of methemoglobinemia.

P_{50}. The PO_2 at which hemoglobin is 50% saturated is known as the P_{50}. It is an indicator of the horizontal position of the oxyhemoglobin dissociation curve and hence the affinity of O_2 for hemoglobin. P_{50} can be measured by equilibrating blood at two or more PO_2 and plotting the resulting saturation at each PO_2. This tonometric method is cumbersome, however, and is not frequently employed. Instead, P_{50} is usually calculated using theoretically or empirically derived formulas. For example, the Hill equation (see earlier) can be solved for P_{50}. A simple formula based on proportionality has been shown to yield accurate results with a standard deviation of ± 1.0 torr when specimens with saturations between 20 and 90% are used:[121]

$$P_{50} = 26.6 \frac{PO_2std}{PO_2sat}$$

where PO_2std is the measured PO_2 standardized to pH 7.40, a PCO_2 of 40 torr, and a temperature of 37°C; PO_2sat is the PO_2 corresponding to the measured saturation, derived graphically or mathematically from the oxyhemoglobin dis-

sociation curve; and 26.6 is the normal P_{50}. Accurate nomograms have been developed to simplify these calculations.[118] When PO_2std is used, the P_{50} result is referred to as the *in vitro* P_{50}. If measured PO_2 is corrected to body temperature (see later) and used directly in the equation, the result reflects the P_{50} at the prevailing conditions of temperature, pH, and PCO_2 in the patient and is termed the *in vivo* P_{50}.[114] For a given specimen, the difference between in vivo P_{50} and in vitro P_{50} is principally a function of 2,3-diphosphoglycerate concentration.

The oxyhemoglobin dissociation curve is essentially flat at usual levels of oxygenation found in arterial blood. Hence, P_{50} values calculated from arterial blood specimens are inaccurate. Mixed venous blood is positioned at the steep portion of the dissociation curve and should therefore yield reliable results.

Bicarbonate and CO_2 Content. Bicarbonate concentration is not generally measured in the clinical chemistry or blood gas laboratory. Instead, it is routinely calculated from blood pH and PCO_2 using the Henderson-Hasselbalch equation:

$$pH = pK' + \log \left(\frac{[HCO_3{}^-]}{sPCO_2} \right)$$

which can be rearranged as

$$[HCO_3{}^-] = sPCO_2{}^{(pH - pK')}$$

where s is the solubility coefficient of CO_2 in plasma (approximately 0.03 mmol/L/torr) and pK' is the apparent dissociation constant for carbonic acid (approximately 6.1).[122, 123]

Although the terms *bicarbonate* and *CO_2 content* (CCO_2) are frequently used as though they were identical, they are not actually interchangable. CCO_2 refers to the total concentration of several forms of CO_2 in plasma or serum, including bicarbonate, carbonate, carbonic acid, dissolved CO_2 gas, and CO_2 bound to proteins as carbamino groups. For this reason it is sometimes referred to as *total CO_2*. Bicarbonate makes the greatest contribution, accounting for about 95% of total CCO_2. CO_2 gas that is physically dissolved in plasma water is the next most abundant form but accounts for less than 5% of the total. The other forms contribute negligibly. Therefore, CCO_2 may be calculated as

$$CCO_2 = [HCO_3{}^-] + sPCO_2$$

The solubility coefficient s converts PCO_2 expressed as a gas tension in torr to concentration units of millimoles per liter. Alternatively, rearrangement of this equation allows bicarbonate to be calculated from measured CCO_2 and measured PCO_2. At a normal bicarbonate concentration of 24 mmol/L and PCO_2 of 40 torr, CCO_2 would be 25.2 mmol/L. The contribution of dissolved CO_2 to CCO_2 is more apparent, but still not striking, in the patient with severe hypercapnia. For example, with a bicarbonate level of 28 mmol/L and PCO_2 of 100 torr, CCO_2 would be 31 mmol/L.

Direct measurement of CCO_2 is routinely done in the evaluation of serum electrolytes. The accuracy and precision of calculated bicarbonate and CCO_2 depend on the accuracy and precision of the pH and PCO_2 measurements used in the equations. Their accuracy is also dependent on the constancy of pK'. Although the constancy of pK' has been called into question in patients who are severely ill or acutely unstable, several studies have demonstrated that pK' is, in fact, sufficiently constant to allow accurate calculation of bicarbonate and total CO_2.[124-126] Despite the high level of agreement and correlation between measured and calculated CCO_2 values (Fig. 19–12), occasional discrepancies are observed in clinical practice. As shown earlier, a bicarbonate value reported by the blood gas laboratory should be slightly

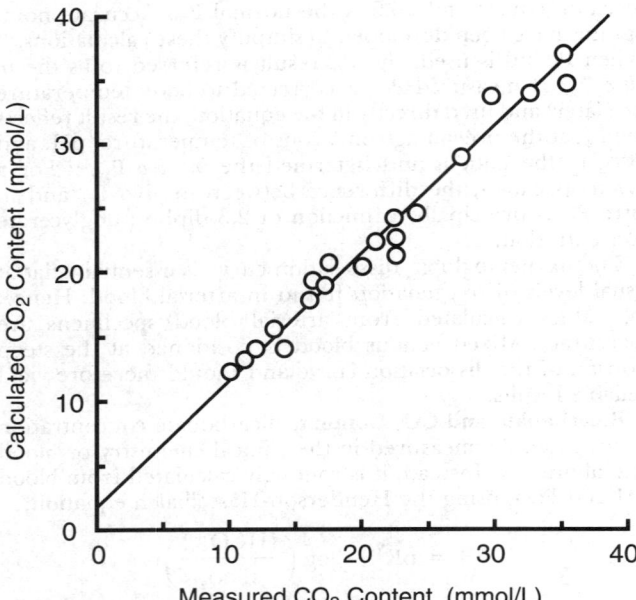

Figure 19–12. Graph of measured Cco_2 versus Cco_2 calculated from blood gas results using the Henderson-Hasselbalch equation. Blood specimens were obtained from patients undergoing cardiopulmonary resuscitation. The close correlation ($r = .99$; $P < .0001$) illustrates the constancy of carbonic acid pK′ and validity of calculating bicarbonate or Cco_2, even in critically ill patients. (From Kruse JA, Hukku P, Thill-Baharozian MC, et al: Constancy of blood carbonic acid pK′ in patients during cardiopulmonary resuscitation. Chest 93:1221, 1988.)

lower than a corresponding Cco_2 result from an electrolyte analyzer. Electrolyte profiles are typically obtained with venous blood samples, whereas the calculated values are most often obtained with arterial blood gas specimens. The acid-base status of arterial blood is different from that of venous blood. With respect to bicarbonate, this difference is small under normal conditions, being about 2 mmol/L higher in venous than in arterial blood.[127] However, these differences can be magnified in critically ill patients.[128] Because Cco_2 is usually measured in the clinical chemistry laboratory and blood gas analysis is often performed in a separate laboratory, differences in specimen handling and laboratory technique may be a factor. As noted previously, heparin dilution can lead to such discrepancies. Blood gas specimens are usually delivered to the laboratory on ice, and great pains are often taken to minimize the time between obtaining the sample and performing the assay. Analysis of samples for Cco_2 may not occur as promptly, yet CO_2 can escape from these specimens during storage and specimen handling. In fact, under certain conditions, losses of up to 8 mmol/L may occur.[129] Unless it is known for certain that the same blood specimen was used for both blood gas and Cco_2 analysis, there is always the possibility that the samples were obtained at different times. The times given on clinical reports may indicate the time the requisition was filled out, the time the specimen was sent or received by the laboratory, or the time the assay was performed; they do not necessarily indicate the time the specimen was drawn. Even small differences in timing between Cco_2 samples and blood gas samples can be critical if the patient is unstable. Consider, for example, the patient who has a grand mal seizure during the interval between the two sampling times or the patient with severe ketoacidosis who receives intravenous bicarbonate and/or insulin. Accuracy of Cco_2 assays may suffer in the presence of high plasma glucose concentrations, with

alterations in plasma water content, or when the total CO_2 level is severely abnormal.[130] These effects have prompted some investigators to conclude that bicarbonate and Cco_2 values calculated from blood gas results using the Henderson-Hasselbalch equation are more accurate indicators of actual plasma concentrations.[131]

Base Excess. Base excess is defined as the alkali concentration of blood expressed in milliequivalents per liter.[132] It is measured by titration with a strong acid to pH 7.40 at a temperature of 37°C and Pco_2 of 40 torr. If the blood pH is less than 7.40 to begin with, the titration is carried out using a strong alkali and the result is termed *base deficit* or expressed as a negative base excess. Because the actual measurement is cumbersome, base excess is calculated in practice. Calculation is also cumbersome, however, and can involve iteration procedures using complicated equations.[114, 133] One noniterative empirical equation is[134]

$$\text{Base excess} = \frac{1}{2} \left[\left(\frac{8a - 0.919}{a} \right) + \sqrt{ \left(\frac{0.919 - 8a}{a} \right)^2 - 4 \left(\frac{24.47 - HCO_3(40)}{a} \right) } \right]$$

where

$$a = 0.00404 + 0.000264 Hb$$

$$HCO_3(40) = 0.0306 \times 40 \times 10^{[(pH(40) - 6.161)/0.9524]}$$

$$pH(40) = \left(\frac{pH(Hb) - pH}{\log [Pco_2 (Hb)] - \log (Pco_2)} \right) \times [\log (40) - \log (Pco_2)] + pH$$

$$\log [Pco_2(Hb)] = -0.010968 Hb + 3.4046 + 2.12 \times 10^{(-0.09407 Hb)}$$

$$pH(Hb) = 0.0252 Hb + 5.980 - 1.920 \times 10^{(-0.10034 Hb)}$$

Base excess has been commonly employed as a single numeric value that quantitates the extent of metabolic, as opposed to respiratory, acid-base disturbances. In this application, a base excess of 0 ± 2 mEq/L is considered normal, with values above 2 representing metabolic alkalosis and values below -2 representing metabolic acidosis. This concept is founded on the assumption that changes in Pco_2 have the same effect on blood in vitro as in the intact organism.[135] Unfortunately, whole body titration experiments subsequently established that this assumption is invalid.[135, 136] Consider a patient with chronic hyperventilation and no other underlying acid-base pathology, who presents with a Pco_2 of 20 torr. With this degree of hypocapnia, this patient's bicarbonate concentration would be approximately 15 mmol/L, because of physiologic renal compensation, and the pH would be 7.5. Base excess in this case is -5.0, even though there is no pathologic metabolic acid-base disturbance.[135, 137] Thus, although widely touted as a reflection of nonrespiratory acid-base status, base excess is flawed if interpreted without considering this limitation. Most modern blood gas instruments nevertheless provide the automatic calculation of base excess.

Specimen Temperature Correction. In a closed system, blood Po_2 and Pco_2 vary directly and pH varies inversely with temperature. These changes are physical phenomena resulting principally from temperature-dependent changes in gas solubility. Such changes would therefore be expected to occur not only within a specimen syringe but also within the patient, barring any competing physiologic derangements of gas exchange or acid-base balance. Blood gas results for a hypo- or hyperthermic subject (who is otherwise completely normal) might be expected to reflect these changes. Remember, however, that the specimen is equilibrated to 37°C in the blood gas machine before performance of the assays. The results thus reflect pH, P_{O_2}, and P_{CO_2} at 37°C and not at the patient's actual body temperature.

A number of formulas have been developed to allow calculation of the in vivo blood gas values from those measured at standard temperature.[138, 139] For example,

$$pH = mpH - 0.0146(T - 37)$$

$$P_{CO_2} = mP_{CO_2} \times 10^{[0.019(T - 37)]}$$

$$P_{O_2} = mP_{O_2} \times 10^{\{0.0252/[0.243(P_{O_2}/100)^{3.88} + 1] + 0.00564\}(T - 37)}$$

where m stands for the values measured at 37°C. Modern blood gas instruments can automatically perform these calculations if the patient's body temperature is entered into the machine. Consider a normal subject who suddenly becomes hypothermic to a body temperature of 30°C. If pH were 7.40, P_{O_2} 80 torr, and P_{CO_2} 40 torr as measured at 37°C, the actual in vivo values would be pH 7.50, P_{O_2} 51 torr, and P_{CO_2} 29 torr, using the foregoing equations. Because appreciable differences in blood gas results for hypothermic patients can occur, depending on whether or not the values are temperature corrected, it is important for the clinician to know whether a particular laboratory routinely reports corrected or uncorrected results. On the other hand, O_2 saturation, C_{O_2}, C_{CO_2}, and bicarbonate concentration are nearly independent of temperature.[29, 84, 122, 138–140]

It might seem logical to assume that the actual in vivo blood gas results would be desirable clinically. However, as noted, changes in blood temperature alter pH, P_{CO_2}, and P_{O_2} even when there are no other physiologic or pathologic abnormalities in acid-base balance, pulmonary gas exchange, C_{O_2}, or C_{CO_2}. Thus, the "normal" ranges for blood gases and pH are temperature dependent. Rather than being familiar with the normal ranges at every degree of pathologic body temperature, it is far simpler to report the blood gas results at 37°C and employ the usual physiologic normal ranges.[29, 123, 138, 141–144]

IN VIVO BLOOD GAS MONITORING

Rapid and accurate blood gas measurements are frequently of crucial importance in the management of the critically ill patient. The growing use of noninvasive methods, such as end-tidal exhaled air analysis, pulse oximetry, and transcutaneous measurements, attests to the value clinicians place on continuous feedback of gas exchange parameters in certain critical situations. But these methods have certain shortcomings, at least in specific circumstances, and cannot completely substitute for conventional blood gas analysis (see Chapter 17).

Application of Conventional Measurement Techniques. One approach has been to simplify the blood gas instrument, making it physically smaller and easier to operate, so that it can be used at the point of care, that is, at the patient's bedside in the intensive care unit or in the operating suite. Such portable, cartridge-based devices are available for bedside use by clinical personnel who are not necessarily laboratory technicians. They can be used for rapid (less than 2 minutes) determinations of blood gases, pH, and electrolytes, including sodium, potassium, and calcium, from small (less than 1 mL) sample volumes.[86, 98, 145–147] Although they facilitate frequent measurements, these instruments do not offer true continuous monitoring. Similar portable systems are available for blood gas and pH monitoring by direct connection to an extracorporeal circuit, such as that used during cardiac surgery.[148, 149] These offer true continuous monitoring, but the requirement for an extracorporeal circuit obviously limits clinical utility.

Major strides have been made in perfecting the technology necessary to achieve continuous blood gas monitoring using intravenous and intra-arterial catheter systems that allow automatic and continuous or near-continuous measurements of pH, P_{CO_2}, P_{O_2}, and saturation. In vivo monitoring of mixed venous saturation using specialized indwelling pulmonary arterial catheters equipped for fiberoptic oximetry has been perfected and is currently widely used for assessing the adequacy of systemic oxygenation. However, until recently the prospect of on-line monitors for intra-arterial pH and gas tensions has been an elusive goal.[150] The ideal invasive device would allow all standard blood gas parameters to be monitored continuously with the same accuracy as conventional in vitro analysis, be sufficiently miniaturized to fit within standard-sized vascular catheters, provide stable readings for the duration of catheterization, have a rapid response, be inexpensive, and not place the patient at higher risk (e.g., for thrombosis) than with presently used intra-arterial catheters.

Conventional electrodes, miniaturized and contained within vascular catheters, have been used for in vivo pH,[151] P_{CO_2},[151–153] and P_{O_2}[154–157] determinations with varying degrees of success. Like their larger counterparts, these polarographic and ion-selective electrode–based devices are initially calibrated by exposure to solutions of known pH and gas tensions. After they are inserted into the patient, however, this process cannot be readily repeated. The problem of subsequent electrode output drift has proved to be a major technical hurdle, especially with prolonged use. Mass spectrometry[158–162] and gas chromatography[150, 163–165] methodologies have also been used. These techniques involve continuous vacuum extraction of gases from the blood through a small-diameter, gas-permeable, indwelling catheter. Analysis is semicontinuous with updated results displayed every few minutes. Although this approach is promising, the performance of most of these devices has, to date, fallen short of being acceptable for routine clinical use.

Ion-Selective Field Effect Transistor Technology. Advances in semiconductor technology have led to the development of transistors that can be used as sensors for ion activity determinations. Transistors may be thought of as electronic valves in which a small control current can be used to regulate a much larger electric current, with the strength of the output current being proportional to the control signal. Transistors can be fabricated to very small dimensions. Field effect transistors are highly sensitive devices in which extremely weak signals may be used for this control current. An extremely weak electrical signal applied to the gate of a field effect transistor controls the total current flowing from the source terminal to the drain terminal. The regulating signal at the gate can also be generated by an ion. Ion-selective field effect transistors (ISFETs) are field effect transistors covered by ion-selective membranes so that they respond only to one particular ionic species. ISFETs can be used to detect and accurately quantify the activity of specific ions, and the ion's activity is closely related to its concentration. Using this technology, solid-state measuring devices small enough to be mounted inside a standard indwelling vascular catheter have been developed and used experimentally for in vivo monitoring of pH, P_{CO_2}, sodium, potassium, and calcium in humans and laboratory animals.[153, 166, 167] Because of their small size, multiple different ISFETs may be mounted within the same catheter, allowing the prospect for continuous in vivo monitoring of several analyte concentrations simultaneously. The application of ISFET technology to routine bedside use in the intensive care unit awaits further development.

Fluorescent Optodes. Fluorescence is the emission of light by certain substances after stimulation with light of a differ-

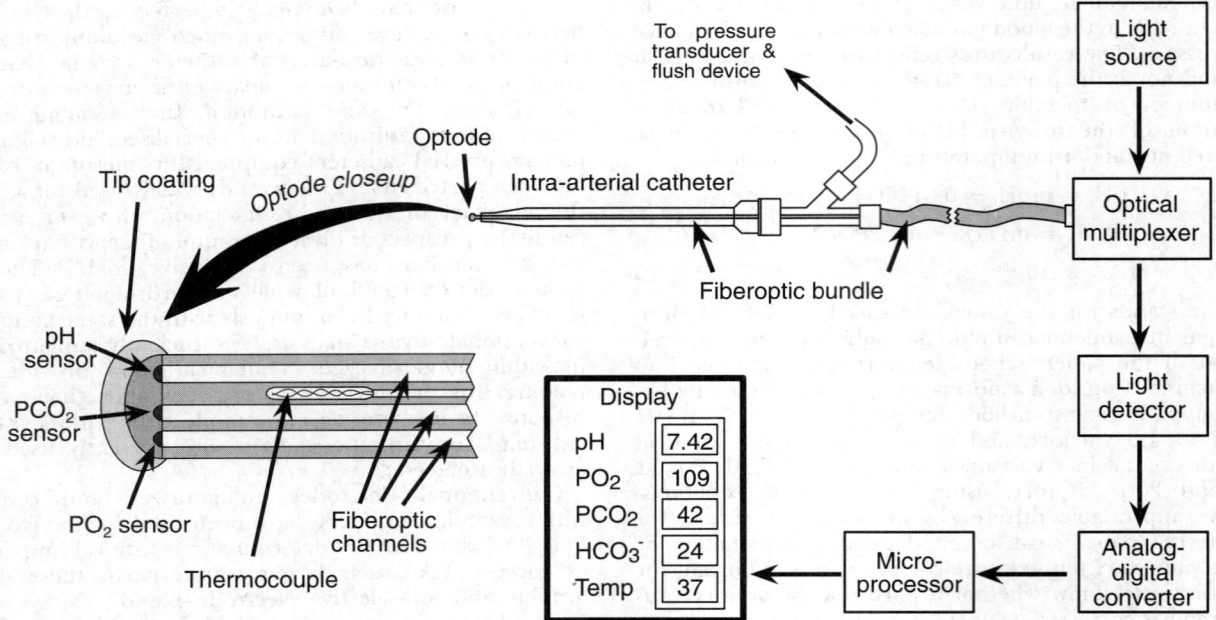

Figure 19–13. Simplified block diagram of multichannel intra-arterial blood gas analyzer for continuous in vivo blood gas monitoring using fluorescent optode technology.

ent wavelength. The process is initiated by an incident photon that excites an electron within a substance, boosting the electron to a higher energy level.[81, 87, 168] After discontinuation of the incident light, the electron decays to a lower energy level and energy is released. For most substances this energy is released in the form of heat; for fluorescing substances it is released as photons. Alternatively, the high-energy electron may interact with a nearby molecule, such as O_2, raising it to a higher vibrational state. Inhibition of the fluorescent response by this mechanism is called *quenching* and is the basis for fluorescence-based optode technology. The degree of quenching is indicative of the concentration of the analyte in question. This methodology has been used for in vitro and in vivo assays of O_2, pH, CO_2, osmolality, and ions of potassium, sodium, calcium, chloride, and cyanide.[169, 170] Using enzyme- or antibody-linked techniques, hormones, metabolites, and drugs could also be measured, at least in vitro.

Fluorescent optical electrodes, or *optodes*, for pH, P_{CO_2}, and P_{O_2} have been fabricated within thin (0.6 mm), flexible, disposable probes that surround three separate fiberoptic channels. The probe can be inserted through standard intra-arterial catheters and still permit pressure monitoring and intermittent blood sampling (Fig. 19–13). A light source transmits photons to the tips of the three optical fibers, which contain specific photoluminescent dyes. After photoexcitation, the resulting fluorescent emissions are conducted back to the bedside instrument, where they are quantitated by a photodetector and associated electronics. Analog-to-digital and microprocessor circuitry then generates a numeric display of the three measurements. Because the process is temperature dependent, a temperature sensor is also contained in the probe assembly for continuous blood temperature monitoring. This instrumentation has been tested in clinical trials and shown to have good accuracy, precision, and agreement when compared to simultaneous in vitro blood gas analysis by conventional laboratory instruments.[171–174] Thrombus formation and contact of the optode with the vessel wall have caused technical problems and loss of accuracy. Although these devices are reliable for only a

limited period (about 24 hours), refinements may lengthen this interval to several days.

Further technical developments and testing of these and other technologies are being actively pursued, and disposable catheter systems allowing continuous blood gas, pH, and electrolyte analyses will likely become part of routine intensive care monitoring in the near future.

References

1. Severinghaus JW, Astrup PB: pH and acid-base balance measurements. Int Anesthesiol Clin 25:27, 1987.
2. Itano M: CAP blood gas survey—First year's experience. Am J Clin Pathol 74:535, 1980.
3. Sachner MA, Avery WG, Sokolowski J: Arterial puncture by nurses. Chest 59:97, 1971.
4. Fleming WH, Bowen JC: Complications of arterial puncture. Milit Med 139:307, 1974.
5. Lindensmith LA, Winga ER, Goodnough DE, et al: Arterial puncture by inhalation therapy personnel. Chest 61:83, 1972.
6. Felix WR, Sigel B, Popki GL: Doppler ultrasound in the diagnosis of peripheral vascular disease. Semin Roentgenol 10:315, 1975.
7. Allen EV: Thromboangiitis obliterans: Methods of diagnosis of chronic occlusive arterial lesions distal to the wrist with illustrative cases. Am J Med Sci 178:237, 1929.
8. Greenhow DE: Incorrect performance of Allen's test: Ulnar artery flow erroneously presumed inadequate. Anesthesiology 37:356, 1972.
9. Richards RL: Peripheral Arterial Disease, a Physician's Approach. London, E & S Livingstone, p 47, 1970.
10. Ryan J, Raines J, Dalton BC, et al: Arterial dynamics of radial artery cannulation. Anesth Analg 52:1017, 1973.
11. Barker WJ, Wyte SR: Arterial puncture and cannulation. In: Roberts JR, Hedges JR (eds): Clinical Procedures in Emergency Medicine. Philadelphia, WB Saunders, p 352, 1985.
12. Rozenberg B, Rosenberg M, Birkhan J: Allen's test performed by pulse oximeter. Anaesthesia 43:515, 1988.
13. Mangano DT, Hickey RF: Ischemic injury following uncomplicated radial artery catheterization. Anesth Analg 58:55, 1979.
14. Gaspar MR: Arterial trauma. In: Gaspar MR, Barker WF (eds): Peripheral Arterial Disease. 3rd ed. Philadelphia, WB Saunders, p 124, 1981.
15. Williams T, Schenken JR: Radial artery puncture and the Allen test. Ann Intern Med 106:164, 1987.
16. Miller WC: The ABCs of blood gases. Emerg Med 16:37, 1984.
17. Peters KR, Chapin JW: Allen's test—positive or negative. Anesthesiology 53:85, 1980.
18. Messick JM: Allen's test—Neither positive nor negative. Anesthesiology 54:523, 1981.

19. Centers for Disease Control: Recommendations for prevention of HIV transmission in the health-care settings. MMWR 36:3S, 1987.
20. Centers for Disease Control: Update: Universal precautions for prevention of transmission of human immunodeficiency virus, hepatitis B virus, and other bloodborne pathogens in health-care settings. MMWR 37:377, 1988.
21. Brown HI, Goldiner PL, Turnbull AD: The reliability of the 25-gauge needle for arterial blood sampling. Anesthesiology 37:363, 1972.
22. Sabin S, Taylor JR, Kaplan AI: Clinical experience using a small-gauge needle for arterial puncture. Chest 69:437, 1976.
23. Petty TL, Bailey D, Best C: A new device for arterial blood gas sampling. JAMA 239:2016, 1978.
24. Bageant RA: Variations in arterial blood gas measurements due to sampling techniques. Respir Care 20:565, 1975.
25. Glauser FL, Morris JF: Accuracy of routine arterial puncture for the determination of oxygen and carbon dioxide tensions. Am Rev Respir Dis 106:776, 1972.
26. Morgan EJ, Baidwan B, Petty TL, et al: The effects of unanesthetized arterial puncture on P_{CO_2} and pH. Am Rev Respir Dis 120:795, 1979.
27. Miller WF, Gast LR: The technique of arterial blood gas sampling via needle puncture. Steps that ensure safe and reliable assessment of gas exchange. J Crit Illness 4:67, 1989.
28. Ansel G, Douce FH: Quantitative study of the effects that syringe material and needle size exert on minimum filling pressures of arterial blood gas syringes. Respir Care 25:1234, 1980.
29. Shapiro BA, Harrison RA, Cane RD, et al: Clinical Application of Blood Gases. 4th ed. Chicago, Year Book Medical Publishers, 1989.
30. Winkler JB, Huntington CG, Wells DE, et al: Influence of syringe material on arterial blood gas determinations. Chest 66:518, 1974.
31. Fan LL, Dellinger KT, Mills AL, et al: Potential errors in neonatal blood gas measurements. J Pediatr 97:650, 1980.
32. Hansen JE, Simmons DH: A systematic error in the determination of blood P_{CO_2}. Am Rev Respir Dis 115:1061, 1977.
33. Yoshimura H: Effects of anticoagulants on the pH of the blood. J Biochem (Tokyo) 22:297, 1935.
34. Petty TL, Bigelow DB, Levine BE: The simplicity and safety of arterial puncture. JAMA 195:181, 1966.
35. Mortensen JD: Clinical sequelae from arterial needle puncture, cannulation, and incision. Circulation 35:1118, 1967.
36. Bergentz SE, Hansson LO, Norbäck B: Surgical management of complications to arterial puncture. Ann Surg 164:1021, 1966.
37. Eriksen HC, Sörenson R: Arterial injuries. Iatrogenic and non-iatrogenic. Acta Chir Scand 135:133, 1969.
38. Bedford RF: Radial arterial function following percutaneous cannulation with 18- and 20-gauge catheters. Anesthesiology 47:37, 1977.
39. Bedford RF: Wrist circumference predicts the risk of radial artery occlusion after cannulation. Anesthesiology 48:377, 1978.
40. Matthews JI, Gibbons RB: Embolization complicating radial artery puncture. Ann Intern Med 75:87, 1971.
41. Luce EA, Futrell JW, Wilgis EF, et al: Compression neuropathy following brachial arterial puncture in anticoagulated patients. J Trauma 16:717, 1976.
42. Macon WL, Futrell JW: Median-nerve neuropathy after percutaneous puncture of the brachial artery in patients receiving anticoagulants. N Engl J Med 288:1396, 1973.
43. Neviaser RJ, Adams JP, May GI: Complications of arterial puncture in anticoagulated patients. J Bone Joint Surg [Am] 58A:218, 1976.
44. Ladenson JH: Nonanalytical sources of variation in clinical chemistry results. In: Sonnenwirth AC, Jaret L (eds): Gradwohl's Clinical Laboratory Methods and Diagnosis. 8th ed St Louis, CV Mosby, p 149, 1980.
45. Oeseburg B, Kwant G: Inaccuracy of oxygen electrode systems. Anesthesiology 51:368, 1979.
46. Walton JR, Shapiro BA, Wine C: Pre-analytical error in arterial blood gas measurement. Respir Care 26:1136, 1981.
47. Biswas CK, Ramos JM, Agroyannis B, et al: Blood gas analysis: Effect of air bubbles in syringe and delay in estimation. Br Med J 284:923, 1982.
48. Mueller RG, Lang GE, Beam JM: Bubbles in samples for blood gas determinations. Am J Clin Pathol 65:242, 1976.
49. Mueller RG, Lang GE: Blood gas analysis: Effects of air bubbles and delay in estimation (letter). Br Med J 285:1659, 1982.
50. Ishikawa S, Fornier A, Borst C, et al: The effects of air bubbles and delay on blood gas analysis. Ann Allergy 33:72, 1974.
51. Mueller RG, Lang GE, Daskam JM, et al: Phase equilibria of oxygen in blood-gas control samples. Clin Chem 21:165, 1975.
52. Madiedo G, Sciacca R, Hause L: Air bubbles and temperature effect on blood gas analysis. J Clin Pathol 33:864, 1980.
53. Harsten A, Berg B, Inerot S, et al: Importance of correct handling of samples for the results of blood gas analysis. Acta Anaesthesiol Scand 32:365, 1988.
54. Nanji AA, Whitlow KJ: Is it necessary to transport arterial blood samples on ice for pH and gas analysis? Can Anaesth Soc J 31:568, 1984.
55. Bloom SA, Canzanello VJ, Strom JA, et al: Spurious assessment of acid-base status due to dilutional effect of heparin. Am J Med 79:528, 1985.
56. Goodwin NM, Schreiber MT: Effects of anticoagulants on acid-base and blood gas estimation. Crit Care Med 7:473, 1979.
57. Bradley JG: Errors in the measurement of blood P_{CO_2} due to dilution of the sample with heparin solution. Br J Anaesth 44:231, 1972.
58. Siggard-Anderson O: Sampling and storing of blood for determination of acid-base status. Scan J Clin Lab Invest 13:196, 1961.
59. Hamilton RD, Crockett AJ, Alpers JH: Arterial blood gas analysis: Potential errors due to the addition of heparin. Anaesth Intensive Care 6:251, 1978.
60. Ng RH, Dennis RC, Yeston N, et al: Factitious cause of unexpected arterial blood gas results (letter). N Engl J Med 310:1189, 1984.
61. Smoller BR, Kruskall MS: Phlebotomy for diagnostic laboratory tests in adults: Pattern of use and effect on transfusion requirements. N Engl J Med 314:1233, 1986.
62. Bhaskaran NC, Lawler PG: How much blood for a blood gas? Anaesthesia 43:811, 1988.
63. Brown DR, Fenton LJ, Tsang RC: Blood sampling through umbilical catheters. Pediatrics 55:257, 1975.
64. Al-Ameri MW, Kruse JA, Carlson RW: Blood sampling from arterial catheters: Minimum discard volume to achieve accurate laboratory results. Crit Care Med 14:399, 1986.
65. Scott PV, Horton JN, Mapleson WW: Mechanism and magnitude of leakage from blood and water samples stored in plastic syringes. Br J Anaesth 43:717, 1971.
66. Scott PV, Horton JN, Mapleson WW: Leakage of oxygen from blood and water samples stored in plastic and glass syringes. Br Med J 3:512, 1971.
67. Evers W, Racz GB, Levy OA: A comparative study of plastic (polypropylene) and glass syringes in blood gas analysis. Anesth Analg 51:92, 1972.
68. Tokessy N, Ooi DS, Fleming KS: Evaluation of four polyethylene blood gas syringes. Clin Chem 36:1063, 1990.
69. Shohat M, Schonfeld T, Zaizoz R, et al: Determination of blood gases in children with extreme leukocytosis. Crit Care Med 16:787, 1988.
70. Schuch CS, Price JG: Determination of time required for blood gas homeostasis in the intubated, post–open heart surgery adult following a ventilator change. Heart Lung 5:314, 1986.
71. McHugh RD, Epstein RM, Longnecker DE: Halothane mimics oxygen in oxygen microelectrodes. Anesthesiology 50:47, 1979.
72. Dent JG, Netter KJ: Errors in oxygen tension measurements caused by halothane. Br J Anaesth 48:195, 1976.
73. Douglas IHS, McKenzie PJ, Ledingham I McA, et al: Effect of halothane on Po₂ electrode. Lancet 2:1370, 1978.
74. Maekawa T, Okuda Y, McDowall DG: Effect of low concentrations of halothane on the oxygen electrode. Br J Anaesth 52:585, 1980.
75. Hood LC, Noble WE, Smith E: Negligible halothane carryover in the IL-813 blood gas analyzer. Clin Chem 26:675, 1980.
76. Pruden EL, Siggard-Andersen O, Tietz NW: Blood gases and pH. In: Tietz NW (ed): Textbook of Clinical Chemistry. Philadelphia, WB Saunders, p 1191, 1986.
77. Lapinski M: Collection, processing, and measurement of blood gases. In: Henry JB (ed): Clinical Diagnosis and Management by Laboratory Methods. 16th ed, Philadelphia, WB Saunders, p 110, 1979.
78. Sorensen SPL: Enzymstudien. II. Mitteilung uber die Messung und die Bedeutung der Wasserstoffionenkonzentration bei enzymatischen Prozessen. Biochem Z 21:131, 1909.
79. Severinghaus JW, Astrup PB: Development of electrochemistry. Int Anesthesiol Clin 25:1, 1987.
80. Haber F, Klemensiewicz Z: Uber elektrische Phasengrezkrafte. Z Phys Chem 67:385, 1909.
81. Skoog DA, West DM: Fundamentals of Analytical Chemistry. 2nd ed. New York, Holt, Rinehart & Winston, 1969.
82. MacInnes DA, Dole M: Tests of a new type of glass electrode. Ind Eng Chem Anal Ed 1:57, 1929.
83. Maron SH, Prutton CF: Principles of Physical Chemistry. 3rd ed. New York, Macmillan, p 560, 1958.
84. Cohen JJ, Kassirer JP, Gennari FJ, et al: Acid-Base. Boston, Little, Brown, 1982.
85. Clark LC Jr: Monitor and control of blood and tissue oxygen tensions. Trans Am Soc Artif Intern Organs 2:41, 1956.
86. Meyerhoff ME: New in vitro analytical approaches for clinical chemistry measurements in critical care. Clin Chem 36:1567, 1990.
87. Willard HH, Merritt LL, Dean JA, et al: Instrumental Methods of Analysis. 6th ed. Belmont, CA, Wadsworth Publishing, 1981.
88. Demko PR, Welch R, Bellino L, et al: Simultaneous determination of urea, glucose, sodium, potassium, chloride, and total carbon dioxide in undiluted human serum using an electrode based automated analyzer. Clin Chem 35:1091, 1989.
89. Bertholf RL, Savory MG, Winborne KH, et al: Lithium determined in serum with an ion-selective electrode. Clin Chem 34:1500, 1988.
90. Gouget B, Lacour B, Gourmelin Y, et al: Lithium I.S.E. measurement on whole blood with the CIBA-Corning 654. Clin Chem 36:1068, 1990.
91. Bachas LG, Daunert S, Wotring VJ, et al: Design and development of anion-selective electrodes using principles of host-guest chemistry. Clin Chem 36:1066, 1990.
92. Osawa H, Yoshino F, Yamada A: Rapid determination of bromide ion in body fluid using a cyclicvolammetric method. Clin Chem 36:1064, 1990.
93. Csosz M, Bartalits L, Simon W, et al: Calibration and measurement with Mg-ionselective electrode in serum samples. Clin Chem 36:1065, 1990.
94. Yasuda K, Miyagi H, Hamada Y, et al: Determination of urea in whole

blood using a urea electrode and immobilized urease membrane. Analyst 109:61, 1984.

95. Willems D, Steenssens W: Ammonia determined in plasma with a selective electrode. Clin Chem 34:2372, 1988.

96. Gourmelin Y, Gouget B, Truchaud A: Electrode measurement of glucose and urea in undiluted samples. Clin Chem 36:1646, 1990.

97. O'Connell KM: Use of enzyme electrodes in whole blood measurements. Clin Chem 35:1233, 1989.

98. Burritt MF: Current analytical approaches to measuring blood analytes. Clin Chem 36:1562, 1990.

99. Elser RC: Quality control of blood gas analysis: A review. Respir Care 31:807, 1986.

100. Van Kessel AL, Eichhorn JH, Clausen JL, et al: Inter-instrument comparison of blood gas analyzers and assessment of tonometry using fresh heparinized whole human blood. Chest 92:418, 1987.

101. Eichhorn JH: Accuracy and comparisons in blood gas measurements. Chest 94:1, 1988.

102. Hansen JE, Feil MC: Blood gas quality control materials compared to tonometered blood in examining interinstrument bias in P_{O_2}. Chest 94:49, 1988.

103. Hansen JE, Jensen RL, Casaburi R, et al: Comparison of blood gas analyzer biases in measuring tonmetered blood and a fluorocarbon-containing, proficiency-testing material. Am Rev Respir Dis 140:403, 1989.

104. Hansen JE, Clausen JL, Levy SE, et al: Proficiency testing materials for pH and blood gases. The California Thoracic Society experience. Chest 89:214, 1986.

105. Ong ST, David D, Snow M, et al: Effects of variations in room temperature on measured values of blood gas quality-control materials. Clin Chem 29:502, 1983.

106. Feil MC, Cormier AD, Legg KD: Perfluorocarbon emulsions as pH/blood gas controls. Clin Chem 28:2187, 1982.

107. Hansen JE, Clausen JL, Mohler JG, et al: Blood gas proficiency-testing materials: A multilaboratory comparison of an aqueous solution and a fluorocarbon-containing emulsion. Clin Chem 28:1818, 1982.

108. Ehrmeyer SS, Laessig RH, Garber CC: Monthly interlaboratory pH and blood-gas survey. Establishing accuracy based on interlaboratory performance. Am J Clin Pathol 81:224, 1984.

109. Burki NK: Arterial blood gas measurement. Chest 88:3, 1985.

110. Cane RD, Harrison RA, Shapiro BA, et al: The spectrophotometric absorbance of Intralipid. Anesthesiology 53:53, 1980.

111. Adair GS: The hemoglobin system. VI. The oxygen dissociation curve for hemoglobin. J Biol Chem 63:529, 1925.

112. Aberman A, Cavanilles JM, Trotter J, et al: An equation for the oxygen hemoglobin dissociation curve. J Appl Physiol 35:570, 1973.

113. Ruiz BC, Tucker WK, Kirby RR: A program for calculation of intrapulmonary shunts, blood-gas and acid-base values with a programmable calculator. Anesthesiology 42:88, 1975.

114. Gabel RA: Algorithms for calculating and correcting blood-gas and acid-base variables. Respir Physiol 42:211, 1980.

115. Kelman GR: Digital computer subroutine for the conversion of oxygen tension into saturation. J Appl Physiol 21:1375, 1966.

116. Woodson RD: O_2 transport: DPG and P_{50}. Basics of RD 5:1, 1977.

117. Thomas HM, Lefrak SS, Irwin RS, et al: The oxyhemoglobin dissociation curve in health and disease. Role of 2,3-diphosphoglycerate. Am J Med 57:331, 1974.

118. Canizaro PC, Nelson JL, Hennessy JL, et al: A technique for estimating the position of the oxygen-hemoglobin dissociation curve. Ann Surg 180:364, 1974.

119. Kelman GR, Nunn JF: Nomograms for correction of blood P_{O_2}, P_{CO_2}, pH, and base excess for time and temperature. J Appl Physiol 21:1484, 1966.

120. Willford DC, Hill EP, Moores WY: Theoretical analysis of optimal P_{50}. J Appl Physiol 52:1043, 1982.

121. Aberman A, Cavanilles JM, Weil MH, et al: Blood P_{50} calculated from a single measurement of pH, P_{O_2}, and S_{O_2}. J Appl Physiol 38:171, 1975.

122. Burnett RW, Noonan D: Calculations and correction factors used in determination of blood pH and blood gases. Clin Chem 20:1499, 1974.

123. Swain JA: Hypothermia and blood pH. Arch Intern Med 148:1643, 1988.

124. Kruse JA, Hukku P, Carlson RW: Constancy of blood carbonic acid pK' in patients during cardiopulmonary resuscitation. Chest 93:1221, 1988.

125. Kruse JA, Hukku P, Carlson RW: Relationship between the apparent dissociation constant of blood carbonic acid and severity of illness. J Lab Clin Med 114:568, 1989.

126. Karlowicz MG, Simmons MA, Brusilow SW, et al: Carbonic acid dissociation constant (pK_1) in critically ill newborns. Pediatr Res 18:1287, 1984.

127. Relman AS: "Blood gases": Arterial or venous? N Engl J Med 315:188, 1986.

128. Weil MH, Rackow EC, Trevino R, et al: Differences in acid-base state between venous and arterial blood during cardiopulmonary resuscitation. N Engl J Med 315:153, 1986.

129. Bandi ZL: Estimation, prevention, and quality control of carbon dioxide loss during aerobic sample processing. Clin Chem 27:1676, 1981.

130. Halperin ML, Goldstein MB, Pichette C, et al: Evaluation of the bicarbonate buffer system. Am J Nephrol 3:245, 1983.

131. Pichette C, Chen CB, Goldstein M, et al: Influence of solutes in plasma on the total CO_2 content determination: Implications for clinical disorders. Clin Biochem 16:91, 1983.

132. Andersen OS, Astrup P, Bates RG, et al: Report of Ad Hoc Committee on Acid-Base Terminology. Ann NY Acad Sci 133:251, 1966.

133. Gershwin R, Smith NT, Suwa K: An equation system and programs for obtaining base excess using a programmable calculator. Anesthesiology 40:89, 1974.

134. Radiometer: ABL300 Acid-Base Laboratory User's Manual. Copenhagen, Radiometer, p 138, 1984.

135. Schwartz WB, Relman AS: A critique of the parameters used in the evaluation of acid-base disorders. N Engl J Med 268:1382, 1963.

136. Cohen JJ, Brackett NC Jr, Schwartz WB: The nature of the carbon dioxide titration curve in the normal dog. J Clin Invest 43:777, 1964.

137. Kruse JA: Metabolic acidosis in severe acute asthma, acid-base nomenclature. Crit Care Med 16:1255, 1988.

138. Ashwood ER, Kost G, Kenny M: Temperature correction for blood-gas measurements. Clin Chem 29:1877, 1983.

139. Andritsch RF, Muravchick S, Gold MI: Temperature correction of arterial blood-gas parameters: A comparative review of methodology. Anesthesiology 55:311, 1981.

140. Rahn H: Body temperature and acid-base regulation. Pneumonologie 151:87, 1974.

141. Hansen JE, Sue DY: Should blood gas measurements be corrected for the patient's temperature? N Engl J Med 303:341, 1980.

142. Ream AK, Reitz BA, Silverberg G: Temperature correction of P_{CO_2} and pH in estimating acid-base status: An example of the Emperor's new clothes? Anesthesiology 56:41, 1982.

143. Sivarajan M: Temperature correction of arterial blood-gas values. Anesthesiology 56:329, 1982.

144. Blume P: Blood gas measurements. Am J Clin Pathol 70:440, 1978.

145. Zaloga GP, Hill TR, Strickland RA, et al: Bedside blood gas and electrolyte monitoring in critically ill patients. Crit Care Med 17:920, 1989.

146. Strickland RA, Hill TR, Zaloga GP: Bedside analysis of arterial blood gases and electrolytes during and after cardiac surgery. J Clin Anesthesiol 1:248, 1989.

147. Misiano DR, Lowenstein E: Performance characteristics of the Gem-Stat monitor. Proc Int Fed Clin Chem Stresa Italy 10:239, 1988.

148. Fogt EJ: Continuous ex vivo and in vivo monitoring with chemical sensors. Clin Chem 36:1573, 1990.

149. Claremont DJ, Pagdin TM, Walton N: Continuous monitoring of blood P_{O_2} in extracorporeal systems. Anaesthesia 39:362, 1984.

150. Eberhart RC: Continuous blood gas analysis: An elusive ideal. Crit Care Med 8:418, 1980.

151. Coon RL, Lai NCJ, Kampine JP: Evaluation of a dual-function pH and P_{CO_2} in vivo sensor. J Appl Physiol 40:625, 1976.

152. Neumark J, Bardeen A, Sulzer E, et al: Miniature intravascular P_{CO_2} sensors in neurosurgery. J Neurosurg 43:172, 1975.

153. Kohama A, Nakamura Y, Nakamura M, et al: Continuous monitoring of arterial and tissue P_{CO_2}. Crit Care Med 12:940, 1984.

154. Pfeifer PM, Pearson DT, Clayton RH: Clinical trial of the Continucath intra-arterial oxygen monitor. Anaesthesia 43:677, 1988.

155. Gold MI, Diaz PM, Feingold A, et al: A disposable in vivo oxygen electrode for the continuous measurement of arterial oxygen tension. Surgery 78:245, 1975.

156. Bratanow N, Polk K, Bland R, et al: Continuous polarographic monitoring of intra-arterial oxygen in the perioperative period. Crit Care Med 13:859, 1985.

157. Nilsson E, Edwall G, Larsson R, et al: Polarographic P_{CO_2} sensors with heparinized membranes for in vitro and continuous in vivo registration. Scand J Clin Lab Invest 41:557, 1981.

158. Mapleson WW, Willis BA, Williams B: Blood-gas tension measurement in anaesthesia by bubble equilibration and mass spectrometry. Br J Anaesth 52:1061, 1980.

159. Lundsgaard JS, Groenlund J, Einer-Jensen N: In vivo calibration of flow-dependent blood gas catheters. J Appl Physiol 44:124, 1978.

160. Brantigan JW, Dunn KL, Albo D: A clinical catheter for continuous blood gas measurement by mass spectrometry. J Appl Physiol 40:443, 1976.

161. Lundsgaard JS, Jensen B, Gronlund J: Fast-responding flow-independent blood gas catheter for oxygen measurement. J Appl Physiol 48:376, 1980.

162. Brantigan JW: Catheters for continuous in vivo blood and tissue gas monitoring. Crit Care Med 4:239, 1976.

163. Hall JR, Poulton TJ, Downs JB, et al: In vivo arterial blood gas analysis: An evaluation. Crit Care Med 8:414, 1980.

164. Richman KA, Jobes DR, Schwalb AJ: Continuous in-vivo blood gas determination in man: Reliability and safety of a new device. Anesthesiology 52:313, 1980.

165. Moffitt EA, McLaren RG, Imrie DD, et al: Inline blood gas analysis by gas chromatography in patients during and after coronary artery surgery. Can Anaesth Soc J 26:157, 1979.

166. McKinley BA, Houtchens BA, Janata J: Continuous monitoring of interstitial fluid potassium during hemorrhagic shock in dogs. Crit Care Med 9:845, 1981.

167. McKinley BA, Wong KC, Janata J, et al: In vivo continuous monitoring

of ionized calcium in dogs using ion sensitive field effect transistors. Crit Care Med 9:333, 1981.
168. Barker SJ, Tremper KK: Intra-arterial oxygen tension monitoring. Int Anesthesiol Clin 25:199, 1987.
169. Opitz N, Lubbers DW: Theory and development of fluorescence-based optochemical oxygen sensors: Oxygen optodes. Int Anesthesiol Clin 25:177, 1987.
170. Bachas LG, Blair TL, Freeman MK: Ion-selective fiber optic sensing devices using immobilized chromoionophores. Clin Chem 36:1066, 1990.
171. Miller WW, Yafuso M, Yan CF, et al: Performance of an in-vivo, continuous blood-gas monitor with disposable probe. Clin Chem 33:1538, 1987.
172. Shapiro BA, Cane RD, Chomka CM, et al: Preliminary evaluation of an intra-arterial blood gas system in dogs and humans. Crit Care Med 17:455, 1989.
173. Tremper KK, Barker SJ: The optode: Next generation in blood gas measurement. Crit Care Med 17:481, 1989.
174. Halbert SA: Intravascular monitoring: Problems and promise. Clin Chem 36:1581, 1990.

CHAPTER 20

Arterial Pressure Monitoring

Lisa L. Kirkland
Christopher Veremakis

With the sophisticated physiologic monitoring systems available today, the critical care physician is compelled to maintain a high level of expertise in the appropriate utilization and interpretation of the data generated by these systems. Intermittent noninvasive measurements of arterial pressure are easily obtained and are accurate in healthy persons. However, these measurements are rendered inaccurate by cardiovascular decompensation and are inadequate in patients who may require minute-to-minute hemodynamic surveillance. Consequently, invasive modalities are indicated for immediate recognition of physiologic aberrations in unstable patients. Unfortunately, these modalities have significant limitations and may deliver erroneous data. Comparisons of the noninvasive and invasive means of blood pressure assessment reveal the indications and drawbacks of each method and underscore the importance of quality control to ensure the acquisition of accurate information.

INDIRECT OR NONINVASIVE ARTERIAL PRESSURE MONITORING

Noninvasive arterial pressure monitoring is adequate for the majority of patients, because most do not require continuous assessment of hemodynamic parameters. Current methods of intermittent noninvasive blood pressure measurement include auscultation, oscillometry, and Doppler probe. In addition, photoplethysmography is a new noninvasive method that provides a continuous read-out of arterial components.

Manual Method

Auscultation is the most commonly used manual method of blood pressure monitoring and is accurate in hemody-namically stable patients when performed correctly. Auscultation of Korotkoff sounds (K_1 to K_5) depends on displacement of the partially occluded vessel wall by turbulent blood flow. A pneumatic cuff is placed just proximal to the point of arterial auscultation and inflated until flow through that artery ceases; at that point cuff pressure exceeds systolic pressure. The cuff is gradually deflated and, as the external pressure falls below systolic pressure, pulses of blood intrude under the cuff and emerge as turbulent flow. The initial tapping sounds are termed K_1 sounds[1] and the corresponding manometric pressure is recorded as the *systolic pressure*. As cuff pressure is further reduced, flow persists through an increasing portion of the cardiac ejection cycle until the artery is no longer compressed. K_2 is defined by the transition to an audible murmur or swish.[1] Thereafter, turbulence decreases, although there may still be some deformation of the arterial wall. K_3 marks the point at which sounds increase in clarity, followed by abrupt muffling of sounds, termed K_4.[1] In low-peripheral-resistance states, K_4 marks the attainment of diastolic pressure, as sounds may persist well below this point when flow is rapid because of high run-off.[2] However, in healthy adults or high-resistance states, vascular sounds disappear entirely at diastolic pressure, a point termed K_5.[1]

Auscultation has been demonstrated to be inaccurate in patients with high-vascular-resistance states caused by shock or vasoconstrictive therapy. Although there is a correlation between auscultation and direct measurements of blood pressure in low-vascular-resistance states and hypotension,[3] the auscultatory method does not provide the continuous surveillance required in unstable patients.

Automatic Noninvasive Methods

Automatic noninvasive devices have gained popularity because of their relatively low cost, reasonable accuracy, and capacity for frequent measurements.

Oscillometry is an indirect method of blood pressure determination based on the measurement of manometric oscillations induced by arterial pulsations during cuff deflation. A cuff attached to a mercury manometer is inflated above systolic pressure and gradually deflated. When pressure waves first intrude under the cuff, oscillations appear on the manometer, corresponding to systolic pressure. Of note, K_1 (the initial auscultated sound) is not yet audible; this point is termed 0.[1] As cuff pressure declines, oscillations increase to a maximal intensity that corresponds well with direct measurements of mean arterial pressure.[4, 5] Diastolic pressure is determined when oscillations vanish.[6]

Doppler technology has also been applied to measurement of systemic blood pressure. A Doppler probe placed over an artery emits a short burst of sound waves and subsequently receives the waves as they reflect back from the blood vessel. The reflected wave is analyzed for frequency shift, an indication of vessel wall motion or blood flow.[5, 6] When combined with a blood pressure cuff, intermittent systolic and diastolic pressures[6] may be determined with acceptable accuracy. Significant deficiencies in clinical applicability are related to interference caused by movement of the patient and probe displacement.

Photoplethysmography permits indirect blood pressure measurements through the application of a finger cuff containing an infrared light source and photodetector cell.[2] Blood volume is monitored by analyzing infrared reflections. Cuff pressure is increased until the external pressure surrounding the digit maintains a constant blood volume. This external pressure is equivalent to mean arterial pressure. As this device is capable of measuring pressure with each cardiac cycle, continuous recordings of systolic and diastolic pressures may also be made. However, peripheral vasoconstriction may result in inaccurate readings.[2]

Comparative Accuracy: Noninvasive Versus Invasive

Comparative studies of auscultation, oscillometry, and the invasive methods have yielded variable results.[4, 7–10] In healthy patients with steady-state hemodynamics, noninvasive techniques may underestimate systolic blood pressure and overestimate diastolic blood pressure by up to 15% of simultaneous direct readings.[4, 7] Oscillometry may provide the most accurate approximation of systolic pressure among the noninvasive methods.[2] When an indirectly measured systolic pressure exceeds that measured by an intra-arterial catheter, technical error involving cuff size or the monitoring equipment should be suspected. Additional factors that may introduce errors include speed of cuff deflation, cuff size and positioning, arm circumference, sensor displacement, and interobserver variation.[11] Frequent cuff inflation may result in damage to the ulnar nerve.[6, 11] Noninvasive methods may fail in the presence of cardiac arrhythmias and wide beat-to-beat pressure swings.[5, 11] Also, diminished arterial compliance occurring in severe arteriosclerosis may impair arterial occlusion, resulting in noninvasive systolic pressure readings that are higher than those measured by arterial catheter.[5, 6] Nonetheless, automatic noninvasive techniques provide an effective method for monitoring relatively stable patients who require frequent blood pressure checks for brief periods.

In labile hemodynamic states, however, indirect methods are much less accurate, as well as being hampered by slow response times and limited frequency of repetition.[5, 7] Auscultation consistently underestimates systolic pressure[10] and oscillometry and Doppler methods are inconsistent in unstable patients.[11] Indirect errors of over 30 mm Hg are common in postoperative patients. For patients requiring vasoactive medications there may be even greater discrepancies.[12] Direct intra-arterial pressure monitoring is indicated in hemodynamically unstable patients, patients with severe peripheral vasoconstriction, patients requiring intravenous vasoactive medications, and patients whose condition merits continuous surveillance of blood pressure. Intra-arterial catheters are also indicated when frequent sampling of arterial blood is anticipated.

INVASIVE OR DIRECT ARTERIAL PRESSURE MONITORING

When managing ill or unstable patients, constant surveillance of hemodynamic parameters is essential for rapid assessment of cardiovascular decompensation or efficacy of therapeutic maneuvers. Invasive arterial monitoring provides continuous real-time physiologic data, but for this information to be interpreted and applied correctly, its limitations must be understood. Often, too much emphasis is placed on the numbers without proper consideration of the principles underlying the data or potential sources of error. A peripheral arterial waveform is not an exact replica of pressure characteristics in the proximal aorta or the peripheral vascular tree. The inotropic state of the left ventricle, the impedance within the aorta and peripheral vasculature, and the dynamics of the monitoring system all contribute to producing the waveform displayed on the monitor (Table 20–1). The monitoring system itself may generate artifacts, producing a waveform not at all reflective of the actual physiology in the systemic circulation. Correct interpretation of the information generated by invasive monitoring requires a level of expertise capable of recogniz-

TABLE 20–1

COMMON WAVEFORM VARIATIONS

Waveform	Physiology	Possible Causes
Blunted	Overdamping	Large air bubbles, clot, loose connections, deflated pressure bag, no fluid under transducer diaphragm
Systolic overshoot	Underdamping	Small bubbles, excessive tubing
	High initial vascular frequencies approaching system resonant frequency	Heart rate > 120 beats/min, increased inotropic state
	Resonance of vascular tree	Noncompliant vasculature (atherosclerosis)
	Low system resonant frequency (<7.5 Hz)	Compliant or excessive tubing, small air bubbles, small-bore catheter
Depressed volume displacement wave	Low cardiac output	Hypovolemia, vasoconstriction, depressed left ventricular function
Rapid down-slope	Rapid run-off, low peripheral resistance	Vasodilatation
Reflected wave (C)* lost or shifted to right	Low flow state	Hypotension, vasoconstriction

*See Figure 20–5.

ing unreliable data. Erroneous data analysis may result in incorrect and potentially adverse therapeutic decisions.

Equipment

An invasive arterial monitoring system typically consists of the hydraulic or fluid-filled elements, a fluid-mechanical interface, the transducer, and the electrical equipment including the amplifier, monitor, oscilloscope, and strip chart recorder (Fig. 20–1). The hydraulic component of the monitoring system includes a catheter, noncompliant connection pressure tubing, stopcocks, a flush device, and the transducer dome. A Teflon or polyethylene intra-arterial catheter provides the initial interface between the vascular tree and the monitoring system. Although short large-bore catheters maximize accurate replication of physiologic data, catheter size is limited because the incidence of vessel thrombosis is increased with larger-diameter catheters. Noncompliant pressure tubing connects the catheter to the transducer and should be no longer than 18 to 24 inches. A stopcock is placed close to the patient for blood sampling. A second stopcock may be positioned adjacent to the transducer to facilitate zeroing. The flush device is pressurized to 300 mm Hg and delivers a continuous infusion of heparinized saline (1 to 3 mL/h) to ensure patency of the system and reduce thrombotic complications.

Intravascular pressure changes are transmitted through the fluid-filled tubing to the strain gauge transducer, where mechanical displacement is converted into an electrical signal proportional to the applied pressure. This signal is amplified and then filtered to remove high-frequency noise. A waveform is then displayed on the monitor, which provides both graphic and digital read-outs. Calibrated strip chart record-

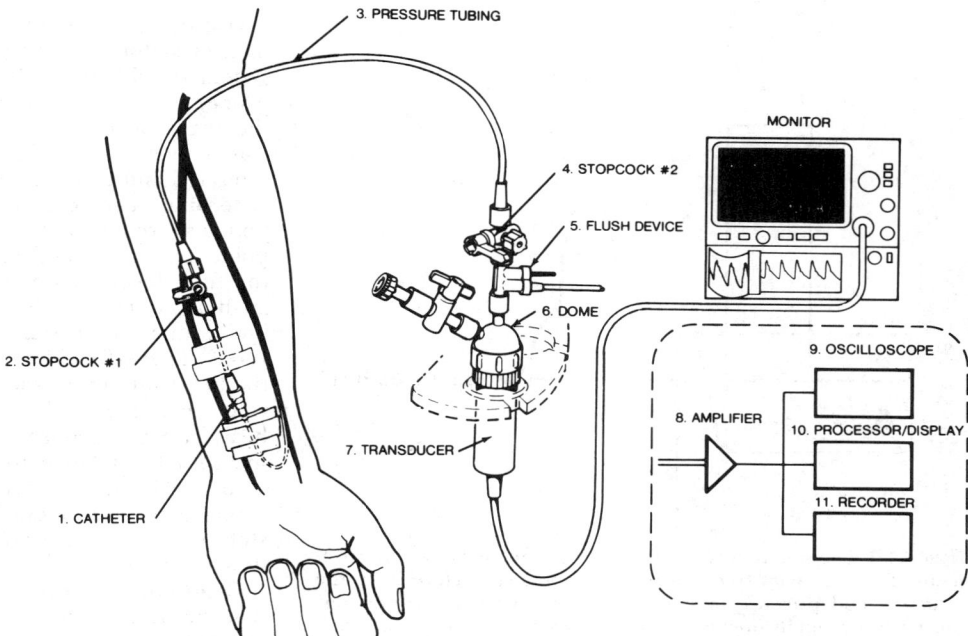

Figure 20–1. The 10 components used to monitor direct blood pressure. The monitoring components are nearly the same whether the catheter is in an artery (radial, brachial, or femoral) or in the pulmonary artery. (Size of transducer and plumbing components were enlarged for illustration purposes.) (From RM Gardner, KW Hollingsworth, Optimizing the electrocardiogram and pressure monitoring, Crit Care Med, 14, 7, 651–658, © by Williams & Wilkins, 1986.)

ings of the waveform assist in ascertaining the accuracy of digital information.

Accurate pressure readings are dependent on the ability of the entire system to acquire and translate correctly physiologic data. The technical specifications of standard monitoring equipment far exceed the requirements for accurate signal reproduction. However, the hydraulic components are not as sophisticated as the electrical components and often prove to be the weak link in the monitoring system.

Dynamic Response of the Monitoring System

Frequency Response. The dynamic characteristics of the system may be tested by mechanically applying an alternating pressure signal of constant amplitude at increasing frequencies.[11] The resulting pressure readings may be graphed to yield a frequency response curve representative of the dynamic reproductive accuracy of the monitoring system. Faithful reproduction of a spectrum of varying frequencies yields a straight or flat frequency response curve, which reflects the ability of the monitoring system to reproduce signal input without distortion, that is, augmentation or compression. To ensure such accuracy, the system response must be flat within a range five to eight times that of the original frequency. Frequencies in the vascular tree directly correspond to heart rate. Therefore, the frequency of the normal vasculature is 60 to 180 cycles/min or 1 to 3 cps (Hz).[2] Hence, an arterial monitoring system must have a flat frequency response of at least 5 to 20 Hz to allow accurate signal reproduction.

Resonant Frequency. All fluid-filled monitoring systems have a tendency to vibrate or oscillate when stimulated. In addition, each system has a unique natural or resonant frequency (Fig. 20–2). On stimulation at or near the resonant frequency, a system "rings," amplifying the magnitude of the original stimulus. Ringing may produce artifactually high pressure readings in arterial monitoring systems. Physiologic vascular frequencies may approach 10 to 15 Hz in some settings;[2] therefore, the monitoring system should have a resonant frequency greater than 15 Hz and preferably greater than 25 Hz.[13] Unfortunately, the resonant frequency of fluid-filled tubing is between 5 and 20 Hz.[14] Hence, its

frequency response curve is not always flat within the physiologic vascular frequency range. Consequently, systolic pressure amplification is a common artifact.

Damping. After excitation, frictional forces opposing oscillation eventually extinguish the response and return the system to zero baseline. This tendency also depends on viscosity[2] and compliance[15] of the system and is termed *damping*. Damping characteristics are expressed by the damping coefficient. Coefficients approaching 0 permit excessive oscillation, whereas those approaching 1 prevent any oscillation even at the resonant frequency.[2, 15] Theoretically, the optimal damping coefficient is between 0.6 and 0.7.[6] Hydraulic monitoring systems are generally underdamped, which preserves high-frequency responsiveness but contributes to signal augmentation. Overdamped systems respond sluggishly and diminish or obscure pressure waves generated in the vascular tree.

Optimizing the Dynamic Response. The resonant fre-

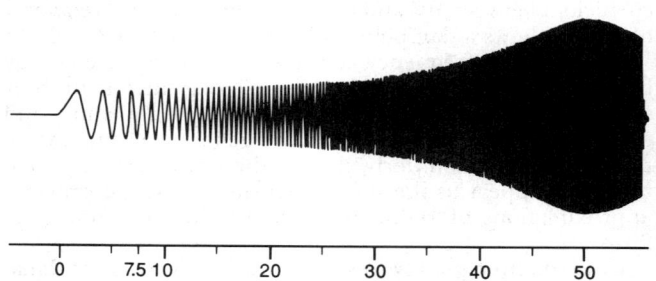

Figure 20–2. Pressure recorded by an arterial pressure monitoring system. With increasing frequencies at constant amplitude, the system begins to oscillate at 30 Hz, exaggerating the signal input. Maximal oscillations occur at 50 Hz, defining the resonant frequency of this system. As the frequency response is flat within the physiologic range, this system is acceptable for clinical use without additional damping. However, most arterial pressure monitoring systems have resonant frequencies of 10 to 20 Hz; therefore, damping is necessary to avoid signal distortion. Resonant frequencies less than 7.5 Hz are not acceptable for clinical use. (Modified from Gravenstein JS, Paulus DA: Clinical Monitoring Practice. 2nd ed. Philadelphia, JB Lippincott, 1987.)

Time

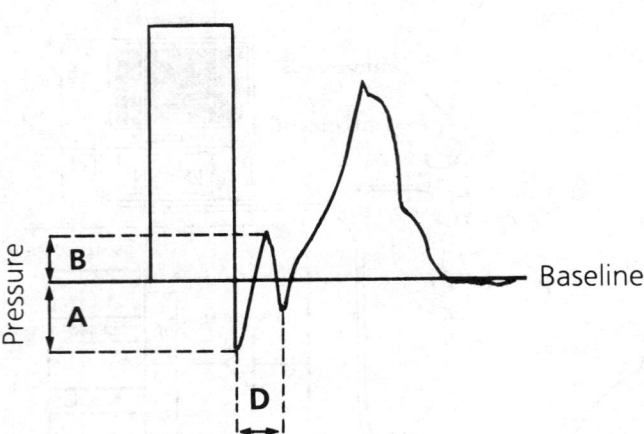

Figure 20–3. The square wave or fast-flush technique allows measurement of the resonant frequency and damping characteristics of the arterial blood pressure monitoring system. When the continuous flush valve is rapidly opened and closed, a square wave is generated. As the oscillations return to baseline, they provide the information necessary for quantification of resonant frequency and damping coefficient. The resonant frequency (in hertz) equals 25/D, where D signifies the distance in millimeters between two successive peaks or troughs (paper speed is 25 mm/s). The damping coefficient is estimated by calculating the amplitude ratio of two successive half-cycle oscillations (B/A). An amplitude ratio of 0.3 or less ensures adequate damping if the resonant frequency is between 10 and 20 Hz; a ratio of 0.3 to 0.6 indicates adequate damping with a resonant frequency greater than 20 Hz. (From Veremakis C, Halloran TH: The technique of monitoring arterial blood pressure. J Crit Illness 4[10]:82, 1989.)

quency and damping characteristics determine the accuracy of the monitoring system. An ideal system requires a resonant frequency in excess of that usually encountered in the clinical setting.[9] There is little distortion regardless of the damping coefficient if the resonant frequency of an arterial pressure-monitoring system exceeds 30 Hz.[14] Conversely, at resonant frequencies below 7.5 Hz, signal amplification results regardless of the system's damping characteristics.[13] Typical clinical monitoring systems have a resonant frequency between 10 and 20 Hz and require a damping coefficient between 0.5 and 0.7. A system resonant frequency of 25 Hz allows a damping coefficient as low as 0.2 to 0.3.[13]

The resonant frequency and damping characteristics may be ascertained at the bedside by employing the fast-flush or square wave technique (Fig. 20–3). Rapid opening and closing of the continuous flush valve generate a square wave tracing. Information derived from the characteristic oscillations that appear as the system returns to baseline provides approximations of resonant frequency and damping (Fig. 20–4).

Underdamping, a low resonant frequency, or a combination of the two produces systolic overshoot and overestimates true systolic pressure. Maneuvers that increase resonant frequency while optimizing damping include use of short noncompliant tubing and transducers,[15–18] meticulous extraction of air bubbles,[15–17, 19] and minimization of injection sites and stopcocks.[13] Simple preassembled kits may reduce technical problems.[20] If ringing persists despite efforts to increase resonant frequency, insertion of a damping device may be necessary.[20, 21] Insertion of air bubbles is not recommended. Small bubbles lower resonant frequency and contribute to signal amplification.

Overdamping blunts the arterial waveform and underestimates systolic pressure. If overdamping is present, the system should be carefully inspected for poor fittings, improper pressure bag inflation, and absence of fluid under the transducer dome. Large air bubbles increase system compliance and overdamp the signal. The system should be aspirated and carefully flushed to eliminate clots.[20]

Zeroing. The accuracy of the blood pressure determination also requires the establishment of a zero reference point. This is accomplished by opening a stopcock to expose the transducer to atmospheric pressure while aligning the air-fluid interface at the level of the right atrium (midaxillary line, fourth intercostal space) and adjusting the monitor to zero.[20] Thereafter, the position of the transducer relative to the heart influences the blood pressure readings,[21] yielding values erroneously high when the transducer is below the heart and erroneously low when above it. The position of the catheter relative to the heart does not affect system accuracy. Failure to zero the transducer leads to significant errors of measurement. Zeroing should be repeated every shift or whenever significant changes in blood pressure develop, as monitoring systems tend to drift with time.[21]

Calibration. The transducer requires calibration to ensure that the strain gauge accurately reflects pressure gradations in mechanical displacement. Calibration is accomplished at the bedside by opening the transducer to a predetermined pressure from a column of water. The fixed degree of mechanical displacement of the transducer diaphragm and equivalent electrical signals result in the corresponding pressure displayed on the monitor. If a discrepancy exists, malfunction of the transducer is the most common etiology, as the electrical components are usually reliable.

Arterial Waveforms

The arterial waveform is a confluence of multiple waveforms and may be divided into three basic functional phases: inotropic phase, volume displacement phase, and run-off and reflection (Fig. 20–5). The inotropic phase reflects acceleration of blood into the aorta after aortic valve opening and is a function of the contractile state of the left ventricle. This narrow peaked pressure wave represents the initial impact of the pressure jet of blood on the low-velocity blood in the aorta.[22] The shoulder of the arterial wave is formed by the balance of the stroke volume as it is added to the aorta and is termed the volume displacement wave. Under normal conditions the peak of the inotropic spike and the volume displacement wave are essentially equal. However, in patients with good contractility, marked vasoconstriction, and low cardiac output, volume displacement may be significantly reduced. The shoulder of the waveform then falls far below the initial inotropic spike.[22] In other instances,

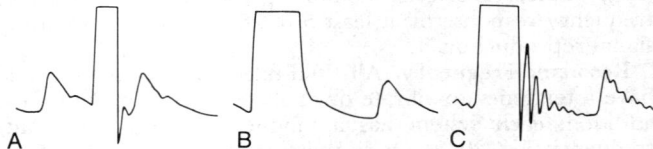

Figure 20–4. Rapid evaluation of the square wave resulting from a fast-flush test qualitatively describes the frequency response and damping characteristics of the arterial pressure monitoring system to a trained observer. The tracing in *A* illustrates a normal square wave and waveform configuration, signifying adequate damping. The square wave and waveform in *B* demonstrate overdamping; those in *C* represent underdamping. (From Veremakis C, Halloran TH: The technique of monitoring arterial blood pressure. J Crit Illness 4[10]:82, 1989.)

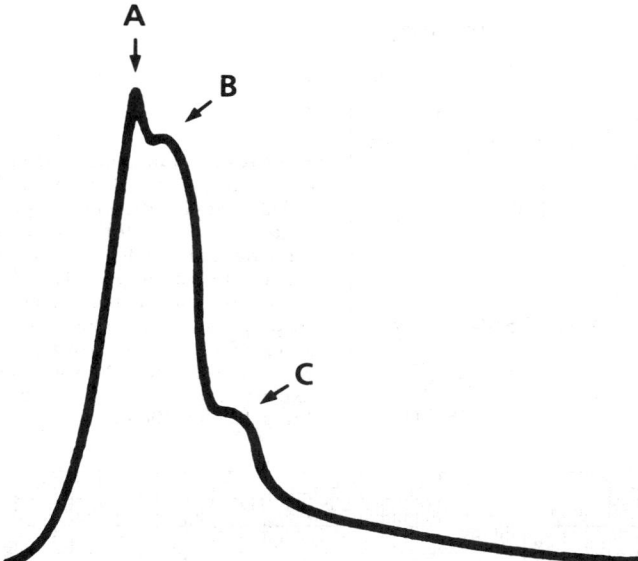

Figure 20–5. A series of electronically interpreted signals creates the visual configuration of the arterial pressure waveform. Contraction of the left ventricle and acceleration of blood flow are demonstrated by the inotropic spike (A). The shoulder of the wave represents volume displacement (B), and the declining slope illustrates peripheral circulatory tone. The dicrotic notch reflects aortic closure; thus it is rarely seen with peripheral monitoring. A secondary hump on the down-slope (C) occurs as a time-delayed echo pattern or a reflection of the volume displacement wave. (From Veremakis C, Halloran TH: The technique of monitoring arterial blood pressure. J Crit Illness 4[10]:82, 1989.)

marked discrepancies between the two peaks represent technical artifacts resulting from system hyper-resonance.

As volume displacement declines, run-off into the periphery reduces aortic root pressure. The rate of run-off determines the downward slope of the waveform and reflects peripheral circulatory tone. Undulations in this phase are the result of changes in impedance as the pressure pulse moves distally.[22] The dicrotic notch present in centrally measured pressures is rarely demonstrated in the peripheral arterial waveform. Instead, a time-delayed reflection of the volume displacement wave creates a secondary hump that varies in position along the down-slope relative to cardiac output and peripheral vascular tone.[23]

Site. The site of arterial cannulation and pressure measurement affects the configuration of the arterial waveform. Aortic pressure perfuses the major organs through short, large-diameter arteries.[24] Cannulation of these vessels would reveal true central pressure but usually is not feasible. Tracings obtained from more accessible sites such as the radial, brachial, femoral, and dorsalis pedis arteries are assumed to reflect accurately central arterial pressures. Such assumptions may be incorrect.

For example, tracings obtained from the axillary artery closely resemble aortic waveforms[25] (Fig. 20–6). However, radial arterial pressures are generally 10 to 15% higher than axillary pressures[23] and may exceed femoral arterial recordings, although comparative studies are lacking. Dorsalis pedis pressures may be 20 mm Hg higher than radial pressures,[26] significantly exceeding central pressures. Therefore, interpretation of arterial pressure waveforms may require consideration of the site from which the data arise.

The pulse wave encounters increasing impedance as it travels distally through progressively narrower vessels.[10] Increasing impedance acts to increase pressure wave ampli-

tude. Consequently, systolic pressure is augmented and diastolic pressure decreased as the cannulation site moves peripherally.[10] The perceived rise in systolic pressure primarily reflects an increase in the inotropic phase of the waveform, exaggerating the discrepancy between the systolic spike and the volume displacement wave. Despite the change in waveform configuration, the area under the arterial waveform is not significantly altered. Monitoring systems derive mean arterial pressure by integrating the area under the waveform. Hence, peripheral mean arterial pressures are similar to those in the central circulation and may be used in determining therapy.

Common Variations in Arterial Waveforms. In addition to overdamping, systolic overshoot is one of the most common artifacts of arterial waveforms seen in clinical practice. Peripheral arterial measurements commonly display a systolic spike 10 to 15 mm Hg higher than the volume displacement wave and central pressure. However, overshoot of 20 to 40 mm Hg is often noted in patients during the first 48 hours after cardiac and major vascular surgery. This phenomenon is similar to that seen in the noncompliant vascular tree of patients with generalized atherosclerosis.[23] Cuff systolic pressures frequently correspond to the peak of the volume displacement wave and are identical with cuff pressures obtained before surgery. Systolic overshoot also occurs in patients with high inotropic states and at heart rates greater than 120 beats/min. In this setting, the summation of the high-frequency components of the pressure signal with the resonant frequency of the monitoring system and/or the vascular tree may be responsible.

The arterial waveform in low-cardiac-output states associated with hypovolemia, vasoconstriction, and good contractility may demonstrate a marked divergence of the inotropic spike and the volume displacement wave (Fig. 20–7). Augmentation of the inotropic phase, possibly affected by altered vascular resonance, combined with diminution of volume displacement resulting from poor stroke volume may contribute to the waveform distortion. Systolic digital read-outs may indicate hypertension. Misinterpretation of this waveform may lead to inappropriate and potentially dangerous therapy.

Augmented inotropic spikes may also develop after the administration of pharmacologic agents. Vasoconstrictors may increase pressure wave reflection by 100%, dramatically increasing waveform amplitude and thereby systolic peak while diminishing downstream flow.[23] In contrast, vasodilating agents abolish reflections, decreasing pressure and enhancing flow.[23] Waveforms resulting from these alterations in peripheral vascular tone may not be reflective of central physiology or pressures.

It is important to realize that in the presence of systolic overshoot, mean arterial pressure remains accurate. Inotropic spikes contribute little to the area under the arterial waveform, regardless of their height. Therefore, in these situations, surveillance, monitor alarms, and parameters for therapeutic intervention should be predicated on mean arterial pressure rather than on digital systolic pressure.[14]

Reversal of the usual relationships between peripheral and central arterial pressures has been reported immediately after cardiopulmonary bypass.[24, 27, 28] Systolic pressures 10 to 30 mm Hg below central aortic pressures lasting up to 60 minutes after bypass have been noted.[27] Alterations in forearm vascular resistance[27] and vasoconstriction-induced waveform damping[28] are purported mechanisms. Hence, vasopressor therapy may not be necessary in this setting as central pressures may be adequate.

Changes in intrapleural pressures may affect arterial pressure tracings and provide diagnostic clues for management of the patient. In normal respiration, arterial pressure drops

Blood Pressure

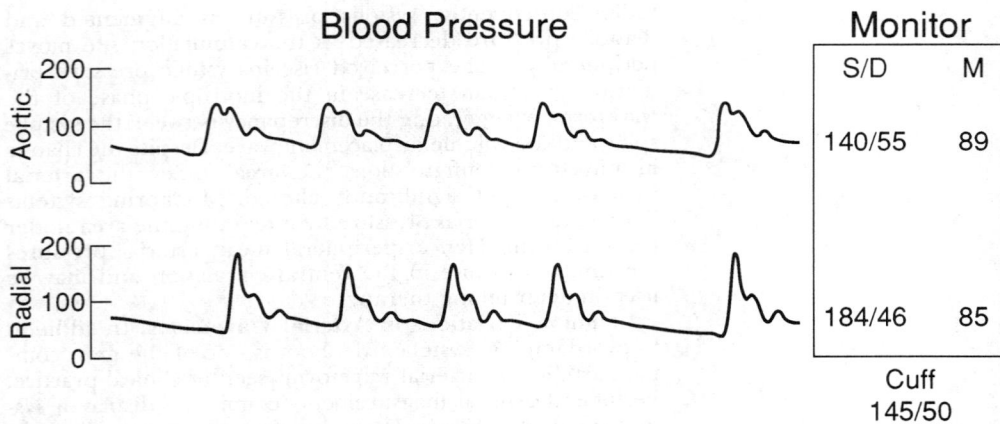

Monitor

	S/D	M
Aortic	140/55	89
Radial	184/46	85

Cuff
145/50

Figure 20–6. Simultaneous tracings from axillary arterial (aortic) and radial arterial catheters. Both catheters and monitoring systems are identical. The tracing is slightly underdamped. On the right are shown the monitor readings and cuff blood pressures. (From Bryan-Brown CW, Kwun KB, Lumb PD, et al: The axillary artery catheter. Heart Lung 12:492, 1983.)

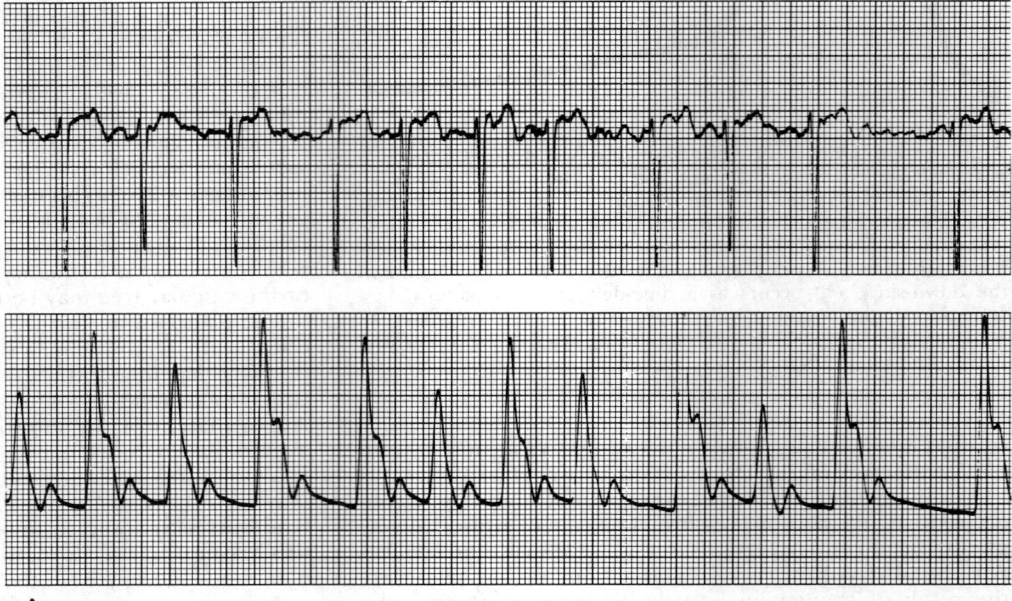

A

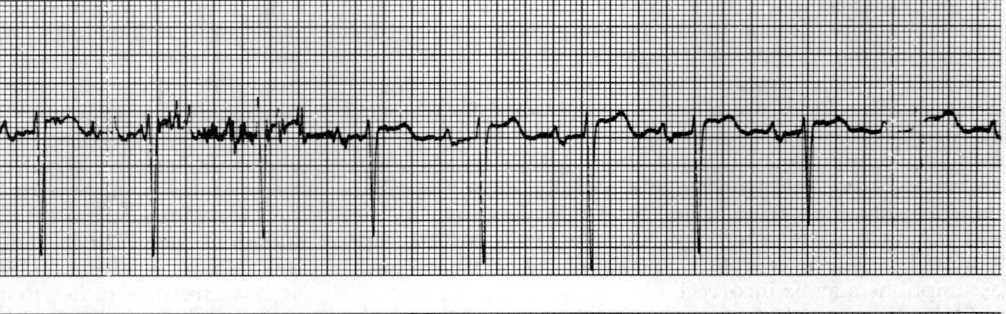

Figure 20–7. Arterial pressure tracing from a patient with hypovolemia, low cardiac output, and vasoconstriction. Blood pressure by digital read-out is 210/49, mean arterial pressure 79 mm Hg (A). Systolic pressure at the shoulder of the waveform averages approximately 148 mm Hg. After the addition of volume and restoration of normal sinus rhythm (B), cardiac output is improved, and the waveform has much less systolic overshoot. The volume displacement wave is unchanged. Arterial pressure now reads 144/45, mean arterial pressure 71 mm Hg.

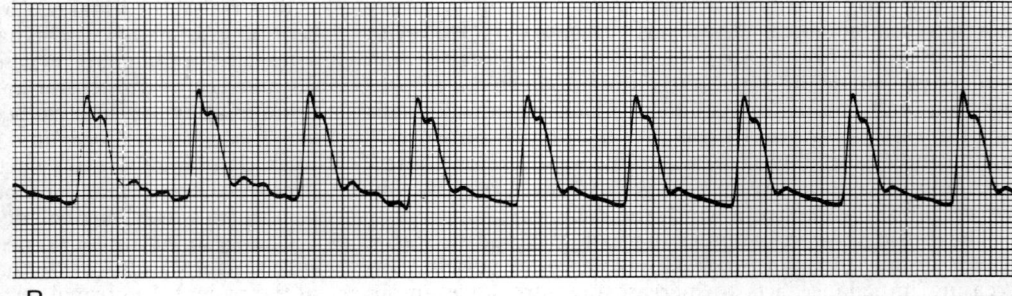

B

slightly during inspiration and rises with expiration because of alterations in left ventricular afterload and ventricular interdependence.[29-31] Increased respiratory efforts exaggerate these mechanisms and are responsible for the pulsus paradoxus seen in cardiac tamponade and severe asthma.[29] Positive pressure ventilation may increase pulse pressure, particularly in patients with poor left ventricular function by reducing left ventricular afterload.[32] However, blood pressure drops transiently in hypovolemic patients placed on positive pressure ventilation. Observation of changes in arterial waveforms with the respiratory cycle may provide important clues to the ongoing cardiopulmonary pathophysiology in critically ill patients.

CONCLUSION

The measurement of arterial blood pressure is a vital part of hemodynamic assessment and therapeutic decisions. Assumptions about perfusion of major organs and myocardial workload are based on data from arterial blood pressure measurements. The clinician must realize, however, that arterial pressure measurements may not reflect true pressures in the aorta or major organs and that tissue perfusion may not be adequate despite seemingly adequate pressures. Lack of correlation between modalities exists even in stable patients, and changing physiologic states significantly affect information generated from a single system at any given moment. Correct interpretation and appropriate therapy require understanding the limitations of each method.

References

1. Finnie KJC, Watts, DG, Armstrong PW: Biases in the measurement of arterial pressure. Crit Care Med 12:965, 1984.
2. Carroll GC: Blood pressure monitoring. Crit Care Clin 4:411, 1988.
3. Cohn JN: Blood pressure measurement in shock. JAMA 199:118, 1967.
4. Davis RF: Clinical comparison of automated auscultatory and oscillometric and catheter-transducer measurements of arterial pressure. J Clin Monit 1:114, 1985.
5. Paulus DA: Noninvasive blood pressure measurement. Med Instrum 15:91, 1981.
6. Gravenstein JS, Paulus, DA: Clinical Monitoring Practice. 2nd ed. Philadelphia, JB Lippincott, 1987.
7. Hutton P, Dye J, Prys-Roberts C: An assessment of the Dinamap 845. Anaesthesia 39:261, 1984.
8. Nystrom E, Reid KH, Bennett R, et al: A comparison of two automated indirect arterial blood pressure meters: With recordings from a radial arterial catheter in anesthetized surgical patients. Anesthesiology 62:526, 1985.
9. Bruner JMR, Krenis LJ, Kunsman JM, et al: Comparison of direct and indirect methods of measuring arterial blood pressure. Part III. Med Instrum 14:182, 1981.
10. Bruner JRM, Krenis LJ, Kunsman JM, et al: Comparison of direct and indirect methods of measuring arterial blood pressure. Med Instrum 15:11, 1981.
11. Johnson CJH, Kerr JH: Automatic blood pressure monitors. A clinical evaluation of five models in adults. Anaesthesia 40:471, 1985.
12. Harrington DP: Disparities between direct and indirect arterial systolic blood-pressure measurements. Cardiovasc Pulmonary Technol 6:4, 1978.
13. Gardner RM: Direct blood pressure measurement—Dynamic response requirements. Anesthesiology 54:227, 1981.
14. Veremakis C, Halloran TH: The technique of monitoring arterial blood pressure. J Crit Illness 4(10):82, 1989.
15. Shapiro GG, Krovetz LJ: Damped and undamped frequency responses of underdamped cathether manometer systems. Am Heart J 80:226, 1970.
16. Gibbs NC, Gardner RM: Dynamics of invasive pressure monitoring systems: Clinical and laboratory evaluation. Heart Lung 17:43, 1988.
17. Boutros A, Albert S: Effect of dynamic response of transducer-tubing system on accuracy of direct blood pressure measurement in patients. Crit Care Med 11:124, 1983.
18. Rothe CF, Kim KC: Measuring systolic arterial blood pressure. Possible errors from extension tubes of disposable transducer domes. Crit Care Med 8:683, 1980.
19. Shinozaki T, Deane RS, Mazuzan JE: The dynamic responses of liquid-filled catheter systems for direct measurements of blood pressure. Anesthesiology 53:498, 1980.
20. Gardner RM, Chapman RH: Trouble-shooting pressure monitoring sys-
tems: When do the numbers lie? In: Fallat RJ, Luce JM (eds): Clinics in Critical Care Medicine, Cardiopulmonary Critical Care Management. New York, Churchill Livingstone, p 145, 1988.
21. Gardner RM, Hollingsworth KW: Optimizing the electrocardiogram and pressure monitoring. Crit Care Med 14:651, 1986.
22. Bruner JMR: Handbook of Blood Pressure Monitoring. Littleton, MA, PSG Publishing, 1978.
23. O'Rourke MF, Yaginuma T: Wave reflections and the arterial pulse. Arch Intern Med 144:366, 1984.
24. Bazaral MG, Nacht A, Petre J, et al: Radial artery pressures compared with subclavian artery pressure during coronary artery surgery. Cleve Clin J Med 55:448, 1988.
25. Bryan-Brown CW, Kwun KB, Lumb PD, et al: The axillary artery catheter. Heart Lung 12:492, 1983.
26. Youngberg JA, Miller ED: Evaluation of percutaneous cannulations of the dorsalis pedis artery. Anesthesiology 44:80, 1976.
27. Stern DH, Gerson JI, Allen FC, et al: Can we trust the direct radial artery pressure immediately following cardiopulmonary bypass? Anesthesiology 62:557, 1985.
28. Gallagher JD, Moore RA, McNicholas KW, et al: Comparison of radial and femoral arterial blood pressures in children after cardiopulmonary bypass. J Clin Monit 1:168, 1985.
29. McGregor M: Pulsus paradoxus. N Engl J Med 301:480, 1979.
30. Yeston NS, Niehoff JM: Important procedures in the intensive care unit. In: Civetta JM, Taylor RW, Kirby RR (eds): Critical Care. Philadelphia, JB Lippincott, p 243, 1988.
31. Ellis DM: Interpretation of beat-to-beat blood pressure values in the presence of ventilatory changes. J Clin Monit 1:65, 1985.
32. Wise R: Effect of alterations of pleural pressure on cardiac output. South Med J 78:423, 1985.

CHAPTER 21

Imaging the Chest

Kathleen A. McCarroll

Patients in an intensive care unit (ICU) require the full range of modern medical technology for appropriate diagnosis and therapy. Unfortunately, only a fraction of the sophisticated modalities available in the hospital can come to the bedside. This seriously limits the input that imaging specialists can have on these patients' complicated problems. The irony is that the patients most in need of sophisticated technology are those for whom only the basic imaging modalities are consistently available.

The anteroposterior (AP) chest radiograph obtained at the bedside is the mainstay of imaging in the ICU. Although the radiograph can be obtained quickly with portable units, is inexpensive, and is (questionably) easy to perform, accurate interpretation is infinitely more difficult than for many of the technically more sophisticated studies performed at substantially greater cost. Some observers have taken the position that chest radiographs obtained in the ICU should be used for evaluating catheter locations only. Others, most notably Milne and colleagues,[1-6] developed a sophisticated approach to the interpretation of the ICU chest radiograph and reported success in distinguishing cardiogenic, noncardiogenic, and capillary permeability edema.[7] For most radiologists and intensivists, working with real-world limitations, the true value of the ICU chest radiograph lies somewhere between these extremes. This chapter reviews portable chest radiography, as well as other commonly employed imaging techniques utilized for patients in the ICU. Examples of abnormalities that are commonly encountered, together with guidelines for their interpretation, are given.

IMAGING SYSTEMS

At major teaching hospitals, bedside studies have constituted more than half of all inpatient chest x-ray films for nearly the past decade, with the volume of these examinations increasing by 7 to 15% yearly.[8] The design of modern ICUs has been directed to facilitate this trend. Ideally, an ICU could be built with overhead tracks and a movable x-ray tube, which can travel to each patient's bed, as necessary. Significant progress has been made in the development of digital radiographic systems. Current limitations include cost, prohibitive archival requirements, and slow transmission speed.[9] Currently, most ICUs use mobile x-ray machines and standard 14 × 17 inch acetate films. The transmission of reports of the examinations to the ICU via hospital computer lines is, however, an increasingly attainable goal, even in hospitals of modest means.

PORTABLE CHEST RADIOGRAPHY

Whether the hardware is sophisticated or simple, certain principles apply to ICU imaging. First, the quality of the interpretation of the study is always linked to the quality of the film. Several technical factors contribute substantially to the diagnostic quality of the study. An optimally exposed chest radiograph obtained with a portable unit allows evaluation of the lung parenchyma without use of a "hot light" but is not sufficiently underexposed (light) to obscure visualization of catheter tips in the heart and the great vessels. The details of techniques that produce the best possible film should be accessible to all of the radiologic technicians so that consistency is achieved in both film density and contrast. One effective method of achieving technically consistent films is to place a sticker, with the technique recorded on it, on each patient's bed. The distance of the tube from the patient should be as great as practicable. More important, this distance should be the same from study to study. If possible, the patient's position (upright, semiupright, or supine) should be the same from study to study and must be clearly marked on the radiograph. The best and most experienced technicians and the best mobile equipment should be sought for ICU studies.

The value of daily chest radiographs in the ICU has been studied extensively, but it is common sense that daily radiographs are desirable in critically ill patients who undergo frequent changes in therapy (catheters, ventilatory support, and medications). As a patient's condition stabilizes and the number of manipulations decreases, the number of films necessary should also decrease. In one analysis of ICU chest x-ray studies, a new finding or a significant change was identified on 65% of films.[10] These included catheter and tube position changes. Other radiographic changes have been documented in 47% of patients who were otherwise clinically stable.[11] Bekemeyer and colleagues identified findings that warranted alterations in management of patients on 23.7% of routine daily films.[12]

There is no single, correct rule regarding the frequency of filming, but generally, the number of studies necessary increases as more diagnostic and therapeutic manipulations are performed in a given patient. In one report, one half of ICU patients had more than 0.7 chest radiographs per day.[10] During daily review with the ICU staff, the ICU radiologist can often assist the intensivist to determine the frequency of studies appropriate for assessing the problem in question so that standing orders for daily bedside radiography are not necessary. The overall severity of illness in different ICUs varies greatly, and this should be reflected in film usage.

Systems that are relatively easy to institute can improve not only patient care but also other important derivatives, such as education and interdepartmental cooperation. A designated alternator in the ICU or radiology department is, ideally, the fixed location of the ICU patients' films. Films should be maintained in this area. If possible, each patient needs to be allotted at least two panels (eight 14 × 17 inch spaces) on which sequential films can be easily viewed for comparison. The entire film jacket must also be readily accessible.

RADIOLOGY CONFERENCES

At least daily, the intensivists and a designated radiologist should meet and discuss the clinical and roentgenographic findings for each case. At this time, plans for additional studies can be discussed and their risks, costs, and benefits can be evaluated. This procedure should eliminate the mistake of subjecting critically ill patients and support staff to studies that are dangerous, inappropriate, or of little benefit. Transportation of critically ill patients is a well-known cause of complications.[13]

ICU radiology conferences are an efficient forum for evaluation of ICU patients' multiple indwelling catheters. The various complications of tube placement have been described by several authors.[14-26] In addition to assessment of each chest radiograph for potential catheter problems, ICU radiology rounds are an excellent opportunity for discussion of new or different devices in use in the ICU. Any unusual line projected over the patient must be identified, and occasionally this is accomplished only by a trip to the bedside (Fig. 21–1). It is of utmost importance that every catheter approved for use in the hospital be evaluated for the presence and adequacy of its radiopaque marker. A poorly radiopaque catheter, if lost in the patient, may be impossible to retrieve.

VERIFYING CATHETER POSITION

Evaluation of the placement of all the tubes and catheters used in the ICU and their potential complications can be a formidable task. In the obtunded or comatose mechanically ventilated ICU patient, the potential for life-threatening complications from malpositioned tubes is magnified. A thorough knowledge of the complications and procedures unique to each specific device is essential.[16]

Central Venous Catheters

The most common catheter used in many ICUs is the triple-lumen central venous catheter. The insertion sites are usually radiographically identifiable as subclavian (horizontal and below the clavicle), internal jugular (medial and relatively vertical in the neck), and external jugular (obliquely oriented in the neck) (Fig. 21–2). During examination of the films, the continuity of the central venous catheter should be ascertained from its origin, through the expected course, to its desired termination, which is usually to the right of, and parallel to, the spine in the area of the superior vena cava. It is a good practice for the individual performing the catheter check to place the index finger on the film at the catheter origin and trace it manually to its tip. The eye has fooled the mind many times while checking catheter position and the finger trace eliminates most oversights.

Misplaced catheters tend to occur (1) in the neck, when they turn into the jugular vein instead of the vena cava (Fig. 21–3A); (2) in the subclavian vein, where they fold back on themselves; (3) in the superior vena cava, where they can

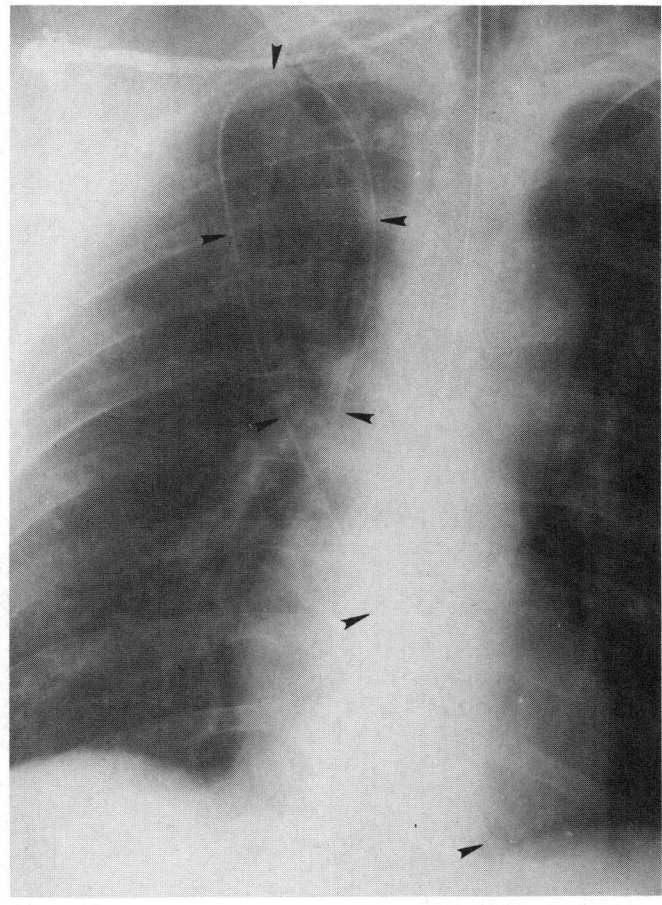

Figure 21–1. An unusual catheter projects over the right chest and left upper abdomen (*arrowheads*). One end appears to lie in the superior vena cava. Examination of the patient and his medical history indicated prior placement of a portacaval shunt.

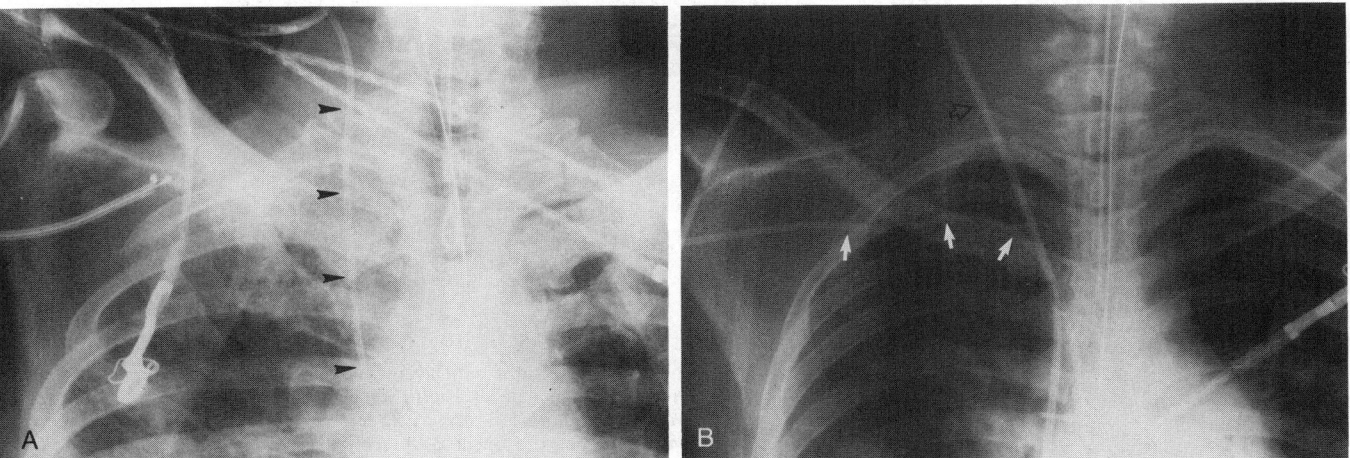

Figure 21–2. *A.* Internal jugular central venous catheter. This catheter (*arrowheads*) parallels the cervical spine and lies in a vertical orientation. *B.* External jugular and subclavian catheters. The external jugular catheter can be identified by its oblique orientation in the neck (*open arrows*); the subclavian route is identified by a horizontal orientation inferior to the clavicle (*white arrows*).

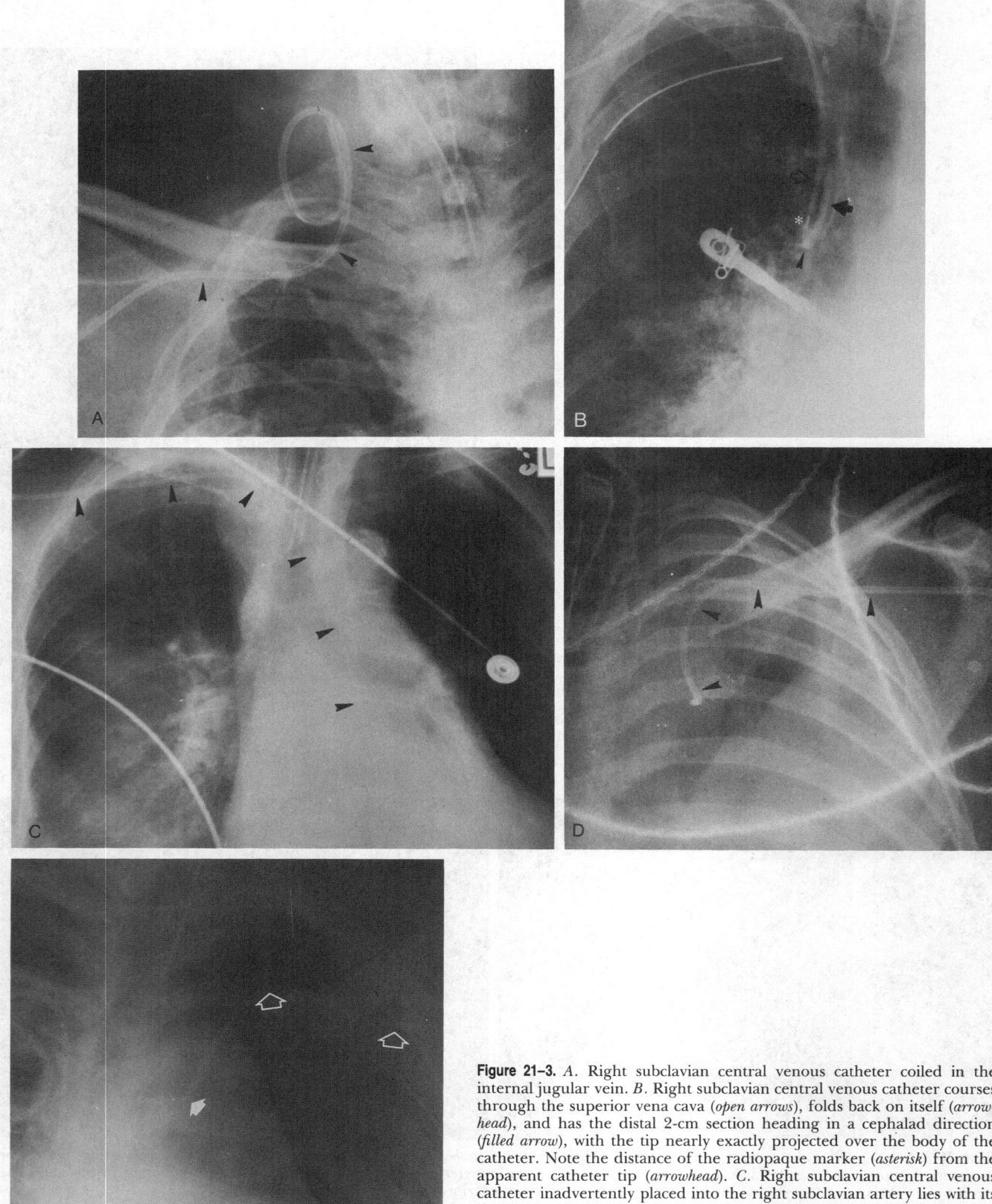

Figure 21–3. *A.* Right subclavian central venous catheter coiled in the internal jugular vein. *B.* Right subclavian central venous catheter courses through the superior vena cava (*open arrows*), folds back on itself (*arrowhead*), and has the distal 2-cm section heading in a cephalad direction (*filled arrow*), with the tip nearly exactly projected over the body of the catheter. Note the distance of the radiopaque marker (*asterisk*) from the apparent catheter tip (*arrowhead*). *C.* Right subclavian central venous catheter inadvertently placed into the right subclavian artery lies with its tip in the descending thoracic arota (*arrowheads*). *D.* Left subclavian central venous catheter lies with its tip in an extravascular location (*arrowheads*). *E.* Left subclavian central venous catheter (*open arrows*) lies with its tip (*arrow*) in an uncertain location.

cause pressure on the vessel wall or fold back on themselves (see Fig. 21–3*B*); (4) in the carotid, subclavian, or other artery (see Fig. 21–3*C*); or worse, (5) when they are not in an intravascular location at all (see Fig. 21–3*D*). Often, the exact location of the catheter tip is not known (see Fig. 21–3*E*). Arterial puncture is reported to occur in 3% of subclavian insertions and in 3 to 10% of attempted jugular insertions.[27] Sznajder and associates reported misplaced lines in 4% of subclavian or jugular placements, 30% of external jugular insertions, and 47% of attempted basilic placements.[27] The appearance of an unusual mass on the chest radiograph, especially if it is in the mediastinum or lung apex, should be considered to be a possible hematoma resulting from catheter placement (even if the catheter appears to be in an appropriate location). This suspicion can often be confirmed by comparison of the current study with previous films obtained before catheter insertion (Figs. 21–4 to 21–6).

Pulmonary Arterial Catheters

Pulmonary arterial catheters are more difficult to place properly, but far fewer placement problems are identified on films compared with central venous catheters. Overall, however, arterial and pulmonary arterial catheters are associated with more frequent complications than are central venous catheters.[26] This reflects that incorrect positioning provides instantaneous hemodynamic feedback, allowing for immediate correction. Correct identification of pulmonary arterial catheter tip location requires an understanding of heart and great vessel anatomy in the coronal plane (chest radiography, magnetic resonance imaging) and in cross-section (computed tomography [CT], magnetic resonance imaging).

The catheter may be inserted via the superior or inferior vena cava. Its entry into the right atrium and its subsequent course through the right ventricle, the pulmonary outflow

track, and the main pulmonary artery should be characterized by smooth, gentle curves in expected locations (Fig. 21–7). When wedge readings are not being obtained, the pulmonary arterial catheter tip should lie in a relatively proximal pulmonary arterial location.

Aortic Catheters

Intra-aortic counterpulsation balloon catheters should be optimally placed with the balloon just distal to the origin of the left subclavian artery, below the apex of aortic arch. Abnormally high placement can occlude the arch vessels, causing cerebrovascular compromise. The tip of the catheter can move up to 5 cm with changes in patient position, making frequent monitoring mandatory. As with any vascular catheter, a change in mediastinal contours should raise the suspicion of perforation.[28]

Endotracheal and Tracheostomy Tubes

Endotracheal tubes should be evaluated for proximity to the carina, angulation, and cuff inflation. Conrardy and colleagues[29] provided a detailed discussion of this subject, emphasizing that the tube diameter should be one half to two thirds of the tracheal lumen to provide adequate flow without producing excessive resistance and without causing pressure necrosis of the tracheal wall (Fig. 21–8). The latter condition also occurs with cuff overinflation. The optimal diameter of the inflated cuff should not be significantly greater than that of the tracheal lumen (Fig. 21–9). The tube tip should reside approximately 4 to 5 cm above the carina, unless the patient's head was abnormally flexed or extended at the time the film was obtained. An abnormally high location of the endotracheal tube not only predisposes to unintentional extubation, but also increases the chance of pressure necrosis of the vocal cords resulting from cuff inflation. An abnormally low endotracheal tube is a well-

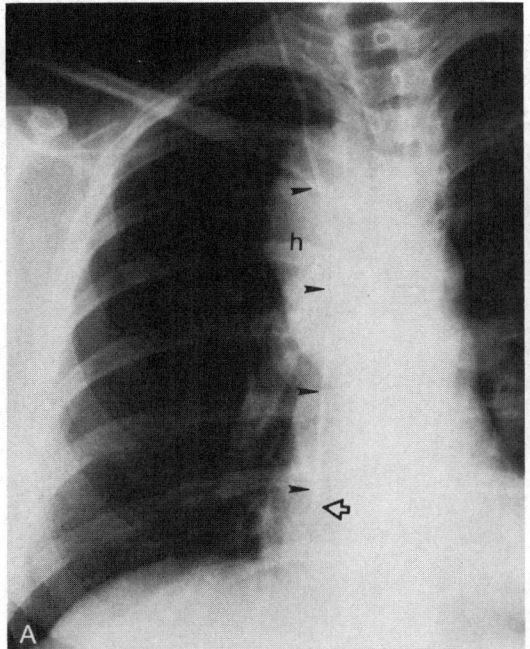
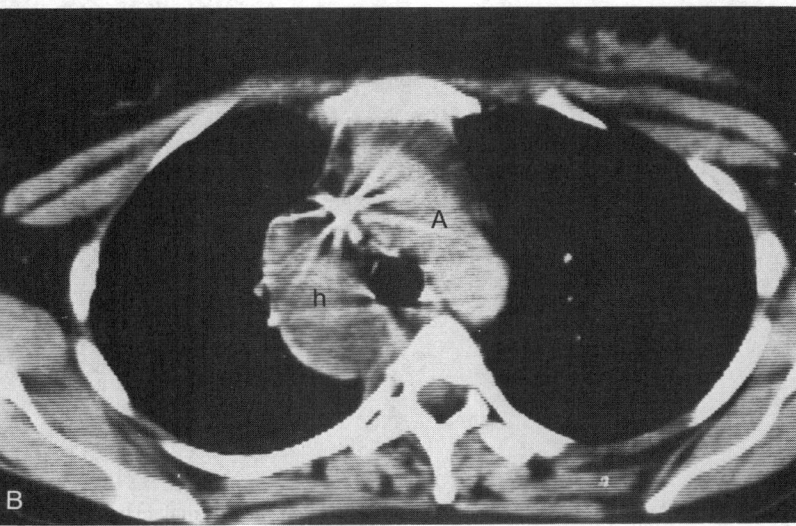

Figure 21–4. *A.* Internal jugular central venous catheter (*arrowheads*) lies with its tip (*open arrow*) in the area of the right atrium. Twenty-four hours after insertion, a right mediastinal mass (h) appeared, compatible with a line insertion hematoma. *B.* Computed tomographic scan of the thorax reveals the mediastinal mass to represent a low-density hematoma (h) seen at the level of the aortic arch (A). The star artifact is secondary to a subsequently placed Swan-Ganz catheter.

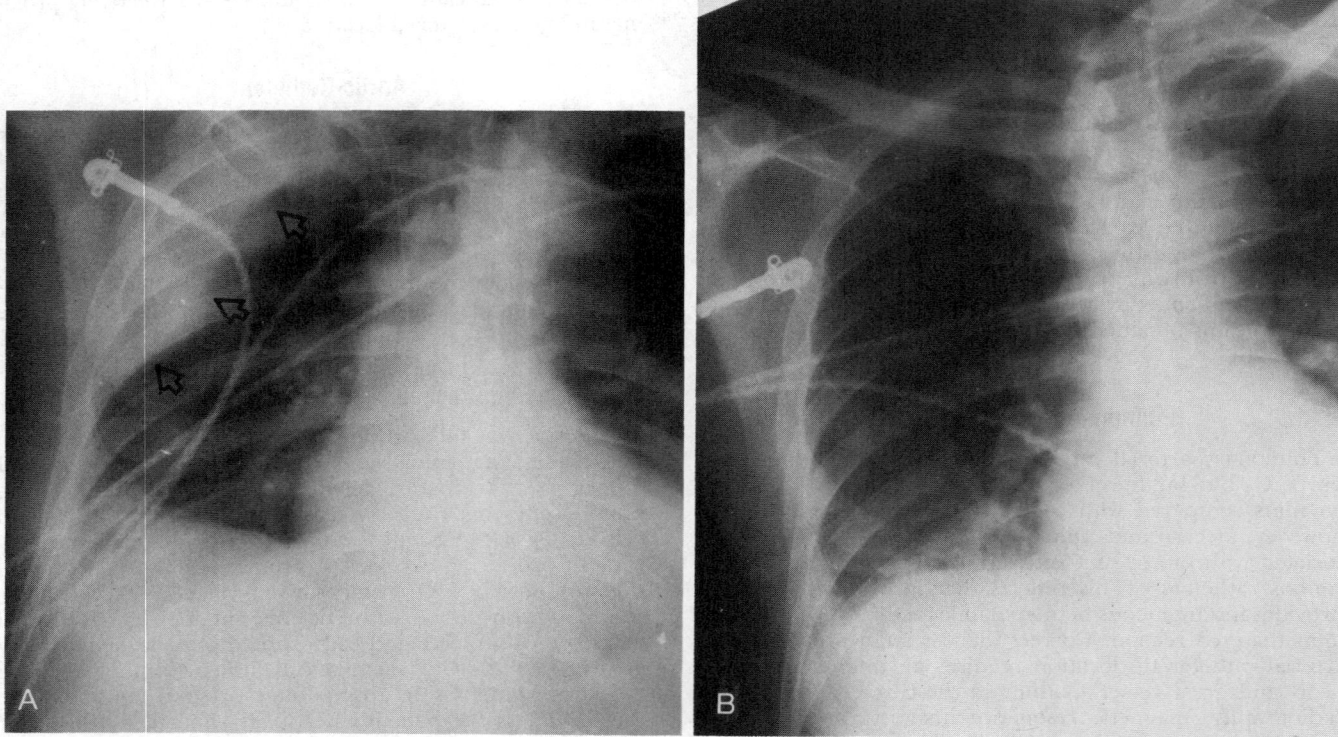

Figure 21–5. Extrapleural hematoma after placement of a right central venous catheter. *A.* A large pleura-based hematoma (*open arrows*) appeared. *B.* The film obtained immediately after line placement (24 hours earlier) reveals no pre-existing abnormality.

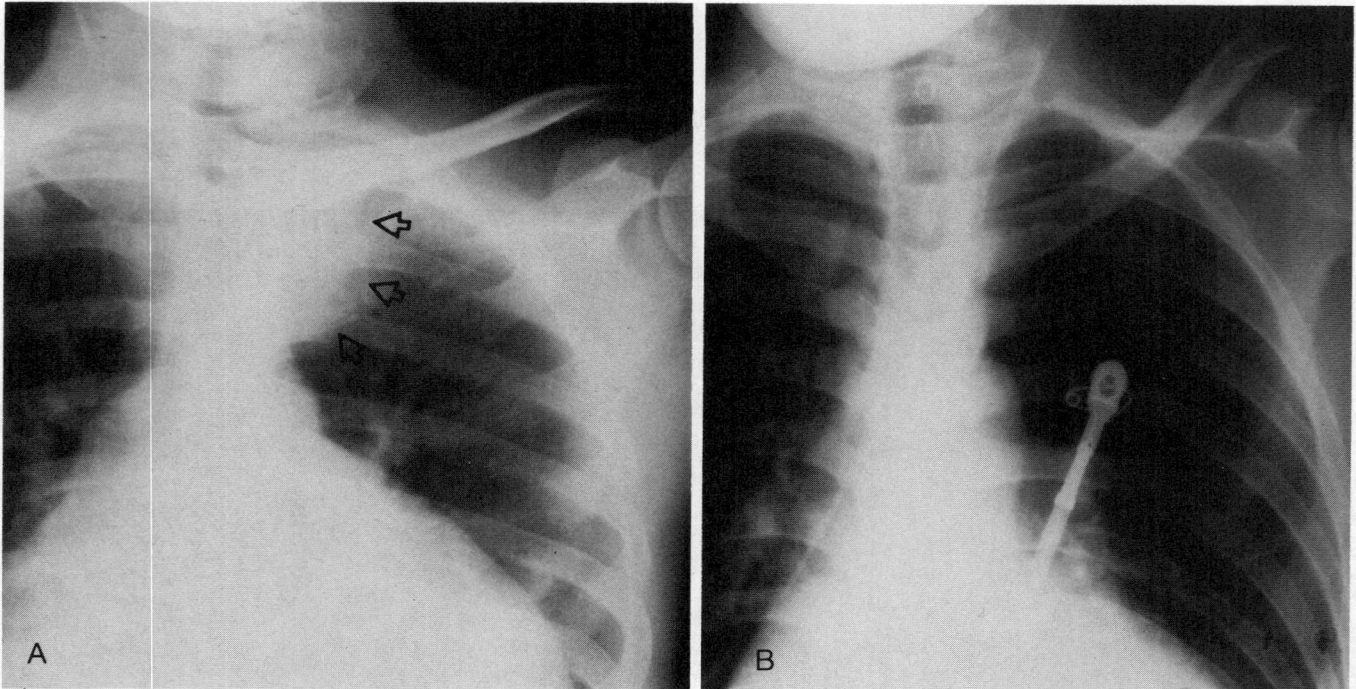

Figure 21–6. *A.* Mediastinal hematoma. A left superior mediastinal mass (*open arrows*) was believed to represent a line hematoma after a difficult placement of a central venous catheter. *B.* The immediately previous film study reveals the mediastinum to be normal.

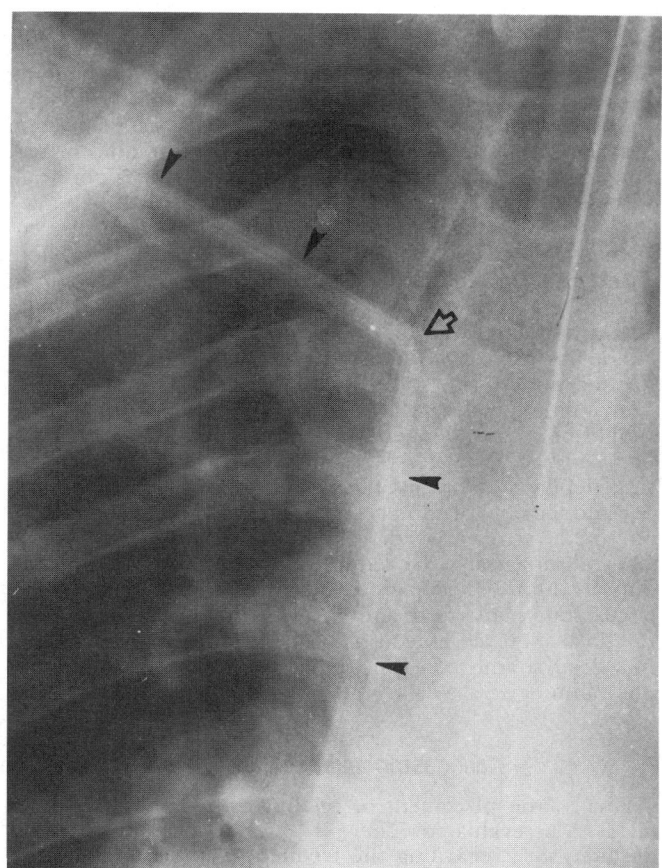

Figure 21-7. Right subclavian Swan-Ganz catheter (*arrowheads*) is kinked at the site where the catheter exits the introducer (*open arrow*).

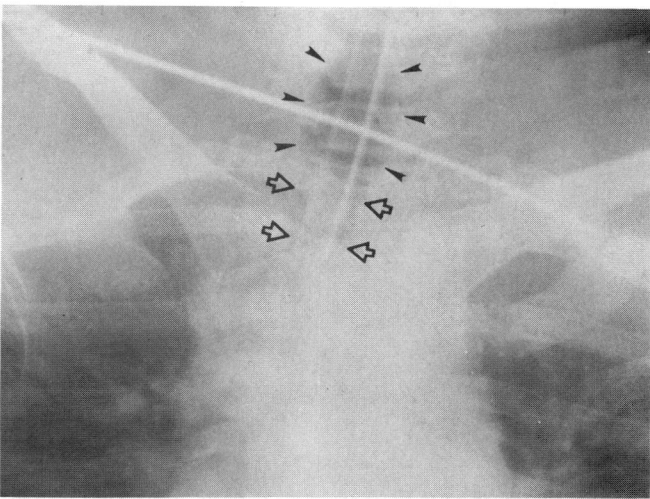

Figure 21-9. Mildly overinflated endotracheal balloon cuff (*arrowheads*) when compared with the diameter of the tracheal lumen (*open arrows*). Note also the appropriate width of the endotracheal tube compared with the luminal diameter.

tubation can closely simulate tracheal intubation and may be indistinguishable radiographically. If secondary signs of esophageal intubation such as gross gastric distention and esophageal air are present, confirmation of endotracheal tube location should be vigorously sought. Occasionally, the endotracheal tube or its cuff projects lateral to, and may deviate, the trachea. If there is any question of its location, radiographic confirmation of the endotracheal tube's position can be performed with an oblique film. In a large series by Smith and coworkers, the trachea and esophagus were superimposed in 96% of patients in AP or left posterior

known cause of atelectasis, usually left sided (Fig. 21-10). Finally, the endotracheal tube should be in the trachea, not in the esophagus.

The trachea and the esophagus overlie each other on the nonrotated frontal chest film. Consequently, esophageal in-

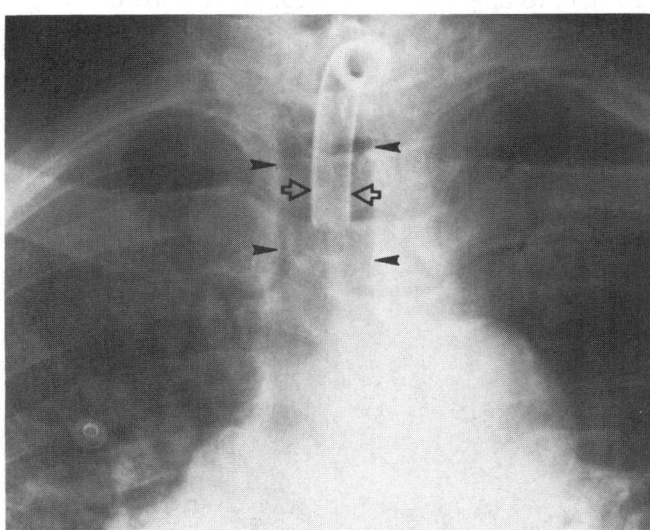

Figure 21-8. Small tracheostomy tube. The tracheostomy tube diameter (*open arrows*) is less than 50% of the tracheal diameter (*arrowheads*).

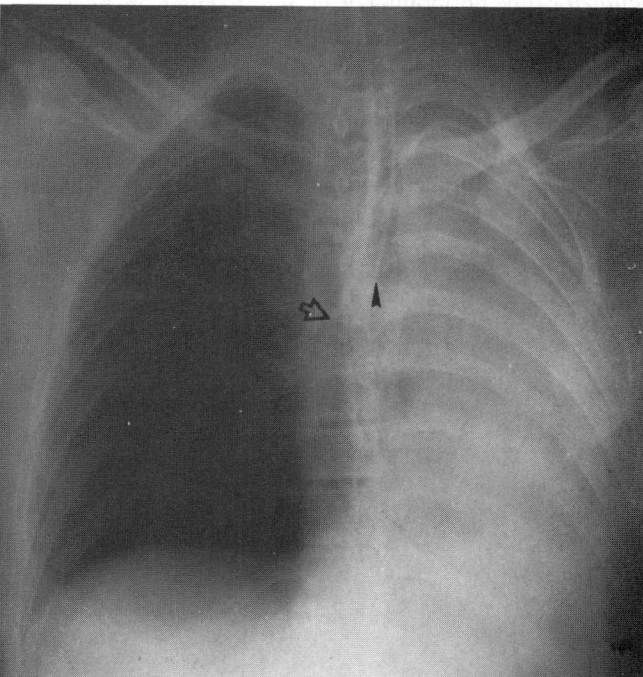

Figure 21-10. The endotracheal tube tip (*open arrow*) lies in the right mainstem bronchus, beyond the carina (*arrowhead*). Note extensive opacification of the left hemithorax, with ipsilateral shift of the heart and mediastinum secondary to complete left lung atelectasis. The endotracheal tube is ventilating the right lung only.

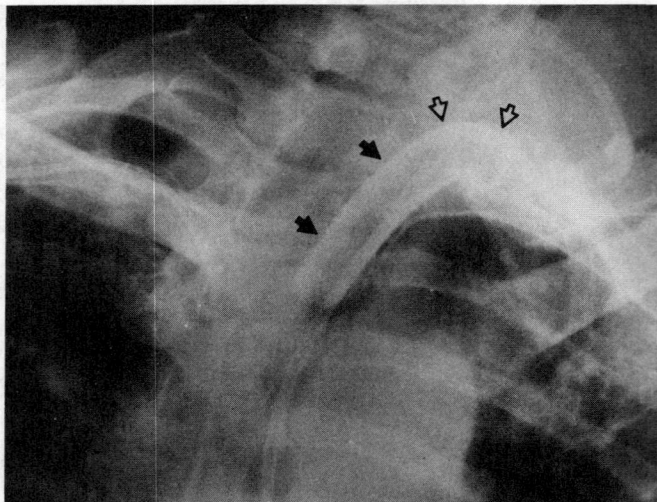

Figure 21–11. Normal tracheostomy tube position. Approximately one third of the tracheostomy tube lies in a horizontal orientation (*open arrows*) and two thirds of the tube lies in a vertical orientation (*filled arrows*).

oblique projections.[14] The 25° right posterior oblique view with rightward mandible position, however, avoided superimposition in 93% and the AP projection with rightward mandible position avoided superimposition in 76%.[14] In some institutions, the slightly oblique film is routinely obtained.

Tracheostomy tubes should also be evaluated for location at regular intervals. The tube should lie with one third of the tube horizontally oriented and two thirds of the tube vertically situated in the trachea (Fig. 21–11). If this ratio is reversed, extubation may be imminent (Fig. 21–12). A frequent observation is the angled tracheostomy tube, in which the tip is touching the tracheal wall. This may be caused by ventilator tube positioning or by an off-center tracheostomy. Persistent angulation of the tube leads to erosion, hemorrhage, or scarring of the tracheal wall.

Thoracostomy Tubes

Thoracostomy tubes are difficult to evaluate accurately with a single AP chest film. Two films that are obtained

from perpendicular directions (e.g., AP and lateral) are necessary for accurate assessment of the location of an object or structure anywhere in the body. Unfortunately, obtaining a lateral view on an ICU patient is an arduous task. Although a thoracostomy tube may lie in the pleural space, its position has a profound impact on its ability to remove fluid or gas. For example, an anteriorly placed chest tube does not drain a posterior fluid collection.

CT has revealed a much higher incidence of intraparenchymal chest tube placement than was previously suspected. A chest tube that has no curvature on the frontal radiograph should be suspected to reside within the major fissure or in an intraparenchymal location (Fig. 21–13). An oblique or lateral film or even CT may therefore be necessary to identify the location of the tube, particularly if the tube is not functioning properly. The anatomy of the pleural spaces should be well understood so that an aberrant location can be identified (Fig. 21–14). Optimal function of the chest tube depends on correct placement (Fig. 21–15). The number and location of thoracostomy tube side holes should also be noted and compared from study to study (Fig. 21–16). Chest drainage may be reduced or absent if a side hole lies outside the thoracic cage or near the skin surface. In this circumstance, the drainage includes air that has been aspirated through the hole at or near the surface. This air leak may lead to the conclusion that there is a disruption of pleural integrity.

Nasogastric and Feeding Tubes

Finally, the placement of feeding and nasogastric tubes needs to be evaluated. There is considerable controversy in the literature regarding the frequency, cause, and severity of complications related to the various types of feeding tubes.[15-22] The most frequent problem is insertion of these tubes into the tracheobronchial tree with possible perforation into the pleural space[16] (Figs. 21–17 and 21–18). Nasogastric tubes frequently coil in the esophagus or the pharynx (Fig. 21–19).

Woodall and associates' series of 17 adult patients in whom feeding tubes had been placed in the lung identified a variety of complications, including pneumothorax, hydropneumothorax, empyema, and pneumonitis.[15] Penetration of the pleural space occurred in patients in whom a small-diameter (2.7-mm) feeding tube was placed, whereas use of a larger

Text continued on page 269

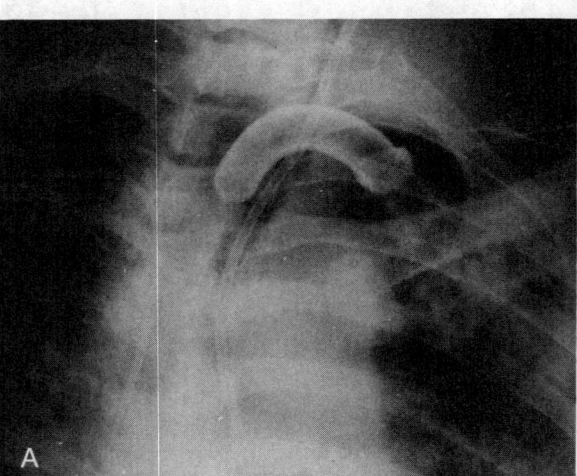

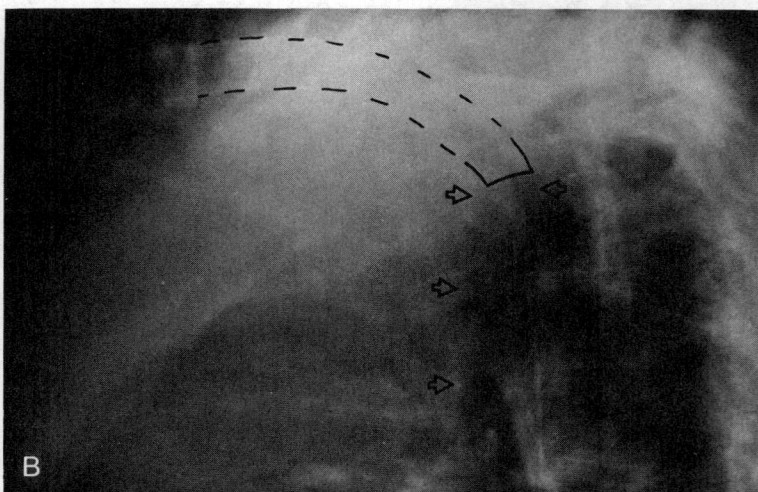

Figure 21–12. Imminent extubation. Posteroanterior (*A*) and lateral (*B*) views of the chest reveal an endotracheal tube that has almost completely exited the tracheal lumen. Note two thirds of the endotracheal tube lies horizontally and one third lies vertically. On the posteroanterior film the vertical portion is presumed to be intratracheal.

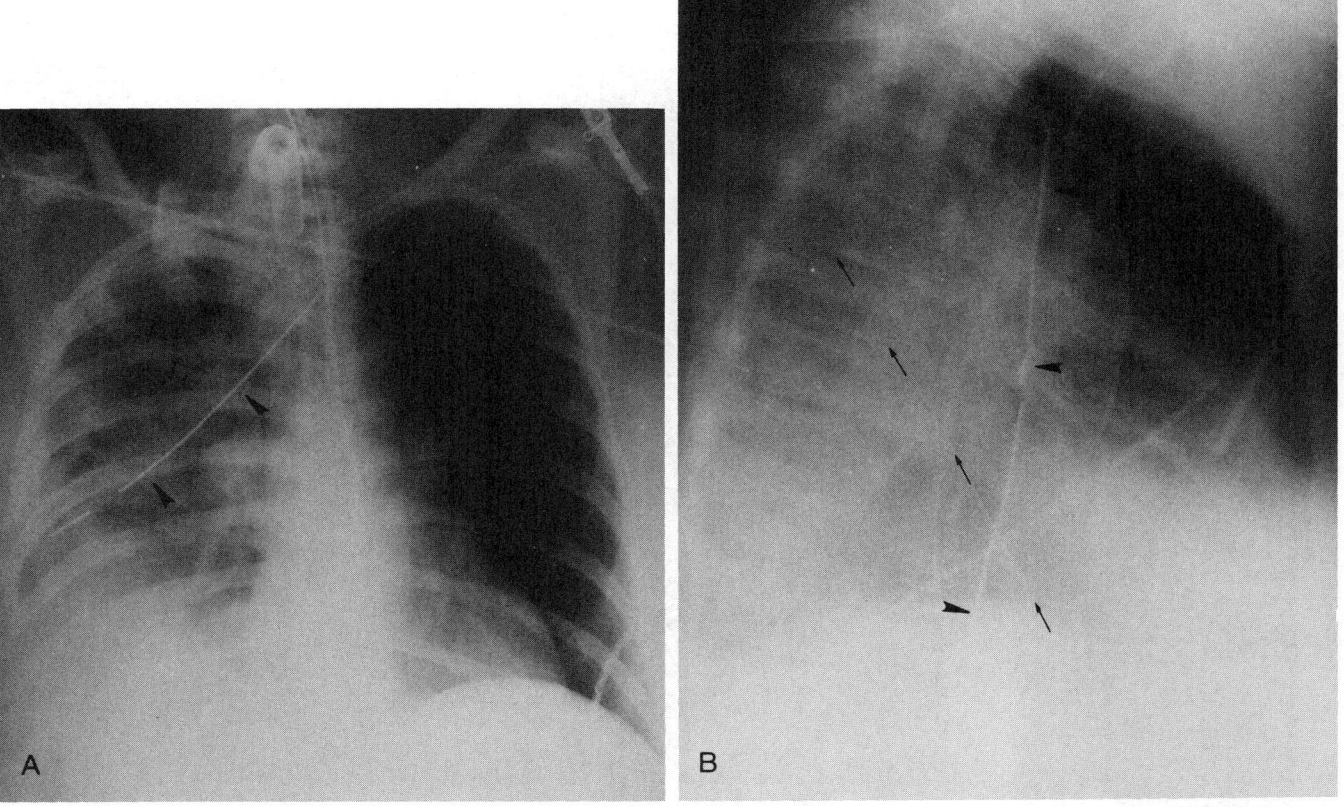

Figure 21–13. Intraparenchymal chest tube. In both posteroanterior (*A*) and lateral (*B*) projections, this chest tube (*arrowheads*) lies in the mid-hemithorax. The expected course of the fissure is shown on the lateral view (*small arrows*).

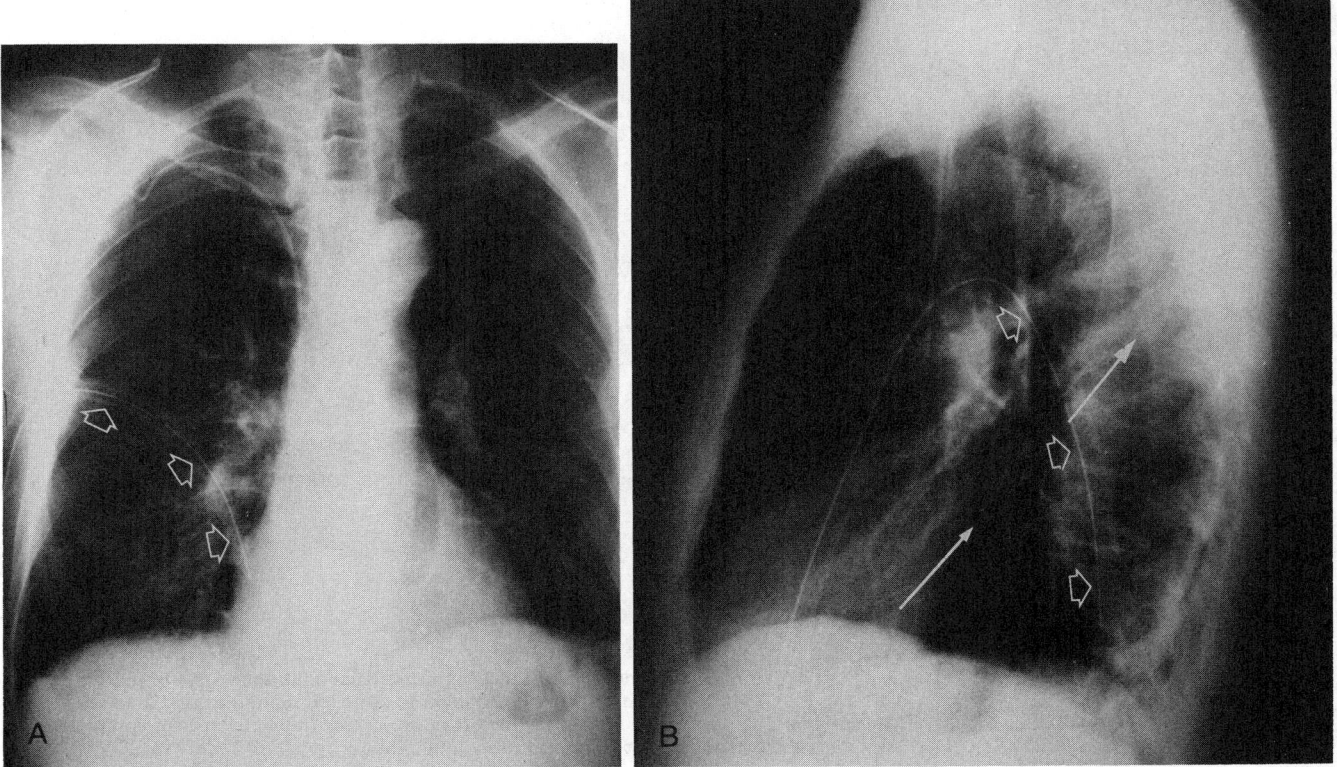

Figure 21–14. *A*. Intraparenchymal chest tube. On the posteroanterior projection the chest tube (*open arrows*) appears to lie in satisfactory position, as did the chest tube in Figure 21–13*A*. *B*. In the lateral view, the chest tube (*open arrows*) follows in an unusual course, nearly perpendicular to the expected course of the major fissure marked (*filled arrows*).

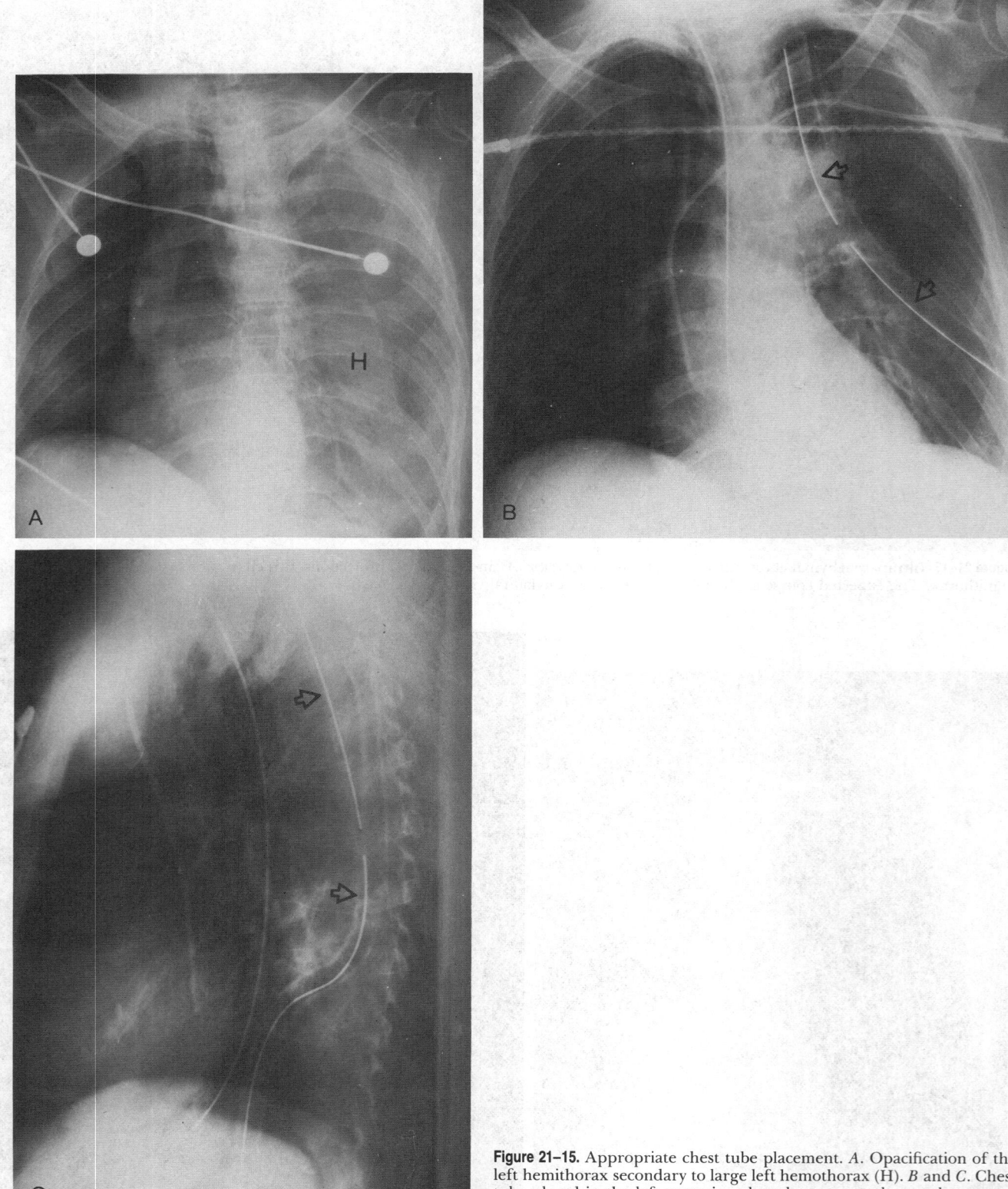

Figure 21–15. Appropriate chest tube placement. *A.* Opacification of the left hemithorax secondary to large left hemothorax (H). *B* and *C.* Chest tube placed in the left posterior pleural space reveals complete evacuation of the posterior hemothorax.

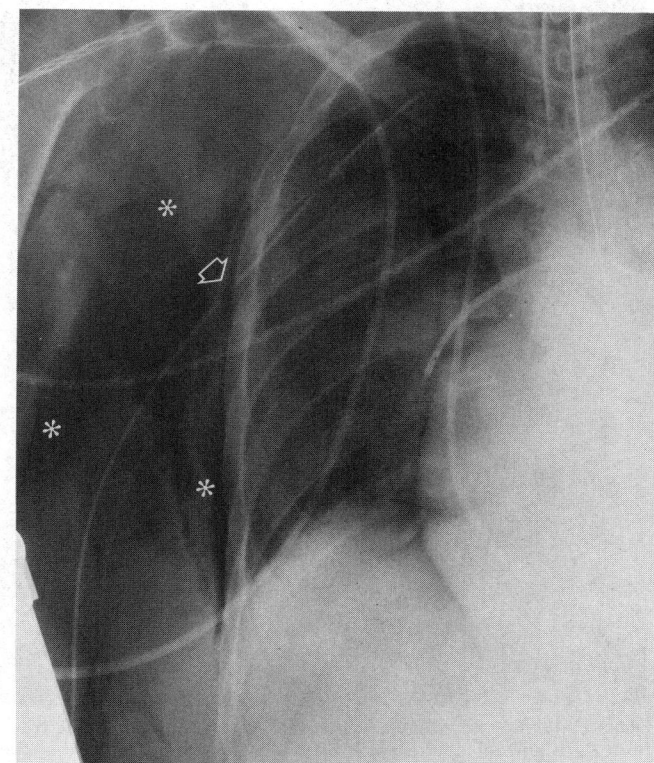

Figure 21–16. Right chest tube placed with the most distal side hole (*open arrow*) located outside the thoracic cage. Notice extensive subcutaneous emphysema (*asterisks*).

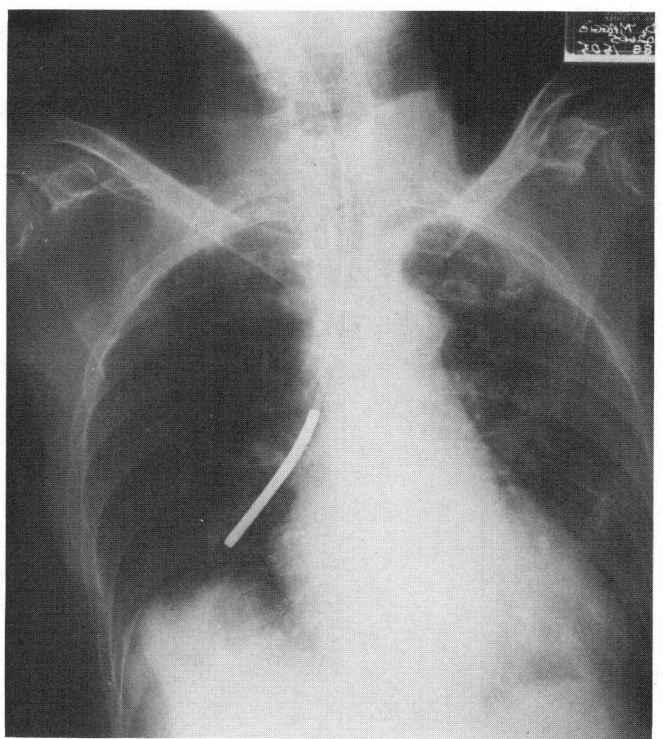

Figure 21–17. The Dobbhoff tube has been inserted into the tracheobronchial tree and now lies in the right lower lobe.

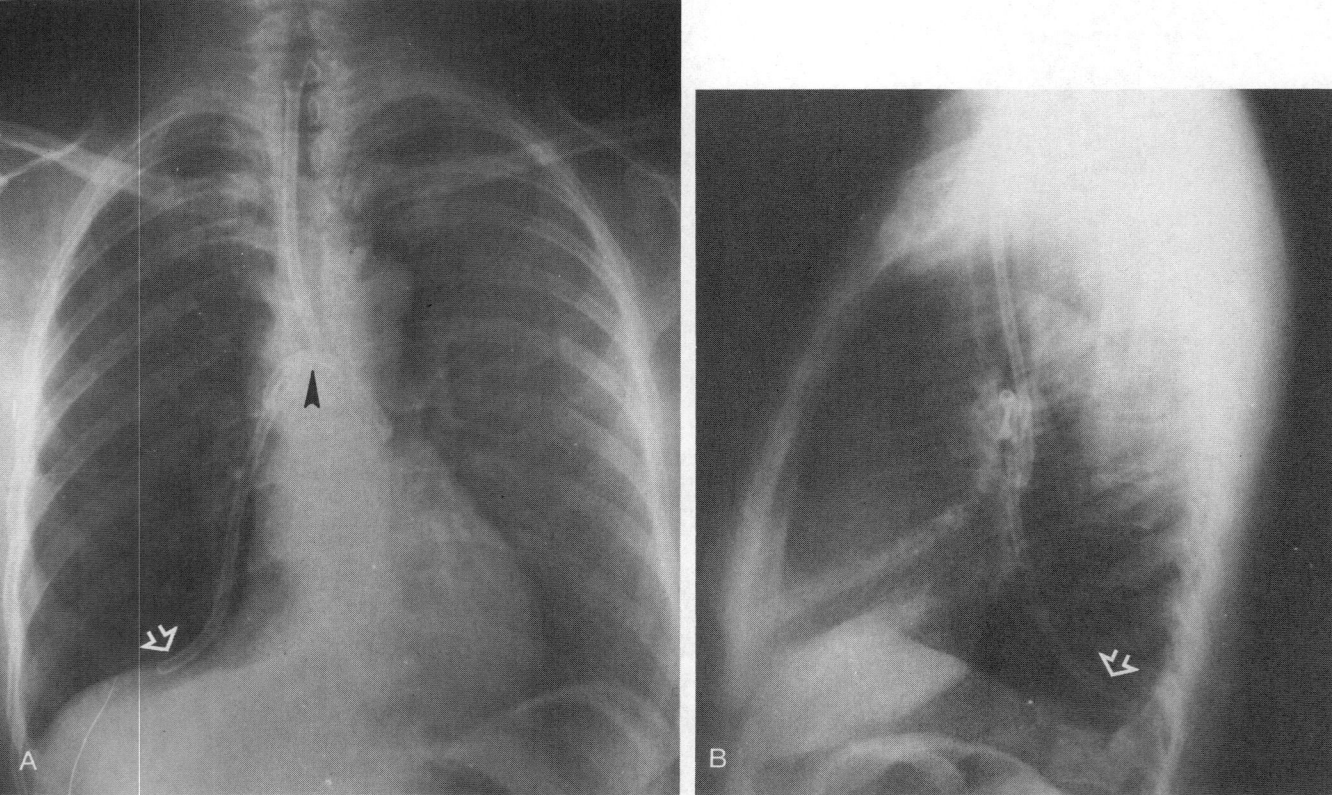

Figure 21–18. *A.* A feeding tube has been inserted through the trachea, is draped over the carina (*arrowhead*), and is folded back on itself in both right and left mainstem bronchi. Its tip lies at the base of the right lung (*open arrow*). *B.* A lateral view reveals the feeding tube to lie in the lower lobe (*open arrow*).

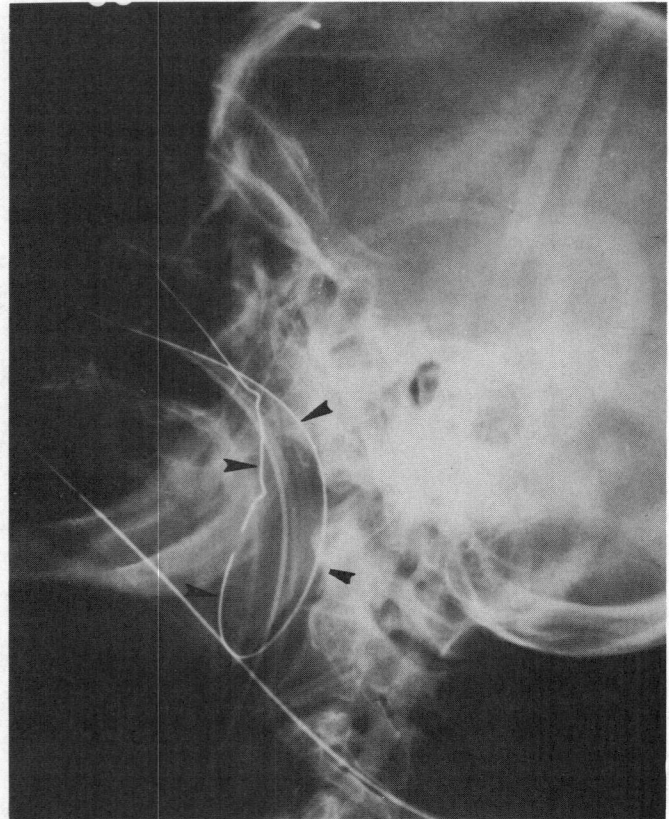

Figure 21–19. Coiled nasogastric tube. The tube folds back on itself in the hypopharynx (*arrowheads*) and lies with its tip high in the nasal cavity.

(4.3-mm) tube did not cause pneumothorax. All of the patients had impaired cough, gag, or swallowing reflexes or were sedated during the procedure. The overall risk of complications appears to be lessened by the use of larger-tip-diameter feeding tubes, but peripheral tracheobronchial placement of even the larger-tip-diameter (5.9-mm) Dobbhoff tube does occur,[18] and pleural perforation may result.

The roentgenographically identifiable complications of nasogastric tube placement such as pneumothorax and tension pneumothorax may not occur until removal of the malpositioned catheter.[17] Close clinical and radiographic evaluation should follow correction of a malpositioned tube.

The accidental placement of Entriflex, Dobbhoff, Flexiflow, Cantor, or other tubes into the airway is not, in itself, a major problem if perforation does not occur. However, infusion of liquid diets into the lungs may lead to serious and potentially fatal lung injury. This complication should never occur if (1) the postinsertion film is checked before feeding and (2) the course of the feeding tube is carefully evaluated. Tracing the tube with the index finger is far more accurate than visual tracking alone. A feeding tube in the right mainstem bronchus is an easily recognizable problem. However, location in a deep left costophrenic sulcus may be easily mistaken to be intragastric, as the opaque tip marker may be projected over the region of the stomach. The tube tip must not only be in the expected location of the stomach, but the catheter must also traverse the expected course of the esophagus and the gastroesophageal junction, not the left tracheobronchial tree (Fig. 21–20). It is important for the intensivist to recall that the location of the gastroesophageal junction is several centimeters below the left hemidiaphragm on the plain film. All feeding and nasogastric tubes must pass through this area before proper placement can be assumed. It might be argued that a nasogastric tube in the distal esophagus is not particularly harmful, but several hundred milliliters of CT contrast medium instilled through a nasogastric tube in this position could be aspirated into the lung, leading to fatal respiratory failure.

The intra-abdominal course of the nasogastric or the feeding tube is greatly influenced by gastric anatomy. The fundus of the stomach is located posteriorly in the left upper quadrant. As it crosses the midline, the body of the stomach extends several centimeters anteriorly before the antrum is directed posteriorly and joins the duodenal bulb. The second portion of the duodenum becomes retroperitoneal, where it remains until it passes the ligament of Treitz and the jejunum becomes intraperitoneal.

Passage of a feeding tube to the duodenum may be difficult to achieve in the supine patient. When a weighted catheter tip is in the posteriorly located fundus, it is difficult for the tip to proceed anteriorly to cross the midline and then descend toward the duodenum. For this reason, positioning the patient in the right lateral decubitus position during insertion and for at least 2 hours thereafter encourages gravity to carry the tube to its desired location.

Specialized guidable enteric feeding tubes, such as the Frederick-Miller tube (Cook, Bloomington, IN), are available. These are specifically designed for placement under fluoroscopy. An increased margin of safety can be obtained by utilizing direct visualization for catheter placement as suggested by Gelfand and Ott[23] and Ghahremani and Gould.[21] However, a rigid internal stylet increases the risk of perforation if malposition occurs, with or without fluoroscopic guidance. The McLean-Ring enteral feeding tube set (Cook, Bloomington, IN) has been designed to use a soft guidewire system, with the aim of eliminating perforations resulting from stiffening devices.[24]

In the vast majority of patients, neither fluoroscopy nor guidewires are needed, although they are useful techniques when necessary. The procedure should be performed by a physician experienced in both tube placement and fluoroscopy.[25] The risk and the expense of transporting the critically ill patient with support devices and staff to the radiology department for guided catheter placement must, in such circumstances, be weighed against the potential benefit.

Pacemaker Wires and Power Generators

Transvenous endocardial pacing devices are commonly seen on the radiographs of ICU patients. Evaluation of the wire placement and integrity on basis of the AP chest radiograph is potentially inaccurate because it is restricted to a single projection and is therefore incomplete. Nevertheless, an educated attempt at assessment of electrode placement should be made.

Ideally, the pacemaker catheter tip is positioned in the apex of the right ventricle. The tip should not be curved up, and there should not be significant folds, kinks, or sharp angles throughout the course of the wire. Tracing the wire from the power generator to its tip should be performed regularly to assess for lead fracture. Bipolar pacemakers have come into more frequent use. With these devices, one lead is in the usual location in the right ventriclar apex, while a second lead is projected over the right atrium.

The most common problem identified on the radiograph is aberrant location of the pacemaker tips, rather than electrode fracture. The pacemaker tips may be located anywhere along the vascular course from the site of insertion through the peripheral pulmonary arteries. Placement of

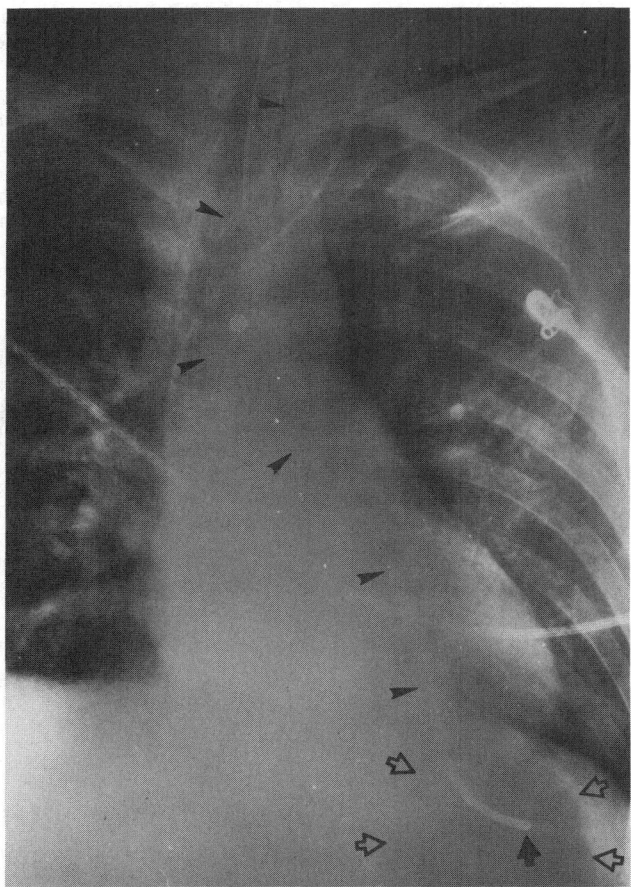

Figure 21–20. Dobbhoff tube tip (*filled arrow*) projects over the gastric air bubble (*open arrows*). Careful inspection of the course of the catheter reveals that it follows the left tracheobronchial tree (*arrowheads*) and that its true position is deep in the left posterior costophrenic sulcus.

the tip in the wrong chamber of the heart is usually easy to identify on the AP radiograph. Somewhat more difficult to assess radiographically is the placement of the tip in the coronary sinus. The catheter may appear to be in normal position on the frontal projection, but if a lateral view is available, the tip is seen to be directed posteriorly. The most helpful finding on the frontal radiograph in this instance of malposition is that the tip often curves upward. If this suspicion is raised, a lateral view is confirmatory.

Pacing wires can perforate vessels or the myocardium. An obvious extravascular or extracardiac location of the pacer tip is easily identified. However, partial myocardial perforation may be virtually impossible to identify radiographically. Fortunately, this condition usually does not result in significant bleeding complications.

Assessment of the power generator (battery pack) radiographically has not met with practical success. Direct measurement of battery output is believed to be more reliable.

NORMAL CHEST FINDINGS

The normal AP chest radiograph obtained with a portable unit is characterized by lung parenchyma that should be easily recognized as clear. The basics of chest radiographic interpretation are the same for supine and upright patients. Only minor differences, usually in measurements, pertain for supine and upright positions. The vascular distribution is more nearly equal from top to bottom in the supine patient, whereas a greater vascular distribution from superior to inferior lung zones is seen in the upright position. A relatively poor inspiration causes widening of the cardiac silhouette and increased prominence of the pulmonary veins and mediastinum. This mediastinal widening is usually a reflection of engorgement of the right-sided superior vena cava but can be due to tortuosity of other vessels or the presence of fat. Apparent cardiac enlargement occurs with a limited inspiratory effort as the heart assumes a more transverse orientation. In addition, there is enlargement of the heart and the mediastinum attributable to the geometric factors relative to the AP projection and the shortened distance between the x-ray tube and the film.

A limited inspiration, which is frequently present in the supine patient, also crowds the vessels and lung parenchyma at the bases of the thoracic cage, occasionally simulating air space disease. Regardless of inspiratory status, the hemidiaphragms should always be clearly visible from the lateral through the medial costophrenic angles. Careful inspection of the retrocardiac region should reveal the left hemidiaphragm, even in a relatively underexposed film.

Surrounding Structures

The ICU chest radiograph often demonstrates many cardiopulmonary abnormalities, which distract the viewer from a systematic approach to film evaluation. Periodically, a thorough evaluation of the bones and soft tissues of the chest, the neck, the abdomen, the shoulder girdle, and the spine should be undertaken.

The rib cage should be evaluated for symmetry as well as the presence and integrity of all ribs. Absence or deformity of a rib may result from prior surgery or be due to direct extension or distant metastasis of a malignancy. Rib resection or deformity may be the only clue to a previous major thoracic surgical procedure, such as lobectomy. Removal of a lobe significantly alters the lung anatomy, and unless this history is known, pathologic alterations may be sought where there are none. Postlobectomy chest findings have been reviewed in detail by Holbert and colleagues.[30] Rib fracture may be the cause of a pleural mass, pleural fluid collection, or pneumothorax. Similar findings should be sought in the

shoulder girdle, but special attention must be directed to shoulder dislocation and proximal humeral fracture, both of which can be easily overlooked in the ICU patient.

An optimally exposed chest film should permit visualization of the thoracic vertebral bodies. Scoliosis not only distorts the intrathoracic structures, making the heart and mediastinum difficult to evaluate, but also, if severe, may compromise cardiorespiratory function. Vertebral body density abnormalities and vertebral body collapse may be seen with malignant, infectious, metabolic, or traumatic conditions. Radionuclide bone scan is highly sensitive for detection of additional occult skeletal lesions. It is limited, however, by poor specificity. Focal radiographs of an area identified on bone scan should reveal the cause of increased uptake. This study is not customarily available at the bedside.

Soft tissues of the neck should be assessed for mass or swelling. Deviation of the trachea at the thoracic inlet (clavicles) is most frequently due to the presence of a thyroid mass. In the evaluation of a thyroid mass, ultrasonography is preferred, as CT with contrast enhancement floods the body's iodine pool, making radionuclide iodine thyroid scan impossible for several weeks. The diaphragm should be seen in its entirety, with the right hemidiaphragm lying no more than one vertebral body higher than the left. Abnormal elevation of the diaphragm on either side may be due to subpulmonic effusion (in the upright patient), phrenic nerve paralysis, or anatomic variant. Less frequent causes include subphrenic abscess and traumatic diaphragmatic hernia. Lateral decubitus positioning for radiography enables diagnosis of subpulmonic effusion, and chest fluoroscopy (sniff test) can clearly demonstrate diaphragmatic paralysis. Ultrasonography is diagnostic for subphrenic fluid collections, whereas contrast radiography remains the most useful modality for hernia assessment.

The portion of the abdomen present on the chest film should be inspected for bowel gas patterns (e.g., obstruction, ileus, and esophageal intubation), clips and sutures (e.g., vagotomy), and pneumoperitoneum.

No discussion of ICU imaging, however brief, would be complete without a few comments on pneumoperitoneum. This is a diagnosis that would elude few if the patient is upright (Fig. 21–21). As with pleural effusion, however, the

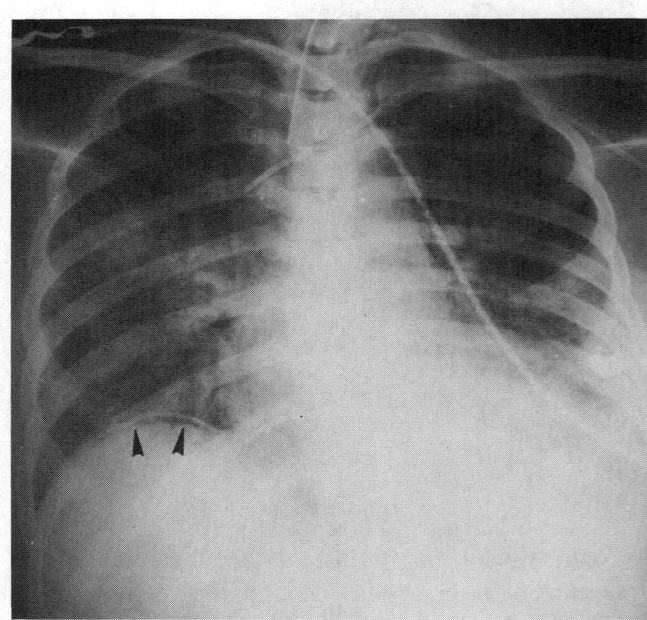

Figure 21–21. Pneumoperitoneum. A small radiolucent crescent (*arrowheads*) represents free intraperitoneal air collecting beneath the hemidiaphragm.

supine position creates diagnostic difficulty. To overcome this problem, the patient should be filmed in the left lateral decubitus position. When the patient's left side is down, the liver forms a homogeneous, dense backdrop for the lucent gas, which collects between the liver and the abdominal wall. The liver also acts to displace radiographically confusing bowel loops from this area. It is important to remember that the pneumoperitoneum is often present on supine abdomen or chest films obtained before the definitive film. On the supine film, free air collects in the most anterior part of the abdomen.[31] This area extends from the anterior axillary lines and across the costochondral junction to the xiphoid. This is the site of attachment of the anterior leaflet of the diaphragm and is the place to look for pneumoperitoneum in the supine or semierect patient. The finding to seek is a subtle radiolucent triangle, which appears to extend above the diaphragm in the midline (Fig. 21–22). If this finding is present, identification of the falciform ligament (Fig. 21–23) should be sought. Left lateral decubitus or upright films are confirmatory.

Last, all areas on the film should be scrutinized for foreign bodies, surgical and otherwise (Fig. 21–24). Evidence of previous thoracotomy for lung resection, prosthetic cardiac valve insertion, coronary artery bypass graft, or open lung biopsy may provide valuable information not necessarily available by history. The airway should be considered a potential location for teeth or dental prostheses as well as edible material. Loose teeth can be easily dislodged and aspirated during intubation (Fig. 21–25). Psychiatric patients may ingest or insert into their skin a variety of foreign bodies.

ABNORMAL CHEST FINDINGS
Atelectasis

Atelectasis results from a variety of causes in the patient receiving intensive care. Two common factors are tube location and poor inspiration. An endotracheal tube that has been advanced beyond its desired mid-tracheal location tends to follow the straighter pathway of the right mainstem bronchus. This effectively precludes ventilation of the entire left lung and results in atelectasis, which progresses from the left lower lobe to the entire lung (Fig. 21–26). If the endotracheal tube is advanced into the intermediate bronchus, the right upper lobe is subject to collapse. By further distal tube placement, the right middle lobe can also collapse.

Occasionally, the endotracheal tube enters the left main bronchus, predisposing to complete right lung atelectasis. It should be kept in mind that there is an approximately 1-cm septum extending upward from the radiographically visible carina. When the endotracheal tube is within 1 cm of the carina, it can be presumed that ventilation is occurring predominantly in one lung. The tube should be retracted immediately.

The radiographic findings of atelectasis have been well described.[32] The characteristic diagnostic points include (1) relatively homogeneous opacification of the lung in the appropriate distribution for a collapsed lobe and (2) signs of volume loss (shift of the heart and mediastinum ipsilaterally, elevation of diaphragm, and narrowing of the adjacent intercostal spaces).

A helpful finding in identifying atelectasis is intermittent, spontaneous resolution and recurrence on successive films. It is also important to note that the dense, homogeneous opacity of atelectasis may contain air bronchograms, with occasional evidence of compression of the air-filled bronchi resulting from overall volume loss.[33]

The upper lobes characteristically collapse upward and medially (Fig. 21–27), so that they lie adjacent to the superior mediastinum on the AP view and form a retrosternal opacity on the lateral view. Similarly, the lower lobes collapse medially, although downward, forming dense triangles at the medial lung bases (Figs. 21–28 and 21–29). On the lateral view, the abnormal opacity is posterior. The middle lobe collapses medially, coming to lie adjacent to the right-sided heart border. These patterns are quite characteristic and well known.

Interpretive difficulties arise when combinations of adjacent lobes collapse together.[34] Coincident right middle and lower lobe atelectasis produces a typical pattern on the chest radiograph (Fig. 21–30), which closely simulates a pleural effusion. Indeed, atypical atelectasis leads to substantial problems in diagnosis.[35–37] The use of CT[9, 38–43] may clarify the anatomy but may delay diagnosis. Although less reliable than CT, ultrasonography can be used at the bedside. However, the accuracy of ultrasound images in establishing the correct diagnosis is highly operator dependent. Ultrasonography is widely regarded by radiologists as the most difficult study to perform well and also the most difficult to interpret. These limitations are compounded in the bedside examination. Commonly encountered limitations include the patient's inability to suspend respiration or change position; the presence of catheters and dressings at a desired imaging

Text continued on page 277

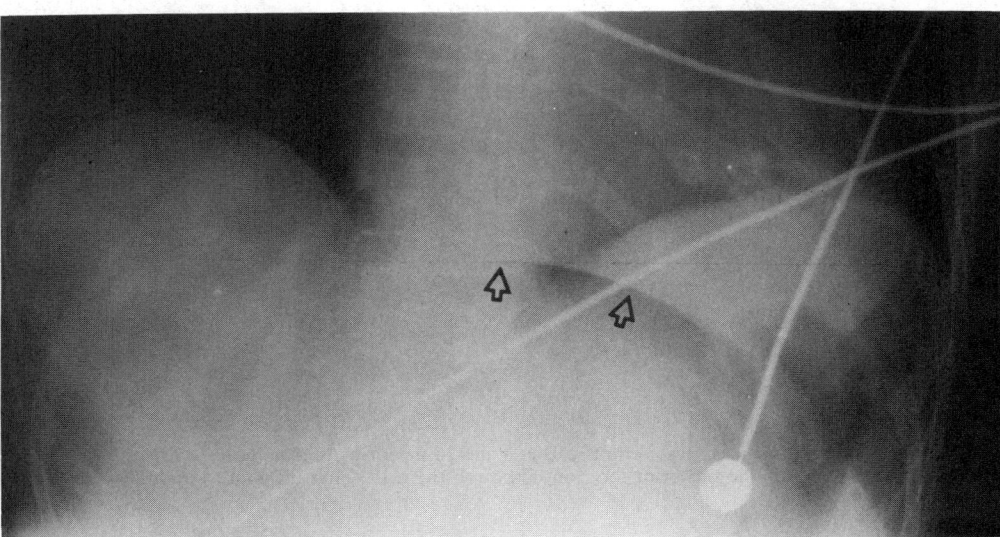

Figure 21–22. Pneumoperitoneum. A curvilinear lucency (*open arrows*) in the upper midline of the abdomen should be suspected to be pneumoperitoneum in a supine patient.

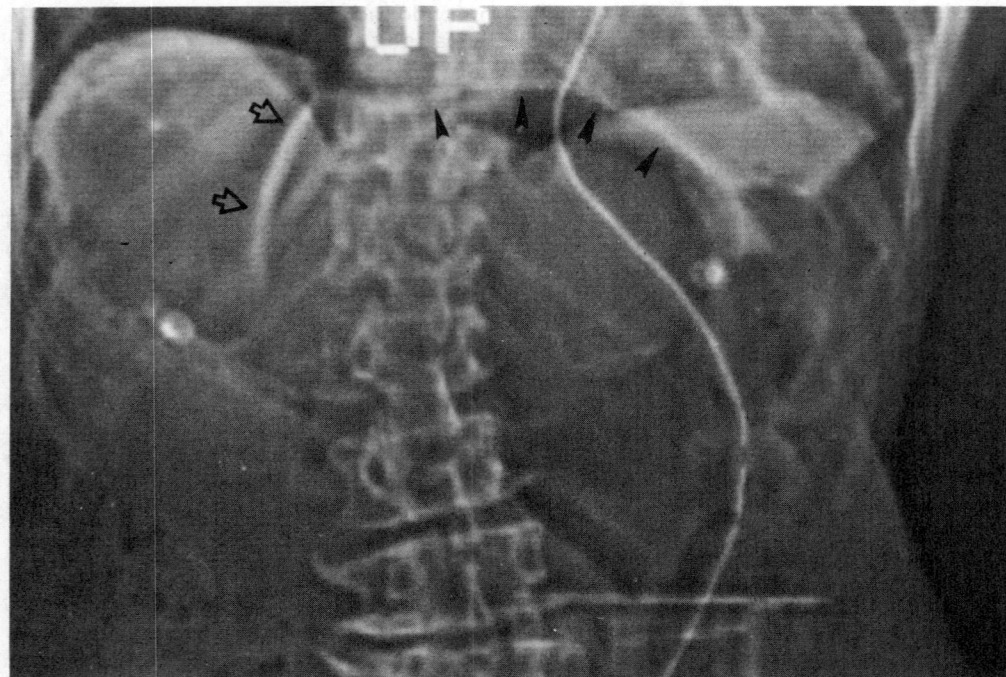

Figure 21–23. Pneumoperitoneum. This preliminary CT image reveals gross free air under the diaphragm anteriorly (*arrowheads*) and outlines the falciform ligament (*open arrows*).

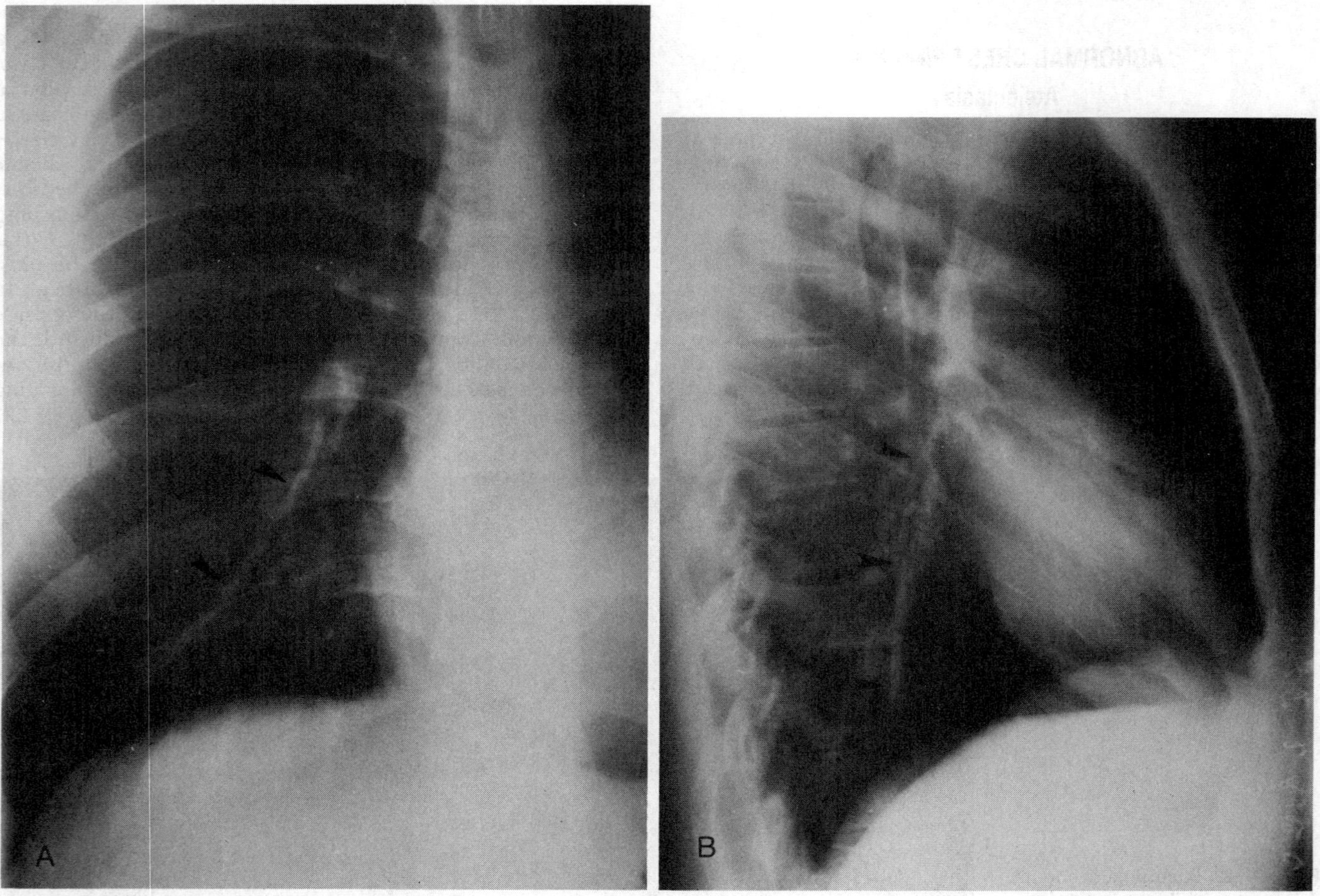

Figure 21–24. *A.* A fractured central venous catheter lies in an intravascular location in the right lower lobe (*arrowheads*). *B.* Lateral view of the same patient reveals the posterior location, although the catheter is difficult to identify because of a poorly radiopaque marker.

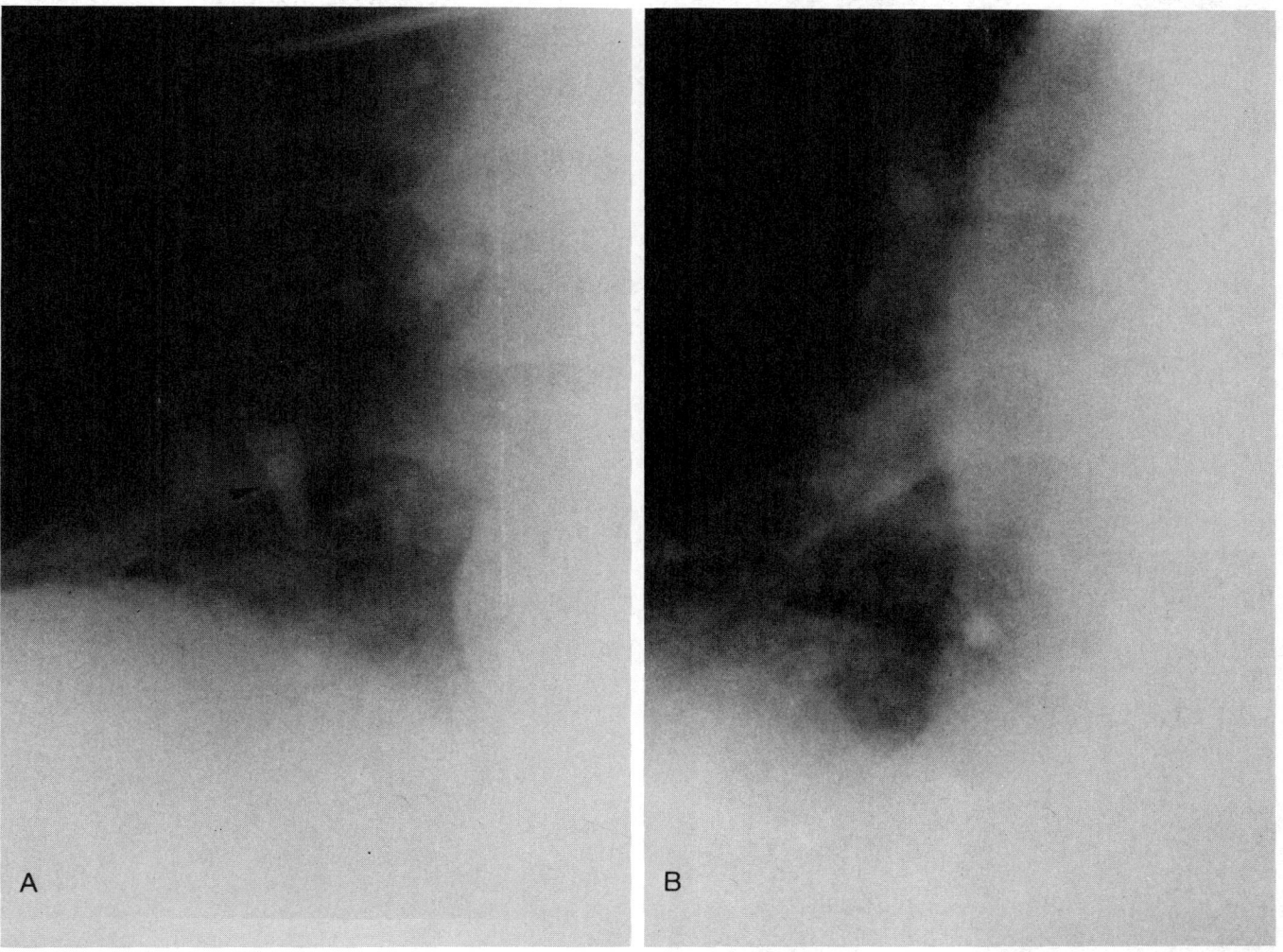

Figure 21–25. *A*. A coned-down view of the medial right lung base reveals a tooth (*arrowhead*). *B*. No tooth is present on the study from the preceding day.

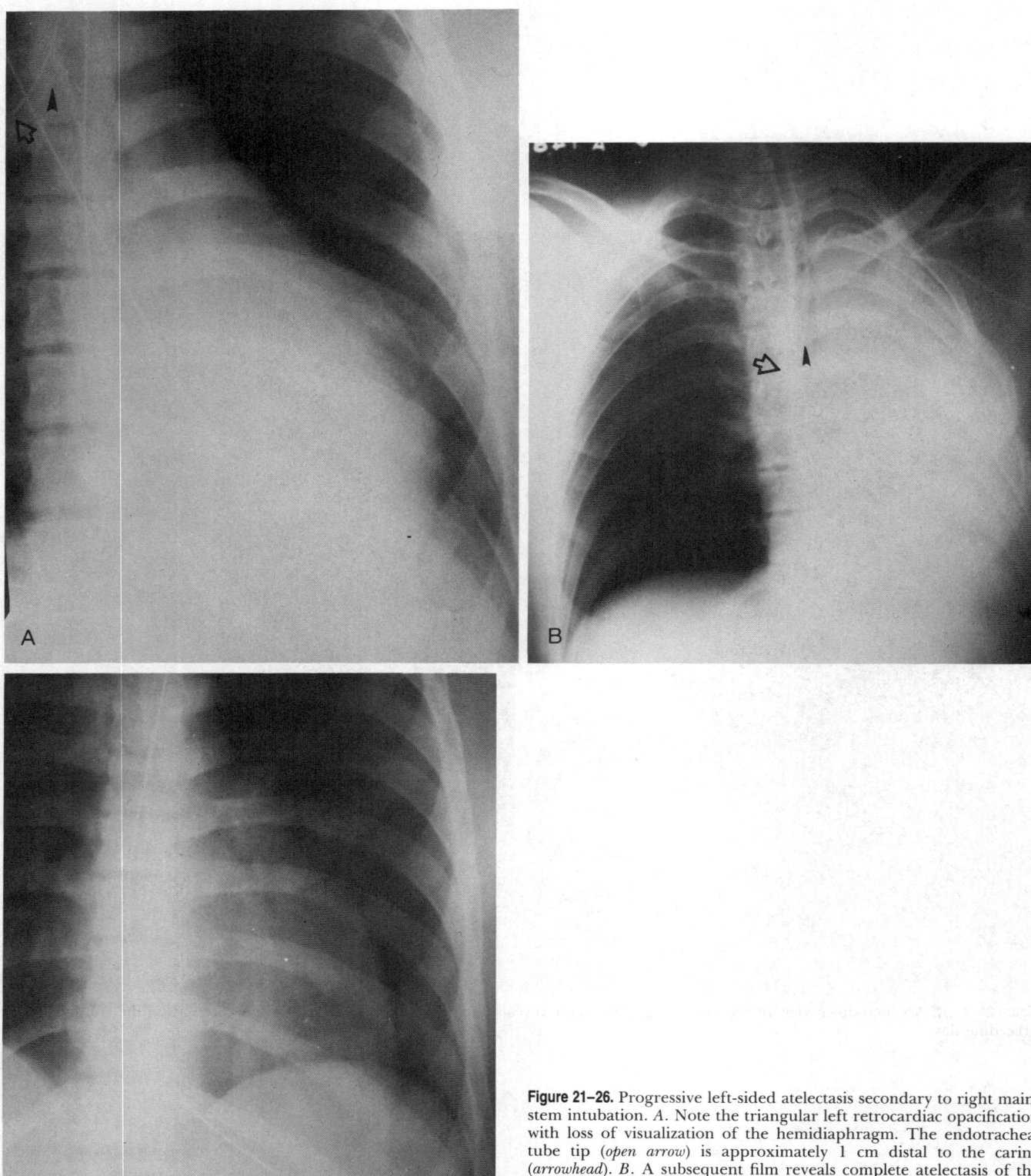

Figure 21–26. Progressive left-sided atelectasis secondary to right main-stem intubation. *A.* Note the triangular left retrocardiac opacification with loss of visualization of the hemidiaphragm. The endotracheal tube tip (*open arrow*) is approximately 1 cm distal to the carina (*arrowhead*). *B.* A subsequent film reveals complete atelectasis of the left lung after failure to reposition the endotracheal tube. *C.* Retraction of the endotracheal tube allows re-expansion of the left lung. Note the visualization of the retrocardiac vessels and the hemidiaphragm when compared with *A.*

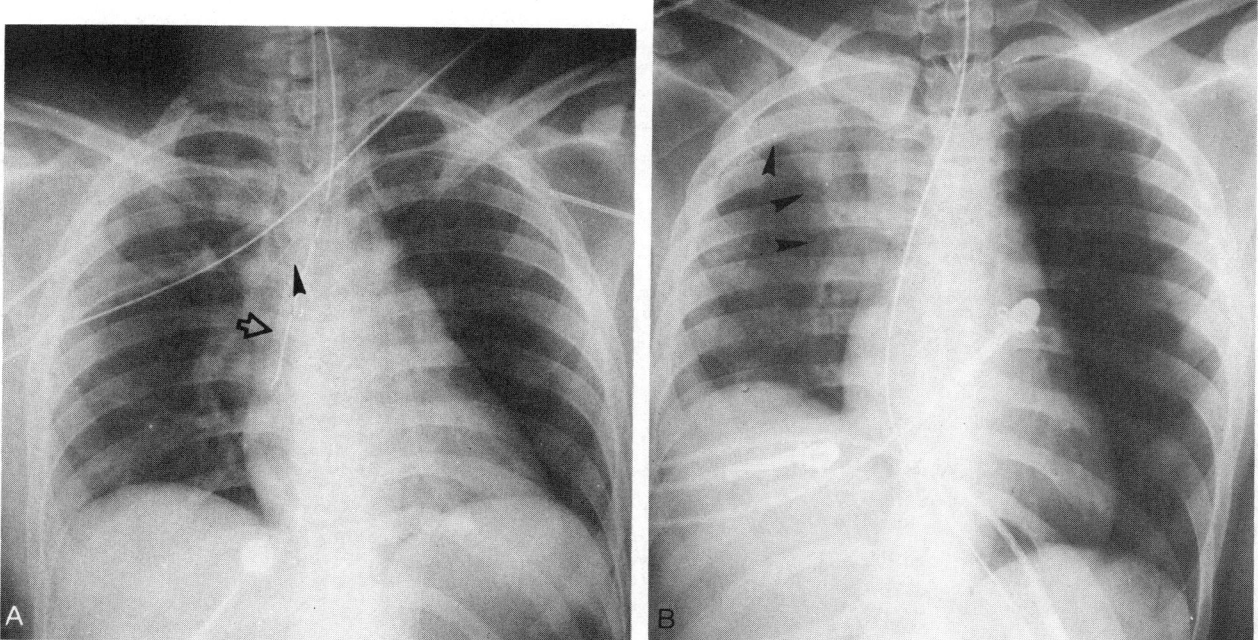

Figure 21–27. Right upper lobe atelectasis. *A.* A nasogastric tube (*open arrow*) has been passed into the intermediate bronchus, several centimeters distal to the carina (*arrowhead*). *B.* A subsequent film, after removal of the nasogastric tube, reveals collapse of the right upper lobe with elevation of the minor fissure (*arrowheads*).

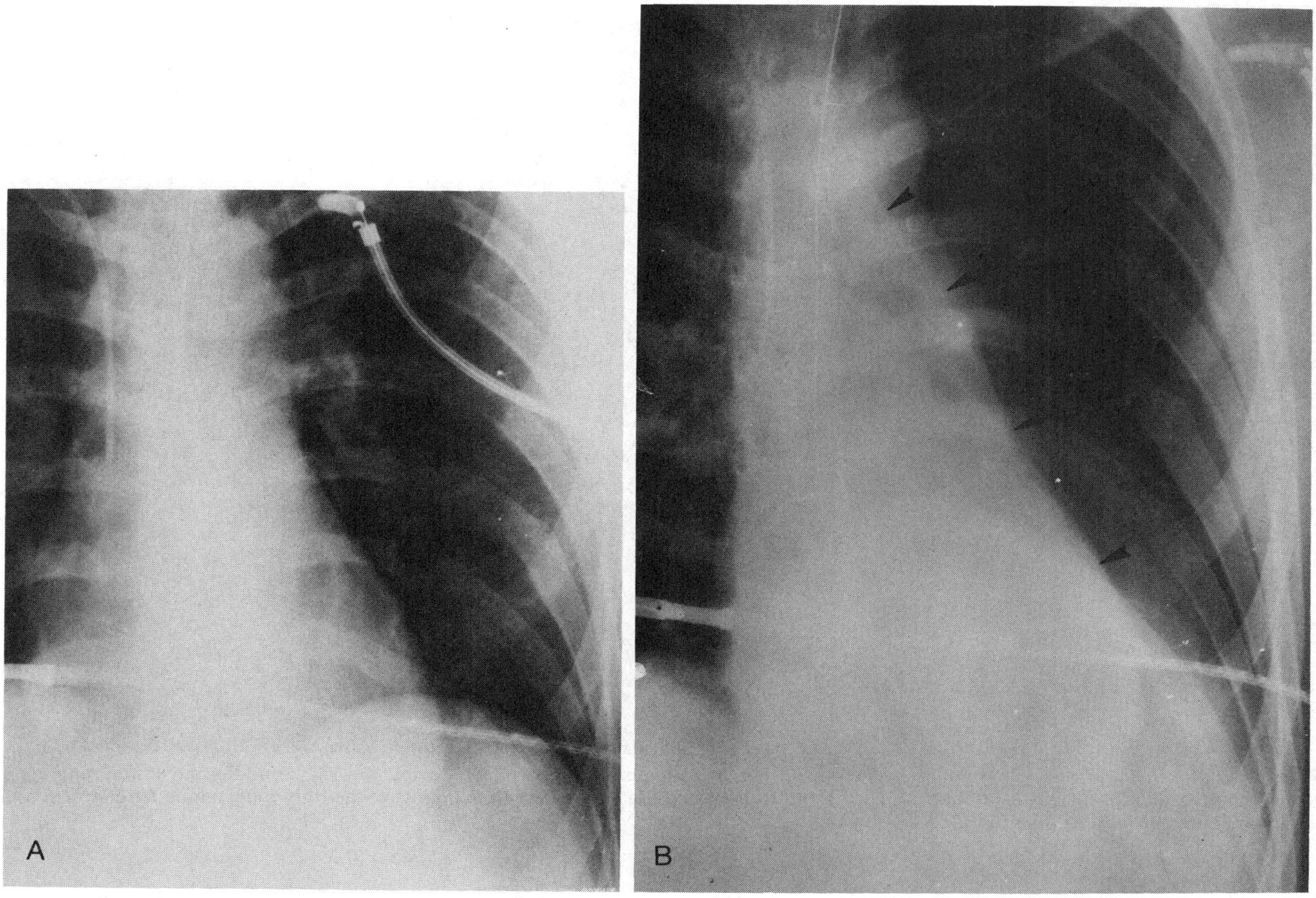

Figure 21–28. Left lower lobe atelectasis. *A.* Normal left lung base reveals clearly identified lung markings through the left side of the heart and a well-defined left hemidiaphragm. *B.* There is increased left retrocardiac opacity forming a radiopaque triangle (*arrowheads*) conforming to the cardiac contour, typical of left lower lobe atelectasis. Note also typical silhouetting of the left hemidiaphragm and ipsilateral shift of the heart.

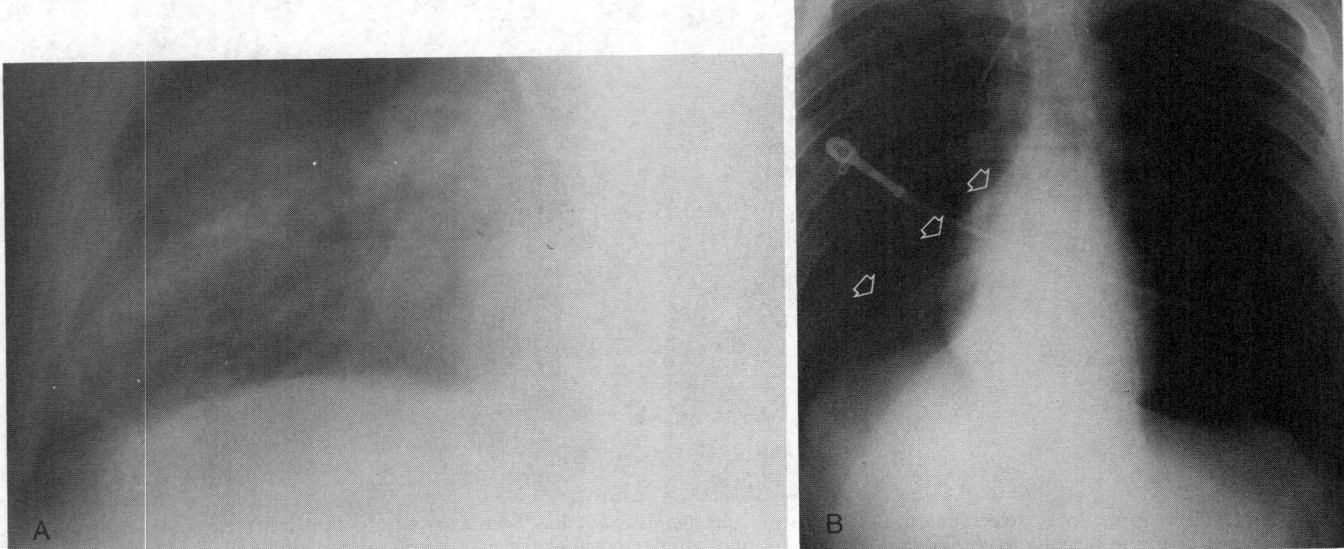

Figure 21–29. Right lower lobe atelectasis. *A.* Relatively normal right base with slight increased triangular opacity at the right medial base. The diaphragm, however, continues to be clearly seen. *B.* There is a right retrocardiac opacity that is triangular (*open arrows*), obscures the normal retrocardiac markings, and silhouettes the right hemidiaphragm. Note the symmetry with left lower lobe atelectasis (Fig. 21–28).

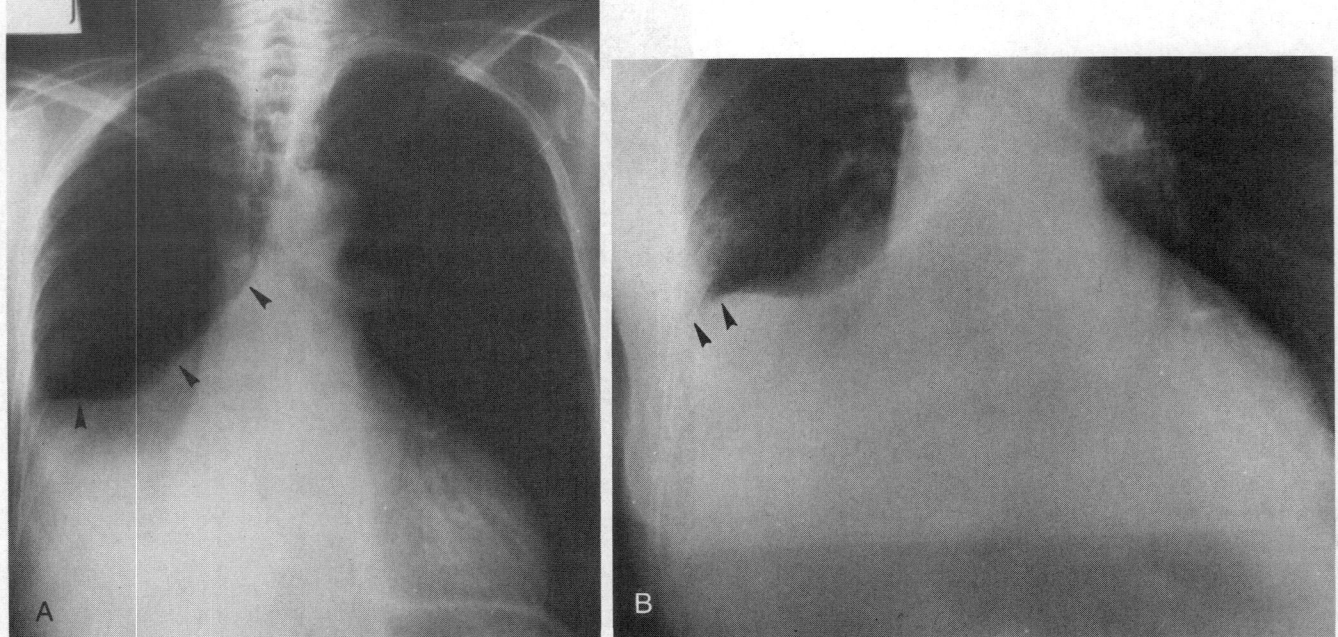

Figure 21–30. Right middle and lower lobe atelectasis. *A.* There is an unusual opacity occupying the right middle and lower lung zones (*arrowheads*), simulating a right pleural effusion. *B.* Note the downward lateral curve of the opacity at the right medial lung base (*arrowheads*), which differentiates atelectasis from pleural effusion.

site; space restrictions in the ICU, which limit access by the technologist to the patient; and the presence of excessive ambient light. In spite of these problems, ultrasonography has been shown to be useful in the differentiation of pleural and air space disease.[44] CT studies are also helpful in this regard.[43, 45–47] CT is also useful to identify the cause of atelectasis,[48, 49] which may simulate pleural fluid.

Complete lung atelectasis is less frequent than lobar collapse and, as described earlier, often complicates a misplaced endotracheal tube. Frequently, a lobe is obstructed by a mucous plug. Occasionally, an entire lung may have the ventilation interrupted by a mucous plug, with subsequent complete lung atelectasis.

Acute bronchial obstruction may present atypical roentgenographic findings. Immediately after a major bronchus has been obstructed, but before resorption of alveolar air, the lung appears normal on the chest x-ray film. However, there is no air exchange. The patient may then manifest dyspnea, hypoxemia, and respiratory alkalosis, suggesting pulmonary embolism as the cause of acute, severe respiratory decompensation. Pulmonary angiography is likely to be entirely normal, and the chest x-ray film may reveal significantly less disease than is anticipated by the patient's clinical status (Fig. 21–31). However, the ventilation-perfusion scan is diagnostic[50] and reveals relatively normal perfusion but a complete absence of ventilation in the affected lobes.

The well-known appearance of complete lung atelectasis is that of total opacification of a hemithorax. The differential diagnosis includes massive pleural fluid collection and dense parenchymal consolidation. Confirmatory findings for atelectasis include ipsilateral heart, mediastinal, and diaphragmatic displacement and narrowing of the ipsilateral intercostal spaces (Fig. 21–32). Massive pleural effusion acts as a large space-occupying lesion, with contralateral displacement of the heart and the mediastinum (Fig. 21–33). The diaphragm is typically silhouetted, and if the effusion is left sided, caudal displacement of gastric air may be present. Owing to the mass effect, the intercostal spaces are usually widened. In contrast, complete lung consolidation fails to displace any of the intrathoracic, chest wall, or abdominal

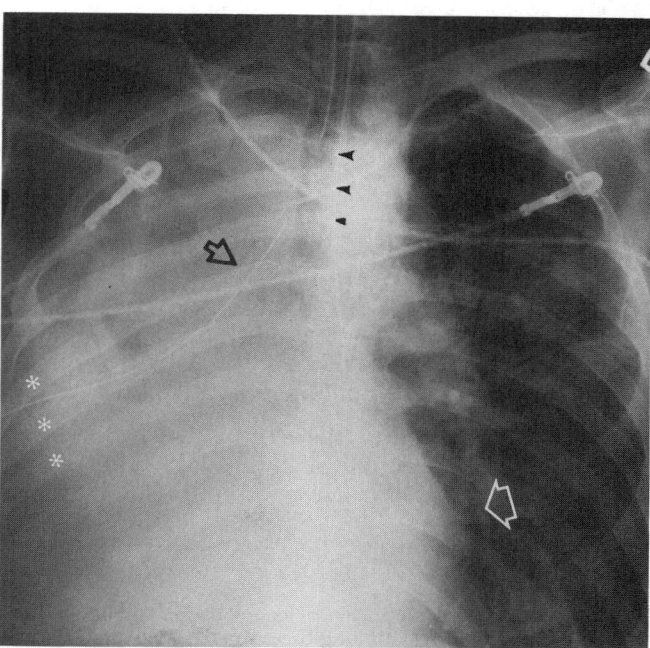

Figure 21–32. Right lung atelectasis. Complete opacification of the right hemithorax with a shift of the trachea (*arrowheads*) and heart (*white open arrow*), as well as narrowing of the intercostal spaces (*asterisks*), all indicated right-sided atelectasis. Nevertheless, the erroneous assumption that these results represented a massive pleural effusion resulted in thoracostomy tube placement (*black open arrow*).

structures (Fig. 21–34). A diagnostic dilemma occurs when atelectasis and pleural effusion coexist. The mass effect of the fluid may compensate for the signs of volume loss produced by the atelectasis. Subtle differences in density between peripheral pleural fluid and the central lung zone

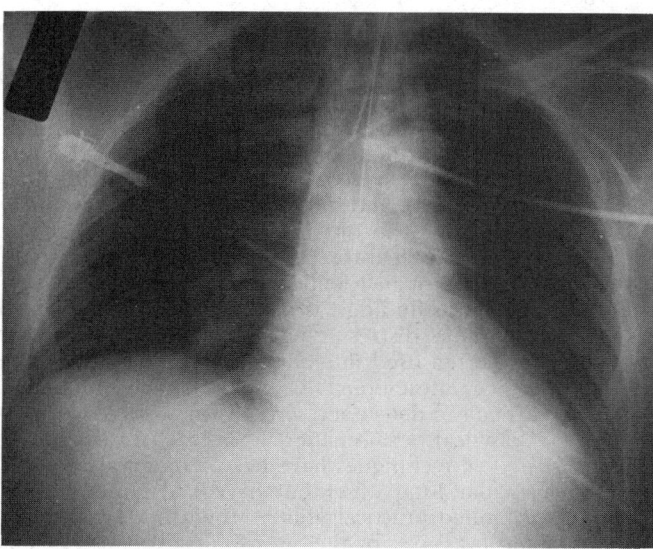

Figure 21–31. Acute left bronchial obstruction. The chest radiograph revealed only left lower lobe atelectasis in this patient who had acutely decompensated with a suspected clinical diagnosis of massive pulmonary embolism. A radionuclide ventilation-perfusion scan revealed normal perfusion with complete absence of ventilation of the left lung. Pulmonary angiography results were normal.

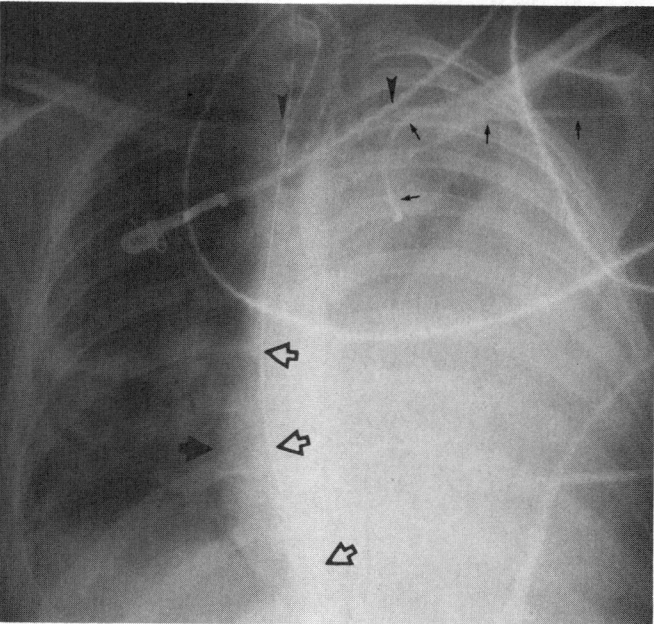

Figure 21–33. Massive left hemothorax. The patient is rotated to the left, as seen by the location of the clavicular heads (*arrowheads*). Nevertheless, the border of the right side of the heart (*filled arrow*) is still seen in the right hemithorax. The endotracheal tube tip is in the midline and the nasogastric tube (*open arrows*) is displaced to the right. An aberrant left central venous catheter placement (*small arrows*) was the cause of the massive hemothorax.

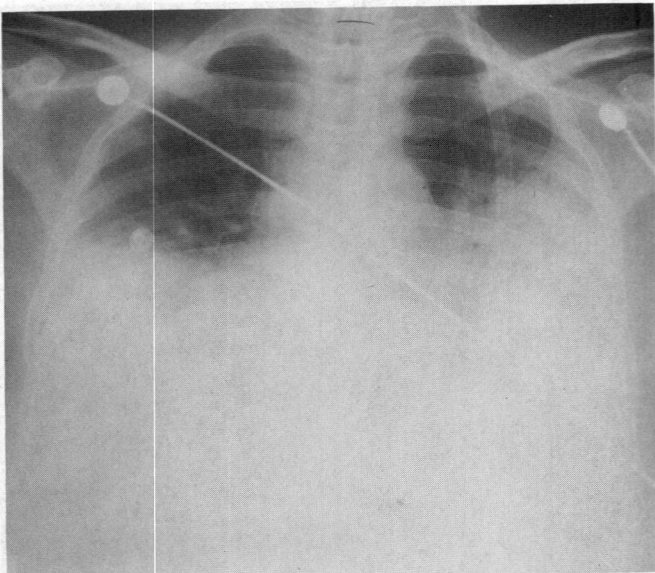

Figure 21–34. Bilateral parenchymal consolidation. Bilaterally symmetric opacification of both lung bases simulates pleural effusions. No layering was identified on decubitus films, and ultrasonography confirmed the presence of consolidation and lack of pleural fluid.

may be of some help, but this distinction may necessitate the use of ultrasonography or CT (Fig. 21–35). These three entities (pleural effusion, parenchymal consolidation, and atelectasis) necessitate quite divergent therapies, and only in the rarest of circumstances should these diagnoses be confused.

Rounded atelectasis is an unusual type of pulmonary collapse that may be seen after resolution of a pleural effusion. Rounded atelectasis can closely mimic a lung mass on plain films.[51, 52] Comparison with old films reveals a mass that has developed rapidly and the presence of an intercur-

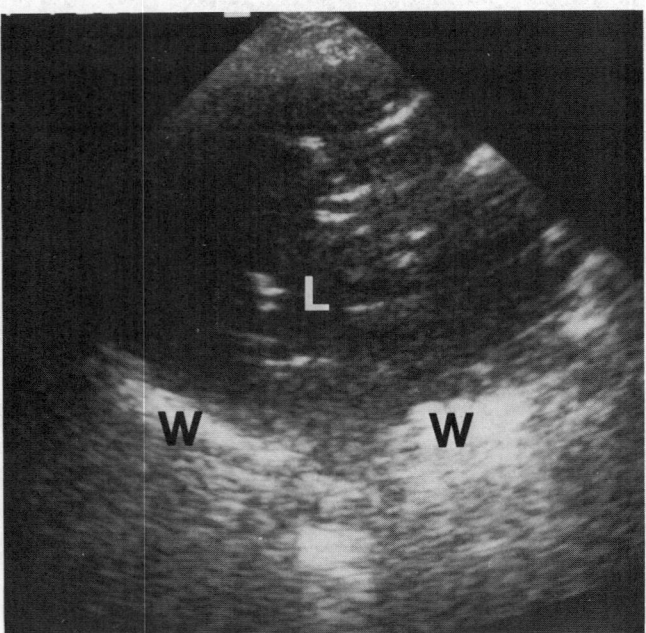

Figure 21–35. Pulmonary consolidation. Sonogram of the patient whose basilar opacity is seen in Figure 21–34 reveals consolidated lung (L) extending to the chest wall (W) with no intervening pleural fluid.

rent pleural effusion or other pleural disease. Typical features include a "comet tail" of compressed vessels entering the mass and proximity to a pleural surface. This type of collapse has been extensively studied with CT, which allows improved identification of the known radiographic findings.[53–55]

Air Space Disease

The most frequent condition confused with atelectasis is pneumonitis. Those who practice intensive care medicine or radiology are well aware that parenchymal consolidation can, and does, occur in nearly every shape, size, distribution, and severity. However, atelectasis is characteristically limited to a (collapsed) lobar distribution with distinct borders and displaced pleural surfaces. Pneumonia tends to be more random in distribution, is less homogeneous, and may be characterized by cavitation. If pneumonia is lobar, the shape, size, and location of the lobe are normal. If the patient has sustained significant trauma to the thorax, the possibility of pulmonary contusion or laceration should be entertained. The roentgenographic findings of pulmonary contusion may closely simulate those of pneumonic consolidation. These findings have been described and classified by Wagner and associates.[56] CT has been shown to increase the sensitivity of detection of traumatic pulmonary parenchymal lesions,[56, 57] as well as pulmonary edema[58] and causes of hemoptysis.[59]

Various organisms have been widely reported to cause specific patterns of consolidation on the chest radiograph. However, in practice, pattern recognition is highly unreliable. An exception to this general rule is *Pneumocystis carinii* pneumonia, which produces a reliable, bilaterally symmetric interstitial pattern that may progress to a diffuse, ground-glass parenchymal opacity.[60] Even this pattern is subject to a large number of atypical appearances that may be unilateral and/or nodular. In the critically ill, human immunodeficiency virus–positive patient, difficulty may arise in distinguishing severe *P. carinii* pneumonia from adult respiratory distress syndrome.[61, 62] Indeed, the two may coexist. Other difficulties arise in patients with chronic underlying diseases that may significantly complicate both the chest pathologic changes and film interpretation.[63–65]

Pulmonary Edema and Adult Respiratory Distress Syndrome

A frequent diagnostic challenge is the differentiation of the various types of pulmonary edema: cardiogenic, volume overload (attributable to renal failure or aggressive fluid resuscitation of shock), and increased capillary permeability caused by a variety of insults that result in damage to the pulmonary microvasculature.[66, 67] Permeability pulmonary edema, when present in a patient with a well-known constellation of clinical findings, is also commonly referred to as adult respiratory distress syndrome[68] (Fig. 21–36). The two terms are often used interchangeably in describing the radiographic manifestations. Early interstitial pulmonary edema is difficult to detect and virtually impossible to quantitate by physical examination. Several invasive and noninvasive[67, 69–76] techniques have been attempted to measure extravascular lung water but have had either limited accuracy or limited practical utility. Monitoring of left ventricular filling pressures by the Swan-Ganz catheter remains the single most common technique to assess pulmonary microvascular hydrostatic pressure but has limitations related to cost, invasiveness, and possibility of interpretative error. Sampling endobronchial fluid may be possible in selected patients to measure protein concentration in edema fluid as a method of distinguishing high-pressure

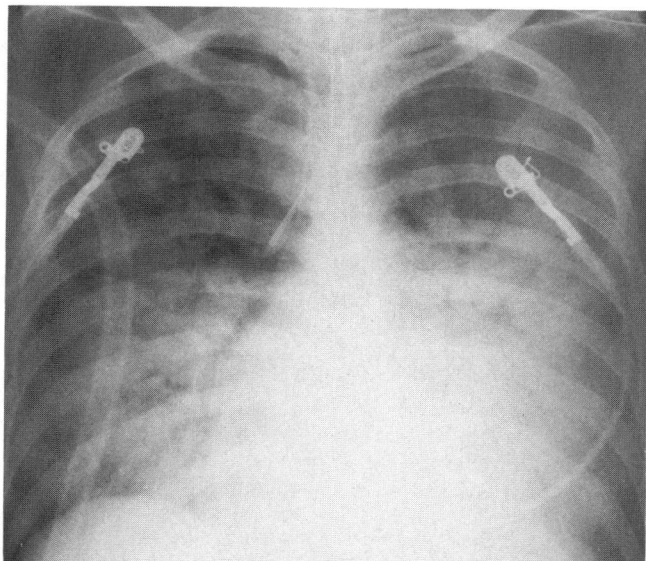

Figure 21–36. Adult respiratory distress syndrome. Note diffuse bilateral parenchymal opacities that are relatively symmetric, which is typical of capillary permeability edema.

cardiac permeability edema.[76] However, the mainstay of diagnosing pulmonary edema continues to be the chest radiograph.[1–7, 61, 62, 77]

The chest radiograph, however, is also an imperfect technique for this purpose.[78–80] Halperin and coworkers reported a linear correlation between the findings of pulmonary edema on supine and portable chest films and extravascular lung water measured by the thermal dye indicator dilution technique.[81] Respiratory maneuvers may influence the interpretation of edema on the radiograph. Wegenius and colleagues found that positive end-expiratory pressure renders the chest x-ray film unreliable in the evaluation of adult respiratory distress syndrome and useful only for identification of complications (e.g., pneumothorax, atelectasis, and pleural effusion).[82]

The relationship between positive end-expiratory pressure therapy and imaging of inflammatory pulmonary edema has also been studied in detail by Gattinoni and associates.[83] They concluded that CT is a useful method of evaluating extravascular lung water, but its interpretation is greatly complicated by external changes in thoracic physiology (e.g., with positive end-expiratory pressure). In this series, increased positive end-expiratory pressure caused decreased lung opacities by recruitment of previously collapsed pulmonary units. However, there was an associated decrease in pulmonary arterial pressure.

Pulmonary edema is classically described as "batwing" in appearance on chest radiographs. There are multiple causes for a chest x-ray film to demonstrate an acute perihilar infiltrate pattern, including adult respiratory distress syndrome, cardiac decompensation, cerebral injury, aspiration, pneumonia, fluid overload, pulmonary thromboembolism, renal failure, and sepsis. Less common causes include cardiopulmonary bypass, the effects of various drugs, fat embolism, pulmonary hemorrhage, rapid re-expansion of the lung, and transfusion reactions.[84] Myriad causes of adult respiratory distress syndrome exist, including trauma, sepsis, shock, and pancreatitis. The problem of interpreting the chest x-ray film is that all of the various causes of pulmonary edema may produce an acute, bilaterally symmetric pattern of pulmonary air space disease, the so-called butterfly or batwing appearance. Although the radiographic appearance

of the bilateral infiltrates may be the same, the composition of the edema fluid and the causative pathophysiology of the various types are widely divergent. Permeability edema fluid is caused by damage to the pulmonary microvascular membrane and has a high protein content, similar to that of plasma. Cardiac and volume overload (renal) edema fluid is characterized by low protein content.[85, 86] The radiologist is usually unable to identify the cause of pulmonary edema without appropriate clinical information.

Some authors have suggested that it is possible to classify pulmonary edema by radiographic findings. Milne and coworkers,[1, 3–7, 8] Pistolesi and associates,[2, 74] and Miniati and colleagues[88] identified radiographic criteria to distinguish cardiac, renal (volume overload), and injury lung edema and reported accuracy of 86 to 100% in differentiating these three types of edema.[7, 88] They assessed several variables, including heart shape and size, vascular pedicle width, hilar abnormalities (increased size or density, blurring, nonvisualization), pulmonary blood flow distribution and volume, peribronchial and perivascular cuffing, septal (Kerley's) lines, lung density increase (qualitative distribution and extension), air bronchograms, and the presence or absence of pleural effusion. The distribution of findings for each of the three types of edema is shown in Table 21–1.

The presence of cardiac enlargement was not found to be a significant variable. However, as expected, the heart size was more frequently normal in injury edema (55% of cases) as opposed to cardiac (45%) and renal (42%) edema. A normal width (less than 43 mm) or enlarged vascular pedicle width (greater than 63 mm)[1, 2] is a reliable feature to differentiate cardiac and renal edema from microvascular injury. The pedicle width was usually normal in the latter (Fig. 21–37). Hilar enlargement or increased hilar density or blurring were helpful features to separate cardiac and renal causes from injury edema. The distribution of pulmonary blood flow to superior and inferior lung zones was another factor that helped to distinguish these forms of edema. In injury edema, flow was normal (greater in the inferior regions), whereas flow was balanced in renal edema and inverted in cardiac edema. In injury edema, pulmonary blood volume was normal in 75% of cases and increased in 20% of cases, whereas an opposite pattern was observed for renal edema. Cardiac edema blood volume was decreased in

---

TABLE 21–1

RADIOGRAPHIC FINDINGS IN THREE TYPES OF PULMONARY EDEMA

Injury Lung Edema
Normal heart shape
Few hilar abnormalities
Normal pulmonary blood flow distribution
Absence of septal lines
Rare peribronchovascular cuffs
Rare pleural effusion
Frequent air bronchograms
Patchy increased lung density
Peripheral increased lung density

Renal (Volume Overload) Lung Edema
Enlarged vascular pedicle
Balanced pulmonary blood flow distribution
Increased pulmonary blood volume
Central distribution of increased lung density

Cardiac Lung Edema
Base-to-apex blood flow inversion
Even distribution of increased lung density

Data from Miniati M, Pistolesi M, Paoletti P, et al: Objective radiographic criteria to differentiate cardiac, renal and lung injury edema. Invest Radiol 23:433, 1988.

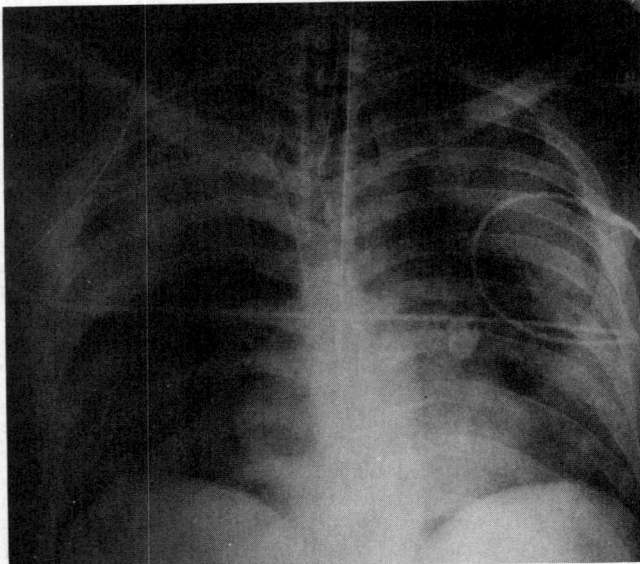

Figure 21–37. Capillary permeability edema. Patchy peripheral infiltrates typical of injury edema are present in patients with adult respiratory distress syndrome.

13%, normal in 48%, and increased in 39%. The presence of peribronchial and perivascular cuffing was also helpful for distinguishing cardiac and renal from injury edema, in which it was less frequently present. Septal lines were present in only cardiac (32%) and renal (21%) edema. Increased lung density was patchy in injury edema and homogeneous for the other two categories (Fig. 21–38). Distribution of the increased density was nearly always bilateral in all patients,

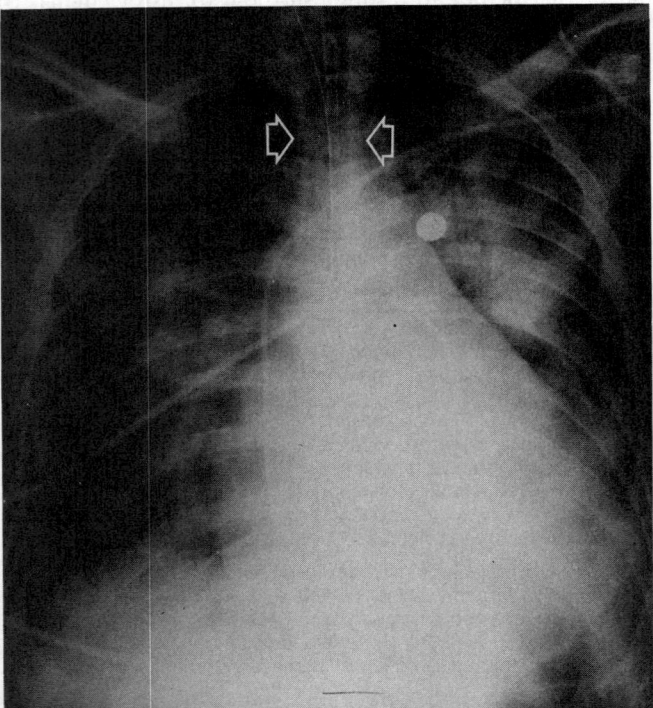

Figure 21–38. Volume overload pulmonary edema. Central, homogeneous perihilar infiltrates are present with a normal vascular pedicle (*open arrows*) in this patient with edema secondary to volume overload. The presence of cardiac enlargement is inaccurate as a predictor of the type of edema.

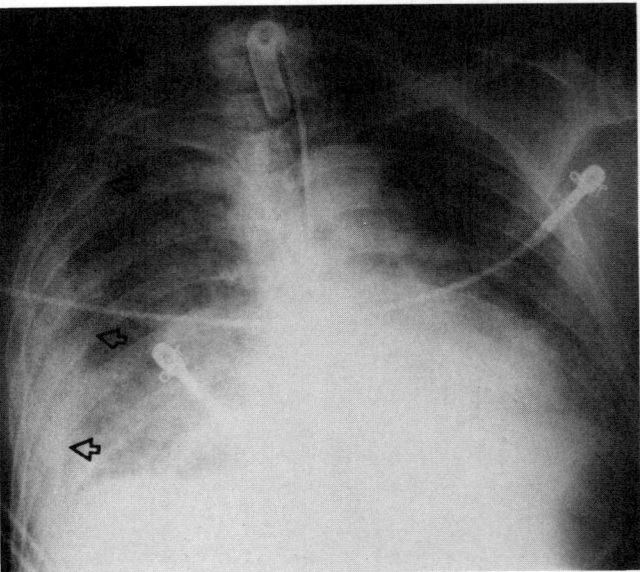

Figure 21–39. Cardiogenic pulmonary edema. Diffuse bilateral parenchymal opacities, cardiac enlargement, and right pleural effusion (*open arrows*) are seen in this radiograph of a patient with cardiogenic pulmonary edema.

except in 20% of patients with injury to the microcirculation. Air bronchograms were most often seen in patients with injury edema, whereas pleural effusions were most common in patients with cardiac edema (Fig. 21–39).

Therefore, a variety of techniques can be utilized in analyzing the radiograph to classify pulmonary edema. These findings may be helpful to separate the three most common types of diffuse pulmonary parenchymal opacities in ICU patients. However, uncommon causes of lung opacities, such as pulmonary hemorrhage and pulmonary alveolar proteinosis,[89, 90] should also be considered, especially when the clinical, biochemical, microbiologic, and radiographic data are atypical. For example, Panicek reported a case of widened mediastinum and interstitial edema attributable not to cardiac or renal disease, but rather to hemorrhage from aortic rupture.[91] Diffuse pulmonary hemorrhage can be difficult to differentiate from diffuse pneumonia or pulmonary edema and may not present with classic hemoptysis and anemia. Albelda and coworkers provided an excellent review and classification of pulmonary hemorrhage.[92] A detailed knowledge of the patient's history before and subsequent to admission may be helpful. Recent bronchoalveolar lavage has been reported to cause areas of consolidation, which can simulate pulmonary edema, aspiration, pneumonitis, or hemorrhage on postprocedure radiographs.[93] The appropriate diagnosis, in many instances, can be suggested by thorough integration of historical and procedural information.

Pleural Disease

Two major conditions that affect the pleural space and are exceedingly common in the ICU patient are pleural effusion and pneumothorax. Pleural effusion is the most common manifestation of pleural pathologic change.[94] Pneumothorax is seen more frequently in the ventilator-dependent ICU patient. The adverse effects of these conditions are potentiated in the patient whose status is already compromised.

Pleural disease is characterized by a homogeneous opacity that usually does not have sharply defined borders. A mobile density from lung base to apex. Massive effusion is a cause for unilateral "whiteout." If the quantity of fluid is large, the lung is displaced from the costal cage (see Fig. 21–39, open arrows). This may be seen at the lateral bases or, occasionally, at the apices. This radiographic pattern is so typical and reproducible that decubitus films often are not necessary for confident diagnosis in most instances. Obtaining additional views, decubitus and semisupine oblique,[97] increases the sensitivity and specificity of supine radiographs, reported to be 67 and 70%, respectively.[98] The use of additional films should be reserved for evaluation of atypical opacities, assessment of fluid mobility, or detection of small fluid collections[99, 100] (Fig. 21–41). Experience with the appearance of layering effusions on supine films should, in most cases, obviate the need for decubitus films to quantify the amount of fluid.

Difficulty arises in the diagnosis of the atypical pleural opacity, which is most often a loculated effusion. Loculation of fluid suggests hemothorax or empyema (Fig. 21–42). However, infected fluid can be mobile (especially early) and sterile fluid can be loculated, but these are less frequent occurrences. If the loculated collection is in the anterior or posterior pleural space, overlying the lung fields, the characteristics of subtle homogeneous opacity without borders should suggest the pleural space as the site of abnormality. However, if visualization is limited by the overlying heart, differentiation of atelectasis and pneumonitis from loculated pleural fluid is often difficult (Fig. 21–43). CT scans, sonograms, or horizontal beam radiographs often clarify the finding (Figs. 21–44 to 21–46).

Ultrasonography is useful for the detection of pleural fluid. However, it is not recommended as a screening test for loculated collections or for small amounts of fluid. Ultrasonography is useful to assess the potential for percutaneous image-guided catheter drainage or tube thoracostomy for a known collection. The size, the location, and the presence or absence of multiple septations may suggest the appropriate mode of therapy. Hirsch and colleagues found

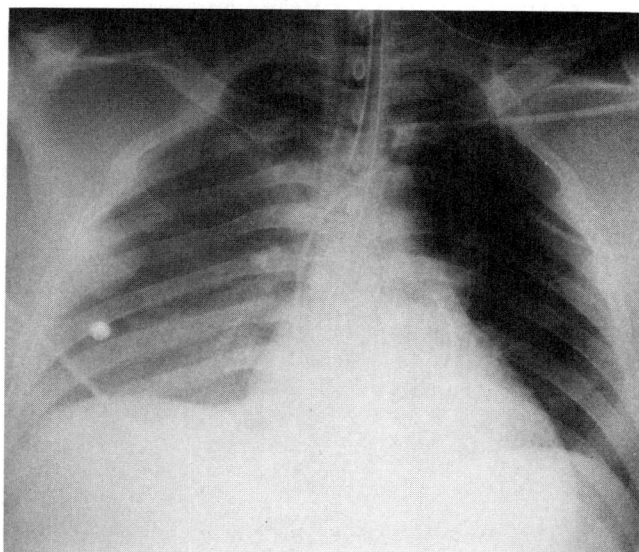

Figure 21–40. Right pleural effusion. Freely layering pleural fluid in the supine patient is characterized by relatively homogeneous opacity, without borders, that fades imperceptibly from base to apex.

pleural effusion has an easily identified meniscus sign on the upright chest radiograph.[95, 96] However, the appearance of a layering effusion in the supine patient is less well known. Therefore, pleural effusion is frequently overlooked on the ICU chest film. Pleural effusion in the supine or semierect patient presents as a homogeneous density, which is greatest at the lung base and fades imperceptibly toward the apex (Fig. 21–40). The density is the same from medial to lateral but typically decreases gradually from caudad to cephalad. The larger the effusion is, the less the decrease in

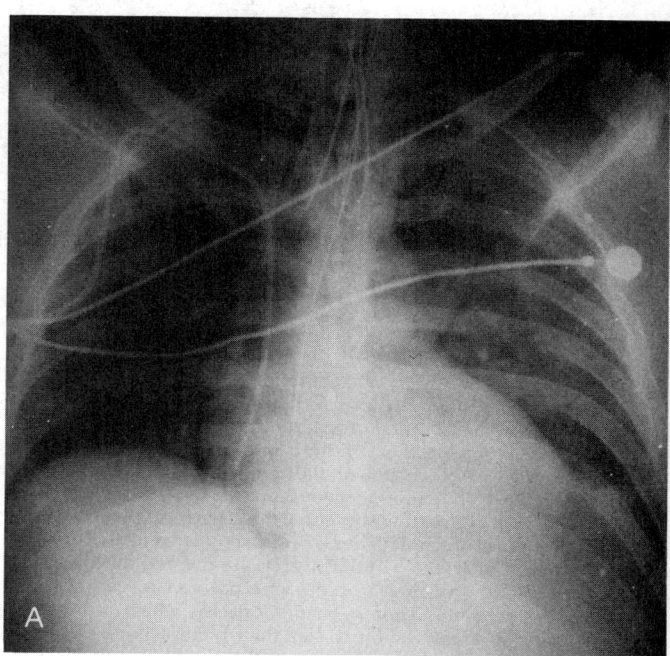
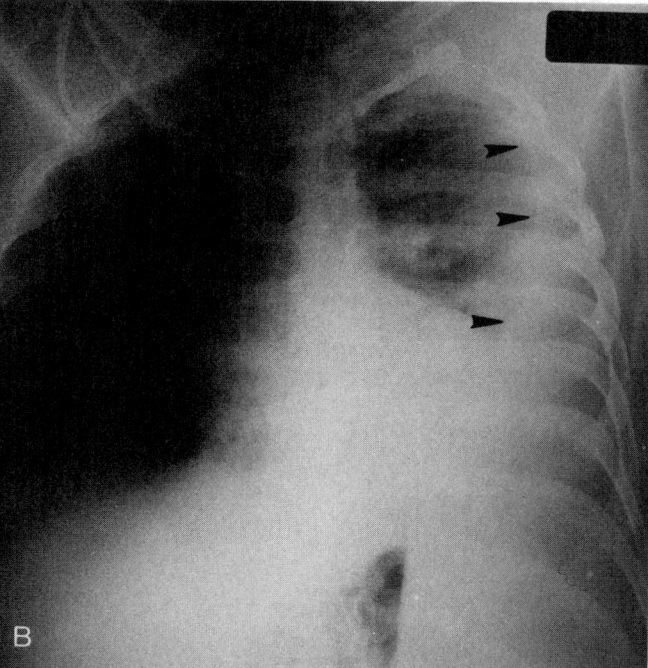

Figure 21–41. Left pleural effusion. *A.* In the supine patient, a pleural effusion on the left presents as a relatively homogeneous unilateral opacity. *B.* Left lateral decubitus film reveals layering of the pleural effusion (*arrowheads*).

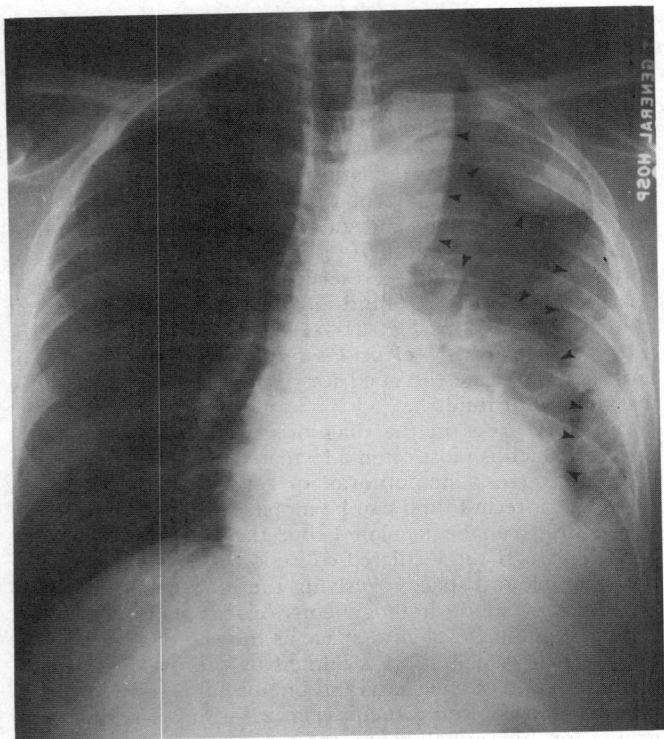

Figure 21–42. Empyema. Multiple lobulated pleura-based masses are identified (*arrowheads*) secondary to empyema caused by pneumococcal pneumonia.

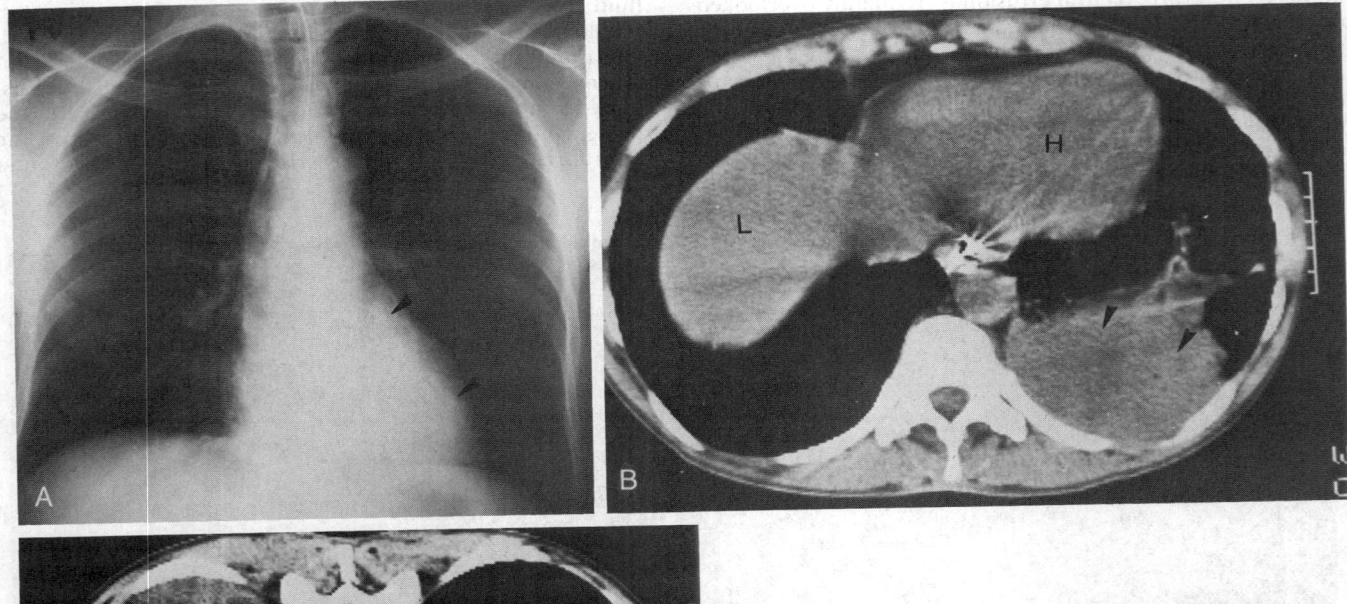

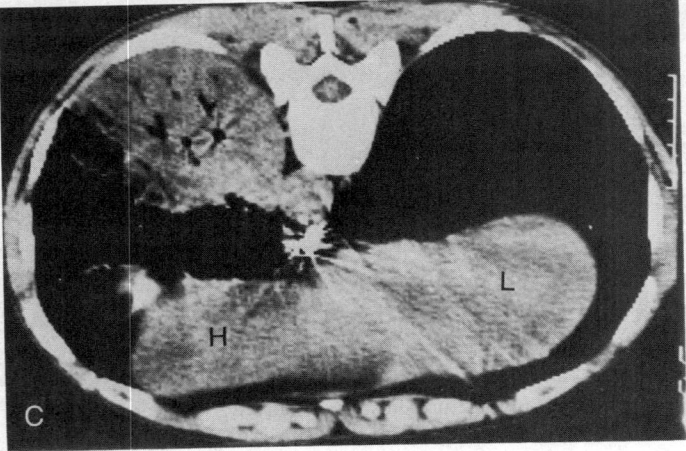

Figure 21–43. Left lower lobe consolidation. *A.* There is increased left retrocardiac opacity (*arrowheads*) suggestive of left lower lobe atelectasis. The absence of silhouetting of the hemidiaphragm raises the suspicion that infiltrate rather than atelectasis may be the cause. *B.* A CT scan of the left hemithorax in the supine position reveals a homogeneous opacity at the left lung base (*arrowheads*), which may be either air space or pleural disease. Renal failure precluded use of intravenous contrast for differentiation. The liver (L) and heart (H) are marked for orientation. *C.* A CT scan obtained in the prone position reveals air within the previously seen homogeneous opacity, which indicates the presence of consolidation rather than pleural fluid. There is a relatively normal distance between the air-filled bronchi, which suggests that consolidation rather than atelectasis is the likely cause.

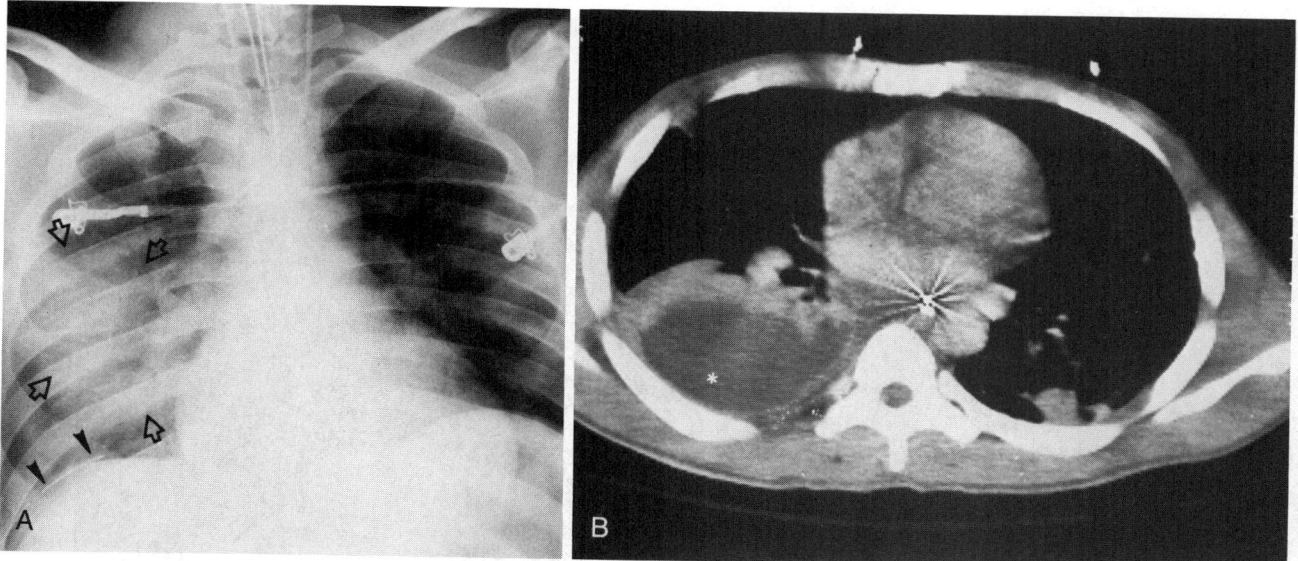

Figure 21–44. Empyema. *A.* A poorly defined opacity without clearly defined borders is seen in the right hemithorax (*open arrows*). Note a chest tube in place at the right base (*arrowheads*). *B.* A CT scan reveals a loculated right posterior empyema (*asterisk*) as a cause for the poorly defined opacity in the right hemithorax seen on the chest radiograph.

that approximately three quarters of septated collections contained exudative fluid; the presence of anechoic fluid did not, however, accurately predict the frequency of an exudate or a transudate.[101] Multiseptated collections are frequently excluded from percutaneous catheter management because of the need for a separate catheter for each space that does not communicate with others. (The interventional radiologist may, however, elect to place several catheters in selected patients.) For similar reasons, tube thoracostomy may fail to achieve adequate drainage, and the patient may require a thoracotomy. Before assigning tube thoracostomy failure to the nature of the pleural fluid collection, accurate identification of the tube position is necessary. If a technically adequate lateral chest x-ray film cannot be obtained, CT may be necessary.[102] A patient for whom thoracotomy is contraindicated or undesirable may be treated by infusion of streptokinase or urokinase into the pleural space. Several studies demonstrated good results with treatment of empyema by this technique.[103–105] Ultrasonography has been accurate in distinguishing pleural from parenchymal disease[44, 106, 107] (see Figs. 21–34, 21–35, and 21–40). However, pleural ultrasonography is laden with pitfalls,[108–110] making accurate diagnosis extremely difficult.

CT is the "gold standard" for the assessment of pleural disease. Nevertheless, there are instances in which differentiation of pleural and parenchymal disease by CT is difficult. Appropriate CT technique (e.g., positioning and contrast medium administration) frequently remedies the problem.[43] It must be emphasized that, in complicated cases, consultation with the radiologist before the examination is essential. The technical adjustments necessary to optimize accurate diagnosis of the specific problem in question should be made so that examination is tailored to the patient. This avoids the necessity of a repeated examination if the technique for the initial study is not suitable to the patient's problem. CT should therefore be used selectively.

Direct physician-to-physician communication is essential when planning such studies. The question of desirability of CT-guided percutaneous catheter drainage should also be discussed in advance with the radiologist. In certain institutions, this may occur through a formal consultation with the interventional radiology service. The interdisciplinary patient management conference should include all of the patient's films and clinical data. CT is a powerful modality

for evaluating pleural disease, but it entails the risks associated with transporting the patient to the CT suite. The desired outcome and potential change in therapy should be carefully assessed before the examination is requested.

Pleural collections on CT are relatively homogeneous, but they may contain air if a gas-forming organism is present. Other causes of gas in a pleural fluid collection include bronchopleural fistula and recent tube thoracostomy or thoracentesis. CT is much less sensitive than ultrasonography for the detection of septations and internal debris within pleural fluid collections. Other CT characteristics of pleural fluid include a lenticular or crescentic shape, forming obtuse angles with the pleural surface and a sharp interface with the lung parenchyma.[45] In addition, pleural fluid does not enhance with intravenous contrast medium administration, although lung parenchyma does enhance.[43] Pleural disease tends to compress the adjacent lung parenchyma (bronchi and vessels) rather than destroy it.[46] The split pleura sign of empyema is caused by visceral and parietal pleural thickening, separation,[46] and contrast enhancement (Fig. 21–47). Intraparenchymal fluid-filled bullae and lung cysts may present difficulties in diagnosis, as their CT appearance may closely simulate that of pleural disease.[47]

Magnetic resonance imaging will likely have a role in evaluation of pleural disease in the future. At this time, however, two factors preclude its use in the critically ill patient. The first is the need for special nonferromagnetic devices to support the patient during image acquisition. The second is significantly increased image acquisition times compared with those for CT. The long data acquisition times not only lead to image degradation because of respiratory motion, but also markedly prolong the duration of the study. This, in turn, increases the time that the patient must be away from the ICU. Nevertheless, with anticipated decreases in acquisition times and development of new monitoring devices, magnetic resonance imaging may hold great promise for future imaging in the ICU patient.

Pneumothorax and Barotrauma

Pneumothorax is also a common finding on the ICU chest radiograph. Pneumothorax occurs in 4.2% of all patients receiving assisted ventilation[111] and in 17% of those receiving positive end-expiratory pressure ventilation.[112] The ICU pa-

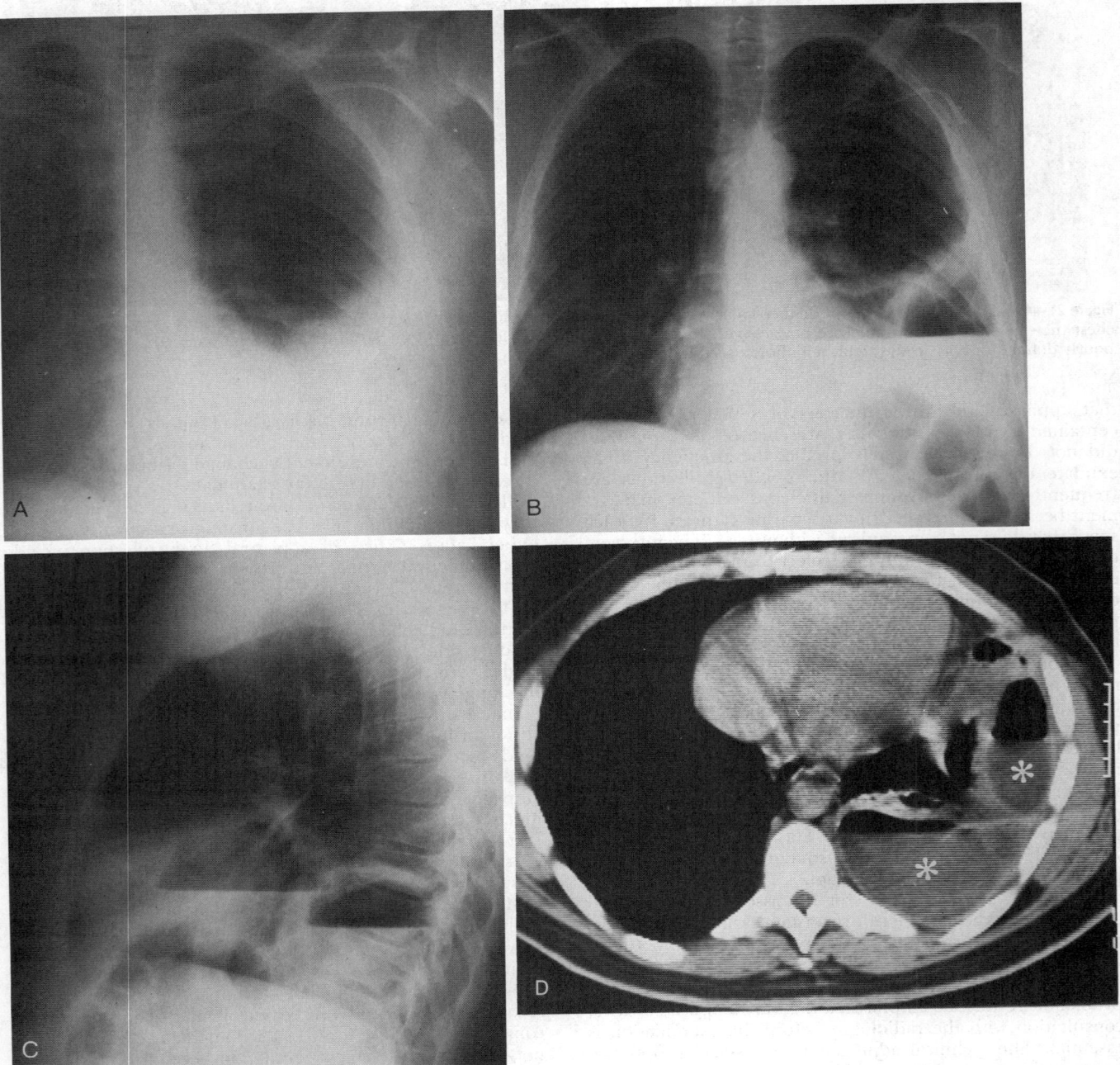

Figure 21–45. Multiloculated empyema. *A.* Homogeneous opacity at the left lung base representing pleural fluid. *B* and *C.* Upright posteroanterior and lateral views of the chest reveal the multiloculated nature of the empyema with multiple clearly defined air-fluid levels. *D.* A CT scan of the left hemithorax defines the multiloculated gas and fluid-containing collections (*asterisks*).

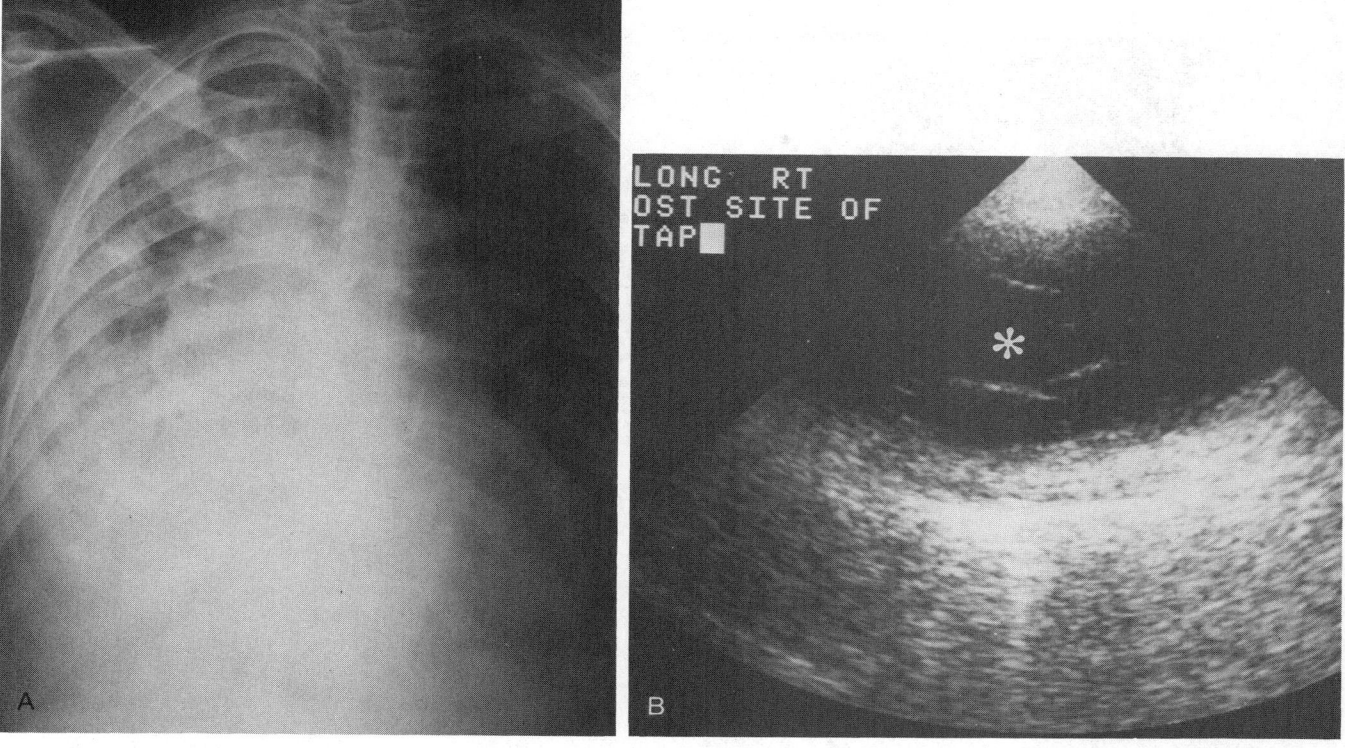

Figure 21–46. *A*. Loculated right pleural effusion. Homogeneous and inhomogeneous opacities in the right hemithorax in a rotated patient make differentiation among pleural fluid, atelectasis, and air space disease impossible. *B*. A real-time ultrasound image of the right chest reveals a significant multiseptated pleural fluid collection (*asterisk*).

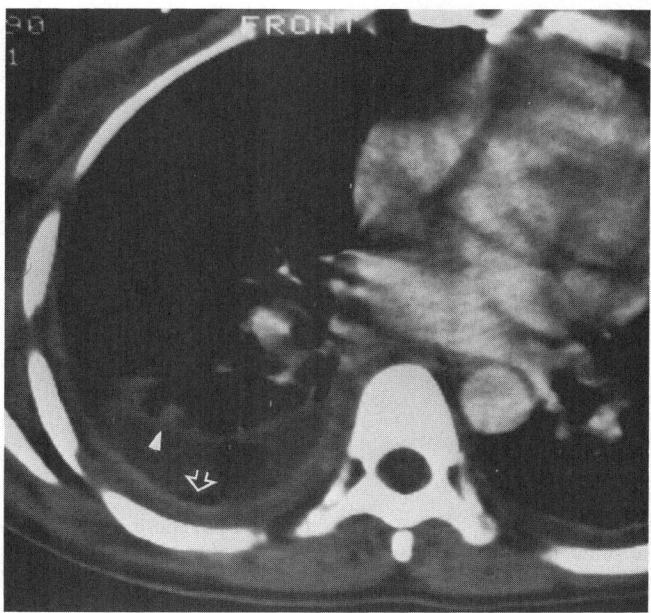

Figure 21–47. The split pleura sign of empyema. Inflamed visceral (*arrowhead*) and parietal (*open arrow*) pleura appear split or separated by the infected pleural fluid.

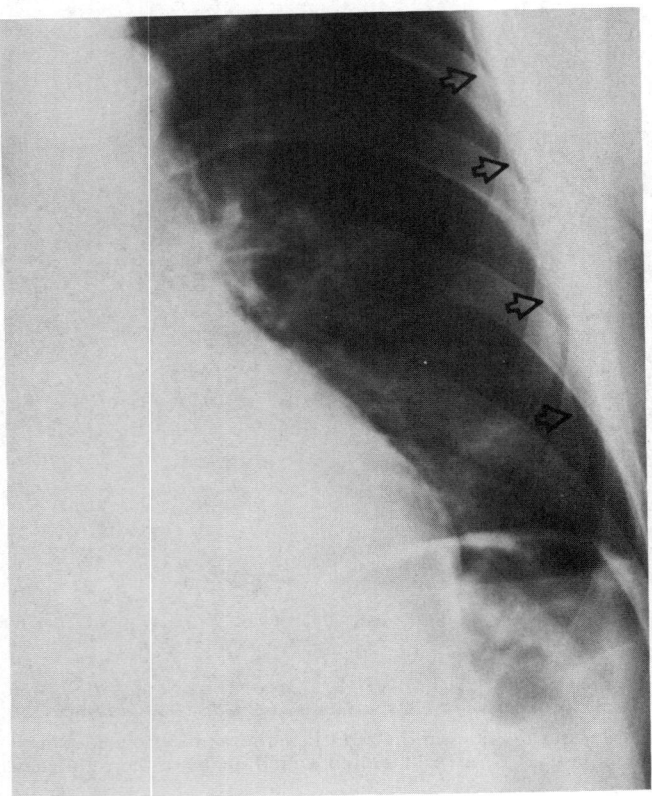

Figure 21–48. Spontaneous pneumothorax. Note the thin white line of the visceral pleura (*open arrows*) that marks this left pneumothorax.

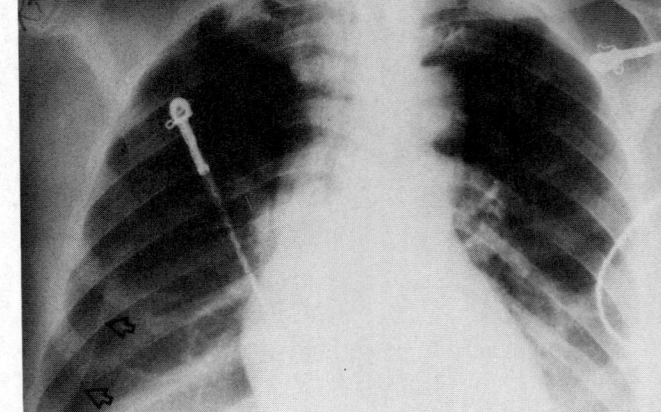

Figure 21–49. Hydropneumothorax. In the supine position the typical air-fluid level is not present. Only subtle density change and the visceral pleura line (*open arrows*) may be seen.

tient is predisposed to pneumothorax by the frequency of catheter placement as well as by barotrauma. In the upright chest film, the findings of pneumothorax are well known. A reliable indicator of pneumothorax is the presence of a thin white line marginating the lung. The thin white line is caused by tangential imaging of the visceral pleura. It can be clearly seen as a white line (less than 1 mm), which courses through the expected path of the collapsed lung margin and is outlined by air in the pneumothorax space peripherally and air in the lung centrally (Fig. 21–48). The thin white line (the visceral pleura) disappears when the pneumothorax is so great that the alveoli are collapsed and all air has been excluded from the adjacent lung. In such a case, the lung is small and dense, and the pneumothorax space is large and lucent. The relative lucency peripheral to the visceral pleural line may be absent in the supine film if pleural fluid coexists

with the pneumothorax (Fig. 21–49). In radiographs obtained with the patient in the upright position, hydropneumothorax is identified by the presence of an air-fluid level in the pleural space.

The frequency of pneumothorax in the supine patient in the ICU is greater than the frequency with which it is identified by portable chest radiography. It is not unusual to detect an abnormal collection of air on the chest film and have its cause undetermined for several days before its characteristics become such that the correct diagnosis is suggested. The increasing use of thoracic CT has revealed many previously unsuspected pneumothoraces, some of which are quite large (Fig. 21–50). CT shows unusual air collections to be clearly pleural or parenchymal, and it also demonstrates collections of gas not identified at all on the chest x-ray film. Curiosity as to the location of an unusual

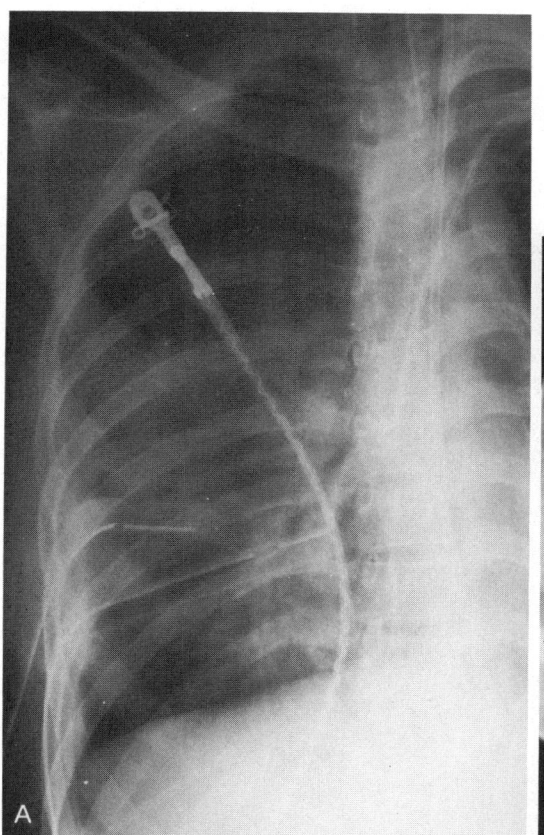
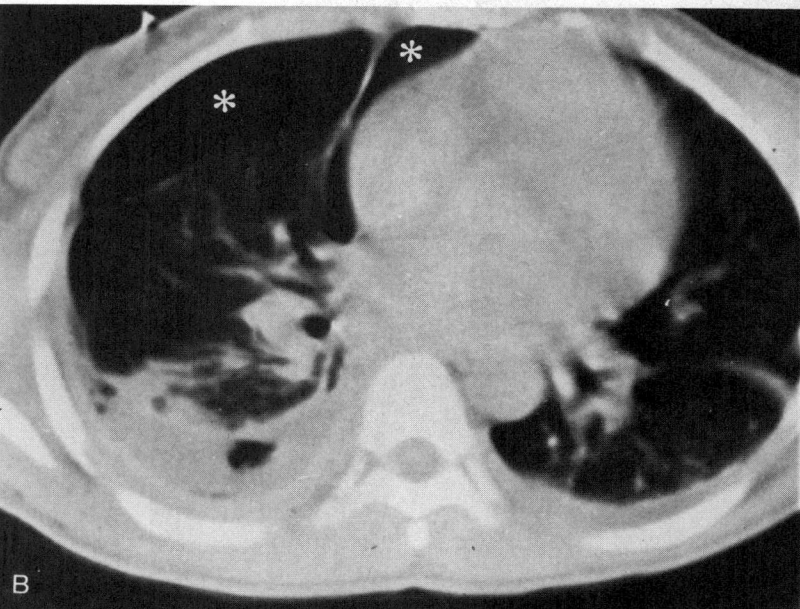

Figure 21–50. *A.* Imperceptible pneumothorax. With two thoracostomy tubes in place, the supine film fails to reveal evidence of pneumothorax. *B.* A large anterior pneumothorax is identified on the CT scan (*asterisks*) of the patient in *A.*

lucency is, however, a doubtful indication for CT, except in selected cases. The radiologist is able to answer the majority of questions raised by the plain film without the use of cross-sectional imaging. Familiarity with the appearance of atypical pneumothoraces increases the frequency of accurate diagnosis from the chest film.

In the supine view, the classic radiographic findings of pneumothorax are unchanged, but the location of the pneumothorax is different from that on the upright film. This may cause problems in the identification of the pneumothorax. The radiographic anatomy and appearance of pneumothorax in a supine patient have been clearly described by Tocino.[113] In the supine position, the most anterior (highest) portion of the thorax is near the lung bases (Fig. 21–51) and the sternum (Fig. 21–52). Because pneumothorax air rises to the highest location in the chest, the lung bases and

medial paracardiac locations should be closely scrutinized for a thin white line and a paucity of lung markings. The air may layer over the anterior lung surface, just deep to the anterior costal cage, similar to posterior layering of pleural fluid. Unfortunately, an anterior collection of air projected over air-filled lung is often virtually imperceptible. Lateral, cross-table lateral, or supine oblique lateral films may be helpful, as may CT,[114] to make the diagnosis in this setting (Fig. 21–53).

Because most chest tubes are in the posterior portion of the chest, the thoracostomy tube often does not drain anterior air. When unsuspected pneumothorax exists, an unsuspected tension pneumothorax may also exist. For this reason, evaluation of the location of the heart, the mediastinum, and the diaphragm is essential on every film, even if there is no evidence of pneumothorax. It must be emphasized

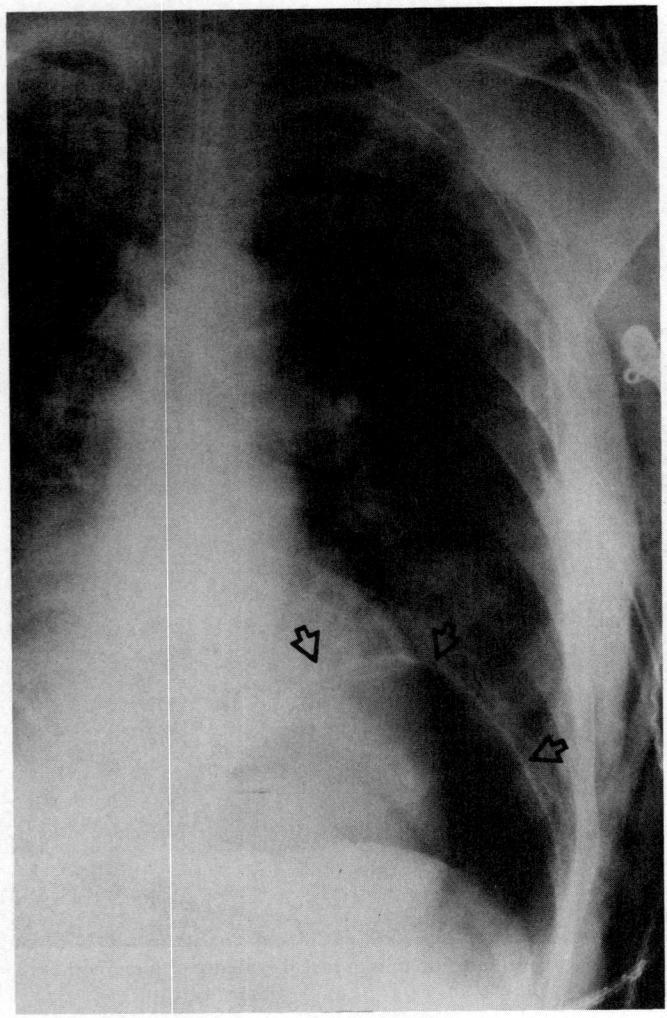

Figure 21–51. Basilar pneumothorax. Large radiolucent collection is identified at the left base and is bounded by a thin white line (*open arrows*) identifying a large left basilar pneumothorax.

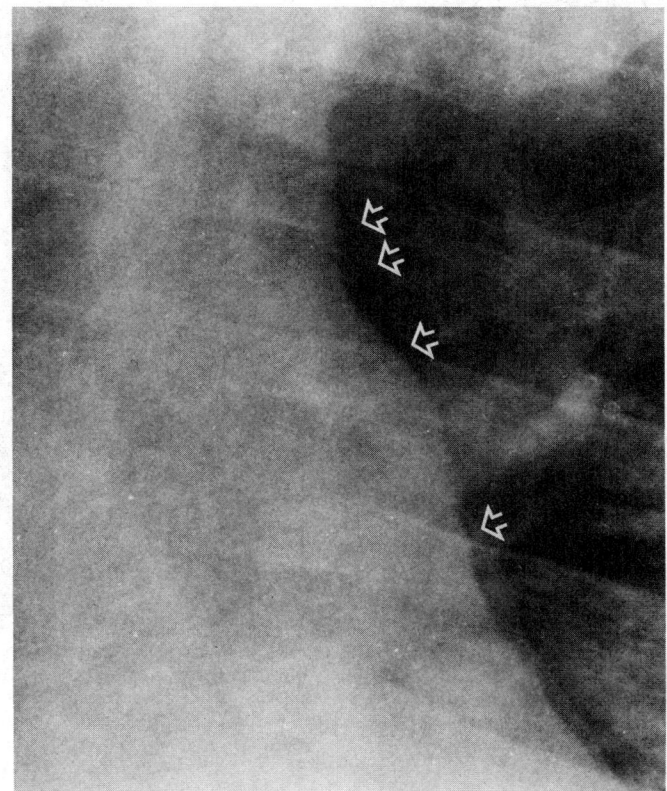

Figure 21–52. Medial pneumothorax. Coned-down view of the area of the aortic arch reveals a paucity of markings medially and a thin white line (*open arrows*) indicating a small medial pneumothorax.

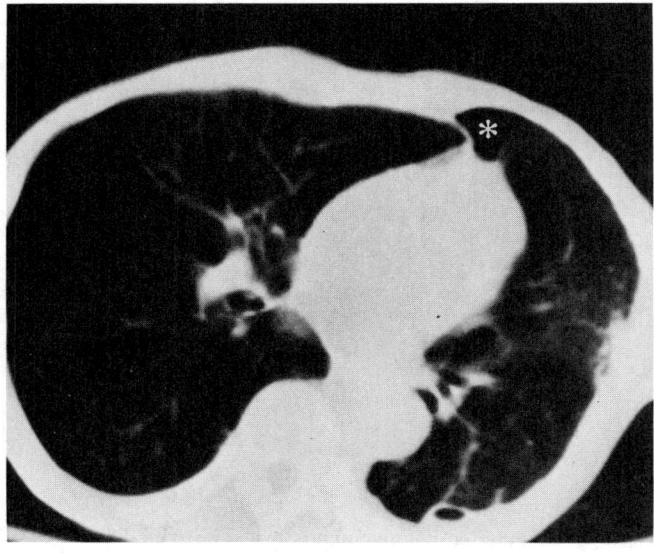

Figure 21–53. Medial pneumothorax. There is a radiolucent region anteromedially on the left (*asterisk*) indicating a small medial pneumothorax. Note the thin white line adjacent to the pneumothorax.

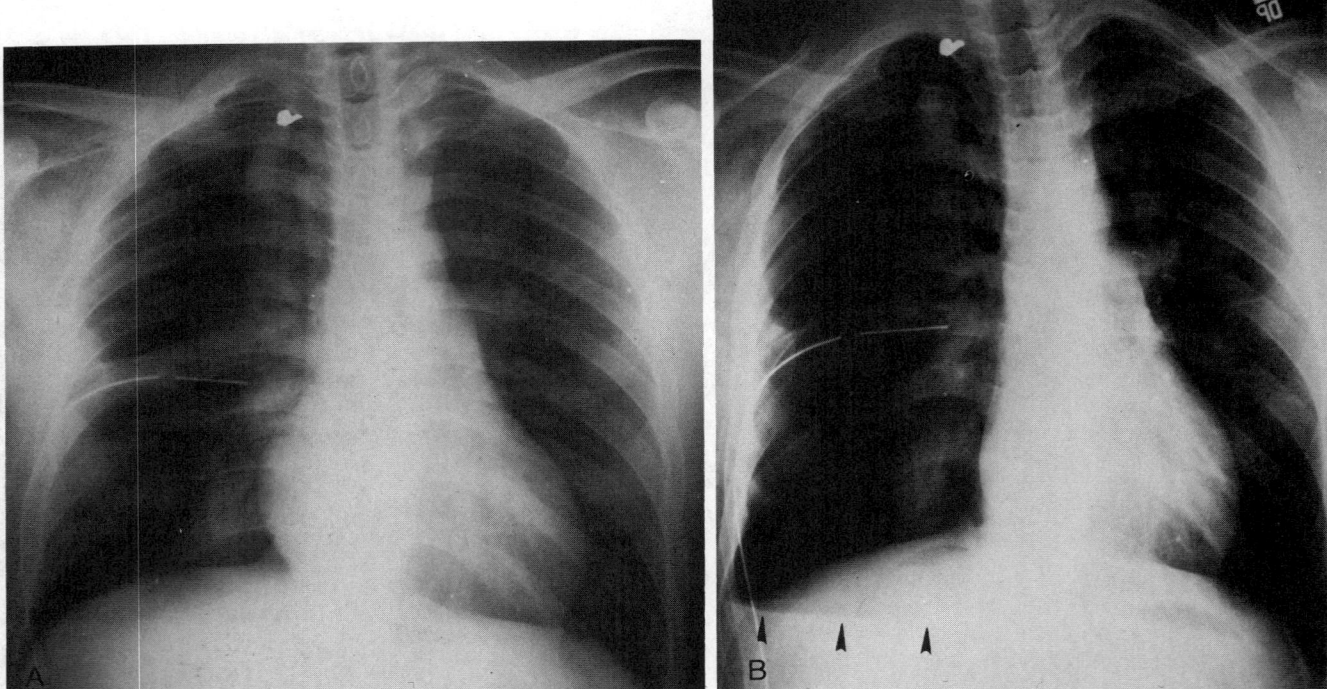

Figure 21–54. Tension hydropneumothorax. *A.* With a right thoracostomy tube in place, there is no evidence of pneumothorax or hydrothorax. Only subtle depression of the right hemidiaphragm and shift of the heart to the left are evident. *B.* In the upright position the air-fluid level left at the right base (*arrowheads*) indicates the presence of hydropneumothorax. There is an increased shift of the heart and mediastinum to the left in spite of the patient's being rotated to the right.

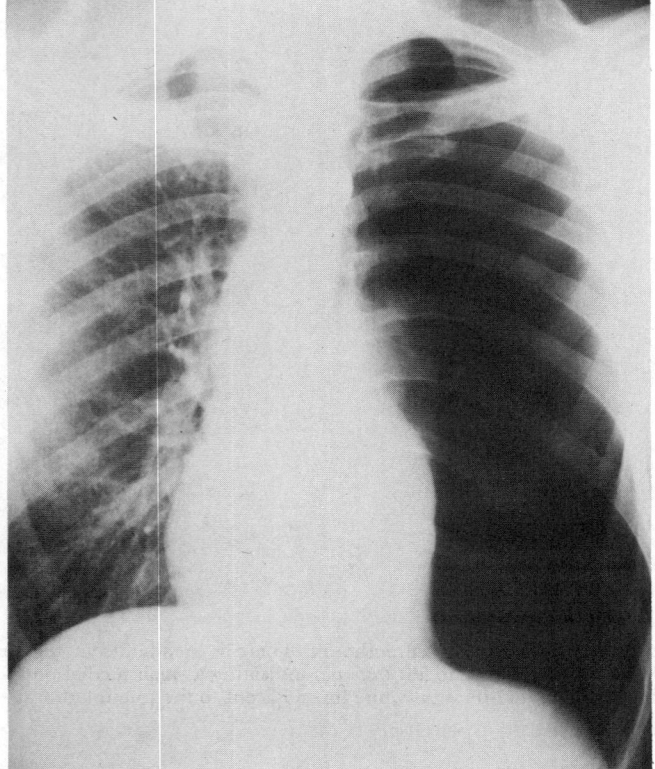

Figure 21–55. Left tension pneumothorax. The typical findings of tension pneumothorax include depression of the hemidiaphragm and shift of the heart and the mediastinum contralaterally. Note also the ipsilateral splaying of the ribs.

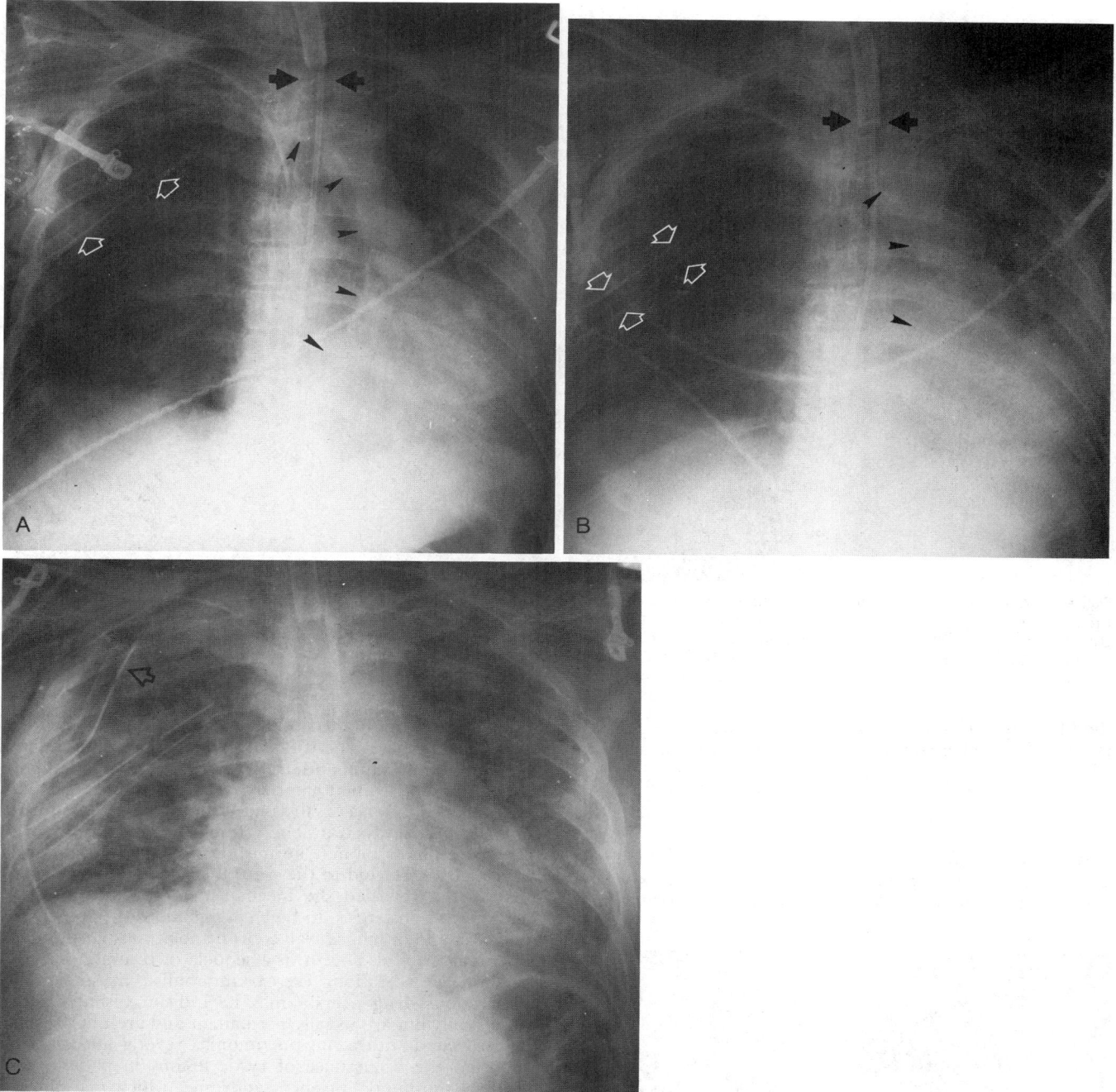

Figure 21–56. Tension pneumothorax. *A.* With a right chest tube (*open arrows*) in place, shift of the heart and the mediastinum (*filled arrows*) to the left, increased lucency over the right diaphragm, and herniation of the right lung across the midline (*arrowheads*) are noted. *B.* After placement of a second chest tube, there is no change. *C.* Resolved tension pneumothorax. A lateral view revealed the two initial right thoracostomy tubes to reside in the major fissure (note their straight configuration). After insertion of an anterior thoracostomy tube (*open arrow*), the right hemidiaphragm, heart, trachea, and right lung have returned to normal.

that the presence of multiple thoracostomy tubes does not preclude the presence of life-threatening tension pneumothorax (Fig. 21–54). It is noted that tension pneumothorax is first and foremost a clinical diagnosis in an unstable patient. If there is a strong suspicion of a tension pneumothorax on the basis of clinical criteria, the intensivist should insert chest tubes before radiographic confirmation is obtained.

The radiographic findings of tension pneumothorax are similar to those of massive pleural effusion, except that a mass effect is exerted by the radiolucent air instead of the radiopaque pleural fluid. The heart and the mediastinum are shifted contralaterally, and the ipsilateral diaphragm is displaced downward (Fig. 21–55). The heart size is often decreased beyond the 1-cm difference in cardiac diameter that occurs between systole and diastole. It is important to note that the pneumothorax itself need not be seen and that the presence of chest tubes does not exclude the presence of tension pneumothorax (Fig. 21–56). If tension pneumothorax is present, it is more likely to be near the lung bases or the heart. Owing to depression of the adjacent diaphragm by the mass effect, the diaphragm may not be included on

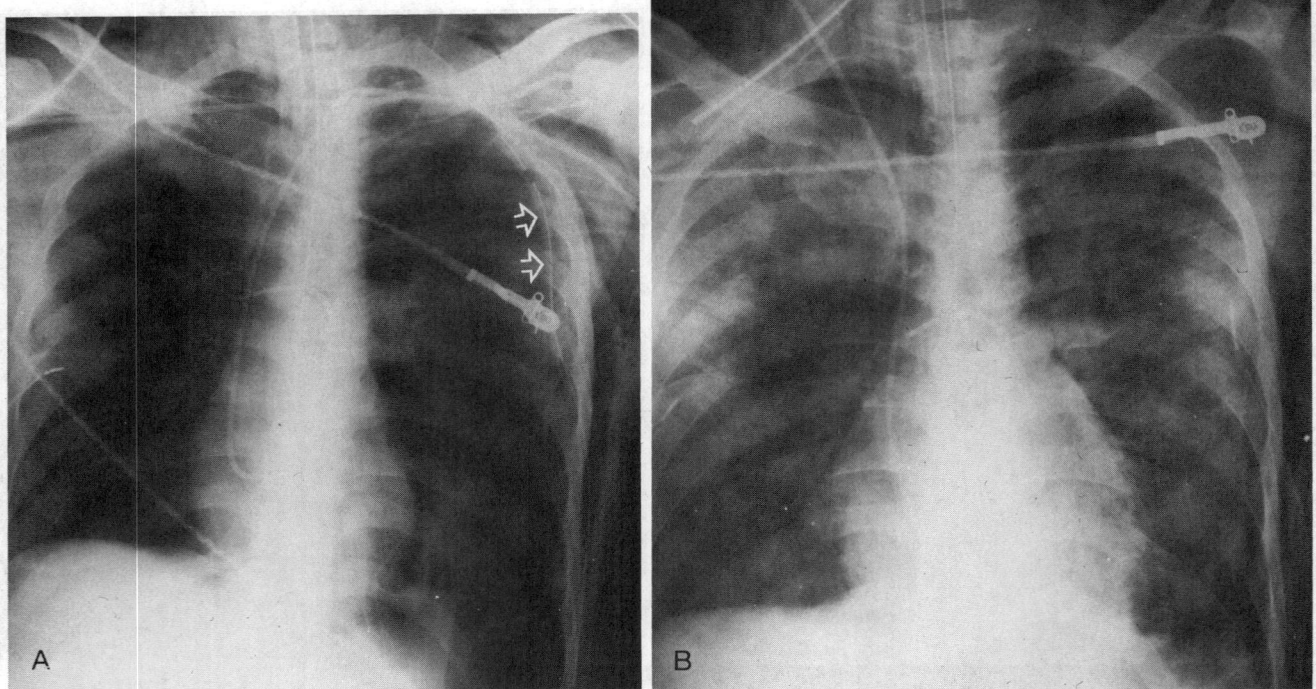

Figure 21–57. Tension pneumothorax. *A.* With a left thoracostomy tube in place (*open arrows*), depression of the hemidiaphragm and shift of the heart and mediastinum to the right are seen. Note also the compressed heart. This patient presented with signs of pericardial tamponade. *B.* After manipulation of the left thoracostomy tube, the left hemidiaphragm returns to a more normal location. The heart and mediastinum are now also in a normal location and the heart size has also returned to normal.

the film (Fig. 21–57). Tension effect may also be seen from large bullae, which trap air by a ball valve mechanism (Fig. 21–58).

Pneumatocele

Whenever an unusual lucency is projected over the lungs, the question of its location should be raised. A thick-walled cavitary lesion may be clearly parenchymal in origin, but

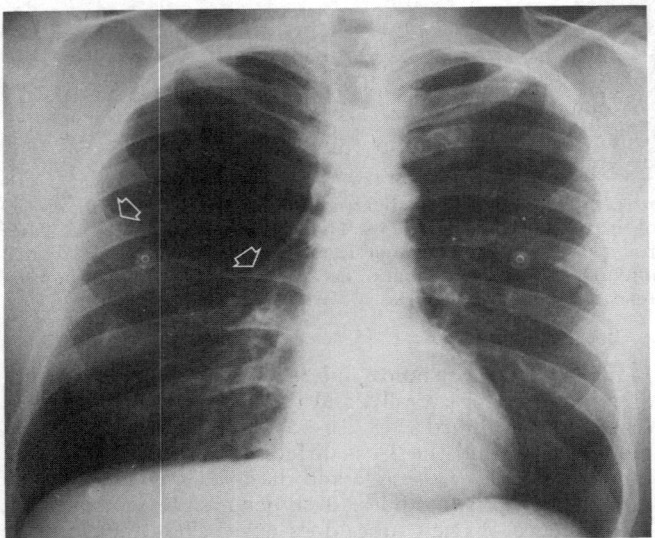

Figure 21–58. Tension effect caused by a large bulla. There is a large bulla in the right upper lobe with a white line forming its inferior margin (*open arrows*). Note the shift of the heart to the left despite mild rightward patient rotation.

other round, thin-walled pulmonary cystic lesions may present greater diagnostic difficulty. They may be thought to be pleural in location and, thus, are briefly mentioned here.

A pulmonary pneumatocele is a thin-walled, gas-filled space that usually occurs in association with acute pneumonia and is almost always transient.[115] It may be overlooked during the acute illness or may be misinterpreted as an abnormal air collection related to the pleural space. Pathologic examination has revealed the mechanism of production, in at least certain instances, to be a combination of parenchymal necrosis and/or check valve bronchiolar obstruction.[116–119] Pneumatoceles also occur as a sequela of trauma, especially pulmonary laceration. Pre-existing bullae in smokers or intravenous drug users[120] may be indistinguishable radiographically but are usually permanent and are not necessarily associated with acute pneumonia. Several authors have reported the occurrence of cystic lesions in patients with acquired immunodeficiency syndrome, which may or may not be related to *P. carinii* pneumonia.[121–124]

Unusual rounded or irregular lucencies may be projected over the lung fields. They may represent loculated areas of pneumothorax or collections of gas within the parenchyma. If the location of such a collection critically affects therapy, CT is often necessary.

CONCLUSION

Common pathologic changes cause reproducible and understandable radiographic findings. Thoughtful consideration of the pathologic change suspected and the susceptible anatomy makes it possible to anticipate the radiographic appearance. The vital link between physics and radiology is that gravity and wave theory always act consistently. Just as a systematic approach to the clinical condition of the patient is a reflex action at the bedside, a systematic, careful approach to the film is the sine qua non of accurate diagnosis.

References

1. Milne ENC, Pistolesi M, Miniati M, et al: The vascular pedicle of the heart and the vena azygous. I. The normal subject. Radiology 152:1, 1984.
2. Pistolesi M, Milne ENC, Miniati M, et al: The vascular pedicle and the vena azygous. II. In cardiac failure. Radiology 152:9, 1984.
3. Milne ENC, Burnett K, Aufrichtig D, et al: Evaluating cardiac size on portable films (abstract). Invest Radiol 17:52, 1982.
4. Milne ENC: Physiologic interpretation of the chest radiograph. In: Margulis A, Gooding CA (eds): Diagnostic Radiology. San Francisco, University of California Press, p 201, 1980.
5. Milne ENC: Pulmonary patterns in heart disease. In: Partridge JA (ed): A Textbook of Radiologic Diagnosis, Volume 2, The Cardiovascular System. London, HK Lewis, 1985.
6. Milne ENC: Chest radiology in the surgical patient. Surg Clin North Am 60:1503, 1980.
7. Milne ENC, Pistolesi M, Miniati M, et al: The radiologic distinction of cardiogenic and non-cardiogenic edema. AJR 144:879, 1985.
8. Spirin PW: Chest radiography of intensive care patients. Presented at Radiological Society of North America, Chicago, IL, December 1990.
9. Goodman LR, Foley WD, Wilson CR, et al: Pneumothorax and other lung diseases: Effect of altered resolution and edge enhancement on diagnosis with digitized radiographs. Radiology 167:83, 1988.
10. Henschke GI, Pasternak GS, Schroeder S, et al: Bedside chest radiography: Diagnostic efficacy. Radiology 149:23, 1983.
11. Janower ML, Jennas-Nocera Z, Mukai J: Utility and efficacy of portable chest radiographs. AJR 142:265, 1984.
12. Bekemeyer WB, Crapo RO, Calhoon S et al: Efficacy of chest radiography in a respiratory intensive care unit. A prospective study. Chest 88:691, 1985.
13. Braman SS, Dunn SM, Amico CA: Complications of intrahospital transport in critically ill patients. Ann Intern Med 107:469, 1987.
14. Smith GM, Reed JC, Choplin RH: Radiographic detection of esophageal malposition of endotracheal tubes. AJR 154:23, 1990.
15. Woodall BH, Winfield DF, Bissett GS III: Inadvertent tracheobronchial placement of feeding tubes. Radiology 165:727, 1987.
16. Wheeler PS: Feeding tubes that pierce the lung: A case study in risk prevention and quality assurance (editorial). Radiology 165:861, 1987.
17. Ziess J, Woldenberg LS: Letter to the editor. Radiology 168:874, 1988.
18. Ghahremani GG: Complications due to inadvertent tracheobronchial placement of feeding tubes (letter). Radiology 167:875, 1988.
19. Ghahremani GG: Complications of gastrointestinal intubation. In: Meyers MA, Ghahremani GG (eds): Iatrogenic Gastrointestinal Complications. New York, Springer-Verlag, p 65, 1981.
20. Gould RJ, Ghahremani GG: Radiographic spectrum of complications associated with enteral feeding tubes (abstract). Invest Radiol 19:476, 1984.
21. Ghahremani GG, Gould RJ: Nasoenteric feeding tubes: Radiographic detection of complications. Dig Dis Sci 31:574, 1986.
22. Miller KS, Tomlinson JR, Sahn SA: Pleuropulmonary complications of enteral feeding tube feedings: Two reports, review of the literature, and recommendations. Chest 88:320, 1985.
23. Gelfand DW, Ott DJ: Inadvertent pulmonary placement of feeding tubes (letter). Radiology 167:283, 1988.
24. McLean GK, Meranze SG, Burke DR: Enteric alimentation: A radiologic approach. Radiology 160:555, 1986.
25. McLean GK, Meranze SG, Burke DR: Inadvertent tracheobronchial placement of feeding tubes (letter). Radiology 170:278, 1989.
26. Puri VK, Carlson RW, Bander JJ, et al: Complications of vascular catheterization in the critically ill: A prospective study. Crit Care Med 8:495, 1980.
27. Sznajder JI, Zveibil FR, Bitterman H: Central vein catheterization, failure and complication rates by three percutaneous approaches. Arch Intern Med 146:259, 1986.
28. Hyson EA, Ravin CE, Kelley MJ, et al: Intra-aortic counterpulsation balloon: Radiographic considerations. AJR 128:915, 1977.
29. Conrardy PA, Goodman LR, Lainge F, et al: Alteration of endotracheal tube position. Flexion and extension of the neck. Crit Care Med 4:8, 1986.
30. Holbert JM, Libshitz HI, Chasen MH, et al: The postlobectomy chest: Anatomic considerations. Radiographics 7:889, 1987.
31. Kleinman PK, Raptopoulos V: The anterior diaphragmatic attachments: An anatomy and radiologic study with clinical correlates. Radiology 155:289, 1985.
32. Felson B: Chest Roentgenology. Philadelphia, WB Saunders, 1973.
33. Marini JJ, Pierson DJ, Hudson LD: Acute lobar atelectasis: A prospective comparison of fiberoptic bronchoscopy and respiratory therapy. Am Rev Respir Dis 119:971, 1979.
34. Don C, Desmarais R: Peripheral upper lobe collapse in adults. Radiology 170:657, 1989.
35. Felson B: Lung torsion: Radiographic findings in nine cases. Radiology 162:631, 1987.
36. Moser ES, Proto AV: Lung torsion: Case report and literature review. Radiology 162:639, 1987.
37. Morimoto S, Takeuchi N, Imanaka H, et al: Gravity-dependent atelectasis: Radiologic, physiologic and pathologic correlation in rabbits on high-frequency oscillation ventilation. Invest Radiol 24:522, 1989.
38. Adler J, Cameron DC: CT correlation in peripheral right upper lobe collapse. J Comput Assist Tomogr 12:510, 1988.
39. Saterfiel JL, Virapongse C, Clore FC: Computed tomography of combined right upper and middle lobe collapse. Comput Assist Tomogr 12:383, 1988.
40. Paling MR, Griffin GK: Lower lobe collapse due to pleural effusion: A CT analysis. J Comput Assist Tomogr 9:1079, 1985.
41. Federle MP, Mark AS, Guillaumin ES: CT of subpulmonic pleural effusions and atelectasis: Criteria for differentiation from subphrenic fluid. AJR 146:685, 1986.
42. Malmgren N, Laurin S, Ivancev K, et al: Mediastinal pseudomass: Pneumonia and atelectasis behind the left pulmonary ligament. Pediatr Radiol 17:451, 1987.
43. Bressler EL, Francis IR, Glazer GM, et al: Bolus contrast medium enhancement for distinguishing pleural from parenchymal lung disease. J Comput Assist Tomogr 11:436, 1987.
44. Acunas B, Celik L, Acunas A: Chest sonography. Differentiation of pulmonary consolidation from pleural disease. Acta Radiol 30:273, 1989.
45. Pugatch RD, Faling LJ, Robbins AH, et al: Differentiation of pleural and pulmonary lesions using computed tomography. J Comput Assist Tomogr 2:601, 1978.
46. Starr DD, Federle MP, Goodman PC, et al: Differentiating lung abscess and empyema: Radiography and computed tomography. AJR 141:163, 1983.
47. Zinn WL, Naidich DP, Whelan CA, et al: Fluid within preexisting pulmonary air-spaces: A potential pitfall in the CT differentiation of pleural from parenchymal disease. J Comput Assist Tomogr 11:441, 1987.
48. Woodring JH: Determining the cause of pulmonary atelectasis: A comparison of plain radiography and CT. AJR 150:757, 1988.
49. Glazer HS, Anderson DJ, Sagel SS: Bronchial impaction in lobar collapse: CT demonstration and pathologic correlation. AJR 153:485, 1989.
50. Pham DH, Huang D, Korwan A, et al: Acute unilateral pulmonary nonventilation due to mucous plugs. Radiology 165:135, 1987.
51. Schneider HJ, Felson B, Gonzales LL: Rounded atelectasis. AJR 134:225, 1980.
52. Woodring JH: Round atelectasis. Australas Radiol 31:144, 1987.
53. Doyle TC, Lawler GA: CT features of rounded atelectasis of the lung. AJR 143:225, 1984.
54. McHugh K, Blaquiere RM: CT features of rounded atelectasis. AJR 153:257, 1989.
55. Ren H, Hruban RH, Kuhlman JE, et al: CT of rounded atelectasis. J Comput Assist Tomogr 12:1031, 1989.
56. Wagner RB, Crawford WO, Schimpf PP: Classification of parenchymal injuries of the lung. Radiology 167:77, 1988.
57. Shild HH, Strunk H, Weber W, et al: Pulmonary contusion: CT versus plain radiograms. J Comput Assist Tomogr 13:417, 1989.
58. Hedlund LW, Vock P, Effmann EL, et al: Hydrostatic pulmonary edema. An analysis of lung density changes by computed tomography. Invest Radiol 19:254, 1984.
59. Haponic EF, Britt EJ, Smith PL, et al: Computed chest tomography in the evaluation of hemoptysis. Chest 91:80, 1987.
60. DeLorenzo LJ, Huang CT, Maguire GP, et al: Roentgenographic patterns of Pneumocystis carinii pneumonia in 104 patients with AIDS. Chest 91:323, 1987.
61. Joffe N: Roentgenologic findings in post shock and postoperative pulmonary insufficiency. Radiology 94:369, 1970.
62. Greene RE: Acute respiratory failure and the adult respiratory distress syndrome. In: Taveras J, Ferrucci JT (eds): Radiology, Volume 1. Philadelphia, JB Lippincott, p 1, 1986.
63. Rubin SA: Radiology of immunologic diseases of the lung. J Thorac Imaging 3(2):21, 1988.
64. van Buchem MA, Wondergem JH, Kool LJS, et al: Pulmonary leukostasis: Radiologic-pathologic study. Radiology 165:739, 1987.
65. Silver SF, Grymaloski MR, Bosken CH, et al: Clinico-radiologic pathologic conference: Pulmonary consolidation with an air crescent sign in an immunocompromised woman. J Can Assoc Radiol 40:167, 1989.
66. Bachofen H, Bachofen M, Weibel ER: Ultrastructural aspects of pulmonary edema. J Thorac Imaging 3(3):1, 1988.
67. Staub NC: New concepts about the pathophysiology of pulmonary edema. J Thorac Imaging 3(3):8, 1988.
68. Greene R: Adult respiratory distress syndrome: Acute alveolar damage. Radiology 163:57, 1987.
69. Basran GS, Hardy JG: Monitoring pulmonary vascular permeability using radiolabelled transferrin. J Thorac Imaging 3(3):28, 1988.
70. Giuntini C, Pistolesi M, Miniati M, et al: Theoretical and practical considerations of measuring extravascular lung water. J Thorac Imaging 3(3):34, 1988.
71. Petty TL, Silvers GW, Paul GW, et al: Abnormalities in lung elastic properties and surfactant function in adult respiratory distress syndrome. Chest 75:571, 1979.

72. Fein A, Grossman RF, Jones JG, et al: Evaluation of transthoracic electrical impedance in the diagnosis of pulmonary edema. Circulation 60:1156, 1979.
73. Gamsu G, Kauffman L, Swann SJ, et al: Absolute lung density in experimental canine pulmonary edema. Invest Radiol 14:261, 1979.
74. Pistolesi M, Giuntini C: Assessment of extravascular lung water. Radiol Clin North Am 16:551, 1978.
75. Lewis FR, Elings VB, Sturm JA: Bedside measurement of lung water. J Surg Res 27:250, 1979.
76. Carlson RW, Schaffer RC, Michaels GS, et al: Pulmonary edema fluid: Spectrum of features in 37 patients. Circulation 60:1161, 1979.
77. Milne ENC: A physiological approach to reading critical care unit films. J Thorac Imaging 1(3):60, 1986.
78. Aberle DR, Wiener-Kronish JP, Webb WR, et al: Hydrostatic versus increased permeability pulmonary edema: Diagnosis based on radiographic criteria in critically ill patients. Radiology 168:73, 1988.
79. Milne ENC: Hydrostatic versus increased permeability pulmonary edema (letter). Radiology 170:891, 1989.
80. Aberle DR, Wiener-Kronish JP, Mattay MA, et al: Hydrostatic versus increased permeability pulmonary edema (letter). Radiology 170:892, 1989.
81. Halperin BD, Feley TW, Mihm FG, et al: Evaluation of the portable chest roentgenogram for quantitating extravascular lung water in critically ill adults. Chest 88:649, 1985.
82. Wegenius G, Erikson U, Borg T, et al: Value of chest radiography in adult respiratory distress syndrome. Acta Radiol [Diagn] 25:177, 1984.
83. Gattinoni L, Pesenti A, Baglioni S, et al: Inflammatory pulmonary edema and positive end-expiratory pressure: Correlations between imaging and physiologic studies. J Thorac Imaging 3(3):59, 1988.
84. Wells GA: Gamut: Pulmonary edema and other causes of a butterfly pattern in the postoperative chest. Semin Roentgenol 23:4, 1988.
85. Carlson RW, Schaeffer RC, Michaels SG, et al: Pulmonary edema fluid. Spectrum of features in 37 patients. Circulation 60:1161, 1979.
86. Carlson RW, Schaefe RC, Carpio M. et al: Edema fluid and coagulation changes during fulminant pulmonary edema. Chest 79:43, 1981.
87. Milne ENC: Correlation of physiologic findings with chest roentgenology. Radiol Clin North Am 11:17, 1973.
88. Miniati M, Pistolesi M, Paoletti P, et al: Objective radiographic criteria to differentiate cardiac, renal and lung injury edema. Invest Radiol 23:433, 1988.
89. Ramirez J: Pulmonary alveolar proteinosis—A roentgenologic analysis. AJR 92:571, 1964.
90. Murch CR, Carr DH: Computed tomography appearances of pulmonary alveolar proteinosis. Clin Radiol 40:240, 1989.
91. Panicek DM, Ewing DK, Markarian B, et al: Interstitial pulmonary hemorrhage from mediastinal hematoma secondary to aortic rupture. Radiology 162:165, 1987.
92. Albelda SM, Gefter WB, Epstein DM, et al: Diffuse pulmonary hemorrhage: A review and classification. Radiology 154:289, 1985.
93. Gurney JW, Harrison WC, Sears K, et al: Bronchoalveolar lavage: Radiographic manifestations. Radiology 163:71, 1987.
94. Henschke CI, Davis SD, Romano PM, et al: The pathogenesis, radiologic evaluation, and therapy of pleural effusions. Radiol Clin North Am 27:1241, 1989.
95. Davis S, Gardner Q: The shape of a pleural effusion. Br Med J 26:436, 1963.
96. Fleischner FG: Atypical arrangement of free pleural effusion. Radiol Clin North Am 1:347, 1963.
97. Moller A: Pleural effusion: Use of the semi-supine position for radiographic detection. Radiology 150:245, 1984.
98. Ruskin JA, Gurney JW, Thorsen MK: Detection of pleural effusions on supine chest radiographs. AJR 148:681, 1987.
99. Rigler LG: Roentgen diagnosis of small pleural effusions. JAMA 96:104, 1931.
100. Rigler LG: Errors in diagnosis of free pleural effusions. AJR 30:410, 1933.
101. Hirsch JH, Rogers JV, Mack LA: Real-time sonography of pleural opacities. AJR 136:297, 1981.
102. Stark DD, Federle MP, Goodman PC. CT and radiographic assessment of tube thoracostomy. AJR 141:253, 1983.
103. Willsie-Ediger SK, Salzman G, Reisz G, et al: Use of intrapleural streptokinase in the treatment of thoracic empyema. Am J Med Sci 300:296, 1990.
104. Bergh NP, Ekroth R, Larsson S, et al: Intrapleural streptokinase in the treatment of hemothorax and empyema. Scand J Thorac Cardiovasc Surg 11:265, 1977.
105. Moulton JS, Moore PT, Mencini RA: Treatment of loculated pleural effusions with transcatheter intracavitary urokinase. AJR 153:941, 1989.
106. Dorne HL: Differentation of pulmonary parenchymal consolidation from pleural disease using the sonographic fluid-bronchogram. Radiographics 158:41, 1986.
107. Doust BD, Baum JK, Maklad NF, et al: Ultrasonic evaluation of pleural opacities. Radiology 14:135, 1975.
108. Laing FC, Filly RA: Problems in the application of ultrasonography for the evaluation of pleural opacities. Radiology 126:211, 1978.
109. Landay MJ, Conrad MR: Lung abscess mimicking empyema on ultrasonography. AJR 133:731, 1979.
110. Shin MS, Gray PW Jr. Pitfalls in ultrasonic detection of pleural fluid. J Clin Ultrasound 6:421, 1978.
111. Zwillich CW, Pierson DJ, Creagh CE, et al: Complications of assisted ventilation. A prospective study of 354 consecutive episodes. Am J Med 57:161, 1974.
112. Steier M, Ching N, Roberts EB, et al: Pneumothorax complicating continuous ventilatory support. J Thorac Cardiovasc Surg 67:17, 1974.
113. Tocino IM: Pneumothorax in the supine patient: Radiographic anatomy. Radiographics 5:557, 1985.
114. Glazer HS, Anderson DJ, Wilson BS, et al: Pneumothorax: Appearance on lateral chest radiographs. Radiology 173:707, 1989.
115. Tuddenham WJ: Glossary of terms for thoracic radiology: Recommendations of the Nomenclature Committee of the Fleischner Society. AJR 143:509, 1984.
116. Quigley MJ, Fraser RS: Pulmonary pneumatocele: Pathology and pathogenesis. AJR 150:1275, 1988.
117. Caffey D: Regional obstructive pulmonary emphysema in infants and children. Am J Dis Child 60:586, 1940.
118. Conway DD: Origin of lung cysts in childhood. Arch Dis Child 26:504, 1951.
119. Flaherty KA, Keegan JM, Sturtevant HN: Postpneumonic pulmonary pneumatoceles. Radiology 74:50, 1960.
120. O'Donnell AE, Pappas LS: Pulmonary complications of intravenous drug abuse,: Experience at an inner-city hospital. Chest 94:251, 1988.
121. Kuhlman JE, Knowles MC, Fishman EK, et al: Premature bullous pulmonary damage in AIDS: CT diagnosis. Radiology 173:23, 1989.
122. Sandhu JS, Goodman PC: Pulmonary cysts associated with *Pneumocystis carinii* pneumonia in patients with AIDS. Radiology 173:33, 1989.
123. Gurney JW, Bates FT: Pulmonary cystic disease: Comparison of *Pneumocystis carinii* pneumatoceles and bullous emphysema due to intravenous drug abuse. Radiology 173:27, 1989.
124. Panicek DM: Cystic pulmonary lesions in patients with AIDS (editorial). Radiology 173:12, 1989.

SECTION THREE

The Septic Syndrome

Section Editor

Robert A. Balk

CHAPTER 22

The Septic Syndrome and Septic Shock

Robert A. Balk
Roger C. Bone

A systemic response to an infection and bacteremia has traditionally been referred to as sepsis.[1] The terminology and definitions used in describing the systemic inflammatory response to infection or sepsis have been the source of confusion in clinical practice and in the literature.[2] A consensus conference, cosponsored by the American College of Chest Physicians and the Society of Critical Care Medicine, has proposed that sepsis be described as the systemic inflammatory response resulting from a documented infection.[2] The gradations or stages of sepsis as well as the approach to multiple-organ dysfunction were also addressed by this consensus conference.[2]

The incidence of sepsis and bacteremia and its various sequelae has been on the rise.[2, 3] The exact numbers and the full ramifications of this increase are largely unknown because sepsis is not a reportable disease. Data concerning the incidence of bacteremia reveal that there has been a marked increase in reported episodes of bacteremia during the past three decades.[2, 3] There has been a 139% increase in reported instances of bacteremia in the United States during the past 10 years.[3] It is logical to conclude that there must be an accompanying increase in the incidence of sepsis. Past estimates of 70,000 to 300,000 cases of sepsis each year in the United States have been revised up to 300,000 to 500,000 cases per year.[1, 4]

There are many reasons behind this alarming increase in the incidence of sepsis[1–5] (Table 22–1). The average age of the U.S. population has increased, and the ever-expanding number of elderly individuals are at an increased risk for the development of sepsis.[2] The septicemia rate for patients 65 years and older rose by 162% between 1979 and 1987.[3] There has been greater use of invasive procedures in the diagnosis and management of disease.[5] These procedures frequently result in a disturbance of the natural protective barriers against infection and may predispose to the subsequent development of sepsis. There has also been a more aggressive approach to a variety of disease processes, such as malignancy and collagen-vascular disease, which has resulted in an increased use of immunosuppressive and cytotoxic therapies.[4, 5] The greater prevalence of organ transplantation and its requisite immunosuppression has also enhanced the likelihood of infectious complications.[4, 5] The ever-expanding number of patients with the acquired immunodeficiency syndrome is also instrumental in the dramatic increase in the incidence of sepsis during the past decade.[4, 5]

It is no surprise that the current predictions are for a continued increase in the number of patients with sepsis. Significant morbidity and mortality are associated with the septic process, and efforts need to be directed at the prevention of sepsis, as well as its treatment. The overall mortality associated with sepsis is highly variable and dependent on the patient's underlying health status and the subsequent development of adverse sequelae (e.g., septic shock, multiple organ system failure [MOSF], and adult respiratory distress syndrome [ARDS]). Mortality rates of 5 to 90% in patients with sepsis have been reported, with the higher mortality occurring in those patients with the various adverse sequelae.[1, 4, 5] Sepsis is reported to be the most common cause of death in the noncoronary intensive care unit.[5, 6]

This section is concerned with the current body of knowledge concerning the septic syndrome. This chapter defines the clinical problem, and Chapter 23 discusses the pathophysiology of the septic process. The pivotal role of the various cytokines (e.g., tumor necrosis factor and interleukins) in the pathogenesis of the septic process is discussed in Chapter 24. Among the adverse sequelae of sepsis that deserve special emphasis are cardiovascular dysfunction, MOSF, and abnormalities in oxygen delivery and utilization.

TABLE 22–1

FACTORS ASSOCIATED WITH INCREASED INCIDENCE OF SEPSIS

Increased numbers of aged individuals
Expanded use of invasive procedures
Greater use of immunosuppressive agents
Increased numbers of immunosuppressed individuals
Aggressive management of malignant conditions
Increased use of transplantation
Advances in technology

TABLE 22-2

DIAGNOSTIC CRITERIA FOR SEPTIC SYNDROME

Clinical evidence of infection
Fever or hypothermia
Tachycardia (>90 beats/min)
Tachypnea (>20 breaths/min)
Evidence of inadequate organ system function or perfusion (one
   of the following):
     Altered mental status
     Unexplained hypoxemia
     Elevated plasma lactate level
     Decreased urine output (<0.5 mL/kg/h)
     Unexplained coagulopathy
     Hypotension (despite adequate volume replacement)

Adapted from RC Bone, CJ Fisher Jr, TP Clemmer, et al, Sepsis syndrome: A valid clinical entity. Methylprednisolone Severe Sepsis Study Group, Crit Care Med, 17, 389–393, © by Williams & Wilkins, 1989.

These issues are addressed in Chapters 25, 26, and 27, respectively. Finally, Chapter 28 presents an in-depth discussion of the current recommendations for the treatment of the septic patient, with an emphasis on the rationale behind some of the new and currently experimental therapeutic interventions.

DEFINITIONS

The traditional definition of sepsis incorporated the presence of bacteremia with the systemic response to infection.[1, 7, 8] In some cases, authors went so far as to require the presence of shock before the patient was classified as having sepsis. The major problem with these definitions is that they delay the diagnosis and require laboratory confirmation, which typically entails an additional 24 to 48 hours. Studies have targeted the early identification of patients with sepsis to allow the early initiation of therapeutic intervention.[9–11] The clinical criteria listed in Table 22–2, fever or hyperthermia, tachycardia, tachypnea, and evidence of inadequate organ system function and/or perfusion in the clinical setting of infection, were used to diagnose the septic syndrome. The septic syndrome diagnosis does not require the presence of positive blood or other cultures.[1]

It is apparent that there may be a great deal of confusion regarding what constitutes the septic process, depending on the definitions used. In an attempt to eliminate some of the confusion, a plea has made been to adopt uniform terminology and definitions.[12] As previously stated, *sepsis* is defined as the systemic response to an infection.[1] Not all infectious processes, even if bacteremia is present, give rise to a systemic response. *Bacteremia* is merely the documentation of microorganisms in the blood stream. In certain situations, bacteremia has been found to have a significant impact on the morbidity and mortality of the infectious process.[13, 14] When sepsis is accompanied by evidence of organ dysfunction or inadequate organ perfusion, the *septic syndrome* is present.[12] *Hypotension* is defined by a decrease in the systolic blood pressure to less than 90 mm Hg or a greater than 40 mm Hg decrease in the systolic blood pressure from baseline readings.

There is still a great deal of controversy over the exact definition of *shock* and *septic shock*. The shock state implies that there is organ system dysfunction and an impairment in the normal cellular process of oxidative metabolism.[15] The traditional diagnosis of shock is based on the finding of hypotension and an otherwise unexplained metabolic or lactic acidosis. There have been attempts in the past to characterize the severity or the duration of the shock by the clinical descriptors warm and cold shock.[16] Warm shock was an early (hyperdynamic) phase during which the patient manifested an elevated cardiac output and a reduction in the systemic vascular resistance.[16] Cold shock was a late (hypodynamic) phase during which there was a reduction in cardiac output and a return to normal systemic vascular resistance.[5] Currently, there is an attempt to reclassify shock on the basis of the response to therapeutic interventions. In the volume-responsive phase, the hypotension responds to fluid volume replacement and/or the administration of low doses of dopamine. The pressor-dependent, or volume-unresponsive, shock state is characterized by requirements for higher doses of vasopressor agents.

VALIDITY OF THE SEPTIC SYNDROME

The concept of the septic syndrome was developed to allow the early identification and initiation of directed therapy in septic patients.[1] Because the definition is based on clinical criteria (see Table 22–2) and not the presence of positive culture results, the diagnosis is easily made in a relatively short time. The validity of the septic syndrome was established by a large prospective study of the use of high-dose methylprednisolone in the treatment of sepsis and septic shock in which the control population was analyzed with regard to the presence or absence of bacteremia.[11] The population of patients studied was initially referred to as having "severe sepsis" and would be similar to the severe sepsis group as currently defined in the proposal from the consensus conference of the American College of Chest Physicians and the Society of Critical Care Medicine mentioned earlier.[2, 9] Forty-five percent of the 191 control patients were bacteremic. In comparing the admission demographic data for bacteremic and nonbacteremic patients (Table 22–3), the only significant differences were in patient age and initial platelet count.[11] These statistical differences are not of clinical importance. The only significant difference in the clinical courses of bacteremic and nonbacteremic patients was a greater incidence of shock development (47% versus 29.6%, $P < .05$) in the bacteremic patients.

The septic syndrome population in this large multicenter study had a 25.6% mortality rate. Overall, 36% of the patients were in shock at study entry, and in an additional 23%, shock developed during their subsequent hospital course. The presence or the absence of shock was a major determinant of patient survival. The mortality rate for patients who did not experience shock was 13%, and the mortality rates increased to 27.5% and 43.2% for patients who presented with shock or who subsequently experienced shock, respectively. When shock developed during the course of the septic process, 70% of the time it manifested within the initial 24 hours. It is also worth noting that, in bacteremic patients, gram-positive and gram-negative bacteremias were associated with a similar incidence of shock development and shock reversal. ARDS developed in 25% of the septic syndrome population. The incidence and outcome of both shock and ARDS were similar to those in previous reports of sepsis and bacteremia.[11]

Clinical Manifestations of Sepsis

As the definitions of sepsis and septic syndrome imply, these are systemic processes and can have a variety of clinical manifestations. The complex pathophysiology of sepsis, which is discussed in detail in subsequent chapters, illustrates the vast potential for involvement of various organ systems. The clinical manifestations of sepsis (Table 22–4) lack specificity when assessed individually. However, when multiple clinical manifestations are present, the clinician's suspicion

TABLE 22–3

CLINICAL DATA IN BACTEREMIC VERSUS NONBACTEREMIC PATIENTS

Variable	Nonbacteremic	Bacteremic
Age (y)	55.8 ± 1.6	51.1 ± 1.6*
Temperature (°F)	101.6 ± 0.3	101.5 ± 0.3
Respiratory rate (breaths/min)	30.1 ± 0.8	31.0 ± 1.0
Heart rate (beats/min)	118 ± 1.8	123 ± 2.2
Systolic blood pressure (mm Hg)	103 ± 3	103 ± 3
Diastolic blood pressure (mm Hg)	59 ± 2	57 ± 2
Mean blood pressure (mm Hg)	72 ± 26	82 ± 20
Hemoglobin (g/dL)	11.7 ± 0.2	11.5 ± 0.3
White blood cell count (cells/mm³)	15,070 ± 890	14,920 ± 1,010
Platelet count (cells/mm³)	233,850 ± 15,440	195,910 ± 13,640†
Prothrombin time (s)	22 ± 3.2	17 ± 1.9
pH	7.41 ± 0.01	7.39 ± 0.01
Pao_2 (torr)	80 ± 3	93 ± 11
$Paco_2$ (torr)	35 ± 1	33 ± 1
Plasma lactate (mg/dL)	3.3 ± 0.4	4.5 ± 1
Total protein (g/dL)	5.7 ± 0.1	5.6 ± 0.2
Albumin (mg/dL)	2.9 ± 0.1	2.87 ± 0.1
Glucose (mg/dL)	171 ± 9.9	173 ± 11.9
Blood urea nitrogen (mg/dL)	29 ± 2	31 ± 2.4
Creatinine (mg/dL)	2.2 ± 0.2	2.0 ± 0.2
Total bilirubin (mg/dL)	1.6 ± 0.2	2.6 ± 0.5
Serum glutamic-oxaloacetic transaminase (U/mL)	214 ± 91	147 ± 73
Alkaline phosphatase (U/mL)	169 ± 16	159 ± 19
HCO_3 (mEq/L)	22 ± 0.6	21 ± 0.7
K^+ (mEq/L)	4.1 ± 0.1	4.0 ± 0.1
Na^+ (mEq/L)	137 ± 0.7	136 ± 0.9
Cl^- (mEq/L)	102 ± 0.9	102 ± 0.9

*$P < .05$.
†$P < .001$.
From RC Bone, CJ Fisher Jr, TP Clemmer, et al, Sepsis syndrome: A valid clinical entity. Methylprednisolone Severe Sepsis Study Group, Crit Care Med, 17, 389–393, © by Williams & Wilkins, 1989.

of the presence of sepsis should be heightened. It is important to emphasize that a necessary component of the diagnosis of sepsis and the septic syndrome is the clinical suspicion of an infectious process. A variety of illnesses can manifest the clinical aspects of the septic syndrome.

TABLE 22–4

CLINICAL MANIFESTATIONS OF SEPSIS

Fever
Tachycardia
Mental status changes
Seizures
Hypoglycemia
Lactic acidosis
Disseminated Intravascular coagulation
Proteinuria
Hypothermia
Tachypnea
Stupor
Hyperglycemia
Hypoferremia
Thrombocytopenia
Anemia
Liver function abnormalities
Hypoxemia
Leukocytosis
Coma
Coagulopathy
Shock
ARDS
Leukopenia

Modified from Harris RL, Musher DM, Bloom K, et al: Manifestations of sepsis. Arch Intern Med 147:1895–1906, 1987. Copyright 1987, American Medical Association.

Fever

An alteration in the thermoregulatory function of the patient is one of the most common clinical manifestations of sepsis.[16] Fever or hyperthermia is more commonly found than hypothermia.[16] The febrile response is most probably related to the elaboration of various pyrogens, such as endotoxin, and various cytokines (see Chapters 23, 24) that act on the thermoregulatory centers in the hypothalamus.[16, 17] The fever is a part of the acute-phase reaction typical of the septic process. Hypothermia is most commonly found in patients at the extremes of age (young and old) or those who have chronic debilitating or immunosuppressing conditions (such as chronic renal failure, hepatic failure, and alcoholism).[18] A large retrospective study found 13% incidence of hypothermia in sepsis, and the inability of a patient to generate a body temperature greater than 99.6°F in the initial 24 hours of the clinical illness has been associated with an increased mortality rate.[19]

Pulmonary Manifestations of Sepsis

Tachypnea and hyperventilation are two of the most common pulmonary manifestations of the septic process[16, 20] (Table 22–5). Tachypnea is one of the earliest indicators and may be the direct result of the various mediators of sepsis[16, 20, 21] (see Chapter 23). The tachypnea may also be the direct effect of sympathetic discharge, be caused by the presence of circulating endotoxin, or result from central respiratory stimulation related to the increase in extravascular lung water stimulating the pulmonary stretch receptors.[20, 21] It does not appear that the tachypnea and hyperventilation are related to the fever, and the degree of

TABLE 22–5

RESPIRATORY DYSFUNCTION IN SEPSIS

Tachypnea
Hyperventilation
Hypoxemia
Respiratory muscle dysfunction
Pulmonary hypertension
Bronchoconstriction
ARDS
Hypercapnic respiratory failure
Nosocomial infection

hyperventilation outstrips the respiratory compensation for the increased lactic acid or carbon dioxide production.[16]

Septic patients frequently manifest hypoxemia.[16, 20, 21] An imbalance in the ventilation-perfusion relationship appears to be the major mechanism involved in the production of hypoxemia and may be present even with normal chest x-ray findings.[16, 20, 21] Additional mechanisms include shunt, especially in patients with an underlying pneumonia or ARDS.[22] Animal models of sepsis have demonstrated an increase in the airway resistance and pulmonary vascular hypertension, in addition to the decrease in compliance that is typical of the lung injury of sepsis.[23] Persistent pulmonary hypertension in the setting of sepsis-induced lung injury has been shown to be a poor prognostic sign.[24] The pathophysiologic mechanisms of these alterations are complex and probably involve the interaction of multiple potential mediators (see Chapter 23).

Experimental studies in animal models of septic shock also supported a role for early initiation of mechanical ventilatory support to aid the increased work of breathing and treat the respiratory muscle fatigue.[25] Respiratory muscle support lessens the likelihood of hypercapnic respiratory failure and helps maintain adequate oxygenation. There are also theoretic advantages of preventing MOSF by providing improved oxygen delivery to other organ systems. Respiratory muscle fatigue, hypercapnic respiratory failure, and eventually death were found in spontaneously breathing dogs that were injected with *Escherichia coli* endotoxin.[25] In contrast, similarly injected dogs that were supported with mechanical ventilation had significantly improved survival. There was also a fourfold decrease in blood flow to the respiratory muscles and an increase in blood flow to the gastrointestinal tract, the brain, and the skeletal muscles in the latter dogs.[25]

From 5 to 40% of patients with sepsis experience ARDS.[26–30] The noncardiogenic pulmonary edema characteristic of this syndrome is thought to be one of the earliest manifestations of the generalized capillary leak that results from the endothelial cell injury characteristic of the septic process. This same panendothelial injury may be involved, at least to some extent, in the subsequent development of MOSF, which is also a complication of sepsis. Some researchers consider ARDS to be an early manifestation of MOSF.

In the lung, the endothelial cell injury results in the loss of intravascular fluid into the interstitial and alveolar space and leads to stiff noncompliant lungs, increased dead space ventilation, and an increase in the shunt fraction.[26, 31] Clinically, the patient manifests respiratory distress with tachypnea and labored breathing.[31, 32] Auscultation of the chest reveals diffuse crackles, and the chest roentgenogram demonstrates diffuse interstitial and/or alveolar infiltrates. The shunt physiology is exemplified by persistent hypoxemia, despite the administration of high concentrations of supplemental oxygen. The pathophysiology and clinical ramifications of ARDS are beyond the scope of this chapter but are reviewed in more detail in Chapters 23, 26, and 27.

The development of ARDS can add significantly to the morbidity and mortality associated with sepsis.[26–30] Unfortunately, at this time, there is no specific therapy for ARDS.[26–30] Efforts are directed at treating the underlying or predisposing process and providing supportive care to the patient in an attempt to allow repair of the lung injury and prevent the development of complications, such as MOSF.[27] The overall mortality rate for patients with ARDS continues to be 50 to 70%, despite the advances in medical knowledge, technology, and therapeutics.[32] The development of ARDS in patients with gram-negative sepsis has been associated with a 90% mortality in one large retrospective review.[26]

Cardiovascular Manifestations of Sepsis

The cardiovascular manifestations of sepsis are reviewed in detail in Chapter 25. As stated earlier, tachycardia is an early, nonspecific indicator of sepsis.[16] Early in the septic process, the patient has a normal blood pressure but an elevated cardiac output and a decreased systemic vascular resistance.[33] This phase of sepsis is termed the *hyperdynamic phase*. The subsequent development of shock may be related to alterations in vascular tone.[33] Initially, there is hyperdynamic cardiac function with an increase in cardiac output and a persistence of the low systemic vascular resistance characteristic of this hyperdynamic phase of sepsis.[16, 33–36] Fluid or volume replacement may correct the alterations in blood pressure in patients who do not manifest refractory shock. In persistent hypotension (refractory shock), vasopressors are required for therapy.

Hypodynamic cardiac function characterized by a reversible decrease in biventricular ejection fraction and an increase in end-diastolic volume has been reported to occur commonly in patients with septic shock.[37] The mechanism for this cardiac dysfunction is currently under investigation and is reviewed in detail in Chapter 25.

Gastrointestinal and Hepatic Manifestations of Sepsis

Patients with sepsis are at risk for several different gastrointestinal complications, including stress ulceration and gastrointestinal bleeding.[16, 38] The risk of stress ulceration is further increased when additional complications, such as the need for mechanical ventilatory support, hepatic dysfunction, and coagulopathy, exist.[38, 39] The pathophysiologic alterations that may be responsible for the development of stress ulceration include altered mucosal blood flow, altered permeability of the gastric mucosa, hypoxia of the gastric mucosal cells, release of mucosal lysozyme, disruption of the gastric mucosal barrier, the irritative effects of acid and/or bile on the hypoxic gastric mucosa, and some unknown mechanism. The incidence of stress-related gastrointestinal bleeding is variable, affecting up to 85% of patients with ARDS in one study.[40] There has also been a great deal of controversy regarding the best approach to this potential problem.[41, 42] The use of antacid, cytoprotective agents, and histamine H_2–blocking therapy has created confusion over the potential risks and benefits of each of these maneuvers.[41] Antacid and H_2-blocker therapy have been incriminated as potential risk factors for nosocomial pneumonia in critically ill patients.[41, 42] This risk appears to be related to increasing the gastric pH and allowing colonization with colonic bacteria that eventually migrate to the hypopharynx and are aspirated into the tracheobronchial tree.[42, 43]

Ischemia and direct mucosal injury have been implicated in the process of translocation of enteric bacteria and endotoxin that occurs in the critically ill.[44–46] The bacteria-endotoxin translocation process has been described as the fuel for the eventual development of MOSF and can be a factor in maintaining a hypermetabolic clinical course.[45] It appears that a normal enteral diet is the best means to prevent the development of translocation.[44] Other important aspects of prevention include the administration of complete enteral nutritional support, including fiber and glutamine.[45, 47] These findings add new evidence in support of early initiation of enteral nutrition in the care of septic and critically ill patients.

Hepatic dysfunction is frequently encountered in sepsis.[16] The liver is an important part of the reticuloendothelial system to help detoxify the translocated bacteria and endotoxin that evade the mesenteric lymph nodes.[48] The Kupffer cells of the liver may then be stimulated to elaborate acute-phase reactants, such as tumor necrosis factor, interleukin-1, interleukin-6, and other potential mediators of the septic process.[45, 48–51] Some of these mediators are directly toxic to the hepatocytes. Abnormalities of liver function can have profound effects on patient survival.[52, 53] In patients with ARDS that was predominantly from a septic insult, Schwartz and coworkers reported an increased mortality rate in those who had pre-existing hepatic dysfunction.[53] The liver's ability to detoxify and neutralize potentially toxic by-products appears to be an important mechanism for the preservation of the critically ill patient.

Renal Manifestations of Sepsis

Renal abnormalities in sepsis may take a variety of forms. Oliguria is one of the organ perfusion or dysfunction manifestations that herald the development of the septic syndrome.[11] The oliguria and other renal manifestations may develop in the absence of documented shock or hypotension.[16] Other renal manifestations include azotemia, active urinary sediment, proteinuria, acute tubular necrosis, glomerulonephritis, and interstitial nephritis.[16] Acute renal failure may result from the septic insult or, more commonly, from a variety of factors. These factors may include acute tubular necrosis related to a period of hypoperfusion of the renal tubules, the administration of nephrotoxic medications and antibiotics, and immune complex deposition related to the underlying disease state or an infectious process.[16]

Hematologic Manifestations of Sepsis

The most common hematologic manifestation of sepsis is leukocytosis, which is frequently accompanied by a shift to the left.[16] Some patients may not manifest leukocytosis initially and may even have leukopenia.[16] Patients who have neutropenia related to underlying disorders of their bone marrow are at increased risk for gram-negative infections and may be unable to increase their neutrophil count in response to the infectious process.[16] An examination of the peripheral smears of septic patients frequently reveals increased numbers of hypersegmented polymorphonuclear leukocytes and band or immature forms of polymorphonuclear leukocytes. Typically, there is also evidence of toxic granulations, vacuolization, and Döhle's bodies in the polymorphonuclear leukocytes.

The septic process may result in decreased maturation and/or survival of red blood cells.[16, 54] Unless the septic process is of long duration, this abnormality does not result in anemia. There is a well-characterized decrease in serum iron concentration in sepsis that is related to iron uptake by the reticuloendothelial system.[55]

Thrombocytopenia and clotting abnormalities are commonly encountered in septic patients.[16, 26, 28] Up to 66% of septic patients with ARDS have been reported to have thrombocytopenia.[26, 28] The mechanism for this abnormality is unclear and is probably multifactoral. Animal models of sepsis typically demonstrate a reduction in the platelet and white blood cell counts early after the septic insult.[56] There are increased platelets and polymorphonuclear leukocytes in the microvasculature of the lung in these models of sepsis, which may partially explain the mechanism of the ensuing lung injury as well as the observed leukopenia and thrombocytopenia.[57]

Abnormalities of coagulation are frequently encountered in septic patients.[16, 58] This may take the form of elevations in the prothrombin time or the partial thromboplastin time or disseminated intravascular coagulation.[58] Approximately 66% of septic children and adults have been reported to have abnormalities in their vitamin K–dependent coagulation factors and prolonged prothrombin time.[59] Septic patients have been found to have reductions in levels of antithrombin III, which may be responsible for intravascular coagulation and possibly involved in the development of MOSF and disseminated intravascular coagulation.[60]

Sepsis is the most common cause of disseminated intravascular coagulation.[61] The diagnosis of disseminated intravascular coagulation includes thrombocytopenia, prolonged prothrombin time and partial thromboplastin time, increased fibrin split products (or fibrin degradation products), and decreased levels of fibrinogen, factor V, factor VIII, and antithrombin III. The clinical sequelae of the disseminated intravascular coagulation may be predominantly a laboratory phenomenon or may take the form of a bleeding diathesis. The presence of disseminated intravascular coagulation adds significantly to the morbidity and mortality associated with the septic episode.[61]

Neurologic Manifestations of Sepsis

The most common neurologic manifestation of sepsis is a change in mental status.[16, 62] The altered mentation may manifest as confusion, disorientation, lethargy, obtundation, agitation, coma, and even seizures.[16, 62] The mechanism for this change in mental status is thought to be related to alterations in cerebral perfusion or to the cerebral metabolism of certain amino acids.[63] Mizock reported that septic patients with an encephalopathy had elevated levels of the amino acid phenylethylamine and its metabolite phenylacetic acid in the cerebrospinal fluid and blood.[63] This defect is similar to that seen in patients with end-stage liver disease and hepatic encephalopathy. Elderly patients who may have pre-existing cerebrovascular disease or structural changes in the brain may be particularly susceptible to these alterations during the septic process.[63]

The syndrome of critical illness polyneuropathy has also been described in septic patients with evidence of MOSF.[64] This syndrome is characterized by impaired deep tendon reflexes, muscle weakness, and muscle wasting related to the primary axonal degeneration of both the sensory and motor fibers. Prolonged requirement for ventilatory assistance and delayed weaning from the mechanical ventilator may result from this disorder. It is reported that 3 to 6 months may be required for a complete recovery.[64]

Metabolic and Endocrine Manifestations of Sepsis

Septic patients may exhibit a variety of endocrine and metabolic disturbances. Sepsis can trigger a hypermetabolic phase, with the inability to utilize glucose as an energy source in the skeletal muscles.[65] This can lead to hyperglycemia, glucose intolerance, and relative insulin resistance in as many as 40% of septic patients.[65] There are also reports of hypoglycemia as a manifestation of severe sepsis, and this may exacerbate any neurologic impairment that is present.[66]

Hypoglycemia is most commonly found in patients with underlying protein deficiency or severe liver injury.[66] Adding to the increased glucose load is the skeletal muscle protein catabolism and increased hepatic gluconeogensis.[65] The pyruvate produced by the glycolytic pathway is not able to enter the tricarboxylic acid (Krebs') cycle and there is thus a build-up of lactate, which is responsible for the lactic acidosis of sepsis.[65]

The stress hormone levels are also elevated during the septic process and may contribute to some of the glucose and other metabolic derangements that characterize this clinical state.[16] There are elevations in the concentrations of catecholamines, epinephrine and norepinephrine, growth hormone, cortisol, and glucagon.[16, 65] Some patients manifest hypocalcemia during sepsis, and others with a prolonged illness may have the euthyroid sick syndrome.[66–68] Rarely, patients may manifest adrenal insufficiency related to hemorrhagic infarction of the adrenal glands. This has been most commonly seen in patients with disseminated meningococcemia, fungal disease, or tuberculosis. Pituitary infarction is a rare complication of sepsis.

Adverse Sequelae of Sepsis

A number of adverse sequelae can complicate the course of sepsis and increase the morbidity and mortality associated with the injury state. Included in this list is the development of septic shock, ARDS, and MOSF. Septic shock occurs in approximately 40% of septic patients and is associated with a mortality rate of 40 to 60%.[4] The subsequent development of shock during the septic course was associated with a greater mortality rate (43%) as compared with that for patients who presented with shock (27.5% mortality rate) or patients who never developed shock (13% mortality rate) in a review of 191 patients with septic syndrome.[11]

ARDS and MOSF also significantly increase the mortality associated with the diagnosis of sepsis. The mortality rate of ARDS associated with gram-negative sepsis has been reported to be as high as 90%.[26] Sepsis is the most frequent predisposing condition for the development of ARDS, and the mortality rate for sepsis-related ARDS is higher than for most other causes of ARDS.[30] ARDS develops in 5 to 40% of septic patients, and it occurs more frequently when multiple risk factors are present.[27, 28, 30, 31, 69] Some investigators believe that the ARDS may be just the initial manifestation of the MOSF syndrome. MOSF adversely influences survival in critically ill patients.[32, 48, 49] Both the number of involved organs and the duration of the MOSF are important determinants of the impact of MOSF on eventual survival.[70] A large study of more than 2800 patients with MOSF found that there was 100% mortality rate when three or more organ systems were dysfunctional for more than 5 days.[70]

Prognosis

The septic syndrome has been associated with mortality rates of approximately 25%.[11] This mortality is consistent with past mortality reports derived from investigations using a variety of definitions of sepsis.[9–11] The 25% mortality rate is quite impressive considering the advances in supportive care and specific treatment options during the past decade. For improved survival, it is important to avoid complications, including shock, ARDS, and MOSF, which increase the morbidity and mortality rates. The treatment of sepsis and septic shock is discussed in greater detail in Chapter 28.

SUMMARY

This chapter emphasizes the importance of using clinical criteria to identify the septic syndrome early in its course, before the results of cultures and other sophisticated laboratory examinations are known. It is hoped that early identification will lead to early treatment and potentially modify some of the adverse sequelae of the septic syndrome. Kreger and coworkers showed that the early institution of appropriate antibiotic therapy is associated with lower incidence of septic shock and improved survival.[19] Sepsis can affect any and all of the organ systems of the body. The clinical manifestations are often nonspecific. However, in the setting of a high clinical suspicion of infection, the clinical criteria of the septic syndrome should alert the clinician to perform the proper diagnostic tests, obtain appropriate cultures, and institute empirical therapy.

References

1. Balk RA, Bone RC: The septic syndrome: Definition and clinical implications. Crit Care Clin 5:1, 1989.
2. American College of Chest Physicians/Society of Critical Care Medicine Consensus Conference Committee: Definitions for sepsis and organ failure and guidelines for the use of innovative therapies in sepsis. Chest. In press.
3. Increase in national hospital discharge survey rates for septicemia—United States, 1979–1987. MMWR 39:31, 1990.
4. Parker MM, Parrillo JE: Septic shock: Hemodynamics and pathogenesis. JAMA 250:3324, 1983.
5. Parrillo JE, Parker MM, Natanson C, et al: Septic shock: Advances in the understanding of pathogenesis, cardiovascular dysfunction, and therapy. Ann Intern Med 113:227, 1990.
6. Manship L, McMillin RD, Brown JJ. The influence of sepsis and multisystem and organ failure on mortality in the surgical intensive care unit. Am Surg 50:94, 1984.
7. Shubin H, Weil MH: Bacterial shock. JAMA 235:421, 1976.
8. Kreger BE, Craven DE, Carling PC, et al: Gram-negative bacteremia III. Reassessment of etiology, epidemiology, and ecology in 612 patients. Am J Med 68:332, 1980.
9. Bone RC, Fisher CJ Jr, Clemmer TP, et al: A controlled clinical trial of high-dose methylprednisolone in the treatment of severe sepsis and septic shock. N Engl J Med 317:653, 1987.
10. The Veterans Administration Systemic Sepsis Cooperative Study Group: Effect of high-dose glucocorticoid therapy on mortality in patients with clinical signs of systemic sepsis. N Engl J Med 317:659, 1987.
11. Bone RC, Fisher CJ Jr, Clemmer TP, et al: Sepsis syndrome: A valid clinical entity. Methylprednisolone Severe Sepsis Study Group. Crit Care Med 17:389, 1989.
12. Bone RC: Sepsis, the sepsis syndrome, multi-organ failure: A plea for comparable definitions. Ann Intern Med 114:332, 1991.
13. Bryant RE, Hood AF, Hood CE, et al: Factors affecting mortality of gram-negative rod bacteremia. Arch Intern Med 127:120, 1971.
14. Phair JP, Bassaris HP, Williams JE, et al: Bacteremic pneumonia due to gram-negative bacilli. Arch Intern Med 143:2147, 1983.
15. Dantzker D: Oxygen delivery and utilization in sepsis. Crit Care Clin 5:81, 1989.
16. Harris RL, Musher DM, Bloom K, et al: Manifestations of sepsis. Arch Intern Med 147:1895, 1987.
17. Atkins E: Fever: The old and the new. J Infect Dis 149:339, 1984.
18. Gleckman R, Hibert D: Afebrile bacteremia: A phenomenon in geriatric patients. JAMA 248:1478, 1982.
19. Kreger BE, Craven DE, McCabe WR: Gram-negative bacteremia IV. Reevaluation of clinical features and treatment in 612 patients. Am J Med 68:344, 1980.
20. Balk RA: The spectrum of pulmonary manifestations of sepsis. Hosp Phys 26:24–1, 1990.
21. Clowes GHA Jr: Pulmonary abnormalities in sepsis. Surg Clin North Am 54:993, 1974.
22. Lee RM, Balk RA, Bone RC: Ventilatory support in the management of septic patients. Crit Care Clin 5:157, 1989.
23. Snapper JR, Hutchinson AA, Ogletree ML, et al: Effects of cyclooxygenase inhibitors on the alterations in lung mechanics caused by endotoxemia in the unanesthetized sheep. J Clin Invest 72:63, 1983.
24. Zapol WM, Snider MT: Pulmonary hypertension in severe acute respiratory failure. N Engl J Med 296:476, 1977.
25. Hussain SNA, Simkus G, Roussos C: Respiratory muscle fatigue: A cause of ventilatory failure in septic shock. J Appl Physiol 58:2033, 1985.
26. Kaplan RL, Sahn SA, Petty TL: Incidence and outcome of the respiratory distress syndrome in gram-negative sepsis. Arch Intern Med 139:867, 1979.
27. Balk RA, Bone RC: The adult respiratory distress syndrome. Med Clin North Am 67:685, 1983.
28. Fein AM, Lippmann M, Holtzman H, et al: The risk factors, incidence, and prognosis of ARDS following septicemia. Chest 83:40, 1983.

29. Pepe PE, Potkin RT, Reus DH, et al: Clinical predictors of the adult respiratory distress syndrome. Am J Surg 144:124, 1982.
30. Fowler AA, Hamman RF, Good JT, et al: Adult respiratory distress syndrome: Risk with common predispositions. Ann Intern Med 98:593, 1983.
31. Petty TL: Adult respiratory distress syndrome: Definition and historical perspective. Clin Chest Med 3:3, 1982.
32. Bersten A, Sibbald WJ: Acute lung injury in septic shock. Crit Care Clin 5:49, 1989.
33. Cunnion RE, Parrillo JE: Myocardial dysfunction in sepsis. Crit Care Clin 5:99, 1989.
34. Luce JM: Pathogenesis and management of septic shock. Chest 91:883, 1987.
35. Suffredini AF, Fromm RF, Parker MM, et al: The cardiovascular response of normal humans to the administration of endotoxin. N Engl J Med 321:280, 1989.
36. Abraham E, Shoemaker WC, Bland RD, et al: Sequential cardiorespiratory patterns in septic shock. Crit Care Med 11:799, 1983.
37. Parker MM, McCarthy KE, Ognibene FP, et al: Right ventricular dysfunction and dilatation, similar to left ventricular changes, characterize the cardiac depression of septic shock in humans. Chest 97:126, 1990.
38. Zuckerman GR, Cort D, Shuman RB: Stress ulcer syndrome. J Intensive Care Med 3:21, 1988.
39. Schuster DP, Rowley H, Feinstein S, et al: Prospective evaluation of the risk of upper gastrointestinal bleeding after admission to a medical intensive care unit. Am J Med 76:623, 1984.
40. Harris SK, Bone RC, Ruth WE: Gastrointestinal hemorrhage in patients in a respiratory intensive care unit. Chest 72:301, 1977.
41. Driks MR, Craven DE, Celli BR, et al: Nosocomial pneumonia in intubated patients given sucralfate as compared with antacids or histamine type 2 blockers. N Engl J Med 317:1376, 1987.
42. Peura DA, Johnson LF: Cimetidine for prevention and treatment of gastroduodenal mucosal lesions in patients in an intensive care unit. Ann Intern Med 103:173, 1985.
43. Zinner MJ, Zuidema GD, Smith PL, et al: The prevention of upper gastrointestinal tract bleeding in patients in an intensive care unit. Surg Gynecol Obstet 153:214, 1981.
44. Alexander JW: Nutrition and translocation. JPEN 14:170S, 1990.
45. Cerra FB: Hypermetabolism–organ failure syndrome: A metabolic response to injury. Crit Care Clin 5:289, 1989.
46. Marshall JC, Christou NV, Horn R, et al: The microbiology of multiple organ failure: The proximal gastrointestinal tract as an occult reservoir of pathogens. Arch Surg 123:309, 1988.
47. Souba WW, Herskowitz K, Klimberg S, et al: The effects of sepsis and endotoxemia on gut glutamine metabolism. Ann Surg 211:543, 1990.
48. Pinsky MR, Matuschak GM: Multiple systems organ failure: Failure of host defense homeostasis. Crit Care Clin 5:199, 1989.
49. Pinsky MR: Multiple systems organ failure: Malignant intravascular inflammation. Crit Care Clin 5:195, 1989.
50. Dominioni L, Dionigi R, Zanello M, et al: Sepsis score and acute-phase protein response as predictors of outcome in septic surgical patients. Arch Surg 122:141, 1987.
51. Kelly J: State of the art: Cytokines of the lung. Am Rev Respir Dis 141:765, 1990.
52. Matuschak GM, Martin DJ: Influence of end-stage liver failure on survival during multiple systems organ failure. Transplant Proc 19:40, 1987.
53. Schwartz DB, Bone RC, Balk RA, et al: Hepatic dysfunction in the adult respiratory distress syndrome. Chest 95:871, 1989.
54. Cartwright GE: The anemia of chronic disorders. Semin Hematol 3:351, 1966.
55. Beisel WR: Trace elements in infectious processes. Med Clin North Am 60:831, 1976.
56. Tate RM, Repine JE: State of the art: Neutrophils and the adult respiratory distress syndrome. Am Rev Respir Dis 128:552, 1983.
57. Meyrick B, Brigham KL: Acute effects of *Escherichia coli* endotoxin on the pulmonary microcirculation of anesthetized sheep: Structure:function relationships. Lab Invest 48:458, 1983.
58. Bone RC, Francis PB, Pierce AK: Intravascular coagulation associated with the adult respiratory distress syndrome. Am J Med 61:585, 1976.
59. Corrigan JJ Jr: Vitamin K–dependent coagulation factors in gram-negative septicemia. Am J Dis Child 138:240, 1984.
60. Emerson TE Jr, Fournel MA, Redens TB, et al: Efficacy of antithrombin III supplementation in animal models of fulminant *Escherichia coli* endotoxemia or bacteremia. Am J Med 87:27S, 1989.
61. Mant MJ, King EG: Severe, acute disseminated intravascular coagulation: A reappraisal of its pathophysiology, clinical significance and therapy based on 47 patients. Am J Med 67:557, 1979.
62. Mizock BA, Sabelli HC, Dubin A, et al: Septic encephalopathy. Arch Intern Med 150:443, 1990.
63. Mizock BA: Branched-chain amino acids in sepsis and hepatic failure. Arch Intern Med 145:1284, 1985.
64. Zochodne DW, Bolton CF, Wells GA, et al: Critical illness polyneuropathy: A complication of sepsis and multiple organ failure. Brain 110:819, 1987.
65. Mizock B: Septic shock: A metabolic perspective. Arch Intern Med 144:579, 1984.
66. Miller SI, Wallace RJ Jr, Musher DM, et al: Hypoglycemia as a manifestation of sepsis. Am J Med 63:649, 1980.
67. Zaloga GP, Chernow B: Divalent ions: Calcium, magnesium, and phosphorous. In: Chernow B (ed): The Pharmacologic Approach to the Critically Ill Patient. 2nd ed. Baltimore, Williams & Wilkins, p 610, 1988.
68. Burman KD: Thyroid hormones. In: Chernow B (ed): The Pharmacologic Approach to the Critically Ill Patient. 2nd ed. Baltimore, Williams & Wilkins, p 671, 1988.
69. Marks JO, Marks CB, Luce JM, et al: Plasma tumor necrosis factor in patients with septic shock: Mortality rate, incidence of adult respiratory distress syndrome, and effects of methylprednisolone administration. Am Rev Respir Dis 141:94, 1990.
70. Knaus WA, Wagner DP: Multiple systems organ failure: Epidemiology and prognosis. Crit Care Clin 5:221, 1989.

CHAPTER 23

Pathophysiology of Sepsis

Matthew A. Ivanovich
Robert A. Balk

Sepsis is common in today's hospital setting and has been increasing in frequency during the past several decades. Sepsis can be defined as the systemic inflammatory response to the intrusion of microorganisms or their noxious products into the blood stream. Septic shock is a syndrome of inadequate tissue perfusion, leading to organ dysfunction in the setting of the septic response. Shock attributable to sepsis can be manifested in three syndromes: hypotension, shock, and refractory shock. Hypotension is not synonymous with shock but reflects a decrease in systolic blood pressure, as measured by a cuff manometer, to less than 90 mm Hg. The decrease in systolic blood pressure in the setting of sepsis occurs frequently. Septic shock is evident in approximately 40% of septic patients and adversely affects the patients' course. The hypotension associated with sepsis can usually be corrected with infusion of fluids and, when necessary, intravenous vasopressors. When these measures fail, one is faced with refractory shock, and all its attendant complications and high mortality. Although classically described as separate clinical entities, sepsis and septic shock can be considered phases of a spectrum consisting of infection, blood stream invasion, early sepsis, late sepsis, and the various adverse sequelae of sepsis, such as shock, multiple organ system failure, and death (Fig. 23–1).

This chapter addresses the exceedingly complex pathophysiology of sepsis and septic shock, with particular emphasis on some of the various implicated mediators.

INCIDENCE AND EPIDEMIOLOGY

The past 40 years have seen a marked increase in the incidence of sepsis and septic shock.[1–6] Sepsis has become a major clinical problem encountered in both medical and surgical specialties.[1–4] Data concerning the exact incidence and mortality are not readily available because sepsis is not a reportable disease.[1] However, a number of studies noted an increase in the incidence and mortality from gram-negative bacteremia among patients admitted to hospitals.[2–4] From frequency rates at a university hospital, a projection was made that there may be up to 300,000

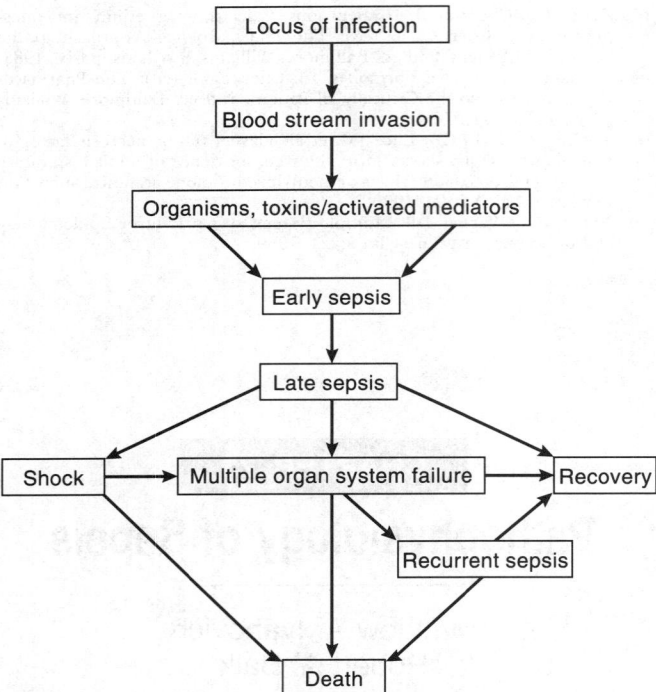

Figure 23–1. Pathogenesis of sepsis, septic shock, and its sequelae, beginning with a locus of infection. See text for details.

episodes of gram-negative bacteremia, resulting in more than 100,000 fatalities per year in the United States.[5] Gram-negative rods are by no means the sole etiologic agents of septic shock; gram-positive bacteria, fungi, parasites, and viruses may be involved. Taking this into account, the current annual incidence of sepsis, septic shock, and death from sepsis in the United States has been estimated at 400,000, 200,000, and 100,000, respectively.[6] What is disturbing is the remarkably high mortality associated with sepsis and its various sequelae. When septic shock is present, mortality rates as high as 80% have been reported, with an average of 40%, and vary depending on the underlying host factors.[1, 7, 8]

In spite of the great number of advances in the diagnostic and therapeutic arenas in medicine, sepsis and septic shock remain serious clinical problems, often appearing as complications of otherwise successful procedures. Septic shock is the leading cause of death in patients admitted to a surgical intensive care unit with a nontraumatic illness and to the noncoronary intensive care unit.[9–11]

ETIOLOGY

Numerous and various organisms have been implicated as the etiologic agents of septic shock.[12–14] These include viruses, fungi, protozoa, spirochetes, rickettsiae, chlamydiae, and bacteria (both gram-negative and gram-positive). Past studies have demonstrated that approximately two thirds of septic shock cases are caused by gram-negative organisms and about one third are caused by gram-positive organisms.[15] Research regarding gram-negative enteric rods remains at the forefront of scientific investigation, in part related to the ability of researchers to study the effects of certain cell wall components, such as lipopolysaccharide (endotoxin). The most frequently encountered gram-negative bacilli include *Escherichia coli*, *Klebsiella* species, *Pseudomonas aeruginosa*, *Serratia marcescens*, and *Enterobacter* and *Proteus* species. The

mortality seen in *Pseudomonas* species infections is by far the highest, up to 70%. By contrast, *E. coli* is associated with mortality rates of approximately 40%.[2, 4, 16] There has been an increase in sepsis related to gram-positive organisms, especially streptococci and staphylococci. In some institutions, the incidences of gram-positive and gram-negative infections are equal.

Potential sources of bacteremia abound in the hospitalized and critically ill patient. The gastrointestinal tract, with its large population of aerobic gram-negative bacilli, is a readily identifiable reservoir. Genitourinary infections, including pyelonephritis, presumably result from fecal contamination. Colonization of the oropharynx by gram-negative rods, which is present in up to 57% of critically ill patients, also serves as a possible source of sepsis.[17] In patients with respiratory failure who require endotracheal intubation and mechanical ventilation, the artificial airway bypasses normal protective mechanisms and the tracheobronchial tree is subject to colonization by gram-negative bacteria. This may act as a potential locus for pneumonia and the subsequent development of sepsis. In patients with nasotracheal intubation, a maxillary sinusitis secondary to obstructed drainage has been shown to be an often-overlooked source of sepsis.[18]

It is clear that septic shock can be due to organisms other than the gram-negative enteric rods; earlier investigators were concerned with differences in the clinical picture and hemodynamic profiles of patients with bacterial shock in relation to the type of infecting organism. Gram-negative sepsis was found to produce shock with a markedly decreased cardiac output and an increased peripheral vascular resistance as the major hemodynamic derangements. Shock attributable to gram-positive bacteria, on the other hand, was noted to have a reduced arterial resistance, with only a small degree of cardiac output impairment.[7, 12, 14, 19, 20] Earlier observations stressed a distinct clinical entity of gram-negative bacteremia and shock, with the host response dependent on the type of organism. It is currently accepted that the manifestations of septic shock are independent of the specific pathogenic microorganism and are dependent instead on the response of the host.[21–24]

RISK FACTORS

Among the risk factors for the development of sepsis are extremes of age; the young and the elderly have a greater predisposition to sepsis.[3, 4] Certain underlying diseases carry an increased risk of infection and at times a significantly worse outcome. Other risk factors include alterations in immune function (congenital or acquired), alterations in neutrophil numbers or function, absence or dysfunction of the spleen, aggressive chemotherapeutic treatment of malignant and inflammatory disease states, and invasive procedures. Alcoholism, chronic steroid administration, hepatic cirrhosis regardless of cause, and diabetes mellitus are also associated with an increased incidence of infection.[4] A multitude of invasive procedures and iatrogenic complications ranging from such simple actions as transmission of bacteria by health care workers via unwashed hands to urinary bladder catheterization and manipulation predisposes patients to infections and sepsis.[19, 25–27] Trends in the overall increase in the acuteness of illness in hospitalized patients may contribute to enhanced infection susceptibility.

PATHOGENESIS

Although the exact pathogenesis of sepsis remains incompletely understood,[1, 6, 28] it seems that the first step in the chain of events toward the development of sepsis and its various sequelae is the infection of a patient by a causative

---

TABLE 23–1

POTENTIAL MEDIATORS OF SEPSIS

Activated complement
Intrinsic coagulation cascade
Fibrinolysis activation
Bradykinin system
Arachidonic acid metabolites
Cytokines (TNF, interleukins)
Myocardial depressant factor or substance
Polymorphonuclear leukocytes
Endorphins
Platelet-activating factor
Toxic oxygen radicals
Tissue macrophages and monocytes
Histamine
Platelets
Lysosomal enzymes and elastase

---

organism. Common inciting conditions are urinary tract infections, pneumonias, and an abdominal catastrophe, such as an abscess or peritonitis.[2–4, 29] Subsequently, the nidus of infection can lead to invasion of the blood stream by the offending microorganism or its toxic products (e.g., endotoxin, exotoxin, and toxic shock syndrome toxin 1). The mere presence of microbes in the blood stream is not sufficient to trigger the development of the septic process as illustrated by the common occurrence of transient bacteremia during dental and urinary tract manipulation.[19] What *is* required is the initiation of the host response, which involves the activation of a number of potential endogenous mediators[1, 6, 28] and the initiation of various cascades, which may be self-escalating and self-modulating or merely the defense mechanisms gone awry.

The proposed endogenous mediators of the septic process are complex and numerous and include the following: intrinsic coagulation cascade, activated complement, kinins, various cytokines (the interleukins and tumor necrosis factor [TNF]), products of arachidonic acid metabolism, myocardial depressant factor or substance, polymorphonuclear leukocytes, endorphins, histamine, macrophages, lysosomal enzymes, platelets, platelet-activating factor (PAF), and toxic oxygen radicals (Table 23–1). The mediators and cascades involved are difficult to classify as initiators, propagators, or innocent bystanders in this process. An analogy with this reaction is a riot, in which it may be difficult to distinguish the instigators from the perpetuators or spectators involved in the melee.

Efforts to discern the exact mechanisms are hampered by a lack of animal models that precisely mimic human sepsis in all of its attributes. For example, endotoxin administration in a canine model causes vasomotor collapse, high fever, and bloody diarrhea, presumably owing to the unique lack of gastrointestinal collateral circulation in dogs.[12] This hypodynamic sepsis is in contrast to the more typical hyperdynamic sepsis that is seen in human patients.[12] However, in spite of the inherent differences between human and animal models, it has been possible to gain insight into potential mechanisms involved in the pathogenesis of the septic process by utilizing various experimental models.[6, 28]

As mentioned earlier, a nidus of infection seems to be necessary and may be accompanied by the intravascular release of various toxins and microbial by-products. These substances may be exotoxins, cell wall components, endotoxin, or the microorganism itself. These microbial products may then stimulate release of various other endogenous mediators from target cells within the body. The major target cells are neutrophils, monocytes, tissue macrophages, and endothelial cells. These cells are in various stages of activation, and they can be up-regulated and down-regulated through further interaction with the various mediators.

Endotoxin

Endotoxin, more specifically the lipid A moiety of lipopolysaccharide, is found in the outer wall of gram-negative bacteria and has been extensively studied in relationship to the manifestations of infections caused by gram-negative bacilli.[1, 5] Initially postulated as the cause of shock in gram-negative infections in 1951,[12] endotoxin is the principal exogenous mediator in sepsis attributable to gram-negative organisms.[30] Gram-negative bacterial outer membranes consist of endotoxin (Fig. 23–2), which in turn is composed of three parts: a surface O antigen side chain; the outer and inner R core; and the innermost component, lipid A.[1, 6] The highly variable O antigen, a serologically specific polysaccharide, is heat stable and has been used for somatic typing of bacteria.[1] The R core antigen has been shown to be an acidic hetero-oligosaccharide, also termed core glycolipid, which is more constant among the various gram-negative organisms.[1] Lipid A is the component that elicits the common endotoxin responses of pyrogenicity, hemodynamic collapse, and inflammation.[1, 6, 30]

Endotoxin possesses numerous properties and has been shown to cause or participate in the activation of factor XII (Hageman's factor), disseminated intravascular coagulation, activation of various kinins (bradykinin), production of fever, complement consumption, endothelial injury, release of cytokines (TNF and interleukins) from monocytes and activated macrophages, hypotension, and shock.[1, 6, 31, 32] Studies of canine mesenteric vasculature after the infusion of E. coli endotoxin revealed endothelial cell thickening, leukocyte margination, and sluggish flow.[33] There is also thrombosis of the small vessels, which is followed by subsequent clot lysis and pronounced extravasation of erythrocytes into the interstitial spaces. This is associated with a marked and rapid fall in systemic arterial pressure.[33] The direct damage to endothelial cell membranes and the microvasculature by endotoxin, as well as clotting system activation, [33] is part of the malignant intravascular inflammation and the panendothelial injury that are present in the septic process. This process may be further amplified in patients with adverse sequelae of sepsis, especially multiple organ system failure.

The hemodynamic effects of endotoxin administration were studied in sheep, by utilizing pulmonary arterial and thoracic aortic catheters. In addition, cannulation of the thoracic caudal lymphatic duct was performed to monitor lung lymph flow (an indicator of lung permeability abnormalities).[34] The investigators noted a triphasic response to intravenous E. coli endotoxin: an initial fall in the cardiac output with a rise in both peripheral vascular resistance and pulmonary arterial pressure, with an associated significant increase in hematocrit. Within 2 hours, these changes returned to baseline values, with the exception of a continued elevation in the hematocrit and sustained pulmonary arterial hypertension, roughly twice the control values.[34] The third phase of endotoxin response was characterized by a gradual decline in cardiac output. Lymph flow was noted to be increased, with an increase in the lymph-to-serum protein ratio, suggesting a permeability defect.[34] Significant fluid shifts occurred in this ovine model, resulting from elevated microvascular pressure and increased membrane permeability, which led to intravascular hypovolemia and subsequent reduction in cardiac output. Diminished cardiac work was not due to hypovolemia solely, as a 50% fall in stroke work in the face of an essentially unchanged arterial pressure was observed. Thus, endotoxin not only possesses peripheral

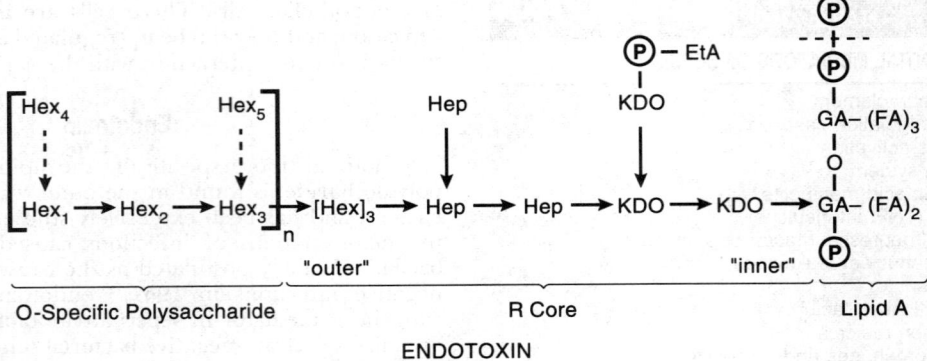

Figure 23-2. Biochemical structure of endotoxin: O-antigen specific side chain composed of repeating units of hexose (Hex); an R core of hexose, heptose (Hep), 2-keto-3-deoxyoctonate (KDO), phosphate (P), and ethanolamine (EtA); and lipid A, consisting of phosphate, glucosamine (GA), and fatty acid (FA). (Modified from Parillo JE, Parker MM, Natanson C, et al: Septic shock in humans. Advances in the understanding of pathogenesis, cardiovascular dysfunction, and therapy. Ann Intern Med 113:227, 1990.)

vascular effects but also causes depression of myocardial contractility, as supported by this work and that of many others.[34] (For further discussion, refer to Chapter 25.)

More recently, the cardiovascular response to the infusion of endotoxin was studied in human volunteers, revealing hemodynamic changes similar to those observed in septic shock.[30] The injection of a small dose of endotoxin was followed by the appearance of fever and chills, approximately 1 hour after infusion. An increased heart rate and an increased cardiac index associated with a reduced systemic vascular resistance was noted at 3 hours. The volunteers were found to have a significant decrease in both mean arterial pressure and left ventricular stroke work when compared with those in controls. There was also evidence of endotoxin-induced depression of myocardial contractility.[30] In addition, endotoxin infusion was followed by elevated serum levels of TNF, a cytokine implicated as a mediator of the septic response. Although elevations in pulmonary arterial pressures were not seen, there were significant changes in gas exchange. An increase in mixed venous oxygen tension, alveolar-arterial oxygen gradient, and alveolar epithelial cell permeability in conjunction with a decreased arterial oxygen tension and oxygen extraction were noted in an earlier study.[6] Endotoxin administration in humans is accompanied by activation of the fibrinolytic system. This is characterized by an early release of tissue plasminogen activator, followed by an increase in plasminogen activator inhibitor activity.[6]

These studies and many others have given weight to the suggestion that endotoxin has a prominent role as a mediator in septic shock caused by gram-negative organisms as well as non–gram-negative infections.[2, 6, 30, 35] Additional support for endotoxin involvement in the production of sepsis syndrome and septic shock is the frequent detection of endotoxemia, despite lack of a documented gram-negative infection.[36] Endotoxemia was correlated with shock and organ injury and depressed myocardial contractility.[36] Multiple organ system failure was more likely to occur with endotoxemia than with shock and no endotoxemia.

Arachidonic Acid Metabolites

The products of arachidonic acid metabolism also appear to have a role as possible mediators of the septic process.[37] Elevated serum levels of the arachidonic acid metabolites prostacyclin (PGI$_2$) and thromboxane A$_2$ (TXA$_2$) have been demonstrated in patients with septic shock.[38] Attention has been focused on the eicosanoids, which are fatty acids with

vasoactive properties. Cell membranes, specifically the phospholipid components, serve as stored precursors of the eicosanoids. Initially, the action of lysosomal enzymes phospholipase A$_2$, C, and D on the cell membrane releases arachidonic acid. This fatty acid is, in turn, metabolized by the monooxygenase, cyclooxygenase, or lipoxygenase enzymatic pathways.[39] The by-products of these reactions are a number of eicosanoids: epoxides, leukotrienes, and prostaglandins (PGs)[39, 40] (Fig. 23–3). The PGs are metabolites of the cyclooxygenase pathway and have been found to be involved in various disease states, including inflammation, peptic ulcer disease, platelet dysfunction, diarrhea, fever, and shock.[41] These eicosanoids are degraded in part by enzymes in the kidney, the liver, or the lung.[42]

In the cyclooxygenase pathway, the catalytic action of cyclooxygenase on arachidonic acid leads to the formation of the endoperoxides PGG$_2$ and PGH$_2$. Subsequent action by prostacyclin synthetase forms PGI$_2$, whereas thromboxane synthetase, found in platelets, lung tissue, and lung fibroblasts, metabolizes the endoperoxides to TXA$_2$.[40]

PGI$_2$, released from vascular endothelial cells, has been shown to be responsible for arachidonate-induced vasodilation, the stimulation of renin release from the kidney, inhibition of thrombus formation, and disaggregation of platelets in vitro.[39, 40] TXA$_2$ is a potent vasoconstrictor, acting especially on the pulmonary, coronary, splanchnic, and renal beds. TXA$_2$ is generated by cells in the lung, with a substantial contribution to peak plasma levels coming from circulating leukocytes.[43] Other biologic actions of TXA$_2$ include platelet and neutrophil aggregation, increase in cell membrane permeability, and pulmonary bronchoconstriction. Diverse clinical conditions such as preeclampsia, cerebrovascular accidents, transient ischemic attacks, unstable angina pectoris, acute myocardial infarction, peripheral vascular disease, pulmonary hypertension in sepsis, and bronchoconstriction in gram-negative sepsis and anaphylaxis may involve initiation, mediation, or amplification by TXA$_2$[44] (see Fig. 23–3). Additional cyclooxygenase products, PGE$_2$ and PGD$_2$, can potentiate the effects of histamine and bradykinin on vascular permeability and contribute to the inflammatory-septic response.[39]

The lipoxygenase pathway of arachidonic acid metabolism yields a number of leukotrienes, some of which have been implicated as mediators in a number of inflammatory disease and microcirculatory changes.[39] Leukotriene B$_4$ is a potent chemoattractant for both eosinophils and neutrophils, in addition to a lymphocyte activator.[39] Some of the leukotrienes seem to have a role in the modification of membrane function and composition; 15-hydroperoxyeicosatetraenoic

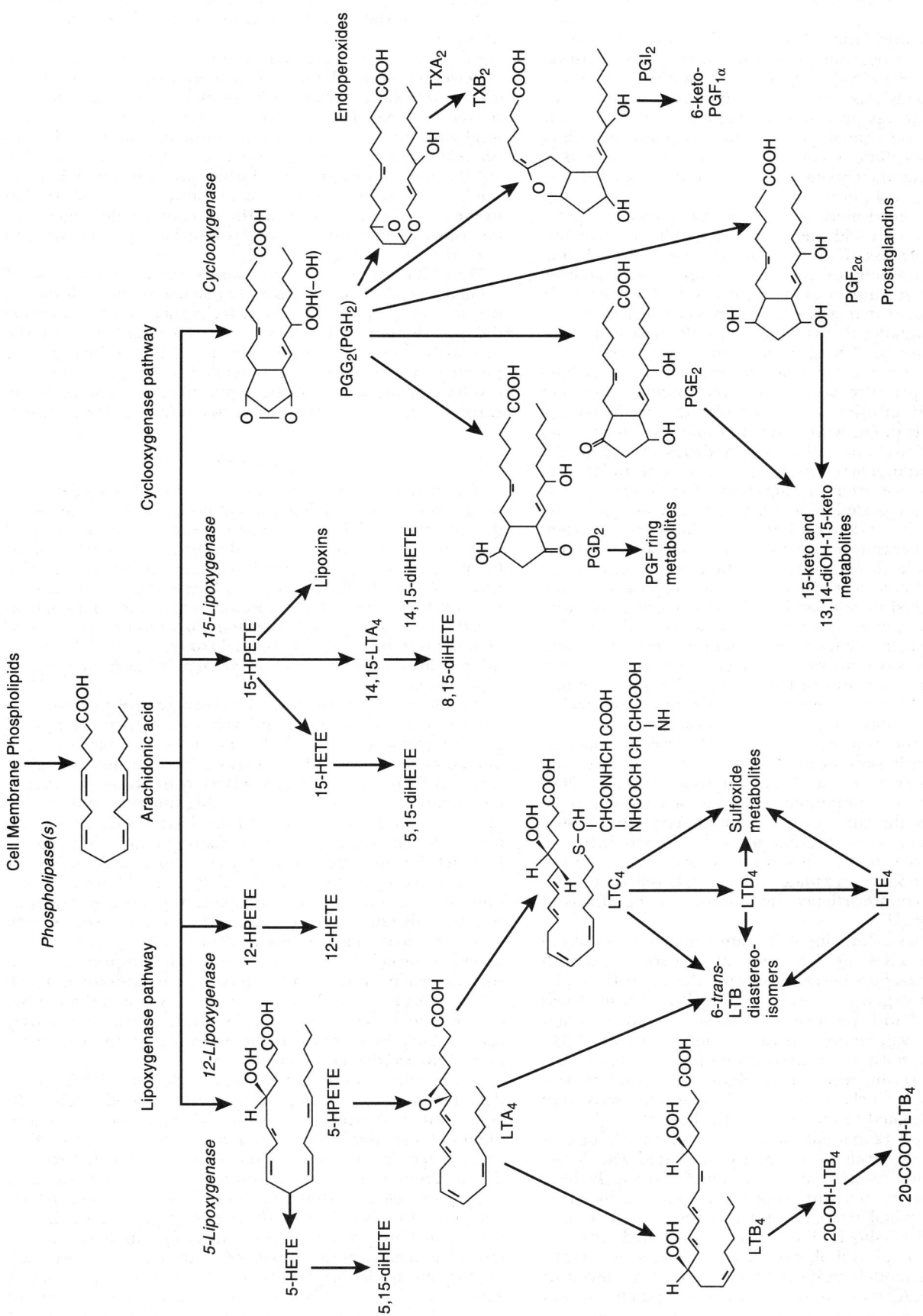

Figure 23–3. The arachidonic acid cascade. Eicosanoids that are important biologically and their degradation products are indicated: HPETE, hydroperoxyeicosatetraenoic acid; HETE, hydroxyeicosatetraenoic acid; LTA$_4$, LTB$_4$, LTC$_4$, LTD$_4$, LTE$_4$, leukotrienes A$_4$, B$_4$, C$_4$, D$_4$, and E$_4$, respectively; PGD$_2$, PGE$_2$, PGF$_{2\alpha}$, PGF$_{1\alpha}$, PGG$_2$, PGH$_2$, and PGI$_2$, prostaglandins D$_2$, E$_2$, F$_{2\alpha}$, F$_{1\alpha}$, G$_2$, H$_2$, and I$_2$, respectively; TXA$_2$ and TXB$_2$, thromboxanes A$_2$ and B$_2$, respectively. (Adapted from Henderson WR Jr: Eicosanoids and lung inflammation. Am Rev Respir Dis 135:1176, 1987.)

305

acid metabolites demonstrate inhibition of natural killer cell activity.[39]

Arachidonic acid from phospholipids can also be metabolized via the cytochrome P-450 monooxygenase pathway (not shown in Fig. 23–3). Products include the epoxyeicosatetraenoic acids (epoxides), with significant actions demonstrated in vitro; peptide hormone release; cellular calcium mobilization; and changes in sodium and potassium transport.[39] However, little is known about the in vivo effects of monooxygenase metabolites; this remains as an area of continued investigation.

Numerous animal models of sepsis have implicated products of arachidonic acid metabolism as potential mediators of the septic process. The ovine preparation with a chronic lymph fistula draining the mediastinal lymph nodes has been utilized in a large number of these studies.[34, 40, 43, 45] Endotoxin infusion produces an increase in pulmonary arterial pressure and airway resistance that is associated with an early increase in thromboxane B_2 (TXB_2) levels.[43] Sheep rendered leukopenic via nitrogen mustard showed less increase in pulmonary arterial pressure and pulmonary vascular resistance after endotoxin infusion, compared with that in the control group.[43] Pretreatment with ibuprofen, meclofenamate, and other nonsteroidal anti-inflammatory drugs prevented the increase in pulmonary arterial pressure and pulmonary vascular resistance after the injection of endotoxin. These investigations suggested that TXA_2 was at least partly responsible for the endotoxin-induced pulmonary hypertension. The mechanisms for the increase in pulmonary arterial pressure include direct vasoconstriction of the pulmonary vasculature[38, 47] and microthrombi in small capillaries secondary to enhanced platelet and neutrophil aggregation, with a resultant decrease in vascular cross-sectional area.[38, 47] Hypoxemia, which occurs in endotoxin-induced shock and causes hypoxic vasoconstriction, theoretically can be implicated in the pathogenesis of endotoxin-induced pulmonary hypertension. However, sepsis is typically associated with a loss of hypoxic pulmonary vasoconstriction.

Additional studies indicate that the PG cyclic endoperoxide PGH_2 is an important mediator of pulmonary vasoconstriction in the ovine model.[46] The opposing effects of PGI_2 and TXA_2 on the pulmonary arterial bed may also be responsible for the changes in the pulmonary circulation.[44] Both substances were present after endotoxin infusion. Their respective vasodilating and vasoconstricting properties affect the pulmonary vasculature. The PGI_2 release may be an attempt to counterbalance the vasoconstricting effects of TXA_2 and $PGF_{2\alpha}$.[44]

Clinical studies in humans with gram-negative sepsis found that PGI_2 and TXB_2 were released at an early stage, with plasma concentration correlating with the severity of the sepsis-induced organ failure.[48] Elevated PGI_2 serum levels were associated with preserved organ system function and improved survival, whereas patients with significant TXB_2 elevations had more organ dysfunction and increased mortality.[48] TXB_2 serum levels were elevated in patients with sepsis and septic shock, but 6-keto-$PGF_{1\alpha}$ serum levels were significantly elevated in only those with shock.[49]

In a study of 12 patients with septic shock, circulating phospholipase A_2 levels were directly correlated with hypotension, in both severity and duration.[50] Extremely high levels were assayed in serum while the patient was hypotensive, with a gradual decrease and clearing with treatment and resolution of shock. The authors concluded that, because exogenous phospholipase A_2 administered to experimental animal models induces hypotension, high levels of phospholipase A_2 may contribute to the hypotension and cardiovascular instability in human septic shock.[50] This is not surprising; the source of phospholipase A_2 is activated neutrophils. The phospholipase A_2 is one of the phospholipases necessary for the release of arachidonic acid from membrane phospholipids.

Ibuprofen, a nonsteroidal anti-inflammatory agent, is a cyclooxygenase inhibitor with preferential blocking effects on thromboxane synthetase.[40] Animal studies have demonstrated the beneficial effects of thromboxane synthetase inhibition on the hemodynamic instability induced by endotoxin.[40] Rats rendered hypotensive by endotoxin had significantly improved survival when pretreated with ibuprofen (81% versus 8% for controls).[51] Ibuprofen administration in the ovine model improved the physiologic derangements described earlier but did not prevent later pulmonary and hemodynamic changes.[43, 45]

When ibuprofen was given before the administration of small doses of E. coli endotoxin to normal human volunteers, the clinical symptoms of fever, tachypnea, and tachycardia did not develop.[52] There was also an attenuation of the increase in stress hormone production.[52] The cyclooxygenase products of arachidonic acid metabolism are most certainly involved as mediators in the septic process, at least in the early phase; however, their exact role remains to be clarified.

Endorphins

Endogenous opiates, or endorphins, have been extensively researched since their initial isolation in 1976, 3 years after the discovery of specific opiate receptors in the central nervous system.[53] Intravenous administration of endorphins to rats is followed by profound hypotension and tachycardia, producing a shock-like state.[53] These symptoms can be blocked by the use of the specific opiate antagonist naloxone.[54] This, coupled with the demonstration of reversal of endotoxin-induced shock by naloxone,[54] has sparked an interest in the possible role of endorphins as a mediator of septic shock.

β-Endorphin is formed by the cleavage of β-lipotropin (a polypeptide with a common parent of corticotropin) and pro-opiotropin (a molecule found in the pituitary gland).[55] Simultaneous release of the endogenous opiates and corticotropin from the pituitary is effected by stressors, such as endotoxin.[56] Several studies utilizing murine and canine models of endotoxin-induced shock have shown that pituitary endorphins are involved as pathophysiologic factors.[54] Hypotension induced by the injection of E. coli endotoxin was reversed by naloxone in the early phase.[54] However, 24-hour survival ratios were not significantly improved in rats treated with saline infusion alone versus those treated with saline and naloxone. On the other hand, dogs subjected to a similar protocol did show a significant improvement in survival when treated with naloxone for endotoxin shock (83% versus 21%).[54] The investigators postulated that, in the canine model, naloxone primarily increased the mean arterial pressure by reversal of the endotoxin-induced depression of myocardial contractility.[54]

Subsequent studies in the canine endotoxin shock model demonstrated up to a fivefold increase in blood levels of β-endorphin.[56] Pretreatment with naloxone blocked endotoxin-induced hypotension and depression of the cardiac index,[56] lending support to the theory that endotoxin-induced hypotension is, at least in part, mediated through endorphin release. After hypotension is established, naloxone administration is also effective in improving cardiovascular function, with significant increases in both cardiac index and mean arterial pressure.[57] This reflects an increased cardiac output, increased stroke volume, and improved left ventricular function. Naloxone treatment, however, did not reverse the lactic acidosis, despite the improvements in blood pressure and cardiac index.[57]

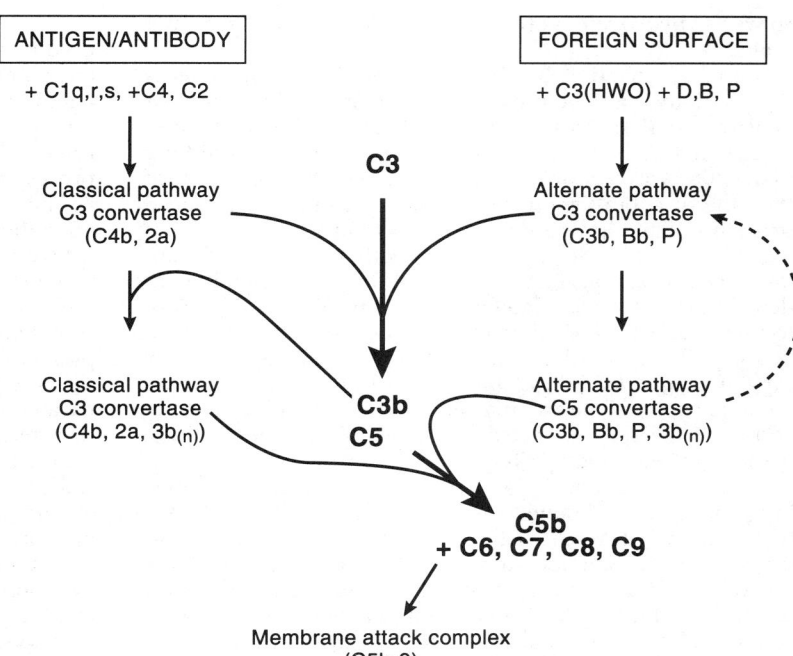

ANTIGEN/ANTIBODY

+ C1q,r,s, +C4, C2

C3

Classical pathway
C3 convertase
(C4b, 2a)

FOREIGN SURFACE

+ C3(HWO) + D,B, P

Alternate pathway
C3 convertase
(C3b, Bb, P)

Classical pathway
C3 convertase
(C4b, 2a, 3b$_{(n)}$)

C3b
C5

Alternate pathway
C5 convertase
(C3b, Bb, P, 3b$_{(n)}$)

C5b
+ C6, C7, C8, C9

Membrane attack complex
(C5b-9)

Figure 23–4. Schema of reactions of complement activation, both classic and alternative pathways. (From Taetle R, Rapaport SI: Inflammation and phagocytosis. In: West JB [ed]: Best and Taylor's Physiological Basis of Medical Practice. 12th ed. Baltimore, Williams & Wilkins, p 363, 1990. © 1990, the Williams & Wilkins Co., Baltimore.)

A series of patients in septic shock were given intravenous naloxone, with a demonstrable improvement of hypotension occurring in 8 of 13.[55] This anecdotal report was followed by several studies in humans, which failed to show a clear, beneficial effect of naloxone on hypotension and survival. In fact there have been associated side effects of profound hypotension, seizures, and pulmonary edema.[58] Citing differences in timing of administration and dosage as possible critical factors in efficacy, a group of investigators carefully monitored the hemodynamic response of 13 hypotensive septic patients to a continuous 1-hour infusion of naloxone.[59] The authors noted a significant increase in mean arterial pressure after naloxone administration, in addition to an increase in systolic arterial pressure. Although no adverse side effects were observed in this series of patients, presumably owing to the lower dosages administered, there was no improvement in mortality or survival.[59]

The exact role of the β-endorphins in the pathophysiologic response of sepsis is unknown. The complex pathophysiology of sepsis makes the likelihood of a single agent, such as naloxone, with actions on one possible mediator, unlikely to be a consistently effective therapeutic agent. Data to date do not support a prominent role for β-endorphins in the pathogenesis or a major role for naloxone in the treatment of sepsis and septic shock.

Activated Complement

The complement system, via both the classic and alternative pathways, is one of the earliest cascades to be activated in sepsis and septic shock.[32] The classic pathway is initiated by the binding of complement component C1 to antibodies (immunoglobulin G or M) that have reacted to corresponding antigens, in this case antibody-coated bacteria.[32, 60] Endotoxin, functioning as a particulate activator, stimulates the alternative pathway[32, 60] (Fig. 23–4). Complement components, of which complement fragment C5a is the most biologically potent, enhance the nonspecific host defenses. This is done in part by promoting bacterial phagocytosis and acting as a chemoattractant for activated neutrophils.[1, 32, 61] C5a also functions as an anaphylatoxin, producing mediator release from mast cells, in addition to inducing neutrophil aggregation.[62]

A murine model of systemic complement activation produced hemodynamic changes similar to those seen in clinical sepsis.[61] Zymosan, a potent activator of the alternative pathway of complement, is a glucopolysaccharide found in the cell walls of yeast. Administration of zymosan in increasing doses produced a spectrum of hemodynamic changes as the degree of complement activation increased. Low doses were associated with tachycardia, elevated cardiac outputs, and mild hypertension.[61] Circulatory collapse marked by hypotension, tachycardia, and systemic hypoperfusion was induced by high doses of zymosan. Endotoxin administered to rats produces a similar hemodynamic pattern; both endotoxin and zymosan are potent activators of the alternative pathway of complement.[61] The authors concluded that complement activation is an early occurrence in sepsis and is probably involved in the cascade of events leading to hemodynamic collapse.

The effects of systemic complement activation have been studied in a variety of animal models, with a focus on pulmonary changes.[62–64] Intravascular activation of complement causes neutrophil stimulation and aggregation and sequestration of neutrophils in capillaries, with resultant endothelial cell damage, presumably from the release of highly reactive toxic oxygen metabolites.[62] Complement fragment C5a has been shown to induce these actions, aggregating neutrophils, which act as leukocytic emboli or microemboli, affecting the pulmonary circulation and other tissues.[65]

In an attempt to elucidate the roles of complement, neutrophils, and toxic oxygen metabolites in lung injury, intravascular complement activation induced by purified cobra venom factor was studied in rats.[62] Acute lung injury after cobra venom factor injection, as manifested by changes in lung vascular permeability, was determined by leakage of ^{125}I-labeled rat immunoglobulin G into the extravascular lung compartment. Neutrophil-depleted animals and animals given specific enzymes, superoxide dismutase or catalase, were studied. Superoxide dismutase converts the superoxide ion to hydrogen peroxide, whereas catalase converts hydrogen peroxide to molecular oxygen and water.[64]

Animals injected with cobra venom factor demonstrated a threefold increase in lung vascular permeability, whereas neutropenic (less than 500 neutrophils per cubic millimeter blood) animals had a marked reduction in the extent of lung injury (68% protection).[62] Rats treated with both enzymes at the time of cobra venom factor injection showed enhanced protection from lung injury, more so than when each agent was administered alone. However, both superoxide dismutase and catalase protect the lungs from neutrophil-dependent injury after complement activation (53 and 66% protection, respectively).[62] The authors suggested that activated neutrophil aggregation, with subsequent intrapulmonary capillary sequestration, is initiated by intravascular complement activation. The vascular endothelial cell injury may be related to the release of toxic oxygen radicals from complement-activated neutrophils.[62]

Additional evidence of the role of complement in septic lung injury was obtained from the study of C5-sufficient (C5$^+$) and C5-deficient (C5$^-$) mice strains.[63] Sepsis was induced by cecal ligation and puncture, with survival time noted, in addition to lung studies: the pulmonary air-blood barrier thickness, pulmonary intracapillary granulocyte count, and arterial blood gas values. In comparison to C5$^-$ mice, the C5$^+$ animals demonstrated a significant increase in the air-blood barrier thickness, increased intracapillary granulocyte count, and a decrease in the arterial oxygen tension (59.2 versus 85.7 mm Hg). The mean survival time for the C5$^+$ septic animals was 40 hours, whereas the C5$^-$ septic animals had a survival time more than twice as long (87.8 hours).[63] Activated complement, especially C5a, seems to be involved in the pathogenesis of septic lung injury.

Investigations of complement activation and septic lung injury, especially the adult respiratory distress syndrome (ARDS), in patients have yielded confusion and at times apparently contradictory results. In a series of 61 patients thought to be at risk for ARDS, polymorphonuclear granulocyte aggregation induced by activated complement was determined at various intervals throughout their clinical course.[65] Thirty-three patients developed ARDS; abnormally elevated plasma C5a levels were noted in 31, either on the day of diagnosis or during the preceding 72 hours.[65] The authors found that neutrophil aggregation induced by activated complement reflects plasma C5a activity, which in turn was highly correlated with the development of ARDS in their series of patients.[65]

Additional studies of the role of complement activation in acute lung injury in sepsis yielded conflicting results.[66–68] Although plasma levels of C5a were elevated in patients who were hypotensive and/or acidotic, no correlation was found with initial severity or with prediction of development of acute lung injury.[66] In a separate series of 50 patients, of whom 36 developed ARDS, elevated plasma C5a activity was found in 86% of patients with ARDS.[67] However, the authors noted that intense complement activation is also associated with a number of clinical conditions, such as multiple traumatic injuries, acute pancreatitis, severe burns, and disseminated intravascular coagulation, which predispose patients to the development of ARDS. The investigators concluded that C5a-like activity is not always related to the development of ARDS and is of no predictive value.[67]

Complement pathway determination and C3 and C4 levels were determined in a study of 59 patients in septic shock.[68] ARDS occurred in 27 patients at some time during their clinical course. No consistent correlation with the plasma levels of C3 or C4 or pathway activation and the development of acute lung injury was found.[68] Although complement activation, via either the classic or the alternative pathway,

was noted in 76% of the septic patients, no clinically valuable predictors were found. Possible explanations for the different observations include various methods of C5a determination (e.g., neutrophil aggregation and radioimmunoassay), the presence of septic shock, medication (e.g., corticosteroids), the time of blood sampling, and the method of processing samples.

The terminal C5b,6,7,8,9 complement complex (TCC) was quantified in 87 septic patients, during a 2-year prospective study.[69] The presence of TCC, a stable complement byproduct of the cleavage of C5 by convertase, in plasma indicates that the complement cascade has been activated to completion.[69] In the 22 patients who developed ARDS, plasma TCC concentrations were markedly elevated (average increase, 110%) 2 days before the onset of lung injury. In parallel determinations of C3, C4, and C5a, it was found that plasma TCC concentrations were more sensitive in measuring the acute septic lung injury.[69] The authors concluded that plasma TCC concentrations were able to differentiate between septic ARDS patients and septic non-ARDS patients.

TCC may be involved in the pathogenesis of ARDS via two possible mechanisms: (1) direct endothelial damage resulting from the direct deposition of TCC on the pulmonary vascular endothelium and (2) the stimulation of arachidonic acid metabolites and release of toxic oxygen metabolites by TCC.[69] Another study of septic patients could not confirm the specific or temporal relationship of TCC and the eventual development of ARDS.[70] What is evident is the complex pathophysiology of acute lung injury in sepsis. It is most certainly not due to solely complement activation;[71] a number of other cascades and cellular elements are involved, the exact role of each being unresolved at this time.

Serum C3b levels are known to be decreased in patients with gram-negative bacteremia, especially those patients whose course was complicated by shock and eventual death.[31, 72] Septic shock patients more frequently had elevated plasma levels of C5a than of other complement components.[72] In this same study, the C5a level was negatively correlated with the decrease in systemic vascular resistance index, that is, high C5a levels were associated with a significant depression in systemic vascular resistance index, reflecting hemodynamic alteration in sepsis.[72] Mast cell induction by C5a with elaboration of vasodilatory mediators is presumed to be one of the major mechanisms of depressed peripheral vascular resistance, contributing to the hypotension associated with sepsis.[72]

High plasma levels of C3a and C4a were found to be associated with a fatal outcome in patients with sepsis.[73] Plasma levels of C3a and C4a, in addition to C1–C1-inhibitor complexes, were determined in 48 septic patients and correlated with clinical events such as shock, ARDS, and eventual outcome. Plasma C3a levels were elevated in all but one patient at the time of hospital admission. Septic shock was evident in 23 patients, the mean of the highest C3a levels was 38 nmol/L compared with 18 nmol/L in patients without shock. In the 15 patients who had ARDS, there was an increased level of C3a when compared with that in other septic patients; however, this did not reach statistical significance. When plasma C3a levels were related to clinical outcome, a high level of correlation was seen. The mean highest level was 36 nmol/L in nonsurvivors as compared with 18 nmol/L in those who did survive. The higher the level of plasma C3a, the higher the mortality rate was. In addition, a prognostic relationship was found: all patients whose C3a levels dropped to normal survived, whereas 86% of patients in whom the levels did not decrease to 9 nmol/L or less died.[73] The authors concluded that complement activation via the classic pathway is involved in the development of fatal complications of sepsis.

Cytokines

Cytokines have been the subject of intense study, not only in the area of endothelial cell biology, but also with regard to their actions in pathologic processes, such as acute inflammation, vascular leakage, allograft rejection, and sepsis.[74, 75] Previously known as lymphokines, these polypeptide products of activated cells have been found to be elaborated by monocytes and macrophages, in addition to the originally described lymphoid cells.[74] There are numerous cytokines, called interleukins, previously named according to various biologic actions (e.g., TNF and interferon). At this time, at least 10 interleukins have been characterized by amino acid sequences.

Cytokines have been implicated as mediators of sepsis and septic shock. Infusion of small amounts of *E. coli* endotoxin in human volunteers causes an increase in TNF levels.[30] Another cytokine, interleukin-6, has been shown to be present in the plasma of septic patients.[76] Moreover, increased levels of interleukin-6 were significantly correlated with plasma lactate level and heart rate and inversely correlated with mean arterial pressure and platelet counts. The level of interleukin-6 had prognostic significance: low levels on hospital admission were associated with survival, whereas high levels, exceeding 7500 U/mL, were associated with a fatal outcome in 89% of patients.[76] At this time, however, it is unclear whether interleukin-6 is directly involved in the pathophysiology of sepsis or merely the result of endothelial cell injury caused by other mediators. An in-depth discussion of the role of cytokines in the pathophysiology of sepsis is provided in Chapter 24.

Activated Neutrophils

The polymorphonuclear leukocyte has been implicated in the pathophysiology of sepsis, especially the complication of acute lung injury (ARDS).[71] Insights into the possible role of polymorphonuclear leukocytes came from the clinical observation of sudden neutropenia associated with hemodialysis using cuprammonium cellulose membranes.[77] It was found that this neutropenia was due to complement activation (see earlier), with subsequent sequestration of aggregated polymorphonuclear leukocytes in the pulmonary vasculature, causing mild pulmonary dysfunction.[77]

In an attempt to elucidate the actions of endotoxin in shock and lung injury, neutrophils and their function were studied in a canine model.[78] Endotoxemia resulted in leukopenia and increased leukocyte adherence in the vasculature. Treatment with ibuprofen after endotoxin administration improved hemodynamic alterations but did not affect improvement in the lung, either histologically or morphometrically.[78] Although ibuprofen decreased leukocyte adherence, its administration after endotoxin injection was unable to ameliorate the effects of toxic products released by activated granulocytes.[78]

Sheep rendered granulocytopenic with hydroxyurea were studied after endotoxin infusion.[79] Lung lymph protein clearance, a measure of pulmonary vascular permeability, was increased after the infusion of *E. coli* endotoxin. In granulocyte-depleted animals, the increase in lung vascular permeability was significantly lower (10.4 ± 1 mL/h) when compared with that in controls (21.4 ± 1.4 mL/h). The authors concluded that circulating granulocytes are required for endotoxin-induced increases in lung vascular permeability.[79]

These and other studies suggested that neutrophils are involved in mediating acute lung injury in ARDS. However, the role of polymorphonuclear leukocytes in the pathogenesis of septic lung injury is yet to be clarified. One example

of the inherent difficulty in elucidating these mechanism is the occurrence of ARDS in neutropenic patients.[80] At this time, it is clear that the activated neutrophil is involved in the septic response. Various neutrophil products, such as toxic oxygen radicals, elastase, PGs, and leukotrienes, have been implicated as mediators; however, the precise roles and relationships are yet to be determined.

Platelet-Activating Factor

PAF is an ether phospholipid known to be an important proinflammatory mediator. Released from cells after physiologic stimulation or injury, this mediator has been found in platelets, macrophages, vascular endothelium, leukocytes, kidneys, and lungs.[81] Gram-negative sepsis and endotoxemia cause PAF elaboration from injured cells. In animals given PAF, pathophysiologic derangements of decreased peripheral vascular resistance, systemic arterial hypotension, pulmonary arterial hypertension, and death occur.[81] These effects are quite similar to endotoxin- and PG-induced changes.

A murine model of severe endotoxemia was used to determine the effects of a specific PAF antagonist (BN 52021) on eicosanoid production and hemodynamic response.[81] Endotoxin-induced hypotension was associated with increased production of TXB_2 and PGE_2. Rats pretreated with the PAF receptor antagonist demonstrated no hypotension after endotoxin infusion. The production of TXB_2 and PGE_2 was significantly attenuated by BN 52021, with values one fourth of those measured after endotoxin infusion alone.[81] The authors concluded that a relationship between PAF and the eicosanoids may exist, and at least in endotoxemia, the effects of PAF may be mediated via the cyclooxygenase pathway.[81]

Further evidence of a relationship between PAF and the products of arachidonic acid metabolism came from a study of murine isolated lung preparations.[82] PAF produced pulmonary edema in this model, which can be prevented by blocking the cyclooxygenase pathway. Increases in pulmonary vascular resistance secondary to PAF, which had been demonstrated previously in the ovine model, were attenuated by lipoxygenase inhibition.[83] This study demonstrated an increase in leukotriene C_4, a potent pulmonary vasoconstrictor, after the infusion of PAF and cyclooxygenase inhibition by indomethacin.[82] Other work with septic patients also demonstrated a link between leukotriene C_4 and PAF, especially in ARDS.[84] There may be a role played by PAF in the pathogenesis of septic ARDS. At this time, one may presume that PAF is involved in the pathogenesis of sepsis, its role being intertwined with that of the eicosanoids; however, definite evidence is lacking.

ADVERSE SEQUELAE

The end result of mediator activation and initiation of this complex septic host response is the involvement of a variety of cascades with diverse effects. The most significant effects are centered on the blood vessels, especially the arterioles, and may lead to the development of hypotension related to loss of vascular tone and a decrease in the systemic vascular resistance.

The vascular endothelial cell is also affected and may be damaged, with a resultant loss of vessel integrity. This can lead to increased permeability of the capillary beds. The loss of vascular tone coupled with membrane damage leads to a distributive form of shock.[6] Shock is a well-known complication of sepsis, occurring on average in 40% of patients.[6, 85]

ARDS is associated with many noninfectious insults; however, sepsis is the most common risk factor for its development. Of septic patients, 5 to 40% experience ARDS.[38, 86] Multiple organ system failure is a dreaded complication of ARDS, with sepsis being a major risk factor. The greater the number of systems involved and the longer the duration of failure, the greater is the mortality rate.[87] Recurrent sepsis and multiple organ system failure are now the major causes of mortality in patients with sepsis. New and aggressive modes of treatment have prolonged the survival of septic patients, increasing the appearance of these late sequelae.

SUMMARY

The pathogenesis of sepsis and septic shock seems to require an infecting organism. Subsequent activation and initiation of various cascades, with release of active mediators, result in a diffuse intravascular endothelial injury. The use of antibiotics has resulted in a remarkable advance in treating infections because they decrease mortality. Unfortunately, antibiotics, even those with proven activity against a susceptible causative organism, do not halt the septic response and mediator cascade. Treatment therefore continues to be supportive, with early and aggressive support of the cardiopulmonary system to maintain organ perfusion. Fluids and antibiotics remain the cornerstones of therapy, supplemented with judicious use of vasopressors and inotropic agents when necessary. Attention to correcting metabolic and electrolyte derangements, while optimizing blood flow to organs, is an important part of the treatment plan.

Adjunctive therapy in sepsis and septic shock is continuing to be an area of research. Corticosteroids have been shown not to improve survival in septic patients.[88, 89] In fact, certain patients with impaired renal function or ARDS seem to have a worse outcome when treated with steroids.[88, 90] In the absence of adrenal insufficiency, corticosteroids should not be used in the treatment of sepsis or septic shock.

Another avenue of research has been adjunctive immunotherapy using antibodies to endotoxin, specifically the core determinants of lipopolysaccharide, derived from the J5 mutant *E. coli*.[35] Patients with gram-negative septic shock receiving antiserum prepared from volunteers inoculated with heat-inactivated J5 *E. coli* demonstrated a marked benefit. Overall mortality was significantly decreased, as was the mortality associated with profound shock requiring vasopressor support.[35] Widespread use of this form of preventive therapy is not practical, owing to the difficulty in preparation of the vaccine and the inherent risk of transmission of diseases such as viral hepatitis and the acquired immunodeficiency syndrome. New technology utilizing monoclonal antibodies has been tested in a multicenter clinical trial in patients with sepsis and septic shock.[91] Other areas of research have been the modulation and inhibition of the various mediators of the septic response. A more detailed discussion of the approach to treatment can be found in Chapter 28.

References

1. Young LS: Gram-negative sepsis. In: Mandel GL, Douglas G Jr, Bennett JE (eds): Principles and Practice of Infectious Diseases. 3rd ed. New York, Churchill Livingstone, p 611, 1990.
2. Kreger BE, Carven DE, Carling P, et al: Gram-negative bacteremia III. Reassessment of etiology, epidemiology, and ecology in 612 patients. Am J Med 68:332, 1980.
3. McGowan JE Jr, Barnes MW, Finland MW: Bacteremia at Boston City Hospital. Occurrence and mortality during 12 selected years (1935–1972), with special reference to hospital-acquired cases. J Infect Dis 132:316, 1975.
4. DuPont HL, Spink WW: Infections due to gram-negative organisms; An analysis of 860 patients with bacteremia at the University of Minnesota Medical Center, 1958–1966. Medicine 48:307, 1969.
5. McCabe WR, Kreger BE, Johns ME: Type-specific and cross-reactive antibodies in gram-negative bacteremia. N Engl J Med 287:261, 1972.
6. Parrillo JE, Parker MM, Natanson C, et al: Septic shock in humans. Advances in the understanding of pathogenesis, cardiovascular dysfunction, and therapy. Ann Intern Med 113:227, 1990.
7. McCabe WR, Jackson GG: Gram-negative bacteremia II. Clinical, laboratory, and therapeutic observations. Arch Intern Med 110:856, 1962.
8. Kreger BE, Craven DE, McCabe WR: Gram-negative bacteremia IV. Re-evaluation of clinical features and treatment in 612 patients. Am J Med 68:344, 1980.
9. Machiedo GW, LoVerme PJ, McGovern PJ Jr, et al: Patterns of mortality in a surgical intensive care unit. Surg Gynecol Obstet 152:757, 1981.
10. Thibault GE, Mulley AGE, Barnett GO, et al: Medical intensive care: Indications, interventions, and outcomes. N Engl J Med 302:938, 1980.
11. Thibault GE: The medical intensive care unit: A five-year perspective. In: Parrillo JE, Ayers SM (eds): Major Issues in Critical Care Medicine. Baltimore, Williams & Wilkins, p 9, 1984.
12. Waisbren BA: Gram-negative shock and endotoxin shock. Am J Med 36:819, 1964.
13. McCabe WR, Treadwell TL, De Maria A Jr: Pathophysiology of bacteremia. Am J Med 75:7, 1983.
14. Kwaan HM, Weil MH: Differences in the mechanisms of shock caused by bacterial infections. Surg Gynecol Obstet 128:37, 1969.
15. Hoeprich PD, O'Grady LF: Manifestations of infectious diseases. In: Hoeprich PD, Jordan MC (eds): Infectious Diseases. 4th ed. Philadelphia, JB Lippincott, p 83, 1989.
16. Singer C, Kaplan MH, Armstrong D: Bacteremia and fungemia complicating neoplastic disease. A study of 364 cases. Am J Med 62:731, 1977.
17. Johanson WC, Pierce AK, Sanford JP: Changing pharyngeal bacterial flora of hospitalized patients. Emergence of gram-negative bacilli. N Engl J Med 281:1137, 1969.
18. Caplan ES, Hoyt NJ: Nosocomial sinusitis. JAMA 247:639, 1982.
19. Gunnar RM, Loeb HS, Winlow EJ, et al: Hemodynamic measurements in bacteremia and septic shock in man. J Infect Dis 128:S295, 1973.
20. MacLean LD, Mulligan WG, McLean APH, et al: Patterns of septic shock in man—A detailed study of 56 patients. Ann Surg 166:543, 1967.
21. Wiles JB, Cerra FB, Siegal JH, et al: The systemic septic response: Does the organism matter? Crit Care Med 8:55, 1980.
22. Parker MM, Parrillo JE: Septic shock. Hemodynamics and pathogenesis. JAMA 250:3324, 1983.
23. Deutschman CS, Konstantinides FN, Tsai M, et al: Physiology and metabolism in isolated viral septicemia. Further evidence of an organism-independent host-dependent response. Arch Surg 122:21, 1987.
24. Marshall J, Sweeny D: Microbial infection and the septic response in critical surgical illness. Sepsis, not infection, determines outcome. Arch Surg 125:17, 1990.
25. Band JD, Maki DG: Infections caused by arterial catheters used for hemodynamic monitoring. Am J Med 67:735, 1979.
26. Nelson N, Singh S, Check F, et al: Colonization and cathether-related sepsis pulmonary and arterial catheters. Crit Care Med 9:144, 1981.
27. Maki DG, Goldman DA, Rhame FS: Infection control in intravenous therapy. Ann Intern Med 79:867, 1973.
28. Luce JM: Pathogenesis and management of septic shock. Chest 91:883, 1987.
29. Shubin H, Weil MH: Bacterial shock. JAMA 235:421, 1976.
30. Suffredini AF, Fromm RE, Parker MM, et al: The cardiovascular response of normal humans to the administration of endotoxin. N Engl J Med 321:280, 1989.
31. McCabe WR: Serum complement levels in bacteremia due to gram-negative organisms. N Engl J Med 288:21, 1973.
32. Fearon DT, Ruddy S, Schur PH, et al: Activation of the properdin pathway of complement in patients with gram-negative bacteremia. N Engl J Med 292:937, 1975.
33. Baris C, Guest MM, Frazer ME: Direct effects of endotoxin on the microcirculation. Adv Shock Res 4:153, 1980.
34. Traber TL, Adair T, Adams T Jr: Hemodynamic consequences of endotoxemia in sheep. Adv Shock Res 4:153, 1980.
35. Ziegler EJ, McCutchan JA, Fierer J, et al: Treatment of gram-negative bacteremia and shock with human antiserum to a mutant *Escherichia coli*. N Engl J Med 307:1225, 1982.
36. Danner RL, Elin RJ, Hosseini JM, et al: Endotoxemia in human septic shock. Chest 99:169, 1991.
37. Fletcher JR: The role of prostaglandins in sepsis. Scand J Infect Dis [Suppl] 31:55, 1982.
38. Bersten A, Sibbald WJ: Acute lung injury in septic shock. Crit Care Clin 5:49, 1989.
39. Holtzman MJ: Arachidonic acid metabolism. Implications of biological chemistry for lung function and disease. Am Rev Respir Dis 143:188, 1991.
40. Petrak RA, Balk RA, Bone RC: Prostaglandins cyclooxygenase inhibitors, and thromboxane synthetase inhibitors in the pathogenesis of multiple systems organ failure. Crit Care Clin 5:303, 1989.
41. Fletcher JR, Ramwell WR: Prostaglandins in shock: To give or to block? Adv Shock Res 3:57, 1980.
42. Henderson WR Jr: Eicosanoids and lung inflammation. Am Rev Respir Dis 135:1176, 1987.
43. Huttemeier PC, Watkins WD, Peterson MB, et al: Acute pulmonary hypertension and lung thromboxane release after endotoxin in normal and leukopenic sheep. Circ Res 50:688, 1982.

44. Ogletree ML: Overview of physiological and pathophysiological effects of thromboxane A_2. Fed Proc 46:133, 1987.
45. Demling RH, Smith M, Gunther R, et al: Pulmonary injury and prostaglandin production during endotoxemia in conscious sheep. Am J Physiol 240:H348, 1981.
46. Bowers RE, Ellis EF, Brigham KL, et al: Effects of prostaglandin cyclic endoperoxides on the lung circulation of unanesthetized sheep. J Clin Invest 63:131, 1979.
47. Parratt JR, Pacitti N, Rodger IW: Mediators of acute lung injury in endotoxaemia. Prog Clin Biol Res 308:357, 1989.
48. Oettinger W, Berger D, Beger HG: The clinical significance of prostaglandins and thromboxane as mediators of septic shock. Klin Wochenschr 65:61, 1987.
49. Yellin SA, Nguyen D, Quinn JV, et al: Prostacyclin and thromboxane A_2 in septic shock: Species differences. Circ Shock 20:291, 1986.
50. Vadas P, Pruzanski W, Stefanski E, et al: Pathogenesis of hypotension in septic shock: Correlation of circulating phospholipase A_2 levels with circulatory collapse. Crit Care Med 16:1, 1988.
51. Wise WC, Cook JA, Halushka PV: Implications for thromboxane A_2 in the pathogenesis of endotoxic shock. Adv Shock Res 6, 1981.
52. Revhaug A, Michie HR, Manson JM, et al: Inhibition of cyclo-oxygenase attenuates the metabolic response to endotoxin in humans. Arch Surg 123:162, 1988.
53. Krieger DT: Endorphins and enkephalins. Dis Mon 28(10):1, 1982.
54. Faden AI, Holaday JW: Experimental endotoxin shock: The pathophysiologic function of endorphins and treatment with opiate antagonists. J Infect Dis 142:229, 1980.
55. Peters WP, Johnson MW, Friedman PA, et al: Pressor effects of naloxone in septic shock. Lancet 1:529, 1981.
56. Bone RC, Jacobs ER, Potter DM, et al: Endorphins in endotoxin shock. Microcirculation 1:285, 1981.
57. Jacobs ER, Bone RC, Wilson FJ Jr, et al: Naloxone blockade of endorphins in canine endotoxin shock. Microcirculation 2:19, 1982.
58. Rock P, Silverman H, Plump D, et al: Efficacy and safety of naloxone in septic shock. Crit Care Med 13:28, 1985.
59. Hackshaw KV, Parker GA, Roberts JW: Naloxone in septic shock. Crit Care Med 18:47, 1990.
60. Schifferli JA, Na YC, Peters DK: The roles of complement and its receptor in the elimination of immune-complexes. N Engl J Med 292:937, 1975.
61. Schirmer WJ, Schirmer JM, Naff GB, et al: Systemic complement activation produces hemodynamic changes characteristic of sepsis. Arch Surg 123:316, 1988.
62. Till GO, Johnson KJ, Kunkel R, et al: Intravascular activation of complement and acute lung injury. Dependency on neutrophils and toxic oxygen metabolities. J Clin Invest 69:1126, 1982.
63. Olson LM, Moss GS, Baukus O, et al: The role of C5 in septic lung injury. Ann Surg 202:771, 1985.
64. Till GO, Ward PA: Systemic complement activation and acute lung injury. Fed Proc 45:13, 1986.
65. Hammerschmidt DE, Weaver LJ, Hudson LD, et al: Association of complement activation and elevated plasma-C5a with adult respiratory distress syndrome. Pathophysiological relevance and possible prognostic value. Lancet 1:947, 1980.
66. Weinberg PF, Matthay MA, Webster RO, et al: Biologically active products of complement and acute lung injury in patients with the sepsis syndrome. Am Rev Respir Dis 130:791, 1984.
67. Duchateau J, Haas M, Schregen H, et al: Complement activation in patients at risk of developing the adult respiratory distress syndrome. Am Rev Respir Dis 130:1058, 1984.
68. Schein RMH, Bergman R, Marcial EH, et al: Complement activation and corticosteroid therapy in the development of the adult respiratory distress syndrome. Chest 91:850, 1987.
69. Langlois PF, Gawryl MS: Accentuated formation of the terminal C5b–9 complement complex in patient plasma precedes development of the adult respiratory distress syndrome. Am Rev Respir Dis 138:368, 1988.
70. Parsons PE, Giclas PC: The terminal complement complex (sC56-g) is not specifically associated with the development of ARDS. Am Rev Respir Dis 137:230, 1988.
71. Tate RM, Repine JE: Neutrophils and the adult respiratory distress syndrome. Am Rev Respir Dis 128:552, 1983.
72. Parker MM, Ognibene F, Natanson C, et al: Elevated C5a levels in patients with septic shock. Crit Care Med 13:303, 1985.
73. Hack CE, Nuijens JH, Felt-Bersma RJF, et al: Elevated plasma levels of the anaphylatoxins C3a and C4a are associated with a fatal outcome in sepsis. Am J Med 86:20, 1989.
74. Dinarello CA, Mier JW: Lymphokines. N Engl J Med 319:940, 1987.
75. Pober JS, Cotran RS: Cytokines and endothelial cell biology. Physiol Rev 70:427, 1990.
76. Hack CE, DeGroot ER, Felt-Bersma RJF, et al: Increased plasma levels of interleukin-6 in sepsis. Blood 74:1704, 1989.
77. Craddock PR, Fehr J, Brigham KL, et al: Complement and leukocyte-mediated pulmonary dysfunction in hemodialysis. N Engl J Med 296:764, 1977.
78. Balk RA, Jacobs RF, Tryka AF, et al: Effects of ibuprofen on neutrophil function and acute lung injury in canine endotoxin shock. Crit Care Med 16:1121, 1988.
79. Heflin AC, Brigham KL: Prevention by granulocyte depletion of increased vascular permeability of sheep lung following endotoxemia. J Clin Invest 68:1253, 1981.
80. Maunder RJ, Hackman RC, Riff E, et al: Occurrence of the adult respiratory distress syndrome in neutropenic patients. Am Rev Respir Dis 133:313, 1986.
81. Fletcher JR, DiSimone AG, Earnest MA: Platelet-activating factor receptor antagonist improves survival and attenuates eicosanoid release in severe endotoxemia. Ann Surg 211:312, 1990.
82. Davidson D, Singh M, Wallace GF: Role of leukotriene C_4 in pulmonary hypertension: Platelet-activating factor vs. hypoxia. J Appl Physiol 68:1628, 1990.
83. Toyofuku T, Kobayashi T, Koyama S, et al: Pulmonary vascular response to platelet-activating factor in conscious sheep. Am J Physiol 255:H434, 1988.
84. Fink A, Geva D, Zung A, et al: Adult respiratory distress syndrome: Roles of leukotriene C_4 and platelet activating factor. Crit Care Med 18:905, 1990.
85. Bone RC, Fisher CJ, Clemmer TP, et al: Sepsis syndrome: A valid clinical entity. Crit Care Med 17:389, 1989.
86. Fowler AA, Hamman RF, Zerbe GO, et al: Adult respiratory distress syndrome. Am Rev Respir Dis 132:472, 1985.
87. Knaus WA, Wagner DP: Multiple systems organ failure: Epidemiology and prognosis. Crit Care Clin 5:221, 1989.
88. Bone RC, Fisher CJ Jr, Clemmer TP, et al: A controlled clinical trial of high-dose methylprednisolone in the treatment of severe sepsis and septic shock. N Engl J Med 317:653, 1987.
89. The Veterans Administration Systemic Sepsis Cooperative Study Group: Effect of high-dose glucocorticoid therapy on mortality in patients with clinical signs of systemic sepsis. N Engl J Med 317:659, 1987.
90. Bone RC, Fisher CJ Jr, Clemmer TP, et al: Early methylprednisolone treatment for septic syndrome and the adult respiratory distress syndrome. Chest 92:1032, 1987.
91. Ziegler EJ, Fisher CJ, Sprung CL, et al: Treatment of gram-negative bacteremia and septic shock with HA-1A human monoclonal antibody against endotoxin. N Engl J Med 324:431, 1991.

CHAPTER 24

Cytokines, Tumor Necrosis Factor, and Other Mediators of Sepsis

Thomas J. Fahey III
Kevin J. Tracey

Critically ill patients frequently succumb to sepsis and its complications. The hemodynamic and metabolic derangements that commonly develop as the result of invasive bacterial infection are often irreversible, causing death even after the underlying infection has been identified and treated. Despite continued advances in antibiotic therapy and intensive care technology, mortality attributable to septic shock has remained in excess of 30%.[1–5] Moreover, mortality exceeds 90% when septic shock occurs with adult respiratory distress syndrome (ARDS). Because the incidence of septic shock has continued to increase, this catastrophic illness represents a major problem in intensive care medicine.[6]

The apparent temporal dissociation of the progressive failure of multiple-organ systems from the underlying infection raised speculation about the identity of the mediators underlying the pathogenesis of the septic shock syndrome. Initially, these effects were attributed to the direct effects of

TABLE 24–1

ABRIDGED HISTORY OF CURRENT UNDERSTANDING OF THE PATHOGENESIS OF SEPTIC SHOCK

Date	Reference	Event
1892	Pfeiffer[7a]	Coined the term *endotoxin*.
1941	Shear[7b]	Bacterial lipopolysaccharide (LPS) caused hemorrhagic necrosis in some tumors.
1944	Franke[7]	LPS infusion caused shock in dogs and guinea pigs.
1953	Bennett and Beeson[8]	Polymorphonuclear leukocyte extracts mediated fever in otherwise healthy animals.
1973	Kampschmidt et al.[9]	Coined the term *leukocyte endogenous mediator*.
1975	Carswell et al.[29]	Identified tumor necrosis factor (TNF), an LPS-induced serum factor that caused hemorrhagic necrosis in some tumors.
1977	Dinarello et al.[10]	Identified interleukin-1 as a leukocyte endogenous mediator.
1985	Beutler et al.[30]	Purified cachectin, an LPS-induced polypeptide, and recognized its identity to TNF.
1986	Tracey et al.[32]	Demonstrated the ability of TNF to induce shock and tissue injury in vivo.

the invasive pathogens and their associated endotoxins and enterotoxins. More recently, it has become clear that these exogenous products do not directly account for all of the pathophysiologic derangements that are observed clinically and that many of these effects are mediated by endogenous factors produced (or overproduced) by the septic host.

Although these mediators are beneficial when produced in small, timely quantities, an excess may be lethal. In this way, septic shock is somewhat analogous to other examples of immune-mediated over-responsiveness (e.g., anaphylactic shock) that may be ultimately deleterious to the host. The identification of these endogenous mediators and their po-

TABLE 24–2

CYTOKINE MEDIATORS OF SEPSIS AND SEPTIC SHOCK

Abbreviation*	Synonyms	Molecular Weight	Principal Cell Sources
TNF-α	Tumor necrosis factor α Cachectin	17,000	Circulating monocytes Tissue macrophages 　Alveolar 　Peritoneal 　Kupffer's cells Polymorphonuclear leukocytes Mast cells Lymphocytes Astrocytes Paneth's cells
IL-1	Interleukin-1α Interleukin-1β Endogenous pyrogen B cell–stimulating factor Lymphocyte-activating factor Osteoclast-activating factor	17,000	Circulating monocytes Tissue macrophages Lymphocytes Polymorphonuclear leukocytes Endothelial cells Keratinocytes Fibroblasts
IL-2	T cell growth factor	15,500	Lymphocytes
IL-6	Hepatocyte-stimulating factor B cell differentiation factor Interferon-β₂ Hybridoma growth factor	23,000–30,000 >45,000	Fibroblasts Circulating monocytes Tissue macrophages Keratinocytes Endothelial cells
IL-8	Neutrophil-activating factor Neutrophil-activating peptide	8,000	Fibroblasts Monocytes Tissue macrophages Keratinocytes Endothelial cells Lymphocytes
IFN-γ	Interferon-γ	55,000	Lymphocytes Tissue macrophages
CSFs	Macrophage-CSF Granulocyte-CSF Granulocyte-macrophage CSF Interleukin-3	35,000–45,000 18,000–22,000 14,000–35,000 14,000–28,000	Fibroblasts Endothelial cells Monocytes Macrophages Lymphocytes
TGF-β	Transforming growth factor β	25,000	Almost all cell types

*TNF-α = tumor necrosis factor α; IL-1 = interleukin-1; IL-2 = interleukin-2; IL-6 = interleukin-6; IL-8 = interleukin-8; IFN-γ = interferon-γ; CSF = colony-stimulating factor; TGF-β = transforming growth factor β.

TABLE 24-3
STIMULI KNOWN TO INDUCE PRODUCTION OF TUMOR NECROSIS FACTOR

Organism	Specific Stimuli
Bacteria	Gram-negative bacteria
	Gram-positive bacteria
	Endotoxin or lipopolysaccharide
	Toxic shock syndrome toxin
	Pertussis toxin
Mycoplasma	*Mycoplasma pneumoniae*
	Acholeplasma laidlawii
Mycobacteria	*Mycobacterium tuberculosis*
	(lipoarabinomannan)
Rickettsiae	*Rickettsia conorii*
	Israeli spotted fever
Fungi and yeast	*Coccidioides immitis*
	Candida albicans
Viruses	Sendai virus
	Newcastle disease virus
Parasites	*Plasmodium falciparum*
	Leishmania
	Trypanosoma

tential toxicity has led to exciting advances in understanding the pathogenesis of sepsis and septic shock.

This chapter gives a brief review of the developments in the study of the endogenous mediators of sepsis. Although the extensive work published in this field cannot be completely covered in a single chapter, an overview of the complex cascade of mediators involved in the pathogenesis of the septic shock syndrome is provided here.

HISTORY

The ability of bacterial cell wall products to induce septic shock has been recognized for decades.[7] However, it has only recently become apparent that cytokines, synthesized and secreted in response to infectious stimuli, mediate the deleterious consequences of overwhelming infection (Table 24–1). The presence of endogenous mediators of infection was suggested by Bennett and Beeson, who found that fever could be induced by the administration of polymorphonuclear leukocyte extracts.[8] Subsequent investigators (in the 1970s) attributed these effects to interleukin-1 (IL-1), a polypeptide secreted by activated leukocytes that proved to be an endogenous pyrogen and mediator of infection.[9, 10] Although most of the pathogenesis of sepsis was initially attributed to lipopolysaccharide (LPS) and IL-1, more recent studies have demonstrated that another mediator, cachectin, or tumor necrosis factor α (TNF-α), is a principal mediator of sepsis and lethal septic shock.

Cytokines, such as TNF-α and IL-1 (Table 24–2), can be defined as inducible proteins or glycoproteins, secreted by a variety of host cells, that are capable of mediating the function of diverse target cells at minute concentrations.[11] They function by binding to specific receptors both locally, at sites of injury or infection, and at distant target organs. At local tissue sites, the release of cytokines and other inflammatory mediators leads initially to warmth, redness, and fluid extravasation. Although these responses are normally beneficial and protect the host from infection or invasion, the continued production of these mediators may lead to progressive local tissue injury. Systemic release of these inflammatory mediators causes fever, generalized fluid extravasation, widespread tissue injury, and shock. Thus, the systemic consequences of the locally adaptive responses initiated by cytokines may be catastrophic.

BIOSYNTHESIS AND RELEASE OF TUMOR NECROSIS FACTOR α

TNF-α, a 17,000-dalton polypeptide secreted principally by activated leukocytes and immunoregulatory cells (see Table 24–2), is induced in response to a variety of infectious stimuli, including gram-negative and gram-positive bacteria, yeasts, rickettsiae, viruses, and parasites[12] (Table 24–3). The gene for human TNF-α lies on chromosome 4 and is close to the gene for lymphotoxin (tumor necrosis factor β [TNF-β]), with which it shares considerable homology.[13] LPS is an extremely potent stimulus for systemic TNF-α secretion, and monocytes and tissue macrophages apparently represent the principal cell source of secreted TNF-α during infection.

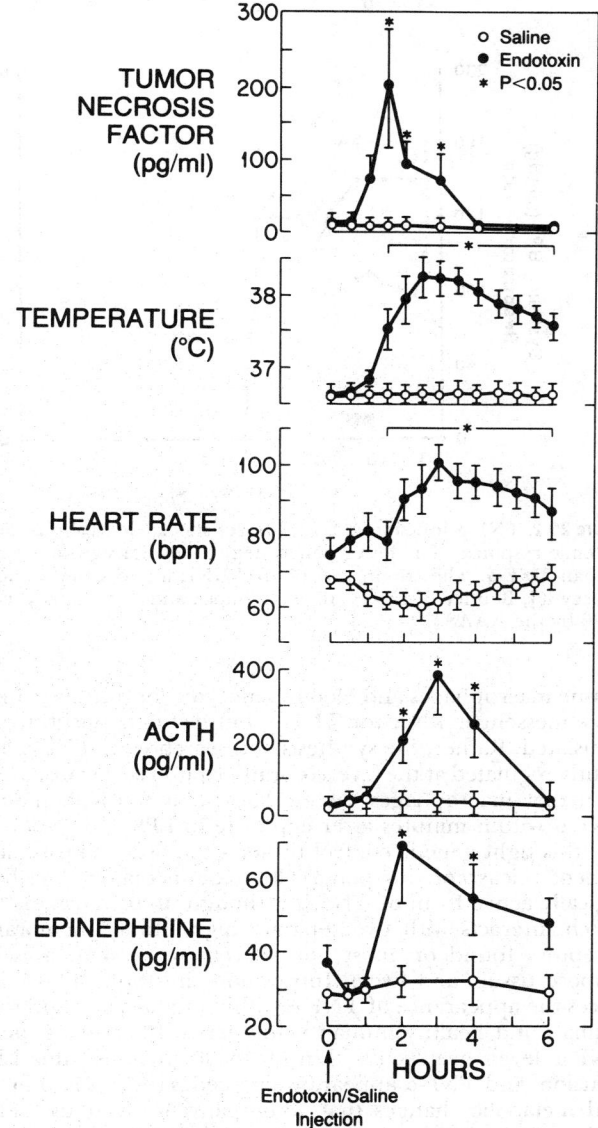

Figure 24-1. Endotoxin induces appearance of circulating TNF-α. Intravenous infusion of a low dose of endotoxin results in peak appearance of circulating TNF-α within 60 to 90 minutes. Detection of circulating TNF-α occurs before the onset of fever or changes in heart rate and precedes stress hormone responses. (From Michie HR, Manogue KR, Spriggs DR, et al: Detection of circulating tumor necrosis factor after endotoxin administration. Reprinted with permission from the New England Journal of Medicine, 318, 1481–1486, 1988.)

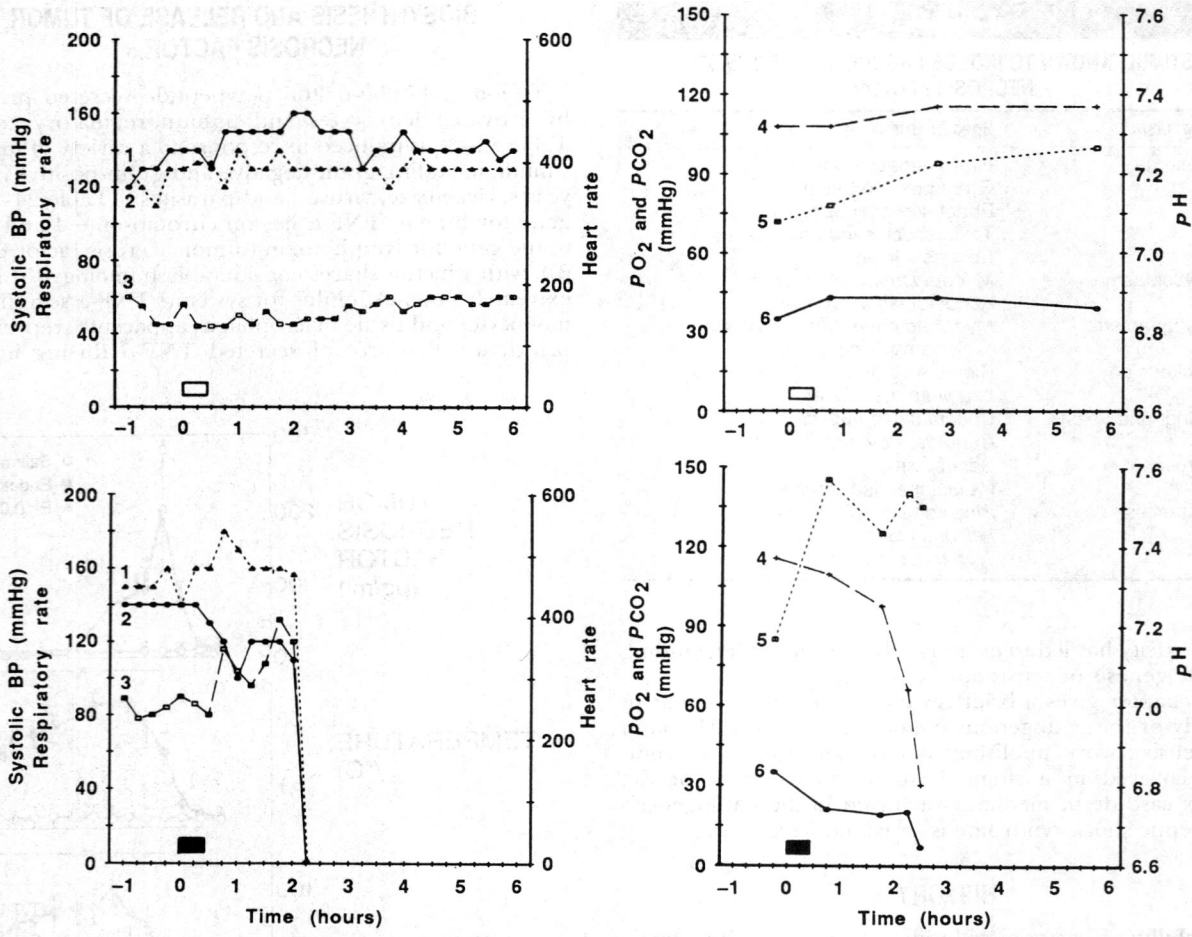

Figure 24–2. TNF-α infusion into rats causes shock. Control rats *(top)* received an infusion of isotonic saline and did not exhibit any significant systemic response. The lower panels depict the vital signs and arterial blood gas results for rats administered a single dose of recombinant human TNF-α. The administration of TNF-α induces shock and respiratory compromise that lead to death. BP = blood pressure. (From Tracey KJ, Beutler B, Lowry SF, et al: Shock and tissue injury induced by recombinant human cachectin. Science 234:470, 1986. Copyright 1986 by the AAAS.)

Tissue macrophages and blood monocytes constitutively produce messenger RNA for TNF-α, but it is not constitutively translated. Rather, the synthesis and secretion of TNF-α are tightly regulated at the levels of transcription and translation, such that macrophages secrete large quantities of mature TNF-α within minutes after exposure to LPS.[14, 15] Presumably, this tight genetic control protects the host against inadvertent release of this potentially toxic mediator. The biologically active form of TNF-α is thought to be a trimer,[16, 17] which interacts with two separate high-affinity membrane receptors found on most normal cells (e.g., skin, muscle, adipose tissue, and liver). Intravenous infusion of LPS induces the appearance of TNF-α within minutes in laboratory animals and healthy human volunteers.[18] In humans, peak TNF-α levels are seen within 60 to 90 minutes after LPS infusion, and TNF-α appearance precedes the onset of fever and metabolic changes that accompany intravenous endotoxin infusion[19] (Fig. 24–1). Because of its short serum half-life (14 to 18 minutes), serum TNF-α levels return to baseline within 180 minutes. Rapid clearance of TNF-α from the circulation is due largely to TNF-α binding to high-affinity receptors present on a variety of diverse target cells.[20–23] Circulating inhibitors of TNF-α, thought to be TNF-α receptor fragments, may also partially account for rapid TNF-α clearance and reduced ability to detect circulating levels of TNF-α.[24–28]

EVIDENCE IMPLICATING TUMOR NECROSIS FACTOR α AS A MEDIATOR OF SEPSIS AND SEPTIC SHOCK

TNF-α was initially isolated for its ability to induce hemorrhagic necrosis in some solid tumors.[29] Some years later, Beutler and Cerami identified an LPS-inducible protein secreted by macrophages (cachectin) as a mediator of cellular cachexia and weight loss.[30] The identity of TNF-α and cachectin was established by subsequent cloning of the gene for cachectin, and it was then recognized that TNF-α may not be specifically tumoricidal.[31] Early studies by Tracey and coworkers revealed that TNF-α infusion into rats[32] and dogs[33] triggered a syndrome of physiologic and metabolic derangements that was characterized by the rapid onset of shock, followed by the development of acute pulmonary edema, renal failure, and death (Fig. 24–2). Histopathologic examination of organs from animals receiving TNF-α infusions revealed neutrophil plugging of pulmonary capillaries and hemorrhagic necrosis of the lungs, kidneys, and gastrointestinal tract. These effects were nearly indistinguishable from those associated with endotoxic or septic shock and indicated that this single endogenous mediator was capable of initiating the diverse sequelae of sepsis with multiple-organ failure. Subsequent studies confirmed that TNF-α infusion is capable of reproducing a syndrome of lethal multiple-organ injury in mice, rats, rabbits, and sheep.[34–36] More recently, accumulated evidence has indicated that TNF-α toxicity appears to be potentiated by the presence of LPS and that the presence of trace quantities of LPS may markedly enhance the metabolic derangements mediated by TNF-α.[37]

Although these early studies demonstrated that TNF-α infusion was capable of inducing hemodynamic and metabolic derangements that paralleled those characteristic of septic shock, the pivotal nature of TNF-α in the host response to invasive infection was identified using anti–TNF-α antibodies in a model of lethal, gram-negative septic shock in primates.[38] Pretreatment of baboons with a monoclonal antibody to TNF-α before infusion with a lethal dose of live *Escherichia coli* bacteria provided complete protection against the development of shock, septic multiple organ system failure, and death (Fig. 24–3). In this model, all animals received lethal numbers of bacteria, but no antibiotics were given for 10 hours after infusion of *E. coli*. Nonimmunized controls succumbed to septic shock within hours, but animals passively immunized against TNF-α did not develop shock and survived. Although anti–TNF-α therapy had no effect on the numbers of bacteria cultured from the blood, the injurious effects of systemic infection were prevented.

The ability to prevent septic shock by administration of anti–TNF-α antibodies has been independently confirmed by several investigators. Mathison and colleagues showed that anti–TNF-α antibody administration protected rabbits from lethal endotoxin-induced shock.[35] Silva and colleagues demonstrated that anti–TNF-α antibodies protected mice from the consequences of gram-negative bacteremia when given either prophylactically or therapeutically.[39] Hinshaw and coworkers reported 100% survival of baboons given a lethal dose of *E. coli*, even when TNF-α antibody was given 30 minutes after starting the *E. coli* infusion.[40]

In addition to these studies, further evidence indicating a pivotal role for TNF-α in the initiation of the cascade of toxic mediators stimulated by systemic infection was obtained from serum analysis for IL-1 and interleukin-6 (IL-6) from baboons that received anti–TNF-α antibody pretreatment.[41] Anti–TNF-α pretreatment almost completely abrogated the IL-1 and IL-6 responses to live bacterial infusion, suggesting that TNF-α appearance is a requirement for massive production of IL-1 and IL-6 in septic states (Fig. 24–4). This was somewhat surprising, as IL-1 and IL-6 had previously been thought to be produced directly in response to LPS. It seems that TNF-α triggers production of IL-1 and IL-6, which then propagate and amplify a cascade of other humoral mediators. Although *E. coli* or endotoxin infusion may not exactly mimic clinical septicemia, these studies have demonstrated that lethal septic shock is dissociable from the presence of the organisms themselves. Furthermore, they directly implicate TNF-α as the trigger for the cascade of toxic host mediators that result in organ and tissue injury.

TUMOR NECROSIS FACTOR α AND THE PATHOPHYSIOLOGY OF SEPSIS AND SEPTIC SHOCK

The mechanisms by which TNF-α mediates the pathophysiology of sepsis and septic shock remain under active investigation. It has become clear that TNF-α is able to induce the synthesis and release of a variety of secondary mediators, including other cytokines, arachidonic acid metabolites, complement components, and superoxides, that possess toxic properties, either alone or in conjunction with TNF-α. Among cytokines induced by TNF-α, IL-1 is notable for its independent capacity to induce many of the same

secondary mediators, as well as augment TNF-α toxicity[42, 43] (Fig. 24–5). In addition, TNF-α has significant toxic properties of its own, and the mechanisms of direct cellular toxicity related to TNF-α are under active investigation.[44, 45]

TNF-α–induced biochemical and molecular changes that affect the complex interactions between endothelial cells and circulating blood components underlie many of the known toxic effects of TNF-α. Much of the end-organ damage that accompanies sepsis and septic shock (clinically manifested as ARDS or renal tubular necrosis, for example) is due to TNF-α–enhanced neutrophil chemoattraction and activation and the development of widespread and inappropriate clotting. TNF-α enhances neutrophil adherence to endothelium largely through the induction and expression of endothelium-leukocyte adhesion molecules and intercellular cell adhesion molecules on both endothelial cells and neutrophils.[46–48] Studies in this rapidly advancing field have demonstrated that TNF-α, as well as IL-1 and LPS, induces the expression of the CD11/CD18 family of integrins on neutrophil cell membranes and the induction of intercellular and endothelium-leukocyte adhesion molecules, some of which have not yet been purified, on endothelial cells.[49–51] In addition, TNF-α and IL-1 are both capable of inducing interleukin-8 (IL-8), a potent neutrophil chemoattractant and activator produced by a variety of cell types, including fibroblasts, keratinocytes, type II pneumocytes, and hepatocytes.[52] Finally, TNF-α stimulates neutrophils to generate and release toxic oxygen radicals[53] and to cause nonspecific degranulation.[54] In addition to augmenting endothelial cell adhesive properties for neutrophils, TNF-α also enhances endothelial cell procoagulant effects and increases the expression of cell surface tissue factor.[55–56] TNF-α is capable of generating thrombin and decreasing activated protein C,[57] which probably acts to induce capillary stasis and thrombosis. The induction of plasminogen-activator inhibitor and the simultaneous suppression of tissue-type plasminogen activator probably act to stabilize capillary thrombi locally.[58, 59] The net result predisposes to local hemorrhagic necrosis and the development of disseminated intravascular coagulation. Direct effects of TNF-α on vascular endothelium lead to increased endothelial permeability through the rearrangement of endothelial actin filaments and decreased transepithelial resistance leading to increased solute flow across the endothelium.[60, 61] In addition, TNF-α has been shown to be mildly cytotoxic to cultured endothelial cells, and this may further contribute to the development of a vascular leak.[62] Moreover, sheep infused with TNF-α had morphologic changes in pulmonary capillary endothelium similar to those seen in vitro.[63] These alterations in endothelium-neutrophil interactions, release of toxic neutrophil products, increased propensity for clotting, and altered vascular permeability contribute to the biochemical basis for the commonly recognized clinical entities of ARDS, acute tubular necrosis, and generalized organ dysfunction that occur during sepsis and septic shock.

METABOLIC EFFECTS OF TUMOR NECROSIS FACTOR α

In addition to its role in mediating the acute tissue effects of septic shock just noted, TNF-α is capable of initiating the complex metabolic state of catabolism that complicates chronic sepsis and leads to protein-calorie malnutrition (Table 24–4). It is well known that chronic infection can lead to a wasting diathesis characterized by weight loss, anorexia, anemia, and net losses of body stores of protein and lipid. When administered chronically, TNF-α is capable of reproducing this catabolic state. Studies of these catabolic effects on adipocytes and myocytes have provided a better under-

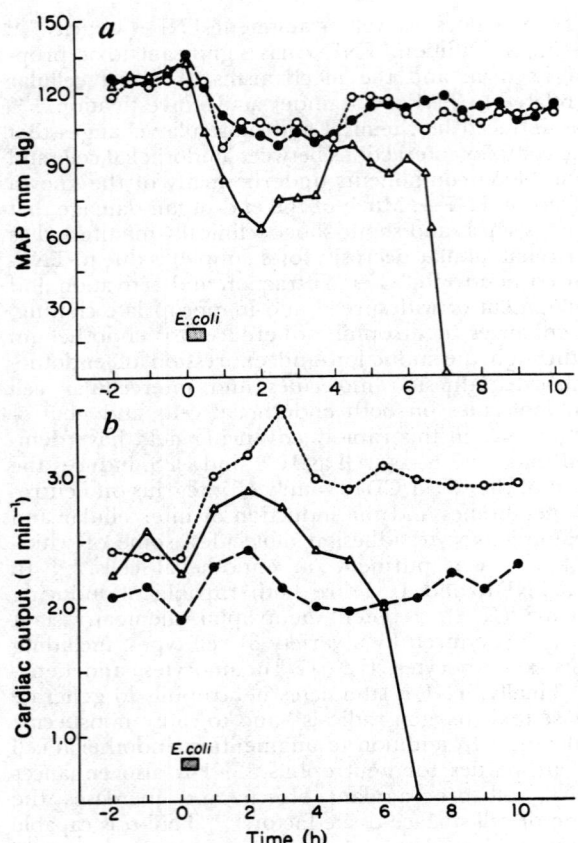

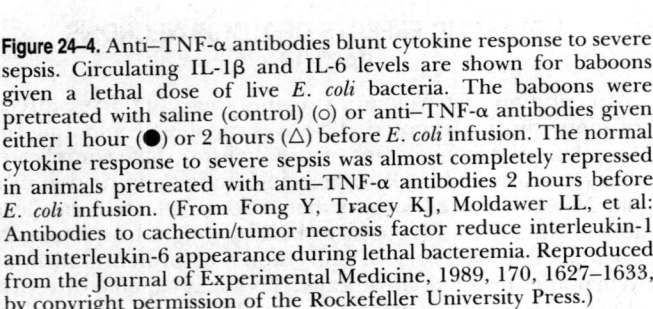

Figure 24-3. Anti-TNF-α antibodies protect against shock and vital organ dysfunction. Mean arterial blood pressure (MAP) (a) and cardiac output (b) in three individual baboons pretreated with saline (control) (△) or anti–TNF-α antibody administered either 1 hour before (o) or 2 hours before (●) an infusion of a lethal dose of live *E. coli* bacteria. Anti–TNF-α antibodies confer complete protection from hemodynamic derangements normally observed with lethal bacteremia. (From Tracey KJ, Fong Y, Hesse DG, et al: Anti-cachectin/TNF monoclonal antibodies prevent septic shock during lethal bacteremia in baboons. Reprinted by permission from Nature Volume 330, 662–664, 1987. Copyright 1987 Macmillan Magazines Limited.)

Figure 24-4. Anti–TNF-α antibodies blunt cytokine response to severe sepsis. Circulating IL-1β and IL-6 levels are shown for baboons given a lethal dose of live *E. coli* bacteria. The baboons were pretreated with saline (control) (o) or anti–TNF-α antibodies given either 1 hour (●) or 2 hours (△) before *E. coli* infusion. The normal cytokine response to severe sepsis was almost completely repressed in animals pretreated with anti–TNF-α antibodies 2 hours before *E. coli* infusion. (From Fong Y, Tracey KJ, Moldawer LL, et al: Antibodies to cachectin/tumor necrosis factor reduce interleukin-1 and interleukin-6 appearance during lethal bacteremia. Reproduced from the Journal of Experimental Medicine, 1989, 170, 1627–1633, by copyright permission of the Rockefeller University Press.)

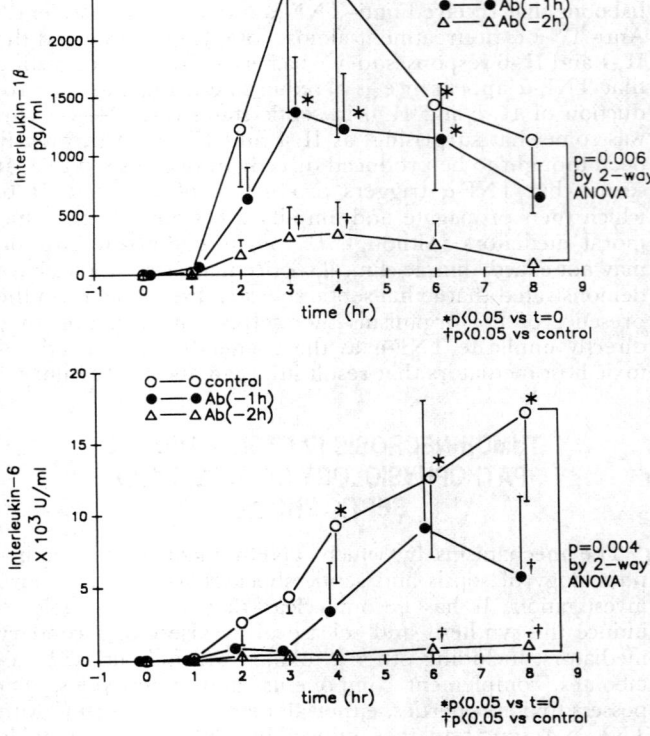

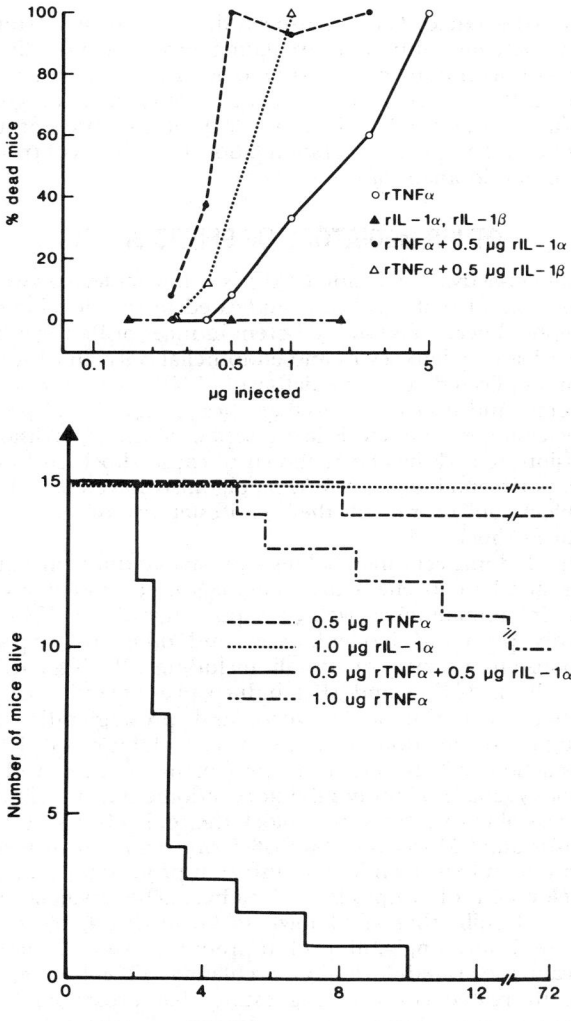

Figure 24–5. IL-1 augments TNF-α toxicity. *(Top)* The lethality for mice given injections of TNF-α alone (○), IL-1α or IL-1β alone (▲), TNF-α plus IL-1α (●), or TNF-α plus IL-1β (△) is shown. *(Bottom)* The survival curves of four groups of mice given various combinations of TNF-α and IL-1 during 72 hours are shown. The synergistic toxicity of TNF-α with IL-1 can be seen. (From Waage A, Espevik T: Interleukin 1 potentiates the lethal effect of tumor necrosis factor/cachectin in mice. Reproduced from the Journal of Experimental Medicine, 1988, 167, 1987–1992, by copyright permission of the Rockefeller University Press.)

standing of the cellular basis for the catabolism that often accompanies the septic syndrome.

Early studies indicated that TNF-α suppresses adipocyte lipoprotein lipase, effectively reducing adipocyte uptake of exogenous lipid and causing a decreased clearance of extracellular lipids.[30] TNF-α has also been shown to inhibit the transcription of key lipogenic enzymes, which prevents the incorporation of glucose into lipid and contributes to a net depletion of stored triglycerides.[64] In vivo studies demonstrated that administration of TNF-α to animals or humans results in cachexia with hypertriglyceridemia, mobilization of stored body fat, and increased free fatty acid turnover.[65, 66]

TNF-α also initiates a catabolic state in myocytes. Exposure of L6 myoblasts to TNF-α induces the release of lactate into the medium and causes a rapid depletion of intracellular glycogen stores.[67] Chronic administration of TNF-α to experimental animals causes whole body protein catabolism,

with a decrease in the transcription of genes encoding for the structural proteins myosin and actin.[65, 68] TNF-α infusion in humans is similarly associated with a net release of amino acids from skeletal muscle,[66] and this has been theorized to contribute to whole body losses of protein and nitrogen associated with chronic inflammation.

The metabolic effects of TNF-α on hepatocellular function also resemble the responses associated with chronic inflammation. Hepatocytes exposed to TNF-α in vitro increase the synthesis of acute-phase proteins and decrease the production of albumin through specific down-regulation of albumin gene transcription.[69] In vivo, TNF-α mediates increased amino acid uptake by hepatocytes via glucagon-dependent pathways,[70] which may serve to facilitate the synthetic increases in acute-phase protein synthesis and ureagenesis. In addition, TNF-α stimulates hepatic lipogenesis,[71] which probably contributes to observed elevations in circulating triglycerides during catabolic states.

These observations indicate that TNF-α is capable of directly or indirectly mediating the metabolic sequelae of chronic sepsis. The role of TNF-α as a regulator of other systemic effects (e.g., in the central nervous, immunologic, and hematologic systems) is beyond the scope of this chapter, but understanding these interactions may one day facilitate the management of critically ill patients with chronic septic syndrome.

OTHER CYTOKINES IMPLICATED IN THE PATHOGENESIS OF SEPSIS AND SEPTIC SHOCK

Like TNF-α, IL-1 is a 17,000-dalton polypeptide secreted by inflammatory cells in response to stimulation with endo-

TABLE 24–4
METABOLIC EFFECTS OF TUMOR NECROSIS FACTOR ON SELECTED TISSUES

System or Tissue	Effect
Central nervous system	Fever
	Anorexia
	Sympathetic discharge
	Increased corticotropin release
	Decreased thyrotropin release
Liver	Stimulates acute-phase protein synthesis
	Decreases albumin synthesis
	Stimulates lipogenesis
	Promotes glucagon-mediated amino acid uptake
	Increases hepatic size and DNA content
Muscle	Decreases glycogen content
	Increases membrane-bound hexose transporters
	Increases lactate efflux
	Suppresses structural protein synthesis
	Increases protein catabolism and induces net release of amino acids
	Decreases resting transmembrane potential
Adipose tissue	Induces net insulin resistance
	Suppresses lipoprotein lipase
	Suppresses lipogenesis
	Increases cellular lipolysis
	Causes free fatty acid and triglyceride release, which results in hypertriglyceridemia and hyperlipemia

toxin, and it has been implicated in the pathogenesis of sepsis and septic shock.[42] IL-1 production is also stimulated in a variety of cell types by exposure to TNF-α,[72, 73] and its effects on target cells overlap extensively with those of TNF-α. In addition, IL-1 is a potent stimulus for the synthesis and release of interleukin-2, which is another cytokine thought to mediate toxicity in the septic shock syndrome.[74] Experimental studies indicate that IL-1 administration is associated with transient hypotension and a modest fluid requirement, but IL-1 does not by itself induce shock or tissue injury.[75] However, IL-1 is capable of markedly potentiating the toxic effects of TNF-α. In both mice and rabbits, TNF-α toxicity occurred at significantly lower doses when TNF-α was coadministered with IL-1.[43] Analysis of IL-1 appearance in patients with meningococcal sepsis demonstrated that IL-1 was detected only in those patients with high levels of TNF-α and IL-6 who had a rapidly fatal course.[76] Furthermore, blockade of the IL-1 receptor in rabbits with endotoxin-induced shock appears to decrease associated mortality.[77] Thus, IL-1 is an important mediator of septic shock because of its ability to augment TNF-α–induced toxicity.

IL-6 is a TNF-α–inducible cytokine that has been detected at high levels in the circulation during a variety of inflammatory states and appears to function primarily as a mediator of the acute-phase response.[78] More recently, IL-6 has been found to function as a thrombopoietic factor by increasing platelet number through the enhancement of megakaryocyte maturation.[79] There is little evidence that IL-6 is inherently toxic, but it has been suggested that anti–IL-6 antibodies may improve survival in severe sepsis.[80] Thus, although IL-6 is an important pleiotropic mediator, its role in the pathogenesis of septic shock is unknown.

IL-8 is another TNF-α– and IL-1–inducible cytokine that has been identified as a potent chemoattractant for neutrophils, and it is probably the principal neutrophil chemoattractant secreted by activated macrophages.[52, 81] Experimental studies have demonstrated that IL-8 is synthesized and secreted by fibroblasts and pneumocytes in response to stimulation with LPS, TNF-α, or IL-1, although it is not detected until 4 to 8 hours after stimulation in vitro.[82, 83] Its appearance in serum after septic challenge seems to follow a similar time course; it is detected relatively late after endotoxin administration to baboons and, like IL-6, has a prolonged period during which serum levels remain elevated.[84] Macrophage inflammatory protein 2 is a small peptide secreted by LPS-stimulated macrophages that also has potent neutrophil chemoattractant properties and is a member of the IL-8 family of proteins.[85] Experimental studies have shown that macrophage inflammatory protein 2 is a mediator of the inflammatory response in meningitis and healing wounds,[86, 87] but like IL-8, its role in the pathogenesis of sepsis and septic shock is currently speculative and is under study.

Interferon-γ (INF-γ), or macrophage-activating factor, is a 55,000-dalton protein secreted principally by activated lymphocytes that is known to increase macrophage antimicrobial activity and to enhance macrophage secretion of inflammatory mediators, including TNF-α.[88, 89] Studies have documented that IFN-γ is capable of overriding the suppressive effects of steroids on macrophage TNF-α production in response to LPS stimulation.[90] The effects of glucocorticoids, which act to inhibit TNF-α production by suppressing synthesis of TNF-α messenger RNA, are overcome by exposure to IFN-γ as much as 48 hours before treatment with dexamethasone and LPS. Whether IFN-γ is able to override the suppressive effects of transforming growth factor β, a cytokine postulated to function as an antiinflammatory mediator in sepsis, on TNF-α release[91] remains

to be determined. IFN-γ has been detected in the serum of septic patients; although circulating levels do not directly correlate with outcome in patients with gram-negative septicemia, they do correlate with the severity of meningococcemia in children.[92, 93] It is unclear at the present time whether macrophage overstimulation by IFN-γ contributes to the development of septic shock.

OTHER MEDIATORS OF SEPTIC SHOCK

Platelet-activating factor (PAF) is a low-molecular-weight phospholipid that has been implicated in the development of septic shock.[94] TNF-α is a potent inducer of PAF synthesis and release by leukocytes and endothelial cells, and PAF has been implicated as a mediator of TNF-α–induced bowel ischemia and necrosis, as well as endotoxin-induced pulmonary changes characteristic of septic shock.[95–97] Although infusion of PAF has been shown to cause shock and death in experimental animals, PAF antagonists have been shown to block only some of the manifestations of endotoxin-induced shock.[98–101]

Arachidonic acid metabolites—prostaglandins, thromboxanes, and leukotrienes—are well recognized as mediators of local inflammation as well as septic shock.[94, 102] They are rapidly produced by leukocytes and other cell types in response to a variety of stimuli, including LPS, TNF-α, and IL-1. Both TNF-α and IL-1 induce prostaglandin E_2 production by fibroblasts in vitro, and prostaglandin E_2 is thought to function as a feedback inhibitor of TNF-α production.[103, 104] In one study, pretreatment of rats with the cyclooxygenase pathway inhibitors indomethacin or ibuprofen was able to substantially block the toxic effects of TNF-α infusion.[105] Moreover, ibuprofen pretreatment of healthy young men before endotoxin infusion protected against the development of symptoms such as headache, myalgias, nausea, and chills that are known to be mediated by TNF-α release. Interestingly, ibuprofen-pretreated subjects had significantly elevated levels of circulating TNF-α compared with untreated controls, suggesting that prostaglandin E_2 release perhaps functions as a negative feedback inhibitor in vivo.[104]

TNF-α also enhances neutrophil generation of leukotriene B_4, a potent mediator of vascular permeability, and augments chemotaxis of neutrophils to leukotriene B_4.[106] Inhibition of 5-lipoxygenase, the enzyme responsible for the generation of the leukotrienes, before endotoxin administration in experimental animals has been shown to partially block the hypotension and hemoconcentration characteristic of endotoxin-induced shock. Blocking 5-lipoxygenase activity also prevents pulmonary sequestration of neutrophils and leukocyte congestion in small-bowel capillary villi.[107]

The complement cascade, with generation of the anaphylatoxins C3a and C5a, is activated in both experimental and clinical septic shock.[108–111] C3a and C5a modulate neutrophil-endothelial adhesiveness, mediate increased vascular permeability,[112] and contribute to the development of hemodynamic changes that are similar to those seen in septic shock.[113] Furthermore, pretreatment of nonhuman primates with anti-C5a antibodies before E. coli infusion reduced systemic hypotension and attenuated the development of ARDS.[114] Work indicates that TNF-α mediates toxicity related to activated complement components by increasing complement receptors on neutrophils.[115, 116]

Studies of the mechanisms underlying hypotension during septic shock have focused on the role of endothelium-derived relaxing factor or nitric oxide as a mediator of hypotension during endotoxemia. N-Methyl-L-arginine, a competitive inhibitor of L-arginine (the precursor for nitric oxide synthesis), has been found to block TNF-α-induced hypotension, suggesting that nitric oxide may mediate the effects of TNF-α on systemic vascular resistance and blood pressure.[117] Although the role of nitric oxide in sepsis and septic shock and its relationship to TNF-α appearance remain to be fully characterized, nitric oxide blockade may offer a potential strategy for ameliorating hypotension during septic shock.

It is clear that PAF, arachidonic acid metabolites, complement, and other factors contribute to the development of sepsis and septic shock. Additional mediators not discussed here include the glucose counter-regulatory hormones (epinephrine, cortisol, and glucagon), kinins, and endogenous opiates. However, of the known endogenous mediators of sepsis and septic shock, only TNF-α has been found capable of inducing the entire clinical spectrum of the septic shock syndrome. The systemic release of TNF-α appears to function as a trigger leading to the induction of other factors that together mediate the catastrophic sequelae of invasive infection.

DETECTION OF TUMOR NECROSIS FACTOR α IN SEPTIC PATIENTS

Detection of TNF-α in the serum of critically ill patients has been hampered by the rapid time course of TNF-α appearance and clearance after invasive stimuli. It is likely that peak TNF-α levels are missed in some patients entered into clinical studies on the basis of the development of shock. Although initial efforts to detect TNF-α in human serum were also hindered by the lack of sensitive assays, the availability of double-antibody enzyme-linked immunosorbent assays has allowed better characterization of TNF-α appearance in septic patients.

Data have indicated that TNF-α can be detected in the serum of patients with sepsis or septic shock and that elevated levels tend to correlate with poorer outcome (Table 24–5). Marks and colleagues examined plasma TNF-α levels from patients in a trial on the effects of methylprednisolone administration during septic shock and found that patients with elevated TNF-α levels had a higher incidence of ARDS and a increased mortality.[118] Similarly, Offner and coworkers found that TNF-α levels were elevated in intensive care unit patients with sepsis compared with intensive care unit patients who were not septic, and early mortality correlated with high levels of circulating TNF-α in septic patients.[119] Despite these studies and others[120–125] that indicate a correlation between circulating TNF-α levels and the severity and outcome of sepsis, serum TNF-α levels are not universally elevated in patients with sepsis.

It has become apparent that the paracrine actions exerted by TNF-α and other inflammatory mediators may be more predictive of their net effects than circulating levels. Furthermore, persistent local production in affected organs after a septic insult may perpetuate end-organ injury. Experimental observations corroborate this hypothesis. In a model using a TNF-α–secreting cell line in mice, we found that local tissue production of TNF-α was the predominant determinant of the cumulative metabolic effects of TNF-α and not the circulating TNF-α levels[126] (Table 24–6). Clinical observations by Waage and colleagues indicate that cerebrospinal fluid levels of TNF-α are more predictive of outcome than are serum TNF-α levels in patients with meningococcal meningitis.[127] Furthermore, preliminary studies of TNF-α or IL-1 appearance in bronchoalveolar lavage fluid in intensive care unit patients suggest that continued pulmonary production of TNF-α or IL-1 correlates with the development and/or presence of ARDS in the absence of circulating TNF-α levels or ongoing systemic infection.[128, 129] Although these latter reports are based on small numbers of patients, they

TABLE 24–5
DETECTION OF TUMOR NECROSIS FACTOR IN SEPTIC PATIENTS

Reference	Finding*
Waage et al.[120]	Serum TNF levels were associated with fatal outcome in patients with meningococcal sepsis.
Damas et al.[121]	Serum TNF levels, but not IL-1β, correlated with sepsis severity score and mortality.
Offner et al.[119]	Serum TNF levels correlated with APACHE score, and extremely high TNF levels predicted early mortality.
Debets et al.[122]	Serum TNF detected in only 25% of patients in this study, but TNF-positive patients had twice the mortality of TNF-negative patients.
Calandra et al.[92]	Elevated serum TNF and IL-1β levels were associated with poorer outcome.
Marks et al.[118]	Plasma TNF levels were elevated in patients with gram-negative and gram-positive septic shock, and higher TNF levels were associated with a higher incidence of ARDS and increased mortality.
Marano et al.[123]	TNF levels correlated with the presence of infection and associated mortality in burn patients.
Mustafa et al.[124]	Peak CSF levels of TNF correlated with mortality.
Giradin et al.[125]	Serum TNF levels were elevated in 91% of patients with severe infectious purpura.
Millar et al.[128]	TNF levels were elevated in BAL from five patients with ARDS in the absence of ongoing systemic infection.
Roberts et al.[129]	TNF levels were elevated in BAL from three of four patients with ARDS, despite undetectable plasma levels.
Waage et al.[127]	CSF levels of TNF were a better predictor of outcome than serum levels in patients with meningococcal sepsis.

*APACHE = Acute Physiology and Chronic Health Evaluation; CSF = cerebrospinal fluid; BAL = bronchoalveolar lavage.

corroborate data suggesting that localized production of TNF-α may adversely affect outcome by initiating or sustaining detrimental inflammatory responses. Thus, the net effects of TNF-α and other cytokine mediators may in a sense be dissociated from their measured blood levels.[126]

FUTURE DIRECTIONS IN SEPTIC SHOCK RESEARCH

Early recognition of clinical sepsis remains essential to successful treatment. Advances in understanding the pathophysiology of the septic shock syndrome have permitted the development of new treatment strategies, some of which are currently undergoing clinical trials. Because gram-negative bacteria are the most common causative organisms of septic shock and LPS is a principal stimulus for production of host endogenous mediators responsible for the development of septic shock, the use of antiendotoxin antibodies offers a mechanism of interrupting the systemic release of toxic host mediators before they are produced. Furthermore, because LPS potentiates the toxicity of TNF-α, neutralization of circulating LPS could theoretically be beneficial even after

TABLE 24–6

DISSOCIATION OF TUMOR NECROSIS FACTOR EFFECT FROM SERUM LEVELS IN MICE WITH TNF-SECRETING TUMORS*

Metabolic Parameter	Metabolic Effect of TNF Production in	
	Peripheral Tissue	Brain
Food intake	Mild anorexia over 6 wk	Severe anorexia within days
Catabolic state	Lipid and protein loss (cachexia)	Protein loss with lipid sparing (starvation)
Hematopoiesis	Anemia developing within 10 d	No anemia developing
Brain histology	Normal brain tissue	Significant inflammation with evidence of neovascularity
Hair growth	No hair growth	Hypertrichosis
Survival	Alive at 6 wk	Dead within 2 wk

*Nude mice were implanted with a tumor genetically engineered to secrete TNF constitutively either in the thigh (peripheral tissue) or in a neurologically silent area of the forebrain (brain). Although circulating levels of TNF were not different between the two groups, marked metabolic effects were noted.[126]

TNF-α release has already occurred. Clinical trials of antiendotoxin antibodies have been under way for more than a decade.[130–132] The most recent study by Ziegler and colleagues reported that administration of an immunoglobulin antiendotoxin antibody, designated HA-1A, reduced mortality associated with gram-negative septic shock from 49 to 30%.[133] However, the majority of the patients in the study did not benefit from antiendotoxin antibody treatment, possibly because only 37% of patients had documented gram-negative infections. In addition, antiendotoxin antibodies would not be expected to protect against septic shock produced in response to organisms other than gram-negative bacteria, which were apparently the majority in the HA-1A trial. Thus, although the use of antiendotoxin antibodies offers promise for the treatment of gram-negative septic shock, other strategies for interfering with host responses to invasive infections remain necessary.

The ability of anti–TNF-α antibodies to protect against the development of septic shock and death in experimental animal models of lethal bacteremia and endotoxemia has stimulated interest in these agents for therapy in human septicemia. Clinical trials of the use of anti–TNF-α antibodies in septic shock are currently in progress. Preliminary results from one phase I trial indicate that anti–TNF-α antibody administration is both safe and associated with increases in the mean arterial blood pressure of patients in shock.[134] Future therapies for controlling the systemic release of TNF-α in response to invasive infection may also lie in blocking TNF-α production (e.g., pentoxifylline[135, 136]) or controlling its release (e.g., cyclosporine[137]). Interrupting TNF-α–induced secondary mediators of septic shock represents another alternative for inhibiting TNF-α toxicity. As noted previously, compounds that block the synthesis and release of a number of these secondary mediators, including cyclooxygenase and lipoxygenase inhibitors, PAF antagonists, competitive inhibitors for TNF-α–induced nitric oxide production, and inhibitors of the coagulation cascade, possess the ability to attenuate some of the injurious effects seen as a result of septicemia. Furthermore, recognition of the importance of local production of TNF-α, as well as other cytokines, may lead to novel treatment strategies, such as the administration of aerosolized anti–TNF-α antibodies or TNF-α–binding proteins to interdict persistent TNF-α–induced lung injury in septic ARDS.

During the past decade, tremendous insight into the mechanisms underlying the pathogenesis of sepsis and septic shock has been gained. The task of translating these advances in our understanding of the host response to overwhelming infection into clinically efficacious treatment strategies remains. Although the treatment of septic shock will continue to require advances in antibiotic therapy and intensive care technology, it is likely that antiendotoxin antibodies

and antagonists of the endogenous mediators of sepsis, of which TNF-α is the prototype, will have a role in the standard treatment of septicemia in the near future. Further investigation of the complex relationships between TNF-α and other cytokines, as well as other mediators of sepsis, is needed to continue to advance the treatment of catastrophic infection.

References

1. van Deventer SJH, Buller HR, ten Cate JW, et al: Endotoxemia: An early predictor of septicemia in febrile patients. Lancet 1:605, 1988.
2. Bone RC, Fisher, CJ Jr, Clemmer TP, et al: Sepsis syndrome: A valid clinical entity. Crit Care Med 17:389, 1989.
3. Ziegler EJ, McCutchan JA, Fierer J, et al: Treatment of gram-negative bacteremia and shock with human antiserum to a mutant *Escherichia coli.* N Engl J Med 307:1225, 1982.
4. Groenveld ABJ, Bronsveld W, Thijs, LG: Hemodynamic determinants of mortality in human septic shock. Surgery 99:140, 1986.
5. Luce JM, Montgomery AB, Marks JD, et al: Ineffectiveness of high-dose methylprednisolone in preventing parenchymal lung injury and improving mortality in patients with septic shock. Am Rev Respir Dis 138:62, 1988.
6. Parrillo JE, Parker MM, Natanson G, et al: Septic shock in humans: Advances in the understanding of pathogenesis, cardiovascular dysfunction, and therapy. Ann Intern Med 113:227, 1990.
7. Franke FR: Action of toxic doses of the polysaccharide from *Serratia marcescens (Bacillus prodigiosus)* in the dog and guinea pig. J Natl Cancer Inst 5:185, 1944.
7a. Pfeiffer R: Untersuchungen über das Cholera Gift. V Hyg Infektion SKR 14:190, 1892.
7b. Shear MJ: Effect of a concentrate from *B. prodigiosus* on subcutaneous primary induced mouse tumor. Cancer Res 1:731, 1941.
8. Bennett IL, Beeson PB: Studies on the pathogenesis of fever. J Exp Med 98:477, 1953.
9. Kampschmidt, RF, Upchurch HF, Eddington CL, et al: Multiple biological activities of a partially purified leukocytic endogenous mediator. Am J Physiol 224:530, 1973.
10. Dinarello CA, Renfer L, Wolff SM: Human leukocytic pyrogen purification and development of a radioimmunoassay. Proc Natl Acad Sci USA 74:4624, 1977.
11. Tracey KJ, Vlassara H, Cerami A: Cachectin / TNF (tumour necrosis factor). Lancet 1:1122, 1989.
12. Beutler B, Cerami A: Cachectin: More than a tumor necrosis factor. N Engl J Med 316:379, 1987.
13. Nedwin GE, Naylor SL, Sakaguchi AY, et al: Human lymphotoxin and tumor necrosis factor genes: Structure, homology and chromosomal localization. Nucleic Acids Res 13:6361, 1985.
14. Beutler B, Krochin N, Milsark IW, et al: Control of cachectin (tumor necrosis factor) synthesis: Mechanisms of endotoxin resistance. Science 232:977, 1986.
15. Jue D-M, Sherry B, Luedke C, et al: Processing of newly synthesized cachectin / tumor necrosis factor in endotoxin-stimulated macrophages. Biochemistry 29:8371, 1990.
16. Smith RA, Baglioni C: The active form of tumor necrosis factor is a trimer. J Biol Chem 262:6951, 1987.
17. Jones EY, Stuart DI, Walker NP: Structure of tumor necrosis factor. Nature 338: 225, 1989.
18. Hesse DG, Tracey KJ, Fong Y, et al: Cytokine appearance in human endotoxemia and primate bacteremia. Surg Gynecol Obstet 166:147, 1988.
19. Michie HR, Manogue KR, Spriggs DR, et al: Detection of circulating

tumor necrosis factor after endotoxin administration. N Engl J Med 318:1481, 1988.

20. Beutler B, Milsark IW, Cerami A: Cachectin / tumor necrosis factor: Production, distribution, and metabolic fate in vivo. J Immunol 135:3972, 1985.

21. Shalaby MR, Sundan A, Loetscher H, et al: Binding and regulation of cellular functions by monoclonal antibodies against human tumor necrosis factor receptors. J Exp Med 172:1517, 1990.

22. Schall TJ, Lewis M, Koller KJ, et al: Molecular cloning and expression of a receptor for human tumor necrosis factor. Cell 61:361, 1990.

23. Thoma B, Grell M, Pfizenmaier K, et al: Identification of a 60-kD tumor necrosis factor (TNF) receptor as the major signal transducing component in TNF responses. J Exp Med 172:1019, 1990.

24. Brockhaus M, Schenfeld H-J, Schlager E-J, et al: Identification of two types of tumor necrosis factor receptors on human cell lines by monoclonal antibodies. Proc Natl Acad Sci USA 87:3127, 1990.

25. Heller RA, Song K, Onasch MA, et al: Complementary DNA cloning of a receptor for tumor necrosis factor and demonstration of a shed form of the receptor. Proc Natl Acad Sci USA 87:6151, 1990.

26. Seckinger P, Isaaz S, Dayer JM: Purification and biologic characterization of a specific tumor necrosis factor alpha inhibitor. J Biol Chem 264:11966, 1989.

27. Engelmann H, Aderka D, Rubinstein M, et al: A tumor necrosis factor–binding protein purified to homogeneity from human urine protects cells from tumor necrosis factor toxicity. J Biol Chem 264:11974, 1989.

28. Lantz M, Gullberg U, Nilsson E, et al: Characterization in vitro of a human tumor necrosis factor–binding protein: A soluble form of a tumor necrosis factor receptor. J Clin Invest 86:1396, 1990.

29. Carswell EA, Old LJ, Kassel RL, et al: An endotoxin-induced serum factor that causes necrosis of tumors. Proc Natl Acad Sci USA 72:3666, 1975.

30. Beutler B, Mahoney J, Le Trang N, et al: Purification of cachectin, a lipoprotein lipase–suppressing hormone secreted by endotoxin-induced RAW 264.7 cells. J Exp Med 161:984, 1985.

31. Beutler B, Greenwald D, Hulmes JD, et al: Identity of tumour necrosis factor and the macrophage-secreted factor cachectin. Nature 316:552, 1985.

32. Tracey KJ, Beutler B, Lowry SF, et al: Shock and tissue injury induced by recombinant human cachectin. Science 234:470, 1986.

33. Tracey KJ, Lowry SF, Fahey TJ III, et al: Cachectin/tumor necrosis factor induces lethal shock and stress hormone responses in the dog. Surg Gynecol Obstet 164:415, 1987.

34. Schirmer WJ, Schirmer JM, Fry DE: Recombinant human tumor necrosis factor produces hemodynamic changes characteristic of sepsis and endotoxemia. Arch Surg 124:445, 1989.

35. Mathison JC, Wolfson E, Ulevitch RJ: Participation of tumor necrosis factor in the mediation of gram negative bacterial lipopolysaccharide-induced injury in rabbits. J Clin Invest 81:1925, 1988.

36. Redl H, Schlag G, Lamche H: TNF-and LPS-induced changes of lung vascular permeability: Studies in unanesthetised sheep. Circ Shock 31:183, 1990.

37. Rothstein JL, Schreiber H: Synergy between tumor necrosis factor and bacterial products causes hemorrhagic necrosis and lethal shock in normal mice. Proc Natl Acad Sci USA 85:607, 1988.

38. Tracey KJ, Fong Y, Hesse DG, et al: Anti-cachectin / TNF monoclonal antibodies prevent septic shock during lethal bacteremia in baboons. Nature 330:662, 1987.

39. Silva AT, Bayston K, Cohen J. Prophylactic and therapeutic effects of a monoclonal antibody to tumor necrosis factor-α in experimental gram-negative shock. J Infect Dis 162:421, 1990.

40. Hinshaw LB, Tekamp-Olson P, Chang ACK, et al: Survival of primates in LD100 septic shock following therapy with antibody to tumor necrosis factor (TNFα). Circ Shock 30:279, 1990.

41. Fong Y, Tracey KJ, Moldawer LL, et al: Antibodies to cachectin/tumor necrosis factor reduce interleukin-1β and interleukin-6 appearance during lethal bacteremia. J Exp Med 170: 1627, 1989.

42. Dinarello CA: Biology of interleukin 1. FASEB J 2:108, 1988.

43. Waage A, Espevik T: Interleukin 1 potentiates the lethal effect of tumor necrosis factor/cachectin in mice. J Exp Med 167:1987, 1988.

44. Laster SM, Wood JG, Gooding LR: Tumor necrosis factor can induce both apoptic and necrotic forms of cell lysis. J Immunol 141:2629, 1988.

45. Scanlon M, Laster SM, Wood JG, et al: Cytolysis by tumor necrosis factor is preceded by a rapid and specific dissolution of microfilaments. Proc Natl Acad Sci USA 86:182, 1989.

46. Pober JS, Gimbrone MA Jr, Lapierre LA, et al: Overlapping patterns of activation of human endothelial cells by interleukin 1, tumor necrosis factor, and immune interferon. J Immunol 137:1893, 1986.

47. Tonnesen MG: Neutrophil-endothelial cell interactions: Mechanisms of neutrophil adherance to vascular endothelium. J Invest Dermatol 93 (suppl):53S, 1989.

48. Munro JM, Pober JS, Cotran RS: Tumor necrosis factor and interferon-gamma induce distinct patterns of activation and associated leukocyte accumulation in skin of *Papio anubis*. Am J Pathol 135:121, 1989.

49. Lo SK, Van Seventer GA, Levin SM, et al: Two leukocyte receptors (CD11a/CD18 and CD11b/CD18) mediate transient adhesion to endothelium by binding to different ligands. J Immunol 143:3325, 1989.

50. Dobrina A, Schwartz BR, Carlos TM: CD11CD18-independent neutro-

phil adherence to inducible endothelial-leukocyte adhesion molecules (E-LAM) in vitro. Immunology 67:502, 1989.

51. Leeuwenberg JF, Jeunhomme GM, Buurman WA: Adhesion of polymorphonuclear cell to human endothelial cells: Adhesion-molecule–dependent, and Fc receptor–mediated adhesion-molecule–independent mechanisms. Clin Exp Immunol 81:496, 1990.

52. Matsushima K, Oppenheim JJ: Interleukin 8 and MCAF: Novel inflammatory cytokines inducible by IL 1 and TNF. Cytokine 1:2, 1989.

53. Nathan CF: Neutrophil activation on biological surfaces: Massive secretion of hydrogen peroxide in response to products of macrophages and lymphocytes. J Clin Invest 80:1550, 1987.

54. Willems J, Joniau M, Cinque S, et al: Human granulocyte chemotactic peptide (IL-8) as a specific neutrophil degranulator: Comparison with other monokines. Immunology 67:540, 1989.

55. Bevilacqua, MP, Pober JS, Majeau GR, et al: Recombinant tumor necrosis factor induces procoagulant activity in cultured human vascular endothelium: Characterization and comparison with the actions of interleukin 1. Proc Natl Acad Sci USA 83:4533, 1986.

56. Conway EM, Bach R, Rosenberg RD, et al: Tumor necrosis factor enhances expression of tissue factor mRNA in endothelial cells. Thromb Res 53:231, 1989.

57. Naworth PP, Stern DM: Modulation of endothelial cell hemostatic properties by tumor necrosis factor. J Exp Med 163: 740, 1986.

58. Schleef RR, Bevilacqua MP, Sawdey M, et al: Cytokine activation of vascular endothelium: Effects on tissue-type plasminogen activator and type I plasminogen activator inhibitor. J Biol Chem 263:5797, 1988.

59. Medcalf RL, Kruithof EKO, Schleuning WD: Plasminogen activator inhibitor 1 and 2 are tumor necrosis factor/cachectin-responsive genes. J Exp Med 168:751, 1988.

60. Stolpen AH, Guinan EC, Fiers W, et al: Recombinant tumor necrosis factor and immune interferon act singly and in combination to reorganize human vascular endothelial monolayers. Am J Pathol 123:16, 1986.

61. Mullin JM, Snook KV: Effect of tumor necrosis factor on epithelial tight junctions and transepithelial permeability. Cancer Res 50:2172, 1990.

62. Sato N, Goto T, Haranaka K, et al: Actions of tumor necrosis factor on cultured vascular endothelial cells: Morphologic modulation, growth inhibition, and cytotoxicity. J Natl Cancer Inst 76:1113, 1986.

63. Hockin DC, Phillips PG, Ferro TJ, et al: Mechanisms of pulmonary edema induced by tumor necrosis factor-α. Circ Res 67:68, 1990.

64. Torti FM, Dieckmann B, Beutler B, et al: A macrophage factor inhibits adipocyte gene expression: An in vitro model of cachexia. Science 229:867, 1985.

65. Tracey KJ, Wei H, Manogue KR, et al: Cachectin/tumor necrosis factor induces cachexia, anemia and inflammation. J Exp Med 167:1211, 1988.

66. Starnes HF, Warren RS, Jeevanadam M, et al: Tumor necrosis factor and the acute metabolic response to tissue injury in man. J Clin Invest 82:1321, 1988.

67. Lee MD, Zentella A, Pekala PH, et al: Effect of endotoxin-induced monokines on glucose metabolism in the muscle cell line L6. Proc Natl Acad Sci USA 84:2590, 1987.

68. Fong Y, Moldawer LL, Marano MA, et al: Cachectin / TNF or IL-1α induces cachexia with redistribution of body proteins. Am J Physiol 256:R659, 1989.

69. Perlmutter DH, Dinarello CA, Punsal PI, et al: Cachectin/tumor necrosis factor regulates hepatic acute phase gene expression. J Clin Invest 78:1349, 1986.

70 Warren RS, Donner DB, Starnes HF, et al: Modulation of endogenous hormone action by recombinant human tumor necrosis factor. Proc Natl Acad Sci USA 84:8619, 1987.

71. Feingold KR, Grunfeld C: Tumor necrosis factor-alpha stimulates hepatic lipogenesis in the rat in vivo. J Clin Invest 80:184, 1987.

72. Yamato K, El-Hajjaoui Z, Koeffler HP: Regulation of levels of IL-1 mRNA in human fibroblasts. J Cell Physiol 139:610, 1989.

73. Nawroth PP, Bank I, Handley D, et al: Tumor necrosis factor/cachectin interacts with endothelial cell receptors to induce the release of interleukin 1. J Exp Med 163:1363, 1986.

74. Fraker DL, Langstein HN, Norton JA: Passive immunization against tumor necrosis factor partially abrogates interleukin-2 toxicity. J Exp Med 170:1015, 1989.

75. Okusawa S, Gelfand JA, Ikejima T, et al: Interleukin 1 induces a shock-like state in rabbits: Synergism with tumor necrosis factor and the effect of cyclooxygenase inhibitor. J Clin Invest 81:1162, 1988.

76. Waage A, Brandtzaeg P, Halstensen A, et al: The complex pattern of cytokines in serum from patients with meningoccoal septic shock: Association between interleukin 6, interleukin 1 and fatal outcome. J Exp Med 169:333, 1989.

77. Ohlsson K, Bjork P, Bergenfeldt M, et al: Interleukin-1 receptor antagonist reduces mortality from endotoxin shock. Nature 348:550, 1990.

78. Kishimoto, T. The biology of interleukin 6. Blood 74:1, 1989.

79. Ishibashi T, Kimura H, Shikama Y, et al: Interleukin-6 is a potent thrombopoietic factor in vivo in mice. Blood 74:1241, 1989.

80. Yim JH, Tewari A, Pearce MK, et al: Monoclonal antibody against murine interleukin-6 prevents lethal effects of *Escherichia coli* sepsis and tumor necrosis factor challenge in mice. Surg Forum 41:114, 1990.

81. Yoshimura T, Matsushima K, Oppenheim JJ, et al: Neutrophil chemotactic factor produced by lipopolysaccharide (LPS)-stimulated human

blood mononuclear leukocytes: Partial characterization and separation from interleukin 1 (IL 1). J Immunol 139:788, 1987.

82. Standiford TJ, Kunkel SL, Basha MA, et al: Interleukin-8 gene expression by a pulmonary epithelial cell line: A model for cytokine networks in the lung. J Clin Invest 86:1945, 1990.

83. Thornton AJ, Strieter RM, Lindley I, et al: Cytokine-induced gene expression of a neutrophil chemotactic factor/IL-8 in human hepatocytes. J Immunol 144:2609, 1990.

84. Van Zee KJ, DeForge LE, Fischer E, et al: IL-8 in septic shock, endotoxemia, and after IL-1 administration. J Immunol 146:3478, 1991.

85. Wolpe SD, Sherry B, Juers D, et al: Identification and characterization of macrophage inflammatory protein 2. Proc Natl Acad Sci USA 86:612, 1989.

86. Saukkonen K, Sande S, Cioffe C, et al: The role of cytokines in the generation of inflammation and tissue damage in experimental gram-positive meningitis. J Exp Med 171:439, 1990.

87. Fahey TJ III, Sherry B, Tracey KJ, et al: Cytokine production in a model of wound healing: The appearance of MIP-1, MIP-2, cachectin/TNF, and IL-1. Cytokine 2:92, 1990.

88. Nathan CF, Murray HW, Wiebe ME, et al: Identification of interferon-gamma as the lymphokine that activates human macrophage oxidative metabolism and antimicrobial activity. J Exp Med 158:670, 1983.

89. Nedwin GE, Svedersky LP, Bringman TS, et al: Effect of interleukin 2, interferon-gamma, and mitogens on the production of tumor necrosis factors alpha and beta. J Immunol 135:2492, 1985.

90. Leudke CE, Cerami A: Interferon-γ overcomes glucocorticoid suppression of cachectin/tumor necrosis factor biosynthesis by murine macrophages. J Clin Invest 86:1234, 1990.

91. Tsunawaki S, Sporn M, Ding A, et al: Deactivation of macrophages by transforming growth factor-beta. Nature 334:260, 1988.

92. Calandra T, Baumgartner J-D, Grau GE, et al: Prognostic values of tumor necrosis factor/cachectin, interleukin-1, interferon-α and interferon-γ in the serum of patients with septic shock. J Infect Dis 161:982, 1990.

93. Girardin E, Grau GE, Dayer J-M, et al: Tumor necrosis factor and interleukin-1 in the serum of children with severe infectious purpura. N Engl J Med 319:397, 1988.

94. Feuerstein G, Hallenbeck JM: Prostaglandins, leukotrienes, and platelet-activating factor in shock. Annu Rev Pharmacol Toxicol 27:301, 1987.

95. Camussi G, Bussolino F, Salvidio G, et al: Tumor necrosis factor/cachectin stimulates peritoneal macrophages, polymorphonuclear neutrophils, and vascular endothelial cells to synthesize and release platelet-activating factor. J Exp Med 166:1290, 1987.

96. Sun X, Hsueh W: Bowel necrosis induced by tumor necrosis factor in rats is mediated by platelet-activating factor. J Clin Invest 81:1328, 1988.

97. Chang SW, Feddersen CO, Henson PM, et al: Platelet-activating factor mediates hemodynamic changes and lung injury in endotoxin-treated rats. J Clin Invest 79:1498, 1987.

98. Lefer AM, Muller HF, Smith JB: Pathophysiological mechanisms of sudden death induced by platelet activating factor. Br J Pharmacol 83:125, 1984.

99. Adnot S, Lefort J, Braquet P, et al: Interference of the PAF-acether antagonist BN 52021 with endotoxin-induced hypotension in the guinea-pig. Prostaglandins 32:791, 1986.

100. Casals-Stenzel J: Protective effect of WEB 2086, a novel antagonist of platelet activating factor, in endotoxin shock. Eur J Pharmacol 135:117, 1987.

101. Toyofuku T, Kubo K, Kobayashi T, et al: Effects of ONO-6420, a platelet-activating factor antagonist, on endotoxin shock in unanesthetized sheep. Prostaglandins 31:271, 1986.

102. Flynn JT: The role of arachidonic acid metabolites in endotoxic shock, II. Involvement of prostanoids and thromboxanes. In: Hinshaw LB (ed): Handbook of Endotoxin: Pathophysiology of Infection. New York: Elsevier Science Publishers, 1985.

103. Dayer JM, Beutler B, Cerami A: Cachectin/tumor necrosis factor stimulates collagenase and prostaglandin E$_2$ production by human synovial cells and dermal fibroblasts. J Exp Med 162:2163, 1985.

104. Spinas GA, Bloesch D, Keller U, et al: Pretreatment with ibuprofen augments circulating tumor necrosis factor-α, interleukin-6 and elastase during acute endotoxemia. J Infect Dis 163:89, 1991.

105. Kettelhut IC, Fiers W, Goldberg AL: The toxic effects of tumor necrosis factor in vivo and their prevention by cyclooxygenase inhibitors. Proc Natl Acad Sci USA 84:4273, 1987.

106. Meyer JD, Yurt RW, Duhaney R, et al: Tumor necrosis factor–enhanced leukotriene B$_4$ generation and chemotaxis in human neutrophils. Arch Surg 123:1454, 1988.

107. Matera G, Cook JA, Hennigar RA, et al: Beneficial effects of a 5-lipoxygenase inhibitor in endotoxic shock in the rat. J Pharmacol Exp Ther 247:363, 1988.

108. Smedegard G, Cui L, Hugli TE: Endotoxin-induced shock in the rat: A role for C5a. Am J Pathol 135:489, 1989.

109. Sprung CL, Schultz DR, Marcial E, et al: Complement activation in septic shock patients. Crit Care Med 14:525, 1986.

110. Solomkin JS, Cotta LA, Satoh PS, et al: Complement activation and clearance in acute illness and injury: Evidence for C5a as a cell-directed

111. mediator of the adult respiratory distress syndrome in man. Surgery 97:668, 1985.

111. Hack CE, Nuijens JH, Felt-Bersma RJF, et al: Elevated plasma levels of the anaphylatoxins C3a and C4a are associated with a fatal outcome in sepsis. Am J Med 86:20, 1989.

112. Tonnesen MG, Smedly LA, Henson PM: Neutrophil–endothelial cell interactions. Modulation of neutrophil adhesiveness induced by complement fragments C5a and C5a des arg and formyl-methionyl-leucyl-phenylalanine in vitro. J Clin Invest 74:1581, 1984.

113. Schirmer WJ, Schirmer JM, Naff GB, et al: Systemic complement activation produces hemodynamic changes characteristic of sepsis. Arch Surg 123:316, 1988.

114. Stevens JH, O'Hanley P, Shapiro JM, et al: Effects of anti-C5a antibodies on the adult respiratory distress syndrome in septic primates. J Clin Invest 77:1812, 1986.

115. Berger M, Wetzler EM, Wallis RS: Tumor necrosis factor is the major monocyte product that increases complement receptor expression on mature human neutrophils. Blood 71:151, 1988.

116. Reed D, Moore, FD Jr: Recombinant human tumor necrosis factor increases granulocyte cell-surface complement receptor number. Arch Surg 123:1333, 1988.

117. Kilbourn RG, Gross SS, Jubran A, et al: N^G-Methyl-L-arginine inhibits tumor necrosis factor-induced hypotension: Implications for the involvement of nitric oxide. Proc Natl Acad Sci USA 87:3629, 1990.

118. Marks JD, Marks CB, Luce JM, et al: Plasma tumor necrosis factor levels in patients with septic shock. Am Rev Respir Dis 141:94, 1990.

119. Offner F, Philippe J, Vogelaers D, et al: Serum tumor necrosis factor levels in patients with infectious disease and septic shock. J Lab Clin Med 116:100, 1990.

120. Waage A, Halstensen A, Espevik T: Association between tumour necrosis factor in serum and fatal outcome in patients with meningococcal disease. Lancet 1:355, 1987.

121. Damas P, Reuter A, Gysen P, et al: Tumor necrosis factor and interleukin-1 serum levels during severe sepsis in humans. Crit Care Med 17:975, 1989.

122. Debets JMH, Kampmeijer R, van der Linden M, et al: Plasma tumor necrosis factor and mortality in critically ill septic patients. Crit Care Med 17:489, 1989.

123. Marano MA, Fong Y, Moldawer LL, et al: Serum cachectin / TNF in critically ill burn patients correlates with infection and mortality. Surg Gynecol Obstet 170:32, 1990.

124. Mustafa MM, Lebel MH, Ramilo O, et al: Correlation of interleukin-1 beta and cachectin concentrations in cerebrospinal fluid and outcome from bacterial meningitis. J Pediatr 115:208, 1989.

125. Giradin E, Grau GE, Dayer DM, et al: Tumor necrosis factor and interleukin-1 in the serum of children with severe infectious purpura. N Engl J Med 319:397, 1988.

126. Tracey KJ, Morgello S, Koplin B, et al: Metabolic effects of cachectin/TNF are modified by its site of production: Cachectin/tumor necrosis factor–secreting tumor in skeletal muscle induces cachexia, while implantation in the brain induces primarily anorexia. J Clin Invest 86:2014, 1990.

127. Waage A, Halstensen A, Shalaby R, et al: Local production of tumor necrosis factor alpha, interleukin 1, and interleukin 6 in meningococcal meningitis: Relation to the inflammatory response. J Exp Med 170:1859, 1989.

128. Millar AB, Foley NM, Singer M, et al: Tumour necrosis factor in bronchopulmonary secretions of patients with adult respiratory distress syndrome. Lancet 2:712, 1989.

129. Roberts DJ, Davies JM, Evans CC, et al: Tumour necrosis factor and adult respiratory distress syndrome. Lancet 2:1043, 1989.

130. Ziegler EJ, McCutchan JA, Fierer J, et al: Treatment of gram-negative bacteremia and shock with human antiserum to a mutant *Escherichia coli*. N Engl J Med 307:1225, 1982.

131. Baumgartner JD, Glauser MP, McCutchan JA, et al: Prevention of gram-negative shock and death in surgical patients by antibody to endotoxin core glycolipid. Lancet 2:59, 1985.

132. Calandra T, Glauser MP, Schellekens J, et al: Treatment of gram-negative septicemia with human IgG antibody to *Escherichia coli* J5: A prospective, double-blind, randomized trial. J Infect Dis 158:312, 1988.

133. Ziegler EJ, Fisher CJ Jr, Sprung CL, et al: Treatment of gram-negative bacteremia and septic shock with HA-1A human monoclonal antibody against endotoxin. N Eng J Med 324:429, 1991.

134. Exley AR, Cohen J, Buurman W, et al: Monoclonal antibody to TNF in severe septic shock. Lancet 1:1275, 1990.

135. Strieter RM, Remick DG, Ward PA, et al: Cellular and molecular regulation of tumor necrosis factor-alpha production by pentoxifylline. Biochem Biophys Res Commun 155:1230, 1988.

136. Schlade UF. Pentoxifylline increases survival in murine endotoxin shock and decreases formation of tumor necrosis factor. Circ Shock 31:171, 1990.

137. Remick DG, Nguyen DT, Eskandari MK, et al: Cyclosporine A inhibits TNF production without decreasing TNF mRNA levels. Biochem Biophys Res Commun 161:551, 1989.

CHAPTER 25

Cardiovascular Dysfunction in Septic Shock

Andrew C. Dixon
Joseph E. Parrillo

The rising prevalence of sepsis and septic shock in the intensive care unit (ICU)[1, 2] has sparked increasing interest in the epidemiologic, pathogenic, and clinical features of this disease.[3] The early clinical studies were often hampered by inability to study the entire spectrum of a disease that produces abrupt and profound physiologic disturbances that require immediate treatment. The natural history remained unknown because of the clinical need for early institution of therapy. In addition, until the past decade the use of intravascular hemodynamic monitoring devices, particularly the indwelling pulmonary arterial catheter, was not routine, and knowledge of hemodynamic and cardiac performance was limited by the lack of an accurate and reproducible measure of left ventricular filling pressure (preload). Lastly, it is difficult to differentiate between the effects of sepsis and pertubations from underlying disease states, which often have effects of their own on the cardiovascular system.

The description of clinical signs that constitute the septic syndrome has allowed investigators to identify patients likely to have sepsis early in their clinical course, before microbiologic results are available.[4] In addition to providing a better picture of the natural history of this disease, the identification of this syndrome has made possible early institution of therapies aimed at modulating the cascade of potent circulating mediators thought to mediate many of the effects of sepsis.

A number of human and animal models have been developed to study the cardiovascular responses to sepsis. Initial investigations relied on animal models and live *Escherichia coli* or other organisms; however, since the isolation and purification of bacterial endotoxin, this agent has been administered intravenously as a simpler method of reproducing many of the hemodynamic effects of sepsis as seen in humans. It must be remembered, however, that although animal models with either live bacteria or endotoxin simulate some of the changes seen in humans. They differ in several important respects. These are addressed in this chapter.

In this chapter we review both the historical and up-to-date features of the hemodynamic and cardiovascular consequences of sepsis and septic shock. We concentrate on human data when available but will supplement them with large-animal data when applicable. Lastly, we identify what is known at present about the role of the cytokines and other substances in mediating the cardiovascular alterations in sepsis.

HISTORICAL FEATURES

Our current understanding of the hemodynamic findings in sepsis and septic shock reflect our improved ability to make accurate measurements of preload (pulmonary capillary wedge pressure [PCWP]), afterload (mean arterial pressure [MAP] and calculated systemic vascular resistance [SVR]), and cardiac output (CO). For only the last 20 or so years has the PCWP been used to assess preload. Before this the central venous pressure (CVP) was the "gold standard" of volume assessment. Because of this, many of the early studies of sepsis were flawed, often including patients with hypovolemic or combined hypovolemic and septic shock.

Approximately 40 years ago patients with sepsis were characterized as having one of two distinct types of septic shock, either warm (hyperdynamic) or cold (hypodynamic) shock, based on examination of skin temperature.[5] Those with cold septic shock were described as having a reduced CO resulting from heart failure, a form of cardiogenic shock, and those with warm shock were thought to have either an elevated CO or a reduced SVR, a distributive form of shock (Table 25–1). In the 1960s it began to be understood that this classification was overly simplified and did not accurately reflect the cardiovascular status of the septic patient.

At this time, several investigations identified and addressed the hemodynamic picture of septic shock using colorimetric methods to measure the CO and indwelling catheters to monitor the CVP. In 1965 Wilson and coworkers demonstrated in humans that septic shock was best characterized by a low SVR and a normal or high CO.[6] These patients were contrasted with those with hypovolemic or cardiogenic shock, both of which groups demonstrated a high SVR and low CO.

The concept of inadequate effective blood flow was first raised by Udhoji and Weil in 1965 when they studied a series of bacteremic patients.[7] Two groups of patients were identified on the basis of hemodynamic findings: a group with hypotension resulting from a reduced CO and high peripheral vascular resistance and a group with a high or normal CO and a reduced peripheral vascular resistance. Although these septic patients probably still had an element of hypovolemia, this study and that of Wilson and colleagues set the tone for future research into the pathophysiology of the vasodilation and cardiovascular depression seen in human sepsis.

Not until the early 1970s was aggressive volume resuscitation used in managing patients with sepsis. Before that time, clinicians thought that volume therapy would aggravate

TABLE 25–1	
CLASSIFICATION OF SHOCK STATES	
Cardiogenic	Myopathic (reduced systolic function)
	Acute myocardial infarction
	Dilated cardiomyopathy
	Myocardial depression in septic shock
	Mechanical
	Mitral regurgitation
	Ventricular septal defects
	Ventricular aneurysm
	Left ventricular outflow obstruction (aortic stenosis, idiopathic hypertrophic subaortic stenosis, asymmetric septal hypertrophy)
	Arrhythmias
Extracardiac obstructive	Pericardial tamponade
	Constrictive pericarditis
	Pulmonary embolism (massive)
	Severe pulmonary hypertension
	Coarctation of the aorta
Oligemic	Hemorrhage
	Fluid depletion
Distributive	Septic shock
	Toxic products (e.g., overdose)
	Anaphylaxis
	Neurogenic
	Endocrinologic

Adapted from Abboud FM: Shock. In: Wyngaarden JB, Smith LH Jr, Bennett JC (eds): Cecil Textbook of Medicine. 17th ed. Philadelphia, WB Saunders, p 211, 1985.

the capillary leak seen particularly in the lungs and would therefore worsen oxygenation and perhaps hasten the development of adult respiratory distress syndrome (ARDS) in these patients. With the development and common clinical use of the pulmonary arterial catheter in the early 1970s, it was found that many of these patients had low left-sided heart filling pressures and that these pressures showed little correlation with the CVP. Thus, routine use of the PCWP as a more accurate measure of left ventricular preload became commonplace and led to the use of more liberal volume infusion. This in turn allowed studies of the effects of sepsis on the cardiovascular system to proceed unhampered by the influence of volume depletion.

We now know that sepsis is characterized most frequently by an elevated CO with a reduced SVR; however, the development of newer modalities of evaluating myocardial performance has allowed a number of investigators to address better the individual responses of the left and right ventricles to sepsis. It is now known that myocardial performance is significantly impaired in sepsis. Both ventricles become reversibly dilated and hypocontractile.[8] This response is associated with a fall in the ejection fraction, while both stroke volume and cardiac index (CI) are maintained or elevated.[8]

HEMODYNAMIC CHARACTERISTICS OF SEPTIC SHOCK

Sepsis and septic shock are separate yet overlapping processes, and understanding the distinction between the two is essential for a discussion of the subject. In fact, these syndromes are best viewed as representing two points on a continuous spectrum from infection with only mild host responses, such as fever and chills, to unrelenting hypotension and/or multiple organ system failure culminating in the death of the patient.

Sepsis is best defined as a constellation of signs and symptoms, all of which are caused by the host response to an infectious agent. Although gram-negative organisms are among the most common causes of sepsis, gram-positive bacteria, fungi, parasites, and viruses can all incite the host responses that we call sepsis. The presence in the blood stream of these organisms or their by-products, such as endotoxin in the case of gram-negative organisms, stimulates a host response. This response is clinically manifested by numerous signs and symptoms, including fever or hypothermia, chills or rigors, tachycardia, tachypnea, and often neurologic changes. Metabolic abnormalities are also common and include early respiratory alkalosis or later onset of a lactic acidosis when disturbances of blood flow to the tissues become manifest. Most noteworthy, however, the presence of positive blood cultures or evidence of a localized infection is not a prerequisite in most definitions of sepsis. It is now well established that bacteremia is often hard to demonstrate during the course of sepsis in many patients, usually because of its intermittent nature. Rather the signs and symptoms mentioned earlier, which represent the host response to the infectious agent, constitute the most commonly used definition of sepsis.

The septic syndrome, as discussed elsewhere in this text, is perhaps one of the more thoroughly researched clinical definitions of sepsis and is often used for investigative work in which early identification of patients allows the institution of experimental therapy at a time when the disease may be most amenable to therapy. This definition uses criteria that reflect impaired organ perfusion or function without specific criteria for blood pressure, CO, or other data obtained invasively. When this definition is applied clinically, approximately 45% of patients eventually develop positive blood cultures. Mortality in the septic syndrome approaches 30%, similar to that in many studies in which positive blood cultures are required to establish the diagnosis.[4]

When systemic hypotension is superimposed on the foregoing criteria, the patient is said to have septic shock. In our ICU, we require an MAP of less than 60 mm Hg to establish this diagnosis. Although clearly an important and easily measured clinical sign used in the management of the septic patient, blood pressure alone does not accurately reflect the delivery of oxygen at the tissue level. However, because it is difficult to measure blood flow and oxygen delivery continuously, most clinicians monitor the blood pressure continuously, usually with an indwelling catheter, to help identify trends that should prompt the determination of more accurate measurements of blood flow. An indwelling arterial catheter provides the advantage of a continuous reading of the MAP, which we use preferentially because it takes into account both the systolic and diastolic measurements, each of which can influence blood flow.

Before common use of the pulmonary arterial catheter for the management of septic patients, clinicians depended on secondary evidence of diminished organ perfusion. A metabolic marker of this is the serum lactate level, which is a reasonable measure of organ perfusion and rapidly reflects improvements in blood flow to lactate-producing tissues. A reduction of urine output was and remains a good indicator of poor renal blood flow; cold, clammy, cyanotic skin suggests a redistribution of blood flow away from the skin and subcutaneous structures. A reduction of flow to the brain leads to impaired cognitive function, ranging from mild confusion to coma. Lastly, reduced perfusion of the liver and lung may contribute to the failure of these organs, resulting in hyperbilirubinemia, hypoxemia, and on occasion the development of ARDS.

With the common use of the pulmonary arterial catheter came better hemodynamic variables that could be followed in patients with sepsis. Most of the studies began to use the CI as the standard measure of cardiac function. The advantages of its use are the ease of bedside measurements and the reproducibility of the results.

Most studies of the hemodynamic findings in sepsis agree that the CI is elevated and the SVR is reduced early in the course of sepsis. This combination of findings in a patient, when accompanied by evidence of infection, is sufficiently specific for sepsis to necessitate the initiation of appropriate therapy including antibiotics and volume resuscitation if hypotension intervenes.

There are several disadvantages of using the CI as a primary estimate of cardiac performance, however. First, the CI is significantly affected by the preload, afterload, and heart rate, all of which may change significantly during the course of sepsis. Many of the older studies that used CI as an indicator of myocardial function did not provide accompanying hemodynamic data, including measures of preload, afterload, and heart rate, that would allow a full interpretation of the myocardial response to this complex disease. Second, the CI is a measure of flow, not intrinsic myocardial function, and is therefore often insensitive to the changes in contractility and ventricular volume that occur during sepsis.

A final concern about using the CI as a measure of cardiac failure is that it is unreliable in prospectively differentiating between survivors and nonsurvivors of a septic episode. Early studies suggested that a low or falling CI, often with the development of acidosis, was characteristic of impending demise.[6, 9-11] In an effort to further clarify this, Winslow and coworkers reported that their data on 50 patients with septic shock and positive blood cultures, noting that no significant hemodynamic differences existed between the patients who survived and those who died from sepsis.[12] Only a higher serum lactate level was predictive of mortality (63 versus 31 mg/dL, $P < .02$). In a later study of 48 patients with septic shock and positive blood cultures, Parker and coworkers identified the heart rate (<106 beats/min) as the only hemodynamic variable that could significantly predict survival on initial evaluation.[13] Both survivors and nonsurvivors demonstrated a hyperdynamic picture on presentation. Twenty-four hours after the onset of shock, both a return of the heart rate toward normal (<95 beats/min) and a rise in the systemic vascular resistance index (SVRI) (>1529 dyne•s/cm[5]) predicted subsequent survival. The CI was predictive of survival only when it fell more than 0.5 L/min/m[2] between the initial recording and one obtained 24 hours later. Mortality during the first week in this study was most commonly the result of a persistently low and poorly responsive SVRI, whereas the patients who died after 1 week succumbed to multiple organ system failure.[13]

From this discussion, it is clear that the characteristic hemodynamic profile of septic shock in humans is one of hyperdynamic circulation, with an elevated CI and a depressed SVR. From the data of Wiles and colleagues we also know that this is true whether the causitive agent is a gram-positive, gram-negative, anaerobic, or even fungal organism.[14]

MYOCARDIAL PRESSURE-VOLUME RELATIONSHIPS IN SEPSIS

It has long been thought that there is an element of myocardial depression in human sepsis. Early studies often detected a low CO despite a normal or high CVP, which was taken as evidence of significant myocardial depression. We now understand that the CVP has little correlation with left ventricular preload, suggesting these studies may have been flawed by the concomitant presence of an element of hypovolemic shock. Because the use of adequate volume resuscitation has become routine, several sensitive techniques for determining the ventricular response to sepsis in humans have been employed, including the effects of volume loading, radionuclide angiography, and echocardiography. These are individually discussed in the following.

The left ventricular stroke work index (LVSWI) is a measure of cardiac performance that contains both a pressure and a volume measurement. Weisul and colleagues used the change of the LVSWI in response to volume administration to characterize the difference in myocardial performance between survivors and nonsurvivors of septic shock.[15] With volume loading that changed the PCWP from 5 to 12 mm Hg, the survivors demonstrated a significantly greater increase in LVSWI than did the nonsurvivors. Although it uncovered a significant difference in the myocardial response to volume infusion between the groups, this study relied on the PCWP as an accurate measure of left ventricular preload in sepsis. This is frequently not the case[16, 17] because left ventricular preload is best measured by the amount of stretch on the myocardium, which is best estimated by ventricular volume (not pressure). Thus the characteristics of the pressure-volume relationship (compliance) determine whether PCWP reflects volume changes and accurately reflects myocardial stretch or preload. This issue was later addressed by Ognibene and coworkers, who studied the response to volume infusion in patients with septic shock compared to patients with sepsis but without shock and to critically ill control patients.[18] Patients with septic shock showed less change in LVSWI after volume infusion than did control patients (Fig. 25–1). To evaluate the ventricular compliance, these authors used radionuclide cineangiography to determine the relationship between the LVSWI and the end-diastolic volume index. The plot of this pressure-

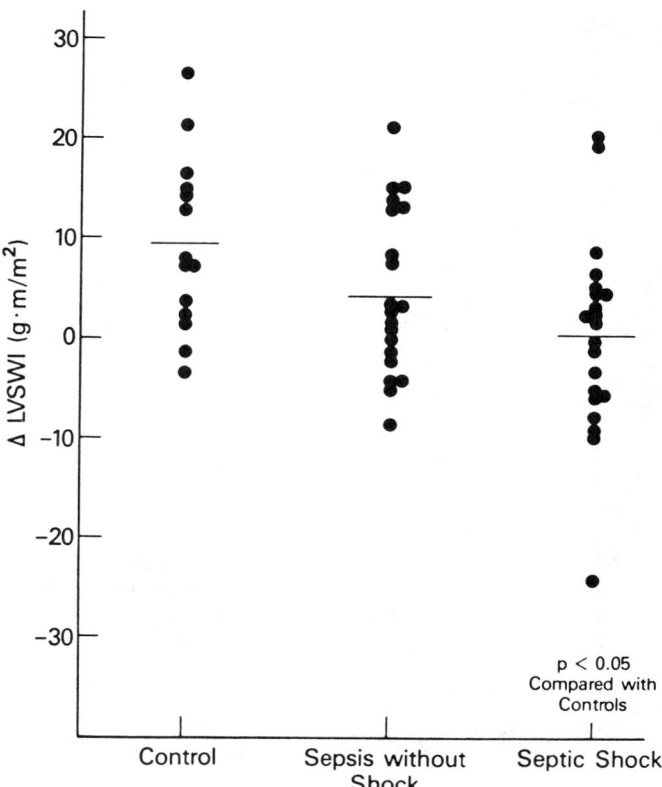

Figure 25–1. Effects of volume infusion on LVSWI in three groups. The horizontal line represents the mean for each group. (From Ognibene FP, Parker MM, Natanson C, et al: Depressed left ventricular performance: Response to volume infusion in patients with sepsis and septic shock. Chest 93:903, 1988.)

volume relationship represents the Frank-Starling curve for each individual patient. These data, presented in Figure 25–2, demonstrate that in patients with septic shock a similar quantity of volume infusion resulted in only small increments in LVSWI and end-diastolic volume index. This suggests a fall in both ventricular compliance and contractility and therefore evidence of severe myocardial depression.

Closer scrutiny of the individual responses of the patients in this study shows that some patients failed to increase LVSWI in response to volume infusion but were able to increase their end-diastolic volume index. This suggests a failure of myocardial contractility. At baseline, most septic shock patients had an increased end-diastolic volume (dilated ventricle) that did not respond normally to volume infusion; this indicates a compliance abnormality. One wonders how the response to inotropic therapy (not specifically studied to date) would differ in these two groups of patients. Rackow and coworkers have also constructed ventricular performance curves for a series of 18 patients with septic shock.[19] They too found that the LVSWI was not elevated as much in the patients with septic shock as in the nonseptic control patients, again evidence of depressed left ventricular performance.

In the study by Ognibene and colleagues, patients with sepsis but without shock also had a reduced myocardial response to volume, but not to the same extent as the group with septic shock (see Fig. 25–2).[18] The control group of critically ill nonseptic patients had a normal left ventricular response to intravascular volume expansion. These data demonstrate that the cardiac response seen in patients with sepsis or septic shock is ventricular dilatation with a fall in left ventricular contractility.

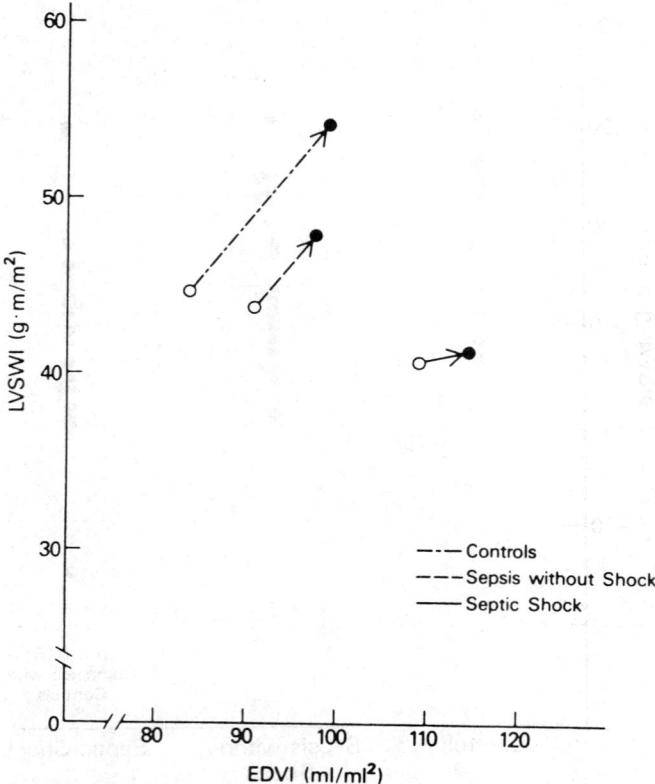

Figure 25–2. The Frank-Starling relationship for each of three patient groups. Open circles represent the mean value for each group before volume infusion; filled circles represent the mean values after volume infusion. (From Ognibene FP, Parker MM, Natanson C, et al: Depressed left ventricular performance: Response to volume infusion in patients with sepsis and septic shock. Chest 93:903, 1988.)

RADIONUCLIDE CINEANGIOGRAPHY IN SEPSIS

Calvin and coworkers were the first to use radionuclide cineangiography in the study of myocardial responses to sepsis.[20] In 1981 they used this technique to evaluate the left ventricular ejection fraction (LVEF) in 20 patients with sepsis but no evidence of shock. The mean LVEF for the group as a whole was normal, but 5 of the 20 patients were noted to have an increase in the left ventricular end-diastolic volume and a fall in ejection fraction.

Subsequently, Parker and coworkers used radionuclide cineangiography with simultaneous thermodilution cardiac outputs to identify the serial responses of 20 patients with septic shock.[8] These investigators used a volume measurement of preload, the end-diastolic volume index, which is obtained by dividing the stroke volume index by the ejection fraction. They identified the expected hemodynamic profile of septic shock (elevated CI and depressed SVRI) in both survivors (13 patients) and nonsurvivors (7 patients). The surprising finding of this study was that several days after the onset of shock the survivors demonstrated a fall in LVEF associated with a markedly increased end-diastolic volume index. This is the picture of a dilated, hypocontractile ventricle. These changes persisted for several days and then returned toward normal by follow-up study after 7 to 10 days (Figs. 25–3 and 25–4) Thus survivors of septic shock showed reversible left ventricular dilatation and depression of contractility. This picture has since been confirmed by other investigators.[21]

In the same study,[8] nonsurvivors of septic shock behaved

somewhat differently. Whereas 10 of the 13 survivors had an initial LVEF of less than 40%, none of the nonsurvivors did. Therefore, an initially depressed LVEF tended to predict survival and patients who did not develop a fall in LVEF more often died of sepsis. The reason for this is unknown, but several mechanisms have been postulated.[22] The nonsurvivors in this study had a lower SVRI than the survivors, reflecting a decreased afterload, which could have unloaded the left ventricle and caused a relative rise in LVEF. Alternatively, perhaps because they had a more severe capillary leak, the nonsurvivors could have developed myocardial edema, causing a reduction in ventricular compliance. Pathologically, this has been demonstrated in animal models of hyperdynamic sepsis.[23] If it occurred in humans, this would be expected to reduce the ability of the ventricle to dilate in response to an undefined stimulus during sepsis, a response that appears to be adaptive in nature.

It appears most likely that one or several of the mediators of sepsis can act as a myocardial depressant factor and can directly decrease myocardial contractility, resulting in the abnormal contractile performance. Preliminary work has shown that tumor necrosis factor (TNF), but not endotoxin, interleukin-1 (IL-1), or interleukin-2 (IL-2), causes a depression of in vitro myocardial cell contraction.[24] Others have shown that adrenergic receptors become down-regulated in animal models of sepsis, which could contribute to a reduced ventricular contractile response to the high levels of circulating catecholamines seen in this syndrome.[25, 26]

RIGHT VENTRICULAR RESPONSE TO SEPSIS

The asymmetric and variable geometry of the right ventricle considerably increases the difficulty encountered in studying its responses to sepsis. This, as well as technical difficulties encountered in critically ill patients, who are often receiving positive pressure ventilation, has limited the utility of echocardiography for estimating the right ventricular ejection fraction (RVEF) in patients with sepsis. The most

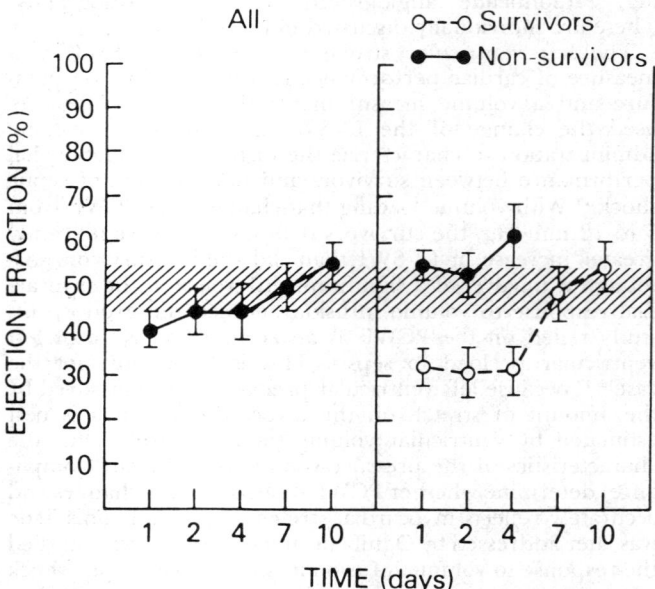

Figure 25–3. Mean (± SE) ejection fraction plotted against time for septic shock patients. The plot on the left represents all patients combined; the plot on the right shows the mean values for survivors and nonsurvivors. The hatched area represents the normal range. (Reproduced, with permission, from Parker MM, Shelhamer JH, Bacharach SL, et al, Profound but reversible myocardial depression in patients with septic shock. Ann Intern Med 1984; 100:483–490).

ACUTE PHASE OF SEPTIC SHOCK

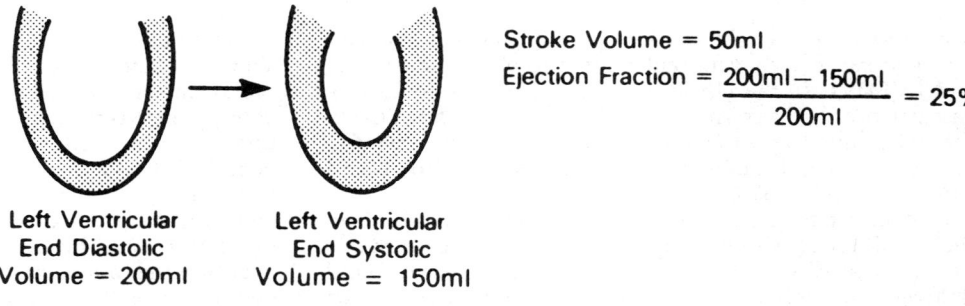

Left Ventricular
End Diastolic
Volume = 200ml

Left Ventricular
End Systolic
Volume = 150ml

Stroke Volume = 50ml

Ejection Fraction = $\dfrac{200ml - 150ml}{200ml}$ = 25%

Figure 25–4. Schematic representation of the volume and contractility changes that occur in the left ventricle in patients with septic shock. These changes are more characteristic of survivors than of nonsurvivors. (Reproduced, with permission, from Parker MM, Shelhamer JH, Bacharach SL, et al, Profound but reversible myocardial depression in patients with septic shock. Ann Intern Med 1984; 100:483–490).

RECOVERY PHASE OF SEPTIC SHOCK

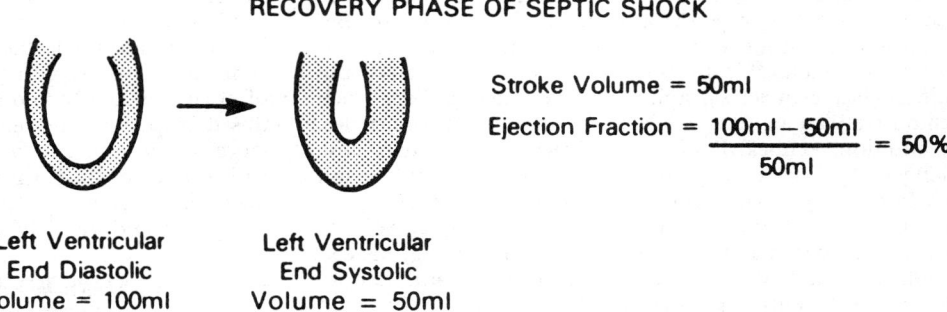

Left Ventricular
End Diastolic
Volume = 100ml

Left Ventricular
End Systolic
Volume = 50ml

Stroke Volume = 50ml

Ejection Fraction = $\dfrac{100ml - 50ml}{50ml}$ = 50%

reliable currently available technique for measuring the RVEF is radionuclide ventriculography.[27, 28] This has been used by several investigators to study the performance and volumes of the right ventricle in sepsis.

Kimchi and colleagues in 1984 were the first to investigate the RVEF in sepsis, when they studied 25 patients with blood culture–positive septic shock.[29] By performing simultaneous thermodilution CO measurements, they were able not only to identify the RVEF but also to calculate the right and left ventricular volumes. A depressed RVEF (<38%) was present in 13 patients at the outset of the study; 8 of these 13 patients also had an abnormal LVEF (<48%) and 5 had a normal LVEF. This suggests that right and left ventricular functions are unrelated in sepsis. Right ventricular impairment occurred regardless of the hemodynamic state of the patient or the presence of elevated right ventricular afterload (pulmonary hypertension). In the 17 patients who survived, the RVEF improved in 6 and was unchanged in 11. The authors concluded that right ventricular performance abnormalities in sepsis are more common than was previously suspected and that interventions to decrease right ventricular afterload and increase contractility might be appropriate for patients with a reduced RVEF.[29] Hoffman and coworkers, in a study of 16 patients with hypovolemic or septic shock, also found that a depressed RVEF occurred in some patients with sepsis and that when it occurred the right ventricular function appeared to be independent of that of the left ventricle.[30] In that study, which was flawed by the lack of repeated scans in several patients, mortality correlated with the failure of improvement in right ventricular performance.[30]

Biventricular responses to fluid loading were studied by Schneider and coworkers,[31] in much the same way as others have studied the left ventricular response to volume infusion.[15, 18, 19] In 18 patients with septic shock accompanied by pulmonary hypertension, the responses to the infusion of 500 mL of plasma were studied using both hemodynamic and radionuclide ventriculography techniques. The 13 patients who responded showed an increase in stroke volume index, right ventricular end-diastolic volume index and stroke work index, and left ventricular end-diastolic volume index (LVEDVI) and stroke work index after the administration of fluid. Nonresponders (n = 5) had no increase in stroke volume index and actually had a decrease in right ventricular stroke work index despite a mild (7%) increase in right ventricular end-diastolic volume index. Both groups showed a significant fall in RVEF (from 45 ± 3% to 41 ± 2%, $P < .01$) and no change in LVEF in response to the increase in intravascular volume. The authors concluded that in some patients with septic shock, volume loading fails to improve forward flow because of the right ventricular dysfunction.[31]

Using a modified pulmonary arterial catheter equipped with a fast-response thermistor in 127 critically ill patients, Vincent and colleagues were able to demonstrate a fall in RVEF during the development of septic shock (from 35.1 ± 9.8 to 24.2 ± 10.4%, $P < .01$) and an increase during recovery (from 25.0 ± 7.6 to 29.8 ± 8.5%, $P < .05$) in 14 patients.[32] They also found that the RVEF was significantly lower in septic shock (23.8 ± 8.2%) than in sepsis without shock (30.3 ± 10.1%) or in patients with no evidence of either sepsis or cardiopulmonary impairment (32.5 ± 7.1%). Lastly, their septic shock patients who did not survive had a more severely impaired RVEF than the survivors (20.9 ± 6.7 and 27.8 ± 8.6%, respectively; $P < .02$). The effect of sepsis on the left ventricle could not be assessed with this technique, which, although easily used at the bedside, remains to be validated by comparison to a gold standard.

Parker and coworkers evaluated the relation of biventricular performance to survival using concomitant hemodynamic and radionuclide ventriculography studies in 39 patients with septic shock.[33] By using serial examinations (within 24 hours of death for the nonsurvivors), they demonstrated that both hemodynamic and cardiac performance indices returned toward normal in survivors (n = 22), including a rise in MAP, RVEF, LVEF, and right ventricular stroke work index and a fall in CVP, PCWP, mean pulmonary artery pressure, right ventricular end-diastolic volume index, and LVEDVI. In the nonsurvivors (n = 17) the only cardiovascular profile that significantly changed from the initial to the final study was an increase in heart rate. Thus, persistence of the myocardial depression seen in sepsis correlated with a poor prognosis.

In contrast to the studies of Kimchi and Hoffman and their colleagues,[29, 30] the study by Parker and coworkers[33] evaluated serial changes in ventricular function and found that right and left ventricular performance changed in the same direction in 82% of their patients, demonstrating that both ventricles are similarly affected in septic shock. Others have suggested that leftward shift of the interventricular septum can occur in sepsis associated with pulmonary hypertension, resulting in a reduction of left ventricular volume and preload.[34] This would appear unlikely from the radionuclide ventriculography data presented earlier, which demonstrate an increase in the dimensions of both ventricles. In addition, echocardiographic studies suggest that these changes of ventricular geometry are not persistent enough to affect left ventricular filling.[35] Vasodilator therapy, which would be expected to be beneficial if right ventricular volume overload caused a failure of left ventricular filling, instead results in a fall of right ventricular preload and fails to improve left ventricular diastolic function or to augment oxygen delivery.[36, 37] This again argues for a common mechanism for both left and right ventricular dysfunction in septic shock.

OXYGEN TRANSPORT IN SEPSIS

In addition to the impairment in cardiac function, septic patients have abnormalities in tissue oxygen delivery and utilization (see Chapter 27). Although sepsis is characterized by a hyperdynamic state, with an elevated CI and oxygen delivery ($\dot{D}O_2$), it has been found that oxygen consumption ($\dot{V}O_2$) becomes pathologically dependent on $\dot{D}O_2$ in sepsis and ARDS.[38–49] This relationship is shown in Figure 25–5. The reasons for this remain unknown but it may be related to inability at a cellular level to unload and utilize oxygen appropriately or to impaired $\dot{D}O_2$ at the capillary level secondary to microvascular occlusion and the loss of autoregulatory tone.[50, 51] The importance of the presence of pathologic oxygen supply dependence is underscored by the work of Gutierrez and Pohil, who showed that critically ill patients with pathologic oxygen supply dependence had a

mortality of 70%, whereas those who did not manifest this abnormal state had a 30% mortality.[38]

Shoemaker and colleagues have also looked at the relationship between oxygen delivery and supply in patients with sepsis as well as nonseptic critically ill surgical patients.[52–55] They, too, found that $\dot{D}O_2$ and $\dot{V}O_2$ were greater in survivors than nonsurvivors of septic shock as well as high-risk surgical patients.[52, 53] In an effort to see whether this effect could be overcome, they then studied prospectively whether augmentation of $\dot{D}O_2$ and $\dot{V}O_2$, predominantly by the use of fluids and inotropic therapy, could improve survival in these patients. The therapeutic goals for the protocol groups in these studies were the mean oxygen transport values that had been found in survivors of sepsis or high-risk surgery.[52, 53] The mortality of the protocol group in each of several studies was significantly less than that of controls whose oxygen transport values were in the range of normal values for non–critically ill patients.[54, 55] Although this therapeutic intervention remains to be confirmed in a large multicenter trial and in medical (nonsurgical) patients with septic shock, many centers are now making efforts to maximize oxygen transport values in septic patients by use of volume and inotropic therapy.

A CANINE MODEL THAT SIMULATES THE CHANGES SEEN IN HUMAN SEPSIS

Numerous animal models of septic shock have been employed in an effort to better define the pathogenesis of this exceedingly complex disease. Since purified endotoxin became commercially available, many investigators have relied on either bolus injections or infusions of this lipopolysaccharide to simulate sepsis as seen in humans. Although these models have provided a large volume of data on the biochemistry and pathology of this disease, they have failed to reproduce reliably the hemodynamic and cardiac manifestations seen in humans.

When endotoxin is administered to a large animal, the most common response is a reduced CI and an elevated SVR. This pattern is more typical of either cardiogenic or hypovolemic shock than of the distributive form of shock that characterizes human sepsis. In the absence of volume infusions, the animals usually die of a progressive fall in CI with hypotension and metabolic acidosis.

Natanson and colleagues have perfected a canine peritonitis model that closely simulates the cardiovascular variables seen in human septic shock.[56] To create a nidus of infection, a fibrin clot, which contains a known concentration of bacteria, is surgically implanted in the peritoneal cavity of a dog. This causes a chronic bacteremia that can be studied by the use of indwelling arterial and pulmonary artery catheters, as well as radionuclide cineangiography, in a fashion similar to the human clinical studies described earlier. Besides the obvious benefit of having a model of chronic bacteremia, an additional benefit is that the serial hemodynamic and radionuclide scans can be performed in conscious unsedated animals, eliminating the need for anesthetic agents or sedatives that often have confounding cardiovascular effects of their own.

Both myocardial compliance and contractility are affected in this model of sepsis. Initial evaluation of the dogs 24 hours after the surgical clot implantation shows a reduced pressure measurement of preload (PCWP), a low MAP, a decreased CI, and usually a normal SVRI. On administration of fluid to normalize the preload, all of these parameters return to nearly normal. This suggests that at this stage of canine sepsis there is a preload-dependent hyperdynamic state.[22]

When fluid challenged before clot implantation, the ani-

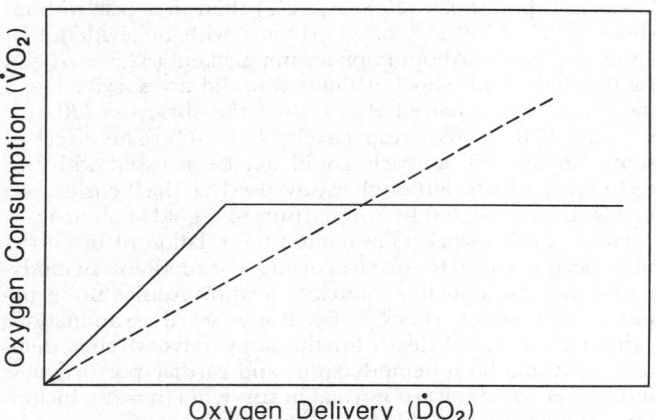

Figure 25–5. Relationship between $\dot{D}O_2$ and $\dot{V}O_2$ in normal patients (*solid line*) and patients with either septic shock or ARDS (*dashed line*).

mals develop a greatly increased LVSWI with a small increase in LVEDVI. At days 1 and 2 of sepsis, fluid loading studies showed a considerable increase in LVEDVI with normal PCWP, suggesting an increase in ventricular compliance. Concomitant radionuclide scans demonstrated a profound fall in LVEF relative to baseline. Recovery of this depressed LVEF and normal function took 2 to 4 weeks. To summarize, in this model there is a change in both myocardial compliance and contractility. As in the human studies by Parker and colleagues, both ventricular dilatation and a reduction of systolic performance are observed.[8]

By implanting progressively more bacterial organisms, these investigators were able to construct a dose-response curve for the cardiovascular abnormalities observed.[57] As increasing numbers of live *E. coli* were implanted, they observed a dose-dependent decrease in myocardial function with a reduction in systolic performance and an increase in ventricular volume (LVEDVI). The dogs that survived extremely high doses of bacterial inoculum had more compliant ventricles and a higher LVSWI than the nonsurvivors. This suggests that the ability to increase ventricular volume in response to sepsis is necessary for survival.

The influence of various types of bacterial organisms has also been investigated in this model.[58, 59] This was done to determine the role of endotoxin production in modulating the cardiovascular abnormalities observed and to identify other virulence factors that might provide insight into the pathophysiology of sepsis. When quantitatively similar amounts of *Staphylococcus aureus* (a gram-positive organism not containing endotoxin) and *E. coli* (a gram-negative organism containing endotoxin) were implanted intraperitoneally in a fibrin clot, the dogs that received *S. aureus* had a more profound reduction in LVEF than those receiving *E. coli*. When formalin-killed organisms were used in this experiment, the dogs that received formalin-killed *E. coli* developed more severe myocardial dysfunction than those that received formalin-killed *S. aureus*. Elevated endotoxin levels were detected in the serum of animals that received live or formalin-killed *E. coli* but not those that received either form of *S. aureus*.[58] These results suggest that organism viability plays an important role in *S. aureus* but not *E. coli* sepsis–related cardiovascular dysfunction in dogs. They confirm that both gram-negative and gram-positive organisms can elicit the cardiovascular manifestations of sepsis and that there is probably a common pathway independent of endotoxin that mediates these abnormalities.

To further understand the roles of various organisms in the development of septic shock, these investigators used the same model to study the differences between *E. coli*– and *Pseudomonas aeruginosa*–induced sepsis.[59] Both organisms produced concordant hemodynamic patterns of septic shock; however, endotoxin concentrations were 10-fold lower in the animals that received *P. aeruginosa*. Despite the lower endotoxin concentrations, *P. aeruginosa*–infected animals had significantly higher mortality, more severe hypotension, and a greater reduction of LVEF than the dogs that received *E. coli*. This demonstrates that bacterial organisms have different virulence factors, independent of endotoxin, that contribute to the development of the clinical manifestations of septic shock.

In response to bacteremia, mammals including humans produce TNF, a cytokine produced by mononuclear cells that has received much attention and is postulated to be a central mediator of the septic syndrome.[60] To determine whether TNF mediates the cardiovascular dysfunction of sepsis, Natanson and coworkers separately administered both this agent and endotoxin to dogs and found that they reliably reproduced the findings described earlier.[61] A similar infusion of IL-1, another cytokine produced by white

blood cells, caused only transient hypotension but failed to produce the cardiovascular dilation and reduced ejection fraction seen with live organisms, endotoxin, or TNF.[62]

The canine peritonitis model has also proved useful for evaluating therapies in septic shock. In the first of two studies, it was hypothesized that plasmapheresis might effectively remove the mediators discussed earlier, as well as others responsible for the clinical manifestations of septic shock. The same investigators studied this in their canine bacteremia model.[63] Three groups of dogs were studied: a group that received plasmapheresis at 5 and 24 hours with reinfusion of fresh frozen plasma, a group that received plasmapheresis in a similar fashion but with reinfusion of their own infected plasma, and a control group that received only the antibiotics given to each of the other two groups. The results were surprising; removal of plasma with plasma exchange in this model increased mortality compared to that in the two control groups. Even cardiovascular variables such as the LVEF failed to improve with plasmapheresis. This suggests that removal of mediators by this method fails to improve outcome and may even increase mortality.

In the second study, the effects of two conventional therapies, antibiotics and cardiovascular support, were investigated.[64] Animals were randomized to receive antibiotics and no cardiovascular support, cardiovascular support with no antibiotics, or a combination of both therapies. Antibiotic therapy consisted of a 5-day course of both gentamicin and cefoxitin, and the cardiovascular support consisted of 3 days of fluids and dopamine to maintain a normal MAP. The cardiovascular therapy was guided by the use of chronic indwelling catheters. Mortality correlated closely with the type of therapy delivered. Dogs that received both therapies had a 43% survival rate, whereas the dogs that were treated with either therapy alone had a 13% survival rate regardless of which therapy was received. Control dogs that received neither form of therapy had 0% survival. Thus, antibiotics and cardiovascular support appear to be synergistic, with each therapy contributing to the effectiveness of the combined regimen.[63] These studies suggest that cardiovascular support can allow the patient to survive long enough for antibiotics to eradicate the responsible organisms.

This chronic bacteremic canine model closely simulates the hemodynamic and cardiovascular changes seen in human sepsis. Studies with this model have provided an improved understanding of the cardiovascular host responses, the impact of therapy, and the role of bacterial virulence factors in modulating the outcome of sepsis. Because of marked species differences in response to mediator effects, some studies are best performed in humans to determine responses in humans.

CHARACTERIZATION OF RESPONSES TO INTRAVENOUS ADMINISTRATION OF ENDOTOXIN TO HUMAN VOLUNTEERS

The ability of endotoxin, a lipopolysaccharide associated with the outer membrane of gram-negative organisms, to induce the release of multiple mediators thought to play a role in the development of septic shock has been known for years. The precise role of endotoxin in the development of the cardiovascular manifestations of human sepsis was more fully elucidated by Suffredini and colleagues, who administered small intravenous boluses of purified endotoxin to normal human volunteers.[65] Each individual was monitored with radial and pulmonary arterial catheters and serial radionuclide ventriculograms. The patients were monitored for 3 hours, after which they each received an infusion of volume to simulate the clinical management of sepsis. In doing this the investigators were also able to assess ventricular performance in response to an increase in preload. Control patients received saline in place of endotoxin but underwent similar evaluation and volume resuscitation.

Core temperatures of the experimental subjects rose quickly and peaked at 3 to 4 hours.[65] Also at 3 hours, the CI and heart rate had increased by 53 and 36%, respectively, and the SVRI had decreased by 46%. The LVEF fell below baseline at the completion of the volume infusion, whereas control patients demonstrated a rise in the LVEF (Fig. 25–6) Both left ventricular end-diastolic and end-systolic volume indices increased, with a reduction of the pressure-to-volume ratio, suggesting that ventricular compliance had increased.

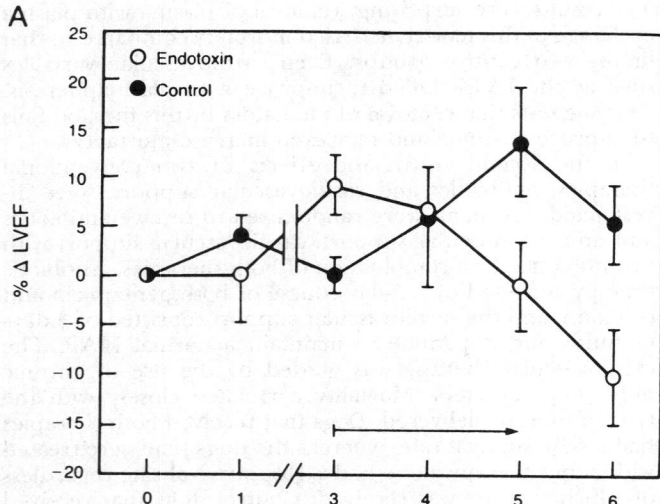

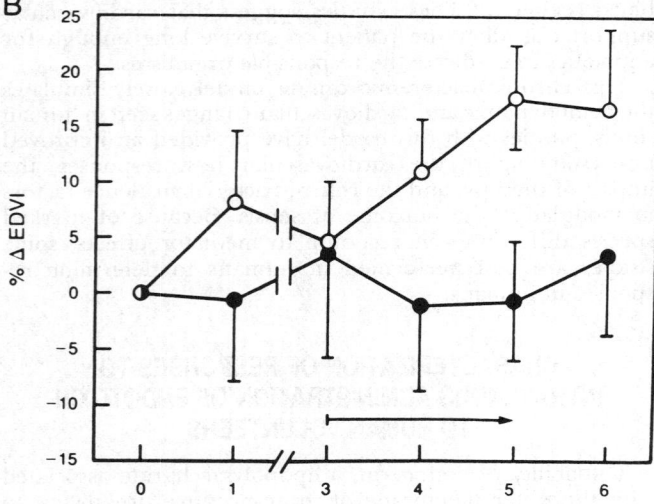

Hours from Base Line

Figure 25–6. Percent change (± SEM) from baseline for LVEF (*A*) and left ventricular end-diastolic volume index (EDVI) (*B*) in response to endotoxin or placebo infusion. At 3 and 5 hours the values for LVEF were significantly different between the two groups. Although the EDVI of the endotoxin group rose above that of the controls between 4 and 6 hours, this difference did not reach significance. (From Suffredini AF, Fromm RE, Parker MM, et al: The cardiovascular response of normal humans to the administration of endotoxin. Reprinted, by permission of the New England Journal of Medicine, 321; 280–287, 1989.)

In addition to the fall in LVEF, systolic function was found to be abnormal, as evidenced by the fall in SVI and rise in LVSWI when normalized to the end-diastolic volume index. This confirms that preload and afterload changes were not responsible for the altered ventricular performance. Lastly, a load-independent variable, the ratio of peak systolic pressure to end-systolic volume index, fell in the endotoxin group but increased by a small amount in normal controls.

These changes demonstrate that in normal humans a small intravenous bolus of endotoxin produces a rise in compliance and a fall in contractility of the left ventricle. Follow-up echocardiographic studies at 24 and 48 hours after endotoxin administration demonstrated no residual abnormalities.[65] With the exception of the rapid resolution of the changes, these findings qualitatively matched the changes observed in clinical septic shock, specifically a dilated and depressed left ventricle associated with a hyperdynamic circulatory state.

MECHANISMS OF THE CARDIOVASCULAR DYSFUNCTION IN SEPSIS

Over the years two predominant hypotheses have emerged to explain mechanistically the cardiovascular depression that occurs in septic patients. The first, which was until recently thought to be the more accurate, was that myocardial ischemia resulting from either a reduction or a maldistribution of coronary blood flow led to the reduced contractile function. This theory was supported by a number of animal studies that demonstrated global myocardial hypoperfusion resulting in depressed myocardial performance.[66–70]

Two human studies have evaluated the adequacy of myocardial perfusion during sepsis by using coronary sinus catheters. Cunnion and coworkers used coronary sinus thermodilution catheters to assess serially coronary blood flow and myocardial metabolism in patients with septic shock.[71] As can be seen in Figure 25–7, the coronary sinus blood flow of patients with septic shock (n = 7) was either equal to or higher than that of normal controls. Metabolic studies demonstrated that no patient had net myocardial lactate production and that, in comparison with the controls, the septic patients had a narrowed difference between arterial and coronary sinus oxygen content and a diminished oxygen extraction in the coronary circulation.[71] The latter two findings are similar to those related to the systemic circulation, where disrupted autoregulation results in a pattern suggesting arteriovenous shunting. Overall, the findings of normal or elevated coronary blood flow, lack of lactate production, and increased oxygen availability to the myocardium suggest that global myocardial ischemia is not the primary mechanism of the ventricular dysfunction.

A subsequent study by Dhainaut and coworkers confirmed these findings in a larger series of septic shock patients.[72] They also demonstrated a shift in myocardial substrate utilization away from free fatty acids, glucose, and ketones toward the consumption of lactate. When they attempted to correlate exogenous substrate utilization with myocardial oxygen consumption, a discrepancy was found, suggesting that during sepsis the myocardium consumes endogenous substrates. Thus a reduction of endogenous energy substrates, with concomitant failure of cellular consumption of exogenous substrates, could contribute to the performance abnormalities observed. This hypothesis remains to be more thoroughly investigated. In the meantime it is clear that global ischemia as a result of reduced coronary blood flow is not a major pathogenic mechanism of myocardial dysfunction in human sepsis.

The second hypothesis used to explain the myocardial depression of septic shock is the presence of one or more

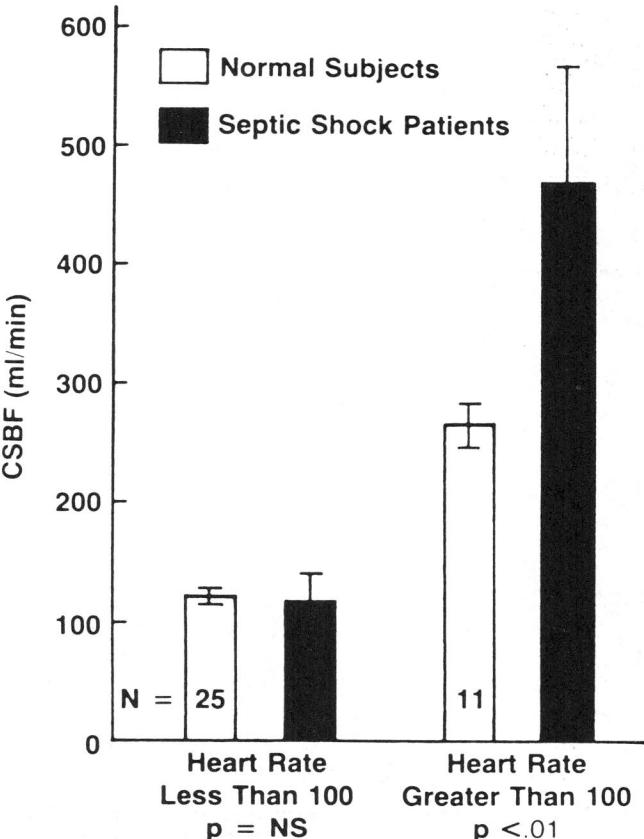

Figure 25–7. Effect of sepsis on coronary sinus blood flow (CSBF) in patients with septic shock (n = 7) and normal controls. Flow measurements were stratified into heart rates above and below 100 beats/min. (From Cunnion RE, Schaer GL, Parker MM, et al: The coronary circulation in human septic shock. Circulation 73:637, 1986. Reproduced with permission. Circulation. Copyright 1986 American Heart Association.)

circulating substances capable of reducing myocardial contractility. In 1966 Brand and Lefer reported the presence of a myocardial depressant factor in the blood of cats that had been subjected to hemorrhagic shock and later in animals with endotoxic shock.[73, 74] Concluding in 1970 that the myocardial depressant factor was produced primarily by the ischemic pancreas, Lefer and Martin helped initiate the modern search for the origins, mechanisms, and structures of what are now commonly called myocardial depressant substances (MDSs).[75]

Several experimental models have been used to help identify the presence of MDSs in various disease states. Lovett and colleagues used the isolated papillary muscle from cats to demonstrate MDS activity in 11 of 14 surgical patients with circulatory shock; however, assays for several patients without shock also displayed activity.[76] In an isolated perfused whole heart preparation Maksad and coworkers found MDS activity, evidenced by a reduction of myocardial work index, in the plasma of septic shock patients.[77] Patients with sepsis without shock and critically ill patients receiving dopamine infusions did not have MDS activity in that study.

In 1985 Parrillo and colleagues reported a highly reproducible assay for MDS using an in vitro spontaneously beating isolated rat myocyte preparation.[78] In this assay, newborn rat myocytes are grown in cell culture until they beat spontaneously at rates of 30 to 100 beats/min. By using videodensitometry focused either on the edge of an individual myocyte or on a Sepharose bead embedded in the myocyte membrane (Fig. 25–8), a quantitative recording of the extent and velocity of shortening of an individual cell can be obtained. This is then printed on a strip chart recorder. By placing serum from septic shock and control patients onto the myocytes, the amount of MDS activity can be quantitated. Figure 25–9 shows representative tracings for several patients in the acute phase of septic shock. As depicted, these cells demonstrate a significant reduction in the extent and velocity of contraction when the septic serum is placed on them and a return to normal after the substitution of control serum.

This assay was used to compare serum from patients in the acute phase of septic shock with serum from the same patients drawn before they developed sepsis or after recovery.[78] Three control groups comprising normal volunteers, critically ill nonseptic patients, and patients with impaired left ventricular function resulting from structural heart disease were also studied. As shown in Figure 25–10, the control groups all had no change in the extent of myocyte shortening. Patients in the acute phase of septic shock (but not the presepsis or recovery phase) had a reduction in the extent of myocyte shortening. Importantly, the percent change in the extent of myocyte shortening in this in vitro assay correlated significantly with the LVEF determined in vivo by radionuclide ventriculography during the acute phase of septic shock. These findings strongly support the hypothesis that a circulating factor is responsible for the abnormalities in myocardial performance seen in patients with sepsis.

In a subsequent study, serum samples from 34 patients with septic shock were evaluated for the presence or absence of MDS activity and the results were compared with clinical characteristics.[79] The patients with high levels of MDS activity (n = 14) had a higher mean PCWP, a larger LVEDVI, and a higher peak serum lactate level than patients with lower or undetectable MDS activity. Although the population size was

Figure 25–8. Artist's rendition of the technique used to track an individual rat myocardial cell in vitro. This system is capable of determining small changes in both the extent and velocity of shortening of the cell. (From Parrillo JE, Burch C, Shelhamer JH, et al: A circulating myocardial depressant substance in humans with septic shock: Septic shock patients with a reduced ejection fraction have a circulating factor that depresses in vitro myocardial cell performance. Reproduced from the Journal of Clinical Investigation, 1985, volume 76, pp 1539–1553 by copyright permission of the American Society of Clinical Investigation.)

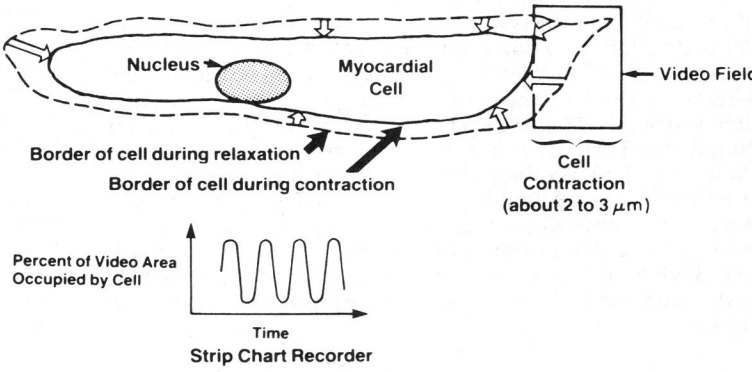

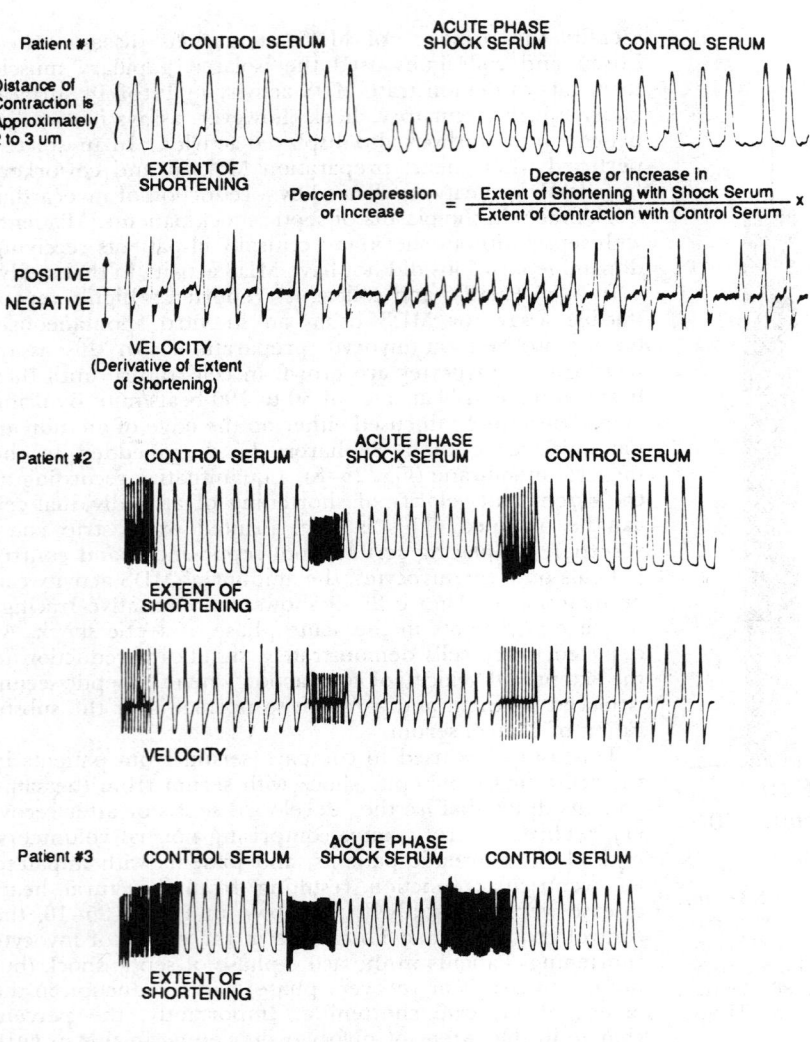

Figure 25–9. Representative tracings obtained from three patients with septic shock. The extent and velocity of shortening when the serum from these patients is applied to the contracting myocyte result in a 30 to 70% reduction from the values obtained with control serum. (From Parrillo JE, Burch C, Shelhamer JH, et al: A circulating myocardial depressant substance in humans with septic shock: Septic shock patients with a reduced ejection fraction have a circulating factor that depresses in vitro myocardial cell performance. Reproduced from the Journal of Clinical Investigation, 1985, volume 76, pp 1539–1553 by copyright permission of the American Society of Clinical Investigation.)

insufficient for the results to reach significance, there was a trend toward higher mortality in the patients with high MDS activity than in those with low levels or no MDS activity (36% versus 10%, respectively). These findings suggest that MDS has important depressant effects on the myocardium during sepsis and these abnormalities may be associated with a higher mortality. The high lactate level suggests that MDS may also have a peripheral vascular effect.

Relatively little is known about the structure and identity of this MDS. Its effects in this assay system are concentration dependent, and it is thought to be a moderate-sized molecule of at least 10,000 daltons.[78, 79] In an effort to determine whether several of the more recently described mediators demonstrate MDS activity, Hollenberg and associates studied endotoxin, TNF, IL-1, and IL-2 in their in vitro assay.[24] Of these, only TNF produced a significant reduction in myocyte contractility. Subsequently, it was shown that TNF can produce a concentration- and time-dependent depression of myocardial cell shortening in vitro.[80] These results suggest that TNF is one of several circulating depressant molecules that contribute to the myocardial depression evident during sepsis.

MECHANISMS OF PERIPHERAL VASOREGULATORY CONTROL ABNORMALITIES

Systemic vasodilation best characterizes the peripheral vascular response to sepsis; despite this, evidence of tissue hypoxia and lactate production is common in patients with severe sepsis. The most likely cause is a maldistribution of blood flow, with some arteriolar-capillary-venular beds vasoconstricted, some vasodilated, and some occluded by microthrombi. This leads to foci of organ ischemia resulting in organ dysfunction, lactate production, and evidence of arteriovenous shunting. Three closely integrated systems are involved in these complex events, including activation of the coagulation cascade, abnormalities of white blood cell function, and the effects of mediators on the vascular endothelium and the underlying vascular smooth muscle. Most of these are thought to be initiated and modulated by the release of mediators from a variety of cell types, such as polymorphonuclear neutrophils, mononuclear cells including macrophages and mast cells, and injured endothelial cells. Several of the mediators postulated to play a role in

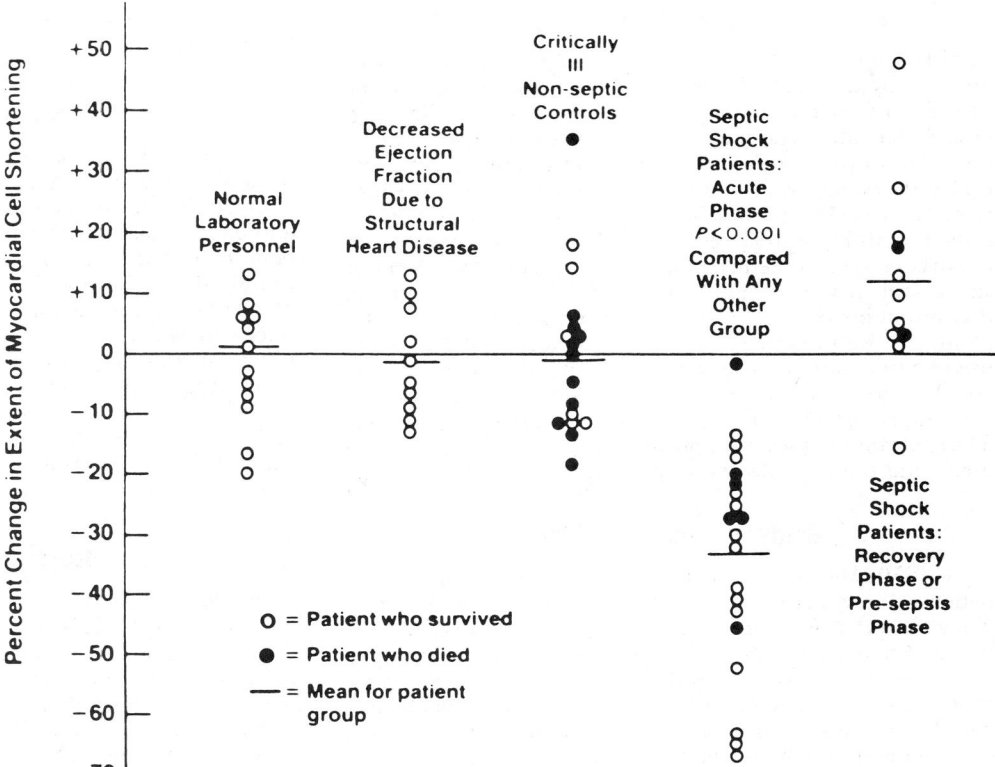

Figure 25–10. Effect of serum from several groups of patients on the extent of myocardial cell shortening in vitro. (From Parrillo JE, Burch C, Shelhamer JH, et al: A circulating myocardial depressant substance in humans with septic shock: Septic shock patients with a reduced ejection fraction have a circulating factor that depresses in vitro myocardial cell performance. Reproduced from the Journal of Clinical Investigation, 1985, volume 76, pp 1539–1553 by copyright permission of the American Society of Clinical Investigation.)

the cardiovascular dysfunction in sepsis are individually described in the following.

Endotoxin and Other Bacterial Products

Of the exogenous mediators, defined as products directly derived from the invading microorganism, endotoxin is by far the most extensively studied and characterized. Endotoxin is a lipopolysaccharide that constitutes a portion of the outer cell membrane of gram-negative bacteria. It is composed of three separate sections capable of stimulating differing host responses. The lipid A moiety is thought to be the most toxic and is able to activate the classic pathway of complement, as well as stimulating TNF release.[81] The variable O-specific polysaccharide side chain is what is used to identify the serotype of various organisms and is also able to activate complement via the alternative pathway.[82] The final portion of the endotoxin molecule is the R core region, which is less active and varies little between organisms.

Data related to the role of endotoxin in mediating the consequences of sepsis have been obtained over a number of years. As described earlier, in animal models endotoxin given either as an infusion or as a bolus can cause cardiovascular dysfunction that closely simulates that seen clinically in humans. Endotoxin also has a direct inhibitory effect on vascular smooth muscle contraction in vitro, an effect that is in large part endothelium dependent.[83] Endotoxin administration can initiate the release of many secondary mediators, including TNF, IL-1, IL-2, IL-6, and platelet-activating factor, many of which are themselves thought to be important mediators in sepsis. Lastly, endotoxin enhances endothelial cell adhesiveness for leukocytes[84] and can cause the development of disseminated intravascular coagulation.

The most compelling argument for the involvement of endotoxin as a mediator in gram-negative septic shock is the decrease in mortality seen when monoclonal antibodies against either the lipid A or core portion of endotoxin are administered. An improved outcome after this form of monoclonal antibody therapy is well established in animals.[85] Subsequent human studies have confirmed these findings and are discussed elsewhere. Numerous other bacterial products from both gram-negative and gram-positive organisms may be involved in the pathogenesis of sepsis.[81]

Activated Complement Fragments

Several types of white blood cells are involved in this sequence of events, including the polymorphonuclear neutrophil and the monocyte-macrophage line. The former are thought to contribute primarily to direct cellular injury, and the latter are thought to play a central role in the process of antigen presentation and to produce soluble mediators capable of activating the entire inflammatory cascade.[86] Much attention has focused on the activated complement fragment C5a as a potential mediator because of its ability to activate and cause the aggregation of polymorphonuclear neutrophils and therefore initiate the development of multiple microemboli.[87] Studies have demonstrated that complement activation occurs with gram-negative bacteremia and that C5a plays a role in the pathogenesis of ARDS.[88–90] C5a also has the ability to activate mast cells, which can synthesize and secrete a variety of vasoactive compounds. Therefore, Ognibene and colleagues measured C5a activity, using a neutrophil aggregation assay, in septic shock patients.[91, 92] They found a significant negative correlation between elevated C5a levels and decreased SVR in septic patients, suggesting that C5a may play a role in the pathogenesis of vasodilation, most likely through activation of mast cells with subsequent production and release of vasodilatory substances.

Histamine

Histamine, a well-known compound produced in large quantity by the mast cell, is capable of causing many of the vasodilatory effects observed in sepsis. Early studies suggested that antihistamines could partially reverse some of the effects of endotoxin administration to animals.[93–95] Several authors have reported some success in the treatment of circulatory shock in animals using a combination of antagonists to both H₁ and H₂ receptors.[93, 96–98] This led Jacobs and coworkers to examine histamine levels in patients with septic shock and in appropriate controls.[99] They not only found that histamine concentrations were normal in sepsis but also identified the presence of several inhibitors of the enzymes used in the histamine assay. Even with correction of the assay by removal of the inhibitor, the serum histamine concentrations of septic shock patients remained normal. Thus histamine does not appear to play a significant role in mediating the vasodilatory state of sepsis.

Bradykinin and Other Kinins

In 1970 Mason and associates evaluated septic shock patients for evidence of activation of the kinin system.[100] They found activation of this system, evidenced by low prekallikrein and kallikrein levels, in patients with septic shock but not in controls with hemorrhagic or cardiogenic shock. They suggested that bradykinin, a potent vasodilator, had been released in the septic patients and may have contributed to the vasodilation. Endotoxin administration to normal humans has been shown to activate the kallikrein-kinin system.[101] Further studies are needed to define the precise role of this system in sepsis pathogenesis.

Prostaglandins and Leukotrienes

Much of the information about the role of arachidonic acid metabolites, including those of the cyclooxygenase (prostaglandins and thromboxane) and lipoxygenase (leukotrienes and hydroxyeicosatetraenoic acid compounds) pathways, has come from animal models. It is known that levels of the enzyme phospholipase A₂, which helps synthesize arachidonic acid in platelets, neutrophils, and endothelium, are elevated in patients with sepsis.[102] It has also been shown by several studies that both cyclooxygenase and lipoxygenase metabolites are elevated in the lymph of animals given endotoxin infusions.[103]

The bulk of the information on the role of these products in the pathogenesis of sepsis has come from studies in which one or the other pathway has been inhibited pharmacologically. Ibuprofen, an agent that reversibly inhibits the cyclooxygenase pathway but also has effects on leukocytes and some cytokines, has been most extensively investigated. In the animal studies that specifically addressed survival or prolongation of life, all but one demonstrated a beneficial effect of ibuprofen.[104] This has led to its use experimentally in one pilot study of humans with the septic syndrome.[105] Patients in that study received three 800-mg doses of ibuprofen or placebo administered as an enema. Those who received ibuprofen demonstrated a reversal of shock more frequently than did controls. Improvements in heart rate, temperature, blood pressure, minute ventilation, and airway pressures were also noted in response to the ibuprofen therapy. Despite significant concerns, renal toxicity did not occur within the 5-day study period. These encouraging results have led to the organization of a larger multicenter trial of ibuprofen for the treatment of sepsis.

These studies suggest that products of arachidonic acid metabolism, long known to have effects on vasoregulation, are involved in the vascular and microvascular manifestations of septic shock.

Platelet-Activating Factor

Platelet-activating factor is a phospholipid that is produced by and interacts with a number of cell types, including neutrophils, eosinophils, monocyte-macrophages, platelets, and endothelial cells.[106] It is produced in response to bacteremia or endotoxemia in animal models and has also been found to be elevated in human sepsis.[107, 108] Infusions of platelet-activating factor into dogs cause hypotension, reduced coronary flow, impaired cardiac contractility, reduced renal function, hemoconcentration, and metabolic acidosis, mimicking many of the changes seen in sepsis.[106] Platelet-activating factor antagonists have been shown to reduce mortality in bacteremic or endotoxemic shock in a number of animal models. Human trials of platelet-activating factor inhibitors in sepsis can be expected in the next few years.

Tumor Necrosis Factor

In 1985 Beutler and colleagues demonstrated that passive immunization to TNF was able to protect mice from lethal doses of endotoxin.[109] Since then there has been a wealth of published data demonstrating a significant role of TNF in the cascade of cytokines that mediate the cardiovascular abnormalities of sepsis. When administered as an infusion to animal models, TNF is capable of causing vasodilation and myocardial depression. In the canine model studied by Natanson and colleagues, the falls in MAP and ejection fraction caused by TNF closely approximated those seen in bacterial septic shock.[110] Furthermore, the recovery of these changes required a 7- to 10-day period, much as human sepsis.

Attempts to identify a correlation between serum levels of TNF and clinical symptoms or outcome have provided conflicting and contradictory results, depending on study design and entry timing. A striking exception to this is in acute meningococcal disease, in which TNF levels on hospital admission correlate closely with outcome.[111] Several explanations for the failure of this correlation in other septic populations exist, but the most likely of these is the rapid clearance and short half-life of TNF in the circulation. Michie and associates found that TNF activity peaked within 90 to 180 minutes after the administration of endotoxin to normal volunteers.[112] Levels then became undetectable within 4 hours after endotoxin administration. This would explain the wide variability of TNF levels in patients with sepsis, who are often studied at various times in relation to the development of their disease process.

The strongest argument for the involvement of TNF in the pathophysiology of sepsis is the protection conveyed in animal models by passive immunization to TNF.[109, 113] This has led to the development of monoclonal antibodies to TNF, currently under study in multicenter human trials.

Interleukins

Eleven interleukins have been identified, of which three, IL-1, IL-2, and IL-6, have received intensive evaluation regarding their role in sepsis.

IL-1 was initially called endogenous pyrogen because of its role in mediating the febrile response to endotoxin.[114] It is also thought to play a large role in mediating the inflammatory effects of sepsis, particularly in causing the neutrophil migration induced by endotoxin.[115] Several in vitro models have shown a significant reduction of vascular contractility when IL-6 was applied to vascular smooth muscle preparations.

Administration of IL-1 in vivo to animals produces immunologic and hemodynamic abnormalities similar to those seen in sepsis. In a rabbit model it was found that when IL-1 and TNF were administered simultaneously, hemodynamic effects were seen at doses that produced no effect when only one agent was given.[116] This implies a synergistic effect between TNF and IL-1. Furthermore, the cyclooxygenase inhibitor ibuprofen inhibited the IL-1 response, suggesting that IL-1 exerts its hemodynamic effects by activating either prostaglandins or leukotrienes.[116]

IL-2, with and without lymphocyte-activated killer cells, has been used as adjuvant immunologic therapy in the treatment of several types of malignancies.[117] To identify its cardiovascular effects, Ognibene and coworkers studied patients who received this therapy with invasive monitoring and radionuclide ventriculography.[118] IL-2 was found to produce a fall in blood pressure, SVR, and LVEF and a rise in heart rate, CO, and left ventricular end-diastolic volume, a pattern identical to that found in patients with septic shock. This suggests that IL-2 may be one of the many mediators contributing to the cardiovascular findings in sepsis.

Like TNF, IL-1, and IL-2, IL-6 is rapidly released into the circulation in both volunteers who have received an intravenous bolus of endotoxin and patients with meningococcal shock.[119, 120] It is thought to play an important role in the synthesis of acute-phase proteins, particularly those from the liver, in sepsis and other inflammatory states. Data regarding the role of IL-6 in mediating the cardiovascular effects in sepsis, however, remain incomplete.

Endothelial Cells and Their Products

Sepsis is characterized by an intense inflammatory state associated with disseminated intravascular thrombosis and deposition of microthrombi in small vessels and capillaries. Activation of endothelial cells and abnormalities of the coagulation cascade occur, with the initial release of endogenous plasminogen activator, a product of endothelial cells. After this, the synthesis and release of plasminogen activator inhibitor occur, leading to a prothrombotic state, with microthrombi obstructing capillaries and a resulting inequality of perfusion through tissue beds leading to anaerobic metabolism and lactate production.[121] A cellular deficit in oxygen extraction ability is also thought to contribute to the anerobic metabolism commonly seen in these patients. The role of the individual cell and its products in modulating local flow characteristics remains poorly defined and is the subject of intense research.

Other endothelial cell products, including antithrombin III and von Willebrand's factor, are deranged in sepsis, perhaps contributing to the prothrombotic state. Because of the fall in antithrombin III level in sepsis, studies using replacement therapy are under way in the United States and Europe. In contrast to antithrombin III, levels of which are probably reduced by consumption, von Willebrand's antigen and activity are elevated in sepsis, and particularly high levels have been reported to correlate with the development of ARDS in nonpulmonary septic syndrome.[122]

Lastly, two classes of mutually antagonistic endothelial products, endothelins 1, 2, and 3 and endothelium-derived relaxing factor, may also contribute to aberrations in flow regulation in small vessels and capillaries. The role of these compounds in sepsis has not yet been elucidated.

PRINCIPLES OF MANAGING THE CARDIOVASCULAR DYSFUNCTION OF SEPTIC SHOCK

Role of Prevention

Any discussion of the management of septic shock would be incomplete without a statement regarding the role of prevention. The increasing prevalence of sepsis is due in large part to the widespread use of invasive catheters and immunosuppressive agents. Simple measures, including meticulous care of catheters, regular catheter changes to new sites using sterile technique, and prompt discontinuation of all indwelling devices when no longer needed, can be expected to reduce the rate of nosocomial line infections. Prophylactic antibiotics can at times reduce the rate of sepsis, particularly in patients who have received bone marrow transplantation or patients with acquired immunodeficiency syndrome at risk for *Pneumocystis carinii* pneumonia.

Selective decontamination of the oropharynx and the gut is the subject of many research protocols but is not yet routinely done in most ICUs. Along the same line, maintenance of the acidic environment in the stomach (using agents such as sucralfate and avoiding the use of histamine blockers or antacids) is thought to prevent overgrowth of bacterial flora, which predisposes to the development of nosocomial pneumonias when aspirated. Lastly, a Veterans Administration cooperative trial sponsored by the National Institutes of Health is under way to evaluate the role of prophylactic active immunization against a number of gram-negative organisms in critically ill patients. If effective, this would be an exciting, albeit expensive, addition to the currently available methods for reducing the rate of nosocomial sepsis in ICUs.

The Intensive Care Unit Environment and Invasive Monitoring

The impact of the modern ICU with its invasive monitoring capabilities has been largely underemphasized in many reviews. We believe that all hemodynamically unstable patients with sepsis are best cared for in this environment, where rapid identification and correction of laboratory and hemodynamic abnormalities can be performed by appropriately trained intensive care staff. One retrospective study has confirmed this point by evaluating the mortality resulting from sepsis in a community hospital before and after the addition of a dedicated ICU physician staff.[123] In the 1-year period before the addition of a full-time ICU physician staff the mortality resulting from sepsis was 92%, compared with 61% ($P < .05$) after the addition of this staff. A subsequent study, performed in a university hospital, found a similar reduction in mortality when ICUs with trained intensive care physicians were used.[124]

On the basis of these studies, we aggressively utilize invasive monitoring with indwelling arterial and pulmonary arterial catheters. Indwelling arterial catheters not only allow easy access for blood sampling, including frequent arterial blood gas measurements, but also give continuous recording of the blood pressure, including the MAP, which provides a better estimate of flow because it takes into account both the systolic and diastolic blood pressures. Although they are not yet available, in the future indwelling arterial catheters will also provide continuous recordings of the blood pH, Pco_2, Po_2, and arterial oxygen saturation, reducing the need for frequent arterial blood gas measurements.

It is well documented that clinical examination alone is

often insufficient for accurate prediction of left and right ventricular filling pressures and the CI of critically ill patients. The use of pulmonary arterial catheters clearly influences therapy in this population of patients; however, critics of these catheters correctly point out that survival benefits have not yet been demonstrated. Despite this, we believe that when these catheters are placed and used by experienced personnel in the closely monitored environment that an ICU provides, the benefits gained outweigh the risks. These benefits include not only measurements of filling pressures and cardiac performance but also accessibility for sampling the mixed venous blood to provide data on $\dot{D}o_2$ and $\dot{V}o_2$. Data from the surgical literature suggest that augmenting $\dot{D}o_2$ and $\dot{V}o_2$ may enhance survival in certain groups of patients.[54, 55]

Antibiotics in Sepsis

The ICU provides not only an environment for monitoring and hemodynamic therapy but also an opportunity for physicians to obtain quickly and scrutinize data regarding the diagnosis and response to therapy of critically ill patients. With respect to sepsis, perhaps the most important therapeutic step is the establishment of the correct diagnosis followed by a thorough search for a source of infection.

In most non-neutropenic patients, a nidus of infection can be found by a complete physical examination and routine radiographic and laboratory testing. In patients with neutropenia, the lack of an easily identified inflammatory response complicates the search for the nidus of infection, a situation that should compel the physician to take an even more thorough and often invasive approach to the diagnostic strategy.

When the source of infection is established, appropriate antibiotic therapy must be instituted immediately. In a review of gram-negative bacteremia, Kreger and colleagues demonstrated a marked increase in mortality when inappropriate antibiotic therapy was used (the organism was resistant to the antibiotics employed).[125] This suggests that the physician must not only determine the site and likely identity of the infecting organisms but also be familiar with the sensitivities and resistances of these organisms at his or her own hospital. In the case of neutropenic patients or patients whose source of sepsis remains unknown, broad-spectrum agents covering both gram-positive and gram-negative organisms must be instituted initially and later tailored when the results of cultures and diagnostic tests become available.

Hemodynamic Goals for the Septic Shock Patient

The primary goal in the management of the septic patient is restoration and maintenance of adequate tissue and organ perfusion. Blood flow to most organs is difficult to assess clinically, and instead we rely on direct measurements of CO, $\dot{D}o_2$, and $\dot{V}o_2$. As described earlier an MAP of 60 mm Hg usually provides adequate coronary and cerebral blood flow and is therefore an initial goal of therapy. Once placement of a pulmonary arterial catheter has been accomplished, CO, CI, stroke work index, and SVR can be determined using the thermodilution technique. By using simultaneous arterial and mixed venous blood gas measurements and knowing the blood hemoglobin value, one can calculate $\dot{D}o_2$ and $\dot{V}o_2$ (Appendix 25–1). These determinations should be followed closely to assess the clinical course of the patient, as well as the response to therapy.

Table 25–2 shows the therapeutic goals we and others use to guide our volume, inotropic, and pressor therapy in patients with septic shock.

TABLE 25–2
THERAPEUTIC GOALS IN THE TREATMENT OF SEPTIC SHOCK
MAP greater than 60 mm Hg
Normalization of blood lactate level
PCWP greater than 12 mm Hg (or up to 18 mm Hg when there is evidence of reduced organ perfusion)
Optimize oxygen delivery ($\dot{D}o_2$)*
Hemoglobin value greater than 10 g/dL
O_2 saturation greater than 92%
CI greater than 4.0 L/min/m²
Reversal and/or normalization of organ dysfunction
Renal: blood urea nitrogen, creatinine, urine output
Hepatic: bilirubin
Pulmonary: alveolar-arterial gradient
Cardiovascular: MAP, CI
Central nervous system: mental status

*Data for critically ill postoperative patients suggest that optimal survival occurs with a CI > 4.5 L/min/m², $\dot{D}o_2$ > 600 mL/min/m², and $\dot{V}o_2$ > 170 mL/min/m² (see ref 54).

Volume Support of the Septic Patient

The most characteristic hemodynamic findings in patients with septic shock who have been adequately volume resuscitated are a low SVR and an elevated CO. In the absence of volume resuscitation, a reduced CO is not uncommon. During the initial stabilization period of a patient with septic shock, the primary goals are re-establishment of an MAP greater than 60 mm Hg and maintenance of adequate organ and tissue perfusion. These are best accomplished initially by the administration of intravenous volume. Most clinicians appropriately choose crystalloids as the volume expander; however, when severe anemia (hematocrit < 28%) or hypoalbuminemia (serum albumin value < 2.0 g/dL) coexists, one should choose as the volume expander packed red blood cells or albumin infusions, respectively.

Once a pulmonary arterial catheter has been placed to guide therapy, we continue to use volume expansion of the persistently hypotensive patient until the PCWP exceeds 12 mm Hg. At this point one should begin to construct a bedside Starling curve to determine the effects of subsequent volume therapy. A patient whose cardiac performance continues to improve (indicated by a rise in CI, stroke work index, $\dot{D}o_2$, and $\dot{V}o_2$) in response to volume therapy should continue to receive volume until either a PCWP of 18 mm Hg is reached or no further improvement in cardiac performance is identified. Patients should not receive volume expansion past a PCWP of 18 mm Hg because of the risk of pulmonary edema resulting from both hydrostatic forces and the leaky capillaries and noncardiogenic edema that often accompany severe sepsis.

Most patients continue to respond to the administration of volume with a rise in CI and stroke work index; however, occasional patients do not show this response because of profound abnormalities of ventricular compliance and/or contractility. These patients may benefit from additional tests to better define their reduced myocardial performance. Both echocardiography and radionuclide cineangiography can be used. Where available, the latter used with simultaneous thermodilution CO determination provides quantitative information about cardiac performance that can be followed and compared with subsequent scans done after either clinical improvement or the institution of inotropic therapy.

Vasopressors in the Management of the Septic Patient

Many patients with severe septic shock remain hypotensive despite volume resuscitation. These patients usually have either a severely reduced SVR or extremely reduced systolic cardiac performance. The distinction between these two types of patients is important; the former have severe distributive shock, and the latter have cardiogenic shock superimposed on their distributive shock.

The vasopressor initially used in hypotensive septic patients is dopamine at a dose of 2 to 5 μg/kg/min, a range that provides both a modest inotropic effect and a direct vasodilating effect on the renal and mesenteric arteries. If this is ineffective in increasing the MAP to 60 mm Hg, the dose is titrated upward to as much as 20 μg/kg/min, which provides both alpha- and beta-adrenergic stimulation. Although most patients respond to this agent alone, those with severe sepsis may require the addition of intravenous norepinephrine for more potent vasoconstriction. If this is required, we recommend reducing the dopamine to the renal vasodilating dose range of 2 to 5 μg/mg/kg, which has been shown in an animal model to maintain renal perfusion despite high levels of norepinephrine.[126]

Occasional patients may not respond to either of these agents. As can be expected, this corresponds to an exceedingly poor prognosis. In that situation, one can occasionally achieve an adequate pressor response by using either phenylephrine, a pure alpha-adrenergic agonist, or epinephrine, a combined alpha- and beta-agonist.

Use of Inotropic Therapy in Sepsis

Maintenance of an adequate blood pressure is important in the management of sepsis, but it is equally important to ensure adequate organ perfusion. Patients who have inadequate organ flow require augmentation of Do_2 by using blood, volume expansion, improved oxygenation, inotropic therapy, or a combination of these. If a patient demonstrates reduced organ perfusion despite these maneuvers, we begin inotropic therapy.

In hypotensive patients, the agents (with the exception of phenylephrine) described in the preceding section can be used because they all have inotropic effects. Additional useful agents include both dobutamine and amrinone, which are potent inotropic agents but have little pressor effect. Dobutamine is the preferred inotrope in our ICU because of its potent and long-lasting inotropic effect with minimal side effects. Amrinone has similar potent inotropic effects, but it is also a vasodilator and can precipitate hypotension in patients who may already have a reduced SVR. The use of either of these agents requires careful observation of the blood pressure, especially at the initiation of the infusion, as well as frequent determinations of CO by thermodilution.

CONCLUSIONS

Developments of the past two decades, including the use of pulmonary arterial catheters, echocardiography, and radionuclide cineangiography, have provided an enhanced understanding of the cardiovascular responses to sepsis. We now know that the characteristic hemodynamic findings of an elevated CO and a reduced systemic venous resistance are accompanied by biventricular dilatation and abnormalities of both myocardial compliance and contractility. These changes have been shown to result from one or several circulating myocardial depressant factors.

The next decade should see better definition of not only the clinical manifestations of sepsis but also the mediators and mechanisms responsible for these changes. The development and clinical use of inhibitors of mediators, including monoclonal antibodies to endotoxin and TNF, will provide opportunities to inhibit selectively several of the pathogenic pathways involved in sepsis. These advances, combined with attempts to reduce the prevalence of sepsis, should result in a significantly improved outcome in this highly fatal disease.

References

1. Parker MM, Parrillo JE: Septic shock: Hemodynamics and pathogenesis. JAMA 250:3324, 1983.
2. National Center for Health Statistics: Increase in national hospital discharge survey rates for septicemia—United States, 1979–1987. JAMA 263:937, 1990.
3. Parrillo JE, Parker MM, Natanson C, et al: Septic shock in humans: Advances in the understanding of pathogenesis, cardiovascular dysfunction, and therapy. Ann Intern Med 113:227, 1990.
4. Balk RA, Bone RC: The septic syndrome: Definition and clinical implications. Crit Care Clin 5:1, 1989.
5. Cunnion RE, Parrillo JE: Myocardial dysfunction in sepsis. Crit Care Clin 5:99, 1989.
6. Wilson RF, Thal AP, Kindling PH, et al: Hemodynamic measurements in septic shock. Arch Surg 91:121, 1965.
7. Udhoji VN, Weil MH: Hemodynamic and metabolic studies on shock associated with bacteremia. Observations on 16 patients. Ann Intern Med 62:966, 1965.
8. Parker MM, Shelhamer JH, Bacharach SL, et al: Profound but reversible myocardial depression in patients with septic shock. Ann Intern Med 100:483, 1984.
9. Clowes GHA, Vucinic M, Weidner MG: Circulatory and metabolic alterations associated with survival or death in peritonitis. Ann Surg 163:866, 1966.
10. Kwaan HM, Weil MH: Differences in the mechanism of shock caused by bacterial infections. Surg Gynecol Obstet 128:37, 1969.
11. Nishijima H, Weil MH, Shubin H, et al: Hemodynamic and metabolic studies on shock associated with gram negative bacteria. Medicine 52:287, 1973.
12. Winslow EJ, Loeb HS, Rahimtoola SH, et al: Hemodynamic studies and results of therapy in 50 patients with bacteremic shock. Am J Med 54:421, 1973.
13. Parker MM, Shelhamer JH, Natanson C, et al: Serial cardiovascular variables in survivors and nonsurvivors of human septic shock: Heart rate as an early predictor of prognosis. Crit Care Med 15:923, 1987.
14. Wiles JB, Cerra FB, Siegel JR, et al: The systemic septic response: Does the organism matter? Crit Care Med 8:55, 1980.
15. Weisul RD, Vito L, Dennis RC, et al: Myocardial depression during sepsis. Am J Surg 133:512, 1977.
16. Calvin JE, Driedger AA, Sibbald WJ: Does the pulmonary capillary wedge pressure predict left ventricular preload in critically ill patients? Crit Care Med 9:437, 1981.
17. Packman MI, Rackow EC: Optimum left heart filling pressure during fluid resuscitation of patients with hypovolemic and septic shock. Crit Care Med 11:165, 1983.
18. Ognibene FP, Parker MM, Natanson C, et al: Depressed left ventricular performance: Response to volume infusion in patients with sepsis and septic shock. Chest 93:903, 1988.
19. Rackow EC, Kaufman BS, Falk JL, et al: Hemodynamic response to fluid repletion in patients with septic shock: Evidence for early depression of cardiac performance. Circ Shock 22:11, 1987.
20. Calvin JE, Driedger AA, Sibbald WJ: An assessment of myocardial function in human sepsis utilizing ECG gated cardiac scintigraphy. Chest 80:579, 1981.
21. Ellrodt AG, Riedinger MS, Kimchi A, et al: Left ventricular performance in septic shock: Reversible segmental and global abnormalities. Am Heart J 110:402, 1985.
22. Cunnion RE, Parrillo JE: Myocardial dysfunction in sepsis. Crit Care Clin 5:99, 1989.
23. Hersch M, Troster M, Gnidec A, et al: Histopathologic evidence of tissue ischemia in a hyperdynamic and non-hypotensive septic animal model (abstract). Crit Care Med 16:421, 1988.
24. Hollenberg SM, Cunnion RE, Lawrence M, et al: Tumor necrosis factor depresses myocardial cell function: Results using an in vitro assay of myocyte performance (abstract). Clin Res 37:528A, 1989.
25. Baker CH, Wilmoth FR: Microvascular responses to E. coli endotoxin with altered adrenergic activity. Circ Shock 12:165, 1984.
26. Cadden S, Philp RB, Sibbald WJ: Cardiac beta receptor dysfunction in an animal model of the sepsis syndrome (abstract). Crit Care Med 15:439, 1987.
27. Berger HJ, Matthay RA, Loke J, et al: Assessment of cardiac performance with quantitative radionuclide angiocardiography: Right ventricular ejection fraction with reference to findings in chronic obstructive pulmonary disease. Am J Cardiol 41:897, 1978.
28. Maddahi J, Berman DS, Matsuoka DT, et al: A new technique for assessing right ventricular ejection fraction using rapid multiple-gated equilibrium cardiac blood pool scintigraphy: Description, validation, and findings in coronary artery disease. Circulation 60:581, 1979.
29. Kimchi A, Ellrodt AG, Berman DS, et al: Right ventricular performance in septic shock: A combined radionuclide and hemodynamic study. J Am Coll Cardiol 4:945, 1984.

30. Hoffman MJ, Greenfield LJ, Sugerman HJ, et al: Unsuspected right ventricular dysfunction in shock and sepsis. Ann Surg 198:307, 1988.
31. Schneider AJ, Teule GJJ, Groeneveld ABJ, et al: Biventricular performance during volume loading in patients with early septic shock, with emphasis on the right ventricle: A combined hemodynamic and radionuclide study. Am Heart J 116:103, 1988.
32. Vincent JL, Reuse C, Frank N, et al: Right ventricular dysfunction in septic shock: Assessment by measurements of right ventricular ejection fraction using the thermodilution technique. Acta Anaesthesiol Scand 33:34, 1989.
33. Parker MM, McCarthy KE, Ognibene FP, et al: Right ventricular dysfunction and dilatation, similar to left ventricular changes, characterize the cardiac depression of septic shock in humans. Chest 97:126, 1990.
34. Jardin F, Farcot JC, Boisante L, et al: Influence of positive end-expiratory pressure on left ventricular performance. N Engl J Med 304:387, 1981.
35. Chin D, Melendez L, Wells G, et al: Determinants of interventricular septal position in ARDS (abstract). Am Rev Respir Dis 129:A98, 1984.
36. Sibbald WJ, Driedger AA, McCallum D, et al: Nitroprusside infusion does not improve biventricular performance in patients with acute hypoxemic respiratory failure. J Crit Care 1:197, 1986.
37. Sibbald WJ, Bersten A, Rutledge F: Inotropes or vasodilators treatment of an O2 debt in hyperdynamic sepsis (abstract). Crit Care Med 16:395, 1988.
38. Gutierrez G, Pohil RJ: Oxygen consumption is linearly related to O2 supply in critically ill patients. J Crit Care 1:45, 1986.
39. Kaufman BS, Rackow EC, Falk JL: The relationship between oxygen delivery and consumption during fluid resuscitation of hypovolemic and septic shock. Chest 85:336, 1984.
40. Haupt MT, Gilbert EM, Carlson RW: Fluid loading increases oxygen consumption in septic patients with lactic acidosis. Am Rev Respir Dis 131:912, 1985.
41. Wolf YG, Cotev S, Perel A, et al: Dependence of oxygen consumption on cardiac output in sepsis. Crit Care Med 15:198, 1987.
42. Nelson DP, Samsel RW, Wood LDH, et al: Pathologic supply dependence of systemic and intestinal O2 uptake during endotoxemia. J Appl Physiol 64:2410, 1988.
43. Gilbert EM, Haupt MT, Mandanas RY, et al: The effect of fluid loading, blood transfusion, and catecholamine infusion on oxygen delivery and consumption in patients with sepsis. Am Rev Respir Dis 134:873, 1986.
44. Vincent JL, Roman A, De Backer D, et al: Oxygen uptake/supply dependency. Effects of short-term dobutamine infusion. Am Rev Respir Dis 142:2, 1990.
45. Astiz ME, Rackow EC, Falk JL, et al: Oxygen delivery and consumption in patients with hyperdynamic septic shock. Crit Care Med 15:26, 1987.
46. Danek SJ, Lynch JP, Weg JG, et al: The dependence of oxygen uptake on oxygen delivery in the adult respiratory distress syndrome. Am Rev Respir Dis 122:387, 1980.
47. Mohsenifar Z, Goldbach P, Tashkin DP, et al: Relationship between O2 delivery and O2 consumption in the adult respiratory distress syndrome. Chest 84:267, 1983.
48. Kariman K, Burns SR: Regulation of tissue oxygen extraction is disturbed in the adult respiratory distress syndrome. Am Rev Respir Dis 132:109, 1985.
49. Russell JA, Ronco JJ, Lockhat D, et al: Oxygen delivery and consumption and ventricular preload are greater in survivors than in nonsurvivors of the adult respiratory distress syndrome. Am Rev Respir Dis 141:659, 1990.
50. Cain SM: Supply dependency of oxygen uptake in ARDS: Myth or reality. Am J Med Sci 288:119, 1984.
51. Groeneveld ABJ, Kester ADM, Nauta JJP, et al: Relation of arterial blood lactate to oxygen delivery and hemodynamic variables in human shock states. Circ Shock 22:35, 1987.
52. Abraham E, Bland RD, Cobo JC, et al: Sequential cardiorespiratory patterns associated with outcome in septic shock. Chest 85:75, 1984.
53. Bland RD, Shoemaker WC, Abraham E, et al: Hemodynamic and oxygen transport values in surviving and nonsurviving postoperative patients. Crit Care Med 13:85, 1985.
54. Shoemaker WC, Appel PL, Waxman K, et al: Clinical trial of survivors' cardiorespiratory patterns as therapeutic goals in critically ill postoperative patients. Crit Care Med 10:398, 1982.
55. Shoemaker WC, Appel PL, Kram HB, et al: Prospective trial of supranormal values of survivors as therapeutic goals in high-risk surgical patients. Chest 94:1176, 1988.
56. Natanson C, Fink MP, Ballantyne HK, et al: Gram-negative bacteremia produces both severe systolic and diastolic cardiac dysfunction in a canine model that simulates human septic shock. J Clin Invest 78:259, 1986.
57. Natanson C, Danner RL, Fink MP, et al: Cardiovascular performance with E. coli challenges in a canine model of human sepsis. Am J Physiol 254:H558, 1988.
58. Natanson C, Danner RL, Elin RJ, et al: The role of endotoxemia in cardiovascular dysfunction and mortality. Escherichia coli and Staphylococcus aureus challenges in a canine model of human septic shock. J Clin Invest 83:243, 1989.
59. Danner RL, Natanson C, Elin RJ, et al: Pseudomonas aeruginosa compared with Escherichia coli produces less endotoxemia but more cardiovascular dysfunction and mortality in a canine model of septic shock. Chest 98:1480, 1990.
60. Tracey KJ, Fong Y, Hesse DG, et al: Anti-cachectin/TNF monoclonal antibodies prevent septic shock during lethal bacteremia. Nature 330:662, 1987.
61. Natanson C, Eichenholz PW, Danner RL, et al: Endotoxin and tumor necrosis factor challenges in dogs simulate the cardiovascular profile of human septic shock. J Exp Med 169:823, 1989.
62. Natanson C, Eichacker PQ, Hoffman WD, et al: Human recombinant interleukin-1 produced minimal effects on canine cardiovascular function (abstract). Clin Res 37:346A, 1989.
63. Natanson C, Hoffman WD, Danner RL, et al: A controlled trial of plasmapheresis fails to improve outcome in an antibiotic canine model of human septic shock (abstract). Clin Res 37:346A, 1989.
64. Natanson C, Danner RL, Reilly MM, et al: Antibiotics versus cardiovascular support in a canine model of human septic shock. Am J Physiol 259:H1440, 1990.
65. Suffredini AF, Fromm RE, Parker MM, et al: The cardiovascular response of normal humans to the administration of endotoxin. N Engl J Med 321:280, 1989.
66. Elkins RC, McCurdy JR, Brown PP, et al: Effects of coronary perfusion pressure on myocardial performance during endotoxin shock. Surg Gynecol Obstet 137:991, 1973.
67. Hinshaw LB, Archer LT, Spitzer JJ, et al: Effects of coronary hypotension and endotoxin on myocardial performance. Am J Physiol 227:1051, 1974.
68. Peyton MD, Hinshaw LB, Greenfield LJ, et al: The effects of coronary vasodilation on cardiac performance during endotoxin shock. Surg Gynecol Obstet 143:533, 1976.
69. Hess ML, Soulsby ME, Davis JA, et al: The influence of venous return on cardiac mechanical and sarcoplasmic reticulum function during endotoxemia. Circ Shock 4:143, 1977.
70. Bruni FD, Komwatana P, Soulsby ME, et al: Endotoxin and myocardial failure: Role of the myofibril and venous return. Am J Physiol 235:H150, 1978.
71. Cunnion RE, Schaer GL, Parker MM, et al: The coronary circulation in human septic shock. Circulation 73:637, 1986.
72. Dhainaut JF, Huyghebaert MF, Monsallier JF, et al: Coronary hemodynamics and myocardial metabolism of lactate, free fatty acids, glucose, and ketones in patients with septic shock. Circulation 75:533, 1987.
73. Brand ED, Lefer AM: Myocardial depressant factor in plasma from cats in irreversible post-oligemic shock. Proc Soc Exp Biol Med 122:200, 1966.
74. Wangensteen SL, Geissinger WT, Lovett WL, et al: Relationship between splanchnic blood flow and a myocardial depressant factor in endotoxin shock. Surgery 69:410, 1971.
75. Lefer AM, Martin J: Origin of the myocardial depressant factor in shock. Am J Physiol 218:1423, 1970.
76. Lovett WL, Wangensteen SL, Glenn TM, et al: Presence of a myocardial depressant factor in patients in circulatory shock. Surgery 70:223, 1971.
77. Maksad KA, Cha JC, Stuart CR, et al: Myocardial depression in septic shock: Physiologic and metabolic effects of a plasma factor on an isolated heart. Circ Shock 1(suppl):35, 1979.
78. Parrillo JE, Burch C, Shelhamer JH, et al: A circulating myocardial depressant substance in humans with septic shock. J Clin Invest 76:1539, 1985.
79. Reilly JM, Cunnion RE, Burch-Whitman C, et al: A circulating myocardial depressant substance is associated with cardiac dysfunction and peripheral hypoperfusion (lactic acidemia) in patients with septic shock. Chest 95:1072, 1989.
80. Kumar A, Dimou C, Hollenberg SM, et al: Tumor necrosis factor produces a concentration-dependent depression of myocardial cell contraction in vitro (abstract). Clin Res 39:321A, 1991.
81. Danner RL, Suffredini AF, Natanson C, et al: Microbial toxins: Role in the pathogenesis of septic shock and multiple organ failure. In: Cerra FB, Bihari DE (eds): New Horizons: Multiple Organ Failure. Fullerton, CA, Society of Critical Care Medicine, p 151, 1989.
82. Danner RL: Mediators and endotoxin inhibitors. Ann Intern Med 113:227, 1990.
83. Beasley D, Cohen RA, Levinsky NG: Endotoxin inhibits contraction of vascular smooth muscle in vitro. Am J Physiol 258:H1187, 1990.
84. Cybulsky MI, Chan MKW, Movat HZ: Acute inflammation and microthrombosis induced by endotoxin, interleukin-1, and tumor necrosis factor and their implication in gram-negative infection. Lab Invest 58:365, 1988.
85. Larrick JW: Antibody inhibition of the immunoinflammatory cascade. J Crit Care 4:211, 1989.
86. Jacobs RF, Tabor DR: Immune cellular interactions during sepsis and septic injury. Crit Care Clin 5:9, 1989.
87. Frank MM: Complement in the pathophysiology of human disease. N Engl J Med 316:1525, 1987.
88. McCabe WR: Serum complement levels in bacteremia due to gram-negative organisms. N Engl J Med 288:21, 1973.
89. Fearon DT, Ruddy S, Schur PH, et al: Activation of the properdin pathways of complement in patients with gram-negative bacteremia. N Engl J Med 292:937, 1975.

90. Hammerschmidt DE, Weaver LJ, Hudson LD, et al: Association of complement activation and elevated plasma C5a with adult respiratory distress syndrome. Lancet 1:947, 1980.
91. Ognibene FP, Parker MM, Burch-Whitman C, et al: Neutrophil aggregation activity and septic shock in humans: Neutrophil aggregation by a C5a-like material occurs more frequently than complement component depletion and correlates with depression of systemic vascular resistance. J Crit Care 3:103, 1988.
92. Parker MM, Ognibene F, Natanson C, et al: Elevated C5a levels in patients with septic shock. Crit Care Med 13:303, 1985.
93. Halevy S, Altura BM: H1 and H2 histamine receptor antagonists and protection against endotoxic shock. Proc Soc Exp Biol Med 154:453, 1977.
94. Krause SM, Hess ML: Diphenhydramine protection of the failing myocardium during gram-negative endotoxemia. Circ Shock 6:75, 1979.
95. Brigham KL, Padove SJ, Bryant D, et al: Diphenhydramine reduces endotoxin effects on lung vascular permeability in sheep. J Appl Physiol 49:516, 1980.
96. Lowry P, Blanco T, Santiago-Delphin EA: Histamine and sympathetic blockade in septic shock. Am Surg 43:12, 1977.
97. Wittig HJ, Cook TJ, Tittmanic T: Protection against fatal endotoxin shock in mice by antihistamines. Allergol Immunopathol 6:409, 1978.
98. Kaliner M, Shelhamer JH, Ottesen E: Effects of infused histamine: Correlation of plasma histamine levels and symptoms. J Allergy Clin Immunol 69:283, 1982.
99. Jacobs R, Kaliner M, Shelhamer JH, et al: Blood histamine concentrations are not elevated in humans with septic shock. Crit Care Med 17:30, 1989.
100. Mason JW, Kleesberg U, Dolan P, et al: Plasma kallikrein and Hageman factor in gram-negative bacteremia. Ann Intern Med 75:545, 1970.
101. de la Cadena RA, Suffredini AF, Kaufman N, et al: Activation of the kallikrein-kinin system after endotoxin administration to normal human volunteers (abstract). Clin Res 38:346A, 1990.
102. Vadas P, Pruzanski W, Stefanski E, et al: Pathogenesis of hypotension in septic shock: Correlation of circulating phospholipase A₂ levels with circulatory collapse. Crit Care Med 16:1, 1988.
103. Bersten A, Sibbald WJ: Acute lung injury in septic shock. Crit Care Clin 5:49, 1989.
104. Metz CA, Sheagren JN: Ibuprofen in animal models of septic shock. J Crit Care 5:206, 1990.
105. Bernard GR, Reines HD, Metz CA, et al: Effects of a short course of ibuprofen in patients with severe sepsis (abstract). J Am Thorac Soc 137:1543, 1988.
106. Hosford D, Braquet P: The potential role of platelet-activating factor in shock and ischemia. J Crit Care 5:115, 1990.
107. Bussolino F, Porcellini MG, Varese L, et al: Intravascular release of platelet-activating factor in children with sepsis. Thromb Res 48:619, 1987.
108. Lopez-Diez F, Nieto ML, Fernandez-Gallardo S, et al: Occupancy of platelet receptors for platelet-activating factor in patients with septicemia. J Clin Invest 83:1733, 1989.
109. Beutler B, Milsaark IW, Cerami AC: Passive immunization against cachectin/tumor necrosis factor protects mice from lethal effects of endotoxin. Science 229:869, 1985.
110. Natanson C, Eichenholz PW, Danner RL, et al: Endotoxin and tumor necrosis factor challenges in dogs simulate the cardiovascular profile of human septic shock. J Exp Med 169:823, 1989.
111. Waage A, Halstensen A, Espevik T: Association between tumor necrosis factor in serum and fatal outcome in patients with meningococcal disease. Lancet 1:355, 1987.
112. Michie HR, Manogue KR, Spriggs DR, et al: Detection of circulating tumor necrosis factor after endotoxin administration. N Engl J Med 318:1481, 1988.
113. Tracey KJ, Fong Y, Hesse DG: Anti-cachectin/TNF monoclonal antibodies prevent septic shock during lethal bacteremia. Nature 330:662, 1987.
114. Dinarello CA: Biology of interleukin 1. FASEB J 2:108, 1988.
115. Cybulsky MI, Chan MKW, Movat HZ: Acute inflammation and microthrombosis induced by endotoxin, interleukin-1, and tumor necrosis factor and their implication in gram-negative infection. Lab Invest 58:365, 1988.
116. Okusawa S, Gelfand JA, Ikejima T, et al: Interleukin 1 induces a shock-like state in rabbits. J Clin Invest 81:1162, 1988.
117. Rosenberg SA, Lotze MT, Mulé JJ: NIH conferences. New approaches to the immunotherapy of cancer using interleukin-2. Ann Intern Med 108:853, 1988.
118. Ognibene FP, Parker MM, Natanson C, et al: Interleukin-2 infusion produces cardiovascular dysfunction with decreased ejection fraction and ventricular dilatation. Chest 94:750, 1988.
119. Fong Y, Moldawer LL, Marano MA, et al: Endotoxemia elicits increased circulating B2-IFN/IL-6 in man. J Immunol 142:2321, 1989.
120. Waage A, Brandtzaeg P, Halstensen A, et al: The complex pattern of cytokines in serum from patients with meningococcal septic shock. J Exp Med 169:333, 1989.
121. Suffredini AF, Harpel PC, Parrillo JE: Promotion and subsequent inhibition of plasminogen activation after administration of endotoxin to normal subjects. N Engl J Med 320:1165, 1989.
122. Rubin DB, Wiener-Kronish JP, Murray JF, et al: Elevated von Willebrand factor antigen is an early plasma predictor of acute lung injury in nonpulmonary septic syndrome. J Clin Invest 86:474, 1990.
123. Li TCM, Phillips M, Shaw L, et al: The impact of tertiary physicians on a community hospital intensive care unit. JAMA 252:2023, 1984.
124. Reynolds HN, Haupt MT, Thill-Baharozian MC, et al: Impact of critical care physician staffing on patients with septic shock in a university hospital medical intensive care unit. JAMA 260:3446, 1988.
125. Kreger BE, Craven DE, McCabe WR: Gram-negative bacteremia: IV. Re-evaluation of clinical features and treatment in 612 patients. Am J Med 68:344, 1980.
126. Schaer GL, Fink MP, Parrillo JE: Norepinephrine alone versus norepinephrine plus low-dose dopamine: Enhanced renal blood flow with combination pressor therapy. Crit Care Med 13:492, 1985.

Appendix 25–1

Mean arterial pressure (MAP):

$$MAP = \tfrac{1}{3}(\text{systolic BP} - \text{diastolic BP}) + \text{diastolic BP}$$

where BP = blood pressure

Systemic vascular resistance (SVR):

$$SVR = \frac{MAP - CVP}{CO} \times 79.9$$

Pulmonary vascular resistance (PVR):

$$PVR = \frac{\text{mean pulmonary arterial pressure} - PCWP}{CO} \times 79.9$$

Arterial O₂ content (CaO₂):

$$CaO_2 = (Hb \times 1.34)SaO_2 + (PaO_2 \times 0.0031)$$

where Hb = hemoglobin
SaO₂ = % saturation of arterial blood

Mixed venous O₂ content (C$\bar{v}$O₂):

$$C\bar{v}O_2 = (Hb \times 1.34)\,S\bar{v}O_2 + (P\bar{v}O_2 \times 0.0031)$$

where S$\bar{v}$O₂ = % saturation of mixed venous blood
P$\bar{v}$O₂ = partial pressure of oxygen in mixed venous blood

Oxygen delivery ($\dot{D}$O₂):

$$\dot{D}O_2 = CO \times CaO_2 \times 10$$

where CaO₂ = arterial oxygen concentration

Oxygen consumption ($\dot{V}$O₂):

$$\dot{V}O_2 = (CaO_2 - C\bar{v}O_2) \times CO \times 10$$

Extraction ratio (ER):

$$ER = \frac{\dot{V}O_2}{\dot{D}O_2}$$

Stroke volume (SV):

$$SV = \frac{CO}{HR}$$

where HR = heart rate

End-diastolic volume (EDV)

$$EDV = \frac{SV}{EF}$$

where EF = ejection fraction as determined by radionuclide angiography

Left ventricular stroke work index (LVSWI):

$$LVSWI = \frac{(MAP - PAD)SV \times 0.0136}{BSA}$$

where PAD = pulmonary arterial diastolic pressure
BSA = body surface area

Right ventricular stroke work index (RVSWI):

$$RVSWI = \frac{(PAM - CVP)SV \times 0.0136}{BSA}$$

where PAM = mean pulmonary arterial pressure

CHAPTER 26

Multiple Organ System Failure in Sepsis

William J. Sibbald
William C. Darrah

Progressive dysfunction and eventual failure of multiple organs and organ systems increasingly complicate the management of patients admitted to the intensive care unit (ICU). This syndrome, known as multiple organ system failure (MOSF), results from the critically ill state and is considered a common but nonspecific final pathway in the progression of a critical illness. The emergence of MOSF as a major threat to the survival of patients in the ICU has followed improvements in the ability to support organ function during and immediately after life-threatening illnesses that would previously have been associated with death in the short term. Although this syndrome was described by Tinley[1] and Baue[2] in the 1970s, considerable gaps remain in the knowledge base for MOSF, in part because of a lack of agreement on when individual organs or systems should be defined as dysfunctional or failed. In this chapter, MOSF is defined as a process that is acute in onset and in which dysfunction of more than one organ or organ system complicates a critical illness.

In the 1970s, acute hypoxemic respiratory failure was recognized as a major complication of serious illnesses. This adult respiratory distress syndrome (ARDS) complicated insults to the patient that are now recognized as common antecedents to MOSF. When it was also recognized that late death in ARDS patients was associated with severe infection and the development of MOSF,[3] it became apparent that this syndrome might simply reflect the beginning of a more generalized process in which failure of nonpulmonary organs followed the acute hypoxemic respiratory failure in a sequential process. The clinical grouping of dysfunctional organ systems complicating a critical illness into the MOSF syndrome recognized the likelihood that a common sequence of events underlies the failure of individual organs in this patient population.

Sepsis describes the clinical syndrome that encompasses the host's response to severe infection and other insults and includes the process now referred to as MOSF. MOSF is the final step in a process that usually includes a well-defined insult to the host (Fig. 26–1). The principal characteristics of sepsis and MOSF include a hyperdynamic and hypermetabolic state,[2] as well as many of the features typical of the inflammatory response. When organ dysfunction complicates sepsis, it is often thought to be the result of an uncontrolled and systemic activation of the inflammatory response.[4, 5] The progression from a state of organ *dysfunction*, where recovery is possible, to organ *failure* is a continuum, with the clinical demarcation between organ dysfunction and failure poorly defined. Throughout the process by which organs and organ systems are injured in sepsis, secondary insults continuously amplify the progression of the MOSF process.[6]

This chapter characterizes the epidemiology of MOSF including the criteria employed to define organ dysfunction and subsequent failure. The pathology and pathogenesis of MOSF are emphasized, illustrating the complexity of the interactions among mediators, cellular components of the immune response, and the decompensation of normal physiologic responses precipitating dysfunction and ultimately failure of organ systems. The review of management strategies will focus on the therapeutic modalities important in the prevention and/or limitation of the MOSF process. For detailed reviews of supportive therapy for individual organs, the reader is referred to the relevant chapters in this text.

EPIDEMIOLOGY OF MULTIPLE ORGAN SYSTEM FAILURE

Definitions and Incidence

Defining MOSF as an acute to subacute process characterized by dysfunction or failure of more than one organ or organ system distinguishes this syndrome from the chronic organ failure produced by slowly progressive disease states. The word *process* is emphasized in this definition because MOSF follows a course of events that result in a common injury to many organs. MOSF is also considered a *syndrome* because it describes a set of symptoms that occur together and that likely have a common pathophysiologic mechanism.

Criteria to objectively define MOSF are vital to a better understanding of the incidence, progression, and outcome of this syndrome in critically ill patients. Knaus and colleagues[7] proposed a uniform set of definitions for failure of the five organs most commonly involved in MOSF. Based on objective and reproducible physiologic and biochemical variables indicative of organ dysfunction, these quantitative criteria initially lacked a quantitative description of both gut and liver dysfunction in MOSF. Table 26–1 summarizes the Knaus criteria for the diagnosis of individual organ failures that constitute the MOSF syndrome, to which markers of hepatic and gut dysfunction have been added.[7] In recognition that MOSF is a continuum representing a process of organ dysfunction progressing to organ failure, other tabular definitions of MOSF have categorized the severity of this syndrome according to mild versus marked categories.[6] Conceptually, organ dysfunction becomes organ failure at the often imperceptible point where supportive therapies of

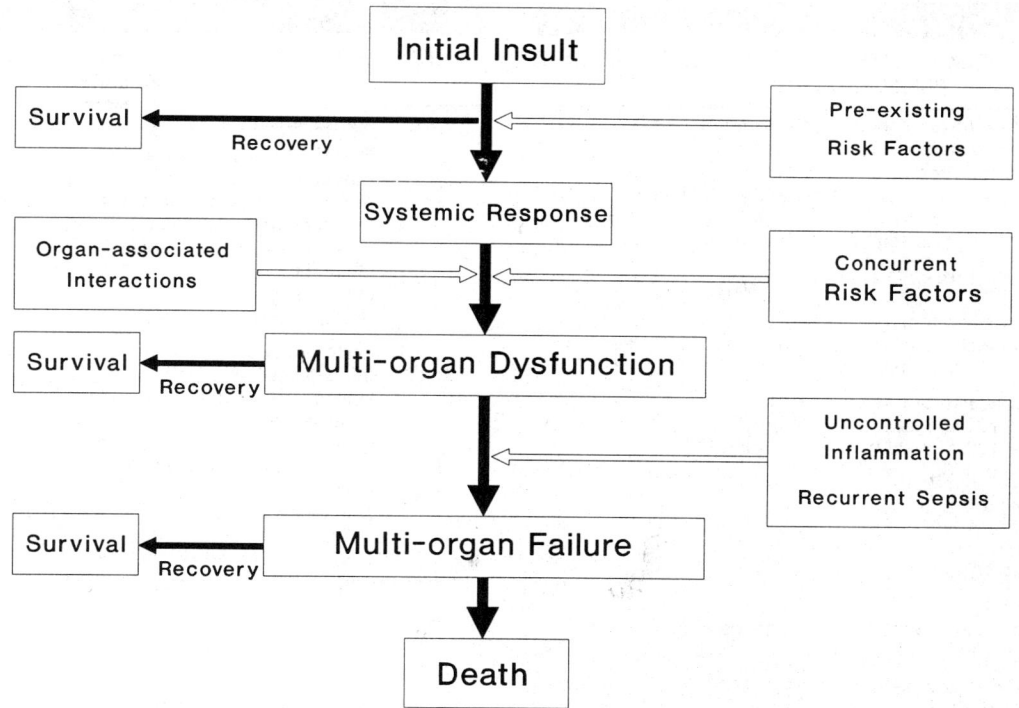

Figure 26–1. The process of MOSF.

organ dysfunction are maximized, the possibility of reversal of organ failure is unlikely, and death is imminent. The need to describe MOSF using a range of objective measurements to separate milder from more severe forms is similar to proposals that ARDS be quantitatively described according to different stages of severity.[8]

The lack of standardized criteria differentiating organ dysfunction from organ failure results in ambiguity when defining the incidence and outcome of MOSF. The incidence of MOSF also varies between individual ICUs by virtue of differences in the patient groupings admitted to each unit. For example, incidence figures derived from large, tertiary, and teaching units may not be applicable to describing the epidemiology of MOSF in smaller, nonteaching hospitals. Given these caveats and recognizing that milder forms of organ dysfunction in critically ill patients have not been defined as MOSF in large, epidemiologic studies, the most comprehensive definition of incidence was provided by the Knaus study of 5248 patients admitted to ICUs in the United States and France.[7] In that study, 49% of patients admitted to ICUs demonstrated evidence of failure of one organ before discharge, whereas 15% of total admissions demonstrated failure of more than one organ.

Clinical Patterns and Host Insults That Precede Multiple Organ System Failure

MOSF has been reported to follow a number of insults sustained by critically ill patients, including severe infection, prolonged hypotension, pancreatitis, major trauma with devitalization of tissue, gut ischemia, and massive blood transfusions.[9–11] These insults, which predispose a patient to the development of MOSF, are similar to those previously described as antedating the onset of ARDS.[3, 12]

Different patterns of onset have also been reported to follow various insults leading to MOSF. Faist concluded that MOSF occurred in two time frames after major trauma. In the first, MOSF was recognized immediately after initial

resuscitation; in the second, MOSF developed after a more protracted period of life support during which sepsis frequently developed.[9] This early versus late pattern in the development of MOSF is similar to that described in ARDS patients, where early mortality after ARDS was correlated with severity of the initial insult and late mortality was accompanied by the development of nosocomial infection and MOSF.[3]

There may also be distinct patterns to the order in which specific organs fail in the MOSF process. Failure of the lungs (i.e., ARDS) is invariably the first evidence of altered organ function in sepsis, and the cardiovascular system is usually the next most frequent system to be affected. Later, the liver, kidneys, and gut fail. Recognizing that distinct patterns characterize organ system failures, Goris described three clinical stages in the progression of MOSF[13] (Table 26–2). Perhaps more important than describing a unique sequence of organ dysfunction in MOSF is recognizing that dysfunction of one organ has an impact on the functional reserve of other organs in a process of poorly understood organ-organ interactions. The principle here is that pre-existing organ dysfunction or organ dysfunction complicating early MOSF may amplify or stimulate the processes underlying this syndrome.

Risk Factors and Prognosis

A number of factors have been identified as conferring increased risk for the development of MOSF. These factors may be categorized according to whether they precede the insult that leads to MOSF, occur at the same time as the insult, and/or complicate the natural progression as well as the treatment of MOSF[2] (Table 26–3).

Risk factors that precede the insult include advancing age, the presence of chronic disease, pre-existing malnutrition, and alcohol abuse. Malnutrition and alcohol abuse are risk factors in the development of MOSF by virtue of their ability to depress the patient's host defense systems, thus increasing

---

TABLE 26–1

DEFINITIONS OF ORGAN SYSTEM FAILURE (FRENCH DEFINITION WHEN DIFFERENT)*

Cardiovascular Failure (presence of one or more):
  Heart rate ≤ 54 beats/min
  Mean arterial blood pressure ≤ 49 mm Hg
  Occurrence of ventricular tachycardia and/or ventricular
    fibrillation
  Serum pH ≤ 7.24 with a $Paco_2$ of ≤ 49 mm Hg

Respiratory Failure (presence of one or more):
  Respiratory rate ≤ 5 or ≥ 49
  Pao_2 ≥ 50 mm Hg with pH <7.35
  Dependent on mechanical ventilation or CPAP on the second
    day of OSF (e.g., not applicable for the initial 24 h of OSF).

Renal Failure (presence of one or more):†
  Urine output ≤ 479 mL/24 h or ≤ 159 mL/8 h
  Serum BUN ≥ 100 mg/100 mL (>36 μmol/L)
  Serum creatinine > 350 μmol/L

Hematologic Failure
  WBC ≤ 1000/mm³
  Platelets ≤ 20,000/mm³
  Hematocrit ≤ 0.20

Neurologic Failure
  Glasgow Coma Scale score ≤ 6 (in absence of sedation or
    neuromuscular blocking agents)

The presence of one or more of the above during a 24-h period
  (regardless of other values), organ system failure (OSF)
  existed on that day.

*WBC = white blood cell count; BUN = blood urea nitrogen; Pao_2 = partial arterial pressure of oxygen; CPAP = continuous positive airway pressure.
†Excluding patients on chronic dialysis before hospital admission.
From Knaus WA, Wagner DP: MSOF: Epidemiology and prognosis. Crit Care Clin 5:221, 1989.

the likelihood of nosocomial infection complicating life-support treatments required by the critically ill patient. This may perpetuate existing organ dysfunction when sepsis results. The presence of chronic disease unquestionably confers increased risk to patients sustaining insults that result in MOSF, and involvement of certain organs may also be of particular importance. For example, by virtue of its central role in supporting host defense, pre-existing hepatic dysfunction (i.e., alcoholic liver disease) is believed to be a particularly important risk factor in MOSF development.[14] Pre-existing ischemic heart disease limits the hyperdynamic state typically found in MOSF, further conferring increased risk to both onset and eventual outcome of MOSF in critical illness by limiting tissue oxygen delivery.

TABLE 26–2

PROPOSED CLINICAL STAGES OF THE PROGRESSION OF MULTIPLE ORGAN SYSTEM FAILURE

Stage	Clinical Manifestations
I	Sepsis and acute respiratory failure and depressed whole body oxygen extraction
II	Hepatic failure
III	Biventricular cardiac failure

Adapted from Goris RJ, Boekhorst PA te, Nuytinck JK, et al: Multiple-organ failure. Generalized autodestructive inflammation? Arch Surg 120:1109–1115, 1985. Copyright 1985, American Medical Association.

TABLE 26–3

RISK FACTORS IN THE DEVELOPMENT OF MULTIPLE ORGAN SYSTEM FAILURE

Age (especially >65 y)

Pre-Existing Disease States
Diabetes mellitus
Atherosclerosis/ischemic heart disease
Inflammatory/autoimmune disease
Cirrhosis/hepatic dysfunction
Malnutrition
Malignancy
Renal impairment

Acute Insults
Infection/sepsis
Nosocomial sepsis
Multiple trauma
Complex surgical procedures
Multiple transfusions of blood
Pancreatitis
Neurologic injury
  Trauma
  Vascular injury

Sepsis is perhaps the most important risk factor that both precedes the development of and contributes to the progression of MOSF. Sepsis and severe infection are important issues in patients who ultimately develop MOSF. Marshall emphasized the importance of distinguishing infection from sepsis in patients at risk for MOSF development.[16] Infection describes the effect of invading microorganisms on normally sterile tissue in the host, whereas sepsis is the host's response to infection.[16] In this context, infection may be either primary or nosocomial. The importance of this distinction is that sepsis seems to be the important risk factor for MOSF development and not infection per se. For example, some epidemiologic studies have concluded that infection leading to MOSF is present in less than 50% of the population studied, whereas criteria defining the presence of clinical sepsis is simultaneously present in over 90%. Thus, not all patients who develop MOSF are infected, yet the majority of patients with MOSF demonstrate the clinical criteria of sepsis: hyperthermia or hypothermia; neutropenia or neutrophilia; and hyperdynamic circulatory state. Therefore, MOSF is thought to simply represent an extension of the septic process, albeit one of the more severe components in the clinical spectrum of sepsis.

Another issue that may be particularly germane to the development and progression of MOSF is the presence of organ dysfunction itself. For example, dysfunction of the circulatory system represented by shock has been described as an independent risk factor for the development of MOSF when compared with sepsis alone.[17] Circulatory dysfunction represented by failure to maintain a "supranormal" systemic oxygen delivery in acute illnesses has also been associated with increased risk for development of MOSF.[18, 19] Renal dysfunction complicating ARDS has been noted to increase the risk of MOSF development,[3] and hepatic dysfunction preceding or occurring early in the course of ARDS has been reported to be another added risk factor for MOSF development and progression.[20] The importance placed on the presence of chronic disease and previous organ dysfunction, as well as the severity of the insult preceding the development of MOSF, is evident in epidemiologic studies

TABLE 26-4

DATA RESULTS FROM 5248 INTENSIVE CARE UNIT ADMISSIONS WITH MULTIPLE ORGAN SYSTEM FAILURE IN 40 FRENCH AND U.S. HOSPITALS

Parameter	Day of Failure		
	1	3	7
Failure of one organ system			
Age <65 y			
No. deaths/no. patients	440/2297	248/1036	145/542
% mortality	19%	24%	27%
Age >65 y			
No. deaths/no. patients	488/1323	309/672	179/353
% mortality	37%	46%	51%
Failure of two organ systems			
Age <65 y			
No. deaths/no. patients	313/718	291/415	126/217
% mortality	44%	53%	58%
Age >65 y			
No. deaths/no. patients	267/419	153/214	87/105
% mortality	64%	71%	83%
Failure of three or more organ systems			
All ages			
No. deaths/no. patients	404/491	209/223	103/105
% mortality	82%	93%	98%

Adapted from Knaus WA, Wagner DP: MSOF: Epidemiology and prognosis. Crit Care Clin 5:221, 1989.

demonstrating that age and severity of disease at admission are significant factors in MOSF development.[21] Therefore, although MOSF may be considered an acute and potentially reversible process in its early stages, the progression of this syndrome is significantly influenced by the depressed physiologic reserve of organ-specific systems that complicate antecedent chronic disease and the aging process.

The prognosis for patients developing MOSF is directly correlated with the number of failed organ systems and concommitant risk factors. Both retrospective and prospective studies have identified age, illness severity, and the presence of sepsis as the most common factors correlated with outcome.[21, 23] Of these factors, the impact of age on outcome is particularly impressive. For patients older than 65 years of age with failure of fewer than three organ systems, mortality rates are approximately double those of patients less than 65 years of age[24] (Table 26–4). The number and duration of dysfunctional or failed organ systems directly modify outcome, and Knaus has reported that failure of some organ systems disproportionately modifies outcome. For example, the combination of an encephalopathy with failure of another organ system was reported to carry a greater mortality rate than the failure of any other organs or two organ systems.[10]

Other investigators have attempted to predict outcome from analyzing the clinical course of MOSF. Emphasizing liver function tests, Cerra described three clinical scenarios of MOSF onset from which he reasoned that outcome might be defined.[25] More recently, a retrospective analysis of patients with ARDS demonstrated a correlation between systemic oxygen delivery, the alveolar-arterial oxygen tension gradient on the third day, and the progression to MOSF.[26] Despite these latter data, there is not yet sufficient information to quantify outcome on the basis of specific patterns, other than using the number and duration of organs failed.

The lack of unanimity on the definition of organ system dysfunction or failure continues to hamper studies of outcome. Nonetheless, available studies allow the following conclusions:

- Mortality in patients with MOSF is directly related to the number of failed organs and organ systems.
- Pre-existing organ dysfunction that limits overall physiologic reserve reduces the patient's capacity to tolerate further acute insults; therefore, MOSF is more common in patients with organ dysfunction antedating a critical illness.
- The longer organ system dysfunction or failure is evident, the less likelihood of either recovery of organ function or survival of the patient.
- Extrapolation of population-based data to a prediction of outcome in individual patients must be avoided, as none of the available scoring models are yet sensitive enough to subserve such a purpose.

PATHOLOGY OF MULTIPLE ORGAN SYSTEM FAILURE

Despite the potential for clarifying mechanisms involved in the development of MOSF in critically ill patients, there have been comparatively few detailed pathologic reviews of this syndrome. ARDS may be viewed as one component of the MOSF syndrome, so insight into the mechanisms underlying MOSF may be obtained from a review of the histologic characteristics of ARDS.[27] Indeed, lessons gained from study of the lung in ARDS and nonpulmonary tissues in MOSF suggest that separating these syndromes into distinct clinical entities may no longer be appropriate.[28]

In ARDS, injury to the alveolocapillary barrier membrane separating the intravascular from the interstitial and alveolar spaces is accompanied by evidence of an increased transmicrovascular flux of protein-rich fluid into the interstitium and alveoli.[29, 30] The endothelium is therefore a particular target of the many processes capable of initiating ARDS.[31] ARDS is also typically characterized by evidence for diffuse activation of the inflammatory response, as evidenced by an accumulation of neutrophils in the interstitium and activation of pulmonary macrophages.[32] Similarly, extrapulmonary organ injury in MOSF is accompanied by a panendothelial injury, as protein-rich interstitial edema is observed in the microcirculation of all organs in this syndrome.[33] Electron microscopy has demonstrated that, remote from an inflammatory focus, injury to nonpulmonary organs includes a loss of cell volume regulation and mitochondria.[33] When hypotension complicated a standardized insult that evoked ARDS, an infiltration of neutrophils into nonpulmonary microcirculations was also demonstrated,[34] thereby highlighting the involvement of cellular constituents of the inflammatory response in the nonpulmonary organ injury that underlies MOSF.

Although a number of autopsy studies of ARDS and MOSF have also been reported, therapies used in the premorbid state render it difficult to describe any direct or unique effect of processes leading to MOSF. For example, when exogenous sympathomimetics are used to support arterial pressures and oxygen delivery before death, endothelial injury related to prolonged sympathomimetic infusion alone may obscure a description of changes in endothelial structure related to septic MOSF. Nevertheless, despite the inherent limitations of autopsy studies, a number of clues about the epidemiology and the pathogenesis of MOSF may be found in such work. First, common to all autopsy studies is the finding of variable degrees of residual infection, which may or may not have been recognized before death.[1, 35] In patients dying early after the onset of ARDS, unrecognized infection was most frequently found intra-abdominally, whereas in ARDS patients dying after a protracted course, unsuspected infection was most frequent in the lungs.[12] Although the incidence of residual infection in patients dying with MOSF varies among clinical reports, the message is similar. Invasive infection is the most frequent event both preceding the onset and complicating the progression of MOSF. Finally, an autopsy review by Nuytinck and colleagues of 35 patients dying after trauma demonstrated that the syndrome of MOSF complicating a critical illness had many of the features of a systemic and uncontrolled inflammatory response.[4] In addition to emphasizing the importance of unrecognized infection as an antedating event in MOSF, this study demonstrated widespread organ edema with infiltration of neutrophils in the nonpulmonary microcirculation.

The pathology of MOSF has provided a number of important lessons. First, the pivotal lesion underlying the tissue injury in MOSF, and which may occur remote from the initiating process, is a panendothelial injury. This microcirculatory lesion involves both the lung and nonpulmonary organs. The functional result is an increase in protein-rich intravascular fluid in the interstitium, producing pulmonary and systemic edema. By virtue of the infiltration of neutrophils in both pulmonary and nonpulmonary interstitium, simultaneous evidence for a widespread activation of the inflammatory response is noted in MOSF. In Nuytinck's study,[4] the systemic panendothelial injury, characterized by infiltration of inflammatory effector cells at sites considerably remote from the initiating process, represented an unchecked and inappropriate systemic expression of the normal inflammatory response. This process has been referred to as "malignant intravascular inflammation."[4] As will be described in the pathophysiology section of this chapter, the functional effect of the many structural changes noted in MOSF is to depress the cellular oxygen availability at all levels of the circulation normally responsible for this process.

The paradox in the concept that an unchecked and systemically expressed inflammatory response is the important process underlying tissue injury in MOSF is that inflammation is the anticipated response to insults that cause devitalization of tissue, such as through the invasion of bacteria into normally sterile areas. Inflammation normally serves to contain, neutralize, and subsequently initiate healing in infected sites. What precipitates the transition from an organized and appropriate inflammatory response to one that is no longer contained and thus results in an unrestrained systemic response is uncertain. For this to occur, the normal regulation of the inflammatory process must be disrupted so that mechanisms of containment are no longer operative. Another means by which the inflammatory response could be continuously stimulated would be the development of nosocomial infection, a complication particularly common to this class of patients by virtue of their depressed host defense, the use of intravascular lines, and other life-support technologies. As will subsequently be discussed, dysfunction of the gut may also serve to perpetuate and/or amplify the host's inflammatory response by virtue of endotoxin and bacterial translocation from the gut to the liver, and perhaps then to the systemic circulation. Finally, in contrast to excessive or protracted stimulation of the normal inflammatory response, inadequate anti-inflammatory responses at the level of individual tissues in MOSF may also promote the continued systemic expression of the inflammatory reaction (Fig. 26–2).

PATHOGENESIS OF MULTIPLE ORGAN SYSTEM FAILURE

Hypermetabolism in Multiple Organ System Failure

The progression of sepsis and MOSF is associated with significant changes in the metabolic requirements of all

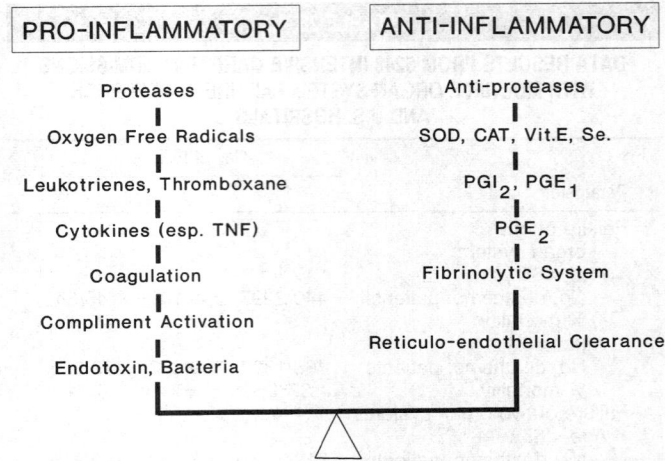

Figure 26–2. Control of the inflammatory process. TNF = tumor necrosis factor; SOD = superoxide dismutase; CAT = catalase; PGI_2 = prostaglandin I_2; PGE_1, PGE_2 = prostaglandins E_1 and E_2.

organ systems. Generally, resuscitation of a critically ill patient can be categorized into two distinct clinical stages: the "ebb" phase and the "flow" phase. The ebb phase is that period of resuscitation during which treatment restores core perfusing pressures. During the flow phase of resuscitation, tissue oxygen and nutrient needs are increased, hypermetabolism is a consistent feature, and treatment is directed at supporting the increased nutrient requirements, thereby affording the best chance of recovery.

As evidenced by an increase in both oxygen uptake and carbon dioxide excretion, energy expenditure is augmented during the hypermetabolism or flow phase of the septic MOSF syndrome. This increase in both visceral and peripheral metabolic demands in sepsis has a number of causes.[36] Tissue injury is characterized by an obligate increase in oxygen requirements to subserve the normal inflammatory response (e.g., energy-dependent neutrophil chemotaxis and phagocytosis). Remote from the inflammatory focus, augmented metabolic demands may be influenced by associated pyrexia, increased hepatic biosynthetic activity, elevated heart work, maintenance of cellular osmotic integrity, and support of increased substrate breakdown in striated muscle to maintain hepatic amino acid flux. Although current data remain controversial, inefficient mitochondrial utilization of oxygen may be an added mechanism explaining the elevated tissue oxygen requirements in the septic MOSF process.

Arguments for Tissue Hypoxia Complicating the Septic Multiple Organ System Failure Syndrome

Despite a hyperdynamic circulatory state, presumably to facilitate maintenance of an appropriate oxygen supply to satisfy augmented oxygen needs within the periphery, tissue ischemia contributing to cell injury and ultimately organ dysfunction in the septic MOSF syndrome has been suggested. Arguments to support the likelihood of tissue ischemia in the septic MOSF syndrome include the observation that both sepsis and ARDS are accompanied by a functional microcirculatory lesion, clinically described as pathologic oxygen supply dependency. This is a situation in which the dependence of oxygen uptake on oxygen delivery occurs at a point sooner than would be observed in health and is accompanied by a depression in the maximal ability of tissues to extract oxygen. The demonstration of a positive correlation between arterial lactate and death in septic patients with ARDS and MOSF is further evidence of tissue hypoxia in this syndrome.[37] Furthermore, pharmacologically vasodilating the microcirculations has uncovered a covert oxygen debt.[38] Some clinical studies have demonstrated that maintaining a supranormal oxygen delivery favored survival in both retrospective[39] and prospective[40] analyses. Therefore, protracted tissue hypoxia may be an important link in the sequence of events by which MOSF complicates a septic state.

Metabolic Changes in Multiple Organ System Failure

During the hypermetabolic stage of MOSF, the respiratory quotient varies between 0.78 and 0.82, reflecting utilization of a mixed fuel source. The metabolic profile of the patient's response to increased nutrient needs in sepsis is different from other types of energy expenditure (i.e., starvation) in that a greater proportion of amino acids are used as fuel substrates. Total body catabolism is increased significantly, a process that has been referred to as autocannibalism.[41] In this process, total body protein synthesis is increased relative to that found with starvation, but it remains significantly less than the rate of catabolism. The clinical correlate is a rapid loss of skeletal muscle mass, increased urinary nitrogen excretion, and hyperglycemia, the latter often characterized by insulin intolerance. This provides a metabolic profile that has been related with outcome. The catabolism of skeletal muscle yields glutamine and alanine as the major nitrogen carriers from muscle to core organs. This catabolism of skeletal muscle serves many purposes, providing amino acids to support the synthesis of acute phase reactants in the liver and protein synthesis in inflammatory foci and/or wounds, as well as substrate for hepatic gluconeogenesis and ammonia production in the kidney. Finally, the breakdown of skeletal muscle also provides an essential substrate for both the gut and immune system (Fig. 26–3).

Mediators in Multiple Organ System Failure

The normal host response to infection and devitalized tissue involves activation of the coagulation, kinin, complement, and cytokine systems (see Chapter 24). These processes attempt to limit the adverse effects of the insult and simultaneously promote the process of tissue repair. Of these various systems, the cytokine system occupies a prominent role in the control of the normal inflammatory response. This is of particular importance in the process of MOSF, where there appears to be loss of the poorly understood mechanisms governing cytokine metabolism. The prominent role of cytokines and other mediators in the pathogenesis of MOSF is reflected in previous descriptions of MOSF as a disease of mediators.[6] Although considerable gaps remain in current understanding of how specific cytokines induce the tissue injury underlying MOSF, tumor necrosis factor (TNF) has been implicated in initiating not only the normal inflammatory response but also the remote and generalized evidence of inflammation that characterizes sepsis and MOSF.

TNF has multiple effects on cellular function and may be a proximal mediator in the processes by which sepsis and MOSF complicate acute host insults. TNF is released by macrophages and circulating polymorphonuclear leukocytes in response to the lipopolysaccharide component of gram-negative organisms, and its elevation in the circulation is short-lived, with clearance through binding receptors present in the liver, kidney, and lung.[43] In the microcirculation, TNF promotes interaction between endothelial cells and the cellular components of the immune response. TNF-induced changes in the endothelium include increased expression of surface adhesion molecules, release of cytokines (including

TNF), and decreased thromboglobulin secretion. Consequences of these TNF-induced effects include generation of reactive oxygen species and the development of ischemia-reperfusion injury within the microcirculation. Reactive oxygen species can further augment a destructive cascade in tissue through direct cellular injury and macrophage priming. The activated macrophage/neutrophil-endothelial interactions in the various microcirculations create a microenvironment into which lysosomal contents are discharged by neutrophils and macrophages, a process that further contributes to increasing microvascular permeability in septic MOSF. Proteases released from macrophages may also interact with plasma proteins, leading to dysregulation of the coagulation, fibrinolytic, kinin, and complement systems. The septic MOSF process includes positive feedback mechanisms that perpetuate a cycle of mediator release, recruitment and activation of immunocytes to the inflammatory response, and tissue injury. The apparent dysregulation and chaos of what is normally an appropriate host response is the basis for the reference to the process of *malignant inflammation*.[4]

Mediator activation in the pathogenesis of sepsis is considered an appropriate and beneficial host response to invasive infection, devitalized tissue, and other insults that can be contained only with an appropriate inflammatory response. However, when systemically expressed in tissues remote from the primary insult, the dysregulated mediator cascade, with built-in amplification mechanisms, induces the microvascular lesion in both lung and nonpulmonary organs. The tissue edema that follows increases the diffusion distance for oxygen from the microcirculation to cell, and a process is established whereby cellular hypoxia may progress to ischemic cell injury and death. Therefore, the final pathway by which malignant inflammation complicates sepsis may result in MOSF through a disruption of the normal circulatory control of tissue oxygen delivery in a syndrome where oxygen needs are demonstrably increased.

DYSFUNCTION AND FAILURE OF INDIVIDUAL ORGANS AND ORGAN SYSTEMS

The process by which MOSF complicates an insult to critically ill patients and eventuates in multiple-organ failure and death has been likened to a domino effect.[44] Organs and organ systems appear to be interrelated such that the development of dysfunction or overt failure in one organ predisposes another to a similar fate. The process gathers increased momentum as more organs are recruited into the process. The final outcome is death, unless progression in this organ-associated phase of sepsis can be interrupted. The discussion of dysfunction and failure of the individual organ systems collectively defining the MOSF syndrome is limited here to the circulation, the neurologic system, and the organs that constitute the splanchnic system. ARDS and renal failure are discussed in Chapters 73 and 107, respectively.

The Circulation

When MOSF complicates a critical illness, deranged patterns of oxygen delivery and tissue oxygen uptake exist in the setting of increased oxygen demands. Although local metabolic regulation normally couples blood flow to tissue oxygen demands, there is apparent circulatory dysfunction in MOSF, a process that may lead to a significant imbalance between the tissue oxygen demands of MOSF and actual tissue oxygen delivery.

Abnormalities in the circulatory regulation of tissue oxygen availability can be found at all of the central, regional, and microcirculatory levels in MOSF. Some of the many

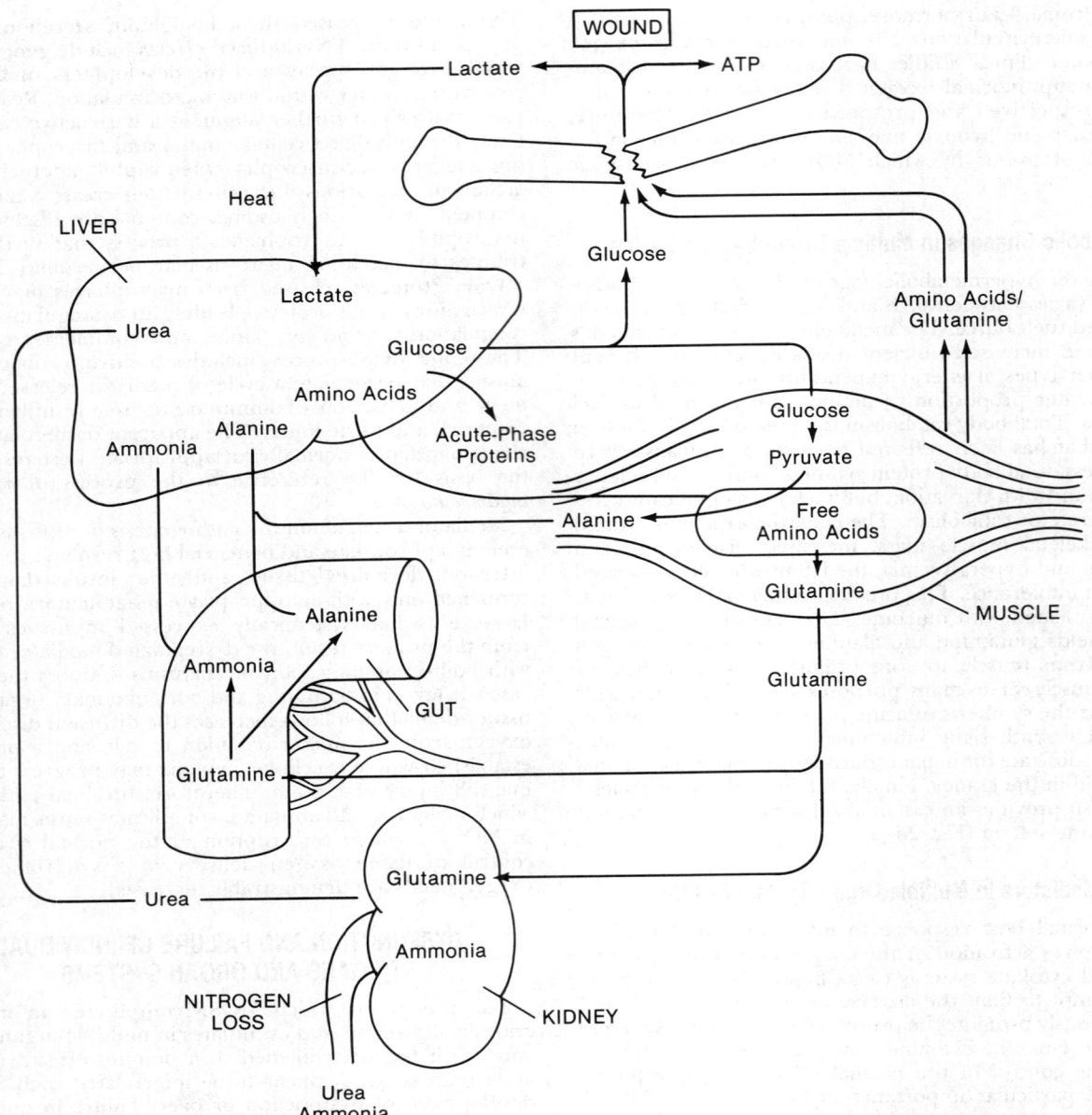

Figure 26–3. The development of the host's response to an insult and the subsequent progression into organ dysfunction and MOSF result from the balance between activators and inhibitors of the inflammatory response. (Adapted from Bessey PO: Metabolic response to critical illness. In: Wilmore DW, Brennan MF, Harken AH, et al [eds]: Care of the Surgical Patient, Volume I, Section II, Subsection 11. New York, Scientific American, p 11.11, 1989. © 1989 Scientific American, Inc. All rights reserved.)

arguments supporting the existence of a tissue oxygen debt in nonpulmonary organs in the early phases of sepsis have already been noted. Normally, local blood flows, tissue oxygen demand, and tissue oxygen delivery are closely linked.[45] With the onset of tissue hypoxia, both central and local mechanisms govern central and local compensation to ensure that adequate oxygen exists within the periphery to subserve essential cellular metabolic functions. Table 26–5 lists the various circulatory features of sepsis and MOSF that may restrict the normal increase in tissue oxygen availability required to support elevated tissue oxygen demand in this syndrome.

The Central Circulation. A depression in the normal systemic flow reserve is typical of sepsis and MOSF. Changes in both systolic and diastolic ventricular performance accompany sepsis and therefore restrict the available increase in

cardiac output that would normally underwrite the increases in systemic oxygen delivery required by a hypermetabolic state.[46] These functional myocardial abnormalities in sepsis likely have a multifactorial cause (Fig. 26–4). First, depressed biventricular contractility may accompany the presence of circulating myocardial depressant substances in sepsis.[47] In addition, the panendothelial injury characteristic of sepsis results in increased myocardial edema, which is also associated with depressed systolic and diastolic function. Alpha- and beta-adrenoreceptor dysfunction may also contribute to depressed contractility. Because of the pulmonary hypertension that can accompany ARDS, right ventricular dilatation may interfere with normal left ventricular performance. Finally, patients with ischemic heart disease have an added limitation on the ability to augment cardiac output and subsequent oxygen delivery in the septic MOSF syndrome.[15]

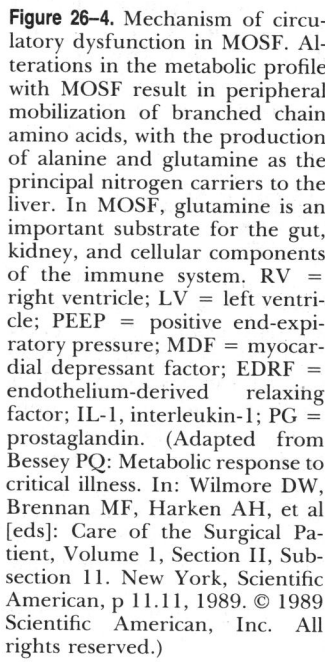

TABLE 26-5

CAUSES OF CIRCULATORY DYSFUNCTION IN THE SEPTIC MULTIPLE ORGAN SYSTEM FAILURE SYNDROME

Central Circulation
Reduced preload
Myocardial contractile depression
Pulmonary hypertension
Pre-existing disease (e.g., coronary artery disease)
Anemia
Oxygen desaturation secondary to ventilation-perfusion mismatch

Regional Circulation
Altered vascular responsiveness
Inability to redistribute blood flow to vital organs

Microcirculation
Endothelial cell damage and interstitial edema
Microembolism
Increased spatial and temporal heterogeneity of capillary perfusion

The Regional Circulations. A number of abnormalities modify the normal control of tissue oxygen delivery at the level of the regional circulations in the hypermetabolic septic MOSF syndrome. For example, sepsis is accompanied by significant alterations in the normal distribution of blood flow between core and peripheral organs. Some organs receive a greater fraction of an increase in oxygen delivery than others (e.g., the myocardium), perhaps because of the increased oxygen need of these organs in sepsis. On the other hand, animal models of sepsis have demonstrated that some organs sustain an absolute depression in blood flow (e.g., the pancreas). In this latter instance, ischemic injury might therefore supervene, and if pancreatitis results, further amplification of the septic MOSF process must be anticipated.

The flow reserve of the regional circulations is also depressed in sepsis. When tissue hypoxia complicates sepsis, for whatever reason, a redistribution in blood flow is an important compensatory mechanism to support organs such as the heart, which has little oxygen extraction reserve compared with the gut. However, sepsis depresses the ability to shunt blood from nonvital to vital organs.[49] This has also been demonstrated when burns complicate hemorrhagic hypotension.[48] The inability to appropriately redistribute flow among organs of varying oxygen need may be due to depressed vascular responsiveness in sepsis.[50] A restricted ability to redistribute flows from the gut to the myocardium further depresses the myocardial oxygen availability reserve, thereby accentuating any process that might establish a hypoxic-ischemic insult. Depressed vascular reactivity complicating sepsis could be explained by alpha- and beta-adrenoreceptor dysfunction or an imbalance between vasodilator and constrictor factors. This imbalance may involve products of the cyclooxygenase pathway, angiotensin II, vasopressin, and endothelium-derived relaxing factor.

The Microcirculation. A number of issues are apparent in the systemic microcirculations in the septic MOSF syndrome, and all have the potential to further disrupt the ability to support the increased tissue oxygen requirements. As previously discussed, the septic MOSF process induces a panendothelial cell injury that results in tissue edema and an increased diffusion distance for cellular nutrients. In addition, these changes are associated with reduced capillary luminal diameter, which impedes red blood cell transit.[51] The normal spatial and temporal heterogeneity of capillary perfusion may also be disturbed in sepsis and MOSF. The resulting maldistribution in the normal pattern of flow at the microcirculatory level amplifies the supply-demand mismatch already increased by dysfunction of both the regional and central circulations. Although increases in total blood flow will tend to decrease the heterogeneity of flow dispersion among capillaries,[52] the observed increase in systemic

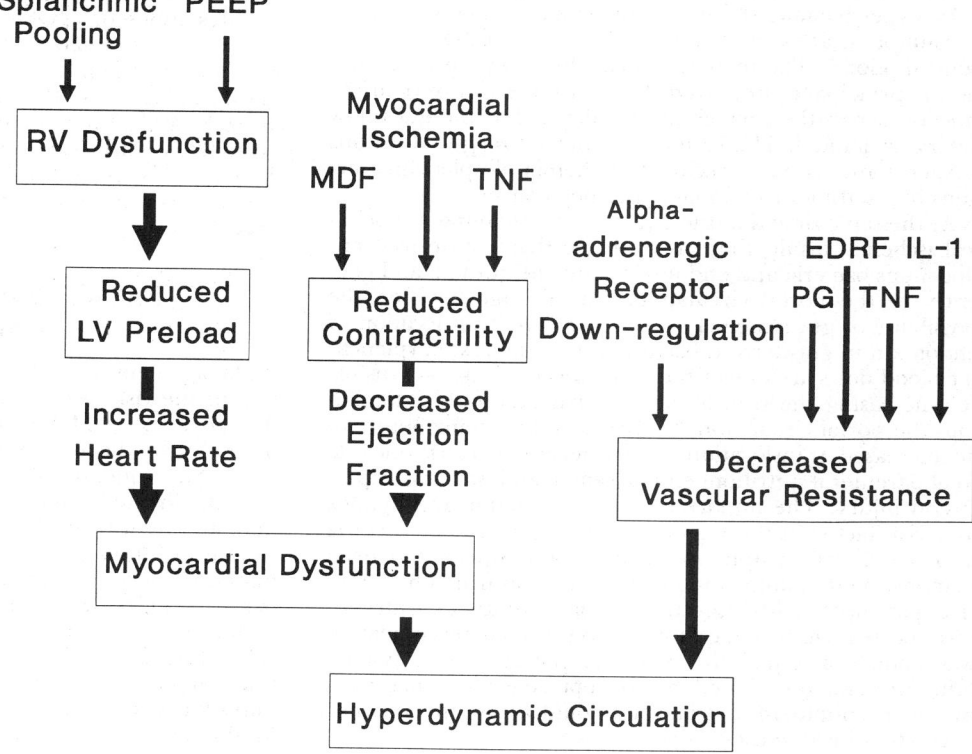

Figure 26-4. Mechanism of circulatory dysfunction in MOSF. Alterations in the metabolic profile with MOSF result in peripheral mobilization of branched chain amino acids, with the production of alanine and glutamine as the principal nitrogen carriers to the liver. In MOSF, glutamine is an important substrate for the gut, kidney, and cellular components of the immune system. RV = right ventricle; LV = left ventricle; PEEP = positive end-expiratory pressure; MDF = myocardial depressant factor; EDRF = endothelium-derived relaxing factor; IL-1, interleukin-1; PG = prostaglandin. (Adapted from Bessey PQ: Metabolic response to critical illness. In: Wilmore DW, Brennan MF, Harken AH, et al [eds]: Care of the Surgical Patient, Volume 1, Section II, Subsection 11. New York, Scientific American, p 11.11, 1989. © 1989 Scientific American, Inc. All rights reserved.)

flows in the sepsis and MOSF does not appear to redress the concurrent alterations in the microcirculation.

In summary, sepsis-induced alteration in the normal autoregulation of tissue oxygen delivery with the elevated tissue oxygen needs in this syndrome are demonstrable at all of the central, regional, and microregional levels of the circulation (see Table 26–5). The net result is a depression in tissue oxygen availability below tissue oxygen needs and a hypoxic-ischemic process that may lead to cellular injury and eventual death. In a cumulative sense, the longer the situation in which tissue oxygen availability is less than need continues, the greater the likelihood that organ failure will complicate the organ dysfunction that initially described the onset of the MOSF syndrome.

The Splanchnic Organs

In the 1950s, Lillehei and MacLean[53] proposed that the gastrointestinal tract was an important target organ in shock, and injury to the gut secondarily amplified injury related to shock itself. In the early 1970s, Fine[54] proposed that the gut was a source of "noxious" substance, which could be released into the circulation and thereby amplify organ injury. Renewed interest in the role of the gastrointestinal tract in the hypermetabolic septic MOSF syndrome has focused primarily on its ability to not only initiate but also potentiate the MOSF syndrome.

Two principal issues relating to the gastrointestinal tract may underscore its importance in the septic MOSF syndrome. First, the gut becomes colonized with anaerobic bacilli and candida early in the course of treating critically ill patients. This may be augmented by use of H_2-receptor blockers. Subclinical aspiration of this altered gut flora may colonize the oropharynx and subsequently lead to colonization of the lower respiratory tract and eventually to the development of nosocomial pneumonia. Second, if the previously discussed tissue oxygen supply-demand imbalance in sepsis occurs at the level of the gut, increased permeability of the gut wall may lead to the translocation of both endotoxin and bacteria into the portal and systemic circulations.

In hyperdynamic sepsis, an increased splanchnic oxygen consumption accounts for 45 to 55% of total body oxygen consumption.[55] The increased splanchnic oxygen consumption is principally supported through increased oxygen extraction across the splanchnic vascular bed as the gut's flow reserve is limited. The resulting reduction of portal venous oxygen tensions may precipitate ischemia of splanchnic organs in a setting of regional hypermetabolism.

At the same time that the gut may be sustaining a subclinical ischemic insult, there is evidence that gut-derived endogenous bacteria and endotoxin cross the gut wall and gain entry to the portal circulation. The linkage between the possibility of gut ischemia in sepsis and the translocation of endotoxin in gut-derived bacteria is that depressed splanchnic blood flows are one of the many mechanisms responsible for increasing the translocation of bacteria and endotoxin into the portal circulation.[56, 57] Other factors contributing to an increased translocation of gut-derived bacteria include total parenteral nutrition, endotoxemia, and ischemic-reperfusion injury. The importance of resuscitation from shock as a risk factor in the translocation of gut-derived bacteria into mesenteric lymph nodes, liver, and spleen has been demonstrated in animal models[56–58] and confirmed hypotensive patients.[59] Although the primary route of entry of translocated bacteria in endotoxin to the systemic circulation was initially assumed to be by the portal venous system, other work has questioned this concept. Alternative pathways by which endotoxin and bacteria could access the systemic circulation include the thoracic duct.[60]

In addition to serving as a source of endogenous bacteria and endotoxin, the gastrointestinal tract releases cytokines into the splanchnic vascular bed. After an infusion of endotoxin, the release of TNF in normal volunteers was approximately 25 to 50% of the total body TNF response.[61] This amplification process may also be an important modulator of hepatic cytokine production. Restoration of arterial perfusion pressures in the treatment of septic shock may also cause an ischemic reperfusion hepatic injury, resulting in elevated TNF levels and subsequent pulmonary injury. In the presence of an excessive endotoxin load, as with splanchnic hyperperfusion, saturation of hepatic function may occur with a spillover of endotoxin into the pulmonary systemic circulation, thereby causing the nonbacteremic syndrome. Therefore, endotoxin, bacteria, and TNF from the splanchnic circulations may contribute to the pulmonary and systemic manifestations of sepsis in MOSF.

Central and Peripheral Nervous Systems

Involvement of the central nervous system in the process of MOSF is a frequent and early finding. Neurologic manifestations in MOSF include altered sensorium of encephalopathy and a peripheral neuropathy. The encephalopathy occurs in 23% of septic patients[62] and is associated with high mortality (49%). Higher mortality is also conferred by pre-existing altered mental status,[62] possibly reflecting reduced physiologic reserve from pre-existing chronic disease. Factors important in the development of encephalopathy include hypotension, thrombocytopenia, and temperature extremes.[63] Young and colleagues confirmed that hypotension is a significant correlate with encephalopathy.[64] The pathogenesis of the encephalopathy of MOSF is ill-defined, and an autopsy study[63] by Young's group has not conclusively improved understanding. Although a high incidence of brain microabscesses was noted, they questioned the significance of brain infection as the principal mechanism because of the considerable heterogeneity in the observed pathologic findings.

Peripheral neuropathy is also a feature of the neurologic manifestations of MOSF in up to 43% of patients and is frequently associated with an encephalopathy.[65] The combination of muscle proteolysis resulting from the hypermetabolism of MOSF and the neuropathy has a significant impact on respiratory function and weaning from respiratory support. This complication will delay recovery from critical illness and increase the likelihood of developing recurrent nosocomial infection, thereby potentiating the septic MOSF process.

MANAGEMENT OF MULTIPLE ORGAN SYSTEM FAILURE

Management of MOSF is directed primarily at identification of the risk factors that, with modification, may reduce the incidence of MOSF complicating a critical illness. Early measures in the prevention of MOSF are given in Table 26–6. Subsequently, management of established MOSF is broadly directed toward five concerns: eradication, prevention, and treatment of infection; support of the circulation; support of nutritional status and immunologic function; minimization of the impact of organ dysfunction on other organs; and innovative therapies. The majority of therapeutic interventions applicable to the management of the critically ill have already been discussed in this text under the relevant subsection. The treatment modalities of particular importance to the prevention and/or limitation of the septic MOSF process are discussed here.

TABLE 26–6

EARLY MANAGEMENT IN THE PREVENTION OF MULTIPLE ORGAN SYSTEM FAILURE

Rapid, definitive management of all treatable injuries
Immediate cardiovascular and respiratory resuscitation
Optimization of tissue oxygen delivery (and consumption)
Early implementation of nutritional support (preferably enteral)
Prevention or rapid eradication of infectious complications

Eradication, Prevention, and Treatment of Infection

Initial management of MOSF is directed at the elimination of actual or potential pathology, principally infective, that could initiate or fuel the systemic responses that culminate in sequential organ dysfunction and failure. Therefore, appropriate surgical intervention with débridement of wounds, abscess drainage, and control of injuries are essential in patients with sepsis. Monitoring for signs of sepsis in the postresuscitation or postoperative period is essential, as MOSF is a component of the host's septic response to infection, pancreatitis, major surgery, massive transfusions, aspiration, and other insults. Recognition of a septic response in a patient at risk requires careful work-up, particularly for the remediable causes of sepsis. The cause of sepsis may not be obvious, particularly in critically ill patients for whom a good history and physical examination may be difficult. In pursuit of the source, intravascular lines must be recognized as a frequent cause of nosocomial infection in critically ill patients. Early in the course of a septic illness, the abdomen may be a site of unrecognized infection, whereas later in the course, the lungs are the most frequent site of nosocomial infection. Other causes of infection in critically ill patients include acalculous cholecystitis, sinusitis, and prostatitis.

Nosocomial infections are a particular risk in critically ill patients. The predisposition to nosocomial infection results from the necessity for endotracheal intubation, insertion of intravascular lines, and indwelling urinary catheters in patients whose host defense system is depressed by either the primary illness or the complicating critical illness itself. Nosocomial infection may perpetuate a septic response to the initial host insult and thereby perpetuate or amplify the processes by which MOSF complicates sepsis. Organisms particularly responsible for nosocomial infections include *Staphylococcus epidermidis*, gram-negative organisms that colonize the proximal gastrointestinal tract and oropharynx (including *Pseudomonas* species, *Escherichia coli*, *Enterobacter*, and *Acinetobacter*), and other opportunistic pathogens, especially *Candida albicans*. Growth of these potentially pathogenic organisms in the already immunologically compromised patient is further promoted by the use of broad-spectrum antibiotics and the practice of alkalization of the upper gastrointestinal tract for stress ulcer prevention. Selective decontamination of the gastrointestinal tract (SDD) has been proposed to reduce such endogenous infections. By using combinations of topical, nonabsorbable antibiotics and brief systemic antibiotic prophylaxis, it has been proposed that SDD reduces nosocomial infection in the lungs and the translocation of gut-derived bacteria by preventing colonization of the gastrointestinal tract. A commonly employed antibiotic combination in the SDD process includes an aminoglycoside (usually tobramycin), polymyxin E, and amphotericin B. Essential for the success of SDD is effective bacteriologic surveillance of both patients and the ICU environment. This allows early detection of resistant organisms, although the emergence of such organisms has not been found to be of significance.[67] Although reduction in the rates of infection in most SDD studies has been impressive, only one study has demonstrated a significant reduction in overall mortality resulting from nosocomial infections.[68] Therefore, before widespread implementation of SDD as a prophylaxis for sepsis and MOSF, several concerns must be addressed, particularly the role of systemic antibiotic prophylaxis, the cost/benefit ratio, and the effects of long-term application of SDD on the epidemiology of nosocomial infections.

Support of Circulation

Although eradication of primary or secondary infection is important in the prevention and therapy of MOSF, appropriate resuscitation of both macro- and microcirculations is essential because tissue oxygen availability represents an important variable in the development of MOSF.[69] (The principles of resuscitating the circulation are discussed in Chapter 28.) By manipulating determinants of the cardiac output (Table 26–7), elevated systemic oxygen delivery to supranormal levels may minimize development of an oxygen debt and thereby influence outcome.[40] At this time, no specific therapies can be directed at the regional and/or microregional levels of the circulation to improve tissue oxygen availability. As there is little in the way of clinical technique to monitor specific and/or regional microcirculations, clinical objectives in treating sepsis and preventing MOSF are focused on determinants of tissue oxygen delivery within the central circulation.

Although maintaining a supranormal systemic oxygen delivery is a reasonable therapeutic goal, monitoring the adequacy of tissue oxygen availability to meet oxygen needs remains most effectively monitored by measuring changes in arterial lactate level. An elevated arterial lactate concentration may imply flow dependency of tissue oxygen.[69] In this circumstance, systemic oxygen delivery should be increased by augmenting any or all of oxygen-carrying capacity, preload, and myocardial performance. Inotropic agents are used to increase cardiac output. There may be some benefit to using sympathomimetics that may have unique effects on specific regional circulations. For example, adding dobutamine has been demonstrated to improve tissue oxygenation and reduce lactic acidemia in sepsis.[69] Alternatively, dopexamine, a new inodilator that may preferentially improve splanchnic oxygen delivery, may be of benefit if ischemia in the organ is demonstrated to be an important component of the septic process.[71, 72] Reduced splanchnic ischemia may limit hepatic dysfunction and reduce bacterial translocation from the gut.

A similar argument has been used to advance the concept of vasodilator therapy in sepsis and MOSF. Prostacyclin has been used to improve tissue oxygen uptake in critically ill

---

TABLE 26–7

HEMODYNAMIC GOALS FOR THE PREVENTION AND TREATMENT OF MULTIPLE ORGAN SYSTEM FAILURE

Parameter	Goal
Blood volume	500 mL above normal
Cardiac index	>4.5 L/min/m² (50% above normal)
Oxygen delivery	>600 mL/min/m²
Oxygen consumption	>170 mL/min/m² (30% above normal)
Pulmonary vascular resistance	<250 dyne · s/cm⁵/m²
Arterial blood pressure	Normal

patients,[38] although this was not correlated with survival. The duration of prostacyclin infusion was limited and changes in arterial lactate levels were not reported.[38] Other vasodilatory agents have been proposed to be of benefit in sepsis and ARDS, but multicenter trials have not shown such therapy to improve outcome.[73]

Nutritional and Immunologic Support

As previously noted, septic MOSF is associated with increased metabolic requirements. The importance of fuel availability is as significant as adequate oxygen delivery to the support of cellular metabolism and tissue function. In addition, nutritional status influences immunologic function. A more recently introduced concept in the treatment of MOSF is that of metabolic support, which aims to minimize organ dysfunction or failure from substrate-limited metabolism. Metabolic support aims to utilize the immunomodulating effects of micro- and macronutrients (e.g., the free radical scavenging actions of vitamin E and selenium or the influence of certain polyunsaturated fatty acids) on mediator balance.

Optimal nutritional support includes providing adequate nonprotein calories and amino acids, with the goal of achieving positive nitrogen balance. Although achieving a positive nitrogen balance is likely not attainable in the septic patient, minimizing the degree of nitrogen loss is an important therapeutic goal. The concepts of nutritional support reviewed in Chapter 136 of this text are applicable to treating the septic MOSF patient. Briefly, minimizing nitrogen loss can be achieved through the administration of 35 to 40 nonprotein cal/kg/d with 2 to 4 g/kg/d of amino acids and further titration according to measured resting expenditure. Branched chain amino acids may offer advantages over conventional amino acid preparations by improving nitrogen balance during the hypermetabolic phase, as well as limiting the increase in aromatic amino acids. However, no large clinical trial has yet shown such benefit in the septic MOSF syndrome, and the routine use of these amino acids in this syndrome cannot be recommended at this time. Providing high caloric loads in septic patients may be detrimental because of respiratory decompensation related to excessive carbon dioxide generation, hyperglycemia, and hyperosmolar complications.

It is apparent that adequate metabolic support of the increased tissue substrate needs is important in the survival of critically ill patients. Certain research has focused on differences in survival that accompany different routes of administering nutrition. Compared with enteral nutrition, parenteral nutrition may be associated with increased bacterial and endotoxin translocation in the splanchnic organs, increased risk of acalculous cholecystitis, and increased risk of nosocomial infection complicating the use of central intravascular catheters. Enteral nutrition, particularly when initiated at an early stage of a critical illness, may reduce the onset and/or progression of sepsis and MOSF. For example, enteral nutrition may minimize the loss of gut integrity in a critical illness and thereby reduce the degree of bacterial translocation into the portal and systemic circulations. Enteral nutrition may also prevent gut bacterial overgrowth and thereby reduce the incidence of nosocomial pneumonias.

Present methods of specific support for the immune system are limited; however, appropriate metabolic support may improve both the responsiveness of the elements of the immune system and the immunologic profile associated with the process of MOSF. In addition, the route chosen for nutritional support can modify gut immune function. Interventions that reduce the catabolic response also improve immunologic function, including early and aggressive treatment of infection, débridement of devitalized tissue, and enteral nutrition. Serotherapy and immunoprophylaxis may be of value in selected patient groups[74] and include active immunization against pneumococcal infection in trauma patients requiring splenectomy or the use of monoclonal antibodies to endotoxin.[75] Future therapeutic interventions appear to hold the promise of directly modifying the immunologic process in MOSF.

Innovative Therapies

Currently available therapeutic interventions in MOSF are directed at organ support, with the principal aim of opti-

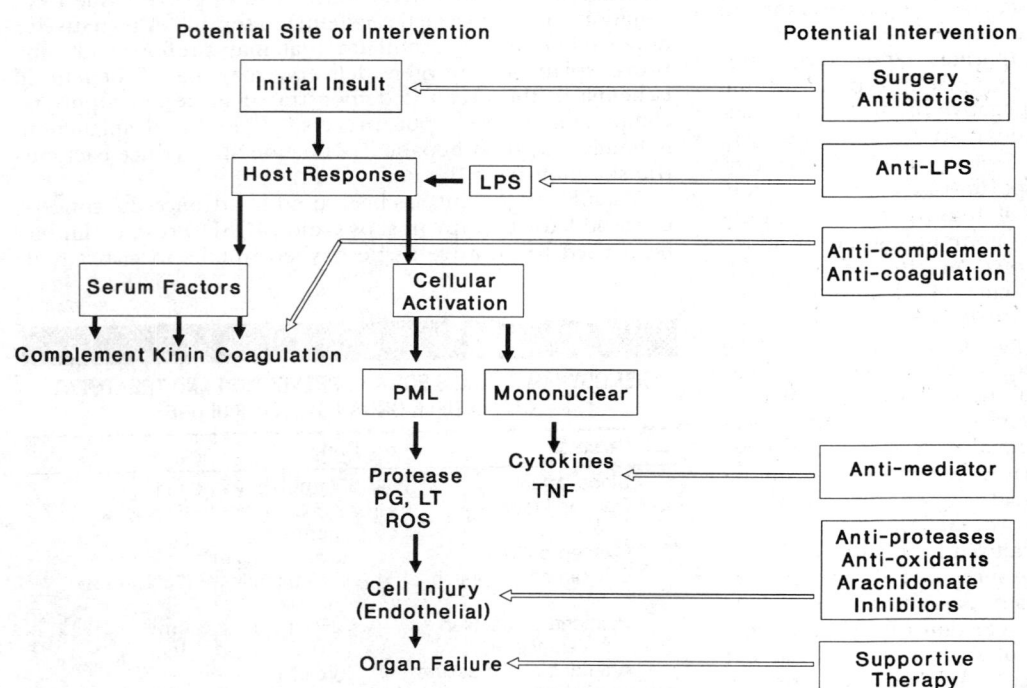

Figure 26–5. Potential management strategies in MOSF. LPS = lipopolysaccharide; PML = polymorphonuclear leukocyte; PG = prostaglandin; LT = leukotriene; ROS = reactive oxygen species. (Adapted from Niederman MS, Fein AM: Sepsis syndrome, ARDS and nosocomial pneumonia. Clin Chest Med 11:633, 1990.)

mizing tissue oxygen delivery and consumption, cellular metabolism, and organ function (Fig. 26–5). On the therapeutic horizon, however, are an array of proposed interventions, some of which offer the potential to modify processes implicated in the development and perpetuation of septic MOSF. These include reduction in the mediator load through ultrafiltration and/or dialysis[76, 77] or plasma exchange.[78] Alternatively, neutralization of endotoxin[79, 80] or cytokines such as TNF through the use of specific antibodies may ameliorate the systemic response and potentially reduce distant organ dysfunction and/or failure. These techniques may significantly contribute to the therapeutic armament necessary to combat sepsis and MOSF. The concept of therapeutically modified expression of the inflammatory response in sepsis is exciting, yet at the same time not without concern. Because it is now understood that sepsis progressing to MOSF is a process characterized by an excessive and unchecked inflammatory process occurring remote from an inflammatory site, it is tempting to use whatever tools are possible to interrupt this process. In so doing, caution must be expressed about the potential for therapy directed at the host's inflammatory response to ameliorate the beneficial effects of the process, such as that in inflammatory focus. For a more detailed review of the newer concepts in the management of MOSF, the reader is referred to Chapter 28 of the current text.

Since Baue initially recognized multiple-organ dysfunction as a clinical entity, numerous therapeutic and management strategies have attempted to attenuate or reverse the observed progressive decline in organ function. However, the process of MOSF, once initiated, becomes increasingly refractory to these measures and thus remains a major source of mortality in the critically ill. Although the therapeutic horizon appears promising, the most effective treatment remains prevention of those factors that initiate the development of sepsis and subsequent progression to MOSF.

References

1. Tilney NL, Bailey GL, Morgan AP, et al: Sequential system failure after rupture of abdominal aortic aneurysms. Ann Surg 178:117, 1973.
2. Baue AE: Multiple, progressive or sequential systems failure: A syndrome of the 1970s. Arch Surg 110:779, 1975.
3. Montgomery AB, Stager MA, Carrico CJ, et al: Changes of mortality in patients with the adult respiratory distress syndrome. Am Rev Respir Dis 132:485, 1985.
4. Nuytinck JKS, Goris RJA, Weerts JGE, et al: Acute generalised microvascular injury by activated compliment and hypoxia: The basis of adult respiratory distress syndrome and multiple organ failure? Br J Exp Pathol 67:537, 1986.
5. Fry DE, Pearlstein L, Fulton RL, et al: Multiple system organ failure. Arch Surg 115:136, 1980.
6. Marshall JC, Meakins JC: Multiorgan failure. In: Wilmore DW, Brennan MF, Harken AH, et al (eds): Care of the Surgical Patient, Volume 1, Section II. Care in the ICU. New York, Scientific American, p 13.1, 1989.
7. Knaus WA, Wagner DP: MSOF: Epidemiology and prognosis. Crit Care Clin 5:221, 1989.
8. Murray JF, Matthay MA, Luce J, et al: An expanded definition of the adult respiratory distress syndrome. Am Rev Respir Dis 138:720, 1988.
9. Faist E, Baue AE, Dittmer H, et al: Multiple organ failure in polytrauma patients. J Trauma 23:775, 1982.
10. Pine RW, Wertz MJ, Lennard ES, et al: Determinants of organ malfunction or death in patients with intra-abdominal sepsis: A discriminant analysis. Arch Surg 118:242, 1983.
11. Fry DE, Garrison RN, Hertsch RC, et al: Determinants of death in patients with intra-abdominal abscesses. Surgery 88:517, 1980.
12. Seidenfeld JJ, Pohl DF, Bell RC, et al: Incidence, site and outcome of infections in patients with adult respiratory distress syndrome. Am Rev Respir Dis 134:121, 1986.
13. Goris RJA, Boekholtz DF, van Bebber IPT, et al: Multiple-organ failure and sepsis without bacteria. Arch Surg 121:897, 1986.
14. Matuschak GM, Rinaldo JE, Pinsky MR, et al: Effect of end-stage liver failure on the incidence and resolution of the adult respiratory distress syndrome. J Crit Care 2:162, 1987.
15. Raper RF, Sibbald WJ: The effects of coronary artery disease on cardiac function in nonhypotensive sepsis. Chest 94:507, 1988.
16. Marshall JC, Sweeney D: Microbial infection and the septic response in critical illness: Sepsis, not infection, determines outcome. Arch Surg 125:17, 1990.
17. Bone RC, Fisher CJ Jr, Clemmer TP, et al: A controlled clinical trial of high dose methylprednisolone in the treatment of severe sepsis and septic shock. N Engl J Med 311:653, 1987.
18. Abraham E, Bland RD, Cobo JC, et al: Sequential cardiorespiratory patterns associates with outcome in septic shock. Chest 85:75, 1984.
19. Fowler AA, Hamman RF, Zerbe GO, et al: Adult respiratory distress syndrome. Am Rev Respir Dis 132:472, 1985.
20. Matuschak GM, Rinaldo JE: Organ interactions in the adult respiratory distress syndrome during sepsis: Role of liver in host defense. Chest 94:400, 1988.
21. Knaus WA, Draper EA, Wagner DP, et al: APACHE II: A severity of disease classification system. Crit Care Med 13:818, 1985.
22. Stevens LE: Gauging the severity of surgical sepsis. Arch Surg 118:1190, 1988.
23. Elebute EA, Stoner HB: The grading of sepsis. Br J Surg 70:29, 1983.
24. Cerra FB, Negro F, Eyer S: Multiple organ failure syndrome: Patterns and effect of current therapy. In: Vincent JL (ed): Update in Intensive Care and Emergency Medicine. Berlin, Springer-Verlag, p 22, 1990.
25. Cryer HG, Richardson JD, Longmire-Cook S, et al: Oxygen delivery in patients with adult respiratory distress syndrome who underwent surgery: Correlation with multiple-system organ failure. Arch Surg 124:1378, 1990.
26. Tomashefski JF: Pulmonary pathology of the adult respiratory distress syndrome. Clin Chest Med 11:593, 1990.
27. Matthay MA: The adult respiratory distress syndrome: New insights into diagnosis, pathophysiology and treatment. West J Med 150:187, 1989.
28. Dorinsky PM, Gadek JE: Mechanisms of multiple non-pulmonary organ failure in ARDS. Chest 96:885, 1989.
29. Orell SR: Lung pathology in respiratory distress following shock in the adult. Acta Pathol Microbiol Scand [A] 79:65, 1971.
30. Craig I, Judges D, Gnidec A, et al: Pulmonary permeability edema in a large animal model of non-pulmonary sepsis: A morphologic analysis. Am J Pathol 128:241, 1987.
31. Riede UN, Joachim H, Hassenstein J, et al: The pulmonary air blood barrier of human shock lungs (a clinical, ultrastructural and morphometric study). Pathol Res Pract 162:41, 1978.
32. Bachofen M, Weibel ER: Alterations of the gas exchange apparatus in adult respiratory insufficiency associated with septicemia. Am Rev Respir Dis 116:589, 1977.
33. Hersch M, Gnidec AA, Bersten AD, et al: Histologic and ultrastructural changes in nonpulmonary organs during early hyperdynamic sepsis. Surgery 107:397, 1990.
34. Mizer L, Weisbrode S, Dorinsky PM: Neutrophil accumulation and structural changes in non-pulmonary organs following phorbol myristate acetate-induced acute lung injury. Am Rev Respir Dis 139:1017, 1989.
35. Bell RC, Coalson JJ, Smith JD, et al: Multiple organ system failure and infection in adult respiratory distress syndrome. Ann Intern Med 99:293-298, 1983.
36. Watters JM, Bessney PQ, Dinarello CA, et al: Both inflammatory and endocrine mediators stimulate host responses to sepsis. Arch Surg 121:179, 1986.
37. Babbier J, Coffernails M, Leon M, et al: Blood lactate levels are superior to oxygen-derived variables in predicting outcome in human septic shock. Chest 99:986, 1991.
38. Bihari D, Smithies M, Gimson A, et al: The effects of vasodilation with prostacyclin on oxygen delivery and uptake in critically ill patients. N Engl J Med 317:397, 1987.
39. Shoemaker WC, Montgomery ES, Kaplan E, et al: Physiological patterns in surviving and nonsurviving shock patients. Arch Surg 106:630, 1973.
40. Shoemaker WC, Appel PL, Kram HB, et al: Prospective trial of supranormal values of survivors as therapeutic goals in high-risk surgical patients. Chest 94:1176, 1988.
41. Cerra FB: Hypermetabolism, organ failure and metabolic support. Surgery 191:1, 1987.
42. Bessey PQ: Metabolic response to critical illness. In: Wilmore DW, Brennan MF, Harken AH, et al (eds): Care of the Surgical Patient, Volume 1, Section II, Care in the ICU. New York, Scientific American, p 11.11, 1989.
43. Palladino MA, Shalaby MR, Kramer SM, et al: Characterization of the anti-tumor activities of human tumor necrosis factor alpha and the comparison with other cytokines: Induction of tumor specific immunity. J Immunol 138:4023, 1987.
44. Eiserman B, Beart R, Norton L: Multiple organ failure. Surg Gynecol Obstet 144:323, 1977.
45. Sherherd AP, Granger HJ, Smith EE, et al: Local control of tissue oxygen delivery and its contribution to the regulation of cardiac output. Am J Physiol 225:747, 1973.
46. Parker MM, Shelhamer JH, Bacharach SL, et al: Profound but reversible myocardial depression in patients with septic shock. Ann Intern Med 100:483, 1984.
47. Parrillo JE, Burch C, Shelhamer JH, et al: A circulating myocardial depressant substance in humans with septic shock. J Clin Invest 76:1539, 1983.
48. Raper RF, Rutledge FS, Hobson J, et al: Regional blood flow distribution

in high output normotensive sepsis. Clin Invest Med 9:A23, 1988. Abstract.

49. Carter EA, Tompkins RG, Yarmush ML, et al: Redistribution of blood flow after thermal injury and hemorrhagic shock. J Appl Physiol 65:1782, 1988.

50. Baker CH, Wilmoth FR: Microvascular responses to E. coli endotoxin with altered adrenergic activity. Circ Shock 12:165, 1984.

51. Hersch M, Bersten AD, Neal A, et al: Quantitative evidence of microcirculatory compromise in skeletal muscle of normotensive, hyperdynamic sepsis. Crit Care Med 17:S60, 1989. Abstract.

52. Tyml K: Redistribution of RBC flow in skeletal muscle in response to altered metabolism (abstract). Int J Microcirc Clin Exp 8(suppl I):20, 1989.

53. Lillehei RC, MacLean LD: The intestinal factor in irreversible endotoxic shock. Ann Surg 148:513, 1958.

54. Fine J, Frank ED, Ravin HA, et al: The bacterial factor in traumatic shock. N Engl J Med 260:214, 1989.

55. Dahn MS, Lange P, Lobdell K, et al: Splanchnic and total body oxygen consumption differences in septic and injured patients. Surgery 101:69, 1987.

56. Deitch EA, Bridges RM: Effect of stress and trauma on bacterial translocation from the gut. J Surg Res 42:536, 1987.

57. Deitch EA, Berg R, Specian R: Endotoxin promotes the translocation of bacteria from the gut. Arch Surg 122:185, 1987.

58. Mainous MR, Tso P, Berg RD, et al: Studies of the route, magnitude and time course of bacterial translocation in a model of systemic inflammation. Arch Surg 126:33, 1991.

59. Baker JW, Deitch EA, Berg RD, et al: Hemorrhagic shock induced bacterial translocation from the gut. J Trauma 28:896, 1988.

60. Olofsson P, Nylander G, Olsson P: Endotoxin: Routes of transport in experimental peritonitis. Am J Surg 151:443, 1986.

61. Fong YM, Marano MA, Moldawer LL, et al: The acute splanchnic and peripheral tissue metabolic response to endotoxin in humans. J Clin Invest 85:1896, 1990.

62. Sprung CL, Peduzzi PN, Shatney CH, et al. Impact of encephalopathy on mortality in the sepsis syndrome. Crit Care Med 18:801, 1990.

63. Jackson AC, Gilbert JJ, Young GB, et al: The encephalopathy of sepsis. Can J Neurol Sci 12:303, 1985.

64. Young GB, Bolton CF, Auston TW, et al: The encephalopathy associated with septic illness. Clin Invest Med 13:297, 1990.

65. Witt NJ, Zochodne DW, Bolton CF, et al: Peripheral nerve function in sepsis and multiple organ failure. Chest 99:176, 1990.

66. Niederman MS, Fein AM: Sepsis syndrome, ARDS and nosocomial pneumonia. Clin Chest Med 11:633, 1990.

67. Stoutenbeck CP, Van Saene HKF, Zandstra DF: Effect of organ nonabsorbable antibiotics on the emergency of resistance ICU patients. J Antimicrob Chemother 19:513, 1987.

68. Ulrich C, Harrick de Weerd JE, Bakker NC, et al: Selective decontamination of the digestive tract with norfloxacin in the prevention of ICU-acquired infections: A prospective randomized study. Intensive Care Med 15:424, 1989.

69. Gutierrez G, Pohil RJ: Oxygen consumption is linearly related to O₂ supply in critically-ill patients. J Crit Care 1:45, 1986.

70. Vincent JL, Roman A, Kahn RJ: Dobutamine administration in septic shock: Addition to a standard protocol. Crit Care Med 18:689, 1990.

71. Brown RA, Farmer JB, Hall JC, et al: The effects of dopexamine on the cardiovascular system of the dog. Br J Pharmacol 85:609, 1987.

72. Vincent JL, Reuse C, Kahn RJ: Administration of dopexamine, a new adrenergic agent, in cardiorespiratory failure. Chest 96:1233, 1989.

73. Holdcroft JW, Vassar MJ, Webber CJ, et al: Prostaglandin E₁ and survival in patients with adult respiratory distress syndrome. Ann Surg 203:371, 1986.

74. Young LS: Immunoprophylaxis and serotherapy of bacterial infections. Am J Med 76:664, 1984.

75. Zeigler EJ, McCutchan JA, Fierer J, et al: Treatment of gram negative bacteremia and shock with human antiserum to a mutant Escherichia coli. N Engl J Med 307:1225, 1982.

76. DiCarlo JV, Dudley TC, Sherbotie JR, et al: Continuous arteriovenous hemofiltration/dialysis improves pulmonary gas exchange in children with multiple organ system failure. Crit Care Med 18:872, 1990.

77. Gomez A, Wang R, Unruh H, et al: Hemofiltration reverses left ventricular dysfunction during sepsis in dogs. Anesthesiology 73:671, 1990.

78. Barzilay E, Kessler D, Berlot G, et al: Use of extracorporeal supportive techniques as additional treatment for septic-induced multiple organ failure patients. Crit Care Med 17:634, 1989.

79. Ziegler EJ, Fisher CJ, Sprung CL, et al: Treatment of gram-negative bacteremia and septic shock with HA-1A human monoclonal antibody against endotoxin. N Engl J Med 324:429, 1991.

80. Danner RL, Jorner KA, Parillo JE: The inhibition of endotoxin induced priming of humans neutrophils by lipid X and 3-Aza-lipid X. J Clin Invest 80:605, 1987.

CHAPTER 27

Abnormalities of Oxygen Delivery and Uptake in Sepsis

Guillermo Gutierrez
Kristen Price

Sepsis is a significant cause of morbidity and death in critically ill patients; however, we lack a clear understanding of the basic mechanisms that lead to the full-blown expression of this syndrome. In addition to its well-recognized systemic and hemodynamic alterations, sepsis is associated with alterations in peripheral tissue oxygenation and perhaps also with impairments in cellular energy metabolism. The former may occur with decreases in cardiac output produced by an endotoxin-mediated depression of myocardial contractility.[1] Decreases in local O_2 utilization also may occur by microcirculatory alterations that lead to the formation of functional arteriovenous peripheral shunts. Furthermore, there is compelling evidence that sepsis is the systemic manifestation of a cytokine-mediated defect in cellular energy metabolism.

In this chapter we review the abnormalities of O_2 transport ($\dot{T}O_2$) and utilization by the tissues during sepsis, placing special emphasis on cellular metabolic dysfunction.

TRANSPORT OF OXYGEN TO THE TISSUES: AN EVOLUTIONARY PERSPECTIVE

During the early development of life on earth, primitive organisms developed anaerobic biochemical reactions to produce energy in the form of ATP. One such metabolic pathway is anaerobic glycolysis, in which ATP is produced from the fermentation of glucose into lactate. The energy liberated from the hydrolysis of ATP allowed these organisms to evolve organs for locomotion and endowed membranes with selective permeability. A major evolutionary advance was the appearance of unicellular organisms capable of using solar energy to produce ATP. This took place in organelles called chloroplasts that consumed CO_2 but produced O_2, a highly toxic substance that cells learned to tame with endogenous antioxidants such as superoxide dismutase. By an unknown symbiotic process, these unicellular organisms incorporated into their cytoplasm an organelle, thought to be a bacterium, that not only consumed O_2 and generated CO_2 in almost equimolar amounts but also could produce huge quantities of ATP. Of course, this was the mitochondrion, in which reducing equivalents ($NADH^+$) produced by the metabolism of different substrates (glucose, fats, or proteins) are carried down an electric gradient in the cytochrome chain until the final reaction with molecular oxygen results in the formation of water. During this process three ATP molecules are produced by the oxidation of each $NADH^+$. This was a most fortunate development, because the proliferation of photosynthetic bacteria had brought about the pollution of the earth's atmosphere with O_2. Furthermore, the wealth of ATP produced by the mitochondria allowed these cells to encode different proteins, promoting differentiation, increased cellular complexity, and growth. Eventually, cellular proliferation led to the formation of multicellular organisms, an event preceded by the evolution of cytokines that enabled neighboring cells to communicate with each other.

With larger size came increased protection against predators, which in turn promoted further growth. Eventually, these multicellular organisms grew so large that diffusion of O_2 dissolved in the primeval oceans was not sufficient to provide the innermost cells with the rate of O_2 transport required by the membrane-associated pumps and energy-consuming organelles, placing a severe restriction on growth. This situation provided the impetus for the development of a series of proteins capable of binding molecular O_2 in a reversible manner, along with a transport system that could shuttle these hemoproteins back and forth from the peripheral regions to the interior of the organism. After the passing of millions of years, this has evolved into a hydraulic system of marvelous complexity (the cardiovascular system) that carries O_2 bound to a hemoprotein (hemoglobin) inside a protected environment (the red blood cell) from a gas-exchanging organ (the lung) to every cell in the body. Given the complexity of the O_2 transport process and our somewhat primitive understanding of this system, it is not surprising that there is much controversy about the functional alterations that occur with disease, especially during sepsis.

HEMODYNAMIC ALTERATIONS DURING SEPSIS

Sepsis is a condition characterized by impaired vascular control leading to profound alterations in peripheral vascular resistance and cardiac output.[2] At least two different hemodynamic states have been described during sepsis. A hyperdynamic state is seen early in the development of the syndrome, with high cardiac output and low peripheral vascular resistance.[3–6] This is often followed by a hypodynamic picture, with decreases in cardiac output and hypotension. There is some argument, however, about whether the hyperdynamic septic picture is the result of fluid infusion and catecholamines administered to the septic patient. Animals injected with live bacteria or endotoxin usually present a hypodynamic picture,[7–10] but there are reports of hyperdynamic sepsis in well-hydrated animal models.[4, 11] Therefore, it is possible that the initial presentation in sepsis is a hypodynamic one, as a direct result of depressed myocardial contractility.[12, 13] Decreases in cardiac output during sepsis have been attributed to inhibition of mitochondrial respiration by endotoxin,[14] decreased adrenergic responsiveness in myocytes,[15] the action of prostaglandins,[16, 17] and a myocardial depressant substance.[1]

MICROCIRCULATORY ALTERATIONS IN SEPSIS

The orderly function of the microcirculation appears to be impaired in sepsis, resulting in edema formation and decreases in the rate of O_2 diffusion from the capillaries to the mitochondria. Infusion of endotoxin in sheep increases the lymphocyte and neutrophil population in the microvasculature.[18] Degranulation of these cells produces endothelial injury and the formation of intercellular gaps in the capillaries. These gaps allow protein and fluid to move into the tissues, promoting edema formation. Furthermore, plasma concentrations of cyclooxygenase and lipoxygenase metabolites are increased after endotoxin infusion. It is thought that small amounts of endotoxin activate neutrophils,[19, 20] resulting in the release of superoxide anion radicals and lysozymes. These highly reactive metabolites produce endothelial damage and activate the arachidonic acid cascade,[21] altering local microvascular control and inducing platelet aggregation and microembolization. The aggregate result of these changes is an increase in microcirculatory heterogeneity and a mismatch of perfusion to cellular O_2 need in the tissues—in other words, the formation of functional peripheral shunts.

There is convincing evidence that endotoxin and tumor necrosis factor stimulate the release of nitric oxide (NO), an endothelium-derived relaxing factor formed in the endothelial cells from the amino acid L-arginine. The release of NO relaxes resistance vessels, and this may be the mechanism responsible for the hypotension that often accompanies sepsis.[22–24] Beasley and coworkers[25] found depressed vascular smooth muscle contractions in response to phenylephrine, an alpha-adrenoreceptor agonist, in rings of thoracic aorta from rats previously exposed to *Escherichia coli* endotoxin. On the other hand, Wylam and associates[26] noted impaired relaxation in response to acetylcholine in arteries removed from septic dogs, indicating that persistent vascular muscle contraction was the cause of a loss of microvascular control and increased microcirculatory heterogeneity. It is possible, however, that the contradictory results of Beasley and Wylam and their associates are related to species differences in response to endotoxin.

Gutierrez and colleagues[27] examined the effect of *E. coli* endotoxin administration on rabbit hind limb skeletal muscle oxygenation measured with surface P_{O_2} microelectrodes.[28] Although the frequency distribution of the tissue P_{O_2} readings does not permit direct quantification of microvascular heterogeneity, it offers qualitative information on the presence of microvascular disturbances. The distribution of tissue P_{O_2} values depends on the relationship of capillary perfusion to cellular O_2 demand and, as shown by Lund and colleagues,[29] reflects changes in microvascular control. When the microcirculation is disturbed, the histogram becomes irregular with a dispersion of P_{O_2} values. The highest readings most likely represent overperfused areas, where functional O_2 shunts may occur, and the lowest P_{O_2} values probably correspond to regions of tissue with the lowest levels of O_2 supply. Gutierrez and colleagues[27] found that endotoxin decreased O_2 transport and in turn this resulted in tissue hypoxia. However, the distribution of P_{O_2} readings, as shown by the series of histograms in Figure 27–1, did not change. Furthermore, as shown by the clear bar in the figure, the venous P_{O_2} from the hind limb was substantially greater than the mean tissue P_{O_2}, suggesting some type of functional peripheral shunting at the organ level. However, the distribution of the tissue P_{O_2} histograms remained constant for 2 hours after the infusion of *E. coli* endotoxin, implying that increases in skeletal muscle microcirculatory heterogeneity did not take place. These findings agree with those of Kopp and coworkers[30] who measured muscle P_{O_2} in pigs and concluded that microcirculatory changes do not take place during the first 2 hours of septic shock. These findings raise a reasonable doubt about the role of microvascular heterogeneity as the primary mode of action of endotoxin on O_2 transport disturbances.

CELLULAR ENERGY METABOLISM: A REVIEW

Before discussing the metabolic alterations that may take place during sepsis, it is appropriate to review the most salient aspects of cellular energy metabolism. The process of cellular energy transduction, that is, the conversion of energy stored in foodstuffs into a form readily usable by the various cellular organelles, depends not only on a steady supply of O_2 and substrates but also on intact metabolic machinery. Under normal conditions of O_2 and substrate supply, cells derive their energy from aerobically generated ATP. Under conditions of O_2 deprivation there are anaerobic sources of ATP that help maintain normal levels of

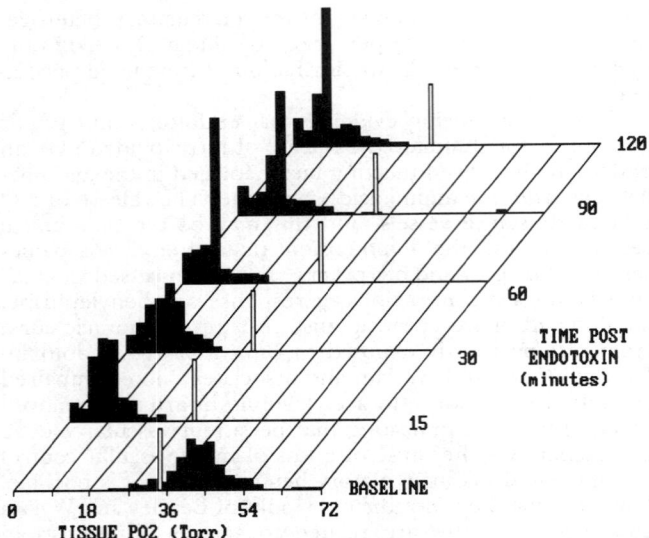

Figure 27–1. Combined hind limb skeletal muscle Po₂ histograms from seven rabbits injected with *E. coli* endotoxin. The data were obtained before and 15, 30, 60, 90, and 120 minutes after the infusion of endotoxin. The histograms shift to regions of lower Po₂ with sepsis. Moreover, the limb venous Po₂ (open bar) was greater than most tissue Po₂ readings during sepsis. (From Gutierrez G, Lund N, Palizas F: Rabbit skeletal muscle Po₂ during hypodynamic sepsis. Chest 99:224, 1991.)

cellular activity. A fundamental question in the study of sepsis is: does sepsis decrease the cellular supply of O₂ and substrate, or does it directly impair the cellular bioenergetic machinery? A brief review of the various bioenergetic pathways and the possible role of endotoxin in producing the cellular manifestations of sepsis follows.

The Aerobic Energy Cycle

Figure 27–2 is a schematic representation of the aerobic energy cycle. O₂ dissociates from hemoglobin and is released into plasma as the erythrocytes traverse the capillaries. From the capillaries O₂ diffuses into the inner mitochondrial membrane, where ATP is produced by oxidative phosphorylation. The process of oxidative phosphorylation is composed of a series of reactions in which electrons derived from the metabolism of the various substrates (glucose, fat, or protein) are transferred to O₂. ATP diffuses out of the mitochondria into the cytosol, where it provides the cells with readily available energy. The process of intracellular ATP transport is complex and more is said about it later.

ATP is hydrolyzed to ADP, inorganic phosphate (P_i), and hydrogen ions (H^+), liberating large quantities of energy in the process:

$$ATP \rightarrow ADP + P_i + H^+ + energy$$

The energy derived from ATP is used to maintain cell membrane integrity through the various membrane ionic pumps, provide contractile force, and allow protein synthesis. ADP, P_i, and H^+ are reutilized in the mitochondria as the aerobic cycle closes. Accumulation of the by-products of ATP hydrolysis provides the cell with a powerful signal to increase the rate of cellular respiration. The phosphate potential (PP), defined as

$$PP = \frac{[ATP]}{[ADP][P_i]}$$

appears to be a major controlling parameter of oxidative

phosphorylation.[31] Increases in the rate of cellular respiration are inversely proportional to PP. In other words, when PP decreases (corresponding to the accumulation of ADP and P_i) the rate of oxidative phosphorylation increases, producing a rise in substrate and O₂ consumption ($\dot{V}o_2$). This occurs during exercise, in which O₂ is plentiful and decreases in PP result in increases in aerobic ATP production. During hypoxia, however, decreases in PP do not increase aerobic ATP production, because the rate of oxidative phosphorylation is limited by the supply of O₂. Therefore, the rate of aerobic ATP production becomes less than the rate of cellular ATP utilization.

Anaerobic Sources of Energy

As illustrated schematically in Figure 27–3, the hypoxic cell has various recourses to supplement aerobic ATP production. A universal response to hypoxia is an increase in the rate of glucose utilization, the Pasteur effect. Glycolysis is the preferred metabolic pathway during hypoxia because the complete metabolism of glucose yields more ATP per molecule of O₂ than the metabolism of fat or protein. This allows the cell to maximize the utilization of the scarce O₂ molecules. Furthermore, the metabolism of glucose to lactate produces ATP, albeit less than is produced by oxidative phosphorylation. There is controversy regarding the contribution of glycolysis to cellular acidosis. It appears that one H^+ is produced per molecule of lactate generated.[32, 33] The major source of cellular acidosis during hypoxia is the hydrolysis of ATP, because the H^+ generated during this reaction is not reutilized by the mitochondria and accumulates in the cytosol.

Another readily available source of energy is the creatine kinase reaction, in which a high-energy phosphate bond in phosphocreatine (PCr) is used to generate ATP and creatine:

$$PCr + ADP + H^+ \rightleftharpoons ATP + creatine$$

This reaction occurs in organs that require a steady supply of energy, such as the brain, heart, and contracting skeletal muscle. The creatine kinase reaction also may play a major role in the intracellular transport of high-energy phosphates by the PCr energy shuttle.[34] An obvious advantage of the creatine kinase reaction, in addition to that of generating ATP anaerobically, is the utilization of cytosolic H^+ and ADP, thus providing a buffer for these by-products of ATP hydrolysis.

The creatine kinase reaction is not found in every organ; furthermore, the supplies of PCr are limited. However, most cells can use the adenylate kinase reaction to produce energy from the accumulated ADP:

$$ADP + ADP \rightarrow ATP + AMP$$

AMP can be converted to adenosine, a potent vasodilator, by the 5'-nucleotidase reaction. This provides the tissue with a metabolic feedback loop, allowing it to increase flow in response to hypoxia. AMP also can be deaminated to inosine monophosphate (IMP), with concurrent production of ammonia. Deamination of AMP to IMP is an important metabolic step that attenuates the loss of adenine nucleotides from the cell. This allows the cell to resynthesize AMP from IMP during recovery from exercise. Otherwise, adenine nucleotides would have to be created de novo, a relatively slow metabolic process.

The Hypoxia Theory of Sepsis

Tissue hypoxia during sepsis may be the end result of myocardial depression or may be due to local alterations in microvascular perfusion.[35] Endotoxin, or a mediator such as

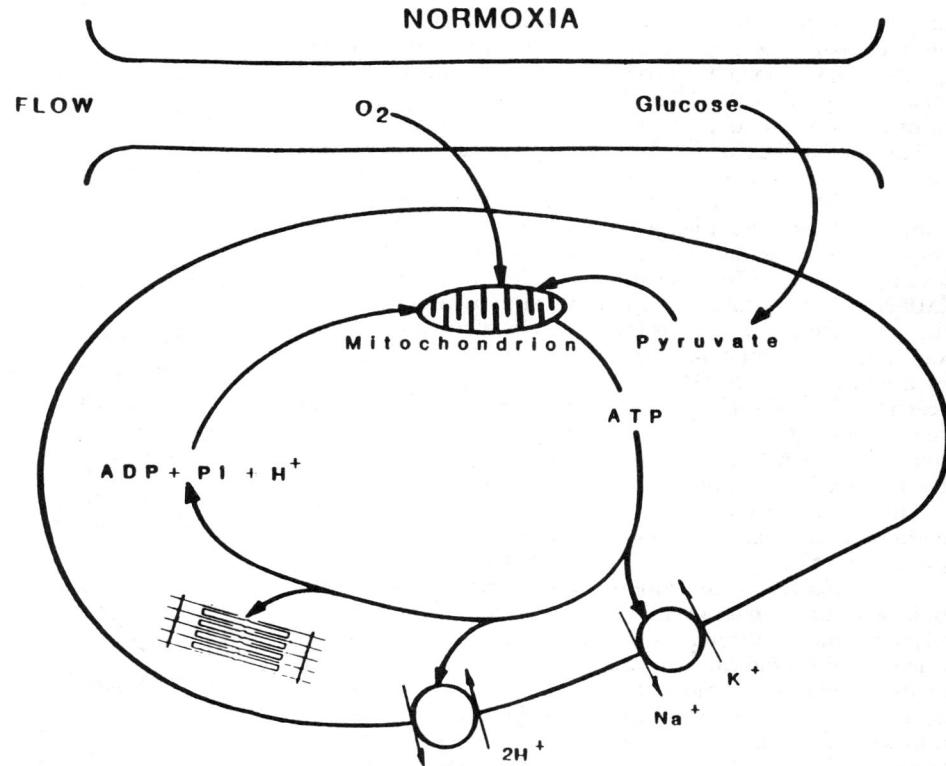

Figure 27–2. The aerobic energy cycle. ATP is generated in the mitochondria using O_2 and substrates that diffuse from the capillaries. ATP in turn is hydrolyzed to produce energy to drive the various cellular functions. The products of ATP hydrolysis, ADP, P_i, and H^+, are reutilized by the mitochondria as long as the flux of O_2 from the capillaries to the cell continues. (From Gutierrez G, Lund N, Bryan-Brown CW: Cellular oxygen utilization during multiple organ failure. Crit Care Clin 5:271, 1989.)

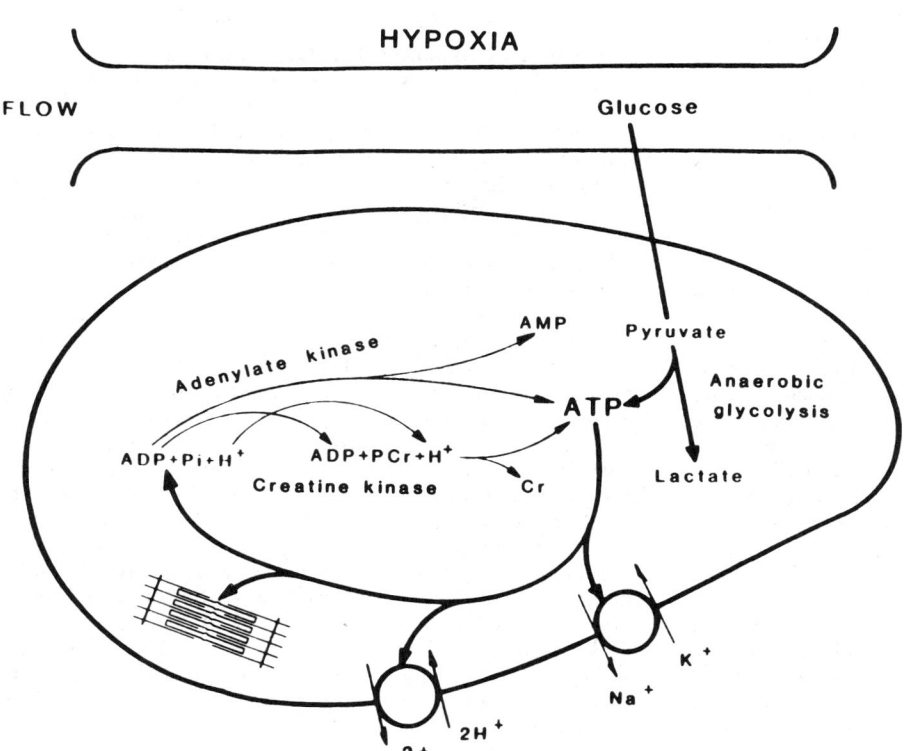

Figure 27–3. Anaerobic sources of energy. During hypoxia, glycolysis, the creatine kinase reaction, and the adenylate kinase reaction provide the cell with additional ATP. See text for details. (From Gutierrez G, Lund N, Bryan-Brown CW: Cellular oxygen utilization during multiple organ failure. Crit Care Clin 5:271, 1989.)

tumor necrosis factor, could initiate this process by increasing metabolic rate and cellular ATP requirements to levels greater than maximal aerobic ATP production. Cellular anaerobic sources of ATP are marshaled, with resulting intracellular accumulation of H^+, P_i, ADP, and AMP.

The metabolism of AMP to adenosine can produce increased microcirculatory heterogeneity and local hypoxia. These microcirculatory alterations may be compounded by endotoxin-mediated release of NO from the endothelial cells. AMP accumulation promotes its deamination to IMP, leading to irreversible catabolism of adenine nucleotides as IMP is further metabolized to inosine and hypoxanthine. In the presence of O_2, hypoxanthine is in turn converted to xanthine by xanthine oxidase, a reaction that is accompanied by the production of O_2 free radical species.[36] These highly reactive metabolites attack the endothelial membrane and release into the circulation arachidonic acid metabolites, some of which are potent vasoactive agents, producing further microcirculatory disruption.

The activation of neutrophils, in addition to the degradation of adenine nucleotides, can result in O_2 radical production during sepsis.[36] Grisham and coworkers[19] found increased activity of myeloperoxidase (a marker of neutrophil activation) in dogs injected with endotoxin. Using a hypodynamic model of sepsis, Morgan and associates[37] found evidence of O_2 radical formation, manifested by an increase in the products of lipid peroxidation. This was prevented by prior administration of the antioxidants superoxide dismutase and catalase but not by depletion of activated neutrophils. They concluded that O_2 radical formation in sepsis occurs in the xanthine oxidase reaction as a result of tissue hypoxia. However, Novotny and coworkers[38] found no beneficial hemodynamic effects in dogs given O_2 radical scavengers during endotoxemia. Furthermore, prior exposure to endotoxin may protect cells against hyperoxia, possibly by the induction of manganese superoxide dismutase.[39]

ALTERATIONS IN CELLULAR METABOLISM DURING SEPSIS

Numerous metabolic alterations have been reported to occur in sepsis. These range from increases in the rate of glycolysis to inhibition of mitochondrial ATP production. It is clear, however, that sepsis is accompanied by cellular acidosis, lactate and alanine production, and altered organ function. In this section we review the major impact of sepsis on metabolism.

Glucose Utilization

The effects of sepsis on glucose metabolism are complex. Endotoxin administration results in increases in cellular glucose utilization by an unknown mechanism, probably involving the action of a cytokine, such as tumor necrosis factor or interleukin-1. Increases in skeletal muscle glucose uptake occur when muscle is exposed to endotoxin in plasma but not when it is exposed to endotoxin alone.[40] The initial response to endotoxin administration is an immediate rise in blood glucose, followed by a steady decrease as glucose is consumed.[41, 42] Increased glucose utilization leads to hypoglycemia[43] and decreases in muscle glycogen[44] in rabbits. Romanosky and coworkers[45] found decreases in arterial glucose concentration after endotoxemia, which were accompanied by increases in the skeletal muscle glucose level despite normal levels of plasma insulin. These findings suggest that endotoxin has an "insulin-like" effect[46] or potentiates the sensitivity of tissues to insulin. Kober and coworkers[47] also noted an increase in blood insulin levels and marked hypoglycemia in septic dogs.

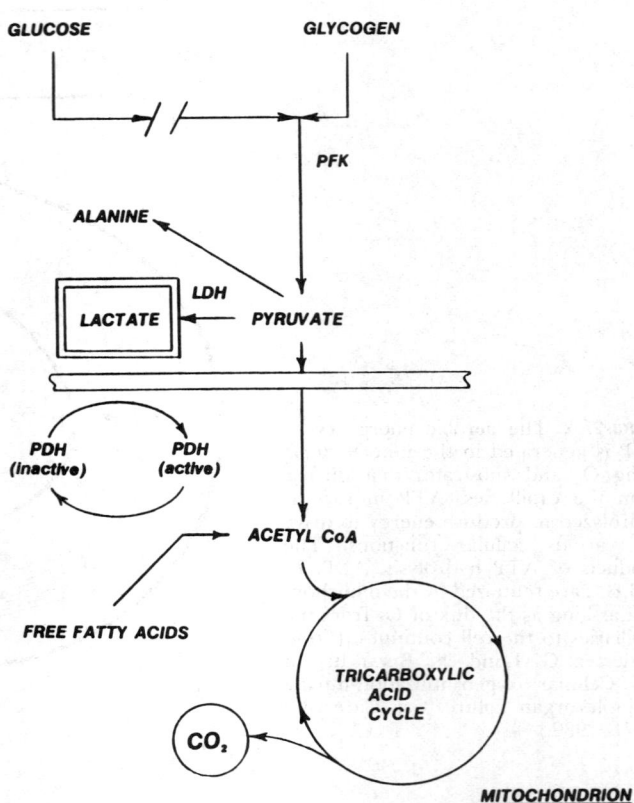

Figure 27–4. The metabolism of glucose and glycogen. Shown are two of the key control points of glycolysis, the PFK and PDH reactions. Accumulation of pyruvate results in the formation of lactate and alanine.

Control of Glycolysis and Lactate Production

Phosphofructokinase (PFK) is an important glycolytic regulatory enzyme that is activated by ADP, AMP, and P_i and inhibited by ATP and PCr (Fig. 27–4). It is possible that increases in glycolytic flux produced by the activation of PFK result in pyruvate accumulation and lactate and alanine production during sepsis.[48] To date, however, this theory has not been supported by experimental evidence. In fact, the opposite is true, as shown by Lundsgaard-Hansen and colleagues,[49] who found that PFK was inhibited in rabbits injected with endotoxin.

Another possible metabolic target of endotoxin is the enzyme that regulates the rate of pyruvate oxidation by the mitochondria, pyruvate dehydrogenase (PDH). Pyruvate is converted to acetyl coenzyme A (see Fig. 27–4) in this reaction, which serves to control the utilization of glucose or glycogen by the mitochondria. There are two isozymes of PDH, an active and an inactive one. Active PDH is phosphorylated to the inactive form by PDH kinase, a reaction promoted by high ATP/ADP and $NADH^+$/NAD ratios. The converse reaction is promoted by PDH phosphatase, a step facilitated by Ca^{2+} and Mg^{2+} and low levels of intramitochondrial ATP. It has been proposed that endotoxin stimulates the conversion of the active to the inactive form of PDH,[50] resulting in accumulation of pyruvate and formation of lactate by a mass action phenomenon. Vary and associates[50] found a threefold increase in inactive PDH in sepsis, and Kilpatrick-Smith and Erecinska[51] noted a 54% decrease in PDH activity in endotoxin-treated neuroblastoma

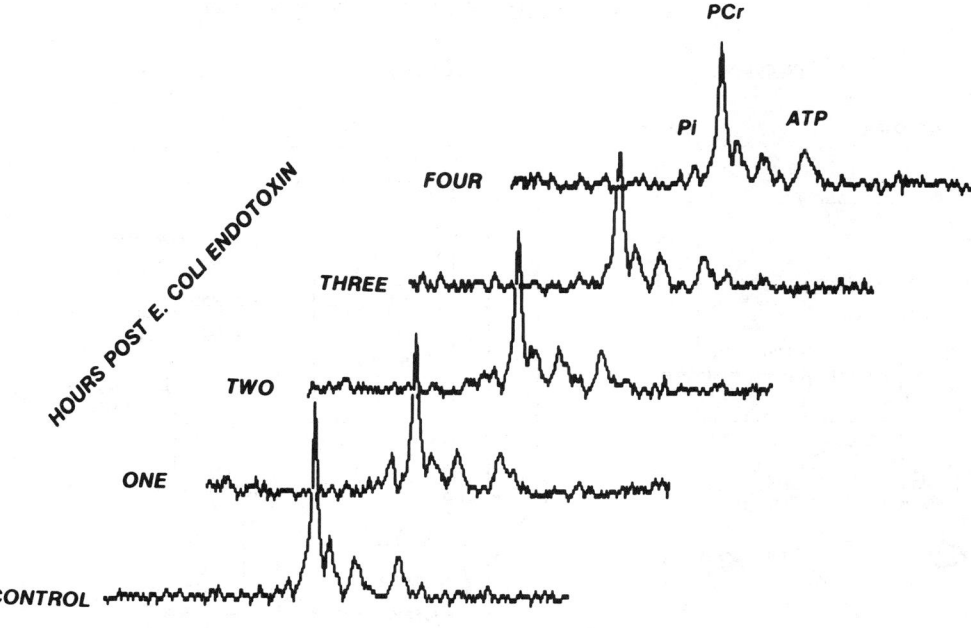

Figure 27–5. Sequential ^{31}P nuclear magnetic resonance spectra from a rabbit hind limb skeletal muscle during 4 hours of *E. coli* endotoxemia. No significant changes in the relative concentration of high-energy phosphates were noted during that time. (From Gutierrez G, Dubin A: Cellular metabolism in sepsis. In: Gutierrez G, Vincent JL [eds]: Update in Intensive Care and Emergency Medicine, Volume 12, Tissue Oxygen Utilization. New York, Springer-Verlag, p 227, 1990.)

SEQUENTIAL 31-PHOSPHORUS MAGNETIC RESONANCE SPECTRA

FROM A RABBIT HINDLIMB DURING E. COLI ENDOTOXEMIA

cells. Dichloroacetate promotes the formation of active PDH and decreases the lactic acidosis of sepsis,[52] although its beneficial effects on cellular function are less clear.[53]

Results of a study by Fink and coworkers[54] support the hypothesis that the lactic acidosis of sepsis is not related to a state of cellular anaerobiosis. Using an intestinal PCO_2 Silastic tonometer, they measured intraluminal pH in pigs after injection of *E. coli* endotoxin. The intestinal mucosa pH was calculated by the method of Fiddian-Green and coworkers.[55, 56] They found that the intestinal mucosa pH increased after the administration of endotoxin, although intestinal $\dot{V}O_2$ remained constant.

Control of Mitochondrial Respiration

A lower turnover rate of the tricarboxylic acid cycle has been implicated as the cause of decreased $\dot{V}O_2$ during sepsis.[3, 7, 57] However, Hotchkiss and colleagues,[58] using ^{31}P nuclear magnetic resonance spectroscopy and fluorometric enzymatic methods, found no differences in tricarboxylic acid cycle intermediates or high-energy phosphates between septic rat myocardium and a nonseptic control.

It has been hypothesized that endotoxin inhibits mitochondrial respiration,[59] and defective skeletal muscle mitochondrial $\dot{V}O_2$ has been noted in patients with septic shock.[60] On the other hand, Dawson and coworkers[61] found enhanced respiration in rat liver mitochondria after lethal doses of *E. coli* endotoxin.

Changes in Adenine Nucleotides and Cellular Energetics

Sepsis affects the levels of $\dot{V}O_2$ and organ function, but the cellular concentrations of high-energy phosphates, ATP, ADP, AMP, PCr, and P_i, remain unaltered. Pappova and associates[44] found no changes in the concentration of adenine nucleotides in rabbits given endotoxin intravenously. Chaudry and coworkers[62] also measured tissue adenine nu-

cleotides in liver, kidney, diaphragm, and skeletal muscle from rats in which sepsis was produced by cecal ligation. They found no changes in blood flow or in adenine nucleotides in early sepsis, 10 hours after cecal ligation. During late sepsis, 16 to 24 hours, ATP and ADP levels were decreased in liver and kidney but not in diaphragm or gastrocnemius muscle. Pasque and coworkers[63] noted an increase in myocardial ATP in rats 18 hours after cecal ligation, which was attributed to an increase in energy production by a sepsis-stimulated myocardium. Myrvold and colleagues[64] also found increases in skeletal muscle ATP in endotoxin-treated dogs and concluded that tissue hypoxia does not occur during the initial period of endotoxemia.

The foregoing studies have been complemented by experiments in septic animals using ^{31}P magnetic resonance spectroscopy. This technique allows the measurement of high-energy phosphates ATP, PCr, and P_i in a noninvasive manner. Therefore, sequential measurements can be taken in the same experimental preparation. Jepson and coworkers[65] found decreases in blood flow and $\dot{V}O_2$ in skeletal muscle of rats given *E. coli* endotoxin but no changes in the levels of high-energy phosphate. The lack of effect of endotoxin on skeletal muscle ATP and PCr levels was corroborated by Gutierrez and Dubin[66] in rabbit skeletal muscle (Fig. 27–5). Hotchkiss and associates[67] examined the brain of septic rats and found that severe neurologic depression was not due to changes in the levels of brain high-energy phosphates or brain acidosis.

HYPOTHESIS OF CELLULAR METABOLIC DYSFUNCTION DURING SEPSIS

As discussed earlier, the specific intracellular mechanisms of action of endotoxin are still unknown. Possible sites of action are shown by the thick arrows in Figure 27–6. This figure is a schematic representation of the relationship between glycolysis, oxidative phosphorylation, and intracellular ATP transport and utilization. Endotoxin, or a media-

POSSIBLE SITES OF ACTION OF E. COLI ENDOTOXIN

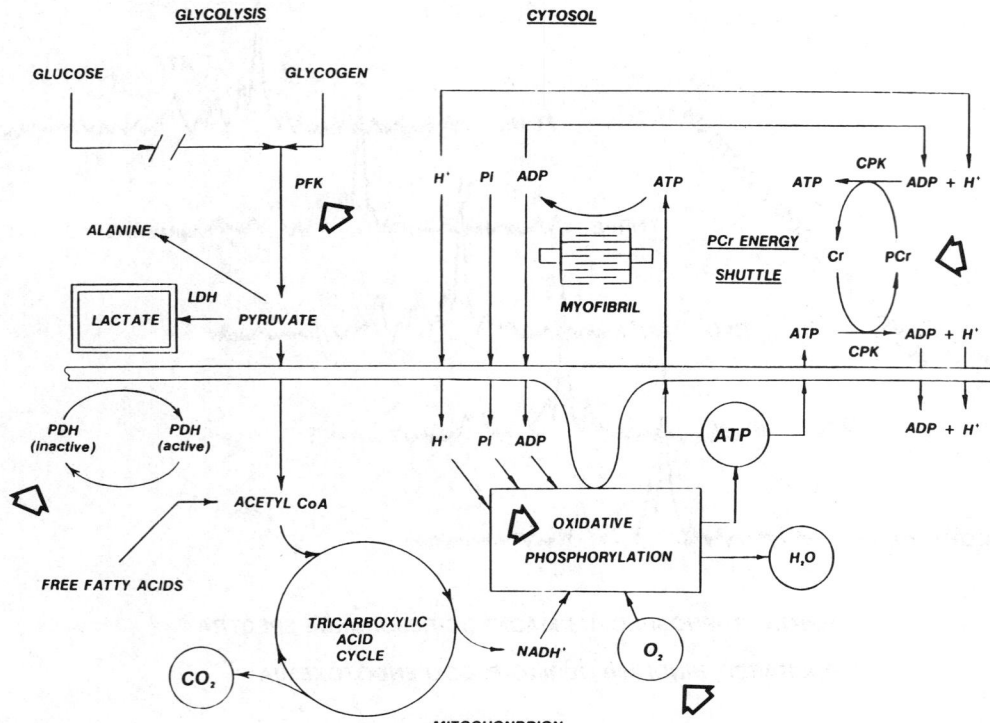

Figure 27–6. Schematic representation of the various metabolic pathways of glycolysis, oxidative phosphorylation, and the transport of ATP from the mitochondrion to the cytosol. Shown as thick arrows are the possible sites of action of endotoxin. These include inhibition of the enzymes PFK and PDH, decreases in the cellular availability of O_2, inhibition of oxidative phosphorylation, and interference with the creatine kinase energy shuttle. (From Gutierrez G, Dubin A: Cellular metabolism in sepsis. In: Gutierrez G, Vincent JL [eds]: Update in Intensive Care and Emergency Medicine, Volume 12, Tissue Oxygen Utilization. New York, Springer-Verlag, p 227, 1990.)

tor, may affect glucose or glycogen metabolism, resulting in increases in lactate production by the induction of glycolytic enzymes, such as PFK, or by decreasing pyruvate utilization by the inhibition of PDH.

Endotoxin also could affect oxidative phosphorylation, resulting in decreased mitochondrial ATP production, or interfere with the transfer of ATP from the mitochondria to the cytosol. Transport of ATP across the mitochondrial membrane takes place by the action of the ATP:ADP translocases. In the cytosol, ATP can diffuse to the sites of utilization or can transfer a high-energy phosphate bond to creatine to form PCr, which in turn diffuses to the myofibrils, where the creatine kinase reaction is reversed and ATP is regenerated from PCr and ADP. This transport mechanism is the creatine kinase energy shuttle[34] (Fig. 27–7). The advantages of PCr as an energy carrier are its small size in comparison with ATP, which allows easier diffusion through the cytosol, and less need for large concentrations of adenine nucleotides.

Endotoxin may disrupt the intracellular transport of ATP by inhibiting the ATP:ADP translocases or may interfere with the creatine kinase energy shuttle. In either case, the cytosolic concentration of ATP would decrease but ATP could accumulate in the mitochondria. The low cytosolic ATP concentration would not be enough to satisfy cellular energy requirements and glycolysis would be needed to supplement ATP production, resulting in lactate production and acidosis. Furthermore, increased levels of ATP in the mitochondria would inhibit PDH, as increased levels of ATP normally would be expected to occur. This imbalance between cytosolic and mitochondrial ATP pools might not be apparent from measures of the total cellular ATP concentration, which could be normal or slightly decreased.

To summarize, the bulk of the evidence so far presented suggests that endotoxin, either directly or via a cellular mediator, disrupts cellular energy metabolism by the action of one, or several, of the following mechanisms:

1. Decreases in regional $\dot{T}O_2$, resulting in tissue hypoxia
2. Alterations in the rate of glucose and glycogen utilization
3. Decreases in pyruvate oxidation by the inhibition of PDH
4. Changes in mitochondrial respiratory control
5. Decreases in the pool of adenylate precursors produced by the degradation of AMP, which also may result in the production of O_2 radical species
6. Disruption of ATP transport from the mitochondria to the cytoplasm

PHYSIOLOGICAL ASPECTS OF OXYGEN TRANSPORT IN SEPSIS

Many of the possible mechanisms of cellular metabolic dysfunction with sepsis are difficult, if not impossible, to detect in the septic patient. On the other hand, we have the clinical means of monitoring changes in systemic $\dot{T}O_2$ and $\dot{V}O_2$ in the septic patient. These parameters at times are useful in characterizing the adequacy of aerobic energy metabolism; however, much controversy surrounds their use for patients with sepsis. A good place to begin our discussion of the abnormalities of $\dot{T}O_2$ during sepsis is with a description of the normal functioning of the $\dot{T}O_2$ system. As shown in Figure 27–8, O_2 moves down a pressure gradient from the atmosphere to the mitochondria by several complex processes. These include convection of O_2 into the alveoli, diffusion across the alveolar capillary membrane and the red blood cell sarcolemma, chemical reaction and binding to hemoglobin, bulk transport in blood by the pumping action of the heart, dissociation from hemoglobin in the peripheral capillaries, and finally diffusion across the endothelium into the cell mitochondria. These are interrelated processes, carefully controlled by multiple layers of interacting feedback control mechanisms whose function is to ensure that every cell in the body has an adequate O_2 supply.

The pressure gradient of the $\dot{T}O_2$ process from the at-

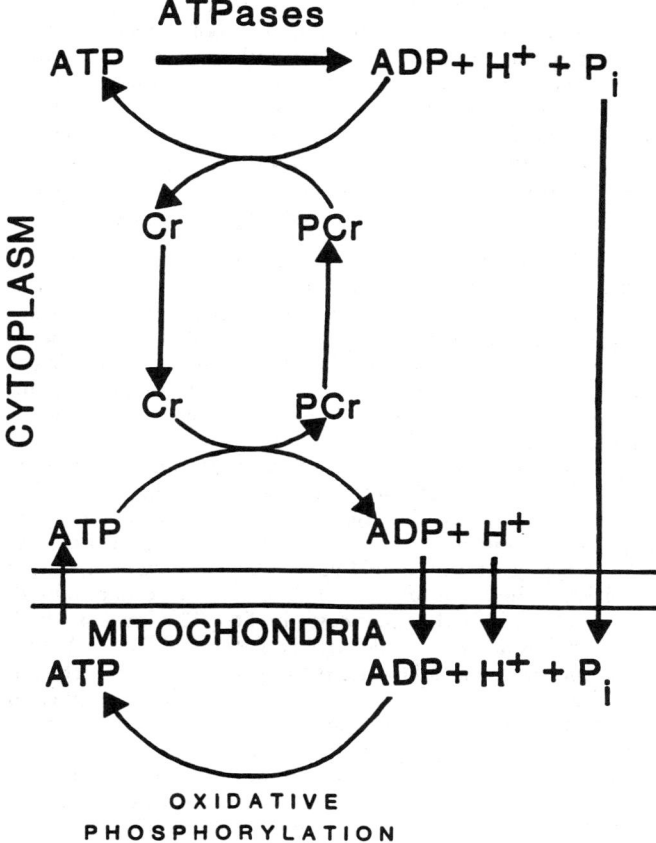

Figure 27–7. The creatine kinase energy shuttle. ATP leaves the mitochondria and PCr is formed by a membrane-associated creatine kinase isoenzyme. PCr diffuses to the sites of energy utilization, where the creatine kinase reaction is reversed.

mosphere to the mitochondria is extremely large. It can be calculated by noting that the partial pressure of oxygen in air is

$$(Po_2)_{atm} = 0.209(\text{atmospheric pressure} - \text{vapor pressure})$$

At sea level $(Po_2)_{atm}$ is 149 torr.* The mitochondria require less than 1 torr for respiration.[31] This is the $(Po_2)_{atm}$ thought to exist during the early stages of evolution.

PHYSIOLOGIC DESCRIPTION OF THE OXYGEN TRANSPORT SYSTEM

The process of systemic $\dot{T}o_2$ can be characterized without a precise knowledge of the mechanisms that regulate the movement of O_2 from the capillaries into the tissues. This can be accomplished by using a "black box" analysis, as illustrated in Figure 27–9, where the relationship between systemic $\dot{T}o_2$ and tissue $\dot{V}o_2$ is shown.

Systemic $\dot{T}o_2$ to the tissues is defined as the product of the cardiac output ($\dot{Q}$), usually measured by the thermodilution method, and the arterial O_2 content (Cao_2).

$$\dot{T}o_2 = \dot{Q} \times Cao_2 \tag{1}$$

*After Evangelista Torricelli (1608–1647), the Italian discoverer of the barometer. Europeans prefer to use the unit kilopascal, after the French mathematician Blaise Pascal (1623–1662); 1 kPa = 13.3 torr.

where

$$Cao_2 = 1.34[Hb] \times Sao_2 + 0.003Pao_2 \tag{2}$$

[Hb] represents the concentration of hemoglobin in arterial blood (g/100 mL), Sao_2 is the fraction of hemoglobin saturated with O_2, and Pao_2 is the partial pressure of O_2 in arterial blood. Here a denotes arterial blood, v venous blood, and $\bar{v}$ mixed venous blood.

The preferred way to measure systemic $\dot{V}o_2$ is by directly measuring the inspired and expired fractions of O_2 and CO_2 and minute ventilation. A warning: the error of this measurement increases in direct proportion to the fraction of inspired oxygen and is generally considered unreliable at a fraction greater than 0.60. The technique usually used in clinical practice to measure $\dot{V}o_2$ is based on Fick's equation. A pulmonary arterial catheter is used to obtain measures of $\dot{Q}$ by thermodilution and $C\bar{v}o_2$. An arterial blood gas measurement yields the information necessary to calculate Cao_2. Then

$$\dot{V}o_2 = \dot{Q}(Cao_2 - C\bar{v}o_2) \tag{3}$$

Another parameter that can be of use in defining the state of tissue oxygenation is the O_2 extraction ratio (ERo_2):

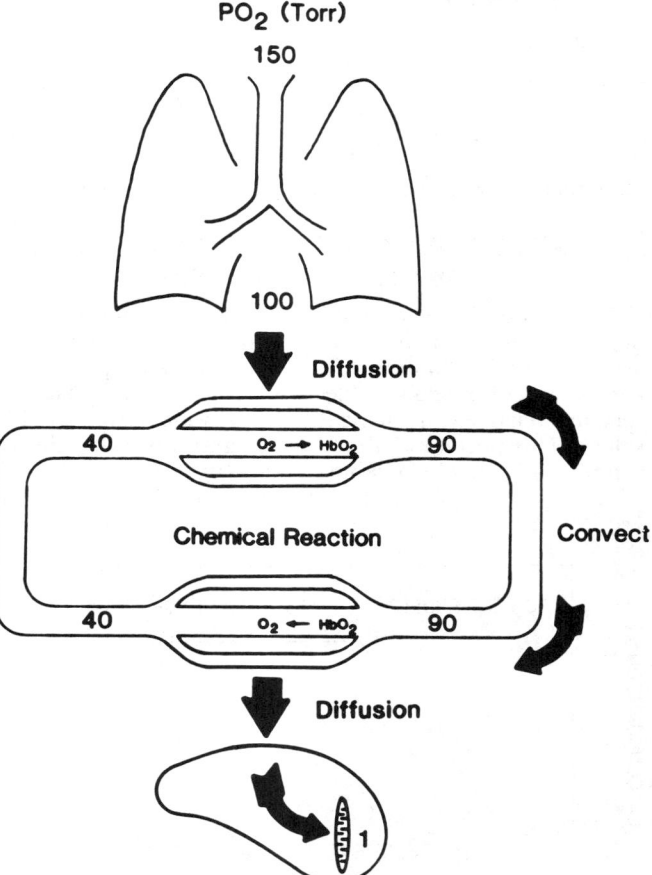

Figure 27–8. The transport of O_2 from the atmosphere to the mitochondria requires a series of complex processes including convection of air into the alveoli; diffusion into the pulmonary capillaries and chemical reaction with hemoglobin; bulk flow transport to the tissue capillaries, where O_2 dissociates from hemoglobin; and diffusion into the cellular mitochondria. The O_2 gradient for this process is approximately 149 torr. (From Gutierrez G: Peripheral delivery and utilization of oxygen. In: Dantzker DR [ed]: Cardiopulmonary Critical Care. New York, Grune & Stratton, p 169, 1986.)

PHYSIOLOGICAL OUTLOOK OF

O₂ UTILIZATION

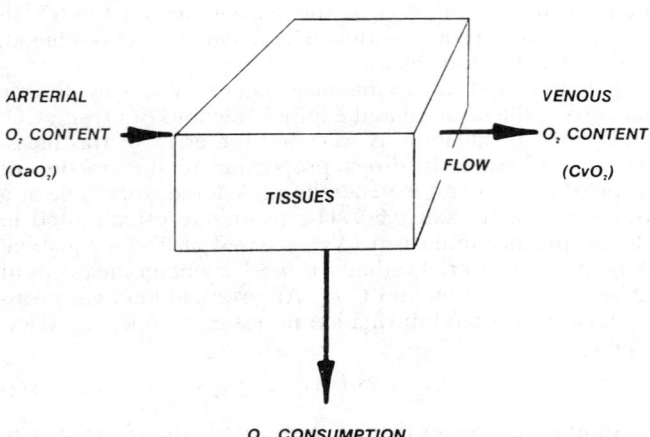

O₂ TRANSPORT TO₂ = FLOW X CaO₂

O₂ CONSUMPTION VO₂ = FLOW X (CaO₂ -CVO₂)

Figure 27–9. The black box approach to tissue O_2 delivery.

$$ERO_2 = \frac{\dot{V}O_2}{\dot{T}O_2} = \frac{CaO_2 - C\bar{v}O_2}{CaO_2} \qquad (4)$$

Note that ERO_2 can be calculated without knowing $\dot{Q}$.

RELATIONSHIP OF OXYGEN TRANSPORT TO OXYGEN CONSUMPTION

The relationship between $\dot{T}O_2$ and $\dot{V}O_2$ and the relevance of this relationship to the management of critically ill patients are subjects of continuing debate. If we take an experimental animal and progressively decrease $\dot{T}O_2$, we find that $\dot{V}O_2$ remains relatively unchanged over a wide range of $\dot{T}O_2$ values. This portion of the $\dot{T}O_2$-$\dot{V}O_2$ graph is called the O_2 supply–independent region (Fig. 27–10).

The constancy of $\dot{V}O_2$ is due to the vasculature adapting

to hypoxia by redistributing cardiac output from overperfused organs to those with high metabolic needs and by increasing the number of open capillaries in a particular tissue bed, thus decreasing the diffusion distance from capillary to cell. As more capillaries are perfused, the intercapillary distances shorten and it takes lower levels of PO_2 to maintain a constant O_2 flux into the tissues. This can be put in terms of the following equation:

$$\dot{V}O_2 = \text{cellular } O_2 \text{ flux} = K(PcO_2 - PmO_2) \qquad (5)$$

where K is a diffusion term accounting for tissue composition and geometry, PcO_2 is the capillary PO_2, and PmO_2 is the PO_2 in the mitochondria. By recruiting capillaries, the tissues increase the diffusion term K, allowing smaller PO_2 gradients to provide the same O_2 flux. Wagner[68] has combined Equations 3 and 5 into a simple, yet ingenious, model of peripheral O_2 exchange that helps describe limitations in tissue O_2 diffusion during exercise.

In systemic terms, these vascular adaptations to hypoxia are reflected in progressive increases in ERO_2, a term that can be visualized as the slope of a line drawn from the origin to a point in the $\dot{T}O_2$-$\dot{V}O_2$ curve (see Fig. 27–10). As $\dot{T}O_2$ decreases, the slope of this line becomes steeper until a point is reached where constant $\dot{V}O_2$ cannot be maintained, and it falls with further decreases in $\dot{T}O_2$. The level at which $\dot{V}O_2$ becomes a function of $\dot{T}O_2$[69] is the critical $\dot{T}O_2$.[69] At that point microvascular adaptations to hypoxia are not sufficient to maintain a constant flux of O_2 into the cells. The portion of the $\dot{T}O_2$-$\dot{V}O_2$ diagram where $\dot{V}O_2$ decreases as a function of $\dot{T}O_2$ is the O_2 supply–dependent region.[69]

In the supply-independent region, $\dot{V}O_2$ can be assumed to equal the rate of aerobic ATP production, as long as we neglect the small but measurable fraction of O_2 consumed by nonoxidative reactions (Fig. 27–11). Furthermore, $\dot{V}O_2$ is a measure of cellular energy requirements as long as the system is in aerobic equilibrium, meaning that all ATP molecules hydrolyzed in the cell are derived from the mitochondria. This, of course, is the resting, normoxic condition. However, in the supply-dependent region, aerobic ATP production declines in proportion to the decreases in $\dot{V}O_2$ and the tissues must resort to anaerobic sources of ATP production, which results in lactate production, cellular acidosis, and, if not reversed, in the death of the organism. Therefore, in the supply-dependent region we cannot assume that $\dot{V}O_2$ is a measure of cellular energy requirements, because anaerobic metabolism accounts for a significant portion of ATP production.

A biphasic $\dot{T}O_2$-$\dot{V}O_2$ relationship has been observed under different experimental conditions of tissue hypoxia, including hypoxemia (low PaO_2), hemorrhage, isovolemic anemia,

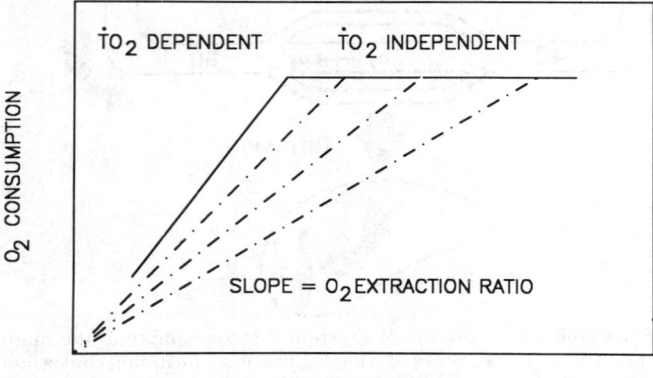

Figure 27–10. The relationship of $\dot{T}O_2$ to $\dot{V}O_2$ found in experimental animals. $\dot{V}O_2$ remains constant until a critical level of $\dot{T}O_2$ is reached. Shown as a series of dashed lines is the progressive increase that occurs in O_2 extraction ratio, the slope of a curve drawn from the origin to any point along the $\dot{T}O_2$-$\dot{V}O_2$ curve.

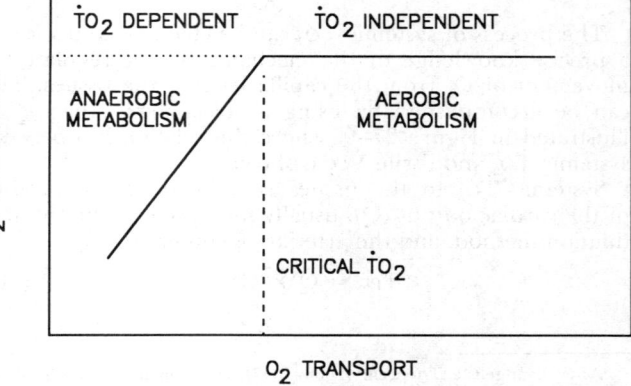

Figure 27–11. The $\dot{T}O_2$-$\dot{V}O_2$ relationship. See text for details.

carbon monoxide poisoning, and myocardial dysfunction. Furthermore, this relationship provides us with a useful index, the critical $\dot{T}_{O_2}$, the level of O_2 supply associated with the onset of anaerobic metabolism.

PATHOLOGIC OXYGEN SUPPLY DEPENDENCE

The development of the pulmonary arterial (PA) catheter in the early 1970s gave clinicians a tool with which to measure changes in PA and capillary wedge pressures. This information has proved to be of inestimable value in differentiating cardiogenic pulmonary edema from the adult respiratory distress syndrome. The PA catheter also provided easy access to mixed venous blood and made possible the determination of $\dot{Q}$ by thermodilution. This information, along with Ca_{O_2} measured in blood drawn through arterial catheters, allows routine measurement of systemic $\dot{T}_{O_2}$ and $\dot{V}_{O_2}$.

The development of the PA catheter, along with a greater understanding of the $\dot{T}_{O_2}$-$\dot{V}_{O_2}$ relationship, held great promise for clinicians treating critically ill patients. It was thought that measurements of $\dot{T}_{O_2}$ and $\dot{V}_{O_2}$ in the intensive care unit would provide an index to guide therapeutic interventions aimed at preventing anaerobiosis by maintaining patients in the supply-independent portion of the $\dot{T}_{O_2}$-$\dot{V}_{O_2}$ curve. Increases in $\dot{T}_{O_2}$ can be accomplished by optimizing $\dot{Q}$, hemoglobin concentration, and hemoglobin O_2 saturation.

However, measures of $\dot{V}_{O_2}$ and $\dot{T}_{O_2}$ in patients with sepsis and adult respiratory distress syndrome did not display a biphasic curve with a clearly defined critical $\dot{T}_{O_2}$. Instead, a linear $\dot{T}_{O_2}$-$\dot{V}_{O_2}$ relationship was found, a behavior that was called pathologic supply dependence. The linear nature of the $\dot{T}_{O_2}$-$\dot{V}_{O_2}$ function observed in critically ill patients, as opposed to the biphasic function observed in experimental animals, has been a subject of lengthy and heated debate. Three possible explanations exist. The first is that linearity is the result of mathematic coupling, because both $\dot{T}_{O_2}$ and $\dot{V}_{O_2}$ are calculated variables that include $\dot{Q}$. Therefore, random errors in the measurement of $\dot{Q}$ would result in spurious linear functions. This problem was analyzed mathematically by Moreno and colleagues,[70] who concluded that mathematic coupling, although present, probably plays a minor role in the genesis of the linear $\dot{T}_{O_2}$-$\dot{V}_{O_2}$ function. Several authors have recommended independent measurement of $\dot{V}_{O_2}$ using the method of expired gases. Preliminary data seem to suggest that supply dependence disappears when independent measurements of $\dot{T}_{O_2}$ and $\dot{V}_{O_2}$ are used.[71]

A second possibility is that the linear $\dot{T}_{O_2}$-$\dot{V}_{O_2}$ relationship merely reflects changes in O_2 requirements at the time when measurements are obtained, which in patients may vary with the clinical condition. For example, $\dot{V}_{O_2}$ and $\dot{T}_{O_2}$ are lower when the patient is sleeping or sedated, increase in the awake state, and increase even further with agitation and fever. As a result, a straight line could be drawn through these points but not as a result of O_2 supply dependence; on the contrary, it would represent the dependence of O_2 supply on O_2 demand, the normal state of affairs. In contrast, in the laboratory, decreases in $\dot{T}_{O_2}$ occur during a relatively short time in anesthetized, ventilated animals, in which energy needs are not likely to change.

A third hypothesis was developed by Cain,[69] who reasoned that two separate factors combine in these patients to produce a straight-line relationship: (1) higher cellular energy needs as the result of fever, inflammation, and the like, which raise the basal $\dot{V}_{O_2}$ levels above normal, and (2) impaired ability of the tissues to extract O_2 from blood. Among the possible mechanisms for impaired ER_{O_2} in sepsis are maldistribution of $\dot{Q}$ to organs with low O_2 requirements,

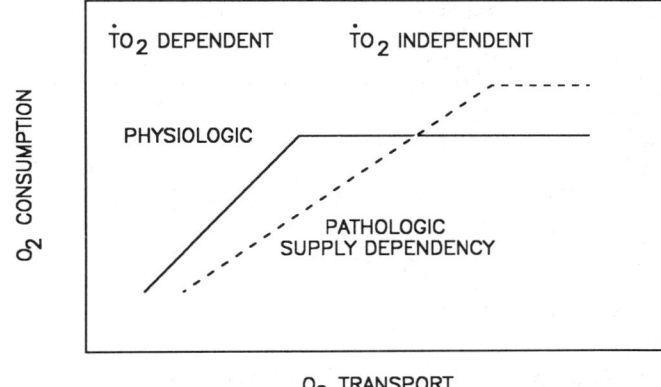

Figure 27–12. Comparison of the physiologic behavior of the $\dot{T}_{O_2}$-$\dot{V}_{O_2}$ relationship in experimental animals *(solid line)* to that thought to occur in patients with sepsis and the adult respiratory distress syndrome. The pathologic curve is characterized by a flatter O_2 extraction slope and a higher $\dot{V}_{O_2}$ plateau. This combination results in a wider range of $\dot{T}_{O_2}$ where the tissues are O_2 supply dependent.

opening of arteriovenous anastomoses, and the development of functional peripheral shunts. The last may occur as microcirculatory heterogeneity increases, resulting in a local mismatch in the levels of capillary O_2 delivery and cellular O_2 requirements. The combination of greater O_2 requirements and decreased critical ER_{O_2} results in the curve shown in Figure 27–12, along with a curve representing the normal response of the system. This theory suggests that, by increasing $\dot{T}_{O_2}$, patients can reach the supply-independent region, and it has served as the basis of numerous studies aimed at eliminating supply dependence in critically ill patients.

The clinical basis of the pathologic supply dependence hypothesis can be found in the work of Gutierrez and Pohil,[72] who measured $\dot{T}_{O_2}$ and $\dot{V}_{O_2}$ in a series of critically ill patients and found that the patients could be divided into two groups, those who maintained $\dot{V}_{O_2}$ constant in the presence of changing $\dot{T}_{O_2}$ (supply independent; 30% mortality) and those whose $\dot{V}_{O_2}$ decreased with decrease in $\dot{T}_{O_2}$ (supply dependent; 70% mortality). In a subsequent study, Bihari and coworkers[73] found that infusion of the vasodilator prostacyclin resulted in increased $\dot{V}_{O_2}$ in a subset of critically ill patients, all of whom died. This was taken as evidence that inadequate oxygenation of the peripheral tissues is often unrecognized. These authors proposed the use of an oxygen flux test whereby acute increases in $\dot{T}_{O_2}$ are used to unmask covert tissue hypoxia. Increases in $\dot{V}_{O_2}$ in response to the O_2 flux test suggest that the patient is in a supply-dependent state and may benefit from sustained increases in $\dot{T}_{O_2}$.

The idea that septic patients may be in the supply-dependent portion of the $\dot{T}_{O_2}$-$\dot{V}_{O_2}$ relationship has been supported by animal experiments showing that *E. coli* endotoxin administration to anesthetized dogs impairs their ability to extract O_2 from blood.[74, 75] On the other hand, Astiz and coworkers[76] using a model of rat peritonitis, found that $\dot{V}_{O_2}$ was maintained by increases in ER_{O_2}.

CHANGES IN OXYGEN CONSUMPTION AND OXYGEN TRANSPORT DURING SEPSIS

The direct consequence of myocardial depression during sepsis is a decrease in $\dot{T}_{O_2}$. The effects of sepsis on $\dot{V}_{O_2}$ have not been well established; $\dot{V}_{O_2}$ in sepsis has been reported to be elevated, normal, or decreased.[77, 78] Clowes and associates[3] found no changes in pig hind limb $\dot{V}_{O_2}$ in high- or low-flow sepsis, although increases in $\dot{V}_{O_2}$ with endotoxin

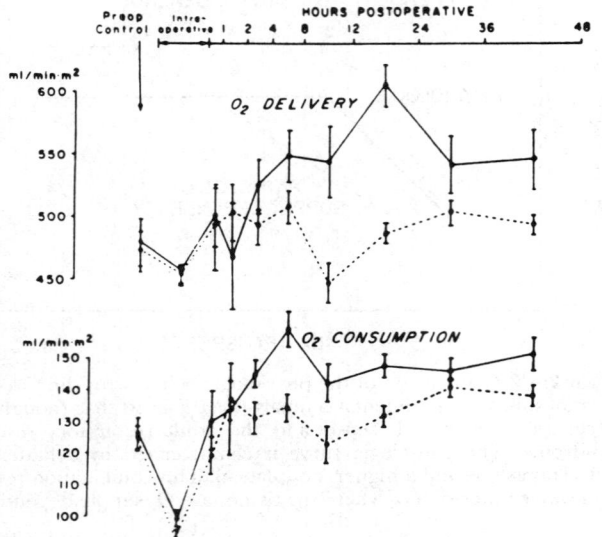

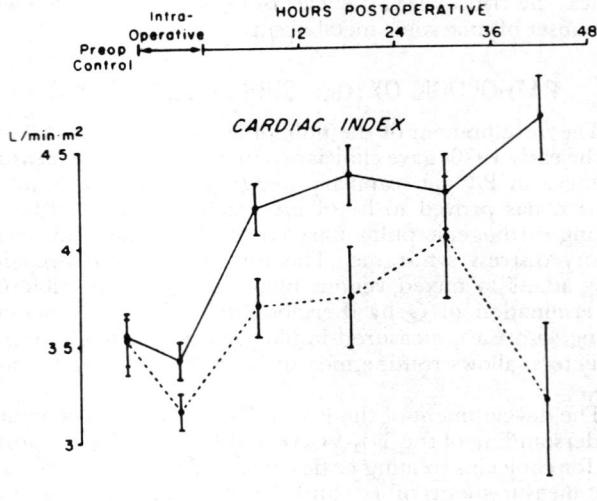

Figure 27–13. Changes in $\dot{T}O_2$, $\dot{V}O_2$, and cardiac index in a group of patients in whom $\dot{T}O_2$ was maximized with fluids and dobutamine, as compared with a control group. (From Shoemaker W, Appel P, Kram H, et al: Prospective trial of supranormal values of survivors as therapeutic goals in high risk surgical patients. Chest 94:1176, 1988.)

have been noted in the canine hind limb.[79] Using primates, Houtchens and Westenskow[80] found no changes in $\dot{V}O_2$ during hyperdynamic sepsis and depressed $\dot{V}O_2$ in hypodynamic sepsis.

Tissue O_2 requirements appear to increase during sepsis[81, 82] to levels beyond those provided by aerobic metabolism. The difference between cellular ATP requirements and aerobic ATP supply is made up by anaerobic sources, such as glycolysis, resulting in increased lactate production and cellular acidosis. Perhaps the discrepancy noted in published $\dot{V}O_2$ values during sepsis is related to variable utilization of glycolysis as an energy source by the tissues. It is clear that we need an independent index of cellular aerobic metabolism to help us determine the end points of resuscitation from compensated shock, a state characterized by inadequate perfusion of the organs with the lowest threshold for hypoxic damage.

Many studies have focused on increasing $\dot{T}O_2$ beyond the normal physiologic levels as a therapeutic maneuver in sepsis. As discussed earlier, the rationale behind this therapy is the prevention of an O_2 deficit in the tissues as the patient moves up the $\dot{T}O_2$-$\dot{V}O_2$ curve toward a $\dot{V}O_2$ plateau. The impetus for much of this work stems from the observation of Shoemaker and coworkers,[83] who found better postoperative survival rates in patients in whom PA catheters were used to help maximize $\dot{Q}$, $\dot{V}O_2$, and $\dot{T}O_2$. This was a prospective, randomized study comparing three groups: a group treated according to information derived from central venous lines (central venous pressure control), a group in which PA catheters were used to achieve normal values of oxygenation parameters as therapeutic goals (PA control), and a protocol group of patients with PA catheters who were treated with fluids and catecholamines (mainly dobutamine) in efforts to reach supranormal levels of $\dot{V}O_2$ and $\dot{T}O_2$ as therapeutic end points (PA protocol). Figure 27–13 shows changes in $\dot{T}O_2$, $\dot{V}O_2$, and cardiac index during the study for the PA control and PA protocol groups. $\dot{T}O_2$ was greater in the PA protocol group beginning at approximately 4 hours after operation. Hospital mortalities were 38, 23, and 4% for the central venous pressure control, PA control, and

PA protocol groups, respectively. An important lesson to be derived from this seminal study is that prevention of an O_2 debt improved survival. This concept was further explored by these investigators in a follow-up study of 100 high-risk surgical operations in which the magnitude and duration of a $\dot{V}O_2$ deficit were greater in nonsurvivors.[84]

This concept has been applied to critically ill patients with variable success. Russell and colleagues[85] studied 29 patients with adult respiratory distress syndrome. They found that survivors (n = 13) had higher levels of $\dot{T}O_2$ and $\dot{V}O_2$ within the first 24 hours of onset of the syndrome, although no effort was made to increase $\dot{T}O_2$ to supranormal levels in this study. In a retrospective analysis of patients with sepsis, Tuchschmidt and colleagues[86] found similar levels of $\dot{V}O_2$ but higher cardiac index and $\dot{T}O_2$ values in survivors 48 hours after admission to the intensive care unit. Other investigators have found increases in $\dot{V}O_2$ in response to catecholamines and fluid loading in septic patients,[87–90] but the effect on mortality of increasing $\dot{V}O_2$ could not be assessed from these studies.

Increased levels of serum lactate have been used as an index of anaerobiosis in sepsis and taken as proof of the inadequacy of $\dot{V}O_2$ for a given level of $\dot{T}O_2$. There are those who believe that a normal lactate level indicates that $\dot{T}O_2$ is appropriate to meet the energy requirements of the tissues in a given patient. However, others disagree, because the level of serum lactate depends on the balance of hepatic and renal production and its consumption by the heart and other tissues. Haupt and coworkers[91] used fluid loading to increase $\dot{T}O_2$ and found that $\dot{V}O_2$ increased in a group of patients with high initial lactate levels. They found, however, that $\dot{T}O_2$ and $\dot{V}O_2$ decreased in response to fluid loading in another group of patients who also had high lactate levels, suggesting that fluid loading may be detrimental in a subpopulation of patients with high lactate levels. In subsequent studies, these investigators corroborated the utility of a high serum lactate concentration as a marker of anaerobic metabolism in septic patients.[92, 93] In a study by Vincent and associates,[94] dobutamine was administered to septic patients with hyperlactatemia. They observed a marked increase in cardiac index, stroke index, and $\dot{T}O_2$. There was a concurrent increase in $\dot{V}O_2$, although the association between this finding and mortality was not reported. At this time, much controversy remains about the value of serum lactate as a measure of the adequacy of $\dot{T}O_2$. However, clinicians should be concerned by a sudden increase in serum lactate concentration because more often than not it signifies the onset of anaerobic metabolism; its causes should be carefully sought out and, when appropriate, treated vigorously with increases in O_2 supply.

In addition to dobutamine, other pharmacologic agents have been tried in efforts to induce increases in $\dot{T}O_2$. Bollaert and colleagues[95] found that $\dot{T}O_2$ and $\dot{V}O_2$ were both increased after epinephrine infusion in septic patients who were still hypotensive despite administration of fluids and dopamine. In addition, there was a strong correlation between baseline lactic acidemia and the increase in $\dot{V}O_2$. Similarly, in a case report by Bouffard and coworkers,[96] cardiac index and $\dot{V}O_2$ were both increased after infusion of norepinephrine in a septic patient unresponsive to dopamine and dobutamine as well as plasma volume expansion. Dopexamine hydrochloride is a new synthetic catecholamine with beta$_2$-adrenergic and dopaminergic properties. Doses up to 5 μg/kg/min result in significant increases in cardiac index and decreases in systemic vascular resistance. The hemodynamic effects of intravenous dopexamine hydrochloride in sepsis are still not well defined. Colardyn and colleagues[97] studied a group of 10 septic patients and found a dose-dependent increase in cardiac index and heart rate and a decrease in systemic vascular resistance. In the long term, however, these effects seemed to wane, implying tolerance to this drug.

OTHER THERAPEUTIC AND MONITORING OPTIONS

It is evident that manipulation of $\dot{T}O_2$ affects O_2 consumption. However, it is not clear whether such manipulation alters survival in septic patients. It can be seen from this review that perhaps the clinical monitoring of septic patients should shift from global measures of $\dot{T}O_2$ and $\dot{V}O_2$ to measures of cellular oxygenation and metabolism. Furthermore, knowledge of basic cellular mechanisms of sepsis may allow us to intervene early in the course of this syndrome, before the onset of multiple organ system failure.

One such therapeutic strategy is the use of antibodies to endotoxin or to tumor necrosis factor, with the aim of preventing the interaction of these mediators with the target cell. Ziegler and associates[98] reported on the results of a multicenter prospective trial of the treatment of gram-negative bacteremia and septic shock with a human monoclonal antibody against endotoxin. They found that patients with proven gram-negative bacteremia had a significantly lower mortality rate when treated with this antibody. However, there were no significant differences in mortality between the groups when all the patients treated with the monoclonal antibody were compared. Further studies are needed in this promising area of therapy. Also, there is great interest in the role of cytokines as mediators of the host's response to sepsis. Cytokines are produced by macrophages that have been stimulated by the toxins produced by microorganisms. These cytokines may be responsible for many of the physiologic responses associated with sepsis. Tumor necrosis factor, or cachectin, is thought to be the primary cytokine involved in these responses. Michie and coworkers[99] found increased plasma levels of tumor necrosis factor 90 to 180 minutes after infusion of *E. coli* endotoxin in 13 healthy men. Subsequent physiologic responses seemed to be associated with peak concentrations of this cytokine. Large clinical trials are under way to determine whether antibody to tumor necrosis factor alters survival in septic patients.

The measurement of global indices of tissue oxygenation, such as $\dot{T}O_2$ and $\dot{V}O_2$, is helpful in establishing the presence of a hypodynamic state; however, this type of monitoring appears to have limited utility in the everyday management of the septic patient. A more rational approach may be to follow changes in tissue metabolism, in particular in the organs most vulnerable to hypoxia and sepsis, such as the gut and the kidneys. One such monitoring method is the measurement of gut mucosa pH by tonometry. In a study by Doglio and colleagues,[100] levels of gastric pH$_i$ below 7.35 measured on admission to the intensive care unit and again 12 hours later were highly predictive of mortality. Similar findings have been reported by Fiddian-Green and Baker[101] and Gys and coworkers[102] regarding complications in postoperative patients. Gutierrez made sequential measurements of gastric mucosa pH and compared them to concurrent measures of $\dot{T}O_2$, $\dot{V}O_2$, and ERO_2.[103] Mortality and clinical status were closely associated with changes in gastric mucosa pH but not with systemic oxygenation parameters.

Other monitoring modalities include the use of magnetic resonance spectroscopy and near-infrared spectroscopy to follow changes in high-energy phosphate levels and cytochrome aa_3 redox state, respectively. However, further refinement of these techniques will be required before they can be used in the intensive care unit setting.

CONCLUSIONS

A reasonable approach to the oxygenation of the septic patient is to try to avoid hypoxia at all costs. Although there is controversy regarding the use of supramaximal levels of $\dot{T}O_2$ transport in septic patients, no one argues with the idea that the combination of sepsis with hypoxia is a deadly condition. To avoid hypoxia, we suggest that hemoglobin level be maintained above 10 mg/dL, arterial O_2 saturation above 90%, and cardiac index above 4.0 mL/min/m^2.

It is clear from this review that, to better understand and treat sepsis, the clinical monitoring of septic patients should shift from global measures of $\dot{T}O_2$ and $\dot{V}O_2$ to organ-specific measures of cellular oxygenation and metabolism. This knowledge may allow us to intervene early in the course of this syndrome and perhaps prevent the onset of multiple organ system failure.

Acknowledgments. Supported in part by National Institutes of Health grant HL41415–01 and an American Lung Association Career Investigator Award.

References

1. Parrillo JE, Burch C, Shelhamer JH, et al: A circulating myocardial depressant substance in humans with septic shock. J Clin Invest 76:1539, 1985.
2. Ayres SM: Sepsis and septic shock. A synthesis of ideas and proposals for the direction of future research. In: Sibbald WJ, Sprung CL (eds): Perspectives in Sepsis and Septic Shock. Fullerton, CA, Society of Critical Care Medicine, p 375, 1986.
3. Clowes GHA, O'Donnell TF, Ryan NT, et al: Energy metabolism in sepsis: Treatment based on different patterns in shock and high output stage. Ann Surg 179:684, 1974.
4. Fink MP, Fiallo V, Stein KL, et al: Systemic and regional hemodynamic changes after intraperitoneal endotoxin in rabbits. Circ Shock 22:73, 1987.
5. Parker MM, Shelhamer JH, Natason C, et al: Serial cardiovascular variables in survivors and nonsurvivors of human septic shock: Heart rate as an early predictor of prognosis. Crit Care Med 15:923, 1987.
6. Shoemaker WC, Appel PL, Kram HB: Role of oxygen transport patterns in the pathophysiology, prediction of outcome, and therapy of shock. In: Bryan-Brown CW, Ayres SM (eds): New Horizons. Oxygen Transport and Utilization, Volume 2. Fullerton, CA, Society of Critical Care Medicine, p 65, 1987.

7. Finley RJ, Duff JH, Holiday RL, et al: Capillary muscle blood flow in human sepsis. Surgery 78:87, 1975.
8. Goldfarb RD, Tambolini W, Wiener SM, et al: Canine left ventricular performance during LD_{50} endotoxemia. Am J Physiol 244:H370, 1983.
9. Hess M, Hastillo A, Greenfield L: Spectrum of cardiovascular function during gram-negative sepsis. Prog Cardiovasc Dis 23:279, 1981.
10. Pass JL, Schloerb PR, Pearce FJ, et al: Cardiopulmonary response of the rat to gram-negative bacteremia. Am J Physiol 246:H344, 1984.
11. Lang CH, Bagby GJ, Ferguson JL, et al: Cardiac output and redistribution of organ blood flow in hypermetabolic sepsis. Am J Physiol 246:P331, 1984.
12. Adams HR, Parker JL, Laughlin MH: Intrinsic myocardial dysfunction during endotoxemia: Dependent or independent of myocardial ischemia? Circ Shock 30:63, 1990.
13. Reilly JM, Cunnion RE, Burch-Whitman C, et al: A circulating myocardial depressant substance is associated with cardiac dysfunction and peripheral hypoperfusion (lactic acidemia) in patients with septic shock. Chest 95:1072, 1989.
14. Raffa J, Trunkey DD: Myocardial depression in sepsis. J Trauma 18:617, 1978.
15. Shepherd RE, McDonough KH, Burns AH: Mechanisms of cardiac dysfunction in hearts from endotoxin-treated rats. Circ Shock 19:371, 1986.
16. Carmona RH, Tsao TC, Trunkey DD: The role of prostacyclin and thromboxane in sepsis and septic shock. Arch Surg 119:189, 1984.
17. Peevy KJ, Reed T, Chartrand SA, et al: The comparison of myocardial dysfunction in three forms of experimental septic shock. Pediatr Res 20:1240, 1986.
18. Meyrick B, Brigham KL: Acute effects of *Escherichia coli* endotoxin on the pulmonary microcirculation of anesthetized sheep structure: function relationships. Lab Invest 48:458, 1983.
19. Grisham MB, Everse J, Janssen HF: Endotoxemia and neutrophil activation in vivo. Am J Physiol 254:H1017, 1988.
20. Korthuis RJ, Grisham MB, Granger DN: Leukocyte depletion attenuates vascular injury in postischemic skeletal muscle. Am J Physiol 254:H823, 1988.
21. Brigham KL, Meyrick B: Endotoxin and lung injury. Am Rev Respir Dis 133:913, 1986.
22. Kilbourn RG, Gross SS, Jubran A, et al: N^G-Methyl-L-arginine inhibits tumor necrosis factor–induced hypotension: Implications for the involvement of nitric oxide. Proc Natl Acad Sci USA 87:3629, 1990.
23. Kilbourn RG, Jubran A, Gross SS, et al: Reversal of endotoxin-mediated shock by N^G-methyl-L-arginine, an inhibitor of nitric oxide synthesis. Biochem Biophys Res Commun 172:1132, 1990.
24. Julou-Schaeffer G, Gray G, Fleming I, et al: Loss of vascular responsiveness induced by endotoxin involves L-arginine pathway. Am J Physiol 259:H1038, 1990.
25. Beasley D, Cohen R, Levinsky N: Endotoxin inhibits contraction of vascular smooth muscle in vitro. Am J Physiol 258:H1187, 1990.
26. Wylam M, Samsel R, Umans J: Endotoxin in vivo impairs endothelium dependent relaxation of canine arteries in vitro. Am Rev Respir Dis 142:1263, 1990.
27. Gutierrez G, Lund N, Palizas F: Rabbit skeletal muscle Po_2 during hypodynamic sepsis. Chest 99:224, 1991.
28. Gutierrez G, Lund N, Acero AL, et al: Relationship of venous Po_2 to muscle Po_2 during hypoxemia. J Appl Physiol 67:1093, 1989.
29. Lund N, Damon DH, Damon DN, et al: Capillary grouping in hamster tibialis anterior muscles: Flow patterns and physiological significance. Int J Microcirc Clin Exp 5:359, 1987.
30. Kopp KH, Sinagowitz E, Muller H: Oxygen supply of skeletal muscle in experimental septic shock. In: Lubbers DW, Acker H, Leniger-Follert E, et al (eds): Oxygen Transport to Tissue, Volume V. New York, Plenum Publishing, p 467, 1984.
31. Chance B, Leigh JS, Clark BJ, et al: Control of oxidative metabolism and oxygen delivery in human skeletal muscle: A steady-state analysis of the work/energy cost transfer function. Proc Natl Acad Sci USA 82:8384, 1985.
32. Gevers W: Generation of protons by metabolic processes in heart cells. J Mol Cell Cardiol 9:864, 1977.
33. Mainwood GW, Renaud JM: The effect of acid base balance on fatigue of skeletal muscle. Can J Physiol Pharmacol 63:403, 1985.
34. Bessman SP: The creatine–creatine phosphate energy shuttle. Annu Rev Biochem 54:831, 1985.
35. Gutierrez G, Lund N, Bryan-Brown CW: Cellular oxygen utilization during multiple organ failure. Crit Care Clin 5:271, 1989.
36. Granger DN, Hollwarth MA, Parks DA: Ischemia reperfusion injury: Role of oxygen derived free radicals. Acta Physiol Scand [Suppl 548] 126:47, 1986.
37. Morgan RA, Manning PB, Coran AG, et al: Oxygen free radical activity during live *E. coli* septic shock in the dog. Circ Shock 25:319, 1988.
38. Novotny MJ, Laughlin MH, Adams HR: Evidence for lack of importance of oxygen free radicals in *Escherichia coli* endotoxemia in dogs. Am J Physiol 254:H954, 1988.
39. Shiki Y, Meyrick BO, Brigham KL, et al: Endotoxin increases superoxide dismutase in cultured bovine pulmonary endothelial cells. Am J Physiol 252:C436, 1987.
40. Amaral J, Shearer J, Mastrofrancesco B: The effect of endotoxin on glucose metabolism in skeletal muscle requires the presence of plasma. Arch Surg 124:727, 1989.
41. Wolfe RR, Dariush E, Spitzer JJ: Glucose and lactate kinetics after endotoxin administration in dogs. Am J Physiol 232:E180, 1977.
42. Merril, GF, Spitzer JJ: Glucose and lactate kinetics in guinea pigs following *Escherichia coli* endotoxin administration. Circ Shock 5:11, 1978.
43. Hinshaw LB, Beller BK, Archer LT, et al: Hypoglycemic response of blood to live *Escherichia coli* organisms and endotoxin. J Surg Res 21:141, 1976.
44. Pappova E, Urbaschek B, Heitmann L, et al: Energy-rich phosphates and glucose metabolism in early endotoxin shock. J Surg Res 11:506, 1971.
45. Romanosky AJ, Bagby GJ, Bockman EL, et al: Increased muscle glucose uptake and lactate release after endotoxin administration. Am J Physiol 239:E311, 1980.
46. Raymond RM, Harkema JM, Emerson TE, et al: Insulin like action of *E. coli* in promoting skeletal muscle glucose uptake in the dog. Adv Shock Res 6:141, 1981.
47. Kober PM, Thomas JX, Filkins JP: Glucose dyshomeostasis and cardiovascular failure in endotoxic dogs. Am J Physiol 249:R570, 1985.
48. Marrou A, Turner D, Oglethorpe N: Fructose 1,6-diphosphate: An agent for treatment of experimental endotoxin shock. Surgery 90:482, 1981.
49. Lundsgaard-Hansen P, Pappova E, Urbaschek B, et al: Circulatory deterioration as the determinant of oxygen energy metabolism in endotoxin shock. J Surg Res 13:282, 1972.
50. Vary TC, Siegel JH, Nakatani T, et al: Effect of sepsis on activity of PDH complex in skeletal muscle and liver. Am J Physiol 250:E634, 1986.
51. Kilpatrick-Smith L, Erecinska M: Cellular effects of endotoxin in vitro. I. Effect of endotoxin on mitochondrial substrate metabolism and intracellular calcium. Circ Shock 11:85, 1983.
52. Park R, Arieff AI: Treatment of lactic acidosis with dichloroacetate in dogs. J Clin Invest 70:853, 1982.
53. Vary TC, Siegel JH, Tall BD, et al: Metabolic effect of partial reversal of pyruvate dehydrogenase activity by dichloroacetate in sepsis. Circ Shock 24:3, 1988.
54. Fink MP, Cohn SM, Lee PC, et al: Effect of lipopolysaccharide on intestinal mucosal hydrogen concentration in pigs: Evidence of gut ischemia in a normodynamic model of septic shock. Crit Care Med 17:641, 1989.
55. Fiddian-Green R, Pittenger G, Whitehouse WM: Back-diffusion of CO_2 and its influence on the intramural pH in gastric mucosa. J Surg Res 33:39, 1982.
56. Fiddian-Green RG: Studies in splanchnic ischemia and multiple organ failure. In: Marston A, Bulkley GB, Fiddian-Green RG, et al (eds): Splanchnic Ischemia and Multiple Organ Failure. St Louis, CV Mosby, p 349, 1989.
57. Wright CJ, Duff JH, McLean APH, et al: Regional capillary blood flow and oxygen uptake in severe sepsis. Surg Gynecol Obstet 132:637, 1971.
58. Hotchkiss R, Long R, Hall J: An in vivo examination of rat brain during sepsis with ^{31}P-NMR spectroscopy. Am J Physiol 257:C1055, 1989.
59. Mela L, Bacalzo LV, Miller LD: Defective oxidative metabolism of rat liver mitochondria in hemorrhagic and endotoxin shock. Am J Physiol 220:571, 1971.
60. Poderoso JJ, Boveris A, Jorge MA, et al: Function mitochondrial en el shock septico. Medicina 38:371, 1978.
61. Dawson KL, Geller ER, Kirkpatrick JR: Enhancement of mitochondrial function in sepsis. Arch Surg 123:241, 1988.
62. Chaudry IH, Wichterman KA, Baue AE: Effect of sepsis on tissue adenine nucleotide levels. Surgery 85:205, 1979.
63. Pasque MK, Murphy CE, Van Tright P, et al: Myocardial adenosine triphosphate levels during early sepsis. Arch Surg 118:1437, 1983.
64. Myrvold HE, Enger E, Haljamae H: Early effects of endotoxin on tissue phosphagen levels in skeletal muscle and liver of the dog. Eur Surg Res 7:181, 1975.
65. Jepson M, Cox P, Bates N: Regional blood flow and skeletal muscle energy status in endotoxemic rats. Am J Physiol 252:E581, 1987.
66. Gutierrez G, Dubin A: Cellular metabolism in sepsis. In: Gutierrez G, Vincent JL (eds): Update in Intensive Care and Emergency Medicine, Volume 12, Tissue Oxygen Utilization. New York, Springer-Verlag, p 227, 1990.
67. Hotchkiss RS, Long RC, Hall JR, et al: An in vivo examination of rat brain during sepsis with ^{31}P-NMR spectroscopy. Am J Physiol 257:C1055, 1989.
68. Wagner PD: An integrated view of the determinants of maximum oxygen uptake. Adv Exp Med Biol 227:245, 1988.
69. Cain SM: Supply dependency of oxygen uptake in ARDS: Myth or reality? Am J Med Sci 288:119, 1984.70.
70. Moreno LF, Stratton HH, Newell JC, et al: Mathematical coupling of data: Correction of a common error for linear calculations. J Appl Physiol 60:335, 1986.
71. Ronco JJ, Phang PT, Wiggs B, et al: Does oxygen consumption depend on delivery in patients who have the adult respiratory distress syndrome (ARDS)? Am Rev Respir Dis 141:A584, 1990.
72. Gutierrez G, Pohil RJ: Oxygen consumption is linearly related to O_2 supply in critically ill patients. J Crit Care 1:45, 1986.

73. Bihari D, Smithies M, Gimson A, et al: The effects of vasodilation with prostacyclin on oxygen delivery and uptake in critically ill patients. N Engl J Med 317:397, 1987.
74. Samsel RW, Nelson DP, Sanders WN, et al: Effect of endotoxin on systemic and skeletal muscle O_2 extraction. J Appl Physiol 65:1377, 1988.
75. Nelson DP, Samsel RW, Wood L, et al: Pathological supply dependence of systemic and intestinal O_2 uptake during endotoxemia. J Appl Physiol 64:2410, 1988.
76. Astiz ME, Rackow EC, Falk JL, et al: Oxygen delivery and consumption in patients with hyperdynamic septic shock. Crit Care Med 15:26, 1987.
77. Bronsveld WA, van Lambalgen AA, van den Bos GC, et al: Regional blood flow and metabolism in canine endotoxin shock before, during, and after infusion of glucose-insulin-potassium (GIK). Circ Shock 18:31, 1986.
78. Duff JH, Groves AC, McLean APH, et al: Defective oxygen consumption in septic shock. Surg Gynecol Obstet 128:1051, 1969.
79. Broadie TA, Homer L, Herman CM, et al: Effect of endotoxin on oxygen consumption by a flow-controlled canine hindlimb preparation. Surgery 88:566, 1980.
80. Houtchens BA, Westenskow DR: Oxygen consumption in septic shock: Collective review. Circ Shock 13:361, 1984.
81. Cain SM: Assessment of tissue oxygenation. Crit Care Clin 2:536, 1986.
82. Kreuzer F, Cain SM: Regulation of the peripheral vasculature and tissue oxygenation in health and disease. Crit Care Clin 1:453, 1985.
83. Shoemaker W, Appel P, Kram H, et al: Prospective trial of supranormal values of survivors as therapeutic goals in high risk surgical patients. Chest 94:1176, 1988.
84. Shoemaker W, Appel P, Kram H: Tissue oxygen debt as a determinant of lethal and non lethal postoperative organ failure. Crit Care Med 16:1117, 1988.
85. Russell JA, Ronco JJ, Lockhat D, et al: Oxygen delivery and consumption and ventricular preload are greater in survivors than in nonsurvivors of the adult respiratory distress syndrome. Am Rev Respir Dis 141:659, 1990.
86. Tuchschmidt J, Fried J, Swinnery R, et al: Early hemodynamic correlates of survival in patients with septic shock. Crit Care Med 17:719, 1989.
87. Kaufman BS, Rackow EC, Falk JL: The relationship between oxygen delivery and consumption during fluid resuscitation of hypovolemic and septic shock. Chest 85:336, 1984.
88. Wolf YG, Cotev S, Perel A, et al: Dependence of oxygen consumption on cardiac output in sepsis. Crit Care Med 15:198, 1987.
89. Edwards JD, Brown GC, Brown S, et al: Use of survivors' cardiorespiratory values as therapeutic goals in septic shock. Crit Care Med 17:1098, 1989.
90. Lucking S, Williams T, Chaten F, et al: Dependence of oxygen consumption on oxygen delivery in children with hyperdynamic septic shock and in oxygen extraction. Crit Care Med 18:1316, 1990.
91. Haupt M, Gilbert E, Carlson R: Fluid loading increases oxygen consumption in septic patients with lactic acidosis. Am Rev Respir Dis 131:912, 1985.
92. Gilbert E, Haupt M, Mandanas R, et al: The effect of fluid loading, blood transfusion, and catecholamine infusion on oxygen delivery and consumption in patients with sepsis. Am Rev Respir Dis 134:873, 1986.
93. Kruse J, Haupt M, Puri V, et al: Lactate levels as predictors of the relationship between oxygen delivery and consumption in ARDS. Chest 98:959, 1990.
94. Vincent JL, Reman A, Kahn R: Dobutamine administration in septic shock: Addition to a standard protocol. Crit Care Med 18:689, 1990.
95. Bollaert P, Bauer P, Audibert G, et al: Effects of epinephrine on hemodynamics and oxygen metabolism in dopamine resistant septic shock. Chest 98:949, 1990.
96. Bouffard Y, Tissot S, Viale J, et al: The effects of norepinephrine infusion on oxygen consumption in a patient with septic shock. Intensive Care Med 16:133–134, 1990.
97. Colardyn NF, Vandenbogaerde J, Vogelaers D, et al: Use of dopexamine hydrochloride in patients with septic shock. Crit Care Med 19:999, 1989.
98. Ziegler E, Fisher C, Sprung C, et al: Treatment of gram negative bacteremia and septic shock with HA-1A human monoclonal antibody against endotoxin. N Engl J Med 324:429, 1991.
99. Michie H, Manogue K, Spriggs D, et al: Detection of circulating tumor necrosis factor after endotoxin administration. N Engl J Med 318:1481, 1988.
100. Doglio G, Pusajo J, Egurrola M, et al: Gastric mucosa pH as a prognostic index of mortality in critically ill patients. Crit Care Med. In press.
101. Fiddian-Green R, Baker S: Predictive value of the stomach wall pH for complications after cardiac operations: Comparison with other monitoring. Crit Care Med 15:153, 1987.
102. Gys T, Hubens A, Neus H, et al: Prognostic value of gastric intramural pH in surgical intensive care patients. Crit Care Med 16:1222, 1988.
103. Gutierrez G, Bismar H, Dantzker DR, et al: Comparison of gastric intramucosal pH to measures of oxygen transport and consumption in critically ill patients. Crit Care Med 20:451, 1992.

CHAPTER 28

Treatment of Sepsis and Septic Shock: Standard and Experimental Therapies

Michael A. Solomon
Charles Natanson

You know that medicines when well used restore health to the sick: they will be well used when the doctor together with his understanding of their nature shall understand also what man is, what life is, and what constitution and health are. Know these well and you will know their opposites; and when this is the case you will know how to devise a remedy.

Leonardo da Vinci, Codice Atlantico, 270

EPIDEMIOLOGY

Sepsis and septic shock account for a significant portion of the morbidity and mortality in critical care units in the United States.[1, 2] Hospital-acquired infections are responsible for annual health care expenditures of $5 billion to $10 billion in the United States.[3, 4] The National Hospital Discharge Survey recorded 2.57 million discharge diagnoses of septicemia from 1979 through 1987. During the 9 years reviewed by this survey, the hospital discharge diagnosis of septicemia increased 139%, from 73.6 to 175.9 per 100,000 persons discharged.[4] This increased rate of septicemia occurred over all geographic regions and age groups analyzed.[4] The incidence of septicemia will probably continue to rise because of the increasing number of immunodeficient patients and the more prevalent use of invasive medical technology. Furthermore, the increased use of intensive life-support procedures and broad-spectrum antibiotics has created a large hospital-based population at risk for nosocomial infections by resistant microorganisms. The mortality rate of patients with the septic syndrome, treated with standard therapy (antibiotics and intensive life support), has been estimated at 25 to 65%.[4–7] Thus, effective new therapies integrated with current standard regimens are needed.

PATHOGENESIS

The pathogenesis of sepsis and septic shock is complex and not completely understood. Sepsis and septic shock may begin with the entry of microorganisms (bacteria, fungi, or protozoa) or their toxins (endotoxin, exotoxins, and cell wall and membrane components) into the blood stream, usually from a nidus of infection (Fig. 28–1). These events trigger host cells (neutrophil, monocyte-macrophage) to release a variety of interacting cytokines (tumor necrosis factor [TNF], interleukins, and interferons). This results in the activation of several pathways (complement, coagulation, fibrinolytic, and hormonal) and the increased production of numerous endogenous mediators (C5a, eicosanoids, endorphins, toxic oxygen radicals, nitric oxide, and platelet-activating factor [PAF]).[1, 7–17] The reader is referred to Chapter 23 for a more in-depth discussion of these processes.

The ensuing peripheral and pulmonary vascular effects,

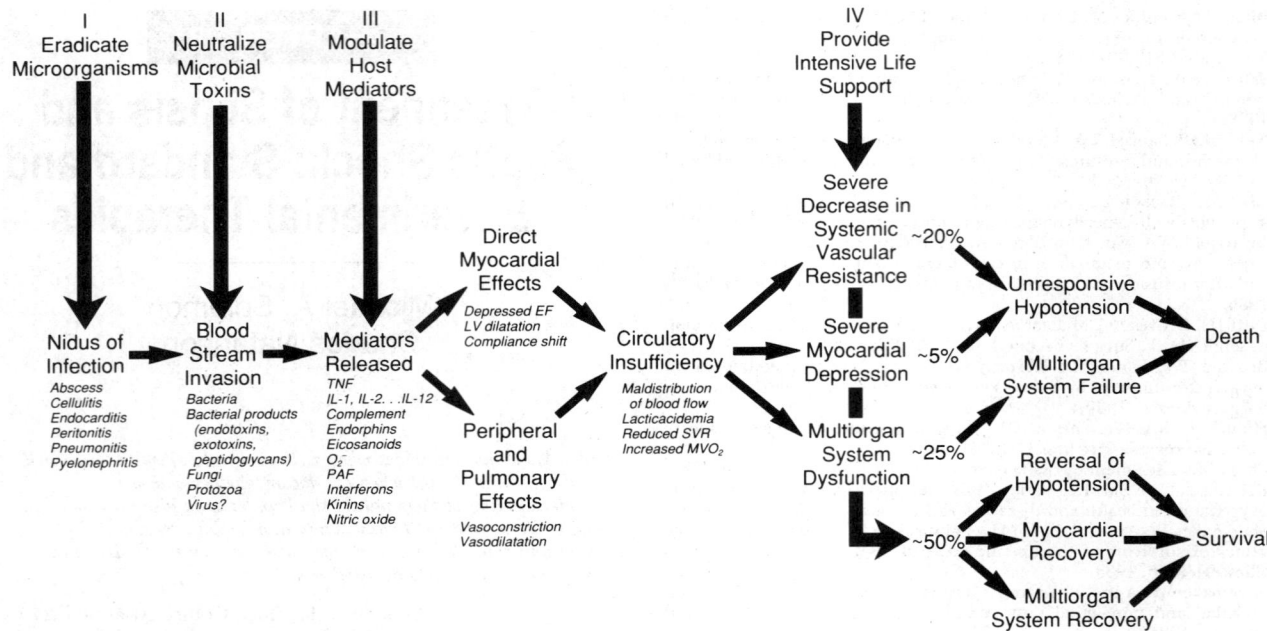

Figure 28–1. An integrated four-step approach to the treatment of sepsis and septic shock based on the pathogenesis of the disease, from the nidus of infection to unresponsive hypotension and multisystem dysfunction. Invading microorganisms release toxic bacterial products into the blood stream, triggering the activation of host mediators leading to direct myocardial, peripheral, and pulmonary vascular effects that result in circulatory insufficiency. These events can cause death through either refractory hypotension or multiple organ system failure. Treatment is designed to prevent and reverse these deleterious effects at multiple points in the pathogenesis of septic shock: (1) eradicate microorganisms to sterilize foci of infection; (2) neutralize microbial toxins to prevent their deleterious effects; (3) modulate host mediators to limit and reverse harmful endogenous responses; and (4) provide intensive life support to maintain vital organ functions. TNF = tumor necrosis factor; IL-1 = interleukin-1; IL-2 = interleukin-2; IL-12 = interleukin-12; O_2^- = toxic oxygen radicals; PAF = platelet-activating factor; EF = ejection fraction; SVR = systemic vascular resistance; MVO_2 = myocardial oxygen consumption. (Modified from Natanson C, Hoffman WD: Septic shock and other forms of distributive shock. In: Parrillo JE [ed]: Current Therapy in Critical Care Medicine. 2nd ed. Philadelphia, BC Decker, p 62, 1991.)

together with direct myocardial effects, may cause a distributive shock characterized by decreased mean arterial pressure (MAP), decreased left ventricular (LV) filling pressure, reduced total peripheral resistance, and normal to increased cardiac output (CO) (Table 28–1, Fig. 28–2). In addition, the LV ejection fraction is depressed.[5, 6, 18–21] With adequate

volume resuscitation, the left ventricle dilates and stroke volume is maintained by Frank-Starling mechanisms. In survivors, these abnormalities in cardiac function resolve in 7 to 10 days[5, 18–20, 22] (Fig. 28–3). In nonsurvivors, the septic syndrome progresses to refractory hypotension, with insufficient tissue oxygen delivery resulting in multiple organ system failure and death.

To be most efficacious, the treatment strategy for sepsis and septic shock should be an integrated, four-step approach (see Fig. 28–1) consisting of (1) eradicating microorganisms; (2) neutralizing microbial toxins; (3) modulating host mediators; and (4) providing intensive life support (Table 28–2). Standard therapies address primarily the initial and final phases of this paradigm. Experimental therapies aim at attenuating the effects of microbial toxins and harmful host mediators.

FOUR-STEP THERAPEUTIC APPROACH

Step 1: Eradicate Microorganisms

Eradicating microorganisms involves prompt antibiotic administration and judicious drainage of infected sites (see Table 28–2). The history and physical examination, along with preliminary roentgenograms and laboratory data, should guide the clinician in obtaining cultures and locating sites of pus or loculated fluid for immediate drainage or further definition by radiologic studies. When the septic syndrome is suspected, blood cultures should be obtained from at least two different sites, and if indicated, additional cultures should be obtained from sputum, urine, and other

---

TABLE 28–1

CLASSIFICATION OF SHOCK

Distributive
Septic
Anaphylactic
Endocrinologic (e.g., thyroid storm, adrenal insufficiency)
Neurogenic
Toxic/drug

Cardiogenic
Myopathic (infarction, cardiomyopathy)
Mechanical (valvular disease, ventricular septal defect, ventricular aneurysm)
Dysrhythmic

Extracardiac Obstructive
Pericardial tamponade
Pulmonary emboli (massive)

Oligemic
Hemorrhage
Fluid depletion (protracted vomiting, diarrhea)

Modified from Natanson C, Hoffman WD: Septic shock and other forms of distributive shock. In: Parrillo JE (ed): Current Therapy in Critical Care Medicine. 2nd ed. Philadelphia, BC Decker, p 62, 1991.

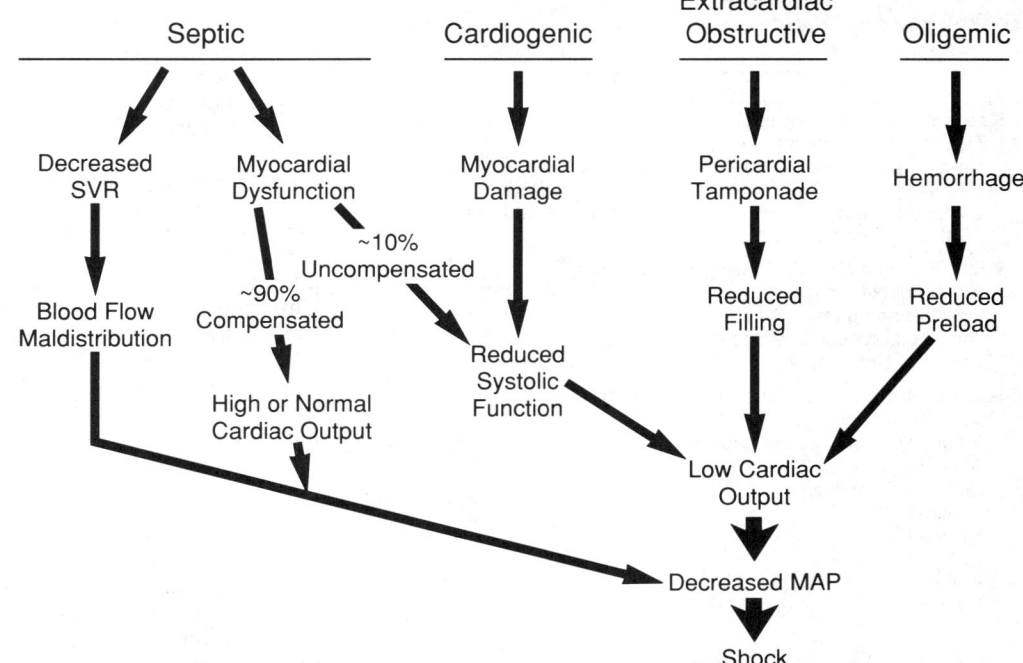

Figure 28–2. The different types of shock. Cardiogenic shock, extracardiac obstructive shock, and oligemic shock are characterized by a low-CO state causing hypotension, whereas in septic shock approximately 90% of the patients have a normal to high CO with a severe decrease in systemic vascular resistance (SVR), leading to hypotension. (Modified from Natanson C, Hoffman WD: Septic shock and other forms of distributive shock. In: Parrillo JE [ed]: Current Therapy in Critical Care Medicine. 2nd ed. Philadelphia, BC Decker, p 62, 1991.)

possible sites of infection (i.e., abscesses, loculated fluids, transcutaneous drains).

Initial antibiotic therapy is usually empirical, even though the site of infection may be clinically apparent, because identification of causative organisms and sensitivity testing may take several days. Treatment must be directed toward all possible pathogens indicated by a careful history and physical examination. For hospitalized patients, it is important to consider the profile of pathogens found at that institution.

Sepsis or septic shock can exist with no identifiable source of infection and with negative blood culture results. Such states are commonly seen in neutropenic patients and may represent microscopic foci of infection with transient release of microbial toxins or bacteria into the blood stream. In addition, patients who received antibiotics before cultures were obtained are less likely to have a causative organism identified.

For patients with sepsis or septic shock, an empirical antimicrobial regimen should have a broad spectrum. We

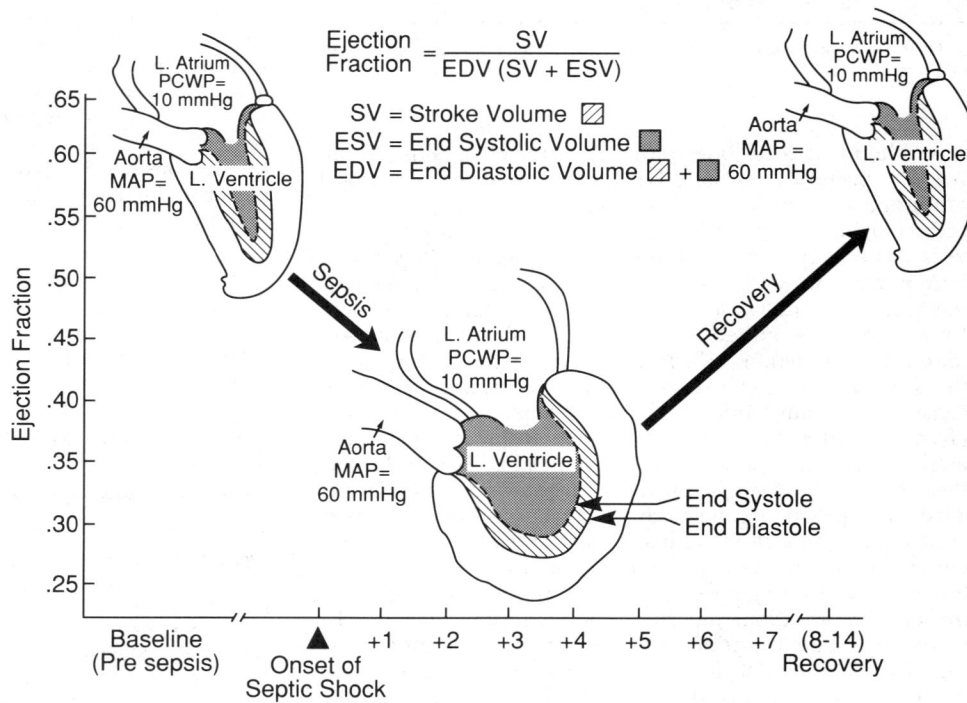

Figure 28–3. Serial changes in LV size and function during the first 2 weeks after the onset of septic shock. PCWP = pulmonary capillary wedge pressure. (Modified from Natanson C, Hoffman WD, Parrillo JE: Septic shock: The cardiovascular abnormality and therapy. J Cardiothorac Anesth 3:215, 1989.)

TABLE 28–2

THERAPY FOR SEPSIS AND SEPTIC SHOCK: AN INTEGRATED, FOUR-STEP APPROACH

Step 1. Eradicate Microorganisms
  Obtain necessary cultures
  Start empirical antibiotic adminstration (broad spectrum)
  Perform preliminary laboratory and radiologic studies
  Eliminate source of infection (drain abscesses and remove infected foreign bodies)

Step 2. Neutralize Microbial Toxins (Investigational)
  Antiendotoxin antibodies
  Lipid A analogues
  Cationic polypeptide antibiotics
  Plasma detoxification

Step 3. Modulate Host Mediators (Investigational)
  Anti-TNF antibodies
  Interleukin-1 receptor antagonists
  Anti-C5a antibodies
  Eicosanoid inhibitors
  Anticoagulants
  Pentoxifylline
  PAF antagonists
  Antioxidants
  Naloxone
  Corticosteroids

Step 4. Provide Intensive Life Support
  Critical care setting
  Patient monitoring
    Right-sided heart catheterization
    Intra-arterial blood pressure monitoring
    Cardiac rhythm monitoring
    Metabolic and hemodynamic profiles
  Cardiovascular support
    Correct anemia, hypoxemia, acidosis, and electrolyte abnormalities
    Volume resuscitation
      If MAP* < 60 mm Hg, use volume expanders to obtain a PCWP of 12–15 mm Hg
    Vasopressor therapy
      If MAP < 60 mm Hg despite a PCWP of 12–15 mm Hg, use pressor agents (see Table 28–4 and Fig. 28–7 for specific pressor agents)

*MAP = mean arterial pressure; PCWP = pulmonary capillary wedge pressure.

recommend at least one antibiotic directed against gram-positive bacteria and another antibiotic directed against gram-negative bacteria, or a single antibiotic with broad activity against both gram-positive and gram-negative bacteria. If indicated, specific antimicrobials against *Streptococcus faecalis* and *Streptococcus faecium, Staphylococcus epidermidis,* methicillin-resistant *Staphylococcus aureus,* anaerobes, and fungi should be added. If the patient is immunocompromised or if infection with *Pseudomonas* species is suspected, therapy directed against gram-negative organisms should consist of two antibiotics of different classes (i.e., an aminoglycoside and a third-generation cephalosporin, or an aminoglycoside and a semisynthetic penicillin). Not only may these drugs act synergistically, but they also provide "insurance" against an organism that may be resistant to either antibiotic. After culture and sensitivity results are available, empirical therapy can be tailored, but caution is required because culture-negative sepsis and septic shock may be present. In addition, all causative organisms may not be recovered. The duration of antimicrobial treatment may vary from 10 days to more than 6 weeks and depends on the location, extent, and source of the infection and the underlying clinical condition of the patient.

In summary, eradicating microorganisms entails prompt institution of broad-spectrum antimicrobials and, when appropriate, drainage of specific foci of infection and removal of necrotic tissue and infected foreign bodies. However, despite aggressive standard therapy, the morbidity and mortality associated with sepsis and septic shock remain high. This severe, acute toxicity may be caused by the antibiotic-unresponsive interactions between circulating microbial toxins and the multiple endogenous mediators they invoke. Certain animal and human data suggest that although bactericidal antibiotics can reduce the levels of bacteremia, the plasma levels of free endotoxin may continue to rise.[23–25] This may partly explain the continuing deterioration of some patients despite appropriate antimicrobial therapy. Thus, experimental therapies have focused on supplementing standard therapies with properly timed new strategies that neutralize microbial toxins and modulate harmful host mediators.

New Therapies

The therapies described in the next two sections focus on neutralizing microbial toxins and modulating host mediators. Some of the agents have shown efficacy in large multicenter clinical trials (antiendotoxin monoclonal antibodies), others only in animal models (monoclonal antibodies to TNF). To date, no therapy of sepsis aimed at reversing the effects of bacterial toxins or harmful endogenous mediators has gained widespread clinical acceptance. However, these new agents offer promise in reducing the high mortality of sepsis and septic shock, and they are presented in detail to offer the reader insight into the investigative path leading to their possible U.S. Food and Drug Administration approval and clinical acceptance.

Step 2: Neutralize Microbial Toxins

Gram-negative bacteria are frequent etiologic agents of sepsis and septic shock. A major toxic component of gram-negative bacteria is endotoxin, a lipopolysaccharide (LPS) found in the outer membrane. Endotoxin can be conceptualized as having three parts[9, 26, 27] (Fig. 28–4). The O-specific side chain is a hypervariable hydrophilic polysaccharide that is specific for bacterial species and serotype. The R core region is a less variable oligosaccharide that bridges the O-specific side chain and lipid A region. The lipid A region is embedded within the bacterial membrane and is highly conserved across different genera of gram-negative bacteria. Lipid A is considered to be the toxic moiety of endotoxin.

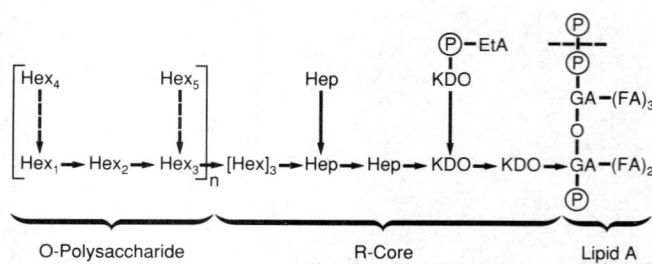

Figure 28–4. Schematic of the tripartite structure of endotoxin (lipopolysaccharide [LPS]). Hex = hexose; Hep = heptose; KDO = 2-keto-3-deoxyoctonate; P = phosphate; EtA = ethanolamine; GA = glucosamine; FA = fatty acid. (Modified, with permission, from Danner RL: Mediators and endotoxin inhibitors, p 235. In: Parrillo JE [moderator]: Septic shock in humans: Advances in the understanding of pathogenesis, cardiovascular dysfunction, and therapy. Ann Intern Med 1990; 113:227–242.)

Several lines of evidence suggest a primary role for endotoxin in gram-negative bacterial sepsis and septic shock.[21, 28–31] Endotoxin, when administered to canines or healthy human volunteers, produces cardiovascular changes similar to those observed in human septicemia.[21, 29] Endotoxemia in human sepsis and septic shock has been correlated with important clinical outcomes, including lactic acidemia, renal insufficiency, adult respiratory distress syndrome, myocardial dysfunction, multiple organ system failure, and death.[30, 31] Experimental therapies attempting to attenuate or neutralize microbial toxins are primarily directed at limiting endotoxemia (see Table 28–2).

Antiendotoxin Antibodies

Antibodies against O-specific polysaccharide side chains of a particular gram-negative strain confer a survival advantage.[32, 33] Unfortunately, the wide-ranging antigenic diversity inherent in the O-specific side chain limits the practicality of this type of therapy. It has been known for some time that chemical degradation of O-specific polysaccharide side chains of gram-negative bacteria exposes the highly conserved core–lipid A region.[34] In the 1960s, investigators hypothesized that antibodies against the core–lipid A region of gram-negative bacteria may bind and neutralize a wide range of gram-negative organisms with serologically unrelated O-specific side chains.[34] The past two decades have seen considerable scientific progress in this area.

Investigators examining acute-phase serum specimens from patients with gram-negative bacteremia showed that high titers of naturally occurring antibody to the core–lipid A region were associated with a lower frequency of shock and death.[35] Thus, human polyclonal immune serum directed against endotoxin core–lipid A determinants was developed by immunizing volunteers with the heat-inactivated rough mutant *Escherichia coli* J5 (a gram-negative bacterium with an exposed core–lipid A region).[36] In a randomized controlled human trial, J5 antiserum, when given at the onset of gram-negative bacteremia, substantially lowered mortality (22% [23 of 103] vs. 39% [42 of 109], P = .011). The identity of the protective factor in this antiserum was never satisfactorily determined.[37, 38]

Monoclonal antiendotoxin antibodies with defined specificity have the potential to be a more potent therapy while posing less risk of transmitting infectious agents than the polyclonal antiserum. Monoclonal antibodies have been developed against both the O-specific polysaccharide and core–lipid A regions of endotoxin.[33, 39, 40] Monoclonal antiendotoxin antibodies have been shown to be protective in animal models of gram-negative sepsis and septic shock.[33, 39, 41] A murine immunoglobulin M (E5) and a human immunoglobulin M (HA-1A) monoclonal antibody to the J5 mutant's lipid A region of endotoxin have already been used in and are continuing to undergo clinical trials. They were found to be safe in human volunteers without gram-negative bacteremia, as well as in patients with gram-negative bacteremia.[42–45] In a large, multicenter, prospective, double-blind, randomized, placebo-controlled clinical trial, standard therapy plus E5 at a dose of 2 mg/kg given once daily for 2 days did not confer a survival advantage in the overall population of 316 documented gram-negative infections, but in a subpopulation of 137 patients with gram-negative bacteremia without "severe" shock, mortality was significantly reduced.[46] In a separate large, multicenter, prospective, double-blind, randomized, placebo-controlled clinical trial, standard therapy plus a single 100-mg dose of HA-1A significantly reduced mortality in the subpopulation of patients with gram-negative bacteremia and shock (33% [18 of 54] vs. 57% [27 of 54], P = .017).[47] The conflicting results in the two studies

have not been resolved. U.S. Food and Drug Administration approval is pending.

At present, the clinical data in support of monoclonal antibodies reactive with the lipid A region of endotoxin are based on subgroup analysis, and although they are suggestive of efficacy, they are not confirmatory. Furthermore, the exact mechanisms by which monoclonal antibodies lower lethality (i.e., enhanced bacterial/LPS clearance, attenuation of LPS-induced host reactions, nonspecific immunomodulation) are unclear. Also antiendotoxin therapies offer no proven benefit to patients with fungal, gram-positive bacterial, and blood culture–negative sepsis, which in total represents a large portion of the cases of sepsis.[47] Even in patients with documented gram-negative bacteremia and shock who are treated with antiendotoxin antibodies, the mortality is still relatively high. This further serves to emphasize the need for a more comprehensive approach to the treatment of sepsis and septic shock.

Lipid A Analogues

Another area of active investigation relates to lipid A analogues, which are compounds structurally similar to the toxic lipid A moiety of endotoxin. To be therapeutic, lipid A analogues should maintain beneficial immunostimulatory activities but lack toxicity. Several lipid A analogues have been investigated. Of these, deacylated lipopolysaccharide (deacylated LPS), lipid X (2,3-diacylglucosamine-1-phosphate), and monophosphoryl lipid A have shown the most therapeutic potential.[26, 48–53]

Deacylated LPS is formed from endotoxin by the hydrolysis of certain acyloxyacyl bonds.[52, 54] Acyloxyacyl hydrolases are found in vivo in neutrophils and may be important in detoxifying endotoxin and modulating the organisms' response to gram-negative sepsis.[54, 55] In vitro, deacylated LPS maintains some of the potential beneficial immunostimulatory properties of endotoxin (B cell mitogenicity) while having greatly reduced tissue toxicity (dermal Shwartzman's reaction).[54] Deacylated LPS inhibits the ability of endotoxin to augment endothelial cell–mediated neutrophil adherence, plasminogen activator inhibitor-1 expression, and prostaglandin production.[55, 56]

Lipid X is a monosaccharide precursor of the disaccharide glucosamine lipid A[27, 48, 50, 57] (Fig. 28–5). In an in vitro neutrophil system, lipid X prevents LPS-induced enhancement of the production of toxic oxygen radicals. These inhibitory effects of lipid X are dose and time dependent. The structural similarity between lipid X and lipid A, as well as this pattern of inhibition, suggests that lipid X functions as a competitive inhibitor of some LPS properties.[58] In vivo lipid X was protective in small animals even when given after a lethal dose of endotoxin.[59] In a large-animal model of endotoxemia, lipid X reduced pulmonary hypertension, pyrogenicity, and mortality.[60] Despite these promising antiendotoxin effects of lipid X, a controlled large-animal septic shock study using viable *E. coli* failed to show any beneficial effects comparing standard therapy (antibiotic and volume resuscitation) alone with standard therapy plus lipid X.[61]

Monophosphoryl lipid A was isolated from *Salmonella* mutants. In vitro, monophosphoryl lipid A inhibits endotoxin-induced enhancement of neutrophil superoxide production.[62] Rats challenged with monophosphoryl lipid A do not exhibit the hemodynamic derangements seen with endotoxin challenges.[53] In animal endotoxin challenges, monophosphoryl lipid A attenuates the adverse cardiovascular effects[63, 64] and improves short-term survival.[64]

Lipid A analogues are still in an early research stage. They may eventually be useful as supplemental therapy for gram-negative bacterial infections, but such adjunctive therapy is

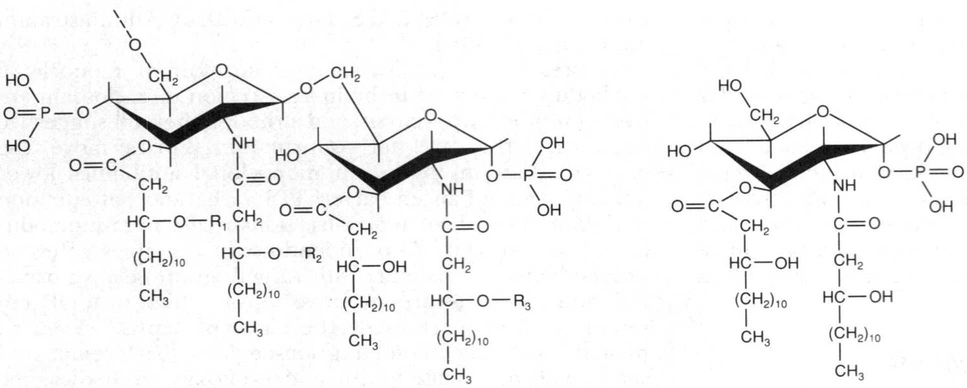

Lipid A

Lipid X

Figure 28–5. The chemical structures of the lipid A (the toxic moiety of endotoxin) and lipid X (a proposed competitive inhibitor of endotoxin) molecules. (Modified, with permission, from Danner RL: Mediators and endotoxin inhibitors, p 235. In: Parrillo JE [moderator]: Septic shock in humans: Advances in the understanding of pathogenesis, cardiovascular dysfunction, and therapy. Ann Intern Med 1990; 113:227–242.)

unlikely to be the complete answer. It is important to remember that the septic syndrome is probably not the result of one single constituent but rather the interaction of several factors. A multiple-phase therapeutic arsenal is still needed.

Cationic Polypeptide Antibiotics

The polycationic antibiotics polymyxin B and colistin, and their closely related derivatives polymyxin B nonapeptide and colistin nonapeptide, have antiendotoxin properties.[65–71] Polymyxin B, the best studied of the group, is thought to exert its anti-LPS effects by tightly binding to endotoxin.[72] In small-animal endotoxic shock models, polymyxin B reduced lethality when given prophylactically, simultaneously with, or temporally close to endotoxin challenge.[70, 73, 74] However, in a large-animal endotoxin challenge model, pretreatment with intramuscular polymyxin B (at doses that were protective in mice) was toxic and ineffective in preventing death.[70] In animal models in which viable gram-negative organisms are used, polymyxin B infusion plus an appropriate nonpolycationic antibiotic also did not significantly reduce mortality;[74, 75] however, polymyxin B therapy did improve morbidity as represented by amelioration of hypotension and acidosis.[74]

Because the polycationic antibiotics have antiendotoxin properties[65, 67, 70, 71, 74] but significant toxicities[70, 76] limiting their therapeutic usefulness, less toxic derivatives were developed and studied. One such derivative, polymyxin B nonapeptide, is without the in vivo toxicities of the parent compound but still possesses antiendotoxin properties in vitro. Unfortunately, it is a much weaker antiendotoxin than the parent compound and is probably still hindered by the need to be given before or simultaneously with endotoxin to be effective.[69] Another method of reducing polymyxin B tissue toxicity uses extracorporeal hemoperfusion with polymyxin B immobilized on a filter. This technique was protective in a large-animal model using an intravenous challenge of live gram-negative bacteria.[77]

Although toxicity, dosage, and timing have been problematic, polycationic antibiotics have intriguing therapeutic potential. Ameliorating endotoxemia in patients is likely to be beneficial. Thus, further in vivo efficacy studies using polycationic antibiotics to attenuate the toxic effects of endotoxin are continuing.

Plasma Detoxification

Besides polymyxin B, other materials can adsorb endotoxin. In vitro, activated charcoal, bentonite, and Kaopectate are more efficient at removing endotoxin from plasma than is polymyxin B bound to Sepharose beads.[78] In a large-animal endotoxic challenge model, extracorporeal activated charcoal hemoperfusion removed the majority of circulating endotoxin from the blood within an hour.[79] There are also case reports indicating that exchange whole blood transfusion in neonates may affect survival by clearing endotoxin.[80]

Several experimental plasma detoxification therapies focus not only on removing endotoxin but also on nonselectively removing all harmful products from the plasma. The rationale for plasma detoxification strategies comes from retrospective and anecdotal evidence in infants and children that exchange blood transfusion as an adjunct to standard antibiotic and volume therapy mitigates the abnormalities of disseminated intravascular coagulation[81] and may improve survival in severe sepsis.[82–84] There are also case reports showing that plasmapheresis combined with standard sepsis therapy improves coagulation parameters and may decrease mortality in patients with severe meningococcal and pneumococcal sepsis.[84–86] It must be emphasized that these reports are anecdotal, and controlled laboratory and prospective clinical trials are needed. A cautionary note is evident from a controlled large-animal bacteremic shock model, which found plasmapheresis to be harmful. Plasmapheresis with plasma exchange worsened hemodynamics and increased mortality in septic animals.[87] A similarly designed large-animal septic shock study using continuous arteriovenous hemofiltration also failed to show any beneficial effect.[88]

The septic syndrome results from complex interactions between bacterial toxins and host responses. As many host mediators are immunomodulators, their actions may range from beneficial to harmful. It is possible that nonselective plasma detoxification schemes (exchange transfusion, hemoperfusion, plasmapheresis, continuous arteriovenous hemofiltration), in addition to removing bacterial toxins, also remove host mediators to the extent that various beneficial effects may be compromised. This lack of selectivity in current plasma detoxification schemes limits their therapeutic utility. One successful plasma detoxification strategy might be to preferentially eliminate microbiologic toxins while regulating the host's endogenous responses so as to leave intact their beneficial immunomodulating properties. Modulation of host mediators is discussed in detail in the next section.

Step 3: Modulate Host Mediators

Endotoxin alone is sufficient but not necessary to produce most of the derangements of the septic syndrome.[29, 89] Gram-positive organisms that lack endotoxin can induce the same cardiovascular abnormalities as gram-negative organisms.[89] Various bacterial products can initiate the syndrome; also, cytokines like TNF and interleukin-1 (IL-1), when infused into animals, produce a shock-like state.[29, 90] Cytokines may act alone or synergistically to induce hemodynamic changes characteristic of septic shock.[90, 91] These findings support the concept that the sequential and concerted action of endogenous mediators, induced by microbial products from various structurally and functionally discrete microorganisms, is the common pathway that produces the typical cardiovascular profile of septic shock.[29] This hypothesis has led investigators to actively research therapies that modulate host mediators (see Table 28–2).

Anti-TNF Antibodies

TNF, also known as cachectin,[92, 93] is secreted primarily by monocyte-macrophages.[94, 95] There is considerable evidence that TNF is a mediator of sepsis and septic shock.[96] In human volunteers, after low intravenous doses of endotoxin, serum TNF levels increase and peak in approximately 90 minutes.[11, 97, 98] In animals, intravenous TNF infusions can cause metabolic acidosis, hypotension, extensive tissue injury, cardiovascular collapse, and death.[13, 29, 96, 99] In patients with septicemia, markedly elevated serum TNF levels were associated with severity of disease.[97, 100] In one clinical study, nonsurvivors of septic shock had elevated serum TNF levels for several days.[101]

In small-animal models of septic shock, polyclonal anti-TNF immune serum[102, 103] and monoclonal anti-TNF antibody,[13] when given prophylactically, protect against the lethal effect of either endotoxin or TNF infusion. However, a marked decrement in the protective ability of polyclonal anti-TNF immune serum was evident when it was given several hours after endotoxin administration.[102] In nonhuman primate shock models in which lethal intravenous infusions of live *E. coli* were used, murine immunoglobulin G monoclonal anti-TNF antibody fragments (F(ab')$_2$) given prophylactically (2 hours before)[104] or complete murine monoclonal anti-TNF antibody[105] given concurrently protected against organ dysfunction and death. A randomized multicenter clinical trial using anti-TNF antibodies to treat patients with septic shock is currently being designed in the United States and Europe (Silverman M, personal communication, 1992).

Clinical enthusiasm for anti-TNF therapy is tempered by the results of a study that compared the efficacy of anti-TNF immunoglobulin G using two different types of toxic challenges.[106] In one model, the animals received an intravenous challenge of endotoxin, whereas in the other model the animal's peritoneum was inoculated with viable *E. coli*. Prophylactic anti-TNF immunoglobulin G improved survival in the intravascular endotoxin challenge model but not in the viable *E. coli* peritonitis model. The peritonitis model may be more representative of the natural course of clinical infection. It is possible that intermittent release of endotoxin by a localized gram-negative bacterial infection results in host cytokine levels and effects different from those observed with intravenous endotoxin challenges. Thus, anti-TNF therapies may not be therapeutic in clinical infections occurring over time, despite being efficacious in intravenous endotoxin challenges.

Host cytokines like TNF possess a wide array of activities. As an immunomodulator, TNF probably has both beneficial and harmful effects.[107, 108] At some level, TNF's enhancement of inflammation may become detrimental. New agents that modulate rather than completely neutralize TNF responses may offer an exciting new therapeutic approach.

Interleukin-1 Receptor Antagonist

IL-1, like TNF, is an immunomodulator that is secreted primarily by monocyte-macrophage cells. IL-1 causes fever, neutrophil activation (chemotaxis, aggregation, and degranulation), B cell and T cell activation, fibroblast proliferation, prostaglandin production, and acute-phase protein synthesis.[14] Intravascular injection of IL-1 into animals produces hypotension, leukopenia, and thrombocytopenia.[90] Clinical studies detect elevated IL-1 levels in the plasma of both normal volunteers given endotoxin infusions[97] and patients with gram-negative sepsis and shock.[12, 101]

A monocyte-derived IL-1 receptor antagonist (IL-1ra) has been isolated and purified.[109] Its DNA has been sequenced,[109, 110] cloned,[110] and expressed in *E. coli*.[110] In vitro, IL-1ra appears to be a pure IL-1 receptor antagonist, with approximately the same affinity as IL-1 for the receptor.[109] In an animal endotoxic shock model, repeated administration of IL-1ra, starting at the time of or up to 2 hours after endotoxin injection, reduced lethality in a dose-dependent manner.[111] Further in vivo studies with animal models more analogous to human sepsis and septic shock are necessary to assess whether IL-1ra will be therapeutically beneficial and practical. Nonetheless, phase II trials have been completed in humans and suggest therapeutically beneficial effects. (Fisher C, personal communication, 1992).

During infection, IL-1 release follows TNF release.[12] The toxicities of IL-1 and TNF are synergistic.[90] However, probably not all of their interactions are deleterious.[108] Clinical data show higher plasma IL-1 levels in survivors compared with nonsurvivors of septic shock.[97] These cytokines also likely have beneficial effects; therefore, new therapies for sepsis may need to modulate rather than completely neutralize cytokine interactions.

Anti-C5a Antibodies

In patients with gram-negative bacteremia, there is activation of both classic[112] and alternative pathways of complement.[112, 113] C5a, an anaphylatoxin, can aggregate and activate neutrophils,[114, 115] increase circulating levels of arachidonic acid metabolites,[116] stimulate monocyte-macrophage secretion of IL-1 and TNF in vitro,[117] and induce increased vascular permeability, systemic vasodilatation, and hypotension in vivo.[116] C5a has also been associated with the adult respiratory distress syndrome.[118]

In vitro, polyclonal anti-C5a antibodies prevent endotoxin-induced leukocyte aggregation.[119] In nonhuman primates, polyclonal anti-C5a antibodies given concurrently with viable *E. coli* protected against early hypotension and impairment of pulmonary gas exchange.[119] In this primate study, the observation period lasted only 4 hours; therefore, no statement on long-term efficacy can be made. Currently, there are no human clinical trial data concerning polyclonal anti-C5a antibodies, but a panel of murine monoclonal anti-C5a antibodies has been developed and is being tested in vitro.[120]

Eicosanoid Inhibitors

Arachidonic acid is liberated from cell membranes by the action of phospholipases. The lipoxygenase and cyclooxygenase enzymes rapidly oxygenate arachidonic acid to produce substrates for a wide range of eicosanoids (leukotrienes [LTs], thromboxane [TX], and prostaglandins). These eicosanoids have diverse pharmacologic activities.[121] Many of their activities promote inflammation. The LTs enhance vascular permeability. LTB$_4$ is a powerful leukocyte chemotactic agent. LTC$_4$, LTD$_4$, and LTE$_4$ cause vasoconstriction, TX promotes platelet aggregation, and prostaglandins E$_2$ and I$_2$ cause vasodilatation.[122] These varied interactions may enhance vascular injury and maldistribution of blood flow, resulting in worsening tissue ischemia. New experimental therapies are focusing on inhibiting eicosanoid production or antagonizing eicosanoid receptors.

The lipoxygenase pathway is responsible for LT production. In vitro, endotoxin can increase the release of LTs from stimulated macrophages and neutrophils.[16, 17] LTD_4 infusions can produce hypotension, hypoxia, and acidosis.[123] These qualities further suggest the importance of LTs as mediators of some of the harmful effects of bacterial products. In a murine endotoxic shock model, coadministration of endotoxin and various lipoxygenase inhibitors attenuates serum TNF levels.[124] The LT inhibitor diethylcarbamazine and the LT antagonist FPL 55712 protected mice against endotoxin-induced lethality.[125] Other LT inhibitors (BW 755C, a dual lipoxygenase and cyclooxygenase inhibitor) and antagonists (LY 171883) have also shown efficacy in small-animal endotoxin challenges.[122, 125–127]

The intrinsic diversity of the LTs and their respective receptors poses a practical problem.[127] Further research is necessary before these LT inhibitors and antagonists can be used selectively and beneficially to modulate the host's response to sepsis.

Like the lipoxygenase pathway, the cyclooxygenase pathway's activity is also probably enhanced during sepsis and septic shock. The cyclooxygenase pathway is responsible for prostaglandin and TX production. The plasma levels of TXB_2 (the stable metabolite of TXA_2) and 6-keto-prostaglandin $F_{1\alpha}$ (the stable metabolite of prostacyclin) rise after infusion of endotoxin in rats[128] or infusion of live *E. coli* in nonhuman primates.[129] Nonsteroidal anti-inflammatory agents like ibuprofen and indomethacin inhibit the cyclooxygenase enzyme and suppress prostaglandin and TX synthesis. In a small-animal model, pretreatment with intravenous ibuprofen can prevent IL-1 and TNF challenges from inducing a shock-like state.[90] In rat endotoxic shock models, pretreatment with intravenous ibuprofen[128] or the thromboxane synthetase inhibitor 7-(1-imidazolyl)-heptanoic acid[130] reduced the rise in TXB_2 plasma levels and improved survival rate. In large-animal endotoxic shock models, the intravenous administration of either aspirin or indomethacin was shown to improve survival.[131] In a canine peritonitis shock model, treatment with either intravenous indomethacin or ibuprofen (24 hours after the onset of infection) restored normal hemodynamics.[132] In normal human volunteers, pretreatment with oral ibuprofen can attenuate endotoxin-induced metabolic responses (fever, tachycardia, hypermetabolism).[11, 133] In a small (29 patients) prospective, multicenter, randomized, double-blind, placebo-controlled clinical trial, standard therapy plus ibuprofen (600 mg [n = 11] or 800 mg [n = 5] intravenously within 4 hours of diagnosis followed by three 800-mg retention enemas on a 6-hour dosing schedule) did not significantly alter hemodynamic and respiratory paramaters or alter survival in patients with the septic syndrome.[133a] A larger clinical trial using a purely intravenous route of administration is being considered.

As with other experimental therapies, caution is advisable. In human volunteers given low doses of endotoxin, inhibition of prostanoids by ibuprofen has resulted in significant increases in plasma TNF levels, despite blunting the LPS-induced clinical responses (i.e., fever, chills, myalgias, headache, and nausea).[134] In septic patients, markedly elevated TNF levels have been associated with increased severity of disease.[97, 100] Furthermore, nonsteroidal anti-inflammatory agents can harm kidney function. Eicosanoids, like the many other possible mediators of sepsis and septic shock, possess a broad spectrum of activities. A deeper understanding of the molecular and cellular pathogenesis of sepsis and septic shock may eventually allow preferential inhibition of the harmful and not the beneficial actions of mediators.

Anticoagulants

Abnormalities of the coagulation and fibrinolytic systems may be prominent early in sepsis and septic shock. These abnormalities may progress to the syndrome of disseminated intravascular coagulation. In the setting of sepsis, the appearance of this syndrome is a poor prognostic sign. The resulting microvascular clotting contributes to blood flow maldistribution and tissue ischemia. Furthermore, procoagulant and platelet consumption, together with accelerated fibrinolysis, can lead to diffuse bleeding. Regulation of the coagulation and fibrinolytic systems during sepsis and septic shock is an area of important investigation. Research has focused on the native anticoagulants antithrombin III (AT-III) and protein C.

AT-III inactivates thrombin and other serine proteases of the coagulation system. Studies suggest that AT-III plasma levels are abnormally decreased in patients with sepsis and disseminated intravascular coagulation.[135–137] In small animals receiving an endotoxin challenge and nonhuman primates receiving a bacterial challenge, prophylactic AT-III infusions (sufficient to increase AT-III plasma levels above premorbid levels) significantly increased survival.[138–141]

Protein C is a potent anticoagulant that inactivates clotting factors Va and VIIIa and enhances fibrinolysis. In nonhuman primates receiving a bacterial challenge, coadministration of activated protein C prevents coagulopathic and lethal effects. Furthermore, if native protein C activation is antagonized, sublethal bacterial challenges become lethal unless exogenous activated protein C is infused in sufficient quantities to prevent the coagulopathic response.[142]

The anticoagulants AT-III and protein C may be important endogenous and therapeutic regulators of the coagulation system in gram-negative sepsis and septic shock. Clinical data on the efficacy of these anticoagulant regimens in sepsis and septic shock are too limited to be conclusive.[143–145] Controlled prospective clinical trials are needed.

Pentoxifylline

Pentoxifylline (a xanthine derivative) is currently used in treating peripheral arterial insufficiency, as it reportedly augments erythrocyte pliability and thus improves capillary blood flow. Data suggest that pentoxifylline may also have anti-inflammatory properties. In vitro, pentoxifylline inhibits platelet aggregation[146] and moderates activated neutrophil inflammatory actions (migration, adherence, degranulation, and superoxide production).[147] In normal human volunteers, treatment with intravenous pentoxifylline prevents the endotoxin-induced increases in plasma TNF levels.[148] In a murine endotoxic shock model, treatment with intravenous pentoxifylline as early as 24 hours before or as late as 7 hours after endotoxin infusion improves survival in a dose-dependent manner.[149] In a large-animal fecal peritonitis sepsis model, pentoxifylline pretreatment attenuated lung, liver, and spleen microvascular and cellular injury.[150] No prospective, controlled clinical trial data are available.

Platelet-Activating Factor Antagonists

PAF is a natural phospholipid found in several cell populations (platelets, neutrophils, monocyte-macrophages, and endothelial cells). Several studies suggest that PAF may be an endogenous mediator of sepsis and septic shock.[151–158] Within 20 minutes after endotoxin challenge in rats, blood PAF levels significantly increase.[151] Patients with either gram-negative or gram-positive sepsis and septic shock have a marked increase in platelet-associated PAF, compared with critically ill patients without sepsis or normal subjects.[152]

Synthetic PAF infused into animals can cause intravascular platelet aggregation,[153] thrombocytopenia,[153, 154] elevation of plasma TXB_2 levels,[154, 155] increased vascular permeability with hemoconcentration,[154–156] hypotension,[153–158] and circulatory collapse.[155]

Several specific PAF receptor antagonists have been studied in animal models. These include kadsurenone,[157] CV-3988,[151, 158, 159] and SRI 63–441.[151, 156] In vitro, CV-3988 inhibits the binding of PAF to the PAF receptor on human platelets and prevents PAF-induced platelet aggregation.[159] In endotoxin- or PAF-challenged rats, kadsurenone and CV-3988 can reverse hypotension.[151, 157, 158] CV-3988 has also been shown to prolong survival in endotoxin-challenged rats.[151, 158] SRI 63–441 can prevent hypotension and hemoconcentration in various animals challenged with PAF.[156]

PAF, through its varied interactions, may promote tissue damage in patients with sepsis and septic shock. PAF receptor antagonists may attenuate tissue injury and prolong survival in sepsis and septic shock. To better evaluate PAF receptor antagonists, further controlled animal studies with models more analogous to human infection are needed.

Antioxidants

Toxic oxygen radicals (i.e., superoxide, hydrogen peroxide, and hydroxyl radical) are capable of damaging compounds of diverse biochemical classes (proteins, carbohydrates, lipids, and nucleic acids). Oxygen radicals can alter cellular gene expression, membrane function, and metabolism.[160] Oxygen radicals are thought to mediate tissue injury in several disease processes, including sepsis and septic shock. In vitro, endotoxin-induced neutrophils exhibit enhanced release of superoxide.[58, 161] In vivo, animals challenged with endotoxin showed increased peroxidation of lipids.[162, 163] Lipid peroxidation may damage the cell membrane and adversely affect cellular function.

Antioxidant therapies under investigation include enzymatic scavengers (superoxide dismutase, catalase[164–168]), chemical quenchers (vitamin E, reduced glutathione[163, 166–168]), chelators (deferoxamine, diethyldithiocarbamate[165, 168]), and the xanthine oxidase inhibitor allopurinol.[163, 165–167] In animal endotoxin challenges, pretreatment with superoxide dismutase, vitamin E, reduced glutathione, or allopurinol limited the increase in hepatic lipoperoxidase concentrations[163, 166] but did not improve long-term survival or consistently improve short-term survival.[164–167] In an animal bacterial challenge model, various combinations of antioxidant agents (superoxide dismutase, vitamin E, deferoxamine, diethyldithiocarbamate) did not significantly alter hypotension or survival.[168]

Toxic oxygen radicals damage cellular membranes, resulting in microvascular injury, increased vascular permeability, and tissue ischemia. Antioxidant therapies have met with limited success in animal models of sepsis and septic shock. Further investigation into tissue damage by toxic oxygen radicals and methods of antagonizing such injury are needed.

Naloxone

Naloxone is an opiate antagonist. The plasma level of β-endorphin, an endogenous opiate, is elevated in nonhuman primates with shock[169] and in patients with septicemia.[170] Investigators have hypothesized that endorphin systems become activated in septic shock and contribute to the cardiovascular derangements of septic shock through their opiate receptors.[171, 172]

Endotoxic shock models using early naloxone therapy showed various degrees of hypotension reversal. However, most studies failed to show an improved long-term survival rate.[169, 171–173] Large-animal bacteremic (viable gram-negative organism) shock models in which antibiotic and early naloxone therapy was used also showed conflicting results with respect to improvement in mortality.[174] Early clinical studies of naloxone in septic shock were uncontrolled.[175, 176] These studies showed improvement in MAP in naloxone-treated patients but failed to show improvement in long-term survival rate. In a prospective, double-blind, randomized, placebo-controlled clinical trial, septic shock patients treated with naloxone (0.4 to 1.2 mg intravenously) and standard therapy showed no significant benefit in terms of reversal of hypotension and survival rate.[177] The dose of naloxone used in this study has been criticized as being considerably below that shown to have beneficial effects on nonhuman primate survival.[169] Naloxone therapy remains controversial and without widespread clinical acceptance.

Corticosteroids

Corticosteroids have anti-inflammatory properties. Animal studies had suggested that high doses of these agents might be beneficial in septic shock,[178, 179] but clinical data from the early 1980s were controversial.[180–184] Several of these early clinical trials were criticized for faulty experimental design (i.e., lack of optimal and consistent conventional support and corticosteroid treatment). Two large, multicenter, prospective, randomized, double-blind, placebo-controlled clinical trials evaluating high-dose glucocorticoid treatment as an adjunct to standard therapy in severe sepsis have helped settle the issue.[185, 186] One study compared placebo with four boluses of methylprednisolone (30 mg/kg) given every 6 hours, starting within 2 hours of diagnosis.[185] The other study, a Veterans Administration Cooperative Study, compared placebo with a single bolus of methylprednisolone (30 mg/kg) followed by a 9-hour infusion (5 mg/kg/h).[186] Again, an attempt was made to start treatment within 2 hours of diagnosis. Both studies concluded that in patients with severe sepsis and septic shock, the use of high doses of corticosteroids neither improves survival nor confers any substantial beneficial effects. In fact, in a subpopulation of septic patients with elevated serum creatinine values (>2 mg/dL), adjunctive high-dose corticosteroids were found to be harmful.[185] Thus, high-dose corticosteroids cannot at present be generally recommended as part of a therapeutic regimen for sepsis and septic shock.

There are, however, specific indications for moderate-to-low doses of steroids in sepsis and septic shock. Adrenal-insufficient septic patients should receive stress doses of corticosteroids. In infants and children with *Haemophilus influenzae* meningitis, dexamethasone (0.15 mg/kg every 6 hours for 4 days) has been shown to help prevent hearing loss.[187] In patients with acquired immunodeficiency syndrome and moderate-to-severe *Pneumocystis carinii* pneumonia, early adjunctive corticosteroid treatment (40 mg of methylprednisolone every 6 hours or 40 mg of prednisone every 12 hours) can improve survival.[188, 189]

Step 4: Provide Intensive Life Support

Intensive life support (see Table 28–2) involves careful monitoring of patients in a critical care unit setting. Metabolic derangements should be aggressively corrected, as they can worsen the hemodynamic abnormalities of septic shock. Volume resuscitation and vasopressor therapy are vigorously pursued to avoid circulatory collapse and tissue injury. The goal is to maintain vital functions while previously discussed therapies eradicate microorganisms, neutralize microbial toxins, and limit harmful host responses.

Critical Care Unit Setting

A basic tenet of critical care units is the concentration of critically ill patients into a setting where urgent care can be provided. These units are equipped with specialized intravascular and extravascular monitoring systems (e.g., systemic and pulmonary arterial pressure monitors, cardiac rhythm monitors, pulse oximeters, and capnometers) and specific organ support devices (e.g., mechanical ventilators, dialysis equipment, and cardiac pacemakers). A full-time staff of nurses, physicians, and technicians trained to use and maintain monitoring systems and support devices should be continuously available. Retrospective analyses of septic shock patients in a critical care setting showed a significant decrease in mortality when full-time, on-site physicians were present[190] and when specially trained, full-time critical care physicians attended.[191] The septic syndrome is a dynamic and life-threatening state. Optimal therapy requires careful full-time monitoring by trained personnel in a critical care setting to facilitate therapeutic decisions and expedite antimicrobial treatment, volume resuscitation, and pharmacologic support.

Monitoring of Patients

The septic syndrome is a systemic illness. To treat patients properly, multiple physiologic and metabolic parameters must be evaluated. Laboratory monitoring is essential and when feasible should consist of assays of coagulation parameters, serum electrolytes, calcium, phosphorus, magnesium, glucose, blood urea nitrogen, creatinine, and arterial and mixed venous blood gases, complete blood counts, and liver function tests. These simple tests aid in identifying and correcting electrolyte and mineral imbalances, metabolic disturbances, bleeding abnormalities, anemia, and impending adrenal, renal, liver, and pulmonary dysfunction. Adult respiratory distress syndrome, acute tubular necrosis, and disseminated intravascular coagulation are serious complications of the septic syndrome. Acute adrenal insufficiency can be characterized by fever, hypotension, and a hyperdynamic cardiovascular profile mimicking septic shock.[192] Thus, the pituitary-adrenal axis should be evaluated in patients with poorly responsive hypotension or those with relevant historical and physical findings. Similar circumstances should also prompt an evaluation of thyroid function. The frequency of obtaining core laboratory parameters should be guided by the stability of the patient.

Noninvasive monitoring in a modern critical care unit consists of pulse oximetry, cardiac rhythm monitoring, input and output measurements, and automated blood pressure cuffs. Pulse oximetry provides information on tissue oxygenation. Rhythm monitoring is essential, as many patients have intracardiac catheters and receive potent cardiac stimulants. Input and output assessments aid in evaluating the patient's fluid balance and renal function. Automated blood pressure cuffs, although useful in stable and improving patients, are not recommended for labile and critically ill patients. An intra-arterial cannula is preferred because it can provide reproducible and continuous blood pressure readings.

Invasive hemodynamic monitoring requires systemic and pulmonary intra-arterial catheters.[193] These catheters have been instrumental in diagnosing and managing septic shock. Intra-arterial catheters provide beat-to-beat analysis, allowing therapy to keep pace with rapidly changing clinical parameters. Balloon flotation pulmonary arterial catheters allow simultaneous assessment of right ventricular and LV filling pressures by measuring central venous pressure and pulmonary capillary wedge pressure (PCWP), respectively. The thermistor port permits determination of cardiac output (CO),[195] systemic vascular resistance, and LV stroke work.

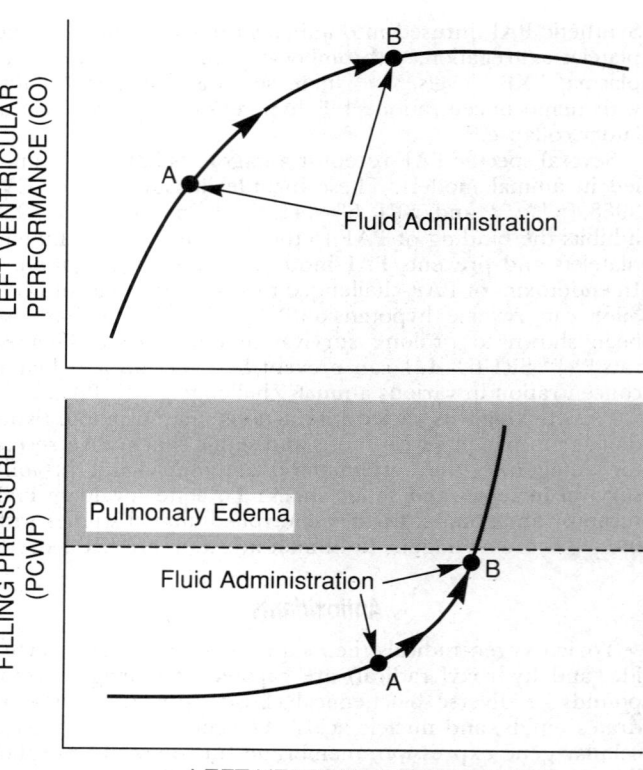

Figure 28–6. Use of right-sided heart catheter for fluid management. The upper graph depicts the Frank-Starling relationship, which is LV performance versus LV volume (EDVI, end diastolic volume index). As volume is increased from point A to B, there is a corresponding increase in LV performance. The lower graph shows the LV pressure-volume relationship at end diastole. As LV volume increases from point A to B, there is a corresponding increase in LV filling pressure. Further increases in LV volume beyond point B do not substantially increase ventricular performance and lead to a sharp rise in LV filling pressure and pulmonary edema. Thus, CO and PCWP measurements can safely guide fluid administration in optimizing LV performance while avoiding pulmonary edema *(shaded area)*. (Modified from Natanson C, Hoffman WD: Septic shock and other forms of distributive shock. In: Parrillo JE [ed]. Current Therapy in Critical Care Medicine. 2nd ed. Philadelphia, BC Decker, p 62, 1991.)

Therapy can then be based on Frank-Starling principles relating cardiac filling pressures and ventricular performance.[195] Thus, PCWP, an indicator of LV preload, together with MAP and CO, can safely guide the physician when volume resuscitation requires rapid and extensive fluid infusions (Fig. 28–6). Pulmonary arterial catheters also contain multiple infusion ports. Multiple infusion ports allow simultaneous administration of a variety of crucial fluids and medications (e.g., antibiotics, resuscitation fluids, vasopressors, and parenteral nutrition).

A complete hemodynamic profile consists of measures of MAP, central venous pressure, PCWP, CO, and systemic vascular resistance. The initial profile aids the physician in distinguishing septic shock from other forms of shock (Table 28–3). It also helps define the severity of the illness. Subsequent profiles track the progression of the illness and guide further treatment. As with core laboratory parameters, the frequency of a complete hemodynamic profile should be governed by the dynamics of the patient's illness. In a labile, critically ill shock patient, it is reasonable to obtain a complete hemodynamic profile every 2 hours and more frequently

TABLE 28–3

USE OF RIGHT-SIDED HEART CATHETERIZATION TO DIAGNOSE ETIOLOGY OF SHOCK

Type of Shock	Pulmonary Capillary Wedge Pressure*	Cardiac Output*	Comments
Cardiogenic			
Myocardial dysfunction	↑ ↑	↓ ↓	Usually occurs with evidence of extensive myocardial infarction, severe cardiomyopathy, or myocarditis
Acute ventricular septal defects	↑ or N	↓ ↓	Oxygen saturation "step-up" in right ventricle with left-to-right shunt
Acute mitral regurgitation	↑ ↑	↓ ↓	V waves in pulmonary capillary wedge pressure tracing
Right ventricle infarction	↓ or N	↓ ↓	Elevated right atrial and right ventricular filling pressures
Extracardiac Obstructive			
Pericardial tamponade	↑ ↑	↓ or ↓ ↓	Mean right atrial, right ventricular end-diastolic, and pulmonary capillary wedge pressure are all within 5 mm Hg
Pulmonary embolism (massive)	↓ or N	↓ ↓	Right-sided heart pressures may be elevated
Oligemic (Hypovolemia)	↓ ↓	↓ ↓	
Distributive			
Septic shock	↓ or N	↑ ↑ or N (rarely ↓)	High mixed venous oxygen saturation
Anaphylactic shock	↓ or N	↑ or N	

* ↑ ↑ or ↓ ↓ = moderate-to-severe increase or decrease; ↑ or ↓ = mild-to-moderate increase or decrease; N = normal.
Modified from Parrillo JE. Septic shock: clinical manifestations, pathogenesis, hemodynamics, and management in a critical care unit. In: Parrillo JE, Ayres SA (eds): Major Issues in Critical Care. Baltimore, Williams & Wilkins, p 111, 1984. © 1984, the Williams & Wilkins Co., Baltimore.

during rapid volume infusions to prevent fluid overload and pulmonary edema (see Fig. 28–6). As the patient's status improves, monitoring frequency is similarly adjusted.

Intensive Supplemental Organ Support

Cardiovascular support is the cornerstone of organ support. A large-animal bacteremic shock model simulating the human disease emphasized the need for both early antibiotic therapy and cardiovascular support. The study showed combined antibiotic and cardiovascular support regimens to significantly decrease mortality compared with either therapy alone or no therapy. The increase in survival exhibited by combined therapy proved to be synergistic. The authors concluded that cardiovascular support is essential to bridge the time gap until antibiotics and the host immune system are able to eradicate the invading microorganisms and neutralize their toxins.[196]

Cardiovascular support consists primarily of volume resuscitation and vasopressor therapy. Volume resuscitation can be accomplished with crystalloid, colloid, or blood products. The class of fluid is controversial, but the underlying principle of rapid volume resuscitation guided by MAP and PCWP is sound. In anemic, hypoxic, and hypotensive patients, it is reasonable to administer red blood cells to raise the hematocrit to approximately 30 to 35% in an attempt to improve oxygen-carrying capacity. In most situations, crystalloids and colloids are easier to obtain and without the risk of transmissible organisms. Of these two agents, crystalloids are safer and less expensive; colloids stay in the intravascular space longer.

Volume resuscitation is the initial cardiovascular treatment of choice in a septic shock patient with a MAP of less than 60 mm Hg and a low LV preload (i.e., a low PCWP). LV preload must be optimized so as to increase CO and raise MAP enough to prevent tissue ischemia of vital organs. To accomplish this in the face of an extremely low systemic vascular resistance, it may be necessary to administer large quantities of fluid in the first 24 hours, raising CO to

supranormal levels. Initially, rapid fluid boluses of 500 to 1000 mL during 15 minutes to 1 hour may be necessary. As the septic syndrome is associated with depressed myocardial function[5, 6, 197] and an abnormal LV response to volume infusion,[22] arterial and pulmonary catheters are advantageous. They safely guide therapy and help avoid such therapeutic misadventures as pulmonary edema (see Fig. 28–6).

Treatment of septic shock patients should include maintenance of MAP at 60 mm Hg or more to avoid limiting coronary artery and cerebral autoregulation and to prevent inadequate tissue perfusion. Volume is rapidly infused to maximize ventricular performance. Generally, this can be obtained at a PCWP of 12 to 15 mm Hg.[198, 199] An occasional patient may benefit from a PCWP as high as 18 mm Hg, but patients with PCWP of 20 mm Hg or more carry a substantial risk of developing pulmonary edema. It should be emphasized that the use of central venous pressure to guide volume therapy in the critically ill septic shock patient is discouraged. In this patient population, changes in PCWP and central venous pressure may not significantly correlate.[199]

Generally, if MAP remains below 60 mm Hg when PCWP is above 15 mm Hg, it is prudent to start vasopressors. Pharmacotherapy with vasoactive agents is based on the patient's hemodynamic profile, and the cardiac inotropic and peripheral vasculature effects of the specific drugs available (Fig. 28–7, Table 28–4). The majority of septic shock patients have normal or increased CO, with low systemic vascular resistance and low MAP. Initial therapy in these patients is best accomplished with low doses of dopamine (2 to 4 μg/kg/min). At these doses, there are enhanced cardiac chronotropic and inotropic responses and increased renal perfusion. If MAP remains below 60 mm Hg, dopamine is titrated upward to a maximal dose of 20 μg/kg/min. At high doses of dopamine (>10 μg/kg/min), the vasodilating effects disappear and the alpha-adrenergic vasoconstricting properties are dominant. At doses higher than 20 μg/kg/min,

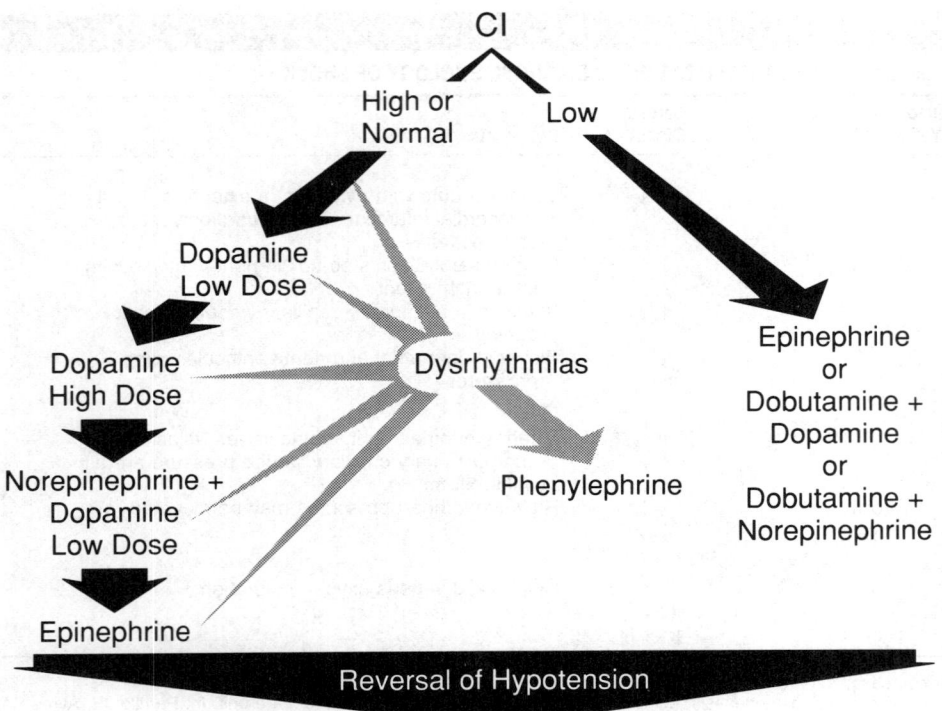

Figure 28–7. An algorithm for selecting vasopressors in septic shock. The goal is reversal of hypotension (MAP > 60 mm Hg with a PCWP of 12 to 15 mm Hg) (see also Table 28–4). CI = cardiac index. (Modified from Natanson C, Hoffman WD: Septic shock and other forms of distributive shock. In: Parrillo JE [ed]. Current Therapy in Critical Care Medicine. 2nd ed. Philadelphia, BC Decker, p 62, 1991.)

deleterious side effects such as atrial and ventricular dysrhythmias become more frequent.[200]

If, despite maximal dopamine therapy (20 μg/kg/min), the patient's MAP is persistently below 60 mm Hg, norepinephrine should be the next vasopressor applied. This agent has potent alpha-adrenergic vasoconstricting properties, along with beta-adrenergic cardiac inotropic properties. As norepinephrine is a powerful vasoconstrictor, its use in treating septic shock patients who are unresponsive to dopamine has been controversial. It is feared that the vasoconstriction may worsen tissue ischemia in vital organs. However, a clinical study in septic shock patients showed that norepinephrine can improve MAP and urine flow in hypotensive patients unresponsive to dopamine and volume therapy.[201] Clinical experience at the National Institutes of Health critical care unit has been similar, with norepinephrine doses of 2 to 10 μg/min usually being sufficient to treat the dopamine-unresponsive episodes of sepsis-induced hypotension.[20, 202] In conjunction with escalating norepinephrine doses, it is recommended that dopamine be tapered to a low dose (2 to 4 μg/kg/min). An animal model suggests that the renal vasodilating abilities of low doses of dopamine endures despite high pressor doses of norepinephrine.[203] If dysrhythmias recur, the vasopressor phenylephrine is recommended instead of norepinephrine. As phenylephrine is a pure alpha-adrenergic vasoconstrictor, direct cardiac stimulatory activity is avoided. In persistently hypotensive patients, the possibility of thyroid or adrenal dysfunction should be considered.[192]

A small percentage of septic shock patients (<10%) have a concurrent, sepsis-induced cardiogenic shock characterized by low CO and low MAP. In these patients, vasopressor regimens possessing potent beta-adrenergic cardiac stimulatory and alpha-adrenergic vasoconstrictive properties are recommended. Suitable therapy consists of epinephrine alone or dobutamine in combination with either norepinephrine or dopamine.

TABLE 28–4

SEPTIC SHOCK VASOPRESSOR THERAPY*

Pressor	Dose μg/kg/min (μg/min)	Cardiac Stimulation (Beta$_1$)	Vasoconstriction (Alpha$_1$)	Vasodilatation (Beta$_2$)	Dopaminergic	Indication (MAP <60 mm Hg, PCWP ≥12–15 mm Hg)
Dopamine	1–10	++	+	++	+++	↑ or normal CO
	10–20	+++	+++	+	0	
Norepinephrine	(2–10)	+++	++++	0	0	Dopamine failure
Phenylephrine	(20–200)	0	++++	0	0	Dysrhythmias
Epinephrine	(1–8)	++++	++++	++	0	↓ CO, norepinephrine failure
Dobutamine	1–10	++++	+	++	0	↓ CO, combine with norepinephrine therapy

*+ = mild increase; ++ = moderate increase; +++ = large increase; ++++ = very large increase; 0 = no significant change. See also Figure 28–7.
Modified from Natanson C, Hoffman WD: Septic shock and other forms of distributive shock. In: Parrillo JE (ed): Current Therapy in Critical Care Medicine. 2nd ed. Philadelphia, BC Decker, p 62, 1991.

High doses of potent alpha-adrenergic vasoconstrictors threaten the kidneys with increased ischemic injury. Volume therapy may worsen lung injury and hypoxemia by increasing lung water content. The diffuse capillary leak that usually accompanies septic shock serves only to further this concern. In septic shock, as with most systemic critical care illnesses, there is a fine line between organ preservation and organ injury. The above-mentioned guidelines, based on careful monitoring of patients and Frank-Starling mechanisms of ventricular performance, should optimize blood flow to vital organs while minimizing the risk of pulmonary edema. In the event of severe pulmonary or renal injury, the physician should not hesitate to institute mechanical ventilation or dialysis. Many critical care units can now perform continuous arteriovenous hemofiltration. This procedure uses the patient's arterial blood pressure as the driving force and thus produces less hemodynamic perturbations than a dialysis machine. By running a countercurrent dialysate, this technique can also be a means of temporary dialysis.

Providing intensive life support will occupy most of the clinician's time in treating sepsis and septic shock. Neutralizing bacterial toxins and modulating host mediators are intriguing; however, it is in life support that the true clinical art lies: the physician at the bedside anticipating, reacting, and interacting.

SUMMARY

The septic syndrome is a common systemic illness with a high mortality. Various microorganisms can induce the syndrome through complex interactions between bacterial toxins and host mediators. Standard therapy calls for promptly eradicating microorganisms and providing intensive life support. Therapy to eradicate microorganisms aims at sterilizing foci of infection with antibiotics and drainage techniques. Empiric antibiotics should be broad in spectrum and made specific when culture results are available. Intensive life support requires careful and continuous monitoring to guide volume resuscitation and vasopressor therapy. To safely sustain tissue perfusion to vital organs, the physician should strive to maintain an MAP of 60 mm Hg or more, with PCWP of 12 to 15 mm Hg. Intensive life-support therapy maintains vital functions, and antibiotics and host immune responses neutralize the microorganisms. Novel therapies seek to neutralize bacterial toxins and modulate host responses. In the latter, modulation rather than neutralization is emphasized, because a specific host mediator may have both beneficial and harmful effects.

Caution is warranted in reviewing the newer therapies because most of the beneficial data are derived from brief endotoxin and bacterial challenges in anesthetized animals. However, gram-negative infections in patients, unlike brief endotoxin and bacterial challenges, may be characterized by persistent endotoxemia and bacteremia lasting hours to several days.[31] It is conceivable that in infected patients the pathogenesis of sepsis and septic shock on cellular and molecular levels may be different from that in animal models. Until these new agents are shown to be safe and beneficial in both controlled animal models and controlled, prospective clinical trials, these therapies must be considered experimental. The most promising novel therapies are antiendotoxin antibodies and anti-TNF antibodies, both of which are currently undergoing clinical trials.

One vision of a future sepsis and septic shock regimen is an integrated, four-step approach (see Fig. 28–1) consisting of eradicating microorganisms to sterilize foci of infection, neutralizing microbial toxins to prevent their deleterious effects, modulating host mediators to limit and reverse harmful endogenous responses, and providing intensive life support to maintain vital organ functions. Although these steps were discussed separately, we envision an integrated approach in which many if not all of these steps will be applied simultaneously and repeatedly.

As research progresses, physicians gain greater insight into the body's response to sepsis. To paraphrase Leonardo da Vinci: we need to understand what constitution and health are. When we know these well, we will begin to understand where in the spectrum a response shifts from being beneficial to harmful. The offspring of this knowledge will be better therapeutic regimens. As always, the ultimate goal remains lower mortality with improved quality of life.

Acknowledgments. The authors wish to thank Darlene McCullough, MSN CCRN for help in preparing this manuscript; William D. Hoffman, MD, and Robert L. Danner, MD, for their critical reviews of this manuscript; and Matthew W. Pollack, MD, Uniformed Services University of the Health Sciences, for allowing us to review a preprint of his manuscript: New therapeutic strategies in gram-negative sepsis and septic shock based on molecular mechanisms of pathogenesis. In: Mandell GL, Douglas RG, Bennett JE (eds): Principles and Practice of Infectious Diseases. Update 8. New York, Churchill Livingstone, 1991.

References

1. Hoffman WD, Natanson C: Bacterial septic shock. Anesthesiol Clin North Am 7:845, 1989.
2. Wilson RF, Thal AP, Kindling PH, et al: Hemodynamic measurements in septic shock. Arch Surg 91:121, 1965.
3. Wenzel RP: Nosocomial infections, diagnosis-related groups, and study on the efficacy of nosocomial infection control: Economic implications for hospitals under the prospective payment system. Am J Med 78 (suppl 6B):3, 1985.
4. Centers for Disease Control. Increase in national hospital discharge survey rates for septicemia—United States, 1979–1987. MMWR 39:31, 1990.
5. Parker MM, Shelhamer JH, Bacharach SL, et al: Profound but reversible myocardial depression in patients with septic shock. Ann Intern Med 100:483, 1984.
6. Parker MM, McCarthy KE, Ognibene FP, et al: Right ventricular dysfunction and dilatation, similar to left ventricular changes, characterize the cardiac depression of septic shock in humans. Chest 97:126, 1990.
7. Natanson C, Hoffman WD: Septic shock and other forms of distributive shock. In: Parrillo JE (ed): Current Therapy in Critical Care Medicine. 2nd ed. Philadelphia, BC Decker, p 62, 1991.
8. Luce JM: Pathogenesis and management of septic shock. Chest 91:883, 1987.
9. Dannner RL, Suffredini AF, Natanson C: Microbial toxins: Role in the pathogenesis of septic shock and multiple organ failure. In: Cerra FB (ed): New Horizons: Multiple Organ Failure. Fullerton, CA, Society of Critical Care Medicine, p 151, 1989.
10. Parrillo JE: Pathogenesis of human septic shock, p 228. In: Parrillo JE (moderator): Septic shock in humans: Advances in the understanding of pathogenesis, cardiovascular dysfunction, and therapy. Ann Intern Med 113:227, 1990.
11. Michie HR, Manogue KR, Spriggs DR, et al: Detection of circulating tumor necrosis factor after endotoxin administration. N Engl J Med 318:1481, 1988.
12. Waage A, Halstensen A, Shalaby R, et al: Local production of tumor necrosis factor α, interleukin 1, and interleukin 6 in meningococcal meningitis. J Exp Med 170:1859, 1989.
13. Tracey JK, Beutler B, Lowry SF, et al: Shock and tissue injury induced by recombinant human cachectin. Science 234:470, 1986.
14. Dinarello CA: Interleukin-1 and the pathogenesis of the acute-phase response. N Engl J Med 311:1413, 1984.
15. Guthrie LA, McPhail LC, Henson PM, et al: Priming of neutrophils for enhanced release of oxygen metabolites by bacterial lipopolysaccharide. J Exp Med 160:1656, 1984.
16. Aderem AA, Cohen DS, Wright SD, et al: Bacterial lipopolysaccharides prime macrophages for enhanced release of arachidonic acid metabolites. J Exp Med 164:165, 1986.
17. Doerfler ME, Danner RL, Shelhamer JH, et al: Bacterial lipopolysaccharides prime human neutrophils for enhanced production of leukotriene B₄. J Clin Invest 83:970, 1989.
18. Natanson C, Fink MP, Ballantyne HK, et al: Gram-negative bacteremia produces both severe systolic and diastolic cardiac dysfunction in a

canine model that simulates human septic shock. J Clin Invest 78:259, 1986.

19. Natanson C, Danner RL, Fink MP, et al: Cardiovascular performance with E. coli challenges in a canine model of human sepsis. Am J Physiol 254:H558, 1988.
20. Natanson C, Hoffman WD, Parrillo JE: Septic shock: The cardiovascular abnormality and therapy. J Cardiothorac Anesth 3:215, 1989.
21. Suffredini AF, Fromm RE, Parker MM, et al: The cardiovascular response of normal humans to the administration of endotoxin. N Engl J Med 321:280, 1989.
22. Ognibene FP, Parker MM, Natanson C, et al: Depressed left ventricular performance response to volume infusion in patients with sepsis and septic shock. Chest 93:903, 1988.
23. Shenep JL, Mogan KA: Kinetics of endotoxin release during antibiotic therapy for experimental gram-negative bacterial sepsis. J Infect Dis 150:380, 1984.
24. Shenep JL, Barton RP, Morgan KA: Role of antibiotic class in the rate of liberation of endotoxin during therapy for experimental gram-negative bacterial sepsis. J Infect Dis 151:1012, 1985.
25. Shenep JL, Flynn PM, Barrett FF, et al: Serial quantitation of endotoxemia and bacteremia during therapy for gram-negative bacterial sepsis. J Infect Dis 157:565, 1988.
26. Ganalos C, Lehmann V, Lüderitz O, et al: Endotoxic properties of chemically synthesized lipid A part structures. Eur J Biochem 140:221, 1984.
27. Danner RL: Mediators and endotoxin inhibitors, p 235. In: Parrillo JE (moderator): Septic shock in humans: Advances in the understanding of pathogenesis, cardiovascular dysfunction, and therapy. Ann Intern Med 113:227, 1990.
28. van Deventer SJH, Cate JWT, Buller HR, et al: Endotoxemia: An early predictor of septicaemia in febrile patients. Lancet 1:605, 1988.
29. Natanson C, Eichenholz PW, Danner RL, et al: Endotoxin and tumor necrosis factor challenges in dogs simulate the cardiovascular profile of human septic shock. J Exp Med 169:823, 1989.
30. Brandtzaeg P, Kierulf P, Gaustad P, et al: Plasma endotoxin as a predictor of multiple organ failure and death in systemic meningococcal disease. J Infect Dis 159:195, 1989.
31. Danner RL, Elin RJ, Hosseini JM, et al: Endotoxemia in human septic shock. Chest 99:169, 1991.
32. Pollack M, Young LS: Protective activity of antibodies to exotoxin A and lipopolysaccharide at the onset of Pseudomonas aeruginosa septicemia in man. J Clin Invest 63:276, 1979.
33. Stoll BJ, Pollack M, Young LS, et al: Functionally active monoclonal antibody that recognizes an epitope on the O side chain of Pseudomonas aeruginosa immunotype-1 lipopolysaccharide. Infect Immun 53:656, 1986.
34. Chedid L, Parant M, Parant F, et al: A proposed mechanism for natural immunity to enterobacterial pathogens. J Immunol 100:292, 1968.
35. McCabe WR, Kreger BE, Johns M: Type-specific and cross-reactive antibodies in gram-negative bacteremia. N Engl J Med 287:261, 1972.
36. Ziegler EJ, McCutchan JA, Fierer J, et al: Treatment of gram-negative bacteremia and shock with human antiserum to a mutant Escherichia coli. N Engl J Med 307:1225, 1982.
37. Greisman SE, Johnston CA: Failure of antisera to J5 and R595 rough mutants to reduce endotoxemic lethality. J Infect Dis 157:54 1988.
38. Ziegler EJ: Protective antibody to endotoxin core: The emperor's new clothes? J Infect Dis 158:286, 1988.
39. Teng NNH, Kaplan HS, Hebert JM, et al: Protection against gram-negative bacteremia and endotoxemia with human monoclonal IgM antibodies. Proc Natl Acad Sci USA 82:1790, 1985.
40. Pollack M, Raubitschek AA, Larrick JW: Human monoclonal antibodies that recognize conserved epitopes in the core-lipid A region of lipopolysaccharides. J Clin Invest 79:1421, 1987.
41. Hoffman WD, Pollack M, Banks SM, et al: Monoclonal anti-endotoxin antibodies as therapy in a canine model of human septic shock (abstract). Clin Res 38:454A, 1990.
42. Wedel NI, Gorelick KJ, Saria EA, et al: Pharmacokinetics and safety of antiendotoxin antibody E5 in normal subjects (abstract). Crit Care Med 18:S212, 1990.
43. Gorelick KJ, Wedel NI, Kunz AY, et al: E5 antiendotoxin antibody in gram-negative sepsis: Report of a phase II study (abstract). Crit Care Med 18:S261, 1990.
44. Khazaeli MB, Rogers KJ, LoBuglio AF: Initial evaluation of a human IgM monoclonal antibody (HA-1A) in man. J Biol Response Mod 9:178, 1990.
45. Fisher CJ Jr, Zimmerman J, Khazaeli MB, et al: Initial evaluation of human monoclonal anti-lipid A antibody (HA-1A) in patients with sepsis syndrome. Crit Care Med 18:1311, 1990.
46. Gorelick KJ, RMH Schein, MacIntyre NR, et al: Multicenter trial of antiendotoxin antibody E5 in the treatment of gram negative sepsis (abstract). Crit Care Med 18:S253, 1990.
47. Ziegler EJ, Fisher CJ, Sprung CL, et al: Treatment of gram-negative bacteremia and septic shock with HA-1A human monoclonal antibody against endotoxin: A randomized, double-blind, placebo-controlled trial. N Engl J Med 324:429, 1991.
48. Ray BL, Painter G, Raetz CRH: The biosynthesis of gram-negative endotoxin: Formation of lipid A disaccharides from monosaccharide precursors in extracts of Escherichia coli. J Biol Chem 259:4852, 1984.

49. Kiso M, Ishida H, Hasegawa A: Synthesis of biologically active, novel monosaccharide analogs of lipid A. Agric Biol Chem 48:251, 1984.
50. Takayama K, Qureshi N, Mascagni P, et al: Fatty acyl derivatives of glucosamine-1-phosphate in Escherichia coli and their relation to lipid A. J Biol Chem 258:7379, 1983.
51. Tanamoto K, Zähringer U, McKenzie GR, et al: Biological activities of synthetic lipid A analogs: Pyrogenicity, lethal toxicity, anticomplement activity, and induction of gelation of Limulus amoebocyte lysate. Infect Immun 44:421, 1984.
52. Munford RS, Hall CL: Uptake and deacylation of bacterial lipopolysaccharides by macrophages from normal and endotoxin-hyporesponsive mice. Infect Immun 48:464, 1985.
53. Astiz ME, Rackow EC, Kim YB, et al: Hemodynamic effects of monophosphoryl lipid A compared to endotoxin. Circ Shock 27:193, 1989.
54. Munford RS, Hall CL: Detoxification of bacterial lipopolysaccharides (endotoxins) by a human neutrophil enzyme. Science 234:203, 1986.
55. Riedo FX, Munford RS, Campbell WB, et al: Deacylated lipopolysaccharide inhibits plasminogen activator inhibitor-1, prostacyclin, and prostaglandin E_2 induction by lipopolysaccharide but not by tumor necrosis factor-α. J Immunol 144:3506, 1990.
56. Pohlman TH, Munford RS, Harlan JM: Deacylated lipopolysaccharide inhibits neutrophil adherence to endothelium induced by lipopolysaccharide in vitro. J Exp Med 165:1393, 1987.
57. Raetz CRH: The enzymatic synthesis of lipid A: Molecular structure and biologic function of monosaccharide precursors. Rev Infect Dis 6:463, 1984.
58. Danner RL, Joiner KA, Parrillo JE: Inhibition of endotoxin-induced priming of human neutrophils by lipid X and 3-aza-lipid X. J Clin Invest 80:605, 1987.
59. Proctor AR, Will JA, Burhop KE, et al: Protection of mice against lethal endotoxemia by a lipid A precursor. Infect Immun 52:905, 1986.
60. Golenbock DT, Will JA, Raetz CRH, et al: Lipid X ameliorates pulmonary hypertension and protects sheep from death due to endotoxin. Infect Immun 55:2471, 1987.
61. Danner RL, Natanson C, Doerfler ME, et al: Lipid X fails to reverse lethal septic shock in a canine model. Clin Res 36:799A, 1988.
62. Heiman DF, Astiz ME, Rackow EC, et al: Monophosphoryl lipid A inhibits neutrophil priming by lipopolysaccharide. J Lab Clin Med 116:237, 1990.
63. Rackow EC, Astiz ME, Kim YB, et al: Monophosphoryl lipid A blocks hemodynamic effects of lethal endotoxemia. J Lab Clin Med 113:112, 1989.
64. Carpati C, Astiz ME, Rackow EC, et al: Monophosphoryl lipid A attenuates septic shock in pigs (abstract). Crit Care Med 18:S260, 1990.
65. Rifkind D, Palmer JD: Neutralization of endotoxin toxicity in chick embryos by antibiotics. J Bacteriol 92:815, 1966.
66. Bannatyne RM, Harnett NM, Lee KY, et al: Inhibition of the biologic effects of endotoxin on neutrophils by polymyxin B sulfate. J Infect Dis 136:469, 1977.
67. Vaara M, Vaara T: Polycations sensitize enteric bacteria to antibiotics. Antimicrob Agents Chemother 24:107, 1983.
68. Warren HS, Kania SA, Siber GR: Binding and neutralization of bacterial lipopolysaccharide by colistin nonapeptide. Antimicrob Agents Chemother 28:107, 1985.
69. Danner RL, Joiner KA, Rubin M, et al: Purification, toxicity, and antiendotoxin activity of polymyxin B nonapeptide. Antimicrob Agents Chemother 33:1428, 1989.
70. Craig WA, Turner JH, Kunin CM: Prevention of the generalized Shwartzman reaction and endotoxin lethality by polymyxin B localized in tissues. Infect Immun 10:287, 1974.
71. Stokes DC, Shenep JL, Fishman M, et al: Polymyxin B prevents lipopolysaccharide-induced release of tumor necrosis factor-α from alveolar macrophages. J Infect Dis 160:52, 1989.
72. Morrison DC, Jacobs DM: Binding of polymyxin B to the lipid A portion of bacterial lipopolysaccharides. Immunochemistry 13:813, 1976.
73. Rifkind D: Prevention by polymyxin B of endotoxin lethality in mice. J Bacteriol 93:1463, 1967.
74. Flynn PM, Shenep JL, Stokes DC, et al: Polymyxin B moderates acidosis and hypotension in established, experimental gram-negative septicemia. J Infect Dis 156:706, 1987.
75. Corrigan JJ Jr, Kiernat JF: Effect of polymyxin B sulfate on endotoxin activity in a gram-negative septicemia model. Pediatr Res 13:48, 1979.
76. Vinnicombe J, Stamey TA: The relative nephrotoxicities of polymyxin B sulfate, sodium sulfomethyl-polymyxin B, sodium sulfomethyl colistin (Coly-Mycin) and neomycin sulfate. Invest Urol 6:505, 1969.
77. Hanasawa K, Tani T, Oka T, et al: Selective removal of endotoxin from the blood by extracorporeal hemoperfusion with polymyxin B immobilized fiber. Prog Clin Bio Res 264:337, 1988.
78. Bysani GK, Shenep JL, Hildner WK, et al: Detoxification of plasma containing lipopolysaccharide by adsorption. Crit Care Med 18:67, 1990.
79. Bende S, Bertók L: Elimination of endotoxin from the blood by extracorporeal activated charcoal hemoperfusion in experimental canine endotoxin shock. Circ Shock 19:239, 1986.
80. Togari H, Mikawa M, Iwanaga T, et al: Endotoxin clearance by exchange blood transfusion in septic shock neonates. Acta Paediatr Scand 72:87, 1983.
81. Gross S, Melhorn DK: Exchange transfusion with citrated whole blood for disseminated intravascular coagulation. J Pediatr 78:415, 1971.

82. Töllner U, Pohland TF, Heinze F, et al: Treatment of septicaemia in the newborn infant: Choice of initial antimicrobial drugs and the role of exchange transfusion. Acta Paediatr Scand 66:605, 1977.

83. Vain NE, Mazlumian JR, Swarner OW, et al: Role of exchange transfusion in the treatment of severe septicemia. Pediatrics 66:693, 1980.

84. Bjorvatn B, Bjertnaes L, Fadnes HO, et al: Meningococcal septicaemia treated with combined plasmapheresis and leucapheresis or with blood exchange. Br Med J [Clin Res] 288:439, 1984.

85. Brandtzaeg P, Sirnes K, Folsland B, et al: Plasmapheresis in the treatment of severe meningococcal or pneumococcal septicemia with DIC and fibrinolysis. Scand J Clin Lab Invest 45:53, 1985.

86. Scharfman WB, Tillotson JR, Taft EG, et al: Plasmapheresis for meningococcemia with disseminated intravascular coagulation (letter). N Engl J Med 300:1277, 1979.

87. Natanson C, Hoffman WD, Danner RL, et al: A controlled trial of plasmapheresis fails to improve outcome in an antibiotic treated canine model of human septic shock (abstract). Clin Res 37:346A, 1989.

88. Yatsiv I, Koev LA, Hoffman WD, et al: A controlled trial of continuous arterial-venous hemofiltration fails to improve outcome in a canine model of human septic shock (abstract). Clin Res 39:264A, 1991.

89. Natanson C, Danner RL, Elin RJ, et al: Role of endotoxemia in cardiovascular dysfunction and mortality. *Escherichia coli* and *Staphylococcus aureus* challenges in a canine model of human septic shock. J Clin Invest 83:243, 1989.

90. Okusawa S, Gelfand JA, Ikejima T, et al: Interleukin 1 induces a shock-like state in rabbits: Synergism with tumor necrosis factor and the effect of cyclooxygenase inhibition. J Clin Invest 81:1162, 1988.

91. Waage A, Espevik T: Interleukin 1 potentiates the lethal effect of tumor necrosis factor α/cachectin in mice. J Exp Med 167:1987, 1988.

92. Wang AM, Creasey AA, Ladner MB, et al: Molecular cloning of the complementary DNA for human tumor necrosis factor. Science 228:149, 1985.

93. Pernica D, Nedwin GE, Hayflick JS, et al: Human tumour necrosis factor: Precursor structure, expression and homology to lymphotoxin. Nature 312:724, 1984.

94. Beutler B, Mahoney J, Le Trang N, et al: Purification of cachectin, a lipoprotein lipase–suppressing hormone secreted by endotoxin-induced RAW 264.7 cells. J Exp Med 161:984, 1985.

95. Beutler B, Greenwald D, Hulmes JD, et al: Identity of tumor necrosis factor and the macrophage-secreted factor cachectin. Nature 316:552, 1985.

96. Tracey KJ, Lowry SF, Cerami A: Cachectin: A hormone that triggers acute shock and chronic cachexia. J Infect Dis 157:413, 1988.

97. Cannon JG, Tompkins RG, Gelfand JA, et al: Circulating interleukin-1 and tumor necrosis factor in septic shock and experimental endotoxin fever. J Infect Dis 161:79, 1990.

98. Hesse DG, Tracey KJ, Fong Y, et al: Cytokine appearance in human endotoxemia and primate bacteremia. Surg Gynecol Obstet 166:147, 1988.

99. Tracey KJ, Lowry SF, Fahey TJ III, et al: Cachectin/tumor necrosis factor induces lethal shock and stress hormone responses in the dog. Surg Gynecol Obstet 164:415, 1987.

100. Waage A, Halstensen A, Espevik T: Association between tumour necrosis factor in serum and fatal outcome in patients with meningococcal disease. Lancet 1:355, 1987.

101. Calandra T, Baumgartner JD, Grau GE, et al: Prognostic values of tumor necrosis factor/cachectin interleukin-1, interferon-α, and interferon-γ in the serum of patients with septic shock. Swiss-Dutch J5 Immunoglobulin Study Group. J Infect Dis 161:982, 1990.

102. Beutler B, Milsark IW, Cerami AC: Passive immunization against cachectin/tumor necrosis factor protects mice from lethal effect of endotoxin. Science 229:869, 1985.

103. Mathison JC, Wolfson E, Ulevitch RJ: Participation of tumor necrosis factor in the mediation of gram-negative bacterial lipopolysaccharide-induced injury in rabbits. J Clin Invest 81:1925, 1988.

104. Tracey KJ, Fong Y, Hesse DG, et al: Anti-cachectin/TNF monoclonal antibodies prevent septic shock during lethal bacteremia. Nature 330:662, 1987.

105. Hinshaw LB, Tekamp-Olson P, Chang ACK, et al: Survival of primates in LD$_{100}$ septic shock following therapy with antibody to tumor necrosis factor (TNFα). Circ Shock 30:279, 1990.

106. Bagby GJ, Plessala KJ, Wilson LA, et al: Divergent efficacy of antibody to tumor necrosis factor-α in intravascular and peritonitis models of sepsis. J Infect Dis 163:83, 1991.

107. Beutler B, Cerami A: Cachectin: More than a tumor necrosis factor. N Engl J Med 316:379, 1987.

108. Cross AS, Sadoff JC, Kelly N, et al: Pretreatment with recombinant murine tumor necrosis factor α/cachectin and murine interleukin 1α protects from lethal bacterial infection. J Exp Med 169:2021, 1989.

109. Hannum CH, Wilcox CJ, Arend WP, et al: Interleukin-1 receptor antagonist activity of a human interleukin-1 inhibitor. Nature 343:336, 1990.

110. Eisenberg SP, Evans RJ, Arend WP, et al: Primary structure and functional expression from complementary DNA of a human interleukin-1 receptor antagonist. Nature 343:341, 1990.

111. Ohlsson K, Björk P, Bergenfeldt M, et al: Interleukin-1 receptor antagonist reduces mortality from endotoxin shock. Nature 348:550, 1990.

112. Morrison DC, Kline LF: Activation of the classical and properdin pathways of complement by bacterial lipopolysaccharides (LPS). J Immunol 118:362, 1977.

113. Fearon DT, Ruddy S, Schur PH, et al: Activation of the properdin pathway of complement in patients with gram-negative bacteremia. N Engl J Med 292:937, 1975.

114. Sacks T, Moldow CF, Craddock PR, et al: Oxygen radicals mediate endothelial cell damage by complement-stimulated granulocytes: An in vitro model of immune vascular damage. J Clin Invest 61:1161, 1978.

115. Craddock PR, Hammerschmidt DE, White JG, et al: Complement (C5a)-induced granulocyte aggregation in vitro: A possible mechanism of complement-induced leukostasis and leukopenia. J Clin Invest 60:260, 1977.

116. Hammerschmidt DE, Weaver LJ, Hudson LD, et al: Association of complement activation and elevated plasma C5a with adult respiratory distress syndrome: Pathophysiological relevance and possible prognostic value. Lancet 1:947, 1980.

117. Okusawa S, Yancey KB, van der Meer JWM, et al: C5a stimulates secretion of tumor necrosis factor from human mononuclear cells in vitro. Comparison with secretion of interleukin 1β and interleukin 1α. J Exp Med 168:443, 1988.

118. Lundberg C, Marceau F, Hugli TE: C5a-induced hemodynamic and hematologic changes in the rabbit: Role of cyclooxygenase products and polymorphonuclear leukocytes. Am J Pathol 128:471, 1987.

119. Stevens JH, O'Hanley P, Shapiro JM, et al: Effects of anti-C5a antibodies on the adult respiratory distress syndrome in septic primates. J Clin Invest 77:1812, 1986.

120. Larrick JW, Wang J, Fendly BM, et al: Characterization of murine monoclonal antibodies that recognize neutralizing epitopes on human C5a. Infect Immun 55:1867, 1987.

121. Marcus AJ: Eicosanoids as bioregulators in clinical medicine. Am J Med 78:805, 1985.

122. Lefer AM: Leukotrienes as mediators of ischemia and shock. Biochem Pharmacol 35:123, 1986.

123. Lux WE Jr, Feuerstein G, Faden AI: Thyrotropin-releasing hormone reverses the hypotension and bradycardia produced by leukotriene D$_4$ in unanesthetized guinea pigs. Prostaglandins Leukotrienes Med 10:301, 1983.

124. Schade UF, Ernst M, Reinke M, et al: Lipoxygenase inhibitors suppress formation of tumor necrosis factor in vitro and in vivo. Biochem Biophys Res Commun 159:748, 1989.

125. Hagmann W, Denzlinger C, Keppler D: Role of peptide leukotrienes and their hepatobiliary elimination in endotoxin action. Circ Shock 14:223, 1984.

126. Keppler D, Hagmann W, Rapp S: Role of leukotrienes in endotoxin action in vivo. Rev Infect Dis 9:S580, 1987.

127. Fleisch JH, Rinkema LE, Marshall WS: Pharmacologic receptors for the leukotrienes. Biochem Pharmacol 33:3919, 1984.

128. Wise WC, Cook JA, Eller T, et al: Ibuprofen improves survival from endotoxic shock in the rat. J Pharmacol Exp Ther 215:160, 1980.

129. Camporesi EM, Oda S, Fracica PJ, et al: Eicosanoids and the hemodynamic course of live *Escherichia coli*–induced sepsis in baboons. Circ Shock 29:229, 1989.

130. Wise CW, Cook JA, Halushka PV, et al: Protective effects of thromboxane synthetase inhibitors in rats in endotoxic shock. Circ Res 46:854, 1980.

131. Fletcher JR, Ramwell PW: Modification, by aspirin and indomethacin, of the haemodynamic and prostaglandin releasing effects of *E. coli* endotoxin in the dog. Br J Pharmacol 61:175, 1977.

132. Fink MP, MacVittie TJ, Casey LC: Inhibition of prostaglandin synthesis restores normal hemodynamics in canine hyperdynamic sepsis. Ann Surg 200:619, 1984.

133. Revhaug A, Michie HR, Manson JM, et al: Inhibition of cyclo-oxygenase attenuates the metabolic response to endotoxin in humans. Arch Surg 123:162, 1988.

133a. Haupt MT, Jastremski MS, Clemmer TP, et al: Effect of ibuprofen in patients with severe sepsis: A randomized, double-blind, multicenter study. The ibuprofen study group. Crit Care Med 19:1339, 1991.

134. Spinas GA, Bloesch D, Keller U, et al: Pretreatment with ibuprofen augments circulating tumor necrosis factor-α, interleukin-6, and elastase during acute endotoxinemia. J Infect Dis 163:89, 1991.

135. Mammen EF, Miyakawa T, Phillips TF, et al: Human antithrombin concentrates and experimental disseminated intravascular coagulation. Semin Thromb Hemost 11:373, 1985.

136. Bick RL, Bick MD, Fekete LF: Antithrombin III patterns in disseminated intravascular coagulation. Am J Clin Pathol 73:577, 1978.

137. Lämmle B, Tran TH, Ritz R, et al: Plasma prekallikrein, factor XII, antithrombin III, C$_1^-$-inhibitor and α_2-macroglobulin in critically ill patients with suspected disseminated intravascular coagulation (DIC). Am J Clin Pathol 82:396, 1984.

138. Triantaphyllopoulos DC: Effects of human antithrombin III on mortality and blood coagulation induced in rabbits by endotoxin. Thromb Haemost 51:232, 1984.

139. Emerson TE Jr, Fournel MA, Leach WJ, et al: Protection against disseminated intravascular coagulation and death by antithrombin-III in the *Escherichia coli* endotoxemic rat. Circ Shock 21:1, 1987.

140. Taylor FB Jr, Emerson TE Jr, Jordan R, et al: Antithrombin-III prevents

the lethal effects of *Escherichia coli* infusion in baboons. Circ Shock 26:227, 1988.

141. Emerson TE Jr, Fournel MA, Redens TB, et al: Efficacy of antithrombin III supplementation in animal models of fulminant *Escherichia coli* endotoxemia or bacteremia. Am J Med 87 (suppl 3B):27S, 1989.

142. Taylor FB Jr, Chang A, Esmon CT, et al: Protein C prevents the coagulopathic and lethal effects of *Escherichia coli* infusion in the baboon. J Clin Invest 79:918, 1987.

143. Hellgren M, Javelin L, Hägnevik K, et al: Antithrombin III concentrate as adjuvant in DIC treatment: A pilot study in 9 severely ill patients. Thromb Res 35:459, 1984.

144. Hanada T, Abe T, Takita H, et al: Antithrombin III concentrates for treatment of disseminated intravascular coagulation in children. Am J Pediatr Hematol Oncol 7:3, 1985.

145. Blauhut B, Kramar H, Vinazzer H, et al: Substitution of antithrombin III in shock and DIC: A randomized study. Thromb Res 39:81, 1985.

146. Hammerschmidt DE, Kotasek D, McCarthy T, et al: Pentoxifylline inhibits granulocyte and platelet function, including granulocyte priming by platelet activating factor. J Lab Clin Med 112:254, 1988.

147. Sullivan GW, Carper HT, Novick WJ Jr, et al: Inhibition of the inflammatory action of interleukin-1 and tumor necrosis factor (alpha) on neutrophil function by pentoxifylline. Infect Immun 56:1722, 1988.

148. Zabel P, Schönharting MM, Wolter DT, et al: Oxpentifylline in endotoxaemia. Lancet 2:1474, 1989.

149. Schade UF, Bosch JVD, Schönharting M: Pentoxifylline increases survival of mice in endotoxic shock. Prog Clin Biol Res 301:223, 1988.

150. Tighe D, Moss R, Hynd J, et al: Pretreatment with pentoxifylline improves the hemodynamic and histologic changes and decreases neutrophil adhesiveness in a pig fecal peritonitis model. Crit Care Med 18:184, 1990.

151. Chang SW, Feddersen CO, Henson PM, et al: Platelet-activating factor mediates hemodynamic changes and lung injury in endotoxin-treated rats. J Clin Invest 79:1498, 1987.

152. Diez FL, Nieto ML, Fernandez-Gallardo S, et al: Occupancy of platelet receptors for platelet-activating factor in patients with septicemia. J Clin Invest 83:1733, 1989.

153. McManus LM, Hanahan DJ, Demopoulos CA, et al: Pathobiology of the intravenous infusion of acetyl glyceryl ether phosphorylcholine (AGEPC), a synthetic platelet-activating factor (PAF), in the rabbit. J Immunol 124:2919, 1980.

154. McManus LM, Pinckard RN, Fitzpatrick FA, et al: Acetyl glyceryl ether phosphorylcholine: Intravascular alterations following intravenous infusion into the baboon. Lab Invest 45:303, 1981.

155. Bessin P, Bonnet J, Apffel D, et al: Acute circulatory collapse caused by platelet-activating factor (PAF-acether) in dogs. Eur J Pharmacol 86:403, 1983.

156. Handley DA, Tomesch JC, Saunders RN: Inhibition of PAF-induced systemic responses in the rat, guinea pig, dog and primate by the receptor antagonist SRI 63–441. Thromb Haemost 56:40, 1986.

157. Doebber TW, Wu MS, Robbins JC, et al: Platelet activating factor (PAF) involvement in endotoxin-induced hypotension in rats. Studies with PAF-receptor antagonist kadsurenone. Biochem Biophys Res Commun 127:799, 1985.

158. Terashita Z, Imura Y, Nishikawa K, et al: Is platelet activating factor (PAF) a mediator of endotoxin shock? Eur J Pharmacol 109:257, 1985.

159. Terashita Z, Imura Y, Nishikawa K: Inhibition by CV-3988 of the binding of [³H]-platelet activating factor (PAF) to the platelet. Biochem Pharmacol 34:1491, 1985.

160. Cross CE, Halliwell B, Borish ET, et al: Oxygen radicals and human disease. Ann Intern Med 107:526, 1987.

161. Guthrie LA, McPhail LC, Henson PM, et al: Priming of neutrophils for enhanced release of oxygen metabolites by bacterial lipopolysaccharide: Evidence for increased activity of the superoxide-producing enzyme. J Exp Med 160:1656, 1984.

162. Morgan RA, Manning PB, Coran AG, et al: Oxygen free radical activity during live *E. coli* septic shock in the dog. Circ Shock 25:319, 1988.

163. Ogawa R, Morita T, Kunimoto F, et al: Changes in hepatic lipoperoxidase concentration in endotoxemic rats. Circ Shock 9:369, 1982.

164. Broner CW, Shenep JL, Stidham GL, et al: Effect of scavengers of oxygen-derived free radicals on mortality in endotoxin-challenged mice. Crit Care Med 16:848, 1988.

165. Novotny MJ, Laughlin MH, Adams HR: Evidence for lack of importance of oxygen free radicals in *Escherichia coli* endotoxemia in dogs. Am J Physiol 254:H954, 1988.

166. Kunimoto F, Morita T, Ogawa R, et al: Inhibition of lipid peroxidation improves survival rate of endotoxemic rats. Circ Shock 21:15, 1987.

167. McKechnie K, Furman BL, Parratt JR: Modification by oxygen free radical scavengers of the metabolic and cardiovascular effects of endotoxin infusion in conscious rats. Circ Shock 19:429, 1986.

168. Broner CW, Shenep JL, Stidham GL, et al: Effect of antioxidants in experimental *Escherichia coli* septicemia. Circ Shock 29:77, 1989.

169. Gurll NJ, Reynolds DG, Holaday JW: Evidence for a role of endorphins in the cardiovascular pathophysiology of primate shock. Crit Care Med 16:521, 1988.

170. Weissglas IS: The role of endogenous opiates in shock: Experimental and clinical studies in vitro and in vivo. Adv Shock Res 10:87, 1983.

171. Holaday JW, Faden AI: Naloxone reversal of endotoxin hypotension suggests role of endorphins in shock. Nature 275:450, 1978.

172. Reynolds DG, Gurll NJ, Vargish T, et al: Blockade of opiate receptors with naloxone improves survival and cardiac performance in canine endotoxic shock. Circ Shock 7:39, 1980.

173. Fettman M, Hand M, Chandrasena L, et al: Effects of naloxone (N) therapy and lethality, hemodynamic, and metabolic parameters in awake endotoxemic yucatan minipigs. Circ Shock 9:185, 1982.

174. Hinshaw LB, Beller BK, Chang ACK, et al: Evaluation of naloxone for therapy of *Escherichia coli* shock. Arch Surg 119:1410, 1984.

175. Peters WP, Johnson MW, Friedman PA, et al: Pressor effect of naloxone in septic shock. Lancet 1:529, 1981.

176. Groeger JS, Graziano CC, Howland WS: Naloxone in septic shock. Crit Care Med 11:650, 1983.

177. DeMaria A, Heffernan JJ, Grindlinger GA, et al: Naloxone versus placebo in treatment of septic shock. Lancet 1:1363, 1985.

178. Hinshaw LB, Archer LT, Beller-Todd BK, et al: Survival of primates in lethal septic shock following delayed treatment with steroid. Circ Shock 8:291, 1981.

179. Hinshaw LB, Beller-Todd BK, Archer LT: Current management of the septic shock patient: Experimental basis for treatment. Circ Shock 9:543, 1982.

180. Schumer W: Steroids in the treatment of septic shock. Ann Surg 184:333, 1976.

181. Kreger BE, Craven DE, McCabe WR: Gram-negative bacteremia. IV: Re-evaluation of clinical features and treatment of 612 patients. Am J Med 68:344, 1980.

182. Schumer W: Controversy in shock research. Pro: The role of steroids in septic shock. Circ Shock 8:667, 1981.

183. Blaisdell FW: Controversy in shock research. Con: The role of steroids in septic shock. Circ Shock 8:673, 1981.

184. Sprung CL, Caralis PV, Marcial EH, et al: The effects of high-dose corticosteroids in patients with septic shock. N Engl J Med 311:1137, 1984.

185. Bone RC, Fisher CJ Jr, Clemmer TP, et al: A controlled clinical trial of high-dose methylprednisolone in the treatment of severe sepsis and septic shock: The Methylprednisolone Severe Sepsis Study Group. N Engl J Med 317:653, 1987.

186. Hinshaw L, Peduzzi P, Young E, et al: Effect of high-dose glucocorticoid therapy on mortality in patients with clinical signs of systemic sepsis: The Veterans Administration Systemic Sepsis Cooperative Study Group. N Engl J Med 317:659, 1987.

187. Lebel MH, Freij BJ, Syrogiannopoulos GA, et al: Dexamethasone therapy for bacterial meningitis. N Engl J Med 319:964, 1988.

188. Gagnon S, Boota AM, Fischl MA, et al: Corticosteroids as adjunctive therapy for severe *Pneumocystis carinii* pneumonia in the acquired immunodeficiency syndrome. N Engl J Med 323:1444, 1990.

189. Bozzette SA, Sattler FR, Chiu J, et al: A controlled trial of early adjunctive treatment with corticosteroids for *Pneumocystis carinii* pneumonia in the acquired immunodeficiency syndrome. N Engl J Med 323:1451, 1990.

190. Li TCM, Phillips MC, Shaw L, et al: On-site physician staffing in a community hospital intensive care unit. JAMA 252:2023, 1984.

191. Reynolds HN, Haupt MT, Thill-Baharozian MC, et al: Impact of critical care physician staffing on patients with septic shock in the university hospital medical intensive care unit. JAMA 260:3446, 1988.

192. Martinez A, Levine SJ, Parker MM, et al: Hemodynamic changes in acute adrenal insufficiency (abstract). Clin Res 38:766A, 1990.

193. Swan HJ, Ganz W, Forrester J, et al: Catheterization of the heart in man with use of a flow-directed balloon-tipped catheter. N Engl J Med 283:447, 1970.

194. Ganz W, Donoso R, Marcus HS, et al: A new technique for measurement of cardiac output by thermodilution in man. Am J Cardiol 27:392, 1971.

195. Glower DD, Spratt JA, Snow ND, et al: Linearity of the Frank-Starling relationship in the heart: The concept of preload recruitable stroke work. Circulation 71:994, 1985.

196. Natanson C, Danner RL, Reilly JM, et al: Antibiotics versus cardiovascular support in a canine model of human septic shock. Am J Physiol 259:H1440, 1990.

197. Parker MM, Suffredini AF, Natanson C, et al: Responses of left ventricular function in survivors and non-survivors of septic shock. J Crit Care 4:19, 1989.

198. Rackow EC, Kaufman BS, Falk JL, et al: Hemodynamic response to fluid repletion in patients with septic shock: Evidence for early depression of cardiac performance. Circ Shock 22:11, 1987.

199. Packman MI, Rackow EC: Optimum left heart filling pressure during fluid resuscitation of patients with hypovolemic and septic shock. Crit Care Med 11:165, 1983.

200. Goldberg LI, Hsich YY, Risnekov L: Newer catecholamines for treatment of heart failure and shock. Prog Cardiovasc Dis 19:327, 1977.

201. Desjars P, Pinaud M, Potel G, et al: A reappraisal of norepinephrine therapy in human septic shock. Crit Care Med 15:134, 1987.

202. Ognibene FP: Management of septic shock, p 239. In: Parrillo JE (moderator): Septic shock in humans: Advances in the understanding of pathogenesis, cardiovascular dysfunction, and therapy. Ann Intern Med 113:227, 1990.

203. Schaer GL, Fink MP, Parrillo JE: Norepinephrine alone versus norepinephrine plus low-dose dopamine: Enhanced renal blood flow with combination pressor therapy. Crit Care Med 13:492, 1985.

Infectious Diseases

Section Editor

Jack D. Sobel

Control and Prevention of Infection

Jeffrey D. Band

During the past 20 years, remarkable progress has been made in the medical care of critically ill adults. Specialized centers for care of patients and intensive care units (ICUs) have emerged to provide care to severely ill patients who often have markedly compromised host defenses and are in need of continuous invasive monitoring and life-support equipment. ICUs have contributed greatly to improved survival of selected subsets of patients.[1, 2] However, mortality in ICUs remains high, often exceeding 25%.

One major factor contributing to added morbidity and mortality in ICU patients is nosocomial infection. In contrast to general wards, where an average nosocomial rate of 5 to 10% has been observed, the incidence of nosocomial infections in ICUs may exceed 20 to 30%.[4–9] The rates of nosocomial infection among patients after 1 week of advanced life support in an ICU are threefold to fivefold higher than the rates among patients in non-ICU units.[6, 9–11] Clearly, critically ill patients are at very high risk for developing nosocomial infection, and its occurrence has catastrophic consequences.

PREDISPOSING FACTORS

Factors predisposing a critically ill patient to an increased risk of infection are generally well understood. Patients with life-threatening illnesses are particularly susceptible because of the nature of their underlying disease, multiple comorbid conditions, impaired host defenses, and intensive exposures to invasive devices and necessary therapeutic interventions. Intensive exposure to medical personnel also occurs, as well as indirect exposure to other critically ill and often infected patients. Not surprisingly, most outbreaks of nosocomial infections have occurred in ICUs, even though less than 10% of hospitalized patients ever require treatment in an ICU.[6] Infections with selected pathogens such as *Serratia*, *Acinetobacter*, enterococci, *Candida* species, and antibiotic-resistant gram-negative bacilli also occur more commonly in an ICU setting.[12–15] The ICU may become an "epicenter" for subsequent spread of these organisms to outside units as colonized or infected patients no longer in need of intensive care monitoring are transferred to general wards.[16, 17] Colonized medical personnel may also transmit these and other organisms to patients hospitalized elsewhere.

Because many of these nosocomial infections are causally related to invasive procedures and devices, surgery, intravascular catheters, urethral catheters, or endotracheal tubes,[18, 19] or to organisms transmitted between patients on the hands of medical personnel,[12, 20, 21] infection control practices can potentially prevent many such infections.[22] Nosocomial infection in critically ill patients must never be assumed to be an inevitable consequence. Measures to prevent the spread of infection within ICUs and to limit its occurrence must be given high priority.

EPIDEMIOLOGY OF NOSOCOMIAL INFECTIONS

Magnitude of the Problem

The incidence of nosocomial infections among patients hospitalized in an ICU varies markedly, depending on the type of unit and intensive care population studied as well as methods of surveillance (Table 29–1). In general, rates of nosocomial infection appear to be highest in specialized units such as burn and trauma centers. In these units, rates of nosocomial infection often exceed 50%.[5, 6, 8] Rates of nosocomial infection in surgical units have varied from 8% to as much as 62%;[4, 6–9, 23–27] rates observed in medical ICUs are appreciably lower, ranging from 7 to 36%.[6, 8, 9, 25–27] The lowest rates of nosocomial infection have been reported from coronary care units, where rates from 4 to 7% have been noted.[8, 28]

It is difficult to compare studies from different institutions because of inherent differences in populations studied, local practices regarding usage of invasive devices and antibiotics, and surveillance techniques. Length of stay, another important factor in determining effect on rates of nosocomial infections, can also vary in different institutions. More units are beginning to appreciate the impact of these factors and are correcting their overall crude infection rates by use of a time-weighted denominator (patient-days of risk) and further adjusting their data for severity of illness.[29] Because the majority of nosocomial infections observed in ICUs are procedure related,[18, 19] calculation of device-specific rates may assist infection control personnel in better focusing their prevention efforts on high-risk procedures.

TABLE 29–1

NOSOCOMIAL INFECTION RATES IN ADULT INTENSIVE CARE UNITS

Author	Type of Unit	Infection Rate*	Patients with Nosocomial Infection (%)
Chandrasekar et al[8]	Burn	29.8	12.8
Wenzel et al[6]	Burn	64.0	—
Caplan et al[5]	Trauma	50.9	30.4
McGuckin and Kelsen[23]	Surgical	—	10.3
Northy et al[4]	Surgical	27.3	23.4
Daschner et al[24]	Surgical	—	27.6
Kollish et al[25]	Surgical	—	36.0
Munzinger et al[7]	Surgical	42.5	28.2
Chandrasekar et al[8]	Surgical	35.2	13.6
Wenzel et al[6]	Surgical	8.0	—
Craven et al[9]	Surgical	61.6	30.9
Kollish et al[25]	Medical	—	23.0
Chandrasekar et al[8]	Medical	13.9	10.9
Wenzel et al[6]	Medical	7.0	—
Craven et al[9]	Medical	35.4	23.8
Preston et al[26]	Mixed	—	11.7
Donowitz et al[11]	Mixed	—	18.0
Brown et al[27]	Mixed	11.2	—
Wenzel et al[6]	Mixed	5.0	—
Chandrasekar et al[8]	Coronary	6.6	1.9
Schandorf et al[28]	Coronary	4.7	4.0

*Rate expressed as number of infections per 100 admissions (a patient may have more than one nosocomial infection).

Sites of Infection

The most commonly reported sites of infection in patients in adult ICUs are the lower respiratory tract (tracheobronchitis, pneumonia), urinary tract, blood stream, and wounds (Table 29–2). The majority of these infections appear to be causally related to medical devices. For example, lower respiratory tract infections usually account for at least 25% of all nosocomial infections in adult ICUs. Patients needing mechanical ventilation are at 5 to 23 times increased risk for development of a nosocomial pneumonia.[30-32] The vast majority of urinary tract infections occur in patients with an indwelling urethral catheter.[33] (Please refer to Chapter 44.) Wenzel and colleagues[19] found that 33 to 45% of all nosocomial blood stream infections occurred in patients residing in ICUs. It has been estimated that close to 80% of primary bacteremias in these patients are associated with indwelling vascular devices.[34] (Please refer to Chapters 16 and 123.)

Pathogens

The spectrum of pathogens responsible for ICU-associated infections is shown in Table 29–3. More than half of infections documented in adult ICUs are due to aerobic gram-negative bacilli.[8, 9, 28, 35] *Klebsiella, Enterobacter,* and *Serratia* species usually account for the majority of both urinary and lower respiratory tract infections. *Staphylococcus aureus* also remains an important cause of nosocomial pneumonia and wound infection and, along with *Staphylococcus epidermidis,* is the major cause of primary blood stream infections. In fact, data collected by the Centers for Disease Control (CDC) suggest that the incidence of blood stream infections with coagulase-negative staphylococci has increased from 10% in 1980 to more than 30% in 1989.[36] Besides the emergence of *S. epidermidis* as a major nosocomial pathogen, enterococci and members of the *Candida* species (and *Torulopsis*) have become important nosocomial pathogens.[37]

ICUs in particular are often reservoirs of antibiotic-resistant bacteria. Several studies have found that antibiotic resistance is more prevalent in the ICU setting.[38] In a study by Wenzel and coworkers, ICU patients represented a large proportion (31%) of patients with infection with gram-negative rods whose infecting organisms were resistant to commonly used aminoglycoside antibiotics.[19] There are many reasons for this, but it may be due in part to the

TABLE 29–2

NOSOCOMIAL INFECTIONS IN ADULT INTENSIVE CARE UNITS BY SITE OF INFECTION

Author	Type of Unit	Infection Site (%)				
		Respiratory Tract	Urinary Tract	Blood	Wound	Other
Craig and Connelly[35]	Medical	33	29	11	11	16
Daschner et al[24]	Surgical	16	27	22	7	28
Donowitz et al[11]	Mixed	25	25	29	8	13
Wenzel et al[6]	Surgical	31	21	19	13	16
	Medical	36	29	14	7	14
	Mixed	30	30	20	12	8
	Coronary	33	20	33	7	7
Chandrasekar et al[8]	Mixed	26	17	26	16	16
Craven et al[9]	Surgical	35	25	12	22	6
	Medical	46	28	13	12	1

TABLE 29–3

DISTRIBUTION OF ORGANISMS RESPONSIBLE FOR NOSOCOMIAL INFECTIONS IN INTENSIVE CARE UNITS*

| | Patients (%) | | | | | | | |
| | Urinary Tract Infection | | Pneumonia | | Wound Infection | | Blood Stream | |
Organism	MICU†	SICU‡	MICU	SICU	MICU	SICU	MICU	SICU
Gram negative								
E. coli	23	21	7	8	0	17	28	17
Klebsiella, Enterobacter, Serratia sp.	34	34	30	38	9	29	12	27
Pseudomonas	11	15	16	27	27	23	4	9
Other	7	11	51	53	9	21	20	11
Gram positive								
S. aureus	0	1	19	36	36	20	16	15
S. epidermidis	5	4	2	18	18	14	0	17
Enterococci	7	5	0	0	0	6	4	21
Other	0	3	0	0	9	14	16	5
Candida species	20	16	8	0	0	6	0	5

*In some infections more than one organism was isolated.
†MICU = medical ICU.
‡SICU = surgical ICU.
Modified from Craven DE, Kunches LM, Lichtenberg DA, et al: Nosocomial infection and fatality in medical and surgical intensive care unit patients. Arch Intern Med 148:1161–1168, 1988. Copyright 1988, American Medical Association.

selective pressures exerted by the intensity of use of broad-spectrum antibiotics in ICUs.

Epidemics

Most epidemics of hospital-acquired infections occur in ICUs. During a 5-year period of study, Wenzel and coworkers[6] identified 11 major outbreaks of nosocomial infection at the University of Virginia Hospital. Ten of the outbreaks occurred in ICUs. The reservoirs of the outbreaks included devices in five instances, contaminated medication in one, probably blood products in another, and other roommates in three instances. Eight of the 10 outbreaks occurring in the ICU involved blood stream infections. More than one third of the 97 outbreaks of epidemic bacteremias occurring between 1965 and 1978 stemmed from some aspect of infusion therapy.[39] Two thirds of these outbreaks occurred in closed populations of patients, most commonly adults in ICUs. An ICU setting consisting of severely ill individuals, congregated together and requiring life-sustaining devices and continuous supportive or therapeutic interventions, not infrequently becomes an epicenter for certain types of microorganisms and for epidemic nosocomial infections.

Risk Factors

Many studies have examined the risk factors associated with nosocomial infection. However, few investigations have specifically addressed the ICU population. Patients in ICUs are particularly vulnerable to nosocomial infections because of three major factors: (1) compromised host factors; (2) therapy for underlying diseases and concomitant comorbidities; and (3) paradoxically, the lifesaving ICU technology, especially the numerous invasive devices—endotracheal tubes, urethral catheters, intravascular cannulas, and others. These invasive devices often amplify colonization by nosocomial organisms, increasing vulnerability to infection and providing a direct portal of entry for organisms.[12]

Host Factors

A major determinant of host susceptibility to infection is the nature and degree of the patient's underlying disease.

Certain disease states are associated with specific defects in host defenses (Table 29–4). Patients with chronic debilitating disorders and patients with fatal and ultimately fatal illnesses are at high risk for developing infection.[40, 41] Craven and associates found 23 variables associated univariately with nosocomial infection.[9] These included demographic variables such as age and sex, the severity of acute illness on admission (as measured by shock or coma on admission and the acute physiologic score of the Acute Physiology and Chronic Health Evaluation [APACHE] I method, described by Knaus and associates[42]), the admission diagnosis, evidence of renal failure or acidosis, and the use of invasive devices for more than 3 days. When invasive devices were excluded

TABLE 29–4

HOST FACTORS PREDISPOSING PATIENTS TO INFECTIONS

Demographic variables
  Age, sex, race
Underlying disease state
  Damage of anatomic barriers
    Skin, e.g., trauma, burns
    Gastrointestinal, e.g., surgery, inflammatory conditions, mucositis
  Obstruction of natural passages
    Bronchus, e.g., obstructive lung disease, tumor
    Urinary tract, e.g., stone, tumor
  Humoral immune deficiency
    Congenital immune deficits
    Multiple myeloma
    Splenectomy
  Cellular immune deficiency
    Lymphomas
    Malnutrition
    Acquired immunodeficiency syndrome
    Immunosuppressive drugs
  Granulocytopenia
    Leukemia, aplastic anemia
    Cancer chemotherapy
  Severity of acute illness
    Coma, shock, multiorgan failure
Medical interventions
  Chemotherapy, steroids
  Antibiotics

from the stepwise logistic regression model, five factors (days in ICU, shock on admission, hospitalization in the surgical ICU, administration of steroids or chemotherapy, and renal failure) were associated with the development of nosocomial infection.

Medical Therapy

At times, the therapy for the disease itself rather than the underlying illness increases susceptibility to infection. Chemotherapeutic agents used to treat myeloproliferative disorders, cancer, and certain immunologic disorders may have locally toxic effects on the mucosal lining of the gastrointestinal tract and permit organisms to invade damaged barriers. Neutropenia, especially counts of 500 cells per cubic millimeter or less, greatly increases risk of infection.[43] Such neutropenic states are commonly associated with use of chemotherapy for myeloproliferative disorders, lymphoproliferative disorders, solid tumors, and organ transplantation. Cytotoxic agents may also depress both humoral and cellular immunity.[44] Corticosteroids also have profound influences on host defenses, affecting neutrophil function, monocyte function, the activity of the reticuloendothelial system, and lymphocyte function.[45]

Antimicrobial agents may have direct adverse effects on host defenses as well as greatly influencing the ecologic flora of the host.[38, 46] Antibiotic pressure appears to be one of the most important factors predisposing patients to epidemic infection with resistant organisms.[38]

Many other drugs or biologic products may have direct or indirect adverse effects on the host. For example, antacids or histamine H_2 receptor antagonists, by elevating gastric pH, may promote the growth of microorganisms in the stomach normally inhibited by gastric acid.[47]

Nosocomial infections including outbreaks have been traced to contaminated medications, infusion fluids, blood products, inhalation therapy equipment, and dialysis machines.[48–52]

Exposure to Medical Devices

Exposure to invasive medical devices and procedures greatly increases the risk of nosocomial infection and appears to be at least as important in susceptibility to nosocomial infection as underlying diseases. The ICU patient frequently is in need of multiple medical devices, including peripheral intravenous catheters, arterial catheters, central venous catheters, Swan-Ganz catheters, endotracheal tubes, nasogastric tubes, urinary catheters, surgical drains, and intracranial pressure-monitoring devices. Each of these devices breaches the body's normal physical barriers and provides an avenue for entry of endogenous or exogenously acquired colonizing organisms. Many of these devices are attached to reservoirs that may permit further multiplication of colonizing organisms, increasing the chance of infection. In general, the longer such devices are required, the higher the risk of infection. Patients requiring mechanical ventilation are at 5- to 23-fold higher risk for developing nosocomial pneumonia than the nonventilated patient.[30–32] The risk is especially increased if mechanical ventilation is required beyond 3 days.[9] Indwelling bladder catheters are associated with high rates of nosocomial urinary tract infections. ICU patients requiring an indwelling bladder catheter for more than 10 days have a threefold higher incidence of infections than patients requiring shorter-term catheterization.[9] Likewise, patients in need of continuous arterial pressure monitoring are at higher risk of infection if monitoring is needed at the same site beyond 4 days.[53]

Exposure to Personnel

Health care workers may transfer potential pathogens to susceptible patients. Hand carriage of gram-positive cocci, gram-negative bacilli, fungi, and viruses has been implicated in outbreaks of nosocomial infection.[12, 20, 21, 54] Health care workers have also been responsible for transmitting such infections as tuberculosis, measles, mumps, rubella, and hepatitis B to susceptible patients.[55–59]

Miscellaneous Exposures

Exposure to potential pathogens may also occur within the hospital via contaminated common vehicles (hospital equipment), contaminated air or water supplies, and food sources.[60] The topics of exposures to personnel and the environment are covered in later sections of this chapter.

PATHOGENESIS OF NOSOCOMIAL INFECTION

One of the most important principles in epidemiology and infection control is the chain of infection. Three interrelated factors—the agent, the host, and the transmission of the agent—make up the chain of infection.[61] The chain of infection may be interrupted by attacking any of these links. For example, colonization of the host with the implicated pathogen—a prerequisite to infection—can be eliminated. This can be done either by eradicating the source of the agent or, more commonly, by interrupting transmission. Reversal of host defense defects and immune enhancement may also serve as effective means of interrupting the chain.

Susceptibility of the Host

The importance of the nature of the patient's underlying disease in influencing susceptibility has already been discussed. Length of stay in an ICU, a marker of degree of illness of the patient, also greatly influences susceptibility to infection.[9] Patients with serious underlying diseases are frequently colonized by microbial flora that differs significantly from that of healthy hosts. For example, the microbial flora of the oropharynx is replaced by aerobic gram-negative bacilli in critically ill patients.[62, 63] This may be due in part to the elevated salivary protease activity with resulting decreases in fibronectin observed in debilitated patients.[64] Loss of fibronectin results in increased adherence of gram-negative bacilli to epithelial cells and decreased adherence of gram-positive cocci.[65–67] Intestinal and cutaneous colonization may also be altered in disease states, and new strains of organisms may be acquired. Rapid reversal of underlying disease states or measures to augment host defenses may help prevent nosocomial infections.

Source of Microorganisms

Organisms that cause nosocomial infections come from either endogenous (autogenous) or exogenous sources. Endogenous infections are caused by the patient's own microflora; exogenous infections result from transmission of organisms from a source outside the patient. Endogenous organisms may be part of the patient's flora before hospitalization or may become colonizers after hospitalization. The term *autogenous infection* indicates that the infection was derived from the patient, whether or not the infecting organism was acquired before or after hospitalization.

Autogenous Flora

It has been estimated that up to half of nosocomial infections in critically ill patients are due to their autogenous flora.[68, 69] Disruptions of normal mechanical barriers by trauma, surgery, or invasive devices can result in the patient's autochthonous strains causing infection. As discussed earlier, advanced age and underlying disease may predispose the host to gram-negative pharyngeal colonization and cutaneous colonization with *S. aureus*, streptococci, gram-negative bacilli, and fungi.[62, 63, 70] These microorganisms may then gain entrance to sites that were previously sterile, such as the catheterized urinary tract, blood stream, or lung. Endogenous infections are best prevented by preserving the patient's host defenses, but measures of asepsis designed primarily to limit exogenous organisms to susceptible sites may be important as well. Antimicrobial therapy has a profound influence on the autogenous flora and can rapidly result in the replacement of existing flora with more resistant ones.[38]

Exogenous Flora

Hospitalized patients can acquire new organisms from other patients, the hospital staff, and the inanimate environment. The most important source is the hands of medical personnel.[12, 20, 21] Cross-colonization occurs commonly, especially if hands are not adequately washed between contacts with patients. Failure to change gloves between patients may also result in nosocomial infections.[71, 72] Health care workers may periodically shed *S. aureus*, *S. epidermidis*, and group A streptococci from their nares or perineum.[12] Infected patients also serve as direct disseminators of infectious agents.

Nosocomial infection may be linked to inanimate objects. Contaminated medical equipment has been responsible for exogenously acquired organisms, infection, and outbreaks. Respiratory therapy equipment,[51] inhaled or parenterally administered medications,[48] contaminated infusates,[49] pressure transducers,[73] dialysis machines,[52] water baths,[74] ice machines,[75] ice baths for thermodilution measurements of cardiac outputs,[76] mattresses and air-fluidized beds,[77] bandages,[78] and other contaminated devices[79] have all resulted in outbreaks of nosocomial infections.

Outbreaks of nosocomial infection (and sporadic cases) have been associated with airborne pathogens spread directly or indirectly by contaminated ventilation systems. *Aspergillus*, *Rhizopus*, *Legionella*, and *Pseudomonas* infections have resulted. Airborne spread of other pathogens such as varicella, measles, influenza, and parainfluenza viruses or *Mycobacterium tuberculosis* may also result from infected patients.

Food and water are less common sources of infection, although outbreaks traced to these vehicles have occurred.[60]

Reservoirs of Organisms

Reservoirs are places where organisms maintain their presence, metabolize, and replicate. The reservoir and source may be one and the same, or the source may become contaminated from the reservoir. For example, infected or colonized patients frequently serve as the reservoir and source of certain bacterial and viral infections. Gram-positive bacteria, especially *S. aureus*, *S. epidermidis*, and group A streptococci, frequently derive from patients or personnel. Gram-negative bacilli may derive from either a human reservoir or the inanimate environment and the source and reservoir may differ. In an outbreak of *Pseudomonas cepacia* infections, the source of the organism was a contaminated pressure transducer but the reservoir was a disinfectant harboring the organism.[73] *Legionella pneumophila* may be spread via a contaminated cooling tower (airborne) but the reservoir is often contaminated potable water.[80]

Modes of Transmission

There are three major routes of nosocomial transmission of organisms: contact, common vehicle, and airborne. An organism may have more than one route of transmission.

Contact transmission may be direct, indirect, or by respiratory droplets. Direct-contact transmission is the major route of spread of exogenous organisms within the ICU setting, with the hands (or gloves) of hospital personnel serving as the mechanism. Direct contact is also responsible for many autogenous infections. For example, a patient's surgical wound may become colonized from organisms transmitted into the wound directly by the patient.

Indirect spread may occur if the source of contamination is an inanimate object. An example would be spread of pathogens to an individual patient via a contaminated endoscope. In contrast, droplet spread occurs when large respiratory droplets are inadvertently spread from a colonized health care worker or a hospitalized roommate to the patient, as in nosocomial transmission of *M. tuberculosis*.

Common vehicle transmission occurs when a contaminated inanimate vehicle is the medium for the transmission to multiple exposed patients. Examples of this mechanism of spread include the delivery of intrinsically contaminated infusion fluid to patients with resulting gram-negative sepsis or use of blood products originally derived from a patient infected with hepatitis C.

Airborne transmission occurs with some pathogens capable of being disseminated by small droplet nuclei or dust particles. These particles may remain suspended for many hours; examples are varicella, *Aspergillus*, and *M. tuberculosis*.

CONTROL AND PREVENTION

Infection control practices, if applied consistently and regularly, can significantly reduce the burden of nosocomial infections. In the ICU setting, where many such infections are associated with procedures or devices, the possibilities for reduction are great. Unfortunately, at the time of the study on the efficacy of nosocomial infection control, only half of U.S. hospitals were following less than a third of the CDC-recommended control practices, and the other half were following more than a third of the practices.[81] Hospitals with intensive infection control programs reduced nosocomial infection by an average of 32%. Still, infections in critically ill patients are not entirely preventable, in part because many arise endogenously.[69, 82]

Surveillance and Control

The backbone of an infection control program is surveillance. Monitoring provides information about endemic rates and types of infection, magnitude of antibiotic resistance, early warning signs of an outbreak, and whether or not there are problems associated with specific devices or procedures. Feedback of this information to medical personnel is essential. Surveillance is best conducted by appropriately trained infection control personnel. Guidelines for performing surveillance may be obtained from the CDC, the Association of Practitioners in Infection Control, or the Society for Hospital Epidemiology of America.

Policies and procedures for the prevention of infection must be individualized for the specific type of ICU. Guidelines for reducing device- or procedure-related infections must be adhered to and modified as newer information becomes available.[83–87] Programs to educate the staff on infection control must be provided regularly and compliance with established procedures monitored.

Structural and Staffing Considerations

Considerations in the design of a well-functioning and safe environment for critically ill patients are reviewed elsewhere in this text, and standards have been published.[88] ICUs generally are best placed in cul-de-sacs to limit traffic control to essential personnel. Some studies have suggested that single-patient rooms offer better protection to patients than open units.[89, 90] Single-patient rooms decrease the chance for exposure to other colonized or infected patients and may be most important for severely compromised hosts. Adequate space with convenient hand-washing facilities is essential to permit access to the patient and the life-support equipment and lessens the chance of contact transmission. Ventilation must be monitored to ensure proper handling and filtration of air; units must be cleaned regularly to lessen the chances of airborne spread of pathogens. At least some of the individual rooms in the ICU setting must be equipped to handle patients infected with airborne communicable diseases. These rooms should be able to provide negative pressures and air exhausted directly to the outside.

Specialized isolation units containing life islands of complete laminar flow may help reduce infections in a subset of severely compromised hosts when combined with antibiotic decontamination of the patient.[91–94] These units are extremely costly and their efficacy has not been established for the average adult ICU.

Specially trained staff well versed in the needs of critically ill patients is required for ICUs. Although the optimal nurse-to-patient ratio is not known, elevated rates of infection and outbreaks have been documented when staffing is reduced. One-to-one nurse-to-patient ratios 24 hours a day may significantly reduce cross-infection.[6]

Hospital staff may transmit infections to susceptible hosts as well as become colonized or infected through exposure to patients if proper precautions are not utilized. Detailed guidelines for infection control in hospital personnel have been published.[95] Hospital staff should always engage in proper hand washing before and after each contact with a patient and understand the proper techniques of asepsis. They should be fully up to date with their immunizations to reduce the chance of acquiring or transmitting a vaccine-preventable disease. These immunizations must include measles, rubella, and hepatitis B. Workers with potentially transmissible infections should be relieved of work unless the infection is under adequate treatment or its potential for spread is limited by barriers. Employees exposed to potentially transmissible agents (e.g., varicella-zoster virus) should receive prompt evaluation and treatment. All health care workers must practice "universal precautions"[96] or modified body substance barrier precautions[97] when caring for their patients. The elements to be addressed in an infection control program are summarized in Table 29–5.

TABLE 29–5

ELEMENTS OF AN INFECTION CONTROL PROGRAM FOR EMPLOYEES

Placement evaluations
Personnel health and safety education
Immunization programs
Protocols for surveillance and management of occupational illnesses and exposures
Counseling services
Guidelines for work restriction because of infectious diseases and illnesses
Maintenance of health records

Isolation, Hand Washing, and Environmental Control

In general, the modes of transmission of an infectious agent should determine the level of precautions or isolation needed to prevent transmission to other patients and health care workers. The CDC has published extensive guidelines for isolation precautions in hospitals.[98] Types of precautions include

- *Category-specific isolation precautions.* Under this system, patients with known or suspected infections are placed in one or more of the seven isolation categories, based on the agent, its mode(s) of transmission, and the site and extent of infection. The seven basic categories are strict isolation, respiratory isolation, tuberculosis (acid-fast bacilli) isolation, contact isolation, drainage/secretion precautions, enteric precautions, and universal precautions (formerly blood and body fluid precautions). The specifications for each category and representative processes are summarized in Table 29–6.
- *Disease-specific isolation.* Patients with known or suspected diseases are managed with precautions known to interrupt the transmission of the specific agent. Only the precautions that interrupt transmission of that agent are recommended. Barrier placements are more specifically tailored under this system, but most hospitals have found the development of specific guidelines for each disease overwhelming.

Many institutions have developed their own modifications of the foregoing systems or have combined them in various manners. For example, some centers have developed category-specific isolation precautions called myelo/immunosuppressive precautions. Patients at high risk for infection, such as granulocytopenic patients, are placed in private rooms, and hand washing *with an antiseptic soap* is required before and after contact with these patients. Health care workers with potentially communicable diseases are excluded from care of the patients, and masks are required, especially if a health care worker has an unexplained cough. In many ICUs, this type of precaution would be utilized for all critically ill patients. More elaborate precautions—protective isolation—have been adopted by some ICUs as the standard of care. With protective isolation, patients are generally cared for in single-bed rooms and all personnel are required to use, at a minimum, disposable high-barrier gowns and gloves for all contacts with the patients. (Some persons also favor routine use of masks.) The value of protective isolation for all ICU patients remains uncertain because of the conflicting results of published studies.[82, 91–94]

The basic barrier to hand-contact transmission is hand washing (and the appropriate use of gloves). Hands (and gloves) of hospital personnel are a major means of transmitting pathogenic organisms.[12, 20, 21, 54] Up to 80% of hospital personnel working in ICUs carry large numbers of methicillin-resistant, coagulase-negative staphylococci on their hands[99] and more than 50% harbor gram-negative bacilli.[100] Hands should always be washed before and after each contact with the patient. Gloves worn by health care workers for personal protection (universal precautions) or for protection of the patient must be discarded after use and the hands must be washed. Gloves may pose additional hazards to other patients if they are not changed after each use. An antiseptic-containing hand-washing agent is generally recommended in ICUs. Maki and Hecht demonstrated a nearly 50% reduction in nosocomial infection when an antiseptic-containing hand-washing agent was used instead of nongermicidal soap by hospital staff.[101] Unfortunately, studies in ICUs have demonstrated that most personnel wash their hands less than 50% of the time that is indicated.[82, 102–105]

TABLE 29–6

SUMMARY OF CENTERS FOR DISEASE CONTROL CATEGORY-SPECIFIC ISOLATION PRECAUTIONS

Category	Private Room	Masks	Gown	Gloves	Hand Washing	Representative Diseases
Strict	Yes	Yes	Yes	Yes	Yes	Varicella, disseminated zoster, zoster in compromised host, pneumonic plague
Respiratory	Yes	Yes	No	No	Yes	Meningococcal or *Haemophilus influenza* B infection, measles, mumps, pertussis
Acid-fast bacilli	Yes	Yes, if patient is coughing	No	No	Yes	Pulmonary or laryngeal tuberculosis
Contact	Yes, unless cohorted	Yes, close contact	Yes, if contact likely	Yes, if contact likely	Yes	Major wound infections, multiply resistant bacteria, pneumonia caused by *S. aureus* (or *S. pyogenes*), pediculosis
Drainage/ secretion	No	No	Yes, if contact likely	Yes, if contact likely	Yes	Minor wound infection, skin infection, conjunctivitis
Enteric	No, unless hygiene poor	No	No, unless soiling likely	No, unless contact likely	Yes	Infective gastroenteritis, enterovirus infection, viral meningitis, poliomyelitis
Universal	No	No	No, unless soiling with blood or body fluids likely	No, unless contact with blood or body fluids likely	Yes	All patients

Hand-washing practices must be monitored continuously, especially in ICU settings, and programs to improve compliance must be encouraged.

As recommended by the policy of universal precautions, all health care workers should routinely use appropriate barrier precautions to prevent skin and mucous membrane exposure when contact with blood or other body fluids of any patient is anticipated. Gloves should be worn for touching blood or body fluids, mucous membranes, or nonintact skin for all patients, for handling items or surfaces soiled with blood or body fluids, and for performing venipuncture and other vascular access procedures. Gloves should be changed after tasks involving body fluid contact and after each patient. Masks and protective eyewear or face shields should be worn during procedures likely to generate droplets of blood or other body fluids. Gowns or protective garments should be worn during procedures that are likely to generate splashes of blood or other body fluids. Other recommendations of the policy of universal precautions are as follows:

1. Needles should not be recapped, purposely bent or broken by hand, removed from disposable syringes, or otherwise manipulated by hand.
2. Disposable syringes and needles, scalpel blades, and other sharps should be placed in puncture-resistant containers for disposal.
3. Mouth-to-mouth resuscitation should be discouraged if possible. Instead, mouthpieces, resuscitation bags, and other ventilation devices should be readily available.

Effective cleaning, disinfection, and sterilization of equipment used in care of patients are of critical importance in preventing nosocomial infection. Objects that enter sterile tissue or the vascular system must be completely sterile. Most of these items should be purchased sterile or should be sterilized by heat (steam under pressure). If heat labile, the object must be treated with gas (ethylene oxide) or, if other methods are unsuitable, a chemical sterilant such as glutaraldehyde, stabilized hydrogen peroxide, or demand-release chlorine dioxide. Objects that come in contact with mucous membranes or nonintact skin should also be free of all microorganisms, with the exception of bacterial spores. Examples of these items are endoscopes, respiratory therapy equipment, and anesthesia breathing circuits. These items—commonly referred to as semicritical devices—require high-level disinfection. This can be accomplished by using either wet pasteurization or chemical germicides. Objects that come into contact with intact skin, such as blood pressure cuffs, stethoscopes, and electrocardiographic leads, need not be sterile but must be clean. This can be accomplished with germicidal soaps or low-level disinfectants. Two excellent guidelines to assist with environmental control have been developed by the CDC and the Association for Practitioners in Infection Control.[106, 107]

Routine sampling of the environment in the ICU including the air, water, or environmental surfaces is not recommended, nor is the use of special shoe covers or "antimicrobial" floor mats.[108, 109]

Control of Medical Devices

It has been estimated that more than 850,000 device-associated infections occur annually in the United States and that epidemics of device-related infections continue to rise.[19] Use of devices in ICUs is increasing rapidly. Guidelines for the use of medical devices are periodically updated by the CDC.[83–86] The reader is also encouraged to consult the many other excellent chapters in this textbook dealing with device-related infections. Advancing technology is resulting in exciting developments in the design of existing devices to minimize potential infectious sequelae. For example, newer endotracheal tubes may be developed that are less damaging to the mucosa and coated with colonization-resistant polymer. Newer mechanical ventilators may be able to eliminate the humidifying cascade, a source of contaminated condensate, by use of a heat-moisture exchanger. Intravascular devices are being made with newer polymers that are less thrombogenic and less irritating to the vessel wall. The device itself may be coated with an antimicrobial-containing substance. Subcutaneous cuffs, made of biodegradable collagen and impregnated with bactericidal silver ion, may lower the incidence of central venous catheter infections.[110] Newer indwelling bladder catheters may be constructed of polymers resistant to encrustation and colonization or coated with broad-spectrum antimicrobials. Existing infection control measures can greatly reduce the frequency of device-associated infections. These specific measures must be adhered to whenever medically feasible. Most important, medical devices should never be inserted unless they are clearly indicated for definite therapeutic or diagnostic purposes and asepsis is carefully maintained at all times. Medical devices must be removed as soon as they are no longer medically needed.

Control of Endogenous Flora

Much of the focus of infection control programs has been on minimizing acquisition of nosocomial flora by eliminating exogenous (environmental) sources or by preventing cross-infections. Strict adherence to asepsis, another well-recognized aspect of infection control, also limits opportunities for endogenous flora to cause nosocomial infections. For example, because most intravenous catheter–related infections result from contamination of the cannula wound by the patient's own microflora,[111–113] control measures are aimed at preventing such contamination. These include hand washing and gloving by personnel before cannula insertion, preparation of the insertion site with an antiseptic, and often application of an antibiotic or antiseptic ointment to the catheter wound after insertion. Other measures for reducing the likelihood of contamination of the catheter wound include use of sterile dressings and reapplication of antibiotic or antiseptic ointments. We found that topical antibiotic ointment containing polymyxin, neomycin, and bacitracin may help prevent peripheral venous catheter infection and that povidone-iodine ointment is best suited for care of central venous catheters and for arterial catheters.[114] Similarly, most surgical wound infections are caused by endogenous organisms. Preoperative bathing or showering with antiseptic soaps, washing the operative site and applying an antimicrobial preoperative skin preparation, and selectively using parenteral antimicrobial prophylaxis have helped reduce rates of surgical wound infections. Infections after bowel surgery have also been reduced by careful preparation of the gastrointestinal tract via mechanical cleansing and antibiotic decontamination.[115]

Selective decontamination of the digestive tract has also been widely used in immunocompromised granulocytopenic patients in attempts to prevent infection.[91–94, 116–118] Although various oral, nonabsorbable antibiotics have been used, the regimen of gentamicin, vancomycin, and nystatin has been most thoroughly studied. In all studies, bacterial counts in the stool were significantly reduced within the first 1 to 2 weeks of use. However, not all studies demonstrated reductions in nosocomial infections, especially if patients were not simultaneously cared for in a protected environment.[116, 119, 120]

Investigators have begun to examine the effect of selective decontamination of the gastrointestinal tract on the incidence of nosocomial infections in the ICU patient. Studies have shown that oropharyngeal colonization precedes nosocomial pneumonia; the source of oropharyngeal colonization is frequently organisms found in the patient's oropharynx at admission or in the patient's stomach.[121] It was postulated that effective decontamination of the oropharynx and digestive tract by the use of topically administered antimicrobics might reduce nosocomial infections. Several studies have shown that a regimen of topical polymyxin, tobramycin, and amphotericin suspension and paste (often, supplemented with a short course of parenterally administered antibiotic such as cefotaxime) results in fewer nosocomial infections, particularly of the respiratory tract.[122–126] Other investigators failed to demonstrate a reduction in nosocomial infections with this or similar regimens or witnessed the emergence of resistant organisms.[127, 128] Further well-designed studies in ICUs are needed to define the role and consequences of selective decontamination.

Control of Antibiotics

Pathogens causing nosocomial infections in ICUs may be significantly influenced by use of antimicrobial agents in these patients. McGowan has reviewed evidence linking antibiotic usage and antibiotic resistance in hospital bacteria.[38] This includes the following:

1. Antimicrobial resistance is more prevalent in bacterial strains that cause nosocomial infections.
2. During outbreaks, patients with resistant strains were more likely to have received prior antibiotics than controls.
3. Changes in antimicrobial usage lead to parallel changes in prevalence of resistance.
4. Areas within the hospital having the highest usage of antimicrobial, such as ICUs, also have the highest prevalence of resistant bacteria.
5. Patients exposed to antibiotics for longer durations are more likely to become colonized or infected with resistant organisms.
6. Increasing dosage of antimicrobials leads to greater likelihood of superinfection or colonization with resistant organisms.
7. Antibiotic therapy has marked effects on the endogenous flora of patients and can select preferentially for organisms resistant to the drug.

Antibiotics may result in replacement of susceptible strains with resistant ones or induction of drug resistance.[16, 129]

TABLE 29–7

INVESTIGATION OF A SUSPECTED OUTBREAK

1. Determine the nature, magnitude, and gravity of the suspected problem and initiate preliminary control measures. Develop a case definition.
2. Confirm the existence of an epidemic. Seek additional cases by review of available data and by surveillance.
3. Characterize the cases of disease according to time, place, and person.
4. Formulate tentative epidemiologic hypothesis about likely cause-effect relationship.
5. Identify appropriate control group(s).
6. Test the epidemiologic hypothesis (case-control study, cohort study, or prospective intervention study) and conduct more systematic studies.
7. Attempt to confirm the epidemiologic hypothesis microbiologically.
8. Institute further infection control measures as needed.
9. Determine the impact of these control measures. Document actual control by reduction of rates.
10. Summarize your findings in a written report. Provide feedback to key individuals and to members of the infection control committee.

Careful selection and control of antimicrobial agents are essential in minimizing the spread of resistant nosocomial pathogens and superinfection with *Candida* species.

Outbreak Investigation

When an outbreak is suspected (an unusual, statistically significant increase in the incidence of a particular disease or pathogen), an immediate investigation is warranted. Table 29–7 summarizes the basic steps in outbreak investigation. Cooperation between the ICU staff and the infection control or hospital epidemiology department is essential. The infection control effort must also have adequate administrative and laboratory support.

References

1. Campion EW, Malley AG, Goldstein RL, et al: Medical intensive care for the elderly. JAMA 246:2052, 1981.
2. Paneth N, Kiely JL, Wallenstein S, et al: Newborn intensive care and neonatal mortality in low-birth weight infants: A population study. N Engl J Med 307:149, 1982.
3. Abramson NS, Silvasy K, Grenvik AN, et al: Adverse occurrences in intensive care units. JAMA 244:1582, 1980.
4. Northy D, Adess ML, Hartsuck JM, et al: Microbial surveillance in a surgical intensive care unit. Surg Gynecol Obstet 139:321, 1974.
5. Caplan ES, Hoyt N, Conley RA: Changing patterns of nosocomial infections in severely traumatized patients. Am Surg 45:204, 1979.
6. Wenzel RP, Thompson RL, Landry SM, et al: Hospital-acquired infections in intensive care unit patients: An overview with emphasis on epidemics. Infect Control 4:371, 1983.
7. Munzinger J, Buhler M, Geroulanos S, et al: Nosokomiale Infektionen in einem Universitatsspital. Schweiz Med Wochenschr 113:1787, 1983.
8. Chandrasekar PH, Kruse JA, Mathews MF: Nosocomial infection among patients in different types of intensive care units at a city hospital. Crit Care Med 14:508, 1986.
9. Craven DE, Kunches LM, Lichtenberg DA, et al: Nosocomial infection and fatality in medical and surgical intensive care unit patients. Arch Intern Med 148:1161, 1988.
10. Caplan ES, Hoyt N: Infection surveillance and control in the severely traumatized patient. Am J Med 70:638, 1981.
11. Donowitz LG, Wenzel RP, Hoyt JW: High risk of hospital-acquired infection in the ICU patient. Crit Care Med 10:355, 1982.
12. Maki DG: Control of colonization and transmission of pathogenic bacteria in the hospital. Ann Intern Med 89:777, 1978.
13. Daschner F, Langmaack H, Wiedemann B: Antibiotic resistance in intensive care unit areas. Infect Control 4:382, 1983.
14. Archer GL, Kietrick DR, Johnston JL: Molecular epidemiology of transmissible gentamicin resistance among coagulase-negative staphylococci in a cardiac surgery unit. J Infect Dis 151:243, 1985.
15. Shlaes DM, Currie-McCumber C, Eanes M, et al: Gentamicin resistance plasmids in an intensive care unit. Infect Control 7:355, 1986.
16. Weinstein RA, Kabins SA: Strategies for prevention and control of multiple drug–resistant nosocomial infection. Am J Med 70:449, 1981.
17. Gaynes RP, Weinstein RA, Smith J, et al: Control of aminoglycoside resistance by barrier precautions. Infect Control 4:221, 1983.
18. Stamm WE: Infections related to medical devices. Ann Intern Med 89:764, 1978.
19. Wenzel RP, Osterman CA, Donowitz LG, et al: Identification of procedure-related nosocomial infections in high-risk patients. Rev Infect Dis 3:701, 1981.
20. Steere A, Mallison GF: Handwashing practices for the prevention of nosocomial infection. Ann Intern Med 83:683, 1975.
21. Larson E: A causal link between hand washing and risk of infection? Examination of the evidence. Infect Control Hosp Epidemiol 9:28, 1988.
22. Haley RW, Culver DH, White JW, et al: The efficacy of infection surveillance and control programs in preventing nosocomial infections in U.S. hospitals. Am J Epidemiol 121:182, 1985.
23. McGuckin MB, Kelsen SG: Surveillance in a surgical intensive care unit: Patient and environment. Infect Control 2:21, 1981.
24. Daschner FD, Frey P, Wolff G, et al: Nosocomial infections in intensive care ward: A multicenter prospective study. Intensive Care Med 8:5, 1982.
25. Kollish NR, Kunches LM, Craven DE: A prospective analysis of nosocomial infections occurring in the intensive care units at Boston City Hospital. In: Proceedings of the Ninth Annual Conference of the Association for Practitioners in Infection Control, New Orleans, LA, May 1982.
26. Preston GA, Larson EL, Stamm WE: Effect of private isolation rooms on patient care practices: Colonization and infection in an intensive care unit. Am J Med 70:641, 1981.
27. Brown RB, Hosmer D, Chen HC, et al: A comparison of infections in different ICUs within the same hospital. Crit Care Med 13:472, 1985.
28. Schandorf WA, Brown RB, Sands M, et al: Infections in a coronary care unit. Am J Cardiol 56:757, 1985.
29. Freeman J, McGowan JE Jr: Differential risks of nosocomial infection. Am J Med 70:245, 1981.
30. Haley RW, Hooton TM, Culver DH, et al: Nosocomial infections in U.S. hospitals, 1975–1976: Estimated frequency by selected characteristics of patients. Am J Med 70:947, 1981.
31. Cross AS, Roup B: Role of respiratory assistance devices in endemic nosocomial pneumonia. Am J Med 70:681, 1981.
32. Celis R, Torres A, Gatell JM, et al: Nosocomial pneumonia: A multivariate analysis of risk and prognosis. Chest 93:318, 1988.
33. Stamm WE: Guidelines for prevention of catheter-associated urinary tract infections. Ann Intern Med 82:386, 1975.
34. Maki DG: Nosocomial bacteremia: An epidemiologic overview. Am J Med 70:719, 1981.
35. Craig CP, Connelly S: Effect of intensive care unit nosocomial pneumonia on duration of stay and mortality. Am J Infect Control 12:233, 1984.
36. Banerjee S, Emori G, Culver D, et al: Trends in nosocomial bloodstream infections (BSI) in the United States, 1980–1989. In: Proceedings of the Third International Conference on Nosocomial Infections, Atlanta, GA, July 31–August 3, 1990, p 25.
37. Schaberg DR: Major trends in nosocomial bacterial pathogens. In: Proceedings of the Third International Conference on Nosocomial Infections, Atlanta, GA, July 31–August 3, 1990, p 20.
38. McGowan JE Jr: Antimicrobial resistance in hospital organisms and its relation to antibiotic use. Rev Infect Dis 5:1033, 1983.
39. Bennett JV: Incidence and nature of endemic and epidemic nosocomial infections. In: Bennett JV, Brachman PS (eds): Hospital Infections. Boston, Little, Brown, p 233, 1979.
40. Britt MR, Schleupner CJ, Matsomiya S: Severity of underlying disease as a predictor of nosocomial infection. JAMA 239:1047, 1978.
41. Tran DD, Groeneveld J, Van Der Meulen J, et al: Age, chronic disease, sepsis, organ system failure, and mortality in a medical intensive care unit. Crit Care Med 18:474, 1990.
42. Knaus WA, Zimmerman JE, Wagner DT, et al: APACHE: Acute physiology and chronic health evaluation: A physiologically-based classification system. Crit Care Med 9:591, 1981.
43. Bodey GP, Buckley M, Sathe YS, et al: Quantitative relationships between circulating leukocytes and infections in patients with acute leukemia. Ann Intern Med 64:328, 1966.
44. Santos GW, Owens AH Jr, Sensenbrenner LL: Effects of selected cytotoxic agents on antibody production in man; A preliminary report. Ann NY Acad Sci 114:404, 1964.
45. Fauci AS, Dale DC, Balow JE: Glucocorticosteroid therapy: Mechanisms of action and clinical considerations. Ann Intern Med 84:304, 1976.
46. Hauser WE, Remington JS: Effect of antibiotics on the immune system. Am J Med 72:711, 1982.
47. Ruddell WS, Axon AT, Bartholomew BA, et al: Effect of cimetidine on the gastric bacterial flora. Lancet 1:672, 1980.
48. Mertz JJ, Scharer L, McClement JH: A hospital outbreak of *Klebsiella pneumoniae* from inhalation therapy with contaminated aerosol solutions. Am Rev Respir Dis 95:454, 1967.
49. Maki DG, Rhame FS, Mackel DC, et al: Nationwide epidemic of septicemia caused by contaminated intravenous products. I. Epidemiologic and clinical features. Am J Med 60:471, 1976.
50. Rhame FS, Root RK, MacLowry JD, et al: Salmonella septicemia from platelet transfusions. Study of an outbreak traced to a hematogenous carrier of *Salmonella choleraesuis*. Ann Intern Med 76:633, 1973.
51. Ringrose RE, McKown B, Felton FG, et al: A hospital outbreak of *Serratia marcescens* associated with ultrasonic nebulizers. Ann Intern Med 69:719, 1988.
52. Band JD, Ward JI, Fraser DW, et al: Peritonitis caused by a *Mycobacterium chelonei*–like organism associated with intermittent chronic peritoneal dialysis. J Infect Dis 45:9, 1982.
53. Band JD, Maki DG: Infections caused by indwelling arterial catheters used for hemodynamic monitoring. Am J Med 67:635, 1979.
54. Larson E: Handwashing and skin physiologic and bacteriologic aspects. Infect Control 6:14, 1985.
55. Catanzaro A: Nosocomial tuberculosis. Am Rev Respir Dis 125:559, 1982.
56. Williams WW, Preblud SR, Reichelderfer PS, et al: Vaccines of importance in the hospital setting: Problems and developments. Infect Dis Clin North Am 3:701, 1989.
57. Wharton M, Cochi SL, Hutcheson RH, et al: Mumps transmission in hospitals. Arch Intern Med 150:47, 1990.
58. Polk BF, White JA, DeGirolami PC, et al: An outbreak of rubella among hospital personnel. N Engl J Med 303:541, 1980.
59. Snydmen DR, Hindman SH, Wineland MD: Nosocomial viral hepatitis B: A cluster among staff with subsequent transmission to patients. Ann Intern Med 85:573, 1976.
60. Rutala WA, Weber DJ: Environmental issues and nosocomial infections. In: Farber BF (ed): Infection Control in Intensive Care. New York, Churchill Livingstone, p 131, 1987.
61. Garner JS: Isolation techniques in critical care units. Crit Care Q 3:29, 1980.

62. Johanson WG, Pierce AK, Sanford JP: Changing pharyngeal bacterial flora of hospitalized patients: Emergence of gram-negative bacilli. N Engl J Med 281:1137, 1969.

63. Johanson WG, Pierce AK, Sanford JP, et al: Nosocomial respiratory infections with gram-negative bacilli: The significance of colonization of the respiratory tract. Ann Intern Med 77:701, 1972.

64. Woods DE, Straus DC, Johanson WG Jr, et al: Role of salivary protease activity in adherence of gram-negative bacilli to mammalian buccal epithelial cells in vivo. J Clin Invest 68:1435, 1981.

65. Johanson WG Jr, Woods DE, Chaudhuri T, et al: Association of respiratory tract colonization with adherence of gram-negative bacilli to epithelial cells. J Infect Dis 139:667, 1979.

66. Woods DE, Straus DC, Johanson WG Jr, et al: Role of fibronectin in the prevention of adherence of *Pseudomonas aeruginosa* to buccal cells. J Infect Dis 143:784, 1981.

67. Abraham SN, Beachey EH, Simpson WA: Adherence of *Streptococcus pyogenes*, *Escherichia coli*, and *Pseudomonas aeruginosa* to fibronectin-coated and uncoated epithelial cells. Infect Immun 41:1261, 1983.

68. Schimpff SC, Young VM, Greene WH, et al: Origin of infection in acute nonlymphocytic leukemia: Significance of hospital acquisition of potential pathogens. Ann Intern Med 77:707, 1972.

69. Kerver AJH, Rommes JH, Mevissen-Verhage EAE, et al: Colonization and infection in surgical intensive care patients, a prospective study. Intensive Care Med 13:347, 1987.

70. Aly R, Maibach HI, Rahman R, et al: Correlation of human in vivo and in vitro cutaneous antimicrobial factors. J Infect Dis 131:579, 1975.

71. Doebbeling BN, Pfaller MA, Houston AK, et al: Removal of nosocomial pathogens from the contaminated glove: Implications for glove reuse and handwashing. Ann Intern Med 109:394, 1988.

72. Patterson JE, Pantelick E, Farrell P, et al: *Acinetobacter* outbreak in surgical intensive care unit linked to gloves used for universal precautions. In: Proceedings of the Twenty-eighth Interscience Conference on Antimicrobial Agents and Chemotherapy, Los Angeles, CA, October 23–26, 1988, p 358.

73. Weinstein RA, Emori TG, Anderson RL, et al: Pressure transducers as a source of bacteremia after open heart surgery. Chest 69:338, 1976.

74. Abrutyn E, Goodhart GL, Roos K, et al: *Acinetobacter calcoaceticus* outbreak associated with peritoneal dialysis. Am J Epidemiol 107:328, 1978.

75. Newsom SWB: Hospital infection from contaminated ice. Lancet 2:620, 1968.

76. Pien FD, Bruce AE: Nosocomial *Ewingella americana* bacteremia in an intensive care unit. Arch Intern Med 146:111, 1986.

77. Vesley D, Hankinson SE, Lauer JL: Microbial survival and dissemination associated with an air-fluidized therapy unit. Am J Infect Control 14:35, 1986.

78. Keys TF, Haldorson AM, Rhodes KH, et al: Nosocomial outbreak of *Rhizopus* infections associated with Elastoplast wound dressings—MN. MMWR 27:33, 1978.

79. Earnshaw JJ, Clark AW, Thorn BT: Outbreak of *Pseudomonas aeruginosa* following endoscopic retrograde cholangiopancreatography. J Hosp Infect 5:371, 1984.

80. Band JD, LaVenture M, David JP, et al: Epidemic legionnaires' disease: Airborne transmission down a chimney. JAMA 245:2404, 1981.

81. Haley RW, Culver DH, White JW, et al: The efficacy of infection surveillance and control programs in preventing nosocomial infections in U.S. hospitals. Am J Epidemiol 121:183, 1985.

82. Preston GA, Larson EL, Stamm WA: The effect of private isolation rooms on patient care practices, colonization and infection in an intensive care unit. Am J Med 70:285, 1981.

83. Simmons B, Wong ES: Guidelines for prevention of nosocomial pneumonia. Infect Control 3:327, 1982.

84. Simmons B, Hooton TM, Wong E, et al: Guidelines for Prevention of Intravascular Infections. Washington, DC, US Government Printing Office, p 61, 1981. US Department of Health and Human Services manual.

85. Simmons B, Hooton TM, Wong E, et al: Guideline for Prevention of Infections Related to Intravascular Pressure-Monitoring Systems. Washington, DC, US Government Printing Office, p 68, 1981. US Department of Health and Human Services manual.

86. Wong ES, Hooton TM: Guideline for Prevention of Catheter-Associated Urinary Tract Infections. Washington, DC, US Government Printing Office, p 1, 1981. US Department of Health and Human Services manual.

87. Garner JS: Guideline for Prevention of Surgical Wound Infections. Washington, DC, US Government Printing Office, p 2, 1985. US Department of Health and Human Services manual.

88. US Department of Health and Human Services: Guidelines for Construction and Equipment of Hospital and Medical Facilities. Washington, DC, US Government Printing Office, 1984. US Department of Health and Human Services publication (HRS-M-HF) 84.

89. Laufman H: The infection hazard of intensive care. Surg Gynecol Obstet 139:413, 1974.

90. Smylie HG, Davidson AIG, MacDonald A, et al: Ward design in relation to postoperative wound infection. Part I. Br Med J 1:67, 1971.

91. Dietrich M, Gaus W, Vossen J, et al: Protective isolation with antimicrobial decontamination in patients with high susceptibility to infection. Infection 5:107, 1977.

92. Pizzo PA, Levine AS: The utility of protected environmental regimens for the compromised host: A clinical reassessment. Prog Hematol 10:311, 1977.

93. Rodriguez V, Bodey GP, Freireich EG, et al: Randomized trial of protected environment–prophylactic antibiotics in 145 adults with acute leukemia. Medicine 57:253, 1978.

94. Navari RM, Buckner CD, Cleft RA, et al: Prophylaxis of infection in patients with aplastic anemia receiving allogeneic marrow transplants. Am J Med 76:564, 1984.

95. Williams WW: Guidelines for infection control in hospital personnel. Am J Infect Control 12:34, 1984.

96. Centers for Disease Control: Recommendations for prevention of HIV transmission in health care settings. MMWR 36: No 2S, 1987.

97. Lynch P, Jackson MM, Cummings MJ, et al: Rethinking the role of isolation practices in the prevention of nosocomial infections. Ann Intern Med 107:243, 1987.

98. Garner JS, Simmons BP: Guideline for isolation precautions in hospitals. Am J Infect Control 12:103, 1984.

99. Maki DG, Alvarado C, Hassemer C: Comparison of organisms carried on the hands of hospital personnel and nonmedical control personnel: Methicillin-resistant coagulase-negative staphylococcus is a common organism. In: Proceedings of the Twenty-fourth Interscience Conference on Antimicrobial Agents and Chemotherapy, Washington, DC, October 1984.

100. Knittle MA, Eitzman DV, Baer H: Role of hand contamination of personnel in the epidemiology of gram-negative nosocomial infections. J Pediatr 86:433, 1975.

101. Maki DG, Hecht J: Antiseptic-containing handwashing agents reduce nosocomial infections—A prospective study. In: Proceedings of the Twenty-second Interscience Conference on Antimicrobial Agents and Chemotherapy, Miami Beach, October 1982, p 303.

102. Albert RK, Condie F: Handwashing patterns in medical intensive care units. N Engl J Med 304:1465, 1981.

103. Kaplan LM, McGuckin M: Increasing handwashing compliance with more accessible sinks. Infect Control 7:408, 1986.

104. Conly JM, Hill S, Ross J, et al: Handwashing practices in an intensive care unit: The effects of an educational program and its relationship to infection rates. Am J Infect Control 17:330, 1989.

105. Simmons B, Bryant J, Neiman K, et al: The role of handwashing in prevention of endemic intensive care unit infections. Infect Control Hosp Epidemiol 11:589, 1990.

106. Garner JS, Favero MS: Guideline for handwashing and environmental control, 1985. Am J Infect Control 14:110, 1986.

107. Rutala WA: APIC guideline for selection and use of disinfectants. Am J Infect Control 18:99, 1990.

108. Ayliffe GAF, Collins BJ, Lowburg EJL, et al: Ward floors and other surfaces as reservoirs of hospital infections. J Hyg 65:515, 1967.

109. Maki DG, Alvarado CJ, Hassemer C, et al: Relation of the inanimate hospital environment to endemic nosocomial infection. N Engl J Med 307:1562, 1982.

110. Maki DG, Cobb L, Garman JK: An attachable silver-impregnated cuff for prevention of infection with central venous catheters: A prospective randomized multicenter trial. Am J Med 85:307, 1988.

111. Maki DG, Weise CE, Sarafini HW: A semi-quantitative culture method for identifying intravenous catheter–related infection. N Engl J Med 296:1305, 1977.

112. Bjornson HS, Colley R, Bower RH, et al: Association between microorganism growth at the catheter site and colonization of the catheter in patients receiving total parenteral nutrition. Surgery 92:720, 1982.

113. Snydman DR, Pober BR, Murray SA, et al: Predictive value of surveillance skin cultures in total-parenteral nutrition–related infection. Lancet 2:1385, 1982.

114. Maki DG, Band JD: A comparative study of polyantibiotic and iodophor ointments in prevention of vascular catheter–related infection. Am J Med 70:739, 1981.

115. Clarke JS, Condon RE, Bartlett JG, et al: Preoperative oral antibiotics reduce septic complications of colon operations: Results of prospective randomized, double-blind clinical study. Ann Surg 186:251, 1977.

116. Yates JW, Holland JF: A controlled study of isolation and endogenous microbial suppression in acute myelocytic leukemia patients. Cancer 32:1490, 1972.

117. Schimpff SC, Greene WH, Young VM, et al: Infection prevention in acute nonlymphocytic leukemia: Laminar air flow room reverse isolation with oral nonabsorbable antibiotic prophylaxis. Ann Intern Med 82:351, 1975.

118. Bodey GP, Rodriguez V, Cabanillas F, et al: Protected environment–prophylactic antibiotic program for malignant lymphoma: Randomized trial during remission induction chemotherapy. Am J Med 66:74, 1979.

119. Levine AS, Siegel SE, Schriber AD, et al: Protected environment and prophylactic antibiotics: A prospective controlled study of their utility in the therapy of acute leukemia. N Engl J Med 288:477, 1973.

120. Lohner D, Debusscher L, Prevost JM, et al: Comparative randomized study of protected environment plus oral antibiotics versus oral antibiotics alone in neutropenic patient cancer treatment. Cancer Treat Rep 63:363, 1979.

121. Sanderson PJ: The sources of pneumonia in ITU patients. Infect Control 7:104, 1986.

122. Stoutenbeek CP, van Saene HKF, Miranda DR, et al: The effect of selective decontamination of the digestive tract on colonization and infection in multiple trauma patients. Intensive Care Med 10:185, 1984.
123. Ledingham McAI, Alcock SR, Eastaway AT, et al: Triple regimen of selective decontamination of the digestive tract, systemic cefotaxime, and microbiological surveillance for prevention of acquired infection in intensive care. Lancet 1:785, 1988.
124. Kerver AJH, Rommes JH, Verhage EAE, et al: Prevention of colonization and infection in critically ill patients: A prospective randomized study. Crit Care Med 16:1087, 1988.
125. Flaherty J, Nathan C, Kabins SA, et al: Pilot trial of selective decontamination for prevention of bacterial infection in an intensive care unit. J Infect Dis 162:1393, 1990.
126. Rodriguez-Roldan JM, Altona-Cuesta A, Lopez A, et al: Prevention of nosocomial lung infection in ventilated patients: Use of an antimicrobial pharyngeal nonabsorbable paste. Crit Care Med 18:1239, 1990.
127. Feeley TW, DuMoulin GC, Hedley-Whyte J, et al: Aerosol polymyxin and pneumonia in seriously ill patients. N Engl J Med 293:471, 1975.
128. Brun-Boisson C, Legrand P, Rauss A, et al: Intestinal decontamination for control of nosocomial multiresistant gram-negative bacilli. Study of an outbreak in an intensive care unit. Ann Intern Med 110:873, 1989.
129. Murray BE, Moellering RC Jr: Patterns and mechanisms of antibiotic resistance. Med Clin North Am 62:899, 1978.

CHAPTER 30

Fulminant Viral Infections

Michael J. Borucki
Richard B. Pollard

More than 400 different viruses can infect humans, but only a limited number cause significant morbidity and mortality in the noncompromised host. Specifically, agents that cause hepatitis, involve the central nervous system (CNS), produce hemorrhagic fevers, or cause pneumonia may be associated with significant disease in the normal host (Table 30–1). Diagnosis is usually achieved through the identification of disease syndromes combined with confirmatory viral cultures (Table 30–2), serologic study results, or histopathologic findings.

In the immunocompromised host, a number of additional agents become significant pathogens: herpes simplex virus (HSV), human cytomegalovirus (CMV), varicella-zoster virus (VZV), and the agents associated with progressive multifocal leukoencephalopathy. Progressive varicella, for example, may occur in up to 30% of childhood leukemias.

The human herpesviruses are sufficiently pathogenic, however, to cause disease in the absence of severe compromise. Herpes simplex encephalitis occurs in patients without demonstrable immunodeficiency. Pregnant women appear to be at increased risk for mortality from varicella pneumonia. Cigarette smokers more frequently have complications of viral pneumonic processes, particularly varicella pneumonia.

VIRAL RESPIRATORY INFECTIONS

The average adult experiences three or four respiratory illnesses each year, most of which are of viral origin. Although viral infections caused by a variety of agents of the respiratory tract are common (Table 30–3), serious morbidity and fatal disease rarely occur. Respiratory infections caused by viruses typically present as one of five clinical syndromes: upper respiratory tract infection, pharyngitis, influenza-like disease, bronchitis, and pneumonia.

A number of host factors may be protective, including physical barriers: mucociliary clearance, filtration, and large-particle deposition in the nasopharynx. Specific immunity, including antibody and cytotoxic T cell responses, and nonspecific immune responses, such as alveolar macrophages and complement, also contribute to the control of respiratory pathogens.

A pulse-temperature deficit may be seen with viral pneumonias, and the patient may exhibit few abnormalities on physical examination in spite of prominent radiographic abnormalities.

The differential diagnostic considerations should include a variety of potentially treatable conditions, including mycoplasmosis, Q fever, psittacosis, and legionnaires' disease in immunocompetent hosts and cryptococcosis, histoplasmosis, strongyloidiasis, toxoplasmosis, pneumocystosis, and respiratory syncytial and herpesvirus infections in immunocompromised hosts. Noninfectious disorders that may be amenable to therapy also result in interstitial pneumonitides: sarcoidosis, vasculitis, and hypersensitivity pneumonitis.

Influenza Virus

Influenza virus is a frequent cause of epidemic and pandemic respiratory tract disease. The pandemic of 1918 to 1919 may have been responsible for more than 0.5 million fatalities in the United States and more than 20 million deaths worldwide. The organism of influenza A was first isolated after inoculation of ferrets[1] and the agent of influenza B was isolated shortly thereafter.[2]

Influenza virus types A and B have been well characterized, with the most interesting biologic features of the virus being harbored in two surface glycoproteins (hemagglutinin and neuraminidase). The virus additionally codes for a matrix protein that lies immediately subjacent to the host cell–derived lipid envelope bilayer, three polymerases involved in viral RNA transcription, and a duplex helicoid nucleoprotein that associates with the viral RNA. The antigenic drift or antigenic shift results from changes in the surface glycoproteins hemagglutinin and neuraminidase.[3, 4] Three distinct hemagglutinins (H_1, H_2, and H_3) and two antigenically distinct neuraminidase proteins (N_1 and N_2) have been described. Each subtype is further classified by the site and year of isolation of the strain; for example, influenza A/Texas/77 H_3N_2 is an influenza serotype A virus isolated in Texas in 1977 bearing the major antigens H_3 and N_2.

Clinical studies of the 1957 influenza A pandemic suggest that four distinct patterns of pulmonary disease may arise as complications of influenza infection:[5] influenza with physical signs of lower respiratory tract disease but without radiographic signs of pneumonia, influenza complicated by secondary bacterial pneumonia, primary influenzal pneumonia, and combined influenza virus and bacterial pneumonia. The first entity is thought to represent influenzal bronchiolitis, with the patients exhibiting high fever, pleurisy, dyspnea, and prostration. Signs of local consolidation were absent, and these patients recovered without antibiotic therapy.

Primary influenzal pneumonia occurred in patients with established heart disease. After a typical influenzal prodrome of fevers, chills, sore throat, dry cough, muscle aches, and prostration, the principal complaint of increasing respiratory distress brought the patients to medical attention, typically within 24 to 36 hours of the onset of symptoms. All patients

TABLE 30–1		
VIRAL INFECTIONS THAT MAY CAUSE SEVERE MORBIDITY IN HUMANS		
Family	**Genus**	**Pathogens***
Arenaviridae	*Arenavirus*	Lassa fever virus
		Lymphocytic choriomeningitis virus
		Junin virus (Argentine HF)
		Machupo virus (Bolivian HF)
Bunyaviridae	*Bunyavirus*	California encephalitis virus
		La Crosse encephalitis virus
	Phlebovirus	Rift Valley fever virus
		Sandfly fever virus
		Punta Toro virus
	Nairovirus	Congo-Crimean HF virus
	Hantavirus	Hantaan virus
	Not assigned	Seoul virus
		Puumala virus (nephropathia epidemica)
Filoviridae		Ebola HF virus
		Marburg HF virus
Hepadnaviridae	*Hepadnavirus*	Human hepatitis B virus
Herpesviridae		Human
		Herpes simplex virus type 1
		Herpes simplex virus type 2
		Varicella-zoster virus
		Epstein-Barr virus
		Human cytomegalovirus
		Human herpesvirus type 6
		Nonhuman
		Cercopithecine herpesvirus 1 (B virus)
Paramyxoviridae	*Paramyxovirus*	Mumps virus
	Morbillivirus	Measles virus
Picornaviridae	*Rhinovirus*	Poliovirus 1–3
	Enterovirus	Coxsackievirus A1–24
		Coxsackievirus B1–6
		Echoviruses 1–34
		Enterovirus serotypes 68 and upward
		Enterovirus type 72, hepatitis A virus
Poxviridae	*Orthopoxvirus*	Smallpox virus
		Vaccinia virus
Rhabdoviridae	*Lyssavirus*	Rabies virus
Togaviridae	*Alphavirus* (arbovirus group A)	Eastern equine encephalitis virus (M)
		Venezuelan equine encephalitis virus 1–4 (M)
		Western equine encephalitis virus (M)
		Semliki Forest virus (M)
	Flavivirus (arbovirus group B)	Yellow fever virus (M)
		Dengue HF virus serotypes 1–4 (M)
		Japanese B virus (M)
		St. Louis encephalitis virus (M)
		Rocio virus (? M)
		Murray Valley virus (M)
		West Nile virus (M)
		Omsk HF virus (T)
		Powassan virus (T)
		Kyasanur Forest disease virus (T)
	Rubivirus	Rubella virus

*HF = hemorrhagic fever; (M) = mosquito-borne; (T) = tick-borne.

in this group appeared seriously ill, with respiratory rates of 36 to 54 breaths/min and cyanosis. Diffuse fine inspiratory rales associated with scattered inspiratory wheezes were noted. Chest roentgenograms were characterized by diffuse infiltrates, which mimicked cardiogenic pulmonary edema. Mortality occurred frequently in this group.

Ribavirin (1β-D-ribofuranosyl-1*H*-1,2,4-triazole-3-carbox-amide) aerosol has been effective in lessening the duration of fever and decreasing viral shedding in trials against both influenza A and B in college students.[6]

Human Cytomegalovirus

Human CMV infections occur frequently and cause significant morbidity and mortality in predisposed populations.

TABLE 30–2
VIRUS ISOLATION IN DIAGNOSTIC VIROLOGY

Virus Isolation	Permissive Cells	Other
Echovirus	Primary monkey kidney Human diploid cell lines	
Influenza	Primary monkey kidney	Embryonated egg

Paramyxovirus
  Respiratory syncytial virus
  Measles
  Mumps
  Parainfluenza
	Primary monkey kidney
	Primary human embryonal kidney	

Herpesvirus
  Herpes simplex
  Human cytomegalovirus
  Varicella-zoster virus
	Human diploid fibroblast	

Equine encephalitis viruses
  Eastern equine encephalitis
  Western equine encephalitis
  St. Louis encephalitis
  California encephalitis
		Suckling mouse

Poliovirus	Primary monkey kidney Primary human embryonal kidney Human diploid fibroblast	

Primary infection in the immunocompetent adult host, when symptomatic, typically results in a mild, self-limited disease similar to Epstein-Barr virus–associated mononucleosis or hepatitis.[7] Characteristic of the human herpesviruses, life-long latent infection typically follows primary infection and severe disease may result if host immunity is sufficiently compromised to permit reactivation.[8] Infections with human CMV-like agents occur in a variety of animal species, but CMV infections and disease are highly host specific such that human CMV disease and transmission occur only in and between humans. In addition to the morbidity and mortality attributable to human CMV, primary CMV infections have also been reported to increase the risk of bacterial superinfections.[9] CMV may cause disease in a number of target organs,[10] including the retina, the gastrointestinal tract, the brain, the adrenal glands, and the lungs (Table 30–4).

CMV has been called the "troll of transplantation"[11] because human CMV disease so frequently complicates the post-transplant clinical course of solid organ and bone marrow transplant recipients. CMV frequently causes life-threatening infection in profoundly immunocompromised populations, including patients with the acquired immunodeficiency syndrome (AIDS)[12] and bone marrow transplant recipients.[13] Solid organ transplant recipients of livers,[14] kidneys,[15] and hearts[16] are also at risk for severe disease

attributable to human CMV infection. CMV infection may be associated with up to 30% of the post-transplant febrile illnesses, 25% of post-transplant deaths, and 20% of graft failure caused by rejection.[15] Although 60% of patients may have a fourfold increase in human CMV antibody, cell-mediated responses, particularly lymphocyte transformation, are typically diminished.[17] Seroconversion, a fourfold increase in anti–human CMV titer, often accompanies acute CMV infection, but the failure to achieve seroconversion may be observed and is considered a poor prognostic sign.

Since the original description of CMV infection in patients after bone marrow transplantation,[18] human CMV continues to be a major concern and a frequent cause of death in this highly immunocompromised population. CMV pneumonia often occurs in association with graft-versus-host disease and is characterized by fever, cyanosis, a nonproductive cough, and dyspnea. Hypoxemia and bilateral interstitial infiltrates are typical, and a decreased arterial oxygen tension often precedes the roentgenographic abnormalities.

In a large, retrospective review of 545 patients who had undergone bone marrow transplantation, 16.7% (91 patients) experienced CMV pneumonia at a median onset of 62 days.[13] The overall mortality rate was 84.6%. Only 53%

TABLE 30–3
VIRAL INFECTIONS INVOLVING THE LUNGS

Influenza A
Adenovirus infection
Varicella
  Disseminated zoster
Human cytomegalovirus infection
Herpes simplex
  Pharyngitis
  Tracheobronchitis
  Pneumonia (less commonly)
Respiratory syncytial virus infection

TABLE 30–4
ORGAN INVOLVEMENT BY CYTOMEGALOVIRUS IN BONE MARROW TRANSPLANT RECIPIENTS AT AUTOPSY

Frequency (%)	Disease Limited to Single Organ (%)	Organ System
80	28	Lung
72	10	Adrenal gland
41	3	Retina
28		Gastrointestinal tract
15		CNS
10		Spleen
10		Liver
8		Pancreas
8		Genitourinary tract
5		Lymph nodes

of the cases were diagnosed ante mortem, with the lung being the most common site of recovery of human CMV at autopsy. A variety of risk factors for the development of CMV pneumonia were identified, including the presence of graft-versus-host disease, anti–human CMV seropositive status before bone marrow transplantation, and the presence of viremia. The isolation of human CMV from the blood was associated with a 2.5-fold increased risk of disease.

In one series, symptomatic human CMV disease occurred in more than 20% (22 of 101) of liver transplant recipients, most commonly presenting with neutropenia, fever, and thrombocytopenia a mean of 37 days after transplantation.[14] Disseminated disease attributable to human CMV occurred in 6 of 22 patients and most commonly was diagnosed at postmortem examination. One patient with CMV gastritis, and without associated pneumonitis, survived. Ante mortem, the six patients had been treated with OKT3 for graft rejection and four of the six had a clinical picture consistent with adult respiratory distress syndrome.

CMV infection in heart transplant recipients has been associated with an increased risk of graft rejection, graft atherogenesis, and mortality.[19] Since the introduction of cyclosporine, human CMV infection occurs in 30% of patients undergoing cardiac transplantation. Half of those infected have symptoms referable to CMV infection, and 10% experience life-threatening infections.[19] Infectious complications were typically more frequent before the introduction of cyclosporine,[20] with reactivation of CMV described in up to 100% of CMV-seropositive patients undergoing heart transplantation. Human CMV–seronaive individuals may have primary infection, which is more frequently symptomatic.

Pretransplant anti–human CMV complement fixation antibody status correlates with increasing age and with the occurrence of CMV infection after kidney transplantation.[15] The risk of CMV infection remains modest during the first 3 weeks after kidney transplantation, approximates 50% by 7 weeks after transplantation, and continues to rise linearly until more than 80% of patients have infection by week 14. Leukopenia and fever are the most typical associated signs of CMV infection. The onset of CMV infection not uncommonly accompanies the onset of renal graft rejection.[15]

In a prospective study of human CMV disease in 141 kidney transplant recipients,[21] 44 (31%) experienced overt CMV-related disease at a median onset of 46 days. Twelve patients had lethal CMV disease, all had pulmonary involvement. Overall, 25 patients had pulmonary manifestations, and hypoxemia developed 10 days into the course of the illness. Of 13 patients requiring ventilatory support, only 1 survived. A variety of clinical conditions were associated with an increased risk of human CMV disease, including the presence of anti–human CMV antibody in the donor, a cadaveric transplant donor (two- to threefold increased risk), and the presence of transplant rejection. Human leukocyte antigen–identical matched recipients had the lowest risk of symptomatic disease attributable to CMV.

The diagnosis of CMV pneumonia depends on the demonstration of the typical CMV cytopathologic finding: cytomegaly with intranuclear "owl's eye" inclusions. Viral cultures appear to be useful for monitoring the response to antiviral therapy,[13, 22, 23] as well as for distinguishing between CMV and other herpesviruses, particularly HSV.

Ganciclovir (9-[1,3-dihydroxy-2-propoxymethyl]guanine [DHPG], Cytovene), given for an induction course of 14 to 21 days at a dose of 5 mg/kg every 12 hours, has significant activity against CMV and is the current therapy of choice for sight- or life-threatening CMV infections. Foscarnet (trisodium phosphonoformate, Foscavir) appears to be active in the therapy of some infections caused by CMV. Contro-

versy surrounds the use of human CMV immune globulin, however; two reports examined its utility in combination with ganciclovir.[24, 25] One study found that all of 10 patients undergoing treatment for CMV pneumonia in the setting of bone marrow transplantation treated with the combination of passive immunotherapy and ganciclovir responded and that 7 of them survived without disease recurrence.[24] By contrast, none of the 11 patients treated with either agent alone survived.

Varicella-Zoster Virus

VZV infections occur commonly as the childhood infection chickenpox, typically affecting those 2 to 8 years of age. The disease is highly contagious and is readily transmitted by aerosolized droplets. Viremic spread to the endothelial cells of the epidermis results in the characteristic widespread vesicular exanthem. The attack rate varies from a minimum of 60 to 70% after moderate exposure (as little as 2 hours of exposure is sufficient to transmit chickenpox) to 87% for heavily exposed household contacts. The incubation period has been explicitly defined; in 99% of cases, a rash develops between 11 and 20 days after exposure. The patient is highly infectious for at least 2 days before the onset of the rash and for at least 5 days after the eruption. Virus can be readily isolated from the skin lesions during the first 3 days and occasionally on the fourth day of the eruption. In the compromised host, the skin lesions may contain viable virus for 10 days or longer. Localized zoster may transmit primary varicella to approximately 6% of susceptible individuals, and the risk of transmission increases with dissemination. Although varicella is typically a benign, self-limited disease, the estimated 3 to 3.5 million cases result in 364,000 physician office visits and 4000 hospitalizations in the United States annually.[26] By age 20 years, only about 8% of the population have not been infected with VZV.

After infection, a prodrome of fevers and chills, myalgias, and arthralgias occurs commonly and may last for several days in the adult. The eruption begins on the scalp or trunk and spreads centrifugally, with new lesions continuing to appear for 3 to 4 days. Lifelong latent infection follows primary infection, and the risk of reactivation increases with age and with the presence of immune suppression. Reactivation from the dorsal root ganglia typically presents as zoster (shingles), with a painful vesicular eruption occurring in the cutaneous distribution of a single nerve root dermatome. Zoster occurs with increasing frequency with advancing age. More than one recurrence of zoster is rare, occurring in from 3 to 5% of patients.

Varicella has an associated mortality of less than 1%; however, most deaths from varicella are related to pulmonary involvement. Pulmonary involvement occurs in 267 of 100,000 cases and is the most common complication in adults, resulting in approximately one hospitalization per 400 adult cases of varicella. An increased risk of pulmonary complications of varicella occurs in cigarette smokers. If varicella is untreated, the mortality with pulmonary involvement may approximate 10% in otherwise healthy adults, 30% in pregnant women, and perhaps higher in the immunocompromised host.

Immunocompromised hosts may have progressive varicella, characterized by the development of new lesions continuing into the second week of illness and associated with temperatures greater than 40°C. The mortality with progressive varicella approximates 20%. Zoster recurrences may occur with increased frequency in patients with lymphoreticular malignancies, solid tumors, surgical or nonsurgical trauma, or medical immunosuppressive regimens. Widespread cutaneous dissemination in immunocompromised patients may occur in up to 30 to 45% of cases. Visceral dissemination occurs rarely and typically in association with widespread cutaneous dissemination. In approximately 1% of cases, the initial presentation is with cutaneous disseminated disease; in about 11%, widespread cutaneous dissemination follows a typical zosteriform presentation.[27] Patients with AIDS may have more frequent recurrences and a more protracted duration of cutaneous disease.

Manifestations of pulmonary involvement typically occur within 72 hours of the onset of the rash. Auscultation of the chest reveals few abnormalities. Chest radiography demonstrates diffuse interstitial to nodular infiltrates. These infiltrates are frequently peribronchial and clustered near the hilum and may occur in 16% of young adults, although only 2 to 4% of these experience dyspnea or cough. Abnormalities in diffusion capacity occur early and may remain abnormal for as long as 1 year after recovery.[28] Occasionally, healing of varicella pneumonia leads to diffuse nodular calcifications replacing areas of focal necrosis. Tzanck's smears of skin lesions readily demonstrate multinucleate giant cells and confirm the herpesvirus nature of the exanthem. Rapid differentiation from HSV may be achieved by counterimmunoelectrophoresis to confirm the presence of VZV-specific antigens in the vesicle fluid. Tzanck's smears of expectorated sputum may occasionally be positive and provide a rapid noninvasive means of diagnosis.[29] Immunoglobulin M (IgM) responses can be assayed by enzyme-linked immunosorbent assay and appear as early as the second day of the illness, allowing for the rapid diagnosis of primary varicella as well as zoster infections.

Acyclovir (Zovirax) is active against VZV with a median effective dose (ED_{50}) of 0.08 to 1.2 mg/L; however, VZV is 4- to 30-fold less sensitive to acyclovir than is HSV. When otherwise normal adults who were hospitalized with varicella pneumonia were examined retrospectively, acyclovir treatment appeared to promote more rapid clinical improvement.[30] When acyclovir is administered intravenously at a dose of 5 mg/kg, the peak plasma concentration approximates 10 mg/L. Doses of 10 mg/kg every 8 hours, and occasionally greater,[31] are more appropriate for immunocompromised adults with serious lung or CNS involvement attributable to VZV. To control the nosocomial spread of infection, respiratory isolation of an exposed susceptible patient should be started 10 days after the first known exposure to varicella and be continued until 21 days after the last known exposure to the index case.

VIRAL INFECTIONS OF CENTRAL NERVOUS SYSTEM

Viral infections involving the CNS may be grouped into four classes (meningitis, encephalitis, poliomyelitis, and leukoencephalitis) on the basis of symptoms primarily referable to the meninges, the cerebral cortex, the anterior horns of the spinal cord, and demyelinating processes, respectively (Table 30–5). Overlaps in the symptom complexes do occur (e.g., meningoencephalitis).

Meningitis

Acute meningitis refers to the symptom complex of the abrupt onset of fevers, headache, neck stiffness,[32] and photophobia with obvious progression within a 24-hour period. Vomiting may be an associated symptom. The acute meningitis syndrome is most often caused by pyogenic bacterial infections. More commonly, the presentation of meningitis is subacute, with symptoms and signs evolving during 24 to 48 hours. Subacute meningitis results from diverse processes, with the infectious causes including viral, bacterial, myco-

TABLE 30–5

VIRAL INFECTIOUS AGENTS INVOLVING THE CENTRAL NERVOUS SYSTEM

Aseptic Meningitis
Frequent
  Coxsackievirus A9
  Coxsackievirus B1–5
  Echovirus 4, 6, 9, 11, 14, 18, 30, 31
  Mumps virus
Occasional
  Measles virus
  Lymphocytic choriomeningitis virus
  Adenoviruses
  Human immunodeficiency virus (HIV)
Rare
  VZV
  HSV
  Epstein-Barr virus
  Human CMV
  St. Louis encephalitis virus
  Western equine encephalitis virus
  California encephalitis virus

Aseptic Meningitis with Paralysis
Poliovirus 1–3
Coxsackievirus A7
Enterovirus 71

Encephalitis
Frequent
  Arboviruses
    Alphaviruses
    Bunyaviruses
    Flaviviruses
  HSV
  Rabies virus
Occasional
  VZV
  HIV
Rare
  Measles virus
  Enterovirus 71
  Epstein-Barr virus
  Human CMV
  Herpes B virus

bacterial, and fungal agents. Enteroviruses are the most frequent cause of viral meningitis, with a yearly peak in incidence during May through December;[33] however, a broad range of viral agents may occasionally be implicated in the etiology of viral meningitis. Virtually all patients with viral meningitis and three quarters of those with bacterial meningitis have a subacute presentation.[34]

Examination of the cerebrospinal fluid (CSF) often proves to be the critical determinant in differentiating bacterial from aseptic meningitis. Pleocytosis in excess of 1000 white blood cells per cubic millimeter or significant hypoglycorrhachia rarely accompanies viral meningitis. The presence of a mononuclear cell predominance also strongly supports a viral cause; however, a polymorphonuclear cell predominance early in the course of the infection may occur in two thirds of patients. In support of a viral origin, a repeated lumbar puncture may demonstrate a shift to a mononuclear cell predominance in 87% of patients in as little as 6 to 8 hours, and in 94% when performed after 12 hours.[35] Awareness of a community-based viral epidemic may also suggest the possibility of a viral cause of meningitis. Although prior antibiotic therapy decreases the likelihood of isolation of responsible bacterial organisms, cultures recover the organism in 50 to 68% of cases despite prior therapy.[36]

Enteroviruses

Enteroviruses are members of the picornavirus family and infect humans via a fecal-oral route of spread. Enteroviral meningitis exhibits seasonal variation, with attack rates that are 10-fold greater in August to September when compared with those during the winter months (approximately 1 case per 100,000 versus 0.1 per 100,000). After an incubation period of 4 to 8 days, the symptoms of subacute meningitis begin, and occasionally, associated symptoms of pleuritis, abdominal pain, or an exanthem may suggest the viral cause. Echovirus type 9 infection may produce an exanthem that mimics that of meningococcal meningitis. Aseptic meningitis attributable to enteroviral infection usually resolves spontaneously without sequelae within 5 to 7 days. Chronic enteroviral infections occur in patients with humoral immunodeficiency, in children with hypogammaglobulinemia, and rarely in adults with multiple myeloma.

Care must be taken to avoid treating pyogenic or granulomatous meningitis as aseptic meningitis. Unlike mycobacterial or fungal meningitides in which a basilar exudate may be seen on computed tomographic (CT) scans, in viral meningitis no abnormality of the basal nonventricular CSF space is demonstrable.[37] Because the exudate associated with the basilar meningitides may be hypodense, isodense, or hyperdense, it is most readily demonstrated after enhancement by contrast tomography.

The ingested virus attaches to the mucosa of the gastrointestinal tract, undergoes local replication, spreads to the regional and then more distant lymphoid tissue, and then gives rise to a transient viremia. In most patients, the course of the infection is aborted at this point. Those patients who clinically manifest disease have a heavy viral burden in tissues of the reticuloendothelial system after the initial viremia and then develop a more profound viremia as productive infection of the reticuloendothelial system tissues progresses. With the second viremia, visceral dissemination to other target tissues, especially the CNS, occurs. Enteroviral infections with associated meningitis occur in the acute and infectious stage of the illness, with virus recoverable from the stool for a week after the onset of clinical meningitis. Neutralizing antibody responses appear to be critical for the limitation of disease after enteroviral infection, and IgM and IgG class antibodies can be detected in the serum as soon as 3 days after enteroviral infection.

Enteroviruses from serotype 68 upward are numbered sequentially without regard to whether they more closely resemble echoviruses, coxsackievirus serogroup A, coxsackievirus serogroup B, or polioviruses. Nonpoliovirus enterovirus surveillance in the United States suggests that isolates from March through May predict the serotypes that will be isolated during the peak enterovirus season, which begins in midsummer.[38] Enterovirus 71 has been an infrequent cause of CNS disease and exanthems and is unique in that it is the first nonpoliovirus enterovirus associated with epidemic paralytic disease.[39]

Polioviruses

Poliomyelitis describes the syndrome of painful flaccid paralysis with associated aseptic meningitis. After a prodromal period of 1 to 2 days typified by a clinical syndrome consistent with aseptic meningitis, the characteristic pain, spasms, and paralysis ensue. Paralytic poliomyelitis is typically associated with one of three serotypes (1, 2, and 3) and is rarely due to other enteroviruses. The case fatality rate for paralytic poliomyelitis approximates 10%. Subclinical infections caused by polioviruses are common; only 1 in 50 to 1 in 1000 of those infected develop paralytic poliomyelitis.

Poliovirus serotypes 1, 2, and 3 may also produce aseptic meningitis without associated paralysis, so-called nonparalytic poliomyelitis.

The pathogenesis of poliovirus infection has been well characterized because these agents grow readily in nonhuman primates. Each of the three serotypes has four major structural viral proteins labeled VP1, VP2, VP3, and VP4. VP1 appears to contain the major antigenic determinant.[40] Poliovirus may be shed in the stool for 4 to 7 weeks.

After the introduction of the Salk (inactivated virus) vaccine in 1955 and the Sabine vaccine (live attenuated oral poliovirus) vaccine in 1961, the attack rate in the United States underwent a profound decline. Before vaccine availability, 16,000 cases per year occurred in the United States and 10.4 paralytic cases per 100,000 population but declined to 7 cases per year and 0.02 paralytic cases per 100,000 population after the introduction of routine poliovirus vaccination. Only 335 cases of poliomyelitis were reported in the Americas in 1988.[41] The risk of paralytic poliomyelitis after oral poliovirus vaccinations with all three serotypes is less than one case per 3 million doses distributed among both vaccinees and their contacts. Most vaccinees excrete all three serotypes after oral poliovirus vaccination and exhibit seroconversion to all three serotypes within 1 month of vaccination. An enhanced potency inactivated poliovirus vaccine appears to have an efficacy approximating 89%.[42]

Coxsackieviruses

These enteroviruses are named after Coxsackie, New York, where a cluster of clinical diseases resembling poliomyelitis was first recognized in children. Coxsackievirus A produces generalized inflammation of skeletal muscle, whereas the coxsackievirus serogroup B tends to cause more widespread involvement, affecting the myocardium, the pericardium, the CNS, and the pancreas.[43] Coxsackievirus A7 occasionally causes aseptic meningitis with paralysis resembling poliomyelitis.

Mumps Virus

Mumps has an incubation period of 14 to 21 days, is spread by airborne droplets, and typically comes to medical attention in the infectious phase of the illness. Mumps may be readily transmitted for 2 days before and 4 days after the onset of meningitis. Accompanying parotitis is present in two thirds of cases and suggests the diagnosis. However, many other viral pathogens may cause parotid swelling, most notably lymphocytic choriomeningitis virus, parainfluenza virus, and the enteroviruses. Mumps may also manifest with symptoms and signs of encephalitis, and diagnostic confusion often arises in the one third of cases with meningitis in the absence of parotitis. Subclinical involvement of the CNS may be demonstrated by the frequent finding of CSF pleocytosis, but clinical meningoencephalitis is a rare complication of mumps, occurring in 0.5 to 1% of cases. Adults who contract mumps may have a threefold greater risk of associated meningitis than do affected children. Aseptic meningitis attributable to mumps usually resolves spontaneously without sequelae within 5 to 7 days. Rarely, mumps meningoencephalitis may be fatal or result in slowly resolving CNS disease with ataxia, electroencephalographic abnormalities, and CSF pleocytosis.

Lymphocytic Choriomeningitis Virus

Lymphocytic choriomeningitis virus causes viral meningitis infrequently; however, unlike other viral agents, it may cause marked pleocytosis in the CSF (white blood cell count greater than 1000/mm³) and marked hypoglycorrhachia (glucose level less than 40 mg/dL). Fortunately, a characteristic lymphocytic predominance occurs from the onset of symptoms, and so lymphocytic choriomeningitis virus is not readily confused with bacterial causes of meningitis.

Human Immunodeficiency Virus

Human immunodeficiency virus (HIV) infections may produce aseptic meningitis as part of the acute phase of infection with HIV. CSF abnormalities after the acute phase of infection with HIV do occur but are often quite modest. Pleocytosis tends to be scant, 5 to 12 white blood cells per cubic millimeter, typically with a lymphocytic predominance. The CSF protein level tends to be mildly elevated, ranging from 40 to 58 mg/dL, with a mean of 45 mg/dL in patients with neuropsychiatric manifestations of disease.[44] Mild abnormalities of the CSF may be attributable solely to HIV infection; pleocytosis in the range of 5 to 44 white blood cells per cubic millimeter occurs in one third of HIV-infected individuals, and a CSF protein level in the range of 48 to 117 mg/dL may be seen in approximately one fourth.[45] More profound abnormalities should prompt a search for alternative causes.

Encephalitis

A diverse group of bunyaviruses, flaviviruses, and alphaviruses may cause clinical encephalitis in humans. They are generally referred to as arboviruses because each involves an arthropod vector for transmission, either via ticks (*Ixodes, Dermacentor,* and *Haemaphysalis*) or culicine mosquitoes (*Culex, Culiseta,* and *Aedes*). Vertical transmission may occur via transovarian (St. Louis or California serogroups) or transstadial transmission. Birds, chipmunks, and tree squirrels typically constitute the reservoir for these viruses. Sufficient viremia exists in these reservoirs to allow the vector to become infected. After infection of the vector occurs, a 1- to 3-week period of extrinsic incubation occurs before sufficient virus is shed in the salivary glands of the vector for the vector to transmit disease (Fig. 30–1).

The alphaviruses that cause encephalitis include eastern equine encephalitis (EEE), western equine encephalitis (WEE), and Venezuelan equine encephalitis (VEE) viruses. Japanese B encephalitis, St. Louis encephalitis, Rocio, Murray Valley, West Nile, Powassan, and Kyanasur Forest viruses are examples of the flaviviruses. St. Louis encephalitis accounts for more than half of all arboviral encephalitis and the California serogroup, particularly La Crosse encephalitis, accounts for nearly another third (Table 30–6).

The initial symptoms include temperatures of up to 39°C, chills, and headache associated with nausea and vomiting. Confusion and somnolence can follow within 2 days and may progress rapidly to coma. Seizures may be seen with more advanced stages of encephalitis. The various agents of arboviral encephalitis have subtle epidemiologic and clinical differences; however, EEE, WEE, St. Louis encephalitis, and California encephalitis cannot be distinguished on clinical grounds alone. The specific diagnosis depends on serologic confirmation in the setting of clinically compatible disease. Comparison of acute and convalescent serum titers demonstrates a fourfold or greater rise in antibody by hemagglutinin inhibition or complement fixation techniques. Specific neutralizing antibody studies are available to diagnose encephalitis attributable to the California serogroup. In fatal cases of alphavirus encephalitis, virus may be isolated from the brain at postmortem examination; however, virus is not typically present in the CSF.

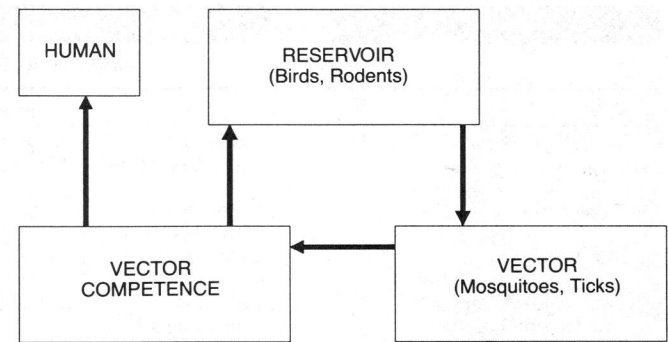

Figure 30–1. Life cycle of encephalitis-causing agents. The arboviral encephalitides maintain a life cycle in which humans are a coincidental participant. The usual reservoirs of the agents are birds and small mammals, particularly waterfowl and rodents. The vector may include ixodid ticks or any of a wide variety of mosquitoes. After ingestion of a blood meal from an infected reservoir species, an extrinsic incubation period follows. The extrinsic incubation period consists of the time required for the virus to multiply within the vector until enough virus is present to allow transmission to the end host or to another reservoir host. The extrinsic incubation period varies widely depending on the size of the blood meal, the ambient temperature, and the ability of the vector to multiply its viral burden. An abortive infection of the vector, or one that results in modest viral replication, or that does not present the virus at a suitable site for transmission (salivary glands of the vector) may be termed vector incompetence. The vector must be competent for the cycle to continue uninterrupted.

California Serogroup

The California serogroup includes bunyaviruses that account for approximately 30% of arboviral encephalitis, of which the La Crosse agent is the most medically important, accounting for 87 cases and one fatality in 1987.[46] The disease occurs endemically in the northern Midwest, an area centered on Wisconsin and Minnesota. *Aedes triseriatus* is the principal vector and squirrels and chipmunks are the principal reservoir. *A. triseriatus* is most active in the midsummer and uses tree holes that retain water as its principal habitat, accounting for the prominence of this species in heavily wooded areas.[47] In addition to infecting naive mosquitoes after blood meals from infected mammals, the La Crosse agent can also be transmitted from mosquito to mosquito either by vertical (transovarian) or sexual transmission. La Crosse encephalitis may be diagnosed in a patient with clinically compatible illness by the demonstration of a fourfold or greater rise in titer between acute and convalescent sera by immunofluorescent antibody technique, in preference to the less sensitive complement fixation technique.

Eastern Equine Encephalitis Virus

EEE virus causes the most severe of the North American encephalitides and occurs across a broad area of the United States, from the Eastern seaboard to the Great Lakes to the Gulf Coast. Birds form the reservoir for EEE, mosquitoes serve as the vector, and horses are the usual end host. The case fatality rate in horses approximates 90%, but they are not an important reservoir of disease because the duration of viremia is limited. Humans are only coincidentally involved in the life cycle of EEE virus and person-to-person transmission does not occur. A mosquito that breeds in freshwater swamps and feeds on wild birds, *Culiseta melanura,* is the principal vector. Peak mosquito activity occurs in the evening hours, and peak disease activity is associated with

TABLE 30–6

ARBOVIRAL ENCEPHALITIDES

Agent	%	Vector	Geography	Reservoir
St. Louis	61	Culex pipiens	Texas	Chickens
		Culex quinquefasciatus	Mississippi and Ohio river valleys	
California	30			
California		Aedes melanimon	California to Texas	Squirrels
		Aedes dorsalis		
La Crosse		Aedes triseriatus	Minnesota to Northeastern United States	Mammals
Jamestown Canyon		Culiseta inorata	Alaska to Florida	White-tailed deer
Snowshoe hare virus		Aedes implicatus		Snowshoe hares and ground squirrels
		Aedes canadensis		
		Culiseta inorata		
WEE	7	Culex tarsalis	Western United States, Saskatchewan to South America	Ducks
		Other Culex spp.		
EEE	2	Culiseta melanura	East central United States, South America, and Caribbean	Quails, pheasants
		Aedes spp.		
		Coquillettidia spp.		
VEE		Culex taeniopus	South America to Texas	Rodents
		Aedes spp.		
		Psorophora spp.		
Japanese B encephalitis		Culex tritaeniorhynchus	Southeast Asia	Black heron
		Culex gelidus	India and China	
Murray Valley		Culex annulirostris	Australia	Birds
Everglades		Culex spp.	Florida	Rodents
Tahyna virus		Culiseta annulata	Czechoslovakia, Mozambique	Hares
West Nile		Culex univittatus	Africa, Asia, and Europe	Birds
		Culex antennatus		
		Culex modestus		
		Culex vishnui		
Tick-borne encephalitis		Ixodid ticks	Europe and the former U.S.S.R.	Rodents, birds, and domestic livestock
Louping-ill		Idodid ticks	Great Britain	Rodents and sheep
Powassan		Ixodid ticks	United States and Canada	Squirrels, chipmunks

the movement of migratory birds in the fall. EEE virus may cause fatal disease in susceptible birds and epornitic surveillance may provide clues to EEE virus activity.[48] Mosquito control remains critical in the control of this infection.

The incubation period ranges from 5 to 15 days, and clinical disease is characterized by the rapid onset of high fevers, drowsiness, meningism, and vomiting. Children more frequently develop generalized, facial, and periorbital edema. The course progresses rapidly, such that coma may supervene by the second day of illness. Paralysis and autonomic dysfunction occur occasionally. Disturbed respiration, profound lethargy, excessive salivation, and airway congestion all contribute to compromised ventilation and may be a factor in the 30 to 70% case fatality rate. Significant neurologic sequelae may persist in 30% of survivors and further contribute to the overall morbidity with EEE.

Increased pressure of the CSF accompanied by lymphocytic pleocytosis is typical. Viral isolation of EEE virus may be accomplished by intracerebral inoculation of suckling mice or by inoculation onto Vero or other cell lines. Direct viral isolation from clinical specimens is of limited utility because viremia occurs for only a brief period. The diagnosis is typically made by demonstrating a fourfold rise in antibody titer by one of three methods: complement fixation, hemagglutination inhibition, and plaque reduction neutralization.

Therapy for EEE is largely supportive, often requiring an intensive care unit level of support, intubation, and ventilatory support combined with the use of careful fluid balance monitoring and osmotic diuresis for the management of increased intracranial pressure. A human vaccine is under investigation.

Venezuelan Equine Encephalitis Virus

VEE occurs endemically from South America through Central America, occasionally reaching the southern United States. Unlike the agents of EEE and WEE in which horses are an end host and have no role in transmission of disease, the agent of VEE undergoes amplification in equine reservoirs. Mosquitoes of five different genera have been implicated in the transmission of VEE, including Aedes and Culex species. An outbreak in Venezuela in the early 1960s was associated with over more than 30,000 human cases, with an overall case fatality rate of 0.6%. Although horses are an important intermediary in the life cycle of VEE, significant disease may occur in horses as well. Spread of the VEE agent to Texas in 1971 was associated with the loss of more than 10,000 horses.

Western Equine Encephalitis Virus

WEE was first isolated in 1930 from horses in California with fatal encephalitis and was the first virus isolated in the United States. Culex tarsalis is the principal vector, and it prefers to inhabit irrigated farmlands. Rare, sporadic cases of WEE have been reported east of the Mississippi River. Concurrent equine epizootics may help suggest the diagnosis.[46] An increased risk of WEE with male sex and advanced age has been noted with most outbreaks, and the overall case fatality rate approximates 10%. Human-to-human transmission has not been reported.

St. Louis Encephalitis Virus

St. Louis encephalitis is caused by a flavivirus that may produce clinical disease, which varies from mild headaches

---

TABLE 30–7

DISEASES THAT MAY MIMIC FOCAL ENCEPHALITIS

HSV encephalitis
Bacterial meningitis
Brain abscess
Subdural empyema, hematoma
Embolic encephalitis accompanying subacute bacterial
    endocarditis
Tuberculous meningitis
Fungal meningitis
Cerebral malaria
Plague
Diphtheria
Rickettsiosis
Botulism
Toxoplasmosis
Behçet's syndrome
Guillain-Barré syndrome
Multiple sclerosis
Reye's syndrome
Systemic lupus erythematosus with cranial arteritis

---

and fevers to aseptic meningitis to overt encephalitis. *C. tarsalis* is the principal vector for St. Louis encephalitis as well as for WEE, and combined outbreaks may occur, with St. Louis encephalitis cases lagging in time of onset behind WEE cases. The incubation period is typically 4 to 21 days and is followed by a nonspecific prodrome of fevers, headaches, myalgias, and malaise. The more severe fever (greater than 40°C) and longer duration of fever (more than 1 week) correlate with a poorer prognosis. Convulsions occur in 10% and also connote a poor prognosis. Up to 30% of cases may be further complicated by the syndrome of inappropriate antidiuretic hormone. Objective neurologic residua after recovery occur uncommonly.

Herpes Simplex Virus

HSV is the most common cause of severe sporadic encephalitis in the United States.[49, 50] Without treatment, the mortality exceeds 70% and survivors experience significant morbidity. Despite advances in diagnostics, the ready availability of neuroimaging studies, and effective antiviral therapy, significant morbidity and mortality attributable to HSV encephalitis still occur.

HSV encephalitis typically involves the frontotemporal cortex,[51] with associated necrosis and hemorrhage. In neonates, a more diffuse encephalitis is more typically observed. The clinical course is often that of a subacute meningoencephalitis, with symptoms evolving during several hours to a few days. The most common symptoms are headaches, fever, and progressive obtundation. Focal cortical signs, such as localized weakness, seizures, dysphasia, and personality changes support HSV encephalitis but other infections of the CNS may occasionally present with focal signs or symptoms (Table 30–7). The CT appearance of a pyogenic brain abscess in the first 2 to 4 days of evolution has been described as a poorly demarcated area of "acute focal encephalitis,"[37] which may mimic HSV encephalitis.

Controversy exists regarding the necessity of establishing the diagnosis of HSV encephalitis through brain biopsy. This hinges on the potential morbidity and mortality associated with biopsy of the brain as the only definitive diagnostic method[52] contrasted with noninvasive neuroimaging studies, which can provide supportive evidence for the diagnosis of HSV encephalitis; the safety and efficacy profile of acyclovir therapy; and the perceived paucity of alternative, treatable, diagnostic considerations. The National Institute

of Allergy and Infectious Diseases Collaborative Antiviral Study Group conducted clinical trials during a 10-year period to evaluate the natural history of, and antiviral therapy for, HSV encephalitis. The group evaluated 432 patients who had uniform clinical features supportive of the diagnosis of HSV encephalitis: mental status changes, focal neurologic symptoms or signs, and electroencephalographic or neuroradiologic (CT or radionuclide brain scan) demonstration of focality.[53] Brain biopsy was routinely required for study inclusion and 193 patients (45%) had biopsy-confirmed HSV, whereas 239 (55%) were biopsy-negative for HSV encephalitis. Of the latter, 95 had alternative disorders demonstrated on biopsy specimen, many of which (38 of 95, or 40%) were amenable to specific treatment.

The authors developed an estimate of the probability of HSV encephalitis based on five clinical criteria: focal uptake on brain technetium scanning, focal abnormalities on CT, focal abnormalities on electroencephalogram, age greater than 30 years, and more than five leukocytes per cubic millimeter in the CSF. If all five criteria were present, the probability that the biopsy specimen would demonstrate HSV was greater than 90%. With the expectation that radionuclide brain scans would not be routinely performed in addition to CT in clinical practice, a second estimate involved only the remaining four criteria. If the patient was more than 30 years old, had CSF pleocytosis, and had typical focal abnormalities on both electroencephalographic and CT evaluations (and a radionuclide brain scan was not performed), the probability of the biopsy specimen's demonstrating HSV encephalitis was greater than 70%. If none of the criteria were present, the model predicted a likelihood of HSV encephalitis of less than 2%.

Because of the potential morbidity associated with biopsy of intracranial lesions, a number of alternative diagnostic methods have been evaluated: intrathecal antibody production, the presence of HSV antigen in the CSF, and the detection of HSV genomic material in the CSF after amplification by polymerase chain reaction. Polymerase chain reaction was examined in 43 patients with biopsy- or autopsy-proven disease (13 of 43) or with intrathecal antibody production supportive of the diagnosis of HSV encephalitis (40 of 43). Three patients had HSV encephalitis proved only by tissue diagnosis.[54] Samples were taken at 1 to 30 days after the onset of symptoms in 76% and after 31 days to 7 years in 24%. Polymerase chain reaction detected HSV DNA in 42 of 43 patients.

CT provides a readily accessible means to evaluate for HSV encephalitis. Typically, CT demonstrates unilateral or bilateral hypodensity characteristically located in the temporal lobe. Associated hemorrhage, although not often visualized radiographically, may be hyperdense. Some controversy exists regarding whether technetium radionuclide scanning or CT is more sensitive, with a bias toward radionuclide scanning being of somewhat better sensitivity.[37] Unilateral or bilateral hyperperfusion associated with focal uptake supports the diagnosis of HSV encephalitis.

The treatment course of choice consists of 10 days of parenteral acyclovir, although vidarabine (adenine arabinoside [ara-A]) is also efficacious.[55] Relapses of HSV encephalitis after intravenous therapy with 10 mg/kg every 8 hours occur rarely,[56, 57] but may be seen from 4 to 11 days after the completion of a standard 10-day course of therapy. In one instance, the relapse was confirmed by the recovery of HSV from the CSF. The HSV remained sensitive to acyclovir,[57] prompting recommendations to extend therapy to 14 to 21 days.

Cercopithecine Herpesvirus 1 (B Virus)

The B virus is an alphaherpesvirus whose natural hosts include various Old World monkeys, especially macaques, but not New World monkeys.[58] In macaques, such as *Macaca mulatta* (rhesus) and *Macaca fascicularis* (cynomolgus), the B virus tends to produce long-standing latent infections, probably harbored in neural ganglia, which may be reactivated by stress or immunosuppression. Seroprevalence data suggest that B virus infections may be present in up to 80 to 100% of monkeys in captivity.[59] Human infection by the B virus most commonly follows a monkey bite and produces a distinct, often fulminant clinical presentation.

Human disease was first recognized in 1932 when a physician was bitten by an apparently normal rhesus monkey; local signs of infection 3 days later were followed by more systemic complaints and death from encephalitis.[60] Since the original description, approximately 30 additional cases have been reported,[59, 61] including one case of human-to-human spread.[62]

Early symptoms routinely include fever, myalgias, fatigue, and headaches. Sensations of numbness or pruritus localized to the wound site may lead to more generalized neurologic signs and symptoms, which herald progressive disease and include agitation, ataxia, diplopia, and an ascending flaccid paralysis. Survivors commonly have long-term neurologic sequelae.

One series of four patients with B virus infection included three patients with vesicular skin lesions suggestive of a herpesvirus infection that developed at the wound site after an incubation period of 2 to 5 days. Overall, herpetic vesicles have been recorded in only 6 of the 29 reported cases.

Definitive diagnosis depends on the demonstration of herpesvirus-like nuclear inclusions or viral isolation in an appropriate clinical setting, preferably with supportive serologic data. Because of the similarity of B virus to human HSV, some serologic cross-reactivity may be expected, does occur, and may be marked.[63] It has been suggested that the degree of overlap in serologic identity precludes serologic testing with *Herpesvirus hominis* or B virus preparations alone. Specific B virus serologic tests include a dot immunobinding assay after herpes simplex antigen absorption, which offers specificity and rapid identification.[64] Restriction endonuclease DNA analysis and polyacrylamide gel electrophoretic polypeptide profiles are sufficiently distinctive to unambiguously differentiate B virus from HSV[65, 66] and related isolates.[67] None of these analyses are routinely available.

No controlled trials of therapy exist and the data on individual treatment modalities are limited, but in vitro and clinical data suggest that acyclovir is the most active agent available. One report described four patients with B virus infection treated with acyclovir, two with only cutaneous vesicles and two with neurologic manifestations at the time acyclovir administration was started. The two patients with cutaneous disease responded to intravenous acyclovir, whereas the other two had progressive disease and were subsequently treated with parenteral ganciclovir.[62] One individual had intrathecal anti–B virus antibodies, supporting the diagnosis of B virus encephalitis, and was successfully treated with 15 mg/kg of acyclovir every 8 hours for 3 days followed by ganciclovir at a dosage of 5 mg/kg every 12 hours.[68] Although the available data do not allow specific recommendations regarding the optimal dosage or duration of treatment, early and aggressive therapy appears warranted.

Measles Virus

Measles has an overall annual incidence of 1.4 cases per 100,000 population, with the peak incidence occurring May through June. Case definition includes temperature of 38°C, generalized rash lasting at least 3 days, and at least one additional symptom: cough, conjunctivitis, or inflammation of or discharge from the mucous membranes of the sinuses, eyes, or nares (coryza). The 1988 provisional total for the United States was 3411 cases; however, by June of 1989 more than 8500 cases had been reported to the Centers for Disease Control, with more than 90 outbreaks occurring at secondary schools and on college campuses.[69] More than half of the cases in 1988 occurred in six major outbreaks of more than 100 cases each. An increased incidence was noted in the 15- to 19-year-old and 20- to 24-year-old age categories. Despite a history of prior vaccination in the majority of those infected, the highest rate of infection was noted in 15- to 19-year-old persons, with an incidence of 5.8 per 100,000. Epidemiologic data suggest that persons vaccinated before 1980 are at increased risk for clinical disease. The progressive cognitive and motor dysfunction associated with subacute sclerosing panencephalitis follows infection with the measles virus. The CT scan demonstrates hypodense lesions of the white matter, which occasionally enhance with contrast.

Rabies Virus

Rabies is caused by a *Lyssavirus* (Greek *lyssa,* meaning rage), which is typically transmitted through the bite of an infected animal and results in about one human case per year in the United States. The rate in the United States was higher before the introduction of canine vaccination circa 1950. Unvaccinated animals in the United States may be readily infected from feral animal reservoirs. In contrast to popular notions of the route of exposure to rabies, the reported incidence of rabid animals in the United States approximates 4000 cases per year, of which less than 200 occur in dogs. Rabies in dogs in Mexico remains a considerable problem, with Mexico reporting more than 14,000 cases of rabies for 1987, almost all of them occurring in dogs. The majority of United States rabies cases for a typical year (1987) revealed more than 2000 rabid skunks, more than 1300 cases in raccoons, and more than 600 infected bats.[70] In the United States, a case of acquired human rabies was related to a bat bite.[71] The numbers of domestic animal cases (170 dogs, 166 cats, and 174 cattle) were modest by comparison. Arctic, red, and gray foxes can also be infected. Regional variations exist in the incidence of rabid animals within the United States, but only the state of Hawaii is rabies free. Because of the large wild animal reservoir of rabies, continued diligence regarding domesticated animal vaccination provides the best protection against rabies.[72]

After the bite of an infected animal, a 30- to 90-day incubation period ends with a prodrome that is consistent with a number of benign, nondescript conditions. The risk of clinical rabies after the bite of a rabid animal ranges from 5 to 80%, but best estimates are 5 to 15%.[73] The symptoms that occur in the prodromal phase include fevers, headaches, malaise, fatigue, anorexia, abdominal pain, nausea, vomiting, and occasionally upper respiratory tract infection–like symptoms. The second phase of the illness is dominated by neurologic symptoms: anxiety, hallucinations, photophobia, and neuralgias (related to the area of the bite). Hydrophobia occurs in about one fifth of patients and is a characteristic symptom related to the development of painful laryngopharyngeal contractions, which frequently result in choking or aspiration. Focal or generalized seizures occur and may directly contribute to fatality in one quarter of cases.

The clinical presentation may occasionally have striking abdominal complaints, delaying recognition of the true cause.[74] Given the protean manifestations present during the prodrome, diagnosis depends on a high degree of suspicion for rabies. The diagnosis can be made by three methods: histopathologic study, virus isolation, and serologic study.

TABLE 30-8

SEROLOGIC FINDINGS IN ACUTE HEPATITIS*

IgM Anti-HAV	HBsAg	IgM Anti-HBc	Anti-HCV	Anti-HDV	Disease
+	−	−	−	−	Acute HAV
−	+	+	−	−	Acute HBV
−	+	−	−	−	Chronic HBV
−	−	−	+ or −	−	Acute HCV
−	+	+	−	+	Acute HBV and HDV
−	+	−	−	+	Acute HDV
−	−	−	−	−	HEV, CMV, other

*HBc = hepatitis B core; HCV = hepatitis C virus; HDV = hepatitis delta virus; HEV = hepatitis E virus.

Viral antigen detection methods provide the most rapid means of definitive diagnosis.

A postexposure trial of a combination of human rabies immune globulin and a five-dose regimen of a human diploid cell vaccine (W-HDCV, Wyeth-Ayerst Laboratories) appeared to confer significant protection to 21 patients known to be bitten by rabid animals.[73]

There has been considerable debate regarding the occurrence of rabies in patients without an apparent exposure history, and a variety of explanations have been offered: trivial injuries, exposure to aerosols, and a prolonged period of incubation. Three immigrants to the United States experienced animal exposures in their native country between 11 months and 6 years before the development of clinical rabies, and these three patients' rabies isolates were studied using monoclonal antibody serologic categorization and DNA analysis. Rabies isolates from these patients were consistent with isolates endemic to their countries of origin and not with those seen in the United States, supporting a prolonged incubation period between exposure and clinical disease.[74]

VIRAL HEPATITIS

Hepatitis has long been recognized as a distinct clinical entity with significant morbidity and mortality. With clinical disease (icterus), type A hepatitis has a mortality of less than 0.5%, and type B hepatitis has a mortality of about 1%. The incidence of hepatitis is on the order of 0.5 to 2 cases per 1000 population per year. Serologic testing of random population samples suggest that, by age 50 years, 70% of persons have antibody against hepatitis A and 7% have antibody against hepatitis B.

The clinical presentations of acute disease attributable to hepatitis A, hepatitis B, hepatitis C, and hepatitis delta viruses are generally similar. After infection, a symptom-free incubation period follows: for hepatitis A, 15 to 45 days (mean of 30 days); for hepatitis B, 30 to 180 days (mean of 70 days); for hepatitis C, 15 to 150 days (mean of 50 days); and unknown for delta hepatitis.

The most common symptoms begin 3 to 10 days before the onset of icterus and include malaise (95%), anorexia (90%), nausea and vomiting (80%), and right upper quadrant pain (60%). A 1- to 3-week icteric phase follows in which bilirubinuria is the most consistent complaint, as some patients fail to note the icteric skin coloration despite marked bilirubinemia. Fever, if present, is low grade and diarrhea is not a prominent complaint.

On physical examination, the patient is usually afebrile, and bradycardia may be noted when bilirubinemia is pronounced. Jaundice may first be appreciated by discoloration of the patient's sclera (at about a bilirubin level of 2.5 mg/dL) and, at increasingly higher levels (2.5 to 3 mg/dL), may be observed in the sublingual mucous membranes, skin, and tympanic membranes.

Spider angiomas, although small in size and few in number, are usually found, as is a tender, mildly enlarged liver. A spleen tip may be felt in 5 to 25% of cases. The presence of ascites, edema, prominent splenomegaly, or caput medusae should prompt a search for causes of chronic liver injury.

The levels of hepatic transaminases, serum glutamic-oxaloacetic transaminase (aspartate aminotransferase) and serum glutamic-pyruvic aminotransferase (alanine aminotransferase), are characteristically 8- to 10-fold increased when measured when jaundice appears. The transaminase levels become abnormal during the late incubation period and are invariably abnormal after symptoms occur. They normalize with recovery but remain abnormal for several weeks after symptoms have abated.

The bilirubin level may be elevated in both direct and indirect fractions, in a ratio of about 1:1. A much higher indirect than direct fraction (greater than 4:1) suggests hemolysis, and patients with glucose-6-phosphate dehydrogenase deficiency or thalassemia minor are predisposed to exaggerated hemolysis in association with viral hepatitis. Prothrombin time abnormalities suggest serious hepatic dysfunction and, in combination with acute hepatitis, are a grave finding. Specific serologic tests allow diagnosis of the acute and chronic viral hepatitides (Table 30-8) and historical information often suggests alternative diagnoses (Table 30-9).

No specific treatment exists for fulminant acute viral

TABLE 30-9

AGENTS OF HEPATITIS

Type of Etiology	Agent
Infectious	
Viral	Epstein-Barr virus, human CMV, HSV, VZV, coxsackievirus B, rubella, adenoviruses, rubeola, mumps, yellow fever
Bacterial	Pneumococcal pneumonia, leptospirosis, syphilis, brucella
Noninfectious	
Drugs	Antituberculous therapy (e.g., isoniazid and rifampin), acetaminophen, antiseizure therapy
Hepatotoxins	Carbon tetrachloride, beryllium, vinyl chloride
Miscellaneous	Shock, right-sided congestive heart failure, Wilson's disease, hemochromatosis, α_1-antitrypsin deficiency

hepatitis and the management is largely supportive; maintaining caloric intake, ensuring fluid and electrolyte homeostasis, managing coagulopathy and bleeding, monitoring for hypoglycemia, and caring for the comatose patient may all be necessary. Caution is warranted in the use of drugs that are hepatotoxins or that undergo significant hepatic metabolism. A high-calorie diet, which is restricted in protein, is desirable. Lactulose or neomycin may be used to moderate the effects of hepatic encephalopathy. A variety of heroic measures have been attempted and found to be largely ineffectual, among them massive doses of corticosteroids, plasmapheresis, and exchange transfusions.

Hepatitis A Virus

Hepatitis A virus (HAV) also known as infectious hepatitis virus, is a highly contagious agent, which is usually spread via the fecal-oral route. The source of outbreaks can often be traced to a single person, often with spread of the illness occurring during the asymptomatic, incubation period of the virus. HAV is now classified as enterovirus 72.

Among the common means of spread identified are via ingestion of contaminated food or drink, through exposure to improper sanitation associated with flooding and hurricanes, via ingestion of raw shellfish from contaminated waters, via travel in areas with poor hygiene, among institutionalized persons, by exposure to primates imported from areas of endemic disease, among children in day care centers, and through sexual promiscuity.

Although HAV may be cultured from the stool during the asymptomatic, prodromal phase of the illness, viral cultures of the stool are usually not helpful in establishing the diagnosis because of decreased shedding when icterus supervenes. Anti-HAV antibodies are routinely present at the onset of clinical illness. Within 3 to 12 months, anti-HAV antibody levels of the IgM class decrease to undetectable levels. Anti-HAV antibody levels of the IgG class remain elevated at high titers and confer lifelong immunity to reinfection.

Hepatitis B Virus

Hepatitis B virus (HBV) is the prototype virus of the Hepadnaviridae. In 1970, Dane used electron microscopic techniques to view and describe the large spheric particles (hence Dane particles) that are now known to represent the complete hepatitis B virion. Treatment of these complete virions with detergent yielded two separate particles, the core and surface components (the latter was subsequently identified as the Australia antigen, now known as hepatitis B surface antigen [HBsAg]).

Well-recognized risk factors include intravenous drug abuse, intravenous administration of blood products to hemophiliacs, renal hemodialysis, sexual promiscuity, accidental needle sticks, and institutionalization of children for mental retardation. The prevalence of hepatitis B is higher in foreigners, in those of lower socioeconomic class, in patients with HIV infection, in Eskimos, and in health care workers than in the general population.

Ninety-two percent of patients with acute hepatitis B have self-limited clinical illness and recover after a period of several weeks to several months. Approximately 1% of patients have acute fulminant HBV infection and the remaining 7% have chronic hepatitis B. Hepatitis B has significant associated morbidity and is ranked second only to alcoholism as a cause of cirrhosis. Worldwide, as many as 176 million people are currently infected with HBV, and 5 to 9% evidence a chronic carrier state, of whom 2% may develop hepatocellular carcinoma.

The outcome of patients with chronic hepatitis B has been studied by various groups. The largest study examined 379 patients who were being examined for possible therapeutic intervention. By examining patients who had liver biopsies and hepatitis B markers, it was possible to separate patients into those with chronic persistent, chronic active, and chronic active hepatitis with underlying cirrhosis. The predicted 5-year survival rate was 97% for those with chronic persistent hepatitis, 86% for those with chronic active hepatitis, and 55% for those patients who had cirrhosis with chronic active hepatitis. In a randomized, controlled trial comparing interferon alfa-2b therapy with prednisone withdrawal followed by interferon alfa-2b for the treatment of chronic hepatitis B, biochemical, histologic, and virologic improvements were significantly more commonly seen in patients treated with 5 million units of interferon alfa-2b daily.[75] Approximately one third of patients had normal hepatic transaminase levels after therapy, and about 10% resolved hepatitis B e antigenemia.

When administered into the lateral deltoid area of the arm, immunization as determined by antibody response is successful in excess of 90% with three serial injections. The response is approximately 10% poorer when the vaccine is administered to the gluteal region, presumably owing to erratic absorption from the highly adipose tissue in this area. Assuming a relatively low yearly risk for infection (0.5 to 1%), vaccination of 100,000 persons might be expected to prevent two or three deaths from acute hepatitis B, 37 to 73 cases of chronic active hepatitis, and 448 to 887 cases of icteric hepatitis. With a more realistic incidence rate for a general internist of 2 to 4% per year, the aforementioned rates can be quadrupled. In three particular circumstances, the risk of HBV infection is known to be high enough to warrant preventive measures: perinatal exposure of an infant born to an HBsAg-positive mother, percutaneous or mucosal exposure to HBsAg-positive blood, and sexual exposure to an HBsAg-positive person. Transmission of HBV infection from a mother who is HBsAg- and hepatitis B e antigen–positive to a neonate occurs with a frequency of about 85%, of which as many as 90% become chronic carriers of HBV. The scenario is less ominous if the mother is positive for only HBsAg, with some 10 to 20% of infants becoming infected.

Hepatitis C Virus

Hepatitis C virus was first suspected when, after the advent of routine screening of donor blood for the HBsAg in the United States, it was thought that a marked decrease in the incidence of post-transfusion hepatitis would be realized, but post-transfusion hepatitis still occurred in approximately 12% of blood recipients. Of this group, a portion represented HBsAg-negative blood that harbored HBV; nonetheless, type B hepatitis accounted for a minority (about 10%) of cases; non-A, non-B hepatitis constituted most of the remainder. The agent responsible for non-A, non-B post-transfusion hepatitis has subsequently been defined; it is now known as hepatitis C virus.[76, 77]

Well-recognized risk factors include intravenous drug abuse (42%), blood transfusions (6%), renal hemodialysis (0.6%), sexual promiscuity (6%), and accidental needle sticks (2%).

Post-transfusion hepatitis, or hepatitis C virus infection, clinically resembles type B hepatitis rather closely and lacks truly distinctive clinical or biochemical characteristics. On average, it is a somewhat milder illness than hepatitis B, with an insidious onset and a prolonged, relapsing course. Abnormalities of serum transaminase levels often persist for several months in those who appear to have an uneventful recovery. Abnormalities of serum transaminase levels may display wide fluctuations, including distinct elevations surrounding apparent periods of biochemical remission. About two to three times as many cases of hepatitis C are anicteric when compared with cases of hepatitis B (estimated that 50% of hepatitis B cases experience icterus, whereas approximately 20 to 25% of hepatitic C patients become clinically icteric). Serum glutamic-oxaloacetic transaminase and serum glutamic-pyruvic transaminase levels usually peak at 10 to 20 times normal versus the 20- to 50-fold elevations seen in hepatitis B.

Hepatitis C appears to have a strong tendency for chronicity, with three large studies of post-transfusion hepatitis suggesting persistent elevations in hepatic transaminase levels at 6 to 10 months in 36 to 55% of patients.

Hepatitis Delta Virus

The delta agent was first identified in 1977 as an incomplete RNA virus, which requires HBsAg for replication. Delta hepatitis has not been found in persons who are HBsAg-negative and therefore need not be considered in an HBsAg-negative patient. As a consequence, it is seen in only three known circumstances: acute delta hepatitis superimposed on chronic hepatitis B, acute delta hepatitis superimposed on acute hepatitis B, and chronic delta hepatitis superimposed on chronic hepatitis B.

In patients who acquire HBV and delta agent infections concurrently, the fate of the delta infection is largely dependent on the progression or resolution of the HBV infection. Most commonly, delta infection is limited by the brief period of excessive production of HBsAg and results in an illness that appears similar to acute hepatitis B. Occasionally, a more severe episode of hepatitis occurs, and some data suggest that as much as one third of what has been thought to be fulminant hepatitis B may represent coinfection with HBV and hepatitis delta virus. Acute hepatitis after HBV and hepatitis delta virus coinfection causes a biphasic illness in 25%,[78] with an average interval from initial infection to relapse of 2 weeks (range, 1.5 to 4 weeks). The state of chronicity with both agents appears to connote the greatest risk for progressive hepatic disease.

The HBsAg coat apparently serves to protect the hepatitis delta virus RNA from hydrolysis. The delta antigen is a protein of approximately 68,000 daltons and is resistant to heating as well as to a variety of chemicals. Anti–delta virus antibody appears early in the clinical stage of the disease but drops to undetectable levels in as short a time as 3 to 6 months.

An evaluation of 106 consecutive chronic HBV carriers revealed that 20 had serum and/or liver expression of anti–delta virus antibody.[79] All 20 of these patients were symptomatic, and all underwent biopsy. Those with anti–delta virus antibodies had chronic active hepatitis on biopsy in 45%, and active cirrhosis was noted in the remainder (55%). In a histologic study of delta hepatitis appearing in the face of HBsAg carriage in 31 patients, 24 of 31 developed chronic progressive hepatitis delta virus infection as determined by serologic markers and intrahepatic staining of biopsy specimens for hepatitis delta virus antigen. Cirrhosis was frequently demonstrated in this group, with 30% of biopsy specimens demonstrating evidence of either active or inactive cirrhosis. The overall case fatality rate was 23%; fulminant hepatitis caused 17 of 29 (59%) deaths.

VIRAL HEMORRHAGIC FEVER

The viral hemorrhagic fever syndrome is caused by related agents that occur endemically across Eurasia and result in clinically similar disease. The syndrome is characterized by the triad of fevers, hemorrhagic manifestations, and renal dysfunction.

Dengue Hemorrhagic Fever

Dengue was first recognized in Southeast Asia in the 1960s, and it continues to be a frequent cause of hospitalization and death in many children in Southeast Asia. Dengue is an acute viral illness caused by one of four dengue serotypes (types 1 to 4). Disease activity in the United States has been largely due to imported disease, and disease attributable to all four serotypes has been confirmed.[80] The acute illness is manifested by fevers, headaches, myalgias, nausea, and vomiting. The epidemiologic characteristics of dengue in the Americas appear to be changing, with a continued increase in the distribution of multiple dengue virus serotypes coupled with the introduction of the *Aedes albopictus* vector into the Western Hemisphere. *A. albopictus* is a frequent dengue vector in Asia; however, *A. aegypti* occurs in the southeastern United States and dengue transmission in the United States has been via this vector. The total number of reported dengue cases in the Americas had increased to nearly 89,000 for 1986, more than twice the number of cases reported just 2 years earlier.[81] The actual number of cases appears to be largely under-represented from several areas. Brazilian authorities estimated that the total number of dengue infections in Brazil in 1986 may actually have been closer to 400,000 cases. Disease activity in Mexico, the Caribbean, and Puerto Rico also reached high levels in 1986.

Korean Hemorrhagic Fever

Korean hemorrhagic fever, also known as hemorrhagic fever with renal syndrome, occurs endemically in Eurasia, with the greatest incidence in China north of the Himalaya Mountains. In the People's Republic of China, more than 100,000 cases of Korean hemorrhagic fever may occur annually. Smaller numbers of cases with related agents have been reported from Europe. The prototype virus was isolated in 1978 and named after a Korean river, Hantaan.[82–84] Approximately 3000 United Nations troops had Korean hemorrhagic fever during the Korean conflict.

The clinical presentation has been divided into five phases: febrile, shock, oliguric, polyuric, and convalescent; however, the stages are not always discrete. The initial clinical signs commonly include fever, facial flushing, periorbital edema, and palatal petechiae. Laboratory abnormalities frequently include an elevated hematocrit (reflecting hemoconcentration), thrombocytopenia, and proteinuria. Frank hemorrhage is not typical of Korean hemorrhagic fever; however, mortality may relate to the hemorrhagic complications, particularly intracranial hemorrhage. The overall mortality approximates 3 to 7%.

Rodents are silently and persistently infected and shed large quantities of virus throughout their life. High titers of infectious virus are found in the rodent lungs and kidneys. The infected rodents most commonly implicated as reservoirs of disease include *Apodemus agrarius*, *Rattus rattus*, and *Clethrionomys glariolus* (vole). Transmission is thought to occur through contact of abraded skin with rodent excrement and perhaps though exposure to aerosols.

An outbreak of 14 cases of Korean hemorrhagic fever in U.S. Marines included 10 who were hospitalized and 2 who expired.[85] The 10 who were hospitalized initially had an influenza-like illness characterized by fevers, fatigue, and headache (100%). Most had conjunctival injection on examination (90%). Thrombocytopenia and proteinuria were seen in all hospitalized patients. All fifteen were Hantaan virus IgM–reactive by enzyme-linked immunosorbent assay at titers of 1:3000 or greater. Thirteen of the 15 were subsequently confirmed by immunofluorescent antibody and plaque reduction assay methods. Plaque reduction methods are useful in distinguishing Hantaan virus from the related Seoul virus.

Ribavirin is highly active against Hantaan virus, with an ED_{50} of 15 μg/mL.[86] Mortality in untreated patients ranges from 15 to 50%; with the best supportive care, particularly careful volume management and renal dialysis, the mortality may be reduced to 5 to 30%. In a prospective, placebo-controlled trial, ribavirin was given as a loading dose of 33 mg/kg followed by 16 mg/kg every 6 hours for 4 days and then by 8 mg/kg every 8 hours for 3 additional days. Ten of 118 placebo recipients expired, whereas only 3 of 126 treated patients expired (P = .04) when therapy was begun before the fourth day of illness.[86] In addition to survival advantages, significant improvements in oliguria and in the serum creatinine level were also noted. The only significant adverse effect was a reversible anemia. Some survival advantage may occur in patients begun on therapy after the fourth day, but the benefits may be more modest.

Congo-Crimean Hemorrhagic Fever

Congo-Crimean hemorrhagic fever was first recognized and reported from areas of Crimea, the former U.S.S.R., Bulgaria, and the Middle East. Seroprevalence studies in regions of the Middle East suggest that the infection occurs with a frequency of 3 to 29%.[87, 88] Congo-Crimean hemorrhagic fever is a tick-borne disease, with the aggressive *Hyalomma* tick being the principal vector. Peak tick, and disease, activity occurs from June to September.

After a 3- to 12-day incubation period, the sudden onset of severe headaches associated with fevers and rigors marks the onset of clinical disease. The fever typically persists for a week and may be biphasic in about one half of patients. Lumbar myalgias, sore throat, photophobia, abdominal pain, and diarrhea may be seen. The characteristic hemorrhagic complications appear 3 to 6 days into the course of the illness. A petechial rash accompanied by epistaxis, hematemesis, melena, and laboratory abnormalities consistent with disseminated intravascular coagulation occur.

Findings on physical examination may include bradycardia, a temperature-pulse deficit, a flushed facies with chemotic conjunctivae, hepatomegaly, and a petechial rash.

Nosocomial transmission to health care workers occurs and appears to result in disease with a higher fatality rate than native, tick-borne disease. Strict blood and body fluid precautions and respiratory isolation are recommended. The mortality with nosocomial transmission approximates 40%.[89]

Death may occur 6 to 14 days into the illness, and the case fatality rate has been reported to be 13 to 50%. A variety of laboratory abnormalities have been correlated with a poorer prognosis: white blood cell count greater than 10,000/mm³, platelet count less than 20,000/mm³, serum glutamic-oxaloacetic transaminase level greater than 200 IU/dL, activated partial thromboplastin time greater than 60 seconds, and a fibrinogen level less than 110 mg/dL.[90]

The use of immune sera as therapy has been suggested; however, this is controversial and not currently recommended. No therapy has proved efficacious; however, in vitro studies demonstrating the activity of ribavirin and the high rate of morbidity and mortality in untreated Congo-Crimean hemorrhagic fever have prompted some to suggest that a trial of ribavirin is warranted in high-risk patients. An intravenous loading dose of 2 g of ribavirin followed by 1 g intravenously every 8 hours for 4 days is recommended. Postexposure prophylaxis with ribavirin consists of 400 mg orally every 6 hours for 24 hours followed by 400 mg orally every 8 hours for 6 additional days.[91]

Ribavirin is highly active against Congo-Crimean hemorrhagic fever virus in vitro, and efficacy was reported in a suckling mouse model from the former U.S.S.R.[86] A single report in humans suggested that ribavirin may help moderate the clinical course of Congo-Crimean hemorrhagic fever. Six of nine health care workers who experienced percutaneous injuries with Congo-Crimean hemorrhagic fever–contaminated blood received prophylaxis with ribavirin. One of these six had seroconversion and had mild clinical disease; the other five did not. Two of the three who went untreated developed severe disease.

Rift Valley Fever

Rift Valley fever virus is endemic to sub-Saharan Africa, where it was first isolated in association with an epizootic of hepatitis, abortion, and fatalities in sheep. In addition to producing pathogenicity in sheep, cattle, and goats, the agent also causes significant, occasionally fatal (1%), disease in humans. This highly infectious virus may be transmitted by aerosols but the principal vectors are *Aedes*, *Culex*, and *Anopheles* mosquitoes. After a 2- to 6-day incubation period, illness characterized by prostration, myalgias, and fever supervenes. The physical examination may show conjunctival suffusion and pharyngeal injection. The virus may be readily recovered by culture of the blood, in which the concentration of virus in the acute phase of the illness approximates 1 million to 100 million infectious particles per milliliter. The diagnosis can also be confirmed serologically.

In mouse or hamster models of Rift Valley fever, infection typically results in death 4 to 6 days after inoculation. Ribavirin at high dose, and begun at the time of inoculation, prevents death in 100% of animals. In mice treated with lower doses of ribavirin, death typically resulted from encephalitis and not from hepatic necrosis, which is the typical cause of death in untreated animals. Delays of up to 36 hours may still allow for effective treatment as measured by increased survival. After intracerebral inoculation, ribavirin was not effective in decreasing mortality. Because of the sporadic, unpredictable nature of epidemics attributable to Rift Valley fever, clinical trials of ribavirin have not been attempted.

Sandfly fever, a related, self-limited illness, occurs endemically across large areas of Europe, Africa, and Asia and may serve as a useful model in humans.

Lassa Fever

Lassa fever occurs endemically in western Africa where it exists enzootically in the rat *Mastomys natalensis*. In endemic areas, Lassa fever may be responsible for as many as 300,000 infections and 5000 deaths annually. Transmission occurs primarily through contact with contaminated rat urine. The incubation period varies from 7 to 18 days, and modern intercontinental travel allows infected persons to travel widely during this period. Secondary, person-to-person transmission occurs through unprotected contact with the infected patient's body fluids: through sexual contacts, via contact with the patient's saliva (kissing or sharing eating utensils), or by contact with the patient's blood through medical instrumentation. Unprotected contact with body fluid or blood-contaminated surfaces places one at intermediate risk, and unprotected contact with the patient in the absence of body fluid contact is considered to impose a low risk of infection.[92] In contrast to earlier recommendations, data suggest that secondary spread of Lassa fever virus can be prevented through the use of barrier techniques. Universal precautions surrounding all body fluids are advised with particular care in the handling of blood, human excrement, and respiratory secretions (in the setting of mechanical ventilation).

Ribavirin treatment in Lassa fever–inoculated monkeys appeared beneficial when treatment was begun before the fifth day, whereas a delay to day 8 resulted in 50% mortality.[93] Data in humans treated with 2 g intravenously followed by 1 g intravenously every 6 hours for 4 days, then 0.5 g intravenously every 8 hours for an additional 6 days,[94] when compared with historical controls, suggested a survival advantage. Patients who had a median tissue culture infective dose of greater than $10^{3.6}$/mL of blood had a mortality less than half that of historical controls (32% versus 76%). Similar to the data garnered in animals, treatment of humans before day 7 was critically associated with outcome. Ten days of ribavirin therapy given four times daily, at an oral dose of 600 mg in adults or 400 mg in children aged 6 to 9 years, has been recommended as prophylaxis.[92, 94]

Yellow Fever

Yellow fever remains a serious endemic disease in tropical areas of South America and Africa. The vector for yellow fever is the mosquito *Aedes aegypti*, which has a cosmopolitan distribution. Yellow fever was the first viral disease and the first arthropod-borne disease identified. After a blood meal from an infected individual, a susceptible mosquito enters an extrinsic incubation period, which ends when the yellow fever virus reaches high enough titers in the mosquito's salivary glands to allow yellow fever transmission. An infected mosquito remains infected for life. Three to 6 days after a bite by an infected mosquito, the intrinsic incubation period ends, with the abrupt onset of fevers, chills, and headache. Myalgias, facial flushing, and conjunctival suffusion follow, and after a short period of remission, fevers, hemorrhagic manifestations, and jaundice ensue. Widespread organ involvement may be seen in individuals who come to autopsy, but the characteristic pathologic effects are seen in the liver. Yellow fever virus appears to be quite resistant to ribavirin, with an ED_{50} that is 10-fold greater than against Lassa fever virus, Korean hemorrhagic fever virus, or Rift Valley fever virus.[86] Animal models of therapy with ribavirin have also been disappointing.

ANTIVIRAL THERAPEUTICS

A limited number of antiviral agents have been approved for clinical use in the United States. With the exception of ribavirin and the interferons, antivirals have a limited spectrum of activity, for example, methisazone (3-methylisatin-β-thiosemicarbazone) is useful only as prophylaxis against smallpox.

Vidarabine

Vidarabine is an analogue of adenine deoxyriboside, which is approved for the treatment of HSV encephalitis and neonatal herpes infections. The toxicity of this agent has been substantial, with dose-dependent gastrointestinal and CNS toxicities, as well as reports of myelosuppression, hepatotoxicity, and nephrotoxicity. Vidarabine is sparingly soluble in conventional intravenous solutions, obligating large amounts of fluids for administration of this agent. It is active in HSV encephalitis and severe mucocutaneous HSV infection and protects against dissemination of VZV. The usefulness of vidarabine has been limited by its toxicologic profile

and the introduction of acyclovir, which is less toxic and more active.

Acyclovir

Acyclovir is an acyclic analogue of guanosine, which is triphosphorylated to its active form, acyclovir triphosphate, within the cell. A herpes simplex–coded thymidine kinase is responsible for the phosphorylation of acyclovir to acyclovir monophosphate. Subsequent steps in the phosphorylation process are undertaken by cellular kinases. The oral bioavailability approximates 20%. After a 400-mg oral dose, peak plasma levels of 1.2 mg/L are attained, with a serum half-life of 3 hours. Acyclovir is highly effective and nontoxic against HSV but has limited activity against human CMV, with an ED_{50} of 10 μg/mL.[95] Topical acyclovir exhibits marginal benefits in the therapy of recurrent herpes labialis, but oral therapy appears highly effective, and long-term suppressive therapy is well tolerated.[96] Intravenous acyclovir at a dose of 10 mg/kg every 8 hours is the treatment of choice for HSV encephalitis and higher doses are being investigated for poor-prognosis HSV encephalitis. Intravenous doses in excess of 5 mg/kg, which reach peak plasma levels in excess of 10 mg/L, may be more frequently associated with azotemia, phlebitis, gastrointestinal irritation, or confusion. High-dose oral acyclovir, 4000 mg/d, may help ameliorate the course of zoster in the normal host and is well tolerated. Acyclovir is also useful for the treatment of disseminated HSV and primary HSV infections.

Ganciclovir

Ganciclovir is an acyclic nucleoside analogue of acyclovir, which is 10 to 100 times more active against human CMV than is acyclovir.[97] After it is in the cell, ganciclovir is triphosphorylated and completely inhibits human CMV DNA polymerase by chain termination. After a 1-hour infusion of 5 mg/kg of ganciclovir, a peak plasma concentration of 6.6 μg/mL is reached.[98, 99] Trough levels, measured at 11 hours, approximate 1 μg/mL. The serum half-life approximates 3.6 hours. Ganciclovir is excreted in the urine, largely as the unmetabolized parent compound. Ganciclovir clearance correlates with the creatinine clearance,[99] and decreased doses are required in patients with renal insufficiency.[100] Open-label studies suggested an overall efficacy of 85 to 97% after a course of induction therapy for acute human CMV retinitis in patients with AIDS. Resolution typically begins 1 to 2 weeks into treatment. Virologic responses occur in 92% of CMV infections overall.[12, 22] Ganciclovir is licensed for the therapy of sight-threatening CMV retinitis in patients with AIDS and is the most active drug for other life-threatening human CMV infections.[101, 102] Ganciclovir, when given as a standard induction course, 5 mg/kg every 12 hours, frequently causes significant neutropenia. By the 14th day of treatment, one third of patients may experience neutropenia.[12] Other toxicities have been reported (Table 30–10) but occur much less frequently.[22, 103] Other myelosuppressive therapies may need to be discontinued when ganciclovir is administered, most notably zidovudine.[104]

Ribavirin

Ribavirin does not have the complete six-membered ring of guanosine and has a modified five-membered (triazole) ring. X-ray diffraction studies support structural similarity with guanosine, and antagonism of antiviral action by guanosine in vitro supports its role as a guanosine analogue.[105] After it is inside the cell, ribavirin is sequentially phosphor-

TABLE 30-10

REPORTED TOXICITIES OF GANCICLOVIR THERAPY

Neutropenia
    30% with induction
    38–42% on maintenance
Inhibition of spermatogenesis
Thrombocytopenia
Phlebitis
Peripheral edema
Urticarial rash
Progressive neuropathy
Anemia
Elevated alkaline phosphatase level
Gastrointestinal mucosal atrophy or ulceration
Anorexia
Diarrhea
Fever

ylated to the monophosphate, then to the diphosphate, and finally to the triphosphate, which is the dominant intracellular metabolite. Ribavirin appears to have several possible mechanisms of action;[106] it competes with guanosine for phosphorylation and decreases the intracellular pool of guanosine triphosphate, the monophosphate inhibits inosine 5'-monophosphate dehydrogenase,[105] and the triphosphate inhibits guanosine triphosphate–dependent 5'-RNA capping. The multiple sites of action may help to explain the two unique features of ribavirin among antivirals: it has an extremely broad in vitro range of antiviral effect and resistance to its antiviral effect has been difficult to demonstrate.

Aerosolized ribavirin is licensed for the treatment of children with severe pneumonitis attributable to respiratory syncytial virus and has proved effective in infections caused by influenza virus strains A/H_1N_1 and B/Texas/1/84 in adults and against parainfluenza type 3 in immunocompromised children. Ribavirin has demonstrable in vitro activity against the Arenaviridae, Bunyaviridae, Filoviridae, and the mosquito-borne Flaviviridae. Animal studies in susceptible monkeys suggest that activity may be realizable in vivo for Junin virus and Machupo virus; however, animals that survived the acute hemorrhagic illness appear to succumb more often to a later manifestation, neurologic disease, and this may be related to the poor penetration of ribavirin into the CNS. Oral and intravenous ribavirin is also effective for the treatment of Lassa fever virus.[94]

The principal toxicity of ribavirin is a reversible anemia that appears related to increased red blood cell distribution. Decreased reticulocytosis and bone marrow erythroid hypoplasia may also contribute. Thrombocytosis may also be seen, but neither leukopenia nor leukocytosis have been described. Ribavirin appears not to affect red blood cell osmotic or mechanical fragility; however, red blood cells avidly sequester ribavirin.

Foscarnet

Foscarnet is a virustatic agent that inhibits reverse transcription in all human herpesviruses by selective inhibition of viral DNA polymerases. The agent is licensed for the treatment of CMV retinitis in patients with AIDS.

In a study of 31 AIDS patients treated openly with foscarnet,[107] complete resolution of CMV retinitis occurred in 19 (61%) and a partial response was seen in 10 more (32%). The patients were treated with a 20 mg/kg initial bolus followed by the continuous infusion of 0.16 mg/kg/min for 3 to 5 weeks. Two of 31 patients had treatment stopped after 10 to 16 days of treatment owing to acute renal failure

necessitating dialysis. Anemia or aberrations in serum calcium and phosphorus levels occurred commonly. All of 25 patients who were not given maintenance therapy relapsed within 3 weeks.

In another study, 20 patients with AIDS and CMV retinitis were treated with a 20 mg/kg bolus followed by the continuous infusion of 230 mg/kg/d of foscarnet.[108] Of the 14 patients who completed the initial 21 days of therapy, a beneficial clinical response occurred in 95%. Azotemia and anemia occurred commonly (50%), and 10% developed thrombocytopenia. The median time to recurrence was 78 days for a 90 mg/kg/d maintenance dose, and a lower maintenance dose was less successful.

The current recommendations support lower induction doses, 60 mg/kg every 8 hours, combined with higher maintenance doses, 120 mg/kg/d, to improve the toxicity profile of induction and the efficacy of maintenance therapy as well. Foscarnet may also favorably affect the course of severe and prolonged mucocutaneous herpes simplex lesions attributable to acyclovir-resistant HSV in patients with AIDS.

References

1. Smith W, Andrewes CH, Laidlow PP: A virus obtained from influenza patients. Lancet 2:66, 1933.
2. Francis T Jr: A new type of virus from epidemic influenza. Science 92:405, 1940.
3. Laver WG, Webster RG: Selection of antigenic mutants of influenza viruses. Isolation and peptide mapping of their hemagglutinin proteins. Virology 34:193, 1968.
4. Lai C-J, Markoff LJ, Sveda MM, et al: Genetic variation of influenza A viruses as studied by recombinant DNA techniques. Ann NY Acad Sci 354:162, 1980.
5. Louria DB, Blumenfeld HL, Ellis JT, et al: Studies on influenza in the pandemic of 1957–1958. II. Pulmonary complications of influenza. J Clin Invest 38:213, 1959.
6. McClung HW, Knight V, Gilbert BE, et al: Ribavirin aerosol treatment of influenza B virus infection. JAMA 249:2671, 1983.
7. Horwitz CA, Henle W, Henle G, et al: Clinical and laboratory evaluation of cytomegalovirus-induced mononucleosis in previously healthy individuals. Report of 82 cases. Medicine 65:124, 1986.
8. Jordan MC: Latent infection and the elusive cytomegalovirus. Rev Infect Dis 5:205, 1983.
9. Rand KH, Pollard RB, Merigan TC: Increased pulmonary superinfections in cardiac-transplant patients undergoing primary cytomegalovirus infection. N Engl J Med 298:951, 1978.
10. Wallace JM, Hannah J: Cytomegalovirus pneumonitis in patients with AIDS. Findings in an autopsy series. Chest 92:198, 1987.
11. Balfour HH Jr: Management of cytomegalovirus disease with antiviral drugs. Rev Infect Dis 12:S849, 1990.
12. Buhles WC Jr, Mastre BJ, Tinker AJ, et al: Ganciclovir treatment of life- or sight-threatening cytomegalovirus infection: Experience in 314 immunocompromised patients. Rev Infect Dis 10(suppl 3):S495, 1988.
13. Meyers JD, Flournoy N, Thomas ED: Risk factors for cytomegalovirus infection after human marrow transplantation. J Infect Dis 153:478, 1986.
14. Kusne S, Dummer JS, Singh N, et al: Infections after liver transplantation: An analysis of 101 consecutive cases. Medicine 67:132, 1988.
15. Marker SC, Howard RJ, Simmons RL, et al: Cytomegalovirus infection: A quantitative prospective study of three hundred twenty consecutive renal transplants. Surgery 89:660, 1981.
16. Pollard RB, Rand HK, Arvin AM, et al: Cell-mediated immunity to cytomegalovirus infection in normal subjects and cardiac transplant patients. J Infect Dis 137:679, 1978.
17. Pollard RB, Arvin AM, Gamberg P, et al: Specific cell-mediated immunity and infections with herpes viruses in cardiac transplant recipients. Am J Med 73:679, 1982.
18. Neiman PE, Wasserman PB, Wentworth BB, et al: Interstitial pneumonia and cytomegalovirus infection as complications of human marrow transplantation. Transplantation 15:478, 1973.
19. Grattan MT, Morenocabral CE, Starnes VA, et al: Cytomegalovirus infection is associated with cardiac allograft rejection and atherosclerosis. JAMA 261:3561, 1989.
20. Preiksaitis JK, Rosno S, Grumet C, et al: Infections due to herpesviruses in cardiac transplant recipients: Role of the donor heart and immunosuppressive therapy. J Infect Dis 147:974, 1983.
21. Peterson PK, Balfour HH Jr, Marker SC, et al: Cytomegalovirus disease in renal allograft recipients: A prospective study of the clinical features, risk factors and impact on renal transplantation. Medicine 59:283, 1980.
22. Collaborative DHPG Treatment Study Group: Treatment of serious

cytomegalovirus infections with 9-(1,3-dihydroxy-2-propoxymethyl) guanine in patients with AIDS and other immunodeficiencies. N Engl J Med 314:801, 1986.

23. Jennens ID, Lucas CR, Sandland AM, et al: Cytomegalovirus cultures during maintenance DHPG therapy for cytomegalovirus (CMV) retinitis in acquired immunodeficiency syndrome (AIDS). J Med Virol 30:42, 1990.

24. Emmanuel D, Cunningham I, Jules-Elysee K, et al: Cytomegalovirus pneumonia after bone marrow transplantation successfully treated with the combination of ganciclovir and high-dose intravenous immune globulin. Ann Intern Med 109:777, 1988.

25. Reed EC, Bowden RA, Dandliker PS, et al: Treatment of cytomegalovirus pneumonia with ganciclovir and intravenous cytomegalovirus immunoglobulin in patients with bone marrow transplants. Ann Intern Med 109:783, 1988.

26. Guess HA, Broughton DD, Melton LJ III, et al: Population-based studies of varicella complications. Pediatrics 78:723, 1986.

27. Rusthoven JJ, Ahlgren P, Elhakim T, et al: Varicella-zoster infection in adult cancer patients: A population study. Arch Intern Med 148:1561, 1988.

28. Johanson WG Jr, Pierce AK, Sanford JP: Pulmonary function in uncomplicated influenza. Am Rev Respir Dis 100:141, 1969.

29. Schlossberg D, Littman M: Varicella pneumonia. Arch Intern Med 148:1630, 1988.

30. Haake DA, Zakowski PC, Haake DL, et al: Early treatment with acyclovir for varicella pneumonia in otherwise healthy adults: Retrospective controlled study and review. Rev Infect Dis 12:788, 1990.

31. Janier M, Hillion B, Baccard M, et al: Chronic varicella zoster infection in acquired immunodeficiency syndrome (letter). J Am Acad Dermatol 18:584, 1988.

32. Verghese A, Gallemore G: Kernig's and Brudzinski's signs revisited. Rev Infect Dis 9:1187, 1987.

33. Karandanis D, Shulman JA: Recent survey of infectious meningitis in adults: Review of laboratory findings in bacterial, tuberculosis, and aseptic meningitis. South Med J 69:449, 1976.

34. Carpenter RR, Petersdorf RG: The clinical spectrum of bacterial meningitis. Am J Med 33:262, 1962.

35. Feigin RD, Shackelford PG: Value of repeat lumbar puncture in the differential diagnosis of meningitis. N Engl J Med 289:571, 1973.

36. Jarvis CW, Saxena KM: Does prior antibiotic treatment hamper the diagnosis of acute bacterial meningitis? An analysis of a series of 135 childhood cases. Clin Pediatr 11:201, 1972.

37. Sarwar M, Falkoff G, Naseem M: Radiologic techniques in the diagnosis of CNS infections. Neurol Clin 4:41, 1986.

38. Enterovirus surveillance—United States, 1989. MMWR 38:563, 1989.

39. Moore M: Enteroviral disease in the United States, 1970–1979. J Infect Dis 146:103, 1982.

40. Racaniello VR, Baltimore D: Molecular cloning of poliovirus cDNA and determination of the complete nucleotide sequence of the viral genome. Proc Natl Acad Sci USA 78:4887, 1981.

41. Current trends: Progress toward eradicating poliomyelitis from the Americas. MMWR 38:532, 1989.

42. Paralytic poliomyelitis—Senegal, 1986–1987: Update on the N-IPV efficacy study. MMWR 37:257, 1988.

43. Melnick JL, Shaw EW, Curnen EC: A virus from patients diagnosed as non-paralytic poliomyelitis or aseptic meningitis. Proc Soc Exp Biol Med 71:344, 1949.

44. McArthur JC, Cohen BA, Farzedegan H, et al: Cerebrospinal fluid abnormalities in homosexual men with and without neuropsychiatric findings. Ann Neurol 23:S34, 1988.

45. Chalmers AC, Aprill BS, Shepard H: Cerebrospinal fluid and human immunodeficiency virus: Findings in healthy, asymptomatic, seropositive men. Arch Intern Med 150:1538, 1990.

46. Arboviral infections of the central nervous system—United States, 1987. MMWR 37:506, 1988.

47. Epidemiologic notes and reports: La Crosse encephalitis in West Virginia. MMWR 37:79, 1988.

48. Eastern equine encephalitis—United States, 1989. MMWR 38:619, 1989.

49. Miller JK, Hesser F, Tompkins VN: Herpes simplex encephalitis: Report of 20 cases. Ann Intern Med 64:92, 1966.

50. Rawls WE, Dyck PJ, Klass DW, et al: Encephalitis associated with herpes simplex virus. Ann Intern Med 64:104, 1966.

51. Davis LE, Johnson RT: An explanation for the localization of herpes simplex encephalitis? Ann Neurol 5:2, 1979.

52. Whitley RJ, Soong S-J, Linneman C Jr, et al: Herpes simplex encephalitis: Clinical assessment. JAMA 247:317, 1982.

53. Soong S-J, Watson NE, Caddell GR, et al: Use of brain biopsy for diagnostic evaluation of patients with suspected herpes simplex encephalitis: A statistical model and its clinical implications. J Infect Dis 163:17, 1991.

54. Aurelius E, Johansson B, Skoldenberg B, et al: Rapid diagnosis of herpes simplex encephalitis by nested polymerase chain reaction assay of cerebrospinal fluid. Lancet 337:189, 1991.

55. Whitley RJ, Soong S-J, Dolin R, et al: Adenine arabinoside therapy of biopsy-proved herpes simplex encephalitis: National Institute of Allergy and Infectious Diseases Collaborative Antiviral study. N Engl J Med 289:571, 1973.

56. VanLandingham KE, Marsteller HB, Ross GW, et al: Relapse of herpes simplex encephalitis after conventional acyclovir therapy. JAMA 259:1051, 1988.

57. Rothman AL, Cheeseman SH, Nusinoff-Lehrman S, et al: Herpes simplex encephalitis in a patient with lymphoma: Relapse following acyclovir therapy. JAMA 259:1056, 1988.

58. Kalter SS, Heberling RL: B virus (Herpesvirus simiae) infection. ASM News 54:71, 1988.

59. Palmer AE: B virus, Herpesvirus simiae: Historical perspective. J Med Primatol 16:99, 1987.

60. Sabin AB, Wright AM: Acute ascending myelitis following a monkey bite, with the isolation of a virus capable of reproducing the disease. J Exp Med 59:115, 1934.

61. Perspectives in disease prevention and health promotion: Guidelines for prevention of Herpesvirus simiae (B virus) infection in monkey handlers. MMWR 36:680, 1987.

62. Epidemiologic notes and reports: B virus infection in humans—Pensacola, Florida. MMWR 36:289, 1987.

63. Hutt R, Guajardo JE, Kalter SS: Detection of antibodies to Herpesvirus simiae and Herpesvirus hominis in nonhuman primates. Lab Anim Sci 31:184, 1981.

64. Heberling RL, Kalter SS: A dot-immunobinding assay on nitrocellulose with psoralen inactivated Herpesvirus simiae (B virus). Lab Anim Sci 37:304, 1987.

65. Hilliard JK, Eberle R, Lipper SL, et al: Herpesvirus simiae (B virus): Replication of the virus and identification of viral polypeptides in infected cells. Arch Virol 93:185, 1987.

66. Hilliard JK, Munoz RM, Lipper SL, et al: Rapid identification of Herpesvirus simiae (B virus) DNA from clinical isolates in nonhuman primate colonies. J Virol Methods 13:55, 1986.

67. Wall LVM, Zwartouw HT, Kelly DC: Discrimination between 20 isolates of Herpesvirus simiae (B-virus) by restriction enzyme analysis of the viral genome. Virus Res 12:283, 1989.

68. Epidemiologic notes and reports: B virus infections in humans—Michigan. MMWR 38:453, 1989.

69. Current trends: Measles—United States, 1988. MMWR 38:601, 1989.

70. Fishbein DB, Dobbins JG, Bryson JH, et al: Rabies surveillance, United States, 1987. MMWR 37:1, 1988.

71. Human rabies—Texas, 1990. MMWR 40:132, 1991.

72. The National Association of State Public Health Veterinarians, Inc: Compendium of Animal Rabies Control, 1989. MMWR 37:789, 1989.

73. Anderson LJ, Sikes RK, Langkop CW, et al: Post-exposure trial of a human diploid cell rabies vaccine. J Infect Dis 142:133, 1980.

74. Smith JS, Fishbein DB, Ruprecht CE, et al: Unexplained rabies in three immigrants in the United States: A virologic investigation. N Engl J Med 324:205, 1991.

75. Perrillo RP, Schiff ER, Davis GL, et al: A randomized, controlled trial of interferon alfa-2b alone and after prednisone withdrawal for the treatment of chronic hepatitis B. N Engl J Med 323:295, 1990.

76. Kuo G, Choo Q-L, Alter HJ, et al: An assay for circulating antibodies to a major etiologic virus of human non-A, non-B hepatitis. Science 244:362, 1989.

77. Choo Q-L, Kuo G, Weiner AJ, et al: Isolation of a cDNA clone derived from a blood-borne non-A, non-B viral hepatitis genome. Science 244:359, 1989.

78. DeCock KM, Govindarajan S, Chin KP, et al: Delta hepatitis in the Los Angeles area: A report of 126 cases. Ann Intern Med 105:108, 1986.

79. Lok A, Lindsay I, Scheuer PJ, et al: Clinical and histological features of delta infection in chronic hepatitis B carriers. J Clin Pathol 38:530, 1985.

80. Current trends: Imported dengue—United States, 1987. MMWR 38:463, 1989.

81. Dengue and dengue hemorrhagic fever in the Americas, 1986. MMWR 37:129, 1988.

82. Schmaljohn CS, Hasty SE, Dalrymple JM, et al: Antigenic and genetic properties of viruses linked to hemorrhagic fever with renal syndrome into a newly defined genus of Bunyaviridae. Science 227:1041, 1985.

83. World Health Organization: Hemorrhagic fever with renal syndrome: Memorandum from a WHO meeting. Bull WHO 61:269, 1983.

84. Cohen MS: Epidemic hemorrhagic fever revisited. Rev Infect Dis 4:992, 1982.

85. International notes: Korean hemorrhagic fever. MMWR 37:87, 1988.

86. Huggins JW: Prospects for treatment of viral hemorrhagic fevers with ribavirin, a broad-spectrum antiviral drug. Rev Infect Dis 11(Suppl 4):S750, 1989.

87. Al-Nakib W, Lloyd G, El-Mekki A, et al: Preliminary report on arbovirus-antibody prevalence among patients in Kuwait: Evidence of Congo/Crimean virus infection. Trans Soc Trop Med Hyg 78:474, 1984.

88. Al-Tikriti SK, Hassan FK, Moslih IM, et al: Congo/Crimean haemorrhagic fever in Iraq: A seroepidemiological survey. J Trop Med Hyg 84:117, 1981.

89. Donchev A, Kebedzhiev G, Rusakiev M: Hemorrhagic fever in Bulgaria. Bulgar Akad Nauk Mikrobiol Inst, 1 Kongr Mikrobiol 1:777, 1965.

90. Swanepoel R, Gill GE, Shepherd AJ, et al: The clinical pathology of Crimean-Congo hemorrhagic fever. Rev Infect Dis 11(suppl 4):S794, 1989.

91. Oldfield EC III, Wallace MR, Hyams KC, et al: Endemic infectious diseases of the Middle East. Rev Infect Dis 13(suppl 3):S197, 1991.

92. Holmes GP, McCormick JB, Trock SC, et al: Lassa fever in the United States: Investigation of a case and new guidelines for management. N Engl J Med 323:1120, 1990.
93. Jahrling PB, Hesse RA, Eddy GA, et al: Lassa fever infection of rhesus monkeys: Pathogenesis and treatment with ribavirin. J Infect Dis 141:580, 1980.
94. McCormick JB, King IJ, Webb PA, et al: Lassa fever: Effective therapy with ribavirin. N Engl J Med 314:20, 1986.
95. Plotkin SA, Drew WL, Felsenstein D, et al: Sensitivity of clinical isolates of human cytomegalovirus to 9-(1,3-dihydroxy-2-propoxy-methyl) guanine. J Infect Dis 152:833, 1985.
96. Kaplowitz LG, Baker D, Gelb L, et al: Prolonged continuous acyclovir treatment of normal adults with frequently recurring genital herpes simplex virus infection. JAMA 265:747, 1991.
97. Hennis HL, Scott AA, Apple DJ: Cytomegalovirus retinitis. Surv Ophthalmol 34:193, 1989.
98. Matthews T, Boehme R: Antiviral activity and mechanism of action of ganciclovir. Rev Infect Dis 10(suppl 3):S490, 1988.
99. Sommadossi J-P, Bevan R, Ling T, et al: Clinical pharmacokinetics of ganciclovir in patients with normal and impaired renal function. Rev Infect Dis 10(suppl 3):S507, 1988.
100. Snydman DR: Ganciclovir therapy for cytomegalovirus disease associated with renal transplants. Rev Infect Dis 10(suppl 3):S554, 1988.
101. Erice A, Jordan MC, Chace BA, et al: Ganciclovir treatment of cytomegalovirus disease in transplant recipients and other immunocompromised hosts. JAMA 257:3082, 1987.
102. Thomson MH, Jeffries DJ: Ganciclovir therapy in iatrogenically immunosuppressed patients with cytomegalovirus disease. J Antimicrob Chemother 23:61, 1989.
103. D'Amico DJ, Talamo JH, Felsenstein D, et al: Ophthalmoscopic and histologic findings in cytomegalovirus retinitis treated with BW-B759U. Arch Ophthalmol 104:1788, 1986.
104. Hochster H, Dietrich D, Bozzette S, et al: Toxicity of combined ganciclovir and zidovudine for cytomegalovirus disease associated with AIDS. An AIDS Clinical Trials Group study. Ann Intern Med 113:111, 1990.
105. Streeter DG, Witkowski JT, Kahre GP, et al: Mechanism of action of 1-beta-D-ribofuranosyl-1,2,4-triazole-3-carboxamide (Virazole), a new broad-spectrum antiviral agent. Proc Natl Acad Sci USA 70:1174, 1974.
106. Gilbert BE, Knight V: Minireview. Biochemistry and clinical applications of ribavirin. Antimicrob Agents Chemother 30:201, 1986.
107. Lehoang P, Girard B, Robinet M, et al: Foscarnet in the treatment of cytomegalovirus retinitis in acquired immune deficiency syndrome. Ophthalmology 96:865, 1989.
108. Fanning MM, Read SE, Benson M, et al: Foscarnet therapy of cytomegalovirus retinitis in AIDS. J Acquir Immune Defic Syndr 3:472, 1990.

CHAPTER 31

Gram-Positive Bacterial Sepsis

James J. Gordon
Dennis R. Schaberg

Although gram-negative bacteria have become increasingly important as etiologic agents in nosocomial sepsis, gram-positive organisms continue to play a significant role. *Staphylococcus aureus* is the predominant gram-positive pathogen responsible for the septic syndrome, but other bacteria such as enterococci, streptococci, and more unusual organisms may occasionally be responsible. Although viridans streptococci and those belonging to the *Streptococcus milleri* group (*S. intermedius*, *S. anginosus*, *S.* MG, and *S. constellatus*) are often recovered from blood culture specimens, they rarely result in the septic syndrome. These organisms are most commonly associated with subacute endocarditis and pyogenic infections and are discussed in Chapter 40. This chapter reviews the pathophysiologic and epidemiologic characteristics of and therapy for gram-positive sepsis, as the causative pathogens are particular to certain clinical settings and offer different therapeutic challenges.

STAPHYLOCOCCI
Microbiology

There are approximately 20 currently recognized species of staphylococci, although only 3 are responsible for the majority of clinical infections. *Staphylococcus epidermidis* is an important pathogen in infections of intravenous catheters and prosthetic devices. This pathogen is responsible for 27% of positive blood cultures in hospitalized patients[1] and is discussed later. *Staphylococcus saprophyticus* is an important cause of acute cystitis, primarily in young, otherwise healthy women.[2] *S. aureus* causes a variety of clinical syndromes, including sepsis.

Staphylococci are gram-positive cocci, which grow predominantly in clusters but can also be found in singlets, pairs, and chains. They are nonmotile, are facultative anaerobes, and only rarely form spores. On sheep blood agar, *S. aureus* forms yellow colonies and often causes beta-hemolysis, whereas coagulase-negative staphylococci usually form white colonies.

A variety of laboratory tests aid in differentiating *S. aureus* from other gram-positive cocci. Staphylococci are differentiated from streptococci primarily by the production of catalase, an enzyme that catalyzes the breakdown of hydrogen peroxide. *S. aureus* also produces coagulase, which allows it to act on fibrinogen via a cell-bound enzyme called clumping factor. This reaction differentiates *S. aureus* from the remainder of staphylococci. *S. aureus* ferments mannitol and produces deoxyribonuclease. Surface protein A, which binds the Fc portion of immunoglobulin G, is rather specific for *S. aureus* and forms the basis for a rapid assay under development.

The Species *Staphylococcus aureus*
History

S. aureus is frequently touted as a persistent and hardy organism.[3] Throughout the years, it has been capable of altering its antibiotic susceptibility patterns and maintaining its virulence to remain a common and dangerous pathogen. *S. aureus* is the second most frequently identified isolate from positive blood cultures in the hospital setting, after coagulase-negative staphylococci (usually *S. epidermidis*).[1] It consistently accounts for 10 to 40% of nosocomial infections, with this variance dependent on the institution and the patient population surveyed.

The first effective antimicrobial therapeutic agents for staphylococcal infections were the benzylpenicillins, which were released in 1943. Although sulfonamide antibiotics had been available for clinical use since the late 1930s, acquisition of resistance by staphylococci to these agents is rapid and their activity in pus, a common milieu for infection caused by staphylococci, is severely limited. Initially, only 5 to 7% of *S. aureus* isolates were resistant to penicillin, but by 1949, 59% were resistant, and by 1960, 82% were resistant, primarily a result of the production of β-lactamase.[4] By the late 1950s, nosocomial staphylococcal infections attributable to strains resistant to virtually all available antibiotics, except vancomycin, became prevalent. However, this agent was used with much caution, as impurities in the earlier preparations resulted in excessive toxicity.

In 1959, semisynthetic penicillins resistant to the action of penicillinase became available, with an associated dramatic improvement in therapy. However, by 1961 there were reports of methicillin resistance in Europe,[5] and in 1968, 18 cases were reported at Boston City Hospital.[6] This resistance mechanism, which rendered all available β-lactam antibiotics ineffective, was ultimately shown to be due to alteration of penicillin-binding proteins (PBPs). During the next 10 years, this intrinsic resistance became more widespread, and in the late 1970s, intrinsically resistant isolates that were also resistant to non–β-lactam agents became more prevalent. Fortunately, these isolates remained uniformly sensitive to the glycopeptide vancomycin.

Epidemiology

S. aureus accounts for approximately 10% of nosocomial infections, and 15 to 20% of all bacteremias.[1] Sixty percent of these bacteremias are nosocomial.[3] Sources of bacteremia are varied, but the most often implicated source is an intravenous catheter. Other less common sources include primary infections of wounds, skin and soft tissues, bones, and joints, and endocarditis.

Colonization and interpersonal transmission are central to understanding the epidemiology of infection with *S. aureus.* Approximately 20 to 40% of healthy persons are colonized with this organism in their anterior nares and/or intertriginous regions at any point in time.[7] It is estimated that over the course of several years, 30% of individuals have prolonged carriage and 50% have intermittent carriage.[7] The remaining 20% of individuals probably never become colonized.[7] Persons with certain underlying conditions are at exceedingly high risk for staphylococcal carriage.[3] These include intravenous drug abusers (40%), insulin-requiring diabetics (50%), patients receiving allergy injections (50%), patients undergoing long-term hemodialysis (75%), and those with chronic dermatologic conditions such as psoriasis or cutaneous T cell lymphoma (up to 100%).

It is unclear why certain healthy individuals become colonized with *S. aureus,* whereas others do not. It most likely relates to a certain combination of genetic and environmental factors. Among hospitalized patients, risk factors for staphylococcal acquisition and infection include hospitalization in a tertiary care center, prolonged hospital stay, illness necessitating care in a burn or intensive care unit, surgical wounds, prolonged intravenous access, and advanced age.

As patients become colonized, they may also act as reservoirs for infection. Transmission is most often mediated by carriage on hospital staff members' hands, although airborne transmission from heavy shedders may occur. Of interest, physicians and nurses carry this organism 50 and 70% of the time, respectively.[8] Hospital ward workers may harbor the organism as much as 90% of the time. In that health care workers are frequently transient carriers, and environmental contamination is unusual, judicious hand washing is essential in curtailing the spread of this organism within the hospital environment.

Pathogenesis

S. aureus has received much attention with regard to virulence factors. A variety of factors (discussed later) have been found to aid in the pathogenesis of illness. Additionally, three toxins, exfoliatin, enterotoxins, and toxic shock syndrome toxin 1 (TSST-1), have been associated with specific disease syndromes. To gain an understanding of the roles of various enzymes and toxins, one must first appreciate the spectrum of events in the genesis of human infection.

Staphylococcal infection is invariably associated with an initial breach of the first line of defense (skin and mucous membranes), followed by disruption and avoidance of humoral and phagocytic defense mechanisms. The phagocytic component of immunity is of supreme importance in the eradication of staphylococcal infections, as most staphylococci are not susceptible to the host's extracellular bactericidal mechanisms. Furthermore, in some instances, staphylococci are capable of surviving within polymorphonuclear leukocytes, where they multiply and eventually kill the cells.[9] This may be in part due to the production of catalase, an enzyme that inactivates potentially bactericidal hydrogen peroxide.

After staphylococci have invaded tissues, a variety of enzymes and toxins assist in propagation of the infectious process. For instance, hyaluronidase breaks down the hyaluronic acid component of connective tissue, and lipase helps disrupt lipid tissue integrity. α-Toxin is a protein capable of inducing tissue necrosis, although its role in the pathogenesis of human infection is still not clear.[10] Similarly, β-, γ-, and δ-toxins may be important virulence factors in the pathogenicity of staphylococcal infection, although their precise roles remain to be determined.

Proteins capable of inhibiting polymorphonuclear leukocyte function and complement activity are also elaborated by *S. aureus.* Leukocidin, in addition to its cytolytic activity, inhibits chemotaxis of polymorphonuclear leukocytes and monocytes.[11] Protein A inhibits opsonization and subsequently interferes with phagocytosis.[12] This is achieved by its ability to bind to the Fc receptor of immunoglobulin G, which prevents binding of the opsonic antibody molecule to the Fc receptor on the membrane of the phagocyte.

After *S. aureus* reaches the blood stream, the peptidoglycan/teichoic acid component of the bacterial cell wall appears to be capable of initiating endogenous mediators of sepsis, with a resultant syndrome identical to that elicited by gram-negative pathogens. This has been confirmed in animal models, although 10 to 100 times more peptidoglycan/teichoic acid is required than is lipopolysaccharide (endotoxin).[13] In any event, the activation of endogenous mediators, such as interleukin-1, tumor necrosis factor (cachectin), interleukin-6, and interferon-α, stimulates a network of secondary mediators. This results in the septic syndrome, with hyperthermia or hypothermia, hypotension, increased cardiac output with depressed systemic vascular resistance, and subsequently, impaired end-organ function caused by hypoperfusion and direct toxic effects.

As mentioned earlier, three groups of toxins produced by staphylococci have been associated with specific disease syndromes: Exfoliatin is an epidermolytic toxin responsible for staphylococcal scalded skin syndrome. TSST-1 results in the clinical syndrome recognized as toxic shock syndrome (TSS). Last, enterotoxins produced by some strains of *S. aureus* are important causes of toxin-mediated gastroenteritis. Enterotoxin F may be responsible for some cases of TSS in which TSST-1 is not identified.[14]

Clinical Presentation

Staphylococcal infections may present in myriad fashions, depending on the mode of entry, the virulence, and the quantity of organisms and the integrity of the host's defenses. Some strains of staphylococci produce toxins that mediate clinical syndromes, whereas most produce disease via direct invasion of organisms.

The typical sequence of septicemic staphylococcal infection begins with colonization, followed by integumentary penetration, tissue invasion, abscess formation, bacteremia, and systemic seeding. Abscess formation may occur in solid organs such as the brain, the kidney, the liver, and the adrenal gland. In these situations, the clinical scenario is dictated by the location of primary and metastatic infection. A vasculitic reaction attributable to staphylococcal infection, which may resemble Rocky Mountain spotted fever or disseminated meningococcal infection, has been reported.[15, 16]

Staphylococcal sepsis frequently begins with chills and sometimes with frank rigors. Patients often experience mental status changes, arthralgias, and myalgias. The patient appears to be acutely ill, and careful physical examination may uncover a suspected focus. In the hospitalized individual, an intravascular device or surgical wound may be implicated. Left unchecked, staphylococcal bacteremia carries an ominous prognosis, with sepsis and death occurring. This was evident in the preantibiotic era, when the presentation of staphylococcal sepsis was somewhat uniform.[17] The patients were typically young and without underlying illness. Metastatic foci were common and mortality was greater than 80%. Currently, the young and elderly seem to be at highest risk.[18] In the latter group, mortality is greater than 60%. Associated conditions include kidney and liver disease, cardiovascular compromise, underlying malignancy, intravenous drug abuse, and loss of cutaneous integrity.[18, 19]

It is useful to separate patients clinically into groups on the basis of whether a primary source can be identified. For those in whom a focus can be identified, endocarditis and secondary infection are unusual, being observed in less than 5% of cases.[20] In contrast, patients who clinically have an occult source of bacteremia frequently have endocarditis and a course complicated by secondary bacterial seeding. In one study, 57% of patients without an identifiable source of bacteremia had endocarditis and more than 90% had secondary foci of infection.[20] Conversely, in those in whom a source could be easily identified, endocarditis and secondary bacterial seeding were less common, occurring in 3 and 10% of patients, respectively.

Resolution of fever and clinical improvement of staphylococcal sepsis may appear as early as 8 hours after the initiation of appropriate therapy.[21] However, patients most frequently begin to defervesce after approximately 24 hours, with complete resolution of fever observed at a mean of 60 hours. There is a tendency toward an increase in response time in those cases complicated by the presence of prosthetic material or endocarditis. In patients with staphylococcal infection failing to respond to apparently appropriate therapy, a sequestered focus of infection must be suspected.

Therapy

Basic components of therapy for all infectious processes include (1) eradication of the source of infection, (2) aggressive supportive care, and (3) appropriate antimicrobial therapy.

In the case of staphylococcal sepsis, a source should be sought and eradicated, if at all possible. In the case of soft tissue infection or infection at the site of a foreign body, such as an intravascular catheter, this may be readily accomplished. Septic joints and deep abscesses should be drained. However, in many instances, such as endocarditis or pulmonary infections, this may not be possible.

Supportive care, including the maintenance of adequate oxygenation and vital organ perfusion are of ultimate importance in the management of these patients. These principles are addressed in great detail elsewhere in this text.

Antimicrobial therapy is based on in vitro susceptibility testing of the isolated organism (Table 31–1). Staphylococci are capable of a number of resistance mechanisms, which render many antimicrobial agents ineffective. The most important of these are β-lactamase production and the alteration of PBPs.

The majority of S. aureus strains produce β-lactamase (at least 85% of community-acquired and 90 to 100% of nosocomial organisms), and an isolate should be assumed to be a β-lactamase producer until proved otherwise. Semisynthetic penicillins (nafcillin or oxacillin), first-generation cephalosporins (cefazolin), agents that contain β-lactamase inhibitors (ampicillin-sulbactam and ticarcillin-clavulanate), and imipenem-cilastatin all have excellent activity against these strains. However, strains with alterations of the PBPs, commonly referred to as methicillin-resistant S. aureus, are resistant to these agents. In that these organisms are resistant to the action of all β-lactam agents, they are more accurately referred to as intrinsically resistant S. aureus (IRSA). IRSA is a common pathogen in certain populations such as intravenous drug abusers, nursing home residents, and patients hospitalized where it is endemic. Whereas β-lactamase production is generally plasmid mediated, the trait for intrinsic resistance to β-lactam antibiotics is carried on the bacterial chromosome.[22] This chromosomal trait results in an alteration of the structure of PBP-2a, with resultant decreased affinity for all β-lactam agents.

Vancomycin is the drug of choice for the therapy of infections caused by IRSA (see Table 31–1). This agent's three mechanisms of action, inhibition of RNA synthesis, inhibition of cell wall synthesis via inhibition of steps not involving PBPs, and lethal membrane effects, are probably responsible for the fact that no isolate of S. aureus resistant to this agent has been reported. Vancomycin is generally well tolerated. Impurities in earlier preparations contributed to a high incidence of nephrotoxicity with this agent. Preparations are now more pure, and nephrotoxicity is unusual unless vancomycin is combined with an aminoglycoside or other nephrotoxic agent. The red man syndrome results from vancomycin's inherent ability to directly induce degranulation of histamine from cell-bound mast cells. It is strongly correlated with excessively rapid administration of the drug and, in most instances, can be avoided by slower infusion. Clinical characteristics of this syndrome include tingling and flushing of the face, the neck, and the thorax; diaphoresis; and occasionally, hypotension with shock. Bone marrow toxicity, ototoxicity, and true allergic reactions are less common side effects. Monitoring serum levels of vancomycin helps prevent toxicity and ensures adequate blood levels for therapeutic efficacy.

Occasionally, patients do not tolerate vancomycin owing to true allergic reactions or toxicity. In this instance, other agents must be utilized. Trimethoprim-sulfamethoxazole is active against approximately 95% of clinical isolates of IRSA and can be useful. However, its efficacy in therapy for staphylococcal endocarditis has been disappointing. Quinolones, such as ciprofloxacin, pefloxacin, and ofloxacin, act via disruption of the activity of bacterial DNA gyrase. These agents are often active against IRSA strains and are promising. However, extensive clinical experience is still lacking, and rapid emergence of resistance has been seen. Alternative agents being evaluated include teicoplanin, daptomycin, and fosfomycin.

The tolerance phenomenon refers to the property of certain strains of S. aureus that display a significant disparity between their minimal inhibitory concentrations (MIC) and the minimal bactericidal concentration.[23] In general, the ratio of MIC to minimal bactericidal concentration in tolerant strains is greater than 1:32, although the ratio may be much greater. This discrepancy is thought to be caused by the antibiotic's failure to activate staphylococcal autolytic enzymes in these strains, resulting in bacteriostatic rather than bactericidal activity.[24] Many investigators believe that organisms that display tolerance have a high incidence of treatment failure in infections requiring bactericidal activity, such

TABLE 31–1			
DRUGS OF CHOICE FOR SELECTED GRAM-POSITIVE BACTERIA			
Organism	Drug of Choice	Alternative Agents	Comments
Staphylococcus aureus			Consider addition of rifampin or aminoglycoside for tolerant species.
Intrinsically sensitive	Semisynthetic penicillin Nafcillin or oxacillin First-generation cephalosporins Cefazolin	Erythromycin, clindamycin Ampicillin-sulbactam, ticarcillin-clavulanate, imipenem-cilastatin	
Intrinsically resistant	Vancomycin	Trimethoprim-sulfamethoxazole, ciprofloxacin	
Staphylococcus epidermidis	Vancomycin	Trimethoprim-sulfamethoxazole, ciprofloxacin	
Enterococcus spp.	Ampicillin, penicillin, or vancomycin *plus* gentamicin		
Highly gentamicin resistant	Ampicillin or penicillin or vancomycin		Streptomycin effective in up to one third of cases.
Vancomycin resistant	Ampicillin or penicillin *plus* gentamicin		If high-level, inducible vancomycin resistance, addition of vancomycin may increase susceptibility to penicillin.
β-Lactamase–producing	Ampicillin-sulbactam or vancomycin *plus* gentamicin		
Beta-hemolytic streptococci	Penicillin or ampicillin	Erythromycin, vancomycin	Under certain circumstances, addition of an aminoglycoside is appropriate (see text).
Streptococcus pneumoniae	Penicillin or ampicillin	Vancomycin	Penicillin resistance prevalent in some regions.
Viridans streptococci	Penicillin or ampicillin	Vancomycin	See text for therapeutic strategies.
Corynebacterium group JK	Vancomycin		
Listeria monocytogenes	Ampicillin or penicillin	Trimethoprim-sulfamethoxazole	

as endocarditis and meningitis.[23] Thus, for severe infections caused by *S. aureus,* it is generally recommended that all isolates be assessed for this property. If the isolate proves tolerant, a second agent, such as an aminoglycoside or rifampin, may be added.

Determination of the appropriate duration of antimicrobial therapy is a key component in the management of patients with staphylococcal bacteremia. Of primary concern is the risk of occult endocarditis or metastatic infection if the treatment course is too short. As a rule, all patients with positive blood cultures for *S. aureus* should be treated for a minimum of 2 weeks. If the host has no cardiac valvular lesions, prosthetic joints, or other artificial devices and has intact immunity, the source of infection (e.g., central venous catheter) is rapidly removed; there is prompt response to therapy; the initial antimicrobial agent is active against the organism isolated; and there is no evidence of complications during the initial 2 weeks of therapy, then this short course may be considered (Table 31–2). All other patients should be treated for a full 4 to 6 weeks with antistaphylococcal antibiotics.

Even under the best of circumstances, short-course therapy (2 weeks) results in a relapse rate of approximately 5%.[25] On the basis of this information, some researchers have advocated that an additional 2-week course of oral therapy follow parenteral therapy in those treated for only 2 weeks.[25]

If the patient fails to meet all of the earlier-mentioned criteria, a full 4- to 6-week course of parenteral antibiotics is required.

Prevention of Nosocomial Infection

Control of nosocomial infections caused by *S. aureus* is a difficult undertaking. Indeed, in that it has remained an important pathogen throughout the antibiotic era, it appears

TABLE 31–2
CHARACTERISTICS OF PATIENTS WITH *STAPHYLOCOCCUS AUREUS* BACTEREMIA WHO QUALIFY FOR SHORT-COURSE THERAPY

1. The host has
    No valvular heart lesions
    No other obvious seedable sites
    Normal humoral and cellular defenses
2. The primary source of infection is obvious and easily managed.
3. There is prompt and complete response to initial therapy.
4. The causative *S. aureus* organism is fully sensitive to the antibiotics chosen initially.
5. There is no evidence of metastatic infectious complications during the 14-d period of therapy.

that at best we may be able to curtail the course of *S. aureus* infections. Several measures have been proposed in an effort to control outbreaks of *S. aureus* infection. The most important of these remains careful, repeated, and compulsive hand washing by hospital personnel. Hands should be washed with an approved bactericidal cleanser for at least 15 to 20 seconds. Although it may appear trivial, this measure has repeatedly been shown to be the single most important factor in controlling and preventing outbreaks.

Outbreaks of staphylococcal infection should be promptly recognized and efficiently evaluated by an infection control team. If a source is identified, measures should be taken to eradicate the focus. For instance, if a caregiver is the focus owing to asymptomatic carriage of the organism, measures can be taken to eradicate the carrier state. If an association is made with a particular form of instrumentation, appropriate measures should be taken. Some investigators support isolation of all patients with staphylococcal infections, particularly IRSA infections, with institution of barrier precautions. Patients thus identified may be discharged from the hospital as soon as is medically feasible and be appropriately identified so that they may receive isolation as indicated for subsequent hospital admissions. With strict adherence to these measures, many institutions have been able to keep their hospitals reasonably free from IRSA. However, under certain circumstances, this approach may not be feasible, as is the case in some institutions that serve areas where the organism is endemic.

Toxin-Mediated Staphylococcal Disease

Staphylococcal Scalded Skin Syndrome. Staphylococcal scalded skin syndrome is a disorder characterized by severe exfoliative dermatitis. It typically begins as a perioral erythematous eruption, and during 2 to 3 days, it spreads to include the entire body surface. What initially appears as a diffuse erythroderma, rapidly evolves into diffuse bullae formation and desquamation. Nikolsky's sign, the wrinkling and displacement of apparently normal skin with gentle pressure, is typical at this stage. Patients can be quite ill, akin to a burn patient, with nearly 100% of their total body surface involved. During the ensuing 3 to 5 days, desquamation is complete, and within 10 days of onset, replacement with new epidermis is generally complete.

S. aureus is typically isolated from cutaneous sites, although bacteremia is not typical. The illness is mediated by exfoliative toxin. Exfoliative toxin is composed of exfoliatins A and B, which are chromosome and plasmid mediated, respectively.[10] This toxin causes splitting of desmosomes within the stratum granulosum, resulting in desquamation. It can be neutralized by antibodies, perhaps explaining its preponderance in infants.

Therapy of staphylococcal scalded skin syndrome is primarily supportive and directed toward the prevention of dehydration and secondary infection.

Toxic Shock Syndrome. TSS is a multisystemic illness mediated in most instances by a staphylococcus-produced toxin called TSST-1. Although it was initially described in menstruating women using tampons, in 1989 greater than one fourth of cases were not menses related.[26] It is now recognized that TSS may be seen as a complication of any type of staphylococcal infection in which TSST-1 (or another as yet unidentified toxin) is produced. TSS has been described as a complication of soft tissue infections, infections of nasal packing, respiratory infections, and postoperative wound infections.[27] The latter may be quite deceiving, in that classic findings of postoperative wound infection, such as erythema, tenderness, and purulent discharge, are most often mild or lacking altogether.[28]

TABLE 31-3

DIAGNOSTIC CRITERIA FOR TOXIC SHOCK SYNDROME*

1. Temperature > 38.9°C
2. Systolic blood pressure < 90 mm Hg
3. Rash with subsequent desquamation, especially on palms and soles
4. Involvement of three or more of the following organ systems:
   Gastrointestinal: vomiting, profuse diarrhea
   Muscular: severe myalgias or greater than fivefold increase in creatine kinase level
   Mucous membranes (vagina, conjunctivae, or pharynx): frank hyperemia
   Renal insufficiency: blood urea nitrogen or creatinine level at least twice the upper limit of normal, with pyuria in the absence of urinary tract infection
   Liver: hepatitis, bilirubin, serum glutamic-oxaloacetic transaminase, and serum glutamic-pyruvic transaminase levels at least twice the upper limit of normal
   Blood: thrombocytopenia < 100,000/mm^3
   Central nervous system: disorientation without focal neurologic signs
5. Negative results of the serologic tests for Rocky Mountain spotted fever, leptospirosis, and measles

*TSS is present if three or more major criteria are met in the presence of desquamation, or five major criteria in its absence.

Whereas TSST-1–producing strains of *S. aureus* are isolated from 91 to 100% of menstrual isolates, only 40 to 64% of nonmenstrual isolates produce it.[29] Of note, finding TSST-1–producing strains of *S. aureus* in uncomplicated staphylococcal infections is not unusual. Most individuals infected with these strains produce protective antibody and do not have an illness suggestive of TSS.[30] However, in patients who lack protective antibody titers, TSS occurs at a higher rate (25% in one study).[30]

Findings in TSS include high fever, hypotension, diffuse erythroderma of the skin and mucous membranes, headache or confusion, and evidence of multiple-organ involvement (Table 31-3). This may be manifest as myalgias with elevated creatine kinase values, renal dysfunction, hepatic abnormalities, thrombocytopenia, cardiac abnormalities, nausea and vomiting, severe watery diarrhea, and electrolyte abnormalities such as hypocalcemia and hypophosphatemia. Later, desquamation, especially of the hands and feet, may occur.

Of note is the acute onset and rapidly progressive nature of this illness. It is not unusual for a previously healthy patient to progress to florid shock within a matter of hours. Hypotension is the result of decreased vasomotor tone in association with a rapid, nonhydrostatic leakage of high-protein fluid into the interstitium. The multiple-organ involvement observed in TSS is the result of the direct action of toxins and secondary mediators, as well as impaired tissue perfusion. In this regard, the clinical scenario may resemble that seen in sepsis of any cause.

Diagnosis of TSS is established with the combination of a high index of clinical suspicion and confirmation of staphylococcal infection in the appropriate clinical setting. TSS should be in the differential diagnosis of all septic syndromes associated with multiple-organ involvement.

Therapy of TSS is reasonably straightforward and primarily supportive. Early and aggressive fluid replacement is a key component of therapy. Pulmonary arterial catheters are often helpful in managing fluid resuscitation, as large volumes are frequently required, and patients may experience impaired myocardial contractility as a result of profound hypocalcemia and other factors. Of interest, this hypocalcemia, which may be due to excessive calcitonin secretion, is largely uncorrectable.[31] Fortunately, it has not been associated with cardiac arrhythmias. The source of staphylococci must be eradicated.

Antistaphylococcal therapy is primarily utilized to reduce the risk of recurrence. In untreated menses-associated disease, some patients have experienced as many as 6 to 12 recurrences.[32] There is no usual pattern to these recurrences, and several normal menses may occur between episodes. Administration of antistaphylococcal antibiotics and discontinuation of tampon use are often effective in reducing or eradicating recurrences. Fortunately, recurrences after nonmenstrual TSS are unusual.

Coagulase-Negative Staphylococci

Epidemiology

Coagulase-negative staphylococci (most often *S. epidermidis*) are currently the most commonly reported etiologic agents of nosocomial bacteremia, accounting for 27% of cases.[1] This is a sharp increase from the 10% value reported in 1980. The reason for this dramatic increase is not entirely clear but is most likely due to increased utilization of intravascular devices in concert with greater appreciation of the role of this organism as a nosocomial pathogen.

Those at greatest risk for bacteremia caused by *S. epidermidis* are patients with implanted foreign bodies, such as intravascular catheters, prosthetic heart valves, mechanical joints, transvenous cardiac pacemakers, and ventriculoperitoneal shunts. Also at risk are those with neutropenia, those receiving antibiotics or long-term ambulatory peritoneal dialysis, and neonates. Outside of these populations, bacteremia attributable to *S. epidermidis* is distinctly unusual.

Pathogenesis

Coagulase-negative staphylococci are ubiquitous colonizers of the skin. In the competent host, they are appropriately considered nonpathogenic. However, in the patient with any of the aforementioned risk factors, especially those with implanted foreign bodies, they are apt to cause serious infection.

As with *S. aureus*, *S. epidermidis* follows a sequential process of adherence, colonization, and infection. Foreign devices are key to the development of infection caused by *S. epidermidis*, and microbial adherence to these devices has received much attention. Nonspecific electrostatic and hydrophobic interactions are important in the initial attachment of *S. epidermidis* to foreign bodies.[33] Of note, many catheters and other prostheses most susceptible to infection are often produced from biopolymers, which have hydrophobic properties. Teflon-coated catheters, in that they are less amenable to bacterial adherence, seem to be less prone to infection.[34]

Clinical isolates often produce a viscous polysaccharide extracellular substance referred to as slime. Many investigators have suggested that this is an important virulence factor. Slime augments bacterial binding to the bioprosthesis and acts as a mechanical barrier to the host's defenses and antimicrobial penetration.[35]

Virulence factors not related to bacterial adherence have been less well studied. Nevertheless, there is evidence that coagulase-negative staphylococci owe at least part of their virulence to their ability to elaborate many of the exoproteins produced by *S. aureus*.[36] Toxins and enzymes such as hemolysins, cytotoxins, deoxyribonuclease, fibrinolysin, proteinase, and lipase-esterase have been identified.[36, 37] Their respective roles in the pathogenesis of coagulase-negative staphylococcal bacteremia remain to be determined.

Clinical Presentation

The most common clinical presentation of coagulase-negative staphylococcal bacteremia is low-grade fever in the absence of systemic toxicity. Thus, it is essential that blood cultures be obtained in patients who have unexplained fever and are at risk for infection attributable to this organism. In one study, coagulase-negative staphylococcal bacteremia after coronary arterial bypass grafting was associated with a 59% incidence of underlying wound infection.[38] Clinical evidence of a sternal wound infection would often be inapparent until several days after the positive blood culture was obtained. Similarly, infections originating from intravascular sites, long-term ambulatory peritoneal dialysis catheters, or ventriculoperitoneal shunts may be occult early on, with the exception of fever and bacteremia.

Coagulase-negative staphylococci are the most common cause of bacterial endocarditis of prosthetic valves and rarely may infect native valves as well. Prosthetic valve endocarditis has been divided into early- and late-onset endocarditis, depending on the timing of the clinical presentation in relationship to surgery. Traditionally, early-onset endocarditis occurs within 2 months of surgery. However, this has been challenged, as the typical manifestations of early-onset endocarditis may occur as long as 1 year postoperatively.[39, 40] Early-onset endocarditis is usually a rapid and fulminant illness, carrying a case fatality rate of greater than 50%. Coagulase-negative organisms are responsible for up to two thirds of these cases. It is believed that the etiologic agents are acquired in the hospital, most often intraoperatively. Late-onset endocarditis typically occurs longer than 1 year postoperatively. Coagulase-negative staphylococci are implicated in only one fourth of these cases. The course of late-onset prosthetic valve endocarditis is most typical of that observed in subacute endocarditis.

Neonates and patients who are neutropenic may experience spontaneous infection and bacteremia.[41] In neonates, impaired opsonic defenses are in part responsible for this finding. Apnea and feeding difficulties are the most common signs of sepsis in these patients.

The mortality associated with coagulase-negative staphylococcal bacteremia is quite high, with crude mortality ranging from 18 to 57%.[42] Nevertheless, in that it has traditionally been considered an organism of low virulence, its direct contribution to mortality has been questioned. That is because patients who acquire infection caused by this pathogen typically have severe underlying disease. However, one study indicated that patients with coagulase-negative staphylococcal bacteremia have an attributable mortality of 13.6%, with a risk ratio of dying of 1.8.[42] In addition, the average length of hospital stay in patients infected with this organism was 22.7% greater than that of matched controls.

Therapy

Therapy of coagulase-negative staphylococcal bacteremia is dependent on the severity of infection, the suspected anatomic site, the presence of a foreign body, and the in vitro susceptibility of the isolate.

Owing to the frequency of coagulase-negative staphylococci in occult infections and their high frequency as blood culture contaminants, it is often difficult to determine the validity of positive culture results. Certainly, patients with previously discussed risk factors must be seriously evaluated for infection when this organism is isolated from blood cultures. Features suggestive of true bacteremia include growth within 48 hours, multiple positive cultures within a short period, and growth in both aerobic and anaerobic bottles. Patients who are not septic or febrile, have no risk factors for acquisition of this organism, and have only a single positive blood culture may simply be carefully observed. Follow-up blood cultures should be obtained. Those with evidence of infection or risk factors and those with multiple positive blood cultures warrant therapy.

The recommended agent for empirical therapy of infections attributable to *S. epidermidis* is vancomycin, as intrinsically β-lactam–resistant isolates are common. Vancomycin susceptibility is near universal for coagulase-negative staphylococci, although resistant isolates of *Staphylococcus haemolyticus* have been reported.[43] For susceptible strains, semisynthetic penicillins or cephalosporins such as cefazolin and cefamandole are recommended. The management of catheter-associated bacteremia and prosthetic valve endocarditis are comprehensively discussed in Chapters 51 and 40, respectively.

ENTEROCOCCI

Enterococci have traditionally been classified within the Lancefield classification scheme as group D streptococci. Despite this, they have long been recognized as a unique clinical entity, primarily owing to their property of relative antibiotic resistance. However, soon after the edition of Bergey's Manual of Systematic Bacteriology[43a] was published in 1984, Schleifer and Kilpper-Balz suggested that *Enterococcus* species be placed within a unique genus on the basis of DNA and RNA homology studies.[44] This has generally been accepted within the scientific community.

The enterococcus is an important cause of community-acquired and nosocomial bacteremia, with an increase in frequency during the past several years. According to a report produced by the National Nosocomial Infection Study in 1984, it was responsible for 7.1% of nosocomial bacteremias,[45] and in a more recent report, it had increased to 8%.[1] Of all nosocomial infections, it is responsible for 12%, an increase from 11% in the 1984 report.[1] It is capable of causing a wide variety of infectious processes, including bacteremia with or without sepsis, endocarditis, and urinary tract infections. It is also commonly associated with intra-abdominal, pelvic, bone, and soft tissue infections.

Microbiology

A multitude of *Enterococcus* species have been described, including *E. faecalis*, *E. faecium*, *E. durans*, *E. avium*, *E. casseliflavus*, and *E. gallinarum*. However, *E. faecalis* is responsible for approximately 85% of human infections, with *E. faecium* being responsible for the majority of the remainder. Enterococci are gram-positive facultative anaerobes, which are particularly hardy organisms. They are capable of growing in hypertonic saline (6.5% sodium chloride), 40% bile, and 0.1% methylene blue. They are capable of surviving, and even proliferating, at extremes of both temperature and pH.

Epidemiology

Enterococcal organisms can be readily isolated as normal flora of various body sites, particularly the colon, but also the vagina, the urethral meatus, and the oral cavity.[46] In patients with wounds or decubitus ulcers, they are frequently identified, even in the absence of clinical infection. Enterococcal bacteremia has traditionally been thought to arise exclusively from the host's endogenous flora. In that bacteremia is frequently preceded by urinary tract instrumentation, gynecologic infections, and intra-abdominal sepsis, in most cases this contention is probably true. However, in a series of studies utilizing plasmid analysis for strain identi-

fication, the potential for nosocomial acquisition was confirmed.[47, 48] These studies were strongly suggestive that intrahospital person-to-person spread of enterococcus occurs, most likely via transient carriage on the hands of hospital personnel. In fact, interhospital transmission was also documented, most likely via the hands of hospital personnel who worked at more than one hospital. Outbreaks of enterococcal bacteremia have since been documented in neonatal intensive care units, further supporting the role of this organism as a nosocomial pathogen.

It is often helpful to separate enterococcal bacteremia on the basis of whether the infection was acquired in the community or in the hospital. Most importantly, community-acquired enterococcal bacteremia is highly associated with endocarditis. In one large review of enterococcal bacteremia, approximately one third of community-acquired cases had evidence of endocarditis.[49] This is in sharp contrast to the situation with hospital-acquired infection, in which endocarditis is a rare occurrence.[49] Other features commonly associated with endocarditis include previous genitourinary tract instrumentation or infection, recent pelvic inflammatory disease, postpartum endometritis, and postoperative pelvic infections. On the basis of these risk factors, it is not surprising that those populations most commonly acquiring endocarditis are elderly men and younger women of childbearing age. Patients who experience endocarditis most often have underlying valvular pathologic changes, although normal valves may become infected. Vegetations are invariably left sided.

Nosocomial infections are more likely than community-acquired infections to have an obvious extracardiac focus. Recognized sources of bacteremia in these patients include burn wounds, intra-abdominal or surgical wounds, the genitourinary or biliary systems, intravascular catheters, and rarely, decubitus ulcers.[49, 50] In that many of these sites are commonly infected with multiple pathogens, it is not surprising that the enterococcus is the most commonly cited gram-positive pathogen in polymicrobial bacteremia.[51] Those at greatest risk for nosocomial acquisition of infection are those who have spent a long time in the hospital, frequently in intensive care areas, having received previous antibiotics. Cephalosporins are often cited as predisposing agents, because they have no appreciable activity against enterococci.

Clinical Presentation

The presentation of enterococcal bacteremia is highly dependent on the clinical setting in which it occurs. For instance, enterococcal endocarditis, which is almost always encountered in community-acquired infection, most often presents in a fashion akin to subacute endocarditis attributable to viridans streptococci. Typical signs and symptoms include low-grade fever, weight loss, fatigue, and malaise, which may have been present for several months. A murmur is almost always present, and splenomegaly, petechiae, Osler's nodes, and splinter hemorrhages may occasionally be appreciated. Laboratory findings may include leukocytosis, an active urinary sediment, and a positive rheumatoid factor finding. Major embolic phenomena occur in approximately one third of patients, and blood cultures are positive more than 95% of the time.[49] Rarely, enterococcal endocarditis may be acute in onset, presenting with clinical sepsis and rapid progression of heart failure. Survival from enterococcal endocarditis, in patients receiving combination therapy with a β-lactam agent and an aminoglycoside, is approximately 90%.

Nosocomial enterococcal bacteremia typically occurs in the setting of a prolonged hospitalization, as described earlier. Its associated mortality is lower than that from community-

TABLE 31–4

REPRESENTATIVE MINIMAL INHIBITORY CONCENTRATIONS (μg/mL) FOR ROUTINE ENTEROCOCCAL ISOLATES

Antimicrobial Agent	E. faecalis MIC Range	E. faecalis MIC₉₀	E. faecium MIC Range	E. faecium MIC₉₀
Penicillin	1–2	2	8–32	32
Ampicillin	0.5–1	1	4–16	16
Mezlocillin	1–2	2	16–64	64
Piperacillin	2–4	4	8–128	128
Cefoperazone	8–32	32	>128	>128
Cefotaxime	<0.5–>128	>128	32–>128	>128
Imipenem	1–2	2	16–64	64
Vancomycin	1–4	2	0.5–2	2
Teicoplanin	0.12–0.5	0.5	0.25–1	0.5
Daptomycin	1–8	4	0.25–8	8
Ciprofloxacin	0.5–2	2	1–16	8

acquired infection, primarily owing to the virtual absence of endocarditis in these patients. One instance in which enterococcal bacteremia takes a more aggressive stance is in the setting of polymicrobial bacteremia, especially when gram-negative pathogens are involved. In this situation, mortality approaches 60%.[51]

Therapy

Enterococci present a multitude of therapeutic difficulties because of the infections they cause in conjunction with their ability to resist the bactericidal actions of most antibiotics. This has been most important for the therapy of endocarditis, an infection in which bactericidal action is highly desirable. Fortunately, other infections necessitating bactericidal activity, such as meningitis or neutropenia, are unusual manifestations of enterococcal infection.

Enterococci are intrinsically tolerant to all β-lactam antibiotics. Only a few penicillins and imipenem are capable of inhibiting bacterial growth at clinically achievable concentrations. This intrinsic tolerance is most marked in isolates of *E. faecium*, although it is seen in *E. faecalis* as well. The reason for this relative resistance to β-lactam agents is not antimicrobial degradation or impaired bacterial penetration, but rather a decreased affinity of enterococcal PBPs.[52] It is of historical interest that tolerance to β-lactams may actually be an acquired trait.[53] Investigators studying isolates of *E. faecalis* that had not been exposed to antibiotics, which had been collected from the Solomon Islands, found these strains to be quite sensitive to the lytic effects of penicillin. However, when exposed to pulses of penicillin, they rapidly acquired tolerance characteristics typical of clinical isolates encountered in practice (Table 31–4).

Despite the phenomenon of intrinsic tolerance, β-lactams, such as penicillin and ampicillin (see Table 31–1), play a central role in the therapy of enterococcal infections. Their bacteriostatic activity is adequate for the therapy of many infectious processes. In circumstances in which bactericidal therapy is desirable, the addition of an aminoglycoside (e.g., gentamicin and streptomycin) to a β-lactam agent most often yields a bactericidal combination. For those patients allergic to penicillins, vancomycin may be substituted. Vancomycin is also bacteriostatic for enterococcal organisms when used alone but has synergistic and bactericidal activity in combination with an aminoglycoside.

In addition to the phenomenon of intrinsic tolerance to β-lactam agents described earlier, a variety of other antimicrobial resistance mechanisms have become increasingly important. These include the production of β-lactamase, van-comycin resistance, and most importantly, high-level gentamicin resistance.

β-Lactamase production in isolates of *E. faecalis* was first discovered in 1983[54] and remains a rather unusual property. These enzymes render normally active β-lactams, such as penicillin, ampicillin, and piperacillin, inactive, although imipenem remains effective. From DNA hybridization techniques with a β-lactamase probe, it has been determined that the gene probably originated from *S. aureus* and has been transmitted via conjugation.[55] Fortunately, this problem can be easily overcome with the addition of β-lactamase inhibitors, such as sulbactam and clavulanic acid.

High-level resistance to the glycopeptides vancomycin and teicoplanin has been described in both *E. faecalis* and *E. faecium*. This is distinctly unusual for gram-positive isolates; the only other gram-positive organisms reported to be resistant to vancomycin have been *Leuconostoc* species, *Lactobacillus* species, *Pediococcus* species, and a rare strain of *S. haemolyticus*.[43, 56] It is plasmid mediated, inducable, transferable by conjugation, and associated with a new surface protein that remains to be fully characterized.[57]

Aminoglycoside activity against enterococcal species is predicated on their use in combination with a cell wall–active agent, which enhances intracellular uptake. Penicillin-streptomycin combinations were the first to be utilized clinically, leading to marked improvements in the therapeutic outcome of patients with enterococcal endocarditis. However, by the late 1970s, high-level resistance to streptomycin (MIC greater than 2000 μg/mL) became prevalent, rendering this agent ineffective. The mechanism of resistance was most often a streptomycin-adenylating enzyme,[58] but in some strains ribosomal resistance was reported.[59] *E. faecalis* was often resistant to streptomycin alone,[60] whereas a chromosomally mediated 6′-aminoglycoside–acetylating enzyme in *E. faecium* was also capable of inactivating kanamycin, tobramycin, netilmicin, and sisomicin.[60, 61] Some strains of *E. faecalis* and *E. faecium* also contained the plasmid-mediated enzyme 3′-phosphotransferase, which confers resistance to kanamycin and amikacin.[62] Fortunately, most of these strains remained highly sensitive to the effects of gentamicin, despite the loss of activity of other aminoglycosides. However, in 1979, strains resistant to high levels of gentamicin were first recognized[63] and are now highly prevalent in some centers.

High-level resistance to gentamicin relates to the presence of a plasmid-mediated 2′-phosphorylating enzyme that inactivates the drug.[65] This same enzyme exhibits 6′-acetylating activity, rendering kanamycin, tobramycin, netilmicin, and sisomicin ineffective. The majority of these isolates also demonstrate 3′-phosphotransferase and streptomycin-adenylating activity, yielding high-level resistance to streptomycin and other available aminoglycosides. In less than one third of isolates, the streptomycin-adenylating enzyme is absent, allowing streptomycin to remain active.[66] Thus, the presence of high-level gentamicin resistance frequently serves as a marker for complete aminoglycoside resistance and the unavailability of bactericidal therapy for these organisms.

In the absence of aminoglycoside activity, the best one can hope to achieve is adequate bacteriostatic activity. Concurrent use of two cell wall–active agents has been studied (e.g., ampicillin plus vancomycin), with the result being no better than that with either agent being used alone. The one caveat to this is the unusual circumstance in which certain strains of vancomycin-resistant enterococci may actually be primed to be more sensitive to penicillin by the concurrent use of vancomycin.[67] Although the efficacy of therapy for endocarditis is far superior with the use of an aminoglycoside plus a cell wall–active agent, cure has been achieved with single-agent therapy. Ampicillin or penicillin is the preferred agent. In the penicillin-allergic patient, vancomycin is a potential alternative.

A variety of other agents may be useful in therapy for enterococcal infections, including teicoplanin, daptomycin, and newer fluoroquinolones. Teicoplanin is a glycopeptide antibiotic similar to vancomycin, although it is not yet available in the United States. This agent appears to be two to four times more active than vancomycin against enterococci.[68] Daptomycin is a cyclic lipopeptide that is currently under investigation. It is active against enterococci, especially *E. faecalis*, and may actually have some bactericidal activity. The fluoroquinolones currently available (norfloxacin and ciprofloxacin) are not sufficiently active against enterococci to be considered effective alternatives for life-threatening infections, although some agents under investigation appear to be quite promising.

Prevention

Prevention of nosocomial transmission of enterococcal infections is of vital importance, especially with regard to isolates with a high level of gentamicin resistance, which may be exceedingly difficult to treat. Effective control measures are similar to those utilized for staphylococci or highly resistant gram-negative pathogens, including diligent hand washing, careful use of antibiotics, barrier precautions and cohorting of patients when appropriate, and efficient surveillance mechanisms.

STREPTOCOCCI

In the preantibiotic era, streptococci were extremely common causes of bacteremia and sepsis. This is no longer the case. In fact, in a National Nosocomial Infections Study, streptococcal species collectively accounted for only approximately 4% of all bacteremias.[1]

Of the Lancefield groups of streptococci, groups A, B, C, D, and G seem to be the most prevalent. *Streptococcus pneumoniae* is an important cause of community-acquired sepsis and is also discussed. As mentioned earlier, enterococcal species are no longer classified within the genus of streptococci and are discussed earlier. In that each group of streptococci has varying epidemiologic and clinical features, they are considered individually.

Group A Streptococci

Group A beta-hemolytic streptococci (e.g., *Streptococcus pyogenes*) are most commonly recognized as a frequent cause of pharyngitis and soft tissue infections. Although the incidence of septicemic events attributable to this organism has decreased in the antibiotic era, there has been an increased incidence of bacteremias in intravenous drug abusers and the suggestion that some strains may now be more virulent, resulting in a syndrome similar to staphylococcal TSS.

Epidemiology

The epidemiology of group A beta-hemolytic streptococci has been well studied. This organism is rather ubiquitous in the pediatric population, with school-aged children carrying it in their posterior pharynx as much as 30 to 40% of the time.[69] The cumulative annual incidence of carriage is at least 60 to 80%. This is in sharp contradistinction to the situation in adults, in whom only approximately 5% carry the organism, even with symptomatic infection.[70, 71] In addition to the pharyngeal carriage common to pediatric populations, colonization of the rectum, the vagina, or the skin

can be found under certain circumstances. These include transient skin carriage in patients with upper respiratory tract infections and in the setting of epidemic streptococcal impetigo.[72, 73]

Group A streptococcal bacteremia has been reported by some to occur most commonly in the fall and winter, but this has been disputed by others.[74] Those affected most often have significant underlying disease, such as chronic renal failure, alcohol or intravenous drug abuse, diabetes mellitus, connective tissue diseases, loss of cutaneous integrity, and malignancy, especially solid tumors.[75] Among pediatric patients, it may be seen in neonates during epidemics in nurseries, or in children with underlying diseases, as noted earlier. Rarely, group A beta-hemolytic streptococcal bacteremia may occur in otherwise healthy individuals. The source of bacteremia is most often the skin and the soft tissues, but it may rarely arise from primary infections of the lungs, the joints, or the pharynx.

Pathogenesis

A variety of virulence factors have been evaluated in group A beta-hemolytic streptococci. The lipid moiety of lipoteichoic acid, found on fimbriae, is surface structures that enable the organisms to adhere to epithelial cells.[76] There is considerable variability not only in the number and type of receptors on epithelial cells, but also in adherence determinants of certain strains. This may account for the clinical observation that some strains result primarily in pharyngeal infection, whereas others affect primarily cutaneous sources.[77]

The M protein is a surface protein that was first believed to be responsible for bacterial adherence to epithelial cells. It is now recognized that its true virulence trait is the result of its antiphagocytic properties. As a result of passive mechanical blockade of complement receptors, it helps inhibit opsonization. Another less important function of the M protein is its ability to protect the organism from infection attributable to bacteriophage, by masking phage receptors.

Hyaluronic acid production by streptococci also seems to play a role in survival and multiplication. It has an inhibitory effect on phagocytosis, although to a less pronounced degree than does the M protein.

Group A beta-hemolytic streptococci produce a variety of toxins that contribute to the development of clinical sepsis. Erythrogenic toxins, perhaps owing to a hypersensitivity mechanism, induce the rash of scarlet fever and may have other systemic effects akin to those of the lipopolysaccharide (endotoxin) moiety of gram-negative bacteria. These toxins, primarily pyrogenic exotoxin A, have also been implicated as possible mediators of the newly recognized toxic strep syndrome.[78] Streptolysins O and S lyse leukocytes, erythrocytes, and other cells and cellular components. The peptidoglycan component of the bacterial cell wall has many of the properties of endotoxin. Lipoteichoic acid is important in the adherence of group A streptococci to fibronectin on epithelial surfaces.[79] Enzymes such as hyaluronidase and streptokinase facilitate spread of infection by disrupting hyaluronic acid and fibrinous clots.

Clinical Presentation

Clinical bacteremia is heralded by the abrupt onset of spiking fevers and rigors, often associated with nonspecific gastrointestinal symptoms and mental status changes. Patients clinically appear to be toxic and have associated shock in 30 to 40% of cases.[80] Although the source is often obvious at presentation, at times it may not be discernible.

Different patient populations seem to have varying clinical

courses. For instance, although intravenous drug abusers may often have a septic clinical picture, mortality is extremely low. Some investigators reported a high incidence of endocarditis, a complication of group A streptococcal bacterial infection that is distinctly unusual in the antibiotic era, in intravenous drug abusers.[81] Elderly individuals often follow a rapidly progressive clinical course, with mortality rates approaching 50%. These patients, who often have significant underlying disease, have traditionally represented the majority of patients with this illness.

It has been suggested that the virulence of group A beta-hemolytic streptococci may be increasing, perhaps owing to an increased prevalence of strains producing pyrogenic exotoxin A. Previously healthy individuals have experienced a rapidly fatal illness manifested by sepsis, shock, and multiple organ system failure, in association with a diffuse erythroderma reminiscent of that caused by staphylococcal TSS. This illness has been termed the *toxic strep syndrome*.[82]

Therapy

As with any systemic infection, therapy combines supportive care with antimicrobial therapy. Group A beta-hemolytic streptococci remain uniformly sensitive to penicillin (see Table 31–1). For those with immunoglobulin E–mediated allergic reactions to penicillins, vancomycin is an alternative agent. Neither tolerance nor development of resistance during therapy has been documented with this organism.

Group B Streptococci

Group B streptococci (e.g., *Streptococcus agalactiae*) are well-recognized causes of neonatal and puerperal sepsis. These organisms also are responsible for bacteremic events in elderly and otherwise debilitated individuals. In one study of group B streptococcal bacteremia in a community teaching hospital, 61% of group B streptococcal bacteremias occurred in elderly patients.[83]

Group B streptococci are frequent inhabitants of the gastrointestinal and genitourinary tracts. Occasionally, it may be isolated from the pharynx of healthy individuals. Six different serotypes are currently recognized, including Ia, Ib/c, Ia/c, II, III, and IV. Among neonates who develop septicemia, strains I, II, and III are seen with equal frequency. Serotype III is the predominant form isolated from infants who go on to have delayed sepsis with meningitis.[84] This may be due to increased invasiveness and selective affinity for the meninges of this serotype.

Neonatal sepsis has been separated into two types depending on the timing of onset. Early-onset neonatal sepsis refers to that with an onset within 5 days of birth, although the mean onset is approximately 20 hours.[85] In these patients, the illness is generally the result of intrapartum transmission of the organism from mother to infant. Maternal obstetric complications are present in more than half of the cases, including prolonged labor and premature rupture of membranes. Early-onset disease is most often characterized by multisystem involvement, including bacteremia, pneumonia, and meningitis, and is associated with a high mortality. Late-onset disease generally occurs from 6 days to 3 months of life.[85] This variant has a lower mortality rate than does early-onset disease but also has a high incidence of meningitis.

The rate of asymptomatic vaginal carriage of group B streptococci in pregnant women has been estimated to be 25 to 35%; approximately 50% of babies born to these women become colonized during delivery.[86] Despite this, neonatal septicemia attributable to group B streptococci is a rather unusual event. It has been suggested that the mothers of children who experience serious group B streptococcal sep-

ticemia frequently lack neutralizing antibody to the serotype with which their children have become infected. Conversely, those neonates who do not have symptomatic infection generally have antibody titers to the serotype with which they are colonized.

The majority of adult infections caused by group B streptococci occur in postpartum women. It most commonly causes endometritis, with symptom onset generally within 48 hours of delivery. Patients who have undergone cesarean section are at greatest risk. Bacteremia and sepsis attributable to this infection are unusual, occurring in less than 2% of patients.[87]

In adults, bacteremia is most common in elderly, debilitated individuals. These patients typically have significant underlying illness, including malignancy, diabetes mellitus, diffuse atherosclerotic vascular disease, and chronic renal failure, or have been given corticosteroids or cytotoxic agents.[83, 88] The clinical onset of bacteremia is generally subacute in affected patients, and overt sepsis is rare. Nevertheless, mortality is exceedingly high, approaching 70% in one study.[83] Most patients die of their underlying illness rather than the bacteremia itself. Endocarditis has also been reported, frequently in individuals who have underlying valvular heart disease.[83]

Group B streptococci are uniformly susceptible to penicillins in vitro. However, MICs for this organism are 4- to 10-fold higher than those observed with group A streptococci.[89] Furthermore, especially in neonates, the inoculum load may be exceedingly high, approaching 10^7 to 10^8 organisms per milliliter in the cerebrospinal fluid.[90] Therefore, large initial doses of ampicillin or penicillin are recommended. In the case of the neonate, it is recommended that an aminoglycoside be part of the initial regimen in cases of bacteremia and meningitis until a confirmed microbiologic diagnosis is achieved. Therapy may then be completed with penicillin alone. For patients allergic to penicillin, vancomycin is a reasonable alternative. Other effective agents include most first- and second-generation cephalosporins, ceftriaxone and cefotaxime, and imipenem-cilastatin.

Group C Streptococci

Group C streptococci are unusual causes of bacteremia, accounting for only 0.1% of positive blood cultures. There are four group C *Streptococcus* species: *S. equisimilis, S. zooepidemicus, S. equi,* and *S. dysgalactiae.* Most human infections are caused by *S. equisimilis* and *S. zooepidemicus.* Infection attributable to *S. zooepidemicus* can be traced to animal exposure in most instances, a feature shared with an occasional case of bacteremia caused by *S. equisimilis.* This characteristic is unique to group C streptococci among the beta-hemolytic streptococci.[91]

Infections are generally community acquired, as is the case with group A and group G streptococcal infections. Approximately 75% of patients have significant underlying disease, including malignancy, cardiovascular disease, diabetes mellitus, immunosuppression, and chronic renal or hepatic disease.[91] The portals of entry for infection include primarily the skin and the upper respiratory and gastrointestinal tracts.

The clinical presentation is not unlike that of sepsis caused by other pathogens, with fever, chills, and prostration commonly being seen. Endocarditis is present in almost 30% of patients and has an associated mortality of 33%.[91] Major embolic events in these patients are common, occurring in 37.5% of individuals. The overall mortality of group C streptococcal bacteremia in the largest series of patients reported was greater than 25%.[91]

Group C streptococci are generally exquisitely sensitive to

penicillin G, with MICs of less than 0.1 μg/mL in most instances. Alternative agents include most cephalosporins and vancomycin. Some investigators have alleged that tolerance is an issue with this organism, with one study reporting 16 of 17 isolates to be tolerant to penicillin.[92] Others have not confirmed this finding.[93] Until this issue is further clarified, it is reasonable to administer penicillin plus an aminoglycoside for life-threatening infections, such as endocarditis and meningitis.

Group D Streptococci

The group D streptococci have traditionally been separated into enterococcal and nonenterococcal species on the basis of the former's ability to grow in broth with 6.5% sodium chloride. This has been a significant distinction for clinical reasons as well. The enterococcal streptococci have a much greater role in human infection and necessitate different management strategies with regard to antimicrobial therapy. However, on the basis of studies of DNA homology and certain other features, the enterococci have been reclassified as a separate genus. Therefore, only *Streptococcus bovis* and *Streptococcus equinus* remain within the group D classification of streptococcal organisms.

S. bovis and *S. equinus* are present in the stool of 5 to 10% of healthy adults. *S. bovis* is an unusual cause of bacteremia, occurring perhaps 25% as frequently as *E. faecalis* in neonatal septicemia and much less so in adults. If *S. bovis* is isolated from the blood of an adult, colonic pathologic changes, including carcinoma, must be strongly suspected.[94]

As opposed to *Enterococcus* species, *S. bovis* and *S. equinus* are extremely sensitive to relatively low concentrations of penicillin, as well as cephalothin and clindamycin.[95] Rarely, these organisms are relatively resistant to these agents, so in vitro testing should be performed on all clinical isolates.

Group G Streptococci

Group G streptococci are unusual causes of bacteremia, accounting for less than 1% of bacteremic episodes in most studies. These organisms have also been reported as a cause of endocarditis, meningitis, pneumonia, arthritis, pharyngitis, and soft tissue infections.[96] They are occasionally included in the normal flora of the vagina, the pharynx, the gastrointestinal tract, and the skin. In patients with bacteremia caused by this organism, the skin is the implicated source in 70 to 80% of cases, whereas the source of the remainder frequently remains unknown. The majority of patients with group G streptococcal bacteremia have severe underlying disease, including malignancy, alcoholism, diabetes mellitus, and connective tissue disease, or have undergone prolonged corticosteroid administration.[97–99] Dermatologic disease and/or local stasis also place a patient at increased risk.

The reported frequency of endocarditis attributable to this pathogen is somewhat controversial. Venezio and colleagues reported a 47% incidence of endocarditis,[99] whereas other investigators reported an incidence of 0 to 25%.[96–98] Both native and prosthetic valves may be involved with approximately equal frequency. The incidence of metastatic suppurative infections caused by bacteremia with this organism is low, although arthritis, meningitis, peritonitis, and seeding of foreign bodies have been reported.

The vast majority of group G streptococci are exquisitely sensitive to the bactericidal action of penicillin, although some investigators reported varying degrees of in vitro tolerance.[100] Additionally, with large inocula, killing caused by penicillin may be impaired despite apparently low MICs.[98] On the basis of this information, it has been proposed that combined β-lactam–aminoglycoside therapy be utilized in patients with severe infections such as sepsis, endocarditis, and perhaps, septic arthritis. Those who fail to respond favorably to therapy should be evaluated for the possibility of a sequestered focus of infection. Otherwise, it must be recognized that, because this infection most typically affects those with severe underlying disease and an immunocompromised state, impaired clearance of infection is not unexpected.

The Species *Streptococcus pneumoniae*

S. pneumoniae remains the most frequently identified cause of community-acquired bacterial pneumonia and the second most frequent cause of bacterial meningitis in the United States. Bacteremia caused by this organism is an important problem in that it is associated with 20 to 30% of each of these infections.

There are currently 84 recognized serotypes of *S. pneumoniae*, classified according to capsular types. However, the majority of clinical infections are due to fewer than 20 of these serotypes. The pneumococcus is a frequent colonizer of the oropharynx, being present in 5 to 70% of individuals.[101] Healthy adults carry the organism only 5 to 10% of the time, whereas in closed populations, such as orphanages and schools, the carriage rate may be significantly higher.

Certain populations are at particular risk for increased morbidity and mortality from pneumococcal disease. Those who have undergone splenectomy for any reason and those who are functionally asplenic as a result of sickle cell anemia are less capable of clearing the organism and of generating appropriate neutralizing antibodies.[102] Additionally, those with sickle cell disease also appear to have impaired function of the alternative complement pathway.[103] Owing to these defects, pneumococcal sepsis often results in a rapidly progressive and fatal course in these patients. Similarly, individuals with congenital agammaglobulinemia or hematologic malignancies such as multiple myeloma and acute or chronic lymphocytic leukemia are at increased risk because of impaired primary antibody responses.[104] Patients infected with human immunodeficiency virus contract pneumococcal bacteremia 100 times more frequently than would be expected, probably as a result of their impaired de novo antibody response.[105] Also at risk are the elderly and otherwise debilitated, as well as those with disorders that result in loss of respiratory mucosal integrity. This is particularly evident in cases of bacterial superinfection of influenza virus–induced pulmonary disease, in which the pneumococcus is the most common etiologic agent, followed closely by *S. aureus*.

Pulmonary infections generally begin with aspiration of upper respiratory tract secretions that contain the organism; it is not primarily an airborne disease. Therefore, any factor that promotes increased aspiration of oropharyngeal contents, such as altered consciousness, decreased cough reflexes, and impaired ciliary motion, may increase the risk of pneumococcal pneumonia. Owing to this mode of infection, respiratory isolation is not required in the hospital setting, except for the unusual situation of epidemic pneumococcal infection.

A variety of pathogenesis factors are active in the development of pneumococcal disease. As noted earlier, pneumococci are coated with a polysaccharide capsule, which is effective in impairing phagocytosis and forms the basis of its serotyping scheme. It has been well demonstrated that encapsulated organisms are capable of inducing disease, whereas nonencapsulated organisms are not. A variety of toxins are produced by pneumococci, although their contribution to infection is unknown. These include pneumolysin, which results in hemolysis and dermatotoxicity in experimental animals, as well as beta-hemolysis on sheep blood agar. Neuraminidase is thought to play a role in the tissue-invasive properties of the organism. Purpura-producing principle is capable of inducing purpuric lesions in experimental animals, although its role in human disease remains to be determined.

Pneumococci are capable of producing a large variety of infections, such as pneumonia, otitis media, sinusitis, meningitis, endocarditis, arthritis, and spontaneous bacterial peritonitis. With regard to bacteremia and sepsis, pneumonia, meningitis, and endocarditis are the most significant infections. As noted earlier, there is a high association of bacteremia with pneumonia and meningitis. Of course, bacteremia is the sine qua non of endocarditis.

Clinical features depend on the source of the primary infection and the immune status of the host. The onset of the illness is often abrupt, associated with shaking chills, disseminated intravascular coagulation, and generalized systemic toxicity. Specific features of pneumonia and meningitis are dealt with in other chapters. Of note, although pneumococci were associated with 10% of cases of endocarditis in the preantibiotic era, this is no longer the case; they now account for less than 1% of all cases. However, this disease tends to follow a highly aggressive course with frequent destruction of heart valves, often necessitating valve replacement.

Penicillin G is the antimicrobial agent of choice in the therapy of pneumococcal bacteremia (see Table 31–1). In septic patients, or those with meningitis, endocarditis, or septic arthritis, 20 million U/d is recommended. Patients who have an uncomplicated pneumonia require substantially less. However, as opposed to the beta-hemolytic streptococci, which are almost uniformly sensitive to penicillin, moderate and highly resistant pneumococci have been isolated throughout the world.[106] As with intrinsically resistant staphylococci, penicillin-resistant pneumococci tend to be endemic to certain areas. For instance, in 1987, Istre and coworkers reported a 12.2% incidence of resistant pneumococci in infected patients residing in Oklahoma City.[107] In most areas, penicillin-resistant pneumococci are not yet a significant problem. However, this problem mandates antimicrobial susceptibility testing of all significant clinical isolates.

The mechanism of pneumococcal resistance to penicillin is not related to the production of β-lactamase. Hence, this resistance is generally applicable to all β-lactam agents and is not reversed by the addition of a β-lactamase inhibitor. The mechanism is similar to that observed in intrinsically resistant staphylococci and enterococci, via alterations of PBPs.[108] Fortunately, these pneumococci remain susceptible to vancomycin, which is also a reasonable therapeutic choice for those with significant penicillin allergy.

Pneumococcal vaccination was first commercially licensed in the United States in 1978, and consisted of 14 different capsular polysaccharides, which accounted for approximately 80% of all bacteremic pneumococcal infections.[109] This formulation was revised in 1983 to include 23 different capsular polysaccharides, now covering approximately 90% of bacteremic infections.[109] This vaccine is highly effective when given to immunocompetent individuals older than 2 years of age. However, individuals with significant immune dysfunction often may not develop a protective immune response. The Centers for Disease Control does not recommend routine revaccination for those who have previously received the 14-valent vaccine.[109a] However, those at risk for rapid decline of antibody titer (i.e., patients with chronic renal failure, patients with nephrotic syndrome, and organ transplant recipients) or for fatal pneumococcal infections (i.e., asplenic patients) should be strongly considered for revaccination every 6 years.

DIPHTHEROIDS

Diphtheroids are common contaminants of blood cultures in that they are part of the normal skin flora. However, a few species warrant careful consideration as pathogens, and under certain circumstances, they may result in the septic syndrome. Species associated with the septic syndrome include primarily *Corynebacterium pseudodiphtheriticum*, *Rhodococcus equi*, and group JK corynebacteria, although a host of other *Corynebacterium* species have been rarely implicated in human blood stream infections.

C. pseudodiphtheriticum is a component of the normal oral flora of humans. This organism has been reported in several instances of endocarditis, primarily involving prosthetic heart valves.[110] Antimicrobial susceptibility is unpredictable, so in vitro antibiotic susceptibility testing is essential in patients infected with this organism.

R. equi infections most typically occur in patients with animal exposure and conditions associated with defects in cell-mediated immunity, such as lymphoreticular tumors, human immunodeficiency virus infection, and corticosteroid administration.[111–113] The most frequently implicated site of infection is the lung; infection is acquired via the aerosolized route. Clinical findings include systemic toxicity in association with a necrotizing pneumonia, which may form upper lobe nodules or cavitary lesions. In this clinical scenario, it may easily be confused with tuberculosis. *R. equi* may also result in brain abscesses and cutaneous lesions suggestive of nocardiosis. Active antibiotics include vancomycin, chloramphenicol, erythromycin, and aminoglycosides. Surgery in conjunction with prolonged medical therapy may be required to optimize clinical response. Mortality is approximately 30%.

Corynebacteria group JK are a cause of sepsis primarily in patients with underlying neoplasia.[114] Other risk factors include neutropenia, prolonged hospitalization and administration of antibiotics, use of central venous catheters, and previous cardiac surgery.[115, 116] In addition to causing primary bacteremia, this organism may be responsible for endocarditis, pneumonia, and infection of ventriculoperitoneal shunts. It is a frequent colonizer of the skin of hospitalized patients and is thought by some investigators to be transmitted from person to person within the hospital setting, akin to the situation with *S. aureus* and enterococci.[117] Corynebacteria group JK are typically resistant to most antibiotics, although they are uniformly sensitive to vancomycin.[118]

LISTERIA MONOCYTOGENES

Listeria monocytogenes is a gram-positive aerobic rod that has been associated with a variety of clinical syndromes, including sepsis, meningitis, granulomatosis infantiseptica, and peripartum infections. Infections caused by *L. monocytogenes* occur in several defined risk groups and situations, including (1) peripartum women and neonates; (2) immunosuppressed individuals, particularly those with defects in cell-mediated immunity; (3) epidemics related to food-borne outbreaks in which immunocompetent hosts are commonly affected; and (4) immunologically normal individuals with no known risk factors.

Infections occurring during pregnancy may occur at any time, although they most typically occur during the final trimester. These patients typically have a nonspecific febrile illness that may subside spontaneously.[119] Subsequently, blood cultures reveal *L. monocytogenes*. In unfortunate circumstances, it may precipitate preterm labor with resultant fetal wastage or infection. Transplacental transmission of infection to the fetus results in an illness referred to as granulomatosis infantiseptica.[119] This illness is characterized by disseminated abscesses and granulomas involving the lungs, the brain, the liver, the spleen, the kidneys, and other sources. Papular lesions may appear on the skin. Mortality in some studies has approached 100%, although it appears that with prompt initiation of appropriate antimicrobial therapy some children survive.

Sepsis of unknown origin is a common presentation of listeriosis. In this instance, most infected adults are immunocompromised with ineffective function of cell-mediated immunity.[120] However, it is not unusual for sepsis to occur in a previously immunocompetent host.[121] Those at highest risk appear to be patients with leukemia or lymphoma and transplant recipients. Also at risk are the elderly and neonates. Neonates who develop *L. monocytogenes* bacteremia most likely acquire their infection during or after birth rather than in utero. Patients infected with the human immunodeficiency virus are at surprisingly low risk for listeriosis, suggesting that CD4+ lymphocytes may not play a significant role in immunity for this organism. Those human immunodeficiency virus–infected patients who have listeriosis frequently have concomitant colonic pathologic changes, supporting this mode of entry.[122]

Meningoencephalitis caused by *L. monocytogenes* occurs in the same patient populations as does sepsis.[123] These patients, in that they are frequently otherwise immunocompromised, do not display typical findings of meningitis. The clinical onset is commonly subacute, and a mild fever or personality change may be the lone clinical finding. Meningitis is a frequent complication of *L. monocytogenes* bacteremia, prompting some investigators to suggest that lumbar puncture be performed in all these patients.

The therapeutic agents of choice in listerial infection are ampicillin or penicillin (see Table 31–1). However, trimethoprim-sulfamethoxazole is active and also achieves excellent central nervous system penetration.[124] For central nervous system infections, the addition of intrathecal and systemic gentamicin may be considered in an attempt to achieve synergistic activity. Other agents that are active in vitro include cephalothin, tetracyclines, erythromycin, and chloramphenicol, although clinical experience with these agents is limited. The appropriate duration of therapy is not well established, but as recurrences occur with 2-week courses of therapy, it is recommended that a 3- to 6-week course be utilized.

References

1. Schaberg DR, Culver DH, Gaynes RP: Major trends in the microbial etiology of nosocomial infection. Am J Med. 91(suppl 3B):72S, 1991.
2. Hovelius B, Mardh PA, Bygren P: Urinary tract infections caused by *Staphylococcus saprophyticus*. J Urol 122:645, 1979.
3. Sheagren JN: *Staphylococcus aureus*. The persistent pathogen. N Engl J Med 310:1368, 1437, 1984.
4. Hughes GB, Chidi CC, Macon WL IV: Staphylococci in community-acquired infections: Increased resistance to penicillin. Ann Surg 183:355, 1976.
5. Jevons MP: Celbenin-resistant staphylococci (letter). Br Med J 1:124, 1961.
6. Barrett FF, McGehee RF Jr, Finland M: Methicillin-resistant *Staphylococcus aureus* at Boston City Hospital: Bacteriologic and epidemiologic observations. N Engl J Med 279:441, 1968.
7. Fekety FR Jr: The epidemiology and prevention of staphylococcal infection. Medicine 43:593, 1964.
8. Godfrey ME, Smith IM: Hospital hazards of staphylococcal sepsis. JAMA 166:1197, 1958.
9. Mandell GL, Vest TK: Killing of intraleukocytic *Staphylococcus aureus* by rifampin: In vitro and in vivo studies. J Infect Dis 125:486, 1972.
10. Rogolsky M: Nonenteric toxins of *Staphylococcus aureus*. Microbiol Rev 43:320, 1979.
11. Arvidson SO: Extracellular enzymes from *Staphylococcus aureus*.: In: Easmon CSF, Admal C (eds): Staphylococci and Staphylococcal Infections, Volume 2. New York, Academic Press, p 745, 1983.
12. Peterson PK, Quie PG: Bacterial surface components and the pathogenesis of infectious diseases. Annu Rev Med 32:29, 1981.
13. Sheagren JN: Inflammation induced by *Staphylococcus aureus*. In: Gallin JI, Goldstein IM, Snyderman R (eds): Inflammation: Basic Principles and Clinical Correlates. New York, Raven Press, p 329, 840, 1988.
14. Parsonnet J: Mediators in the pathogenesis of toxic shock syndrome. Rev Infect Dis 11 (suppl 1):S263, 1989.
15. Milunski MR, Gallis HA, Fuekerson WJ: *Staphylococcus aureus* septicemia mimicking fulminant Rocky Mountain spotted fever. Am J Med 83:801, 1987.
16. Murray HW, Tuazon CU, Sheagren JN: Staphylococcal septicemia and disseminated intravascular coagulation. Arch Intern Med 137:844, 1977.
17. Skinner D, Keefer CS: Significance of bacteremia caused by *Staphylococcus aureus*. A study of one hundred and twenty-two cases and a review of the literature concerned with experimental infection in animals. Arch Intern Med 68:851, 1941.
18. Cluff LE, Reynolds RC, Page DL, et al: Staphylococcal bacteremia and altered host resistance. Ann Intern Med 69:859, 1968.
19. Musher DM, McKenzie SO: Infections due to *Staphylococcus aureus*. Medicine 56:383, 1977.
20. Nolan CM, Beaty HN: *Staphylococcus aureus* bacteremia. Current clinical patterns. Am J Med 60:495, 1976.
21. Walters S, Griffith GE: Resolution of fever in *Staphylococcus aureus* septicemia—Retrospective analysis by means of Cusum plot. J Infect 12:57, 1986.
22. Hackbarth CJ, Chambers HF: Methicillin-resistant staphylococci: Genetics and mechanisms of resistance. Antimicrob Agents Chemother 33:991, 1989.
23. Sabath LD: Mechanisms of resistance to beta-lactam antibiotics in strains of *Staphylococcus aureus*. Ann Intern Med 97:339, 1982.
24. Best GK, Best NH, Kovac AV: Evidence for participation of autolysins in bactericidal action of oxacillin on *Staphylococcus aureus*. Antimicrob Agents Chemother 6:825, 1974.
25. Rahal JJ: Preventing second-generation complications due to *Staphylococcus aureus*. Arch Intern Med 149:503, 1989.
26. Reduced incidence of menstrual toxic-shock syndrome—United States, 1980–1990. MMWR 39:421, 1990.
27. Reingold AL, Shands KN, Dan BB, et al: Toxic-shock syndrome not associated with menstruation. Lancet 1:1, 1982.
28. Bartlet P, Reingold AL, Graham DR: Toxic shock syndrome associated with surgical wound infections. JAMA 247:1448, 1982.
29. Broome CV. Epidemiology of toxic shock syndrome in the United States: Overview. Rev Infect Dis 11(suppl 1):S14, 1989.
30. Jacobson JA, Kasworm E, Daly JA: Risk of developing toxic shock syndrome associated with toxic shock syndrome toxin 1 following nongenital staphylococcal infection. Rev Infect Dis 11(Suppl 1):S8, 1989.
31. Chapman-Winokur R, Ospina L, Lauter C: Hypocalcemia of toxic shock syndrome (abstract). Rev Infect Dis 11(suppl 1):S329, 1989.
32. Davis JP, Osterholm MT, Helms CM, et al: Tristate toxic-shock syndrome study. II. Clinical and laboratory findings. J Infect Dis 145:441, 1982.
33. Hogt AH, Dankert J, deVries JA, et al: Adhesion of coagulase-negative staphylococci to biomaterials. J Gen Microbiol 129:2959, 1983.
34. Sheth NK, Franson TR, Rose HD, et al: Colonization of bacteria on polyvinyl chloride and Teflon intravascular catheters in hospitalized patients. J Clin Microbiol 18:1061, 1983.
35. Peters G, Gray ED, Regelmann, et al: Effect of extracellular slime-substance (ESS) on the human cellular immune response (abstract 764). In: Program and Abstracts of the 23rd Interscience Conference on Antimicrobial Agents and Chemotherapy. Washington, DC, American Society for Microbiology, p 225, 1983.
36. Pfaller MA, Herwaldt LA: Laboratory, clinical, and epidemiologic aspects of coagulase-negative staphylococci. Clin Microbiol Rev 1:281, 1988.
37. Gummel CG: Virulence characteristics of *Staphylococcus epidermidis*. J Med Microbiol 22:287, 1986.
38. Kohman LJ, Coleman MJ, Parker FB Jr: Bacteremia and sternal infection after coronary artery bypass grafting. Ann Thorac Surg 49:454, 1990.
39. Calderwood SB, Swinski LA, Waterhause CM, et al: Risk factors for the development of prosthetic valve endocarditis. Circulation 82:31, 1985.
40. Karchmer AW, Archer GL, Dismukes WE: *Staphylococcus epidermidis* prosthetic valve endocarditis: Microbiological and clinical observations as a guide to therapy. Ann Intern Med 98:447, 1983.
41. Wade JC, Schimpff SC, Newman KA, et al: *Staphylococcus epidermidis*: An increasing cause of infection in patients with granulocytopenia. Ann Intern Med 97:503, 1982.
42. Martin MA, Pfaller MA, Wenzel RP: Coagulase-negative staphylococcal bacteremia. Mortality and hospital stay. Ann Intern Med 110:9, 1989.
43. Schwalbe RS, Stappleton JT, Gilligan PH: Emergence of vancomycin resistance in coagulase-negative staphylococci. N Engl J Med 316:927, 1987.
43a. Krieg NR, Holt JG (eds): Bergey's Manual of Systematic Bacteriology. Volume 1. Baltimore, Williams & Wilkins, 1984.
44. Schleifer KH, Kilpper-Balz R: Transfer of *Streptococcus faecalis* and *Streptococcus faecium* to the genus *Enterococcus* nom. rev. as *Enterococcus faecalis* comb. nov. and *Enterococcus faecium* comb. nov. Int J Sys Bacteriol 34:31, 1984.
45. Centers for Disease Control: Nosocomial infectious surveillance. MMWR CDC Surveill Summ 35:17, 1984.

46. Chenoweth C, Schaberg DR: The epidemiology of enterococci. Eur J Clin Microbiol 9:80, 1990.
47. Zervos MJ, Mikesell TS, Schaberg DR: Heterogeneity of plasmids determining high-level resistance in clinical isolates of *Streptococcus faecalis*. Antimicrob Agents Chemother 30:78, 1986.
48. Zervos MJ, Dembinski S, Mikesell T, et al: High-level resistance to gentamicin in *Streptococcus faecalis;* Risk factors and evidence for exogenous acquisition of infection. J Infect Dis 153:1075, 1986.
49. Maki DG, Agger WA. Enterococcal bacteremia: Clinical features, the risk of endocarditis, and management. Medicine 67:248, 1988.
50. Shlaes DM, Levy J: Enterococcal bacteremia without endocarditis. Arch Intern Med 141:578, 1981.
51. Reuben AG, Musher DM, Broucke I, et al: Polymicrobial bacteremia: Clinical and microbiologic patterns. Rev Infect Dis 11:161, 1989.
52. Fontana R, Canepari P, Lleo MM, Satta G: Mechanisms of resistance of enterococci to beta-lactam antibiotics. Eur J Clin Microbiol 9:103, 1990.
53. Eliopoulos GM, Eliopoulos CT: Therapy of enterococcal infections. Eur J Clin Microbiol 9:118, 1990.
54. Murray BE, Mederski-Samoraj B: Transferable beta-lactamase. A new mechanism for in vitro penicillin resistance in *Streptococcus faecalis*. J Clin Invest 72:1168, 1983.
55. Murray BE, Mederski-Samoraj B, Foster SK, et al: In vitro studies of plasmid-mediated penicillinase from *Streptococcus faecalis* suggest a staphylococcal origin. J Clin Invest 77:289, 1986.
56. Colman G, Efstration A: Vancomycin-resistant leuconostocs, lactobacilli, and now pediococci. J Hosp Infect 10:1, 1987.
57. Nicas TI, Wu CYE, Hobbs JN Jr: Characterization of vancomycin resistance in *Enterococcus faecium* and *Enterococcus faecalis*. Antimicrob Agents Chemother 33:1121, 1989.
58. Krogstad DJ, Korfhagen TR, Moellering RC, et al: Aminoglycoside-inactivating enzymes in clinical isolates of *Streptococcus faecalis*. An explanation for resistance to antibiotic synergism. J Clin Invest 62:480, 1978.
59. Eliopoulos GM, Farber BF, Murray BE, et al: Ribosomal resistance of clinical enterococcal isolates to streptomycin. Antimicrob Agents Chemother 25:398, 1984.
60. Moellering RC, Jorzeniowski OM, Sande MA, et al: Species-specific resistance to antimicrobial synergism in *Streptococcus faecium* and *Streptococcus faecalis*. J Infect Dis 140:203, 1979.
61. Wennersten CB, Moellering RC: Mechanisms of resistance to penicillin and aminoglycoside synergism in *Streptococcus faecium*. In: Nelson JD, Grassi C (eds): Current Chemotherapy and Infectious Disease, Volume I. Washington DC, American Society for Microbiology, p 710, 1980.
62. Combes T, Carlier C, Courvalin P: Aminoglycoside-modifying enzyme content of a multiply resitant strain of *Streptococcus faecalis* subspecies *zymogenes*. J Antimicrob Chemother 11:41, 1983.
63. Horodniceanu T, Boubvueleret L, El-Solh N, et al: High-level, plasmid-borne resistance to gentamicin in *Streptococcus faecalis* subspecies *zymogenes*. Antimicrob Agents Chemother 16:686, 1979.
64. Zervos MJ, Kauffman CA, Therasse PM, et al: Nosocomial infection by gentamicin-resistant *Streptococcus faecalis*. An epidemiologic study. Ann Intern Med 106:687, 1987.
65. Courvalin P, Carlier C, Collatz E: Plasmid-mediated resistance to aminocyclitol antibiotics in group D enterococci. J Bacteriol 143:541, 1980.
66. Nachamkin I, Axelrod P, Talbot GH, et al: Multiply high-level-aminoglycoside-resistant enterococci isolated from patients in a university hospital. J Clin Microbiol 26:1287, 1988.
67. Gutmann L, Al-Obeid S, Billot-Klein D: Vancomycin (Van) resistance and synergy between van and penicillin (Pen) involve an inducible carboxypeptidase (CDPase) in Van-resistant enterococci (abstract). In: 30th Interscience Conference on Antimicrobial Agents and Chemotherapy, Atlanta, GA, October 21–24, 1990.
68. Greenwood D: Microbiological properties of teicoplanin. J Antimicrob Chemother 21(suppl A):1, 1988.
69. Peter G, Smith AL: Group A streptococcal infections of the skin and pharynx. N Engl J Med 297:311, 365, 1977.
70. Commission for Acute Respiratory Diseases: The role of Lancefield groups of beta-hemolytic streptococci in respiratory infections. N Engl J Med 236:157, 1947.
71. Walsh BT, Brookheim WW, Johnson RC, et al: Recognition of streptococcal pharyngitis in adults. Arch Intern Med 135;493, 1975.
72. Ferrieri P, Dajani AS, Wannamaker LW, et al: Natural history of impetigo. I. Site sequence of acquisition and familial patterns of spread of cutaneous streptococci. J Clin Invest 51:2851, 1972.
73. Colebrook L, Maxted WR, Johns AM: The presence of haemolytic and other streptococci on human skin. J Pathol Bacteriol 4:5521, 1935.
74. Bibler MR, Rouan GW: Cryptogenic group A streptococcal bacteremia: Experience at an urban general hospital and review of the literature. Rev Infect Dis 8:941, 1986.
75. Duma RJ, Weinberg AN, Medrek TF, et al: Streptococcal infections: A bacteriologic and clinical study of streptococcal bacteremia. Medicine 48:87, 1969.
76. Ellen RP, Gibbons RJ: M protein–associated adherence of *Streptococcus pyogenes* to epithelial surfaces: Prerequisite for virulence. Infect Immun 5:826, 1972.
77. Alkan M, Ofek I, Beachey EH: Adherence of pharyngeal and skin strains of group A streptococci to human skin and oral epithelial cells. Infect Immun 18:555, 1977.

78. Stevens DL, Tanner MH, Winship J, et al: Severe group A streptococcal infections associated with a toxic shock–like syndrome and scarlet fever toxin A. N Engl J Med 321:1, 1989.
79. Simpson WA, Courtney HS, Ofek I: Interactions of fibronectin with streptococci: The role of fibronectin as a receptor for *Streptococcus pyogenes*. Rev Infect Dis 9(suppl 4):351, 1987.
80. Ispahani P, Donald FE, Aveline AJD: *Streptococcus pyogenes* bacteremia: An old enemy subdued, but not defeated. J Infect 16:37, 1988.
81. Borg HL, Kish MA, Kauffman CA, et al: Group A streptococcal bacteremia in intravenous drug abusers. Am J Med 78:569, 1985.
82. Cone LA, Woodard DR, Schlievert PM: Clinical and bacteriologic observations of a toxic shock–like syndrome due to *Streptococcus pyogenes*. N Engl J Med 317:146, 1987.
83. Gallagher PG, Watanakunakorn C: Group B streptococcal bacteremia in a community teaching hospital. Am J Med 78:795, 1985.
84. Baker CJ, Barrett FF: Group B streptococcal infection in infants: The importance of various serotypes. JAMA 230:1158, 1974.
85. Baker CJ: Group B streptococcal infections. Adv Intern Med 25:475, 1980.
86. Yow MD, Leeds LJ, Thompson PK, et al: The natural history of group B streptococcal colonization in the pregnant woman and her offspring. I. Colonization studies. Am J Obstet Gynecol 137:34, 1980.
87. Duff P: Pathophysiology and management of postcesarean endomyometritis. Obstet Gynecol 67:269, 1986.
88. Verghese A, Mireault K, Arbeit RD: Group B streptococcal bacteremia in men. Rev Infect Dis 8:912, 1986.
89. Baker CN, Thornsberry C, Facklam RR: Synergistic killing kinetics, and antimicrobial susceptibility of group A and B streptococci. Antimicrob Agents Chemother 19:716, 1981.
90. Feldman WE: Concentrations of bacteria in cerebrospinal fluid of patients with bacterial meningitis. J Pediatr 88:549, 1976.
91. Bradley SF, Gordon JJ, Baumgartner DD, et al: Group C streptococcal bacteremia: Analysis of 87 cases. Rev Infect Dis. 13:270, 1991.
92. Portnoy D, Prentis J, Richards GK: Penicillin tolerance in human isolates of group C streptococci. Antimicrob Agents Chemother 20:235, 1981.
93. Rolston KV, LeFrock JL, Schell RF: Activity of nine antimicrobial agents against Lancefield group C and G streptococci. Antimicrob Agents Chemother 22:930, 1982.
94. Klein RS, Picco RA, Calalano MT: Association of *Streptococcus bovis* with carcinoma of the colon. N Engl J Med 297:800, 1977.
95. Moellering RC Jr, Watson BK, Kunz LJ: Endocarditis due to group D streptococci. Am J Med 57:239, 1974.
96. Vartian C, Lerner PI, Schlaes DM, et al: Infections due to Lancefield group G streptococci. Medicine 64:75, 1985.
97. Auckenthaler R, Hermans PE, Washington JA: Group G streptococcal bacteremia: Clinical study and review of the literature. Rev Infect Dis 5:196, 1983.
98. Lam K, Bayer AS: Serious infections due to group G streptococci. Am J Med 75:561, 1983.
99. Venezio FR, Westenfelder GO, Cook FV, et al: Infective endocarditis in a community hospital. Arch Intern Med 142:789, 1982.
100. Noble JT, Tyburski MB, Berman M, et al: Antibiotic tolerance in group G streptococci. Lancet 2:982, 1980.
101. Hendley JO, Sande MA, Stewart PM, et al: Spread of *Streptococcus pneumoniae* in families. I. Carriage rates and distribution of types. J Infect Dis 132:55, 1975.
102. Bohnsack JF, Brown EJ: The role of the spleen in resistance to infection. Annu Rev Med 37:49, 1986.
103. Zarkowsky HS, Gallagher MS, Gill FM, et al: Bacteremia in sickle hemoglobinopathies. J Pediatr 109:579, 1986.
104. Chou MY, Brown AE, Blevins A, et al: Severe pneumococcal infection in patients with neoplastic disease. Cancer 51:1546, 1983.
105. Redd SC, Rutherford GW III, Sande MA: The role of human immunodeficiency virus in pneumococcal bacteremia in San Francisco residents. J Infect Dis 162:1012, 1990.
106. Applebaum PC: World-wide development of antibiotic resistance in pneumococci. Eur J Clin Microbiol 6:367, 1987.
107. Istre GR, Tarpay M, Anderson M, et al: Invasive disease due to *Streptococcus pneumoniae* in an area with a high rate of relative penicillin resistance. J Infect Dis 156:732, 1987.
108. Jacobs MR, Koornhof HJ, Robins-Browne RM, et al: Emergence of multiply resistant pneumococci. N Engl J Med 299:735, 1978.
109. Bolan G, Broome CV, Facklam RR, et al: Pneumococcal vaccine efficacy in selected populations in the United States. Ann Intern Med 104:1, 1986.
109a. Centers for Disease Control: Update on adult immunization. Recommendations of the Immunization Practices Advisory Committee (ACIP). MMWR 40:42, 1991.
110. Lipsky BA, Goldberger AC, Tompkins LS, et al: Infections caused by non-diphtheria corynebacteria. Rev Infect Dis 4:1220, 1982.
111. MacGregor IH, Samuelson WM, Sane DC, et al: Opportunistic lung infection caused by *Rhodococcus (Corynebacterium) equi*. Radiology 160:83, 1986.
112. Samies JH, Hathaway BN, Echols RM, et al: Lung abscess due to *Corynebacterium equi*. Am J Med 80:685, 1986.
113. Weingarter JS, Huang DY, Jackman JD Jr: *Rhodococcus equi* pneumonia—An unusual early manifestation of the acquired immunodeficiency syndrome (AIDS). Chest 94:195, 1988.

114. Pearson TA, Braine HG, Rathbun HK: *Corynebacterium* sepsis in oncology patients. JAMA 238:1737, 1977.
115. Young VM, Meyers WF, Moody MR, et al: The emergence of coryneform bacteria as a cause of nosocomial infections in compromised hosts. Am J Med 70:646, 1981.
116. Riebel W, Frantz N, Adelstein D, et al: Corynebacterium JK: A cause of nosocomial device-related infection. Rev Infect Dis 8:42, 1986.
117. Kerry-Williams SM, Noble WC: Plasmids in group JK coryneform bacteria isolated in a single hospital. J Hyg (Lond) 97:255, 1986.
118. Gill VJ, Manning C, Lamson M, et al: Antibiotic-resistant group JK bacteria in hospitals. J Clin Microbiol 13:472, 1981.
119. Bejsen-Moller J: Human listeriosis: Diagnostic, epidemiological and clinical studies. Acta Pathol Microbiol Scand 229(suppl):1, 1972.
120. Simpson JF, Leddy JP, Hare JD: Listeriosis complicating lymphoma: A report of four cases and interpretive review of pathogenetic factors. Am J Med 43:39, 1967.
121. Cielsielski CA, Hightower AW, Parsons SK, et al: Listeriosis in the United States: 1980–1982. Arch Intern Med 148:1416, 1988.
122. Real FX, Gold JW, Krown SE, et al: *Listeria monocytogenes* bacteremia in the acquired immunodeficiency syndrome. Ann Intern Med 101:883, 1984.
123. Lavetter A, Leedom JM, Mathies AW, et al: Meningitis due to *Listeria monocytogenes*. A review of 25 cases. N Engl J Med 285:585, 1971.
124. Spitzer PG, Hammer AM, Karchmer AW: Treatment of *Listeria monocytogenes* infection with trimethoprim-sulfamethoxazole: Case report and review of the literature. Rev Infect Dis 8:427, 1986.

CHAPTER 32

Tuberculosis and Other Mycobacterial Infections

Laurel C. Preheim

Increasing numbers of patients who require intensive care for any reason have concurrent mycobacterial infection. After decades of decline, numbers of new cases of tuberculosis have increased in recent years. Nontuberculous mycobacteria, once thought harmless, are now recognized as formidable pathogens in patients who have compromised local or systemic host defenses. In many instances, mycobacterial infections themselves precipitate the need for intensive care. Although usually slowly progressive, mycobacterial infections (especially tuberculosis) can be acute or evolve rapidly into life-threatening disease involving virtually any organ system.

Mycobacteria are acid- and alcohol-fast, aerobic, non–spore-forming, nonmotile, slender, rod-shaped organisms. The major distinguishing features among different species of mycobacteria include nutritional and temperature requirements, growth rates, pigments, and range of pathogenicity in experimental animals.[1] Nineteen mycobacterial species are associated with human disease, classically producing slowly developing, destructive granulomas. This chapter confines itself to the species responsible for tuberculosis and the other nontuberculous (or atypical) mycobacterial infections.

TUBERCULOSIS

Pathophysiology

Tuberculosis is a necrotizing infection caused by two species of mycobacteria, *Mycobacterium tuberculosis* and *Myco-*

bacterium bovis. With control of bovine tuberculosis, *M. bovis* has become a rare cause of human infection in the United States. Nearly all *M. tuberculosis* infections are acquired by inhalation of droplet nuclei containing tubercle bacilli. In most cases, this entails repeated or prolonged contact with a person who has cavitary disease and whose sputum contains many tubercle bacilli. However, coughing once or talking for 5 minutes can produce 3000 infectious droplet nuclei.[2]

The initial infection is usually localized to the well-ventilated lower two thirds of the lungs. Tubercle bacilli are ingested by phagocytes. Infected macrophages transport organisms to hilar and mediastinal lymph nodes. In nonimmune individuals, the infection spreads from there to the blood stream. This silent dissemination can establish distant, dormant foci in virtually any organ. Upper lobe pulmonary disease (especially within apical posterior segments) is the most common manifestation of secondary, or reactivation, tuberculosis. Tubercle bacilli continue to multiply in the lung as well as in extrapulmonary foci until their growth is limited by an immune response. Disease may progress directly to involve the lung apices or other organs, or infection may be reactivated after decades of latency.

Specific immunity develops within several weeks of the primary infection and involves a series of interactions among macrophages, T lymphocytes, and B lymphocytes. At this stage, the tuberculin skin test result becomes positive and pulmonary infiltrates occur. These changes are due to activation of macrophages and tissue hypersensitivity. In the lung and other tissues, especially the hilar lymph nodes, the bacilli are contained within small granulomas. These tubercles may heal with fibrosis, or they can undergo central necrosis. The enlarging lesion has a cheese-like consistency and is termed caseous necrosis. A Ghon complex represents the combination of tubercles in the lung and caseation in lymph nodes.

Epidemiology

In the United States, the number of new cases per 100,000 persons had dropped steadily from 100 in 1930 to 9 in 1984. In 1986, the trend reversed, with an increase to 9.4 new cases per 100,000 persons. In 1989, 23,495 tuberculosis cases were reported (9.5 per 100,000 U.S. population), a 4.7% increase from 1988 (Fig. 32–1). Twice as many cases occurred in males as in females. Case rates varied geographically (Fig. 32–2) and by population groups (Fig. 32–3). Compared with non-Hispanic whites, minority groups had higher rates of infection that peaked in early adulthood rather than in old age [3] (Fig. 32–4).

Epidemiologic studies have identified other growing segments of the United States population that are at increased risk for tuberculosis.[4] These include persons with acquired immunodeficiency syndrome (AIDS),[5, 6] the elderly,[6, 7] and the homeless.[8] Immigrants and refugees from underdeveloped countries are another reservoir.[6] Currently in the United States, an estimated 10 million persons are infected with the tubercle bacillus. Worldwide, an estimated 10 million new cases occur annually. Thus, despite renewed efforts to eradicate the disease, the survival of tuberculosis appears ensured well into the 21st century.

Pulmonary Tuberculosis

Pathophysiology

Primary tuberculosis, the initial pulmonary infection of a nonimmune person, has classically been a disease of children. It is occurring with increased frequency, however, in the growing U.S. population of nonimmune adults. Most indi-

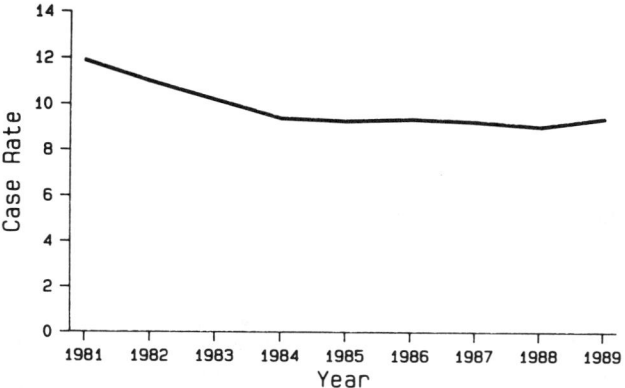

Rate per 100,000 population.

Figure 32–1. Tuberculosis case rates, United States, 1981 to 1989. (From Centers for Disease Control: Summary of notifiable diseases, United States, 1989. MMWR 38:43, 1989.)

viduals remain asymptomatic. Self-limited nonspecific symptoms and low-grade fever may occur in approximately 4 weeks. Rarely, erythema nodosum can be seen. Occasionally, the initial pneumonia progresses directly to cavitary pulmonary disease. Massive hematogenous dissemination is uncommon but most likely to occur in recently infected young children. Approximately 5 to 10% of adults go on to have clinical tuberculosis. Pneumonitis may occur in any part of the lung. Unlike children, however, adults rarely have marked hilar adenopathy. In the elderly, new tuberculosis in tuberculin-negative individuals may occur as nonspecific, unresolving pneumonitis involving the lower or middle lobes or the anterior segments of the upper lobes, similar to the clinical picture of primary infection of childhood.[9]

Chronic, or reactivation, pulmonary tuberculosis commonly follows a period of latency that can last longer than 60 years. It classically begins as a patch of pneumonitis in the subapical posterior segment of an upper lobe. Occasionally, it appears in the apical portion of a lower lobe. With disease progression, the lesion evolves into an area of caseous necrosis, granulation tissue, and fibrosis. Cavitation occurs when the caseous center liquefies and drains into the bronchial tree. At this point, tubercle bacilli are readily spread

by coughing. As mycobacteria are aerosolized, they are also inhaled and distributed throughout the lung, a process termed *bronchogenic spread*. The organisms thrive within cavities where they may multiply to numbers of 10^9 to 10^{11}. Acquired immunity or therapy may arrest the disease before cavity formation. However, viable organisms are retained in granulomas surrounded by fibrous tissue. These lesions may be reactivated later if the patient's local or systemic defenses are impaired by surgery or disease. Individuals with untreated cavitary disease are highly contagious and generally experience slow but gradual progression of signs and symptoms.

Clinical Features

Most individuals remain asymptomatic early in the disease. Many cases are detected serendipitously through a routine chest roentgenogram or during the examination of elderly patients with persistent bronchitis or presumed pneumonia. Nonspecific symptoms gradually evolve, including malaise, fatigue, anorexia, weight loss, and afternoon fevers. Night sweats, when patients defervesce and perspire enough to soak their bedclothes, are common as the disease progresses. Cough is frequent, generally producing mucopurulent sputum, which may become blood tinged. Massive hemoptysis is rare but can occur if an advancing cavity erodes into a pulmonary artery (Rasmussen's aneurysm). Occasionally, the course of tuberculosis can mimic that of bacterial pneumonia with a relatively sudden onset of fever, productive cough, or pleuritic pain. Acute respiratory failure, an uncommon complication, may necessitate intensive care.[10] Patients may have clinical and radiologic features of adult respiratory distress syndrome.[11, 12] Affected patients usually require ventilatory assistance, and disseminated intravascular coagulation may develop. Mortality rates are high despite antituberculous and steroid therapy.

Diagnosis

Radiographic Studies. The most common abnormality seen on chest roentgenogram is a multinodular, cavitary infiltrate in the apical or subapical posterior areas of the upper lobes. The superior segment of a lower lobe may also be involved. Bronchogenic spread of tubercle bacilli pro-

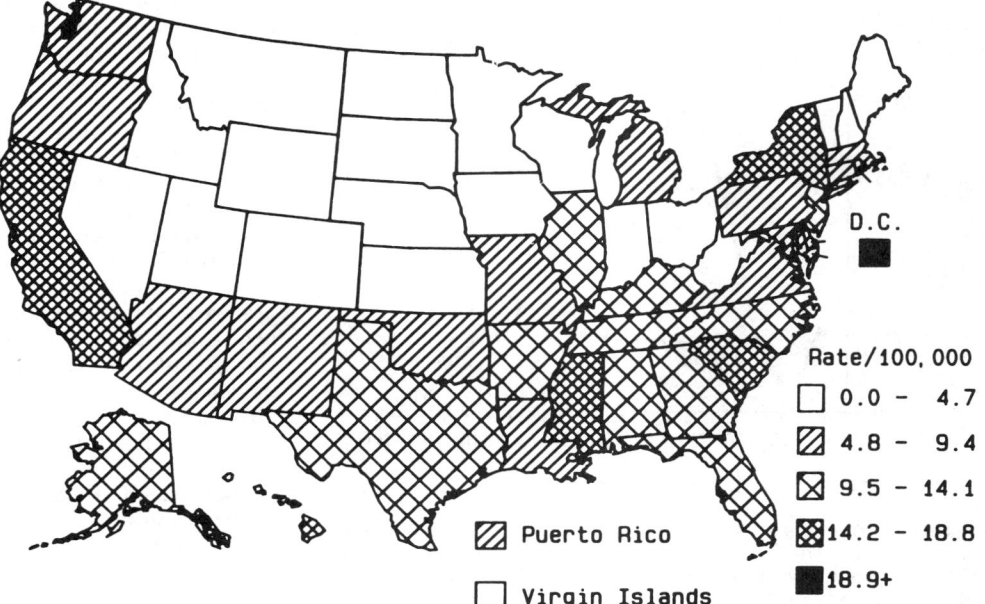

Figure 32–2. Tuberculosis rates by state, United States, 1989. (From Centers for Disease Control: Summary of notifiable diseases, United States, 1989. MMWR 38:43, 1989.)

Rate/100,000

□ 0.0 – 4.7
▨ 4.8 – 9.4
⊠ 9.5 – 14.1
▩ 14.2 – 18.8
■ 18.9+

▨ Puerto Rico

□ Virgin Islands

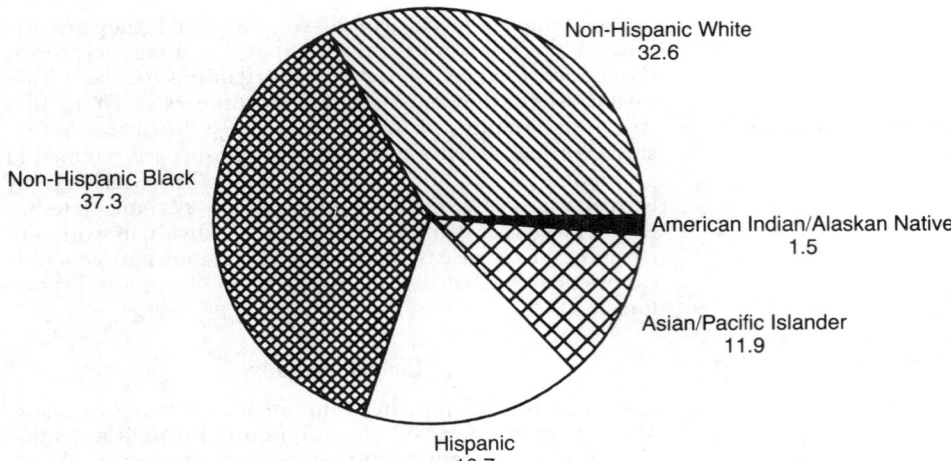

Figure 32–3. Percentage of tuberculosis cases by race and ethnicity, United States, 1989. (From Centers for Disease Control: Summary of notifiable diseases, United States, 1989. MMWR 38:43, 1989.)

duces multiple, discrete fluffy infiltrates. Pleural effusions may be present. Hilar adenopathy may be prominent in children but is often absent in adults. Isolated tuberculosis in the lower lung fields occurs in 1 to 18% of patients and is often mistaken for viral or bacterial pneumonia.[13, 14] Findings more common in tuberculosis involving lower lung fields include cavities larger than 3 cm, pleural effusion, hilar adenopathy, and confluent consolidations.[15] Apical-lordotic views and specialized techniques such as computed tomography and magnetic resonance imaging may help detect or define pulmonary lesions.

Tuberculin Skin Test. Delayed cutaneous skin reactivity to tuberculin, a protein fraction of tubercle bacilli, develops 2 to 10 weeks after the initial infection. The American Thoracic Society and Centers for Disease Control revised their guidelines for the interpretation of Mantoux's tests.[16] A reaction with induration of 5 mm or greater is considered positive in the following:

1. Persons with human immunodeficiency virus (HIV) infection or persons in groups at special risk for HIV infection
2. Persons who have had recent close contact with infectious tuberculosis cases

3. Persons who have chest roentgenograms consistent with old healed tuberculosis

A reaction of 10 mm or greater is considered positive in persons who do not meet these criteria but who have other risk factors for tuberculosis. These include

1. Foreign-born persons from high-prevalence countries in Asia, Africa, and Latin America
2. Intravenous drug users
3. Medically underserved low-income populations, including high-risk racial and ethnic minority groups
4. Residents of long-term care facilities (e.g., nursing homes, correctional facilities, and mental institutions)
5. Persons with medical conditions reported to increase the risk of tuberculosis, such as silicosis, gastrectomy, jejunoileal bypass, body weight of 10% or more below ideal values, chronic renal failure, diabetes mellitus, high-dose corticosteroid and other immunosuppressive therapy, leukemia, lymphoma, and other malignancies
6. Persons belonging to other high-risk populations as defined by individual community or institutional circumstances.

A reaction of 15 mm or greater is classified as positive in all other persons.[16]

False-negative reactions occur in up to 20% of persons with known tuberculosis on first testing. False-negative reactions may be due to severe illness or to immunosuppressive infections, diseases, or drugs. Cutaneous delayed hypersensitivity to purified protein derivative antigen may weaken with time. Applying a second tuberculin skin test 1 week after the first test can enhance dormant hypersensitivity and yield a true-positive reaction. This booster effect is usually a recall of reactivity established by distant prior infection rather than a new conversion caused by recent exposure. False-positive test results are due to infection with nontuberculous mycobacteria.

Microbiologic Studies. The diagnosis of tuberculosis depends on the isolation of *M. tuberculosis* from clinical specimens. Sputum smears reveal acid-fast bacilli in 50 to 80% of patients with pulmonary tuberculosis. For patients who have difficulty producing sputum, inhalation of aerosolized hypertonic saline may stimulate a productive cough. This procedure may induce uncontrolled coughing and should be performed using a hood or other air control device. Gastric aspirates of about 50 mL obtained after overnight fast are suitable for studies in patients unable to produce sputum. Fiberoptic bronchoscopy with transbronchial biopsy,[17] bronchoalveolar lavage, bronchial washings, and post-

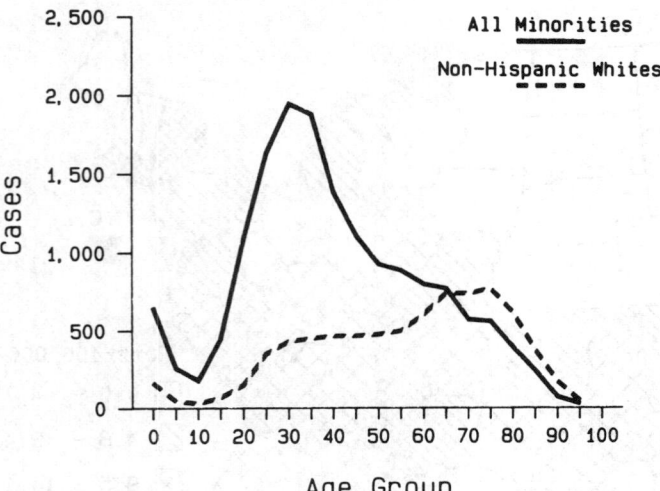

Figure 32–4. Frequency distribution of tuberculosis cases by age, race, and ethnicity, United States, 1989. (From Centers for Disease Control: Summary of notifiable diseases, United States, 1989. MMWR 38:43, 1989.)

TABLE 32–1
TUBERCULOSIS THERAPY FOR ADULTS AND CHILDREN

Drug	Dosage Forms	Daily Dose Adults	Daily Dose Children	Maximal Daily Dose*	Major Adverse Reactions
Isoniazid	Tablets: 100 mg, 300 mg Syrup: 50 mg/5 mL Vials: 1 g	5 mg/kg† PO or IM	10–20 mg/kg† PO or IM	300 mg	↑ hepatic enzymes, hepatitis, peripheral neuropathy, hypersensivity
Rifampin	Capsules: 150 mg, 300 mg Syrup: made from capsules, 10 mg/mL Vials: 600 mg	10 mg/kg PO or IV	10–20 mg/kg PO or IV	600 mg	Orange discoloration of urine and secretions; nausea, vomiting, hepatitis, fever, purpura (rare)
Pyrazinamide	Tablets: 500 mg	15–30 mg/kg PO	15–30 mg/kg PO	2 g	Hepatotoxicity, hyperuricemia, arthralgias, rash, gastrointestinal upset
Ethambutol	Tablets: 100 mg, 400 mg	15–25 mg/kg‡ PO	15–25 mg/kg‡ PO	2.5 g	Optic neuritis (↓ red-green color discrimination, ↓ visual acuity), rash
Streptomycin	Vials: 1 g, 4 g	15 mg/kg§ IM	20–40 mg/kg IM	1 g§	Ototoxicity (vestibular, acoustic), nephrotoxicity

*For both children and adults.
†Give pyridoxine 25–50 mg/d to prevent peripheral neuropathy.
‡Risk of optic neuritis is higher for doses greater than 15 mg/kg.
§In persons older than 60 years of age, limit daily dose to 10 mg/kg with a maximal dose of 750 mg.

bronchoscopy sputum smears[18] may help establish the diagnosis when sputum is unobtainable or unrevealing. Pleural biopsy specimens obtained for culture and histologic studies have a high diagnostic yield in patients with tuberculous pleural effusions.

Diagnostic Advances. Radiometric culture systems have increased the speed of recovery, identification, and susceptibility testing of *M. tuberculosis* from smear-positive and smear-negative clinical specimens. Utilizing a ^{14}C-labeled palmitic acid mycobacterial substrate, the BACTEC system rapidly grows (average, 9 days), identifies (5 days), and tests the antimicrobial susceptibility (5 days) of *M. tuberculosis* from smear-positive specimens.[19]

Enzyme-linked immunosorbent assays (ELISAs) show promise for the serodiagnosis of tuberculosis.[20] ELISA can detect antibodies against *M. tuberculosis* in bronchial washings[21] and mycobacterial antigen in BACTEC bottles.[22]

Genetic probes specific for the mycobacteria that cause tuberculosis as well as for nontuberculous mycobacterial species are available. These probes can speed detection and identification of pathogenic mycobacteria in culture[23] and may ultimately prove useful when applied to clinical specimens as well.

Polymerase chain reaction dramatically enhances the sensitivity of detection of microbe-specific DNA sequences. Polymerase chain reaction has been used to detect and identify species of mycobacterial isolates from cultures[24] and clinical specimens.[25, 26] Future refinements of polymerase chain reaction techniques will likely revolutionize existing approaches to the diagnosis of mycobacterial infections.

Treatment

The current treatment recommendations[27] are based on two fundamental principles: (1) any regimen must contain multiple drugs to which the organisms are susceptible and (2) therapy must continue for a sufficient time. Bactericidal agents are preferred, and at least two new drugs should be included in any regimen used in cases of treatment failure. Three first-line agents (isoniazid [INH], rifampin, streptomycin [STM]) can be given parenterally if gastrointestinal absorption of drugs is in doubt. Several agents have impor-

tant interactions with other drugs commonly used for patients who require intensive care.

First-Line Drugs. Table 32–1 summarizes dosage information and major adverse reactions for first-line antituberculous agents.

Isoniazid. INH is bactericidal against both intracellular and extracellular organisms. It is well absorbed from the gastrointestinal tract but also can be given parenterally.[28] INH penetrates well into all body fluids and cavities, and concentrations approximate those achieved in serum. It is acetylated and oxidized in the liver and excreted by the kidneys.

Hepatitis is the major toxic effect. The risk of hepatitis increases with age to 65 years and is reported as 0% for those aged 20 years or younger, 0.3% at 20 to 34 years of age, 1.2% at 35 to 49 years of age, and 2.3% at 50 to 64 years of age.[29] INH interference with pyridoxine metabolism can result in peripheral neuropathy. Pyridoxine supplement of 25 to 50 mg/d should be given to persons with diabetes, uremia, alcoholism, malnutrition, pregnancy, or seizure disorders. INH inhibits the metabolism of phenytoin, carbamazepine, anticoagulants, benzodiazepines, and vitamin D.[30] When INH and phenytoin are given concomitantly, the serum level of phenytoin should be monitored.

Rifampin. Rifampin is bactericidal against both intracellular and extracellular organisms. Like INH, it is well absorbed from the gastrointestinal tract, with peak serum concentrations occurring 1 to 2 hours after administration. A parenteral form is available. Rifampin penetrates well into tissues and cells, and therapeutic concentrations are obtained in cerebrospinal fluid (CSF) when the meninges are inflamed. Rifampin is generally well tolerated. Gastrointestinal upset is the most common adverse reaction. Infrequent reactions include skin eruptions, hepatitis, and thrombocytopenia. Intermittent therapy with doses larger than 10 mg/kg may cause hypersensitivity reactions associated with an influenza-like syndrome, thrombocytopenia, hemolytic anemia, and acute renal failure.

Rifampin is a potent inducer of the hepatic microsomal system and may accelerate clearance of drugs metabolized by the liver.[31, 32] Consequently, rifampin may decrease the efficacy of a number of drugs used to treat patients who are acutely ill (Table 32–2). For each of these drugs, caution is

---

TABLE 32–2

DRUGS WITH REDUCED EFFICACY DURING RIFAMPIN THERAPY

Anticoagulants (oral)	Digitoxin
Contraceptives (oral)	Digoxin
Theophylline	Beta-blockers
Glucocorticoids	Verapamil
Cyclosporine	Quinidine
Chloramphenicol	Phenytoin
Ketoconazole	Methadone
Sulfonylureas	

---

advised when starting or discontinuing rifampin therapy. Whenever possible, serum levels should be obtained to help guide appropriate therapeutic dosing of drugs during concomitant rifampin therapy.[32] The excretion of rifampin into urine, tears, sweat, and other body fluids colors them orange and can permanently stain soft contact lenses.

Pyrazinamide. Pyrazinamide (PZA) is bactericidal in an acid environment and kills extracellular and intracellular organisms. It is well absorbed from the gut, and peak serum levels occur approximately 2 hours after ingestion. Liver injury, an important adverse reaction, is uncommon. With usual daily doses, PZA does not increase risks of hepatotoxicity when used with INH and rifampin during the initial 2 months of treatment.[33] Hyperuricemia also occurs, but acute clinical gout is rare.

Ethambutol. Ethambutol (EMB) is bacteriostatic at conventional doses. Gastrointestinal absorption is excellent, and peak levels occur 2 hours after ingestion. EMB is excreted mainly in the urine and accumulates in persons with renal insufficiency. Adverse reactions with EMB are infrequent. Optic neuritis is the most common and serious adverse effect. It occurs in less than 1% of patients at daily doses of 15 mg/kg, increasing to approximately 3% at 30 mg/kg/d. The risk is greater in patients with renal failure. Symptoms include red-green color blindness, blurred vision, and central scotomata followed by decreased visual acuity. EMB should be used with caution in children too young to allow accurate assessment of visual acuity and red-green color discrimination.

Streptomycin. STM has bactericidal activity in an extracellular alkaline environment. Poorly absorbed from the gut, it must be given parenterally. Excretion is almost entirely renal, so dosage reductions and extreme caution are required in patients with renal insufficiency. Tissue penetration is good, but CSF penetration occurs only with inflamed meninges. Ototoxicity is the most common and serious adverse effect. Vertigo is more common than hearing loss, and both are potentiated by concomitant use of other ototoxic drugs. Renal toxicity may be increased in patients who have coexisting renal insufficiency or are receiving other nephrotoxic agents. The risks of ototoxicity and nephrotoxicity are related both to cumulative dose and to peak serum concentrations.

Initial Treatment Regimens. In the past decade, the recommended course of therapy has been reduced from 18 to 24 months to a minimum of 6 months.[27] The initial phase of a 6-month regimen must consist of at least a 2-month period of daily INH, rifampin, and PZA administration. EMB should be added when INH resistance is suspected. The next phase consists of INH and rifampin given daily or twice weekly for 4 months. Nine-month regimens using INH and rifampin are equally effective. These generalizations do not apply if the organisms are resistant. The prevalence of initial drug resistance remains low in the United States and Canada. Rates vary geographically, and outbreaks of multi-

drug-resistant tuberculosis can occur within communities[34] and institutions.[35] Drug resistance is more likely in persons with a history of prior antituberculous therapy and in recent emigrants from parts of the world where drug-resistant tuberculosis occurs frequently, such as Latin America and Asia.[36]

Second-Line Drugs. Second-line antituberculous agents, dosages, and major adverse effects are listed in Table 32–3. As a group, they are less active and more toxic than the first-line drugs. *M. tuberculosis* isolates may be susceptible to other agents used to treat nontuberculous mycobacterial infections (see later).

Prevention. The purposes of preventive therapy are to prevent (1) progression of latent infection to clinical disease, (2) initial infection, and (3) recurrence of past disease. In the United States, persons with any of the following six risk factors should be considered candidates for preventive therapy, regardless of age, if they have not been treated previously. The criterion for a positive reaction to a skin test (in millimeters of induration) for each group is given. The groups are

1. Persons with risk factors for HIV infection who are either known or suspected to be infected with HIV (≥ 5 mm).
2. Close contacts of persons with newly diagnosed infectious tuberculosis (≥ 5 mm). In addition, children and adolescents who are tuberculin-negative (<5 mm) and who have been close contacts of infectious persons within the past 3 months are candidates for preventive therapy until a repeated tuberculin skin test is performed 12 weeks after contact with the infectious source.
3. Those who evidence seroconversion, as indicated by a tuberculin skin test (≥ 10 mm increase within a 2-year period for those younger than 35 years old; ≥ 15 mm increase for those 35 years of age or older).
4. Persons with abnormal chest radiographs that show fibrotic lesions likely to represent old healed tuberculosis (≥ 5 mm).
5. Intravenous drug users known to be HIV-seronegative (≥ 10 mm).
6. Persons with medical conditions (see earlier) that have been reported to increase the risk of tuberculosis (≥ 10 mm).

In addition, in the absence of any of the six risk factors, persons younger than 35 years of age in the following high-incidence groups are appropriate candidates for preventive therapy if their reaction to a tuberculin skin test is 10 mm or greater:

1. Foreign-born persons from high-prevalence countries
2. Medically underserved low-income populations, including high-risk racial and ethnic minority populations, especially black, Hispanic, and Native American persons
3. Residents of facilities for long-term care (e.g., correctional institutions, nursing homes, and mental institutions)[37]

The usual preventive therapy regimen is INH (10 mg/kg daily for children, up to a maximal adult dose of 300 mg daily). The recommended duration of INH preventive treatment varies from 6 to 12 months of continuous therapy. Twelve months of therapy is recommended for persons with HIV infection and persons with stable abnormal chest radiographs consistent with past tuberculosis. The other groups should receive a minimum of 6 months of continuous therapy.[37]

Extrapulmonary Tuberculosis

Pathophysiology. Extrapulmonary tuberculosis is a consequence of the lymphohematogenous dissemination of tu-

TABLE 32–3

SECOND-LINE ANTITUBERCULOUS DRUGS

Drug	Dosage Forms	Usual Daily Dose*	Maximal Daily Dose*	Major Adverse Reactions
Capreomycin	Vials: 1 g	15–30 mg/kg IM	1 g	Auditory, vestibular, and renal toxicity
Kanamycin	Vials: 75 mg, 500 mg, 1 g	15–30 mg/kg IM or IV	1 g	Auditory and renal toxicity, rarely vestibular toxicity
Ethionamide	Tablets: 250 mg	15–20 mg/kg PO	1 g	Gastrointestinal intolerance, neuritis, mental depression, hypersensitivity, hepatitis
Cycloserine	Capsules: 250 mg	15–20 mg/kg PO	1 g	Psychosis, seizures, rash
Aminosalicylic acid	Tablets: 500 mg, 1 g	150 mg/kg	12 g	Gastrointestinal intolerance, hypersensitivity, hematologic toxicity

*For both children and adults. Doses based on weight should be adjusted as weight changes.

bercle bacilli throughout the body that accompanies primary pulmonary infection. The progression from pulmonary infection to nonpulmonary manifestations of clinical disease can be rapid. In most cases, however, extrapulmonary tuberculosis occurs at a variable but commonly long period of latency after the primary infection.

Epidemiology. In past decades, the decline in extrapulmonary cases has not paralleled that seen for pulmonary tuberculosis. As a consequence, extrapulmonary tuberculosis is responsible for an increasing proportion of all reported tuberculosis cases in the United States.[38] In 1987, of 22,517 patients with tuberculosis reported to the Centers for Disease Control, 4056 (18%) had an extrapulmonary site reported as the major locus of disease.[4] A study found that the age group with the largest proportion of extrapulmonary tuberculosis cases was children younger than age 15 years.[38] By race and ethnicity, Native Americans and Alaskan natives were most likely to have extrapulmonary tuberculosis. Rates among blacks and Asians and Pacific Islanders also exceeded those among non-Hispanic whites. Women had higher rates than men, and foreign-born persons were more likely than persons born in the United States to have extrapulmonary tuberculosis.[38] AIDS also increases the risk of extrapulmonary disease.[39]

Clinical Features. The most commonly reported sites of extrapulmonary tuberculosis are given in Table 32–4.

Treatment. In general, antituberculous regimens recommended for pulmonary tuberculosis are used to treat extrapulmonary infections as well (see Table 32–1). The use of steroids as adjunctive therapy remains controversial. They may be beneficial for selected patients with miliary, central nervous system, or pericardial tuberculosis. Physiologic doses of corticosteroids are necessary if adrenal gland involvement results in adrenocortical insufficiency (Addison's disease).

TABLE 32–4

REPORTED EXTRAPULMONARY TUBERCULOSIS CASES BY ANATOMIC SITE, UNITED STATES, 1987

Anatomic Site	Number of Cases	Percentage
Lymphatic	1143	28.2
Pleural	1044	25.7
Genitourinary	505	12.5
Bone and/or joint	374	9.2
Miliary	305	7.5
Meningeal	200	4.9
Peritoneal	140	3.5
Other	345	8.5

Adapted from Bloch AB, Reider HL, Kelly GD, et al: The epidemiology of tuberculosis in the United States. Clin Chest Med 10:297, 1989.

Surgical intervention is rarely indicated but may prove useful in some patients with tuberculous spondylitis (Pott's disease), constrictive pericarditis, or central nervous system involvement.

Miliary Tuberculosis

Pathogenesis. Miliary tuberculosis derives its name from the millet seed–like appearance of the disseminated granulomas characteristic of this disease. The numerous lesions are approximately the same age and size and usually progress to necrosis and caseation in multiple organs. Classically, a diffuse miliary pattern is visible in chest roentgenograms at some time of the disease.[40] The lesions are usually not visible for several weeks and, when present, frequently accompany pulmonary infiltrates and/or effusions.[41]

Miliary tuberculosis may develop shortly after the lymphohematogenous dissemination of primary tuberculosis. Historically, this acute form occurred mainly in children and was commonly associated with meningitis. Nonimmune adults may experience a similarly rapid course, but generally their illness is less acute. Miliary disease can also follow reactivation of old primary lesions that chronically discharge tubercle bacilli into the blood stream. The foci responsible are usually extrapulmonary and often clinically silent. This chronic form may progress to acute illness resembling early postprimary miliary tuberculosis. More commonly, however, illness evolves slowly or even episodically over time, particularly in elderly people.

Epidemiology. Risk factors for miliary tuberculosis include age and race. In 1986, most United States cases reported to the Centers for Disease Control occurred in patients younger than 15 years or older than 65 years of age.[38] Rates among blacks and Native Americans and Alaskan natives exceeded those in non-Hispanic whites. No significant differences were seen between male and female patients or between patients born in the United States and the foreign born.[38] Previous clinical series identified alcoholism, diabetes, pregnancy, malignancies, and immunosuppressive therapy as commonly associated or underlying conditions.[40–42] Except for a history of prior tuberculosis, however, most patients have no defined predisposing condition.

Clinical Features. The nonspecific symptoms of weakness, cough, anorexia, fatigue, weight loss, fever, and night sweats are insidious and commonly evolve for weeks or even months before the diagnosis is considered. As a consequence, miliary tuberculosis remains an important cause of fever of unknown origin. Headache correlates with the presence of meningitis, and abdominal pain is often associated with peritonitis.[40, 41] Rarely, patients with miliary tuberculosis may have adult respiratory distress syndrome or experience respiratory failure during antituberculous therapy.[43, 44]

Diagnosis. Physical findings and laboratory abnormalities are generally nonspecific. Hematologic abnormalities are frequently seen. Anemia is common and may be associated with a leukemoid reaction, leukopenia, lymphopenia, thrombocytosis, thrombocytopenia, and rarely, disseminated intravascular coagulation.[42] Mild hyponatremia and elevated serum alkaline phosphatase levels are frequently reported. The tuberculin skin test reaction is negative in one quarter or more of patients. Miliary lesions on chest rentgenogram are characteristic of the disease. This classic pattern, however, does not develop until several weeks after acute hematogenous dissemination.[45] Similarly, chest roentgenograms are frequently normal and tuberculin skin test results are commonly negative in chronic miliary tuberculosis. This clinical picture is especially prevalent among elderly patients, who may die of miliary disease before the characteristic radiographic pattern develops.[46, 47] Miliary tuberculosis should also be considered in patients with adult respiratory distress syndrome of unknown cause.

The diagnosis of miliary tuberculosis requires a high degree of suspicion. Gastric aspirate, urine, blood, and CSF cultures may be positive. Tissue biopsy for histologic studies, acid-fast staining, and mycobacterial culture is usually required. Lymph nodes may show involvement. Liver biopsy or bone marrow biopsy reveals granulomas in more than 80% of patients.[42] Fiberoptic bronchoscopy can yield the diagnosis via transbronchial lung biopsy, bronchial brushing, and/or lavage.[17, 42]

Treatment. The prognosis in miliary tuberculosis correlates with how quickly the diagnosis is made and antituberculous therapy begun. The same rules of therapy used for pulmonary tuberculosis apply to patients with miliary tuberculosis.[27] The standard regimen includes INH and rifampin and should be continued for a minimum of 6 months. Adjunctive steroid therapy (60 to 80 mg of prednisone daily, tapered over 2 weeks) may be beneficial for patients with adult respiratory distress syndrome and disseminated intravascular coagulation or in those with accompanying tuberculous meningitis or pericarditis.

Tuberculous Meningitis

Pathogenesis. Tubercle bacilli reach the brain or meninges during the hematogenous dissemination that accompanies primary or, less commonly, chronic tuberculosis. After a latent period of weeks to decades, meningitis can develop via rupture of a subependymal tubercle into the subarachnoid space.[48] The pathologic picture is that of a meningoencephalitis primarily involving the base of the brain. Communicating hydrocephalus may result from exudative obstruction of the basal cisterns or adhesive leptomeningitis.[49]

Epidemiology. Tuberculous meningitis accounts for less than 0.5% of all new tuberculosis cases but composes 5 to 8% of extrapulmonary tuberculosis cases.[38, 41] More than 30% of patients with the diagnosis of miliary tuberculosis have meningeal involvement, which is often asymptomatic early in the disease.[40] In the United States, patient populations with increased likelihood of tuberculous meningitis include children under the age of 15 years, women, Hispanic and Native American and Alaskan native racial and ethnic groups, and patients who were born in the United States.[38]

Clinical Features. The signs and symptoms are diverse and frequently subtle early in the illness. Classically, patients have an insidious, subacute prodrome associated with fever, malaise, and intermittent headache. This is followed by meningeal signs and severe headache with progression to altered consciousness, cranial nerve palsies, and long tract signs.[50] Occasionally, it presents acutely, mimicking bacterial meningitis. Seizures can occur at any stage and may be the presenting symptom. They tend to be focal in adults and generalized in children.[51]

Uniform criteria have been established to classify patients' neurologic status on hospital admission.[52] In stage 1, patients have meningeal irritation but are fully conscious, are rational, and lack focal neurologic signs. Stage 2 is characterized by the presence of confusion and/or focal neurologic signs or hemiparesis. In stage 3, patients are unresponsive owing to stupor or delirium and/or have complete hemiplegia or paraplegia. Patients whose disease is diagnosed and treated in stage 1 have the best prognosis.

Diagnosis. The diagnosis of tuberculous meningitis depends on a high degree of clinical suspicion. It should be suspected in all cases of miliary tuberculosis. However, at least 25% of patients lack clinical or radiographic evidence of current or prior pulmonary or extrapulmonary tuberculosis.[53] A positive tuberculin skin test result supports the diagnosis, but a negative test result does not exclude it.

CSF studies are critical to establishing the diagnosis. Classic findings include an elevated protein level, decreased glucose concentration, and lymphocytosis. More than three fourths of patients have less than 400 cells per cubic millimeter, more than 50% of which are lymphocytes. Early in the course of disease, however, polymorphonuclear cells can predominate.[49, 50] Serial CSF samples generally reveal this shift from neutrophils to lymphocytes during days to weeks, accompanied by gradually rising protein and falling glucose levels. Although hypoglycorrhachia develops in the majority of cases, depression of CSF glucose level may not be evident in hyperglycemic patients. Simultaneous blood and CSF glucose levels should be determined in all patients. A CSF/blood glucose ratio of less than 0.5 should arouse suspicion. The finding of high CSF protein levels associated with xanthochromia carries a poor prognosis and suggests subarachnoid block, which may be due to spinal meningitis.[50]

Most publications report positive CSF acid-fast smears in 10 to 40% of patients. Careful examination of CSF from serial spinal taps can increase the yield to 87%.[54] Optimally, 10 to 20 mL of CSF should be sampled and centrifuged, and the sediment should be stained and cultured for acid-fast bacilli.[55] The combination of smears and cultures generally yields true-positive findings in more than 80% of patients. A 2-to four-week period is required for conventional mycobacterial cultures. Thus, culture results cannot help guide early treatment decisions.

Serodiagnostic techniques show great promise for rapid, accurate detection of tuberculous meningitis. ELISA can detect mycobacterial antigen or antibody[56–58] in CSF in a few hours. False-negative results were seen with ELISA studies of CSF. However, in areas of low prevalence, a negative ELISA result could prove useful in excluding tuberculous meningitis and reduce the number of unnecessary CSF mycobacterial cultures.[59] Preliminary studies indicate that latex particle agglutination methods can detect mycobacterial antigen in infected fluids, including CSF.[60] Polymerase chain reaction assay of CSF appears successful for the diagnosis of tuberculous meningitis.[61]

Computed tomography can provide supportive, although nonspecific, information for the diagnosis of tuberculous meningitis.[62] The two most common lesions (each seen in approximately 60 to 80% of patients) are hydrocephalus and meningeal enhancement with contrast. Tuberculomas are detectable in 22 to 28% of patients with tuberculous meningitis. Cerebral infarction, more common in children than in adults, is found in 20 to 50% of patients. The finding of an entirely normal computed tomographic scan performed with contrast enhancement in a drowsy patient appears to be strong evidence against a diagnosis of tuberculous meningitis.

Routine laboratory tests are not helpful in diagnosing tuberculous meningitis. A moderate anemia is common, and the erythrocyte sedimentation rate is elevated in more than 50% of cases. The white blood cell count is usually normal. Hyponatremia and hypochloremia may occur and are secondary to syndrome of inappropriate antidiuretic hormone.

Antimicrobial Therapy. Once uniformly fatal, tuberculous meningitis can be treated successfully with antimicrobial agents. The degree of success depends largely on how soon therapy is begun. Antimicrobials should be administered empirically *as soon as the disease is suspected.* Therapy should not be withheld until the diagnosis is confirmed.

The currently recommended regimen for children and adults is a combination of INH, rifampin, and PZA. Treatment guidelines follow those for pulmonary tuberculosis[27] (see Table 32–1). If a resistant isolate is suspected, EMB or STM should be added and then discontinued if the isolate proves susceptible. Duration of therapy should be at least 6 months, or longer depending on isolate susceptibility and clinical response.

For immunocompromised hosts, a four-drug regimen that includes INH and rifampin is recommended during the initial 2 months of therapy. Supplemental initial therapy should also include maximal doses of either PZA or EMB. The other supplemental agent can be STM, rifabutin (300 mg/d; currently investigational), or clofazimine (300 mg/d). The supplemental drugs are discontinued after 2 months if the isolate proves susceptible and the clinical response is favorable. The duration of therapy is a minimum of 6 months, or longer depending on isolate susceptibility and clinical response.

In addition to the drugs listed earlier, kanamycin, ethionamide, and cycloserine achieve concentrations in CSF, which are above the minimal inhibitory concentration for *M. tuberculosis.*[63] These agents, rarely used for tuberculous meningitis, may be more useful to treat meningitis caused by nontuberculous mycobacteria. There is no indication for intrathecal therapy of tuberculous meningitis.

Steroid Therapy. Although controversial, the use of steroids in patients with stage 2 or 3 tuberculous meningitis is supported by limited trials and general consensus. Prednisone is given at a dosage of 60 to 80 mg/d in adults and 1 to 3 mg/kg/d in children. Depending on clinical response, the dose can be reduced after 1 or 2 weeks, tapered gradually, and discontinued entirely in 4 to 6 weeks.[63]

Surgical Therapy. Surgical procedures are directed primarily at relief of hydrocephalus. They are most commonly required in patients with stage 3 disease.[62] Ventricular shunts may relieve signs and symptoms as well as improve sensorial and neurologic deficits. They can be inserted safely despite active disease, but subsequent revisions may be necessary because of the high protein content of the CSF.[49] Intracranial tuberculomas usually respond to antimicrobial therapy, and surgical excision is rarely required.[64]

The outcome of tuberculous meningitis depends on a number of factors, including delay in diagnosis or treatment, the severity of illness at time of hospital admission, the presence of miliary disease, extremes of age, and the presence of underlying medical conditions. Studies from Scotland and the United States reported overall mortality rates of 15 to 42%.[49, 53, 54] In one small pediatric series, therapy with INH and rifampin reduced mortality to 5%.[65] Mortality increases with age[49, 53] and can reach 60% in patients older than 60 years.[54] Residual neurologic deficits are present in approximately 25% of survivors. They are more common among infants and children and in patients whose therapy was delayed. Chronic brain syndrome, hemiparesis, paraplegia, optic atrophy with blindness, oculomotor palsy, deafness, seizures, and various symptoms of hypothalamic or pituitary dysfunction have been reported.[50]

Tuberculous Pericarditis

Pathophysiology. Tuberculous pericarditis usually develops by spread of tubercle bacilli from mediastinal lymph nodes directly adjacent to the pericardium. Occasionally, it results from lymphohematogenous dissemination or direct spread from a contiguous lung focus. The infected pericardium releases an exudative effusion, develops granulomas, and ultimately undergoes fibrosis.

Epidemiology. Currently, approximately 1% of persons with tuberculosis experience pericarditis. This may increase as more persons with AIDS contract the disease.[66, 67]

Clinical Features. The onset may be gradual or abrupt with fever, pericardial pain, and cardiac tamponade. The most common presenting symptoms include dyspnea, cough, night sweats, weight loss, orthopnea, chest pain, and ankle edema.[68–70] Additional findings may include a pericardial friction rub, cardiomegaly, fever, tachycardia, pulsus paradoxus, and hepatomegaly.

Diagnosis. Pericardial effusions are easily detected by a variety of techniques, including echocardiography and computed tomography. The tuberculin skin testing result may be negative in up to 40% of cases. Pericardial fluid findings are nonspecific. Cultures are positive in only 40 to 60% of cases, and smears are negative in the majority. New diagnostic techniques (e.g., BACTEC, ELISA, and polymerase chain reaction) may ultimately increase this yield. Currently pericardial biopsy for histologic study and culture is the procedure most likely to reveal the diagnosis.

Treatment. All patients should receive antituberculous agents as recommended for pulmonary tuberculosis. The use of steroids remains controversial. However, in a double-blind study, 5 mg of prednisolone taken daily during the initial 11 weeks of therapy reduced the risk of death from pericarditis and the need for repeat pericardiocentesis.[71] Adequate drainage of pericardial fluid is essential in cases with tamponade. A pericardial window procedure may be both diagnostic and therapeutic in patients with suspected effusive pericarditis.[69] Early pericardiectomy is indicated for the minority of patients who have cardiac tamponade unrelieved by pericardiocentesis. The majority of patients who do not require early pericardiectomy respond well to medical therapy alone.[71] A few patients require late pericardiectomy for constrictive pericarditis.

Tuberculosis and Pregnancy

All pregnant women with tuberculosis should receive therapy appropriate for their infection. Tuberculosis is not an indication for a therapeutic abortion.[72] The initial treatment regimen should consist of INH and rifampin. EMB should be added if INH resistance is suspected. All three drugs cross the placenta but have not been demonstrated to have teratogenic effects. Pyridoxine supplementation should accompany INH therapy in pregnant women. The routine use of PZA is discouraged owing to inadequate teratogenicity data. STM may cause congenital deafness and should be avoided. There is little information regarding the toxic or teratogenic potential of kanamycin, capreomycin, cycloserine, and ethionamide. They should be avoided if possible.[27] Preventive therapy should be given during the second and third trimesters of pregnancy to selected patients at high risk for progressive disease.[72]

Tuberculosis and Acquired Immunodeficiency Syndrome

Tuberculosis is one of the few contagious respiratory tract diseases that occur in patients with HIV infection. The diagnosis of tuberculosis usually precedes but may follow or be made simultaneously with the diagnosis of AIDS. Diagnosis is often delayed by an unusual clinical presentation. The tuberculin skin test result is negative in about 60% of patients with AIDS and tuberculosis. Diffuse or miliary infiltrates are more common than focal infiltrates and/or cavitation,[5, 73] and extrapulmonary disease occurs more frequently.[39] Multiple sputum samples should be obtained for acid-fast smears and cultures.[74, 75] The absence of acid-fast bacilli and granulomas in tissue specimens does not exclude the diagnosis of tuberculosis.[76]

Because the presentations of tuberculosis and nontuberculous mycobacterial infections are similar, antituberculous chemotherapy should be started whenever acid-fast bacilli are found in a specimen from a patient with AIDS or suspected HIV infection. The standard regimens for initial therapy of tuberculosis apply, and most patients respond well. However, treatment should be continued for a minimum of 9 months and for at least 6 months after documented culture conversion. If either INH or rifampin is not in the regimen, treatment is continued for a minimum of 18 months and at least 12 months after culture conversion.[76] Twelve months of INH preventive therapy should be considered in persons with a positive tuberculin skin test result who are HIV-seropositive.

NONTUBERCULOUS MYCOBACTERIAL INFECTIONS

Microbiology. In the 1950s, Timpe and Runyon established that nontuberculous mycobacteria could cause disease in humans and classified these organisms into four broad groups on the basis of pigment production, growth rate, and colonial characteristics.[77, 78] Table 32–5 lists the major species for each group.

Epidemiology. The rate of isolation of nontuberculous mycobacteria is increasing and has surpassed that for *M. tuberculosis* in some areas.[79] Ubiquitous in nature, many have been isolated from water, soil, and domestic and wild animals and birds. Despite their wide distribution, some species are more common in certain geographic locations. Most infections, including those that are hospital acquired, result from inhalation or direct inoculation from environmental sources. These infections are not considered contagious because person-to-person transmission is extremely rare.

Pathophysiology. The pathogenic potential for human disease varies among nontuberculous mycobacteria. As a group, these organisms are less virulent for humans than *M. tuberculosis* and may colonize body surfaces or secretions without causing disease. The existence of a predisposing condition frequently is required for tissue invasion to occur. In general, disease is slowly progressive, and histopathologic findings resemble those seen in tuberculosis.

Diagnosis. The steps taken to diagnose tuberculosis generally apply to nontuberculous mycobacterial infections as well. However, colonization of asymptomatic individuals and environmental contamination of specimens can yield positive cultures in the absence of clinical disease. Diagnostic guidelines are helpful.[80] Nontuberculous mycobacterial disease can be considered present in patients with a cavitary infiltrate on chest radiograph when (1) two or more sputum samples (or sputum and a bronchial washing) are smear-positive for acid-fast bacilli and/or yield moderate-to-heavy growth on culture and (2) other reasonable causes of the disease process have been excluded, (e.g., fungal disease, tuberculosis, and malignancy). An additional criterion, (3) failure of the sputum cultures to convert to negative with either bronchial hygiene or 2 weeks of specific mycobacterial drug therapy, is applied in the presence of a noncavitary infiltrate not known to be due to another disease.

The diagnosis is also established if transbronchial, percutaneous, or open lung biopsy tissue reveals mycobacterial histopathologic changes and yields the organism. If the lung biopsy specimen has a negative culture but shows mycobacterial histologic features, a diagnosis of nontuberculous lung disease can be made when (1) two or more sputum samples (or sputum and a bronchial washing) are culture-positive for nontuberculous mycobacteria and (2) other reasonable causes of granulomatous disease have been excluded.

The diagnosis of extrapulmonary or disseminated disease is established by isolation of the organism from normally sterile body fluids, closed sites, or lesions and when environmental contamination of specimens is excluded.

Clinical Disease. Nontuberculous mycobacteria are capable of causing a broad spectrum of diseases.[81–83] The following discussion includes infections caused by selected species most likely to be encountered in intensive care settings.

Mycobacterium avium-intracellulare Infection

M. avium and *M. intracellulare* strains are so similar that most laboratories group them together. They are commonly referred to as *M. avium-intracellulare* or *M. avium* complex. These organisms are distributed worldwide and rank first among nontuberculous isolates in the United States.[79] Pulmonary infection usually occurs in individuals with underlying pulmonary disease and generally follows an indolent or slowly progressive course.[84] Differentiation between colonization and true infection may be difficult initially. Extrapulmonary or disseminated disease, seen infrequently in immunocompetent patients, is extremely common among individuals with AIDS.[85–88] In the United States, *M. avium-intracellulare* is the most common mycobacterial species isolated from AIDS patients. Infection almost invariably presents as disseminated disease. Persistent or intermittent fever is characteristic, and other suggestive symptoms include weight loss of greater than 20 lb, anorexia, abdominal pain, and diarrhea.[89] Other findings may include hepatospleno-

TABLE 32–5
RUNYAN'S CLASSIFICATION OF NONTUBERCULOUS *MYCOBACTERIUM* SPECIES

I. Photochromogens
   M. kansasii
   M. marinum
   M. simiae
   M. asiaticum
II. Scotochromogens
   M. flavescens
   M. gordonae
   M. scrofulaceum
   M. szulgai
III. Nonchromogens
   M. avium-intracellulare
   M. gastri
   M. haemophilum
   M. malmoense
   M. terrae
   M. ulcerans
   M. xenopi
IV. Rapid growers
   M. chelonae
   M. fortuitum

megaly and generalized lymphadenopathy, including mediastinal adenopathy. Diagnosis of disseminated disease is made by culture of the organism from blood, bone marrow, and/or stool. Rarely, biopsy of other tissues may be needed to demonstrate the organism.

The treatment of *M. avium-intracellulare* disease remains controversial. Most conventional antituberculous agents have little or no activity against these organisms, and no controlled therapeutic trials have been conducted. Most regimens employ multiple drugs, and the risk of drug toxicity is high. Current guidelines for the initial treatment of pulmonary disease suggest use of the following four-drug regimen: INH (300 mg), rifampin (600 mg), EMB (25 mg/kg for the first 2 months, then 15 mg/kg), with STM for the initial 3 to 6 months of therapy.[80] Daily therapy or five times per week is recommended for patients who have normal renal function and who are younger than 70 years of age. After the initial 6 to 12 weeks, maintenance doses of STM are given twice or thrice weekly for an additional 3 to 4 months. In both initial and maintenance stages, STM dosing must be based on the patient's age, weight, and renal function.[80] All patients must be monitored for signs or symptoms of STM toxicity.

Patients who experience treatment failure with this four-drug regimen require therapeutic agents that are associated with higher incidences of side effects and toxicity. Intensive therapy with multiple drugs, including cycloserine (250 mg twice daily), ethionamide (250 mg twice daily, then increased to three times daily as tolerated), and prolonged use of STM (three to five times per week), is recommended. Other oral drugs with potential use in this setting include clofazimine (100 mg once daily) and ciprofloxacin (500 mg twice daily).

Disseminated *M. avium-intracellulare* infections in patients without AIDS are often successfully treated with multiple-drug regimens recommended for pulmonary disease. In AIDS patients, however, the response rate generally has been poor. The impact of disseminated *M. avium-intracellulare* on survival in AIDS patients remains controversial, although one large study found disseminated disease to correlate with earlier death.[88] Multiple-drug therapy with rifabutin (300 to 600 mg daily), clofazimine (100 mg daily), EMB (15 mg/kg daily), and INH (300 mg daily) appears effective in clearing mycobacteremia and may improve quality of life.[90, 91]

Other drugs used in this setting include rifampin, cycloserine, ciprofloxacin, and amikacin (7.5 to 10.0 mg/kg once daily with monitoring of serum levels). No specific regimen has emerged as superior in this setting, and the optimal duration of therapy remains unknown.

Mycobacterium kansasii Infection

M. kansasii, the most important photochromogen, often appears beaded or cross-barred on acid-fast stain and produces rough buff-colored colonies that become yellow on exposure to light. It ranks second among nontuberculous mycobacteria in causing human infections.[79] Most disease occurs in the Midwest and South of the United States. Pulmonary infection resembling tuberculosis is the usual clinical presentation. Although adult white men are most commonly affected, infection can occur in individuals of any age, sex, or race. Extrapulmonary disease can involve any organ system, and risks of dissemination are increased in immunocompromised patients.[92–95]

The current recommendation for standard treatment of pulmonary disease is INH (300 mg), rifampin (600 mg), and EMB (15 mg/kg) given daily for 18 months.[80] In patients who are unable to tolerate INH, the administration of rifampin and EMB with or without STM for the first 3

months is an alternative regimen. PZA is unacceptable as an alternative or third drug because *M. kansasii* isolates are resistant to this agent.

For patients with isolates resistant to rifampin, a regimen of daily high-dose INH (900 mg), pyridoxine (50 mg), high-dose EMB (25 mg/kg), and sulfamethoxazole (3 g) for 18 to 24 months has been proposed. The oral therapy has been combined with STM or amikacin given daily or five times per week for 2 to 3 months followed by intermittent STM or amikacin for a total of at least 6 months.[96]

Treatment regimens for patients who have pulmonary infection also apply to those with extrapulmonary disease. The optimal therapy for disseminated disease in patients with AIDS is unknown. Current recommendations suggest that the standard three-drug regimen be used with consideration of the addition of 1 g of STM twice weekly for the first 3 months.[80]

Infection with Rapidly Growing Mycobacteria

Rapidly growing mycobacteria are acid-fast rods that resemble diphtheroids on Gram's stain. Growth is rapid on subculture (1 to 3 days), but primary isolation from clinical specimens may require 2 to 30 days. Unlike other mycobacteria, they grow well on many routine noninhibitory laboratory media. *Mycobacterium fortuitum* and *Mycobacterium chelonae* are the major pathogens in this group. They rank third and fourth among nontuberculous mycobacteria in causing human disease in the United States.[79] Sporadic, community-acquired infections have been reported from most areas of the United States. The spectrum of diseases ranges from localized to disseminated, with cutaneous involvement being most common.[97] Most infections are acquired by inoculation after accidental trauma, surgery, or injection. Nosocomial epidemics or clusters have been reported in numerous settings, including augmentation mammaplasty,[98] hemodialysis,[99] plastic surgery,[100] long-term venous catheterization,[101] cardiac surgery,[102] and jet injector use.[103]

These mycobacteria are highly resistant to conventional antituberculous drugs but may be sensitive to traditional antibiotics. Susceptibility testing of individual isolates is important, as resistance patterns vary by and within species subgroups.[104] *M. fortuitum* isolates are usually susceptible to amikacin, ciprofloxacin, sulfonamides, cefoxitin, and imipenem and occasionally doxycycline. *M. chelonae* subspecies *abscessus* isolates are generally susceptible to amikacin and cefoxitin and occasionally erythromycin. In contrast, *M. chelonae* subspecies *chelonae* isolates are most likely to be susceptible to tobramycin, amikacin, or erythromycin and occasionally doxycycline.

Current guidelines suggest intravenous amikacin (given in doses to yield peak serum levels of 20 to 25 μg/mL) plus intravenous cefoxitin (12 g/d) for initial therapy of severe infections caused by all subgroups except *M. chelonae* subspecies *chelonae*.[80] Considerations of changing to oral therapy depend on clinical improvement and susceptibility testing results. Oral agents may include ciprofloxacin (500 mg twice daily), sulfamethoxazole (1 g three times daily), and doxycycline (100 mg twice daily). Because development of resistance has been reported during single-drug therapy with ciprofloxacin,[105] the use of two agents should be considered. Treatment duration should be a minimum of 3 months for serious disease and 6 months for bone infections. Any regimen should include surgical débridement or excision of infected wounds or foreign bodies whenever possible.

Other Nontuberculous Mycobacterial Infection

Mycobacterium gordonae, also known as the tap water bacillus, has been implicated in pseudo-outbreaks associated with contamination of bronchoscopy specimens[106, 107] and an ice machine.[108] Usually considered a saprophyte, this organism can cause a variety of infections, including pulmonary,[109] cutaneous,[110] and disseminated disease.[111-113] Patients with confirmed infection usually respond to therapy with INH, rifampin, and EMB. Amikacin and trimethoprim-sulfamethoxazole also may prove useful.[110]

Other *Mycobacterium* species—*M. xenopi*,[114, 115] *M. malmoense*,[116] *M. szulgai*,[117] *M. simiae*,[118] *M. haemophilum*,[119] and *M. terrae*[120]—are being reported with increasing frequency as causes of pulmonary or disseminated infections, especially in AIDS patients.[79] Initial therapy for infections attributable to these nontuberculous mycobacteria should consist of INH, rifampin, and EMB with or without STM. Optimal duration of therapy is unknown, but at least 18 to 24 months is recommended.[80]

References

1. Sherris JC, Plorde JJ: Mycobacteria. In: Sherris JC (ed): Medical Microbiology. An Introduction to Infectious Diseases. 2nd ed. New York, Elsevier Science Publishing, p 443, 1990.
2. Rouillon A, Perdrizet S, Parrot R: Transmission of tubercle bacilli. The effects of chemotherapy. Tubercle 57:275, 1976.
3. Centers for Disease Control: Summary of notifiable diseases, United States, 1989. MMWR 38:43, 1989.
4. Bloch AB, Reider HL, Kelly GD, et al: The epidemiology of tuberculosis in the United States. Clin Chest Med 10:297, 1989.
5. Chaisson RE, Schecter GF, Theuer CP, et al: Tuberculosis in patients with acquired immunodeficiency symdrome. Clinical features, response to therapy, and survival. Am Rev Respir Dis 136:570, 1987.
6. Rieder HL, Cauthen GM, Kelly GD, et al: Tuberculosis in the United States. JAMA 262:385, 1989.
7. Stead WW, Lofgren JP, Warren E, et al: Tuberculosis as an endemic and nosocomial infection among the elderly in nursing homes. N Engl J Med 312:1483, 1985.
8. Schieffelbein CW Jr, Snider DE: Tuberculosis control among homeless populations. Arch Intern Med 148:1843, 1988.
9. Stead WW: Pathogenesis of a first episode of chronic pulmonary tuberculosis in man: Recrudescence of residuals of the primary infection or exogenous reinfection? Am Rev Resp Dis 95:729, 1967.
10. Frame RN, Johnson MC, Eichenhorn MS, et al: Active tuberculosis in the medical intensive care unit. A 15-year retrospective analysis. Crit Care Med 15:1012, 1987.
11. Dyer RA, Potgieter PD: The adult respiratory distress syndrome and bronchogenic pulmonary tuberculosis. Thorax 39:383, 1984.
12. Levy H, Kallenbach JM, Feldman C, et al: Acute respiratory failure in active tuberculosis. Crit Care Med 15:221, 1987.
13. Tytle TL, Johnson TH: Changing patterns in pulmonary tuberculosis. South Med J 10:1223, 1984.
14. Khan MA, Kovnat DM, Bachus B, et al: Clinical and roentgenographic spectrum of pulmonary tuberculosis in the adult. Am J Med 62:31, 1977.
15. Berger HW, Granada MG: Lower lung field tuberculosis. Chest 65:522, 1974.
16. American Thoracic Society/Centers for Disease Control: Diagnostic standards and classification of tuberculosis. Am Rev Respir Dis 142:725, 1990.
17. Willcox PA, Potgieter PD, Bateman ED, et al: Rapid diagnosis of sputum-negative miliary tuberculosis using the flexible fiberoptic bronchoscope. Thorax 41:681, 1986.
18. de Gracia J, Currull V, Vidal R, et al: Diagnostic value of bronchoalveolar lavage in suspected pulmonary tuberculosis. Chest 93:329, 1988.
19. Siddiqi SH, Libonati JP, Middlebrook G: Evaluation of a rapid radiometric method for drug susceptibility testing of *Mycobacterium tuberculosis*. J Clin Microbiol 13:908, 1981.
20. Daniel TM, Debanne SM: The serodiagnosis of tuberculosis and other mycobacterial diseases by enzyme-linked immunosorbent assay. Am Rev Respir Dis 135:1137, 1987.
21. Levy H, Wadee AA, Feldman C, et al: Enzyme-linked immunosorbent assay for the detection of antibodies against *Mycobacterium tuberculosis* in bronchial washings and serum. Chest 93:762, 1988.
22. Friedman LN, Filderman AE, D'Aquila TG, et al: ELISA analysis of BACTEC bottles for the earlier diagnosis of tuberculosis. Am Rev Respir Dis 140:668, 1989.
23. Ellner PD, Kiehn TE, Cammarata R, et al: Rapid detection and identification of pathogenic mycobacteria by combining radiometric and nucleic acid probe methods. J Clin Microbiol 26:1349, 1988.
24. Eisenach KD, Cave MD, Bates JH, et al: Polymerase chain reaction amplification of a repetitive DNA sequence specific for *Mycobacterium tuberculosis*. J Infect Dis 161:977, 1990.
25. Hermans PW, Schuitema AR, Van Soolingen D, et al: Specific detection of *Mycobacterium tuberculosis* complex strains by polymerase chain reaction. J Clin Microbiol 28:1204, 1990.
26. Pao CC, Yen TSB, You JB, et al: Detection and identification of *Mycobacterium tuberculosis* by DNA amplification. J Clin Microbiol 28:1877, 1990.
27. American Thoracic Society/Centers for Disease Control: Treatment of tuberculosis and tuberculosis infection in adults and children. Am Rev Respir Dis 134:355, 1986.
28. Koestner JA, Jones LK, Polk WH, et al: Prolonged use of intravenous isoniazid and rifampin. Drug Intell Clin Pharm 23:48, 1989.
29. Kopanoff DE, Snider DE, Caras GJ: Isoniazid related hepatitis. Am Rev Respir Dis 117:991, 1978.
30. Baciewicz AM, Self TH: Isoniazid interactions. South Med J 78:714, 1985.
31. Baciewicz AM, Self TH: Rifampin drug interactions. Arch Intern Med 144:1667, 1984.
32. Baciewicz AM, Self TH, Bekemeyer WB: Update on rifampin drug interactions. Arch Intern Med 147:565, 1987.
33. Girling DJ: The hepatic toxicity of antituberculosis regimens containing isoniazid, rifampicin and pyrazinamide. Tubercle 59:13, 1978.
34. Centers for Disease Control: Outbreak of multidrug-resistant tuberculosis—Texas, California and Pennsylvania. MMWR 39:369, 1990.
35. Centers for Disease Control: Nosocomial transmission of multidrug-resistant tuberculosis to health-care workers and HIV-infected patients in an urban hospital. MMWR 39:718, 1990.
36. Barnes PF: The influence of epidemiologic factors on drug resistance rates in tuberculosis. Am Rev Respir Dis 136:325, 1987.
37. Centers for Disease Control: The use of preventive therapy for tuberculous infection in the United States. MMWR 39(RR-8):9, 1990.
38. Rieder HL, Snider DE Jr, Cauthen GM: Extrapulmonary tuberculosis in the United States. Am Rev Respir Dis 141:347, 1990.
39. Braun MM, Byers RH, Heyward WL, et al: Acquired immunodeficiency syndrome and extrapulmonary tuberculosis in the United States. Arch Intern Med 150:1913, 1990.
40. Munt PW: Miliary tuberculosis in the chemotherapy era: With a clinical review in 69 American adults. Medicine 51:139, 1971.
41. Alvarez S, McCabe WR: Extrapulmonary tuberculosis revisited: A review of experience at Boston City and other hospitals. Medicine 63:25, 1984.
42. Maartens G, Willcox PA, Benatar SR: Miliary tuberculosis: Rapid diagnosis, hematologic abnormalities, and outcome in 109 treated adults. Am J Med 89:291, 1990.
43. Huseby JS, Hudson LD: Miliary tuberculosis and adult respiratory distress syndrome. Ann Intern Med 85:609, 1976.
44. Dyer RA, Chappell WA, Potgeiter PD: Adult respiratory distress syndrome associated with miliary tuberculosis. Crit Care Med 13:12, 1985.
45. Sahn SA, Neff TA: Miliary tuberculosis. Am J Med 56:495, 1974.
46. Proudfoot AT, Akhtar AJ, Douglas AC, et al: Miliary tuberculosis in adults. Br Med J [Clin Res] 2:273, 1969.
47. Bobrowitz ID: Active tuberculosis undiagnosed until autopsy. Am J Med 72:650, 1982.
48. Auerback O: Tuberculous meningitis: Correlation of therapeutic results with the pathogenesis and pathologic changes. I. General considerations and pathogenesis. Am Rev Tuberc 64:408, 1951.
49. Clark WC, Metcalf JC Jr, Muhlbauer MS, et al: *Mycobacterium tuberculosis* meningitis: A report of twelve cases and a literature review. Neurosurgery 18:604, 1986.
50. Sheller JR, Des Prez RM: CNS tuberculosis. Neurol Clin 4:143, 1986.
51. Molavi A, LeFrock JL: Tuberculous meningitis. Med Clin North Am 69:315, 1985.
52. Medical Research Council Report: Streptomycin treatment of tuberculosis meningitis. Lancet 1:582, 1948.
53. Ogawa SK, Smith MA, Brennessel DJ, et al: Tuberculous meningitis in an urban medical center. Medicine 66:317, 1987.
54. Kennedy DH, Fallon RD: Tuberculous meningitis. JAMA 214:264, 1979.
55. Stewart SM: Technical methods: The bacteriological diagnosis of tuberculous meningitis. J Clin Pathol 6:241, 1953.
56. Sada E, Ruiz-Palacios GM, Lopez-Vidal Y, et al: Detection of mycobacterial antigens in cerebrospinal fluid of patients with tuberculous meningitis by enzyme-linked imunosorbent assay. Lancet 2:651, 1983.
57. Kalish SB, Radin RC, Levitz D, et al: The enzyme-linked immunosorbent assay method for IgG antibody to purified protein derivative in cerebrospinal fluid of patients with tuberculous meningitis. Ann Intern Med 99:630, 1983.
58. Watt G, Zaraspe G, Bautista S, et al: Rapid diagnosis of tuberculous meningitis by using an enzyme-linked immunosorbent assay to detect mycobacterial antigen and antibody in cerebrospinal fluid. J Infect Dis 158:681, 1988.
59. Crowson TW, Rich EC, Woolfrey BF, et al: Overutilization of cultures of CSF for mycobacteria. JAMA 251:70, 1984.
60. Krambovitis E, McIllmurray MB, Lock PE, et al: Rapid diagnosis of tuberculous meningitis by latex particle agglutination. Lancet 2:1229, 1984.
61. Shankar P, Manjunath N, Mohan KK, et al: Rapid diagnosis of tuberculous meningitis by polymerase chain reaction. Lancet 337:5, 1991.
62. Teoh R, Humphries MJ, Hoare RD, et al: Clinical correlation of CT

changes in 64 Chinese patients with tuberculous meningitis. J Neurol 236:48, 1989.

63. Holdiness MR: Management of tuberculosis meningitis. Drugs 39:224, 1990.
64. Mayers MM, Kaufman DM, Miller MH: Recent cases of intracranial tuberculomas. Neurology 28:256, 1978.
65. Visudhipan P, Chiemchanya S: Evaluation of rifampin in the treatment of tuberculosis meningitis in children. J Pediatr 87:983, 1975.
66. Dalli E, Quesada A, Juan G, et al: Tuberculous pericarditis as the first manifestation of acquired immunodeficiency syndrome. Am Heart J 114:905, 1987.
67. D'Cruz IA, Sengupta EE, Abrahams C, et al: Cardiac involvement, including tuberculous pericardial effusion, complicating acquired immune deficiency syndrome. Am Heart J 112:1100, 1986.
68. Larrieu AJ, Tyers GFO, Williams EH, et al: Recent experience with tuberculous pericarditis. Ann Thorac Surg 29:464, 1980.
69. Quale JM, Lipschik GY, Heurich AE: Management of tuberculous pericarditis. Ann Thorac Surg 43:653, 1987.
70. Long R, Younes M, Patton N, et al: Tuberculous pericarditis: Long term outcome in patients who received medical therapy alone. Am Heart J 117:1133, 1989.
71. Strang JIG, Gibson DG, Mitchison DA, et al: Controlled clinical trial of complete open surgical drainage and of prednisolone in treatment of tuberculous pericardial effusion in Transkei. Lancet 2:759, 1988.
72. Snider D: Pregnancy and tuberculosis. Chest 86:10S, 1984.
73. Centers for Disease Control: Tuberculosis and acquired immunodeficiency syndrome—New York City. MMWR 36:785, 1987.
74. Modilevsky T, Sattler FR, Barnes PF: Mycobacterial disease in patients with human immunodeficiency virus infection. Arch Intern Med 149:2201, 1989.
75. Kramer F, Modilevsky T, Waliany AR, et al: Delayed diagnosis of tuberculosis in patients with human immunodeficiency virus infection. Am J Med 89:451, 1990.
76. American Thoracic Society/Centers for Disease Control: Mycobacterioses and the acquired immunodeficiency syndrome. Am Rev Respir Dis 136:492, 1987.
77. Timpe A, Runyon EH: The relationship of "atypical" acid-fast bacteria to human disease. J Lab Clin Med 44:202, 1954.
78. Runyon EH: Anonymous mycobacteria in pulmonary disease. Med Clin North Am 43:273, 1959.
79. O'Brien RJ, Geiter LJ, Snider DE: The epidemiology of nontuberculous mycobacterial diseases in the United States. Am Rev Respir Dis 135:1007, 1987.
80. American Thoracic Society: Diagnosis and treatment of disease caused by nontuberculous mycobacteria. Am Rev Respir Dis 142:940, 1990.
81. Wolinsky E: Nontuberculous mycobacteria and associated diseases. Am Rev Respir Dis 119:107, 1979.
82. Woods GL, Washington JA II: Mycobacteria other than Mycobacterium tuberculosis: Review of microbiologic and clinical aspects. Rev Infect Dis 9:275, 1987.
83. Sanders WE Jr, Horowitz EA: Other mycobacterium species. In: Mandell GL, Douglas RG Jr, Bennett JE (eds): Principles and Practice of Infectious Diseases. 3rd ed. New York, Churchill Livingstone, p 1914, 1990.
84. Rosenzweig DY, Schlueter DP: Spectrum of clinical disease in pulmonary infection with Mycobacterium avium-intracellulare. Rev Infect Dis 3:1046, 1981.
85. Zakowski P, Fligiel S, Berlin OGW, et al: Disseminated Mycobacterium avium-intracellulare infection in homosexual men dying of acquired immunodeficiency. JAMA 248:2980, 1982.
86. Macher AM, Kovacs JA, Gill V, et al: Bacteremia due to Mycobacterium avium-intracellulare in the acquired immunodeficiency syndrome. Ann Intern Med 99:782, 1983.
87. Horsburgh CR Jr, Mason UG, Farhi DC, et al: Disseminated infection with Mycobacterium avium-intracellulare. Medicine 64:36, 1985.
88. Horsburgh CR Jr, Selik RM: The epidemiology of disseminated nontuberculous mycobacterial infection in the acquired immunodeficiency syndrome (AIDS). Am Rev Respir Dis 139:4, 1989.
89. Wallace JM, Hannah JB: Mycobacterium avium complex infection in patients with the acquired immunodeficiency syndrome. Chest 93:926, 1988.
90. Agins BD, Berman DS, Spicehandler D, et al: Effect of combined therapy with ansamycin, clofazimine, ethambutol, and isoniazid for Mycobacterium avium infection in patients with AIDS. J Infect Dis 159:784, 1989.
91. Hoy J, Mijch A, Sandland M, et al: Quadruple-drug therapy for Mycobacterium avium-intracellulare bacteremia in AIDS patients. J Infect Dis 161:801, 1990.
92. McGeady SJ, Murphey SA: Disseminated Mycobacterium kansasii infection. Clin Immunol Immunopathol 20:87, 1981.
93. Bennett C, Vardiman J, Golomb H: Disseminated atypical mycobacterial infection in patients with hairy cell leukemia. Am J Med 80:891, 1986.
94. Lillo M, Orengo S, Cernoch P, et al: Pulmonary and disseminated infection due to Mycobacterium kansasii: A decade of experience. Rev Infect Dis 12:760, 1990.
95. Sherer R, Sable R, Sonnenberg M, et al: Disseminated infection with Mycobacterium kansasii in the acquired immunodeficiency syndrome. Ann Intern Med 105:710, 1986.
96. Ahn CH, Wallace RJ Jr, Steele LC, et al: Sulfonamide-containing regimens for disease caused by rifampin-resistant Mycobacterium kansasii. Am Rev Respir Dis 135:10, 1987.
97. Wallace RJ Jr, Swenson JM, Silcox VA, et al: Spectrum of disease due to rapidly growing mycobacteria. Rev Infect Dis 5:657, 1983.
98. Clegg HW, Foster MT, Sanders WE Jr, et al: Infection due to organisms of the Mycobacterium fortuitum complex after augmentation mammaplasty: Clinical and epidemiologic features. J Infect Dis 147:427, 1983.
99. Bolan G, Reingold AL, Carson LA, et al: Infections with Mycobacterium chelonei in patients receiving dialysis and using processed hemodialyzers. J Infect Dis 152:1013, 1985.
100. Safranek TJ, Jarvis WR, Carson LA, et al: Mycobacterium chelonae wound infections after plastic surgery employing contaminated gentian violet skin-marking solution. N Engl J Med 317:197, 1987.
101. Hoy JF, Rolston KVI, Hopfer RL, et al: Mycobacterium fortuitum bacteremia in patients with cancer and long-term venous catheters. Am J Med 83:213, 1987.
102. Wallace RJ Jr, Musser JM, Hull SI, et al: Diversity and sources of rapidly growing mycobacteria associated with infections following cardiac surgery. J Infect Dis 159:708, 1989.
103. Wenger JD, Spika JS, Smithwick RW, et al: Outbreak of Mycobacterium chelonae infection associated with use of jet injectors. JAMA 264:373, 1990.
104. Swenson JM, Wallace RJ Jr, Silcox VA, et al: Antimicrobial susceptibility of five subgroups of Mycobacterium fortuitum and Mycobacterium chelonae. Antimicrob Agents Chemother 28:807, 1985.
105. Wallace RJ Jr, Bedsole G, Sumter G, et al: Activities of ciprofloxacin and ofloxacin against rapidly growing mycobacteria with demonstration of acquired resistance following single-drug therapy. Antimicrob Agents Chemother 34:65, 1990.
106. Steere AC, Corrales J, von Graevenitz A: A cluster of Mycobacterium gordonae isolates from bronchoscopy specimens. Am Rev Respir Dis 120:214, 1979.
107. Stine TM, Harris AA, Levin S, et al: A pseudoepidemic due to atypical mycobacteria in a hospital water supply. JAMA 258:809, 1987.
108. Panwalker AP, Fuhse E: Nosocomial Mycobacterium gordonae pseudoinfection from contaminated ice machines. Infect Control 7:67, 1986.
109. Kumar UN, Varkey B: Pulmonary infection caused by Mycobacterium gordonae. Br J Dis Chest 74:189, 1980.
110. McIntyre P, Blacklock Z, McCormack JG: Cutaneous infection with Mycobacterium gordonae. J Infect 14:71, 1987.
111. Kurnik PB, Padmanabh U, Bonatsos C, et al: Mycobacterium gordonae as a human hepato-peritoneal pathogen, with a review of the literature. Am J Med Sci 285:45, 1983.
112. Chan J, McKitrick JC, Klein RS: Mycobacterium gordonae in the acquired immunodeficiency syndrome. Ann Intern Med 101:400, 1984.
113. Turner DM, Ramsey PG, Ojemann GA, et al: Disseminated Mycobacterium gordonae infection associated with glomerulonephritis. West J Med 142:391, 1985.
114. Simor AE, Salit IE, Vellend H: The role of Mycobacterium xenopi in human disease. Am Rev Respir Dis 129:435, 1984.
115. Contreras MA, Cheung OT, Sanders DE, et al: Pulmonary infection with nontuberculous mycobacteria. Am Rev Respir Dis 137:149, 1988.
116. Warren NG, Body BA, Silcox VA, et al: Pulmonary disease due to Mycobacterium malmoense. J Clin Microbiol 20:245, 1984.
117. Maloney JM, Gregg CR, Stephens DS, et al: Infections caused by Mycobacterium szulgai in humans. Rev Infect Dis 9:1120, 1987.
118. Bell RC, Higuchi JH, Donovan WN, et al: Mycobacterium simiae. Clinical features and follow-up of twenty-four patients. Am Rev Respir Dis 127:35, 1983.
119. Rogers PL, Walker RE, Lane HC, et al: Disseminated Mycobacterium haemophilum in two patients with the acquired immunodeficiency syndrome. Am J Med 84:640, 1988.
120. Krisher KK, Kallay MC, Nolte FS: Primary pulmonary infection caused by Mycobacterium terrae complex. Diagn Microbiol Infect Dis 11:171, 1988.

CHAPTER 33

Candida Infections

Jack D. Sobel

Advances in medical technology, chemotherapeutics, cancer therapy, and organ transplantation have had a major impact on reducing the morbidity and mortality of life-threatening disease. Accompanying these benefits have been a variety of opportunistic infections frequently caused by relatively avirulent organisms. Critically ill patients in medical and surgical intensive care have been the prime targets for opportunistic, nosocomial fungal infections, primarily attributable to *Candida* species. Studies suggest that the problem is worsening. On a daily basis, virtually all physicians are confronted with a positive *Candida* isolate obtained from one or more of various anatomic sites. High-risk areas for *Candida* infections include neonatal, pediatric, and adult intensive care units (ICUs), both medical and surgical. *Candida* infections may involve any anatomic structure (Table 33–1); however, this chapter emphasizes clinical syndromes that the intensivist will encounter on a frequent basis.

DISSEMINATED CANDIDIASIS AND CANDIDEMIA
Epidemiology

Clinical and autopsy studies have confirmed the marked increase in the incidence of disseminated candidiasis, reflecting a parallel increase in the frequency of candidemia.[1-6] This increase is multifactorial in origin and reflects increased recognition, a growing population of patients at risk (e.g., patients undergoing complex surgical procedures and those with indwelling vascular devices), and the improved survival of patients with underlying neoplasms and collagen-vascular disease, as well as immunosuppressed patients.[7-10] Candidiasis is the cause of more case fatalities than any other systemic mycosis.[10] Between 1977 and 1981, estimates of nosocomial blood stream infections caused by *Candida* species increased in the United States from 0.5 to 1.5 per 10,000 admissions (National Nosocomial Infections Study data[3]). In some university tertiary care medical centers, *Candida* is now the third or fourth most common blood stream isolate and represents 10% of all nosocomial blood stream infections.[11] In many centers, the increase in *Candida* blood stream infections increased 10-fold between 1977 and 1984.

The economic impact of serious *Candida* infections in hospitalized patients is enormous.[11] Fungemia has been associated with considerable prolongation of the hospital length of stay (70 versus 40 days in comparable matched nonfungemic patients).

The patients at highest risk of acquiring life-threatening *Candida* infections include seriously ill postoperative patients; granulocytopenic hosts, particularly those with hematologic malignancies; and post-transplantation patients.[6] The widespread use of indwelling vascular catheters has dramatically increased the frequency of candidemia[12-14] (Table 33–2). A case-control study of candidemia in patients without hematologic disease identified the following predisposing factors: recent use of central line, use of Foley's catheter, administration of two or more antibiotics, azotemia, diarrhea, candiduria, and transfer from other hospitals.[15] Invasive candidiasis and candidemia are most frequently seen after organ transplantation, primarily bone marrow transplants, and in

patients with hematologic malignancies.[6, 16-19] In a study of nosocomial candidemia, 30% of patients with candidemia had underlying malignancies,[20] but this figure is even higher in cancer centers. Systemic candidiasis is also reported with increased frequency in burn and surgical patients[21] and in newborns. Clinical data suggest that it is possible to identify a population of patients who may become acutely susceptible

---

TABLE 33–1
CLINICAL SYNDROMES ASSOCIATED WITH *CANDIDA* INFECTIONS

Cutaneous Infection
  Metastatic nodules
  Intertrigo
  Wound infection
  Burns

Gastrointestinal Tract Infection
  Oral thrush/stomatitis
  Esophagitis
  Gastric perforation
  Peritonitis (peritoneal dialysis, nondialysis, surgical)
  Abdominal abscess
  Cholecystitis

Respiratory Tract Infection
  Laryngitis, epiglottitis
  Pneumonia (hematogenous; rarely, bronchogenic)

Vulvovaginal Infection

Candiduria
  Catheter related
  Uncatheterized

Candidemia
  Catheter associated
  Persistent
  Suppurative thrombophlebitis
  Endocarditis
  Disseminated candidiasis

Disseminated Candidiasis
  Renal
  Hepatosplenic
  Central nervous system
  Endophthalmitis
  Arthritis
  Myositis
  Osteomyelitis
  Myocarditis

Hepatosplenic Candidiasis

Chronic Mucocutaneous Candidiasis

TABLE 33–2
PATHOGENESIS OF LIFE-THREATENING *CANDIDA* INFECTIONS

Underlying Diseases	Additional Risk Factors
Organ transplantation	Intravascular lines, monitoring devices
Granulocytopenia	
Severe trauma	Corticosteroids
Hematologic malignancies	Broad-spectrum antibiotics
Solid neoplasms	Parenteral hyperalimentation
Burns	Foley's catheter
Postoperative patient	Recent chemotherapy or radiation
Diabetes mellitus	
Collagen-vascular disease	Duration of hospitalization
Acquired immunodeficiency syndrome	Previous bacterial infection
Severe pancreatitis	
Chronic renal failure	
Premature infant or neonate	

to invasive fungal infection. The two most common case profiles that have emerged are (1) the debilitated surgical patient after 1 or 2 weeks of hospitalization, who has received broad-spectrum antibiotics and prolonged parenteral hyperalimentation and has undergone surgical procedures (often more than one) that have violated the integrity of the alimentary canal; (2) the granulocytopenic patient with underlying hematologic malignancy, who has received mucosa-disrupting chemotherapy and broad-spectrum antibiotics during a prolonged period of severe neutropenia.

In the febrile neutropenic patient who dies of sepsis, there exists a 20 to 40% chance of finding evidence of invasive candidiasis at autopsy.[17] Bodey has noted that 21% of fatal infections in leukemic patients were the result of invasive fungal disease, compared with 13 and 6% in patients with lymphoma and solid tumors, respectively.[1, 2] Systemic candidiasis was described in 20 to 30% of patients undergoing bone marrow transplantation.[6, 22, 23] Epidemiologic studies are hampered because most septic patients dying in an ICU do not undergo an autopsy examination. Autopsy studies indicate that invasive candidiasis is frequently not diagnosed and treated before the patient's death.[24]

Although oral thrush and Candida esophagitis are extremely common in patients with acquired immunodeficiency syndrome (AIDS), candidemia and disseminated candidiasis have been extremely infrequent findings. However, there have been more recent anecdotal reports of candidemia in AIDS patients. This increased prevalence of candidemia is the consequence of increased use of Hickman's catheters and parenteral hyperalimentation. Other contributing factors include zidovudine-induced neutropenia and other causes of severe granulocytopenia.

Microbiology

The numerous species of Candida include C. albicans, C. tropicalis, C. pseudotropicalis, C. guilliermondii, C. krusei, C. parapsilosis, and C. stellatoidea and the related species Torulopsis glabrata. C. albicans and C. tropicalis account for approximately 80% of yeast species isolated from patients with invasive candidiasis. Another rarely found isolate is C. lusitaniae, important because of a high frequency of amphotericin B resistance that may also develop during therapy.[25, 26] Candida species are mostly confined to the human and animal reservoir; however, they are frequently recovered from the hospital environment, including food, counter tops, air-conditioning vents, floors, respirators, and medical personnel. Candida species rarely colonize normal skin but rapidly colonize damaged skin and breaks in the integument.[27] Oropharyngeal colonization is found in 30 to 55% of healthy, young adults, and Candida may be detected in fecal flora in 40 to 65% of subjects.[26] The dominant pathogen at all anatomic sites remains C. albicans, although there has been a marked increase in the isolation of C. tropicalis from the blood stream of granulocytopenic patients with hematologic malignancies.[28] At Harper Hospital, Detroit Medical Center, C. tropicalis was identified in blood cultures from leukemic patients more frequently than was C. albicans (57% vs. 30%) from 1986 to 1988.[29] C. parapsilosis is almost invariably associated with intravascular lines, particularly when used for parenteral hyperalimentation and transducer monitors. Although C. parapsilosis fungemia is associated with a lower mortality than that for other Candida species, this is a result of the involvement of patients who are less ill and who have an underlying disease that has a more favorable prognosis. In contrast, T. glabrata fungemia is associated with a higher mortality rate. Komshian and coworkers reported a 100% mortality in 12 patients with T. glabrata fungemia.[29] A high mortality was also associated with blood cultures positive for

more than one fungal species simultaneously (i.e., polymicrobial fungemia). Surveillance cultures for fungi usually identify C. albicans from at least one anatomic site in most patients undergoing bone marrow transplantation, and the predictive value of a single positive surveillance culture is relatively low. In contrast, positive surveillance cultures of C. tropicalis in this population may have a higher predictive value.[30]

The lack of a simple, reliable typing system to identify more specifically the numerous strains of C. albicans has hampered the understanding of the exact source and spread of C. albicans isolates. Nevertheless, it is apparent that the majority of serious infections are nosocomial, and it is relatively rare for patients to be admitted with initial blood cultures positive for Candida species. Several reports of clusters or local miniepidemics related to C. albicans or one of the non-albicans species have been traced to a common source in the ICU (e.g., contaminated transducer or intravenous fluid).[12, 13] The availability of DNA homology techniques and gene probes allows the implementation of strain typing and the generation of useful epidemiologic studies.[31, 32] The first molecular techniques used restriction enzyme analysis of genomic DNA; however, given the large size of Candida chromosomal DNA, additional methods using pulsed-field gel electrophoresis provide better discrimination among strains of C. albicans.[33] Investigators in France described a marked change in the distribution of serotypes of C. albicans associated with AIDS, with increased prevalence of serotype B.[34] However, more reliable typing methods indicate that the distribution frequency of Candida strains is similar in patients with and without AIDS.[35]

Host Defense Mechanisms

The intact skin constitutes a highly effective, impermeable barrier to Candida penetration. Disruption of the skin such as that occurring with burns, wounds, and ulceration permits invasion by the opportunistic, colonizing organisms. Similarly, indwelling intravascular devices provide an efficient conduit for bypassing the skin barrier.[12] Intact epithelial and mucosal surfaces are relatively resistant to fungal invasion. The major defense mechanisms operative at the mucosal level, tolerating colonization but preventing invasion, include the normal protective bacterial flora and cell-mediated immunity. The importance of the latter mechanism is highlighted by chronic mucocutaneous candidiasis, with a congenital Candida antigen-specific immunodeficiency, manifested by chronic, intractable, and severe mucocutaneous infection; however, candidemia and disseminated candidiasis are extremely rare because of an intact humoral and phagocytic system. Similarly, T helper cell deficiency in AIDS manifests uniquely as a profound predisposition to frequent and severe mucosal surface candidiasis. How the intact cell-mediated immune system prevents Candida mucositis and mucosal invasion is still unclear.

The critical defense mechanism in preventing Candida invasion of deep tissues, limiting candidemia, and preventing dissemination is an effective phagocytic system.[36, 37] Leukocyte failure includes quantitative reduction, usually as a result of acute leukemia, bone marrow failure, or chemotherapy and marrow transplantation. Both polymorphonuclear and monocytic cells can ingest and kill both blastospores and hyphal phases of Candida, and this process is enhanced by serum complement and specific immunoglobulins.[36] Similarly, severe leukocyte qualitative dysfunction (e.g., as in chronic granulomatous disease) is associated with disseminated and often life-threatening candidal infection. Myeloperoxidase deficiency also results in increased susceptibility to invasive infection.

Pathogenesis

The first step in the development of *Candida* infections is colonization of the oropharynx and gastrointestinal tract.[23] Numerous factors are associated with increased colonization[27, 36, 38, 39] (see Table 33–2). Once the colonized but intact oropharyngeal mucosal surface is disrupted by chemotherapy or trauma, organisms that have already increased in number penetrate injured areas and gain access to the blood stream.[40] Although the blastospore phase of *Candida* can penetrate intact mucosal cells, the relatively more virulent hyphal phase is more frequently associated with tissue invasion.[40, 41]

It has been noted that a frequent route of blood stream invasion appears to be via indwelling catheters.[12, 13, 29] This route is thought to account for at least 20% of cases of candidemia.[3] In prospective studies, fungemia has been found in 10 to 20% of all patients receiving intravenous hyperalimenation by way of central replaceable lines.[12, 41–45] Hyperalimentation constitutes an independent risk factor adding to the risk of the central intravenous line. The risk of fungemia is increased with prolonged duration of catheterization, which also increases the risk of local phlebitis, occasionally progressing to suppurative thrombosis that may not only occlude the blood vessel but also cause persistent candidemia long after the removal of the central intravascular catheter.[46] The latter is a particular problem in victims of severe burns.

In contrast, the use of Hickman's and Broviac's catheters is only rarely the source of candidemia, but the intravascular portion may become colonized and infected as the result of candidemia originating from a second, independent focus or portal of entry. Fungal invasion from colonized wounds rarely occurs,[45] except in patients with extensive burns. Similarly, the respiratory tract, although frequently colonized, is not a common site for *Candida* invasion and rarely is a source of dissemination. Tissue invasion and candidemia are further facilitated by factors that alter the host's immune status (Table 33–3). Several authors have noted the association among numbers of sites colonized with *Candida*, quantitative cultures obtained from these sites, and the occurrence of invasive *Candida* infections in granulocytopenic patients.[47] After invasion of the blood stream, efficient phagocytic cell function rapidly clears the invading organisms, especially when the inoculum is small. More prolonged candidemia is likely in granulocytopenic patients, especially when diagnosis and treatment are delayed, which results in an increased risk of hematogenous spread and metastatic seeding of multiple visceral sites, primarily kidney, eyes, liver, skin, and central nervous system. Manifestations of metastatic infection may be apparent immediately or may be delayed several weeks or even months, long after predisposing factors (e.g., granulocytopenia) have resolved.

A third route for blood stream invasion is persorption via the gastrointestinal wall after massive colonization with a high titer of organisms that pass directly into the blood stream.[40, 45] Candidemia and disseminated candidiasis almost invariably follow serious bacterial infections often characterized by bacteremia. Although simultaneous bacteremia and fungemia are occasionally reported and are associated with a high mortality, the sequential relationship between the two infections is unexplained. Antimicrobial agents have no direct effect on the invasive capacity of *Candida*, but they do enhance mucosal and skin colonization.

In contrast to candidemia and systemic candidiasis, a more localized form of visceral candidiasis involving only the liver or spleen is frequently observed. This syndrome has been called focal hepatic (hepatosplenic) candidiasis and is most often seen in association with acute myeloblastic leukemia, particularly after cytosine arabinoside therapy.[48] Hepatic involvement is thought to follow gastrointestinal ulceration induced by chemotherapy in individuals with bowel colonization by *Candida* species, and the yeast reach the liver via the portal venous system. Autopsy studies indicate that the focal visceral syndrome is not nearly as focal as originally thought, with more than 50% of cases exhibiting disseminated, extrahepatosplenic, visceral involvement.[2, 8]

Clinical Manifestations
Candidemia

Candidemia presents a diverse clinical picture.[36] On the one hand, the clinical picture may be indistinguishable from that of bacteremia with acute onset of high fever, chills, rigors, tachycardia, tachypnea, and hypotension rapidly progressing to frank septic shock. Conversely, low-grade fever may be the only manifestation. Often, the clinical features are overshadowed by the manifestations of the underlying disease. The clinical picture is also determined by the duration of fungemia and the concentration of the circulating organisms. The candidemia persists for a variable period depending on the underlying cause and portal of entry, and thereafter the clinical features of candidemia merge with and are replaced by those of disseminated candidiasis. The outcome of candidemia is variable. It frequently resolves spontaneously (especially when it results from a removable source) and no further clinical sequelae occur. However, the patient may succumb to overwhelming sepsis, or focal metastatic invasive disease may develop even if the patient survives the initial fungemia.

Disseminated Candidiasis

Similarly, in disseminated candidiasis there is no characteristic constellation of clinical signs and symptoms. Often, the only manifestation is persistent fever in a deteriorating patient who is unresponsive to antibacterial chemotherapy and who has negative blood culture results. Because many patients have pre-existing bacteremia, it is difficult to determine when the fungal infection began. Any fever pattern is possible, including hypothermia.[16] The presence of oral thrush or esophagitis is not a reliable indicator of disseminated candidiasis.

Cutaneous Lesions

Skin lesions are most frequently encountered in leukemic individuals. Approximately 10% of such patients with sys-

---

TABLE 33–3

HOST DEFENSE MECHANISMS AGAINST *CANDIDA* INFECTION

Defense Mechanism	Defect Altering Immune Status
Intact mucocutaneous barriers	Burns, ulceration, wounds, intravascular catheter
Phagocytic cells	Granulocytopenia
Polymorphonuclear leukocytes	Chronic granulomatous disease
Monocytic cells	Myeloperoxidase deficiency
Complement	Hypocomplementemia
Immunoglobulins	Hypogammaglobulinemia
Cell-mediated immunity	Chronic mucocutaneous candidiasis
	Cyclosporine
	Corticosteroids
	AIDS
Mucocutaneous protective bacterial flora	Broad spectrum antibiotics

temic disease have cutaneous lesions, usually firm, raised nodules, pink to red, and widely variable in number. *Candida* organisms are identified in the dermis by histologic studies and are cultured from about half of the biopsy samples.[17] Myalgias, often severe and accompanied by tender muscles, are frequently seen and tend to be most pronounced in the lower extremities; they are often found in association with cutaneous dissemination. Diagnosis of myositis is made by muscle biopsy.[49]

Endophthalmitis

Of all the targets of hematogenous *Candida* spread, a unique site is involvement of the eyes.[50] Endophthalmitis is usually unilateral and may be asymptomatic or present with acute visual abnormalities from scotomata to complete blindness. The importance of endophthalmitis is the high correlation between eye lesions and multiorgan infection. The most common physical finding on fundal examination is that of single or multiple, fluffy white exudates that represent small abscesses rather than infarcts and result from the focal infiltration of leukocytes attempting to localize the invading organisms. Accordingly, neutropenic patients lacking leukocytes rarely have identifiable eye lesions.[50, 51] In prospective studies of surgical patients undergoing parenteral hyperalimentation, eye lesions were identified in 10 to 15% of the patients,[52] and in one series, 11 of 21 candidemic patients had detectable eye lesions.[53]

Central Nervous System Involvement

Candida species constitute the most frequent cause of central nervous system mycosis.[54] As with other visceral sites of hematogenous infection, the incidence of central nervous system candidiasis has increased markedly in more recent years and often occurs simultaneously with systemic candidiasis at other active sites. Central nervous system involvement includes meningitis, diffuse cerebritis with micro- and macroabscesses, mycotic aneurysms, fungus ball formation, and parenchymal hemorrhage. A variable clinical and cerebrospinal fluid picture is found, depending on the site of infection. Lipton has emphasized the lack of specificity of findings that develop in already critically ill patients, and the fungal manifestations are mistakenly thought to represent cerebrovascular accidents.[54] Not surprisingly, the diagnosis is frequently delayed, and this is reflected in the poor response to chemotherapy. In meningitis, low numbers of organisms are found in the cerebrospinal fluid, and less than half the patients have yeast identified on Gram's stain. One third of the patients have hypoglycorrhachia, and a variable cell count is found.

Endocarditis

Endocarditis caused by *Candida* species is uncommon and is suggested by persistent candidemia.[55] A relatively characteristic feature of left-sided endocarditis is the formation of large vegetations and thus large emboli that tend to occlude proximal peripheral arteries (e.g., femoral artery). Fortunately, fungal endocarditis of natural heart valves is rare, and the majority of cases are associated with prosthetic heart valves that require surgical replacement and antifungal chemotherapy to achieve cure. For unexplained reasons, only 50% of patients with autopsy-proven *Candida* endocarditis were found to have positive cultures. Similar results were obtained in the animal model of experimental *Candida* endocarditis.[36]

Pulmonary Involvement

In spite of the frequency with which *Candida* is cultured from the sputum and from lower respiratory tract secretions obtained during bronchoscopy (25%), bronchogenic spread of *Candida* species to the lung parenchyma and resultant pneumonia are inexplicably rare. Occasionally, after aspiration in debilitated subjects, bronchopneumonia, cavitation, and lung abscess may occur.[56–59] More frequently but still by no means common, lung involvement occurs as the result of hematogenous spread and usually develops in severely neutropenic leukemia patients. In all circumstances, the diagnosis is difficult to establish because isolation of *Candida* from respiratory secretions is extremely common and by no means establishes the diagnosis, even when the patient fails to respond to antibacterial agents. Diagnosis of interstitial pneumonia or bronchopneumonia requires histologic confirmation obtained by biopsy. Unfortunately, all too frequently the patient is too ill to undergo a biopsy. Upper respiratory tract *Candida* infection involving the larynx or epiglottis may occur frequently. Superficially invasive bronchial infection attributable to *Candida* species has been described in AIDS patients. In general, bronchial candidiasis in patients with AIDS is usually asymptomatic, with mucosal plaques and mucositis often found coincidentally at the time of bronchoscopy for non-*Candida*–related pulmonary infiltrative disease. Occasionally, bronchogenic spread of *Candida* organisms may result in pneumonia in patients with AIDS.

Musculoskeletal Involvement

Candida septic arthritis is uncommon, usually involves the knee joint, and, as with the majority of disseminated sites of *Candida* infection, is usually caused by *C. albicans* and results from hematogenous spread.[60] Most patients have underlying hematologic malignancy, trauma, and chronic articular disease. Diagnosis is made by aspiration and culture of the purulent synovial fluid. *Candida* osteomyelitis is similarly reported, with increased frequency in the past decade. The pattern of spread is hematogenous, resembling that of bacterial osteomyelitis,[61] and *Candida* osteomyelitis similarly presents with pain and local tenderness. Not infrequently, acute osteomyelitis manifests weeks or months after discharge from hospital. In adults the most frequent site of infection is the vertebral region, and bone biopsy is required not only to confirm the diagnosis but also to identify the microbial cause. Other sites of disseminated infection include pericardium, liver, and spleen.

Nosocomial Candidemia

Crude mortality rates associated with nosocomial candidemia range from 13 to 90%, with a median of 55%.[11, 14, 21, 28, 29] Several studies indicated the absence of a trend to lower mortality in the past decade. The single dominant factor influencing mortality is the severity of the underlying disease. In a case-control study, Wey and coworkers analyzed nosocomial candidemia in their institution and reported an overall crude mortality of 57% and an attributable mortality rate of 38%.[11]

Diagnosis and Management

Although a single positive blood culture for *Candida* species may reflect contamination, it is never appropriate to assume this in the neutropenic patient, for whom the positive predictive value of a single positive blood culture exceeds 80% and failure to act on this information may have disastrous sequelae. A similar approach appears reasonable in other severely immunocompromised patients and other high-risk patients, especially after major surgery. Likewise, although candidemia may be transient and uncomplicated, it is equally inappropriate to disregard a single positive blood culture until the patient has been carefully evaluated. The initial evaluation of the candidemic patient includes determining whether the patient is febrile or septic, has clinical evidence of disseminated disease, is neutropenic, is an immunocompromised host, and has had recent surgery.[23] Consideration should be given to the number of positive blood cultures in relation to the number of blood cultures obtained. It is apparent that the more cultures that are positive, the greater the significance of this finding. When necessary, additional blood cultures should be done before initiation of antifungal therapy.

Initial management should include removal of possible foci of infection, including removal of intravascular lines, and consideration should be given to removal of Hickman's catheters. In the presence of a clinical picture of sepsis or evidence of invasive or disseminated *Candida* infection, neutropenia (regardless of the number of positive blood cultures), a severely immunocompromised host, or recent surgery, and particularly when multiple blood cultures are positive, intravenous therapy with amphotericin B should be initiated. Pending the results of additional blood cultures, the only patients requiring further observation before initiating therapy are afebrile subjects without a history of recent surgery and who are not in any way immunocompromised. Even in this latter group, although subsequent blood cultures may be negative, delayed manifestations such as endophthalmitis or osteomyelitis occasionally occur several weeks later.

Once a decision has been made to initiate therapy with amphotericin B, it is apparent that a dosage regimen should be selected to rapidly achieve serum fungicidal levels of amphotericin B. This usually requires administration of amphotericin B at a dose of at least 0.3 mg/kg within 24 hours. After a test dose of 1 mg of amphotericin B, the candidemic immunocompromised patient should receive therapeutic concentrations of amphotericin B administered during 3 to 6 hours in a glucose infusion. In less ill patients, the amphotericin B can be initially given as a 5-mg infusion and repeated every 8 hours, with progressive 5-mg increments until 0.3 mg/kg has been reached. In all immunocompromised patients with candidemia, a therapeutic daily dose of 0.5 to 1.0 mg/kg should be rapidly achieved and continued until a total dose of at least 1.0 g has been administered. Many authorities recommend even higher total doses of 2 to 3 g of amphotericin B during a 4- to 6-week period. The total dose should be influenced by the duration of fungemia before therapy, the response to antifungal therapy, the underlying status of the patient, and whether evidence of disseminated visceral disease is documented. Because the clinical response rate of fungemic patients with persistent neutropenia is uniformly poor,[11, 28] attempts have been made to improve survival by earlier diagnosis and initiation of fungicidal therapy, as well as by the use of combination therapy of amphotericin B and flucytosine at 100 to 150 mg/kg/d. Combination therapy should be considered for all granulocytopenic and other severely immunocompromised patients with candidemia, although data about improved survival are still scant.

The status of combination therapy with amphotericin B and one of the azoles (ketoconazole, itraconazole, or fluconazole) remains controversial. Initial animal studies suggested lack of synergy and possible antagonism in vivo.[62] This observation has not been confirmed, and in vitro studies show an absence of antagonism. Currently, no clinical evidence exists of the beneficial effect of using this form of combination therapy.

In selecting a dosage regimen for amphotericin B or other antifungal agents, little attention has been directed at the *Candida* species involved. Similarly, antifungal therapy is not conventionally based on in vitro susceptibility tests, nor are levels of antifungal agents measured, except to prevent flucytosine toxicity. Accordingly, a great deal of empiricism remains even after a decision is made to use an antifungal agent. Not all *Candida* species are equally susceptible to the various antifungal agents, including amphotericin B. *C. tropicalis, C. lusitaniae, T. glabrata*, and *C. parapsilosis* all have higher minimal inhibitory concentrations than does *C. albicans*. Thus, it seems reasonable to use higher doses of antifungal agents for these organisms. Minimal inhibitory concentrations of amphotericin B observed with blood isolates in bone marrow transplant patients were significantly higher than those observed with blood, sputum, and skin isolates from nonimmunocompromised hosts (P < .02).[63] Moreover, the mortality rate for candidemic individuals with organisms having higher in vitro minimal inhibitory concentrations was significantly higher than that when candidemia was caused by more susceptible strains.[63] Currently, in vitro testing of fungal susceptibility to antimycotic tests are not yet standardized. Nevertheless, it should be recognized that no standard dosage regimen can be recommended. Higher doses should be considered for non-*albicans* species and in patients who are severely immunocompromised.

Catheter-Related Candidemia

The common problem of catheter-related candidemia requires special consideration. In the past, if removal of the central line and portal of *Candida* entry was accompanied by prompt defervescence and conversion of positive blood cultures to negative in a stable patient, no additional antifungal therapy was recommended.[5] In most patients, this expectant approach is usually satisfactory. However, transient catheter-associated candidemia is no longer perceived as benign as previously considered. Numerous anecdotal reports indicate that it is by no means uncommon to see patients with recent untreated transient candidemia experience devastating sequelae such as endophthalmitis, brain abscess, and the like. Komshian and coworkers, in a retrospective analysis of 135 cases of nosocomial candidemia, observed a mortality of 47% for patients with candidemia associated with intravascular catheters.[29] There is growing agreement that catheter-associated candidemia is frequently not transient and is by no means benign. Accordingly, most authorities recommend treatment of transient catheter-related candidemia with daily low doses of amphotericin B at 15 to 30 mg/d until a total dose of 250 to 500 mg has been administered.

In the recent past, candidemia in patients with indwelling Hickman/Broviac-type catheters was treated by immediate removal of the catheter and amphotericin therapy. Given the frequency of candidemia in these subjects and the fact that these subcutaneous catheters are infrequently the primary source or portal of entry for candidemia, attempts have been made to salvage these catheters in candidemic patients. No reliable method currently exists of predicting whether the catheter is infected (primary or secondary), although studies comparing quantitative cultures obtained simultaneously through the suspect catheter and from peripheral blood before and after antifungal therapy are in progress. In patients in whom the Hickman catheter is not immediately removed because of paucity of alternative vascular access sites, persistent candidemia despite therapy or relapsing candidemia mandates catheter removal.

Disseminated candidiasis merits a higher total dosage regimen of amphotericin. For visceral disease, a total dose of 1.5 to 2 g is recommended. A higher total dose is recommended for a more immunosuppressed host. As with candidemia in neutropenic subjects, combination therapy with flucytosine is now recommended for central nervous system disease and endophthalmitis (in addition to local therapy) and usually for more compromised hosts. Renal disease is most resistant to therapy.

In general, oral ketoconazole therapy has no place in the treatment of life-threatening systemic candidiasis, particularly in the compromised host. Similarly, parenteral miconazole is rarely used because of toxicity and lack of predictable efficacy. The use of the newer antifungal triazoles, intraconazole and fluconazole, is under investigation.[64] These oral and intravenous agents appear to be safer than ketoconazole and are severalfold more active in vitro. In experimental animal models of disseminated candidiasis, both agents have demonstrated encouraging results in systemic fungal disease.[65, 66] In septic arthritis, systemic amphotericin B is administered and frequent joint aspiration is performed.[60] Failure to achieve therapeutic progress should merit combination antifungal therapy or synovectomy, meniscectomy, and intra-articular amphotericin B. A similar approach with parenteral amphotericin B is required for *Candida* osteomyelitis. For both forms of soft tissue infection after completion of parenteral amphotericin B, it may be reasonable to continue oral ketoconazole or fluconazole as suppressive chemoprophylaxis for several months if the patient remains immunosuppressed.

Although not all positive blood cultures for *Candida* indicate disseminated infection,[28] a greater problem is the inability to culture *Candida* from the blood stream of patients with *Candida* sepsis or endocarditis and in the majority of patients with disseminated candidiasis (70 to 80%). This failure results in considerable delay in diagnosis and initiation of potentially lifesaving therapy. Hart and coworkers found positive blood cultures in approximately 50% of patients with disseminated candidiasis, and even lower recovery rates have been observed for leukemic individuals with autopsy evidence of dissemination.[67]

Although candiduria has been observed in 38 to 80% of patients with disseminated infection,[18, 53, 56, 67, 68] most patients with candiduria do not have renal or disseminated candidiasis.[16, 24] *C. tropicalis* in the urine in one study did have a higher positive predictive value.[47] Similarly, isolation of *Candida* from other anatomic and especially mucosal sites is unreliable in the diagnosis of systemic infection because of the high frequency of colonization by *Candida*, especially after antibiotic therapy. Nevertheless, positive cultures for *Candida* obtained from multiple body sites in high-risk neutropenic and surgical patients should at least increase the clinician's suspicion about the likelihood of *Candida* infection.[16, 69]

To date, serologic tests have been of little value in diagnosing systemic candidiasis. Numerous methods for measuring antibodies to *Candida* species have been introduced and have been particularly unhelpful in differentiating *Candida* colonization from infection.[17] Another problem has been the inability of severely immunocompromised hosts to mount a detectable humoral response.[17] Accordingly, investigators have turned to alternative methods to facilitate the early diagnosis of invasive *Candida* infections.[70] *Candida* antigen detection by using enzyme-linked immunosorbent assay techniques appears to be most promising in this regard, but these techniques still require careful investigation and they are not yet available for routine clinical use.[70, 71] Evaluation of the *Candida* antigen detection tests using latex agglutination has shown a high incidence of false-negative results.[70] Similarly, the measurement of serum arabitol levels remains controversial and unsubstantiated. The availability of the lysis-centrifugation technique for earlier and higher yield of positive blood cultures has resulted in approximately a 10 to 20% improvement in microbiologic confirmation. Thus, invasive techniques to obtain tissue biopsies and histologic confirmation continue to be the cornerstone of diagnosis.

Nevertheless, it is apparent that given the nonspecific signs and symptoms of invasive *Candida* infections and the problem of differentiating colonization from infection, clinicians are required to act definitively and early on the basis of a high index of suspicion. In the past, the majority of patients with life-threatening candidiasis died without receiving antifungal therapy.[16, 21] To be effective, therapy must be given early and, regrettably, empirically in the febrile at-risk patient. Empirical therapy with amphotericin B is especially indicated in the granulocytopenic patient with persistent fever after 4 to 7 days of antibiotic therapy, even in the absence of microbiologic confirmation. This aggressive approach, which is now widely advocated, appears to be reducing the high mortality of invasive *Candida* infection.[17,72] However, it should also be emphasized that new antifungal agents and regimens are required because of the continued high mortality still observed, particularly in patients with serious or rapidly fatal underlying disease.

Oral and Esophageal Candidiasis

Candida colonization of the oropharynx is present in 20 to 55% of normal adults and increases dramatically in debilitated and immunocompromised hosts.[67] Symptomatic thrush is readily recognized by the white exudative reaction and resultant pseudomembranous lesions on the gingival margins, tongue, and buccal mucosa. Other clinical manifestations include an atrophic reaction characterized by a diffuse or patchy erythematous lesion, as well as angular cheilosis. Management in the past relied predominantly on the use of nystatin at 200,000 to 500,000 U every 4 hours. Newer approaches with improved response include the use of clotrimazole troches of 10 mg five times daily or oral ketoconazole at 200 mg daily and fluconazole at 100 mg daily.[64]

The most common symptoms of esophageal candidiasis are dysphagia and odynophagia, often precipitated by drinking either hot or cold liquids. Symptoms of esophageal candidiasis may be absent in severely debilitated patients and those with mild infection and particularly in patients with AIDS and chronic mucocutaneous candidiasis. The disease usually affects the distal half of the esophagus. Superficial ulcerations are responsible for the characteristic radiologic feature of the disease, the "shaggy" appearance of the esophagus. When edema accompanies ulceration, a cobblestone-like appearance results. Deep ulceration may also occur, as well as disturbed motility in the form of esophageal spasm. *Candida* esophagitis may present in the absence of signs and symptoms of oral candidiasis. Moreover, although the barium swallow has conventionally been the first diagnostic procedure performed, in the majority of cases of mild to moderately severe esophagitis no abnormality is detected on barium swallow.[73] Accordingly, fiberoptic esophagoscopy has replaced radiology as the method providing the best means of diagnosing the cause and extent of esophagitis. Direct observation of the esophageal mucosa accompanied by smears and esophageal brushing and biopsy where appropriate allows the differentiation of *Candida* esophagitis from herpetic or cytomegaloviral infection, as well as from other infiltrative and inflammatory lesions (e.g., reflux esophagitis). Lesions observed include patchy white plaques surrounded by hyperemia, variable edema, ulceration, and a friable mucosa. Endoscopy and direct smear allow the quickest and most accurate means of diagnosing *Candida* esophagitis. Cultures are useful in establishing the presence of *Candida* but may be positive in the absence of clinical involvement and by themselves are not diagnostic of *Candida* esophagitis. The presence of fungal mycelia on smears or demonstration of tissue invasion by esophageal biopsy is considered diagnostic of *Candida* esophagitis. Radiologic and endoscopic findings of herpetic and cytomegaloviral esophagitis may closely resemble those of *Candida* esophagitis; these infections may frequently coexist as concomitant. Biopsy, cytologic, and culture studies facilitate the differential diagnosis.

Although mild esophagitis frequently responds to oral nystatin at 200,000 to 500,000 U (2 mL) every 2 to 4 hours, several studies have shown improved results with oral ketoconazole at 200 mg once daily[74] and clotrimazole troche of 10 mg, five times daily.[75] Ketoconazole and fluconazole have produced highly satisfactory results in more severe grades of esophagitis and are alternatives to low-dosage intravenous amphotericin B at 15 to 20 mg/d given for 10 to 14 days. The low-dose amphotericin regimen usually results in rapid clinical improvement and is associated with little risk of toxicity. Ketoconazole, although occasionally associated with hepatotoxicity, has proved both effective and safe in this condition. After eradication of *Candida* esophagitis, long-term suppressive maintenance prophylaxis with oral azoles (ketoconazole, intraconazole, and fluconazole) taken daily is recommended in patients in whom the risk factors for recurrent esophagitis persist (e.g., patients with AIDS).

HEPATOSPLENIC CANDIDIASIS

Although hepatic candidiasis is usually part of a systemic infection, a marked increase in cases has been observed in which the infection is confined to the liver, the spleen, or both.[48, 76, 77] This variant of disseminated candidiasis is unusual in its clinical presentation and is characterized by delay in diagnosis and resistance to conventional amphotericin B therapy. Most patients have underlying acute leukemia, most frequently granulocytic. Lesions in the liver include microabscesses and are probably secondary to intestinal candidal colonization, ulceration, and portal fungemia. The microabscesses may advance to granuloma formation after the granulocyte count returns to normal and occasionally the granuloma may calcify, often when the patient is in clinical remission. This process is analogous to that described for *Candida* in chronic granulomatous disease.

During the neutropenic phase, the patient presents with relatively nonspecific features of fever, right hypochondrial pain, nausea, vomiting, abdominal distention, and rarely, jaundice. Liver function tests are mildly abnormal, particularly an elevated alkaline phosphatase value. Radionuclide studies and ultrasound and computed tomography scans are usually negative, but the last is occasionally helpful.[48] Blood and liver biopsy cultures are also usually negative, and antemortem diagnosis is made by histopathologic examination of liver biopsy material. The diagnosis is often made only when the neutropenia resolves and the imaging techniques are more likely to show positive results. Several patients have failed to be cured by conventional doses of 2 to 3 g of amphotericin B and may require a total dose of two- to threefold the usual dose to achieve cure. Preliminary studies have indicated that liposomal preparations of amphotericin B appear to be highly successful in eradicating hepatic candidiasis.[78] On an optimistic note, several cases have been described in which patients failed to experience defervescence with amphotericin B but responded dramatically to fluconazole therapy.[79]

Most cases of splenic infection simultaneously involve the liver and respond to antifungal therapy. Nevertheless, occasionally patients with a large splenic abscess or multiple abscesses present with persistent fever, intermittent candidemia, and even hypersplenism.[80] Only these latter complications necessitate splenectomy.

CANDIDA PERITONITIS

In nonsurgical patients, *Candida* peritonitis has emerged as a problem in patients undergoing peritoneal dialysis, especially continuous ambulatory peritoneal dialysis.[81, 82] Risk factors include hospitalization, recent prior episodes of peritonitis, and antibacterial therapy. Clinically, *Candida* peritonitis cannot be differentiated from bacterial peritonitis except by Gram's stain and culture of dialysate. In contrast to bacterial peritonitis, therapy tends to be delayed, because clinicians usually consider a positive fungal culture as resulting from contamination. Likewise, in contrast to bacterial peritonitis, fungal infection invariably requires removal of the indwelling Tenckhoff's or other permanent catheters, together with systemic amphotericin B to achieve cure.[83] Occasionally, for patients without life-threatening disease who are metabolically and hemodynamically stable or in whom vascular access sites are scarce, and particularly in the early phases of infection, a trial of systemic antifungal therapy is reasonable before removal of the catheter. In these infrequent, selected cases, retaining the catheter is accompanied by intraperitoneal amphotericin B therapy and continued peritoneal dialysis. Even when cure is achieved, only a small percentage of patients are suitable for continued long-term peritoneal dialysis because of peritoneal fibrosis.[82, 83] Several patients undergoing continuous ambulatory peritoneal dialysis who had fungal peritonitis have been successfully treated with fluconazole, a therapy exploiting the favorable pharmacokinetic properties of this agent.[84]

It is in seriously ill surgical patients that isolation of *Candida* species after abdominal surgery has presented a diagnostic and therapeutic dilemma. Some surgeons remain unconvinced of the significance of *Candida* isolated from the peritoneal cavity, even in the presence of peritonitis.[85]

Other investigators have presented convincing data that *Candida* species have the potential as pure isolates or as part of a polymicrobial flora to cause peritonitis, intraperitoneal abscesses, and subsequent candidemia.[86, 87] Most cases of *Candida* peritonitis (>80%) are polymicrobial and usually follow perforation of peptic ulcers or are a sequela to colonic surgery, including anastomotic leaks. Clinically, *Candida* peritonitis and abscess formation are identical to those seen with bacterial process. The infection usually remains confined to the peritoneal cavity, but if treatment is inadequate with delay in initiation of systemic antifungal therapy, fungemia may result in widespread dissemination and almost predictable fatal outcome. Survival and response to amphotericin therapy are contingent on early diagnosis and initiation of parenteral therapy and usually correlate with the administration of 375 to 500 mg of amphotericin B, particularly when the infection remains confined to the peritoneal cavity. Thus, relatively low doses of daily amphotericin B (approximately 0.3 mg/kg) for 10 to 14 days are well tolerated by patients and are accompanied by good results, in contrast to a mortality of 50 to 70% for patients in whom therapy is delayed and fungemia supervenes.[86, 87] Antifungal therapy is always accompanied by appropriate surgical intervention to repair bowel perforation and drainage of suppurative collections.

Thus, the dominant clinical view today is aggressive early therapy of all intraperitoneal isolates of *Candida* species in symptomatic patients with peritonitis. The patient presenting with an abdominal abscess who undergoes surgical drainage, whose fever is promptly reduced, who remains well, and whose culture result 24 to 48 hours later reveals a polymicrobial flora including *Candida* species remains the object of controversy. In this latter context, many surgeons would observe the now afebrile, improving patient and treat expectantly.[88] Nevertheless, there is a growing acceptance of treatment of all intraperitoneal isolates of *Candida* with at least low-dosage amphotericin B, 375 to 500 mg during 7 to 14 days. Current experience with systemic azole agents (fluconazole, itraconazole, ketoconazole) in treating fungal peritonitis is limited but may be a reasonable alternative to amphotericin. The isolation of *Candida* species from wound or drainage sites, such as with a Penrose drain, is common, particularly in patients receiving antibiotics. Under these circumstances, therapy is not mandatory, but the patient requires careful evaluation.

PREVENTION OF INFECTION

Because of the frequency of nosocomial, often life-threatening *Candida* infections, numerous attempts have been made to prevent the establishment of fungal infection.[88, 91] The prognosis for these infections remains extremely poor, especially in cancer patients. Preventive strategies are best categorized by two groups of patients: cancer patients with neutropenia and critically ill surgical patients. In neutropenic patients, because candidemia most frequently originates from endogenous flora in the patient's gastrointestinal tract, attempts to prevent infection have been directed at reducing *Candida* colonization of the gastrointestinal tract.[92] Although many prophylactic regimens, including nonabsorbable polyenes (nystatin, amphotericin B) and imidazoles (ketoconazole, clotrimazole), have been shown to reduce fungal colonization of the gastrointestinal tract as well as symptomatic mucositis, evidence confirming their efficacy in preventing candidemia, disseminated candidiasis, febrile morbidity, and overall mortality has not been forthcoming.[89, 90] Reduced colonization should not be confused with fungal sterilization because the latter cannot be achieved over the long term with any antifungal regimen. Not only have the data been disappointing, but the results in neutropenic patients have been conflicting. Few studies have documented reduction of serious invasive fungal infections, and although ketoconazole at 600 mg daily appeared efficacious, the toxicity was not acceptable.[88, 90] No single regimen can be recommended at this time for prevention of invasive candidiasis, although preliminary studies with more potent triazoles (e.g., itraconazole and fluconazole) appear encouraging. Bodey reported the successful use of fluconazole at 50 mg daily in preventing oropharyngeal candidiasis in cancer patients, and additional studies with neutropenic patients are in progress.[93] However, the potential emergence of fungal strains resistant to polyenes and azoles is a real danger.[94] *T. glabrata* is prominent in causing fungal superinfection in patients receiving imidazole prophylaxis.[91]

There is remarkably little information regarding the efficacy of antimycotic prophylaxis in the seriously ill surgical patient. In the absence of neutropenia, the portal of entry in these patients is also frequently intravascular lines, as well as burn wounds and peritoneal fluid colonization after bowel perforation. In these patients, nonabsorbable antimycotics may reduce the development of oral and esophageal disease but are unlikely to reduce the incidence of fungemia related to portals of entry other than the gastrointestinal tract. In a randomized study, Slotman and Burchard showed reduced *Candida* sepsis in critically ill surgical patients receiving ketoconazole at 200 mg daily as prophylaxis.[95] As expected, multisite colonization was reduced but not prevented; however, invasive candidiasis was not observed, and reduced stay in the surgical ICU was accomplished. This result requires additional confirmation, and it must be remembered that ketoconazole must be administered in an acid environment to achieve adequate absorption. This property may be problematic in patients receiving H_2 blockers and antacids. Similarly, studies designed to identify superinfection with resistant strains are also essential.

CANDIDURIA

Candida organisms are not normally found in urine and are detected in less than 1% of clean-voided urine specimens.[96, 97] The overall prevalence of candiduria is 0.2 to 4.8%,[98] and the highest risk area for the hospitalized patient is the ICU.

The majority of patients in the ICU setting who develop candiduria have indwelling Foley's catheters. This factor significantly complicates the clinical significance of finding yeast in the urine. The likelihood of finding candiduria in catheterized patients increases with the duration of catheterization. Other risk factors include diabetes mellitus, concomitant antibiotic administration, urinary tract instrumentation, and previous bacteriuria.[98]

Candiduria may indicate contamination of the urine specimen, may reflect benign saprophytic colonization of the catheter and lower urinary tract, or may indicate true invasive infection of the upper and/or lower urinary tract. In the ICU, the majority of patients with candiduria are asymptomatic and have no symptoms referable to the urinary tract, although invasive cystitis occasionally results in pain, discomfort, and hematuria in the catheterized patient. In noncatheterized subjects, true *Candida* cystitis is rare and presents with typical symptoms of frequency of micturition, dysuria, suprapubic pain, and the like. Rare complications of bladder infection include pneumaturia and fungus ball formation in the bladder lumen. Occasionally, retrograde ascending infection occurs, resulting in renal parenchymal infection or pyelonephritis; this is most likely to occur in the presence of obstruction. Renal invasion by *Candida* species (renal candidiasis) is, however, most often the result of hematogenous spread complicating candidemia, as part of the syndrome of disseminated candidiasis. The kidney is the most frequently involved organ in systemic candidiasis (90%).[99]

Renal candidiasis, regardless of the route of infection, is frequently asymptomatic, but clinical manifestations include fever and unexplained deterioration in renal function, as well as the classic features of acute pyelonephritis. Complications of renal involvement include intrarenal and perinephric abscess formation. Upper urinary tract infection may also be complicated by the development of fungus balls in the kidney drainage system, particularly when associated with renal papillary necrosis, which may act as a nidus for fungus ball formation. The development of fungus balls is more common in the presence of partial or complete bladder or ureteral obstruction and may act as an independent mechanism of ureteral or pelvic outflow obstruction, further reducing renal function.

Candiduria is also frequently observed in patients with internal stents placed to overcome severe ureteric obstruction. As with patients with indwelling Foley's catheters, most such patients are asymptomatic, but complicated ascending symptomatic infections occasionally occur. Similarly, critically ill subjects with obstructive uropathy in whom nephrostomy tubes are inserted for external urinary diversion frequently develop candiduria.

Management

Although candiduria in a hospitalized patient may reflect improper collection and sample processing and is most often the result of catheter colonization, this finding may nevertheless be an important clue as to the cause of overwhelming sepsis, including renal involvement with *Candida* or invasive bladder disease. Therefore, all cases require careful evaluation.

Management of candiduria requires localization of the source of the candiduria and distinguishing contamination or colonization from true infection. In the asymptomatic patient or one in whom fever alone is present, no clinical picture or pattern accurately localizes the site of *Candida* infection. Serologic tests are not at all useful in localization, and in contrast to bacterial infections the antibody-coating test is of no localizing value, as *Candida* species are often antibody coated regardless of the site of infection.

Blood cultures, when positive, are useful in identifying renal candidiasis but are positive in less than half the patients with metastatic renal infection. Similarly, radiographic techniques are of little value in localization. Quantitative urine cultures for *Candida* species are of limited value. A colony count of less than 10^4 colony-forming units/mL mitigates against renal candidiasis;[96] however, colony counts tend to be diagnostically invalid in the presence of an indwelling Foley's catheter because it may be heavily colonized and accompanied by titers higher than 10^5 colony-forming units/mL. In the absence of an indwelling catheter, a titer higher than 10^4 colony-forming units/mL obtained from a midstream urine specimen is highly suggestive of infection rather than colonization. Although previously considered useful, the presence of pseudohyphae or hyphae or examination of the urine by Gram's stain is of no value in localizing the site of infection or in differentiating between colonization and infection. Of considerable value when present is the finding on urine microscopy of hyaline renal tubular casts containing *Candida* organisms, particularly with pseudohyphae. Bladder irrigation or washout with amphotericin B (50 µg/mL) not only serves as adequate therapy for bladder infection in the catheterized patient but is also a useful diagnostic localization test. Candiduria persisting after 5 days of daily bladder washouts strongly suggests renal candidiasis. Diagnosis and evaluation of candiduria require consideration of multiple factors; particularly, the recognition of renal candidiasis includes attention to factors predisposing to disseminated candidiasis. Another clue in the diagnosis of renal candidiasis is unexplained renal function deterioration. In the catheterized patient with persistent candiduria after bladder irrigation, radiologic studies should be performed to rule out a fungus ball in the renal drainage system. Intravenous pyelography misses at least one third of ureteric fungus balls, compared with retrograde pyelography, which is more reliable for detecting the filling defects.[100]

Management of asymptomatic candiduria in the catheterized patient for whom there is no indication of either renal candidiasis or renal obstruction requires only change of the indwelling catheter and observation.[68] Symptomatic cystitis requires therapeutic bladder washouts or irrigation with amphotericin B. In the presence of a nephrostomy tube or urinary stents, local irrigation with amphotericin B can be performed through the nephrostomy tube. Successful eradication of lower urinary tract *Candida* infection has also been reported with 5-fluorocytosine, oral ketoconazole,[101] and a single intravenous dose (0.3 mg/kg) of amphotericin B.[98] Fluconazole achieves considerably higher concentrations in the urine than ketoconazole and offers greater assurance for clinical success in lower urinary tract candidiasis. The excellent safety profile and clinical efficacy of fluconazole in eradicating candiduria have resulted in a situation in which therapeutic advances have overtaken the standard diagnostic and localization methods, allowing for potential abuse in fluconazole prescription for every canduric patient.

In patients with proven or suspected renal candidiasis, parenteral amphotericin B is required and usually prescribed in doses generally used for systemic candidiasis (i.e., 0.5 to 0.7 mg/kg/d and a total dose of 1 to 2 g), usually administered during several weeks. Some authors have reported anecdotal experience with successful eradication of renal candidiasis with considerably lower dosage regimens of amphotericin B not exceeding 140 mg and divided over 5 successive days.[102] If renal candidiasis represents one of many sites of *Candida* infection as the result of candidemia, the role of low-dosage abbreviated therapy with amphotericin B remains to be proved and should be viewed in this light. Fungus balls obstructing the ureters or renal pelvis usually require surgical removal.

REFERENCES

1. Bodey GP, Bolwar R, Fainstain V: Infectious complications in leukemic patients. Semin Hematol 19:193, 1982.
2. Bodey GP: Candidiasis in cancer patients. Am J Med 77(suppl 4D): 13, 1986.
3. Centers for Disease Control: National Nosocomial Infections Study Report. Annual Summary 1979. Atlanta, Centers for Disease Control, March 1982.
4. Hammerman KJ, Powell KE, Tosh FE: The incidence of hospitalized cases of systemic mycotic infections. Sabouraudia 12:33, 1974.
5. Young RC, Bennett JE, Geelhoed G, et al: Fungemia with compromised host resistance: A study of 70 cases. Ann Intern Med 80:605, 1974.
6. Meyers JD: Fungal infections in bone marrow transplant patients. Semin Oncol 17:10, 1990.
7. MacMillan BG, Law EJ, Holder IA: Experience with *Candida* infections in the burn patient. Arch Surg 104:509, 1972.
8. Bodey GP, Rodriguez V, Chang HY, et al: Fever and infection in leukemic patients. A study of 494 consecutive patients. Cancer 41:1610, 1978.
9. Rifkind D, Marchioro TL, Schreck SA, et al: Systemic fungal infections complicating renal transplantation and immunosuppressive therapy: The clinical, microbiological, neurological and pathological features. Am J Med 43:28, 1967.
10. Reingold AL, Lu XD, Plikaytis BD, et al: Systemic mycoses in the United States, 1980–1982. J Med Vet Mycol 24:433, 1986.
11. Wey SB, Mora M, Pfaller MA, et al: Hospital-acquired candidemia. The attributable mortality and excess length of stay. Arch Intern Med 148:2642, 1988.
12. Band JD, Maki DG: Infections caused by arterial catheters used for hemodynamic monitoring. Am J Med 67:735, 1979.
13. Rose HD: Venous catheter-associated candidemia. Am J Med 275:265, 1978.
14. Harvey RL, Myers JP: Nosocomial candidemia in a large community teaching hospital. Arch Intern Med 147:2117, 1987.
15. Bross J, Talbot GH, Maislin G, et al: Risk factors for nosocomial candidemia: A case control study in adults without leukemia. Am J Med 87:614, 1989.
16. Bodey GP: Fungal infections complicating acute leukemia. J Chronic Dis 19:667, 1966.
17. Bodey GP, Fainstein V: Systemic candidiasis. In: Bodey GP, Fainstein V (eds): Candidiasis. New York, Raven Press, p 135, 1985.
18. DeGregorio MW, Lee WM, Linker CA, et al: Fungal infections in patients with acute leukemia. Am J Med 73:543, 1982.
19. Krick JA, Remington JS: Opportunistic invasive fungal infections in patients with leukaemia and lymphoma. Clin Haematol 5:249, 1976.
20. Miller PJ, Wenzel RP: Etiologic organisms as independent predictors of death and morbidity associated with bloodstream infections. J Infect Dis 153:471, 1987.
21. Gaines JD, Remington JS: Disseminated candidiasis in the surgical patient. Surgery 72:730, 1972.
22. Winston DW, Gale RP, Meyer DV, et al: Infectious complications of human bone marrow transplantation. J Clin Invest 58:1, 1979.
23. Ellis CA, Spivack ML: The significance of candidemia. Ann Intern Med 67:511, 1967.
24. Myerowitz RL, Pazin GJ, Allen CM: Disseminated candidiasis. Changes in incidence, underlying diseases, and pathology. Am J Clin Pathol 68:29, 1977.
25. Hadfield TL, Smith MB, Winn RE, et al: Mycoses caused by *Candida lusitaniae*. Rev Infect Dis 5:1006, 1987.
26. Pappaginnis D, Collins MB, Hecter R, et al: Development of resistance to amphotericin B in *Candida lusitaniae* infecting a human. Antimicrob Agents Chemother 2:123, 1979.
27. Louria DB: Pathogenesis of candidiasis. Antimicrob Agents Chemother 5:417, 1965.
28. Meunier-Carpentier F, Kiehn TE, Armstrong D: Fungemia in the immunocompromised host: Changing patterns, antigenemia, high mortality. Am J Med 71:363, 1981.
29. Komshian SV, Uwaydah AK, Sobel JD, et al: Fungemia caused by

Candida species and *Torilopsis glabrata* in hospitalized patients. Frequency, characteristics and evaluation of factors influencing outcome. Rev Infect Dis 3:379, 1989.

30. Wingard JR, Merz WG, Saral R: *Candida tropicalis*: A major pathogen in immunocompromised patients. Ann Intern Med 91:539, 1979.

31. Burnie JP, Matthews R, Lee W: Four outbreaks of nosocomial systemic candidiasis. Epidemiol Infect 99:201 211, 1987.

32. Fox BC, Mobley HLT, Wade JC: The use of a DNA probe for epidemiological studies of candidiasis in immunocompromised hosts. J Infect Dis 159:488, 1989.

33. Vazquez J, Beckley A, Sobel JD, et al: Comparison of restriction enzyme analysis versus pulsed-field gradient gel electrophoresis as a typing system for *Candida albicans*. J Clin Microbiol 29:962, 1991.

34. Drouhet E, Dupont B: Mycoses in AIDS patients: An overview. In: Third International Symposium on Mycoses in AIDS, Paris, November 21, 1989. New York, Plenum Publishing, p 27, 1990

35. Whelan WL, Kirsch DR, Kwon-Chung KJ, et al: *Candida albicans* in patients with the acquired immunodeficiency syndrome: Absence of a novel of hypervirulent strain. J Infect Dis 162:513, 1990.

36. Edwards JE, Lehrer RI, Stiehm ER, et al: Severe candidal infections: Clinical perspective, immune defense mechanisms, and current concepts of therapy. Ann Intern Med 89:91, 1978.

37. Letiner RI, Cline MJ: Leukocyte candidacidal activity and resistance to systemic candidiasis in patients with cancer. Cancer 27:1211, 1971.

38. Ruddell WSJ, Axon ATR, Findlay JM, et al: Effect of cimetidine on the gastric bacterial flora. Lancet 1:672, 1980.

39. Seelig MS: The role of antibiotics in the pathogenesis of candida infections. Am J Med 40:887, 1966.

40. Krause W, Matheis H, Wulf K: Fungemia and funguria after oral administration of *Candida albicans*. Lancet 1:598, 1969.

41. Rogers TJ, Balish E: Immunity to *Candida albicans*. Microbiol Rev 44:660, 1980.

42. Currie CR, Quie PG: Fungal septicemia in patients receiving parenteral hyperalimentation. N Engl J Med 285:1221, 1971.

43. Ashcroft KW, Leape LL: *Candida* sepsis compicating parenteral feeding. JAMA 212:454, 1970.

44. Montgomerie JZ, Edwards JE: Association of infection due to *Candida albicans* with intravenous hyperalimentation. J Infect Dis 137:197, 1978.

45. Stone HH, Kolb LD, Currie CA, et al: *Candida* sepsis: Pathogenesis and principles of treatment. Ann Surg 179:697, 1974.

46. Walsh TJ, Bustamente CI, Vlahoir D, et al: Candidal suppurative peripheral thrombophlebitis: Recognition, prevention and management. Infect Control 7:16, 1986.

47. Sandford GR, Merz WG, Wingard JR, et al: The value of fungal surveillance cultures as predictors of systemic fungal infections. J Infect Dis 142:503, 1980.

48. Thaler M, Pastakia B, Shawker TH, et al: Hepatic candidiasis in cancer patients: The evolving picture of the syndrome. Ann Intern Med 108:88, 1988.

49. Jarowski CI, Failk MA, Murray HW: Fever, rash and muscle tenderness. A distinctive clinical presentation of disseminated candidiasis. Arch Intern Med 138:544, 1978.

50. Edwards JE, Foos RY, Montogerie JZ, et al: Ocular manifestations of *Candida* septicemia: Review of seventy-six cases of hematogenous *Candida* endophthalmitis. Medicine 53:47, 1974.

51. Henderson DK, Hockey LJ, Vukalcic LT: Effect of immunosuppression on the development of experimental hematogenous *Candida* endopthalmitis. Infect Immun 27:628, 1980.

52. Henderson DK, Edwards JE, Montgomerie JZ: Hemotogenous *Candida* endopthalmitis in patients receiving parenteral hyperalimenation fluids. J Infect Dis 143:655, 1981.

53. Klein JJ, Watanakunakorn C: Hospital-acquired fungemia. Its natural course and clinical significance. Am J Med 67:51, 1979.

54. Lipton SA, Hickey WF, Morris JH, et al: Candidal infection in the central nervous system. Am J Med 76:101, 1984.

55. Ihde DC, Roberts WC, Marr KC: Cardiac candidiasis in cancer patients. Cancer 41:2364, 1978.

56. Louria DB, Stiff DP, Bennett B: Disseminated moniliasis in the adult. Medicine 41:307, 1962.

57. Rosenbaum RB, Barber JV, Stevens DA: *Candida albicans* pneumonia. Am Rev Respir Dis 109:373, 1974.

58. Schiffman RL, Johnson SJ, Weinberger SR, et al: *Candida* lung abscess: Successful treatment with amphotericin B and 5-flucytosine. Am Rev Respir Dis 125:766, 1982.

59. Sickles EA, Young VM, Greene WH, et al: Pneumonia in acute leukemia. Ann Intern Med 79:528, 1973.

60. Fainstain V, Gilmore C, Hopfer RL, et al: Septic arthritis due to *Candida* species in patients with cancer: Report of five cases and review of the literature. J Infect Dis 4:78, 1982.

61. Edwards JE, Turkel SB, Elder HA, et al: Hematogenous *Candida* osteomyelitis. Report of three cases and review of the literature. Am J Med 59:89, 1975.

62. Polak A: Combination therapy of experimental candidiasis, cryptococcosis, aspergillosis and wangiellosis in mice. Chemotherapy 33:381, 1987.

63. Powderly WG, Kobayashi G, Herzig GP, et al: Amphotericin B resistant yeast infection in severely immunocompromised patients. Am J Med 84:826, 1988.

64. Meunier F: Fluconazole treatment of fungal infections in the immunocompromised host. Semin Oncol 17:19, 1990.

65. Walsh TJ, Aoki S, Mechinaud F, et al: Effects of preventative, early and late antifungal chemotherapy with fluconazole in different granulocytopenic models of experimental disseminated candidiasis. J Infect Dis 161:755, 1990.

66. Fisher MA, Lee PG, Tarry WF: Fluconazole treatment of candidiasis in normal and diabetic rats. Antimicrob Agents Chemother 7:1042, 1989.

67. Hart PD, Russell E, Remington JS: The compromised host and infection. II. Deep fungal infection. J Infect Dis 120:169, 1969.

68. Rivett AG, Perry JA, Cohen J: Urinary candidiasis: A prospective study in hospitalized patients. Urol Res 14:153, 1986.

69. Martino P, Gurmenia C, Venditti M, et al: *Candida* colonization and systemic infection in neutropenic patients. Cancer 64:2030, 1989.

70. Phillips P, Dowrd A, Jewesson P, et al: Non-value of antigen detection immunoassays for diagnosis of candidemia. J Clin Microbiol 28:2320, 1990.

71. Mathews R, Burnie J: Diagnosis of systemic candidiasis by an enzyme-linked dot immunobinding assay for a circulating immunodominant 47-kilodalton antigen. J Clin Microbiol 26:459, 1988.

72. EORTC International Antimicrobial Therapy Cooperative Group: Empiric antifungal therapy in febrile granulocytopenic patients. Am J Med 56:668, 1989.

73. Jones JM: The recognition and management of *Candida* esophagitis. Hosp Pract 16:64, 1981.

74. Fazio RA, Wickremesinghe PC, Arsura EL: Ketoconazole treatment of *Candida* esophagitis: A prospective study of 12 cases. Am J Gastroenterol 78:261, 1983.

75. Ginzburg CH, Braden GL, Tauber AI, et al: Oral clotrimazole in the treatment of esophageal candidiasis. Am J Med 71:891, 1981.

76. Haron E, Feld R, Tuffnel P, et al: Hepatic candidiasis: An increasing problem in immunocompromised patients. Am J Med 83:17, 1987.

77. Tashjian LS, Abramson JS, Peacock JE: Focal hepatic candidiasis: A distinct variant of candidiasis in immunocompromised patients. Rev Infect Dis 6:689, 1984.

78. Lopez-Berestein G, Bodey GP, Frankel LS, et al: Treatment of hepatosplenic candidiasis with liposomal-amphotericin B. J Clin Oncol 5:310, 1987.

79. Kauffman CA, Bradley SF, Ross SC, et al: Successful treatment of hepatic candidiasis with fluconazole. Am J Med 91:137, 1991.

80. Bodey GP, DeJongh D, Isassi A, et al: Hypersplenism due to disseminated candidiasis in a patient with acute leukemia. Cancer 26:417, 1969.

81. Bayer AS, Blumenkrantz MJ, Montgomerie JZ, et al: *Candida* peritonitis. Report of 22 cases and review of the English literature. Am J Med 61:832, 1976.

82. Eisenberg ES, Leviton I, Soeiro R: Fungal peritonitis in patients receiving peritoneal dialysis: Experience with 11 patients and review of the literature. Rev Infect Dis 8:309, 1986.

83. Bastani B, Westervelt FB Jr: Persistence of *Candida* despite seemingly adequate systemic and intraperitoneal amphotericin B treatment in a patient on CAPD. Am J Kidney Dis 8:265, 1986.

84. Levine J, Bernard DB, Idelson BA, et al: Fungal peritonitis complicating continous ambulatory peritoneal dialysis: Successful treatment with fluconazole, a new orally active antifungal agent. Am J Med 86:825, 1989.

85. Rutledge R, Mandel SR, Wild RE: *Candida* species. Insignificant contaminant or pathogenic species. Am Surg 52:299, 1986.

86. Marsh PK, Tally FP, Kellum J, et al: *Candida* infections in surgical patients. Ann Surg 198:42, 1983.

87. Solomkin JS, Flohr AB, Quie PG, et al: The role of candida in intra-peritoneal infections. Surgery 88:524, 1980.

88. Cauwenbergh G: Prophylaxis of mycotic infections in immunocompromised patients: A review of 27 reports and publications. Drugs Exp Clin Res 12:419, 1986.

89. Estey E, Maksymiuk A, Smith T: Infection prophylaxis in acute leukemia: Comparative effectiveness of trimethoprim, sulfamethoxazole, ketoconazole, and trimethoprim-sulfamethoxazole and ketoconazole as infection prophylaxis in acute leukemia. Arch Intern Med 144:1562, 1984.

90. Meunier F: Prevention of mycoses in immunocompromised patients. Rev Infect Dis 9:408, 1987.

91. Young LS: Antimicrobial prophylaxis against infection in neutropenic patients (editorial). J Infect Dis 147:611, 1983.

92. Wingard JR, Dick JD, Merz WG, et al: Pathogenicity of *Candida tropicalis* and *Candida albicans* after gastrointestinal inoculation in mice. Infect Immun 29:808, 1980.

93. Bodey GP, Samonis G, Rolston K: Prophylaxis of candidiasis in cancer patients. Semin Oncol 17:24, 1990.

94. Dick JD, Merz WG, Saral R: Incidence of polyene-resistant yeasts recovered from clinical specimens. Antimicrob Agents Chemother 18:158, 1980.

95. Slotman GJ, Burchard KW: Ketoconazole prevents *Candida* sepsis in critically ill surgical patients. Arch Surg 122:147, 1987.

96. Kozinn PJ, Taschdjian CL, Goldberg PK, et al: Advances in the diagnosis of renal candidiasis. J Urol 119:184, 1978.

97. Schoneback J, Ansehn S: The occurrence of yeast like fungi in the urine under normal conditions and in various types of urinary tract pathology. Scand J Urol Nephrol 6:123, 1972.

98. Fisher JF, Chew WH, Shadomy S, et al: Urinary tract infections due to *Candida albicans*. Rev Infect Dis 4:1107, 1982.
99. Lehner T: Systemic candidiasis and renal involvement. Lancet 1:1414, 1964.
100. Gerle RD: Roentgenographic features of primary renal candidiasis fungus ball of the renal pelvis and ureter. AJR 119:731, 1973.
101. Graybill JR, Galgiani JN, Jorgensen JH, et al: Ketoconazole therapy for fungal urinary tract infections. J Urol 129:68, 1983.
102. Gentry LO, Price MF: Urinary and Genital *Candida* Infections in Candidiasis. New York, Raven Press, p 169, 1985.

CHAPTER 34

Fungal Infections

Rebecca E. Martin
Robert W. Bradsher

The most common fungal infection diagnosed in patients in an intensive care unit is candidiasis (see Chapter 33). However, other types of fungal infections are increasingly being found in patients hospitalized in intensive care units, because there are greater numbers of immunocompromised patients, who become infected with unusual organisms or have reactivation of infection with organisms that were previously controlled by the host defense. This review focuses on the more unusual presentations by relatively common fungi and on the more common presentations of opportunistic organisms in immunosuppressed patients.

Histoplasma capsulatum, Blastomyces dermatitidis, Coccidioides immitis, Paracoccidioides brasiliensis, Penicillium marneffei, and *Sporothrix schenckii* represent dimorphic fungi that exist in nature as mycelia and convert to a parasitic phase at body temperature. These organisms most often cause asymptomatic or mildly symptomatic pulmonary infection. Paracoccidioidomycosis and penicilliosis occur in South America and China, respectively, and are not discussed further here. Sporotrichosis occurs after cutaneous inoculation, manifests as local infection, and only rarely disseminates to cause pulmonary involvement that tends to cavitate.

COCCIDIOIDOMYCOSIS, HISTOPLASMOSIS, AND BLASTOMYCOSIS

Coccidioidomycosis, histoplasmosis, and blastomycosis occur in specific geographic areas, with up to 90% of the populations of hyperendemic areas infected with the particular organism.[1-3] The presentation to the intensivist would most likely be overwhelming infection leading to multiorgan involvement, including the adult respiratory distress syndrome. Diagnosis is suggested by detecting the organism in direct smears of sputum or exudate after potassium hydroxide digestion of the human tissue on a microscope slide or in fungal stains of biopsy material (lung, bone marrow, bone, or other tissue). Diagnosis is confirmed by culture. Unlike the case with *Candida* or *Aspergillus*, if one of these dimorphic fungi is identified, infection is confirmed; contamination or colonization does not occur.

Coccidioidomycosis is observed in patients from California, Arizona, Texas, New Mexico, and Mexico.[3, 4] Asians (particularly Filipinos) and to a lesser degree blacks and Native Americans are at more risk for progressive, life-threatening disease.[3] In addition, pregnancy increases the potential for fatal outcome. Meningitis is not infrequent with disseminated coccidioidomycosis and cerebrospinal fluid should be examined in selected patients.[4]

Histoplasmosis is found in patients who have lived in the southern and central portions of the United States at some point in their life. Chronic pulmonary histoplasmosis is related more to the structural abnormality of bullous or centrilobular emphysema than to the immune defects considered to be the cause of progressive disseminated histoplasmosis.[5] Oral mucosa, adrenal glands, cardiac valves, and the meninges may be sites of focal destructive lesions associated with the progressive disseminated form of this infection. Infection with human immunodeficiency virus, which is discussed in Chapter 50, adds to the severity of these two fungal infections.[6, 7]

Blastomycosis is diagnosed in patients from states on either side of the Mississippi River, as well as a few other areas of the southern and central United States. Even though a few immunosuppressed patients (e.g., those with human immunodeficiency virus infection or chronic lymphocytic leukemia, and kidney transplant recipients) have had this fungal infection, most cases occur in normal hosts.[2] Intensivists will most likely see blastomycosis patients who have had adult respiratory distress syndrome. One postulate for the mechanism of this disease is rupture of carinal lymph nodes containing the organisms into the trachea, although progressive alveolar involvement may also occur.[8]

The treatment of choice for the overwhelmingly ill patient with dimorphic fungal infection continues to be amphotericin B.[2, 6, 9] Trials with ketoconazole, itraconazole, and fluconazole have excluded this type of patient. Doses of amphotericin B should rapidly escalate in these extremely ill patients to 0.5 to 0.6 mg/kg/d and should be continued until clinical response is noted. After partial recovery, a switch to oral agents for completion of therapy can be considered. No advantages have been noted in the simultaneous administration of azole antifungal agents, such as ketoconazole, itraconazole, or fluconazole.[10]

CRYPTOCOCCOSIS

Cryptococcus neoformans, found throughout the United States, is a saprophytic yeast that causes subclinical pneumonia. Dissemination may occur subsequently, particularly to the central nervous system, which results in meningitis. Diseases associated with altered cell-mediated immunity (Hodgkin's disease, sarcoidosis, steroid therapy, renal transplantation, human immunodeficiency virus infection) are usually present when disseminated cryptococcal infection is detected.[11, 12] *C. neoformans* may cause pneumonia in normal hosts and may even colonize the respiratory tract without disease. However, this fungus may also cause severe pneumonia with reticulonodular infiltrates, mass lesions, or cavitary disease; pleural effusions have been described.[13] Diagnostic help is provided by detection of cryptococcal antigen by latex agglutination in serum or cerebrospinal fluid. Measurement of the titer depends on presence of the polysaccharide capsule of the organism and not on development of host immunity.

Two therapeutic options have been approved by the U.S. Food and Drug Administration for treatment of cryptococcal meningitis and have been suggested for other forms of severe systemic infections with this yeast. Oral fluconazole has been used successfully for this infection in patients with acquired immunodeficiency syndrome, although initial reports have suggested a higher early mortality rate than in patients treated with amphotericin B.[14] Amphotericin B, either with or without flucytosine, has been the "gold standard" of therapy for this infection. Flucytosine is excreted exclusively by renal mechanisms and can accumulate in patients who are simultaneously treated with amphotericin B, which is nephrotoxic. Unless serum level results of flucytosine can be rapidly obtained, flucytosine therapy should be used with great caution because of the leukopenia that accompanies high serum concentrations.[10]

MUCORMYCOSIS

Mucormycosis is the name given to disease caused by fungi of the order Mucorales. The terms zygomycosis and phycomycosis have also been applied to this infection. The pathogenic Mucorales reproduce asexually and can grow in both aerobic and microaerophilic conditions.[15] Because growth in tissue and the environment is in the hyphal form, they are classified as molds. The agents of mucormycoses are found throughout nature, particularly in soil or decaying organic material.[16] Disease is usually initiated via inhalation or inoculation into previously traumatized skin. Fulminant infection is most likely to develop in patients with hematologic malignancies and diabetics with acidosis, but it has also been described in patients with organ transplants, renal failure, burns, and malnutrition, and in those having prolonged hospitalization or receiving immunosuppressive drugs, especially corticosteroids.[16, 17] Normal hosts are rarely infected, which suggests that a defect of macrophage or neutrophil function is responsible for the development of invasive disease.[16] Many common medical interventions that are lifesaving to the patient may also predispose to infection with the Mucorales. Nosocomial mucormycosis has been reported in patients whose only risk was advanced life-support care in an intensive care setting.[17] Prolonged use of broad-spectrum antibiotics, hyperalimentation, and systemic corticosteroids have been implicated as factors possibly related to nosocomial mucormycosis.

Rhinocerebral mucormycosis, seen in patients with diabetic ketoacidosis and hematologic malignancies, is usually rapidly progressive and disfiguring.[18] Because of the characteristic thrombosis and hemorrhagic infarction seen in tissue sections, the lesions commonly have a black, necrotic exudate. Entry of the fungi through the palate or nasal mucous membranes, with spread through the sinuses into the orbit, is characteristic, and direct invasion of the brain may occur. Spread may also occur through either the cavernous sinus or the cribriform plate. Most patients present with ocular or facial pain, followed by cellulitis with necrotic ulcers and a black nasal discharge.[19] As the disease progresses, proptosis and loss of extraocular muscle function may occur and cause diplopia. Thrombosis of the retinal artery may lead to sudden blindness.

Pulmonary invasion by Mucoraceae is most commonly seen in patients with hematologic malignancies, and mortality rates are quite high. Thrombosis and infarction of vessels are also seen with pulmonary infection. Pleuritic pain is a frequent complaint.[20] The most common radiographic presentation is a necrotizing, nodular pneumonia resulting from vascular invasion by the fungus. Pleural effusions and fungus balls have been described, as have miliary, wedge-shaped, and cavitary lesions.[15, 20]

Invasion of the gastrointestinal tract by Mucorales is unusual and occurs mainly in severely malnourished patients. Contaminated food is often the source, but infection has also been associated with nasogastric intubation.[21] The stomach is most frequently involved, but mucormycosis has been documented throughout the gastrointestinal tract. Dissemi-

nation from the gastrointestinal tract is most likely to happen in children with malabsorption or diarrhea, in adults with a bowel defect arising from surgery for trauma or from inflammatory bowel disease, or in patients with underlying liver disease.[22]

Mucormycosis of the skin can be a primary, localized phenomenon or the manifestation of disseminated disease. Localized disease may be seen in diabetics as a superficial ulcer or in severely burned or traumatized wounds as gangrenous cellulitis.[16] Primary cutaneous infection has also been seen in cancer patients, typically at the insertion site of an intravenous catheter, as an erythematous, macular lesion that can progress quickly to purpura and eventually to ulcer with eschar formation. Survival is related to resolution of chemotherapy-associated neutropenia.[23] Nosocomial acquisition of cutaneous mucormycosis has also been associated with the use of contaminated elastic adhesive bandages. The majority of these cases occurred in the 1970s, but similar infections are still occasionally reported.[24] If primary cutaneous mucormycosis is detected early, débridement can result in cure. When the infection is allowed to progress, however, the fungal growth can extend into subcutaneous tissue and muscle and invade the vasculature, with subsequent hematogenous spread. Cutaneous mucormycosis may also represent hematogenous dissemination resembling ecthyma gangrenosum, so that cutaneous lesions should prompt a search for infection in other organs in an immunocompromised host.

Primary central nervous system mucormycosis is rare and most often seen in intravenous drug users, although cases have been described in patients with head trauma, renal insufficiency, and human immunodeficiency virus infection.[16] Fever, headache, lethargy, hemiparesis, and speech disturbances are the usual presenting features. Infection apparently develops from direct inoculation of spores contained in the street drugs. Therefore, central nervous system mucormycosis should be considered as a potential cause of rapidly deteriorating neurologic status in a drug abuser.

As with specific organ infection, disseminated mucormycosis is most often found in patients with hematologic malignancies, and only a few survive this devastating illness. Pneumonia, cerebrovascular accident, subarachnoid hemorrhage, brain abscess, and skin manifestations are the clinical signs most often seen with dissemination.[22] Wide dissemination, however, may occur, including spread to the spleen, kidney, pancreas, and heart.[15] Mucormycosis has been reported with increasing frequency among hemodialysis patients receiving deferoxamine for aluminum and iron overload states.[25, 26] More than 90% of disseminated mucormycosis cases are diagnosed at autopsy.

Biopsy of infected material is necessary for diagnosis, and samples should be obtained at the margin of a lesion. Touch preparations of biopsy specimens after potassium hydroxide digestion on a glass slide may be helpful, but the most useful means for identification of the fungus are hematoxylin and eosin, Gomori's methenamine silver, and periodic acid–Schiff stains done on fixed tissue. Frozen sections should be examined to avoid delay in diagnosis. Broad (10 to 20 nm in diameter), nonseptate, thick-walled hyphae that branch at right angles are characteristically seen.[15] The hallmark of the histopathology examination is vascular invasion with resultant thrombosis, hemorrhage, and necrotic infarction. Tissue invasion must be demonstrated because Mucorales can colonize without causing infection. The Mucoraceae grow well on Sabouraud's agar at 37°C but require immediate inoculation of the biopsy tissue. Sufficient growth for identification usually occurs in 1 day. Noninvasive diagnostic tests have not been helpful.

Early diagnosis, aggressive surgery, and amphotericin B

are the mainstays of treatment for mucormycosis.[16] Rhino-orbital mucormycosis often requires exenteration with removal of the total contents of the orbit. Daily irrigation and packing are essential, along with systemic antifungal therapy. Repeated débridement may be necessary. In uncontrolled studies with a small number of patients, hyperbaric oxygen has been successfully used.[16] Success also depends largely on correction of the underlying medical problem.

Amphotericin B is the only effective antifungal agent for mucormycosis. High doses (1.0 to 1.5 mg/kg/d) are recommended. In vitro synergy between amphotericin B and rifampin has been demonstrated, but the addition of rifampin is controversial and should be considered only when conventional therapy is failing.

ASPERGILLOSIS

Aspergillosis describes a wide range of illness caused by the fungus *Aspergillus*. Manifestations of disease range from tissue invasion to colonization to host hypersensitivity to the fungus. Invasive disease is more likely to occur in the immunocompromised host and is often fatal. Colonization may lead to fungus ball formation and massive hemoptysis. Host hypersensitivity to *Aspergillus* can produce severe asthma. Each problem requires careful medical management, often in an intensive care setting.

The name *Aspergillus* was coined by an 18th century priest and botanist, Micheli, who noted the similarity between the microscopic appearance of a fungus and the aspergillum, a religious vessel used to sprinkle holy water during mass.[27] More than 200 species of the genus *Aspergillus* have been identified, but four species of *Aspergillus* (*fumigatus, flavus, niger,* and *terreus*) are responsible for most human disease. Invasive disease is usually caused by *A. fumigatus*.[28]

Aspergilli are widespread in nature, frequently found in soil, decaying organic matter, water, and hay.[27] Disease is usually caused by inhalation of *Aspergillus* spores or inoculation of traumatized skin or corneal tissue. Rarely, implantation of contaminated prosthetic devices has resulted in infection. Airborne spread of *Aspergillus* during hospital renovation has resulted in outbreaks of aspergillosis in immunosuppressed patients.[29]

Invasive aspergillosis rarely occurs in a normal host. Patients who are immunosuppressed from hematologic malignancies, organ transplants, or use of corticosteroids or cytotoxic drugs are predisposed to invasive disease. The hallmark of invasive aspergillosis is spread into the vasculature, with resultant tissue hemorrhage, necrosis, and infarction, such as in mucormycosis.[28] An effective host response depends on an intact phagocytic system, with macrophages acting first to kill the conidia of the *Aspergillus*, followed by neutrophils destroying the mycelia.[30] Oxidative killing probably plays a role in containing this fungus because patients with chronic granulomatous disease have an increased incidence of *Aspergillus* infection.[28] Vascular dissemination of *Aspergillus* is not prominent in these patients.

Colonization by aspergilli can occur at almost any body site. Ectatic bronchi and cavitary lung lesions in patients with chronic debilitating pulmonary disease are common manifestations. Proliferation of the saprophytic mycelia can lead to fungus ball or aspergilloma formation. The aspergilloma may enlarge the pre-existing cavity but does not invade surrounding tissue. Recurrent, blood-streaked sputum and rarely, massive hemoptysis may occur, but more often the patient has symptoms only of the underlying disease.[28] A chest roentgenogram usually reveals a mass surrounded by a crescent of air in a cavity. Diagnosis is confirmed by demonstration of immunoglobulin (Ig) G antibodies to *A. fumigatus*.

Hypersensitivity to *Aspergillus* antigens causes episodic bronchial obstruction in predisposed individuals, leading to the syndrome of allergic bronchopulmonary aspergillosis.[31] Hyphae colonize the respiratory passages and stimulate production of IgE, IgG, and IgA and possibly sensitized lymphocytes. Eosinophils, mononuclear cells, fibrin, Charcot-Leyden crystals, and Curschmann's spirals are found histologically in the mucus of patients with the allergic syndrome.[31] The patient usually has episodic asthma, blood eosinophilia, transient pulmonary infiltrates, serum-precipitating antibodies to *A. fumigatus*, and markedly elevated IgE levels. Sputum cultures occasionally grow *Aspergillus*. The syndrome is one of intermittent exacerbations that can eventually lead to corticosteroid-dependent asthma.

Allergic *Aspergillus* sinusitis refers to pathologic findings similar to those with allergic bronchopulmonary aspergillosis in patients with recurrent allergic rhinitis and sinusitis.[32] Colonization of the sinuses and external ear by *Aspergillus* is usually a benign process; a black, fungal growth caused by the species *A. niger* occludes the canal, although the middle ear and mastoids are usually spared. Rarely, the fungus causes a malignant external otitis similar to that caused by *Pseudomonas aeruginosa*. Because *Aspergillus* is commonly a saprophytic inhabitant of the ear, diagnosis is often missed or delayed. In a patient with neutrophil dysfunction and poor response to broad-spectrum antibiotics, recovery of *Aspergillus* from the ear should prompt aggressive investigation.

Invasive aspergillosis of the sinuses may have a clinical course similar to that of rhinocerebral mucormycosis.[33] Vascular invasion, necrosis, and spread from the sinuses into the orbit and brain may occur. Headache, edema, unilateral proptosis, and nasal discharge are the most common manifestations.[33] Blindness, extraocular muscle palsies, and stroke may also occur.[27]

Ocular aspergillosis occurs in three primary circumstances.[27, 28] Trauma to the cornea with resultant fungal keratitis may follow cataract surgery or accidental injury. A second mechanism is contiguous spread into the orbit from invasive paranasal aspergillosis. Third, hematogenous dissemination may occur in a patient with pneumonia or endocarditis.

Invasive pulmonary aspergillosis has been called a disease of medical progress.[34] Between 50 and 70% of cases occur in patients with acute leukemia.[35] Neutropenia is the primary predisposing factor, with each day of neutropenia resulting in a corresponding rise in risk for *Aspergillus* infection. Other factors, such as underlying sinus or lung disease, length of antibiotic therapy, or number of relapses of leukemia, are not specific risks for development of pulmonary aspergillosis. Cases of invasive pulmonary aspergillosis in nonimmuno-compromised hosts (e.g., patients after influenza, alcoholics, and others with no apparent risk) have been reported in the literature.[36]

Clinical findings of invasive pulmonary aspergillosis are subtle and easily missed. Common early symptoms include pleuritic pain, cough, and sinus congestion. Chest crackles are usually present; hemoptysis occurs less frequently. Fever that continues despite aggressive antibiotic therapy suggests fungal infection. Chest roentgenograms demonstrating early pulmonary aspergillosis are usually interpreted as normal.[37] Initial findings include consolidation, cavitary lesions, and nodular infiltrates.[38] The oxygen level often remains relatively preserved despite diffuse involvement.[34]

Bone marrow recovery is necessary for survival, but granulocyte return may cause cavitation of the pulmonary *Aspergillus* lesions. Massive hemoptysis is not seen in patients who remain granulocytopenic[35] but may be a complication of this semi-invasive form of aspergillosis. Extrapulmonary dissemination occurs in up to 25% of neutropenic patients with invasive pulmonary aspergillosis.[38] Unusual complications include pleural involvement, Pancoast's syndrome, and necrotizing bronchitis.[27, 28] A pseudomembrane composed of *Aspergillus* hyphae covering the lower trachea was described in a patient with acquired immunodeficiency syndrome who had episodic asthma unresponsive to bronchodilators and steroid therapy and rapid respiratory failure.[39]

Cutaneous aspergillosis is rare and is usually a manifestation of primary infection rather than dissemination.[23] Fungal infection has been associated with skin breakdown resulting from adhesive tape, arm boards, and long-term use of intravascular catheters involving both the cutaneous tunnel and the exit site. Lesions begin as erythematous, maculopapular eruptions and progress to pustules and black eschars. Cutaneous aspergillosis is usually found on extremities.[38]

Aspergillus is known to infect both native and prosthetic heart valves, although the latter is a bit more common.[27] The vegetation is large, friable, and prone to embolization, although peripheral blood cultures are rarely positive.[40] Myocardial abscesses and invasion of adjacent tissue may occur. Contamination at the time of surgery is thought to be the most likely etiology.[34] Onset of symptoms is frequently delayed postsurgery. Pericarditis, tamponade, and tension pneumopericardium are complications of contiguous spread.

Infection of the central nervous system by *Aspergillus* is usually rapidly fatal. Vascular invasion and infarction are particularly common. Dissemination from the lung is most common, but contamination at surgery and injection of spores by intravenous drug abusers has also been the cause. *Aspergillus* meningitis complicating transsphenoidal surgery has been reported.[27]

Most patients with widely disseminated disease are immunosuppressed. The organs most commonly involved are lung, intestines, and brain. Recovery from disseminated disease is rare and depends on granulocyte recovery. Unusual sites of dissemination include the thyroid gland and pancreas.[38] Vascular invasion of the hepatic veins by *Aspergillus* can cause an insidious onset of a Budd-Chiari syndrome with pain, hepatomegaly, ascites, and death.

Definitive diagnosis depends on culture results and microscopic examination of tissue. Histopathology demonstrates septate hyphae that branch at 45° angles. The mycelia are 3 to 4 nm in diameter and are uniform in size. Tissue specimens can be homogenized, mounted on a slide with 10 to 20% potassium hydroxide, and examined directly.[28] Histologic examination is best done with Gomori's methenamine silver stain. Biopsy specimens are necessary for certain diagnosis, but isolation of *Aspergillus* from respiratory secretions in neutropenic patients strongly suggests the presence of invasive pulmonary aspergillosis. This is not true for patients with solid tumors or those with normal neutrophil function.[41] Serologic tests for antibodies to *Aspergillus* are not of value for disseminated disease, however, because patients who are immunosuppressed lack the ability to make antibodies.[42]

Invasive aspergillosis should be treated with amphotericin B at high daily doses (1.0 to 1.5 mg/kg) after rapid advancement from test doses.[28] Addition of other agents such as 5-fluorocytosine or rifampin is a controversial point but may be tried in fulminant cases. Itraconazole, an oral triazole, has been effective in a group of patients with invasive aspergillosis,[43] and further studies are planned. Significant hemoptysis from an aspergilloma requires resection, but otherwise the patient should be managed conservatively. Aggressive surgical débridement is necessary in invasive head and neck infection, central nervous system infection, or endocarditis. Cutaneous lesions in the immunocompromised host have better healing with antifungal therapy alone.[44]

Because early diagnosis and institution of antifungal therapy are critical to survival of patients, intensive care physicians should be familiar with the type of host who is predisposed to fungal infection and the clinical features suggesting infection. Immunocompromised patients, particularly those with acute leukemia during profound neutropenia, are at highest risk of infection with opportunistic fungi. Subtle findings of dimorphic fungal infection must be aggressively investigated and treated. The intensivist should recognize and appropriately treat these systemic fungal infections.

References

1. Goodwin RA, Loyd JE, DesPrez RM: Histoplasmosis in the normal hosts. Medicine 60:231, 1981.
2. Bradsher RW: Blastomycosis. Infect Dis Clin North Am 2:877, 1988.
3. Pappagianis D. Epidemiology of coccidioidomycosis. In: Stevens DA (ed): Coccidioidomycosis: A Text. New York, Plenum Publishing, p 63, 1980.
4. Drutz DJ, Cantanzaro A: Coccidioidomycosis. Am Rev Respir Dis 117:559, 1978.
5. Goodwin RA, DePrez RM: Histoplasmosis. Am Rev Respir Dis 117:929, 1978.
6. Wheat LJ: Histoplasmosis. Infect Dis Clin North Am 2:841, 1988.
7. Galgiani JN, Ampel NM: Coccidioidomycosis in human immunodeficiency virus–infected patients. J Infect Dis 162:1165, 1990.
8. Evans ME, Haynes JB, Atkinson JB, et al: *Blastomyces dermatitidis* and the adult respiratory distress syndrome. Am Rev Respir Dis 126:1099, 1982.
9. Knoper SR, Galgiani JN: Coccidioidomycosis. Infect Dis Clin North Am 2:861, 1988.
10. Sarosi GA, Bates JH, Bradsher RW: Chemotherapy of the pulmonary mycoses. ATS position paper. Am Rev Respir Dis 138:1078, 1988.
11. Diamond RD, Bennett JE: Prognostic factors in cryptococcal meningitis. A study of 111 cases. Ann Intern Med 80:176, 1974.
12. Zuger A, Louie E, Holzman RS, et al: Cryptococcal disease in patients with the acquired immune deficiency syndrome. Diagnostic features and outcome of treatment. Ann Intern Med 104:234, 1986.
13. Kerkering TM, Duma RJ, Shadomy S: The evolution of pulmonary cryptococcosis. Ann Intern Med 94:611, 1981.
14. Larsen RA, Leal MAE, Chan LS: Fluconazole compared with amphotericin B plus flucytosine in the treatment of cryptococcal meningitis. Ann Intern Med 113:183, 1990.
15. Lehrer RI, Howard DH, Sypherd PS, et al: Mucormycosis. Ann Intern Med 93:93, 1980.
16. Sugar AM: Agents of mucormycosis and related species. In: Mandell GL, Douglas RG, Bennett JE (eds): Principles and Practice of Infectious Diseases. 3rd ed. New York, Churchill Livingstone, p 1962, 1990.
17. Agger WA, Maki DG: Mucormycosis: Complication of critical care. Arch Intern Med 138:925, 1978.
18. Parfrey NA: Improved diagnosis and prognosis of mycormycosis. Medicine 65:113, 1986.
19. Meyers BR, Wormser G, Hirschman SZ, et al: Rhinocerebral mucormycosis: Premortem diagnosis and therapy. Arch Intern Med 139:557, 1979.
20. Bigby TD, Serota ML, Tierney LM, et al: Clinical spectrum of pulmonary mucormycosis. Chest 89:435, 1986.
21. Kahn LB. Gastric mucormycosis: Report of a case and review of literature. S Afr Med J 37:1265, 1965.
22. Ingram CW, Sennesh J, Cooper JN, et al: Disseminated zygomycosis: Report of four cases and review. Rev Infect Dis 11:741, 1989.
23. Khardori N, Hayat S, Rolston K: Cutaneous rhizopus and aspergillus infections in five patients with cancer. Arch Dermatol 125:952, 1989.
24. Patterson JE, Barden GE, Bia FJ: Hospital-acquired gangrenous mucormycosis. Yale J Biol Med 59:453, 1986.
25. Eiser AR, Slifkin RF, Neff MS: Intestinal mucormycosis in hemodialysis patients following deferoxamine. Am J Kidney Dis 10:71, 1987.
26. Windus DW, Stokes TJ, Julian BA, et al: Fatal *Rhizopus* infections in hemodialysis patients receiving deferoxamine. Ann Intern Med 107:678, 1987.
27. Rinaldi MG: Invasive aspergillosis. Rev Infect Dis 5:1061, 1983.
28. Bennett JE: Aspergillus species. In: Mandell GL, Douglas RG, Bennett JE (eds): Principles and Practice of Infectious Diseases. 3rd ed. New York, Churchill Livingstone, p 1958, 1990.
29. Lentino JR, Rosenkranz MA, Michaels JA, et al: Nosocomial aspergillosis: A retrospective review of airborne disease secondary to road construction and contaminated air conditioners. Am J Epidemiol 116:430, 1982.
30. Diamond RD: Inhibition of monocyte-mediated damage to fungal hyphe by steroid hormones. J Infect Dis 147:160, 1983.
31. Ricketti AJ, Greenberger PA, Mintzer RA, et al: Allergic bronchopulmonary aspergillosis. Arch Intern Med 143:1553, 1983.
32. Katzenstein AA, Sale SR, Greenberger PA: Pathologic findings in allergic aspergillus sinusitis. Am J Surg Pathol 7:439, 1983.
33. Lowe J, Bradley J: Cerebral and orbital *Aspergillus* infection due to invasive aspergillosis of ethmoid sinus. J Clin Pathol 39:774, 1986.

34. Herbert PA, Bazer AS: Fungal pneumonia: Invasive pulmonary aspergillosis. Chest 80:220, 1981.
35. Albelda SM, Talbot GH, Gerson SL, et al: Pulmonary cavitation and massive hemoptysis in invasive pulmonary aspergillosis. Am Rev Respir Dis 131:115, 1985.
36. Karam GH, Griffin FM: Invasive pulmonary aspergillosis in nonimmunocompromised, nonneutropenic hosts. Rev Infect Dis 8:357, 1986.
37. Gerson SL, Talbot GH, Lusk E, et al: Invasive pulmonary aspergillosis in adult acute leukemia: Clinical clues to its diagnosis. J Clin Oncol 3:1109, 1985.
38. Young RC, Bennett JE, Vogel CL, et al: Aspergillosis: The spectrum of the disease in 98 patients. Medicine 49:147, 1970.
39. Pervez NK, Klunerman J, Kattan M, et al: Pseudomembranous necrotizing bronchial aspergillosis. Am Rev Respir Dis 131:961, 1985.
40. Barst RJ, Prince AS, Neu HC: Aspergillus endocarditis in children. Pediatrics 68:73, 1981.
41. Yu VL, Muder RR, Poorsattar A: Significance of isolation of Aspergillus from respiratory tract in diagnosis of invasive pulmonary aspergillosis. Am J Med 81:249, 1986.
42. Bennett JE: Rapid diagnosis of candidiasis and aspergillosis. Rev Infect Dis 9:398, 1987.
43. Denning DW, Tucker RW, Hanson LH, et al: Treatment of invasive aspergillosis with itraconazole. Am J Med 86:791, 1989.
44. Allo MD, Miller J, Townsend J: Lethal primary cutaneous aspergillosis associated with Hickman intravenous catheters. N Engl J Med 317:1105, 1987.

CHAPTER 35

Life-Threatening Skin and Soft Tissue Infections

W. Lance George

Skin and soft tissue infections are relatively frequent and may constitute the primary illness or may be a significant cause of comorbidity in the patient who is severely ill from other medical or surgical diseases. The presence and significance of these infections may be overshadowed either by the coexistence of other infections or by the presence of life-threatening, noninfectious conditions. Because the skin and soft tissues can easily be assessed on examination (in comparison to the abdominal viscera or lungs, for example), evidence of clinically important infection of these tissues should be sought on a routine basis. It is important to appreciate that life-threatening skin and soft tissue infections may develop outside the hospital or after admission in a nonsurgical or surgical patient. In the last instance, the infection may or may not be related directly to the surgical procedure itself.

The purpose of this chapter is to describe skin and soft tissue infections that may develop in the intensive care unit or that may lead to admission to the intensive care unit from either the community or the hospital inpatient ward.

PATHOPHYSIOLOGY

The number and type of soft tissue infections that may threaten the patient are diverse; they arise either endogenously from the patient's own normal body bacterial flora or exogenously from environmental flora.

Endogenous bacterial infections of the skin and soft tissue commonly involve anaerobic bacteria. A typical antecedent of such infections is devitalization or significant ischemia of tissues (related to either trauma or progression of vascular insufficiency), which produces a low tissue oxidation-reduction potential (oxygen-poor state) that facilitates the growth of anaerobic bacteria. The causes of lowered oxidation-reduction potential may not always be obvious to the clinician. These include devitalization of tissue, such as might occur after major trauma; loss of blood supply to an extremity, attributable either to trauma or to progressive arterial insufficiency; pressure-induced ischemia, such as that occurring during the development of a sacral decubitus ulcer; and the relative ischemia that can occur at the site of a surgical incision during a prolonged or complicated operation. An additional predisposing factor for anaerobic infections is the existence of a nonanaerobic infection, as might occur at the site of a sacral decubitus ulcer or a surgical incision. The nonanaerobic process itself can lower the oxidation-reduction potential such that any anaerobic bacteria present may begin to proliferate and extend the infectious process.

The skin serves as a barrier that is relatively resistant to penetration by microorganisms. Inoculation of bacteria through breaks in the skin that occur because of accidental trauma (motor vehicle accidents or thermal burns, for example) or because of hospital procedures (venipuncture, insertion of central venous lines, or operative incisions, for example) represent mechanisms by which both local and systemic infections may arise. Soft tissue hematomas provide an excellent medium in which bacteria may grow, and trauma to soft tissues may impair the ability of host defenses to eradicate bacteria inoculated into the tissue.

Finally, the overall immunologic (and nutritional) status of the patient is an exceedingly important factor in determining predisposition to life-threatening skin and soft tissue bacterial infections. These immunologic factors include immunosuppressive therapy, severe granulocytopenia, impaired T lymphocyte function, and solid organ or bone marrow transplantation. Serious, nonbacterial infections caused by certain viruses (such as herpesviruses) and fungi may involve the skin or soft tissue; these processes are typically associated with significant immunodeficiency and are discussed in other chapters.

EPIDEMIOLOGY

The types and numbers of organisms involved in skin and soft tissue infections depend to a large extent on the pathogenesis of the infectious process. A convenient way to group these organisms for therapeutic purposes is as follows: (1) community- or hospital-acquired infections involving anaerobes; (2) community-acquired nonanaerobic infections; and (3) hospital-acquired nonanaerobic infections.

There are three major endogenous sources of anaerobic bacteria: the normal flora of the oropharynx, the female genital tract, and the large intestine. The normal flora of these sites is complex and also contains a variety of species of nonanaerobes, including streptococci and (in the case of the female genital tract and the large intestine) enteric (or facultative) gram-negative bacilli such as Escherichia coli. Infections involving anaerobic bacteria are typically mixed anaerobic-aerobic infections from which three or four species of anaerobes and two or three (or more) species of nonanaerobes can be isolated by rigorous microbiologic techniques. The exceptions to this rule are actinomycosis and certain clostridial diseases.

The taxonomy of anaerobic bacteriology has become complex and not easily dealt with for routine clinical purposes. In general, the anaerobic gram-negative bacilli (previously

TABLE 35–1

CATEGORIES OF SKIN AND SOFT TISSUE INFECTIONS

Infections Involving Primarily Skin	Infections Involving Subcutaneous Tissue with or Without Skin Involvement	Infections Involving Primarily Fascia	Infections Involving Primarily Muscle
Cellulitis*	Cutaneous and subcutaneous	Necrotizing fasciitis†‡	Clostridial myonecrosis
Infected cutaneous ulcers*†	abscesses*†	Fournier's gangrene†‡	(gas gangrene)†‡
Infected sebaceous or inclusion cyst	Diabetic foot infection*†	Clostridial fasciitis†‡	Anaerobic streptococcal myositis
Hidradenitis suppurativa	Infected decubitus ulcer*†	Postoperative wound infection	Synergistic nonclostridial
Pyoderma	Bite wound infection*†		myonecrosis (synergistic
Paronychia	Anaerobic cellulitis, gas abscess,		necrotizing cellulitis)†‡
Tropical ulcer	and clostridial cellulitis†		Infected vascular gangrene*†
Ecthyma gangrenosum	Bacterial synergistic gangrene		Muscle abscess or pyomyositis
Postoperative wound infection*	Infected visceral sinus tract*†		Postoperative wound infection
	Noma (cancrum oris)†		
	Infected pilonidal sinus/cyst		
	Meleney's ulcer		
	Burn wound infection		
	Postoperative wound infection*		

*This type of infection is relatively common.
†Anaerobic bacteria are frequently involved.
‡This infection may have a rapidly lethal course.
Modified from George WL: Other infections of skin, soft tissue and muscle. In: Finegold SM, George WL (eds): Anaerobic Infections in Humans. San Diego, CA, Academic Press, p 485, 1989.

belonging to the genera *Bacteroides* and *Fusobacterium*) are the most prevalent anaerobic pathogens and possess the greatest degree of antimicrobial resistance. Unfortunately, these two genera have been split into several others. In the clinical setting, it may be most reasonable to consider anaerobic gram-negative bacilli as the most important group of anaerobic pathogens and to recognize that the *Bacteroides fragilis* group constitutes the most resistant of the anaerobic gram-negative bacilli.

The second most important group of anaerobic bacteria is the gram-positive cocci. Previously, these were classified in the genera *Peptococcus* and *Peptostreptococcus*; because taxonomic changes have complicated the issue, it is practical to consider these organisms simply as anaerobic gram-positive cocci.

The only other important group of anaerobes is the genus *Clostridium*. A number of different species of clostridia can be recovered from mixed skin and soft tissue infections, but they are typically not responsible (at least as the sole pathogen) for severe disease. *Clostridium perfringens* and occasionally other species (*Clostridium septicum, Clostridium novyi, Clostridium fallax, Clostridium histolyticum*, and *Clostridium bifermentans*) produce the devastating syndrome known as gas gangrene or more appropriately, clostridial myonecrosis. In such instances, the *Clostridium* species is usually the sole pathogen.

In general, the potentially pathogenic component of the normal oral flora includes gram-negative anaerobic bacilli (but not the *B. fragilis* group), anaerobic gram-positive cocci, and streptococci. Nonanaerobic gram-negative bacilli such as *E. coli* are normally not present in the oropharyngeal flora. The potentially pathogenic flora of the large intestine consists of anaerobic, gram-negative bacilli, including members of the *B. fragilis* group, anaerobic gram-positive cocci, clostridia, streptococci, and enteric bacilli such as *E. coli* and *Klebsiella* species. The normal flora of the female genital tract undergoes complex cyclic changes but may often contain many or all of the important pathogens found in the colon.

It is exceedingly important to realize that the description just given of normal flora refers to a healthy individual who has neither received recent antimicrobial therapy nor been hospitalized recently. Chronic illness, antimicrobial therapy, and hospitalization tend to alter the normal flora such that the patient may become colonized with nosocomial or hospital-associated pathogens such as *Staphylococcus aureus* (both methicillin susceptible and resistant strains), *Pseudomonas aeruginosa*, and *Serratia marcescens*.

CLINICAL SYNDROMES

The skin and soft tissue infections given in Table 35–1 provide the reader with a relatively complete list of such infections. Only those that are potentially life threatening are discussed in this chapter. The interested reader is referred to relevant chapters in this text and to other reference sources.[1–3]

Cellulitis

Cellulitis is an infection of the skin and superficial layers of the subcutaneous tissues. The classic picture of cellulitis is that of an infection of intact skin characterized by redness, warmth, tenderness, and a tense appearance because of edema. The etiologic agents usually implicated are either *S. aureus* or *Streptococcus pyogenes* (group A beta-hemolytic streptococcus), and it is presumed that inoculation of the tissues occurs via a minute break in the skin. A variety of other organisms (*E. coli, Aeromonas* species, anaerobic bacteria, and group B and group G beta-hemolytic streptococci, for example) have also been implicated. The potential for lesser-known agents to produce significant disease should underscore the need for an etiologic diagnosis when cellulitis is extensive or rapidly progressive.

The complications of cellulitis can be life threatening and include bacteremia and certain other severe systemic processes. Cellulitis attributable to *S. aureus*, particularly in children, can cause toxic epidermal necrolysis or staphylococcal scalded skin syndrome, which is characterized by extensive epidermal exfoliation. Although toxic shock syndrome has classically been associated with use of vaginal tampons colonized by toxigenic *S. aureus*, it can be caused by any type of localized staphylococcal infection. Reports have also shown that *S. pyogenes* can produce a lethal toxic shock–like process that may begin as a cellulitis or pyoderma.[4]

Postoperative Surgical Wound Infection

A postoperative wound infection may involve primarily the skin or deeper soft tissues, including muscle. Exogenously acquired wound infections frequently involve *S. aureus* or, less frequently, gram-negative bacilli and streptococci, particularly *S. pyogenes*. Infections arising after incision through mucous membranes (such as the oral cavity) or the mucosa of a viscus (such as the colon) are likely to involve the normal flora of that site, and the infection is therefore likely to be a mixed anaerobic-aerobic process.

Because most surgical wound infections do not become clinically manifest within the first 48 to 72 hours postoperatively, signs of wound infection in this period should suggest infection caused by *S. pyogenes* (group A beta-hemolytic streptococcus) or myonecrosis related to *C. perfringens*.

Cutaneous and Subcutaneous Abscesses

Cutaneous and subcutaneous abscesses are usually thought to be due to *S. aureus*. Although this organism does account for a significant proportion of abscesses, a variety of other aerobic and anaerobic bacteria have been recovered from such abscesses in both adults[5, 6] and children.[7] Because an abscess is a localized process, it is not in itself life threatening. If untreated, however, a soft tissue abscess can progress and cause a potentially lethal soft tissue infection (see Table 35–1) or bacteremia. In certain areas of the body, particularly in obese individuals, the diagnosis of soft tissue abscess may be difficult to make by physical examination alone; these areas include the flanks, the perineum, and the buttocks.

Diabetic Foot Infections

Diabetes mellitus is responsible for the loss of thousands of limbs annually as a consequence of either vascular insufficiency or infection or both. Generally, there is a tendency to underestimate the extent and severity of the infection. Because neuropathy is common in diabetic patients, breaks in the skin of the sole of the foot may not be noticed by the patient and a progressively enlarging ulcer forms. Early in the course of infection, the process is usually mild, typically caused by *S. aureus*, and relatively easily treated. Frequently, the infection goes unnoticed for several weeks, during which time there is spread of infection from the superficial ulcer into subcutaneous tissues and even to bone. During this period, anaerobic bacteria and nonanaerobic gram-negative bacilli may also have become involved; a putrid odor often develops (documenting the presence of anaerobes). At this juncture, the patient may be hyperglycemic and ketotic and bacteremia may have developed. Examination may reveal a plantar ulcer with modest surrounding inflammation and swelling of the forefoot or midfoot or both. The presence of a rather mild local response may reflect vascular insufficiency and an inadequate host response rather than a mild infection; in other words, a potentially lethal infection may be overlooked because of the poor local host response. This type of infection may suddenly progress to one of the rapidly lethal soft tissue infections, such as necrotizing fasciitis. Gas may be detectable by examination or radiograph at any point in the course of a diabetic foot infection. The detection of soft tissue gas should prompt an urgent surgical evaluation.

Infected Decubitus Ulcer

Decubitus ulcers, or bedsores, can develop rapidly in immobilized patients. Infection of a decubitus ulcer may precipitate hospitalization or may arise during hospitalization. The areas most frequently involved are the sacrum, the greater trochanters, and the heels. Decubitus ulcers around the pelvic girdle are extremely likely to become infected unless there is meticulous local care. This type of infection is invariably a polymicrobial, mixed anaerobic-aerobic infection; grossly necrotic tissue with purulent drainage and a foul odor are commonly present. One group reported that 79% of 24 septic patients with infected decubitus ulcers had bacteremia and that anaerobes, particularly members of the *B. fragilis* group, were recovered from blood in 50% of the 24 patients.[8] Bacteremia was polymicrobial in a substantial proportion of these subjects.

Anaerobic Cellulitis

The term anaerobic cellulitis is not accurate because the process is not simply a cellulitis caused by anaerobes. It is synonymous with gas abscess and is sometimes termed clostridial cellulitis, the latter term being used when clostridia have been isolated from the infection.[1, 2] The clinical picture of clostridial cellulitis does not appear to be distinct from similar lesions in which anaerobes other than clostridia are present. In other words, clostridial cellulitis does not appear to be a clostridial toxin–induced process but rather a process in which clostridia play a role similar to the other anaerobic bacteria that are present. In fact, it is important to recognize that the recovery of clostridia from an infection is not diagnostic for gas gangrene or clostridial myonecrosis; that diagnosis can only be made clinically and confirmed histopathologically.

Anaerobic cellulitis involves the epifascial soft tissues of the neck, thorax, hip, buttocks, retroperitoneum, abdominal wall, perineum, and extremities. Predisposing factors include contamination of the subcutaneous tissues of an accidental or operative wound, pre-existing localized infection, and contamination of an injection site (often with saliva) at the time of injection in an illicit drug user.

The onset is usually mild and systemic symptoms are limited, particularly when compared with necrotizing fasciitis, synergistic nonclostridial anaerobic myonecrosis, and clostridial myonecrosis. Although necrotizing features and rapid spread may occur, they are not typical. However, delay in diagnosis and therapy may permit progression of disease with an attendant increase in toxemia, morbidity, and mortality.

The infectious process tends to be *relatively* superficial; the deep fascia is not involved, nor are the structures deep to it. Anaerobic cellulitis is an inflammation of the subcutaneous tissues that progresses to necrosis with crepitation within 2 to 5 days of onset. The skin may be grossly uninvolved unless the process started as a wound infection.

Pain may be the first symptom, but it is mild in comparison with necrotizing fasciitis or clostridial myonecrosis. Soon after, swelling and redness of the overlying skin occur, followed by tenderness to palpation and development of crepitation. Although soft tissue gas may be readily detected by palpation or radiography, the extent of the infection is *not* reflected by the extent of soft tissue gas. At surgery, the usual findings include a putrid odor (diagnostic of anaerobic infection), gas, variable amounts of pus, and shreds of devitalized, subcutaneous tissue. By definition, muscle necrosis is absent, although there may be muscle edema with long-standing infection. The usual bacterial flora includes anaerobic gram-negative bacilli, gram-positive cocci, and streptococci. Enteric gram-negative bacilli, *S. aureus*, and other facultative bacteria may also be recovered.

Necrotizing Fasciitis

Necrotizing fasciitis is an uncommon infection that typically has an abrupt onset. The mortality approaches or exceeds 50% without appropriate therapy.[1, 2] The infection usually begins in a traumatic musculoskeletal wound but may develop at an operative wound site, at a site of lesser infection, or even after trivial trauma. The pathognomonic feature of necrotizing fasciitis is subcutaneous and fascial necrosis, with undermining of the skin. The process begins with sudden onset of local pain and swelling. Chills and fever may be absent initially; later, prostration may become severe. Within 24 hours, there may be considerable phlegmon and erythema or cellulitis. Bluish-to-brownish, ecchymotic skin discoloration is often present and may progress to cutaneous gangrene later in the disease. Pain is gradually replaced by cutaneous anesthesia as a result of compression and destruction of cutaneous nerves as they pass through the edematous fascia. Obstruction of nutrient vessels as they pass through deeper tissues results in cutaneous necrosis that begins with the appearance of bullae in the area of involvement and progresses to cutaneous gangrene. The most striking diagnostic feature of necrotizing fasciitis is the extensive undermining of the skin and subcutaneous tissues. This can be demonstrated in the operating room by the ease with which a sterile instrument can be passed along the plane just superficial to the deep fascia because of the extensive necrosis of the epifascial and subcutaneous tissues. This maneuver cannot normally be done, nor can it be done with other types of infection.

Gas is frequently present in the soft tissues but is difficult to detect by examination. In one series, crepitation was detectable in only 19% of patients, whereas gas could be detected in 81% by radiography.[9] Although *S. aureus*, hemolytic streptococci, and enteric gram-negative bacilli have been considered to be the causes of necrotizing fasciitis,[10] more recent studies have indicated that anaerobic gram-negative bacilli and anaerobic gram-positive cocci are also important pathogens and are present more often than not.[11]

Fournier's Gangrene

Fournier's gangrene is a necrotizing fasciitis that begins in the scrotum and usually extends to involve the subcutaneous tissues and fascia of the perineum, penis, abdominal wall, and flanks.[1, 2, 12] Although the origin of many cases is idiopathic, trauma, antecedent surgery, and perianal infection can be inciting events. Diabetes mellitus, obesity, or both are often predisposing factors. As is the case with necrotizing fasciitis arising in other parts of the body, the infection may spread extremely rapidly and be rapidly fatal. The infection is almost invariably a mixed anaerobic-aerobic process.

Clostridial Fasciitis

Clostridial fasciitis is a poorly described entity that appears to be distinct from necrotizing fasciitis on the one hand and clostridial myonecrosis on the other hand. This syndrome is said to be caused by one of several species of clostridia (*C. septicum, Clostridium ramosum*, and *C. histolyticum*). It begins locally as a consequence of trauma, tumor invasion, or antecedent infection, and there is rapid spread of infection along fascial planes and death within 48 hours. Clinical manifestations include toxemia, hemolysis, and increased capillary permeability that produces extensive fluid exudation.[13] This entity is reminiscent of the rapidly disseminated infection that can be seen with *C. septicum* bacteremia.[14]

Clostridial Myonecrosis (Clostridial Gas Gangrene)

Use of the term *gas gangrene* should be limited to cases of clostridial infection in which muscle necrosis (myonecrosis) is present. The mere presence of gangrene (dead tissue) or the presence of gas in tissue or both does not necessarily imply a severe illness, whereas muscle necrosis caused by a *Clostridium* (clostridial myonecrosis) is a potentially lethal process that requires emergent surgical intervention.[1, 2, 15]

The typical picture of clostridial myonecrosis is that of sudden onset of pain at the site of a traumatic or surgical wound. Occasionally, clostridial myonecrosis may occur (apparently spontaneously) as a consequence of clostridial bacteremia and is often referred to as metastatic clostridial myonecrosis; the onset is manifested by sudden progressive pain in the absence of a wound or trauma. The pain, when clostridial myonecrosis occurs in an extremity, may appear so suddenly as to suggest the occurrence of a complete vascular occlusion. The pain steadily increases in severity but remains localized to the infected areas, spreading as the infection spreads. Local swelling, edema, and a hemorrhagic exudate from the wound then develop. There is often a rapid pulse, the degree of pulse elevation being out of proportion to the degree of fever. The skin is tense and white (often with areas of bluish discoloration) and is colder than normal; the edematous area is exquisitely tender. The pain may become so severe as to cause the patient to plead with the physician to perform an amputation. Bronze discoloration of the skin may develop, the swelling and toxemia increase rapidly, the serous discharge becomes profuse (sometimes so profuse that the wound dressings become soaked almost immediately), the skin becomes duskier, and bullae filled with dark red or purplish fluid may appear. The appearance of bullae in association with significant localized pain is extremely suggestive of clostridial myonecrosis, especially if the bullous fluid is hemorrhagic. In the case of metastatic clostridial myonecrosis, exudate from the affected site occurs only after rupture of the bullae. Gas may be present in the tissues but typically is not abundant in the early stages and may be quite difficult to demonstrate.

Several aspects of mentation may be rather striking. Some patients may be alert and oriented and have a clear understanding of the gravity of the disease; this may manifest as a profound terror or sense of impending doom. Others may manifest a toxic delirium before any visible changes in the wound. The patient may at any point become incoherent, disoriented, and obstreperous.

The extent of change in involved muscle is usually appreciated only at operation. Hence, it is essential that surgical exploration be done whenever the clinical findings are consistent with clostridial myonecrosis. Early changes in the muscle are edema and pallor; later, there is change in the color of the muscle (progressive reddening and purple mottling), its blood supply is lost, contractile ability disappears, and gas may be demonstrable. The consistency may be pasty or mucoid; still later, the muscle may become liquefied.

As disease advances, there may be multiorgan involvement and failure, including respiratory, renal, neurologic, and cardiovascular dysfunction. Hemolysis is usually seen only with uterine myonecrosis and is associated with bacteremia.

Eighty to 95% of cases are caused by *C. perfringens*;[16] the most frequent causes of civilian clostridial myonecrosis are *C. perfringens* and *C. septicum*.

Major predisposing causes of clostridial myonecrosis are extensive laceration or devitalization of muscles, particularly large muscle groups of the buttocks or lower extremity; impaired blood supply to a limb or muscle group; contamination of a muscle wound by foreign material; and delay in prompt management of a contaminated wound. Compound fractures in particular predispose because bacteria can gain direct access to the soft tissues and because invariably there is muscle injury, development of hematomata, and impairment of blood supply to the muscle. These conditions all favor the growth of clostridia. Abdominal wall myonecrosis usually follows surgery involving the gallbladder or colon. Myonecrosis involving an extremity may also follow injection of medications or of illicit drugs.

Metastatic (spontaneous) clostridial myonecrosis is due to either *C. septicum* or *C. perfringens* and results from hematogenous seeding of the involved muscle. This form of myonecrosis is frequently associated with carcinoma of the colon, particularly cecal carcinoma. Other processes that alter the integrity of the gut mucosa, such as cancer chemotherapy, may also be responsible. The clinical picture is identical to that of wound-associated myonecrosis. The diagnosis may be missed, however, because of the lack of a wound. The development of bullae associated with severe local pain, however, is quite suggestive of clostridial myonecrosis.

Anaerobic Streptococcal Myositis

Myositis and myonecrosis may also be caused by organisms other than clostridia, including the "anaerobic" streptococci.[1-3] These organisms are not all true anaerobes but are extremely fastidious and are likely to be recovered by techniques used for the isolation of anaerobic bacteria. Anaerobic streptococcal myositis is uncommon and may resemble clostridial myonecrosis, but it has a more subacute course. The usual incubation period is 3 to 5 days after an injury, and the presenting signs are edema and purulent or seropurulent wound exudate. Pain develops later in the course of illness; this feature is distinctly different from clostridial myonecrosis. The pain may later become severe. After pain has become established as a symptom, the illness tends to progress relatively rapidly, although not as rapidly as with clostridial disease. Edema progresses diffusely and gas is present both inter- and intramuscularly, but it is not abundant. The involved muscle is at first pale and soft and later becomes bright red, with a typical regular purple barring. Later, the muscle becomes markedly swollen, dark purple, friable, and then gangrenous. There is a peculiar sour odor to the wound.

Patients with fatal disease die after 1 week or longer with toxemia, mild delirium or disorientation, and shock as preterminal events. Although the condition is termed anaerobic streptococcal myositis, the anaerobic streptococci are invariably found in association with other organisms, particularly *S. pyogenes* and *S. aureus*. The character of the illness depends on the coinfecting organisms.[1] Myositis associated with *S. pyogenes* tends to be more acute and to be associated with cutaneous erythema, bright red discoloration of the muscle, and a terminal bacteremia. When staphylococci are present, the disease tends to be more insidious and the muscles are paler and more edematous.

A distinct difference from clostridial myonecrosis is that the edematous and discolored muscle (early in the course of disease) is reactive to stimuli and is viable.

Synergistic Nonclostridial Anaerobic Myonecrosis

This infection of muscle has been known by several names, including synergistic necrotizing cellulitis, gram-negative anaerobic cutaneous gangrene, and necrotizing cutaneous myositis.[1] The term *synergistic nonclostridial anaerobic myonecrosis* is most appropriate because this highly virulent mixed anaerobic soft tissue infection is characterized by involvement of muscle and the tissues superficial to the muscle. The disease occurs most commonly in the lower extremities and perineum.[1, 17]

The presence of large, discrete, blue-gray areas of skin necrosis separated by normal skin is a unique feature of this infection. The extent of disease is much greater than can be appreciated by cutaneous findings, however. There is extensive confluent necrotic liquefaction or gangrene of the subcutaneous tissues, fascia, and muscle. The wound drainage is foul smelling and is often referred to as *dishwater pus*. Severe systemic toxicity is usual and is sudden in onset; before this, however, the extensive subcutaneous necrosis has developed. Exquisite local tenderness and severe pain are evident. Soft tissue gas can be detected in approximately 25% of patients, but it is usually not pronounced. Predisposing factors include malnutrition, obesity, chronic renal dysfunction, and advanced age. Diabetes is present in approximately 75% of cases. Anaerobic and nonanaerobic gram-negative bacilli, anaerobic streptococci, or both are present in almost all cases. Bacteremia attributable to one or more of these organisms occurs in approximately 30% of cases.

Infected Vascular Gangrene

Infected vascular gangrene is a condition in which anaerobic bacteria (and nonanaerobes) are commonly found in soft tissue and muscle. In this condition, the limb or part of the limb has died because of circulatory insufficiency and the bacteria act as saprophytes. There is a tendency for the infection to remain confined to the dead tissue, and there is seldom toxemia. There is often an extremely foul odor to the wound, and there may be substantial gas in the devitalized tissue. If the condition is neglected, the process may begin to spread proximally to involve healthy tissue and cause serious complications.

Muscle Abscess

Muscle abscess related to illicit drug injection has been reported; such cases almost invariably involve anaerobes.[1, 2] A more common but still relatively rare muscle infection in the United States is pyomyositis, a primary muscle infection.

Pyomyositis is an infection of muscle that occurs as a consequence of bacteremic seeding rather than penetrating trauma. Bacteremia is present in less than 5% of patients at the time of presentation, however.[3] Most cases of pyomyositis occur in the tropics and approximately 95% are caused by *S. aureus*. A wide variety of other organisms have been implicated on rare occasion. Only a small number of cases have been reported in the United States,[3] whereas an apparently identical infection in the tropics (tropical pyomyositis) occurs with a much greater frequency than does the process in temperate climates. There is no convincing evidence to relate the higher incidence of pyomyositis in the tropics causally to factors unique to the tropics.[3]

In 25 to 50% of cases of pyomyositis, there is a history of blunt trauma to the affected muscles. The onset of illness is usually subacute, with pain, swelling, induration, and tenderness evolving over several days. The most frequent sites of involvement are the muscles of the lower extremities and trunk; in the majority of instances a single muscle group is involved. Because the muscle abscess is contained by the surrounding fascia, there may be little cutaneous evidence of infection. Early on, there may be little pain or tenderness to palpation. Eventually, however, the process extends to superficial tissues, and localized findings suggest the site of the infection. In one series of 18 patients, the duration of symptoms ranged from 1 day to 1 year, with a majority of patients being symptomatic for 2 to 8 weeks before diagnosis.[18]

On rare occasion, *S. pyogenes* may produce a fulminant pyomyositis associated with toxemia, bacteremia, and a high mortality rate.

DIAGNOSIS

Diagnosis of skin and soft tissue infections requires exercise of certain basic principles of clinical infectious practice and recognition that a wide variety of such infections exist and that some of these infections may be rapidly fatal.

An accurate, focused history and physical examination help determine whether a necrotizing disease of fascia or muscle is likely. Gram's stain of smears of wound exudate may suggest the etiologic agent(s), such as *S. aureus, C. perfringens*, or a mixed anaerobic process. In addition, cultures of wound exudate, tissue aspirates, and blood should be performed. Cultures for anaerobic bacteria are expensive and difficult for most clinical laboratories to perform; however, anaerobic bacteria play a prominent role in many soft tissue infections. Anaerobic cultures should be done (using appropriate collection and transport techniques[1, 2]) whenever the diagnosis is in doubt or a potentially life-threatening infection is a consideration. It is particularly important that tissue samples and exudates obtained at operation be cultured for anaerobes (and nonanaerobes).

With many of the entities listed in Table 35–1, the only means by which a potentially rapidly lethal soft tissue infection can be distinguished from some of the more milder processes is by surgical exploration, which may thus provide a diagnosis (or tissue samples for microbiologic and histologic diagnosis) and be an important aspect of treatment. It is essential that the clinician appreciate the crucial diagnostic role of surgical exploration in many of the skin and soft tissue infections.

Repeated evaluation of the affected site is prudent, and whenever there is concern about the accuracy of the working diagnosis, infectious disease and surgical consultations should be obtained.

TREATMENT

Treatment of the processes discussed in this chapter can be divided into two basic categories: antimicrobial therapy and surgical therapy. For some infections, antimicrobial therapy alone will suffice, as in the case of an uncomplicated cellulitis. In general, oxacillin (or an equivalent penicillin), a first-generation cephalosporin (such as cefazolin), and vancomycin are effective against *S. aureus*; however, only the last agent is active against methicillin-resistant *S. aureus*. Most streptococci are susceptible to penicillin G or a first-generation cephalosporin. Anaerobic bacteria are susceptible to a variety of agents, depending on the particular anaerobe being considered. Oral anaerobes are usually susceptible to high-dose penicillin G (10 million U daily) and are virtually always susceptible to clindamycin, cefoxitin, metronidazole, imipenem plus cilastatin, and the combination of a penicillin plus β-lactamase inhibitor (such as ampicillin plus sulbactam or ticarcillin plus clavulanate). Anaerobes from the colon and female genital tract may be more resistant than oral anaerobes, but they are virtually always susceptible to metronidazole, imipenem plus cilastatin, and the penicillin plus β-lactamase inhibitor combinations. Metronidazole is the agent with the greatest antianaerobic activity; however, unlike the other agents mentioned, it has no activity against nonanaerobes. Empirical therapy for gram-negative nonanaerobic bacilli should probably involve an aminoglycoside (regardless of the degree of renal dysfunction), such as gentamicin or amikacin, until susceptibility data are available. The agent of choice for clostridial myonecrosis is penicillin G (approximately 20 million U daily if renal function is normal); metronidazole is appropriate when penicillin cannot be given.

In general, empirical antimicrobial therapy should be based on the results of Gram's stain of infected material and an understanding of the pathogens likely to be present in the particular clinical situation being assessed. This empirical therapy should be broad, and the agents given should be active (based on general knowledge and the hospital's antimicrobial susceptibility profile) against the suspected pathogens. As the results of culture and susceptibility tests for nonanaerobes are generated by the laboratory, therapy can be modified to maximize efficacy, minimize toxicity, and limit costs (in that order of priority). Unfortunately, it is quite common for therapy to be initiated before appropriate cultures are taken; in some instances, cultures are simply not done. The likelihood of poor clinical outcome or significant drug toxicity or both is substantial if the appropriate microbiologic evaluation is not initiated.

The key to both diagnosis and therapy of many of the infections discussed here is surgical evaluation and treatment. Devitalized tissues should be débrided; multiple débridements are often needed. This is particularly true for the necrotizing infections of fascia and muscle.

Necrotizing fasciitis, Fournier's gangrene, clostridial myonecrosis, and synergistic nonclostridial anaerobic myonecrosis often cannot be diagnosed by clinical examination, and there are no diagnostic laboratory tests available that will yield an accurate and prompt diagnosis.[1, 2] Therefore, the proper management of the patient in whom one of these syndromes is a consideration is surgical exploration with radical débridement of all injured or devitalized tissues. The surgeon must continue to explore the affected site along fascial planes and muscles until healthy tissue is encountered and all nonviable tissue has been removed. Experience has shown repeatedly that multiple trips to the operating room may be necessary to ensure that the process has been halted by removal of all devitalized tissue. When complete débridement is not possible and the disease is progressing, amputation may be necessary if an extremity is involved. Certain conditions, such as clostridial myonecrosis of the paraspinal muscles or extensive myonecrosis of the abdominal wall musculature, do not permit adequate débridement nor do they afford the possibility of amputation. Hyperbaric oxygen therapy may be considered in such individuals, but it should be recognized that there is no compelling scientific data to support the usefulness of this modality for treatment of bacterial infections of any type. It is important to avoid transfer of a patient with a potentially surgically curable infection for the purpose of obtaining hyperbaric oxygen therapy. These infections progress extremely rapidly and the delay of surgery, even for just a few hours, can be fatal. In the past, gas gangrene antitoxin was used for treatment of clostridial myonecrosis; efficacy of this preparation has not been shown, and the antitoxin preparation has not been available in the United States for several years.

Preventive Aspects of Infection in the Intensive Care Unit

Most of the infections discussed in this chapter are causes for admission to the intensive care unit and are not necessarily preventable.

Obviously, meticulous intravenous catheter care and decubitus ulcer care are important for prevention of infection. Prevention of most of the other infections requires good surgical technique, proper use of prophylactic antibiotics, and aggressive surgical management of traumatic wounds, particularly those that are heavily contaminated with foreign material.

Vigilance and early treatment of lesser infections may prevent progression to some of the more severe, life-threatening infections.

References

1. Finegold SM: Anaerobic Bacteria in Human Disease. New York, Academic Press, 1977.
2. Finegold SM, George WL (eds): Anaerobic Infections in Humans. San Diego, Academic Press, 1989.
3. Mandell GL, Douglas RG Jr, Bennett JE (eds): Principles and Practice of Infectious Diseases. 3rd ed. New York, Churchill Livingstone, 1990.
4. Cone LA, Woodard DR, Schlievert PM, et al: Clinical and bacteriological observations of a toxic shock–like syndrome due to *Streptococcus pyogenes*. N Engl J Med 317:146, 1987.
5. Meislin HW, Lerner SA, Graves MH, et al: Cutaneous abscesses. Anaerobic and aerobic bacteriology and outpatient management. Ann Intern Med 87:145, 1977.
6. Ghoneim ATM, McGoldrick J, Blick PWH, et al: Aerobic and anaerobic bacteriology of subcutaneous abscesses. Br J Surg 68:498, 1981.
7. Brook I, Finegold SM: Aerobic and anaerobic bacteriology of cutaneous abscesses in children. Pediatrics 67:891, 1981.
8. Chow AW, Galpin JE, Guze LB: Clindamycin for sepsis caused by decubitus ulcers. J Infect Dis 135(suppl):S65, 1977.
9. Fisher JR, Conway MJ, Takeshita RT, et al: Necrotizing fasciitis. Importance of roentgenographic studies for soft tissue gas. JAMA 241:803, 1979.
10. Freeman HP, Oluwole SF, Ganepola GAP, et al: Necrotizing fasciitis. Am J Surg 142:377, 1981.
11. Guiliano A, Lewis F Jr, Hadley K, et al: Bacteriology of necrotizing fasciitis. Am J Surg 134:52, 1977.
12. Nickel JC, Morales A: Necrotizing fasciitis of the male genitalia (Fournier's gangrene). Can Med Assoc J 129:445, 1983.
13. Gorbach S: Discussion [of Virulence factors of *Clostridium perfringens*]. Rev Infect Dis 1:261, 1979.
14. Katlic MR, Derkac WM, Coleman WL: *Clostridium septicum* infection and malignancy. Ann Surg 193:361, 1981.
15. MacLennan JD: The histotoxic clostridial infections of man. Bacteriol Rev 26:177, 1962.
16. Altemeier WA, Fullen WD: Prevention and treatment of gas gangrene. JAMA 217:806, 1971.
17. Stone HH, Martin JD Jr: Synergistic necrotizing cellulitis. Ann Surg 175:702, 1972.
18. Hall RL, Callaghan JJ, Moloney E, et al: Pyomyositis in a temperate climate. Presentation, diagnosis, and treatment. J Bone Joint Surg [Am] 72:1240, 1990.

CHAPTER 36

Bacterial Meningitis

Allan R. Tunkel
W. Michael Scheld

The central nervous system (CNS) represents an area in which bacterial infections are frequently devastating. Although the brain possesses several defense mechanisms (e.g., intact cranium and blood-brain barrier [BBB]) to prevent entry of bacterial species, once microorganisms gain entry to the CNS, host defense mechanisms are generally inadequate to control the infection. Antimicrobial therapy is limited by the poor penetration of many agents into the CNS, as well as by the ability of antibiotics to induce further inflammation in the CNS via their bacteriolytic action, thereby contributing to brain damage. This chapter provides a review of bacterial meningitis and emphasizes developments in diagnosis and therapy as they pertain to the care of the critically ill patient.

EPIDEMIOLOGY AND ETIOLOGY

The overall annual attack rate for bacterial meningitis is approximately 3.0 cases per 100,000 population in the United States, although variability exists depending on geographic area, sex, and race.[1] More than 80% of all cases are due to infection with *Haemophilus influenzae*, *Neisseria meningitidis*, or *Streptococcus pneumoniae*. Other bacterial species are more likely to be present depending on the patient's age, underlying disease status, and other predisposing conditions (discussed later).

H. influenzae is isolated in 48.3% of all cases of bacterial meningitis in the United States, with an overall mortality rate of 6.0%.[1] Nearly all cases occur in children less than 6 years of age, with 90% caused by capsular type b strains. Disease is most likely initiated after nasopharyngeal acquisition of a virulent organism, with subsequent systemic invasion.[2] *H. influenzae* represents only about 5% of total cerebrospinal fluid (CSF) isolates after age 6 years, and isolation of the organism in this age group should suggest the presence of certain predisposing factors, including sinusitis, otitis media, epiglottitis, pneumonia, head trauma with CSF leak, diabetes mellitus, alcoholism, splenectomy or asplenic states, and immune deficiency (e.g., hypogammaglobulinemia).[3]

Meningitis caused by *N. meningitidis* is most often found in children and young adults and may occur in epidemics, usually attributable to serogroups A and C. Type B strains are isolated most frequently in sporadic cases accounting for 51.1% of all isolates, and type Y strains may be associated with pneumonia. The meningococcus is isolated in 19.6% of all cases of bacterial meningitis in the United States; the mortality rate is 10.3%.[1] Nasopharyngeal carriage of virulent organisms also accounts for initiation of infection.[4] Infection is more likely in patients who have deficiencies in the terminal complement components (C5b,6,7,8,9, the so-called membrane attack complex), in whom there is a greater than 8000-fold increase in the incidence of neisserial infections, although mortality rates are lower than those in patients with intact complement systems.[5]

Pneumococcal meningitis is most frequently observed in adults older than 30 years of age and accounts for 13.3% of total cases of meningitis, with a mortality rate of 26.3%.[1] Infection is often associated with distant foci of infection such as pneumonia, otitis media, mastoiditis, sinusitis, or endocarditis. Serious pneumococcal infections may be observed in patients with predisposing conditions such as splenectomy or asplenic states, multiple myeloma, hypogammaglobulinemia, and alcoholism.[6] *S. pneumoniae* is the most common meningeal isolate from head trauma patients who have suffered basilar skull fracture with subsequent CSF leak.[7–9]

Listeria monocytogenes represents only about 1.9% of all cases of bacterial meningitis in the United States but carries a high mortality rate (28.5%). Infection with *Listeria* is more likely in neonates, elderly persons, alcoholics, cancer patients, and immunosuppressed adults (e.g., renal transplant patients).[10] However, up to 30% of adults and 54% of children and young adults who have listeriosis have no apparent underlying condition. Listeriosis has been associated with several food-borne outbreaks involving contaminated coleslaw, milk, and cheese.

Meningitis caused by aerobic gram-negative bacilli is observed in specific clinical situations.[11] *Escherichia coli* is isolated from 30 to 50% of infants under 2 months of age with bacterial meningitis. *Klebsiella* species, *E. coli*, and *Pseudomonas aeruginosa* may be isolated from patients after head trauma and neurosurgical procedures, elderly persons, immunosuppressed patients, and patients with gram-negative septicemia. Despite the low frequency of meningitis related to this group of organisms, the mortality rates have been quite high (approximately 84% with *P. aeruginosa*).

Specific clinical situations may predispose to the development of meningitis caused by staphylococcal species.[12] *Staphylococcus epidermidis* is the most common cause of meningitis in patients with CSF shunts. Meningitis attributable to *Staphylococcus aureus* is frequently found in the early postneurosurgical period, as well as in patients with CSF shunts. Underlying diseases in patients with no prior CNS disease and who develop *S. aureus* meningitis include diabetes mellitus, alcoholism, chronic renal failure requiring hemodialysis, and malignancies. Conditions that increase *S. aureus* nasal carriage rates (e.g., in intravenous drug abusers, insulin-requiring diabetics, and hemodialysis patients) may also predispose to staphylococcal infection of the CNS.

Group B streptococcal disease in neonates may occur as an early-onset septicemia associated with premature rupture of the membranes and low-birth-weight infants or as a late-onset (>7 days after birth) meningitis.[13] The early-onset disease is acquired from the maternal genital tract, whereas the source of the organism in late-onset disease is controversial because 40% of affected infants are born to culture-negative mothers. This organism (*Streptococcus agalactiae*) is the most common cause of serious neonatal infection in many large centers. Rare cases have also been reported in postpartum women after vaginal delivery.[14] Although it accounts for only about 3.4% of all cases of meningitis, mortality rates (approximately 22.5%) in the United States remain high.

Bacterial meningitis also remains a significant problem in other parts of the world. A review of all cases of meningitis in an isolation-fever hospital in Salvador, Brazil, for the decade 1973 to 1982 revealed an approximately 10-fold higher incidence than that in the United States.[15] The average annual incidence was 45.8 cases per 100,000 population, with an overall mortality rate of 33%. The three common meningeal pathogens (*N. meningitidis*, *H. influenzae*, and *S. pneumoniae*) accounted for 72% of all cases and 70% of the deaths. The case fatality rates for *H. influenzae* and *S. pneumoniae* were 38 and 59%, respectively, much higher than those seen in the United States. The mortality caused by the Enterobacteriaceae was 86%, with more than half of these cases in children younger than 24 months of age caused by *Salmonella* species.

PATHOGENESIS AND PATHOPHYSIOLOGY
Mucosal Colonization, Systemic Invasion, and Bacteremia

A critical first step in the initiation of bacterial meningitis is host acquisition of a new organism by nasopharyngeal colonization. An important virulence factor in this regard is bacterial capsule. The type b capsular strains of *H. influenzae* are the most virulent, and the intranasal inoculation of *H. influenzae* type b often leads to invasive disease in infant animal models.[16] Serum antibodies to polyribosyl-ribitol phosphate, the capsular polysaccharide of type b isolates, confer protection against invasive disease.[17] Organism adhesion is an important factor allowing nasopharyngeal colonization. Elegant experiments utilizing *N. meningitidis* have shown that meningococci bind to nasopharyngeal epithelial cells through fimbriae, or pili, to a specific cell surface receptor,[18] with subsequent transport across nonciliated columnar nasopharyngeal cells within a phagocytic vacuole.[19] Adhesion of microorganisms to mucosal cells may be blocked by natural antibodies, such as immunoglobulin A, found in mucosal secretions, although high concentrations of circulating immunoglobulin A antibodies to *N. meningitidis* may paradoxically permit the development of invasive disease by preferentially binding to these organisms, inhibiting the beneficial effects of bactericidal antibodies to immunoglobulins M and G.[20]

After nasopharyngeal colonization and mucosal invasion, bacteria gain access to the blood stream, where they must overcome host defense mechanisms for survival. Bacterial capsule is an important virulence factor that facilitates development of high-grade bacteremia through its ability to resist classic complement pathway bactericidal activity and inhibit neutrophil phagocytosis. The host possesses several defense mechanisms to counteract the antiphagocytic activity of bacterial capsule.[9] One is the alternative complement pathway that is activated by the capsular polysaccharides of *S. pneumoniae*, which results in cleavage of C3 with attachment of C3b to the bacterial surface, facilitating opsonization, phagocytosis, and intravascular clearance of the organism.

Meningeal Invasion

After the microorganism evades the systemic host defenses, there is meningeal invasion and bacterial multiplication within the subarachnoid space (SAS). The site and mechanism of meningeal invasion by bacteria, however, are poorly understood. Early studies of *H. influenzae* meningitis in an experimental infant rat model suggested that the route of CNS invasion was through the dural venous sinus system.[21] Other studies, however, suggested that during bacteremia, a nonspecific, sterile, focal inflammation above the cribriform plate facilitated CNS invasion at this site. Additional studies with infant rats and primates have demonstrated that bacteria enter the CSF via the choroid plexus because of its exceptionally high rate of blood flow, suggesting that more bacterial organisms are delivered to this site per unit time than to many other anatomic locations in the body. Studies have shown that cells in the choroid plexus and/or cerebral capillaries possess receptors mediating adherence of meningeal pathogens with subsequent transport into the SAS. For example, *E. coli* strains expressing S fimbriae bind to the luminal surface of the vascular endothelium and to the epithelium lining the choroid plexus and brain ventricles.[22]

Survival in the Subarachnoid Space

After bacteria enter the SAS, host defense mechanisms are inadequate to control the infection. Assays for complement components in CSF are usually negative or reveal only minimal concentrations. Although CSF complement concentrations are increased with meningeal inflammation,[23, 24] they remain low, and this local complement deficiency impedes opsonization of encapsulated meningeal pathogens, precluding efficient phagocytosis. It has been suggested that during bacterial meningitis, leukocyte proteases degrade complement components crossing the BBB, resulting in inefficient opsonic activity at the site of infection.[25] Immunoglobulin concentrations are also low in normal CSF, and CSF immunoglobulin concentrations remain lower than simultaneous serum concentrations, even in the presence of bacterial meningitis.[25, 26] Low concentrations of immunoglobulins, in concert with the local complement deficiency, contribute to the regional host deficiency in the CSF during bacterial meningitis.

A CSF neutrophilic pleocytosis is a major hallmark of SAS inflammation during bacterial meningitis. The pathway of neutrophil traversal into the CSF, however, is unknown. Adherence of neutrophils to vascular endothelial cells may be a necessary prerequisite for this traversal. Pretreatment of endothelial cells in tissue culture with various inflammatory cytokines induces formation of specific adhesion molecules (e.g., endothelial leukocyte adhesion molecule-1),[27] although these adhesion molecules have not yet been demonstrated in cerebral endothelium. Studies of experimental meningitis in a rabbit model have suggested that the intravenous inoculation of a monoclonal antibody (IB4) against the CD18 family of receptors on leukocytes blocks the accumulation of leukocytes in CSF, despite intracisternal challenge with *H. influenzae* type b, *N. meningitidis, S. pneumoniae*, pneumococcal cell wall, or lipopolysaccharide (LPS).[28] Although the site of leukocyte traversal into the SAS is unknown, purulent CSF is chemotactic for leukocytes in vitro.[29, 30] Experimental models of pneumococcal meningitis have identified one putative chemotactic substance as C5a, and the intracisternal inoculation of C5a into rabbits causes a rapid, early influx of leukocytes into CSF.[31] This effect is decreased by the CSF administration of prostaglandin E₂ (PGE₂) in a dose-related fashion, suggesting that PGE₂ may exert an anti-inflammatory action in meningitis.

Subarachnoid Space Inflammation

The induction of SAS inflammation is a critical event leading to many of the pathophysiologic consequences of bacterial meningitis. Despite the fact that bacterial capsule is crucial for intravascular and SAS survival of meningeal pathogens, capsular polysaccharides are remarkably noninflammatory. Studies of *S. pneumoniae* meningitis in an experimental rabbit model have shown that the pneumococcal cell wall is the most potent inducer of CSF inflammation.[32] Furthermore, independent intracisternal injection of the major components of the pneumococcal cell wall, teichoic acid and peptidoglycan, also induced CSF inflammation.[33] These findings suggested that bacterial lytic products (e.g., cell wall) released by antibiotic-induced autolysis during treatment of bacterial meningitis contributed to the host inflammatory response in the SAS, resulting in significant morbidity and mortality. SAS inflammation is also induced by intracisternal inoculation of purified *H. influenzae* type b LPS,[34, 35] an effect that was blocked by polymyxin B (a cationic antibiotic that binds to the lipid A region of the LPS molecule) and neutrophil acyloxyacyl hydrolase (which removes nonhydroxylated fatty acids from the lipid A region of the LPS), indicating that the lipid A region of LPS contributes to its inflammatory properties. Similar CSF inflammatory changes are invoked after the intracisternal inoculation of *H. influenzae* type b outer membrane vesicles,[36, 37] which serve as relevant nonreplicating vehicles for the delivery of the toxic moieties of LPS to host cells, supporting the concept that LPS carried via outer membrane vesicles leads to induction of SAS inflammation.

Evidence suggests that pneumococcal cell wall and *H. influenzae* type b LPS elicit SAS inflammation through CSF release of inflammatory mediators such as interleukin-1 (IL-1) and/or tumor necrosis factor (TNF). Intact pneumococci and pneumococcal cell walls induce human peripheral monocytes in vitro to produce large amounts of IL-1 but not TNF.[38] In addition, the intracisternal inoculation of *H. influenzae* type b LPS into rats leads to increased CSF concentrations of both IL-1 and TNF within 30 to 120 minutes.[39] Elevated CSF concentrations of TNF have also been observed in rabbits after intracisternal inoculation of LPS;[40] simultaneous analyses of serum samples for TNF activity were negative, indicating that the TNF was principally produced within the CNS. In addition, these increased CSF TNF concentrations may be specific for bacterial meningitis because TNF concentrations, measured in mice and humans

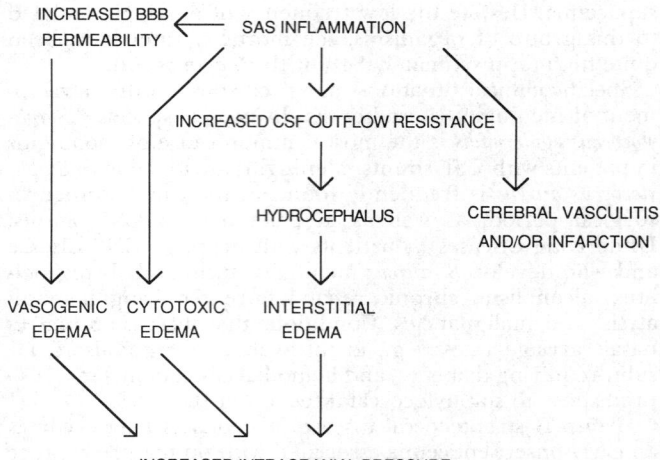

Figure 36–1. Pathophysiologic consequences of SAS inflammation. (From Tunkel AR, Wispelwey B, Scheld WM: Pathogenesis and pathophysiology of meningitis. Infect Dis Clin North Am 4:555, 1990.)

with either bacterial or viral meningitis, were elevated in the CSF only during bacterial meningitis.[41–43] However, the absence of TNF did not exclude a bacterial etiology. The role of other inflammatory cytokines in the induction of SAS inflammation is less clear. Although interleukin-6 activity has been documented in the CSF of patients with bacterial meningitis,[44] additional studies are necessary to precisely define its contribution in this disease. Elevated CSF concentrations of platelet-activating factor have also been observed in children with *H. influenzae* meningitis that correlated with bacterial density and with CSF LPS and TNF concentrations;[43] these increased concentrations of TNF and platelet-activating factor were associated with severity of disease.

Alterations in the Blood-Brain Barrier

The induction of SAS inflammation by bacterial virulence factors and/or inflammatory cytokines has important pathophysiologic consequences in the patient with bacterial meningitis, as depicted in Figure 36–1. One of the major pathophysiologic consequences of bacterial meningitis is increased permeability of the BBB, which leads to the production of vasogenic cerebral edema. An adult rat model has been utilized to investigate the propensity for bacterial meningitis to induce functional and morphologic alterations in the BBB.[45] After the intracisternal inoculation of *E. coli, S. pneumoniae*, or *H. influenzae*, there was a uniform host response to experimental meningitis with all three encapsulated pathogens at the level of the cerebral capillary endothelium, characterized morphologically by an early and sustained increase in pinocytotic vesicle formation and a progressive increase in separation of intercellular tight junctions. These morphologic alterations correlated with the functional penetration of albumin across the BBB. In addition, significant increases in BBB permeability occurred in the near absence of CSF leukocytes,[46] although the presence of CSF leukocytes augmented changes in permeability late in the disease course. To determine the bacterial virulence factors responsible for increased BBB permeability, permeability was assessed after the intracisternal inoculation of rats with *H. influenzae* type b LPS.[35] Functional increases in BBB permeability were observed after the intracisternal inoculation of LPS in a dose- and time-dependent manner (peak at 4 hours). Similar changes were observed after the intracisternal inoculation of *H. influenzae* type b outer membrane vesicles.[37] Intracisternal inoculation of the inflammatory cytokine human recombinant IL-1, but not TNF, also induced permeability changes, suggesting that LPS may alter BBB permeability via production of cytokines.[47] It appears, however, that IL-1 and TNF may act synergistically because inoculation with submaximal doses of IL-1 plus TNF (at concentrations that produced no changes individually) enhanced BBB permeability.[39]

Increased Intracranial Pressure

Another pathophysiologic consequence of bacterial meningitis is the development of increased intracranial pressure, primarily related to the development of cerebral edema that may be vasogenic, cytotoxic, and/or interstitial in origin. Vasogenic cerebral edema is primarily a consequence of increased BBB permeability; cytotoxic cerebral edema results from swelling of the cellular elements of the brain, most likely caused by release of toxic factors from neutrophils and/or bacteria; and interstitial cerebral edema occurs secondary to obstruction of normal CSF pathways, as in hydrocephalus. Studies of pneumococcal and *E. coli* meningitis in the experimental rabbit model have shown that the CSF outflow resistance (defined as factors that inhibit the flow of CSF from the SAS to the major dural sinuses) was markedly elevated, which suggests that attenuation of the normal CSF absorptive mechanisms during meningitis may decrease the ability of the brain to compensate in situations of increased intracranial pressure.[48] Subsequent studies attempted to solidify these concepts in greater detail by measuring the brain water content (indicative of cerebral edema, if elevated), CSF lactate level, and CSF pressure in animals with pneumococcal meningitis.[49] All three parameters were elevated in infected animals. Antibiotic therapy normalized CSF pressure and brain edema within 24 hours, but CSF lactate concentrations remained elevated. A pathway responsible for the increased brain water content was subsequently identified in an experimental rabbit model of *E. coli* meningitis.[50] Treatment with either cefotaxime or chloramphenicol was effective in reducing CSF bactericidal titers, but only treatment with cefotaxime was associated with an increase in brain water content that correlated with CSF LPS concentrations, which suggests that antimicrobial therapy with bacteriolytic antibiotics and subsequent release of bacterial cell surface constituents may be important in the pathogenesis of cerebral edema in bacterial meningitis.

Alterations in Cerebral Blood Flow

Cerebral blood flow alterations may also be seen in patients with bacterial meningitis. In an infant rhesus monkey model of *H. influenzae* meningitis, certain areas of the cortex (postcentral, temporal, and occipital) were hypoperfused relative to the hypothalamus and midbrain while the brain stem was hyperperfused, which suggests that one of the initial physiologic changes in *H. influenzae* meningitis is cerebral cortical hypoperfusion, with resultant relative cerebral anoxia.[21] One study has demonstrated loss of cerebral autoregulation in an experimental rabbit model of pneumococcal meningitis.[51] Even minor fluctuations of mean arterial blood pressure may have adverse consequences for patients with meningitis, with risk of brain injury from either transient hypotension or hypertension. Blood flow alterations may lead to regional hypoxia, increased brain lactate concentration secondary to utilization of glucose by anaerobic glycolysis, and CSF acidosis, which may be a precursor to encephalopathy.

CLINICAL PRESENTATION

The classic clinical presentation in adults with bacterial meningitis includes fever, headache, meningism, and signs of cerebral dysfunction;[6, 52] these are found in more than 85% of patients. The meningism may be subtle or marked or accompanied by Kernig's and/or Brudzinski's signs.[53] Kernig's sign is elicited by flexing the thigh on the abdomen with the knee flexed; the leg is then passively extended and when there is meningeal inflammation, the patient resists leg extension. Brudzinski's sign is positive when passive flexion of the neck leads to flexion of the hips and knees. However, these signs are elicited in only about 50% of cases of bacterial meningitis in adults, and their absence does not rule out this possibility. Cerebral dysfunction is manifested by confusion, delirium, or a declining level of consciousness ranging from lethargy to coma. Cranial nerve palsies (especially involving cranial nerves III, IV, VI, and VII) and focal cerebral signs are uncommon (10 to 20% of cases), manifesting as visual field defects, dysphasia, and hemiparesis. Seizures occur in about 30% of cases. Cranial nerve palsies likely develop as the nerve becomes enveloped by exudate in the arachnoid sheath surrounding the nerve. Alternatively, cranial nerve palsies may be a sign of increased intracranial pressure; the presence of bilateral sixth cranial nerve palsies, manifested as weakness of the lateral rectus muscles, is a well-recognized sign of increased intracranial pressure. Focal neurologic deficits and seizure activity arise from cortical and subcortical ischemia and infarction (bland and hemorrhagic), which are the result of inflammation and thrombosis in arteries and veins. However, hemiparesis may also be a sign of the presence of a large subdural effusion, which arises when infection in the adjacent SAS leads to an increase in permeability of the thin-walled capillaries and veins in the inner layer of the dura. This process is usually self-limited, and fluid in the subdural space is resorbed,[54] although an enlarging effusion can lead to mass effect with resultant hemiparesis. Papilledema is rare (<1%) and should suggest an alternative diagnosis (e.g., an intracranial mass lesion). Later in the disease course, patients may develop signs of increased intracranial pressure, including coma, hypertension, bradycardia, and third cranial nerve palsy; these findings are ominous prognostic signs.

Certain symptoms and signs may suggest an etiologic diagnosis in patients with bacterial meningitis. Meningococcemia, with or without meningitis, presents with a prominent rash, principally on the extremities, in about 50% of cases.[55, 56] Early in the disease course, the rash may be erythematous and macular, but it typically quickly evolves into a petechial phase with further coalescence into a purpuric form. The rash often matures rapidly, with new petechial lesions appearing during the physical examination. A petechial, purpuric, or ecchymotic rash may also be seen in other forms of meningitis (related to echovirus type 9, *Acinetobacter* species, *S. aureus*, and rarely *S. pneumoniae* or *H. influenzae*), Rocky Mountain spotted fever, *S. aureus* endocarditis, and rapidly overwhelming sepsis (caused by *S. pneumoniae* or *H. influenzae*) in splenectomized patients. An additional suppurative focus of infection (e.g., otitis media, sinusitis, or pneumonia) may be seen in 30% of patients with pneumococcal or *H. influenzae* meningitis. In patients who have suffered basilar skull fractures in which a dural fistula is produced between the subarachnoid space and the nasal cavity, paranasal sinuses, or middle ear, meningitis is usually caused by *S. pneumoniae*.[8] These patients commonly present with rhinorrhea or otorrhea related to a CSF leak, and a persistent defect is a common explanation for recurrent bacterial meningitis.

Certain subgroups of patients may not manifest many of the classic signs and symptoms of bacterial meningitis.[57] Neonates usually do not demonstrate meningism or fever, and the only clinical clues to meningitis are listlessness, high-pitched crying, fretfulness, refusal to feed, or irritability.[58]

Elderly patients, especially those with underlying conditions such as diabetes mellitus or cardiopulmonary disease, may present insidiously with lethargy or obtundation, variable signs of meningeal irritation, and without fever.[59] In this subgroup of patients, an altered mental status should not be ascribed to other causes until bacterial meningitis has been excluded by CSF examination. The postneurosurgical patient or the patient who has undergone head trauma also presents a unique clinical situation because these patients already have many of the symptoms and signs from their underlying disease process that are similar to those seen in patients with meningitis.[8, 60] A low threshold for CSF examination is needed in these patients should they develop any clinical deterioration.

DIAGNOSIS

The diagnosis of bacterial meningitis rests on the CSF examination after lumbar puncture. Although a relatively safe procedure, lumbar puncture carries risks ranging in severity from mild to fatal.[61] The most common complication is headache (10 to 25%), which can persist for several days. Minor neurologic complications, including painful or persistent paresthesias and cranial nerve palsies, have been reported infrequently, with the risk of 0.19 to 0.43% for disabling complications. Local bleeding and infection are even rarer complications. The most feared complication is tonsillar herniation in patients with increased intracranial pressure. The true incidence of this complication is unknown, although there is a high frequency of fatal outcome if it develops. Therefore, if increased intracranial pressure is suspected (e.g., related to the presence of an intracranial mass lesion), a computed tomographic (CT) scan of the head should be performed before lumbar puncture. An algorithm for the initial diagnostic approach in the patient with bacterial meningitis is shown in Figure 36–2.

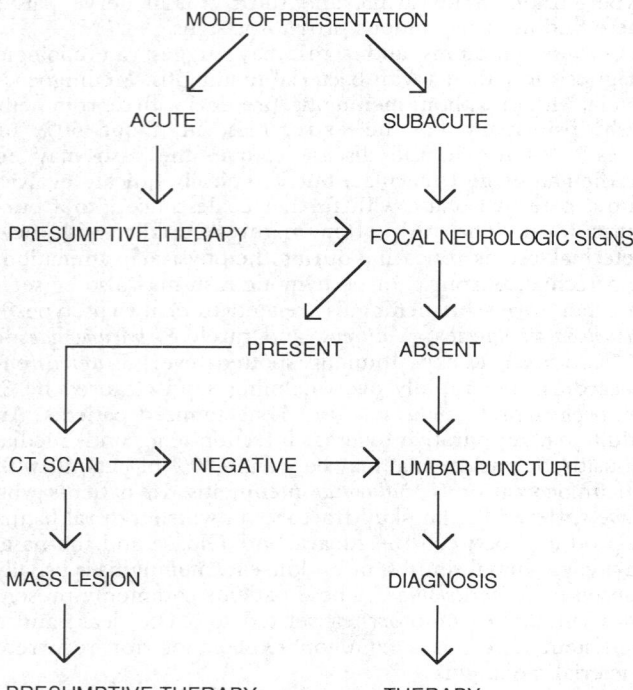

Figure 36–2. Algorithm for the initial diagnostic approach in patients with bacterial meningitis. (From Roos KL, Scheld WM: The management of fulminant meningitis in the intensive care unit. Crit Care Clin 4:375, 1988.)

TABLE 36–1	
TYPICAL CEREBROSPINAL FLUID FINDINGS IN ACUTE BACTERIAL MENINGITIS	
Test	**Finding**
Opening pressure	200–300 mm H$_2$O
White blood cell count	1000–5000 × 10^6/L (range, <100 to >10,000)
Percentage of neutrophils	≥80%
Protein	1–5 g/L (100–500 mg/dL)
Glucose	≤2.2 mmol/L (40 mg/dL)
Gram's stain	Positive in 60–90%
Culture	Positive in 70–85%
Bacterial antigens	Positive*
Lactate	Positive (≥3.9 mmol/L)
C-reactive protein	Positive
Limulus lysate	Positive†

*Complete description of bacterial antigen tests available for specific infecting microorganisms is in the text.
†Positive in ≥90% of cases of gram-negative meningitis.

The typical CSF findings in acute bacterial meningitis are shown in Table 36–1. The opening pressure is elevated in virtually all cases. Values over 600 mm H$_2$O suggest cerebral edema, the presence of intracranial suppurative foci, or communicating hydrocephalus. The appearance of the fluid may be cloudy or turbid if the white blood cell count is elevated (>200 × 10^6/L). With traumatic lumbar puncture, the CSF may initially appear bloody but should clear as flow continues. Xanthochromia, a pale pink to yellow-orange color of the supernatant of centrifuged CSF, is found in the CSF of patients with subarachnoid hemorrhage, usually within 2 hours posthemorrhage.[62]

The CSF white blood cell count is usually elevated in patients with untreated bacterial meningitis, ranging from 100 to 10,000 × 10^6/L, with a neutrophilic predominance.[62] About 10% of patients present with a predominance (>50%) of lymphocytes in CSF.[63] Occasionally, patients may have a low CSF white blood cell count (0 to 20 × 10^6/L) despite high bacterial concentrations in CSF, a finding usually with a poor prognosis. Therefore, a Gram stain and culture should be performed on all CSF specimens, even those with a normal cell count. A CSF glucose concentration of less than 2.2 mmol/L (40 mg/dL) is found in about 60% of patients with bacterial meningitis, and a CSF/serum glucose ratio of less than 0.31 is present in about 70% of patients.[61] The CSF glucose concentration must always be compared to a simultaneously obtained serum glucose concentration. The CSF protein concentration is elevated in virtually all cases of bacterial meningitis, presumably because of disruption of the BBB.[45] One analysis found that a CSF glucose level of less than 1.9 mmol/L (34 mg/dL), a CSF/blood glucose ratio of less than 0.23, a CSF protein level of greater than 2.2 g/L (220 mg/dL), more than 2000 × 10^6/L CSF leukocytes, and more than 1180 × 10^6/L CSF neutrophils were individual predictors of bacterial compared with viral meningitis, with 99% or higher certainty.[64]

CSF examination by Gram's stain permits a rapid, accurate identification in 60 to 90% of cases of bacterial meningitis.[61] The probability of detecting the organism correlates with bacterial concentrations in CSF; CSF bacterial concentrations of up to 10^3 colony-forming units/mL are associated with poor microscopic results (organisms seen 25% of the time), whereas microscopy is positive in 97% of cases when CSF bacterial concentrations are 10^5 colony-forming units/mL or more.[65] False-positive findings may occur as a result of contamination in either the collection of tubes or staining. CSF cultures are positive in 70 to 85% of cases. The probability of identifying an organism may decrease in patients who have received prior antimicrobial therapy.

Several rapid diagnostic tests have been developed to aid in the diagnosis of bacterial meningitis.[66, 67] Counterimmunoelectrophoresis detects specific antigens in CSF caused by meningococci (serogroups A and C), *H. influenzae* type b, pneumococci (representing 83 serotypes), type III group B streptococci, and *E. coli* K1. The sensitivity ranges from 62 to 95%, although the test is highly specific. Newer tests using staphylococcal coagglutination or latex agglutination are more rapid and sensitive than counterimmunoelectrophoresis, with the ability to detect bacterial antigen concentrations of approximately 1 ng/mL. However, none of the tests detects the antigens of group B meningococci. One of these rapid diagnostic tests (preferably latex agglutination) should be performed on all CSF specimens from patients in whom bacterial meningitis is suspected when the Gram stain result is negative. However, it must be emphasized that a negative test does not rule out infection related to a particular meningeal pathogen. The *Limulus* lysate test is useful in suspected cases of gram-negative meningitis in which a positive test is due to the presence of endotoxin, although it does not distinguish between the types of gram-negative organisms that may be present (low specificity).[68, 69]

Neuroimaging techniques have little role in the diagnosis of acute bacterial meningitis except to rule out the presence of other pathologic conditions or to identify a parameningeal source of infection.[70, 71] However, CT or magnetic resonance imaging may be useful for patients with prolonged fever several days after initiation of antimicrobial therapy, prolonged obtundation or coma, new or recurrent seizure activity, signs of increased intracranial pressure, or focal neurologic deficits. Magnetic resonance imaging is better than CT for evaluation of subdural effusions, cortical infarctions, and cerebritis, although it is more difficult to obtain a magnetic resonance imaging scan in a critically ill patient, which limits its usefulness in many patients with meningitis.

DIFFERENTIAL DIAGNOSIS

Multiple infections and noninfectious processes may be responsible for an acute meningitis syndrome. Parameningeal foci of infection (e.g., brain abscess, subdural empyema, and epidural abscess) are often suggested by the clinical setting, but each has similarities with and features that distinguish it from bacterial meningitis. The most common symptom of brain abscess is headache, present in more than 70% of patients.[72, 73] Other findings include nausea and vomiting (approximately 50% of cases), nuchal rigidity (approximately 25%), and papilledema (approximately 25%). The majority of patients have mental status changes ranging from lethargy to coma. Seizures, usually generalized, occur in 25 to 35% of patients. Only one half of patients present with the classic triad of fever, headache, and focal neurologic deficit. Subdural empyema can present as a rapidly progressive, life-threatening clinical condition, with symptoms and signs related to the presence of increased intracranial pressure, meningeal irritation, or focal cortical inflammation.[74, 75] Headache, initially localized to the infected ear or sinus, is a prominent complaint and can become generalized as the infection progresses. Temperature above 39°C is present in most cases. Focal neurologic signs appear in 24 to 48 hours and progress rapidly, with involvement of the entire cerebral hemisphere. About one half of patients have altered mental status early in infection that can progress to obtundation if the patient is not treated. Seizures are observed in more than 50% of cases. The onset of symptoms in cranial epidural abscess, compared with subdural empyema, may be insidious

and overshadowed by the primary focus of infection (e.g., sinusitis or otitis media).[75] Because the dura is closely apposed to the inner surface of the cranium, the abscess usually enlarges too slowly to produce sudden major neurologic deficits unless there is deeper intracranial extension. Without treatment, papilledema and other signs of increased intracranial pressure develop as the abscess enlarges. CT or magnetic resonance imaging is useful in the diagnosis of these conditions[76] and should be used before lumbar puncture if a focal mass lesion is suspected.

Patients with viral meningitis usually present with fever, headache, lethargy, myalgias, and nuchal rigidity.[77] Compared with bacterial meningitis, viral meningitis has a more insidious onset and slower progression. Patients with viral meningitis often complain of an incapacitating headache but are otherwise awake and alert, and although generalized malaise may be present, stupor, obtundation, and coma are rare. CSF findings are typically a lymphocytic pleocytosis, elevated protein concentration, and normal glucose level, although a study found that viral meningitis elicits a neutrophilic leukocytosis in CSF with a striking frequency (median of 70%).[64] Isolation of virus should be attempted by culture of throat, stool, and CSF specimens; however, CSF cultures are rarely positive.[78] Herpes simplex virus type 1 infection of the CNS usually produces a progressive, often fatal encephalitis,[79] whereas herpes simplex virus type 2 presents as a benign aseptic meningitis in normal adults.[80] Meningitis in the human immunodeficiency virus–infected patient usually occurs in the asymptomatic seropositive patient, although it may manifest before seroconversion or in patients with full-blown acquired immunodeficiency syndrome.[81] The CSF typically shows a mononuclear pleocytosis with normal glucose and slightly elevated protein levels.

Spirochetes may invade the CNS and produce a meningitis syndrome. Acute meningitis may be the first clue to CNS syphilis in about 25% of cases.[82] CSF analysis reveals the characteristics of the aseptic meningitis syndrome, although hypoglycorrhachia is present in 55% of cases. Serologic tests for syphilis should be performed on serum and CSF samples in all patients with the aseptic meningitis syndrome. Lyme disease, caused by *Borrelia burgdorferi*, may produce meningitis during its second stage (weeks to several months after the initial infection) in which patients have symptoms of headache, stiff neck, nausea, vomiting, malaise, and fever of several weeks' duration that may alternate with periods of milder symptoms.[83–85] Serum tests for antibodies to *B. burgdorferi* are usually positive in the majority of cases during this stage.

Tuberculous meningitis usually presents in a subacute or chronic aseptic form, although an acute presentation may occur with a CSF neutrophilic pleocytosis in immunosuppressed hosts or during the course of miliary tuberculosis.[86, 87] Cranial nerve palsies are common because of the predominantly basilar exudate. The CSF protein level may be high and hypoglycorrhachia is usual. Smears of CSF for acid-fast bacilli are usually negative. Cultures are eventually positive in the majority of cases (≥80%) but are not helpful in the acute situation. Therefore, other diagnostic tests (tuberculin skin test, chest radiograph, and bone marrow or liver biopsy) may be needed to secure the diagnosis. Several rapid diagnostic tests are under development; the presence of tuberculostearic acid is the most promising.[88] High CSF concentrations of adenosine deaminase support the diagnosis.[89]

Meningitis caused by fungi may also have acute, subacute, or chronic presentations. In the acute situation, the CSF findings may be indistinguishable from those of bacterial or tuberculous meningitis, but usually a lymphocytic pleocytosis is predominant. Certain epidemiologic features may point

TABLE 36–2

EMPIRICAL THERAPY OF PURULENT MENINGITIS

Age	Standard Therapy	Alternative Therapies
0–3 wk	Ampicillin plus cefotaxime	Ampicillin plus an aminoglycoside*
4–12 wk	Ampicillin plus a third-generation cephalosporin†	Ampicillin plus chloramphenicol
3 mo–18 y	Third-generation cephalosporin†	Ampicillin plus chloramphenicol; cefuroxime
18–50 y	Penicillin G or ampicillin plus or minus a third-generation cephalosporin†‡	Third-generation cephalosporin†
>50 y	Ampicillin plus a third-generation cephalosporin†	Ampicillin plus an aminoglycoside,* trimethoprim-sulfamethoxazole

*Gentamicin, tobramycin, or amikacin.
†Cefotaxime or ceftriaxone.
‡See text for specific indications.

to a fungal cause. For example, cryptococcal meningitis may be seen in patients with acquired immunodeficiency syndrome or lymphoma, after organ transplantation, and in patients receiving corticosteroids.[90, 91] Cryptococci may be seen on India ink stains of CSF in about 50 to 60% of cases. CSF cryptococcal polysaccharide antigen can be detected in more than 90% of cases.

Bacterial endocarditis may produce an acute meningitis syndrome with a culture-negative, purulent CSF.[92] This may represent the cerebritis that is common in acute staphylococcal endocarditis. The diagnosis may be established by the presence of other manifestations of endocarditis such as heart murmurs or splenomegaly.

Headache, fever, rash, and altered mental status are symptoms of rickettsial infections. Rocky Mountain spotted fever, caused by *Rickettsia rickettsii*, characteristically produces a macular rash initially noted on the wrists and ankles, with spread centrally to the face, chest, and abdomen.[93, 94] Mucous membranes are spared. Petechial lesions are also often seen in the axillae and around the ankles. Diagnosis can be made by biopsy of the lesions and staining of the specimen with fluorescent antibodies to *R. rickettsii* (sensitivity 70%) or by serologic testing.

Several noninfectious neurologic disorders may also have clinical presentations similar to meningitis. These disorders include neoplasia, cerebral vasculitis, granulomatous angiitis, sarcoidosis, chemical meningitis (e.g., related to drugs, radiocontrast agents, or anesthetics), cyst-related meningitis, subarachnoid hemorrhage, neuroleptic malignant syndrome, and various poorly understood chronic or recurrent syndromes (e.g., Mollaret's meningitis). These conditions are rarely confused with acute bacterial meningitis.

TREATMENT
Antimicrobial Therapy

The initial approach to the patient with suspected bacterial meningitis is to perform a lumbar puncture to determine whether the CSF formula is consistent with that diagnosis. Patients should receive emergent empirical, antimicrobial therapy based on their age and underlying disease status if no etiologic agent is identified by Gram's stain or rapid diagnostic tests and the diagnosis of bacterial meningitis is likely.[95, 96] In patients with a focal neurologic examination, a CT scan should be performed immediately to exclude an intracranial mass lesion because lumbar puncture is relatively contraindicated in that setting. However, if there is any delay in obtaining a CT scan, empirical antimicrobial therapy should be started immediately and before the lumbar puncture because of the high mortality rate in patients with bacterial meningitis in whom antimicrobial therapy is delayed (see Fig. 36–2). Our choices for empirical antibiotic therapy based on age in patients with presumed bacterial

meningitis are shown in Table 36–2.[96] For neonates (ages 0 to 3 weeks), the most likely infecting organisms are *E. coli*, *S. agalactiae*, or *L. monocytogenes*. For infants 4 to 12 weeks of age, infection may additionally be due to either *H. influenzae* or *S. pneumoniae*. In both of these age groups, empirical therapy with ampicillin plus a third-generation cephalosporin (cefotaxime or ceftriaxone) should be initiated. Cefotaxime is the third-generation agent of choice in neonates (0 to 3 weeks) because of the effects of ceftriaxone on bilirubin metabolism in this age group. In patients 3 months to 6 years of age, *H. influenzae* is by far the most common etiologic agent of bacterial meningitis, and from ages 6 to 18 years, pneumococci or meningococci are also possibilities; empirical therapy with a third-generation cephalosporin should be used in these age groups pending culture results. In adults 18 to 50 years of age, most cases of meningitis are due to *N. meningitidis* and *S. pneumoniae*, and penicillin G or ampicillin should be empirically utilized. However, in adults with certain predisposing factors (sinusitis, otitis media, epiglottitis, pneumonia, head trauma with CSF leak, diabetes mellitus, alcoholism, splenectomy or asplenic states, or immune deficiency), there is an increased risk of meningitis caused by *H. influenzae*, and a third-generation cephalosporin should be included in the empirical regimen. In older adults (50 years of age and older), meningococci or pneumococci are possible, as well as *L. monocytogenes* or gram-negative bacilli. Empirical therapy should consist of ampicillin in combination with a third-generation cephalosporin, because of the increased frequency of aerobic gram-negative bacillary meningitis in this age group.

One other situation deserves comment. In postneurosurgical patients or patients with CSF shunts or foreign bodies, likely infecting organisms include staphylococci (either *S. epidermidis* or *S. aureus*), diphtheroids, and gram-negative bacilli (including *P. aeruginosa*). Empirical antimicrobial therapy in these situations should consist of vancomycin plus ceftazidime pending culture results.

After an infecting microorganism has been isolated, antimicrobial therapy can be modified for optimal treatment.[96] Antibiotics of choice are shown in Table 36–3. Dosages for children and adults are given in Table 36–4. For bacterial meningitis caused by *S. pneumoniae* or *N. meningitidis*, penicillin G or ampicillin is equally efficacious. However, certain developments may modify these recommendations. In the past, pneumococci have been uniformly susceptible to penicillin (minimal inhibitory concentration ≤ 0.06 µg/mL). Reports from several centers have documented relatively resistant and highly resistant strains of pneumococci with minimal inhibitory concentrations of 0.1 to 1.0 and 2 or more µg/mL, respectively.[97, 98] The mechanism underlying penicillin resistance in pneumococci involves alterations in the structure and molecular size of the penicillin-binding proteins. These patterns of alterations are, in addition,

TABLE 36–3

ANTIMICROBIAL THERAPY FOR BACTERIAL MENINGITIS

Organism	Standard Therapy	Alternative Therapies
Neisseria meningitidis	Penicillin G or ampicillin	Third-generation cephalosporin;* cefuroxime; chloramphenicol
Streptococcus pneumoniae	Penicillin G or ampicillin	Third-generation cephalosporin;* cefuroxime; chloramphenicol
Haemophilus influenzae		
β-Lactamase–negative	Ampicillin	Third-generation cephalosporin;* cefuroxime; chloramphenicol
β-Lactamase–positive	Third-generation cephalosporin*	Chloramphenicol; cefuroxime
Enterobacteriaceae	Third-generation cephalosporin*	Extended-spectrum penicillin† plus an aminoglycoside; aztreonam;‡ quinolones‡
Pseudomonas aeruginosa	Ceftazidime (plus an aminoglycoside)	Extended-spectrum penicillin† plus an aminoglycoside; aztreonam;‡ quinolones‡
Streptococcus agalactiae	Penicillin G or ampicillin (plus an aminoglycoside)	Third-generation cephalosporin;* chloramphenicol
Listeria monocytogenes	Ampicillin or penicillin G (plus an aminoglycoside)	Trimethoprim-sulfamethoxazole
Staphylococcus aureus		
Methicillin sensitive	Nafcillin or oxacillin	Vancomycin
Methicillin resistant	Vancomycin	Trimethoprim-sulfamethoxazole; quinolones‡
Staphylococcus epidermidis	Vancomycin (plus rifampin)	Teicoplanin;‡ daptomycin‡

*Cefotaxime, ceftizoxime, and ceftriaxone have received the most scrutiny and are recommended. Cefoperazone and moxalactam are not indicated. Ceftazidime should be reserved for suspected or proven *P. aeruginosa* meningitis.

†Piperacillin or azlocillin.

‡The effectiveness of these antibiotics in bacterial meningitis has not been clearly documented.

Reproduced, with permission, from Tunkel AR, Wispelwey B, Scheld WM, Bacterial meningitis: Recent advances in pathophysiology and treatment. Ann Intern Med 1990; 112:610–623.

genetically stable, which allows these proteins to be used to identify particular isolates for epidemiologic purposes.[99] In view of these trends, susceptibility testing should be performed on all CSF pneumococcal isolates. For relatively resistant strains, a third-generation cephalosporin (e.g., cefotaxime or ceftriaxone) should be used,[100] and vancomycin is the antimicrobial agent of choice for highly resistant strains. In geographic locales where relatively resistant strains of pneumococci are prevalent, empirical antimicrobial therapy with a third-generation cephalosporin should be utilized in age groups in which *S. pneumoniae* is a likely pathogen. Meningococcal strains have also been reported from several areas (particularly Spain) that are relatively resistant to penicillin.[101] These strains do not produce β-lactamase, and the relative resistance appears to be mediated by a reduced affinity for penicillin-binding protein 3.[102] However, most patients harboring these strains have re-

covered with standard penicillin therapy, so their clinical significance is unclear.

Treatment of *H. influenzae* type b meningitis has been hampered by the emergence of β-lactamase–producing strains, first reported in 1974, which now account for approximately 25% of all isolates overall in the United States, although there is geographic variability.[1] Chloramphenicol resistance is rare in the United States (<1% of isolates),[103] although more than 50% of isolates from Spain are chloramphenicol resistant.[104] In addition, chloramphenicol has been found to be bacteriologically and clinically inferior to certain β-lactam antibiotics (ampicillin, ceftriaxone, and cefotaxime) in childhood bacterial meningitis in which the majority of cases were due to *H. influenzae* type b.[105] On the basis of the findings just noted and studies documenting that the third-generation cephalosporins (cefotaxime or ceftriaxone) are as efficacious as ampicillin plus chloramphen-

TABLE 36–4

RECOMMENDED DOSES OF ANTIBIOTICS FOR INTRACRANIAL INFECTIONS IN CHILDREN AND ADULTS WITH NORMAL RENAL FUNCTION

Antibiotic	Total Daily Dose in Children (Dosing Interval)	Total Daily Dose in Adults (Dosing Interval)
Penicillin G	250,000 U/kg (q 6 h)	24 million U (q 4 h)
Ampicillin	150–200 mg/kg (q 6 h)	12 g (q 4 h)
Nafcillin, oxacillin	100–150 mg/kg (q 6 h)	9–12 g (q 4 h)
Chloramphenicol	100 mg/kg (q 6 h)	4–6 g* (q 6 h)
Cefotaxime	200 mg/kg (q 6 h)	8–12 g (q 4 h)
Ceftriaxone	100 mg/kg (q 12 h)	4–6 g† (q 12 h)
Ceftazidime	150 mg/kg (q 8 h)	6–12 g‡ (q 8 h)
Vancomycin	50 mg/kg (q 6 h)	2 g (q 12 h)
Gentamicin, tobramycin	5 mg/kg (q 8 h)	3–5 mg/kg (q 8 h)
Amikacin	20 mg/kg (q 8 h)	15 mg/kg (q 8 h)
Trimethoprim-sulfamethoxazole	10 mg/kg§ (q 12 h)	10 mg/kg§ (q 12 h)
Metronidazole	15 mg/kg (q 12 h)	30 mg/kg (q 6 h)

*Higher dose is recommended for pneumococcal meningitis.

†Actual dose studied was 50 mg/kg q 12 h.

‡Not enough patients were studied to make firm recommendations.

§Dose is based on the trimethoprim component.

icol for therapy of *H. influenzae* meningitis, the American Academy of Pediatrics has endorsed the use of the third-generation cephalosporins as empirical therapy in children with bacterial meningitis.[106] Cefuroxime, a second-generation cephalosporin, has also been evaluated for the therapy of *H. influenzae* meningitis. Although initial studies documented efficacy similar to ampicillin plus chloramphenicol, later case reports have shown delayed CSF sterilization and the development of epiglottitis in patients receiving cefuroxime for meningitis.[107] In addition, a prospective, randomized study comparing ceftriaxone to cefuroxime for the treatment of childhood bacterial meningitis has documented the superiority of ceftriaxone, with patients having milder hearing impairment and more rapid CSF sterilization than the patients receiving cefuroxime.[108] We recommend a third-generation cephalosporin for empirical therapy when *H. influenzae* is considered a likely infecting pathogen.

The treatment in adults of bacterial meningitis caused by gram-negative enteric bacilli has been revolutionized by the third-generation cephalosporins.[109, 110] Cure rates of 78 to 94% have been obtained with these agents, compared with mortality rates of 40 to 90% with previous standard therapy (usually an aminoglycoside with or without chloramphenicol). One agent, ceftazidime, is also active against *P. aeruginosa* meningitis, and this agent alone or in combination with an aminoglycoside resulted in cure of 19 of 24 patients with *Pseudomonas* meningitis in one report.[111] Intrathecal or intraventricular aminoglyoside therapy should be considered if there is no response to systemic therapy, although this mode of administration is rarely needed at present. The quinolones (e.g., ciprofloxacin or pefloxacin) have been used in some patients with gram-negative bacillary meningitis[112, 113] but at this time can be considered only for adult patients with meningitis related to multidrug resistant gram-negative bacilli or in patients failing to respond to conventional therapy.

The third-generation cephalosporins are, however, inactive against meningitis caused by *L. monocytogenes*, an important meningeal pathogen. Therapy in this situation should consist of ampicillin or penicillin G, and addition of an aminoglycoside for the first several days should be considered in documented infection.[10] Alternatively, trimethoprim-sulfamethoxazole, which is bactericidal against *Listeria* in vitro, can be used.[114] Patients with *S. aureus* meningitis should be treated with nafcillin or oxacillin, with vancomycin reserved for patients allergic to penicillin or for patients with disease caused by methicillin-resistant organisms.[12] Infections with *S. epidermidis*, the most likely isolate in patients with CSF shunts, should be treated with vancomycin; rifampin is added if the patient fails to improve.[115] Shunt removal is often essential to optimize therapy.

The duration of therapy for bacterial meningitis should be 10 to 14 days for most causes of nonmeningococcal meningitis and 3 weeks for meningitis caused by gram-negative enteric bacilli. Newer studies have led to some modifications in these recommendations. Seven days of therapy appears adequate for meningococcal meningitis, and several reports have suggested that 1 week of therapy is also efficacious for *H. influenzae* meningitis. However, the standards for duration of treatment in meningitis have been based primarily on clinical experience, not rigidly standardized prospective studies.[116] Therefore, therapy must be individualized, and some patients may require longer courses of treatment based on clinical response.

Adjunctive Therapy

Despite the availability of effective antimicrobial therapy, the morbidity and mortality from bacterial meningitis remain unacceptably high. Studies have focused on the pathogenesis and pathophysiology of bacterial meningitis in the hopes of developing innovative strategies for the treatment of this disorder.[96, 117]

Anti-inflammatory Agents. Several studies of meningitis in experimental animal models have reported the usefulness of anti-inflammatory agents (e.g., corticosteroids or nonsteroidal anti-inflammatory agents) in decreasing the inflammatory response in the SAS, which may be responsible for development of neurologic sequelae in this disorder. In the rabbit model of experimental pneumococcal meningitis, the generation of pneumococcal cell wall components after therapy with bacteriolytic antibiotics increased the SAS inflammatory response, which correlated with increased CSF concentrations of PGE_2.[33] This CSF inflammatory response was reduced by inhibitors of the cyclooxygenase pathway of arachidonic acid metabolism (especially oxindanac), whereas an inhibitor of the lipoxygenase pathway (nordihydroguaiaretic acid) was ineffective in preventing cell wall–induced inflammation.[118] Another cyclooxygenase inhibitor, indomethacin, was effective in decreasing both brain water content and PGE_2 concentrations in another study of experimental pneumococcal meningitis;[119] however, there was no reduction in intracranial pressure.

Several corticosteroid agents have also been evaluated in experimental models of meningitis. Methylprednisolone has been shown to significantly reduce the mass of leukocytes within the meninges of rabbits with pneumococcal meningitis.[120] CSF outflow resistance is also reduced after methylprednisolone therapy and to a greater extent than in untreated or penicillin-treated animals.[48] Additional experimental studies have examined the effects of methylprednisolone or dexamethasone on brain water content, CSF pressure, and CSF lactate concentrations.[49] Both agents completely reversed the development of brain edema, whereas only dexamethasone reduced the increase in CSF pressure and lactate concentration in experimental pneumococcal meningitis. However, neither agent was superior to ampicillin alone in reducing cerebral edema or intracranial pressure. In a subsequent study of experimental lapine *H. influenzae* meningitis, dexamethasone plus ceftriaxone was compared with ceftriaxone alone; the combination consistently reduced brain water content, CSF pressure, and CSF lactate level to a greater extent than did ceftriaxone alone, although the differences were not statistically significant.[121] The efficacy of dexamethasone for bacterial meningitis may be in its ability to reduce CSF concentrations of TNF and the indices of meningeal inflammation.[122]

Adjunctive dexamethasone therapy has been evaluated in a double-blind, placebo-controlled trial in 200 infants and children with bacterial meningitis.[123] The patients who received dexamethasone and antibiotics, compared with those who received antibiotics plus placebo, became afebrile sooner and were significantly less likely to acquire moderate to severe bilateral sensorineural hearing loss. CSF examination 24 hours after the initiation of therapy revealed a more rapid increase in glucose and decrease in lactate and protein concentrations in the patients receiving dexamethasone. These findings, however, were significant only for meningitis caused by *H. influenzae* type b. Another study from Egypt documented significant reduction in case fatality rates and overall neurologic sequelae in children and adults with pneumococcal meningitis who received dexamethasone in addition to antibiotics.[124] However, no significant differences were observed in time to afebrility or improvement of CSF parameters.

Concerns have been raised about the routine use of dexamethasone therapy in all patients with bacterial meningitis,[125, 126] although it appears likely that dexamethasone will prove to be useful adjunctive therapy in children and possibly in adults, pending results of ongoing studies. If dexamethasone is to be used, however, it should be administered concomitant with or just before antibiotic therapy to attenuate the CSF inflammatory response. Close monitoring of the hematocrit and stool guaiac for occult blood is essential during therapy because gastrointestinal hemorrhage has been described.

The mechanism of the beneficial effect of dexamethasone is incompletely defined. Elevated CSF concentrations of IL-1β have been shown to correlate significantly with outcome from neonatal gram-negative bacillary meningitis in which patients with concentrations of 500 pg/mL or higher were more likely to develop neurologic sequelae.[127] Dexamethasone therapy led to a more rapid reduction in CSF IL-1β concentrations than that observed with antibiotics alone, which suggests that dexamethasone may exert its anti-inflammatory effects in the SAS by inhibiting IL-1β gene expression. No correlation was observed between CSF concentrations of TNF and outcome in patients with bacterial meningitis.

Reduction of Intracranial Pressure. Other adjunctive therapies may be useful in critically ill patients with bacterial meningitis.[128] Patients with signs of increased intracranial pressure (e.g., altered level of consciousness, dilated poorly reactive or nonreactive pupils, and ocular movement disorders) and who are stuporous or comatose, precluding assessment of worsening neurologic function, may benefit from the insertion of an intracranial pressure-monitoring device.[129–131] Pressures exceeding 20 mm Hg are abnormal and should be treated. Significant increases in intracranial pressure are observed by turning the head to the side (particularly the left); hyperextension of the neck (secondary to presence of an endotracheal tube), which can increase the jugular venous pressure or block the flow of CSF; suctioning; or vigorous chest physiotherapy. There is also rationale for treating smaller elevations in intracranial pressure (>15 mm Hg) to avoid the large elevations or so-called plateau waves that can lead to cerebral herniation and irreversible brain stem injury.[132]

Intracranial pressure can be reduced by the following measures: (1) elevation of the head of the bed to 30° to maximize venous drainage with minimal compromise of cerebral perfusion; (2) hyperventilation (maintain $Paco_2$ between 27 and 30 mm Hg), which causes cerebral vasoconstriction with reduction in cerebral blood volume, although this beneficial effect is of short (e.g., approximately 24 hours) duration; (3) use of hyperosmolar agents such as mannitol (dose of 1 g/kg during 10 to 15 minutes or in doses of 0.25 g/kg every 2 to 3 hours), which makes the intravascular space hyperosmolar to the brain with movement of water from brain tissue into the intravascular compartment; (4) use of intravenous lidocaine, which blocks the reflex increase in intracranial pressure after endotracheal suctioning; and (5) use of corticosteroids. However, corticosteroid use may decrease antibiotic penetration into CSF[133] and is thus not routinely recommended for the management of cerebral edema in bacterial meningitis, pending the results of clinical trials. If steroids are to be used, they should be continued for only about 4 days at most and then rapidly tapered.[134]

High-dose barbiturate therapy may be useful when hyperventilation and hyperosmolar agents have failed to decrease intracranial pressure.[128, 130, 135] These agents decrease the cerebral metabolic oxygen demands and therefore decrease cerebral blood flow. Barbiturates can also protect the brain from ischemic insult, in part by causing vasoconstriction in normal tissue and thus shunting of blood to ischemic brain tissue. Pentobarbital (initial dose of 5 to 30 mg/kg, then 1.0 to 1.5 mg/kg/h) is administered and the patient is monitored to measure decreases in intracranial pressure

(<20 mm Hg). Alternatively, the dose of pentobarbital is titrated to the development of a burst-suppression pattern on the electroencephalogram. Because of the risk of cardiac toxicity (e.g., decreased cardiac output, decreased contractile force, arrhythmias) with high-dose barbiturate therapy, Swan-Ganz catheters should be utilized to monitor cardiac parameters. After the intracranial pressure is reduced to below 20 mm Hg for 24 hours, the dose of pentobarbital is slowly tapered to prevent a rebound increase in intracranial pressure. Fever increases the brain's metabolic demands, resulting in increased cerebral blood flow; temperatures greater than 38°C should be reduced with antipyretic agents and/or cooling blankets.[128]

Treatment of Seizures. Seizures must be treated promptly to avoid status epilepticus, which may lead to anoxic brain injury.[128, 136] Initially, a short-acting anticonvulsant (e.g., lorazepam or diazepam) should be used, followed immediately by a long-acting anticonvulsant, usually phenytoin. Lorazepam is administered at dosages of 1 to 4 mg in adults (0.05 mg/kg in children) and diazepam in a dose of 0.25 to 0.4 mg/kg at a rate of 1 to 2 mg/min (maximum of 10 mg). The 10-mg dose of diazepam can be administered up to three times at intervals of 15 to 20 minutes. Phenytoin is administered at a rate no faster than 50 mg/min for a total loading dose of 18 to 20 mg/kg; if this dose fails to control seizure activity, an additional dose of 500 mg of phenytoin can be given. Patients must be carefully monitored for hypotension and arrhythmias (secondary to a prolonged QT interval). With continued seizure activity, the patient should be intubated, receive mechanical ventilation, and be treated intravenously with phenobarbital (loading dose of 20 mg/kg at a rate of 100 mg/min in adults and 30 mg/min in children). These maneuvers control seizure activity in the majority of patients, although if seizure activity continues, general anesthesia with pentobarbital (3.5 mg/kg loading dose, then 1 to 2 mg/kg/h) can be utilized.

Fluid Restriction. Another important adjunctive measure in children with bacterial meningitis is fluid restriction to combat excess secretion of antidiuretic hormone,[134] although this is not appropriate in patients with severe shock or dehydration because hypotension may predispose to cerebral ischemia. A majority of children with bacterial meningitis are hyponatremic (serum sodium level < 135 mEq/L) on presentation, and the degree and duration of hyponatremia may contribute to neurologic sequelae. If the patient is not hypotensive, fluids should be restricted to one half of maintenance levels and the serum sodium concentration will normalize in most patients. The management of hyponatremia is discussed in greater depth in Chapter 99.

PREVENTION

The rationale for the use of chemoprophylaxis for prevention of secondary disease is eradication of nasopharyngeal carriage of the bacterial pathogen. Therefore, transmission to contacts is prevented, as well as the development of disease in those already colonized. In addition, the index case must receive prophylaxis because the usual antibiotics given for invasive disease do not necessarily eliminate nasopharyngeal carriage. For contacts of a patient with meningococcal meningitis, chemoprophylaxis is administered to only intimate contacts (e.g., family, roommates) and is usually not indicated for other groups (e.g., office workers, classmates) unless there has been intimate contact.[56] However, one study has suggested that school-aged children may be at increased risk of secondary meningococcal infection in crowded classrooms, when contact during lunch or recess or both is frequent.[137] Prophylaxis is not necessary for medical personnel unless there has been intimate contact (e.g., mouth-to-mouth resuscitation). Contacts of a case of *H. influenzae* meningitis should receive chemoprophylaxis if exposure has occurred in a household or day care center containing children 4 years of age or younger (other than the index case), providing that the exposure to *H. influenzae* type b was in the week before prophylaxis.[138, 139] The drug of choice for chemoprophylaxis for contacts of both types of meningitis is rifampin. For contacts of patients with *H. influenzae* meningitis, rifampin at a daily dose of 20 mg/kg (not exceeding 600 mg) for 4 consecutive days is most effective. For contacts of meningococcal cases, one rifampin dose of 10 mg/kg (not exceeding 600 mg) twice a day for 2 days is effective. One dose of ciprofloxacin (500 or 750 mg) may also be efficacious in eradication of the meningococcal nasopharyngeal carrier state.[140] Ceftriaxone, given once intramuscularly at a dosage of 250 mg in adults and 125 mg in children less than 15 years of age, also shows promise for eradication of the meningococcal carrier state.[141]

Acknowledgments. We gratefully acknowledge Mona Bernhardt for secretarial assistance. This work was supported in part by a research grant (RO1 Al17904) and a training grant (T32 Al07046) from the National Institute of Allergy and Infectious Diseases. WMS is an established investigator of the American Heart Association.

References

1. Schlech WF, Ward JI, Band JD, et al: Bacterial meningitis in the United States, 1978 through 1981. The National Bacterial Meningitis Surveillance Study. JAMA 253:1749, 1985.
2. Moxon ER, Smith AL, Averill DR, et al: *Haemophilus influenzae* meningitis in infant rats after intranasal inoculation. J Infect Dis 129:154, 1974.
3. Spagnuolo PT, Ellner JJ, Lerner PI, et al: *Haemophilus influenzae* meningitis: The spectrum of disease in adults. Medicine 61:74, 1982.
4. McGee ZA, Stephens DS, Hoffman LH, et al: Mechanisms of mucosal invasion by pathogenic *Neisseria*. Rev Infect Dis 5:S708, 1983.
5. Ross SC, Densen P: Complement deficiency states and infection: Epidemiology, pathogenesis and consequences of neisserial and other infections in an immune deficiency. Medicine 63:243, 1984.
6. Geiseler PJ, Nelson KE, Levin S, et al: Community-acquired purulent meningitis: A review of 1,316 cases during the antibiotic era, 1954–1976. Rev Infect Dis 2:725, 1980.
7. Hand WL, Sanford JP: Posttraumatic bacterial meningitis. Ann Intern Med 91:835, 1979.
8. Tunkel AR, Scheld WM: Acute infectious complications of head trauma. In: Braakman R (ed): Handbook of Clinical Neurology, Head Injury. Amsterdam, Elsevier Science Publishers, p 317, 1990.
9. Scheld WM: Pathogenesis and pathophysiology of pneumococcal meningitis. In Sande MA, Smith AL, Root RK (eds): Bacterial Meningitis. London, Churchill Livingstone, p 37, 1985.
10. Gellin BG, Broome CV: Listeriosis. JAMA 261:1313, 1989.
11. Cherubin CE, Marr JS, Sierra MF, et al: *Listeria* and gram-negative bacillary meningitis in New York City, 1972–1979. Frequent causes of meningitis in adults. Am J Med 71:199, 1981.
12. Schlesinger LS, Ross SC, Schaberg DR: *Staphylococcus aureus* meningitis: A broad-based epidemiologic study. Medicine 66:148, 1987.
13. Edwards MS, Baker CJ: *Streptococcus agalactiae* (group B streptococcus). In Mandell GL, Douglas RG Jr, Bennett JE (eds): Principles and Practice of Infectious Diseases. 3rd ed. New York, Churchill Livingstone, p 1554, 1990.
14. Aharoni A, Potasman I, Levitan Z, et al: Postpartum maternal group B streptococcal meningitis. Rev Infect Dis 12:273, 1990.
15. Bryan JP, de Silva HR, Tavares A, et al: Etiology and mortality of bacterial meningitis in northeastern Brazil. Rev Infect Dis 12:128, 1990.
16. Moxon ER, Vaughn KA: The type b capsular polysaccharide as a virulence determinant of *Haemophilus influenzae*: Studies using clinical isolates and laboratory transformants. J Infect Dis 143:517, 1981.
17. Anderson P, Johnston RB, Smith DH: Human serum activities against *Haemophilus influenzae* type b. J Clin Invest 51:31, 1972.
18. Stephens DS, McGee ZA: Attachment of *Neisseria meningitidis* to human mucosal surfaces: Influence of pili and type of receptor cell. J Infect Dis 143:525, 1981.
19. Stephens DS, Hoffman LH, McGee ZA: Interaction of *Neisseria meningitidis* with human nasopharyngeal mucosa: Attachment and entry into columnar epithelial cells. J Infect Dis 148:369, 1983.
20. Griffis JM, Bertram MA: Immunoepidemiology of meningococcal disease in military recruits. II. Blocking of serum bactericidal activity by circulating IgA early in the course of invasive disease. J Infect Dis 136:733, 1977.
21. Smith AL, Daum RS, Scheifele D, et al: Pathogenesis of *Haemophilus influenzae* meningitis. In Sell SH, Wright PF (eds): *Haemophilus influenzae*: Epidemiology, Immunology, and Prevention of Disease. New York, Elsevier Science Publishers, p 89, 1982.
22. Parkkinen J, Korhonen TK, Pere A, et al: Binding sites in the rat brain for *Escherichia coli* S fimbriae associated with neonatal meningitis. J Clin Invest 81:860, 1988.
23. Rahal JJ Jr, Simberkoff MS: Host defense and antimicrobial therapy in adult gram-negative bacillary meningitis. Ann Intern Med 96:468, 1982.
24. Simberkoff MS, Moldover HN, Rahal JJ Jr: Absence of detectable bactericidal and opsonic activities in normal and infected human cerebrospinal fluids. A regional host defense deficiency. J Lab Clin Med 95:362, 1980.
25. Whittle HC, Greenwood BM: Cerebrospinal fluid immunoglobulins and complement in meningococcal meningitis. J Clin Pathol 30:720, 1977.
26. Smith H, Bannister B, O'Shea MJ: Cerebrospinal fluid immunoglobulins in meningitis. Lancet 1:591, 1973.
27. Bevilacqua MP, Stengelin S, Gimbrone MA Jr, et al: Endothelial leukocyte adhesion molecule 1: An inducible receptor for neutrophils related to complement regulatory proteins and lectins. Science 243:1160, 1989.
28. Tuomanen EI, Saukkonen K, Sande S, et al: Reduction of inflammation, tissue damage, and mortality in bacterial meningitis in rabbits treated with monoclonal antibodies against adhesion-promoting receptors of leukocytes. J Exp Med 170:959, 1989.
29. Greenwood BM: Chemotactic activity of cerebrospinal fluid in pyogenic meningitis. J Clin Pathol 31:213, 1978.
30. Wyler DJ, Wasserman SI, Karchmer AW: Substances which modulate leukocyte migration are present in CSF during meningitis. Ann Neurol 5:322, 1979.
31. Kadurugamuwa JL, Hengstler B, Bray MA, et al: Inhibition of complement-factor-5a-induced inflammatory reactions by prostaglandin E_2 in experimental meningitis. J Infect Dis 160:715, 1989.
32. Tuomanen E, Tomasz A, Hengstler B, et al: The relative role of bacterial cell wall and capsule in the induction of inflammation in pneumococcal meningitis. J Infect Dis 151:535, 1985.
33. Tuomanen E, Liu H, Hengstler B, et al: The induction of meningeal inflammation by components of the pneumococcal cell wall. J Infect Dis 151:859, 1985.
34. Syrogiannopoulos GA, Hansen EJ, Erwin AI, et al: *Haemophilus influenzae* type b lipooligosaccharide induces meningeal inflammation. J Infect Dis 157:237, 1988.
35. Wispelwey B, Lesse AJ, Hansen EJ, et al: *Haemophilus influenzae* lipopolysaccharide-induced blood brain barrier permeability during experimental meningitis in the rat. J Clin Invest 82:1339, 1988.
36. Mustafa MM, Ramilo O, Syrogiannopoulos GA, et al: Induction of meningeal inflammation by outer membrane vesicles of *Haemophilus influenzae* type b. J Infect Dis 159:917, 1989.
37. Wispelwey B, Hansen EJ, Scheld WM: *Haemophilus influenzae* outer membrane vesicle-induced blood-brain barrier permeability during experimental meningitis. Infect Immun 57:2559, 1989.
38. Riesenfeld-Orn I, Wolpe S, Garcia-Bustos JF, et al: Production of interleukin-1 but not tumor necrosis factor by human monocytes stimulated with pneumococcal cell surface components. Infect Immun 57:1890, 1989.
39. Wispelwey B, Long WJ, Castracane JM, et al: Cerebrospinal fluid interleukin-1 activity following intracisternal inoculation of *Haemophilus influenzae* lipopolysaccharide into rats. In: Program and Abstracts of the 28th Interscience Conference on Antimicrobial Agents and Chemotherapy, Los Angeles, CA, October 1988, p 265.
40. Mustafa MM, Ramilo O, Olsen KD, et al: Tumor necrosis factor in mediating experimental *Haemophilus influenzae* type b meningitis. J Clin Invest 84:1253, 1989.
41. Leist TP, Frei K, Kam-Hansen S, et al: Tumor necrosis factor alpha in cerebrospinal fluid during bacterial, but not viral meningitis. Evaluation in murine model infections and in patients. J Exp Med 167:1743, 1988.
42. Nadal D, Leppert D, Frei K, et al: Tumor necrosis factor-alpha in infectious meningitis. Arch Dis Child 64:1274, 1989.
43. Arditi M, Manogue KR, Caplan M, et al: Cerebrospinal fluid cachectin/tumor necrosis factor-alpha and platelet-activating factor concentrations and severity of bacterial meningitis in children. J Infect Dis 162:139, 1990.
44. Waage A, Halstensen A, Shalaby R, et al: Local production of tumor necrosis factor alpha, interleukin 1, and interleukin 6 in meningococcal meningitis. Relation to the inflammatory response. J Exp Med 170:1859, 1989.
45. Quagliarello VJ, Long WJ, Scheld WM: Morphologic alterations of the blood-brain barrier with experimental meningitis in the rat. Temporal sequence and role of encapsulation. J Clin Invest 77:1084, 1986.
46. Lesse AJ, Moxon ER, Zwahlen A, et al: Role of cerebrospinal fluid pleocytosis and *Haemophilus influenzae* type b capsule on blood brain barrier permeability during experimental meningitis in the rat. J Clin Invest 82:102, 1988.
47. Quagliarello VJ, Long WJ, Scheld WM: Human interleukin-1 modulates blood-brain barrier injury in vivo. In: Program and Abstracts of the 27th Interscience Conference on Antimicrobial Agents and Chemotherapy, New York, October 1987, p 204.
48. Scheld WM, Dacey RG, Winn HR, et al: Cerebrospinal fluid outflow

resistance in rabbits with experimental meningitis. Alterations with penicillin and methylprednisolone. J Clin Invest 66:243, 1980.

49. Täuber MG, Khayam-Bashi H, Sande MA: Effects of ampicillin and corticosteroids on brain water content, cerebrospinal fluid pressure, and cerebrospinal lactate levels in experimental pneumococcal meningitis. J Infect Dis 151:528, 1985.

50. Täuber MG, Shibl AM, Hackbarth CJ, et al: Antibiotic therapy, endotoxin concentration in cerebrospinal fluid, and brain edema in experimental Escherichia coli meningitis in rabbits. J Infect Dis 156:456, 1987.

51. Tureen JH, Dworkin RJ, Kennedy SL, et al: Loss of cerebrovascular autoregulation in experimental meningitis in rabbits. J Clin Invest 85:577, 1990.

52. Carpenter RR, Petersdorf RG: The clinical spectrum of bacterial meningitis. Am J Med 33:262, 1962.

53. Verghese A, Gallemore G: Kernig's and Brudzinski's signs revisited. Rev Infect Dis 9:1187, 1987.

54. Klein JO, Feigin RD, McCracken GH: Report of the task force on diagnosis and management of meningitis. Pediatrics 78S:959, 1986.

55. Swartz MN, Dodge PR: Bacterial meningitis—A review of selected aspects. I. General clinical features, special problems and unusual meningeal reactions mimicking bacterial meningitis. N Engl J Med 272:725, 1965.

56. Scheld WM: Meningococcal diseases. In: Warren KS, Mahmoud AAF (eds): Tropical and Geographical Medicine. 2nd ed. New York, McGraw-Hill, p 798, 1990.

57. Geiseler PJ, Nelson KE: Bacterial meningitis without clinical signs of meningeal irritation. South Med J 75:448, 1982.

58. Baumgartner ET, Augustine A, Steele RW: Bacterial meningitis in older neonates. Am J Dis Child 137:1052, 1983.

59. Gorse GJ, Thrupp LD, Nudleman KL, et al: Bacterial meningitis in the elderly. Arch Intern Med 144:1603, 1984.

60. Schoenbaum SC, Gardner P, Shillito J: Infections of cerebrospinal fluid shunts: Epidemiology, clinical manifestations, and therapy. J Infect Dis 131:543, 1975.

61. Marton KI, Gean AD: The spinal tap: A new look at an old test. Ann Intern Med 104:840, 1986.

62. Conly JM, Ronald AR: Cerebrospinal fluid as a diagnostic body fluid. Am J Med 75:102, 1983.

63. Powers WJ: Cerebrospinal fluid lymphocytosis in acute bacterial meningitis. Am J Med 79:216, 1985.

64. Spanos A, Harrell FE Jr, Durack DT: Differential diagnosis of acute meningitis. An analysis of the predictive value of initial observation. JAMA 262:2700, 1989.

65. La Scolea LJ, Dryja D: Quantitation of bacteria in cerebrospinal fluid and blood of children with meningitis and its diagnostic significance. J Clin Microbiol 19:187, 1984.

66. Martin WJ: Rapid and reliable techniques for the laboratory detection of bacterial meningitis. Am J Med 75:119, 1983.

67. Hoban DJ, Witwicki E, Hammond GW: Bacterial antigen detection in cerebrospinal fluid of patients with meningitis. Diagn Microbiol Infect Dis 3:373, 1985.

68. Saubolle MA, Jorgensen JH: Use of the Limulus amebocyte lysate test as a cost-effective screen for gram-negative agents of meningitis. Diagn Microbiol Infect Dis 7:177, 1987.

69. Dwelle TL, Dunkle LM, Blair L: Correlation of cerebrospinal fluid endotoxin-like activity with clinical and laboratory variables in gram-negative bacterial meningitis in children. J Clin Microbiol 25:856, 1987.

70. Kline MW, Kaplan SL: Computed tomography in bacterial meningitis of childhood. Pediatr Infect Dis J 7:855, 1988.

71. Mathews VP, Kuharik MA, Edwards MK, et al: Gd-DTPA-enhanced MR imaging of experimental bacterial meningitis: Evaluation and comparison with CT. AJR 152:131, 1989.

72. Wispelwey B, Scheld WM: Brain abscess. Clin Neuropharmacol 10:483, 1987.

73. Chun CH, Johnson JD, Hofstetter M, et al: Brain abscess. A study of 45 consecutive cases. Medicine 65:415, 1986.

74. Kaufman DM, Miller MH, Steigbigel NH: Subdural empyema: Analysis of 17 recent cases and review of the literature. Medicine 54:485, 1975.

75. Silverberg AL, DiNubile MJ: Subdural empyema and cranial epidural abscess. Med Clin North Am 69:361, 1985.

76. Zimmerman RD, Haimes AB: The role of MR imaging in the diagnosis of infections of the central nervous system. In: Remington JS, Swartz MN (eds): Current Clinical Topics in Infectious Diseases. New York, McGraw-Hill, p 82, 1989.

77. Ratzan KR: Viral meningitis. Med Clin North Am 69:399, 1985.

78. Rubin SJ: Detection of viruses in spinal fluid. Am J Med 75:124, 1983.

79. Whitley RJ: Viral encephalitis. N Engl J Med 323:242, 1990.

80. Corey L, Spear PG: Infections with herpes simplex viruses. N Engl J Med 314:749, 1986.

81. Hollander H, Stringari S: Human immunodeficiency virus-associated meningitis. Clinical course and correlations. Am J Med 83:813, 1987.

82. Katzman M, Ellner JJ: Chronic meningitis. In: Mandell GL, Douglas RG Jr, Bennett JE (eds): Principles and Practice of Infectious Diseases. 3rd ed. New York, Churchill Livingstone, p 755, 1990.

83. Reik L, Steere AC, Bartenhagen NH, et al: Neurologic abnormalities of Lyme disease. Medicine 58:281, 1979.

84. Pachner AR: Neurologic manifestations of Lyme disease, the new "great imitator." Rev Infect Dis 11:S1482, 1989.

85. Steere AC: Lyme disease. N Engl J Med 321:586, 1989.

86. Klein NC, Damsker B, Hirschman SZ: Mycobacterial meningitis. Retrospective analysis from 1970 to 1983. Am J Med 79:29, 1985.

87. Ogawa SK, Smith MA, Brennessel DJ, et al: Tuberculous meningitis in an urban medical center. Medicine 66:317, 1987.

88. Daniel TM: New approaches to the rapid diagnosis of tuberculous meningitis. J Infect Dis 155:599, 1987.

89. Ribera E, Martinez-Vazquez JM, Ocana I, et al: Activity of adenosine deaminase in cerebrospinal fluid for the diagnosis and follow-up of tuberculous meningitis in adults. J Infect Dis 155:603, 1987.

90. Perfect JR: Cryptococcosis. Infect Dis Clin North Am 3:77, 1989.

91. Chuck SL, Sande MA: Infections with Cryptococcus neoformans in the acquired immunodeficiency syndrome. N Engl J Med 321:794, 1989.

92. Pruitt AA, Rubin RH, Karchmer AW, et al: Neurologic complications of bacterial endocarditis. Medicine 57:329, 1978.

93. Kaplowitz LG, Fischer JJ, Sparling PF: Rocky Mountain spotted fever: A clinical dilemma. In: Remington JS, Swartz MN (eds): Current Clinical Topics in Infectious Diseases. New York, McGraw-Hill, p 89, 1981.

94. Kirk JL, Fine DP, Sexton DJ, et al: Rocky Mountain spotted fever: A clinical review based on 48 confirmed cases, 1943–1986. Medicine 69:35, 1990.

95. Tunkel AR, Scheld WM: Therapy of bacterial meningitis: Principles and practice. Infect Control Hosp Epidemiol 10:565, 1989.

96. Tunkel AR, Wispelwey B, Scheld WM: Bacterial meningitis: Recent advances in pathophysiology and treatment. Ann Intern Med 112:610, 1990.

97. Simberkoff MS, Lukaszewski M, Cross A, et al: Antibiotic-resistant isolates of Streptococcus pneumoniae from clinical specimens: A cluster of serotype 19A organisms in Brooklyn, New York. J Infect Dis 153:78, 1986.

98. Appelbaum PC: World-wide development of antibiotic resistance in pneumococci. Eur J Clin Microbiol 6:367, 1987.

99. Jabes D, Nachman S, Tomasz A: Penicillin-binding protein families: Evidence for the clonal nature of penicillin resistance in clinical isolates of pneumococci. J Infect Dis 159:16, 1989.

100. Viladrich PF, Gudiol F, Linares J, et al: Characteristics and antibiotic therapy of adult meningitis due to penicillin-resistant pneumococci. Am J Med 84:839, 1988.

101. Van Esso D, Fontanals D, Uriz S, et al: Neisseria meningitidis strains with decreased susceptibility to penicillin. Pediatr Infect Dis J 6:438, 1987.

102. Mendelman PM, Campos J, Chaffin DO, et al: Relative penicillin G resistance in Neisseria meningitidis and reduced affinity of penicillin-binding protein 3. Antimicrob Agents Chemother 32:706, 1988.

103. Givner LB, Abramson JS, Wasilauskas B: Meningitis due to Haemophilus influenzae type b resistant to ampicillin and chloramphenicol. Rev Infect Dis 11:329, 1989.

104. Campos J, Garcia-Tornel S, Gairi JM, et al: Multiply resistant Haemophilus influenzae type b causing meningitis: Comparative clinical and laboratory study. J Pediatr 108:897, 1986.

105. Peltola H, Anttila M, Renkonen OV, et al: Randomized comparison of chloramphenicol, ampicillin, cefotaxime, and ceftriaxone for childhood bacterial meningitis. Lancet 1:1281, 1989.

106. Committee on Infectious Diseases, Academy of Pediatrics: Treatment of bacterial meningitis. Pediatrics 81:904, 1988.

107. Arditi M, Herold BC, Yogev R: Cefuroxime treatment failure and Haemophilus influenzae meningitis: Case report and review of the literature. Pediatrics 84:132, 1989.

108. Schaad UB, Suter S, Gianella-Borradori A, et al: A comparison of ceftriaxone and cefuroxime for the treatment of bacterial meningitis in children. N Engl J Med 322:141, 1990.

109. Landesman SH, Corrado ML, Shah PM, et al: Past and current roles for cephalosporin antibiotics in the treatment of meningitis. Emphasis on use in gram-negative bacillary meningitis. Am J Med 71:693, 1981.

110. Cherubin CE, Corrado ML, Nais SR, et al: Treatment of gram-negative bacillary meningitis. Role of new cephalosporin antibiotics. Rev Infect Dis 4:S453, 1982.

111. Fong IW, Tomkins KB: Review of Pseudomonas aeruginosa meningitis with special emphasis on treatment with ceftazidime. Rev Infect Dis 7:604, 1985.

112. Segev S, Barzilai A, Rosen N, et al: Pefloxacin treatment of meningitis caused by gram-negative bacilli. Arch Intern Med 149:1314, 1989.

113. Scheld WM: Quinolone therapy for infections of the central nervous system. Rev Infect Dis 11:S1194, 1989.

114. Levitz RE, Quintiliani R: Trimethoprim-sulfamethoxazole for bacterial meningitis. Ann Intern Med 100:881, 1984.

115. Gombert ME, Landesman SH, Corrado ML, et al: Vancomycin and rifampin therapy for Staphylococcus epidermidis meningitis associated with CSF shunts. J Neurosurg 55:633, 1981.

116. Radetsky M: Duration of treatment in bacterial meningitis. A historical inquiry. Pediatr Infect Dis J 9:2, 1990.

117. Saez-Llorens X, Ramilo O, Mustafa MM, et al: Molecular pathophysiology of bacterial meningitis: Current concepts and therapeutic implications. J Pediatr 116:671, 1990.

118. Tuomanen E, Hengstler B, Rich R, et al: Nonsteroidal anti-inflammatory agents in the therapy for experimental pneumococcal meningitis. J Infect Dis 155:985, 1987.

119. Tureen JH, Stella FB, Clyman RI, et al: Effect of indomethacin on

brain water content, cerebrospinal fluid white blood cell response and prostaglandin E_2 levels in cerebrospinal fluid in experimental pneumococcal meningitis. Pediatr Infect Dis J 6:1151, 1987.

120. Nolan CM, McAllister CK, Walters E, et al: Experimental pneumococcal meningitis. IV. The effect of methylprednisolone on meningeal inflammation. J Lab Clin Med 91:979, 1978.

121. Syrogiannopoulos GA, Olsen KD, Reisch JS, et al: Dexamethasone in the treatment of experimental *Haemophilus influenzae* type b meningitis. J Infect Dis 155:213, 1987.

122. Mustafa MM, Ramilo O, Mertsola J, et al: Modulation of inflammation and cachectin activity in relation to treatment of experimental *Haemophilus influenzae* type b meningitis. J Infect Dis 160:818, 1989.

123. Lebel MH, Freij BJ, Syrogiannopoulos GA, et al: Dexamethasone therapy for bacterial meningitis. Results of two double blind placebo controlled trials. N Engl J Med 319:964, 1988.

124. Girgis NI, Farid Z, Mikhail IA, et al: Dexamethasone treatment for bacterial meningitis in children and adults. Pediatr Infect Dis J 8:848, 1989.

125. Kaplan SL: Dexamethasone for children with bacterial meningitis. Should it be routine therapy? Am J Dis Child 143:290, 1989.

126. Täuber MG, Sande MA: Dexamethasone for bacterial meningitis: Increasing evidence for a beneficial effect. Pediatr Infect Dis J 8:842, 1989.

127. Mustafa MM, Lebel MH, Ramilo O, et al: Correlation of interleukin-1β and cachectin concentrations in cerebrospinal fluid and outcome from bacterial meningitis. J Pediatr 115:208, 1989.

128. Roos KL, Scheld WM: The management of fulminant meningitis in the intensive care unit. Crit Care Clin 4:375, 1988.

129. Dacey RG: Monitoring and treating increased intracranial pressure. Pediatr Infect Dis J 6:1161, 1987.

130. Lyons MK, Meyer FB: Cerebrospinal fluid physiology and the management of increased intracranial pressure. Mayo Clin Proc 65:684, 1990.

131. Rebaud P, Berthier JC, Hartemann E, et al: Intracranial pressure in childhood central nervous system infections. Intensive Care Med 14:522, 1988.

132. Ropper AH: Raised intracranial pressure in neurologic disease. Semin Neurol 4:397, 1984.

133. Scheld WM, Brodeur JP: Effect of methylprednisolone on entry of ampicillin and gentamicin into cerebrospinal fluid in experimental pneumococcal and *Escherichia coli* meningitis. Antimicrob Agents Chemother 23:108, 1983.

134. Kaplan SL, Fishman MA: Supportive therapy for bacterial meningitis. Pediatr Infect Dis J 6:670, 1987.

135. Trauner DA: Barbiturate therapy in acute brain injury. J Pediatr 5:742, 1986.

136. Delgado-Escueta AV, Wasterlain C, Treiman DM, et al: Current concepts in neurology. Management of status epilepticus. N Engl J Med 306:1337, 1982.

137. Feigin RD, Baker CJ, Herwaldt LA, et al: Epidemic meningococcal disease in an elementary-school classroom. N Engl J Med 307:1255, 1982.

138. Broome CV, Mortimer EA, Katz SL, et al: Use of chemoprophylaxis to prevent the spread of *Haemophilus influenzae* b in day-care facilities. N Engl J Med 316:1226, 1987.

139. Peter G: Treatment and prevention of *Haemophilus influenzae* type b meningitis. Pediatr Infect Dis J 6:787, 1987.

140. Dworzack DL, Sanders CC, Horowitz EA, et al: Evaluation of single-dose ciprofloxacin in the eradication of *Neisseria meningitidis* from nasopharyngeal carriers. Antimicrob Agents Chemother 32:1740, 1988.

141. Schwartz B, Al-Tobaiqi A, Al-Ruwais A, et al: Comparative efficacy of ceftriaxone and rifampicin in eradicating pharyngeal carriage of group A *Neisseria meningitidis*. Lancet 1:1239, 1988.

CHAPTER 37

Ophthalmic Infections

Martin Mayers
Michael H. Miller

Patients in intensive care units (ICUs) are at risk of acquiring infections of the eye and orbit. The most severe infections include conjunctivitis, keratitis or corneal ulcers, endophthalmitis, and periocular infections. Ocular and periocular infections in the ICU may be endemic or occur in clusters and may result in loss of sight and life. A retrospective study from our institution showed the incidence of ocular infection in adults in the medical-surgical ICU to be 1.3%.[1] The true incidence is probably much higher. In a prospective study 7% of pediatric ICU nosocomial infections involved the eye, an incidence similar to that of skin and postoperative infections.[2] Patients with acquired immunodeficiency syndrome may develop a variety of ophthalmic opportunistic infections.

Risk factors for ocular infection in the ICU can be divided into those related to the patient and those attributable to the patient's environment. Personal risk factors include systemic diseases such as acquired immunodeficiency syndrome, diabetes mellitus, and septicemia, as well as local ocular conditions such as dry eye syndrome, exposure keratopathy (Fig. 37–1), contact lens wear, and topical corticosteroid use. Environmental risk factors include inadequate infection control measures, which may result in epidemic keratoconjunctivitis outbreaks, nosocomial microbial conjunctivitis, and corneal ulceration.

CONJUNCTIVITIS

The conjunctiva is the moist translucent mucous membrane that begins at the lid margin mucocutaneous junction posterior to the meibomian gland orifices, covers the posterior aspect of the eyelids (tarsal or palpebral conjunctiva), extends over the upper and lower cul-de-sac (forniceal conjunctiva), reflects over the anterior surface of the globe (bulbar conjunctiva), and terminates at the sclera-cornea junction (limbus) (Fig. 37–2). Proper assessment of the conjunctivae therefore requires careful examination. The

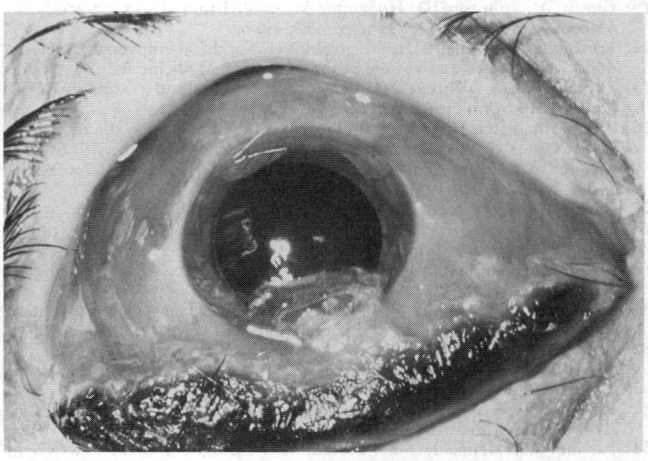

Figure 37–1. Exposure keratoconjunctivitis with corneal ulceration.

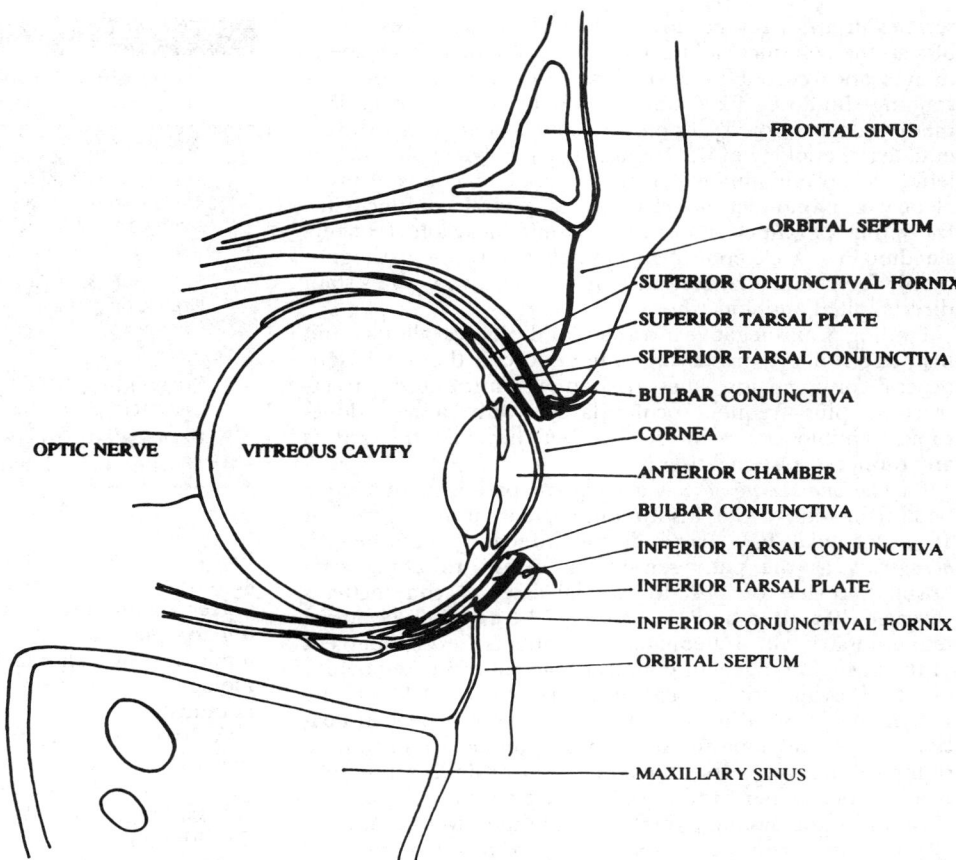

FRONTAL SINUS

ORBITAL SEPTUM

SUPERIOR CONJUNCTIVAL FORNIX

SUPERIOR TARSAL PLATE

SUPERIOR TARSAL CONJUNCTIVA

BULBAR CONJUNCTIVA

CORNEA

ANTERIOR CHAMBER

BULBAR CONJUNCTIVA

INFERIOR TARSAL CONJUNCTIVA

INFERIOR TARSAL PLATE

INFERIOR CONJUNCTIVAL FORNIX

ORBITAL SEPTUM

MAXILLARY SINUS

OPTIC NERVE   VITREOUS CAVITY

Figure 37–2. Anatomy of the eye and orbit.

lower tarsal and forniceal conjunctivae can be examined by pulling down the lower eyelids. Placing an applicator stick horizontally just above the upper tarsal plate and everting the lid allow examination of the upper tarsal conjunctivae. Conjunctivitis is differentiated and graded on the basis of the tarsal conjunctival findings. Lymph from the upper lid and temporal aspect of the lower lid drains into the preauricular nodes. The nasal lower lid drains to submandibular nodes. Preauricular lymphadenopathy is more prominent in viral infections than in bacterial infections.

Papillary conjunctivitis is a nonspecific inflammation. Papillae are small (<1.0 mm), slightly elevated polygonal structures with a central vascular tuft that develop on the tarsal conjunctivae. The bulbar conjunctivae concurrently display variable degrees of hyperemia and chemosis. Although nonspecific, papillary conjunctivitis is the clinical appearance of most bacterial conjunctivitis. Common pathogens include *Staphylococcus aureus*, group A streptococci, *Streptococcus pneumoniae*, *Haemophilus influenzae*, and *Neisseria gonorrhoeae*.[3] Acute bacterial conjunctivitis often produces a purulent discharge and may progress to corneal ulceration.

Follicular conjunctivitis is a more specific inflammatory response. Follicles are 0.2- to 2.0-mm round, elevated, lymphoid germinal centers. Associated papillary hypertrophy and bulbar hyperemia are common. Acute follicular conjunctivitis usually begins in one eye, with the contralateral eye being involved within a week. The differential diagnosis includes adenoviral keratoconjunctivitis (epidemic keratoconjunctivitis, pharyngoconjunctival fever), primary herpes simplex virus [HSV] keratitis, Newcastle's disease, acute hemorrhagic conjunctivitis, inclusion conjunctivitis, molluscum contagiosum, and *Moraxella* conjunctivitis.

In the neonate, conjunctivitis generally presents nonspe-cifically with eyelid edema and erythema, conjunctival hyperemia and chemosis, and discharge. The agents that classically produce a follicular response do not elicit one in newborns. The differential diagnosis includes chemical irritation (e.g., silver nitrate instillation), *Chlamydia trachomatis*, HSV, *N. gonorrhoeae*, and various gram-positive and gram-negative bacteria.

Pseudomembranous conjunctivitis appears as a coagulum of protein and fibrin on the tarsal and forniceal conjunctivae. It can be due to adenoviral keratoconjunctivitis, beta-hemolytic streptococcal conjunctivitis, primary HSV keratoconjunctivitis, gonococcal conjunctivitis, diphtherial conjunctivitis, inclusion conjunctivitis in newborns, and candidal conjunctivitis.

Bacterial conjunctival cultures should be taken from the lower forniceal and tarsal conjunctivae with a trypticase soy broth–moistened calcium alginate or cotton-tipped applicator and plated onto blood and chocolate agar. Viral cultures should be taken with a dry cotton-tipped applicator rubbed over the upper and lower tarsal and forniceal conjunctivae and then transferred into viral transport media. Chlamydial cultures are best obtained with a dry calcium alginate swab rubbed over the upper and lower tarsal and forniceal conjunctivae and transferred promptly in chlamydial transport media. Topical anesthetics may interfere with microbial recovery and should not be instilled before culture.[4]

A topical ophthalmic anesthetic may be instilled before scraping for Gram's, Giemsa's, or microimmunofluorescence testing. Microorganisms are more likely to be obtained from conjunctival scrapings with a spatula than from cotton-tipped swabs of a discharge. With the tarsal conjunctiva appropriately exposed, the ophthalmologist holds the rounded tip of the spatula perpendicular to the tarsal conjunctiva and scrapes in a horizontal movement with enough pressure to blanch the conjunctiva but not induce bleeding. Each specimen is smeared onto a clean glass slide. Slides for Giemsa's staining should be fixed immediately by immersion in 95% methyl alcohol for 5 minutes. Giemsa's stain helps differentiate the etiology of the conjunctivitis. Polymorphonuclear leukocytes predominate in acute bacterial infections. A prevalence of mononuclear cells typifies a viral conjunctivitis. Basophilic paranuclear intracytoplasmic inclusions (Halberstaedter-Prowazek bodies) in epithelial cells are pathognomonic for chlamydial conjunctivitis. A positive Gram's stain directs initial antibiotic therapy.

Finding gram-negative intracellular diplococci allows rapid institution of eye-preserving antigonococcal therapy.[4] Gonococcal conjunctivitis is best treated with intramuscular ceftriaxone plus frequent ocular lavage with saline. Alone, topical antibiotics are ineffective, but they may be used as an adjunct to systemic therapy.

Pseudomonas aeruginosa is a frequent pathogen that must be anticipated. In our institution, evaluation of a cluster of 10 nosocomial ICU bacterial eye infections identified *P. aeruginosa* as the pathogen in six cases.[1] In a pediatric hospital, review of 114 nosocomial cases of conjunctivitis revealed 30 caused by *P. aeruginosa*, 70% of which occurred in pulmonary ICU or neonatal ICU patients. Seventy percent of the nasopharyngeal or endotracheal cultures taken before onset of conjunctivitis yielded *P. aeruginosa*. All but one patient had preceding tracheostomy, endotracheal intubation, oxygen by hood, or suctioning.[5] Immediate institution of topical therapy is essential because corneal ulceration may result in ocular perforation in less than 24 hours.

In an infant, systemic therapy in addition to topical therapy should be considered for any severe purulent bacterial conjunctivitis. In mild presumptive bacterial conjunctivitis, in the absence of a diagnostic Gram's stain, patients of any age can be treated with any of the available broad-spectrum ophthalmic antibiotics (Tables 37–1 and 37–2), pending the culture and sensitivity report.

Chlamydial conjunctivitis in the adult should be treated with a 3-week course of systemic tetracycline or erythromycin. In the infant, chlamydial conjunctivitis requires a 2-week course of systemic erythromycin.

No specific antiadenoviral therapy is available. Management is supportive and aimed at preventing further transmission. In cases with pseudomembrane formation, gentle lysis with a glass rod may prevent formation of cicatrizing scars. Topical corticosteroids can diminish the conjunctival inflammatory response and decrease the corneal infiltrates

TABLE 37–1
COMMERCIALLY AVAILABLE SINGLE OPHTHALMIC ANTIBIOTICS

Antibiotic	Strength	Formulation
Bacitracin	500 U/g	Ointment
Chloramphenicol	0.5%	Solution
	1.0%	Ointment
Ciprofloxacin	0.3%	Solution
Erythromycin	0.5%	Ointment
Gentamicin	0.3%	Solution
		Ointment
Norfloxacin	0.3%	Solution
Sulfacetamide	10, 15, 30%	Solution
	10%	Ointment
Sulfisoxazole	4.0%	Solution
Tetracycline	1.0%	Solution
		Ointment
Tobramycin	0.3%	Solution
		Ointment

TABLE 37–2
COMMERCIALLY AVAILABLE OPHTHALMIC ANTIBIOTIC COMBINATIONS

Contents	Formulation	Brand Name
Polymyxin B, 10,000 U/g Bacitracin, 400 U/g Neomycin, 3.5 mg/g	Ointment	Neosporin Ak-Spore Ocutricin Ocu-Spor-B
Polymyxin B, 10,000 U/mL Gramicidin, 0.025 mg/mL Neomycin, 1.75 mg/mL	Solution	Neosporin Ak-Spore Ocutricin Ocu-Spor-G
Polymyxin B, 10,000 U/mL Bacitracin, 500 U/mL	Ointment	Polysporin
Polymyxin B, 10,000 U/mL Trimethoprim, 1.0 mg/mL	Solution	Polytrim

(see the section on keratitis), but they exacerbate all other actively infective keratitis.

Herpes simplex therapy is aimed at preventing the blinding complications of corneal involvement. In the ICU, systemic acyclovir should be instituted with frequent ophthalmologic examination of the cornea (see the section on keratitis).

Although in a healthy population acute bacterial conjunctivitis is generally self-limiting, this is not the case in the ICU. Untreated conjunctivitis may lead to severe conjunctival scarring, corneal ulceration and perforation, and endophthalmitis.

Prevention of nosocomial conjunctivitis is of paramount importance. The obtunded ICU patient often has an exposure keratoconjunctivitis. Normal tear production and normal blink reflex allow one to flush away potential pathogens. An exposed eye rapidly desiccates and allows normally present nonpathogenic flora to gain a foothold. Simple lubrication is often insufficient to prevent complications. For the short term, the upper and lower eyelids should be closed and taped together with paper tape, making sure that the eyeball is not exposed. Partial suturing of the upper and lower eyelids together with a temporary tarsorrhaphy can be performed at the bedside by an ophthalmologist while ocular examinations are done as indicated. Suctioning should not be performed in such a way that droplets inadvertently fall onto the eye. A study at our institution showed that routine suctioning of patients with copious sputum production was likely to produce high bacterial counts on periocular settle plates. In a series of 10 bacterial nosocomial eye infections in our ICUs, the sputum and eye cultures revealed identical organisms in 9 cases.[1] Ophthalmic dropper tips or ointment tube tips should not come in direct contact with the eye. Touching the dropper or tube tip to the eye can result in retrograde flow and contamination of the bottle or tube. Hands should be washed or new gloves used before separating the eyelids for instillation of medications.

Although most patients with adenoviral keratoconjunctivitis shed virus from their eyes for 2 weeks, desiccated adenovirus can maintain its infectivity on fomites for up to 35 days.[6]

KERATITIS AND CORNEAL ULCERS

The cornea is the clear refracting surface on the front of the eyeball that allows images to be focused on the retina. The cornea is normally covered by a three-layered tear film composed outwardly of an oily layer sandwiching a watery layer against the inner mucous layer. The normal blink pattern allows the eyelids to resurface the cornea continually with a stable tear film. When there is a deficiency of tears or absence of a normal blink pattern, as is common in obtunded ICU patients, the surface becomes desiccated and open to microbial invasion. Tears contain secretory immunoglobulins A, G, and E; lysozyme; β-lysin; and lactoferrin, which function as antimicrobial surface defenses. The cornea is composed of five layers. The outer epithelial layer is continuous with the conjunctival epithelium at the limbus. Even microscopic trauma to the epithelium is sufficient to allow *P. aeruginosa* to gain a generally unyielding foothold. *N. gonorrhoeae, Listeria monocytogenes, Corynebacterium diphtheriae*, and *Haemophilus* species are epithelial parasites that can infect an intact epithelium. Beneath the epithelium is Bowman's layer, a compact layer of collagen. The stroma is the central layer of collagen fibrils composing the bulk of the cornea. Descemet's membrane is a resilient layer posterior to the stroma on which the endothelial cells lie. Severe ulceration and loss of stroma result in a ballooning forward of Descemet's membrane, called a descemetocele.

Keratitis refers to corneal inflammation, whereas corneal ulceration indicates an epithelial defect with loss of stroma. In cases that are due predominantly to exposure, ulceration often involves the inferior cornea at the 6 o'clock limbus (see Fig. 37–1). The adjacent exposed conjunctiva is generally desiccated with underlying hyperemia and chemosis. On penlight examination, the cornea lacks its normal luster. Areas of opacity must be considered possible infectious infiltrates. Fluorescein staining indicates an overlying epithelial defect. The virulence of the infecting organism determines the likelihood of ulceration developing. Although purulent discharge, dense inflammatory cell infiltration, and extensive stroma loss are poor prognostic signs, any corneal ulceration can lead to perforation and loss of the globe. Because the cornea is highly innervated, corneal inflammation is generally associated with photophobia and pain in the noncomatose patient. Keratitis is generally accompanied by circumlimbal hyperemia.

The keratitis of adenoviral keratoconjunctivitis (e.g., epidemic keratoconjunctivitis) is preceded by and initially concurrent with an acute follicular conjunctivitis. Both eyes are usually affected, the first eye more severely. The originally diffuse biomicroscopic superficial punctate epithelial keratopathy coalesces during the second week to form focal lesions. The conjunctivitis resolves after the second week, and central corneal subepithelial infiltrates develop. After the fourth week the subepithelial infiltrates, which can reduce vision, generally begin to resolve spontaneously.

HSV keratitis can accompany primary HSV acute follicular conjunctivitis or can be recurrent corneal disease. Recurrent HSV keratitis is commonly associated with decreased corneal sensation and is generally unilateral. The risk factors that can trigger viral reactivation, such as stress, trauma, fever, surgery, infection, and immune suppression, are common in the ICU. Active epithelial keratitis can manifest in a dendritic or geographic pattern epithelial defect. Disciform keratitis refers to the diffuse central stromal edema associated with a delayed-type hypersensitivity reaction.

Herpes zoster ophthalmicus is due to a breach of immune surveillance with activation of latent varicella-zoster virus involving the first division of the trigeminal nerve. Although Hutchinson's sign (involvement of the tip or mid-portion of the nose) is often reliable in warning of ocular involvement via the nasociliary nerve, the intensivist should note that ocular involvement may occur without Hutchinson's sign in up to 61% of patients.[7]

All corneal ulcers are presumed infected until proved otherwise. Although specific microorganisms have "classic"

presentations, because any bacteria may be pathogenic in a debilitated ICU patient, one should avoid empirical therapy solely on the basis of clinical appearance. Frequently, rapidly fulminant and necrotic-appearing ulcers with a hypopyon and purulent discharge are due to *P. aeruginosa*. Of six nosocomial ICU eye infections with *P. aeruginosa*, corneal ulceration occurred in all and perforation occurred in two.[1] *P. aeruginosa* can cause a descemetocele or frank perforation within 24 hours. Staphylococci tend to form round, localized grayish white ulcers. *Mycobacterium fortuitum* infections often have a cracked windshield appearance. *S. pneumoniae* can create a serpiginous path across the cornea. *Acanthamoeba* is associated with a ring abscess. *Streptococcus viridans* is a common cause of crystalline keratopathy. Fungal ulcers can form satellites and may have an intact overlying epithelium. The most commonly isolated fungi are *Candida, Aspergillus*, and *Fusarium* species.

Before scraping corneal ulcers, trypticase soy broth–moistened cotton-tipped swabs should be used to obtain conjunctival cultures. If necessary, after the conjunctival cultures have been obtained, topical proparacaine 0.5% provides adequate anesthesia for corneal scraping. Under optimal visualization, the ophthalmologist sequentially scrapes the ulcer bed and rim with a sterile Kimura platinum spatula and inoculates a single medium or glass slide. The following media should be inoculated: blood agar, chocolate agar, Sabouraud's agar, thioglycolate broth, brain-heart infusion broth, and an anaerobic medium. Glass slides should be fixed and processed for Gram's and Giemsa's staining. In suspected fungal keratitis, deep scrapings and débridement from the base of the ulcer are more productive than superficial scrapings. Although the hypopyon found in bacterial corneal ulcers is routinely sterile because of the Descemet membrane's barrier effect, this is not true in deep fungal infections. Paracentesis of a suspected fungal hypopyon may be necessary to obtain adequate material for cytologic studies and culture.

Viral keratitis is commonly diagnosed on a clinical basis alone. Laboratory verification may be required in suspected cases of adenoviral or HSV epithelial keratitis. Débridement is an effective adjunct in the treatment of HSV epithelial keratitis, and the débrided epithelium can be inoculated into viral transport media for culture and can be used for Giemsa's or Papanicolaou's staining or fluorescent-antibody studies. Adenoviral isolation should be from the conjunctiva as discussed earlier.

Suspected bacterial corneal ulcers are often initially treated with a "shotgun" approach consisting of topical cefazolin at 50 mg/mL alternating every 30 minutes with gentamicin at 13.6 mg/mL. Vancomycin at 50 mg/mL can be substituted for cefazolin in patients known to be allergic to penicillin. These antibiotics must be compounded by the pharmacy because they are not commercially available in these concentrations. In more severe bacterial corneal ulcers, initial subconjunctival injections of cefazolin at 100 mg and gentamicin at 40 mg are often warranted. Commercially available ciprofloxacin eye drops have been approved by the U.S. Food and Drug Administration for the treatment of corneal ulcers.

If after 24 to 48 hours the sensitivity tests indicate a bacterial isolate resistant to the instituted antibiotics and if there is clinical deterioration or lack of substantial improvement, a change in antibiotic therapy may be warranted. For a deteriorating ulcer infected with *P. aeruginosa* it may be beneficial to switch to topical fortified tobramycin alternated with ticarcillin or pipercillin, plus subconjunctival injections of tobramycin and ticarcillin or pipercillin. For a deteriorating staphylococcal corneal ulcer it may be beneficial to change to topical bacitracin solution plus a subconjunctival injection of vancomycin.

Severe ulceration may require cyanoacrylate gluing to prevent further ulceration or occasionally corneal transplantation to salvage the eye should perforation occur or be imminent. Systemic antibiotics are not indicated for bacterial corneal ulceration unless perforation has occurred or is imminent.

Natamycin 5%, the only commercially available antifungal ophthalmic preparation, is the initial drug of choice for the treatment of *Fusarium* keratitis. It is frequently active against *Candida* and *Aspergillus*. Amphotericin B has been used effectively in topical concentrations from 0.1 to 0.5% in the therapy of *Candida* and *Aspergillus* keratitis. Several of the imidazoles (clotrimazole, miconazole, econazole, and ketoconazole) have been used topically for treating various keratomycoses. Therapy is best withheld until fungus has been identified by either cytologic studies or culture. Topical antifungal penetration is enhanced by removal of the corneal epithelium.

Trifluridine solution and vidarabine ointment are the most effective anti-HSV ophthalmic preparations available in the United States. Acyclovir ophthalmic ointment is available in Europe. Idoxuridine is the least effective and most toxic. Simple epithelial débridement is an accepted adjunctive therapy for recurrent epithelial keratitis. The ICU patient with primary HSV keratoconjunctivitis or recurrent active keratitis resistant to topical trifluridine or vidarabine may benefit from systemic acyclovir. Acyclovir is the only effective anti–varicella-zoster virus antiviral agent available and has been shown to reduce ocular morbidity when instituted within 48 to 72 hours of onset. No antiviral agent is known to be clinically effective in the treatment of adenoviral keratoconjunctivitis.

Bacterial and fungal corneal ulceration leads to corneal scarring, which, if in the visual axis, reduces vision. Often, the progressive ulceration leads to perforation with the potential for endophthalmitis and loss of the eye.

The corneal scarring of HSV keratitis is the leading cause of corneal blindness in developed countries. The neurotrophic cornea resulting from HSV keratitis or herpes zoster ophthalmicus is predisposed to epithelial breakdown, stromal ulceration, and secondary infection.

Subepithelial infiltrates of adenoviral keratoconjunctivitis usually resolve spontaneously. In some cases, perhaps more commonly in those treated initially with topical corticosteroids, the infiltrates persist or recur, causing diminished vision and steroid dependence.

Because microbial conjunctivitis and corneal ulceration are more frequently found in ICU patients undergoing suctioning, preventive steps should be emphasized. Morbidity is more severe and more common in the obtunded patients with untreated exposure keratoconjunctivitis. A temporary tarsorrhaphy can easily be performed at the bedside by an ophthalmologist. Paper tape can be used in the short term to maintain eyelid closure, but if improperly applied the tape can abrade the cornea. Nurses should be cautioned to ensure that during suctioning the eyes are fully closed and covered and that the suction catheter does not pass over the eyes. In general, recommendations for prevention of conjunctivitis are applicable for the prevention of keratitis.

ICU patients should not wear contact lenses. Daily-wear soft contact lenses worn overnight increase risk of ulcerative keratitis ninefold. Wearing extended-wear soft contact lenses on an extended-wear schedule increases the risk 10- to 15-fold. Each additional night of wearing daily-wear soft contact lenses increases the risk by an additional 46%.[8] Patients requiring a visual aid in the ICU should use spectacles rather than contact lenses.

INFECTIONS OF THE INNER EYE: UVEITIS AND ENDOPHTHALMITIS

Endophthalmitis is a broad term referring to inflammation of the inner eye. Uveitis refers to inflammation of the uveal tract. Inflammation may be anterior (iritis, iridocyclitis); in the intermediate region including ciliary body, peripheral choroid, and retina (pars planitis); posterior (choroiditis or chorioretinitis, retinitis or retinochoroiditis); or diffuse (pan-uveitis). Most uveitis is of endogenous origin. As a result of bacteremia, viremia, or fungemia, organisms may infect any ocular structure and cause focal destruction. Post-traumatic infectious endophthalmitis is an example of exogenous uveitis. Signs and symptoms depend on the site of infection. Accurate diagnosis requires an adequate history and ophthalmic examination. Prompt diagnosis and therapy may prevent further, often irreparable, loss of vision.

Anterior Uveitis

The classic symptoms of acute iridocyclitis include pain, photophobia, blurred vision, redness, and tearing. Ophthalmic examination reveals reduced vision, blepharospasm, circumlimbal flush, keratic precipitates, aqueous white blood cells and proteinaceous flare (hypopyon if severe), and a miotic sluggish pupil. Although most cases of anterior uveitis are not infectious in origin, infectious etiologies include HSV keratouveitis, herpes zoster keratouveitis, syphilitic uveitis, tuberculous uveitis, and lepromatous uveitis. Infection originating posteriorly, if severe, may extend into the anterior chamber.

Intermediate Uveitis

Initial symptoms tend to be minimal; the patient may note more prominent floaters and intermittent blurring of vision. Inflammation restricted to the regions of the peripheral choroid and retina, ciliary body, and adjacent vitreous humor is rarely of infectious etiology but can be due to tuberculosis, syphilis, Lyme disease, or toxocariasis.

Posterior Uveitis

Reduced vision is common, especially with macular involvement. Pain and conjunctival erythema, if present, are minimal. Infectious agents that preferentially target the retina include *Toxoplasma gondii*, cytomegalovirus, *Toxocara canis*, HSV, *Treponema pallidum*, *Mycobacterium tuberculosis*, *Candida* species, and other fungi. However, any systemic bacterial infection can lead to retinitis. A Roth spot is a white-centered retinal hemorrhage that may be seen in septic embolic retinitis. It is due to focal nerve fiber layer infarction, causing retinal edema and necrosis of the retina and vessel wall. If left untreated, microbial extension may result in suppurative endophthalmitis.

Panophthalmitis

Diffuse inflammation of the eye causes pain, reduced vision, and redness. The anterior inflammation may obscure visualization of the posterior segment. Hence, the finding of a severe anterior uveitis must raise suspicion of endophthalmitis when the posterior segment cannot be directly visualized.

Candida Endophthalmitis

Infectious endophthalmitis may be of exogenous or endogenous etiology. Accurate data regarding the relative incidence of infectious endophthalmitis in critically ill patients are lacking, but it is likely that endogenous fungal endophthalmitis is the most common entity seen by intensivists. *Candida albicans* and other *Candida* species are the most common nosocomial blood stream fungal isolates known to involve the eye by hematogenous spread. In the past several decades there has been a marked increase in the prevalence of fungemia associated with intravenous devices, hyperalimentation, widespread use of antibiotics, surgical and nonsurgical trauma, and both therapeutic and acquired immunosuppression (see Chapter 33). The most common portals of entry for *Candida* are the gastrointestinal tract and intravenous devices. In 1990 there were 111 patients at our institution with nosocomial septicemia associated with intravenous lines; *C. albicans* was the second most frequent isolate (19%) after *Staphylococcus epidermidis* (34%). A prospective study found that 28% of 32 candidemic patients manifested ophthalmologic findings consistent with *Candida* endophthalmitis.[9] In another study of 131 postoperative patients receiving parenteral hyperalimentation, half of whom were candidemic, 9.9% had clinical findings consistent with *Candida* endophthalmitis.[10] Endogenous fungal endophthalmitis can be due to other fungi such as *Aspergillus* species and may not be clinically differentiable.

Endogenous *Candida* endophthalmitis develops more insidiously than bacterial endophthalmitis. Initially patients may have no ocular symptoms. Signs and symptoms of anterior uveitis are uncommon. Vitreous cells and snowballs may be seen overlying chorioretinitis. Inflammatory lesions may persist after complete eradication of the fungus.[11] Neutropenia may further attenuate the clinical ophthalmoscopic appearance.[12]

If patients at risk are not diagnosed early by indirect ophthalmoscopy, *Candida* endophthalmitis may present subacutely with pain, photophobia, floaters, and reduced vision. The clinical diagnosis is presumptive and usually supported by positive blood cultures. Some patients with *Candida* endophthalmitis are not candidemic. There is at present no serologic test that reliably diagnoses deep invasive *Candida* infections.

Ophthalmologic consultation is of paramount importance in the diagnosis of fungal endophthalmitis. Ophthalmologic examination requires pharmacologic pupillary dilation for both direct and indirect ophthalmoscopy because the lesions may be few in number and peripheral in location. Characteristic vitreous lesions are off-white "snowballs" with surrounding vitreous haze. Hemorrhage surrounding the chorioretinal lesions and Roth's spots may be seen. Less commonly, fungal lesions can be seen on the iris or ciliary body. No ocular finding is pathognomonic for *Candida* and, as noted earlier, it is not possible to distinguish between fungi clinically. Cytomegalovirus and toxoplasmosis are included in the differential diagnosis, especially in immunosuppressed patients (see Chapter 50).

In the absence of a positive blood culture, diagnostic vitreous aspiration or vitrectomy may provide cytologic or culture confirmation; however, vitreal cultures may be negative in histologically proven fungal endophthalmitis. Aspiration of aqueous humor from the anterior chamber in the absence of findings at this site is unlikely to yield useful information.

The treatment of early mild endogenous *Candida* chorioretinitis, unlike that of bacterial endophthalmitis, may not require immediate therapeutic vitrectomy. Although chorioretinal lesions may resolve without therapy, all patients should be treated. Many patients can be managed initially with systemic amphotericin B despite its poor penetration into the vitreous. In one study of 64 patients, 67.2% improved with systemic antifungal therapy.[13] For patients with normal renal function, we suggest treatment with amphotericin B combined with 5-fluorocytosine because this combination may be synergistic and 5-fluorocytosine shows excellent penetration into the vitreous humor of experimental animals[14] and humans.[15] In *Candida* endophthalmitis that is initially diagnosed in a more severe stage including macular involvement, in patients whose condition is deteriorating despite systemic antifungal therapy, or in patients who are unable to tolerate systemic amphotericin B, intravitreal injection of amphotericin B usually with vitrectomy is indicated. The duration of antifungal therapy has not been established. There have been no studies of the efficacy of the new fungistatic azoles (fluconazole and itraconazole) in human *Candida* endophthalmitis, but both drugs significantly and equally decrease the number of organisms in a rabbit model of *Candida* endophthalmitis despite the fact that fluconazole penetrates to a much greater degree than itraconazole.[16]

Bacterial Endophthalmitis

Although most cases of endophthalmitis occur after intraocular surgery, in the ICU bacterial endophthalmitis is more likely to be secondary to hematogenous dissemination or exogenous spread after local trauma or perforating corneal ulcer. In a retrospective review of 114 patients with endophthalmitis in which bacteria were isolated in 74 cases, 10 of the 74 were due to penetrating trauma, 5 were due to hematogenous dissemination, 3 were secondary to periocular infection, and the majority (53 of 74) occurred after ocular surgery.[17] The prevalence of hematogenous bacterial endophthalmitis is not known, but common pathogens include pneumococci (30%), staphylococci (15%), and meningococci (15%).[18] Facultative gram-negative bacilli also commonly cause hematogenous endophthalmitis.[17] Primary systemic infections in patients with hematogenous endophthalmitis include meningitis, vascular access infection, abdominal infections, endocarditis, and pneumonia.[19] *Bacillus* species cause a particularly aggressive panophthalmitis, often with fever and leukocytosis.[20] *Bacillus* endophthalmitis can develop hematogenously in intravenous drug abusers but more commonly occurs as an exogenous endophthalmitis after perforating ocular trauma. In addition to *Bacillus* species (20 to 27%), *S. epidermidis* (20 to 29%) and gram-negative bacteria (20%) are common pathogens in post-traumatic endophthalmitis.[17, 21]

Regardless of the route of infection, bacterial endophthalmitis is a rapidly progressing infection associated with acute and rapid changes in signs and symptoms. Alert patients generally complain of reduced vision, pain, and photophobia. Because ICU patients are often obtunded or sedated, a high index of suspicion is necessary. Clinical findings include eyelid edema; conjunctival hyperemia and chemosis; corneal edema or infiltrates; anterior chamber cells, fibrin, or hypopyon; vitritis; and retinitis. Bacterial endophthalmitis, unlike fungal endophthalmitis, tends to present acutely; however, the clinical course depends on both the organism's virulence and the patient's immune status. *Bacillus* endophthalmitis follows a particularly fulminant course and irreversibly destroys an eye within 72 hours. Suspicion of endophthalmitis warrants immediate ophthalmologic consultation and intervention. The differential diagnosis includes all of the entities that can cause uveitis (see earlier).

The bacterial cause must be identified both to confirm the diagnosis and to provide optimal antibiotic therapy. Empirical regimens conventionally used for postoperative endophthalmitis may not be appropriate for the different microorganisms associated with post-traumatic or endogenously spread endophthalmitis. All patients with suspected endophthalmitis should have a diagnostic vitreous tap or vitrectomy; vitreous samples are more often positive than aqueous fluid samples.

Currently recommended treatment of bacterial endophthalmitis includes pars plana vitrectomy in conjunction with intravitreal and systemic antibiotics. However, the precise role of each therapeutic modality is unclear for several reasons. The ocular penetration of many antibiotics is considered marginal after systemic administration, so the importance of systemic administration of antibiotics is uncertain. Moreover, because most antibiotics instilled directly into the vitreous distribute freely, the role of vitrectomy is uncertain. For the highly virulent organisms associated with post-traumatic and hematogenous bacterial endophthalmitis, rapid identification of the causative organisms is of paramount importance. Two therapeutic approaches may be considered based on clinical severity. In less severe cases, after obtaining vitreous samples via paracentesis for culture and cytologic studies, systemic and intravitreal antibiotics are administered empirically but guided by Gram's and Giemsa's stains. The treatment for the more severe case—and we believe the preferable approach for the ICU patient, who is more likely to be infected with a highly virulent organism(s)—includes forthwith vitreous tap with intravitreal antibiotic injection and systemic antibiotics followed by a pars plana vitrectomy. In the absence of a helpful Gram's or Giemsa's stain, the initial intravitreal injections should include amikacin, 400 μg, or gentamicin, 100 μg in 0.1 mL, and either vancomycin, 1 mg in 0.1 mL, or a β-lactam. When Gram's stain or clinical history is suggestive of *Bacillus* endophthalmitis, we recommend gentamicin in combination with vancomycin, although clindamycin has been used. Subconjunctival antibiotic injections and topical antibiotic drops are common adjuncts and can contribute to antibiotic levels in the aqueous humor, although they do not result in measurable vitreous levels when given alone. Intravitreal steroids may help suppress inflammation and thereby limit retinal destruction and salvage some visual function. However, Smith and associates found that the combination of intravitreal vancomycin with dexamethasone in a rabbit model is associated with lower intraocular levels of vancomycin than when vancomycin is administered alone.[21a] Intravitreal antibiotic injection may be repeated at 48 hours or as clinically indicated.

The prognosis for preservation of sight is dependent on the concomitant medical conditions, the presence or absence of trauma, and the intrinsic virulence of the infecting organism. *S. epidermidis*, a relatively common but mild pathogen, is associated with the best prognosis, whereas *Bacillus* species commonly destroy the eye. Unfortunately, the overall prognosis for a visual acuity of 20/400 or better after traumatic endophthalmitis is approximately 20%.

ACQUIRED IMMUNODEFICIENCY SYNDROME

Ocular infections associated with acquired immunodeficiency syndrome are common.[22] Cytomegalovirus infection, the most common visually debilitating ocular infection associated with the syndrome, appears as a hemorrhagic necrotic retinopathy spreading along the vascular arcades. HSV and herpes zoster virus can cause a peripheral confluent acute retinal necrosis. *Toxoplasma* chorioretinitis and accompanying vitritis may appear as a "headlight in the fog." *Pneumocystis carinii* causes a choroiditis that appears as creamy white round lesions deep to the retina, even when the patient is receiving aerosolized pentamidine prophylaxis.[23] Syphilitic retinitis and choroiditis are usually more severe and refractory to treatment in patients with acquired

immunodeficiency syndrome. The diagnosis and therapy of these infections are discussed in Chapter 50.

PERIOCULAR INFECTIONS

Periocular infection in ICU patients may occur after facial trauma or spread from a sinusitis. The ethmoid sinus is separated from the orbital space by a paper-thin bone. In children spread of infection into the orbit usually occurs from the ethmoid sinuses, whereas spread from the frontal sinuses is more common in adults. Nosocomial sinusitis usually occurs in association with nasotracheal intubation, nasal packing, or trauma and represents 5 to 10% of bacterial infections in ICU patients.[24] Hematogenous spread to the periocular space, although rare, may occur in children with *H. influenzae* or *S. pneumoniae* bacteremia. Periocular bacterial infections may involve soft tissues anterior or posterior to the orbital septum (see Fig. 37–2). On the basis of temporal, clinical, and anatomic considerations, Chandler and colleagues[25] have differentiated five posterior clinical entities: subperiosteal abscess, orbital cellulitis, orbital abscess, superior orbital fissure syndrome, and cavernous sinus thrombosis.[26]

Preseptal Cellulitis

Infection of the soft tissue anterior to the orbital septum is called preseptal cellulitis. Clinical manifestations of preseptal cellulitis include hyperemia, edema, and warmth of the lid and face; a purulent discharge may also be present. Although local soft tissue findings are often dramatic, preseptal cellulitis is not associated with proptosis determined by exophthalmometry, pupillary changes, or limitations of ocular motility. Trauma and skin infection are common risk factors in cases of *S. aureus* and *Streptococcus pyogenes* preseptal cellulitis. If the history suggests a human or animal bite or trauma involving the mouth, anaerobes such as *Peptococcus*, *Peptostreptococcus*, and *Bacteroides* species must be considered. In children under 6 years of age *H. influenzae* type b and *S. pneumoniae* are typical in the absence of other risk factors. Facultative gram-negative bacilli may also be isolated in association with trauma.

The differential diagnosis of preseptal cellulitis includes maxillary sinusitis, allergy, facial trauma without infection, myositis, and angioneurotic edema. Thin-section orbital computed tomographic (CT) or magnetic resonance scanning of the orbit is generally helpful to ensure that infection is limited to the preseptal space. Empirical antibiotic therapy should be based on Gram's stain results for purulent discharge. Susceptibility testing allows modification of antimicrobial therapy. Surgical drainage may be necessary in patients with abscess formation.

Nonsuppurative preseptal cellulitis in children under the age of 6 without evidence of trauma or skin infection is thought to be due to vascular or lymphatic spread of *H. influenzae* or *S. pneumoniae* from an upper respiratory tract infection. The involved skin in *H. influenzae* infection has a classic purplish discoloration.[27]

Orbital Cellulitis

Orbital cellulitis is an acute bacterial infection of the retroseptal orbital contents before abscess formation. Ocular findings are pain, proptosis measured by exophthalmometry, eyelid edema and erythema, limitation of ocular mobility, conjunctival hyperemia and chemosis, and congestion of retinal veins. Visual loss may be due to infectious or compressive optic neuropathy. Systemic signs of septicemia are generally present.

Orbital abscesses are a late manifestation of orbital cellulitis and often cause proptosis, chemosis, ophthalmoplegia, and visual impairment. A fluctuant mass may also be noted.

Subperiosteal Abscess

Subperiosteal abscesses occur when pus from a contiguous sinus erodes through the orbital wall and collects beneath the periosteum. Fever, erythematous and edematous eyelids, conjunctival chemosis, and local tenderness are common. Because the most common primary sites of infection are the ethmoid and frontal sinuses, the orbital contents may be displaced laterally or inferiorly, respectively.

Orbital Apex Syndrome

The orbital apex syndrome can occur acutely or subacutely. It manifests with visual loss (cranial nerve II) and ophthalmoplegia (cranial nerves III, IV, and VI). If the presentation is subacute, signs of infection may be absent. This syndrome is often due to chronic ethmoid or sphenoid sinusitis. Orbital apex syndrome is indistinguishable from anterior cavernous sinus syndromes because the same cranial nerves traverse both locations.

Cavernous Sinus Thrombosis

Cavernous sinus thrombosis is one of the most serious complications of preseptal and orbital cellulitis. Both the superior and inferior ophthalmic veins drain the orbit and communicate with the cavernous sinus. Cavernous sinus thrombosis can occur when infection spreads by means of septic thrombophlebitis into the cavernous sinuses. *S. aureus* is the most common pathogen, although facultative gram-negative bacilli and anaerobes may also be seen in the ICU. Most patients are bacteremic, and metastatic foci of infection are frequent. Early clinical findings include unilaterality, edema of the forehead and eyelid, proptosis, conjunctival chemosis, episcleral venous dilation, and engorgement of the retinal vessels. Complete external and internal ophthalmoplegia may occur. Infection and thrombophlebitis may spread to the contralateral cavernous sinus, causing bilateral ophthalmoplegia. Late complications include disk edema and retinal hemorrhage. Central nervous system extension with meningitis commonly occurred in the preantibiotic era and is still a danger.

Prognosis and therapy vary among these infectious periorbital syndromes. CT and magnetic resonance scanning help differentiate these conditions. Air-fluid levels in the sinuses visible on orbit or sinus x-ray films may be due to trauma or infection and are therefore nonspecific. Sonography is helpful but less reliable than CT scanning. CT scans reliably show the extent of orbital involvement and frequently distinguish between cellulitis and abscess formation. The CT scan also permits better assessment of bone involvement. Magnetic resonance studies provide superior visualization of the cavernous sinus and cranial nerves.

The differential diagnosis includes benign lymphoepithelial lesions, Wegener's granulomatosis, midline lethal granuloma, Tolosa-Hunt syndrome, inflammatory pseudotumor, trichinosis, echinococcosis, posterior scleritis, endophthalmitis, and tumors.

Purulent material should be obtained for Gram's staining and culture and susceptibility testing. Needle aspiration of orbital material is not indicated except when abscesses are present. In patients with sinusitis, infected sinus material should be obtained by antral puncture or by surgical drainage. Because routine cultures of nasal secretions are not reliable in predicting organisms responsible for invasive disease, blood cultures should be obtained in all patients.

Parenterally administered antibiotics are indicated for all periorbital infections. The initial empirical coverage should be based on Gram's stain results and susceptibility patterns of facultative gram-negative bacilli and staphylococci endemic to the ICU. Extended-spectrum cephalosporins or imipenem with or without an aminoglycoside or vancomycin might be used until the results of culture and susceptibility tests become available. If there is poor response to the initial empirical therapy, susceptibility data direct changes in treatment. Anaerobes occurring in association with mouth trauma are generally susceptible to penicillins and cephalosporins. Surgical intervention is indicated for subperiosteal and orbital abscesses. Sinus infection should be surgically drained, particularly if a rapid clinical response is not forthcoming.

RHINO-ORBITOCEREBRAL MUCORMYCOSIS

Mucormycosis (zygomycosis) is an invasive fungal infection caused by saprophytic fungi of the class Zygomycetes that may involve the orbit, the periorbital space, and the central nervous system. The factors that cause these normally saprophytic molds to become invasive are not fully understood, but most patients with mucormycosis are diabetics in ketoacidosis. Metabolic acidosis of a variety of causes also predisposes to mucormycosis, as do leukemia and corticosteroid therapy. Mucormycosis can be seen even in well-controlled diabetics and transplant recipients.

Mucormycosis generally begins in the mucous membranes of the soft palate, nose, or sinuses and invades the face, orbit, and occasionally the central nervous system by direct extension or retrograde spread through blood vessels. Zygomycetes show a marked predilection for blood vessel invasion, causing tissue invasion and ischemic necrosis.

Clinical manifestations may initially be subtle. A high index of suspicion in predisposed patients is required to permit early diagnosis and therapy. Initial symptoms are often limited to the nose or mouth. The presence of black necrotic material on the palatine or nasal mucosa suggests the diagnosis, but this finding may be absent, particularly when a sinus is the primary focus. Early findings include nasal discharge or epistaxis, lacrimation, eye or periorbital pain or numbness, and headache, which may be unilateral. Thereafter adjacent structures are invaded and symptoms and signs involving the sinuses, orbit, and central nervous system follow. Cavernous sinus thrombosis and/or orbital or central nervous system invasion is associated with internal and external ophthalmoplegia, ptosis, proptosis, and blindness. Cranial nerves II through VII may be involved. The globe may be invaded. Thrombosis of the internal carotid artery associated with contralateral hemiplegia also occurs in approximately one third of patients. Involvement of the central nervous system is associated with focal neurologic findings or coma and occurs by direct extension or retrograde spread through blood vessels. The diagnosis of mucormycosis requires the demonstration of characteristic fungi with nonseptate hyphae in a biopsy specimen. Culture results are less reliable and may be negative even when invasive fungal elements are found in tissue specimens. Moreover, cultures may take several days to yield positive results and any delay in diagnosis can be disastrous. Sinus abnormalities or bone destruction may be noted radiographically. Angiography often shows occlusive disease of the carotid or ophthalmic arteries, and CT or magnetic resonance scanning demonstrates the extent of sinus, orbital, or central nervous system involvement.

Treatment consists of amphotericin B and extensive surgical débridement. Most clinicians suggest that after a test dose, full therapeutic doses should be achieved during the first 12 to 24 hours of therapy (1 mg/kg/d). Control of metabolic acidosis is necessary but not sufficient for the eradication of infection. Even with combined medical and surgical management, the mortality approaches 50% and surviving patients are often left with permanent neurologic deficits and blindness. Prevention is truly more important than treatment and consists of rigorous control of diabetes and acidosis in critically ill patients.

Acknowledgment. This work was supported in part by a grant from Research to Prevent Blindness.

References

1. Hilton E, Adams AA, Uliss A, et al: Nosocomial bacterial eye infections in intensive-care units. Lancet 1:1318, 1983.
2. Milliken J, Tait GA, Ford-Jones EL, et al: Nosocomial infections in a pediatric intensive care unit. Crit Care Med 16:233, 1988.
3. Seal DV, Barrett SP, McGill JI: Aetiology and treatment of acute bacterial infections of the external eye. Br J Ophthalmol 66:357, 1982.
4. Jones DB, Liesegang TJ, Robinson NM: Laboratory diagnosis of ocular infections. In: Washington JA (ed): Cumitech. Washington, DC, American Society for Microbiology, p 11, 1981.
5. King S, Devi SP, Mindorff C, et al: Nosocomial *Pseudomonas aeruginosa* conjunctivitis in a pediatric hospital. Infect Control Hosp Epidemiol 9:77, 1988.
6. Nauheim RC, Romanowski EG, Araullo-Cruz T, et al: Prolonged recoverability of desiccated adenovirus type 19 from various surfaces. Ophthalmology 97:1450, 1990.
7. Jones DB: Herpes zoster ophthalmicus. In: Golden B (ed): Ocular Inflammatory Disease. Springfield, IL, Charles C Thomas, p 198, 1974.
8. Schein OD, Glynn RJ, Poggio EC, et al: The relative risk of ulcerative keratitis among users of daily-wear and extended-wear soft contact lenses. N Engl J Med 321:773, 1989.
9. Brooks RB: Prospective study of *Candida* endophthalmitis in hospitalized patients with candidemia. Arch Intern Med 149:2226, 1989.
10. Henderson DK, Edwards JE Jr, Montgomerie JZ: Hematogenous *Candida* endophthalmitis in patients receiving parenteral hyperalimentation fluids. J Infect Dis 143:665, 1981.
11. Demant E, Easterbrook M: An experimental model of *Candida* endophthalmitis. Can J Ophthalmol 12:304, 1977.
12. Henderson DK, Hockey LJ, Vukalcic LJ, et al: Effect of immunosuppression on the development of experimental hematogenous *Candida* endophthalmitis. Infect Immun 27:628, 1980.
13. Odds FC: *Candida* and Candidosis. Baltimore, University Park Press, 1979.
14. Walsh JA, Haft DA, Miller MH, et al: Ocular penetration of 5-fluorocytosine. Invest Ophthalmol Vis Sci 17:691, 1978.
15. Jones BR: Principles in the management of oculomycosis. Am J Ophthalmol 79:719, 1975.
16. Savani DA, Perfect JR, Cobo LM, et al: Penetration of new azole compounds into the eye and efficacy in experimental candidal endophthalmitis. Antimicrob Agents Chemother 31:9, 1987.
17. Shrader SK, Band JD, Lauter CB, et al: The clinical spectrum of endophthalmitis: Incidence, predisposing factors, and features influencing outcome. J Infect Dis 162:115, 1990.
18. Gamel JW, Allansmith MR: Metastatic staphylococcal endophthalmitis presenting as chronic iridocyclitis. Am J Ophthalmol 77:454, 1974.
19. McDonnell PJ, Green WR: Endophthalmitis. In: Mandell GL, Douglas RG Jr, Bennett JE (eds): Principles and Practice of Infectious Diseases. 3rd ed. New York, Churchill Livingstone, p 987, 1990.
20. O'Day DM, Smith RS, Gregg CR, et al: The problem of *Bacillus* species infection with special emphasis on the virulence of *Bacillus cereus*. Ophthalmology 88:833, 1981.
21. Affeldt JC, Flynn HW, Forster RK, et al: Microbial endophthalmitis resulting from ocular trauma. Ophthalmology 94:407, 1987.
21a. Smith MA, Sorenson JA, Smith C, et al: Effects of intravitreal dexamethasone on concentration of intravitreal vancomycin in experimental methicillin-resistant *Staphylococcus epidermidis* endophthalmitis. Antimicrob Agents Chemother 35:1298, 1991.
22. Culbertson WW: Infections of the retina in AIDS. Int Ophthalmol Clin 29:108, 1989.
23. Dugel PU, Rao NA, Forster DJ, et al: *Pneumocystis carinii* choroiditis after long-term aerosolized pentamidine therapy. Am J Ophthalmol 110:113, 1990.
24. Caplan ES, Hoyt NJ: Nosocomial sinusitis. JAMA 247:639, 1982.
25. Chandler JR, Langenbrunner DJ, Stevens ER: The pathogenesis of orbital complications in acute sinusitis. Laryngoscope 80:1414, 1970.
26. Kutnick SL, Kerth JD: Acute sinusitis and otitis: Their complications and surgical treatment. Otolaryngol Clin North Am 9:689, 1976.
27. Jones DB, Steinkuller PG: Strategies for the initial management of acute preseptal and orbital cellulitis. Trans Am Ophthalmol Soc 86:94, 1989.

CHAPTER 38

Upper Respiratory Tract Infections

Carol V. Garner
Ann Sullivan Baker

Upper respiratory tract infections are relatively uncommon in the intensive care setting, either as primary admitting diagnoses or as nosocomial complications. When they are identified, it is often because of the development of septicemia or other serious sequelae resulting from lack of earlier recognition and therapy. The major upper respiratory tract infections encountered in the adult intensive care unit (ICU) are epiglottitis, sinusitis, oropharyngeal space infections, and complications of these processes.

EPIGLOTTITIS (SUPRAGLOTTITIS)

Epiglottitis has long been recognized as a life-threatening disease in children and is now known to be a serious disease in adults as well.[1-4] The usual causative organism in children is *Haemophilus influenzae*, and it has been speculated by some authors that use of the *H. influenzae* type b vaccine in children gradually may transform epiglottitis from a primarily pediatric to an adult disease. Although some cases of adult epiglottitis are caused by *H. influenzae*, various other organisms have been isolated from throat cultures in adults with this disease, including other *Haemophilus* species, pneumococci and other streptococci, staphylococci, and *Klebsiella pneumoniae*. The role of viruses is unclear. One report[3] attempted to distinguish the non–*H. influenzae* adult variety of supraglottitis from the classic childhood epiglottitis, but most of the literature makes no such distinction.

The pathophysiology is that of inflammation and edema of the supraglottic structures including the epiglottis, arytenoid cartilages, aryepiglottic folds, and false vocal cords. Because the generalized cellulitis involves the entire supraglottic area and rarely even may spare the epiglottis, *supraglottitis* is the term preferred by some authorities.[5] The inflammation may progress explosively, with development of complete airway obstruction within 30 minutes of symptom onset. It is the standard of care for a person with acute supraglottitis to be observed for at least 24 to 48 hours in an intensive care setting where, if not established prophylactically, an artificial airway can be placed quickly as needed.

Adult supraglottitis is often less dramatic in presentation than its pediatric counterpart. Sore throat is a prominent symptom, often associated with fever, dysphagia, hoarseness, stridor, drooling, and respiratory distress ranging from mild to severe. The diagnosis is made when visualization of the supraglottic area reveals the characteristic erythema and edema. The findings in adults may be mild, contrasting with the cherry red supraglottic tissues seen in children. The differential diagnosis includes other supraglottic inflammatory processes such as peritonsillar abscess and severe tonsilloadenitis. Lateral neck roentgenograms are useful and may reveal generalized tissue swelling or the classic "thumb sign"[6] of the enlarged epiglottis, but negative films should not exclude the diagnosis.[7] The patient should be accompanied at all stages of the evaluation in case of sudden respiratory deterioration.

Although direct visualization of the inflamed epiglottis may precipitate airway obstruction in children, this has not been found true in adults.[2, 3] Adults have larger, more rigid airways with proportionately less lymphoid tissue. The examination is accomplished most safely with a laryngoscope or bronchoscope in an operating room where an artificial airway can be established if needed. In children, immediate airway provision is recommended and has reduced mortality from more than 6% to less than 1%.[8] Controversy exists over the need for prophylactic airway intervention in adults with supraglottitis, who often do not require intubation when observed closely in an ICU. In one study, adults presenting within 8 hours of onset of symptoms were more likely to require airway intervention than those presenting more than 8 hours after onset of symptoms.[1] Another study found that patients with positive blood cultures were more likely to have severe respiratory compromise.[2] Unfortunately, there are no presenting features that enable reliable identification of the subset of patients who go on to develop acute respiratory obstruction, and decisions regarding prophylactic airway placement must be made individually for each patient. Pediatric studies favor endotracheal tube placement over tracheostomy, citing as advantages the ease of removal in 48 to 72 hours when edema has subsided, the relative noninvasiveness of intubation compared with surgical tracheostomy, and complication rates equal to or lower than those for tracheostomy.[9, 10]

When supraglottic and blood cultures have been obtained, intravenous antibiotics effective against *H. influenzae*, other gram-negative organisms, and staphylococci should be administered. Because of the increasing prevalence of β-lactamase–producing strains, intravenous cefuroxime or a third-generation cephalosporin active against *H. influenzae* is recommended until culture results are available to guide therapy. Most patients improve within 48 hours, but therapy should be continued for 10 to 14 days. High-dose corticosteroids are often advocated to reduce edema, but no randomized trials exist to support their efficacy in supraglottitis.[5]

SINUSITIS

Sinusitis is not a usual cause for admission to an ICU, but the physical proximity of the sinuses to the orbits and to intracranial neurovascular structures predisposes to life-threatening complications warranting intensive care (Table 38–1). Instrumentation with nasotracheal or nasogastric tubes may result in nosocomial sinusitis, a diagnosis that should always be considered in the febrile ICU patient.

Underlying all cases of sinusitis is the collection of secretions in the sinus cavities. The pathophysiologic mechanisms leading to retained secretions include (1) mucosal edema with obstruction of sinus ostia and impaired drainage, (2) quantitative and qualitative ciliary transport abnormalities,

TABLE 38–1

SERIOUS COMPLICATIONS OF SINUSITIS

Site	Complication
Contiguous spread	Osteomyelitis Subperiosteal abscess
Orbital	Orbital cellulitis Orbital abscess
Intracranial	Subdural empyema Cerebral epidural abscess Dural vein thrombosis/thrombophlebitis Meningitis

and (3) excessive secretion production.[11] Oxygen exchange in the sinuses is an important contributing factor. The reduction in sinus cavity oxygen tension accompanying ostial obstruction enhances growth of anaerobic and facultative bacteria and impairs normal phagocytic cell functions.[12, 13]

The maxillary sinuses are the most common site of sinusitis, followed in frequency by the ethmoid, frontal, and sphenoid sinuses.[14–16] An antecedent viral, allergic, or vasomotor rhinitis is common, and the associated nasal mucosal hyperemia allows proliferation of the normal nasopharyngeal microbes, which eventually spread to the sinus cavities. Pharyngeal and odontogenic infections may also serve as foci for spread to the sinuses. Chemical irritants, barotrauma, or other traumatic injuries altering anatomy may impair secretion clearance and foster microbial proliferation. Less common predisposing conditions include disorders of mucociliary function (e.g., dyskinetic ciliary syndromes, cystic fibrosis, Young's syndrome), chronic granulomatous disease (e.g., Wegener's granulomatosis, sarcoid), and midline granuloma.[14]

Nosocomial sinusitis has been recognized as a significant source of sepsis in the ICU. One study found sinusitis to account for 5% of all nosocomial infections in a trauma unit.[17] The single greatest risk factor for development of nosocomial sinusitis is prolonged (>48 hours) intubation with a nasotracheal or nasogastric tube.

The frequency of sepsis resulting from purulent sinusitis in nasotracheally intubated patients varies in reports from 2.3%[18] to 26%.[19] One study looked at the incidence of maxillary sinusitis in ill adult patients with nasogastric tubes and more than 48 hours of mechanical ventilatory support. Sinusitis occurred in 1 of 53 (1.9%) patients with orotracheal tubes and in 25 of 58 (43.1%) patients with nasotracheal tubes.[20] Disease occurred on the side of the nasogastric tube in the orally intubated patient and was frequently bilateral in the nasally intubated group, reflecting the influence of the nasogastric tube. One report found rhinitis in 75% of patients with nasogastric tubes and noted lessening of the inflammation within hours after tube removal.[21] In addition to nasal tubes, other factors implicated as predisposing to nosocomial sinusitis are nasal packing, craniofacial injuries, corticosteroid therapy, diabetes mellitus, prolonged mechanical ventilation, and broad-spectrum antibiotic therapy.[17, 22]

Nosocomial sinusitis differs significantly from the community-acquired disease.[23] The usual outpatient symptoms of headache, facial pain, nasal congestion, and discharge are infrequently recognized in the critically ill, and the diagnosis of sinusitis in these patients requires a high index of suspicion coupled with awareness of the aforementioned risk factors. Fever is more common in the nosocomial than in the community-acquired disease, but other aspects of the physical examination rarely aid the diagnosis. Bedside radiographic procedures often yield unsatisfactory results in ICU patients, and a computed tomographic (CT) scan should be obtained when sinusitis is considered. Sinus puncture by an otolaryngologist may be useful for drainage and to obtain material for culture. Pus from an ostium is helpful for Gram's stain and culture.

Nosocomial sinusitis is usually polymicrobial, caused by some combination of *Staphylococcus aureus*, Enterobacteriaceae, *Pseudomonas aeruginosa*, and other gram-negative organisms as well as anaerobes. Phycomycetes, *Aspergillus*, atypical mycobacteria, *Fusarium*, and other unusual pathogens have been isolated from immunosuppressed patients.[24] Sinusitis in the critically ill is treated with removal of all nasal tubes and with broad-spectrum antimicrobial agents to cover the usual causative organisms. Acceptable regimens include nafcillin and a third-generation cephalosporin, nafcillin and chloramphenicol, or ampicillin and sulbactam.

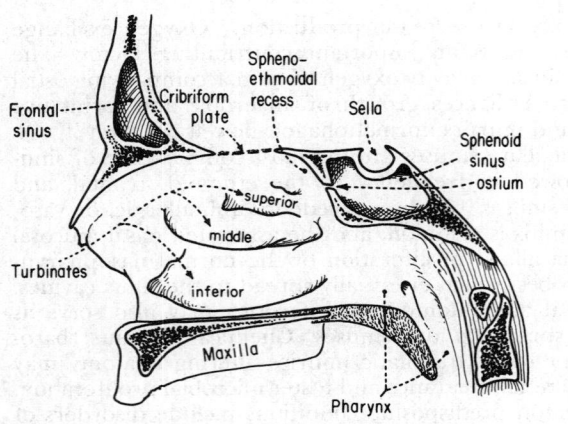

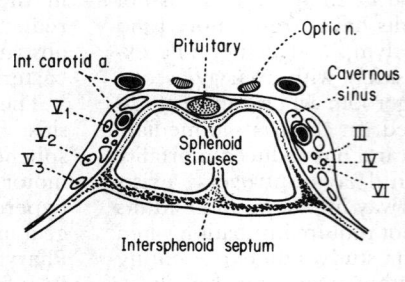

Figure 38–1. Sagittal and coronal sections of the sphenoid sinus. *A.* The sagittal section shows the relation of the sphenoid sinus to the sella turcica, cribriform plate, and nasopharynx. *B.* The coronal section of the posterior aspect of the sphenoid sinus shows its proximity to the cavernous sinuses and pituitary gland. (From Lew D, Southwick FS, Montgomery WW, et al: Sphenoid sinusitis: A review of 30 cases. Reprinted with permission from the New England Journal of Medicine, 309, 1149–1154, 1983.)

Antibiotic regimens are simplified when culture results are available. Vasoconstricting agents such as oxymetazoline hydrochloride may be sprayed on the nasal mucosa twice daily to aid in sinus drainage by decreasing edema. More aggressive surgical drainage is advocated early in cases of associated overwhelming sepsis but is not generally performed until medical therapy has failed.

Complications of Sinusitis

Inadequately treated sinusitis may result in life-threatening conditions requiring ICU care. These complications of sinusitis may be classified as resulting from local or contiguous spread, involving the orbit, or involving intracranial structures.[5]

Osteomyelitis

Contiguous spread to the periosteum is most frequently seen with frontal sinusitis. External spread of infection to the anterior bony table may produce a subperiosteal abscess or Pott's puffy tumor.[25] Inferior extension may cause periosteal abscess of the upper ethmoid cells or orbital roof. Posterior extension may result in an epidural abscess, most commonly subdural abscess, or even may progress to a frontal lobe brain abscess.[26]

The microbiology of sinusitis-associated osteomyelitis is that of chronic sinusitis and includes staphylococci, streptococci, anaerobes, and gram-negative organisms. Diagnosis requires clinical suspicion, which can be confirmed with a CT scan.[27] A bone scan is usually not helpful because of the diffuse inflammatory changes in the contiguous sinus. Recommended initial empirical therapies are ampicillin and sulbactam or nafcillin plus metronidazole and a third-generation cephalosporin; intravenous antibiotics should be continued for 4 weeks. Surgical débridement and obliteration of the frontal sinus may be required in refractory cases.

Orbital Complications

Contiguous spread from the ethmoid and/or frontal sinus is the usual route of orbital involvement. Five stages of orbital involvement are described:[28] inflammatory edema, orbital cellulitis, subperiosteal abscess, orbital abscess, and cavernous sinus thrombosis. Inflammatory edema involves nontender swelling of the eyelids without impairment of visual acuity or extraocular movement. Treatment is directed at the primary sinus infection. In orbital cellulitis, fever, lid edema, headache, orbital pain, and tenderness are present. As infection progresses, the eyelids become deeply red and warm and proptosis with axial displacement of the globe

may occur, but there is no lateral or vertical globe displacement. The diagnosis is made primarily by clinical features, although a CT scan is helpful. It is difficult but critical to differentiate orbital cellulitis from cavernous sinus thrombosis. This far more lethal condition is characterized by headache, nausea, vomiting, fever, chills, and altered consciousness. Venous congestion produces chemosis, proptosis, and a purplish, cyanotic discoloration of the eyelids and upper face. Compression of cranial nerves III, IV, and VI causes ophthalmoplegia, which, if bilateral, is virtually diagnostic of cavernous sinus thrombosis.[29, 30] Immediate intravenous antibiotics and surgical drainage of any accessible orbital or sinus infectious foci are essential. The use of steroids is controversial but anticoagulants are not recommended.

Subperiosteal abscesses are usually associated with ethmoid or frontal sinusitis. Downward or lateral displacement of the globe is a helpful clinical clue. Orbital abscess usually follows untreated orbital cellulitis. Ethmoid sinusitis and frontal sinusitis are the most common sources; molar abscess may also be a precipitating condition. Ophthalmoplegia and severe, progressive vision loss suggest orbital abscess. Subperiosteal and orbital abscesses are treated with antibiotics and surgical drainage. Antibiotics should cover staphylococci and gram-negative organisms until specific culture results are available.

Intracranial Complications

The three major localized intracranial suppurative lessons include cerebral epidural abscess, subdural empyema, and cerebral abscess. Thrombosis of the large dural sinuses and cortical thrombophlebitis are less common. Most of these entities are discussed elsewhere in this text. The bacteriology of these complications is that of the initiating sinusitis and includes streptococci, *S. aureus*, anaerobes, and, less commonly, aerobic gram-negative organisms. Therapy of cerebral epidural abscess and subdural empyema requires drainage of the abscess and initial sinus focus as well as antibiotics. Cerebral abscess may respond to antibiotics alone. Dural sinus thrombosis may involve the cavernous, lateral, and superior sagittal sinuses. As discussed in the preceding section, cavernous sinus thrombosis may progress from an orbital complication of sinusitis; most commonly the focus is the sphenoid sinus[30] (Fig. 38–1). Lateral sinus thrombosis is usually a complication of otitis or mastoiditis, rather than sinusitis. Superior sagittal sinus thrombosis occurs by contiguous spread from a frontal sinusitis–associated osteomyelitis. *S. aureus* is a common pathogen, with streptococci and anaerobic gram-negative organisms also playing important roles.

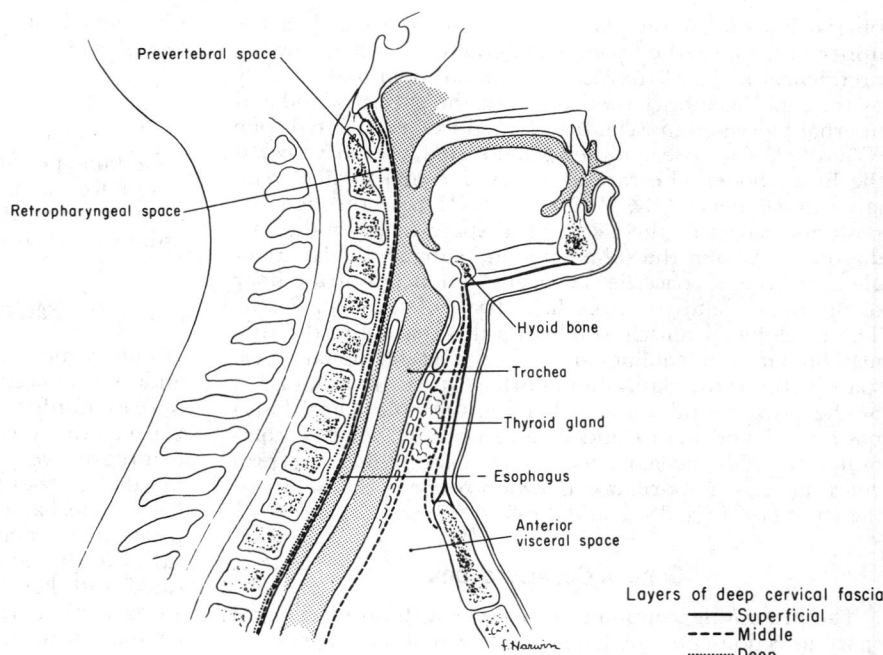

Figure 38–2. Midsagittal section of the neck illustrating the anterior visceral space, retropharyngeal space, and prevertebral space. (From Levitt GW: Cervical fascia and deep neck infections. Laryngoscope 80:409, 1970.)

OROPHARYNGEAL SPACE INFECTIONS

Deep neck infections usually result from extension of dental, tonsillar, or pharyngeal infection. They have become rare in the antibiotic era but may be extremely serious, requiring aggressive medical intervention.[31]

Anatomy

A basic understanding of cervical fascial anatomy is essential to the diagnosis and management of these infections (Figs. 38–2 and 38–3). The deep cervical fascial planes define three major spaces of clinical importance. The para-

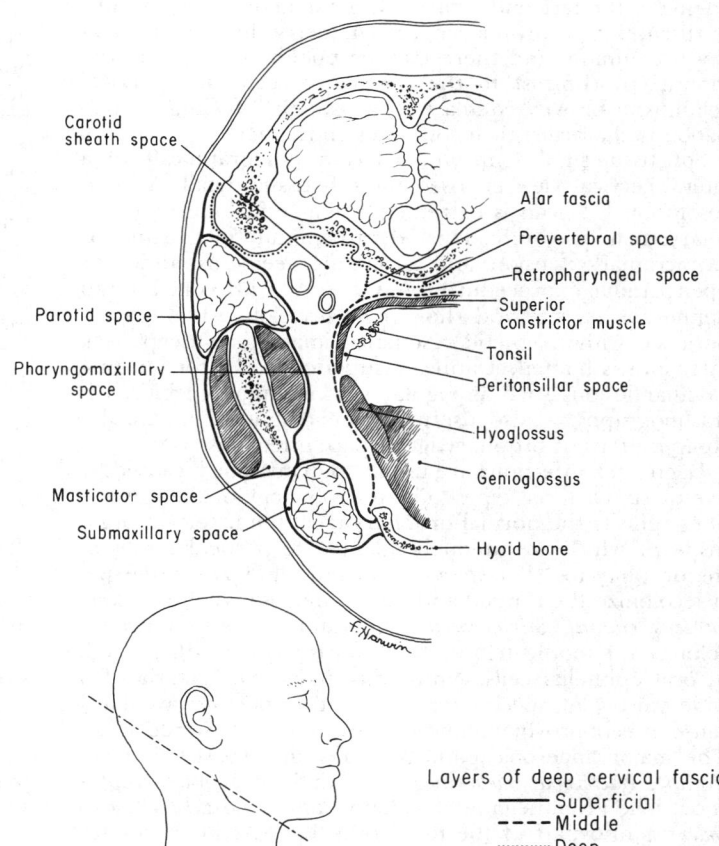

Figure 38–3. Oblique section through the head. (From Langenbrunner D, Dajani S: Pharyngomaxillary space abscess with carotid artery erosion. Arch Otolaryngol 94:447–457, 1971. Copyright 1971, American Medical Association.)

pharyngeal (or lateral pharyngeal) space is located in the upper neck above the hyoid bone, bounded medially by the pretracheal fascia of the visceral compartment and laterally by the superficial fascia, which invests the parotid gland and internal pterygoid muscle. It is shaped like an inverted cone with the skull as base and the apex directed inferiorly toward the hyoid bone. The carotid artery, internal jugular vein, and cranial nerves IX, X, XI, and XII pass through the posterior aspect of the pharyngeal space to enter the mediastinum. Within the submental and submandibular triangles, the second space lies between the mucosa of the floor of the mouth and the superficial layer of the deep fascia. The myelohyoid muscle subdivides this space into the submandibular and sublingual spaces. The retropharyngeal space is the third clinically important space. It is bounded by the prevertebral fascia anteriorly, the pretracheal fascia posteriorly, and the carotid sheaths laterally, where it communicates with the parapharyngeal space. This space provides the most important connection between the neck and the chest (see Figs. 38–2 and 38–3).

General Considerations

The presenting symptoms of patients with oropharyngeal space infections provide clues to the extent and severity of the infection. Sore throat is common and nonspecific, but trismus indicates involvement of the masticator muscles or the motor branch of the trigeminal nerve. Dysphagia and odynophagia are secondary to inflammation around the cricoarytenoid joints. Involvement of cranial nerve X may cause hoarseness and dysphonia; lingual paresis indicates cranial nerve XII involvement. Stridor and dyspnea may result from obstructing local inflammation or mediastinal spread.

Physical examination commonly reveals erythematous edema of the face and/or neck. Inflammation usually results in disruption of oropharyngeal symmetry. Lymphadenopathy is common, and there may be pooling of saliva in the mouth. In contrast to the fluctuance seen in superficial cellulitis, a brawny edema with a "doughy" feeling on palpation is characteristic of pus deep in the neck.

Soft tissue swelling may be detected radiographically on a lateral cervical view exposed for soft tissue detail. A high-resolution CT scan is extremely valuable in localizing oropharyngeal space infections, identifying any mediastinal or extracranial extension, and facilitating needle aspiration or open drainage procedures. A CT scan with contrast can define abscess size and show bone invasion. Although experience with magnetic resonance imaging in deep neck infections is limited, it appears superior to CT for imaging vascular lesions such as jugular vein thrombophlebitis. Ultrasonography is also useful in the diagnosis of vascular complications of oropharyngeal space infections.[32, 33]

Deep neck infections are usually polymicrobial, caused by five or six bacterial types. The microbiology of these infections reflects the normal oropharyngeal flora, certain organisms of which are uniquely adapted to particular sites in the oropharynx.[34] *Streptococcus salivarius* and *Veillonella* species colonize the tongue and buccal mucosa, whereas *Streptococcus mutans*, *Streptococcus mitis*, and *Actinomyces viscosus* colonize the tooth surface. *Streptococcus pyogenes* adheres well to oral epithelial cells. Numerous anaerobic bacteria of a wide variety of species reside in the upper airway. They cause infections when allowed access to usually sterile areas. The major anaerobic pathogens include *Fusobacterium nucleatum*, *Bacteroides melaninogenicus*, and anaerobic streptococci. The gram-negative facultative anaerobe *Eikenella corrodens* is also part of the usual oral flora. Actinomyces are filamentous, branching gram-positive coccobacilli that colo-

nize dental plaque and may contribute to oropharyngeal infections.[35–38]

SPECIFIC INFECTIONS

Certain specific oropharyngeal infections are particularly relevant to intensive care as they may cause airway compromise or other life-threatening complications such as mediastinitis, carotid sheath infections, or intracranial infections.

Peritonsillar Abscess (Quinsy Throat)

This is the most common deep head and neck infection and usually occurs as a complication of bacterial tonsillitis. Spread of infection outside the tonsillar capsule to the space between the tonsil and the superior constrictor muscle leads to progressive pharyngeal pain, trismus, dysarthria, and a muffled or "hot potato" voice. Examination reveals an exudative tonsillar mass with surrounding edema, medial soft palate displacement, and shift of the uvula to the opposite side. Needle aspiration and parenteral antibiotics are indicated, with later change to oral antibiotics for a total 10- to 14-day course. Extension of infection beyond the peritonsillar space with penetration of the muscle bed of the tonsillar fossa creates a parapharyngeal space infection. Necrotizing fasciitis is a rare but lethal complication of peritonsillar abscess.[39–41]

Submandibular Space Infections (Ludwig's Angina)

Ludwig's angina is a rapidly spreading cellulitis of the mouth floor and the tissue above and below the myelohyoid muscles. A precipitating gingival or dental infection can be found in 85% of cases.[42, 43] The cellulitis may penetrate the deep cervical fasciae and spread over the neck and face. The fulminant syndrome is characterized by edema and brawny induration of the floor of the mouth with displacement of the tongue, trismus, dysphagia, dyspnea, spiking fevers, and evidence of sepsis. Therapy is first directed at securing the airway, which may require intubation, tracheostomy, or surgical decompression.[44] Intravenous penicillin G and clindamycin, chloramphenicol, or metronidazole are traditionally recommended, as streptococci and anaerobes are the organisms most frequently isolated from soft tissue cultures. Rarely, however, other organisms such as *S. aureus*, *H. influenzae*, and *P. aeruginosa* have been isolated. Because the fulminant form of the disease leaves little margin for error, broad-spectrum antibiotic therapy with nafcillin and a third-generation cephalosporin plus clindamycin or metronidazole is reasonable until culture results are available. Without adequate drainage, infection may spread to the parapharyngeal space, retropharyngeal space, or superior mediastinum.

Parapharyngeal Abscess

This occurs most commonly as a complication of a peritonsillar abscess, but pharyngeal infections, parotitis, or dental infections may also spread to the parapharyngeal space. The triad of (1) tonsillar prolapse with lateral pharyngeal wall edema, (2) trismus, and (3) parotid swelling is indicative of an abscess in this space. Fever, odynophagia, and dyspnea are frequently present. An abscess in the posterior neurovascular compartment of the parapharyngeal space is associated with cranial nerve findings such as Horner's syndrome, hoarseness, and unilateral lingual paresis. A CT or magnetic resonance imaging scan assists in defining the infection when the clinical diagnosis has been made; therapy consists of antibiotics and external drainage.[45]

Carotid sheath infection is a serious and frequent complication of parapharyngeal abscess. Before antibiotics were available, fatal hemorrhage resulting from carotid artery erosion was a major cause of death from this infection. Spread to the jugular vein may produce the syndrome of postanginal sepsis, characterized by anaerobic bacteremia, septic thrombophlebitis, and septic pulmonary emboli.[46–49] Ultrasound examination may aid in diagnosing jugular venous thrombosis, and therapy is targeted at anaerobic gram-negative bacilli such as *Fusobacterium* species.[50] The role of anticoagulation, surgical thrombectomy, or venous ligation has not been clearly established. Intracranial involvement may occur via the infected jugular vein or by superior extension of the abscess to the base of the skull. Spread to the pyriform sinus inferiorly may cause airway obstruction.

Retropharyngeal Space Infections

These infections may localize between the pharyngeal wall and visceral fascia, between the visceral and alar fasciae, or in the "danger space" between the alar and prevertebral fasciae. Lymphatic spread of pharyngeal or sinus infection to retropharyngeal lymph nodes with subsequent suppuration and abscess formation is the usual mode of development. These infections are more common in children and may be precipitated by trauma or a trapped foreign body.[51] Anaerobes, streptococci, and staphylococci are the usual pathogens of these polymicrobial processes.[52] In adults pharyngitis, dysphagia, chills, fever, neck pain or stiffness, dyspnea, and regurgitation are common presenting symptoms. Dysphonia and drooling may progress to tachypnea and stridor as swelling increases. Examination of the hypopharynx may reveal bulging of the posterior pharyngeal wall to one side of the midline. Neck tenderness, lymphadenopathy, and hyperextension are common. A lateral cervical roentgenogram of the soft tissues is important in diagnosis and is examined for increased thickness of prevertebral soft tissues, air or air-fluid levels, and foreign bodies. Mediastinal extension may be identified on chest x-ray films. Treatment consists of prompt abscess drainage and antibiotic therapy with intravenous high-dose penicillin and other agents as guided by culture results.

Spontaneous rupture of a retropharyngeal abscess with aspiration of pus may lead to pneumonia and empyema. The danger space lying immediately anterior to the prevertebral fascia provides a direct route from the retropharyngeal area to the mediastinum. Descent of a retropharyngeal space infection through this area results in mediastinitis. Extension of infection to adjacent vascular structures may cause serious hemorrhage or thrombophlebitis with sepsis.[45, 53–55]

PREVENTION

Early recognition and appropriate therapy of upper respiratory tract infections are essential if serious complications are to be avoided. Many severe oropharyngeal space infections are odontogenic and preventable by regular dental hygiene.

The major nosocomial upper respiratory tract infection is sinusitis, which can be prevented by using oral rather than nasal routes of endotracheal or gastric intubation. The critically ill, mechanically ventilated patient gradually replaces the normal oropharyngeal microflora with hospital-acquired organisms, including *S. aureus* and a variety of gram-negative bacteria. The oropharynx and the rest of the digestive tract become a reservoir of nosocomial organisms that can cause serious infections. There is much interest in the use of topical antibiotics as digestive tract decontaminants to prevent nosocomial repopulation and subsequent infections. This selective decontamination of the digestive tract with various regimens (polymyxin B sulfate, neomycin sulfate, and vancomycin hydrochloride; polymyxin E, tobramycin, and amphotericin B) has shown particular promise in reducing the incidence of nosocomial pneumonia and bacteremia.[56, 57] Because the microbiology of sinusitis reflects that of the oropharynx, one might speculate that oropharyngeal decontamination would be useful in reducing the incidence of nosocomial sinusitis.

References

1. Deeb ZE, Yensen AC, DeFries HO: Acute epiglottitis in the adult. Laryngoscope 95:289, 1985.
2. Mayosmith MF, Hirsch PJ, Wodzinski SF, et al: Acute epiglottitis in adults: An eight year experience in the state of Rhode Island. N Engl J Med 314:1133, 1986.
3. Shapiro J, Eavey RD, Baker AS: Adult supraglottitis: A prospective analysis. JAMA 259:563, 567, 1988.
4. Mace SE: Acute epiglottis in adults. Am J Emerg Med 3:543, 1985.
5. Baker AS, Eavey RD: Adult supraglottitis (epiglottitis). N Engl J Med 314:1185, 1986.
6. Podgore JK, Bass JW: The "thumb sign" and "little finger sign" in acute epiglottitis. J Pediatr 88:154, 1976.
7. Schumaker HM, Doris PE, Birnbaum G: Radiographic parameters in adult epiglottitis. Ann Emerg Med 13:588, 1984.
8. Cantrell RW, Bell RA, Morioka WT: Acute epiglottitis: intubation versus tracheostomy. Laryngoscope 88:994, 1978.
9. Crockett DM, Healy GB, McGill TJ, et al: Airway management of acute supraglottitis at the Childrens' Hospital, Boston: 1980–1985. Ann Otol Rhinol Laryngol 97:114, 1988.
10. Oh TH, Motoyama ED: Comparison of nasotracheal intubation and tracheostomy in management of acute epiglottitis. Anesthesiology 46:214, 1977.
11. Slavin RG: Sinusitis in adults. J Allergy Clin Immunol 81:1028, 1988.
12. Carenfelt C, Lundberg C: Purulent and non-purulent maxillary sinus secretions with respect to pO$_2$, pCO$_2$ and pH. Acta Otolaryngol 84:138, 1977.
13. Daley CL, Sande M: The runny nose: Infection of the paranasal sinuses. Infect Dis Clin North Am 2:131, 1988.
14. Baker AS: Sinusitis. Med Grand Rounds 3:154, 1984.
15. Evans FD, Sydnor JB, Moore WEC, et al: Sinusitis of the maxillary antrum. N Engl J Med 293:735, 1975.
16. Lew D, Southwick FS, Montgomery WW, et al: Sphenoid sinusitis: A review of 30 cases. N Engl J Med 309:1149, 1983.
17. Caplan ES, Hoyt NJ: Nosocomial sinusitis. JAMA 247:639, 1982.
18. Aebert H, Hiinefeld G, Regel G: Paranasal sinusitis and sepsis in ICU patients with nasotracheal intubation. Intensive Care Med 15:27, 1988.
19. O'Reilly MJ, Reddick EJ, Black W, et al: Sepsis from sinusitis in nasotracheally intubated patients: A diagnostic dilemma. Am J Surg 147:601, 1984.
20. Salord F, Gaussorgues P, Marti-Flich J, et al: Nosocomial maxillary sinusitis during mechanical ventilation: A prospective comparison of orotracheal versus the nasotracheal route for intubation. Intensive Care Med 16:390, 1990.
21. Desmond P, Ramou R, Idikula J: Effect of nasogastric tubes on the nose and maxillary sinus. Crit Care Med 19:509, 1991.
22. Kronberg FG, Goodwin WJ: Sinusitis in intensive care unit patients. Laryngoscope 95:936, 1985.
23. Humphrey MA, Simpson GT, Grindlinger GA: Clinical characteristics of nosocomial sinusitis. Ann Otol Rhinol Laryngol 96:687, 1987.
24. Berlinger NT: Sinusitis in immunodeficient and immunosuppressed patients. Laryngoscope 95:29, 1985.
25. Tudor RB, Carson JP, Puzziam MN, et al: Pott's puffy tumor, frontal sinusitis, frontal bone osteomyelitis and epidural abscess secondary to a wrestling injury. Am J Sports Med 9:390, 1981.
26. Wenig BL, Goldstein MN, Abramson AL: Frontal sinusitis and its intracranial complications. Int J Pediatr Otorhinolaryngol 5:285, 1983.
27. Wells RG, Sty JR, Landers AD: Radiological evaluation of Pott puffy tumor. JAMA 255:1331, 1986.
28. Chandler JR, Langenbrunner DJ, Stevens ER: The pathogenesis of orbital complications in acute sinusitis. Laryngoscope 80:1414, 1970.
29. Maniglia AJ, Kronberg FG, Culbertson W: Visual loss associated with orbital and sinus disease. Laryngoscope 94:1050, 1984.
30. Southwick F, Richardson EP Jr, Swartz MN: Septic thrombosis of the dural venous sinuses. Medicine 65:82, 1986.

31. Baker AS, Montgomery WW: Oropharyngeal space infections. In: Remington JS, Swartz MN (eds): Current Clinical Topics in Infectious Diseases, Volume 7. New York, McGraw-Hill, p 227, 1987.
32. Mancuso AA, Dillon WP: The neck. Radiol Clin North Am 27:407, 1989.
33. Council on Scientific Affairs of the AMA: Magnetic resonance imaging of the head and neck region. Present status and future potential. JAMA 260:3313, 1988.
34. Gibbons RJ, VanHoute J: Bacterial adherence in oral microbiological ecology. Annu Rev Med 29:19, 1975.
35. Busch DF: Anaerobes in infections of the head, neck, ear, nose and throat. Rev Infect Dis 6(suppl):S115, 1984.
36. Newman MG: Anaerobic oral and dental infections. Rev Infect Dis 1(suppl):S107, 1984.
37. Bartlett JG, O'Keefe P: The bacteriology of perimandibular space infections. J Oral Surg 37:407, 1979.
38. Tami TA, Parker GS: *Eikenella corrodens:* An emerging pathogen in head and neck infections. Arch Otolaryngol 110:752, 1984.
39. Brodsky L, Sobie SR, Korwin D, et al: A clinical prospective study of peritonsillar abscess in children. Laryngoscope 98:780, 1988.
40. Spires JR, Owens JJ, Woodson GE, et al: Treatment of peritonsillar abscess. A prospective study of aspiration vs. incision and drainage. Arch Otolaryngol Head Neck Surg 113:984, 1987.
41. Herbild O, Barding P: Peritonsillar abscess: Recurrence rate and treatment. Arch Otolaryngol 107:540, 1981.
42. Moreland LW, Corey J, McKenzie R: Ludwig's angina. Report of a case and review of the literature. Arch Intern Med 148:461, 1988.
43. Juang YC, Cheng DL, Wang LS, et al: Ludwig's angina: An analysis of 14 cases. Scand J Infect Dis 21:121, 1989.
44. Allen D, Loughnan TE, Ord RA: A re-evaluation of the role of tracheostomy in Ludwig's angina. J Oral Maxillofac Surg 43:436, 1985.
45. de Marie S, Richenel TO, Tham TA, et al: Clinical infections and nonsurgical treatment of parapharyngeal space infections complicating throat infections. Rev Infect Dis 11:975, 1989.
46. Alexander DN, Leonard JR, Trail ML: Vascular complications of deep neck abscesses. Laryngoscope 78:361, 1968.
47. Goldhagen J, Alford BA, Prewitt LH, et al: Suppurative thrombophlebitis of the internal jugular vein: Report of three cases and review of the pediatric literature. Pediatr Infect Dis J 7:410, 1988.
48. Cepikel TH, Mhuthuswamy PP: Septic pulmonary emboli secondary to internal jugular vein phlebitis (post anginal sepsis) caused by *Eikenella corrodens*. Am Rev Respir Dis 130:510, 1984.
49. Bach MC, Roediger JH, Rinder HM: Septic anaerobic jugular phlebitis with pulmonary embolism: Problems in management. Rev Infect Dis 10:424, 1988.
50. Seidenfeld SM, Sutker WL, Luby JP: *Fusobacterium necrophorum* septicemia following oropharyngeal infection. JAMA 248:1348, 1982.
51. Barrat GE, Koopman CF Jr, Coulthard SW: Retropharyngeal abscess—a ten year experience. Laryngoscope 94:455, 1984.
52. Brook I: Microbiology of retropharyngeal abscess in children. Am J Dis Child 141:202, 1987.
53. Pearse HE: Mediastinitis following cervical suppuration. Ann Surg 108:588, 1938.
54. Howell HS, Prinz, RA, Pickelman JR: Anaerobic mediastinitis. Surg Gynecol Obstet 143:353, 1976.
55. Salinger S, Pearlman SJ: Hemorrhage from pharyngeal and peritonsillar abscesses. Arch Otolaryngol 18:464, 1933.
56. Stoutenbeek CP, van Saene HKF: Infection prevention in intensive care by selective decontamination of the digestive tract. J Crit Care 5:137, 1990.
57. Pugin J, Auckenthaler R, Lew DP, et al: Oropharyngeal decontamination decreases incidence of ventilator-associated pneumonia. JAMA 265:2704, 1991.

CHAPTER 39

Pneumonia

Steven L. Berk
David W. Allen

EPIDEMIOLOGY

Pneumonia is a leading cause of death and extended morbidity in the intensive care unit (ICU). The incidence of nosocomial pneumonia is about 10 cases per 1000 admissions in community hospitals and general medicine[1-3] wards but may be as high as 120 to 220 cases per 1000 admissions in the ICU.[4] A study at Beth Israel Hospital in Boston between 1967 and 1969 found that 21.6% of all ICU patients had pneumonia.[4] About half of these patients came to the unit with pneumonia, and half developed pneumonia while in the ICU. The overall mortality of patients with pneumonia was 50%, whereas only 3.8% of ICU patients without pneumonia died.

Such early studies may overestimate the true incidence of ICU pneumonia, because clinical diagnostic criteria are increasingly noted to be inaccurate. However, Craven and associates,[5] using well-defined clinical criteria for pneumonia, studied mechanically ventilated patients in an ICU and found a 21% (49 of 233) incidence and a 55% mortality rate. Fagan and coworkers[6] determined the incidence of ventilator-associated pneumonia in an ICU in Paris. Diagnosis of bacterial pneumonia was made by protected specimen bronchoscopy, defining pneumonia with quantitative counts of bacteria greater than 10^3. The incidence of pneumonia was 6.3% after 10 days on a ventilator and 19% at 20 days. Nine percent of all ventilated patients developed pneumonia, and 71% of patients with pneumonia died. Coalson[7] found the incidence of pneumonia to be greater than 70% for patients with adult respiratory distress syndrome for whom necropsy studies were performed.

The true incidence of pneumonia in ICUs is uncertain and varies markedly, depending on the patients' severity of illness and the diagnostic criteria for the disease. Clearly, pneumonia is the most common infectious cause of hospital mortality,[8] and the ICU is the setting in which many such life-threatening infections occur and are treated.[9]

PATHOGENESIS OF PNEUMONIA IN THE INTENSIVE CARE UNIT

In the normal host, various defense mechanisms keep the lower respiratory tract sterile.[10] These include filtration of inspired air in the upper respiratory tract, intact cough reflex, secretion of mucus in the tracheobronchial tree, pulmonary macrophage clearing of bacteria that escape initial defense mechanisms, and intact humoral immunity. Pneumonia occurs in the ICU patient when host defenses break down or when there is a large inoculum of virulent organism. The latter may be responsible for pneumonia, for example, in the young patient admitted to the ICU from the community for pneumococcal pneumonia. In general, however, pneumonia in the ICU is caused by breakdown of host defenses of a debilitated or traumatized patient. The etiologic agent is often a relatively nonvirulent organism, for instance, an opportunistic bacterium such as a gram-negative bacillus.

Conditions known to interfere with host defense mechanisms are common in the critically ill individual. Lethargy or coma in the patient admitted for stroke, seizure, or drug intoxication compromises epiglottic closure and cough and results in aspiration of oropharyngeal bacteria.[11] Endotracheal intubation or tracheostomy bypasses upper respiratory filtration defenses.[10] Impaired pulmonary macrophage function is secondary to hypoxemia,[12] uremia, malnutrition, and heart failure.[13]

In the ICU, bacteria may gain access to the lung by one of three mechanisms: (1) hematogenously (e.g., *Staphylococcus aureus* may cause pneumonia when an infected intravenous line results in bacteremia and pulmonary seeding); (2) by aerosolization, as may occur during respiratory therapy, particularly with reservoir nebulizers (e.g., *Pseudomonas aeruginosa* pneumonia); and (3) by aspiration of endogenous bacteria colonizing the oropharynx.

Most nosocomial, and particularly ICU-acquired, pneumonia is caused by gram-negative bacilli that colonize the upper respiratory tract. Johanson and coworkers[14-16] have delineated the pathophysiology of gram-negative bacillary pneumonia. The prevalence of oropharyngeal gram-negative colonization increases with severity of illness and is highest in the ICU patient. Coma, hypotension, acidosis, azotemia, and endotracheal intubation have been shown to increase colonization.[15] Host factors such as fibronectin on cell surfaces and reduced protease levels facilitate gram-negative colonization.[17] Respiratory pathogens rapidly colonize the oropharynx, and colonization predicts risk of respiratory infection. In one study, 22 of 95 ICU patients who were colonized with gram-negative bacilli developed pneumonia (23%), compared with 4 of 118 (3%) not colonized.[15] Aspiration is common during sleep in the normal individual. A larger inoculum is likely to be aspirated in the sedated or comatose individual. Pulmonary macrophages are unable to cope with this unexpected bacterial load, particularly if they are compromised by an unfavorable metabolic milieu.

DIAGNOSIS OF PNEUMONIA IN THE INTENSIVE CARE UNIT

The evaluation of a patient with pneumonia in the ICU remains controversial. Methods of specimen recovery range from sputum sampling (via endotracheal suctioning) to open lung biopsy. Diagnostic methodology has become an area of extensive research since Andrews and coworkers[18] emphasized that clinical suspicion alone was inadequate for the diagnosis of pneumonia in the mechanically ventilated patient. Andrews and coworkers defined pneumonia as involving (1) the presence of a new or progressive asymmetric infiltrate, (2) fever, (3) leukocytosis or leukopenia, and (4) purulent tracheal secretions. These criteria, although useful and highly sensitive in the patient with community-acquired pneumonia, are less reliable in the ICU, where a 29% incidence of misdiagnosis was found.[15] Of ICU patients *without* pneumonia, 80% had fever and leukocytosis, 70% had purulent tracheal secretions, and 30% had a new asymmetric infiltrate (compared with only 57% of patients with proven pneumonia). Subsequent studies have confirmed the difficulty of this diagnosis and reported false-negative rates as high as 66%.[5, 19] Fagan and colleagues[20] evaluated 147 patients, of whom more than 90% met at least three of the criteria of Andrews and coworkers but only 31% actually had pneumonia. Likewise, Bryant and coworkers[21] estimated that 60 of 111 patients had pneumonia by clinical criteria. Definitive studies showed that only 18 of the 60 patients actually had an infectious infiltrate. It is also important to note that of the 60 patients with suspected pneumonia, 58 had fever, leukocytosis, an infiltrate, and positive tracheal

TABLE 39–1
NONINFECTIOUS PROCESSES THAT CAN MIMIC PNEUMONIA
Congestive heart failure
Chemical aspiration
Pleural effusions
Adult respiratory distress syndrome
Atelectasis
Malignancy
Blood or medication reactions
Oxygen toxicity
Pulmonary embolus
Pulmonary contusion
Hemorrhage

cultures with potential pathogens present. Misdiagnosis was most commonly attributed to atelectasis and pulmonary edema. Craven and associates[5] attempted to increase the sensitivity of clinical diagnosis by using the Andrews criteria plus the specifications that the sputum (or endotracheal secretions) has more than 25 leukocytes and less than 10 epithelial cells per low-power field and that a significant pathogen is recovered by stain or culture. Because of colonizing pathogens, this approach has been of little value.

ICU patients are also at risk for a variety of conditions that can mimic pneumonia. Table 39–1 lists other noninfectious causes of pulmonary infiltrates. Atypical pulmonary edema secondary to left ventricular failure must always be considered.[22-24] Fagan and coworkers[20] studied 15 clinical variables and found that no specific variable or combination of variables was consistently reliable in the differentiation of infectious from noninfectious infiltrates.

We must first determine the need for achieving a diagnosis of pneumonia. Would it not be much easier and reasonable to begin empirical antibiotic treatment of all patients with a new infiltrate, fever, leukocytosis, and purulent tracheal secretions? Empirical antibiotics should not hamper the further diagnosis or treatment of a noninfectious infiltrate. Then why must we differentiate between infectious and noninfectious infiltrates? The most convincing argument for proper diagnosis before treatment is the possibility of development of superinfection and increased mortality with antibiotic-resistant organisms.[3, 6, 20, 21, 24-26] Fagan and coworkers[6] reported that prior antibiotic therapy increased the incidence of pneumonia caused by *P. aeruginosa* and *Acinetobacter calcoaceticus* (65% versus 19%) and methicillin-resistant *S. aureus* (100% versus 33%). Of the patients who developed a superinfecting pneumonia after antibiotic therapy, 87% died, compared with 55% mortality with all other pneumonias.[6] Another study[21] found that only 28 of 40 patients had pathogenic organisms sensitive to the described antibiotic regimen. Six patients receiving antibiotics developed a superinfecting pneumonia and five of them died. All six of the patients developed a gram-negative resistant colonizer after prior antibiotic therapy. Additional arguments against the use of empirical antibiotics for ICU patients are listed in Table 39–2.

Evaluation for the presence and etiology of pneumonia must begin, of course, with a thorough history (Table 39–3) and physical examination. The age of the patient, the presence of underlying disease, and the epidemiology of the region are all important in the formulation of a differential for a new chest infiltrate.

The chest x-ray film can offer further clues, but the clinician must remember that any pathogen or noninfectious process can lead to a variety of different patterns on the chest film. For that reason, Joshi and colleagues[27] recommend vigorous chest physiotherapy for new infiltrates, fol-

TABLE 39–2

ARGUMENTS AGAINST USE OF EMPIRICAL ANTIBIOTICS

Empirical antibiotics lead to superinfection with resistant organisms such as *Pseudomonas* and *S. aureus* and subsequently to increased morbidity and mortality.
Empirical antibiotics compromise efforts to document infection and recover a causative organism.
There is a risk of drug reactions, as well as drug-drug interactions, that can also lead to an increase in morbidity and mortality.
There is a risk of *Clostridium difficile* infection and its associated diarrhea, which leads to weakness and a poor nutritional state.
Treating all suspected pneumonias in the ICU with a long course of empirical antibiotics is an unnecessary and inefficient use of financial resources.

lowed by a another chest x-ray study in 4 to 8 hours. They found that with chest physical therapy, 80% of all infiltrates cleared and did not require antibiotics. Another study[20] found that infectious infiltrates tended to persist for days or weeks, whereas atelectasis resolved in less than 48 hours. In addition, the presence or location of a pleural effusion has low sensitivity for a noninfectious process or organism. It can present as readily with congestive heart failure or malignancy as with an infectious pneumonia.

Laboratory results are also nonspecific because the degree of leukocytosis is not helpful, although a white blood cell count greater than 50,000/mm³ may implicate miliary tuberculosis, which is known to cause a leukemoid reaction. Infections caused by *Legionella* are associated with an elevation of the liver function tests and an increase of creatine kinase (secondary to myositis) with associated myoglobinuria. The diagnostic value of these findings with *Legionella* infection has been questioned.[28] Blood cultures are positive in 10 to 30% of patients with pneumonia.[20, 29, 30] Thoracentesis should be performed on any patient with an undiagnosed pleural effusion. A pH less than 7.0 or a glucose concentration less than 40 mg/dL suggests a parapneumonic process that may require a thoracostomy.[31]

Appropriate specimen recovery is the area of greatest controversy in the diagnosis and differential diagnosis of pneumonia.

Sputum

With suspected community-acquired pneumonia, a good sputum sample that is examined by Gram's stain for bacterial organisms, KOH for fungal disease, Ziehl-Neelsen stain for evidence of tuberculosis, and, when appropriate, silver methenamine stain for *Pneumocystis carinii* may be all that is needed, along with culture results, to establish the cause of pneumonia.[32] Sputum can also be tested for direct fluorescent antibodies to *Legionella,* and the quellung anticapsular antiserum reaction can be performed if pneumococcal pneumonia is suggested by Gram's stain. A 90% correlation has been shown between the quellung reaction and culture results.[33] Sputum is unfortunately often of poor quality, more consistent with saliva or contaminated with epithelial cells, oropharyngeal flora, and yeast. Because it is often misinterpreted, the initial evaluation of the sputum specimen should rarely be the reason for narrowed antibiotic coverage. Instead, it should be used as a guide to ensure that antibiotic coverage is broad enough for all suspected pathogens.

It is well accepted that a high percentage of mechanically ventilated patients, in the ICU more than 72 hours, become colonized with a variety of pathogens such as *Pseudomonas* and *S. aureus.* This colonization makes the examination of sputum or tracheal secretions difficult.[3, 34, 35] Barrett-Conner[34] found that sputum was only 45% accurate in the recovery of *Streptococcus pneumoniae* in patients with bacteremic pneumonia. Johanson and coworkers[15] examined the use of quantitative sputum cultures and found that they had no correlation with the presence of pneumonia. One study[35] attempted not only to grade the Gram stain by the number of leukocytes and bacteria but also to evaluate for the presence of elastin fibers. Elastin-positive specimens had 100% specificity and 52% sensitivity. They were most helpful in the diagnosis of necrotizing pneumonias secondary to gram-negative organisms or *S. aureus.* When a high-grade Gram's stain was combined with the presence or absence of elastin fibers, 96% probability of infection was achieved. Other approaches that bypass the oropharynx and attempt to recover uncontaminated secretions from the lower respiratory tract for examination and culture are listed in Table 39–4.

Transtracheal Aspiration

Transtracheal aspiration (TTA) is rarely used, mainly because the procedure is not commonly taught and there is a risk when it is done by an unskilled operator. The procedure cannot be performed in the mechanically ventilated patient. Pratter and Irwin[36] gave four criteria that should be met in each patient before TTA: (1) the patient must be cooperative, (2) a well-defined cricothyroid membrane must

TABLE 39–3

ELEMENTS OF THE HISTORY PERTINENT FOR PNEUMONIA

Agent	History
Streptococcus pneumoniae	Rusty, blood-streaked sputum; single shaking chill
Klebsiella pneumoniae	Dark red, mucoid sputum (currant jelly); pleuritic chest pain
Staphylococcus aureus	Purulent, blood-streaked sputum; multiple shaking chills
Pseudomonas aeruginosa	Thick, yellow-green sputum; persistent cough
Chlamydia psittaci	Bird handler (chickens, parakeets)
Histoplasma capsulatum	Travel to the southeast United States; nonproductive cough
Adenovirus	Recent military work; few systemic symptoms
Respiratory syncytial virus	Day care worker
Bacteroides species (anaerobic infection)	Foul-smelling sputum; poor dentition (recent toothache)
Legionella species	Diarrhea; delirium; ? epidemic
Mycoplasma pneumoniae	Gradual onset; persistent nonproductive cough
Coxiella burnetii (Q fever)	Exposure to cattle; high fever; myalgia
Mycobacterium tuberculosis	History of prior exposure to tuberculosis

TABLE 39–4

PROCEDURES USED TO OBTAIN RESPIRATORY SECRETIONS

Technique	Advantages	Disadvantages
Transtracheal aspiration	Reduced oropharyngeal contaminants Cultures can be obtained	Uncomfortable Requires skilled hands Requires a cooperative patient Cannot be done on the intubated patient
Percutaneous needle aspiration	Valid for peripheral, cavitary lesions Valid for anaerobic cultures Can diagnose mixed infections No risk of contamination	Uncomfortable Requires skilled hands Cannot be done if patient is mechanically ventilated High risk of pneumothorax and hemorrhage
Open lung biopsy	Most definitive procedure (gold standard) Valid for aerobic and anaerobic cultures Can diagnose mixed infections No risk of contamination	Uncomfortable Requires skilled hands 10% risk of complications (hemorrhage, pneumothorax) Pain of surgery can lead to splinting and thus atelectasis
Bronchoalveolar lavage	Performed at the bedside Low complication rate Can be performed on the intubated patient Allows immediate results (Gram's stain, cell count) Valid for diagnosis of cytomegalovirus and *Pneumocystis*	Cultures do not appear useful because of contaminants Limited in definitive diagnosis of bacterial pathogens
Protected specimen bronchoscopy	Excellent culture results Valid for aerobic and anaerobic cultures, mixed infections No risk of contamination Valid results regardless of prior antibiotic therapy Valid results regardless of which area is sampled Cost-effective in ICU	24- to 48-h delay while awaiting results of cultures Many centers are not equippped to perform PSB and quantitative cultures Results are helpful only in association with quantitative culture techniques

be felt, (3) the Po_2 should be greater than 70 mm Hg, and (4) there should be no evidence of clotting problems. If these criteria are met and TTA is performed by a person properly skilled in the procedure, the risks are quite low. Otherwise, subcutaneous emphysema and bleeding can occur and can be fatal.[24] Finally, the accuracy of TTA has been questioned. Many studies[37–40] support the accuracy of TTA, but they were performed on the premise that pneumonia was present on clinical grounds. Johanson and associates[41] found that more than 40% of organisms recovered by TTA were not present in the lower respiratory tract. Because of the availability of newer bronchoscopy methods, TTA is rarely performed today.

Percutaneous Needle Aspiration

Percutaneous needle aspiration is contraindicated in the mechanically ventilated patient. Needle aspiration can be accurate in the diagnosis of a peripheral cavitary lesion or an anaerobic lung abscess, but otherwise it provides a small inoculum of a small sampling area and thus is prone to a high rate of false-negatives.[42, 43] Its most important drawback is a high rate of complications. Studies have found a 10 to 30% incidence of pneumothorax and a 3 to 18% incidence of hemorrhage in even the most skilled hands;[42–44] hence this procedure is reserved for specific cases, such as diagnosis of a peripheral mass lesion or probable anaerobic lung abscess.

Bronchial Washings

Bronchial washings have been of little use in the diagnosis of pneumonia in the ICU patient. Although little risk is involved, bronchial washings recover specimens that are confined to focal large airways. Because washings are performed in a nonwedged manner, smaller volumes are involved, which raises the question of whether the lower respiratory tract is adequately sampled. Krieger and colleagues[45] have shown bronchial washings to be of no help in the diagnosis of pneumonia in the ICU patient.

Transbronchial Biopsy

Transbronchial biopsy is useful in the diagnosis of a central mass lesion that can easily be reached with the bronchoscope, but its diagnostic utility with pneumonic infiltrates is unproved. This procedure, like that of transthoracic needle aspiration, samples only an extremely small area (less than 25 alveolar spaces) and has a risk of pneumothorax in the 6 to 19% range.[46–49]

Open Lung Biopsy

Open lung biopsy, the most invasive procedure, has long been regarded as the "gold standard" in the diagnosis of pneumonia.[50–52] Rossiter and coworkers[53] found open lung biopsy to have 97% accuracy and a complication rate of 9.6% (no deaths were reported), and the results led to antibiotic changes in more than 50% of patients. Many clinical studies use open lung biopsy via a limited thoracotomy as their gold standard for the presence or absence of pneumonia. Despite the accuracy of this procedure, it cannot be performed quickly and easily in most patients (especially those on ventilators in the ICU), and the complication rate of 10% is too high to justify it on a routine basis. Open lung biopsy should be reserved for patients in whom other methods of specimen recovery have failed.

Bronchoalveolar Lavage

Bronchoalveolar lavage (BAL) requires a wedged bronchoscope through which 20 to 60 mL of saline is instilled to a total of 100 to 400 mL of saline. It samples more than 1 million alveoli, has been shown to be safe, and is the method of choice at many institutions.[45, 54, 55] Johanson and coworkers[41] compared BAL sampling with the other methods described in 35 mechanically ventilated baboons and found 74% recovery for all organisms. They stated that "BAL is the best reflection of the lung's bacterial burden" on the basis of a large sampling area and good recovery rate. Chastre and colleagues[56] and other investigators[57, 58] have found BAL cultures to be of little value because of the high rate of contamination with colonizing bacteria. Some investigators[59, 60] have attempted to screen BAL samples by examination with Gram's stain for epithelial cells and bacteria, but this screening process needs further study to demonstrate its usefulness. Although Chastre and colleagues[56] do not find BAL cultures useful, they support the use of BAL samples in conjunction with protected specimen brushing. They recognize the 24- to 48-hour delay that occurs while waiting for bronchoscopic brushing cultures and propose that BAL fluid be obtained at the same time, sent for cytocentrifugation, and examined with Gram's stain. If more than 25% of cells contain intracellular organisms, antibiotics should be given pending the culture results. If less than 15% of cells have intracellular organisms, it is safe to observe the patient until culture results are available.

Rouby and associates[61] proposed a method of protected BAL sampling via the endotracheal tube of ICU patients (without the use of bronchoscope). They found positive BAL results in 80% of patients with known pneumonia (20% false-negative rate) and 34% of control patients (as a result of contamination). This gave 80% sensitivity and 66% specificity. They also reported a 74% recovery rate for all organisms via protected BAL sampling. These results are not much different from those obtained with bronchial washings and, as with that procedure, contamination is a major problem. In addition, the 20% false-negative rate is unacceptable because it implies that one fifth of patients would be thought not to have pneumonia and would therefore not receive antibiotics.

BAL sampling is attractive because it is easily performed at the bedside, allows immediate results (Gram's stain and cell count), and has a low element of risk (only a rare episode of hempotysis or pneumothorax).[56, 55] In addition, it is an excellent method for the diagnosis of *P. carinii*, with 90 to 97% sensitivity.[62–64] Rankin[55] suggests that if BAL fluid is cytocentrifuged and then cultured in a viral medium, a positive culture (for cytomegalovirus) can be achieved. Although BAL cultures may have limited usefulness in the mechanically ventilated patient, the procedure does have certain advantages and should probably be used, in conjunction with the protected specimen brush, for an initial screen and also as aid in the diagnosis of cytomegalovirus and *P. carinii* pneumonia.

Protected Specimen Bronchoscopy

Protected specimen bronchoscopy (PSB) is done with a plugged double-catheter system that allows an internal catheter and brush to extend 3 to 4 cm beyond the end of the bronchoscope. Because of the outer structure, the internal brush is protected from contaminated secretions that may pool on the outside of the bronchoscope.[65–68] Most studies suggest that PSB samples be sent for quantitative cultures and that more than 10^3 colony-forming units/mL be used as the cutoff for the presence or absence of infection. With 10^3 as the dividing line, excellent results can be obtained with essentially no false-negatives.[6, 19, 20, 54, 56, 69] Fagan,[6, 20] Chastre and coworkers,[19, 56] and others[69, 70] achieved almost 100% sensitivity and specificity with the 10^3 colony-forming units/mL limit. The organism recovery rate with PSB is found to be greater than 75% in all studies.[6, 19, 20, 54, 56, 69, 70] One of the most interesting studies was that of Chastre and associates,[19] who performed PSB, as well as limited thoracotomy, on 26 patients at the time of death (before the ventilator was turned off). Every patient with histologically proven pneumonia was identified by PSB, and no patient with a culture growth rate of less than 10^3 colony-forming units/mL was shown by histology to have pneumonia. The most important point to focus on is the lack of false-negative results with PSB. A low degree of false-positive results can be tolerated, because without any diagnostic investigation the patient would most likely receive conservative treatment with antibiotics. What cannot be tolerated is a procedure that has a sensitivity of 75, 80, or even 90%. As stated before, 80% sensitivity suggests that one of every five pneumonias is missed. The lack of false-negatives is one of the greatest strengths of PSB.

Arguments against the use of PSB include reduced accuracy after prior use of antibiotics, the delay before obtaining culture results, the concern that PSB samples only a small area of the lung, and the cost of an invasive procedure. One study[66] suggested that prior antibiotic treatment decreased the recovery rate of PSB and affected its sensitivity. Since that time, both Chastre[19] and Fagan[20] and their coworkers have effectively shown that prior antibiotics have little, if any, effect on PSB specimen recovery. Because of the inherent delay with cultures, Pollock and coworkers[70] evaluated the use of Gram's stain with PSB sampling. They found 78% sensitivity and stated that the Gram stain is a "good predictor of culture results." The sensitivity and specificity of PSB in this study approached 100%. In addition, the use of BAL fluid for initial evaluation may prove to be the bridge between PSB and culture results.[56] Although PSB may sample only a small area, the sensitivity of the procedure (compared with that of open lung biopsy) is high. Winterbauer and colleagues[69] similarly reported identical results with PSB regardless of whether the involved lung or the contralateral lung was examined. The argument of cost was most effectively evaluated by Fagan and coworkers.[20] PSB and quantitative cultures were initially more expensive, but the results kept more than two thirds of all patients with suspected pneumonias from receiving a long course of antibiotics. When the expense of PSB, quantitative cultures, and antibiotics in one third of patients was compared to that of a course of antibiotics in all patients suspected of having pneumonia, the use of PSB was much more cost-efficient. Fagan and coworkers showed that the fifth day of antibiotics was the point at which PSB gained the upper hand in cost-efficiency. The cost of empirical antibiotics in terms of superinfection and increased mortality has already been addressed.

The major weakness of PSB and quantitative cultures is that many centers are not yet equipped to perform these procedures. We consider PSB in conjunction with quantitative cultures to be necessary for most ICU patients who are suspected of having a pneumonia on clinical grounds. At the least, PSB should be performed on immunosuppressed patients, patients who have failed antibiotic trials, and patients in whom other diagnostic methods have been unable to give definitive results.[69] In addition, BAL fluid should be examined for intracellular organisms and decisions about

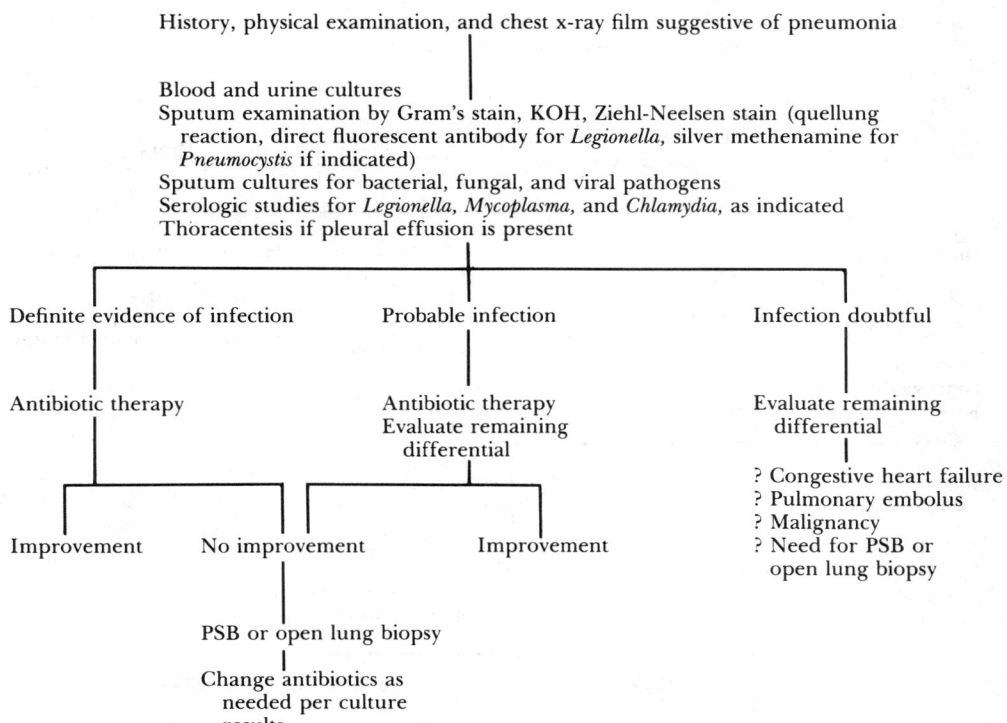

Figure 39–1. Algorithm for the diagnosis of community-acquired pneumonia. PSB = protected specimen bronchoscopy.

initial antibiotic therapy should be made on the basis of these results. Although superinfection with resistant organisms and increased mortality caused by these organisms have been shown to occur with unnecessary empirical antibiotic therapy, further investigation of the effects on mortality with such diagnostic procedures is needed to resolve the existing controversy.

Other attempts have been made to increase the yield from BAL or PSB specimens. Winterbauer and colleagues[69] evaluated recovered bacteria for the presence of antibody coating. They found that colonizing bacteria were not coated with antibody, whereas lower respiratory tract pathogens stimulated the immune system and were coated with immunoglobulin. Although future variations on this technique may prove helpful, at present there are two major weaknesses. First, Winterbauer and colleagues found that only about 50% of bacteria are coated with antibody during the first 7 days of infection. Smith and coworkers[71] found similar results in pyelonephritis, with antibody coating requiring between 8 and 11 days. Therefore, bacterial antibody coating does not appear to be helpful in the diagnosis of a new infiltrate. Second, a high rate of false-negatives is expected if the patient is immunocompromised or has an underlying illness that suppresses antibody formation. Other methods of evaluation have included the use of latex agglutination and counterimmunoelectrophoresis for *S. pneumoniae, Haemophilus influenzae,* and *P. aeruginosa* with disappointing results. Counterimmunoelectrophoresis for pneumococci has been shown to have lower sensitivity than either the quellung reaction or culture results.[72]

Algorithms for the diagnosis of community-acquired and nosocomial pneumonias are proposed in Figures 39–1 and 39–2.

ETIOLOGIC AGENTS IN INTENSIVE CARE UNIT PNEUMONIA

The spectrum of microorganisms known to cause nosocomial pneumonia has rapidly increased. These include low-virulence bacteria such as *Staphylococcus epidermidis, Corynebacterium,* nontypable *H. influenzae, Moraxella (Branhamella) catarrhalis,* and others.[73] Fungi including *Candida* and *Aspergillus* and viruses including influenza and respiratory syncytial virus are all capable of causing nosocomial infection and pneumonia. However, the etiologic agents responsible for pneumonia in the ICU, as reported in the current literature, are usually gram-negative bacilli and *S. aureus.* Table 39–5 summarizes etiologic agents that cause pneumonia in an ICU setting.

These studies confirm that the gram-negative bacilli are the most common etiologic agents in ICU pneumonia. In the five studies tabulated, gram-negative bacilli were present in bronchoscopy specimens or tracheal aspirates of 55 to 85% of patients. The incidence of *P. aeruginosa* pneumonia was in the range 17 to 27% of all ICU pneumonias. *S. aureus* was the next most common cause of pneumonia in the ICU, accounting for 8 to 20% of cases. The incidence and type of streptococcal pneumonia in the ICU were variable. Seidenfeld and associates[30] found either *H. influenzae* or *M. (B.) catarrhalis* in 12% of patients. *Candida* species occurred in 2 to 6% of cases. *Legionella* was looked for in most studies but was noted in only one case. However, *Legionella* has been an important cause of nosocomial and ICU pneumonia in some hospitals.

In one study[74] the etiologic agents in ICU community-acquired versus nosocomial pneumonia were compared (Table 39–6). As expected, *S. pneumoniae* was by far the most common cause of community-acquired ICU pneumonia, responsible for 34% of all cases. *S. aureus* was the next most common pathogen.[14, 75] In the hospital-acquired ICU pneumonias, *P. aeruginosa* was responsible for 31% of cases and gram-negative bacilli in general accounted for 83%.

The etiologic agents responsible for pneumonia in an ICU setting depend on several variables.

1. The percentage of cases of pneumonia occurring in ventilated patients (usually *S. aureus* and gram-negative ba-

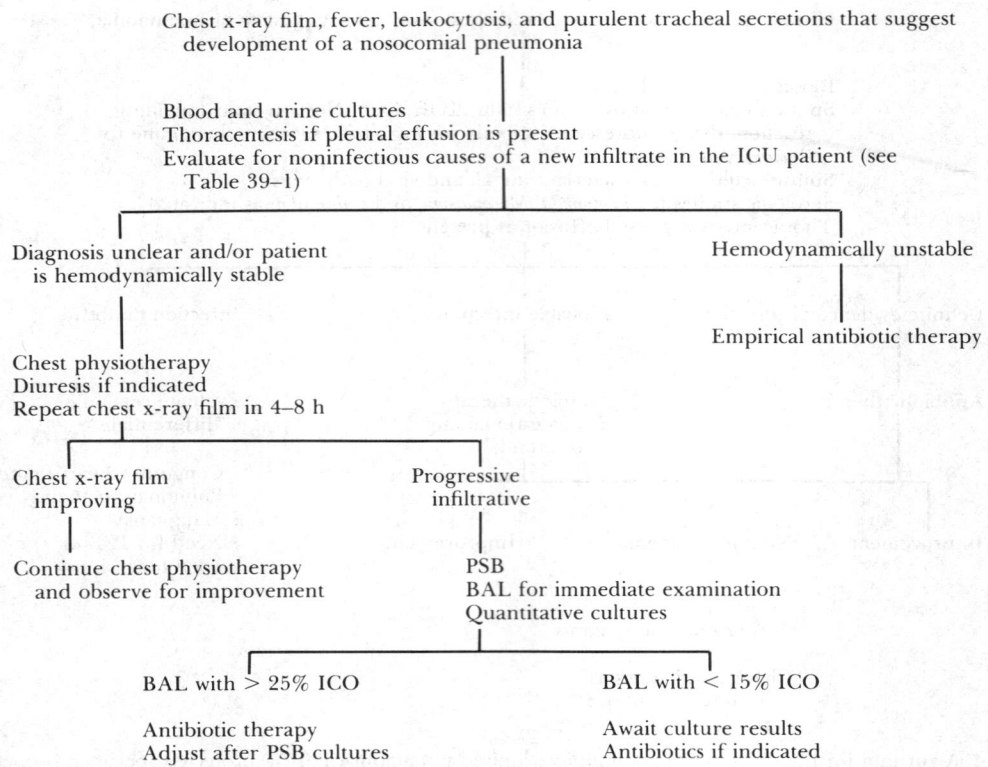

Chest x-ray film, fever, leukocytosis, and purulent tracheal secretions that suggest development of a nosocomial pneumonia

Blood and urine cultures
Thoracentesis if pleural effusion is present
Evaluate for noninfectious causes of a new infiltrate in the ICU patient (see Table 39–1)

Diagnosis unclear and/or patient is hemodynamically stable

Hemodynamically unstable

Empirical antibiotic therapy

Chest physiotherapy
Diuresis if indicated
Repeat chest x-ray film in 4–8 h

Chest x-ray film improving

Progressive infiltrative

Continue chest physiotherapy and observe for improvement

PSB
BAL for immediate examination
Quantitative cultures

BAL with > 25% ICO

BAL with < 15% ICO

Antibiotic therapy
Adjust after PSB cultures

Await culture results
Antibiotics if indicated

Figure 39–2. Algorithm for the diagnosis of a nosocomial pneumonia. PSB = protected specimen bronchoscopy; BAL = bronchoalveolar lavage; ICO = intracellular organisms.

cilli) versus those admitted from the community with overwhelming pneumonia (mainly *S. pneumoniae*).

2. Populations of patients and underlying diseases. Patients with acquired immunodeficiency syndrome develop more *P. carinii*, fungal, and mycobacterial infections.

3. The hospital's unique indigenous flora, reflecting the pattern of antibiotic usage and variable incidence of antibiotic-resistant gram-negative bacilli, methicillin-resistant staphylococci, and *Legionella*.

4. Appropriateness of the work-up and availability of specialized studies. These affect the diagnosis of less common pathogens such as influenza, respiratory syncytial virus, and fungi.

SPECIFIC ETIOLOGIC AGENTS IN PNEUMONIA
Pneumonia Caused by *Streptococcus pneumoniae*

Pneumococcal pneumonia was called the "Captain of the Men of Death" by Osler in 1892. Despite the availability of penicillin and the pneumococcal vaccine, pneumococcal disease remains an important cause of death in the United States. The case mortality rate from bacteremic pneumococcal pneumonia is about 25%[76] and is as high as 60% in adults older than the age of 70.[77] The risk of death is also high in patients with certain underlying diseases such as sickle cell anemia, asplenia, multiple myeloma, and, to a lesser extent, chronic obstructive pulmonary disease and congestive heart

TABLE 39–5

ETIOLOGIC AGENTS IN INTENSIVE CARE UNIT PNEUMONIA

Agent	Frequency (%)*				
	Salata et al;[35] Intubated Patients, TA	Craven et al;[9] All Medical ICU Patients, TA	Fagan et al;[6] ICU Patients, Intubated, PSB	Chastre et al;[19] ICU Patients, Intubated, PSB	Seidenfeld et al;[30] ICU Patients with ARDS, TA
P. aeruginosa	27	16	19	24	17
Other gram-negative bacilli	52	69	28	44	39
S. aureus	19	16	20	8	11†
S. epidermidis	8	—	—	—	—†
Streptococci	—	18	13	10	20‡
Candida	4	2	—	6	—
H. influenzae	—	9	6	2	—
Legionella	—	—	6	—	—
M. (B.) catarrhalis	—	—	6	—	—
Anaerobes	—	—	2	—	5

*TA = tracheal aspirate; PSB = protected specimen bronchoscopy; ARDS = adult respiratory distress syndrome.
†No distinction between made *aureus* and *epidermidis*.
‡15% were enterococci.

TABLE 39-6

TABLE 39-6
DISTRIBUTION OF ORGANISMS CAUSING HOSPITAL- AND COMMUNITY-ACQUIRED PNEUMONIAS

Organism	Hospital Acquired			Community Acquired		
	Total No. (%)*	Definitive No.	Probable No.	Total No. (%)*	Definitive No.	Probable No.
Streptococcus pneumoniae	10 (5.6)	4	6	16 (34)	11	5
Streptococcus viridans				1 (2.1)		1
Staphylococcus aureus	14 (7.8)	6	8	7 (14.9)	1	6
Other gram-positive aerobes	2 (1.1)	2		3 (6.4)	2	1
Pseudomonas aeruginosa	56 (31.1)	10	46	1 (2.1)		1
Other *Pseudomonas* spp.	6 (3.3)	2	4	1 (2.1)		1
Proteus mirabilis	15 (8.3)	4	11	2 (4.3)	1	1
Serratia marcescens	13 (7.2)	6	7	2 (4.3)	1	1
Other *Serratia* spp.	2 (1.1)		2	1 (2.1)		1
Escherichia coli	14 (7.8)	12	2	1 (2.1)		1
Klebsiella pneumoniae	13 (7.2)	10	3	1 (2.1)	1	
Enterobacter sp.	11 (6.1)	6	5	2 (4.3)	1	1
Haemophilus influenzae	8 (4.4)	3	5	4 (8.6)		4
Other gram-negative aerobes	12 (6.6)	4	8	4 (8.6)	1	3
Bacteroides fragilis	1 (0.6)	1		1 (2.1)	1	
Bacteroides sp.	1 (0.6)	1				
Other gram-negative anaerobes	1 (0.6)	1				
Fungi	1 (0.6)		1			
Classified pneumonias	180 (100)	72	108	47 (100)	20	27

*Percentages are given in parentheses.
From S Ruiz-Santana, A Garcia-Jiminez, A Esteban, et al, ICU pneumonias: A multi-institutional study, Crit Care Med, 15, 930–932, © by Williams & Wilkins, 1987.

failure. Penicillin therapy has not changed the mortality for this disease during the first 5 days of hospitalization. Patients with predisposing disease may present with shock and disseminated intravascular coagulation.[78] In these critically ill patients, organisms are sometimes seen on peripheral blood smears.[79]

Pneumococcal pneumonia is the most common community-acquired pneumonia, characteristically manifesting with a single shaking chill, rusty sputum, pleuritic chest pain on the side of the pneumonia, and consolidation on chest x-ray films. With appropriate therapy defervescence is often rapid but may take a week or more.[80] Infiltrates may not resolve for 6 to 8 weeks.[81]

In patients who remain febrile, septic complications such as meningitis, pericarditis, and empyema must be considered. Superinfection with gram-negative bacilli commonly occurs, particularly when the patient has been treated with high-dose penicillin. *S. pneumoniae* has been increasingly reported as a cause of nosocomial pneumonia, particularly in elderly patients with chronic obstructive pulmonary disease.[82]

Penicillin G remains the antibiotic of choice for pneumococcal infection. For uncomplicated pneumonia, low-dose regimens such as procaine penicillin, 600,000 U every 12 hours intramuscularly, can be used. When extrapulmonary sites of infection are suspected, much higher doses of penicillin are needed. In patients with endocarditis or meningitis, 10 million to 24 million U of procaine penicillin is recommended. If patients are critically ill and hypotensive, some authorities also recommend higher-dose penicillin.[83]

Pneumonia Caused by *Staphylococcus aureus*

S. aureus is an extremely important cause of pneumonia in the ICU patient. Community-acquired infection may occur after influenza or may be secondary to hematogenous seeding.[84, 85] Nosocomial pneumonia may be secondary to aspiration or to hematogenous spread, particularly via infected catheters and other intravenous access lines.[86] Staph-

ylococcus produces a necrotizing pneumonia with cavities and thin-walled abscesses or pneumatoceles.

Appropriate therapy requires administration of oxacillin, nafcillin, or a first-generation cephalosporin. Intravenous therapy is required for at least 2 weeks, and many recommend 3 to 4 weeks. Doses of 9 to 12 g of oxacillin or nafcillin are used in adults. Vancomycin is the drug of choice for methicillin-resistant *S. aureus*, an increasingly common pathogen in the ICU setting. Risk factors include tertiary setting, length of stay, and prior antibiotic therapy.[87]

Pneumonia Caused by Gram-Negative Bacilli

Gram-negative bacilli are now the leading cause of bacteremia in the United States[88] and the leading cause of nosocomial and ICU-acquired pulmonary infection in most studies.[89] The National Nosocomial Infection Study between 1980 and 1983 found *P. aeruginosa* to be the most common nosocomial respiratory pathogen,[90] followed by *Klebsiella, Enterobacter, Escherichia coli, Proteus,* and *Serratia marcescens*.

Although the gram-negative bacilli share a common pathophysiology, there are probably clinical and epidemiologic differences among species. *P. aeruginosa* pneumonia is most likely to occur in patients with neutropenia or cystic fibrosis and patients who are receiving broad-spectrum antibiotics. Pneumonia may be acquired by aspiration of oropharyngeal flora or secondarily by inhalation from reservoir nebulizers. It is characterized as fulminant with high fever, severe dyspnea, and hypoxia. Chest x-ray films reveal a bilateral bronchopneumonia with nodular infiltrates and small pleural effusions.[91] Microabscesses and focal hemorrhages are seen on autopsy.

Klebsiella pneumoniae is also commonly associated with life-threatening lower respiratory tract infection, particularly in alcoholics or nursing home patients in addition to those who are hospitalized. Classic features include right upper lobe consolidation with sagging fissure, necrotizing pneumonia with production of "currant jelly" sputum, and slow response to therapy. For life-threatening infections, a cephalosporin-aminoglycoside combination is generally preferred.[75]

E. coli pneumonia is a serious infection, particularly when associated with bacteremia. It is often a consequence of intra-abdominal or genitourinary tract infection with seeding to the lung.[92] *E. coli* is usually sensitive to a variety of antimicrobial agents, but antibiotic therapy must be guided by sensitivity patterns. The organism may be resistant to broad-spectrum antibiotics such as piperacillin or ampicillin plus sulbactam.

S. marsescens is a ubiquitous organism in the ICU setting. In our pneumonia study, it was the second most common gram-negative organism to cause bacteremic pneumonia.[75] The clinical features of *S. marcescens* pneumonia are difficult to distinguish from those of other gram-negative pneumonias. Red-pigmented strains have rarely turned sputum red, leading to a clinical picture of pseudohemoptysis.[93] Outbreaks of nosocomial infection have occurred, and intrahospital spread is documented.[94] Contaminated nebulizers and fiberoptic bronchoscopes have been responsible for some outbreaks. Antibiotic treatment is complicated by the high frequency of multiple drug resistance. Amikacin is usually the aminoglycoside of choice used in combination with third-generation cephalosporins, imipenem plus cilastatin, or parenteral quinolones.

Streptococcal Species Pneumonia

In addition to *S. pneumoniae*, other streptococci, particularly group A and group B beta-hemolytic streptococci, are responsible for pneumonia in the ICU.

Pneumonia caused by group B beta-hemolytic streptococci is increasingly reported in the elderly.[95] It often presents as a mixed infection with *S. aureus*. Necrotizing bronchopneumonia is seen on chest x-ray films. The disease has a high mortality rate. It can occur as a community-acquired or nosocomial infection. Pneumonia caused by *Streptococcus pyogenes* (group A) is less common in the antibiotic era but still occurs in association with preceding viral infections, in military recruits,[96, 97] and in nursing home residents.[98] Streptococcal infection of the upper respiratory tract precedes the pneumonia in about one third of cases. Empyema is particularly common, having been reported in 30 to 40% of cases. The fluid is serosanguineous and usually must be drained with a chest tube. Morbidity is low because patients tend to be less debilitated than with other pneumonias. Penicillin is the drug of choice for both group A and group B beta-hemolytic streptococcal pneumonia.

Enterococci (group D streptococci) have been implicated in pneumonia relatively recently,[99] although they have long been associated with hospital-acquired bacteremia, urinary tract infection, and endocarditis. Patients with enterococcal pneumonia have almost always been previously treated with broad-spectrum antibiotics. Enteral feeding tubes may also be a predisposing factor. Seidenfeld and associates reported enterococcus as a cause of pneumonia in 15% of patients with pneumonia and adult respiratory distress syndrome.[30]

H. influenzae is an important respiratory pathogen in patients with chronic obstructive pulmonary disease. The organism is almost always nontypable. In ICUs in which patients have end-stage chronic lung disease, *H. influenzae* is frequently responsible for bronchopneumonia precipitating respiratory failure.[100] *H. influenzae* was responsible for 9% of ICU pneumonia in the study by Craven and colleagues[9] and 6% of ICU pneumonia in the study by Fagan and colleagues.[6] Bacteremia and empyema are extremely rare. About 10% of *H. influenzae* organisms produce β-lactamase; therefore initial therapy with a second-generation cephalosporin or ampicillin plus sulbactam is indicated.

M. (B.) catarrhalis, long considered a commensal of the oropharynx, is now clearly recognized as an important pathogen in pneumonia and bronchitis.[101] The organism may be reported only as "normal throat flora" by some microbiology laboratories. Most patients with *M. (B.) catarrhalis* pneumonia have underlying lung disease, and many are receiving corticosteroids. The clinical picture is similar to that of *H. influenzae* pneumonia. β-Lactamase is produced by 80% of *M. (B.) catarrhalis* strains, and second-generation cephalosporin or ampicillin plus sulbactam is the drug of choice. Fagan and coworkers[6] found *M. (B.) catarrhalis* in 6% of ICU patients with pneumonia.

COMPLICATIONS OF PNEUMONIA

Empyema

Empyema may be a complication of pneumonia in the critically ill patient. Although some patients with empyema may have a severe infection, in others the presentation is more subtle. Frequently a first clue is the inability of the pneumonia patient to respond to appropriate antimicrobial therapy. When pleural fluid is noted on physical examination or chest x-ray film in the patient with pneumonia, thoracentesis is necessary to rule out pleural space infection. Pleural fluid studies differentiate benign parapneumonic effusions from early empyema. Several studies have used pleural fluid pH to predict which patients will require chest tube drainage. Patients with a pleural fluid pH of 7.0 or less and a glucose level below 40 mg/dL usually require chest tube placement.[102]

When thoracentesis reveals gross pus in the pleural space, chest tube drainage is mandatory. When pleural fluid is exudative and bacteria are present but fluid is thin, repeated thoracentesis may be adequate for drainage.[103]

S. aureus is the organism most prone to cause pleural space infection. However, gram-negative bacilli, anaerobes, *H. influenzae*, *S. pneumoniae*, and beta-hemolytic streptococci can all produce empyema. Appropriate antibiotic therapy should continue for several weeks in patients with empyema. As stated, total drainage by closed tube thoracotomy is needed when infected fluid becomes thick. Duration of drainage varies with the amount of fluid. When the fluid volume decreases to less than 50 mL, the tube is gradually withdrawn.

Purulent Pericarditis

Purulent pericarditis, a common complication of pneumococcal pneumonia in the preantibiotic era, is now rarely seen as a complication of pneumonia. Pleuropulmonary infection is the leading predisposing factor in the development of purulent pericarditis. It is most likely to occur in the critically ill patient, particularly after thoracic surgery. Purulent pericarditis is now most commonly associated with pneumonia caused by *S. aureus* or gram-negative bacilli.[104] Pneumococcal pericarditis secondary to pneumonia still occurs and is often misdiagnosed.[105] Purulent pericarditis should be considered in the pneumonia patient who has not responded to antibiotic therapy and has signs of an expanding cardiac silhouette, atrial arrhythmias, chest pain, or signs of cardiac tamponade. Pericardial fluid is demonstrated by emergency echocardiography, and prompt drainage of the pericardial space is almost always required. A pericardial window or pericardiectomy is usually necessary to prevent the development of chronic constrictive pericarditis.

Bacterial Meningitis

Severely ill patients with pneumonia may present with concomitant meningitis or develop meningitis as a complication of their pneumonia. In the elderly, pneumococcal

TABLE 39–7

DRUG REGIMENS OF CHOICE FOR ETIOLOGIC AGENTS IN PNEUMONIA

Agent	Drug of Choice	Alternative
S. pneumoniae	Penicillin G	Erythromycin
H. influenzae	Cephalosporin, second generation (cefuroxime, cefonicid, cefamandole) or third generation (cefotaxime, ceftizoxime, ceftriaxone)	Ampicillin (if β-lactamase–negative)
	Ampicillin-sulbactam	
S. aureus		
Methicillin sensitive	Oxacillin, nafcillin, cephalosporin, first generation	Imipenem-cilastatin
Methicillin resistant	Vancomycin	Imipenem-cilastatin
Gram-negative bacilli		
K. pneumoniae	Cephalosporin, third generation, with or without aminoglycoside	Aztreonam, imipenem
P. aeruginosa	Antipseudomonal penicillin plus aminoglycoside	Ceftazidime
	Ceftazidime plus aminoglycoside	Aztreonam
		Imipenem (depends on hospital sensitivity pattern)
S. marcescens	Cephalosporin, third generation, plus aminoglycoside	Imipenem
		Aztreonam
Legionella	Erythromycin, may add rifampin	
P. carinii	Trimethoprim-sulfamethoxazole (steroids may be indicated for life-threatening infection)	Pentamidine

pneumonia is the most common predisposing factor in the development of pneumococcal meningitis. In patients with pneumonia, abnormal mental status or coma is sometimes attributed to hypoxia or sepsis, and central nervous system infection is not considered. Carpenter and Petersdorf[106] stated that "in pneumonia it is particularly dangerous to ascribe confusion to age or toxic depression of the central nervous system." Hence, lumbar puncture must be performed in the patient with pneumonia who is seen with coma or a rapid change in mental status even if meningeal signs are not present.

Superinfection

Superinfection is likely to occur in the ICU patient being treated for pneumonia. Narrow-spectrum antibiotic therapy probably lessens the likelihood of a secondary pneumonia. When the ICU patient with pneumonia deteriorates after initial improvement, becomes febrile, or develops a new pulmonary infiltrate, one must consider the possibility of pneumonia with a new (secondary) organism. A repeated sputum Gram's stain or bronchoscopy specimen distinguishes progressive primary pneumonia from a new infection.

TREATMENT OF PNEUMONIA IN THE INTENSIVE CARE UNIT
Antimicrobial Therapy

As previously noted, the first step in choosing an antimicrobial agent is to obtain a history and physical examination in conjunction with a Gram-stained smear of respiratory secretions. In patients ill enough to require ICU admission, it is often necessary to use bronchoscopy or a protected brush catheter to determine an etiologic agent. If a good expectorated sputum sample can be obtained and a presumptive diagnosis made on the basis of a Gram-stained smear, further diagnostic study is not usually pursued. The treatment of gram-negative pneumonia depends in part on the antibiotic sensitivity patterns at the particular hospital. P. aeruginosa is an important pathogen in almost all ICUs. Hence, treatment of pneumonia in the extremely ill patient

with gram-negative bacilli detected in a smear requires initial antipseudomonal coverage until culture and sensitivity results are available. Ticarcillin or piperacillin plus an aminoglycoside is the commonly used regimen for the ICU patient. Ceftazidime, aztreonam, and imipenem plus cilastatin have been used successfully as monotherapy, depending again on known susceptibility patterns. When staphylococci are suspected in a Gram-stained smear, the incidence of methicillin-resistant staphylococci in the ICU becomes a critical issue. Suspicion of methicillin-resistant S. aureus pneumonia requires initial therapy with vancomycin. A patient suspected of having H. influenzae pneumonia (small pleomorphic gram-negative bacilli) or M. (B.) catarrhalis pneumonia (gram-negative diplococci) should be treated initially with a second- or third-generation cephalosporin. Trimethoprim-sulfamethoxazole is the treatment of choice for presumed P. carinii pneumonia and should be initiated for interstitial pneumonia in patients with acquired immunodeficiency syndrome. Pentamidine has also been used effectively and may be necessary because of the high incidence of allergic reactions to sulfa among acquired immunodeficiency syndrome patients.[107] Table 39–7 lists the most common causes of pneumonia in ICU patients and the treatments of choice.

TREATMENT OF PNEUMONIA
Supportive Measures

Physiotherapy, including postural drainage, percussion, and tracheal suctioning, has been used to mobilize purulent secretions. In acute bacterial pneumonia, these measures have not affected the clinical course of the disease.[108] However, in patients who have thick and copious secretions (e.g., in bronchiectasis) such measures may improve air exchange.

Intermittent positive pressure breathing has been used to increase lung inflation for many types of lung disease including pneumonia. However, it has no proven role in pneumonia, and one study found that the procedure had no value in resolving the infection.[56] Similarly, routine use of aerosol or humidity therapy is not indicated in the treatment of pneumonia.

Supplemental oxygen therapy is critical in patients with pneumonia and documented hypoxemia. The use of oxygen, however, cannot be indiscrimate and oxygen toxicity must be avoided.

Adequate analgesia is sometimes needed in the pneumonia patient to allow deeper breathing and coughing. Codeine is usually adequate, but parenteral meperidine has also been used.

Intracostal nerve block may relieve pleurisy without depressing respiratory drive. Aspirin should be avoided so that temperature can be followed. Sporadic use of antipyretics can increase the patient's discomfort by causing periods of heavy sweating. If antipyretics are used, they should be given around the clock.

Some patients, particularly those with pneumococcal pneumonia, may develop gastric distention and ileus. Nasogastric suction should be instituted until bowel sounds return.

References

1. Centers for Disease Control: Nosocomial infection surveillance, 1984. MMWR CDC Surveill Summ 35(1SS):17, 1986.
2. Barrett FF, Casey JI, Finland M: Infections and antibiotic use among patients at Boston City Hospital, February 1967. N Engl J Med 278:5, 1968.
3. Gross PA, Neu HC, Aswapokee P, et al: Deaths from nosocomial infection: Experience in a university and community hospital. Am J Med 68:219, 1980.
4. Stevens RM, Teres D, Skillman JJ, et al: Pneumonia in an intensive care unit. A 30 month experience. Arch Intern Med 134:106, 1974.
5. Craven DE, Kunches LM, Kilinsky V, et al: Risk factors for pneumonia and fatality in patients receiving continuous mechanical ventilation. Am Rev Respir Dis 133:792, 1986.
6. Fagan JY, Chastre J, Domart Y, et al: Nosocomial pneumonia in patients receiving continuous mechanical ventilation. Am Rev Respir Dis 139:877, 1989.
7. Coalson JJ: Pathophysiologic features of respiratory distress in the infant and adult. In: Shoemaker WC, Thompson WL (eds): Critical Care. State of the Art, Volume III (A). Fullerton, CA, Society of Critical Care Medicine, p 1, 1982.
8. Graybill JR, Marshall LW, Charache P, et al: Nosocomial pneumonia. A continuing major problem. Am Rev Respir Dis 108:1130, 1973.
9. Craven DE, Kunches LM, Lichtenberg DA, et al: Nosocomial infection and fatality in medical and surgical intensive care unit patients. Arch Intern Med 148:1161, 1988.
10. Green GM: The J. Burns Amberson lecture—A defense of the lung. Am Rev Respir Dis 102:691, 1970.
11. Huxley EJ, Viroslav J, Gray WR, et al: Pharyngeal aspiration in normal adults and patients with depressed consciousness. Am J Med 64:564, 1978.
12. Green GM, Kass EH: The influence of bacterial species on pulmonary resistance to infection in mice subjected to hypoxia, cold stress and ethanolic intoxication. Br J Exp Pathol 46:360, 1965.
13. LaForce FM, Mullane JF, Boehme RF, et al: The effect of pulmonary edema on antibacterial defenses of the lung. J Lab Clin Med 82:634, 1973.
14. Johanson WG, Pierce AK, Sanford JP: Changing pharyngeal bacterial flora of hospitalized patients: Emergence of gram-negative bacilli. N Engl J Med 281:1137, 1969.
15. Johanson WG Jr, Pierce AK, Sanford JP, et al: Nosocomial respiratory infections with gram-negative bacilli. The significance of colonization of the respiratory tract. Ann Intern Med 77:701, 1972.
16. Johanson WG Jr, Woods DE, Chaudhuri T: Association of respiratory tract colonization with adherence of gram-negative bacilli to epithelial cells. J Infect Dis 139:667, 1979.
17. Abraham SN, Beachey EH, Simpson WA: Adherence of Streptococcus pyogenes, Escherichia coli, and Pseudomonas aeruginosa to fibronectin-coated and uncoated epithelial cells. Infect Immun 41:1261, 1983.
18. Andrews CP, Coalson JJ, Smith JD, et al: Diagnosis of nosocomial bacterial pneumonia in acute, diffuse lung injury. Chest 80:254, 1981.
19. Chastre J, Viau F, Brun P, et al: Prospective evaluation of the protected specimen brush for the diagnosis of pulmonary infections in ventilated patients. Am Rev Respir Dis 130:924, 1984.
20. Fagan JY, Chastre J, Hance AJ, et al: Detection of nosocomial lung infection in ventilated patients: Use of a protected specimen brush and quantitative culture techniques in 147 patients. Am Rev Respir Dis 138:110, 1988.
21. Bryant LR, Mobin-Uddin K, Dillon ML, et al: Misdiagnosis of pneumonia in patients needing mechanical respiration. Arch Surg 106:286, 1973.
22. Sladen A, Laver MB, Pontoppidan H: Pulmonary complications and water retention in prolonged mechanical ventilation. N Engl J Med 279:448, 1968.
23. Bahl OP, Oliver GC, Rockoff SD: Localized unilateral pulmonary edema: An unusual presentation of left heart failure. Chest 60:277, 1971.
24. Hublitz UF, Shapiro JH: Atypical pulmonary patterns of congestive failure in chronic lung disease. Radiology 93:995, 1969.
25. Laforce FM: Hospital-acquired gram-negative rod pneumonias: An overview. Am J Med 70:664, 1981.
26. Tillotson JR, Finland M: Bacterial colonization and clinical superinfection of the respiratory tract complicating antibiotic treatment of pneumonia. J Infect Dis 119:597, 1969.
27. Joshi M, Ciesla N, Caplan E: Diagnosis of pneumonia in critically ill patients. Chest 94:45, 1988.
28. Yu VL, Kroboth FJ, Shonnard J, et al: Legionnaire's disease: New clinical perspective from a prospective pneumonia study. Am J Med 73:357, 1982.
29. Graybill JR, Marshall LW, Charache P, et al: Nosocomial pneumonia. A continuing major problem. Am Rev Respir Dis 108:1130, 1973.
30. Seidenfeld JJ, Pohl DF, Bell RC, et al: Incidence, site, and outcome of infections in patients with the adult respiratory distress syndrome. Am Rev Respir Dis 134:12, 1986.
31. Light RW, Girard WM, Jenkinson SG, et al: Parapneumonic effusions. Am J Med 69:507, 1980.
32. Murray PR, Washington JA III: Microscopic and bacteriologic analysis of expectorated sputum. Mayo Clin Proc 50:339, 1975.
33. Merrill CW, Gwaltney JM Jr, Hendley JO, et al: Rapid identification of pneumococci. N Engl J Med 288:510, 1973.
34. Barrett-Conner E: The nonvalue of sputum culture in the diagnosis of pneumococcal pneumonia. Am Rev Respir Dis 103:845, 1971.
35. Salata RA, Lederman MM, Shlaes DM, et al: Diagnosis of nosocomial pneumonia in intubated, intensive care unit patients. Am Rev Respir Dis 135:426, 1987.
36. Pratter MR, Irwin RS: Transtracheal aspiration. Guidelines for safety. Chest 76:518, 1979.
37. Verghese A, Berk SL: Bacterial pneumonia in the elderly. Medicine 62:271, 1983.
38. Hahn HH, Beaty HN: Transtracheal aspiration in the evaluation of patients with pneumonia. Ann Intern Med 72:183, 1970.
39. Kalinske RW, Parker RH, Brandt D, et al: Diagnostic usefulness and safety of transtracheal aspiration. N Engl J Med 276:604, 1967.
40. Ries K, Levison ME, Kaye D: Transtracheal aspiration in pulmonary infection. Arch Intern Med 133:453, 1974.
41. Johanson WG Jr, Seidenfeld JJ, Gomez P, et al: Bacteriologic diagnosis of nosocomial pneumonia following prolonged mechanical ventilation. Am Rev Respir Dis 137:259, 1988.
42. Gherman CR, Simon HJ: Pneumonia complicating severe underlying disease: A current appraisal of transthoracic lung puncture. Dis Chest 48:297, 1965.
43. Zavala DC, Schoell JE: Ultrathin needle aspiration of the lung in infectious and malignant disease. Am Rev Respir Dis 123:125, 1981.
44. Moser KM, Maurer J, Jassy L, et al: Sensitivity, specificity and risk of diagnostic procedures in a canine model of Streptococcus pneumoniae pneumonia. Am Rev Respir Dis 125:436, 1982.
45. Krieger B, Blinder L, Inchausti BC: Clinical utility of bronchoalveolar lavage in a general hospital. Arch Intern Med 149:1605, 1989.
46. Feldman NT, Pennington JE, Ehrie MG: Transbronchial lung biopsy in the compromised host. JAMA 238:1377, 1977.
47. Nishio JN, Lynch JP III: Fiberoptic bronchoscopy in the immunocompromised host: The significance of a "nonspecific" transbronchial biopsy. Am Rev Respir Dis 121:307, 1980.
48. Poe RH, Utell MU, Israel RH, et al: Sensitivity and specificity of the nonspecific transbronchial lung biopsy. Am Rev Respir Dis 119:25, 1979.
49. Cunningham JH, Zavala DC, Corry RJ, et al: Trephine air drill, bronchial brush, and fiberoptic transbronchial lung biopsies in immunosuppressed patients. Am Rev Respir Dis 115:213, 1977.
50. Cockerill FR III, Wilson WR, Carpenter HA, et al: Open lung biopsy in immunocompromised patients. Arch Intern Med 145:1398, 1985.
51. Dijkman JH, van der Meer JWM, Bakker W, et al: Transpleural lung biopsy by the thoracoscopic route in patients with diffuse interstitial pulmonary disease. Chest 82:76, 1982.
52. McCabe RE, Brooks RG, Mark JBD, et al: Open lung biopsy in patients with acute leukemia. Am J Med 78:609, 1985.
53. Rossiter SU, Miller C, Chung AM, et al: Open lung biopsy in the immunosuppressed patient. Is it really beneficial? J Thorac Cardiovasc Surg 77:338, 1979.
54. Torres A, Puig de laBellacasa J, Xaubet A, et al: Diagnostic value of quantitative cultures of bronchoalveolar lavage and telescoping plugged catheters in mechanically ventilated patients with bacterial pneumonia. Am Rev Respir Dis 140:306, 1989.
55. Rankin JA: Role of bronchoalveolar lavage in the diagnosis of pneumonia. Chest 95:187S, 1989.
56. Chastre J, Fagon JY, Soler P, et al: Diagnosis of nosocomial bacterial pneumonia in intubated patients undergoing ventilation: Comparison of the usefulness of bronchoalveolar lavage with the protected specimen brush. Am J Med 85:499, 1988.

57. Bartlett JG, Alexander J, Mayhew J, et al: Should fiberoptic bronchoscopy aspirates be cultured? Am Rev Respir Dis 114:73, 1976.

58. Fossieck BE Jr, Parker RH, Cohen MH, et al: Fiberoptic bronchoscopy and culture bacteria from the lower respiratory tract. Chest 72:5, 1977.

59. Thorpe JE, Baughman RP, Frame PT, et al: Bronchoalveolar lavage for diagnosing acute bacterial pneumonia. J Infect Dis 155:855, 1987.

60. Kahn FW, Jones JM: Diagnosing bacterial respiratory infection by bronchoalveolar lavage. J Infect Dis 155:862, 1987.

61. Rouby JJ, Rossignon MD, Nicolas JH: A prospective study of protected bronchoalveolar lavage in the diagnosis of nosocomial pneumonia. Anesthesiology 71:679, 1989.

62. Clement MJ, Luce JM, Hopewell PC: Diagnosis of pulmonary diseases. Clin Chest Med 9:497, 1988.

63. Broaddus C, Dake MD, Stulbarg MS, et al: Bronchoalveolar lavage and transbronchial biopsy for the diagnosis of pulmonary infections in the acquired immunodeficiency syndrome. Ann Intern Med 102:747, 1985.

64. Golden JA, Hollander H, Stulbarg MS, et al: Bronchoalveolar lavage as the exclusive diagnostic modality for *Pneumocystis carinii* pneumonia: A prospective study among patients with acquired immunodeficiency syndrome. Chest 90:18, 1986.

65. Wimberley N, Faling LJ, Bartlett JG: A fiberoptic bronchoscopy technique to obtain uncontaminated lower airway secretions for bacterial culture. Am Rev Respir Dis 119:337, 1979.

66. Wimberley NW, Bass JB Jr, Boyd BW, et al: Use of a bronchoscopic protected catheter brush for the diagnosis of pulmonary infections. Chest 81:556, 1982.

67. Higuchi JH, Coalson JJ, Johanson WG Jr: Bacteriologic diagnosis of nosocomial pneumonia in primates. Usefulness of the protected specimen brush. Am Rev Respir Dis 125:53, 1982.

68. Villers D, Derriennic M, Raffi F, et al: Reliability of the bronchoscopic protected catheter brush in intubated and ventilated patients. Chest 88:527, 1985.

69. Winterbauer RH, Hutchinson JF, Reinhardt GN, et al: The use of quantitative cultures and antibody coating of bacteria to diagnose bacterial pneumonia by fiberoptic bronchoscopy. Am Rev Respir Dis 128:98, 1983.

70. Pollock HM, Hawkins EL, Bonner JR, et al: Diagnosis of bacterial pulmonary infections with quantitative protected catheter cultures obtained during bronchoscopy. J Clin Microbiol 17:255, 1983.

71. Smith JW, Jones SR, Kaijser B: Significance of antibody-coated bacteria in urinary sediment in experimental pyelonephritis. J Infect Dis 135:577, 1977.

72. Guzzetta P, Toews GB, Robertson KJ, et al: Rapid diagnosis of community-acquired bacterial pneumonia. Am Rev Respir Dis 128:461, 1983.

73. Berk SL, Verghese A: Emerging pathogens in nosocomial pneumonia. Eur J Clin Microbiol Infect Dis 8:11, 1989.

74. Ruiz-Santana S, Garcia Jiminez A, Esteban A, et al: ICU pneumonias: A multi-institutional study. Crit Care Med 15:930, 1987.

75. Karnad A, Alvarez S, Berk SL: Pneumonia caused by gram-negative bacilli. Am J Med 79(suppl 1A):61, 1985.

76. Austrian R, Gold J: Pneumococcal bacteremia with special reference to bacteremic pneumococcal pneumonia. Ann Intern Med 60:759, 1964.

77. Mufson MA, Kruss DM, Wasil RE, et al: Capsular types and outcome of bacteremic pneumococcal disease in the antibiotic era. Arch Intern Med 134:505, 1974.

78. Bisno AL, Freeman JC: The syndrome of asplenia, pneumococcal sepsis and disseminated intravascular coagulation. Ann Intern Med 72:389, 1970.

79. Torres J, Bisno AL: Hyposplenism and pneumococcemia. Visualization of *Diplococcus pneumoniae* in the peripheral blood smear. Am J Med 55:851, 1973.

80. Fekety FR Jr, McDaniel E: The fever index in evaluation of the course of infectious diseases, with special reference to pneumococcal pneumonia. Yale J Biol Med 41:282, 1968.

81. Jay SJ, Johanson WG, Pierce AK: The radiographic resolution of *Streptococcus pneumoniae* pneumonia. N Engl J Med 293:798, 1975.

82. Alvarez S, Guarderas J, Shell CG, et al: Nosocomial pneumococcal bacteremia. Arch Intern Med 146:1509, 1986.

83. Mufson MA: Streptococcus pneumoniae. In: Mandell GL, Douglas RG Jr, Bennett JE (eds): Principles and Practice of Infectious Disease. 3rd ed. New York, Churchill Livingstone, p 1547, 1990.

84. Rebhan AW, Edwards HE: Staphylococcal pneumonia: A review of 329 cases. Can Med Assoc J 82:513, 1960.

85. Lindsay MI Jr, Herrmann EC Jr, Morrow GW Jr, et al: Hong Kong influenza: Clinical, microbiologic, and pathologic features in 127 cases. JAMA 214:1825, 1970.

86. Cross AS, Steigbigel RT: Infective endocarditis and access site infections in patients on hemodialysis. Medicine 55:453, 1976.

87. Haley RW, Hightower AW, Khabbaz RF, et al: The emergence of methicillin-resistant *Staphylococcus aureus* infections in United States hospitals. Ann Intern Med 97:297, 1982.

88. Kreger BE, Craven DE, Carling PC, et al: Gram-negative bacteremia. III: Reassessment of etiology, epidemiology and ecology in 612 patients. Am J Med 68:332, 1980.

89. Gross PA, Neu HC, Aswapokee P, et al: Deaths from nosocomial infections: Experience in a university and a community hospital. Am J Med 68:219, 1980.

90. Centers for Disease Control: Nosocomial infection surveillance: 1983. MMWR CDC Surveill Summ 33(2SS):9, 1984.

91. Tillotson JR, Lerner AM: Characteristics of nonbacteremic *Pseudomonas* pneumonia. Ann Intern Med 68:295, 1968.

92. Berk SL, Neumann P, Holtsclaw S, et al: *Escherichia coli* pneumonia in the elderly. With reference to the role of *E. coli* K1 capsular polysaccharide antigen. Am J Med 72:899, 1982.

93. Yu VL: *Serratia marcescens*. Historical perspective and clinical review. N Engl J Med 300:887, 1979.

94. Schaberg DR, Alford RH, Anderson R, et al: An outbreak of nosocomial infection due to multiple resistant *Serratia marcescens:* Evidence of inter-hospital spread. J Infect Dis 134:181, 1976.

95. Verghese A, Berk SL, Boelen LJ, et al: Group B streptococcal pneumonia in the elderly. Arch Intern Med 142:1642, 1982.

96. Basiliere JL, Bistrong HW, Spence WF: Streptococcal pneumonia: Recent outbreaks in military recruit populations. Am J Med 44:580, 1968.

97. Tuazon CU: Gram-positive pneumonias. Med Clin North Am 64:343, 1980.

98. Ruben FL, Norden CW, Heisler B, et al: An outbreak of *Streptococcus pyogenes* infections in a nursing home. Ann Intern Med 101:494, 1984.

99. Berk SL, Verghese A, Holtsclaw SA, et al: Enterococcal pneumonia. Occurrence in patients receiving broad spectrum antibiotic regimens and enteral feeding. Am J Med 74:153, 1983.

100. Berk SL, Holtsclaw SA, Khan A, et al: Transtracheal aspiration in the severely ill elderly patient with bacterial pneumonia. J Am Geriatr Soc 29:228, 1981.

101. Nicotra B, Rivera M, Luman JI, et al: *Branhamella catarrhalis* as a lower respiratory tract pathogen in patients with chronic lung disease. Arch Intern Med 146:890, 1986.

102. Miller KC, Sahn SA: Chest tubes. Indications, technique, management and complications. Chest 91:258, 1987.

103. Renzetti AD: Current treatment of nontuberculous empyema. Pulmonary Perspectives 3(4):1, 1986.

104. Klacsmann PG, Bulkley BH, Hutchins GM: The changed spectrum of purulent pericarditis. An 86 year autopsy experience in 200 patients. Am J Med 63:666, 1977.

105. Berk SL, Rice PA, Reynholds CA, et al: Pneumococcal pericarditis: A persisting problem in contemporary diagnosis. Am J Med 70:247, 1981.

106. Carpenter RR, Petersdorf RG: The clinical spectrum of bacterial meningitis. Am J Med 33:262, 1962.

107. Gordin FM, Simon GL, Wofsy CB, et al: Adverse reactions to trimethoprim-sulfamethoxazole in patients with the acquired immunodeficiency syndrome. Ann Intern Med 100:495, 1984.

108. Graham WG, Bradley DA: Efficacy of chest physiotherapy and intermittent positive-pressure breathing in the resolution of pneumonia. N Engl J Med 299:624, 1978.

CHAPTER 40

Endocarditis

Marla J. Gold
Oksana M. Korzeniowski

With the advent of antibiotics, eradication of infection in nearly all cases of endocarditis has become possible, provided the diagnosis is made and treatment is begun sufficiently early. When fatalities do occur, they are often the result of irreversible anatomic injury such as heart failure or cerebral hemorrhage.[1-3]

Patients with infective endocarditis (IE) often present to the physician's office or emergency room with generalized complaints such as fatigue, fever, and weight loss. There are no pathognomonic physical or laboratory findings. The diagnosis and therapy of this potentially life-threatening medical and surgical problem thus reside in awareness of the populations susceptible to disease, the predisposing cardiac lesions, and the potential infecting agent.

DEFINITIONS

IE most often refers to bacterial or fungal infection within the heart. Chlamydial and rickettsial infections occur less commonly. Infection of the extracardiac endothelium, termed *endarteritis,* can produce a clinical syndrome indistinguisable from that of IE.[4, 5]

Before the availability of antibiotics, IE was classified as acute or subacute, as determined by clinical course.[6] When the disease occurred on a normal valve with virulent organisms such as *Staphylococcus aureus* or *Streptococcus pyogenes,* it resulted in rapid valvular damage and widespread metastatic foci and often caused death in less than 6 weeks. Such a fulminant clinical course was regarded as acute bacterial endocarditis. Subacute endocarditis denoted infection on an abnormal valve (usually caused by rheumatic valvulitis) by a relatively avirulent microorganism such as a viridans streptococcus. Infection was indolent and metastatic foci were uncommon.

Currently, parenteral drug users, patients with prosthetic valves, and patients with mitral valve prolapse (MVP) or other nonrheumatic abnormalities account for the majority of cases of IE. Their clinical presentations rarely follow the classic patterns of the preantibiotic era. Nosocomial endocarditis, defined as endocarditis occurring 72 hours or more after hospital admission or infection directly related to a procedure performed during hospitalization, is increasing.[7, 8]

Thus classifications that refer to underlying cardiac lesions and to the etiologic agent responsible for infection are more useful guides for the management of patients with IE.

EPIDEMIOLOGY

Children. The incidence of IE in infancy and childhood is generally low. Most cases in the neonatal period are in high-risk infants under intensive care management.[9] Predisposing factors are believed to be damage to the endothelium (with establishment of nonbacterial thrombotic endocarditis) and bacteremia resulting from instrumentation. Cardiac structural abnormalities are uncommon. The predominant pathogens have been staphylococci and fungi.

In children infected after the neonatal period, 75 to 100% have identifiable predisposing lesions.[10] Ventricular septal defect, patent ductus arteriosus, and tetralogy of Fallot are the most common abnormalities. Other congenital lesions predisposing to IE include ostium primum atrial septal defect, coarctation of the aorta, Marfan's syndrome, subaortic stenosis, and common atrioventricular valve.[11, 12] Viridans streptococci and group D streptococci cause about 40 to 50% of pediatric cases after the neonatal period. *S. aureus* is responsible for about 25% of pediatric endocarditis cases. Less common causes include beta-hemolytic streptococci, enterococci, pneumococci, gram-negative bacilli, and fungi.

Adults. Improvement in cardiac diagnostic techniques and a decline in the incidence of rheumatic heart disease have changed the spectrum of recognized cardiac lesions underlying IE in adults.[13] MVP is the most common underlying predisposing cardiac lesion in nonaddict patients with native valve endocarditis (NVE).[13-15] MVP is a common condition with prevalence estimates ranging from 2.5 to 5.0% in general, healthy populations and up to 20% among young women.[16] Among patients with MVP, male sex, the presence of a systolic murmur, and age above 45 years appear to characterize patients at highest risk for IE. The risk for IE with MVP with no murmur is 0.0046% per year, compared with 0.0520% per year in persons with MVP and a systolic murmur.[17, 18]

Rheumatic heart disease now accounts for about 30% of heart lesions in patients with IE.[19] The mitral valve is most commonly affected.

Congenital heart disease is the underlying lesion in 10 to 20% of adult patients.[13] Common predisposing lesions include patent ductus arteriosus, ventricular septal defect, bicuspid aortic valve, coarctation of the aorta, and pulmonic stenosis. Approximately 5% of patients with idiopathic hypertrophic subaortic stenosis develop IE.[20] A high peak systolic pressure gradient enhances the risk of infection.

The Elderly. There is a significant trend toward increasing age in patients with IE.[21] In series of patients seen between 1976 and 1985, the percentage of patients older than 60 years ranged from 26% of those treated in a Veterans Administration hospital to 23% in a university center to 60% of patients treated in a community hospital (the last institution having the lowest proportion of intravenous drug abusers [IVDAs]).[22] The most common factor predisposing to IE in those older than 65 years of age is a prosthetic intravascular device. In elderly patients with native valve infection, degenerative cardiac lesions are gaining prominence.[23, 24] Some patients may in fact have no structural defects but may have nosocomially acquired endocarditis related to intravenous catheters (23% in one series).[22] Rheumatic heart disease is uncommon in the elderly. Overall, the mitral valve is involved more commonly than the aortic valve. Right-sided lesions are uncommon and are usually associated with transvenous lines.

Diabetes Mellitus. Diabetes mellitus has been shown to be associated with IE.[22] Metabolic, immunologic, and vascular abnormalities in diabetes may have a significant impact on the susceptibility of patients to infection. Accelerated atherosclerosis results in a high incidence of calcific valvular nodular lesions.[25] Urinary tract and soft tissue infections are common in diabetes and can serve as sources of bacteremia.[26]

Pregnancy. In pregnancy, IE is an important but uncommon complication.[27] Based on data from earlier eras (1950s to 1970s), the calculated incidence of IE is 0.03 to 0.14 cases per 1000 deliveries and 5.5 to 9 cases per 1000 for patients with underlying cardiac disease. The true incidence, incorporating improved management of obstetric complications, legalization of abortion, falling incidence of rheumatic heart disease, and increasing use of intravenous drugs by women, is unknown. In pregnancy, bacteria appear to enter most commonly during dental procedures.

PATHOGENESIS

The development of IE involves a complex interaction among host vascular endothelium, host hemostatic response, and circulating bacteria. Three hemodynamic factors predispose patients to the development of infection: a high-velocity jet stream, flow from a high- to a low-pressure chamber, and a comparatively narrow orifice separating the two chambers that creates a pressure gradient.[28, 29] Lesions of IE form just beyond the narrowed orifice through which the high-velocity jet stream passes, and satellite lesions can also grow where the jet stream strikes the endocardium. The force of the jet stream denudes the endothelium and promotes the deposition of clumps of fibrin and platelets, which form sterile vegetations termed *nonbacterial thrombotic endocarditis.*[30, 31] Noninfectious vegetations of the endocardium can also occur in patients with malignancies and other debilitating diseases, in patients with collagen-vascular disease (e.g., systemic lupus erythematosus), in areas surrounding foreign bodies such as intracardiac catheters, and at surgical implant sites.[31] In the event of bacteremia or fungemia, organisms are deposited onto the sterile vegetations. Platelets and fibrin are deposited over the bacteria, forming a site protected from the host immune ~~...~~ The morphology of vegetations can vary dependi ~~...~~ nature of the infecting organism and the activity ~~...~~ sease. Unimpaired growth results in extremely hig ~~...~~ counts of bacteria.

Organisms with little inherent pathogenicity, such as viridans streptococci, usually adhere only on sites with pre-existing nonbacterial thrombotic endocarditis; more virulent organisms such as *S. aureus* can infect apparently normal valves.

Transient bacteremias are most commonly associated with dental extraction; periodontal surgery; and oropharyngeal, gastrointestinal, urologic, and gynecologic invasive diagnostic or surgical procedures. Spontaneous bacteremia may occur with lung or skin infections and in patients with severe periodontal disease. Most cases of IE cannot be related to iatrogenic procedures.[32]

CLINICAL PRESENTATION OF INFECTIVE ENDOCARDITIS

The symptoms and signs of IE are highly variable. Clinical features of the disease result from the local valvular infection and its attendant complications, embolization of fragments of vegetation to any organ, constant bacteremia with metastatic seeding of organisms, and the development of immune complex disease.[29]

Symptoms

Symptoms of IE generally begin within 2 weeks of the precipitating bacteremia.[30] The patient often has numerous, nonspecific complaints such as weakness, fatigue, night sweats, anorexia, and weight loss. One third of patients have neurologic symptoms.[33, 34] The most common complaint is headache. Nonspecific complaints are more prominent in patients infected with organisms of low pathogenicity (e.g., viridans steptococci). The onset of infection with organisms of high pathogenicity (e.g., *S. aureus*) is often explosive. Almost all patients with IE have fever. Other common complaints include back pain, rashes, and cough. In obtaining the patient's history, a search should be made for an event resulting in bacteremia. Patients should be questioned about recent dental, genitourinary, or gastrointestinal procedures. A history of a predisposing cardiac lesion should be sought. Up to 85% of cases of IE have no identifiable inciting event.[19, 35]

Physical Examination

Depending on the infecting organism and predisposing cardiac lesion, patients with IE can present with a wide range of physical findings. They may be acutely ill with hemodynamic decompensation or appear relatively well and have a new murmur noted on examination. Symptomatic predominance of extracardiac sites of infection can mimic other diseases such as influenza, tuberculosis, collagen-vascular diseases, congestive heart failure (CHF), stroke, or carcinoma. Valvular murmurs are almost always present except in acute infections or with right-sided infection. A new regurgitant murmur or changes in a pre-existing murmur suggest acute staphylococcal disease and correlate with development of CHF. IE must be considered in any febrile patient known to have a heart murmur.[22]

Splenomegaly tends to occur in disease of long duration.[36] The spleen is usually soft and nontender. Splenic infarctions have been reported in 44% of autopsies but are rarely detected clinically. Clubbing of the fingers occurs in 10 to 20% of patients with disease of long duration. Cutaneous lesions, especially petechiae, can frequently be found. Petechiae may be embolic or vasculitic and are located on the conjunctivae, palate, buccal mucosa, and skin above the clavicles. Splinter hemorrhages may occur spontaneously on the fingers and toes and appear as subungual dark red streaks. They are more commonly related to trauma. Osler's nodes, most frequently found on the finger or toe pads, are small, tender nodules that persist for hours to days. They occur in 10 to 25% of patients and are nonspecific. On the basis of histopathology it appears that Osler's nodes are due to endothelial deposition of immune complexes, but occasional recovery of bacteria after aspiration suggests that they may also result from septic emboli.[37, 38] Janeway's lesions are 1 to 4 mm, nontender, hemorrhagic areas on the palms and soles. They occur in 5% of patients or less and are most commonly seen in acute infection. Janeway's lesions are caused by septic emboli. Retinal hemorrhages (Roth's spots) are presumed to result from microemboli to the retina and are found in less than 5% of patients. They are also found in connective tissue disease and hematologic disorders.[39] Joint pain and swelling may mimic those in rheumatologic disorders. Systemic emboli may occur at any time during the course of IE. Pulmonary emboli are common in parenteral drug abusers with tricuspid valve endocarditis, and pneumonia is frequently the presenting illness in this population. Neurologic findings in patients with IE include stroke, seizures, meningitis, and cranial nerve palsies. Mycotic aneurysms account for 2.5 to 6.2% of all intracranial aneurysms.[40, 41] Severe, unremitting, localized headache should strongly suggest the possibility of a mycotic aneurysm; however, most intracranial mycotic aneurysms are silent. The diagnosis is usually made after an acute cerebral hemorrhage.[41] The most common cardiac complication of IE is CHF. Metastatic infection can occur and is most frequently seen with *S. aureus* infections. Bacterial seeding can result in pyogenic meningitis, splenic abscess, pyelonephritis, osteomyelitis, and diskitis.

Differential Diagnosis

Definitive diagnosis of IE requires isolation of the infecting organism from blood, from an embolus, or from a vegetation at surgery or autopsy.[14, 36] The diagnosis of IE should be considered in any patient with a significant murmur and unexplained fever, in a febrile IVDA regardless of the presence of a murmur, and in a young person with a stroke.[42] Patients with prosthetic valves who have fever and/or valvular dysfunction should also be evaluated for IE. In the absence of positive blood cultures, a search must be made for other causes of fever. The differential diagnosis includes atrial myxoma, nonbacterial thrombotic endocarditis, systemic lupus erythematosus, sickle cell disease, and acute rheumatic fever.

The diagnosis of IE in a febrile patient with positive blood cultures depends in part on three factors: the nature of the bacteremia, the identity of the organism, and exclusion of other causes of bacteremia. IE produces sustained bacteremia and serial blood cultures obtained even hours apart remain positive.[43, 44] Enteric gram-negative bacilli are rare causes of IE despite sustained bacteremia, whereas when bacteremia with viridans streptococci is sustained an intravascular focus is almost always present. Extracardiac sites, such as a pulmonary infection or deep-seated abscess, may result in sustained bacteremia. Often, combinations of these factors must be analyzed to determine the risk for IE.

Laboratory Assays

In the absence of previous antibiotic therapy, blood cultures are positive in more than 95% of patients. It is preferable to obtain three sets of cultures, 1 hour apart. Because bacteremia is continuous, cultures do not have to be obtained at any particular time or body temperature. At least 10 mL of blood should be obtained per culture. Arterial blood offers no advantage over venous blood. Blood cultures may be negative in infections with fastidious organisms such as nutritionally deficient streptococci,[45] *Haemophilus parainfluenzae*, *Rickettsia*, *Brucella* sp., or anaerobes. The yield of positive blood cultures is increased by instructing the clinical laboratory to observe the samples over 3 weeks with periodic Gram's stains and subcultures. Chlamydiae and fungi can also result in "culture-negative endocarditis." A more common cause of negative blood cultures is antecedent administration of antimicrobial agents. When a history of recent antibiotic therapy is obtained, it may be prudent to withhold antibiotics if the patient is clinically stable and continue to obtain blood cultures periodically.

Other laboratory findings include a normochromic, normocytic anemia and elevated sedimentation rate. The white blood cell count is often normal. A positive rheumatoid factor is present in 50% of patients with chronic disease.[46] Circulating immune complexes can be detected in virtually all patients with IE. Renal abnormalities include microscopic hematuria and/or pyuria and proteinuria. The cerebrospinal fluid is often abnormal with pleocytosis, elevated protein concentration, and normal glucose concentration.

Imaging Studies

Two-dimensional echocardiograms demonstrate the vegetation in up to 80% of patients with NVE.[47–49] Vegetations under 3 mm are usually missed. M-mode echocardiograms are less sensitive (40 to 50%) than two-dimensional studies, and transesophageal echocardiograms have further increased sensitivity for detection of vegetations. Echocardiography can provide valuable information about the degree of valvular destruction and its hemodynamic effects and whether myocardial or valve ring abscess or aneurysm of the sinus of Valsalva is present. However, thickened valves, noninfected thrombi, nodules, tumors, and flail leaflets can be misinterpreted as vegetations.[48, 49] There is no definitive evidence that increasing vegetation size correlates with risk of embolization, but it seems likely that vegetations 10 mm in size or larger are associated with a greater risk of emboli.[50, 51] Prosthetic valve endocarditis (PVE) is more commonly evaluated with cineradiography, which can show abnormal rocking movements indicative of valve dehiscence.

Complications

CHF is the most common complication of IE. Heart failure may be due to valve destruction, myocarditis, coronary artery emboli with infarction, or myocardial abscesses.[52, 53] Aortic insufficiency with heart failure is associated with a higher mortality than is CHF with mitral valve infection.[54] Rupture of an abscess into the pericardial space can result in acute tamponade. Arrhythmia may be the earliest indication that the infection has spread to the conduction system. Conduction abnormalities imply involvement of the aortic valve.

Distal embolization may involve any organ system.[33] Embolization can result in metastatic infection, mycotic aneurysms, or distal infarction. Mycotic aneurysms may remain asymptomatic, cause local discomfort, or rupture unexpectedly with catastrophic hemorrhage.

Cerebral infarctions occur in up to 30% of patients with IE. The majority of infarcts involve the middle cerebral artery. Meningeal involvement in IE ranges from aseptic meningitis to frank purulent central nervous system infection.

CLINICAL SYNDROMES
Native Valve Endocarditis

Most patients with NVE have an identifiable, predisposing cardiac le███ ▓P is a common underlying lesion and tends to ███ ██ patients younger than age 40.[3, 13] The frequency of rheumatic heart disease is decreasing. Most patients with rheumatic heart disease and IE are middle-aged or older. Congenital heart disease is the underlying lesion in 10 to 20% of patients. Other underlying diseases include degenerative valve disease and idiopathic hypertrophic subaortic stenosis. The mitral valve is most commonly involved, followed by the aortic valve.

Streptococci (50 to 70%), enterococci (10%), and staphylococci (25%) account for the majority of cases of endocarditis on native valves.[13, 14, 22, 23] Viridans streptococci account for up to two thirds of cases[55] of IE on native valves. Most are highly sensitive to penicillin and cause infections primarily on abnormal valves. Enterococci normally inhabit the gastrointestinal tract and anterior urethra and are capable of infecting normal or damaged valves. Most cases are in elderly men who have undergone recent urologic manipulation or younger women who have undergone abortion, pregnancy, or cesarean section. *Streptococcus bovis* IE occurs primarily in the elderly and is strongly associated with colonic polyps or colonic malignancy.[56] The finding of *S. bovis* in blood cultures should prompt an evaluation of the gastrointestinal tract for malignancy even in the absence of other signs and symptoms. Other Lancefield group streptococci account for less that 5% of cases. Diabetics are particularly at risk for group B organisms.

Staphylococci cause 25% of NVE.[57] *S. aureus* accounts for most isolates. *S. aureus* IE is often acute with multiple metastatic abscesses. Valvular destruction can be rapid and mortality rates are high.

Streptococcus pneumoniae, *Neisseria gonorrhoeae*, *Haemophilus* sp., gram-negative rods, diphtheroids, and fungi are unusual causes of NVE in the non-IVDA.

Endocarditis in Intravenous Drug Abusers*

IVDAs with IE are usually male and young. The presentation of IE in IVDAs differs from that of both NVE and prosthetic valve infection. The tricuspid valve is infected in approximately 54%, aortic in 25%, and mitral in 20%. *S. aureus* is isolated in 60% of cases, reflecting the source of bacteremia, the patient's skin. Gram-negative bacilli account for up to 10% of cases, and fungi (usually *Candida*) cause disease in 5% of IVDAs. *S. aureus* accounts for 80% of clinical isolates in tricuspid valve endocarditis. The frequency of audible tricuspid murmurs in endocarditis is quite low. The majority (70 to 100%) of addicts with tricuspid disease develop septic pulmonary emboli with resultant pneumonia. A chest radiograph may aid in diagnosis. Patients with a syndrome compatible with tricuspid IE may actually have an extracardiac site of infection, that is, septic thrombophlebitis involving the femoral vein rather than IE.[58]

Prosthetic Valve Endocarditis

Infections of prosthetic valves account for 10 to 20% of all cases of IE. Early PVE denotes infection occurring within 60 days of valve placement, and late infection occurs after that time. The overall incidence in patients with prosthetic valves is 1 to 4%.[59, 60]

Early PVE is thought to result from infection arising in the perioperative period. Infection can occur intraopera-

---

*See Chapter 48.

tively via direct inoculation of organisms into the operative site or through contamination of the bypass machine. Bacteremia may also be caused by use of intravenous catheters, urethral catheters, cardiac pacing wires, and endotracheal tubes. Staphylococcal infections account for 45 to 50% of early PVE. *Staphylococcus epidermidis* is the most common organism isolated, with an average incidence of 25 to 30%. *S. aureus* is the second most common pathogen. Less common causes include gram-negative organisms, fungi, streptococci, enterococci, and diphtheroids. A positive blood culture in a patient with a prosthetic valve should never be regarded as a false-positive without a thorough evaluation.

Late PVE has been estimated to occur at an incidence of 0.2 to 0.5% per patient-year. The microbiology of late PVE resembles that of NVE. Viridans streptococci predominate (25 to 30%), with staphylococci, gram-negative bacilli, fungi, and diphtheroids occurring less commonly.[59]

In contrast to NVE, in PVE the aortic prosthetic valve is most commonly infected. Currently, there does not seem to be a difference in the overall incidence of PVE between tissue and mechanical valves. The incidence of PVE after replacement of an infected native valve is approximately 4%. Black race, male sex, and longer time of bypass have all been associated with an increased incidence of PVE.[61]

Infection often begins in the securing ring and may extend into an abscess. The prosthetic valve may tear from the ring with a resultant paravalvular leak. Early on, dehiscence of the valve may be noted only in imaging studies, but frank valvular insufficiency may result. Burrowing abscesses may result in conduction defects or purulent pericarditis if the abscess ruptures into the pericardium.[59] Tears and perforations of the valve leaflets also occur, resulting in valve dysfunction and new or changing cardiac murmurs. Early PVE is associated with a high mortality rate, whereas late PVE is often clinically indistinguishable from endocarditis occurring in patients without a prosthesis.

Nosocomial Endocarditis

In several large series of patients with IE, 10 to 29% of the episodes were acquired in the hospital.[7, 8, 62, 63] Patients with underlying valvular disease or prosthetic heart valves or those undergoing invasive procedures that could potentially damage the right side of the heart (e.g., cardiac catheterization) are particularly at risk of IE during an episode of nosocomial bacteremia.[7, 8, 64] Compared with patients with community-acquired infection, patients with nosocomial IE tend to be older and experience higher mortality. The infecting organisms are predominantly staphylococci and reflect the major source of nosocomial bacteremias—intravascular devices. In one series,[7] nosocomial IE accounted for 14.3% of the total cases of IE seen during a 9-year period. The mean age of the patients was 55 ± 3.2 years. *S. aureus* and coagulase-negative streptococci were responsible for 75% of the cases. Streptococcal infection occurred less commonly. The most important source of the infection was an intravascular device, and frequently the device had been left in place for an excessive length of time. In one half of the cases, surgical procedures or instrumentation of the genitourinary tract, heart, or gastrointestinal tract caused bacteremias that resulted in valvular infection. Less common sources of bacteremias leading to IE include postpartum endometritis, infected intrauterine devices, and ventriculoperitoneal shunt placement. In another survey,[8] 93% of cases of nosocomial IE occurring during a 7-year period had a definable source of bacteremia, usually related to an invasive procedure. The clinical presentation of nosocomial IE does not appear to differ significantly from that of community-acquired disease. Proper care of intravascular devices and administration of antibiotic prophylaxis to appropriate patients may prevent as many as one half of the cases of nosocomial IE.

MANAGEMENT

Hemodynamically stable patients can be admitted to the regular medical unit. Blood should be obtained for assessment of electrolytes, renal and hepatic function tests, and a complete blood count. Three sets of blood cultures should be obtained approximately 1 hour apart. Routine urinalysis should be performed along with urine cultures. If a pulmonary infiltrate is present, sputum should be obtained for cultures. Antibiotics may be withheld while awaiting culture results if patients are clinically stable. Acutely ill patients should receive antibiotic therapy when cultures have been obtained.

Hemodynamically unstable patients, such as those with signs of heart failure, embolic complications, and conduction defects or arrhythmias, may need to be monitored with telemetry or admitted directly to the intensive care unit. Imaging studies should be performed emergently on all unstable, acutely ill patients to help evaluate the need for surgical intervention. Cardiac surgery has evolved into an important adjunct for the management of IE caused by resistant organisms.

Antibiotic Therapy: General Principles

Microorganisms within the vegetation exist at high densities and are protected from host defenses.[65] Thus, bactericidal rather than bacteriostatic agents must be used in high concentrations and for prolonged periods (4 to 6 weeks) to achieve a cure. Parenteral therapy is preferable and should be administered in a peripheral vein, as central venous catheters increase the risk for superinfection of the vegetation. Antimicrobial susceptibility tests should be performed. The minimal inhibitory concentration (MIC) and minimal bactericidal concentration are the two most useful susceptibility measures for managing IE. The MIC is the minimal concentration of antibiotic that inhibits growth of a bacterium in vitro, and the minimal bactericidal concentration is the minimal concentration of antibiotic that results in a 99.9% "kill" within 24 hours. It is useful to save the infecting organism in case further antimicrobial susceptibility testing is needed. A peak serum bactericidal titer (the highest dilution of the patient's serum while the patient is receiving antimicrobial agents that kills a standard inoculum of the patient's organism in vitro) of 1:8 or greater generally indicates adequate therapy.[66] In most cases (e.g., streptococcal, enterococcal, and staphylococcal endocarditis) adequate therapeutic efficacy may be anticipated by using penicillins, cephalosporins, and vancomycin. Routine assays of bactericidal titers are therefore not necessary. Bactericidal titers are most helpful when response to therapy is suboptimal, when the infection is due to an unusual organism, or when an unconventional treatment regimen is used.[67]

In patients with a subacute course who have received antibiotics within 2 weeks of hospitalization, it is usually safe to delay therapy for several days while drawing daily blood cultures, in an attempt to isolate the infecting organism. In acutely ill patients, however, it is imperative to begin therapy within 2 to 3 hours of presentation, regardless of recent therapy, because valvular damage and abscess formation proceed rapidly. Blood cultures should be obtained soon after initiation of therapy to demonstrate eradication of organisms from the blood stream.

TABLE 40–1

TREATMENT OF INFECTIVE ENDOCARDITIS

Streptococci
  Viridans streptococci and *S. bovis*
    Penicillin G susceptible (MIC ≤ 0.1 g/mL)

Regimen A:	Penicillin G, 10–20 million U/d IV in divided doses q 4 h × 4 wk
Regimen B:	Penicillin as in regimen A plus streptomycin, 7.5 mg/kg IM q 12 h, or gentamicin, 1 mg/kg IV q 8 h, both for 2 wk
Regimen C:	Penicillin plus streptomycin or gentamicin × 2 wk as in regimen B with penicillin continued 2 wk longer
*Regimen D:	Cefazolin 1–2 g IV or IM q 8 h × 4 wk
*Regimen E:	Vancomycin, 15 mg/kg IV q 12 h × 4 wk

    Relatively penicillin G resistant (MIC > 0.1 but < 0.5 g/mL)

Regimen F:	Penicillin G, 20 million U/d in divided doses q 4 h plus streptomycin or gentamicin as in regimen B
*Regimen E	

Enterococci and viridans streptococci with MIC ≥ 0.5 g/mL

Regimen G:	Penicillin G, 20–30 million U/d, or ampicillin, 12 g/d IV in divided doses q 4 h plus gentamicin, 1 mg/kg IV q 8 h or streptomycin, 7.5 mg/kg IM q 12 h, both × 4–6 wk
Regimen H:	Vancomycin, 15 mg/kg IV q 12 h, plus gentamicin or streptomycin as in regimen G, both × 4–6 wk

  Prosthetic valve—see text
Staphylococci
  Native valve
    Methicillin susceptible (*S. epidermidis* and *S. aureus*)

Regimen I:	Nafcillin, 2 g IV q 4 h × 4–6 wk with or without gentamicin, 1 mg/kg q 8 h × the first 3–5 d
*Regimen J:	Cefazolin, 2 g IV q 8 h × 4–6 wk with or without gentamicin as in regimen I
*Regimen K:	Vancomycin, 15 mg/kg q 12 h × 4–6 wk

    Methicillin resistant
      Regimen K
  Prosthetic valve
    Methicillin susceptible
      Regimen I, J, or K × 6–8 wk with gentamicin for the first 2 wk
    Methicillin resistant
      Regimen K × 6–8 wk with gentamicin for the first 2 wk; in the presence of *S. epidermidis* add rifampin, 300 mg PO q 8 h × 6–8 wk

*Regimens for penicillin-allergic patients.

Modified from Bisno AL, Dismukes WE, Durack DT, et al: Antimicrobial treatment of infective endocarditis due to viridans streptococci, enterococci and staphylococci. JAMA 261:1471–1477, 1989. Copyright 1989, American Medical Association.

Empirical Antimicrobial Therapy

When treatment must be initiated before the microbiologic and sensitivity studies are completed, therapy should be based on the presenting clinical setting. With a subacute presentation of NVE, therapy should be directed against enterococci, which are the most resistant bacteria that may infect the valve in this setting. Empirical therapy for acute NVE should also cover staphylococci.[67, 68]

Initial therapy for presumed PVE should cover *S. epidermidis*, *S. aureus*, and gram-negative bacilli.[59, 61] Therapy for IE in the IVDAs is directed against *S. aureus* and gram-negative bacilli.[69] In hospital-acquired (nosocomial) IE the initial antimicrobial coverage should be directed against the most resistant nosocomial pathogens, including methicillin-resistant *S. aureus* and *Pseudomonas*.[7, 8]

Specific Antimicrobial Therapy

Once the infecting organism has been isolated, antimicrobial susceptibility tests should guide therapy. The most effective and least toxic therapy should be used. Recommendations for treatment of streptococcal, enterococcal, and staphylococcal IE have been published[67] and are summarized in Table 40–1.

Streptococci

Infections with highly penicillin-susceptible (MIC ≤ 0.1 μg/mL) viridans streptococci can be treated with penicillin G alone for 4 weeks. An added aminoglycoside is synergistic with penicillin and more rapidly sterilizes the vegetation. The 4-week regimen of penicillin alone is preferred for patients likely to manifest side effects with aminoglycosides (i.e., those with age older than 65 years, underlying renal insufficiency, or eighth cranial nerve disease) (regimen A). A 2-week, synergistic regimen consisting of penicillin plus gentamicin can be used in uncomplicated streptococcal infection (short duration of infection, no extracardiac foci of infection) (regimen B). A third regimen that involves 4 weeks of penicillin with an aminoglycoside for the initial 2 weeks is used for nutritionally variant streptococci or a relapse or when complications are present (regimen C). PVE should be treated with 6 weeks of penicillin with an aminoglycoside added for at least the first 2 weeks. Penicillin-allergic patients can be treated with cephalosporins or vancomycin, depending on the nature of the allergy (rash vs. anaphylaxis) (regimen D or E).

Relatively penicillin-resistant (MIC > 0.1 μg/mL and < 0.5 μg/mL) streptococcal infection is treated with a combination of penicillin and aminoglycoside for 2 weeks, followed by penicillin alone for 2 more weeks (regimen F). A cephalosporin or vancomycin may be substituted for penicillin, depending on the patient's allergy.

Infections with enterococci and with viridans streptococci with MIC of 0.5 μg/mL or more are treated for 4 to 6 weeks with a combination of penicillin and aminoglycoside for the full course of treatment (regimen G). A cephalosporin cannot be used to treat the enterococci because of universal resistance to this class of antibiotics. Enterococci resistant to more than 2000 μg/mL gentamicin and other aminoglycosides (termed high-level aminoglycoside resistance) and β-lactamase–producing strains of enterococci have been isolated.[70, 71] Thus, it is important to perform in vitro aminoglycoside susceptibility testing routinely when treating enterococcal endocarditis. It is unlikely that the addition of any aminoglycoside would be of benefit in treating isolates highly resistant to aminoglycosides, and therefore therapy with penicillin, ampicillin, or vancomycin alone should be prolonged to 8 weeks. Relapse is more likely with the 8-week, single-therapy regimen. Vancomycin must be substituted for penicillin for the treatment of β-lactamase–producing strains (regimen H).

Staphylococci

The treatments of choice for most native valve staphylococcal infections are penicillinase-resistant penicillins such as nafcillin or first-generation cephalosporins (regimens I and J). In areas where methicillin resistance among staphylococci is common, vancomycin should be used. Addition of an aminoglycoside for the initial 3 to 5 days of therapy appears to hasten the clearing of bacteremia.[72, 73] The standard duration of therapy is 4 weeks but may be extended to 6 weeks in the presence of extracardiac foci of infection or other complications. Relatively short courses of treatment (nafcillin plus tobramycin for 2 weeks) have been proposed for the IVDA with uncomplicated staphylococcal tricuspid valve infection.[74]

Three antibiotics are usually employed in the treatment of *S. epidermidis* PVE. The most effective regimen consists of vancomycin plus rifampin for 6 to 8 weeks with an aminoglycoside added for the first 2 weeks of therapy[67] (regimen K). Medical failures nevertheless still occur, and valve replacement may be necessary. *S. aureus* PVE is treated within a 6- to 8-week course of a penicillinase-resistant penicillin with gentamicin added during the first 2 weeks (regimens I and J). Vancomycin is used against methicillin-resistant strains (regimen K).

Other Organisms

Less common causes of IE such as gram-negative bacilli and anaerobes are best treated with combinations of penicillins, cephalosporins, or vancomycin with an aminoglycoside administered for 4 to 6 weeks. In vitro susceptibility testing and serum bactericidal titers should be used to guide therapy.

Fungal endocarditis is treated with a combination of an antifungal agent and surgery. Outcome is usually poor.

Culture-Negative Endocarditis

When blood cultures remain negative but the clinical response is good, therapy should be continued as for the usual course of therapy for the suspected organism. When blood cultures are sterile but there is no clinical response after 7 to 10 days of empirical therapy, special cultures and serologic studies should be performed. Organisms to consider include *Brucella*, *Rickettsia*, *Legionella*, *Chlamydia*, and fastidious gram-negative bacilli.[75–77] Often it is helpful to inform the microbiology division that unusual organisms are being considered so that appropriate cultures can be set up and held for a prolonged period.

When a patient with clinical IE but negative cultures has no change in symptoms after several weeks of empirical therapy, consideration should be given to discontinuing the treatment and re-evaluating the patient.

SPECIAL CONSIDERATIONS
Anticoagulation

In most cases, anticoagulants are of no value in the therapy of IE. Anticoagulants do not prevent embolization of pieces of the vegetation, and the risk of bleeding from a mycotic aneurysm, cerebral emboli, or infarction precludes anticoagulation. However, anticoagulation may have to be used in patients with prosthetic valves and in those with extracardiac sources of pulmonary emboli.[78, 79] In such patients, careful control is important to maintain a low therapeutic range of anticoagulation.

Surgery

The decision to replace a valve in patients with IE should be made only when definite indications exist. The major indications include CHF resulting from valvular dysfunction, cardiac abscess requiring drainage, uncontrolled infection, and prosthetic valve dysfunction with dehiscence.[80–83] Mortality in patients with CHF secondary to acute aortic regurgitation exceeds 50%. Immediate valve replacement is essential. Other indications for valve replacement include persistently positive blood cultures, recurrent relapse despite appropriate therapy, and unavailability of appropriate microbicidal therapy, as occurs with infections caused by fungi or certain gram-negative bacilli. Surgery often becomes necessary in PVE caused by organisms other than streptococci.

Persistent bacteremia after at least 1 week of appropriate antimicrobial therapy warrants surgical evaluation. Before any surgery, the organism's antibiotic susceptibilities and the drug levels in the patient's serum should be confirmed. Prompt surgical intervention may be lifesaving in IE complicated by myocardial or valve ring abscess, as can occur in prosthetic valve infection. Persistent bacteremia may also point to an extracardiac focus of infection. Surgical intervention may be required for drainage of such metastatic abscesses.

When a definitive indication for valve replacement exists, surgery should not be delayed. There is less than a 5% incidence of infection with the same organism when a valve is replaced before sterilization of blood cultures. Postoperative antibiotics should be continued long enough to eradicate metastatic foci of infection.

Valve replacement based on vegetation size alone is controversial.[83, 84] Patients with large vegetations and recurrent major arterial emboli may require surgical intervention. The number or type of embolic events that determines at which point to operate is controversial. There are no data to indicate the risk of additional embolic events in patients with recurrent emboli.[83, 84] Surgery is often recommended after two or more emboli.

In cases in which the valve is relatively intact, valvuloplasty with resection of the vegetation may be preferable to total valve replacement. Isolated tricuspid valve IE is frequently seen in IVDAs. It is most often caused by *S. aureus*. When it is caused by resistant gram-negative bacilli or fungi, surgery is often indicated. One approach has been valve resection without replacement. Many patients tolerate absence of the tricuspid valve for prolonged periods. A tricuspid prosthetic valve can be implanted later if the patient's condition deteriorates (e.g., the patient develops pulmonary artery hypertension).

The presence of cardiac arrhythmias or new conduction abnormalities warrants emergent repeated echocardiography, looking for myocardial abscesses. Arrhythmias may also result from myocardial ischemia or infarction. Surgery undertaken to drain a myocardial abscess is associated with extreme morbidity and mortality.[85]

RESPONSE TO THERAPY AND PROGNOSIS

The majority of patients with IE should defervesce by 3 to 7 days after effective antibiotics are begun.[86] Persistence or recurrence of fever may be due to associated myocardial metastatic abscesses, recurrent emboli, superinfection, or febrile reactions to antimicrobial agents.[1-3, 53] Blood cultures generally become negative after several days of therapy. Repeated blood cultures should be obtained 2 to 4 weeks after completion of therapy to monitor for disease relapse. Despite successful antimicrobial therapy, petechiae, Osler's nodes, emboli, rupture of mycotic aneurysms, and heart failure may occur at any time during the course of IE. Blood cultures should be obtained during any new clinical events (such as emboli) to evaluate for ongoing, active infection. Changes in valve size and architecture can occur during therapy with resultant changes in cardiac murmurs.

Aneurysms may form anywhere and are often asymptomatic until they suddenly rupture, requiring emergent surgery. Symptoms of headache or neurologic abnormalities should prompt consideration of a leaking or enlarging cerebral aneurysm.[53, 87] Cerebral angiography is necessary for definitive diagnosis. Surgical intervention should be considered for symptomatic patients with intracranial aneurysms.

The glomerulonephritis associated with IE often improves during therapy. Patients with persistent renal insufficiency despite antibiotic therapy may benefit from corticosteroids, plasma exchanges, and/or cytotoxic chemotherapy.

At least 6% of patients with NVE who are not IVDAs have subsequent episodes of IE.[88] Drug abusers are at particularly high risk for additional episodes. The results of treatment of those with additional episodes of IE on native valves are not different from the results of therapy of first episodes of IE.[88]

The type of cardiac valve, identity of the causative organism, age of the patient, and presence or absence of complications determine the prognosis of IE. Factors predisposing to a poor prognosis are nonstreptococcal disease, development of heart failure, aortic valve involvement, large vegetations, prosthetic valve infection, left- versus right-sided disease, older age, and valve ring or myocardial abscesses. The cure rate is 90% or more for native valve streptococcal IE. Cure rates for *S. aureus* IE in drug abusers exceed 90%, but the same infection carries a 25 to 40% mortality in the nonaddict. Outcome is often poor in fungal and gram-negative IE. Underlying medical conditions can also increase the chance of mortality.

PVE has a worse prognosis than native valve disease. The overall mortality from PVE over the last 10 years averaged 54%. Early disease has a significantly higher mortality than late disease (74% versus 43%).

After cure of IE, the risk of increased mortality remains and is due mainly to heart failure, major emboli, and rupture of mycotic aneurysms.

PREVENTIVE ASPECTS OF INFECTION IN THE INTENSIVE CARE UNIT

Attempts to prevent IE include prophylaxis with antibiotics and reduction of the risk of nosocomial bacteremia.

Although there is no proof that antibiotic prophylaxis reduces the risk of IE, indirect evidence that it should do so is generally accepted.[89-91] However, IE may occur despite appropriate antibiotic prophylaxis. Prophylaxis is recommended for patients with predisposing lesions undergoing procedures known to cause bacteremia. Many of these procedures are commonly performed in the intensive care setting. Conditions for which prophylaxis is recommended included valvular or congenital heart disease (except for uncomplicated secundum atrial septal defects or surgically corrected cardiac lesions without prosthetic implants more than 6 months after operation), intracardiac prostheses (except for pacemakers), and asymmetric septal hypertrophy. Patients with a prior episode of IE are at increased risk of additional episodes and should also receive prophylaxis. In patients with MVP, prophylaxis is recommended only for those with insufficiency (i.e., significant murmur).[89] Recommendations for prophylaxis are published by numerous authoritative groups.[89, 91]

Prophylaxis for dental and other traumatic procedures in the mouth, nose, throat, or esophagus likely to cause bleeding is aimed at the viridans streptococci. Endotracheal intubation is not an indication for antimicrobial prophylaxis. The regimens are tailored to the patient's ability to take oral medications, a history of allergy to penicillin, and the risk of developing IE. Simple oral regimens, whenever possible, ensure better compliance. Amoxicillin (3.0 g orally 1 hour before procedure, then 1.5 g 6 hours after the initial dose) has become the recommended standard oral regimen because it is well absorbed, even in the presence of food, provides blood levels that are bactericidal for most viridans streptococci for many hours, and is more effective than penicillin in reducing bacteremia.[91] For penicillin-allergic individuals, erythromycin (erythromycin stearate, 1.0 g orally 2 hours before procedure, then half the dose 6 hours after the initial dose) is recommended. Patients intolerant to both penicillin and erythromycin can receive clindamycin prophylaxis (300 mg orally 1 hour before procedure and 150 mg 6 hours after the initial dose). Some authorities prefer parenteral prophylaxis (ampicillin, 2.0 g intravenously [or intramuscularly], with or without gentamicin, 1.5 mg/kg intravenously [or intramuscularly] 30 minutes before procedure, followed by amoxicillin, 1.5 g orally 6 hours after the initial dose; for penicillin-allergic patients, a single dose of vancomycin at 1.0 g intravenously administered over 1 hour, starting 1 hour before the procedure, may be substituted) for patients with a previous history of endocarditis or surgically constructed systemic-pulmonary shunts.

For genitourinary and lower gastrointestinal tract procedures likely to cause significant trauma (e.g., urethral catheterization, prostatic surgery, vaginal hysterectomy, colon or gallbladder surgery), prophylaxis is directed against enterococci. Combination parenteral regimens include ampicillin at 2.0 g intravenously (or intramuscularly) plus gentamicin at 1.5 mg/kg intravenously (or intramuscularly) (not to exceed 80 mg) 30 minutes before procedure, followed by amoxicillin at 1.5 g orally 6 hours after the initial dose. Alternatively, the parenteral regimen may be repeated once 8 hours after the initial dose. In penicillin-allergic patients, vancomycin at 1.0 g intravenously administered over 1 hour plus gentamicin at 1.5 mg/kg intravenously (or intramuscularly) (not to exceed 80 mg) 1 hour before the procedure (may be repeated once 8 hours after the initial dose) is recommended except for minor repetitive procedures in patients not at high risk for IE. Fiberoptic endoscopy without biopsy and barium enema involve such low risk that prophylaxis is not justified except possibly in patients at extremely high risk such as those with prosthetic valves.

Prophylaxis for cardiac surgery, including implantation of prosthetic devices, patches, and sutures, is directed against staphylococci and should be of short duration. The usual regimen is cefazolin at 2 g intravenously plus 1.7 mg/kg gentamicin intravenously at induction of anesthesia, followed by repeated doses 8 and 16 hours later. With the emergence of methicillin-resistant *S. epidermidis* (and more recently methicillin-resistant *S. aureus*) as an important nosocomial pathogen, substitution of vancomycin (15 mg/kg intravenously over 1 hour starting 1 hour before the procedure, 10 mg/kg after completion of bypass, and then 7.5 mg/kg every 6 hours for three doses) for cefazolin may be prudent. Vancomycin is also used in patients with hypersensitivity to penicillin and cephalosporins. There are no data supporting routine antibiotic prophylaxis for procedures such as Swan-Ganz or central venous catheter placement and chest tube insertion. Antimicrobial agents should not be administered to prevent infection during the time when invasive devices are present in a patient other than for the previously noted procedures. The practice of "covering" intravascular catheters with antibiotics for prolonged periods often predisposes to superinfection with unusual or resistant organisms. Close care of intravenous catheters and surgical drains is important in preventing both local infection and bacteremia, which can lead to IE.[92] Such invasive devices should be discontinued as early as possible to decrease the risk of infection.

References

1. Lerner PI, Weinstein L: Infective endocarditis in the antibiotic era. N Engl J Med 274:199 (also 259, 323, 388), 1966.
2. Gray IR: Infective endocarditis 1937–1987. Br Heart J 57:211, 1987.
3. Naggar CZ, Forgacs P: Infective endocarditis: A challenging disease. Med Clin North Am 70:1279, 1986.
4. Parkhurst GP, Decker JP: Bacterial aortitis and mycotic aneurysms of the aorta; a report of 12 cases. Am J Pathol 31:821, 1955.
5. Johnson F, Darling RC, Mundth ED, et al: The management of infected arterial aneurysms. J Cardiovasc Surg 18:361, 1977.
6. Kerr A Jr: Subacute Bacterial Endocarditis. Springfield, IL, Charles C Thomas, p 3, 1955.
7. Terpenning MS, Buggy BP, Kauffman CA: Hospital-acquired infective endocarditis. Arch Intern Med 148:1601, 1988.
8. Friedland G, Von Reyn CF, Levy B, et al: Nosocomial endocarditis. Infect Control 5:284, 1984.
9. Millard DD, Shulman ST: The changing spectrum of neonatal endocarditis. Clin Perinatol 15:587, 1988.
10. Sholler GF, Hawker RE, Celermajer JM: Infective endocarditis in childhood. Pediatr Cardiol 6:183, 1986.
11. Saiman L, Prince A: Infections of the heart. Adv Pediatr Infect Dis 4:139, 1989.
12. Johnson CM, Rhodes KH: Pediatric endocarditis. Mayo Clin Proc 57:86, 1982.
13. McKinsey DS, Ratts TE, Bisno AL: Underlying cardiac lesions in adults with infective endocarditis. The changing spectrum. Am J Med 82:681, 1987.
14. Von Reyn CF, Levy BS, Arbeit RD, et al: Infective endocarditis: An analysis based on strict case definitions. Ann Intern Med 94:505, 1981.
15. MacMahon SW, Roberts JK, Kramer-Fox R, et al: Mitral valve prolapse and infective endocarditis. Am Heart J 113:1291, 1987.
16. Lavie CJ, Khandheria BK, Seward JB, et al: Factors associated with the recommendation for endocarditis prophylaxis in mitral valve prolapse. JAMA 262:3308, 1989.
17. Baddour LM, Bisno AL: Infective endocarditis complicating mitral valve prolapse: Epidemiologic, clinical and microbiological aspect. Rev Infect Dis 8:117, 1986.
18. MacMahon SW, Hickey AJ, Wilcken DEL, et al: Risk of infective endocarditis in mitral valve prolapse with and without precordial systolic murmurs. Am J Cardiol 58:105, 1986.
19. Griffin MR, Wilson WR, Edwards WD, et al: Infective endocarditis—Olmstead County, Minnesota, 1950 through 1981. JAMA 254:1199, 1985.
20. Chagnac A, Rudniki C, Loebel H, et al: Infectious endocarditis in idiopathic hypertrophic subaortic stenosis. Report of three cases and a review of the literature. Chest 81:346, 1982.
21. Kaye D: Changing pattern of infective endocarditis. Am J Med 78(suppl 6B):157, 1985.
22. Terpenning MS, Buggy BP, Kauffman CA: Infective endocarditis: Clinical features in young and elderly patients. Am J Med 83:626, 1987.
23. Pomerance A: Cardiac pathology in the elderly. Cardiovasc Clin 12:9, 1981.
24. Applefeld MM, Hornick RB: Infective endocarditis in patients over age 60. Am Heart J 88:90, 1974.
25. Seltzer A: Changing aspects of the natural history of valvular aortic stenosis. N Engl J Med 317:91, 1971.
26. Cooper G, Platt R: *Staphylococcus aureus* bacteremia in diabetic patients. Endocarditis and mortality. Am J Med 73:658, 1982.
27. Cherubin CE, Neu HC: Infective endocarditis at the Presbyterian Hospital in New York City from 1938–1967. Am J Med 51:83, 1971.
28. Rodbard S: Blood velocity and endocarditis. Circulation 27:18, 1963.
29. Weinstein L, Schlesinger JJ: Pathoanatomic, physiologic and clinical correlates in endocarditis. N Engl J Med 291:832, 1122, 1974.
30. Lopez JA, Ross RS, Fishbein MC, et al: Nonbacterial thrombotic endocarditis: A review. Am Heart J 113:773, 1987.
31. Baddour LM, Christensen GD, Lowrance JH, et al: Pathogenesis of experimental endocarditis. Rev Infect Dis 11:452, 1989.
32. Durack DT: Current issues in the prevention of infective endocarditis. Am J Med 78(suppl 6B):149, 1985.
33. Lerner PI: Neurologic complications of infective endocarditis. Med Clin North Am 69:385, 1985.
34. Pruitt AA, Rubin RH, Karchmer AW, et al: Neurologic complications of bacterial endocarditis. Medicine 57:329, 1978.
35. Morris GK: Infective endocarditis: A preventable disease? Br Med J 290:1532, 1985.
36. Weinstein L, Rubin RH: Infective endocarditis—1973. Prog Cardiovasc Dis 16:239, 1973.
37. Albeit JS, Krous HF, Dalen JE, et al: Pathogenesis of Osler's nodes. Ann Intern Med 85:471, 1976.
38. Yee J, McAllister K: The utility of Osler's nodes in the diagnosis of infective endocarditis. Chest 92:751, 1987.
39. Silverberg HH: Roth spots. Mt Sinai J Med 37:77, 1970.
40. Wilson WR, Giuliani ER, Danielson GK, et al: Management of complications of infective endocarditis. Mayo Clin Proc 57:162, 1982.
41. Wilson WR, Lie JT, Houser OW, et al: The management of patients with mycotic aneurysms. Curr Clin Top Infect Dis 2:151, 1981.
42. Robbins MJ, Sveiro R, Fishman WH, et al: Right-sided valvular endocarditis: Etiology, diagnosis, and approach to therapy. Am Heart J 111:128, 1986.
43. Werner AS, Cobbs CG, Kaye D, et al: Studies on the bacteremia of bacterial endocarditis. JAMA 202:199, 1967.
44. Scheld WM: Pathogenesis and pathophysiology of infective endocarditis. In: Sande MA, Kaye D, Root RK (eds): Endocarditis. New York, Churchill Livingstone, p 1, 1984.
45. Stein DS, Nelson KE: Endocarditis due to nutritionally deficient streptococci: Therapeutic dilemma. Rev Infect Dis 9:908, 1987.
46. Williams RC: Rheumatoid factors in subacute bacterial endocarditis and other infectious diseases. Scand J Rheumatol Suppl 75:300, 1988.
47. Melvin ET, Berger M, Lutzker LG, et al: Noninvasive methods for detection of valve vegetations in infective endocarditis. Am J Cardiol 47:271, 1981.
48. Klodas E, Edwards WD, Khandheria BK: Use of echocardiography for improving detection of valvular vegetations in subacute bacterial endocarditis. J Am Soc Echocardiogr 2:386, 1989.
49. Dubois RW, Gizton LE: Role of echocardiography in suspected infective endocarditis in intravenous drug abusers. Am J Cardiol 58:649, 1986.
50. Lutas EM, Roberts RB, Devereux RB, et al: Relation between the presence of echocardiographic vegetations and the complication rate in infective endocarditis. Am Heart J 112:107, 1986.
51. Buda AJ, Zotz RJ, Le Mire MS, et al: Prognostic significance of vegetations detected by two-dimensional echocardiography in infective endocarditis. Am Heart J 112:1291, 1986.
52. DiNubile MJ, Calderwood SB, Steinhaus DM, et al: Cardiac conduction abnormalities complicating native valve active infective endocarditis. Am J Cardiol 58:1213, 1986.
53. Weinstein L: Life-threatening complications of infective endocarditis and their management. Arch Intern Med 146:953, 1986.
54. Griffin FM Jr, Jones G, Cobbs CG: Aortic insufficiency in bacterial endocarditis. Ann Intern Med 76:23, 1972.
55. Roberts RB, Krieger AG, Schiller NL, et al: Viridans streptococcal endocarditis: The role of various species including pyridoxal-dependent streptococci. Rev Infect Dis 1:955, 1979.
56. Leport C, Bure A, Leport J, et al: Incidence of colonic lesions in *Streptococcus bovis* and enterococcal endocarditis. Lancet 1:748, 1987.
57. Karchmer AW: Staphylococcal endocarditis. Laboratory and clinical basis for antibiotic therapy. Am J Med 78(suppl 6B):116, 1985.
58. Barg WL, Supena RB, Fekety R: Persistent staphylococcal bacteremia in an intravenous drug abuser. Antimicrob Agents Chemother 29:209, 1986.
59. Cowgill LD, Addonizio VP, Hopeman AR, et al: Prosthetic valve endocarditis. Curr Probl Cardiol 11:617, 1986.
60. Calderwood SB, Swinski LA,, Waternaux CM, et al: Risk factors for the development of prosthetic valve endocarditis. Circulation 72:31, 1985.
61. Watanakunakorn C: Prosthetic valve infective endocarditis. Prog Cardiovasc Dis 22:181, 1979.

62. Guze LB, Pearce ML: Hospital-acquired bacterial endocarditis. Arch Intern Med 112:56, 1963.
63. Venezio FR, Westenfelder GO, Cook FV, et al: Infective endocarditis in a community hospital. Arch Intern Med 142:789, 1982.
64. Rowley KM, Clubb KS, Smith GJW, et al: Right-sided infective endocarditis as a consequence of flow-directed pulmonary artery catheterization. N Engl J Med 311:1152, 1984.
65. Durack DT, Beeson PB: Experimental bacterial endocarditis II. Survival of bacteria in endocardial vegetations. Br J Exp Pathol 53:50, 1972.
66. Wolfson JS, Swartz MN: Drug therapy: Serum bactericidal activity as a monitor of antibiotic therapy. N Engl J Med 312:968, 1985.
67. Bisno AL, Dismukes WE, Durack DT, et al: Antimicrobial treatment of infective endocarditis due to viridans streptococci, enterococci, and staphylococci. JAMA 261:1471, 1989.
68. Mandell GL, Kaye D, Levison ME, et al: Enterococcal endocarditis; an analysis of 38 patients observed at the New York Hospital–Cornell Medical Center. Arch Intern Med 125:258, 1970.
69. Reisberg BE: Infective endocarditis in the narcotic addict. Prog Cardiovasc Dis 22:193, 1979.
70. Petterson JE, Zervos MJ: Susceptibility and bacterial activity studies of four β-lactamase producing enterococci. Antimicrob Agents Chemother 33:251, 1989.
71. Ingerman M, Pitsakis PG, Rosenberg A, et al: β-Lactamase production in experimental endocarditis due to aminoglycoside resistant *Streptococcus faecalis*. J Infect Dis 155:1226, 1987.
72. Sande MA, Korzeniowski OM: The Antimicrobial Therapy of Infective Endocarditis. New York, Grune & Stratton, p 113, 1981.
73. Korzeniowski OM, Sande MA: The National Collaborative Endocarditis Study Group: Combination antimicrobial therapy for *Staphylococcus aureus* endocarditis in patients addicted to parenteral drugs and in non-addicts: A prospective study. Ann Intern Med 97:496, 1982.
74. Chambers HF, Miller RT, Newman MA: Right-sided *Staphylococcus aureus* endocarditis in intravenous drug abusers: Two-week combination therapy. Ann Intern Med 109:619, 1988.
75. Ellner JJ, Rosenthal MS, Lerner PI, et al: Infective endocarditis caused by slow-growing, fastidious, gram-negative bacteria. Medicine 58:145, 1979.
76. Al-Kasab S, Fagih MR, Al-Yousef S, et al: *Brucella* infective endocarditis: Successful combined medical and surgical therapy. J Thorac Cardiovasc Surg 95:862, 1988.
77. Tobin MJ, Cahill N, Gearty G, et al: Q fever endocarditis. Am J Med 72:396, 1982.
78. Wilson WK, Geraci JE, Danielson GK, et al: Anticoagulant therapy and central nervous system complications in patients with prosthetic valve endocarditis. Circulation 57:1004, 1979.
79. Heimburger TS, Duma RJ: Infections of prosthetic heart valves and cardiac pacemakers. Infect Dis Clin North Am 3:221, 1989.
80. Alsip SG, Blackstone EH, Kirklin JW, et al: Indications for cardiac surgery in patients with active infective endocarditis. Am J Med 78(suppl 6B):138, 1985.
81. Karp RB: Role of surgery in infective endocarditis. Cardiovasc Clin 17:141, 1987.
82. Da Costa Lins RH, Soares DMN, Van Berg L, et al: Surgical treatment of active valvular infective endocarditis. Scand J Thorac Cardiovasc Surg 22:43, 1988.
83. Cobbs CG, Gnann JW: Indications for surgery. In: Sande ME, Kaye D, Root RK (eds): Endocarditis. New York, Churchill Livingstone, p 201, 1984.
84. Mugge A, Daniel WG, Frank G, et al: Echocardiography in infective endocarditis: Reassessment of prognostic implications of vegetation size determined by the transthoracic and the transesophageal approach. J Am Coll Cardiol 14:631, 1989.
85. D'Agostino RS, Miller DC, Stenson EB, et al: Valve replacements in patients with native valve endocarditis; what really determines operative outcome. Ann Thorac Surg 40:429, 1985.
86. Frimodt-Moller N, Espersen F, Rosdahl VT: Antibiotic treatment of *Staphylococcus aureus* endocarditis. A review of 119 cases. Acta Med Scand 222:175, 1987.
87. Nakayama DK, O'Neill JA Jr, Wagner H, et al: Management of vascular complications of bacterial endocarditis. J Pediatr Surg 21:636, 1986.
88. Levison ME, Kaye D, Mandell GL, et al: Characteristics of patients with multiple episodes of bacterial endocarditis. JAMA 211:1355, 1970.
89. Dajani AC, Bisno AL, Chung KJ, et al: Prevention of bacterial endocarditis: Recommendations by the American Heart Association. JAMA 264:2919, 1990.
90. Imperial JF, Horowitz RI: Does prophylaxis prevent postdental infective endocarditis? Am J Med 88:131, 1990.
91. Kaye D: Prophylaxis for infective endocarditis: An update. Ann Intern Med 104:419, 1986.
92. Maki DG, Goldman DA, Rhame FS: Infection control in intravenous therapy. Ann Intern Med 79:867, 1973.

CHAPTER 41

Gastroenteric Infections

Robert Fekety

Patients in the United States infected with one of the common endemic viral or bacterial infections of the gastrointestinal tract are rarely critically ill and therefore are not often admitted to intensive care units (ICUs). When they are, it is usually because of a complication of an underlying disease, such as perforation, abscess formation, peritonitis, massive intestinal hemorrhage, and septic shock. There are two important exceptions to this statement. The first relates to patients with cholera, which is occasionally seen in the United States and is readily treated by vigorous fluid and electrolyte replacement. The second exception concerns pseudomembranous colitis (PMC), which is sometimes the primary disease resulting in admission to ICUs and more often is a serious and potentially fatal complication of antibiotic therapy given for management of underlying serious illnesses that necessitated admission to the ICU. PMC is by far the most common and important gastrointestinal infection in patients in ICUs.

PSEUDOMEMBRANOUS COLITIS

Nonspecific diarrhea is a common side effect of antibiotic therapy. It is often referred to as simple or benign diarrhea. It resolves quickly after antibiotic administration is stopped and is treated supportively. In marked contrast, about 10% of hospitalized patients with antibiotic-associated diarrhea have a more severe disease known as antibiotic-associated colitis (AAC), a form of PMC. In these patients, the colon is inflamed and covered with an adherent exudate, which may be either nodular or diffuse. Pseudomembranes consist of dead leukocytes and mucosal cells enmeshed in mucus and fibrin. Grossly visible pseudomembranes may not be evident in patients with AAC, especially early in the illness, and the process is then likely to be diagnosed as nonspecific colitis or acute self-limited colitis. However, biopsies of these colonic lesions may reveal microscopic pseudomembranes as well as inflammation of the mucosa. Thus, AAC may present as PMC, nonspecific colitis, or acute self-limited colitis. It may also present as an acute abdomen, toxic megacolon, or colonic perforation. It is fortunate that the latter are not common, as they still have a significant mortality rate. Finally, patients with PMC or AAC may have a mild illness that is indistinguishable clinically from nonspecific diarrhea. Therefore, *any* patient with diarrhea after receiving antibiotics, especially in the hospital, should be suspected of having colitis; unlike benign diarrhea, colitis is both serious and treatable with specific antibiotics.[1]

Clostridium difficile and its toxins cause almost all cases of AAC.[1] Rare cases have been attributed to toxigenic *Staphylococcus aureus*, *Salmonella*, *Clostridium perfringens* type C, *Plesiomonas shigelloides*, *Yersinia enterocolitica*, *Shigella*, *Escherichia coli* O127:H7, *Campylobacter*, *Aeromonas*, cytomegalovirus, *Entamoeba histolytica*, and *Listeria monocytogenes*. A pseudomembrane is detected only rarely in association with the enterocolitis caused by most of the latter organisms. Although there is no good evidence that *C. difficile* causes chronic inflammatory bowel diseases such as Crohn's colitis and chronic idiopathic ulcerative colitis, it should be remembered that persons with these conditions can have complicating *C. difficile* colitis. The true frequency of AAC caused by organisms other than *C. difficile* is not known. Because patients with AAC no longer uniformly receive a thorough diagnostic evaluation, failure to implicate *C. difficile* in all cases may occur in cases caused by the unusual organisms mentioned or may be attributable to technical problems with the simple laboratory tests that are often relied on as diagnostic aids.

Historical Aspects

Although antibiotics are the single most important factor in the induction of PMC, they are undoubtedly not the only factor. A serious and often fatal form of this disease was recognized in the preantibiotic era. One of the earliest reports of PMC was in 1893, and many cases were reported, usually by surgeons, between 1900 and 1940.[1] After antibiotics were introduced into hospital practice (1945 to 1960), PMC was attributed to *S. aureus* with some justification, even in retrospect. Antibiotic-resistant *S. aureus* was often found in stools and blood of these patients, and vancomycin given orally was effective in treatment. Some investigators now believe that the implication of staphylococci in those cases was erroneous, because recognition of the etiologic relationship of *C. difficile* and PMC was not made until 1978. Although staphylococcal enterocolitis is now rare, it is probably a real entity. It commonly involves the distal ileum (which is rare with *C. difficile* colitis) and cecum as well as the distal colon. PMC became a relatively frequent complication of antibiotic therapy between 1970 and 1980, and at that time was often and erroneously called clindamycin colitis. *C. difficile* was shown to be the actual etiologic agent in 1978.

In 1976, about 8% of patients at the University of Michigan Hospital who received either ampicillin or clindamycin experienced diarrhea,[2] but only 16% of patients with antibiotic-associated diarrhea had PMC as well. Thus, the overall rate of PMC was about 1%.[3] When investigators challenged hamsters with clindamycin (or other antibiotics) in 1976, they were found to be highly susceptible to development of severe enterocolitis.[4] Next it was found that a cytotoxin neutralizable by *Clostridium sordellii* antitoxin could be detected in the feces of these hamsters and that a similar toxin was also present in the feces of a patient with PMC (who incidentally responded to treatment with oral vancomycin).[5] Her illness was subsequently determined to be caused by toxigenic *C. difficile*. Simultaneously, several groups of investigators from various parts of the world conclusively implicated *C. difficile* in the causation of the disease.[1] It was also shown that isolates of *C. difficile* produced a cytotoxin that was neutralizable by *C. sordellii* antitoxin.[5] *C. difficile* isolates were then found to be highly susceptible to inhibition by vancomycin, metronidazole, or bacitracin, and patients with PMC began to be treated successfully with either oral vancomycin or oral metronidazole, with bacitracin a slightly less desirable alternative.

Pathology

The salient lesion of *C. difficile* colitis is inflammation of the mucosa and submucosa of the colon. Pseudomembranes may not always be present, and in addition, small pseudomembranes may be dislodged during histologic processing. The inflammation usually affects only the epithelium and the lamina propria; but in severe cases, necrosis may occur, deeper tissues may be involved, and secondary infection may be seen. Such patients may require admission to ICUs. Transmural necrosis may result in toxic dilatation of the colon, perforation, and peritonitis; the latter are now rec-

ognized as surgical emergencies and potentially fatal complications of PMC. Lesions can be found throughout the colon but are usually most prominent in the rectosigmoid. In about 10% of cases, lesions may be restricted to the cecum or the transverse colon and patients may have little or no diarrhea, but instead localized abdominal pain, fever, and leukocytosis. These cases tend to follow a severe course.[6]

Although *C. difficile* colitis occurs at all ages, it is most frequent and severe in elderly or debilitated patients. PMC occurs in infants occasionally but is difficult to diagnose, as it is not uncommon for healthy infants to have both the organism and its toxins in their stools. *C. difficile* is believed to be an important cause of the ischemic enterocolitis that complicates Hirschsprung's disease in infants.[2] Oral therapy with vancomycin followed by resolution of symptoms is the only good way to establish the probable diagnosis of PMC in infants, as they rarely undergo endoscopy when they have diarrhea.

Microbiology, Epidemiology, and Pathogenesis

C. difficile is a spore-forming, gram-positive, obligate anaerobic bacillus that is a component of the normal intestinal flora of about 3 to 5% of healthy adults. It is found in soil and water and has been isolated from stools of healthy dogs, cats, and many other domestic and wild animals. Rates of asymptomatic fecal carriage are often much higher than 5% in hospitalized patients. The organism has been found in the stools of 15 to 20% of antibiotic-treated hospitalized adults without diarrhea. It is easy to detect in stools using a selective agar medium containing cycloserine, cefoxitin, and fructose (CCFA).[7] The addition of 0.2% highly purified sodium taurocholate increases the ability of CCFA to detect small numbers of spores in stools of asymptomatic carriers or from contaminated surfaces.[8] The addition of taurocholate is not needed for diagnosis of PMC, as patients with PMC usually have large numbers of the organisms in their stools.

Groups at high risk for PMC include the elderly; patients with cancer, leukemia, uremia, burns, and colonic stasis; those undergoing abdominal surgery or cesarean section; and patients in ICUs. Antibiotics given for even short periods (as for short-course perioperative surgical prophylaxis or for treatment of minor infections) may precipitate AAC, which can follow oral, intramuscular, intravenous, or topical use of antibiotics. More cases occur after parenteral than oral therapy. The list of inciting (or inducing) antimicrobial agents includes practically every antimicrobial used in the treatment of infections in humans, including vancomycin and metronidazole (the two drugs preferred for treatment of the disease). The important deleterious and predisposing consequences of antimicrobial administration consist of poorly understood alterations in the colonic flora. They permit *C. difficile* to multiply and produce large amounts of its toxins within the intestinal lumen. The toxins adhere to the mucosa and cause the disease. The organism rarely invades colonic tissue. The mechanisms of toxin actions are complex and not completely understood. PMC may not begin until after antibiotic administration has been discontinued, because the permissive intestinal flora resulting from antibiotics may remain suitable for colonization of the colon with *C. difficile* for 6 weeks or more *after* antibiotic administration is stopped. As many as 20% of cases of PMC begin after discontinuation of antimicrobials. Such cases are often misdiagnosed initially, thus resulting in more severe illness in many cases. The relative risks of different antimicrobials cannot be stated with confidence, because antibiotic-specific attack rates for induction of PMC in comparable groups of patients have not been determined. However, most cases of

PMC reported within the past two decades have been related to the use of ampicillin, clindamycin, lincomycin, or one of the cephalosporins.[1]

High rates of PMC have been reported from some hospitals. This is not surprising, as *C. difficile* can be acquired nosocomially, transmitted via the hands of personnel, by direct contact with patients who are carriers of the organism, or by contact with contaminated surfaces or objects.[9] *C. difficile* has been isolated from the hands of hospital personnel caring for colonized patients, especially those with diarrhea. Spores of *C. difficile* have been found in abundance in the environment of patients who are carriers, especially when they have diarrhea, and have been shown to persist on fomites and surfaces in hospitals for long periods (i.e., up to 5 months). Antibiotic-treated hamsters given only two viable *C. difficile* colony-forming organisms by nasogastric tube have developed lethal enterocolitis. Spores are resistant to acid and bile, and even a few of them may be enough to colonize the gastrointestinal tract of an antibiotic-treated person. Person-to-person cross-infection related transmission on hands is probably the most important way the organism is spread in hospitals, but other mechanisms may also be significant. When hospital personnel are in contact with patients with PMC, precautions such as hand washing, use of gloves, and enteral isolation precautions designed to prevent transmission are worthwhile.

Prophylaxis with metronidazole or vancomycin is only temporarily effective (if at all) in preventing transmission of the organism to patients and is not recommended. To prevent transmission of *C. difficile* by instruments inserted into the gastrointestinal tract, they should be thoroughly cleaned after use and disinfected with sodium hypochlorite (1600 ppm), glutaraldehyde, or ethylene oxide. Although vegetative forms of the organism are easily killed by most disinfectants commonly used in hospitals, spores are much more resistant. Careful hand washing before and after contact with patients, especially those with diarrhea or PMC, is recommended for control of outbreaks. Enteral or stool precautions and use of gloves when handling stools or other contaminated materials are also recommended.[10] Reports of patients with PMC who had received no antibiotic therapy (mostly in the preantibiotic era) suggest that dietary changes, anesthesia, surgery on the intestinal tract, changes in bowel motility, uremia, and various medications (especially cancer chemotherapeutic agents) may also be important in precipitating the disease, probably by producing changes in the bowel flora similar to those produced by antibiotics.[11]

C. difficile does not produce colitis by invasion of tissues; in fact, it is rarely invasive, except occasionally in neutropenic patients or after injury to the colon. Colitis results from toxin production *within* the intestinal lumen. Isolates from patients with colitis produce two or more toxins. About 25% of *C. difficile* isolates are nontoxigenic, and these isolates do not cause colitis or diarrhea. The most important toxins of *C. difficile* are toxin A (the enterotoxin) and toxin B (the cytotoxin).[12, 13] These toxins attack the membranes and microfilaments of the mucosa, producing cytoplasmic contraction, hemorrhage, necrosis, inflammation, and loss of protein into the lumen. Toxin B also interferes with mucosal protein synthesis, and toxin A also stimulates granulocyte chemotaxis. Isolates producing toxin A or B almost invariably produce the other toxin as well, but not necessarily to the same degree, which may account for some variation in the manifestations and severity of the illness in different patients. The titer of toxin B detected in individual patient's stools does not correlate well with the severity of their illness, although when patients are grouped, higher titers of toxin B tend to be associated with more severe disease. The lack of a simple quantitative assay for toxin A has hampered study of the relation between its titers in stools and disease severity. Other toxins of *C. difficile* increase intestinal myoelectric responses and peristalsis, but their clinical importance in causation of diarrhea of abdominal pain has not been established.

When patients undergo colonoscopy, diarrhea caused by *C. difficile* has usually been associated with demonstrable colitis, although sometimes the lesions are minimal and easily overlooked. Biopsy of minor lesions characterized simply by erythema and friability may reveal PMC.

Paradoxically, healthy newborns may be colonized with toxigenic *C. difficile* and may also have large amounts of both toxin A and B in their stools. Various mechanisms have been proposed to account for the apparent resistance of the intestines of newborns to the adverse effects of these toxins. The most attractive explanation is that the toxins do not bind to the immature mucosa of newborns because it has few receptors for the toxins. Rates of infant colonization with *C. difficile* as high as 50 to 60% have been reported from some nurseries. The environment appeared to harbor the strains obtained from infants in one study, and it was also the main source of the organism. In another study, transmission of organisms from infant to infant by hands of nursery personnel seemed responsible for most of the subsequent colonization of infants; the introduction into a nursery of a heavily colonized infant from an ICU was followed by spread of that infant's strain to other infants in the nursery.[14] As newborn infants gradually acquire a normal intestinal flora, the rate of isolation of *C. difficile* from their stools declines toward the rates characteristic of adults.

Clinical Manifestations

The symptoms of PMC are highly variable. Reports of PMC in the preantibiotic era consisted mostly of severe cases found at the time of emergency colectomy or autopsy. Using the many tests now available to aid in diagnosis of PMC, mild or self-limited cases are found to be frequent, and severe PMC is infrequent. Not surprisingly, recognition of a severely ill patient may be followed by a heightened index of suspicion for the disease, with subsequent recognition of many mild cases. There may appear then to be an outbreak (actually a pseudoepidemic), which all too commonly results in the unnecessary institution of expensive and cumbersome control measures.

The typical patient with PMC has profuse watery or mucoid, green, foul-smelling stools along with cramping abdominal pain. The illness most often begins 3 to 9 days after starting antibiotic administration. There is wide variation, however, and a few cases have been recognized only a day or two after starting antibiotics. In about 20% of cases, diarrhea does not begin until up to 6 weeks after antibiotic administration has been discontinued. The latter cases are especially likely to go undiagnosed initially. The diarrheal stools often contain small amounts of blood but are rarely grossly bloody unless the patient has a coagulopathy. Increased numbers of leukocytes are found in stained smears of stools from 50% of patients with AAC; finding them suggests colitis but is not specific for *C. difficile*. In a patient with antibiotic-associated diarrhea beginning in the hospital who has a positive test result for fecal leukocytes, AAC is probably present. However, a negative test result for fecal leukocytes does not rule out AAC. The test for fecal leukocytes is nonspecific, but it is a simple, rapid, and useful screening tool for excluding the diagnosis of benign diarrhea (which is *never* associated with increased numbers of leukocytes in stools). Viewed in this way, many consider it the best initial diagnostic test in patients with antibiotic-associated diarrhea. It is easily performed. Although clostridia are rarely prominent in stained smears of diarrheal stools from patients with AAC, staphylococci may occasionally be abundant, which then suggests both the diagnosis of staphylococcal enterocolitis and initial therapy with oral vancomycin or bacitracin, *not* metronidazole.

High fever (103 to 105°F), marked crampy abdominal pain and tenderness, a peripheral leukocyte count as high as 35,000 to 50,000/mm³, and hypoalbuminemia are common with PMC and point strongly to the diagnosis of colitis rather than benign or simple diarrhea. Sometimes patients with AAC have little or no diarrhea, but an acute abdomen with localized abdominal pain or toxic megacolon, colonic perforation, or peritonitis.[6] These patients may have their disease restricted to the cecum and proximal colon, and they often pursue a fulminant course.

The clinical picture may be confused with that of Ogilvie's syndrome, or pseudo-obstruction of the colon.[15] AAC was in fact associated with colonic pseudo-obstruction in two reported cases. This severe form of the disease with little or no diarrhea appears to be relatively frequent in women given prophylactic antibiotics at the time of a cesarean section.[16] The altered colonic motility of pregnancy along with use of morphine or other opiates for postoperative pain is contributory to the development of toxic dilatation without diarrhea. Unfortunately, stool studies for the presence of *C. difficile* or its toxins usually take too long to be of much use in patients with an acute surgical abdomen. This atypical, nondiarrheal form of the illness is difficult to diagnose unless colonoscopy is performed, or unless it is strongly suggested by an abnormal [33]In scan or an abnormal computed tomographic (CT) scan of the abdomen.[17, 18] The CT scan is useful and may show distention and thickening of the wall of the colon, along with pericolonic inflammation and peritonitis (Figs. 41–1 and 41–2). The presence of concomitant toxic megacolon and/or ileus greatly interferes with effective oral antibiotic therapy of colitis, and many of these patients require emergency colectomy.

Some patients with leukemia or granulocytopenia who are receiving antibiotics or antineoplastic chemotherapy have ileocecitis or typhlitis similar to the disease process occasion-

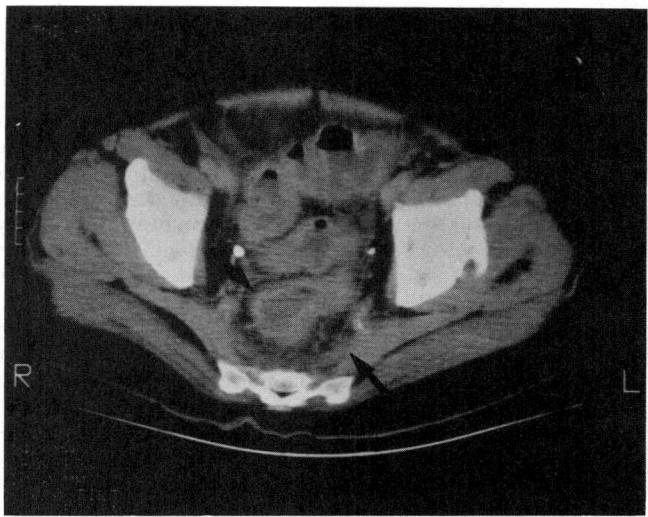

Figure 41–2. CT scan at another level of patient with postoperative PMC described in Figure 41–1. Arrow on left points to thickening of the rectal mucosa. Arrow on right points to edema and inflammation in the perirectal soft tissues.

ally caused by *C. difficile*.[11] Some but not all of these are caused by *C. difficile*. A staphylococcal cause should be suspected when there is involvement primarily of the distal ileum or when results of tests for *C. difficile* are negative. In these patients, oral vancomycin is preferred in treatment, as metronidazole has no antistaphylococcal activity. In some patients, diarrhea attributed erroneously to cancer chemotherapeutic agents has actually been caused by *C. difficile* colitis, and treatment with vancomycin or metronidazole has stopped the diarrhea and permitted continuation of antineoplastic chemotherapy.[11]

If *C. difficile* colitis goes unrecognized and untreated despite severe diarrhea, the outcome may be fatal. Mortality rates of 10 to 20% have been reported in untreated elderly or chronically debilitated patients with PMC. Hypovolemic shock, hypoproteinemia, edema, cecal perforation, secondary sepsis, and hemorrhage are the most serious complications of severe PMC.

C. difficile colitis can occur in patients with chronic inflammatory bowel diseases and can cause symptoms that may be erroneously interpreted as an acute exacerbation of the underlying disease. This presentation may begin during or several weeks after treatment with antibiotics, which then makes PMC difficult to think of and, therefore, to diagnose. This is an important problem in patients admitted to ICUs because of chronic inflammatory bowel disease or its complications.

As mentioned earlier, *C. difficile* is an important cause of the ischemic enterocolitis that complicates Hirschsprung's disease in infants and young children.[15] When such patients show signs of colitis, even if they have not recently received antibiotics, *C. difficile* should be suspected and treatment with oral vancomycin should be begun promptly after appropriate diagnostic tests have been ordered or results obtained.

Clinical Diagnosis

When patients, especially those in ICUs, with antibiotic-associated diarrhea have unexplained high fever, leukocytosis, severe abdominal pain and tenderness, and large numbers of leukocytes in their stools, benign diarrhea is safely ruled out, and *C. difficile* colitis is probably present.

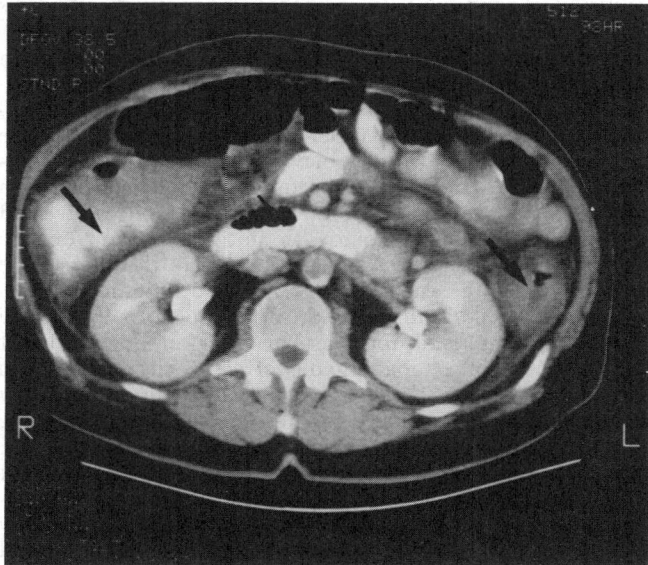

Figure 41–1. CT scan of abdomen in an elderly neurosurgical patient with fever and diarrhea postoperatively. Stools were positive for *C. difficile* cytotoxin. Arrow on left indicates irregularly thickened cecal mucosa. Arrow on right indicates lumenal narrowing, mucosal thickening, and edema of the descending colon.

Almost all of these patients should be treated promptly with antibiotics specific for *C. difficile* after appropriate diagnostic testing. The diagnosis of PMC is most rapidly and certainly established in mild as well as severe cases by performing endoscopy, which detects inflammation (colitis) and/or pseudomembranous lesions and is an especially useful diagnostic measure in patients in ICUs. The nodules and plaques characteristic of *C. difficile* colitis are usually most numerous in the distal colon, the sigmoid, and the rectum, where they are easily detected by sigmoidoscopy. In about 10% of cases of PMC, lesions are present only in the cecum or the transverse colon.[19] This form of the illness is difficult to detect without performing colonoscopy or a CT scan and is often, but not always, mild. One problem is that many physicians prefer not to perform colonoscopy or a CT scan in patients with a mild illness. This presentation is common when patients with colitis have an acute abdomen or neutropenic typhlitis. Right-sided colonic disease should be suspected when patients with antibiotic-associated diarrhea and toxin-positive stools have no lesions visualized during proctosigmoidoscopy. It should be remembered that the lesions of *C. difficile* colitis may be atypical and consist grossly only of edema, hyperemia, and friability. Such lesions are worthy of biopsy, which may reveal colitis with a minute pseudomembrane. Although a diarrheal illness without colitis and caused by *C. difficile* has been postulated, such has not been proved conclusively, because normal colonoscopic findings plus normal biopsy results for all minor lesions would be required for its documentation. Fever, leukocytosis, and fecal leukocytes strongly suggest that colitis is present. Four types of pseudomembranous lesions are recognized: (1) large adherent pseudomembranes; (2) small (2- to 4-mm) nodular or plaque-like elevated lesions; (3) small faint, flat, circular or ring-like whitish yellow lesions on an erythematous background; and (4) pseudomembranes that are not seen by the naked eye but are visualized in biopsy specimens by using microscopy. Colonic biopsy is not needed when typical gross lesions are seen, but biopsies may aid in diagnosis of clostridial colitis when lesions are atypical or when so-called nonspecific colitis is visualized, because a biopsy may reveal pseudomembranes that suggest *C. difficile* as the etiologic agent.

In the differential diagnosis of nonspecific colitis associated with antibiotic usage beginning outside of the hospital, it is important also to consider Crohn's disease, idiopathic ulcerative colitis, ischemic colitis, gold-induced colitis, chemical colitis, and infection with other intestinal pathogens such as *S. aureus*, *C. perfringens* type C, *Salmonella*, *Edwardsiella*, *Shigella*, *E. coli* (especially the O157:H7 serotype if the colitis is hemorrhagic), *P. shigelloides*, *E. histolytica*, *Campylobacter*, *Yersinia*, *Strongyloides*, cytomegalovirus, and *L. monocytogenes*. Other organisms that cause diarrhea, usually without colitis, include enterotoxigenic *E. coli*, *Bacillus cereus*, *Aeromonas*, *Vibrio*, other Enterobacteriaceae, *Pseudomonas*, *Candida*, and human immunodeficiency virus. When a patient develops diarrhea after admission to the hospital and after antibiotics have been given, stool cultures for these pathogens are probably not indicated unless results of tests for *C. difficile* are normal and the diarrhea is severe and persistent.

Air-contrast barium enema studies can show thumbprinting and other signs of PMC in patients with diarrhea, but these findings are not specific and, more important, are often absent in early cases. In addition, barium studies may precipitate toxic megacolon, perforation, or other complications and are therefore best avoided. As mentioned earlier, CT scans may be useful for making the diagnosis of probable PMC rapidly and noninvasively.

Laboratory Diagnosis

The laboratory tests most useful for aiding in diagnosis of *C. difficile* colitis include stool cultures for *C. difficile* and tests on stools for the presence of *C. difficile* toxins. A search for fecal leukocytes is a simple screening test, because a positive test result excludes the benign form of antibiotic diarrhea. However, no more than 50% of patients with *C. difficile* colitis have positive fecal leukocyte test results.

Anaerobic incubation of stools cultured on selective media (such as CCFA, which contains cefoxitin and cycloserine to inhibit most other stool organisms) can detect as few as 100 colony-forming units of *C. difficile* per gram of stool, and patients with active colitis usually carry many more organisms than that. Few fecal organisms that closely resemble *C. difficile* grow on CCFA.[7] Rare isolates of *C. difficile* may fail to grow on CCFA. Using CCFA, it is possible to isolate and identify *C. difficile* presumptively in just a few days. A toxin test done using a colony transferred from CCFA to a cell culture with a toothpick has been used for rapid identification of *C. difficile*. Almost all patients with PMC are culture-positive if their stools are processed properly, but vegetative forms of the organism are easily killed by exposure to air or other adverse conditions. Spores are hardier but less numerous and therefore harder to detect. Asymptomatic carriers may have only a few spores per gram of stool. For detection of asymptomatic stool carriers, CCFA containing highly purified sodium taurocholate or broth cultures after heat shock are needed.[8]

The isolation of *C. difficile* from stools of a patient with diarrhea does not prove that the patient has colitis caused by *C. difficile*. There are several reasons for this. First, about 25% of isolates of *C. difficile* from humans are nontoxigenic and also nonpathogenic. Second, 3% or more of healthy adults are asymptomatic carriers of the organism, and in hospitals where PMC is frequent, 15 to 30% (or more) of asymptomatic adults treated with antibiotics have been found to be carriers. Nevertheless, a positive culture may be useful in making management decisions. For example, because the cytotoxin is both heat and acid labile, stools from patients with PMC may be (falsely) toxin-negative (but culture-positive) if the specimen is not transported to the laboratory under ideal conditions. In my hospital, about 85% of adults with antibiotic-associated diarrhea and positive stool cultures for *C. difficile* had colitis. Cultures can also be useful in detecting post-treatment carriers, who appear to be at increased risk for relapse. However, they are not done routinely, because there is as yet no effective treatment of the carrier state. Stool cultures may be useful during an outbreak, when carriers may be sequestered or grouped as a cohort in an attempt to interrupt transmission, or treated with vancomycin or metronidazole until discharge from the hospital to prevent spread of the organism to others. The efficacy of such measures has not been documented.

Tests to detect *C. difficile* toxin B in stools usually employ monolayer cultures of fibroblasts or other cell lines to detect its characteristic cytopathogenic effect. Cell cultures are difficult to maintain, and the test is expensive and not readily available in most hospitals. Furthermore, in actual practice, cytotoxin assays usually require a day or two for completion. A parallel test to determine whether antitoxin will prevent the cytopathogenic effect is needed for proving the specificity of the cytopathogenic effect. Nonspecific cytotoxicty may mask the presence of toxin B unless stool filtrates are diluted to overcome nonspecific cytotoxicity. Transport of specimens to reference laboratories (with or without the use of Dry Ice or refrigeration) can result in false-negative toxin test results, as the toxin is both heat and acid pH labile. Various medications (such as lactulose) can inactivate toxin B. Staphylococcal enterotoxins produce cytopathic effects in Walker rat carcinoma cell cultures (as do *C. difficile* toxins), but staphylococcal toxins are not neutralized by *C. difficile* antitoxin and are not cytopathic in most of the fibroblast monolayers used to detect *C. difficile* toxins. These differences may be useful in diagnosis of staphylococcal enterocolitis (as are stool cultures). Finally, *C. difficile* toxin B is cytopathic in Vero cells, which are often used to detect *Shigella* and *E. coli* toxins causing hemorrhagic colitis and/or the hemolytic-uremic syndrome.[20]

Demonstration of the presence of *C. difficile* cytotoxin B in stools of adults is helpful to clinicians but does not prove beyond doubt that the patient with diarrhea has colitis. Occasional asymptomatic adults (and many colonized infants) may have the toxin in stools and yet remain asymptomatic. However, a good test for the presence of toxin B is at present the best laboratory aid in diagnosis of PMC. At least 95% of adults with antibiotic-associated diarrhea and *C. difficile* cytotoxin–positive stools have documentable colitis. When proctosigmoidoscopy performed on patients with toxin B titers greater than 1:10 is normal, it is likely that they have colitis at a proximal site, such as the cecum, or mild so-called nonspecific colitis without pseudomembranes. Colonoscopy, CT scans, or radionuclide scans using indium-labeled leukocytes may be helpful in detecting and localizing colitis in these patients.[17, 19]

Both toxins A and B produced by *C. difficile* can almost always be found in stools of patients with PMC. Until recently, toxin A has required a rodent bioassay for its reliable detection; this is cumbersome, and consequently, the test was rarely performed outside of research laboratories. Enzyme-linked immunosorbent assays or radioimmunoassays for toxin A have been developed. Some of them may be rapid, reliable, and simple, but caution with them is indicated until more studies are reported. Fortunately, both toxins A and B are present in stools of patients with colitis. Therefore, a positive toxin B assay indicates that the stool is positive for toxin A as well, and vice versa. Thus, the test for toxin B is a reliable surrogate test for toxin A.[13]

C. difficile produces several other soluble antigenic substances in addition to toxins A and B.[13] One of these is a protein that is immunologically similar to proteins produced by other microbial species. This creates a problem with respect to some of the newer rapid immunologic tests for *C. difficile* toxins. Counterimmunoelectrophoresis has been used as a rapid method for detection of toxin B in fecal extracts. Because this test uses nonspecific antisera, it may detect these other antigens and is therefore subject to frequent false-positive results, especially with toxin-negative isolates of *C. difficile*. False-negative results also occur. It is no longer used often.

A rapid and inexpensive latex agglutination test is now widely used for the diagnosis of colitis caused by *C. difficile*. The test takes less than an hour, is inexpensive, and can be done in most hospital laboratories. Originally thought to detect toxin A, it is now known to actually detect an antigen that is distinct from toxin A and of no apparent pathogenetic significance. Unfortunately, nontoxigenic isolates of *C. difficile* also produce this antigen. They account for up to 25% of all clinical isolates, and they seem to be particularly common in newborns. Several other species of organisms found in the intestinal tract also produce a cross-reactive antigen. Consequently, both false-negative and false-positive latex agglutination results occur; the latter are more common. The sensitivity and specificity of the latex agglutination test have been estimated at about 90%, but its positive predictive value ranged from a low of 17% (when the prevalence of the disease was low) to a high of 95% (when

the prevalence was high), with a mean of about 50%. In my laboratory, there was overall agreement between the toxin B and the latex agglutination results about 90% of the time. However, when specimens positive in either the toxin B test or in the latex agglutination test were analyzed, there was agreement in my laboratory between them in only 50% of specimens. Thus, the clinical significance of a positive latex agglutination test result is roughly equivalent to that of a positive culture for *C. difficile*. As compared with cultures, it is useful primarily as a rapid, inexpensive screening test to aid in management. The latex agglutination test is not sensitive enough for reliably detecting asymptomatic carriers.

Treatment of *Clostridium difficile* Colitis

Antibiotics

Oral antimicrobials are always preferred for treatment of AAC, being more reliable by far than parenteral therapy. This is especially important to note in ICUs, where patients are always seriously ill even when they do not have colitis. Because susceptibility tests on *C. difficile* isolates are rarely performed as a guide to treatment of individual patients, treatment is empirical and based on published data from study of large numbers of isolates. In critically ill patients, empirical therapy should be begun while awaiting results of tests designed to implicate *C. difficile*, especially if the patient is elderly, debilitated, or likely to have a severe form of the disease. Empirical therapy is designed to prevent hypovolemia, hypoproteinemia, edema, toxic colonic dilatation, colonic perforation, and other complications. Vancomycin or metronidazole is recommended for empirical therapy, but vancomycin given orally is preferred in ICUs. *C. difficile* is always susceptible to vancomycin, usually susceptible to metronidazole and rifampin, and often susceptible to bacitracin.[16] The minimal inhibitory concentration of these antimicrobials for most isolates of *C. difficile* is about 5 mg/L or less. Thus, isolates are susceptible at the high concentrations found in stools when therapy is administered orally. Isolates resistant to metronidazole and bacitracin have been reported, but vancomycin-resistant isolates have not. This is the main reason why vancomycin is the drug of choice for critically ill patients. Because resistance to rifampin can develop rapidly, this drug should not be used alone in treatment of AAC. Although *C. difficile* is also often susceptible to tetracycline, erythromycin, ampicillin, cefamandole, and cefazolin, none of these have been useful in treatment of the disease.

Not all patients with AAC need to be treated with specific antimicrobials. When patients have only mild or moderately severe diarrhea, it may be sufficient to discontinue administration of the precipitating antibiotic and to give supportive therapy with fluid and electrolyte replacement. If the patient improves within a few days, supportive therapy can be continued and the diarrhea usually subsides completely within 7 to 10 days. If not, specific antibiotic therapy should be given. Antibiotics need not be prolonged for more than 7 to 10 days in most cases after improvement. To facilitate return of the normal fecal flora and colonization resistance, the duration of antibiotic treatment should be *short* rather than long. Both vancomycin and metronidazole can induce PMC in humans and hamsters; they do this by altering the fecal flora in a way that favors overgrowth by *C. difficile*. If the inducing antibiotic is needed and *must* be continued during treatment of AAC, specific oral antimicrobial treatment with vancomycin or metronidazole as well as supportive therapy should be started *promptly*, even if the symptoms of colitis are mild. All patients suspected of having PMC who have high fever, marked leukocytosis, profuse diarrhea, severe abdominal pain, and signs of peritoneal inflammation should be treated promptly with oral vancomycin (or metronidazole), as should patients who are severely ill, elderly, toxic, debilitated, or unresponsive to supportive therapy or cholestyramine. Discontinuation of administration of the inducing antibiotic after recognition of colitis is probably not essential if specific therapy for AAC is given. The antibacterial effects of vancomycin on C. *difficile* in vitro are not antagonized by other antimicrobials, and vancomycin can stop multiplication and toxin production by the organism in humans despite continuation of antimicrobials favoring the overgrowth of C. *difficile*. Switching to an alternative antibiotic regimen in patients treated with oral vancomycin has not been appreciably harmful, even though many of the antibiotics chosen as alternatives were capable of inducing AAC. Nonetheless, it is a good idea to change to another appropriate antimicrobial regimen for treating the original infection when possible, if only for medicolegal reasons.

Vancomycin. Vancomycin given orally is relatively expensive (compared with metronidazole) but much less so than in the past. Most experts consider it the treatment of choice for severe AAC. The efficacy of vancomycin has been so well documented in so many parts of the world that it must be considered the most reliable treatment for the disease.[21-24] No isolates of C. *difficile* have been shown resistant to it; furthermore, it is the drug of choice for oral therapy for the rare cases of staphylococcal enterocolitis. Metronidazole and bacitracin are alternatives if the illness is mild or moderately severe or when vancomycin is unavailable or not tolerated. Vancomycin was compared with metronidazole or bacitracin in a few studies (see later) and appeared at least as effective as they were in the treatment of AAC.

C. *difficile* isolates are almost always susceptible to vancomycin at concentrations of less than 5 mg/L, and no isolate has ever been identified that necessitated more than 16 mg/L. Because vancomycin is poorly absorbed systemically when it is given orally, it is relatively nontoxic and concentrations far exceeding 16 mg/L are easily achieved in stools. When a dose of 500 mg is given orally four times per day, stool concentrations have averaged 2000 mg/L or more; when 125 mg is given four times daily, concentrations have been in the range of 300 to 1000 mg/L. All of these are far above the necessary concentrations. Even patients with profuse diarrhea achieve adequate concentrations of vancomycin in stools with these regimens. Although vancomycin is poorly absorbed from the gastrointestinal tract even in the presence of colitis, small amounts are absorbed, and it has been detected in low concentrations in the urine of patients with PMC who were treated orally. Vancomycin is usually undetectable in serum during oral treatment of colitis, but concentrations ranging from 5 to 30 mg/L (therapeutic serum concentrations) have been reported, usually in patients with severely impaired renal function. Serum levels should be monitored in such patients. Toxic serum concentrations have never been reported with oral therapy. Therefore, it is not surprising that systemic side effects have been rare or nonexistent after oral use of vancomycin, even in patients with an inflamed colonic mucosa.

When oral vancomycin was evaluated in one controlled study, it was found to be significantly better than placebo for treatment of C. *difficile* toxin–positive postoperative diarrhea.[22] The dose used was usually 125 mg every 6 hours for 5 days. As expected, vancomycin-treated patients who had C. *difficile*–negative antibiotic-associated diarrhea fared no better than did placebo-treated patients. In uncontrolled studies, many additional patients with C. *difficile* colitis have been treated with oral vancomycin. Their clinical responses almost invariably were excellent unless the disease was far

advanced when treatment was begun or unless oral therapy was not possible because of ileus or vomiting (but vomiting is rarely caused by PMC). Good antibacterial activity within colonic tissues does not appear necessary for success in treatment of PMC; instead, cessation of toxin production within the lumen or at the mucosal surface seems sufficient and indeed essential. Thus, C. *difficile* colitis should be considered a colonic intoxication more than an infection.

Patients treated with oral vancomycin usually show improvement in fever, diarrhea, abdominal cramps, and malaise within 48 to 72 hours, and toxin titers in stools begin to decline shortly after treatment is begun. Diarrhea and fever may require a week or two to resolve completely, especially if the patient is severely ill and has extensive lesions. Treatment should continue for at least 7 to 10 days but is rarely needed for more than 14 days. Some investigators believe that therapy should not be discontinued until the toxins are no longer detectable in stools. Routine tests to detect toxin B in stools of patients who are doing well are generally believed unnecessary and are rarely done. Stools often (25%) remain culture-positive for C. *difficile* after successful treatment, but because there is no reliable treatment of the asymptomatic carrier state, routine cultures for detecting C. *difficile* in stools of asymptomatic patients are unnecessary.

The major disadvantages of oral treatment with vancomycin are its expense ($8 to $16 or more per day), its short supply in some parts of the world, and its bitter taste. A relatively inexpensive capsule (pulvule) form of vancomycin for oral use has been made available in the United States. It is well tolerated and appears as efficacious as the powder used to prepare solutions of vancomycin. If transit time is rapid, some clinicians worry that the capsule may not dissolve completely before its excretion in the diarrheal stool, and the liquid preparation given by mouth in 500-mg doses is therefore preferred for patients with impending ileus.

In about 50 patients entered into a randomized study of treatment with two different doses of vancomycin, no statistically significant differences were found in the overall clinical or bacteriologic responses of those treated with oral vancomycin in dosages of either 125 or 500 mg every 6 hours.[23] Although diarrhea in ill patients ceased slightly sooner on the average with the higher dose, the difference was clinically and statistically insignificant. The 125 mg per dose regimen is considerably less expensive and is therefore preferable, except for treatment of extremely ill patients or those with vomiting, impending ileus, or megacolon. For treatment of infants and children with colitis, a dose of 500 mg/1.73 m² every 6 hours orally has been recommended. Because the diagnosis of C. *difficile* colitis is extremely difficult to establish in infants, a therapeutic trial with vancomycin is often used to confirm the diagnosis in infants with protracted diarrhea after antibiotic therapy. Metronidazole should probably not be used for treatment of infants or pregnant women because of its toxic potential.

Vancomycin is the drug of choice for treatment of staphylococcal enterocolitis, which may be suspected when smears of stools show gram-positive cocci and leukocytes. A dosage of 500 mg four times per day is preferred in this setting. The possibility of staphylococcal enterocolitis is another advantage of vancomycin over metronidazole for treatment of PMC.

Patients who are unable to take vancomycin orally may be given it via a nasogastric tube (along with intermittent suction if needed), but patients with ileus still may not achieve adequate concentrations of vancomycin within the colonic lumen, where it is needed to stop toxin production. These patients tend to be admitted to ICUs and pose a formidable therapeutic problem; most investigators believe that there is no completely reliable parenteral regimen for treatment of

PMC. When healthy adults are given intravenous vancomycin, their subsequent stool concentrations range from 0 to 100 mg/L, and most patients treated parenterally for PMC have little or no vancomycin in stools unless they are bleeding from colonic lesions. Thus, most patients with colitis treated intravenously with vancomycin do not achieve therapeutic concentrations within the bowel lumen. Although a few patients with colitis appear to have responded to intravenous vancomycin, other seriously ill patients have failed to respond.[25] Therefore, reliance on intravenous vancomycin (or any other antimicrobial given intravenously) for treatment of AAC, to the exclusion of oral therapy, is *not* recommended.

When parenteral therapy is essential or unavoidable (as in patients with paralytic ileus), I recommend treatment with *both* intravenous vancomycin and intravenous metronidazole (see later), supplemented by vancomycin given via nasogastric tube or a long intestinal tube passed to the ileocecal valve (500 mg four times per day for adults), or into ileostomies, into colostomies, or by enema. Oral metronidazole plays no role in this setting, because if small amounts pass down the intestinal tract, they are probably completely absorbed systemically from the small intestine, and none reaches the colon. Passage under fluoroscopic control of a long intestinal tube to the distal ileum or through the ileocecal valve has been shown to be possible within a few hours in many patients and may permit perfusion of the colon with vancomycin solutions in a concentration of 500 to 1000 mg/L. This has been successful therapy for a few patients with PMC and ileus. The same concentrations may be used for vancomycin enemas or for rectal or colonoscopic perfusion. It has been suggested that intravenous erythromycin be given, not because of its antibacterial activity, but because it stimulates peristalsis.

Metronidazole. This inexpensive antimicrobial is usually active against *C. difficile*, and it is effective in treatment of most patients with AAC.[24] However, metronidazole is inactive against staphylococci and thus is of no value in treatment of the rare case of staphylococcal enterocolitis. In a randomized comparative study of treatment of diarrhea and/or colitis in adult men, oral metronidazole (250 mg every 6 hours) was associated with a cure rate (within 7 days) of 92%, whereas the rate was 100% with oral vancomycin (500 mg every 6 hours). Although this difference was not statistically significant, it may be clinically significant. Patients who failed to respond to metronidazole were switched to vancomycin and responded to it. Metronidazole was well tolerated, significantly less expensive than vancomycin, and associated with about the same rate of post-treatment carriage, relapse, and side effects (which were uncommon). The usual oral dose of metronidazole for colitis is 500 to 750 mg three times daily or 250 mg four times daily for 7 to 10 days. This drug is so well absorbed from the small intestine that concern has been raised about whether the concentrations achieved within the colonic lumen are adequate in all patients, especially when they are seriously ill. Fortunately, systemic absorption of metronidazole is probably impaired when patients have diarrhea. However, 5 to 10% of patients with PMC have been reported to fail to respond to metronidazole.[24, 26] Metronidazole also has a number of potentially serious side effects, and it is not recommended for use in pregnant women or in children. Several cases of colitis after treatment with oral or parenteral metronidazole have been reported, at least one of them with a metronidazole-resistant organism.[27] Therefore, metronidazole is recommended only for patients who are mildly or moderately ill with AAC.

Studies in animals and humans suggested that metronidazole given intravenously may be transported across the colonic mucosa into the lumen of the bowel.[28–30] They have encouraged some clinicians to use intravenous metronidazole for treatment of patients with AAC who have ileus or who are too ill to be treated via the oral route. The usual intravenous dose was 500 mg every 6 to 8 hours. These brief studies are best considered preliminary and unconfirmed. It is true that metronidazole given intravenously has been detected in stools of patients and in intestinal tissues of animals. However, it is possible that excretion of metronidazole via the hepatobiliary route was responsible for the drug's reaching the intestinal lumen and for the clinical improvement noted in these patients, most of whom apparently did not have ileus or impaired intestinal motility. Furthermore, failure of intravenous metronidazole to treat AAC successfully has been reported at least twice.[31, 32] Evidence supporting the transport of metronidazole across the mucosa and into the colonic lumen of humans in concentrations adequate to treat severe PMC is not yet convincing. Speculation that metronidazole given intravenously may get into the colon in some patients because of bleeding into the colon associated with PMC is not reassuring to those dealing with a critically ill patient. In my opinion, *neither* intravenous metronidazole nor vancomycin is reliably effective in treatment of severe PMC. If they must be used, I recommend giving both of them together; there is no reason to worry about antagonism between them.

Because no form of parenteral therapy has yet proved reliable in treatment of AAC, parenteral therapy should be used only when oral therapy is not practical, and even then only to supplement other therapy or to tide the patient over until a surgical attack on the disease can be done. In such patients, both metronidazole and vancomycin may be given intravenously. Vancomycin (500 mg four times per day for adults) should also be given via nasogastric tube or a long intestinal tube (with intermittent clamping if suction is needed), and vancomycin can also be given by enema or by direct instillation through an ileostomy or a colostomy in concentrations ranging from 500 to 1000 mg/L. This is far more than is needed for inhibition of all isolates of *C. difficile* and is comparable to those concentrations achieved when the drug is given orally to treat AAC. Serum concentrations should be monitored when vancomycin is given in these multiple ways, especially in patients with renal failure. Many of these patients require an emergent colectomy as a lifesaving measure.

Teicoplanin and Daptomycin. Teicoplanin is a glycopeptide that resembles vancomycin and is active against *C. difficile*. Although it has been used successfully in an oral dose of 200 mg two or three times per day in therapy of patients with PMC, it does not appear to have any advantages over vancomycin.[33] Daptomycin is a lipopeptide resembling vancomycin. Although active against most strains of *C. difficile*, it has not yet been used in treatment of PMC.

Bacitracin. Several groups of investigators reported that patients with PMC could be treated successfully with oral bacitracin, and there is little doubt that bacitracin can be an effective alternative to vancomycin and metronidazole.[34–36] The oral dosage used most often was 25,000 U (about 500 mg) four times per day for 7 to 19 days. The response to bacitracin was somewhat slower and less certain than that to vancomycin; furthermore, carriage rates and stool toxin titers declined less rapidly and less often than with vancomycin. Some patients relapsed after bacitracin administration and were then treated successfully with vancomycin. Most isolates of *C. difficile* are susceptible to bacitracin, but some require more than 20 U/mL (about 1000 mg/L) for inhibition.[16] These concentrations may indicate resistance, because they may not be achieved in the stools of every patient with diarrhea. Bacitracin has an extremely bitter taste and is nauseating. In addition, some absorption of bacitracin may occur when it is given orally. The possibility of systemic toxicity of bacitracin in patients with an inflamed intestinal mucosa, as well as the frequency of relapse, indicates that it needs additional evaluation for use in PMC. Furthermore, bacitracin for oral administration is often unavailable and it is now as expensive as vancomycin. However, like vancomycin, it is also active against staphylococci. Bacitracin seems to be a useful alternative to vanocomycin or metronidazole but is not a primary treatment for the disease.

Other Antibiotics. Fusidic acid is highly active against *C. difficile* and staphylococci; it has been used successfully for the oral treatment of 15 patients with AAC. Tetracycline and erythromycin have been used occasionally in treatment of AAC of unknown cause, but many isolates of *C. difficile* are resistant to them and their use is not recommended. Fluoroquinolone antimicrobials such as ciprofloxacin and norfloxacin are not considered to have good anaerobic antibacterial activity, because when *C. difficile* isolates were tested (using *serum* concentration breakpoints) they were resistant. However, when these antimicrobials are given orally, much higher concentrations than those used in ordinary susceptibility tests are found in stools, with levels ranging from 100 to 900 mg/L. *C. difficile* is usually susceptible to ciprofloxacin and norfloxacin at these high concentrations. Thus, is it possible that, when used for empirical treatment of bacterial diarrhea, they may have some beneficial effects in treatment of PMC. Furthermore, it has been suggested that ciprofloxacin administered intravenously may provide high fecal concentrations as a result of its transport across the colonic mucosa and that intravenous ciprofloxacin might be useful in treatment of patients with ileus and AAC. However, much more evidence needs to be brought forth before the administration of fluoroquinolones by any route can be recommended for treatment of antibiotic-associated diarrhea and colitis.

Cholestyramine and Colestipol

These anion-exchange–binding resins were used in treatment of PMC before the cause of the disease was known. Their use was based on speculation that secretory bile acids might be responsible for antibiotic-associated diarrhea or colitis. Subsequent studies suggested that secretory bile acids were an unlikely cause of antibiotic-associated diarrhea, and attention turned to other causes, such as *C. difficile*. Cholestyramine binds *C. difficile* toxin B, which is its presumed mechanism of beneficial action in PMC. It has no demonstrable inhibitory effects on *C. difficile,* and there is no proof as yet that it can bind toxin A. Because many patients with AAC respond slowly or not at all to cholestyramine and often require a change to oral treatment with antibiotics, it is usually reserved for patients with a mild illness. The usual oral dose of cholestyramine for treatment of PMC in adults is 4 g three or four times per day. Obstipation is the most serious side effect of these anion-binding resins. They can also bind vancomycin, so the simultaneous use of cholestyramine and low doses of vancomycin should be avoided. Anecdotal case reports suggested that cholestyramine may be useful when given for a short period after long courses of antibiotic therapy for multiple relapses of *C. difficile* colitis have been completed, but this has not been substantiated in controlled studies.

Antidiarrheal Agents

Antiperistaltic agents should be avoided in patients with AAC.[36, 37] This statement has important implications for patients in ICUs. Although these agents often provide symptomatic relief of diarrhea, they may do this simply by causing pooling of toxin-laden fluid within the intestinal lumen. Diphenoxylate with atropine (Lomotil) is especially dangerous in infants because of this and other side effects. The condition of some patients with AAC became worse after being given antiperistaltic drugs. They may improve the diarrhea but promote more severe damage to the colon because of toxin retention, with toxic dilatation of the colon the possible result. Although there is no scientific proof that these agents are dangerous in adults with colitis, their lack of proven value in the face of possible serious side effects provides no encouragement for their use. The antiperistaltic effects of morphine and related opiates given postoperatively for relief of pain may also decrease the signs of diarrhea that would alert one to the possibility of PMC and may predispose to severe colitis and toxic megacolon.

Corticosteroids

These are of no proven value in PMC. Mortality may be higher in patients who received steroids, but such patients tended to be sicker on the average before treatment with steroids, which were given because of the severity of PMC.

Surgical Measures

Before specific antibiotic therapy was available for AAC, diversion of the fecal stream or resection of the diseased bowel was often necessary. These drastic measures are rarely performed except in life-threatening situations, such as with toxic megacolon or cecal perforation. Sometimes a colostomy or ileostomy is needed to facilitate instillation of vancomycin or metronidazole into the colonic lumen of patients with ileus.

Treatment of Relapse or Recurrence

Although most patients who are post-treatment carriers of *C. difficile* never experience a relapse, more than one episode of colitis has been observed in 10 to 20% of patients treated with vancomycin, metronidazole, or bacitracin. Recurrences occur at about the same rate after all forms of treatment for PMC. Recurrences should not be considered treatment failures if the patient previously responded to specific antibiotic therapy. Recurrences usually respond promptly to retreatment with vancomycin, metronidazole, or bacitracin. Recurrences may be caused either by germination of spores persisting in the colon (relapse) or by reinfection of the permissive colon by organisms from environmental or human contacts. On the basis of typing studies, persistence appears much more common than reinfection, but both can occur. The *C. difficile* carrier state cannot be reliably eradicated with antimicrobials or any other regimen yet available. Most recurrences are spontaneous and occur within a few weeks or months after treatment of the initial episode. Some occur after reinstitution of antibiotics.[38–41]

Little is known about local, humoral, or cellular immune responses to the toxins, the organism, or the disease and about their relationship to recurrences. Serum antibodies to the toxins have been detected in most healthy adults, but only in a minority of patients who recovered from the disease or who experienced recurrences. One of my patients developed neutralizing antibodies to toxin B in serum after eight episodes of colitis. He had no further recurrences, despite the presence of large amounts of toxin in his stools.

Patients who experience relapse may be treated again with oral vancomycin, metronidazole, or bacitracin for only 7 to

10 days or until their diarrhea ceases. Longer courses of therapy are popular but do not appear more efficacious in prevention of recurrences. Indeed, short courses of antibiotics may be preferable, as they may permit more rapid restoration of the normal fecal flora, which is presumed to suppress growth of *C. difficile.*

Although most patients with PMC have only one recurrence, some unfortunate persons have multiple recurrent attacks. No entirely satisfactory way to manage them is known; anecdotal observations and experiences have led to management of them with long courses (4 to 6 weeks) of oral vancomycin, metronidazole, or bacitracin followed by gradual tapering of the dose; by intermittent short periods (5 to 7 days) of treatment alternating with periods without antibiotics (pulsing); or with postantibiotic therapy with cholestyramine to suppress symptoms by binding toxins, presumably while a normal flora is being re-established. Oral vancomycin plus rifampin has also been used for multiple relapses with apparent success in a small uncontrolled study.[38–41]

Theoretically, the best way to prevent relapses is by restoration of the normal flora. Patients with multiple relapses have been treated with oral or rectal administration of organisms designed to suppress *C. difficile* and facilitate restoration of the normal fecal flora. Direct attempts at recolonization of the colon have been done in uncontrolled studies by administering oral lactobacillus preparations, especially as *Lactobacillus* GG,[42] by giving enemas with feces from healthy persons,[43] by giving enemas with mixtures of bacterial isolates obtained from the stools of persons who have recovered from PMC (bacteriotherapy),[44] or by administering orally a nonpathogenic yeast, *Saccharomyces boulardii.*[45, 46] *S. boulardii* given orally was protective in the hamster model of antibiotic-induced enterocolitis and was also shown to significantly reduce the frequency of antibiotic-associated diarrhea in patients. It was also demonstrated that the frequency of *C. difficile*–associated diarrhea after antibiotic administration was reduced from 31% (placebo) to 9.4% with *S. boulardii* administration, but this difference was not statistically significant.[47] *S. boulardii* given by mouth to patients did appear beneficial in preventing relapses in uncontrolled studies.[45] Recolonization attempts using a non-toxigenic strain of *C. difficile* have been effective in the hamster model, and in two patients with relapsing colitis.[46] Results with oral *Lactobacillus* GG or *S. boulardii* in prevention of recurrences have been especially promising and are the subject of controlled studies.

Prevention

It may eventually be possible to immunize patients against the toxins and/or other virulence factors of *C. difficile,* but this is not yet the case. Passive immunization of hamsters with *C. sordellii* antitoxin, which cross-reacts with toxins A and B of *C. difficile,* protected them against clindamycin-induced colitis. This antitoxin is not available for use in humans. Ordinary immune serum globulin does not appear effective in prevention of AAC. Immunization of hamsters with toxoids prepared from toxins A and B protected them from challenge with antibiotics and the organism. However, many experts doubt that there is sufficient clinical need for development of *C. difficile* toxoids for human use. More work is needed with these toxoids; they could be used to immunize all children, high-risk persons, or those experiencing multiple relapses. Prophylaxis with antibiotics such as vancomycin or metronidazole in patients at high risk for AAC is not of proven value, is expensive, and is theoretically undesirable because it may induce susceptibility to intestinal colonization and disease with *C. difficile* or other pathogens

after administration of the drugs is discontinued. It may also encourage development and spread of organisms, other than *C. difficile,* that are resistant to vancomycin or metronidazole. Treatment of hospitalized carriers with oral vancomycin until discharge from a patient unit where there was a high rate of PMC may have been useful (along with environmental decontamination) in terminating a few outbreaks. Use of sodium hypochlorite diluted to 1600 ppm for disinfection of contaminated surfaces has been recommended for control of nosocomial outbreaks. Careful hand washing by staff after contact with affected patients or carriers is also beneficial. Wearing gloves is strongly encouraged when dealing with contaminated surfaces or objects. Bacteriophage-bacteriocin typing systems, as well as immunologic, DNA, protein, or plasmid profile systems for detecting or typing *C. difficile,* have become available, and their use in epidemiologic studies may lead to the development of new or better preventive measures.[48, 49]

STAPHYLOCOCCAL TOXIC SHOCK SYNDROME

An infectious disease syndrome in seven children with high fever, profound and refractory shock, profuse diarrhea, a sunburn-like rash resembling scarlet fever, renal failure, and confusion was described by Todd and Fishaut in 1978.[50] The entity was related to *S. aureus* infections and was later named the toxic shock syndrome. In 1980, this syndrome was observed in young adult women, primarily during menstruation and was associated with production of the responsibile toxin by staphylococci colonizing the cervix, the vagina, and hyperabsorbable tampons.[51] With better understanding of the factors responsible for toxin production and the syndrome, and altering usage of tampons, the disease has become relatively infrequent. However, it still occurs and has a significant case fatality rate (approximately 3%). Cases in women have been observed after cesarean section or vaginal deliveries or with prolonged use of diaphragms. Cases have also been reported in association with relatively minor staphylococcal postoperative wound infections, often in association with various types of cotton packs used at the site of the procedure. Cases have also been associated with staphylococcal osteomyelitis, abscesses, or postinfluenza pneumonia.[52] The syndrome is surprisingly uncommonly associated with severe staphylococcal wound infections or severe staphylococcal sepsis. Various partial forms of the syndrome have been recognized, and it is now apparent that not all patients with the syndrome have a severe illness or exhibit all its manifestations. Diarrhea, myalgia, vomiting, and fever are the most frequent symptoms, but sore throat, conjunctivitis, decreased mentation, and peripheral edema associated with an erythroderma are common. The syndrome may occur without an erythroderma, and it is then difficult to recognize. The majority of patients with the fully developed syndrome have abnormal renal function, thrombocytopenia, hypocalcemia, hyperbilirubinemia, elevated hepatic and muscle enzyme levels, and leukocytosis with a shift to the left. An erythematous mucosal rash and vaginal hyperemia are common. Blood cultures are usually negative. Renal failure is usually reversible and is of both oliguric and nonoliguric types. Desquamation of the mucocutaneous lesions occurs toward the end of the first week of the illness. It is important to recognize that the primary focus of the staphylococcal infection is often inconspicuous, but cultures from the focus are usually positive for *S. aureus.*

Pathogenesis. *S. aureus* is almost invariably isolated from the presumed site of the infection and the unique toxins (most often toxic shock syndrome toxin 1) it produces have been identified, especially in association with menstrual toxic shock syndrome. Although the prevalence of antibodies to toxic shock syndrome toxin 1 is high in the general population, patients with the syndrome usually have undetectable antibodies to it at the onset of disease. A significant percentage of isolates not associated with the menstrual syndrome do not produce toxic shock syndrome toxin 1 but produce other enterotoxins. Evidence suggests indeed that some cases may be related to one or more toxins produced by group A beta-hemolytic streptococci that are similar to the staphylococcal toxins.[53]

Management. The most important aspect of the immediate management of a patient with the toxic shock syndrome is aggressive fluid replacement with saline and/or colloid. Antibiotics have relatively little role in the immediate management of a patient with the toxic shock syndrome, although they may help to prevent recurrences of the disease, especially in menstrually associated cases. Antibiotics are useful in helping to control the staphylococcal infection that is sometimes associated with the syndrome. Surgical drainage and removal of foreign bodies at the infected site play a most important role. Antibiotic therapy should be parenteral and should consist of a good β-lactamase–resistant antistaphylococcal antibiotic, such as oxacillin, nafcillin, and vancomycin. Antibiotic treatment usually is given for 10 to 14 days.

CHOLERA

In certain areas in Southeast Asia, particularly in areas with poor sanitation, cholera is an endemic cause of severe and often fatal watery diarrhea. Isolated cases of cholera have occurred in the United States, but well-nourished and otherwise healthy Americans are relatively immune to cholera, and especially to severe cholera. Outbreaks in the United States are rare, tend to occur in southeastern coastal areas, and are usually traced to contaminated water or undercooked or raw shellfish. Any patient who has severe dehydration and watery diarrhea in an endemic area or with a history of recent travel to a cholera endemic area should be suspected of having cholera. Cholera is diagnosed clinically and confirmed by stool examination and bacteriologic studies. Cholera vibrios can be seen and reliably recognized in stools using darkfield or phase microscopy because of their characteristic motility, which has been likened to shooting stars. Addition of a specific antiserum to the stool result in immobilization of the *Vibrio* and lead to a specific diagnosis.[54] Cultures can be made directly from rectal swabs or stools. Thiosulfate-citrate-bile salts agar and MacConkey's agar media are widely available in the United States and suitable for isolation of *V. cholerae*. The disease can cause fulminant diarrhea, hypovolemic shock, and death from the outpouring of fluid into the upper small intestine. The cholera toxin stimulates active secretion of chloride in the small intestine by increasing the activity of adenylate cyclase in the intestinal mucosa, with resultant increase in levels of adenosine 3′,5′-cyclic monophosphate. Cholera appears to be related to the potent effects of the cholera enterotoxin on the intestinal adenylate cyclase system, with resultant outpouring of salt and water.[55] Therapy consists of fluid replacement, either orally or intravenously with isotonic or hypotonic fluids. Hypertonic fluids should *not* be used to replace salt losses in patients with cholera. Glucose-containing solutions given orally are useful in the treatment of cholera, because glucose absorption is unaffected by changes in the adenylate cyclase system and glucose absorption is accompanied by obligatory salt and water absorption. It is now known that *E. coli* can produce a toxin that is similar to the cholera toxin in structure and mode of action. A previously healthy person with diarrhea can die from cholera because of massive diarrheal fluid loss within 2 or 3 hours if no treatment is provided, but more commonly shock occurs within 4 to 12 hours after onset, with death following in 1 day or longer. After the illness is well advanced, the stools take on the typical appearance of rice water and do not have any odor. When cholera is treated appropriately with fluid and electrolyte replacement, diarrhea may continue but all the other serious manifestations of the disease subside. It should be noted that cholera may occur as a mild diarrhea. Severe hypoglycemia is occasionally seen in cholera, as are other electrolyte imbalances, especially hypokalemia. Water intoxication, acidosis, and renal failure may also occur.

As mentioned, the cornerstone of treatment of cholera is a replacement of water and salts lost in the choleraic stools. This can often be done, even in severe cases, via the oral route. Intravenous replacement therapy is necessary in patients ill enough to be in an ICU. Lactated Ringer's solution is a readily available replacement solution that can be used for intravenous therapy. Large volumes may need to be given. About a liter of fluid can be given within the first 10 to 20 minutes, and adequate initial hydration usually can be accomplished within an hour. Tetracycline or its analogues given by mouth shorten the duration of the infection and diarrhea and thereby reduce fluid losses and hasten recovery. The usual dosage is 250 mg every 6 hours for 3 to 5 days. Ampicillin may be used during pregnancy. Other effective antimicrobials include trimethoprim-sulfamethoxazole, furazolidone, fluoroquinolones, and chloramphenicol. Blood glucose, potassium, and other electrolyte levels should be monitored frequently during therapy and corrections made whenever possible.

ACUTE DYSENTERY

The term *dysentery* refers to the passage of frequent small bowel movements accompanied by blood and mucus, with pain and tenesmus on defecation. The syndrome results from an inflammatory process caused by microorganisms that invade the colonic mucosa. It may result from a variety of different infectious agents. Pathologic changes of this inflammatory colitis range from a superficial severe exudative process involving the mucosa, and commonly caused by *Shigella*, to deep penetrating flask-shaped ulcers that have undermined edges and are caused by amebae. The etiologic agents to be considered in the differential diagnosis of acute dysentery and enterocolitis are listed in Table 41–1. Cytotoxic products of some of these organisms may contribute to the inflammatory process. Many fecal polymorphonuclear or mononuclear cells may be seen on microscopic examination of stools from these patients. The etiologic organisms may spread readily to persons contacting patients with the disease. Organisms are commonly transmitted via the fecal-oral route, especially in endemic areas where sanitation is poor. Culture of fresh stools or rectal swabs on appropriate

TABLE 41–1

DIFFERENTIAL DIAGNOSIS OF INFLAMMATORY ENTEROCOLITIS AND ACUTE DYSENTERY

Bacillary dysentery (*Shigella*, invasive *E. coli*)	Gonococcal proctitis
Campylobacteriosis	Herpetic proctitis
Amebic dysentery	Chlamydial proctitis
Vibriosis	Syphilitic proctitis
Salmonellosis	Enteritis necroticans
Typhoid fever	Pseudomembranous colitis (*C. difficile*)
Balantidium coli infection	Idiopathic ulcerative colitis
Yersiniosis	Crohn's colitis

media is important in the isolation of *Shigella*, *Campylobacter*, and other agents causing this syndrome. *Shigella* isolation rates are higher using rectal swabs than with stools, probably because this is an adherent, invasive organism. Sigmoidoscopy is often useful in diagnosis. Acute shigellosis is often associated with widespread, shallow ulcers ranging from 3 to 7 mm in diameter and having an intense inflammatory exudate. Discrete small ulcerations with undermined edges in the midst of relatively normal mucosa are characteristic of amebic colitis, which also can be suspected when there are few polymorphonuclear leukocytes in the dysenteric stool.

Shigellosis is treated with the replacement of fluid and electrolyte losses, which can often be done by the oral route. Antibiotics are also useful in the management of shigellosis. With susceptible strains, ampicillin or tetracycline shortens the course of the illness and decreases the period of fecal excretion and infectivity of the organism; when susceptibility is unknown, trimethoprim-sulfamethoxazole, ciprofloxacin, norfloxacin, and ceftriaxone are useful. Antidiarrheal (antiperistaltic) drugs are best avoided in the treatment of bacillary dysentery, as they could increase the likelihood of development of toxic dilatation of the colon.

Shigella organisms are the most important causes of acute bloody dysentery with high fever and marked systemic manifestations. The incubation period is usually less than 72 hours and the organism is usually spread by ingestion of relatively small numbers of the organism in contaminated food or water. Bacteremia and disseminated infection are uncommon in acute shigellosis, but PMC, the hemolytic-uremic syndrome, or a leukemoid reaction may be seen in severe cases. Seizures may occur, especially in children. An arthritis similar to that seen in Reiter's syndrome may occur after the dysenteric illness. *E. coli* may occasionally produce a syndrome similar to acute shigellosis. The invasivity of these strains of *E. coli* can be demonstrated if they are present in HeLa cells or the guinea pig conjunctivae or if they carry the plasmid associated with invasiveness.[20, 54]

Acute enterocolitis or gastroenteritis is the most common clinical manifestation of acute *Salmonella* infection. The incubation period is 6 to 48 hours after ingestion of contaminated food or water. Nausea, vomiting, myalgia, and headache are common. The cardinal manifestation of the disease is diarrhea, which may vary from a few loose stools to profuse watery diarrhea. Tenesmus and gross blood may be seen occasionally. Patients have fever, increased bowel sounds, and abdominal tenderness. Stools contain numerous polymorphonuclear leukocytes. Diarrhea usually is self-limited and persists for less than 7 days, although it may be more prolonged. Localization of pain in the right lower quadrant of the abdomen may lead to surgical exploration; the findings at operation are usually not remarkable, but there may be cecitis and local adenopathy. Most patients with acute salmonellal gastroenteritis infection have colitis. Electrolyte and water depletion may be severe and toxic dilatation of the colon may occur. Bacteremia occurs in less than 5% of adults with salmonellal gastroenteritis but may be more frequent in children and in persons with serious underlying diseases. Antimicrobial therapy is not indicated in the vast majority of patients with salmonellal enterocolitis, as antibiotics do little to shorten the duration of the illness but they may prolong the carrier state. However, it has been shown that ciprofloxacin and norfloxacin given orally appear to shorten the duration of the clinical illness, although the carrier state may still be prolonged.[56] Patients with bacteremia or signs of severe sepsis may benefit from treatment with trimethoprim-sulfamethoxazole, ceftriaxone or other third-generation cephalosporins, ampicillin, chloramphenicol, ciprofloxacin, or another fluoroquinolone.

AMEBIC DYSENTERY

E. histolytica cysts pass through the acid stomach contents after ingestion and their capsule is subsequently digested in the small bowel. Trophozoites invade the distal intestinal mucosa and produce shallow undermining ulcers. The organisms may seed the liver via the portal vein and disseminate to other parts of the body. Severe illness appears more commonly in undernourished patients and in those being treated with steroids or immunosuppressive medication, during late pregnancy, and in association with carcinoma or other severe systemic disease.[57]

The diagnosis of intestinal amebiasis is made by identifying either trophozoites or cysts of *E. histolytica* in stools. There is great variation among laboratories in their ability to diagnosis amebiasis. Warm stool specimens uncontaminated with laxatives, barium, soaps, enema solutions, antibiotics, and other medications are preferred. Stools should arrive in the laboratory warm and fresh unless an appropriate transport medium is used. An aspirate obtained during sigmoidoscopy or a scraping from the edge of an ulcer is useful in diagnosis. At least three good stool specimens should be submitted before excluding the diagnosis of amebiasis. A warm saline-purged specimen may increase the likelihood of diagnosis. At endoscopy, amebic colitis appears as punctate hemorrhagic areas or small ulcers with exudative centers and hyperemic borders. Pseudomembranous changes can be seen. In the early stages of the disease, endoscopic findings may be normal. Amebic disease may be localized to the cecum or the ascending colon. Serologic studies are useful in the diagnosis of invasive intestinal amebiasis. There is no unanimity about the preferred treatment regimens for amebic enteritis.

Invasive and symptomatic amebic colitis should be treated with either metronidazole or tinetazole. Metronidazole can be given in a dosage of 750 mg three times a day for 5 to 10 days. Tetracycline plus chloroquine hydrochloride or phosphate is an alternative treatment. In any case, metronidazole should be followed by treatment with an agent such as tetracycline that is known to eradicate the extraluminal encysted organisms.

ENTEROHEMORRHAGIC COLITIS CAUSED BY *ESCHERICHIA COLI*

E. coli belonging to serotype O157:H7 was implicated in a multistate outbreak of acute, self-limited hemorrhagic colitis in 1982.[58] Contaminated undercooked ground beef was the source of the organism. Organisms or toxins they produce appear to adhere primarily to the cecum and the proximal colon, the major sites of lesions.[20, 57] The toxins are similar to Shiga's toxins and are cytotoxic for Vero cells. No invasion or inflammation of the mucosa is produced by the organisms or its toxins. Typically, the patient is a child or a young adult, but the disease can occur and lead to death in the elderly. Patients are typically afebrile and complain primarily of massive bloody diarrhea. Sigmoidoscopy usually reveals no abnormalities. Diagnosis is confirmed by finding the organism or its toxin in stool cultures, using a sorbitol fermentation test for identification of the organism. The hemolytic-uremic syndrome has been associated with this illness. Treatment is supportive, with replacement of blood loss as needed. The illness is usually self-limited.

ACQUIRED IMMUNODEFICIENCY SYNDROME AND DIARRHEA

Diarrhea is a common presenting complaint of patients with acquired immunodeficiency syndrome (AIDS). Most patients with AIDS in the United States have prolonged diarrhea at one time or another during their illness. In some patients, it becomes life-threatening and at least presents major problems in their lives. Although it is possible that some of the diarrhea associated with AIDS is related to a primary human immunodeficiency virus infection of the gut, enteral pathogens are frequently isolated from patients with AIDS and diarrhea.[58, 59] Infections with *Giardia, Entamoeba, Campylobacter, Shigella, Chlamydia,* or *Neisseria gonorrheae* or proctitis caused by herpes simplex viruses can be responsible for the diarrhea, especially in sexually promiscuous homosexual males. Other common etiologic agents found in AIDS patients with diarrhea are *Cryptosporidium,* cytomegalovirus, *Vibrio, Mycobacterium,* and *Isospora.* Eradicative treatment of these organisms is difficult in most patients, although many of them respond at least transiently to specific antimicrobial therapy. *Cryptosporidium* infection is a common cause of gastrointestinal infection in patients with AIDS, but it responds poorly to all forms of antimicrobial therapy tried. Most patients with AIDS and diarrhea end up being treated with supportive and symptomatic therapy with antiperistaltic agents, after which they come to some level of cautious acceptance of the diarrheal problem. Somatostatin may be useful in treating the diarrhea in some patients with AIDS, but it is expensive.

References

1. Bartlett JG: Antibiotic-associated pseudomembranous colitis. Rev Infect Dis 1:530, 1979.
2. Brearly S, Armstrong GR, Nairn R, et al: Pseudomembranous colitis: A lethal complication of Hirschsprung's disease unrelated to antibiotic usage. J Pediatr Surg 22:257, 1987.
3. Lusk RH, Fekety FR, Silva J, et al: Gastrointestinal side effects of clindamycin and ampicillin therapy. J Infect Dis 135(suppl):111, 1977.
4. Lusk RH, Fekety FR, Silva J, et al: Clindamycin-induced enterocolitis in hamsters. J Infect Dis 137:464, 1978.
5. Rifkin GD, Fekety FR, Silva J, et al: Antibiotic-induced colitis: Implications of a toxin neutralized by *Clostridium sordellii* antitoxin. Lancet 2:1103, 1977.
6. Drapkin MS, Worthington MG, Chang TW, et al: *Clostridium difficile* colitis mimicking acute peritonitis. Arch Surg 120:1321, 1985.
7. George WL, Sutter VL, Citron D, et al: Selective and differential medium for isolation of *Clostridium difficile.* J Clin Microbiol 9:214, 1979.
8. Wilson KH, Kennedy MJ, Fekety FR: Use of sodium taurocholate to enhance spore recovery on a medium selective for *Clostridium difficile.* J Clin Microbiol 15:443, 1982.
9. Fekety, FR, Kim K-H, Brown D, et al: Epidemiology of antibiotic-associated *Clostridium difficile* diarrhea with oral vancomycin. J Pediatr 97:151, 1980.
10. Johnson S, Gerding DN, Olson MM, et al: Prospective, controlled study of vinyl glove use to interrupt *Clostridium difficile* nosocomial transmission. Am J Med 88:137, 1990.
11. Cudmore MA, Silva J, Fekety R, et al: *Clostridium difficile* colitis associated with cancer chemotherapy. Arch Intern Med 142:333, 1982.
12. Taylor NS, Thorne GM, Bartlett JG: Comparison of two toxins produced by *Clostridium difficile.* Infect Immun 34:1036, 1981.
13. Lyerly DM, Krwan HC, Wilkins TD: *Clostridium difficile:* Its disease and toxins. Clin Microbiol Rev 1:1, 1988.
14. Bacon AE, Fekety R, Schaberg DR, et al: Epidemiology of *Clostridium difficile* colonization in newborns: Results using a bacteriophage and bacteriocin typing system. J Infect Dis 158:349, 1988.
15. Fekety FR, Silva J, Kauffman C, et al: Treatment of antibiotic-associated *Clostridium difficile* colitis with oral vancomycin: Comparison of two dosage regimens. Am J Med 86:15, 1989.
16. Arsura EL, Fazio RA, Wickremesinghe PC: Pseudomembranous colitis following prophylactic antibiotic use in primary caesarean section. Am J Obstet Gynecol 151:87, 1985.
17. Yankes JR, Baker ME, Cooper C, et al: CT appearance of fecal pseudomembranous colitis. J Comput Assist Tomogr 12:394, 1988.
18. Brunner D, Feifarek C, McNeely D, et al: CT of pseudomembranous colitis. Gastrointest Radiol 9:73, 1984.
19. Tedesco FJ, Corless JK, Brownstein RE: Rectal sparing in antibiotic-associated pseudomembranous colitis: A prospective study. Gastroenterology 83:1259, 1982.
20. Riley LW: The epidemiologic, clinical and microbiologic features of hemorrhagic colitis. Annu Rev Microbiol 41:383, 1987.
21. Tedesco F, Markham R, Gurwith M, et al: Oral vancomycin for antibiotic-associated pseudomembranous colitis. Lancet 2:226, 1978.
22. Keighley MRB, Burdon DW, Arabi Y, et al: Randomized controlled trial of vancomycin for pseudomembranous colitis and postoperative diarrhea. Br Med J 2:1667, 1978.
23. Peikin SR, Galdibini J, Bartlett JG: Role of *Clostridium difficile* in a case of nonantibiotic-associated pseudomembranous colitis. Gastroenterology 79:948, 1980.
24. Teasley DG, Gerding DN, Olson MN, et al: Prospective randomized trial of metronidazole versus vancomycin for the treatment of *Clostridium difficile* associated diarrhea and colitis. Lancet 2:1043, 1983.
25. Oliva SL, Guglielmo BJ, Jacobs R, et al: Failure of intravenous vancomycin and intravenous metronidazole to prevent or treat antibiotic-associated pseudomembranous colitis. J Infect Dis 159:1154, 1989.
26. Cherry RD, Portnoy D, Jabbari M, et al: Metronidazole: An alternate therapy for antibiotic-associated colitis. Gastroenterology 82:849, 1982.
27. Saginur R, Hawley CR, Bartlett JG: Colitis associated with metronidazole therapy. J Infect Dis 141:772, 1980.
28. Bolton RF, Culshaw MA: Faecal metronidazole concentrations during oral and intravenous therapy for antibiotic-associated colitis due to *Clostridium difficile.* Gut 27:1169, 1986.
29. Kleinfeld DI, Sharpe RJ, Donta ST: Parenteral therapy for antibiotic-associated pseudomembranous colitis. J Infect Dis 157:389, 1988.
30. Bergan T, Solhaug JH, Søreide O, et al: Comparative pharmacokinetics of metronidazole and tinidazole and their tissue penetration. Scand J Gastroenterol 20:945, 1985.
31. Guzman R, Kirkpatrick J, Forward K, et al: Failure of parenteral metronidazole in treatment of pseudomembranous colitis. J Infect Dis 158:1146, 1988.
32. Oliva SL, Guglielmo BJ, Jacobs R, et al: Failure of intravenous vancomycin and intravenous metronidazole to prevent or treat antibiotic-associated pseudomembranous colitis. J Infect Dis 159:1154, 1989.
33. de Lalla F, Privitera G, Rinaldi E, et al: Treatment of *Clostridium difficile*–associated disease with teicoplanin. Antimicrob Agents Chemother 33:1125, 1989.
34. Chang T-W, Gorbach SL, Bartlett JG, et al: Bacitracin treatment of antibiotic-associated colitis and diarrhea caused by *Clostridium difficile* toxin. Gastroenterology 78:1584, 1980.
35. Tedesco FJ: Bacitracin therapy in antibiotic-associated pseudomembranous colitis. Dig Dis Sci 25:783, 1980.
36. Dudley MN, McLauglin JC, Carrington G, et al: Oral bacitracin vs vancomycin therapy for *Clostridium difficile*–induced diarrhea. A randomized double-blind trial. Arch Intern Med 146:1101, 1986.
37. Novak E, Lee JG, Seckman E, et al: Unfavorable effect of atropine-diphenoxylate (Lomotil) therapy in lincomycin-caused diarrhea. JAMA 235:1451, 1976.
38. George WL, Volpicelli NA, Stiner DB, et al: Relapse of pseudomembranous colitis after vancomycin therapy. N Engl J Med 301:414, 1979.
39. Barlett JG, Tedesdo FJ, Shull S, et al: Symptomatic relapse after oral vancomycin therapy of antibiotic-associated pseudomembranous colitis. Gastroenterology 78:431, 1980.
40. Walters BAJ, Roberts R, Stafford R, et al: Relapse of antibiotic-associated colitis: Endogenous persistence of *Clostridium difficile* during vancomycin therapy. Gut 24:206, 1983.
41. Tedesco FJ: Treatment of recurrent antibiotic-associated pseudomembranous colitis. Am J Gastroenterol 77:220, 1982.
42. Gorbach SL, Chang TW, Golden B: Successful treatment of relapsing *Clostridium difficile* colitis with *Lactobacillus* GG (letter). Lancet 2:1519, 1987.
43. Schwan A, Sjolin S, Trottestan U: Relapsing *Clostridium difficile* enterocolitis cured by rectal infusion of homologous faeces. Lancet 2:845, 1983.
44. Tvede M, Rask-Madsen B: Bacteriotherapy for chronic relapsing *Clostridium difficile* diarrhoea in six patients. Lancet 1:1156, 1989.
45. Surawicz CM, McFarland LV, Elmer G, et al: Treatment of recurrent *Clostridium difficile* colitis with vancomycin and *Saccharomyces boulardii.* Am J Gastroenterol 84:1285, 1989.
46. Barclay FE, Borriello SP: *Clostridium difficile* and colonization resistance. In: Borriello SP (ed): Antibiotic Associated Diarrhoea and Colitis. Boston, Martinus Nijhoff Publishers, p 79, 1984.
47. Surawicz CM, Elmer GW, Speelman P, et al: Prevention of antibiotic-associated diarrhea by *Saccharomyces boulardii:* A prospective study. Gastroenterology 96:981, 1989.
48. Wust J, Sullivan NM, Hardegger U, et al: Investigation of an outbreak of antibiotic-associated colitis by various typing methods. J Clin Microbiol 16:1096, 1982.
49. Sell TL, Schaberg DR, Fekety FR: Bacteriophage and bacteriocin typing scheme for *Clostridium difficile.* J Clin Microbiol 17:1148, 1983.
50. Todd J, Fishaut M: Toxic-shock syndrome associated with phage-group-I staphylococci. Lancet 2:1116, 1978.
51. Davis JP, Chesney PJ, Wand PJ, et al: Toxic shock syndrome. N Engl J Med 303:1429, 1980.
52. Reingold AL, Hargrett NT, Dan BB, et al: Non-menstrual toxic shock syndrome. A review of 130 cases. Ann Intern Med 96:871, 1982.
53. Cone LA, Woodard DR, Schlievert PM, et al: Clinical and bacteriologic observations of a toxic shock–like syndrome due to *Streptococcus pyogenes.* N Engl J Med 317:146, 1987.
54. Benenson AS, Islam MR, Greenough WB: Rapid identification of *Vibrio cholerae* by darkfield microscopy. Bull WHO 30:827, 1964.
55. Kimberg DV, Field M, Johnson J, et al: Stimulation of intestinal mucosal

adenylate cylase by cholera enterotoxin and prostaglandins. J Clin Invest 50:1218, 1971.

56. Neill MA, Opal SM, Heelan J, et al: Failure of ciprofloxacin to eradicate convalescent fecal excretion after acute salmonellosis: Experience during an outbreak in health care workers. Ann Intern Med 114:195, 1991.
57. Blacklow NR, Dolin R, Fedson DS, et al: Acute infectious nonbacterial gastroenteritis. Ann Intern Med 76:933, 1972.
58. Bean BH: Venereal amoebiasis. NY State J Med 76:930, 1967.
59. Keystone JS, Keystone DL, Proctor LM: Intestinal parasitic infections in homosexual men. Can Med Assoc J 123:512, 1980.

CHAPTER 42

Abdominal Infections

Steven M. Steinberg
Ronald Lee Nichols

Concepts concerning the mechanisms of abdominal infections have undergone radical change during the past decade. Identification of the source of abdominal infections in critically ill patients is no longer simply a matter of determining what part of the gastrointestinal tract has perforated or infarcted. Other factors such as bacterial translocation and alterations in the host's defense mechanisms attributable to trauma, burns, malignancy, and even blood transfusions have been discovered and all may play roles in the development and progression of abdominal infections. Significant improvement in survival occurred early in this century, with mortality rates falling from 90% to 40 to 50%, with the understanding that surgical intervention was necessary to cure most intra-abdominal infections.[1] However, the mortality rate has only minimally decreased during the past 50 years, despite the discovery and use of effective antibiotics and the advent of modern critical care. It is hoped that with increasing knowledge of the pathophysiology of abdominal infections, including such factors as bacterial translocation, alteration of the host's immune function, and the septic syndrome, another major improvement in survival will be possible.

PERITONEAL MEMBRANE

The adult peritoneal membrane is made up of a single layer of mesothelial cells and measures approximately 1.7 m², closely approaching the size of the total cutaneous surface. This membrane lines the peritoneal cavity and viscera within this space, forming the largest preformed extravascular space in the body. Normally, this space is lubricated with about 20 to 50 mL of clear yellow transudate, which has been reported to possess some intrinsic antibacterial activity.[2, 3] Normally, this peritoneal fluid contains less than 300 cells per cubic millimeter, most of which are macrophages and lymphocytes. However, when inflammation or infection is present, rapid increases in the total fluid volume and cell counts occur, with a shift in cell type to predominantly neutrophils.

The ability of the peritoneal membrane to participate in fluid exchange and absorption is well documented. Bacterial peritonitis can result in a rapid inflow of 300 to 500 mL of fluid per hour into the peritoneal space, which can lead to hypovolemia unless therapy is promptly initiated. Some have likened the fluid losses in acute generalized peritonitis to those of a burn involving 50% of body surface area.

It should be realized that, although the entire peritoneal membrane participates in fluid and solute exchange, lymphatic vessels, which are capable of absorbing particulate matter, underlie the peritoneum only on the undersurface of the diaphragm.[4] Stomas, 8 to 12 μm in diameter, take up particulate matter less than 10 μm in diameter, including red blood cells and bacteria. It has been demonstrated that passive stretching of the diaphragm during exhalation causes a rapid influx of fluid into the diaphragmatic lymphatics via the stomas and that contraction of the diaphragmatic muscle fibers during inhalation causes this fluid to move into the efferent lymphatics. Bacteria injected into the peritoneal cavity have been found in thoracic lymph within 6 minutes of injection and in the blood stream within 12 minutes, indicating that peritoneal clearance is extremely rapid.[5] Such factors as increased intra-abdominal pressure and possibly the head-down position increase the rate of clearance of material from the peritoneal cavity, whereas general anesthetics, head-up position (Fowler's position), and possibly positive pressure ventilation decrease the rate of bacterial clearance from the abdomen.[6, 7]

Experimental investigations have shown that the peritoneal mesothelium sloughs readily even after brief exposure to air or saline, with rapid regeneration beginning within hours of these insults and being completed within 1 week of the injury.[8] It is probable that these new mesothelial cells arise either from the proliferation of local macrophages or fibroblasts, which differentiate into mesothelial cells, or from mesothelial cells from the opposing peritoneal edges that seed the denuded surface.

In addition to the body's commonly recognized humoral and cellular immune system, the peritoneal cavity has other defense mechanisms against infection. One of the most studied and possibly the most important of these mechanisms is the so-called peritoneal circulation, which tends to clear the peritoneal cavity of bacteria or at least to wall them off in certain defined areas where they may become abscesses instead of causing diffuse suppurative peritonitis. Autio reported in 1964 that contrast media placed in the peritoneal cavity did not spread haphazardly but followed definite paths.[9] He found that the contrast medium began moving shortly after its placement into the peritoneal cavity and by 3 hours had begun to arrive in the spaces where it would eventually accumulate. After being introduced into the ileocecal region in patients undergoing appendectomy, contrast medium rapidly accumulated in the pelvis and then moved along the right paracolic gutter into the right subhepatic space. From the subhepatic space, the contrast material frequently migrated to the subphrenic space. In patients undergoing cholecystectomy and having contrast instilled in the right subhepatic space, much of the dye remained in the subhepatic space but some was transported to the right subphrenic space and some to the pelvis. Interestingly, even though contrast material was introduced at the foramen of Winslow, the only anatomic opening into the lesser sac, no dye ever entered the lesser sac. In addition, although the subhepatic space opens into the infracolic (interloop) space, no dye crossed over the transverse colon and entered that space. This peritoneal circulation seems to allow the rapid clearance of bacteria from the peritoneal cavity via lymphatics.

PATHOPHYSIOLOGY

The establishment of abdominal infection is a complex phenomenon that requires the interaction of several elements, including the many host defense mechanisms and the virulence factors of the potential pathogens. As in other types of infections, it is unusual for microorganisms to establish an invasive infection within the abdomen of a normal host. Usually, there is a perturbation in the host, which may involve alterations in immune status, foreign body, injured or dead tissue, or substances that act as adjuvants to bacteria.

Hemoglobin, ascitic fluid, fibrin clots, necrotic tissue, bile, and barium sulfate have all been demonstrated to promote the establishment of intra-abdominal bacterial infection.[10–13]

Hemoglobin, when injected intraperitoneally with bacteria into experimental animals, has been noted to increase mortality substantially.[14] Although it seems certain that hemoglobin acts locally within the peritoneal cavity, the exact mechanism by which it potentiates infection has not been elucidated. It has been postulated that hemoglobin may impair local host defenses, stimulate bacterial growth, or stimulate bacterial toxin production. It has been demonstrated that, in the presence of hemoglobin, *Escherichia coli* organisms produce alpha-hemolysin, which impedes neutrophil chemotaxis. Crystalline hemoglobin preparations have been shown by Lee and coworkers to interfere with chemotaxis, phagocytosis, and bacterial killing by human neutrophils.[15]

It is well known that fluid in the peritoneal cavity increases the likelihood of primary bacterial peritonitis and worsens the prognosis in secondary peritonitis. Cirrhotic patients with ascites are at significantly greater risk for primary peritonitis than are cirrhotic patients without ascites.[16] Under normal conditions, bacteria are cleared from the peritoneal cavity rapidly and without the establishment of infection. When free fluid is present in the peritoneal cavity, this process does not occur as readily. The mortality rate in experimental animals increases when saline is infused along with an otherwise sublethal dose of *E. coli.*[17] The intraperitoneal fluid probably acts by both diluting opsonins and interfering with the ability of nonadherent white blood cells to optimally phagocytize bacteria.

The basis for radical débridement of the peritoneal cavity is found in the observation that fibrin clots harbor bacteria. Fibrin may actually act as a double-edged sword. It may cause localization of bacteria but then shield the bacteria from phagocytosis. It has been reported in a canine model that the intraperitoneal administration of heparin decreased mortality in a model of intra-abdominal infection, implying that by preventing fibrin clot formation one could minimize mortality.[18] Ahrenholz and Simmons demonstrated that fibrin clots decreased the early mortality in an animal model of lethal peritonitis.[19] The mortality rate at 24 hours in rats who had fibrin clots impregnated with *E. coli* implanted intraperitoneally was 0% compared with 100% in rats who had the same number of *E. coli* organisms instilled in similar volumes of saline. However, 100% of those animals had intra-abdominal abscesses by day 10 and 90% died. Operative débridement of the fibrin clots prevented the formation of abscesses and improved survival.

Although barium is known to be a rather benign substance in some areas of the body, such as the tracheobronchial tree, perforation of the gastrointestinal tract during the course of a radiologic procedure utilizing barium sulfate is a dreaded occurrence. Even sterile barium, when injected into the peritoneal cavity of experimental animals, results in a significant mortality rate and causes a hemorrhagic peritonitis with adhesions and granulomas in survivors.[20] Other experimental models demonstrated that the combination of barium and intestinal contents produces a more virulent peritonitis than that with either alone.[21, 22] It is thought that the water-insoluble barium tenaciously binds with the intestinal

bacteria. This mixture is difficult, if not impossible, to remove surgically and often results in multiple abscesses.

MICROBIOLOGY

The polymicrobial nature of intra-abdominal infections was first noted by Altemeier in 1938 in patients with perforated appendicitis.[23] It was reported that the average number of bacterial isolates in patients with abdominal infections caused by gastrointestinal tract diseases ranged from 2.5 to 5.[24, 25] In 1942, Altemeier also noted the pathogenicity of anaerobic bacteria in patients with peritonitis.[26] The primary conclusions of this study were (1) the great majority of the bacteria did not produce a fatal peritonitis when injected in pure culture; (2) many avirulent strains of bacteria, particularly *E. coli,* became highly virulent in the presence of dead sterile tissue within the peritoneal cavity; (3) in mixed culture, these bacteria show a synergistic action, producing a high degree of pathogenicity; and (4) acute perforated appendicitis–related peritonitis appears to be an infection resulting from the synergistic activities of the various bacterial symbionts present in a given case. These important studies were not elaborated on for nearly three decades until modern techniques for the isolation and growth of anaerobic bacteria were introduced, thereby allowing their better classification in both normal flora and postoperative infection studies.[27–29]

Intestinal Microflora

The numbers and types of microorganisms increase progressively down the gastrointestinal tract. In the normal human, the stomach and the proximal small intestine support a rather sparse bacterial flora of both aerobes and anaerobes ($<10^4$/mL).[30] Acidity and motility appear to be the major factors that inhibit the growth of bacteria within the stomach. Diseases of the stomach and the duodenum may compromise these defense mechanisms. Thus, in cases of obstructing peptic ulcer, gastric ulcer or carcinoma, or alkalization of the stomach, the microflora of the stomach usually increases, being composed principally of anaerobes from the oral cavity and aerobic coliforms.

The microflora of the distal small bowel represents a transitional zone between the microflora of the upper and lower gastrointestinal tract; modest numbers of aerobic and anaerobic microorganisms (up to 10^8/mL) are usually present.[31, 32] The largest concentrations of microorganisms are located in the colon, where up to 10^{11} anaerobes per gram of stool or per milliliter of intestinal aspirate can be identified.[33] Coliforms are also present in the colon in concentrations of 10^8/g. In all organs of the gastrointestinal tract, obstruction or stasis from ileus allows multiplication of bacteria and significant increases in their concentrations.

Microbiology of Intra-abdominal Infections

The number of aerobic and anaerobic bacteria isolated from sites of intra-abdominal infections depends on the nature of the microflora of the diseased or traumatized organ. A complex polymicrobial flora results from contamination of the gastrointestinal tract. The polymicrobial nature of the pathogens in patients with intra-abdominal infection is evident from several reports, which, when combined, showed that the average number of isolates of microorganisms from the infected sites ranged from 2.5 to 5.[34–36] These figures included an average of 1.4 to 2 aerobes and 2.4 to 3 anaerobes per infection. One or more anaerobic species were isolated from 65 to 94% of the patients.

The type of microflora isolated from abdominal infections

depends on the microflora of the diseased or injured organ. The most commonly isolated aerobic bacteria are *E. coli, Klebsiella* species, *Proteus* species, *Streptococcus* species, and *Enterobacter* species. The anaerobes isolated most frequently include *Bacteroides* species, *Peptostreptococcus* species, and *Clostridium* species. *Bacteroides fragilis* is the most frequently isolated anaerobe and, together with other *Bacteroides* species, accounts for 30 to 60% of all anaerobic isolates. Purely anaerobic intra-abdominal infection is reported in less than 15% of the cases, whereas purely aerobic infections have been noted in about 10%. Both aerobes and anaerobes are involved in more than 75% of the cases of intra-abdominal infections.

In addition, highly antibiotic-resistant strains, such as *Pseudomonas aeruginosa, Serratia marcescens,* and *Providentia* species, are frequently isolated from patients who have an intra-abdominal infection within the hospital setting.[37] Persistent peritonitis in patients with long hospitalizations, repeated courses of antibiotics, multiple operations, and/or admissions to the critical care unit favor the growth of breakthrough microorganisms such as *Staphylococcus aureus, Enterococcus* species, and *Candida* species.[38, 39]

CLINICAL ASPECTS

Secondary bacterial peritonitis occurs primarily after the leakage of endogenous microflora from a diseased or traumatized intraperitoneal hollow viscus. The extent of dissemination and the severity of the infection within the peritoneal cavity depend on a number of factors, including the source of contamination, the duration of contamination, the presence of adjuvant substances, and the host response. The presence of adhesions from previous operations and a well-functioning omentum help to confine the infection.

Abdominal pain is present in almost all cases of peritonitis. In patients with intra-abdominal abscesses, the pain, as well as the physical findings of involuntary guarding and tenderness, is localized to the area of the abscess. In generalized peritonitis, the pain and tenderness are diffuse and are worsened by any movement, including coughing or jarring of the hospital bed. Abdominal distention results from the accumulation of peritoneal fluid and increased intraluminal bowel gas and liquid. Bowel sounds are usually diminished or absent. Patients with peritonitis also have fever and other symptoms and signs related to hypovolemia attributable to fluid sequestration in the peritoneal cavity. With adequate fluid resuscitation, the patient manifests the typical hyperdynamic state associated with sepsis, with an elevated cardiac output, decreased systemic vascular resistance, and hypermetabolism.

DIAGNOSIS

The diagnosis of diffuse or localized peritonitis is usually based on the clinical history and typical physical examination findings. Associated increases of the peripheral leukocyte count frequently exceed 15,000/mm³, with a shift to the left often observed. Plain or contrast radiologic examinations of the abdomen and the chest may be helpful in demonstrating perforations, obstruction, or ileus. Specialized radiologic procedures such as ultrasonography and computed tomography are most helpful in searching for localized intra-abdominal fluid collections. In patients with ascites, paracentesis may be helpful. If gross pus, bile, or feces are aspirated, the diagnosis is confirmed. In patients without ascites and with borderline physical examination findings, peritoneal lavage may be extremely helpful. The technique was first described in a clinical setting by Richardson and colleagues in 1983.[40] The procedure requires placing a catheter intra-

TABLE 42–1
CLASSIFICATION OF ABDOMINAL INFECTIONS

Primary Peritonitis
  Childhood
  Adulthood
  Tuberculous

Secondary Peritonitis
  Localized
    Intra-abdominal abscess
    Early gastrointestinal tract ischemia or infarction
  Diffuse
    Suppurative peritonitis caused by
      Gastrointestinal tract perforation
      Late gastrointestinal tract ischemia or infarction
    Peritonitis in patients with continuous ambulatory peritoneal dialysis catheters

peritoneally by small cutdown or percutaneously and then instilling 1 L of saline. The fluid is then drained, and an aliquot is examined. The diagnosis of peritonitis is made if there is gross pus, bile, or feces in the fluid; if the polymorphonuclear leukocyte cell count is greater than 500/mm³; or if bacteria or food fibers are seen on microscopic examination. It is important to culture the fluid from both peritoneal lavage and paracentesis.

Frequently, the exact cause of the peritonitis is not ascertained until abdominal exploration, at which time definitive treatment is rendered. Delay in surgery is more common with immunosuppressed patients, as they frequently do not manifest the abdominal symptoms and signs of peritonitis or the systemic manifestations of sepsis. This almost certainly contributes to these patients' poorer prognosis, regardless of the cause of peritonitis.

CLINICAL SYNDROMES

Owing to significant differences in treatment, it is helpful to categorize peritonitis as to whether it is primary or secondary and localized or diffuse (Table 42–1). One must remember that not all peritonitis is associated with infection. Examples include acute pancreatitis and early perforated peptic ulcer.

Primary Peritonitis

Primary peritonitis in children usually occurs in those with pneumococcal pneumonia. This was not unusual before the widespread use of penicillin. In these instances, it is thought that *Streptococcus pneumoniae* peritonitis results from hematogenous spread. The diagnosis was made by finding neutrophils and gram-positive cocci in pairs in the peritoneal fluid and finding a pure growth of *S. pneumoniae* on culture. Since the advent of the use of penicillin for pneumococcal pneumonia, this disease has all but disappeared.

Spontaneous peritonitis now occurs most commonly in patients with ascites. The most frequently affected are cirrhotic, but patients with nephrotic syndrome and other causes of ascites also occasionally have primary peritonitis. Correia and Conn reported that 18% of cirrhotic patients with ascites had primary peritonitis.[16] These patients typically have atypical clinical pictures. It is not infrequent that patients with primary peritonitis, particularly cirrhotic individuals, exhibit only a worsening of their underlying disease and no abnormal peritoneal findings on physical examination. Cirrhotic patients may simply have hepatic failure or decreased mental status as a result of hepatic encephalopathy.

Gram-negative bacilli, primarily *E. coli,* are responsible for 70% of all cases.[41] It is unclear how the bacteria gain access to the ascitic fluid. It is likely that bacteria originate in the gastrointestinal tract, but whether they reach the ascitic fluid by bacterial translocation, hematogenous spread, or some other process is unclear. Virtually all patients with primary peritonitis have defects in the areas of serum bactericidal activity, chemotaxis, opsonic function, and impaired neutrophil and macrophage function. As with pneumococcal peritonitis, the diagnosis is made by inspecting the ascitic fluid. The peritoneal fluid should be examined for cell count and differential count, pH, and lactate level and with Gram's stain. If the cell count is greater than 250/mm³ and more than one third are polymorphonuclear leukocytes, ascitic fluid pH is less than 7.35, and the ascitic fluid lactate level is greater than 30 mg/dL, there is a great likelihood of peritonitis.[42-44] Gram's stain of a centrifuged sample of ascitic fluid is helpful if positive, but 60 to 80% of ascitic fluid samples from patients with primary peritonitis are negative for bacteria.

The administration of antibiotics directed at aerobic gram-negative bacilli should be started without waiting for the culture report if primary peritonitis is suspected. A pure culture of bacteria should grow in culture. It is important to distinguish between primary and secondary peritonitis. If the ascitic fluid aspirate demonstrates gross feces, bile, or blood or if more than one type of bacteria is seen on Gram's stain or grows in culture, one must assume that the patient does not have primary peritonitis and has peritonitis resulting from some other intra-abdominal process. Although surgery is the cornerstone of the treatment of most types of secondary peritonitis, surgical therapy offers little to patients with primary peritonitis. The mortality of laparotomy in patients with primary peritonitis may be as high as 80%.[16] In patients with cirrhosis treated with antibiotics, the mortality rate is approximately 50%, with most patients dying of liver failure. It is noteworthy that, in cirrhotic patients who survive primary peritonitis, there is a 74% incidence of recurrence within 2 years.[45]

In otherwise healthy adults, group A streptococcus may rarely cause primary peritonitis.[46] This type of primary peritonitis occurs almost exclusively in women and is thought to arise from streptococci present in the vagina that ascend to the peritoneal cavity via the cervix, the uterus, and the fallopian tubes. In the few males in whom streptococcal primary peritonitis has been reported, the organisms are thought to have seeded the peritoneal cavity hematogenously. Patients usually have complaints of nausea, vomiting, and abdominal pain. Physical examination usually reveals abdominal tenderness with peritoneal signs, and examination of peritoneal fluid demonstrates high polymorphonuclear leukocyte counts with gram-positive cocci in chains. Treatment with penicillin is usually curative.

Tuberculous peritonitis is a variant of primary peritonitis that is rarely seen in the United States anymore but still is relatively common in developing countries. The diagnosis of tuberculous peritonitis may be more problematic than that of other types of primary peritonitis because mycobacteria are not seen on Gram's stain, and even when acid-fast stain is used, bacteria are frequently not detected. Tuberculous peritonitis is best diagnosed by laparoscopy and peritoneal biopsy with culture and acid-fast stain.[47] Tuberculous peritonitis is best treated with two- or three-drug regimens, including isoniazid, rifampicin, ethambutol, pyrazinamide, and streptomycin, for 6 to 9 months.

Secondary Peritonitis

For therapeutic purposes, it is helpful to divide secondary abdominal infections into diffuse and local types. Those that

TABLE 42–2
INTRA-ABDOMINAL ABSCESS LOCATION

Subphrenic space	Interloop
Subhepatic space	Pelvic area
Paracolic gutters	Parenchyma

are localized are amenable to local therapy, including resection, surgical drainage, and percutaneous drainage. Diffuse suppurative processes are not particularly amenable to these types of treatment and other approaches such as open abdominal packing, radical peritoneal débridement, peritoneal lavage, and planned repeated abdominal explorations have been utilized.

Common examples of localized abdominal infectious processes include all intra-abdominal abscesses (Table 42–2), gangrenous appendicitis or cholecystitis, acute diverticulitis with walled-off perforation, and strangulated hernias. Most of these diagnoses are relatively easily made by obtaining a history and performing physical examination. Appendicitis, cholecystitis, diverticulitis, and strangulated hernias are all examples of processes that may be amenable to resection. Although it is clear that not all the bacteria are removed with the involved organ, removing the offending organ, limiting ongoing peritoneal soilage, and treating the patient with appropriate antibiotics allows the patient the opportunity to eliminate the remaining bacteria.

One particular type of secondary peritonitis shares many qualities with primary peritonitis and that is peritonitis associated with indwelling peritoneal catheters, particularly continuous ambulatory peritoneal dialysis catheters. As in patients with ascites who have primary peritonitis, the manifestations of peritonitis may be vague and nonspecific and may include fever, mild abdominal pain, and tenderness. Vas defined peritonitis to include at least two of the following criteria: (1) the presence of organisms on Gram's stain or culture of the peritoneal fluid, (2) cloudy peritoneal fluid containing polymorphonuclear leukocytes, and (3) symptoms of peritoneal inflammation.[48] The most common organisms recovered from the peritoneal fluid are *Staphylococcus epidermidis, Pseudomonas* species, and *Candida* species.

Treatment consisting of continuous dialysis to prevent fluid loculation and parenteral and intraperitoneal antibiotic administration is initiated. Dialysis is maintained continuously until culture results are negative for 3 days and the patient is asymptomatic. Oral administration of antibiotics is continued for 1 to 3 additional weeks. It is unnecessary, except for *Candida* infection, to remove the catheter unless an infection of the subcutaneous tunnel occurs. On occasion, the dialysis catheter erodes through the bowel wall. This situation is distinguished from catheter-associated peritonitis in that it is usually polymicrobial and involves coliforms. This occurrence mandates immediate laparotomy with repair of the bowel perforation and placement of a new catheter.

TREATMENT

The most critical aspect of treatment of secondary peritonitis is early diagnosis and prompt surgical intervention. Pitcher and Musher found a strong correlation of the interval between presentation and treatment with morbidity and mortality.[49] Antibiotics, treatment in critical care units, and other adjunctive modalities cannot make up for delays in definitive surgical treatment. Preoperative, intraoperative, and postoperative care of these patients demands rapid restitution of intravascular volume and other measures de-

TABLE 42–3
PARENTERAL ANTIBIOTIC AGENTS FOR ABDOMINAL INFECTIONS

Combination Therapy
Aerobic coverage—to be combined with a drug having anaerobic activity

Amikacin	Cefotaxime
Aztreonam	Gentamicin
Ceftriaxone	Tobramycin
Cefoperazone	

Anaerobic coverage—to be combined with a drug having aerobic activity

Carbenicillin	Metronidazole
Chloramphenicol	Mezlocillin
Clindamycin	Ticarcillin

Single-Drug Therapy
Aerobic-anaerobic coverage—single agents

Ampicillin-sulbactam	Imipenem-cilastatin
Cefotetan	Moxalactam
Cefoxitin	Piperacillin
Ceftizoxime	Ticarcillin-clavulanic acid

signed to maximize oxygen delivery to tissues. In some instances, this may necessitate invasive monitoring with arterial and Swan-Ganz catheters. Because sepsis, and intra-abdominal infection in particular, is commonly associated with the adult respiratory distress syndrome, the patient may require endotracheal intubation and mechanical ventilation, even in the preoperative period. Preoperative placement of a nasogastric tube is recommended to decompress the accumulated gastrointestinal fluid and gas, which helps to minimize the risk of aspiration as well as to relieve pressure on the diaphragm. Administration of analgesics and antibiotics should be initiated only after the diagnosis of peritonitis has been made and definitive therapy has been planned.

Nutritional requirements for septic patients differ greatly from those for normal patients. Caloric requirements may be increased by as much as 25 to 35% over basal requirements and protein requirements may be as high as 2 to 4 g/kg/d. Placement of a nasojejunal feeding tube fluoroscopically or intraoperatively is strongly recommended, as the enteral route of nutrition seems to correlate strongly with improvement of sepsis.[50]

Antibiotic Selection

Unlike patients with superficial wound abscesses in whom surgical drainage alone suffices, those with intra-abdominal infections are best managed by a combination of surgical repair, excision, diversion, or drainage with appropriately chosen, parenterally administered antibiotics. The antibiotic therapy should be initiated as soon as the diagnosis is made preoperatively and continued during the operation and into the postoperative period. The choice of the ideal agent or agents and the necessary length of the therapeutic course remain controversial. On the basis of early experimental and clinical studies, the chosen antibiotics must have activity against both the colonic aerobes and anaerobes, including *B. fragilis*.[37, 51–53] Conventionally, antibiotic regimens for peritonitis have included an aminoglycoside and either clindamycin or metronidazole, but more recently, the use of single antibiotics with both aerobic and anaerobic activity has been espoused. Table 42–3 lists antibiotics that are commonly used singly or in combination.

Many studies of the treatment of peritonitis have utilized the abundant data obtained regarding patients with penetrating trauma. Efficacy of treatment in this setting of acute

contamination in healthy young males does not necessarily translate into success in therapy for severe intra-abdominal infections that occur after organ perforation in older, frequently immunosuppressed patients. These studies emphasized the importance of utilizing antibiotic agents with efficacy against both gastrointestinal aerobic and anaerobic bacterial species.[53] A prospective study of 100 patients with abdominal trauma reported in 1973 revealed a significantly increased rate of anaerobic bacteremia and intra-abdominal infections in the group of patients treated with cephalothin plus kanamycin (aerobic coverage) as compared with those treated with clindamycin plus kanamycin (aerobic and anaerobic coverage).

In 1984, Hofstetter and coinvestigators reported a prospective study of 119 patients who sustained abdominal trauma.[54] Results in this heterogeneous group appeared to indicate that a short-term course with a single drug, cefoxitin, was as safe and effective as the use of a triple-drug regimen of an aminoglycoside, ampicillin, and clindamycin. The authors also suggested that it might be prudent to consider leaving the skin and subcutaneous tissues open in patients who had hollow viscus injury because of the high incidence of localized wound infection in this clinical setting. Additional prospective randomized studies of purely penetrating abdominal trauma reached similar conclusions regarding the efficacy of antibiotic therapy.[55–57] The use of cefoxitin alone was found to be equal to combination therapy and superior to cefamandole alone. The differences in efficacy of single cephalosporin agents was thought to be due to the varying activity of these agents against *B. fragilis*. The antibiotics used in these studies generally lacked efficacy against enterococci, which were frequently isolated from infected sites in mixed cultures. Despite their isolation, rarely is it necessary to alter the original antibiotic therapy to achieve a successful outcome. However, a similar study stressed the potential for broad-spectrum cephalosporins to result in enterococcal overgrowth in patients with abdominal trauma.[58] The results of the initial peritoneal culture in penetrating abdominal trauma are thought to have no predictive value for the development of postoperative infection or for the eventual pathogen identified from such infections when they occurred.[59] This is distinctly different from the value of culture in cases of established peritonitis.[60]

The duration of antibiotic therapy in cases of established peritonitis is controversial. Data from Lennard and coworkers indicate that, if a patient still has leukocytosis without fever at the conclusion of the antibiotic course, the risk of having ongoing or recurrent intra-abdominal infection was 33%.[61] Seventy-nine percent of patients who were febrile at the conclusion of their antibiotic course experienced recurrent infection. No patient who was both afebrile and had a normal white blood cell count had recurrent intra-abdominal infection. We believe that, in patients with established intra-abdominal infections, antibiotics should be continued for a minimum of 7 to 10 days and it may be appropriate to continue antibiotics until both fever and leukocytosis have resolved. The use of antibiotics in patients with penetrating abdominal trauma is somewhat different. Although antibiotics in patients with gastrointestinal tract injuries lower the risk of postoperative wound infection compared with that in patients who have not received antibiotics, the antibiotics do not need to be continued for more than 48 hours.

Treatment Methods for Localized Infection
Resection

Resectional therapy for diseases such as gangrenous appendicitis or cholecystitis, infarcted bowel, or perforated diverticulitis is the standard of care today. Perforated diverticulitis used to be and, on occasion, still is treated in three surgical stages: drainage of abscess with diverting colostomy, resection of the involved colon, and finally, closure of colostomy. Most surgeons today combine the first and second stages. However, with the ability to drain abscesses percutaneously, there have been suggestions that another potential approach would be first to drain the peridiverticular abscess percutaneously and then to allow the patient's acute symptoms and signs of infection and obstruction to resolve.[62] This would be followed by mechanical and antibiotic colon preparation and then resection of the involved colon with primary anastomosis. It remains to be seen whether this approach will be widely applicable.

Drainage

The optimal method of treating abscesses continues to be incision and drainage. Today, there are more techniques available for drainage of abscesses.

Percutaneous drainage of intra-abdominal abscesses was first reported by Grønvall and colleagues in 1977.[63] Since that time, there has been a marked increase in percutaneous drainage of various intra-abdominal fluid collections using both ultrasonic and computed tomographic techniques for the visualization of the collection. Comparisons of percutaneous and surgical drainage of abdominal abscesses are extremely variable and lack prospective, randomized studies comparing the two drainage approaches.

Gerzof and associates reported in 1981 their experience with percutaneous drainage of intra-abdominal abscesses.[64] They achieved an overall cure rate of 86% in 67 patients, with a 15% complication rate and a 16% mortality rate. Six of the 11 deaths were due to ongoing sepsis (related to either inadequate drainage or progression to multiple organ system failure) and one was due to a complication of the choice of the percutaneous technique (postoperative death after splenectomy following percutaneous drainage of a clostridial splenic abscess). The technique had the best success rate in simple, unilocular abscesses located either within a solid organ or contiguous to one. They reported a 90% success rate with subphrenic, subhepatic, intrahepatic, and intrarenal abscesses, but a lower success rate with more complex types of abscesses. They reported a 40% success rate with pancreatic abscess and a 75% success rate with mid-abdominal (interloop, lesser sac) and pelvic abscesses. The mortality rates associated with these two groups were 20% and 25%, respectively.

In a similar later study, Gerzof and colleagues reported a success rate with simple abscesses of 82%, whereas it was only 45% with complex abscesses.[65] They defined complex abscesses as those that were "loculated, ill-defined or extensive, containing viscous pus or semisolid material, or having an enteric communication." The size of the abscess, the distance from the abdominal wall, whether the abscess was spontaneous or postoperative, and whether the abscess was single or multiple had little bearing on the success of the procedure. Aeder and colleagues, in a retrospective study, reported a 69% success rate with percutaneous drainage.[66] They suggested criteria to determine which abscesses were amenable to percutaneous drainage: (1) less than two abscess cavities or loculations; (2) a drainage route not traversing bowel, uncontaminated organs, or uncontaminated peritoneal or pleural spaces; (3) the absence of a source of continuous contamination; and (4) the absence of fungi as causative organisms.

Olak and coworkers reported a case-control study comparing 27 patients who had percutaneously drained abscesses with 27 patients matched for age, sex, diagnosis, and abscess

TABLE 42-4		
PERCUTANEOUS DRAINAGE OF ABSCESSES		
Author	**Type of Abscess (Number of Patients)**	**Success Rate (%)**
Brolin et al.[87]	All (24)	92
vanSonnenberg et al.[88]	All (250)	84
Pruett et al.[89]	All (55)	47
	Simple, nonfungal, nonfistulous (26)	96
	With fistula (9)	28
	With fungi (9)	0
Lang et al.[90]	All (136)	77
Lamaris et al.[91]	All (112)	74
	Multiple abscesses (16)	50
	Pancreatic abscess (8)	50
	Complex intraparenchymal abscess (7)	57
Civardi et al.[92]	All (50)	70

cause and location who underwent operative drainage.[67] They found no difference in outcome between the two groups and suggested that percutaneous drainage is a reasonable initial approach to the drainage of selected intra-abdominal abscesses if early and frequent reassessments of the patient's clinical condition are made and that abscesses that do not respond promptly to percutaneous drainage should be drained operatively. Table 42-4 summarizes the overall results of several studies on abdominal abscess drainage.

Barakos and colleagues[68] and Nunez and associates[69] reported on the utility of draining periappendiceal abscesses percutaneously and found 90% (9 of 10) and 100% (5 of 5) success rates in treating well-localized abscesses. Hiatt and coworkers reported that percutaneous aspiration of peripancreatic fluid collections was also helpful diagnostically.[70] They found the technique to be 94% (17 of 18) accurate and without complications.

On the basis of current data, we believe that percutaneous drainage of intra-abdominal abscesses is not advisable under any of the following circumstances:

1. Complex abscesses defined as those with more than two septations, in continuity with the gastrointestinal tract, filled with thick debris, containing primarily fungi
2. More than two abscesses
3. Pancreatic abscesses
4. Drainage paths that necessitate traversing bowel or uncontaminated body cavities.

If abscesses do not fall within these criteria, the success rate of percutaneous drainage should be in the range of 80 to 90%. The technique of abscess localization, ultrasonography versus computed tomography, is not considered an important consideration and the choice depends on the radiologist's experience.

Treatment Methods for Diffuse Infections

Although the overriding principle in the management of localized purulent collections is incision and drainage and the major controversies are over differences in technique, the same cannot be said for the treatment principles for diffuse suppurative peritonitis. Several different alternatives are available (Table 42-5).

Simple Drainage

Simple drainage of the peritoneal cavity in the setting of diffuse suppurative peritonitis is totally ineffective. This is

TABLE 42–5

TREATMENT APPROACHES TO DIFFUSE PERITONEAL INFECTIONS

Continuous postoperative peritoneal lavage
Intraoperative irrigation and closure
Radical surgical débridement
Packing the peritoneal cavity open
Etappenlavage: planned repetitive operations

possibly because drains are rapidly walled off by fibrin deposition along the drain track.[71, 72]

Continuous Postoperative Peritoneal Lavage

Continuous peritoneal lavage refers to the placement of irrigation catheters in the peritoneal cavity *at the time of operation* to irrigate the peritoneal cavity with fluid to dilute and/or wash away bacteria and other toxic substances. It is extremely important to note that the use of this technique has been proposed only as a therapeutic adjunct after exploratory laparotomy has controlled the inciting factors in the development of peritonitis and has no utility when used by itself. The technique usually involves instilling a liter of fluid during 5 to 10 minutes, allowing it to remain in the peritoneal cavity for approximately 30 minutes, and then draining the fluid during the subsequent 20 to 25 minutes.[73] This process is continuously repeated until either the effluent remains totally clear or an arbitrary time point has been reached. The choice of fluid and any additives varies widely among the proponents of this technique. Standard peritoneal dialysis fluids, normal saline, and lactated Ringer's solution have all been used. Common additives include antibiotics (most commonly first-generation cephalosporins) and heparin, but many other substances, including povidone-iodine and hydrogen peroxide, have been used. In experimental animals, the addition of substances such as povidone-iodine and hydrogen peroxide have been demonstrated to increase mortality when used with continuous postoperative peritoneal lavage.[74, 75] Results reported have been mixed. Many of the nonrandomized retrospective studies showed a survival advantage using continuous postoperative peritoneal lavage; of the six prospective studies in the literature, five show no improvement with lavage. The results of several studies are summarized in Table 42–6.

Although continuous postoperative peritoneal lavage has

the theoretic advantage of washing out bacteria and can be used as a method to deliver high concentrations of antibiotics, it also has the theoretic disadvantages of diluting opsonins and reducing the leukocytes' ability to phagocytize bacteria and debris. Because this technique has not convincingly been demonstrated to improve survival, it should be used only in selected instances such as in patients with peritonitis and renal failure who require dialysis anyway.

Intraoperative Irrigation

Although intraoperative irrigation with crystalloid solutions has not been shown to decrease either mortality or recurrent abscesses, virtually all studies have supported the use of intraoperative peritoneal irrigation with antibiotic-containing solutions in patients with bacterial peritonitis. Schumer and colleagues demonstrated that crystalloid irrigation reduced the number of bacteria remaining in the peritoneal cavity.[76] Although Rosato and coworkers also demonstrated a reduction in the concentration of adjuvant substances, they were unable to show improvement in either mortality or abscess formation.[77] Various antibiotics, including cephalothin (1 g/L), kanamycin (1 g/L), and bacitracin (50,000 U/L), chloramphenicol, and other aminoglycosides, have all been used successfully and have been shown to decrease the incidence of recurrent intra-abdominal infection.[78–81]

Radical Peritoneal Débridement

In 1975, Hudspeth introduced the concept of radical peritoneal débridement for the treatment of generalized peritonitis.[82] The technique involves the complete exposure of the entire peritoneal cavity. Initially, all free peritoneal fluid and pus are suctioned out of the abdomen and then the entire peritoneal cavity is meticulously débrided. All fibrin peels are removed from the serosal surfaces of the bowel. Hudspeth stated that in his experience this procedure added 2 to 3 hours of operative time. In the only study comparing radical peritoneal débridement with standard therapy, Polk and Fry reported an absence of difference in outcome.[83]

Leaving the Peritoneal Cavity Open

The concept of treating the peritoneal cavity as a large abscess and managing generalized bacterial peritonitis by widely draining it by packing the abdomen open was revived by Steinberg in 1979.[84] He reported on 14 patients with generalized peritonitis with only one death and one case of recurrent intra-abdominal infection. Since that time, there have been several reports of use of this technique or modifications of the technique. The combination of use of polypropylene mesh to avoid evisceration and planned repeated return to the operating room (termed *etappenlavage*) has been widely adopted and practiced in the specific group of patients with severe generalized bacterial peritonitis. The decision is made at the initial operation, based on the operative findings, whether to return the patient to the operating room daily to break up loculations and débride dead tissue. The abdomen is closed only when no further fluid collections or necrotic debris can be found. There are no published prospective, randomized clinical studies comparing the technique of packing the abdomen open or any of its variations with any other form of treatment.

Wittman and colleagues reported their mortality results in patients treated with mesh closure and etappenlavage compared with expected mortality rates using Acute Physiology and Chronic Health Evaluation (APACHE) II scor-

TABLE 42–6

MORTALITY ASSOCIATED WITH CONTINUOUS POSTOPERATIVE PERITONEAL LAVAGE

	Lavage		Control	
	n	Mortality (%)	n	Mortality (%)
Prospective Studies				
Del Carmen Nieto and Nava[93]	40	10	20	40
Olesen et al.[94]	20	0	10	0
Shweni et al.[95]	20	20	19	10.5
Hunt[96]	15	33	29	27.6
Kumar et al.[97]	20	35	30	26.6
Retrospective Studies				
Bhushan et al.[98]	30	20	30	60
Gjessing and Tomlin[99]	72	15.3	106	5.7
Uden et al.[100]	181	0.6	188	0.5
Washington et al.[101]	50	14	44	9.1

ing.[85] Each patient underwent an average of 6.1 procedures (initial operation plus 5.1 re-explorations). An actual mortality rate of 25% was found compared with an expected median mortality rate of 47%. Additional pathologic changes necessitating treatment were found in 57% of patients at the subsequent re-explorations. Bradley similarly used the open packing technique to successfully treat pancreatic abscesses.[86] In a series of 28 patients, only 3 (11%) died, and none died of sepsis.

This open type of treatment has been proposed to have the following real and theoretic advantages: decreased intra-abdominal pressure, improving blood flow to the abdominal viscera; daily elimination of purulent and necrotic material to maintain control over infection; prompt recognition of intra-abdominal complications; and the ability to get the patient out of bed and in the upright position, both of which have been demonstrated to improve pulmonary function in sepsis. The complications associated specifically with the procedure appear to be related to an increased risk of bowel perforation and fistula formation.

References

1. Wittmann D: Intraabdominal infections—Introduction. World J Surg 14:145, 1990.
2. Ahrenholz D, Simmons R: Peritonitis and other intraabdominal infections. In: Howard RJ, Simmons RL (eds): Surgical Infectious Diseases. 2nd ed. East Norwalk, CT, Appleton & Lange, p 605, 1988.
3. Bercovici B, Michel J, Miller J, et al: Antimicrobial activity of human peritoneal fluid. Surg Gynecol Obstet 141:885, 1975.
4. Tsilibary E, Wissig S: Absorption from the peritoneal cavity: SEM study of the mesothelium covering the peritoneal surface of the muscular portion of the diaphragm. Am J Anat 149:127, 1977.
5. Steinberg B: Infections of the Peritoneum. New York, Hoeber, 1944.
6. Forey H: Reactions of, and absorption by, lymphatics, with special reference to those of the diaphragm. Br J Exp Pathol 8:479, 1927.
7. Last M, Kurtz L, Stein T, et al: Effect of PEEP on the rate of thoracic duct flow and bacterial clearance from the peritoneal cavity. Am J Surg 145:126, 1983.
8. Watters W, Buck R: Scanning electron microscopy of mesothelial regeneration in the rat. Lab Invest 26:604, 1972.
9. Autio V: The spread of intraperitoneal infection: Studies with roentgen contrast medium. Acta Chir Scand 321(suppl):4, 1964.
10. Hau T, Hoffman R, Simmons R: Mechanisms of the adjuvant effect of hemoglobin in experimental peritonitis. I. In vivo inhibition of peritoneal leukocytosis. Surgery 83:223, 1978.
11. Dunn D, Rotstein O, Simmons R: Fibrin in peritonitis. IV. Synergistic intraperitoneal infection caused by Escherichia coli and Bacteroides fragilis within fibrin clots. Arch Surg 119:139, 1984.
12. Onderonk A, Kasper D, Mansheim B, et al: Experimental animal models for anaerobic infections. Rev Infect Dis 1:291, 1979.
13. Scheierson S, Amsterdam D, Perlman E: Enhancement of intraperitoneal staphylococcal virulence for mice with different bile salts. Nature 190:829, 1961.
14. Yull A, Abrams J, Davis J: The peritoneal fluid in strangulation obstruction. The role of the red blood cell and E. coli bacteria in producing toxicity. J Surg Res 2:223, 1962.
15. Lee J, Ahrenholz D, Nelson D, et al: Mechanisms of the adjuvant effect of hemoglobin in experimental peritonitis. V. The significance of the coordinated iron component. Surgery 86:41, 1979.
16. Correia J, Conn H: Spontaneous bacterial peritonitis in cirrhosis: Endemic or epidemic? Med Clin North Am 59:963, 1975.
17. Dunn D, Barke R, Ahrenholz D, et al: The adjuvant effect of peritoneal fluid in experimental peritonitis. Ann Surg 199:37, 1984.
18. Hau T, Simmons R: Heparin in the treatment of experimental peritonitis. Ann Surg 187:294, 1978.
19. Ahrenholz D, Simmons R: Fibrin in peritonitis: I. Beneficial and adverse effects of fibrin in experimental E. coli peritonitis. Surgery 88:41, 1980.
20. Cochran DQ, Almond CH, Shucart WA: An experimental study of the effects of barium and intestinal contents on the peritoneal cavity. Am J Roentgenol 89:883, 1963.
21. Bartlett J, Onderonk A, Louie T, et al: A review: Lessons from an animal model of intra-abdominal sepsis. Arch Surg 113:853, 1978.
22. Nichols R, Smith J, Balthazar E: Peritonitis and intraabdominal abscess: An experimental model for the evaluation of human disease. J Surg Res 25:129, 1978.
23. Altemeier W: The bacterial flora of acute perforated appendicitis: a bacteriologic study based upon one hundred cases. Ann Surg 107:517, 1938.
24. Stone H, Kolb L, Geheber C: Incidence and significance of intraperitoneal anaerobic bacteria. Ann Surg 181:705, 1975.
25. Lorber B, Swenson R: The bacteriology of intra-abdominal infections. Surg Clin North Am 55:1349, 1975.
26. Altemeier W: The pathogenicity of the bacteria of appendicitis peritonitis: An experimental study. Surgery 11:374, 1942.
27. Nichols R, Smith J: Modern approach to the diagnosis of anaerobic sepsis. Surg Clin North Am 55:21, 1975.
28. Bentley D, Nichols R, Condon R, et al: The microflora of the human ileum and intra-abdominal colon: Results of direct needle aspiration at surgery and evaluation of the techniques. J Lab Clin Med 79:421, 1972.
29. Nichols R: Intraabdominal sepsis: Characterization and treatment. J Infect Dis 135(suppl):S54, 1977.
30. Nichols R, Smith J: Intragastric microbial colonization in common disease states of the stomach and duodenum. Ann Surg 182:557, 1975.
31. Gorbach S, Bartlett J: Anaerobic infections (first of three parts). N Engl J Med 290:1177, 1974.
32. Nichols R, Condon R, Bentley D, et al: Ileal microflora in surgical patients. J Urol 105:351, 1971.
33. Nichols R, Condon R, Gorbach S, et al: Efficacy of preoperative antimicrobial preparation of the bowel. Ann Surg 176:227, 1972.
34. Altemeier W, Culbertson W, Fullen W, et al: Intra-abdominal abscesses. Am J Surg 125:701, 1973.
35. Swenson R, Lorber B, Michaelson T, et al: The bacteriology of intra-abdominal infections. Arch Surg 109:398, 1974.
36. Gorbach S, Thadepalli H, Norsen J: Anaerobic microorganisms in intraabdominal infections. In: Balows A, DeHaan R, Dowell V, et al (eds): Anaerobic Bacteria: Role in Disease. Springfield, IL, Charles C Thomas, p 399, 1974.
37. Tally F, McGowan K, Kellum J, et al: A randomized comparison of cefoxitin with or without amikacin and clindamycin in surgical sepsis. Ann Surg 193:318, 1981.
38. Rotstein O, Pruett T, Simmons R: Microbiologic features and treatment of persistent peritonitis in patients in the intensive care unit. Can J Surg 29:247, 1986.
39. Nichols R, Musik A: Enterococcal infections in surgery—The mystery continues! Rev Infect Dis. In press.
40. Richardson J, Flint L, Polk H: Peritoneal lavage: A useful diagnostic adjunct for peritonitis. Surgery 94:826, 1983.
41. Crossley I, Williams R: Spontaneous bacterial peritonitis. Gut 26:325, 1985.
42. Runyon B, Umland E, Merlin T: Inoculation of blood culture bottles with ascitic fluid: Improved detection of spontaneous bacterial peritonitis. Arch Intern Med 147:73, 1987.
43. Garcia-Tsao F, Conn H, Lerner E: The diagnosis of bacterial peritonitis: Comparison of pH, lactate concentration, and leukocyte count. Hepatology 5:91, 1985.
44. Yang C, Liaw Y, Chu C, et al: White count, pH, and lactate in ascites in the diagnosis of spontaneous bacterial peritonitis. Hepatology 5:85, 1985.
45. Tito L, Rimola A, Llach J: Recurrence of spontaneous bacterial peritonitis in cirrhosis: Frequency and predictive factors. Hepatology 8:27, 1988.
46. Casadevall A, Pirofski L, Catalano M: Primary group A streptococcal peritonitis in adults. Am J Med 88:63, 1990.
47. Sherman S, Rohwedder J, Ravikushnan K, et al: Tuberculous enteritis and peritonitis. Report of 36 general hospital cases. Arch Intern Med 140:506, 1980.
48. Vas S: Peritonitis during CAPD: A mixed bag. Perit Dial Bull 1:47, 1981.
49. Pitcher W, Musher D: Critical importance of early diagnosis and treatment of intra-abdominal infection. Arch Surg 117:328, 1982.
50. Border J, Hassett J, LaDuca J, et al: The gut origin septic states in blunt multiple trauma (ISS = 40) in the ICU. Ann Surg 206:427, 1987.
51. Weinstein W, Onderonk A, Bartlett J, et al: Antimicrobial therapy of experimental intraabdominal sepsis. J Infect Dis 132:282, 1975.
52. Nichols R, Smith J, Fossedal E, et al: Efficacy of parenteral antibiotics in the treatment of experimentally induced intraabdominal sepsis. Rev Infect Dis 1:302, 1979.
53. Thadepalli H, Gorbach S, Broido P, et al: Abdominal trauma, anaerobes, and antibiotics. Surg Gynecol Obstet 173:270, 1973.
54. Hofstetter S, Pachter H, Bailey A, et al: A prospective comparison of two regimens of prophylactic antibiotics in abdominal trauma: Cefoxitin versus triple drug. J Trauma 24:307, 1984.
55. Gentry L, Feliciano D, Lea A, et al: Perioperative antibiotic therapy for penetrating injuries of the abdomen. Ann Surg 200:561, 1984.
56. Nichols R, Smith J, Klein D, et al: Risk of infection after penetrating abdominal trauma. N Engl J Med 311:1065, 1984.
57. Jones R, Thal E, Johnson N, et al: Evaluation of antibiotic therapy following penetrating abdominal trauma. Ann Surg 201:576, 1985.
58. Feliciano D, Gentry L, Bitondo C, et al: Single agent cephalosporin prophylaxis for penetrating abdominal trauma—Results and comment on the emergence of the enterococcus. Am J Surg 152:674, 1986.
59. Nichols R, Smith J, Klein D, et al: Risk of infection after penetrating abdominal trauma. N Engl J Med 311:1065, 1984.
60. Browder W, Smith J, Vivoda L, et al: Nonperforative appendicitis: A continuing surgical dilemma. J Infect Dis 159:1088, 1989.

61. Lennard E, Dellinger E, Wertz M, et al: Implications of leukocytosis and fever at conclusion of antibiotic therapy for intra-abdominal sepsis. Ann Surg 195:19, 1982.
62. Sparks F, Strauss E, Corey J: Percutaneous drainage of a diverticular abscess can make colostomy unnecessary in selected cases. Conn Med 54:305, 1990.
63. Grønvall J, Grønvall S, Hegedüs V: Ultrasound-guided drainage of fluid-containing masses using angiographic catheterization techniques. AJR 131:323, 1977.
64. Gerzof S, Robbins A, Johnson W, et al: Percutaneous catheter drainage of abdominal abscesses: A five-year experience. N Engl J Med 305:653, 1981.
65. Gerzof S, Johnson W, Robbins A, et al: Expanded criteria for percutaneous abscess drainage. Arch Surg 120:227, 1985.
66. Aeder M, Wellman J, Haaga J, et al: Role of surgical and percutaneous drainage in the treatment of abdominal abscesses. Arch Surg 118:273, 1983.
67. Olak J, Christou N, Stein L, et al: Operative vs. percutaneous drainage of intra-abdominal abscesses. Comparison of morbidity and mortality. Arch Surg 121:141, 1986.
68. Barakos J, Jeffrey R, Federle M, et al: CT in the management of periappendiceal abscess. AJR 146:1161, 1986.
69. Nunez D, Huber J, Yrizarry J, et al: Nonsurgical drainage of appendiceal abscesses. AJR 146:587, 1986.
70. Hiatt J, Fink A, King W, et al: Percutaneous aspiration of peripancreatic fluid collections: A safe method to detect infection. Surgery 101:523, 1987.
71. Hermann G: Intraperitoneal drainage. Surg Clin North Am 49:1279, 1969.
72. Yates J: An experimental study of the local effects of peritoneal drainage. Surg Gynecol Obstet 1:473, 1905.
73. Stephen M, Loewenthal J: Continuing peritoneal lavage in high-risk peritonitis. Surgery 85:603, 1979.
74. Lagarde M, Bolton J, Cohn I: Intraperitoneal povidone-iodine in experimental peritonitis. Ann Surg 187:613, 1978.
75. Lawson K, Lavery I: Hydrogen peroxide vs. normal saline lavage in experimental fecal peritonitis. Cleve Clin J Med 54:279, 1987.
76. Schumer W, Lee D, Jones B: Peritoneal lavage in postoperative therapy of late peritoneal sepsis. Surgery 55:841, 1964.
77. Rosato E, Oram-Smith J, Mullis W, et al: Peritoneal lavage treatment in experimental peritonitis. Ann Surg 175:384, 1972.
78. Noon G, Beall A, Jordan G, et al: Clinical evaluation of peritoneal irrigation with antibiotic solution. Surgery 62:73, 1967.
79. Rambo W: Irrigation of the peritoneal cavity with cephalothin. Am J Surg 123:192, 1972.
80. Sherman J, Luck S, Borger J: Irrigation of the peritoneal cavity for appendicitis in children: A double-blind study. J Pediatr Surg 11:371, 1976.
81. Nomikos I, Katsouyanni K, Papaioannou A: Washing with or without chloramphenicol in the treatment of peritonitis: A prospective clinical trial. Surgery 99:20, 1986.
82. Hudspeth A: Radical surgical debridement in the treatment of advanced generalized bacterial peritonitis. Arch Surg 110:1233, 1975.
83. Polk H, Fry D: Radical peritoneal debridement for established peritonitis: The results of a prospective randomized clinical trial. Ann Surg 192:350, 1980.
84. Steinberg D: On leaving the peritoneal cavity open in acute generalized suppurative peritonitis. Am J Surg 137:216, 1979.
85. Wittmann D, Aprahamian C, Bergstein J: Etappenlavage: Advanced diffuse peritonitis managed by planned multiple laparotomies utilizing zippers, slide fastener, and Velcro analogue for temporary abdominal closure. World J Surg 14:218, 1990.
86. Bradley E: Management of infected pancreatic necrosis by open drainage. Ann Surg 206:542, 1987.
87. Brolin R, Nosher J, Leiman S, et al: Percutaneous catheter versus open surgical drainage in the treatment of abdominal abscesses. Am Surg 50:102, 1984.
88. vanSonnenberg E, Mueller P, Ferrucci J: Percutaneous drainage of 250 abdominal abscesses and fluid collections. Part I: Results, failures, and complications. Radiology 151:337, 1984.
89. Pruett T, Rotstein O, Crass J, et al: Percutaneous aspiration and drainage for suspected abdominal infection. Surgery 96:731, 1984.
90. Lang E, Springer R, Glorioso L, et al: Abdominal abscess drainage under radiologic guidance: Causes of failure. Radiology 159:329, 1986.
91. Lamaris J, Bruining J, Jeekel J: Ultrasound-guided percutaneous drainage of intra-abdominal abscesses. Br J Surg 74:620, 1987.
92. Civardi G, Fornari F, Cavanna L, et al: Ultrasonically guided percutaneous drainage of abdominal fluid collections: A long-term study of its therapeutic efficacy. Gastrointest Radiol 15:245, 1990.
93. Del Carmen Nieto R, Nava C: Continuous peritoneal lavage: Its employment in the treatment of diffuse peritonitis. Invest Clin 27:107, 1975.
94. Olesen A, Jorgensen F, Bilde T, et al: Peritoneal lavage in diffuse peritonitis originating from perforated appendix. Ugeskr Laeger 142:1415, 1980.
95. Shweni P, Pitsoe S, Mokgokong E: Continuous antibiotic peritoneal lavage compared with simple drainage for severe intraperitoneal sepsis of gynaecological and obstetric origin. S Afr Med J 57:117, 1980.
96. Hunt J: Generalized peritonitis: To irrigate or not to irrigate the abdominal cavity. Arch Surg 117:209, 1982.
97. Kumar G, Smile S, Sibal R: Postoperative peritoneal lavage in generalised peritonitis. A prospective analysis. Int Surg 74:20, 1989.
98. Bhushan C, Mital V, Elhence I: Continuous postoperative peritoneal lavage in diffuse peritonitis using balanced saline antibiotic solution. Int Surg 60:526, 1975.
99. Gjessing J, Tomlin P: Continuous peritoneal lavage. Acta Chir Scand 140:124, 1974.
100. Uden P, Eskilsson P, Brunes L, et al: A clinical evaluation of postoperative peritoneal lavage in the treatment of perforated appendicitis. Br J Surg 70:348, 1983.
101. Washington B, Villalba M, Lauter C, et al: Cefamandole-erythromycin-heparin peritoneal irrigation: An adjunct to the surgical treatment of diffuse bacterial peritonitis. Surgery 94:576, 1983.

CHAPTER 43

Burns

Karen A. Mello
Jeffrey A. Gelfand

Each year in the United States, 12,000 people die of burn injury, and more than 100,000 are hospitalized. Infection remains the leading cause of mortality in hospitalized burn patients, accounting for approximately 75% of deaths.[1] Sepsis is the most common infection resulting in mortality, and although the incidence has decreased with improved wound care and isolation techniques, mortality from sepsis in burn patients remains at least twice that from sepsis in general. Burn wound infection, pneumonia, and intestinal microflora are all points of origin contributing to the generation of the septic syndrome, and the pathophysiologic distinction between clear-cut septic death and multiple organ system failure without positive blood cultures has become increasingly blurred.[1] It is clear that burn trauma–initiated activation of inflammatory mechanisms results in immune dysregulation and inadequate defenses against infection (Table 43–1).

PATHOPHYSIOLOGY OF INFECTIONS WITH BURNS

Burn Disruption of Normal Skin Barrier Function

The skin acts as a mechanical barrier to penetration through the rather impermeable keratinized layers (Table 43–2). Desiccation, produced by the relatively dry skin, is inhibitory to the growth of gram-negative organisms. Desquamation quite literally sweeps organisms away, and the elaboration of unsaturated free fatty acids is thought to play a role in inhibiting a number of microorganisms, particularly the group A streptococci.

Bacterial interference, or the inhibition of pathogen proliferation by a nonpathogenic resident flora, also appears to play a significant role in controlling cutaneous colonization of normal and burned skin. Finally, the Langerhans cell, a bone marrow–derived immunocompetent cell that migrates to the skin, may play an important role in immune function in the skin.

Burn injury obviously destroys the skin and thereby de-

TABLE 43–1

IMMUNOLOGIC ABNORMALITIES IN BURN PATIENTS

Phagocytic Cells
Granulocytopenia, common
Diminished chemotactic responsiveness
Partial degranulation
Decreased superoxide and hydrogen peroxide production (stimulated)
Some impairment of bactericidal activity
Polymorphonuclear neutrophil aggregation

Humoral
Immunoglobulins: are decreased proportional to burn size; depression is moderate (rarely <60% of normal): nadir 2–5 d after burn; B cell response to old antigens is almost normal, but there is decreased response to new antigens
Complement: massive alternative pathway activation by burn produces active cleavage products and deficient function; extravasation and depressed synthesis also occur; by comparison, classic pathway moderately depressed, then rebounds
Fibronectin: is markedly depressed after burn injury

Cellular Immune Function
Anergy; markedly delayed allograft rejection
Decreased mitogen and antigen responses
Total lymphocyte count usually normal, but decreased T helper cells, increased T suppressor cells
Normal lymphocytes suppressed by several circulating serum immunosuppressive factors in burn serum

---

stroys a major organ of host defense. In the burn wound, the barrier becomes culture media, normal flora is destroyed, and an ischemic wound is created, which prevents the delivery of plasma proteins such as antibody and complement, white blood cells, and even antibiotics.[2]

Humoral Immune Dysfunction in Burn Patients

Complement System

The complement system plays an essential role in the host's defenses against bacteria, fungi, and viruses. Complement may act as a recognition system, being activated by foreign or altered host structures and generating critical host defense responses. These responses include the development of vascular permeability (permitting egress of yet more antibody and complement), chemotaxis of inflammatory cells, opsonization, and bacteriolysis.

There are two major pathways of complement activation. The classic pathway is typically activated by the interaction of antigen with immunoglobulin (Ig) G or IgM antibody and thus usually requires a specific immunologic response. The alternative complement pathway may be initiated by the polysaccharide moiety of bacterial endotoxin, fungi, thermally damaged cells, or serum proteins. When activated, complement proteins are usually fixed or covalently bound to activating surfaces, whereas low-molecular-weight cleavage products (such as C3a and C5a) are released into

---

TABLE 43–2

ROLE OF SKIN IN DEFENSE AGAINST INFECTION

Physical barrier to penetration (keratin layers)
Desquamation
Antibacterial substances—unsaturated free fatty acids
Bacterial interference from normal flora (colonization resistance)
Antigen presentation to T lymphocytes (Langerhans' cells)

---

surrounding tissue and/or the blood stream, where they act as chemotactic peptides.

As expected from the mechanisms by which the complement pathways are activated, the alternative pathway appears to play a critical function in limiting infection with bacteria for which prior humoral immunity does not exist. Thus, this pathway serves as a first line of defense and is phylogenetically older than the classic pathway. With the appearance of specific antibody in evolution as well as in individual development, the classic pathway is recruited. This pathway is activated more rapidly than the alternative pathway, providing an efficient defense mechanism.

A number of investigators noted hypocomplementemia after burn injury, both in animals and in humans.[3–8] One study of complement in burn patients found that all patients whose complement levels were less than 50% of normal had positive blood cultures.[9]

Although it has been known for some time that burn injury is associated with abnormalities of complement and complement activity, this was previously attributed to serum protein loss and negative nitrogen balance. Work in our laboratory and in other laboratories has demonstrated that, in fact, the complement system is activated by thermal injury, resulting in the release of a number of biologically potent activation products and the depletion of this critical host defense mechanism.

More recently, we demonstrated that thermally injured cells, remaining in the wound, act as an additional complement-activating stimulus, adding to local and systemic immune dysfunction and lending additional scientific support for the clinical practice of early, extensive débridement of burned tissue.[10]

The generation of complement cleavage products such as C5a by burn injury may be critical in the development of immune dysfunction, as well as burn shock, adult respiratory distress syndrome, and multiple organ system failure. Animal studies have documented C5a generation by burns;[7] evidence is harder to come by in human burns, because C5a is rapidly bound by neutrophils and hence cleared from the circulation, usually within 15 to 30 minutes of injury—too soon for most patients to be adequately studied. Nonetheless, the indirect evidence of C5a generation in burn injury is overwhelming. C5a bound to neutrophils first stimulates, then down-regulates chemotactic and respiratory burst functions. Furthermore, C5a, alone or in concert with otherwise substimulatory levels of lipopolysaccharide, stimulates monocytes and macrophages to produce interleukin-1 (IL-1) and tumor necrosis factor α (TNF-α). TNF-α and IL-1 are presumed to be critical mediators in the septic shock syndrome, adult respiratory distress syndrome, and multiple organ system failure.[11]

Fibronectin

Fibronectin is a glycoprotein found in plasma and in the extracellular matrix of most tissues. It appears to be necessary for normal reticuloendothelial cell function and is opsonic for *Staphylococcus aureus,* an important pathogen in burn patients. Clinical studies have shown that fibronectin levels are low with burn injury, that low fibronectin levels often precede sepsis, and that infusion of fibronectin-rich cryoprecipitate may improve the clinical course of infections in burn patients.[12, 13]

Immunoglobulins

Ig levels are depressed early by burn injury, with the nadir at 2 to 5 days after the burn. In general, IgG levels are the most depressed, with little early change in IgM levels.[14–16]

Burn blister fluid contains all the serum Igs, and one cause of the drop in Ig levels may be the extravasation of previously intravascular IgG into tissue through the increasingly permeable capillary endothelium. Increased tissue levels of IgG in deeper layers of burned skin have been demonstrated.[16]

Mild depression of serum antibody concentrations correlates poorly with the incidence of infection, but IgG levels of less than 5 mg/mL are associated with a high risk of sepsis. The secondary humoral response to antigens appears intact, whereas the Ig response to new antigens is variable, being depressed for some antigens and intact for others.[17]

Neutrophil Function

Granulocytopenia is common in the few days after burn injury and has been shown to correlate with burn surface area.[18] Neutrophil function from patients with burns involving greater than 25% of body surface area has been shown to be impaired for as long as several months after burn injury.[19] In addition to the loss of complement activity and the resultant deficiency of opsonization, chemotaxis, and bacteriolysis, burn-associated complement activation suddenly floods the immune system with anaphylatoxins C3a and C5a. This may have multiple opposing but nonetheless profound effects on other immune functions. Liberation of C3a may produce increased suppressor T cell activity and may, in turn, inhibit both polyclonal B lymphocyte activation and the response to specific T cell–dependent antigens. Other C3 cleavage products have been shown to have inhibitory effects.[20]

C5a also activates neutrophils; after being activated, neutrophils may ultimately become less responsive, a phenomenon known as down-regulation. Evidence suggests that neutrophils from burn patients have, in fact, become partially deactivated, as manifested by partial degranulation.[21] Chemotactic activity and random migration are markedly depressed during the first 2 weeks after injury, and sepsis is seen in patients in whom chemotaxis is most depressed. In addition, the severity of the defect is a function of burn wound area.[21] Solomkin and colleagues,[22] Alexander and associates,[23] and others noted diminished chemotaxis and poor bactericidal activity in severely burned patients. They observed that the opsonic index of serum was depressed soon after the burn but returned to near-normal values by the 4th to the 14th postburn day. Warden and coworkers studied neutrophil chemotaxis in 46 burn victims.[24] Leukocyte chemotaxis was inversely correlated with burn size during the first 72 hours after injury. After 72 hours, leukocyte chemotaxis directly correlated with the clinical state and was highly predictive of ultimate survival. Furthermore, serum from burn patients inhibited the chemotaxis of normal donor neutrophils. The level of lysozyme in neutrophil-specific granules was reduced in the patients with neutrophils that were least responsive to chemotactic stimuli, and the degree of neutrophil lysozyme reduction was related to the extent of thermal injury. The investigators concluded that peripheral blood neutrophils from burn patients had degranulated their specific granule contents and that such degranulation resulted in decreased chemotaxis. These defects are comparable with in vivo exposure to C5a before in vitro testing.[25]

A number of investigators described serum factors associated with burns and trauma suppressive of leukocyte function.[26–28] Finally, it was reported that fluid-phase C3b, generated in the course of complement activation by burn injury, inhibits neutrophil opsonophagocytosis and bactericidal activity.[29]

Cell-Mediated Immunity

Absolute levels of both monocytes and lymphocytes fall significantly in the first 72 hours after burn injury. These two variables have each been independent predictors of survival. Persistent monocytopenia and lymphopenia are grave prognostic signs, which precede septicemia by several days.[18]

Many investigators reported abnormalities of cell-mediated immunity and lymphocyte function in burn patients. Anergy, delayed allograft rejection, decreased number of T cells, increased ratio of suppressor to helper T cells, and decreased antigen and mitogen responsiveness have been described by a number of groups, reviewed in articles by Miller and colleagues[30] and Ninnemann.[31] Complement cleavage fragments and high plasma prostaglandin levels may be causes of this suppression, and several circulating inhibitory factors have been identified.[32, 33] Thus, in addition to the enormous defects in the anatomic barriers that permit microorganisms access to deeper structures, there are major defects of humoral, cellular, and phagocytic immune function. The burn patient is therefore the archetypical immunosuppressed host.

Cytokines

Tissue injury is thought to result in the generation of the cytokines TNF-α and IL-1β, with profound effects on host defense, immunologic, and metabolic functions. After burns, patients have elevated plasma levels of TNF-α and IL-1β.[34] Levels of the acute-phase proteins, such as C-reactive protein (CRP), then increase dramatically. In vitro studies of thermally killed cells suggest that these cells in turn bind CRP. CRP bound to dead cells leads to further complement activation and deposition, in turn opsonizing dead cells for ingestion by phagocytic neutrophils and monocytes. Monocyte ingestion of CRP-opsonized cells stimulates TNF-α secretion, which further elevates CRP levels.[35] Thus, with tissue injury, cytokine generation and acute-phase protein synthesis result in a system enhancing cellular débridement and promoting repair, perpetuated by the persistence of damaged tissue. Furthermore, CRP may play a critical role in an inflammatory amplification system in which cytokine-induced CRP is bound to damaged or necrotic cells, stimulating yet more cytokine synthesis.[35] These events are offered as an explanation for the frequent clinical observation that immunologic and metabolic homeostasis is not restored until damaged tissue is removed, and the wound has healed.

Whatever the stimuli for cytokine production (C5a, endotoxin, dead cells, and so on) in burns, the levels of TNF-α are among the highest we have measured in any disease state.[34] IL-1β levels are also high, especially initially after the burn. In our studies, TNF-α levels correlated directly with disease severity as measured by Acute Physiology and Chronic Health Evaluation (APACHE) II score, whereas IL-1β levels were actually less elevated in the more seriously injured. In addition, we found that climbing TNF-α levels heralded clinical deterioration.[34] We found that monocytes of burn patients in vitro spontaneously (without stimulation) produced abnormally high IL-1β and TNF-α levels and, when stimulated, produced less than normal increments of IL-1β. This improved with time as patients recovered, approaching normal levels with healing.[36] This would help to explain the paradox of increased levels of cytokines after injury, associated with inadequate cellular immune responses to new antigens.

TABLE 43–3

TYPES OF INFECTION IN BURN PATIENTS

Burn wound invasion	Suppurative thrombophlebitis
Burn wound sepsis	Suppurative chondritis
Cellulitis	Pyelonephritis
Pneumonia	Endocarditis
Septicemia	Miscellaneous

Adapted from Pruitt BA Jr, McManus AT: Opportunistic infections in severely burned patients. Am J Med 76(suppl 3A):146, 1984.

The elevated plasma cytokine levels certainly contribute to the development of both burn and septic shock, adult respiratory distress syndrome, and multiple organ system failure; cytokine abnormalities undoubtedly play a major role in the immune, inflammatory, and metabolic abnormalities of burn injury.

CLINICAL INFECTIONS IN BURN PATIENTS

The risk of burn infection is a function of burn surface area, depth of burn, and age of the patient. Burn depth determines how much vascular supply remains, and this is a critical determinant of infection. Partial-thickness wounds rarely become severely infected with good supportive care, whereas full-thickness wounds, being avascular, are readily infected. In addition, life-threatening burn wound infection is uncommon with full-thickness burns of less than 30% body surface area. Mortality is also directly proportional to age. In general, the older the adult burn patient is, the poorer the prognosis. A list of the types of infections typically seen in severely burned patients is seen in Table 43–3. The peak incidence of infection is in the second and third weeks after injury.

Microbiology of Burn Wounds

Bacterial colonization of the burn wound occurs early. In a study of children with burn injuries, burn wound colonization began in perioral and perianal areas. Surface cultures of these burn areas were predominantly anaerobic in the first week, with aerobic gram-negative isolates thereafter. However, burn wounds provide a milieu for anaerobic organisms, with an associated risk of tetanus and gas gangrene.

Burn wound pathogens reflect colonization from the patient's endogenous flora and the hospital environment. Pronounced variations in the incidence of certain pathogens are seen in any particular burn unit, depending on local antibiotic use and resistance patterns. Most wounds harbor multiple organisms, including *Staphyloccus* species, *Streptococcus* species, *Bacteroides* species, *Enterobacter* species, *Escherichia coli* species, *Pseudomonas aeruginosa* species, *Acinetobacter* species, *Proteus* species, *Klebsiella* species, and *Serratia* species. The large reservoir of bacteria in the gut has been postulated to be the source of gram-negative sepsis in severely burned patients. Bacterial translocation from the gut to reticuloendothelial organs has been demonstrated in an animal model of cutaneous thermal injury.[38, 39]

In one report of invasive burn wound infections, *P. aeruginosa* was cultured in almost 50% of burn wounds.[40] The overall incidence of invasive burn wound infection in this series was 12.7%, with a mortality rate of 90%.[40] Pathogenic features of this organism include antibiotic resistance, production of extracellular proteases, and motility enabling it to penetrate the burn wound and invade surrounding tissue. The Enterobacteriaceae isolated from burn wounds

also display a high level of antibiotic resistance. Infections with methicillin-resistant *S. aureus* have been a significant problem in certain burn units.[41]

The nature of burn wound infections is also influenced by microbial selection pressures attributable to the use of antibacterial agents and the prolonged survival of patients in a hospitalized setting. Opportunistic infections with fungi and the herpesviruses are seen more frequently in patients who are surviving longer in the hospital environment.[41] Fungal infections with *Candida, Mucor,* and *Aspergillus* species are occurring with increased frequency.[42–44]

Contributing factors to the development of candidemia in the burn patient include the use of multiple broad-spectrum antibiotics, central venous catheters, and parenteral nutrition. *Candida* colonization of wounds occurs in approximately 10 to 30% of burn wounds. Most series report an incidence of candidemia of 1.8 to 5.4%, with mortality rates of 70% or more. Uncontrolled investigations using aggressive treatment with amphotericin B and topical antifungal agents have reported markedly lower mortality rates.[45] The use of topical wound therapy with mafenide acetate and the use of enteral antifungal agents such as nystatin appear to decrease the incidence of invasive fungal inections in certain burn units.[46] Earlier diagnosis and treatment are the key to reduced mortality from this complication.

Surveillance surface cultures of the burn wound provide information on the patient's flora and its antimicrobial sensitivity. Weekly surveillance cultures of wounds, urine, and the respiratory tract should be obtained. Blood cultures should be routinely obtained after extensive surgical débridement, or with the development of fever, hypothermia, altered mentation, hypotension, hypoglycemia, acidosis, respiratory distress, oliguria, or ileus (all cardinal signs of burn wound invasion or sepsis). Routine wound biopsy with quantitative culture is controversial, and the reliability of the technique has been questioned.[37]

Specific Infections

Burn Wound Sepsis. A change in the margins of the wound, with ischemic, hemorrhagic, or violaceous discoloration; extension of the necrotic area; or the sudden spontaneous separation of the eschar suggests of burn wound sepsis. A sudden change in the clinical status of the patient should prompt a close inspection of the entire burn wound for this possibility. The development of mental confusion, metabolic acidosis, hyperpnea, deteriorating renal function, and hypothermia, as well as fever or hypotension, should prompt a careful examination for infection. Rapid diagnosis of suspected burn wound sepsis by biopsy and examination by frozen section for both bacteria and fungi, followed by reexamination of permanent sections coupled with culture, is an alternative to quantitative culture.[37] Invasion of unburned tissue by bacteria and fungi is the cardinal sign of burn wound sepsis.

Pneumonia. Improvements in wound care in specialized burn units have resulted in the emergence of pneumonia as the most common origin of sepsis. Bronchopneumonia originating from colonization of the airways predominates and is especially likely in the presence of inhalation injury, intubation, or aspiration. Hematogenous seeding of the lungs also occurs, frequently producing nodular infiltrates, but is less common. Two pathogens require special note when considering burn-associated pneumonias—*S. aureus* and *Pseudomonas*. Both commonly cause pneumonia in these patients. Of course, other pathogens must also be considered.

Suppurative Chondritis. Auricular cartilage is easily destroyed by thermal injury to the ear and in turn is readily

TABLE 43-4
TOPICAL AGENTS FOR BURN WOUND CARE*

Activity and Side Effects	Silver Sulfadiazine 1% Cream (Silvadine)	Mafenide Acetate (Sulfamylon)	Silver Nitrate 0.5% Soaks
Antimicrobial Spectrum			
Gram-positive cocci	+ +	+	+ + +
Gram-negative rods	+ + +	+ + +	+ + +
Fungi	+ + +	+ +	+ + +
Development of resistance	+ +	–	–
Eschar penetration	+/–	+ +	–
Side Effects			
Pain on application	–	+	–
Hypersensitivity	+	+ + +	–
Neutropenia	+ +	–	–
Metabolic acidosis	–	+ + +	+ +
Hyponatremia	–	–	+
Methemoglobinemia	+	–	–

*+ + + = strong effect; + + = substantial effect; + = some effect; +/– = minimal effect; – = no effect.

infected, frequently by *Pseudomonas.* Infected cartilage must be excised.[41]

Suppurative Thrombophlebitis. This should be suspected when a site of sepsis cannot be found or when hematogenous pneumonia develops. It is especially common when cutdown venotomies are used for access, or the catheter site lies near a burn wound. When this entity is suspected, diagnostic venotomy should be performed. If the diagnosis is confirmed, surgical excision is necessary.

Bacterial Endocarditis. The requirement for prolonged pulmonary arterial catheters and central intravenous lines makes burn patients more susceptible to bacterial endocarditis; again, this diagnosis should be suspected in patients with signs of sepsis or bacteremia in the absence of another source.

THERAPY
General Measures

Complete sterility of the burn wound is practically impossible. Ward nursing procedures, wound excision, and grafting, as well as topical therapy, are all carried out with the aim to keep wound colonization at low levels (≤100 colony-forming units per gram of tissue). In contrast, lethal burn wound sepsis is usually seen with colony counts of 100,000 colony-forming units or more per gram of tissue.

With modern resuscitation and physiologic monitoring, improved survival from burns has resulted from the creation of specialized burn units.[37] The combination of a physical environment designed to isolate patients from exposure to bacteria in the environment and intensive care by both nurses and surgeons experienced in dealing with burns and their complications has vastly improved survival figures. Thus, the first step in management of burn patients after resuscitation ought to be transfer to a specialized burn unit. The bacteria-controlled nursing unit, in which patients are barrier isolated in a plastic film–contained area with positive pressure and bacteria-free filtered air to prevent cross-contamination, has resulted in a marked reduction in burn infections. Aggressive fluid and nutritional support, as well as early excision of full-thickness wounds and early wound closure with skin grafts, is crucial. Wound closure is truly the definitive therapy of burn infection.

Prophylactic Measures

A tetanus booster, using the adult combined tetanus and diphtheria toxoids (0.5 mL), is given to all patients without a history of immunization in the past year. If the state of tetanus immunity is unknown, or if the wound has been grossly contaminated, human tetanus immune globulin (250 to 500 U) is administered intramuscularly at a site distant from the tetanus and diphtheria toxoid booster injection.

Topical therapy is begun immediately.[46] The aim of topical therapy is not sterility but reduction of wound colony counts. A list of the major agents in wide use in topical burn care is given in Table 43–4, along with attributes and side effects.

In the Massachusetts General Hospital Burn Unit, we use primarily silver nitrate 0.5%, which has a wide antibacterial spectrum and is bacteriostatic for gram-positive and gram-negative organisms, as well as fungi. Resistance is extremely rare but has been reported. It does not cause pain on application and is also relatively inexpensive. There are some major drawbacks, however. Silver nitrate 0.5% penetrates the eschar poorly, making it more useful in preventing wound infection than in treating established wound infection. We do not use silver nitrate on the face and perineum (where we use 1% silver sulfadiazene [Silvadene]). Silver nitrate discolors everything it contacts (skin, dressings, linen, floors), and dressings must be rewetted with silver nitrate every 2 hours to maintain bacteriostatic activity at the wound surface. The dressing is soaked every 2 hours because if the silver nitrate evaporates and concentrates to greater than 1%, then it actually damages the skin. At a concentration of less than 0.5%, it is not bacteriostatic. Dressings are changed every 12 hours. This restricts the utility of the agent to burn units prepared to deal with these considerable logistic drawbacks. Hyponatremia is a significant threat but is readily detectable and preventable. Methemoglobinemia is a rare complication.

Silver sulfadiazine 1% cream is the most commonly used topical burn agent. It is active against gram-negative rods, gram-positive cocci, and fungi. However, the development of resistance, especially by *Staphylococcus* species, *Providencia*, *Pseudomonas* species, and *Enterobacter* species, has been described. Silver sulfadiazine penetrates the eschar, although not as well as mafenide, is painless on application, and does not discolor skin or linen. Transient leukopenia, appearing usually between days 3 and 5 and resolving despite continued use of the agent, is common. It is advisable to discontinue administration of the drug when the leukocyte count falls below 3000/mm³. Hypersensitivity reactions, methemoglobinemia, and crystalluria are also potential side effects.

Mafenide acetate is bacteriostatic against gram-positive cocci, many anaerobes such as clostridia, and gram-negative bacilli. It has minimal activity against fungi. Superinfection by resistant gram-negative bacteria and fungi occurs with significant frequency. Mafenide readily penetrates the burn wound and is therefore most useful for treating established wound infection. This results in its being absorbed, where its action as a carbonic anhydrase inhibitor can cause bicarbonate loss, hyperchloremic metabolic acidosis, and compensatory hyperventilation, sometimes leading to respiratory exhaustion. Extreme caution must be used when treating large burns with this agent. An additional, serious drawback is pain on application. This, coupled with the metabolic side effects, limits its use by most burn centers to short-term prophylaxis, management of smaller wounds, or treatment of developing infection.

Polymyxin B-neomycin (Neosporin) ointment is costly and difficult to apply but is useful for small burns and in specific regions such as the periorbital area.

Systemic prophylactic antibiotics are useful for two additional situations. Beta-hemolytic streptococci may inhabit hair follicles and persist despite topical therapy. We routinely use penicillin G (4 million U intravenously every 6 hours) for 2 or 3 days in all patients; however, this remains controversial. Most centers treat children, especially with scalds, with penicillin.

Bacteremia is common during wound débridement. Prophylactic antibiotics are advocated immediately before, during, and after such surgery. The choice of drugs should be guided by wound cultures; in general, both gram-negative rods and staphylococci should be covered. A reasonable empirical regimen is an aminoglycoside (gentamicin or amikacin if there is resistance, as well as nafcillin or vancomycin). Prophylaxis is initiated immediately before surgery and usually spans 24 hours.

Treatment of Invasive Infection

Differentiating colonization from invasion clinically has been previously discussed, as has the issue of surveillance surface cultures versus biopsy and quantitative culture. Mafenide affords penetration of wounds and may be helpful in topical therapy of invasive infection. Surveillance cultures, with sensitivity patterns, should certainly guide systemic therapy. Initial therapy should cover both gram-negative organisms and staphylococci. A reasonable regimen might be to start with gentamicin or amikacin with piperacillin, as well as nafcillin or vancomycin, and to discontinue administration of the latter if staphylococci are not isolated. Gentamicin can be used if sensitivities permit. There are no studies in burn patients comparing newer agents such as ceftazidime, imipenem, and timentin with established combinations. Although these are theoretically attractive, both ceftazidime alone and timentin alone have had notably equivocal results in some studies involving patients undergoing chemotherapy for malignancies. *Pseudomonas* isolates resistant to imipenem have been obtained from several burn patients.

It is important to emphasize that serum levels of drugs must be monitored especially carefully in burn patients to prevent toxicity and ensure efficacy. Aminoglycoside and vancomycin half-lives are substantially reduced in burn patients with normal renal function, for example.[47] Higher than normal doses may thus be required but should be based on monitoring of serum levels.

References

1. Deitch EA: The management of burns. N Engl J Med 323:1249, 1990.
2. Gelfand JA: Infections in burn patients: A paradigm for cutaneous infection in the patient at risk. Am J Med 76(suppl):S158, 1984.
3. Heideman M: Complement activation in vitro induced by endotoxin and injured tissue. J Surg Res 26:670, 1979.
4. Bjornson AB, Altemeier WA, Bjornson HS: Host defense against opportunistic microorganisms following trauma. II. Changes in complement and immunoglobulins in patients with abdominal trauma and in septic patients without trauma. Ann Surg 188:102, 1978.
5. Alexander JW, Stinnett D, Ogle CK, et al: A comparison of immunologic profiles and their influence on bacteremia in surgical patients with a high risk of infection. Surgery 86:94, 1979.
6. Bjornson AB, Bjornson HS, Altemeier WA: Reduction in alternative complement pathway mediated C3 conversion following burn injury. Ann Surg 194:224, 1981.
7. Gelfand JA, Donelan MB, Hawiger A, et al: Alternative complement pathway activation as a cause of mortality from burns in a murine model. J Clin Invest 70:1170, 1982.
8. Gelfand JA, Donelan MB, Burke JF: Preferential activation and depletion of the alternative complement pathway by burn injury in humans. Ann Surg 198:58, 1983.
9. Heideman M, Saravis C, Clowes GHA: The effect of nonviable tissue and abscesses on complement depletion and the development of bacteremia. J Trauma 22:527, 1982.
10. Yamada Y, Hefter K, Burke JF, et al: An in vitro model of the wound microenvironment: Local phagocytic cell abnormalities associated with in situ complement activation. J Infect Dis 155:998, 1987.
11. Okusawa S, Gelfand JA, Ikejima T, et al: Interleukin-1 induces a shock-like state in rabbits: Synergism with tumor necrosis factor and the effect of cyclooxygenase inhibition. J Clin Invest 81:1162, 1988.
12. Saba TM, Blumenstock FA, Scovill WA, et al: Cryoprecipitate reversal of opsonic α_2 surface binding glycoprotein deficiency in septic surgical and trauma patients. Science 201:622, 1978.
13. Robbins AB, Doran JE, Reese AC, et al: Clinical response to cold insoluble globulin replacement in a patient with sepsis and thermal injury. Am J Surg 142:636, 1981.
14. Munster AM, Hoagland HC, Pruitt BA Jr: The effect of thermal injury on serum immunoglobulin. Ann Surg 172:965, 1970.
15. Daniels JC, Larson DL, Abston S, et al: Serum protein profiles in thermal burns. I. Serum electrophoretic patterns, immunoglobulins and transport proteins. J Trauma 14:137, 1974.
16. Daniels JC, Fukushima M, Larson DL, et al: Tissue levels of various globulins in burned patients. J Trauma 11:699, 1971.
17. Alexander JW, Moncrief JJ: Alterations of the immune response following severe thermal injury. Arch Surg 93:75, 1966.
18. Peterson V, Murphy J, Haddix T, et al: Identification of novel prognostic indicators in burned patients. J Trauma 28:632, 1988.
19. Ogle C, Alexander J, Nagy H, et al: A long term study and correlation of lymphocyte and neutrophil function in the patient with burns. J Burn Care Rehabil 11:105, 1990.
20. Gelfand JA: How do complement components and fragments affect cellular immunological function? J Trauma 9(suppl):S118, 1984.
21. Davis JM, Dineen P, Gallin JI: Neutrophil degranulation and abnormal chemotaxis after thermal injury. J Immunol 127:1467, 1980.
22. Solomkin JS, Nelson RD, Chenoweth DE, et al: Regulation of neutrophil migratory function in burn injury by complement activation products. Ann Surg 200:742, 1984.
23. Alexander JW, Stinnett D, Ogle CK, et al: A comparison of immunologic profiles and their influence on bacteremia in surgical patients with a high risk of infection. Surgery 86:94, 1979.
24. Warden JD, Mason AD Jr, Bruitt BA Jr: Evaluation of leukocyte chemotaxis in vitro in thermally injured patients. J Clin Invest 54:1001, 1974.
25. Wolach B, Coates TD, Hugli TE, et al: Plasma lactoferrin reflects granulocyte activation via complement in burn patients. J Lab Clin Med 103:284, 1984.
26. Altman LC, Furukawa CT, Klebanoff SJ: Depressed mononuclear chemotaxis in thermally injured patients. J Immunol 119:199, 1977.
27. Warden G, Mason AD Jr, Pruitt BA Jr: Suppression of leukocyte chemotaxis in vitro by chemotherapeutic agents used in the management of thermal injuries. Ann Surg 181:363, 1975.
28. Ward PA: Chemotactic mechanisms in thermal injury. In: Ninnemann JL (ed): The Immune Consequences of Thermal Injury. Baltimore, Williams & Wilkins, p 119, 1981.
29. Ogle JD, Ogle CK, Alexander JW: Inhibition of neutrophil function by fluid phase C3b of complement. Infect Immun 40:967, 1983.
30. Miller SE, Miller CL, Trunkey DD: The immune consequences of trauma. Surg Clin North Am 62:167, 1982.
31. Ninnemann JL: Suppression of lymphocyte response following thermal injury. In: Ninnemann JL (ed): The Immune Consequences of Thermal Injury. Baltimore, Williams & Wilkins, p 66, 1981.
32. Ninnemann JL, Fisher JC, Wachtel TL: Thermal injury–associated immunosuppression: Occurrence and in vitro blocking effect of recovery serum. J Immunol 122:1746, 1979.
33. Wolfe JHN, Saporoschetz I, Young AE, et al: Suppressive serum, suppressor lymphocytes, and death from burns. Ann Surg 193:513, 1981.
34. Cannon JG, Gelfand JA, Tompkins RG, et al: Plasma IL-1β and TNFα levels in humans following cutaneous injury. In: Dinarello CA, Kluger MJ, Powanda MC, et al (eds): The Physiological and Pathological Effects of Cytokines. New York, Wiley-Liss, p 301, 1990.
35. Yamada Y, Kimball K, Okusawa S, et al: Cytokines, acute phase proteins, and tissue injury: C-reactive protein opsonizes dead cells for debridement and stimulates cytokine production. Ann NY Acad Sci 587:351, 1990.

36. Wakabayashi G, Cannon JG, Bellavia ES, et al: Impaired cytokine production by mononuclear cells of burn patients. In: Proceedings of the American Burn Association 21:145A, 1989.
37. Demling RH: Burns. N Engl J Med 313:1389, 1985.
38. Deitch EA, Maejima K, Berg R: Effects of oral antibiotics and bacterial overgrowth on the translocation of the GI tract microflora in burned rats. J Trauma 25:385, 1985.
39. Deitch EA: Intestinal permeability is increased in burn patients shortly after injury. Surgery 107:411, 1990.
40. McManus WF, Goodwin CW, Mason AD Jr, et al: Burn wound infection. J Trauma 21:753, 1981.
41. Pruitt B, McManus W, Mason A: Opportunistic infections in severely burned patients. Am J Med 76(suppl 3A):146, 1984.
42. Bruck HM, Nash G, Foley FD, et al: Opportunistic fungal infection of the burn wound with phycomycetes and aspergillus: A clinicopathologic review. Arch Surg 102:476, 1971.
43. Bruck HM, Nash G, Stein JM, et al: Studies on the occurrence and significance of yeast and fungi in the burn wound. Ann Surg 108, 1972.
44. Prasad J, Feller I, Thompson P: A ten year review of *Candida* sepsis and mortality in burn patients. Surgery 101:213, 1987.
45. Grube B, Marvin J, Heimbach D: Candida: A decreasing problem for the burned patient? Arch Surg 123:194, 1988.
46. Monafo WW, Freedman B: Tropical therapy for burns. Surg Clin North Am 67:133, 1987.
47. Glew RH, Moellering RC, Burke JF: Gentamicin dosage in children with extensive burns. J Trauma 16:819, 1976.

CHAPTER 44

Nosocomial Urinary Tract Infections

John W. Warren

Urinary tract infections (UTIs) are the most common infections occurring in hospitals. About 80% of nosocomial UTIs are associated with the use of urethral catheters[1] and another 5 to 10% occur after other genitourinary manipulations. The emphasis of this chapter is on catheter-associated bacteriuria, by far the most common type of nosocomial UTI in the intensive care unit (ICU).

PATHOPHYSIOLOGY

For centuries, a urethral catheter system was a tube inserted into the bladder that drained urine into an open container. The universal development of bacteriuria from these open catheters elicited in the 1950s a major advance in design, the closed catheter system.[2] This system is composed of an indwelling bladder catheter inserted into a collection tube that is fused to a collection bag on its distal end. This arrangement allows drainage so that the urine is always contained within a lumen protected from the contaminating environment. The onset of universal bacteriuria was 4 days with open catheters[3] but is more than 30 days with closed catheter systems.[2] Although no well-designed controlled trials comparing open with closed catheters have been performed, reports have been sufficiently persuasive so that the closed system has become the standard for patients requiring indwelling urethral catheters. However, the closed catheter system has only postponed and has not eliminated catheter-associated bacteriuria.

The majority of organisms causing catheter-associated bacteriuria are from the patient's own colonic flora, either brought in from the community or acquired in the hospital.[4] These bacteria may migrate across the perineum to colonize the periurethral area. In addition, exogenous organisms may directly colonize the periurethral area or catheter equipment.[5-7] Organisms may be transferred to the patient by the hands of health care personnel[5-7] or, infrequently, by contaminated products or containers.[5]

After organisms are in or on the patient or on the catheter system surface, they may enter the bladder through one of three ways. The normal urethra is colonized with bacteria, particularly in its distal portion, and the insertion of a catheter may carry some of these organisms into the bladder, the first method of entry. Catheter insertion is associated with rates of bacteriuria ranging from less than 1% in healthy individuals to 20% in elderly hospitalized patients.[8] Overall, the incidence of bacteriuria in hospitalized patients undergoing a single catheter insertion and removal is about 3%.

The second method of entry is through the lumen of the catheter, bacteria having gained access there via the catheter–collection tube junction or the drainage bag. The junction between the catheter and the collection tube may be disconnected, inappropriately, for catheter irrigation or urine collection; bacteriuria is associated with such interruptions.[9, 10] The drainage tube of the collection bag must be opened periodically to drain urine from the bag. If the lumen of the drainage tube is contaminated with bacteria (e.g., from an unwashed container previously used to collect urine from a bacteriuric patient[5]), organisms may enter the drainage bag and before the next emptying multiply to high concentrations. Even after the bag is drained, organisms may persist in the urine film coating the inside of the collection bag and multiply as the bag refills with urine. Bacteria in the bag may ascend the collection tube and catheter through the urine itself[5] or by growth of organisms along the internal surface.[11]

The closed catheter system is successful because it has greatly limited intraluminal entry of organisms. However, even with meticulous attention to maintenance of this system, the opportunity for bacterial entry exists in the space between the catheter surface and the urethral mucosa.[12] Furthermore, Schaeffer and Chmiel[13] and Kunin and Steele[14] demonstrated progressive uropathogen colonization of the urethra in catheterized patients, particularly women. At present, with appropriate catheter hygiene, the third and now most common site of bacterial entry is through the urethra, external to the catheter.

Even after removal of the catheter, the patient may remain at risk for bacteriuria for an unknown period. Hartstein and colleagues found that 11% of patients developed bacteriuria within 24 hours after catheter removal, a rate higher than on any single day during the actual catheterization.[15]

The catheterized urinary tract appears to be a hospitable environment for bacteria, and the majority of bacterial strains that enter are able to multiply quickly to high concentrations.[16] The bacteria may maintain themselves in the catheterized urinary tract by specific and nonspecific adherence mechanisms. Specific adhesions include fimbria binding to uroepithelial cells or the catheter surface.[17-19] Among nonspecific mechanisms, glycocalyx, or biofilm, which covers and secures the bacteria against a catheter or mucosal surface, has been demonstrated on drainage bags, catheters, and uroepithelium.[11, 20] Organisms contained within the biofilm appear to be well-protected from the mechanical flow of urine, possibly other host defense mechanisms, and even antibiotics.[20] The biofilm may allow the contained sessile organisms to establish a microenvironment from which some may move into the urine; these planktonic microbes are those that are voided and enumerated as bacteriuria by the clinical laboratory.

With time, the presence of bacteria elicits an inflammatory response resulting in acute and chronic cystitis with pyuria and production of antibody.[21, 22] Organisms may move up the ureter to one or both kidneys where a similar biofilm microenvironment may develop within the pelvis and/or the tubular system. Perturbation of the unicellular epithelium there may elicit an inflammatory response, which is recognized pathologically as acute pyelonephritis.[23] Bacteremia may develop from this renal site and possibly from inflamed bladder mucosa as well.

DIAGNOSIS

Escherichia coli is the bacteriuric species most frequently isolated from catheterized hospital patients. Other common organisms are *Pseudomonas aerguinosa, Klebsiella pneumoniae, Proteus mirabilis, Staphylococcus epidermidis,* and enterococci.[10, 24] Particularly when antibiotics are in use, yeasts may be isolated as well.[10, 24] Many investigators have required organism concentrations of 100,000 colony-forming units or more per milliliter of urine for diagnosis,[25] whereas others have selected lower concentrations to diagnose UTI.[26]

EPIDEMIOLOGY

Between 15 and 25% of patients in acute care hospitals, and an even greater percentage of patients in ICUs, have a catheter in place sometime during their hospital stay.[27, 28] The indications for catheterization may be grouped into four main categories: (1) urine output measurement, (2) surgical procedure, (3) urine retention, and (4) urinary incontinence. Most catheters are in place for only a short time; up to one third are removed in less than 1 day.[9] The mean and median durations of hospital catheterization are between 2 and 4 days.[9, 10, 15] Nevertheless, between 10 and 30% of catheterized patients experience bacteriuria,[2, 8, 27] significantly greater than the 1% found among noncatheterized patients.[27] Because of the large number of patients catheterized, catheter-associated bacteriuria is the most common hospital-acquired infection, representing about 40% of such infections and constituting the majority of the 900,000 cases of nosocomial bacteriuria in American hospitals each year.[29]

Several multivariate analyses have clarified risks of catheterization.[24, 30] These risks include patient factors such as diabetes mellitus, renal dysfunction, indications for catheter use other than surgery or urine output measurement, and female sex. In addition, catheter factors such as duration in place, errors in catheter care, microbial colonization of the drainage bag, and absence of a urinometer and of antibiotic administration are important.[24] The mean incidence of bacteriuria ranges between 3 and 10% per day; prolonged catheterization makes bacteriuria inevitable.[2, 9, 15, 24, 30]

PREVENTION OF CATHETER-ASSOCIATED BACTERIURIA

Studies of risk factors have led to preventive techniques. After a urethral catheter is in place, two principles are universally recommended for prevention of bacteriuria: (1) maintain the closed catheter system and (2) minimize the duration of catheterization.[31, 32]

Maintain Closed System. Urine specimens should be obtained without opening the catheter–collection tube junction.[9, 10] The use of a presealed junction diminishes the incidence of bacteriuria.[33] The system should be opened only at the bag drainage tube; personnel must avoid touching the end of the drainage tube to potentially contaminated containers.[5] Communication of these techniques to caregivers has been a largely successful effort of infection control teams.[34]

Minimize Duration. If the catheter can be removed before bacteriuria develops, postponement becomes prevention. Hartstein and colleagues, using a predetermined list of durations appropriate for each indication, found that the duration of catheterization averaged one-third longer than necessary.[15] Importantly, the majority of bacteriuria cases occurred after the catheter would have been removed had the appropriate catheter durations been observed.

Additional Efforts. Efforts beyond these two preventive techniques have been, for the most part, superfluous. Numerous antibacterial compounds have been applied at the catheter-urethra interface in attempts to block this most common site of bacterial entry. Most such studies have shown little if any clinical usefulness of this procedure.[35, 36] An intriguing variation of this theme is the use of silver-coated catheters, which have been evaluated in several controlled trials.[37–39] The largest of these trials showed no difference between the groups with and without the silver-coated catheters. However, analysis of subsets of patients revealed that women who received no antibiotics during their catheterization (a group composing only 9% of the study population) were significantly less likely to have bacteriuria if a silver-coated catheter was used.[39] How these findings may affect clinical care is unclear and may depend on economic considerations.

Attempts have been made to kill organisms that have entered the interior of the closed system or at least to prevent their proximal movement. Several methods of irrigating the catheter with antibacterial solutions have been developed but have not been effective in postponing bacteriuria.[10, 40, 41] Such practices have necessitated either another catheter junction (for continuous irrigation) or frequent opening of the closed system (for intermittent irrigation). These modifications have offered additional opportunities for entry of bacteria; bacteria that survive are often resistant to the irrigating antibiotic.[10] Likewise, most controlled studies of antibacterial compounds in the collection bag have generally demonstrated no effectiveness in curtailing bacteriuria.[42–44] (One that did show effectiveness reported a bag contamination rate that was two to four times higher than that of other trials.[45]) Another strategy directed at the drainage bag includes the use of devices that ensure a discontinuous column of urine in the catheter-collection tube, thus presumably obstructing bacterial movement toward the bladder. Certain catheter vents and urinometers might be worth further study in some situations.[46, 47]

Because of underlying disease or procedures, up to 80% of catheterized patients are administered antibiotics during but not because of catheterization. Comparisons of these patients with those not receiving antibiotics have generally shown that antibiotic use is associated with a lower incidence of bacteriuria.[9, 12, 15, 24, 30, 34] Furthermore, several trials of antibiotic prophylaxis have found that antibiotic recipients have lower incidences of bacteriuria than controls.[22, 48–51] Nevertheless, the studies that have observed patients for sufficient time have revealed that antibiotics are effective in postponement but not prevention of bacteriuria.[9, 15, 22, 24, 30, 48, 50] Antibiotics appear to be effective for the first several days of use and then resistant organisms begin to appear in the urine.[22, 48, 49, 52] Most authorities believe that the use of antibiotics to postpone bacteriuria is not indicated because of side effects, cost, and the emergence of antibiotic-resistant bacteria in the patient and the medical unit.[31, 32, 53]

CLINICAL SYNDROMES

The majority of episodes of catheter-associated bacteriuria are asymptomatic.[15, 27, 34] However, fevers and other symptoms of UTI occur in 10 to 30% of patients with catheter-associated bacteriuria.[15, 27, 34] Fortunately, only 1 to 5% of patients with catheter-associated bacteriuria have clinical bacteremia.[1, 23, 34, 54, 55] Men appear to be at greater risk for bacteremia than women.[1] In some reports, certain bacteriuric organisms (e.g., *Serratia marcescens*) may be more likely than others to cause bacteremia.[1, 54] The mortality directly attributed to bacteremia from nosocomial bacteriuria has been reported to be approximately 13%.[55] Even without overt evidence of systemic infection, catheter-associated bacteriuria appears to be related to an increased risk of death.[56] At autopsy examination of patients with catheter-associated bacteriuria who died in a hospital, there may be evidence of acute pyelonephritis, urinary stones, or perinephric abscesses.[23, 55]

Patients who have long-term catheters in place, who are usually admitted from nursing homes, present special problems in that most have polymicrobial bacteriuria.[57, 58] Like patients with short-term catheters, these individuals can have symptomatic UTIs, including fever, acute pyelonephritis, and bacteremia.[59, 60] In addition, catheter obstruction can be a problem and appears to be associated with *P. mirabilis*, an organism that produces urease causing ammonia production. This results in precipitation of struvite and apatite crystals in the catheter lumen.[61] The same process causes urinary stones;[62] these may be merely a crust around the balloon in the bladder or may develop as masses in the ureters or pelvis. In these latter situations, stones may be associated with acute pyelonephritis, bacteremia, chronic pyelonephritis, and renal dysfunction.[22, 63, 64] Particularly in men, periurethral infections may develop. These include urethritis, urethral fistulas, epididymitis, prostatitis, and abscesses in the scrotum or prostate.[63]

TREATMENT

Symptomatic Catheter-Associated Bacteriuria. If a patient has fever or signs of bacteremia, the clinician should rule out sources outside the urinary tract, catheter obstruction, and especially among men, periurethral infection. Cultures of urine and blood should be obtained. Many clinicians empirically treat such patients with parenteral antibiotics at doses high enough to achieve concentrations in the serum adequate to treat bacteremia by a known or suspected bacteriuric species. The selection of antibiotics should be based on knowledge of organisms common in the ICU and Gram's stain of the patient's urine at the time of the fever. Not surprisingly, survival of patients with bacteremia from nosocomial UTIs is related to the administration of antibiotics that are active against the bacteremic strain.[55]

The catheterized patient with lower abdominal pain, and without fever or other evidence of systemic infection, may benefit from an enteral antibiotic active in vitro in the same doses used for non–catheter-related UTIs. Appropriate durations of parenteral or enteral therapies have not been well established. For patients with increasing renal dysfunction or evidence of recalcitrant or recurring bacteremia, a search for urinary stones may be helpful in anticipation of surgical intervention.[55]

Asymptomatic Catheter-Associated Bacteriuria. A study of Garibaldi and colleagues is instructive in addressing the value of antibiotic therapy of asymptomatic bacteriuria in the prevention of symptomatic infection in catheterized patients.[34] This group studied 608 catheterized patients in hospital. Seventy-six patients acquired bacteriuria, of which

25 had symptoms, including 2 with bacteremia. Of these 25, 15 had symptoms on the first day of bacteriuria. The investigators speculated that prevention of symptomatic UTI by treating bacteriuria would be possible in only the 10 patients who had late symptoms. The results indicated that 250 urine cultures would be necessary to prevent one symptomatic UTI and more than 1000 cultures would be needed to prevent one episode of bacteremia. Other studies tend to confirm these findings.[15, 27] These data therefore do not support the routine treatment of asymptomatic catheter-associated bacteriuria to prevent symptomatic infection.[31, 32, 53]

However, after bacteriuria has developed in the catheterized ICU patient, its consequences may extend beyond the individual patient. The urine[31] and surfaces of the catheter system[5, 7] (as well as the skin[65] and feces[66] of the patient) are sources for contamination of the hands of medical personnel who may carry the bacteria to other patients.[5, 7, 67] Such patient-to-patient transmission leads to clusters of nosocomial bacteriuria, particularly with nonfecal isolates such as *Serratia*, *Pseudomonas*, and *Citrobacter* species. These organisms also tend to be resistant to many antibiotics.[7, 68] Schaberg and associates found that 15% of cases of nosocomial bacteriuria occurred in such clusters.[68] Further, patients transferred from one institution to another have been the source of subsequent outbreaks in the second institution.[69] This is a particular problem in ICUs.

Efforts to stop clusters of catheter-associated bacteriuria can be divided into three categories: (1) diminishing the number of bacteria in reservoirs; (2) diminishing contact spread; and (3) modifying risk factors.[6] To diminish the role of urine in the collection bag as a reservoir, consideration might be given to systemic or bag antibiotics[31, 42, 45] or to systemic methenamine with urine acidification.[32] Enteral nonabsorbable antibiotics might be considered for intestinal colonization.[6] For limiting contact spread, the caregiver should view the catheterized urinary tract as an open wound.[6] The most important procedure is hand washing between patients, including those in whom only skin surfaces are touched.[67] Other steps include use of gloves and segregation of catheterized patients,[70] particularly those infected from those uninfected. Many of the risk factors for bacteriuria are patient features that cannot be modified.[24] Of those that can be, the two most critical are errors of closed catheter hygiene and prolonged catheterization.

In addition, antibiotic therapy of asymptomatic bacteriuria may be useful if certain bacterial strains in the institution are known to cause a high incidence of bacteremia. As noted, some investigators have reported that *S. marcescens* may be such an organism.[1, 54] In this regard, it is interesting that Krieger and associates reported a prolonged period between the onset of bacteriuria caused by *S. marcescens* and the development of bacteremia, a delay that may allow antibiotic therapy in an effort to prevent bacteremia by this species.[1]

Asymptomatic Bacteriuria and Catheter Removal. Evidence is accumulating that the patient with catheter-associated bacteriuria whose catheter is removed, ironically, may be an appropriate recipient of antibiotic therapy. Harding and colleagues identified women with catheter-associated bacteriuria that persisted 48 hours beyond catheter removal.[71] By that time, 26% were already symptomatic and thus were treated with antibiotics. Of those still asymptomatic, an additional 16% left untreated developed symptomatic UTI by 14 days. Women randomly assigned to receive either single-dose or 10-day courses of trimethoprim-sulfamethoxazole experienced significantly greater clearance of bacteriuria (81 and 79%, respectively) than women who received no antibiotics (36%). Importantly, the authors pointed out a substantial difference between young and old.

Of women 65 years of age or younger, 74% spontaneously cleared their bacteriuria; the single-dose and 10-day course of trimethoprim-sulfamethoxazole showed somewhat higher clearance rates (94 and 84%, respectively). Among women older than 65 years of age, only 4% cleared their bacteria spontaneously; antibiotic therapy yielded 56 and 71% clearance with single-dose and 10-day therapy, respectively. The authors recommended antibiotic therapy for all women with catheter-associated bacteriuria that is still present 48 hours after catheter removal. They suggest single-dose trimethoprim-sulfamethoxazole for those women 65 years of age and younger. For older women, while recommending antibiotic therapy, they indicated that the appropriate dose and duration are yet to be determined. They cautioned that these findings should not be extrapolated to the management of men with bacteriuria persisting after catheter removal.

CATHETER USE

Obviously, the most direct method to prevent catheter-associated bacteriuria is to prevent catheterization. The past several decades have seen major advances in understanding complications of catheterization, in weighing its risks and benefits, and in determining appropriate indications for catheter use.[31, 32, 53] Clearly, if patients can be managed without a catheter or other urine collection device, the incidence of bacteriuria and its complications will be minimized. If this is not possible, urine collection devices other than the indwelling urethral catheter may be associated with lower incidences of bacteriuria and should be recommended.

For many patients in ICUs, condom catheters are not particularly useful because urine retention and easy removal may preclude accurate measurement of urine output. However, if used, the condom catheter avoids the problem of a tube in the urinary tract and offers the probable advantage of a lower incidence of bacteriuria than that observed with urethral catheters. Condom catheters, however, are associated with colonization of organisms on the skin of the penis; bladder bacteriuria may develop, particularly in patients who frequently manipulate the condom.[72] Careful collection of urine in a new condom by properly trained individuals is necessary to distinguish bladder bacteria from skin or condom contamination.[73]

Intermittent catheterization is an option for some patients. Many patients with spinal cord injury or with neurogenic bladders can use their bladders as containers for urine storage, yet cannot initiate urination. Insertion of a sterile or clean catheter every 3 to 6 hours by caregivers or the patient, with drainage of urine followed by immediate removal of the catheter, provides periodic bladder emptying.[74] However, bacteriuria develops in the majority of such patients, although with a lower incidence than that normally seen with long-term indwelling catheters.[75]

Suprapubic catheterization is based on the concept that the lower density of bacteria on the anterior abdominal skin yields lower rates of bacteriuria than that associated with catheters in the urethra. Another advantage not shared with urethral catheters is that clamping of the suprapubic catheter allows testing of voiding per urethra. Suprapubic catheters have been used in gynecologic, urologic, and other types of surgery and may postpone bacteriuria in some patients.[76] Complications include cellulitis, leakage, and hematoma at the puncture site and occasional catheter prolapse through the urethra. For comfort and convenience, patients and caregivers may prefer suprapubic over indwelling catheters.[76]

SUMMARY

Catheter-associated bacteriuria is a frequent acquired infection in ICUs and would be much more common without the use of the closed catheter system. The closed system protects luminal urine from the contaminating environment. Although many modifications have been attempted, none have markedly improved on it. However, primarily because of bacterial entry through the urethra, even excellent catheter hygiene does not prevent bacteriuria forever. Consequently, removing the catheter as soon as possible represents excellent medical care.

Catheter-associated bacteriuria places the patient at risk for fever, acute pyelonephritis, and bacteremia. Furthermore, in the ICU, the infected urine is a reservoir for organisms that may be transmitted to other patients with subsequent colonization or infection inside or outside their urinary tract. The fact that many of these organisms are resistant to commonly used antibiotics compounds the problem. Consequently, the urinary catheter system and urine might be perceived as an open wound, necessitating proper attention to the use of gloves and hand washing.

Although antibiotics are commonly used in these seriously ill patients for a variety of other indications, the urinary catheter or its associated bacteriuria are rarely indications for such use. For those patients who are not yet bacteriuric, systemic antibiotics postpone but do not prevent bacteriuria and, when bacteriuria develops, the organisms likely are resistant to the antibiotics. For the patient who is bacteriuric, pyuric, or febrile and in whom no other site of infection is apparent, invasive UTI and bacteremia should be suspected and appropriately treated with antibiotics and supportive measures. For patients with bacteriuria but who are asymptomatic, antibiotics generally are not indicated. A few exceptions to this tenet may pertain. The first is when antibiotic administration is part of an overall attempt to control an epidemic within the unit. The second might be to treat organisms or strains reported or known locally to result in a high incidence of bacteremia; *S. marcescens* might be an example. The third might be treatment of asymptomatic bacteriuria persisting in the patient whose catheter has been removed.

There are two overriding tenets to the use of the uretheral catheter: (1) maintain the closed catheter system closed and (2) remove the catheter as soon as the indication no longer pertains. Attention to the first postpones bacteriuria; attention to the second may allow removal of the catheter before bacteriuria develops and thus postponement becomes prevention of bacteriuria.

References

1. Krieger JN, Kaiser DL, Wenzel RP: Urinary tract etiology of bloodstream infections in hospitalized patients. J Infect Dis 148:57, 1983.
2. Kunin CM, McCormack RC: Prevention of catheter-induced urinary-tract infections by sterile closed drainage. N Engl J Med 274:1155, 1966.
3. Kass EH: Asymptomatic infections of the urinary tract. Trans Assoc Am Physicians 69:56, 1956.
4. Daifuku R, Stamm W: Association of rectal and urethral colonization with urinary tract infection in patients with indwelling catheters. JAMA 252:2028, 1984.
5. Rutala WA, Kennedy VA, Loflin HB, et al: *Serratia marcescens* nosocomial infections of the urinary tract associated with urine measuring containers and urinometers. Am J Med 70:659, 1981.
6. Schaberg DR, Weinstein RA, Stamm WE: Epidemics of nosocomial urinary tract infection caused by multiply resistant gram-negative bacilli: Epidemiology and control. J Infect Dis 133:363, 1976.
7. Maki DG, Hennekens CG, Phillips CW, et al: Nosocomial urinary tract infection with *Serratia marcescens:* An epidemiologic study. J Infect Dis 128:579, 1973.
8. Turck M, Goffe B, Petersdorf RG: The urethral catheter and urinary tract infection. J Urol 88:834, 1962.
9. Garibaldi RA, Burke JP, Dickman ML, et al: Factors predisposing to bacteriuria during indwelling urethral catheterization. N Engl J Med 291:215, 1974.
10. Warren JW, Platt R, Thomas RJ, et al: Antibiotic irrigation and catheter-associated urinary-tract infections. N Engl J Med 299:570, 1978.

11. Nickel JC, Grant SK, Costerton JW: Catheter-associated bacteriuria, an experimental study. Urology 26:369, 1985.
12. Garibaldi RA, Burke JP, Britt MR, et al: Meatal colonization and catheter-associated bacteriuria. N Engl J Med 303:316, 1980.
13. Schaeffer AJ, Chmiel J: Urethral meatal colonization in the pathogenesis of catheter-associated bacteriuria. J Urol 130:1096, 1983.
14. Kunin CM, Steele C: Culture of the surface of urinary catheters to sample urethral flora and study the effect of antimicrobial therapy. J Clin Microbiol 21:902, 1985.
15. Hartstein AI, Garber SB, Ward TT, et al: Nosocomial urinary tract infection: A prospective evaluation of 108 catheterized patients. Infect Control 2:380, 1981.
16. Stark RP, Maki DG: Bacteriuria in the catheterized patient. What quantitative level of bacteriuria is relevant? N Engl J Med 311:560, 1984.
17. Daifuku R, Stamm W: Bacterial adherence to bladder uroepithelial cells in catheter-associated urinary tract infection. N Engl J Med 314:1208, 1986.
18. Mobley HLT, Chippendale GR, Tenney JH, et al: Expression of type 1 fimbriae may be required for persistence of *Escherichia coli* in the catheterized urinary tract. J Clin Microbiol 25:2253, 1987.
19. Mobley HLT, Chippendale GR, Tenney JH, et al: MR/K hemagglutination of *Providencia stuartii* correlates with adherence to catheters and with persistence in catheter-associated bacteriuria. J Infect Dis 157:264, 1988.
20. Nickel JC, Ruseska I, Wright JB, et al: Tobramycin resistance of *Pseudomonas aeruginosa* cells growing as a biofilm on urinary catheter material. Antimicrob Agents Chemother 27:619, 1985.
21. Kostiala AAI, Nyren P, Jokinen EJ, et al: Prospective study on the appearance of antibody-coated bacteria in patients with an indwelling urinary catheter. Nephron 30:279, 1981.
22. Nyren P, Runeberg L, Kostiala AI, et al: Prophylactic methenamine hippurate or nitrofurantoin in patients with an indwelling urinary catheter. Ann Clin Res 13:16, 1981.
23. Gordon D, Bune A, Grime B, et al: Diagnostic criteria and natural history of catheter-associated urinary tract infections after prostatectomy. Lancet 1:11269, 1983.
24. Platt R, Polk BF, Murdock B, et al: Risk factors for nosocomial urinary tract infection. Am J Epidemiol 124:977, 1986.
25. US Department of Health and Human Services: NNIS Manual: National Nosocomial Infections Surveillance System. US Public Health Service. Atlanta, Centers for Disease Control, p XIII-5, 1988.
26. Warren JW, Muncie HL Jr, Bergquist EJ, et al: Sequelae and management of urinary infection in the patient requiring chronic catheterization. J Urol 125:1, 1981.
27. Haley RW, Hooton TM, Culver DH, et al: Nosocomial infections in U.S. hospitals, 1975–1976: Estimated frequency by selected characteristics of patients. Am J Med 70:947, 1981.
28. Garibaldi RA: Hospital acquired urinary tract infection. In: Wenzel RP (ed): Handbook of Hospital Acquired Infections. Boca Raton, FL, CRC Press, p 513, 1981.
29. Haley R, Culver D, White J, et al: The nationwide nosocomial infection rate: A new need for vital statistics. Am J Epidemiol 121:159, 1985.
30. Hooton TM, Haley RW, Culver DH, et al: The joint associations of multiple risk factors with the occurrence of nosocomial infection. Am J Med 70:960, 1981.
31. Kunin CM: Detection, Prevention and Management of Urinary Tract Infections. 4th ed. Philadelphia, Lea & Febiger, p 245, 1987.
32. Garibaldi RA: Hospital-acquired urinary tract infections: Epidemiology and prevention. In: Wenzel RP (ed): Prevention and Control of Nosocomial Infections. Baltimore, Williams & Wilkins, p 335, 1987.
33. Platt R, Murdock B, Polk BF, et al: Reduction of mortality associated with nosocomial urinary tract infection. Lancet 1:1893, 1983.
34. Garibaldi RA, Mooney BR, Epstein BJ, et al: An evaluation of daily bacteriologic monitoring to identify preventable episodes of catheter-associated urinary tract infection. Infect Control 3:466, 1982.
35. Burke J, Jacobson J, Garibaldi R, et al: Evaluation of daily meatal care with polyantibiotic ointment in prevention of urinary catheter-associated bacteriuria. J Urol 129:331, 1983.
36. Burke JP, Garibaldi RA, Britt MR, et al: Prevention of catheter-associated urinary tract infections. Efficacy of daily meatal care regimens. Am J Med 70:655, 1981.
37. Schaeffer AJ, Story KO, Johnson SM: Effect of silver oxide/trichloroisocyanuric acid antimicrobial urinary drainage system on catheter-associated bacteriuria. J Urol 139:69, 1988.
38. Lundberg T: Prevention of catheter-associated urinary-tract infections by use of silver-impregnated catheters. Lancet 1:1031, 1986.
39. Johnson JR, Roberts PL, Olsen RJ, et al: Prevention of catheter-associated urinary tract infection with a silver oxide–coated urinary catheter: Clinical and microbiologic correlates. J Infect Dis 162:1145, 1990.
40. Bastable JRG, Peel RN, Birch DM, et al: Continuous irrigation of the bladder after prostatectomy: Its effect on post-prostatectomy infection. Br J Urol 49:689, 1977.
41. Savage JE, Phillips B, Lifshitz S, et al: Bacteriuria in closed bladder drainage versus continuous irrigation in patients undergoing intracavitary radium for treatment of gynecologic cancer. Gynecol Oncol 13:26, 1982.
42. Gillespie W, Jones J, Teasdale C, et al: Does the addition of disinfectant to urine drainage bags prevent infection in catheterized patients? Lancet 1:1037, 1983.
43. Sweet DE, Goodpasture HC, Holl K, et al: Evaluation of H_2O_2 prophylaxis of bacteriuria in patients with long-term indwelling Foley catheters: A randomized controlled study. Infect Control 6:263, 1985.
44. Thompson RL, Haley CE, Searcy MA, et al: Catheter-associated bacteriuria. Failure to reduce attack rates using periodic instillations of a disinfectant into urinary drainage systems. JAMA 251:747, 1984.
45. Maizels M, Schaeffer AJ: Decreased incidence of bacteriuria associated with periodic instillations of hydrogen peroxide into the urethral catheter drainage bag. J Urol 123:841, 1980.
46. Blenkharn JJ: Prevention of bacteriuria during urinary catheterization of patients in an intensive care unit: Evaluation of the "Ureofix 500" closed drainage system. J Hosp Infect 6:187, 1985.
47. Monson TP, Macalalad FV, Hamman JW, et al: Evaluation of a vented drainage system in prevention of bacteriuria. J Urol 117:216, 1977.
48. Britt MR, Garibaldi RA, Miller WA, et al: Antimicrobial prophylaxis for catheter-associated bacteriuria. Antimicrob Agents Chemother 11:240, 1977.
49. Mountokalakis T, Skounakis M, Tselentis J: Short-term versus prolonged systemic antibiotic prophylaxis in patients treated with indwelling catheters. J Urol 134:506, 1985.
50. Polk BF, Tager IB, Shapiro M, et al: Randomized clinical trial of perioperative cefazolin in preventing infection after hysterectomy. Lancet 1:437, 1980.
51. Bivens MD, Neufeld J, McCarthy WD: The prophylactic use of Keflex and Keflin in vaginal hysterectomy. Am J Obstet Gynecol 122:169, 1975.
52. Warren JW, Anthony WC, Hoopes JM, et al: Cephalexin for susceptible bacteriuria in afebrile, long-term catheterized patients. JAMA 248:454, 1982.
53. Warren JW: Catheter-associated urinary tract infections. Infect Dis Clin North Am 1:823, 1987.
54. Stamm WE, Martin SM, Bennett JV: Epidemiology of nosocomial infections due to gram-negative bacilli: Aspects relevant to development and use of vaccines. J Infect Dis 136(suppl):S151, 1977.
55. Bryan C, Reynolds K: Hospital-acquired bacteremic urinary tract infection: Epidemiology and outcome. J Urol 132:494, 1984.
56. Platt R, Polk BF, Murdock B, et al: Mortality associated with nosocomial urinary tract infection. N Engl J Med 307:637, 1982.
57. Warren JW, Tenney JH, Hoopes JM, et al: A prospective microbiologic study of bacteriuria in patients with chronic indwelling urethral catheters. J Infect Dis 146:719, 1982.
58. Steward DK, Wood GL, Cohen RL, et al: Failure of the urinalysis and quantitative urine culture in diagnosing symptomatic urinary tract infections in patients with long-term urinary catheters. Am J Infect Control 13:154, 1985.
59. Warren JW, Damron D, Tenney JH, et al: Fever, bacteremia, and death as complications of bacteriuria in women with long-term urethral catheters. J Infect Dis 155:1151, 1987.
60. Warren JW, Muncie HL Jr, Hall-Craggs M: Acute pyelonephritis associated with the bacteriuria of long-term catheterization: A prospective clinico-pathological study. J Infect Dis 158:1341, 1988.
61. Mobley HLT, Warren JW: Urease-positive bacteriuria and obstruction of long-term urinary catheters. J Clin Microbiol 25:2216, 1987.
62. Takeuchi H, Takayama H, Konishi T, et al: Scanning electron microscopy detects bacteria within infection stones. J Urol 132:67, 1984.
63. Tribe CR, Silver JR: Renal failure in paraplegia. London, Pitman Medical Publishing, p 35, 1969.
64. Nikakhtar B, Vaziri ND, Khonsari F, et al: Urolithiasis in patients with spinal cord injury. Paraplegia 19:363, 1981.
65. Stratford B, Gallus AS, Matthiesson AM, et al: Alteration of superficial bacterial flora in severely ill patients. Lancet 1:68, 1968.
66. Selden R, Lee S, Wang WLL, et al: Nosocomial *Klebsiella* infections: Intestinal colonization as a reservoir. Ann Intern Med 74:657, 1971.
67. Casewell M, Phillips I: Hands as route of transmission for *Klebsiella* species. Br Med J 2:1315, 1977.
68. Schaberg DR, Haley RW, Highsmith AK, et al: Nosocomial bacteriuria: A prospective study of case clustering and antimicrobial resistance. Ann Intern Med 93:420, 1980.
69. Schaberg DR, Alford RH, Anderson R, et al: An outbreak of nosocomial infection due to multiply resistant *Serratia marcescens:* Evidence of inter-hospital spread. J Infect Dis 134:181, 1976.
70. Maki D, Hennekens C, Bennet J: Prevention of catheter-associated urinary tract infection. JAMA 221:1270, 1972.
71. Harding GKM, Nicolle LE, Ronald AR, et al: How long should catheter-acquired urinary tract infection in women be treated? A randomized controlled study. Ann Intern Med 114:713, 1991.
72. Hirsh DD, Fainstein V, Musher DM: Do condom catheter collecting systems cause urinary tract infection? JAMA 242:340, 1979.
73. Ouslander JG, Greengold BA, Silverblatt FJ, et al: An accurate method to obtain urine for culture in men with external catheters. Arch Intern Med 147:286, 1987.
74. Guttmann L, Frankel H: The value of intermittent catheterization in the early management of traumatic paraplegia and tetraplegia. Paraplegia 4:63, 1966.
75. Mohler JL, Cowen DL, Flanigan RC: Suppression and treatment of urinary tract infection in patients with an intermittently catheterized neurogenic bladder. J Urol 138:336, 1987.

76. Andersen JT, Heisterberg L, Hebjørn S, et al: Suprapubic versus trans-urethral bladder drainage after colposuspension/vaginal repair. Acta Obstet Gynecol Scand 64:139, 1985.

CHAPTER 45

Infections in Granulocytopenic Patients*

Thomas J. Walsh
Philip A. Pizzo

Granulocytopenia (defined as an absolute neutrophil count of less than 500/mm³) may complicate the course of cytotoxic chemotherapy, radiation therapy, aplastic anemia, human immunodeficiency virus infection, drug reactions, and other conditions.[1-3] Patients with granulocytopenia may be admitted to the intensive care unit (ICU) for hemodynamic, pulmonary, or gastrointestinal complications caused by life-threatening infections. Many granulocytopenic cancer patients also are admitted to the ICU for the respiratory, cardiac, metabolic, or renal complications of cytotoxic chemotherapy[2] or radiation therapy. Patients treated aggressively for potentially curable neoplastic diseases are often admitted to the ICU with multiple deficits in host defense: persistent profound granulocytopenia, diffuse gastrointestinal mucosal erosions, impaired cell-mediated immunity, and other defects.

Successful management of such granulocytopenic patients by the intensive care team requires a structured and rational approach to treating infections. The purpose of this chapter, therefore, is to review approaches to the diagnosis and management of infections in granulocytopenic patients who are admitted to ICUs.

HOST DEFECTS AND ASSOCIATED INFECTIONS
Granulocytopenia

Granulocytopenia is the leading factor predisposing to infection in patients treated with cytotoxic chemotherapy.[4-7] The frequency and the severity of infections increase progressively as total granulocyte counts continue to decline from less than 1000/mm³ to less than 100/mm³. The greatest frequency of severe infections occurs in patients with total granulocyte counts of less than 100/mm³ (profound granulocytopenia) persisting for more than 3 weeks. Cytotoxic chemotherapy also damages mucosal epithelial surfaces, creating extensive portals of entry for endogenous microflora along the alimentary and respiratory tracts.[8]

The absence of granulocytes attenuates or completely eliminates the classic signs of inflammation at infected foci.[9] Fever is frequently the only sign of infection. However, meticulous repeated physical examinations and routine laboratory evaluation may reveal the source of fever in approximately 60% of febrile granulocytopenic patients.[10, 11] Findings from our patients indicate that earlier diagnosis and treatment may be preventing clinically overt sites from developing. However, patients admitted to the ICU may be more likely to have defined foci.

The most common overt sites of infection in febrile granulocytopenic patients are (1) the alimentary tract, including the periodontium, the oropharynx, the esophagus, and the anorectal region; (2) the respiratory tract, including the paranasal sinuses and the lungs; and (3) the skin, especially at points of vascular catheter insertion, catheter tunnel tracks, and other puncture wounds (Table 45–1). These sites are associated commonly with particular patterns of infecting microorganisms summarized in Table 45–1.

The most common causes of infection in granulocytopenic patients are aerobic bacteria, which include *Escherichia coli*, *Klebsiella pneumoniae*, *Enterobacter* species, *Pseudomonas aeruginosa*, *Staphylococcus aureus*, and *Staphylococcus epidermidis* (Table 45–2). These bacteria originate from the endogenous flora of the host or from the hospital environment.[12-18] Historically, Enterobacteriaceae and *P. aeruginosa* were the most common isolates recovered from granulocytopenic patients. During the past decade, however, gram-positive bacteria, particularly coagulase-negative *Staphylococcus*, have equalled or exceeded the aerobic gram-negative bacteria as the principal agents of proven infection in granulocytopenic patients.[19-22]

Bacteria are usually the initial cause of documented infection; fungi are often the cause of subsequent infections in granulocytopenic patients.[23, 24] The most common opportunistic fungi are *Candida* and *Aspergillus* species. However, the Mucoraceae, *Trichosporon*, *Fusarium*, and *Pseudallescheria boydii* are being increasingly recognized as causes of invasive fungal infection in granulocytopenic patients.[25, 26]

Impaired Cell-Mediated Immunity

Granulocytopenic patients almost invariably have other immunologic and mechanical deficits that further predispose them to infections. Effective cell-mediated immunity is dependent on an intact repertoire of T helper, T suppressor, and effector lymphocytes. The most profound deficits in cell-mediated immunity commonly encountered in the ICU occur in patients with the acquired immunodeficiency syndrome (AIDS). Patients with AIDS may also become granulocytopenic owing to azidothymidine given for human immunodeficiency virus infection, trimethoprim-sulfamethoxazole for *Pneumocystis carinii* pneumonia, or cytotoxic chemotherapy for Kaposi's sarcoma or for diffuse large-cell lymphomas. Neoplastic diseases associated with impaired cell-mediated immunity include Hodgkin's lymphoma, non-Hodgkin's lymphoma, hairy cell leukemia, T cell leukemia, and chronic lymphocytic leukemia. Solid organ transplant recipients receiving cyclosporine, prednisone, and azathioprine may be neutropenic owing to the latter compound. Neutropenic patients receiving corticosteroids must also be assumed to have an increased risk of infections associated with impaired cell-mediated immunity.

T cell–dependent immunity confers host defense against protozoa (*P. carinii*, *Toxoplasma gondii*, *Cryptosporidium*), viruses (cytomegalovirus, herpes simplex virus, varicella-zoster virus, adenovirus), helminths (*Strongyloides stercoralis*), certain fungi (*Cryptococcus neoformans*, *Histoplasma capsulatum*, *Coccidioides immitis*), and certain bacteria (e.g., *Legionella* species, *Listeria monocytogenes*, *Mycobacterium tuberculosis*, *Mycobacterium kansasii*, and *Mycobacterium avium-intracellulare*). Certain neoplastic and immunodeficiency diseases appear to be associated with threats from these pathogens. For example, patients with AIDS have a high risk of *Pneumocystis* and cytomegalovirus pneumonia, cryptococcosis, and disseminated mycobacterial infections. Those with Hodgkin's lymphoma have an especially increased risk of tuberculosis and

---

*All material in this chapter is in the public domain, with the exception of any borrowed figures or tables.

TABLE 45-1

COMMON SITES AND AGENTS OF INFECTIONS IN GRANULOCYTOPENIC PATIENTS*

Site	Aerobic Gram-Positive	Aerobic Gram-Negative	Anaerobic Gram-Positive	Anaerobic Gram-Negative	Fungi Yeasts	Fungi Filamentous	Viruses	Protozoa
Alimentary Tract								
Periodontitis	−	+	+	+	+	−	−	−
Stomatitis	+	+	−	−	+	−	+	−
Pharyngitis	+	+	−	−	+	−	+	−
Esophagitis	+	+	±	−	+	+	+	−
Enteritis	+	+	+	+	+	+	+	−
Typhlitis	+	+	+	+	+	+	+	−
Colitis (*Clostridium difficile*)	−	−	+	−	−	−	+	−
Perianal cellulitis	+	+	+	+	−	−	±	−
Perirectal abscess	+	+	+	+	±	−	−	−
Respiratory Tract								
Sinusitis	+	+	+	+	+	+	−	−
Epiglottiditis	±	+	−	−	+	−	±	−
Tracheobronchitis	+	+	−	−	+	+	+	−
Pneumonia	+	+	+	+	+	+	+	+
Skin								
Axillary lesions	+	+	+	−	+	−	−	−
Venipuncture sites	+	±	−	−	+	+	−	−
Venous catheter infections								
Exit site	+	+	−	−	±	+	−	−
Tunnel site	+	+	−	−	−	+	−	−
Entrance site	+	+	−	−	−	+	−	−
Bone marrow aspirate site	+	+	−	−	+	+	−	−

*+ = associated; ± = occasionally associated; − = not associated.

recurrent varicella-zoster infections. Patients with chronic lymphocytic leukemia have an increased risk of *Pneumocystis* pneumonia. Hairy cell leukemia has been strongly associated with infections caused by atypical mycobacteria, especially *M. kansasii* and *M. avium-intracellulare*.[27]

B Cell–Dependent Immunity

B cell–mediated immunity confers protection especially against encapsulated bacteria by means of opsonizing antibodies. These encapsulated bacteria include *Haemophilus influenzae*, *Streptococcus pneumoniae*, and *Neisseria meningitidis*. Conditions associated with impaired B cell–mediated immunity that may occur in granulocytopenic hosts include multiple myeloma,[28] hypogammaglobulinemia, chronic lymphocytic leukemia, and AIDS. Apparently as the result of disordered immunoregulation of new antibody formation, patients with AIDS, especially children, are especially susceptible to life-threatening recurrent infections caused by encapsulated bacteria.

As the spleen has an important role in the formation of new opsonizing antibody, the synthesis of complement, the production of tuftsin, and reticuloendothelial clearance, patients undergoing splenectomy have an increased risk of fulminant bacterial sepsis, especially that caused by *S. pneumoniae*, *H. influenzae*, and *N. meningitidis*. Children and adolescents undergoing splenectomy have a higher risk of this uncommon but devastating septic complication, which invariably necessitates aggressive ICU management. Patients with Hodgkin's lymphoma and hairy cell leukemia may have undergone splenectomy as part of their staging procedure.

Mechanical Defects

Penetration of cutaneous barriers by vascular catheters increases the risk of infection attributable to bacteria and fungi.[29–31] Puncture sites, such as those related to diagnostic procedures (e.g., bone marrow aspiration), also create portals of entry. Mucosal epithelial barriers along the alimentary tract are also disrupted by radiation injury and by cytotoxic chemotherapeutic agents, such as high-dose methotrexate, anthracyclines, cytosine arabinoside, and 5-fluorouracil. Enteric bacteria and endotoxins gain access to the portal venous system through these disrupted mucosal surfaces.

Combined Deficits in Host Defense

Cytotoxic chemotherapy–induced granulocytopenia in cancer patients seldom if ever exists as an isolated immunologic deficit. For example, oral mucocutaneous infections with herpes simplex virus are common in granulocytopenic patients receiving cytotoxic chemotherapy. In addition to being granulocytopenic, patients receiving cyclophosphamide also acquire deficits in T cell–dependent immunity. Deficits in the cell-mediated immunity and mechanical barriers occur frequently in granulocytopenic patients and must be anticipated in formulating a strategy for treating their infections.

EMPIRICAL ANTIBIOTIC THERAPY
Combination Antibiotic Therapy

The new onset of fever in a granulocytopenic cancer patient constitutes a medical emergency. In contrast to the management of a febrile but otherwise stable nongranulocytopenic patient in the ICU, in whom antibiotics are initiated only for identifiable sites of infection,[32] broad-spectrum antibiotics must be initiated empirically in the granulocytopenic patient with a new fever.[25] Clinically stable but febrile granulocytopenic patients who do not receive broad-spectrum antibiotics may have rapid hemodynamic deterioration

TABLE 45–2

IMMUNOLOGIC DEFICIENCIES, MECHANICAL DEFECTS, AND COMMONLY ASSOCIATED PATHOGENS AMONG GRANULOCYTOPENIC PATIENTS

Granulocytopenia
Bacteria
  Gram-negative bacilli
    Escherichia coli
    Klebsiella pneumoniae
    Enterobacter spp.
    Pseudomonas aeruginosa
  Gram-positive cocci
    Staphylococcus epidermidis and other coagulase-negative
      staphylococci
    Staphylococcus aureus
    Group D streptococci, alpha-hemolytic streptococci
      (especially *Streptococcus mitis*), *Corynebacterium* spp.
      (especially *C. jeikeium*)
Fungi
  Yeast-like fungi
    Candida spp. (increased risk of disseminated candidiasis)
    Torulopsis glabrata
    Trichosporon beigelii
  Filamentous fungi
    Aspergillus spp.
    Mucorales (especially *Rhizopus* spp., *Cunninghamella*)
    Fusarium spp.

Cellular (T Lymphocyte) Immune Deficiency or Dysfunction
Bacteria
  Listeria monocytogenes
  Salmonella spp.
  Mycobacterium spp.
  Nocardia asteroides
  Legionella spp.
Fungi
  Candida spp. (increased risk of mucosal candidiasis)
  Cryptococcus neoformans
  Histoplasma capsulatum
  Coccidioides immitis
Viruses
  Varicella-zoster virus
  Herpes simplex virus
  Cytomegalovirus
  Epstein-Barr virus
Protozoa
  Pneumocystis carinii
  Toxoplasma gondii
  Cryptosporidium
Helminths
  Strongyloides stercoralis

Humoral (B Lymphocyte) Immune Deficiency
Bacteria
  Streptococcus pneumoniae
  Haemophilus influenzae

Invasive Procedures
Bacteria and fungi (colonizing respiratory tract and skin)

Neoplastic Obstruction of Hollow Visci
Bacteria and fungi (colonizing gastrointestinal and urinary tracts)

---

and intractable septic shock. Empirical initiation of antibiotics decreases the mortality rates, the frequency of bacteremias, and clinically evident foci of infection.[33–36]

Combination antibiotic therapy with a β-lactam antibiotic and an aminoglycoside historically has been the treatment of choice in the febrile granulocytopenic patient. These combinations have been discussed elsewhere[33–36] and are summarized in Table 45–3. Acceptable combinations include an aminoglycoside and a β-lactam antibiotic (an antipseudomonal cephalosporin or an antipseudomonal penicillin)

or a double β-lactam combination (an antipseudomonal cephalosporin and an antipseudomonal penicillin). The rationale for such combinations includes (1) providing broad-spectrum activity against all likely initially infecting pathogens, (2) improving serum bactericidal activity through a synergistic interaction, and (3) preventing emergence of resistance to one antibiotic by the use of at least one other antibiotic active against the same bacteria. Several studies indicate that synergistic combinations of antibiotics in granulocytopenic patients control a greater proportion of gram-negative bacteremias than do nonsynergistic combinations.[35–37]

The combination of antibiotics depends most importantly on particular ICU's epidemiologic trends of prevalent bacteria and patterns of antibiotic resistance.[38] A combination of gentamicin and ticarcillin, for example, may be appropriate as an initial empirical therapy in febrile granulocytopenic patients in a unit with predominantly susceptible nosocomial gram-negative bacilli.[39] Addition of cefazolin or cephalothin to this combination provides added activity against susceptible *S. aureus* and *K. pneumoniae*. However, many ICU environments have indigenous multiply resistant gram-negative bacteria. Depending on the prevalent patterns of bacterial susceptibility within those ICUs, a combination of amikacin and mezlocillin or piperacillin might be warranted. Vancomycin should be added when methicillin-resistant *S. aureus* is a problem within an ICU, especially in postoperative cancer patients with open wounds. Vancomycin, however, need not be added routinely in newly febrile granulocytopenic patients.[20] The relatively new monobactam aztreonam, which has activity restricted only to aerobic gram-negative bacilli, should be combined with vancomycin.[38]

Single-Agent Antibiotic Therapy

The advent of ceftazidime and the imipenem-cilastatin combination has permitted the use of a single agent (monotherapy) initially for empirical therapy of newly febrile granulocytopenic patients. As single agents, the aminoglycosides and earlier β-lactam antibiotics generally lacked a sufficiently broad spectrum, bactericidal activity, or the stability against β-lactamase degradation necessary to be useful as single agents. Ceftazidime and imipenem, however, possess the broad spectrum and serum bactericidal activity provided by traditional synergistic combinations.[40, 41] Their low minimal inhibitory concentrations are associated with potent serum bactericidal activity.

A study from the National Cancer Institute demonstrated that ceftazidime was equivalent to a combination of cephalothin, gentamicin, and carbenicillin as the initial empirical antibiotic regimen in 550 febrile episodes in granulocytopenic cancer patients.[41] The selection of a single antibiotic such as ceftazidime or imipenem-cilastatin versus a combination of antibiotics for empirical treatment should depend on the patterns of antimicrobial susceptibility of pathogenic bacteria within the ICU. Ceftazidime now is used as the initial antibiotic at the National Cancer Institute in newly febrile granulocytopenic patients who are not eligible for clinical study protocols; when resistant bacteria are suspected or isolated, ceftazidime administration is discontinued, and the combination of vancomycin, piperacillin, and gentamicin is instituted.

Modification of Initial Empirical Antibacterial Therapy

The accepted monotherapy and traditional combinations of antibiotics used for the initial empirical treatment of febrile granulocytopenic patients obviously do not possess

TABLE 45–3

EMPIRICAL COMBINATION AND SINGLE-AGENT ANTIBACTERIAL THERAPY FOR CRITICALLY ILL, FEBRILE GRANULOCYTOPENIC PATIENTS

Aminoglycosides with	Penicillins* or	Cephalosporins* or	Monobactam* or	Carbapenem
Gentamicin	Ticarcillin	Cephalothin	Aztreonam†	Imipenem‡
Tobramycin	Mezlocillin	Cefazolin		
Amikacin	Piperacillin	Cefotaxime		
Netilmicin	Azlocillin	Cefoperazone§		
		Ceftazidime‡§		

*β-Lactam antibiotics.
†Spectrum of activity is limited to aerobic gram-negative bacilli and must be combined with vancomycin for gram-positive bacteria.
‡Ceftazidime and imipenem may each be used for single-agent empirical antibacterial therapy.
§Antipseudomonal cephalosporins.

activity against the entire spectrum of resistant bacteria, fungi, viruses, mycobacteria, protozoa, and other pathogens to which the granulocytopenic host is susceptible. Protracted profound granulocytopenia is associated with a greater frequency of new febrile episodes during the initial antibiotic course. Granulocytopenic patients admitted to the ICU are generally those in higher-risk groups with long-term (7 to 14 days or longer) and profound (less than 100/mm³) granulocytopenia. New febrile episodes in these patients may be due to fungal, viral, or resistant bacterial infections.

Table 45–4 summarizes frequently implemented modifications of the initial empirical antibiotic regimen in febrile granulocytopenic patients. Such modifications are needed because of the inevitable appearance of new infections in patients with protracted granulocytopenia rather than nec-

essarily because of a failure of the empirical regimen. New infections appear with the same frequency in patients receiving appropriate, initial single-agent therapy and those receiving traditional combination therapy.[42]

Empirical administration of amphotericin B is among the most important modifications of initial therapy in the granulocytopenic patients. When administered empirically to persistently febrile granulocytopenic patients already receiving broad-spectrum antibiotics, amphotericin B reduced the frequency and mortality of invasive fungal infections, especially those caused Candida, in two randomized studies.[24, 43] Granulocytopenic patients at the National Cancer Institute who have persistent or recurrent fever on or after the seventh day of initial antibiotic therapy empirically receive amphotericin B (0.5 mg/kg/d). In the absence of a proven

TABLE 45–4

MODIFICATIONS OF EMPIRICAL ANTIBIOTIC THERAPY OF CRITICALLY ILL, FEBRILE GRANULOCYTOPENIC PATIENTS

Infection	Organism	Modifications
Breakthrough bacteremia	S. epiderimidis, other coagulase-negative staphylococci, enterococcus, Corynebacterium group JK	Add vancomycin.
	Resistant gram-negative bacillus (e.g., Enterobacter spp., Serratia spp., Citrobacter spp., Pseudomonas aeruginosa, X. maltophilia)	Change antibiotics according to susceptibility patterns of new organism.
Catheter-associated infection*	S. epidermidis, Corynebacterium JK, Bacillus, gram-negative bacilli (Klebsiella, Enterobacter, Pseudomonas)	Add vancomycin and where appropriate, change gram-negative coverage according to susceptibility patterns of new organisms.
	Candida spp.	Amphotericin B.
Severe oral mucositis or necrotizing gingivitis	Peptococci, peptostreptococci, alpha-hemolytic streptoccoci, Bacteroides spp. (including B. melaninogenicus)	Clindamycin (antianaerobic), vancomycin (for alpha-hemolytic streptococci).
	Herpes simplex	Add IV acyclovir.
	Candida spp.	Add oral clotrimazole, fluconazole, or IV amphotericin B.
Esophagitis	Candida spp.	Add IV amphotericin B.
	Herpes simplex	Add IV acyclovir.
	Resistant gram-positive bacteria	Add vancomycin.
Perianal cellulitis	Bacteroides, resistant gram-negative bacilli	Add specific antianaerobic agent: clindamycin or metronidazole; culture for resistant gram-negative bacteria.
Pneumonia Diffuse or interstitial	P. carinii, Mycoplasma, L. pneumophila	Trial of trimethoprim-sulfamethoxazole and erythromycin (continue empirical antibiotics).
Focal infiltrate	Enterobacteriaceae, P. aeruginosa, X. maltophilia, Aspergillus, Mucoraceae, Fusarium spp.	If granulocyte count is not rising, biopsy for diagnosis; if biopsy cannot be done, empirically add amphotericin B. If granulocyte count is rising and patient is stable, monitor carefully.
Persistent fever and granulocytopenia	Candida spp., Aspergillus spp.	Add amphotericin B empirically.

*Remove catheter for infection caused by Candida spp. or Bacillus spp.

fungal infection, amphotericin B is continued with other antibiotics until recovery from granulocytopenia. The rationale for such use is to provide early control of clinically occult invasive fungal infections and to prevent the development of a fatal disseminated mycosis.

Although empirically administered amphotericin is clearly effective in reducing the frequency and morbidity of invasive fungal infections in cancer patients, it is not entirely protective against all invasive mycoses. Among the invasive fungal infections developing during empirical amphotericin B therapy are pulmonary aspergillosis,[44] disseminated trichosporosis,[45, 46] and systemic fusariosis.[47] Invasive pulmonary aspergillosis may emerge during empirical amphotericin B treatment as the new onset of fever and pulmonary infiltrates during granulocytopenia.[44] Disseminated trichosporosis occurs during empirical amphotericin B therapy as fever, new cutaneous lesions, renal failure, and refractory fungemia.[45, 46] Systemic *Fusarium* infection may emerge as pulmonary infiltrates and cutaneous lesions.[47] When such infections develop, the dosage of amphotericin B should be increased to 1 to 1.5 mg/kg/d.[48, 49]

Other frequently implemented modifications of empirical antibiotic therapy include the addition of clindamycin to ceftazidime for periodontal and perianal infections, the administration of acyclovir for herpes simplex mucocutaneous infections, and the inclusion of vancomycin for emergence of a β-lactam–resistant *S. epidermidis* bacteremia associated with a Hickman catheter. Vancomycin has been suggested as part of the initial antibacterial regimen; however, as previously noted, vancomycin need not be part of the initial antibiotic treatment with ceftazidime or imipenem plus cilastatin.[90] It may be safely added after isolation of coagulase-negative *Staphylococcus* from a clinically significant culture.

Duration of Antibiotic Therapy

Patients who have been febrile on or after day 7 of initial antibiotic administration and are also receiving amphotericin B should continue this therapy until they recover from granulocytopenia. Antibiotic administration should not be discontinued in persistently febrile granulocytopenic patients because of the risk of septic shock.[42] Some persistently granulocytopenic patients with or without a documented focus of infection who respond to 14 days of antibiotics and are afebrile may have the antibiotic regimen discontinued even while they remain granulocytopenic. However, continuation of antibiotics for the duration of granulocytopenia is often the more prudent and inevitable choice for critically ill pancytopenic patients in the ICU.

Unexplained Fever in Granulocytopenic Patient

Granulocytopenic patients with unexplained fever may be classified as low risk and high risk.[42] Low-risk patients with unexplained fever by definition recover from granulocytopenia within 1 week of initiating antibiotics. These patients generally have an excellent outcome when their antibiotic therapy is continued until restoration of their granulocyte count to more than 500/mm³.

High-risk granulocytopenic patients with unexplained fever continue to have granulocytopenia for more than 1 week. These patients may be further stratified according to whether they defervesce or remain febrile after the initiation of antibiotic administration. The management of these patients has been the subject of a series of investigations by Pizzo and colleagues.[23, 24, 50, 51] Among the patients who had unexplained fever and whose antibiotics were discontinued on day 7, 41% had recrudescence of fever within 3 days.

Bacteria recovered from these patients remained susceptible to the initial antibiotics. No infections developed in those patients who continued to receive antibiotics. Antibiotics should not be discontinued in persistently febrile granulocytopenic patients, as bacteremia and septic shock may ensue. A subsequent study among granulocytopenic patients with unexplained fever that resolved with a regimen of antibiotics demonstrated that, regardless of whether antibiotics were discontinued on day 14 or continued beyond day 14, approximately one third in both study arms become febrile again. Thus, granulocytopenic patients with unexplained fever should receive antibiotics for a full 14-day course. Antibiotics may then be discontinued in such patients if their fever has resolved, bearing in mind that approximately one third become febrile again. Continuation of antibiotics in such granulocytopenic patients may result in increased frequency of invasive candidiasis.

DEFINED SITES OF INFECTION
Vascular Catheter–Associated Infections

Febrile granulocytopenic patients admitted to the ICU often have an indwelling Silastic central venous catheter of the Hickman or the Broviac type. Infections related to these catheters include bacteremias, tunnel infections, and exit site infections.[30, 52–55] Bacteremias associated with Hickman's catheters are often caused by coagulase-negative staphylococci. Because these organisms are frequently resistant to β-lactam antibiotics, vancomycin is necessary. Catheters in granulocytopenic patients with coagulase-negative staphylococcal bacteremia or gram-negative bacteremia usually do not require removal. However, if the bacteremia persists for more than 48 hours after the initiation of appropriate antibiotics or recurs after 10 to 14 days of antibiotic administration, the catheter should be removed.

Catheter-associated fungemia caused by *Candida* or bacteremia attributable to *Bacillus* generally necessitates removal of the catheter.[56–58] Subcutaneous tunnel infections of Hickman's or Broviac's catheters are virtually always refractory to antibiotic therapy unless the catheter is removed. By contrast, catheter exit site infections usually respond to antibiotics without removal of the catheter.

Coagulase-negative staphylococci and other gram-positive bacteria, including *Clostridium* species,[22, 59–61] *Bacillus* species,[56] *Propionibacterium*,[62] alpha-hemolytic streptococci, and enterococci, have been recognized with increased frequency during the past decade as causes of infection in granulocytopenic patients.[19, 21, 50, 63, 64] This trend is attributable not only to the use of indwelling catheters but also to the broad spectrum and potent activity of antimicrobial regimens against gram-negative bacteria.

Respiratory Tract Infections
Pulmonary Infiltrates

The lungs are the single most common tissue site of proven infection in the granulocytopenic patient. Most episodes of pneumonia in granulocytopenic patients are due to aspiration of the microbial flora of the upper airways. A gram-negative bacillary pneumonia or respiratory failure necessitating mechanical ventilation in a granulocytopenic patient carries an ominous prognosis.[65, 66] Appropriate early antimicrobial therapy, which is paramount for successful management, is predicated on understanding the likely pathogens in these complicated disorders.

Pulmonary infiltrates and fever are the initial hallmarks of pneumonia in granulocytopenic patients. Pulmonary infiltrates in these patients may be classified as localized and

TABLE 45–5

APPROACHES TO DIAGNOSIS OF PULMONARY INFILTRATES IN GRANULOCYTOPENIC PATIENTS*

| Diagnostic Approach | Localized Infiltrates | | | Diffuse Infiltrates |
	Early	Refractory	Late	
Cultures of blood, urine, and sputum†	+	+	+	+
Chest radiographs	+	+	+	+
CBC	+	+	+	+
Serum chemistry	+	+	+	+
O₂ saturation‡ or PaO₂	+	+	+	+
PT, PTT§	+	+	+	+
CT scan	−	+‖	+‖	+‖
Bronchoalveolar lavage	−	+	+	+
Open lung biopsy	−	+¶	+¶	+**

*CBC = complete blood count; PT = prothrombin time; PTT = partial thromboplastin time; CT = computed tomography; + = indicated; − = not indicated.
†Although sputum usually is not produced by granulocytopenic patients, any induced or spontaneously produced samples should be studied.
‡Arterial oxygen saturation (pulse oximeter).
§Prothrombin time and partial thromboplastin time are indicated when patient is being evaluated for bronchoscopy or open lung biopsy.
‖Where appropriate, baseline and follow-up computed tomographic scans of focal infiltrates.
¶Open lung biopsy is usually pursued in granulocytopenic patients with persistent fever and focal pulmonary infiltrates, if bronchoscopy has not revealed the cause of infiltrates.
**Open lung biopsy is usually pursued in granulocytopenic patients with persistent fever and diffuse pulmonary infiltrates, if bronchoscopy has not revealed the cause of infiltrates and/or if the patient has not responded to empirical antimicrobial therapy.

diffuse. Localized pulmonary infiltrates in granulocytopenic patients may be further characterized as early, refractory, and late. Early pulmonary infiltrates develop concurrently with the first onset of fever in a granulocytopenic patient. Refractory pulmonary infiltrates are early pulmonary infiltrates that are clinically unresponsive to the initial empirical antimicrobial therapy. Late pulmonary infiltrates are defined as infiltrates that develop on or after day 7 of empirical antimicrobial therapy in granulocytopenic patients. Tables 45–5 and 45–6 summarize this classification, concomitant organisms, and suggested approaches to these pulmonary infiltrates.

Localized Pulmonary Infiltrates. *Early Localized Pulmonary Infiltrates.* Localized pulmonary infiltrates that develop with the initial fever in granulocytopenic patients are usually due to bacteria and less commonly due to fungi, viruses, and protozoa. The most common bacterial causes of early pulmonary infiltrates in granulocytopenic patients include *Klebsiella* species, other Enterobacteriaceae, and *P. aeruginosa.* Concomitant corticosteroid therapy increases the risk of *Pneumocystis* pneumonia and pulmonary fungal infections. Noninfectious causes of early pulmonary infiltrates include cytotoxic chemotherapy, acute radiation pneumonitis, and progression of neoplastic disease.

The initial evaluation of granulocytopenic cancer patients with new onset of fever and pulmonary infiltrates is directed toward elucidating the cause of fever. This examination entails history, physical examination, two sets of blood cultures, a urine culture, serum biochemistry studies, and a complete blood count and a review of chest radiographs. Because granulocytopenia reduces the inflammatory response, physical findings may be relatively minimal; cough, sputum production, rales, and bronchial breath sounds may be delayed in development or absent.

An arterial blood gas analysis or calibrated pulse oximeter reading is warranted in granulocytopenic patients with new pulmonary infiltrates. Hypoxemia may be more severe than that which would be anticipated from the chest radiograph. Arterial blood gas analysis can be safely performed in granulocytopenic patients, provided the compression to the radial artery puncture site is maintained and the platelet count can be supported. A pulse oximeter measurement is more appropriate for children and for those adults whose platelet count cannot be maintained.

Although most granulocytopenic patients are not able to expectorate sputum, any sample that can be induced should be examined by Gram's stain and cultured. Sputum expectoration may be induced by aerosolized hypertonic saline. This method has been used increasingly for diagnosis of *Pneumocystis* pneumonia and may be useful for diagnosis of other causes of pneumonia. Febrile granulocytopenic patients with early onset of pulmonary infiltrates usually do not immediately require invasive diagnostic procedures. Instead, such patients are generally given a trial of empirical broad-spectrum antibacterial therapy. If there is clinical improvement within 48 to 72 hours after initiation of antibiotics, a course of 2 to 3 weeks of antibiotic therapy is administered.[23] If there is no response within 48 to 72 hours, bronchoscopy or open lung biopsy is necessary.

Refractory Focal Pulmonary Infiltrates. The lack of clinical response within 48 to 72 hours of empirical antibacterial therapy in a granulocytopenic patient with fever and new pulmonary infiltrates suggests that a pneumonia may be present that may require modification of antibiotics for less common etiologic agents, such as *Legionella pneumophila, Mycoplasma pneumoniae, P. carinii, C. neoformans, Aspergillus* species, *Candida albicans, H. capsulatum, Nocardia asteroides, M. tuberculosis,* atypical mycobacteria, cytomegalovirus, and helminthic infections, especially *S. stercoralis,* as well as gram-positive or gram-negative bacteria that are resistant to the initial antibiotic regimens. Noninfectious causes also must be considered in the evaluation of putatively refractory pulmonary infiltrates in granulocytopenic patients.

Repeated history, physical examination, and blood cultures, as well as additional studies, are indicated in patients who apparently have not responded to the empirical regimen. If induced sputum does not reveal a respiratory pathogen (e.g., *P. carinii*), more invasive diagnostic procedures are warranted.[67–74] These include bronchoscopy, usually with bronchoalveolar lavage, and when appropriate, transbronchial brushing and biopsy. If bronchoscopy is not diagnostic, an open lung biopsy may be necessary. A mini-thoracotomy (for diffuse pneumonic processes) or a major thoracotomy (for more focal or localized infiltrates) may be performed.

Invasive procedures, of course, should not be undertaken without due consideration of the ability to support a patient who may be thrombocytopenic and who may also have a

TABLE 45–6

PULMONARY INFILTRATES IN GRANULOCYTOPENIC PATIENTS: CLASSIFICATION, ASSOCIATED ORGANISMS, AND APPROACHES TO TREATMENT

Infiltrate	Organisms*	Treatment*
Localized		
Early	*Klebsiella* spp. Other Enterobacteriaceae *Pseudomonas aeruginosa*	Empirical antibacterial therapy
Refractory	Resistant Enterobacteriaceae and *P. aeruginosa* *Xanthomonas maltophilia* *Pneumocystis carinii*† *Legionella* spp.† *Mycoplasma* spp. *Mycobacterium tuberculosis* *Nocardia asteroides*† *Cryptococcus neoformans*† *Histoplasma capsulatum*‡ *Aspergillus* spp.§	Modify according to susceptibility TMP-SMX TMP-SMX Erythromycin ± rifampin Erythromycin INH, rifampin, and PZA TMP-SMX Amphotericin B Amphotericin B HD ampho B ± 5-FC
Late	*Aspergillus* spp. *Candida* spp. *Pneumocystis carinii*† *Trichosporon beigelii* *Fusarium* spp. Zygomycetes Resistant Enterobacteriaceae and *P. aeruginosa* *Xanthomonas maltophilia* *Legionella* spp.† *N. asteroides*† *M. tuberculosis* *H. capsulatum*‡ *Coccidioides immitis*‡	HD ampho B‖ ± 5-FC Amphotericin B¶ ± 5-FC TMP-SMX HD ampho B‖ ± 5-FC HD ampho B‖ ± 5-FC HD ampho B Modify according to susceptibility TMP-SMX Erythromycin ± rifampin TMP-SMX INH, rifampin, and PZA Amphotericin B Amphotericin B
Diffuse	*P. carinii* *Legionella* spp. *Candida* spp. *M. tuberculosis* *H. capsulatum* Cytomegalovirus Empirical therapy**	TMP-SMX Erythromycin ± rifampin Amphotericin B ± 5-FC INH + rifampin Amphotericin B Ganciclovir Erythromycin and TMP-SMX

*TMP-SMX = trimethoprim-sulfamethoxazole; INH = isoniazid; PZA = pyrazinamide; HD ampho B = high-dose amphotericin B (1–1.5 mg/kg/d); 5-FC = 5-fluorocytosine.

†Granulocytopenic patients who have concomitant defective cell-mediated immunity or who are receiving corticosteroids carry a particularly high risk of these infections.

‡Granulocytopenic patients from endemic areas who have concomitant defective cell-mediated immunity or who are receiving corticosteroids carry a particularly high risk of these infections.

§Granulocytopenic patients with a previous episode of pulmonary aspergillosis have a high risk of recurrent pulmonary aspergillosis early in the course of a subsequent course of cytotoxic chemotherapy.

‖Pulmonary aspergillosis, trichosporonosis, and fusariosis often develop in patients who are already receiving empirical amphotericin B (0.5 mg/kg/d); studies indicate that these mycoses are more responsive to higher doses of amphotericin B (1–1.5 mg/kg/d). Although the role of flucytosine in pulmonary aspergillosis is controversial, we administer this compound to selected patients, as described in the text.

¶Amphotericin B is initiated for uncomplicated fungemia in granulocytopenic patients at 0.5 mg/kg/d. However, several conditions warrant a higher dosage of amphotericin B (1 mg/kg/d): fungemia developing during empirical amphotericin B; sustained fungemia; fungemia attributable to *Candida tropicalis;* or fungemia plus end-organ infection (e.g., pulmonary candidiasis). We also administer flucytosine for these conditions, as described in the text.

**If diagnostic procedure is not possible, empirical antifungal therapy is initiated.

deficit in coagulation proteins, as reflected in elevated prothrombin and partial thromboplastin times. In general, the platelet count should be maintained at 60,000/mm³ or greater during and after the procedure. Patients who are alloimmunized may require donor-specific platelets. Abnormal prothrombin and partial thromboplastin times should be correctable with administration of fresh frozen plasma. The risks of bronchoscopy and open lung biopsy in granulocytopenic, thrombocytopenic, and possibly hypoxic patients must be balanced thoughtfully against the diagnostic information that may beneficially alter the course of therapy. Complications, including bleeding, pneumothorax, and other cardiopulmonary events, have complicated transbronchial biopsy, percutaneous needle aspiration and biopsy, and open lung biopsy.[73, 74] Bronchoalveolar lavage appears to be associated with fewer complications.

When the bronchoalveolar lavage fails to yield a specific diagnosis, an open lung procedure should be performed. A major thoracotomy using either a lateral or a mediastinal approach is required for diagnosis of a localized infiltrate. As the distribution of organisms in infected lesions varies substantially, the surgeon should obtain biopsy tissue from the peripheral and central areas of abnormal lung.

Few studies have compared one diagnostic modality with another for evaluation of pulmonary infiltrates in granulocytopenic patients. A study by Burt and associates evaluated transthoracic needle aspiration and biopsy as well as transbronchial brush procedure and biopsy in patients undergoing open lung biopsy.[75] The open biopsy established a diagnosis in 94%, transbronchial biopsy in 59%, and closed aspiration in 30%. This relatively low yield of transbronchial biopsy as well as the high risk of postbiopsy hemorrhage has been noted by several investigators. Although the risks of postbiopsy hemorrhage and pneumothorax are present in each of the invasive procedures, they tend to be better controlled with open procedures. The diagnostic yield of open biopsy also has its limitations, especially late in the course of pulmonary infiltrates or when the patient has received an extended course of antibiotics and amphotericin B.[71] Nevertheless, invasive aspergillosis, neoplastic infiltrates, and cytomegalovirus infection may still be diagnosed by open biopsy in granulocytopenic patients with pulmonary infiltrates refractory to empirical therapy.[76]

Modification of the initial empirical antibiotic regimen depends on new microbiologic and pathologic findings. For example, strains of *Enterobacter* species, *Serratia marcescens*, and *Citrobacter freundii* may potentially have stably derepressed inducible β-lactamase. Recovery of such isolates in patients receiving monotherapy necessitates the addition of an aminoglycoside. *Xanthomonas (Pseudomonas) maltophilia* resistant to imipenem is usually treated with trimethoprim-sulfamethoxazole. *P. carinii*, when recovered from granulocytopenic patients, such as those with aggressively treated non-Hodgkin's lymphoma, also necessitates the addition of trimethoprim-sulfamethoxazole.[77]

Late Onset of Focal Pulmonary Infiltrates.
The probability of the emergence of pathogens unresponsive to the initial empirical antibiotic therapy increases[42] as the duration of granulocytopenia increases. Fungal pathogens have an increasingly prominent role in pulmonary infections arising in persistently granulocytopenic patients.

New focal pulmonary infiltrates developing after the first week of empirical antibiotic therapy most commonly are due to invasive fungi, resistant bacteria, viruses, and protozoa. Invasive mycoses, particularly with *Aspergillus fumigatus* and *Aspergillus flavus* and *Candida* species (attributable to either hematogenous pulmonary candidiasis or, less commonly, *Candida* bronchopneumonia) are especially important to recognize. Less common fungal pathogens including *Trichosporon beigelii*, *Fusarium* species, and the Zygomycetes (e.g., *Rhizopus* species and *Cunninghamella*) may emerge during empirical amphotericin B therapy. Resistant bacteria (e.g., *P. aeruginosa*, *Enterobacter* species, and *X. maltophilia*), *N. asteroides* and *P. carinii*, and cytomegalovirus may also be causes of late pulmonary infiltrates.

Late focal pulmonary infiltrates may develop during persistent granulocytopenia or during recovery from granulocytopenia.[79] A new pulmonary infiltrate that appears during recovery from granulocytopenia usually represents a focus of previously unrecognized and radiographically inapparent pulmonary infection owing to the absence of granulocytes. During careful follow-up, most of these infiltrates usually resolve without complications. A new focal pulmonary infiltrate developing in a persistently febrile granulocytopenic patient who is already receiving broad-spectrum antibiotic therapy represents a more ominous finding that is most consistent with fungal pneumonia, especially invasive pulmonary aspergillosis.

Development of pleuritic pain, a pleural friction rub, production of blood-streaked sputum, or hemoptysis in febrile granulocytopenic patients with late-onset pulmonary infiltrates should suggest invasive pulmonary aspergillosis.[81, 82] Panos and colleagues found that invasive pulmonary aspergillosis was the most common cause of fatal hemoptysis in patients with hematologic malignancies.[82] This study identified two mechanisms of mycosis-related pulmonary hemorrhage: (1) pulmonary infarction attributable to angioinvasion during granulocytopenia and (2) mycotic aneurysm formation during recovery from granulocytopenia. Development of a focal neurologic deficit in febrile granulocytopenic patients with new pulmonary infiltrates is also an ominous sign and is consistent with central nervous system aspergillosis.[83]

Diagnostic Approach. A microbiologically and/or histopathologically defined diagnosis ideally should be sought in persistently febrile granulocytopenic patients who have new pulmonary infiltrates. The administration of high nephrotoxic dosages of amphotericin B (1 to 1.5 mg/kg/d) should be based on a *proven* infection. Such dosages are seldom justified on empirical grounds. The early initiation of appropriate doses of amphotericin B also is an important factor for improved survival from invasive pulmonary aspergillosis. Isolation of *Aspergillus* species from respiratory tract cultures of febrile granulocytopenic patients with pulmonary infiltrates should be considered a priori evidence of pulmonary aspergillosis.[84] Multivariate analysis demonstrated that granulocytopenia and absence of smoking were the most significant predictors of invasive aspergillosis in patients with respiratory tract cultures growing *Aspergillus* species. Bronchoscopy and bronchoalveolar lavage or open lung biopsy should be considered in the absence of positive respiratory tract cultures for *Aspergillus* species.

Computed tomographic scans often demonstrate multiple lesions of invasive aspergillosis when such lesions are less discernible by chest radiograph. Thoracic computed tomographic scanning may contribute to an early diagnosis of pulmonary aspergillosis and afford a noninvasive means of following pulmonary infiltrates during the course of antifungal therapy. Detection of a crescent sign in pulmonary lesions on computed tomographic scan in febrile granulocytopenic patients also should suggest invasive pulmonary aspergillosis.

Pulmonary aspergillosis, trichosporosis,[60] fusariosis,[61] and other mycoses may develop despite the administration of empirical amphotericin B (0.5 mg/kg/d). If an invasive pulmonary mycosis is proved during empirical amphotericin B administration, the dosage of amphotericin B is increased to 1 to 1.5 mg/kg/d. Flucytosine may be added to the amphotericin B, provided peak serum levels are maintained between 40 and 60 μg/mL. This approach was effective in achieving a survival rate in 13 of 15 cases (87%) of invasive aspergillosis in patients with acute leukemia.[48] Merz and coworkers also found a similar survival rate in granulocytopenic patients with pulmonary and disseminated *Fusarium* infection.[49] These encouraging findings need confirmation in randomized trials. High dosages of amphotericin B require close attention to appropriate hydration, which may prevent significant azotemia but not hypokalemia or renal tubular acidosis.

Interstitial or Diffuse Infiltrates.
P. carinii, cytomegalovirus, *L. pneumophila*, and *M. pneumoniae* are leading infectious causes of diffuse pulmonary infiltrates in granulocytopenic patients. Less common causes of diffuse pulmonary infiltrates in patients include *Streptococcus mitis* infection, mycobacterial infection, varicella-zoster, influenza A, respiratory syncytial virus infection, disseminated hematogenous candidiasis, and *S. stercoralis* infection. Among the important noninfectious causes of diffuse pulmonary infiltrates in cancer patients are the adult respiratory distress syndrome, cytotoxic chemotherapy, radiation, pulmonary edema, and lymphangitic metastases. Granulocytopenic patients who are receiving concomitant corticosteroids have an increased risk of having diffuse miliary pulmonary infiltrates caused by pulmonary tuberculosis, histoplasmosis, and cryptococcosis.

Diffuse pulmonary infiltrates may develop at any time point during the course of induction or recovery from granulocytopenia. When the cause of diffuse pulmonary infiltrates is *Pneumocystis* pneumonia, the non-AIDS patient with cancer commonly demonstrates progressive fever, tachypnea, tachycardia, and hypoxia. Although the classic radiographic pattern of pneumocystis pneumonia is one of diffuse alveolar-interstitial infiltrates, localized infiltrates also may occur. *S. stercoralis* may cause a syndrome of autoinfection and dissemination (hyperinfection) characterized by fever, diffuse pulmonary infiltrates, abdominal pain, meningitis, polymicrobial bacteremia, and septic shock during larval invasion of intestinal mucosal blood vessels. Cytomegalovirus pneumonia is especially common in allogeneic bone marrow transplant recipients but may also occur in other populations of granulocytopenic patients.

The diagnostic approach to the granulocytopenic patient with diffuse pulmonary infiltrates entails a careful review of the patient's clinical course, including status of the primary neoplastic disease, usage of pulmonary toxic medications, and history of radiation therapy. An induced sputum specimen should be examined with toluidine blue for *P. carinii*, direct fluorescent antibody for *Legionella* species, Kinyoun and fluorochrome stains for acid-fast bacilli, and calcofluor white with potassium hydroxide for fungi. The specimen should be cultured for bacteria (including *Legionella* species on charcoal yeast extract agar), mycobacteria, and fungi. Serum should be evaluated when appropriate for antibodies to *M. pneumoniae* and cryptococcal polysaccharide antigen. If initial examination of induced sputum is not diagnostic, bronchoalveolar lavage should be performed. The specimen is concentrated and examined as noted for induced sputum. The bronchoalveolar lavage specimen is cultured for bacteria (including *Legionella* species), fungi, mycobacteria, and selected viruses, including cytomegalovirus, adenovirus, and respiratory syncytial virus. If no definitive microbiologic diagnosis is established from these measures and if a favorable response is not obtained to empirical therapy, an open lung biopsy should be performed. A minithoracotomy with biopsy of the lingula may yield sufficient tissue for diagnosis of the cause of diffuse pulmonary infiltrates.

Empirical treatment with trimethoprim-sulfamethoxazole and erythromycin can be initiated pending the performance of bronchoalveolar lavage and the results of diagnostic studies. Treatment of *P. carinii* pneumonia in patients without human immunodeficiency virus infection necessitates trimethoprim-sulfamethoxazole (20 mg/kg/d of trimethoprim) for 2 weeks. If trimethoprim-sulfamethoxazole is not tolerated, pentamidine (4 mg/kg/d) intravenously may be used as an alternative.

Granulocytopenic patients who have diffuse pulmonary infiltrates and whose platelet counts cannot be maintained for invasive diagnostic procedures or who are too unstable may be treated empirically with trimethoprim-sulfamethoxazole and erythromycin. If a favorable response is obtained, a complete course of antimicrobial therapy of 2 weeks of trimethoprim-sulfamethoxazole and 3 weeks of erythromycin should be completed. Isolation of *M. tuberculosis* initially warrants isoniazid, rifampin, and pyrazinamide. Patients who are found to have disseminated strongyloidiasis should be treated with thiabendazole for at least 3 weeks or longer if immunosuppression persists. Histoplasmosis or cryptococcosis in immunocompromised cancer patients initially requires a course of intravenous amphotericin B.

Cytomegalovirus, which may also cause diffuse pulmonary infiltrates in granulocytopenic patients, has been a major cause of morbidity and mortality in allogeneic bone marrow transplant recipients. Two studies in allogeneic bone marrow transplant recipients indicated that administration of ganciclovir and intravenous immunoglobulin significantly improved survival and response in comparison to other antiviral regimens.[85, 86] Although the role of ganciclovir with anticytomegalovirus activity is relatively certain, the effect of the immunoglobulin component is less certain. Preliminary findings suggest that the intravenous immunoglobulin may have an immunomodulatory effect, possibly in relation to graft-versus-host disease, rather than a direct anticytomegalovirus effect, although this latter mechanism cannot be excluded. Ganciclovir alone may be sufficient for treatment of cytomegalovirus pneumonia in non–allogeneic bone marrow transplant recipients. Ganciclovir is administered in a 1-hour infusion at 2.5 mg/kg every 8 hours for 2 weeks. The dosage of ganciclovir is decreased for renal insufficiency and for ganciclovir-induced granulocytopenia, which is the principal dose-limiting side effect of this compound. Single-agent prophylactic administration of ganciclovir (without intravenous immunoglobulin) is currently undergoing study in randomized clinical trials.

The value of open lung biopsy versus empirical therapy for diffuse pulmonary infiltrates in nongranulocytopenic cancer patients was evaluated prospectively at the National Cancer Institute.[76] *P. carinii* pneumonia was the most common diagnosis by open biopsy. The study found that initial empirical treatment with trimethoprim-sulfamethoxazole and erythromycin was as effective as an immediate open biopsy in the management of diffuse pulmonary infiltrates in nongranulocytopenic patients.

Pancytopenic patients with diffuse pulmonary infiltrates may have low platelet counts that cannot be supported for invasive diagnostic procedures or may be too unstable clinically. Such patients may be treated empirically with trimethoprim-sulfamethoxazole and erythromycin. If a response is obtained with empirical therapy for a diffuse pneumonic process, a complete course of antimicrobial therapy is required (e.g., trimethoprim-sulfamethoxazole, 2 to 3 weeks intravenously; and erythromycin, 3 weeks total).

Another cause of diffuse pulmonary infiltrates in granulocytopenic patients in the ICU is the adult respiratory distress syndrome. The pathogenesis of adult respiratory distress syndrome has been related to complement-mediated granulocyte aggregation and degranulation in the pulmonary microvasculature. However, a study identified 11 critically ill granulocytopenic patients during a 2.5-year period who also fulfilled the clinical and pathologic criteria for adult respiratory distress syndrome.[87]

Sinusitis

The paranasal sinuses of granulocytopenic patients may be the focus of infection caused by aerobic and anaerobic bacteria or to filamentous fungi such as *Aspergillus*,[88] the Mucoraceae,[89] *Fusarium, Bipolaris,* and *Pseudallescheria boydii.* The granulocytopenic host with maxillary sinusitis is often devoid of tenderness over the maxillary facial region. Instead, the patient may have only fever and persistent anterior or posterior nasal discharge and/or sinus congestion.

Diagnosis of infectious sinusitis is corroborated by radiographs of the paranasal sinuses and by smears and culture of sinus aspirates. Sinusitis related to nasotracheal or nasogastric intubation in patients in ICUs has been well defined.[90] Thus, such intubation should also be avoided in granulocytopenic patients to prevent nosocomial sinusitis.

Epiglottiditis

Candida epiglottiditis is a probably underdiagnosed upper respiratory tract complication in granulocytopenic patients.[91,&92] Initial complaints include odynophagia and persistent pain in the hypopharyngeal region. Diagnosis is corroborated by indirect laryngoscopy with direct culture and smear of the epiglottis. These patients may have respiratory stridor and require evaluation for possible endotracheal intubation. Early initiation of amphotericin B may avert the need for endotracheal intubation for *Candida* epiglottiditis. Although *H. influenzae* is the most common cause of epiglottiditis in nongranulocytopenic patients, this organism is seldom a pathogen in granulocytopenic hosts.

Infections of Alimentary Tract

Stomatitis, periodontitis, esophagitis, enteritis, typhlitis, colitis, perirectal abscesses, and perianal cellulitis are the principal infectious complications of the alimentary tract in granulocytopenic patients in the ICU. Although the majority of these infections may be managed medically, typhlitis and perirectal abscess should be evaluated by a surgical consultant.

Stomatitis

Local oral infections were found in 32% of 38 febrile patients receiving treatment for acute nonlymphocytic leukemia;[93] more than half of these oral infections were thought to be the source of fever. Stomatitis frequently follows administration of high-dose cytotoxic chemotherapy, especially with methotrexate, cytosine arabinoside, and 5-fluorouracil. *S. mitis* bacteremia, septic shock, and adult respiratory distress syndrome have been recognized as a complication of severe mucosal erosions attributable to cytotoxic chemotherapy or herpes simplex virus. Oral quinolones may increase the risk of superinfection caused by viridans streptococci.[94] As *S. mitis* tends to be resistant to penicillin, vancomycin is the preferred antibiotic treatment. Treatment of antecedent herpes simplex infection may prevent *S. mitis* bacteremia in patients with oral mucositis.

Because oral anaerobic bacteria may contribute to the superimposed polymicrobial infection, clindamycin is added to the initial empirical therapy for severe or refractory stomatitis. Herpes simplex is a frequent concurrent infection in radiotherapy- or chemotherapy-associated stomatitis. Reactivation of orolabial herpes infections may be the predominant cause of stomatitis. Isolation of the virus by cultures from mucocutaneous ulcerations in granulocytopenic patients in the ICU warrants intravenous administration of acyclovir. A 7-day course (250 mg/m^2 every 8 hours with adjustment for renal insufficiency) significantly attenuates viral shedding, accelerates resolution of ulcers, and decreases pain.[98, 99] Acyclovir, 500 mg/m^2 intravenously every 8 hours, is also effective against varicella-zoster infections in immunocompromised hosts.[90, 91] Oral candidiasis in the granulocytopenic patient may respond to oral clotrimazole troches (10 mg five times per day)[100] or to a short course of amphotericin B (0.1 to 0.5 mg/kg daily for 7 days). Oral ketoconazole or fluconazole may also be used for oropharyngeal candidiasis in cancer patients.[93] The role of fluconazole in systemic candidiasis in neutropenic patients, however, remains investigational. Ketoconazole is clearly not an alternative to amphotericin B in treating systemic mycoses in granulocytopenic patients.[101]

Periodontitis

The periodontium is a common source of oral infection in granulocytopenic patients.[15,93, 102] Necrotizing marginal gingivitis develops in the setting of existing chronic periodontitis. Severe oral infections are generally best treated with combined antibiotics with broad-spectrum aerobic and anaerobic activity, such as ceftazidime plus clindamycin. Severe periodontal infections and possible root abscesses warrant an evaluation by a dentist experienced with these complications in granulocytopenic patients.

Esophagitis

Infective esophagitis is a frequent complication in granulocytopenic hosts.[103–106] Suspicion of esophagitis should be raised by patient complaints of retrosternal burning, dysphagia, or odynophagia. Controversy prevails concerning diagnosis and treatment. Endoscopy, which carries risks of hemorrhage, bacteremia, and hypotension, should be performed only by endoscopists skilled in working with granulocytopenic patients and only in patients whose platelet counts are maintained at greater than 60,000/mm^3. Nevertheless, granulocytopenic patients in the ICU who have persistent symptoms of esophagitis should be approached, if possible, with endoscopy for a definitive microbiologic and histopathologic diagnosis. Endoscopy with brushings and biopsy in granulocytopenic patients may reveal herpes simplex virus, *Candida* species, bacteria, cytomegalovirus, or a combination of these organisms. A finding of herpes simplex virus necessitates intravenous acyclovir. Isolation of *Candida* warrants intravenous amphotericin B, especially because invasive esophageal candidiasis may be indicative of clinically occult distal gastrointestinal candidiasis and early disseminated candidiasis. Bacterial esophagitis may necessitate modification of current antibiotic therapy such as starting vancomycin administration for the presence of resistant gram-positive bacteria identified on esophageal biopsy and culture.[106]

Some pancytopenic patients with esophagitis, such as those who are thrombocytopenic and alloimmunized to random donor platelets, are not candidates for esophagoscopy. At the National Cancer Institute, such patients are treated empirically with an initial course of clotrimazole. If there is no resolution of symptoms within 48 hours, a 7-day course of intravenous amphotericin B and acyclovir is administered. Most patients respond to this combination.

Typhlitis

Examination of the abdomen in a critically ill febrile granulocytopenic patient may reveal few localized findings because of the paucity of abscess formation or of the suppression of inflammation by concomitant corticosteroids. When evaluating a granulocytopenic patient with fever and abdominal pain, acute appendicitis, intestinal perforation, or typhlitis must be considered.[107–111] Typhlitis is a necrotizing infection of the cecum, which may be evident in granulocytopenic patients as fever, right lower quadrant abdominal pain, and rebound tenderness, suggesting occult appendicitis or an acute abdomen.[100, 101] Usually, the patient is already receiving antibiotics. If the infection progresses, a medical and surgical emergency of septic shock and gastrointestinal hemorrhage may rapidly evolve.

The management of typhlitis in granulocytopenic patients is controversial.[112–113] Granulocytopenic patients with typhlitis are managed at the National Cancer Institute with broad-spectrum antibiotics active against aerobic and anaerobic organisms and by prompt surgical intervention, including resection of necrotic cecum and other involved tissues. Postoperative ICU antibiotic management should include a combination of an acylureidopenicillin (e.g., piperacillin), an aminoglycoside, and clindamycin or the single agent imipenem-cilastatin. Occasionally, symptoms of typhlitis may appear in patients with *Clostridium difficile*–associated diarrhea.

Medical treatment of the diarrhea may be sufficient for resolution of fever and symptoms in such cases.

Antibiotic-Associated Colitis

During the course of ICU management, granulocytopenic patients often have diarrhea. *C. difficile* colitis is an important cause of antibiotic-associated diarrhea.[115, 116] Samples of diarrheal stool should be submitted for toxin assay to confirm the presence of cytotoxin-producing organisms. After this organism is confirmed as the cause of the diarrhea, enteral precautions are required, as the organism can be transmitted by hospital personnel as a nosocomially acquired pathogen to other patients,[116] especially within an ICU where beds are close together.

Discontinuation of antibiotic administration is often sufficient treatment for antibiotic-associated colitis. However, this measure usually is not feasible in critically ill granulocytopenic patients. Oral vancomycin (500 mg four times per day) or oral metronidazole (250 mg four times per day) for a 10- to 14-day course is often effective in patients receiving parenteral antibiotics. Should a relapse of toxin-positive clostridial diarrhea develop, a second course of vancomycin or metronidazole is usually successful. Vancomycin is our preferred regimen, but this may not be readily administered to critically ill patients, thus warranting intravenous metronidazole.

Strongyloidiasis

Patients from tropical or subtropical climates, including the southern United States, may harbor endogenous *S. stercoralis* in the gastrointestinal tract. During immunosuppression, rhabditiform larvae invade the intestinal mucosa. Filariform larvae may disseminate hematogenously to invade multiple tissues.[117] This autoinfection syndrome in an immunocompromised host develops with high spiking fevers, generalized abdominal pain, gastrointestinal hemorrhage, diffuse pulmonary infiltrates, septic shock, and bacteremia. The bacteremia associated with disseminated strongyloidiasis is often polymicrobial, apparently owing to translocation of enteral bacteria with the filariform larvae. Stool samples from patients who have lived in endemic areas should be screened for *S. stercoralis* before initiation of immunosuppressive therapy. Infected patients are treated with thiabendazole (25 mg/kg twice per day for 2 days).

Anorectal Infections

Anorectal infections in granulocytopenic patients are most frequently mixed bacterial infections.[11] Early initiation of a combination of an antianaerobic antibiotic such as clindamycin or metronidazole with a standard agent against aerobic gram-negative bacteria usually prevents progression of a perianal cellulitis to gluteal or ischiorectal infections, which usually require surgical intervention. Surgery may increase survival in far-advanced anorectal lesions in selected granulocytopenic patients.[118] However, early initiation and continuation of appropriate parenteral antibiotics usually prevent such advanced disease.

Central Nervous System Infections

Bacterial infections of the central nervous system are unusual causes of fever in the granulocytopenic patient. *L. monocytogenes* has been reported to be the most common cause of bacterial meningitis in patients with neoplastic disease.[119] The presence of gram-positive bacilli or coccobacillary forms in the cerebrospinal fluid should suggest the possibility of central nervous system *Listeria* infection. Ampicillin plus gentamicin is considered the combination of choice. However, vancomycin, imipenem-cilastatin, and chloramphenicol may be considered as individual alternatives.

Patients with defective B cell–mediated immunity, such as those with multiple myeloma, lymphoma and hypogammaglobulinemia, or chronic lymphocytic leukemia, and postsplenectomy patients, have an increased risk of central nervous system infection caused by *S. pneumoniae* and *H. influenzae*. Aqueous penicillin G and ceftazidime are appropriate if the patient is granulocytopenic. Otherwise, either cefotaxime or chloramphenicol is effective if the patient is nongranulocytopenic.

However, bacterial infections of the central nervous system in granulocytopenic patients are most likely to develop as a complication of the use of Ommaya reservoirs or cerebrospinal fluid shunts. *Propionibacterium acnes, Corynebacterium,* and coagulase-negative staphylococci are the most common organisms found in those appliances.[62] Thus, the presence of fever and an Ommaya reservoir, ventricular drain, or ventricular shunt, or a history of recent neurosurgery warrants inclusion of vancomycin, 1 g every 12 hours.

Lumbar puncture is warranted, however, when headache, confusion, or focal neurologic deficits are present in febrile granulocytopenic patients in the ICU. If there are focal deficits or evidence of increased intracranial pressure, a computed tomographic scan should be performed for evaluation of a mass lesion. If a space-occupying mass and midline shift have been excluded, lumbar puncture may be performed with platelet transfusion support in thrombocytopenic patients.

The new onset of a focal neurologic defect in a febrile, profoundly granulocytopenic patient is often the presenting manifestation of central nervous system aspergillosis.[120] By comparison, candidiasis of the central nervous system is usually a clinically occult process of multiple subcortical microabscesses that seldom induce a focal deficit. *C. neoformans* and *T. gondii* are rarely seen in granulocytopenic patients unless there is a concomitant cellular immune deficit conferred by corticosteroids or underlying immunodeficiency.

PREVENTION OF INFECTION IN GRANULOCYTOPENIC PATIENTS

Most granulocytopenic patients admitted to the ICU already have or soon have fever for which they receive systemic antibiotics. Prophylactic administration of oral quinolones such as ciprofloxacin may reduce the frequency of bacterial infections and preserve colonization resistance of the alimentary tract. Critically ill granulocytopenic patients require parenteral antibiotics that have proved effective in granulocytopenic patients. Oral or parenterally administered quinolones alone have yet to be proved equivalent to agents such as ceftazidime, imipenem, or the combination of a potent β-lactam plus an aminoglycoside for empirical therapy of febrile, granulocytopenic patients. Administration of parenteral antibiotics obviously abrogates the intended effects of prophylactic antibacterial agents.[121]

The use of empirical amphotericin B as outlined for febrile granulocytopenic patients may also obviate oral antifungal prophylaxis, especially because most of these oral regimens have only marginal efficacy in preventing systemic fungal infections.[122] Ketoconazole has not proved effective in preventing invasive candidiasis in granulocytopenic patients. Fluconazole, a new bis-triazole oral and parenteral antifungal agent, has in vivo activity in the prevention of disseminated candidiasis.[123] Clinical trials are currently being pursued to investigate the utility of fluconazole in prevention of invasive fungal infections. Unfortunately, fluconazole has little antifungal activity against invasive aspergillosis at currently approved dosages of 400 mg/d or less. Itraconazole, which is an investigational antifungal triazole, may be effective in neutropenic patients for prevention of invasive aspergillosis. Again, randomized clinical trials are currently being initiated to investigate this question.

Protected laminar airflow environments are expensive and often deter the frequent bedside contact required for managing granulocytopenic patients.[124] These environments have no role for most critically ill granulocytopenic patients, with the possible exception of allogeneic bone marrow transplant recipients. Prophylactic ganciclovir has been effective in prevention of cytomegalovirus pneumonia in allogeneic bone marrow transplant recipients with asymptomatic infection.[125]

AUGMENTATION OF IMMUNE HOST DEFENSES

Granulocyte Transfusions. Granulocyte transfusions have been administered both therapeutically and prophylactically to granulocytopenic patients in clinical trials.[125–127] As the result of advances achieved in antimicrobial therapy as well as the problems of alloimmunization, transmission of cytomegalovirus, pulmonary reactions, and the need for frequent leukapheresis from a single donor, prophylactic granulocyte transfusions are seldom recommended. The role of transfusion of elutriated monocytes for refractory infections is undergoing investigation.

Immunoglobulins. Varicella-zoster immunoglobulin preparation is effective in preventing disseminated varicella-zoster in immunocompromised patients who may have been recently exposed.[128] Intravenous immunoglobulin (400 mg/kg) administered every 3 weeks for 1 year to patients with chronic lymphocytic leukemia, which is associated with a high frequency of hypogammaglobulinemia, significantly reduced the frequency of bacterial infections in comparison with those treated with a saline placebo.[129] Pooled immunoglobulins administered to allogeneic bone marrow transplant recipients, however, have decreased the incidence of cytomegalovirus pneumonitis[130] and may decrease the frequency of bacterial infections in such patients.

Clinical trials administering human antibody against the core glycolipid of Enterobacteriaceae to patients with gramnegative bacteremia and septic shock demonstrated improved survival, but these results require confirmation in neutropenic patients.[131–133]

Recombinant Cytokines. Several clinical trials have demonstrated that human recombinant colony-stimulating factors, particularly granulocyte-macrophage colony-stimulating factor or granulocyte colony-stimulating factor, have decreased the duration and depth of granulocytopenia in patients treated with cytotoxic chemotherapy.[134–137] It is hoped that the appropriate use of these promising agents will translate into a meaningful reduction in the frequency and severity of infections in granulocytopenic patients.

Acknowledgments. We thank Ms. Patricia Andrews for her expert secretarial assistance in preparation of the manuscript.

References

1. Pizzo PA, Young RC: Infections in the cancer patient. In: DeVita VT, Helman S, Rosenberg SA (eds): Cancer: Principles and Practice of Oncology. 2nd ed. Philadelphia, JB Lippincott, p 1963, 1985.
2. Kaufman D, Rosen N, Young RC: Clinical consequence and management of antineoplastic agents. In: Parillo JE, Masur H (eds): The Critically Ill Immunosuppressed Patient. Rockville, MD, Aspen Publishers, p 265, 1987.
3. Bader JL, Glatstein E: Radiation therapy: Issues in the critically ill immunosuppressed patient. In: Parillo JE, Masur H (eds): The Critically Ill Immunosuppressed Patient. Rockville MD, Aspen Publishers, p 305, 1987.
4. Bodey GP, Buckley M, Sathe YS, et al: Quantitative relationship between circulating leukocytes and infection in patients with acute leukemia. Ann Intern Med 64:328, 1966.
5. Bodey GP, Bolivar R, Fainstein V, et al: Infectious complications in leukemia patients. Semin Hematol 19:193, 1982.
6. Gerson SL, Talbot GH, Hurwitz S, et al: Prolonged granulocytopenia: The major risk factor for invasive pulmonary aspergillosis in patients with acute leukemia. Ann Intern Med 100:345, 1984.
7. Hersh EM, Gutterman JV, Mavligit GM: Effect of haematological malignancies and their treatment on host defense factors. Clin Haematol 5:425, 1976.
8. Slavin RE, Dias MA, Saral R: Cytosine arabinoside–induced gastrointestinal toxic alterations in sequential chemotherapeutic protocols: A clinical-pathologic study of 33 patients. Cancer 42:1747, 1978.
9. Schimpff SC: Diagnosis of infection in patients with cancer. Eur J Cancer 11:S29, 1975.
10. EORTC International Antimicrobial Therapy Project Group: Three antibiotic regimens in the treatment of infection in febrile granulocytopenic patients with cancer. J Infect Dis 137:14, 1978.
11. Schimpff SC, Wiernik PH, Block JB: Rectal abscesses in cancer patients. Lancet 2:844, 1971.
12. Albert RK, Condie F: Handwashing patterns in medical intensive care units. N Engl J Med 304:1465, 1981.
13. Schimpff SC, Moody MM, Young VM: Relationship of colonization with Pseudomonas aeruginosa to development of Pseudomonas bacteremia in cancer patients. Antimicrob Agents Chemother 10:240, 1970.
14. Fainstein V, Rodriguez W, Turk M, et al: Patterns of oropharyngeal and fecal flora in patients with leukemia. J Infect Dis 144:10, 1981.
15. Greenberg MS, Cohen SG, McKitrick JC, et al: The oral flora as a source of septicemia in patients with acute leukemia. J Oral Surg 53:32, 1982.
16. Johanson WG, Pierce AK, Sanford JP: Changing pharyngeal flora of hospitalized patients: Emergence of gram-negative bacilli. N Engl J Med 281:1137, 1969.
17. Kramer BK, Pizzo PA, Robichaud KJ, et al: Role of serial microbiological surveillance in cancer patients with fever and granulocytopenia. Am J Med 72:561, 1982.
18. Schimpff SC, Young VM, Greene WH, et al: Origin of infection in acute nonlymphocytic leukemia: Significance of hospital acquisition of potential pathogens. Ann Intern Med 77:707, 1972.
19. Pizzo PA, Ladisch SL, Gill F, et al: Increasing incidence of gram-positive sepsis in cancer patients. Med Pediatr Oncol 5:241, 1978.
20. Rubin M, Hathorn J, Gress J, et al: Gram-positive infections and use of vancomycin in 550 episodes of fever and neutropenia. Ann Intern Med 108:30, 1988.
21. Wade JC, Schimpff SC, Newman KA, et al: Staphylococcus epidermidis: An increasing cause of infection in patients with granulocytopenia. Ann Intern Med 97:507, 1982.
22. Thaler M, Gill V, Pizzo PA: The emergence of Clostridium tertium as a pathogen in neutropenic patients. Am J Med 81:596, 1986.
23. Pizzo PA, Robichaud KJ, Gill FA, et al: Duration of empiric antibiotic therapy in granulocytopenic cancer patients. Am J Med 67:194, 1979.
24. Pizzo PA, Robichaud KJ, Gill FA, et al: Empiric antibiotic and antifungal therapy for cancer patients with prolonged fever and granulocytopenia. Am J Med 72:101, 1982.
25. Walsh TJ, Schimpff SC: Treatment of infection in immunocompromised hosts. In: Brain MC, Carbone P (eds): Current Therapy in Hematology-Oncology—3. Philadelphia, BC Decker, p 243, 1988.
26. Anaissie E, Bodey GP, Kantarjian H, et al: New spectrum of fungal infections in patients with cancer. Rev Infect Dis 11:369, 1989.
27. Weinstein RA, Golomb HM, Grumet G, et al: Hairy cell leukemia: Association with disseminated atypical mycobacterial infection. Cancer 43:380, 1981.
28. Norden CW: Infections in patients with multiple myeloma. Arch Intern Med 140:1150, 1980.
29. Maki DG, McCormick RD, Uman SJ, et al: Septic endarteritis due to intraarterial catheters for cancer chemotherapy. Cancer 44:1228, 1979.
30. Press OW, Ramsey PG, Larsen EB, et al: Hickman catheter infections in patients with malignancies. Medicine 63:189, 1984.
31. Puri VK, Carlson RW, Bander JJ, et al: Complications of vascular catheterization in the critically ill. Crit Care Med 8:495, 1980.
32. Walsh TJ, Caplan E: Use of antibiotics in the traumatized and critically ill patient. In: Cowley RA, Conn A, Dunham M (eds): Trauma Care: Medical Management, Volume 2. Philadelphia, JB Lippincott, p 51, 1987.
33. Love JL, Schimpff SC, Schiffer CA, et al: Improved prognosis for granulocytopenic patients with gram-negative bacteremia. Am J Med 68:643, 1980.
34. Walsh TJ, Schimpff SC: Antibiotic combinations for the empiric treatment of the febrile neutropenic patient. Schweiz Med Wochenschr 113:58, 1983.
35. Klastersky J, Cappel RA, Daneau D: Clinical significance of in vitro synergism between antibiotics in gram-negative infections. Antimicrob Agents Chemother 2:470, 1972.

36. Klastersky J, Meunier-Carpentier F, Provost JM: Significance of antimicrobial synergism for outcome of gram-negative sepsis. Am J Med Sci 273:157, 1977.

37. Donowitz LG, Wenzel RP, Hoyt JW: High risks of hospital infection in the ICU patient. Crit Care Med 10:355, 1982.

38. Jones P, Rolston KV, Fainstain V, et al: Aztreonam therapy in neutropenic patients with cancer. Am J Med 81:243, 1986.

39. Anderson ET, Young LS, Hewitt WL: Antimicrobial synergism in the therapy of gram-negative rod bacteremia. Chemotherapy 24:45, 1978.

40. Barza M: Imipenem: First of a new class of beta-lactam antibiotics. Ann Intern Med 103:552, 1985.

41. Pizzo PA, Hathorn J, Hiemenz J, et al: A randomized trial comparing ceftazidime alone with combination antibiotic therapy in cancer patients with fever and neutropenia. N Engl J Med 315:552, 1986.

42. Pizzo PA: After empiric therapy or what to do until the granulocyte count comes back. Rev Infect Dis 9:214, 1987.

43. EORTC International Antimicrobial Therapy Cooperative Group: Empiric antifungal therapy in febrile granulocytopenic patients. Am J Med 86:668, 1989.

44. Navarro E, Lecciones J, Witebsky F, et al: Invasive aspergillosis developing during empirical antifungal therapy. In: Abstracts of the Annual Meeting of the American Society for Microbiology, 1990, p 420.

45. Walsh TJ, Newman KR, Moody M, et al: Trichosporonosis in patients with neoplastic disease. Medicine 65:268, 1986.

46. Walsh TJ: Trichosporonosis. Infect Dis Clin North Am 3:43, 1989.

47. Anaissie E, Kantarjian H, Ro J, et al: The emerging role of *Fusarium* infections in patients with cancer. Medicine 67:77, 1988.

48. Burch PA, Karp JE, Merz WG, et al: Favorable outcome of invasive aspergillosis in patients with acute leukemia. J Clin Oncol 5:1985, 1987.

49. Merz WG, Karp J, Hoagland M: Diagnosis and successful treatment of fusariosis in the compromised host. J Infect Dis 158:1046, 1988.

50. Pizzo PA, Commers JR, Cotton DJ, et al: Approaching the controversies in the antibacterial management of cancer patients. Am J Med 76:436, 1984.

51. Pizzo PA, Robichaud KJ, Wesley R, et al: Fever in the pediatric and young adult patient with cancer. A prospective study of 1001 episodes. Medicine 61:153, 1982.

52. Hiemenz J, Skelton J, Pizzo PA: Perspective on the management of catheter-related infections in cancer patients. Pediatr Infect Dis 5:6, 1986.

53. Press OW, Ramsey PG, Larsen EB, et al: Hickman catheter infections in patients with malignancies. Medicine 63:189, 1984.

54. Begala JE, Maher K, Cheryy JD: Risk of infection associated with the use of Broviac and Hickman catheters. Am J Infect Control 10:17, 1981.

55. Johnston P, Lee J, Demanski M, et al: Late recurrent *Candida* endocarditis. Chest. 99:1531, 1991.

56. Cotton DJ, Gill VJ, Marshall DJ, et al: Clinical features and therapeutic interventions in 17 cases of *Bacillus* bacteremia in an immunosuppressed patient population. J Clin Microbiol 25:672, 1987.

57. Lecciones J, Witebsky F, Marshall D, et al: Vascular catheter-associated fungemia in cancer patients: Analysis of 155 episodes. Rev Infect Dis (In press).

58. Dato VM, Dajani AS: Candidemia in children with central venous catheters: Role of catheter removal and amphotericin B therapy. Pediatr Infect Dis J 9:309, 1990.

59. Tikko SJ, Distenfield A, Davidson M: *Clostridium septicum* septicemia with identical metastatic myonecroses in a granulocytopenic patient: Infectious disease emergency. Am J Med 79:256, 1985.

60. Kornbluth AA, Danzey JB, Bernstein LH: *Clostridium septicum* infection and associated malignancy: Report of 2 cases and review of the literature. Medicine 68:30, 1989.

61. Bretzke ML, Bubrick MP, Hitchcock CR: Diffuse spreading *Clostridium septicum* infection, malignant disease, and immune suppression. Surg Gynecol Obstet 166:197, 1988.

62. Browne MJ, Dinndorf PA, Perek D, et al: Infectious complications of intraventricular reservoirs in cancer patients. Pediatr Infect Dis J 6:182, 1987.

63. Kilton KJ, Fossieck BE, Cohen MH, et al: Bacteremia due to gram-positive cocci in patients with neoplastic diseases. Am J Med 66:596, 1979.

64. McGowan JE Jr: Changing etiology of nosocomial bacteremia and fungemia and other hospital-acquired infections. Rev Infect Dis 7(suppl 3):S357, 1985.

65. Johnson MH, Gordon PW, Fitzgerald FT: Stratification of prognosis in granulocytopenic patients with hematologic malignancies using the APACHE-II severity of illness score. Crit Care Med 14:693, 1986.

66. Schuster DP, Marion JM: Precedents for meaningful recovery during treatment in a medical intensive care unit: Outcome in patients with hematologic malignancy. Am J Med 75:402, 1983.

67. Cordonnier C, Bernaudin JF, Fleury J, et al: Diagnostic yield of bronchoalveolar lavage in pneumonitis occurring after allogeneic bone marrow transplantation. Am Rev Respir Dis 132:1118, 1985.

68. Cheson BK, Samlowski WE, Tang TT, et al: Value of open-lung biopsy in 87 immunocompromised patients with pulmonary infiltrates. Cancer 55:453, 1985.

69. Canham BM, Kennedy TC, Merick TA: Unexplained pulmonary infiltrates in the compromised patient: An invasive investigation in a consecutive series. Cancer 52:325, 1983.

70. Hiatt JR, Gong H, Mulder DG, et al: The value of open lung biopsy in the immunosuppressed patient. Surgery 92:285, 1982.

71. McCabe RE, Brooks RG, Mark JBD, et al: Open lung biopsy in patients with acute leukemia. Am J Med 78:609, 1985.

72. Stover MB, Zaman Ll, Hajdu Sl, et al: Bronchoalveolar lavage in the diagnosis of diffuse pulmonary infiltrates in the immunosuppressed host. Ann Intern Med 101:1, 1984.

73. Webster J, Clarke J: A doctor's dilemma—1980 (editorial). Chest 78:417, 1980.

74. Tenholder MF: Pulmonary infections in the immunocompromised host. Chest 94:676, 1988.

75. Burt ME, Fly MW, Webber BL, et al: Prospective evaluation of aspiration needle, cutting needle, transbronchial, and open lung biopsy in patients with pulmonary infiltrates. Ann Thorac Surg 32:146, 1981.

76. Singer C, Armstrong D, Rosen PP, et al: Diffuse pulmonary infiltrates in immunosuppressed patients: Prospective study of 80 cases. Am J Med 66:110, 1979.

77. Browne M, Hubbard S, Longo DL, et al: Excess prevalence of *Pneumocystis* pneumonia in lymphoma patients with chemotherapy. Ann Intern Med 104:338, 1986.

78. Potter D, Pass Hl, Brower S, et al: Prospective randomized study of open lung biopsy versus empiric antibiotic therapy for acute pneumonitis in non-neutropenic cancer patients. Ann Thorac Surg 40:422, 1985.

79. Commers J, Robichaud KJ, Pizzo PA, et al: New pulmonary infiltrates in granulocytopenic patients being treated with antibiotics. Pediatr Infect Dis 3:423, 1984.

80. Kugler JW, Armitage JO, Helms CM, et al: Nosocomial Legionnaires' disease: Occurrence in recipients of bone marrow transplants. Am J Med 74:281, 1983.

81. Albelda SM, Talbot GH, Gerson SL, et al: Pulmonary cavitation and massive hemoptysis in invasive pulmonary aspergillosis. Am Rev Respir Dis 131:115, 1985.

82. Panos RJ, Barr LF, Walsh TJ, et al: Factors associated with fatal hemoptysis in cancer patients. Chest 94:1008, 1988.

83. Walsh TJ, Caplan LR, Hier DB: Aspergillus infections of the central nervous system: A clinicopathologic analysis. Ann Neurol 18:574, 1985.

84. Yu VL, Mader RR, Poorsatter A: Significance of isolation of *Aspergillus* from the respiratory tract in diagnosis of invasive pulmonary aspergillosis. Results from a three-year prospective study. Am J Med 81:249, 1986.

85. Emmanuel D, Cunningham I, Jules-Elysee K, et al: Cytomegalovirus pneumonia after bone marrow transplantation successfully treated with combination of ganciclovir and high-dose intravenous immune globulin. Ann Intern Med 109:777, 1988.

86. Reed EC, Bowden RA, Dandliker PS, et al: Treatment of cytomegalovirus pneumonia with ganciclovir and intravenous cytomegalovirus immunoglobulin in patients with bone marrow transplants. Ann Intern Med 109:783, 1988.

87. Ognibene FP, Martin SE, Parker MM, et al: Adult respiratory distress syndrome in patients with severe neutropenia. N Engl J Med 315:547, 1986.

88. Violler AF, Person DE, de Jongh CA, et al: *Aspergillus* sinusitis in cancer patients. Cancer 58:366, 1986.

89. Meyer RD, Rosen P, Armstrong D: Phycomycosis complicating leukemia and lymphoma. Ann Intern Med 77:871, 1972.

90. Caplan ES, Hoyt NJ: Nosocomial sinusitis. JAMA 247:639, 1982.

91. Cole S, Zawin M, Lundberg B, et al: *Candida epiglottitis* in an adult with acute nonlymphocytic leukemia. Am J Med 82:662, 1987.

92. Walsh TJ, Gray W: *Candida epiglottitis* in immunocompromised patients. Chest 91:482, 1987.

93. Peterson DG, Overholser CD: Increased morbidity associated with oral infections in patients with acute nonlymphocytic leukemia. Oral Surg 51:390, 1981.

94. Classen DC, Burke JP, Ford CD, et al: *Streptococcus mitis* sepsis in bone marrow transplant patients receiving oral antimicrobial prophylaxis. Am J Med 89:441, 1990.

95. Gluckman E, Lotsberg J, Devergie A, et al: Prophylaxis of herpes infections after bone marrow transplantation by oral acyclovir. Lancet 2:705, 1983.

96. Meyers JD, Wade JC, Mitchell CD, et al: Multicenter collaborative trial of intravenous acyclovir for treatment of mucocutaneous herpes simplex virus infection in the immunocompromised host. Am J Med 73:229, 1982.

97. Saral R, Burns WH, Laskin OL, et al: Acyclovir prophylaxis of herpes simplex virus infections: A randomized double-blind controlled trial in bone marrow transplant recipients. N Engl J Med 305:63, 1983.

98. Balfour HH Jr, Bean B, Laskin OL, et al: Acyclovir halts the progression of herpes zoster in immunocompromised patients. N Engl J Med 308:1448, 1983.

99. Prober CG, Kirk LE, Keeney RE: Acyclovir therapy of chicken pox in immunosuppressed children—A collaborative study. J Pediatr 101:622, 1982.

100. Shechtman LB, Funaro L, Robin T, et al: Clotrimazole treatment of oral candidiasis in patients with neoplastic disease. Am J Med 76:91, 1984.

101. Walsh TJ, Rubin M, Hathorn J, et al: Amphotericin B versus high-dose ketoconazole empirical antifungal therapy among febrile granulocyto-

penic cancer patients: A prospective randomized study. Arch Intern Med 151:765, 1991.

102. Overholser CD, Peterson DE, Williams LT, et al: Periodontal infections in patients with acute non-lymphocytic leukemia: Prevalence of acute exacerbations. Arch Intern Med 142:551, 1982.
103. Walsh TJ, Hamilton S, Belitsos N: Esophageal candidiasis. Diagnosis and treatment of an increasingly recognized fungal infection. Postgrad Med 84:193, 1988.
104. Buss DH, Scharyj M: Herpes virus infection of the esophagus and other visceral organs in adults: Incidence and clinical significance. Am J Med 66:457, 1979.
105. McDonald GB, Sharma P, Hackman RC, et al: Esophageal infections in immunosuppressed patients after marrow transplant. Gastroenterology 88:1111, 1985.
106. Walsh TJ, Belitsos N, Hamilton SR: Bacterial esophagitis in immuno-compromised patients. Arch Intern Med 146:1345, 1986.
107. Abramson SJ, Berdon WE, Baker DH: Childhood typhlitis: Its increasing association with acute myelogenous leukemia. Radiology 146:61, 1983.
108. Exelby PR, Ghandchi A, Lansigan N, et al: Management of the acute abdomen in children with leukemia. Cancer 35:826, 1984.
109. Ikard RW: Neutropenic typhlitis in adults. Arch Surg 116:943, 1981.
110. Jones GT, Abramson N: Gastrointestinal necrosis in acute leukemia: A complication of induction therapy. Cancer Invest 1:315, 1983.
111. Matolo NM, Garfinkle SE, Wolfman EF: Intestinal necrosis and perforation in patients receiving immunosuppressive drugs. Am J Surg 132:753, 1976.
112. Shaked A, Shinar E, Freund H: Neutropenic typhlitis: A plea for conservatism. Dis Colon Rectum 26:351, 1983.
113. Varki AP, Armitage JO, Feagler JR: Typhlitis in acute leukemia: Successful treatment by early surgical intervention. Cancer 43:695, 1979.
114. Bartlett JG, Chang TW, Gurwith M, et al: Antibiotic-associated pseudomembranous colitis due to toxin-producing clostridia. N Engl J Med 298:531, 1978.
115. Kim KH, Fekety R, Batts DH, et al: Isolation of Clostridium difficile from environment and contacts of patients with antibiotic-associated colitis. J Infect Dis 143:42, 1981.
116. Larson HE, Price AB, Honour P, et al: Clostridium difficile and the aetiology of pseudomembranous colitis. Lancet 1:1063, 1978.
117. Scowden EB, Schaffner W, Stone WJ: Overwhelming strongyloidiasis: An unappreciated opportunistic infection. Medicine 57:527, 1978.
118. Barnes S, Sattler F, Ballard J: Perirectal infections in acute leukemia: Improved survival after incision and debridement. Ann Intern Med 100:510, 1984.
119. Chernik NL, Armstrong D, Posner JB: Central nervous system infections in patients with cancer: Changing patterns. Cancer 40:268, 1977.
120. Walsh TJ, Hier DB, Caplan LR: Fungal infections of the central nervous system: Analysis of risk factors and clinical manifestations. Neurology 35:1654, 1985.
121. Pizzo P, Robichaud KJ, Edwards BK, et al: Oral antibiotic prophylaxis in patients with cancer: A double blind randomized placebo-controlled study. J Pediatr 102:125, 1983.
122. DeGregorio MW, Lee W, Ries C: Candida infections in patients with acute leukemia: Ineffectiveness of nystatin prophylaxis and relationship between oropharyngeal and systemic candidiasis. Cancer 50:2780, 1983.
123. Walsh TJ, Lee J, Aoki S, et al: Experimental basis for use of fluconazole for preventive or early treatment of disseminated candidiasis in granulocytopenic hosts. Rev Infect Dis 12(suppl 3):S307, 1990.
124. Armstrong D: Symposium on infectious complications of neoplastic disease (part II). Protected environments are discomforting and expensive and do not offer meaningful protection. Am J Med 76:685, 1984.
125. Schmidt GM, Horak DA, Niland JC, et al: A randomized, controlled trial of prophylactic ganciclovir for cytomegalovirus pulmonary infection in recipients of allogeneic bone marrow transplants. N Engl J Med 324:1005, 1991.
126. DiNubile MJ: Therapeutic role of granulocyte transfusions. Rev Infect Dis 7:232, 1985.
127. Wright DG, Robichaud KJ, Pizzo PA, et al: Lethal pulmonary reactions associated with the combined use of amphotericin B and leukocyte transfusions. N Engl J Med 304:1185, 1981.
128. Stevens DA, Merigan TC: Zoster immune globulin prophylaxis of disseminated zoster in compromised hosts: A randomized trial. Arch Intern Med 140:52, 1980.
129. Cooperative Group for the Study of Immunoglobulin in Chronic Lymphocytic Leukemia: Intravenous immunoglobulin for the prevention of infection in chronic lymphocytic leukemia: A randomized, controlled, clinical trial. N Engl J Med 319:902, 1988.
130. Winston DJ, Ho WG, Lin C-H, et al: Intravenous immunoglobulin for modification of cytomegalovirus infections associated with bone marrow transplantation. Am J Med 76(suppl 3A):128, 1984.
131. Ziegler EJ, McCutchan JA, Fierer JA, et al: Treatment of gram-negative bacteremia and shock with human antiserum to mutant Escherichia coli. N Engl J Med 307:1225, 1982.
132. Baumgartner J-D, Glauser MP, McCutchan JA: Prevention of gram-negative shock and death in surgical patients by antibody to endotoxin core glycolipid. Lancet 1:59, 1985.
133. Ziegler EJ, Fisher CJ Jr, Sprung CL, et al: Treatment of gram-negative bacteremia and septic shock with HA-1A human monoclonal antibody against endotoxin. A randomized, double-blind, placebo-controlled trial. The HA-1A Sepsis Study Group. N Engl J Med 324:429, 1991. (Comment in: N Engl J Med 324:486, 1991.)
134. Morstyn G, Campbell L, Souza L, et al: Effect of granulocyte colony stimulating factor on neutropenia induced by cytotoxic chemotherapy. Lancet 2:667, 1988.
135. Bronchud MH, Scarffe JH, Thatcher N, et al: Phase I/II study of recombinant human granulocyte colony-stimulating factor in patients receiving intensive chemotherapy for small cell lung cancer. Br J Cancer 56:809, 1987.
136. Antman KS, Griffin JD, Elias A, et al: Effect of recombinant human granulocyte-macrophage colony-stimulating factor on chemotherapy-induced myelosuppression. N Engl J Med 319:593, 1988.
137. Brandt SJ, Peters RA, Waters K, et al: Effect of recombinant human granulocyte-macrophage colony stimulating factor on hematopoietic reconstitution after high dose of chemotherapy and autologous bone marrow transplantation. N Engl J Med 318:869, 1988.

CHAPTER 46

Infections in Cancer Patients

Pranatharthi Chandrasekar

A large number of patients admitted to the intensive care unit (ICU) are cancer patients with documented or suspected infection. They may also develop infection during their stay in the ICU or are admitted to the ICU with hemodynamic, pulmonary, renal, or gastrointestinal complications secondary to infection. Underlying malignancy and its treatment cause multiple defects in the host defenses, increasing the host's susceptibility to infection. Noteworthy organisms of low virulence frequently assume pathogenic importance in the immunodeficient host. Consequently, infections caused by usual and unusual pathogens are more common and more severe in patients with malignancies than in those with normal defenses. Optimal management requires a thorough knowledge of the risk factors predisposing the cancer patient to infection and the infectious syndromes that occur in this population.

Among the various defects in the host defenses, a reduction in the circulating granulocyte count is the most serious, induced either by the underlying malignant state (e.g., acute leukemia) or cancer therapy.[1-4] A peripheral granulocyte (neutrophils plus band forms) count of less than 500/mm³ is associated with a high risk of developing life-threatening infection. On the other hand, infections in nongranulocytopenic cancer patients are not usually associated with rapid lethality, and routine practice of therapeutic empiricism is often not necessary. The widespread practice of immediate administration of a combination regimen of an antipseudomonal β-lactam and an aminoglycoside for suspected infection in all cancer patients is clearly inappropriate. Instead, as in infected patients without cancer, appropriate diagnostic measures should be undertaken and a reasonable diagnosis made before initiation of therapy. In serious situations, however, early empirical therapy directed against the most probable causative pathogen(s) is justified.

The first part of this chapter deals with the defects in host defenses and associated infections. The second part deals with the management of specific infectious syndromes seen in the nongranulocytopenic cancer patient.

IMPAIRED HOST DEFENSES AND ASSOCIATED INFECTIONS

Multiple risk factors exist in the intensive care setting, and the contributory role of each requires careful assessment. Factors predisposing to infection in the cancer patient are listed in Table 46–1. The defensive role of neutrophils and the effects of neutropenia are discussed in Chapter 23.

Defective Cell-Mediated Immunity

A functional cell-mediated immune system requires macrophages, and suppressor T cells, and effector lymphocytes. Impaired cell-mediated immunity (CMI) is seen in Hodgkin's and non-Hodgkin's lymphoma, hairy-cell leukemia, and chronic lymphatic leukemia. Cytotoxic chemotherapy, corticosteroids, and radiation treatment also profoundly impair CMI. This type of immunity is the major defense against a broad range of obligate intracellular microorganisms (Table 46–2).[5] Infections attributable to these pathogens represent reactivation of a latent or dormant process and, in contrast to those in the normal host, are more likely to disseminate and become life threatening in the immunodeficient host. Except for reactivation of tuberculosis and varicella-zoster virus (VZV) infection, other infections are infrequent. Patients with Hodgkin's lymphoma tend to have recurrent VZV infection and are at high risk of developing tuberculosis. Infections caused by atypical mycobacteria and *Pneumocystis carinii* have frequently been documented in hairy-cell leukemia[6] and chronic lymphatic leukemia, respectively.

Infections in patients with defective CMI involve the lung, central nervous system, gastrointestinal tract, and skin. As the list of possible etiologic agents is extensive, prompt diagnostic procedures, frequently including tissue biopsy, should be performed to determine appropriate treatment. Unlike the granulocytopenic host, there usually are no major contraindications for a diagnostic invasive procedure in patients with defective CMI. Failure to aggressively pursue the diagnosis early in the management may later require empirical polypharmacy.

Defective Humoral Immunity

Humoral immunity is mediated through antibodies (immunoglobulins) produced by B lymphocytes. The antibodies promote phagocytosis and destruction of microorganisms via opsonization, toxin neutralization, and lysis of susceptible organisms.[7] Pathogens frequently observed include encapsulated pyogenic bacteria such as *Streptococcus pneumoniae*, *Haemophilus influenzae*, and rarely, *Neisseria meningitidis*. Multiple myeloma, chronic lymphatic leukemia, and Waldenström's macroglobulinemia are common disease states associated with humoral immunodeficiency.[8, 9] In multiple myeloma, normal antibody levels are decreased, impairing the activity of all phagocytic cells, including granulocytes, monocytes, and macrophages. Deficiency in functional complement activity is also seen. In chronic lymphatic leukemia, the level of serum immunoglobulin (immunoglobulin G) is normal in early stages but gradually falls with disease progression; unlike the situation in multiple myeloma, antibody levels do not revert to normal after chemotherapy. Common bacterial infections in patients with chronic lymphatic leukemia involve the paranasal sinuses, upper and lower respiratory tract, urinary tract, and skin.

Splenectomy

Splenectomy is most commonly performed as a staging procedure for lymphoreticular malignancy. Because the spleen has at least two major anti-infective roles, namely, formation of opsonizing antibody and reticuloendothelial sequestration of organisms from the blood stream, splenectomy is associated with rapidly fatal infections.[10, 11] Septicemia is mainly caused by *S. pneumoniae* and *H. influenzae* and occasionally by *N. meningitidis*, *Staphylococcus aureus*, DF-2 bacillus, or *Babesia*.[12–17] The bacteremia-associated mortality rate varies with age and the underlying condition. Overwhelming pneumococcal septic syndrome is more common in splenectomized children than in adults. Risk of serious infection in those undergoing splenectomy for trauma is about 1.5%, whereas the risk rises to about 25% in asplenic patients with thalassemia.[18] Administration of prophylactic oral penicillin to all splenectomized hosts has been recommended, but convincing proof of therapeutic efficacy is lacking. Because of the rapid progression of illness, the splenectomized patient may be advised to take 1 g of oral amoxicillin plus clavulanate at the onset of fever and chills and then seek medical attention. Alternatively, trimetho-

---

TABLE 46–2

PATHOGENS COMMONLY FOUND IN CANCER PATIENTS WITH CELLULAR IMMUNE DYSFUNCTION

Bacteria
Listeria monocytogenes
Salmonella
Mycobacterium tuberculosis
Atypical mycobacteria
Legionella pneumophila

Viruses
Varicella-zoster virus
Herpes simplex virus
Cytomegalovirus
Epstein-Barr virus

Helminths
Strongyloides stercoralis

Fungi
Cryptococcus neoformans
Histoplasma capsulatum
Coccidioides immitis
Candida sp.

Protozoa
Pneumocystis carinii
Toxoplasma gondii
Cryptosporidium

TABLE 46–1

FACTORS PREDISPOSING TO INFECTION IN THE CANCER PATIENT

Granulocytopenia
Defect in cell-mediated immunity
Defect in humoral immunity
Obstruction to natural passages
Splenectomy
Breach in mucosa and integument
Central nervous system dysfunction
Parenteral nutrition
Alteration in microflora
Tissue necrosis
Chemotherapy or radiation

prim-sulfamethoxazole may be useful in penicillin-allergic patients.

Susceptibility to infection in patients with a history of splenectomy is often overlooked in the ICU. The possibility of overwhelming sepsis must be considered when examining moribund febrile cancer patients with a left upper abdominal surgical scar indicative of prior splenectomy. Sudden onset of fever and chills with no obvious cause should prompt immediate hospitalization, careful examination, and institution of appropriate intravenous antibiotics active against *S. pneumoniae* and *H. influenzae* until blood culture results become available.

Adverse Effects of Chemotherapy and Radiation

Damage to mucosal surfaces, in particular gastrointestinal mucosa, is frequently caused by cytotoxic chemotherapeutic agents such as high-dose methotrexate, cytosine arabinoside, and 5-fluorouracil. The loss of intestinal mucosal integrity promotes local infection and possible systemic invasion by alimentary canal flora. In patients with oral mucositis, reactivation of herpes simplex virus (HSV) infection and oropharyngeal candidiasis is common, and these infections may occur simultaneously. Besides causing mucositis, antineoplastic agents profoundly impair defense mechanisms, primarily via myelosuppression. CMI and humoral immunity are impaired by many chemotherapeutic drugs, even at small nonmyelosuppressive doses. Experimental studies involving dogs and mice exposed to 6-mercaptopurine, methotrexate, or cyclophosphamide have demonstrated an increased incidence of infectious mortality. Extravasation of intravenous drugs such as doxorubicin and vincristine produces severe tissue necrosis, providing an ideal site for microbial proliferation. More recently, interleukin-2 used in the treatment of renal cell carcinoma, melanoma, and lymphoma has been shown to predispose patients, particularly those with intravascular catheters, to an increased incidence of toxic skin reactions and staphylococcal bacteremias, with substantial morbidity.[19] Adrenal corticosteroids widely used in antitumor chemotherapy are known to cause multiple defects in host defense mechanisms. Corticosteroids suppress acute and chronic inflammatory responses, impair phagocytosis and killing by neutrophils and macrophages, depress CMI, and decrease antibody production and interferon synthesis. In humans, the use of corticosteroids has been associated with an enhanced susceptibility to infection caused by *P. carinii* and *Aspergillus* species, an increased incidence of oropharyngeal candidiasis, and a reactivation of tuberculosis. Radiation treatment also leads to mucositis, enteritis, and myelosuppression. Late skin changes include atrophy, fibrosis, hyper- or hypopigmentation, ulceration, and necrosis that may disrupt the integument and allow microbial invasion. Irradiation of lymph node areas can depress CMI and antibody production. Total body radiation results in profound suppression of CMI for months to years. In patients undergoing radiation therapy for head or neck cancer, decreased salivary flow, decreased salivary antibacterial immunoglobulin A levels, and occasionally, mandibular osteonecrosis are seen.[20, 21] Sequelae include gingivitis, increased risk of dental caries, and in some cases mandibular osteomyelitis.

Breach in Natural Host Barriers

Skin and mucosal surfaces, the primary host defenses against invading microorganisms, are often breached by the neoplastic process and even more frequently during invasive procedures. In the past decade, there has been a dramatic increase in the use of long-term intravascular catheters, such as Hickman's catheters and implantable catheters (Infus-A-Ports, Port-A-Cath), in cancer patients. The increased use of catheters has contributed to a marked rise in infections caused by microflora colonizing the skin.[22-26] Vascular catheters remain in the same location for prolonged periods ranging from several weeks to months and serve as excellent conduits for the cutaneous organisms to reach the blood stream. Gram-positive cutaneous flora, usually of low virulence (e.g., *Staphylococcus epidermidis*, *Corynebacterium*, and *Bacillus* species), most commonly cause catheter-associated infection. Less frequently, enteric gram-negative bacilli and fungi, particularly *Candida* species, are involved. Cancer patients, like other critically ill patients, undergo procedures such as venipuncture, catheterization with arterial and Swan-Ganz catheters, skin biopsy, and bone marrow aspiration. Meticulous skin cleansing and measures to prevent hematoma at the puncture site are essential, as extravasated blood into the surrounding tissues provides an ideal growth medium for microorganisms. Urinary catheterization should be avoided if at all possible. Wherever feasible, urinary drainage by condoms is preferable to indwelling Foley's catheters. The presence of any drainage device (e.g., biliary drains, Ommaya reservoirs, thoracostomy tubes, and stents) is clearly associated with an increased risk of infection with microorganisms colonizing the adjacent skin.[27, 28]

Alterations in Microflora

Alterations in indigenous microflora are regularly seen in critically ill patients. In cancer patients after hospitalization, there is a decrease in the normal aerobic gram-positive oral flora, with concomitant colonization of the oropharynx and lower gastrointestinal tract with aerobic gram-negative bacteria. Of the various influences, the use of broad-spectrum antimicrobial agents has the most dramatic effect on colonization. Antibiotics suppress growth of noninvasive normal flora, which allows increased binding of aerobic gram-negative bacteria to the epithelial cell surface receptors (colonization), with consequent infection. With systemic antibiotic use, the anaerobic population in the large intestine is gradually replaced by pathogenic aerobic enteric bacteria and fungi. Because of their increased virulence, certain colonizing organisms such as *Pseudomonas aeruginosa* and *Candida tropicalis* are more likely to be invasive than others.[29, 30]

Because most cancer patients spend a substantial amount of time in the hospital or outpatient clinic, exposure to and subsequent colonization by potential pathogens in the environment are unavoidable. Microorganisms in the hospital or clinic tend to be multiresistant, and acquisition of such flora leads to infections that are difficult to treat. Resistant microflora is most common in the ICU because of selective pressure induced by the high-volume use of broad-spectrum antibiotics.

Obstruction to Natural Body Passages

Natural passages such as the bronchus and the biliary or urinary tract can become partially blocked by solid tumors or lymphomas or as a consequence of fibrosis after surgery or radiation, resulting in stasis of body secretions distal to the site of obstruction. Such postobstructive sites provide an appropriate milieu for organisms nearby to thrive and cause infection. Primary or metastatic lung tumors predispose to postobstructive pneumonia and lung abscesses, usually caused by oropharyngeal aerobic and anaerobic microflora.[31] Patients with head, neck, or esophageal tumors have difficulty in handling oral secretions, frequently aspirate their oropharyngeal contents, and develop pneumonia.[32] Urinary tract infection caused by aerobic gram-negative rods commonly occurs after obstruction of the bladder or ureters by prostatic, ovarian, cervical, or rectal carcinoma. Frequent complications include hydronephrosis, pyonephrosis, and chronic pyelonephritis. Obstruction of the biliary tract secondary to lymphoma or intra-abdominal malignancies (e.g., pancreatic tumor) may result in ascending cholangitis. Common pathogens involved are enteric gram-negative bacilli and anaerobic bacteria. Gastrointestinal neoplasms (e.g., colonic carcinoma) cause luminal obstruction leading to perforation, peritonitis, septicemia, and death.

Hospital microflora replaces normal colonizing flora at the site of obstruction and cause infection in patients with a history of prior hospitalization or prior exposure to broad-spectrum antibiotics. Antimicrobial therapy must be chosen empirically in many instances, as the sites of infection may be inaccessible to obtaining specimens for testing. Use of appropriate antibiotics is critical for controlling systemic effects of acute infection, but cure cannot be achieved unless relief of obstruction and adequate drainage are established. Unfortunately, mechanical or anatomic abnormalities cannot always be corrected, particularly in patients with advanced cancer. In such cases, palliative procedures and long-term suppressive antimicrobial therapy may be the only available options.

Transfusion-Related Infections

Cancer patients are the major users of blood and blood products. Routine screening of blood donors for hepatitis B, hepatitis C (non-A, non-B), and human immunodeficiency viruses has largely reduced transfusion-related infections caused by these viruses. Transmission of cytomegalovirus via transfusions remains a major concern, and cytomegalovirus infection should be suspected in patients with unexplained fever who have had multiple transfusions.[33-35] Infection caused by cytomegalovirus can lead to hepatitis, pneumonitis, myelosuppression, and enterocolitis. In selected conditions, such as bone marrow transplantation, use of cytomegalovirus-seronegative blood for seronegative recipients is appropriate.[36] Less commonly, transfusions have been responsible for transmission of infections related to Epstein-Barr virus, human T cell lymphotropic virus types I and II, *Toxoplasma, Trypanosoma, Babesia*, plasmodia, and treponemes. Currently, blood donors in the United States are routinely screened for human T cell lymphotropic virus type I, the agent associated with adult T cell leukemia/lymphoma and tropical spastic paraparesis.

Usually, transfusion-associated fever is of noninfectious origin and is caused by the interaction of preformed agglutinating antibodies in the recipient's serum with antigens on the surfaces of leukocytes present in the transfused blood. Administration of leukocyte-poor blood or blood products helps eliminate such reactions. In addition to fever, immunosuppressive changes have been associated with blood transfusion, notably in patients undergoing dialysis, in those with thalassemia or hemophilia with long-term transfusion regimens, and in those requiring transfusions perioperatively.[37-42] Common immune alterations include depressed lymphocyte responses to antigens and mitogens, inversion of the helper-to-suppressor T cell ratio, and reduced natural killer cell cytotoxicity. Such changes in immunity may potentially result in increased infectious complications.

Central Nervous System Dysfunction

Altered consciousness related to brain tumors or administration of medications (e.g., narcotic analgesics) often leads to poor respiratory effort and atelectasis. Loss or diminution of the gag reflex may predispose to serious complications,

such as aspiration pneumonia. Impaired micturition, complicating neurologic dysfunction, may result in urinary retention and secondary infection. Infections occurring as a consequence of neurologic deficits are difficult to treat unless the underlying cause is corrected. Such complications are common in the ICU among ventilated patients and those treated with potent sedatives.

Tissue Necrosis

Solid tumors have a disorganized growth pattern; some areas within the tumor outgrow their own blood supply. Nonvascularized areas die and form a necrotic area, whereas the less vascularized areas become damaged. Ischemia and tissue anoxia may also result from compression of blood vessels by the tumor mass. Such poorly vascularized areas, commonly seen with tumors of the breast and female genital tract, serve as suitable sites for microbial invasion and proliferation. At times, the presence of infection in a necrotic tumor mass is difficult to diagnose because specimens for microbiologic verification are needed from sites not readily accessible. In such instances, empirical antibiotic treatment may need to be used. Infection in necrotic areas frequently does not respond to antibiotics unless therapy includes surgical débridement.

Nutritional Deficiency

Malnutrition is a frequent complication of cancer therapy. Both chemotherapy and radiation therapy are associated with nausea and vomiting, which result in loss of appetite. In addition, mucositis and secondary oropharyngeal infections with HSV and *Candida* contribute to symptoms such as sore mouth and odynophagia, which diminish food intake. Furthermore, chronic malnutrition leads to reduced immunocompetence. Phair and colleagues demonstrated that bacteremia occurred significantly more frequently in cancer patients with evidence of malnutrition.[43] Nutritional repletion can restore immune function.[44]

Often, cancer patients are fed via gastrostomy or jejunostomy tubes or depend on total parenteral nutrition for prolonged periods. Available data suggest that parenteral nutrition is associated with increased intraluminal bacterial count and impaired local defenses within the intestine that ultimately lead to bacterial translocation and perhaps systemic infection.[45, 46]

INFECTIONS RELATED TO ORGAN SYSTEMS
Bacteremia and Catheter-Associated Infections

In contrast to bacteremia in profoundly granulocytopenic patients, bacteremia in nongranulocytopenic cancer patients is usually accompanied by signs of infection related to the involved site. Common infected sites are those involving the neoplasm itself or those close to it. Examples include infected cutaneous malignancies, postobstructive pneumonia in lung cancer, urinary tract infection in obstructive genitourinary malignancies, and liver abscesses in pancreatic carcinoma with biliary obstruction. The most common causative pathogens are aerobic gram-negative bacteria. In a study of 364 episodes of bacteremia and fungemia in cancer patients, *Escherichia coli, P. aeruginosa, Klebsiella pneumoniae*, and *S. aureus* were commonly isolated from patients with hematologic malignancies, whereas *E. coli, S. aureus, Bacteroides* species, and *Candida* species were most frequently seen in those with solid tumors.[47] High mortality was associated with pulmonary and intra-abdominal infections and with *P. aeruginosa, K. pneumoniae*, or polymicrobial sepsis. Although most bacteremic episodes may be successfully treated with antibiotic therapy for 10 to 14 days, prolonged therapy may be necessary with persistent infection. Management should include relief of obstruction or débridement of infected necrotic tumor whenever necessary.

The clinical utility of intravenous immunoglobulins and specific antibodies directed against endotoxin and tumor necrosis factor is currently under evaluation in the treatment of gram-negative sepsis.[48–51] Although used empirically in "septic" cancer patients, polyclonal intravenous immunoglobulins have not been proved to be of benefit in gram-negative sepsis. More promising are monoclonal antibodies (antiendotoxin antibodies) of mouse or human origin against *E. coli* (J5 mutant), which appear to reduce mortality in gram-negative bacteremia.[52, 53]

Catheter-related bacteremia has become exceedingly common with the increased use of intravascular catheters (Hickman's, Port-A-Cath) in the cancer population. In febrile patients, an indwelling intravascular catheter must be a suspected source, particularly in the absence of another apparent focus of infection. The types of catheter-associated infection include infection at the exit site, "tunnel" infection (tenderness, erythema, and induration along the subcutaneous track of the catheter from the exit site to its insertion into vein), and catheter-related bacteremia or fungemia. Careful inspection of the catheter exit site, subcutaneous tunnel in Hickman's catheters, or the subcutaneous reservoir site in Port-A-Cath catheters is helpful for diagnosis, but lack of signs of inflammation does not rule out catheter-related infection. If the catheter is suspected to be clotted, clot lysis may be attempted with urokinase or streptokinase. In the absence of local signs, the diagnosis of catheter-related bacteremia can be confirmed by documenting positive blood cultures obtained simultaneously from the catheter and from the peripheral venous site. Multiple blood cultures are often necessary to distinguish true pathogens from contamination of cultures or catheters. The rate of infection appears to be equal in Hickman's or Broviac's and implantable catheters.

Most cases of catheter-associated bacteremia are caused by coagulase-negative staphylococci that may be treated with a 10-day course of intravenous antibiotic without mandatory removal of the catheter. Vancomycin is usually the antibiotic of choice, as most hospital-acquired coagulase-negative staphylococci are methicillin resistant. The antibiotic should be infused via all lumens of the catheter.[54] Exit site infections are most amenable to antibiotic therapy alone. If tunnel infection is noted or if there is persistent bacteremia and fever despite 2 to 3 days of intravenous antibiotic therapy, removal of the catheter may be necessary. Catheter removal may also be required if the infection is due to pathogens such as *Acinetobacter* species, *Bacillus* species, non-*aeruginosa* *Pseudomonas* species, or *Candida* species. Persistently positive blood cultures of *S. aureus* or *Candida* after removal of the catheter should raise the possibility of endocarditis or local suppurative thrombophlebitis. Unusual causes of catheter-related bacteremia or fungemia in cancer patients include *Malassezia furfur (Pityrosporum orbiculare)*, *Aspergillus*, and atypical mycobacteria.[56, 57]

Respiratory Tract Infections
Sinusitis

Obstruction of the sinus passages attributable to carcinoma of the maxillary sinus or nasopharynx leads to acute or chronic sinusitis. *S. pneumoniae*, *H. influenzae*, and *Moraxella (Branhamella) catarrhalis* cause acute infection,[58] and anaerobic bacteria are involved in cases with prolonged duration

---

TABLE 46–3

PULMONARY INFILTRATES IN CANCER PATIENTS

Noninfectious Causes
Tumor
  Spread
  Lysis
  Obstruction → distal atelectasis
Pulmonary emboli or hemorrhage
Transfusion-associated leukoagglutinin reaction
Drug-induced damage
Radiation-induced damage

Infectious Causes
Pathogens (common in all populations)
  S. pneumoniae, Mycoplasma, Legionella, H. influenzae
Related to anatomic changes caused by tumor or therapy
  Head or neck cancer
  Tracheostomy → aspiration pneumonia
  Lung cancer → postobstructive pneumonia
  Lung resection → lung abscess or empyema
Related to immunosuppression caused by
  Tumor or tumor therapy
  P. carinii pneumonia, cytomegalovirus
  Atypical mycobacteria

---

of symptoms. Also, aerobic gram-negative bacteria must be considered as potential pathogens in compromised hosts. Use of appropriate antibiotics may resolve some cases of sinusitis, but when obstruction is related to tumor masses, an antral window for adequate drainage may be required for a sustained favorable outcome.

Not infrequently, surgery involving paranasal sinuses in cancer patients leads to colonization of the sinus cavities with fungi such as *Aspergillus*. Isolating *Aspergillus* from sinuses may not portend a poor prognosis as in granulocytopenic patients. Careful evaluation to distinguish colonization from true infection is essential. If invasive infection into bone is detected by computed tomography and/or multiple biopsies, use of high-dose intravenous amphotericin B in combination with surgical débridement must be seriously considered. If no invasion is present, symptomatic therapy with or without surgical evacuation of fungal mass may suffice.

Pneumonitis

Pneumonia of infectious or noninfectious origin is one of the most common reasons for admission of cancer patients to the ICU. Table 46–3 lists the various predisposing factors for the development of pulmonary infiltrates. Etiology of pneumonia may be predicted on the basis of rapidity of onset of symptoms and whether the infiltrate is localized or diffuse (Table 46–4).[59] Patients with pneumonitis attributable to fungi, mycobacteria, and tumors have subacute onset of symptoms with minimal ventilation-perfusion mismatch and maintain satisfactory oxygenation until late in the clinical course. In contrast, those with rapidly progressive bacterial or viral infections and chemical or radiation-induced lung damage exhibit a large shunt, with significantly impaired oxygenation. The clinical picture may be further confusing in the presence of chronic pulmonary disease or congestive heart failure. Although some etiologies of pneumonia are identifiable with a thorough history, physical examination, radiologic appearance, and sputum findings, tissue biopsy is often required for an accurate diagnosis.

Patients with bacterial pneumonia should have sputum examined by Gram's stain and cultures. Patients with postobstructive pneumonia may be unable to expectorate sputum unless the obstruction is relieved with chemotherapy,

---

TABLE 46–4

DIFFERENTIAL DIAGNOSIS OF PULMONARY INFILTRATES IN NON-NEUTROPENIC CANCER PATIENTS

Onset of Illness	Focal Infiltrate	Diffuse (Interstitial) Infiltrate
Acute	Bacteria: *S. pneumoniae* *Legionella* Pulmonary embolism Pulmonary hemorrhage	Pulmonary edema Leukoagglutinin reaction Miliary tuberculosis *Legionella*

Subacute	Fungi: *Cryptococcus, Histoplasma,*
	    Coccidioides
	Tuberculosis
	Tumor
		Viruses: cytomegalovirus, adenovirus,
		    HSV, VZV, influenza
		Pneumocystis, Toxoplasma
		Radiation, chemotherapy, tumor

Adapted from Rubin RH, Greene R: Etiology and management of the compromised patient with fever and pulmonary infiltrates. In: Rubin RH, Young LS (eds): Clinical Approach to Infection in the Compromised Host. New York, Plenum Publishing, p 131, 1988.

---

radiation, or brachytherapy. At times, bronchoscopy may be required to facilitate expectoration. Empirical antibiotic therapy for postobstructive pneumonia should include the antibiotics active against gram-negative bacilli and oral anaerobes. Aspiration pneumonia, often seen in patients with head or neck tumors and in tracheotomized patients, is commonly due to hospital-acquired gram-negative bacilli and oropharyngeal anaerobic bacteria. During management of patients with pneumonia in the ICU, the utility of daily chest x-ray films for assessing progress is greatly hampered by the patient's changing fluid status and the suboptimal quality of bedside radiographs. Continued treatment must be based on judicious interpretation of a combination of bedside, hemodynamic, and laboratory assessments.

Among the opportunistic organisms causing pneumonia in the nongranulocytopenic, nontransplant cancer patient, *P. carinii* and mycobacteria are the most significant.

Pneumocystis carinii. *Pneumocystis* pneumonia in cancer patients, as in those with acquired immunodeficiency syndrome (AIDS), most often represents reactivation of latent infection. However, clustering of cases of *Pneumocystis* infection has been noted, suggestive of person-to-person transmission of this organism.[60–63] Patients at risk for *Pneumocystis* infection are those receiving corticosteroids for underlying acute lymphatic leukemia or lymphoma. A history of recent tapering of the corticosteroid dose is common. Also at high risk are those with solid tumors exposed to radiation of the thorax and receiving corticosteroids (e.g., breast carcinoma). Data suggest an increasing frequency of this type of pneumonia in patients with solid tumors.[64] In contrast to infection in patients with AIDS, the disease runs a more rapid and fulminant course, with clinical features of fever, dry cough, increasing hypoxemia, and bilateral alveolar infiltrates spreading from the hilum to the periphery.[65] Pleural effusions are uncommon; if they are present, another etiology must be suspected. Diagnosis requires demonstration, with special stains, of characteristic cysts or trophozoites in expectorated sputum, bronchoalveolar lavage fluid, or lung tissue obtained by fiberoptic bronchoscopy or open lung biopsy. Diagnostic yield from sputum or bronchoalveolar lavage fluid may be limited in view of the relatively small burden of organisms in cancer patients. If the patient's clinical condition does not permit an invasive diagnostic procedure to evaluate bilateral pulmonary infiltrates, an empirical trial of therapy with trimethoprim-sulfamethoxazole plus erythromycin (for *Legionella*) is justified. Because chemical or drug-induced pneumonitis cannot be ruled out in many instances, empirical addition of corticosteroids may also be necessary. If no improvement is seen within 4 to 5 days of therapy, intravenous pentamidine isethionate may be attempted as alternative therapy. For a definitive diagnosis, open lung biopsy is the preferred procedure. Al-

though use of trimethoprim-sulfamethoxazole is not widely accepted, some physicians would consider using this agent for *Pneumocystis* prophylaxis in cancer patients, particularly those receiving high-dose corticosteroids as part of an intense, prolonged chemotherapy regimen.

Mycobacterium. The incidence of tuberculosis is on the rise with the AIDS epidemic, and this may contribute to its increased occurrence in cancer patients as well.[66] The disease becomes manifest in cancer patients after immunosuppressive therapy. Tuberculin skin testing should be performed before cancer therapy, and if the result is positive, administration of isoniazid prophylaxis to prevent reactivation is appropriate. However, the test may be of limited value in anergic patients. Reactivation tuberculosis should be a diagnostic consideration when upper lobe lung involvement is seen in patients with alcoholism and head or neck tumors or in patients with lymphoma. In the latter, acute tuberculous pneumonia or disseminated infection associated with a high mortality rate is occasionally seen. The diagnosis of tuberculosis may be missed when fever, weight loss, night sweats, pulmonary infiltrates, and hepatosplenomegaly are mistakenly believed to be due to underlying malignancy.[67, 68] In the ICU, failure to maintain a high index of suspicion may lead to rapid spread of infection from the index case to other critically ill patients. During active infection, smears and cultures of sputum or bronchoscopic specimens for acid-fast bacilli are helpful for diagnosis. Response to treatment with the standard combination of isoniazid and rifampin by the oral route is usually satisfactory, and intramuscular isoniazid and an intravenous formulation of rifampin are useful in patients with paralytic ileus. In critically ill patients with overwhelming tuberculosis, use of corticosteroids may be of benefit in controlling the inflammatory process.

Nontuberculous mycobacteria *Mycobacterium kansasii* and *Mycobacterium avium–intracellulare* cause disseminated infection or pulmonary disease in patients with hairy-cell leukemia.[69] *Mycobacterium fortuitum* and *Mycobacterium chelonei* have been reported to cause pneumonia and bacteremia secondary to infections with central venous catheters.[57, 70] No effective therapy is available to treat such infections. Antimicrobial agents that may have activity against atypical mycobacteria include ciprofloxacin, amikacin, cefoxitin, erythromycin, doxycycline, rifabutin, clofazimine, and sulfonamides.

Although other organisms causing pneumonia in the compromised host are uncommon in the nongranulocytopenic, nontransplant cancer patient, they include HSV, cytomegalovirus, *Aspergillus,* and *Nocardia.* It must be cautioned that *Candida* cultured from the sputum sample most often represents colonization. A definitive diagnosis of *Candida* pneumonia requires histopathologic confirmation.

Gastrointestinal Tract Infections

Chemotherapeutic agents such as methotrexate, cytosine arabinoside, and 5-fluorouracil produce ulceration along the entire gastrointestinal tract. Radiation therapy produces similar mucositis. Occasionally, extreme oral soreness from severe stomatitis leads to malnutrition in patients treated with chemotherapy or radiation for advanced head and neck malignancies. Ulcerations in the oral mucosa are in turn invaded by the indigenous aerobic and anaerobic flora, resulting in local or systemic infections. Concurrent infections caused by reactivated HSV and *Candida* are frequent. Because clinical examination often does not reveal typical findings of specific pathogens, evaluation with the direct fluorescent antibody test for HSV, potassium hydroxide smear, and viral and fungal cultures are necessary before treatment. In patients intubated via the orotracheal route, evaluation becomes difficult, and HSV may spread from the mouth into the trachea or lung, causing life-threatening illness. Frequently, therapy in ICU patients requires an intravenous route of delivery of antiviral or antifungal drugs.

Esophagitis must be suspected when symptoms of retrosternal burning pain and dysphagia or odynophagia are present. In non-neutropenic patients, esophagitis is usually of noninfectious origin, related to radiation or chemotherapy. Infectious causes include HSV, *Candida*, cytomegalovirus, and oropharyngeal bacteria. Because radiologic findings with barium swallow examination are nonspecific and of low sensitivity, upper gastrointestinal tract endoscopy with biopsy for histologic studies and cultures is necessary to identify the pathogen(s) in patients with persistent symptoms. In extremely ill patients in whom esophagoscopy may be contraindicated, empirical treatment with a short course of intravenous amphotericin B or fluconazole followed by acyclovir is justified.

Infectious complications in the abdomen tend to be secondary to the underlying malignancy or its treatment. Signs of peritoneal inflammation, such as guarding and rebound tenderness, may be minimized or masked by corticosteroids; hence, even minor findings must be viewed with caution. Use of vinca alkaloids may lead to severe paralytic ileus and obstipation. Obstruction caused by tumors may result in cholangitis, liver abscesses, splenic infarcts, fistulas, perforated viscera, and fatal peritonitis. Complications from radiation therapy include scarring, enteritis, strictures, and fistula formation. Unique to neutropenic cancer patients are typhlitis (neutropenic enterocolitis), clostridial peritonitis, and perirectal or perianal cellulitis.[71–73]

Diarrhea is a common side effect of antitumor agents, radiation therapy, and antibiotics. Risk for antibiotic-associated *Clostridium difficile* colitis is increased by use of antitumor agents and antibiotics such as clindamycin, ampicillin and broad-spectrum β-lactam antibiotics. All cancer patients with diarrhea should be evaluated with *C. difficile* toxin assay. The organism may be isolated from stool cultures in asymptomatic oncologic patients, as it frequently colonizes individuals exposed to multiple courses of antibiotics.[74] Treatment of *C. difficile* colitis consists of oral metronidazole or vancomycin for 10 days, with discontinuation of the offending agent whenever possible.

Hepatic inflammation indicated by elevation of serum transaminase levels may be due to infection or cancer chemotherapy. The anicteric form of hepatitis is common. Among infectious causes of hepatitis, hepatitis A, B, and C (non-A, non-B) and the delta agent viruses primarily infect the liver, whereas HSV, cytomegalovirus, Epstein-Barr virus, coxsackievirus B, adenovirus, and toxoplasma cause secondary hepatic involvement. Infections related to hepatitis C and less commonly hepatitis B may be encountered in cancer patients who have had multiple transfusions. Clinical or biochemical evidence of hepatitis warrants serum tests for anti–hepatitis A virus (immunoglobulin M), hepatitis B surface and e antigens, hepatitis B core antibody, hepatitis B DNA polymerase, and hepatitis C antibody. If active hepatitis is present, potentially hepatotoxic cancer chemotherapy may be substantially delayed. Immunosuppressive or cytotoxic treatment increases the risk of hepatitis and also may reactivate quiescent liver disease related to hepatitis B.[75–77] Fulminant hepatic failure requiring liver transplantation has been known to occur as a consequence. Treatment for hepatitis B is primarily supportive. Specific therapies include acyclovir for HSV hepatitis and interferon alfa for chronic hepatitis B and C infections.[78]

Cutaneous Infections

The cutaneous barrier to infection in ICU patients is frequently breached with invasive procedures involving hemodynamic monitoring devices and intravascular catheters. In addition, cancer patients undergo skin biopsy, radiation, and chemotherapy that may damage the skin. Secondary bacterial infections at the damaged skin sites are common. Skin overlying tumors (e.g., breast cancer and sarcoma) may become ulcerated, which provides a portal of entry for microorganisms. Staphylococci are the initial pathogens, but colonization and superinfection with gram-negative bacilli follow and lead to septicemia, particularly when patients undergo myelosuppressive chemotherapy. Successful therapy includes use of antibiotics and wide excision of infected, necrotic tumors, but removal of malignancies fixed to the underlying tissues is not always easily accomplished.

Reactivated HSV and VZV are commonly encountered in the non-neutropenic, nontransplant cancer patient. HSV causes painful vesicular lesions commonly on the lips and oral mucosa, less often in the genital and perianal areas. Associated features include severe mucositis and at times superinfection of the ulcerated areas with bacteria or fungi. In patients with Hodgkin's lymphoma, the viral infection may become disseminated. Diagnosis is made by specific immunofluorescence testing (direct fluorescent antibody) and viral culture of scrapings from the base of vesicles. For therapy, acyclovir by the oral or the intravenous route is extremely effective.[79, 80] VZV infection occurs as unilateral vesicular rash with a dermatomal distribution, most commonly in patients with Hodgkin's disease, non-Hodgkin's lymphoma, or lung carcinoma of the small-cell type. Chances of reactivation of VZV increase with intensity of immunosuppression. VZV lesions occur close to the site of tumor or radiation. Ophthalmic zoster involves the ophthalmic branch of the trigeminal nerve and may result in corneal scarring and blindness. The infection is usually self-limited, but use of corticosteroids, radiation, or antitumor chemotherapy may predispose to widespread cutaneous or visceral dissemination affecting the lung, liver, or brain. Encephalitis occurs by direct viral invasion or as a postinfectious manifestation. Diagnosis of infection caused by VZV, as with HSV, can be made with the direct fluorescent antibody test and cultures of scrapings from the base of the vesicular lesions.[81] The mortality rate, even with the disseminated form, is low, and the treatment with acyclovir shortens the duration of symptoms and viral shedding and reduces the incidence of visceral dissemination.[82, 83] Occasionally, viral cultures are required to distinguish between HSV and VZV infections; such a distinction is important because infection control precautions are more rigorous for VZV[84] than for HSV and the dose of acyclovir needed against VZV is twice as much as that utilized for HSV. Other microorganisms that cause systemic infection with skin lesions include bacteria such as *Pseudomonas*, *Aero-*

monas, and *Serratia* and fungi such as *Candida, Aspergillus, Mucor, Trichosporon,*[85] and *Fusarium.*[86] All new skin lesions must be aspirated or submitted to biopsy, and the material must be cultured and examined with Gram's stain, Tzanck's preparation, potassium hydroxide smear, methylene blue, and modified acid-fast stain. Noninfectious causes of skin lesions include pyoderma gangrenosum and Sweet's syndrome.[87–89]

Central Nervous System Infections

Central nervous system infections can be easily missed as the increased use of narcotics and sedatives in the ICU tends to obscure significant neurologic findings. Those involving the intraventricular shunts and the Ommaya reservoirs are particularly common.[28, 90, 91] Infection usually results from failure to observe stringent aseptic techniques during the use of these devices. Symptoms of infection may be minimal or absent; the diagnosis requires a high index of suspicion. Clinical features, when present, include fever, headache, neck stiffness, and altered mentation. Usual pathogens include skin flora, especially staphylococci, corynebacteria, and gram-negative bacilli. As blood cultures are seldom positive, cultures of cerebrospinal fluid (CSF) obtained through the shunt or reservoir are necessary to identify the pathogen. Treatment includes appropriate intravenous antibiotics without removal of the device. If the response to treatment is poor, however, the device may require removal.

Meningitis in patients with defective CMI is usually caused by *Listeria monocytogenes* or *Cryptococcus neoformans. Listeria,* an intracellular gram-positive bacillus, can cause meningitis, encephalitis, septicemia, or endocarditis.[92–94] The clinical course of *Listeria* meningitis is subacute, with low-grade fever. CSF findings include pleocytosis with mononuclear or polymorphonuclear predominance, elevated protein and lowered glucose levels, and a positive culture. Appropriate antibiotics are intravenous penicillin or ampicillin and an aminoglycoside. Alternative agents include trimethoprim-sulfamethoxazole, vancomycin, and imipenem-cilastatin.

The fungus *C. neoformans,* acquired by inhalation, has a predilection for the meninges.[95] The clinical course of meningitis is indolent, with chronic headache and low-grade fever, with or without altered mentation. Occasionally, a focal neurologic deficit may be present. Characteristic CSF findings are lymphocytic pleocytosis, elevated protein and lowered glucose levels, and the presence of budding yeast cells. In all suspected cases of meningitis, the latex agglutination test to detect cryptococcal antigen in CSF must be performed because the organism may not always be visualized on Gram's stain or with India ink preparation. Disseminated cryptococcal infection is not uncommon in cancer patients and involves lymph nodes, liver, spleen, adrenal glands, kidneys, bone, prostate, and skin. Treatment includes the combination of intravenous amphotericin B and oral 5-flucytosine for 4 to 6 weeks.[96] Fluconazole may be considered as an effective, less toxic alternative, as it has been demonstrated to be effective in the treatment of cryptococcal meningitis in AIDS patients.[97–101] In contrast to treatment for AIDS patients, maintenance treatment with fluconazole or amphotericin B has not been proved to be necessary in cancer patients. In patients with defective B cell–mediated immunity, *S. pneumoniae* and *H. influenzae* may cause meningitis and disseminated fatal infections. If septicemia or meningitis is suspected in such patients, empirical therapy with intravenous antibiotics must be promptly administered, even before lumbar puncture.

Encephalitis attributable to HSV or VZV may be seen in patients with depressed CMI. Disease process confined to the temporal lobe, as detected by computed tomography of the brain or electroencephalogram, suggests HSV involvement. Cutaneous manifestations are absent in HSV encephalitis, whereas vesicular skin eruptions are commonly associated with VZV encephalitis. CSF findings are nonspecific, with lymphocytic pleocytosis, mildly elevated protein level, and normal glucose level. HSV encephalitis, unlike that caused by VZV, is hemorrhagic and carries a more serious prognosis. Definitive diagnosis can be made only by brain biopsy, and, therefore, in patients strongly suspected of having HSV encephalitis, an empirical trial of therapy with high-dose intravenous acyclovir is justified.[101]

Cancer patients with solitary or multiple focal lesions in the brain should not be assumed to have cerebral metastases, and the possibility of brain abscess must be entertained. Organisms causing focal infections in the brain are aerobic and anaerobic bacteria, mycobacteria, fungi, *Nocardia,* and parasites such as toxoplasma. Possible etiologic considerations in patients with focal neurologic deficits in combination with radiographic abnormalities in the lung should include *Nocardia, Aspergillus,* and *Mucor.* In all cases, brain biopsy is required for a definitive diagnosis. Early diagnostic intervention is crucial in most cases for a favorable outcome.

Urinary Tract Infections

In the ICU, cancer patients develop urinary tract infection after urethral catheterization or secondary to obstructive ovarian, bladder, or prostatic malignancies. Other predisposing factors are urinary retention related to spinal cord damage or medication (e.g., narcotics and vinca alkaloids) and local anatomic changes produced by surgery or radiation. The presence of nephrostomy tubes often leads to renal infection. Common pathogens are *E. coli, Proteus, Klebsiella,* and *Streptococcus.* In recurrent infections, resistant hospital flora, namely *Serratia, Enterobacter,* and *Pseudomonas,* may be involved. Among the fungi, *Candida* and *Torulopsis* frequently colonize the urinary tract and at times cause infection. Successful management of urinary tract infection in cancer patients depends on appropriate antimicrobial therapy and removal of the predisposing cause. Sterile hemorrhagic cystitis, a noninfectious entity, is occasionally seen in patients treated with cancer chemotherapeutic agents (e.g., cyclophosphamide).

Cardiovascular Infections

Persistent bacteremia or fungemia suggests an endovascular focus of infection. Endocarditis may occur after intravascular catheter-related bacteremia. Clinical features and management of endocarditis are identical with those in patients without cancer. Common pathogens are staphylococci and streptococci; however, fungi and aerobic gram-negative bacilli should also be considered. Among staphylococci, *S. aureus* can damage previously healthy native cardiac valves, whereas coagulase-negative staphylococci usually establish infection in abnormal or prosthetic cardiac valves. As poor dentition predisposes to serious infections and increased risk of bacteremia in neutropenic hosts, oral hygiene should be improved before chemotherapy or radiation to head and neck regions.

Osteomyelitis

Osteomyelitis in cancer patients may follow extensive surgical resections involving bone. Occasionally, radionecrosis and subsequent osteomyelitis of the mandible occur in patients treated with radiation for head or neck malignancies. Complications include persistent severe pain, nonhealing sinus tracts, and chronic drainage.

TABLE 46–5
NONINFECTIOUS ENTITIES MIMICKING INFECTION*

Features Suggestive of Infection	Drug Induced	Radiation Induced	Primary Disease
Fever	+	+	+
Mucositis	+	+	–
Rash	+	+	+
Diarrhea	+	+	–
Peritonitis	+	+	+
Hepatitis	+	+	–
Pulmonary infiltrates	+	+	+
Pulmonary cavitation	–	–	+
Meningitis or encephalitis	+	–	+
Bone destruction	–	+	+
Necrosis in tumor	+	+	+

*+ = yes; − = no.

NONINFECTIOUS ENTITIES PRODUCING SYMPTOMS AND SIGNS RESEMBLING INFECTION

Cancer patients, as a result of depressed immunity, often fail to exhibit signs of inflammation during infection. A high index of suspicion is thus required for early and accurate diagnosis of infection. Conversely, clinical features suggestive of infection may be produced by several noninfectious etiologies. Lack of awareness of infection mimickers leads to missed diagnoses and inappropriate or unwarranted therapy. Table 46–5 gives the symptoms and signs of infection caused by noninfectious entities. Among these, chemotherapy-induced toxic reactions resembling infection are the most common.

INFECTION PREVENTION

Prevention of infection may be considered under four categories: (1) prevention of acquisition of new organisms; (2) suppression of endogenous microflora; (3) reduction of procedures that increase risk of infection; and (4) restoration of immune competence.

Prevention of Acquisition of New Organisms

Despite numerous studies evaluating measures to prevent or reduce infection, the most effective technique remains careful hand washing among health care personnel.[102] Simple hand washing removes most transient microflora, which prevents transfer of organisms from person to patient or from inanimate objects such as respirators, water sinks, and bed sheets to patients. Other maneuvers to prevent acquisition of organisms from environmental sources include the use of well-cooked foods devoid of microorganisms, avoidance of fresh fruits and salads that are naturally contaminated with gram-negative bacteria, use of air filtration systems, and use of various isolation procedures for patients.[102–105] Such laborious and expensive measures may help to reduce the infection rate in profoundly granulocytopenic patients but are not necessary for other patients.

Suppression of Endogenous Microflora

About 80 to 85% of aerobic gram-negative bacillary infections in cancer patients originate from the alimentary canal flora. Thus, suppression or elimination of aerobic organisms with preservation of protective anaerobic flora (selective decontamination) in the gastrointestinal tract has led to a reduction in the frequency of infection in patients with prolonged granulocytopenia.[106] This technique has been somewhat successfully applied using oral nonabsorbable antibiotics or trimethoprim-sulfamethoxazole or quinolones in profoundly myelosuppressed patients.[106–112] Disadvantages include poor patient compliance, increase in fungal colonization and infection, prolongation of neutropenia, and possible emergence of drug-resistant microflora. Prophylactic antibiotic trials conducted among patients in the ICU have produced conflicting results.[113–117] The potential selection of resistant microorganisms consequent to the widespread use of antibiotics remains a major concern. Because most patients with lymphoma or solid tumors do not become granulocytopenic or have short-term granulocytopenia (less than 7 days) after chemotherapy, no antibacterial prophylaxis is required.

Because invasive fungal infections in cancer patients have become increasingly common in the past two decades, antifungal prophylaxis has been investigated. *Candida* has been the most common pathogen studied, and trials evaluating the efficacy of antifungal prophylaxis with nystatin, clotrimazole, or ketoconazole have aimed at reducing infection caused by *Candida* species. These drugs do not have any impact on the frequency of infections related to other fungi such as *Aspergillus* or *Mucor*.[118] Use of clotrimazole or fluconazole in patients with solid tumors who have received antitumor chemotherapy has shown a significant reduction in the incidence of oropharyngeal candidiasis.[119, 120] Patients at risk include those receiving antibiotics or adrenal corticosteroids or those with *Candida* species isolated from initial throat cultures. However, long-term consequences such as emergence of resistance from widespread antifungal prophylaxis are unknown.

Reactivation of HSV stomatitis in high-risk patients can be prevented with oral or intravenous acyclovir.[121, 122] Prolonged use of the drug has led to selection of clinically significant acyclovir-resistant HSV strains.[123] For prophylaxis against *Pneumocystis*, use of trimethoprim-sulfamethoxazole twice or three times weekly must be reserved for high-risk patients, such as those with leukemia undergoing intense immunosuppression in centers where the infection is common.[124] In instances of myelosuppression associated with trimethoprim-sulfamethoxazole, aerosolized pentamidine may prove to be an effective alternative.

Reduction of Procedures That Increase Risk of Infection

In ICU patients, device-related infections caused by organisms colonizing the adjacent skin are extremely common. Every effort should be made to minimize the use of intravascular monitoring and therapeutic devices. Invasive procedures including urinary catheterization should be avoided and stringent aseptic techniques observed when they are performed. Removal of all devices at the earliest possible opportunity reduces the frequency of nosocomial infections.

Restoration of Immune Competence

Intravenous immunoglobulins, in polyclonal or hyperimmune form, have been useful in selected groups of compromised hosts. Passive immunization via monthly administration of pooled intravenous immunoglobulin to patients with hypogammaglobulinemia and chronic lymphatic leukemia has been associated with a significant reduction in the frequency of major bacterial infections.[128–130] In neutropenic patients with fever, however, preliminary studies with intravenous immunoglobulin have been disappointing. Zoster immunoglobulin is useful in seronegative immunosuppressed patients when administered within 72 hours of exposure to a potentially infectious source. Another advance in immune restoration has been the development of colony-stimulating factors (granulocyte-macrophage and granulocyte) that can significantly shorten the duration of neutropenia, thereby reducing the at-risk period for infection.

Active immunization with vaccines has been only partially successful because protective immunity may not be sustained in cancer patients subjected to repeated courses of immunosuppressive therapy. In splenectomized hosts, immunization with polyvalent pneumococcal vaccine is advised in view of the increased risk of pneumococcal infection. The vaccine must be administered before splenectomy to obtain an optimal immune response.

Often, infection in a cancer patient is the reason for admission to the ICU, or more commonly it occurs as a preterminal event in many critically ill cancer patients. Sepsis continues to be the "final common pathway" before death among ICU patients. Aggressive therapeutic regimens currently used for most types of cancer, combined with invasive technology of intensive care management, have vastly contributed to an increase in the frequency of infection. Many such infections are preventable and an even larger number can be successfully treated with early diagnosis and appropriate therapeutic intervention.

References

1. Bodey GP, Buckley M, Sathe YS, et al: Quantitative relationships between circulating leukocytes and infection in patients with acute leukemia. Ann Intern Med 64:328, 1966.
2. Bodey GP, Bolivar R, Fainstein V, et al: Infectious complications in leukemia patients. Semin Hematol 19:193, 1982.
3. Hersh EM, Gutterman JU, Mavligit GM: Effect of haematological malignancies and their treatment on host defence factors. Clin Haematol 5:425, 1976.
4. Browder AA, Hoff JA, Petersdorf RG: The significance of fever in neoplastic disease. Ann Intern Med 55:932, 1961.
5. Hahn H, Kaufman SHE: The role of cell mediated immunity in bacterial infections. Rev Infect Dis 3:1221, 1981.
6. Weinstein RA, Golomb HM, Grumet G, et al: Hairy cell leukemia: Association with disseminated atypical mycobacterial infection. Cancer 43:380, 1981.
7. Cooper MD: B lymphocytes: Normal development and function. N Engl J Med 317:1452, 1987.
8. Norden CW: Infections in patients with multiple myeloma. Arch Intern Med 140:1150, 1980.
9. Fahey JL, Scoggins R, Utz JP, et al: Infection, antibody response and gamma globulin components in multiple myeloma and macro globulinemia. Am J Med 35:698, 1973.
10. Bohnsack JF, Brown EJ: The role of the spleen in resistance to infection. Annu Rev Med 37:49, 1986.
11. Rosse WF: The spleen as a filter. N Engl J Med 317:705, 1987.
12. Schimpff SC, O'Connell MJ, Greene WH, et al: Infections in 92 splenectomized patients with Hodgkin's disease. A clinical review. Am J Med 59:695, 1975.
13. Weitzman S, Aisenberg AC: Fulminant sepsis after the successful treatment of Hodgkin's disease. Am J Med 62:47, 1977.
14. Donaldson SS, Glatstein E, Vosti KL: Bacterial infections in pediatric Hodgkin's disease. Relationship to radiation, chemotherapy and splenectomy. Cancer 41:1949, 1978.
15. Chilcote RR, Baehner RL, Hammond D, et al: Septicemia and meningitis in children splenectomized for Hodgkin's disease. N Engl J Med 295:798, 1976.
16. Bisno AL, Freeman JC: The syndrome of asplenia, pneumococcal sepsis, and disseminated intravascular coagulation. Ann Intern Med 72:389, 1970.
17. Sun T, Tenenbaum MJ, Greenspan J, et al: Morphologic and clinical observations in human infection with Babesia microti. J Infect Dis 148:239, 1983.
18. Wilson SA, Johnson WO: Infections complicating surgical or functional splenectomy. In: Greco MH (ed): Infections in the Abnormal Host. New York, Yorke Medical, p 848, 1980.
19. Snydman DR, Sullivan B, Gill M, et al: Nosocomial sepsis associated with interleukin-2. Ann Intern Med 112:102, 1990.
20. Eneroth CM, Henrikson CO, Jakobsson PA: Effects of fractionated radiotherapy on salivary gland functions. Cancer 30:1147, 1972.
21. Jonis ST: Oral complications of cancer therapy. In: DeVita VT, Hellman S, Rosenberg SA (eds): Cancer. Principles and Practice of Oncology. 2nd ed. Philadelphia JB Lippincott, p 2014, 1985.

22. Lowder JN, Lazarus HM, Herzig RH: Bacteremias and fungemias in oncologic patients with central venous catheters. Changing spectrum of infection. Ann Intern Med 142:1456, 1982.
23. Pizzo PA, Ladisch SL, Gill F, et al: Increasing incidence of gram-positive sepsis in cancer patients. Med Pediatr Oncol 5:241, 1978.
24. EORTC International Antimicrobial Therapy Cooperative Group: Gram-positive bacteremia in granulocytopenic cancer patients. Eur J Cancer 26:569, 1990.
25. Cotton DJ, Gu V, Hiemenz J, et al: Bacillus bacteremias in an immunocompromised patient population: Clinical features, therapeutic interventions, and relationship to chronic intravascular catheters in sixteen cases. J Clin Microbiol 25:672, 1987.
26. Banerjee C, Bustamanke CI, Wharton R, et al: Bacillus infections in patients with cancer. Arch Intern Med 148:1769, 1988.
27. Szabo S, Mendelson MH, Mitty HA, et al: Infections associated with transhepatic biliary drainage devices. Am J Med 82:921, 1987.
28. Obbens EAMT, Leavens ME, Beal JW, et al: Ommaya reservoirs in 387 cancer patients. A 15 year experience. Neurology 35:1274, 1985.
29. Schimpff SC, Greene WH, Young VM, et al: Significance of Pseudomonas aeruginosa in the patient with leukemia or lymphoma. J Infect Dis 130(suppl):S24, 1974.
30. Wingard JR, Merz WG, Saral R: Candida tropicalis: A major pathogen in immunocompromised patients. Ann Intern Med 91:539, 1979.
31. Hagan JL, Hardy JD: Lung abscess revisited—A survey of 186 cases. Ann Surg 197:755, 1983.
32. Crane LR: Infection in patients with head and neck cancer. In: Al-Sarraf M, Crissman JD, Jacobs JR, Valeriote F (eds): Head and Neck Cancer: Scientific Perspectives in Management and Strategies for Cure. New York, Elsevier, p 145, 1987.
33. Winston DJ, Winston GH, Howell CL, et al: Cytomegalovirus infections associated with leukocyte transfusions. Ann Intern Med 93:671, 1980.
34. Yeager AS, Grumet FC, Hafleigh EB, et al: Prevention of transfusion-acquired cytomegalovirus infections in newborn infants. J Pediatr 98:281, 1981.
35. Fiala M, Payne JE, Berne TV, et al: Epidemiology of CMV infection after transplantation and immunosuppression. J Infect Dis 132:421, 1975.
36. Bowden RA, Sayers M, Flournoy N, et al: Cytomegalovirus immune globulin and sero-negative blood products to prevent primary cytomegalovirus infection after marrow transplantation. N Engl J Med 314:1006, 1986.
37. Kerman RH, Van Buren CT, Payne W: Influence of blood transfusions on immune responsiveness. Transplant Proc 14:335, 1982.
38. Fischer E, Lenhard V, Seiffert P, et al: Blood transfusion–induced suppression of cellular immunity in man. Hum Immunol 1:187, 1980.
39. Proud G, Shenton BU, Smith BM: Blood transfusion and renal transplantation. Br J Surg 66:678, 1966.
40. Gascon P, Zoumbos NC, Young NS: Immunologic abnormalities in patients receiving multiple blood transfusion. Ann Intern Med 100:172, 1984.
41. Kaplan J, Sarnalk S, Gitlin J, et al: Diminished helper-suppressor lymphocyte ratios and natural killer activity in recipients of repeated blood transfusions. Blood 64:308, 1984.
42. Wang W, Herrod H, Presbury G, et al: Immunologic studies in chronically transfused children (abstract). Blood 62:241, 1983.
43. Phair JP, Riesing KS, Metzger E: Bacteremic infection and malnutrition in patients with solid tumors. Investigation of host defense mechanisms. Cancer 45:2702, 1980.
44. Law DK, Dudrick SJ, Abdaub NI: Immunocompetence of patients with protein-calorie malnutrition: The effects of nutritional repletion. Ann Intern Med 79:545, 1973.
45. Alverdy JC, Aoys E, Moss GS: Total parenteral nutrition promotes bacterial translocation from the gut. Surgery 104:185, 1988.
46. Alverdy J, Chi HS, Sheldon GF: The effect of parenteral nutrition on gastrointestinal immunity. The importance of enteral stimulation. Ann Surg 202:681, 1985.
47. Singer C, Kaplan MH, Armstrong D: Bacteremia and fungemia complicating neoplastic disease. A study of 364 cases. Am J Med 62:731, 1977.
48. Calandra T, Glauser MP, Schellekens J, et al: Treatment of gram-negative septic shock with human IgG antibody to Escherichia coli J5: A prospective, double-blind, randomized trial. J Infect Dis 158:312, 1988.
49. Young LS, Gascon R, Alam S, et al: Monoclonal antibodies for the treatment of gram-negative infections. Rev Infect Dis 11(suppl 7):S1564, 1989.
50. Ziegler EJ, McCutchan JA, Fierer J, et al: Treatment of gram-negative bacteremia and shock with human antiserum to a mutant Escherichia coli. N Engl J Med 307:1225, 1982.
51. Silva AT, Bayston KF, Cohen J: Prophylactic and therapeutic effects of a monoclonal antibody to tumor necrosis factor-α in experimental gram-negative shock. J Infect Dis 162:421, 1990.
52. MacIntyre NR, Emmanuel G, Wedel NI, et al: E5 antibody improves outcome from multi-organ failure in survivors of gram-negative sepsis. Crit Care Med 19(suppl 14):4, 1991.
53. Ziegler EJ, Fisher CJ, Sprung CL, et al: Treatment of gram-negative bacteremia and septic shock with HA-1A human monoclonal antibody against endotoxin: A randomized, double-blind, placebo-controlled trial. N Engl J Med 324:429, 1991.

54. Pizzo PA: Diagnosis and management of infectious disease problems in the child with malignant disease. In: Rubin RH, Young LS (eds): Clinical Approach to the Infection in the Compromised Host. New York, Plenum Publishing, p 439, 1988.

55. Rolston KVI, Guen Z, Bodey GP, et al: *Acinetobacter calcoaceticus* septicemia in patients with cancer. South Med J 78:647, 1985.

56. Allo MD, Miller J, Towsend T, et al: Primary cutaneous aspergillosis associated with Hickman intravenous catheters. N Engl J Med 317:1105, 1987.

57. Hoy JF, Rolston KVI, Hopfer RL, et al: *Mycobacterium fortuitum* bacteremia in patients with cancer and long-term venous catheters. Am J Med 83:213, 1987.

58. Wald ER, Milmoe GJ, Bowen AD, et al: Acute maxillary sinusitis in children. N Engl J Med 304:749, 1982.

59. Rubin RH, Greene R: Etiology and management of the compromised patient with fever and pulmonary infiltrates. In: Rubin RH, Young LS (eds): Clinical Approach to Infection in the Compromised Host. New York, Plenum Publishing, p 131, 1988.

60. Jacobs JL, Libby DM, Winters RA, et al: A cluster of *Pneumocystis carinii* pneumonia in adults without predisposing illnesses. N Engl J Med 324:246, 1991.

61. Ruebush TK, Weinstein RA, Baehner RL, et al: An outbreak of *Pneumocystis* pneumonia in children with acute lymphocyte leukemia. Am J Dis Child 132:143, 1978.

62. Singer C, Armstrong D, Rosen PP, et al: *Pneumocystis carinii* pneumonia: A cluster of eleven cases. Ann Intern Med 82:772, 1975.

63. Chusid MJ, Heyrman KA. An outbreak of *Pneumocystis carinii* pneumonia at a pediatric hospital. Pediatrics 62:1031, 1967.

64. Sepkowitz KA, Gottlieb S, Brown AE, et al: *Pneumocystis carinii* pneumonia among non-AIDS patients at a cancer hospital. In: Abstracts, Sixth International Symposium on Infections in the Immunocompromised Host, Peebles, Scotland, June 3–6, 1990.

65. Kovacs JA, Hiemenz JW, Macher AM, et al: *Pneumocystis carinii* pneumonia: A comparison of clinical features in patients with acquired immune deficiency syndrome and patients with other immune diseases. Ann Intern Med 100:663, 1984.

66. Centers for Disease Control: Tuberculosis and acquired immunodeficiency syndrome: New York City. MMWR 36:785, 1987.

67. Feld R, Bodey GP, Groschel D: Mycobacteriosis in patients with malignant disease. Arch Intern Med 136:67, 1976.

68. Ludmerer KM, Kissnae JM: Fulminant pneumonia and death in an immunocompromised woman. Am J Med 75:1043, 1983.

69. Bennett C, Vardiman J, Golomb H: Disseminated atypical mycobacterial infection in patients with hairy cell leukemia. Am J Med 80:891, 1986.

70. Rolston KVI, Jones PG, Fainstein V, et al: Pulmonary disease caused by rapidly growing mycobacteria in patients with cancer. Chest 87:503, 1985.

71. Skibber JM, Matler GJ, Lotze MT, et al: Right lower quadrant complications in young patients with leukemia: A surgical perspective. Ann Surg 206:711, 1987.

72. Wynne JW, Armstrong D: Clostridial septicemia. Cancer 29:215, 1972.

73. Glenn J, Cotton D, Wesley R, et al: Anorectal infections in patients with malignant diseases. Rev Infect Dis 10:42, 1988.

74. Elstner CL, Lindsay AN, Book LS, et al: Lack of relationship of *Clostridium difficile* to antibiotic-associated diarrhea in children. Pediatr Infect Dis 2:364, 1983.

75. Flowers MA, Heathcote J, Wanless IR, et al: Fulminant hepatitis as a consequence of reactivation of hepatitis B. Infection after discontinuation of low-dose methotrexate therapy. Ann Intern Med 112:381, 1990.

76. Lam KC, Lai CL, Trepo C, et al: Deleterious effect of prednisone in HBsAg-positive chronic active hepatitis. N Engl J Med 304:380, 1981.

77. Hanson CA, Sutherland DE, Snover DC: Fulminant hepatic failure in an HBsAg carrier renal transplant patient following cessation of immunosuppressive therapy. Transplantation 39:311, 1985.

78. DiBisceglie AM, Martin P, Kassianides C, et al: Recombinant alpha interferon therapy for chronic hepatitis C. A randomized, double-blind, placebo-controlled trial. N Engl J Med 321:1506, 1989.

79. Whitley RJ, Levin M, Barton N, et al: Infections caused by herpes simplex virus in the immunocompromised host: Natural history and topical acyclovir therapy. J Infect Dis 150:323, 1984.

80. Meyers JD, Wade JC, Mitchell CD, et al: Multicenter collaborative trial of intravenous acyclovir for the treatment of mucocutaneous herpes simplex virus infection in the immunocompromised host. Am J Med 73(suppl):229–235, 1982.

81. Drew WL, Mintz L: Rapid diagnosis of varicella-zoster virus infection by direct immunofluorescence. Am J Clin Pathol 73:699, 1980.

82. Balfour HH, Bean B, Laskin OL, et al: Acyclovir halts progression of herpes zoster in immunocompromised patients. N Engl J Med 308:1448, 1983.

83. Shepp DH, Dandliker PS, Meyers JD: Treatment of varicella-zoster virus infection in severely immunocompromised patients: A randomized comparison of acyclovir and vidarabine. N Engl J Med 314:208, 1986.

84. Garner JS, Simmons BP: Guideline for isolation precautions in hospitals. Infect Control 4:245, 1983.

85. Hoy J, Hsu K, Rolston KVI, et al: *Trichosporon beigelli* infection: A review. Rev Infect Dis 8:959, 1986.

86. Anaissie E, Kantarjian H, Ro J, et al: The emerging role of *Fusarium* infections in patients with cancer. Medicine 67:77, 1988.

87. Hay CRM, Messenger AG, Cotton DWK, et al: Atypical bulous pyoderma gangrenosum associated with myeloid malignancies. J Clin Pathol 40:387, 1987.

88. Kanel KT, Kroboth FJ, Swartz WM: Pyoderma gangrenosum with myelofibrosis. Am J Med 82:1031, 1987.

89. Cohen PR, Kurzrock R: Sweet's syndrome and malignancy. Am J Med 82:1220, 1987.

90. Browne M, Dinndorf P, Perek D, et al: Infectious complications of intraventricular reservoirs in cancer patients. Pediatr Infect Dis 6:182, 1987.

91. Lishner ML, Perrin RG, Feld R, et al: Complications associated with Ommaya reservoirs in patients with cancer. The Princess Margaret Hospital experience and a review of the literature. Arch Intern Med 150:173, 1990.

92. Louria DB, Henselec T, Armstrong D, et al: Listeriosis complicating malignant disease. Ann Intern Med 67:261, 1967.

93. Lavetter A, Leedom JM, Mathies AE, et al: Meningitis due to *Listeria monocytogenes*. N Engl J Med 285:598, 1971.

94. Gordon RC, Barrett FF, Yow MD: Ampicillin treatment of listeriosis. J Pediatr 77:1067, 1970.

95. Kaplan MS, Rosen PP, Armstrong D: Cryptococcosis in a cancer hospital: Clinical and pathological correlates in forty-six patients. Cancer 39:2265, 1977.

96. Dismukes WE, Cloud G, Gallis HA, et al: Treatment of cryptococcal meningitis with combination amphotericin B and flucytosine for four as compared with six weeks. N Engl J Med 317:334, 1987.

97. Galgiani JN. Fluconazole, a new antifungal agent (editorial). Ann Intern Med 113:177, 1990.

98. Jones PD, Marriot D, Speed BR: Efficacy of fluconazole in cryptococcal meningitis. Diagn Microbiol Infect Dis 12:235S, 1989.

99. Tozzi V, Bordi E, Galgani S, et al: Fluconazole treatment of cryptococosis in patients with acquired immunodeficiency syndrome. Am J Med 87:353, 1989.

100. Larsen RA, Leal MA, Chan LS: Fluconazole compared to amphotericin B plus flucytosine for the treatment of cryptococcal meningitis: A prospective study. Ann Intern Med 113:183, 1990.

101. Whitley RJ, Alford CA, Hirsch MS, et al: Vidarabine versus acyclovir therapy in herpes simplex encephalitis. N Engl J Med 314:144, 1986.

102. Albert RK, Condie F: Handwashing patterns in medical intensive care units. N Engl J Med 304:1465, 1981.

103. Remington JS, Schimpff SC: Please don't eat the salads. N Engl J Med 304:433, 1981.

104. Pizzo PA, Purvis D, Waters CW: Microbiological evaluation of food items for patients undergoing gastrointestinal decontamination and protected isolation. J Am Diet Assoc 81:272, 1982.

105. Pizza PA: Do results justify the expense of protected environments? In: Wiernik P (ed): Controversies in Oncology. New York, John Wiley & Sons, p 267, 1982.

106. Schimpff SC, Young VM, Greene WH, et al: Origin of infection in acute nonlymphocytic leukemia: Significance of hospital acquisition of potential pathogens. Ann Intern Med 77:707, 1972.

107. Pizzo PA: Antibiotic prophylaxis in the immunosuppressed patient with cancer. In: Remington JS, Swartz MN (eds): Current Clinical Topics in Infectious Diseases. 4th ed. New York, McGraw-Hill, p 153, 1983.

108. Kauffman CA, Leipman MJ, Bergman AG, et al: Trimethoprim-sulfamethoxazole prophylaxis in neutropenic patients: Reduction of infections and effect on bacterial and fungal flora. Am J Med 74:599, 1983.

109. Wade JC, DeJongh CA, Newman KA, et al: Selective antimicrobial modulation as prophylaxis against infection during granulocytopenia: Trimethoprim-sulfamethoxazole versus nalidixic acid. J Infect Dis 147:624, 1983.

110. Wilson JM, Guinery DG: Failure of oral trimethoprim-sulfamethoxazole prophylaxis in acute leukemia: Isolation of resistant plasmids from strains of enterobacteriaceae causing bacteremia. N Engl J Med 306:16, 1982.

111. Karp JE, Merz WG, Hendricksen C, et al: Oral norfloxacin for prevention of gram-negative bacterial infections in patients with acute leukemia and granulocytopenia. Ann Intern Med 106:1, 1987.

112. Dekker AW, Rozenberg-Arska M, Verhoef J: Infection prophylaxis in acute leukemia: A comparison of ciprofloxacin with trimethoprim-sulfamethoxazole and colistin. Ann Intern Med 106:7, 1987.

113. Condon RE. Selective bowel decontamination. Less enthusiasm and more study is in order. Arch Surg 125:1537, 1990.

114. Ledingham I, Alcock SR, Eastaway AT, et al: Triple regimen of selective decontamination of the digestive tract, systemic cefotaxime, and microbiological surveillance for prevention of acquired infection in intensive care. Lancet 1:785, 1988.

115. Thulig B, Hartenauer U, Diemer W, et al: Selective flora suppression for control of infection in surgical intensive care medicine. Anasth Intensivther Notfallmed 24:345, 1989.

116. Ulrich C, Harinck-de Weerd JE, Bakker NC, et al: Selective decontamination of the digestive tract with norfloxacin in the prevention of ICU-acquired infections: A prospective randomized study. Intensive Care Med 15:424, 1989.

117. Tetteroo GWM, Wagenvoort JHT, Castelein A, et al: Selective decontamination to reduce gram-negative colonisation and infections after oesophageal resection. Lancet 335:704, 1990.

118. Meunier F: Prevention of mycoses immunocompromised patients. Rev Infect Dis 9:408, 1987.
119. Yeo E, Alvarado T, Fainstein V, et al: Prophylaxis of oropharyngeal candidiasis with clotrimazole. J Clin Oncol 3:1668, 1985.
120. Bodey GP, Samonis G Rolston KVI: Prophylaxis of candidiasis in cancer patients. Semin Oncol 17(suppl 6):24, 1990.
121. Saral R, Bruns WH, Laskin OL, et al: Acyclovir prophylaxis of herpes simplex virus infections: A randomized, double-blind controlled trial in bone marrow transplant recipients. N Engl J Med 305:63, 1981.
122. Saral R, Ambinder RF, Burns WH, et al: Acyclovir prophylaxis against herpes simplex virus infection in patients with leukemia. Ann Intern Med 99:773, 1983.
123. Englund JA, Zimmerman ME, Swierkosz EM, et al: Herpes simplex virus resistant to acyclovir. A study in a tertiary care center. Ann Intern Med 112:416, 1990.
124. Hughes WT, Rivera GK, Schnell MJ, et al: Successful intermittent chemoprophylaxis for *Pneumocystis carinii* pneumonitis. N Engl J Med 316:1627, 1987.
125. Cooperative Group for the Study of Immunoglobulins in Chronic Lymphocytic Leukemia: Intravenous immunoglobulin for the prevention of infection in chronic lymphocytic leukemia. N Engl J Med 319:902, 1988.
126. Gershon AA, Steinberg S, Brunnell PA: Zoster immune globulin. A further assessment. N Engl J Med 290:243, 1975.
127. Centers for Disease Control: Varicella-zoster immune globulin for the prevention of chicken pox: Recommendations of the immunization practices advisory committee. Ann Intern Med 100:859, 1984.
128. Groopman JE: Status of colony-stimulating factors in cancer and AIDS. Semin Oncol 17:31, 1990.
129. Groopman JE, Molina J, Scadden DT: Hematopoietic growth factors. Biology and clinical applications. N Engl J Med 321:1449, 1989.
130. Gabrilove JL, Jakubowski A, Scher H, et al: Effect of granulocyte colony-stimulating factor on neutropenia and associated morbidity due to chemotherapy for transitional-cell carcinoma of the urothelium. N Engl J Med 318:1414, 1988.

CHAPTER 47

Infections in the Multitrauma Patient

Donna I. Whittle
Ellis S. Caplan

Trauma remains a leading cause of morbidity, mortality, and health care expenditure in the United States each year. In 1987, 5.5% of U.S. deaths were caused by traumatic injury. Accidents are the prime cause of death for persons 15 to 34 years old and are the fourth most common cause of death for the whole population.[1] An estimated 9 to 14% of motor vehicle accident victims require hospitalization.[2, 3] Firearm injuries also result in substantial yearly hospitalization; in 1984, estimated hospitalizations for firearm injuries totaled 62,075, with a minimal cost of $429 million.[4]

The majority of traumatically induced deaths occur in the first week after injury and are due to severe central nervous system (CNS) damage, hemorrhage, or respiratory failure.[5-7] Fatal infection is more common in patients who survive the first 5 days after injury and is the cause of 6 to 44% of all mortality after trauma.[6-8] Infection develops in 14 to 62% of trauma victims, with the higher rates affecting the more severely injured.[8, 9] The infections are predominantly nosocomial, the most common being urinary tract infections (17 to 47% of detected infections), pneumonia (15 to 18%), wound infections (12 to 16%), and bacteremias related to vascular catheter access (10 to 16%).[8-11] Nosocomial infection risk increases with the patient's length of hospitalization and with the use of a ventilator, tracheostomy, urinary catheter, or intravenous device.[12, 13] Colonization with pathogenic bacteria commonly precedes the development of nosocomial infection and is found in as many as 95% of the patients 10 days after admission.[12] Although the increased severity of injury among the patients susceptible to infection accounts for some portion of their prolonged care, there is no doubt that superimposed infection substantially augments the duration and cost of hospitalization.[14]

The victim of blunt or penetrating trauma is in jeopardy of acquiring an infection for many reasons. First, injuries break the skin and mucosal barriers, which allows entry of bacteria. Additional barrier disruption results from surgery, débridement, invasive monitoring, and skin breakdown from prolonged immobility. Second, artificial devices are foci that are not subject to the host's immune mechanisms and thus serve as portals of colonization and infection. Third, the traumatized patient's immunity may be impaired from both the primary injury and therapeutic interventions such as steroid administration. Fourth, despite hyperalimentation, the patient is often nutritionally deficient. Fifth, care in the intensive care unit results in exposure to virulent bacterial strains, which in spite of rigorous attempts to control infection are often spread from patient to patient during routine daily care. Finally, transfusion places the patient at risk for infections with cytomegalovirus, Epstein-Barr virus, and hepatitis virus, for example.

The diagnosis of infection in the multiply traumatized patient is complicated because many standard signs of infection are altered by traumatic injury. Although infection is unusual in the first 3 days after injury, fever, leukocytosis, and a hyperdynamic state are frequently present. In a prospective study of patients with postoperative temperatures greater than 38.5°C, documented infection was found in only 27%.[15] Furthermore, a white blood cell count of higher than 12,000/mm³ was found in more than 33% of patients without documented infection.[15] Conditions that may simulate infection include CNS injury with "central fever," atelectasis, pulmonary hemorrhage, pneumothorax, hematoma, tissue necrosis, deep venous thrombosis, hypovolemia, alcohol withdrawal, drug fever, and transfusion reactions. Diagnostic efforts by the physician are hampered by a physical examination that is limited by the patient's immobility and pain, difficulty in obtaining standard diagnostic interventions in a setting of critical illness, and the patient's inability to communicate. Scoring systems have yet to succeed in predicting infection accurately enough to be of diagnostic use.[16] The diagnosis of infection continues to rest on the clinician's careful assessment of physical findings, clinical course, and laboratory data, integrated with the judicious use of the many diagnostic modalities currently available.

IMMUNODEFICIENCY IN TRAUMA

A variety of normal immune defenses are significantly disrupted after trauma. Macrophage antigen presentation and monokine production are subnormal.[17-20] Elevated levels of prostaglandin E_2 and decreased levels of interferon-γ have been associated with these changes in macrophage function.[17, 20] T lymphocytes, which normally respond to these macrophage functions, have decreased responsiveness to mitogenic stimuli for up to 20 days after injury when studied in vitro.[21] Evidence also suggests that circulating serum factors and/or inadequate monokine production may disrupt T lymphocyte function.[17, 22–24] The production of immunoglobulins, especially immunoglobulin M, is diminished for weeks after trauma.[25–28] The addition of normal T cells to in vitro suspensions of B cells from the post-trauma patient results in normal antibody production and thus suggests that T lymphocyte dysfunction plays a role in the immunoglobulin insufficiency.[25] Other lymphocytes such as natural killer cells also function poorly in the trauma patient.[29]

Activation of the complement cascade, especially the alternative pathway, after trauma may deplete selected factors.[27, 30] This depletion probably partially contributes to the inadequate polymorphonuclear leukocyte chemotaxis and phagocytosis. Complement activation also results in inappropriate activation, deactivation, and auto-oxidation of neutrophils.[31] In addition, serum factors have been shown to alter neutrophil chemotaxis and adherence.[32] Skin test anergy has been correlated with these neutrophil derangements and portends a worse outcome.[32–34] Mortality rates as high as 75 to 100% have been seen in persistently anergic patients.[34]

Reticuloendothelial system function, as measured by clearance of circulating particulate markers, is curtailed after trauma.[35, 36] Post-trauma decreases in plasma levels of fibronectin, an α_2-glycoprotein with significant opsonic activity, have been correlated with the change in the function of the reticuloendothelial system.[36, 37]

The immunosuppression related to trauma is compounded by further deficits induced by hemorrhage, allogeneic transfusion, steroid administration, anesthesia, and surgery. Hemorrhage impairs macrophage proliferation, interleukin-2 production, and antigen presentation; suppresses the inflammatory response by polymorphonuclear leukocytes; decreases B cell numbers and immunoglobulin levels; and reduces the efficiency of phagocytosis by the reticuloendothelial system.[22, 38, 39] Blood product transfusion can disrupt lymphocyte blastogenesis, alter the T4/T8 ratio, and impair natural killer cell activity.[40] Post-transfusion increases in prostaglandin and thromboxane levels may also be immunosuppressive.[41]

Antigen presentation by macrophages and chemotaxis by lymphocytes and polymorphonuclear cells are decreased postoperatively.[42, 43] Complement activation occurs during surgery and may partially explain the altered chemotaxis. The phagocytic function of the reticuloendothelial system is also suboptimal postoperatively. The role of anesthesia in immune suppression is less defined. Animals with experimentally induced *Escherichia coli* peritonitis have decreased survival rates after undergoing general anesthesia without surgery.[40]

MICROBIOLOGY OF INFECTIONS IN THE TRAUMA PATIENT*

The microbial pathogens responsible for infection in the traumatized patient have changed in recent decades, presumably in response to the broader-spectrum antibiotics and altered modes of care used. Although gram-positive infections are still encountered frequently, gram-negative organisms have become increasingly prevalent as causes of significant infection.[8, 9] In addition, with the extensive use of broad-spectrum antibiotics, more drug-resistant pathogens such as fungi, *Staphylococcus aureus* (methicillin resistant), enterococcal species (aminoglycoside resistant), and gram-negative rods (multidrug resistant) are proving to be more common. Among the 2310 infections occurring in a 7-year period at the Shock Trauma Center of the Maryland Insti-

*Please refer to Chapter 138.

tute for Emergency Medical Services System, the most commonly isolated organisms were *S. aureus* (25%), *E. coli* (13%), *Pseudomonas aeruginosa* (10%), *Enterobacter* species (10%), and *Klebsiella* species (9%).[8] Others have found a marked prevalence of *Staphylococcus epidermidis*, *Serratia* species, enterococci, and *Candida* species among identified pathogens.[13] It is clear that the relative importance of a given pathogen varies among hospitals, geographic areas, and even types of patients. Familiarity with the local environment is of considerable value when one is forced to initiate empirical therapy in the potentially infected host. For this reason, some physicians, including the staff at the Maryland Institute for Emergency Medical Services System, advocate the use of routine surveillance cultures of critically ill trauma patients. It should be noted, however, that the impact of routine surveillance cultures on outcome and cost has yet to be objectively evaluated.

Sepsis, Bacteremia, and Multiple Organ System Failure

Although infection occurs commonly in trauma victims, only an unfortunate few have fulminant sepsis or multiple organ system failure (MOSF). Sepsis and MOSF are both recognized sequelae of infection, but either may also precede recognition of infection or occur in the absence of infection. The relationships between these entities are poorly defined, and studies have often failed to distinguish between the different conditions. For example, Goris and Draaisma defined sepsis as the "failure of two or more organ systems synchronous with or following the clinical onset of infection."[6] Not suprisingly, this study found death caused by organ failure to be closely associated with infection. For purposes of this discussion, the term *bacteremia* refers to the demonstrable presence of bacteria in the blood, *infection* is the demonstrable presence of bacteria from a site that also has signs of local inflammation or is normally sterile, and *sepsis* is defined as a physiologic state marked by increased metabolism, increased cardiac output, and decreased systemic vascular resistance. As noted by Marshall and colleagues, "while infection is a microbial phenomenon, sepsis is the consequence of the host immunologic response and can occur in the absence of ongoing infection."[44] The term *multiple organ system failure* is the failure, determined by objective measures, of two or more organ systems. To make this assessment, the pulmonary, hepatic, renal, gastrointestinal, CNS, cardiovascular, hematologic, metabolic, immunologic, and coagulation systems are evaluated.[44–46]

In one study, primary bacteremia occurred in 196 (8%) of 2310 infected trauma patients and carried a mortality rate of 13%.[8] In these same patients, secondary bacteremia was observed in 704 (33%) of the other 2114 infections. The overall mortality rate associated with any bacteremia was 21%, but the number of patients developing concomitant MOSF or sepsis was undocumented.[8] Vascular infections (22%), pneumonias (10%), empyema (9%), intra-abdominal infections (10%), and wound infections (8%) accounted for the majority of secondary bacteremias. The primary cause of bacteremia in this series was *S. aureus*, which was responsible for 35% of all bacteremias. Other significant causes were *Klebsiella* (12%), *Enterobacter* (10%), *P. aeruginosa* (8%), and *E. coli* (9%).[8] High rates of infection with *Pseudomonas* species, coagulase-negative staphylococci, *Candida* species, enterococci, and methicillin-resistant *S. aureus* have been reported in other series.[9, 44, 45]

Astute clinical acumen is often needed to distinguish sepsis and early MOSF from the events commensurate with traumatic injury. Temperature higher than 38.5°C is one of the most common signs of infection and sepsis; however, steroids, paralytic agents, and age may blunt the temperature response. Hypothermia may also be a harbinger of early infection. Additional markers include a hyperdynamic state; hypotension; altered mental status; lactic acidemia with decreased oxygen consumption; hypoxemia relative to the fraction of inspired oxygen; hypercapnia; an increasing white blood cell count with a shift to the left; mild thrombocytopenia; rising lactate dehydrogenase, bilirubin, or alkaline phosphatase level; or worsened glucose tolerance. Unfortunately, therapy with vasoactive amines, oxygen, sedatives, and total parenteral nutrition often confounds the interpretation of these signals of infection. Diligent evaluation for infection, including cultures, is appropriate when these signs are recognized. If no clear focus of infection is found and the patient is hemodynamically stable, careful observation without antibiotic therapy may be continued. When infection is identified, directed surgical and antibiotic therapy should be initiated immediately.

Empirical therapy with broad-spectrum antibiotics should be started in the hemodynamically unstable patient, even in the absence of demonstrable infection. The use of routine surveillance cultures can be helpful when empirical therapy is necessary. In this setting, a combination of an aminoglycoside, vancomycin, and ceftazidime is recommended. Alternatively, vancomycin with imipenem is also effective empirical coverage. The former regimen is preferable in the patient with substantial head injury because ceftazidime and other third-generation cephalosporins have been demonstrated to reach clinically effective levels in the CNS. In addition, patients with cerebral injury may be at increased risk of developing seizures when treated with imipenem. In patients with significant intra-abdominal injury, either metronidazole or clindamycin should be added to the first regimen to cover anaerobes, or the second regimen should be used. Regardless of antibiotic choice, the search for a focus of infection should continue and empirical antibiotic coverage should be re-evaluated daily. As further diagnostic information is obtained, the antibiotics should be tailored to treat all recognized infections while minimizing the risk of side effects or superinfection.

Allgower and colleagues documented septicemia, as defined earlier, in 25 of 300 (8.3%) polytraumatized patients.[9] These septic patients had a mortality rate of 65%, but in all fatal cases the infection was complicated by respiratory failure.[9] Using a more liberal definition of sepsis, Fry and colleagues found that 123 of 566 patients undergoing emergency surgery developed septicemia and that MOSF complicated septicemia in 34 instances.[46] The mortality rate among the septic patients was 28%, but in the subpopulation with MOSF it increased to 70%.[46] Retrospective reviews of mortality in trauma patients have found sepsis complicated by MOSF to account for 22 to 88% of late deaths.[6, 7] The mortality rate of MOSF rises as the number of organs involved increases: the rates were 30 and 100% for failure of one and four organs, respectively.[46] Underlying organ dysfunction, hypovolemic shock, massive transfusion, and infection are all risk factors for the development of MOSF.[45, 46] Poor nutrition, steroid use, and splenectomy have also been implicated.

Although sepsis or MOSF may be the first evidence of occult infection in a patient, not all septic episodes are due to infection.[44] The recognition of culture-negative sepsis has led to the concept of sepsis as a host response to either an infectious or an inflammatory stimulus, regardless of culture results. Mediators of the host response include prostaglandins, hormones, tumor necrosis factor, and many other substances.[47] As more is learned about the immunologic mechanisms acting in sepsis and MOSF, the therapeutic emphasis may shift from infection control and supportive care to the use of directed immunologic interventions.

In some cases of culture-negative sepsis, the gastrointestinal tract may be the hidden reservoir of pathogenic agents. Translocation of bacteria across the gastrointestinal tract, a postulated etiology of MOSF in trauma victims, has been demonstrated in animal models and in patients with intestinal obstruction.[48, 49] Alteration of the normal intestinal microflora, defective host immunity, and physical disruption of the gastrointestinal mucosa are all necessary for bacterial translocation to occur.[50] Altered intestinal microflora results from prolonged fasting, altered gastrointestinal motility, changes in pH of the gastrointestinal tract, and antibiotic usage. Mucosal disruption is caused by ischemia, immunologic injury, fasting, and possibly, inadequate availability of nutrients (such as glutamine) and hormones.[50]

Attempts to modify potential gut-originating septic states by using selective decontamination of the gastrointestinal tract have met with mixed results.[50] At present, few documented therapeutic interventions are available to limit bacterial translocation. Efforts should be made to limit antibiotic usage, begin enteral feedings as early as possible, maintain gastrointestinal motility, and bolster the host's immune function. Border and colleagues suggested that comprehensive surgery performed at the time of admission may limit the likelihood of MOSF developing from a gut origin, because it allows earlier extubation, mobilization, and enteral feeding of patients.[51] Further recommendations will depend on the results of ongoing research in this area.

Given the high mortality rates of patients with sepsis and MOSF in spite of aggressive supportive care, it is clear that more effective preventive and therapeutic strategies of care must be developed. It is hoped that these goals will be realized as more is learned about the pathogenesis of these conditions.

CENTRAL NERVOUS SYSTEM INFECTIONS

CNS infections are uncommon among trauma victims. In one series, only 4% of 2310 infections occurring among multiply traumatized patients were due to CNS infection.[8] Diagnoses in these patients were meningitis (67%), ventriculitis (17%), or brain abscess (15%).[8] Patients having dural disruption (with or without cerebrospinal fluid [CSF] leak), either by penetrating head trauma or by surgical intervention, are at greatest risk of developing infection of the CNS.

Intracranial pressure monitors may be placed in the extradural area (the hollow bolt or the Camino fiberoptic system), in the subdural or subarachnoid spaces (the subarachnoid screw or the subdural catheter), or into the cerebral ventricle (the intraventricular catheter). Although infection rates for epidural devices are not documented, clinical experience suggests that the rates are low. Infection rates per placed device are otherwise reported to be 1.0 to 14.9% for subdural catheters, 0 to 7.5% for subarachnoid screws, and 3.6 to 26.8% for intraventricular catheters.[52] The lack of standardization of prophylactic antibiotic usage, populations of patients, definitions of infection, and surgical technique may explain the variability in rates.

Some investigators report increased infection risk associated with intracranial monitors used in patients with intracerebral hemorrhage, open head trauma, or intraventricular hemorrhage.[53-55] Age is also variably implicated as a risk factor.[52, 55] Although the effects of prophylactic antibiotics and the insertion environment (intensive care unit versus operating room) have been evaluated repeatedly, no studies have found that either factor affects subsequent infection rates.[52-54] Almost all series have shown infection risk to be increased if the catheter is irrigated (even with an antibiotic-containing solution) or is maintained in place for more than 3 to 5 days.[52-55] The risk is also increased in proportion to the number of in-line stopcocks and the frequency of opening them.[52] On the basis of these observations, many clinicians now recommend using rigorous aseptic technique during placement of monitors, limiting opening of the system, avoiding irrigation of the catheters, and scheduling changes of the catheter every 3 to 5 days.

The diagnosis of monitor-related ventriculitis or meningitis is suggested by fever, peripheral leukocytosis, CSF pleocytosis, and bacteriologic growth in CSF cultures obtained via lumbar puncture or shunt. However, fever and peripheral leukocytosis are unreliable indices of CNS infection.[53] In one study, CSF pleocytosis was significantly correlated with infection, but 4 of 18 patients with CNS infection had no CSF pleocytosis and 23% of patients with negative cultures had CSF pleocytosis.[53] The diagnosis depends on microbiologic demonstration of bacterial growth in CSF, thus necessitating the judicious use of CSF sampling. In the absence of associated symptoms of infection, a positive culture may be due to contamination but warrants further evaluation. Another CSF culture and cell count should be obtained before beginning any antibiotic therapy. Contamination of the initial cultures is suggested if additional cultures are negative, but if the same pathogen is persistently present, the existence of a monitor-related infection must be assumed. In some series, gram-positive and gram-negative organisms have been equally prevalent.[8, 54]

Infection is treated by removing the catheter when present and administering intravenous antibiotics based on available in vitro sensitivities of the pathogen. If continued monitoring is necessary, a new device should be placed at a different site. The integrity of the blood-brain barrier may prevent penetration of adequate levels of antibiotics into the CSF after intravenous dosing, particularly in settings in which there is minimal meningeal inflammation. Intraventricular antibiotic therapy is occasionally necessary but is complicated by the need for continued ventricular access, the risk of secondary infection, and the potential CNS toxicity of antimicrobial agents. For these reasons, intraventricular antibiotics should be used only if infection fails to clear after removal of the monitor and treatment with systemic antibiotics capable of attaining adequate levels in the CSF. There is little pharmacokinetic information about intraventricular antibiotic administration, but recommendations are available.[56] The preparations for intraventricular usage must not contain preservatives in any component used.

Osteomyelitis and local wound infection occur in up to 5.4 and 17.6% of patients with intracranial pressure monitors, respectively.[54] The pathogenic flora in these infections consists predominantly of gram-positive organisms. When these infections are recognized, CSF cultures should be obtained, the monitor should be removed, and systemic antibiotics should be initiated.

Basilar skull fractures constituted 15 and 24% of all skull fractures in two retrospective series with more than 1000 cases.[57, 58] Of the patients with basilar skull fractures in these series, 21 to 40% had CSF otorrhea or rhinorrhea. Meningitis develops in 2 to 25% of patients with basilar skull fractures.[57] In the majority of cases, meningitis develops within 2 weeks of trauma.[59] However, post-traumatic meningitis related to CSF fistulas may occur many years after injury. The diagnosis of meningitis in a patient with head trauma should trigger a renewed search for a basilar fracture and CSF leak if such an injury has not been previously recognized. After head trauma, *Streptococcus pneumoniae* is the most common meningeal pathogen, although resistant gram-negative rods are also found, particularly if the patient has received antibiotic therapy.[59, 60] In one early study, no infections occurred among patients treated with prophylactic antibiotics for CSF leaks, but an 18% infection rate was seen among the untreated group.[57] Since then, multiple retrospective and prospective series have failed to show a significant difference in infection between prophylactically treated and untreated patients.[57–60] Furthermore, Ignelzi and VanderArk found that the natural oropharyngeal flora was rapidly altered from gram-positive to multiply resistant gram-negative flora under antibiotic pressure.[60] The use of prophylactic antibiotics cannot be recommended in view of the currently available data and the risk of potentially devastating CNS superinfection. Systemic antibiotics that penetrate the blood-brain barrier are usually adequate to treat meningitis. Until diagnostic culture or CSF latex agglutination results are available, coverage should begin with broad-spectrum antibiotics that are known to achieve reasonable levels in the CSF.

Brain abscess in trauma patients occurs predominantly after penetrating head injuries with retained fragments, after postoperative scalp wound infections, and in patients with undrained sphenoid, ethmoid, or frontal sinusitis. Among patients who had war-related injuries, the risk of brain abscess with a penetrating bullet was 3%.[61] Most abscesses develop within 1 month of injury and can be diagnosed with computed tomography (CT) or magnetic resonance imaging. Removal of foreign debris and drainage of the abscess are usually indicated, along with administration of systemic antibiotics. Microbiologic cultures should ideally be obtained before antibiotic use because mixed flora and exotic organisms have been identified in abscesses associated with penetrating injury. The mortality rate may be as high as 54%, and morbidity may be even higher.[61]

SINUSITIS

Sinusitis can be an occult source of cryptic fever in the trauma patient. At the Shock Trauma Center of the Maryland Institute for Emergency Medical Services System, 168 of 2310 infections occurring during 7 years were caused by nosocomial sinusitis.[8] Humphrey and colleagues surveyed 208 head-injured patients admitted to an intensive care unit and diagnosed nosocomial sinusitis in 24.[62] Prospective surveys of critically ill medical patients have documented an even higher incidence of sinusitis after nasotracheal intubation for more than 8 days.[63] Risk factors for nosocomial sinusitis include nasotracheal intubation, nasal packing, nasogastric tubes, steroid usage, facial fractures, immunosuppression, antibiotic usage, and sedation.[64, 65]

Clinical symptoms of sinusitis in the trauma patient may include purulent sinus drainage, but more often the presentation includes fever and leukocytosis without an identifiable cause. Caplan and Hoyt reported purulent nasal discharge in only 9 of 32 patients with proven sinusitis, but all had leukocytosis (white blood cell count > 10,500/mm^3) and fever (temperature > 38.3°C).[64] A tentative diagnosis depends on radiographic study, a daunting task in the immobilized trauma patient. In cooperative outpatients, the accuracy of plain films with five views is 88% but falls to 24% when only four views are available.[65] In the sedated trauma patient, portable x-ray studies are often attempted and five views are rarely obtained; therefore, the diagnostic yield of plain films is often quite low. The presence of air-fluid levels or opacification in a sinus is strongly suggestive of infection. A CT scan of the paranasal sinuses using bone window settings at thin (2- to 4-mm) sections is more sensitive and can better reveal sphenoid sinusitis.[66] All sinuses may be affected, but unilateral maxillary sinusitis is the most common finding.[65] Sinus hematoma, mucosal thickening, and serous filling of the sinuses may give false-positive radiologic results. For this reason and to obtain cultures, the sinuses should be aspirated. Aspirated material should be examined with Gram's stain and cultured on media for both aerobic and anaerobic organisms. The presence of both neutrophils and bacteria in this material is considered to be diagnostic for sinusitis.

Although most community-acquired sinusitis is generally due to pneumococci or *Haemophilus influenzae*, nosocomial sinusitis is largely caused by gram-negative organisms and anaerobes.[62-64] Polymicrobial infections are common. These nosocomial pathogens are also frequently isolated from respiratory secretions. The co-occurrence of sinusitis and pulmonary infection has been noted.[62, 63] Bacteremia presumed secondary to sinusitis has been reported by Humphrey and colleagues[62] in 2 of 24 patients and by Guerin and coworkers[63] in 3 of 52 patients. In the trauma patient, the simplest "therapy" for sinusitis is to prevent it by consistently avoiding the use of nasogastric and nasotracheal tubes. Otherwise, treatment consists of administration of decongestants and of systemic antibiotics based on culture results and removal of all tubes or packing obstructing the nasal ostia. Further irrigation procedures or surgery for drainage may be needed if the patient does not respond to medical management or if sphenoid sinusitis is present.

RESPIRATORY TRACT AND INTRATHORACIC INFECTIONS

Respiratory infection with either pneumonia or empyema is a significant risk for trauma patients. Pulmonary infection has been reported to be the cause of up to 31% of late deaths after motor vehicle accidents.[67] The clinical diagnosis of pneumonia was made by Langer and associates in 27.8% of 180 trauma victims hospitalized in intensive care for more than 48 hours.[68] The mortality rate was 36% among patients with pneumonia and 23.9% among those without it. Excess hospitalization necessitated by nosocomial pneumonia ranged from 5 to 13 days.[69] Nosocomial pneumonia is the origin of 14 to 36% of episodes of bacteremia for trauma patients.[8, 9]

Pneumonia developing in the trauma patient in the first few days of hospitalization often represents a community-acquired pneumonia caused by aspiration of oropharyngeal secretions. Pathogens most commonly encountered in this setting include oral anaerobes, pneumococcus, and *H. influenzae*. Conversely, nosocomial pneumonia is a hospital-acquired infection that is neither present nor incubating at the time of admission. Gram-negative pathogens are the cause of 50 to 60% of nosocomial pneumonias and are associated with a higher mortality than the 30 to 40% of infections with gram-positive organisms.[8, 69] Nosocomial pneumonia pathogens include *S. aureus*; *Pseudomonas, Klebsiella, Enterobacter, Serratia*, and *Acinetobacter* species; and *E. coli*.[8, 9, 70, 71] Polymicrobial infections are frequently encountered. Fungal pathogens and atypical organisms such as *Legionella* are reported rarely.[70]

In 1972, Johanson and associates noted the strong correlation between gram-negative colonization of the respiratory tract and development of nosocomial pneumonia in critically ill patients.[72] In that series, factors associated with gram-negative colonization included underlying respiratory disease, coma, hypotension, tracheal intubation, acidosis, azotemia, and either leukocytosis or leukopenia.[72] Identified risk factors for gram-negative colonization include (1) contamination of respiratory equipment, particularly ventilator tubing; (2) suppression of normal flora by broad-spectrum antibiotic use; and (3) alterations of the mucosal epithelium during serious illness.[73] The stomach has been shown to be a reservoir of gram-negative organisms, which are readily aspirated even by the intubated patient. Overgrowth of the stomach with gram-negative rods occurs both after surgery

and when the acidity of the stomach is reduced.[74, 75] Finally, the incidence of nosocomial pneumonia clearly rises with increasing duration of intubation.[68]

The diagnosis of pneumonia is suggested by the presence of a temperature above 38°C, leukocytosis, increased pulmonary secretions, worsening hypoxemia and/or hypercapnia, the radiographic finding of a new pulmonary infiltrate that does not clear after chest physiotherapy, and results of a Gram stain of sputum consistent with infection (more than 25 leukocytes and less than 10 squamous epithelial cells per low-power field with pathogenic organisms present). However, these clinical indices may be misleading, particularly in patients with diffuse lung injury. Andrews and coworkers looked at the utility of clinical parameters for the diagnosis of pneumonia in 24 patients with acute diffuse lung injury.[76] At postmortem histologic examination, 20% of patients thought to have pneumonia had only diffuse lung disease, and 36% of patients thought to have only diffuse lung disease actually had pneumonia. In the nonpneumonia group, 80% had fever and leukocytosis, 70% had pulmonary pathogens, and 30% had asymmetry of the chest film.[76] Pulmonary contusion, pulmonary hemorrhage, atelectasis, pulmonary embolus, pulmonary edema, aspiration, infection at other sites, and adult respiratory distress syndrome may all mimic the symptoms of pneumonia to varying degrees.

Colonization of the respiratory tract without concomitant pulmonary infection also confounds attempts to diagnose pneumonia in ventilated patients.[77] Routine surveillance cultures and Gram's stains of the sputum may provide useful information by demonstrating an increasing bacterial burden and inflammatory response preceding the onset of clinical symptoms of pneumonia.[8] Collection of respiratory specimens through the fiberoptic bronchoscope by using either the protected specimen brush or bronchoalveolar lavage has been proposed as a strategy for diagnosing pneumonia. Quantitative culture techniques are then used for these specimens. Bacterial species with more than 10^3 colony-forming units per milliliter in protected brush specimens are regarded as pathogenic. Although these techniques have been useful in the diagnosis of opportunistic infections in the neutropenic patient or the patient with acquired immunodeficiency syndrome, there is only limited experience with them in the diagnosis of bacterial infection in the traumatized patient or in patients receiving antibiotics.[78, 79] Furthermore, there is no evidence that survival is improved by using these diagnostic modalities. The risk of worsened hypoxemia, a reported complication of bronchoalveolar lavage, must be weighed in assessing the risk/benefit ratio of this technology for a patient. Until more experience accumulates, the use of these invasive procedures should be evaluated on a case-by-case basis. Until there are new discoveries, the diagnosis of pneumonia must still rest largely on the admittedly imperfect clinical evaluation.

The ideal management of nosocomial pneumonia consists of prevention by paying meticulous attention to infection control procedures, encouraging extubation as soon as possible, limiting antibiotic usage, and considering the need for altered gastric acidity. Attempts to prevent infection by using nebulized antibiotics have decreased the overall infection rate but have selected for a more resistant population of pathogens.[78] Gut decontamination by using nonabsorbable antibiotics along with oropharyngeal application of antibiotics has been shown to decrease the incidence of infection in a few preliminary studies, but overall survival in these studies has not been reported.[78] When preventive efforts fail, treatment of pneumonia should consist of antibiotic therapy directed against pathogens identified by Gram's stain and culture. In vitro sensitivities should guide therapy, which should be given for 10 to 14 days. In general, therapy of gram-negative infections necessitates combination antibiotic therapy, preferably with a β-lactam and an aminoglycoside.

Empyema is an ominous complication for the trauma patient. Stillwell and Caplan reported it as the cause of 7% of diagnosed infections in patients with predominantly blunt trauma.[8] The mortality rate for patients with empyema was 18% compared with 7% for patients with other infections.[8] Notably, Villalba and colleagues identified no episodes of empyema after blunt chest trauma in 900 patients.[80] The reported risk of developing empyema after penetrating chest trauma has varied with the era of the study, the type of injury, and the use of prophylactic antibiotics.[81] Several investigators have documented rates of empyema formation as low as 0.5 to 1.3% after penetrating chest trauma.[80, 82] However, Grover and colleagues reported a rate of 16.2% after penetrating trauma.[81] Predisposing conditions for empyema development include large hemothorax, lower respiratory tract infection, chest tube placement, diaphragmatic perforation, lung contusion, obstruction of the chest tube, residual pneumothorax, associated extrapleural chest wall hematoma, and severe head or chest injury.[8, 80]

The most frequent isolates from empyemas are *S. aureus*, *Pseudomonas*, anaerobes, *Enterobacter*, *E. coli*, and *Klebsiella*.[8] CT of the thorax in 37 trauma victims is 80% sensitive and 65% specific for the diagnosis of empyema.[83] Bedside ultrasonography may be useful for the patient who cannot be transported.[8] If empyema is detected while fluid is free flowing, chest tube drainage and antibiotic therapy may effectively clear the infection. If loculated fluid or signs of ongoing infection persist, more aggressive surgical intervention may be necessary.[80] Attempts to prevent empyema by using prophylactic antibiotics have met with mixed results. In a prospective double-blind study of clindamycin versus placebo, Grover and colleagues noted a trend toward decreased rates of respiratory and pleural space infection, but statistical significance was not achieved.[81] However, Villalba and coworkers found no advantage to the use of prophylactic antibiotics in 3000 chest trauma patients.[80] Furthermore, in 734 patients with penetrating chest trauma reported anecdotally by Bryant and coworkers, no difference in infection rates was seen with prophylactic antibiotic use.[77]

On occasion, lung abscess or secondary infection of a posttraumatic pulmonary cavity may develop after lung trauma. CT is 87% sensitive and 96% specific for this diagnosis.[83] Bronchoscopy can be used to obtain cultures to guide antibiotic therapy. A minimum of 4 weeks of systemic antibiotics is usually needed for lung abscess therapy.

INTRA-ABDOMINAL INFECTIONS

Abscess formation, peritonitis, and acalculous cholecystitis are some of the serious infectious complications that occur in the abdomen after trauma. Among civilians with penetrating injuries of the abdomen, the rate of intra-abdominal abscess formation is 2.4 to 11%.[84–86] Blunt abdominal trauma resulted in intra-abdominal abscesses in 4.6% of 325 patients reported by Goins and associates.[87] Investigators who have focused on patients with liver injury have reported intra-abdominal abscess formation rates of 1.8 to 7% for penetrating trauma and 2.9 to 16% for blunt trauma.[88, 89] Gunshot wounds are associated with a higher likelihood of abscess formation than are stab wounds.[89] Other risk factors for abscess formation are voluminous blood transfusion, increased age, injury to multiple organs, splenectomy, packing of the liver, and colon injury necessitating colostomy formation.[85, 87, 89]

The relative importance of open drainage with respect to abscess formation remains disputed. In one evaluation, an 11% incidence of abscess formation was noted in patients with a Penrose drain, compared with no abscesses in 82 patients without drains.[89] Noyes and coworkers reported a 1.2% incidence of abscess formation with either no drainage or closed suction drainage but a 14% incidence when open drainage was used.[90] However, Trunkey and colleagues reported a series in which abscess formation occurred in only 2.1% of the patients in spite of the fact that almost all of them were treated with open drainage.[88] The precise importance of open drainage to subsequent abscess formation cannot be determined in the absence of multivariate analysis of these populations.

In essentially all reported series, the predominant locations of abscesses are in the upper quadrants of the abdomen bilaterally.[86, 87] Multiple abscesses are found in 8 to 46% of patients.[87, 91] Polymicrobial infection is common, with enteric gram-negative rods predominating. *Klebsiella pneumoniae*, *E. coli*, and *Enterobacter* are the most frequently reported gram-negative organisms, but *Serratia*, *Pseudomonas*, *Acinetobacter*, *Proteus*, and *Citrobacter* have been recovered from these abscesses. Anaerobes are assumed to play a role in abscess formation, but most investigators have not assessed anaerobic cultures. Eleven to 42% of isolated pathogens are nonenterococcal gram-positive organisms, especially coagulase-negative staphylococci.[87, 89] Enterococci are frequently isolated in mixed infections.[87, 89] Bacteremia associated with an abscess occurs in 20 to 37% of the patients.[87, 90, 91]

The diagnosis of an intra-abdominal abscess is suggested on clinical grounds by fever, leukocytosis, abdominal distention, peritoneal signs, purulent drainage from any drains, wound infection or dehiscence, or other signs of sepsis. Symptoms may occur as early as 2 days postoperatively.[87] Leukocytosis was noted in at least 80% of patients with abscess in a series reported by Fry and associates, but only 36% had localized abdominal tenderness.[91] Pleural effusions and lower lobe atelectasis are also frequently reported findings and should raise the suspicion of an abscess in a febrile patient.[91]

Noninvasive evaluation with CT or ultrasonography can be useful. CT sensitivity for detection of an intra-abdominal abscess is 80 to 90% with high (more than 90%) specificity.[92] Ultrasonography complements the sensitivity of CT by optimizing the view of the perihepatic region.[87, 89] With radiographic guidance, percutaneous drainage of some intra-abdominal abscesses can be achieved. Conditions for optimal results with percutaneous drainage include (1) a single abscess cavity, (2) no loculations in the abscess, (3) direct access to the lesion from a percutaneous entry position, (4) no fistula formation or other evidence for ongoing contamination, and (5) no evidence of fungal infection. Success rates as high as 96% have been reported in treating such clearly defined lesions; with increasing experience, good responses are also being achieved by using percutaneous drainage for more complex abscesses.[92] If successful percutaneous drainage is not feasible, operative drainage is imperative. At the time of any drainage procedure, separate cultures for aerobic and anaerobic organisms should be obtained in appropriate transport media. Broad-spectrum antibiotics with coverage for anaerobes and enteric gram-negative rods should be administered systemically until in vitro sensitivities are available to guide therapy. Protracted courses of therapy and repeated drainage may be necessary because infection recurs in up to 41.6% of cases.[87, 89]

Mortality rates among patients with intra-abdominal abscesses have ranged from 7 to 30%.[84, 86, 87, 89] Most patients succumb to MOSF. Fatal outcome is correlated with organ failure, lesser sac or subhepatic abscess, positive blood cultures, recurrent or persistent abscess, multiple abscesses, age greater than 50, and multiple organisms per abscess.[87, 91]

Many studies have demonstrated a decrease in the intra-abdominal infection rate when prophylactic antibiotics are administered urgently to the patient with penetrating abdominal trauma.[93, 94] Effective prophylactic antibiotic regimens target anaerobes and Enterobacteriaceae. Recovery of enterococci in large numbers from abdominal infections has led some surgeons to favor additional enterococcal coverage.[85, 94] Others have advocated increased staphylococcal coverage because of a rising incidence of both *S. aureus* and coagulase-negative staphylococci in abdominal infections.[8] Optimal duration of therapy is not known. Most recommendations are for 2 to 5 days of therapy if peritoneal soiling is present during the initial laparotomy.[8, 86, 94] If no bowel perforation or fecal spillage is found, antibiotics should be discontinued.

Diffuse peritonitis results from intra-abdominal dissemination of colonic or biliary contents, either at the time of injury or as a result of uncorrected lesions. Of 14 patients with diffuse peritonitis found on re-exploration, all had a persistent defect including anastomotic leak (six patients), ischemic bowel (four), acute acalculous cholecystitis (two), or bile leakage (two).[95] Mortality with diffuse peritonitis varies widely, with estimates of 30 to 80%.[96] An absence of distinguishing clinical symptoms in the postoperative patient often results in a delay in diagnosing this disease. This delay, combined with technically limited therapeutic options, results in unacceptable mortality. A high index of suspicion and a low threshold for re-exploration of the abdomen are needed to make the diagnosis. Antibiotic therapy combined with surgical débridement of devitalized tissue, repair of injured structures, and copious irrigation are the crucial interventions for successful recovery. Repeated intra-abdominal therapy is often needed to control infection.

Acute acalculous cholecystitis is recognized as an uncommon but serious complication in trauma victims. The patients are postulated to be at increased risk because of tissue ischemia resulting from hypovolemic shock, increased bile acid load caused by massive transfusion, and relative biliary stasis induced by opiates, positive end-expiratory pressure ventilation, and total parenteral nutrition.[97–100] The onset of symptoms may be as early as 3 days after injury or as late as 6 weeks.[97, 98] Fever (88 to 100% of affected patients) and leukocytosis (79 to 94%) are the most common findings. Nausea, vomiting, right upper quadrant pain, diffuse abdominal pain, or liver function abnormalities may be found in as few as half of the patients.[99, 100] Radionuclide scanning has been reported to have a sensitivity of 78 to 100% for acalculous cholecystitis, but its specificity can be as low as 38%.[98, 100] Ultrasound and CT criteria for the diagnosis include (1) gallbladder wall thickness of 4 mm or more, (2) pericholecystic fluid or subserosal edema without ascites, (3) intramural gas, and (4) a sloughed mucosal membrane. Sensitivity approximates 70 to 90% with either of these modalities, and specificities are 96 and 100%, respectively.[98, 100]

Once the diagnosis is made or strongly suspected, emergent drainage of the gallbladder is indicated. Cholecystectomy is the favored procedure because almost half of the patients have necrosis, gangrene, and possibly perforation of the gallbladder.[100] Percutaneous drainage has been used successfully in some patients for whom surgery was not feasible, but experience with this technique is still limited.[99, 101] Cultures are often negative at the time of drainage; when pathogens are isolated, the most common are *E. coli*, *Klebsiella*, *Pseudomonas*, *Enterobacter*, *Streptococcus*, and *Clostridium*.[99] Among early studies of acalculous cholecystitis, the mortality rate reached as high as 75%. With earlier detection and aggressive therapy, mortality has decreased to the range of 7 to 30%.[98, 100]

Splenectomy poses additional risk for the development of serious infection in the trauma patient. Subphrenic abscess after splenectomy has been reported in 2.3 to 14% of patients.[8, 102] The frequency of severe late infection after splenectomy ranges from 2.1 to 2.5%.[103–105] However, these series have had both incomplete and short-term follow-up of patients. For these reasons, some clinicians now advocate splenorrhaphy when splenic injury and associated intra-abdominal injuries are of limited magnitude.[102] When splenectomy is necessary, immunization with a polyvalent pneumococcal vaccine should be administered immediately to decrease the risk of subsequent overwhelming infection.[106] The trauma patient's immunologic response to the vaccine is similar to the normal host's response.[107]

CATHETER-ASSOCIATED INFECTIONS

Both bacteremia and local infection are complications of the use of vascular access devices. In one series, 196 (22%) of 900 episodes of bacteremia were related to infection of a vascular access device.[8] Among seriously ill patients, catheter-related sepsis complicates 2.4 to 5% of central venous catheterizations, and local infection may occur in as many as 11%.[108–110] Likewise, an incidence of bacteremia of up to 4% has been associated with use of arterial catheters; local infection may occur in as many as 18% of these devices.[111] The most commonly cited risk factor for development of infection is duration of cannulation exceeding 3 days.[110, 111] The exception may be the hyperalimentation line, which is placed under sterile technique and is manipulated only once a day by a trained team.[110] Additional risk factors include insertion by cutdown, number of catheter manipulations, use of multilumen catheters, use of transparent occlusive dressings, and violations of aseptic technique.[111, 112]

This diagnosis should be suspected in any febrile patient with an indwelling vascular catheter. The presence of purulence at any catheter site is strongly correlated with infection; the catheter should be removed and the indwelling end sent for quantitative culture. For patients with fever only, blood cultures should be obtained and all lines should be changed and cultured. Ideally, intravenous lines should be reinserted at a new site in these patients. When this is not technically feasible, the catheter should be changed aseptically over a wire and the tip cultured. If the catheter tip cultures are subsequently positive, the new line must be changed to a new site, because reinfection has been documented to occur after insertion of the catheter over a wire.[112] Quantitative cultures may be performed by using the rolling method described by Band and Maki or by plating serial dilutions of broth used to flush the catheter.[111, 112] Catheter infection is correlated with more than 15 colonies per plate by the rolling method or more than 10^3 colony-forming units when serial dilutions of broth are plated.[111, 112] Catheter-associated bacteremia is diagnosed when both blood and catheter cultures grow the same organism. *S. aureus* and coagulase-negative staphylococci are the most common isolates, but enterococci, *Klebsiella*, *Enterobacter*, and *Candida* are also frequent.[8, 109, 111]

Removal of all catheters is central to the treatment of these infections. Secondary seeding of a catheter with subsequent perpetuation of infection can follow bacteremia.[112] Appropriate antibiotic therapy should be administered for a minimum of 10 to 14 days. Although endocarditis is uncommon after line infection, a longer duration of therapy should be considered in the patient with underlying cardiac valvular disease or an intravascular prosthetic device. If clinical improvement is slow after line removal and antibiotic therapy, additional blood cultures should be obtained. Positive blood cultures after removal of all lines should prompt an urgent search for a persistent intravascular focus of infection. Septic thrombophlebitis generally necessitates surgical intervention to débride residual infection. Fortunately, these complications are unusual, and mortality from line-associated sepsis is infrequent.

WOUND INFECTIONS

Among 10,308 traumatized patients, wound infections accounted for 12% of the 2310 observed infections.[8] Bacteremia occurred in 80 (30%) of these 267 patients, but mortality associated with wound infection was only 1.5%. In a group of 300 polytrauma victims, Allgower and associates noted a 4% incidence of infection of surgical wounds but a 45% incidence in traumatic wounds.[9] This is consistent with a survey of 62,936 general surgical wounds in which the infection rates were 1.5, 7.7, 15.2, and 40% for clean, clean-contaminated, contaminated, and dirty wounds, respectively.[113] All traumatic wounds should be considered to be dirty.

Risk factors for traumatic wound infection include the amount of bacterial contamination, shock, blood loss, the number of organs injured, and time in the operating room.[8] Cruse and Foord identified preoperative shaving, length of preoperative hospital stay, duration of surgery, and hematoma formation at the operative site as risk factors for the development of infection in operative wounds.[113] Although mortality related to these infected wounds is low, they cause substantial morbidity and have been shown to increase the duration of hospital stay by as much as 10.1 days.[113]

Wound infection is suggested by erythema, warmth, and increased drainage at the wound site. Fever and leukocytosis are often present. Gram-positive and gram-negative organisms both occur with significant frequency in these wounds. Gram-positive organisms are more commonly the offending pathogen when infection occurs early after admission.[9] Wounds subsequently become contaminated with nosocomial gram-negative bacteria, and these cause many of the late wound infections. Frequently reported pathogens include *S. aureus, Enterobacter, Pseudomonas, E. coli, Acinetobacter, Klebsiella,* and *Proteus.*[8, 9] Anaerobic cultures have not been routinely reported in the literature, but in one series such cultures were positive for 11% of wounds.[8] *Aeromonas hydrophila* and *Vibrio* species can cause severe wound infections and are associated with exposure to fresh and salt water, respectively.[114] Therapeutic intervention for all wound infections consists of opening and draining the wound, débriding necrotic tissue, culturing for aerobes and sometimes anaerobes, and broad-spectrum antibiotic coverage until culture results are available.

Clostridial myonecrosis (gas gangrene) is an uncommon but devastating infection among trauma victims. Caplan and Kluge reported 32.3% mortality among 34 patients with gas gangrene.[115] Elevated levels of urea nitrogen, creatinine, and serum bilirubin, as well as neutropenia and thrombocytopenia, were associated with a poor prognosis. Amputation was necessary in 17 of the 22 cases involving an extremity. *Clostridium perfringens* was recovered from the wounds in 79% and the blood in 15% of these 34 patients.[115] Mixed infections, including aerobic pathogens, occurred in 29 of the 34 patients. Clinical symptoms of gas gangrene include intense local wound pain, confusion, tachycardia, and tachypnea.[116] At the wound, there is mild erythema, woody induration, and minimal discoloration. Crepitus is often but not always present. Gram's stains of the wound exudate have visible gram-positive bacilli without spores but rare neutrophils. Immediate therapy is indicated when this diagnosis is suspected. Therapy consists of vigorous débridement of necrotic tissue; amputation when necessary; use of broad-spectrum antibiotics, including penicillin; and adequate volume support. Hyperbaric oxygen therapy may provide some benefit but should not delay the fundamental therapy just noted.[117]

Necrotizing fasciitis is a rapidly advancing infection causing necrosis of the fascial plane with or without concomitant cellulitis. The site of origin may be a trivial lesion. Pain may be the earliest indication of infection. Dermal edema and minimal erythema follow. The infection progresses over hours to leave the skin purple-gray and without sensation because of disruption of nerves and blood vessels.[116] A thin, gray exudate may be seen in the wounds. Eventually the epidermis may blister. Gas formation is rare.[116] Diagnosis depends largely on the finding of necrotic fascial planes at the time of surgery. Group A streptococci infection or synergistic infections with aerobes and anaerobes are common in these wounds.[118] Both *Aeromonas* and *Vibrio* species can also cause necrotizing fasciitis.[114, 116] Fluid rescusitation, extensive surgical débridement, and broad-spectrum antibiotics are therapeutic. Optimal antibiotic regimens combine penicillin, clindamycin or metronidazole, and an aminoglycoside. If there is a history of water exposure, coverage for *Aeromonas* or *Vibrio* species, as appropriate, should be added during any empirical therapy. A worse outcome is found with underlying diabetes, truncal or perineal involvement, a delay in diagnosis, or inadequate débridement at initial surgery.[115] The mortality rate among 272 reported patients was 38.5%.[115]

Wounds associated with open fractures are particularly vulnerable to infection; the severity of injury is the single greatest risk factor.[119–121] According to a modified classification of open fracture, infection rates have been reported at 1.4 to 4.2% for class I, 3.6 to 8% for class II, and 22 to 41% for class III fractures.[119–122] Further subdivision of class III fractures into those with adequate soft tissue coverage of bone (class IIIA) versus those with extensive soft tissue and neurovascular injury (class IIIB and IIIC) revealed respective infection rates of 4.4 and 48.6%.[121] Controversy persists regarding the infection risk associated with internal fixation of the fracture, primary wound closure, blood transfusion, and delayed antibiotic administration.[119, 120] In 1974, Patzakis and colleagues reduced the overall rate of open fracture infection from 13.9 to 2.3% by administering prophylactic cephalothin.[123] At that time *S. aureus* was the predominant pathogen, but more recent studies have shown an increasing incidence of gram-negative infections, particularly among patients with extensive soft tissue injury.[119, 120] For this reason, a few physicians now advocate using third-generation cephalosporins or the combination of cephalothin and an aminoglycoside for prophylaxis.[121] The appropriate duration of prophylaxis is disputed; some studies have shown no deleterious results from limiting therapy to 24 hours.[119, 120]

Appropriate tetanus prophylaxis must be administered to all trauma victims with more than minor open wounds. For the patient who has completed a primary immunization series, recommendations are based on the timing of the last booster dose of the vaccine as follows: (1) if less than 1 year since the last booster, no further therapy is needed; (2) if less than 10 years, administer 0.5 mL of tetanus toxoid; (3) if more than 10 years, give 0.5 mL of tetanus toxoid and 250 U of tetanus immune globulin (human). In the absence of a history of primary immunization, 250 to 500 U of tetanus immune globulin (human) should be given and primary immunization should be initiated.[124]

URINARY TRACT INFECTIONS

Urinary tract infections are frequent infectious complications in the trauma patient. Allgower and associates reported a 32% incidence of such infections among 300 trauma patients.[9] Bacteremia associated with urinary tract infection occurs in 4.2 to 17% of patients, but mortality caused by infection of the urinary tract is uncommon.[9, 125] Antecedent antibiotic therapy and urethral catheterization are risks for development of urinary tract infections.[125] Clinical symptoms include fever, dysuria, frequency, urgency, and cloudy urine. If there is an indwelling catheter, cultures of the urine may often be positive because of colonization. In the absence of neutropenia, concomitant pyuria is advocated as the criterion for distinguishing infection from colonization of the urinary tract.[8, 9] Screening surveillance cultures and urinalysis at regular intervals can be helpful for recognizing early infection in the critically ill population.[8] Gram-negative pathogens are more common, and *E. coli* is the leading culprit in most series, followed by *Klebsiella* and *Enterobacter*. Other pathogens include *Pseudomonas, Proteus, Serratia,* enterococci, and *Candida*. The last two organisms tend to be more prevalent among patients with prior antibiotic exposure.[125] Asymptomatic bacteriuria, or colonization, is not an indication for antibiotic treatment.

Therapeutic guidelines for urinary tract infections include the administration of renally excreted antibiotics based on in vitro sensitivities and removal of any indwelling catheter as soon as adequate bladder emptying can be achieved spontaneously or with limited intermittent straight catheterization. The optimal duration of antibiotic therapy is unknown. Some clinicians have suggested that as few as 3 days is effective if the catheter is removed.[125] A conservative recommendation is treatment for 7 days after catheter removal. In the absence of catheter removal, treatment failure is highly likely and intermittent suppressive therapy may be all that is achievable.

ACQUIRED IMMUNODEFICIENCY SYNDROME IN THE TRAUMA PATIENT

By current estimates, between 1 and 1.5 million people in the United States are infected with the human immunodeficiency virus type 1 (HIV-1), and more than 100,000 have been diagnosed with the acquired immunodeficiency syndrome.[126] The presence of HIV infection among trauma victims reflects the geographic variability in disease prevalence.[127] Series of trauma patients from Illinois, Wisconsin, and San Antonio, Texas have had less than 1% prevalence of HIV infection.[128–130] However, other studies in Baltimore and Miami have reported seroprevalence rates between 1.67 and 7.8%.[131–133] Risk of HIV infection among trauma patients has been shown to be increased for black patients, victims between 25 and 34 years of age, and patients with penetrating trauma.[131, 133] The possibility that a trauma patient may suffer from HIV-induced defects of cell-mediated immunity must be considered. Such defects would render the patient susceptible to opportunistic infections that are not readily discovered by using standard diagnostic evaluations of the infected trauma patient. Clinicians must therefore maintain an appropriate level of suspicion for the possibility of HIV infection and be ready to initiate relevant diagnostic studies when warranted.

The Centers for Disease Control now recommends the routine use of universal precautions for the care of all patients. Universal precautions consist of meticulous care when handling sharp objects and the use of barrier precautions to prevent skin and mucous membrane contact with blood and body fluids. In the setting of trauma, barrier precautions include protective eyewear, masks, gowns and/or aprons, and gloves. Others have encouraged the use of ankle and leg coverings also.[132, 134] Only 16% compliance with strict universal precautions was found during the initial emergency room management of trauma victims in Miami.[132]

Ready availability of protective barrier items and verbal reminders to use universal precautions improved compliance to 62% in the same setting. At present, less than 1% of exposed health care workers have seroconverted when tested for HIV, but duration of follow-up has been limited.[134, 135] Vigilant efforts by health care workers are needed to limit transmission of the disease during the events associated with care of the trauma patient.

CONCLUSION

Patients with multiple trauma are at risk for a variety of infections as a result of underlying immunosuppression and overt injuries. Iatrogenic interventions further increase the risk of infection. The optimal "therapy" is to prevent infection by carefully practicing infection control (especially hand washing), limiting the use of empirical antibiotics, and weighing the infection risk against the perceived benefit for each planned intervention. Ongoing surveillance for infection must be vigorous and sustained because signs of infection may be subtle or obscured by other processes. Early therapeutic intervention and diligent prevention offer the best outcomes in the management of infection in the trauma patient.

References

1. National Center for Health Statistics: Advance report of final mortality statistics, 1987. Monthly Vital Stat Rep 38(suppl):1, 1989.
2. Mortality from leading types of accidents. Stat Bull Metrop Insur Co 59:10, 1978.
3. Trunkey DD: Overview of trauma. Surg Clin North Am 62:3, 1982.
4. Martin MJ, Hunt TK, Hulley SB: The cost of hospitalization for firearm injuries. JAMA 260:3048, 1988.
5. Baker CC, Oppenheimer L, Stephens B, et al: Epidemiology of trauma deaths. Am J Surg 140:144, 1980.
6. Goris RJA, Draaisma J: Causes of death after blunt trauma. J Trauma 22:141, 1982.
7. Shackford SR, Mackersie RC, Davis JW, et al: Epidemiology and pathology of traumatic deaths occurring at a level I trauma center in a regionalized system: The importance of secondary brain injury. J Trauma 29:1392, 1989.
8. Stillwell M, Caplan ES: The septic multiple trauma patient. Infect Dis Clin North Am 3:155, 1989.
9. Allgower M, Durig M, Wolff G: Infection and trauma. Surg Clin North America 60:133, 1980.
10. Schimpff SC, Miller RM, Polakavetz S, et al: Infection in the severely traumatized patient. Ann Surg 179:352, 1974.
11. Caplan ES, Hoyt N, Cowley RA: Changing patterns of nosocomial infections in severely traumatized patients. Am Surg 45:204, 1979.
12. Northey D, Adess ML, Hartsuck JM, et al: Microbial surveillance in a surgical intensive care unit. Surg Gynecol Obstet 139:321, 1974.
13. Wenzel RP, Osterman CA, Hunting KJ: Hospital-acquired infections. Am J Epidemiol 104:645, 1976.
14. McLean APH, Boulanger MA: Epidemiology of infection in the surgical intensive care unit. In: Meakins JL (ed): Surgical Infection in Critical Care Medicine. Edinburgh, Churchill-Livingstone, p 46, 1985.
15. Freischlag J, Busuttil RW: The value of post-operative fever evaluation. Surgery 94:358, 1983.
16. Dellinger EP: Use of scoring systems to assess patients with surgical sepsis. Surg Clin North Am 68:123, 1988.
17. Faist E, Mewes A, Strasser T, et al: Alteration of monocyte function following major injury. Arch Surg 123:287, 1988.
18. Stephan RN, Saizawa M, Conrad PJ, et al: Depressed antigen presentation function and membrane interleukin-1 activity of peritoneal macrophages after laparotomy. Surgery 102:147, 1987.
19. Rodrick ML, Wood JJ, O'Mahony JB, et al: Mechanisms of immunosuppression associated with severe nonthermal traumatic injuries in man: Production of interleukin 1 and 2. J Clin Immunol 6:310, 1986.
20. Livingstone DH, Appel SH, Wellhausen SR, et al: Depressed interferon gamma production and monocyte HLA-DR expression after severe injury. Arch Surg 123:1309, 1988.
21. O'Mahoney JB, Palder SB, Wood JJ, et al: Depression of cellular immunity after multiple trauma in the absence of sepsis. J Trauma 24:869, 1984.
22. Abraham E: Host defense abnormalities after hemorrhage, trauma, and burns. Crit Care Med 17:934, 1989.
23. Constantian MB, Menzoian JO, Nimberg RB, et al: Association of

circulating immunosuppressive polypeptide with operative and accidental trauma. Ann Surg 185:73, 1977.

24. Abraham E, Regan RF: The effects of trauma and hemorrhage on interleukin 2 production. Arch Surg 120:1341, 1985.
25. McRitchie DI, Girotti MJ, Rotstein OD, et al: Impaired antibody production in blunt trauma. Arch Surg 125:91, 1990.
26. Ertel W, Faist E, Nestle C, et al: Dynamics of immunoglobulin synthesis after major trauma. Arch Surg 124:1437, 1989.
27. Bjornson AB, Altemeier WA, Bjornson HS: Host defense against opportunistic microorganisms following trauma. Ann Surg 188:102, 1978.
28. Faist E, Ertel W, Baker CC, et al: Terminal B-cell maturation and immunoglobulin (Ig) synthesis in vitro in patients with major injury. J Trauma 29:2, 1989.
29. Morrison G, Cunningham-Rundles S, Stahl WM, et al: Augmentation of NK cell activity by a circulating peptide isolated from the plasma of trauma patients. Ann Surg 203:21, 1986.
30. Kapur MM, Jain P, Gidh M: Estimation of serum complement and its role in management of trauma. World J Surg 12:211, 1988.
31. Maderazo EG, Woronick CL, Albano SD, et al: Inappropriate activation, deactivation, and probable autooxidative damage as a mechanism of neutrophil locomotory defect in trauma. J Infect Dis 154:471, 1986.
32. Christou NV, McLean APH, Meakins JL, et al: Host defense in blunt trauma: Interrelationships of kinetics of anergy and depressed neutrophil function, nutritional status, and sepsis. J Trauma 20:833, 1980.
33. Meakins JL, McLean APH, Kelley R, et al: Delayed hypersensitivity and neutrophil chemotaxis: Effect of trauma. J Trauma 18:240, 1978.
34. Pietsch JB, Meakins JL: Predicting infection in surgical patients. Surg Clin North Am 59:185, 1979.
35. Schildt B, Gertz I, Wide L: Differentiated reticuloendothelial system (RES) function in some critical surgical conditions. Acta Chir Scand 140:611, 1974.
36. Altura BM, Hershey SG: RES phagocytic function in trauma and adaptation to experimental shock. Am J Physiol 215:1414, 1968.
37. Saba TM, Jaffe E: Plasma fibronectin (opsonic glycoprotein): Its synthesis by vascular endothelial cells and role in cardiopulmonary integrity after trauma as related to reticuloendothelial cell function. Am J Med 68:577, 1980.
38. Stephan RN, Ayala A, Harkema JM, et al: Mechanism of immunosuppression following hemorrhage: Defective antigen presentation by macrophages. J Surg Res 46:553, 1989.
39. Ayala A, Perrin MM, Wagner MA, et al: Enhanced susceptibility to sepsis after simple hemorrhage. Arch Surg 125:70, 1990.
40. Waymack JP, Warden GD, Alexander JW, et al: Effect of blood transfusion and anesthesia on resistance to bacterial peritonitis. J Surg Res 42:528, 1987.
41. Shelby J, Hisatake G: Effect of ibuprofen and interleukin 2 on transfusion-induced suppression of cell mediated immunity. Arch Surg 123:1397, 1988.
42. Christou NV, Meakins JL: Delayed hypersensitivity in surgical patients: A mechanism for anergy. Surgery 67:78, 1979.
43. Stephan RN, Saizawa M, Conrad PJ, et al: Depressed antigen presentation function and membrane interleukin-1 activity of peritoneal macrophages after laparotomy. Surgery 102:147, 1987.
44. Marshall JC, Christou NV, Horn R, et al: The microbiology of multiple organ failure. Arch Surg 123:309, 1988.
45. Manship L, McMillin RD, Brown JJ: The influence of sepsis and multi system and organ failure on mortality in the surgical intensive care unit. Am Surg 50:94, 1984.
46. Fry DE, Pearlstein L, Fulton RL, et al: Multiple system organ failure: The role of uncontrolled infection. Arch Surg 115:136, 1980.
47. Fry DE: Multiple system organ failure. Surg Clin North Am 68:107, 1988.
48. Deitch EA: Simple intestinal obstruction causes bacterial translocation in man. Arch Surg 124:699, 1989.
49. Baker JW, Deitch EA, Berg RD, et al: Hemorrhagic shock induces bacterial translocation from the gut. J Trauma 28:896, 1988.
50. Deitch EA: The role of intestinal barrier failure and bacterial translocation in the development of systemic infection and multiple organ failure. Arch Surg 125:403, 1990.
51. Border JR, Hassett J, LaDuca J, et al: The gut origin septic states in blunt multiple trauma (ISS=40) in the ICU. Ann Surg 206:427, 1987.
52. Hickman KM, Mayer BL, Muwaswes M: Intracranial pressure monitoring: Review of risk factors associated with infection. Heart Lung 19:84, 1990.
53. Mayhall CG, Archer NH, Archer Lamb V, et al: Ventriculostomy-related infections: A prospective epidemiologic study. N Engl J Med 310:553, 1984.
54. Aucoin PJ, Kotilainen HR, Gantz NM, et al: Intracranial pressure monitors: Epidemiologic study of risk factors and infections. Am J Med 80:369, 1986.
55. Clark WC, Muhlbauer MS, Lowrey R, et al: Complications of intracranial pressure monitoring in trauma patients. Neurosurgery 25:20, 1989.
56. Fan-Havard P, Nahata NC: Treatment and prevention of infections of cerebrospinal fluid shunts. Clin Pharm 6:866, 1987.
57. Frazee RC, Mucha P Jr, Farnell MB, et al: Meningitis after basilar skull fracture: Does antibiotic prophylaxis help? Postgrad Med 83:267, 1988.
58. Dagi TF, Meyer FB, Poletti CA: The incidence and prevention of meningitis after basilar skull fracture. Am J Emerg Med 3:295, 1983.
59. Applebaum E: Meningitis following trauma to the head and face. JAMA 173:1818, 1960.
60. Ignelzi RJ, VanderArk GD: Analysis of the treatment of basilar skull fractures with and without antibiotics. J Neurosurg 43:721, 1975.
61. Rish BL, Caveness WF, Dillon JD, et al: Analysis of brain abscess after penetrating craniocerebral injuries in Vietnam. Neurosurgery 9:535, 1981.
62. Humphrey MA, Simpson GT, Grindlinger GA: Clinical characteristics of nosocomial sinusitis. Ann Otol Rhinol Laryngol 96:687, 1987.
63. Guerin JM, Meyer P, Barbotin-Larrieu F, et al: Nosocomial bacteremia and sinusitis in nasotracheally intubated patients in intensive care (letter). Rev Infect Dis 10:1226, 1988.
64. Caplan E, Hoyt N: Nosocomial sinusitis. JAMA 247:639, 1982.
65. Miner JD, Elliott CL, Johnson CW, et al: Nosocomial sinusitis. Indiana Med 81:684, 1988.
66. Carter BL, Bankoff MS, Fisk JD: Computed tomographic detection of sinusitis responsible for intracranial and extracranial infections. Radiology 147:739, 1983.
67. Fife D, Kraus J: Infection as a contributory cause of death in patients hospitalized for motor vehicle trauma. Am J Surg 155:278, 1988.
68. Langer M, Mosconi P, Cigada M, et al: Long term respiratory support and risk of pneumonia in critically ill patients. Am Rev Respir Dis 140:302, 1989.
69. Leu HS, Kaiser DL, Mori M, et al: Hospital-acquired pneumonia: Attributable mortality and morbidity. Am J Epidemiol 129:1258, 1989.
70. Machiedo GW, Suval WD: Detection of sepsis in the postoperative patient. Surg Clin North Am 68:215, 1988.
71. Jimenez P, Torres A, Rodriguez-Roison R, et al: Incidence and etiology of pneumonia acquired during mechanical ventilation. Crit Care Med 17:882, 1989.
72. Johanson WG Jr, Pierce AK, Sanford JP, et al: Nosocomial respiratory infections with gram-negative bacilli. The significance of colonization of the respiratory tract. Ann Intern Med 77:701, 1972.
73. Johanson WG, Higuchi JH, Chaudhuri TR, et al: Bacterial adherence to epithelial cells in bacillary colonization of the respiratory tract. Am Rev Respir Dis 121:55, 1980.
74. Atherton ST, White DJ: Stomach as source of bacteria colonising respiratory tract during artificial ventilation. Lancet 2:968, 1978.
75. Craven DE, Kunches LM, Kilinsky V, et al: Risk factors for pneumonia and fatality in patients receiving continuous mechanical ventilation. Am Rev Respir Dis 133:792, 1986.
76. Andrews CP, Coalson JJ, Smith JD, et al: Diagnosis of nonocomial bacterial pneumonia in acute, diffuse lung injury. Chest 80:254, 1981.
77. Bryant LR, Trinkle JK, Mobin-Uddin K, et al: Bacterial colonization profile with tracheal intubation and mechanical ventilation. Arch Surg 104:647, 1972.
78. Pingleton SK: Complications of acute respiratory failure. Am Rev Respir Dis 137:1460, 1988.
79. Guerra LF, Baughman RP: Use of bronchoalveolar lavage to diagnose bacterial pneumonia in mechanically ventilated patients. Crit Care Med 18:69, 1990.
80. Villalba M, Lucas CE, Ledgerwood AM, et al: The etiology of post-traumatic empyema and the role of decortication. J Trauma 19:414, 1979.
81. Grover FL, Richardson JD, Fewel JG, et al: Prophylactic antibiotics in the treatment of penetrating chest wounds. J Thorac Cardiovasc Surg 74:528, 1977.
82. Oparah SS, Mandal AK: Penetrating stab wounds of the chest: Experience with 200 consecutive cases. J Trauma 16:868, 1976.
83. Mirvis SE, Rodriguez A, Whitley NO, et al: CT evaluation of thoracic infections after major trauma. AJR 144:1183, 1985.
84. Dawidson I, Miller E, Litwin MS: Gunshot wounds of the abdomen: A review of 277 cases. Arch Surg 11:862, 1976.
85. Nichols RL, Smith JW, Klein DB, et al: Risk of infection after penetrating abdominal trauma. N Engl J Med 311:1065, 1984.
86. Gibson DM, Felicians DV, Mattox KL, et al: Intraabdominal abscess after penetrating abdominal trauma. Am J Surg 142:699, 1981.
87. Goins WA, Rodriguez A, Joshi M, et al: Intra-abdominal abscess after blunt abdominal trauma. Ann Surg 212:60, 1990.
88. Trunkey DD, Shires GT, McClelland R: Management of liver trauma in 811 consecutive patients. Ann Surg 179:722, 1974.
89. Bender JS, Geller ER, Wilson RF: Intra-abdominal sepsis following liver trauma. J Trauma 29:1140, 1989.
90. Noyes LD, Doyle DJ, McSwain NE: Septic complications associated with the use of peritoneal drains in liver trauma. J Trauma 28:337, 1988.
91. Fry DE, Garrison RN, Heitsch RC, et al: Determinants of death in patients with intraabdominal abscess. Surgery 88:517, 1980.
92. Pruett TL, Simmons RL: Status of percutaneous catheter drainage of abscesses. Surg Clin North Am 68:89, 1988.
93. Fullen WD, Hunt J, Altemeier WA: Prophylactic antibiotics in penetrating wounds of the abdomen. J Trauma 12:282, 1972.
94. Sacks T: Prophylactic antibiotics in traumatic wounds. J Hosp Infect 11(suppl A):251, 1988.
95. Driver T, Kelly GL, Eiseman B: Reoperation after abdominal trauma. Am J Surg 135:747, 1978.
96. Walsh GL, Chiasson P, Hedderich G, et al: The open abdomen: The Marlex mesh and zipper technique: A method of managing intraperitoneal infection. Surg Clin North Am 68:25, 1988.

97. DuPriest RW, Khaneja SC, Cowley RA: Acute cholecystitis complicating trauma. Ann Surg 189:84, 1979.

98. Frazee RC, Nagorney DM, Mucha P Jr.: Acute acalculous cholecystitis. Mayo Clin Proc 64:163, 1989.

99. Long TN, Heimbach DM, Carrico CJ: Acalculous cholecystitis in critically ill patients. Am J Surg 136:31, 1978.

100. Cornwell EE, Rodriguez A, Mirvis SE: Acute acalculus cholecystitis in critically injured patients. Ann Surg 210:52, 1989.

101. Berger H, Pratschke E, Arbogast H: Percutaneous cholecystostomy in acute acalculous cholecystitis. Hepatogastroenterology 36:346, 1989.

102. Feliciano DV, Spjut-Patrinely V, Burch JM, et al: Splenorraphy: The alternative. Ann Surg 211:569, 1990.

103. Schwartz PE, Sterioff S, Mucha P, et al: Postsplenestomy sepsis and mortality in adults. JAMA 248:2279, 1982.

104. Malangoni MA, Dillon LD, Klamer TW, et al: Factors influencing the risk of early and late serious infection in adults after splenectomy for trauma. Surgery 96:775, 1984.

105. Sekikawa T, Shatney CH: Septic sequelae after splenectomy for trauma in adults. Am J Surg 145:667, 1983.

106. Ammann AJ, Addiego J, Wara DW, et al: Polyvalent pneumococcal-polysaccharide immunization of patients with sickle-cell anemia and patients with splenectomy. N Engl J Med 297:897, 1977.

107. Caplan ES, Boltansky H, Snyder MJ, et al: Response of traumatized splenectomized patients to immediate vaccination with polyvalent pneumococcal vaccine. J Trauma 23:801, 1983.

108. Van Berge Henegouwen DP, Leguit P, Boissevain ACH, et al: The risk of central venous catheter-related sepsis in patients with surgical infection. Neth J Surg 34–5:201, 1982.

109. Snydman DR, Murray SA, Kornfield SJ, et al: Total parenteral nutrition–related infections. Am J Med 73:695, 1982.

110. Pinilla JC, Ross DF, Martin T, et al: Study of the incidence of intravascular catheter infection and associated septicemia in critically ill patients. Crit Care Med 11:21, 1983.

111. Band JD, Maki DG: Infections caused by arterial catheters used for hemodynamic monitoring. Am J Med 67:735, 1979.

112. Hampton AA, Sherertz RJ: Vascular-access infections in hospitalized patients. Surg Clin North Am 68:57, 1988.

113. Cruse PJE, Foord R: The epidemiology of wound infection. A 10-year prospective study of 62,939 surgical wounds. Surg Clin North Am 60:27, 1980.

114. Semel JD, Trenholme G: *Aeromonas hydrophila* water-associated traumatic wound infections: A review. J Trauma 30:324, 1990.

115. Caplan ES, Kluge RM: Gas gangrene: A review of 34 cases. Arch Intern Med 136:788, 1976.

116. Ahrenholz DH: Necrotizing soft-tissue infections. Surg Clin North Am 68:199, 1988.

117. Cohn GH: Hyperbaric oxygen therapy: Promoting healing in difficult cases. Postgrad Med 79:89, 1986.

118. Giuliano A, Lewis F, Hadley K, et al: Bacteriology of necrotizing fasciitis. Am J Surg 134:52, 1977.

119. Dellinger EP, Miller SD, Wertz MJ, et al: Risk of infection after open fracture of the arm or leg. Arch Surg 123:1320, 1988.

120. Patzakis MJ, Wilkins J: Factors influencing infection rate in open fracture wounds. Clin Orthop 243:36, 1989.

121. Gustilo RB, Mendoza RM, Williams DN: Problems in the management of type III (severe) open fractures: A new classification of type III open fractures. J Trauma 24:742, 1984.

122. Chapman MW, Mahoney M: The role of early internal fixation in the management of open fractures. Clin Orthop 138:120, 1979.

123. Patzakis MJ, Harvey JP, Ivler D: The role of antibiotics in the management of open fractures. J Bone Joint Surg 56A:532, 1974.

124. Yurt RW, Shires GT: Prophylaxis and treatment of infection in trauma. In: Mandell GL, Douglas RG, Bennett JE (eds): Principles and Practice of Infectious Diseases. New York, Churchill Livingstone, p 827, 1990.

125. Asher EF, Oliver BG, Fry DE: Urinary tract infections in the surgical patient. Am Surg 54:466, 1988.

126. Centers for Disease Control: HIV prevalence, projected AIDS case estimates: Workshop, October 31–November 1, 1989. JAMA 263:1477, 1990.

127. St. Louis ME, Rauch KJ, Petersen LR, et al: Seroprevalence rates of human immunodeficiency virus infection at sentinel hospitals in the United States. N Engl J Med 323:213, 1990.

128. Orr M, Hoos A, Riester DE, et al: HIV-1 infection in patients with penetrating trauma in San Antonio, Texas (letter). JAMA 262:1629, 1989.

129. Aprahamian C, Olson D, Gottschall JL, et al: Potential risk of human immunodeficiency virus in critially injured patients (abstract). J Trauma 281:1081, 1988.

130. Zeman MG, Mayhue FE: Human immunodeficiency virus (HIV) seropositivity in a midwestern community trauma population (abstract). Ann Emerg Med 17:409, 1988.

131. Soderstrom CA, Furth PA, Glasser D, et al: HIV infection rates in a trauma center treating predominantly rural blunt trauma victims. J Trauma 29:1526, 1989.

132. Hammond JS, Eckes JM, Gomez GA, et al: HIV, trauma, and infection control: Universal precautions are universally ignored. J Trauma 30:555, 1990.

133. Kelen GD, Fritz S, Qaquish B, et al: Substantial increase in human immunodeficiency virus (HIV-1) infection in critically ill emergency patients: 1986 and 1987 compared. Ann Emerg Med 18:378, 1989.

134. Centers for Disease Control: Recommendations for prevention of HIV transmission in health-care settings. MMWR 36:3S, 1987.

135. Gerberding JL, Bryant-LeBlanc CE, Nelson K, et al: Risk of transmitting human immunodeficiency virus, cytomegalovirus, and hepatitis B virus to health care workers exposed to patients with AIDS and AIDS-related conditions. J Infect Dis 156:1, 1987.

CHAPTER 48

Infections in Intravenous Drug Abusers

Donald P. Levine

In any modern intensive care unit one is likely to care for patients who are intravenous drug abusers (IVDAs). The drug user is susceptible to all the serious infectious diseases that affect the general population. Despite appearing debilitated, drug users tend to handle many serious infections as well as, or in some cases better than, others with similar diseases. This may be due in part to the relative youth of the IVDA. Nevertheless, a variety of infections, some with serious consequences, are seen quite frequently in drug users, and these infections are discussed in this chapter. Drug users constitute one of the major groups at risk of acquiring human immunodeficiency virus (HIV) infections and are thus likely to have acquired immunodeficiency syndrome (AIDS); infections unique to that syndrome are discussed elsewhere in this book (see Chapter 50). This chapter discusses the infectious diseases that are typically a direct result of the injection of illicit substances and that are most likely to necessitate admission of an IVDA to the intensive care unit.

CENTRAL NERVOUS SYSTEM

Drug users may present with serious abnormalities of the central nervous system (CNS) that may or may not be infectious. The noninfectious complications include a variety of disorders that are directly related to the injection of illicit substances. Among these are coma, postanoxic encephalopathy, delirium or acute confusional states, seizures, and cerebral edema or compromise of the neurovascular system (e.g., cerebral infarction or hemorrhage). The etiology of these lesions may not be readily apparent, and a thorough work-up may be necessary to exclude infectious causes. In contrast, when an infection is the primary problem, the patient usually presents with focal findings and frequently has a fever. In addition, the presence of focal findings raises the possibility of a mass lesion in need of immediate intervention. It is helpful to construct a differential diagnosis including both infectious and noninfectious etiologies and then to further differentiate between a purely local process and a neurologic complication of a distant primary infection (Table 48–1).

TABLE 48–1

NEUROLOGIC MANIFESTATIONS OF INFECTION IN INTRAVENOUS DRUG ABUSERS

Intracranial Lesions Manifesting with Focal Findings
Noninfectious
    Subdural hematoma
    Intracranial hemorrhage
    Ischemic infarct
Infectious
    Meningitis
    Brain abscess
        Primary
        Secondary to infection elsewhere
    Subdural empyema
    Encephalitis or cerebritis
        Viral
        Bacterial (secondary to infectious endocarditis)
    AIDS related
        Toxoplasma encephalitis
        Cryptococcal meningoencephalitis
        Tuberculoma
        Progressive multifocal leukoencephalopathy

Extracranial Lesions Manifesting with Focal Findings
Spinal epidural abscess
Spinal disk infection
Local abscess

Nonfocal Involvement of Nervous System
Tetanus
Wound botulism

Brain Abscess and Subdural Empyema

Localized CNS infection in IVDAs includes brain abscess and subdural empyema. Brain abscess is the most common and is usually caused by pyogenic bacteria (mainly *Staphylococcus aureus*), although fungi, including *Aspergillus* species,[1, 2] *Nocardia* species,[1] and *Mucor*,[1, 3–7] have also been seen. Another potential complication of drug abuse is loss of consciousness leading to the development of a lung abscess and a secondary brain abscess. Infectious endocarditis may also cause brain abscesses secondary to infected cerebral emboli, particularly in patients with mitral or aortic valve infection.[8–11] Infection may also result if the addict unintentionally introduces pathogens directly into the arterial system during an attempted jugular vein injection. Alternatively, infected arterial emboli that originate in or travel through the pulmonary circulation may also arise, particularly with *S. aureus* infections.[12] Subdural empyema may be the result of direct extension from a local infectious process or may arise in a fashion similar to that of brain abscess in these patients.[2, 13]

Meningitis is an occasional complication of drug abuse but is usually secondary to infectious endocarditis.[9]

AIDS in addicts may be associated with dramatic CNS findings. Most notable are the multifocal abscesses attributable to *Toxoplasma gondii* and the lesions caused by *Cryptococcus* and *Mycobacterium tuberculosis*, which are more often solitary findings (see Chapter 50).

Infectious Endocarditis

In addicts, CNS manifestations of endocarditis in addition to brain abscess are numerous. In my medical center, neurologic abnormalities were present in almost 25% of addicts with endocarditis.[10] In another study that focused on patients with *S. aureus* infection (which in addicts is more likely to occur on the tricuspid valve and thereby reduce the likelihood of neurologic involvement), CNS complications were less frequent in drug users than in others.[8] Not only is endocarditis the most common cause of CNS disease in drug users, but it is responsible for the most serious complications, including meningitis, brain abscess, and hemorrhage from ruptured mycotic aneurysms.[10] However, encephalitis and cerebritis must also be considered in a drug user with focal CNS findings.

Drug addicts are as susceptible as the general population to the usual viral causes of encephalitis. More often, however, the addict presenting with signs of diffuse cerebral infection has cerebritis attributable to the high-grade, sustained bacteremia that is associated with endocarditis.[10]

Spinal Epidural Abscess

Spinal epidural abscess is usually accompanied by focal findings depending on the area of the spinal cord involved.[14, 15] These abscesses may result from the direct extension of infection from an infected intervertebral disk or infected vertebral body or from bacteremia with subsequent seeding of the epidural space. Most often such lesions are reported in the thoracic or lumbar region and affect the posterior spinal cord. In the upper thoracic and cervical regions, the anterior cord may be involved. The usual presentation is relatively sudden onset of limb weakness or paralysis associated with spinal ache, fever, and point tenderness (often severe) over the involved area of the spine. Neurologic symptoms may be dramatic when the patient is first seen, but frequently the disease process progresses because of delayed recognition of the infection. In such cases, the lack of immediate drainage and antibiotic therapy may lead to permanent neurologic impairment.

Approach to the Patient with Focal Neurologic Findings

The patient's history may provide useful information about whether local trauma to the affected region or attempted injection into the neck veins has occurred. It is also worthwhile to determine if self-medication with antibiotics has been attempted because their use may hinder the ability to recover organisms from the blood or other infected sites.[16] Physical examination should be conducted with scrupulous attention to locate the lesion site (i.e., intracerebral, spinal cord, or peripheral). Examination should include evaluation of the conjunctiva and ocular fundus for hemorrhages and Roth's spots indicative of endocarditis.

If an intracranial lesion is suspected, computed tomography (CT) of the head is mandatory, initially without contrast to exclude an intracranial hemorrhage and then followed by contrast enhancement to detect abscesses or other mass lesions. If no space-occupying lesion is found and there is no evidence of elevated intracranial pressure, a lumbar puncture is indicated to assess the possibility of meningitis. Caution is necessary in the interpretation of the cerebrospinal fluid findings because a high percentage of patients with endocarditis have pleocytosis or even positive cerebrospinal fluid cultures caused by endocarditis alone.[10, 17]

If a mass lesion is detected by CT, if the patient is known to have HIV infection, and especially if there are multiple ring-enhancing lesions, toxoplasmosis is highly likely and empirical therapy for that disease may be started. If there is a brain abscess considered to be secondary to endocarditis, further CNS work-up may not be necessary because blood cultures are likely to identify the responsible pathogen. Otherwise, brain biopsy or aspiration of the lesion is imperative to determine the microbiologic etiology and to ensure effective therapy.

For lesions of the spinal cord, especially if there is evidence of cord compression, CT or magnetic resonance imaging of the spinal cord may establish the site of pathology, although myelography may still be necessary to establish the upper and lower limits of the lesion. Urgent surgical decompression not only prevents permanent neurologic damage but also provides material for Gram's stain and culture. Use of the former test increases the likelihood of appropriate initial empirical therapy.

Blood cultures should be obtained in all cases and must always precede the administration of antibiotics. Organisms most likely to be associated with bacteremia in the drug addict, regardless of the underlying focus of infection, are *S. aureus* and *Streptococcus pyogenes*, followed by gram-negative bacilli and mixed organisms.[10] The rate of positive blood cultures in addicts is quite high, which facilitates selection of antibiotics. Empirical therapy should, with rare exception, always be deferred until after appropriate material, including tissue specimens, has been obtained for culture. Unanticipated and unusual organisms are recovered with high frequency in addicts, which emphasizes a need to obtain cultures before therapy to avoid a prolonged course of potentially toxic but ineffective therapy.

Wound Botulism and Tetanus

Wound botulism and tetanus, although rare, are seen in addicts, particularly among those with poor venous access who resort to "skin popping" (i.e., intentionally injecting drugs into the subcutaneous tissues rather than intravenously), which often results in numerous skin ulcerations. Patients who have multiple skin abscesses and ulcerations related to failed intravenous injections are also at risk.[18–21] These skin lesions become colonized by either *Clostridium tetani* or *Clostridium botulinum*, which then elaborate the neurotoxins responsible for the distinctive clinical syndromes. However, disease can also occur in patients who have no obvious skin lesions, such as a heavy user of intranasal cocaine.[22] Two additional cases of botulism in addicts are noteworthy because the patients shared needles, which may have facilitated transfer of *C. botulinum* from one patient to the other.[20]

The symptoms of botulism are similar to those seen in nonaddicts, except for the usual history of long-term intravenous drug use. The patient may have progressive dysphonia, dysarthria, dysphagia, dry mouth, dyspnea, and weakness. Ptosis and ocular paralysis may be found in addition to other evidence of facial nerve palsies. Cerebrospinal fluid examination is usually normal.[22–24] The differential diagnosis should include toxic neuropathy, descending variant of Guillain-Barré syndrome, and myasthenia gravis. A negative cerebrospinal fluid examination and a negative Tensilon test are helpful in making the distinction. Any wounds should be cultured anaerobically because recovery of the organism helps to confirm the diagnosis. Serum toxin assays are unlikely to be positive. A high index of suspicion is essential because antitoxin, to be of benefit, must be given within the first 24 hours of illness.[20] Supportive care, primarily to ensure adequate ventilation, is also critical because the neurotoxin reverses over time and full recovery is expected. A previous bout of botulism does not produce immunity; therefore, even patients with a history of botulism should be evaluated and treated for the disease if they have a compatible clinical picture.

Although addicts no longer constitute the majority of patients in the United States who contract tetanus, drug abuse remains a risk factor and, in the proper clinical setting, the disease must still be considered.[25] In the past, the tetanus-prone addict was a female with multiple skin lesions related to skin popping.[21, 26] Perhaps because of a decline in the popularity of this technique, the incidence of tetanus in

addicts has similarly declined.[25] The previously observed predominance of tetanus in women was the result of their being more likely to resort to this subcutaneous method of injection; this predominance no longer exists.[18, 19, 25, 27]

The clinical pattern of tetanus is similar in addicts and nonaddicts, although the former have almost double the mortality rate.[18, 19, 28] One explanation is that large amounts of toxin are produced because of the number and severity of the skin lesions from which the addict may suffer, each potentially colonized by *C. tetani*.[27] Early symptoms of tetanus, seizures and muscle rigidity, may be dismissed as side effects of illicit drug use. Furthermore, some of the other characteristic features of tetanus, such as sweating, hyperpyrexia, fluctuating tachycardia, episodic hypertension and hypotension, cardiac arrhythmias, pallor, and hyperglycemia, may be mistakenly attributed to narcotic withdrawal.[29] This misconception may lead to a delay in diagnosis and initiation of appropriate management, which is directed at treating and limiting these life-threatening complications. If therapy is successful, the patient should be provided with a primary series of tetanus immunization because, similar to the case with botulism, previous disease does not afford protection from future attacks.[29] It is worthwhile to give a tetanus booster to any addict who is seen for any medical reason to prevent future tetanus.

PULMONARY INFECTIONS
Septic Pulmonary Embolism

Drug abusers are prone to developing life-threatening pulmonary infections (Table 48–2), the most common of which is septic pulmonary embolism. These emboli can arise from several sites but most commonly arise from the tricuspid valve in patients with infectious endocarditis. Additional foci are infected venous thrombi, particularly the large clots that are found in patients with septic thrombophlebitis of the femoral veins.[30–33] These infections arise after injury of the vein and introduction of bacteria in the process of nonsterile injection. As with any deep venous thrombosis, significant pulmonary embolism is a complication. More confusing are patients who have septic pulmonary embolism with no evidence of endocarditis or thrombophlebitis. Many of these patients have large abscesses of the groin that erode into nearby vessels and initiate thrombus formation and, ultimately, septic pulmonary emboli.[10] Mycotic arterial or venous aneurysms may coexist with suppurative thrombophlebitis.[10] Regardless of the underlying pathology and source of emboli, the clinical picture is dominated by the pulmonary involvement.

TABLE 48–2

PULMONARY COMPLICATIONS OF INTRAVENOUS DRUG ABUSE

Infectious Diseases
Septic pulmonary embolism
Empyema
Bacterial pneumonia
Lung abscess
Mycotic aneurysm
Tuberculosis
Opportunistic infections (AIDS related)
   Pneumocystis carinii pneumonia
   Toxoplasma pneumonia

Acute Noninfectious Diseases That Mimic Infection
Pneumothorax
Pneumomediastinitis
Acute respiratory failure
Drug-induced noncardiogenic pulmonary edema

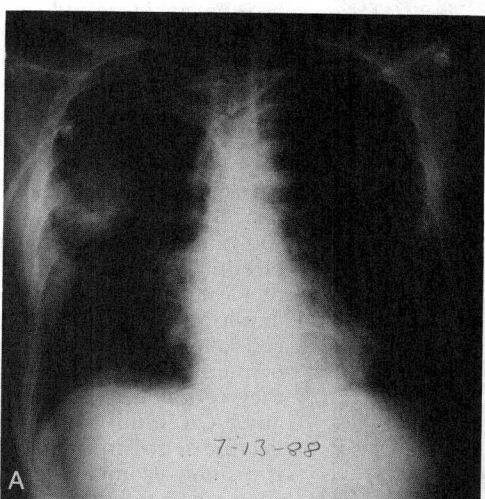
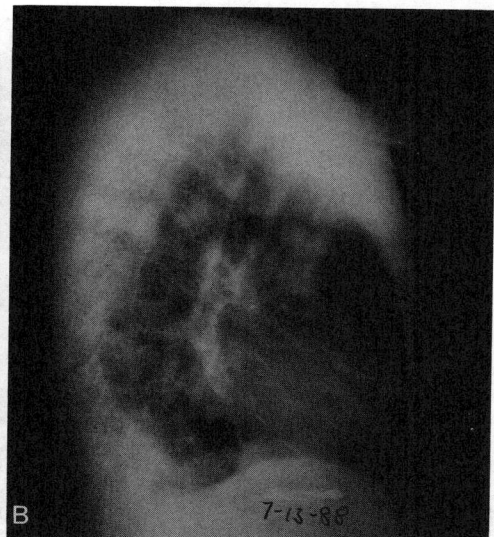

Figure 48–1. Posteroanterior *(A)* and lateral *(B)* chest roentgenograms showing multiple, bilateral pleural-based opacities. Figures 48–1 to 48–3 show progression of septic pulmonary emboli in an IVDA. (From Greville HW: Pulmonary infections in intravenous drug abusers. In: Levine DP, Sobel JD [eds]: Infections in Intravenous Drug Abusers. New York, Oxford University Press, p 215, 1991.)

Patients with septic pulmonary embolism present with a broad spectrum of clinical findings; however, most are extremely ill. Typically, patients have sudden onset of fever, chills, dyspnea, and chest pain that is often pleuritic. Cough is a frequent accompaniment and may be nonproductive or associated with blood-streaked sputum. Occasionally, patients present with septicemia and shock. Severe respiratory compromise may ensue and may necessitate mechanical ventilation.

Physical examination may not reveal the full extent of the pulmonary involvement. Evidence of pneumonia, with or without signs of pleural involvement or empyema, is found. The presence of murmurs is a clue to underlying endocarditis, although murmurs are frequently absent or unimpressive in addicts with endocarditis. Similarly, the classic peripheral signs such as Roth's spots, Osler's nodes, and Janeway's lesions are frequently absent in this population of patients.[10]

A diagnosis of septic pulmonary embolism is suggested in the setting of endocarditis or bacteremia with multiple ill-defined densities scattered throughout the lungs on chest x-ray films. These infiltrates tend to be localized in the periphery of the lungs and usually in the lower lobes. Frequently, they appear as rounded or wedge-shaped areas of consolidation (Fig. 48–1). The diagnosis may be difficult if only a single lesion is found, which suggests bronchial pneumonia. Multiple lesions may coalesce to form larger areas of consolidation. If *S. aureus* is the offending pathogen, cavitation within the infiltrates may occur, leading to thin-walled cavities that may contain air-fluid levels. Such a progression usually takes several days but can occur as early as 24 hours[34, 35] (Figs. 48–2 and 48–3). Additional complications of septic emboli are pleural effusion, empyema, bronchopleural fistula, and pneumothorax. Pulmonary infiltrates gradually resolve with antimicrobial therapy, but it is not unusual for showers of emboli to produce new lesions, even after the patient has been started on effective therapy. In some cases, there is no evidence of septic emboli on admission to the hospital, but infiltrates develop several days into the hospital course. It may be difficult to distinguish septic pulmonary embolism from bacterial pneumonia. The Gram's stain and culture of sputum specimens are important because blood cultures are less likely to be positive in pneumonia.

The differential diagnosis of the septic IVDA who has hypoxemia must now be broadened to include the serious pulmonary complications found in patients with AIDS. If HIV infection is unlikely, either because of a recent negative serologic test or a history of high-risk behavior that is too brief to allow time for immunosuppression to develop despite HIV infection, an opportunistic infection is not likely. If AIDS is a consideration, an illness with a history of a gradual onset and slow progression for several weeks makes opportunistic infection more likely than acute bacterial infection. In contrast, acute onset and a cough producing purulent sputum argue in favor of a bacterial infection, including septic pulmonary embolism. When the diagnosis of infectious endocarditis or septic thrombophlebitis is obvious, the characteristic clinical pattern of septic pulmonary embolism is enough to secure the diagnosis. In the absence of an apparent cause for pulmonary embolism, a radioisotope lung scan or pulmonary angiogram may help to establish the diagnosis.[30, 36] Tomograms have been used to find emboli that are not apparent on plain x-ray films.[37]

Therapy consists primarily of antibiotic administration. Blood and sputum cultures invariably provide a microbiologic diagnosis. The usual pathogens that cause infection in IVDAs, notably *S. aureus*,[10, 38] *Pseudomonas aeruginosa*,[10, 38–41] and streptococci, are also the most common in this setting.

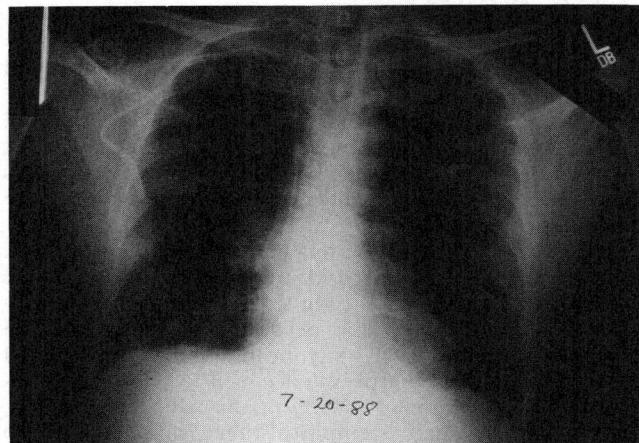

Figure 48–2. Same patient as that in Figure 48–1, 7 days later. New infiltrates are present despite therapy. Note the presence of cavitation. (From Greville HW: Pulmonary infections in intravenous drug abusers. In: Levine DP, Sobel JD [eds]: Infections in Intravenous Drug Abusers. New York, Oxford University Press, p 216, 1991.)

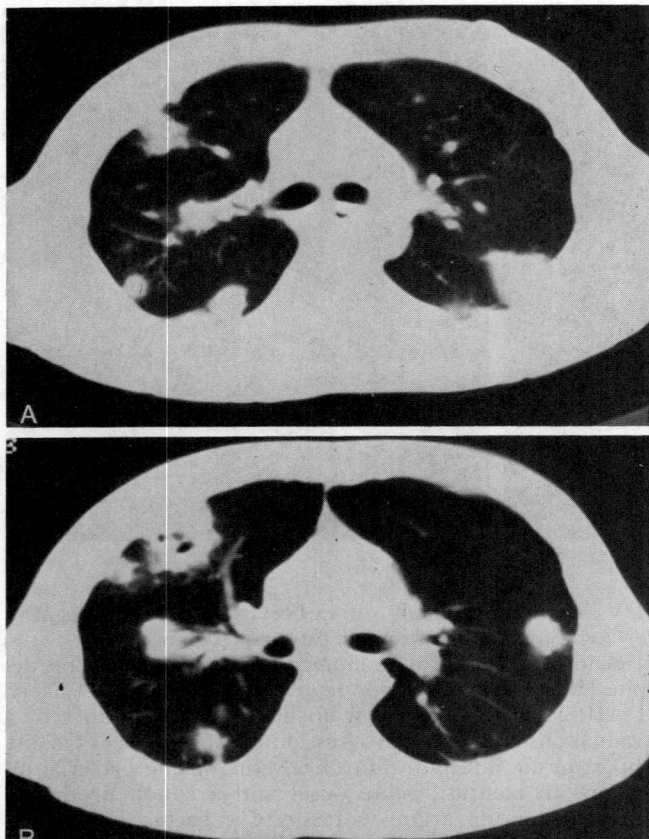

Figure 48–3. CT scans at two levels *(A and B)*. CT was performed 1 day after the initial roentgenogram. A number of emboli not seen on the first roentgenogram are present, some of which show cavitation. (From Greville HW: Pulmonary infections in intravenous drug abusers. In: Levine DP, Sobel JD [eds]: Infections in Intravenous Drug Abusers. New York, Oxford University Press, p 217, 1991.)

Among the streptococci, groups A and G are most frequently implicated,[10, 42, 43] but even *Streptococcus viridans* and *Streptococcus pneumoniae* have been reported to produce septic pulmonary embolism.[30, 44] Less common causes are *Pseudomonas cepacia*,[45] *Serratia marcescens*,[30, 46] and enterococci.[44] The initial antibiotic selection is generally directed at the most likely pathogens: *S. aureus* and streptococci. Empirical therapy against gram-negative organisms is not recommended unless there is a known predilection in the community for infection caused by a specific pathogen. It has been argued that the standard doses of aminoglycosides needed to treat most gram-negative isolates are generally higher than doses one chooses to use empirically and that after the organism is identified, specific therapy can be instituted.

Although some data indicate a combination of a β-lactam antibiotic plus an aminoglycoside allows for a 2-week course of therapy for addicts with right-sided staphylococcal endocarditis,[47] it is doubtful that delaying the addition of an aminoglycoside 1 or 2 days significantly alters the eventual outcome. Because of the prevalence of infection with methicillin-resistant *S. aureus* (MRSA) in the addict population, vancomycin is selected as empirical therapy and a switch to nafcillin is made when susceptibility data are available. There is mounting evidence that vancomycin is inferior to β-lactam antibiotics in the treatment of methicillin-susceptible *S. aureus*, at least with respect to rapid resolution of bacteremia;[48] thus, it is important to change to nafcillin as soon as antibiotic

susceptibilities are known. However, because MRSA cannot be predictably treated with any currently available antibiotics other than vancomycin, it is imperative to initiate therapy with this agent if MRSA is a consideration.

The use of heparin in the setting of septic pulmonary embolism has been the subject of considerable debate. Thus far, there are no controlled studies evaluating the use of anticoagulants in patients with emboli that arise from either tricuspid endocarditis or other infected peripheral venous foci. Some authors have concluded that anticoagulation is contraindicated because it may induce massive pulmonary bleeding.[49] Others have raised concerns about the possibility of local bleeding from a mycotic aneurysm or, of greater importance, intracranial hemorrhage from a cerebral mycotic aneurysm. Some favor anticoagulation when the source of pulmonary emboli is the peripheral vessels, especially if they continue to occur despite appropriate antibiotic therapy.[50] Given this uncertainty and because severe respiratory insufficiency is relatively uncommon,[10] routine use of heparin is not recommended until more information is available concerning safety and efficacy of anticoagulants. When the emboli originate in peripheral vessels, ligation of the affected vessel remains an option, although one that is seldom used.

Empyema

Empyema is also frequently seen in the critically ill IVDA. This complication may be the result of septic pulmonary embolism or an extension of a primary pneumonia. In either case, the infecting organism should be identified to facilitate appropriate antibiotic therapy. This identification can be accomplished by a diagnostic thoracentesis, with the fluid evaluated by Gram's stain and culture, as well as by the usual chemical analysis. The generally accepted indications for chest tube drainage include a low pH or glucose level and high lactate dehydrogenase level.[51] Chest tube drainage should also be given strong consideration when organisms are visualized by Gram's stain. Streptokinase has been used to lyse loculating membranes[51] but is generally reserved for highly refractory cases.

Bacterial Pneumonia and Lung Abscess

Bronchogenic pneumonia unrelated to septic pulmonary embolism also appears to have an increased incidence in IVDAs.[21, 52] The usual bacterial causes of pneumonia predominate, particularly *S. pneumoniae*.[53] Because of the effects of the narcotics and the tendency for loss of consciousness or suppression of the cough reflex, aspiration pneumonia is also common.[54] Lung abscess may result from aspiration pneumonia and is occasionally difficult to differentiate from a large septic pulmonary embolus that has progressed to cavitation. The Gram's stain of sputum is often useful in making the distinction because a polymicrobial flora is anticipated in primary lung abscess (aspiration pneumonia), whereas a single organism (usually *S. aureus*) is seen in patients with septic pulmonary embolism. In addition, patients with emboli usually have other evidence of an underlying focus of infection. Furthermore, unlike patients with lung abscess, those with septic pulmonary embolism invariably have positive blood cultures.

The clinical picture of pneumonia or lung abscess in addicts is similar to that in nonaddicts, and the principles of therapy are identical. Therapy is based on the results of a Gram-stained sputum specimen, and final antibiotic selection is based on the results of blood and sputum cultures. It is important to remember that *S. pneumoniae* (although still the most frequently found organism[53]) may not be isolated unless the sputum is cultured immediately by using scrupulous techniques. Also, because aspiration pneumonia and lung abscess are primarily polymicrobial anaerobic infections, sputum culture is of little value unless bronchial specimens are obtained via transtracheal aspiration.

Mycotic Aneurysm

Mycotic aneurysm of the pulmonary vessels, although an infrequent complication in the IVDA, is important because the outcome may be fatal. The first indication of the presence of pulmonary mycotic aneurysm may be massive hemoptysis. Because there are few reports describing this entity, it is difficult to completely characterize the typical patient; however, there may be an association with methylphenidate abuse.[31, 55] The radiologic appearance is frequently confused with that of septic pulmonary embolism. Although aneurysms may be seen in conjunction with right-sided endocarditis, this is by no means a prerequisite.[56, 57] Suspicion of the diagnosis may be aroused when the borders of the lesion become more sharply defined radiologically during antibiotic therapy. Definitive diagnosis can be made only by pulmonary angiogram. The lesions usually resolve with antibiotic administration alone,[55] although a single accessible lesion may be treated surgically.

Pulmonary Tuberculosis

Drug abuse is recognized as an independent risk factor for the development of tuberculosis (TB),[58] a disease that is now seen with increased frequency.[21, 59] With the increasing prevalence of HIV infection among IVDAs and the strong association between HIV and TB, it is likely that TB will become more common among drug users.[60] In a prospective study of TB among IVDAs, addicts with HIV infection were far more likely to develop TB than HIV-seronegative addicts ($P < .002$), especially if the addict had a prior history of a positive purified protein derivative test ($P < .0001$).[61] Frank TB may precede the development of AIDS by months to years in HIV-positive individuals.[62] TB is often much more aggressive in the HIV-infected addict than in the nonaddict. Extrapulmonary and disseminated disease is common, with an incidence of 72% in HIV-infected patients, compared with only 16% in the general population.[63] Although lymphatic TB and hematogenous TB are common in addicts, CNS involvement, including brain abscess, also occurs with increased frequency. The latter condition may be especially difficult to diagnosis in the HIV-infected patient in view of the prevalence of CNS toxoplasmosis and cryptococcal meningitis, which may present with similar findings and may also occur in conjunction with TB.[64] The diagnosis is easier to confirm with pulmonary rather than CNS involvement because the acid-fast stain of a sputum specimen may be positive and the organism will likely be cultured, albeit after a delay of several weeks. A positive purified protein derivative test strongly supports the diagnosis in the IVDA, however. In HIV-infected patients, both the purified protein derivative test and the acid-fast smear of sputum[65] are unlikely to be positive. Furthermore, the chest roentgenogram seldom displays the typical findings generally associated with TB (e.g., right upper lobe infiltrates with cavities).[62, 65] Rather, the disease is more often found in the middle and lower lung fields.[65] When cavitation occurs, there may also be air-fluid levels, a finding that is unusual among non-AIDS patients with TB.[63] Mediastinal lymphadenopathy and hilar lymphadenopathy are present in as many as half of patients with AIDS and TB.[65, 66] Both pleural and pericardial effusions are common, and the latter are occasionally responsible for cardiac tamponade.[63]

In view of the similarities between other serious pulmonary infections and TB in addicts with HIV infection, when the acid-fast stain of a sputum sample is negative, early bronchoalveolar lavage (BAL) with transbronchial biopsy may be necessary to establish the diagnosis. The absence of granulomas does not exclude the diagnosis because these histologic findings are frequently absent in patients with coexisting HIV infection and tuberculosis. The tissue stain for acid-fast bacilli is therefore imperative.[67]

The IVDA with TB is occasionally admitted to the hospital with overwhelming infection. Adult respiratory distress syndrome may develop in the IVDA with pulmonary TB, even after appropriate therapy has been started. Nevertheless, even when coinfected with HIV and TB, most patients have a satisfactory and rapid response to therapy. No specific therapeutic recommendations pertaining to the IVDA with TB (whether HIV infected or not) exist. Standard therapy with isoniazid at 300 mg/d and rifampin at 600 mg/d may be initiated; however, most clinicians add pyrazinamide at 20 to 30 mg/kg/d for the first 2 months.[67, 68] Fortunately, both isoniazid and rifampin are available in parenteral forms and can thus be used in the critically ill patient, even in the presence of intestinal ileus or other gastrointestinal complications that preclude oral therapy.

Opportunistic Infections

Unlike TB, which is common among addicts even without HIV infection, several pulmonary infections are limited almost exclusively to IVDAs with AIDS. Most notable among these is *Pneumocystis carinii* pneumonia (PCP), which accounts for 85% of all pulmonary infections in AIDS patients and will occur in at least 80% at some time during the course of the illness.[69] Two additional facts are noteworthy: PCP is more common among addicts than among homosexuals,[70, 71] and PCP is associated with another opportunistic infection in approximately one third of patients[66] (see Chapter 50).

As the IVDA without a previous diagnosis of HIV infection is unlikely to seek routine medical attention, it is not unusual for addicts with PCP to present with advanced disease. Drug users with PCP frequently present with severe respiratory failure, including adult respiratory distress syndrome, as the first indication of HIV infection. When the differential diagnosis includes PCP and adult respiratory distress syndrome, the presence of fever strongly suggests the former and may be the first clue that leads to the diagnosis of AIDS unless associated findings, such as oropharyngeal candidiasis or severe herpetic infection, are also present.

In the critically ill IVDA with respiratory failure in whom the differential diagnosis of the pulmonary infiltrate is broad, empirical therapy is hazardous. Definitive diagnosis mandates obtaining a respiratory specimen for appropriate staining and culture, either via BAL or lung biopsy.[69, 72, 73] When BAL is performed, it is important to include a transbronchial biopsy because the diagnostic yield is improved from 79 to 95% by using the combined techniques.[66] These results are further improved if touch imprints are made of biopsies and fixed tissue sections.[69]

It is particularly risky to delay a BAL or biopsy while awaiting the results of a therapeutic drug trial. Often, the patient's respiratory condition deteriorates, which necessitates high fraction of inspired oxygen and positive end-expiratory pressure and makes diagnostic procedures such as bronchoscopy or open lung biopsy exceptionally hazardous, if not impossible. If such deterioration occurs in the patient in whom a definite diagnosis has been made and for whom appropriate therapy has been prescribed, the clinician is secure in the knowledge that nothing more can be done other than to continue to support the patient and wait for clinical improvement. In contrast, the febrile addict with undiagnosed pulmonary infiltrates who is too ill to undergo diagnostic procedures should be given a large number of antibacterial, antiprotozoan, and antifungal agents, analogous to the neutropenic host.

T. gondii pneumonia, although rare, is included among the opportunistic infections that addicts acquire as a result of HIV infection.[74–76] Although the incidence is still well below that of PCP, the ratio of toxoplasma pneumonia to PCP increased from approximately 1:300 in 1984 to almost 1:40 in 1988. In one study of patients with AIDS, toxoplasma infections were more common in IVDAs than in other risk groups with HIV infection,[74] although in another study of T. gondii pneumonia, only 2 of 13 patients were addicts.[75] In each case, the patient had symptomatic HIV infection before the onset of T. gondii pneumonia; 8 of 13 patients met the Centers for Disease Control case definition for AIDS. Several patients had antecedent PCP and one had a prior history of visceral toxoplasmosis. In each case, the underlying HIV infection was far advanced, with CD4$^+$ cell counts being less than 1000/mm^3 and p24 antigen being positive.

In 11 of 13 patients, the clinical features of T. gondii pneumonia were similar to those seen in PCP except for a rapid onset with a mean delay to diagnosis of only 11 days. Fever was universal and dyspnea was almost as common. An unproductive cough and hemoptysis were also seen. All patients had diffuse bilateral pulmonary infiltrates, occasionally with nodular features. The patients also had severe hypoxemia, with a mean arterial oxygen tension of 47 mm Hg. In two cases, the clinical presentations differed slightly. Both patients presented with acute respiratory failure, shock, metabolic acidosis, and disseminated intravascular coagulation. In both cases, the diagnosis was made at postmortem examination. The diagnosis in the other patients was established by performing BAL and finding T. gondii tachyzoites in the transbronchial fluid. Cytologic examination of the fluid was also helpful and revealed increased numbers of both neutrophils and eosinophils. Several patients also had P. carinii coinfection. In a single case, BAL was not helpful, but an open lung biopsy revealed the correct diagnosis. Serologic evidence of previous infection with the organism may contribute to the diagnosis because almost all patients have immunoglobulin G antibodies against toxoplasma. Extrapulmonary toxoplasmosis is also common in these patients and may provide a clue to the diagnosis.

Drugs used to treat toxoplasma encephalitis and brain abscess are effective in pneumonia. The most frequently used regimen has been a combination of sulfadiazine (4 to 6 g/d) plus pyrimethamine (50 to 100 mg/d). The regimen of clindamycin (4800 mg/d) plus pyrimethamine (100 mg/d) has also been used with success. Fewer data exist regarding the use of trimethoprim-sulfamethoxazole, but it appears to be less effective than either choice just mentioned, an observation that is of critical importance. If a drug user who is either known or suspected to have HIV infection presents with a typical clinical picture, many clinicians make a presumptive diagnosis of PCP and treat accordingly. If the diagnosis is T. gondii pneumonia rather than PCP and trimethoprim-sulfamethoxazole is chosen as empirical therapy, there is a substantial risk that the patient will fail to respond. If pentamidine is used, the patient will not receive marginally effective treatment. In view of the severity of the disease and the probability of death if treatment is less than optimal, it is clear that empirical therapy without first attempting a diagnostic procedure is to be discouraged.

Noninfectious Disease That Mimics Infection

An important noninfectious cause of acute respiratory disease in the IVDA is acute pulmonary edema. This complication is most often associated with drug overdose or drug intoxication and may present with dramatic consequences. In addition to heroin, a variety of substances have been implicated, including chlordiazepoxide,[77] cocaine,[78] codeine,[79] ethchlorvynol,[80] methadone,[81] paraldehyde,[82] propoxyphene,[83] and propylhexedrine.[84] The usual presentation is mental obtundation of varying severity; coma is common. There is also marked depression of respiration, with cyanosis. The chest x-ray film shows a variety of abnormalities ranging from mild congestion to florid pulmonary edema, and the changes are usually bilateral. When the radiographic findings are not typical, revealing unilateral changes or abnormalities of only one area of the lung, the diagnosis may be missed. Furthermore, these changes may be absent on admission but develop after several hours of hospitalization.[85, 86] The arterial blood gas assays reflect the severity of the process with profound hypoxemia, hypercapnia, and acidosis.[87]

Although the etiology of the syndrome is obscure, it represents a form of noncardiac pulmonary edema characterized by increased permeability of the pulmonary capillaries, which leads to the leak of a protein-rich fluid into the alveoli. It has been suggested that the release of histamine induced by narcotics may be responsible for the excessive capillary permeability,[88] although aspiration of gastric contents with resulting chemical pneumonitis may also be involved.[89] Occasionally, some patients with this characteristic picture are septic, and adult respiratory distress syndrome is a direct consequence of infection.

The management of these patients is supportive. Many require extensive resuscitative measures, including mechanical ventilation, positive end-expiratory pressure, and the full spectrum of vasoactive drugs needed to maintain homeostasis. Antibiotic therapy is critical if infection is diagnosed as the underlying cause. Even with appropriate management, the mortality rate is high. Those who survive frequently have complete recovery,[89] although some have residual impairment of pulmonary function.[87, 90–92]

INFECTIOUS ENDOCARDITIS

Infectious endocarditis is the most common cause of bacteremia in the IVDA.[10] The microbial etiology of infectious endocarditis has shifted since it was first recognized as a common complication of drug abuse. Today, S. aureus and S. pyogenes (group A, B, or G) account for approximately 75% of cases, the remainder being due to either gram-negative bacilli (most notably P. aeruginosa and S. marcescens) or polymicrobial infection (often S. aureus plus gram-negative bacilli).[10] Fungal endocarditis accounts for 5% of cases in addicts and is almost always caused by Candida species, although rarely Candida albicans.

Pathophysiology

The pathophysiology of endocarditis in addicts is incompletely understood. Unlike patients with subacute bacterial endocarditis who usually have underlying valvular abnormalities, it is unusual for addicts to have a history of cardiac disease.[10, 39] Most likely some combination of factors is responsible, including the possibility that the injection of impure substances leads to an altered valve surface that permits adherence of bacteria after they enter the blood stream. The reason that some organisms predominate and the mechanism by which they enter the blood stream have been well studied. It is now generally accepted that the bacteria are part of the patient's own flora,[10, 93] although in the case of P. aeruginosa, contamination of the paraphernalia used for injection has also been implicated.[40, 94, 95] Regardless of the variations in disease acquisition, there are similarities among patients that depend on the infecting organism. Many more IVDAs have right-sided infection than left-sided disease.[96, 97] When the right side (predominantly the tricuspid valve) is involved, *S. aureus* is the most likely pathogen. *S. aureus* may also be the cause of aortic or mitral valve infection, but streptococci are found almost exclusively on the left side of the heart.[10] *S. marcescens*[98] and enterococci[99] are also predominantly left-sided pathogens. Ultimately, the shared contributions of the bacteria causing the disease and of the valve involved account for the clinical pattern of endocarditis in the addict.

Clinical Aspects

Most addicts with endocarditis present within the first week of illness with signs and symptoms of acute infection.[100] Constitutional symptoms are common. Indeed, every organ system is affected to some degree by the persistent and high-grade bacteremia (Table 48–3). The severity of the clinical picture varies depending on the valve or valves infected; whether there is additional cardiac damage such as a valve ring abscess or valve perforation; the location and number of metastatic abscesses; and the pathogens involved, with *P. aeruginosa* being far more likely than other bacteria to be associated with refractory bacteremia and neurologic complications.[10] The most frequent significant complication of endocarditis that brings the addict to the attention of the intensive care specialist is septic pulmonary embolism, which has already been discussed.

Cardiovascular System

Cardiovascular complications, although less frequent, may be life threatening. When cardiac signs or symptoms dominate the clinical picture, they are usually a poor prognostic sign, especially if valve destruction leads to congestive heart failure and pulmonary edema. Acute left-sided heart failure that is unresponsive to medical management necessitates immediate resuscitative efforts and surgical intervention.[10, 38, 39, 43, 44, 101, 102] The presence of pathogens with a predilection for infecting the aortic or the mitral valve, such as streptococci, enterococci, and *Serratia* species, should alert the clinician to the possible development of rapid deterioration of cardiac function.[10, 98] Pericarditis is another potential complication of left-sided endocarditis and can be life threatening. Immediate drainage may be lifesaving.[44, 103] Arterial emboli, especially to the cerebral circulation, are of great clinical importance.[10, 103] In unusual cases of right-sided *S. aureus* endocarditis, systemic emboli can arise from the pulmonary circulation,[12] so the clinician must carefully assess the patient's heart before making decisions based solely on the presence of such emboli. Fungi and *Serratia* species are also common causes of emboli to major vessels, especially the carotid, femoral, brachial, and renal arteries.[98, 104, 105] The patient with such emboli experiences sudden vascular occlusion. In the case of a cerebral embolism, the patient suddenly has a cerebrovascular accident, which may have severe neurologic consequences, although frequently of short duration. When an embolus affects a distal extremity, prompt removal of the clot may be possible, with full recovery of normal circulation. In fact, in culture-negative endocarditis, extraction followed by histologic examination and culture of such an embolus may confirm the diagnosis. This is especially true of fungal endocarditis, which is frequently associated with negative blood cultures. Some patients, especially those with overwhelming sepsis, develop ischemia or necrosis of the distal digits with no evidence of a clot, presumably related to vasculitis.

TABLE 48–3
CLINICAL FINDINGS OF ENDOCARDITIS

Central nervous system
  Headache
  Focal neurologic deficits
    Hemiplegia
    Aphasia
    Facial paresis
    Homonymous hemianopia
  Mycotic aneurysms
    Intracerebral hemorrhage
  Toxic encephalopathy
  Meningeal irritation
    Meningism
    Meningitis
  Brain abscesses and microabscesses
Respiratory tract
  Pulmonary embolism
  Cavitary pneumonia
  Empyema
  Pulmonary artery aneurysm
Cardiovascular system
  Valvular defects and destruction
  Heart failure
  Pericarditis
  Myocarditis
  Arterial emboli
  Peripheral ischemia and necrosis
Gastrointestinal tract
  Nausea, vomiting, and diarrhea
  Acute abdominal pain
    Ileus
    Splenic infarct or abscess
    Bowel infarction
    Gastrointestinal hemorrhage
    Hepatomegaly
    Splenomegaly
Renal system
  Renal impairment (glomerulonephritis)
  Hematuria
  Proteinuria
  Renal abscess
Musculoskeletal system
  Arthralgia
  Arthritis
  Myalgia
  Osteomyelitis
  Myositis
Integumentary system
  Conjunctival petechial hemorrhages
  Osler's nodes and Janeway's lesions
  Subungual splinter hemorrhages
Reproductive system
  Intrauterine fetal death
  Intrauterine growth retardation

Adapted from Levine DP. Infectious endocarditis in intravenous drug abusers. In: Levine DP, Sobel JD (eds): Infections in Intravenous Drug Abusers. New York, Oxford University Press, p 261, 1991.

Gastrointestinal System

Involvement of the gastrointestinal tract may be revealed by gastrointestinal hemorrhage, which at times is life threatening.[10, 101] An acute surgical abdomen may be suspected in patients suffering from acute abdominal pain related to ileus, splenic infarct or abscess, infarcted bowel, or peritonitis.[8, 17, 43, 103, 106] The recognition of a splenic abscess is important because it may be the source of prolonged bacteremia, despite appropriate antibiotic therapy. In such cases, if a cardiac source is suspected rather than the spleen, the patient may be subjected to unnecessary valve surgery.

Noninvasive tests, including ultrasonography and CT, are helpful in detecting such lesions.[107] In my medical center, a splenic abscess is routinely excluded before subjecting any patient to valve surgery if the sole indication is persistent bacteremia. Furthermore, because patients requiring valve replacement for other reasons may have an infected prosthetic valve if there is bacteremia from a noncardiac source, the spleen deserves preoperative evaluation in all patients with endocarditis who are undergoing elective valve replacement.

Skeletal Involvement

Bone and joint involvement attributable to immune complex deposition is fairly common in IVDAs with endocarditis,[8, 17, 38, 103] as is septic arthritis.[8, 10, 38, 44, 101, 103] These complications are generally not critical and often respond to the usual therapeutic measures, such as drainage of infected joints.

Renal Involvement

Involvement of the kidney, by direct infection with microabscesses, by septic emboli to the renal artery, or by immune complex disease, is extremely common in addicts with endocarditis.[10, 38, 103] When *Pseudomonas* is the etiologic agent, more than two thirds of the patients have altered renal function at some time during their disease.[39] Glomerulonephritis has also been noted in 40% of patients with MRSA endocarditis;[38] an incidence of up to 60% has been reported by others, usually in patients with *S. aureus* infection.[108] Microscopic hematuria occurs in nearly half of all patients,[8, 39, 41, 101] and gross hematuria is also seen.[17, 39, 43] When pyuria occurs, it may indicate metastatic kidney infection.[8, 17, 43]

Renal failure is usually mild; the severity may be reflected by the degree of complement depression. Although renal failure may be of short duration, some patients require dialysis. From a therapeutic standpoint, it is important to determine whether the renal failure is due to the disease itself or to toxic effects of therapy. Although most antibiotics used to treat endocarditis are minimally nephrotoxic, thereby allowing continuation of therapy with the same agent, it is important to remember that dosage adjustments may be required.

Central Nervous System

CNS involvement is related to occlusion of the cerebral arteries; expansion, leakage, or rupture of mycotic aneurysms; or direct infection (meningitis or brain abscess).[9] The initiating event is one or more emboli to the cerebral circulation. As noted earlier, this occurs almost exclusively with left-sided infection, although rarely right-sided disease has been implicated. When an addict presents with an altered level of consciousness, it is possibly due to toxic effects of the illicit drug used, but frequently it is a consequence of endocarditis. The symptoms are usually mild; headache, for example, may occur in up to 40% of patients.[8, 17, 43, 103] Cerebral embolism may result in hemiplegia, aphasia, facial paralysis, or homonymous hemianopia.[101, 109] The symptoms are usually transient, although permanent defects do occur and can be devastating after a ruptured cerebral mycotic aneurysm[10, 39, 110] and subarachnoid hemorrhage.[10, 109, 110]

Toxic encephalopathy, which typically affects patients who are critically ill with high-grade fever and toxemia, results in severely altered mentation and is observed in almost 30% of patients at the initial presentation.[8, 10, 17, 38, 103, 109] Fortunately, with antibiotic therapy and supportive care, the encephalopathy tends to resolve. Meningeal irritation, which is often associated with meningism or frank meningitis, is an occasional complication of addict-related endocarditis.[8, 17, 39, 103] The cerebrospinal fluid findings indicate a parameningeal focus, even though the cerebrospinal fluid culture may be positive for the etiologic agent.[10, 17, 111] Generally, therapy directed at the endocarditis is adequate to control the neurologic process.

Finally, brain abscesses can complicate endocarditis in addicts.[98, 109] These lesions may be large and multiple, although microabscesses are more common. Fortunately, these lesions respond to antibiotic therapy and seldom require surgical drainage. Serial CT scans help to assess progress and ensure resolution.

Complications of endocarditis affecting other organ systems are important but seldom have implications for the intensive care specialist. However, some features (e.g., conjunctival petechial hemorrhages) that are present in 50% of patients[109] (and that are easily missed unless the examiner is careful to fully retract the lower eyelid) are extremely helpful at suggesting the diagnosis. In a critically ill patient, this information may prove to be lifesaving. The classic physical findings of endocarditis, such as Osler's nodes and Janeway's lesions, can be equally helpful but are observed in the minority of addicts with endocarditis.[8, 38, 39, 103] Arthralgia and true septic arthritis are frequent accompaniments of the bacteremia and circulating immune complexes associated with endocarditis but are managed in fashion similar to that for patients without endocarditis.

Diagnosis

Unlike many other diseases in which there may be a specific laboratory test or a constellation of abnormalities that lead to the proper diagnosis, in endocarditis, with virtually every organ in the body affected, almost every laboratory test provides an abnormal result (Table 48–4). The single most important test, and the one that leads to both the diagnosis and the etiologic agent, is the blood culture. Because 80 to 100% of blood cultures are positive in addicts with endocarditis, the diagnosis is generally not difficult.[8, 17, 38, 39, 41, 44, 101–103] Indeed, even after several days of appropriate antibiotic therapy, the bacteremia may persist.[8, 10, 38] Because addicts frequently take oral antibiotics before hospital admission, it is theoretically possible for initial blood cultures to be negative.[16] However, I rarely, if ever, have

---

TABLE 48–4

LABORATORY TESTS WITH ABNORMAL RESULTS IN ENDOCARDITIS

Hematologic assays
  Anemia
  Leukocytosis
  Neutropenia
  Thrombocytopenia
  Elevated erythrocyte sedimentation rate
Chemistry assays
  Hyponatremia
  Elevated hepatic enzyme levels
  Hypoalbuminemia
  Elevated serum immunoglobulin values
  Elevated blood urea nitrogen values
  Elevated serum creatinine levels
Urine tests
  Pyuria
  Hematuria
  Albuminuria

been faced with negative blood cultures despite the patient's admission to recent antibiotic use. Inappropriately, the most widely used test to confirm the diagnosis of endocarditis is echocardiography: both M-mode echocardiography and two-dimensional echocardiography are frequently not helpful and may in some cases be misleading.[10] On the other hand, echocardiography is useful in assessing cardiac function after the diagnosis has been made.

Confirming the diagnosis of endocarditis is difficult. Many authors believe that direct visualization of the valve, either at surgery or at autopsy, is required to prove the diagnosis. Von Reyn and coworkers have published diagnostic criteria that are widely used;[112] however, these criteria depend heavily on the finding of new and changing murmurs. Use of these criteria requires some knowledge of the patient's previous cardiac condition; this information is seldom available for drug addicts. Most clinicians depend on the finding of sustained bacteremia (I use more than 3 days' duration during which time the patient is receiving appropriate antibiotics) in the absence of any other focus of infection to identify addicts with *S. aureus* endocarditis.[38] As noted earlier, careful physical examination with special attention to external evidence of endocarditis, such as Osler's nodes, Janeway's lesions, Roth's spots, and subconjunctival lesions, may provide the diagnosis before the results of blood cultures and permit antibiotic therapy at an early stage.

Treatment

Addicts with endocarditis who are only moderately ill can safely be observed without antibiotic therapy while waiting for the results of blood cultures. In fact, this practice may ultimately provide far more information than any of the diagnostic tests and procedures just mentioned. In every instance, therapy must be withheld until necessary blood cultures have been obtained. Only then should an empirical regimen be initiated, with the choice of regimen based in part on necessary epidemiologic information (i.e., the organisms most likely to cause endocarditis in that geographic location). For example, in Detroit, therapy is begun with vancomycin because MRSA are quite common. In other settings where MRSA account for few cases, nafcillin or a similar β-lactamase–resistant penicillin is preferred. Even in locations that are notable for a high prevalence of unusual pathogens, such as *Serratia* in Oakland or *Pseudomonas* in Detroit and Chicago, staphylococci are still the predominant organisms and antibiotics with antistaphylococcal activity are a required part of any empirical regimen. Whether any additional coverage (e.g., gram-negative agent) should be added is still an open question. The addition of an aminoglycoside to a β-lactam antibiotic has been shown effective in reducing the duration of bacteremia and the length of therapy in patients with right-sided staphylococcal endocarditis.[47] In the critically ill patient, there may be a role for such combination therapy from the outset. Unfortunately, the standard dose of aminoglycoside used to provide synergy against staphylococci is unlikely to have any effect against the most worrisome gram-negative organisms, especially *Pseudomonas*.[113, 114] After the offending pathogen has been identified, therapy is adjusted to a specific regimen consisting of a bactericidal antibiotic or a combination directed against that organism.

A more difficult situation arises when a patient's condition appears to be worsening despite an antibiotic regimen that is considered to be effective against the offending pathogen. It is useful to note that in some instances the favored drug may have become the therapy of choice not because of its well-studied efficacy but because no other regimen is available. For example, I routinely observe prolonged bacteremia

among patients with MRSA endocarditis who are receiving vancomycin, a drug that has long been the only one used to treat this infection.[115] Almost always, continuation of the same treatment leads to eradication of the bacteremia. When bacteremia persists beyond 10 to 14 days, a second antibiotic, either gentamicin or rifampin, is added. On rare occasions, a four-drug combination (vancomycin, rifampin, gentamicin, and trimethoprim-sulfamethoxazole) is required to eradicate bacteremia.

Gram-negative endocarditis, particularly if caused by *P. aeruginosa*, is often extremely difficult to treat with antibiotics alone. Reyes and coworkers demonstrated that use of a high-dose aminoglycoside (8 mg/kg) plus an antipseudomonal β-lactam antibiotic reduces the mortality associated with *Pseudomonas* to only 25%.[113] Use of a proven synergistic combination seems logical, yet when studied, synergy did not predict a cure. Rather, the lack of synergy was useful to predict failure to respond to antibiotic therapy.[114] There is insufficient information to allow precise recommendations for nonpseudomonal gram-negative endocarditis. Ultimately, if the patient's condition continues to worsen despite appropriate antibiotic therapy, surgical resection of the infected valve or valves is usually required to achieve a cure.

In at least two situations (i.e., *Pseudomonas* infection of either the aortic or the mitral valve and endocarditis caused by fungi, regardless of the valve involved), immediate surgical intervention is recommended because there are virtually no instances of successful management by antibiotics alone.[116, 117] Other than these two circumstances and the setting of persistent bacteremia, surgical intervention is generally recommended to prevent life-threatening complications. Foremost among these is the need to replace a perforated or ruptured aortic or mitral valve. Failing to do so invariably results in progressive heart failure and death.[118] The same applies to patients whose endocarditis causes heart failure that is unresponsive to medical management. Surgery is also recommended for patients who suffer a second major arterial embolus. Some authors have recommended surgery for patients with tricuspid endocarditis and persistent fever with echocardiographic evidence of large vegetations (larger than 1 cm), even if bacteremia has cleared,[119, 120] although others have disagreed.[121] Likewise, some authors have advocated surgery for any patient with left-sided *S. aureus* endocarditis (with the possible exception of IVDAs because they tend to respond well to antibiotics alone[122]). More emphasis is being placed on nonsurgical approaches, with operation being reserved for those who meet the criteria cited.[123]

SKIN AND SOFT TISSUE INFECTIONS
Cellulitis and Skin Abscesses

Drug abusers are subject to a host of skin and soft tissue infections, but few achieve significance for the intensive care specialist (Table 48–5). Cellulitis, abscesses, and skin ulcers are so common that they are almost considered to be normal findings among those who have used drugs for a substantial

TABLE 48–5

SKIN AND SOFT TISSUE INFECTIONS IN INTRAVENOUS DRUG ABUSERS

Cellulitis
Abscesses
Skin ulcers
Septic thrombophlebitis
Necrotizing fasciitis and myositis

period. Indeed, cellulitis may be the most common reason that drug addicts seek medical attention.[124] Abscesses are seen with almost equal frequency and are often encountered in conjunction with cellulitis.[10, 125–128] Infrequently, an abscess may spread to adjacent tissues, with devastating consequences.[126, 128] Abscesses of the femoral triangle may tunnel beneath muscle layers to the distal thigh or proximally into the retroperitoneal space. Cervical abscesses can extend into the mediastinum, leading to mediastinitis. Those in the carotid triangle can dissect into the carotid arteries, resulting in massive hemorrhage.[129] Thrombosis of the internal jugular vein causing septic shock has also been described as a possible complication.[130] In addition, a cervical abscess can produce laryngeal edema or extrinsic tracheal compression that may lead to upper airway obstruction. Pneumothorax and pneumomediastinum are additional complications that should be considered in a patient who develops dyspnea, cyanosis, cervical crepitance, and distended neck veins.[131]

These lesions are caused by injection of illicit substances without benefit of sterile technique through skin that is colonized with potential pathogens.[19, 127] S. aureus is the most likely pathogen,[10, 27, 127–129, 132–135] followed by streptococci alone[10, 128, 133] or in combination with other bacteria.[135] Coagulase-negative staphylococci and alpha-hemolytic streptococci are seen,[127, 128, 133] as are gram-negative bacilli.[133, 134] Some patients have been infected by mixed oral flora, including S. pneumoniae,[132, 136] presumably as a result of the practice of licking their needles before injection in an effort to facilitate drug administration.[132, 137, 138] Anaerobes may also play a major role.[10, 44, 127, 134, 139]

The symptoms associated with these abscesses are variable. In some published series, the majority of patients appeared septic and required hospitalization;[53] in others, the minority were seriously ill, with findings that included a rapid, thready pulse, low blood pressure, and bacteremia.[1, 43, 133, 136] Approximately 10% of deep abscesses extend to adjacent arteries and lead to the formation of mycotic pseudoaneurysms.[128, 140] These lesions carry a high risk of rupture, which leads to sudden and severe blood loss.

The diagnosis of an abscess can be difficult. CT is especially useful for cervical abscesses[129–131] and may also be effective for detecting abscesses in the femoral region, although confirming studies have yet to be published. Ultrasonography is useful but of variable accuracy for diagnosing lesions in the groin.[141, 142]

Treatment of abscesses in addicts is no different from the management of similar lesions in the general population. Cultures of blood and any purulent material are necessary to determine the causative organism or organisms so that the correct antibiotic is used. As with any other abscess, surgical drainage is often required. In fact, in drug addicts, it is not unusual for multiple drainage procedures to be required before a lesion is eradicated.[128, 133]

Skin Ulcerations

Skin ulcerations are extraordinarily common among IVDAs. They may be the end result of superficial abscesses that cause necrosis and ulceration of the overlying skin or a direct result of necrosis induced by the illicit substances that are injected.[143–147] Regardless of the pathophysiology, these lesions, although chronic and important, do not themselves cause critical illness, except to the extent that they serve as a focus of dissemination of potential pathogens or toxins, such as tetanus or botulinus toxin.

Septic Thrombophlebitis

Septic thrombophlebitis, particularly of the femoral vein, is another common condition that is rarely a direct cause of critical illness. Bacteremia is common and may result in distant infection. The most important complication, especially when large vessels of the femoral triangle are affected, is septic pulmonary embolism,[10, 30] which was discussed earlier. When septic pulmonary emboli occur, it can be difficult to distinguish between tricuspid or pulmonic valve endocarditis and deep venous thrombosis. Ultrasonography may support the diagnosis if it reveals a dilated and anechoic vein with irregular margins, and in conjunction with the characteristic clinical picture (usually a markedly edematous, tender extremity), it may be considered to be diagnostic.[141] Gallium scans and CT have also been used to identify an infected thrombus, but there are insufficient data to permit a recommendation for the use of either.[148, 149] Venography is the most sensitive test but is understandably difficult to accomplish in addicts who tend to have marked peripheral edema and a paucity of accessible veins.

The therapy for septic thrombophlebitis is controversial. The dilemma is whether to use anticoagulant therapy. There are arguments in favor of[30] and against[147, 149] anticoagulation. Because of the concern about the possibility of massive hemorrhage in the event of a concomitant but possibly unknown mycotic aneurysm, most investigators do not currently recommend heparinization. Parenteral therapy with antibiotics to which the organism is susceptible, plus bed rest and elevation of the involved extremity, constitutes my preferred regimen. Nonsteroidal anti-inflammatory agents and warm compresses to the affected area have been advocated by others.[150]

Necrotizing Fasciitis

Necrotizing fasciitis, with or without myositis, is perhaps the single infection of drug users that is most likely to require immediate intervention. Unfortunately, the clinical picture is often subtle and rarely invokes the kind of urgent response that is necessary. The initial impression may be that of mild cellulitis with a complete absence of bullae, crepitance, high fever, and skin necrosis.[151] The primary indicators of the true nature of the infection are signs and symptoms, such as local pain and hemodynamic instability, that are disproportionate to the apparent extent of the local process.[151] Addicts are often viewed as complainers who attempt to manipulate physicians into providing analgesics for what may be viewed as insignificant lesions. In necrotizing fasciitis, in which severe pain is the most important finding, adopting such an attitude may make the physician oblivious to the true emergency and gravity of the situation.[152]

Gram-positive cocci are present in most infections. The predominant pathogens are beta-hemolytic streptococci, which account for 50% of cases, but S. aureus and alpha-hemolytic streptococci (approximately 25%) and coagulase-negative staphylococci (20%) are also frequently isolated. Gram-negative organisms are seen less often and are usually represented by enteric organisms, especially Escherichia coli (24%), Klebsiella, Proteus mirabilis, Pseudomonas, and Enterobacter. Anaerobes are found in approximately 12% of patients,[151–154] and even Candida may be seen.[27] In view of the polymicrobial nature of the infection, it appears that the infection is a form of synergistic gangrene that ultimately results in liquefaction of the fascia and diffuse spread into the adjacent tissues.[126] Once initiated, the process is characterized by rapid progression and serious systemic effects.[152]

As noted earlier, severe pain is the most important clinical finding. Fever is common,[152, 153] but hypothermia also occurs and may be an ominous sign.[152] Laboratory investigations are not revealing and provide only nonspecific indications of a disease in progress.[152] Soft tissue x-ray films may or may not demonstrate gas in the tissues[152-154] and must not be relied on to confirm the diagnosis. Diagnosis can be made only if there is a high index of suspicion on the part of the physician.

Immediate surgical exploration is mandatory if the diagnosis is suspected. Up to 75% of patients who are initially managed by antibiotics alone experience a progression of infection. During the first 24 hours, advancing cellulitis, skin blebs, ulceration, and skin necrosis can be expected. Thus, any addict who presents with an extremely painful lesion, generally in an extremity and particularly if accompanied by cellulitis, local skin changes, or crepitance, should be rapidly taken to the operating suite.[152] If necrotizing fasciitis is present, a blunt instrument (or hand) can be passed freely along what are usually adherent fascial planes, thereby demonstrating the dissolution of the fascia and confirming the diagnosis.[152] As part of the disease process, necrosis of adjacent fat and tendons is expected.[153] It is also common for adjacent muscle to be involved, and this should be tested with electrical stimulation for viability. Wide débridement is vital, including all necrotic skin, fat, fascia, and muscle. Some authors advocate re-exploration at 24 hours and as often as necessary after that to completely remove all necrotic tissue and to arrest the disease process.[152] Delay in débridement or inadequate débridement is associated with considerable morbidity and mortality.[151] Not to be overlooked, however, is the need for prolonged parenteral antibiotic therapy, which is also an essential component of the treatment plan. In addition, aggressive parenteral or enteral nutrition and early soft tissue coverage improve the outcome.[152] Drug addicts, who tend to be young and relatively free of underlying disease, have the lowest mortality rate among patients with this disease.[154]

References

1. Caplan LR, Chinnamma T, Banks G: Central nervous system complications of addiction to "T's and blues." Neurology 32:623, 1982.
2. Leeds NE, Malhotra V, Zimmerman RD: The radiology of drug addiction affecting the brain. Semin Roentgenol 18:227, 1983.
3. Addman LS, Aronson SM: The neuropathologic complications of narcotics addiction. Bull NY Acad Med 45:225, 1969.
4. Masocci EF, Farara JA, Saini N, et al: Cerebral mucormycosis (phycomycosis) in a heroin addict. Arch Neurol 39:304, 1982.
5. Pierce PF Jr, Solomon SK, Kaufman L, et al: Zygomycetes brain abscesses in narcotic addicts with serological diagnosis. JAMA 248:2881, 1982.
6. Stave GM, Heimberger T, Kerkering TM: Zygomycosis of the basal ganglia in intravenous drug users. Am J Med 86:115, 1989.
7. Woods KF, Hanna BJ: Brain stem mucormycosis in a narcotic addict with eventual recovery. Am J Med 80:126, 1986.
8. Chambers HF, Korzeniowski OM, Sande MA: Staphylococcus aureus endocarditis: Clinical manifestations in addicts and non-addicts. Medicine 62:170, 1983.
9. Lerner PI: Neurologic complications of infective endocarditis. Med Clin North Am 69:385, 1985.
10. Levine DP, Crane LR, Zervos MJ: Bacteremia in narcotic addicts at the Detroit Medical Center. II. Infectious endocarditis: A prospective comparative study. Rev Infect Dis 8:374, 1986.
11. Pruitt AA, Rubin RH, Karchmer AW, et al: Neurologic complications of bacterial endocarditis. Medicine 57:329, 1978.
12. Reisberg BF: Infective endocarditis in the narcotic addict. Prog Cardiovasc Dis 22:193, 1979.
13. Pierog S, Nigam RE, Ruiz N: Male adolescent with subdural parietal abscess: A probable complication of substance abuse. J Adolesc Health Care 3:180, 1982.
14. Chandrasekar PH, Mehta R: Spinal epidural abscess in intravenous drug abusers. In: Program and Abstracts of the 26th Interscience Conference on Antimicrobial Agents and Chemotherapy, American Society for Microbiology, New Orleans, LA, 1986.
15. Baker AS, Ojemann RG, Swarta MN, et al: Spinal epidural abscess. N Engl J Med 293:463, 1975.
16. Pazin GJ, Saul S, Thompson ME: Blood culture positivity, suppression by out-patient antibiotic therapy in patients with bacterial endocarditis. Arch Intern Med 142:263, 1982.
17. Tuazon CU, Cardella TA, Sheagren JN: Staphylococcal endocarditis in drug users. Arch Intern Med 135:1555, 1975.
18. Blake PA, Feldman RA: Tetanus in the United States, 1970–1971. J Infect Dis 131:745, 1975.
19. Cherubin CE: Epidemiology of tetanus in narcotic addicts. NY State J Med 70:267, 1970.
20. MacDonald KL, Rutherford GW, Friedman SM, et al: Botulism and botulism-like illness in chronic drug abusers. Ann Intern Med 102:616, 1985.
21. Rho YM: Infections as fatal complications of narcotism. NY State J Med 72:823, 1972.
22. Kudrow DB, Haake DA, Mathisen GE: Botulism associated with clostridium botulism sinusitis after intranasal cocaine abuse. Ann Intern Med 109:984, 1988.
23. Centers for Disease Control: Wound botulism associated with parenteral cocaine abuse—New York City. MMWR 31:87, 1982.
24. MacDonald KL, Cohen ML, Blake PA: The changing epidemiology of adult botulism in the United States. Am J Epidemiol 124:794, 1986.
25. Centers for Disease Control: Annual summary 1984: Reported morbidity and mortality in the United States. MMWR 33:6, 1986.
26. Butterfield WC: Surgical complications of narcotic addiction. Surg Gynecol Obstet 134:237, 1972.
27. Louria DB: Infectious complication of non-alcoholic drug abuse. Annu Rev Med 25:219, 1974.
28. Hagen DP: Public health and preventive medicine. J Am Osteopath Assoc 73:1012, 1974.
29. Redmond J, Stritch M, Blaney P: Severe tetanus in a narcotic addict. Ir Med J 77:325, 1984.
30. Hussey HH, Katz S: Infections resulting from narcotic addiction. Am J Med 9:186, 1950.
31. Jaffe RB, Koschmann EB: Intravenous drug abuse: Pulmonary, cardiac and vascular complications. AJR 109:107, 1970.
32. Jaffe RB, Koschmann EB: Septic pulmonary emboli. Radiology 96:527, 1970.
33. Joseph WL, Fletcher HS, Giordani JM, et al: Pulmonary and cardiovascular implications of drug addiction. Ann Thorac Surg 15:263, 1973.
34. Briggs JH, McKerron CG, Souhami RL, et al: Severe systemic infections complicating "mainline" heroin addiction. Lancet 2:1227, 1967.
35. Koval JC, Tenholder MF, Derderian SS: Rapidly cavitating nodules in a young man. Chest 88:625, 1985.
36. Fred HL, Harle TS: Septic pulmonary embolism. Dis Chest 55:483, 1969.
37. Williams MH Jr: Pulmonary complications of drug abuse. In: Fishman AP (ed): Pulmonary Diseases and Disorders. New York, McGraw-Hill, p 1465, 1988.
38. Levine DP, Cushing RD, Jui J, et al: Community-acquired methicillin-resistant Staphylococcus aureus endocarditis in the Detroit Medical Center. Ann Intern Med 97:330, 1982.
39. Reyes MR, Palutke WA, Wylin RF, et al: Pseudomonas endocarditis in the Detroit Medical Center. Medicine 53:173, 1973.
40. Shekar R, Rice TW, Zierdt CH, et al: Outbreak of endocarditis caused by Pseudomonas aeruginosa serotype O11 among pentazocine and tripelennamine abusers in Chicago. J Infect Dis 151:203, 1985.
41. Archer G, Fekety FR, Supena R: Pseudomonas aeruginosa endocarditis in drug addicts. Am Heart J 88:570, 1974.
42. Lam K, Bayer AS: Serious infection due to group G streptococci. Report of 15 cases with in vitro–in vivo correlations. Am J Med 75:561, 1983.
43. Barg NL, Kish MA, Kauffman CA, et al: Group A streptococcal bacteremia in intravenous drug abusers. Am J Med 78:569, 1985.
44. Banks T, Fletcher R, Ali N: Infective endocarditis in heroin addicts. Am J Med 55:444, 1973.
45. Cohen PS, Maguire JH, Weinstein L: Infective endocarditis caused by gram-negative bacteria: Review of the literature, 1945–1977. Prog Cardiovasc Dis 22:205, 1980.
46. Chiu CL, Roelofs JD: Acute bacterial endocarditis with septic emboli. J Iowa Med Soc 64:434, 1974.
47. Chambers H, Miller RT, Newman MD: Right-sided Staphylococcus aureus endocarditis in intravenous drug abusers: Two-week combination therapy. Ann Intern Med 109:619, 1988.
48. Small PM, Chambers HF: Vancomycin for Staphylococcus aureus endocarditis in intravenous drug abusers. Antimicrob Agents Chemother 34:1227, 1990.
49. Vidal E, LeVeen HH, Yarnoz M, et al: Lung abscess secondary to pulmonary infection. Ann Thorac Surg 11:557, 1971.
50. MacMillan JC, Milstein SH, Samson PC: Clinical spectrum of septic pulmonary embolism and infarction. J Thorac Cardiovasc Surg 75:670, 1978.
51. Light RW: Parapneumonic effusions and empyema. Clin Chest Med 6:55, 1985.
52. Blanck RR, Ream NW, Deleese JS: Infectious complications of illicit drug use. Int J Addict 19:221, 1984.
53. Louria DB, Hensle T, Rose J: The major medical complications of heroin addiction. Ann Intern Med 67:1, 1967.
54. Warnock ML, Ghahremani GG, Rattenborg C, et al: Pulmonary complications of heroin intoxication: Aspiration pneumonia and diffuse bronchiectasis. JAMA 219:1051, 1972.
55. SanDretto MA, Scanlon GT: Multiple mycotic pulmonary artery aneurysms secondary to intravenous drug abuse. AJR 142:89, 1974.
56. Morgan JM, Morgan AD, Addis BM, et al: Fatal haemorrhage from mycotic aneurysm of the pulmonary artery. Thorax 41:70, 1986.

57. Navarro C, Dickinson PCT, Kowdalapoodi P, et al: Mycotic aneurysms of the pulmonary arteries in intravenous drug addicts: Report of three cases and review of the literature. Am J Med 76:1124, 1984.

58. Reichman LB, Felton CP, Edsall JR: Drug dependence, a possible new risk factor for tuberculosis disease. Arch Intern Med 139:337, 1979.

59. Sapira JD: The narcotic addict as a medical patient. Am J Med 45:555, 1968.

60. Handwerger S, Mildvan D, Senie R: Tuberculosis and the acquired immunodeficiency syndrome at a New York City hospital: 1978–1985. Chest 91:176, 1987.

61. Selwyn PA, Hartel D, Lewis VA, et al: A prospective study of the risk of tuberculosis among intravenous drug users with human immunodeficiency virus infection. N Engl J Med 320:545, 1989.

62. Maayon S, Wormser GP, Hewlett D, et al: Acquired immunodeficiency syndrome (AIDS) in an economically disadvantaged population. Arch Intern Med 145:1607, 1985.

63. Sunderam G, McDonald RJ, Maniatis T, et al: Tuberculosis as a manifestation of the acquired immunodeficiency syndrome. JAMA 256:362, 1986.

64. Fischl MA, Pitchenik AE, Spira TJ: Tuberculosis brain abscess and Toxoplasma encephalitis in a patient with the acquired immunodeficiency syndrome. JAMA 253:3428, 1985.

65. Pitchenik AE, Burr J, Suarez M, et al: Human T-cell lymphotropic virus-III (HTLV-III) seropositivity and related disease among 71 consecutive patients in whom tuberculosis was diagnosed. Am Rev Respir Dis 135:875, 1987.

66. Murray JF, Felton CP, Garay SM, et al: Pulmonary complications of the acquired immunodeficiency syndrome: Report of a National Heart, Lung and Blood Institute workshop. N Engl J Med 310:1682, 1984.

67. American Thoracic Society Position Paper: Mycobacterioses and the acquired immunodeficiency syndrome. Am Rev Respir Dis 136:492, 1987.

68. Centers for Disease Control: Diagnosis and management of mycobacterial infection and disease in persons with human T-lymphotrophic virus type III/lymphadenopathy associated virus infection. MMWR 35:448, 1986.

69. Murray JF, Garay SM, Hopewell PC, et al: Pulmonary complications of the acquired immunodeficiency syndrome: An update. Am Rev Respir Dis 135:504, 1987.

70. Rothenberg R, Woelfel M, Stoneburner R, et al: Survival with the acquired immunodeficiency syndrome: Experience with 5833 cases in New York City. N Engl J Med 317:1297, 1987.

71. Wormser GP: AIDS in prisons. In: Wormser GP, Stahl RE, Bottone EJ (eds): AIDS-Acquired Immune Deficiency Syndrome and Other Manifestations of HIV Infection. Park Ridge, NJ: Noyes Publications, p 48, 1987.

72. Stover DE, White DA, Romano PA, et al: Diagnosis of pulmonary disease in acquired immune deficiency syndrome (AIDS). Role of bronchoscopy and bronchoalveolar lavage. Am Rev Respir Dis 130:659, 1984.

73. Masur H, Lane HC, Kovacs JA, et al: Pneumocystis pneumonia: From bench to clinic. Ann Intern Med 111:813, 1989.

74. Ambros RA, Lee E-Y, Sharer LR, et al: The acquired immunodeficiency syndrome in intravenous drug abusers and patients with a sexual risk: Clinical and postmortem comparisons. Hum Pathol 18:1109, 1987.

75. Oksenhendler E, Cadranel J, Sarfati C, et al: Toxoplasma gondii pneumonia in patients with the acquired immunodeficiency syndrome. Am J Med 88:18N, 1990.

76. Berk SL, Verghese A: Parasitic pneumonia. Semin Respir Infect 3:172, 1988.

77. Richmann S, Harris RD: Acute pulmonary edema associated with librium use. Radiology 103:57, 1972.

78. Allred RJ, Ewer S: Fatal pulmonary edema following intravenous "freebase" cocaine use. Ann Emerg Med 10:441, 1981.

79. Sklar J, Timms RM: Codeine-induced pulmonary edema. Chest 72:230, 1977.

80. Glauser FL, Smith WR, Caldwell A, et al: Ethchlorvynol (placidyl)–induced pulmonary edema. Ann Intern Med 84:46, 1976.

81. Presant S, Knight L, Klassen G: Methadone-induced pulmonary edema. Can Med Assoc J 113:966, 1975.

82. Mountain R, Ferguson S, Fowler A, et al: Noncardiac pulmonary edema following administration of paraldehyde. Chest 82:371, 1982.

83. Fisch HP, Wands J, Yeung J, et al: Pulmonary edema and disseminated intravascular coagulation after intravenous abuse of d-propoxyphene (Darvon). South Med J 65:493, 1972.

84. Anderson RJ, Garza HR, Garriot JC, et al: Intravenous propylhexedrine (Benzedrez) abuse and sudden death. Am J Med 67:15, 1979.

85. Stern WZ: Roentgenographic aspects of narcotic addiction. JAMA 236:963, 1976.

86. Stern WZ, Subbarao K: Pulmonary complications of drug addiction. Semin Roentgenol 18:183, 1983.

87. Light RW, Dunham TR: Severe slowly resolving heroin-induced pulmonary edema. Chest 67:63, 1975.

88. Katz S, Aberman A, Frand VR, et al: Heroin pulmonary edema: Evidence for increased pulmonary capillary permeability. Am Rev Respir Dis 106:472, 1972.

89. Duberstein JL, Kaufman DM: A clinical study of an epidemic of heroin intoxication and heroin-induced pulmonary edema. Am J Med 51:704, 1971.

90. Frand UI, Shim CS, Williams H: Heroin-induced pulmonary edema: Sequential studies of pulmonary function. Ann Intern Med 77:29, 1972.

91. Karlinger JS, Steinberg AD, Williams MH: Lung function after pulmonary edema associated with heroin overdose. Arch Intern Med 124:350, 1969.

92. Leechawengwong M, Berger HW, Jaymanne DS: Long-term serial follow-up after two episodes of heroin-induced adult respiratory distress syndrome. Mt Sinai J Med 46:119, 1979.

93. Tuazon CU, Sheagren JN: Staphylococcal endocarditis in parenteral drug abusers: Source of the organism. Ann Intern Med 82:788, 1975.

94. Botsford KB, Weinstein RA, Nathan CR, et al: Selective survival in pentazocine and tripelennamine of Pseudomonas aeruginosa serotype O11 from drug addicts. J Infect Dis 151:209, 1985.

95. Rajashekaraiah KR, Rice TW, Kallick CA: Recovery of Pseudomonas aeruginosa from syringes of drug addicts with endocarditis. J Infect Dis 144:482, 1981.

96. Roberts WC, Buchbinder NA: Right-sided valvular infective endocarditis. A clinicopathologic study of twelve necropsy patients. Am J Med 53:7, 1972.

97. Buchbinder NA, Roberts WC: Left-sided valvular active infective endocarditis. A study of forty-five necropsy patients. Am J Med 53:20, 1972.

98. Mills J, Drew D: Serratia marcescens endocarditis: A regional illness associated with intravenous drug abuse. Ann Intern Med 84:29, 1976.

99. El-Khatib MR, Wilson FM, Lerner AM: Characteristics of bacterial endocarditis in heroin addicts in Detroit. Am J Med Sci 271:197, 1976.

100. Garvey GJ, Neu HC: Infective endocarditis—An evolving disease. Medicine 57:105, 1978.

101. Menda KB, Gorbach SL: Favorable experience with bacterial endocarditis in heroin addicts. Ann Intern Med 78:25, 1973.

102. Pelletier LL Jr, Petersdorf RG: Infective endocarditis: A review of 125 cases from the University of Washington Hospitals, 1963–72. Medicine 56:287, 1977.

103. Neufeld GK, Branson CG, Marshall LW, et al: Infective endocarditis as a complication of heroin use. South Med J 69:1148, 1976.

104. Harris PD, Yeoh CB, Breault J, et al: Fungal endocarditis secondary to drug addiction. J Thorac Cardiovasc Surg 63:980, 1972.

105. Rubinstein E, Noriega EB, Simberkoff MS, et al: Fungal endocarditis: Analysis of 24 cases and review of the literature. Medicine 54:331, 1975.

106. Stimmel B, Donoso E, Dack S: Comparison of infective endocarditis in drug addicts and nondrug users. Am J Cardiol 32:924, 1973.

107. Balthazar EJ, Hilton S, Naidich D, et al: CT of splenic and perisplenic abnormalities in septic patients. AJR 144:53, 1985.

108. Neugarten J, Baldwin DS: Glomerulonephritis in bacterial endocarditis. Am J Med 77:297, 1984.

109. Dreyer NP, Fields BN: Heroin-associated infective endocarditis. A report of 28 cases. Ann Intern Med 78:699, 1973.

110. Reiner NE, Gopalakrishna KV, Lerner PI: Enterococcal endocarditis in heroin addicts. JAMA 235:1861, 1976.

111. Neu HC, Garvey GJ, Beach MP: Successful treatment of Pseudomonas cepacia endocarditis in a heroin addict with trimethoprim-sulfamethoxazole. J Infect Dis 128(suppl):S768, 1973.

112. Von Reyn CF, Levy BS, Arbeit RD, et al: Infective endocarditis: An analysis based on strict case definitions. Ann Intern Med 94:505, 1986.

113. Reyes MP, Brown WJ, Lerner AM: Treatment of patients with pseudomonas endocarditis with high dose aminoglycoside and carbenicillin therapy. Medicine 57:57, 1978.

114. Reyes MP, El-Khatib MR, Brown WJ, et al: Synergy between carbenicillin and an aminoglycoside (gentamicin or tobramycin) against Pseudomonas aeruginosa isolated from patients with endocarditis and sensitivity of isolates to normal human serum. J Infect Dis 140:192, 1979.

115. Levine DP, Fromm BS, Reddy BR: Slow response to vancomycin or vancomycin plus rifampin therapy among patients with methicillin-resistant Staphylococcus aureus endocarditis. Ann Intern Med 115:674, 1991.

116. Wieland M, Lederman MM, Kline-King, C, et al: Left-sided endocarditis due to Pseudomonas aeruginosa. A report of 10 cases and review of the literature. Medicine 65:180, 1986.

117. Rubinstein E, Noriega ER, Simberkoff MS, et al: Tissue penetration of amphotericin B in candida endocarditis. Chest 66:376, 1974.

118. Weinstein L: Life-threatening complications of infective endocarditis and their management. Arch Intern Med 146:953, 1986.

119. Robbins MJ, Frater RWM, Soeiro R, et al: Influence of vegetation size on clinical outcome of right-sided infective endocarditis. Am J Med 80:165, 1986.

120. Robbins MJ, Soeiro R, Frishman WH, et al: Right-sided valvular endocarditis: Etiology, diagnosis, and an approach to therapy. Am Heart J 111:128, 1986.

121. Bayer AS, Blomquist IK, Bello E, et al: Tricuspid valve endocarditis due to Staphylococcus aureus. Correlation of two-dimensional echocardiography with clinical outcome. Chest 93:247, 1988.

122. Richardson JV, Karp RB, Kirklins JW, et al: Treatment of infective endocarditis: A 10-year comparative analysis. Circulation 58:589, 1978.

123. DiNubile M: Surgery for addiction-related tricuspid valve endocarditis: Caveat emptor. Am J Med 82:811, 1987.

124. Organ CH: Surgical procedures upon the drug addict. Surg Gynecol Obstet 134:947, 1972.
125. Vollum DI: Skin lesions in drug addicts. Br Med J 2:647, 1970.
126. Geelhoed GW: Surgical (and medical) sequelae of drug addiction. Med Ann DC 43:307, 1974.
127. Fullarton GM: Soft tissue infections in drug abusers presenting to an accident and emergency department. Health Bull 41:296, 1983.
128. Wallace JR, Lucas CE, Ledgerwood A: Social, economic, and surgical anatomy of a drug-related abscess. Am Surg 52:398, 1986.
129. Merhar GL, Colley DP, Clark RA: Cervicothoracic complications of intravenous drug abuse. Comput Tomogr 5:271, 1981.
130. Tom MB, Rice DH: Presentation and management of neck abscess: A retrospective analysis. Laryngoscope 98:877, 1988.
131. Myers EM, Kirkland LK, Mickey R: The head and neck sequelae of cervical intravenous drug abuse. Laryngoscope 98:213, 1988.
132. O'Sullivan M, Beatie T, Keane CT: A review of drug addict abscesses. Ir Med J 77:68, 1984.
133. Hasan SB, Albu E, Gerst PH: Infectious complications in IV drug abusers. Infect Surg 7:218, 1988.
134. Webb D, Thadepalli H: Skin and soft tissue polymicrobial infections from intravenous abuse of drugs. West J Med 130:200, 1979.
135. Petrie PW, Lamb DW: Severe hand problems in drug addicts following self-administered injections. Hand 5:130, 1973.
136. Lewis RJ, Richmons AS, McGrory JP: *Diplococcus pneumoniae* cellulitis in drug addicts. JAMA 232:54, 1975.
137. Tennont FS: Complications of propoxyphene abuse. Arch Intern Med 132:191, 1973.
138. Zeplenyi J, Colman MF: Deep neck abscess is secondary to methylphenidate (Ritalin) abuse. Head Neck Surg 6:858, 1984.
139. Gorbach SL, Thadepalli H: Isolation of clostridium in human infections: Evaluations of 114 cases. J Infect Dis 131(suppl):S81, 1975.
140. Sander B: Carotid triangle abscess secondary to heroin injection. J Oral Med 31:88, 1976.
141. Gitschlag KF, Sandler MA, Madrazo BL, et al: Disease in the femoral triangle: Sonographic appearance. AJR 139:515, 1982.
142. Yiengpruksawan A, Ganepola AP, Freeman HP: Acute soft tissue infection in intravenous drug abusers: Its differential diagnosis by ultrasonography. J Natl Med Assoc 78:1193, 1986.
143. Hahn HH, Schweid AI, Beaty HN: Complications of injecting dissolved methylphenidate tablets. Arch Intern Med 123:656, 1969.
144. Seymour R, Raynor C: Extensive leg ulceration from intravenous use of pentazocine. Am Surg 40:671, 1974.
145. Palestine RF, Millins JD, Spigel GT, et al: Skin manifestations of pentazocine abuse. J Am Acad Dermatol 2:47, 1980.
146. Padilla RS, Becker LE, Hoggman H, et al: Cutaneous and venous complications of pentazocine abuse. Arch Dermatol 115:975, 1979.
147. Kirchenbaum SE, Midenberg ML: Pedal and lower extremity complications of substance abuse. J Am Podiatry Assoc 72:380, 1982.
148. Merhar GL, Colley DP, Clark RA, et al: Computed tomographic demonstration of cervical abscess and jugular vein thrombosis. A complication of intravenous drug abuse in the neck. Arch Otolaryngol 107:313, 1981.
149. Ford PV, Parker HG: Unsuspected deep venous thrombophlebitis detected by gallium-67 imaging. Clin Nucl Med 12:556, 1987.
150. Stuck RM, Doyle D: Superficial thrombophlebitis following parenteral cocaine abuse. A case report. J Am Podiatry Assoc 77:351, 1987.
151. Schecter W, Meyer A, Schecter G, et al: Necrotizing fasciitis of the upper extremity. J Hand Surg [Am] 7:15, 1982.
152. Sunarsky LA, Laschinger JC, Coppa GF, et al: Improved results from a standardized approach in treating patients with necrotizing fasciitis. Ann Surg 206:661, 1987.
153. Jacobson JM, Hirschmann SZ: Necrotizing fasciitis complicating intravenous drug abuse. Arch Intern Med 142:634, 1982.
154. Clark DD: Surgical management of infections and other complications resulting from drug abuse. Arch Surg 101:619, 1970.

CHAPTER 49

Infections in the Organ Transplant Recipient

Robert H. Rubin

Each year in the United States approximately 17,000 organ transplantations are carried out, with an equal number being performed in the rest of the world. At present, there is an 80 to 85% chance that the allograft will be functioning at the end of 1 year, whether the organ be a heart, a liver, or a kidney (and the results of lung and pancreas transplantation are rapidly improving to reach the same level). These results represent a improvement from a mere decade ago, when the 1-year graft survival was only slightly better than 50%. Despite this striking improvement, infection continues to threaten both short-term and long-term survival of the transplant patient; at least 75% of patients have some form of clinically significant infection after transplantation, and infection, often accompanied by allograft rejection, is the leading cause of death in this population of patients.[1]

The infectious disease problems of the organ transplant patient present a unique challenge to the clinician for several reasons: the range of infections is broad, including a group of pathogens that rarely cause disease in normal hosts; many of these pathogens, because of the exogenous immunosuppressive therapy that is required to maintain allograft function, produce chronic and/or relapsing infection that has clinical effects far beyond those observed in other populations of patients; the clinical manifestations of the infection are often quite subtle until the disease is far advanced; and therapy, often with potentially toxic drugs that can interact adversely with the immunosuppressive drugs, usually must be prolonged.[1-3] In view of these challenges, the purpose of this chapter is to present an approach to the prevention and management of the infectious disease problems of the organ transplant recipient, particularly as they apply to the intensive care unit.

RISK FACTORS IN THE DEVELOPMENT OF INFECTION IN THE TRANSPLANT PATIENT

The risk of infection in general, and of opportunistic infection in particular, in organ transplant patients is due to the interaction of two major factors: the *epidemiologic exposures* the individual encounters and the patient's *net state of immunosuppression*. If the exposure is great enough, even minimally immunosuppressed individuals become infected; conversely, if the net state of immunosuppression is great enough, microorganisms that normally produce little or no disease may cause life-threatening infection. Indeed, the term opportunistic infection is meant to connote either the occurrence of significant infection with organisms unable to produce such infection in the normal host (e.g., disseminated aspergillosis) or the occurrence of clinical syndromes of a type and severity unknown in the normal host, although clinically trivial infections with such organisms may be observed (e.g., disseminated visceral candidiasis vs. vaginal candidiasis).[1-4]

The epidemiologic exposures that are of importance in the transplant patient can be divided into three general categories:[1-4]

1. Remote exposures to tuberculosis, the geographically restricted endemic mycoses (*Coccidioides immitis, Histoplasma capsulatum,* and *Blastomyces dermatitidis*), and *Strongyloides stercoralis.*

2. Recent exposures within the community to such pathogens as influenza, tuberculosis, the endemic mycoses, and such organisms as *Listeria monocytogenes* and nontyphoidal salmonellae that can contaminate foodstuffs.

3. Nosocomial exposures to such pathogens as *Aspergillus* and *Legionella* species.

From this list it is clear that exposure to both *Mycobacterium tuberculosis* and the systemic endemic mycoses can occur at two points in the transplant patient's life that could have clinical consequences. On the one hand, exposure in the remote past could lead to smoldering infection capable of being reactivated, resulting even in disseminated infection, with the initiation of immunosuppressive therapy. On the other hand, individuals who encounter these organisms for the first time after transplantation can develop progressive, primary infection, resulting again in disseminated disease. Finally, because of the immunosuppressed state, an individual with past experience with one of these microbial agents, and thus apparently rendered immune to reinfection, may be superinfected if sufficient exposure occurs.[1-4]

S. stercoralis represents a special problem. Because of its unique autoinfection cycle, asymptomatic carriage in the gastrointestinal tract may persist for decades after an individual leaves an endemic region. Initiation of immunosuppressive therapy can result in two major clinical syndromes: a hyperinfection syndrome, which is an exaggerated form of the usual manifestations of this infection, resulting in hemorrhagic pneumonia and/or colitis; and a disseminated infection syndrome, in which these helminths migrate throughout the body, carrying with them normal gastrointestinal flora, so that the clinical syndrome may include gram-negative bacteremia and/or meningitis. Because routine ova and parasite testing before transplantation has a low diagnostic yield, we usually treat "on an epidemiologic basis" before transplantation individuals with histories of residence in Southeast Asia, Latin America, Africa, and other developing areas of the world. Such pre-emptive therapy with thiabendazole is far easier to accomplish than the management of one of the disastrous post-transplantation syndromes.[1, 5, 6]

Community-wide influenza outbreaks can have a significant impact on transplant populations, resulting in a high incidence of both influenzal and secondary bacterial pneumonias. Although both influenza and pneumococcal vaccines can be given to transplant patients without harm to the allograft, efficacy is far less than that in the normal population, and consideration should be given to the initiation of amantadine prophylaxis to these patients in the setting of community influenza outbreaks.[7]

Of greatest epidemiologic concern are the exposures that occur within the hospital environment. Two types of epidemics have been well documented to occur: *domiciliary* epidemics, in which air contaminated with such organisms as *Aspergillus fumigatus, Legionella pneumophila,* or *Pseudomonas aeruginosa* is aerosolized into the rooms in which patients reside in the hospital, such as the transplant unit or the intensive care unit; and *nondomiciliary* epidemics, in which the exposure occurs at a central location within the hospital environment to which the patient is taken for an essential procedure, examples being radiology suites or operating rooms. Whereas domiciliary epidemics are usually identified rather easily on the basis of clustering of cases in time and space, the nondomiciliary epidemics are far more difficult to identify. Typically, problems arise in the hospital environment in association with hospital construction (in the case of *Aspergillus*) or contamination of some part of the water system (in the case of *Legionella* infection). The point to be emphasized is that the immunosuppressed transplant patient is like a "sentinel chicken" who reflects any and all excessive traffic in microbes, particularly within the hospital environment. Within the hospital, especially in the intensive care unit, consideration should be given to protecting the patient against undue environmental exposures with such measures as providing high-efficiency particulate air–filtered rooms.[3, 8]

The net state of immunosuppression is a rather complex function determined by a numbers of factors:[1-3]

1. The dose, duration, and temporal sequence of deployment of immunosuppressive agents.

2. The presence of granulocytopenia.

3. The presence of significant injury to the primary mucocutaneous barrier to infection or of foreign bodies such as intravenous catheters, endotracheal tubes, and/or bladder and biliary tract catheters that bypass or render inefficient this critical host defense. (It is clear that this factor is of particular importance in the intensive care unit, where invasive monitoring and therapeutic interventions are the rule.)

4. A variety of incompletely understood metabolic abnormalities such as protein malnutrition, uremia, and hyperglycemia.

5. The presence of infection with one or more of the immunomodulating viruses: human immunodeficiency virus, hepatitis B and C viruses, Epstein-Barr virus (EBV), and, most important, cytomegalovirus (CMV). The importance of this factor is underlined by the following observation: at Massachusetts General Hospital during a 5-year period, renal transplant patients with opportunistic infection could be divided into two general categories—those with underlying viral infection (the vast majority) and those who had suffered an unusually intense epidemiologic exposure. Indeed, the presence of opportunistic infection in the absence of immunomodulating viral infection in organ transplant patients should initiate a search for an unsuspected environmental exposure.[1-3]

From the preceding discussion, it is apparent that the infectious disease problems of particular importance can be divided into three general categories (Table 49–1): those related to technical mishaps, those related to particular epidemiologic exposures, and those related to certain viruses that chronically infect (often latently) many individuals and are then activated by immunosuppressive therapy. Whereas immunosuppression is a contributory factor in the first two categories, it is the prime mover of the viral infections.

EFFECTS OF IMMUNOSUPPRESSIVE THERAPY ON THE OCCURRENCE OF INFECTION IN TRANSPLANT PATIENTS

Clearly, the major identifiable factor in the pathogenesis of infection in the transplant patient is the antirejection therapy that is administered. The following general principles should be kept in mind as one approaches this issue:

1. As with cancer chemotherapy, the strategy that has emerged thus far involves the deployment of multiple drugs to achieve the desired antirejection effect to minimize the toxicity from any one agent. Because of this, rather than relating risk of infection to any one agent, the net effects of the entire program must be defined.[1-3]

2. Different immunosuppressive agents administered at doses with equal antirejection effects can have different

TABLE 49–1

CLASSIFICATION OF INFECTIONS OCCURRING IN TRANSPLANT PATIENTS

Infections related to technical complications*
    Transplantation of a contaminated allograft
    Anastomotic leak or stenosis
    Wound hematoma
    Intravenous line contamination
    Urinary or biliary catheter contamination
    Iatrogenic damage to the skin
Infections related to excessive nosocomial hazard
    Aspergillus spp.
    Legionella spp.
    P. aeruginosa and other gram-negative bacilli
    Nocardia asteroides
Infections related to particular exposures within the community
    Systemic mycotic infections in certain geographic areas
        H. capsulatum
        C. immitis
        B. dermatitidis
    Community-acquired opportunistic infection resulting from
        ubi quitious saprophytes in the environment†
        Cryptococcus neoformans
        Aspergillus spp.
        N. asteroides
        Pneumocystis carinii
    M. tuberculosis
    S. stercoralis
    Respiratory infections circulating in the community
        Influenza
        Adenoviruses
    Infections acquired by ingestion of contaminated food or water
        Salmonella spp.
        L. monocytogenes
Viral infections of particular importance in transplant patients
    Herpes group viruses
    Hepatitis viruses
    Papovaviruses
    Human immunodeficiency virus (the causative agent of
        acquired immunodeficiency syndrome)
    Adenoviruses

*All lead to infection with gram-negative bacilli, *Staphylococcus* spp., and/or *Candida* spp.

†The incidence and severity of these infections and, to a lesser extent, the other infections listed are directly related to the net state of immunosuppression in a particular patient.

Modified from Rubin RH: Infection in the renal and liver transplant patient. In Rubin RH, Young LS (eds): Clinical Approach to Infection in the Compromised Host. 2nd ed. New York, Plenum Publishing, p 557, 1988.

effects on the progress of certain forms of infection. For example, whereas antilymphocyte antibodies (either polyclonal, such as antithymocyte globulin, or monoclonal, such as OKT3) are extremely potent at reactivating latent CMV infection, they are only moderately active in promoting replicating viral infection. In contrast, other drugs such as cyclosporine have no ability to reactivate latent viral infection but are extremely potent in promoting replicating viral infection because of their profound effect on virus-specific cytotoxic T cells, the critical host defense against viral infection. From the point of view of infection, the worst possible strategy is to use a regimen in which an antilymphocyte antibody is given that reactivates virus, followed by a drug such as cyclosporine that blocks the host's ability to respond to this virus. Recognizing this, means of countering such events must be incorporated in the therapeutic program whenever antirejection considerations dictate such a strategy (discussed later).[9, 10]

3. The daily dose of immunosuppressive drugs is less important in determining the net immunosuppressive effect than the cumulative doses over time, the "area under the curve." This is perhaps best illustrated by the observation that whereas the highest daily doses of immunosuppressive drugs are administered in the first 2 weeks after transplantation, opportunistic infection is virtually unknown during this time. Another way of stating this is to make an analogy to buying goods via credit card: increasing immunosuppressive therapy is likely to result in immediate benefit in terms of allograft function; the bill, in terms of significant infection, does not come due for several weeks.[1–3]

4. Every immunosuppressive agent or program that has been or is being developed increases the risk of one or another form of infection. This almost assuredly will remain true until the goal of specific tolerance can be achieved on a regular basis and nonspecific immunosuppression is no longer necessary. The strategy that has emerged to make immunosuppressive therapy safer is to define the types and incidence of given infectious disease problems. One then prescribes an antimicrobial program concomitantly with the immunosuppressive program to allow the patient to enjoy the benefits of the antirejection therapy, while minimizing the infectious disease consequences of such therapy. For example, low-dose trimethoprim-sulfamethoxazole prophylaxis effectively protects the transplant patient against *Pneumocystis carinii*, *L. monocytogenes*, and *Nocardia asteroides* infection. Also, various strategies are now emerging for preventing serious CMV and EBV disease in transplant patients (discussed later), based on immunosuppression-triggered antiviral prophylaxis. Thus, it has been suggested that the therapeutic program for the transplant patient should include both antirejection and anti-infection prophylaxis.[10]

TIMETABLE OF INFECTION AFTER ORGAN TRANSPLANTATION

As already emphasized, both the duration and the temporal sequence of immunosuppressive therapy have an important effect on the net state of immunosuppression and the occurrence of different infections in the transplant patient. This concept can be translated into a practical "timetable" that presents the differential diagnosis in transplant patients who present with such infectious disease clinical syndromes as pneumonia or unexplained fever at different time points in the post-transplantation course (Fig. 49–1). In organ transplant recipients, the post-transplantation course can be divided into three separate periods: the first month after transplantation, the period 1 to 6 months after transplantation, and the late period, more than 6 months after transplantation.[1, 2]

Infection in the First Month After Transplantation

Three categories of infection may occur in the first month after transplantation. (1) Infection present in the recipient before transplantation that is exacerbated by the surgical procedure, general anesthesia, and/or initiation of immunosuppressive therapy. It is axiomatic that every effort must be made to eradicate or prevent infection before transplantation. This is particularly important in liver transplant candidates, who, because of an acceleration in the gravity of their liver disease while they await transplantation, develop such complications as aspiration pneumonia or spontaneous bacterial peritonitis. Transplantation in the presence of such processes is doomed to failure. (2) Infection conveyed with the allograft. Of particular concern is acute bacterial contamination of the organ with gram-negative bacteria, especially *P. aeruginosa*, *Staphylococcus aureus*, or *Candida* species, during the terminal stages of a potential cadaveric donor's illness because of the intravenous lines, catheters, and endotracheal

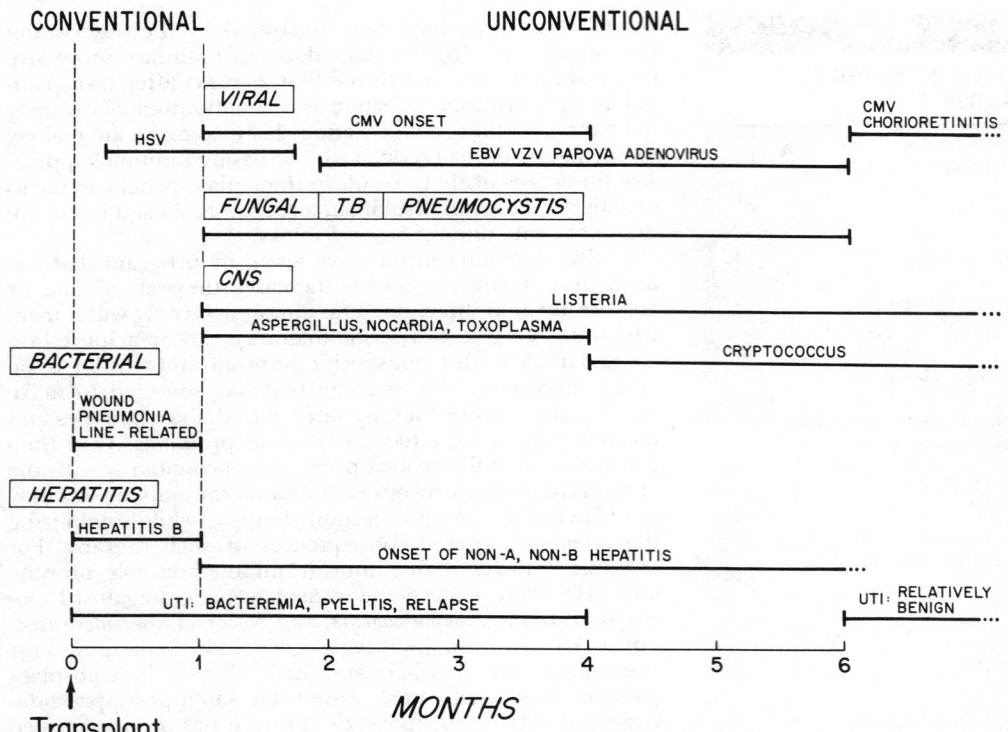

Figure 49–1. Timetable for occurrence of infection in the organ transplant recipient. Exceptions to this timetable should initiate a search for an unusual environmental hazard. CMV = cytomegalovirus; HSV = herpes simplex virus; EBV = Epstein-Barr virus; VZV = varicella-zoster virus; CNS = central nervous system; UTI = urinary tract infection. (Modified from Rubin RH, Wolfson JS, Cosimi AB, et al: Infection in the renal transplant recipient. Am J Med 70:405, 1981.)

tube that are part of such care. Less commonly, microbial contamination may occur during the organ procurement procedure. Transplantation of contaminated organs results in disseminated infection, as well as such major local complications as disrupted suture lines and mycotic aneurysms. (3) The usual postoperative wound, urine, catheter-related, or pulmonary infections that occur after comparable surgery in nonimmunosuppressed patients. This category accounts for more than 90% of infections occurring in this period. Although the incidence of such infections can probably be decreased with a short course of peritransplantation antibiotics, the major factors determining the occurrence of these complications are the technical skill involved in the surgical procedure, the management of the endotracheal tube, and the use of lines, drains, and catheters. A technical mishap in this population of patients virtually guarantees a clinically significant infection.[1, 2]

Infection 1 to 6 Months After Transplantation

The highest incidence of clinically important infection occurs in this period. By far the most important are the infections with viruses—CMV, EBV, the hepatitis viruses, and (if the donor was infected) primary human immunodeficiency virus. These infections are important in themselves and because of their contribution to the net state of immunosuppression. Because of these immunomodulating viruses, and because the duration of immunosuppression has now been long enough to lower host defenses significantly, opportunistic infections with such organisms as *A. fumigatus*, *L. monocytogenes*, and *P. carinii* are not uncommon during this time. Recognizing that these patients are particularly vulnerable to these pathogens at this time, special attention should be directed toward protecting them from environmental hazards (e.g., providing care in high-efficiency particulate air–filtered environments) and providing effective anti-*Pneumocystis* prophylaxis (discussed later).[1-3]

Infection More than 6 Months After Transplantation

Organ transplant patients who receive maintenance immunosuppression to maintain long-term allograft function can be divided into three categories in terms of infectious disease problems: (1) Patients with chronic viral infection with CMV, EBV, hepatitis B and viruses C, and human immunodeficiency virus have progressive disease because of these infections. Thus, progressive CMV chorioretinitis, EBV-induced lymphoproliferative disease, progressive liver disease and/or hepatocellular carcinoma, and overt acquired immunodeficiency syndrome are the eventual results of the interaction between chronic viral infection and chronic immunosuppressive therapy. Such patients account for approximately 10 to 15% of the transplant population who reach this stage in their post-transplantation course. (2) Patients with good allograft function, who are receiving baseline immunosuppressive therapy, are at risk for the same infections that affect the general community—influenza, pneumococcal pneumonia, urinary tract infection, and so forth. They are at relatively low risk of opportunistic or overwhelming infection. Fortunately, this category includes the majority of patients who reach this time point. (3) Patients with poor allograft function, who have received too much acute and chronic immunosuppressive therapy and who often have chronic viral infection with CMV, hepatitis B or C virus, or human immunodeficiency virus. These patients, although relatively few in number, are at the highest risk of opportunistic infection, particularly with *Cryptococcus neoformans*, *P. carinii*, *A. fumigatus*, *L. monocytogenes*, and *N. asteroides*.[1-4]

INFECTIOUS DISEASE SYNDROMES OF PARTICULAR IMPORTANCE IN THE TRANSPLANT RECIPIENT
Fever of Unclear Origin

The differential diagnosis of fever in the transplant recipient is quite broad, including both noninfectious and infectious etiologies. The two major noninfectious causes of fever in the transplant patient are thromboembolic disease and drug reactions.

Thromboembolic disease refers particularly to deep venous thrombophlebitis and pulmonary emboli but also includes thrombosis of the vascular anastomosis to the allograft resulting in tissue infarction (usually, particularly in the liver transplant patient, followed by secondary bacterial and candidal infection). Venous thromboembolic disease at one time was common in the first few weeks after transplantation, related to surgical manipulation of pelvic vessels and postoperative restrictions on ambulation. Occlusion of the vascular anastomosis is a particular issue in liver transplantation, especially pediatric liver transplantation, in which the size of the vessels to be anastomosed can represent a major challenge. Fortunately, as surgical technique has improved and experience has been gained, thromboembolic causes of fever have become quite uncommon.

Transplant patients are administered a wide variety of medications, with varying potential for inducing febrile reactions. Classic drug reactions to antimicrobial agents, especially β-lactam and sulfonamide drugs, anticonvulsants, and antiarrhythmic agents, do occur in transplant recipients but, presumably because of the immunosuppressive therapy, less commonly than in the normal population. Administration of the antilymphocyte antibodies, both the equine and rabbit polyclonal preparations (e.g., antilymphocyte serum and antithymocyte globulin) and the murine monoclonal antibody OKT3, to treat rejection is frequently associated with febrile reactions. Typically, the first infusion is associated with the highest temperature response, with lesser elevations occurring with the subsequent two or three doses, after which the patient has little response to this therapy. Not infrequently, however, after 10 to 14 days of such therapy fevers reappear because of an immunologic response to the foreign protein. Such a response often is associated with accelerated clearing of the antibody, as well as decreased antirejection potency, as shown by evidence of decreased clearance of T lymphocytes from the circulation by flow cytometric measurement. Either the dose of the antibody preparation has to be increased to achieve the desired antirejection effect or alternative immunosuppressive therapies must be employed.[11, 12]

The infectious causes of fever in the transplant patient vary according to the timetable in Figure 49–1. In the first month, virtually all microbial processes causing fever are due to technical aspects of the transplantation procedure and the postoperative management. Thus, the evaluation of such patients includes chest x-ray films to rule out aspiration pneumonia, blood cultures to rule out line sepsis, urinalysis and urine culture to rule out urosepsis, and ultrasonography of the surgical wound to rule out deep wound infection. In contrast, in the period 1 to 6 months after transplantation CMV alone accounts for more than two thirds of febrile episodes;[13, 14] the differential diagnosis in the late period is far broader, reflecting more closely the patient's epidemiologic exposures and how they interact with the patient's net state of immunosuppression.

While the febrile patient is being evaluated, the critical question that the clinician must answer is whether empirical antimicrobial therapy should be instituted while awaiting culture data and, if so, what this should include. In general, emergent institution of antiviral or antifungal therapy is usually not necessary before the culture results are obtained. In contrast, antibacterial therapy may be necessary. The three considerations that should be kept in mind in approaching this issue are whether the patient is leukopenic, whether he or she appears toxic, and whether true rigors have been noted. If the answer to any one of these questions

is yes, broad-spectrum antimicrobial therapy aimed at both gram-positive and gram-negative pathogens should be instituted after adequate cultures have been obtained.

Pneumonia

Pneumonia is the most common form of life-threatening infection encountered in the transplant patient. Although the timetable in Figure 49–1 presents a useful general overview of the differential diagnosis of pneumonia in transplant patients, further information can be gained by paying attention to four other types of clue: the clinical and epidemiologic setting in which the pulmonary process is occurring, the rate of progression of the illness, the pattern of radiologic abnormality produced on chest radiography, and the effect of the pneumonitis on pulmonary function tests and arterial blood gas measurements.[15]

Perhaps the most useful clue to the correct diagnosis comes from an assessment of the mode of onset and rate of progression of the pulmonary process. Thus, an acute onset during less than 24 hours of symptoms severe enough to bring the patient to medical attention suggests conventional bacterial infection (and, of the noninfectious causes, pulmonary embolic disease, pulmonary edema, a leukoagglutinin reaction, or pulmonary hemorrhage). A subacute onset during a few days to a week suggests viral or *Pneumocystis* infection or, in some instances, fungal or *Nocardia* infection. A more chronic course during 1 week or more suggests fungal, nocardial, or tuberculous infection. When the mode of clinical presentation is combined with the radiologic finding, the range of etiologic possibilities becomes considerably more limited and much more manageable for the clinician[15] (Table 49–2).

Additional useful information may be obtained by measuring the arterial blood gases while the patient is breathing room air. Most of the causes of the acute pneumonias, as well as such causes of the subacute pneumonias as viral and *Pneumocystis* infection, are associated with significant impairment in oxygenation early in the clinical course (room air $PaO_2 < 65$ mm Hg). By contrast, most patients with pulmonary disease caused by fungi, tuberculosis, and *Nocardia* have relatively well-maintained oxygenation, despite even extensive consolidation on x-ray films, until late in the clinical course. Although a rare patient with these three forms of infection has an acute overwhelming pneumonia resembling acute bacterial infection in both clinical presentation and arterial blood gas findings, the great majority have subacute or chronic presentations associated with well-preserved oxygenation.[15]

Organ transplant patients with pneumonia differ in one important respect from such other immunocompromised patients with pneumonia as those with acquired immunodeficiency syndrome or leukemia: whereas the other patients have a limited prognosis even if they recover from the current episode of pulmonary infection, the organ transplant patient has the potential for many years of useful and comfortable life. Therefore, the obligation of the clinician to make a specific diagnosis and effect prompt therapy is particularly important in this population of patients. This is especially true because the use of cyclosporine-based immunosuppression makes the possibility of drug interactions and toxicities important (discussed later). Hence, we take an aggressive approach to diagnosis rather than relying just on empirical therapy. In the first month after transplantation, induced sputum specimens or bronchoscopy is the usual basis of diagnosis, as is the case later in the course for patients with postinfluenzal pneumonias. In other situations, more invasive procedures are usually employed. In the patient with rapidly evolving disease who represents a ther-

TABLE 49–2

DIFFERENTIAL DIAGNOSES OF FEVER AND PULMONARY INFILTRATES IN THE ORGAN TRANSPLANT RECIPIENT ACCORDING TO ROENTGENOGRAPHIC ABNORMALITY AND RATE OF PROGRESSION OF THE SYMPTOMS[a]

Chest Radiographic Abnormality	Etiology According to Rate of Progression of the Illness*	
	Acute	*Subacute-Chronic*
Consolidation	Bacterial	Fungal
	Thromboembolic	Nocardial
	Hemorrhagic	Tuberculous
	(Pulmonary edema)	(Viral, *Pneumocystis*)
Peribronchovascular ("interstitial") infiltrate	Pulmonary edema	Viral
	Leukoagglutinin reaction	*Pneumocystis*
	(Bacterial)	(Fungal, nocardial, tuberculous)
Nodular infiltrate	(Bacterial, pulmonary edema)	Fungal
		Nocardial
		Tuberculous
		(*Pneumocystis*, viral)

*An acute illness is one developing and requiring medical attention in a relatively few hours (<24 h). A subacute-chronic process develops during several days to weeks. Unusual causes of a process are placed in parentheses here.

Modified from Rubin RH, Greene R: Etiology and management of the compromised patient with fever and pulmonary infiltrates. In Rubin RH, Young LS (eds): Clinical Approach to Infection in the Compromised Host. 2nd ed. New York, Plenum Publishing, p 131, 1988.

apeutic emergency, open lung biopsy should be considered. In the patient who represents more of a diagnostic dilemma, either brochoscopy with lavage and transbronchial biopsy or percutaneous aspiration under radiologic guidance should be employed—utilizing the bronchscopic techniques for diffuse lung disease and percutaneous aspiration for focal, particularly cavitary, disease.[15]

Central Nervous System Infection

Between 5 and 10% of organ transplant recipients have central nervous system (CNS) infection after transplantation, with four distinct clinical syndromes being observed: (1) acute meningitis primarily caused by *L. monocytogenes*, the most common cause of bacterial CNS infection in the transplant patient; (2) subacute to chronic meningitis usually caused by *C. neoformans*, although occasionally, in patients with the appropriate epidemiologic background, *M. tuberculosis* and *C. immitis* also cause this clinical syndrome; (3) focal brain infection with focal neurologic abnormalities occasionally caused by *Listeria*, *Toxoplasma gondii*, or *N. asteroides*, but most commonly by *Aspergillus* metastatic from a site of active pulmonary infection; and (4) progressive dementia resulting from progressive multifocal leukoencephalopathy caused by the papovavirus JC virus.[16]

The presentation of CNS infection in the renal transplant patient may be quite different from that in the normal host. In particular, the anti-inflammatory effects of the immunosuppressive therapy being administered may obscure the signs of meningeal irritation usually associated with meningitis in the normal patient or delay the appearance of mass lesions on computed tomographic scan. For this reason, the indication for a neurologic evaluation, including lumbar puncture, in this population of patients is an unexplained headache, and a magnetic resonance scan should be considered if there is substantial suspicion of a focal intracranial process.[16]

Finally, CNS infection usually occurs in the setting of disseminated disease. Two other organ systems that are commonly involved are the lungs (particularly with such organisms as *Aspergillus*, *Nocardia*, and *Cryptococcus*) and the skin (20 to 30% of disseminated fungal and nocardial infection involves the skin as well, often giving the first clue to the presence of disseminated opportunistic infection). Thus, evaluation of the CNS is obligatory when extracranial infec-

tion with these organisms is diagnosed; on the other hand, these other more accessible sites may provide a source for diagnosing occult causes of CNS infection.[1]

PARTICULAR INFECTIONS OF MAJOR CONCERN IN THE TRANSPLANT RECIPIENT

Cytomegalovirus

CMV is the single most important cause of infectious disease morbidity and mortality in the organ transplant patient in the period 1 to 6 months after transplantation, with documented evidence of infection in approximately two thirds of transplant recipients. In all forms of organ transplantation, clinically overt disease is clustered in this period, with the initial manifestations of the disease occurring as early as 3 weeks and as late as 4 months after transplantation. The major difference in clinical manifestations in the different transplant groups is not in the systemic effects of the infection but rather in the effects of the virus on the organ transplanted. Thus, clinically important hepatitis is primarily a problem in liver allograft recipients, myocarditis is recognized only in heart transplant recipients, and pneumonitis is a particular problem in lung transplant recipients. There are probably several reasons for this: in many cases the allograft itself is the site of viral reactivation and thus harbors the greatest amount of virus initially; the key host defense in the recovery of individuals from CMV infection consists of virus-specific, major histocompatibility complex–restricted cytotoxic T lymphocytes, and thus elimination of the virus from allograft tissue may be impaired; and, finally, allogeneic reactions, such as occur with the rejection process, promote CMV infection. Thus, the transplanted organ appears to be a relatively privileged site for CMV replication.[1, 9, 17, 18]

That CMV is such an effective pathogen in transplant patients is well explained by three of its characteristics: latency, cell association, and ability to be disseminated throughout the body, infecting virtually all tissue in the immunocompromised host.[17] The term latency connotes that after primary infection CMV, like other herpes group viruses, persists in an inactive form for the lifetime of the host, the laboratory marker for this being the presence of antibody to CMV in the individual's serum. Latency of CMV infection is reasonably stable (in contrast to that of EBV, discussed later), with viral reactivation occurring only with the administration of certain immunosuppressive agents (antilymphocyte antibodies and cytotoxic drugs such as cyclophosphamide and azathioprine being particularly potent CMV reactivators), the rejection process, and pregnancy. Thus, viral reactivation would be expected to be the rule in transplant recipients.[9] Once active, replicating CMV infection is present; the virus is highly cell associated, rendering humoral immunity inefficient and cell-mediated immunity, the host defense most affected by antirejection immunosuppressive therapy, critical in the control of this infection. It is not surprising that when active, replicating CMV infection is present in the transplant patient, disseminated infection can ensue. One other characteristic of herpes group viruses is, at present, only a theoretic concern: herpesviruses should be considered as potentially oncogenic. Whether CMV infection is involved in the development of one or more of the malignant processes that occur at an increased rate in transplant recipients remains to be determined.[1, 9, 17]

Three patterns of CMV transmission are observed, each with a different risk for symptomatic disease:[1, 2, 9]

1. *Primary* CMV infection occurs when a CMV-seronegative individual receives latently infected cells from a CMV-seropositive donor. More than 90% of the time, those cells are found within the allograft (whether it be kidney, heart, lung, liver, or pancreas); in the remaining patients, viable leukocytes in transfused blood products can transmit the virus. Approximately 10% of transplant recipients are at risk of primary CMV infection, and approximately 60% of these individuals become ill with symptomatic CMV disease.[17, 19, 20]

2. *Reactivation* CMV infection occurs when a CMV-seropositive individual reactivates endogenous latent virus. Approximately 50 to 70% of patients coming to transplantation are seropositive before transplantation, and an estimated 20% of these develop symptomatic disease.[17, 19, 20]

3. *Superinfection* with CMV occurs when a seropositive individual receives an allograft from a seropositive donor and the virus that is activated after transplantation and disseminates is of donor rather than endogenous origin. Superinfection, as opposed to endogenous reactivation, may occur in as many as 50% of these individuals. It is unclear whether individuals with superinfection have a higher incidence of clinical disease than those with reactivation infection, although several lines of evidence suggest that seropositive patients receiving allografts from seropositive donors have a significantly worse clinical outcome than patients receiving allografts from seronegative organs.[9, 21–23]

The clinical effects of CMV infection can be grouped into three categories:[1–3, 9]

1. Direct causation of infectious disease syndromes (Table 49–3).

2. Production of a net state of immunosuppression far greater than that caused by the immunosuppressive therapy itself, and which predisposes to potentially lethal superinfection with such pathogens as *P. carinii*, *L. monocytogenes*, and *Aspergillus*.[24]

3. Participation of the virus in the pathogenesis of allograft injury. Two types of mechanisms have been proposed to explain this "indirect consequence" of CMV infection: in molecular mimicry an immune response directed against a CMV antigen damages the allograft because of homology between the CMV antigen and cell surface antigens in the allograft tissue; alternatively, cytokines, such as interferon-γ, elaborated in response to the CMV infection up-regulate the display of antigens on the allograft, triggering an immune response. Although this effect of CMV infection should be considered hypothetic, there is extensive epidemiologic evidence linking CMV with accelerated coronary atherosclerosis in heart transplant recipients, bronchiolitis obliterans in lung transplant recipients, the disappearing bile duct syndrome in liver transplant recipients, and a unique form of glomerular lesion in renal transplant patients.[24, 25]

Considering this array of effects of CMV infection, it is not surprising that a major effort has been made to control it. Extended prophylactic courses of CMV hyperimmune globulin,[26, 27] as well as high-dose oral acyclovir (approximately 3200 mg/day in an adult with normal renal function),[28] appear to be approximately 50% effective in preventing primary CMV disease. Ganciclovir has been effective in treating CMV disease;[29] in addition, in the most challenging form of CMV disease, CMV pneumonia in bone marrow transplant recipients, the combination of hyperimmune globulin and ganciclovir has been more effective than either agent alone.[30, 31] Because there have been similar findings in a murine model of CMV infection,[32] our policy is to use such combined therapy in all organ transplant patients with serious consequences of CMV infection, recognizing that studies supporting this practice are not yet available. Finally, other data suggest that pre-emptive therapy might be possible. In a study of CMV-seropositive renal transplant patients, it was observed that if OKT3 antirejection therapy was added to the cyclosporine-based immunosuppression program, the incidence of symptomatic disease increased from 20 to 60%. In a pilot study in which ganciclovir was administered concomitantly with the OKT3 therapy, the incidence of symptomatic disease was decreased to 10%.[33] Thus, adjusting antiviral strategies to the needs and effects of immunosuppressive therapy appears to be feasible.

Epstein-Barr Virus

EBV is an increasingly important pathogen in the transplant patient. It has occasionally caused a heterophil-negative mononucleosis syndrome in transplant patients that mimics many of the clinical effects of CMV infection. However, its major importance is as an oncogenic agent, initiating the process that results in B cell lymphoproliferative disease, which is particularly likely to occur in children who are seronegative before transplantation and manifest primary EBV infection. More than 90% of the adult population is EBV seropositive and hence harbors latent virus. The attack rate for lymphoproliferative disease is far lower in seropositive individuals, but because of the larger percentage of adults receiving transplants, lymphoproliferative disease in

TABLE 49–3

DIRECT CLINICAL MANIFESTATIONS OF CYTOMEGALOVIRUS INFECTION IN THE ORGAN TRANSPLANT RECIPIENT*

Early†	Late‡
Fever	Chorioretinitis
Pneumonia	
Hepatitis	
Gastrointestinal ulcerations	
Leukopenia	
(Atypical lymphocytosis)	
Thrombocytopenia	
Arthralgias, myalgias	
(Encephalitis, transverse myelitis, rash)	

*Unusual manifestations are listed in parentheses.
†Occurring 1–4 mo after transplantation.
‡Occurring >4 mo after transplantation.

seropositive individuals is the predominant pattern observed. Unlike CMV latency, EBV latency is not stable, and at any one time 20% of seropositive adults excrete the virus in their pharyngeal secretions. Immunosuppressive therapy with antilymphocyte antibodies increases the rate of viral reactivation. Secondary infection of B lymphocytes follows active viral replication, and these EBV-infected lymphocytes are transformed and immortalized—the cellular equivalent of oncogenesis. In normal individuals seropositive for EBV, circulating cytotoxic T lymphocytes specific for EBV-induced antigens on the surface of infected B lymphocytes prevent the outgrowth of virally induced, transformed cells that initiate the oncogenic process. Immunosuppressive therapy has two effects: it not only reactivates virus from its latent state but also blocks the surveillance mechanism. The greatest impairment of this surveillance mechanism occurs with cyclosporine, which inhibits the EBV-specific cytotoxic T cell response in a dose-dependent fashion. When this was recognized and cyclosporine doses were decreased, the incidence of this problem fell off sharply.[1, 34–45]

Unfortunately, there has been an increase in EBV-associated lymphoproliferative disease related to the use of other immunosuppressive agents given in addition to full-dose cyclosporine, azathioprine, and prednisone. In particular, the addition of OKT3 to such regimens has been associated with a 10-fold increase in the incidence of lymphoproliferative disease.[46] Again, it is the net state of immunosuppression created by the entire regimen, not a single agent, that is responsible.

The clinical impact of EBV-associated lymphoproliferative disease can be diverse, with transformed cells invading the brain, bowel, liver, spleen, and even the allograft. Unlike the situation in other forms of lymphoproliferative disease, lymph node involvement that can be perceived on chest or abdominal computed tomographic scans and thus lead to early diagnosis is the exception and not the rule. Far more common is the discovery of this entity when investigating a gastrointestinal hemorrhage, gut perforation, liver biopsy because of deteriorating liver function tests, or the development of seizures or other findings of focal brain disease. Unfortunately, such events usually signal advanced disease. Because it is hypothesized that this condition evolves from a benign, polyclonal form to a highly malignant, monoclonal neoplasm, early diagnosis is at a premium, and an accurate laboratory marker of early events is badly needed. Currently available radiologic, virologic, or serologic techniques are not useful for this purpose. At present, the diagnosis can be made only pathologically.[47–51]

The current cornerstone of therapy of this entity is to decrease drastically immunosuppressive therapy[52] with or without adding antiviral therapy (as with high-dose intravenous acyclovir).[53] Conventional lymphoma chemotherapy or radiation therapy for the 50 to 75% of individuals who do not respond to such measures has not been successful. Clearly, earlier diagnosis is necessary to effect useful therapy. Again, the utility of pre-emptive antiviral therapy at times of intensive immunosuppressive therapy bears study.

Hepatitis B and Hepatitis C Viruses

Both of these viruses have an impact on transplant patients, 10 to 15% of whom develop chronic liver disease, the consequences of which are several.[1, 54]

Acute hepatitis B, acquired in the peritransplantation period from the allograft or from blood products, is fortunately rare today, as it carries a high risk of fulminant hepatic failure in these immunosuppressed patients. A more common problem is the hepatitis B carrier who comes to transplantation already infected. Data for kidney transplant

recipients (which are presumably applicable to heart and lung transplant recipients as well) suggest that in the first 12 to 24 months after transplantation chronic hepatitis B contributes to the net state of immunosuppression. After this period, the combination of chronic hepatitis B and chronic immunosuppression leads inexorably to end-stage hepatic disease with cirrhosis and/or hepatocellular carcinoma, a process that may take many years, however. Thus, hepatitis B is regarded as a relative contraindication to transplantation.[54–61]

Hepatitis B in patients with end-stage liver disease who require liver transplantation is a special problem. Recurrence of hepatitis B after transplantation is the rule, particularly if there is evidence of active viral replication at the time of the transplantation, with progressive damage to the allograft. Whether prolonged administration of hepatitis B hyperimmune globulin can help ameliorate this problem is not yet clear. Antiviral therapy for hepatitis B, as with interferon-γ, is in its infancy, particularly in the transplant patient.[54]

Non-A, non-B hepatitis (presumably virtually all related to hepatitis C infection) is the major cause of post-transplantation hepatic dysfunction. Typically, asymptomatic anicteric hepatitis is observed 1 to 4 months after transplantation and is followed by chronic infection that may continue asymptomatically for prolonged periods. The only sign of the chronic infection is persistent elevation of aminotransferase levels. After a period of 4 to 10 years, patients may present abruptly with ascites, hepatic encephalopathy, spontaneous bacterial peritonitis, or hemorrhage from esophageal varices—all manifestations of end-stage liver disease. Again, antiviral therapy with interferon-γ in these patients is, at best, only a stopgap measure.[54, 62–65]

PRINCIPLES OF ANTIMICROBIAL THERAPY IN THE ORGAN TRANSPLANT RECIPIENT

A cardinal rule in the transplant patient is that prevention of infection is far more desirable than treatment of infection, and, as outlined in Table 49–4, there are clear-cut indications for antimicrobial prophylaxis. Typically, prophylactic regimens involve the administration of a nontoxic drug, often with less than ideal antimicrobial activity, for a prolonged period (as opposed to therapeutic regimens, which employ the most effective medications, often at toxic doses, for shorter periods). More recently, the concept of pre-emptive therapy has been put forth.[66]

Pre-emptive therapy combines the most desirable aspects of prophylactic and therapeutic regimens—administration of highly effective therapy over a short period to a relatively small number of patients who have evidence of being at risk of serious infection. The short duration of therapy reduces the potential toxicity and makes it possible to use the most effective antimicrobial regimen available. The example of pre-emptive therapy with ganciclovir in CMV-seropositive patients receiving OKT3 has already been cited. A 14-day course of this more potent, although potentially more toxic, drug appears to be more effective than prolonged prophylactic regimens of acyclovir or hyperimmune globulin therapy.[46] Similarly, the early use of fluconazole to eradicate asymptomatic candiduria in kidney transplant recipients and prevent progression to urinary tract obstruction and pyelonephritis and the use of fluconazole in association with surgical manipulation of a pulmonary nodule caused by *Cryptococcus* to prevent CNS infection are other examples of pre-emptive therapy.[66]

The advent of cyclosporine-based immunosuppressive regimens has placed a premium on prophylactic and pre-emptive strategies, as the occurrence of adverse interactions with antimicrobial agents given in full therapeutic doses is

TABLE 49-4

PROPHYLACTIC REGIMENS IN ORGAN TRANSPLANT RECIPIENTS

Treatment	Infection Treated
Of proven value	
Trimethoprim-sulfamethoxazole, ciprofloxacin	Urinary tract infection and urosepsis in kidney transplant patients
Trimethoprim-sulfamethoxazole	*P. carinii* pneumonia
Pyrimethamine plus sulfonamide*	Primary toxoplasmosis in heart transplant patients
Of probable value	
Trimethoprim-sulfamethoxazole	*L. monocytogenes*
	N. asteroides
Oral clotrimazole, oral nystatin	Mucosal candidal infection
High-dose oral acyclovir	CMV
	Herpes simplex virus
CMV hyperimmune globulin	CMV
Perioperative antibiotics or other cephalosporins (e.g., cefazolin at time of transplantation)	Wound infection

*Useful in heart transplant recipients who are seronegative for toxoplasmosis before transplantation and who receive a heart allograft from a seropositive donor. Without prophylaxis, there is a high rate of disseminated toxoplasmosis after transplantation.

quite common (Table 49–5). Thus, whereas low-dose trimethoprim-sulfamethoxazole prophylaxis is usually tolerated in the presence of cyclosporine therapy, full-dose anti-*Pneumocystis* therapy has a high rate of adverse reactions, including oliguric renal failure. Hence, the search is continuing for clinical, epidemiologic, and/or laboratory markers connoting risk of serious infection that can justify the deployment of effective therapies to abort the process and minimize the chances for toxicity associated with prolonged therapeutic courses.

The therapeutic program of the future for the transplant patient will include "epidemiologic protection" from excessive hazards, effective antirejection therapy, and directed antimicrobial therapy to prevent the infectious disease consequences of antirejection therapy. It is as true today as it was when transplantation began that infection and rejection are closely intertwined: any intervention that decreases the risk of infection permits more effective use of antirejection

therapy; conversely, any intervention that decreases the need for immunosuppressive therapy decreases the risk of infection. The clinician, particularly in the intensive care setting, must keep both aspects of this equation firmly in mind if the potential benefits of organ transplantation are to be brought to the increasing numbers of patients who need such therapy.

References

1. Rubin RH: Infection in the renal and liver transplant patient. In Rubin RH, Young LS (eds): Clinical Approach to Infection in the Compromised Host. 2nd ed. New York, Plenum Publishing, p 557, 1988.
2. Rubin RH, Wolfson JS, Cosimi AB, et al: Infection in the renal transplant recipient. Am J Med 70:405, 1981.
3. Rubin RH, Tolkoff-Rubin NE: Infection: The new problems. Transplant Proc 21:1440, 1989.
4. Rubin RH, Tolkoff-Rubin NE: Opportunistic infections in renal allograft recipients. Transplant Proc 20(suppl 8):12, 1988.
5. Scowden EB, Schaffner W, Stone WJ: Overwhelming strongyloidiasis: An unappreciated opportunistic infection. Medicine 57:527, 1978.
6. Morgan JS, Schaffner W, Stone WJ: Opportunistic strongyloidiasis in renal transplant recipients. Transplantation 42:518, 1986.
7. Hibberd PL, Rubin RH: Approach to immunization in the immunosuppressed host. Infect Dis Clin North Am 4:123, 1990.
8. Hopkins CC, Weber DJ, Rubin RH: Invasive aspergillus infection: Possible non-ward common source within the hospital environment. J Hosp Infect 13(1):19, 1989.
9. Rubin RH: Impact of cytomegalovirus infection on organ transplant recipients. Rev Infect Dis 12(suppl 7):S754, 1990.
10. Rubin RH, Cosimi AB: Therapy, both immunosuppressive and antimicrobial, for the transplant patient in the 1990's. In Brent L, Sells RA (eds): Organ Transplantation—Current Clinical and Immunological Concepts. London, Bailliere Tindall, p 71, 1989.
11. Cosimi AB: Antilymphocyte globulin—A final (?) look. In Morris PJ, Tilney NL (eds): Progress in Transplantation, Volume 2. Edinburgh, Churchill Livingstone, p 167, 1986.
12. Cosimi AB: OKT3 in organ transplantation. In Grant DR, Wall WJ (eds): First Canadian Symposium on Multi-Organ Transplantation. London, Canada, Scitex Publications, p 33, 1989.
13. Peterson PK, Balfour HH Jr, Marker SC, et al: Cytomegalovirus disease in renal allograft recipients: A prospective study of the clinical features, risk factors, and impact on renal transplantation. Medicine 59:283, 1980.
14. Peterson PK, Balfour HH Jr, Fryd DS, et al: Fever in renal transplant recipients: Course, prognostic significance and changing patterns at the University of Minnesota Hospital. Am J Med 71:345, 1981.
15. Rubin RH, Greene R: Etiology and management of the compromised patient with fever and pulmonary infiltrates. In Rubin RH, Young LS (eds): Clinical Approach to Infection in the Compromised Host. 2nd ed. New York, Plenum Publishing, p 131, 1988.
16. Conti DJ, Rubin RH: Infection of the central nervous system in organ transplant recipients. Neurol Clin North Am 6:241, 1988.
17. Ho M: Cytomegalovirus: Biology and Infection. 2nd ed. New York, Plenum Publishing, 1981.
18. Rook AH, Quinnan G, Fredrick J, et al: Importance of cytoxic lympho-

TABLE 49-5

ANTIMICROBIAL AGENT–CYCLOSPORINE INTERACTIONS OF IMPORTANCE IN THE ORGAN TRANSPLANT RECIPIENT

1. Antimicrobial agent *up-regulates* hepatic cytochrome P-450 function, thus increasing the rate of cyclosporine metabolism. This results in decreased cyclosporine blood levels and increased chances of allograft rejection unless the administered dose is increased.

   Example: rifampin

2. Antimicrobial agent *down-regulates* hepatic cytochrome P-450 function, thus decreasing the rate of cyclosporine metabolism. This results in increased cyclosporine blood levels, increasing the chances of both cyclosporine nephrotoxicity and overimmunosuppression unless the administered dose is decreased.

   Examples: erythromycin, ketoconazole, fluconazole

3. Antimicrobial agent *interacts idiopathically* with cyclosporine to produce accelerated nephrotoxicity.

   Examples: amphotericin, aminoglycosides, vancomycin, systemic pentamidine, high-dose trimethoprim-sulfamethoxazole*

*Low-dose trimethoprim-sulfamethoxazole (one or two single-strength or double-strength tablets per day) is usually well tolerated. In contrast, full-dose anti-*Pneumocystis* therapy with this drug is associated with a high rate of renal toxicity.

cytes during cytomegalovirus infection in renal transplant recipients. Am J Med 76:385, 1984.

19. Betts RF, Freeman RB, Douglas RH Jr, et al: Transmission of cytomegalovirus infection with renal allograft. Kidney Int 8:385, 1975.

20. Ho M, Suwansirikul S, Dowling JN, et al: The transplanted kidney as a source of cytomegalovirus infection. N Engl J Med 293:1109, 1975.

21. Chou S: Acquisition of donor strains of cytomegalovirus by renal transplant recipients. N Engl J Med 314:1418, 1986.

22. Grundy JE, Super M, Lui S, et al: The source of cytomegalovirus infection in seropositive renal allograft recipients is frequently the donor kidney. Transplant Proc 19:2126, 1987.

23. Grundy JE, Lui SF, Super M, et al: Symptomatic cytomegalovirus infection in seropositive kidney recipients: Reinfection with donor virus rather than reactivation of recipient latent virus. Lancet 2:132, 1988.

24. Rubin RH: The indirect effects of cytomegalovirus infection on the outcome of organ transplantation. JAMA 261:3607, 1989.

25. Grattam MT, Moreno-Cabral CE, Starnes VA, et al: Cytomegalovirus infection is associated with cardiac allograft rejection and atherosclerosis. JAMA 261:3561, 1989.

26. Snydman DR, Weiner BC, Heinze-Lacey B, et al: Use of cytomegalovirus immune globulin to prevent cytomegalovirus disease in renal transplant recipients. N Engl J Med 317:1049, 1987.

27. Snydman DR, Weiner BG, Tilney NL, et al: A further analysis of primary cytomegalovirus disease prevention in renal transplant recipients with a cytomegalovirus immune globulin: Interim comparison of a randomized and an open-label trial. Transplant Proc 20(suppl 8):24, 1988.

28. Balfour HH Jr, Chace BA, Stapleton JT, et al: A randomized, placebo-controlled trial of oral acyclovir for the prevention of cytomegalovirus disease in recipients of renal allografts. N Engl J Med 320:1381, 1989.

29. Rubin RH: Impact of cytomegalovirus infection on organ transplant recipients. Rev Infect Dis 12(suppl 7):S754, 1990.

30. Reed EC, Bowden RA, Dandliker PS, et al: Treatment of cytomegalovirus pneumonia with ganciclovir and intravenous cytomegalovirus immunoglobulin in patients with bone marrow transplants. Ann Intern Med 109:783, 1988.

31. Emmanuel D, Cunningham I, Jules-Elysee K, et al: Cytomegalovirus pneumonia after bone marrow transplantation successfully treated with the combination of ganciclovir and high-dose intravenous immune globulin. Ann Intern Med 109:777, 1988.

32. Rubin RH, Lynch P, Pasternack MS, et al: Combined antibody and ganciclovir treatment of murine cytomegalovirus-infected normal and immunosuppressed BALB/c mice. Antimicrob Agents Chemother 33:1975, 1989.

33. Hibberd PL, Tolkoff-Rubin NE, Cosimi AB, et al: Symptomatic cytomegalovirus disease in the cytomegalovirus antibody seropositive renal transplant recipient treated with OKT3. Transplantation 53:68, 1992.

34. Cheeseman SH, Henle W, Rubin RH, et al: Epstein-Barr virus infection in renal transplant recipients: Effects of antithymocyte globulin and interferon. Ann Intern Med 93:39, 1980.

35. Grose C, Henle W, Horwitz MS: Primary Epstein-Barr virus infection in a renal transplant recipient. South Med J 70:1276, 1977.

36. Marker SC, Ascher NL, Kalis JM, et al: Epstein-Barr virus antibody responses and clinical illness in renal transplant recipients. Surgery 85:433, 1979.

37. Crawford DH, Swany P, Edwards JMB, et al: Long-term T-cell mediated immunity to Epstein-Barr virus in renal allograft recipients receiving cyclosporin A. Lancet 1:10, 1981.

38. Bird AG, McLachlin SM, Britton S: Cyclosporin A promotes spontaneous outgrowth in vitro of Epstein-Barr virus–induced B-cell lines. Nature 289:300, 1981.

39. Crawford DH, Edwards JM, Sweny P, et al: Studies on long-term T-cell–mediated immunity to Epstein-Barr virus in immunosuppressed renal allograft recipients. Int J Cancer 28:705, 1981.

40. Yao QY, Rickinson AB, Gastron JS, et al: In vitro analysis of the Epstein-Barr virus: Host balance in long-term renal allograft recipients. Int J Cancer 35:43, 1985.

41. Strauch B, Andrews L, Miller G, et al: Oropharyngeal excretion of Epstein-Barr virus by renal transplant recipients and other patients treated with immunosuppressant drugs. Lancet 1:234, 1974.

42. Chang RS, Lewis JP, Reynolds RD, et al: Oropharyngeal excretion of Epstein-Barr virus by patients with lymphoproliferative disorders and by recipients of renal homografts. Ann Intern Med 88:34, 1978.

43. Calne RY, Rolles K, White DJ, et al: Cyclosporin A initially as the only immunosuppressant in 34 recipients of cadaveric organs: 32 kidneys, 2 pancreases, and 2 livers. Lancet 2:1033, 1979.

44. Bia MJ, Flye MW: Immunoblastic lymphoma in a cyclosporine-treated renal transplant recipient. Transplantation 39:673, 1985.

45. Ho M, Miller G, Atchison RW, et al: Epstein-Barr virus infections and DNA hybridization studies in post-transplantation lymphoma and lymphoproliferative lesions: The role of primary infection. J Infect Dis 152:876, 1985.

46. Swinnen LJ, Costanzo-Nordin MR, Fischer SG, et al: Increased incidence of lymphoproliferative disorder after immunosuppression with the monoclonal antibody OKT3 in cardiac transplant recipients. N Engl J Med 323:1723, 1990.

47. Hanto D, Frizzera G, Purtilo DT, et al: Clinical spectrum of lymphoproliferative disorders in renal transplant recipients and evidence for the role of Epstein-Barr virus. Cancer Res 41:4253, 1981.

48. Frizzera G, Hanto DW, Gajl-Peczalska KJ, et al: Polymorphic diffuse B-cell hyperplasias and lymphomas in renal transplant recipients. Cancer Res 41:4253, 1981.

49. Hanto D, Sakamoto K, Purtilo DT, et al: The Epstein-Barr virus in the pathogenesis of post-transplant lymphoproliferative disorders. Surgery 90:204, 1981.

50. Hanto D, Frizzera G, Gajl-Peczalska K, et al: Epstein-Barr virus–induced B-cell lymphoma after renal transplantation. N Engl J Med 306:913, 1982.

51. Hanto DW, Gajl-Peczalska KJ, Frizzera G, et al: Epstein-Barr virus (EBV) induced polyclonal and monoclonal B-cell lymphoproliferative disease occurring after renal transplantation. Clinical, pathologic, and virologic findings and implications for therapy. Ann Surg 198:356, 1983.

52. Starzl TE, Nalesnik MA, Porter KA, et al: Reversibility of lymphomas and lymphoproliferative lesions developing under cyclosporin-steroid therapy. Lancet 1:583, 1984.

53. Hanto DW, Frizzera G, Gajl-Peczalska KJ, et al: Acyclovir therapy of Epstein-Barr virus–induced post-transplant lymphoproliferative diseases. Transplant Proc 17:89, 1985.

54. Katkov WN, Rubin RH: Liver disease in the organ transplant recipient: Etiology, clinical impact, and clinical management. Transplant Rev 5:200, 1991.

55. London WT, Drew JS, Blumberg BS, et al: Association of graft survival with host response to hepatitis B infection in patients with kidney transplant. N Engl J Med 296:241, 1977.

56. Pirson Y, Alexandre GPJ, van Ypersele de Strihou C: Long-term effect of HB$_s$ antigenemia on patient survival after renal transplantation. N Engl J Med 296:194, 1977.

57. Toussaint C, Dupont E, Vanherweghem JL, et al: Liver disease in patients undergoing hemodialysis and kidney transplantation. Adv Nephrol 8:269, 1979.

58. Hillis WD, Hillis A, Walker WG: Hepatitis B surface antigenemia in renal transplant recipients; increased mortality risk. JAMA 242:329, 1979.

59. Parfrey PS, Forbes RD, Hutchinson TA, et al: The clinical and pathological course of hepatitis B liver disease in renal transplant recipients. Transplantation 37:461, 1984.

60. Parfrey PS, Forbes RDC, Hutchinson TA, et al: The impact of renal transplantation on the course of hepatitis B liver disease. Transplantation 39:610, 1985.

61. Busuttil RW, Goldstein LI, Danovitch G, et al: Liver transplantation today. Ann Intern Med 104:377, 1986.

62. Ware AJ, Luby JP, Eigenbrodt EH, et al: Spectrum of liver disease in renal transplant recipients. Gastroenterology 68:755, 1975.

63. Kirkman RL, Strom TB, Weir MR, et al: Late mortality and morbidity in recipients of long-term renal allografts. Transplantation 34:347, 1982.

64. Weir MR, Kirkman RL, Strom TB, et al: Liver disease in recipients of long-functioning renal allografts. Kidney Int 28:839, 1985.

65. LaQuaglia MP, Tolkoff-Rubin NE, Dienstag JL, et al: Impact of hepatitis on renal transplantation. Transplantation 32:504, 1981.

66. Rubin RH: Preemptive therapy in immunocompromised hosts. N Engl J Med 324:1057, 1991.

CHAPTER 50

Human Immunodeficiency Virus Infection and the Acquired Immunodeficiency Syndrome

Lawrence R. Crane
Paula C. Schuman

During the summer of 1981, the Centers for Disease Control published two brief reports of *Pneumocystis carinii* pneumonia (PCP) and/or disseminated Kaposi's sarcoma occurring in gay men residing in New York City or California.[1, 2] By the end of that year, it was clear that a syndrome characterized by profound, unexplained immunodeficiency and opportunistic infections and aggressive malignancies was occurring among gay American men. During the following year, clinicians became aware that this syndrome, now termed *acquired immunodeficiency syndrome* (AIDS), was also occurring in intravenous drug users, infants, recipients of blood products, and residents of emerging nations. The past decade has seen an explosion of our understanding of this disease. Its etiology, a novel group of human retroviruses, human immunodeficiency virus types 1 and 2 (HIV-1 and -2), has been established. Its transmission has been defined. The pathogenesis of the infection is being solved. Treatment and prevention are available, and vaccine development is now a reality. HIV infection and AIDS have significantly affected the intensive care unit. A new group of patients is now utilizing intensive care. Our general approach to infection control in the intensive care unit has changed. Finally, the AIDS pandemic has forced us to re-examine our priorities in terms of allocation of resources, personnel policies, and medical ethics. AIDS has truly been a paradigm for the problems of health care in the United States. This chapter reviews the general principles of AIDS care in the intensive care milieu.

PATHOPHYSIOLOGY

A broad spectrum of illness occurs in HIV-infected persons, ranging from the carrier state to full-blown AIDS. Clinical features vary from an acute infectious mononucleosis–like illness to chronic fever, weight loss, malaise, diarrhea, lymphadenopathy, and, finally, AIDS in individuals whose cellular immune systems are unable to defend against opportunistic infections and malignancies. HIV viruses also target the central nervous system; thus, dementia can also develop. Although the role of HIV in the development of this spectrum of diseases is not completely understood, there is increasing evidence that virus–host cell interactions result in the disease states observed by clinicians.

Virology

HIVs are retroviruses. Retroviruses are enveloped RNA viruses that have an RNA-dependent DNA polymerase (reverse transcriptase). The three subfamilies of Retroviridae include the Oncovirinae, comprising the RNA tumor viruses (including the human T cell lymphotropic viruses), the Spumavirinae, and the Lentivirinae. HIV, the etiologic agent of AIDS, belongs to the Lentivirinae subfamily. The first isolates of the virus that is now termed HIV-1 were designated as lymphadenopathy-associated virus,[3] human T cell lymphotropic virus type III,[4] and AIDS-associated retrovirus[5] by their discoverers. With the isolation in West Africa of a second class of AIDS virus initially called lymphadenopathy-associated virus type 2,[6] there are now two main classes of AIDS virus, HIV-1 and HIV-2.

The mature virus is lipid encoated and 100 to 120 nm in diameter. Its internal protein capsid contains a single strand of RNA that is 9300 nucleotide bases long. Virus genetic segments encode structural and regulatory proteins and a virus replication promoter region termed the *long terminal repeat*. Protein-encoding regions that have been identified include the following:

1. The *gag* gene, which encodes the structural proteins p17, p24, and p15.
2. The *pol* gene, which encodes the reverse transcriptase enzyme (p53, p66) that transcribes virus RNA into proviral DNA. A protease gene, *pr*, is located at the 5' end of the *pol* gene and cleaves *gag* and *pol* precursors.
3. The *env* gene, which encodes the envelope glycoprotein gp160. gp160 is processed to form a transmembrane segment, gp41, and an external segment, gp120.

The *gag*, *pol*, and *env* genes are common to all retroviruses. In addition, HIV-1, like other lentiviruses, contains a complex array of other genes that are central to up- and down-regulation of virus replication.[7] It is likely that these genes also account for the profound pathogenicity of HIV-1.[8] These include *tat, rev,* and *nef*. Little is known about the nonstructural genes *vif, vpu,* and *vpr*. These, too, are probably genes for regulatory proteins.

Cells infected with HIV contain two major forms of the virus: proviral DNA, a DNA copy of the entire HIV genome permanently integrated into the host cell DNA, and a double-stranded linear DNA copy present in the host cell cytoplasm. Only a small fraction of cells are infected with HIV—on the order of 1 in 400 peripheral blood mononuclear cells in seropositive individuals or about 7000 infectious particles per milliliter of blood.[9]

The structural and nonstructural proteins of HIV are central to its pathogenesis. The envelope glycoprotein (*env* gene product) is the most important protein class for HIV infectivity.[10] The gp120 portion of the envelope glycoprotein binds cells expressing CD4 (Leu-3 or T4) on their surface. The killing of the CD4+ subset of human lymphocytes as a result of HIV-1 infection causes the significant immune suppression that is the hallmark of advanced AIDS.[11] These cells are essential as regulators and effectors of the human immune response. The virus also infects the monocytes and macrophages but has less cytopathogenic effect. In fact, infected macrophages probably serve as the reservoir for HIV, facilitating spread to the central nervous system. HIV-1 also infects glial cells, dendritic cells, gut epithelium, and bone marrow progenitor cells.[12] In addition, gp120 may be directly toxic to neuronal cells.[13] It is possible that there are gp120 binding sites on neuronal and other cells that lack CD4 antigen, but evidence is still indirect.[14] Similarly, cells lacking the CD4 receptor may become infected by interaction with the gp41 segment of the envelope glycoprotein.[15]

Once bound to the receptor, HIV-1 virions are probably brought inside the cell by virus-mediated membrane fusion.[16] In the cytoplasm, the virion rapidly uncoats and a double-stranded DNA replica of the original RNA genome is synthesized under the direction of viral reverse transcriptase.

	TABLE 50-1		
LIKELIHOOD OF DEVELOPING OPPORTUNISTIC DISEASES IN PERSONS WITH HUMAN IMMUNODEFICIENCY VIRUS INFECTION			
Immune Function Level	**Likelihood of Opportunistic Disease**	**Comments**	
Good or slightly low (CD4$^+$ > 400 cells/mm^3)	Very low	Kaposi's sarcoma possible; recurring vaginal candidiasis; thrush; oral hairy leukoplakia. Other opportunistic infections and malignancies rare.	
Moderately low (CD4$^+$ 200–400 cells/mm^3)	Low	Kaposi's sarcoma, lymphoma. Nonspecific pneumonitis, HIV cardiomyopathy can occur; increased rate of pulmonary tuberculosis, histoplasmosis, coccidioidomycosis in certain geographic areas; community-acquired bacterial pneumonia may be more severe. Candida esophagitis may occur. *P. carinii* infection may be seen in pediatric patients.	
Low (CD4$^+$ < 200 cells/mm^3)	High	All opportunistic infections and malignancies possible.	
Very low (CD4$^+$ < 50 cells/mm^3)	High	Fatal opportunistic infections and malignancies possible.	

The proviral DNA then inserts into the host genome, establishing a latent or persistent infection.[8] Factors that activate HIV-1 replication in a persistently infected CD4$^+$ lymphocyte are not completely understood, but T cell activation seems to be an important stimulus to virus expression. Thus, antigens, mitogens, cytokines, and gene products of different viruses such as cytomegalovirus, human herpesvirus type 6, Epstein-Barr virus, hepatitis B virus, or herpes simplex virus result in a cellular environment that promotes a high level of HIV-1 replication.[8] In practical terms, physicians advise HIV-infected patients to avoid possible cofactors that might lead to heightened HIV-1 replication and early expression of disease. Epidemiologic studies have suggested that certain cofactors may be important in rapid disease progression. For example, continued injection by HIV-1–infected intravenous drug users results in a significant acceleration of CD4$^+$ cell loss.[17] When the cellular milieu is favorable, replication begins first with expression of the regulatory genes *tat, rev,* and *nef.* Transcription of new HIV-1 RNA is regulated by these gene products. Translation of structural and enzymatic genes then occurs, followed by assembly of virus and then budding through the plasma membrane, where the lipid membrane is acquired.

Productive HIV-1 infection results in cytopathic effects in the CD4$^+$ lymphocyte. The precise mechanism of HIV-1 cytopathogenicity is not clear, but it is probably multifactorial. HIV Env protein, present on the surface of infected cells, can result in cell fusion and syncytium formation with uninfected CD4$^+$ lymphocytes that come in contact with the infected cells.[18] The multinucleated syncytial cell eventually dies. Other mechanisms of cytopathogenicity, reviewed by Greene, include host cell membrane injury, accumulation of unintegrated HIV-1 DNA, altered host membrane permeability, and autoimmune destruction of CD4$^+$ lymphocytes by antibody- and cell-dependent cytotoxicity.[8]

Immunology

Absolute lymphopenia, as a result of destruction of CD4$^+$ lymphocytes, is the earliest and most reproducible finding in persons with established HIV infection. A subset of CD4$^+$ lymphocytes, the inducer or TQ1/Leu-8$^+$ subset, is affected earliest.[19] As infection progresses, the absolute CD4$^+$ cell count typically falls below 500/mm^3 and the ratio of CD4$^+$ to CD8$^+$ lymphocytes falls to 0.85 or less (normally the ratio is 2:1). Opportunistic infections and malignancies usually occur in a hierarchic pattern, often corresponding to the absolute CD4$^+$ count (Table 50–1 and Fig. 50–1). In contrast to their CD4$^+$ cell counts, patients exhibit a varying CD8$^+$ (suppressor lymphocyte) count. The absolute count may be normal, depressed, or elevated. In patients with elevated CD8$^+$ cell counts, the majority of cells are of the cytotoxic (CD8$^+$Leu$^-$) subset.[20] Elevated counts of CD8$^+$ cytotoxic cells may play a role in preventing infection of uninfected CD4$^+$ cells and appear to be important in long-term survival of certain HIV-1–infected persons.[21] Many in vitro tests of T cell function are impaired in persons with HIV infection. Profound decreases in mitogen and antigen response occur, even with correction for lymphopenia.[22] Clonal expansion of T cells and generation of effective cytotoxic cells are impaired. The inability of T lymphocytes to respond to neoantigens translates to an impaired ability of B lymphocytes to respond as well. Therefore, impaired vaccine response and infections with encapsulated bacteria are also seen in persons with HIV disease.

The macrophage/monocyte system is impaired in several important areas: phagocytosis of immune complexes,[23] chemotaxis,[22] cytokine production,[24] and responsiveness to antigenic challenge.[25] A summary of immune activation impairments after HIV-1 infection is given in Table 50–2.[26]

Host Responses

An idealized pathogenetic course of HIV infection is shown in Figure 50–2. Shortly after infection, intense replication of HIV-1[9] and a transient decrease in absolute CD4$^+$

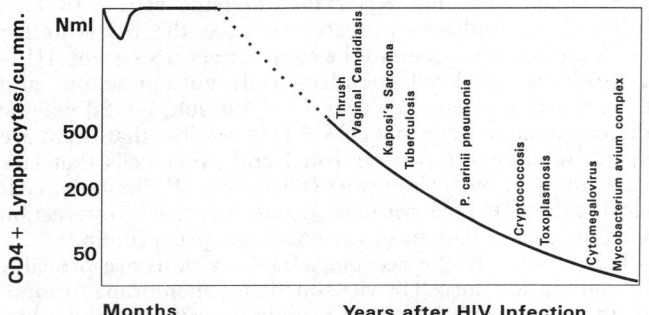

Figure 50–1. Hierarchic appearance of opportunistic diseases in HIV infection.

TABLE 50–2

IMMUNE IMPAIRMENTS OBSERVED IN PERSONS WITH HUMAN IMMUNODEFICIENCY VIRUS TYPE 1 INFECTION

Cell	Defect	Clinical Effect
CD4+ cell	Decreased antigen response Decreased lymphokine production Loss of stimulus for B and T cell activation	Decreased CD4+/CD8+ ratio Decreased delayed hypersensitivity
CD8+ cell	Impaired cytotoxicity Impaired feedback	Lymphopenia
Macrophage	Decreased chemotaxis and phagocytosis Diminished interleukin-1 production Impaired presentation of antigen to T cells	Increased susceptibility to infection, malignancy
B cell	Diminished antibody response to antigen Deregulated immunoglobulin production	Increased serum immunoglobulin

Modified with permission. Selwyn PA: AIDS: What is now known. I. History and immunovirology. Hospital Practice Volume 21, issue 5, page 72, 1986.

cell counts occur. Virus burden begins to decline as neutralizing antibodies to HIV-1 appear. Generally, 85% of infected persons have evidence of cellular and humoral immune responses to HIV viruses within 3 months after exposure. As the immune response occurs, there is recovery of the absolute CD4+ cell count toward normal. After recovery from the acute retroviral syndrome, there is a variable period of asymptomatic infection. Virus burden is low, CD4+ cell counts are relatively normal, and effective cellular and humoral immunity is present. This asymptomatic period varies with age. Symptomatic HIV disease develops in as little as 18 months in neonatal and pediatric AIDS. In contrast, the average asymptomatic period in adults is estimated to be approximately 9 years. Signs and symptoms of HIV disease are preceded by a rise in virus burden and a fall in absolute CD4+ lymphocyte counts and immune responses to the HIV virus. Studies have shown that the virus burden begins to increase at about the time the absolute CD4+ count is 500 cells/mm³; this is generally considered the point at which antiretroviral therapy should be given.[9]

EPIDEMIOLOGY

Transmission

HIV is transmitted by three routes: sexual contact with infected partners; direct exposure to contaminated blood, blood products, or tissues; and perinatal transmission from infected mothers to their offspring. The efficiency of sexual transmission ranges between 0.1 and 1.0%, with the highest risk of transmission occurring with receptive anal inter-

course.[27] Male-to-female transmission and female-to-male transmission via receptive anal or vaginal intercourse have also been well documented.[28] Transmission may be possible by other sexual practices such as fellatio, but such cases are not well documented. Globally, 70 to 80% of persons with HIV infection are estimated to have become infected by sexual routes (Table 50–3). In contrast, the efficiency of transmission of HIV via blood products is as high as 90%.[29] HIV has also been transmitted by artificial insemination and through kidney, liver, heart, pancreas, bone, and probably skin transplantation.[30] The World Health Organization estimates that in about 3 to 5% of HIV cases worldwide the virus was transmitted by transfusion. This high rate is due to the unavailability of established screening procedures for donated blood and blood products in developing nations. Maternal transmission of HIV is the primary cause of pediatric AIDS. Approximately 30% of infants of HIV-infected mothers become infected.[31] Rare cases of transmission to infants through infected breast milk have been reported.[32] The risk of transmission from an infected patient to a health care worker by needle stick exposure is discussed in the infection control section of this chapter. A number of studies demonstrate that HIV is not transmitted through household or other casual contact. At least 12 studies have been done in the United States and Europe to evaluate the risk of nonsexual transmission of HIV infection.[32] None of these studies found serologic or virologic evidence of HIV transmission among household members who lack other risk factors for infection. If HIV is not transmitted between household members whose exposures are repeated, prolonged, and often unsanitary, it is even less likely that this virus is transmitted in the workplace. There is no evidence

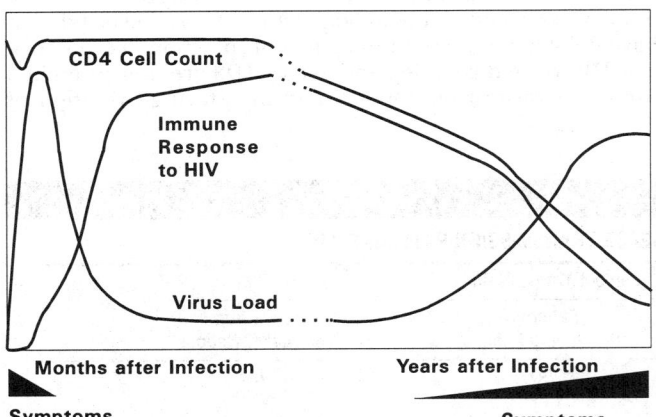

Figure 50–2. Idealized course of HIV infection in adults.

TABLE 50–3

HUMAN IMMUNODEFICIENCY VIRUS TRANSMISSION, GLOBAL SUMMARY, 1991

Exposure Type	Efficiency of Single Exposure (%)	Percentage Infected Globally
Blood transfusion	>90	3–5
Perinatal	30	10–20
Sexual intercourse	0.1–1.0	70–80
Vaginal		60–70
Anal		5–10
Injecting drug use	0.5–1.0	5–10
Health care worker, accidental injection	<0.5	<0.01

Number of Cases

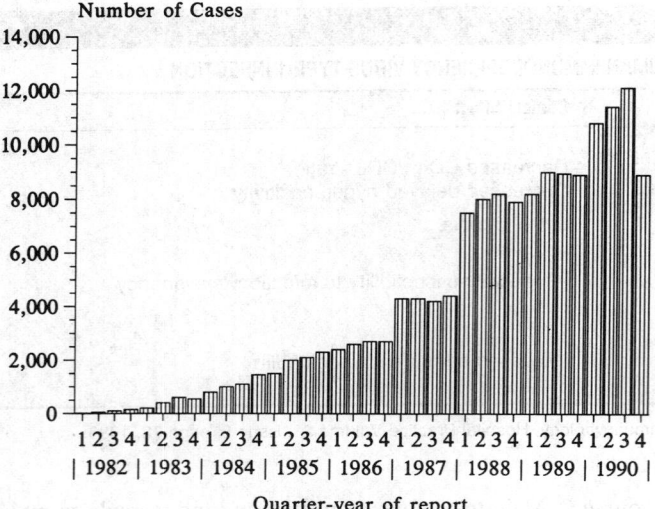

Figure 50–3. Epidemic curve of AIDS, United States, 1982 to 1990.

that blood-borne or sexually transmitted infections such as HIV are transmitted during food preparation. U.S. Public Health Service guidelines state that HIV-infected workers should not be prevented from working because they are infected, nor should they be prevented from using telephones, office equipment, toilets or showers, eating facilities, or drinking fountains.[33]

Incidence and Prevalence

In addition to persons with AIDS, 1 million persons in the United States are estimated to have asymptomatic HIV infection.[34] Figure 50–3 shows the epidemic curve for AIDS in the United States. It is noteworthy that it took approximately 18 months for the first 1000 cases of AIDS to be reported in the United States. Today, roughly 1000 cases are reported to the Centers for Disease Control every 8 days. Between 1983 and 1987, the doubling time for reported cases of AIDS was approximately 14 months.[35] Since 1987, the number of AIDS cases reported has begun to level off. It has been suggested that the main reason for this is a decrease in reported cases of AIDS among urban gay men, reflecting the availability of antiretroviral therapy that delays progression to an AIDS-defining illness.[36] The earliest case of AIDS in the United States occurred in 1968 in a 15-year-old boy from St. Louis, who died of aggressive disseminated Kaposi's sarcoma.[37] However, seroprevalence studies show that the epidemic began in the United States in 1978.[38] The World Health Organization estimated that reported cases of AIDS will level off in pattern I countries, including the United States, during the mid-1990s.[39] Cases will continue

to rise in pattern II and pattern III countries in the foreseeable future.

In 1991, the World Health Organization estimated that 8 million to 9 million persons worldwide are infected, or 1 in 400 adults.[8] There is evidence for a slowing of the increase in AIDS incidence among transfusion recipients and homosexual or bisexual men.[40] Compilation of AIDS incidence data from around the world has led to recognition of three distinct geographic patterns of transmission[41] (Table 50–4):

Pattern I is characterized by high numbers of cases among homosexual or bisexual men and intravenous drug users; roughly 80 to 90% of reported cases of AIDS belong to these categories. Transmission by blood and blood products occurred between the late 1970s and 1985 but is now rare because of self-deferral of persons at risk and routine screening of donated blood. Pattern I countries—including North America, parts of Latin America, Western Europe, Australia, and New Zealand—have reported large numbers of AIDS cases and show a small percentage of heterosexual transmission cases; male-to-female ratios are typically 10:1 to 15:1. Seroprevalence studies generally show less than 1% of the general population to be infected but greater than 50% seroprevalence in selected populations in certain geographic areas.

Pattern II countries are typically developing nations—central, southern, and eastern Africa and some Caribbean countries—with high numbers of cases among heterosexual persons. Perinatal transmission is common. Transmission through blood and blood products remains a problem in countries that have not yet implemented a donor-screening program. If transmission by intravenous drug abuse or homosexual activity occurs at all, it is rare. Seroprevalance studies generally show that over 1% of the general population is infected and prevalence may be as high as 25% in the general population in certain urban areas.

Pattern III is generally restricted to countries that have had very few AIDS cases—Eastern Europe, the Middle East, Asia, and most of the Pacific. HIV-1 was probably introduced into these areas in the early to mid-1980s. Most of these cases are linked to imported contaminated blood or blood products or sexual contact with persons from pattern I or II countries.

CLINICAL SYNDROMES

HIV disease progresses from latent or asymptomatic infection identified only by laboratory evidence in otherwise healthy persons to severely impaired immunologic function in persons with AIDS. Understanding of the spectrum of HIV infection has become increasingly sophisticated as laboratory tests and epidemiologic studies have evolved that have delineated the natural course of infection. Terms such as AIDS-related complex and even AIDS are now of limited use in characterizing patients and monitoring evolution of

TABLE 50–4			
GLOBAL ACQUIRED IMMUNODEFICIENCY DISEASE TRANSMISSION PATTERNS, 1991			
	Percent Transmission		
Risk Group	**Pattern I** (Industrial Nations)	**Pattern II** (Developing Nations)	**Pattern III** (Other Nations)
Heterosexual	5	80	Varies
Drug addicts	20	1	Varies
Homosexual	70	5	Varies
Transfusion	1	10	>50

this disease.[42] The term AIDS-related complex is vague with respect to prognosis and does not adequately describe the severity of immune system derangement. Similarly, the term AIDS is of limited value because there is significant prognostic variation within the subset of patients who fulfill the Centers for Disease Control case definitions of AIDS. Furthermore, it focuses attention away from the remainder of the spectrum of HIV disease. At present, the term HIV infection should be used, as this term encompasses the entire spectrum of clinical states associated with this virus.

Acute Retroviral Syndrome

It is estimated that as many as two thirds of individuals with acute HIV infection present with an infectious mononucleosis–like syndrome or, less commonly, an acute neurologic illness such as meningitis, encephalitis, myelopathy, or polyneuropathy. The interval from infection to disease onset in the acute retroviral syndrome ranges from 1 to 6 weeks.[43] The disease is heralded by the abrupt onset of nonspecific symptoms, which include fever, sweats, muscle aches and pains, headaches, and gastrointestinal disturbances. Sore throat occurs in as many as two thirds of patients. Exudates have been reported.[43] A macular rash is seen in up to 50% of patients.[43] Generalized lymphadenopathy, splenomegaly, and hepatomegaly with liver function abnormalities have also occurred.[43] Various neurologic syndromes may be seen during acute illness, including aseptic meningitis, an encephalitic picture, or even transverse myelopathy. HIV is recovered in blood culture and frequently in a culture of cerebrospinal fluid. HIV antigenemia occurs in up to two thirds of individuals. Lymphopenia occurs with the onset of symptoms. After this, there is a marked proliferation of suppressor T cells, reaching a maximum approximately 2 weeks after the onset of illness. This results in a reversal of the CD4+/CD8+ ratio. At the same time, a typical lymphocytosis is seen. This constellation of symptoms mimics that in infections with Epstein-Barr virus, cytomegalovirus, *Toxoplasma gondii*, or *Treponema pallidum*. These agents should be considered in the differential diagnosis of the acute retroviral syndrome. Seroconversion generally occurs within 3 months of the acute infection.[43]

Asymptomatic Interval

After seroconversion, patients generally make a complete recovery and are asymptomatic. Many patients, however, have clinical signs of persistent generalized lymphadenopathy. The Centers for Disease Control defines HIV-related persistent generalized lymphadenopathy as palpable lymphadenopathy (lymph nodes of 1 cm or greater) at two or more extrainguinal sites persisting for more than 3 months and the absence of other illness or conditions that could explain these findings.[44] Lymph node biopsy is generally not recommended to confirm this diagnosis. Biopsy usually shows benign reactive changes. Adenopathy is unlikely to be found at the later stages of HIV infection. Indeed, in some patients the disappearance of long lasting adenopathy is generally followed by progression of HIV disease.[45]

Symptomatic Disease

It is beyond the scope of this chapter to describe fully the enormous range of clinical signs and symptoms observed in people with HIV disease. Instead, the clinical syndromes that are germane to the management of persons with HIV infection in the intensive care unit are discussed. The reader is referred to standard textbooks on infectious diseases or AIDS for a more encyclopedic discussion. A basic principle

in the management of persons with HIV infection is an appreciation of the appearance of certain opportunistic infections or malignancies in a hierarchic fashion associated with declining CD4+ lymphocyte counts. This hierarchy of complications of HIV infection is illustrated in Figure 50–1. The earliest clinical syndromes or infections seen are thrush, recurring vaginal candidiasis, and oral hairy leukoplakia. All of these conditions can be seen in persons with absolute CD4+ lymphocyte counts in the range 400 to 600/mm³. The first serious opportunistic infection to occur with increased frequency is tuberculosis, which may be seen with CD4+ cell counts in the range 300 to 400/mm³. The clinical presentation of tuberculosis in persons with HIV depends on the degree of immune suppression. In those with relatively intact immunity, pulmonary disease is the rule. As immunity wanes, disseminated or extrapulmonary tuberculosis is seen with increasing frequency. It is noteworthy that the lifetime risk of developing tuberculosis disease in persons with tuberculous infection—that is, asymptomatic persons with a positive tuberculin skin test—is 10%. In contrast, the annual risk of developing tuberculosis disease in HIV-infected persons who are tuberculosis infected is estimated to be 10%.[46] As with tuberculosis, Kaposi's sarcoma is often seen initially in persons with relatively intact CD4+ lymphocyte counts again in the range 300 to 400/mm³. Similarly, non-Hodgkin's lymphoma may be seen initially in persons with these CD4+ cell counts. PCP is generally seen when CD4+ cell counts are about 200/mm³.[47] PCP is a frequently occurring AIDS-defining illness in persons not receiving prophylaxis against this agent. It is estimated that in the absence of prophylaxis, as many as 85% of persons with CD4+ lymphocyte counts less than 200/mm³ eventually develop this infection either as their AIDS-defining illness or after another AIDS-defining illness.[48] Toxoplasmic encephalitis, usually presenting as brain abscesses, is seen with increasing frequency when the CD4+ cell count is 100/mm³ or less. The risk of developing toxoplasmosis is extremely high in persons with pre-existing antibodies to *Toxoplasma*. In one series, one of every three patients with HIV infection and pre-existing antibodies to *Toxoplasma* developed central nervous system disease.[49] When the absolute CD4+ cell count reaches 50/mm³ or less, the risk of disseminated cytomegalovirus disease of the retina, gastrointestinal tract, or other organs increases significantly. Similarly, there is a high rate of infection with so-called atypical mycobacteria, particularly *Mycobacterium avium* complex. Studies have shown that most deaths in persons with advanced symptomatic HIV disease occur when the CD4+ cell count is 50/mm³ or less.[50] Table 50–1 outlines the CD4+ cell counts, risk of infection, and long-term prognosis in persons with HIV disease.

TREATMENT OF HUMAN IMMUNODEFICIENCY VIRUS INFECTION

The life cycle of HIV makes it vulnerable to interruption by therapeutic agents. Vulnerable points include virus attachment, virus entry into the cell, transcription of viral genome, integration into host cell DNA, translation of virus products, and assembly and release. Drugs that inhibit transcription are now available and are discussed later. Drugs that act at other points in the life cycle are under development. Drugs under development are discussed next.

Drugs That Inhibit Virus Attachment and Penetration

Recombinant soluble CD4 molecules bind to the HIV outer coat gp120, blocking its attachment to host cells. First-generation soluble CD4 was safe when given to patients but failed to demonstrate antiretroviral activity.[51, 52] A recombinant CD4–immunoglobulin G chimeric molecule has greater activity in vitro than either molecule alone[53] and appears to have favorable pharmacokinetics in vivo.[54] Trials are under way. A recombinant CD4–*Pseudomonas aeruginosa* exotoxin A hybrid selectively kills host cells expressing gp120.[55] Clinical trials are likewise under way.

Drugs That Inhibit Virus Translation

HIV produces large polyproteins that are precursors of its individual protein components. It also produces a protease that cleaves the polyproteins, for example, the *gag-pol* precursor. Various HIV protease inhibitors have been developed;[56–58] clinical trials are under way. A benzodiazepine compound has been identified that inhibits *tat* activity.[59] Phase I pharmacokinetic trials are under way.

Drugs That Inhibit Virus Assembly

Not as much is known about HIV assembly and release as about attachment, penetration, transcription, and translation. Interferon-α appears to interfere with assembly of HIV. Given alone, injectable interferon-α appears to have modest antiretroviral activity.[60] It has demonstrated synergistic activity when combined with zidovudine (ZDV) in persons with HIV infection.[61] Large-scale trials are beginning to look at this combination.

Drugs That Inhibit Virus Transcription

Many compounds inhibit HIV transcription, particularly by reverse transcriptase inhibition. The first effective reverse transcriptase inhibitors to be developed were nucleoside derived. Two, ZDV and didanosine (formerly dideoxyinosine), are now available by prescription. A third, dideoxycytidine, is expected to be available by prescription soon. Many other nucleoside agents are at various stages of development. In addition, a series of pyridinone reverse transcriptase inhibitors have been developed that exhibit potent in vitro activity versus HIV-1 but not HIV-2. Unfortunately, HIV-1 rapidly becomes resistant to these agents in vitro.[62] Their efficacy in human trials is being investigated.

ZDV is the most successful antiretroviral drug to date. Observations of a significant decrease in mortality after treatment with ZDV compared with placebo in persons with AIDS or advanced symptomatic HIV disease with CD4+ cell counts less than or equal to 200/mm³ led to its licensure in 1987.[63] More recent data demonstrated its efficacy in reducing progression to late symptomatic disease in persons with CD4+ cell counts greater than or equal to 500/mm³.[64, 65] These trials also established the dosage of ZDV, which is now 500 to 600 mg daily in divided doses. The major toxicities are hematologic and occur more frequently in persons with late or advanced symptomatic disease. Regimens for AIDS-associated opportunistic infections are often associated with hematologic toxicity. For that reason, most clinicians deem it prudent to withhold therapy and reintroduce ZDV after the patient has recovered. This is particularly cogent in the intensive care setting. The emergence of HIV strains resistant to ZDV has been described[66] and may correlate with failure of ZDV to maintain remission of HIV disease.[67]

Didanosine is now available by prescription, despite lack of data from ongoing large-scale clinical trials. Antiretroviral activity has been demonstrated in several phase I or phase II clinical trials.[68–70] Its major toxicities are peripheral neuropathy and pancreatitis. It is generally given to patients who are ZDV intolerant or who have developed recurrent major opportunistic infections or malignancies while receiving ZDV. Dideoxycytidine has demonstrated antiretroviral activity in phase I or phase II trials.[71] Its toxicity profile is similar to that of didanosine. Both didanosine and dideoxycytidine are active against ZDV-resistant HIV-1 isolates.[66]

INTENSIVE CARE IN PERSONS WITH HUMAN IMMUNODEFICIENCY VIRUS INFECTION

The complications of late or advanced HIV infection typically involve multiple organ systems. This involvement can produce severe dysfunction that may be life threatening or fatal.[72] Intensive care may be required for persons with AIDS for a variety of reasons. Most major series suggest that the most common reason for intensive care is respiratory failure. However, hypotension and central nervous system disorders are also relatively common. Finally, persons with AIDS may require intensive care for reasons unrelated to AIDS per se, such as drug overdose, trauma, or asthma.[48, 72] Table 50–5 lists the usual indications for intensive care unit admission in two large metropolitan units: San Francisco General Hospital[73] and the Detroit Medical Center. The most common reason for admission is respiratory failure caused by PCP. Surgical intensive care follows, usually for patients who have had brain biopsy surgery. Shock, often related to bacteremia, is third. The next section describes PCP in detail.

PNEUMOCYSTIS CARINII PNEUMONIA
Epidemiology, Microbiology, and Pathogenesis

PCP is the most common life-threatening opportunistic infection in AIDS patients,[48, 72] although, with the widespread use of PCP prophylaxis, PCP as the index disease in AIDS diagnosis decreased to 49% by 1990.[74] As previously noted, the risk of PCP increases substantially when the CD4+ cell count is 200/mm³ or less.[47]

P. carinii was long deemed a protozoan, but studies of its ribosomal RNA showed greater homology with fungi, suggesting that it should be reclassified.[75] The organism has both intracystic (sporozoite) and extracystic (trophozoite) forms. Cysts are oval or round, 5 to 8 μm in diameter, and contain four to eight nucleated sporozoites. The trophozoites are 2 to 5 μm and are pleomorphic with an eccentric nucleus. In lavage and tissue specimens, trophozoites and cysts are associated with an eosinophilic and faintly periodic acid–Schiff–positive "foamy" exudate; as cysts are faintly periodic acid–Schiff–positive, they are poorly seen. Cysts are best demonstrated with Gomori's methenamine-silver or toluidine O stain. Trophozoites and sporozoites can be seen with Giemsa's, Gram's, or Wright's stains.

The life cycle and reservoir of *P. carinii* are not known. Because antibodies to *P. carinii* are seen during childhood,

	San Francisco General 1981–1985 (N = 86)	Detroit Medical Center 1987–1990 (N = 64)
TABLE 50–5		
USUAL INDICATIONS FOR INTENSIVE CARE ADMISSION		
Indication		
PCP requiring intubation and mechanical ventilation	45 (52%)	35 (55%)
PCP, no intubation	9 (10%)	3 (5%)
Surgical procedure	9 (10%)	10 (16%)
Sepsis or hypotension	8 (9%)	6 (9%)
Cardiac arrhythmia	2 (2%)	0 (0%)
Other	13 (15%)	10 (16%)

it is thought that the organisms reside in the lungs as latent infection. Although it is presumed that active disease occurs as a result of reactivation of latent infection, primary infection or reinfection may occur. During early PCP, there are small numbers of cysts and a minimal or absent inflammatory response. Findings are limited to the alveolar spaces. With progression, more alveoli become filled with organisms and exudate, resulting in pulmonary function defects. Hypertrophy of type 1 and type 2 alveolar cells appears. Mononuclear cell infiltrate predominates. Eventually, the alveolar cells desquamate, resulting in increased permeability of the alveolar capillary membrane with consequent pulmonary edema.[76]

Clinical and Laboratory Findings

Symptoms correlate with the pathologic findings. During early PCP, the patient experiences few or no symptoms. As organisms proliferate, symptoms occur.[77] It is instructive to contrast the clinical findings related to PCP in persons with AIDS and those with other immunocompromising diseases. An abrupt onset of illness (<36 hours) and an associated high fever (92% of patients) are hallmarks of PCP in immunocompromised patients without AIDS. In persons with AIDS, PCP is typically characterized by an insidious onset (2 to 3 weeks). Almost one quarter of patients are afebrile. Both groups of patients have dry cough, dyspnea, and clear lungs on auscultation.[78] The cough is typically nonproductive; a thin, watery sputum may be produced. The patient appears acutely ill, febrile, and tachypneic. Despite tachypnea and often florid roentgenographic findings, chest findings are minimal. Rhonchi or wheezes should suggest other etiologies. Extrapulmonary pneumocystosis may occur, particularly in patients receiving pentamadine aerosol for primary or secondary prophylaxis; the rate of occurrence at one institution was reported to be 2.5% in patients with AIDS-associated PCP.[79] Various sites have been involved, including skin, thyroid, ear, marrow, spleen, liver, eye, and adrenals.[79]

Complete blood counts and sedimentation rates are not helpful; aside from elevated serum lactate dehydrogenase levels, reflecting pulmonary injury, serum chemistry assays are not helpful. Elevated serum lactate dehydrogenase levels may correlate with poor outcome,[80] although this needs confirmation. Arterial blood gas measurements typically show uncompensated respiratory alkalosis with increased arterial-alveolar oxygen tension difference. The PaO_2 may exceed 80 mm Hg in one quarter of patients.[78] In PCP, oxygenation is the best indicator of prognosis; generally arterial-alveolar oxygen tension differences greater than 35 mm Hg or a PaO_2 less than 70 mm Hg is associated with decreased survival.[78] The most consistent pulmonary function abnormality is impaired diffusing capacity for carbon monoxide. Volume reductions may occur but not to the same degree as diffusion reductions. Usually, x-ray films show bilateral, interstitial infiltrates, which eventually progress to alveolar filling. However, normal chest x-ray films may be seen 5 to 10% of the time,[81] and various atypical findings have been described, including abscesses, cavitation, consolidation, nodular lesions, effusions, and pneumothorax.[82] In patients with suspected PCP and normal chest x-ray films, gallium scanning of the lungs is positive with 90% specificity.[83]

Diagnosis

Diagnostic algorithms have been developed for the evaluation of PCP. Generally, if PCP is suspected in a person with a normal chest x-ray film, a diffusing capacity test or

TABLE 50–6
PULMONARY DISORDERS IN PATIENTS WITH ACQUIRED IMMUNODEFICIENCY SYNDROME
P. carinii pneumonia (approximately one third of cases associated with coexisting infection, usually cytomegalovirus or *M. avium* complex) *M. avium* complex Cytomegalovirus Encapsulated bacteria (*H. influenzae* or *S. pneumoniae*) *Mycobacterium tuberculosis* *Legionella* sp. Fungi (*Cryptococcus neoformans, Histoplasma capsulatum, Coccidioides immitis*) Kaposi's sarcoma Nonspecific pneumonitis

gallium scan is done; if the results are abnormal, a bronchoscopy with bronchoalveolar lavage is done. In the case of abnormal chest x-ray films, the tempo of the work-up is dictated by the severity of illness; minimal findings dictate less invasive procedures. Although the yield is low (60%) examination of induced sputum for PCP should be tried first to avoid more invasive procedures in mild to moderately ill patients.[84, 85] Today, transbronchial biopsy and bronchoalveolar lavage using the fiberoptic bronchoscope are the standards by which other diagnostic procedures are evaluated. The sensitivity of transbronchial biopsy ranges from 66 to 98% and the sensitivity of bronchoalveolar lavage from 55 to 98%.[86] As a rule, transbronchial lung biopsy is done if PCP is suspected and a bronchoalveolar lavage is negative. In addition, transbronchial lung biopsy should be done in patients who have received pentamidine aerosol prophylaxis or in centers where yields of bronchoalveolar lavage are lower than those reported in the literature.

Other pathogens or conditions may also cause respiratory failure in AIDS; a differential diagnosis is outlined in Table 50–6. A few points are noteworthy. Because of profound perturbations in B cell function, encapsulated bacteria, particularly *Haemophilus influenzae* and *Streptococcus pneumoniae*, can cause severe, bilateral pneumonia in persons with AIDS.[87] A national resurgence of tuberculosis has occurred because of AIDS.[88] Bilateral, diffuse noncavitary infiltrates and respiratory failure can occur. All persons with AIDS and bilateral infiltrates should be in respiratory isolation until tuberculosis is ruled out. Nonspecific pneumonitis is common in pediatric AIDS but rare in adult AIDS; its etiology is not known.[89]

Often, a coexisting infection, as with cytomegalovirus or *M. avium* complex, is present.[3]

Therapy

Data suggest that pentamidine is more efficacious for the treatment of PCP in AIDS than trimethoprim-sulfamethoxazole (TMP-SMX).[90] However, TMP-SMX is used most often as initial therapy for PCP. Pentamidine is nephrotoxic and can produce irreversible, fatal hypoglycemia.[91] Intravenous use can result in shock. The drug is given as a slow (1 hour or longer) 4 mg/kg infusion once daily. Mild cases (first episode, PO_2 > 55 mm Hg) can be treated with a lower dose (3 mg/kg).[92] Aerosolized pentamidine, 300 to 600 mg/d, has shown promise in mild cases in pilot studies.[93] The dose of TMP-SMX is 15 to 20 mg/kg/d (as TMP component) intravenously (four doses). There are high incidences of rash (50%), leukopenia (40%), thrombocytopenia (20%), and hepatotoxicity (20%) in AIDS patients with PCP treated with TMP-SMX. The rate of adverse reactions is directly related to the dose of drug and duration of therapy. Oral dapsone-trimethoprim elicits responses similar to those to TMP-SMX or pentamidine; many consider this a first-line treatment for mild cases.[94] The combination of primaquine and clindamycin, which was equivalent to TMP-SMX in PCP animal models,[95] has been shown to be equivalent to dapsone-trimethoprim in the treatment of mild-to-moderate PCP (AIDS Clinical Trials Group Protocol,[108] unpublished).

Alternative therapy for patients who do not respond to conventional therapy includes trimetrexate, a potent anti-folate (1500 times more potent than TMP) with leucovorin rescue.[96] Agents under study include several 8-aminoquinolines developed as antimalarials by the Walter Reed Army Institute for Research. These agents, which include WR 6026, WR 238,605, and WR 242,511, exhibit potent activity in animal models of PCP.[97] A novel hydroxynaphthoquinone, 566C80, exhibits in vitro and in vivo activity against *P. carinii, Toxoplasma,* and malaria. Clinical trials are under way for PCP and toxoplasmosis.[98]

Several studies have demonstrated that corticosteroid therapy reduces mortality in the hypoxic patient with PCP.[99–101] A National Institutes of Health–sponsored consensus panel recommended routine administration of corticosteroids within 72 hours of beginning therapy for AIDS patients with PCP with a Po_2 less than 70 mm Hg or an arterial-alveolar oxygen difference greater than 35 mm Hg.[102] High-dose corticosteroid therapy has also been tried in unresponsive cases;[103] many clinicians give salvage or rescue doses of corticosteroids to intubated patients with PCP, even though that treatment is unproved.

Confusion abounds as to when to determine that a patient with PCP is not responding to treatment. Most would agree that 1 to 2 days is too soon and 3 weeks is too late.[104] Compared with that in other immunosuppressive states, the clinical and x-ray evidence of response to therapy is delayed in AIDS; typically in non-AIDS patients a response is seen in 3 to 5 days, in AIDS patients in 7 to 10 days.[78] Generally, we consider a change in therapy if there is no response within 5 to 7 days. Recurrence rates are 20 to 40% within 6 months in AIDS, compared to 15% in 15 months in children with acute lymphocytic leukemia.[105] Overall mortality for first-episode PCP is 26%; mortality rises to 40 to 60% with the second or third episode.[106] Mortality rates of 10% have

been reported.[107] Table 50–7 summarizes therapeutic options for the management of PCP.

Prognosis

Wachter and Luce have succinctly reviewed the three changes in the approach to intensive care for persons with AIDS and PCP that have occurred during the first decade of the epidemic.[108] During the early years of the epidemic, physicians lacked the information to make an appropriate decision regarding mechanical ventilation and intensive care for PCP. Intensive care utilization and costs were high.[73] In series reported during the mid-1980s survival rates were 10 to 13%.[73, 109] As a result, patients and physicians often rejected intensive care.[73] In the late 1980s and early 1990s several reports of improved short-term survival, ranging from 40 to 50%,[110, 111] have forced physicians and their patients to reconsider the role of intensive care in PCP and in AIDS. One-year survival, regardless of when the series was published, remains dismal—often less than 15%. The reasons for the remarkable improvement in short-term survival are not clear but probably include such factors as corticosteroids, antiretrovirals, and PCP prophylaxis.[112] Predictors of survival in the mechanically ventilated patient with AIDS and PCP have been examined by several investigators. Several small retrospective series[113–115] have failed to identify risk factors that might predict adverse outcomes at the time of admission to critical care, including such variables as Acute Physiology and Chronic Health Evaluation (APACHE) II scores, HIV risk factors, gender, and various laboratory values. In these retrospective studies, the development of metabolic acidemia, widened alveolar-arterial gradients, or prolonged use of positive end-expiratory pressure occurred significantly more often in nonsurvivors. Le and coworkers have examined several scoring systems for the severity of disease in predicting outcome for patients with PCP-related respiratory failure who require intensive care.[116] Of the scores, including the APACHE II score,[117] the multiple organ system failure score,[118] and the adult respiratory distress score,[119] the multiple organ system failure score and an AIDS prognostic score developed by Justice and coworkers[120] were best in predicting survival of patients with PCP-related acute respiratory failure admitted to intensive care. Table 50–8 summarizes the salient features of the scoring system of Justice and coworkers.

INFECTION CONTROL

This section covers three broad areas of concern related to HIV and infection control in intensive care: transmission issues, ZDV postexposure prophylaxis, and the HIV-infected health care worker.

Transmission Issues

Since the first case report of occupational HIV infection in 1984,[121] some have argued against admitting patients to the intensive care unit because of concerns about exposure of and transmission of HIV-1 to personnel. Essential to allaying these concerns is an understanding of the routes of transmission of HIV-1, which were well established months before the causative agent was isolated. Less sophisticated health care workers often focus on reports of HIV-1 being cultured from virtually every body secretion, including blood, semen, vaginal fluid, amniotic fluid, tears, saliva, breast milk, and cerebrospinal fluid. These observations seemingly imply that extraordinary isolation procedures are needed to protect the health care worker. Transmission by these body fluids is of theoretic concern, but no case of HIV

TABLE 50–7

THERAPEUTIC OPTIONS FOR *PNEUMOCYSTIS CARINII* PNEUMONIA

Critically ill patient
  Trimethoprim-sulfamethoxazole, 20 mg/kg/d (as trimethoprim, four divided doses) *or*
  Pentamidine, 4 mg/kg/d IV daily
If $Po_2 \leq 70$ mm Hg, or alveolar-arterial oxygen tension difference ≥ 35 mm Hg
  Give prednisone, 40 mg orally twice daily days 1–5; 40 mg daily days 6–10; 20 mg daily days 11–21. May give methylprednisolone IV at 75% of oral prednisone doses.
Mild to moderately ill patient
  Dapsone, 100 mg/d, plus trimethoprim, 20 mg/kg/d, four divided doses *or*
  Oral trimethoprim-sulfamethoxazole, 20 mg/kg/d, four divided doses = four tablets q.i.d. in 70-kg patient *or*
  Pentamidine, 3 mg/kg/d IV *or*
  Primaquine, 15 mg (as base) daily, and clindamycin, 300–600 mg four times daily, *or*
  Pentamidine aerosol, 300–600 mg/d
Patient unresponsive to conventional therapy
  Consider experimental therapy (call 1-800-TRIALS-A, the national AIDS hotline)
  Consider high-dose corticosteroids

TABLE 50-8

PROGNOSTIC STAGING SYSTEM FOR ACQUIRED IMMUNODEFICIENCY SYNDROME

Assign 1 point for each of these seven variables, if present:
Nutritional
   Albumin ≤ 2.0 g/dL and/or diarrhea ≥ 2 wk preceding admission
Respiratory
   Po_2 ≤ 50 mm Hg
Neurologic
   Any of the following: lethargy or confusion, new paralysis, stiff neck, seizures, dementia, photophobia, dysarthria, aphasia
Hematologic
   Lymphocytes < 150/mm³
   Hematocrit < 30%
   White blood cells < 2500/mm³
   Platelets < 140,000/mm³
The maximal point score is 7. Stages as follows:
Stage I 0 points total, 1-y survival 50%
Stage II 1 point total, 1-y survival 30%
Stage III ≥2 points total, 1-y survival 8%

Adapted from information appearing in Justice AC, Feinstein AR, Wells CK: A new prognostic staging system for the acquired immunodeficiency syndrome. N Engl J Med 320:1388–1393, 1989.

infection by external body fluids other than semen has been documented. Blood and semen have been directly implicated in transmission of HIV-1, and breast milk and vaginal fluid transmission probably occurs.[32] Transmission data have established that exposure occurs by sexual intercourse, by inoculation of contaminated blood or blood products, and by perinatal routes. Thus, exposure to blood is of primary concern to the health care worker.

Occupational transmission of HIV happens. Worldwide, as of mid-1990, 27 cases of proven occupational transmission of HIV have been reported.[122, 123] Twenty-one were caused by needle stick exposure,[121, 123–131] one by exposure to a laceration,[132] three by mucocutaneous exposure,[133] and two by exposure to high concentrations of HIV in laboratory accidents.[134] Furthermore, a mother who provided the equivalent of intensive nursing care for her infant with AIDS without practicing infection control apparently seroconverted.[135] Prospective studies of exposure of health care workers to persons with HIV infection have now been reported, including over 4000 workers and over 1200 sharp instrument and needle stick incidents. These studies show that seroconversion occurs after needle stick exposure, but the rate of occurrence is low, in the neighborhood of 0.4% or 1:250.[122, 132, 134, 136–140] This rate is substantially lower than the 12 to 17% seroconversion rate after needle stick inoculation from a patient with hepatitis B virus infection.[141, 142] This is illustrated by the report of a bronchoscopy assistant who contracted hepatitis B but not HIV-1 infection after an accidental needle stick exposure to a person infected with both viruses.[143]

These results strongly support the axiom that inoculum size is important in transmission of viruses, including HIV-1. During most of the course of infection, there are 10 or fewer HIV-1 infected mononuclear cells per 10^7 cells in experimental primate infection,[144] perhaps 1 to 10% of CD4⁺ cells.[145] This is an extremely low titer; in contrast, titers as great as 10^8/mL of blood occur in patients with hepatitis B antigenemia.[146]

Except for intense, repeated exposures of nongloved persons to blood,[133] close, nonparenteral contact with infected patients does not result in seroconversion. To date, prospective studies have failed to show seroconversion after mucocutaneous exposures. This is supported by the observation that the incidence of AIDS in health care workers, 5.8%, is no greater than the proportion of Americans in the U.S. labor force employed in the health care professions. The question of isolation of HIV-1 from saliva remains a concern to many health care workers. Several well-designed household contact studies, summarized by Friedland and Klein,[32] have failed to show transmission of virus by salivary routes. Also, the frequency of isolation of virus from saliva is small. To put this in perspective, Ho and coworkers have shown that in 71 men infected with HIV-1, virus could be isolated in 28 of 50 blood samples but in only 1 of 83 saliva specimens.[147]

These data suggest that standard infection control practices, particularly blood precautions, minimize the risk of transmission of HIV-1 to the health care worker. It is noteworthy that 40% of accidental exposure to HIV-1 is preventable.[135] The problem in intensive care, and, for that matter, in all health care areas, is that medical history and physical examination cannot reliably identify all patients who are HIV-1 infected. After infection, expression of disease is silent for months to years. There is, therefore, a large reservoir of infected but clinically silent people. For example, in a prospective HIV-1 serologic study of critically ill patients seen in a emergency facility, six (3% of the total) actively bleeding seropositive patients were identified. All six required multiple invasive procedures. Only two of the six had a history or physical evidence of intravenous drug abuse.[148] The best estimates of seroprevalence in hospitals are provided by the Sentinel Hospital Surveillance Study, a blind seroprevalence study of HIV in patients of all age groups and both sexes with "low-risk" admitting diagnoses. Overall, the national HIV seroprevalence rate of such low-risk hospitalized patients is 0.77%.[149] In any given community, the incidence of unsuspected HIV-1 infection in critically ill patients varies directly with the prevalence of clinically recognized disease. Incidence is highest in the 20- to 45-year age group.

These observations have led the Centers for Disease Control to recommend that blood and body fluid precautions be used consistently for all patients. Universal precautions have been supported by the American Hospital Association and several individual state health departments and are now a Joint Commission on Accreditation of Hospitals standard. The Occupational Safety and Health Administration has mandated universal blood and body fluid precautions for all health care facilities. Universal precautions are summarized in Table 50–9.

Despite the use of universal precautions, some physicians advocate routine screening of patients for HIV-1 antibodies and would make HIV serologic testing routine. The HIV antibody test is in no way routine.[150] Loss of jobs, insurance, housing, schooling, and family support; suicide attempts; and major depressive disease after test disclosure have been described.[150, 151] Because of the important medical, psychologic, legal, and social implications of a positive test, Bayer and coauthors urged consent of the patient and counseling before and after testing.[152] Even though medical leadership has strongly supported these principles, it is disturbing to see that hospital physicians rarely adhere to them. In a study reported from a university hospital,[153] nearly half of the patients tested for HIV-1 antibody had no recognized medical risk factor in their chart and only 10% gave consent or were counseled. Even in the case of a comatose, critically ill patient, all efforts must be made to meet these guidelines. In general, serologic testing for HIV-1 in the intensive care unit should be considered when (1) testing the patient will benefit public health and safety, for example, when the patient is a candidate for organ donation; (2) testing the

TABLE 50–9

PRECAUTIONS TO PREVENT TRANSMISSION OF HUMAN IMMUNODEFICIENCY VIRUS IN THE HEALTH CARE SETTING

Use barrier precautions when there is contact with blood or body fluid of any patient:
  Gloves
    During venipuncture, providing care involving mucous membranes, handling blood- or body fluid–soiled items
  Mask, eye shields
    During procedures likely to result in visible bleeding
  Gowns, aprons
    If procedure likely to result in splashes of blood or body fluids
Discard gloves; wash hands between contact with all patients.
Dispose of sharp devices in puncture-resistant containers; never recap needles.
Minimize the need for mouth-to-mouth resuscitation (although salivary transmission is unproved); ensure accessible ventilation devices.
Health care workers with exudative lesions or dermatitis must refrain from direct care of patients.
Pregnant workers can continue to provide care for patients using these guidelines.

patient will benefit another, most commonly because the patient is source of occupational exposure to a health care worker; and (3) testing the patient will influence medical management (in most instances knowledge of HIV test results does not influence intensive care management but obviously does alter the medical management of a stable patient).

Postexposure Prophylaxis

Studies of the efficacy of prophylactic ZDV after exposure to HIV have been hampered by the lack of an animal model of HIV infection. Early animal model experiments with other retroviral infections suggested that prompt initiation of a brief course of ZDV might successfully abort retroviral infections.[154–156] Furthermore, in an HIV SCID-hu mouse model, postexposure prophylaxis did not prevent HIV infection.[157] The logistics and large numbers required to conduct a double-blind, placebo-controlled trial in health care workers prohibit proving the efficacy of ZDV in a clinical trial. Indeed, there are case reports of failure of ZDV to prevent transmission after accidental parenteral exposures.[158–160] Nevertheless, many institutions are now providing postexposure prophylaxis with ZDV in an effort to prevent HIV infection in health care workers exposed to the virus. Most institutions recommend relatively high doses of ZDV, 1200 mg/d for 4 to 6 weeks. The initial dose should be given as early as possible, preferably within 4 hours after exposure. The exposure must be adequately evaluated to ensure that the drug is not given for trivial reasons. Screening for pregnancy must be done. The exposed health care worker must be counseled about the risks and benefits of prophylactic ZDV and about safe sex practices, and follow-up care must be provided. Psychologic support may be needed.[161]

The Human Immunodeficiency Virus–Infected Health Care Worker

The first report suggesting than an HIV-infected health care worker transmitted the virus to patients appeared in 1990. Five patients of a Fort Lauderdale dentist were found to be infected with strains of HIV-1 that were closely related genetically to the strain infecting the dentist.[162, 163] The strains were distinct from viruses obtained from control patients living in the same area. The route of possible transmission was not known, but all patients had had invasive procedures performed by the dentist. The cause of HIV transmission in this setting is not clear, but the transmission is thought to be related to failure to follow proper infection control procedures. During the first decade of the epidemic, this represented the first possible transmission of HIV to patients by a health care worker. The Centers for Disease Control estimated the risk of acquiring HIV infection from an infected surgeon or dentist to range from 1:42,000 to 1:420,000.[164] Other reports suggested that the risk of HIV transmission from surgeon to patient is considerably lower.[165] To place these risks in greater perspective, they might be compared to the 1:10,000 risk of death of patients undergoing general anesthesia or the 1:100,000 risk of a fatal anaphylactic reaction to penicillin.[166] Should health care workers be required to disclose their HIV infection to patients? Such a policy would discourage health care workers at risk for HIV from being tested. Mandatory testing and disclosure would result in loss of services of noninfected health care workers because of fear of seroconversion. HIV-infected patients would have their limited access to care limited even further. Mandatory testing of health care workers would divert millions of scarce health care dollars from effective HIV prevention activities.[167] Because of the low risks of transmission and the high costs of mandatory testing and disclosure, prudent policy centers on practice of universal precautions, training in proper techniques, development of safe medical devices, voluntary testing and counseling of health care workers, and individual and periodic evaluation of infected health care workers by competent panels of experts.[166]

References

1. Centers for Disease Control: *Pneumocystis* pneumonia—Los Angeles. MMWR 30:250, 1981.
2. Centers for Disease Control: Kaposi's sarcoma and *Pneumocystis* pneumonia among homosexual men—New York City and California. MMWR 30:305, 1981.
3. Barre-Sinoussi F, Chermann JC, Rey F, et al: Isolation of a T-lymphotropic retrovirus from a patient at risk for acquired immune deficiency syndrome (AIDS). Science 220:868, 1983.
4. Popovic M, Sarngadharan MG, Read E, et al: Detection, isolation, and continuous production of cytopathic retroviruses (HTLV-III) from patients with AIDS and pre-AIDS. Science 224:497, 1984.
5. Levy JA, Hoffman AD, Kramer SM, et al: Isolation of lymphocytopathic retroviruses from San Francisco patients with AIDS. Science 225:840, 1984.
6. Brun-Vezinet F, Rey MA, Katlama C, et al: Original articles: Lymphadenopathy-associated virus type 2 in AIDS and AIDS-related complex: Clinical and virological features in four patients. Lancet 1:128, 1987.
7. Haseltine WA: Replication and pathogenesis of the AIDS virus. J Acquir Immune Defic Syndr 1:217, 1988.
8. Greene WC: The molecular biology of human immunodeficiency virus type 1 infection. N Engl J Med 324:308, 1991.
9. Ho DD, Moudgil T, Alam M: Quantitation of human immunodeficiency virus type 1 in the blood of infected persons. N Engl J Med 321:1621, 1989.
10. Mazeika GG, McGrath MS: HIV viral proteins: Structure and function. In: Cohen PT, Sande MA, Volberding PA (eds): The AIDS Knowledge Base. Waltham, MA, Medical Publishing Group, p 3.1.7.1, 1990.
11. Fauci AS: The human immunodeficiency virus: Infectivity and mechanisms of pathogenesis. Science 239:617, 1988.
12. Castro BA, Cheng-Mayer C, Evans LA, et al: HIV heterogeneity and viral pathogenesis. AIDS 2(suppl 1):S17, 1988.
13. Brenneman DE, Westbrook GL, Fitzgerald SP, et al: Neuronal cell killing by the envelope protein of HIV and its prevention by vasoactive intestinal peptide. Nature 335:639, 1988.
14. Kaiser PK, Offerman JT, Lipton SA: Neuronal injury due to HIV-1 envelope protein is blocked by anti-gp120 antibodies but not by anti-CD4 antibodies. Neurology 40:1757, 1990.
15. Gallaher WR: Detection of a fusion peptide sequence in the transmembrane protein of human immunodeficiency virus. Cell 50:327, 1987.
16. Bedinger P, Moriarty A, von Borstel RC, et al: Internalization of the

human immunodeficiency virus does not require the cytoplasmic domain of CD4. Nature 334:162, 1988.

17. DesJarlais DC, Friedman SR, Marmor M, et al: Development of AIDS, HIV seroconversion, and potential co-factors for T4 cell loss in a cohort of intravenous drug users. AIDS 1:105, 1987.

18. Sodroski J, Goh WC, Rosen C, et al: Role of the HTLV-III/LAV envelope in syncytium formation and cytopathicity. Nature 322:470, 1986.

19. Nicholson JK, McDougal JS, Spira TJ, et al: Immunoregulatory subsets of the T helper and T suppressor cell populations in homosexual men with chronic unexplained lymphadenopathy. J Clin Invest 73:191, 1984.

20. Stites DP, Casavant CH, McHugh TM, et al: Flow cytometric analysis of lymphocyte phenotypes in AIDS using monoclonal antibodies and simultaneous dual immunofluorescence. Clin Immunol Immunopathol 38:161, 1986.

21. Levy JA: Changing concepts in HIV infection: Challenges for the 1990s. AIDS 4:1051, 1990.

22. Lane HC, Fauci AS: Immunologic abnormalities in the acquired immunodeficiency syndrome. Annu Rev Immunol 3:477, 1985.

23. Bender BS, Quinn TC, Lawley TJ, et al: Acquired immune deficiency syndrome: A defect in Fc-receptor specific clearance. Clin Res 32:511, 1984.

24. Cox RA, Anders GT, Cappelli PJ, et al: Production of tumor necrosis factor-alpha and interleukin-1 by alveolar macrophages from HIV-1–infected persons. AIDS Res Hum Retroviruses 6:431, 1990.

25. Smith PD, Ohura K, Masur H, et al: Monocyte function in the acquired immune deficiency syndrome. Defective chemotaxis. J Clin Invest 74:2121, 1984.

26. Selwyn PA: AIDS: What is now known. I. History and immunovirology. Hosp Pract 21:67, 1986.

27. Winkelstein W Jr, Lyman DM, Padian N, et al: Sexual practices and risk of infection by the human immunodeficiency virus. The San Francisco Men's Health Study. JAMA 257:321, 1987.

28. Osmond D: Heterosexual transmission of HIV. In: Cohen PT, Sande MA, Volberding PA (eds): The AIDS Knowledge Base. Waltham, MA, Medical Publishing Group, p 1.2.4.1, 1990.

29. Medley GF, Anderson RM, Cox DR, et al: Incubation period of AIDS in patients infected via blood transfusion. Nature 328:719, 1987.

30. Osmond D: HIV transmission in transplant recipients and artificial insemination recipients. In: Cohen PT, Sande MA, Volberding PA (eds): The AIDS Knowledge Base. Waltham, MA, Medical Publishing Group, p 1.2.10.1, 1990.

31. Rogers MF, Thomas PA, Starcher ET, et al: Acquired immunodeficiency syndrome in children: Report of the Centers for Disease Control National Surveillance, 1982 to 1985. Pediatrics 79:1008, 1987.

32. Friedland GH, Klein RS: Transmission of the human immunodeficiency virus. N Engl J Med 317:1125, 1987.

33. Centers for Disease Control: Recommendations for prevention of transmission of infection with HTLV-III/LAV virus in the workplace. MMWR 34:681, 1985.

34. Centers for Disease Control: Estimates of HIV prevalence and projected AIDS cases: Summary of a workshop, October 31–November 1, 1989. MMWR 39:110, 1990.

35. Centers for Disease Control: Quarterly report to the Domestic Policy Council on the prevalence and rate of spread of HIV and AIDS in the United States. MMWR 37:223, 1988.

36. Gail MH, Rosenberg PS, Goedert JJ: Therapy may explain recent deficits in AIDS incidence. J Acquir Immune Defic Syndr 3:296, 1990.

37. Garry RF, Witte MH, Gottlieb AA, et al: Documentation of an AIDS virus infection in the United States in 1968. JAMA 260:2085, 1988.

38. Jaffe HW, Darrow WW, Echenberg DF, et al: The acquired immunodeficiency syndrome in a cohort of homosexual men: A six year follow-up study. Ann Intern Med 103:210, 1985.

39. Chin J: HIV epidemiology. In: Abstracts of the VII International Conference on AIDS, Florence, Italy, Istituto Superiore di Santa, June 16–21, 1991, p 55.

40. Centers for Disease Control: Update: Acquired immunodeficiency syndrome—United States, 1989. MMWR 39:81, 1990.

41. Centers for Disease Control: Update: Acquired immunodeficiency syndrome (AIDS)—Worldwide. MMWR 37:286, 1988.

42. Volberding PA, Cohen PT: Clinical spectrum of HIV infection. In: Cohen PT, Sande MA, Volberding PA (eds): The AIDS Knowledge Base. Waltham, MA, Medical Publishing Group, p 4.1.1, 1990.

43. Cooper DA, Gold J, Maclean P, et al: Acute AIDS retrovirus infection: Definition of a clinical illness associated with seroconversion. Lancet 1:537, 1985.

44. Centers for Disease Control: Classification system for human T-lymphocyte virus type III/lymphadenopathy-associated virus infections. MMWR 35:334, 1986.

45. El-Sadr W, Marmor M, Zolla-Pazner S, et al: Four-year prospective study of homosexual men: Correlation of immunologic abnormalities, clinical status, and serology to human immunodeficiency virus. J Infect Dis 155:789, 1987.

46. Barnes PF, Bloch AB, Davidson PT, et al: Tuberculosis in patients with human immunodeficiency virus infection. N Engl J Med 324:1644, 1991.

47. Phair J, Munoz A, Detels R, et al: The risk of *Pneumocystis carinii* pneumonia among men infected with human immunodeficiency virus type 1. N Engl J Med 322:161, 1990.

48. Hopewell PC: *Pneumocystis carinii* pneumonia: Diagnosis. J Infect Dis 157:1115, 1988.

49. Grant IH, Gold JW, Rosenblum M, et al: *Toxoplasma gondii* serology in HIV-infected patients: The development of central nervous system toxoplasmosis in AIDS. AIDS 4:519, 1990.

50. Yarchoan R, Venzon DJ, Pluda JM, et al: CD4 count and the risk for death in patients infected with HIV receiving antiretroviral therapy. Ann Intern Med 115:184, 1991.

51. Schooley RT, Merigan TC, Gaut P, et al: Recombinant soluble CD4 therapy in patients with the acquired immunodeficiency syndrome (AIDS) and AIDS-related complex. A phase I–II escalating dosage trial. Ann Intern Med 112:247, 1990.

52. Kahn JO, Allan JD, Hodges TL, et al: The safety and pharmacokinetics of recombinant soluble CD4 (rCD4) in subjects with the acquired immunodeficiency syndrome (AIDS) and AIDS-related complex. A phase 1 study. Ann Intern Med 112:254, 1990.

53. Traunecker A, Schneider J, Kiefer H, et al: Highly efficient neutralization of HIV with recombinant CD4-immunoglobulin molecules. Nature 339:68, 1989.

54. Collier A, Katzenstein D, Coombs R, et al: Safety and pharmacokinetics of intravenous recombinant CD4 immunoadhesin (RCD4-IGG) (AIDS Clinical Trials Group Protocol 121). In: Sixth International Conference on AIDS, San Francisco, June 1990, p 206.

55. Ashorn P, Englund G, Martin M, et al: Anti-HIV activity of CD4-*Pseudomonas* exotoxin on infected primary human lymphocytes and monocyte/macrophages. J Infect Dis 163:703, 1991.

56. Erickson J, Neidhart DJ, VanDrie J, et al: Design, activity, and 2.8 Å crystal structure of a C2 symmetric inhibitor complexed to HIV-1 protease. Science 249:527, 1990.

57. Roberts NA, Martin JA, Kinchington D, et al: Rational design of peptide-based HIV proteinase inhibitors. Science 248:358, 1990.

58. Ashorn P, McQuade TJ, Thaisrivongs S, et al: An inhibitor of the protease blocks maturation of human and simian immunodeficiency viruses and spread of infection. Proc Natl Acad Sci USA 87:7472, 1990.

59. Nelbock P, Dillon PJ, Perkins A, et al: A cDNA for a protein that interacts with the human immunodeficiency virus *tat* transactivator. Science 248:1650, 1990.

60. Lane HC, Davey V, Kovacs JA, et al: Interferon-alpha in patients with asymptomatic human immunodeficiency virus (HIV) infection: A randomized, placebo-controlled trial. Ann Intern Med 112:805, 1990.

61. Mildvan D, ACTG 068 Collaborative Group: A phase I/II open label trial to evaluate the antiviral potential of combination low dose zidovudine and interferon-α-2A in patients with symptomatic HIV disease. In: Seventh International Conference on AIDS, Florence, Italy, June 1991.

62. Nunberg JA, Schleif WA, Boots EJ, et al: Viral resistance to human immunodeficiency virus type 1-specific pyridinone reverse transcriptase inhibitors. J Virol 65:4887, 1991.

63. Fischl MA, Richman DD, Grieco MH, et al: The efficacy of azidothymidine (AZT) in the treatment of patients with AIDS and AIDS-related complex. A double-blind, placebo-controlled trial. N Engl J Med 317:185, 1987.

64. Volberding PA, Lagakos SW, Koch MA, et al: Original articles: Zidovudine in asymptomatic human immunodeficiency virus infection: A controlled trial in persons with fewer than 500 CD4-positive cells per cubic millimeter. N Engl J Med 322:941, 1990.

65. Fischl MA, Richman DD, Hansen N, et al: The safety and efficacy of zidovudine (AZT) in the treatment of subjects with mildly symptomatic human immunodeficiency virus type 1 (HIV) infection: A double-blind, placebo-controlled trial. Ann Intern Med 112:727, 1990.

66. Larder BA, Darby G, Richman DD: HIV with reduced sensitivity to zidovudine (AZT) isolated during prolonged therapy. Science 243:1731, 1989.

67. Bach MC: Failure of zidovudine to maintain remission in patients with AIDS. N Engl J Med 320:594, 1989.

68. Yarchoan R, Pluda JM, Thomas RV, et al: Long-term toxicity/activity profile of 2′,3′-dideoxyinosine in AIDS or AIDS-related complex. Lancet 336:526, 1990.

69. Cooley TP, Kunches LM, Saunders CA, et al: Once-daily administration of 2′,3′-dideoxyinosine (ddI) in patients with the acquired immunodeficiency syndrome or AIDS-related complex: Results of a phase I trial. N Engl J Med 322:1340, 1990. [Comment in: N Engl J Med 322:1386, 1990.]

70. Lambert JS, Seidlin M, Reichman RC, et al: 2′,3′-Dideoxyinosine (ddI) in patients with the acquired immunodeficiency syndrome or AIDS-related complex: A phase I trial. N Engl J Med 322:1333, 1990.

71. Merigan TC, Skowron G, Bozzette SA, et al: Circulating p24 antigen levels and responses to dideoxycytidine in human immunodeficiency virus (HIV) infections: A phase I and II study. Ann Intern Med 110:189, 1989.

72. Hopewell PC, Chaisson RE: Critical care for persons with AIDS. In: Cohen PT, Sande MA, Volberding PA (eds): The AIDS Knowledge Base. Waltham, MA, Medical Publishing Group, p 9.2.2.1, 1990.

73. Wachter RM, Luce JM, Turner J, et al: Intensive care of patients with the acquired immunodeficiency syndrome. Outcome and changing patterns of utilization. Am Rev Respir Dis 134:891, 1986.

74. Centers for Disease Control: Mortality attributable to HIV infection/AIDS—United States, 1981–1990. MMWR 40:41, 1991.

75. Edman JC, Kovacs JA, Masur H: Ribosomal RNA sequence shows *Pneumocystis carinii* to be a member of the fungi. Nature 334:519, 1988.

76. Leoung GS, Hopewell PC: *Pneumocystis carinii* pneumonia: Epidemiology, microbiology, and pathophysiology. In: Cohen PT, Sande MA, Volberding PA (eds): The AIDS Knowledge Base. Waltham, MA, Medical Publishing Group, p 6.5.1.1, 1990.

77. Hughes WT: *Pneumocystis carinii*. In: Mandel GL, Douglas RG, Bennett JE (eds): Principles and Practice of Infectious Diseases. New York: John Wiley & Sons, p 1549, 1985.

78. Kovacs JA, Hiemenz JW, Macher AM, et al: *Pneumocystis carinii* pneumonia: A comparison between patients with the acquired immunodeficiency syndrome and patients with other immunodeficiencies. Ann Intern Med 100:663, 1984.

79. Talzak EE, Cote RJ, Gold JW, et al: Extrapulmonary *Pneumocystis carinii* infections. Rev Infect Dis 12:380, 1990.

80. Zaman MK, White DA: Serum lactate dehydrogenase levels and *Pneumocystis carinii* pneumonia. Diagnostic and prognostic significance. Am Rev Respir Dis 137:796, 1988.

81. Heron CW, Hine AL, Pozniak AL, et al: Radiographic features in patients with pulmonary manifestations of the acquired immune deficiency syndrome. Clin Radiol 36:583, 1985.

82. DeLorenzo LJ, Huang CT, Maguire GP, et al: Roentgenographic patterns of *Pneumocystis carinii* pneumonia in 104 patients with AIDS. Chest 91:323, 1987.

83. Coleman DL, Hattner RS, Luce JM, et al: Correlation between gallium lung scans and fiberoptic bronchoscopy in patients with suspected *Pneumocystis carinii* pneumonia and the acquired immune deficiency syndrome. Am Rev Respir Dis 130:1166, 1984.

84. Bigby TD, Margolskee D, Curtis JL, et al: The usefulness of induced sputum in the diagnosis of *Pneumocystis carinii* pneumonia in patients with the acquired immunodeficiency syndrome. Am Rev Respir Dis 133:515, 1986.

85. Pitchenik AE, Ganjei P, Torres A, et al: Sputum examination for the diagnosis of *Pneumocystis carinii* pneumonia in the acquired immunodeficiency syndrome. Am Rev Respir Dis 133:226, 1986.

86. Leoung GS, Hopewell PC: *Pneumocystis carinii* pneumonia: Diagnostic tissue examination and diagnostic algorithm. In: Cohen PT, Sande MA, Volberding PA (eds): The AIDS Knowledge Base. Waltham, MA, Medical Publishing Group, p 6.5.3.1, 1990.

87. Polsky B, Gold JW, Whimbey E, et al: Bacterial pneumonia in patients with the acquired immunodeficiency syndrome. Ann Intern Med 104:38, 1986.

88. Centers for Disease Control: Tuberculosis and acquired immunodeficiency syndrome—New York City. MMWR 36:785, 1987.

89. Chayt KJ, Harper ME, Marselle LM, et al: Detection of HTLV-III RNA in lungs of patients with AIDS and pulmonary involvement. JAMA 256:2356, 1986.

90. Wharton JM, Coleman DL, Wofsy CB, et al: Trimethoprim-sulfamethoxazole or pentamidine for *Pneumocystis carinii* pneumonia in the acquired immunodeficiency syndrome. A prospective randomized trial. Ann Intern Med 105:37, 1986.

91. Sattler FR, Waskin H: Pentamidine and fatal hypoglycemia (letter). Ann Intern Med 107:789, 1987.

92. Conte JE, Hollander H, Golden JA: Inhaled or reduced-dose pentamidine for *Pneumocystis carinii* pneumonia. A pilot study. Ann Intern Med 107:495, 1987.

93. Montgomery AB, Debs RJ, Luce JM, et al: Aerosolised pentamidine as sole therapy for *Pneumocystis carinii* pneumonia in patients with acquired immunodeficiency syndrome. Lancet 2:480, 1987.

94. Leoung GS, Mills J, Hopewell PC, et al: Dapsone-trimethoprim for *Pneumocystis carinii* pneumonia in the acquired immunodeficiency syndrome. Ann Intern Med 105:45, 1986.

95. Queener SF, Bartlett MS, Richardson JD, et al: Activity of clindamycin with primaquine against *Pneumocystis carinii* in vitro and in vivo. Antimicrob Agents Chemother 32:807, 1988.

96. Allegra CJ, Chabner BA, Tuazon CU, et al: Trimetrexate for the treatment of *Pneumocystis carinii* pneumonia in patients with the acquired immunodeficiency syndrome. N Engl J Med 317:978, 1987.

97. Bartlett MS, Queener SF, Tidwell RR, et al: 8-Aminoquinolines from Walter Reed Army Institute for Research for treatment and prophylaxis of *Pneumocystis* pneumonia in rat models. Antimicrob Agents Chemother 35:277, 1991.

98. Hughes WT, Kennedy W, Shenep JL, et al: Safety and pharmacokinetics of 566C80, a hydroxynaphthoquinone with anti–*Pneumocystis carinii* activity: A phase I study in human immunodeficiency virus (HIV)–infected men. J Infect Dis 163:843, 1991.

99. Bozzette SA, Sattler FR, Chiu J, et al: A controlled trial of early adjunctive treatment with corticosteroids for *Pneumocystis carinii* pneumonia in the acquired immunodeficiency syndrome. N Engl J Med 323:1451, 1990.

100. Gagnon S, Boota AM, Fischl MA, et al: Corticosteroids as adjunctive therapy for severe *Pneumocystis carinii* pneumonia in the acquired immunodeficiency syndrome—A double-blind, placebo-controlled trial. N Engl J Med 323:1444, 1990.

101. Montaner JSG, Lawson LM, Levitt N, et al: Corticosteroids prevent early deterioration in patients with moderately severe *Pneumocystis carinii* pneumonia and the acquired immunodeficiency syndrome (AIDS). Ann Intern Med 113:14, 1990.

102. The National Institutes of Health University of California Expert Panel for Corticosteroids as Adjunctive Therapy for *Pneumocystis* Pneumonia: Special report: Consensus statement on the use of corticosteroids as adjunctive therapy for *Pneumocystis* pneumonia in the acquired immunodeficiency syndrome. N Engl J Med 323:1500, 1990.

103. MacFadden DK, Edelson JD, Hyland RH, et al: Corticosteroids as adjunctive therapy in treatment of *Pneumocystis carinii* pneumonia in patients with acquired immunodeficiency syndrome. Lancet 1:1477, 1987.

104. Lo B, Raffin TA, Cohen NH, et al: Ethical dilemmas about intensive care for patients with AIDS. Rev Infect Dis 9:1163, 1987.

105. Haverkos, HW: Assessment of therapy for *Pneumocystis carinii* pneumonia. PCP therapy project group. Am J Med 76:501, 1984.

106. Murray JF, Felton CP, Garay SM, et al: Pulmonary complications of the acquired immunodeficiency syndrome: Report of a National Heart, Lung, and Blood Institute workshop. N Engl J Med 310:1682, 1984.

107. Leoung GS, Hopewell PC: *Pneumocystis carinii* pneumonia: Therapy and prophylaxis. In: Cohen PT, Sande MA, Volberding PA (eds): The AIDS Knowledge Base. Waltham, MA, Medical Publishing Group, p 6.5.4.1, 1990.

108. Wachter RM, Luce JM: Intensive care for patients with *Pneumocystis carinii* pneumonia and respiratory failure. Are we prepared for our new success (editorial)? Chest 96:714, 1989.

109. Schein RM, Fischl MA, Pitchenik AE, et al: ICU survival of patients with the acquired immunodeficiency syndrome. Crit Care Med 14:1026, 1986.

110. Wachter RM, Russi MB, Bloch DA, et al: *Pneumocystis carinii* pneumonia and respiratory failure in AIDS. Improved outcomes and increased use of intensive care units. Am Rev Respir Dis 143:251, 1991.

111. El-Sadr W, Simberkoff MS: Survival and prognostic factors in severe *Pneumocystis carinii* pneumonia requiring mechanical ventilation. Am Rev Respir Dis 137:1264, 1988.

112. Luce JM, Wachter RM, Hopewell PC: Intensive care of patients with the acquired immunodeficiency syndrome: Time for a reassessment? Am Rev Respir Dis 137:1261, 1988.

113. Nielsen TL, Guldager H, Pedersen C, et al: The outcome of mechanical ventilation in patients with an AIDS-associated primary episode of *Pneumocystis carinii* pneumonia. Scand J Infect Dis 23:37, 1991.

114. Larpin R, Chave JP, Schaller MD, et al: Survival of HIV-positive patients hospitalized in intensive care for respiratory insufficiency and *Pneumocystis carinii* pneumonia. Schweiz Med Wochenschr 120:1928, 1990.

115. Peruzzi WT, Noskin GA, Shapiro BA, et al: ICU patients with AIDS and *Pneumocystis carinii* pneumonia: Suggested predictors of hospital outcome. In: Seventh International Conference on AIDS, Florence, Italy, June 1991, p 237.

116. Le AN, Quieffin J, Ronco JJ, et al: Performance of commonly used scoring systems in predicting survival to hospital discharge for patients with PCP-related acute respiratory failure requiring ICU admission. In: Seventh International Conference on AIDS, Florence, Italy, June 1991, p 239.

117. Knaus WA, Draper EA, Wagner DP, et al: APACHE II: A severity of disease classification system. Crit Care Med 13:818, 1985.

118. Bihari D, Smithies M, Gimson A, et al: The effects of vasodilation with prostacyclin on oxygen delivery and uptake in critically ill patients. N Engl J Med 317:397, 1987.

119. Murray JF, Matthay MA, Luce JM, et al: An expanded definition of the adult respiratory distress syndrome. Am Rev Respir Dis 138:720, 1988.

120. Justice AC, Feinstein AR, Wells CK: Special article: A new prognostic staging system for the acquired immunodeficiency syndrome. N Engl J Med 320:1388, 1989.

121. Anonymous: Needlestick transmission of HTLV-III from a patient infected in Africa (editorial). Lancet 2:1376, 1984.

122. Beekmann SE, Fahey BJ, Gerberding JL, et al: Risky business: Using necessarily imprecise casualty counts to estimate occupational risks for HIV-1 infection. Infect Control Hosp Epidemiol 11:371, 1990.

123. Looke DFM, Grove DI: Failed prophylactic zidovudine after needlestick injury. Lancet 1:1280, 1990.

124. Stricof RL, Morse DL: HTLV-III/LAV seroconversion following a deep intramuscular needlestick injury (letter). N Engl J Med 314:1115, 1986.

125. Oksenhendler E, Harzic M, Le Roux JM, et al: HIV infection with seroconversion after a superficial needlestick injury to the finger. N Engl J Med 315:582, 1986.

126. Neisson-Vernant C, Arfi S, Mathez D, et al: Needlestick HIV seroconversion in a nurse. Lancet 2:814, 1986.

127. Gerberding JL, Henderson DK: Design of rational infection control policies for human immunodeficiency virus infection. J Infect Dis 156:861, 1987.

128. Weiss SH, Saxinger WC, Rechtman D, et al: HTLV-III infection among health care workers: Association with needlestick injuries. JAMA 254:2089, 1985.

129. Centers for Disease Control: Recommendations for prevention of HIV transmission in health-care settings. MMWR 36(suppl 2):1S, 1987.

130. Maestro CJ, Kernodle DS, Southin JL, et al: Correspondence: When a house officer gets AIDS. N Engl J Med 322:1154, 1990.

131. Serra MA, Nogueira JM, García-Lomas J, et al: A case of transmission of the human immunodeficiency virus type I after accidental puncture in health personnel. Med Clin (Barc) 92:475, 1989.

132. Kuhls TL, Viker S, Parris NB, et al: Occupational risk of HIV, HBV, and HSV-2 infections in health care personnel caring for AIDS patients. Am J Public Health 77:1306, 1987.

133. Centers for Disease Control: Update: Human immunodeficiency virus infections in health-care workers exposed to blood of infected patients. MMWR 36:285, 1987.

134. Weiss SH, Goedert JJ, Gartner S, et al: Risk of human immunodeficiency virus (HIV) infection among laboratory workers. Science 239:68, 1988.

135. Centers for Disease Control: Apparent transmission of human T-lymphotrophic virus type-III/lymphadenopathy-associated virus from a child to a mother providing health care. MMWR 35:76, 1986.

136. Hirsch MS, Wormser GP, Schooley RT, et al: Risk of nosocomial infection with human T cell lymphotropic virus III (HTLV-III). N Engl J Med 312:1, 1985.

137. McCray E: The Cooperative Needlestick Surveillance Group: Occupational risk of the acquired immunodeficiency syndrome among health care workers. N Engl J Med 314:1127, 1986.

138. Henderson DK, Saah AJ, Zak BJ, et al: Risk of nosocomial infection with human T-cell lymphotropic virus type III/lymphadenopathy-associated virus in a large cohort of intensively exposed health care workers. Ann Intern Med 104:644, 1986.

139. Gerberding JL, Bryant-LeBlanc CE, Nelson K, et al: Risk of transmitting the human immunodeficiency virus, cytomegalovirus, and hepatitis B virus to health care workers exposed to patients with AIDS and AIDS-related conditions. J Infect Dis 156:1, 1987.

140. McEvoy M, Porter K, Mortimer P, et al: Prospective study of clinical, laboratory, and ancillary staff with accidental exposures to blood or other body fluids from patients infected with HIV. Br Med J [Clin Res] 294:1595, 1987.

141. Werner BG, Grady GF: Accidental hepatitis-B-surface-antigen-positive inoculations: Use of e antigen to estimate infectivity. Ann Intern Med 97:367, 1982.

142. Seeff LB, Wright EC, Zimmerman HJ, et al: Type B hepatitis after needlestick exposure: Prevention with hepatitis B immune globulin: Final report of the Veterans Administration Cooperative Study. Ann Intern Med 88:285, 1978.

143. Gerberding JL, Hopewell PC, Kaminsky LS, et al: Transmission of hepatitis B without transmission of AIDS by accidental needlestick. N Engl J Med 312:56, 1985.

144. Fultz PN, McClure HM, Swenson RB, et al: Persistent infection of chimpanzees with human T-lymphotropic virus type III/lymphadenopathy-associated virus: A potential model for acquired immunodeficiency syndrome. J Virol 58:116, 1986.

145. Kunze ROF, Koch MA: Immunological detection of HIV-infected peripheral blood lymphocytes. In: Abstracts of the Third International Conference on AIDS, Washington, DC, US Department of Health and Human Services and World Health Organization, 1987, p 232.

146. Shikata R, Karasawa T, Abe K, et al: Hepatitis B e antigens and infectivity of hepatitis B virus. J Infect Dis 136:571, 1977.

147. Ho D, Byington RE, Schooley RT, et al: Infrequency of isolation of HTLV-III virus from saliva in AIDS. N Engl J Med 313:1606, 1985.

148. Baker JL, Kelen GD, Sivertson KT, et al: Unsuspected human immunodeficiency virus in critically ill emergency patients. JAMA 257:2609, 1987.

149. St Louis ME, Rauch KJ, Peterson LR, et al: Seroprevalence rates of human immunodeficiency virus infection at sentinel hospitals in the United States. N Engl J Med 323:213, 1990.

150. Sherer R: Physician use of the HIV antibody test: The need for consent, counseling, confidentiality, and caution. JAMA 259:264, 1988.

151. Nichols SE: Psychosocial reactions of persons with the acquired immunodeficiency syndrome. Ann Intern Med 103:765, 1985.

152. Bayer R, Levine C, Wolf SM: HIV antibody screening: An ethical framework for evaluating proposed programs. JAMA 256:1768, 1986.

153. Henry K, Maki M, Crossley K: Analysis of the use of HIV antibody testing in a Minnesota hospital. JAMA 259:229, 1988.

154. Ruprecht RM, O'Brien LG, Rossoni LD, et al: Suppression of mouse viraemia and retroviral disease by 3'-azido-3'-deoxythymidine. Nature 323:467, 1986.

155. Sharpe AH, Jaenisch R, Ruprecht RM: Retroviruses and mouse embryos: A rapid model for neurovirulence and transplacental antiviral therapy. Science 236:1671, 1987.

156. Tavares L, Roneker C, Johnston K, et al: 3'-Azido-3'-deoxythymidine in feline leukemia virus–infected cats: A model for therapy and prophylaxis of AIDS. Cancer Res 47:3190, 1987.

157. McCune JM, Namikawa R, Shih CC, et al: 3'-Azido-3'-deoxythymidine suppresses HIV infection in SCID-hu mouse. Science 247:546, 1990.

158. Durand E, LeJeunne C, Hugues FC: Correspondence: Failure of prophylactic zidovudine after suicidal self-inoculation of HIV-infected blood. N Engl J Med 324:1062, 1991.

159. Looke DFM, Grove DI: Failed prophylactic zidovudine after needlestick injury. Lancet 335:1280, 1990.

160. Lange JMA, Boucher CAB, Hollak CEM, et al: Failure of zidovudine prophylaxis after accidental exposure to HIV-1. N Engl J Med 322:1375, 1990.

161. Henderson DK, Gerberding JL: Prophylactic zidovudine after occupational exposure to the human immunodeficiency virus: An interim analysis. J Infect Dis 160:321, 1989.

162. Centers for Disease Control: Possible transmission of human immunodeficiency virus to a patient during an invasive dental procedure. MMWR 39:489, 1990.

163. Centers for Disease Control: Epidemiologic notes and reports: Update: Transmission of HIV infection during invasive dental procedures—Florida. MMWR 40:377, 1991.

164. Bell DM, Martone WJ, Culver DH, et al: Risk of endemic HIV and hepatitis B virus transmission to patients during invasive procedures. In: Seventh International Conference on AIDS, Florence, Italy, June 1991, p 60.

165. Lowenfels AB, Wormser GP: Risk of transmission of HIV from surgeon to patient. N Engl J Med 325:888, 1991.

166. Michigan Department of Public Health: Michigan Recommendations on HIV-Infected Health Care Workers. Lansing, Michigan Department of Public Health, October 1991.

167. Gerberding JL: Expected costs of implementing a mandatory human immunodeficiency virus and hepatitis B virus testing and restriction program for health care workers performing invasive procedures. Infect Control Hosp Epidemiol 12:443, 1991.

CHAPTER 51

Infections Associated with Intravascular Devices

U. Frank
F. D. Daschner

Intravascular (IV) devices have become important in the care of critically ill patients. Rapid access to the vascular system is necessary for hemodynamic monitoring, drug administration, fluid replacement, nutritional support, chemotherapy, and hemodialysis. Various types of IV devices are used: peripheral and central venous catheters, arterial lines, pulmonary arterial catheters, long-term indwelling central venous catheters, and totally implanted central venous catheters. More than half of the 40 million patients hospitalized each year in the United States require insertion of an IV catheter, and up to one third of all nosocomial bacteremias are associated with IV catheter use.[1] It is estimated that 176,000 cases of hospital-acquired bacteremia occur annually in the United States; according to this, more than 50,000 cases of bacteremia per year are associated with IV catheters.[2]

Every type of IV device carries the risk of causing both local and systemic infection. Local inflammation, septic thrombophlebitis, and bacteremia are the most important complications. The literature on IV device–related infection has increased considerably, but data generated are highly variable and there is little consensus regarding infection statistics and catheter management techniques.[3] Diverse definitions of IV catheter– and device–related infections, different microbiologic methods, and varying clinical circumstances make it difficult to compare studies.

INCIDENCE OF INFECTIONS ASSOCIATED WITH INTRAVASCULAR DEVICES

The risk of IV device infection appears highly variable and depends on the device used. In a European multicenter

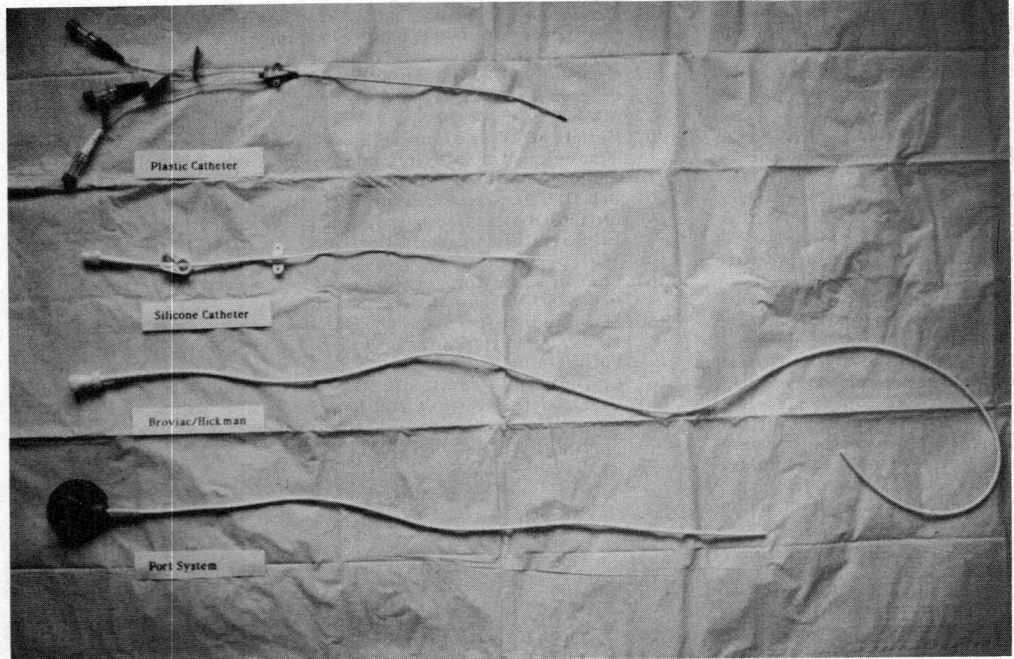

Figure 51–1. Various types of IV devices. (*Top*) Plastic central venous catheter, made of polyethylene, polyvinyl, or polytetrafluoroethylene (Teflon) with single, double, or triple lumens. (*Top middle*) Silicone central venous catheter, made of silicone elastomer, nontunneled or passed through a short subcutaneous tunnel. (*Bottom middle*) Cuffed and tunneled (Broviac's or Hickman's) catheter, made of silicone elastomer; differences in internal diameter: Broviac's, 1.0 mm; Hickman's, 1.6 mm. (*Bottom*) Totally implanted central venous catheter (port system), consisting of a reservoir (port) with a self-sealing septum and a silicone elastomer catheter.

study the risk of bacteremia with peripheral and central venous catheters was investigated in more than 10,000 surgical inpatients, 63% of whom had an IV catheter placed at some time during hospitalization.[4] Nosocomial bacteremia occurred in 0.37% of patients with a peripheral and 4.48% with a central venous catheter, compared with only 0.05% without any IV access. The risk of bacteremia was significantly greater for patients with central than with peripheral intravenous catheters. It should be mentioned, however, that the population of patients requiring central venous access is likely to include a higher proportion of high-risk patients than the population with peripheral catheters.

Central venous catheters commonly used include plastic catheters, silicone catheters, cuffed and tunneled silicone catheters as designed by Broviac or Hickman, and totally implantable catheter systems (Fig. 51–1). With virtually every catheter type, duration of catheterization is the most important risk factor for catheter-related infection. Studies providing statistical catheter life-table analysis suggest that the risk of infection increases linearly with the duration of use.[5] Because the risk per day appears to be constant regardless of duration, different devices may be best compared by

calculating the incidence of infections per day of catheter use (Table 51–1).

Plastic Central Venous Catheters

Plastic central venous catheters, made of polyethylene, polypropylene, polyvinyl, or polytetrafluoroethylene (Teflon), are commonly used in critically ill patients. Infection rates with these catheters vary from 2.8 to 18.8 per 1000 catheter-days.[5] Plastic catheters used for multiple purposes, including prolonged and simultaneous administration of total parenteral nutrition (TPN), have greater infection rates than catheters reserved for TPN only. Because of the multiple hubs and frequent handling of multilumen catheters, the incidence of infection associated with them is presumably higher than that with single-lumen catheters.[5, 6] Several studies suggest that triple-lumen catheters should not be used for nutritional support, because bacterial growth may be promoted by rich nutrient growth media.[7, 8] In two prospective studies, the incidence of infection with triple- and single-lumen catheters was investigated.[9, 10] The infection rates for triple- versus single-lumen catheters were 4.7 versus 0.9 per 1000 catheter-days and 35.7 versus 11.6 per 1000 catheter-days, respectively. In both studies, triple-lumen catheters were associated with significantly higher infection rates than single-lumen catheters. However, not all studies have found this difference.[11, 12] A prospective, randomized trial showed identical infection rates (22.7%) in patients with double-lumen catheters and patients with two separate single-lumen catheters.[11] In another prospective study comparing single-lumen with triple-lumen catheters, no significant differences in the rate of catheter colonization or catheter-related sepsis were found.[12] However, use of TPN or insertion at the femoral vein site increased the rate of catheter colonization significantly, and the duration of catheter use was clearly associated with catheter sepsis, with infection rate increasing from 1.5 to 10% when the period of catheterization exceeded 6 days. A strong correlation between the duration of triple-lumen catheter use and the onset of catheter colonization by microorganisms has been suggested by another study group.[13] Microbial colonization was shown

Device and Review Article	Infections per 1000 Catheter-Days (Range)
TABLE 51–1	
CUMULATIVE EXPERIENCE WITH INTRAVASCULAR DEVICES	
Plastic central venous catheters	
Decker and Edwards, 1988[5]	2.8–18.8
Silicone central venous catheters	
Decker and Edwards, 1988[5]	0.3–5.7
Cuffed and tunneled silicone catheters	
Press et al, 1984[15]	0.0–8.0
Decker and Edwards, 1988[5]	0.0–7.6
Yokoyama et al, 1988[16]	0.3–1.6
Totally implanted central venous catheters	
Decker and Edwards, 1988[5]	0.0–0.7
Toltzis and Goldmann, 1990[21]	0.0–1.0

to be of clinical significance because it preceded subsequent sepsis. The practice of routinely replacing central venous catheters after an arbitrary time interval (e.g., 7 days as recommended in this study), although conceivably lowering the incidence of catheter-related sepsis, would also be expected to increase the incidence of insertion-related mechanical complications.

Silicone (Rubber) Central Venous Catheters

Silicone (rubber) central venous catheters without a fibrous cuff do not have to be passed through a subcutaneous tunnel, although they may be tunneled. These catheters are associated with infection rates comparable to those found with Broviac's catheters. In adult oncology patients, infection rates with percutaneous noncuffed silicone catheters vary from 0.3 to 4.4 per 1000 days.[5] In neonates and infants, a small noncuffed silicone catheter may offer some advantages over the Broviac catheter in terms of the insertion technique;[14] infection rates have ranged from 2.8 to 5.7 per 1000 catheter-days.[5]

Cuffed and Tunneled Silicone Catheters

Cuffed and tunneled silicone catheters as pioneered by Broviac and modified by Hickman are successful devices for the management of patients requiring prolonged central venous access, particularly for chemotherapy or TPN. One or more synthetic fiber (Dacron) cuffs serve as anchors to prevent displacement and as barriers to infection (Fig. 51–2).

One of the first large studies to review infection rates of Hickman's catheters combined the data of 17 articles published between 1979 and 1984 and revealed an incidence of

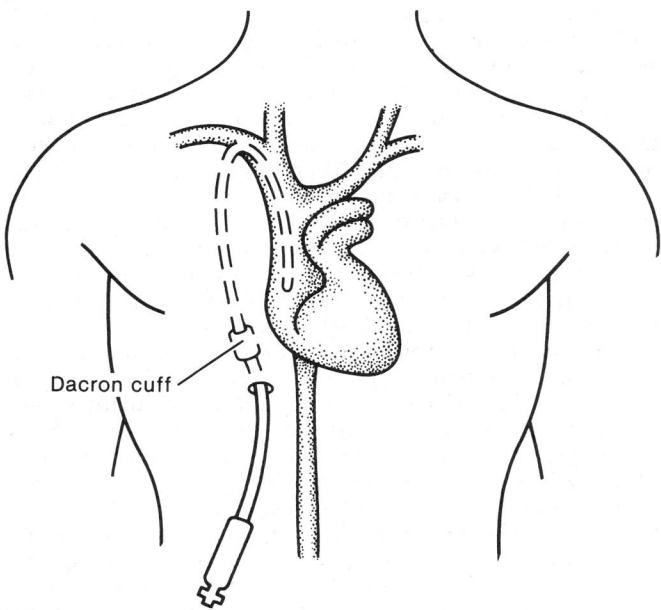

Figure 51–2. Cuffed, tunneled silicone catheter (Broviac's). The original Broviac's catheter, made of silicone rubber, consists of an intravascular and an extravascular segment with an attached synthetic fiber (Dacron) cuff. The intravascular catheter tip is located in the mid-atrial area, and the cuffed extravascular segment is externalized through a long subcutaneous tunnel down the anterior chest wall. After subcutaneous placement, the Dacron cuff promotes tissue fibroblastic ingrowth, preventing accidental catheter dislodgment and forming an anatomic barrier to microorganisms ascending along the outer catheter surface.

Label in figure: Dacron cuff

1.4 catheter-related infections per 1000 catheter-days with a range of 0 to 8.0 infections per 1000 catheter-days for individual series.[15] Another review combining 21 studies published from 1977 to 1986 reported almost identical infection rates with Broviac-type catheters.[5] There were 2339 Broviac-type catheters inserted in 2020 mainly pediatric but also adult patients for 260,578 total days of catheter use. There were 455 septic infections with an infection rate of 1.7 per 1000 catheter-days. However, infection rates varied by study, ranging from 0 to 7.59 per 1000 catheter-days. More recently, a review of five studies published during 1985 to 1987 on Broviac's catheters in children undergoing chemotherapy revealed an incidence of only 0.3 to 1.6 bacteremic episodes per 1000 catheter use days.[16] In the same study, the use of Broviac's or Hickman's catheters for long-term access in pediatric cancer patients was compared with that of tunneled, traditional silicone elastomer (Silastic) catheters; the rate of infection with Broviac's or Hickman's catheters was 0.35 per 1000 catheter-days, compared with 2.6 per 1000 Silastic catheter-days. These studies concluded that for long-term access in pediatric cancer patients, Broviac's or Hickman's catheters appeared to have somewhat lower infection rates than traditional Silastic catheters. However, other smaller studies have reported higher rates of septic infections with Hickman's or Broviac's catheters. A prospective 1 year study of infective episodes in 41 immunocompromised children with 42 indwelling catheters (41 Hickman, 1 Broviac) in place for a total of 4827 days showed an overall rate of bacteremia of 5.18 per 1000 catheter-days, whereas the rate for catheter-related and possible catheter-related bacteremia was 3.94 per 1000 catheter-days.[17]

A higher incidence of Hickman's catheter infection has been reported in patients with acquired immunodeficiency syndrome (AIDS).[18] The rate of Hickman's catheter infection in AIDS patients (4.7 per 1000 catheter-days) was significantly higher than that in patients without AIDS (0.9 infections per 1000 catheter-days). In comparison, only 0.8 infections per 1000 catheter-days were reported for Hickman's catheters used for hemodialysis in patients with end-stage renal failure.[19] As with multilumen plastic central venous catheters, the risk of infection with double-lumen Hickman's catheters appears to be significantly higher than that with single-lumen Hickman's catheters.[20]

Totally Implanted Central Venous Catheters

Totally implanted central venous catheters, consisting of a reservoir (port) with a self-sealing septum and a silicone elastomer catheter, have been reported to reduce the risk of infection by eliminating the exit site of the percutaneous catheter. Results of eight studies of 306 oncology patients with 314 implanted devices in place for 49,918 days revealed 15 septic infections as well as 15 infections localized in the subcutaneous pocket, representing rates of 0.3 per 1000 days each.[5] Another review, including six of these studies, summarized the results of 10 studies published during 1982 to 1988.[21] The infection rate with implantable devices ranged from 0 to 1.0 per 1000 catheter-days, with several investigators reporting rates as low as 0.4 to 0.6 per 1000 catheter-days. In another study, almost identical results were obtained in pediatric and adult patients, representing an infection rate of 0.4 per 1000 catheter-days.[22] However, in a 2-year study of 66 pediatric patients with cancer with 71 ports implanted a higher infection rate of 1.5 episodes of bacteremia per 1000 catheter-days was reported, which appears only slightly lower than that reported for children with Broviac's or Hickman's catheters.[23]

Several additional studies have now suggested that the use of totally implanted central venous catheters is associated with a lower risk of infection than the use of Broviac-type catheters;[24, 25] however, not all studies have found this difference.[26–28] A comparison of complications of totally implantable ports and Broviac's or Hickman's catheters in children with cancer showed that ports had a significantly longer failure-free duration of use than the externalized Broviac's or Hickman's catheters; the greatest risk of infection occurred in the first 100 days of catheter use, particularly for implanted ports.[24] Another study summarized 5 years of experience with Hickman's or Broviac's catheters in mostly adult patients with cancer and reported an overall complication rate for implantable ports of only 0.45 per 1000 catheter-days compared with 4.1 per 1000 catheter-days for Broviac's or Hickman's catheters; infection and suspicion of infection were the most common complications associated with the implantable ports and Broviac's or Hickman's catheters, representing 51.7 and 78% of all complications, respectively.[25] It should be noted, however, that the extensive experience with Broviac's or Hickman's catheters is likely to include a higher proportion of high-risk patients than the experience with implantable ports. Furthermore, the advantage of the implantable port is eliminated if frequent infusion therapy requires permanent access to the port system. In a comparison of infectious complications with totally implanted ports and Broviac's or Hickman's catheters in pediatric oncology patients, no statistically significant difference in the rate of infection could be found; infection rates were 1.4 and 2.1 per 1000 catheter-days with implantable ports and Broviac's or Hickman's catheters, respectively.[26] Other data suggest even higher infection rates, 6.5 per 1000 catheter-days, for implanted devices compared with 3.5 per 1000 days for Broviac's catheters; the difference, however, was not statistically significant.[26] In patients with AIDS who require daily or frequent infusions, no difference in the risk of infection associated with implantable ports and Hickman's catheters has been found.[28] However, the risk of infection associated with indwelling catheters appeared to be significantly higher in patients with AIDS than in patients with non-AIDS immunodeficiencies or immunocompetence; infection rates were 2.02, 0.41, and 0.23 per 1000 catheter-days, respectively.[28]

PATHOGENESIS OF INFECTIONS ASSOCIATED WITH INTRAVASCULAR DEVICES

There are many potential sources and routes of microorganisms causing catheter-associated infections. Skin organisms gain access to the tip of the catheter both at the time of insertion and subsequently by migrating down the interface between catheter surface and tissue. However, IV catheters can also become contaminated by microorganisms on the hands of hospital personnel either at the time of insertion or during subsequent manipulations.[29] It has been emphasized that catheter hub colonization, predominantly with coagulase-negative staphylococci, represents the most common source of organisms causing line-associated infections.[30–32] Other data, however, suggest that the majority of bacteremias associated with IV catheters derive from infection of the percutaneous tract along the external surface of the catheter rather than intraluminally.[33, 34] Subtyping of organisms by plasmid profile analysis has shown that organisms recovered from the catheter tip or blood cultures are more concordant with organisms found on the skin at the insertion site than with organisms recovered from the hub.[35] Possibly transdermal potential differences, moving negatively charged bacteria from the epidermis to the subcutaneous tissue, promote bacterial colonization of IV catheters.[36] Tunneling of the catheter has been shown to reduce the rate of bacterial migration from the skin to the IV catheter, but catheter hub contamination of the tunneled catheter remains an important source of microbial colonization.[37]

An evaluation of surveillance hub and skin cultures in 29 documented cases of catheter sepsis showed sensitivities of 34.5 and 37.9%, respectively.[38] When either the hub or the skin culture result was considered as an indication of catheter sepsis, sensitivity increased to 79.3%. The predictive value of positive superficial cultures for the diagnosis of catheter-related infection was 44.2% and that of negative cultures 93.3%. Comparable data were obtained by another study, demonstrating that contamination of the hub, the skin, or both sites was responsible for catheter infection in 22.6, 56.6, and 15.1% of 53 documented cases, respectively.[39] The positive and negative predictive values in this study were 66.2 and 96.7%. Both studies suggested that simultaneous hub and skin cultures were useful for predicting catheter-related infection. The use of side ports has not been clearly demonstrated as a factor that increases the risk of infection, but contamination of side ports may result from incorrect care and management.[29] Rarely, colonization of IV devices may also arise from hematogenous seeding. Most catheter-related yeast infections and occasionally infections with enteric bacteria appear to be a result of hematogenous dissemination from anatomically distant sites of infection, whereas this is an uncommon route for staphylococci.[40] Although rare, septic infections caused by contaminated infusate are far more likely to be caused by microorganisms introduced during infusate preparation and administration in the hospital than by microorganisms introduced during the manufacturing process.[1]

MICROBIOLOGY

Staphylococci, predominantly coagulase-negative staphylococci but also *Staphylococcus aureus*, are the leading causes of infection of IV devices. A review of 13 studies found that coagulase-negative staphylococci were responsible for 36% and *S. aureus* for 16% of Broviac's catheter–associated sepsis.[5] Another review of five studies revealed almost identical results, reporting that 39% of all Hickman's catheter–associated bacteremias were due to coagulase-negative staphylococci and 9% to *S. aureus*.[41] However, Hickman's catheter infections in patients with AIDS are frequently caused by *S. aureus*, which is isolated in 87% of the cases.[18] In fact, there is an increased incidence of *S. aureus* bacteremia and recurrent staphylococcal infection in AIDS patients, and the presence of an IV catheter has been described as the single most important risk factor for bacteremia in this population of patients (in 73% of the cases).[42]

The predominant role of coagulase-negative staphylococci in device infections has been emphasized in several reviews.[43, 44] Staphylococcal slime, produced by many strains of coagulase-negative staphylococci causing foreign body infections, may mediate and promote persistent colonization of indwelling devices and protect the organisms from clearance by host defense mechanisms and antibiotics.[44] In addition, the association of coagulase-negative staphylococci with device infection appears to be due in part to a capsular polysaccharide adhesin mediating the attachment to catheter surfaces.[44, 45] In vitro, purified capsular polysaccharide adhesin and antibodies against it have been shown to inhibit the adherence of homologous and heterologous adhesin-positive coagulase-negative staphylococcal strains to silicone elastomer catheters.[45] Studies with a rabbit model of IV catheter infection have demonstrated that antibodies against capsular polysaccharide adhesin could protect the animals against staphylococcal colonization and bacteremia in vivo.[46] For *S. aureus*, adherence to catheter materials has been associated with binding to fibronectin or fibrinogen, but the role of these host factors in the adherence of coagulase-negative staphylococci is unclear.[47-49] The risk of coagulase-negative staphylococcal bacteremia in infants in neonatal intensive care units has been investigated and attributed primarily to the intravenous administration of lipid emulsions.[50] Before the onset of coagulase-negative staphylococcal bacteremia, infants were 5.8 times as likely as controls to have received intravenous lipid emulsions and 3.5 times as likely to have had a percutaneous central venous catheter inserted. Presumably, the administration of lipids through a catheter favors rapid staphylococcal proliferation and blood stream infection. If existing protocols for preparation and administration of the infusate are followed, contamination of lipids with coagulase-negative staphylococci is unlikely. However, the occurrence of some of the more uncommon isolates, such as *Enterobacter* species, *Serratia marcescens*, *Pseudomonas cepacia*, or *Citrobacter freundii*, suggests strongly the possibility of sepsis resulting from contaminated infusate.[1]

DIAGNOSIS OF INFECTIONS ASSOCIATED WITH INTRAVASCULAR DEVICES

The diagnosis of a local catheter exit site infection is easy if purulent discharge is found around the catheter insertion site. In this case, a Gram stain and culture of the pus around the insertion site are helpful. The results, however, can also be misleading, particularly if organisms of the normal skin flora are isolated rather than the pathogens responsible for the IV catheter infection. Although a strong correlation between the cutaneous flora and microorganisms recovered from catheter tips has been reported, surveillance skin cultures are unreliable in anticipating or predicting catheter-related infections.[51] More recently, the relationship of surveillance cultures to septic episodes in bone marrow transplant recipients with Broviac's or Hickman's catheters has been investigated.[52] Routine surveillance cultures of the throat, stool, and catheter exit site frequently identified coagulase-negative staphyloccocci that subsequently caused bacteremia. However, for aerobic gram-negative bacilli, diphtheroids, and fungi this correlation was low. Surveillance cultures are of little practical use because they have poor predictive value for subsequent septic infections in catheterized patients. The diagnosis of catheter-related sepsis may be confirmed most accurately by removing the catheter for microbiologic examination. Microscopic examination of an impression smear or direct stain of the catheter may provide more rapid results than are obtained by culture, but unfortunately Gram's or acridine orange staining and direct examination lack sensitivity compared with culture methods.[53] Semiquantitative or quantitative culture techniques applied to IV catheters in correlation with suspected sepsis are more specific, particularly if the same microorganisms are isolated from both the catheter tip and the blood. A semiquantitative method in which the catheter tip was rolled on a blood agar plate showed a good correlation with catheter-related infection.[54] However, the roll plate technique is capable of enumerating fewer than 1000 organisms, and catheter tip cultures growing more than 1000 colonies were lumped into a category of greater than 10^3 organisms. Other culture techniques in which the organisms are flushed from catheters into broth and serially diluted permit quantification with a greater number of organisms than the roll plate technique,[55, 56] and a quantitative sonication method has been described that allows quantification of microorganisms removed from a catheter containing between 10^2 and 10^7 colony-forming units.[57] A major drawback of all these techniques is that the catheter must be removed from the patient before the diagnosis of catheter-related infection can be made.

In certain clinical settings, particularly if long-term venous access is required, it may be necessary to keep the IV catheter in situ even though catheter-related infection is strongly suspected. For diagnosing catheter-related sepsis without catheter removal, comparison of paired quantitative central catheter and peripheral venous blood cultures may be useful. This approach has not yet gained universal acceptance, and additional studies comparing this method with other techniques are needed.[58] A good correlation between semiquantitative cultures of blood taken through the catheter in situ and of the catheter tip after catheter removal has been noted;[59] a bacteriologic study of 149 of 227 TPN catheters from 204 patients during febrile episodes revealed 20 (8.8%) positive semiquantitative cultures of blood taken through the catheter in situ. After removal of the 20 catheters, 8 catheter tip cultures were positive. The remaining 129 catheters with negative semiquantitative blood cultures were left in place and proved to be sterile when removed at the end of TPN (negative predictive value 100%). In comparative quantitative blood cultures, equivalent colony counts of bacteria in catheter blood and peripherally drawn blood are inadequate to determine catheter-related infection, but a fivefold or greater bacterial concentration difference between catheter blood and peripheral blood appears to be a useful criterion for diagnosing catheter-related sepsis.[60-62] The correlation between results of the differential quantitative blood culture technique and the semiquantitative catheter tip culture method has been investigated.[63, 64] One study compared semiquantitative tip cultures and quantitative blood cultures performed by the pour-plate method.[63] Catheter-related sepsis was defined as growth of more than 15 colonies from the catheter tip and a central-to-peripheral bacterial count ratio of more than 7:1. Of nine infected catheters identified by the catheter tip culture, seven had a positive differential culture result, leading to a test sensitivity of 77.8%, specificity of 100%, and overall accuracy of 91.7%. However, because of the extremely small numbers of catheter infections observed in this study, the precision of these estimates is likely to be poor. Another study reported conflicting results and found quantitative blood cultures unreliable for diagnosing catheter-related sepsis.[64] Of 52 catheters studied, 15 were identified as infected by the catheter tip culture but only 7 of these were detected by the quantitative blood culture technique. A high central-to-peripheral bacterial ratio was found in four cases not fulfilling the definition of IV device–related infection, and some catheter blood cultures were positive despite negative cultures of peripheral blood and catheter tips.

A different technique using an intraluminal culture method to identify IV catheter infection without catheter removal has been reported.[65] With the catheter in situ, a sterile plastic obturator is inserted into the lumen of the catheter along its entire length and withdrawn under rotation. The obturator culture seems to represent the bacteriologic status of the entire intravenous line. With this technique, there was a stronger correlation between intraluminal catheter colonization and catheter tip colonization (81.8%) than between growth at the skin puncture site and catheter tip colonization (45.5%). However, the intraluminal culture method does not appear to be practical, and there is a risk of catheter contamination during insertion of the plastic obturator.

PREVENTION AND MANAGEMENT OF INFECTIONS ASSOCIATED WITH INTRAVASCULAR DEVICES

The mechanism of microbial colonization of IV catheters is influenced by many factors, including the type of device, its design, and its composition. Intravenous catheters made of polyvinyl chloride are more susceptible to adherence by coagulase-negative staphylococci than are catheters made of Teflon.[66, 67] Silicone elastomer catheters, particularly when cuffed and tunneled, also appear to have a low infection rate. The development of new catheters consisting of colonization-resistant polymers by binding of substances with antimicrobial activity to the catheter surface or incorporation of such substances in the catheter material may be a promising approach for reducing the risk of catheter-related infection.[68] Results of a prospective randomized multicenter trial of an attachable cuff impregnated with bactericidal silver in 234 catheters showed that catheters with the cuff were three times less likely to be colonized on removal than noncuffed control catheters (28.9% vs. 9.1%) and were nearly four times less likely to produce bacteremia (3.7% vs. 1.0%).[69] The efficacy of the silver-impregnated cuff in preventing IV device infection in intensive care patients receiving additional catheter site care with a polyantibiotic ointment containing polymyxin, neomycin, and bacitracin has been confirmed: catheter colonization developed in 2 of 26 (7.6%) cuffed catheters compared with 10 of 29 (34.5%) noncuffed catheters, and catheter-related sepsis was not observed with cuffed catheters but occurred with 4 of 29 (13.8%) catheters without a cuff.[70] Further research on the production of IV catheters and devices with anti-infectious properties appears warranted.

Application of topical antibiotics to the skin at the catheter insertion site does not prevent catheter-related bacteremia but may have some effect on the colonization of the catheter.[71, 72] In one study, a polyantibiotic ointment containing polymyxin, neomycin and bacitracin reduced the colonization of mostly peripherally inserted catheters by about two thirds.[71] Bacterial colonization was found in 6 of 270 (2.2%) polyantibiotic-treated catheters compared to 18 of 278 (6.5%) nontreated catheters. In another study, mupirocin, a new topical antibiotic with antistaphylococcal activity, was effective in reducing the microbial colonization of internal jugular catheters in cardiothoracic patients.[72] Application of mupirocin ointment to the skin insertion site led to a significant reduction of catheter colonization: only 18 of 110 (16.4%) mupirocin-treated catheters were colonized, compared with 58 of 108 (54%) in the control group. However, neither study documented the efficacy of topical ointments in preventing catheter-related bacteremia. Thus, the utility of antimicrobial skin ointments covering the catheter insertion site remains questionable.

Any time a catheter-related infection is suspected, empirical intravenous antibiotic therapy should be started as soon as blood cultures have been obtained. The catheter should be removed and examined for the presence of microorganisms. The use of a guidewire to place a new line over a pre-existing one is controversial, but a trend toward increased risk of infection has been noticed.[10] If a long-term (silicone) catheter has to be maintained for clinical reasons, antibiotics should be given through the catheter, sequentially using each of the ports in a multilumen catheter. An analogous approach to therapy of catheter-related sepsis has been developed and described as the "antibiotic lock technique."[73] By locking 2 mL of highly concentrated antibiotic solution within a silicone catheter for 12 hours a day, 90% of 22 catheter-related sepsis cases were controlled without catheter removal in 11 patients by the antibiotic lock technique alone for 16 days and in 11 patients by the antibiotic lock technique after a 3-day course of systemic antibiotics for 12 days. Failure of therapy was observed only once in each group of patients and was caused by secondary Candida catheter sepsis. Unfortunately, follow-up of cases was continued for only 1 week after completion of antibiotic treatment. These results, however, indicate a therapeutic improvement, avoiding haz-

ards of catheter change and systemic therapy. The choice of the antibiotic depends on previous culture and antibiotic sensitivity testing results. Because there are great differences in bacterial virulence, antibiotic susceptibility of microorganisms associated with IV catheter infections is difficult to assess. Coagulase-negative staphylococci are the leading cause of IV device–related infections, and attributable bacteremia is associated with excess mortality and prolonged hospital stay. A mortality rate of 30.5% in patients with coagulase-negative bacteremia compared with 16.9% in controls with similar underlying disease alone has been reported.[74] Because 40 to 80% of hospital-associated coagulase-negative staphylococci are resistant to semisynthetic penicillins (e.g., nafcillin and oxacillin), vancomycin (or teicoplanin) may be the drug of choice for treatment of catheter-related infections with coagulase-negative staphylococci.[5, 29, 40] In a noncompromised host, catheter removal or antibiotics for a few (3 to 7) days may be adequate, whereas in neutropenic patients therapy should be continued throughout the period of neutropenia.[5, 40]

S. aureus IV infections always require antibiotic therapy despite catheter removal.[40] Semisynthetic penicillins (e.g., nafcillin and flucloxacillin) are acceptable except in centers where multiresistant strains are present.[29] As a rule, 4 to 6 weeks of therapy is required to treat staphylococcal sepsis, possible endocarditis, and metastatic disease, but a shorter course of therapy may be efficacious if the source of infection is known and removed.[40] A small number of patients with removable sources of infection and S. aureus bacteremia who received antibiotic therapy for 16 days or less were evaluated and the risk of infectious complications with a short course of therapy for S. aureus catheter infections was delineated.[75] The length of intravenous antibiotic therapy in 13 patients with S. aureus catheter infections ranged from 0 to 14 days, with a mean of 9.2 days. As three patients received oral therapy in addition to intravenous therapy for a mean of 8.3 days, total therapy averaged 11.7 days. A single patient relapsed 24 days after completion of therapy with endocarditis. These findings suggest that in the case of S. aureus catheter infections the relapse rate is only 5 to 10% and a short course of therapy may be acceptable. However, this risk may be too high, considering that relapse often means endocarditis or metastatic disease.

Catheter-related Candida infections may be cured without catheter removal, but the outcome is notably worse than that observed with most bacterial line infections.[5] The need for amphotericin B is controversial. Indications for amphotericin B may include positive blood cultures, persistent fever after catheter removal, retinal lesions, and evidence of fungal infection elsewhere or occurrence in an immunocompromised host[40] (see Chapter 33). The duration of amphotericin B therapy should be at least 7 to 14 days in order to suppress any possible metastatic foci such as candidal endophthalmitis.[5]

SUMMARY

Plastic central venous catheters are the most commonly used IV devices in intensive care, but they are also an important source of nosocomial infection. The catheter size is likely to be correlated with an increased risk; similarly, the incidence of infection associated with multilumen catheters appears to be higher than that with single-lumen catheters. Small noncuffed silicone catheters offer some advantages in terms of insertion technique and safety in neonates and infants. Cuffed and tunneled silicone (for example, Broviac's or Hickman's) catheters have become the mainstay for long-term IV therapy, such as chemotherapy or TPN. Compared with external catheters, totally implanted devices seem to have the lowest risk of infection, and because of their versatility and convenience they may be preferable for outpatients.

Standardized insertion and maintenance techniques, including aseptic preinsertion skin preparation, hand washing, and careful management of the insertion site, the catheter hub, the infusion set, and the infusate, can substantially reduce the risk of infection. Whenever a catheter-related infection is suspected, blood should be drawn for cultures. For the treatment of established infections, the catheter should be removed and empirical antibiotic therapy should be started. If a long-term (silicone) catheter has to be maintained in situ, treatment must be individualized for each patient on the basis of clinical presentation and the causative organism.

References

1. Maki DG: Infections due to infusion therapy. In: Bennett JV, Brachman PS (eds): Hospital Infections. 2nd ed. Boston, Little, Brown, p 561, 1986.
2. Bryan CS, Hornung CA, Reynolds KL, et al: Endemic bacteremia in Columbia, South Carolina. Am J Epidemiol 123:113, 1986.
3. Plit ML, Lipman J, Eidelman J, et al: Catheter related infection. A plea for consensus with review and guidelines. Intensive Care Med 14:503, 1988.
4. Nyström B, Larsen SO, Dankert J, et al: Bacteraemia in surgical patients with intravenous devices: A European multicentre incidence study. The European Working Party on Control of Hospital Infections. J Hosp Infect 4:338, 1983.
5. Decker MD, Edwards KM: Central venous catheter infections. Pediatr Clin North Am 35:579, 1988.
6. Rose SG, Pitsch RJ, Karrer FW, et al: Subclavian catheter infections. JPEN 12:511, 1988.
7. Apelgren KN: Triple lumen catheters. Technological advance or setback? Am Surg 53:113, 1987.
8. McCarthy MC, Shives JK, Robison RJ, et al: Prospective evaluation of single and triple lumen catheters in total parenteral nutrition. JPEN 11:259, 1987.
9. Yeung C, May J, Hughes R: Infection rate for single lumen versus triple lumen subclavian catheters. Infect Control Hosp Epidemiol 9:154, 1988.
10. Hilton E, Haslett TM, Borenstein MT, et al: Central catheter infections: Single- versus triple-lumen catheters. Influence of guide wires on infection rates when used for replacement of catheters. Am J Med 84:667, 1988.
11 Powell C, Fabri PJ, Kudsk KA: Risk of infection accompanying the use of single-lumen vs double-lumen subclavian catheters: A prospective randomized study. JPEN 12:127, 1988.
12. Gil RT, Kruse JA, Thill-Baharozian MC, et al: Triple- vs single-lumen central venous catheters. A prospective study in a critically ill population. Arch Intern Med 149:1139, 1989.
13. Ullman RF, Gurevich I, Schoch PE, et al: Colonization and bacteremia related to duration of triple-lumen intravascular catheter placement. Am J Infect Control 18:201, 1990.
14. Leick-Rude MK: Use of percutaneous Silastic intravascular catheters in high-risk neonates. Neonatal Netw 9:17, 1990.
15. Press OW, Ramsey PG, Larson EB, et al: Hickman catheter infections in patients with malignancies. Medicine 63:189, 1984.
16. Yokoyama S, Fujimoto T, Tajima T, et al: Use of Broviac/Hickman catheter for long-term venous access in pediatric cancer patients. Jpn J Clin Oncol 18:143, 1988.
17. Weightman NC, Simpson EM, Speller DCE, et al: Bacteraemia related to indwelling central venous catheters: Prevention, diagnosis and treatment. Eur J Clin Microbiol Infect Dis 7:125, 1988.
18. Raviglione MC, Battan R, Pablos-Mendez A, et al: Infections associated with Hickman catheters in patients with acquired immunodeficiency syndrome. Am J Med 86:780, 1989.
19. Cappello M, DePauw L, Bastin G, et al: Central venous access for haemodialysis using the Hickman catheter. Nephrol Dial Transplant 4:988, 1989.
20. Early TF, Gregory RT, Wheeler JR, et al: Increased infection rate in double-lumen versus single-lumen Hickman catheters in cancer patients. South Med J 83:34, 1990.
21. Toltzis P, Goldmann DA: Current issues in central venous catheter infection. Annu Rev Med 41:169, 1990.
22. Harvey WH, Pick TE, Reed K, et al: A prospective evaluation of the Port-A-Cath^R implantable venous access system in chronically ill adults and children. Surg Gynecol Obstet 169:495, 1989.
23. Becton DL, Kletzel M, Golladay ES, et al: An experience with an implanted port system in 66 children with cancer. Cancer 61:376, 1988.
24. Mirro J Jr, Rao BN, Kumar M, et al: A comparison of placement techniques and complications of externalized catheters and implantable port use in children with cancer. J Pediatr Surg 25:120, 1990.
25. Guenier C, Ferreira J, Pector JC: Prolonged venous access in cancer patients. Eur J Surg Oncol 15:553, 1989.
26. Wurzel CL, Halom K, Feldman JG, et al: Infection rates of Broviac-Hickman catheters and implantable venous devices. Am J Dis Child 142:536, 1988.
27. Kumar A, Brar SS, Murray DL, et al: Central venous catheter infections in pediatric patients—In a community hospital. Infection 16:86, 1988.
28. Skoutelis AT, Murphy RL, MacDonell KB, et al: Indwelling central venous catheter infections in patients with acquired immune deficiency syndrome. J Acquir Immune Defic Syndr 3:335, 1990.
29. Elliott TSJ: Intravascular-device infections. J Med Microbiol 27:161, 1988.
30. Deitel M, Krajden S, Saldanha CF, et al: An outbreak of Staphylococcus epidermidis septicemia. JPEN 7:569, 1983.
31. Sitges-Serra A, Puig P, Linares J, et al: Hub colonization as the initial step in an outbreak of catheter-related sepsis due to coagulase negative staphylococci during parenteral nutrition. JPEN 8:668, 1984.
32. Linares J, Sitges-Serra A, Garau J, et al: Pathogenesis of catheter sepsis: A prospective study with quantitative and semiquantitative cultures of catheter hub and segments. J Clin Microbiol 21:357, 1985.
33. Cooper GL, Hopkins CC: Rapid diagnosis of intravascular catheter-associated infection by direct Gram staining of catheter segments. N Engl J Med 312:1142, 1985.
34. Maki DG, Ringer M: Evaluation of dressing regimens for prevention of infection with peripheral intravenous catheters. Gauze, a transparent polyurethane dressing and an iodophor-transparent dressing. JAMA 258:2396, 1987.
35. Maki DG: Dressing regimens and intravenous catheter–related infections. JAMA 259:1498, 1988.
36. Dealler S, Millar MR, MacKay P: Transdermal potential and bacterial colonisation of intravascular catheters. Lancet 1:703, 1988.
37. De Cicco M, Chiaradia V, Veronesi A, et al: Source and route of microbial colonisation of parenteral nutrition catheters. Lancet 1:1258, 1989.
38. Fan ST, Teoh-Chan CH, Lau KF, et al: Predictive value of surveillance skin and hub cultures in central venous catheters sepsis. J Hosp Infect 12:191, 1988.
39. Cercenado E, Ena J, Rodriguez-Creixems M, et al: A conservative procedure for the diagnosis of catheter-related infections. Arch Intern Med 150:1417, 1990.
40. Hampton AA, Sheretz RJ: Vascular access infections in hospitalized patients. Surg Clin North Am 68:57, 1988.
41. Dugdale DC, Ramsey PG: Staphylococcus aureus bacteremia in patients with Hickman catheters: Am J Med 89:137, 1990.
42. Jacobson MA, Gellermann H, Chambers H: Staphylococcus aureus bacteremia and recurrent staphylococcal infection in patients with acquired immunodeficiency syndrome and AIDS-related complex. Am J Med 85:172, 1988.
43. Pfaller MA, Herwaldt LA: Laboratory, clinical, and epidemiological aspects of coagulase-negative staphylococci. Clin Microbiol Rev 1:281, 1988.
44. Goldmann DA: Coagulase-negative staphylococci: Interplay of epidemiology and bench research. Am J Infect Control 18:211, 1990.
45. Tojo M, Yamashita N, Goldmann DA, et al: Isolation and characterization of a capsular polysaccharide adhesin from Staphylococcus epidermidis. J Infect Dis 157:713, 1988.
46. Kojima Y, Tojo M, Goldmann DA, et al: Antibody to the capsular polysaccharide/adhesin protects rabbits against catheter-related bacteremia due to coagulase-negative staphylococci. J Infect Dis 162:435, 1990.
47. Cheung AL, Fischetti VA: The role of fibrinogen in staphylococcal adherence to catheters in vitro. J Infect Dis 161:1177, 1990.
48. Vaudaux P, Pittet D, Haeberli A, et al: Host factors selectively increase staphylococcal adherence on inserted catheters: A role for fibronectin and fibrinogen or fibrin. J Infect Dis 160:865, 1989.
49. Herrmann M, Vaudaux PE, Pittet D, et al: Fibronectin, fibrinogen, and laminin act as mediators of adherence of clinical staphylococcal isolates to foreign material. J Infect Dis 158:693, 1988.
50. Freeman J, Goldmann DA, Smith NE, et al: Association of intravenous lipid emulsion and coagulase-negative staphylococcal bacteremia in neonatal intensive care units. N Engl J Med 323:301, 1990.
51. Maki DG, Goldmann DA, Rhame FS: Infection control in intravenous therapy. Ann Intern Med 79:867, 1973.
52. Rotstein C, Higby D, Killion K, et al: Relationship of surveillance cultures to bacteremia and fungemia in bone marrow transplant recipients with Hickman or Broviac catheters. J Surg Oncol 39:154, 1988.
53. Coutlee F, Lemieux C, Paradis J-F: Value of direct catheter staining in the diagnosis of intravascular-catheter–related infection. J Clin Microbiol 26:1088, 1988.
54. Maki DG, Weise CE, Sarafin HW: A semiquantitative culture method for identifying intravenous-catheter–related infection. N Engl J Med 296:1305, 1977.
55. Cleri DJ, Corrado ML, Seligman SJ: Quantitative culture of intravenous catheters and other intravascular inserts. J Infect Dis 141:781, 1980.
56. Bjornson HS, Colley R, Bower RH, et al: Association between microorganism growth at the catheter insertion site and colonization of the catheter in patients receiving total parenteral nutrition. Surgery 92:720, 1982.
57. Sherertz RJ, Raad II, Belani A, et al: Three-year experience with sonicated vascular catheter cultures in a clinical microbiology laboratory. J Clin Microbiol 28:76, 1990.

58. Yagupsky P, Nolte F: Quantitative aspects of septicemia. Clin Microbiol Rev 3:269, 1990.
59. Vanhuynegem L, Parmentier P, Potvliege C: In situ bacteriologic diagnosis of total parenteral nutrition catheter infection. Surgery 103:174, 1988.
60. Mosca R, Curtas S, Forbes B, et al: The benefits of Isolator cultures in the management of suspected catheter sepsis. Surgery 102:718, 1987.
61. Flynn PM, Shenep JL, Stokes DC, et al: In situ management of confirmed central venous catheter–related bacteremia. Pediatr Infect Dis 6:729, 1987.
62. Flynn PM, Shenep JL, Barret FF: Differential quantitation with a commercial blood culture tube for diagnosis of catheter-related infection. J Clin Microbiol 26:1045, 1988.
63. Fan ST, Teoh-Chan CH, Lau KF: Evaluation of central venous catheter sepsis by differential quantitative blood culture. Eur J Clin Microbiol Infect Dis 8:142, 1989.
64. Paya CV, Guerra L, Marsh HM, et al: Limited usefulness of quantitative culture of blood drawn through the device for diagnosis of intravascular–device–related bacteremia. J Clin Microbiol 27:1431, 1989.
65. Jakobsen CJB, Hansen V, Jensen JJ, et al: Contamination of subclavian vein catheters: An intraluminal culture method. J Hosp Infect 13:253, 1989.
66. Sheth NK, Rose HD, Franson TR, et al: In vitro quantitative adherence of bacteria to intravascular catheters. J Surg Res 34:213, 1983.
67. Sheth NK, Franson TR, Rose HD, et al: Colonization of bacteria on polyvinyl chloride and Teflon intravascular catheters in hospitalized patients. J Clin Microbiol 18:1061, 1983.
68. Trooskin SZ, Donetz AP, Harvey RA, et al: Prevention of catheter sepsis by antibiotic bonding. Surgery 97:547, 1985.
69. Maki DG, Cobb L, Garman JK, et al: An attachable silver-impregnated cuff for prevention of infection with central venous catheters: A prospective randomized multicenter trial. Am J Med 85:307, 1988.
70. Flowers RH III, Schwenzer KJ, Kopel RF, et al: Efficacy of an attachable subcutaneous cuff for the prevention of intravascular catheter–related infection. A randomized, controlled trial. JAMA 261:878, 1989.
71. Maki DG, Band JD: A comparative study of polyantibiotic and iodophor ointments in prevention of vascular catheter–related infection. Am J Med 70:739, 1981.
72. Hill RLR, Fisher AP, Ware RJ, et al: Mupirocin for the reduction of colonization of internal jugular cannulae—A randomized controlled trial. J Hosp Infect 15:311, 1990.
73. Messing B, Peitra-Cohen S, Debure A, et al: Antibiotic-lock technique: A new approach to optimal therapy for catheter-related sepsis in home–parenteral nutrition patients. JPEN 12:185, 1988.
74. Martin MA, Pfaller MA, Wenzel RP: Coagulase-negative staphylococcal bacteremia. Ann Intern Med 110:9, 1989.
75. Ehni WF, Reller LB: Short-course therapy for catheter-associated *Staphylococcus aureus* bacteremia. Arch Intern Med 149:533, 1989.

CHAPTER 52

Diagnostic Methods and the Laboratory in Intensive Care Unit Patients

John A. Washington

The laboratory diagnosis of any infection requires examination of specimens that are representative of the disease process, that are free of contamination with indigenous flora, and that have been collected before the administration of antibiotics. Exceptions are instances in which culture or serologic procedures are sufficiently selective, sensitive, or specific to provide a diagnosis. These requirements are challenging enough under ordinary circumstances; they are often difficult, if not impossible, to meet in the seriously ill, intubated, cannulated, and catheterized intensive care unit patient.

This chapter focuses on the laboratory aspects of diagnosis of the infections most frequently encountered in patients in intensive care units: blood stream infection, pneumonia, urinary tract infection, and surgical wound infection.

BLOOD STREAM INFECTION

Blood culture is the only method currently available for demonstrating the presence of blood stream infection or septicemia. The effective use of blood cultures requires an understanding of certain principles that have been derived from a number of studies of this subject.

Sensitivity

Because there is no independent, nonculture method for defining septicemia, sensitivity of blood culture is usually estimated as the percentage of positive blood cultures among all blood cultures obtained from patients with clinically significant positive blood cultures.[1] On the basis of roughly equivalent methodologies, Washington[2] and Weinstein and coworkers[3] reported sensitivities of 80 and 91.5%, respectively, for single blood cultures and 89 and 99.3%, respectively, for two blood cultures. The reasons for the small differences in results between these two studies are not readily apparent but may be related to differences in definitions of septic episodes, study populations, and sample sizes. Bacteremia is usually continuous in patients with endocarditis, whereas it is usually intermittent in patients with other types of infection.[3] Sensitivity of the blood culture procedure is, therefore, directly related to the number of blood cultures obtained.

The second and more important variable affecting the sensitivity of blood cultures is the volume of blood collected per culture. In a study of more than 5000 positive blood cultures, Ilstrup and Washington[4] demonstrated that the yields from cultures of 20 and 30 mL of blood per culture were 38 and 62% greater, respectively, than that from 10 mL of blood. The relationship between volume of blood per culture and yield is due to the low order of bacteremia and candidemia in many instances of septicemia in adults. Thus, the number of blood cultures has a bearing on sensitivity because of the frequency with which bacteremias are intermittent, and the volume of blood per culture has a bearing on sensitivity because of the small numbers of organisms per milliliter of blood in many cases of septicemia. It is therefore recommended that a minimum of 10 mL and preferably 20 mL of blood be obtained from adults for each blood culture, regardless of the blood culture system used in the laboratory. A similar relationship between volume and yield occurs in cultures of blood from infants and children, so every effort should be made to maximize the volume of blood obtained per culture. Because the number of blood cultures also affects test specificity, recommendations in this regard are made in the following section on specificity.

Specificity

Guidelines for identifying false-positive blood cultures include the isolation of bacteria normally encountered on the skin (i.e., *Bacillus* species, coagulase-negative staphylococci, diphtheroids), their rare isolation from subsequent cultures in a series of blood cultures, their isolation usually only after prolonged (>48 hours) incubation, a clinical course that is not consistent with sepsis, absence of primary infection with the same microorganism, and absence of predisposing factors.[1]

Use and Interpretation of Blood Cultures

Proper interpretation of negative and positive blood cultures, therefore, is predicated not only on factors influencing sensitivity and specificity but also on the influence of pretest probability of bacteremia on post-test probability of bacteremia.[1] For these reasons Aronson and Bor[1] have published the following guidelines for number of blood cultures to be collected: (1) one blood culture is rarely, if ever, sufficient; (2) two blood cultures are necessary and sufficient to rule out or establish a diagnosis of bacteremia when the anticipated pathogen is different from microorganisms customarily regarded as contaminants and when the pretest probability of bacteremia is low to moderate; (3) three blood cultures should be obtained when the pretest probability of bacteremia is high or when continuous bacteremia is characteristically associated with the suspected diagnosis; and (4) four or more blood cultures should be obtained when the pretest probability is high and the anticipated pathogen is also a common contaminant or when the patient has already received antimicrobial therapy.

It should be apparent that seriously ill, intensive care unit patients with suspected bacteremia usually require three to four blood cultures because bacteremia related to infected intravascular lines or devices with pathogens that are ordinarily considered as contaminants is a frequent occurrence and because such patients are frequently receiving antimicrobial therapy at the time blood cultures are obtained. Confounding the interpretation of blood cultures is the problem created by the practice, despite recommendations to the contrary, of obtaining blood from intravascular lines for multiple purposes, including blood culture. Much attention has, therefore, focused on the distinction between line-related and non–line-related bacteremia. Methods used in the laboratory to make this distinction vary and are the subject of much argument, perhaps because a "gold standard" for the laboratory diagnosis of intravascular catheter–associated sepsis remains unsettled.[5] Controversy exists over whether microorganisms migrate along the external or internal surface of intravascular catheters and therefore, depending on one's persuasion, whether laboratory procedures should entail semiquantitative culture of the external surface or internal lumen of the catheter. The most widely accepted procedure in use today is that described by Maki and colleagues[6] wherein a 2-inch segment of the catheter tip is rolled across the surface of an agar plate and contamination is differentiated from infection on the basis of a break point of 15 colony-forming units (CFU). Because the study involved a limited number of patients and predominantly short, peripheral catheters, suggestions have been made to reduce the break point for defining infection to 5 or more CFU in cultures of long central lines.[5] Suggestions have also been made to culture a 2-inch intradermal segment in addition to the tip of the catheter to increase the sensitivity of the test.

A method for semiquantitative culture of the catheter lumen has been described by Cleri and coworkers[7] in which the interior of the removed catheter segment is flushed with broth and the broth is then cultured quantitatively. In this instance, cultures yielding more than 10^3 CFU are considered positive.

To obtain cultures of catheter segments it is necessary to remove the catheter, and a number of studies have attempted to differentiate between catheter- and non–catheter-related bacteremia without first having to remove the catheter. The major method that has been studied in this regard is quantitative blood culture, wherein the numbers of colony-forming units per milliliter from simultaneously drawn peripheral blood and catheter blood are compared. Although there is not complete agreement on the value of this procedure, a greater number of colony-forming units per milliliter from catheter-drawn blood than from peripherally drawn blood suggests catheter-associated bacteremia.[5] Quantitative blood cultures may readily be made with a commercially available lysis-concentration tube (Isolator, Wampole Laboratories, Cranbury, NJ). Differences in colony-forming units per milliliter between peripherally drawn and catheter-drawn blood may, however, not be detectable unless the blood sample or the lysed concentrate is first serially diluted for culture.

In summary, general guidelines for blood cultures for adults with suspected blood stream infections in the intensive care unit include collection of at least two separate blood specimens with a minimal volume of 10 mL each. Withdrawal of blood from intravascular catheters should be avoided whenever possible to minimize contamination of catheters and cultures. Because selection of a blood culture system by the hospital laboratory is often based on the complementary functions of its components, physicians and nursing personnel should adhere to the guidelines recommended by the laboratory for inoculation of cultures.

Invasive candidiasis occurs most frequently in neutropenic patients and surgical and intensive care unit patients. Diagnosis of invasive candidiasis, however, poses a problem because many *Candida* species colonize the skin and mucous membranes; therefore, the definitive diagnosis of invasive infection requires histopathologic confirmation. Isolation of the organism from blood cultures does not necessarily signify invasive candidiasis. Nonetheless, laboratory procedures should be established to optimize detection of candidemia. As pointed out by Jones[8] in his review of the diagnosis of invasive candidiasis, the varying incidences of candidemia reported for various populations of patients in the literature may reflect both the number of blood cultures and the volume of blood per culture because of the transient nature of candidemia and the small number of yeast cells per milliliter of blood. Jones[8] summarized studies comparing blood culture systems for the recovery of *Candida* species and found that the lysis-centrifugation method (Isolator) was more sensitive than the other methods tested. Lysis-filtration methods have sensitivity equivalent to that of lysis-centrifugation but are not practical or commercially available. One approach to obtaining blood cultures for intensive care unit patients is to use a combination of the lysis-centrifugation method and a broth-based (bottle) system. Again, because these two systems are complementary, both should be used on a routine basis.

Because *Candida* species may take several days to grow in cultures, there has been much interest in the use of rapid immunoassays for *Candida* antigen. In a study of two such tests by Phillips and coworkers,[9] neither reliably identified patients with candidemia.

PNEUMONIA

The diagnosis of pneumonia is complicated by the fact that, with rare exceptions, specimens traverse one of the most heavily colonized areas of the body. The oral cavity and pharynx normally harbor at least 10^6 colonies of aerobic and anaerobic species of bacteria per milliliter of secretions. The composition of this microbial flora may, however, be altered in a variety of situations, such as in chronic alcoholism and leukemia and in patients who have received antibiotics, usually leading to colonization of the oropharynx with gram-negative bacilli. In 1972 Johanson and coworkers[10] observed that gram-negative colonization occurred in approximately 50% of patients within 5 days of admission to an intensive care unit and that nosocomial pneumonias occurred more frequently in colonized than in noncolonized patients. Our understanding of events leading to pharyngeal colonization and pneumonia has evolved through studies demonstrating the importance of gastric colonization after nasogastric intubation and stress ulcer prophylaxis, leading to retrograde colonization of the pharynx and subsequent colonization of the trachea in intubated patients.[11] This sequence of events has been shown to occur in 50% of patients between the second and seventh days of ventilation.[12]

Because tracheal colonization occurs quite rapidly, defining the microbial etiology of pneumonia in the intubated patient is highly problematic. Golden and coworkers[13] found that a positive Gram-stained smear ($\geq 2+$ white blood cells and $\geq 2+$ bacteria of a predominant morphology) and $3+$ growth of one or more pathogenic bacteria from an endotracheal aspirate specimen obtained within 60 minutes of initial intubation successfully distinguished between probable and nonprobable pneumonias in pediatric intensive care unit patients. The presence of gram-negative bacilli in the quantity of $2+$ occurred frequently in the absence of radiographic evidence of pneumonia. Moreover, 5 of 10 pairs of endotracheal aspirates obtained within 18 hours of one another yielded discordant results from cultures. Thus, the distinction between bacteria colonizing the tracheobronchial tree and those causing pneumonia cannot be made readily. In a study of 51 intubated, intensive care unit adult patients, Salata and colleagues[14] examined endotracheal aspirates for elastin fibers, graded Gram-stained smears, and quantitative bacterial cultures along with clinical and radiographic observations to develop criteria for the detection of pneumonia. In the presence of $2+$ bacteria (1 to 10 per oil immersion field) or $3+$ bacteria (>10 per oil immersion field), the odds ratios were, respectively, 36 and 104 and the probabilities 15.1 and 52.4% for definite infection. When the same bacterial gradings were combined with a positive potassium hydroxide preparation for elastin fibers, the odds ratios for infection increased to 156 and 192 and the probabilities to 77.6 and 95.6%, respectively. Elastin fibers were, however, seen in only 52% of patients considered to have definite infection, as well as in 9% of aspirates from colonized patients. Moreover, an association was demonstrated between higher bacterial counts and the appearance of new or progressive infiltrates and clinical manifestations of infection.

On the basis of these two studies of endotracheal aspirates, one might conclude that microscopic examination should be performed and should include a potassium hydroxide preparation for elastin fibers and a graded Gram-stained smear. One might also conclude that the actual bacterial content of the aspirate may be of limited value in establishing the etiology of pneumonia if the specimen was taken more than an hour after intubation. The discordance in bacterial content between paired aspirates should certainly call into question any routine surveillance practice of culturing endotracheal aspirates unless quantitative studies are performed with new or changing pulmonary infiltrates.

Because of the inevitable contamination of endotracheal secretions with oropharyngeal flora, efforts have been made to use fiberoptic bronchoscopy to provide more selective and specific specimen collection and culture techniques for the diagnosis of nosocomial pneumonia. The two techniques in common use today employ the telescoping protected catheter brush and bronchoalveolar lavage. Studies by Chastre and coworkers[15] showed a good correlation between quantitative protected catheter brush cultures and lung biopsy specimens taken immediately post mortem from patients who died while receiving chronic ventilation.

A detailed description of the technique for processing the protected catheter brush has been published by Broughton and colleagues.[16] In essence, the brush is severed from the retracting wire and transported to the laboratory in 1 mL of bacteriostat-free lactated Ringer's solution. After agitation of the specimen container on a mechanical mixer, samples of the solution are removed for Gram-stained smears and, if indicated, smears for acid-fast bacilli and *Legionella* species. Samples of 0.1 mL are cultured for aerobic and anaerobic bacteria. The authors also recommend cultures of diluted sample. Growth in cultures of the 10^{-3} dilution equates to 10^5 to 10^6 CFU/mL, which is considered a positive culture. Widely disparate results with the protected catheter brush have been reported and have been ascribed by Bartlett[17] to instillation of topical anesthetics through the inner channel, the use of nutrient broth for transport of the brush, failure to process the specimen promptly, and failure to culture quantitatively.

Bronchoalveolar lavage fluid is a specimen that has proved to be particularly useful for the diagnosis of pulmonary infections in the immunocompromised patient. Studies of its application to the diagnosis of bacterial pneumonia were initially performed in predominantly immunocompromised patients by Thorpe and coworkers[18] and Kahn and Jones.[19] Both studies concluded that the presence of at least 10^5 CFU/mL correlated well with the presence of pneumonia. Thorpe and coworkers[18] also noted that the presence of at least one bacterium per oil immersion field in a Gram-stained smear of the fluid was highly predictive of a positive culture. Kahn and Jones[19] showed a reasonable correlation ($r = .78$, $P < .001$) between the results of quantitative culture of bronchoalveolar lavage fluid and the brush, with the number of bacteria in the fluid being about 0.5 $\log_{10}$ higher than the number in the brush.

Fagon and colleagues[20] prospectively studied 567 intensive care unit patients for the development of ventilator-associated pneumonia. Protected catheter brush studies were performed for patients demonstrating a new or persistent (>24 hours) infiltrate on chest x-ray film and macroscopically purulent tracheal aspirates. The diagnosis of ventilator-associated pneumonia was retained only when quantitative brush cultures yielded more than 10^3 CFU/mL of at least one organism. On the basis of these criteria, 162 episodes of suspected pneumonia were investigated in 147 patients. Of these, 52 patients had more than 10^3 CFU/mL of brush sample. Of a total of 111 organisms cultured from brushes in the 52 cases, 84 were present in quantities greater than 10^3 CFU/mL (61% gram-negative bacilli, 38% gram-positive organisms, and 1% anaerobic bacteria). Of note was the finding that 14 of the 52 patients had at least two positive blood cultures within the 2 days before and 2 days after the procedure; however, in only 7 did the organism recovered from blood correspond to an organism isolated from the brush.

Another study of intubated patients undergoing ventilation by the same group of investigators in France[21] compared the diagnostic utility of bronchoalveolar lavage and the protected catheter brush. They observed that total and differential counts of lavage cells were not useful in distinguishing between patients with and without bacterial pneumonia. More than 25% of lavage cells in cytocentrifuged smears from five of five patients meeting their criteria for pneumonia contained intracellular organisms. In contrast, less than 1% of lavage cells had intracellular organisms in 9 of 13 patients without pneumonia. The correlation between quantitative cultures of lavage and brush specimens was moderate ($r = .68$, $P < .05$). In a similar study of intubated, mechanically ventilated patients by Torres and associates,[22] quantitative lavage and brush cultures agreed moderately well ($r = .78$, $P < .001$). Bacteremia in the latter study was also infrequent.

If one makes the major assumption that the criteria used in these studies for defining pneumonia are adequate, one might conclude that quantitative cultures of protected catheter brushes are useful in the diagnosis of bacterial pneumonia in the intubated, mechanically ventilated patient. One might also conclude that bronchoalveolar lavage is a useful complementary procedure, particularly when cytocentrifuged smears are examined for the presence of intracellular organisms. Bacteremia appears to occur with low frequency in such patients, so blood cultures are often not helpful and, if positive, often reflect an extrapulmonary site of infection.

Although the protected catheter brush has proved useful in the diagnosis of bacterial pneumonia, its small sample size (approximately 0.001 mL) makes it less useful for the diagnosis of mycobacterial, fungal, viral, and *Pneumocystis carinii* pneumonia, for which bronchoalveolar lavage is recommended.[23] When specimens are obtained from seriously ill immunocompromised patients, the laboratory should follow an established protocol for the lavage fluid to include examination for bacteria, mycobacteria, *Legionella* species, fungi, viruses, and *P. carinii.*[23]

Because *Candida* species are normally present in the oropharynx, the interpretation of their isolation from respiratory secretions has been problematic.[8] The diagnosis of pulmonary candidiasis, therefore, has been established definitively only by histologic examination of lung tissue. Although criteria have been established for the diagnosis of bacterial pneumonia in specimens obtained by the protected catheter brush and bronchoalveolar lavage, insufficient data are available at this time to determine whether the same criteria can be applied to *Candida* species.[8] Similar problems exist with aspergillosis, for which the diagnosis also requires histopathologic confirmation.

URINARY TRACT INFECTION

Urine culture remains the standard method for the laboratory diagnosis of bacteriuria. Urine can be readily obtained from a catheter or a port on the side of the drainage tube of indwelling catheters of intensive care unit patients. As simple as this procedure is, a number of issues related to urine collection, culture procedures, and culture interpretation require emphasis.

Urine is an excellent culture medium; therefore, specimens should be either transported to the laboratory promptly and cultured within 2 hours of collection or refrigerated during storage to prevent bacterial multiplication. The number of colonies per milliliter of refrigerated urine remains stable for long periods. Urine for culture should always be aspirated aseptically from the side port of the drainage tube and not from the drainage bag or by breaking the closed drainage system in any manner. Stark and Maki[24] found that in newly catheterized adult patients, bacteriuria or candiduria of some level developed within 3 days in nearly half of the patients. Low-level ($< 10^5$ CFU/mL) bacteriuria or candiduria was initially identified in 37% of the patients; however, it progressed to high-level ($>10^5$ CFU/mL) bacteriuria or candiduria in more than 90% of cases. Data from this study did not conclusively identify a lower threshold level of colonies that differentiated early infection from contamination. In most cases, however, the culture performed a day later demonstrated a progression from low-level to high-level bacteriuria or candiduria with the same organism.

The microbiologic examination of urine from chronic indwelling urethral catheters is quite complex compared with that of urine from newly inserted catheters in part because bacterial concentrations progressively increase over time. Warren and coworkers[25] followed 20 patients with chronic indwelling urethral catheters for 605 patient-weeks (mean = 30.3 weeks per patient) and found that 98.4% of 619 weekly urine specimens contained at least one strain of bacteria at a concentration of at least 10^5 CFU/mL. Of the specimens, 22% contained a single organism, 35% contained two, 25% contained three, and 16% contained four or more. Thus, polymicrobial bacteriuria was common. Other studies have shown significant changes in species composition, quantitation of organisms, and antibiograms of isolates from urine of patients with chronic indwelling urethral catheters.[26, 27] Moreover, paired urine specimens from "old" and newly replaced catheters can produce divergent results.[28] Although species found in the urine may be associated with bacteremic episodes in such patients, culture of urine from chronic indwelling urethral catheters provides a nonspecific test for organisms causing bacteremia.[26]

For all of the foregoing reasons, the extent of laboratory identification of isolates from catheter urine tends to vary in clinical microbiology laboratories according to the descriptive information provided with the specimen, the number of different species isolated, and the quantity of organisms present in cultures.[29] Most laboratories, therefore, provide definitive identification and perform antimicrobial susceptibility testing of a single isolate in a quantity of at least 10^5 CFU/mL from a catheter urine specimen but might provide only descriptive (morphologic) information if there were two isolates, each at the same concentration.[29] Few laboratories provide more than a descriptive report if three or more morphologic types of bacteria are present in a catheter urine sample, regardless of the quantity of each organism. The interpretation and significance of candiduria are discussed in Chapter 33.

There are numerous rapid screening methods for detecting bacteriuria. These methods range from microscopic examination of uncentrifuged or centrifuged, unstained or stained urine to bioluminescence. The negative predictive value for virtually all available tests (with the exception of the leukocyte esterase-nitrite test) is greater than 95% for bacteriuria at the level of at least 10^5 CFU/mL. Bioluminescence provides a negative predictive value of at least 95% for bacteriuria of at least 10^4 CFU/mL. In many laboratories today, urine specimens with a negative screening test result are not routinely cultured.

Urine culture must always be performed quantitatively. Anaerobic cultures of urine should be restricted to specimens obtained by suprapubic aspiration. Such specimens are the only urine specimens for which broth culture is indicated.

SURGICAL WOUND INFECTION

Surgical wound infections may be acquired exogenously from the operating room environment or personnel; however, most surgical wound infections are of endogenous origin and result from incision, penetration, transection, or perforation of skin, mucous membranes, or a hollow viscus that is normally colonized with bacterial and fungal organisms. Coagulase-negative staphylococci are normally resident on the skin and, as already discussed, pose the greatest problem with intravascular catheter— and implanted prosthetic device—associated infections. *Staphylococcus aureus* may colonize the skin and upper respiratory tract, especially in health care workers and patients with prolonged hospitalizations. The indigenous flora of the oropharynx, ileum, colon, rectum, and vagina consists of a large and diverse collection of aerobic and anaerobic organisms, so infections after surgery in these sites are usually polymicrobial and predominantly anaerobic.

The microbiologic examination of surgical wound infections can be quite complex. Whereas a previously undrained incisional abscess from a sternal wound may yield a pure culture of *S. aureus*, the same sternal wound several days later after spontaneous or surgical drainage may yield not only *S. aureus* but also coagulase-negative staphylococci, diphtheroids, and enterococci, reflecting not only the primary pathogen but also the presence of organisms from the skin and surrounding environment. An intra-abdominal abscess or a wound abscess after elective colon surgery contains a minimum of two or three aerobic bacterial species and a minimum of three anaerobic bacterial species, depending on the extent of anaerobic bacteriology performed. When these abscesses have been opened and drained, changes in the microbiologic composition of further cultures often occur. The point is that the interpretation of cultures representing surgical wound infections is not straightforward and is influenced by whether the site of infection has been previously opened and drained. In chronic infections, such as those in decubitus ulcers, the microbiology is more representative of the patient's fecal flora than of anything else.

Thus it is important, as stated in the introduction to this chapter, to select specimens that are representative of the disease process. The timing of specimen collection is also important (i.e., collection at the time of incision and drainage). Collection technique is another important variable. The amount of specimen must be sufficient to allow adequate examination, and transport of the specimen should ensure survival of both aerobic and anaerobic bacteria. Neither of these requirements is adequately met with a swab, use of which should be limited to sampling the skin and mucous membranes. Abscess material should be aspirated with a syringe and sent directly to the laboratory or injected into an anaerobic transport vial, of which several are commercially available.

A Gram-stained smear offers presumptive evidence of the cause of the infection (e.g., staphylococcal vs. mixed aerobic and anaerobic infection). Cultures should be made aerobically and anaerobically. Although definitive identification of each anaerobic species isolated is probably not necessary for proper clinical care, the laboratory should be able to provide at least presumptive identification of the presence of the *Bacteroides fragilis* group in the specimen. The extent of further identification of anaerobic bacteria may vary according to the source of the specimen, the number of different organisms present in cultures, and the laboratory's interest and expertise. In our laboratory, for example, we would identify definitively an anaerobic gram-negative bacillus isolated from blood or a brain abscess; however, we would simply characterize it morphologically with its β-lactamase reactivity when isolated in mixed culture from a specimen described simply as a "wound," and the remaining isolates would be described as "mixed anaerobic flora."

ANTIMICROBIAL SUSCEPTIBILITY TESTING

Antimicrobial resistance occurs frequently in nosocomial pathogens in general and intensive care unit pathogens in particular;[30] therefore, a major responsibility of the clinical microbiology laboratory is to determine the antimicrobial susceptibility of clinically significant isolates. Methods should be used that accurately detect penicillin and oxacillin resistance in staphylococci, β-lactam resistance in *Pseudomonas aeruginosa* and Enterobacteriaceae, and aminoglycoside resistance in enterococci and *P. aeruginosa*. Specific standards published by the National Committee for Clinical Laboratory Standards[31, 32] provide guidelines for selection of antimicrobial agents for testing and standards for the performance,

quality control, and interpretive criteria for dilution and diffusion susceptibility tests. Strict adherence to these standards optimizes the detection of antimicrobial resistance.

Specific problems exist with the accurate detection of certain types of antimicrobial resistance. Oxacillin has largely supplanted methicillin for in vitro testing purposes because of its greater stability; however, the accurate detection of staphylococci resistant to oxacillin (or methicillin) requires test conditions that induce formation of a penicillin-binding protein (PBP2a) with altered affinity for oxacillin. In most instances, resistance is heterogeneous and is present in only 1 in 10^4 to 1 in 10^8 cells, so detection of the resistant population requires addition of NaCl to the test medium and an incubation temperature of 30 to 35°C. Use of an inoculum standardized to contain approximately 5×10^5 CFU/mL is also important for accurate results with the dilution tests. An agar screen method has also been recommended as a confirmatory test of oxacillin resistance.[32]

Since the introduction of expanded-spectrum cephalosporins and the ureidopenicillins, mutants of *Citrobacter freundii*, *Enterobacter aerogenes*, *Enterobacter cloacae*, *P. aeruginosa*, and, less frequently, *Serratia marcescens* and indole-positive Proteeae that are stably derepressed for type I β-lactamase have been increasingly recognized in nosocomially acquired infections. Such organisms are typically susceptible to expanded-spectrum cephalosporins and ureidopenicillins on initial isolation but may become resistant in as little as 1 or 2 days of therapy with one of these antibiotics through a simple process of elimination of the predominantly susceptible population of cells in the infected site and selection, survival, and multiplication of mutants that are stably derepressed for the chromosomally mediated, type I β-lactamase.[33] Detection of this form of resistance may be difficult unless the inoculum size is properly standardized to contain 5×10^5 CFU/mL and the incubation time exceeds 6 hours.[34] Caution must be exercised in the use of newer, "rapid" susceptibility testing systems that may generate a result in 3 to 5 hours, because false susceptibility or false moderate susceptibility is a frequent occurrence with stably derepressed mutants for type I β-lactamase. This problem is also of special concern with microbroth dilution tests because routine inoculum preparation may fall short of the recommended 5×10^5 CFU/mL concentration.

An additional β-lactamase–related problem is related to plasmid-mediated, broad-spectrum β-lactamases in *Escherichia coli* and *Klebsiella* species that confer resistance to newer β-lactams such as cefotaxime and ceftazidime.[35] Minimal inhibitory concentrations of cefotaxime, ceftriaxone, ceftazidime, and aztreonam vary and may fall within the 8 μg/mL cutoff used to define susceptibility,[31] although they are clearly higher than those of fully susceptible strains that do not harbor these plasmids. In contrast to chromosomal type I β-lactamase, which is unaffected by clavulanate or sulbactam, the novel plasmid-mediated, broad-spectrum cefotaximases and ceftazidimases are inactivated by clavulanate and sulbactam, thereby allowing detection of resistant isolates with a modification of the disk diffusion test.[36] In this test, disks containing cefotaxime or ceftazidime and amoxicillin-clavulanate (Augmentin) are placed approximately 30 mm apart. The presence of the plasmid-mediated β-lactamase is then detected by a synergistic effect in which the zone diameter of inhibition surrounding the cefotaxime or ceftazidime disk bows toward the amoxicillin-clavulanate disk.

High-level streptomycin resistance in enterococci has been recognized for many years; however, high-level resistance of enterococci to gentamicin is of more recent origin and of varying magnitude in hospitals around the country. Because bactericidal activity against enterococci requires a combination of a penicillin or vancomycin with an aminoglycoside, microbiology laboratories should be testing enterococcal isolates from blood, normally sterile body fluids, and tissue for high-level resistance. Lack of inhibition of an enterococcus by 500 μg/mL of gentamicin correlates with lack of synergy and, hence, lack of bactericidal activity of gentamicin in combination with a penicillin or vancomycin. An explanatory note to this effect should be included in the laboratory report. Vancomycin resistance in enterococci has only recently been recognized and is of uncertain incidence and distribution.

Finally, aminoglycoside activity against *P. aeruginosa* is heavily influenced by the cation content of the test medium. More specifically, aminoglycoside activity is inversely related to cation concentration. Because commercially available Mueller-Hinton broth initially contained little or no cation, it was recommended for many years that the broth be supplemented with 50 mg/L Ca^{2+} and 25 mg/L Mg^{2+}. This practice has resulted in two problems. First, a reference lot of Mueller-Hinton agar was chosen by the National Committee for Clinical Laboratory Standards to serve as a performance standard for manufacturers of media to obtain more lot-to-lot consistency in disk diffusion testing, and in many instances thereafter isolates of *P. aeruginosa* proved to be more susceptible by disk diffusion testing than by dilution testing in cation-supplemented broth. Second, clinical data emerged demonstrating that the amount of cation supplementation was associated with a high rate of false resistance and that a lower amount of cation resulted in minimal inhibitory concentrations that were more clinically related to outcome of therapy.[37] Thus, it is currently recommended that dilution testing be performed in broth adjusted to contain 20 to 25 mg/L Ca^{2+} and 10 to 12.5 mg/L Mg^{2+}.[31]

Antimicrobial susceptibility testing of anaerobic bacteria is indicated only in limited circumstances, such as with isolates from blood, brain abscess, vascular grafts, or implanted prosthetic material. At this time, the susceptibility of anaerobic bacteria to metronidazole (except against non–spore-forming gram-positive bacilli), imipenem, chloramphenicol, ampicillin-sulbactam, and ticarcillin-clavulanate remains highly predictable, so testing of isolates against these compounds is rarely indicated.

In conclusion, the microbiology laboratory has an important function in isolating, identifying, and determining the antimicrobial susceptibility of pathogenic organisms. Careful specimen selection and collection are critical steps in this process because interpretation of cultures is only as good as the quality of the specimen received.

References

1. Aronson MD, Bor DH: Blood cultures. Ann Intern Med 106:246, 1987.
2. Washington JA II: Blood cultures: Principles and techniques. Mayo Clin Proc 50:91, 1975.
3. Weinstein MP, Reller LB, Murphy JR: The clinical significance of positive blood cultures: A comprehensive analysis of bacteremia and fungemia in adults. I. Laboratory and epidemiologic observations. Rev Infect Dis 5:35, 1983.
4. Ilstrup DM, Washington JA II: The importance of volume of blood cultured in the detection of bacteremia and fungemia. Diagn Microbiol Infect Dis 1:107, 1983.
5. Collignon PJ, Munro R: Laboratory diagnosis of intravascular catheter associated sepsis. Eur J Clin Microbiol Infect Dis 8:807, 1989.
6. Maki DG, Weise CE, Sarafin HW: A semiquantitative culture method for identifying intravenous catheter–related infection. N Engl J Med 296:305, 1977.
7. Cleri DJ, Corrado ML, Seligman SJ: Quantitative culture of intravenous catheters and other intravascular inserts. J Infect Dis 141:781, 1980.
8. Jones JM: Laboratory diagnosis of invasive candidiasis. Clin Microbiol Rev 3:32, 1990.
9. Phillips P, Dowd A, Jewesson P, et al: Nonvalue of antigen detection immunoassays for diagnosis of candidemia. J Clin Microbiol 28:2320, 1990.
10. Johanson WG, Pierce AK, Sanford JP, et al: Nosocomial respiratory infections with gram-negative bacilli: The significance of colonization of the respiratory tract. Ann Intern Med 77:701, 1972.
11. Craven DE: Nosocomial pneumonia: New concepts on an old disease. Infect Control Hosp Epidemiol 9:57, 1988.
12. Dashner F, Kappstein I, Engels I, et al: Stress ulcer prophylaxis and ventilation pneumonia: Prevention by antibacterial cytoprotective agents? Infect Control Hosp Epidemiol 9:59, 1988.
13. Golden SE, Shehab ZM, Bjelland JC, et al: Microbiology of endotracheal aspirates in intubated pediatric intensive care unit patients: Correlations with radiographic findings. Pediatr Infect Dis J 6:665, 1987.
14. Salata RA, Lederman MM, Shlaes DM, et al: Diagnosis of nosocomial pneumonia in intubated, intensive care unit patients. Am Rev Respir Dis 135:426, 1987.
15. Chastre J, Viau F, Brun P, et al: Prospective evaluation of the protected specimen brush for the diagnosis of pulmonary infections in ventilated patients. Am Rev Respir Dis 130:924, 1984.
16. Broughton WA, Bass JP, Kirkpatrick MB: The technique of protected brush catheter bronchoscopy. J Crit Illness 2:63, 1987.
17. Bartlett JG: Fiberoptic bronchoscopy for diagnosis of pneumonia (editorial). J Crit Illness 2:3, 1987.
18. Thorpe JE, Baughman RP, Frame PT, et al: Bronchoalveolar lavage for diagnosing acute bacterial pneumonia. J Infect Dis 155:855, 1987.
19. Kahn JW, Jones JM: Diagnosing respiratory infection by bronchoalveolar lavage. J Infect Dis 155:862, 1987.
20. Fagon J-Y, Chastre J, Domart Y, et al: Nosocomial pneumonia in patients receiving continuous mechanical ventilation: Prospective analysis of 52 episodes with use of a protected specimen brush and quantitative culture techniques. Am Rev Respir Dis 139:877, 1989.
21. Chastre J, Soler P, Bonnet M, et al: Diagnosis of nosocomial pneumonia in intubated patients undergoing ventilation: Comparison of the usefulness of bronchoalveolar lavage and the protected specimen brush. Am J Med 85:499, 1988.
22. Torres A, De La Bellacasa JP, Kaubet A, et al: Diagnostic value of quantitative sputum cultures of bronchoalveolar lavage and telescoping plugged catheters in mechanically ventilated patients with bacterial pneumonia. Am Rev Respir Dis 140:306, 1989.
23. Bartlett JG, Ryan KJ, Smith TF, et al: Laboratory diagnosis of lower respiratory tract infections. In: Washington JA II (ed): Cumitech 7A. Washington, DC, American Society for Microbiology, p 1, 1987.
24. Stark MP, Maki DG: Bacteriuria in the catheterized patient: What quantitative level of bacteriuria is relevant? N Engl J Med 311:360, 1984.
25. Warren JW, Tenny JH, Hoopes JM, et al: A prospective microbiologic study of bacteriuria in 20 patients with chronic indwelling urethral catheters. J Infect Dis 146:719, 1982.
26. Tenny JH, Warren JW: Bacteriuria in women with long-term catheters: Paired comparison of indwelling and replacement catheters. J Infect Dis 157:199, 1988.
27. Breitenbucher RB: Bacterial changes in the urine samples of patients with long-term indwelling catheters. Arch Intern Med 144:585, 1984.
28. Grahn D, Norman DC, White ML, et al: Validity of urinary catheter specimens for diagnosis of urinary tract infection in the elderly. Arch Intern Med 145:1858, 1985.
29. Clarridge JE, Pezzlo MT, Vosti K: Laboratory diagnosis of urinary tract infections. In: Weissfeld A (ed): Cumitech 2A. Washington, DC, American Society for Microbiology, p 1, 1987.
30. Dashner F: Nosocomial infection in intensive care units. Intensive Care Med 11:284, 1985.
31. National Committee for Clinical Laboratory Standards: Methods for Dilution Antimicrobial Susceptibility Tests for Bacteria That Grow Aerobically—Second Edition; Approved Standard. Villanova, PA, National Committee for Clinical Laboratory Standards, 1990. NCCLS document M7-A2.
32. National Committee for Clinical Laboratory Standards: Performance Standards for Antimicrobial Disk Susceptibility Tests—Fourth Edition; Approved Standard. Villanova, PA, National Committee for Clinical Laboratory Standards, 1990. NCCLS document M2-A4.
33. Livermore DM: Clinical significance of beta-lactamase induction and stable derepression in gram-negative rods. Eur J Clin Microbiol 6:439, 1987.
34. Washington JA II, Knapp CC, Sanders CC: Accuracy of microdilution and the AutoMicrobic System in detection of β-lactam resistance in gram-negative bacterial mutants with derepressed β-lactamase. Rev Infect Dis 10:824, 1988.
35. Phillipon A, Labia R, Jacoby G: Extended spectrum β-lactamases. Antimicrob Agents Chemother 33:1131, 1989.
36. Jarlier V, Nicholas M-H, Fournier G, et al: Extended broad spectrum β-lactamases conferring transferable resistance to newer β-lactam agents in Enterobacteriaceae: Hospital prevalence and susceptibility patterns. Rev Infect Dis 10:867, 1988.
37. Barry AL, Miller GH, Thornsberry C, et al: Influence of cation supplements on activity of netilmicin against *Pseudomonas aeruginosa* in vitro and in vivo. Antimicrob Agents Chemother 3:1514, 1987.

CHAPTER 53

Selection of Antimicrobial Agents: Pharmacokinetic and Pharmacodynamic Principles

Matthew E. Levison

The goal of antimicrobial therapy is clearance of the pathogen from the infected tissues. This is accomplished as a consequence of both the pharmacokinetic and antimicrobial characteristics of the antimicrobial agent and the host defense mechanisms. In severely ill patients, with often debilitating underlying conditions, host defenses may be compromised. In addition, host defenses are not operative in certain types of infection, which include endocarditis,[1] meningitis,[2] and infection in neutropenic patients.[3-5] The effectiveness of antimicrobial therapy in these situations depends mainly on the characteristics of the antimicrobial agent.

ANTIMICROBIAL AGENTS

In severely ill infected patients, antimicrobial therapy has to be initiated promptly, frequently before the pathogen or its antimicrobial sensitivities are known. Use of antimicrobial agents in this way is called empirical therapy and necessitates that the agents (1) have broad spectrum of activity, to cover all the suspected pathogens; (2) have ideally bactericidal action, because host defenses may be compromised; and (3) be used in doses, a route of administration, and a dosing interval that permit a bactericidal action to accumulate at the site of infection with successive doses. To accomplish

Portions of this chapter were adapted from Levison ME, Bush LM: Pharmacodynamics of antimicrobial agents. Infect Dis Clin North Am 3:415, 1989.

this, combinations of antimicrobial agents are frequently used, even at the risk of potential toxicity (e.g., renal dysfunction from the aminoglycosides), because of the likelihood of unacceptable morbidity and mortality from inadequately treated infection. After the clinical microbiology laboratory identifies the pathogen and its sensitivity to antimicrobial agents, the empirical regimen can be modified to the least toxic, least costly agent that has specific activity against the isolated pathogen.

The antimicrobial activity that can be expected from agents used in empirical regimens against commonly encountered pathogens is shown in Table 53–1.

1. Up to 30 to 40% of both community-acquired and nosocomial *Escherichia coli* infections are resistant to ampicillin and first-generation cephalosporins.

2. The commonly encountered nosocomial pathogens *Enterobacter cloacae*, *Serratia marcescens*, *Citrobacter freundii*, *Morganella morganii*, and *Pseudomonas aeruginosa* both produce inducible, chromosome-encoded β-lactamases and exhibit frequent mutational loss of the genetic control of production of these β-lactamases.[6, 7] These stable derepressed mutants, which produce large amounts of β-lactamase, may emerge during therapy with third-generation cephalosporins, including ceftazidime, and are highly resistant to all β-lactams, except imipenem. The β-lactams clavulanic acid and sulbactam are not effective antibiotics but inhibit many commonly occurring β-lactamases, such as the β-lactamases produced by *Staphylococcus aureus*, *E. coli*, *Neisseria gonorrhoeae*, *Haemophilus influenzae*, *Klebsiella pneumoniae*, and *Bacteroides fragilis*. These β-lactamase inhibitors, however, do not inhibit the β-lactamases produced by *Enterobacter*, *Serratia*, *Citrobacter*, *Morganella*, or *P. aeruginosa*. There is no cross-resistance among these strains to quinolones, aminoglycosides, or trimethoprim-sulfamethoxazole.

3. Metronidazole is active against anaerobes, especially anaerobic gram-negative bacilli, but has poor activity against microaerophilic, and some anaerobic, gram-positive cocci. To cover these potentially significant pathogens in mixed anaerobic infection, another antimicrobial agent (e.g., penicillin) is used in combination with metronidazole. In contrast, clindamycin has activity against aerobic, microaerophilic, and anaerobic gram-positive cocci, as well as anaerobic gram-negative bacilli, although resistance has developed among these latter pathogens at some medical centers.

4. Methicillin-resistant staphylococci are resistant to all β-

					Third-Generation Cephalosporins	Ceftazidime	Aztreonam	Amoxicillin Clavulanate, Ampicillin-Sulbactam	Broad-Spectrum Penicillins	Timentin	Imipenem	Aminoglycoside Quinolones
Pathogen	**Ampicillin**	**Cefazolin**	**Cefamandole**	**Cefoxitin**								
Escherichia coli	R	R	S	S	S	S	S	S	S	S	S	S
Proteus mirabilis	S	S	S	S	S	S	S	S	S	S	S	S
Klebsiella	R	S	S	S	S	S	S	S	R	S	S	S
Indole⁺ *Proteus*	R	R	R	S	R§	R§	R§	R	R§	R§	S	S
Enterobacter	R	R	S	R	R§	R§	R§	R	R§	R§	S	S
Serratia	R	R	R	R	R§	R§	R§	R	R§	R§	S	S
Pseudomonas aeruginosa	R	R	R	R	R§	R§	R§	R	R§	R§	S	S
Staphylococci	R	S†	S†	S†	S†	S†	R	S†	R	S†	S†	S
Streptococci	S	S‡	S‡	S‡	S‡	S‡	R	S	S	S	S	R
Bacteroides fragilis	R	R	R	R	R	R	R	S	S	S	S	R

TABLE 53–1

SUSCEPTIBILITY OF CLINICALLY IMPORTANT PATHOGENS TO ANTIMICROBIAL AGENTS IN EMPIRICAL REGIMENS*

*R = clinically significant resistance (>10% of isolates); S = sensitivity.
†Except methicillin-resistant staphylococci.
‡Except enterococci.
§Producers of chromosomal, inducible β-lactamases.

lactam antibiotics. The name derives from the fact that methicillin is the antibiotic frequently used to test for the presence of this type of resistance in the laboratory. Nosocomial infection caused by methicillin-resistant *S. aureus* is encountered frequently in teaching institutions in the United States and in patients in nursing homes. Because the mechanism of high-level methicillin resistance does not involve β-lactamase production, use of a β-lactamase inhibitor, such as clavulanic acid or sulbactam, does not ablate this type of resistance. About half of *Staphylococcus epidermidis* strains are methicillin resistant. *S. epidermidis* organisms are frequent pathogens in the presence of a foreign body (e.g., prosthetic joint, prosthetic cardiac valve, neurosurgical shunt, intravascular access catheter, and bone wax). Alternative agents available for treatment of infection caused by methicillin-resistant staphylococci include the glycopeptides, vancomycin and teicoplanin, trimethoprim-sulfamethoxazole, clindamycin, and possibly the fluorinated quinolones, such as ciprofloxacin, ofloxacin, and temafloxacin. However, methicillin-resistant staphylococci frequently exhibit resistance to multiple other agents, including trimethoprim-sulfamethoxazole, clindamycin, and the fluorinated quinolones.

5. Rifampin has broad-spectrum, bactericidal action, but resistance develops rapidly if this drug is used alone. For this reason, rifampin is never used alone to treat serious infections. It is used as an adjunctive agent, both to enhance the bactericidal action and to prevent the emergence of resistance with another antimicrobial agent, such as one of the antistaphylococcal agents mentioned earlier.

6. Imipenem, aminoglycosides, and the fluorinated quinolones have the broadest spectrum and most reliable activity against common pathogens. Imipenem is inactive against *Xanthomonas (Pseudomonas) maltophilia,* an uncommon nosocomial pathogen. However, unlike imipenem, aminoglycosides and the fluorinated quinolones that are currently available have poor activity against streptococci and anaerobes. If aminoglycosides or the fluorinated quinolones are to be used empirically or for mixed infection, they must be combined with another agent that has activity against streptococci or anaerobes, if these organisms are suspected. Newer fluorinated quinolones have better activity against streptococci (ofloxacin and temafloxacin) and anaerobes (temafloxacin) but are as yet available for oral administration only. Ciprofloxacin currently is the only fluorinated quinolone that can be administered either orally or intravenously. These fluorinated quinolones are absorbed well enough and are sufficiently potent to allow use for systemic infection. Nevertheless, the oral route of administration is often inappropriate in severely ill patients; until a parenteral preparation becomes available, the use of an oral antimicrobial agent is restricted to patients who are initially less severely ill or who have responded sufficiently to prior parenteral antibiotics to allow oral administration of antimicrobial therapy.

Aminoglycosides, despite having the attributes of concentration-dependent bactericidal action, a postantibiotic effect (PAE), and the ability to enhance the bactericidal activity (synergy) of β-lactams (see later) have some well-known problems: (a) Their antimicrobial activity is compromised by in vivo conditions commonly present at the sites of infection (i.e., relatively low pH, anaerobic redox potential, and the presence of calcium ions). (b) The pharmacokinetics are unpredictable (e.g., a third of patients treated with standard doses have peak serum levels [0.5 hour after the end of a 0.5-hour intravenous infusion] outside the therapeutic range, which is 4 to 8 µg/mL for gentamicin or tobramycin and 20 to 30 µg/mL for amikacin. Peak serum levels below the therapeutic range are associated with a poor clinical outcome. (c) Aminoglycosides are potentially nephrotoxic

and ototoxic. (d) The clinical efficacy of aminoglycosides has generally been less than that of β-lactams in noncomparative trials and in at least one controlled comparative trial in severe infection caused by susceptible gram-negative bacilli.[8] For these reasons, aminoglycosides are used for the treatment of severe infections as adjunctive agents in empirical regimens in combination with β-lactams for extension of spectrum and synergistic activity.

PHARMACOKINETICS

Disposition of the drug in the body is usually described in terms of concentration versus time in the serum because of the relative ease of measurement in this body fluid.[9–11] The therapeutic effect, however, depends on the concentration versus time at the site of infection, and concentrations at sites other than blood may not necessarily be equivalent to the serum levels.

Antimicrobial agents are usually administered intermittently. After administration of a dose, an antimicrobial agent is distributed initially throughout the blood volume and the extracellular fluid of highly perfused tissues (heart, lung, liver, and kidneys). The peak level of drug in serum occurs at the completion of an intravenous infusion, after completion of absorption from an intramuscular site of injection, or after absorption from the intestinal tract with oral administration. The peak level in serum is proportional to the size of the dose administered, the amount of drug eliminated during the time of infusion or absorption, and the volume of distribution. If the rate of infusion or absorption is slow, the peak level is correspondingly low and the time to peak level is delayed.

Serum levels that follow the peak concentration decline as a consequence of further diffusion into tissues and elimination from the body by metabolism or excretion. Excretion occurs primarily in bile or urine. The rate of elimination is constant for those drugs that have a constant fraction of the drug eliminated in a given time (e.g., by first-order kinetics). The elimination of these drugs is described by their elimination half-life (i.e., the time it takes to eliminate 50% of the drug present). Most antibiotic agents are administered at a dosing interval equal to about four half-lives. Because about 93% of a dose is eliminated in four half-lives, the subsequent doses do not result in significant accumulation (i.e., each subsequent dose results in serum levels that are identical with those after the initial dose). A progressive increase in serum levels occurs if the dosing interval is less than four half-lives until a steady state is eventually reached. The time required to reach a steady state is also about four half-lives.

Treatment of critically ill patients necessitates that therapeutic antimicrobial levels be established as quickly as possible. Precious time may be lost if therapeutic levels are established only at steady state. In this case, a larger than usual dose (or loading dose) of the agent must be administered initially to rapidly establish therapeutic levels. However, it is customary that loading doses are not used for most antibiotics, because the size of the standard dose is sufficiently large to achieve therapeutic levels after the first dose, and, when used for subsequent dosing, the standard dose yields therapeutic and nontoxic levels at steady state, even for those antimicrobial agents that are customarily given at dosing intervals equal to less than four half-lives.

Loading doses of antimicrobial agents are used in certain situations: If the dose is reduced to compensate for reduced elimination (e.g., renal insufficiency), the initial dose must remain equal to the usual dose that is given to a patient with normal drug elimination, so that the initial serum levels fall within the therapeutic range. A loading dose is also needed if the volume of distribution is initially larger, as may be the case in the presence of ascites.

In patients with decreased drug elimination, the size of the maintenance dose, the dosing interval, or both can be altered to prevent drug accumulation. Extension of the dosing interval to about four times the abnormally prolonged half-life, while maintaining the size of the dose, results in normal peak levels, but possibly long periods with subinhibitory levels. This method may not be effective for agents that fail to exhibit a PAE (e.g., most β-lactams do not have a PAE against gram-negative bacilli [see later]). In an alternative method, lowering the amount of subsequent (maintenance) doses after a standard initial (loading) dose is given, while maintaining the dosing interval, results in normal peak levels, but persistently elevated trough levels. This method, which results in sustained elevated serum levels, may be associated with greater toxicity when used for aminoglycoside dosing.

With renal failure, the daily dose of a drug excreted primarily by glomerular filtration can be decreased to the same extent that the creatinine clearance is diminished, and that dose can be given either as a single daily dose or in divided doses. For example, if the creatinine clearance is 10 mL/min (10% of normal), the daily dose of gentamicin (5 mg/kg) of 300 mg in a 60-kg person can be reduced to 30 mg given at the less frequent than usual 8-hour dosing interval, or 10 mg every 8 hours, after an initial loading dose of 100 mg (1.7 mg/kg). When only the serum creatinine measurement is available, the following formula can be used to estimate the creatinine clearance: males: (weight [kilograms] × 140 − age)/72 × serum creatinine level (mg/dL); females: 0.85 × male value. The amount of drug removed by dialysis can be replaced after dialysis. For example, because about half the body stores of gentamicin are removed when hemodialysis is performed, about half the loading dose should be given after each hemodialysis.

Although with renal failure the creatinine clearance can be used to judge the dose modification for drugs excreted primarily by the kidney, with impairment of hepatic function, no such measure of hepatic function exists for drugs excreted or metabolized by the liver.

Because these recommendations for dose reduction are approximations, they should be confirmed by determination of levels in serum at peak and trough at steady state, whenever the dose is changed, when renal function has changed for drugs whose therapeutic and toxic levels are close (e.g., aminoglycosides), or for drugs that have individual variability in pharmacokinetics (e.g., aminoglycosides).

Drug enters poorly perfused tissues (muscle, skin, and fat) more slowly, as is also the case for closed-space infection, such as an abscess or empyema, in which the ratio of the surface area of the vascular bed that surrounds the abscess to the volume of the abscess is low.[12] Antimicrobial agents move from blood to the extracellular fluid of tissues by passive diffusion along a concentration gradient. Factors that determine the amount of drug transferred from the blood stream into tissues, in addition to blood flow and surface area of the vascular bed, include (1) serum drug levels; (2) serum protein binding (because only that portion of the drug that is not bound to serum protein is free to diffuse into tissues); and (3) the presence of capillary pores. Highly protein-bound drugs, such as nafcillin, cefazolin, and ceftriaxone, have less free drug to diffuse into tissues than do drugs with lower serum protein binding.[13, 14] Tissues such as the lungs are well perfused via capillary beds fenestrated by pores, and the levels of drug in the extracellular fluid of these tissues are similar to free drug levels in serum. Drug levels may be considerably lower than serum levels in those tissues with nonfenestrated capillary beds, such as tissues in

the central nervous system, the eye, and the prostate, in which drug penetration depends on lipid solubility of the drug at the pH of each fluid and the pKa of the drug.[15]

Tissues are mainly cellular, and the volume is mainly intracellular fluid. Only a small portion is extracellular fluid. For drugs that are distributed only in extracellular fluid, such as β-lactams and aminoglycosides, total tissue levels (amount of drug in extracellular plus intracellular fluid) may be only a small fraction of the serum levels of drug that are not bound to serum protein, although the extracellular tissue fluid levels actually may be similar to serum levels of unbound drug. For drugs distributed in both intracellular and extracellular fluid (e.g., fluorinated quinolones, clindamycin, and rifampin), tissue levels may approach levels of the drug in serum not bound to serum protein. Bacteria in tissues may be located in extracellular fluid and within phagocytes. However, the intracellular location of the pathogen may not correspond to the intracellular location of the drug, or the intracellular conditions may not be auspicious, so that an antimicrobial effect may not necessarily occur.

ANTIMICROBIAL EFFECT

Some antimicrobial agents have bactericidal action (Table 53–2). Other antimicrobial agents have only an inhibitory effect on microbial growth. A notable exception is the bactericidal effect of chloramphenicol against pathogens that are frequent causes of meningitis (e.g., *Streptococcus pneumoniae, H. influenzae,* and *Neisseria meningitidis*) and of clindamycin against some strains of *S. aureus.* The type and quantitative assessment of antimicrobial activity are usually determined by the broth dilution technique. With this method, the lowest concentration of the antimicrobial agent that prevents development of turbidity (i.e., allows growth as judged by the naked eye) during overnight incubation of a previously clear suspension of 10^5 to 10^6 organisms per milliliter of broth, in the rapid phase of growth, is called the *minimal inhibitory concentration* (MIC).

The conditions for the in vitro MIC determination (i.e., an 18-hour aerobic incubation, an initial bacterial density of 10^5 to 10^6 colony-forming units per milliliter, organisms in the rapid or logarithmic growth phase, and a protein-free liquid medium at pH 7.2) and conditions at the site of infection may be different and affect the activity of the antimicrobial agents. For example, the activity of many agents may be less against dense microbial populations (10^8 to 10^{10} colony-forming units per gram) that exist in infected tissues. These dense populations may contain small resistant mutant subpopulations that become dominant during antimicrobial therapy. Only assays that use large inocula or

TABLE 53–2	
BACTERICIDAL AGENTS	
Class of Drug	**Agent**
β-Lactams	Penams (e.g., penicillin, ampicillin, nafcillin, ticarcillin)
	Carbapenem (imipenem)
	Cephems (cephalosporins, cefoxitin)
	Monobactam (aztreonam)
Aminoglycosides	Gentamicin, tobramycin, amikacin
Quinolones	Ciprofloxacin
Glycopeptides	Vancomycin, teicoplanin
Other	Trimethoprim-sulfamethoxazole
	Clindamycin
	Metronidazole
	Rifampin

longer incubation times increase the probability of detecting this form of resistance (e.g., β-lactam resistance in staphylococci[16] or third-generation cephalosporin resistance on the basis of stably derepressed β-lactamase production in *Enterobacter* species, *Serratia* species, and *P. aeruginosa*).[6, 7] Furthermore, dense microbial populations may be slow growing and metabolically inactive and thus less susceptible to the activity of β-lactams and aminoglycosides than are logarithmically growing organisms. Dense populations may also produce large amounts of enzymes such as β-lactamase, which are capable of destroying the agent locally and thus protecting sensitive organisms in a mixed infection. This loss of potency of an antimicrobial agent against dense populations (an increase in MIC) is called the *inoculum effect*. Aminoglycoside antibiotics, as well as erythromycin, are much less active at an acid pH, as occurs in an abscess or in infected body fluids). Aminoglycosides are also less active against facultative organisms that are growing under anaerobic conditions, in which the lowered oxygen tension decreases transport of these antimicrobial agents into the bacterial cell.

With antimicrobial agents capable of only bacteriostatic activity, subcultures from broth to antibiotic-free medium show that viable organisms can be recovered from tubes of broth containing antibiotic at the MIC level or higher. With antimicrobial agents that are capable of bactericidal activity, the concentration that prevents the development of turbidity actually may decrease the bacterial count. The extent to which the count is reduced in the clear tubes can be determined by subculturing. The minimal concentration of the drug that reduces the original bacterial count by at least 99.9% (from 10^5 to 10^6 to no more than 10^2 to 10^3 organisms per milliliter) after overnight incubation is defined as the *minimal bactericidal concentration* (MBC). Frequently, the minimal concentration of a bactericidal agent that prevents turbidity (MIC) actually has resulted in at least a 99.9% reduction in the original inoculum after overnight incubation (i.e., the MIC equals the MBC).

The requirement for a 1000-fold reduction of the original inoculum overnight is arbitrary, and there is not much evidence that a 99% (2 log 10/mL) fall in bacterial count after 24 or even 48 hours, rather than the expected 99.9% (3 log 10/mL) fall after overnight incubation is less useful as a definition. Although the clinical significance of a lower rate of in vitro bactericidal action (called tolerance) is a matter of much debate,[17] the ability to demonstrate in vitro tolerance is highly subject to the conditions of the assay system. Nevertheless, cultures of some organisms are not sterilized by otherwise bactericidal agents, no matter how the conditions of the assay system are altered. An example of this type of tolerance (i.e., less than 100% bactericidal action) to a bactericidal agent is the tolerance of enterococcus to penicillin or vancomycin. In the case of enterococcal endocarditis, the clinical significance of this type of tolerance to complete bactericidal action is clear.[1] Unless an aminoglycoside is added to penicillin or vancomycin to increase the rate and extent of bactericidal activity and sterilize bacterial populations in vitro as well as in vegetations in vivo, persistence of enterococci in vegetations is likely to lead to bacteriologic failure of antibiotic therapy.

After a limited exposure of organisms to a bactericidal agent, a portion of the microbial population persists. The size of the residual bacterial population depends on the size of the initial population and the rate and extent of the bactericidal effect. Some antimicrobial agents, such as β-lactams and aminoglycosides, have a bactericidal effect on only exponentially growing bacteria, whereas other agents, such as the quinolones, have a bactericidal effect on both exponentially growing organisms and those organisms in the

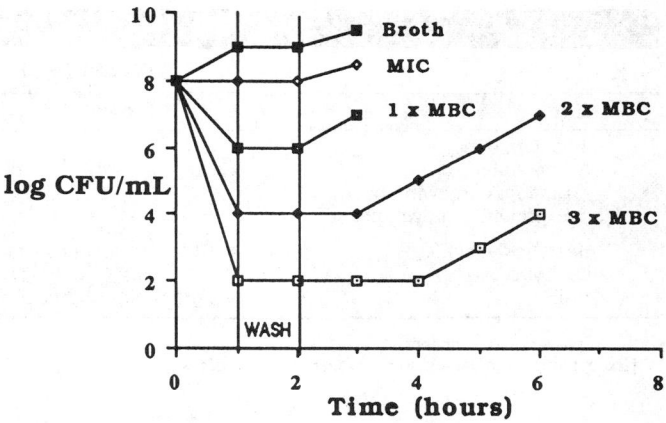

Figure 53–1. Time-kill study in broth containing various concentrations of an antimicrobial agent that exhibits concentration-dependent bactericidal action. A PAE on residual organisms is present after washing these organisms and resuspending them in antibiotic-free broth. CFU = colony-forming unit.

stationary growth phase. Rapidly growing organisms are found in young cultures and early infection. The majority of organisms in maximally dense bacterial populations, as exist in most established infections, are in the stationary growth phase. Only a minor portion of maximally dense bacterial populations are exponentially growing. Therefore, a single exposure to a β-lactam or an aminoglycoside can be expected to cause only a small decrement in maximally dense bacterial tissue populations, as it affects only the minor subpopulation of rapidly growing organisms.

For some antimicrobial agents, the rate and extent of bactericidal activity increase with increasing drug concentration above the MBC up to a point of maximal effect (usually 5 to 10 times the MBC) (Fig. 53–1). Antimicrobial agents that exhibit such concentration-dependent bactericidal action include the aminoglycosides, fluorinated quinolones, and metronidazole. In contrast, the bactericidal action of β-lactam antibiotics is relatively slow and does not increase at concentrations above the MBC; significant bactericidal activity requires continued exposure to concentrations equal to or greater than the MBC (time-dependent bactericidal activity) (Fig. 53–2).

Some antimicrobial agents enhance bacterial susceptibility

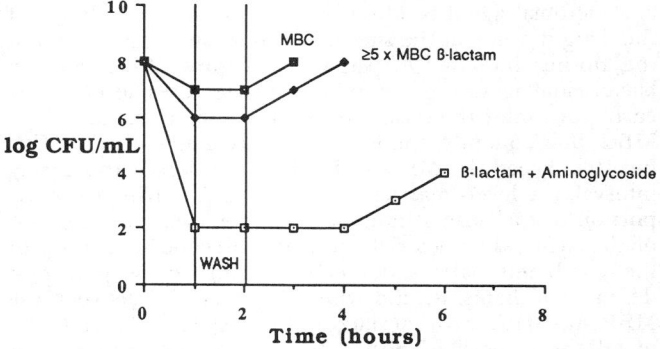

Figure 53–2. Time-kill study in broth containing various concentrations of an antimicrobial agent (i.e., a β-lactam) that exhibits time-dependent bactericidal action against a gram-negative bacillus. No PAE is present on residual organisms after washing and resuspending in antibiotic-free broth. Also shown is the more rapid bactericidal effect from the combination of the β-lactam plus aminoglycoside than would have occurred with the β-lactam used alone or the aminoglycoside used alone. CFU = colony-forming unit.

TABLE 53-3

SUMMARY OF ANTIMICROBIAL EFFECTS*

Effect	β-Lactams	Aminoglycosides	Quinolones
Inoculum effect	+	−	−
Active against			
Stationary growth phase	−	−	+
Exponential growth phase	+	+	+
Bactericidal action	Time dependent	Concentration dependent	Concentration dependent
Low MIC	+ / −	+	+
PAE	− vs. gram-negative bacilli†	+	+

*+ = present; − = absent.
†Except imipenem versus some strains of *P. aeruginosa.*

to host defenses in the presence of subinhibitory concentrations, called the *minimal antibiotic concentration*.[18] After prior exposure of bacteria to inhibitory or bactericidal concentrations, some agents enhance susceptibility of persisting organisms to host defenses, in the absence of residual drug. This has been called the *postantibiotic leukocyte effect*.[19] After a limited prior exposure of bacteria to inhibitory or bactericidal concentrations, antimicrobial agents may cause a persistent suppression of bacterial growth, in the absence of residual drug or host defenses. This has been called the *postantibiotic effect*.[20] A PAE is noted in vitro with most antimicrobial agents versus most pathogens, including imipenem versus *P. aeruginosa*; however, a PAE is not found with other β-lactams against other gram-negative bacilli. Inhibitors of protein or nucleic acid synthesis (aminoglycosides, fluorinated quinolones, tetracyclines, clindamycin, rifampin) induce a long-term PAE against susceptible gram-positive cocci and gram-negative bacilli. However, β-lactams induce a PAE lasting for approximately 2 hours against gram-positive cocci. A summary of antimicrobial effects of the major groups of bactericidal agents is shown in Table 53–3.

PHARMACODYNAMICS

Pharmacodynamics describes the antimicrobial effect at the site of infection during the course of therapy as a consequence of concentrations of the drug in the body versus time. The bacterial count at the site of infection is the result of the antimicrobial effects of the drug, the effectiveness of host defenses, and the rate of microbial growth. When an antimicrobial agent is administered intermittently, levels of the drug develop at the site of infection during a portion of the dosing interval. As shown in Figure 53–3, when a bactericidal agent is given in appropriate doses, levels in the early portion of the dosing interval may be in excess of the MBC. Subsequently, the levels may decline below the MBC but still exceed the MIC. In the later portion of the dosing interval, the levels may be below the MIC. During the early portion of the dosing interval when the levels are in excess of the MBC, the bacterial count may decline as a result of the combined bactericidal effect of the drug plus host defense mechanisms; and when the levels fall between the MBC and MIC, the bacterial count may stabilize (or continue to fall, as a result of host defenses). With a bacteriostatic agent, any decline in bacterial count results from the effectiveness of host defenses. Endocarditis, meningitis, and infections in neutropenic patients necessitate bactericidal agents to clear microorganisms from infected tissues, because of impaired local host defenses.

When drug levels at the site of infection fall below the MIC, the bacterial count may remain stable or fall at a diminished rate, as a result of a minimal antibiotic concentration, postantibiotic leukocyte effect, or PAE. Eventually, these persistent antimicrobial effects wane and the residual organisms may begin to regrow. The rate of regrowth depends on many factors, including the inherent doubling time of the organism, the availability of nutrients in the infected tissues, and the adequacy of host defense mechanisms. In the absence of host defenses (e.g., in endocarditic vegetations or in cerebrospinal fluid), organisms may increase exponentially at a rate similar to that which occurs in vitro. Some regrowth may restore susceptibility of the bacterial population to the bactericidal effect of β-lactams and aminoglycoside antibiotics. However, the next dose is ideally given before clinically significant regrowth occurs.

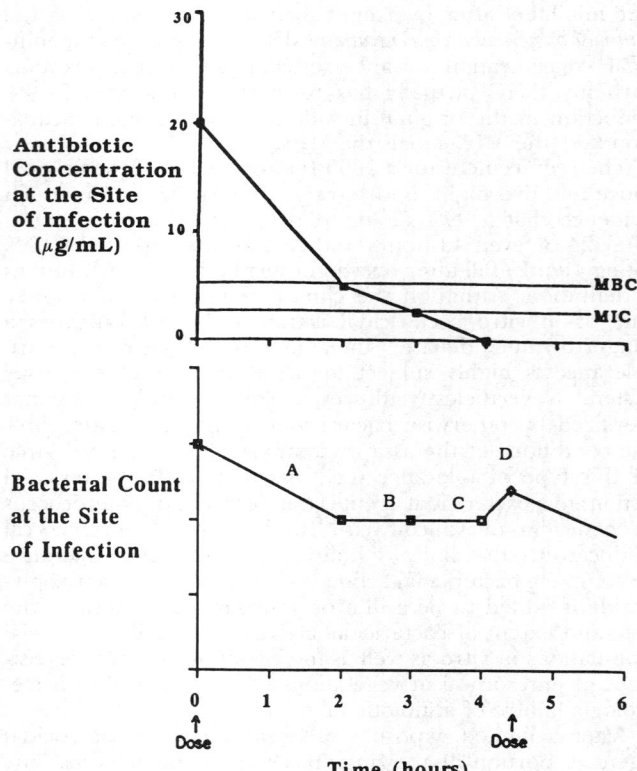

Figure 53–3. Antimicrobial pharmacodynamics. The A indicates time during which drug levels at the site of the infection are in excess of the MBC; the B, time during which the drug levels at the site of infection are less than the MBC but are in excess of the MIC; the C, duration of the minimal antibiotic concentration, postantibiotic leukocyte effect, and PAE when drug levels are less than the MIC; the D, regrowth of residual organisms.

With repeated doses, the bactericidal effect of each dose accumulates, such that the tissue is eventually cleared of the pathogen. If the doses are spaced too far apart, the bacterial count may rise in the later portion of each dosing interval, so that the count is equal to, or even exceeds, the initial count. The factors that allow infrequent dosing without loss of efficacy, especially in the presence of impaired host defenses, include (1) the rate and extent of the bactericidal effect of the drug;[21] (2) the antimicrobial potency of the drug; (3) the half-life of the drug; (4) the duration of any PAE; and (5) the rate of microbial regrowth.

The greater the rate of bactericidal action is, the lower the bacterial count in the residual population and the longer the interval before significant regrowth occurs (Fig. 53–4). With maximally dense bacterial populations in tissues, the extent of bactericidal action from antimicrobial agents that are active against organisms in both the stationary and logarithmic growth phases is expected to be greater than that from drugs active against organisms only in the logarithmic growth phase (see Fig. 53–4). Similar considerations occur with the use of synergistic combinations (i.e., use of two drugs in combination that results in significantly more rapid bactericidal action than occurs with either one of the drugs used alone) (see Fig. 53–2), or with the use of agents with concentration-dependent bactericidal action in doses that result in high peak tissue concentrations (see Fig. 53–4). For example, maximal antibacterial effects may be obtained by administering aminoglycoside so that the total daily dose is given once daily, rather than divided into two or three doses. However, dose-dependent toxicity may limit this goal. In both animal models and several human clinical trials, dosing regimens that provided high peak aminoglycoside concentrations and long subinhibitory concentrations were equally or more effective without excessive toxicity than regimens that provided lower peaks but more persistent inhibitory concentrations.[22–25]

Multiple doses given at relatively short intervals to maintain tissue concentrations in excess of the MIC are necessary for an agent that exhibits time-dependent bactericidal action and no PAE to achieve a bactericidal effect similar to that of an agent exhibiting concentration-dependent effects.[21] In fact, continuous dosing of a β-lactam antibiotic in a human trial was confirmed to be more efficacious than intermittent dosing.[26]

A potent antimicrobial agent with a low MBC has a prolonged time during which the levels of the drug at the site of infection are in excess of the MBC and a more extended time during which bactericidal action can occur.

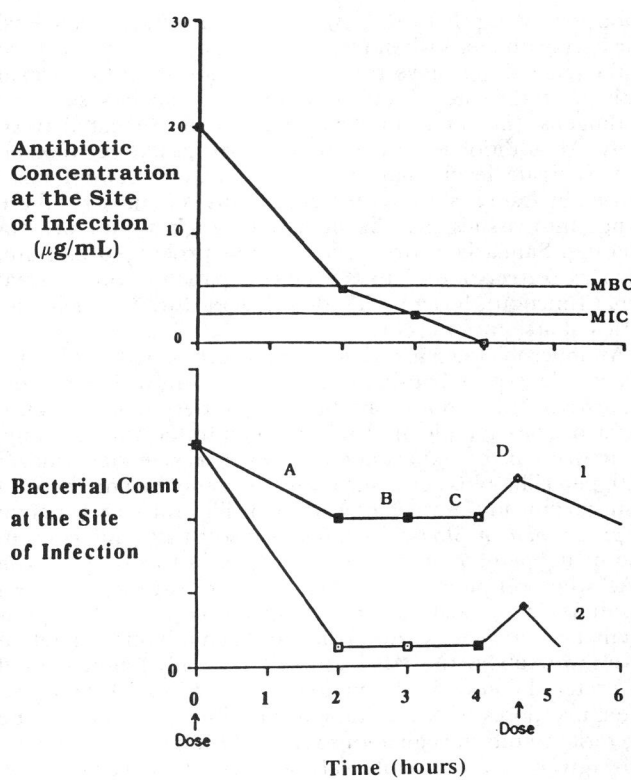

Figure 53–4. Antimicrobial pharmacodynamics for two agents with different rates of bactericidal action. Similarly, antimicrobial pharmacodynamics versus a maximally dense bacterial population of an antimicrobial agent with bactericidal action against only organisms in the logarithmic phase of growth (curve 1) as compared with that of an agent with bactericidal action against organisms in both the logarithmic and stationary phases of growth (curve 2).

However, it should be emphasized that not all sensitive pathogens are equally sensitive to a particular drug. For example, some pathogens may be inhibited by less than 0.1 μg/mL of a third-generation cephalosporin, such as ceftriaxone, whereas other pathogens require up to 10 μg/mL for inhibition. One dose in a 24-hour period may be sufficient to yield drug levels at the site of infection in excess of the MIC for the entire dosing interval (an important consider-

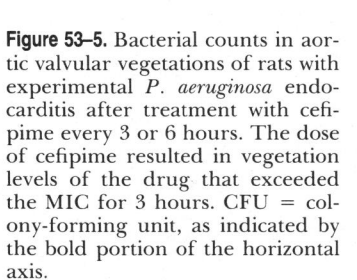

Figure 53–5. Bacterial counts in aortic valvular vegetations of rats with experimental *P. aeruginosa* endocarditis after treatment with cefipime every 3 or 6 hours. The dose of cefipime resulted in vegetation levels of the drug that exceeded the MIC for 3 hours. CFU = colony-forming unit, as indicated by the bold portion of the horizontal axis.

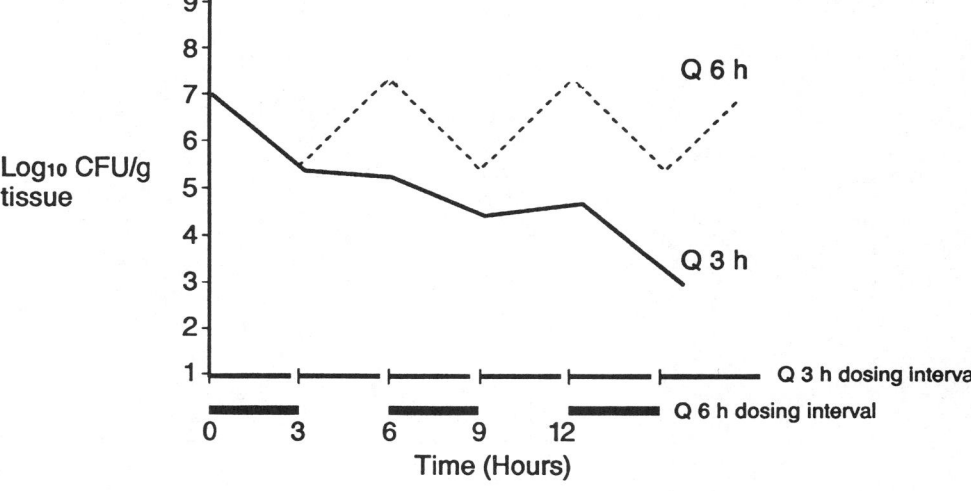

ation for a drug that exhibits no PAE against gram-negative bacillary pathogens when treating infections caused by these pathogens). To achieve the same duration of antimicrobial activity at the site of infection to treat the less sensitive pathogens, the same dose may have to be repeated twice daily. An additional consideration for drugs like ceftriaxone is that tissue levels may be inadequate to treat infection caused by less sensitive pathogens because diffusion of these drugs into tissues may be limited by high serum protein binding. Similarly, a drug with a more prolonged half-life, such as ceftriaxone (6 to 8 hours in patients with normal renal function), has an extended period during which bactericidal action can occur.

Antimicrobial agents that exhibit prolonged PAE also allow widely spaced dosing without loss of efficacy. However, an in vivo PAE is not invariably present despite its presence in vitro. For example, no PAE has been found with cefipime or imipenem for experimental *P. aeruginosa* endocarditis,[27] with penicillin plus gentamicin for experimental enterococcal endocarditis in the rat,[28] or with penicillin for experimental *S. pneumoniae* or *Streptococcus pyogenes* soft tissue infection in the neutropenic mouse.[29] For example, in the absence of a PAE when cefipime, an investigational third-generation ceftazidime-like cephalosporin, was given to rats with experimental *P. aeruginosa* endocarditis so that antibiotic vegetation levels were above the MBC and MIC for only 3 hours, a fall in bacterial counts in vegetations from 10^7 to 10^3 occurred after five doses with a 3-hour dosing interval, whereas the bacterial counts in vegetations remained stable with the same dose given at 6-hour intervals, as a result of bacterial regrowth in the later portion of each 6-hour dosing interval in the absence of a PAE[22] (Fig. 53–5).

References

1. Mandell GL, Kaye D, Levison ME: Enterococcal endocarditis: An analysis of 38 patients observed at the New York Hospital–Cornell Medical Center. Arch Intern Med 125:258, 1970.
2. Scheld WM: Theoretical and practical considerations of antibiotic therapy for bacterial meningitis. Pediatr Infect Dis 4:74, 1985.
3. EORTC International Antimicrobial Therapy Project Group: Three antibiotic regimens in the treatment of infection in febrile granulocytopenic patients with cancer. J Infect Dis 137:14, 1978.
4. Klastersky J, Meunier-Carpenter R, Prevost JM: Significance of antimicrobial synergism for the outcome of gram-negative sepsis. Am J Med Sci 273:157, 1977.
5. Young LS: Empirical antimicrobial therapy in the neutropenic host. N Engl J Med 315:580, 1986.
6. Sanders CC, Sanders WE Jr: Microbial resistance to newer generation β-lactam antibiotics: Clinical and laboratory implications. J Infect Dis 151:399, 1985.
7. Sanders CC, Sanders WE Jr: Type 1 beta-lactamases of gram-negative bacteria: Interactions with beta-lactam antibiotics. J Infect Dis 154:792, 1986.
8. Smith CR, Ambinder R, Lipsky JJ, et al: Cefotaxime compared with nafcillin plus tobramycin for serious bacterial infections. Ann Intern Med 101:469, 1984.
9. Gladtke E, Von Hattinberg HM: Pharmacokinetics: An Introduction. New York, Springer-Verlag, 1979.
10. Greenblatt DJ, Koch-Weser J: Drug therapy: Clinical pharmacokinetics. N Engl J Med 293:707, 964, 1975.
11. Rowland M, Tozer TN: Clinical Pharmacokinetics: Concepts and Applications. Philadelphia, Lea & Febiger, 1980.
12. Van Eita LL, Kravitz GR, Russ TE, et al: The effect of the ratio of surface area to volume on the penetration of antibiotics into extravascular spaces on in vitro model. J Infect Dis 146:423, 1982.
13. Chambers HF, Mills J, Drake TA, et al: Failure of once-daily regimen of cefonicid for treatment of endocarditis due to *Staphylococcus aureus*. Rev Infect Dis 6(suppl 4):S870, 1984.
14. Craig WA, Vogelman B: Changing concepts and new applications of antibiotic pharmacokinetics. Am J Med 77(1 part B):24, 1984.
15. Barza, M, Butler T: The penetration of penicillins and cephalosporins into selected sites of clinical interest. Semin Infect Dis 3:193, 1980.
16. Coudron PE, Jones DC, Dalton HP, et al: Evaluation of laboratory tests for detection of MRSA and MRSE. J Clin Microbiol 24:764, 1986.
17. Kaye D: The clinical of tolerance of *Staphylococcus aureus*. Ann Intern Med 93:924, 1980.
18. Lorian V: Some effects of subinhibitory concentrations of antibiotics on bacteria. Bull NY Acad Med 51:1046, 1975.
19. McDonald PJ, Wetherall BL, Pruul H: Postantibiotic leukocyte enhancement: Increased susceptibility of bacteria pretreated with antibiotics to activity of leukocytes. Rev Infect Dis 3:38, 1981.
20. Bundtzen RW, Gerber AU, Cohn DL, et al: Postantibiotic suppression of bacterial growth. Rev Infect Dis 3:28, 1981.
21. Ingerman MJ, Pitsakis PG, Rosenberg AF, et al: The importance of pharmacodynamics in determining the dosing interval in therapy for experimental *Pseudomonas endocarditis* in the rat. J Infect Dis 153:707, 1986.
22. DeVries PJ, Leguit P, Verkooyen RP, et al: Toxicity of once daily netilmicin in patients with intra-abdominal infections. In: Program and Abstracts of the 27th Interscience Conference on Antimicrobial Agents and Chemotherapy, Washington, DC, American Society for Microbiology, 1987.
23. Feld R, ValDiVieso M, Bodey GP, et al: A comparative trial of sisomicin therapy by intermittent versus continuous infusion. Am J Med Sci 274:179, 1977.
24. Nordstrom L, Crunberg S, Rinberg H, et al: Recent Advances in Chemotherapy. Tokyo, University of Tokyo Press, p 2653, 1985.
25. Powell SH, Thompson WL, Luthe MA, et al: Once daily vs continuous aminoglycoside dosing: Efficacy and toxicity in animal and clinical studies of gentamicin, netilmicin and tobramycin. J Infect Dis 147:918, 1983.
26. Bodey GP, Ketchel SJ, Rodriguez VA: A randomized study of carbenicillin plus cefamandole or tobramycin in the treatment of febrile episodes in cancer patients. Am J Med 67:608, 1979.
27. Hessen MT, Pitsakis PG, Levison ME: Absence of a post antibiotic effect in experimental pseudomonas endocarditis treated with imipenem, with or without gentamicin. J Infect Dis 158:542, 1988.
28. Hessen MT, Pitsakis PG, Levison ME: Postantibiotic effect of penicillin plus gentamicin versus *Enterococcus faecalis* in vitro and in vivo. Antimicrob Agents Chemother 33:608, 1989.
29. Vogelman B, Gudmundsson S, Turnidge J, et al: In vivo postantibiotic effect in a thigh infection in neutropenic mice. J Infect Dis 157:287, 1988.

SECTION FIVE

The Nervous System

Section Editor

Robert P. Lisak

CHAPTER 54

Clinical Neurophysiology in the Intensive Care Unit

A. Robert Spitzer
Patti L. Peterson
Steven D. Ham

In the process of establishing a diagnosis, the physician considers a series of hypotheses to explain available data. The hypotheses are generally considered in terms of their probability or likelihood, although other considerations such as the availability of appropriate diagnostic tests or the availability of effective therapy modify the decision-making process. The primary purpose of diagnostic testing is to identify the likelihood of a hypothetic diagnosis, in a bayesian manner. Individual diagnostic tests themselves are rarely entirely precise in establishing single diagnoses.

The diagnostic evaluation of dysfunction or disease of the nervous system is critically dependent on establishing the precise location of the lesion and its pathophysiologic mechanism. This concept is actually routinely employed by physicians and surgeons evaluating and diagnosing disorders in other organ systems. For example, in considering the diagnosis of epigastric discomfort, one considers diagnoses related to localization in the stomach, the duodenum, the pancreas, the pleura, the myocardium, and the pericardium. In considering neurologic disorders, the concept of anatomic localization and pathophysiologic mechanism is therefore applied with more rigor but is not conceptually different. Neurologists tend to be more explicit about discussing localization. It is most useful in assessing the nervous system to consider localization and identification of mechanism as explicit reasoning steps in establishing the diagnosis. The probabilistic differential diagnosis is arrived at after explicitly considering and listing the reasonable locations and mechanisms for the patient's neurologic problem.

Understanding this process is of considerable aid in helping the clinician use and interpret diagnostic testing of the nervous system appropriately. Although diagnostic testing is usually considered after the clinical examination, it is not always understood that the primary information obtained from diagnostic testing does not usually directly affect the establishment of specific diagnoses. Rather, diagnostic testing provides confirmatory or exclusionary information regarding specific anatomic localizations and pathophysiologic mechanisms. This information is then used to modify directly the hypothetic differential diagnosis list.

This chapter is therefore divided into two sections. The first part follows the traditional organization of discussing individual testing methods. The second part discusses specific clinical problems often encountered in the intensive care unit (ICU) and the appropriate use of the various diagnostic modalities. The emphasis of the first part is therefore somewhat more technical, and the focus of the second part is more clinical. An important purpose of the initial discussion is to help the clinician understand the information obtained from each testing method and, equally importantly, understand its limitations.

METHODOLOGY

Physiology Versus Imaging

Testing methods in general may be broadly divided into two categories. Imaging methods provide information that is primarily anatomic in nature, whereas physiologic techniques provide information that is primarily related to the pathophysiologic mechanism of disease. This distinction is rather arbitrary, in that many methods actually provide some component of both types of information. Nonetheless, distinguishing testing methods on the basis of the primary focus and resulting information is conceptually useful.

Imaging (radiologic) techniques in general provide highly detailed and precise anatomic information. They also tend to have certain other characteristics. In general, the information provided is static rather than dynamic—the condition at a particular time. A significant consideration in the ICU is that the equipment required tends to be cumbersome, large, expensive, and often immobile. Therefore, these images are difficult to obtain and are often widely spaced in time, relative to the rate of physiologic changes that may occur.

Physiologic methods, in contrast, tend to provide dynamic information about disease states, often providing crucial data about the mechanism of disease. These methods tend to require less expensive, portable or bedside equipment and the measurements may be obtained frequently if not continuously. However, the anatomic precision and localization capabilities of these methods are in general less than those of imaging techniques, and in some cases are quite poor.

These methods are therefore complementary. Patient management is greatly enhanced by their coordinated use to investigate neurologic disorders. The essential key to neurologic diagnosis is a detailed history and neurologic examination. In the ICU setting, clinical history and examination are often severely limited. Diagnostic testing cannot replace the history and physical examination but must be used to supplement available clinical findings because of the inadequacy of available clinical information. This chapter does not discuss imaging methods, which are covered elsewhere.

Lumbar Puncture

Lumbar puncture (LP) is a widely familiar method, whose routine techniques need not be addressed. Specific points about LP do merit specific mention. LP is indicated whenever infection of the nervous system is suspected. There are relatively few contraindications, and when LP is diagnostically essential, there is virtually no absolute contraindication. In the presence of a significant bleeding diathesis, LP is relatively contraindicated because of the risk of epidural hemorrhage with compression of the underlying cauda equina. When the procedure is essential, appropriate administration of platelets or fresh frozen plasma or other similar steps should be taken to enable its performance. In some patients, particularly those who are markedly obese or those who have severe degenerative disease of the lumbar spine, LP may be performed in the radiology suite with fluoroscopic visualization. If the lumbar area itself is infected or ulcerated, LP is absolutely contraindicated. Under these circumstances, cerebrospinal fluid (CSF) may be obtained by cervical puncture. This procedure is relatively safe when performed by an experienced radiologist with fluoroscopic guidance.

The CSF obtained is sent for studies depending on the relevant clinical diagnostic considerations. In the ICU setting, the usual primary concern is acute bacterial meningitis and, more rarely, a chronic meningitis or neoplastic infiltration. In this setting, rapidity of accurate diagnosis is often critical. Certain definitive tests, such as culture results, are not available for 24 hours or longer. The intensivist must therefore make early decisions on the basis of results available in the first 4 to 6 hours.

The results that are available immediately include cell count, glucose and protein levels, and counterimmunoelectrophoresis findings. Elevation of the cell count is a key diagnostic marker in infections of the nervous system. The presence of polymorphonuclear lymphocytes in the CSF is strong evidence of a bacterial infection. However, even in the presence of bacterial infection, the earliest taps may yield only a lymphocytic profile. In some cases, a second LP 12 to 24 hours later may be warranted. Counterimmunoelectrophoresis results may be obtained quickly but provide only specific information about the presence or absence of antigens tested. Commonly, *Neisseria meningitidis, Streptococcus pneumoniae, Haemophilus influenzae,* and *Cryptococcus neoformans* are included in the panel. However, any other organisms that can cause meningitis are not ruled out by a normal counterimmunoelectrophoresis study result.

Appropriate cultures are routinely obtained for ICU patients. If clinically warranted, cultures for fungus or various acid-fast bacilli must be requested as well. It is important to note that, in cerebral abscess, cultures and even the cell count often do not yield an answer, if the abscess has not ruptured into the subarachnoid space.

When neoplastic infiltration is suspected, diagnosis is made on the basis of cytologic examination. The yield of any single LP, however, is not extremely high, and several serial taps may be required to discover neoplastic meningeal infiltration.

Certain disease processes have a predilection for a relatively focal infiltration of the meninges at the base of the skull, called basal meningitis. The clinical presentation of these diseases includes multiple isolated cranial nerve palsies. The differential diagnosis of this syndrome is relatively narrow, including lymphoma, direct neoplastic infiltration from nasopharyngeal tumors, tuberculosis, sarcoidosis, and fungal meningitis. Of significance in this setting, the lumbar CSF testing may be nondiagnostic, and cisternal puncture may be required.

A specific entity that is considered frequently in the diagnosis of patients in the ICU is Landry-Guillain-Barré syndrome. The CSF in this syndrome is classically characterized by a significant elevation of the protein level, without pleocytosis, or albuminocytologic dissociation. The CSF protein level may not be significantly elevated in the first specimens obtained early in the course of the disease. Repeated taps after several days may be necessary to confirm a rising protein level. If the protein level is rising extremely rapidly (over hours) and becomes high, consideration should be given to the possibility of an epidural abscess as a cause of the patient's paralysis.

Immunocompromised patients are encountered with increasing frequency in the ICU, and LP is performed frequently to diagnose infections. In these individuals, reactivation of latent syphilis is a significant concern. Central nervous system (CNS) involvement requires the use of the CSF Venereal Disease Research Laboratory or fluorescent treponomal antibody determination, which is frequently not part of the standard battery of studies requested. An additional caveat in these patients is that patients with low peripheral blood counts may fail to manifest a significant pleocytosis, even in the presence of CNS infection.

ELECTROENCEPHALOGRAPHY
Routine Electroencephalography

Electroencephalography (EEG) is readily available in the ICU because the equipment is portable and can be brought to the bedside.[1] Scalp electrodes applied with conductive paste, or rarely scalp needles, are employed. Collodion is best for application of electrodes that must remain in place for considerable periods, but there may be problems related to its flammability and skin irritation. Electrodes that remain in place for a length of time are affected by patient sweating or by drying of the electrolyte, resulting in artifacts, which may render recordings useless. These are significant considerations when it is desired to place long-term electrodes for seizure monitoring, as may be necessary in certain patients in the ICU.

A standard system of 19 electrode placements (the 10–20 system) is commonly used. Modern EEGs generally allow recording from 19 channels or more simultaneously, but some older instruments may allow as few as 6 or 8 channels to be obtained simultaneously. Seizure discharges and other focal abnormalities may be missed if electrodes are not placed over the site of the abnormality. Use of a complete set of electrodes minimizes the chances of missing a focal abnormality.[2]

Modern amplifier design has resulted in instruments that are better able to record the EEG in noisy environments. The amplitude of the EEG is on the order of 10 to 100 μV. Even with the best amplifiers, noise artifact remains a significant problem in the ICU. In part, this is unavoidable because the scalp electrode wires themselves act as antennas and pick up radiated noise from ventilators, infusion pumps, and other sources. Fluorescent lights and electric motors are the worst offenders. This becomes a significant technical limitation in the determination of cerebral death. At times, it is necessary to turn off equipment for a brief time to obtain technically adequate recordings. It should be noted that the use of EEG is considered confirmatory, but it is not required by widely accepted criteria for the diagnosis of brain death.

The routine EEG is interpreted by the technician and the electroencephalographer. Interpretation by the technician is necessary while the recording is being performed because important modifications to the standard recording techniques may be necessary to delineate abnormalities clearly. In particular, the technician frequently changes the arrangement of electrodes from which recording is made (the montage) to delineate a seizure or slow-wave focus. The technician must be skilled in recognizing artifacts in the tracing and taking corrective steps. Such artifacts are much more commonly encountered in the ICU setting than the carefully controlled environment of the EEG laboratory and may render a recording uninterpretable. Some of the artifacts are unique to portable studies and not encountered in routine recordings.

In interpreting the EEG, the electroencephalographer is particularly concerned with certain specific questions, including the following: (1) Are there seizures present? (2) Are there interictal spikes or epileptiform patterns? (3) Are there characteristic abnormal patterns? (4) Is there a normal background rhythm present, or is it absent? (5) Is there abnormal slowing? (6) Is the pattern fluctuating or intermittent, or is it fixed and invariant? The electroencephalographer considers these questions for each particular isolated channel, as well as for groups of channels that provide distribution and localization information. At all times, a critical question that must be considered is whether the abnormality is real or artifact.

The EEG is the sine qua non in the diagnosis of seizures and epilepsy. In the ICU, this is all the more critical, because patients may have clinically unobservable seizures or nonconvulsive status. This may be true even without the use of neuromuscular junction–blocking agents, which are commonly used to aid ventilatory support. In addition, the EEG is frequently abnormal in stroke and becomes abnormal minutes after a vascular event,[4, 5] in comparison with the computed tomographic (CT) scan, which may not show the lesion for several days. Characteristic triphasic waves, when present, are indicative of a metabolic encephalopathy, which is most commonly hepatic or renal.[1] A relatively characteristic increase of fast activity occurs with drug effects, particularly benzodiazepines.[1] A simplistic but useful classification of the patterns of abnormality that may be reported on EEG would be

1. Normal
2. Metabolic encephalopathy
   a. Metabolic encephalopathy strongly suggestive of hepatic or renal encephalopathy
   b. Drug effect
3. Unifocal lesion, asymmetry with slow waves, possibly suggesting a mass lesion
4. Unifocal slowing, asymmetry, or loss of activity, suggestive of focal ischemic event (stroke)
5. Deep midline structural lesion, including brain stem lesions
6. Seizures
   a. Irritative focus (potentially epileptogenic)
   b. Focal seizures
   c. Generalized seizures

   d. Focal or generalized status epilepticus
7. Flattening suggestive of anoxia, barbiturate administration, or severe metabolic disturbance
   a. Burst suppression pattern
   b. Electrocerebral silence
8. Sleep state, or sleep-wave cycles

The utility of this type of information in various clinical settings is discussed later.

Quantitative Electroencephalography

Developments in microprocessor and data acquisition technology have made applications of computer analysis methods to EEG practical. At this time, such methods are still within the domain of research, and established clinical use has not yet been demonstrated. However, new techniques are promising, and the use of quantitative EEG assessment will likely become commonplace during the next decade or two.

The purpose of computer analysis is fourfold. In their simplest application, computer methods allow the presentation and manipulation of standard data, in a manner that is more natural for the electroencephalographer to interpret. A simple example is the presentation of a pattern of electrical activity as a colorful topographic map, which allows easy visualization and localization of an abnormality.[3, 4] A further application of the computer to the EEG allows for quantitative measurement of aspects of the EEG, which can potentially improve the reliability of the technique, compared with current qualitative methods.[3–6, 7] A third use of the computer, is the extraction of additional, new information, which cannot be obtained by routine inspection, from the EEG.[6, 8, 9] A fourth use, the automated detection of transient events, is discussed later.

The application of traditional signal- and image-processing methods has begun to provide additional information from the EEG signal. Most work has been based on the Fourier transform (spectral, frequency analysis), although other mathematic techniques have been employed. A detailed technical discussion of these methods is beyond the scope of this chapter. These methods may allow improved detection and quantitative assessment of encephalopathy, stroke,[4, 5] and focal structural lesions.[6, 7] These methods are of considerable interest in the ICU setting, because they may eventually allow detailed continuous bedside images of brain physiologic processes.

As with any other manipulation of data, manipulation of the EEG by the computer allows the production of meaningless or misleading results. Because the computer allows for considerably greater and more powerful analysis capabilities, it also provides a more powerful tool for producing errors attributable to incorrect input.

Electroencephalographic Monitoring

An important procedural improvement of particular relevance in the ICU is the availability of continuous EEG monitoring capabilities. The clinical application of these methods also remains an important topic of research, but advances in this area suggest that its application may become indicated or even routine within the next decade. This application may be divided into three categories.

The availability of bedside monitors with amplifiers suited to routine EEG recording and display of single channels has its greatest application in the monitoring of seizures and status epilepticus. This technology is currently readily available commercially. This equipment can display EEG activity from scalp electrodes on an oscilloscope, in a manner analogous to traditional ECG and pressure tracings. Monitoring of this type may be used to detect subclinical seizures and guide anticonvulsant therapy. The major drawbacks are that significant expertise in the use and interpretation of the EEG tracings is necessary, and continuous visual monitoring is required.

Another form of available technology is single-channel compressed spectral array monitoring.[10–12] A single channel of EEG is periodically digitized and its Fourier transform computed. The spectrum is displayed in stacked manner that allows easy inspection of the trend. This method has been shown to have some clinical utility in assessing the prognosis of recovery from various forms of global brain injury.[11, 12] It has also been used as a crude automated seizure detector but is probably not sufficiently reliable for this purpose. A claimed advantage is that considerably less experience and skill are required for its use, in part because most compressed spectral array monitors do not record or display the raw EEG signal, which would necessitate expertise for interpretation. In so doing, these devices provide no means for the recognition of artifacts. Because technical artifact is a major consideration in the ICU, ignoring this possibility is a dangerous delusion that can lead to incorrect interpretation. We specifically propose that the use of spectral monitoring can be quite useful for predicting prognosis or monitoring progress in some cases, when provided with the ability to monitor the raw EEG as well and used by appropriately trained individuals. (No clinician would accept automated pressure readings of pulmonary arterial catheter readings without the ability to inspect and verify the waveforms; ignorance is not bliss.)

The third major use of monitoring is in the automated detection of transient events. Transient waveforms present in the EEG that are of most interest include epileptiform patterns, seizure discharges, and sleep-related transients (V waves, spindles, K complexes). To date, no computer methods using traditional signal-processing techniques have been developed that are capable of reliably performing these detection tasks. The background EEG signal is considerably more complex, and the transient waveforms much more poorly defined, than is the case with electrocardiographic processing. Future research in this field using novel processing methods[13, 14] holds some promise for solving this problem.

A combination of detection of transient events, particularly seizures, and assessment of background activity for degree of flattening has also been used to monitor the administration of intensive anticonvulsant therapy, such as intravenous barbiturate infusions to treat status epilepticus.[10] Traditionally, the monitoring has used a standard EEG machine at the bedside, periodically run by the technician, who notes the presence of seizure activity and the flattening of normal activity produced by barbiturates. Automated computer detection of seizures, and quantitative assessment of EEG spectral content, may make such monitoring more readily useful.

EVOKED POTENTIALS

Time-locked responses may be recorded from the nervous system, after the application of specific stimuli. Such responses are called *evoked responses* or *evoked potentials*.[15] Their utility arises because the application of carefully controlled stimuli may be used to excite a specific pathway of known anatomy and physiology selectively. Evoked responses may be grouped as sensory or motor. Technically, peripheral nerve conduction studies are evoked responses but are considered separately.

Sensory evoked responses are produced by the application of visual, auditory, mechanical, or electrical stimuli, and the response in each case is recorded from surface sites overlying specific anatomic structures in the pathways subserving the corresponding modality.[15]

Visual evoked potentials are obtained by the application of bright flashes of light or an alternating checkerboard pattern (pattern reversal visual evoked potentials), which excites the retina. In the ICU, patients are usually unable to cooperate with the technically superior pattern reversal method, which requires a steady gaze at a fixed point on a screen. Responses are recorded from the periocular area, reflecting depolarization of the retina, and from electrodes placed over the occipital lobes. The normal range for flash responses is wide, and the technique is not precise, but it can provide an overall assessment of visual pathway integrity and some information with regard to side-to-side symmetry.

Brain stem auditory evoked responses are induced by the applications of clicks or tones to the ears individually. Responses may be recorded from the external ear canal (the cochlear microphonic) and from the brain stem. Technically, electrodes are placed over the scalp, and far-field potentials projected from the brain stem are recorded. Five distinct reproducible waves are produced by structures including the auditory nerve (cranial nerve VIII) and various locations within the brain stem. Thus, some localization of lesions within the brain stem may be inferred from inspection of each of the individual waves produced by monaural stimulation. Sixth and seventh waves are often produced on the lateral aspects of the hemispheres, arising from temporal auditory processing cortex, but these are less reproducible and are therefore of less diagnostic reliability.

Somatosensory evoked potentials (SSEPs) may be produced by mechanical stimulation of peripheral somatesthetic receptors, but more commonly an electrical stimulus is applied directly to a selected peripheral nerve. The median and tibial nerves produce reliable responses, although ulnar, peroneal, pudendal, and selective dermatomal stimuli have been studied. With median nerve stimulation, responses are recorded from Erb's point, the cervical spine, and the contralateral hemisphere primary sensory gyrus. With tibial nerve stimulation, responses are recorded from the popliteal fossa, the lumbar spine, and the cerebral convexity. Cervical and lumbar responses are variable and, although sometimes useful, cannot be relied on too strongly for localization. The remaining responses are generally quite reliable, can be used to identify lesions along corresponding portions of the somatosensory pathways, and can be particularly useful in identifying side-to-side asymmetries. For example, preservation of Erb's point and popliteal fossa responses, with loss of all cortical responses, can be seen in upper cervical cord lesions. The use of single-channel cerebral recording imposes limitations regarding precise topographic localization. In combination with other factors that influence the latencies of the cortical responses, this can introduce significant uncertainties regarding the interpretation of these studies. Methods that use multichannel cerebral recording may overcome some of these limitations and allow detailed investigations of cortical organizational maps[16–18] but are currently considered research tools.

The primary function and use of SSEPs is to assess the integrity of central sensory pathways. It is not as useful as electromyography (EMG) for the assessment of peripheral abnormalities. In the presence of significant peripheral abnormalities, all responses may be sufficiently affected and further statements about the central pathways, as distinct from the peripheral nerve abnormalities, may be impossible. At times, however, central responses are preserved in the presence of moderate peripheral abnormalities and can help verify that a given disease process is sparing the CNS.

Another limitation of SSEPs is related to the fact that the primary sensory modalities that convey the SSEP have major representation in the dorsal columns, and therefore the responses may be preserved in the presence of a lesion compressing the spinal cord on its ventral surface, such as a herniated disk.

The various sensory evoked response studies require specialized instrumentation, including capabilities for extensive signal averaging to extract small signals from background noise. This equipment is portable, but similar noise constraints apply as discussed with other methods. Because of the electrical noise in the ICU, extremely prolonged recording sessions with extensive and repeated averaging of signals may be necessary to obtain reliable recordings.

Motor evoked responses may also be generated by the application of stimuli to the CNS. Direct stimulation of the nerve roots with needle electrodes, or a magnetic stimulator coil, is feasible using routine EMG equipment and may be quite useful in assessing possible root avulsion or brachial plexus injuries. Methods are now being developed that allow stimuli to be applied to selected portions of the motor cortex.[19, 20] Electrical stimuli of positive polarity, brief duration, and high voltage applied to the scalp can stimulate underlying motor cortex. Magnetic stimulators are also available and may be easier to use. Responses may be recorded from upper and lower extremity limb muscles, having traversed the pyramidal tracts through the capsule, the brain stem, and the spinal cord, to excite anterior horn cells and thereby the peripheral nerves. This stimulation appears safe and well tolerated, although some concern about the exacerbation of existing epileptic foci has been raised.

These methods may be more useful than sensory recordings in diagnosing disorders characterized by motor weakness, including spinal cord compression. However, several methodologic problems exist, particularly with reference to use in the ICU. The responses recorded with motor cortex stimulation are of much greater variability than typical motor conductions. The amplitudes and latencies of the responses are particularly dependent on the level of voluntary activation by the subject, and the responses may disappear under anesthesia. Thus, the reliability of these techniques is not entirely established in a setting in which subject cooperation may be limited, and these methods are still considered investigational.

TRANSCRANIAL DOPPLER ULTRASONOGRAPHY

Transcranial Doppler ultrasonography is relatively new technology that allows noninvasive assessment of the intracranial cerebral circulation.[21, 22] Its established clinical indications include assessment of patterns and extent of intracranial collateral circulation in patients with known regions of severe stenosis or occlusion in the internal carotid arteries, vertebral arteries, or subclavian arteries; detection of hemodynamically significant stenosis in the major intracranial arteries at the base of the brain; assessment and follow-up of patients with vasoconstriction of any cause, especially vasospasm occurring after subarachnoid hemorrhage; and detection of arteriovenous malformations and study of their feeding arteries and the hemodynamic effects of treatment and confirmation of the clinical diagnosis of brain death. Its portability and noninvasive technology allow transcranial Doppler ultrasonography to be used with ease at the bedside; however, it is important that the responsible clinician be well versed in the limitations of its use.

NEAR-INFRARED SPECTROSCOPY

Infrared light from the near-infrared spectroscopy device penetrates the scalp, the skull, and the cerebral parenchyma and is primarily absorbed by several light-absorbing molecules (deoxyhemoglobin and oxyhemoglobin), which play a significant role in cerebral oxygenation and metabolism. The near-infrared spectroscopy device monitors the ratio of absorbance of light at the deoxyhemoglobin and oxyhemoglobin maxima and provides useful information regarding trends in their concentration. The technique is noninvasive and can be used to monitor cerebral oxygenation and blood flow continually.

Near-infrared spectroscopy has proved to be a useful device to monitor physiologic changes noninvasively in the brain.[23-25] It is now available from some commercial suppliers; however, its use remains predominantly in a research capacity.

INTRACRANIAL PRESSURE MONITORING

Increased intracranial pressure (ICP) occurs in three broad categories of CNS disease. It may occur with focal mass lesions, including tumors, infarcts, abscesses, and hematomas. In this category, the focal lesion and the resulting shifts (herniations) are seen on imaging studies. Increased ICP may occur in diseases that affect the resorption of CSF, such as meningitis and subarachnoid hemorrhage. In these cases, there is usually hydrocephalus evident on an imaging study. Increased ICP may also occur in a generalized fashion, often with an underlying metabolic cause that has widespread effects on cellular metabolism. In cases with diffuse increased ICP, including metabolic conditions, the increased ICP may result in a marked decrease in cerebral perfusion, resulting in a secondary ischemic injury. Examples of this category include Reye's syndrome, traumatic brain injury (diffuse axonal injury), hepatic encephalopathy, and anoxia. An idiopathic entity that causes diffuse increased ICP is pseudotumor cerebri. In these latter cases, the imaging study reveals small ventricles and sometimes diffuse cerebral edema.

In each case, particular therapy aimed at the underlying condition is indicated. In the case of focal lesions, it may be necessary to intervene surgically to relieve the herniation, particularly when vital brain stem structures are compromised. In cases of CSF outflow obstruction, shunting may be necessary. In many cases, direct monitoring and therapy of the ICP itself may be required. Although this may be necessary in all of the aforementioned categories, it is particularly true in cases of diffuse increased ICP.

Normal ICP in an adult is less than 15 mm Hg. Therapy is generally instituted if the measured ICP is greater than 20 mm Hg. Medical therapy of increased ICP includes forced hyperventilation, osmotic diuresis, steroids, and in some cases, barbiturates. ICP monitoring is used to determine when therapy is required and to follow the patient's response to therapeutic intervention.

The most accurate monitoring of ICP is obtained by cannulation of the ventricular system. Fiberoptic systems have also proved effective. Older systems, including subarachnoid screws or bolts, and epidural sensors, are often effective if other means are not available. Monitoring requires the active participation of a readily available neurosurgeon to ensure proper placement, continued surveillance of the system for potential complications, and consultation in the treatment of raised ICP.

An ICP monitor or ventriculostomy can be safely placed at the bedside in the ICU, emergency department, CT scan area, recovery room, or hospital room. If the patient is intubated, sedation or paralytic agents may be used to assist placement. When the ICP monitor is in place, antibiotic coverage is usually advised, particularly to cover for hospital-acquired *Staphylococcus aureus* infections. Periodic replacement of the system (e.g., on a weekly basis) may reduce infectious complications and technical artifacts. The patient should be properly restrained or supervised to prevent tampering with the system. Another possible complication of placement of an ICP monitor is hematoma formation at the entry site. If the patient has a significant and persistent elevation of the ICP after placement of a monitor, a CT scan is indicated to evaluate for a possible hematoma. Small hematomas may be managed conservatively, but a large hematoma may necessitate evacuation.

A number of technical factors may affect the validity of measurements obtained from a particular monitoring system. False readings may be obtained if a ventriculostomy is obstructed by debris, blood, brain parenchyma, or clumps of white blood cells or if the tubing is kinked. Subarachnoid screws or bolts may be occluded by brain tissue, particularly when the ICP is high. In the functional ventriculostomy, CSF pulsations and drainage should be apparent. In all systems, jugular compression should result in an immediate rise in measured ICP readings. Fiberoptic ICP monitors may demonstrate a gradual drift during the course of days. This may result in falsely elevated or lowered readings and necessitates clinical correlation or replacement of the system.

It is important to consider elevations of ICP when a patient is transported from the ICU for diagnostic or therapeutic purposes. Portable monitoring devices may alert the transport team to hazardous elevations in ICP. This is a particular problem when the patient is transported for CT and is ventilated manually. The ICP may double or triple because of ineffective ventilation.

ELECTROMYOGRAPHY

Most discussions of neurophysiologic assessment in the ICU neglect careful consideration of peripheral neurophysiologic techniques. In fact, these methods provide essential valuable insights into neurologic dysfunction and disease in the ICU. Modern EMG equipment has also benefitted from improved amplifier technology, and portable ICU recordings can now be made routinely.

Peripheral neurophysiologic techniques actually are a large set of individual methods,[26] and the expression routine, or standard, EMG is misleading. An electrophysiologic investigation is actually a detailed process, conducted at the bedside by a skilled electromyographer. The study is designed to answer specific clinical questions (see later) and varies from patient to patient. The study itself is modified as it is performed; as data are recorded, they are incorporated into a continuously updated diagnostic impression. As each nerve or muscle is studied, certain diagnoses become less likely, whereas new ones may be suggested and the study to be conducted is modified accordingly.

The most basic techniques available include routine motor nerve conductions, sensory nerve conductions, and routine (qualitative) needle EMG.[26] Nerve conduction techniques use a small electric shock to induce depolarization in selected nerves. The responses are then recorded from muscles (in the case of motor nerves) or directly from the nerve (in the case of sensory nerves). The amplitude of the recorded responses is primarily dependent on the integrity of the axons in a nerve. By measuring the time necessary for impulses to traverse a segment of nerve, a velocity of conduction may be computed. This velocity is a measure of the integrity of the myelin sheath of that nerve. Needle EMG uses a small needle, inserted directly into selected muscles, to record the electrical activity in those muscles. Analysis of the potentials generated within an individual muscle at rest or with voluntary contraction allows a determination of whether that muscle is normal or is abnormal

because of myopathy or because of axonal damage to its nerve. By studying numerous individual nerves and muscles, an overall pattern of disease may be determined. In this manner, focal lesions (e.g., a lumbar radiculopathy) may be identified, or an overall pattern of physiologic disturbance may be identified (e.g., demyelinating polyradiculoneuropathy).

Additional techniques are available to address specific physiologic questions. Dysfunction of the neuromuscular junction is readily demonstrated in severe cases by stimulating a nerve repetitively while recording from a corresponding muscle (repetitive stimulation). At low frequencies of stimulation, typically 2 to 5 Hz, neuromuscular junction dysfunction manifests as a progressive decrement in the amplitude of the muscle response with each subsequent stimulus. This finding is not specific for the particular cause of the neuromuscular junction dysfunction and may be seen in severe, active axonal neuropathies, including motor neuron disease, as well as botulism, and myasthenia gravis. A particular pattern of response with high-frequency stimulation in the 20- to 50-Hz range, consisting of a progressive incrementing response, is seen in presynaptic neuromuscular junction dysfunction, and is essentially pathognomonic of Lambert-Eaton syndrome or botulism. This method is of considerable utility in the ICU in the assessment of the diffusely weak or ventilator-dependent patient.

A more advanced technique for assessing the neuromuscular junction, single-fiber EMG, records repeated discharges from neighboring pairs of muscle fibers innervated by the same anterior horn cell (motor unit). Careful analysis of the sequential timing of the discharges can disclose subtle abnormalities (jitter) in neuromuscular junction dysfunction. This is of less utility in the ICU, because an abnormality so subtle as to require this technique for its demonstration is not likely to produce severe clinical weakness.

Patients in the ICU may be weak because of myopathies of numerous causes, including inflammatory, metabolic, endocrine (including steroids), and nutritional causes.[27, 28] Most of these are treatable. The detection of myopathy is enhanced by the quantitative analysis of the EMG (quantitative motor unit potential analysis) recorded from proximal muscles. Identification of a specific cause entails muscle biopsy or specific biochemical investigations. Involvement of proximal respiratory muscles in a disease process can be demonstrated by needle EMG of the intercostal muscles, which is reasonably safe when performed with proper caution.

Another specific study, the blink reflex study, is capable of assessing the integrity of and identifying focal lesions in a pathway comprising afferent sensation in the trigeminal nerve (cranial nerve V), brain stem interconnections, and efferent motor connections via the facial nerve (cranial nerve VII). This study may be useful in distinguishing the relatively benign Bell's palsy from a brain stem lesion or CNS lesion causing unilateral facial paralysis.

Specific technical considerations that affect the reliability of the study are encountered frequently in the ICU. A major consideration is the use of lipid-containing skin protective ointments. These act as high-impedance electrical insulators on the skin, making nerve conduction studies virtually impossible. They must be thoroughly removed before beginning the EMG study. An additional technical consideration is the lack of temperature control in the portable environment. Nerve conduction velocity measurements depend critically on limb temperature, and it is common to encounter extremely cool limbs in ICU patients, because of exposure and peripheral vasoconstriction. This may affect the reliability of these measurements. Electrical noise considerations, similar to the ones encountered with EEG recordings, may also be significant problems at times, even with the best available instrumentation. Signal-averaging capability is essential to allow recording of the extremely small sensory nerve responses (sometimes <1 μV in amplitude). Marked edema of the extremities may also make certain nerve conduction measurements impossible to perform. In the ICU, concentric needles are significantly superior to monopolar needles, because of their markedly reduced sensitivity to environmental electrical noise.

CLINICAL USE OF NEURODIAGNOSTIC METHODS

Acquaintance with the methods of neurophysiologic testing helps one to select and interpret the results of these tests. However, without considerable familiarity with these methods, it is frequently difficult to develop an approach to their proper use in addressing clinical problems. The following discussion demonstrates how these methods may be used to aid in the diagnosis and management of several neurologic problems frequently encountered in the ICU.

Lethargy, Coma, Confusion, and Unresponsiveness

A common and difficult clinical problem facing the clinician in the ICU is the unresponsive patient. Even when this situation results from neuromuscular blocking agents, there are situations in which there is clinical concern about the status of the nervous system. Unresponsiveness can have a number of causes. Appropriate testing can help differentiate among several of these possibilities.

A patient may be unresponsive because of focal hemispheric lesions, brain stem lesions, a metabolic disturbance, or generalized seizures. Patients with focal lesions affecting the speech areas, particularly Wernicke's area (speech comprehension), may seem unresponsive or confused because of the loss of comprehension or expression capabilities. Patients with occipital infarcts may be cortically blind and seem unresponsive or confused. Patients with focal lesions in the brain stem of various causes, such as basilar artery stroke, may become "locked-in" despite being fully mentally alert. Other patients with brain stem lesions or widespread damage to the cerebral hemispheres, as may occur after an episode of anoxia, are in a permanent vegetative state. Subclinical (nonconvulsive) status epilepticus in the ICU may manifest merely as diminished responsiveness. This may occur with generalized and even focal status, particularly when the focus affects the frontal lobes. Metabolic encephalopathy of several types may be sufficiently severe to cause diminished responsiveness. Each of these causes has different prognostic and therapeutic significance.

Imaging techniques are obviously useful in assessing such patients. However, early after stroke, CT scans are frequently normal, and magnetic resonance imaging is often not practical in ventilator-dependent patients. In brain stem lesions, status epilepticus, and metabolic encephalopathy, imaging techniques are frequently not revealing. In this setting, EEG is frequently helpful. It can detect focal and generalized status epilepticus. In metabolic encephalopathies, it reveals widespread disturbance of the normal background rhythm, sometimes with characteristic triphasic waves, whereas in brain stem lesions it is frequently normal or shows rhythmic bifrontal delta activity superimposed on a relatively normal background. With severe anoxic insults, there is marked loss of EEG activity everywhere over the hemispheres, at times with brief bursts of high-voltage activity (burst-suppression pattern). In chronic vegetative states, the EEG may reveal relatively normal sleep-wake cycles. With focal cortical lesions such as left hemispheric lesions causing aphasia or occipital lesions causing cortical blindness, the EEG frequently reveals the focal abnormality, even soon after an acute infarction. A common source of frustration is the expectation that the EEG can establish the diagnosis. When its ability to help distinguish the aforementioned localizations and mechanisms is understood, its utility is more apparent. After one of these localizations or mechanisms is identified, the list of differential diagnoses is narrowed considerably.

Although their usefulness has not been proved, quantitative EEG techniques offer considerable promise in addressing some of the clinical questions that arise in assessing the unresponsive patient. Such methods offer the possibility of more precise, early and reliable detection of focal abnormalities, particularly as occur with cerebrovascular disease. Other potential improvements in this method may allow the quantitative assessment of encephalopathy. Serial determinations using quantitative methods may allow the monitoring of therapy for effectiveness.

Evoked potential studies may be helpful in this setting as well. The most useful studies are brain stem auditory evoked responses to confirm suspected brain stem localization when the patient seems to be locked-in. Other modalities are less commonly employed, although somatosensory studies may be useful in identifying or confirming an asymmetric hemispheric lesion (e.g., stroke) in the presence of other significant abnormalities, such as a marked metabolic encephalopathy that has severely affected the entire EEG. This is particularly true when a stroke is suspected in an encephalopathic patient but the CT scan is normal.

Global cortical dysfunction (encephalopathy) with or without seizures can occur in the setting of infectious diseases, including meningitis and encephalitis. The EEG may be helpful in detecting epileptiform discharges and focal slowing over the temporal lobes in herpes encephalitis. These are seen electroencephalographically before the onset of clinical seizures and well before the appearance of temporal lucency on CT scan. This can be quite helpful in guiding decisions about biopsy or institution of antiviral agents.

LP is important in assessing the encephalopathic patient for possible infection, and this procedure should be performed readily in this setting. Unfortunately, no clinical signs, including the absence of nuchal rigidity, are by themselves sufficiently reliable to exclude infection of the nervous system.

Prolonged Unresponsiveness

After the initial assessment of an unresponsive patient, much information may be gained by ongoing monitoring. In these patients, the neurologic examination is a useful starting point, but in many cases, it does not convey sufficient information for management. In such patients, dynamic bedside information is desired. Although imaging methods can provide an occasional assessment, they are not practical for hour-to-hour monitoring. Furthermore, most imaging methods do not convey the subtle, dynamic physiologic information required.

In following the unresponsive patient, the clinician has certain specific questions that must be answered.

1. Is the patient having unsuspected seizures?
2. Is the patient's condition improving or deteriorating?
3. Has the patient responded to interventional therapy?

Our ability to answer some of these questions is as yet limited. Nonetheless, existing methods do provide some useful information. Periodic routine portable EEG can determine the trend of the patient's condition. If serial EEGs show progressive flattening or loss of activity, the patient's condition is deteriorating, whereas if they show progression from slowing toward a more normal background, the patient is improving. Compressed spectral array monitoring can provide a more continuous picture of cerebral activity. Current methods are limited with respect to the number of channels provided and the inability to detect transient events (e.g., seizures) and artifacts. Technologic progress will enhance our ability to address these clinical questions.

In the unresponsive patient, the only reliable technique for monitoring ICP is with an invasive method, as described earlier. The ability to guide therapy, including the administration of osmotic agents, depends on reliable pressure monitoring.

Jerking, Twitching, Shaking Movements

Use of neurodiagnostic methods to address the problem of adventitious movements is also facilitated by first formulating the problem in terms of specific anatomic localizations and pathophysiologic mechanisms. This formulation can be confused by the application of descriptive terminology without consideration of underlying mechanisms of disease. It is important to remember that terms such as myoclonus are merely descriptive and do not imply a specific cause.

Clinical observation of the movements is often quite helpful, with specific attention to whether the movements are generalized or confined to one limb or segment, rhythmic or irregular, and stereotypic or variable. Movements seen in the ICU generally represent one of the following: shivering, seizures, involuntary (disinhibited) reflexes, asterixis, fasciculations, or reflex or nonreflex subcortical myoclonus. Each of these categories again has quite different implications for possible underlying causes, therapy, and prognosis.

Shivering (rigors) is generally recognized when other causes have been excluded, and it is followed by a rapid rise in temperature. When the movements are prolonged and violent, they may be difficult to distinguish from seizures. An EEG performed while the movement occurs clearly identifies seizures, but interictally the EEG may reveal only spikes or other epileptiform patterns. Fasciculations are due to spontaneous discharges of anterior horn cells, and in cases of severe lower motor neuron disease and reinnervation, the motor units may be large enough to be seen clinically. The diagnosis of fasciculations and lower motor neuron abnormalities is made electromyographically. Involuntary reflexes seen in the ICU are generally diagnosed clinically and can include disinhibition of triple-flexion and tonic neck reflexes, as well as decorticate or decerebrate posturing. Of these, triple flexion may be demonstrated electrophysiologically, but this is rarely necessary.

It is not commonly recognized that appropriate recordings of surface EMG with the EMG instrument can frequently identify asterixis, even when clinically difficult to identify with certainty. Although this is rarely necessary to establish the diagnosis of a metabolic encephalopathy, in selected cases it has proved helpful in assessing the presence and severity of such encephalopathy and guiding management.

The term *myoclonus* is descriptive, referring to any brief isolated twitching movement. It is useful to consider myoclonus in terms of an anatomic and physiologic classification.[29] In the ICU, the important distinction for prognostic and therapeutic reasons is between seizures (cortical-epileptic myoclonus) and subcortical myoclonus. For practical purposes, the EEG is the key to the distinction, which may otherwise be difficult in cases in which the movements are frequent but irregular.

Hemiplegia

Patients in the ICU may be noted to have diminished movements of one side of the body. This includes not only complete hemiplegia but also milder paresis characterized by diminished movements of one side relative to another. Analysis of the causes of hemiplegia, as with other neurologic symptoms or signs, begins with a clinical localization. A critical differentiation is based on the presence or absence of facial asymmetry. If facial asymmetry is present, the lesion is intracranial (above the foramen magnum) and the work-up is directed accordingly. If there is facial sparing (or there is clinical uncertainty about facial involvement), the work-up must be directed at, or include consideration of, lesions of the cervical spine.

The pathophysiology of lesions that cause hemiplegia is diverse, but diagnostic considerations are narrowed considerably by a precise localization. Common localizations include (1) the contralateral middle cerebral artery perfusion territory, with cortical involvement; (2) lesions deep in the hemisphere, involving primarily the internal capsule; (3) lesions confined to the brain stem; and (4) lesions of the cervical spinal cord. This last category is most important, because the pathophysiology of these lesions is quite different. Acute lesions of the cervical cord raise the possibility of epidural abscess or hematoma, disk herniation, compression from spondyloarthropathy, intramedullary hemorrhage, anterior spinal artery infarction, and other rarer conditions. Some of these necessitate emergent surgical intervention, in contradistinction to intracranial lesions, in which large- or small-vessel stroke, hemorrhage, and abscess are the primary considerations. Further differentiation of strokes involving anterior and posterior circulations is often worthwhile, because the prognosis and underlying mechanisms are quite different.

Imaging techniques are most important in helping differentiate among these lesions. Electrophysiologic techniques play a secondary but important role in many cases. Quantitative electrophysiology is likely to play an increased role in the physiologic evaluation of cerebrovascular disorders.[30] EEG may be used both to increase and to decrease the consideration of a cortical localization. Thus, if a stroke involving the middle cerebral artery is the cause of hemiplegia, the EEG is generally abnormal over the appropriate hemisphere and shows asymmetry that is easily distinguished even in the presence of diffuse abnormalities as occur in superimposed metabolic encephalopathies. The EEG shows changes within minutes of the event, days before the CT scan shows changes. Conversely, if the localization is deep in the hemisphere, the EEG may show a different pattern of asymmetry, and if the lesion is in the brain stem or cervical spinal cord, or small deep white matter lesion as in lacunar stroke, the EEG remains normal. Thus, the EEG is most useful and should be obtained early after the onset of a hemiplegia, particularly after the CT scan is normal. The EEG is also useful in this setting, because occasionally the hemiplegia represents a Todd's paralysis from an unobserved focal-onset seizure.

When a brain stem localization is suspected, brain stem auditory evoked responses can confirm this localization. Brain stem auditory evoked responses are abnormal in many cases when the CT scan is normal because the CT scan is limited in assessing the brain stem because of bone-induced artifacts in the posterior fossa. When a cervical spine localization is suspected, upper extremity and lower extremity SSEP studies may be useful in aiding localization. SSEPs are also abnormal if hemispheric lesions are present, but in these cases the abnormality is unilateral, whereas in cervical spine lesions, the abnormality is more frequently bilateral. In some cases, the facial involvement may be prominent, and hemiplegia may not be present. When a facial nerve localization is suspected (Bell's palsy), nerve conduction and EMG studies, including blink reflex studies, may be quite useful.

Upper Extremity Monoplegia

On clinical grounds, a purely localized monoplegia of an upper extremity, without hemiplegia, may be localized to only two possible lesions:

1. A discrete hemispheric lesion of the isolated motor strip of the arm, on the convexity of the hemisphere. This is the most distal perfusion territory of the middle cerebral artery and commonly represents a middle cerebral artery stroke.
2. A peripheral nerve lesion involving cervical nerve roots, the brachial plexus, or single or multiple mononeuropathies in the arm.

As discussed earlier, the EEG is useful to supplement the CT scan in considering middle cerebral artery stroke, particularly soon after onset. It should be noted that immediately after an acute stroke or trauma, the tone of the extremity is frequently flaccid, making differentiation of the central versus peripheral localization difficult. In this case, the other appropriate physiologic study is a nerve conduction and EMG study, which may be done at the bedside. Some important timing considerations apply to the use of EMG. Nerve conduction studies are immediately able to detect neuropractic lesions (demyelination, conduction block), as might occur owing to a traction or compression injury. Thus, radial nerve studies are useful if a wristdrop attributable to compression of the radial nerve in the humeral groove from prolonged outstretched positioning of the arm ("Saturday night" palsy) is suspected. However, axonal changes seen by needle EMG are often necessary for accurate diagnosis or prognostication, and these do not occur immediately after injury. Thus, a study 2 to 3 weeks after the onset of symptoms may be required.

Lower Extremity Paraplegia and Monoplegia

The clinical presentation of monoplegia of a lower extremity, or paraplegia, may be localized to a limited set of possible sites. These sites are (1) the interhemispheric motor cortex, (2) the thoracic spinal cord, (3) compression of the conus medullaris or cauda equina, (4) lumbar plexopathy, and (5) multiple individual nerves. Selective acute lesions of the interhemispheric motor cortex result from stroke in the territory of the anterior cerebral artery or acute ventricular dilatation (obstructive hydrocephalus). Rapidly progressive lesions at the other sites are more likely due to external compression or infiltration. An important clinical clue in the examination of lower extremity weakness is the presence of marked proximal involvement and weakness in the legs, including muscle groups such as quadriceps femoris, the adductors, and gluteii, when the arms are entirely spared both proximally and distally. This clinical pattern localizes the lesion to thoracic cord compression, conus medullaris or cauda equina, or lumbar plexus.

Imaging studies play an important role, particularly in addressing questions of cerebral infarction, hydrocephalus, and thoracic spinal cord compression or lumbar compression of the conus or cauda equina. EEG again proves useful in this setting when considering stroke and when the CT scan is normal. A battery of evoked potentials may be useful in assessing enlarged ventricles for physiologic significance and guiding decisions about shunting.[31] In difficult cases, SSEPs may be helpful in assessing the spinal cord. With thoracic cord compression, median nerve SSEPs are normal, whereas tibial nerve SSEPs show a block of conduction between the periphery and the cortex. Nerve conduction studies and EMG are extremely useful in identifying lesions of the cauda equina, the lumbar roots, the lumbar plexus, and the peripheral nerves, particularly when the problem has been present for several weeks or has been slowly progressive.

Poor Ventilatory Effort, Generalized Paresis

Assessment of generalized abnormality also depends on accurate localization. When the weakness is generalized, localization considerations include

1. Muscle fibers (myopathy)
2. Neuromuscular junction (myasthenia gravis, Lambert-Eaton syndrome, botulism)
3. Sensory and motor axons (sensorimotor polyneuropathy)
4. Motor axons, anterior horn cells (poliomyelitis, motor neuron disease)
5. Myelin sheath (including Guillain-Barré syndrome)
6. Multiple plexopathies; polyradiculopathy (other than Guillain-Barré syndrome)
7. Multifocal disease, including clinically confluent multifocal disease
8. High cervical cord lesions
9. Brain stem lesions
10. Multiple bihemispheric lesions

The last three categories have been discussed earlier, in considering focal monoplegias and hemiplegias. This discussion specifically considers the approach to localizations 1 to 6 and category 7. The role of electrophysiology in assessment of the peripheral nervous system in the ICU is key because the physical examination in this setting is frequently quite limited. Appropriate investigation consists of a series of different techniques that can distinguish and identify lesions and place them in one of these categories.

The most useful methods for determining the physiologic localization of generalized weakness are nerve conduction studies and EMG, in conjunction with specialized techniques. Nerve conduction techniques can demonstrate the presence of demyelinating or axonal neuropathy and distinguish motor and sensory nerve involvement. Needle EMG further adds to the diagnosis of axonal lesions and distinguishes acute and chronic components of the disease. Needle EMG is required to identify the presence of myopathy but is not specific about the particular cause of the myopathy. Repetitive nerve stimulation techniques can identify neuromuscular junction dysfunction. Thus, nerve conduction and EMG study allows the cause of the patient's weakness to be categorized clearly into classes 1 to 5.

Mapping out the anatomy of generalized weakness is critical when multiple focal lesions are suspected. In the common setting of weakness in a patient with neoplasia, involvement of multiple plexus or nerve roots (e.g., meningeal carcinomatosis) may be suspected. It is further essential to differentiate generalized peripheral nervous system disease from multifocal disease. The latter category may be divided into multifocal axonal disease, or mononeuropathy multiplex, and multifocal demyelinating disease. Mononeuropathy multiplex is essentially synonymous with vasculopathy of the peripheral nerves, and specific causes include diabetes, vasculitides (particularly periarteritis nodosa), and collagen-vascular diseases. Multifocal demyelinating neuropathy has been strongly associated with immunologic abnormalities, particularly various paraproteinemias and antibodies against components of peripheral nerve. Both categories may be responsive to appropriate therapy, including immunosuppression, and the demyelinating neuropathies are frequently responsive to plasmapheresis. Thus, the recognition of these multifocal neuropathies has significant diagnostic and therapeutic implications. An appropriately detailed nerve conduction and EMG study can make this critical distinction.

At times, the approach to generalized weakness is improved by obtaining appropriate normal study results. For example, if the lesion is suspected to be in the peripheral nervous system, SSEPs and other CNS evaluation methods may be used to demonstrate that the CNS is intact. Conversely, if the lesion is suspected to be entirely in the CNS, a normal nerve conduction and EMG study result may help confirm that the peripheral nervous system is not involved.

Particular mention should be made of two problems specific to the ICU setting. Zochodne and associates have described a syndrome of an acute, severe axonal sensorimotor polyneuropathy that occurs in septic patients with multiple organ system failure.[32–34] This critical illness polyneuropathy is quite distinct from Guillain-Barré syndrome. The latter is an immunologically mediated demyelinating neuropathy with good prognosis and response to therapy. The etiologic factor responsible for critical illness polyneuropathy is as yet unknown, and the prognosis poor. Both Guillain-Barré syndrome and critical illness polyneuropathy are readily diagnosed by nerve conduction and EMG techniques.

A small but significant number of patients treated successfully in the ICU go on to become ventilator dependent. This failure to wean has been ascribed to numerous factors. It has been shown that, among cases of failure to wean with no evident cause, the most common source of this problem is a severe unsuspected disease of the peripheral nervous system, which can be readily diagnosed by portable nerve conduction and EMG studies.[27] Critical illness polyneuropathy is the single largest category, but clinically unsuspected myopathies, motor neuron disease, Guillain-Barré syndrome, mononeuropathy multiplex, and other potentially treatable conditions are disclosed by EMG evaluation.

Prognosis

Electrophysiologic methods may also be used for prognostication in addition to diagnosis. In this situation, the severity and mechanism of the abnormality are more significant, and the localization or diagnosis is often known. Electrophysiologic methods often provide critical information about prognosis, which is not available from imaging studies.[35, 37]

EEG is often used to assess the severity of an anoxic cerebral insult. Extensive or progressive loss of cortical activity after an anoxic insult implies poor recovery. SSEPs may also be used similarly. If the cortical responses on SSEP studies are absent, the prognosis for recovery is poor. Similar considerations apply to the prognosis of head trauma.[37]

Nerve conduction and EMG techniques may be used to assess the prognosis of peripheral nervous system disease. They are particularly important in detecting the presence of unsuspected axonal components of primarily demyelinating disorders, including Guillain-Barré syndrome. The presence of secondary axonal degeneration implies a significantly worse prognosis. For example, extensive axonal degeneration in the lower extremities may require up to 3 years for regeneration to occur. Conversely, preservation of axons, even in the face of severe demyelination and conduction block, nonetheless carries a good prognosis for rapid recovery, generally in weeks to months. The discovery of critical illness polyneuropathy in an ICU patient carries a prognostic expectation of good but extremely slow recovery, possibly over years.

References

1. Niedermeyer E, Lopes da Silva F: Electroencephalography: Basic Principles, Clinical Applications, and Related Fields. (2nd ed.) Baltimore, Urban & Schwarzenberg, 1987.
2. Goodin DS, Aminoff MJ, Laxer KD: Detection of epileptiform activity by different noninvasive EEG methods in complex partial epilepsy. Ann Neurol 27:330, 1990.
3. Nuwer MR: Quantitative EEG: I. Techniques and problems of frequency analysis and topographic mapping. J Clin Neurophysiol 5:1, 1988.
4. Nuwer MR. Quantitative EEG: II. Frequency analysis and topographic mapping in clinical settings. J Clin Neurophysiol 5:45, 1988.
5. Macdonell RAL, Donnan GA, Bladin PF, et al: The electroencephalogram and acute ischemic stroke: Distinguishing cortical from lacunar infarction. Arch Neurol 45:520, 1988.
6. Duffy FH, Bartels PH, Burchfiel JL: Significance probability mapping: An aid in the topographic analysis of brain electrical activity. Electroencephalogr Clin Neurophysiol 51:455, 1981.
7. Oken BS, Chiappa KH, Salinsky M: Computerized EEG frequency analysis: Sensitivity and specificity in patients with focal lesions. Neurology 39:1281, 1989.
8. Hjorth B, Rodin E: An eigenfunction approach to the inverse problem of EEG. Brain Topogr 1:79, 1988.
9. Hjorth B, Rodin E: Extraction of "deep" components from scalp EEG. Brain Topogr 1:65, 1988.
10. Borel C, Hanley D: Neurologic intensive care unit monitoring. Crit Care Clin 1:223, 1985.
11. Hakkinen VK, Kaukinen S, Heikkila H: The correlation of EEG compressed spectral array to Glasgow coma scale in traumatic coma patients. Int J Clin Monit Comput 5:97, 1988.
12. Cant BR, Shaw NA: Monitoring by compressed spectral array in prolonged coma. Neurology 34:35, 1984.
13. Spitzer AR, Hassoun M, Wang C, et al: Signal decomposition and diagnostic classification of the electromyogram using a novel neural network technique. In: Miller RA (ed): Proceedings of the XIVth Annual Symposium on Computer Applications in Medical Care. Los Alamitos, CA, IEEE, Computer Society Press, p 552, 1990.
14. Rumelhart DE, Hinton GE, Williams RJ: Learning representations by back-propagating errors. Nature 323:533, 1986.
15. Chiappa KH: Evoked Potentials in Clinical Medicine. 2nd ed. New York, Raven Press, 1990.
16. Spitzer AR, Cohen L, Fabrikant J, et al: A method for determining optimal interelectrode spacing for cerebral topographic mapping. Electroencephalogr Clin Neurophysiol 72:355, 1989.
17. Cohen D, Cuffin BN, Yunokuchi K, et al: MEG versus EEG localization test using implanted sources in the human brain. Ann Neurol 28:811, 1990.
18. Cuffin BN, Cohen D, Yunokuchi K, et al: Tests of EEG localization accuracy using implanted sources in the human brain. Ann Neurol 29:132, 1991.
19. Eisen AA, Shtybel W: AAEM minimonograph 35: Clinical experience with transcranial magnetic stimulation. Muscle Nerve 13:995, 1990.
20. Dinner DS (ed): Magnetic stimulation of the nervous system. J Clin Neurophysiol 8:1, 1991.
21. American Academy of Neurology, Therapeutics and Technology Assessment Subcommittee: Assessment: Transcranial Doppler. Neurology 40:680, 1990.
22. Petty G, Wiebers D, Meissner I: Transcranial Doppler ultrasonography: Clinical applications in cerebrovascular disease. Mayo Clin Proc 65:1350, 1990.
23. Jobsis F: Noninvasive infrared monitoring of cerebral and myocardial oxygen sufficiency and circulatory parameters. Science 198:1264, 1977.
24. Chance B, Leigh J, Miyake H: Comparison of time-resolved and unresolved measurements of deoxyhemoglobin in brain. Proc Natl Acad Sci USA 85:4971, 1988.
25. McCormick P, Stewart M, Goetting M, et al: Noninvasive cerebral optical spectroscopy for monitoring cerebral oxygen delivery and hemodynamics. Crit Care Med 19:89, 1991.
26. Kimura J: Electrodiagnosis in Diseases of Nerve and Muscle: Principles and Practice. 2nd ed. Philadelphia, FA Davis, 1989.
27. Spitzer AR, Giancarlo T, Maher L, et al: Neuromuscular causes of prolonged ventilator dependence. Muscle Nerve. In press.
28. Bolton CF: Electrophysiologic studies of critically ill patients. Muscle Nerve 10:129, 1987.
29. Hallett M: Myoclonus: Relation to epilepsy. Epilepsia 26(suppl 1):S67, 1985.
30. Nuwer MR, Jordan SE, Ahn SS: Evaluation of stroke using EEG frequency analysis and topographic mapping. Neurology 37:1153, 1987.
31. Spitzer AR: Assessment of hydrocephalus by a battery of evoked potentials (abstract). Muscle Nerve 14:896, 1991.
32. Zochodne DW, Bolton CF, Gilbert JJ: Polyneuropathy in critical illness: Pathological features. Ann Neurol 18:160, 1985.
33. Zochodne DW, Bolton CF, Wells GA, et al: Polyneuropathy of critical illness: Analysis of etiologic factors. Can J Neurol Sci 12:177, 1985.
34. Zochodne DW, Bolton CF, Wells GA, et al: Critical illness polyneuropathy: A complication of sepsis and multiorgan failure. Brain 110:819, 1987.
35. Anderson DC, Bundlie S, Rockswold GL: Multimodality evoked potentials in closed head trauma. Arch Neurol 41:369, 1984.
36. Rumpl E, Prugger M, Gerstenbrand F, et al: Central somatosensory conduction time and acoustic brainstem transmission time in post-traumatic coma. J Clin Neurophysiol 5:237, 1988.

37. Moulton RJ, Marmarou A, Ronene J, et al: Spectral analysis of the EEG in craniocerebral trauma. Can J Neurol Sci 15:82, 1988.

They become confused and disoriented and may hallucinate as metabolic function within the higher level, polysynaptic pathways becomes compromised.

Coma may result when there is structural impairment of the activating system, either directly within the brain stem or indirectly from a mass effect in the cranial cavity or the posterior fossa; when there is toxic or metabolic dysfunction that diffusely impairs neuronal metabolism; or subsequent to cerebral depression after diffuse neuronal activation, as may occur after a generalized seizure or a concussion.

DIFFERENTIAL DIAGNOSIS

Anatomy and Physiology of the Reticular Activating System

The viral infection responsible for the epidemics of encephalitis lethargica in 1917 and 1927 provided the first structural evidence that focal lesions within the brain stem and the diencephalon could result in disorders of sleep and wakefulness.[2] Later, in 1949, electrical stimulation of the tegmentum of the pons and midbrain was clearly shown in animals to have an effect on the sleep-wake cycle.[3] This represented the first attempt to describe the anatomy and physiology of what was later termed the *reticular activating system* (RAS).

Since the early descriptions, much has been learned about the anatomic basis and physiologic function of the reticular formation. The reticular formation is an extensive, polysynaptic connection of neurons that extends from an interneuronal network of the spinal cord to the level of the hypothalamus and thalamus. The bulk of the reticular formation, however, is located within the central core of the medulla, pons, and midbrain. Within the RAS, the major nuclei include the midline raphe nuclei, which are involved in sleep; laterally located, small cell reticular neurons; and interposed between, the large cell (gigantocellular) reticular neurons. The reticular neurons have widespread and extensive connections throughout the entire central nervous system (CNS) and a profound influence on its function.[4] The reticular formation can influence the processing of sensory information not only at higher centers of the CNS, through its connections to the thalamus and hypothalamus to the cortex, but also at the level of initial sensory input to the spinal cord. The most prominent neurotransmitters within the reticular formation are norepinephrine, serotonin, and acetylcholine.[5] Acetylcholine and norepinephrine appear to influence arousal, whereas norepinephrine and serotonin are involved in the regulation of the sleep-wake cycle. Virtually every cranial and spinal sensory nucleus sends afferent projections to the reticular nuclei, which provide a potent means of responding to the environment. The rostral portion of the reticular formation (caudal diencephalon to the pons) primarily controls wakefulness and receives its blood supply from the long circumferential branches of the basilar artery and branches of the superior cerebellar artery.[6]

In addition to its function as the RAS of the CNS, the reticular formation functions to modulate segmental stretch reflexes and muscle tone via reticulospinal connections to the spinal cord, to control breathing movements and cardiac function, and to modulate the sense of pain by influencing the flow of sensory information through the dorsal horn of the spinal cord.[5]

Dysfunction of the Reticular Activating System

The differential diagnosis of disorders of consciousness is briefly summarized in Table 55–1.

The function of the RAS may be directly disturbed by

CHAPTER 55

Disorders of Consciousness

Patti L. Peterson

Acute alteration of consciousness is a frequently encountered clinical problem in intensive care practice in which the comatose patient is the rule rather than the exception. It is imperative that the intensivist have a comfortable working knowledge of the anatomic substrate of consciousness and of the brain's unique metabolic requirements. This chapter allows the reader to develop a systematic approach to the differential diagnosis and management of patients with disorders of consciousness.

Plum and Posner defined consciousness as the state of awareness of self and one's environment and coma as total absence of this awareness.[1] Between these two extreme states are various levels of consciousness. They further described conscious behavior as composed of two physiologic elements, arousal and content of consciousness. Arousal is associated with the appearance of wakefulness or alertness and is maintained by a primitive, diffuse network of neurons within the brain stem and the diencephalon. Content of consciousness represents the sum of the cognitive and affective mental functions and is a phylogenetically new, higher cortical function of the brain. This has proved to be a useful scheme to help conceptualize how and why alterations of consciousness occur.

In clinical practice, it is useful to think of disorders of consciousness as being due either to a discrete disturbance affecting the arousal or activating system of the brain or to a more diffuse disturbance of neuronal metabolism. Although this concept is not always 100% correct, it provides a useful framework for the practitioner to develop a clinical approach to the patient with an altered level of consciousness.

When only the activating system of the brain stem is affected, the cause is always structural and in adult clinical practice is most often due to a vascular event. The brain stem activating system either may be directly impaired or may be secondarily compromised owing to a mass effect within the cranial vault or the posterior fossa. In the early clinical stages, the disorder of consciousness seen in these patients is predominantly impaired alertness.

Toxic and metabolic disorders are the cause of diffuse disturbances of neuronal metabolism and, unlike structural disorders, may be completely reversible if identified and treated at an early stage in their evolution. Although toxic and metabolic disorders are more difficult to conceptualize, they are far more common in clinical practice and, when rapidly corrected, are eminently more treatable than disorders of consciousness caused by structural defects. Early in the clinical course of toxic and metabolic disorders, patients primarily have a disturbance of content of consciousness.

TABLE 55–1

DIFFERENTIAL DIAGNOSIS OF DISORDERS OF CONSCIOUSNESS

Structural Disorders
Direct impairment of RAS
    Infarction, hemorrhage, trauma, tumor, infection, inflammation, central pontine myelinolysis
Indirect impairment of RAS caused by herniation

Toxic and Metabolic Disorders
Disorders that primarily affect neuronal oxidative metabolism
    Ischemia
    Hypoxia
    Hypoglycemia
    Hyperthermia and hypothermia
    Coenzyme deficiency (vitamins B_1, B_{12}, and B_6; nicotinic acid; pantothenic acid)
Disorders that primarily affect neuronal membrane activity
    Electrolyte disorders
    Acid-base disorders
    Hyperosmolar and hyposmolar states
    Seizure disorders
    Concussion
Disorders that are multifactorial
    Organ failure (hepatic, renal, pancreatic, pulmonary)
    Poisonings, anesthetics
    Infections or intoxications

---

discrete lesions that affect the paramedian tegmentum of the pons or the midbrain immediately ventral to the ventricular system. Damage to the more caudal, medullary portion of the RAS does not produce coma.[1] A clinically useful clue to a structural basis of coma is the presence of abnormal eye movements or abnormalities of the pupils. The third, fourth, and sixth cranial nerve nuclei; the medial longitudinal fasciculus, which interconnects the third and sixth cranial nerve nuclei; and the descending sympathetic fibers are situated directly within the neuronal network of the reticular formation. Damage to these nuclei and tracts is associated with abnormalities of eye movements and the pupils and provides invaluable clinical information that the coma has a structural cause. The most common cause of structural damage to the RAS in the adult is vertebrobasilar insufficiency or hemorrhagic events in this vascular territory. Inflammatory disorders (e.g., encephalitis and abscess), tumors of the brain stem, central pontine myelinolysis, and diffuse axonal injury or hemorrhage after traumatic brain injury may also occur with some frequency.

Herniation Syndromes

The function of the RAS may also be indirectly affected in a process referred to as *herniation*. In herniation, cerebral tissue is displaced by mass effect to a location that it does not normally occupy owing to the bony constraints of the skull. This typically involves passing a rigid septum such as the falx or the tentorium cerebelli with subsequent compression and dysfunction of tissue. The most common form involves the herniation of the cingulate gyrus under the falx (transfalcial herniation) and may result in infarction of the anterior cerebral artery and additional mass effect as edema evolves.

Supratentorial or transtentorial (tissue passes below the tentorium) herniation includes uncal herniation and central herniation. Uncal herniation occurs as a result of a laterally placed mass lesion (e.g., subdural or epidural hematoma, large middle cerebral artery infarction, or temporal lobe tumor) and may be associated with stepwise, progressive compression and dysfunction of adjacent anatomic structures. Initially, the oculomotor nerve is compressed as the

inferomedial portion of the temporal lobe herniates over the tentorium. The posterior cerebral artery may also become compressed and infarction may occur. As the mass effect increases, a greater midline shift of structures occurs, the midbrain is compressed and hemorrhages, and the ascending portion of the RAS is compromised. In central transtentorial herniation, a more centrally located, supratentorial mass lesion (e.g., thalamic hemorrhage) exerts a downward mass effect on the brain stem and diencephalon with subsequent hemorrhage. Progressive, rostrocaudal deterioration of brain stem function may occur.

The most common causes of supratentorial mass lesions in clinical practice are vascular (large middle cerebral or internal carotid artery infarction or hemorrhage, basal ganglia or intraventricular hemorrhage); post-traumatic with extradural or intradural or intraparenchymal collection of blood (subdural, epidural, cerebral contusion or intraparenchymal collection); neoplastic (primary or metastatic); or infectious (abscess, granuloma, or empyema).

Herniation from infratentorial mass lesions may also occur. Mass lesions within the posterior fossa (e.g., cerebellar hemorrhage) may cause the contents of the posterior fossa to herniate upward and compress the midbrain, or there may be herniation of the cerebellar tonsils through the foramen magnum. In the latter situation, the compromise of consciousness is due to anoxic-ischemic encephalopathy as the cerebellar tonsils compress the medulla and result in sudden apnea and cardiac arrest.

Although compromise of the RAS is usually thought to be structural in nature, metabolic disorders may significantly depress the interneuronal, polysynaptic transmission of information within the RAS. Of particular interest, there is evidence that hypoxia and hypoglycemia may actually specifically affect the RAS early in the clinical course as a cerebroprotective mechanism. Depression of the level of consciousness decreases the metabolic demands on the remainder of the CNS and protects the brain from further damage.[7] In addition, in thiamine deficiency, the earliest abnormalities are caused by disturbance of specific brain stem, hypothalamic, and thalamic nuclei, which are particularly rich in the thiamine-dependent enzyme pyruvate dehydrogenase.[8]

Metabolic Considerations of the Central Nervous System

Although the weight of the human brain represents only 2% of the total body weight, its high rate of oxygen consumption accounts for nearly 20% of the body's oxygen consumption. Because there is no significant capacity for anaerobic metabolism within the CNS and little endogenous fuel stores, owing to constraints on the size of the brain imposed by the bony skull, the CNS requires a continual supply of its substrates for oxidative metabolism. This necessitates a high rate of blood flow (15% of the total cardiac output) to meet its metabolic needs. Greater than one third of the total blood glucose delivered to the CNS is extracted. Blood glucose is the major, although not sole, source of cerebral energy. In conditions of stress, the brain has the capacity to oxidize ketone bodies, amino acids, and free fatty acids.

A critical, energy-dependent event in the nervous system is the action of the ATP-driven Na^+-K^+ plasma membrane pump. One third of the ATP consumed by the body at rest is by Na^+,K^+-ATPase. In the CNS, one half of all of the ATP consumed is used by Na^+,K^+-ATPase to re-establish the membrane potential of the cell and render the cell electrically excitable.[8] The other major energy-dependent needs of neurons are to support neurotransmitter metabolism, specific transport within the blood-brain barrier, protein synthesis, and axonal transport.

When there is insufficient ATP available, whatever the cause, the ionic homeostasis of the cell cannot be restored after the neuron discharges. In the excitotoxic hypothesis of cell death, excitatory amino acids (particularly glutamate) allow calcium influx into the cell. Under normal circumstances, when adequate supplies of ATP are available, reuptake of excitatory amino acids terminates their effect at the synapse and calcium and sodium are extruded from the cell to restore the normal ionic gradients so the cell can again become electrically excitable. In the absence of adequate ATP, the cell is unable to regulate the intracellular concentration of electrolytes, particularly calcium, and degradative cell processes are activated. Phospholipases digest the membrane structure of the cell, proteases destroy the cytoskeletal protein structure, and endonucleases damage the DNA of the cell.[9] At present, considerable effort is being expended on the development of therapeutic interventions that prevent the activation of these degradative processes or block their progression.

Toxic and Metabolic Dysfunction

The differential diagnosis of disorders of consciousness due to toxic and metabolic disorders is listed in Table 55–1.

Altered levels of consciousness may result when neuronal oxidative metabolism is compromised. This may occur when delivery of the substrates oxygen and glucose is inadequate, as in global ischemia, or when the substrates themselves are not available in adequate supply, as in hypoxia and hypoglycemia. One of the most important causes from a clinical perspective is global ischemia.

There is normally a delicate balance between provision of a continual supply of nutrients to the brain and satisfaction of its energy demands. The normal cerebral blood flow is 55 mL/100 g/min and is considered critically reduced when it falls below 20 mL/100 g/min. If cerebral blood flow ceases, consciousness is lost within 10 seconds and spontaneous electrical activity ceases within 15 seconds. However, structural brain damage does not occur for 5 minutes or longer.

It is not completely clear why the pathologic events associated with ischemia occur. As ATP levels are depleted, ATP-requiring processes are deprived of their energy supply and calcium-activated degradative processes occur. Adenosine, which is formed from the dephosphorylation of adenine nucleotides, is a potent vasodilator and neuromodulator. Ischemia favors the oxidation of the adenosine metabolite hypoxanthine, which is accompanied by the production of superoxide radicals and hydrogen peroxide and contributes to ischemia-induced membrane pathologic changes. As previously mentioned, calcium activates intracellular phospholipases, which destroy the membrane structure by hydrolyzing phospholipids to free fatty acids and glycerol. Free fatty acids are efficient uncouplers of mitochondrial oxidative phosphorylation. This further impairs ATP production and may be lethal in an already compromised situation.[10] An additional factor to be considered in cerebral ischemia is that toxins formed during cellular metabolism (e.g., lactic acid) are not carried away in the blood stream. These toxins may then have further deleterious effects on cellular metabolism. The most common cause of global ischemia is cardiac arrest (see Chapter 56).

Other causes of clinically significant cerebral ischemia include decreased cerebral blood flow from impaired cardiac function (cardiac arrhythmias, infarction, or failure; aortic stenosis; pulmonary infarction); from a fall in peripheral resistance (shock, vasovagal syncope, carotid sinus hypersensitivity); from increased vascular resistance (hypertensive encephalopathy, subarachnoid hemorrhage); and from disseminated small-vessel vascular occlusion (disseminated intravascular coagulation, fat embolism, subacute bacterial endocarditis).

Hypoglycemia is also a commonly encountered cause of altered consciousness, particularly in the intensive care unit. As the concentration of blood glucose falls, there is progressive compromise of CNS function. Surprisingly, lack of ATP does not account for the CNS dysfunction, which occurs with moderate degrees of hypoglycemia. Impairment of neurotransmitter synthesis and accumulation of toxic products such as ammonia and free fatty acids are more likely the cause.[8]

Most of the initial signs and symptoms of hypoglycemia result from protective physiologic mechanisms triggered by the sympathetic discharge that occurs with a rapid drop in the serum glucose concentration and include tachycardia, diaphoresis, and anxiety. Early symptoms referable to impairment within the CNS include dizziness, headache, and loss of fine motor skills followed by confusion, abnormal behavior, seizures, and eventually coma.

The outcome and neurologic manifestations of hypoglycemia vary in the clinical situation.[11] Patients with preexisting compromise (e.g., cerebrovascular disease, sepsis, liver disease, diabetes, and hypothyroidism) are more likely to be symptomatic at higher blood glucose levels than other patients.[12] In the normal person, acutely lowering the serum glucose level to 50 mg/dL is associated with evidence of autonomic nervous system activation. Blood glucose levels ranging from a mean of 43 mg/dL to a mean of 15 mg/dL have been associated with altered-sensorium-only to coma, respectively.[13] The normal individual responds to hypoglycemia with increased cerebral blood flow to increase the delivery of substrate to the CNS. This response may be impaired in the elderly with cerebrovascular disease, and they may become symptomatic at higher blood glucose levels than other patients. The most common cause of hypoglycemia in the clinical situation is excessive administration of insulin in the diabetic patient. Comparatively, the long-term effects of hypoglycemia are less severe than those of anoxia or ischemia.

Pure hypoxia, uncomplicated by the effects of impaired cerebral blood flow, is actually rare in the clinical situation, although it can occur with anemia (anemic anoxia) and with pulmonary compromise (hypoxic hypoxia). As in hypoglycemia, altered consciousness occurs before depletion of energy stores with moderate degrees of hypoxemia ($Pa_{O_2} > 25$ to 40 mm Hg). As with hypoglycemia, the most likely explanation for this is impaired neurotransmitter metabolism. (Norepinephrine, dopamine, and serotonin are dependent on oxygen for their synthesis. In addition, the amino acid neurotransmitters and acetylcholine are closely coupled to glycolysis and oxidative metabolism.) In severe hypoxemia ($Pa_{O_2} < 25$ mm Hg), the fall in the P_{O_2} to levels that no longer support mitochondrial respiration is the cause of coma.

In the clinical situation, it is imperative to recall that the initial physiologic response to a fall in the Pa_{O_2} is to increase cerebral blood flow twofold.[14] In a patient with a ruptured cerebral aneurysm, intracerebral hemorrhage, or increased intracranial pressure, the effects of this increase in blood flow can be devastating.

Deficiency of enzymatic cofactors (thiamine, niacin, pyridoxine, cyanocobalamin, and folate) may also compromise neuronal oxidative metabolism. The most commonly encountered deficiency in clinical practice, and perhaps the most interesting, is thiamine deficiency. Thiamine is a cofactor for transketolase and α-ketoglutarate, pyruvate, and α-keto acid dehydrogenase. Deficiency of the cofactor impairs enzymatic activity. The characteristic pathologic lesions of Wernicke's disease primarily involve the brain stem; however, the mechanism by which thiamine deficiency results in pathologic damage is unclear. There is evidence that excitatory amino acids are involved in the pathogenesis of the disorder.

Mental status changes are the most common manifestation of thiamine deficiency, and it is relatively uncommon (10% of cases) to see the classic clinical triad of encephalopathy, ataxia, and oculomotor abnormality. In alcoholic patients with thiamine deficiency, horizontal nystagmus, ataxia, and Korsakoff's syndrome result.[15] Standard caloric testing results of vestibular function are always impaired in these patients.

Electrolyte and acid-base balance and hyperosmolar and hyposmolar states may affect neuronal membrane activity in addition to having secondary effects on neuronal metabolism (e.g., alteration in blood flow and respiratory function).

A generalized seizure disorder may acutely affect consciousness by resulting in diffuse neuronal activation. The duration of loss of consciousness or compromise of consciousness (postictal period) is dependent on pre-existing CNS pathologic changes (e.g., cerebrovascular disease, dementia, brain injury) and ongoing toxic or metabolic factors (e.g., drug intoxication, hepatic failure, and uremia). As a rule, the greater the number of factors involved, the more delayed and possibly incomplete the recovery of the patient is.

Concussion has been recognized as a metabolic disorder that can affect consciousness. Although traumatic brain injury is frequently associated with structural change, most commonly diffuse axonal injury, simple concussion may be purely a metabolic compromise. An impact to the head of sufficient severity is associated with diffuse and intense neuronal discharge. The resultant increase in extracellular potassium concentration results in discharge of neurotransmitters, particularly glutamate, and further increase in extracellular potassium level. This massive flux of potassium, as is postulated in spreading depression, results in profound depression of neuronal activity.[16] The duration of loss of consciousness is proportional to the amount of time taken to re-establish the membrane potential. There is typically a 10-day hypometabolic period after concussion.

Space does not permit a detailed discussion of all of the situations described in Table 55–1; however, owing to their clinical significance, hepatic and renal failure are mentioned in brief. Hepatic causes of altered consciousness may be due to acute fulminant hepatic failure or chronic cirrhosis and recurrent hepatic encephalopathy. The latter is more commonly encountered. The metabolic compromise attributable to hepatic encephalopathy is thought to result from toxins that are not appropriately filtered from the circulation, abnormal fatty acid metabolism, abnormalities of neurotransmitter amino acids (glutamate, aspartate), and CNS toxicity caused by ammonia.[10] The latter appears to be the most potent aspect. Ammonia interferes with protein synthesis within the CNS and blocks oxidative metabolism.[17, 18] There is some suggestion that the longer the exposure to elevated levels of ammonia is, the more sensitized the brain becomes to its deleterious effects. In other words, the chronic alcoholic with liver disease is likely to become symptomatic with lower arterial ammonia levels than the patient with no prior history of compromise.[19]

Uremia may be an acute or chronic syndrome, which is characterized by retention of urea, phosphates, proteins, amines, and a number of ill-defined low-molecular-weight compounds. Uremic encephalopathy occurs when the glomerular filtration rate falls below approximately 10% of normal.[8] It is associated with an alteration of the blood-brain barrier, and substantial evidence exists that parathyroid hormone may exert adverse effects on the CNS.[20]

The majority of the conditions listed earlier and in Table 55–1 have a multifactorial effect on CNS metabolism.

COMA

Initial Evaluation and Management

The initial priority in the management of the comatose patient should be to assess and stabilize the patient's vital functions. After this is accomplished, the clinician should make every attempt to identify and treat that which is treatable. This evaluation should proceed as an orderly, systematic review to rapidly identify all pertinent factors and to clarify the cause of the comatose state. In some instances, a cause may appear obvious (witnessed cardiac arrest or generalized seizure); however, it cannot be overstated how essential it is to review the patient's case systematically to determine whether any additional factors may compromise the patient's outcome.

After the patient has been stabilized, a brief neurologic examination is conducted to rapidly identify signs that indicate whether immediate intervention is necessary (e.g., drainage of a subdural hematoma). This screening examination should include brief assessment of the patient's responsiveness to voice or to physical stimuli, examination of the pupils and eye movements, and notation of any abnormal motor movements. If this examination reveals evidence of herniation, immediate diagnostic or therapeutic intervention should be initiated. Hyperventilation, with a goal of PCO_2 of 28 to 32 mm Hg, provides a rapid decrease in intracranial pressure, although the effect is short-lived. Hyperosmolar therapy with mannitol may also provide valuable time to initiate definitive, surgical therapy. The complete neurologic examination is discussed later. If initial evaluation reveals evidence of cranial trauma (scalp contusion or laceration, rhinorrhea or otorrhea, or patterned bruising [raccoon eyes or Battle's sign]), which may have not been appreciated in the emergency department, the patient's neck must be secured in a cervical collar until appropriate x-ray films can be obtained.

Laboratory studies should be performed while the patient is being examined and include complete blood count and differential count, electrolyte (monovalent and divalent) determination, blood glucose determination, assessment of liver and kidney function, and blood gas analysis. An alcohol level, urine screening for therapeutic and abuse drug levels, and anticonvulsant levels may provide useful information when the diagnosis is not immediately obvious. Glucose (25 to 50 g) should be administered in addition to 100 mg of thiamine. The administration of glucose alone to a patient with thiamine deficiency may precipitate the development of florid Wernicke-Korsakoff syndrome. If narcotic intoxication is a consideration, naloxone should be administered. If poisoning becomes a possibility, it may be necessary to aspirate the contents of the stomach for analysis. Emesis should be induced (e.g., with ipecac, 30 mL) only if the patient is alert.

The most valuable information available to help the physician correctly identify and treat the cause of the patient's alteration of consciousness is the history of the illness. The emergency room records, intensive care unit records (particularly any details of previous neurologic complaints, such as headache, weakness, and diplopia), and medication records (particularly sedative dosages) should be reviewed. Those who brought the patient to the emergency room (an emergency medical service, family, or friends) should be carefully questioned. The patient's prior medical and psy-

TABLE 55-2

ABNORMALITIES OF VITAL SIGNS AND THEIR SIGNIFICANCE

Abnormality	Significance
Hyperthermia	Infection (systemic or CNS), hyperthyroidism, drug fever, damage to temperature-regulating centers, heat stroke
Hypothermia	Drug intoxication (alcohol, barbiturates), dehydration, hypothyroidism, hypoglycemia, exposure
Tachycardia	Decreased cerebral perfusion
Bradycardia	Heart block
Hypertension	Hypertensive encephalopathy, increased intracranial pressure
Hypotension	Drug intoxication, shock (septic, cardiogenic, hemorrhagic), cortisol deficiency
Hypopnea	Drug intoxication (morphine, barbiturates), metabolic alkalosis, hypothyroidism, central alveolar hypoventilation
Tachypnea	Respiratory disease (pneumonia), diabetic ketoacidosis, uremia, lactic acidosis, hepatic encephalopathy
Patterned breathing	Cheyne-Stokes respiration, central neurogenic hyperventilation, apneustic breathing, ataxic respiration

chiatric health status, medication history, circumstances of the illness, progress, how the patient was found, and recent stressful events should all be explored.

The patient's temperature, pulse, blood pressure, respiratory rate and depth, and the presence of patterned breathing should be noted (Table 55–2). Bradycardia and systolic hypertension (Cushing's signs) may indicate an attempt to increase cerebral perfusion pressure in the presence of increased intracranial pressure. A careful physical examination of the patient should be performed with attention to the general condition of the patient. Poor dental or nail hygiene suggests the possibility of previous CNS compromise (e.g., an underlying dementia) or a substance abuse problem, which may be significant in predicting outcome. Evidence of urinary or fecal incontinence or laceration or bruising of the tongue is suggestive of a generalized seizure. Resistance to passive forward flexion of the neck may be due to meningitis, subarachnoid hemorrhage, or herniation. Meningism may not be evident in the patient who is deeply comatose. Resistance to movement of the head from side to side is suggestive of bone disease (e.g., cervical fracture and degenerative joint disease).

The skin should be carefully evaluated for evidence of cyanosis of the lips or nail beds (hypoxia), jaundice (hepatic failure), pallor (hypotension), sallow color (pituitary hypofunction), or cherry red color (carbon monoxide poisoning). The patient's breath may have the characteristic odor of acetone, fetor hepaticus, or alcohol. Any rashes should be noted. Generalized petechiae suggest a bleeding diathesis or thrombotic thrombocytopenic purpura. The skin may be sweaty as in hypotension or dry as in diabetic ketoacidosis or uremia. Dry skin and high fever suggest heat stroke or poisoning with anticholinergics. Characteristic stigmata of chronic alcoholism (telangiectasia, spider angioma) or hypothyroidism should be noted. The presence of compression blisters indicates that the patient has been in one position for a prolonged period.

Evaluation of the fundi may also reveal abnormalities that may clarify the cause of the coma. There may be evidence of hypertensive retinopathy, Roth's spots, diabetic retinopathy, retinal ischemia, or a subhyaloid hemorrhage. Papill-

edema suggests an intracranial mass lesion or diffuse increase in intracranial pressure.

Neurologic Examination

The neurologic examination of the comatose patient can be helpful in defining whether the patient's coma is due to a structural or a metabolic condition. There are several excellent descriptions of the neurologic examination of the comatose patient.[1, 21, 22]

It is useful in communication with others to be able to describe accurately the patient's level of consciousness. Consciousness, as stated previously, is the state of awareness of self and the environment. Coma, on the other hand, is characterized by unarousable unresponsiveness, a lack of purposeful responsiveness to sensory stimulation. The comatose patient is unable to communicate in a meaningful manner with the examiner. There are various levels of consciousness between normal consciousness and coma. Sleep is a normal state of physical and mental inactivity from which the individual can be roused to normal consciousness.

In the patient whose altered level of consciousness is due to a toxic or metabolic cause, there is likely to be an interceding state of confusion or delirium before the patient becomes comatose. Delirious patients are typically inattentive, irritable, imperceptive, and disoriented and may hallucinate (usually visually). The stuporous patient is an unresponsive patient who is aroused only by vigorous sensory stimuli and, when left alone, again becomes unresponsive. The terms confusion, delirium, and stupor are useful in describing the patient with an altered consciousness but the best means of communicating a patient's level of consciousness is to describe objectively how he or she responds to a particular sensory stimulus.

Three additional situations may be encountered in caring for and treating patients with altered consciousness. Akinetic mutism describes a state in which the patient appears awake, yet there is no capacity for meaningful communication. Frontal release signs and long tract motor dysfunction may be evident on examination. Damage to the ascending RAS or bilateral medial frontal lesions are usually the anatomic substrate. The most common causes are cerebral infarction (usually of the frontal lobes), trauma, third ventricle mass lesions, and severe acute hydrocephalus.

When there is lack of improvement in the patient's clinical status and the patient's ability to respond is confined to the autonomic system, the situation is referred to as a *chronic vegetative state*.[23]

Patients with "locked-in" syndrome have damage to the ventral portion of the pons and are essentially de-efferented. These patients are alert and aware, are capable of following commands and communicating by blinking or moving their eyes in vertical planes, and have an intact sensory system.[24]

The neurologic assessment of the comatose patient consists of an assessment of spontaneous movements and respiratory pattern, cranial nerve evaluation, and assessment of motor response to sensory stimuli.

Spontaneous Movements

Observation of the patient may reveal restless, spontaneous, purposeful movements such as altering posture or picking at the bedclothes. Abnormal movements such as twitching, myoclonus, and tremor should be noted. Asymmetries in spontaneous movements or posture, such as an externally rotated lower extremity, are suggestive of focal motor deficits. Spontaneous blinking, chewing, and yawning may be seen and indicate that the brain stem component of the RAS is intact.

Respiratory Patterns

The patient's respiratory pattern can be helpful in determining the level of the lesion that is responsible for the patient's altered level of consciousness. The most frequently encountered respiratory pattern is Cheyne-Stokes respiration, which is characterized by a crescendo-decrescendo rate and depth of respiration followed by an apneic period. A rise in the serum PCO_2 initiates the crescendo phase of the respiration and is associated with greater responsiveness of the patient.[25] The pattern may be seen in the awake, alert patient and is characterized by the patient's inability to voluntarily breathe during the apneic period. It is seen with deep, midline, bihemispheric lesions or diffuse cortical impairment and is most useful in documenting clinical deterioration (e.g., incipient herniation) when it appears in a patient who had previously been breathing in a normal fashion.[26] Arterial blood gas values usually reveal a respiratory alkalosis, because the hyperpneic phase of Cheyne-Stokes respiration is usually longer than the apneic period.

Central neurogenic hyperventilation, which is not commonly encountered, is a respiratory pattern characterized by rapid hyperventilation and is associated with structural lesions of the midbrain.[27]

Apneustic respiration and ataxic breathing are not usually recognized in the clinical situation because the patient is generally recognized to be in respiratory distress and rapidly intubated. Apneustic breathing is characterized by a pause after inspiration and is associated with structural lesions of the lateral tegmentum of the mid-caudal pons.[28] In ataxic breathing, there is irregularly irregular respiration and structural dorsomedial medullary dysfunction is associated.

Cranial Nerve Examination

The cranial nerve examination of the patient may reveal asymmetries suggestive of a structural lesion. In general, the comatose patient with normal brain stem reflexes most likely has diffuse cortical impairment of a metabolic source. Corneal reflexes can be elicited and any asymmetries in response noted. A greater degree of stimulation is necessary in the comatose patient, and one must be careful to use aseptic technique to avoid causing a corneal abrasion. If the upper pons and midbrain are intact, stimulation of the cornea causes the eyes to roll upward (Bell's phenomenon).

Examination of the symmetry, size, shape, and response to light of the pupils is useful. The pupillary light reflex should be elicited with a bright light and evaluated with a hand lens when the pupils are miotic. The single most helpful factor in determining whether the cause of the coma is toxic or metabolic is the pupillary response to light, as the light reflex is highly resistant to toxic or metabolic disorders. Glutethimide (Doriden) and atropine may result in unreactive pupils, and inquiry should be made as to their administration or ingestion. Anisocoria, unless previously present, is indicative of a structural lesion. Miosis and anhidrosis may be seen and may be the first evidence of an ipsilateral supratentorial mass effect caused by compression of the hypothalamus. Horner's syndrome, with miosis, ptosis, and anhidrosis, is seen with ipsilateral lateral pontine, medullary, and ventrolateral cervical cord lesions.

Unilateral mydriasis is usually due to supratentorial compression of the oculomotor nerve. Mydriasis occurs before the motor component dysfunction because the parasympathetic sphincter fibers on the exterior of the nerve are involved. Because the sympathetic fibers are unopposed, the pupil becomes widely dilated. Oval pupils may be seen when there is patchy involvement of the fibers innervating the sphincter.

Bilaterally dilated and unreactive pupils are seen with severe midbrain damage or from anticholinergic poisoning. Lesions of the midbrain tegmentum may be associated with pear-shaped pupils owing to irregular constriction of the sphincter of the iris or with displacement of the pupil to one side (corectopia).[29]

Lesions of the tectum of the midbrain are associated with spontaneous oscillations in the size of the pupil, referred to as *hippus*. Pinpoint and reactive pupils are characteristic of pontine lesions and are due to interruption of the descending sympathetic fibers.

Evaluation of eye movements in coma is invaluable in the identification of a structural cause because the RAS and nuclei and tracts subserving eye movements are intermingled. The resting lid tone of the patient may be evaluated by raising the eyelids and noting the rate and completeness of closure of the eyelid. The deeper the coma is, the slower and more incomplete the closure. The position of the eyes and spontaneous movements should be noted. In the drowsy patient, it is normal for the eyes to appear divergent in the horizontal plane. When the patient awakens, the eyes become conjugate. Abduction of one eye at rest associated with pupillary dilatation indicates third cranial nerve compression. Adduction may be due to damage to the sixth cranial nerve or may be a false localizing sign attributable to increased intracranial pressure. Skew deviation (resting dysconjugate vertical gaze) may be seen with damage or dysfunction at various levels of the brain stem and cerebellum.

If the brain stem is intact, the eyes may drift slowly from side to side (roving eye movements).[23] A number of spontaneous eye movements are helpful in localizing lesions in the comatose patient. The majority, for obvious reasons, occur with involvement of the pons. Ocular bobbing is most frequently seen in the clinical situation and is associated with a fast downward phase and a slow return to the resting position. Horizontal eye movements are preserved and damage to the caudal portion of the pons has been described. Ocular dipping is associated with a slow downward phase followed by a rapid return to the resting position and occurs with diffuse anoxic insults. Acute thalamic lesions may cause sustained deviation of the eyes down and in.

Barbiturates, phenytoin, diazepam (Valium), tricyclic antidepressants, and ethanol intoxication may suppress reflex ocular movements; however, the pupillary response to light is intact. Disorder of eye movements can be assessed in the comatose patient by eliciting the oculocephalic reflex (doll's eye maneuver). The oculocephalic reflex requires functional vestibular connections to cranial nerves III, IV, and VI. It cannot be adequately tested in patients who are awake, as voluntary fixation and saccades overcome the vestibulo-ocular response. The comatose patient lacks voluntary saccades, including the quick phase of nystagmus and tracking movements. As a rule, cerebral gaze palsies can be overcome with the doll's eye maneuver, whereas palsies caused by brain stem damage cannot be overcome. The test should never be performed if there is a possibility of cervical trauma, as the cervical spinal cord may be damaged. The test is performed by opening the patient's eyes and rotating the head from right to left and up and down. The normal response is conjugate deviation of the eyes opposite to the direction in which the head is turned. The eyes may be dysconjugate or there may be no movement at all. Both responses are abnormal. The ease with which the response is elicited reflects the degree of inhibition by the cerebral hemispheres. The deeper the metabolic coma is, the easier it becomes to elicit the response. If the response is absent, it is necessary to use a stronger stimulus and caloric stimulation should be performed. Before performing this test, the tympanic membrane must be evaluated and determined to be intact. The head should be elevated 30° from the supine and at least 100 mL of ice water must be irrigated into the ear canal. In the normal response, the eyes conjugately deviate toward the irrigated side with a quick nystagmoid return to midline. The corrective nystagmus is mediated by the cortex. The nystagmus is absent and there is tonic, conjugate deviation in most toxic or metabolic encephalopathies. The test is required in the assessment of brain death (see Chapter 56).

Ping-Pong gaze, in which the eyes rove from side to side in a cyclic fashion, is seen with bilateral cerebral damage. Repetitive conjugate deviation may be seen in focal motor seizures involving the frontal eye fields. Conjugate horizontal deviation of the eyes may be seen in hemispheric frontal lesions, in which case the eyes deviate toward the lesion. The deviation may be overcome with either the oculocephalic or the oculovestibular maneuver. In deep cerebral lesions, the eyes may deviate away from the side of the lesion (wrong way eyes). In lesions affecting the tegmentum of the pons, the eyes deviate away from the side where the lesion is located (toward the hemiparesis) and cannot be overcome with maneuvers. Damage to the tegmental region of the midbrain may abolish vertical gaze.

Motor System Examination

Progressive stimuli, such as calling the patient's name, shouting, gentle shaking, and compressing the nail beds or the supraorbital nerve, are effective methods of evoking a motor response. The response to noxious stimuli is helpful in evaluation. The stimulus is administered and the response observed. The patient may withdraw appropriately, may assume a reflexive position such as decorticate or decerebrate posturing, or may not respond at all. Decorticate and decerebrate posturing may be seen with both toxic or metabolic disorders and structural causes of coma. However, focal motor deficits, with the exception of those related to hypoglycemia, are usually indicative of structural damage. Decorticate posturing is characterized by adduction of the shoulder and arm, flexion at the elbow, and pronation and flexion at the wrist. The lower extremity remains extended at the hip and knee. In decerebrate posturing, there are extension and pronation of the upper extremities and forcible plantar flexion of the foot. In animals, decerebrate posturing is associated with transection at the collicular level below the red nuclei, which leaves intact the pontine reticular formation and vestibular nuclei and removes the normal cerebral inhibition.

Abnormal, adventitious movements such as tremor, asterixis, myoclonus, and seizures are most commonly seen in toxic or metabolic disorders. The tremor seen in metabolic encephalopathies is coarse and irregular and ranges from 8 to 10 Hz. Asterixis is a sudden, brief loss of postural tone that is translated into a flapping movement when the patient's hand is held in dorsiflexion at the wrist and his or her fingers are extended and abducted. Asterixis can be seen in virtually any body part that has the capacity for voluntary movement. Multifocal myoclonus is sudden, nonrhythmic twitching most commonly seen in the facial and proximal limb musculature in uremic and hyperosmolar-hyperglycemic encephalopathy and in carbon dioxide narcosis. Generalized myoclonus, which predominantly involves the axial musculature, occurs with severe anoxic damage.

Clinical Herniation Syndromes

It is important, particularly in an intensive care unit population, to recognize clinical deterioration in a patient with an intracranial mass lesion. In uncal transtentorial herniation, a lateral mass lesion results in herniation of the inferomedial portion of the temporal lobe over the edge of the tentorium. An early indication of impending herniation may be a change in the respiratory pattern to Cheyne-Stokes respiration with development of ipsilateral miosis and anhidrosis. As herniation progresses, there is compression of the oculomotor nerve with dilatation of the pupil. One of the earliest signs may be development of an oval pupil. Compression and infarction of the posterior cerebral artery may result in involvement of the occipital lobe and visual signs and symptoms. Motor deficits may be contralateral or ipsilateral to the lesion. If the lateral aspect of the contralateral midbrain is shifted and compressed against the rigid tentorium, motor deficits that are ipsilateral to the mass lesion may be seen. Consciousness becomes compromised when the midbrain reticular formation becomes compressed or deprived of its blood supply.

In central transtentorial herniation, supratentorial masses have a downward mass effect, which results in compression and distortion of the midbrain and progresses in what is termed rostrocaudal deterioration. It may be possible to identify three stages as the diencephalon, the midbrain and pons, and the pons and medulla are progressively compromised.

1. Diencephalic stage (Cheyne-Stokes respiration, small reactive pupils, tonic deviation of the eyes on caloric testing, decorticate posturing in response to painful stimuli). In the early diencephalic stage, cognition and attention are impaired and frontal release signs such as the grasp and snout reflexes may be seen. In the late diencephalic stage, Cheyne-Stokes respiration, small and reactive pupils, and normal eye movements are seen until late in the course when dysfunction of the tectum may result in restriction of upward gaze. There is decorticate posturing in response to painful stimuli and bilateral extensor plantar responses.

2. Midbrain and upper pontine stage (Cheyne-Stokes respiration or central neurogenic hyperventilation; midposition, fixed, or irregular pear-shaped pupils; conjugate or dysconjugate deviation of the eyes on eye movement examination; decerebrate posturing or no response to painful stimuli). Definitive surgical therapy may allow survival; however, recovery is usually incomplete. Significant alteration in body temperature may be seen.

3. Lower pons and upper medullary stage (ataxic breathing, dilated and fixed pupils, no caloric response, no response to painful stimuli). As herniation progresses, the blood pressure falls, the pulse becomes irregular, and the patient dies. The prognosis for recovery from this stage is exceedingly poor.

Approach to the Comatose Patient

In the most common situation involving coma in the intensive care unit, the patient's case history is well known to those caring for the patient, yet there is either an abrupt or an insidious change in the level of consciousness. The question becomes whether there has been a new pathologic, structural event; whether all of the known metabolic abnormalities are sufficient to account for the patient's level of consciousness; or whether there is an unrecognized toxic or metabolic factor.

The most frequently encountered metabolic abnormalities that produce coma are ischemia or hypoxia, hypoglycemia, electrolyte disorders (particularly of sodium and calcium), elevation of the blood urea nitrogen level, and hepatic dysfunction. The most common mistake is to underestimate the significance of multiple, seemingly mild, metabolic abnormalities. The elderly, diabetic patient with known cerebrovascular disease may have a significant alteration in consciousness with a combination of relatively mild anemia and hypoxia, particularly if it evolves quickly. In addition, the recovery of the patient with compromised CNS reserve (cerebrovascular disease, dementia, long-standing substance abuse) may significantly lag behind correction of the metabolic factors and be incomplete.

Another common error is to accept a small, structural abnormality seen by computed tomography of the brain (e.g., a small rim subdural) as the sole explanation for the patient's alteration in consciousness. It is imperative to systematically review the reasonable diagnostic possibilities.

The first goal of the neurologic examination of the comatose patient is to identify whether there is evidence of structural damage of the CNS. When this information is combined with the history of the evolution of the disorder (insidious development vs. apoplectic onset), the patient's medical history (e.g., diabetes, cerebrovascular disease, and hypertension), and the progress since the onset, it is possible to identify the cause in the majority of cases. As previously mentioned, to explain a comatose state as resulting from a structural lesion, it must either directly affect the RAS in the brain stem or produce a mass effect with secondary impact on the RAS, as in uncal or central transtentorial herniation or herniation of the contents of the posterior fossa. The results of examination of the pupils and the extraocular movements are abnormal. The other diagnostic possibilities are that the patient had an unwitnessed seizure (postictal coma) or had an unwitnessed fall and sustained a traumatic brain injury. Alternatively, the cause of the coma may be toxic or metabolic in origin. An abrupt change in the level of consciousness from a normal, awake, alert state to coma is due to an unwitnessed generalized seizure or head injury, an unwitnessed cardiac arrest, or a posterior circulation vascular event.

Further studies of blood and urine, examination of the cerebrospinal fluid, imaging studies of the brain, and electrophysiologic studies provide confirmation of the diagnostic suspicion.

Lumbar puncture is a useful diagnostic test when infection or inflammatory processes and subarachnoid hemorrhage are diagnostic possibilities. Lumbar puncture should not be performed in the presence of a lesion with significant mass effect unless the information obtained is lifesaving. Electroencephalography is helpful in documenting ongoing, subclinical seizure activity in the comatose patient (most commonly after anoxia or ischemia) who has failed to improve. It is valuable in identifying and assessing the patient with a toxic metabolic insult to determine the severity of the insult. Computed tomographic scanning and magnetic resonance imaging may provide useful information (although magnetic resonance imaging may be difficult to obtain in a critically ill patient), which guides further therapy. The computed tomographic scan may appear deceptively normal in patients with diffuse axonal injury in brain trauma, even though soft tissue swelling is usually apparent. Diffuse cerebral edema or an isodense subdural hematoma may also not be immediately obvious to the untrained observer. Electroencephalography and evoked potentials, lumbar puncture, and imaging studies are described and discussed in detail elsewhere in this text.

Care of the Patient in Coma

Caring for comatose patients is far more challenging than caring for patients who are awake. They are unable to communicate their simplest needs and are completely vulnerable to their environment. The clinician is relied on to anticipate and administer appropriate diagnostic, therapeutic, and rehabilitative care.

The patient's eyes, if incompletely closed, should be lubricated with methylcellulose tears and tape applied to close them. The duration of endotracheal intubation should be carefully monitored owing to the long-term side effects associated with prolonged intubation. Sinusitis should be a consideration in fever of unknown origin in the intubated patient. A nasogastric tube should be inserted. Nutrition should be a primary concern early in the course of the illness because the nutritional needs of the critically ill patient are increased, particularly those with CNS compromise. Stress ulceration is a common complication in patients with CNS lesions and adequate prophylaxis should be undertaken. The CNS temperature-regulating mechanism may be compromised in the comatose patient, and hyperthermia and hypothermia should be rigorously corrected to within 1 to 2°C of normal level. Hyperthermia significantly increases the metabolic demand. Fluid and electrolyte balance should be carefully monitored and the bladder catheterized. Diabetes insipidus, central salt wasting, and inappropriate secretion of antidiuretic hormone may complicate the patient's course. The patient should be carefully positioned to avoid undue risk of aspiration, with care taken to avoid pressure sores, and the urogenital area should be kept clean and dry. Soft restraints may be necessary in some patients to avoid interference with maintenance of invasive catheters and monitors. The lower extremities should be examined daily for any evidence of thrombophlebitis and appropriate prophylactic measures should be taken. In situations in which the coma is prolonged, physical therapy should be administered to ensure full range of movement of the joints. Splints of the upper and lower extremities may be helpful.

Considerable interest has been generated in predicting outcome in comatose patients. The Glasgow Coma Scale, a scoring system based on the patient's best verbal, motor, and eye-opening responses, has some predictive capacity and is useful as a crude monitor of progress.[30] However, it is more informative to objectively document changes in neurologic deficits noted on prior examinations and to describe the patient's response to a particular sensory stimulus. Brain death and outcome after anoxic or ischemic injury are covered in detail in Chapter 56. The prediction of outcome using electrophysiologic measures such as electroencephalography and evoked potentials has shown some predictive capacity (see Chapter 54).

References

1. Plum F, Posner J: The Diagnosis of Stupor and Coma. 3d ed. Philadelphia, FA Davis, 1980.
2. Von Economo C: Encephalitis Lethargica. Its Sequelae and Treatment. New York, Oxford University Press, 1931.
3. Moruzzi G, Magoun H: Brainstem reticular formation and activation of the EEG. Electroencephalogr Clin Neurophysiol 1:455, 1949.
4. Pappas C, Carrion C: Altered levels of consciousness and the reticular activating system. Barrow Neurol Inst Q 5:2, 1989.
5. Kandel E, Schwartz J (eds): Principles of Neural Science. 2nd ed. New York, Elsevier Science Publishing, 1985.
6. Haines D: Neuroanatomy. An Atlas of Structures, Sections and Systems. Baltimore, Urban & Schwarzenberg, 1987.
7. McCandless D: Insulin-induced hypoglycemic coma and regional cerebral energy metabolism. Brain Res 215:225, 1981.
8. McCandless D: Cerebral Energy Metabolism and Metabolic Encephalopathy. New York, Plenum Publishing, 1985.
9. Siesjo B, Bengtsson F: Calcium fluxes, calcium antagonists, and calcium-related pathology in brain ischemia, hypoglycemia, and spreading depression: A unifying hypothesis. J Cereb Blood Flow Metab 9:127, 1989.
10. Siegel G, Agranoff B, Albers R, et al: Basic Neurochemistry. New York, Raven Press, 1989.
11. Malouf R, Brust J: Hypoglycemia : Causes, neurological manifestations and outcome. Ann Neurol 17:421, 1985.
12. Fischer K, Lees JA, Newman JH: Hypoglycemia in hospitalized patients. Causes and outcomes. N Engl J Med 315:1245, 1986.

13. Boyle P, Schwartz NS, Shah SD, et al: Plasma glucose concentrations at the onset of hypoglycemic symptoms with poorly controlled diabetes and in nondiabetics. N Engl J Med 318:1487, 1988.
14. Johannsson J, Siesjo B: Cerebral blood flow and oxygen consumption in the rat in hypoxia. Acta Physiol Scand 93:269, 1975.
15. Charness M, Simon R, Greenberg D: Ethanol and the nervous system. N Engl J Med 321:442, 1989.
16. Katayama Y, Becker D, Tamura T, et al: Massive increases in extracellular potassium and the indiscriminate release of glutamate following concussive brain injury. J Neurosurg 73:889, 1990.
17. Fraser C, Arieff A: Hepatic encephalopathy. N Engl J Med 313:865, 1985.
18. Cooper A, Plum F: Biochemistry and physiology of brain ammonia. Physiol Rev 67:440, 1987.
19. Zieve L: Pathogenesis of hepatic encephalopathy. Metab Brain Dis 2:147, 1987.
20. Fraser C, Arieff A: Nervous system complications in uremia. Ann Intern Med 109:143, 1988.
21. Caronna J, Simon R: The comatose patient: A diagnostic approach and treatment. Int Anesthesiol Clin 17(23):3, 1979.
22. Fisher CM: Neurological examination of the comatose patient. Acta Neurol Scand 45:5, 1969.
23. Brazis P, Masdeu J, Biller J: Localization in Clinical Neurology. Boston, Little, Brown, 1990.
24. Hawkes C: "Locked-in" syndrome: Report of seven cases. Br Med J 4:379, 1974.
25. Cherniak N, Longobardo G: Cheyne-Stokes breathing. An instability in physiologic control. N Engl J Med 288:952, 1973.
26. Brown H, Plum F: The neurologic basis of Cheyne-Stokes respiration. Am J Med 30:848, 1961.
27. Plum F, Swenson A: Central neurogenic hyperventilation in man. AMA Arch Neur Psychiat 81:535, 1959.
28. Plum F, Alvorn E: Apneustic breathing in man. Arch Neurol 10:101, 1961.
29. Selhorst J, Hoyt W, Feinsod M, et al: Midbrain corectopia. Arch Neurol 33:193, 1976.
30. Teasdale G, Jennett B: Assessment of coma and impaired consciousness. A practical scale. Lancet 2:81, 1974.

CHAPTER 56

Brain Damage from Cardiac Arrest: Pathophysiology, Intensive Care Unit Management, and Outcome, Including Brain Death

Michael P. Earnest

Anoxaemia not only stops the machinery but wrecks the machine.

J. S. Haldane[1]

That eloquent insight applies equally to anoxemia and cardiac arrest. When the heart ceases pumping, blood perfusion of the brain ceases. Within 10 seconds, the person loses consciousness, and in 20 seconds, cortical activity seen on the electroencephalogram (EEG) disappears. Four to 8 minutes' absence of cerebral perfusion causes permanent brain injury; longer periods can cause infarction of the entire brain.[2–4]

Cardiopulmonary resuscitation (CPR) has improved sur-

vival from cardiac arrest.[5–7] CPR has also created important medical and ethical problems for physicians treating brain-injured survivors. Even skillful resuscitation produces only partial brain perfusion. Thus, cardiac arrest frequently results in brain injury with clinical deficits ranging from transient mild confusion to deep coma caused by brain death.[8–10]

Conditions other than cardiac arrest also cause anoxic brain injury. Severe, prolonged hypotension, pure hypoxemia, hypoglycemia, status epilepticus, carbon monoxide or cyanide poisoning, and smoke inhalation injure the brain by hypoxic-ischemic mechanisms. The pathophysiology of the injury is different for each condition but the effects on the brain and resultant clinical syndromes are similar to those caused by cardiac arrest. The focus of this chapter is on cardiac arrest but the principles apply to all these related conditions. Important clinical differences are presented when appropriate.

ISCHEMIC-HYPOXIC BRAIN INJURY
Pathophysiology

The brain is composed of gray matter and white matter. The gray matter of the cerebral and cerebellar cortex, the hippocampus, and the deep cerebral and brain stem nuclei is the physiologically effective tissue of the brain. It is composed of neurons and supporting glial cells, mainly astrocytes. White matter of the brain is composed of axons in transit from the gray matter neurons, plus their myelin insulation. Normally, the metabolic rate and blood flow of gray matter are four to five times that of white matter.[11]

The adult human brain constitutes approximately 2% of body weight, but it receives 15% of cardiac output and utilizes 20% of total body oxygen consumption at rest[11] (Table 56–1). Ninety percent of the brain's energy requirement is generated by the oxidation of glucose, which produces the high-energy phosphate bonds necessary for cell metabolism.[12, 13] The brain has negligible stores of other energy sources.[11, 13] Cerebral blood flow depends on adequate cerebral perfusion pressure (i.e., the differential between systemic arterial pressure and intracranial pressure).[11]

At the cellular level, neurons are the most active brain cells. Like many other cells, they maintain large intracellular versus extracellular gradients of ions, especially sodium, potassium, and calcium, and they synthesize proteins for structural and enzymatic use. However, neurons are more

TABLE 56–1

NORMAL PHYSIOLOGIC AND METABOLIC CHARACTERISTICS OF HUMAN BRAIN

Energy process
  Oxidation of glucose to produce high-energy phosphate bonds
Metabolic rate
  Glucose—31 μmol/100 g/min
  Oxygen—156 μmol/100 g/min
  Total—20% of body oxygen consumption
Cerebral blood flow
  Average—55 mL/100 g/min
  Gray/white ratio—78:18 mL/100 g/min
  Total—15% of cardiac output

Data from Ginsberg MD: Cerebral circulation: Its regulation, pharmacology, and pathophysiology. In: Asbury AK, McKhann GM, McDonald WI (eds): Diseases of the Nervous System: Clinical Neurobiology. 2nd ed. Philadelphia, WB Saunders, p 989, 1992; and Plum F, Pulsinelli WA: Cerebral metabolism and hypoxic-ischemic brain injury. In: Asbury AK, McKhann GM, McDonald WI (eds): Diseases of the Nervous System: Clinical Neurobiology. 2nd ed. Philadelphia, WB Saunders, p 1002, 1992.

metabolically active because they also frequently transmit electrical impulses. With each impulse, large transmembrane ion shifts occur, after which the neuron must restore normal gradients. With each discharge, neurons also release and reabsorb neurotransmitters, the chemical messengers that excite or inhibit other neurons. Because of their high metabolic activity, neurons are uniquely susceptible to damage by ischemia, hypoxia, or hypoglycemia.[2]

Pathologic Changes

Of all brain cells, neurons show the greatest pathologic effects of ischemia. Within 15 minutes of total brain ischemia in the rat, visible pathologic changes begin.[14] The earliest change is vasculolation in the cell body cytoplasm. These vacuoles are grossly swollen mitochondria and endoplasmic reticulum.[14] More advanced changes of ischemic neuronal damage include shrinkage and dark staining (with hematoxylin-eosin technique) of the cell body and nucleus.[12, 14, 15] The most severe damage is shown by fragmentation of the nucleus and homogeneous, pale staining of the entire cell.[12, 14] White matter shows pathologic changes only in severe anoxia. Those include cytoplasmic swelling of glial cells and degeneration of myelin.[12]

A characteristic of ischemic-hypoxic brain injury is selective vulnerability of certain groups of neurons. Regions most vulnerable to injury are the hippocampus in the mesial temporal lobes; layers III, V, and VI of the cerebral neocortex; the Purkinje cells of the cerebellum; and portions of the basal ganglia.[12, 14, 16] Other neurons are more resistant to injury, and glial cells, especially in white matter, are the most resistant to injury.

Global ischemia, severe hypoxia, severe hypoglycemia, and status epilepticus produce identical cellular changes and a similar selective vulnerability distribution of injury in the brain.[12, 14, 15] In each clinical condition, the hippocampus and deeper cortical layer neurons show the most severe damage. In hypoglycemia, however, the cerebellar injury is less prominent.[16] Carbon monoxide poisoning has an unusual potency to cause necrosis in the basal ganglia and to cause more severe, widespread white matter injury.[2, 15, 17]

Severe and prolonged global ischemia, hypoxemia, hypoglycemia, and related processes can produce total neuronal destruction throughout the entire cerebral cortex. This pathologic condition and the accompanying clinical syndrome have been called "neocortical death."[18] The most severe result of ischemic-hypoxic injury is total necrosis of the entire brain, including the brain stem. That is the pathologic correlate of the clinical syndrome of brain death.[2, 19]

A different pathophysiology can produce other lesions. Prolonged partial, but inadequate, perfusion of the brain can cause focal brain infarctions (strokes). This is most commonly seen after protracted shock; intraoperative hypotension, especially during cardiopulmonary bypass; and prolonged CPR in elderly patients. In those circumstances, blood perfusion of the brain tissue most distal in the cerebrovascular system falls below the level necessary to maintain tissue viability so infarction occurs. These watershed, or boundary zone, infarcts are usually in the lateral and superior cerebral hemispheres where the most distal anterior, middle, and posterior cerebral artery branches supply the cortex.[8, 12] Watershed lesions often coexist with the more diffuse ischemic-hypoxic neuronal injury. Less commonly, a typical middle cerebral artery or other single-vessel cerebral infarction occurs. That occurs when the hypotension precipitates occlusion or severely impaired perfusion through a previously stenotic atherosclerotic cerebral artery.

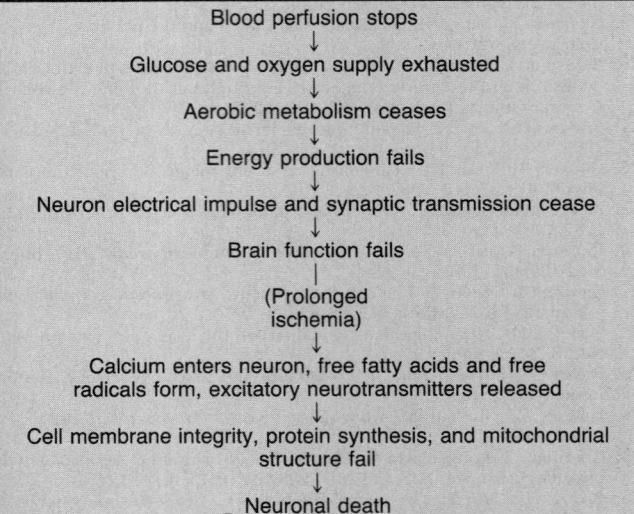

TABLE 56–2

PATHOPHYSIOLOGY OF ISCHEMIC-HYPOXIC NEURONAL INJURY

Blood perfusion stops
↓
Glucose and oxygen supply exhausted
↓
Aerobic metabolism ceases
↓
Energy production fails
↓
Neuron electrical impulse and synaptic transmission cease
↓
Brain function fails
|
(Prolonged ischemia)
↓
Calcium enters neuron, free fatty acids and free radicals form, excitatory neurotransmitters released
↓
Cell membrane integrity, protein synthesis, and mitochondrial structure fail
↓
Neuronal death

Mechanisms of Neuronal Injury

Ischemic injury of the brain is a multiple-mechanism injury. Table 56–2 summarizes the probable major events. In concept, there are two phases of ischemic-hypoxic neuronal injury: (1) failure of membrane potential, neurotransmission, and other physiologic functions and (2) irreversible damage to membrane, protein, nucleotide, and other structures leading to neuronal death.[2, 3] Failure of adequate oxygen and glucose supply leads to exhaustion of the neuron's high-energy phosphate bonds. Transmembrane electrolyte gradients cannot be maintained and so electrical transmission fails and release and reuptake of neurotransmitters cease. Thus, the neuron's physiologic functions halt.[2] If blood perfusion and the oxygen and glucose supply to the cell are restored, the neuron can again generate energy and resume function.

The point at which reversible dysfunction becomes irreversible injury is unknown, and the mechanisms are unclear. The process probably is multifactorial. A likely important factor is intracellular calcium accumulation. Failure of membrane function allows calcium to enter. That, in combination with the release of calcium from the endoplasmic reticulum, produces high cytoplasmic calcium levels. Calcium activates lipid peroxidases, which break down intracellular and membrane lipids, producing toxic free fatty acids and highly reactive free radicals.[4, 20, 21, 52, 54] These in turn produce more free fatty acids and free radicals, which may lead to eventual cell destruction.[4, 13, 20, 21]

Research has also suggested important roles for local tissue lactic acidosis, release of excitatory neurotransmitters, and reactive ferrous iron.[2, 20, 22–25] Other research has identified that irreversible cellular injury probably does not occur immediately.[23, 26] Animal studies suggest that some neuronal functions can survive up to an hour of global ischemia.[2, 26] There is growing evidence that postanoxic events may cause delayed cell death.[2, 24, 27] Delayed hypoperfusion of the cerebral cortex and failure of reopening of the cerebral microvasculature after severe ischemia, the no-reflow phenomenon, have been implicated.[28, 29]

The discovery of prolonged survival of neuronal activity after severe ischemic injury and of delayed, progressive tissue damage has raised hope of intervening to halt or reverse postischemic neuronal damage. Studies have focused on use of barbiturates, calcium channel blockers, excitatory neurotransmitter antagonists, and aggressive improvement of brain perfusion after cardiac arrest.[21, 22, 30-33]

A clinically important secondary consequence of global brain ischemia is brain swelling. Two important pathologic results of ischemia are cellular swelling, probably caused by failure of the membrane to control osmotic ion gradients, and increased permeability of the blood-brain barrier.[2, 14, 34] Thus, severe global ischemia can produce delayed brain swelling, increased intracranial pressure, and brain herniation, leading to further injury and even brain death.

MANAGEMENT OF CARDIAC ARREST

Protection of the Brain During Cardiac Arrest

Preventing or minimizing brain injury during cardiac arrest depends solely on physiologically effective CPR. Maintenance of blood oxygenation and sustained cerebral perfusion are critical to the survival of brain cells. Prompt restoration of normal cardiac rhythm, blood pressure, ventilation, and brain perfusion are essential. Hyperglycemia may aggravate the cellular effects of brain ischemia, so high blood glucose levels (e.g., > 300 mg/dL) probably should be avoided.[2, 35]

General Medical Management

No specific pharmacologic or clinical intervention has been shown to retard or reverse brain injury from global ischemia attributable to cardiac arrest. The best treatment to aid brain recovery is to maintain optimal PaO_2, blood glucose level, and cerebral perfusion (Table 56-3). Careful ventilator and pulmonary management ensures optimal PaO_2 and $PaCO_2$. There is no evidence that hyperoxygenation improves brain recovery, but the author favors maintenance of a high PaO_2 to provide good brain oxygenation at all times. The $PaCO_2$ probably should be maintained in the normal physiologic range. Hypercapnia may increase intracranial pressure and tissue acidosis.[2, 11] Hypocapnia causes intracranial vascular constriction and so may be harmful.[11] Blood glucose concentrations should probably also be maintained in the normal range. Hypoglycemia impairs neuronal function, and hyper-

---

TABLE 56-3

PROTECTION OF THE BRAIN DURING AND AFTER CARDIAC ARREST

During Cardiac Arrest
Perform effective CPR to perfuse the brain
Restore optimal blood oxygenation and glucose

After Cardiac Arrest
Medical Issues
Maintain optimal oxygenation, blood glucose level, and normal $PaCO_2$
Treat hypotension and fever
Avoid brain-depressant drugs
Avoid excessive hydration
Neurologic Issues
Rule out noncardiac causes of cardiac arrest, especially toxins, and intracranial hemorrhage
Follow neurologic signs: level of consciousness, brain stem reflexes, and focal signs
Treat clinically significant increased intracranial pressure with hyperventilation, osmotic diuretics, dexamethasone, and renal diuretics
Treat convulsions and clinically significant myoclonus with phenytoin and other drugs as necessary

---

glycemia has been implicated in aggravating ischemic brain injury.[2, 13, 16, 27]

Prompt treatment of systemic complications may reduce their impact on brain recovery. High fever increases brain metabolism and intracranial pressure, thus further impairing brain function. Many medications depress brain function and so reduce spontaneous ventilation and impair protective cough and gag reflexes. Drugs and dehydration may cause hypotension and reduced brain perfusion. Fluid overload may cause cardiac and pulmonary complications, hypoxia, and further brain injury.

The general management of the unconscious patient after cardiac arrest is the same as that of any patient in coma (see Chapter 55).

Neurologic Management

Patients admitted to an intensive care unit for cardiac arrest generally have an unequivocal history of a sudden cardiac and respiratory arrest. However, other medical conditions may present as apparent cardiac arrest. Any general medical condition severe enough to cause unconsciousness may result in ventilatory failure, hypoxia, hypercapnia, acidosis, and a secondary cardiac arrest. Likewise, drug overdose and carbon monoxide or cyanide poisoning may present as a cardiac arrest. Intracranial hemorrhage, especially subarachnoid, intraventricular, cerebellar, or brain stem hemorrhage, can present with arrhythmias or cardiac arrest. Whenever the clinical history, physical findings, or course of the patient are atypical for primary cardiac arrest, appropriate laboratory tests may yield an unexpected diagnosis.

The most important aspect of neurologic management of the unconscious postarrest patient is repeated careful observation of the neurological signs by intensive care unit physicians and nurses. The most effective system is to have the nurses observe a standard set of neurologic signs regularly (e.g., every 2 to 4 hours). The nurses record those observations on the intensive care unit flow sheet, along with the routine vital signs, cardiac and ventilatory variables, and laboratory values. The physician reviews the neurologic observations and confirms them by examination as necessary.

The first sign to be observed is the patient's level of consciousness. The clinical course of that sign is an important indicator of the patient's prognosis. In addition, any worsening of the level of consciousness may indicate delayed brain swelling or an occult general medical problem that is further impairing brain function. The level of consciousness is best observed in a standardized, reproducible fashion. Terms such as lethargic, semicomatose, and obtunded should not be used. The Glasgow Coma Scale has been widely used in the observation and care of patients with brain trauma.[36] That scale or some similar set of observations can be easily used by intensive care unit nurses. Its basic features include noting the patient's best level of responsiveness to verbal and painful stimuli as indicated by eye opening, vocal responses, and limb movement. Those observations can be reproduced and recorded sequentially throughout the clinical course.

The second set of neurologic observations determines the level of brain stem function by examining the major brain stem reflexes. Those include pupillary light reaction, extraocular movements, corneal blink reflex, facial movement (grimace), and gag and cough reflexes. Table 56-4 describes how to elicit and interpret those signs properly. Other brain stem signs may be noted in patients who are not deeply comatose. Spontaneous roving eye movements, subtle eyelid opening, grimacing, chewing (especially on an endotracheal tube), and tongue protrusion may occur.

Other types of neurologic signs to be sought are focal

TABLE 56–4

BRAIN STEM REFLEX EXAMINATION IN POST–CARDIAC ARREST COMA

Reflex	Cranial Nerves	Active Reflex	Technical Aspects
Pupillary	II, III	Pupil constricts	Bring bright flashlight close to pupil; may use magnifying glass to see reaction of small pupils.
Oculocephalic (doll's eyes)	III, VI, VIII	Eyes lag or drift behind movement	Use brisk full lateral rotation of head to each side.
Oculovestibular (caloric)	III, VI, VIII	Eyes deviate toward the stimulated ear	Infuse 40–50 mL of ice water over 20 s into external ear canal.
Corneal	V, VII	Eyelid closure	Use strong stimulus on cornea and observe closely for ipsilateral and contralateral eyelid movement.
Nasal stimulus	V, VII	Facial grimace or eyelid movement	Use cotton or tissue stimulus to each nostril. If nasal tube is in place, move it briskly.
Facial grimace	V, VII	Grimace or eyelid movement	Induce pain by firm thumbnail pressure on glabella and eyebrow ridges.
Auditory	VII, VIII	Eyelid movement	Use loud clap or other noise close to each ear.
Gag	IX, X	Pharyngeal, tongue, or mouth movement	*Do not perform* if there is possibility of vomiting and aspiration. If done, use strong pharyngeal stimulus, such as moving endotracheal and gastric tubes.
Cough	VII, IX, X, XII	Face, mouth, pharynx, tongue, body movements	Briskly move endotracheal tube or pass suction tube into trachea.
Respiratory	X, somatic (thoracic) nerves	Respiratory effort	See text and Table 56–9.

signs. Those are cranial nerve, limb movement, tone, or reflex signs that are significantly different on one side of the body compared with the other side. In the setting of cardiac arrest, focal signs usually indicate a cerebral infarction, usually of the watershed type.

Management of Intracranial Pressure

The incidence of clinically important brain swelling after cardiac arrest is unknown. However, clinical experience indicates that some patients have delayed deterioration of their level of consciousness, usually 24 to 48 hours after cardiac arrest. Some develop signs of brain stem dysfunction (e.g., dilated, sluggish pupils). In that clinical setting a computed tomographic (CT) scan of the head usually demonstrates severe, diffuse swelling of the cerebral hemispheres with transtentorial brain herniation. That finding is an ominous sign of impending brain stem destruction and subsequent brain death.

Unfortunately, no treatments are known that reliably prevent brain swelling after global ischemic injury. Use of corticosteroids is recommended by some authors.[37] However, others advise against their use.[2] There is no credible medical evidence that steroids prevent postanoxic brain edema. They can complicate the patient's metabolic management and increase infection risk, so the author does not recommend their routine use. Likewise, hyperventilation and osmotic or renal diuretics are not routinely used.

Some clinical measures may decrease the incidence and severity of postanoxic brain edema, but none has been studied specifically. The clinical setting most often foretelling severe brain swelling is the patient who has undergone prolonged CPR, especially when complicated by post–cardiac arrest hypotension, acidosis, or hypoxemia. In such high-risk patients, measures to minimize brain swelling include careful fluid management to keep the patient mildly dehydrated; elevation of the patient's head about 30° to improve venous drainage of the brain; minimal use of tracheal suctioning (tracheal suctioning can cause strong motor reactions that impede venous return); vigorous management of hypercapnia and fever, both of which increase

intracranial pressure; and avoidance of positive end-expiratory pressure, which impedes cerebral venous outflow. Obviously cardiogenic shock, pulmonary edema, or other immediate medical problems may preclude using these measures.

An important measure for managing brain edema is early identification. Careful sequential observation of the neurologic signs is required. If the patient's level of consciousness declines, pupillary or extraocular movement signs worsen, or papilledema appears, a prompt CT scan is required to determine if there is brain swelling. If transtentorial herniation is present, aggressive treatment should be given. Immediate treatment includes hyperventilation to maintain the $Paco_2$ at 25 to 30 mm Hg and administration of an osmotic diuretic, usually mannitol, 0.5 to 1.0 g/kg of body weight by rapid intravenous infusion. A corticosteroid bolus (dexamethasone, 10 mg intravenously) and a renal diuretic (furosemide, 20 to 40 mg intravenously) may also be given. Such aggressive management usually reverses transtentorial herniation for several hours. Repeated doses of mannitol, dexamethasone, and furosemide may be required, usually approximately half of the initial dose every 4 to 8 hours. Nonetheless, brain swelling with increased intracranial pressure after cardiac arrest indicates severe ischemic-anoxic neuronal and white matter injury. Even if the elevated intracranial pressure is reversed, the patient rarely awakens or regains useful cognitive functions.

Management of Seizures and Myoclonus

Occasionally, patients in post–cardiac arrest coma have multifocal, quick, twitching jerks (myoclonus) of the face, eyes, limbs, or trunk. They are asymmetric, asynchronous, and irregular in their timing. Such multifocal myoclonus frequently is accompanied by generalized (grand mal) seizures. The EEG in this setting usually is severely abnormal with multifocal or generalized periodic epileptiform discharges.[38, 39] Seizures and myoclonus may be almost continuous. There is no truly effective treatment for such acute postanoxic seizures and myoclonus.[38, 39] Intravenous lorazepam (2 to 10 mg) in combination with a full phenytoin

(Dilantin) load (15 to 18 mg/kg in 250 mL of normal saline administered during 30 minutes) sometimes reduces or stops the convulsions. Limited clinical experience and theoretic considerations suggest that valproic acid per rectum may be an effective therapy. Some authors recommend high-dose barbiturates, clonazepam, or 5-hydroxytryptophan.[37] However, myoclonus and seizures after cardiac arrest signify widespread, severe cortical injury. The literature and personal experience indicate that survival is uncommon.[38, 39]

A rare syndrome of delayed posthypoxic action myoclonus can be disabling. The striking feature is severe limb, trunk, or even pharyngeal myoclonic jerks precipitated by efforts to move the limb, walk, swallow, or speak.[40, 41] Therapeutic success has been claimed for clonazepam, valproic acid, and 5-hydroxytryptophan.[40]

Use of Neurologic Tests

Laboratory tests have a limited role in the neurologic management of the post–cardiac arrest coma patient. However, selected patients should have some appropriate testing. Patients with suspected intracranial lesions causing the cardiac arrest and those thought to have brain infarcts attributable to the arrest should have a brain imaging test. The most practical imaging test is a CT scan, which reliably demonstrates intracranial hemorrhage and most brain infarctions. The major limitation of the CT scan in this setting is its failure to demonstrate superficial cortical watershed infarcts. A contrast-enhanced CT scan using intravenous contrast medium, done 5 to 7 days after the arrest, may demonstrate the suspected infarctions. A magnetic resonance imaging scan is a more elective, secondary procedure. The magnetic resonance imaging scan more reliably shows superficial cortical infarctions and white matter injury. Magnetic resonance imaging takes more time, requires a medically stable patient, and cannot be done easily on a mechanically ventilated patient.

The EEG has a time-honored history of use in coma from cardiac arrest.[42–44] There is reasonably good correlation between EEG characteristics and clinical outcome. However, it probably does not add any prognostically valuable information to the clinical neurologic examination. The EEG, in the author's opinion, should be used only for cases with seizures and in cases of suspected brain death. Cortical evoked potentials have been studied in coma after cardiac arrest. Some authors claim good correlation with outcome.[45] However, they offer no clear value beyond careful clinical observation of the neurologic signs.

A lumbar puncture often discloses minor nonspecific changes in the cerebrospinal fluid after cardiac arrest, usually elevated protein level and slightly increased white blood cell count. The lumbar puncture has no role in the routine management of cardiac arrest. If subarachnoid hemorrhage or meningitis is suspected as a primary event, a lumbar puncture should be done. Elevated creatine kinase concentration of brain origin has been found in the cerebrospinal fluid of comatose patients after cardiac arrest.[46] The clinical value of that finding has yet to be established.

Carbon Monoxide Intoxication

Carbon monoxide causes brain dysfunction and injury by displacing oxygen from hemoglobin, by reducing oxygen release from hemoglobin, and by impairing biochemical function of the cytochrome oxidase energy system.[15, 17] Patients with severe brain dysfunction, especially those with loss of consciousness, should be treated with hyperbaric hyperoxygenation to reverse acute carbon monoxide effects on the brain and to prevent subsequent postintoxication neuropsychiatric symptoms.[47–50] Some authors recommend treatment of even patients with apparently modest intoxication to prevent the delayed sequelae.[47]

NEUROLOGIC OUTCOME FROM CARDIAC ARREST
Survival

Patients with out-of-hospital cardiac arrest have an in-hospital mortality of 45 to 60%[6, 51] (Table 56–5). In-hospital cardiac arrest patients have better survival rates than those experiencing out-of-hospital cardiac arrest. Increased mortality is related to advanced age, prior congestive heart failure, and noncardiac disease, especially prior neurologic disease.[51, 52] Delay of starting CPR, delay of electrical cardioversion, and prolonged CPR also worsen the prognosis for survival.[51–53] The majority of in-hospital deaths after cardiac arrest are due to general medical complications; they are not primarily neurologic deaths (i.e., brain death). Patients in coma for 6 hours or more after cardiac arrest have a high mortality, 64% at 1 week, 90% at 1 year.[10]

Neurologic Sequelae

Neurologic impairment from the ischemia-anoxia of cardiac arrest can range from no clinical signs to brain death. The severity of the neurologic outcome depends mainly on how long the brain was ischemic (i.e., the time required to

TABLE 56–5

SURVIVAL AND NEUROLOGICAL OUTCOME AFTER CARDIAC ARREST

Reference	Patients*	N	Survival	Best Recovery†
Earnest et al.[9, 16]	Out-of-hospital admitted to intensive care unit	117	45% survived to hospital discharge (at mean of 14.3 d)	21% normal plus 13% did some self-care at discharge from hospital
Levy et al.[10]	Hypoxic-ischemic injury (71% CA) in coma ≥ 6 h	210	36% lived 1 wk; 10%, 1 y	13% regained independent function in 1 y
Mullie et al.[63]	Out-of-hospital CA admitted to intensive care unit	360	31% lived 14 d	17% at "prearrest status," 8% with moderate disability at 14 d
Snyder[64–66]	CA admitted to coronary care unit	63	75% lived 5 d, 40% lived to discharge from hospital	25% fully independent, 13% needed minimal assistance at 6 mo
Willoughby and Leach[67]	In-hospital CA	53	64% lived 2 wk	47% neurologically normal at 2 wk

*CA = cardiac arrest.
†Recovery percentages are based on total number.

effect CPR, achieve cardioversion, and restore adequate cerebral perfusion). Patients in whom the cardiac rhythm and normal blood pressure are restored promptly have brief loss of consciousness and a short period of amnesia for the events of the arrest but usually are neurologically and cognitively intact.

More protracted brain ischemia causes various clinical syndromes. Patients who have modest brain ischemia may have brief (minutes to hours) postarrest unconsciousness and then confusion that can last several days. Some of those patients have a prolonged or even permanent amnestic syndrome, with prolonged post–cardiac arrest (anterograde) and pre–cardiac arrest (retrograde) amnesia, and decreased ability to recall newly presented information.[9, 54, 55] Those deficits may be due to selective injury to the hippocampus. Severe global brain ischemia produces coma, whose duration is directly related to the severity and the duration of reduced cerebral perfusion. Patients who awaken after 12 hours or longer of coma often have a severe, global confusional state that results in a permanent dementia, usually with prominent amnestic features. Those patients also often have bilateral motor signs, including hyperreflexia, hypertonic limbs, severe clumsiness of movements, ataxia, and weakness. Some have signs of parkinsonism, probably resulting from basal ganglia injury. They can rarely function independently and usually require placement in long-term care or support with home health care services.

A more severe form of permanent diffuse brain injury is the persistent vegetative state, also called neocortical death, akinetic mutism, coma vigile, or apallic syndrome.[18, 56] A valid definition and accurate descriptor of this syndrome is eyes-open unresponsiveness. These patients usually are in prolonged coma after cardiac arrest but eventually begin to have eye opening. They may also demonstrate sleep-wake cycles. However, they do not speak, respond to commands, make apparently volitional movements, or show any signs of awareness of their surroundings.[18, 56, 57] They do not respond to rehabilitative therapies and usually require placement in nursing homes. Prognosis for long-term recovery is poor, although there are case reports of late recovery of some mental function.[58, 59] Mortality is more than 70% in 5 years.[58]

The most severely brain-damaged patients never have eye opening or show any signs of awakening. Most of them die in the hospital of cardiac, pulmonary, or infectious complications. Some progress to brain death.

Other neurologic sequelae may be superimposed on the global brain impairments. Focal brain infarctions can be of either the watershed or conventional middle cerebral or other large artery varieties. A typical presentation of watershed infarcts attributable to cardiac arrest occurs as the patient begins to awaken slowly, and he or she cannot move his or her arms or hands. This bibrachial paresis is due to bilateral ischemic infarction of the arm areas of the motor cortex in the boundary zone between the middle and ante-

rior cerebral arteries. Other varieties of focal infarction can occur, including typical middle cerebral artery distribution infarcts.

Seizures are uncommon as a long-term consequence of anoxic injury. Action myoclonus may be disabling but fortunately is rare.[40] A Parkinson's disease–like syndrome can occur, more commonly after carbon monoxide injury.[8, 17] Secondary delayed progressive neurologic deficits have been reported, sometimes associated with degeneration of the cerebral white matter.[60] The course usually is self-limited, but motor and cognitive impairment may be severe. This postanoxic leukoencephalopathy seems to be more common after carbon monoxide poisoning.[17, 50, 60]

Prediction of Neurologic Outcome

The neurologic prognosis after cardiac arrest has been extensively studied[9, 10, 35, 61–67] (see Table 56–5). However, even the largest series do not provide sufficient data to enable accurate prediction of the eventual outcome of most individual patients in coma after cardiac arrest.[68] Moreover, any prediction of neurologic outcome must be tempered by the caveat that medical events, including a second cardiac arrest, hypotension, hypoxia, renal failure, and sepsis, may further damage the brain.

Nonetheless, some basic guidelines can be derived from clinical experience and reported studies (Table 56–6). First, patients who have only brief loss of consciousness or who are awake and talking within a few hours of the cardiac arrest have a high probability (greater than 75%) of a return to normal neurologic function.[61, 64, 67] Many have some confusion for a short period; a small minority have a longer-term amnestic syndrome.[54] Second, patients in coma undergoing ventilation who have absent brain stem functions, including pupillary light reflexes, corneal reflexes, spontaneous or ice water–induced extraocular movements, gag reflex, or cough reflex to tracheal suctioning, at 24 hours have a low chance (probably <1%) of a good recovery.[10, 61, 66] The author and most studies accept as a good recovery the ability to live somewhat independently, including some self-care and the ability to interact with others verbally.[9, 10] Medical conditions such as shock, hypoxemia, hypoglycemia, and drugs that depress nervous system function or cause muscular paralysis must be ruled out before accepting such a morbid prognosis. A third general guideline relies on the duration of unconsciousness. The longer the post–cardiac arrest coma lasts, the higher the mortality and the lower the chance of a good recovery.[10, 61, 64] Unconsciousness (i.e., the absence of eye opening, verbal responses, or voluntary movement) for longer than 48 hours, in the absence of brain edema or complicating systemic medical conditions and medication, denotes a small likelihood (probably <5%) of returning to independent functioning.[61, 64]

For patients whose early recovery falls between prompt awakening and absent brain stem functions at 24 hours or coma at 48 hours, the prediction of neurologic recovery is inexact. The best clinical approach to determining the outcome of those patients is to let the patient's course itself demonstrate the outcome. Table 56–7 summarizes a reasonable clinical management paradigm. Laboratory tests do not enable better prediction in most cases. The EEG has been extensively studied in anoxic encephalopathy, and EEG findings correlate with outcome.[43, 44] However, the EEG activity does not accurately predict outcome in any single patient, except in the setting of clinical brain death. Likewise, abnormalities of cortical evoked potentials correlate with outcome but have not been adequately validated.[45] However, severe abnormalities or absence of EEG or evoked potentials activity can be helpful as physiologic markers of poor out-

TABLE 56-7
PRACTICAL CLINICAL DECISION MAKING ABOUT NEUROLOGIC PROGNOSIS AFTER CARDIAC ARREST
First 48 h
Give all appropriate treatments.
Do not give prognosis (in absence of brain death).
At 48 h
Assess level of consciousness and brain stem signs.
Rule out superimposed metabolic, toxic, or drug processes.
If deep coma is present or brain stem reflexes are absent, probability of good recovery is low.
If patient is in poor prognosis category, discuss limiting care.
If patient is not in poor prognosis state, continue full care.
Beyond 48 h
Assess level of consciousness and brain stem signs daily.
Make daily decision about level of care.

come. The data are complementary to the bedside clinical observations and so increase the confidence in predicting a poor outcome. As with the neurologic evaluation, the presence of central nervous system–depressing medical conditions and drugs must be ruled out before interpreting the EEG and evoked potentials.

BRAIN DEATH

Medical Concept

Brain death is a consequence of medical progress. CPR, mechanical ventilation, and intensive medical care now resuscitate and maintain patients who previously would have experienced cardiorespiratory death. After several decades of clinical research and ethical and legal debate, the concept of brain death is almost universally recognized in the Western world.[19, 69–71] A widely accepted definition is "irreversible cessation of all functions of the entire brain, including the brain stem."[70]

The three primary lesions most commonly causing brain death are severe head trauma, cerebrovascular disease, and anoxic encephalopathy, usually from cardiac arrest.[19, 70–74] Intracranial infections, metabolic disorders, toxins, and tumors are less frequent causes.[19, 72, 74] The clinical syndrome is that of deep coma with total absence of any signs of brain function.[70, 72, 73] The neuropathologic correlate of clinical brain death is complete or almost complete necrosis of all intracranial brain tissue.[19, 71, 72]

The pathophysiology of brain death has not been well defined. Three modes of total brain destruction probably account for most cases. First, the primary condition (e.g., ischemic-hypoxic injury) is so severe that all brain tissue is infarcted. A second mechanism occurs when the primary process (e.g., trauma, hypoxia, and intracranial hemorrhage) causes severe brain edema. The swelling then causes bilateral cerebral infarction and transtentorial herniation with subsequent infarction of the brain stem and the cerebellum. A third mechanism also relates to brain swelling. A severe primary lesion may cause diffuse brain edema, which results in increased intracranial pressure that exceeds cerebral perfusion pressure. At that moment, blood flow to the intracranial space ceases and the whole brain is infarcted. No studies have defined the relative frequencies of these mechanisms. The author believes that the third mechanism is the most common, although frequently it is preceded by signs of transtentorial brain herniation as well.

Brain death must be distinguished from several other forms of severe brain injury.[19, 69, 70] Deep coma with some retained brain stem reflexes is not brain death; the presence of even one brain stem reflex rules out brain death. The persistent vegetative state was described earlier. It is the eyes-open unresponsive state resulting from widespread cerebral cortical destruction.[18, 56, 57] However, deep cerebral structures and the brain stem are functional. Destruction of the brain stem by hemorrhage, infarction, trauma, or pressure from a cerebellar mass lesion can produce deep coma and total absence of brain stem reflexes.[73, 75] However, the cerebral hemispheres are functional, so brain death is not present. Rare patients with these severe but non–brain death conditions have an unexpectedly good recovery.[59, 73] The diagnosis of brain death implies no possibility of any recovery of brain function.

Clinical Diagnosis

The diagnosis of brain death rests on demonstration of two cardinal features: (1) no function of the entire brain, including the brain stem; and 2) an irreversible condition.[70, 73] Table 56–8 summarizes the essential criteria.

Demonstration of absence of function of the brain begins by documentation of deep coma with no responses to multiple stimuli. The initial stimuli are auditory (e.g., loudly calling the patient's name into each ear, then a loud hand clap next to each ear). Next painful stimuli are applied to the face (e.g., with firm thumbnail pressure into the superior orbital rim and bridge of the nose). Similar painful pressure and skin pinching stimuli are applied to each limb and the trunk. The presence of brain activity is shown by eye opening, eyelid blinking, facial grimacing, and head, trunk, or limb movement. Even rudimentary limb or trunk extension movements (so-called decerebrate posturing) or arm flexion plus leg extension movements (decorticate posturing) are signs of brain activity and preclude the diagnosis of brain death.

The one type of motor activity that can persist in brain death is spinal reflex activity.[69, 70, 73] Thus, persisting deep tendon reflexes or the triple-flexion response to painful stimulation of the foot does not preclude a diagnosis of brain death. The triple-flexion reflex, which includes the classic Babinski's toe response plus knee flexion and hip flexion, can appear to be voluntary withdrawal from pain and so may confuse the assessment for brain death. However, the full triple-flexion response usually occurs only with stimuli on the foot and is stereotyped. Voluntary withdrawal can be induced by painful stimuli to multiple sites and is variable (i.e., the movement is appropriate to move the limb away from the painful stimulus).

Skillful evaluation of brain stem reflexes is an essential step in the clinical determination of brain death. Important techniques of the brain stem evaluation (e.g., cranial nerve reflex) include the use of powerful stimuli, bilateral testing methods, and examination of all available cranial nerve reflexes. The reflexes examined and techniques used are

TABLE 56-8
CRITERIA TO DETERMINE BRAIN DEATH
Clinical cause known and sufficient to cause destruction of the entire brain, including the brain stem
Patient in deep coma, no alerting or motor response to any stimulus
Absent brain stem reflexes, including no ventilatory effort
Hypotension, hypothermia, drugs, and other CNS-depressing processes ruled out
Appropriate period of repeated observations to prove irreversible condition
Confirming laboratory tests can be helpful but not required

TABLE 56–9
RIGOROUS TEST FOR APNEA IN DETERMINING BRAIN DEATH

Hyperoxygenate using 100% inspired oxygen for 10 min before test.
Establish normal $Paco_2$ (i.e., do not hyperventilate).
Obtain arterial blood gas measurements to ensure high Pao_2 and normal $Paco_2$.
Disconnect mechanical ventilation.
Place endotracheal cannula to deliver 100% oxygen at 8 L/min.
Observe for ventilatory movements or in-and-out endotracheal airflow.
If ventilatory activity occurs or cardiac arrhythmia or hypotension supervene, terminate test.
If no ventilatory activity occurs in 8 to 10 min, terminate test (apnea is confirmed).
Obtain arterial blood gas values before restoring ventilation to ensure that $Paco_2$ reached 50–60 mm Hg.

Adapted from Schafer JA, Caronna JJ: Duration of apnea needed to confirm brain death. Neurology 28:661, 1978; and Ropper AH, Kennedy SK, Russell L: Apnea testing in the diagnosis of brain death. J Neurosurg 55:942, 1981.

described in Table 56–4. The presence of any reflex at all confirms residual brain stem activity (i.e., brain death has not occurred).

Careful testing for apnea (i.e., absent medullary ventilatory reflexes) is necessary but somewhat controversial.[76–79] Surveys of neurologists and neurosurgeons find that most clinicians identify apnea by simply disconnecting the mechanical ventilator for 3 minutes or less.[76, 77] If no respiratory effort or endotracheal tube airflow is observed, the presence of apnea is considered confirmed. That method probably is adequate for the large majority of cases in which the other signs of brain death have already been established. However, disconnection of the ventilator in some cases induces hypoxemia, bradycardia, and hypotension, risking further brain damage. In such cases and in cases with particular ethical, legal, or medical features, such as those involving children, homicides or other medicolegal issues, and potential organ donors, a more rigorous test should be used (Table 56–9). The more rigorous test ensures adequate blood oxygenation and produces a strong hypercapnic stimulus of the medullary respiratory centers.[78, 79]

Demonstration of irreversibility of the brain injury depends on three factors that require some clinical judgment.[70] The cause of the brain injury must be known and must be sufficient, in the physician's judgment, to cause total, irreversible brain destruction. The diagnosis of brain death should be made with caution in cases in which the cause of brain dysfunction is unknown. The second aspect of irreversibility requires that reversible medical conditions known to depress brain function be ruled out.[69, 70] Drugs that depress central nervous system function, ongoing hypoxia or hypotension, severe metabolic disorders, hypothermia, and medical conditions or drugs that cause total muscular paralysis can obscure residual brain function. These conditions must be ruled out or, if present, reversed before a diagnosis of brain death can be made. Practical clinical experience, however, allows the diagnosis of brain death in the presence of low levels of central nervous system–depressant drugs, hypoxia, hypotension or other medical conditions that cannot be reversed with maximal therapy, or mild hypothermia.[69, 70]

Finally, the absence of clinical signs of brain function should be confirmed during a period of observation.[69, 70] The length of this period is not fixed and depends on the physician's judgment. A second clinical examination 12 to 24 hours after the first is probably best. Shorter periods of observation are appropriate in some cases (e.g., head trauma with obvious physical destruction of most of the brain) or when laboratory tests (e.g., EEG or arteriogram) confirm the diagnosis.[70] Longer periods of observation are warranted when the cause of brain injury is unclear, when the known cause is hypoxia or another metabolic or toxic condition, when there are important legal issues, and when the patient is a child. The diagnosis of brain death in children and infants is more difficult because of the greater resilience of the immature brain.[42, 71] Consultation by a neurologist, neurosurgeon, or other clinician experienced in the determination of brain death is prudent in most cases of suspected brain death.

Confirmatory Laboratory Tests

The EEG has long been viewed as an important test to confirm the absence of cerebral electrophysiologic activity in cases of suspected brain death.[69, 80, 81] The diagnostic finding is electrocerebral silence or a flat line pattern (i.e., no observable cortical activity).[80, 81] However, continuing experience with the EEG in suspected brain death has revealed that it has distinct limitations. In cases fulfilling all other clinical criteria for brain death, rudimentary cortical activity can be seen in up to 20%.[82] In addition, correct performance and interpretation of the EEG require strict adherence to special techniques of recording and knowledge of the many artifacts that may falsely appear to be brain activity or that may obscure true brain activity.[80, 81] Discussions of the diagnosis of brain death view the EEG as an ancillary and helpful test but not required.[70, 73, 81]

Other tests may be helpful. The demonstration of absence of blood flow to the entire brain is believed to confirm brain death. That can be shown by conventional cranial arteriograms, transcranial Doppler ultrasound scans, xenon-flow cranial CT scans, or radionuclide blood flow techniques.[73, 83–87] Cortical evoked potential testing, especially brain stem auditory evoked potentials and somatosensory evoked potentials, have been used as confirmatory tests.[73, 81] However, there are insufficient data to support their routine use.[81]

Confirmatory tests are not required to diagnose brain death.[70] They are especially appropriate and helpful if the clinical signs cannot be elicited (e.g., when facial trauma or edema impair the examination of cranial nerve signs) or if there is concern that the brain stem alone has been damaged, leaving the cerebral hemispheres functional. Confirming tests probably should be used in individuals who are potential organ donors, those whose cases involve important legal issues, and children. Rigorous technique, extensive clinical experience, and expert interpretation are necessary for valid use of any confirmatory test in suspected brain death.

Management After Declaration of Brain Death

After brain death is declared, the general practice is to discontinue all life-support measures, including mechanical ventilation. A reasonable and sensitive practice is to inform the family of the diagnosis and the plan to discontinue support. Nursing staff can remove unnecessary tape, tubes, and monitors and otherwise can improve the patient's physical appearance. The family, if they desire, can make a final visit.

When disconnecting the ventilator it is most appropriate that the family not be present. The physician should be aware, and should warn nursing and resident staff, that in some cases of brain death disconnecting ventilation precipitates active, complex arm, leg, and trunk movements.[88, 89] This Lazarus sign is not voluntary but probably is due to multisegmental motor reflex activity of the upper spinal cord.[88] Such movements create psychologic distress for observers but do not negate the diagnosis of brain death, nor do they necessitate resumption of mechanical ventilation.

Some patients with suspected brain death, especially those who are younger and who have had isolated brain injury (e.g., trauma and intracranial hemorrhage), should be evaluated as potential donors of organs or tissues. There is an urgent need for such donors throughout the United States.[90] Multiple organs and tissues can be used to benefit other patients. After the potential for donation is recognized, and the patient's family is consulted, the proper organ or tissue acquisition program should be contacted, even before brain death is declared. If the case is judged appropriate as a donor and proper consent is obtained, careful management of the hemodynamic, ventilatory, and fluid balance status after the declaration of brain death is required to properly maintain the desired organs.[90]

Legal and Ethical Issues

Brain death is recognized in most Western nations, both by statutes and by scholars, as death of the individual.[70, 73] Thus, physicians may legally and ethically discontinue ventilatory and all other support measures in individuals who are declared brain dead. Concerns about physicians' risking criminal charges are no longer valid. Likewise, the declaration of brain death in cases of brain injury from criminal gunshot wounds or other violence does not protect an assailant from charges of homicide.[91]

Statutes recognizing brain death as personal death usually do not define the criteria by which brain death is diagnosed.[70, 91] Rather, most state that the determination "must be made in accordance with reasonable medical standards."[70, 73] Definition of those standards is left to physicians. Most statutes suggest but do not require confirmatory laboratory tests.

Acknowledgments. Drs. Thomas Neff and Polly Parsons contributed helpful comments and reviews. Ms. Denise Lovator provided excellent secretarial assistance.

References

1. Haldane JS: Quoted by: Barcroft J: Anoxaemia. Lancet 2:485, 1920.
2. Plum F, Pulsinelli WA: Cerebral metabolism and hypoxic-ischemic brain injury. In: Asbury AK, McKhann GM, McDonald WI (eds): Diseases of the Nervous System: Clinical Neurobiology. 2nd ed. Philadelphia, WB Saunders, p 1002, 1992.
3. Schneider M: Survival and revival of the brain in anoxia and ischemia. In: Gastaut H, Meyer JS (eds): Cerebral Anoxia and the Electroencephalogram. Springfield, IL, Charles C Thomas, p 134, 1961.
4. Seisjo BK: Cell damage in the brain: A speculative synthesis. J Cereb Blood Flow Metab 1:155, 1981.
5. Bedell SE, Delbanco TL, Coor EF, et al: Survival after cardiopulmonary resuscitation in the hospital. N Engl J Med 309:569, 1983.
6. Eisenberg MS, Hallstrom A, Bergher L: Long term survival after out-of-hospital cardiac arrest. N Engl J Med 306:1340, 1982.
7. Thompson RG, Hallstrom AP, Cobb LA: Bystander-initiated cardiopulmonary resuscitation in the management of ventricular fibrillation. Ann Intern Med 90:737, 1979.
8. Maiese K, Caronna JJ: Neurological complications of cardiac arrest. In: Aminoff MJ (ed): Neurology and General Medicine—The Neurological Aspects of General Medical Disorders. New York, Churchill Livingstone, p 145, 1989.
9. Earnest MP, Yarnell PR, Merrill SL, et al: Long-term survival and neurologic status after resuscitation from out-of-hospital cardiac arrest. Neurology 30:1298, 1980.
10. Levy DE, Caronna JJ, Singer BH, et al: Predicting outcome from hypoxic-ischemic coma. JAMA 253:1420, 1985.
11. Ginsberg MD: Cerebral circulation: Its regulation, pharmacology, and pathophysiology. In: Asbury AK, McKhann GM, McDonald WI (eds): Diseases of the Nervous System: Clinical Neurobiology. 2nd ed. Philadelphia, WB Saunders, p 989, 1992.
12. Brierley JB, Graham DI: Hypoxia and vascular disorders of the nervous system. In: Adams JH, Corsellis JAN, Duchen LW (eds): Greenfield's Neuropathology. 4th ed. New York, John Wiley & Sons, p 124, 1984.
13. Raichle ME: The pathophysiology of brain ischemia. Ann Neurol 13:2, 1983.
14. Duchen LW: General pathology of neurons and neuroglia. In: Adams JH, Corsellis JAN, Duchen LW (eds): Greenfield's Neuropathology. 4th ed. New York, John Wiley & Sons, p 1, 1984.
15. Schneck SA: Cerebral anoxia. In: Baker AB, Joynt RJ (eds): Clinical Neurology, Volume 2. Philadelphia, Harper & Row, p 1, 1985.
16. Ng T, Graham DI, Adams JH, et al: Changes in the hippocampus and the cerebellum resulting from hypoxic insults: Frequency and distribution. Acta Neuropathol 78:438, 1989.
17. Ginsberg MD: Carbon monoxide intoxication: Clinical features, neuropathology and mechanisms of injury. Clin Toxicol 23:281, 1985.
18. Brierley JM, Adams JH, Graham DI, et al: Neocortical death after cardiac arrest—A clinical, neurophysiological, and neuropathological report of two cases. Lancet 2:560, 1971.
19. Walker AE: Cerebral Death. 2nd ed. Baltimore, Urban & Schwarzenberg, p 97, 1981.
20. Chan PH, Fishman RA: Free fatty acids, oxygen free radicals, and membrane alterations in brain ischemia and injury. In: Plum F, Pulsinelli WA (eds): Cerebrovascular Diseases: Fourteenth Princeton-Williamsburg Research Conference on Cerebrovascular Diseases. New York, Raven Press, p 161, 1985.
21. Seisjo BK, Wieloch T: Molecular mechanisms of ischemic brain damage: CA^{2+}-related events. In: Plum F, Pulsinelli WA (eds): Cerebrovascular Diseases: Fourteenth Princeton-Williamsburg Research Conference on Cerebrovascular Diseases. New York, Raven Press, p 187, 1985.
22. Clark GD: Role of excitatory amino acids in brain injury caused by hypoxia-ischemia, status epilepticus and hypoglycemia. Clin Perinatol 16:459, 1989.
23. Petito CK, Feldman E, Pulsinelli WA, et al: Delayed hippocampal damage in humans following cardiorespiratory arrest. Neurology 37:1281, 1987.
24. Rothman S, Olney JW: Glutamate and the pathophysiology of hypoxic-ischemic brain damage. Ann Neurol 19:105, 1986.
25. Pulsinelli WA, Kraig RP, Plum F: Hyperglycemia, cerebral acidosis and ischemic brain damage. In Plum F, Pulsinelli WA (eds): Cerebrovascular Diseases: Fourteenth Princeton-Williamsburg Research Conference on Cerebrovascular Diseases. New York, Raven Press, p 201, 1985.
26. Hossmann KA, Bodsch W, Ophhoff BG: Recovery of electrophysiological function and protein synthesis in monkey brain after prolonged ischemia. In: Plum F, Pulsinelli WA (eds): Cerebrovascular Diseases: Fourteenth Princeton-Williamsburg Research Conference on Cerebrovascular Diseases. New York, Raven Press, p 173, 1985.
27. Pulsinelli WA, Brierley JB, Plum F: Temporal profile of neuronal damage in a model of transient forebrain ischemia. Ann Neurol 11:491, 1982.
28. Ames A, Wright RL, Kowada M, et al: Cerebral ischemia II. The no-reflow phenomenon. Am J Pathol 52:437, 1968.
29. White BC, Winegar CP, Henderson O, et al: Prolonged hypoperfusion in the cerebral cortex following cardiac arrest and resuscitation in dogs. Ann Emerg Med 12: 414, 1983.
30. Brain Resuscitation Clinical Trial I Study Group: Randomized clinical study of thiopental loading in comatose survivors of cardiac arrest. N Engl J Med 314:397, 1986.
31. Simon RP, Swan JH, Griffiths T, et al: Blockade of N-methyl-D-aspartate receptors may protect against ischemic damage in the brain. Science 226:850, 1984.
32. Kirsch JR, Dean JM, Rogers MC: Current concepts in brain resuscitation. Arch Intern Med 146:1413, 1986.
33. Safar P: Resuscitation after brain ischemia. In: Grenvik A, Safar P (eds): Brain Failure and Resuscitation. New York, Churchill Livingstone, p 155, 1981.
34. Olesen S-P: Rapid increase in blood-brain barrier permeability during severe hypoxia and metabolic inhibition. Brain Res 368:24, 1986.
35. Longstreth WT, Diehr P, Cobb LA, et al: Neurologic outcome and blood glucose levels during out-of-hospital cardiopulmonary resuscitation. Neurology 136:1186, 1986.
36. Teasdale G, Jennett B: Assessment of coma and impaired consciousness: A practical scale. Lancet 2:81, 1974.
37. Adams RD, Victor M: Principles of Neurology. 4th ed. New York, McGraw-Hill, p 850, 1989.
38. Celesia GG, Grigg MM, Ross E: Generalized status myoclonicus in acute anoxic and toxic-metabolic encephalopathies. Arch Neurol 45:781, 1988.
39. Jumao-as A, Brenner RP: Myoclonic status epilepticus: A clinical and electroencephalographic study. Neurology 40:1199, 1990.
40. Fahn S: Post-hypoxic action myoclonus: Review of the literature and report of two new cases with response to valproate and estrogen. Adv Neurol 26:49, 1979.
41. Lance JW, Adams RD: The syndrome of intention or action myoclonus as a sequel to hypoxic encephalopathy. Brain 86:111, 1953.
42. Kohrman MH, Spivack BS: Brain death in infants: Sensitivity and specificity of current criteria. Pediatr Neurol 6:47, 1990.
43. Prior PF: The EEG in Acute Cerebral Anoxia. Amsterdam, Excerpta Medica, 1973.
44. Scollo-Lavizzari G, Bassetti C: Prognostic value of EEG in post-anoxic coma after cardiac arrest. Eur Neurol 26:161, 1987.
45. Brunko E, deBeyl DZ: Prognostic value of early cortical somatosensory evoked potentials after resuscitation from cardiac arrest. Electroencephalogr Clin Neurophysiol 66:15, 1987.

46. Mikell RG, Massey TH: Assessment of neurological damage: Creatine kinase-BB assay after cardiac arrest. Heart Lung 17:247, 1988.
47. Mathieu D, Nolf M, Durocher A, et al: Acute carbon monoxide poisoning—Risk of late sequelae and treatment by hyperbaric oxygen. Clin Toxicol 23:315, 1985.
48. Myers RA, Snyder SK, Emhoff TA: Subacute sequelae of carbon monoxide poisoning. Ann Emerg Med 14:1163, 1985.
49. Raphael J-C, Elkharrat D, Jars-Guincestre M-C, et al: Trial of normobaric and hyperbaric oxygen for acute carbon monoxide intoxication. Lancet 2:414, 1989.
50. Choi IS: Delayed neurologic sequelae in carbon monoxide intoxication. Arch Neurol 40:433, 1983.
51. Hallstrom AP, Cobb LA, Swain M, et al: Predictors of hospital mortality after out-of-hospital cardiopulmonary resuscitation. Crit Care Med 13:927, 1984.
52. Weaver WD, Cobb LA, Hallstrom AP, et al: Considerations for improving survival from out-of-hospital cardiac arrest. Ann Emerg Med 115:1181, 1986.
53. Brain Resuscitation Clinical Trial I Study Group: Neurologic recovery after cardiac arrest: Effect of duration of ischemia. Crit Care Med 13:930, 1985.
54. Finkelstein S, Caronna JJ: Amnestic syndrome following cardiac arrest. Neurology 28:389, 1978.
55. Maiese K, Jennings E, Baynes K, et al: Persistent cognitive impairment in cardiac arrest survivors. Ann Neurol 24:131, 1988.
56. Jennett B, Plum F: Persistent vegetative state after brain damage: A syndrome in search of a name. Lancet 1:734, 1972.
57. Council on Scientific Affairs and Council on Ethical and Judicial Affairs: Persistent vegetative state and the decision to withdraw or withhold life support. JAMA 263:426, 1990.
58. Higashi K, Hatano M, Abiko S, et al: Five-year follow-up study of patients with persistent vegetative state. J Neurol Neurosurg Psychiatry 44:552, 1981.
59. Roenberg GA, Johnson SF, Brenner RP: Recovery of cognition after prolonged vegetative state. Ann Neurol 2:167, 1977.
60. Plum F, Posner JB, Hain RF: Delayed neurological deterioration after anoxia. Arch Intern Med 110:56, 1962.
61. Earnest MP, Breckinridge JC, Yarnell PR, et al: Quality of survival after out-of-hospital cardiac arrest: Predictive value of early neurological evaluation. Neurology 29:56, 1979.
62. Longstreth WI, Diehr P, Inui TS: Prediction of awakening after out-of-hospital cardiac arrest. N Engl J Med 308:1378, 1983.
63. Mullie A, Verstringe P, Buylaert W, et al: Predictive value of Glasgow coma score for awakening after out-of-hospital cardiac arrest. Lancet 1:137, 1988.
64. Snyder BD, Loewenson RB, Gumnit RJ, et al: Neurologic prognosis after cardiopulmonary arrest: II. Level of consciousness. Neurology 30:52, 1980.
65. Snyder BD, Hauser WA, Loewenson RB, et al: Neurologic prognosis after cardiopulmonary arrest: III. Seizure activity. Neurology 30:1292, 1980.
66. Snyder BD, Gumnit RJ, Lappik IE, et al: Neurologic prognosis after cardiac arrest: IV. Brainstem reflexes. Neurology 31:1092, 1981.
67. Willoughby JO, Leach BG: Relation of neurological findings after cardiac arrest to outcome. Br Med J 3:437, 1974.
68. Shewmon DA, DeGiorgio CM: Early prognosis in anoxic coma—Reliability and rationale. Neurol Clin 7:823, 1989.
69. Ad Hoc Committee of the Harvard Medical School to Examine the Definition of Brain Death: A definition of irreversible coma. JAMA 205:337, 1968.
70. Medical Consultants on the Diagnosis of Death to the President's Commission for the Study of Ethical Problems in Medicine and Biomedical and Behavioral Research: Guidelines for the determination of death. JAMA 246:2184, 1981.
71. Task Force for the Determination of Brain Death in Children: Guidelines for the determination of brain death in children. Arch Neurol 44:587, 1987.
72. A Collaborative Study: An appraisal of the criteria of cerebral death. JAMA 237:982, 1977.
73. Black PMcL: Guidelines for the diagnosis of brain death. In: Ropper AK, Kennedy SF (eds): Neurological and Neurosurgical Intensive Care. 2nd ed. Rockville, MD, Aspen Publishers, p 323, 1988.
74. Takeuchi K, Takeshita H, Takakura K, et al: New Japanese criteria of brain death. Neurosurg Rev 12(suppl 1):265, 1989.
75. Ferbert A, Buchner H, Ringelstein EB, et al: Brain death from infratentorial lesions: Clinical neurophysiological and transcranial Doppler ultrasound findings. Neurosurg Rev 12(suppl 1):340, 1989.
76. Black PM, Zervas NT: Declaration of brain death in neurosurgical and neurological practice. Neurosurgery 15:170, 1984.
77. Earnest MP, Beresford HR, McIntyre HB: Testing for apnea in suspected brain death: Methods used by 129 clinicians. Neurology 36:542, 1986.
78. Ropper AH, Kennedy SK, Russell L: Apnea testing in the diagnosis of brain death. J Neurosurg 55:942, 1981.
79. Schafer JA, Caronna JJ: Duration of apnea needed to confirm brain death. Neurology 28:661, 1978.
80. Silverman D, Saunders MG, Schwab RS, et al: Cerebral death and the electroencephalogram: Report of the ad hoc committee of the American Electroencephalographic Society on EEG criteria of cerebral death. JAMA 209:1505, 1969.
81. Chatrian G-E: Coma, other states of altered responsiveness, and brain death. In: Daly DD, Pedley TA (eds): Current Practice of Clinical Electroencephalography. 2nd ed. New York, Raven Press, p 425, 1990.
82. Grigg MM, Kelly MA, Celesia GG, et al: Electroencephalographic activity after brain death. Arch Neurol 44:948, 1987.
83. Darby JM, Yonas H, Gur D, et al: Xenon-enhanced computed tomography in brain death. Arch Neurol 44:551, 1987.
84. Laurin NR, Driedger AA, Hurwitz GA, et al: Cerebral perfusion imaging with technetium-99m HM-PAO in brain death and severe central nervous system injury. J Nucl Med 30:1627, 1989.
85. Patel YP, Gupta SM, Batson R, et al: Brain death: Confirmation by radionuclide cerebral angiography. Clin Nucl Med 13:438, 1988.
86. Petty GW, Molvi JP, Pedley TA, et al: The role of transcranial Doppler in confirming brain death: Sensitivity, specificity, and suggestions for performance and interpretation. Neurology 40:300, 1990.
87. Ropper AH, Kehne SM, Wechsler LS: Transcranial Doppler in brain death. Neurology 37:1733, 1987.
88. Heytens L, Verlooy J, Gheuens J, et al: Lazarus sign and extensor posturing in a brain-dead patient—Case report. J Neurosurg 71:449, 1989.
89. Ropper AH: Unusual spontaneous movements in brain-dead patients. Neurology 34:1089, 1984.
90. Darby JM, Stein K, Grenvik A, et al: Approach to management of the heartbeating "brain dead" organ donor. JAMA 261:2222, 1989.
91. Cranford RE: Minnesota enacts a brain death law. Minn Med 72: 717, 1989.

CHAPTER 57

Cerebrovascular Disease

Steven R. Levine
Nabih M. Ramadan

The pathophysiology of acute human cerebrovascular disease (CVD) has revealed that time is critical for the effective diagnosis and treatment of stroke. This chapter briefly reviews, with particular emphasis to the intensive care specialist, the clinical features of both ischemic and hemorrhagic CVD, including diagnosis, pathophysiology, investigations, and management.

FOCAL CEREBRAL ISCHEMIA IN THE INTENSIVE CARE UNIT

Overview

Cognitive or behavioral change, language dysfunction, acute agitation, delirium, isolated psychiatric disturbance, and visual loss, even in the absence of focal weakness or hemiplegia, may be due to focal brain ischemia.[1-4] Symptoms of CVD depend on the location of the lesion (Table 57–1).

Acute CVD without motor weakness is especially important to recognize in the intensive care unit (ICU) patient, who is generally restrained; who has intra-arterial, intravenous, or central venous indwelling catheters for acute medical or surgical monitoring; and who may be intubated. Several factors should raise suspicion of ischemic CVD. The ICU patient may have several stroke risk factors: hypertension, hyperlipidemia, cigarette smoking, diabetes mellitus, previous stroke, and cardiac disease. Cardiac disease may

TABLE 57–1
MAJOR CLINICAL FEATURES OF STROKE

Left Cerebral Hemisphere	Right Cerebral Hemisphere	Brain Stem
Language disturbance (aphasia)	Hypoarousal, neglect	Dysarthria or dysphagia
Right side of body weakness	Left side of body weakness	Bilateral weakness or ataxia
Right side of body sensory loss	Left side of body sensory loss	Bilateral sensory loss
Right visual field deficit	Left visual field deficit	Vertigo, nystagmus, diplopia
Eyes deviated to left	Eyes deviated to right	Skew deviation
Confusion	Agitation, delirium, confusion	Drowsiness, loss of consciousness

predispose to cerebral embolism or cerebral hypoperfusion secondary to arrhythmia or pump failure. Acutely ill medical or surgical patients are stressed and are therefore at risk for coagulopathy. Hypercoagulable states (including disseminated intravascular coagulation) can lead to an increased tendency for thrombotic stroke.[5, 6] Patients in the ICU are often receiving multiple medications; iatrogenic hypotension can result in hypoperfusion and secondary cerebral ischemia in the setting of fixed atherosclerotic extracranial or intracranial occlusive disease.[7–9]

Clinical Assessment

The term stroke implies an immediate event. Not infrequently, however, the onset of cerebral ischemia can be gradual, fluctuating (wax and wane), stepwise, or steadily progressing.[10–14] Embolization to the brain (predominantly from the heart or the extracranial precerebral vessels) is generally manifested as an acute event. However, up to 30% of patients with a clinical, computed tomographic (CT), or angiographic diagnosis of embolic CVD often have a nonacute onset. Thrombotic occlusion of either large extracranial vessels or small intracranial perforating vessels ("lacunar" stroke) may occur acutely, but it generally presents in a gradual, stepwise, or fluctuating fashion.[12, 14–16] Vertebrobasilar (posterior circulation) ischemia, in contrast to carotid (anterior circulation) territory ischemia, more often has a fluctuating course for a longer period before the patient's neurologic deficit stabilizes.[11, 12, 17] Therefore, it is important to obtain a complete history of the temporal evolution of the symptoms. This may be difficult in the ICU, particularly for a patient who is intubated and has an altered sensorium. It is imperative to question the family, nurses, and other medical personnel to determine the exact time when the patient was last functioning at a baseline status. The nursing notes provide valuable clues to the temporal sequence of events and thus aid in the differential diagnosis.

Because neurologic deterioration from CVD or other causes is not unusual in ICU patients, a thorough baseline neurologic evaluation should be performed, ideally by a neurologist or neurointensivist. Sudden blood pressure changes, especially during or after invasive procedures, may be a vital clue to the cause of cerebral ischemia. A hypotensive episode may significantly impair brain perfusion.[1, 7–10, 18] Hypertensive encephalopathy may also impair cerebral blood flow.[1] CVD may manifest as focal seizures or status epilepticus.[8, 19] Ischemic CVD as a cause of status epilepticus may be more likely in the post–cardiac surgery patient.

Maximal deficit at onset, without a history of transient ischemic attack, suggests that embolism is the most likely mechanism of stroke.[14] In contrast, atherothrombotic strokes are more often preceded by transient ischemic attacks.[16, 20] When symptoms and signs occur serially or stepwise, the diagnosis of stroke in evolution, progressing stroke, or deteriorating stroke may be made.[10, 12] Transient ischemic attacks generally last less than 1 hour.[21]

Although the majority of patients in the ICU cannot leave the bed and walk unassisted as part of the neurologic examination, most of the bedside neurologic examination can be performed to assess the location and severity of the lesion most accurately. Limb-immobilizing restraints should be removed to evaluate range of motion, tone, bulk, reflexes, coordination, strength, and posture in the extremities. Although tedious and at times extremely difficult, proper mental status and cognitive function testing, including orientation, memory, attention, and language, should be performed with all patients with neurologic symptoms who are capable of being tested. Whenever possible, it is extremely useful to have the patient write, draw, and perform tests of visual and spatial perception. These tasks are often ignored on casual, informal, or incomplete tests of higher cognitive functions. Evidence for extensive nondominant or posterior hemisphere damage in the absence of weakness may be provided by a complete assessment of cognitive functions.

The signs and symptoms of clinical stroke syndromes can be easily found in several stroke textbooks.[10, 11, 14] The major features are summarized in Table 57–1, and predominant mechanisms are summarized in Table 57–2. All acute ischemic events in the ICU should be categorized by location and mechanism to identify the most likely pathophysiology and thus treatment. A few important concepts will be briefly reviewed.

Two predominant mechanisms that produce cerebral ischemia in the carotid artery territory are impaired perfusion distal to a stenosed or occluded internal carotid artery, either extracranially or intracranially,[18] and embolic occlusion.[15, 16, 20] Ulceration of an atheromatous plaque with subsequent emboli may occur in the presence of even minimal, nonstenosing atheroma.[14, 22] Carotid artery syndromes are summarized in Table 57–3. At the bedside, an absent common carotid pulse in the neck, prominence of ipsilateral facial pulses, an ipsilateral bounding, superficial, temporal artery pulse, or a bruit may provide evidence for significant stenosis or occlusion of the ipsilateral internal carotid artery.[14]

When collateral flow is compromised or incomplete through pial anastomotic branches or the circle of Willis, the border zones (areas of the brain between territories of the major cerebral vessels) may be involved.[23] These watershed regions are between the middle cerebral artery (MCA) and anterior cerebral artery (anterior border zone), the MCA and posterior cerebral artery (posterior border zone), and the deep and superficial territory of the MCA. Ischemia in

TABLE 57–2
MAJOR MECHANISMS OF ISCHEMIC STROKE

Embolism	Hemodyamic (watershed, distal field)
Cardiac	Vasculopathic
Artery to artery	Hypertension
Paradoxical	Diabetes
Aortic arch	Inflammation
Thrombosis	Dissection
Atherosclerotic	
Coagulopathic	

TABLE 57–3
MAJOR CLINICAL SYNDROMES THAT MAY BE REFERABLE TO THE CAROTID ARTERY
Amaurosis fugax
Ocular infarction
Central retinal artery occlusion
Ischemic optic neuropathy
Hemispheric transient ischemic attacks
Hemispheric infarction
Watershed infarction

TABLE 57–4
MAJOR CAUSES OF IN-HOSPITAL CEREBRAL ISCHEMIA OR HYPOXIA
Systemic hypotension
Acute severe hypertension
Shock
Air embolism
Cardiac disease, including arrest
Thrombosis
Airway obstruction
Obesity
Pulmonary disease
Thoracic cage injury or deformity
Anemia
Systemic hemorrhage
Anesthesia

a border zone area may cause transcortical aphasias (repetition preserved) when present in the dominant hemisphere, among other well-characterized syndromes that occur when other border zones are affected:[14, 23, 24] partial or complete cortical blindness, bilateral arm weakness ("man in the barrel" syndrome), and tetraparesis. These syndromes are most commonly seen after cardiac arrest and secondary to hypotension-induced hypoperfusion, which are not infrequent in the ICU setting. Acute MCA syndromes including isolated aphasia are usually embolic.[10, 25] Primary in situ thrombosis from atherostenosis of the MCA is uncommon;[14, 25] however, coagulopathy may be an alternative mechanism in the ICU.

In-Hospital Strokes

CVDs occurring in the ICU constitute in-hospital strokes. In this category, there is a relatively high incidence of embolic stroke.[7] In-hospital CVD is often associated with invasive diagnostic or surgical procedures, especially related to cardiovascular or peripheral vascular disease.[7, 26, 27] Other causes of in-hospital CVD, particularly in the ICU, are summarized in Table 57–4. Other specific neurovascular complications of anesthesia include hypertensive encephalopathy,[28] transient global amnesia,[29] cerebral subdural hematoma,[30] headache,[30] and spinal cord infarction.[30]

The risk of developing a stroke secondary to diagnostic and surgical procedures may reflect not only the type and quality of the procedure but also the nature and extent of the disease being investigated.[7] Hypotension is a common cause of in-hospital stroke, especially in patients who are chronically hypertensive, with impaired cerebral autoregulation.[10] These patients should *not* have their blood pressure lowered to the normal range when they develop cerebral ischemia associated with increased blood pressure. A stroke that occurs before arrival at the hospital may worsen in the emergency room or in the ICU by overzealous treatment of hypertension. Clinical worsening occurs primarily because cerebral perfusion becomes pressure dependent in ischemic tissue with disrupted cerebral autoregulation.[10] Blood pressure in acute stroke victims generally falls on its own, without treatment, in the first 4 days after the ictus.[31]

The prevention of cerebral ischemia in the ICU may be enhanced by careful attention to hemodynamic, metabolic, and hemostatic parameters. Specific measures to reduce the substantial incidence of in-hospital stroke[7] include careful screening of surgical candidates, avoidance of significant hypotension in patients at risk for stroke (including hypertensive patients), and judicious use of anticoagulant therapy in patients with a cardiac source of embolus. Embolic strokes (Fig. 57–1) are associated with chronic atrial fibrillation, cardioversion, acute myocardial infarction (MI), mitral valve replacement for rheumatic heart disease, mural thrombus, bacterial endocarditis, and cardiac catheterization. There is an association between thrombotic strokes, carotid bruits, and significant carotid stenosis. Patients with in-hospital CVD generally have one or more of the risk factors of stroke: cardiac source of embolus, previous stroke, diagnostic or therapeutic procedures for vascular disease, and chronic hypertension complicated by acute hypotension. One study[7] found that a 30-day case fatality rate for in-hospital stroke was 19% and total mortality at follow-up (average 59 days) was 27%.

Stroke complicating acute MI in 740 consecutive patients admitted to the ICU has been studied.[32] Patients who subsequently suffered stroke had a 61% mortality rate. Patients who did not have a stroke had a 13% mortality rate. Sixty-seven percent of the strokes occurred in the first week after MI, and 90% occurred by the end of the second week. Three

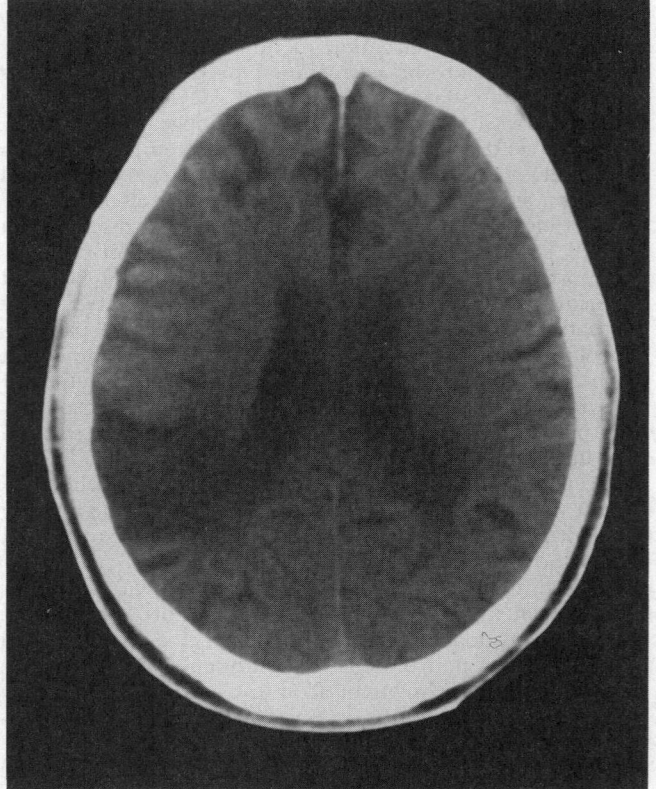

Figure 57–1. CT scan of the head, without contrast infusion, demonstrating a right posterior middle cerebral artery territory cardioembolic infarction.

quarters of the strokes were in the carotid distribution. Most were considered embolic. Risk factors associated with developing stroke in the ICU were *atrial* arrhythmias, cardiac pump failure, apical or anterolateral MI, and history of previous stroke. Ventricular arrhythmias were not significantly associated with the development of stroke.

The median time to the occurrence of stroke after MI ranges from 4 to 8 days.[32, 33] Causes of stroke complicating MI include cardiogenic cerebral emboli, hypotension, simultaneous coronary and cerebrovascular thrombosis secondary to poor perfusion, and coagulopathy.[32–35]

Intensive Care Unit Procedures Associated with Stroke

Several invasive diagnostic and therapeutic procedures have been associated with ischemic strokes.[36–38] These include declotting of Scribner's arteriovenous dialysis shunts with retrograde cerebral embolism and subclavian venipunctures resulting in cerebral embolus, including air embolus. Subclavian venipunctures may result in inadvertent subclavian artery puncture or inadvertent placement of the needle and catheter into the common carotid artery. Cardiac catheterization is a well-documented cause of embolic stroke, including isolated neuro-ophthalmologic syndromes[39] from the aorta, heart, extracranial precerebral vessels, or catheter tip (platelet-fibrin thrombus).

Natural History of Acute Stroke in Patients Admitted to Acute Stroke Unit

Of 1073 consecutive stroke patients admitted to an acute stroke unit, the 30-day mortality rate was 20%.[40] Deaths in the first week were primarily from transtentorial herniation. Deaths in the second through the fourth weeks occurred from pneumonia, pulmonary embolus attributable to the patient's relative immobility, and sepsis. Cardiac causes of death occurred throughout the month. The *degree* of neurologic deficit rather than the *type* of cerebrovascular lesion appeared to be more important in determining short-term outcome.[41]

Three simple bedside tests are predictive of eventual outcome: upper limb motor function, postural function, and proprioception.[42] These three tests compared well to a more detailed examination and may serve as a fairly reliable estimate of outcome.

PATHOPHYSIOLOGY OF FOCAL CEREBRAL ISCHEMIA

Obstruction of a cerebral or precerebral artery by atherothrombotic material or clot is the most common pathologic substrate for focal cerebral infarction. Acute cerebral ischemia has been demonstrated angiographically to be generally caused by thromboembolic occlusion of an intracranial artery.[43] Truly acute clinical and angiographic correlations are much more precise than when angiography is performed days after the ictus. Atherosclerosis is the most common underlying vascular process leading to ischemic stroke. As the brain requires a constant supply of glucose and oxygen, arterial obstruction deprives cerebral tissue of substrate and eventually leads to an area of infarction or cell death. The degree to which the collateral cerebral circulation can supply flow to impaired brain regions determines both the final zone of infarction and the "penumbra," potentially viable region. Neuronal function and viability are highly dependent on the minute-to-minute values of cerebral blood flow (CBF). Potentially reversible clinical deficits have been demonstrated

experimentally to occur when CBF falls below about 23 mL/100 g/min,[44] and electroencephalographic changes occur clinically when CBF falls below about 18 mL/100 g/min.[45] Most data suggest that CBF of approximately 10 to 12 mL/100 g/min causes irreversible damage if prolonged beyond 2 to 3 hours and may cause no or minimal damage if its duration is less than 2 hours. Generally, infarction proceeds when CBF of 18 mL/100 g/min persists for longer than 34 hours, and it may be extremely difficult, if at all possible, to save the brain when cerebral arterial occlusion persists beyond 4 to 6 hours. The longer the arterial occlusion, the more likely the penumbral region surrounding the core of the ischemic zone will also infarct.[46]

Investigations and Approach to Cerebrovascular Disease in the Intensive Care Unit

After a clinical diagnosis of focal CVD has been made, the patient should be evaluated diagnostically to determine the type and cause of the event as rapidly as possible, so that neurologic function can be maximally restored. These diagnostic procedures are given in Table 57–5.

CT scans of the head are generally indicated for all patients suspected of having acute CVD. Angiography is not indicated for all stroke patients and carries a risk of morbidity because of its invasive nature. However, in the current era of intra-arterial digital subtraction techniques, smaller dye loads, and the use of nonionic contrast media, the risks of angiography have improved. Cerebral angiography remains the "gold standard" for assessing extracranial and intracranial cerebral vessel ulceration, stenosis, collateral capacitance, embolic occlusions, and other arteriopathies. Indications for angiography include a young stroke victim, transient ischemic attacks or minor deficits in the absence of a known cardiac embolic source, suspicion of venous stroke, and patients with symptomatic extracranial carotid stenosis who are being considered for carotid endarterectomy. Because arteriography is invasive and does not provide direct cerebral metabolic information, its definite role in the acute stroke has not been ascertained. Unfortunately, the diagnostic yield of angiography is greatest in the acute setting (Fig. 57–2), when arterial occlusion is most likely to be documented. Further, cerebral angiography may not always clarify the etiology of intracranial CVD.

Ultrasonic Doppler studies are becoming routine in the noninvasive investigation of large-vessel disease. Duplex scanning of the carotid arteries combines B-mode ultrasonography and Doppler ultrasonography within a single unit, thus providing both anatomic and flow velocity data. With duplex scanning, a sensitivity greater than 95% and a specificity of 84% (compared with angiography) can be obtained.[47] The greatest accuracy of carotid Doppler studies is when the stenotic lesion is greater than 75% (specificity and sensitivity greater than 95%).[48] The carotid Doppler study is therefore an accurate method to evaluate patients for the presence of hemodynamically significant extracranial disease.

Transcranial Doppler (TCD) testing is gaining wide use for the noninvasive assessment of intracranial CVD.[49, 50] The middle, anterior, and posterior cerebral arteries, ophthalmic arteries, carotid siphon, vertebral arteries, and basilar artery can be studied. Embolic occlusion of the MCA may now be identified and serially studied noninvasively. Blacks, Asians, and females have a higher incidence of intracranial atherosclerotic arterial disease[51] amenable to study with TCD. TCD can be an important noninvasive method for detecting stenosis or occlusion of intracranial vessels, as well as for studying collateral circulation and vasospasm.

TABLE 57–5

INVESTIGATIONS FOR TYPE AND CAUSE OF CEREBROVASCULAR DISEASE

Blood Studies (as Indicated)	Brain Studies	Vascular Imaging
Complete blood count with differential	CT	Doppler studies
Platelet count	Magnetic resonance imaging	Transcranial Doppler studies
Automated serum chemistry assays (SMAC)	Cerebral blood flow (single-photon emission CT, xenon inhalation)	Angiography
Fasting lipid levels	Positron emission tomography	Magnetic resonance imaging
Partial thromboplastin time, prothrombin time, fibrinogen levels	Electroencephalography	Fluorescein retinal angiography
Westergren's erythrocyte sedimentation site	Evoked potentials	
Protein electrophoresis with quantitative immunoglobulin	Cerebrospinal fluid assay	
Antinuclear antibody assay	**Cardiac Studies**	
Platelet function studies	Electrocardiography with rhythm strip	
Specific coagulation factors	Chest x-ray film	
Antithrombin III levels	Echocardiography	
Venereal Disease Research Laboratory test	M-mode	
Fluorescent treponemal antibody absorption test	Two-dimensional	
Proteins S and C assay	Contrast/bubble	
Complement component assay	Transesophageal	
Markers of fibrinolytic system activity	Holter's cardiac monitoring	
Lipoprotein electrophoresis	^{111}In scintigraphy	
Lipoprotein a	Gated CT imaging	
Serum and whole blood viscosity	Gated magnetic resonance imaging	
Circulating immune complexes assay	Multigated angiogram scanning	
Anticardiolipin antibodies assay	Ventriculography	
	Coronary angiography	

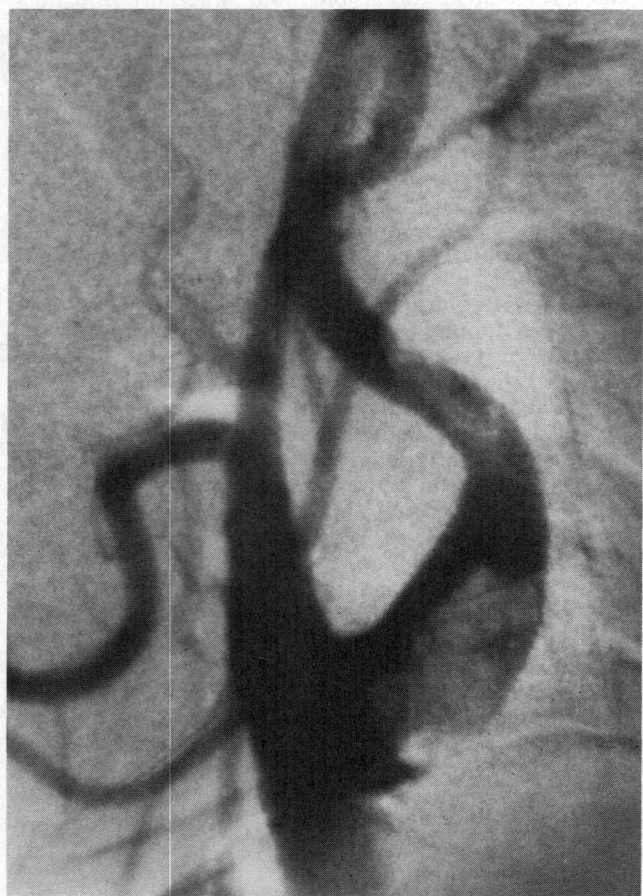

Figure 57–2. Selective right common carotid angiography (subtraction view) demonstrating a large intraluminal clot at the origin of the internal carotid artery.

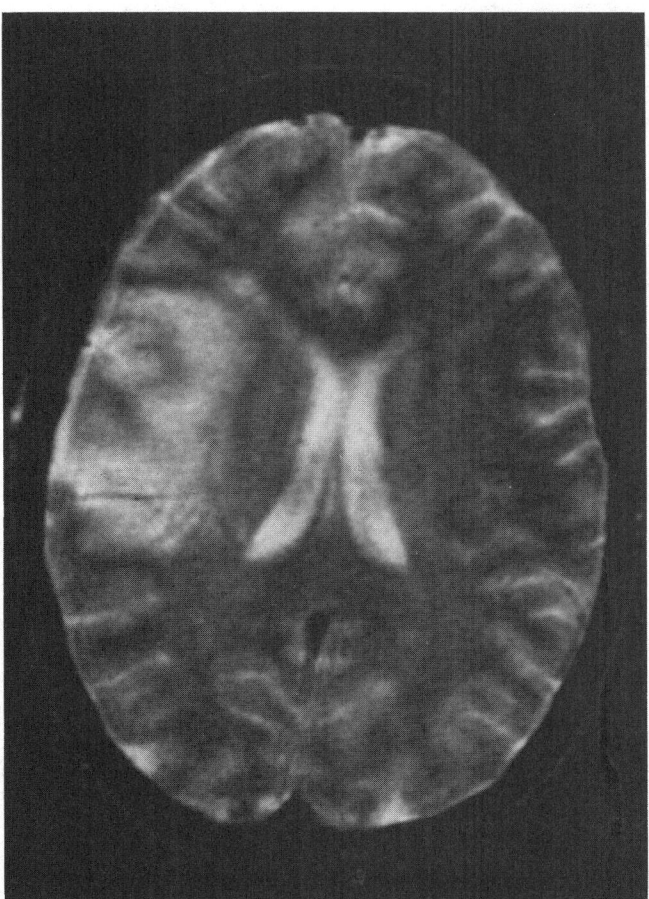

Figure 57–3. MRI scan of the head demonstrating high signal abnormality (ischemia) in the right MCA territory in a patient whose CT scan did not show a definitive stroke.

Basilar artery occlusion may be diagnosed early in the clinical course by magnetic resonance imaging (MRI).[52]

Optimal investigation and subsequent treatment of acute cerebral ischemia may require knowledge of physiologic and metabolic data as well.[48, 53–55] MRI (Figs. 57–3 and 57–4) is more sensitive than a CT scan for diagnosing ischemic stroke;[56] however, the diagnosis of stroke or of a specific stroke syndrome generally relies on the clinical expertise of the examining physician.

Fever in patients with stroke should not be attributed to the vascular process.[57] Twenty-two percent of 104 consecutively and prospectively studied stroke patients (subarachnoid hemorrhage and brain stem stroke excluded) developed a rectal temperature of 101°F or higher within the first 5 days of the ictus. Nineteen of these 23 patients had an identifiable source; 13 were from a pulmonary site. Small lacunar infarcts did not cause fever. Patients with large strokes had fever significantly more often than patients with small or moderately sized strokes.

Fever causes an increase in CBF and cerebral blood volume.[57] Acute increases in intracranial pressure (ICP) also occur with acute temperature elevations.[57] Fever in the wake of stroke should therefore be evaluated and treated aggressively.

Therapy

Care of the acute ischemic CVD patient should be multifactoral. Airway protection and support may include moni-

toring of respiratory rate and arterial blood gas levels, with oxygen provided by nasal cannula, mask, or intubation as needed. Cardiovascular support includes cardiac auscultation, continuous blood pressure and electrocardiographic monitoring for early detection of myocardial ischemia, cardiac arrhythmias, and changes in blood pressure. Central venous lines and Swan-Ganz catheters may supplement more basic monitoring as indicated. ICP monitoring may be appropriate under some circumstances. Careful attention to metabolic balance (i.e., fluid intake and output, glucose and electrolyte values, liver and renal function, and nutrition) is essential. Meticulous bowel and bladder care and prevention of infection and decubitus ulcers via skin protection reduce morbidity and mortality. Ongoing psychologic support and communication with the patient and the family are essential. Frequent neurologic assessments detect both early deterioration and early trends toward improvement.

To date, the treatment of acute ischemic stroke has been largely without significant success in reversing the acute focal ischemic process, cell damage, and clinical neurologic deficit in humans.[58, 59] The disruption of brain energy metabolism caused by ischemia produces neurologic deficit that may be reversible or irreversible, depending on the duration and degree of the insult.[54, 60] Specific therapy should be directed at the underlying mechanism of ischemia.

Fibrinolytic agents are being investigated for truly acute stroke with the aim of lysing the fresh clot that obstructs the artery.[61] Preliminary data provide optimism.[61–63] Pilot studies

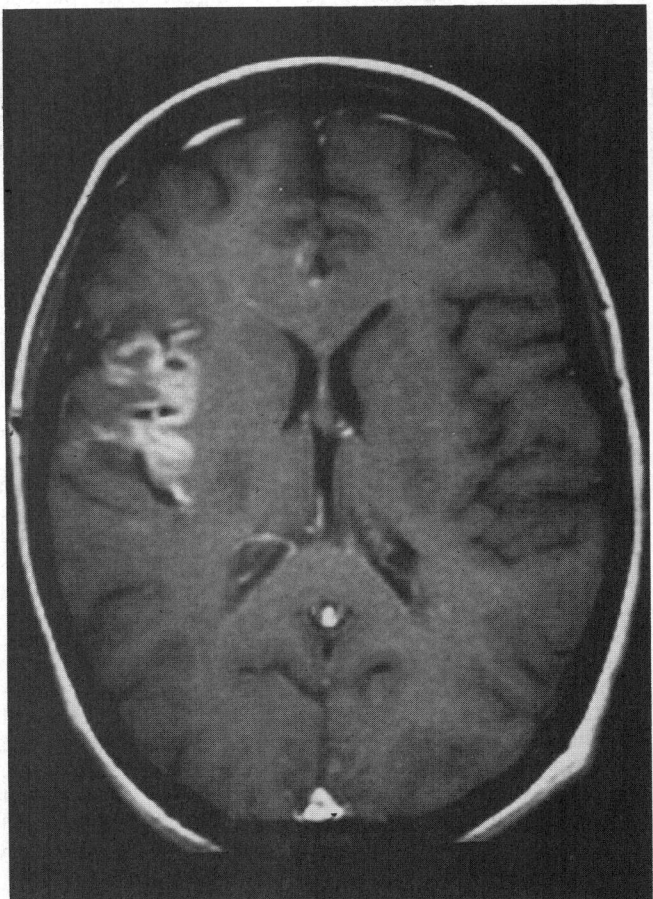

Figure 57–4. MRI scan of the head (T_1-weighted image) demonstrating both high and low signals in the opercular region of the right MCA territory, in a cortical ribbon infarction pattern.

have been completed and randomized studies are under way to determine efficacy. Fifteen of 20 patients with a mean treatment onset interval of 7.6 hours demonstrated complete recanalization. Two thirds of these exhibited varying degrees of clinical improvement by discharge. Twenty percent suffered hemorrhagic transformation of the infarct without clinical worsening.

Hemodilution therapy has received attention because of its ability to increase CBF and tissue oxygenation,[64] although a multicenter randomized trial of hemodilution in acute stroke[65] did not significantly reduce morbidity or mortality. A major reason for the failure of hemodilution therapy in this trial may be that patients with established cerebral infarction were probably included because of the eligibility of patients up to 48 hours after ictus. Specific subgroups, such as those treated truly acutely with elevated or high normal hematocrits, may still benefit.

Calcium channel blocker therapy (nimodipine) in acute (within 48 hours) ischemic stroke was evaluated in the United States in a multicenter trial. Results were disappointing, although patients treated within 12 hours of symptom onset may benefit. A European multicenter, prospective, double-blind, randomized, placebo-controlled trial[66] demonstrated a positive effect of nimodipine (30 mg every 6 hours for 4 weeks) in reducing mortality when given orally within 24 hours of onset of symptoms (8.6% in the nimodipine group vs. 20.4% in the placebo group). The improvement in survival was restricted to men. A 4-week mortality rate of 20% for acute ischemic stroke in the placebo group may be higher than expected. Death from bronchopneumonia and pulmonary embolism was three times higher in the placebo group. An improvement in functional outcome was demonstrated in the nimodipine-treated patients with moderate-to-severe deficits at baseline. However, patients with poor or high baseline scores did not improve with nimodipine. There were no important lasting side effects. Eligibility included an acute persistent neurologic event without progressive deterioration. Concomitant use of antiplatelet agents was not allowed; however, all patients received 10% low-molecular-weight depolymerized dextran, 12 hours daily for 5 days.

The benefit of corticosteroids in acute cerebral ischemia has yet to be proved. The generally accepted explanation is that initial ischemic edema is predominantly cytoxotic (Fig. 57–5) rather than vasogenic, and steroids are primarily effective against the latter. Randomized studies have failed to show a beneficial effect in steroid-treated groups, and steroid-treated patients have fared worse,[43] generally because of the increased morbidity from susceptibility to infection and hyperglycemia.

Anticoagulation remains controversial despite its routine use.[58] Previous studies have been criticized for inadequate design, lack of angiographic data, lack of uniform diagnostic criteria for transient ischemic attacks, and heterogeneous subgroups mixed together.[67] Specific subgroups that may benefit from heparin or warfarin (Coumadin) must be defined. Cardioembolic stroke appears to be the clearest subgroup to date that may benefit from anticoagulation by reducing recurrent emboli.[68, 69] One study found that a significant number of patients with cardiogenic cerebral embolism experience a second brain embolism within the first 2 weeks of the initial event.[67] However, a contemporary, prospective, double-blind, placebo-controlled randomized study of heparin or warfarin for cardioembolic stroke has not yet been achieved. In a patient with presumed cardioembolic stroke (such as after an anterior MI), limited evidence favors anticoagulation with heparin to prevent early recurrent emboli, provided the initial infarct is not significantly hemorrhagic by CT scan or too massive.[68] There is some evidence that an intravenous heparin bolus before the con-

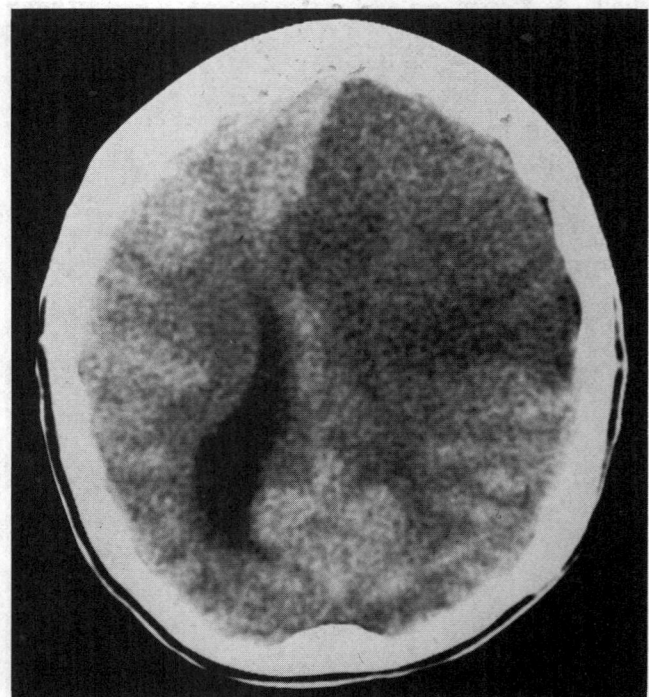

Figure 57–5. CT scan of the head, without contrast infusion, demonstrating ischemic edema with mass effect and midline shift within 72 hours after infarct. The patient died of progressive cerebral herniation.

stant infusion may increase the hemorrhagic complications.[69] Heparin should therefore be initiated as a constant intravenous infusion to maintain the partial thromboplastin time or thrombin clot time at 1.5 to 2.0 times the baseline or control value. Heparin should be continued for 7 to 10 days until warfarin therapy can be initiated—maintaining the prothrombin time 1.3 to 1.5 times the baseline value. More aggressive anticoagulation therapy (i.e., further prolongation of coagulation parameters) may not be more beneficial[70] and may carry a higher hemorrhagic risk.[67] Hemorrhage may occur as a result of lysis of the embolus with subsequent reperfusion, as well as from collateral reperfusion, hypertension, large infarct size, and the presence of blood-brain barrier breakdown.[69, 71] Heparin may also be beneficial for progressing stroke or stroke in evolution, in which the mechanism is probably clot propagation in either the anterior or the posterior circulation.[10–12] Several small, randomized controlled trials (totaling approximately 450 patients) demonstrated a reduction of further stroke or worsening neurologic status during 6 to 15 months of follow-up. Mortality was not significantly changed. Unfortunately, the size of the studies precludes statistical significance and acceptable statistical power. For stroke in evolution, anticoagulation should be empirically continued for 2 to 4 weeks or until the patient is neurologically stable for at least 1 week. Caplan and Stein (see ref 14, p 96) have outlined a rational approach in which heparin or warfarin may be beneficial in various stroke subgroups based on pathophysiology. In view of the hemorrhagic risk, anticoagulation therapy should *not* be routinely used for acute ischemic stroke and should be used with caution when given only after performing a CT scan of the head to exclude hemorrhage. In a controlled study, heparin was not useful in preventing further neurologic deficits in patients with partial ischemic deficits.[72] Full anticoagulation after a completed noncardioembolic cerebral infarct has not proved beneficial and even under optimal control may incur a high bleeding risk. Low-dose heparin initiated shortly after the acute stroke may decrease the complications of deep venous thrombosis[73] and pulmonary embolism, at least in the early postinfarction periods. Subgroups of patients at greatest risk of bleeding from anticoagulation have been identified.[74] Heparinoids have less hemorrhagic risk and are currently being investigated.[75]

The use of carotid endarterectomy is widely debated because of the lack of conclusive guidelines for its application. Randomized, controlled studies with "acceptable" surgical morbidity and mortality are needed to demonstrate efficacy. Furthermore, its utility in the treatment of acute cerebral ischemia has not been clarified. Currently, many patients are undergoing this procedure without appropriate indications.[76] Two current, multicenter, prospective, randomized carotid endarterectomy studies are under way, one for asymptomatic and the other for symptomatic carotid stenosis. Both studies involve a medical component in which aspirin is used.

Although definite recommendations cannot currently be made about the use of glucose or glucose-lowering therapies in acute cerebral ischemia,[77] a growing number of studies are addressing the issue of increased serum glucose level on stroke outcome in both animals and humans.[77–80] Hyperglycemia may predispose to infarction when present at the time of ischemia and to poor recovery from nonlacunar stroke.[77] Careful serum glucose monitoring in patients with acute cerebral ischemia may eventually prove to be necessary, especially in ongoing or incomplete ischemia.[80]

Indicators of poor prognosis and recovery from stroke include dementia, large right cerebral hemisphere infarction, impaired sensory function, and Wernicke's aphasia. The presence of neglect after stroke is a marker for poorer outcome and rehabilitative potential.[10] Fortunately, neglect generally wanes or resolves within several months of the ictus. Functional prognosis should be determined in all acute stroke survivors.[81] A detailed assessment of deficits in the ICU may enhance the coordinated approach to rehabilitation and recovery.

HEMORRHAGIC CEREBROVASCULAR DISEASE

Intracranial hemorrhage, both intracerebral (ICH) and subarachnoid (SAH), accounts for 15 to 25% of CVD. Clinical manifestations of ICH and SAH sometimes overlap, but the pathophysiology, etiology, radiographic findings, and prognosis of the two conditions differ remarkably.

Intracerebral Hemorrhage

ICH refers to acute bleeding into the brain parenchyma. The incidence of ICH is about 10% of all strokes.[82] The incidence of ICH has been declining over the years. In addition, the mortality rate from ICH has significantly declined because of better management of acute ICP, recognition of smaller intracerebral bleeding with the advent of cranial CT and MRI scanning, and improved surgical techniques.

Etiology

Hypertension is the single most common risk factor for ICH. Earlier figures of the incidence of hypertension in spontaneous ICH were 70 to 90%.[82] More recently, Brott and coworkers[83] found that less than 60% of patients with ICH had a history of hypertension or clinical evidence of it (e.g., left ventricular hypertrophy and hypertensive retinopathy). Cigarette smoking, excessive alcohol consumption, and oral contraceptives are independent risk factors for ICH. Among the other nontraumatic causes of ICH (Table 57–6), vascular anomalies, including aneurysms and arteriovenous malformations, and bleeding diatheses, including anticoagulant therapy and thrombocytopenia, account for a significant percentage.

Hypertension. In 1868, Charcot and Bouchard first described microaneurysms as outpouching of the vascular endothelium through areas of weakened media. Those lesions were found in hypertensive patients with ICH. Rupture of these aneurysmal dilatations, which are usually found on end arteries from larger parent arteries (e.g., lenticulostriate from the MCA and thalamoperforator from the posterior cerebral artery), results in ICH at the common sites clinically encountered: putamen, thalamus, subcortical white matter, pons, and cerebellum. Fisher[84] believed that the pathologic process leading to ICH in hypertensive patients is a dynamic one, starting with degeneration of the walls of the penetrating arteries (lipohyalinosis or fibrinoid necrosis) and leading to aneurysmal dilatation and subsequent hemorrhage.

Vascular Anomalies. Saccular aneurysms generally rupture into the subarachnoid space, resulting in SAH; occasionally the blood extends into the brain parenchyma, causing ICH. Rarely, however, an aneurysm ruptures directly into the brain parenchyma (saccular aneurysms are discussed in the section on SAH). Arteriovenous malformations, including venous and cavernous angiomas, can cause ICH. These lesions are often diagnosed by MRI and angiography, although they may sometimes be occult and are found only at autopsy. A complete review is available.[85]

Bleeding Diatheses. Anticoagulant therapy, including heparin and warfarin, has been associated with ICH in less than 3% of treated patients.[86, 87] Although excessive anticoagulation (prolonged prothrombin time and partial throm-

---

TABLE 57–6
CONDITIONS ASSOCIATED WITH NONTRAUMATIC INTRACEREBRAL HEMORRHAGE

Systemic
  Hypertension
  Bleeding diatheses (e.g. thrombocytopenia, hemophilia, anticoagulation, thrombolytic therapy, disseminated intravascular coagulation)

Vascular
  Arteriovenous malformations
  Saccular aneurysms
  Mycotic aneurysms
  Cerebral amyloid angiopathy

Neoplastic
  Primary brain tumors (e.g. glioblastoma, hemangioblastoma, desmoplastic sarcoma, neuroblastoma, pituitary adenoma)
  Metastatic tumors (e.g. melanoma, renal cell carcinoma, choriocarcinoma, lung and breast cancer, medullary thyroid carcinoma)

Inflammatory
  Systemic vasculitis (e.g. systemic lupus erythematosus, periarteritis nodosa, giant cell arteritis)
  Primary central nervous system vasculitis

Toxic
  Amphetamine
  Phenylpropanolamine
  Cocaine and "crack" cocaine

Other
  Moyamoya disease
  Cryptic vascular malformations
  Cerebral venous thrombosis

boplastin time beyond the therapeutic range) has been considered to be the underlying mechanism of bleeding in ICH, some human and animal studies demonstrated that hemorrhage occurs even with subtherapeutic anticoagulation.[88] Elevated blood pressure and large cerebral infarcts have been considered to be risk factors for ICH in patients treated with anticoagulation.[89] Thrombolytic therapy with tissue plasminogen activator, streptokinase, and urokinase has also been associated with ICH.[90] Other bleeding diatheses, such as severe thrombocytopenia (platelet count less than 20,000/mm³), disseminated intravascular coagulation, coagulation factor deficiencies, and idiopathic thrombocytopenic purpura, are occasionally associated with ICH.

Drugs. Use of illicit drugs, including amphetamines and cocaine,[91] and more habitual use of sympathomimetics like phenylpropanolamine (found in some diet pills) are increasingly recognized as causes of ICH. The mechanisms of ICH in association with drug use are probably multiple and include drug-induced vasculitis, transient severe hypertension, incidental vascular anomalies, and possibly a bleeding diathesis.

Vasculopathy. Systemic lupus erythematosus, polyarteritis nodosa, and primary central nervous system vasculitis have all been associated with ICH. Intracranial bleeding in these conditions is probably related to blood leaking from damaged (necrotic or inflamed) blood vessel walls. Cerebral amyloid angiopathy, a vasculopathy occurring predominantly in elderly persons, is a common cause of non–hypertensive-related ICH in the aged population.[92] Amyloid material is deposited in the media and adventitia of small and medium-sized cerebral arteries, predominantly those in the region of the gray matter–white matter junction, which accounts for the more common lobar location of associated ICH. The mechanisms of arterial rupture in cerebral amyloid angiopathy are due to either blood leakage from the damaged and weakened artery or rupture of microaneurysms that develop at sites of amyloid accumulation.[93, 94] A vasculopathy associated with central nervous system aspergillosis has been described in patients with acquired immunodeficiency syndrome who have ICH.[95]

Brain Tumors. Cerebral neoplasms have been found in up to 6% of patients with spontaneous ICH.[96] Likely to bleed are large, malignant, primary neoplasms like glioblastoma, as well as metastatic tumors. Melanoma, choriocarcinoma, and renal cell carcinoma are notorious in their propensity to cause ICH when they metastasize to the brain; broncho-

genic and breast carcinomas are other examples. Hemorrhage is thought to arise from the rapidly growing peripheral portion of the tumor or from adjacent damaged brain tissue.[97]

Others. Rarer causes of ICH include cryptic vascular malformations, moyamoya disease, cerebral venous thrombosis, mucormycosis, hepatic failure, and thrombotic thrombocytopenic purpura, among others.

Clinical Manifestations

General Features. General features include

- Headache
- Nausea and vomiting
- Seizures
- Nuchal rigidity
- Altered mentation

The neurologic symptoms of ICH *usually* begin abruptly and peak in minutes to a few hours.[98] Although such presentation is found in the majority of patients, variation in symptoms is well recognized, and some patients can complain of only mild neurologic dysfunction whereas others present with a rapidly fatal course. The advent of cranial CT scanning has allowed recognition of cases of ICH that overlap in clinical presentation with SAH or cerebral infarction. The extremely early evaluation of ICH with CT scanning has also demonstrated that rebleeding with clinical worsening is not uncommon. Headache, traditionally considered to be a constant feature of ICH, was present at the onset of ICH in only one third of patients in the Harvard Stroke Registry.[78] Headache severity varies from mild to excruciating; it is generally accepted that the larger the hematoma, the more severe the headache. When present, headache usually lateralizes to the side of the bleeding. Nuchal rigidity, nausea, vomiting, and altered mental states occur at variable frequencies. Seizures at the onset of an event are more frequent with cerebral hemorrhages than with cerebral ischemia, excluding venous infarction and probably cerebral embolism. Seizures occurred in 6% of patients in the Harvard Stroke Registry and 2% of the series of Omae and coworkers.[98] Other signs and symptoms of ICH depend on the location of the hematoma.

Signs and Symptoms by Location (Table 57–7).

Putamen. The putamen[99] is the most frequently encountered location of hematoma in hypertensive patients. Putam-

		TABLE 57-7					

CLINICAL MANIFESTATIONS OF INTRACEREBRAL HEMORRHAGE: SYMPTOMS AND SIGNS BY LOCATION*

Location	Onset	Weakness or Ataxia	Sensory Loss	Eye Deviation and Signs	Pupils	Neglect	Aphasia
Putamen	Gradual	Hemiparesis	±	Ipsilateral	Normal	±	±
Thalamus	Abrupt	± hemiparesis	+	Downward	Miotic	±	±
Lobar	Variable	± hemiparesis	±	Ipsilateral	Normal	−	−
Pons (central)	Abrupt	Tetraparesis	−	Ocular bobbing	Miotic	−	−
Pons (lateral)	Variable	Hemiataxia and/or weakness	±	Contralateral	± Horner's	−	−
Cerebellum (central)	Abrupt	Truncal ataxia ± tetraparesis	−	Nystagmus, saccadic or pursuit abnormality	Variable	−	−
Cerebellum (lateral)	Variable	Appendicular ataxia	−	Saccadic or pursuit abnormality	Normal	−	−

*The + denotes generally present; − denotes generally absent; ± denotes variable.

inal hemorrhages develop gradually in about 60% of patients; the symptoms evolve during 6 to 12 hours, with most hemorrhages completed by 6 hours. Focal neurologic symptoms include variable degrees of contralateral hemiparesis or hemi–sensory loss. Homonymous field deficits, both complete and incomplete, have been reported. Left putaminal hemorrhages can be associated with aphasia, whereas right-sided lesions are occasionally associated with contralateral neglect. Conjugate deviation of the eyes to the side of the hematoma is sometimes encountered. Rare cases of putaminal hemorrhage presenting as lacunae ("clumsy hand" dysarthria, pure motor hemiparesis) have been reported.

Thalamus. Thalamic hemorrhage[100] is second to putaminal ICH in frequency of occurrence. The onset of symptoms is usually more abrupt than that in putaminal ICH. Neurologic manifestations vary depending on the location of the bleeding, whether lateral or medial, ventral or dorsal, anterior or posterior. Contralateral hemi–sensory loss and, rarely, hemiparesis are encountered. Altered mental status occurs in more than one third of patients. Pupillary abnormalities and upward gaze restrictions are seen in about 25%. Eyes may be deviated down and in. Miotic pupils in association with thalamic ICH tend to react poorly to light, in contrast to miotic pupils seen in pontine hemorrhage.[101] Hemineglect is occasionally seen with right thalamic ICH, and aphasia has been reported in association with left thalamic ICH. Small thalamic hemorrhage presenting as transient ischemic attack has been reported.[102] Thalamic hematomas have a propensity to rupture into the ventricles, especially when located medially. Weisberg[100] reported intraventricular extension in 21 of 50 patients (42%).

Lobar Hemorrhage. Lobar ICH[103] accounts for about 20% of nontraumatic parenchymal hemorrhages. Often, patients with lobar ICH have no history or physical evidence of hypertension. Underlying structural lesions such as tumors or vascular malformations, drug ingestion, and cerebral amyloid angiopathy are some associated conditions. The clinical manifestations vary according to the site and size of the bleeding. Headache is a frequent complaint; contralateral motor or sensory deficit, visual field defects, neurobehavioral abnormalities (including abulia), apraxia, and aphasia may be encountered.

Brain Stem. Brain stem[104] hematomas are relatively rare. Pontine location[101, 104, 105] is most frequently encountered, followed by the midbrain and the medulla. Before the advent of CT scanning, brain stem hematomas were believed to be invariably fatal. Literature has provided a significant number of reports of patients with brain stem hematoma who present as if they had lacunar strokes. Central pontine hemorrhage manifests with tetraparesis, miotic pupils, ocular bobbing, and rapidly evolving coma. Lateral pontine hematomas cause ipsilateral ataxia, oculomotor abnormalities such as gaze or individual oculomotor nerve palsy, contralateral hemi–sensory loss, and hemiparesis or hemiplegia. Medullary and midbrain hematomas are rare. They can be related to hypertension or more often to underlying vascular malformations.

Cerebellar Hemorrhage. Cerebellar hemorrhage[106] occurs in about 10% of all ICHs. Two distinct clinical presentations have been recognized. Laterally placed lesions cause more appendicular symptoms, with minimal truncal or gait ataxia. In addition, various oculomotor abnormalities are seen related to the saccadic and/or pursuit systems. On the other hand, midline cerebellar hemorrhage presents with a more rapidly evolving course of truncal ataxia, nausea and vomiting, nystagmus leading to tetraparesis, and coma with obstructive hydrocephalus and brain stem compression.

Intraventricular Hemorrhage. This type of hemorrhage[107] accounts for less than 5% of cases of ICH. The clinical manifestations are similar to those of SAH and include sudden headache, impaired consciousness, and memory dysfunction. Focal signs, if present, are minimal. An underlying vascular abnormality is often encountered.

Diagnosis

History and clinical examination are essential in establishing that the patient had an apoplectic event that affected the central nervous system and resulted in focal, generalized, or lateralized deficits. It is important to seek information on hypertension, drug ingestion, history of possible systemic disease, and family history. Cranial CT scanning has revolutionized the diagnosis of ICH by demonstrating the nature of the stroke (i.e., ischemic vs. hemorrhagic, ICH vs. SAH). Acutely, CT scanning demonstrates blood as an area of hyperdensity in the brain parenchyma, surrounded by variable areas of low density reflecting either edema formation or damaged (ischemic) brain tissue (Fig. 57–6). Contrast-infused CT scanning sometimes allows the visualization of underlying structural lesions such as vascular malformations (Fig. 57–7A), aneurysms larger than 0.5 cm in maximal diameter (see Fig. 57–7B), or tumors. CT scanning can miss an intracranial hematoma in the subacute stage (3 weeks to 2 months), when alterations in physiochemical properties of extravascular blood result in a change in the density of the bleeding. In such instances, when the hematoma is isodense (same density as surrounding brain tissue), indirect signs of ICH are edema, mass effect, and peripheral contrast enhancement. MRI is gaining acceptance as an important diagnostic tool in the evaluation of ICH[108, 109] (Fig. 57–8). However, difficulty in identifying hyperacute bleeding, relatively lengthy time of procedure, and lack of widespread resources make the use of MRI unsuitable in the current initial diagnosis of ICH. The evolution of the blood clot on

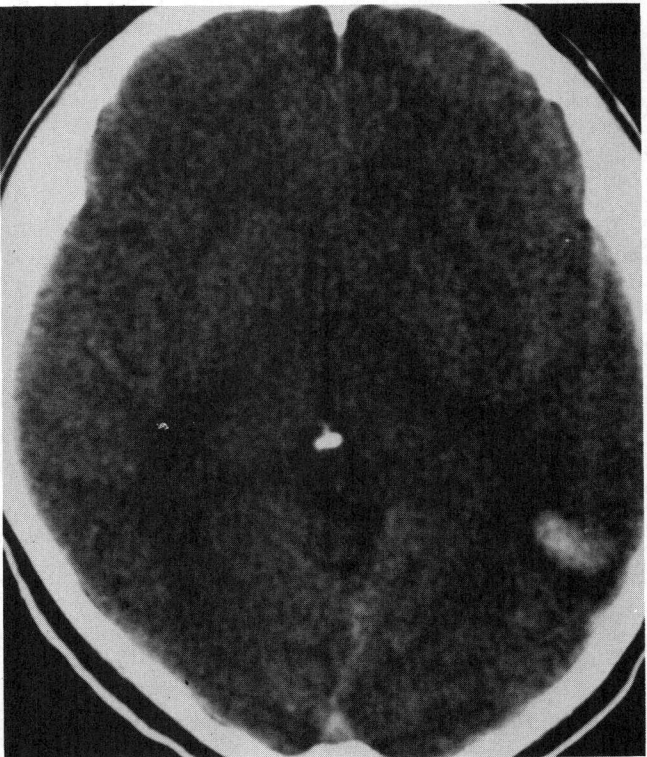

Figure 57–6. CT scan of the head, without contrast infusion, showing a small left parietal ICH with minimal edema surrounding it.

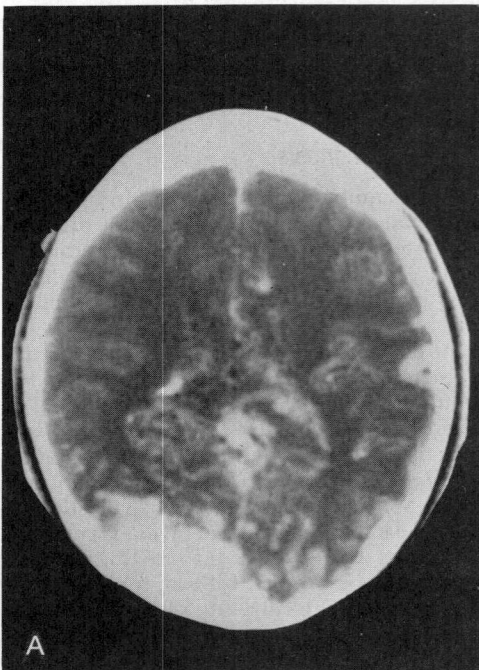
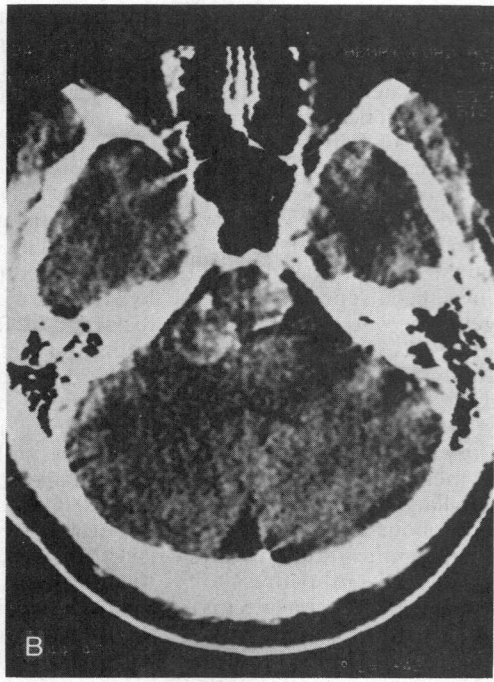

Figure 57–7. *A.* CT scan of the head, after contrast infusion, demonstrating large bilateral cerebral arteriovenous malformations. *B.* CT scan of the head demonstrating a large fusiform basilar artery aneurysm.

MRI is beyond the scope of this discussion but can be reviewed in ref 109. Cerebrospinal fluid analysis has become obsolete in the diagnosis of ICH, unless conditions like vasculitis or infection are suspected. Cerebral angiography should be performed for all young patients with lobar hemorrhage, nonhypertensive patients, and those not devastated by the hematoma. Angiography should be considered in patients with thalamic, pontine, or young nonhypertensive intraventricular hemorrhage, especially when the CT or MRI scan suggests an underlying vascular lesion or tumor. Timing of angiography is variable. It is preferable that the vascular tree be visualized early after the event if the patient's condition is stable and an underlying vascular or neoplastic process is suspected.

Management

General Considerations. Optimal management of patients with ICH includes maintenance of adequate oxygenation, respiratory toilet including frequent nasotracheal suctioning, and prophylactic intubation in selected cases. The management of hypertension should be cautionary. As a general rule, the blood pressure should be managed with short-acting antihypertensive medications, which have rapid onset of action and minimal effect on CBF; nitroprusside is an example. Also, it may be advisable to treat hypertension only when systolic pressure exceeds 180 mm Hg or diastolic pressure exceeds 110 mm Hg. Lowering the blood pressure to normotensive levels can be dangerous in ICH because cerebral autoregulation is largely lost in the affected hemisphere and cerebral perfusion then becomes dependent on the systemic pressure—increasing with raised systemic pressure. Patients should not be fed by mouth, at least in the first 24 to 72 hours, to avoid aspiration. Glucose solutions should be avoided, as there is evidence that they may worsen outcome by increasing edema formation. Hypotonic solutions can worsen cerebral edema and should be avoided. Headache can be managed with narcotics such as codeine or meperidine. Anticonvulsants, especially phenytoin, are used in the management of seizures. Some advocate pro-

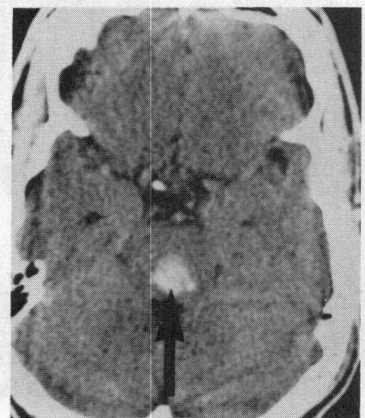
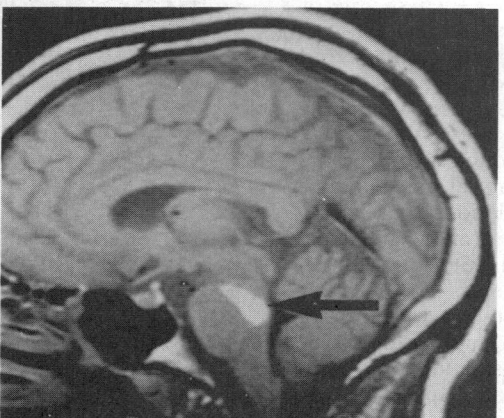
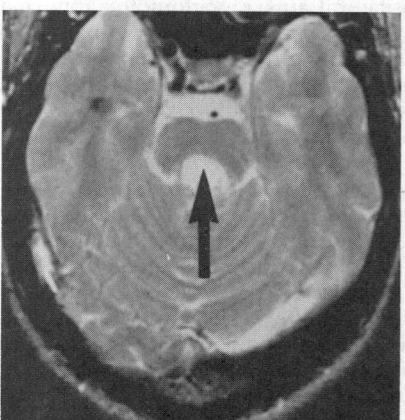

Figure 57–8. CT (*left*) and MRI (*middle:* sagittal; *right:* axial) scans of the head demonstrating an ICH within the dorsal pons (*arrows*).

phylactic use of anticonvulsants in patients with lobar ICH. This management strategy is not universally accepted.

Management of Cerebral Edema and Increased Intracranial Pressure. Bed rest and head elevation (15 to 20°) to facilitate cerebral venous drainage are important measures in the treatment of cerebral edema and increased ICP. Osmotic agents such as mannitol should be used if there is clinical or radiologic evidence of increased ICP. Some centers monitor the ICP directly with subdurally or epidurally placed bolts and administer 0.25 to 0.75 g/kg of a 20% mannitol solution every 4 to 6 hours to keep the ICP below 20 mm Hg or to minimize plateau waves on the ICP monitor. If an ICP-monitoring device is not used, mannitol administration can be gauged by the serum osmolarity, which should be kept in the range 305 to 310 mOsm/L. Hyperventilation to reduce cerebral edema by way of reducing total CBF has a limited role because it has the potential of worsening cerebral ischemia. Nonetheless, it may be used for the initial 10 to 20 minutes when mannitol is being administered (lowering $Paco_2$ to 25 to 30 mm Hg reduces CBF in less than 5 minutes, and mannitol action does not start until 10 to 20 minutes after infusion). Corticosteroids have been advocated for reducing cerebral edema in patients with ICH. Their role remains controversial, and one study[110] has shown no beneficial effect on outcome after ICH.

Surgical Management. To date, there is no clear evidence for superiority of surgical clot evacuation over medical management of ICH. In probably the best controlled prospective study of ICH, published in 1961,[111] there was no difference in morbidity or mortality between the group treated surgically and the one treated medically. Such results have been duplicated in another study.[112] Until further studies are designed, the issue is unresolved. However, there is some evidence that relatively young and stable patients with lobar or cerebellar hemorrhage who show progressive neurologic deterioration should be treated with surgical evacuation of the hematoma. In addition, hydrocephalus can be treated with ventricular drainage if it develops acutely. In all surgically treated patients, the approach should be via an open craniotomy, not needle aspiration of the hematoma.

Prognosis

The prognosis of patients with ICH was reported to be dismal in the pre-CT era. Currently, 40 to 60% of patients with ICH survive and just under 25% can function independently. In general, putaminal hematomas under 3 cm in size, younger age, absence of ventricular extension, absence of hydrocephalus, and intact level of consciousness at presentation are favorable prognostic factors. Central pontine ICH and midline cerebellar ICH usually have a poor prognosis.

Subarachnoid Hemorrhage

Bleeding into the subarachnoid space, most commonly from an arterial source, is referred to as SAH. Traumatic SAH is the most common form and is not discussed here. The incidence of SAH is about 6 to 8% of all strokes, occurring in 15 of 100,000 people annually.[113]

Etiology (Table 57–8)

Nontraumatic or spontaneous SAH occurs secondary to rupture of intracranial aneurysms, bleeding from vascular malformations, tumors, extension of hematomas from ICH into the subarachnoid space, bleeding disorders, infections, vasculopathies, and substance abuse, and in association with

TABLE 57–8

CAUSES OF NONTRAUMATIC SUBARACHNOID HEMORRHAGE

Ruptured Intracranial Aneurysms
  Congenital
  Atherosclerotic
  Mycotic (infectious)
  Oncotic (neoplastic)
  Dissecting

Vascular Malformations
  Arteriovenous malformations
  Cavernous angioma
  Venous angioma
  Capillary telangiectasia

Extension from ICH
Central Nervous System Tumors
  Metastatic (e.g., choriocarcinoma, melanoma, renal cell carcinoma, lung cancer)
  Primary (e.g., hemangioblastoma, glioblastoma, medulloblastoma)

Bleeding Disorders
  Anticoagulant therapy
  Leukemia
  Disseminated intravascular coagulation
  Clotting factor deficiency

Vasculopathies
  Connective tissue disorders (e.g., systemic lupus erythematosus, panarteritis nodosa)
  Primary central nervous system angiitis
  Schönlein-Henoch purpura

Substance Abuse
  Sympathomimetics
  Cocaine

Others
  Sepsis
  Cerebral venous (sinus) thrombosis
  Bacterial endocarditis

cerebral venous thrombosis. Aneurysms are the most common cause of SAH, occurring in more than 50% of cases.[114]

Aneurysms. Congenital, berry, or saccular aneurysms[115] are found mostly at arterial branchings and are believed to be formed when continuous pressure is applied to an artery that has a congenital defect in the medial muscular layer of its wall, with or without focal degeneration of the internal elastic lamina. The congenital theory has been challenged by Stehbners,[116] who claimed that aneurysms result from the hemodynamic stress that caused degeneration in the arterial wall. In order of decreasing frequency, anterior communicating artery, posterior communicating artery, MCA, carotid artery bifurcation, and basilar tip are the most common locations for saccular aneurysms.[117] Most aneurysms are in the anterior circulation tree. Multiple aneurysms are reported in about 10 to 20% of patients.[118] Women have a slightly higher incidence of harboring berry aneurysms. Most aneurysms rupture in the fifth to seventh decade of life. Conventionally, aneurysms are categorized as small (less than 12 mm in largest diameter), large (12 to 25 mm), and giant (more than 25 mm). Aneurysms less than 5 mm in maximal diameter rarely rupture.[119] The average diameter of an aneurysm when it ruptures is about 8 mm.[119] More than 75% of aneurysms are small, and 5% are giant. Giant aneurysms are more likely to present as expanding lesions than hemorrhage. Acquired aneurysms with potential for bleeding into the subarachnoid space include Charcot-Bouchard aneurysms (discussed in the section on ICH), mycotic or septic aneurysms, neoplastic or oncotic aneurysms, and dissecting aneurysms. Charcot-Bouchard aneurysms are found at the junction of penetrating arteries from larger branches, whereas mycotic and neoplastic aneurysms are most frequently seen at cortical branches of the MCA. Mycotic aneurysms are seen most often in the setting of bacterial endocarditis; less frequent causes are pulmonary sepsis and drug abuse. Oncotic aneurysms are rare and are predominantly associated with cardiac myxoma and choriocarcinoma. Dissecting aneurysms are not discussed here (for a comprehensive review, see ref 120).

Clinical Manifestations (Table 57–9)

Patients with SAH can present in coma at onset (21%) or with only mild headache and neck stiffness. Classically, patients develop sudden excruciating and generalized headache (46 to 100%), maximal at onset or in about 1 minute.[121] Lateralized pain, not necessarily to the side of the aneurysm, is reported in one third of patients.[121, 122] Sentinel or warning headaches, probably related to small blood leaks and/or sudden aneurysm expansion, are frequently encountered.[123, 124] Change in mental status occurs frequently in association with SAH and varies from mildly altered sensorium to sudden onset of coma. Neck stiffness, nausea and/or vomiting, photophobia, and neck or back pain occur less frequently. Convulsions occur in about 10 to 15% of patients.[114] Vertigo accompanies posterior circulation aneurysms, including ruptured posterior inferior cerebellar artery aneurysms.[125] Focal or lateralizing symptoms are infrequent and variable depending on the site and size of the aneurysmal rupture. A significant number of patients develop SAH during physical or emotional activity, probably related to transient elevation in blood pressure.[126] Neurologic signs of SAH include (1) altered sensorium; (2) neck stiffness from meningeal irritation and cranial nerve palsies, the third cranial nerve being the most commonly involved by aneurysms arising from the posterior communicating artery or internal carotid artery terminus and manifesting as ptosis with pupillary dilatation; (3) papilledema secondary to increased ICP; (4) various degrees and forms of nystagmus; (5) visual field defects; and rarely (6) focal motor or sensory signs. Non-neurologic signs include retinal subhyaloid hem-

TABLE 57–9
CLINICAL MANIFESTATIONS OF SUBARACHNOID HEMORRHAGE
Sudden severe headache
Altered sensorium (mild confusion → coma)
Nuchal rigidity
Nausea and vomiting
Photophobia
Seizures
Double vision
Ptosis
Dizziness and vertigo
Motor and sensory loss

orrhages, fever, and initial tachycardia followed by bradycardia when ICP is significantly elevated.

Diagnosis

The classic presentation of acute excruciating headache, neck stiffness, and change in mental status in an otherwise healthy middle-aged person poses no difficulty in the diagnosis of SAH. Aside from the history and clinical examination, the diagnosis of SAH is made by cranial CT scanning with or without cerebrospinal fluid analysis. The cranial CT scan reveals blood in the subarachnoid space (Fig. 57–9) in more than 90% of patients with SAH, when they present within 72 hours of symptom onset. Failure to demonstrate SAH can be related to either an extremely thin film of blood, as in small leaks, or in association with reduced hemoglobin. The cranial CT scan also helps to demonstrate an underlying lesion, such as aneurysms larger than 5 mm in diameter or vascular malformations, especially when contrast dye is infused. CT scanning helps to identify hydrocephalus, which occurs frequently, and permits following the course of the hematoma and hydrocephalus and the development of the ischemic complications of vasospasm. MRI is still not as sensitive as CT scanning in detecting SAH. Newer MRI pulse sequences, however, are reported to be highly sensitive. Until more advancement in cranial MRI is seen, CT scanning

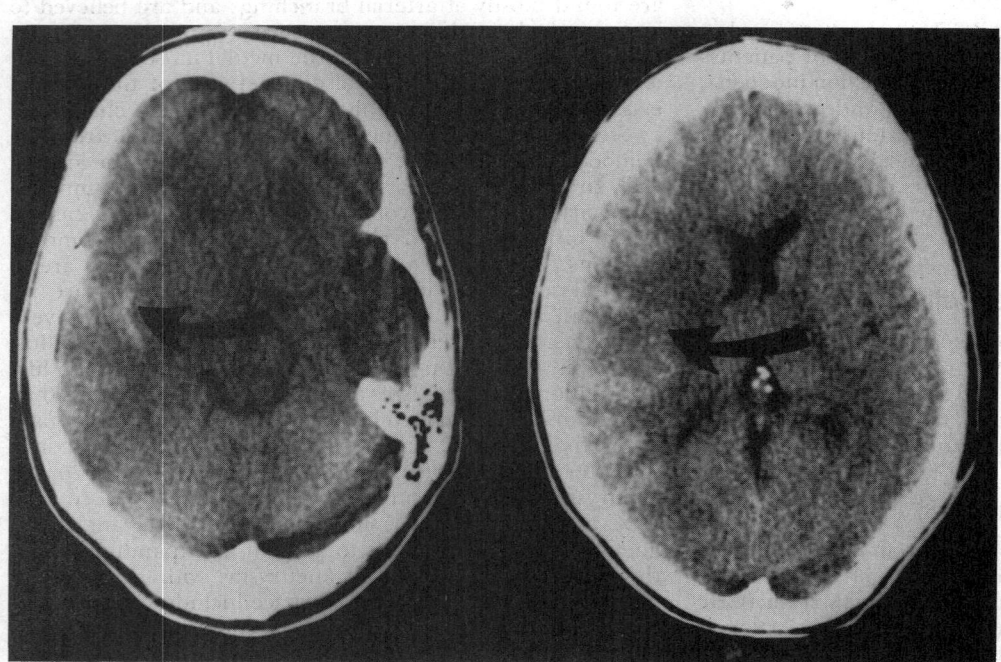

Figure 57–9. CT scans of the head (two axial cuts), without contrast infusion, showing high density in the subarachnoid space (*arrows*), which is diagnostic of SAH.

remains the best diagnostic tool. In patients whose CT scan is normal and SAH is still suspected, lumbar puncture must be performed. A characteristic cerebrospinal fluid formula of SAH is given in Table 57–10. Other laboratory findings in patients with SAH include mild leukocytosis, transient elevation of the erythrocyte sedimentation rate, hyponatremia in those who develop the syndrome of inappropriate antidiuretic hormone secretion, abnormal cardiac rate, ST segment and T wave changes on electrocardiograms, albuminuria, and glycosuria. Cerebral angiography[127] remains the mainstay in diagnosing the underlying etiology of SAH. Cerebral angiography, as well as TCD,[128] helps to identify the vasospastic complications of SAH. The timing of cerebral angiography is variable and depends primarily on the timing of operation.

Management

General Considerations. SAH is an acute neurologic and medical emergency.[129] Patients should be immediately transferred to the nearest facility equipped to manage SAH, both medically and surgically. Complete bed rest, no oral feeding, a dark and quiet room, and stool softeners are essential measures. Patients should be in an ICU where medical staff (nurses or physicians or both) constantly attend to the patient. Respiratory toilet, including prophylactic nasotracheal intubation in selected cases, is of prime importance. Pain killers, preferably codeine or meperidine, laxatives, and deep venous thrombosis prophylaxis with elastic or intermittent pneumatic stockings should be used. Head elevation at 15 to 20° is also advisable to facilitate cerebral venous drainage. Hypertension should be cautiously treated with agents such as nitroprusside, labetolol, or hydralazine to maintain the systolic blood pressure in the range 120 to 150 mm Hg and the diastolic pressure in the range 70 to 90 mm Hg. Such guidelines are used to avoid both rebleeding from hypertension and reduction of CBF with secondary ischemia from hypotension.

Control of Intracranial Pressure. Many authors advocate direct monitoring of ICP by using a dural or an epidural bolt. Osmotic agents such as mannitol should be used as outlined earlier (see ICH management section). Head elevation, sedation, stool softeners, and prevention of straining and pain are general measures that prevent intermittent rise in ICP. Ventricular drainage of cerebrospinal fluid is indicated in patients with acute hydrocephalus. Raised ICP is sometimes associated with neurogenic pulmonary edema, which can be fatal. Such patients should be intubated, receive positive pressure ventilation, and be given diuretics and norepinephrine.

TABLE 57–11

HUNT AND HESS CLASSIFICATION OF SUBARACHNOID HEMORRHAGE

Grade	Characteristics
I	Asymptomatic or minimal headache and slight nuchal rigidity
II	Moderate-to-severe headache, nuchal rigidity, no neurologic deficit other than cranial nerve palsy
III	Drowsiness, confusion, or mild focal deficit
IV	Stupor, moderate-to-severe hemiparesis, possible early decerebrate rigidity and vegetative disturbance
V	Deep coma, decerebrate rigidity, moribund appearance

Cerebral Vasospasm. Cerebral vasospasm occurs in about 40% of patients with SAH.[130] It is the most feared complication and the leading cause of death in patients with SAH who arrive at the hospital alive. The single most important determinant of the occurrence and severity of vasospasm is the amount of blood in the basal cisterns. Cerebral vasospasm is evident on the 3rd or 4th day after an SAH, peaking around the 7th to 10th day. Fifty percent of patients with vasospasm have cerebral ischemic symptoms.[130] Vasospasm is believed to be related to vasoactive substances released (probably by the red blood cell) in the basal cisterns, secondary to hemorrhage. Vasospasm can be detected by angiography or noninvasively by TCD. Vasospasm is best managed by *prevention*. In good surgical candidates, early clipping of the aneurysm and removal of blood has been the most widely accepted form of therapy. Medical prevention of vasospasm and its ischemic complications could be achieved by oral administration of nimodipine;[131] however, the mechanism of action of nimodipine in improving outcome after SAH and in decreasing the incidence of vasospasm is unknown. Management of *established* vasospasm is generally unrewarding. Neurosurgeons recommend ICP reduction, intravascular volume expansion to increase cardiac output, hemodilution, and induced hypertension to improve CBF.

Surgical Management. It is currently the consensus that patients with grades I, II, and III SAH (Table 57–11) should undergo operation as early as possible after SAH from ruptured intracranial aneurysms, provided they are good surgical risks.[132] Aneurysm clipping within 72 hours of SAH has been shown to be associated with decreased incidence of early recurrence of bleeding. In addition, removal of blood from the subarachnoid space prevents the development of vasospasm. Various surgical techniques have been used to manage cerebral aneurysms. Obliteration of the neck of the aneurysm by clipping is the method of choice. Rebleeding occurs in less than 1% of cases. Giant aneurysms are difficult to clip because of their broad neck. Multiple clips, a single clip combined with emptying of the aneurysmal sac, and application of tourniquets are some surgical options. Multiple aneurysms are best treated at one time.[133]

Acknowledgments. Hally Summers provided invaluable assistance in preparing this manuscript. Supported in part by National Institutes of Health grant NS23393, National Institutes of Health contract NO-1-NS-0-2373, and American Heart Association grant-in-aid, Michigan Affiliate.

TABLE 57–10

CHARACTERISTICS OF CEREBROSPINAL FLUID IN SUBARACHNOID HEMORRHAGE

Color: xanthochromia of supernatant fluid (after 2 h of SAH)
Pressure: normal to elevated
Red blood cells (RBCs)
   Elevated in first and last tubes
   1000 RBCs/1 white blood cell (WBC) initially
WBCs
   1 WBC/1000 RBCs initially
   Increased WBC/RBC ratio later
   Neutrophil predominance initially
   Several hundred lymphocytes per cubic millimeter later
Chemistry
   Increased protein level (75–130 mg/dL)
   Normal glucose level (rarely decreased)

References

1. Plum F, Posner JB: Diagnosis of Stupor and Coma. Philadelphia, FA Davis, 1980.
2. Mesulam MM, Waxman SF, Geschwind N, et al: Acute confusional

states with right middle cerebral artery infarctions. J Neurol Neurosurg Psychiatry 29:84, 1976.

3. Hier DB, Mondlock J, Caplan LR: Behavioral abnormalities after right hemisphere stroke. Neurology 33:337, 1983.

4. Boller F: Strokes and behavior: Disorders of higher cortical functions following cerebral disease. Disorders of language and related functions. Stroke 12:532, 1981.

5. Davies-Jones GAB, Preston FE, Timperley WR: Neurologic Complications in Clinical Haematology. Oxford, Blackwell Scientific Publications, 1980.

6. Hart RG, Kanter MC: Hematologic disorders and ischemic stroke. A selective review. Stroke 21:1111, 1990.

7. Kelly RE, Kovacs AG: Mechanism of in-hospital cerebral ischemia. Stroke 17:430, 1986.

8. Ruff RL, Talman WT, Petito F: Transient ischemic attacks associated with hypotension in hypertensive patients with carotid artery stenosis. Stroke 12:353, 1981.

9. Adams JH, Brierley JB, Connor RCR, et al: The effects of systemic hypotension upon the human brain. Clinical and neuropathological observations in 11 cases. Brain 89:235, 1966.

10. Hachinski V, Norris JW: The Acute Stroke. Philadelphia, FA Davis, 1985.

11. Caplan LR: Vertebrobasilar occlusive disease. In: Barnett HJM, Mohr JP, Stein BM, et al (eds): Stroke Pathophysiology, Diagnosis, and Management. New York, Churchill Livingstone, p 549, 1986.

12. Price TR: Progressing ischemic stroke. In: Barnett HJM, Mohr JP, Stein BM, et al (eds): Stroke Pathophysiology, Diagnosis, and Management. New York, Churchill Livingstone, p 1059, 1986.

13. Fisher CM, Pearlman A: The non-sudden onset of cerebral embolism. Neurology 17:1025, 1967.

14. Caplan LR, Stein RW: Stroke: A Clinical Approach. Boston, Butterworth, 1986.

15. Finkelstein S, Kleinman GM, Cunco R, et al: Delayed stroke following carotid occlusion. Neurology 30:84, 1980.

16. Gunning AJ, Pickering GW, Robb-Smith AHT, et al: Mural thrombosis of the internal carotid artery and subsequent embolism. Q J Med 33:155, 1964.

17. Castaigne P, Lhermitte F, Gautier JC, et al: Arterial occlusions in the vertebro-basilar system. A study of 44 patients with postmortem data. Brain 96:133, 1973.

18. Torvik A: The pathogenesis of watershed infarcts in the brain (editorial). Stroke 14:221, 1984.

19. Celesia GG: Modern concepts of status epilepticus. JAMA 235:1571, 1976.

20. Moore WD, Hall AD: Importance of emboli from carotid bifurcation in the pathogenesis of cerebral ischemic attacks. Arch Surg 101:708, 1970.

21. Levy DE: How transient are transient ischemic attacks? Neurology 38:674, 1988.

22. Wechsler LR: Ulceration and carotid artery disease. Stroke 19:650, 1988.

23. Bogousslavsky J, Regli F: Unilateral watershed cerebral infarcts. Neurology 36:373, 1986.

24. Caplan LR, Sergay S: Positional cerebral ischemia. J Neurol Neurosurg Psychiatry 39:385, 1976.

25. Lhermitte F, Gautier JC, Derouesne C: Nature of occlusions of the middle cerebral artery. Neurology 20:82, 1970.

26. Hart R, Hindman B: Mechanisms of perioperative cerebral infarction. Stroke 13:766, 1982.

27. Kelly RE, Kovacs AG: Mechanisms of in-hospital cerebral ischemia. Stroke 17:430, 1986.

28. Pollard JA: Hypertensive encephalopathy following anaesthesia. Br J Anesth 41:640, 1969.

29. Dykes MHM, Sears BR, Caplan LR: Transient global amnesia following spinal anesthesia. Anesthesiology 36:615, 1972.

30. Woodley EJ: Neurologic complications of anesthesia. In: Silverstein A (ed): Neurological Complications of Therapy. Mt. Kisco, NY, Futura Publishing, p 199, 1982.

31. Britton M, Carlsson A, DeFaire V: Blood pressure course in patients with acute stroke and matched controls. Stroke 17:861, 1986.

32. Komrad KS, Coffey CE, Coffey KS, et al: Myocardial infarction and stroke. Neurology 34:1403, 1984.

33. McAllen PM, Marshall J: Cerebrovascular incidents after myocardial infarction. J Neurol Neurosurg Psychiatry 40:951, 1977.

34. Chin PL, Kaminski J, Rout M: Myocardial infarction coinciding with cerebrovascular accidents in the elderly. Age Ageing 6:29, 1977.

35. Fulton RM, Duckett K: Plasma fibrinogen and thromboembolism after myocardial infarction. Lancet 2:1161, 1976.

36. Dawson DM, Fischer EG: Neurologic complications of cardiac catheterization. Neurology 22:496, 1977.

37. Hurwitz BJ, Posner JB: Cerebral infarction complicating subclavian vein catheterization. Ann Neurol 1:253, 1977.

38. Gaan D, Mallick NP, Brewis RAL, et al: Cerebral damage from declotting Scribner shunts. Lancet 2:77, 1969.

39. Kosmorsky G, Hanson MR, Tomsak RL: Neuroophthalmologic complications of cardiac catheterization. Neurology 38:483, 1988.

40. Silver FL, Norris JW, Lewis AJ, et al: Early mortality following stroke: A prospective review. Stroke 15:492, 1984.

41. Britton M, de Faire V, Helmers C, et al: Prognostication in acute cerebrovascular disease. Acta Med Scand 207:37, 1980.

42. Prescott RJ, Garraway WM, Akhtar AJ: Predicting functional outcome following acute stroke using a standard clinical examination. Stroke 13:641, 1982.

43. Solis O, Roberson GR, Taveras JM, et al: Cerebral angiography in acute cerebral infarction. Rev Interam Radiol 2:19, 1977.

44. Jones TH, Morawetz RB, Crowell RM, et al: Thresholds of focal cerebral ischemia in awake monkeys. J Neurosurg 54:773, 1981.

45. Sharbrough FW, Messick JM, Sundt TM: Correlation of continuous electroencephalograms with cerebral blood flow measurements during carotid endarterectomy. Stroke 4:674, 1973.

46. Meyer FB, Anderson RE, Sundt TM, et al: Intracellular brain pH, indicator tissue perfusion, electroencephalography and histology in severe and moderate focal cortical ischemia in the rabbit. J Cereb Blood Flow Metab 6:71, 1986.

47. Wechsler LR, Ropper AH: Management of stroke in the intensive care unit. Semin Neurol 6:324, 1986.

48. Welch KMA, Levine SR, Ewing JR: Viewing stroke pathophysiology: An analysis of contemporary methods. Stroke 17:1071, 1986.

49. Aaslid R, Markwalder TM, Nomes H: Noninvasive transcranial Doppler ultrasound recording of flow velocity in basal cerebral vessels. J Neurosurg 57:769, 1982.

50. Lindegaard KF, Bakke SJ, Grolimund P, et al: Assessment of intracranial hemodynamics in carotid artery disease by transcranial Doppler ultrasound. J Neurosurg 63:890, 1985.

51. Caplan LR, Gorelick PB, Hier DB: Race, sex and occlusive vascular disease. A review. Stroke 17:648, 1986.

52. Biller J, Yuh WTC, Mitchell GW, et al: Early diagnosis of basilar artery occlusion using magnetic resonance imaging. Stroke 19:297, 1988.

53. Powers WJ, Raichle ME: Positron emission tomography and its application to the study of cerebrovascular diseases in man. Stroke 16:361, 1985.

54. Raichle ME: The pathophysiology of brain ischemia. Ann Neurol 12:2, 1983.

55. Wise RJS, Bernardi S, Frackowiak RSJ, et al: Serial observations on the pathophysiology of acute stroke. Brain 106:197, 1983.

56. Kertesz A, Black SE, Nicholson L, et al: The sensitivity and specificity of MRI in stroke. Neurology 37:1580, 1987.

57. Przelomski MM, Roth RM, Gleckman RA, et al: Fever in the wake of a stroke. Neurology 36:427, 1986.

58. Grotta JC: Current medical and surgical therapy for cerebrovascular disease. N Engl J Med 317:1505, 1987.

59. Levine SR: Acute cerebral ischemia in a critical care unit: A review of diagnoses and management. Arch Intern Med 149:90, 1989.

60. Wieloch T, Harris RJ, Siesjo BK: Brain metabolism and ischemia: Mechanism of cell damage and principles of protection. J Cereb Blood Flow Metab 2:S4, 1980.

61. Sloan MA: Thrombolysis and stroke. Past and future. Arch Neurol 44:748, 1987.

62. Zivin JA, Fisher M, DeGirolami U, et al: Tissue plasminogen activator reduces neurological damage after cerebral embolism. Science 230:1289, 1985.

63. Fisher M, Phillips PA, Davis M, et al: Tissue plasminogen activator in a large artery cerebral embolization model (abstract). Stroke 18:280, 1987.

64. Grotta JC: Emerging stroke therapies. Semin Neurol 6:285, 1986.

65. Scandinavian Stroke Study Group: Multicenter trial of hemodilution in acute ischemic stroke. I. Results in the total patient population. Stroke 18:691, 1987.

66. Gelmers HJ, Gorter K, de Weerdt CJ: A controlled trial of nimodipine in acute ischemic stroke. N Engl J Med 318:203, 1988.

67. Miller VJ, Hart RG: Heparin anticoagulation in acute brain ischemia. Stroke 19:403, 1988.

68. Cerebral Embolism Study Group: Immediate anticoagulation of embolic stroke: A randomized trial. Stroke 14:668, 1983.

69. Cerebral Embolism Task Force: Cardiogenic brain embolism. Arch Neurol 43:71, 1986.

70. Hirsh J, Levine MN: The optimal intensity of oral anticoagulant therapy. JAMA 258:2723, 1987.

71. Lyden PD, Zivin JA, Soll M, et al: Intracerebral hemorrhage after experimental embolic infarction. Arch Neurol 44:848, 1987.

72. Duke RJ, Bloch RF, Turpie AG, et al: Intravenous heparin for the prevention of stroke progression in acute partial stable stroke: A randomized, controlled study. Ann Intern Med 105:825, 1986.

73. Gelmers HJ: Effect of low dose subcutaneous heparin on the occurrence of deep vein thrombosis in patients with ischemic stroke. Acta Neurol Scand 61:313, 1980.

74. Landefield CS, Cook EF, Flatley M, et al: Identification and preliminary validation of predictors of major bleeding in hospitalized patients starting anticoagulant therapy. Am J Med 82:703, 1987.

75. Ofosu FA, Gray E: Mechanisms of action of heparin: Applications to the development of derivatives of heparin and heparinoids with antithrombotic properties. Semin Thromb Hemost 14:9, 1988.

76. Winslow CM, Solomon DH, Chasin MR, et al: The appropriateness of carotid endarterectomy. N Engl J Med 318:721, 1988.
77. Helgason CM: Blood glucose and stroke. Current Concepts Cerebrovasc Dis Stroke 23:1, 1988.
78. Pulsinelli WA, Levy DE, Sigsher B, et al: Increased damage after ischemic stroke in patients with hyperglycemia with or without established diabetes mellitus. Am J Med 74:540, 1983.
79. Berger L, Hakim AM: The association of hyperglycemia with cerebral edema in stroke. Stroke 17:865, 1986.
80. Levine SR, Welch KMA, Helpern JA, et al: Prolonged deterioration of ischemic brain energy metabolism and acidosis associated with hyperglycemia: Human cerebral infarction studied serially by 31-P NMR spectroscopy. Ann Neurol 23:416, 1988.
81. Gresham GE: The rehabilitation of the stroke survivor. In: Barnett HJM, Mohr JP, Stein BM, et al (eds): Stroke Pathophysiology, Diagnosis, and Management. New York, Churchill Livingstone, p 1259, 1986.
82. Mohr JP, Caplan LR, Melski JW, et al: The Harvard Cooperative Stroke Registry: A prospective registry. Neurology 28:754, 1978.
83. Brott T, Thalinger K, Hertzberg V: Hypertension as a risk factor for spontaneous intracerebral hemorrhage. Stroke 17:1078, 1986.
84. Fisher CM: Pathological observations in hypertensive cerebral hemorrhage. J Neuropathol Exp Neurol 30:536, 1971.
85. Mohr JP, Stein BM, Hilal SK: Arteriovenous malformations. In: Toole JF (ed): Handbook of Clinical Neurology, Vascular Diseases, Part II, Volume 10. Amsterdam, Elsevier Science Publishers, p 361, 1989.
86. Furlan AJ, Cavalier SJ, Hobbs RE, et al: Hemorrhage and anticoagulation after nonspecific embolic brain infarction. Neurology 32:280, 1982.
87. Ruff RL, Dougherty JH: Evaluation of acute cerebral ischemia for anticoagulant therapy: Computed tomography or lumbar puncture. Neurology 31:736, 1981.
88. Kase CS, Robinson K, Stein RW, et al: Anticoagulant related intracerebral hemorrhage. Neurology 35:943, 1982.
89. Cerebral Embolism Study Group: Cardioembolic stroke, early anticoagulation, and brain hemorrhage. Arch Intern Med 147:636, 1987.
90. Kase CS, O'Neal AM, Fisher M, et al: Intracranial hemorrhage after use of tissue plasminogen activator for coronary thrombolysis. Ann Intern Med 112:17, 1990.
91. Levine SR, Brust JCM, Futrell N: Cerebrovascular complications of the use of the "crack" form of alkaloidal cocaine. N Engl J Med 323:699, 1990.
92. Vinters HV: Cerebral amyloid angiopathy: A critical review. Stroke 18:311, 1987.
93. Okazaki H, Reagan TJ, Campbell RJ: Clinicopathologic studies of primary cerebral amyloid angiopathy. Mayo Clin Proc 54:22, 1979.
94. Kalyan-Raman UP, Kalyan-Raman K: Cerebral amyloid angiopathy causing intracranial hemorrhage. Ann Neurol 16:321, 1984.
95. Walsh TJ, Hier DB, Caplan LR: Aspergillosis of the central nervous system: Clinicopathological analysis of 17 patients. Ann Neurol 18:574, 1985.
96. Little JR, Dial B, Belanger G, et al: Brain hemorrhage from intracranial tumor. Stroke 10:283, 1979.
97. Mandybur TI: Intracranial hemorrhage caused by metastatic tumors. Neurology 27:650, 1977.
98. Omae T, Veda K, Ogata J, et al: Parenchymatous hemorrhage: Etiology, pathology and clinical aspects. In: Toole JF (ed): Handbook of Clinical Neurology, Vascular Diseases, Part II, Volume 10. Amsterdam, Elsevier Science Publishers, p 287, 1989.
99. Hier DB, Davis KR, Richardson EP, et al: Hypertensive putaminal hemorrhage. Ann Neurol 1:152, 1977.
100. Weisberg LA: Thalamic hemorrhage: Clinical-CT correlations. Neurology 36:1382, 1986.
101. Kushner MJ, Bressman SB: The clinical manifestations of pontine hemorrhage. Neurology 35:637, 1985.
102. Weisberg LA: Computerized tomographic abnormalities in patients with hemispheric transient ischemic attacks. South Med J 79:804, 1986.
103. Tanaka Y, Furuse M, Iwasa H: Lobar intracerebral hemorrhage: Etiology and a long-term follow-up study of 32 patients. Stroke 17:51, 1986.
104. Mangiardi JR, Epstein JF: Brainstem hematomas—Review of the literature and presentation of 5 new cases. J Neurol Neurosurg Psychiatry 51:966, 1988.
105. Nakahama K: Clinicopathological study of pontine hemorrhage. Stroke 14:485, 1983.
106. VanderHoop RG, Vermeulen M, van Gijn J: Cerebellar hemorrhage: Diagnosis and treatment. Surg Neurol 1988; 29:6, 1988.
107. Darby DG, Donnan GA, Saling MA, et al: Primary intraventricular hemorrhage: Clinical and neuropsychological findings in a prospective stroke series. Neurology 38:68, 1988.
108. Barkovich AJ, Atlas SW: Magnetic resonance imaging of intracranial hemorrhage. Radiol Clin North Am 1988; 26:801, 1988.
109. Ramadan NM, Deveshwar R, Levine SR: Magnetic resonance and clinical cerebrovascular disease—An update. Stroke 20:1279, 1989.
110. Poungvarin N, Bhoopat W, Viriyavejakul A, et al: Effects of dexamethasone in primary supratentorial intracerebral hemorrhage. N Engl J Med 316:1229, 1987.
111. McKissock W, Richardson A, Taylor J: Primary intracerebral hemorrhage. A controlled trial of surgical and consecutive treatment in 180 unselected cases. Lancet 2:221, 1961.
112. Juvela S, Heiskanen O, Poranen A, et al: The treatment of spontaneous intracerebral hemorrhage. A prospective randomized trial of surgical and conservative treatment. J Neurosurg 70:755, 1989.
113. Garraway WM, Whisnant JP, Drury I: The continuing decline in the incidence of stroke. Mayo Clin Proc 58:520, 1983.
114. Toole JT, Robinson MK, Mercuri M: Primary subarachnoid hemorrhage. In: Toole JF (ed): Handbook of Clinical Neurology, Vascular Diseases, Part III, Volume 10. Amsterdam, Elsevier Science Publishers, p 1, 1989.
115. Ferguson GG: Intracranial arterial aneurysms: A surgical perspective. In: Toole JF (ed): Handbook of Clinical Neurology, Vascular Diseases, Part III, Volume 10. Amsterdam, Elsevier Science Publishers, p 41, 1989.
116. Stehbners WE: Etiology of intracranial berry aneurysms. J Neurosurg 70:823, 1989.
117. Fox JL: Intracranial Aneurysms, Vols. 1–3. New York, Springer-Verlag, 1983.
118. Wilkins RH: Update—Subarachnoid hemorrhage and saccular intracranial aneurysms. Surg Neurol 1981; 15:92, 1981.
119. Kassell NF, Torner JC: Size of intracranial aneurysms. Neurosurgery 12:291, 1983.
120. Hart RG, Easton JD: Dissections of cervical and cerebral arteries. Neurol Clin 1:155, 1983.
121. Fisher CM: Clinical syndromes in cerebral thrombosis, hypertensive hemorrhage and ruptured saccular aneurysm. Clin Neurosurg 22:117, 1975.
122. Fisher CM: Headache in acute cerebrovascular disease. In: Vinken PJ, Bruyn GW (eds): Headaches and Cranial Neuralgias. New York, John Wiley & Sons, p 124, 1968.
123. Gorelick PB, Hier DB, Caplan LR, et al: Headache in acute cerebrovascular disease. Neurology 36:1445, 1986.
124. King RB, Saba MI: Forewarnings of major subarachnoid hemorrhage. NY State J Med 74:638, 1974.
125. Nishizaki T, Tamaki N, Nishida Y, et al: Aneurysms of the distal posterior inferior cerebellar artery: Experience with three cases and review of the literature. Neurosurgery 16:829, 1985.
126. Schievink WI, Karemaker JM, Hageman LM, et al: Circumstances surrounding aneurysmal subarachnoid hemorrhage. Surg Neurol 32:266, 1989.
127. Kwak R, Niizuma H, Ohi T: Angiographic study of cerebral vasospasm following rupture of intracranial aneurysms: Part I. Time of the appearance. Surg Neurol 11:257, 1979.
128. Aaslid R, Huber P, Nornes H: A transcranial Doppler method in the evaluation of cerebrovascular spasm. Neuroradiology 28:11, 1986.
129. Whiting DM, Barnett GH, Little JR: Management of subarachnoid hemorrhage in the critical care unit. Cleve Clin J Med 56:775, 1989.
130. Chyatte D, Sundt TM: Cerebral vasospasm after subarachnoid hemorrhage. Mayo Clin Proc 59:498, 1984.
131. Pickard JB, Murray GD, Illingworth R, et al: Effect of oral nimodipine on cerebral infarction and outcome after subarachnoid haemorrhage: British aneurysm nimodipine trial. Br Med J 298:636, 1989.
132. Solomon RA, Fink ME: Current strategies for the management of aneurysmal subarachnoid hemorrhage. Arch Neurol 44:769, 1987.
133. Yasargil MG, Smith RD: Management of aneurysms of anterior circulation by intracranial procedures. In: Youmans JR (ed): Neurological Surgery, Volume 3, 2nd ed. Philadelphia, WB Saunders p 1663, 1982.

CHAPTER 58

Seizures and Status Epilepticus

Michael R. Sperling

STATUS EPILEPTICUS

The earliest observations that prolonged seizures may be fatal were made 2000 years ago by the Greeks and Romans.[1] However, there was little scientific study of status epilepticus until recent years, and much remains to be learned. Status epilepticus is a common problem, with 60,000 new cases occurring yearly in the United States alone, which often result in death or severe permanent neurologic damage.[2] This chapter reviews the various aspects of status epilepticus, from epidemiology and pathophysiology through treatment.

Definition

Status epilepticus has no universally accepted definition. It is at one end of the spectrum of seizure activity, the other end being the isolated brief seizure. Status epilepticus has been defined as "a condition characterized by an epileptic seizure that is so frequently repeated or so prolonged as to create a fixed and lasting condition."[3] Unfortunately, "frequently repeated" and "prolonged" are terms that lend themselves to various interpretations. Most investigators now define status epilepticus by the duration of seizure activity, the minimum required being 30 minutes, a time limit suggested by animal data indicating that brain damage generally follows seizures that last longer than this.[4] Patients who do not regain consciousness or the ability to follow commands between repeated convulsions have also been considered to have status epilepticus,[5, 6] regardless of how long the seizures last, but these features are probably not significant. However, no one has addressed whether the definition of status epilepticus should differ for various types of seizures. For example, 30 minutes of generalized tonic-clonic activity (convulsions) poses greater risk and warrants more aggressive therapy than 10 hours of isolated finger twitching (focal motor status epilepticus).

With these limitations in mind, the currently favored 30-minute duration of seizure activity is used here as a definition of status epilepticus for all seizure types. This time requirement should not preclude aggressive therapy for individuals whose seizures have not lasted that long. The physician should not wait for a half hour of convulsions before initiating vigorous therapy. However, these individuals should not be formally diagnosed as having status epilepticus. Furthermore, the variability in definitions should be recalled when evaluating various treatments advocated in the literature.

Classification

As with seizures, status epilepticus may be categorized as either partial or generalized.[7, 8] Table 58–1 summarizes the different types of status epilepticus.

Generalized Status Epilepticus

Tonic-clonic (convulsive) status epilepticus is the most life-threatening and common form of the disorder.[7] It accounts for 66 to 100% of patients reported in literature series. It often occurs in patients with pre-existing epilepsy. It may also be caused by tumors and toxic, metabolic, or infectious etiologies in patients without a history of epilepsy. Most often, tonic-clonic seizures, each lasting 3 to 5 minutes, recur at short intervals, and the patient remains comatose between seizures. It is exceedingly rare for convulsive seizures to remain continuous without at least brief interictal periods. Tonic-clonic status epilepticus is particularly dangerous because associated systemic factors, such as hypoxia, hyperthermia, and muscle breakdown, render the brain more susceptible to injury and may damage other organs.[4] Clonic status epilepticus is similar to tonic-clonic status epilepticus but occurs mainly in young children and infants.[7]

Tonic status epilepticus is uncommon, seen largely in individuals with pre-existing tonic seizures, usually children

TABLE 58–1
CLASSIFICATION OF STATUS EPILEPTICUS

Generalized Status Epilepticus
Convulsive
    Tonic-clonic
    Clonic
    Tonic
    Myoclonic
Nonconvulsive
    Absence

Partial Status Epilepticus
Simple
    Motor
    Sensory (somatosensory or special sensory)
    Aphasic
    Autonomic
Complex
    Complex partial

Neonatal

or young adults.[7] These patients are typically mentally retarded and have mixed seizure disorders. Tonic seizures, usually lasting between 10 and 30 seconds, may recur at brief intervals, with interictal obtundation. During seizures, there is stiffening of the extremities and impairment of consciousness. The metabolic consequences of these seizures are not as severe as with convulsive status epilepticus.

Myoclonic status epilepticus is characterized by multifocal or whole body continuous myoclonus.[7] Consciousness is preserved, in contrast to clonic status epilepticus. It is seen mainly in three settings. It occurs in young children with secondary generalized epilepsy. It also occurs in patients with progressive myoclonus epilepsy,[7] late in the course of the disease. These individuals have continuous multifocal myoclonus, the jerks often involving small muscle groups of one limb or the trunk; massive whole body jerks are less frequent. Some degree of consciousness and interaction with the environment is preserved in these unfortunate individuals. Myoclonic status epilepticus also occurs in the setting of anoxic brain damage after cardiac arrest, although some physicians call this status myoclonicus and prefer not to characterize it as epilepsy. Typically, these individuals are comatose and have massive body jerks that last less than 1 to 2 seconds. Myoclonic status epilepticus should be distinguished from other forms of nonepileptic continuous myoclonus, such as Creutzfeldt-Jakob disease or metabolic disorders (Ramsay Hunt syndrome, neurolipidosis). These conditions do not respond to anticonvulsant therapy.

Absence status epilepticus is characterized by a continuous spike-and-wave state in the electroencephalogram (EEG) and clouding of consciousness[9] that may range from subtle cognitive deficits to complete obtundation. This disorder is seen most often in children and adolescents with epilepsy, although it can occur in adult epileptics. It is reported in 5 to 33% of patients in status epilepticus series. A form of absence status epilepticus known as twilight state or spike-wave stupor is seen in elderly persons without a history of seizures.[10] This form of the disorder may be related to cerebrovascular disease.

Partial Status Epilepticus

Simple (elementary) partial status epilepticus may take any form,[7] depending on the location in the brain to which the seizure activity is confined. Hence, seizures arising from the motor cortex may cause continuous jerking of one or both limbs on one side of the body. Seizures in the sensory cortex may produce tingling in the body part subserved by that region of cortex. Occipital seizures may produce unformed or formed visual hallucinations, depending on location in primary or association cortex. Seizures in the speech area may present as isolated aphasia.[11]

Consciousness is preserved during simple partial seizures. This type of status epilepticus is often most difficult to diagnose, and patients may be initially misdiagnosed as having a psychiatric problem when seizures have unusual symptoms, such as visual hallucinations. It is caused by focal encephalitis, acute infarction, tumors, and malformations. Metabolic disturbances, particularly nonketotic hyperglycemia, have been associated with this condition.[12]

Complex partial status epilepticus is an uncommon condition characterized by frequent complex partial seizures repeating every few minutes, with brief interictal periods. Patients exhibit behavioral cycling and experience periods of lessening of and increasing responsiveness that correspond to ictal and postictal states. At times, complex partial status may be due to continuous seizure activity.[13–15] As with absence seizures, the degree of impairment of consciousness varies from partial responsiveness to complete obtundation. This disorder occurs most often in patients with pre-existing complex partial seizures, and the frontal lobes have been implicated in the maintenance of the seizure activity.[16]

Unilateral Status Epilepticus

This entity is usually seen in infants and children younger than 3 years of age.[7] It usually indicates the presence of an acute brain lesion (subdural hematoma, vascular insult, encephalitis) and is associated with high fever. The seizures are hemiclonic and are followed by hemiplegia, which usually resolves over several months' time. This is known as the hemiconvulsions-hemiplegia-epilepsy syndrome, which may lead to partial epilepsy later in childhood.

Neonatal (Erratic) Status Epilepticus

This disorder is characterized by repeated focal seizures, each affecting a restricted part of the body (e.g., chin and face). They may be quite subtle and difficult to recognize.[7] The EEG often shows some electrographic seizures without clinical accompaniment, in addition to the behavioral seizures.

Psychogenic Status (Pseudoseizures)

Prolonged or repetitive psychogenic seizures may be mistaken for status epilepticus, and individuals who have this condition may receive aggressive anticonvulsant therapy.[17, 18] These patients are sometimes found in the intensive care unit after being intubated (perhaps after a respiratory arrest following benzodiazepine injection) or after having had a drug coma induced. Although nonepileptic seizures and epileptic seizures usually produce different behaviors, the distinction is difficult to draw in an emergency room setting, and it often requires an experienced epileptologist to differentiate between the two. Monitoring of the EEG is needed to make a definitive diagnosis. The absence of epileptic activity on the EEG during convulsive activity is diagnostic. The behavior during psychogenic seizures is usually erratic and arrhythmic, with random thrashing. It may be stereotyped from one seizure to the next. In contrast, epileptic seizures are rhythmic and show an orderly progression of motor activity. Individuals with recurrent status epilepticus and intractable seizures should be evaluated for this possibility.

Epidemiology

Acute illnesses account for a substantial proportion of cases in most series (Figs. 58–1 and 58–2). Chronic and cryptogenic neurologic diseases are equally well represented. Epilepsy, trauma, brain tumors, vascular disease, meningitis, encephalitis, high fever (in infants and small children), metabolic derangements (particularly hyponatremia and hypoglycemia), drug withdrawal, and congenital malformations have all been implicated as causes of status epilepticus.[5, 19–21] In one quarter to one third of patients, no cause can be found. Hysteria is an uncommon cause of apparent status epilepticus, with patients experiencing repeated pseudoseizures.[17] Typically, one half of patients with status epilepticus have no history of epilepsy, although one series in children reports no history of epilepsy in 71% of patients.[22] Those with epilepsy who experience status epilepticus often do so during an acute illness. The incidence of each of the above-mentioned causes varies from one series to the next, depending on referral population and whether patients with underlying epilepsy were included. Infectious and febrile causes are more common in infants and children, whereas trauma and cerebrovascular disease are more often seen in

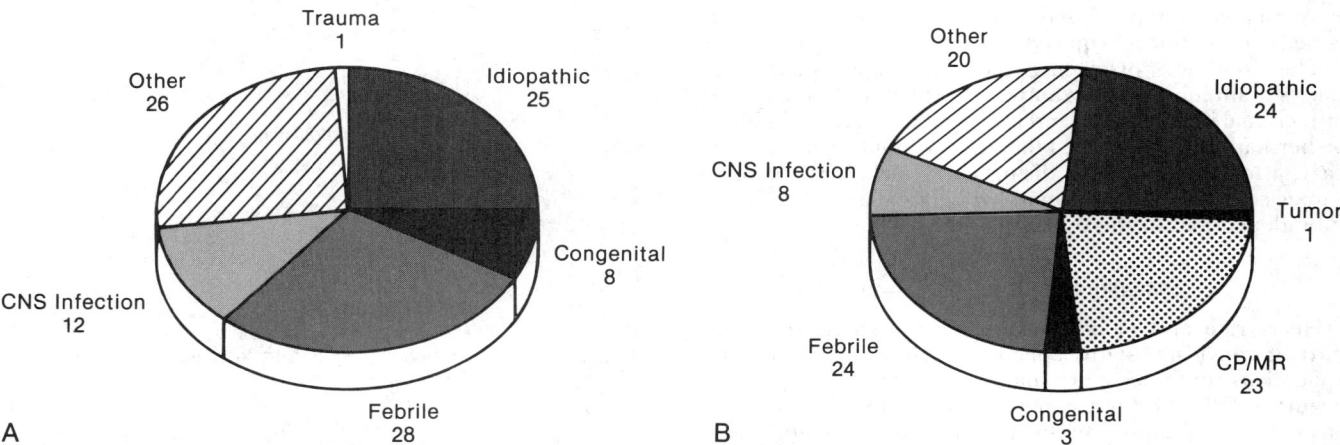

Figure 58–1. Etiology of status epilepticus in children in two series. The numbers represent the percentage for each cause. Different referral patterns probably account for the divergence in findings, although fever appears with the same frequency in each series. (Data in *A* from Aicardi J, Chevrie JJ: Convulsive status epilepticus in infants and children: A study of 239 cases. Epilepsia 11:187, 1970. Data in *B* from Maytal J, Shinnar S, Moshe L, et al: Low morbidity and mortality of status epilepticus in children. Pediatrics 83:323, 1989.)

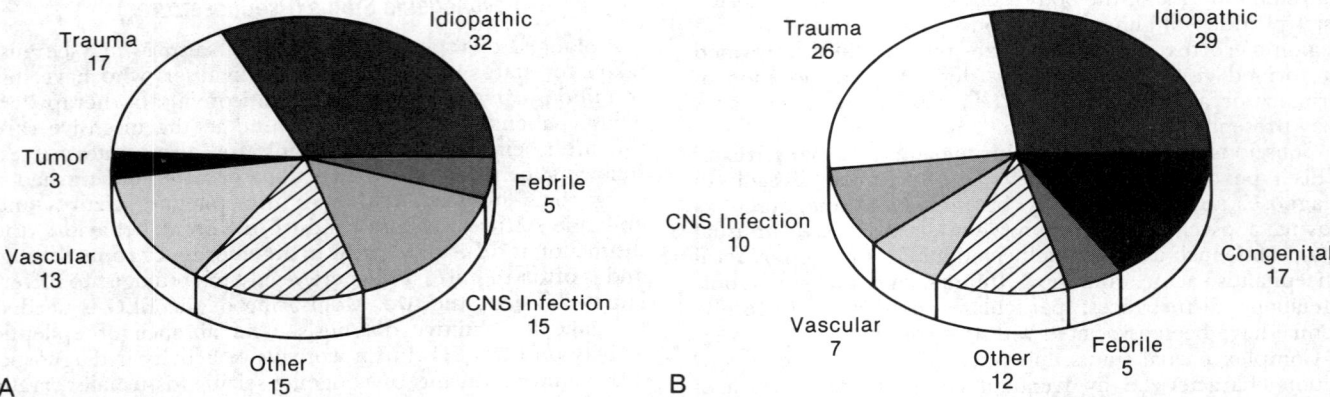

Figure 58–2. Etiology of status epilepticus in adults in two series. Trauma and vascular insults feature more prominently than in the pediatric age group. (Data in *A* from Hauser WA: Status epilepticus: Frequency, etiology, and neurological sequelae. In: Delgado-Escueta AV, Wasterlain CG, Treiman DM, et al. [eds]: Advances in Neurology, Volume 34, Status Epilepticus. New York, Raven Press, p 3, 1983. Data in *B* from Rowan AJ, Scott DF: Major status epilepticus: A series of 42 patients. Acta Neurol Scand 46:573, 1970.)

adults, particularly elderly persons.[23] Although febrile seizures are usually benign,[24] they last more than 30 minutes in approximately 5% of children.[25]

Although estimates vary, some researchers have found that as many as 20% of patients with epilepsy experience status epilepticus within the first 5 years of diagnosis.[2] It is more common in individuals with symptomatic seizures (secondary to an acquired or congenital brain lesion) than in those with idiopathic seizures.[21] Furthermore, epilepsy presents as status epilepticus in as many as 12% of patients,[26] which most often occurs in children, particularly infants. Some types of seizures (e.g., absence seizures) occasionally lead to status epilepticus.

Pathophysiology

Convulsive status epilepticus can cause brain injury or death. Nonconvulsive status epilepticus is not life threatening but may also have permanent deleterious effects. Models of partial and generalized status epilepticus have been created that mimic aspects of human status epilepticus. These permit the careful study and control of physiologic variables and the pathologic consequences. There is evidence that both local and systemic effects contribute to brain damage and that therapy capable of reversing these effects limits injury.[4, 27–30] When systemic factors are controlled (an animal is ventilated and paralyzed, and blood pressure is maintained), more time is required for neuronal injury to occur.[29]

The condition producing the status epilepticus often causes brain injury. For example, encephalitis, brain abscess, intracranial hemorrhage, and tumor all produce brain injury or herniation and may be fatal even without seizures. Similarly, a toxic or metabolic disturbance, such as ingestion of a toxic compound or profound hypoglycemia, may be harmful independent of the seizures.

Systemic Effects (Table 58–2)

Heart rate and blood pressure rise immediately at the start of convulsive status epilepticus. However, after status epilepticus continues more than 30 minutes, blood pressure begins to fall and a normotensive or hypotensive state may ensue.[4, 28–30] Because cerebrovascular autoregulation fails during status epilepticus, cerebral perfusion becomes inadequate during the hypotensive phase, and further brain damage may occur.[31] For this reason, careful attention

should be paid to maintaining systemic blood pressure during status epilepticus.

Fever also occurs, caused by both vigorous muscle activity and central mechanisms. Meldrum and Horton[28] found temperature elevations to 40°C in convulsing baboons, and higher temperature correlated with increased brain damage.

The serum glucose level initially rises secondary to glucagon secretion but then rapidly declines so that hypoglycemia may be found after the first 30 minutes of status epilepticus. Although a moderate degree of hypoglycemia may benefit neurons in animal models,[32] more severe hypoglycemia is harmful and may kill neurons in vulnerable regions of the brain.[4]

Lactate formation and hypercapnia produce acidosis. The pH often falls below 7 within the first few minutes. There is no evidence that diminishing pH increases neuronal injury, however.

TABLE 58–2

SYSTEMIC EFFECTS OF STATUS EPILEPTICUS

Initial Effects (First 30 min)
Hypertension
Hypoxia
Acidosis
Loss of autoregulation
Tachycardia
Hyperglycemia
Hypercapnia

Late Effects (After 30 min)
Hypotension
Hyperthermia
Hyperkalemia
Hypoglycemia
Hypersecretion
Autonomic collapse

Complications
Myoglobinuria, renal failure
Bronchial plugging, atelectasis
Pulmonary edema
Vomiting
Aspiration pneumonia
Dehydration
Cardiac arrhythmia
Electrolyte disturbances

Hypoxia is often seen during convulsive status epilepticus. Apnea and increased respiratory secretions that plug bronchioles may both contribute to this effect. Hypoxia can cause further brain injury[4] and promote harmful systemic effects.

Intracranial pressure increases during status epilepticus because of elevated cerebral blood flow and intravascular volume. Significant brain edema does not accompany this increased pressure.[33]

Pulmonary edema is a rare complication of status epilepticus, as is cardiac arrhythmia. Other systemic complications can also occur, either later in the course of status epilepticus or postictally. Excessive muscle activity may lead to hyperkalemia and myoglobinuria, the latter leading to renal failure. Pulmonary complications include atelectasis and aspiration pneumonia, and late cardiovascular collapse can occur. Excessive sweating and dehydration may follow. Anticonvulsant medications may cause detrimental side effects and idiosyncratic reactions.

Local Effects

Brain damage from status epilepticus is not wholly explained by the derangement of systemic factors. A growing body of evidence indicates that ordinary excitatory neurotransmitters (e.g., glutamate) and their analogues can serve as neurotoxins.[34–37] It has been proposed that excessive amounts of these transmitters released during status epilepticus produce neuronal death (Fig. 58–3). There are several mechanisms by which excitatory neurotransmitters may cause cell death, and research on these continues. The N-methyl-D-aspartate receptor, a glutamate receptor, has been the main subject of study. Excessive calcium influx into neurons through channels activated by agonists of this receptor has been implicated as a primary mechanism of injury. Excess cytosolic calcium can activate a variety of enzymes, including proteases and lipases, and leads to free radical formation. Administration of calcium channel blockers and N-methyl-D-aspartate receptor antagonists attenuates neuronal injury.[35, 38] Excessive sodium influx may play a secondary role in aggravating injury by causing acute swelling of cells, and other harmful intracellular events may be triggered by the calcium influx.

Further evidence for direct neuronal damage from seizures has been provided by models in which systemic effects of status epilepticus do not occur. Kainic acid, an excitatory neurotransmitter, can be administered in doses that produce continuous restricted limbic seizure activity; pathologic lesions similar to those of generalized status epilepticus are seen in the hippocampus.[39] Prolonged electrical stimulation of the hippocampus leads to a form of focal status epilepticus that also causes local neuronal death in the absence of systemic metabolic derangement or local ischemia or hypoxia.[40, 41]

Pathologic Changes

The major pathologic damage from status epilepticus occurs in layers 3, 5, and 6 of the neocortex, Purkinje's and basket cells of the cerebellum, and pyramidal cells of Sommer's sector in the hippocampus, the thalamus, and the amygdala.[42] Early, swelling of neurons is seen; in the chronic state, neuronal cell loss with glial proliferation is present. The pathologic changes may take hours to days to become apparent with conventional light microscopy, and ultrastructural studies are often needed to demonstrate acute changes.

Morbidity and Mortality

The mortality from status epilepticus depends primarily on the type of status epilepticus, the etiology of the condition, and the duration of seizures. Tonic-clonic status epilepticus may be fatal; other types have less serious implications. Studies report widely varying mortality rates, and the past half century has seen steadily improved survival rates.[19–22, 26, 43, 44] Mortality is usually caused by the underlying condition rather than by the seizures themselves and ranges from 2 to 25% acutely, with a 6 to 35% late mortality in tonic-clonic status epilepticus. Neonatal status epilepticus has a mortality of 15%, and mental impairments or motor deficits often remain in survivors.[45]

Morbidity from status epilepticus has been anecdotally reported; no systematic studies have been performed. Assessment of permanent neurologic impairments is confounded because brain damage is produced by both the inciting lesion and the seizures. Reports focus on tonic-clonic status epilepticus, not on other types. Morbidity relates mainly to three factors: type of seizure, etiology, and seizure duration. Seizures that last more than 2 hours convey a poor prognosis in clinical series.[5, 20] Animal data suggest that irreversible brain damage begins after 30 minutes of seizures.[30] Subtle declines in mental ability, chiefly intelligence, and personality changes are the most common adverse effects reported.[5, 20, 44, 46, 47] Systematic studies of recent memory, the function subserved by the hippocampus, have not been performed, and deterioration may be found. Complex partial status epilepticus, with prolonged hippocampal seizure activity, may also cause cognitive decline.

Status epilepticus can lead to the development of epilepsy in a previously nonepileptic individual because both the inciting lesion and the damage produced by prolonged ictal activity may be epileptogenic. Some experimental models of status epilepticus (e.g., frequent electrical hippocampal stimulation technique and use of kainic acid) produce chronic seizure disorders in animals that survive.[41] Careful epidemiologic studies have not been carried out in humans to determine to what extent the status epilepticus itself causes epilepsy or worsens pre-existing epilepsy. It is advisable to treat patients with therapeutic doses of anticonvulsants after a bout of status epilepticus, unless it can be unquestionably attributed to an acute self-limited reversible derangement.

Management

The treatment of status epilepticus depends on the type of seizure that has occurred. Tonic-clonic (convulsive) sei-

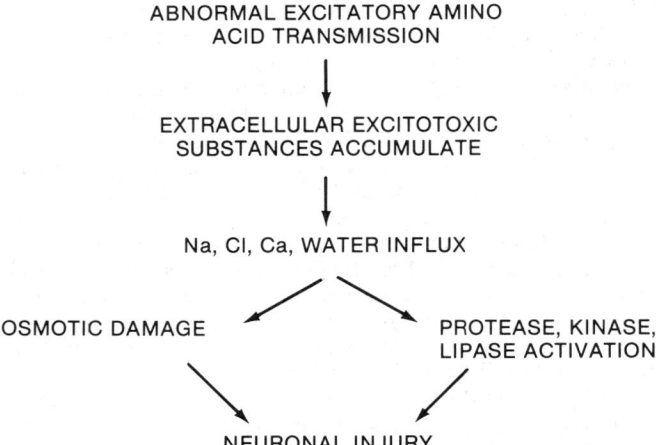

Figure 58–3. Cascade of events leading to cell injury and death resulting from excessive excitatory amino acid release at neural synapses.

zures demand urgent therapy, whereas other seizure types usually warrant a less aggressive approach. Seizure classification is critical because medication choice varies with seizure type. The etiology of the status epilepticus must be determined early because this influences therapy. Because duration of status epilepticus is the other major factor determining prognosis, it is imperative to stop the seizures as quickly as possible.

The objectives in treating status epilepticus are (1) stop seizures, (2) prevent seizure recurrence, (3) correct inciting factors, and (4) prevent systemic complications. Seizures should be terminated as quickly as feasible. Intravenous medication is preferred in life-threatening situations because agents given orally or intramuscularly have a delayed onset of action. However, less risky forms of status epilepticus may be satisfactorily treated with oral or rectal medications, which are safer than intravenous drugs.

Tonic-Clonic Status Epilepticus

It is most important to ascertain that the patient indeed has tonic-clonic status epilepticus and that prolonged or repetitive seizures have occurred. Some patients simply have the misfortune to experience an isolated seizure in the presence of a physician and thus receive aggressive therapy (and suffer complications) unnecessarily. If the patient's history is unavailable, it is often most appropriate to resist the temptation to give drugs for 10 minutes or so and wait for the seizure to stop spontaneously. This medication delay should not prevent preparation of the drugs that may be required, ensuring airway protection, establishing intravenous access, and so forth. Guidelines for treatment are provided in Table 58–3. A series of initial steps must be taken more or less simultaneously. These include (1) maintenance of oxygenation and attention to systemic factors such as cardiac rhythm and blood pressure; (2) assessment of etiology, including history, neurologic examination, and laboratory evaluation; and (3) obtaining intravenous access and initiation of therapy.

The first step is to ensure that the airway is clear; intubation is often not immediately needed. Intubation takes time that is better spent on other measures in the first few minutes and may interfere with prompt institution of appropriate therapy. Blood pressure and cardiac rhythm should be promptly assessed and administration of nasal oxygen begun. It is important to determine if the patient has a history of epilepsy and if antiepileptic medications had been taken. A screening neurologic examination should be performed to assess for a focal intracranial lesion and to exclude herniation. When placing a catheter for intravenous access, blood should be obtained to measure serum electrolytes, blood urea nitrogen, glucose level, complete blood count, toxic substances, and anticonvulsant levels. An isotonic saline infusion should be initiated. Because hypoglycemia occasionally causes status epilepticus and is readily treated with glucose, 50 mL of 50% glucose solution should be given intravenously, along with 100 mg of thiamine intravenously or intramuscularly. A blood gas measurement should be obtained after administration of nasal oxygen is begun, to ensure adequate oxygenation. The pH will be low, but bicarbonate administration should be avoided unless severe acidosis has been present for an extended period. Acidosis is best corrected by stopping seizures, and administration of bicarbonate may cause a rebound metabolic alkalosis when the status epilepticus has ended.

A medical protocol should be adopted that is uniformly applied to all in need of treatment. This leads to a high level of competence and better results. Several protocols have been recommended in the literature, all of which offer

---

TABLE 58–3

TREATMENT PROTOCOL FOR STATUS EPILEPTICUS*

Time: 0 Min
Initiate general systemic support of the airway (insert nasal airway or intubate if needed) and blood pressure; begin nasal oxygen; monitor electrocardiogram and respiration; check temperature frequently; obtain history; perform neurologic examination.
Send sample serum for evaluation of electrolytes, blood urea nitrogen, glucose level, complete blood count, drug screen, and anticonvulsant levels; check arterial blood gas values.
Start intravenous line containing isotonic saline at a low infusion rate.
Inject 50 mL of 50% glucose IV and 100 mg of thiamine IV or IM.
Call EEG laboratory to start recording as soon as feasible.
Administer lorazepam, 0.1–0.15 mg/kg IV (2 mg/min); if seizures persist, administer phenytoin, 18 mg/kg IV (50 mg/min), with an additional 7 mg/kg if seizures continue.
or
Administer diazepam, 0.3 mg/kg IV (5 mg/min); diazepam must be immediately followed by IV phenytoin at the dosage given above.

Time 30–40 Min (If Seizures Persist)
Intubate, insert bladder catheter, start EEG recording, check temperature.
Administer phenobarbital, loading dose of 20 mg/kg IV (100 mg/min).

Time 45–60 Min (If Seizures Persist)
Begin pentobarbital infusion, 5 mg/kg IV initial dose, then push until seizures have stopped using EEG monitoring; continue pentobarbital infusion at 1–3 mg/kg/h; slow infusion rate every 4–6 h to determine if seizures have stopped, with EEG guidance; monitor blood pressure and respiration carefully.
or
Administer paraldehyde 4% solution IV at a rate of 50–100 mL/h, increasing the rate until seizures stop, then maintain infusion; or 0.1–0.2 mL/kg IM with a maximum of 5 mL per injection site; if this fails, use pentobarbital as just noted.
If hyperthermia (>40°C) is present because of convulsive activity, use neuromuscular blockade.
Support blood pressure with pressors if needed.

*Use the infusion rates suggested here only if blood pressure and heart rate are safely maintained.

---

similar results.[48, 49] The protocol recommended in Table 58–3 is typical of those advised.

Several features are desired in any medication used to treat status epilepticus. Ideally, it should reach peak levels quickly in the brain, have a long duration of action to prevent recurrence, have a low incidence of untoward side effects, and be suitable for chronic oral therapy. Regrettably, no agents combine all these features, and combination therapy is usually needed. Benzodiazepines rapidly reach therapeutic levels in the brain and have gained wide acceptance as the first drugs to be used.[6, 49] Phenytoin, phenobarbital, and paraldehyde take longer to achieve therapeutic brain levels, partly because of longer injection times, and they also remain at therapeutic concentrations for many hours. These are preferred as second-line drugs, to be administered after a benzodiazepine. Pharmacokinetic features of the individual drugs are described in Table 58–4.

Diazepam rapidly achieves therapeutic concentrations in the brain but quickly redistributes to adipose tissue, so that brain levels decline by half within 20 minutes.[50] Hence, it has a short effective half-life, despite its long elimination half-life. Diazepam must be immediately followed by an agent with a long effective half-life. Phenytoin is a common

TABLE 58–4

PHARMACOKINETICS OF MEDICATIONS USED TO TREAT STATUS EPILEPTICUS

Feature	Diazepam	Lorazepam	Phenytoin	Phenobarbital	Paraldehyde
Route of administration	IV	IV	IV	IV	IV
Time to enter brain	10 s	2–3 min	1 min	20 min	<2 min
Time to peak brain concentration (min)		30	15–30	30	20
Effective serum concentration (μg/mL)	0.2–0.8	0.2	25	30–40	120–150
Time to stop status epilepticus (min)	1	<5	15–30	20	?
Effective half-life	15–20 min	14 h	22+ h	50–120 h	6 h

Modified from Treiman DM: General principles of treatment: Responsive and intractable status epilepticus in adults. Adv Neurol 34:377–384, 1983.

choice[51] because it depresses respiratory function less than phenobarbital when following diazepam. In some instances, a continuous intravenous infusion of diazepam has been recommended.[48, 52] This should be reserved for patients in whom phenytoin and barbiturates are contraindicated. Diazepam may be given as a constant infusion by diluting 100 mg in 500 mL of 5% dextrose in water and infusing at a rate of 4 mL/h.[48] The major complications of intravenous diazepam are respiratory depression and hypotension.

Although lorazepam peaks later in the brain than diazepam, it still reaches a therapeutic level quickly and does not redistribute substantially to adipose tissue. Consequently, it remains effective for many hours, and it has replaced diazepam in many centers because of this advantage.[49, 50, 53, 54] After lorazepam stops status epilepticus, there is time (8 to 12 hours) to assess the etiology of the status epilepticus, measure any pre-existing anticonvulsant levels, and begin long-term therapy. If chronic therapy with phenytoin is desired, it can be infused more slowly and thereby more safely or given orally. Lorazepam may cause hypotension and respiratory depression. Clinical studies have not demonstrated an advantage of one benzodiazepine over the other,[55] and either may be used.

Intravenous phenytoin should be pushed directly through an intravenous line containing normal saline at a maximal rate of 50 mg/min while cardiac rhythm and blood pressure are monitored.[56] Phenytoin should be started at the same time as diazepam via a separate intravenous line because it takes 15 to 30 minutes for full therapeutic levels to be achieved. Hypotension, probably from the glycol diluent,[57] and arrhythmias are the most common side effects of intravenous phenytoin. QT interval widening is among the earliest findings, and this agent is relatively contraindicated in patients with heart block. Hypotension can be reversed by slowing the rate of infusion. A phenytoin level approaching 30 μg/mL should be reached before concluding that it has failed. Because phenytoin has been reported to exacerbate seizures at extremely high serum levels,[58] some physicians may proceed directly to the use of phenobarbital in an individual receiving this drug chronically if phenytoin levels are not known. However, it is far more likely for status epilepticus to be provoked by subtherapeutic phenytoin levels than supratherapeutic levels, so that most authorities would use phenytoin early in the treatment regimen. Although phenytoin has been shown to be as effective as lorazepam[59] in stopping status epilepticus, its delayed onset of action makes it less desirable. After seizures have stopped, phenytoin should be continued at regular dosage intervals (every 8 to 12 hours) at 5 mg/kg/d to maintain therapeutic levels.

Although phenobarbital is an effective agent, it is sedating, produces respiratory depression, and can cause prolonged unconsciousness after status epilepticus has ceased.[60] These complications are mainly significant at high serum levels.

Phenobarbital takes 10 to 15 minutes to reach effective concentrations, and it does not peak in the brain for approximately 30 minutes. A loading dose of 20 mg/kg produces a serum level of 30 to 40 μg/mL. It has a long half-life, and if seizures stop after the initial bolus, further medication need not be given for the first day. It is the drug of choice for patients with status epilepticus from barbiturate withdrawal or for patients who are allergic to phenytoin. It is preferred for neonatal status epilepticus.

Pentobarbital is the general anesthetic most commonly used to treat status epilepticus that is refractory to benzodiazepines, phenytoin, and phenobarbital.[60–63] The aim is to abolish seizures, and a sufficient amount should be given until that happens; the guidelines in Table 58–3 should not serve to limit the dose of pentobarbital if seizures are not halted. The EEG should be monitored during pentobarbital administration because electrographic seizures may continue despite cessation of motor activity. Some physicians have advocated achieving an EEG state known as burst-suppression as a therapeutic end point.[61, 64] In this state, periods of brain activity alternate with periods of inactivity. However, no controlled studies demonstrate that this state is optimal, and seizures may occur during the burst-suppression state. Thus, only careful clinical and EEG observation can tell when therapy has been effective. A continuous infusion is started after seizures have been stopped. The dosage can be reduced every 4 to 6 hours when the patient and EEG are examined for evidence of seizure recurrence. If no seizures appear, the dosage can be gradually reduced until the continuous infusion is stopped. Thiopental, with an initial intravenous load of up to 200 mg followed by a constant infusion of 1 to 2 mg/min, has also been used as an alternative to pentobarbital.[65]

Lidocaine has anticonvulsant activity at low doses and is a convulsant at higher doses. It has been used for status epilepticus, but pentobarbital is preferred. The dose of lidocaine used ranges from 50 to 100 mg.[66] Valproic acid is not available as an intravenous preparation and is not recommended for tonic-clonic status epilepticus. It has been used rectally at 100 mg/h during intensive monitoring, when more gradual control of frequent seizures (but not status epilepticus) was desired.[67] Inhalational anesthetics such as halothane have been advised if benzodiazepine and phenytoin are ineffective,[48, 68] but pentobarbital is more easily and rapidly given.

Paraldehyde is an older agent that is less often needed. It is mainly used in individuals who do not have immediate intravenous access; who are allergic to phenytoin, benzodiazepines, and barbiturates; or who have renal or hepatic failure (20 to 30% of paraldehyde is exhaled by the lungs). It is also advocated by some physicians in preference to phenytoin for alcohol withdrawal seizures,[66] if benzodiazepines are ineffective. It can be given intramuscularly at a dose of 0.1 to 0.2 mL/kg (maximum of 5 mL per site) or rectally at the same dose as a 2:1 dilution in mineral oil. If the airway is protected to prevent aspiration, it can be also given through a nasogastric tube. Its serum concentration peaks 20 to 60 minutes after intramuscular injection and 2 to 4 hours after rectal insertion.

Neuromuscular blocking agents prevent the muscular contractions but do not alter brain physiology. Consequently, they treat some of the external manifestations of status epilepticus but not the underlying disorder. Their main use is to prevent excessive pyrexia from vigorous muscular contractions and myoglobinuria that may cause renal failure. They are rarely needed before the first 30 minutes of status epilepticus. Partial paralysis can restrict the amount of muscle activity while still allowing clinical observation if the EEG is not available, but this risks abolition of clinical signs and consequent error in diagnosis, and the EEG should be monitored if at all possible to guide therapy.

In addition to using the proper medications, continuous assessment of the physiologic state is necessary during a bout of status epilepticus. Dehydration can occur, and attention should be paid to maintaining intravascular fluid volume, electrolyte balance, and urine outflow. The pH should be assessed, and a sustained severe acidosis merits judicious use of sodium bicarbonate. The physician should target a pH of no more than 7 while seizures continue. Bicarbonate may be followed by metabolic alkalosis after status epilepticus has stopped, so this drug should be used sparingly. Also, acidosis may be neuroprotective. Body temperature should be checked every 10 to 15 minutes, and cooling or neuromuscular blockade should be instituted if temperature reaches 40°C. The creatine kinase value should be checked regularly if muscle contractions continue. Within a few minutes of completion of an intravenous injection of an anticonvulsant, particularly phenytoin, a serum level should be obtained, to help assess medication efficacy and guide therapy.

Although it would be ideal to start EEG recording immediately in all cases of status epilepticus, this is not practical. EEG monitoring is helpful when status epilepticus does not immediately respond to therapy or when the patient does not begin to awaken after apparent cessation of seizure activity. Monitoring also confirms that all epileptic activity has stopped and that therapy has been successful. The EEG also helps to determine where an individual patient is in the course of status epilepticus, which may be of prognostic significance. Treiman and colleagues[69] have shown that a predictable sequence of EEG patterns occurs. Initially, discrete seizures appear with interictal periods of diffuse background slowing. These gradually become more frequent, until continuous ictal activity is present. Next, the continuous seizure discharges begin to be interrupted by brief intervals (several seconds) of suppression. Finally, the EEG shows periodic discharges on a flat background.[70] Diazepam is less effective in the late EEG stages of status epilepticus, and prognosis may be worse in individuals who have progressed this far.[49]

Therapy sometimes fails when it should not. For example, the initial dose of medication may be too low, an extra dose may not be given after the first dose fails, drugs may be given intramuscularly or rectally instead of intravenously, or the underlying cause may not be addressed. It is important to keep these in mind when patients do not respond to treatment.

After seizures have been stopped, maintenance therapy must be given. If the patient had been taking an anticonvulsant previously, this agent can be reinstituted, provided that the status epilepticus did not begin despite therapeutic serum levels of that agent. If no drug was previously taken, and phenytoin or phenobarbital successfully stopped the seizures, one of these drugs may be given chronically.

Recurrent convulsive status epilepticus in children has been treated with rectal diazepam administered at home by the parents.[71, 72] An initial dose of 0.5 mg/kg is recommended, to a maximal total dose of 15 to 20 mg. Seizures typically stop within 5 minutes of treatment, and a test dose should first be given in a physician's office to ascertain the safety of the dose.

Tonic, Clonic, and Myoclonic Status Epilepticus

These conditions should be treated in the same manner as tonic-clonic status epilepticus.

Absence Status Epilepticus

This condition is generally not life threatening, and there is no evidence that prolonged absence seizures cause brain damage. Treatments that pose greater risk than the primary condition should be avoided.

Patients with absence status epilepticus in the setting of childhood or adolescent onset of absence epilepsy respond to either ethosuximide or valproic acid given orally.[73] Valproic acid can be administered rectally at an initial dose of 20 mg/kg, checking levels and increasing to a total of 50 mg/kg/d if there is no response to lower doses. This agent has a short half-life (8 to 12 hours) and wide fluctuations in serum concentrations and should be given on a frequent dosage schedule (every 6 hours). If the condition has persisted for a long time before treatment, intravenous diazepam and valproic acid are effective.[74] General anesthesia is best avoided, unless all other measures have failed.

Adults with absence status epilepticus without a history of absence seizures respond to phenytoin, which can be given orally or intravenously. If that fails, intravenous lorazepam or diazepam can be used. Porter and Penry[9] recommended valproic acid or ethosuximide as an alternative.

Simple Partial Status Epilepticus

This condition is treated with benzodiazepines, phenytoin, carbamazepine, or phenobarbital. Generally, oral therapy is preferred because it carries less risk than intravenous medication and because this condition is not life threatening. The rapidity of response to medical therapy usually depends on the cause of the seizures. Easily reversible causes respond well. If there is a metabolic disturbance (e.g., hyperglycemia), correction of that abnormality will treat the seizures without anticonvulsant medication. More often, simple partial status epilepticus is caused by structural lesions, such as chronic encephalitis,[75] which produce seizures that are resistant to medication and persist for months. When this happens, excision of the epileptic tissue is the only means of stopping the seizures.

Complex Partial Status Epilepticus

This condition should be treated aggressively in the same manner as tonic-clonic status epilepticus in view of the growing body of evidence suggesting that sustained limbic seizures cause permanent brain damage. This condition has a predilection for the frontal lobes and hippocampus[16] and can cause cognitive or personality deterioration.[14]

Unilateral Status Epilepticus

This disorder is treated in the same manner as tonic-clonic status epilepticus. The underlying cause determines response to medication.

TABLE 58-5

DOSES OF AND INDICTIONS FOR ANTICONVULSANT MEDICATIONS

Drug	Seizure Type	Serum Level (μg/mL)	Daily Dose (mg)*
Carbamazepine	All partial, tonic-clonic, tonic, clonic	4–12	600–2400
Ethosuximide	Absence	40–100	500–1500
Phenobarbital	All partial, tonic-clonic, tonic, clonic	15–45	60–300
Phenytoin	All partial, tonic-clonic, tonic, clonic	10–30	300–600
Valproic acid	All generalized, partial†	50–100	750–3000

*Typical daily dose for a 50- to 70-kg individual. Drug metabolism varies, and higher or lower doses may be needed.
†Valproic acid may be effective in partial seizures and tonic-clonic seizures that are secondarily generalized. This is uncertain, and valproic acid is not currently advised for these seizure types unless phenytoin, carbamazepine, and phenobarbital cannot be used.

Neonatal (Erratic) Status Epilepticus

The underlying cause of seizures must be addressed and specific therapy provided. Hypoglycemia should be treated with 25% glucose (2 to 4 mL/kg intravenously). Hypomagnesemia and hypocalcemia should also be treated if present. Phenobarbital is given at a dose of 20 mg/kg/d, with a maintenance dose of 5 mg/kg/d in two divided doses.[45] Diazepam (0.3 to 0.5 mg/kg intravenously), lorazepam (0.1 mg/kg intravenously), phenytoin (20 mg/kg intravenously), and paraldehyde (0.3 to 0.4 mg/kg rectally) can also be given. Because pyridoxine deficiency is a rare cause of neonatal seizures, 50 to 100 mg should also be given intravenously if there is no response to anticonvulsants.

Psychogenic Status (Pseudoseizures)

Anticonvulsants are ineffective for psychogenic seizures. Useless therapy should be avoided; psychiatric or psychologic treatment is indicated for this condition. Some patients with psychogenic seizures also have epilepsy, which may make planning of therapy difficult. This condition is best treated by an experienced epileptologist at an epilepsy facility with appropriate support personnel.

SEIZURES

The treatment of seizures is a complex topic that in itself merits an entire chapter or textbook.[18, 76] Because single seizures are self-limited and fairly benign, the goal of therapy is to prevent further seizures rather than interrupt and shorten a seizure that is presently occurring. The need for prophylaxis depends on etiology and the likelihood of seizure recurrence. Acutely, it is important to ascertain the cause and determine whether the seizure is transient and easily reversible (e.g., metabolic derangement) or whether it is due to a structural brain lesion (e.g., stroke, tumor). The former does not require long-term antiepileptic agents, whereas the latter is treated with chronic therapy.

If more than one seizure has occurred that is not easily explained by a reversible nonepileptic cause, anticonvulsant treatment should be prescribed. For single isolated seizures, the decision to treat can be made jointly in consultation with the patient after he or she has recovered normal mental function and the necessary laboratory tests have been obtained. The need for therapy is rarely urgent, and oral medication is preferred. It is most important to target specific serum anticonvulsant levels rather than a particular oral dose. It makes little sense to give everyone the same 300 mg of phenytoin, to cite a common example, when serum levels can vary from subtherapeutic to toxic levels, depending on body weight and metabolism. The seizure type determines the medication choice; doses and indications are provided in Table 58–5.

In a patient with pre-existing epilepsy, the history and drug levels in the serum should be used to determine the course of action after a seizure has occurred. In the absence of significant symptoms of drug toxicity, the dosage of whatever medication the patient is taking (provided it is appropriate) can be increased as an initial step. If no further increases can be made, a different drug should be prescribed, and the first drug should be discontinued after therapeutic levels of the new agent have been reached.

Some people with epilepsy remain refractory to medication and experience occasional seizures. Should such an individual happen to have a seizure while in the hospital, there is no cause for alarm. Therapeutic medication levels should be established and a neurologist or epilepsy specialist consulted. The specialist can best determine the most suitable course of action. One must also keep in mind that chronic anticonvulsant use induces hepatic microsomal enzymes and that drugs prescribed for other reasons may be metabolized more quickly than usual.

CONCLUSION

Further knowledge about the pathophysiology of seizures and the mechanisms by which they produce brain injury should lead to advances in therapy. Some new therapies currently under evaluation are especially promising. Manipulation of N-methyl-D-aspartate receptors and calcium channels appears to limit neuronal injury and death in experimental models and has the potential to revolutionize the way in which seizures and status epilepticus are treated.

References

1. Temkin O: The Falling Sickness, 2nd ed. Baltimore. The Johns Hopkins University Press, 1971.
2. Hauser WA: Status epilepticus: Epidemiologic considerations. Neurology 40:9, 1990.
3. Gastaut H: Clinical and electroencephalographic classification of epileptic seizures. Epilepsia 11:102, 1970.
4. Meldrum BS: Metabolic factors during prolonged seizures and their relation to nerve cell death. Adv Neurol 34:261, 1983.
5. Rowan AJ, Scott DF: Major status epilepticus: A series of 42 patients. Acta Neurol Scand 46:573, 1970.
6. Sawyer GT, Webster DD, Schutz J: Treatment of uncontrolled seizure activity with diazepam. JAMA 203:913, 1968.
7. Gastaut H: Classification of status epilepticus. Adv Neurol 34:15, 1983.
8. Leppik IE: Status epilepticus: The next decade. Neurology 40:4, 1990.
9. Porter RJ, Penry JK: Petit mal status. Adv Neurol 34:61, 1983.
10. Lee SI: Nonconvulsive status epilepticus: Ictal confusion in later life. Arch Neurol 42:778, 1985.
11. Hamilton N, Matthews T: Aphasia, the sole manifestation of status epilepticus. Neurology 29:745, 1979.
12. Singh BM, Strobos RJ: Epilepsia partialis continua associated with nonketotic hyperglycemia: Clinical and biochemical profile of 21 patients. Ann Neurol 8:155, 1980.
13. Belafsky MA, Carwille S, Miller P, et al: Prolonged epileptic twilight states: Continuous recordings with nasopharyngeal electrodes and videotape analysis. Neurology 28:239, 1978.

14. Engel J Jr, Ludwig BI, Fatell M: Prolonged partial complex status epilepticus: EEG and behavioral observations. Neurology 28:863, 1978.
15. Markand ON, Wheeler GL, Pollack SL: Complex partial status epilepticus (psychomotor status). Neurology 28:189, 1978.
16. Williamson PD, Spencer DD, Spencer SS, et al: Complex partial status epilepticus: A depth electrode study. Ann Neurol 28:647, 1985.
17. Toone BK, Roberts J: Status epilepticus, An uncommon hysterical conversion syndrome. J Nerv Men: Dis 167:548, 1979.
18. Engel J Jr: Seizures and Epilepsy. Philadelphia, FA Davis, 1989.
19. Aicardi J, Chevrie JJ: Convulsive status epilepticus in infants and children: A study of 239 cases. Epilepsia 11:187, 1970.
20. Aminoff MJ, Simon RP: Status epilepticus: Causes, clinical features and consequences in 98 patients. Am J Med 69:657, 1980.
21. Janz D: Conditions and causes of status epilepticus. Epilepsia 2:170, 1961.
22. Phillips SA, Shanahan RJ: Etiology and mortality of status epilepticus in children: A recent update. Arch Neurol 46:74, 1989.
23. Sung CY, Chu NS: Status epilepticus in the elderly: Etiology, seizure type and outcome. Acta Neuro. Scand 80:51, 1989.
24. Annegers JF, Hauser WA, Shirts SB, et al: Factors prognostic of unprovoked seizures after febrile convulsions. N Engl J Med 316:493, 1987.
25. Hauser WA: Epidemiology of febrile seizures. In: Ellenberg J, Nelson D (eds): Febrile Convulsions. New York, Raven Press, p 5, 1982.
26. Hauser WA: Status epilepticus: Frequency, etiology, and neurological sequelae. Adv Neurol 34:3, 1983.
27. Simon RP: Physiologic consequences of status epilepticus. Epilepsia 26(suppl 1):S58, 1985.
28. Meldrum BS, Horton RW: Physiology of status epilepticus in primates. Arch Neurol 28:1, 1973.
29. Meldrum BS, Vigouroux RA, Brierley JB: Systemic factors and epileptic brain damage. Prolonged seizures in paralyzed, artificially ventilated baboons. Arch Neurol 29:82, 1973.
30. Meldrum BS, Brierley JB: Prolonged epileptic seizures in primates. Ischemic cell change and its relation to ictal physiological events. Arch Neurol 28:10, 1973.
31. Ingvar MH, Siesjo BK: Local blood flow and oxygen consumption in the rat brain during sustained bicuculline-induced seizures. Acta Neurol Scand 68:128, 1983.
32. Blennow G, Brierly JB, Meldrum BS, et al: Epileptic brain damage: The role of systemic factors that modify cerebral energy metabolism. Brain 101:687, 1978.
33. Wasterlain CG: Mortality and morbidity from serial seizures: An experimental study. Epilepsia 15:155, 1974.
34. Choi DW, Maulucci-Geddi MA, Kriegstein AR: Glutamate neurotoxicity in cortical cell culture. J Neurosci 7:357, 1987.
35. Dichter MA, Choi DW: Excitatory amino acid neurotransmitters and excitotoxins. In: Appel SH (ed): Current Neurology, Volume 9. Chicago, Year Book Medical Publishers, p 1, 1989.
36. Griffiths T, Evans MC, Meldrum BS: Temporal lobe epilepsy, excitotoxins and the mechanism of selective neuronal loss. In: Fuxe K, Roberts PJ, Schwarcz R (eds): Excitotoxins. London, Macmillan, p 331, 1983.
37. Rothman SM, Olney JW: Excitotoxicity and the NMDA receptor. Trends Neurosci 10:301, 1987.
38. Ford LM, Sanberg PR, Norman AB, et al: MK-801 prevents hippocampal neurodegeneration in neonatal hypoxic-ischemic rats. Arch Neurol 46:1090, 1989.
39. Lothman EW, Collins RC: Kainic acid induced limbic seizures: Metabolic, behavioral, electroencephalographic and neuropathological correlates. Brain Res 218:299, 1981.
40. Lothman EW, Bertram EH, Bekenstein JW, et al: Self-sustaining limbic status epilepticus induced by "continuous" hippocampal stimulation: Electrographic and behavioral characteristics. Epilepsy 3:107, 1989.
41. Lothman E: The biochemical basis and pathophysiology of status epilepticus. Neurology 40:13, 1990.
42. Corsellis JAN, Bruton CJ: Neuropathology of status epilepticus in humans. Adv Neurol 34:129, 1983.
43. Lennox WG. Epilepsy and Related Disorders. Boston, Little, Brown, 1980.
44. Maytal J, Shinnar S, Moshe SL, et al: Low morbidity and mortality of status epilepticus in children. Pediatrics 83:323, 1989.
45. Volpe JJ: Neurology of the Newborn. 2nd ed. Philadelphia, WB Saunders, 1987.
46. Dodrill CB: Correlates of generalized tonic-clonic seizures with intellectual, neuropsychological, emotional, and social function in patients with epilepsy. Epilepsia 27:399, 1986.
47. Dodrill CB, Wilensky AJ: Intellectual impairment as an outcome of status epilepticus. Neurology 40:23, 1990.
48. Delgado-Escueta AV, Wasterlain C, Treiman DM, et al: Management of status epilepticus. N Engl J Med 306:1337, 1982.
49. Treiman DM: The role of benzodiazepines in the management of status epilepticus. Neurology 40:32, 1990.
50. Treiman DM: Pharmacokinetics and clinical use of benzodiazepines in the management of status epilepticus. Epilepsia 30(suppl 2):S4, 1989.
51. Delgado-Escueta AV, Enrile-Bascal F: Combination therapy for status epilepticus: Intravenous diazepam and phenytoin. Adv Neurol 34:477, 1983.
52. Bell DS, Bertino JS Jr: Constant diazepam infusion in the treatment of continuous seizure activity. Drug Intell Clin Pharmacol 18:965, 1984.
53. Homan RW, Walker JE: Clinical studies of lorazepam in status epilepticus. Adv Neurol 34:493, 1983.
54. Walton NY, Treiman DM: Lorazepam treatment of experimental status epilepticus in the rat: Relevance to clinical practice. Neurology 40:990, 1990.
55. Leppik IE, Derivan AT, Homan RW, et al: Double-blind study of lorazepam and diazepam in status epilepticus. JAMA 249:1452, 1983.
56. Wilder BJ, Ramsay E, Wilmore LJ, et al: Efficacy of intravenous phenytoin in the treatment of status epilepticus. Ann Neurol 1:511, 1977.
57. Louis S, Kutt H, McDowell F: The cardiocirculatory changes caused by intravenous Dilantin and its solvent. Am Heart J 74:523, 1967.
58. Rall TW, Schliefer LS: Drugs effective in the therapy of the epilepsies. In: Gilman AG, Goodman LS, Gilman A (eds): Goodman and Gilman's The Pharmacological Basis of Therapeutics. 6th ed. New York, Macmillan Publishing, p 448, 1980.
59. Treiman DM, DiGiorgio CM, Ben-Menachem E, et al: Lorazepam vs. phenytoin in the treatment of generalized convulsive status epilepticus. Report of an ongoing study. Neurology 35(suppl 1):284, 1985.
60. Rashkin MC, Youngs C, Penovich P: Phenobarbitol treatment of refractory status epilepticus. Neurology 37:500, 1987.
61. Goldberg MA, McIntyre HB: Barbiturates in the treatment of status epilepticus. Adv Neurol 34:499, 1983.
62. Osorio I, Reed RC: Treatment of refractory generalized tonic-clonic status epilepticus with pentobarbital anesthesia after high-dose phenytoin. Epilepsia 30:434, 1989.
63. Young GB, Blume WT, Bolton CF, et al: Anesthetic barbiturates in refractory status epilepticus. Can J Neurol Sci 7:291, 1980.
64. Van Ness PC: Pentobarbital and EEG burst suppression in treatment of status epilepticus refractory to benzodiazepines and phenytoin. Epilepsia 31:61, 1990.
65. Brown A, Horton J: Status epilepticus treated by intravenous infusions of thiopentone sodium. Br Med J 1:27, 1967.
66. Browne TR: Paraldehyde, chlormethiazole, and lidocaine for treatment of status epilepticus. Adv Neurol 34:509, 1983.
67. Rosenfeld WE, Leppik I, Gates JR, et al: Valproic acid loading during intensive monitoring. Arch Neurol 44:709, 1987.
68. Opitz A, Marschall M, Degen R, et al: General anesthesia in patients with epilepsy and status epilepticus. Adv Neurol 34:531, 1983.
69. Treiman DW, Walton NY, Kendrick CW: A progressive sequence of electroencephalographic changes during generalized convulsive status epilepticus. Epilepsy Res 5:49, 1990.
70. Snodgrass SM, Tsuburaya K, Ajmone-Marsan C: Clinical significance of periodic lateralized epileptiform discharges: Relationship with status epilepticus. J Clin Neurophysiol 6:159, 1989.
71. Camfield CS, Camfield PR, Smith E, et al: Home use of rectal diazepam to prevent status epilepticus in children with convulsive disorders. J Child Neurol 4:125, 1989.
72. Hoppu K, Santavuori P: Diazepam rectal solution for home treatment of acute seizures in children. Acta Paediatr Scand 70:369, 1981.
73. Vajda FJE: Valproic acid in the treatment of status epilepticus. Adv Neurol 34:519, 1983.
74. Dreifuss FE: Status epilepticus. In: Dreifuss FE (ed): Pediatric Epileptology. Boston, John Wright, p 221, 1983.
75. Rasmussen T: Further observations on the syndrome of chronic encephalitis and epilepsy. Appl Neurophysiol 41:1, 1978.
76. Laidlaw J, Richens A: A Textbook of Epilepsy. New York, Churchill Livingstone, 1982.

CHAPTER 59

Neuromuscular Diseases

Robert P. Lisak

Patients with failure of the motor unit may develop sufficient weakness of the respiratory muscles or the muscles that protect the upper airway to require care in a critical care unit (CCU). In other patients, the symptoms and signs of dysautonomia associated with a neuromuscular illness may precipitate a CCU admission. In some instances, a neurologic disorder is the primary cause for the failure of respiratory and/or bulbar musculature (e.g., Guillain-Barré syndrome, myasthenia gravis, tetanus, and botulism). In other patients, neuromuscular failure may result from generalized metabolic abnormalities (e.g., hypokalemia and hypophosphatemia) or treatment of other disorders (e.g., antibiotic-induced paralysis in nonmyasthenic patients). Not infrequently, more than one factor is important in precipitating sufficient dysfunction of the motor unit to require management in a CCU. For example, a patient with myasthenia gravis with moderate bulbar or respiratory muscle weakness may develop an infection, perhaps pneumonia, to which he or she is more susceptible, which causes a marked increase in weakness. This increased weakness may require intubation and respiratory support (i.e., myasthenic crisis). The use of certain antibiotics with neuromuscular blocking activity, such as the aminoglycosides, may cause further weakness. The importance of searching for multiple factors that have a deleterious effect on the function of the motor unit, especially in a patient who already has a defect in the motor unit, cannot be overemphasized. Modifying and treating these multiple factors are vital for both the diagnosis and the successful treatment of these patients.

ANATOMY AND PHYSIOLOGY OF THE NEUROMUSCULAR SYSTEM
Anatomic Considerations

The principal components of the neuromuscular system are (1) the alpha motor neuron, which is located in the ventral gray matter of the spinal cord, and the somatic and brachial motor neurons of the cranial nerves; (2) the axons, which are the projections of the motor neurons, and the myelin that is wrapped about these large-diameter axons; (3) the neuromuscular junction, which is composed of the specialized ending of the nerve terminal (presynaptic) and the specialized portion of the postsynaptic muscle membrane; and (4) the muscle fibers. The normal function of the motor unit is not only dependent on the integrity of each of the components of this unit but also influenced by sensory input from the periphery, by the effects of smaller (gamma) motor neurons on specialized muscle fibers, and by higher centers within the central nervous system (CNS). Indeed, there are even projections of the alpha motor neuron onto other cells within the CNS that have a feedback influence on the same alpha motor neurons.[1, 2]

Anterior Horn Cell and Axon/Myelin Sheath

Alpha motor neurons have large axons and are therefore myelinated. When an alpha motor neuron discharges, as in a willed volitional movement, the action potentials are conducted down the axon via saltatory conduction. This involves a skipping from one node of Ranvier (where the axon is bare and its membrane and channels are exposed) to the next node of Ranvier. This arrangement allows myelinated axons to conduct at a higher conduction velocity and at a higher frequency than unmyelinated axons, in which conduction is continuous. The myelin sheath, which is the modified Schwann cell membrane, can be thought of as a high-resistance, low-capacitance insulator. At the internodes, depolarization occurs with an influx of sodium (sodium channels open) and an efflux of potassium. Repolarization, with a return of the membrane potential in that region of the axon membrane to approximately baseline, results from an influx of potassium and an efflux of sodium. Current evidence, however, suggests that repolarization does not

involve potassium channels in normal myelinated nerve fibers. Potassium channels are involved in repolarization in unmyelinated axons and may be important in the pathophysiology of myelinated axons during demyelination. In the normal myelinated axon, however, potassium channels may be involved in membrane stabilization.[3, 4]

Neuromuscular Junction

The terminal portion of the axon of the alpha motor neuron is devoid of myelin. The structure of the terminal portion of the axon is modified into a bouton. It is rich in mitochondria, the enzyme choline acetyltransferase, and synaptic vesicles that contain acetylcholine, the neurotransmitter at the neuromuscular junction. Choline acetyl transferase is required for rapid synthesis of acetylcholine from choline and acetate. Some of the vesicles are concentrated in pairs of rows at the presynaptic membrane called active zones. The nerve is separated from the muscle membrane by a 40- to 50-nm space called the synaptic cleft. There is a spontaneous release of acetylcholine, which diffuses through the basilar lamina in the cleft to interact with the specific receptor for acetylcholine (nicotinic acetylcholine receptor) present at the modified postsynaptic muscle membrane.

The postsynaptic muscle membrane is also highly modified into multiple folds, and the acetylcholine receptor is concentrated on the folds closest to the presynaptic nerve membrane. The acetylcholine receptor is a transmembrane protein of approximately 250 kd comprising five peptide chains (alpha$_2$, beta, delta, epsilon at the mature mammalian junction and alpha$_2$, beta, delta, gamma at extrajunctional and in fetal or as yet noninnervated muscle). There is one ligand-binding site on each of the chains. When two molecules of acetylcholine interact with the receptor, which is also a sodium channel, the receptor changes its configuration, resulting in an opening of the channel with an influx of sodium and efflux of potassium. The opening of a few of the receptor-channels as a result of spontaneous release of acetylcholine gives rise to a small depolarization, called miniature end-plate potentials, at the postsynaptic muscle membrane.

When sufficient conducted action potential arrives at the nerve terminal, there is quantal release of acetylcholine through exocytosis, with the vesicles fusing with the nerve membrane. The depolarization of the terminal presynaptic membrane is dependent on presynaptic voltage-gated calcium channels and is therefore sensitive to changes in divalent cations, especially calcium. The quantal release of acetylcholine results in enough open receptor-channels, with resultant influx of sodium and efflux of potassium, to produce an end-plate potential. The end-plate potential results in the muscle membrane's reaching threshold and the firing of an action potential. This action potential is then responsible for initiating changes in the muscle that lead to contraction. Repolarization occurs when sodium exits and potassium re-enters the cell through the channel. There is sufficient release of acetylcholine and sufficient available acetylcholine receptors to provide a safety factor for neuromuscular transmission. Therefore, in the normal situation, even with a decrease in released quanta of acetylcholine because of repeated stimulation or use and normal fluctuations at the junction, the safety factor is more than sufficient to prevent any clinical evidence of failure of transmission and resultant weakness. In disorders of the neuromuscular junction, there is reduction in one or more components of the safety factor, which makes the patient susceptible to anything acting either pre- or postsynaptically that further reduces or blocks transmission. The acetylcholine diffuses away from the receptor and the enzyme acetylcholinesterase cleaves acetylcholine, thus inactivating it. The channels regain their initial closed configuration until they interact with acetylcholine again.[5, 6]

Muscle

The muscle membrane potential, like that of nerve, is achieved in the resting state by actively maintaining a high concentration of sodium outside the cell and a high concentration of potassium inside the cell. When an action potential is propagated along the muscle membrane, there is depolarization, with a shift of sodium into the cell and potassium out. Contraction of the muscle itself results from propagation of the action potential by the transverse tubules. Via a calcium release–dependent series of interactions, there is a change in the relationship between the intracellular contractile proteins that results in the movement of these proteins in a sliding fashion. This causes the shortening of the muscle fiber. Relaxation results from the return of these contractile proteins to their original relationship. These processes are highly energy dependent. Abnormalities in the membrane, in energy metabolism, and in the contractile proteins or the loss of sufficient numbers of muscle fibers lead to a loss of normal muscle function, which could produce weakness, abnormal relaxation, and so forth. It is obvious that all of the presynaptic processes must also be in order for the muscle to work normally.[1, 7]

ASSESSMENT OF THE PATIENT WITH NEUROMUSCULAR FAILURE
General Approach

The first consideration in a patient with failure of the motor unit (lower motor neuron or neuromuscular failure) is to ensure appropriate airway, sufficient oxygenation, and stabilization of any life-threatening cardiovascular problems. Although this may be stating the obvious, it is unfortunately not infrequently forgotten in the attempt to determine a definitive diagnosis in a patient with an as yet undiagnosed neurologic disease or to adjust medications in a patient with a known neurologic disorder to avoid hospitalization, intubation, or CCU transfer. The need for CCU management should be made on the basis of a clinical assessment of the severity of the patient's symptoms and signs and the direction (better, stable, or worse) and rate (rapid or slow) of the patient's course. Testing for strength of bulbar muscles and reflexes and measurement of arterial blood gases, pulse oximetry, end-volume carbon dioxide, vital capacity, and negative inspiratory force are useful and provide baseline numbers, but the decision to admit the patient to the hospital, to transfer the patient to a CCU, to intubate the patient, and to provide ventilator assistance should be based on clinical assessment by physicians experienced in the care of patients with neuromuscular diseases. The decision to discharge a patient from a CCU, whether to a step-down unit, a chronic ventilator unit, or a regular hospital room, should be made on the basis of clinical status and aided by evaluation of laboratory and ventilatory parameters. In general, weaning from a ventilator should be gradual, with particular attention paid to fatigue of ventilatory parameters and the patient's clinical status rather than single measurements of carbon dioxide and oxygen exchange or a single measure of force and volume.

Patients with severe and especially prolonged involvement of the motor unit or neuromuscular system have increased susceptibility to the development of certain problems such as decubitus ulcers, urinary and bowel retention or incontinence (even in the absence of true autonomic involvement because of impairment of lower abdominal wall and external sphincters), exposure of cornea (weakness of eye closure and/or loss of corneal reflex), deep venous thrombosis, aspiration pneumonia, and complications related to enteral tube or parenteral nutrition. In addition, the paralyzed patient needs psychologic support, possibly including psychiatric consultation. Attention should be paid to protein-calorie nutrition; avoidance of hyperthermia (which increases catabolism and can cause temporary worsening of patients with demyelinative neuropathies and defects of neuromuscular transmission); potassium, phosphate, calcium, and magnesium replacement; and physical and occupational therapy to avoid contractures of severely affected muscles and to assist with conditioning of less affected muscle groups. Avoiding the use of drugs with toxic effects on components of the motor unit whenever possible is also an important principle (discussed later). In addition, support groups can help patients and family members; Guillain-Barré Support Group International (215-642-6855), Myasthenia Gravis Foundation (800-541-5454), and the Muscular Dystrophy Association (602-529-2000) are examples of support groups dealing with neuromuscular diseases.

The next issue is to identify any obvious factor that could have led to deterioration of a patient with neuromuscular disease, either previously known or newly evident. Simultaneously with looking for factors that could have led to deterioration of a stable patient or a patient without previous neuromuscular problems, it must be determined whether the patient does indeed have a disorder of the neuromuscular or motor unit system. This is not always easy to do, especially if there is little history available and/or the patient is intubated or has altered levels of consciousness or mentation resulting from another disorder or from complications of the neuromuscular disorder (e.g., hypoxia and ischemia). Several evaluations may be required as the patient becomes more interactive, family members or friends can be interviewed, and the neurologic examination becomes less limited as the patient experiences reduced interference from involvement of higher centers of the nervous system. If a patient is stuporous or comatose, it is difficult to be certain that the patient is weak because of neuromuscular disease. A sensory examination to rule out involvement of the peripheral nerves cannot be reliably performed in such a patient. The flaccid areflexia seen in patients with severe metabolic encephalopathies precludes ascribing such flaccidity and areflexia to neuromuscular failure.

It is not possible to review all aspects of neurologic history and neurologic examination in this chapter. The involvement of a neurologist early in the course of evaluation can shorten the time required to decide if a neuromuscular disease is present and to identify the disorder. This then allows for appropriate specific therapy and better planning for supportive therapy.

Important general guidelines for evaluation are suggested here, with expansion provided in the later sections on individual disorders. Careful history and evaluation of the cranial nerves are important, with close attention to motor, sensory, and special sensory functions. Certain disorders such as myasthenia gravis characteristically affect the muscles in a symmetric fashion and frequently involve the muscles of the eyelids and eyes (this involvement may be asymmetric and variable in degree), but as disorders of the neuromuscular junction they spare sensory and special sensory functions. Special attention to the pupils is also important because loss of reaction to light and/or accommodation would rule out myasthenia, would be possible but unusual in Guillain-Barré syndrome, and would strongly suggest a toxin such as botulin. Asymmetric involvement of the muscles innervated by the cranial nerves is more in keeping with a neuropathy or CNS disease, including motor neuron disease, than a disorder of the neuromuscular junction. Abnormalities of extraocular motion are essentially not seen in polymyositis or dermatomyositis, amyotrophic lateral sclerosis (ALS), or poliomyelitis. Abnormalities of special sensory function such as vision, hearing, or smell suggest that the patient does not have a primary disorder of the neuromuscular system but rather has a disease of the CNS (other than motor neuron disease), has a disorder that can affect both the CNS and the neuromuscular system (such as a collagen-vascular disease), or has a complication of neuromuscular disease.

The motor examination, like that of the cranial nerves, can be difficult in a CCU. It is again important to emphasize certain basic principles related to neurologic history and examination. Although it is classically taught that myopathies result in greater proximal than distal weakness and neuropathies, greater distal than proximal, there are exceptions to this rule, and the magnitude of weakness in a patient who needs critical care may make proximal versus distal distinctions, as well as detection of asymmetry, difficult. In addition, in Guillain-Barré syndrome, the weakness is not infrequently proximal in the lower extremities and even in the upper extremities. Patients with disorders of the neuromuscular junction and muscle have bilateral and basically symmetric weakness. Patients with diseases involving the motor nerves or the anterior horn cells may show asymmetry or symmetry (especially if they are extremely weak or if the disease is of long duration). Severe and rapid muscle atrophy suggests either anterior horn cell disease or a neuropathy. Atrophy in myopathies is more diffuse and is seen in patients with severe disease of longer duration; atrophy in patients with diseases of the neuromuscular junction is extremely rare. Fasciculations may occur in disease of the nerve roots or peripheral nerve but should always suggest anterior horn cell disease when widespread. Normal or decreased tone is common in disorders of the neuromuscular system, but an increase in tone is seen in ALS, in complications of the neuromuscular disorder that involve the CNS, or in involvement of both the CNS and the peripheral nervous system by the same disease process.

Determining if there is a significant history or clinical evidence of sensory system involvement is of great importance. Although patients with inflammatory, metabolic, and ischemic or traumatic muscle diseases may complain of myalgias and patients who are extremely weak from myopathies or neuromuscular diseases may complain of vague aches, especially with activity, severe axial muscle pain is unusual. Sensory symptoms (decreased sensations, paresthesias, or dysesthesias) are seen in disorders of peripheral nerves and their roots or plexus but are not seen in pure degenerative anterior horn cell diseases (acute infections such as poliomyelitis and related disorders are associated with pain because of meningeal involvement) or in most disorders of the neuromuscular junction (patients with Lambert-Eaton syndrome may have myalgias).

Neuromuscular Failure Developing Outside the Hospital

There are four general patterns for patients in this category. One is a patient who has no previous involvement of the neuromuscular system and develops an acute or rapidly evolving syndrome in a nonhospital setting. Examples of these disorders include those related to acute toxins such as organophosphates or botulin; acutely evolving metabolic diseases such as severe hypokalemia, hypophosphatemia, and hypomagnesemia; acute toxin-induced rhabdomyolysis (such as that seen in alcoholics); acute infections (e.g., poliomyelitis, rabies, tetanus); and parainfectious and paraim-

munization disorders such as Guillain-Barré syndrome (acute inflammatory demyelinating polyneuropathy). A second overlapping group comprises patients who have had neurologic symptoms for several weeks to years, who have been diagnosed (sometimes incorrectly) and even treated, and who then decompensate over a relatively short time. Patients with myasthenia gravis commonly present to a CCU in this fashion, especially if they experience an infection, fail to take their medication correctly, or are treated with drugs that impair neuromuscular transmission. Decompensation in patients with myasthenia gravis can also occur for unidentifiable reasons. Occasionally, the condition of patients with Lambert-Eaton myasthenic syndrome, chronic inflammatory demyelinating polyneuropathy, or inflammatory myopathies or of patients with other neuropathies who encounter an additional neurotoxin will worsen to a degree requiring management in a CCU. A third group consists of patients who do not have a primary neuromuscular disorder but instead have a systemic disorder and develop neuromuscular failure, sometimes sufficient to require critical care, as a result of new involvement of the neuromuscular system by that disease or because of treatment of that disease. The development of Guillain-Barré syndrome in a patient with systemic lupus erythematosus is such an example. The fourth group consists of patients who have subclinical neuromuscular disease and are given drugs for another reason; these drugs then bring out the underlying neuromuscular disorder. Rare instances of myasthenia brought to light by treatment with quinine-like agents or phenothiazides are examples of this type of presentation, as are malignant hyperthermia and rhabdomyolysis after use of certain anesthetics and muscle relaxants.

Neuromuscular Failure Developing in the Hospital

This group of patients is quite diverse as well. The simplest management problem is the patient who has a neuromuscular disease requiring neuromuscular management, at first not requiring critical care but then decompensating. Patients with myasthenia gravis and Guillain-Barré syndrome often have this presentation. As pointed out earlier, after the patient's condition is stabilized the critical point is to determine whether the neuromuscular failure is due to natural progression of the disease or whether a superimposed problem, such as an infection or treatment with medication for the infection or for another medical problem, has contributed to or caused the deterioration.

A second group consists of patients who are hospitalized for another condition and who have a neuromuscular disease that is under adequate control but in whom the primary disease or treatment for the primary disease causes worsening of the neuromuscular disease. Once again, the condition of a patient with myasthenia gravis with cardiac, pulmonary, infectious, gastrointestinal, or psychiatric disease may worsen because of the therapeutic agents used for these other disorders. Patients who have subclinical involvement with a neuromuscular disease may have the disease revealed by treatment for another disorder. For example, patients who have preclinical or subclinical myasthenia and are undergoing a thymectomy for thymoma receive standard doses of neuromuscular blocking agents that may lead to prolonged postoperative intubation.

The last and perhaps most diagnostically challenging patients are those who do not have a known neuromuscular disorder and who develop severe weakness with respiratory and/or bulbar failure while hospitalized for another disease not associated with neurologic complications. Some of these patients may already be in the CCU; others are postoperative. They are frequently seen because of failure or difficulty in weaning from the respirator. Among the patients in this category are (1) those who have decreased renal function and receive multiple agents with neuromuscular blocking activity (neuromuscular blocking drugs at surgery or for agitation, anesthetics with blocking activity, certain antibiotics); (2) those with acute neuropathies associated with sepsis and multiple organ system failure (so-called CCU neuropathy); (3) those who develop Guillain-Barré syndrome in the hospital (sometimes postinfectious or postsurgical but often idiopathic); and (4) those who develop severe potassium or phosphate deficiency (although seldom with respiratory insufficiency in those two settings).

DISORDERS OF THE ANTERIOR HORN CELL
Pathophysiology

In response to higher nervous system centers and segmental influences, the alpha motor neuron propagates an electrical impulse in a centrifugal direction, which, as noted earlier in the case of the large myelinated fiber, is propagated by saltatory conduction. These cells influence the response of the muscle via recruitment (motor units are activated individually until a sufficient number are available for the muscle to generate the required force) and by rate coding. Rate coding is defined as making each motor unit fire at a higher frequency as the recruitment continues.[8] Any process that decreases the number of anterior horn cells or their capacity to recruit and rate code results in weakness because fewer motor units (muscle fibers innervated by the same anterior horn cell) will contract. In addition, as neurons fail and/or die, the muscle fiber is deprived of one or more trophic factors, which leads to atrophy of the muscle fibers. Thus, the hallmarks of many disorders involving motor neurons are weakness and atrophy. These are negative symptoms. Reflexes are depressed in proportion to weakness unless there is simultaneous involvement of upper motor neurons (as is seen in many patients with relatively early ALS with hyperreflexia and extensor plantar signs) or of sensory neurons (some hereditary disorders or herpes zoster, in which the primary lesion is in the dorsal root ganglia, with depressed reflexes sometimes noted). Another feature of denervated muscle fibers is a spread of the area rich in acetylcholine receptor to extrajunctional portions of the muscle fiber membrane. In many disorders of the anterior horn cell, as well as disorders of the nerve itself, there is terminal sprouting in which the number of muscle fibers that are innervated by an anterior horn cell increases, thus resulting in extremely large motor units, which unfortunately are not necessarily associated with increased strength. These muscle fibers and motor units are more prone to fire spontaneously, giving rise to fibrillations and fasciculations, respectively. Fibrillations, involving single fibers, are visible only in the tongue, whereas fasciculations can be appreciated in many muscles. Fasciculations are generally associated with anterior horn cell diseases, although they can be seen in disorders of nerve, including nerve roots, and are quite commonly seen in patients with no neurologic disease (benign fasciculations). Both signs of denervation are readily detected with electromyography (EMG) (see Chapter 54). In other disorders of the anterior horn cell, positive symptoms and signs are seen, such as spasms in tetanus or in strychnine poisoning, in which the toxin blocks the inhibition of firing of the anterior horn cell.[8]

Hereditary Diseases

There are several diseases in which the anterior horn cell is exclusively or predominantly affected. Some of these are inherited diseases (hereditary spinal muscular atrophies), or disorders primarily affecting newborns (Werdnig-Hoffmann disease, spinal muscular atrophy type I), slightly older infants (spinal muscular atrophy type II), or adolescents, teen-agers, and rarely adults (Kugelberg-Welander disease, spinal muscular atrophy type III). These patients are unlikely to be cared for in an adult CCU. Indeed, patients with Werdnig-Hoffmann disease seldom survive past 3 years of age, and patients with Kugelberg-Welander disease generally do not require critical care except in the setting of surgery for scoliosis. There are other rarer diseases in this group, including motor neuronopathy associated with hexosaminidase A deficiency (a disorder that must be distinguished from ALS). In addition, several of the hereditary motor-sensory neuropathies, including type II (neuronal Charcot-Marie-Tooth disease), may be neuronopathies (the primary defect is in the neuron cell body rather than in the axon or the myelin), but sensory neuron involvement also occurs, so they cannot be considered purely diseases of the anterior horn cell.[7, 9]

Acquired Motor Neuron Diseases

In this era of immunization against poliovirus, the most common disorder affecting the anterior horn cell is adult motor neuron disease. This disease may represent more than one disorder, although this is still controversial. Clearly, the majority of patients present with or eventually manifest signs of lower motor neuron disease (anterior horn cell disease) and upper motor neuron disease (slowing of coordinated movements, increased tone, and increased reflexes). This common form is called ALS.[7, 9, 10] Although there are some patients in whom the progressive disorder is familial, in most it is sporadic. An association with paraproteinemias with antiganglioside-binding activity has been demonstrated both with and without lymphomas in a small percentage of patients with ALS.[11, 12] At this time, most patients with ALS have a disease of unknown etiology. The syndromic diagnosis of a motor neuron disease is based on the clinical presentation and is confirmed by using EMG plus nerve conduction velocity (NCV) testing. In some instances, imaging studies or lumbar puncture is necessary to rule out a treatable cause of the neurologic dysfunction. Blood studies are important to rule out disorders that may superficially resemble ALS and to identify patients who may have an associated paraproteinemia or lymphoma. It is not clear if all patients need to have determination of antibodies to gangliosides or hexosaminidase A levels. Although many patients with ALS choose not to have treatment for infections (such as pneumonia), respiratory support, or a tracheostomy, some patients do, and therefore patients with ALS may receive care in a critical care setting. As noted earlier, supportive therapy is still one of the most important aspects of critical care management of all diseases of the motor unit (neuromuscular diseases). In most diseases of the motor neuron (anterior horn cell) itself, there is little available specific therapy. No treatment is known to favorably alter the inexorable downhill course of patients with ALS, although it has been reported that immunosuppressive therapy may help some patients with ALS-like syndrome associated with "benign" monoclonal gammopathies and/or lymphomas. No treatment exists for the hereditary disorders.

Infections

Several infections primarily affect the anterior horn cell. Poliomyelitis is the best known but is rarely seen in many countries. It may develop in patients as a result of administration of live vaccine, although this is an exceedingly rare event in nonimmunocompromised hosts. Patients present with typical viremic symptoms that may or may not clear (for 36 to 48 hours) before the second stage. The patient has a rise in temperature, with meningeal signs and symptoms. Patients develop neck and back pain and occasionally changes in level of consciousness, mentation, or mood. Increased weakness and fasciculations may occur before development of weakness. If weakness occurs, it develops 2 to 5 days into the nervous system phase and progresses for 3 to 5 days. The fever may decline before paralysis or during the period of development of weakness. The disease involving the limbs is often quite asymmetric. Some patients develop weakness of bulbar and/or respiratory muscles, which can result in the need for respiratory support, feeding via enteral tubes or parenteral feeding, and tracheostomy for bulbar or respiratory indications. Other enteroviruses may occasionally produce similar syndromes, although severe and lasting weakness is uncommon.[13] A small number of patients who had acute poliomyelitis during the epidemic years may later show slow progression of weakness, generally in limbs that were more severely affected during the original acute disease.[14] This may represent the effect of the natural loss of motor neurons with age in muscles that already have a reduced number of motor neurons rather than reactivation of poliovirus. The relation between this syndrome and ALS is not clear. Although poliomyelitis is preventable, the support of the patient's respiratory and bulbar muscles is the critical issue in the managment of the patient who develops poliomyelitis or polio-like syndromes in association with other enterovirus infections. Physical therapy is helpful in treating the painful muscles and in preventing contractures.

Herpes zoster generally affects the dorsal root ganglia, but if the spinal cord is affected the motor neurons at that level may also rarely be involved and produce segmental lower motor neuron weakness.[12, 15] The therapy of herpes zoster is covered elsewhere (see Chapters 30 and 60).

Rabies infection results in a diffuse encephalitis and myelitis in which changes in levels of consciousness, convulsions, laryngeal spasms and hypersalivation, twitching, and eventually paralysis and coma occur, with death resulting from respiratory paralysis. There is an unusual form of the disease in which the earliest sign is paralysis (paralytic rabies). Rabies can be prevented by prompt immunization with rabies vaccine, but survival after symptoms begin is extremely rare.[12]

Tetanus is caused by the ability of tetanus toxin to presynaptically block the inhibitory synapses between the large afferent sensory fibers and the alpha motor neuron. This lack of inhibition leads to the characteristic spasms of the jaw, face, and back muscles. Generalized seizures may also occur, along with autonomic dysfunction, diaphoresis, hyperthermia, and rhabdomyolysis. Patients develop respiratory failure, inability to swallow, and cardiac arrhythmia and may also develop myoglobinuria and renal failure.[16] Patients with tetanus should receive tetanus immune globulin at 3000 to 6000 U intramuscularly; the concurrent use of intrathecal hyperimmune globulin is suggested by one group.[17] Penicillin or another agent (if the patient is allergic to penicillin) should be given, and if there is a wound it should receive immediate attention by a surgeon. Seizures should be treated by loading with intravenous phenytoin (15 to 20 mg/kg at a rate of 50 mg/min) and maintenance therapy of 300 to 400 mg/d. Muscle spasms can be treated with intravenous diazepam. Because of the laryngeal spasms, intubation followed by tracheostomy is advised. Muscle spasms impairing respiration or causing severe pain or musculoskeletal injury require the use of a neuromuscular blocking agent such as curare or a synthetic substitute. These patients require mechanical ventilation. As in all paralyzed patients, prophy-

laxis with subcutaneous heparin (5000 U every 12 hours) should be considered, along with use of appropriate support stockings.

Metabolic Disorders

A number of metabolic disorders are associated with weakness in which there is some evidence that the motor neuron is affected, although this evidence is controversial in many of these syndromes. These disorders include hypoglycemia from pancreatic tumors, diabetic amyotrophy, an uncommon syndrome of distal weakness associated with uremia, hyperthyroidism, and acromegaly. In each of these syndromes, evidence that the primary problem is related to dysfunction of the anterior horn cells is quite uncertain and even unlikely. However, these disorders must be ruled out in patients with ALS. There is also a group of disorders affecting the nervous system more diffusely in which involvement of the motor neurons is a part and may even be a prominent part. These include Creutzfeldt-Jakob disease (usually accompanied rapidly by dementia, myoclonus, and cerebellar and/or basal ganglia involvement), system degenerations such as the Shy-Drager syndrome (with evidence of other neuronal dysfunction, including autonomic, cerebellar, and basal ganglia dysfunction and changes in mentation), ischemic myelopathies (usually segmental and affecting the lower extremities), radiation injury (generally limited to lower extremities), and electrical injury (often accompanied by sensory abnormalities and almost always limited to one limb, unless there is a concomitant myelopathy with upper motor neuron signs).

Noninfectious Toxins

A number of toxins can cause syndromes in which damage to the alpha motor neuron is responsible for much of the clinical picture. In adults, lead may cause a disorder that resembles ALS, although lead intoxication more often causes a peripheral neuropathy and occasionally an encephalopathy in adults. Subacute mercury intoxication occasionally closely resembles ALS. Most of the other toxic agents cause neuropathy, neuromuscular junction, and muscle or CNS syndromes rather than disease of the anterior horn cells.

DISORDERS OF THE PERIPHERAL NERVES AND NERVE ROOTS
Pathophysiology

As described earlier, the peripheral nerve and nerve roots consist of the axons, which are the cell projections of the motor, sensory, and autonomic neurons; the myelin, which is the modification of the Schwann cell plasma membrane; and supporting structures, including peri-, epi-, and endoneurial cells and blood vessels. The pathologic processes that affect the peripheral nerve can generally be thought of as primarily affecting the nerve cell itself (neuronal or axonal) or the myelin (demyelinating or demyelinative). In some instances, it is possible to distinguish whether the primary insult is to the axon with secondary changes in the perikaryon (peripheral crush being an example) or whether the primary injury is to the perikaryon of the neuron (the dorsal root ganglion in certain inflammatory and inherited diseases; the anterior horn cell as described in an earlier section). By convention, some authors consider pure motor neuronopathies in which the primary defect affects the motor neuron at the level of the perikaryon (within the spinal cord) as anterior horn cell diseases and not peripheral neuropathies. It should be pointed out, however, that in some diseases and in some patients it is not possible to be certain whether the defect affects the perikaryon or the axon. In chronic long-standing diseases, it may not be possible to distinguish axonal and neuronal from demyelinating disorders with clinical, electrophysiologic, or even pathologic examinations. This is because of prominent secondary changes in the myelin sheath that occur in response to axonal atrophy, which is associated with many primary axonal diseases.[18, 19]

However, most of the disorders affecting the peripheral nerves and roots that require management in a CCU are acute or subacute in evolution and can generally be characterized as primarily neuronal/axonal or demyelinating. The symptoms and signs in a patient with a disorder of the peripheral nervous system vary with (1) the types of nerve cells or axons involved (motor, large and/or smaller sensory and/or autonomic); (2) whether the disease process evolves acutely or subacutely (most trauma; inflammatory, vascular, and infectious causes; or certain toxins) or more slowly (entrapment; degenerative and hereditary causes; and certain toxins); and (3) whether the disorder is due to a process that may be expected to cause asymmetric lesions (trauma, entrapment, and vascular and some inflammatory causes) or symmetric lesions (toxins, including medications, and metabolic and hereditary causes).

Patients with a disorder that primarily affects myelin generally have marked motor defects, hyporeflexia or areflexia, and (although they may have prominent sensory complaints) modest sensory loss that chiefly affects large-fiber function, such as defects in proprioception, joint position sense, and vibration. A patient with a process affecting only motor neurons or axons has weakness but no sensory loss and may have relative preservation of reflexes early in the evolution of the disease. Patients with exclusive or predominant sensory neuron or axon disease have decreased sensation, paresthesias, and sensory ataxia with loss of reflexes. Patients who have involvement of the autonomic nervous system may have abnormalities of pulse, blood pressure, temperature, bladder, bowel, sexual function, and pupillary reactions. These may be mild and brought about only by postural challenges, or they may be severe. They may be transient or permanent. It is important to emphasize that other causes for abnormalities of these functions must be sought in each patient before attributing the fever, tachycardia, hypotension, or sphincter impairment to autonomic neuropathy.

The anatomic pattern of deficits depends in large part on the pathogenic mechanism involved in a particular disorder. Vascular disorders (some diabetic neuropathies, certain collagen-vascular diseases with vasculitis, and embolic diseases) would be expected to manifest marked asymmetry, especially early in the evolution of the clinical picture, and often affect individual nerve trunks or elements of a plexus. Most diseases with inflammatory changes not limited to vascular structures have varying degrees of asymmetry, although virtually all (other than herpes zoster) have bilateral effects. Toxins and metabolic disorders and some inflammatory diseases tend to produce quite symmetric deficits and classically depend on fiber length. That is, the longest fibers are affected first and more severely. This explains the involvement of feet and legs before hands. In inflammatory and vascular diseases, symptoms referable to the longer fibers are frequently prominent early in the course of illness, but not invariably so, because a multifocal process need not affect longer fibers first.

Clinical Disorders

Discussion of a number of neurologic diseases and syndromes primarily or exclusively affecting the peripheral

nerves (including cranial nerves III to IX), as well as the peripheral nerve syndromes associated with systemic diseases, toxins, and drugs, is beyond the scope of this book, and the reader is referred to standard neurologic textbooks and specialty texts. The emphasis here is on the diseases that are encountered in the critical care setting. As noted earlier, neuropathies can be classified according to the part of the nerve that seems to be the primary target of the disease process (myelin, distal axon, or neuronal cell body), the anatomic presentation (e.g., symmetric polyneuropathy and mononeuropathy multiplex), evolution of disease (acute, subacute, or chronic progressive), or the more traditional etiologic and pathogenic parameters (e.g., genetic, inflammatory, toxic, metabolic, infectious, and vascular). The correct diagnosis (and therefore the correct specific treatment, when such therapy is available, including withdrawal of a toxin), is more likely if each of these classification is combined.

Mononeuropathies and Mononeuropathy Multiplex

Patients with a mononeuropathy secondary to trauma or entrapment will not be hospitalized in a CCU for that neuropathy, although such a mononeuropathy may become evident in patients who are hospitalized for disorders in which compression of a nerve may result from impaired consciousness (e.g., alcohol- or drug-induced stupor or coma), especially as the patient awakens. A mononeuropathy or plexopathy including cervical radiculopathy may also result from positioning of the limbs or head and neck during surgery and becomes evident when the patient awakens from anesthesia. Patients with a classic mononeuropathy multiplex, whether axonal (diabetic or vasculitic)[20, 21] or demyelinating with conduction block,[22] may be in a CCU, but this is almost invariably because of their primary disease and its effects on other organ systems or on the CNS. In both of these settings, the clinical findings (pattern of weakness, sensory and reflex examinations) depend on which nerve trunks or plexus are involved. Other patients with a mononeuropathy multiplex include those with leprosy and some patients with human immunodeficiency virus (HIV) infection, generally before having fully developed acquired immunodeficiency syndrome. Lead neuropathy may have quite asymmetric effects, generally producing weakness of frequently exercised muscles.

Polyneuropathies

Most patients who require care in a critical care setting for a neuropathy or who develop a neuropathy while in a critical care setting have a polyneuropathy. The neuropathy is generally acute or subacute and is acquired, although patients with more chronic neuropathies and genetic diseases of the peripheral nervous system may be admitted to a CCU for management of other diseases and may show deterioration in their nervous system function at that time. They have bilateral signs with or without some degree of asymmetry. Weakness involves distal as well as proximal muscles in most instances (Guillain-Barré syndrome may involve proximal more than distal muscles or both types equally in many patients). Reflexes are reduced or absent, there are varying degrees of sensory impairment of large-fiber function (proprioception, joint position sense, and vibration) and/or small-fiber function (pinprick sensation, touch, and temperature), and in some patients there is evidence of autonomic dysfunction. There are uncommon neuropathies in which only sensory, motor, or autonomic fibers are affected. It is most important to decide whether the disorder is an axonal or neuronal neuropathy or a demyelinating neuropathy, if possible, on the basis of which fibers seem to be most affected and electrophysiologic results (EMG/NCV).

Demyelinating Neuropathies
Guillain-Barré Syndrome

Guillain-Barré syndrome (e.g., acute inflammatory demyelinating polyradiculoneuropathy and para- or postinfectious demyelinating radiculoneuritis) is the most common neuropathy that results in management in a CCU.[23, 24] The disease evolves during hours or up to 4 weeks. In two thirds to three quarters of patients, the disease follows an intercurrent infection, immunization, or surgical procedure. Guillain-Barré syndrome has been reported in patients who have become infected with HIV, generally when they are asymptomatic, often soon after seroconversion. It has also been associated with systemic lupus erythematosus, Hodgkin's and non-Hodgkin's lymphomas, and perhaps pregnancy. Pain in axial muscles and distal sensory complaints herald the onset, but weakness, often profound, is the major cause of disability. Involvement of the cranial nerves (especially VII, but also V, IX to XII, and occasionally III, IV, and VI, generally but not always sparing the pupillary response) and nerves to muscles responsible for respiration occurs frequently and is one of the reasons for close inpatient observation and management in the CCU. Patients with a vital capacity of 15 mL/kg or less should be intubated. However, elective intubation is better than emergency intubation, and patients with Guillain-Barré syndrome can exhibit rapid deterioration of breathing function. Therefore, even if the patient is being closely observed in a CCU, elective intubation should be strongly considered if there is an indication of progressively falling vital capacity or negative inspiratory force even before hypercapnia or hypoxia become manifest. The other potentially life-threatening manifestation for patients with Guillain-Barré syndrome is autonomic dysfunction, which occurs in approximately 20% of patients, usually relatively early in the course of the disease; it is generally mild or moderate in degree.

Another form of the disease consists of sensory ataxia, ophthalmoplegia, and hyporeflexia or areflexia and is called the Miller Fisher syndrome. With the rare exception of patients who have simultaneous Guillain-Barré syndrome and postinfectious acute disseminated encephalomyelitis, there is no hard evidence of CNS involvement in the Miller Fisher syndrome. These patients should be managed in a manner similar to those with Guillain-Barré syndrome. The pathologic hallmarks of Guillain-Barré syndrome are segmental demyelination and perivascular inflammation with mononuclear cells. Axons are relatively spared, although in many patients both pathologic and physiologic evidence of axon involvement is seen. Extremely rapid evolution of the disease to a respirator-dependent state, a prolonged nadir, electrophysiologic evidence of extensive demyelination early in the course of disease or later evidence of a large amount of denervation, and age at onset older than 60 years are associated with a slower recovery. Extensive denervation is also likely to be associated with a less complete recovery.[25, 26]

The rate of recovery is variable. Generally, patients who are ill enough to require hospitalization at referral centers take several months to recover. As many as 20 to 25% have residual deficits at 1 year; these are severe in 5 to 10% of patients. Further improvement may occur for as long as 2 and even 3 years. About 65% of patients eventually recover with no clinically significant residual effects, another 25% have mild residual findings, and 5 to 10% have significant or severe disability. The relapse rate is about 5%, and fewer than that experience the relapsing form of chronic inflammatory demyelinating neuropathy. The mortality of 1 to 3% is generally associated with pulmonary emboli, infections, and other diseases and in one series was seen, with one exception, in older patients.

The diagnosis is made on the basis of the clinical picture. EMG/NCV studies are useful even early in the course of illness to help support the diagnosis and for prognosis. Lumbar puncture is also helpful. Although only 50% of patients with Guillain-Barré syndrome have the classic elevation of total protein level with no or minimal elevation of cell count in cerebrospinal fluid (CSF) obtained during the first 5 to 7 days, the lack of a high CSF cell count helps to eliminate other disorders such as poliomyelitis and related enteroviral infections, cytomegalovirus infection, or Lyme radiculitis in which the cell count and the protein level are both characteristically elevated. In addition, an abnormal CSF is not seen in tick paralysis or acute intermittent porphyria, which can mimic some aspects of Guillain-Barré syndrome. The etiology of Guillain-Barré syndrome is not known, but it is generally considered to be a immunopathologically mediated, autoimmune disease. The relative role of humoral factors such as antibodies to components of myelin, immune complexes, and T cell–mediated immunity awaits clarification.

The management of patients with Guillain-Barré syndrome consists of careful monitoring of bulbar, respiratory, and autonomic functions. Intubation for pulmonary toilet and for respiratory support may be required, and tracheostomy may eventually be necessary for patients who cannot be weaned from the respirator. Abnormalities of pulse, blood pressure, and thermoregulation are treated if necessary. Hypotension generally poses a greater risk for the Guillain-Barré patient than hypertension; overly aggressive treatment of hypertension should therefore be avoided. Intermittent catheterization is preferable to an indwelling catheter in patients who develop significant urinary retention. Constipation is treated symptomatically. The syndrome of inappropriate antidiuretic hormone is treated with fluid restriction if clinically significant. Neurogenic pain is treated with simple analgesics or nonsteroidal anti-inflammatory agents. If this is not sufficient, amitriptyline can be tried. Muscle pain may also respond to quinine or quinidine. Severe burning paresthesias are rare and can be treated with carbamazepine or phenytoin. Early institution of physical and occupational therapy and speech therapy is important.

The major change in the treatment of patients with Guillain-Barré syndrome is the use of plasma exchange, which has been shown in several controlled studies to speed recovery of patients. In a large multicenter North American trial, patients treated with plasma exchange (200 to 250 mL/kg total in divided treatments) were respirator dependent for a shorter time, required less time to improve one grade of disability, and improved more at 45 days than patients who did not receive plasma exchange.[25-27] Other groups have confirmed these results.[28] The improvement is greatest in patients who receive plasma exchange in the first 2 weeks. It has been suggested that there is a higher incidence of relapse in patients who receive early plasma exchange, so some physicians now prophylactically have the patient undergo another 2 or 3 days of exchange (2.5 to 4.0 L given three times) at 7 to 10 days after the last exchange. The increased rate of relapse is controversial, and no study substantiates a protective or beneficial effect of a prophylactic second series of exchanges. It has also been suggested that infusion of immunoglobulin G (IgG) may have an equally beneficial effect on the course of Guillain-Barré syndrome.[29] As yet, no study shows that it is more effective than reported in the North American study of plasma exchange or that there is any benefit in combining the two forms of therapy or using fresh frozen plasma to reinfuse the cells. Therefore, with the exception of patients who may be endangered by a temporary decrease in clotting factors secondary to pheresis (such as a pregnant woman), replacement should be with albumin and physiologic saline, with potassium chloride as needed. No study shows a beneficial effect of corticosteroids as solitary therapy or in addition to plasma exchange. Some studies currently under way may clarify these points.

Chronic Inflammatory Demyelinating Polyneuropathy

The other relatively common demyelinating neuropathy is chronic inflammatory demyelinating polyneuropathy.[24, 28] It is less likely to be associated with a preceding viral infection or immunization. In some patients, it may be progressive from onset, may develop in a relapsing form, and may rarely develop in the relapsing or chronic progressive form after a typical bout of acute Guillain-Barré syndrome. The relation of this disease to Guillain-Barré syndrome, to which it has similarities in clinical, pathologic, electrophysiologic, and laboratory (CSF) findings, is not known. It is also thought to be immunopathologically mediated, but the exact pathogenic mechanisms are not understood. This disease less frequently paralyzes respiratory or bulbar muscles, so such patients are usually not seen in the critical care setting unless the patient first has Guillain-Barré syndrome. The more typical patient with chronic inflammatory demyelinating polyneuropathy has less cranial nerve, respiratory, and autonomic dysfunction, as well as a slower evolution of the clinical deficits. Most patients with this disease respond to plasma exchange, corticosteroids, and immunosuppressive agents, although perhaps as many as 60 to 70% require continuous therapy to control the disease.

Other Neuropathies

There are patients with predominantly demyelinating neuropathies seen in association with benign monoclonal gammopathies, as well as with osteoclastic myeloma and lymphomas,[30] although most patients with myeloma have cord or root compression and are more likely to have an axonal pattern when they have a neuropathy. Diphtheria may resemble Guillain-Barré syndrome because the toxin seems to affect metabolism or maintenance of myelin. There is prominent early involvement of accommodation, ophthalmoparesis, and weakness of oral and pharyngeal muscles, which is not typical of classic Guillain-Barré syndrome. The neuropathy of acute intermittent porphyria may also resemble Guillain-Barré syndrome, but usually other organs are affected.[23] Patients with genetic demyelinating neuropathies such as hereditary motor-sensory neuropathy type I or Refsum's disease are not discussed here.[31]

Axonal/Neuronal Neuropathies

Axonal/neuronal polyneuropathies constitute the overwhelming majority of diseases of the peripheral nervous system.[18, 19] Many are metabolic (diabetes, nutritional disorders, uremia, porphyria, hypothyroidism) or attributable to toxins such as drugs (isoniazid, hydralazine, nitrofurantoin, vincristine, cisplatin, pyridoxine excess, phenytoin, colchicine, amiodarone, disulfiram, perhexiline maleate, and dapsone), organic compounds (organophosphates, aldrin, dieldrin, acrylamide, hexacarbons, carbon disulfide, and trichloroethylene), or heavy metals (lead, arsenic, mercury, thallium, and gold). Other etiologies for polyneuropathy include hereditary diseases;[3] remote effects of neoplasms, including some associated with plasma cell dyscrasias such as acquired primary amyloidosis; cryoglobulinemia (diffuse polyneuropathy or asymmetric mononeuropathy); sarcoidosis (may be asymmetric, cranial nerve palsies with or without basilar meningitis or diffuse polyneuropathy); and HIV infection (generally when the patient has acquired immunodeficiency syndrome–related complex and especially with acquired immunodeficiency syndrome). In patients with pure sensory neuropathy (sensory neuronopathy) related to Sjögren's syndrome, in association with remote effects of carcinoma, and in an acute idiopathic form (some of which are preceded by banal infections), there is evidence of an inflammatory response in the dorsal root ganglia.[32] Few patients with these neuropathies are cared for in a critical care setting because of the neuropathy, but patients who have these other diseases, who are treated with these drugs, or who are sufficiently exposed to some of these toxins may be hospitalized for the primary problem. However, in some of these situations the neuropathy may be a major problem or the major problem.

Metabolic Neuropathies

Acute intermittent porphyria is a rare disease but one that not infrequently leads to life-threatening problems. Patients almost always give a history of prior episodes of abdominal pain, delirium, or psychotic behavior and/or seizures; these are more common and appear earlier than in acute or subacute polyneuropathy. The abdominal complaints and pain are believed to represent an autonomic neuropathy. The neuropathy may lead to tetraparesis, ophthalmoplegia, and bulbar and respiratory crises and may also be associated with dysautonomia. It is unusual to see a patient with an attack of the neuropathy in the absence of concomitant abdominal pain. The attack may be precipitated by the use of barbiturates. Other drugs have been implicated in triggering attacks, as have menstrual periods. The pathologic changes are modest and the disease is likely a terminal axonopathy. The typical CSF and electrophysiologic studies, which may be normal or show minor axonal abnormalities (although they rarely show unexcitable nerves in severe attacks), differ from the findings of increased protein level and evidence of demyelination seen in Guillain-Barré syndrome. The diagnosis is confirmed during an attack by the demonstration of elevated levels of urinary δ-aminolevulinic acid and porphobilinogen. Treatment consists of supportive care and avoidance of barbiturates and probably phenytoin and carbamazepine as well. Diazepam and its derivatives seem to be acceptable for use. Codeine and meperidine can be used for pain and agitation. Propranolol can be used to control tachycardia and also seems to reduce abdominal pain and agitation. Intravenous hematin given at 4 mg/kg twice a day for 3 days has also been suggested to have a beneficial effect on the neuropathy and the abdominal pain. Patients may have residual neurologic deficits from the neuropathy and may have recurrent attacks. The mortality of major attacks is 15 to 20%.[23, 31, 33]

On occasion, patients with ticks in the scalp present with an acute or subacute motor neuropathy associated with some sensory symptoms but no true sensory findings. This disorder may simulate Guillain-Barré syndrome or porphyria. CSF is normal and physiologic studies suggest an abnormality in terminal axonal function of motor nerves. There is no abnormality similar to that seen in pre- or postsynaptic defects in neuromuscular transmission. Treatment includes removal of ticks and is supportive.[23]

Patients with other non-nutritional metabolic neuropathies (e.g., diabetes, uremia, and hypothyroidism) are seldom hospitalized in a CCU for the neuropathy. The exception is a patient with severe autonomic dysfunction, as is sometimes seen in diabetes mellitus (as part of a mixed neuropathy or occasionally as a pure autonomic neuropathy).

Nutritional Neuropathies

Nutritional neuropathies can be severe but are seldom the cause for admission to a CCU. The most frequent nutritional neuropathies seen in Western society are those associated with alcoholism. Treatment consists of parenteral thiamine (100 mg) given immediately (because of CNS and cardiac problems; see Chapter 62) and then daily for several days, along with multiple B vitamin preparations and followed by oral thiamine and maintenance of the multivitamin preparation. Good nutrition and avoidance of alcohol should be recommended, but this advice is seldom followed. Patients with prolonged fat malabsorption may develop both myopathy and neuropathy related to vitamin E deficiency.

Heavy Metal Toxicity

Neuropathies associated with heavy metal intoxication are also seldom the cause of admission to a CCU. Acute exposure to large amounts of arsenic results in an acutely evolving neuropathy with a 4- to 8-week latency. The acutely poisoned patient often has an acute massive hemorrhagic encephalopathy. Chronic ingestion leads to a more slowly evolving sensorimotor neuropathy. Treatment by chelating agents such as BAL is suggested for acute intoxications but is more controversial in the slowly evolving neuropathy. Lead causes a typically asymmetric neuropathy and may also produce a syndrome that is virtually indistinguishable from ALS. Mercury can cause damage to the CNS and can produce a peripheral neuropathy. Thallium produces a painful sensory and autonomic neuropathy associated with partial or complete alopecia. The autonomic neuropathy may occasionally require monitoring or treatment of tachycardia or hypertension in a CCU or a step-down unit. Although treatment with potassium accelerates thallium excretion, the pain and dysautonomia may temporarily worsen.[34, 35]

Neuropathies Attributable to Medications

Patients with a neuropathy resulting from medication use seldom if ever require treatment of the neuropathy in a CCU. However, the physicians in the unit should recognize the possibility of neuropathy's developing in a patient with neoplastic disease, cardiac disease, urinary infection, tuberculosis, rheumatoid arthritis, and so forth, who is in the unit for treatment of the primary problem.

Neuropathies Attributable to Organic Compounds

Patients with neuropathies associated with organic toxins, other than organophosphates, seldom require care in a CCU. The organophosphates (used as insecticides, in the plastics industry, and in lubricating oils) cause both a depolarizing neuromuscular block (see later) and a polyneuropathy. The neuropathy occurs several weeks after exposure and is generally preceded by an acute neuromuscular syndrome and an autonomic syndrome. Although therapy is helpful in the neuromuscular syndrome, it does not prevent neuropathy. In addition, patients also have abnormalities of the CNS, suggesting spinal cord disease. One agent, tri-o-cresyl phosphate, used in illegal liquor manufacture (ginger jake) and in cooking oil, has been associated with several outbreaks.

Genetic Neuropathies

There are a large number of genetic disorders of the peripheral nervous system, most of which are primarily axonal or neuronal.[31] They are seldom the primary cause for hospitalization in a CCU. Occasionally, a patient with hereditary motor-sensory neuropathy type I who receives an agent such as vincristine may develop severe acute paralysis affecting respiratory muscles.

Inflammatory, Immune, and Paraneoplastic Neuropathies

Several of the immune or inflammatory diseases of the peripheral nervous system are demyelinating and are covered elsewhere in this chapter. There is an acute sensory neuropathy seen after viral infections and a subacute sensory neuropathy seen with Sjögren's syndrome and also in patients with malignancy; it is generally occult and involves breast, gynecologic, or small-cell carcinoma. These are thought to represent an inflammatory disorder primarily affecting cells of the dorsal root ganglion.[32] In addition, axonal neuropathies are seen in patients with other malignancies, including carcinomas, and in patients with dysproteinemias with or without hematologic malignancies. The pathologic mechanisms in these diseases are not known and may involve different processes in different patients. Patients with acquired primary amyloidosis experience a progressive sensorimotor neuropathy that is frequently characterized by early involvement of small-fiber dysfunction leading to a painful neuropathy with prominent autonomic dysfunction. Postural hypotension, urinary difficulties, diarrhea, and arrhythmias occur.[30] Treatment is symptomatic. Some patients with multiple myeloma may have amyloid neuropathy, although the amount of amyloid is seldom as extensive as in primary amyloidosis. As noted elsewhere in this chapter, patients with myeloma also experience a more nonspecific sensorimotor neuropathy and if they have an osteoclastic myeloma may develop a demyelinating neuropathy. Secondary amyloidosis seen with chronic inflammation or infection does not involve the nervous system. There are also several hereditary amyloid neuropathies.[31]

Dysautonomic Neuropathies

Many patients with chronic peripheral neuropathies can be shown to have abnormalities of autonomic function. In most patients, these are of no or minimal clinical importance. There are patients, however, in whom autonomic dysfunction is an important feature of the neurologic picture and a few in whom pure autonomic dysfunction occurs.[36] The neuropathies in which dysautonomia may be the major or sole manifestation of disease of the nervous system have been classified by Low[36] into (1) combined sympathetic and parasympathetic failure (including acute pandysautonomia, paraneoplastic dysautonomia, diabetic autonomic neuropathy, and amyloid neuropathy); (2) cholinergic neuropathy (including Lambert-Eaton syndrome, botulism, Chagas' disease, and acute cholinergic neuropathy); and (3) isolated organ system failure. It should also be noted that autonomic dysfunction occurs in diseases of the CNS such as Shy-Drager syndrome, idiopathic orthostatic hypotension, and other system degenerations, including the familial dysautonomia of Riley-Day syndrome. Simple tests of autonomic dysfunction can be performed at the bedside, including testing for orthostasis, measuring postvoiding residual urine volume, and RR interval recording in response to deep breathing or Valsalva's maneuver. More quantitative and detailed tests can also be performed by laboratories with interest and experience in these other techniques.

In acute pandysautonomia, patients present with an acute or subacute disorder of both sympathetic and parasympathetic systems. They have orthostatic hypotension, anhidrosis, and dry eyes and mouth, as well as sphincter dysfunction, unresponsive pupils, and a fixed heart rate. The etiology is unknown, but an immunologic pathogenesis has been suggested. Treatment is symptomatic and recovery may be complete or incomplete. Some patients with paraneoplastic neuropathies may have a prominent dysautonomia but generally also have evidence of a sensory neuronopathy or a sensorimotor neuropathy. Small-cell carcinoma of the lung has been reported to be the most common tumor, but other carcinomas have also been found.

Critical Care Neuropathy

There have been reports of patients who are hospitalized in CCU settings with sepsis and multiple organ system failure who develop a neuropathy in which motor symptoms predominate and/or sensory examination is difficult to perform. The findings include respiratory failure. These patients generally manifest with a "failure to wean" from a respirator. In many instances, other causes are found (e.g., Guillain-Barré syndrome, porphyria, unsuspected myasthenia gravis, and multiple neuromuscular blocking agents), but in some patients an axonal neuropathy is discovered. Whether this disorder constitutes one or more specific entities is still controversial. It is said that the prognosis for recovery from the neuropathy, if the patient recovers from the sepsis and multiple organ system failure, is good. There is no specific therapy for this syndrome.[37]

DISORDERS OF THE NEUROMUSCULAR JUNCTION
Pathophysiology

As described, the neuromuscular junction consists of specialized presynaptic nerve and postsynaptic muscle structures that allow for the efficient activation of muscle on stimulation by the nerve. The system is organized so that a safety factor for neuromuscular transmission prevents the normal variability and fluctuations in presynaptic and postsynaptic events from becoming clinically manifest. In disorders of the neuromuscular junction, various disease processes compromise synthesis or release of acetylcholine, interaction of acetylcholine with its specific receptor, the normal closing of the receptor channel, or inactivation of acetylcholine by the specific enzyme acetylcholinesterase, which leads to weakness. If the disease process affects a component of the presynaptic system that is shared by autonomic fibers, the pathologic symptoms and signs are not limited to motor symptoms. The autonomic abnormalities seen in patients with botulism and the Lambert-Eaton myasthenic syndrome can be explained by the inhibition of acetylcholine release from autonomic nerve terminals in these two disorders (they are technically not pure disorders of the neuromuscular junction). Conversely, a disorder such as autoimmune myasthenia gravis that specifically affects the postsynaptic nicotinic acetylcholine receptor should produce symptoms that are limited to weakness of skeletal muscle. As noted earlier, once there is a defect in any element of the neuromuscular junction resulting in a reduction in the safety factor for neuromuscular transmission, further reduction occurring either pre- or postsynaptically can lead to clinically manifest failure of the system or to severe worsening in a patient who already has clinical manifestations of neuromuscular failure. Thus, a presynaptically active agent, such as some aminogly-coside antibiotics, can be detrimental to a patient with autoimmune myasthenia gravis, a postsynaptic disorder.

It is useful to determine if the patient has a presynaptic disorder or a postsynaptic disorder because that simplifies the differential diagnosis. Clinical clues can be helpful. As noted earlier, the finding of autonomic dysfunction that is not due to medications or complications of the primary disease (sphincter disturbance, pyrexia, pupillary changes, and bradycardia) suggests a presynpatic disorder in which the disease process affects the motor and autonomic neuron terminal. Hyporeflexia likewise suggests that the patient does not have an isolated postsynaptic disease. The specialized neuromuscular junction testing in conjunction with EMG/NCV, which can be done in the CCU, is critical in establishing the nature of the problem (see Chapter 54).

Toxins

Botulism is the most important presynaptic disorder.[16] Exposure to the toxin may be via oral intake, in which case more than one patient is usually affected in a community, or via a wound. Infantile botulism is believed to result from absorption of toxin from the gastrointestinal tract. The toxin is thought to primarily inhibit the release of acetylcholine rather than to interfere with synthesis or storage. The toxin (there are several types; A, B, and E are the most important in the United States) binds tightly (perhaps irreversibly) to the presynaptic terminal, and eventual recovery may require terminal axonal sprouting. The disease may evolve during 24 hours or may take days to evolve. When the oral ingestion route is the source of the toxin, patients have nausea, vomiting, and dry mouth. Neurologic symptoms may appear simultaneously or may be delayed. Diplopia and blurred vision are usually the first symptoms, and patients have paralysis of the pupillary accommodation and light reflexes and weakness of extraocular muscles. Weakness then involves the other cranial nerves, muscles of respiration, and limb muscles, frequently proximal greater than distal. Autonomic dysfunction also includes ileus, bradycardia, and urinary retention. Although some patients may have mild disease, a patient should be monitored in a critical care setting and intubated if it is obvious that severe bulbar and/or respiratory signs and symptoms are developing. Supportive care including tracheostomy and suctioning is most important. Catheterization for urinary retention may be necessary. It has been suggested that enemas be used to reduce the absorption of toxin from the gastrointestinal tract in food botulism. Antitoxin to all three common types of botulin toxin should be given. Treatment with guanidine hydrochloride, which increases release of acetylcholine, has been advocated by some physicians. Chronic use of guanidine has been associated with bone marrow and renal toxicity. 3,4-Diaminopyridine, which is useful in the treatment of Lambert-Eaton myasthenic syndrome (another presynaptic disorder caused by decreased release of acetylcholine), is an investigational drug at this time.

Lambert-Eaton myasthenic syndrome is a disorder characterized by decreased release of quanta of acetylcholine caused by antibodies to voltage-gated calcium channels located at the presynaptic active zone.[38, 39] The antibodies cause redistribution and decrease in the number of active zones, but because this is not a complement-mediated immunologic reaction there is no membrane lysis or similar changes. Patients complain of weakness and often myalgias, which may improve with effort for a while. The complaints of functional disability are often out of proportion to the weakness noted on formal muscle testing. As noted, patients also have autonomic dysfunction and further differ from patients with autoimmune myasthenia gravis in having much less cranial nerve muscle weakness and in having decreased or absent reflexes. Strength and reflexes may temporarily improve with exercise of the tested muscle. Two thirds of these patients have an associated neoplasm, which is often occult and almost invariably a small-cell carcinoma of the lung. It may take as long as 3 to 4 years to detect the tumor, despite a diligent search. The weakness is milder than that seen in patients with moderate or severe myasthenia gravis. The diagnosis of Lambert-Eaton myasthenic syndrome is made by EMG/NCV. Several research laboratories are able to detect antibodies to voltage-gated calcium channels by using a radioimmunoassay with labeled ω-conotoxin as the ligand for the calcium channel.[40, 41] Therefore, unless an infection, dissemination of the small-cell tumor, or side effects of treatment of the neoplasm occur, patients with Lambert-Eaton myasthenic syndrome do not generally require treatment in a CCU. Therapy is both symptomatic (it is hoped that 3,4-diaminopyridine will be approved) and immunologic (plasma exchange, corticosteroids, and/or cytotoxic immunosuppressive agents) in patients whose disease is severe enough to justify the risks associated with these agents.

Drug- and Toxin-Induced Neuromuscular Junction Defects

A large number of drugs can induce weakness by acting at the neuromuscular junction.[42] Some of these agents are known to act presynaptically and others, postsynaptically. Certain agents act at both sites, and in the case of some agents the exact site of inhibition of neuromuscular transmission is unknown. The actual mechanisms are not well described for most of these agents. Some of these drugs have been reported to cause a myasthenic or myasthenia-like syndrome, generally in patients who have more than one cause of decrease of the normal safety factor for transmission or who have high blood and/or tissue levels of the drug. In other instances, the drug may have unmasked previously unrecognized or undiagnosed myasthenia gravis. Most of these drugs can worsen pre-existent myasthenia gravis.

Organophosphates (including nerve gas) inhibit the action of acetylcholinesterase and result in weakness similar to but longer lasting than that seen in the cholinergic weakness or crisis induced by the shorter-acting cholinesterase inhibitors used in patients with myasthenia gravis. These patients should be intubated with respiratory and other supportive measures. Atropine is useful in reducing the associated muscarinic symptoms. Recovery is generally complete in about 10 days.[43] As noted earlier, some patients may go on to experience a motor neuropathy. Patients with hereditary and sometimes acquired deficiency of pseudocholinesterases may have prolonged apnea after the use of muscle relaxants, especially depolarizing agents. The mechanism is the equivalent of the cholinergic crisis seen with excess inhibitors of cholinesterase. Treatment is supportive. There are a large number of toxins obtained from various animals, including arthropods (e.g., black widow spider), snakes (e.g., kraits, for α-bungarotoxin), and other species (snails, for ω-conotoxin; puffer fish, for tetrodotoxin), which have the ability to bind to presynaptic and postsynaptic structures (generally channels of receptors), as well as to sodium and other channels in nerve and muscle. These toxins are of major use in studies of the motor system but are generally not clinically important in the United States.

Myasthenia Gravis

Several disorders are subsumed under the diagnosis of myasthenia gravis.[5, 44] Some, which are inherited presynaptic or postsynaptic or congenital disorders, might better be termed myasthenic syndromes. These are uncommon, are generally manifested early in life, and usually do not lead a patient to be hospitalized in an adult CCU. The reader is referred elsewhere for details of this interesting and heterogeneous group of disorders, some of which are compatible with a normal life span; an adult intensivist is rarely called on to assist in care of these patients.

The common form of myasthenia gravis is an autoimmune disease caused by antibodies to the muscle nicotinic receptor of acetylcholine. The antibodies reduce the number of available receptors, which in turn reduces the safety factor for transmission below the critical level for normal strength. The weakness characteristically involves the cranial nerves early and with a high frequency, especially the eyelids and the extraocular muscles. The muscles of the arms, legs, and trunk are also frequently affected. The degree of weakness varies from patient to patient, and in the same patient it may vary from muscle to muscle and even from time to time in the same muscle in the same patient. The complaint of weakness worsening with effort and later in the day is classic in patients with myasthenia but may be absent.

The diagnosis is confirmed on the basis of (1) improvement in muscle strength in response to intravenous edrophonium or intramuscular injection of neostigmine; (2) electrophysiologic evidence of a defect in neuromuscular transmission manifested as a decremental response of the compound muscle action potential with repetitive stimulation at slow rates (2 to 5 Hz) or with other specialized techniques (single-fiber EMG is one such example); or (3) elevated serum antibodies to acetylcholine receptor. The pharmacologic electrophysiologic tests should be performed by physicians with experience in interpreting these tests. It is also important to remember that patients with myasthenia gravis often have other associated, immunopathologically mediated diseases. Those reported include hyper- or hypothyroidism, rheumatoid arthritis, systemic lupus erythematosus, idiopathic thrombocytopenia, pernicious anemia, and hemolytic anemia. Myasthenia gravis has also been reported as a complication of bone marrow transplantation, generally not during graft-versus-host disease. Approximately 10 to 15% of patients with autoimmune myasthenia gravis have a thymoma, which is usually benign.

The basic therapy of patients with myasthenia gravis can be divided into symptomatic (attempting to increase the safety factor for neuromuscular transmission) and immunologic.

There are special considerations in managing the patient who is rapidly deteriorating or in crisis, which is the situation for the intensivist. A patient whose condition is deteriorating, especially with increasing bulbar or respiratory complaints, should be admitted and closely monitored, in the CCU if necessary. Much has been made of trying to distinguish between myasthenic crisis (worsening of myasthenia) and cholinergic crisis (increased weakness because of excess acetylcholine at the junction secondary to excessive dosage of a cholinesterase inhibitor). Some authors have advocated the use of intravenous edrophonium to guide the frequency of administration and dose of the oral cholinesterase-inhibiting drugs (pyridostigmine and neostigmine) and to distinguish between myasthenic and cholinergic crisis. In my experience, this is seldom helpful, and trial and error under close observation, including CCU care, is more effective. In particular, patients may show transient response to intravenous edrophonium while receiving optimal or even toxic doses of pyridostigmine. Others have suggested that increasing muscarinic side effects of the cholinesterase inhibitors, such as abdominal cramps, diarrhea, sweating, and bradycardia, mean that the patient is in cholinergic crisis, and that the lack of same indicates myasthenic crisis. In my experience, there is not necessarily a correlation between the muscarinic side effects and a need for more or less activity at the neuromuscular junction, where the receptor is nicotinic. Adjustment of the dose of cholinesterase inhibitor for an outpatient or in the emergency room in a rapidly deteriorating patient with myasthenia gravis, with or without the use of edrophonium as a guide, is inappropriate. It is more important to immediately ensure the patient's bulbar and respiratory function than to immediately decide between myasthenic crisis and cholinergic crisis. In my experience, the former is more common, but in this era of CCUs, the distinction (which is not always possible) is not that important. Although there are injectible forms of pyridostigmine and neostigmine, I generally give the cholinesterase inhibitors orally via a feeding tube or a nasogastric tube, unless there is a problem with the gastrointestinal tract. There is generally little to be gained by high doses of pyridostigmine (>150 to 180 mg per dose), and there is at least a theoretic risk of long-term toxicity to the neuromuscular junction. Withdrawing the patient from all cholinesterase inhibitors, the so-called Mestinon (pyridostigmine) holiday, as the solitary treatment of a patient with myasthenia who is using a respirator has not been of much use in my experience, and with the availability of plasma exchange and corticosteroid therapy (if necessary) it has little to add to the management of myasthenic worsening and crisis.

The second task in managing acute myasthenic deterioration is to determine whether an intercurrent infection, fever, or medication that can reduce the safety factor for transmission may be contributing to the sudden worsening. Even if the downhill course was not induced by an infection, the patient may have an infection, such as aspiration pneumonia, as a consequence of the worsening of the myasthenia, which may cause further deterioration or delay recovery. Much has been made of avoiding medications that can worsen the condition of patients who have myasthenia gravis or who have uncovered latent myasthenia gravis, and certainly a less hazardous substitute should be used if one is available. However, for a patient in the hospital, especially in a CCU or in a step-down unit and using a respirator, there is no reason to avoid using an agent that is clearly the drug of choice, especially for an acute problem such as an infection or transient cardiac abnormality. Prolonged *Pseudomonas* pneumonia is more likely to complicate the management of a patient with myasthenia gravis than is the use of gentamicin for an intubated patient in a CCU.

The use of plasma exchange, along with modern CCU care, has revolutionized the management of patients with myasthenic crisis. A patient who does not rapidly and dramatically respond to a change in cholinesterase inhibitor or corticosteroid medication (if receiving corticosteroids chronically) or who does not dramatically improve with treatment of an infection should undergo a series of plasma exchanges. For patients with crisis or worsening condition severe enough to require hospitalization, I currently recommend three sessions of plasma exchange per week for a total of 12 to 20 L for most adult patients.

Corticosteroids are certainly helpful in the treatment of patients with myasthenia gravis that is refractory to cholinesterase inhibitors and thymectomy. The question of when to use such agents in patients with myasthenia who are not in crisis or in the CCU is not addressed here, although there are many investigators who, if speed is not of the essence, would opt for a well-tolerated cytostatic immunosuppressive agent such as azathioprine instead of corticosteroids. Some patients may require both types of agents. More important, patients with myasthenia gravis who are given high doses of corticosteroids may deteriorate to the point of needing respiratory assistance before they improve. Therefore, even a patient who is not in or near crisis and who is to be given corticosteroids (≥30 mg/d as the starting dose) should be observed in the hospital for at least 7 to 10 days. For a patient who is not receiving corticosteroids but who is in or near crisis, the question of whether to start corticosteroid administration at the same time as plasma exchange or while treating an infection should be individualized. If there is a trigger for the worsening condition, such as an intercurrent infection or failure to take prescribed medications, corticosteroids may not be necessary. In some instances, repeated plasma exchange, manipulation of cholinesterase inhibitors with later outpatient plasma exchange, and institution of immunosuppressive therapy or thymectomy (if not already performed) may be preferable for a particular patient. Infusion of IgG has been reported to result in improvement of patients with myasthenia gravis. However, in many cases it is not clear that other changes in the patient's therapeutic regimen might not also be at least partly responsible for the improvement. A large-scale randomized controlled study in which IgG infusion is the only allowed variable is required to prove or disprove the efficacy of IgG infusions in myasthenia gravis and other disorders.

DISORDERS OF SKELETAL MUSCLE
Pathophysiology

Primary disorders of voluntary muscles are commonly called myopathies. Any disease process in which there is loss of muscle fibers, abnormalities of muscle membrane or elements of the contractile processes, or abnormalities of energy or intermediate metabolism of muscle can result in symptoms such as weakness, muscle aches, pain, and occasionally failure of muscle relaxation, as well as loss of muscle bulk. Because the nerves and the CNS are not involved (unless the patient has a hereditary, toxic, or inflammatory disease process that affects multiple parts of the nervous system or muscle and other organ systems), patients have no sensory signs or symptoms, no autonomic dysfunction, and no changes attributed to spinal cord long tracts or cognitive problems. In many myopathies, muscle weakness tends to occur earliest and is more severe in proximal muscles, although there are notable exceptions. Likewise, electrophysiologic and biopsy studies are compatible with a primary myopathic process. Some myopathies (those that are rapid and/or have considerable necrosis) may have irritative features on an EMG that are similar to those seen in neurogenic diseases, such as increased insertional activity, sharp waves, and fibrillations (but not fasciculations). There is often an elevation of certain serum enzymes such as creatine kinase, attributable to an increase in the MM isoenzyme. However, not all myopathies are associated with increased levels of creatine kinase, and in patients with inactive or end-stage disease this enzyme level is often normal. In addition, modest elevations of serum creatine kinase are seen in some patients with neuropathic processes. An etiologic scheme similar to that for diseases of the peripheral nerve and anterior horn cell can be used to approach a patient who has a myopathy.

Metabolic and Nutritional Disorders[7, 45–47]

There are two general categories of metabolic myopathies. One group includes those in which a genetic defect is involved (e.g., familial periodic paralysis, mitochondrial cytopathies, glycogen storage diseases, lipid storage and metabolism disorders, and malignant hyperthermia) and the other comprises acquired diseases (e.g., hypokalemia, hypophosphatemia, and alcoholic, renal, thyroid, and parathyroid disorders). In many instances, more than one metabolic factor may be involved in producing the weakness (e.g., patients with alcoholic myopathy frequently also are hypokalemic and hypophosphatemic; patients with sporadic hypokalemic periodic paralysis are hyperthyroid). In other instances, the metabolic insult (or drugs) may affect nerve as well as muscle, or the primary site of major pathologic effect is not clear. It is impossible to even outline these different disorders, so the following material highlights the disorders likely to be seen in patients in a CCU, whether they are the cause of admission to the unit or a secondary problem.

Most adult patients with abnormalities of glycogen storage and other carbohydrate metabolic abnormalities do not experience significant weakness to require CCU care. Some patients in whom myoglobinuria occurs, such as those with McArdle's disease, may require CCU care to prevent or treat the occasional renal failure seen in such patients. The degree of weakness in most adult patients with lipid metabolism abnormalities and in patients with mitochondrial cytopathy is seldom severe enough to result in critical care. However, some of these patients have disorders that can also affect the heart (Kearns-Sayre syndrome) or produce seizures or stroke-like syndromes that may require critical care.[48] Treatment of seizures is symptomatic (see Chapter 58). The stroke-like syndromes and muscle weakness have been said to benefit from treatment with corticosteroids (phospholipase inhibition) and perhaps oxygen radical scavengers (vitamins E, K, and C). Other patients experience severe metabolic acidosis and require critical care treatment for that complication.

Malignant hyperthermia is a life-threatening disease of primary concern to anesthesiologists.[49] It is thought to be autosomal dominant with variable penetrance. The symptoms are triggered by anesthetics and muscle relaxants, as well as other agents. Studies suggest that mutation in the calcium channel of the sarcoplasmic reticulum may be the cause of this disorder. Early signs are skin mottling, tachycardia, cyanosis and tachypnea, elevation of body temperature, increased muscle tone, diaphoresis, and fluctuations in blood pressure. If the attack is not aborted, the patient experiences dramatic increases in body temperature over an extremely short time, lactic acidosis, respiratory acidosis, muscle rigidity, hyperkalemia, increased serum creatine kinase level, and myoglobinuria. It is better to avoid the attack by appropriate preoperative screening. Treatment includes body cooling, termination of anesthesia, hydration, respiratory support, maintenance of urine output with diuretics or osmotic diuretics, and the administration of the muscle relaxant dantrolene sodium (1 to 2 mg/kg intravenously, repeated as needed every 5 to 10 minutes to a recommended maximum of 10 mg/kg).

Patients with familial periodic paralysis can become completely paralyzed, especially those with hyokalemic forms. However, in this group of disorders significant involvement of respiratory or cranial muscles is uncommon. There is rarely an associated cardiac arrhythmia.

A large number of acquired metabolic disorders result in myopathic weakness.[45] Patients with alcoholism may develop acute weakness, generally sparing respiratory and bulbar muscles, which may be associated with myoglobinuria. These episodes may be seen with or without other known causes of metabolic myopathies, such as hypokalemia and hypophosphatemia. Some patients have recurrent bouts and others may be left with residual weakness, especially after several bouts. The entity of chronic alcoholic myopathy without acute episodes is less well established. Patients with chronic renal diseases generally have more difficulty with CNS disease (seizures or encephalopathy) and peripheral nervous system disease (uremic neuropathy) than with myopathy. There is, however, a myopathy seen in patients with chronic renal disease. Myopathies occur with a large number of endocrine disorders, including hyperthyroidism, hypothyroidism, hyperadrenocorticism (Cushing's syndrome), hyperaldosteronism, hyperparathyroidism, and hypoparathyroidism. Hypokalemia from any of a number of acquired conditions (including iatrogenic) may cause development of a myopathy and, if acute enough, may have accompanying myoglobinuria. Myopathy has also been reported in patients with severe malnutrition and vitamin E deficiency. A severe myopathy has been seen in patients receiving total parenteral nutrition. The role of changes in phosphate in this entity is unclear. This myopathy may simulate Guillain-Barré syndrome and may require CCU care.

Immune, Inflammatory, and Infectious Disorders[50]

There are a large number of true infectious myopathies, including myositis related to viruses, bacteria, fungi, protozoans, cestodes, and nematodes. Viral myositis is generally benign, although rhabdomyolysis has been rarely observed in some patients. Patients with HIV infection have been reported to experience an inflammatory myopathy, as well as a more nonspecific wasting of muscle as part of end-stage disease. Azidothymidine has been reported to cause a mitochondrial myopathy (see later). The important bacterial infections in the United States are gas gangrene and tetanus. Toxoplasmosis is an important cause of neurologic problems in the CNS, but the myopathy seldom produces weakness—it produces pain instead. Trichinosis produces a painful myopathy but not, in general, clinical weakness from the infestation of muscle. The important inflammatory myopathies likely to be seen in a North American hospital and occasionally in a CCU are the idiopathic disorders such as polymyositis (primary polymyositis or in association with a collagen-vascular disease such as scleroderma, Sjögren's syndrome, or mixed connective tissue disease; in graft-versus-host disease; or possibly in association with occult malignancy), dermatomyositis (with or without associated malignancy), inclusion body myositis, and sarcoidosis. There are other uncommon inflammatory disorders as well. From the point of view of an intensivist, the patients most likely to be seen in a critical care setting (other than those with infections such as gas gangrene or tetanus) are those with polymyositis and dermatomyositis. These patients may rarely have such severe disease that there is rhabdomyolysis requiring attention to renal function. The other circumstance is the unusual patient with respiratory failure or dysphagia severe enough that aspiration results. Of course, side effects from corticosteroid therapy, immunosuppressive therapy, and other problems associated with graft-versus-host disease can also result in care in a CCU. It seems that dermatomyositis is an immune complex–mediated disorder affecting the small vessels of muscle and leading to muscle necrosis, weakness, elevation of serum creatine kinase level, and characteristic EMG and muscle biopsy findings. There is no prospective study to prove that treatment with corticosteroids is effective, but most patients with significant weakness should be treated with 1 mg/kg of oral corticosteroids per day. How long to maintain a high dose, how quickly to taper the dosage, and when to consider treatment a failure are not considered here, but there is a fair amount of controversy related to these issues. Steroids given by pulse dosing (500 mg intravenously during 1 to 4 hours twice daily for 3 to 5 days) has also been suggested for the refractory patient. There is no proof of the efficacy of this treatment, but it can be tried in selected cases. Plasma exchange has also been suggested, but again proof of efficacy is lacking. Azathioprine, cyclophosphamide, and methotrexate have all been used with apparent success in patients refractory to steroid treatment, but there are no randomized prospective studies with these agents.

Genetic Diseases[7]

There are a large number of genetically determined myopathies in addition to the hereditary metabolic disorders already discussed. One large group comprises the muscular dystrophies, in which patients are seemingly normal up to a certain age and then begin to decline. The age at onset and rate of decline vary with the individual dystrophies. The best known and most common is Duchenne's dystrophy, which is X linked and is due to a defect in the gene that codes for a large muscle protein called dystrophin. Other less severe dystrophies include the mild X-linked Becker's dystrophy (also attributable to a defect in dystrophin), facioscapulohumeral dystrophy, limb-girdle dystrophy, ocular pharyngeal dystrophy, and distal muscular dystrophy. Other than for Becker's and Duchenne's dystrophies, the defects are not known, and on the basis of variations in clinical and histologic pictures, several of the other dystrophies may well encompass several different diseases. Because some patients develop kyphoscoliosis, kyphoscoliotic heart disease, cardiomyopathies, and pneumonia, they may require care in a CCU. Unfortunately, treatment at this time is symptomatic, including physical therapy; in certain disorders orthopedic procedures can produce symptomatic improvement. Infections and cardiac disease (cardiac failure and arrhythmias) are treated as needed with the appropriate agents.

Another group of disorders is the heterogeneous congenital myopathies. These diseases are usually manifested from birth or early in life, although some are mild and the onset is recognized in retrospect. These vary from mild and virtually nonprogressive to more severe and slowly progressive. Some are diagnosed by associated characteristic physical findings and others by specific changes found by muscle biopsy. Some of these disorders are associated with respiratory compromise. There is no specific treatment available at this time.

The last group is the hereditary myotonic disorders. Myotonia is manifested by slow relaxation of muscle after use or after percussion. The important disorder for the intensivist is myotonic dystrophy, in which the patient has both myotonia and progressive weakness. It is an autosomal dominant disorder with variable penetrance in which the abnormalities are not limited to skeletal muscle. Patients may have cataracts, gonadal atrophy, and cardiac abnormalities. Other abnormalities include premature frontal balding, mental retardation or dementia, low serum IgG level (because of hypermetabolism of IgG), prolonged elevation of glucose, and high insulin levels, but normal growth hormone levels. The cardiac disease includes bradycardia and any degree of heart block. Complete heart block may develop and require treatment. Sudden death has been reported, as has myocardial dysfunction and decreased cardiac output. There is no specific treatment for the disease. Other diseases of muscle are associated with myotonia, including congenital myotonia (myotonia without weakness or other associated findings) and myotonia in response to cold, with or without accompanying periodic paralysis.

Trauma

Patients with crush injuries experience some weakness but predominantly experience pain related to muscle necrosis. Crush injuries include those related to pressure on a limb because of prolonged periods of unconsciousness and infarcts of large amounts of muscle because of vascular occlusion. Some of the weakness is secondary to simultaneous compression of major nerve trunks as well. The major concern in these patients is the development of myoglobinuria with the attendant risk of renal failure.

Toxins

Several toxins, including saxitoxin and Malayan sea snake toxin, cause weakness and/or rhabdomyolysis. There is also a poorly understood entity called Haff disease. Many other toxins reported to cause rhabdomyolysis do so by producing prolonged unconsciousness or by inducing metabolic changes rather than by direct muscle toxicity, although the definitions can be arbitrary.

Drugs[42, 45]

A large number of drugs can cause myopathy, some related to local injection and others producing a generalized myopathy. In some instances, the myopathy is acute or subacute and has been reported with clofibrate, ε-aminocaproic acid, emetine, and lovastatin combined with gemfibrozil. Emetine myopathy can be quite severe and is reversible but may be associated with cardiomyopathy. Several drugs have been associated with acute rhabdomyolysis. In some instances, this may be a direct toxic or idiosyncratic reaction. In some instances, the injury may be indirect (e.g., crush or hypokalemia). Other medications are associated with a subacute or chronic myopathy that is painless. Corticosteroids are the most common. Weakness is generally subacute or chronic and is seldom severe, although it may cause clinically significant deficits. Rarely, the disease can be acute and severe. Treatment is reduction of steroid dose and supportive therapy. Other drugs associated with myopathy include chloroquine, amiodarone, and azidothymidine (mitochondrial defect, perhaps by affecting mitochondrial DNA). Both polymyositis and myasthenia gravis have been reported in patients treated with penicillamine. The mechanisms here are immunologic.

References

1. Slater CR, Harris JB: The anatomy and physiology of the motor unit. In: Walton JN (ed): Disorders of Voluntary Muscle. 5th ed. Edinburgh, Churchill Livingstone, p 1, 1988.
2. Noback CR, Strominger NL, Demarest RJ: The Human Nervous System: Introduction and Review. 4th ed. Malvern, PA, Lea & Febiger, p 33, 1991.
3. Waxman SG: Normal and abnormal axonal properties. In: Asbury AK, McKhann GM, McDonald WI (eds): Diseases of the Nervous System: Clinical Neurobiology. Philadelphia, WB Saunders, p 36, 1986.
4. Waxman SG: Normal and demyelinated axons. In: Pearlman AL, Collins RC (eds): Neurobiology of Disease. New York, Oxford University Press, p 3, 1990.
5. Lisak RP, Barchi RL: Myasthenia Gravis. Philadelphia, WB Saunders, 1982.
6. Pearlman AL: Neuromuscular junction. In: Pearlman AL, Collins RC (eds): Neurobiology of Disease. New York, Oxford University Press, p 44, 1990.
7. Gilder BF, Brooke MH: Muscle. In: Pearlman AL, Collins RC (eds): Neurobiology of Disease. New York, Oxford University Press, p 62, 1990.
8. Thach WT Jr, Montgomery EB Jr: Motor system. In: Pearlman AL, Collins RC (eds): Neurobiology of Disease. New York, Oxford University Press, p 168, 1990.
9. Campbell MJ: Motor neurone diseases. In: Walton JN (ed): Disorders of Voluntary Muscle. 5th ed. Edinburgh, Churchill Livingstone, p 730, 1988.
10. Williams DB, Windebank AJ: Motor neuron disease (amyotrophic lateral sclerosis). Mayo Clin Proc 66:54, 1991.
11. Shy ME, Rowland LP, Smith T, et al: Motor neuron disease and plasma cell dyscrasia. Neurology 36:1429, 1986.
12. Pestronk A, Adams RN, Cornblath D, et al: Patterns of serum IgM

antibodies to GM1 and GD1a gangliosides in amyotrophic lateral sclerosis. Ann Neurol 25:98, 1989.

13. Jubelt B, Miller JR: Viral infections. In: Rowland LP (ed): Merritt's Textbook of Neurology. 8th ed. Philadelphia, Lea & Febiger, p 96, 1989.
14. Dalakas MC, Elder G, Hallett M, et al: A long-term follow-up study of patients with post-poliomyelitis neuromuscular symptoms. N Engl J Med 314:959, 1986.
15. Kennedy PGE: Neurologic complications of varicella-zoster virus. In: Kennedy PGE, Johnson RT (eds): Infections of the Nervous System. London, Butterworth Publishers, p 177, 1987.
16. Griffin JW: Bacterial toxins: Botulism and tetanus. In: Kennedy PGE, Johnson RT (eds): Infections of the Nervous System. London, Butterworth Publishers, p 76, 1987.
17. Gupta PA, Kapoor R, Goyal S, et al: Intrathecal human immune tetanus immunoglobulin in early tetanus. Lancet 2:439, 1980.
18. Asbury AK, Gilliatt RW: The clinical approach to neuropathy. In: Asbury AK, Gilliat RW (eds): Peripheral Nerve Disorders. London, Butterworth Publishers, p 1, 1984.
19. Griffin JW, Cornblath DR: Peripheral nerve. In: Pearlman AL, Collins RC (eds): Neurobiology of Disease. New York, Oxford University Press, p 22, 1990.
20. Greene DA, Brown MJ: Diabetic polyneuropathy. Semin Neurol 7:18, 1987.
21. Lisak RP, Levinson AI: Neuropathy in connective tissue disorders. In: Asbury AK, Gilliatt RW (eds): Peripheral Nerve Disorders. London, Butterworth Publishers, p 154, 1984.
22. Lewis RA, Sumner AJ, Brown MJ, et al: Multifocal demyelinating neuropathy with persistent conduction block. Neurology 32:958, 1982.
23. Ropper AH, Shahani BT: Diagnosis and management of acute areflexic paralysis with emphasis on Guillain-Barré syndrome. In: Asbury AK, Gilliat RW (eds): Peripheral Nerve Disorders. London, Butterworth Publishers, p 21, 1984.
24. Lisak RP, Brown MJ: Acquired demyelinating polyneuropathies. Semin Neurol 7:40, 1987.
25. McKhann GM, Griffin JW, Cornblath DR, et al: Plasmapheresis and Guillain-Barré syndrome: Analysis of prognostic factors and the effect of plasmapheresis. Ann Neurol 23:347, 1988.
26. Cornblath DR, Mellits ED, Griffin JW, et al: Motor conduction studies in Guillain-Barré syndrome: Description and prognostic value. Ann Neurol 23:354, 1988.
27. The Guillain-Barré Syndrome Study Group: Plasmapheresis and acute Guillain-Barré syndrome. Neurology 35:1096, 1985.
28. French Cooperative Group on Plasma Exchange and Guillain-Barré Syndrome: Efficacy of plasma exchange in Guillain-Barré syndrome: Role of replacement fluids. Ann Neurol 22:753, 1987.
29. Alberts JW, Kelly JJ: Acquired inflammatory demyelinating polyneuropathies: Clinical and electrodiagnostic features. Muscle Nerve 12:435, 1989.
30. Kelly JJ: Polyneuropathies associated with plasma cell dyscrasias. Semin Neurol 7:30, 1987.
31. Harding AE, Thomas PK: Genetically determined neuropathies. In: Asbury AK, Gilliatt RW (eds): Peripheral Nerve Disorders. London, Butterworth Publishers, p 243, 1984.
32. Asbury AK: Sensory neuronopathy. Semin Neurol 7:58, 1987.
33. Rowland LP: Acute intermittent porphyria. In: Rowland LP (ed): Merritt's Textbook of Neurology. 8th ed. Philadelphia, Lea & Febiger, p 544, 1989.
34. LeQuesne PM: Toxic neuropathies. In: Asbury AK, Gilliatt RW (eds): Peripheral Nerve Disorders. London, Butterworth Publishers, p 184, 1984.
35. Sahenk Z: Toxic neuropathies. Semin Neurol 7:9, 1987.
36. Low PA: Autonomic neuropathy. Semin Neurol 7:49, 1987.
37. Zochodine DW, Bolton CF, Wells GA, et al: Critical illness polyneuropathy. A complication of sepsis and multiple organ failure. Brain 110:819, 1987.
38. O'Neill JH, Murray NM, Newsom-Davis J: The Lambert-Eaton myasthenic syndrome. A review of 50 cases. Brain 111:577, 1988.
39. Vincent A, Lang B, Newsom-Davis J: Autoimmunity to the voltage-gated calcium channel underlies the Lambert-Eaton myasthenic syndrome, a paraneoplastic disorder. Trends Neurosci 12:496, 1989.
40. Sher E, Gotti C, Canal N, et al: Specificity of calcium channel autoantibodies in Lambert-Eaton myasthenic syndrome. Lancet 2:640, 1989.
41. Lennon VA, Lambert EH: Autoantibodies to solubilized calcium channel-omega-conatoxin in complexes from small cell lung carcinoma: A diagnostic aid for Lambert-Eaton myasthenic syndrome. Mayo Clinic Proc 64:1498, 1989.
42. Agrov Z, Mastaglia FL: Drug-induced neuromuscular disorders in man. In: Walton JN (ed): Disorders of Voluntary Muscle. 5th ed. Edinburgh, Churchill Livingstone, p 981, 1988.
43. Spenser PS (ed): Possible Long-Term Health Effects of Short-Term Exposure to Chemical Agents, Volume 1, Anticholinesterases and Anticholinergics. Washington, DC, National Academy Press, 1982.
44. Engel AG: Myasthenia gravis. Ann Neurol 16:519, 1984.
45. Layzer RB: Neuromuscular Manifestations of Systemic Disease. Philadelphia, FA Davis, 1985.
46. Rowland LP: Familial periodic paralysis. In: Rowland LP (ed): Merritt's Textbook of Neurology. 8th ed. Philadelphia, Lea & Febiger, p 721, 1989.
47. Rowland LP: Other diseases of muscle. In: Rowland LP (ed): Merritt's Textbook of Neurology. 8th ed. Philadelphia, Lea & Febiger, p 724, 1989.
48. Nelson TE, Flewellen EH: Current concepts: The malignant hyperthermia syndrome. N Engl J Med 309:445, 1983.
49. Peterson PL, Martens ME, Lee CP: Mitochondrial encephalomyopathies. Neurol Clin 6:529, 1988.
50. Dalakas MC (ed): Polymyositis and Dermatomyositis. Stoneham, MA, Butterworth Publishers, 1988.

CHAPTER 60

Viral Encephalitis

Dennis L. Kolson
Francisco Gonzalez-Scarano

Encephalitis is inflammation of the brain parenchyma, which is usually global and, in the case of viral infection, often not accompanied by severe systemic disease. Most primary forms of encephalitis are caused by viruses, and damage to the brain is due to either direct cellular destruction or the effects of the immune system. The clinical manifestations are diverse in severity, onset, and progression but generally include fever, headache, and malaise followed by alteration of mentation. Although the diagnosis always requires a high degree of clinical suspicion, a careful history, including seasonal predominance and geography, and neurologic examination along with appropriate diagnostic tests can often identify the specific etiologic agent and suggest, in some cases, specific treatment. Nonetheless, of all cases of infectious encephalitis reported to the Centers for Disease Control in 1977, 73% were of undetermined etiology, 11% were associated with arboviruses, 6% with exanthematous viruses, 3% with mumps virus, and 7% with other viruses.[1]

APPROACH TO DIAGNOSIS

The symptoms of subacute fever, headache, neck stiffness, and altered sensorium are nearly universal, although nonspecific, and are seen in other toxic, metabolic, and systemic illnesses. However, in this setting focal neurologic signs such as aphasia, focal seizures, and brain stem signs point strongly to infectious encephalitis, and a careful neurologic examination can even suggest specific causes, as discussed in the next section. The evaluation must be directed by geographic and seasonal considerations (*summertime* arboviruses, *sporadic* herpesvirus, and parainfectious reactions) and requires examination of cerebrospinal fluid (CSF) and appropriate specific serum and/or CSF antibody titers, usually immunoglobulin M (IgM). Virus isolation is possible in a few cases, as discussed under the individual encephalitides. Figure 60–1 presents a protocol for evaluating patients with suspected encephalitis. A metabolic or toxic evaluation must begin early, in parallel with the evaluation of appropriate viral titers. CSF examination must also be performed as soon as possible, once clinical and/or neuroimaging evaluations rule out significant intracranial mass effects. However, in cases of suspected bacterial causes, antibiotic therapy should not be delayed while awaiting results of these studies.

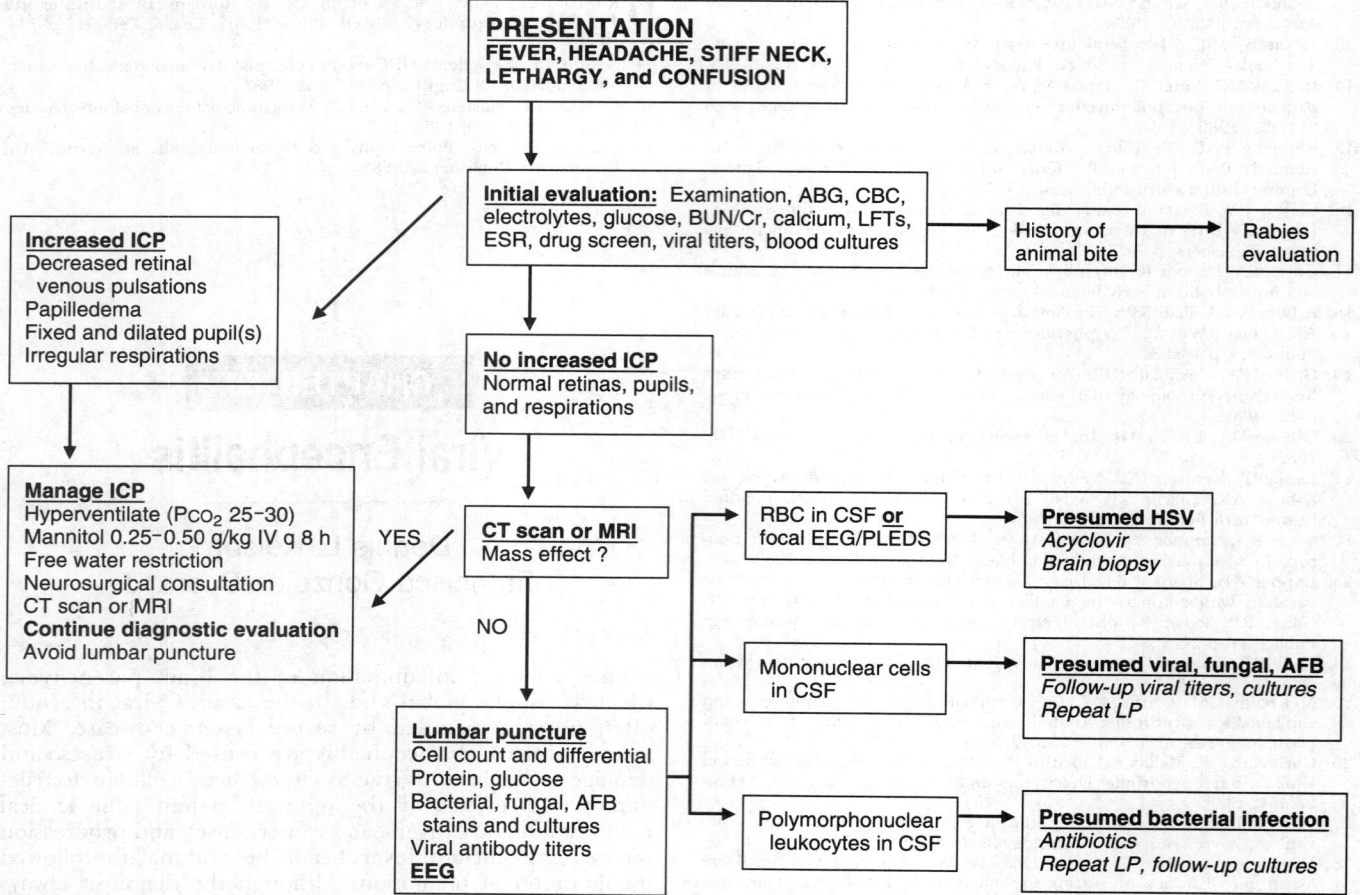

Figure 60–1. Evaluation protocol for clinically suspected encephalitis. In all patients, metabolic and viral studies (dictated by season, geographic location, and clinical factors) should be made, with immediate evaluation for signs of life-threatening increase of intracranial pressure. Management of increased intracranial pressure is discussed in the text. ABG = arterial blood gases; AFB = acid-fast bacilli; BUN = blood urea nitrogen; CBC = complete blood count; ESR = erythrocyte sedimentation rate; HSV = herpes simplex virus; ICP = intracranial pressure; LFT = liver function test; LP = lumbar puncture; MRI = magnetic resonance imaging; PLEDS = paroxysmal lateralized epileptiform discharges; RBC = red blood cell.

SPECIFIC FINDINGS IN THE NEUROLOGIC EXAMINATION

After the initial studies, specific findings can be used to guide the evaluation. In no case are any of these pathognomonic for a specific etiology; *they are merely guides in the setting of specific epidemiologic and serologic observations.* The absence of spontaneous intravenous pulsations in the optic disk indicates elevation of CSF pressure above 190 mm H_2O, often preceding papilledema and diffuse cerebral edema, which are most common in eastern equine encephalitis (EEE) and herpes simplex encephalitis (HSE). In late stages, cerebral edema may be indicated by a Cushing reflex (bradycardia in the setting of hypertension) and herniation syndromes including obtundation, irregular respirations, and hemiparesis with contralateral pupillary dilation. Facial hemiparesis (cranial nerve VII) should alert one to EEE, St. Louis encephalitis (SLE), Venezuelan equine encephalitis (VEE), Japanese B encephalitis (JBE), or HSE. Cutaneous vesicles in the distribution of the trigeminal nerve, especially the ophthalmic division, or in the ear canal suggest varicella-zoster encephalitis (VZE) (zoster ophthalmicus, Ramsay Hunt syndrome, respectively). Multiple cranial nerve palsies indicating brain stem encephalitis are often seen in VZE, rabies, and SLE. Hemiparesis suggests HSE, EEE, and VZE. Tetraparesis suggests EEE and rabies; rabies also includes hyporeflexia in some instances.

MEDICAL MANAGEMENT
Increased Intracranial Pressure

Management of *increased intracranial pressure* should include

1. Elevation of the head of the bed to approximately 45°.
2. Restriction of free water intake to 1000 mL normal saline/m² body surface/d.
3. Hyperventilation to maintain P_{CO_2} at 25 to 30 mm Hg. This decreases cerebral blood flow and intracranial pressure.
4. Use of hyperosmolar agents, such as intravenous mannitol, 0.25 to 0.50 g/kg every 4 to 8 hours as necessary. Steroids are not recommended in viral encephalitis.
5. (Optional) Placement of an intraventricular CSF pressure monitor may be used to keep intracranial pressure less than 20 to 25 cm H_2O by drainage. This depends on the lack of clinical response to hyperosmolar agents and the severity of the mass effect as determined by neuroimaging studies.

Seizures

Seizures can be managed by beginning with a slow intravenous push of phenytoin (Dilantin) at a dose of 18 mg/kg in normal saline at a rate of less than 50 mg/min. Maintenance doses of about 300 to 400 mg/d in three divided doses are used to keep the serum level between 10 and 20 μg/mL. Alternatively, phenobarbital may be loaded at a dose of 5 to 10 mg/kg. Divided daily doses of about 60 to 120 mg are used to maintain serum levels at 20 to 40 μg/mL. This may depress the sensorium. Valproate syrup (250 mg/5 mL) can be administered via clamped rectal tube in a total volume of 30 mL with water, at a dose of 250 to 500 mg every 6 to 8 hours to maintain blood levels of 50 to 100 μg/mL. This may lead to elevated blood ammonia and liver enzyme levels.

The more common clinical viral encephalitides are discussed in the following sections, with specific reference to epidemiology, pathology, symptoms and diagnostic studies, and treatment. Discussion of the encephalitis associated with human immunodeficiency virus is left for other chapters. The encephalitides are grouped as *endemic* (HSE, VZE, and rabies), *epidemic arboviral* (EEE, western equine [WEE], SLE, VEE, JBE, and La Crosse), *epidemic nonarboviral* (influenza, enterovirus, and mumps), and *parainfectious* (measles).

ENDEMIC ENCEPHALITIS
Herpes Simplex Encephalitis

Encephalitis resulting from infection by herpes simplex virus type 1 is the most commonly occurring sporadic viral encephalitis in adults and is estimated to constitute 2 to 10% of all cases.[2] There is no seasonal or geographic predominance and males and females are affected equally. Only one third of all cases are preceded by a history of gingivostomatitis.[3] Untreated, HSE has a mortality rate of 70 to 90%, with only 2.5% of patients surviving without neurologic sequelae.[4]

Pathology

Brain damage caused by herpes simplex virus type 1 is largely confined to the limbic system, which includes the hippocampal formation of the temporal lobe and related deep areas of the brain.[5, 6] Hemorrhagic necrosis commonly involves one or both of the temporal and/or inferior frontal lobes. This focal destruction results in the presence of red blood cells in the CSF and clinical manifestations of focal motor seizures involving the contralateral face and upper extremity. In addition, focal abnormal electrical discharges called periodic lateralized epileptiform discharges are often detectable in electroencephalograms (EEGs).

Symptoms and Diagnosis

In biopsy-proven cases, a typical 4- to 10-day prodromal period of fever and malaise is followed by alteration in consciousness (97%), fever (90%), headache (81%), and personality changes (71%)[7] (Table 60–1). Focal motor seizures affecting the face and upper extremities in this clinical setting are a strong indicator of HSE; other focal neurologic signs including hemiparesis and aphasia are more common in HSE than in other viral encephalitides.

Definitive diagnosis can be made only by brain biopsy, which should be directed by neuroimaging studies to areas of suspected involvement or to the nondominant temporal lobe. Using immunofluorescence staining for viral antigens (sensitivity ~80%, specifity ~95%), a positive result can be obtained in 2 to 3 hours. Viral culture from the brain tissue usually requires at least 48 hours. Electron microscopy is about 98% specific but only about 48% sensitive and therefore is not used routinely.

Computed tomographic (CT) scanning with intravenous contrast shows gyral enhancement, temporal lobe lucencies,

TABLE 60–1

SYMPTOMS AND SIGNS IN PATIENTS WITH CULTURE-POSITIVE HERPES SIMPLEX ENCEPHALITIS

Symptom	Frequency (%)
Altered consciousness	97
Fever	90
Headache	81
Dysphasia	76
Personality change	71
Seizures	67
Vomiting	47
Ataxia	40
Hemiparesis	33
Cranial nerve deficits	32
Memory loss	24
Visual field loss	14
Papilledema	14

These results are from the National Insititute of Allergy and Infectious Diseases (NIAID) Collaborative Antiviral Study Group, summarized by Whitley and coworkers.[4, 5] They summarize the clinical findings in 112 patients in whom the diagnosis of herpes simplex virus type 1 encephalitis was confirmed by virus culture from the brain. Ages ranged from 6 months to more than 60 years, with equal distribution by decade. Males and females were equally represented; whites constituted 86% of patients.

or mass effect in up to 65% of biopsy-proven cases by day 5 or later of clinical symptoms;[8] magnetic resonance scanning may be more sensitive, especially earlier.[9] The EEG is often helpful, showing periodic (2- to 3-second intervals) sharp wave complexes (periodic lateralized epileptiform discharges) unilaterally or bilaterally in the temporal regions as early as 2 days into the course and is localizing in up to 81% of patients.[10]

The CSF typically shows a lymphocytosis of 10 to 400 cells per cubic millimeter (although it is normal in 20% of cases in the first few days), along with an increased protein level (80 to 1000 mg/dL) and up to 1000 red blood cells per cubic millimeter (median ~130/mm³), indicating hemorrhagic necrosis.[2] The CSF glucose level is normal or decreased.

The most sensitive immunologic diagnostic tool is the serum/CSF herpes simplex virus type 1 antibody ratio. Serum/CSF ratios by passive hemagglutination and immunoglobulin G immunofluorescence of less than 20:1 (normal, 100:1 to 300:1) are diagnostic but reach 90% sensitivity only after 2 weeks. Figure 60–2 shows the sensitivity of this test as a function of time in biopsy-positive versus biopsy-negative but clinically suspected cases.[11]

A polymerase chain reaction assay of CSF has been shown to confirm the diagnosis in biopsy-proven cases as early as the first day of neurologic symptoms.[12]

Treatment

Treatment with acyclovir (acycloguanosine) reduces the mortality rate to approximately 19%, if administered early, with up to 38% of survivors showing no significant sequelae.[4, 13] It is administered at an intravenous dose of 10 mg/kg every 8 hours for 10 days. Side effects include reversible elevation in serum creatinine level (10%), local phlebitis (4%), and nausea (2%). Alternatively, vidarabine (ara-A) may be used at an intravenous dose of 15 mg/kg in at least 25 mL of 5% dextrose in normal saline given over 12 hours; estimates of about 28% mortality, with approximately 19% of survivors being normal, have been published.[13]

Supportive care must be directed toward management of cerebral edema and seizures, as outlined earlier.

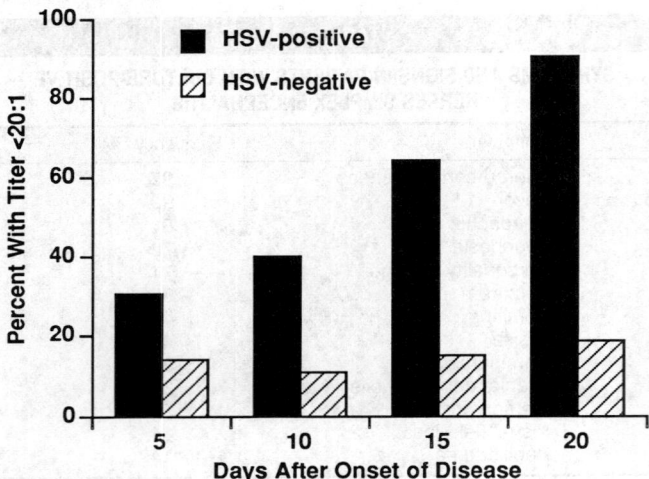

Figure 60–2. Cumulative percentage of patients with clinically suspected HSE with serum/CSF herpes simplex virus type 1 antibody ratios of less than 20:1 (normal, 100:1 to 300:1). This represents the percentage of patients positive by both standard passive hemagglutinin and membrane immunofluorescent immunoglobulin G antibody assays in paired serum and CSF specimens. Patients with brain cultures positive for virus are designated by the filled bars; brain culture–negative patients are designated by hatched bars. (Data are from the National Institute of Allergy and Infectious Diseases [NIAID] Collaborative Antiviral Study Group and are adapted from Nahmias AJ, Whitley RJ, Visintine AN, et al: Herpes simplex virus encephalitis: Laboratory evaluations and their diagnostic significance. J Infect Dis 145:829, 1982.)

Varicella-Zoster Encephalitis

VZE, like HSE, shows no seasonal or geographic predilection. VZE occurs in about 0.05% of childhood chickenpox cases, appearing typically 5 to 6 days after the rash[14] or up to 5 weeks later.[15] It is heralded by fever, headache, and obtundation or delirium and must be distinguished from the more common acute cerebellar ataxia, which develops 1 week after infection, with nystagmus, dysarthria, and ataxia.[16]

VZE is more common in adults after the age of 40, with an incidence of 0.5% after cutaneous zoster eruption.[17] Approximately 35 to 45% of patients have an antecedent cranial nerve (usually trigeminal) or mixed cranial-cervical nerve zoster dermatomal lesion; the average time to occurrence of central nervous system (CNS) symptoms is 9 days, but the time can be as long as 53 days.[15] The average duration of symptoms is 16 to 24 days, and average mortality is about 20% but is much higher in immunosuppressed individuals.[15]

Pathology

No specific or consistent pathologic abnormalities are present in the brain. Subcortical perivascular mononuclear infiltrates, small hemorrhagic foci, and diffuse edema may be seen but are not common. Cowdry's type A inclusion bodies are common but not pathognomonic. Giant cell arteritis and nonspecific arteritis have been demonstrated in cases of herpes zoster ophthalmicus with contralateral hemiparesis.

Symptoms and Diagnosis

Clinical diagnosis depends on the recognition of fever, headache, stiff neck, obtundation, delirium, or personality changes after zoster skin eruptions, especially in immuno-

compromised patients with Hodgkin's disease and chronic lymphocytic leukemia.[15] Seizures are not common. An important association with necrotizing myelitis has been reported in isolated cases.[18] A clinical stroke picture of hemiparesis may develop secondary to varicella-induced vasculitis ipsilateral to ophthalmic involvement of the trigeminal nerve.[19]

Varicella-zoster involving cranial nerve VII may be associated with facial paralysis and vesicles in the external auditory meatus and eardrum (Ramsay Hunt syndrome). This may progress to focal brain stem encephalitis involving cranial nerves V, VI, VIII, IX, and X.[20, 21]

Brain magnetic resonance and CT scans are not generally helpful in the diagnosis of VZE. The EEG shows diffuse slowing in nearly all cases. The CSF white blood cell count is usually less than 500/mm³, but protein levels can vary widely.[15, 22] CSF glucose levels may be low.

Detection of specific antibody to varicella-zoster membrane antigen by indirect membrane immunofluorescence in the CSF from seven of seven patients with clinical encephalitis after zoster infection was reported by Jemsek and coworkers.[15] In another series of 16 patients with zoster-associated encephalitis, 94% had elevated (>1:2) titers in the CSF, whereas none of 25 controls with other CNS pathologic changes had positive CSF titers.[23]

Treatment

No controlled clinical trials of antiviral treatment for VZE have been reported. Controlled trials of intravenous acyclovir in cutaneous zoster infection have demonstrated its efficacy in halting cutaneous dissemination and development of visceral zoster in immunocompromised patients.[24, 25] Reports of improvement of VZE in several patients over several days of treatment with intravenous acyclovir suggest efficacy.[26, 27] A treatment dosage similar to that used in immunocompromised patients (intravenous acyclovir at 500 mg/m² every 8 hours) has been suggested, pending further studies.[20] The usefulness of steroids in VZE has not been demonstrated.

Rabies Encephalitis

Rabies virus causes acute encephalomyelitis after centripetal spread of the virus from peripheral nerve motor end plates to the spinal cord and eventually the brain. All warm-blooded mammals, including birds, are susceptible to the virus, and the disease is present on all continents except Australia and Antarctica. In 1988, approximately 12% of all the total cases in the United States were in domestic animals, cats most commonly (35%), followed by cattle (31%) and dogs (23%). Among wild animals, skunks (38%), raccoons (31%), and bats (14%) account for most cases.[28] The risk of developing rabies from the bite of an affected animal is 5 to 15%;[29] higher risk is associated with bites on the head and face.

The virus gains access to the CNS after entry into peripheral nerves, either at a wound site, through mucous membranes, via aerosolization (laboratory animals and bats), or via transplanted corneas.[30] Typically, nerve entry is heralded by paresthesias at the wound site; the virus enters myocytes, where cytoplasmic replication is followed by extracellular shedding and entry into nerves. Retrograde movement to the spinal cord through the axoplasm occurs at an estimated rate of 3 mm/h, and the virus moves from there to the brain, where extensive virus replication occurs in neurons, especially in the limbic system. The clinical manifestations are thought to follow virus replication in neurons, after which

TABLE 60-2

RABIES POSTEXPOSURE PROPHYLAXIS GUIDE, UNITED STATES, 1991

Animal Type	Evaluation and Disposition of Animal	Postexposure Prophylaxis Recommendations
Dogs and cats	Healthy and available for 10 days of observation	Should not begin prophylaxis unless animal develops symptoms of rabies*
	Rabid or suspected rabid	Immediate vaccination
	Unknown (escaped)	Consult public health officials
Skunks, raccoons, bats, foxes, and most other carnivores; woodchucks	Regarded as rabid unless geographic area is known to be free of rabies or until animal proved negative by laboratory tests†	Immediate vaccination
Livestock, rodents, and lagomorphs (rabbits and hares)	Consider individually	Consult public health officials; bites of squirrels, hamsters, guinea pigs, gerbils, chipmunks, rats, mice, other rodents, rabbits, and hares almost never require antirabies treatment

*During the 10-day holding period, begin treatment with HRIG and HDCV or RVA at first sign of rabies in a dog or cat that has bitten someone. The symptomatic animal should be killed immediately and tested.

†The animal should be killed and tested as soon as possible. Holding for observation is not recommended. Discontinue vaccine if immunofluorescence test results of the animal are negative.

From Centers for Disease Control: Rabies prevention—United States, 1991. Recommendations of the Immunization Practices Advisory Committee (ACIP). MMWR 40:1, 1991.

the virus moves along axoplasmic routes to salivary glands and other tissues. There is no hematogenous spread.

Pathology

Grossly, the brain is congested, and microscopic examination typically shows perivascular inflammatory cells consisting of lymphocytes, macrophages, and plasma cells, with little astrocytosis. These changes are most common in the gray matter of the pons and medulla, thalamus, hypothalamus, basal ganglia, and cervical spinal cord, hence the clinical presentation of brain stem encephalitis (multiple cranial nerve palsies) in some patients. The Negri bodies, which are characteristic and contain viral particles and antigen, are found in 70 to 96% of cases.

Symptoms and Diagnosis

Antemortem diagnosis depends on recognition of the clinical syndrome after exposure, which is difficult in the absence of a history of a recent animal bite. Typically, the incubation period is 30 to 90 days (ranging from 7 days to a year or more),[3] leading to a 2- to 7-day prodrome of fever, headache, myalgia, cough, sore throat, and malaise. An important warning sign is paresthesias around the wound site; they are present in 44 to 50% of cases.[32] Within days of this nonspecific prodrome, one sees either of two clinical courses. The most common course (~80%) is characterized by restlessness, delirium, intolerance to sensory stimuli, and 1- to 5-minute attacks of frenzy, alternating with lucid intervals. Pharyngeal spasms may be precipitated by attempts to drink or by fanning the face. In approximately 20% of patients there is a rapidly progressive ascending paralysis resembling that of the Guillain-Barré syndrome. In either clinical course, progression to stupor, coma, and death occurs in 3 to 7 days. Once clinically established, rabies encephalomyelitis is almost uniformly fatal, although several cases of survival have been reported.[32]

The white blood cell count is often elevated (10,000 to 20,000/mm³) with elevated numbers of polymorphonuclear neutrophils, and the CSF typically has fewer than 125 mononuclear cells per cubic millimeter with mildly elevated protein and normal glucose levels. Brain CT scans are normal and EEGs are diffusely slow.[33]

The most reliable serologic evidence is detection of serum antibody in unvaccinated subjects. In a retrospective study of 22 patients, Anderson and colleagues[34] found that 100% developed positive titers between days 6 and 15 of clinical illness, with mean titers increasing from 1:8 (day 6) to 1:288 (day 15). Virus isolation from either throat swab or saliva was the test found most likely to be positive early in the illness, as early as 2 days in four of four confirmed cases. Rapid antemortem diagnosis can also be made by immunofluorescent staining for virus antigen in corneal scrape specimens or neck skin biopsy,[35] although this is diagnostic in only about 50% of early cases.

Treatment

A decision for treatment must be made before the development of clinical disease. Immediate cleansing of the wound with soap and water, 1 to 2% benzalkonium chloride, or 40 to 70% alcohol is recommended. A decision for postexposure prophylaxis should be based on the animal type and disposition as well as the geographic area (Table 60-2). If prophylaxis is required, human rabies immune globulin (HRIG) at a dose of 20 IU/kg body weight is used, if the patient was not previously vaccinated. One half of the dose is infiltrated around the wound and the remainder is administered intramuscularly in the gluteus (Table 60-3) or in another area away from that of the subsequent vaccine injection. In nonvaccinated patients, 1.0 mL of either human diploid cell vaccine (HDCV) or rabies vaccine adsorbed (RVA) is given intramuscularly in the deltoid (never gluteus) on days 0, 3, 7, 14, and 28. In previously vaccinated persons, this dose is given only on days 0 and 3, after initial wound cleansing.[36] If HRIG was not given before the vaccination, it *can* be administered through the seventh day after the first dose of vaccine. Concomitant use of steroids, immunosuppressants, or antimalarials is contraindicated, as they can interfere with active immunity after vaccination.

Reactions after vaccination with HDCV and RVA are much less common than with earlier vaccines.[36] These include local pain, erythema, and swelling around the injection site in 30 to 74% of patients; and headache, nausea, vomiting, and myalgias in 5 to 40%. Several cases of a reversible Guillain-Barré–like illness have been reported. HRIG has not been associated with significant complications.

TABLE 60–3

RABIES POSTEXPOSURE PROPHYLAXIS SCHEDULE, UNITED STATES, 1991

Status	Treatment	Regimen*
Not previously vaccinated	Local wound cleansing	All postexposure treatment should begin with immediate thorough cleansing of all wounds with soap and water.
	HRIG	20 IU/kg body weight. If anatomically feasible, up to one half the dose should be infiltrated around the wound(s) and the rest should be administered IM in the gluteal area. HRIG should not be administered in the same syringe or into the same anatomic site as vaccine. Because HRIG may partially suppress active production of antibody, no more than the recommended dose should be given.
	Vaccine	HDCV or RVA, 1.0 ml IM (deltoid area†) each on days 0, 3, 7, 14, and 28.
Previously vaccinated‡	Local wound cleansing	All postexposure treatment should begin with immediate thorough cleansing of all wounds with soap and water.
	HRIG	HRIG should not be administered.
	Vaccine	HDCV or RVA, 1.0 mL IM (deltoid area†) each on days 0 and 3.

*These regimens are applicable for all age groups, including children.

†The deltoid area is the only acceptable site of vaccination for adults and older children. For younger children, the outer aspect of the thigh may be used. Vaccine should never be administered in the gluteal area.

‡Any person with a history of pre-exposure vaccination with HDCV or RVA, prior postexposure prophylaxis with HDCV or RVA, or previous vaccination with any other type of rabies vaccine and a documented history of antibody response to the prior vaccination.

From Centers for Disease Control: Rabies prevention—United States, 1991. Recommendations of the Immunization Practices Advisory Committee (ACIP). MMWR 40:1, 1991.

When clinical rabies encephalomyelitis has been established, supportive care is all that can be offered. Respiratory disturbances occur in all cases, requiring intubation for management of secretions as well as respiratiory distress and increased intracranial pressure. Seizures can be expected in two thirds of cases, and cardiac arrhythmias occur almost invariably. Other signs of CNS dysfunction include thermal dysregulation, diabetes insipidus, and autonomic dysfunction.

EPIDEMIC ARBOVIRAL ENCEPHALITIS

The most significant epidemic encephalitides in the United States are caused by the arboviruses (*arthropod-borne viruses*), with the mosquito as the major vector. These viruses include three major groups: (1) the *Togaviridae* alphavirus group, which includes the viruses that cause EEE, WEE, and VEE; (2) the *Togaviridae* flavivirus group, which causes SLE and JBE, among others; and (3) the *Bunyaviridae* California serogroup, which causes La Crosse encephalitis.

Unlike the sporadic encephalitides, arboviral encephalitides have a clear seasonal and geographic pattern of expression, with the appearance of cases in May, peaks in July and August, and a dramatic decrease by the late fall (November), corresponding to infections in the mosquito population. Generally, subclinical infection is widespread, with few individuals showing disease. Of the six major types listed, EEE is the least frequent but most deadly.

St. Louis Encephalitis

SLE accounts for most arboviral cases of adult encephalitis in the United States. First described in 1933, outbreaks of SLE occur at approximately 10-year intervals (the last was in 1985), peaking in August and September primarily in the Ohio-Mississippi Valley, eastern Texas, Florida, Kansas, Colorado, and California. In certain endemic areas, seroprevalence is approximately 3.6% and up to 6% in epidemics, with an estimated ratio of inapparent to apparent infection of 800:1 in children to 80:1 in the elderly. Attack rates are estimated to be 1 to 800 per 100,000 population.[37] The

clinical presentation of encephalitis in an endemic area during July or August should alert one to the diagnosis.

Pathology

Generally, gross changes in the brain are minimal. Microscopic plaques are prominent subcortically (midbrain, substantia nigra, thalamus, striatum, spinal cord, pons, medulla), with perivascular lymphocytes and mononuclear meningeal infiltrates and nerve cell death.[5, 6] The CSF reflects this, with a moderate pleocytosis without red blood cells.

Symptoms and Diagnosis

Clinical manifestations appear on average 4 to 12 days after exposure and are most common in patients more than 60 years of age.[37] Sudden onset of fever (100%), headache (95%), nausea and vomiting (61%), stiff neck (37%), and myalgias is typical, followed in 1 to 4 days by confusion, irritability, disorientation, or apathy. Brain stem and cerebellar findings such as a lower motor neuron deficit, particularly cranial nerve VII (~20%), tremors (~50%), ataxia, nytagmus, and myoclonus may appear.[38] Unusual associated symptoms of urinary urgency, frequency, and incontinence were reported in 25% of patients in one series, as well as the syndrome of inappropriate antidiuretic hormone.[38, 39] Mortality has been estimated at about 10%, and 80% of this occurs in the first 2 weeks. Residual complaints of fatigue may persist for several years in 20% of patients, with no long-term cognitive sequelae.

Rapid, early diagnosis of SLE is best achieved with an IgM-capture enzyme-linked immunosorbent assay (ELISA) on acute-phase and convalescent-phase serum samples.[40] IgM antibodies are detectable in 71% of cases between days 0 and 3 of illness and in 94% between days 4 and 21, gradually decline after the first 10 days of illness, and are generally undetectable at 4 months. There is limited cross-reactivity with related flaviviruses, such as Japanese B virus, which makes this the best serodiagnostic test, replacing the standard hemagglutination inhibition (HI) test, complement fixation (CF) test, and neutralizing antibody test (NT) formerly used.

The CSF shows pleocytosis (average ~100 cells per cubic millimeter) on initial lumbar puncture, with early neutrophil predominance in up to 94% of patients and an elevated protein level (average 78 mg/dL) in more than 80%.[38] By the second week of illness, 75% of the cells are lymphocytes.[39]

Brain CT scans are generally not helpful. In the series of Brinker and colleagues,[38] the EEG showed diffuse abnormalities in all cases, although the severity of the disease did not correlate with the severity of the EEG abnormalities.

Treatment

No effective antiviral treatment is currently available; supportive care is the rule. Particular attention must be paid to fluid management (free water restriction) in cases in which the syndrome of inappropriate antidiuretic hormone secretion develops.

Eastern Equine Encephalitis

EEE is the deadliest arboviral encephalitis, with a mortality rate of 50 to 80%, which is highest in adults. Most cases occur in the Atlantic and Gulf Coast states, upper New York, and western Michigan. Epidemics typically occur in late summer to early fall after a period of heavy rainfall. Of the four major arboviral encephalitides in the United States, EEE has the lowest ratio of inapparent to apparent infection, ranging from 8:1 in infants to 50:1 in young adults.[41] The human infection rate during epidemics is low, estimated at about 2.3%.

Assessments of morbidity and mortality suggest a complete recovery rate of only about 3%. Severe neurologic sequelae, primarily mental retardation but also hemiparesis and aphasia, are seen in up to two thirds of patients, usually children.[42] Infection in adults more often results in death, with fewer patients showing permanent sequelae. Evidence suggests that longer prodromal periods are associated with lower morbidity and mortality.[43]

Pathology

Grossly, the brain is swollen with cloudy leptomeninges.[6] Widespread multifocal microscopic necrosis of the cortical gray matter is common, along with the basal ganglia and substantia nigra, sparing the spinal cord.[6, 20] Polymorphonuclear as well as mononuclear perivascular infiltrates are seen with small-vessel vasculitis and thrombi, and neuronolysis is common. The widespread necrosis and generalized edema account for the CSF findings of red blood cells and markedly elevated opening pressure, resembling those of HSE.

Symptoms and Diagnosis

EEE is a fulminant disease characterized by onset of symptoms 1 to 4 days after infection. These include high temperature (102 to 104°F), lethargy (92%), convulsions (74%), stiff neck (62%), and vomiting (52%), leading to stupor, coma, and death in as little as 24 hours and up to 5 days.[43] Cranial nerve palsies and hemiparesis are sometimes seen (resembling those in HSE), and seizures are seen in about 75% of patients, usually children. In adults, a febrile prodrome may precede the clinical encephalitis by as much as 11 days; in children this is not generally the case.

As with SLE, rapid and early diagnosis of EEE can be made with an IgM-capture ELISA antibody test on serum.[44] In a retrospective series of 20 confirmed cases, positive titers were seen in all patients, one as early as 1 day after onset of clinical disease, with maximum titers seen at 1 to 2 weeks.

There was no cross-reactivity with serum samples from either WEE or VEE patients.[45] As with SLE, this test is replacing the standard HI, CF, and NT serologic tests for diagnosing the equine encephalitides.

The diagnosis has also been made by electron microscopic identification of virus particles in a brain biopsy specimen from an infant.[46] The brain CT scan usually shows generalized edema, and the EEG shows generalized slowing, although periodic lateralized epileptiform discharges resembling those seen in HSE are sometimes seen.[10]

In two series of patients[47, 48] the initial CSF nearly always showed an increased opening pressure and protein level (45 to 100 mg/dL in 62%; >100 mg/dL in 25%) with an average white blood cell count of 900 to 1000/mm³ (60% neutrophils) within 48 hours of the onset of symptoms. Notably, xanthochromia was present in the CSF of more than half of the patients, again as in HSE.

Treatment

No clinically useful pharmacologic therapy is available.[49] Supportive care must be directed toward the control of cerebral edema and seizures, as outlined earlier.

Western Equine Encephalitis

WEE is generally a mild disease, clinically difficult to distinguish from SLE, but nearly always found west of the Mississippi River, particularly the San Joaquin Valley of California, Texas, and Colorado.[20] WEE and SLE epidemics peak slightly earlier in the summer (July and August) than those of EEE (August and September).[50] The ratio of inapparent to apparent infection is estimated to be 60:1 in children and 1100:1 in adults, with increased severity of disease in infants less than 1 year of age. Between 25 and 30% of WEE cases occur in children less than 1 year of age, and 50% of these have severe neurologic sequelae including mental retardation, spasticity, and seizures, because of structural damage to the developing brain.[51, 52] Adults have less than 5% risk of neurologic sequelae. Overall mortality is 2 to 3% but is 10 to 23% in adults over the age of 55 years.[52] Interestingly, the incidence rate in males is twice that in females by age 5 to 9 years, presumably because of increased exposure during outdoor activities.[53]

Pathology

The gross appearance of the brain may resemble the congestion typically seen in EEE. Microscopically, the basal ganglia are most commonly affected, with multifocal necrosis of the gray matter and white matter, although the reactions are milder than those in EEE and there is less polymorphonuclear neutrophil infiltrate. The CSF also shows less cellular reaction (see later). Also, patchy white matter demyelination may be more extensive than in EEE.[5, 6]

Symptoms and Diagnosis

As with each of the equine encephalitides, one must be alert for cases in middle and late summer; WEE particularly occurs in infants less than 1 year of age. The incubation period appears to be about 2 weeks and is followed by a sudden onset of mild headache, fever, nausea, vomiting, and malaise, often with photophobia and vertigo. After several days, the headache progresses in severity and the patient becomes lethargic or even comatose (~15%). In mild cases, these symptoms persist for about 10 days and then subside; in severe cases the fever may reach 105 to 106°F and the lethargy may progress to stupor, coma, and death in 4 to 7 days. Seizures occur in up to 90% of infants and 40% of children 1 to 4 years of age but rarely in adults.[54] Physical examination usually reveals stiff neck and commonly hyporeflexia and weakness. Cranial nerves are spared. Children often exhibit muscular rigidity, involuntary movements, and paralysis.[53]

Again, as with EEE and SLE, rapid and early diagnosis is possible with an IgM-capture ELISA antibody test, although in WEE there is more cross-reactivity with several other, geographically isolated viruses.[44] Fourteen of seventeen (82%) individuals previously confirmed to have WEE by acute and convalescent HI, CF, and NT antibody titers had specific IgM antibody titers, several in the first 2 days of illness.[45] As with EEE, this single determination test was more sensitive and specific for *recent* infection than the standard HI, CF, and NT titers. However, as with EEE, the serodiagnosis can be made by confirmation of a fourfold rise in the standard acute and convalescent titers.

Unlike that in EEE, the CSF in WEE typically shows a normal opening pressure and protein level and a white blood cell count less than 200/mm³, with a mononuclear predominance developing in the first 2 days.

Treatment

There is no specific antiviral treatment; however, aggressive supportive care in these patients often results in complete recovery.

Japanese B Encephalitis

JBE has affected more people and accounts for more morbidity and mortality than any other arboviral encephalitis, resulting in 10,000 cases annually in China and several thousand deaths. The virus is distributed throughout Asia and southeastern Commonwealth of Independent States (formerly the U.S.S.R.), China to India on the west and the Philippines on the east, and may affect travelers to those areas, especially military personnel.[55] Swine are an important source of infection for the species of mosquito that transmit JBE virus to humans.[56] In nonvaccinated populations, children under 15 years of age have the highest incidence of disease.[57] The inapparent-to-apparent infection ratio may be as high as 500:1.[57] In the 1980s the use of inactivated JBE viral vaccine dramatically decreased the morbidity and mortality (estimated at 20 to 50%) of JBE.[58] Both mortality and neurologic sequelae (3 to 32%) are greatest in children, and the latter include psychosis, intellectual impairment, spasticity, and paresis.[20] Rapid appearance of antibodies in the CSF is a predictor of less severe disease.[59]

Pathology

The gray matter of the brain is primarily affected. Perivenous cuffs of mononuclear cells with focal necrotic areas of varying size are most common in the thalamus, substantia nigra, anterior horns of the spinal cord, cerebral cortex, and cerebellum.[5] The damage to the gray matter of the cortex and the spinal cord may cause intellectual impairment and paresis.

Symptoms and Diagnosis

Prodromal symptoms are not common. The 4- to 20-day incubation period is followed by rapid onset of fever (100%), headache (80%), and nuchal rigidity (100%), with altered sensorium, which may range from lethargy to agitation. Interesting features in some include mask-like facies resembling that in parkinsonism; ocular tremors; coarse tremors of the face, lips, and hands; and occasionally a lower motor neuron facial (nerve VII) paresis.[55] In fatal cases, death usually occurs on the fifth to ninth day.

The most useful early test result is the IgM-capture ELISA antibody titer in the CSF. This has confirmed the diagnosis in 68% (day 1) and 100% (day 7) of cases eventually diagnosed by conventional HI assays.[59] Standard CF antibody tests are consistently positive only after weeks of infection. Virus can be cultured from the CSF, but this takes longer than the IgM test.[60] The CSF shows approximately 20 to 400 mixed polymorphonuclear neutrophils and lymphocytes per cubic millimeter in approximately 90% of cases up to day 4, with conversion completely to lymphocytes by day 7.[55] These cell counts may remain elevated for months, although they steadily decline in the majority of cases. Protein levels and opening pressure are minimally elevated.

Isolated case reports suggest no specific findings on brain CT scans or EEGs.

Treatment

There is no effective antiviral treatment.[49] Purified JBE vaccine made from whole virus derived from mouse is estimated to be 91% effective in preventing disease in children.[58]

Venezuelan Equine Encephalitis

VEE in humans is generally a benign disease in adults. It is most common in Central America, South America, and the southern United States, where a major epidemic occurred in 1971.[61] That year there were more than 16,000 cases in Mexico; 75% of the deaths occurred in children under 5 years of age and only 5% in adults over the age of 45 years. Overall, a death rate of 0.2 to 0.6% is estimated. Most infections are thought to lead to systemic disease, although only a fraction have encephalitis. VEE virus is highly infectious by the aerosol route and poses a risk to laboratory personnel.

Pathology

In the fatal cases reviewed by de la Monte and coworkers,[62] the main histopathologic lesions in the brain and other organs were marked congestion and hemorrhage. Mixed cellular infiltrates in the leptomeninges were common. Most striking was the marked depletion of lymphocytes in the lymph nodes, spleen, and gastrointestinal tract, suggesting that the lymphocyte was the primary target for the virus. Thus, VEE virus infection often results in severe systemic disease.

Symptoms and Diagnosis

Disease caused by infection with VEE virus can be categorized into three forms: (1) *influenzal* (most common in adults), manifested by constitutional symptoms including nausea, vomiting, myalgias, and pharyngitis, with a febrile course of 1 to 4 days; (2) *fulminant* (most common in children), characterized by several days of fever followed by shock, coma (2%), and convulsions (6%), and leading to sequelae; and (3) *encephalitic* (~20%, more common in children), characterized by a diphasic febrile course for more than 2 weeks, with CNS manifestations of confusion, drowsiness, hallucinations, or ataxia during the second phase.[54, 61, 63] Of all patients acutely ill with VEE virus, 100% show fever, 43% lethargy, and 22% pharyngitis.

HI antibody titers in acute- and convalescent-phase serum samples remain the standard serologic diagnostic tool, although the IgM-capture ELISA assay shows specificity in the limited number of cases tested.[53] Virus can be isolated from serum during the first 48 hours of illness, as well as from throat swabs by injection into suckling mice.[55] In a small number of cases, the CSF lymphocyte count has been reported to be up to 300+/mm³ by day 3 of disease, with protein levels of about 50 mg/dL. Leukopenia is seen in 75% of patients, unlike the finding in WEE, SLE, and EEE.

Treatment

No effective antiviral therapy is currently available.

La Crosse Encephalitis

In the past two decades, La Crosse encephalitis has been second only to SLE in the number of arboviral cases in the United States (~5% of all viral CNS infections).[64] Most cases (~100 per year) occur in Ohio, Wisconsin, Minnesota, New York, and Indiana, and more than 90% occur in children under 15 years of age, with a peak incidence between ages 4 and 10 years. Most cases occur in August and September. The ratio of inapparent to apparent infection is estimated to be 26:1, and exposure to woodland mosquitoes is a consistent historic risk factor.[65] Fatalities are rare (0.5%) and seizures may persist in up to 19% of patients.[66, 67]

Pathology

Because of the few fatalities, only a few case reports are available. Perivascular infiltrates, degenerated neurons, and patches of necrosis are described in the cerebral cortex and basal ganglia, sparing the white matter.[5, 6]

Symptoms and Diagnosis

The most common presentation is a 2- to 3-day period of fever, headache, malaise, abdominal pain, nausea, and vomiting, followed by signs of meningitis, all of which resolve in approximately 1 week. Less commonly, one sees a more typical encephalitis picture: abrupt onset of fever (100%), disorientation (90%), nuchal rigidity (38%), seizures (50%), tremors (20%), papilledema, and coma, from which most patients recover during a 2-week period.[20, 67] The peripheral blood shows leukocytosis, and the CSF lymphocyte count is less than 300/mm³ in 97% of patients.[65, 68]

An IgM-capture ELISA assay has been developed to diagnose infection in acute-phase serum. In one series of 29 patients, specific IgM was detected in 83% by day 3 after the onset of clinical symptoms.[69] This test is replacing the standard HI, CF, and NT tests formerly used on paired serum samples to make the diagnosis.[70]

EEGs are nearly uniformly abnormal, showing generalized or focal slow waves.[71] Brain CT scans are not diagnostic.

Treatment

There is no effective antiviral treatment. Long-term seizure prophylaxis has been recommended for individuals having seizures during the acute illness.[67]

NONARBOVIRAL EPIDEMIC ENCEPHALITIS
Influenza Encephalitis

Although the frequency of CNS complications with influenza is quite low, varied clinical syndromes may result: acute encephalitis, acute paralysis, and parainfectious processes—encephalomyelitis, acute hemorrhagic leukoencephalopathy, transverse myelitis, acute ataxia of childhood, and Reye's syndrome. A small number of encephalitis cases caused by influenza A virus occur during epidemics and worldwide pandemics. Complete recovery from influenza encephalitis is the rule.

Symptoms and Diagnosis

Diagnosis is difficult and case reports are few. Neurologic signs such as depression of consciousness, disorientation, stupor, coma, and seizures in the setting of fever occur 2 to 7 days after constitutional symptoms of headache, dry cough, and myalgias.[72, 73] Acute psychoses after influenza symptoms have been reported, with recovery occurring for all of these during a 4-week period.

A fourfold rise in serum HI or CF antibody titers in acute-phase and convalescent-phase (day 14 to 21) serum samples or virus isolation from throat swabs is presumptive evidence for acute infection. Alternatively, a single rapid hemolysis test for detection of antibody to influenza virus hemagglutinin may allow more rapid early serologic diagnosis.[74]

Reye's syndrome (encephalopathy with fatty degeneration of the liver) may follow influenza B, influenza A, or varicella-zoster virus infection in children under 14 years of age (90% of cases) and rarely in adults. It is heralded by recurrent vomiting followed by lethargy with markedly elevated serum transaminase levels, ammonia levels, and prothrombin time in the setting of a normal bilirubin level and absence of signs of bacterial CNS infection or focal neurologic deficits. Recognition of the association between salicylate use in children and Reye's syndrome, along with improved therapeutic protocols for reducing intracranial pressure, has decreased the incidence of Reye's syndrome, improved early recognition, and enhanced survival.

Treatment

Amantadine hydrochloride has demonstrated effectiveness in the treatment of influenza A virus infections, but its use in the treatment of influenza encephalitis has not been studied.

General management of Reye's syndrome includes administration of vitamin K and fresh frozen plasma to correct coagulation defects, reduction of elevated serum ammonia levels, and replacement of electrolytes. Aggressive management of elevated intracranial pressure is essential. A successful management protocol reported for a series of patients with nonpurposeful or decorticate responses to pain and serum ammonia levels higher than 300 μg/dL (normal, <150 μg/dL) is as follows:[75]

1. Placement of an intraventricular CSF pressure monitor.
2. Hyperventilation and neuromuscular paralysis (pancuronium bromide, 0.1 mg/kg/h as needed) to maintain P_{CO_2} at 23 to 25 mm Hg.
3. Phenobarbital load (10 mg/kg/d in divided doses) to maintain blood levels at 30 to 40 μg/mL.
4. Dexamethasone, 0.2 mg/kg intravenously every 6 hours.
5. Mannitol boluses of 0.25 to 1.0 g/kg intravenously as needed to keep intracranial pressure less than 20 to 25 cm H_2O if dexamethasone fails.
6. CSF drainage if mannitol boluses fail.

Mortality was reported to be 12% in this retrospective study of 29 children, compared with a rate of about 60% at the same institution before the use of intracranial pressure monitoring to guide therapy.

Enterovirus Encephalitis

The enterovirus group includes the polioviruses, coxsackieviruses A and B, echoviruses, enteroviruses, and hepatitis A virus, all of which infect the human alimentary tract. In patients with clinical presentation, aseptic meningitis is the most frequent neurologic manifestation (35%), followed by encephalitis (11%) and paralysis (1%). Most cases of meningitis or encephalitis occur in July through September, primarily in the 10- to 29-year age group.[76] The outcome of enteroviral encephalitis is usually benign, although a mortality rate of 2.5% has been reported.

Symptoms and Diagnosis

The clinical picture of meningoencephalitis is nonspecific. Enterovirus 70 infection, for example, is often heralded by a self-limiting acute hemorraghic conjunctivitis within 1 to 10 days of infection.[20] In a small number of cases it is followed in 1 to 5 weeks by radicular pain with asymmetric flaccid paralysis, which may be permanent. Coxsackievirus may cause aseptic meningitis associated with herpangina, pleurodynia, pericarditis, and rashes. Enterovirus 71 more commonly causes aseptic meningitis and encephalitis.

In most enteroviral infections, routine serologic screening is impractical, requiring antibody titers against specific viruses because of lack of group-specific antigens. Therefore, emphasis is on virus isolation from throat swabs, stool, blood, and CSF (which was demonstrated in 41% of 111 pediatric cases of meningitis or meningoencephalitis in one report[77]). During specific outbreaks, however, a fourfold increase in antibody against the specific virus is diagnostic.

Treatment

No specific antiviral therapies are available.

Mumps Encephalitis

Before widespread vaccination for mumps began in 1967, mumps encephalitis affected approximately 400 patients per year or about 0.3% of all mumps patients; the total number of encephalitis cases dropped to 26 in 1978, with a concomitant 10-fold decrease in the total number of nonencephalitic mumps cases.[20] Other estimates put the frequency of mumps meningitis with or without signs of encephalitis as high as 11% of mumps cases.[78] As many as one third of mumps infections are asymptomatic, and as many as one half of all clinical mumps cases have CSF pleocytosis, regardless of the presence of neurologic symptoms. The peak incidence in the United States occurs in March and April and is highest in the 5- to 9-year age range; approximately 92% of children acquire mumps antibody by age 15. Although mumps affects males and females equally, males are more susceptible to the development of encephalitis (3:1). Although 0.5 to 2.3% of all mumps encephalitis cases are fatal, most patients show marked clinical improvement within 2 to 4 days and recover fully.[78]

Pathology

A pattern of selective periventricular myelin loss with perivascular mononuclear infiltrates, scattered foci of neuronophagia, and relative sparing of axons is typical, suggesting an autoimmune etiology.

Symptoms and Diagnosis

In general, the incubation period from exposure to the clinical signs of mumps is 18 days. In patients who develop CNS symptoms the distinction between meningitis and encephalitis is blurred. Signs of fever, headache, vomiting, neck stiffness, and lethargy develop about 5 days after the onset of parotitis; of these patients, 20 to 30% have seizures with or without focal neurologic signs. However, only about 50% of encephalitis patients have antecedent parotitis, which occurs in 95% of all mumps patients. Occasionally, encephalitis precedes parotitis.[78]

The EEG is often abnormal but is not diagnostic or predictive of long-term outcome.[79] CSF pleocytosis is present in nearly all encephalitis cases, even in 40 to 50% of all mumps cases without CNS symptoms. Mononuclear cells predominate from the onset of CNS disease, and peak cell counts are seen around day 3 of CNS symptoms (averaging 250/mm³ but as high as 1000/mm³ or more).[78] These cell counts decrease over weeks. Protein concentration is markedly elevated in 60 to 70% of cases, and low CSF glucose levels may be seen on average in one fourth of cases.

Virus can be cultured from the CSF,[80] throat swabs, and testes and identified by electron microscopic analysis of ependymal cells in the CSF.[81]

An IgM-capture ELISA assay has been developed for detection of mumps virus in serum and CSF; positive titers were found in 100% of confirmed cases in at least one series.[82] This will probably prove to be the most sensitive early diagnostic test for CNS infection. Similar results were found for IgM-ELISA assays of acute-phase serum samples, and these IgM tests appear more reliable for early detection than conventional HI, CF, or NT assays.[83]

Treatment

No specific antiviral therapy is available for mumps meningoencephalitis.

PARAINFECTIOUS ENCEPHALITIS

Parainfectious encephalitis is a term describing presumed immune-mediated damage to the CNS arising in temporal relation to overt CNS infection (measles, subacute sclerosing panencephalitis, and others) or after vaccination (rabies and others).

Measles Encephalitis

Measles infection peaks in the 5- to 9-year-old age group, and 99% of subjects have been exposed by age 20 years.

Symptoms and Diagnosis

Typically, 10 to 11 days after exposure one sees a 2- to 4-day prodromal phase of fever, malaise, cough, rhinitis, and conjunctivitis with the characteristic Koplik's spots on the buccal mucosa, which fade in 2–4 days. A distinctive maculopapular rash follows the prodrome, appearing first on the head and face and moving centrifugally in 3 to 4 days to cover the body.[84]

Subacute measles encephalitis occurs in immunosuppressed patients, typically leukemic children undergoing radiation therapy. The incubation period ranges from 5 weeks to 6 months and is followed by focal myoclonic seizures, hemiplegia, stupor, coma, and death after a course of weeks or a few months.

Acute measles postinfectious encephalitis occurs in about 1 in 1000 to 5000 measles cases within 8 days of onset of measles and has a 15% mortality rate. It is characterized by worsening fever, headache, seizures, cerebellar ataxia, and coma. Approximately 20 to 40% of those who recover have permanent neurologic deficits including retardation, seizures, and hemiparesis.

Subacute sclerosing panencephalitis affects 1 in 1 million measles patients approximately 6 to 8 years after acute infection.[84] Approximately 50% of patients have their initial measles attack before the age of 2 years. Generalized intellectual deterioration, psychologic or personality disturbances, and hallucinations lasting weeks or months are followed by dyspraxia, extrapyramidal movement disorders, myoclonus, aphasia, and convulsions. In 75% of cases viral chorioretinitis occurs, which can lead to blindness. Overall, the course is variable and spontaneous remissions occur in only 5% of cases.[85] Death occurs in 1 to 3 years in 70 to 90% of cases. It is thought to result from either slow replication of structurally defective virus in neurons and oligodendrocytes or immune attack on these cells.

Diagnosis of subacute sclerosing panencephalitis can be made in the appropriate clinical setting with demonstration of oligoclonal immunoglobulin G antibody in the CSF. ELISA tests for IgM measles-specific antibody in acute- and convalescent-phase serum samples can provide the diagnosis of measles during the initial illness.[84] HI testing is also commonly used.

The EEG often shows a characteristic burst suppression pattern of high-amplitude slow-wave complexes occurring at a rate of one every 4 to 20 seconds.[10] CT scans may show cortical atrophy and focal or multifocal lucencies in the white matter.

Treatment

Immunosuppressed patients infected with measles viruses should receive human anti-measles gamma globulin 0.25 to 0.5 mL/kg within the first 3 days after exposure. It is ineffective if given 6 or more days after exposure.[84]

Medical therapy in subacute sclerosing panencephalitis is symptomatic. Myoclonus can be treated with benzodiazepines or valproate; seizures can be treated with standard anticonvulsants. The antiviral agent inosiplex (Isoprinosine) at a dose of 100 mg/kg body weight in divided doses every 4 hours by mouth for the course of the disease markedly improved long-term survival and diminished neurologic disability in several nonrandomized trials.[86, 87]

References

1. Downs WG: Arboviruses. In: Evans AS (ed): Viral Infections of Humans: Epidemiology and Control. New York, Plenum Publishing, p 114, 1989.
2. Koskiniemi M, Vaheri A, Taskinen E: Cerebrospinal fluid alterations in herpes simplex virus encephalitis. Rev Infect Dis 6:608, 1984.
3. Longson M: Herpes simplex. In: Zuckerman AJ, Banatvala JE, Pattison JR (eds): Principles and Practice of Clinical Virology. 2nd ed. West Sussex, England, John Wiley & Sons, p 2, 1990.
4. Whitley RJ, Soong SJ, Hirsch MS, et al: Herpes simplex encephalitis: Vidarabine therapy and diagnostic problems. N Engl J Med 304:313, 1981.
5. Lindenberg R: Tissue reactions in the gray matter of the central nervous system. In: Haymaker W, Adams RD (eds): Histology and Histopathology of the Nervous System. Springfield, IL, Charles C Thomas, p 973, 1982.
6. Leetsma JE: Viral infections of the nervous system. In: Davis RL, Robertson DM (eds): Textbook of Neuropathology. Baltimore, Williams & Wilkins, p 704, 1985.
7. Whitley RJ, Soong SJ, Linneman C Jr: Herpes simplex encephalitis: Clinical assessment. JAMA 247:317, 1982.
8. Davis JM, Davis KR, Kleinman GM, et al: Computed tomography of herpes simplex encephalitis, with clinicopathological correlation. Radiology 129:409, 1978.
9. Schroth G, Gawehn J, Thron A, et al: Early diagnosis of herpes simplex encephalitis by MRI. Neurology 37:179, 1987.
10. Aminoff MJ: Electroencephalography: General principles and clinical applications. In: Aminoff MJ (ed): Electrodiagnosis in Clinical Neurology. 2nd ed. New York, Churchill Livingstone, p 21, 1986.
11. Nahmias AJ, Whitley RJ, Visintine AN, et al: Herpes simplex virus encephalitis: Laboratory evaluations and their diagnostic significance. J Infect Dis 145:829, 1982.
12. Aurelius D, Johansson B, Skoldenberg B, et al: Rapid diagnosis of herpes simplex encephalitis by nested polymerase chain reaction assay of cerebrospinal fluid. Lancet 337:189, 1991.
13. Whitley RJ: Herpes simplex virus infections of the central nervous system: A review. Am J Med 85:61, 1988.
14. Tenser RB: Herpes simplex and herpes zoster: Nervous system involvement. Neurol Clin 2:215, 1984.
15. Jemsek J, Greenberg SB, Taber L, et al: Herpes zoster–associated encephalitis: Clinicopathologic report of 12 cases and review of the literature. Medicine 62:81, 1983.
16. Ho DD, Hirsch MS: Acute viral encephalitis. Med Clin North Am 69:415, 1985.
17. Ragozzino MW, Melton LJ III, Kurland LT, et al: Population-based study of herpes zoster and its sequelae. Medicine 61:310, 1982.
18. Hogan EL, Krigman MR: Herpes zoster myelitis. Arch Neurol 29:309, 1973.
19. MacKenzie RA, Forbes GS, Karnes WE: Angiographic findings in herpes zoster arteritis. Ann Neurol 10:458, 1981.
20. Booss J, Esiri ME: Viral Encephalitis: Pathology, Diagnosis, and Management. Boston, Blackwell Scientific Publications, 1986.
21. Aviel A, Marshak C: Ramsay Hunt syndrome: A cranial polyneuropathy. Am J Otolaryngol 3:61, 1982.
22. McKendall RR, Klawans HI: Varicella zoster virus complications. In: Vinken PJ, Bruyn GW (eds): Handbook of Clinical Neurology, Volume 34, Infections in the Nervous System. New York, North Holland, p 161, 1978.
23. Gershon A, Steinberg S, Greenberg S, et al: Varicella zoster–associated encephalitis: Detection of specific antibody in cerebrospinal fluid. J Clin Microbiol 12:764, 1980.
24. Balfour HH, Bean B, Laskin O, et al: Acyclovir halts progression of herpes zoster in immunocompromised patients. N Engl J Med 308:1448, 1983.
25. Shepp DH, Dandliker PS, Meyers JD: Treatment of varicella-zoster infection in severely immunocompromised patients. N Engl J Med 314:208, 1986.
26. Steele RW, Keeney RE, Bradsher RW, et al: Treatment of varicella-zoster meningoencephalitis with acyclovir—Demonstration of virus in cerebrospinal fluid by electron microscopy. Am J Clin Pathol 80: 57, 1983.
27. Hirsch MS, Schooley RT: Drug therapy. Treatment of herpesvirus infections. N Engl J Med 309:963 and 1034, 1983.
28. Eng TR, Hamaker TA, Dobbins JG: Rabies surveillance, United States, 1988. MMWR 38:1, 1988.
29. Applebaum E, Greenberg M, Nelson J: Neurological complications following antirabies vaccination. JAMA 151:188, 1953.
30. Houff SA, Burton RC, Wilson RW, et al: Human-to-human transmission of rabies virus by corneal transplant. N Engl J Med 300: 603, 1979.
31. Chopra JS, Banerjee AK, Murthy JMK, et al: Paralytic rabies: A clinicopathological study. Brain 103:789, 1980.
32. Bernard KW, Fishbein DB: Rabies virus. In: Mandell GL, Doylous RG, Bennett JE (eds): Principles and Practice of Infectious Diseases. 3rd ed. New York, John Wiley & Sons, p 1291, 1990.
33. Maton PN, Pollard JD, Newsom Davis J: Human rabies encephalomyelitis. Br Med J 1:1038, 1976.
34. Anderson LJ, Karl G, Nicholson MB, et al: Human rabies in the United States, 1960 to 1979: Epidemiology, diagnosis, and prevention. Ann Intern Med 100:728, 1984.
35. Bryceson AD, Greenwood BM, Warrell DA, et al: Demonstration during life of rabies antigen in humans. J Infect Dis 131:71, 1975.
36. Centers for Disease Control: Rabies prevention—United States, 1991. Recommendations of the Immunization Practices Advisory Committee (ACIP). MMWR 40:1, 1991.
37. Monath TP: Flaviviruses. In:Fields BN, Knipe DM, Chanock RM, et al (eds): Virology. 2nd ed. New York, Raven Press, p 763, 1990.
38. Brinker KR, Paulson G, Monath T, et al: St Louis encephalitis in Ohio, September 1975. Arch Intern Med 139:561, 1974.
39. Quick DT, Thompson JM, Bond JO: The 1962 epidemic of St. Louis encephalitis in Florida. IV. Clinical features of cases occurring in the Tampa Bay area. Am J Epidemiol 81:415, 1965.
40. Monath TP, Nystrom RR, Bailey RE, et al: Immunoglobulin M antibody capture enzyme-linked immunosorbent assay for diagnosis of St. Louis encephalitis. J Clin Microbiol 20:784, 1984.
41. Johnson RT: Viral Infections of the Nervous System. New York, Raven Press, 1982.
42. Aryes JC, Feemster RF: The sequelae of eastern equine encephalomyelitis. N Engl J Med 240:960, 1949.
43. Feemster RF: Equine encephalitis in Massachusetts. N Engl J Med 257:701, 1957.
44. Calisher CH, el-Kafrawi AO, Al-Deen Mahmud MI, et al: Complex-specific immunoglobulin M antibody patterns in humans infected with alphaviruses. J Clin Microbiol 23:155, 1986.
45. Calisher CH, Berardi VP, Muth DJ, et al: Specificity of immunoglobulin M and G antibody responses in humans infected with eastern and western equine encephalitis viruses: Application to rapid serodiagnosis. J Clin Microbiol 23:369, 1986.
46. Kim JH, Booss J, Manuelidis EE, et al: Human eastern equine encephalitis. Electron microscopic study of a brain biopsy. Am J Clin Pathol 84:223, 1985.

47. Farber S, Connerly ML, Dingle JH: Encephalitis in infants and children. JAMA 114:1725, 1940.
48. Przelomski MM, O'Rourke E, Grady GF, et al: Eastern equine encephalitis in Massachusetts: A report of 16 cases, 1970–1984. Neurology 38:736, 1988.
49. Huggins JW: RNA viruses that cause hemorrhagic, encephalitic, and febrile disease. In: Galasso GJ, Whitley RJ, Merigan TC (eds): Antiviral Agents and Viral Diseases of Man. 3rd ed. New York, Raven Press, p 691, 1990.
50. McGowan JE, Bryan JA, Gregg MB: Surveillance of arboviral encephalitis in the United States, 1955–1971. Am J Epidemiol 97:199, 1973.
51. Finley KH, Fitzgerald LH, Richter RW, et al: Western encephalitis and cerebral ontogenesis. Arch Neurol 16:140, 1967.
52. Earnest MP, Goolishian HA, Calverley JR, et al: Neurologic, intellectual, and psychologic sequelae following western encephalitis. Neurology 21:969, 1971.
53. Peters CJ, Dalrymple JM: Alphaviruses. In: Fields BN, Knipe DM, Chanock RM (eds): Virology. 2nd ed. New York, Raven Press, p 713, 1990.
54. Ho M: Acute viral encephalitis. In: Vinken PJ, Bruyn GW (eds): Handbook of Clinical Neurology, Volume 34, Infections in the Nervous System. New York, North Holland, p 63, 1978.
55. Dickerson RB, Newton JR, Hansen JE: Diagnosis and immediate prognosis of Japanese B encephalitis. Am J Med 12:277, 1952.
56. Rosen L: The natural history of Japanese encephalitis virus. Annu Rev Microbiol 40:395, 1986.
57. Umenai T, Krzysko R, Bektimirov A, et al: Japanese encephalitis: Current worldwide status. Bull WHO 65:625, 1985.
58. Hoke CH, Nisalak A, Sangwhipa N, et al: Protection against Japanese encephalitis by inactivated vaccines. N Engl J Med 319:608, 1988.
59. Burke DS, Nisalak A, Ussery MA, et al: Kinetics of IgM and IgG responses to Japanese encephalitis virus in human serum and cerebrospinal fluid. J Infect Dis 151:1093, 1985.
60. Burke DS, Lorsomrudee W, Leake CJ, et al: Fatal outcome in Japanese encephalitis. Am J Trop Med Hyg 34:1203, 1985.
61. Ehrenkranz NJ, Ventura AK: Venezuelan equine encephalitis in man. Annu Rev Med 25:9, 1974.
62. de la Monte SM, Castro F, Bonella NJ, et al: The systemic pathology of Venezuelan equine encephalitis virus infection in humans. Am J Trop Med Hyg 34:194, 1985.
63. Bowen GS, Fashinell TR, Dean PB, et al: Clinical aspects of human Venezuelan equine encephalitis in Texas. Bull Pan Am Health Organ 10:46, 1976.
64. Porterfield JS: Alphaviruses, flaviviruses and Bunyaviridae. In: Zuckerman AJ, Banatvala JE, Pattison JR (eds): Principles and Practice of Clinical Virology. 2nd ed. New York, John Wiley & Sons, p 435, 1990.
65. Gundersen CB, Brown KL: Clinical aspects of La Crosse encephalitis: Preliminary report. In: Calisher CH, Thompson WH (eds): California Serogroup Viruses. New York, Alan R Liss, p 169, 1983.
66. Gonzalez-Scarano F, Nathanson N: Bunyaviruses. In: Fields BN, Knipe DM, Chanock RM, et al (eds): Virology. 2nd ed. New York, Raven Press, p 1195, 1990.
67. Deering WM: Neurologic aspects and treatment of La Crosse encephalitis. In: Calisher CH, Thompson WH (eds): California Serogroup Viruses. New York, Alan R Liss, p 187, 1983.
68. Chun RWM, Thompson WH, Grabow JD, et al: California arbovirus infection in children. Neurology 18:369, 1968.
69. Jamnback TL, Beaty BJ, Hildreth SW, et al: Capture immunoglobulin M system for rapid diagnosis of La Crosse (California encephalitis) virus infections. J Clin Microbiol 16:577, 1982.
70. Beaty BJ, Jamnback TL, Hildreth SW, et al: Rapid diagnosis of La Crosse virus infections: Evaluation of serologic and antigen detection techniques for the clinically relevant diagnosis of La Crossse encephalitis. In: Calisher CH, Thompson WH (eds): California Serogroup Viruses. New York, Alan R Liss, p 293, 1983.
71. Chun RWM: Clinical aspects of La Crosse encephalitis: Neurological and psychological sequelae. In: Calisher CH, Thompson WH (eds): California Serogroup Viruses. New York, Alan R Liss, p 193, 1983.
72. Sulkava R, Rissanen A, Pyhala R: Post-influenzal encephalitis during the influenza A outbreak in 1979/1980. J Neurol Neurosurg Psychiatry 44:161, 1982.
73. Potter CW: Influenza. In: Zuckerman AJ, Banatvala JE, Pattison JR (eds): Principles and Practice of Clinical Virology. 2nd ed. New York, John Wiley & Sons, p 214, 1990.
74. Schild GC, Pereira MS, Chakraverty P: Single-radial-hemolysis is a new method for the assay of antibody to influenza hemagglutinin. Bull WHO 52:42, 1975.
75. Shaywitz BA, Rothstein P, Venes JL: Monitoring and management of increased intracranial pressure in Reye's syndrome: Results in 29 children. Pediatrics 66:198, 1980.
76. Moore M: Enteroviral diseases in the United States, 1970–1979. J Infect Dis 146:103, 1982.
77. Chunmaitree T, Menegus MA, Powell KR: The clinical relevance of "CSF viral cultures." JAMA 247:1843, 1982.
78. Wolinsky JS, Waxham MN: Mumps virus. In: Fields BN, Knipe DM, Chanock RM (eds): Virology. 2nd ed. New York, Raven Press, p 989, 1990.
79. Gibbs FA, Gibbs EL, Spies HW et al: Common types of childhood encephalitis: Electroencephalographic and clinical relationships. Arch Neurol 10:1, 1964.
80. Bistrian B, Phillips CA, Kaye IS: Fatal mumps meningoencephalitis. JAMA 222:478, 1972.
81. Herndon RM, Johnson RT, Davis LE, et al: Ependymitis in mumps virus meningitis: Electron microscopical studies of cerebrospinal fluid. Arch Neurol 30:475, 1974.
82. Glinkmann G, Pederson M, Mordhorst CH: Detection of specific immunoglobulin M to mumps virus in serum and cerebrospinal fluid samples from patients with acute mumps infection, using an antibody-capture enzyme immunoassay. Acta Pathol Microbiol Immunol Scand 94:145, 1986.
83. Ukkonen P, Vaisanen O, Penttinen K: Enzyme-linked immunosorbent assay for mumps and parainfluenza type 1 immunoglobulin G and immunoglobulin M antibodies. J Clin Microbiol 11:319, 1980.
84. Carter MJ, ter Meulen V: Measles. In: Zuckerman AJ, Banatvala JE, Pattison JR (eds): Principles and Practice of Clinical Virology. 2nd ed. New York, John Wiley & Sons, p 314, 1990.
85. Norrby E: Measles. In: Fields BN, Knipe DM, Chanock RM, et al (eds): Virology. New York, Raven Press, p 1305, 1985.
86. Jones CE, Dyken PR, Huttenlocher PR, et al: Inosiplex therapy in subacute sclerosing panencephalitis. A multicentre, non-randomised study in 98 patients. Lancet 1:1034, 1982.
87. Durant RH, Dyken PR, Swift AV: The influence of inosiplex treatment on the neurological disability of patients with subacute sclerosing panencephalitis. J Pediatr 101:288, 1982.

CHAPTER 61

Hyperpyretic-Rigidity Syndrome (Neuroleptic Malignant Syndrome)

Peter A. LeWitt
Richard C. Berchou

Neuroleptics, known also as "major" tranquilizers, are psychiatric medications capable of producing symptomatic improvement in psychotic states (regardless of their etiology). Drugs of this class are characterized by a wide range of potencies in accomplishing postsynaptic blockade of dopamine receptors (especially the D-2 subtype). In addition to neuroleptic tranquilizers, other medications also in widespread use exert potent inhibition of peripheral and central dopamine D-2 receptors. Among the latter drugs are several antiemetics (including thiethylperazine [Torecan] promethazine [Phenergan], and prochlorperazine [Compazine]) and the gastric motility enhancer metoclopramide (Reglan).

Various untoward effects are known to accompany the use of neuroleptics and related medications. Among their idiosyncratic effects, neuroleptics can cause hypotension, leukopenia, hepatotoxicity, and photosensitivity. Other uncommon but serious side effects include agranulocytosis and sudden cardiovascular collapse. The mechanisms for these problems are incompletely understood. However, the most common adverse effects of the use of dopamine-blocking medications are the direct result of their pharmacologic effects as potent ligands for dopamine D-2 receptors. These drugs often have extrapyramidal effects on the motor system that resemble features of several types of idiopathic movement disorders. Among the outcomes that can be produced are parkinsonism (slowed movement, rigidity of skeletal muscle, resting tremor, and forward flexed posture), dystonia (sustained abnormal muscle contractions and postures, sometimes with a writhing quality), and akathisia (an irresistible urge to remain in movement, manifested as restlessness or pacing). The severity of these movement disorder syndromes is generally related to the dose and potency of the particular neuroleptic medication used. Usually, these movement disorders remit after discontinuation of the causative drugs; they can also respond to the use of antiparkinsonian medications. When administration of a neuroleptic medication results in an acute dystonic reaction (manifesting as a sudden rigid state or an oculogyric "crisis"), injection of an anticholinergic or dopaminergic drug almost always results in prompt relief. Another class of adverse reactions can develop in some individuals as a result of sustained use of dopamine-blocking medication. Once they have evolved, these movement disorders (termed tardive dyskinesia and tardive dystonia) can persist for months or longer.

The topic of this chapter is another rare but serious consequence of dopamine-blocking medication. In this chapter it is designated as the *hyperpyretic-rigidity syndrome* (HRS), although the disorder is most commonly termed the *neuroleptic malignant syndrome*. Neuroleptic malignant syndrome is a misnomer because conditions other than neuroleptic use can cause the same syndrome. Furthermore, the syndrome can have a self-limited course even without the institution of therapy, and with the institution of proper treatment its prognosis is far less "malignant" than it was once thought to be. As an alternative terminology, HRS stresses the appropriate targets for diagnosis and therapy of this syndrome.

HRS can follow a variety of clinical courses, but it usually involves a combination of altered consciousness, abnormal activation of the motor system, and disturbances of autonomic function. The following core features characterize HRS:

1. Encephalopathy, ranging from confusion or agitation to coma, with fluctuating levels of consciousness
2. Potentially fatal elevations of body temperature
3. Blood pressure lability and other elements of autonomic dysregulation (e.g., tachycardia, diaphoresis, pallor)
4. Severe muscle rigidity, sometimes in association with extrapyramidal-type involuntary movements

HRS can result from relatively brief periods of drug exposure or can emerge during more chronic regimens. The various problems can develop whether the inciting therapeutics have been used in high or in conventional dose ranges. Although most cases of HRS have resulted from the use of neuroleptics in psychiatric indications, other pharmacologic manipulations that alter dopaminergic neurotransmission initiate the same clinical syndrome. In just a few hours HRS can evolve from mild, barely recognizable features to a life-threatening state. When it was first described three decades ago, it appeared that this disorder, if untreated, could have a mortality in excess of 20%. Today, even when intensive life-support measures are employed after early detection, HRS is still associated with significant morbidity. Optimal management can, in many instances, result in reversal of much of its symptoms within hours. One of the most important factors in achieving control of this potentially lethal disorder is anticipation of its often unpredictable course. With strong suspicion of HRS, prompt initiation of treatment can be achieved, a critical requirement for averting disastrous outcomes.

CLINICAL FEATURES AND DIAGNOSIS OF HYPERPYRETIC-RIGIDITY SYNDROME

As a syndrome, HRS can appear in a number of guises. The full expression of the classic syndrome—fever, encephalopathy, autonomic abnormalities, elevated creatine kinase (CK) level, and muscle rigidity—may be delayed until a relatively late stage. HRS typically develops during the course of 1 to 3 days in one of several distinct patterns. The earliest features can be autonomic disturbances, such as tachycardia or diaphoresis. In most instances, the early features also come to involve some degree of limb and axial rigidity, slowness of movement (bradykinesia), involuntary movements (dyskinesias), or sustained abnormal postures (dystonia). In some instances, abnormalities of gaze and dysphagia accompany the other motor abnormalities. The rigidity of skeletal muscle can be so severe as to produce extreme pain, seemingly fixed contractures, or stretch injury damage to muscle. Severe tremors or other types of involuntary movement can also contribute to damage to skeletal muscle. At some point, the injury to muscle results in rhabdomyolysis, as recognized by major elevations of the levels of serum CK and other muscle-derived enzymes and myoglobinuria. With sufficiently severe muscle damage, the released muscle protein can produce acute renal failure from damage to the kidneys.

Another common presentation is with mental changes. Prominent alteration of mental status with confusion, agitation, listlessness, or catatonic behaviors (posturing, mute states, and so on[1]) may herald the start of HRS for some patients.[2] Some investigators are of the opinion that some alteration of the mental status almost always accompanies the earliest stages of HRS.[3] Other subjects ultimately found to have HRS present with unexplained fever and nothing else for days. Although elevated body temperature in HRS is most often associated with activation of the motor system in ways that can obviously generate heat, by involuntary movements, agitation, or muscle rigidity, the rise and fall of temperature can also be independent of muscular activity.

Once HRS develops, the related problems commonly mingle into a deteriorating state presenting a number of medical management problems. The onset of fever is an ominous feature of HRS because it can rapidly rise to a range that produces organ and muscle damage. Other types of autonomic dysfunction that can evolve include urine retention, incontinence, rapid respirations, and labile blood pressure. The pulse and blood pressure disturbances can progress to cardiopulmonary failure and shock. Pulmonary congestion has been described with HRS,[4, 5] as has disseminated intravascular coagulation. Even though there appears to be a major central component of the high temperature, the excessive contraction of muscle with rigidity or involuntary movements also contributes to heat production. The reduction in level of consciousness can result from more than fever, because patients with HRS have become encephalopathic even with only relatively minor manifestations of fever. In general, the earliest signs of HRS do not necessarily provide clues to the ultimate severity that will evolve.

Sometimes, clues to HRS are recognized only in retrospect, such as lability of vital signs. HRS can be difficult to recognize in patients who have other medical problems or when it is present only in fragmentary forms. Many neuroleptic-treated patients develop features of parkinsonism, dystonia, or dyskinesia[6] some time in the course of therapy. These features do not necessarily progress to HRS, so instituting treatment for HRS is not appropriate unless additional aspects of the syndrome develop. Prolonged and otherwise unexplained fever with neuroleptic therapy has been reported to occur without rigidity, encephalopathy, or other serious outcomes.[7, 8] Such occurrences raise the possibility that HRS can exist in formes frustes. Although abortive forms of HRS may occur, it is important to regard HRS as an unpredictable syndrome that can rapidly evolve into multiple organ system failure from relatively mild beginnings. Spontaneous recovery of untreated HRS has been described,[2] but high mortality is associated with failure to institute supportive and medical treatment early.

Because HRS can be described in a variety of ways, it is not surprising that many of the definitions and diagnostic criteria proposed by researchers and experienced clinicians differ greatly.[9–15] Some reports have emphasized the concept that HRS represents a spectrum of disorders.[16–18] Other studies have asserted that virtually all cases represent the same disorder.[19, 20] In general, diagnostic definitions that are based on the extent of temperature or serum CK elevation may not be helpful for the goal of recognizing the disorder at its earliest stages.

There is no laboratory study that establishes the diagnosis of HRS. In association with fever, the white blood cell count can be greatly elevated with a shift to the left and can be indistinguishable from that in leukocytosis resulting from infection. Dehydration with HRS is common, resulting in hypernatremia and hyperviscosity of the blood. One of the most common laboratory abnormalities of HRS is the elevation of muscle- and liver-derived enzymes (CK, aldolase, lactate dehydrogenase, alkaline phosphatase, and transaminases) along with myoglobinuria. The elevation of skeletal muscle CK can range from several hundred to more than 10,000 IU/L.[21] Although many patients have an extremely elevated CK level, this laboratory indication of muscle injury is not a requirement for the diagnosis of HRS, especially in its earliest stages. When moderate CK elevations are present, other sources of injury to muscle such as bruises or intramuscular injections should be considered as alternative explanations. Renal impairment is an ominous finding in a patient with HRS, because renal damage can be severe. During episodes of HRS, serum glucose levels can be greatly elevated. Additional laboratory studies can reflect the development of other systemic outcomes, such as metabolic acidosis, the syndrome of inappropriate antidiuretic hormone secretion, pancreatic necrosis, and disseminated intravascular coagulopathy. Apart from indicators of renal failure or myoglobinuria, urinalysis is generally nonrevealing in HRS. Cerebrospinal fluid does not display pleocytosis or other changes.

DIFFERENTIATION OF HYPERPYRETIC-RIGIDITY SYNDROME FROM OTHER DISORDERS

Psychiatric patients constitute the majority of subjects who experience HRS. Such patients may, because of their often psychotic state, present problems for the detection and proper management of HRS. With the occurrence of fever and other features of HRS, the following considerations should enter into the differential diagnosis of HRS.

Fever and Encephalopathy

Fever and an apparent encephalopathy can develop separately or together for reasons other than HRS. With neuroleptic medication use, mild elevations of temperature can occur without activating the full spectrum of other HRS features. These effects are not necessarily related to the mechanism that initiates HRS. Other consequences of use of these drugs include impaired dissipation of body heat, especially if there is agitation causing increased body movements, and decreased water intake. Some of the dopamine-blocking tranquilizers also have prominent anticholinergic

properties and can impair sweating (as can the concomitant use of anticholinergic medications to relieve neuroleptic-induced parkinsonism). Tumors affecting the hypothalamic region can produce changes in body temperature along with other autonomic changes. Patients who have fever with changes in mental status should be evaluated for bacterial, viral, fungal, or parasitic encephalitis and postinfectious encephalopathy.

Heatstroke

Body temperature elevations to the extent encountered in HRS are also found with heatstroke (circulatory collapse resulting from elevated body temperature). This condition can be distinguished from HRS by the absence of rigidity and diaphoresis and by the presence of cutaneous vasodilation.[22] In addition, patients with heatstroke do not have involuntary movements. Although some of the systemic consequences of heatstroke are similar to those of HRS, pharmacologic measures directed against muscle rigidity or central dopaminergic neurotransmission have not been shown to aid in the treatment of heatstroke.[23] Heatstroke is unlikely to be caused by neuroleptic drugs unless the regimen also includes anticholinergic agents that inhibit heat exchange by evaporation of perspiration.[24]

Catatonia

An important alternative diagnosis to HRS is catatonia. Catatonia, a relatively rare schizophreniform disorder, is of unknown pathogenesis. In its most severe manifestation, that of so-called lethal catatonia, a severe rigid state with high fever is associated with virtually the same morbidity and mortality as HRS. Severe catatonic reactions were known to occur before the neuroleptic era. Typical features of catatonia include stereotyped mannerisms, negativistic behaviors, a regressed psychotic state, and involuntary posture maintenance. Patients with lethal catatonia also exhibit many of the features found in HRS: rigidity, fever, and impaired level of consciousness (sometimes with a wakeful but mute state). In the opinion of some observers, lethal catatonia may be a naturally occurring version of HRS.

Differentiation of catatonia from HRS can be challenging. Usually, in catatonia, but not in HRS, there is a prelude of extreme psychotic excitement. Deterioration of the psychiatric state for the preceding 2 weeks can be an important diagnostic clue to catatonia. Sometimes, differentiation can be aided by use of an intravenous benzodiazepine challenge (which reverses catatonic features in some instances),[25] but in general the two disorders are difficult to distinguish.[26, 27] As described later, some patients with HRS also respond to benzodiazepine therapy alone.

Malignant Hyperthermia

The fever of malignant hyperthermia (MH) can resemble the severe elevations of temperature in HRS. MH is a genetically determined (usually autosomal dominant) propensity for skeletal muscle to enter into a hypermetabolic state that can produce fever, hypertonicity, and elevated CK levels, along with other systemic consequences. The generation of fever appears to be entirely peripheral, in contrast to that in HRS. Differentiation of these two disorders should not be difficult because MH is always initiated rapidly after the use of anesthetic medications (succinylcholine, local anesthetics, or halogenated inhalation agents such as halothane). The lack of autonomic and encephalopathic disturbances helps to differentiate the clinical manifestations of the disorders. Whereas one of the most effective medications for HRS, dantrolene, can also lessen muscle hypercontraction in MH, rapid relaxation of muscle by the use of curariform drugs is effective only in HRS.[10]

Most authors have thought that the genetic trait for MH does not confer any risk for the occurrence of HRS. In fact, anesthesia using neuroleptic medication has been successfully applied to persons with a familial risk for MH.[28] The in vitro halothane and caffeine contracture tests with skeletal muscle biopsy specimens are the most reliable methods for identifying susceptibility to MH. When these diagnostic methods were applied to specimens from subjects who had experienced HRS, they were found not be to susceptible,[29] although in another study using similar methods some muscle findings in HRS patients were compatible with abnormalities of MH.[30] Other studies have also suggested similarities between the two disorders.[31]

Central Nervous System Infections

Fever caused by central nervous system infections, such as viral encephalitis or human immunodeficiency virus encephalopathy,[32, 33] can appear abruptly. The neurologic picture can resemble that in HRS in other ways, including agitation and involuntary movements. Such conditions can be overlooked if a febrile patient otherwise fits the diagnostic profile of HRS. Other diagnostic considerations for patients with febrile states and encephalopathy include sepsis, localized infections, vasculitis, and drug allergy. For example, a patient with HRS was initially misdiagnosed as having an "acute abdomen" resulting from intestinal obstruction and septicemia.[34] Concomitant use of neuroleptic medications in the presence of infectious disease may produce ambiguous situations in which HRS should be suspected. In such situations, it may be prudent to initiate treatment appropriate for HRS while awaiting further diagnostic results that can establish whether an infectious cause for fever exists. There is some suspicion[35] that fever produced by an infection might, in some instances, trigger the emergence of HRS.

Other Drug-Induced Syndromes of Hyperpyretic-Rigidity Syndrome or Similar Disorders

Withdrawal of antiparkinsonian medications has been found to initiate a syndrome virtually identical with HRS. Abrupt discontinuation of levodopa in the context of a "drug holiday" has produced hyperthermia and other features of HRS.[36-38] Even the abrupt decline in dopaminergic effect characterizing the wearing off of antiparkinsonian effect has been reported to initiate a lethal outcome with hyperthermia and other impairments.[39] Effective treatment of HRS with dopaminergic therapy supports the idea that HRS is mediated through this neurotransmitter system. During treatment of HRS, discontinuation of amantadine therapy has also been described to result in relapse of HRS.[40] Other studies have cited discontinuation of amantadine as a precipitant of HRS.[41, 42] Cessation of antiparkinsonian medications in the context of lithium and haloperidol treatment[43] or combined use of the monoamine oxidase inhibitor tranylcypromine and L-tryptophan[44] has been associated with initiation of HRS. Burke and colleagues[45] described a case of an HRS-like syndrome developing after combined use of the dopamine depletor tetrabenazine with the dopamine synthesis inhibitor α-methyl-*p*-tyrosine. In other instances, lithium has been implicated as a precipitant of HRS.[46, 47] Among its several neuropharmacologic effects, lithium alters dopamine receptor responsiveness and so may be a factor in triggering HRS.

Several other drug interactions have been described in which febrile states and other encephalopathic features have followed the use of certain psychotropic drugs. With the combination of tricyclic antidepressants (e.g., amitriptyline and imipramine) and monoamine oxidase inhibitors (e.g., tranylcypromine, phenelzine, and isocarboxazid), features similar to those of HRS have developed suddenly.[48, 49] Such conditions could be the result of altered dopaminergic neurotransmission, but an alternative view is that enhanced serotoninergic neurotransmission may have been involved.[44] A potentially fatal syndrome resembling HRS but caused by serotoninergic toxicity (combination of a monoamine oxidase inhibitor with L-tryptophan) has been described.[50] In such instances, rigidity, myoclonic jerks, encephalopathy, agitation, hyperthermia, and convulsions have occurred in a fulminant fashion.[51] Another pharmacologic interaction with features resembling those of HRS results from the combined use of monoamine oxidase inhibitors and meperidine. Dothiepin, an antidepressant, has also been associated with HRS,[52] as has been the use of the antidepressant doxepin in combination with lithium.[53] Discontinuation of the benzodiazepine alprazolam during concomitant amoxopine treatment has been reported to initiate HRS.[54] Fluoxetine taken in combination with selegiline has been reported to cause a manic state, prominent sweating, vasomotor disturbances, and other reactions resembling the early stages of HRS.[55]

The variety of pharmacologic scenarios that have been reported to precede HRS and similar syndromes is such that there are undoubtedly other causes yet to be encountered.

In Table 61-1, these and other diagnostic features are summarized.

INCIDENCE OF HYPERPYRETIC-RIGIDITY SYNDROME

The risk of developing HRS is not easy to define, because it is an idiosyncratic event that sometimes fails to be recognized in the population of psychiatric and medical patients. Susceptibility to HRS is present at all ages.[11, 56] Each of the chemical classes of dopamine-blocking drugs, regardless of their route of administration, has been known to initiate HRS. The one exception seems to be the antiemetic and gastric motility enhancer domperidone (Motilium), a potent systemically acting dopamine blocker that is restricted from crossing the blood-brain barrier. Metoclopramide (Reglan), which resembles domperidone in its peripheral dopamine-blocking actions, enters the central nervous system and so, not surprisingly, can initiate HRS.[57] In several surveys, more than half of HRS cases were associated with the use of haloperidol (Haldol). It seems that, because haloperidol is the most widely used drug for rapid treatment of psychotic or behavioral disturbance, HRS is most likely to emerge with use of this drug. In a review of 115 cases of HRS, haloperidol was associated with 57%, chlorpromazine (Thorazine) with 24%, and fluphenazine (Prolixin) with 16%.[58] Fluphenazine is, like haloperidol, a high-potency neuroleptic, and it is often given in a depot form whose effects last several weeks. Because prompt discontinuation of neuroleptic therapy is an important part of HRS management, use of depot fluphenazine carries special risks for patients who develop HRS.[59]

HRS can occur with all routes of medication administration. It has resulted from use of dopamine-blocking medications in the context of surgery (droperidol intraoperatively and metoclopramide as an antiemetic later).[60] Simultaneous use of several neuroleptic medications does not, in general, appear to be a risk factor, nor does combination of neuroleptics with anticholinergic drugs. However, as mentioned earlier, treatment regimens combining lithium with neuroleptic medications may increase the risk for HRS and a resultant encephalopathy.

TABLE 61–1

DIAGNOSTIC FEATURES OF HYPERPYRETIC-RIGIDITY SYNDROME AND DISORDERS RESEMBLING IT

Feature	Hyperpyretic-Rigidity Syndrome	Malignant Hyperthermia	Viral Encephalitis	Human Immunodeficiency Virus Encephalopathy	Heatstroke
Hyperpyrexia	+	+	+	±	+
Diaphoresis	+	+	−	±	−
Autonomic dysfunction	+	−	−	−	+
Altered consciousness	+	+	+	+	+
Progression during 24–72 h	+	−	±	±	±
Elevated CK level	+	+	−	−	−
Leukocytosis	+	−	−	−	+
Rigidity	+	+	−	−	−
Tremor	±	−	−	±	−
Myoclonus	−	−	±	−	−
Ataxia	−	−	−	−	±

HRS can develop at any time in relation to the start of neuroleptic medication, even during its abrupt reduction.[61] It can emerge during chronic therapy, but most cases follow the start of medication or change of medication dosage. Onset that follows the start of neuroleptic therapy has been described to occur as soon as 45 minutes or as long as 65 days later.[13] Most patients experience development of HRS in the first 10 days after start of neuroleptic medication. A common situation preceding the onset of HRS has been the change from one neuroleptic to another or a significant increase of dose.[62] The rate of loading of medication may be a significant factor in HRS causation.[63]

A 100-fold difference in incidence has been described, largely because of the different populations studied.[64] However, some studies give perspective on the frequency of occurrence of HRS in neuroleptic-treated patients. A 2-year retrospective assessment of patients in a state psychiatric hospital indicated an HRS incidence of 0.9%.[65] Other assessments found its incidence to be 0.5%[66] or less[67] of all neuroleptic treatment episodes. A population survey of neuroleptic-treated psychotic patients in China revealed an annual HRS incidence of 1.23 per 1000 treated patients.[59] The real incidence may be under-reported and under-recognized because the features of HRS can easily be attributed to the coincidence of a parkinsonian state and fever, for which discontinuation of medication may produce remission. If HRS occurs with brief or relatively mild manifestations, its occurrence may be missed and therefore its incidence underestimated.

Most surveys have shown that HRS affects approximately twice as many males as females.[13, 68] In one series, the mean age of incidence was 40 years. In 44% of cases there was a primary diagnosis of schizophrenia, and 26% had bipolar affective disorder in manic phase.[58] In a study of HRS in an Indian population, the syndrome developed earlier in the course of neuroleptic therapy and took longer to resolve in patients diagnosed with schizophrenia rather than other psychiatric disorders.[2] A case-control study matching HRS patients with neuroleptic-treated control patients has been carried out to assess potential risk factors. Those with HRS tended to exhibit more psychomotor agitation. In addition, they received significantly larger doses of neuroleptics and increased rates of advance in dosage. Compared with the controls, subjects developing HRS also had received neuroleptics more often by the intramuscular route.[66]

Initial reports of HRS stressed that subjects with pre-existing central nervous system damage were at greater risk of developing HRS.[4] Later evaluations have confirmed these observations,[69] although it should be considered that this group is also more likely to receive high-dose neuroleptics for behavior control. For example, patients have developed HRS after treatment for agitation caused by closed head injury.[70] Other predisposing factors include pre-existing physical exhaustion and dehydration. One report has suggested that a high exogenous heat load (or elevated body temperature, for whatever reason) may have a role in initiating the development of HRS.[35] However, another disorder in which there are severe increases of body temperature, MH, does not appear to confer a risk for HRS.[71] Other medical conditions that have been associated with the occurrence of HRS are idiopathic hypoparathyroidism,[72] hypothyroidism,[73] Wilson's disease,[74] acquired immunodeficiency syndrome,[32, 75] and Alzheimer's disease.[76]

Risk of death resulting from HRS depends largely on the extent of organ system damage and severity of cardiovascular disturbances during the acute syndrome. During the past decade, the mortality of patients with HRS has decreased by more than half, probably reflecting better recognition and treatment options. Those who die of HRS have an increased incidence (38.5%) of development of organic brain syndrome.[71] Also, the presence of myoglobinuria and renal failure adds significantly to the mortality.

TREATMENT OF HYPERPYRETIC-RIGIDITY SYNDROME

Prompt recognition of HRS and initiation of intensive management, which requires control of several homeostatic disturbances, can significantly reduce mortality and morbidity. Of primary importance is discontinuation (not tapering) of the dopamine receptor antagonist. Although many of the psychotropic and HRS-promoting effects of neuroleptic medications disappear within a few days, some patients must be monitored closely for weeks because of persistent effects from long-acting or depot neuroleptics. A dramatic improvement in patients with HRS can result from immediate withdrawal of the causative medication (or, in the case of HRS initiated by discontinuation of antiparkinsonian drugs, reinstitution of dopaminergic therapy).

With HRS, there should be close monitoring for changes in blood pressure, temperature, or urine output. Myoglobinuria and elevation of the serum CK level should be tested for sequentially. Several types of supportive care should be directed at the extreme and erratic rise in body heat production. Rapid heat reduction can be achieved with measures such as cooling blankets, ice water enemas, antipyretics, and intravenous fluids. Physical measures for reducing body temperature may be insufficient without institution of pharmacotherapy to restore central dopaminergic neurotransmission and alleviate muscle rigidity. Even with only the suspicion of HRS, treatment with cooling and appropriate medications should be initiated promptly. Supportive care should include adequate hydration for possible increased fluid loss and for the renal consequences of rhabdomyolysis.

Other complications that can accompany severe cases of HRS include respiratory distress, arrhythmias, seizures, infection, disseminated intravascular coagulation, and acid-base abnormalities. Although some investigators have thought that monitoring of serum CK offers a guide to the relative severity of HRS,[75, 76] anticipation of worsening HRS may require therapy to be initiated despite no or minimal elevations. HRS is an appropriate indication for admission to an intensive therapy unit for monitoring and institution of immediate care measures.[77–79]

Because of the idiosyncratic and infrequent occurrence of HRS, there has been little opportunity for controlled clinical studies to assess optimal strategies for treatment. There is a growing body of evidence, however, that supports the value of restoring dopaminergic neurotransmission with a centrally acting agent. In addition, there is a major role for lessening rigidity by use of agents that act directly on skeletal muscle. Although no therapy has been proved to be uniformly successful, it appears that combination of these two treatments has the best chance of reversing the peripheral and central mechanisms of HRS pathophysiology.[47] Spontaneous recovery from HRS without the use of drugs has been described.[2] However, with cooling measures alone recovery takes much longer than when medications are also used.[80, 81] The following treatments have been shown to be effective for HRS.

Bromocriptine (Parlodel). High-potency stimulation of dopamine D-2 receptors can be achieved with bromocriptine, an ergot derivative ordinarily used for treatment of parkinsonism (in doses ranging from 7.5 to 100 mg/d). Bromocriptine has been shown to be effective in HRS, presumably by restoring impaired dopaminergic neurotransmission.[78, 82, 83] In several reports, a dose of 5 mg three times a day was started and increased, if tolerated, by 5 mg/d until a positive response was found. For adequate control of HRS, doses of 7.5 to 60 mg/d typically have been required.[84] Addonizio[58] reported that benefits occur in 87 to 100% of patients who receive bromocriptine, although the effect may be less than complete reversal of HRS.[85] In many instances, clinical improvement develops within hours after starting bromocriptine,[86, 87] which can be administered only in an oral form. Another dopaminergic compound, pergolide (Permax), is available in the United States. Pergolide is so similar to bromocriptine that it should accomplish the same outcome, although it has not been formally studied for this purpose. Another dopaminergic ergot derivative, lisuride, has proved effective for treatment of HRS.[88] Lisuride has the practical advantage that it can be administered parenterally.

When an adequate dose has been found, bromocriptine therapy should be continued for 10 days, after which it can be gradually withdrawn. If a depot form of neuroleptic medication has been used, a longer course of bromocriptine is advisable. Recurrence of fever or rigidity during bromocriptine therapy or its withdrawal is grounds for an immediate increase of dosage.[78] HRS and psychosis have been treated with bromocriptine and thioridazine simultaneously, with good control of both problems.[89]

Other Antiparkinsonian Drugs (Amantadine, Anticholin-
ergics, and Levodopa). Medications effective for the symptomatic reversal of parkinsonian features have also been used for treating HRS. Although amantadine and anticholinergic drugs exert less dopaminergic effect than bromocriptine or levodopa, each of these drugs can be effective against HRS. As mentioned earlier, abrupt discontinuation of either amantadine or levodopa has been associated with initiation of HRS.

Amantadine, whose dopaminergic effects appear to involve enhanced release of presynaptic dopamine, has been found to be effective by several investigators.[1, 90–92] In one report, a patient whose HRS did not respond to bromocriptine or levodopa treatment showed improvement with use of amantadine.[56] Anticholinergic drugs, such as trihexyphenidyl (Artane), can reverse parkinsonian rigidity as well as acute dystonic reactions to neuroleptic drugs. When these drugs were used for HRS there were some positive responses,[93, 94] but most clinical experience has been unconvincing about their benefit.[95] Prior use of anticholinergic drugs does not appear to influence the occurrence or outcome of HRS.[67] In one report, a patient who developed both HRS and deep coma rapidly recovered consciousness after injection of an anticholinergic, suggesting that cholinergic hyperactivity might have been responsible for altered consciousness in HRS.[96] Most authorities do not recommend the use of anticholinergics for treating HRS, especially because their actions can also impair consciousness, heat exchange, and other autonomic functions.

Levodopa (the active agent in Sinemet) is the precursor of dopamine, which, unlike dopamine, can cross the blood-brain barrier. It has been reported to reverse HRS in some[97, 98] but not all instances.[99] Like the dopaminergic ergots, levodopa is available only in oral form, although it is somewhat water soluble and can be prepared for intravenous injection.

Dantrolene (Dantrium). Dantrolene, a muscle relaxant generally used for relief of spasticity, is highly effective for the treatment of HRS, sometimes in combination with bromocriptine.[100–102] Dantrolene acts directly on skeletal muscle to produce relaxation by facilitating calcium reabsorption from myoplasm into the sarcoplasmic reticulum. By alleviating the extreme state of muscle contraction in HRS, it can lessen damage to muscle and excessive heat production. Dantrolene is not known to act centrally and so is not known to be beneficial for the autonomic or other CNS effects of HRS. However, cases have been described in which the use of dantrolene monotherapy has been associated with recovery from HRS.[103]

Intravenous therapy with dantrolene can be started at the dose of 0.25 mg/kg twice a day. This dose may be increased to 3 mg/kg four times a day as needed to control rigidity. Normalization or reduction of temperature can be expected in 12 hours or less. When the patient is able to tolerate oral medication, bromocriptine therapy should be initiated. Intravenous dantrolene can be changed to the oral route as symptomatic remission occurs. Oral doses of 25 to 600 mg/d have been used to achieve control of HRS.[104] Dantrolene may be hepatotoxic with continuous use of the drug at greater than 10 mg/kg/d.[105]

Other Treatments of Less Proven Value. Considering the variability of clinical expression and responsiveness to established medication of HRS, it is no wonder that investigation of additional treatments has been done cautiously. As described earlier, even within one class of drugs (those with dopaminergic properties), one can fail to be effective even though another can give benefit.[56] Trials of naloxone, corticosteroids, and curare have not led to symptomatic or definitive relief of HRS. Other treatments have, in some instances, been claimed to be helpful. Individual case reports of benefit from medications outside the classes we have discussed are not necessarily informative, because spontaneous recovery can occur with discontinuation of dopamine-blocking medication. Hence, reports of HRS responsive to diphenhydramine,[106] diazepam,[74, 107] or propanolol[97] should not be used as guides to management of patients.

There are good rationales for using other treatments as supplements to more established therapies. Pridinolum mesylate, a peripherally acting muscle relaxant, was claimed to be useful.[108] Pancuronium, a curariform agent, has also been used successfully to treat HRS.[109] Sodium nitroprusside was used for treatment of HRS in one case and seemingly led to a successful outcome, which was attributed to the drug's enhancing peripheral vasodilation and thereby increasing heat exchange.[110] Administration of lorazepam intravenously seemed to be effective in reversing neuroleptic-induced catatonic reactions,[25] but any role in treating other aspects of HRS was not explored.

Electroconvulsive therapy has been used in a number of HRS cases.[111–113] Experience with electroconvulsive therapy has been limited and in theory it might pose its own hazards in the context of established HRS;[12] excellent outcomes have been reported.

REINSTITUTION OF NEUROLEPTIC THERAPY

One of the dilemmas associated with HRS is that patients who have experienced an episode often have a continuing need for treatment with neuroleptic medication.[114] The risk of recurrence of HRS is difficult to determine. This disorder appears to be idiosyncratic, occurring in some individuals after weeks to years of continued neuroleptic therapy. Certainly, HRS can occur again in the same individual with reinstitution of neuroleptic medications.[85] One study indicated that neuroleptic rechallenge resulted in recurrence of HRS in approximately one third of cases.[104] However, in a number of reported instances, patients have returned to neuroleptic regimens without problem.[11, 47] The difficulty in assessing the risk of recurrence is that the nature of susceptibility to HRS is not well understood. Early diagnosis and effective treatment have reduced the risk of rechallenges with neuroleptics. Two factors appeared to be associated with repeated occurrence of HRS: bipolar affective disorder and reinstitution of neuroleptic therapy while elements of HRS persist.[115] Obviously, patients who have experienced HRS are candidates for exploring alternative medication regimens or, if dopamine-blocking drugs are needed, for close monitoring of possible premonitory HRS features.

Avoidance of high-potency neuroleptics seems to be an appropriate strategy. However, a study of 20 neuroleptic rechallenges after HRS indicated that the choice of a neuroleptic lower in potency and dosage than that which precipitated the original HRS episode was not significantly related to successful outcome.[116] Use of lithium alone has been described to cause a recurrence of HRS features,[116] so this drug probably should be avoided, if possible. Because they are less potent than other neuroleptics, rechallenge with thioridazine[117] or molindone[118] has been proposed for patients who need continuing therapy with major tranquilizers. Although it has been used successfully after HRS, molindone has been linked to causation of HRS.[66] Care should be taken not to discontinue antiparkinsonian therapy given concomitantly with neuroleptic medications, because relapse of HRS has been described with the discontinuation of amantadine.[40]

The risk of recurrence of HRS might be lessened through use of an alternative neuroleptic medication, clozapine (Clozaril). Clozapine, a highly effective antipsychotic agent, has been regarded as an atypical neuroleptic because it does not produce parkinsonian side effects or, with chronic use, tardive dyskinesia. Because clozapine's actions are qualitatively different from those of other antipsychotic drugs, some investigators have considered it a candidate for reducing the risk of HRS recurrence. However, clozapine does act via blockade of dopamine receptors. A single case of HRS has been associated with its use.[15] Further experience is needed to determine whether clozapine is less likely to reinitiate HRS than other available agents.

References

1. Gelenberg AJ, Mandel NR: Catatonic reactions to high-potency neuroleptic drugs. Arch Gen Psychiatry 34:947, 1977.
2. Srinivasan AV, Murugappan M, Krishnamurthy SG, et al: Neuroleptic malignant syndrome. J Neurol Neurosurg Psychiatry 53:514, 1990.
3. Velamoor VR, Fernando ML, Williamson P: Incipient neuroleptic malignant syndrome? Br J Psychiatry 156:581, 1990.
4. Delay J, Deniker P: Drug-induced extrapyramidal syndromes. In: Vinken PJ, Bruyn GW (eds): Handbook of Clinical Neurology, Volume 6. New York, Elsevier/North Holland, p 248, 1968.
5. Levinson DF, Simpson GM: Neuroleptic-induced extrapyramidal symptoms with fever. Heterogeneity of the "neuroleptic malignant syndrome." Arch Gen Psychiatry 43:839, 1986.
6. Haggerty JJ, Gillette GM: Neuroleptic malignant syndrome superimposed upon tardive dyskinesia. Br J Psychiatry 150:104, 1986.
7. Keshavan MS, Kambhampati RK: Prolonged fever without extrapyramidal symptoms during neuroleptic treatment. J Clin Psychopharmacol 9:230, 1989.
8. Bamrah JS: Neuroleptic-induced pyrexia: A benign variant. J Nerv Ment Dis 176:741, 1988.
9. Caroff SN: The neuroleptic malignant syndrome. J Clin Psychiatry 41:79, 1980.
10. Guze BH, Baxter LR: Neuroleptic malignant syndrome. N Engl J Med 313:163, 1985.
11. Levenson JL: Neuroleptic malignant syndrome. Am J Psychiatry 142:1137, 1985.
12. Shalev A, Munitz H: The neuroleptic malignant syndrome: Agent and host interaction. Acta Psychiatr Scand 73:337, 1986.
13. Addonizio G, Susman VL, Roth SD: Neuroleptic malignant syndrome: Review and analysis of 115 cases. Biol Psychiatry 22:1004, 1987.
14. Pope HG, Keck PE, McElroy SL: Frequency and presentation of neuroleptic malignant syndrome in a large psychiatric hospital. Am J Psychiatry 143:1223, 1986.
15. Smego RA, Durack DT: The neuroleptic malignant syndrome. Arch Intern Med 142:1183, 1982.
16. Adityanjee, Singh S, Singh G, et al: Spectrum concept of neuroleptic malignant syndrome. Br J Psychiatry 153:107, 1988.
17. Walker WD: Spectrum concept of neuroleptic malignant syndrome. Br J Psychiatry 153:574, 1988.
18. Levinson DF, Simpson G: Sequelae of neuroleptic malignant syndrome. Biol Psychiatry 22:237, 1987.
19. Shalev A, Hermesh H, Alzenberg D: Neuroleptic malignant syndrome. N Engl J Med 313:1292, 1985.
20. Smego RA, Durack DT: The neuroleptic malignant syndrome. Arch Intern Med 142:1183, 1982.
21. James S: CPK levels and neuroleptic malignant syndrome. Br J Psychiatry 155:567, 1989.
22. Lazarus A: Differentiating neuroleptic-related heatstroke from neuroleptic malignant syndrome. Psychosomatics 30:454, 1989.
23. Vassallo SU, Delaney KA: Pharmacologic effects on thermoregulation: Mechanisms of drug-related heatstroke. Clin Toxicol 27:199, 1989.
24. Lazarus A: Differentiating neuroleptic-related heatstroke from neuroleptic malignant syndrome. Psychosomatics 30:454, 1989.
25. Fricchione GL, Cassem NH, Hooberman D, et al: Intravenous lorazepam in neuroleptic-induced catatonia. J Clin Psychopharmacol 3:338, 1983.
26. Brown CS, Wittkowsky AK, Bryant SG: Neuroleptic-induced catatonia after abrupt withdrawal of amantadine during neuroleptic therapy. Pharmacotherapy 6:193, 1986.
27. Castillo E, Rubin RT, Holsboer-Trachsler E: The neuroleptic malignant syndrome and its differentiation from lethal catatonia. Am J Psychiatry 146:324, 1989.
28. Lofstra F, Linkowski P, Mendlewicz J: General anesthesia after neuroleptic malignant syndrome. Biol Psychiatry 18:243, 1983.
29. Adnet PJ, Krivosic-Horber RM, Adamantidis MM, et al: The association between the neuroleptic malignant syndrome and malignant hyperthermia. Acta Anaesthesiol Scand 33:676, 1989.
30. Araki M, Takagi A, Higuchi I, et al: Neuroleptic malignant syndrome: Caffeine contracture of single muscle fibers and muscle pathology. Neurology 38:297, 1988.
31. Tollefson G: A case of neuroleptic malignant syndrome: In vitro muscle comparison with malignant hyperthermia. J Clin Psychopharmacol 2:266, 1982.

32. Breithart W, Marotta RF, Call P: AIDS and neuroleptic malignant syndrome. Lancet 2:1488, 1988.
33. Manser TJ, Warner JF: Neuroleptic malignant syndrome associated with prochlorperazine. South Med J 83:73, 1990.
34. Lo TC, Unwin MR, Dymock IW: Neuroleptic malignant syndrome: Another medical cause of acute abdomen. Postgrad Med J 65:653, 1989.
35. Shalev A, Hermesh H, Munitz H: The role of external heat load in triggering the neuroleptic malignant syndrome. Am J Psychiatry 145:110, 1988.
36. Toru M, Matsuda O, Makiguchi K: Neuroleptic malignant syndrome–like state following a withdrawal of anti-parkinsonian drugs. J Nerv Ment Dis 169:324, 1981.
37. Sechi GP, Tanda F, Mutani R: Fatal hyperpyrexia after withdrawal of levodopa. Neurology 34:249, 1984.
38. Friedman JH, Feinberg SS, Feldman RG: A neuroleptic malignant–like syndrome due to levodopa therapy withdrawal. JAMA 254:2792, 1985.
39. Pfeiffer R, Sucha EL: "On-off"–induced lethal hyperthermia. Mov Disord 4:338, 1989.
40. Hamburg P, Weilburg JB, Cassem NH, et al: Relapse of neuroleptic malignant syndrome with early discontinuation of amantadine therapy. Compr Psychiatry 27:272, 1986.
41. Simpson DH, Davis GC: Case report of neuroleptic malignant syndrome associated with withdrawal from amantadine. Am J Psychiatry 141:796, 1984.
42. Brown CS, Wittkowsky AK, Bryant SG: Neuroleptic-induced catatonia after abrupt withdrawal of amantadine during neuroleptic therapy. Pharmacotherapy 6:193, 1986.
43. Henderson V, Wooten G: Neuroleptic malignant syndrome: A pathogenic role for dopamine receptor blockade? Neurology 31:132, 1981.
44. Parsa MA, Rohr T, Ramirez LF, et al: Neuroleptic malignant syndrome without neuroleptics. J Clin Psychopharmacol 10:437, 1990.
45. Burke RE, Fahn S, Mayeus R, et al: Neuroleptic malignant syndrome caused by dopamine-depleting drugs in a patient with Huntington disease. Neurology 31:1022, 1981.
46. Cohen WJ, Cohen NH: Lithium carbonate, haloperidol, and irreversible brain damage. JAMA 230:1238, 1974.
47. Ebadi M, Pfeiffer RF, Murrin LC: Pathogenesis and treatment of neuroleptic malignant syndrome. Gen Pharmacol 21:367, 1990.
48. Brennan D, MacManus M, Howe J, et al: "Neuroleptic malignant syndrome" without neuroleptics. Br J Psychiatry 152:578, 1988.
49. Stauffenberg EF, Tantam D: Malingant hyperpyrexia syndrome in combined treatment. Br J Psychiatry 154:577, 1989.
50. Price WA, Zimmer B, Kucas P: Serotonin syndrome: A case report. J Clin Pharmacol 26:77, 1986.
51. Kline SS, Mauro LS, Scala-Barnett DM, et al: Serotonin syndrome versus neuroleptic malignant syndrome as a cause of death. Clin Pharm 8:510, 1989.
52. Grant R: Neuroleptic malignant syndrome. Br Med J 288:1690, 1984.
53. Rosenberg PB, Pearlman CA: NMS-like syndrome with a lithium/doxepin combination. J Clin Psychopharmacol 11:75, 1991.
54. Burch EA Jr, Downs J: Development of neuroleptic malignant syndrome during simultaneous amoxapine treatment and alprazolam discontinuation. J Clin Psychopharmacol 7:55, 1987.
55. Sucherowsky O, deVries J: Interaction of fluoxetine and selegiline. Can J Psychiatry 35:571, 1990.
56. Horikawa M, Ninomiya M, Nishi M, et al: A ten-year-old autistic girl with neuroleptic malignant syndrome caused by neuroleptic agents. No To Hattatsu 21:486, 1989.
57. Samie MR: Neuroleptic malignant–like syndrome induced by metoclopramide. Mov Disord 2:57, 1987.
58. Addonizio G: Neuroleptic malignant syndrome in elderly patients. J Am Geriatr Soc 35:1011, 1987.
59. Deng MZ, Chen GQ, Phillips MR: Neuroleptic malignant syndrome in 12 of 9,792 Chinese inpatients exposed to neuroleptics: A prospective study. Am J Psychiatry 147:1149, 1990.
60. Patel P, Bristow G: Postoperative neuroleptic malignant syndrome. A case report. Can J Anaesth 34:515, 1987.
61. Spivak B, Weizman A, Wolovick L, et al: Neuroleptic malignant syndrome during abrupt reduction of neuroleptic treatment. Acta Psychiatr Scand 81:168, 1990.
62. Shalev A, Hermesh H, Munitz H: The role of loading rate in neuroleptic malignant syndrome. Am J Psychiatry 143:1059, 1986.
63. Kirkpatrick B, Edelsohn GA: Risk factors for the neuroleptic malignant syndrome. Psychiatr Med 2:371, 1985.
64. Caroff SN, Mann SC: Neuroleptic malignant syndrome. Psychopharmacol Bull 24:25, 1988.
65. Keck PE Jr, Sebastianelli J, Pope HG Jr, et al: Frequency and presentation of neuroleptic malignant syndrome in a state psychiatric hospital. J Clin Psychiatry 50:352, 1989.
66. Caroff SN: The neuroleptic malignant syndrome. J Clin Psychiatry 41:79, 1980.
67. Gelenberg AJ, Bellinghausen B, Wojcik JD, et al: A prospective survey of neuroleptic malignant syndrome in a short-term psychiatric hospital. Am J Psychiatry 145:517, 1988.
68. Shalev A, Munitz H: The neuroleptic malignant syndrome: Agent and host interaction. Acta Psychiatr Scand 73:337, 1986.
69. Meltzer HY: Rigidity, hyperpyrexia, and coma following fluphenazine enanthanate. Psychopharmacologia 29:337, 1973.
70. Vincent FM, Zimmerman JE, Van Haren J: Neuroleptic malignant syndrome complicating closed head injury. Neurosurgery 18:190, 1986.
71. Hermesh H, Aizenberg D, Lapidot M, et al: The relationship between malignant hyperthermia and neuroleptic malignant syndrome. Anesthesiology 70:171, 1989.
72. Lim R: Idiopathic hypoparathyroidism presenting as the neuroleptic malignant syndrome. Br J Hosp Med 41:182, 1989.
73. Moore AP, MacFarlane IA, Blumhardt LD: Neuroleptic malignant syndrome and hypothyroidism. J Neurol Neurosurg Psychiatry 53:517, 1990.
74. Kontaxakis VP, Christodoulou GN, Markidis MP, et al: Treatment of a mild form of neuroleptic malignant syndrome with oral diazepam. Acta Psychiatr Scand 78:396, 1988.
75. Bernstein WB, Scherokman B: Neuroleptic malignant syndrome in a patient with acquired immunodeficiency syndrome. Acta Neurol Scand 73:636, 1986.
76. Serby M: Neuroleptic malignant syndrome in Alzheimer's disease. J Am Geriatr Soc 34:895, 1986.
77. Goldwasser HD, Hooper JF, Spears NM: Concomitant treatment of neuroleptic malignant syndrome and psychosis. Br J Psychiatry 154:102, 1989.
78. Dhib-Jalbut S, Hesselbrock R, Mouradian MM, et al: Bromocriptine treatment of neuroleptic malignant syndrome. J Clin Psychiatry 48:69, 1987.
79. Montgomery JN, Ironside JW: Neuroleptic malignant syndrome in the intensive therapy unit. Anaesthesia 45:311, 1990.
80. Shalev A, Hermesh H, Munitz H: Mortality from neuroleptic malignant syndrome. J Clin Psychiatry 50:18, 1989.
81. Rosenberg MR, Green M: Neuroleptic malignant syndrome. Review of response to therapy. Arch Intern Med 149:1927, 1989.
82. Janati A, Webb RT: Successful treatment of neuroleptic malignant syndrome with bromocriptine. South Med J 79:1567, 1986.
83. Verhoeven WMA, Elderson A, Westenberg HGM: Neuroleptic malignant syndrome: Successful treatment with bromocriptine. Biol Psychiatry 20:680, 1985.
84. Granato JE, Stern BJ, Karim RA, et al: Neuroleptic malignant syndrome. Ann Neurol 14:89, 1983.
85. Greenberg LB, Gujavarty K: The neuroleptic malignant syndrome: Review and report of three cases. Compr Psychiatry 26:63, 1985.
86. Mueller PS, Vester JW, Fermaglich J: NMS: Successful treatment with bromocriptine. JAMA 249:386, 1983.
87. Zubenko G, Pope HG: Management of a case of neuroleptic malignant syndrome with bromocriptine. Am J Psychiatry 140:1619, 1983.
88. Rodriguez ME, Luquin MR, Lera G, et al: Neuroleptic malignant syndrome treated with subcutaneous lisuride infusion. Mov Disord 5:170, 1990.
89. Goldwasser HD, Hooper JF, Spears NM: Concomitant treatment of neuroleptic malignant syndrome and psychosis. Br J Psychiatry 154:102, 1989.
90. Jee A: Amantadine in neuroleptic malignant syndrome. Postgrad Med J 63:508, 1987.
91. McCarron MM, Boettger ML, Peck JL: A case of neuroleptic malignant syndrome successfully treated with amantadine. J Clin Psychiatry 43:381, 1982.
92. Lazarus A: The neuroleptic malignant syndrome: A review. Can J Psychiatry 31:670, 1986.
93. Geller B, Greydanus DE: Haloperidol-induced comatose state and hyperthermia and rigidity in adolescence: Two case reports with a literature review. J Clin Psychiatry 40:102, 1979.
94. Itoh M, Ohtsuka N, Ogita K: Malignant neuroleptic syndrome: Its present status in Japan and clinical problems. Folia Psychiatr Neurol Jpn 31:565, 1977.
95. Weinberger DR, Kelly MJ: Catatonia and malignant syndrome: A possible complication of neuroleptic administration. J Nerv Ment Dis 165:263, 1977.
96. Deuschl G, Oepen G, Hermle L, et al: Neuroleptic malignant syndrome: Observations on altered consciousness. Pharmacopsychiatry 20:168, 1987.
97. Kurlan R, Hamill R, Shoulson I: Neuroleptic malignant syndrome. Clin Neuropharmacol 7:109, 1984.
98. Harris M, Nora L, Tanner CM: Neuroleptic malignant syndrome responsive to carbidopa/levodopa: Support for a dopaminergic pathogenesis. Clin Neuropharmacol 10:186, 1987.
99. Tollefson GD, Garvey MJ: The neuroleptic malignant syndrome and central dopamine metabolites. J Clin Psychopharmacol 4:150, 1984.
100. Khan A, Jaffe SH, Nelson WH: Resolution of neuroleptic malignant syndrome with dantrolene sodium: Case report. J Clin Psychiatry 46:244, 1985.
101. Granato JE, Stern BJ, Karim RA: Neuroleptic malignant syndrome: Successful treatment with dantrolene and bromocriptine. Ann Neurol 14:89, 1983.
102. Couns DJ, Hillman FJ, Marshall BW: Treatment of neuroleptic malignant syndrome with dantrolene sodium. Am J Psychiatry 139:944, 1982.
103. Goulon M, de Rohan-Chabot P, Elkharrat D, et al: Beneficial effects of dantrolene in the treatment of neuroleptic malignant syndrome. Neurology 33:516, 1983.
104. Ward A, Chaffman MO, Sorkin EM: Dantrolene: A review of its

pharmacodynamic and pharmacokinetic properties and therapeutic use in malignant hyperthermia, the neuroleptic malignant syndrome and an update of its use in muscle spasticity. Drugs 32:130, 1986.

105. Pearlman CA: Neuroleptic malignant syndrome: A review of the literature. Clin Psychopharmacol 6:257, 1986.

106. Leikin JB, Baron S, Engle J, et al: Treatment of neuroleptic malignant syndrome with diphenhydramine. Vet Hum Toxicol 30:58, 1988.

107. O'Brien P: Neuroleptic malignant syndrome treated with diazepam. Can J Psychiatry 33:780, 1988.

108. Giordani L, Amore M, Montanari A, et al: Pridinolum mesylate and neuroleptic malignant syndrome. Am J Psychiatry 142:389, 1985.

109. Sangal R, Dimitrijevic R: Neuroleptic malignant syndrome: Successful treatment with pancuronium. JAMA 254:2795, 1985.

110. Blue MG, Schneider SM, Noro S, et al: Successful treatment of neuroleptic malignant syndrome with sodium nitroprusside. Ann Intern Med 104:56, 1986.

111. Harland CC, O'Leary MM, Winters R, et al: Neuroleptic malignant syndrome : A case for electroconvulsive therapy. Postgrad Med J 66:49, 1990.

112. Lazarus A: Treatment of neuroleptic malignant syndrome with electroconvulsive therapy. J Nerv Ment Dis 174:47, 1986.

113. Addonizio G, Susman VL: ECT as a treatment for patients with symptoms of neuroleptic malignant syndrome. J Clin Psychiatry 48:102, 1987.

114. Bond WS: Detection and management of the neuroleptic malignant syndrome. Clin Pharmacol 3:302, 1984.

115. Susman VL, Addonizio G: Recurrence of neuroleptic malignant syndrome. J Nerv Ment Dis 176:234, 1988.

116. Rosebush PI, Stewart TD, Gelenberg AJ: Twenty neuroleptic rechallenges after neuroleptic malignant syndrome in 15 patients. J Clin Psychiatry 50:295, 1989.

117. Moysa GD, Anisete LV: Neuroleptic malignant syndrome: Successful rechallenge with thioridazine (letter). DICP 23:712, 1989.

118. Slack T, Stoudemire A: Reinstitution of neuroleptic treatment with molindone in a patient with a history of neuroleptic malignant syndrome. Gen Hosp Psychiatry 11:365, 1989.

CHAPTER 62

Alcoholism

John C. M. Brust

Approximately 10 million Americans are alcoholic, and ethanol abuse accounts for roughly 10% of American mortality.[1, 2] Drinking is an indirect cause of most of these deaths, for example, those resulting from violence (e.g., homicide, suicide, and accidents, especially motor vehicle) or systemic organ damage (e.g., cirrhosis and pancreatitis). Immune suppression by ethanol predisposes drinkers to pneumonia, sepsis, and meningitis,[3] and alcoholics are at increased risk for cancer and stroke (especially hemorrhagic).[4] Heavy drinkers are thus familiar figures in emergency rooms and intensive care units. This chapter focuses on direct consequences of ethanol abuse, namely intoxication and withdrawal, as well as certain potentially life-threatening nutritional and metabolic disturbances. The subject is a complicated one, for ethanol overdose or withdrawal frequently accompanies other ethanol-related diseases as well as overdose or withdrawal from other abused substances. A number of life-threatening illnesses encountered in alcoholics, such as hepatic failure, pancreatitis, and bacterial meningitis, are discussed elsewhere in this volume.

ETHANOL OVERDOSE

Ethanol intoxication is so common that physicians tend to forget that amounts of ethanol only moderately larger than those causing drunkenness can be fatal, especially when additional drugs have been taken[1] (Table 62–1).

Ethanol is rapidly absorbed from the gastrointestinal tract and distributed throughout body water.[5] In a 70-kg man a mildly intoxicating blood ethanol concentration (BEC) of 100 mg/dL follows ingestion of about 50 g (or roughly 2 oz) of 100% ethanol, which would be contained in approximately 4 oz of 90 proof spirits, 14 oz of wine, or 48 oz of beer. In nontolerant individuals, ethanol is metabolized at about 70 to 150 mg/kg body weight/h with a fall in BEC of 10 to 25 mg/dL/h (average 16 mg/dL/h). Most adults therefore take 6 hours to metabolize a 50-g dose. Drinking only an additional 8 g of ethanol per hour maintains the BEC at 100 mg/dL; drinking more rapidly raises it. A controversial report suggested that lower activity of gastric alcohol dehydrogenase in women than in men leads to higher BECs in women.[6]

Ethanol is metabolized by liver alcohol dehydrogenase to acetaldehyde, which is then oxidized by aldehyde dehydrogenase to acetate or acetyl coenzyme A with eventual formation of carbon dioxide and water. Early saturation of alcohol dehydrogenase accounts for the constant rate (zero-order kinetics) of ethanol metabolism.[5] An additional microsomal ethanol-oxidizing system is inducible by ethanol (and other drugs such as barbiturates) and accounts in part for ethanol tolerance, most of which, however, is the result of poorly understood central nervous system adaptive mechanisms, not lower blood levels. Food in the stomach delays ethanol absorption, and alcoholics, who are already often nutritionally compromised, learn that by not eating they can enhance intoxication.

Ethanol is a central nervous system depressant; the euphoria and hyperactivity associated with mild intoxication are the result of cerebral disinhibition, not direct stimulation. At any BEC, intoxication is more severe when the level is rising than when it is falling, when the level is reached rapidly, and when the level has been achieved recently.[7] These factors, plus an individual's degree of tolerance, mean that a single BEC determination is an unreliable indicator of drunkenness; the correlations of Table 62–1 represent broad generalizations.[8] A level of 500 mg/dL would cause fatal coma and respiratory depression in 50% of subjects,

TABLE 62–1	
CORRELATION OF SYMPTOMS WITH BLOOD ETHANOL CONCENTRATION	
Blood Ethanol Concentration (mg/dL)	**Symptoms**
50–150	Euphoria or dysphoria, shyness or expansiveness, friendliness or argumentativeness. Impaired concentration, judgment, and sexual inhibitions
150–250	Slurred speech and ataxic gait, diplopia, nausea, tachycardia, drowsiness, or labile mood with sudden bursts of anger or antisocial acts
300	Stupor alternating with combativeness or incoherent speech, heavy breathing, vomiting
400	Coma
500	Respiratory paralysis, death

TABLE 62–2

TREATMENT OF ACUTE ETHANOL INTOXICATION

For obstreperous or violent patients
    Isolation, calming environment, reassurance—avoid sedatives
    Close observation
For stuporous or comatose patients
    If hypoventilation, artificial respiration in an intensive care unit
    If serum glucose level in doubt, intravenous 50% glucose
    Thiamine, 100 mg, and multivitamins, IM or IV
    Careful monitoring of blood pressure; correction of
       hypovolemia or acid-base imbalance
    Consider hemodialysis if patient severely acidotic, deeply
       comatose, or apneic
    Avoid emetics or gastric lavage
    Avoid analeptics
    Do not forget other possible causes of coma in an alcoholic,
       as well as concomitant drug use

but death has occurred at levels of less than 400 mg/dL, and levels higher than 800 mg/dL have been measured in fully alert subjects.[9, 10]

Low-to-moderate BECs cause slow saccadic eye movements and interrupted, jerky smooth pursuit, which may impair visual acuity. At such levels there is increased electroencephalographic beta activity ("beta buzz").[11, 12] Higher concentrations cause nystagmus, esophoria or exophoria, and diplopia, with electroencephalographic slowing.[13] During sleep there is suppression of the rapid eye movement stage, followed after a few hours by rapid eye movement "rebound." Either low or high BECs can cause hypothermia.[14]

Two unusual forms of ethanol intoxication are poorly understood. Pathologic intoxication, also called idiosyncratic intoxication or acute alcoholic paranoid state, consists of sudden extreme excitement, sometimes with delusions, hallucinations, and even homicidal aggression, lasting minutes to hours and followed by sleep and amnesia for the episode. Some of these episodes probably represent psychologic dissociative reactions; others may represent the kind of paradoxical excitation that can follow barbiturate administration. Alcoholic blackouts are periods of amnesia for intoxication, although at the time the subject appeared fully conscious. Usually associated with frank alcoholism, blackouts sometimes occur in occasional drinkers.[15]

Ethanol intoxication can intensify depressed consciousness of any cause. Although ethanol intoxication alone may adequately explain stupor, especially in patients with "alcoholic breath" and signs of vasodilatation (flushing, tachycardia, hypotension, and hypothermia), it may mask the presence of subdural hematoma, hepatic encephalopathy, meningitis, hypoglycemia, or other drug poisoning.

Serum osmolarity rises about 22 mOsm/L for every 100 mg/dL BEC. Because ethanol freely crosses cell membranes without causing shifts of water, this hyperosmolarity does not cause symptoms, but comatose patients whose serum osmolarity is higher than that predicted by serum sodium, glucose, and urea concentrations should be suspected of having ethanol poisoning.[16]

The treatment of severe ethanol poisoning is similar to that of poisoning by other depressant drugs (Table 62–2). Death results from respiratory depression, so patients require artificial ventilation in an intensive care unit. Hypovolemia, acid-base or electrolyte imbalance, and abnormal temperature require attention, and if a patient's serum glucose level is not known, 50% glucose is given intravenously with parenteral thiamine. Ethanol's rapid gastrointestinal absorption means that gastric lavage is useful only if other drugs have been ingested.[17] The use of sedatives or

neuroleptics in obstreperous or violent patients may push them into coma and respiratory depression. A striking feature of ethanol poisoning is the tendency of patients to appear awake during examination only to lapse into stupor with depressed respirations when stimuli are removed.[18]

A BEC of 400 mg/dL in a nonhabitual drinker takes 20 hours to become zero. The only practical agent that hastens ethanol metabolism is fructose, which, however, causes gastrointestinal upset, lactic acidosis (which may already be present), hyperuricemia, and osmotic diuresis.[9, 15] Hemodialysis or peritoneal dialysis can hasten elimination when the BEC is extremely high (e.g., over 600 mg/dL) and may be indicated for severe acidosis, concurrent ingestion of other drugs (including methanol or ethylene glycol), or severely intoxicated children. Analeptics such as ethamivan, caffeine, or amphetamine are of no value and can precipitate seizures or cardiac arrhythmia. An imidazobenzodiazepine drug that reverses symptoms of mild intoxication but not stupor or respiratory depression has been developed but is not commercially available.[19]

Reports of other therapeutic agents have been conflicting. Low doses of propranolol reduced ethanol-induced depression in mice, but higher doses augmented it, and in humans propranolol increased ethanol "inebriation ratings."[20] Levodopa, aminophylline, and ephedrine have been reported to reduce symptoms of ethanol intoxication in humans, perhaps through norepinephrine pathways;[21] the dopamine agonist apomorphine, however, aggravated ethanol inebriation.[22] Naloxone appears to reverse ethanol-induced coma in a small subset of patients. The mechanism is unclear. Patients most likely to respond are not identifiable before treatment, and there is a strong tendency to relapse after only minutes.[23]

Although alcoholics are often magnesium depleted, magnesium should be replaced with caution during intoxication because magnesium sulfate can further depress consciousness.[17]

Ethanol is often taken with other drugs, recreationally or in suicide attempts.[1] Although there is cross-tolerance for ethanol and barbiturates and other sedatives, when they are taken together the lethal dose for each may be strikingly lowered. Death resulting from respiratory depression occurred with a secobarbital blood level of 50 μg/mL and a BEC of 100 mg/dL.[24] Ethanol combined with chloral hydrate (Mickey Finn) has a particularly notorious reputation.[25]

Additive or synergistic effects can also occur when ethanol is combined with sedating antihistamines, neuroleptics, and other sedatives or tranquilizers such as methaqualone (now a schedule I drug), meprobamate, or benzodiazepines.[26, 27] Agents with half-lives of more than 24 hours, such as diazepam or flurazepam, can aggravate sedation or ataxia when ethanol is taken the next day. Ethanol and opiates can also aggravate each other's effects, and many heroin or methadone users are also alcoholic. Death has occurred when ethanol was taken with propoxyphene. Tricyclic antidepressants have been reported both to antagonize and to potentiate ethanol's effects. The cross-tolerance for ethanol and general anesthetics such as ether, chloroform, or fluorinated agents raises the threshold to sleep induction, but synergistic interaction then increases the depth and length of the anesthetic stage reached.

Ethanol can initially retard or later accelerate phenytoin metabolism, producing either drug toxicity or inadequate seizure control.[28] Ethanol inhibits warfarin metabolism and aggravates postural hypotension in patients taking antihypertensives. A disulfiram-like reaction (flushing, throbbing headache, sweating, dyspnea, palpitations, weakness, vomiting, and hypotension) can occur in subjects who take ethanol with sulfonylurea hypoglycemics or certain antibiotics (chloramphenicol, griseofulvin, quinacrine, metronidazole, isoni-

TABLE 62–3
ETHANOL WITHDRAWAL SYNDROMES
Early symptoms
Tremulousness
Hallucinosis
Seizures
Late symptoms
Delirium tremens

azid); when ethanol is taken with disulfiram itself, the reaction can be fatal.[28]

ETHANOL WITHDRAWAL AND ITS TREATMENT

The familiar symptoms of hangover—headache, malaise, nausea, tremulousness, and sweating—do not require chronic drinking. More severe or prolonged withdrawal symptoms signify physical dependence[11, 29, 30] (Table 62–3).

Tremulousness, more severe than that with simple hangover, is the most common ethanol withdrawal symptom and usually appears after at least several days of drinking. It is promptly relieved by ethanol, but if drinking cannot continue tremor becomes more intense, with easy startling, anxiety, agitation, insomnia, nystagmus, flushing, sweating, anorexia, nausea, vomiting, weakness, tachypnea, tachycardia, and systolic hypertension. There may be inattentiveness, but unless other disturbances are present (e.g., seizures, Wernicke-Korsakoff syndrome, subdural hematoma), mentation is otherwise intact. Tremor is usually distal, coarse, irregular, and worse with movement, interfering with eating or even standing. Without treatment it usually subsides over a few days, although some patients feel "shaky inside" for a few weeks.[13, 15, 29]

About one fourth of these patients develop perceptual disturbances, including vivid dreams, nightmares, illusions, and hallucinations, which can be auditory, visual, tactile, olfactory, or a combination. Visual hallucinations are most common and sometimes occur only with eye closure. Imagery includes insects, animals, or people, sometimes as disembodied heads. Usually fragmentary, the hallucinations tend to last minutes at a time over several days. Insight is variable; the hallucinations may or may not be accompanied by paranoid delusions.[13, 29, 30]

Both transient parkinsonism and transient chorea have occurred during ethanol withdrawal.[13, 32] Parkinsonism affects patients over 50 years of age, beginning usually a few days after the last drink but sometimes while the individual is still drinking. It tends to clear over days or weeks without treatment, and patients followed up for years have not developed Parkinson's disease.[33] Lingual-oral choreiform dyskinesias, sometime spreading to neck or arm muscles, affect younger patients and usually appear 1 to 2 weeks after they stop drinking.[34] Ethanol acutely decreases striatal dopamine release, perhaps accounting for parkinsonian signs. Chorea may be the consequence of dopamine receptor supersensitivity.[13, 35]

The term "rum fits" refers to seizures in alcoholic patients who are not otherwise epileptic.[11, 29] (Ethanol can also precipitate seizures in known epileptics; the amount required is disputed.) In several studies the majority of these seizures occurred between 6 and 48 hours after cessation of chronic drinking, either as single major motor seizures or as clusters over a few hours. Status epilepticus occurs in less than 10%, and focal features, not always attributable to previous head injury or other brain lesions, are observed in up to 25%.[36, 37]

Ethanol-related seizures may occur in otherwise asymptomatic patients or may accompany tremor or hallucinosis.

The amount of ethanol required to provoke such seizures is uncertain. In a case-control study of incident seizures, chronic daily ingestion of 50 g of ethanol raised the odds ratio above 1 and at 200 g daily the odds ratio was 20, but the minimal duration of drinking that conferred increased risk of seizures could not be determined.[38] Moreover, although both human and animal studies have led to general acceptance of the concept of alcohol withdrawal seizures, investigators have frequently observed seizures in subjects either during active drinking or more than a week after cessation. The concepts of "relative" and "protracted" withdrawal have been invoked to explain such seizures; an alternative possibility is that alcohol causes seizures by mechanisms other than withdrawal.[39]

Patients with ethanol-related seizures often have a history of focal brain injury, and periodic lateralizing epileptiform discharges are occasionally observed during ethanol withdrawal.[40, 41] Some studies have found an increased risk of seizures with recurrent ethanol detoxification, compatible with a kindling phenomenon.[42, 43]

The diagnosis of ethanol-related seizures requires that other lesions be excluded, and computed tomographic scanning or magnetic resonance imaging is indicated when such seizures are of new onset. A spinal tap may be necessary if meningitis or subarachnoid hemorrhage is suspected; previous seizures do not exclude the possibility that a recurrent seizure has a more ominous cause. The electroencephalogram in patients with ethanol-related seizures, unlike those with idiopathic epilepsy, is usually normal; a report that photomyclonic or photoconvulsive responses were unusually common in such patients[37] was not borne out by subsequent studies.[44, 45]

In contrast to tremor, hallucinations, and seizures, delirium tremens usually begins 48 to 72 hours after the last drink. Because of the popular misconception that any alcoholic with tremor and hallucinations has delirium tremens, it tends to be overdiagnosed. In fact, delirium tremens consists of not only tremor and disordered sensory perception but also delirium (defined as extreme inattentiveness, usually agitated), autonomic overactivity, and frequently a fatal outcome. In one series the syndrome was present in less than 5% of hospitalized patients with symptomatic ethanol withdrawal.[29] About one third of patients with ethanol-related seizures develop delirium tremens, but seizures during delirium tremens suggest additional diagnoses such as meningitis.

Delirium tremens typically begins and ends abruptly, lasting from hours to a few days.[15] Inattentiveness and confusion may rapidly alternate with lucidity, or symptoms may subside gradually. Infrequently, relapses prolong the illness to a few weeks. The severity and duration of delirium tremens are increased in the presence of concurrent disease such as liver failure, pneumonia, or pancreatitis.[40, 46, 47] Elderly patients also have more severe withdrawal.[48] A typical patient is agitated and grossly tremulous, with fever, tachycardia, and profuse sweating. Tremor may be so widespread as to involve the face, tongue, and pharynx.[13] The patient picks at the bedclothes or stares wildly about, shouting at hallucinated objects or trying to fend them off. Fluid loss can be marked, and heatstroke and myoglobinuria are sometimes complicating features.[47] Less readily diagnosed are patients with "quiet delirium" or those with a single predominant symptom such as confusion, hallucinations, or delusions. Such patients may have striking misperceptions, believing that they are drinking in a bar or, with extreme suggestibility, identifying objects alluded to but not actually seen.[47] In contrast to patients with early withdrawal hallucinosis, who later can

TABLE 62–4

TREATMENT OF ETHANOL WITHDRAWAL

Prevention or reduction of early symptoms
  Diazepam, 10–40 mg PO or IV, repeated hourly until sedation
    or mild intoxication. If successive daily doses are required,
    taper by about one fourth of preceding day's dose with
    resumption of higher dose if withdrawal symptoms recur.
    (Consider short-acting benzodiazepines for patients with
    abnormal liver function.)
  Alternatively, pentobarbital, 200 mg, PO, IM, or IV, and then
    100 mg/h prn. Maintenance dose and duration are
    determined by symptoms. Subsequent tapering at about 100
    mg/d.
  Alternatively, paraldehyde, 5–15 mg, PO or PR, repeated
    hourly prn. Maintenance and tapering are titrated with
    symptoms.
  Thiamine, 100 mg, and multivitamins, IM or IV.
  Magnesium, potassium, and calcium replacement as needed.
Delirium tremens
  Diazepam, 10 mg IV, then 5 mg or more (up to 40 mg) IV or
    IM every 5 min until calming. Maintenance diazepam, 5 mg
    or more IV or IM every 1–4 h prn.
  Pay careful attention to fluid and electrolyte balance; several
    liters of saline per day, or even pressors, may be needed.
  Use cooling blanket or alcohol sponges for high fever.
  Prevent or correct hypoglycemia.
  Use thiamine and multivitamins.
  Consider coexisting illness, e.g., liver failure, pancreatitis,
    sepsis, meningitis, or subdural hematoma.

describe their illusions or hallucinations, those with severe delirium tremens seldom recall the episode.

Reported mortality has been as high as 15%, related to associated disease such as pneumonia or sepsis; patients have often been admitted to the hospital for another reason. Sometimes death follows unexplained shock or occurs suddenly without apparent cause. Fatalities have been variably attributed to cardiac arrhythmia, fat emboli, and heatstroke.

Drug pharmacokinetics can change during ethanol withdrawal. For example, warfarin plasma protein binding was found to decrease, leading to a 20% increase in the free fraction.[49]

Dozens of drugs have been recommended for the treatment of ethanol withdrawal, but it has not always been clear whether the aim of therapy was relief of tremulousness, prevention of delirium tremens, or management of delirium tremens after it started.[9, 50] Some workers believe that early treatment of ethanol withdrawal can prevent delirium tremens, but others doubt that such intervention can either prevent it or reduce its mortality.[15]

It has been suggested that the majority of patients with only mild withdrawal symptoms are satisfactorily managed nonpharmacologically with reassurance, reduced sensory stimuli, rest, hydration, and nutrition.[40, 51, 52] Others recommend sedatives to prevent the appearance of symptoms in recently abstinent heavy drinkers and to relieve early mild withdrawal symptoms[53] (Table 62–4). Obviously, sedatives should be used cautiously in patients with liver disease, head injury, or chronic obstructive pulmonary disease; indeed, hypoxia-induced mental change could be misdiagnosed as worsening withdrawal symptoms.[40, 54] Cross-tolerance with ethanol favors agents such as paraldehyde, barbiturates, or benzodiazepines, and the last (usually diazepam) are currently the drugs of choice.[55] Whatever sedative is used, it should be given in a loading dose sufficient to produce symptoms of mild intoxication (calming, dysarthria, ataxia, fine nystagmus); subsequent doses are adjusted to avoid both intoxication and withdrawal tremulousness. After a few days

dosage is gradually tapered, with reinstitution of intoxicating doses should withdrawal symptoms appear. For benzodiazepines an initial oral dose might consist of 10 to 40 mg diazepam repeated at intervals of one to a few hours, titrated against symptoms; up to 400 mg may be needed on the first day. It can be given intravenously, but intramuscular absorption is unpredictable. Because of its long biologic half-life, diazepam accumulates over days with delayed toxicity (including precipitation of hepatic encephalopathy), so after initial loading subsequent doses are tapered by about 25% per day unless increasing withdrawal symptoms dictate otherwise. Benzodiazepines with short half-lives such as oxazepam or triazolam may be advantageous in such patients.[56] Alternatively, many patients who have received a 60-mg or higher loading dose of diazepam require no further medication.[57] Heavy smokers may require unusually high doses of benzodiazepines.

Reports on the efficacy of neuroleptics in early hallucinosis have been conflicting. There is no cross-tolerance for these agents and ethanol, they can exacerbate seizures, and their side effects include hypotension, hepatic damage, acute dystonia, rash, impaired thermoregulation, and bone marrow suppression. In fact, several studies have found an increased frequency of seizures, delirium tremens, and death in patients receiving phenothiazines compared to those given placebo.[58–63] The recommendation that haloperidol be added to a benzodiazepine for control of hallucinations is therefore controversial at best.[51, 64]

Blood and urinary levels of catecholamines and metabolites are increased during ethanol withdrawal and may contribute to symptoms.[65] Propranolol can decrease tremor and cardiac arrhythmia.[66, 67] It is no more effective than benzodiazepines, however, and in one report side effects included apparent exacerbation of hallucinations.[68] Other workers have reported favorable results with clonidine,[65, 69, 70] atenolol,[71, 72] and lofexidine.[65, 73, 74] One study of clonidine, however, reported high frequencies of hallucinations, seizures, orthostatic hypotension, and drowsiness.[75] In animal and cell culture studies ethanol decreases neuronal calcium flux, with compensatory increases that persist after abstinence.[76, 77] Preliminary reports suggest that calcium channel blockers might have a role in the treatment of ethanol withdrawal.[78–80]

The low therapeutic index of parenteral ethanol makes it potentially dangerous. Oral ethanol (which would be the patient's own treatment were he or she not hospitalized) has the disadvantage of organ toxicity (e.g., liver and possibly central nervous system). Even though most patients resume drinking after discharge, ethanol has no role in the prevention or treatment of withdrawal symptoms.

Because most ethanol-related seizures occur singly or in brief clusters, once they have occurred anticonvulsants are unnecessary unless the diagnosis is doubtful. Both animal and human studies suggest that phenytoin is ineffective in preventing ethanol-related seizures.[47, 81, 82] Valproate and carbamazepine were protective in rat withdrawal seizures;[83–85] carbamazepine also prevented tremor, sweating, gastrointestinal symptoms, irritability, and insomnia in abstinent patients.[86]

Status epilepticus during ethanol withdrawal is treated conventionally; intravenous diazepam and phenobarbital have the advantage over phenytoin of reducing other withdrawal symptoms when the patient awakens. Long-term anticonvulsants in patients with ethanol-related seizures are superfluous; abstainers do not need them and drinkers do not take them. Unfortunately, epileptics whose seizures are precipitated by ethanol do require treatment, even though compliance is unlikely.

Respiratory alkalosis and hypomagnesemia occur during

early ethanol withdrawal, returning to normal before the appearance of delirium tremens (although hyperventilation often recurs as part of that syndrome).[12] Hypomagnesemia may be the result of intracellular shift as well as actual body loss, and it is not considered the primary cause of ethanol-related seizures or other early withdrawal symptoms. It may be a contributing feature, however, so magnesium sulfate should be given to hypomagnesemic patients in early withdrawal.[87] Hypokalemia and hypocalcemia may also be present, and the latter sometimes responds to treatment only after hypomagnesemia is corrected.[88]

Thiamine and multivitamins are given even if there are no clinical signs of their depletion, because glucose can precipitate Wernicke's disease in alcoholics with borderline nutritional deficiency. Because gastrointestinal absorption of thiamine is frequently impaired, it is given parenterally (see later).

In contrast to the symptoms of opiate withdrawal, delirium tremens cannot be abruptly reversed by any agent, and cross-tolerance for a sedative and ethanol is less important during full-blown delirium tremens than during early abstinence (see Table 62–4). In a prospective controlled study comparing parenteral diazepam and rectal paraldehyde in patients with "characteristic advanced delirium tremens," diazepam produced more rapid calming, fewer adverse reactions (e.g., apnea), and lower mortality.[89] Initial diazepam doses (10 mg intravenously followed by 5 mg intramuscularly every 5 minutes as needed) ranged from 15 to 215 mg. Once quieted, patients were maintained with 5 to 10 mg intramuscularly every 1 to 4 hours. Several points regarding benzodiazepine treatment of delirium tremens deserve emphasis. First, the effectiveness of maintenance intramuscular diazepam in this study is perhaps surprising in view of its unpredictable absorption by that route; unsatisfactory responses might call for intravenous administration. Second, doses may be needed that would be fatal in a normal person—sometimes more than 2000 mg of diazepam in the first 24 hours. Third, not only is there great variability in the dose required for calming, but also one cannot predict in an individual patient how high the dose will be. Fourth, liver disease decreases the metabolism of diazepam, and the brain of such a patient is abnormally sensitive to the depressant effect of sedatives; it is not unusual for delirium tremens to be replaced by hepatic encephalopathy.

General medical management in delirium tremens is intensive. Patients should be prone or in the lateral decubitus position and restrained as needed. Oral medicines are avoided. Most patients are dehydrated, some severely so, and many require up to 10 L of intravenous saline daily.[15] Shock may require transfusions or pressors. Patients with liver damage, however, may retain sodium and water. Hyponatremia must be corrected cautiously to avoid central pontine myelinolysis (see later). Cardiac arrhythmias may be secondary to hypokalemia. Fever, with or without infection, is often marked, requiring a cooling blanket or alcohol sponges. Hypoglycemia may be unrecognized, as may other serious coexisting illness such as liver failure, pancreatitis, sepsis, meningitis, or subdural hematoma.

WERNICKE-KORSAKOFF SYNDROME

It is often not appreciated that the mental abnormality associated with acute Wernicke-Korsakoff syndrome consists of more than simply impaired memory and that, untreated, the condition is fatal.[90] Wernicke's and Korsakoff's diseases share the some pathology and etiology—thiamine deficiency—but Wernicke's disease consists of an acute "global confusional state" plus eye movement abnormalities and ataxia of gait and stance, whereas Korsakoff's disease, which most often occurs in patients who have recovered from Wernicke's disease, consists of a chronic and more purely amnestic syndrome.[91]

The mental symptoms of Wernicke's disease evolve during days or weeks and include inattention, psychomotor slowing or abulia (often mistermed apathy or indifference), lethargy, and, when testable, anterograde and retrograde amnesia. Disordered perception is common; a patient might identify the hospital room as his or her apartment or a bar. Untreated patients develop stupor or coma. Abnormal eye movements include nystagmus (horizontal with or without vertical or rotatary), lateral rectus palsy (bilateral but usually asymmetric), and conjugate gaze palsy (horizontal, with or without vertical) progressing to complete ophthalmoplegia. There may be mild anisocoria and sluggish pupillary reactivity to light; more severe pupillary abnormalities are unusual. Small retinal hemorrhages sometimes occur.[91] Truncal ataxia (probably secondary to both vestibular and cerebellar lesions) can be so severe that the patient cannot stand, yet limb ataxia and dysarthria are unusual. Whether Wernicke's disease can occur without mental or eye movement abnormalities is uncertain. The relation of alcoholic pure cerebellar truncal ataxia to Wernicke's disease is uncertain. It is probably nutritional in origin, but the critical deficiency may not be thiamine. Similarly, peripheral neuropathy, although present in the great majority of patients with Wernicke's disease, is not part of the Wernicke-Korsakoff syndrome.

Patients with Wernicke's disease frequently have other signs of nutritional deficiency (skin changes, red tongue, cheilosis) or liver disease (jaundice, ascites, spider angiomas). Autonomic signs are common. Although beriberi heart disease is rare, tachycardia, dyspnea on exertion, and postural hypotension unexplained by hypovolemia are common, and circulatory collapse has followed mild exertion. Hypothermia is less frequent; fever usually indicates infection.

The electroencephalogram may be normal or show diffuse slowing. Cerebrospinal fluid is normal except for occasional mild protein elevation. Computed tomography or magnetic resonance imaging of the head sometimes reveals diencephalic abnormalities.[92, 93] An elevated blood pyruvate level that decreases with treatment is nonspecific. A decreased blood level of transketolase (which requires thiamine pyrophospate as a cofactor) more reliably indicates thiamine deficiency, but the test is unavailable in most hospitals. The diagnosis of Wernicke's disease is usually based on history and examination.

Treatment consists of intravenous thiamine, 50 to 100 mg/d for at least 5 days. Gastrointestinal absorption of thiamine is impaired in many alcoholics, and acute Wernicke's encephalopathy was reported after 12 days of intramuscular thiamine.[94] Particularly at need for high, efficiently delivered thiamine doses is a subgroup of patients with so-called low-affinity transketolase variant.[95] Additional nutritional deficiency is likely, and so multivitamins also are given. Hypomagnesemia, which can retard the response to thiamine, requires early correction.[96] Protein intake must be titrated against possible liver disease. Postural hypotension and tachycardia call for strict bed rest, and associated medical problems often require intensive care. Even among treated patients, mortality is as high as 10%, undoubtedly related in many instances to concurrent liver failure, infection, or delirium tremens.

Animal studies suggest that thiamine deficiency may result in excitatory neurotransmitter neuronal toxicity and that N-methyl-D-aspartate receptor antagonists (e.g., MK-801) might be of therapeutic benefit.[7, 97] Such work does not yet have clinical applicability.

If treated early, the abnormal eye movements of Wernicke's disease begin to improve within a few hours and usually resolve within a week; nystagmus may persist. Mentation may also improve within hours or days and either clear within a few weeks or leave a residual Korsakoff's amnesia. Recovery of ataxia is incomplete in more than half of the patients.

The best approach to Wernicke's disease is preventive. Any alcoholic patient seen in an emergency room should receive thiamine, as should any patient receiving glucose for, say, unexplained seizures or coma. Despite such warnings, Wernicke's disease too often appears in patients hospitalized a few days earlier for some other problem.

PELLAGRA

As noted, nutritional deficiency in alcoholics is not restricted to thiamine, and indeed nicotinic acid deficiency in such patients has produced clinical pellagra, with skin, gastrointestinal, and mental abnormalities.[15] Stomatitis and enteritis can be prominent, with nausea, vomiting, and diarrhea. Central nervous system symptoms include headache, irritability, and insomnia progressing to impaired memory, delusions, hallucinations, dementia, or delirium. Nicotinic acid deficiency may contribute to peripheral neuropathy, and other nutritional deficiency, especially of thiamine and pyridoxine, may contribute to central nervous system or peripheral nerve symptoms.

Treatment of pellagra is with nicotinic acid or nicotinamide, orally at a dose of 50 mg up to 10 times daily or intravenously 25 mg twice or three times daily, plus thiamine and multivitamins. Response is usually rapid; in fact, delirium may clear within hours. As with Wernicke's disease, prevention is preferable to treatment.

HYPOGLYCEMIA

Alcoholics are prone to hypoglycemia for several reasons.[98] They stop eating, and their diseased livers become depleted of glycogen. They also have defective gluconeogenesis, for the metabolism of alcohol by alcohol dehydrogenase and of acetaldehyde by aldehyde dehydrogenase requires NAD, diverting it from the glycolytic pathway. Acute and severe hypoglycemia may interrupt a drinking binge, causing altered behavior, seizures, coma, or, less often, focal neurologic signs with preserved alertness.[99] Therefore, 50% glucose (with thiamine) is given to any patient (alcoholic or not) with unexplained status epilepticus or coma. Although it is true that for any level of coma hypoglycemia is less likely than anoxia and ischemia to cause permanent brain damage, there is no room for complacency; untreated hypoglycemia can result in permanent dementia. Moreover, patients who have responded to glucose require close observation, especially if they are also diabetics taking insulin or oral hypoglycemic drugs, for the blood glucose level may fall again with return of symptoms and potential brain damage. Such patients should not be sent home from emergency rooms but rather should be admitted, preferably to an intensive care unit.[99]

Ethanol stimulates intestinal secretin, which in turn enhances glucose-stimulated insulin release. The result can be severe reactive hypoglycemia, especially in children.[100, 101] Indeed, coma in a small child who has accidentally ingested ethanol is as likely to be secondary to hypoglycemia as to direct intoxication.

CENTRAL PONTINE MYELINOLYSIS

Central pontine myelinolysis is not restricted to alcoholics and is diagnosed more often at autopsy than during life. Magnetic resonance imaging has increased diagnostic accuracy, however.[102] The typical demyelinating lesions in the basis pontis (and, sometimes, in the cerebellum, diencephalon, or cerebral white matter) are thought to result from overvigorous correction of hyponatremia. Whether speed of correction or correction to hypernatremia is the more important factor is disputed; animal studies have suggested a particular hazard in rapidly correcting chronic compared with acute hyponatremia.[103, 104] In any case, central pontine myelinolysis is most often a preventable iatrogenic disease. The earliest symptoms are tetraparesis, dysarthria, and dysphagia; if the lesion extends into the tegmentum there are abnormal eye movements, stupor, or coma. Such signs can, of course, be masked by the underlying condition that produced the hyponatremia in the first place. There is no treatment for central pontine myelinolysis once it has occurred. Most workers agree that prevention includes treating hyponatremia such that serum sodium levels do not exceed 130 mEq/L,[105, 106] with free water restriction and small amounts of hypertonic saline titrated to raise serum sodium levels no more rapidly than 0.55 mEq/L/h or 12 mEq/L/d.[7, 107–109]

MARCHIAFAVA-BIGNAMI DISEASE

Marchiafava-Bignami disease is rare and usually found unexpectedly at autopsy, but its characteristic demyelinating lesions in the corpus callosum have been observed by magnetic resonance imaging.[110] These lesions hardly explain the typically severe symptoms, which include psychosis and dementia, seizures, hemiparesis, aphasia, rigidity, abnormal movements, dysarthria, and ataxia progressing over months to stupor, coma, and death. More chronic courses have been described, and typical lesions have been unexpectedly discovered at autopsy after death from other causes.[15]

The cause of Marchiafava-Bignami disease is unknown, but it seems to be restricted to alcoholics. There is no treatment.

ALCOHOLIC KETOACIDOSIS

Acid-base disturbances in alcoholics can be complex and difficult to interpret. Hyperventilation during ethanol withdrawal or hepatic encephalopaphy causes respiratory alkalosis. Vomiting associated with gastritis or pancreatitis causes metabolic alkalosis. Lactic acidosis can result from seizures, infection, and gastrointestinal or traumatic hemorrhage. (Ethanol intoxication per se does not cause lactic acidosis, although, by inhibiting lactate metabolism, it may prolong it.[111, 112]) These conditions can of course coexist.

Alcoholic ketoacidosis refers to ketosis and an increased anion gap resulting from accumulation of acetoacetate and hydroxybutyrate.[112, 113] Typical patients are young alcoholics who increase their drinking over days or weeks and then stop when overcome by anorexia or vomiting, sometimes caused by gastritis or pancreatitis. Acute starvation for several days is followed by confusion, obtundation, and Kussmaul's respirations, although the depression of consciousness is usually less than occurs with a similar degree of diabetic ketoacidosis. Patients with additional illnesses may have coexisting lactic acidosis. Conversely, coexisting metabolic or respiratory alkalosis can result in a normal or elevated serum pH despite ketosis and anion gap elevation. β-Hydroxybutyrate can predominate over acetoacetate; the nitroprusside test (Acetest) is therefore sometimes negative. The serum glucose level may be low (as a result of starvation and impaired gluconeogenesis) but more often is normal or moderately elevated. Hyperuricemia is common; dehydration increases renal tubular reabsorption of urate and ketones decrease its tubular secretion. The serum potassium level may be normal or low; patients tend to be potassium depleted. Serum insulin levels are often low and serum levels of growth hormone, epinephrine, glucagon, and cortisol are high, yet glucose intolerance usually clears without insulin and is inapparent on recovery. Ethanol is rarely detectable in the blood. Repeated attacks of alcoholic ketoacidosis are common.

The ketosis is caused by increased lipolysis and impaired fatty acid oxidation.[112] Starvation is a major factor; the role of ethanol per se is uncertain. (Normal rat liver slices incubated with ethanol do not display increased ketogenesis, whereas liver slices from rats previously fed ethanol do.[114]) Treatment begins with attention to coexisting serious illness. Ketosis usually responds promptly to intravenous glucose (given with thiamine). Insulin is unnecessary. (On the other hand, if a patient is known to be diabetic, alcoholic ketoacidosis cannot be distinguished from diabetic ketoacidosis, and insulin should be given.[112]) Sodium bicarbonate is also seldom needed, but dehydration and potassium depletion call for saline and potassium salts (including potassium phosphate). Hypocalcemia in excess of hypoalbuminemia may be secondary to hypomagnesemia, which can be corrected with magnesium sulfate.

METHANOL, ETHYLENE GLYCOL, AND ISOPROPANOL INGESTION

Metabolic acidosis with increased anion gap can also occur in alcoholics poisoned by methanol or ethylene glycol. There have been epidemics of methanol poisoning caused by drinking contaminated bootleg spirits; methanol is present in many products, including gasohol, carburetor fluid, duplicator fluid, and windshield washing solution.[115] Although methanol is rapidly absorbed from the gastrointestinal tract, symptoms usually appear only after 12 to 24 hours. Methanol's metabolic products are directly toxic to retinal ganglion cells, and visual blurring, sometimes with yellow spots or central scotomata, can progress to complete blindness and unreactive pupils. Acute optic disk hyperemia and peripapillary edema with engorged retinal veins are then followed by optic atrophy. Other symptoms include headache, dizziness, nausea, vomiting, abdominal pain (often caused by pancreatitis), delirium, seizures, and coma. Respirations become slow, shallow, and gasping. Bradycardia signifies a grave prognosis.[115–117]

Methanol is metabolized by alcohol dehydrogenase to formaldehyde and then to formic acid, which is responsible for the severe anion gap metabolic acidosis.[118] (If hypotension is present, lactic acid contributes.) Treatment is first directed to cardiovascular and respiratory support and gastric emptying. Sodium bicarbonate may have to be given for several days, as acidosis commonly recurs after seemingly successful treatment. Bicarbonate therapy itself can cause hypokalemia. Because the affinity of ethanol for alcohol dehydrogenase greatly exceeds that of methanol, ethanol blocks the conversion of methanol to toxic metabolites. The aim is to achieve a blood ethanol concentration of 100 mg/dL. A usual loading dose is 7.6 to 10 mL/kg 10% ethanol in 5% dextrose intravenously (or 0.8 to 1.0 mL/kg 95% ethanol orally); maintenance dosage is then 1.4 mL/kg/h of 10% ethanol by continuous intravenous drip (or 0.15 mL/kg 95% ethanol orally).[115] Chronic alcoholics and patients receiving hemodialysis require more. Hemodialysis has been recommended for patients with blood methanol levels higher than 50 mg/dL.[115, 116] Folate is also given, as the oxidation of formic acid to carbon dioxide is folate dependent.

Ethylene glycol, found in antifreezes, windshield deicers, and brake fluids, is deliberately drunk as an ethanol substitute.[115] Within a few hours inebriation is followed by nausea,

vomiting, ataxia, nystagmus, ophthalmoparesis, myoclonus, seizures, hypoactive tendon reflexes, and stupor or coma. There may be hypothermia or mild fever. Metabolic acidosis with a marked anion gap is the result of several ethylene glycol metabolites, the most important of which, oxalate, chelates calcium, causing tetany and cardiac symptoms, including pulmonary edema.[115, 116] Calcium oxalate crystals are often (but not always) seen in the urine within a few hours of ethylene glycol ingestion. Their precipitation can lead to renal failure several days later. Treatment begins with gastric emptying and respiratory support. Like methanol, ethylene glycol is metabolized by alcohol dehydrogenase, so ethanol is given. Hemodialysis is recommended for ethylene glycol blood levels higher than 50 mg/dL or when renal failure is present.[115, 116, 119] Forced diuresis can prevent oxalate crystal precipitation, and thiamine and pyridoxine might help to divert ethylene glycol metabolism to products other than oxalate.

Isopropanol, contained in rubbing alcohol as well as household cements, glass cleaners, and windshield deicers, is also an occasional ethanol substitute.[115] Metabolized to acetone, it usually causes ketosis without lactic acidosis.[112] Gastritis, abdominal pain, and vomiting can be prominent, and ataxia, confusion, or coma may ensue. Miosis, decreased tendon reflexes, hypothermia, renal tubular necrosis, myopathy, and hemolytic anemia have been observed. Hypotension is secondary to direct cardiac depression. Treatment is supportive. Gastric emptying is followed by continuous gastric lavage, because isopropanol continues to be secreted into the stomach. Hemodialysis is used for hypotensive or comatose patients.[115, 120] Because isopropanol itself is the major toxin, ethanol is not given.

References

1. Noble EP (ed): Alcohol and Health. Washington, DC, US Government Printing Office, 1978. Third Special Report to the US Congress. Technical Support Document.
2. Ravenholt RT: Addiction mortality in the United States 1980: Tobacco, alcohol, and other substances. Popul Dev Rev 10:697, 1984.
3. Jerrells TR, Eckardt MJ, Weinberg J: Mechanisms of ethanol-induced immunosuppression. In: Seminara D, Watson RR, Pawlowski A (eds): Alcohol, Immunomodulation, and AIDS. New York, Alan R Liss, p 173, 1990.
4. Brust JCM: Drugs and stroke. In: Vinken P, Bruyn CW (ed): Handbook of Clinical Neurology, Volume 45, Cerebrovascular Disease. New York, Elsevier Science Publishers, p 517, 1989.
5. Richie JM: The aliphatic alcohols. In: Gilman AG, Goodman LS, Rall TW, et al (eds): The Pharmacological Basis of Therapeutics. 7th ed. New York, Macmillan Publishing, p 372, 1985.
6. Frezza M, diPadova C, Pozzato G, et al: High blood alcohol levels in women. The role of decreased alcohol dehydrogenase activity and first-pass metabolism. N Engl J Med 322:95, 1990.
7. Charnes ME, Simon RP, Greenberg DA: Ethanol and the nervous system. N Engl J Med 321:442, 1989.
8. Minion GE, Slovis CM, Boutiette L: Severe alcohol intoxication: A study of 204 consecutive patients. J Toxicol Clin Toxicol 27:375, 1989.
9. Koch-Weser J, Sellers EM, Kalant H: Alcohol intoxication and withdrawal. N Engl J Med 294:757, 1976.
10. Davis AR, Lipson AH: Central nervous system depression and high blood ethanol levels. Lancet 1:566, 1986.
11. Isbell H, Fraser HF, Wikler A: An experimental study of the etiology of "rum fits" and delirium tremens. Q J Stud Alcohol 16:1, 1955.
12. Kalant H: Direct effects of ethanol on the nervous system. Fed Proc 34:1930, 1975.
13. Neiman J, Lang AE, Fornazarri L, et al: Movement disorders in alcoholism. A review. Neurology 40:741, 1990.
14. Woodhouse P, Keatings WR, Coleshaw SR: Factors associated with hypothermia in patients admitted to a group of inner city hospitals. Lancet 2:1201, 1989.
15. Victor M: Neurologic disorders due to alcoholism and malnutrition. In: Joynt RJ (ed): Clinical Neurology. Philadelphia, JB Lippincott, p 1, 1986.
16. Loeb JN: The hyperosmolar state. N Engl J Med 290:1184, 1974.
17. Koppanyi T, Canary JJ, Maengwyn-Davis GD: Problems in acute alcohol poisoning. Q J Stud Alcohol 1(suppl):24, 1961.

18. Plum F, Posner JB: The Diagnosis of Stupor and Coma. 3rd ed. Philadelphia, FA Davis, 1980.
19. Suzdak PD, Glowa JR, Crawley JN, et al: A selective imidazobenzodiazepine antagonist of ethanol in the rat. Science 234:1243, 1986.
20. Alkana RL, Parker ES, Cohen HB, et al: Reversal of ethanol intoxication in humans: An assessment of the efficacy of propranolol. Psychopharmacology 51:29, 1976.
21. Alkana RL, Parker ES, Cohen HB, et al: Reversal of ethanol intoxication in humans: An assessment of the efficacy of L-dopa, aminophylline, and ephedrine. Psychopharmacology 55:203, 1977.
22. Alkana RL, Willingham TA, Cohen HB, et al: Apomorphine and amantadine: Interaction with ethanol in humans. Fed Proc 36:331, 1976.
23. Dubocu J: Naloxone and alcohol intoxication. Ann Intern Med 100:618, 1984.
24. Gupta RC, Kofoed J: Toxicological statistics for barbiturates, other sedatives, and tranquilizers in Ontario: A 10-year survey. Can Med Assoc J 94:863, 1966.
25. Gessner PK: Effect of trichloroethanol and of chloral hydrate on the in vivo rate of disappearance of ethanol in mice. Arch Int Pharmacodyn Ther 202:392, 1973.
26. Alcohol-drug interactions. FDA Drug Bull 9:10, 1979.
27. Rada RT, Kellner R, Buckanan JG: Chlordiazepoxide and alcohol: A fatal overdose. J Forensic Sci 20:544, 1975.
28. Interactions of alcohol with drugs. Med Lett 19:47, 1977.
29. Victor M, Adams RD: The effect of alcohol on the nervous system. Assoc Res Nerv Ment Dis 32:526, 1953.
30. Sullivan JT, Sykora K, Schneiderman J, et al: Assessment of alcohol withdrawal: The revised clinical institute withdrawal assessment for alcohol scale (CIWA-Ar). Br J Addict 84:1353, 1989.
31. Victor M, Hope JM: The phenomenon of auditory hallucinations in chronic alcoholism. A critical evaluation of the status of alcoholic hallucinosis. J Nerv Ment Dis 126:451, 1958.
32. Shen WW: Extrapyramidal symptoms associated with alcohol withdrawal. Biol Psychiatry 19:1037, 1984.
33. Carlen PL, Lee MA, Jacob MA, et al: Parkinsonism provoked by alcoholism. Ann Neurol 9:84, 1981.
34. Fornazarri L, Carlen PL: Transient choreiform dyskinesias during alcohol withdrawal. Can J Neurol Sci 9:89, 1982.
35. Balldin J, Alling C, Gottfries CG, et al: Changes in dopamine receptor sensitivity in humans after heavy alcohol intake. Psychopharmacology 86:142, 1985.
36. Earnest MP, Yarnell PR: Seizure admissions to a city hospital: The role of alcohol. Epilepsia 17:387, 1976.
37. Victor M, Brausch CC: The role of abstinence in the genesis of alcoholic epilepsy. Epilepsia 8:1, 1967.
38. Ng SKC, Hauser WA, Brust JCM, et al: Alcohol consumption and withdrawal in new-onset seizures. N Engl J Med 319:666, 1988.
39. Hauser WA, Ng SKC, Brust JCM: Alcohol, seizures, and epilepsy. Epilepsia 29(suppl 2):S66, 1988.
40. Gorelick DA, Wilkins JN: Special aspects of human alcohol withdrawal. Recent Dev Alcohol 4:283, 1986.
41. Chu N-S: Periodic lateralized epileptiform discharges with preexisting focal brain lesion. Role of alcohol withdrawal and anoxic encephalopathy. Arch Neurol 37:551, 1980.
42. Maier DM, Pohorecky LA: The effect of repeated withdrawal episodes on subsequent withdrawal severity in ethanol-treated rats. Drug Alcohol Depend 23:103, 1989.
43. Brown ME, Anton RF, Malcolm R, et al: Alcohol detoxification and withdrawal seizures: Clinical support for a kindling hypothesis. Biol Psychiatry 23:507, 1988.
44. Lechtenberg R, Worner TM: Seizure risk with recurrent alcohol detoxification. Arch Neurol 47:535, 1990.
45. Fisch BJ, Hauser WA, Brust JCM, et al: The EEG response to diffuse and patterned photic stimulation during acute untreated alcohol withdrawal. Neurology 39:434, 1989.
46. Tavel ME, Davidson W, Baterton TD: A critical analysis of mortality associated with delirium tremens. Am J Med 242:18, 1961.
47. Thompson WL: Management of alcohol withdrawal syndromes. Arch Intern Med 138:278, 1978.
48. Liskow BI, Rinck C, Campbell J, et al: Alcohol withdrawal in the elderly. J Stud Alcohol 50:414, 1989.
49. Sandor P, Naranjo CA, Khouw V, et al: Variations in drug free fraction during alcohol withdrawal. Br J Clin Pharmacol 15:481, 1983.
50. Moskowitz G, Chalmers TC, Sacks HS, et al: Deficiencies of clinical trials of alcohol withdrawal. Alcoholism 7:42, 1983.
51. Naranjo CA, Sellers EM: Clinical assessment and pharmacotherapy of the alcohol withdrawal syndrome. Recent Dev Alcohol 4:265, 1986.
52. Whitfield EL, Thompson G. Lamb A, et al: Detoxification of 1024 alcoholic patients without psychoactive drugs. JAMA 293:1409, 1978.
53. Devenyi P, Harrison ML: Prevention of alcohol withdrawal seizures with oral diazepam loading. Can Med Assoc J 132:798, 1985.
54. Greenblatt DJ, Shader RI: Treatment of the alcohol withdrawal syndrome. In: Shader RI (ed): Manual of Psychiatric Therapeutics. Boston, Little, Brown, p 211, 1975.
55. Guthrie SK: The treatment of alcohol withdrawal. Pharmacotherapy 9:131, 1989.
56. Miller JC, McCurdy L: A double-blind comparison of the efficacy and safety of lorazepam and diazepam in the treatment of the acute alcohol withdrawal syndrome. Clin Ther 6:364, 1984.
57. Sellers EM, Naranjo CA, Harrison M, et al: Oral diazepam loading: Simplified treatment of alcohol withdrawal. Clin Pharmacol Ther 34:822, 1983.
58. Thomas DW, Freedman DX: Treatment of the alcohol withdrawal syndrome: Comparison of promazine and paraldehyde. JAMA 188:316, 1964.
59. Muller DJ: A comparison of three approaches to alcohol withdrawal states. South Med J 62:495, 1969.
60. Sereny G, Kalant H: Comparative clinical evaluation of chlordiazepoxide and promazine in treatment of alcohol-withdrawal syndrome. Br Med J 1:92, 1965.
61. Golbert TM, Sanz CJ, Rose HE, et al: Comparative evaluation of treatments of alcohol withdrawal syndromes. JAMA 201:99, 1967.
62. Kaim SC, Klett CJ, Rothfeld B: Treatment of the acute alcohol withdrawal state: A comparison of four drugs. Am J Psychiatry 125:1640, 1969.
63. Kaim SC, Klett CJ: Treatment of delirium tremens: A comparison of four drugs. Q J Stud Alcohol 33:1065, 1972.
64. Sellers EM, Kalant H: Alcohol withdrawal and delirium tremens. In: Pattison EM, Kaufman E (eds): Encyclopedic Handbook of Alcoholism. New York, Gardner Press, p 147, 1982.
65. Linnoila M, Mefford I, Nutt D, et al: Alcohol withdrawal and noradrenergic function. Ann Intern Med 107:875, 1987.
66. Zilm DH, Sellers EM, MacLeod SM, et al: Propranolol effect on tremor in alcohol withdrawal. Ann Intern Med 83:234, 1975.
67. Zilm DH, Jacob MS, MacLeod SM, et al: Propranolol and chlordiazepoxide effects on cardiac arrhythmias during alcohol withdrawal. Alcohol Clin Exp Res 4:400, 1980.
68. Jacob MS, Zilm DH, MacLeod SM, et al: Propranolol-associated confused states during alcohol withdrawal. J Clin Psychopharmacol 3:185, 1983.
69. Bjorkqvist SE: Clonidine in alcohol withdrawal. Acta Psychiatr Scand 52:256, 1975.
70. Wilkins AJ, Jenkins WJ, Steiner JA: Efficacy of clonidine in treatment of alcohol withdrawal state. Psychopharmacology 81:78, 1983.
71. Kraus ML, Gottlieb LD, Horwitz RI, et al: Randomized clinical trial of atenolol in patients with alcohol withdrawal. N Engl J Med 313:906, 1985.
72. Horwitz RI, Gottlieb LD, Kraus ML: The efficacy of atenolol in the outpatient management of the alcohol withdrawal syndrome. Results of a randomized clinical trial. Arch Intern Med 149:1089, 1989.
73. Cushman P Jr, Forbes R, Lerner W, et al: Alcohol withdrawal syndromes: Clinical management with lofexidine. Alcoholism 9:103, 1985.
74. Cushman P Jr, Sowers JR: Alcohol withdrawal syndrome: Clinical and hormonal responses to alpha$_2$-adrenergic agonist treatment. Alcoholism 13:361, 1989.
75. Robinson BJ, Robinson GM, Maling TJ, et al: Is clonidine useful in the treatment of alcohol withdrawal? Alcoholism 13:95, 1989.
76. Lovinger DM, White G, Weight FF: Ethanol inhibits NMDA-activated ion current in hippocampal neurons. Science 243:1721, 1989.
77. Hoffman PL, Rabe CS, Moses F, et al: N-Methyl-D-aspartate receptors and ethanol: Inhibition of calcium flux and cyclic GMP production. J Neurochem 52:1937, 1989.
78. Greenberg DA, Carpenter CL, Messing RO: Ethanol-induced component of ^{45}Ca^{2+} uptake in PC12 cells is sensitive to Ca^{2+} channel modulating drugs. Brain Res 410:143, 1987.
79. Little HJ, Dolin SJ, Halsey MJ: Calcium channel antagonists decrease the ethanol withdrawal syndrome. Life Sci 39:2059, 1986.
80. Koppi S, Eberhardt G, Haller R, et al: Calcium-channel–blocking agent in the treatment of acute alcohol withdrawal—Caroverine versus meprobamate in a randomized double-blind study. Neuropsychobiology 17:49, 1987.
81. Alldredge BK, Lowenstein DH, Simon RP: A placebo-controlled trial of intravenous diphenylhydantoin for the short-term treatment of alcohol withdrawal seizures. Am J Med 87:645, 1989.
82. Alldredge BK, Simon RP: Treatment of alcohol withdrawal seizures with phenytoin. In: Porter RJ, Mattson RH, Cramer JA, et al (eds): Alcohol and Seizures. Basic Mechanisms and Clinical Concepts. Philadelphia, FA Davis, p 290, 1990.
83. Hillbom ME: The prevention of ethanol withdrawal seizures in rats by dipropylacetate. Neuropharmacology 14:755, 1975.
84. Stornebring B: Treatment of alcohol withdrawal seizures with carbamazepine and valproate. In: Porter RJ, Mattson RH, Cramer JA, et al (eds): Alcohol and Seizures. Basic Mechanisms and Clinical Concepts. Philadelphia, FA Davis, p 315, 1990.
85. Chu N-S: Carbamazepine: Prevention of alcohol withdrawal seizures. Neurology 29:1397, 1979.
86. Bjorkqvist SE, Isohanni M, Makela R, et al: Ambulant treatment of alcohol withdrawal symptoms with carbamazepine: A formal multicentre double-blind comparison with placebo. Acta Psychiatr Scand 53:333, 1976.
87. Victor M: The role of hypomagnesemia and respiratory alkalosis in the genesis of alcohol-withdrawal symptoms. Ann NY Acad Sci 215:235, 1973.
88. Meyer JG, Urban K: Electrolyte changes and acid-base balance after

alcohol withdrawal, with special reference to rum fits and magnesium deficiency. J Neurol 215:135, 1977.

89. Thompson WL, Johnson AD, Maddrey WL, et al: Diazepam and paraldehyde for treatment of severe delirium tremens. A controlled trial. Ann Intern Med 82:175, 1975.

90. Reuler JB, Girard DE, Cooney TG: Wernicke's encephalopathy. N Engl J Med 312:1035, 1985.

91. Victor M, Adams RD, Collins GH: The Wernicke-Korsakoff Syndrome. 2nd ed. Philadelphia, FA Davis, 1988.

92. Charness ME, De La Paz RL: Mamillary body atrophy in Wernicke's encephalopathy: Antemortem identification using magnetic resonance imaging. Ann Neurol 22:595, 1987.

93. Mensing JW, Hoogland PH, Sloof JL: Computed tomography in the diagnosis of Wernicke's encephalopathy: A radiological-neuropathological correlation. Ann Neurol 16:363, 1984.

94. Harper CG, Giles M, Finlay-Jones R: Clinical signs in the Wernicke-Korsakoff complex: A retrospective analysis of 131 cases diagnosed at necropsy. J Neurol Neurosurg Psychiatry 49:341, 1986.

95. Jeyasingham MD, Pratt OE, Burns A, et al: The activation of red blood cell transketolase in groups of patients especially at risk from thiamin deficiency. Psychol Med 17:311, 1987.

96. Ross J, Birmingham CL: Wernicke's encephalopathy. N Engl J Med 313:637, 1985.

97. Langlais PJ, Mair RG, McEntee WJ: Acute thiamine deficiency in the rat: Brain lesions, amino acid changes, and MK-801 pretreatment. Soc Neurosci Abstr 14:774, 1988.

98. Isselbacker KJ: Metabolic and hepatic effects of alcohol. N Engl J Med 296:612, 1977.

99. Malouf R, Brust JCM: Hypoglycemia: Causes, neurological manifestations, and outcome. Ann Neurol 17:422, 1985.

100. O'Keefe SJD, Marks V: Lunchtime gin and tonic a cause of reactive hypoglycemia. Lancet 1:1286, 1977.

101. Norris JFB, Robinson A: Post-alcoholic hypoglycemia in a child. Br Med J 1:714, 1976.

102. Miller GM, Baker HL, Okazaki H, et al: Central pontine myelinolysis and its imitators: MR findings. Radiology 168:795, 1988.

103. Norenberg MD, Papendick RE: Chronicity of hyponatremia as a factor in experimental myelinolysis. Ann Neurol 15:544, 1984.

104. Illowsky BP, Laureno R: Encephalopathy and myelinolysis after rapid correction of hyponatremia. Brain 110:855, 1987.

105. Narins RG: Therapy of hyponatremia: Does haste make waste? N Engl J Med 314:1573, 1986.

106. Ayus JC, Krothapalli RK, Arieff AI: Treatment of symptomatic hyponatremia and its relation to brain damage: A prospective study. N Engl J Med 317:1190, 1987.

107. Sterns RH: Severe symptomatic hyponatremia: Treatment and outcome: A study of 64 cases. Ann Intern Med 107:656, 1987.

108. Laureno R, Karp BI: Pontine and extrapontine myelinolysis following rapid correction of hyponatremia. Lancet 1:1439, 1988.

109. Sterns RH, Riggs JE, Schochet SS: Osmotic demyelination syndrome following correction of hyponatremia. N Engl J Med 414:1535, 1986.

110. Kawamura M, Shiota J, Yagishita T, et al: Marchiafava-Bignami disease: Computed tomographic scan and magnetic resonance imaging. Ann Neurol 18:103, 1985.

111. Zaleski J, Bryla J: Ethanol-induced impairment of gluconeogenesis from lactate in rabbit hepatocytes: Correlation with an increased reduction of mitochondrial NAD pool. Int J Biochem 11:237, 1980.

112. Fulop M: Alcoholism, ketoacidosis, and lactic acidosis. Diabetes Metab Rev 5:365, 1989.

113. Goldfrank LR, Starke CL: Metabolic acidosis in the alcoholic. In: Goldfrank LR, Flomenbaum NE, Lewin NA, et al (eds): Toxicologic Emergencies. 3rd ed. Norwalk, CT, Appleton-Century-Crofts, p 435, 1986.

114. Lefevre A, Adler H, Lieber CS: Effect of ethanol on ketone metabolism. J Clin Invest 49:1775, 1970.

115. Litovitz T: The alcohols: Ethanol, methanol, isopropanol, ethylene glycol. Pediatr Clin North Am 33:311, 1986.

116. Goldfrank LR, Flomenbaum NE, Lewin NA, et al: Methanol and ethylene glycol. In: Goldfrank LR, Flomenbaum NE, Lewin NA, et al (eds): Toxicologic Emergencies. 3rd ed. Norwalk, CT, Appleton-Century-Crofts, p 452, 1986.

117. Swartz RD, Millman RP, Billi JE, et al: Epidemic methanol poisoning: Clinical and biochemical analysis of a recent episode. Medicine 60:373, 1981.

118. Sejeersted OM, Jacobsen D, Ovrebo S, et al: Formate concentrations in plasma from patients poisoned with methanol. Acta Med Scand 213:105, 1983.

119. Peterson CD, Collins Aj, Himes JM, et al: Ethylene glycol poisoning: Pharmacokinetics during therapy with ethanol and hemodialysis. N Engl J Med 304:21, 1981.

120. Lacouture PG, Watson S, Abrams A, et al: Acute isopropyl alcohol intoxication: Diagnosis and management. Am J Med 75:680, 1983.

CHAPTER 63

Critical Care Management of Traumatic Brain Injury and Spinal Cord Injury

Fernando G. Diaz

An accurate and complete grasp of the management of the patient with head or spinal injury is essential to anyone interested in critical care. It is fundamental to understand the dynamics of intracranial pressure (ICP) and how it alters cerebral blood flow and cerebral perfusion, the mechanisms of compensation for changes in the ICP and cerebral blood flow, and the different pathologic entities that can affect the brain during or after an injury. Recognition of the different herniation syndromes and management of the patient with craniocerebral trauma are essential in the care of head-injured patients. It is also important to acquire a complete understanding of the mechanisms of injury and pathophysiologic changes that occur during and after an injury to the spinal cord, the associated bone structural abnormalities and their mechanical implications, and the methods of immobilization of the spine and transport of patients. Accurate application of these principles influences the ultimate outcome of patients with a spinal cord injury. A review of these aspects is presented, with emphasis on those of most importance in critical care.

HEAD INJURY

The human skull is a rigid box that contains the brain, cerebrospinal fluid (CSF), and vascular structures. The skull is fully formed and completely fused by 2 years of age, and from then on the only major communication with the extracranial structures is through the foramen magnum. The human brain weighs between 1200 and 1500 g in the adult and has 45 to 60 mL of CSF, including the fluid in the cranial subarachnoid space. The brain is supplied by approximately 1000 to 1200 mL of blood per minute. The brain, blood, and CSF are in a constant state of hemodynamic balance and maintain a constant pressure.[1, 2]

Intracranial Pressure and Blood Flow

The ICP results from the interaction of the static properties of the tissue pressures of the brain, meninges, and vascular structures within the skull; the dynamic forces of the constant blood flow; and the effect that this flow has on the CSF. Under normal basal conditions, the ICP fluctuates between 6 and 10 mm Hg. The amount of blood entering the brain at any given moment is determined by the cerebral perfusion pressure, which can be calculated as the mean systemic arterial pressure minus the mean pressure of the CSF within the ventricles. Under normal conditions, a cerebral perfusion pressure of 50 mm Hg is maintained in spite of fluctuations in the systemic arterial pressure by the mechanism of autoregulation.[1, 2] Autoregulation is mediated by the elastic properties of the arterial vessels, by pH changes in the brain and CSF, and by the response of the vessels to neurogenic sympathetic and parasympathetic influences. Under normal conditions, the autoregulatory mechanisms maintain the cerebral perfusion pressure constant within

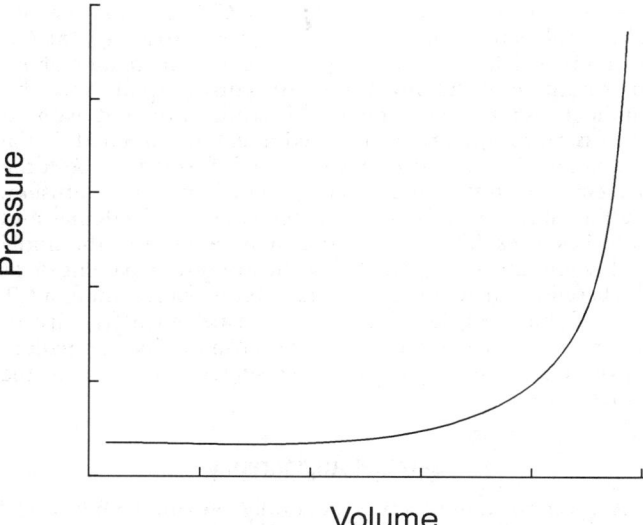

Figure 63–1. Pressure-volume curve. This curve indicates that as long as the volume increases remain within the horizontal portion of the curve, pressure changes are minimal. However, when the changes in volume increase steadily, eventually minor changes in volume produce marked changes in pressure.

ranges of fluctuation of the systemic arterial pressure that extend from 50 to 150 mm Hg mean pressure. Trauma to the central nervous system and other pathologic conditions disrupt the autoregulatory function of the brain and make the changes in perfusion pressure follow in a linear manner the changes in arterial pressure.[1–4] The metabolic component of the autoregulatory function is the most accessible to the clinician because it is tied directly to tissue pH changes. These can easily be influenced by changes in the Pco_2 of the blood. A rise in the Pco_2 is followed by moderate cerebral vasodilatation; conversely, a drop in the Pco_2 causes moderate cerebral vasoconstriction. Local changes in an injured area cause local metabolic acidosis, which in turn renders the area unresponsive to any other systemically induced factors.[1, 2]

Adaptation to Changes in Intracranial Pressure

The intracranial contents are fundamentally brain tissue, blood, and CSF. Any changes in pressure within the skull are compensated by the buffering action of the displacement of CSF out of the cranial cavity. The ability of the brain to accommodate pressure changes is defined by the pressure-volume curve (Fig. 63–1).[2, 3] As a mass develops within the skull, CSF is displaced from the intracranial cavity without much change in ICP; however, when the buffering ability of the CSF is exhausted, similar changes in volume produce drastic changes in ICP. The ability of the brain to accommodate to these changes in volume is also dependent on the time during which the changes occur. Rapidly expanding masses can be accommodated less well than slowly growing ones. This relationship explains why many patients may have large hematomas or tumors and yet be in relatively good clinical condition.[4–7]

Brain Herniation

When all the CSF has been displaced and the accommodating capacity of the brain has been exhausted, shifts of the brain parenchyma take place, leading to the development of herniation syndromes. The most common form of her-

niation is herniation of the cingulate gyrus under the edge of the falx cerebri. A patient with this type of herniation is usually asymptomatic if it does not progress beyond this stage. When the herniation is severe, it can be associated with occlusion of the anterior cerebral artery, which may result in the development of unilateral or bilateral lower extremity paresis. When a laterally placed mass develops on the cerebral cortex, the uncus of the hippocampus may be displaced into and through the edge of the tentorium cerebelli. This is known as transtentorial herniation and is clinically manifested by a progressive decrease in the level of consciousness, ipsilateral dilatation of the pupil, loss of pupillary reflex on the same side, and usually contralateral hemiparesis. In some cases, when the degree of herniation is severe the contralateral cerebral peduncle is compressed on the opposite tentorial edge, producing the "crux phenomenon."[3, 5, 7, 8] This phenomenon is clinically manifested by the development of hemiparesis on the same side as the dilated pupil. When a hemiparesis is found ipsilateral to the side of the mydriasis on a patient suspected of having a space-occupying lesion in the brain, the side of the pupillary dilatation is the diagnostic feature.[3] When the hemiparesis and the pupillary dilatation are on the same side, the intracranial mass is generally on the same side as the dilated pupil.

In some patients with masses that develop in the subtentorial space, the cerebellar tonsils may herniate through the foramen magnum and compress the brain stem. This type of herniation is characteristically rapid in development, manifested by abrupt loss of consciousness, loss of respiration, and rapid development of hypotension. Severe medullary compression may then be followed by cardiac arrest. Some patients present with intermittent events of medullary compression, usually the result of prolonged and gradual intracranial hypertension such as that seen with tumors or chronic subdural hematomas. These patients present with intermittent loss of consciousness and decerebrate posturing, which may be confused with seizure events.[3, 5] It is important not to confuse episodes of decerebration and intermittent loss of consciousness with seizure events. The distinguishing features in episodes of intermittent cerebellar herniation are abrupt loss of consciousness, sudden spontaneous bilateral extensor posturing of the upper and lower extremities, pronator rotation of both upper extremities, and absence of tonic-clonic movements. Intermittent events of cerebellar herniation are grave and should be recognized immediately because they are the harbingers of imminent death caused by medullary compression.

Evaluation of Head Injuries

The initial evaluation of the patient with a head injury can be critical because the outcome of the patient depends on the accuracy with which the initial observations are made and recorded.[3, 5–7] Furthermore, the initial evaluation is frequently the cornerstone of the treatment that is given or withheld from these patients. Depending on the nature of the initial injury, other forms of life-threatening problems may have to be evaluated and treated first. A head injury should take a secondary place to a major thoracoabdominal injury associated with severe blood loss and hypotension. Any form of shock should be thoroughly evaluated and treated first. A rapid neurologic evaluation can easily be conducted even in the most difficult situations, and the extent and possibly the level of neurologic injury can usually be assessed rapidly.

The initial neurologic examination should include a record of the level of consciousness, response to verbal and painful stimuli, ability to use and understand spoken language, and movement of all extremities and a gross assessment of ability to perceive pain and touch throughout the body. All these neurologic functions can be checked in a few minutes; the severity of an injury, as well as the level of neurologic dysfunction, should be documented rapidly.[3, 4] The Glasgow Coma Scale has been used for the initial evaluation and follow-up of head-injured patients in many centers.[3, 4] The scale is based on recording the level of response of the patient in opening his or her eyes, responding verbally, and moving all extremities on command. A scale of 0 to 15 is assigned to rate worst to best responses. The Glasgow Coma Scale is useful as a general screening tool and as a uniform and relatively simple way to record consistently gross neurologic findings. However, because many patients have associated injuries that impair their ability to open their eyes, answer verbally, or move their extremities on command (despite having normal or nearly normal neurologic function), the observations made with the Glasgow Coma Scale must be obtained carefully and must be correlated with associated problems. A prognostic value has been reported for head-injured patients based on the Glasgow Coma Scale; patients with scores lower than 8 are usually considered unlikely candidates for any meaningful recovery.[3, 5–7, 9]

Immediately on admission, all patients with severe traumatic brain injuries require several measures to ensure their survival and safety, including placement of an endotracheal tube, nasogastric tube, Foley's catheter, intravenous lines, and arterial line and all basic laboratory studies, including alcohol and drug screen levels. Care should be taken not to place a nasogastric tube in patients with associated facial injuries because they frequently have fractures of the base of the skull. In patients with such facial injuries, it is necessary to evacuate the stomach contents with an orogastric tube. Further diagnostic studies may be needed to determine the severity and location of possible pathologic problems secondary to the initial injury. Routine skull x-ray and cervical spine films have been criticized because their yield may be limited.[3] However, skull and cervical radiographs should be considered indispensable when a serious neurologic injury is suspected. Many consider that endotracheal intubation should be delayed until good-quality anteroposterior and lateral radiographs of the cervical spine have been obtained to exclude the possibility of a cervical spine fracture or dislocation. In most cases in which the severity of respiratory distress is limited or the need for endotracheal intubation to induce hypocapnia is not urgent, one may wait to place an endotracheal tube until the cervical spine films have been obtained. However, if rapid endotracheal intubation is urgently needed, a decision to place an endotracheal tube must be made and the tube inserted without delay as a lifesaving maneuver. Transnasal intubation can generally be accomplished rapidly, even in an awake and uncooperative patient, with minimal movement of the cervical spine and therefore minimal risk of causing additional injury to the spinal cord. When it becomes necessary to paralyze or to use narcotic or hypnotic medication to accomplish placement of the endotracheal tube, it is generally preferable to wait until the cervical spine films have been obtained and show no evidence of fracture or dislocation including the C-7 to T-1 level.

Computed Tomographic Scan

When the patient is hemodynamically stable and all ancillary forms of support have been instituted, a decision must be made regarding the need for further diagnostic procedures including computed tomographic (CT) scanning, magnetic resonance imaging, and cerebral angiography.[3–5, 7] Usually, any patient who has a head injury that has resulted in

loss of consciousness should have a CT scan to rule out additional pathologic change. The great advantage of CT scanning is that it provides a great deal of information about the condition of the intracranial structures rapidly and with minimal risk to the patient. CT scans with and without contrast infusion are considered ideal for a good initial evaluation. The CT scan may provide information about the presence of intracranial hematomas, cerebral contusion, midline shifts, ventricular symmetry, cerebral edema, and skull fractures. This information may be used in the initial evaluation and treatment of the head-injured patient or as the baseline for follow-up studies. Before performing a CT scan of the head, it is important to rule out a fracture or dislocation of the cervical spine, because placing the patient on the CT scanner generally necessitates movement of the patient's neck.

Cerebral Angiography

A cerebral angiogram is generally obtained after a CT scan, especially for patients in whom a primary vascular injury is considered.[3] When one suspects a carotid dissection or carotid occlusion resulting from direct trauma to the neck or a carotid cavernous fistula or arteriovenous fistula, an angiogram should be obtained. In some centers in which CT scanning is not available, a cerebral angiogram is used as a screening tool to rule out a space-occupying lesion. However, when cerebral angiography is used as the primary diagnostic modality without CT scanning, the accuracy of the diagnosis decreases.[4–6]

Magnetic Resonance Imaging

Magnetic resonance imaging has made it possible to see many lesions that are not observed with conventional CT scanning. Lesions at the level of the brain stem compatible with diffuse axonal injury, multiple small contusions, and diffuse cerebral edema may be appreciated better with magnetic resonance scans. The use of magnetic resonance imaging is limited by the fact that to perform the scan it is necessary not to have any metallic objects in the scanning room. Specially designed respirators are required to allow continued ventilation of the patient in the scanner. Nursing care is difficult when the patient is inside the scanner because the patient is completely covered by the magnetic ring.

Monitoring

Having established the nature and the extent of the intracranial lesion, one may consider the alternatives of medical or surgical management. For patients who do not have a space-occupying lesion and do not urgently need surgical decompression, medical treatment must be conducted in the intensive care unit.[2, 4, 5] These patients are placed under direct hourly supervision by the nursing staff, with continued monitoring of their vital functions and neurologic signs. Monitoring of the arterial blood pressure through an indwelling arterial line and monitoring of cardiac function and cardiopulmonary hemodynamics with a Swan-Ganz catheter are considered essential in most cases.

Monitoring the ICP is also considered fundamental in the management of the severely head-injured patient, although some have questioned its usefulness.[1–5] Many agree that the most reliable form of monitoring ICP is through a ventricular catheter, although other devices such as epidural transducers, subarachnoid bolts or transducers, subarachnoid catheters, cisternal catheters, or intraparenchymal catheters have been used with different degrees of success.

Therapy

A mild degree of dehydration is used in most patients to prevent or control the secondary development of cerebral edema. Dehydrating agents such as mannitol and furosemide are generally used in small but repeated doses in an attempt to control the ICP without producing significant hypovolemia or hemoconcentration.[1, 3, 5, 6] Corticosteroids, which were introduced for the management of patients with cerebral edema secondary to brain tumors, have been used in the management of the head-injured patient. However, their efficacy in reducing cerebral edema or decreasing tissue damage after experimentally induced cerebral injury has not been scientifically supported.[3] Barbiturates have been effective in controlling ICP, but their contribution to the ultimate recovery and survival of patients has not been established through scientific clinical trials.[2] Intravenously administered narcotics, such as small doses of morphine, have been effective not only in controlling agitation and facilitating continued ventilation but also in reducing ICP. The most effective means of controlling the ICP is the use of moderate degrees of hyperventialtion. Maintaining the P_{CO_2} at approximately 31 to 35 mm Hg produces sustained vasoconstriction without causing significant changes in tissue perfusion.[1-4]

Parenteral or enteral nutrition has been added to the management of the severely head-injured patient as a significant factor contributing to recovery.[10] No significant side effects of the additional fluid volume given to these patients have been observed. Parenteral nutrition is considered to provide an increased amount of calories to meet the increased metabolic demands of the patient, to support the patient's immunologic system, to support the continued production of formed elements of the blood, and to provide an anabolic rather than a catabolic state.

Parenteral antibiotics have been recommended for the treatment of patients with compound craniofacial wounds. In most cases a brief course of antibiotics immediately after the injury is considered acceptable. However, the use of prolonged antibiotic coverage in the treatment of patients with fractures involving the paranasal sinuses is not considered acceptable. There is concern that after chronic administration of antibiotics, any secondary infections that developed would be resistant to conventional antibiotics.

Surgical intervention is indicated for patients who have a space-occupying lesion with signs of progressing intracranial hypertension, especially those with shifts in the midline structures or with posterior fossa masses. An operation may also be considered for some patients who have a mass effect secondary to cerebral edema. In these patients, an operation is performed to increase the space in the cranium by removing part of the temporal or frontal pole or to increase space for swelling to expand through a decompressing craniectomy.[3, 5-9] The need for surgical repair of penetrating injuries to the brain, such as those caused by a missile or a puncture wound, should be evident. Likewise, compound fractures of the skull with disruption of the skin overlying the fracture site or penetrating a paranasal sinus demand surgical attention. It is important to note that most cranial injuries with disruption of the skin cause profuse bleeding. However, even though the bleeding may appear to be considerable, this type of hemorrhage is rarely the cause of hypotension or shock. A patient who is in hypovolemic shock with an open cranial wound is considered to have a major thoracoabdominal vascular injury until proved otherwise. The only exceptions to this rule are injuries in infants or in patients with coagulopathies, who may exsanguinate through a cranial wound.[5]

SPINAL TRAUMA

Structure

The length and mobility of the spinal column make it susceptible to injury in many of the activities performed in our daily lives. Flexion-extension forces, acceleration-deceleration forces, and rotational, torque, and compressive forces may play a part individually or in combination in the development of spinal injuries.[11, 12] Fractures and dislocations of the spinal column may occur in many locations but occur most commonly at the arch of the atlas, the dens of the odontoid, the body or dorsal arch of the C-5 and C-6 vertebrae, and the body of the L-1 vertebra. Because the spinal canal and the spinal cord are not matched in length, injuries to the spinal column usually do not correspond anatomically to the level of spinal cord injury.[11] In the cervical region the anatomic levels of the bony landmarks are almost exactly the same as those of the spinal cord, although at the C-7 level there begins to be a tendency for the spinal cord to be shorter than the bony level. In the thoracic spine there is a rapid and progressive mismatch of the anatomic levels for the spinal cord and the vertebrae. The spinal cord ends anatomically at the level of the body of T-12 to L-1. One must be careful when determining the level of injury of the spinal cord, because the neurologic level may not correspond to the vertebral level.[11, 12]

Clinical Evaluation

Determining the level of neurologic dysfunction and the presence or absence of pathologic reflexes is fundamental in evaluating the patient with a spinal injury. In most cases, the level of neurologic injury can be determined in a few minutes by checking the following: presence of spontaneous or induced movement of various muscle groups in the upper and lower extremities, presence of deep tendon reflexes in all four extremities, preservation of pain and tactile sensation throughout the body, preservation of response to deep pain, and preservation of rectal sensation and anal sphincter tone. As general guidelines, the motor levels may be remembered by counting from 1 to 8: S1-2 mark the function of the gastrocnemius, L3-4 the quadriceps femoris, C5-6 the biceps, and C7-8 the triceps. Sensory levels to remember are C-5 at the shoulder, C-6 lateral arm and thumb, C-7 middle finger, C-8 fifth finger, T-4 nipple line, T-10 umbilicus, L-4 anterior thigh, L-5 lateral leg and dorsum of foot, and S-1 lateral foot. Sphincter tone and perianal sensation are controlled by S2-4. A rectal examination is a mandatory part of the neurologic examination, especially in patients with suspected complete spinal cord injuries.[11]

When the level of injury has been determined by clinical examination, spinal radiographs must be obtained to document the presence of fractures or dislocations. Questionable areas of instability may require special dynamic views, which should be obtained only in the presence of a neurosurgeon knowledgeable of the problem. Serial laminograms, CT scans with and without contrast enhancement, and myelograms may be required to document further the level of injury and the possible existence of spinal canal blocks.[11]

Clinical Management

All patients suspected of having a cervical or thoracic spinal cord injury should receive a nasogastric tube and a Foley catheter because the development of gastric atony may be followed by regurgitation and aspiration; loss of bladder function may result from massive dilatation of the bladder wall. All patients should be immediately immobilized on a firm surface, preferably a fracture board.[12] Patients with cervical spine injuries may be temporarily supported with sandbags placed on either side of the neck but preferably should be held by skeletal fixation in the form of Gardner-Wells tongs placed by a neurosurgeon.[12] When the patient has been immobilized by skeletal fixation, the fracture board may be removed and the patient placed either on a rotokinetic bed or a low-pressure bed.

It is important to remember that patients with spinal cord injury frequently experience a period of spinal shock characterized by inability to control all autonomic functions, especially blood pressure. Abrupt and severe episodes of hypotension may be observed in these patients when they are placed in a sitting or a vertical position soon after their injury. Many patients with cervical cord injury develop respiratory insufficiency that requires temporary artificial respiratory assistance. The respiratory insufficiency in these patients results from total loss of function of all respiratory muscles except the diaphragm. Eventually the diaphragm becomes strong enough to take over the entire respiratory function, but this requires a period of training and adaptation. A tracheostomy is frequently necessary for these patients to assist in their respiratory toilet and to decrease the workload associated with the tracheal dead space.

There is no proven medical or surgical therapy of value in the management of the patient with a spinal cord injury. All maneuvers suggested are intended to prevent any further loss of neurologic function caused by inappropriate manipulation of the patient or the development of spinal cord edema or hemorrhage.[11, 12] Some patients may benefit from surgical removal of disk fragments compressing the nerve roots, but in general any surgical procedure used to decompress the spinal cord has been unsuccessful.[11] In a multicenter study it was found that when large doses of methylprednisolone were administered to patients with spinal cord injuries soon after the injury, there was some improvement in some patients when re-evaluated after several months. The improvement was limited and the number of patients who improved was also limited. It is necessary to follow up these patients longitudinally and study larger numbers of patients before we can assume that methylprednisolone is indeed beneficial to all patients with acute spinal cord injuries.[13] Early surgical stabilization is now recommended to facilitate rapid mobilization and early rehabilitation.

The most valuable therapeutic tool is early institution of rehabilitation methods, which are frequently limited by unwillingness of the patient or the family members to accept the irreversibility of most of these devastating injuries. The sooner the patient and the family recognize and accept that the injury is final and that any recovery of function depends on the active process of rehabilitation, the better the long-term result and adaptation.[11]

References

1. Miller JD, Garibe J, North JB, et al: Effects of increased arterial pressure on blood flow in the damaged brain. J Neurol Neurosurg Psychiatry 38:657, 1975.
2. Saul TG, Ducker TB: Effect of intracranial pressure monitoring and aggressive treatment on mortality in severe head injury. J Neurosurg 56:498, 1982.
3. Jane JA, Rimel RW, Pobereskin LH, et al: Outcome and pathology of head injury. In: Grossman RG, Gildenberg PO (eds): Head Injury: Basic and Clinical Aspects. New York, Raven Press, p 229, 1982.
4. Jennett B, Teasdale G: Management of Head Injuries. Philadelphia, FA Davis, p 290, 1981.
5. Becker DP, Miller JD, Ward JD, et al: The outcome from severe head injury with early diagnoses and intensive management. J Neurosurg 47:491, 1977.
6. Egennarelli PA, Spielman GM, Langfitt TW, et al: The influence of the type of intracranial lesion on outcome from severe head injury: A multicenter study. J Neurosurg 56:26, 1982.
7. Jane JA, Rimel RW: Prognoses in head injury. Clin Neurosurg 19:346, 1982.
8. Seelig JM, Becker DP, Miller JD, et al: Traumatic subdural hematoma: Major mortality reduction in comatose patients treated within four hours. N Engl J Med 304:1511, 1981.
9. Langfitt TW: Measuring the outcome from head injury. J Neurosurg 48:673, 1978.
10. Clifton GL, Hodge S, Robertson CS, et al: Nutritional management of patients with severe head injury. In: Dacey RG Jr et al (eds): Trauma of the Central Nervous System. New York, Raven Press, p 350, 1985.
11. Osterholm JL: The Pathophysiology of Spinal Cord Trauma. Springfield, IL, Charles C Thomas, 1978.
12. Rimel RW, Edlich RF, Winn HR, et al: Acute Care of the Head and Spinal Cord Injured Patient at the Site of Injury. Charlottesville, University of Virginia Press, 1978.
13. Bracken MB: Spinal Cord Injury National Cooperative Study. N Engl J Med 255:450, 1990.

SECTION SIX

The Pulmonary System

Section Editor

Mark A. Kelley

Mechanical Properties of the Respiratory System

Michael A. Grippi

Hypercapnic respiratory failure, a clinically important entity in virtually all medical intensive care units, arises when there is disruption of neural or muscular output anywhere along the efferent pathway from the central nervous system to the respiratory pump mechanism.[1, 2] Neuromuscular fatigue is a common underlying etiology that frequently occurs in the setting of severe mechanical alterations of the respiratory system. This chapter focuses on normal respiratory system mechanics. Consideration is also given to important changes that take place in disease states, with emphasis on the concept that mechanical alterations arising from pathologic processes, such as inflammation and fibrosis, infection, and bronchospasm, result in a dissociation between the work demands placed on the respiratory pump and its output capacity. First, an overview of the functional design of the airways is given. Next, important respiratory pressures and pressure gradients are defined in order to provide a basis for understanding the pertinent elastic and flow-resistive properties. Particular attention is devoted to an analysis of the dynamics of airflow, including expiratory airflow limitation. The relevance of regional variations in dynamic lung function is also described. Finally, the concept of work of breathing is highlighted, and its relationship to airway resistance and respiratory system compliance is underscored. All of the principles developed are important in understanding alterations in disease states and the physiologic effects of mechanical ventilation on the respiratory system.

OVERALL DESIGN OF THE AIRWAYS

The airways can be viewed as a series of dichotomously branching tubes in which each parent branch divides into two smaller daughter branches. A number of "generations" of airways is thereby created. The daughter branches in a given generation may differ in diameter or length; that is, the dichotomy is irregular. However, in general, the diameters of the daughter branches are smaller than those of the parent branch.

Mean airway diameter may be expressed mathematically as

$$d(z) = d_0 \times 2^{-z/3} \qquad (1)$$

where $d(z)$ = mean diameter of airways in generation z
 d_0 = diameter of the trachea

According to this scheme,[3] the trachea is considered as generation 0 and each generation of daughter branches is designated successively (Fig. 64–1). Mean airway diameter decreases progressively with each generation until the acinar airways are reached (acinar airways are the respiratory bronchioles, alveolar ducts, alveolar sacs, and alveoli). Thereafter, mean airway diameter decreases less than predicted by this formula, a factor that contributes to enhanced diffusion in the gas-exchanging regions of the lung (Fig. 64–2).

Although individual airway cross-sectional area decreases in successive generations, the total cross-sectional area of each generation increases. This effect is exaggerated in the acinar airways, because the progressive decreases in mean airway diameter are less than for previous generations. A plot of total airway cross-sectional area versus airway generation (Fig. 64–3) demonstrates the so-called trumpet model, the hallmark of which is an expansive increase in area at the end of the gas pathway.[4] As gas movement changes from primarily bulk flow in the larger airways to diffusion in the smaller airways, the greatly increased cross-sectional area and shorter airway lengths facilitate the process. With this simple design in mind, an analysis of the fundamental pressure relationships in the respiratory system forms the basis of understanding normal respiratory mechanics.

PRESSURE RELATIONSHIPS IN THE RESPIRATORY SYSTEM

In a spontaneously breathing subject, the formation of a pressure gradient between alveoli and atmosphere results in gas flow into and out of the alveoli. Similarly, in a mechanically ventilated patient, gas flow develops as a pressure gradient is created between the gas source (the ventilator) and the alveoli. The characteristics of the flow, including flow rate, flow pattern, and gas distribution, depend fundamentally on the mechanical properties of the airways, lungs, and chest wall.

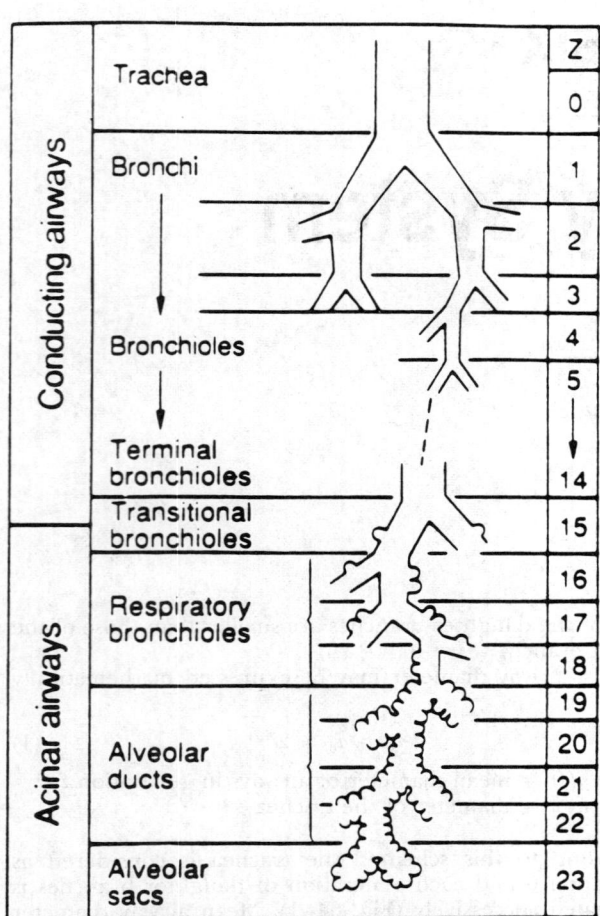

Figure 64–1. Dichotomous branching of human airways. Conducting and acinar airways are depicted; airway generations (z) are designated in the column on the right. (From Weibel EW: Geometry and dimensions of airways of conductive and transitory zones. In: Morphometry of the Human Lung. New York, Springer-Verlag, p 111, 1963.)

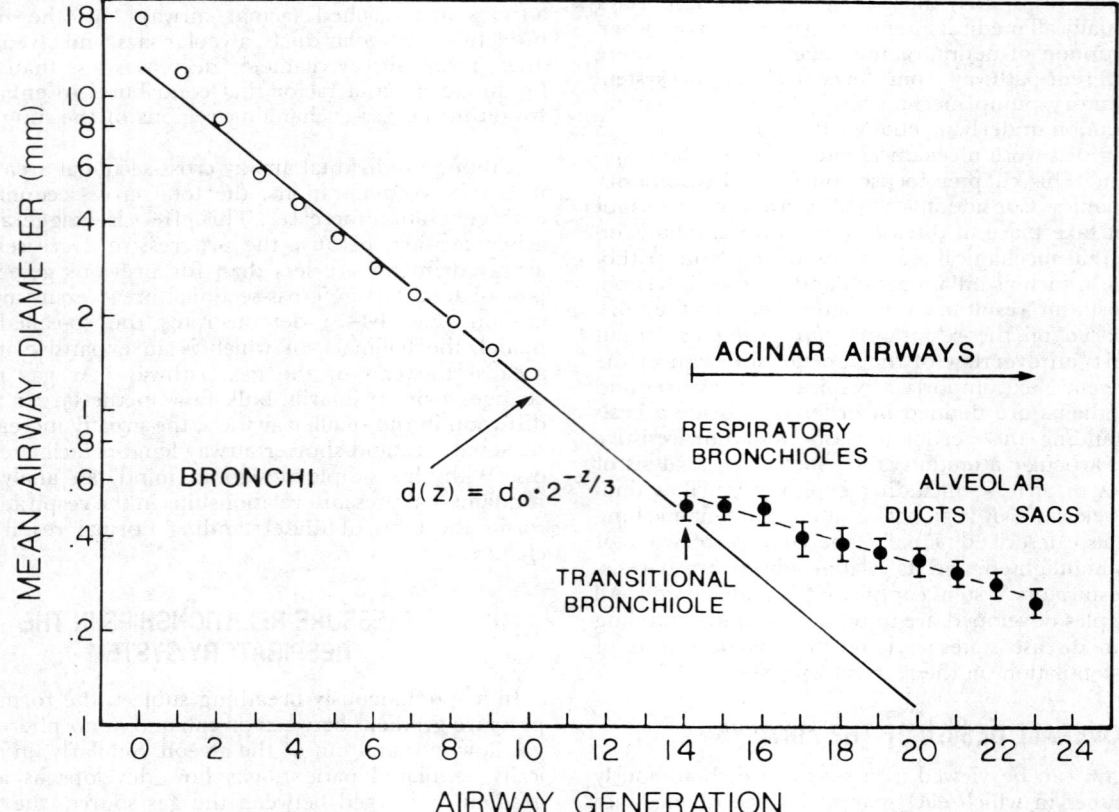

Figure 64–2. Semilogarithmic plot of mean airway diameter versus airway generation. The progressive decrease in mean airway diameter of the acinar airways is less than predicted by the formula given. See text for discussion. (From Haefeli-Bleuer B, Weibel ER: Morphometry of the human pulmonary acinus. Anat Rec 220:413, 1988. Copyright © 1988. Reprinted by permission of Wiley-Liss, a division of John Wiley & Sons, Inc.)

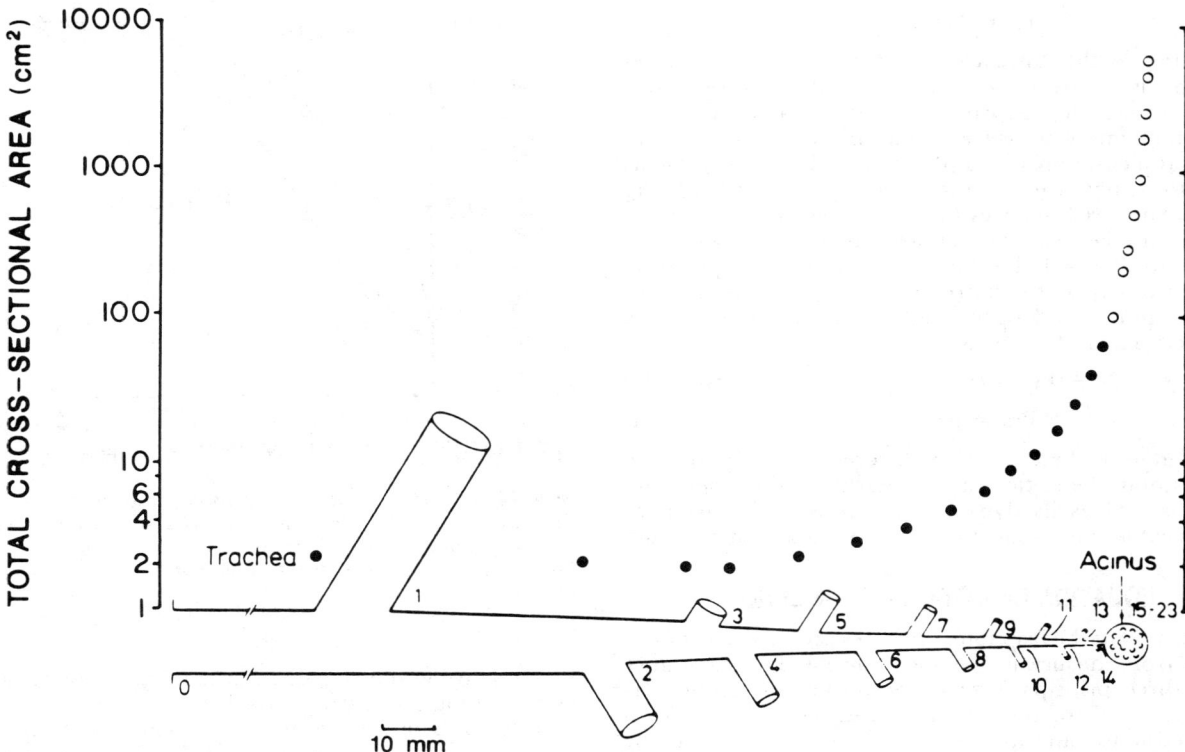

Figure 64–3. Plot of total airway cross-sectional area (logarithmic scale) versus airway generation. Conducting airways are drawn to scale along the abscissa. Filled circles represent the conducting airways; open circles represent the acinar airways. The marked increase in total cross-sectional area at the level of the acinar airways is evident. (From Weibel EW: Design of airways and blood vessels considered as branching trees. In: Crystal RG, West JB [eds]: The Lung: Scientific Foundations. New York, Raven Press, p 717, 1991.)

Figure 64–4 depicts schematically the important pressures and pressure gradients determining flow in the respiratory system. Under normal circumstances, the pressure at the airway opening (Pawo) is atmospheric; that is, Pawo = 0 cm H_2O. Similarly, the pressure surrounding the thoracic cage—the pressure at the body surface (Pbs)—is also atmospheric; Pbs = 0 cm H_2O. The pleural pressure (Ppl) is determined by the magnitudes and directions of forces generated by the elastic lung parenchyma and chest wall. Its measurement can be approximated using an intraesophageal balloon catheter.[5] The elastic recoil pressure of the lung (Pel) is always directed inward, favoring lung deflation. The magnitude of Pel depends on the degree of lung inflation. In contrast, the direction of the chest wall recoil pressure depends on inflation volume; it is directed outward at lung volumes below

two thirds of the inspired vital capacity and inward as total lung capacity (TLC) is approached. The relationship between lung and chest wall elastic recoil pressures at various inflation volumes is discussed in the following.

Alveolar pressure (PA) is the pressure within the alveoli at any time in the respiratory cycle. At end inspiration and end expiration PA is atmospheric; hence, at these times there is no pressure gradient for airflow into, or out of, the lungs. In a spontaneously breathing subject, PA is negative during inspiration and positive during expiration. In a patient on positive pressure mechanical ventilation (without positive end-expiratory pressure), PA ranges from 0 to a positive value, which is maximal at peak inflation. The alveolar pressure is equal to the sum of the elastic recoil pressure of the lung and the pleural pressure:

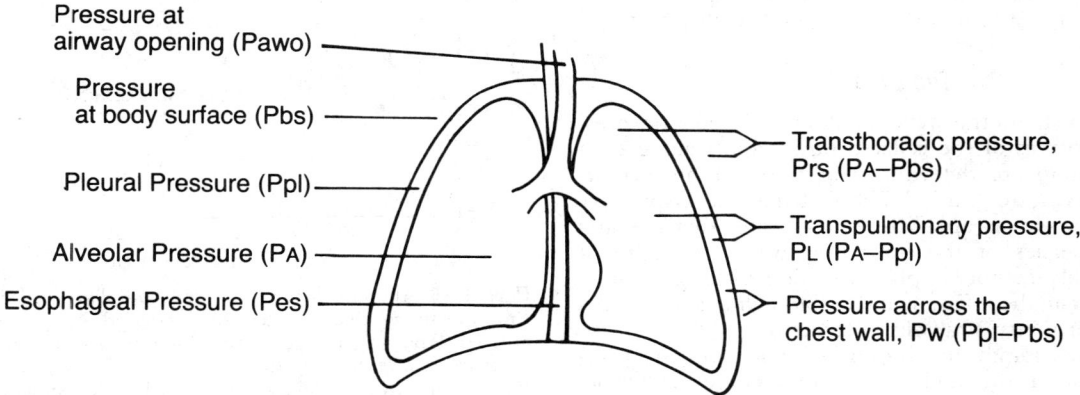

Figure 64–4. Schematic of respiratory system showing pressures and pressure gradients important in respiratory mechanics.

$$PA = Pel + Ppl \qquad (2)$$

In addition to the "primary" pressure measurements depicted in Figure 64–4, several important pressure differences are shown. PL, the pressure difference across the lung, or transpulmonary pressure, is the difference between alveolar and pleural pressures (PL = PA − Ppl). It represents the pressure necessary to maintain a given level of lung inflation. Similarly, the pressure across the chest wall, Pw, is the difference between pleural pressure and pressure at the body surface (Pw = Ppl − Pbs). The transthoracic pressure, or pressure across the entire respiratory system (Prs), is, both conceptually and algebraically, the sum of the pressure differences across the lung and the chest wall:

$$Prs = PL + Pw = (PA − Ppl) + (Ppl − Pbs) \qquad (3)$$

$$Prs = PA − Pbs \qquad (4)$$

Knowledge of these pressure differences is important in understanding the static, elastic behavior of the respiratory system, as well as its dynamic, flow-resistive behavior, as summarized in the so-called equation of motion of the lung.

EQUATION OF MOTION OF THE LUNG

Contraction of the inspiratory muscles produces a pressure gradient from the airway opening to alveoli. For inspiratory airflow, three principal resistances must be overcome: (1) the elastic recoils of the lung and chest wall, (2) frictional airway resistance, and (3) the inertial resistances offered by the gas within the airways and the lung and chest wall. Each of these terms is represented in the equation of motion of the lung:[6]

$$Ptot = (E × V) + (Raw × \dot{V}) + (I × \ddot{V}) \qquad (5)$$

where
Ptot = total pressure generated across the respiratory system
E = elastance
V = inflation volume
Raw = airway resistance
$\dot{V}$ = airflow rate
I = inertance
$\ddot{V}$ = rate of acceleration of airflow

Under normal ambient conditions, inertance (I) is small; hence the last term of the equation is insignificant. The pressure gradient required for lung inflation can then be described in terms of a static, elastic component (E × V), and a dynamic, flow-resistive component (Raw × $\dot{V}$).

Elastic Properties of the Respiratory System

Although the lungs and chest wall are functionally coupled through the pleural space, for analysis of respiratory mechanics it is simplest to first dissociate the two structures.[7, 8]

The Lung

Figure 64–5 shows the static inflation and deflation pressure-volume curves of the isolated lung. Points along each limb of the loop are determined at times of no airflow; hence the curves are "static." The fact that the inspiratory and expiratory curves are different indicates that the mechanical properties of the lung vary with the phase of respiration and are not simply a function of lung volume. The difference in the inflation and deflation limbs represents hysteresis, a property of all elastic structures.

An additional important finding evident from the pressure-volume plot is the nonlinearity of the curves. In particular, the slopes of the curves decrease at higher lung volumes. The slope, a measure of the change in lung vol-

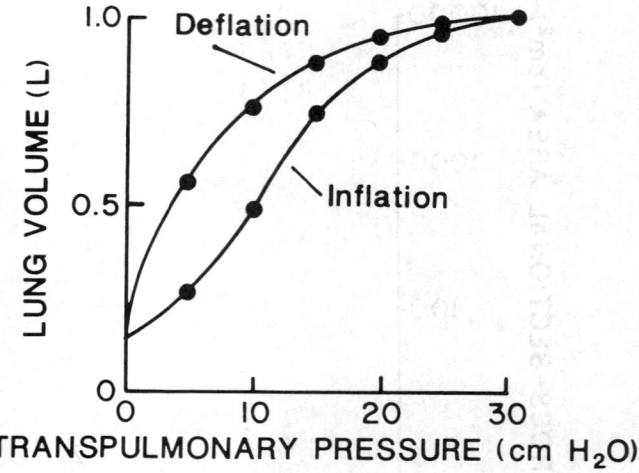

Figure 64–5. Static inflation and deflation pressure-volume curves of the isolated lung. As progressive increases in transpulmonary pressure are applied, lung volume or, more appropriately, changes in lung volume, are measured at times of no airflow. See text for details.

ume relative to the change in distending pressure, is known as static lung compliance, which has a normal value of 0.2 L/cm H_2O. The decline in lung compliance at higher lung volumes indicates decreased distensibility. Generally, compliance is measured on the expiratory limb of the pressure-volume curve over the range of resting lung volume or functional residual capacity (FRC) plus 0.5 L.[9] The reciprocal of static lung compliance is elastance (E), which appears in the equation of motion of the lung.

Various pathologic conditions, including many seen in critically ill patients, produce significant alterations in lung compliance (Fig. 64–6).[10, 11] For example, emphysema, characterized pathologically by destruction of parenchymal connective tissue components, results in a high lung compliance. Conversely, interstitial edema, pulmonary fibrosis, and alveolar filling processes (e.g., lung hemorrhage and pneumonia) produce reduced lung compliance.

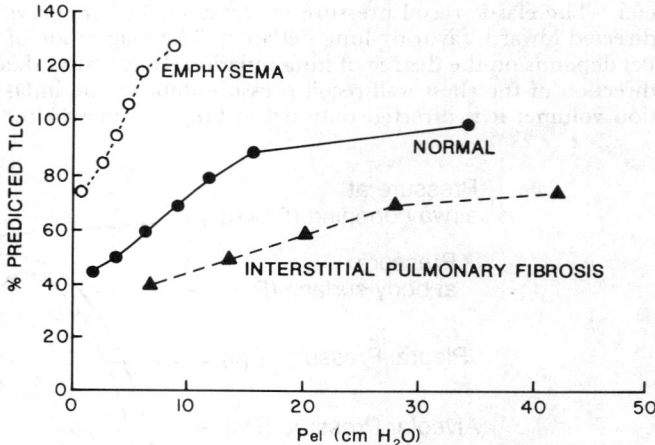

Figure 64–6. Alterations in static lung compliance in disease states. Emphysema is characterized by increased lung compliance (increased slope) and a larger lung volume for a given transpulmonary pressure (curve shifted upward and to the left). With interstitial fibrosis and alveolar filling processes, lung compliance is reduced (decreased slope) and lung volume is diminished for a given transpulmonary pressure (curve shifted downward and to the right).

Under static conditions, with the airway open to the atmosphere, alveolar pressure is zero; consequently, transpulmonary pressure, the distending pressure used in calculating lung compliance, equals the pleural pressure, which, in turn, equals the static elastic recoil pressure. Several factors determine static elastic recoil pressure, including the properties of the connective tissue constituents of the lung parenchyma, surface tension in alveoli, and lung volume. The greater the lung volume, the greater the degree of stretch and, hence, the higher the static elastic recoil pressure.

The Chest Wall

From a mechanics perspective, the chest wall includes the bony thorax, intercostal muscles, overlying soft tissues, parietal pleura, diaphragm, and abdominal wall. At FRC the chest wall generates an outwardly directed recoil pressure which is counterbalanced by the inwardly directed elastic recoil of the lung (see Pressure Relationships in the Respiratory System). The offsetting of these oppositely directed forces results in the respiratory system coming to rest at FRC and remaining at that lung volume until inspiratory or expiratory muscles contract (with the airway open).

With activation of the muscles of inspiration, lung volume expands beyond FRC and the elastic recoil of the chest wall decreases. At approximately 60% of TLC, chest wall elastic recoil drops to zero and, with further inflation, chest wall recoil becomes inwardly directed.[12] In this range, the elastic recoils of the lung and chest wall become additive (i.e., are in the same direction). When expiratory muscles contract and decrease lung volume below FRC, outwardly directed chest wall recoil increases and opposes the lung elastic recoil.

Various clinically significant disorders result in decreases in chest wall compliance. Examples are extreme obesity, kyphoscoliosis, and extensive pleural fibrosis.

The Intact Respiratory System

When the lungs and chest wall are considered in unison, volume changes created by inspiratory or expiratory muscle activity may be related to pressure changes across the entire respiratory system, as noted in Equations 3 and 4. The compliance curve of the respiratory system is the composite of the compliance curves of the lung and chest wall (Fig. 64–7).[7, 8, 12] As noted previously, in the setting of mechanical ventilation it is respiratory system compliance, rather than lung compliance, that is measured. For patients in whom pathologic changes in the lungs develop without coincidental changes in the chest wall, the assumption is that alterations in the measured compliance of the respiratory system represent changes in lung compliance. Normal respiratory system compliance is approximately 0.1 L/cm H_2O.[12] It can be measured easily in a mechanically ventilated patient as the inflation volume divided by the distending pressure, also known as the plateau pressure. The plateau pressure is determined by momentarily interrupting exhalation (e.g., by occluding the exhalation tubing), thereby creating static or no-flow conditions. Reductions in respiratory system compliance are seen in a variety of acute and chronic disorders in patients undergoing mechanical ventilation—for example, progressive adult respiratory distress syndrome, the development of pulmonary edema, and pneumothorax.

Static respiratory system compliance must be distinguished from dynamic compliance (Cdyn), measured as the inflation volume divided by peak inflation pressure. Cdyn depends on airway resistance, as well as the static elastic properties of the respiratory system; consequently, it is affected by a variety of other factors that are potentially operative during

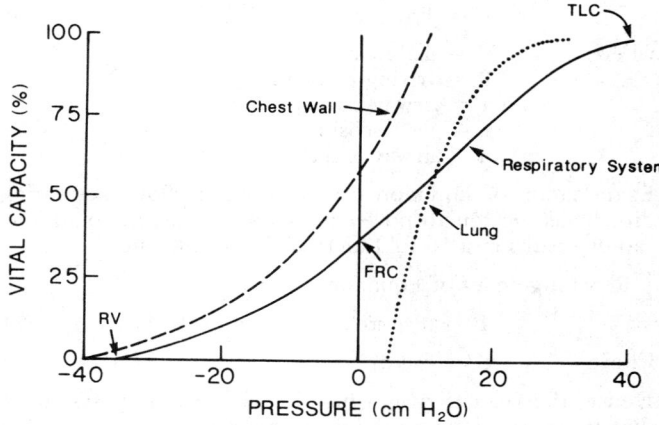

Figure 64–7. Pressure-volume curves for the chest wall, lung, and respiratory system (chest wall and lung). Volume is expressed as percentage of vital capacity. For the chest wall curve, the pressure expressed on the abscissa is the pressure across the chest wall (Ppl − Pbs). For the lung curve, the pressure is transpulmonary pressure (PA − Ppl). For the respiratory system, the pressure is transthoracic pressure (PA − Pbs). RV = residual volume. See text for details.

mechanical ventilation. For example, the development of increased airway resistance as a result of bronchospasm or mucus plugging results in a reduction in Cdyn (reflected in an increased peak inflation pressure).[13]

Flow-Resistive Properties of the Respiratory System

Thus far, only the static mechanical properties of the respiratory system have been considered. However, during inspiration and expiration, the dynamic properties of the airways, lung parenchyma, and chest wall become important in determining lung inflation and deflation. Once again, analysis of the equation of motion of the lung indicates the terms involved:

$$Ptot = (E \times V) + (Raw \times \dot{V}) + (I \times \ddot{V})$$

The second term, $(Raw \times \dot{V})$, denotes the component of the driving pressure for airflow between the airway opening and alveoli necessary to overcome airway resistance (Raw) and to produce airflow at a given rate $(\dot{V})$. In both spontaneously breathing and mechanically ventilated patients, the pressure gradient for expiratory airflow is created by the elastic recoil pressures of the lung and chest wall generated during the previous inspiration.

It is useful to consider the types of airflow seen in the lung and then to analyze, individually, the components of airway resistance.

Types of Airflow in the Lung

Once again the tracheobronchial tree is considered as a system of dichotomously branching tubes, and three patterns of airflow may, at least theoretically, be described: laminar, turbulent, and transitional.[14]

Laminar airflow (Fig. 64–8A) consists of streamlines of gas moving parallel to one another along the long axis of a tube. Because the tube walls offer frictional resistance to the flow of gas, the streamlines in the center of the tube move faster than the lateral ones, creating a parabolic front. Laminar airflow prevails at low flow rates. The velocity of gas in a laminar flow system is calculated according to Poiseuille's law:

$$\dot{V} = (P\pi r^4)/8\eta l \qquad (6)$$

where
$\dot{V}$ = airflow rate
P = driving pressure
r = airway radius
η = gas viscosity
l = airway length

Examination of Equation 6 reveals that airflow rate varies directly as the fourth power of airway radius; doubling the radius results in a 16-fold increase in airflow rate.

Rearrangement of Equation 6 yields

$$P = (8\eta l/\pi r^4) \times \dot{V} = K \times \dot{V} \qquad (7)$$

where
$K = 8\eta l/\pi r^4$

Hence, the velocity of gas flow in a laminar flow system is directly proportional to the driving pressure.

Turbulent airflow (see Fig. 64–8B), typically seen in airways with high airflow rates (e.g., the trachea), is characterized by more disordered movement of gas. In such a system, the driving pressure for gas flow is approximately proportional to the square of the velocity of flow. Gas density is also an important determinant of flow rate in a turbulent flow system. Clinically, advantage is taken of this relationship

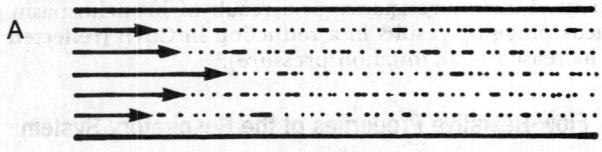

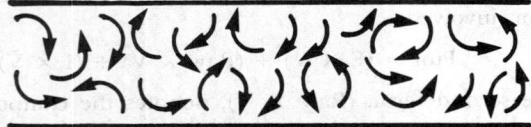

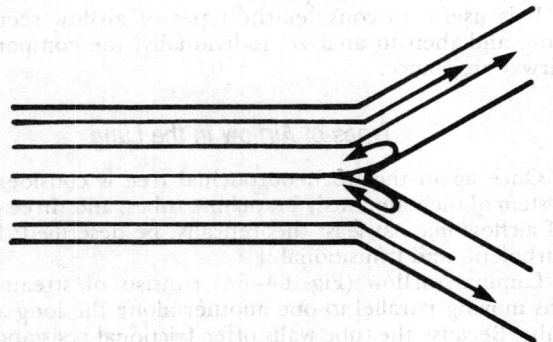

Figure 64–8. Airflow patterns in rigid tubes. *A.* Laminar pattern. The flow profile is parabolic; flow rate is described by Poiseuille's law. *B.* Turbulent pattern. Driving pressure is approximately proportional to the square of velocity of flow. *C.* Transitional pattern. Relatively orderly flow is disrupted at bifurcation points in the system.

with the use of helium-oxygen gas mixtures (heliox) in the management of upper airway obstruction. Because the flow-related pressure drop across a narrowed airway is density dependent (because flow is turbulent), inhalation of heliox, which has a lower density than room air–oxygen mixtures, results in a decrease in the work of breathing and relief of dyspnea.

Whether flow through a system is laminar or turbulent is predicted by calculating the Reynolds number, a unitless measure determined as follows:

$$Re = 2r\dot{V}d/\eta \qquad (8)$$

where
Re = Reynolds number
r = airway radius
$\dot{V}$ = velocity of gas flow
d = gas density
η = gas viscosity

Turbulent airflow is generally observed when the Reynolds number is greater than 2000.

Although this simple categorization of flow patterns in the lung is useful from a conceptual standpoint, the actual patterns are more complicated. Because the airways are a series of branched tubes with asymmetric bifurcations, varying diameters, and irregular walls, eddy formation occurs, creating so-called transitional flow (see Fig. 64–8C). Transitional flow prevails throughout most of the bronchial tree.

Airway Resistance

As indicated in the equation of motion of the lung, airway resistance is a key variable in determining airflow rate in the lung. The normal value for airway resistance is 1.6 cm H_2O/L/s. The two principal components of airway resistance are the frictional component offered by the walls of the tracheobronchial tree and the resistance to convective acceleration. Convective acceleration is the acceleration of a gas as it is funneled through a series of adjoining tubes in which the total cross-sectional area progressively decreases (Fig. 64–9). In such a system, gas must be accelerated during expiration to maintain constancy of airflow rate.[15]

Airway resistance is not homogeneous throughout the respiratory system[16] (Fig. 64–10). With pure nasal breathing, the nose contributes approximately 50% of the total airway resistance. During mouth breathing, the pharynx and larynx contribute about 25% of the resistance. Within the chest, the trachea and lobar and segmental bronchi are responsible for 80% of intrathoracic airway resistance; peripheral airways (<2 mm in diameter) contribute the remaining 20%.[17] Figure 64–10 indicates that airway resistance falls significantly in the periphery of the lung. Although the peripheral airways have smaller diameters and smaller cross-sectional areas than the central airways, the total cross-sectional area progressively increases toward the periphery (see Overall Design of the Airways).

Although airway diameter may be altered significantly in disease states, a number of other factors normally influence this variable. An important one is lung volume[18] (Fig. 64–11). As lung volume increases, airway diameters enlarge because of a tethering effect of the elastic lung parenchyma around the airways. Consequently, airway resistance falls. Figure 64–11 also demonstrates the reciprocal relationship between airway resistance and airway conductance, the latter increasing with increasing lung volume.

Finally, several other variables that influence resistance are worth noting. They include airway length, the presence of airway secretions, and other obstructing endobronchial lesions. In addition, airflow rate itself affects resistance—as flow rate increases, resistance increases.

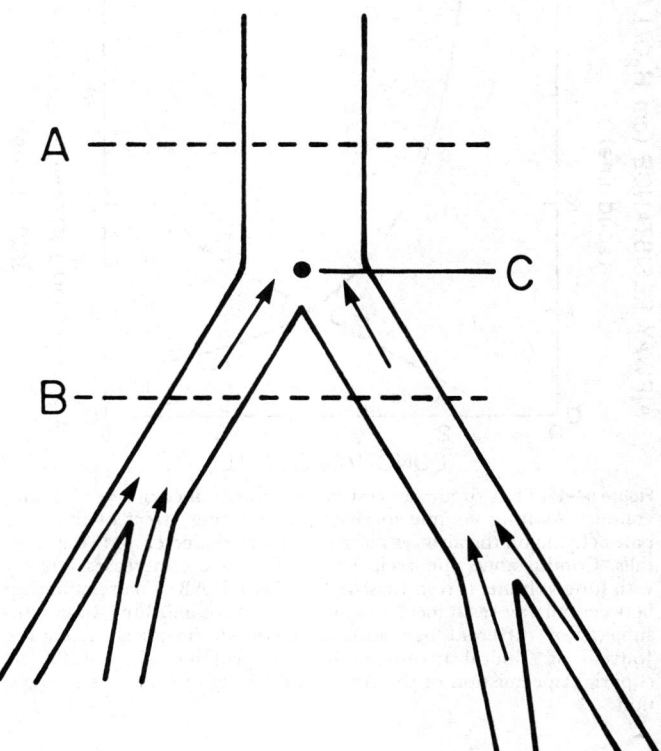

Figure 64–9. Concept of convective acceleration. As gas flow proceeds through a system of adjoining tubes in which total cross-sectional area progressively decreases (total cross-sectional area at level A less than at level B), the gas must be accelerated at junction points (C) to maintain overall constancy of flow rate. An additional pressure drop in the system is thereby created.

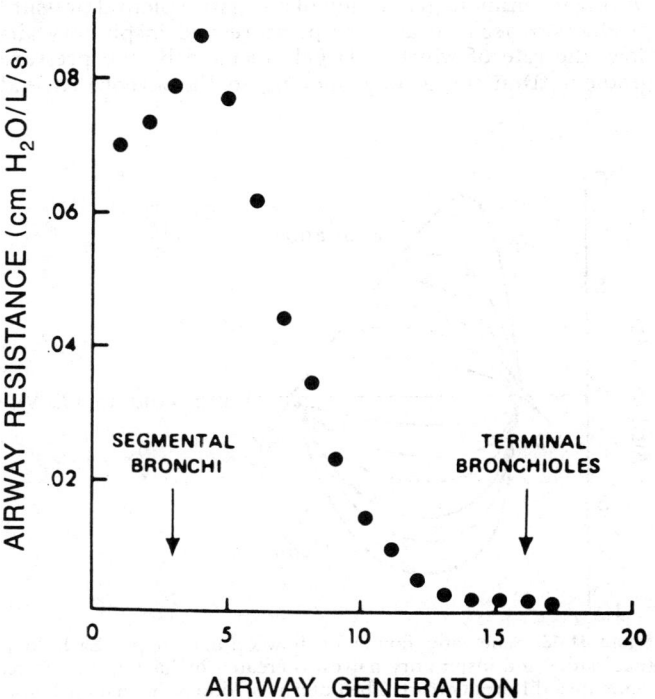

Figure 64–10. Relationship between airway resistance and airway generation. Airway resistance is highest in bronchi of intermediate size and declines progressively as the terminal bronchioles are approached. Small peripheral airways (<2 mm in diameter) contribute little to overall airway resistance. (From Pedley TJ, Schroter RC, Sudlow MF: The prediction of pressure drop and variation of resistance within the human bronchial airways. Respir Physiol 9:391, 1970.)

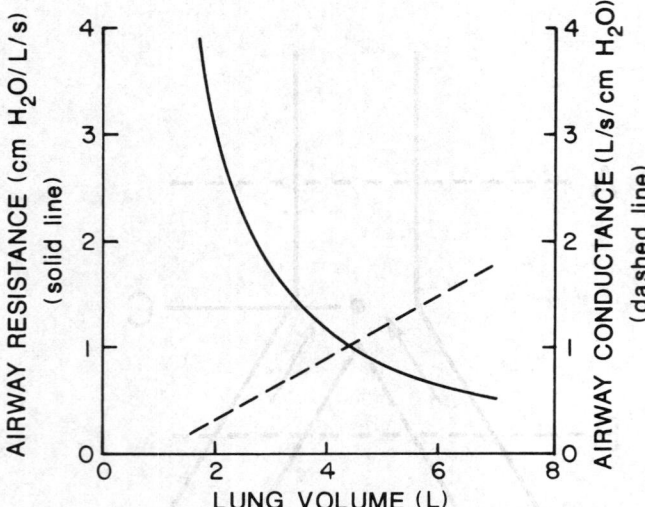

Figure 64–11. Plots of airway resistance and conductance versus lung volume. As lung volume increases, a tethering effect of the lung parenchyma on the airways increases airway diameter and resistance falls. Conductance, the reciprocal of resistance, increases linearly with lung volume. (From Briscoe WA, Dubois AB: The relationship between airway resistance, airway conductance and lung volume in subjects of different age and body size. Reproduced from the Journal of Clinical Investigation, 1958, volume 37, p 1280, by copyright permission of the American Society of Clinical Investigation.)

EXPIRATORY AIRFLOW LIMITATION

One issue not addressed in the previous discussion of airflow patterns and resistance is that these variables are also significantly affected by the phase of the respiratory cycle. In particular, a limitation to expiratory airflow exists, even in normal subjects. Such a limitation assumes importance in spontaneously breathing and mechanically ventilated patients with a variety of disease states. For example, patients with acute asthma or severe chronic obstructive pulmonary disease who require mechanical ventilation have markedly prolonged expiratory times. Failure of the clinician to recognize this and to make appropriate provisions in determining ventilator settings can result in life-threatening hypotension and barotrauma caused by lung hyperinflation (see Chapters 82 and 84).

To understand the basis for expiratory airflow limitation, it is useful to consider several important physiologic constructs: the flow-volume loop, the isovolume pressure-flow curve, equal pressure point theory, and, as an alternative to equal pressure point theory, wave speed theory.

The Flow-Volume Loop

A flow-volume loop (Fig. 64–12) is a plot of inspiratory and expiratory flow rates versus lung volume. Flow is measured by using a pneumotachograph; the flow signal is integrated electronically to determine inhaled and exhaled volumes. After a series of tidal volume breaths, the subject inspires to TLC and then initiates a maximal expiratory effort to residual volume; subsequently, a maximal inspiratory effort back to TLC is made.[9]

Inspection of the flow-volume loop reveals several notable findings. For example, the contours of the inspiratory and expiratory curves are different. Whereas the inspiratory curve is fairly symmetric, peak expiratory flow occurs early in the expiratory phase. In addition, there is a linear rela-

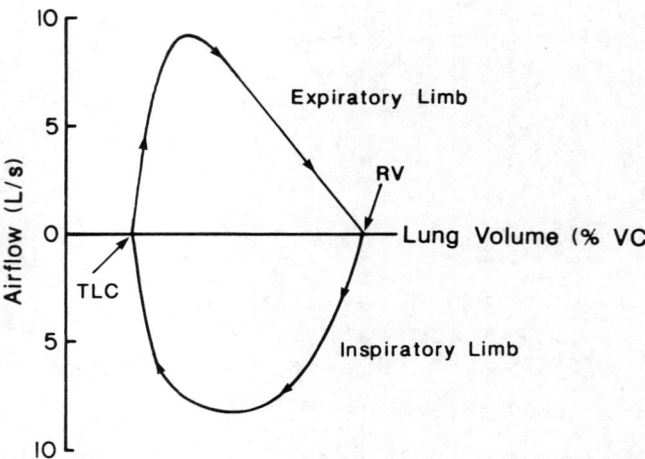

Figure 64–12. Schematic flow-volume loop. Expiratory and inspiratory airflow are plotted against lung volume, expressed as percentage of vital capacity (VC). Lung volume decreases from left (TLC) to right (RV). The loop is generated with the subject using maximal effort. See text for details.

tionship between expiratory flow and lung volume over the lower three quarters of the expiratory vital capacity.

If a family of flow-volume loops (Fig. 64–13) is generated by having the subject use a different level of effort for each loop, another important observation can be made: after the initial 20 to 25% of the vital capacity is exhaled, at any given lung volume, expiratory flow rate is limited. Decreases in effort result in decreases in flow rate, but increases in effort produce no augmentation of flow; that is, an "envelope" of expiratory flow rate is defined. To the extent that airflow cannot be increased beyond the envelope, it is effort independent.

In accounting for these observations, consideration of the pressure relationships depicted in Figure 64–14 is useful. During inspiration, generation of a negative pleural pressure produces a negative alveolar pressure and inspiratory airflow, the rate of which is largely dictated by the pressure gradient from the airway opening to the alveoli. At end

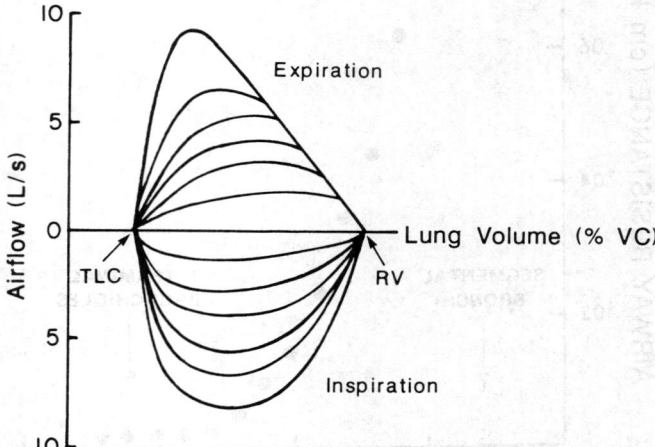

Figure 64–13. Schematic family of flow-volume loops. Each loop (expiratory and inspiratory halves) is created by having the subject generate a different effort. The outermost loop is the maximal flow-volume loop. An "envelope" for expiratory flow rate exists over the lower three quarters of the expiratory vital capacity. See text for details.

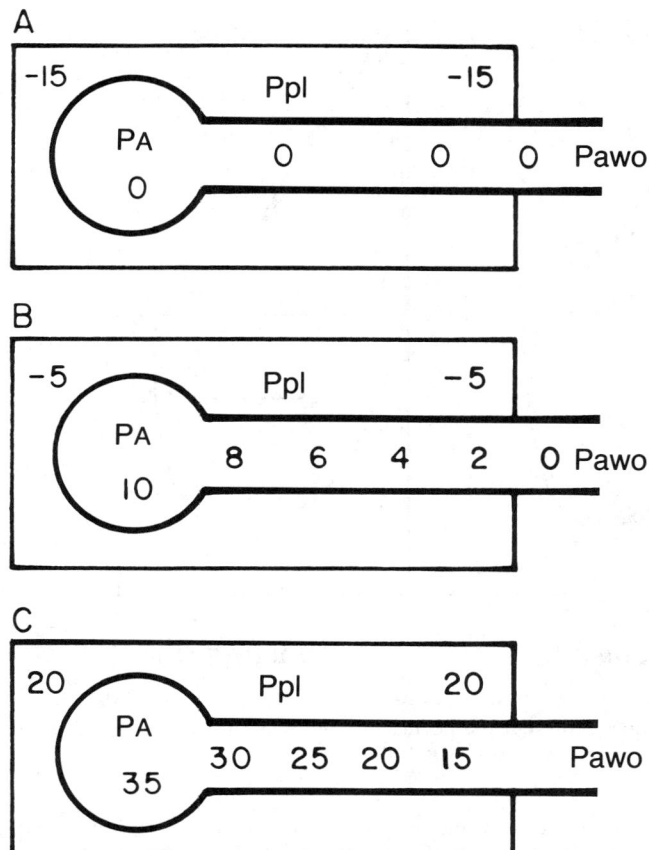

Figure 64–14. Changes in alveolar (PA) and pleural (Ppl) pressures at peak inspiration *(A)*, during quiet expiration *(B)*, and during forced expiration *(C)*. Pawo = pressure at the airway opening. See text for details.

inspiration (see Fig. 64–14A), the pleural and elastic recoil pressures offset one another; alveolar pressure is zero, and inspiratory airflow ceases. During quiet expiration (see Fig. 64–14B), relaxation of the inspiratory muscles allows pleural pressure to decline to a smaller negative value. The lung elastic recoil pressure now exceeds the negative pleural pressure, producing a positive alveolar pressure and, hence, a pressure gradient for expiratory airflow (recall, PA = Pel + Ppl).

With forced expiration (see Fig. 64–14C), activation of expiratory muscles creates a positive pleural pressure that sums with the lung elastic recoil pressure to generate a large positive alveolar pressure. During expiration, relaxed or forced, the driving pressure for airflow is dissipated along the airways by frictional airway and tissue resistances. During a forced maneuver, the intraluminal pressure may fall below the pressure in the surrounding pleural space. If the conducting airways are rigid and capable of withstanding any tendency to narrowing created by this negative transmural pressure, such a development has no physiologic consequences. However, if the airways are collapsible at the point where a negative transmural pressure is created, major effects on expiratory airflow are seen.[19–24]

The flow-volume loop, in addition to highlighting the physiologic principles that underpin expiratory airflow limitation in the lung, is used clinically in cases of suspected upper airway obstruction.[25] Functionally, the upper airway may be defined as the region between the glottis and prox-

imal main bronchi. Upper airway obstructions are categorized as either fixed, in which the overall cross-sectional area of the narrowed airway is independent of the phase of respiration, or variable, in which the cross-sectional area changes with inspiration and expiration. Furthermore, variable obstructions may be classified as either intrathoracic or extrathoracic, depending on whether the narrowing is below or above the suprasternal notch (i.e., whether it is subject to variations in intrathoracic pressure).

With fixed obstructions (e.g., tracheal stenosis resulting from a tracheostomy), both inspiratory and expiratory limbs of the flow-volume loop are flattened (Fig. 64–15A), reflecting proportionately diminished flow rates. With variable intrathoracic obstructions (e.g., a tumor of the lower trachea), the increase in surrounding pleural pressure during expiration potentiates the airway narrowing, limiting expiratory flow rate. However, during inspiration, the negative pleural pressure tends to minimize the obstruction by "tethering open" the airway, thereby preserving inspiratory flow (see Fig. 64–15B). With variable extrathoracic obstructions (e.g., a vocal cord fixed in the midline), the inspiratory fall in intratracheal pressure relative to atmospheric pressure (which surrounds the extrathoracic trachea) enhances the narrowing and results in diminished inspiratory flow. During expiration, the rise in intratracheal pressure minimizes the narrowing, and expiratory flow rate is preserved (see Fig. 64–15C).

The Isovolume Pressure-Flow Curve

Further analysis of the expiratory phase of the normal flow-volume loop reveals that expiratory flow rate depends on lung volume and that, at any given lung volume in the lower three quarters of the vital capacity, the flow rate is independent of effort. Consideration of the relationship between expiratory flow rate and intrapleural pressure at constant lung volume—the isovolume pressure-flow curve—is helpful in understanding this observation.[19]

If airflow is measured by using a pneumotachygraph, lung volume by using a body box, and intrapleural pressure by using an intraesophageal balloon catheter, all three variables may be plotted during timed expiratory maneuvers performed with varying degrees of subject effort. Corresponding points of intrapleural pressure and flow rate at specified lung volumes can then be plotted to construct a series of isovolume pressure-flow curves. Three such curves, corresponding to low, intermediate, and high lung volumes, are shown in Figure 64–16.

Examination of the curves reveals that during expiration, increased intrapleural pressure (increased effort) produces higher flow rates only at high lung volumes; at intermediate and low lung volumes, flow rate is constant despite increasing intrapleural pressure. At these volumes, flow rate is effort independent.

Equal Pressure Point Theory

Based on the previous considerations, two questions then arise: (1) What accounts for the difference in flow rates at different lung volumes at the same level of intrapleural pressure? (2) Why does flow rate reach a plateau at low and intermediate lung volumes?

The answer to the first question lies in an analysis of the maximal flow–static recoil curve (Fig. 64–17). The curve demonstrates the relationship between expiratory flow rate and static elastic recoil pressure (Pel). As Pel increases, so does the flow rate. The primary determinant of Pel is lung volume. Therefore, at a given intrapleural pressure (Ppl), the driving pressure for expiratory airflow, PA − Pawo,

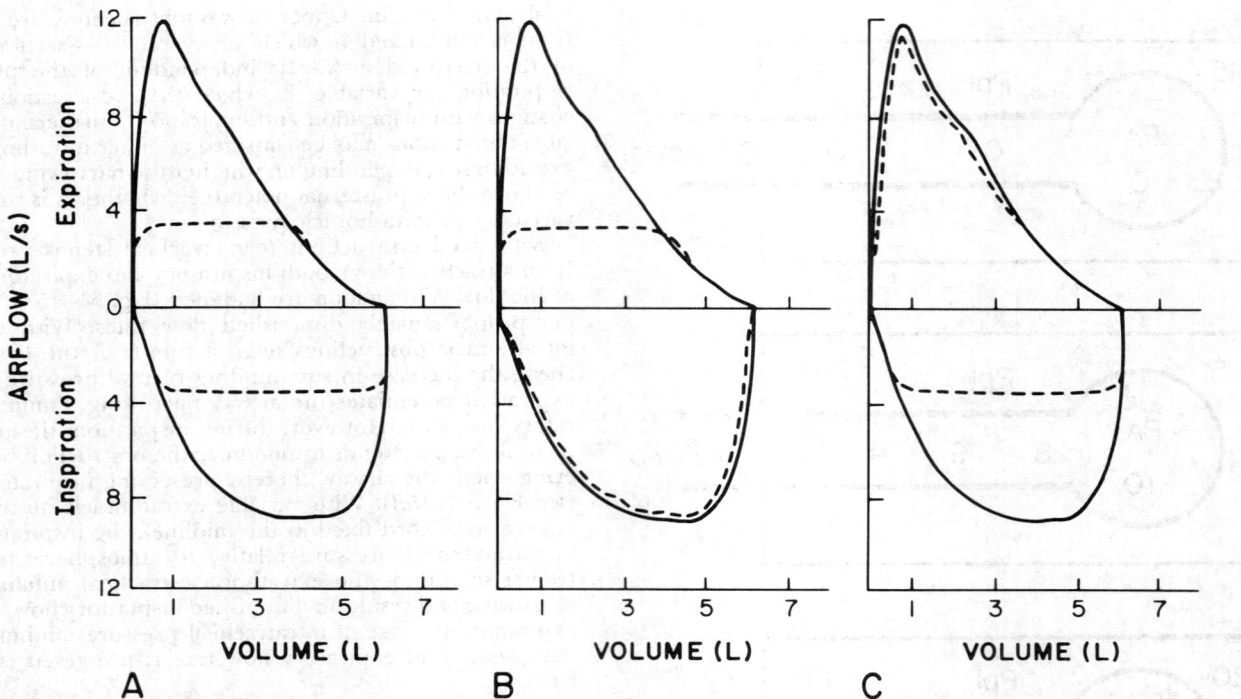

Figure 64–15. Flow-volume loops in upper airway obstruction. The solid lines represent the normal curves. The dashed lines indicate flow rates with obstruction. *A.* Fixed obstruction. *B.* Variable intrathoracic obstruction. *C.* Variable extrathoracic obstruction.

increases as lung volume increases, based on the relationship $P_A = P_{el} + P_{pl}$.

To understand the answer to the second question, consideration of the model depicted in Figure 64–18 is helpful. This model is similar to that shown in Figure 64–14, except that somewhere along the cartilagenous portion of the tracheobronchial tree is interposed a collapsible region, dividing the airway into "upstream" and "downstream" segments (see Fig. 64–18*C*). During forced expiration, positive pleural pressure is applied equally along the airway. The driving pressure is $P_A - P_{awo}$. As noted previously, P_A is the sum of P_{pl} and P_{el}; P_{el} is determined primarily by lung volume, and P_{pl} is determined by effort. As lung volume decreases, P_{el} and, hence, P_A decline. As the driving pressure is dissipated along the airway, a point is reached during forced expiration at which intraluminal pressure falls below pleural, resulting in a negative transmural pressure gradient farther downstream (i.e., toward the airway opening). If the point where the transmural pressure becomes negative lies along the collapsible region, airway narrowing develops.[20, 22–24]

If the collapsible region is completely collapsible, total airway closure would be expected. However, under such circumstances, airway pressure proximal to the closure rises to alveolar, resulting in "popping open" of the airway until occlusion once again develops. What actually occurs is a critical narrowing and creation of a so-called Starling resistor. Under the circumstances prevailing in a Starling resistor, the pressure gradient determining flow rate is $P_A - P_{pl}$, rather than $P_A - P_{awo}$. $P_A - P_{pl}$ represents the pressure gradient across the upstream segment, because the intraluminal pressure at the point of narrowing in the Starling resistor equals the pleural pressure—the equal pressure point. Furthermore, under the conditions of the equal pressure point model, as P_A increases with increases in P_{pl} (achieved through increases in expiratory effort), the driving pressure, $P_A - P_{pl}$, remains constant (and equal to P_{el}). Therefore, expiratory flow rate remains constant and effort independent. In the presence of severe airway obstruction, as in acute asthma, the large pressure drop across obstructed airway segments further enhances the development of neg-

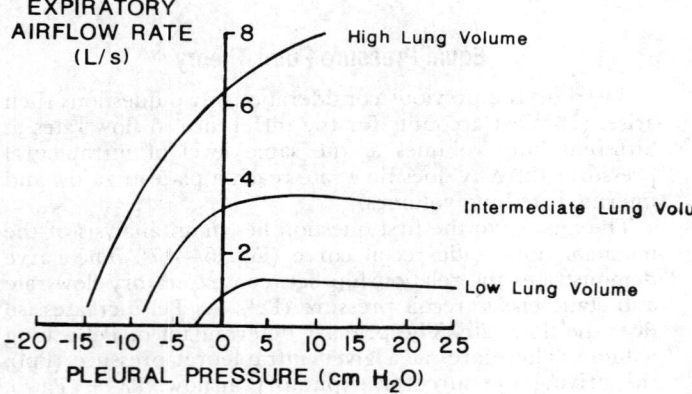

Figure 64–16. Isovolume pressure-flow curves. The curves are generated secondarily by plotting intrapleural pressure and flow rate measured during timed expiratory maneuvers done with varying effort by the subject. In the diagram, pressure and flow at three idealized lung volumes are shown.

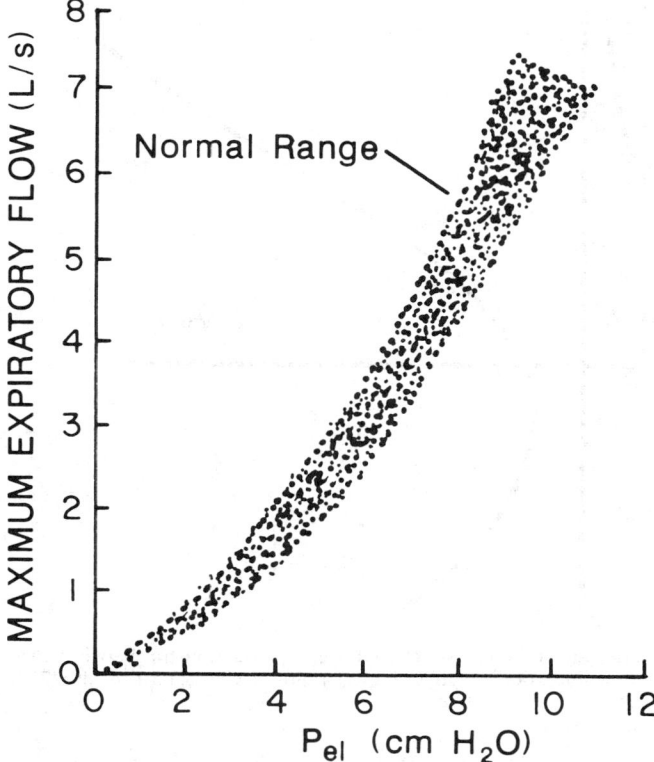

Figure 64–17. Maximal expiratory flow–static recoil curve. The stippled area shows the range of maximal expiratory flow plotted as a function of static elastic recoil pressure. Expiratory flow rate increases in a curvilinear fashion as lung "stretch" increases. (From Macklem PT: Tests of lung mechanics. Reprinted with permission from The New England Journal of Medicine, 293, 342, 1975.)

ative transmural pressure gradients. Consequently, despite increasing expiratory effort, such patients cannot augment the rate of expiratory airflow.

Finally, why is such effort independence of flow rate seen at low and intermediate lung volumes and not at high lung volumes? At high lung volumes Pel is large and the point along the airway where equal pressure points develop is far downstream, in large, cartilaginous airways. As lung volume decreases, Pel falls and equal pressure points move upstream, where airways are collapsible and the Starling resistors develop.

Wave Speed Theory

From the preceding discussion it is evident that, according to the equal pressure point model, airways are considered as completely rigid or completely collapsible. However, conducting airways may have walls that partially resist deformation. Wave speed theory,[24, 26–28] a model less widely appreciated than that of the equal pressure point, has been proposed as an alternative that takes this factor into consideration.

Wave speed is defined as the velocity at which a small disturbance, such as a pressure wave, propagates in a compliant tube that is filled with fluid. In the arteries, wave speed is the velocity of propagation of the pulse. A basic tenet of wave speed theory is that fluid in an elastic tube cannot travel at a velocity greater than that of the pressure head moving along the tube.[26] In addition, the wave speed of such a fluid may be only a theoretic maximal speed; the

actual speed of bulk movement of the fluid may be negligible. As an example, consider a partially fluid-filled tube whose ends are sealed. As the ends of the horizontally oriented tube are alternately raised and lowered, a wave is generated that moves toward the dependent end of the tube. Despite the propagation of the fluid wave within the tube, there is no net movement of the fluid beyond the tube's ends.

Determinants of Wave Speed

The wave speed flow of a fluid moving through an elastic tube may be calculated as

$$\dot{V}ws = (A/\rho \times dPtm/dA)^{0.5} \times A \qquad (9)$$

where $\dot{V}ws$ = wave speed flow
    A = cross-sectional area of the tube
    ρ = fluid density
    Ptm = transmural pressure

The term $(A/\rho \times dPtm/dA)$ is the tube wave speed and includes the reciprocal of tube compliance $(dA/dPtm)$. Tube compliance is the change in cross-sectional area of an elastic tube per unit change in transmural pressure. From Equation 9 it is clear that wave speed flow increases with increases in cross-sectional area, decreases in fluid density, and decreases in tube compliance or increases in tube stiffness. In effect,

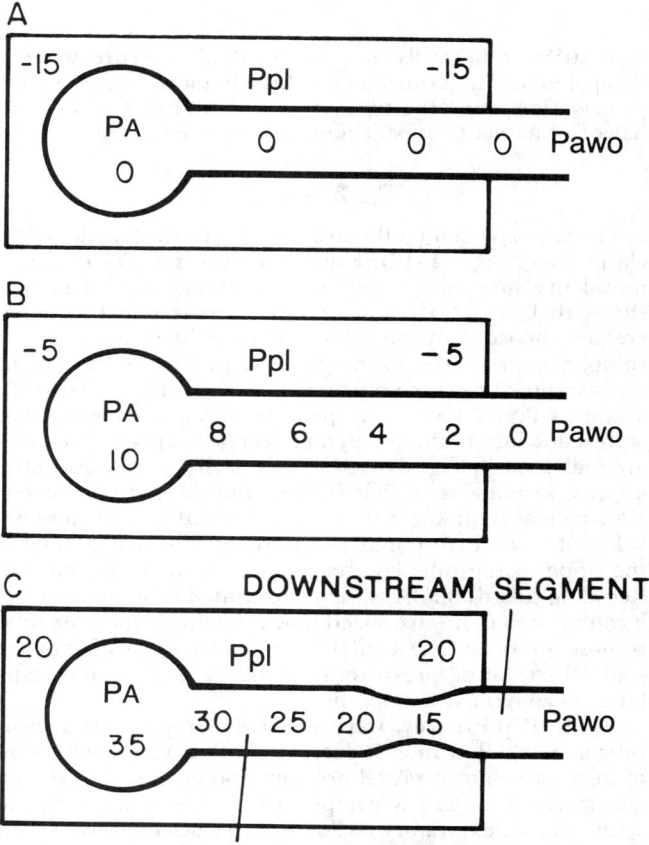

Figure 64–18. Creation of a Starling resistor. The model is similar to that depicted in Figure 64–14 except that a collapsible region divides the airway into upstream and downstream segments. During forced expiration (C), when the intraluminal pressure within the collapsible segment is less than the surrounding pleural pressure, airway narrowing develops. A Starling resistor is created and expiratory flow rate becomes limited. See text for details.

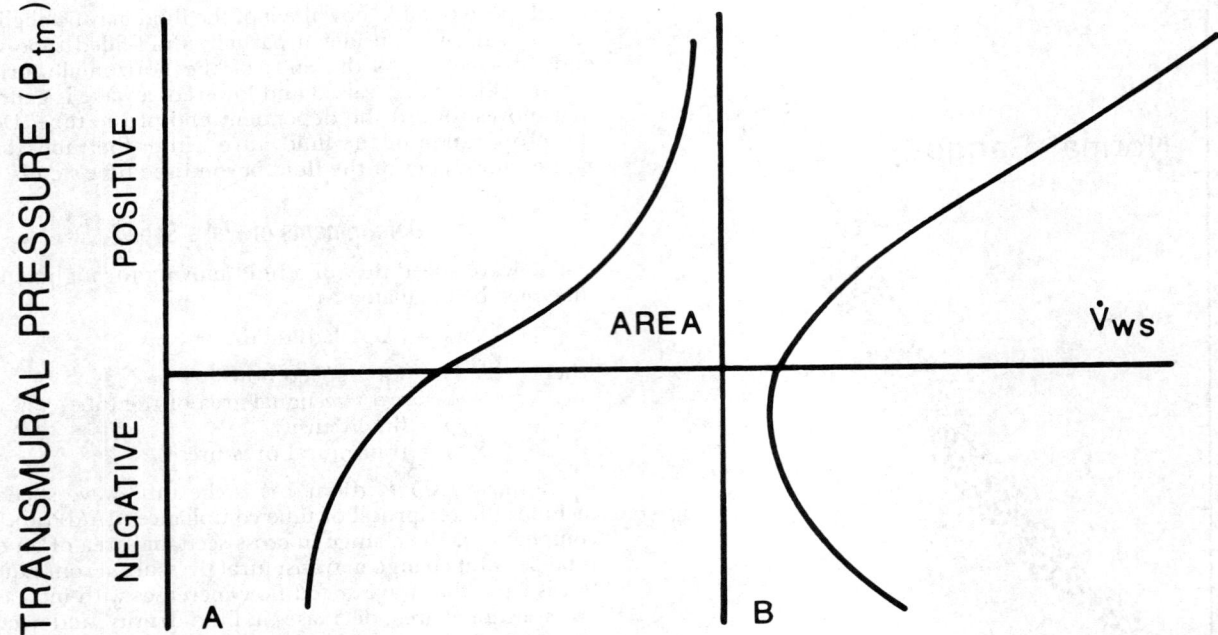

Figure 64–19. The tube law. *A.* Relationship between transmural pressure (Ptm) and tube cross-sectional area. *B.* Relationship between Ptm and wave speed flow (V̇ws). See text for details. (From Mead J: Expiratory flow limitation: A physiologist's point of view. Fed Proc 39:2772, 1980.)

with stiffer tube walls, less of the fluid pressure wave is dissipated in wall distortion, resulting in more effective wave propagation along the tube's longitudinal axis.[27, 28] The behavior of an elastic tube is described by the tube law.

The Tube Law

The tube law defines the distensibility characteristics of an elastic tube (Fig. 64–19). Figure 64–19*A* is a plot of transmural pressure versus tube cross-sectional area. The plot shows that, up to a point, as tube cross-sectional area decreases, the slope of the curve, dPtm/dA, decreases; that is, compliance increases. However, with further reductions in cross-sectional area, compliance decreases. Figure 64–19*B*, a plot of Ptm versus wave speed flow (V̇ws), indicates that with reductions in Ptm related to decreases in cross-sectional area (as seen in Fig. 64–19*A*), V̇ws declines. Subsequently, as cross-sectional area falls further and dPtm/dA increases, V̇ws increases (lower half of Fig. 64–19*B*). The minimal value of V̇ws corresponds to the point at which dPtm/dA, the slope of the tube law curve (Ptm vs. area), is minimal. Recalling that dPtm/dA is the reciprocal of tube compliance, it can be seen that wave speed flow is minimal when the tube is most compliant (least stiff). The determinants of Ptm are static elastic recoil pressure, frictional resistance, and resistance to convective acceleration.[28]

As noted previously, wave speed flow represents a theoretic maximal flow rate. It decreases with expiration because of decreases in transmural pressure and cross-sectional area and increases in airway compliance. During expiration, the actual rate of expiratory airflow approaches the wave speed flow and, when the two are equal, a "choke point" develops, limiting flow rate.

Local Variations in Dynamic Mechanical Properties

Regional variations in the mechanics of airflow have important effects on ventilation and the matching of ventilation and perfusion. In addition to topographic differences, local differences in airway resistance and lung compliance can produce significant inhomogeneity in ventilation.

The filling and emptying characteristics of a lung region may be defined in terms of its mechanical time constant—the time required to fill a unit to approximately two thirds of capacity. Mathematically, the mechanical time constant is the product of resistance (R) and compliance (C). Hence, lung units that are supplied by airways with high resistances or that are extremely compliant take longer to fill (or to empty) than normal units (Fig. 64–20). As long as inspiratory time is significantly greater than the longest local time constant, the tidal volume distribution does not depend on respiratory rate. However, with shorter inspiratory times or with increasing respiratory rate, the tidal volume becomes preferentially distributed to units with shorter time constants. In addition, the same units empty earlier. Such regional variation has major effects on ventilation-perfusion matching and the efficiency of gas exchange.[29] In addition,

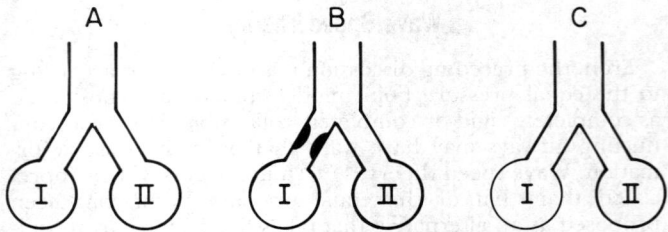

Figure 64–20. Heterogeneity of alveolar filling and emptying. Regional lung ventilation depends on mechanical time constants. The time constant (RC) is the product of airway resistance (R) and lung compliance (C). In *A*, units I and II, which have similar compliances and are supplied by airways with similar resistances, fill and empty symmetrically. In *B*, unit I is supplied by an airway with increased resistance. In *C*, unit I has increased compliance. In both *B* and *C*, unit I takes longer to fill (and empty) than unit II. The heterogeneity is accentuated at rapid respiratory rates, when there is inadequate time for filling and emptying of units with long time constants.

in the setting of high minute ventilatory requirements of some mechanically ventilated patients, marked heterogeneity in the distribution of ventilation may arise. As a common example, consider the patient with severe bullous lung disease. The combination of varying degrees of airway obstruction and the presence of lung units with highly compliant bullae results in marked heterogeneity of ventilation because some lung regions have extremely long time constants (high resistance and high compliance). Furthermore, if insufficient expiratory time is provided during mechanical ventilation, "ball valve" physiology may prevail, resulting in localized hyperinflation and barotrauma.

BACKDROP FOR CLINICAL RELEVANCE OF RESPIRATORY MECHANICS IN CRITICAL ILLNESS: WORK OF BREATHING

All of the previous discussion of respiratory mechanics can be focused on an important clinical concept—the work of breathing.[30–32] Work is done when a force moves through a distance. In a fluid system, work is performed when pressure produces a change in the volume of the system. Because pressure is force applied per unit area and volume is area times length, work is the product of pressure and volume:

$$W = P \times V \qquad (10)$$

where
$$\begin{aligned} W &= \text{work} \\ P &= \text{pressure} \\ V &= \text{volume} \end{aligned}$$

During a dynamic respiratory cycle, the work done by the respiratory muscles is

$$W = \int P \, dV \qquad (11)$$

where dV = change in volume of respiratory system

The work performed is represented as the area under the pressure-volume curve for the respiratory system (Fig. 64–21). During a respiratory cycle, the inspiratory muscles overcome a number of forces already discussed: (1) the elastic recoils of the lung and chest wall, (2) the flow-resistive forces of the airway and lung tissues, (3) the inertial forces of the airway gases and lung and chest wall tissues, (4) gravitational forces, and (5) the chest wall's distorting forces.[31, 32] Under circumstances in which the configuration of the respiratory system remains constant during respiration, the work of breathing performed by the respiratory muscles can be determined from analysis of the pressure-volume diagram, which relates lung volume to pleural pressure.

If the airway is maintained open and lung volume is held constant at different levels of inflation, a static pressure-volume curve for the lung can be generated. In addition, if the inspiratory muscles are relaxed and the airway opening is occluded, the same static measurements of pleural pressure and lung volume can be used to generate a static pressure-volume curve for the relaxed chest wall (see Fig. 64–21A). In Figure 64–21A, the horizontal distance between corresponding points on the lines −Pst(l) and Pst(w) (at any given lung volume) represents the pressure that the respiratory muscles must generate to maintain that lung volume with the airway open. This pressure also corresponds to the pressure-volume curve of the relaxed respiratory system shown in Figure 64–7. The elastic work of breathing done by the inspiratory muscles in inflating the lung from FRC is the area inscribed in Figure 64–21A by ABCA.

During dynamic lung inflation, additional pressure must be generated and work performed to overcome flow resistance (see Fig. 64–21B). In Figure 64–21B the vertically hatched area indicates the additional work required to overcome flow resistance of the airways and lung; the stippled area represents the additional work required to overcome the flow resistance offered by the chest wall.[31]

There has been renewed interest in calculating the work of breathing in various clinical settings, including that of mechanical ventilation. Although, in general, the methodology is cumbersome enough to preclude routine measurements in ventilator-dependent patients, reasonably accurate estimates of the work of breathing can be made. Using ventilators that deliver gas at a constant inspiratory flow rate and recognizing that lung volume is linearly related to inspiratory time under constant flow conditions, one can make measurements of tidal volume and airway pressure to calculate the work of breathing from a pressure-time (volume) plot.[33] Studies indicate that patient-generated work is

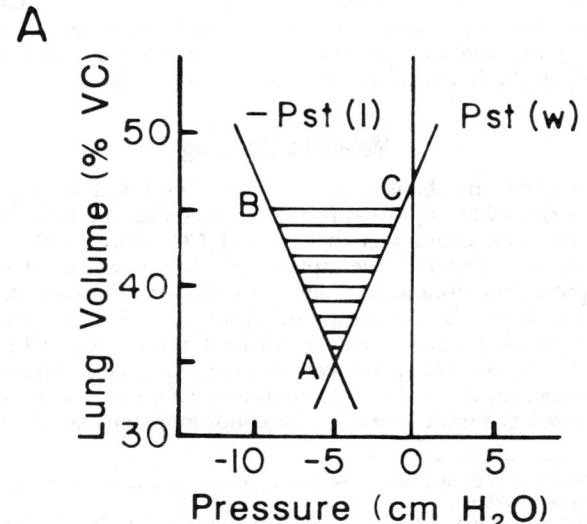

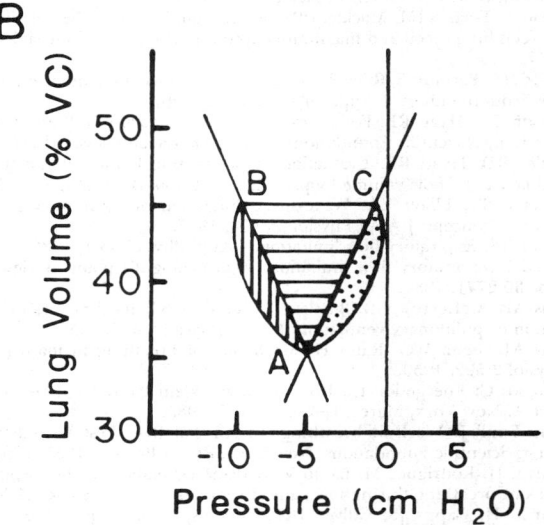

Figure 64–21. Pressure-volume diagrams for the lung and chest wall used in calculating the work of breathing. *A.* Determination of the elastic component. *B.* Determination of the resistive component. See text for details. (Reprinted from Roussos C: Energetics. In: Roussos C, Macklem PT [eds]: The Thorax, Part A. New York, Marcel Dekker, pp 449, 451, 1985 by courtesy of Marcel Dekker, Inc..)

substantial during assisted mechanical ventilation and that it can be adversely affected by inappropriate selection of ventilator flow and sensitivity settings.[34]

References

1. Roussos C, Macklem PT: The respiratory muscles. N Engl J Med 307:786, 1982.
2. Roussos C: Respiratory muscle fatigue and ventilatory failure. Chest 97:89S, 1990.
3. Weibel ER: Morphometry of the Human Lung. New York, Springer-Verlag, p 105, 1963.
4. Paiva M, Engel LA: Model analysis of gas distribution within human lung acinus. J Appl Physiol 56:418, 1984.
5. Milic-Emili J, Mead J, Turner JM, et al: Improved technique for estimating pleural pressure from esophageal balloons. J Appl Physiol 19:207, 1964.
6. Mead J: Mechanical properties of lungs. Physiol Rev 41:281, 1961.
7. Rahn H, Otis AB, Chadwick LE, et al: The pressure-volume diagram of the thorax and lung. Am J Physiol 146:161, 1946.
8. Sharp JT, Hammond MD: Pressure-volume relationships. In: Crystal RG, West JB (eds): The Lung: Scientific Foundations. New York, Raven Press, p 839, 1991.
9. Grippi MA, Metzger LF, Krupinski AV, et al: Pulmonary function testing. In: Fishman AP (ed): Pulmonary Diseases and Disorders. 2nd ed. New York, McGraw-Hill, p 2469, 1988.
10. Fry DL, Ebert RV, Stead WW, et al: The mechanics of pulmonary ventilation in normal subjects and in patients with emphysema. Am J Med 16:80, 1954.
11. Schlueter DP, Immekus J, Stead WW: Relationship between maximal inspiratory pressure and total lung capacity (coefficient of retraction) in normal subjects and in patients with emphysema, asthma, and diffuse pulmonary infiltration. Am Rev Respir Dis 46:656, 1967.
12. Grassino AE, Roussos C, Macklem PT: Static properties of the chest wall. In: Crystal RG, West JB (eds.): The Lung: Scientific Foundations. New York, Raven Press, p 855, 1991.
13. Tobin M: Respiratory monitoring in the intensive care unit. Am Rev Respir Dis 138:1625, 1988.
14. Pedley TJ, Kamm RD: Dynamics of gas flow and pressure-flow relationships. In: Crystal RG, West JB (eds): The Lung: Scientific Foundations. New York, Raven Press, p 995, 1991.
15. Hyatt RE, Wilcox RE: The pressure-flow relationships of the intrathoracic airway in man. J Clin Invest 42:29, 1963.
16. Pedley TJ, Schroter RC, Sudlow MF: The prediction of pressure drop and the variation of resistance within the human bronchial airways. Respir Physiol 9:387, 1970.
17. Macklem PT, Mead J: Resistance of central and peripheral airways measured by a retrograde catheter. J Appl Physiol 22:395, 1967.
18. Briscoe WA, Dubois AB: The relationship between airway resistance, airway conductance and lung volume in subjects of different age and body size. J Clin Invest 37:1279, 1958.
19. Hyatt RE, Schilder DP, Fry DL: Relationship between maximum expiratory flow and degree of lung inflation. J Appl Physiol 13:331, 1958.
20. Jordanoglou J, Pride NB: Factors determining maximum inspiratory flow and maximum expiratory flow of the lung. Thorax 23:33, 1968.
21. Macklem PT, Mead J: The physiologic basis of common pulmonary function tests. Arch Environ Health 14:5, 1967.
22. Mead J, Turner JM, Macklem PT, et al: Significance of the relationship between lung recoil and maximum expiratory flow. J Appl Physiol 22:95, 1967.
23. Pride NB, Permutt S, Riley RL, et al: Determinants of maximal expiratory flow from the lungs. J Appl Physiol 23:646, 1967.
24. Wilson TA, Hyatt RE: Forced expiration. In: Crystal RG, West JB (eds): The Lung: Scientific Foundations. New York, Raven Press, p 1021, 1991.
25. Miller RD, Hyatt RE: Evaluation of obstructing lesions of the trachea and larynx by flow-volume loops. Am Rev Respir Dis 108:475, 1973.
26. Dawson SV, Elliott EA: Wave-speed limitation on expiratory flow—A unifying concept. J Appl Physiol 43:498, 1977.
27. Hyatt RE: Expiratory flow limitation. J Appl Physiol 55:1, 1983.
28. Mead J: Expiratory flow limitation: A physiologist's point of view. Fed Proc 39:2771, 1980.
29. Otis AB, McKerrow CB, Bartlett RA, et al: Mechanical factors in distribution of pulmonary ventilation. J Appl Physiol 8:427, 1956.
30. Otis AB, Fenn WO, Rahn H: Mechanics of breathing in man. J Appl Physiol 2:592, 1950.
31. Roussos C: Energetics. In: Roussos C, Macklem PT (eds): The Thorax, Part A. New York, Marcel Dekker, p 437, 1985.
32. Milic-Emili J: Work of breathing. In: Crystal RG, West JB (eds): The Lung: Scientific Foundations. New York, Raven Press, p 1065, 1991.
33. Marini JJ, Rodriguez M, Lamb V: Bedside estimation of the inspiratory work of breathing during mechanical ventilation. Chest 89:56, 1986.
34. Marini JJ, Capps JS, Culver BH: The inspiratory work of breathing during assisted mechanical ventilation. Chest 87:612, 1985.

CHAPTER 65

Physiology of Gas Exchange

Gary T. Kinasewitz
Barry A. Gray

Respiration at the cellular level is dependent on the ability of the lungs to eliminate CO_2 and add O_2 from the inspired air to the mixed venous blood in the pulmonary capillaries. Ventilation replenishes the O_2 content and removes CO_2 from alveolar gas, while the pulmonary circulation brings mixed venous blood to the alveolar capillary, where it is arterialized. Gas exchange is dependent not only on the absolute levels of ventilation and blood flow but also on their relative distributions within the lung. Optimal gas exchange is attained when the distribution of ventilation is proportionate to the amount of perfusion within the alveolar capillary. Hypoventilation, inadequate perfusion, and diffusion defects that impair gas transfer across the alveolar capillary membrane are all causes of hypoxemia. However, the maldistribution of ventilation relative to perfusion is the most common cause of respiratory failure in the critically ill.

VENTILATION

Normal Requirements

The level of ventilation must be sufficient to maintain partial pressures of O_2 and CO_2 in alveolar gas that are adequate for CO_2 elimination and O_2 uptake by the pulmonary capillary blood. The minute ventilation ($\dot{V}E$, BTPS*) is the amount of gas expired each minute. Because the amount of O_2 taken up across the pulmonary capillary is slightly greater than the amount of CO_2 eliminated, $\dot{V}E$ is slightly less than the volume of air inspired each minute ($\dot{V}I$, BTPS).

The normal ventilatory requirement for gas exchange at rest is approximately 80 mL/kg/min or 5.7 L/min in a 70-kg individual. When metabolic activity is increased in response to a stimulus such as hyperthermia, the minute ventilation increases in proportion to the metabolic demand. O_2 consumption and CO_2 production may increase by more than 50% in the hypermetabolic patient with sepsis.[1]

Metabolic Coupling

Aerobic metabolism at the tissue level utilizes O_2 and generates CO_2 as a by-product of this metabolism. Under steady-state conditions the O_2 and CO_2 stores within the body are constant; the uptake of O_2 across the alveolar capillary membrane is equal to its rate of utilization at the tissue level. O_2 consumption ($\dot{V}O_2$) in a healthy resting individual is approximately 3.5 to 4 mL/kg/min (STPD†). Similarly, the CO_2 produced as a consequence of anaerobic metabolism is equal to the amount of CO_2 eliminated in the expired gas under steady-state conditions, typically 3 to 3.5

---

*BTPS = body temperature, ambient pressure, saturated with water vapor at these conditions.

†STPD = standard temperature and pressure dry (0°C, 760 mm Hg, zero water vapor).

mL/kg/min (STPD) under resting conditions. Because the production of CO_2 is metabolically linked to O_2 utilization, the amount of CO_2 generated increases as the aerobic metabolism of peripheral tissue increases. The respiratory quotient is the amount of CO_2 produced per mole of O_2 consumed. Under steady-state conditions the value of the respiratory quotient is identical with the respiratory exchange ratio (R), that is, the ratio of CO_2 elimination to O_2 uptake across the alveolar capillary membrane. A typical value for R in a person with an average diet is 0.8, but the value varies depending on the relative proportions of fat (R = 0.7), protein (R = 0.82), and carbohydrate (R = 1.0) being utilized for fuel.[2] When the caloric intake is excessive and lipogenesis is occurring, the value of R may exceed 1.0.

CO_2 production per minute ($\dot{V}CO_2$) can be determined by measuring minute ventilation and the fractional concentration of CO_2 in expired air ($FECO_2$). Because the concentration of CO_2 in inspired air is negligible, it follows that

$$\dot{V}CO_2 = 0.863(\dot{V}E \times FECO_2) \quad (1)$$

where 0.863 is a constant that converts liters BTPS to milliliters STPD.

It is more difficult to measure $\dot{V}O_2$ because there is O_2 in the inspired air and the total volume expired is slightly less than that inspired. This difference is due to the fact that more O_2 is taken up from the alveolar gas than CO_2 is added. However, because nitrogen is not exchanged across the lung, the concentration of nitrogen in the expired gas increases and, if the expired volume is known, the inspired volume can be calculated as

$$\dot{V}I = \dot{V}E (FEN_2/FIN_2) \quad (2)$$

where FEN_2 and FIN_2 are the fractional concentrations of nitrogen in expired and inspired gas, respectively. Once $\dot{V}I$ is known, O_2 uptake may be determined as the difference between the O_2 inspired and the amount expired:

$$\dot{V}O_2 = 0.863(FIO_2 \times \dot{V}I - FECO_2 \times \dot{V}E) \quad (3)$$

R is calculated as the ratio $\dot{V}CO_2/\dot{V}O_2$. The availability of metabolic monitoring systems has made it possible to measure $\dot{V}CO_2$ and $\dot{V}O_2$ at the bedside. The major limitation of these systems is the difficulty in accurately measuring FIO_2 and FEO_2 when high concentrations of O_2 are required to support a critically ill patient.[3]

An alternative to monitoring expired gas to measure $\dot{V}O_2$ is to calculate it from the Fick equation. The availability of pulmonary arterial catheters has made it possible to measure the cardiac output (CO, in liters per minute) by thermodilution and obtain samples of mixed venous blood. If the O_2 content of mixed venous blood and that of a simultaneously obtained arterial sample are measured, $\dot{V}O_2$ may be calculated as

$$\dot{V}O_2 = CO \times (CaO_2 - C\bar{v}O_2) \times 10 \quad (4)$$

where CaO_2 and $C\bar{v}O_2$ are the O_2 content (in milliliters per deciliter) of arterial and mixed venous blood, respectively. The O_2 content of blood can be measured in a CO-oximeter or calculated as

$$CaO_2 = 1.39 \times Hb \times \%sat + PO_2 \times 0.003 \quad (5)$$

where Hb is the hemoglobin concentration in grams per deciliter, %sat is the percent O_2 saturation of hemoglobin, and 0.003 is the solubility constant for O_2 in blood.

Dead Space

The volume of air entering the lungs during each breath is the tidal volume (VT). The entire tidal volume does not reach the alveolar spaces; a portion of each tidal breath is retained within the trachea and conducting airways. Because these airways do not participate in gas exchange, the volume of gas they contain is termed anatomic dead space. The volume of the anatomic dead space in milliliters is approximately equal to an individual's body weight in pounds, for example, 150 mL in a 150-lb person. Alveolar ventilation (VA) is the difference between the tidal volume (VT) and dead space (VDS):

$$VA = VT - VDS \quad (6)$$

Because the composition of the gas in the anatomic dead space is essentially the same as that of inspired air, its CO_2 concentration is negligible and CO_2 production is the product of alveolar ventilation and the concentration of CO_2 in alveolar gas. Note that the alveolar CO_2 concentration is higher than the mixed expired CO_2 concentration because the latter sample contains both alveolar and dead space gas. The partial pressure of CO_2 in alveolar gas ($PACO_2$) is the product of its fractional concentration ($FACO_2$) and barometric pressure (PB), that is,

$$PACO_2 = FACO_2 \times PB \quad (7)$$

The diffusion of CO_2 across the alveolar capillary membrane is rapid, so equilibration between alveolar gas and pulmonary capillary blood is usually complete and the PCO_2 of alveolar air may be approximated by the PCO_2 of arterial blood ($PaCO_2$). (The potential error in assuming CO_2 equilibration between alveolar gas and arterial blood is small because the difference between the extremes of mixed venous and arterial PCO_2 is only a few millimeters of mercury). Therefore, at any level of CO_2 production

$$PaCO_2 = \frac{0.863 \times \dot{V}CO_2}{VA} \quad (8)$$

This relationship implies that the $PaCO_2$ is a reflection of the adequacy of alveolar ventilation relative to the patient's metabolic requirements. Doubling the alveolar ventilation at a constant level of $\dot{V}CO_2$ reduces the $PaCO_2$ by 50% (Fig. 65–1). Whenever the $\dot{V}CO_2$ rises, as in a hyperthermic patient, the $PaCO_2$ increases unless ventilation rises proportionately. The $PaCO_2$ may fluctuate considerably in the paralyzed patient who develops a fever while receiving controlled ventilatory support.

The volume of the anatomic dead space increases slightly during inspiration because radial traction on the airways increases their diameter. However, the increase in VDS is insignificant relative to the volume of gas within the lung and for practical purposes the anatomic dead space can be considered constant in any individual.

Far more important in the evaluation of critically ill patients with pulmonary disease is the inspired gas that reaches alveoli that are poorly perfused relative to their ventilation. The excess ventilation is, in effect, alveolar dead space. In the patient with bullous emphysema, a significant proportion of each tidal breath may ventilate alveoli that are poorly perfused. The physiologic consequence of this wasted ventilation is that the patient must increase VE to maintain an adequate level of alveolar ventilation. If the patient is able to compensate for the rise in alveolar dead space by increasing VE, VA and therefore $PaCO_2$ may be normal.

The $PaCO_2$ is an indication of the adequacy of alveolar ventilation. Although we cannot directly measure the amount of alveolar ventilation that is wasted, we can estimate the physiologic dead space (which is the sum of anatomic and alveolar dead space) if the minute ventilation and concentration of CO_2 ($PECO_2$) in expired gas are known. The

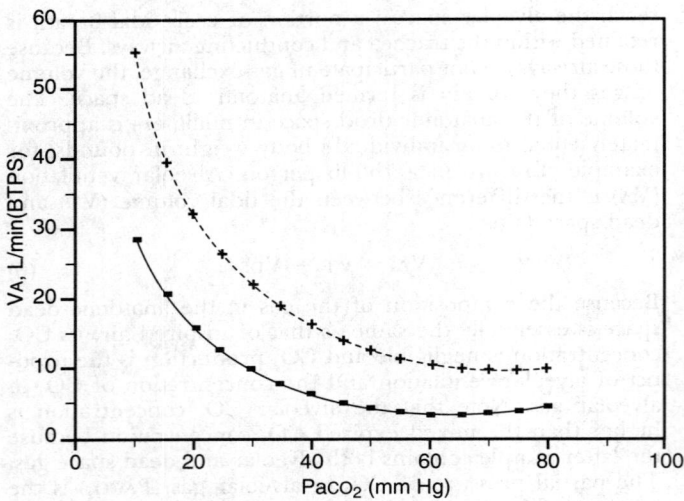

Figure 65–1. Relationship between $Paco_2$ and alveolar ventilation (V_A) at a $\dot{V}co_2$ of 240 mL/min (STPD; filled squares and solid line). When V_A decreases by 50%, the $Paco_2$ doubles. Doubling the $\dot{V}co_2$ to 480 mL/min (STPD; plus signs and dashed line) requires a proportionate increase in V_A to maintain a normal $Paco_2$.

CO_2 in the expired gas all comes from alveolar gas because the concentration of CO_2 in the inspired air filling V_{DS} during each breath is essentially zero. Thus

$$V_T \times Peco_2 = V_A \times Paco_2 + V_{DS} \times Pico_2 \qquad (9)$$

Because $Pico_2 \approx 0$, $V_A = V_T - V_{DS}$ and $Paco_2 \approx Paco_2$,

$$V_T \times Peco_2 = (V_T - V_{DS}) \times Paco_2 \qquad (10)$$

Rearranging yields the modified Bohr equation

$$\frac{V_{DS}}{V_T} = \frac{Paco_2 - Peco_2}{Paco_2} \qquad (11)$$

In a healthy individual the physiologic dead space calculated via the Bohr equation is slightly greater than the anatomic dead space.

The normal V_{DS}/V_T ratio is approximately 0.30 (0.25 to 0.35) at rest. As tidal volume increases, as during exercise, the increase in the volume of the trachea and conducting airways is insignificant relative to the increase in alveolar ventilation, so the V_{DS}/V_T ratio falls and ventilation becomes more efficient.[4] In patients with pulmonary disease a significant portion of the inspired air is distributed to poorly perfused lung units. The V_{DS}/V_T ratio at rest may exceed 0.50 and increase even further when ventilation increases in response to a stimulus such as hypoxia.[5]

The increase in dead space is compounded when a critically ill patient requires mechanical ventilation. The Y of the ventilator circuit is usually placed as close as possible to the endotracheal tube to minimize the effect of the ventilator tubing. However, when pressures within the ventilator circuit increase during inspiration the tubing expands, reducing the volume delivered to the patient. The volume retained within the circuit can be estimated by assuming a tubing compliance of 3 mL/cm H_2O. If the airway pressure increases by 40 cm H_2O during a tidal breath, 120 mL remains in the tubing, increasing the effective dead space. V_{DS}/V_T ratios exceeding 0.6 may be encountered in critically ill patients with respiratory failure.

DISTRIBUTION OF VENTILATION
Normal Distribution

Inspired gas is not uniformly distributed throughout the alveolar volume, even in healthy individuals. This is due to differences in transpulmonary pressure at different heights within the lung. Alveolar pressure is uniformly distributed throughout the normal lung. At the end of expiration alveolar pressure is zero (atmospheric). In contrast, pleural pressure is more negative at the top of the lung than at the bottom. The vertical gradient of pleural pressure, approximately 0.5 cm H_2O/cm distance, is due to the effects of gravity on the lung.[6] As a consequence of this pleural pressure gradient the transpulmonary pressure at the apex is greater than at the base, so apical alveoli operate from a higher position on their pressure-volume curve (Fig. 65–2). The volume of the alveoli at the apex is greater than alveolar volume at the base, but during inspiration, for a given change in pleural pressure, a greater portion of the inspired volume goes to the lung bases, which are operating on a steeper portion of their pressure-volume curve.[7] At low lung volumes the intrapleural pressure at the lung base may exceed airway pressure and compression of alveoli and collapse of airways at the base of the lung may occur. When inspiration is initiated from a low lung volume, ventilation to the bases is impossible until the pleural pressure at the bottom of the lung falls below atmospheric pressure; the initial portion of an inspired breath from a low lung volume is delivered to the apices (see Fig. 65–2).

Airway Closure

During expiration small airways in the periphery of the lung close and trap air in the distal alveoli. Airway closure occurs only at lung volumes below functional residual capacity (FRC) in healthy young individuals. However, aging is associated with a loss of elastic recoil so that airway closure occurs at a higher lung volume.[8] In older individuals airway closure at lung volumes above FRC decreases ventilation to the bases, even during tidal breathing. In the patient with chronic obstructive lung disease airway closure occurs at even higher lung volumes and contributes to the maldistribution of ventilation in these individuals.

Ventilation is more uniformly distributed in the supine subject.[9] In the supine position the difference in pleural pressure between the top and bottom of the lung is minimized. However, FRC is lower in the supine position, so airway closure is more likely to occur during tidal breathing.

LUNG DISEASE

The pleural pressure gradient and airway closure affect the distribution of ventilation in both healthy subjects and patients with pulmonary disease. However, the pattern of

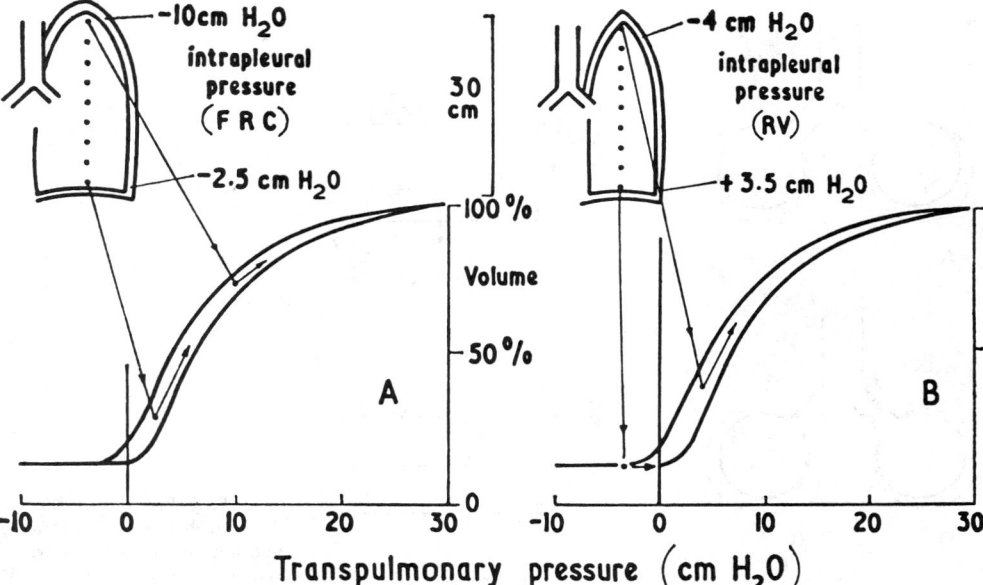

Figure 65–2. Alveoli at the top and bottom of the lung operate on different portions of their compliance curve because of the vertical gradient of intrapleural pressure. A tidal breath from FRC produces a greater increase in alveolar volume at the base of the lung *(A)*, but the apex is better ventilated if the tidal breath begins from residual volume (RV) *(B)*. (From West JB: Ventilation/Blood Flow and Gas Exchange. 5th ed. Oxford, Blackwell Scientific Publications, p 28, 1990.)

ventilation is far more heterogeneous in the diseased lung because of regional differences in the mechanical properties of the lung. If diseases that affect the airways and interstitium were uniformly distributed throughout the entire lung, ventilation would be equally affected in all regions and the overall pattern of distribution of ventilation would not be changed. However, many pulmonary diseases are focal in nature; they may involve one respiratory lobule and spare an adjacent region. This focal involvement produces regional differences in resistance and compliance that have important effects on the inhomogeneity of ventilation.

Resistance, Compliance, and Time Constants

Whenever there are regional differences in resistance or compliance, alveolar inflation occurs in a heterogeneous manner.[10] For example, if two lungs have identical compliance but the airway resistance of one lung is markedly increased, then an identical change in pleural pressure produces an equal driving pressure for inspiratory flow into both lungs but, because of the increased airway resistance, airflow into lung A is slower and it takes longer to fill the same volume as that of lung B (Fig. 65–3). If the duration of inspiration is shortened in the tachypneic patient, then the volume of A is less than that of B. Alternatively, if the resistances of both lungs are equal but the compliance of lung A is increased, then a given decrease in pleural pressure produces similar rates of inspiratory flow into both lungs but, because lung B is less compliant, it reaches its maximal volume more quickly than lung A.

The rate at which different regions of the lung fill and empty is related to their time constants. The time constant of a lung unit is the product of its resistance and compliance. Units with long time constants, because of increased airway resistance or increased lung compliance, take longer to fill and empty than regions with shorter time constants. When the respiratory rate is low, the duration of both inspiration and expiration may be long enough to allow complete filling and emptying of all lung units during each tidal breath. However, at high respiratory rates the ventilation of different lung units may become asynchronous and the regions with high time constants may not completely fill or empty. Respiratory system compliance, which is determined by dividing the tidal volume by the plateau airway pressure in a ventilator patient, may demonstrate a frequency-dependent decrease with increasing respiratory rate and/or decreasing expiratory time.[11, 12]

Regional differences in resistance and compliance are the most important factors leading to a nonuniform distribution of ventilation in the patient with lung disease. To a limited extent regional inhomogeneity is ameliorated by the interdependence of contiguous respiratory units. Because adjacent respiratory units share common connective tissue elements, the expansion of one respiratory unit exerts traction on the adjacent units and facilitates synchronous ventilation within the lung.[13] There is also interdependence between the lung and chest wall. When regional lung filling lags during inspiration, local deformation of the chest wall decreases the adjacent pleural pressure, thereby increasing the transpulmonary pressure gradient promoting alveolar filling in the lung units that are lagging.[14] Ventilation through collateral channels such as the pores of Kohn also contributes to the synchronous ventilation of alveolar units subtended by obstructed airways.[15]

Inhomogeneity in the distribution of ventilation may be detected in the pulmonary function laboratory by the increased slope of phase III during the single-breath nitrogen washout test.[16] During nitrogen washout or inert tracer equilibration, the time to reach steady-state gas concentrations is prolonged in the patient with poorly ventilated units.[17, 18] These regional differences in the distribution of ventilation are an important factor in the overall problem of ventilation-perfusion matching in the critically ill patient with respiratory failure.

PULMONARY BLOOD FLOW

The entire cardiac output courses through the pulmonary capillaries, where it comes into contact with alveolar gas. Pulmonary blood flow generally increases as ventilation rises in response to a metabolic stimulus such as exercise. However, the relative increase in pulmonary blood flow is less than the corresponding increase in ventilation. During maximal exercise $\dot{V}_E$ may increase 30- to 40-fold while the maximal increment in cardiac output is only a 5- to 6-fold rise. Increased O_2 extraction with widening of the arterial–mixed venous O_2 difference also contributes to the increase in O_2 utilization. However, pulmonary blood flow is not

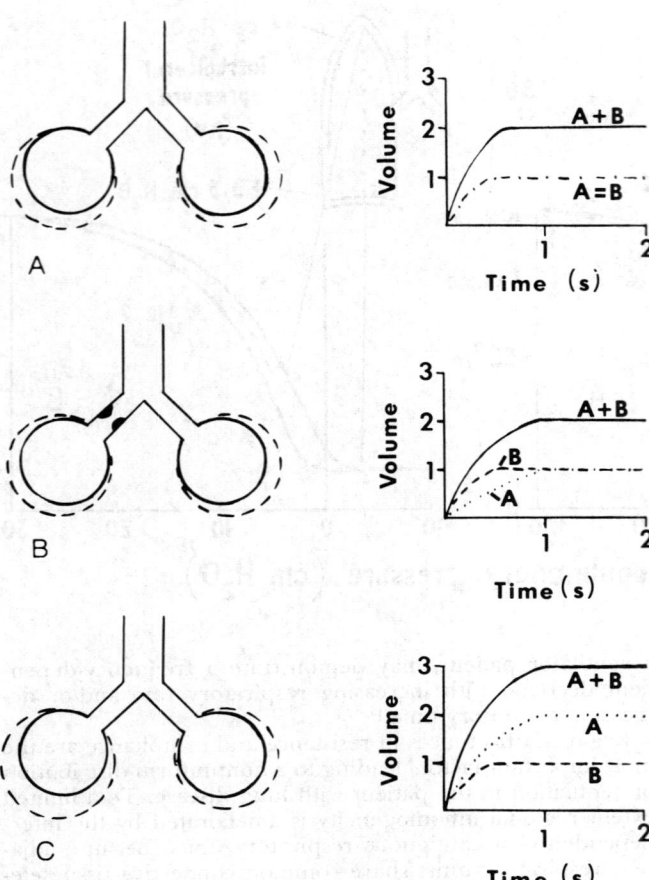

Figure 65–3. Frequency dependence of compliance can occur if either the compliance or resistance of the lung is increased in a nonuniform manner. *A.* Two lungs with equal compliances and resistances fill synchronously (curve A = B) and, as long as the time of inspiration is 0.5 second or greater, the volume within the lungs (curve A + B) and therefore the compliance ($\Delta V/\Delta P$) are constant. *B.* The resistance of the lung on the left is increased so that the time it takes to fill, indicated by the dotted curve A, is prolonged; when the duration of inspiration is less than 1.0 second, the volume of the lungs (curve A + B) and therefore the compliance of A + B fall. *C.* The compliance of the lung on the left is increased so that a greater volume of air must flow into that unit before it is filled to capacity (dotted curve A) and therefore it takes longer to fill. The compliance of A + B also falls when the duration of inspiration is less than 1.0 second. (From Conrad SA, Kinasewitz GT, George RB: Pulmonary Function Testing: Principles and Practice. Churchill Livingstone, New York, p 48, 1984.)

invariably coupled to the level of ventilation. Right ventricular output may be markedly depressed in a patient with acute pulmonary embolism despite a marked rise in ventilation.

Normal Hemodynamics

Pressures in the pulmonary blood vessels are low compared with those in the systemic circulation. The normal pulmonary arterial pressure, 10 to 20 mm Hg, is only one sixth that in a systemic artery. Because pulmonary arterial pressure is low, there is little smooth muscle in the walls of the pulmonary arteries and arterioles. In contrast to the systemic circulation, where most of the pressure drop occurs in muscular arteries, resistance in the pulmonary circulation is relatively evenly divided among the arterial, capillary, and venous segments of the pulmonary circulation.[19, 20] Pulmonary capillary pressure is midway between pulmonary arterial and pulmonary venous pressures, approximately one third of that in a systemic capillary. This low capillary pressure prevents accumulation of fluid in the lung under normal conditions (see Chapter 83).

The paucity of smooth muscle in the wall of the pulmonary arterioles suggests that there is little vasomotor tone in the normal pulmonary circulation. A two- to threefold increase in pulmonary blood flow is accommodated within the pulmonary vessels with little increase in pulmonary arterial pressure. The degree of vasomotor tone in the pulmonary vasculature may be inferred from examination of pressure-flow curves (Fig. 65–4). When left atrial pressure is constant, an increase in vasomotor tone is manifest by a shift to the left in the pressure-flow curve. However, because the differences in pressures may be small, changes in vasomotor tone

are most easily recognized when pressure and flow change in opposite directions; that is, an increased pulmonary arterial pressure and decreased cardiac output reflect an increase in vasomotor tone. In the presence of pulmonary hypertension, muscular hypertrophy develops within the media of pulmonary arterial walls. This hypertrophy encroaches on the vascular lumen and is responsible for a leftward shift of the pressure-flow curve and an exaggerated pressor response to a vasoconstrictor stimulus such as hypoxia.[21]

The pressure difference across the pulmonary circulation—that is, the difference between pulmonary arterial pressure and left atrial pressure—is low, generally about 10 mm Hg. This implies that pulmonary vascular resistance (PVR) is low. Analogous to the calculation of systemic vascular resistance, resistance in the pulmonary circuit can be calculated as

$$PVR = \frac{\text{pulmonary arterial pressure} - \text{left atrial pressure}}{\text{cardiac output}} \qquad (12)$$

Because of the lack of muscle in the pulmonary arterial wall, blood flow is pulsatile down to the level of the capillary. Mean pulmonary arterial pressure is used in the calculation of resistance. Clinically, the left atrial pressure is often approximated by the pulmonary capillary wedge pressure obtained with a balloon occlusion catheter. Normally, PVR is one sixth of that in the systemic circulation. Whereas it makes little difference if one includes the right atrial pressure in the calculation of systemic vascular resistance, the left atrial pressure is a significant fraction of the pulmonary arterial pressure and ignoring it leads to overestimating PVR.

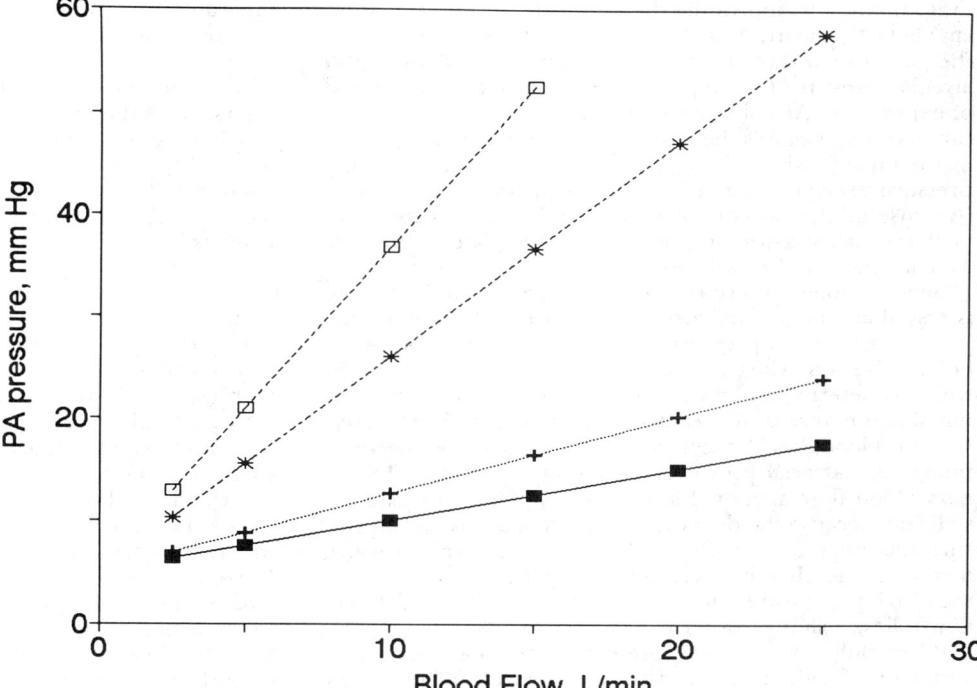

Figure 65–4. Pressure-flow relationships in the pulmonary circulation. In the normal pulmonary circulation the increase in pulmonary arterial (PA) pressure in response to increases in blood flow (at a constant left atrial pressure) is small (filled squares). An increase in vasomotor tone (plus signs) produces a minimal increase in PA pressure. In the patient with pulmonary hypertension the basal pressure-flow curve (asterisks) is shifted to the left and the amount of vasoconstriction that produced little response in the normal pulmonary circulation produces an exaggerated pulmonary pressor response (open squares).

The resistance of a blood vessel varies inversely with the fourth power of its radius. The pulmonary blood vessels are thin walled and easily distended whenever the pressure within them increases relative to the pressure outside them. Increases in pulmonary arterial and pulmonary venous pressure, increases in pulmonary blood flow, and increases in central blood volume all act not only to distend patent pulmonary vessels but also to recruit previously unperfused capillaries, thereby lowering PVR.[22–25] The pressure on the outside of the pulmonary vessels varies depending on whether they are extra-alveolar or alveolar vessels. The pressure surrounding extra-alveolar vessels is subatmospheric, similar to pleural pressure. Decreases in pleural pressure tend to further increase the transmural pressure—that is, the difference between intravascular and surrounding extramural pressures—of the arteries and veins, dilating them and decreasing their resistance. In contrast, the pressure surrounding the alveolar capillaries is probably similar to alveolar pressure. As the lung is inflated these vessels are stretched and compressed by the expanding alveoli so that their resistance increases. Total PVR, which is the sum of the extra-alveolar and alveolar resistances, is minimal at FRC and increases at both higher and lower lung volumes (Fig. 65–5).

DISTRIBUTION OF PERFUSION
Effect of Gravity

Lung inflation and changes in vasomotor tone tend to affect the pulmonary circulation in a uniform manner; that is, they produce similar changes in vascular resistance throughout the lung. However, even in a healthy individual blood flow through the pulmonary circulation is not uniformly distributed. Perfusion is greatest at the lung bases and decreases as the height above the most dependent portion of the lung increases. This vertical gradient in pulmonary blood flow is primarily due to the effect of gravity on pulmonary vascular pressures. Alveolar pressure is identical in all regions of the lung, whereas intravascular pressure

increases or decreases by 1 cm H_2O for each centimeter of distance below or above the level of the heart. The interrelationships of pulmonary arterial, pulmonary venous, and alveolar pressures determine the relative perfusion at different heights in the lung.[26]

The pressures in the pulmonary arteries and pulmonary veins decrease by about 1 cm H_2O for each centimeter of vertical distance the blood ascends toward the apex of the

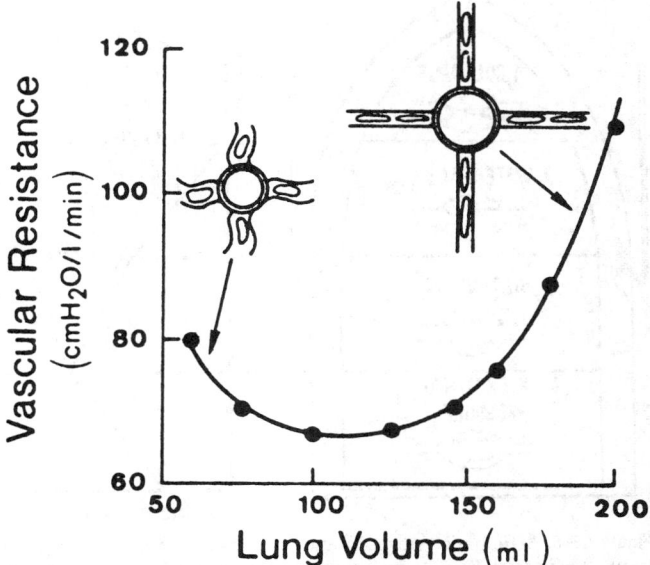

Figure 65–5. Effect of lung volume on PVR when capillary transmural pressure is held constant. At low lung volumes the resistance is high because the extra-alveolar vessels become narrow. At high lung volumes the capillaries are stretched and their caliber is reduced. (Data from a dog lobe preparation.) (From West JB: Respiratory Physiology—The Essentials. 2nd ed. Baltimore, Williams & Wilkins, p 39, 1979. © 1979, the Williams & Wilkins Co., Baltimore.)

lung. In an erect individual the apices are approximately 20 cm above the heart, so that, as the blood rises, at some point the pressure within the pulmonary artery may fall below alveolar pressure (which is zero or atmospheric at the end of expiration). Alveolar pressure exceeds the pressure in the capillaries and causes them to collapse. Zone 1 is the portion of the lung in which there is no perfusion because alveolar pressure exceeds pulmonary arterial pressure (Fig. 65–6). (Because of the pulsatile nature of pulmonary blood flow, peak systolic pressure actually may be adequate to produce a small amount of flow in zone 1.)

Beneath zone 1 there is a region where alveolar pressure is less than pulmonary arterial pressure but greater than pulmonary venous pressure. The vessels within this zone 2 behave like a Starling resistor or thin tube, the diameter of which is determined by the difference between the intraluminal and extramural pressures. The relevant driving pressure for blood flow through zone 2 is the difference between pulmonary arterial pressure and alveolar pressure. Pulmonary blood flow in zone 2 has been compared to a vascular waterfall because the downstream (pulmonary venous) pressure has no effect on flow.[27] Pulmonary arterial pressure increases linearly with descending distance, and therefore the driving pressure for blood flow, Pa − PA, and blood flow follow a similar pattern.

When pulmonary venous pressure exceeds alveolar pressure (zone 3), the relevant driving pressure for blood flow is the difference between pulmonary arterial and pulmonary venous pressure. Both increase equally with decreasing vertical height within zone 3. Even though the driving pressure for blood flow (i.e., the difference between pulmonary arterial and pulmonary venous pressure) remains constant in zone 3, blood flow increases down the lung, although not as rapidly as in zone 2. This increasing blood flow has been attributed to the fact that even though the arteriovenous pressure difference is constant, absolute intravascular pressure increases with decreasing height in zone 3. This increas-

ing transmural pressure produces greater vascular distention and/or recruitment and therefore a progressive decrease in PVR.

At the lung bases blood flow may actually decrease despite the fact that the highest intravascular pressures are encountered at the bottom of the lung. The size of zone 4 increases at low lung volumes and is most pronounced at residual volume.[28, 29] The resistance of the extra-alveolar vessels is increased at low lung volumes, and this is thought to be responsible for the diminution of flow in zone 4.

Hypoxia

Hypoxia is a potent stimulus that induces pulmonary vasoconstriction.[30] Global hypoxia, such as that experienced by high-altitude residents, produces generalized pulmonary vasoconstriction and pulmonary hypertension. The vasoconstrictor response is generalized and therefore has little effect on the overall distribution of resistance in the lung.

Hypoxia at the local level also produces pulmonary vasoconstriction. Regional alveolar hypoxia commonly develops when alveoli are underventilated relative to their perfusion. In contrast to the potentially detrimental pulmonary hypertensive response to global hypoxia, the localized vasoconstriction that develops in response to regional hypoxia can have beneficial effects. Arterial hypoxemia is a consequence of perfusion to underventilated alveoli. A localized increase in PVR as a result of regional hypoxia diverts the pulmonary blood flow to the better-ventilated regions of the lung and improves arterial oxygenation. The extent of pulmonary vasoconstriction in response to alveolar hypoxia varies widely among individuals. Even though pulmonary hypertension may ensue when the parenchymal lung disease is widespread, patients with a strong vasoconstrictive response to alveolar hypoxia generally have better blood gas values than those with a weak response.

Blood Flow in Lung Disease

Hypoxia is just one of many factors that influence pulmonary blood flow and the distribution of perfusion (Table 65–1). When hypoxia persists for more than a few days it stimulates vascular smooth muscle proliferation and leads to the development of muscular hypertrophy within the media of the pulmonary arterial wall.[31] Increases in arterial wall smooth muscle accentuate the vasoconstrictor response to hypoxia and other stimuli and can produce both pulmonary hypertension and a redistribution of blood flow. This vascular remodeling may be associated with localized capillary loss that reduces the effective alveolar capillary surface area available for gas exchange.

Pulmonary embolism is the prototypical example of a pulmonary vascular disease that produces a redistribution of blood flow. However, many parenchymal diseases also affect adjacent blood vessels. Pulmonary fibrosis within the interstitium may obliterate adjacent arterioles and capillaries, leading to pulmonary hypertension. Indeed, the severity of pulmonary hypertension in patients with interstitial disease correlates with the degree of fibrosis as reflected by the reduction in lung volume rather than with the PaO_2.[32] In contrast, pulmonary hypertension and vascular remodeling are more closely related to the PaO_2 in patients with emphysema and chronic bronchitis.[33]

Low-output states resulting from hemorrhage or pump failure may alter the pattern of distribution in the critically ill. Hypovolemia is usually associated with reduced pulmonary vascular pressures and increased amounts of zones 1 and 2.[34] Pulmonary venous hypertension increases the portion of the lung that is zone 3.[35] Intravascular thrombi are

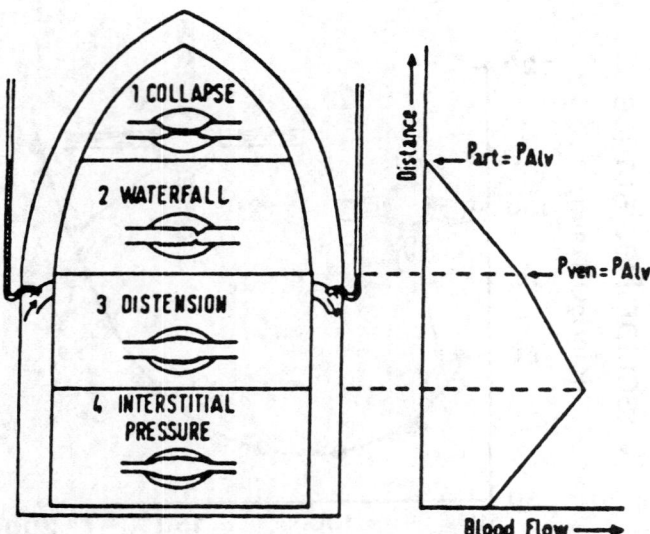

Figure 65–6. Schematic representation of how arterial (Pa [P$_{art}$ on figure]), alveolar (PA [P$_{Alv}$ on figure]), and venous (Pv [P$_{ven}$ on figure]) pressure determine pulmonary blood flow in the different zones of the lung. The diagram on the left shows factors that influence blood flow in zones 1 to 4, and the diagram on the right shows regional blood flow per unit alveolar volume at corresponding levels in the lung. See text for details. (From Hughes JMB, Glazier JB, Maloney JE: Effect of lung volume on the distribution of pulmonary blood flow in man. Respir Physiol 4:70, 1968.)

TABLE 65–1

FACTORS THAT INFLUENCE THE DISTRIBUTION OF PULMONARY PERFUSION

In Health	In Critically Ill Patients
Gravity	Disease related
Pulmonary arterial pressure	Hypoxia
Left atrial pressure	Acidosis
Cardiac output	Vasoactive mediators
Pulmonary blood volume	Thrombi
Lung volume	Therapy related
Alveolar pressure	Positive end-expiratory
Vasomotor tone	pressure
	Inotropic agents
	Vasodilators

another important cause of perfusion maldistribution in the critically ill. Cardiac failure, tissue injury, sepsis, and disseminated intravascular coagulation all predispose to the development of thrombosis. Deep venous thrombosis and catheter-associated thrombi are potential sources of pulmonary emboli.[36–38] However, because the incidence of intravascular thrombi parallels the severity of the parenchymal disease in patients with acute respiratory failure, it is thought that many of these lesions are formed in situ.[39] Vasoactive mediators such as locally produced prostanoids (e.g., thromboxane) and cytokines (e.g., interleukin-1 and tumor necrosis factor) are also potential modulators of pulmonary perfusion.[40–45]

GAS EXCHANGE

The major functions of the respiratory system are to provide O_2 for tissue metabolism and to eliminate CO_2. O_2 moves from a region of high concentration in alveolar gas to a region of low concentration, mixed venous blood, by passive diffusion. Similarly, CO_2 in mixed venous blood escapes into the alveolar gas by diffusion. For O_2 and CO_2 exchange to occur, there must be sufficient ventilation to maintain the O_2 and CO_2 concentration gradients between alveolar gas and mixed venous blood. Pulmonary blood flow must be adequate so that the overall level of O_2 delivery to the tissues is sufficient for the metabolic demand. Moreover, the blood flow must be distributed to ventilated alveoli so that gas exchange can take place.

The simplest measures of the adequacy of gas exchange are the arterial Po_2 and Pco_2. Impaired diffusion across the alveolar capillary membrane and blood flow to nonventilated alveoli are potential causes of hypoxemia. An inadequate level of ventilation can produce hypoxemia and hypercapnia. However, mismatching of ventilation ($\dot{V}$) and perfusion ($\dot{Q}$) is the most common cause of impaired gas exchange encountered clinically.

DIFFUSION

The rate at which a gas diffuses across a membrane is proportional to the partial pressure difference between the two sides and the surface area (SA) of the membrane and is inversely related to the thickness of the membrane:

$$\dot{V}gas = \frac{SA}{T} \times D\,(P_1 - P_2) \qquad (13)$$

where D is the diffusion constant. When diffusion occurs between gas (alveolar air) and liquid (tissue and blood) phases, the value of D is proportional to the solubility of the gas and inversely related to its molecular weight. CO_2 is so

much more soluble than O_2 that its equilibration between pulmonary capillary blood and alveolar gas is extremely rapid and its excretion is relatively unaffected by the diffusing capacity of the lung.[46]

O_2 transfer across the alveolar capillary membrane may be diffusion limited under certain circumstances. Capillary blood flow is pulsatile and red blood cells reside in the pulmonary capillary for about 0.75 second under normal resting conditions. This is sufficient time for the Po_2 in alveolar gas and that in pulmonary capillary blood to equilibrate (Fig. 65–7). However, when pulmonary blood flow increases, the amount of time each red blood cell spends in the pulmonary capillary diminishes. In high-output states, such as exercise or sepsis, O_2 equilibration between alveolar gas and capillary blood may be incomplete.

The diffusing capacity of the lung (DL) for O_2 depends not only on the physical characteristics of the alveolar capillary membrane (i.e., its area and thickness) but also on the rate at which O_2 combines with the hemoglobin in the pulmonary capillaries. The latter is determined by the rate at which O_2 combines with a known quantity of hemoglobin (Θ) and the volume of blood in the pulmonary capillaries (Vc). Because the diffusing capacity is the flow of gas per millimeter of mercury pressure difference, the inverse, $1/DL$, represents the resistance to gas transfer by diffusion. This may be expressed as the sum of two resistances in series:

$$1/DL = 1/Dm + 1/(\Theta \times Vc) \qquad (14)$$

In a normal individual the membrane component, Dm, and $\Theta \times Vc$ contribute equally to DL, so disorders that reduce the surface area or increase the thickness of the barrier to diffusion and those that reduce the capillary blood volume affect the rate at which O_2 diffuses across the alveolar capillary membrane.[47, 48] Diffusion is impaired in diseases that destroy alveolar septa, such as emphysema, and when the functional capillary blood volume is reduced, as in pulmonary embolism.

The rate at which O_2 diffuses also depends on the partial pressure difference between alveolar gas and the mixed

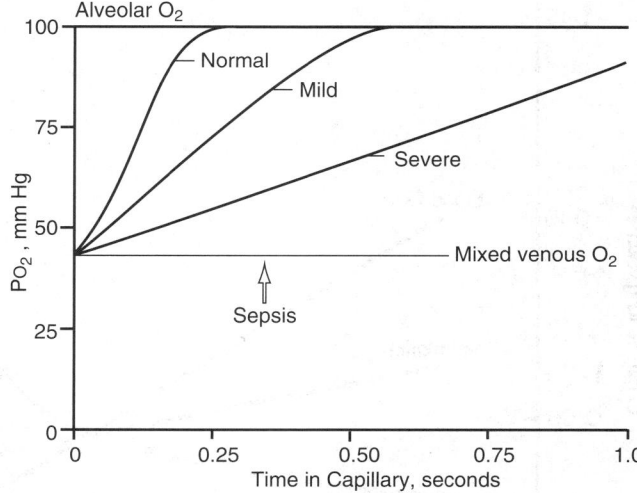

Figure 65–7. Time course of O_2 transfer by diffusion into pulmonary capillary blood. In the normal individual oxygenation is complete within 0.25 second, so the 0.75 second that the red blood cell spends in the pulmonary capillary represents a significant time reserve. Severe diffusion impairment produces hypoxemia at rest, whereas mild impairment may not be evident unless the transit time of the red blood cell through the capillary is decreased, as when the cardiac output increases during sepsis.

venous blood returning to the pulmonary capillary. It is intuitively obvious that a reduction in the P_{O_2} of inspired air, such as occurs at high altitude, reduces the driving pressure for O_2 transfer across the alveolar capillary membrane. An analogous situation can develop at a local level in the poorly ventilated alveolus with a low P_{O_2} resulting from ventilation-perfusion mismatching.

MATCHING OF VENTILATION AND PERFUSION

Normal Ventilation-Perfusion Matching

In a healthy individual alveolar ventilation averages 4 to 6 L/min and cardiac output is approximately 5 to 7 L/min, for an overall $\dot{V}/\dot{Q}$ ratio of 0.8 to 1.0. Alterations in the absolute level of either ventilation or pulmonary blood flow change $\dot{V}/\dot{Q}$ ratios throughout the lung and have an effect on gas exchange. Increasing alveolar ventilation raises the alveolar O_2 content and lowers the alveolar CO_2 content, which produces similar changes in the arterial P_{O_2} and P_{CO_2}. The opposite occurs when ventilation is reduced. Changes in cardiac output primarily affect the mixed venous O_2 and CO_2 contents. A reduction in blood flow is accompanied by a decrease in mixed venous P_{O_2} and an increase in P_{CO_2}. However, under normal conditions mixed venous blood equilibrates with alveolar gas so that the effect of a reduction in blood flow on arterial gas tensions may be minimal. The effect of lowering the mixed venous O_2 content on arterial oxygenation is most noticeable in the patient with pulmonary disease in whom gas transfer may be impaired.

Even though the overall $\dot{V}/\dot{Q}$ ratio in a healthy subject may be 0.9, there is considerable variability in regional $\dot{V}/\dot{Q}$ ratios in the normal lung.[49] Ventilation is not uniformly distributed because of the effect of the gradient in pleural pressure. Recall that alveoli at the top of the lung have a higher resting volume but those at the base receive a relatively greater proportion of each tidal breath. Perfusion is least at the apex of the lung and progressively increases through zones 2 and 3. The relative amounts of ventilation and perfusion to the apex and base of the lung are illustrated

in Figure 65–8. As the vertical height above the lung bases decreases, the amount of perfusion to each alveolar capillary unit increases faster than the amount of ventilation so that the $\dot{V}/\dot{Q}$ ratio falls with progression toward the bottom of the lung.

The pulmonary end-capillary P_{O_2} and P_{CO_2} expected for blood perfusing alveolar capillary units with different $\dot{V}/\dot{Q}$ ratios are illustrated in Figure 65–9. The pulmonary end-capillary P_{O_2} changes significantly as the $\dot{V}/\dot{Q}$ ratio varies above and below the normal mean value of 0.9. However, below a $\dot{V}/\dot{Q}$ ratio of 0.1 the pulmonary end-capillary P_{O_2} is close to the mixed venous P_{O_2} and little further decrease occurs with falling $\dot{V}/\dot{Q}$ ratios below this level. Increasing $\dot{V}/\dot{Q}$ ratios above 10 produce little further increase in pulmonary end-capillary P_{O_2}, which is rapidly approaching that of the inspired air. However, if one examines the O_2 content of end-capillary blood, it can be seen that little additional O_2 is added at $\dot{V}/\dot{Q}$ ratios greater than 1. The normal pulmonary end-capillary P_{CO_2} is so close to the mixed venous P_{CO_2} that it changes very little if the $\dot{V}/\dot{Q}$ ratio falls below 0.8. As the $\dot{V}/\dot{Q}$ ratio increases above this value, the P_{CO_2} of end-capillary blood falls. Because the relationship between the blood P_{CO_2} and its CO_2 content is linear in this range, there is a proportionate fall in the CO_2 content of end-capillary blood.

Despite the presence of $\dot{V}/\dot{Q}$ heterogeneity resulting from regional differences in ventilation and perfusion, $\dot{V}/\dot{Q}$ ratios in a healthy young individual are narrowly dispersed around a mean value of 0.8 to 1.0 (Fig. 65–10). When expressed in terms of absolute ventilation or blood flow, virtually all perfusion and ventilation are unimodally distributed to alveolar capillary units with a $\dot{V}/\dot{Q}$ ratio close to the mean. Deviations from this normal pattern are primarily responsible for the abnormalities in gas exchange that develop in critically ill patients.

VENTILATION-PERFUSION MATCHING IN DISEASE

A wide variety of $\dot{V}/\dot{Q}$ patterns may be present when the distributions of both ventilation and perfusion are altered

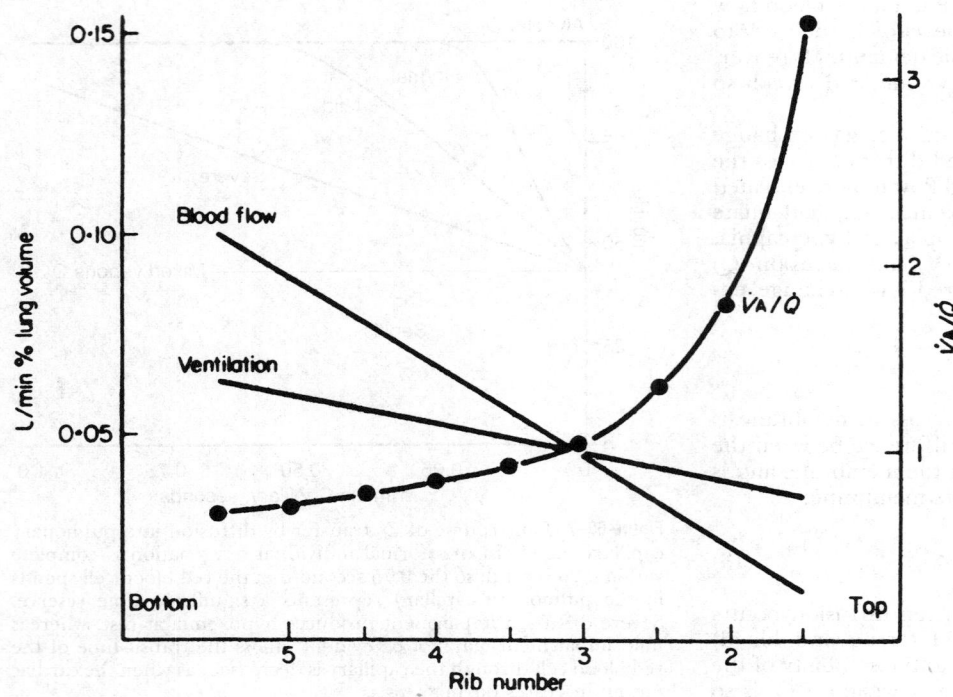

Figure 65–8. Effect of vertical height (expressed as the level of the anterior ends of the ribs) on ventilation and pulmonary blood flow (*left ordinate*) and the ventilation/perfusion ratio (*right ordinate*). (From West JB: Ventilation/Blood Flow and Gas Exchange. 5th ed. Oxford, Blackwell Scientific Publications, p 30, 1990.)

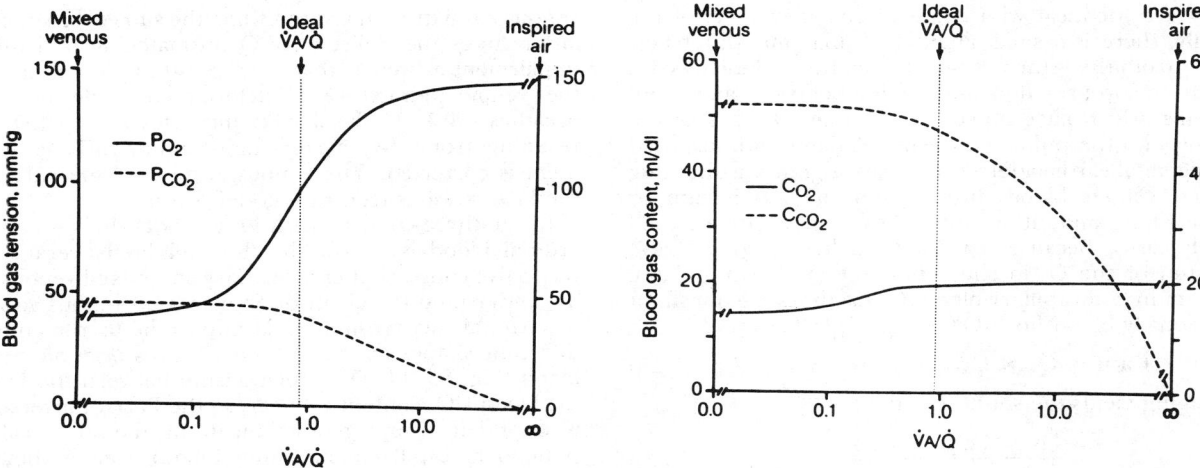

Figure 65–9. Relationship between $\dot{V}/\dot{Q}$ ratio and the end-capillary P_{O_2} and P_{CO_2} *(left)* and O_2 and CO_2 contents *(right)*. The major increment in oxygenation occurs over a relatively narrow range of $\dot{V}/\dot{Q}$ ratios. The P_{CO_2} and CO_2 content of blood continue to fall as the $\dot{V}/\dot{Q}$ ratio increases. (From Fishman AP [ed]: Pulmonary Diseases and Disorders. 2nd ed. New York, McGraw-Hill, p 194, 1988. Reproduced with permission of McGraw-Hill.)

in patients with lung disease. In these patients the local effects of alterations in airway resistance and lung compliance are superimposed on the normal gradient in pleural pressure. This produces a heterogeneous pattern of ventilation in adjacent regions of the lung. Similarly, regional variations in blood flow resulting from alveolar hypoxia, vascular obstruction, and alterations in vasomotor tone caused by mediator release may modify or override the normal gravity-dependent pattern of pulmonary perfusion. Excess ventilation of alveolar capillary units that are underperfused relative to their ventilation (high $\dot{V}/\dot{Q}$ ratios) has

little effect on arterial P_{O_2} but is responsible for an increase in physiologic dead space. Perfusion of poorly ventilated alveoli (low $\dot{V}/\dot{Q}$ units) contributes little CO_2 to the mixed expired gas, but capillary blood from these units has a low P_{O_2} and is primarily responsible for the arterial hypoxemia of many of these patients.

SHUNT

Blood flow through alveolar capillary units that receive no ventilation ($\dot{V}/\dot{Q} = 0$) is shunt flow. Its end-capillary gas

Figure 65–10. Distribution of ventilation (open circles) and perfusion (filled circles) to alveoli with different $\dot{V}/\dot{Q}$ ratios in a normal individual. Note that most of the ventilation and perfusion goes to lung units with $\dot{V}/\dot{Q}$ ratios near 1. (From Wagner PD, Laravuso RB, Uhl RR, et al: Continuous distributions of ventilation-perfusion ratios in normal subjects breathing air and 100% O_2. Reproduced from the Journal of Clinical Investigation, 1974, volume 54, pp 54–68 by copyright permission of the American Society of Clinical Investigation.)

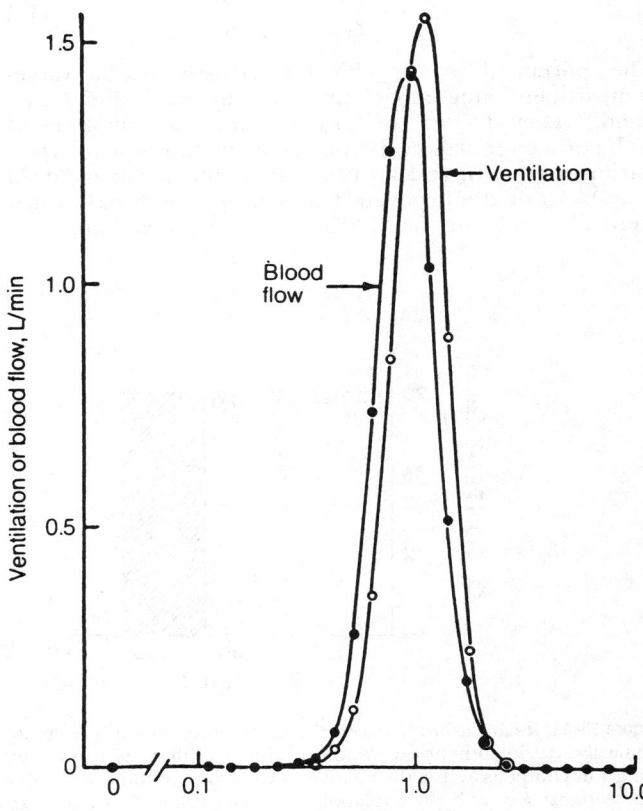

tensions are identical with those of mixed venous blood. Normally, there is a small amount of anatomic shunt flow resulting from the return of blood from the thebesian veins, which drain coronary flow into the left ventricle, and bronchial veins, which have no contact with alveolar gas before emptying into the pulmonary veins. Patients with acquired and congenital cardiac defects can have significant shunting of mixed venous blood directly into the left atrium or ventricle. The amount of shunt flow can be determined relatively easily. Because systemic O_2 delivery, $\dot{Q}_T \times Cao_2$, is the sum of the O_2 in shunt flow ($\dot{Q}s \times C\bar{v}o_2$) and the O_2 content in end-capillary blood ($Cc'o_2$) times the nonshunt or pulmonary blood flow ($\dot{Q}_T - \dot{Q}s$), it follows that

$$\dot{Q}_T \times Cao_2 = \dot{Q}s \times C\bar{v}o_2 + (\dot{Q}_T - \dot{Q}s) \times Cc'o_2 \quad (15)$$

Rearranging yields the shunt equation:

$$\frac{\dot{Q}s}{\dot{Q}_T} = \frac{Cc'o_2 - Cao_2}{Cc'o_2 - C\bar{v}o_2} \quad (16)$$

The O_2 content of end-capillary blood is calculated from the alveolar Po_2. Either the O_2 content of mixed venous blood is measured directly or, if the cardiac output is normal, an estimated arteriovenous O_2 difference of 4.5 mL/dL can be used to calculate the shunt flow. The normal physiologic shunt flow is less than 5%.

Blood flow from unventilated alveoli has a composition identical with that of mixed venous blood. Blood flow from alveoli that are underventilated relative to their perfusion has O_2 and CO_2 contents somewhere between those of mixed venous blood and ideal alveolar gas. One can account for the hypoxemia associated with perfusion of low $\dot{V}/\dot{Q}$ alveoli by calculating the venous admixture, $\dot{Q}va$, that is, the physiologic shunt flow needed to account for the observed depression in arterial O_2 content. Analogous to the calculation of true shunt,

$$\frac{\dot{Q}va}{\dot{Q}_T} = \frac{Cc'o_2 - Cao_2}{Cc'o_2 - C\bar{v}o_2} \quad (17)$$

The concept of venous admixture is based on the three-compartment lung model proposed by Riley and Cournand.[50] They divided the lung into an ideal compartment with normal ventilation and perfusion, an unventilated compartment (shunt), and an unperfused compartment (dead space). All of the hypoxemia present is considered as if it were due to shunt flow through unventilated lung. The venous admixture measured while the subject breathes room air includes the effect of $\dot{V}$-$\dot{Q}$ mismatching and diffusion impairment as well as that of true right-to-left shunt. When the venous admixture is determined while the patient breathes 100% O_2, alveolar Po_2 increases and the hypoxemia resulting from $\dot{V}$-$\dot{Q}$ mismatching and/or diffusion impairment is corrected. The venous admixture measured when the $Fio_2 = 1.0$ is true right-to-left shunt.

In the three-compartment lung model the gas content of arterial blood is simply the flow-weighted average of the respective contents of end-capillary and mixed venous blood. To understand the effect of an increased venous admixture on arterial gas tensions it is important to remember the different shapes of the O_2 and CO_2 dissociation curves in blood (Fig. 65–11). The relationship between the Pco_2 and the blood CO_2 content is linear, so the Pco_2 of arterial blood is essentially the algebraic mean of the Pco_2 values of pulmonary capillary and shunt blood; even if the venous admixture were to increase drastically, a modest increment in alveolar ventilation would maintain a normal $Paco_2$. In contrast, the sigmoid shape of the hemoglobin dissociation curve means that there is little increase in the O_2 content of pulmonary capillary blood with hyperventilation because hemoglobin is almost completely saturated at a Pao_2 of 100 mm Hg. Therefore the Pao_2 must fall as the shunt fraction increases. The effect of increasing the inspired O_2 concentration on Pao_2 at different levels of shunt is illustrated in Figure 65–12.

DEAD SPACE

The opposite extreme is the alveolus that is ventilated but not perfused ($\dot{V}/\dot{Q} = \infty$), that is, alveolar dead space. Because such alveoli are not perfused, they have no direct effect on arterial gas tensions. Pao_2 and $Paco_2$, the alveolar partial pressures of O_2 and CO_2, are identical with those of inspired air, and when expired gas from these alveoli mixes with the effective alveolar ventilation, it reduces the Pco_2 of mixed expired gas. If a minimal amount of perfusion is restored to this alveolus, the amount of O_2 removed from the alveolar gas and the amount of CO_2 added are small because of the limited amount of mixed venous blood available to be arterialized. Alveolar gas tensions change minimally, and the small quantity of capillary blood from this gas exchange unit has little appreciable effect on arterial gas tensions. In terms of the three-compartment lung model, the amount of phys-

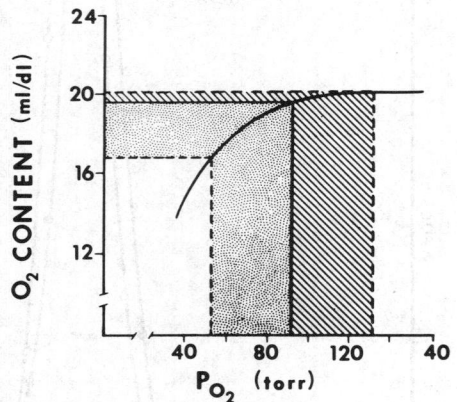
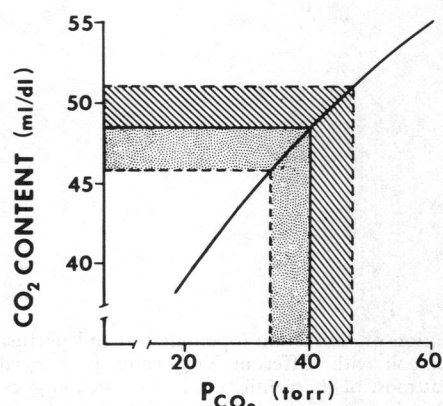

Figure 65–11. Relationship between the partial pressure and content of O_2 and CO_2 in blood over the range of partial pressures encountered clinically. Regional hypoventilation produces a fall in O_2 content and an increase in CO_2 content; hyperventilation in another region of the lung can compensate for the change in CO_2 content, but the small increase in O_2 content produced by hyperventilation does not correct the decrease caused by hypoventilation. (From Conrad SA, Kinasewitz GT, George RB: Pulmonary Function Testing: Principles and Practice. Churchill Livingstone, New York, p 67, 1984.)

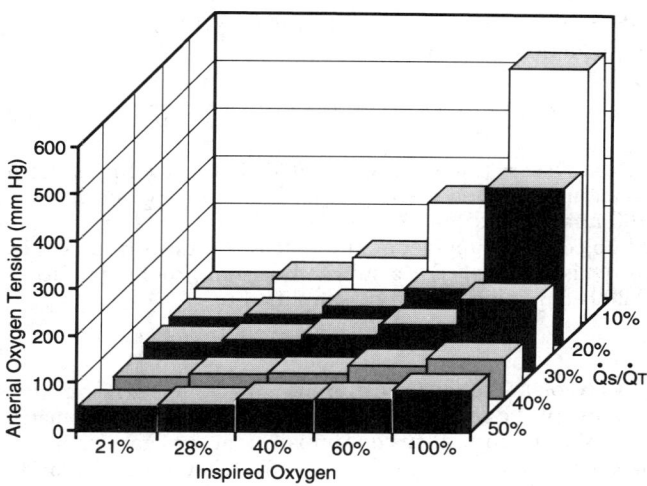

Figure 65–12. Effect of changes in F_{IO_2} on Pa_{O_2} with different-size shunts. Notice that for each of the different-size shunts ($\dot{Q}s/\dot{Q}T$) an increase in F_{IO_2} produces an increase in Pa_{O_2}, but for a $\dot{Q}s/\dot{Q}T$ of 50% the increase is barely perceptible (43 to 57 torr as F_{IO_2} increases from 21 to 100%).

iologic dead space can be quantitated using the Bohr equation (Equation 11).

VENTILATION-PERFUSION HETEROGENEITY

Between the extremes of shunt and dead space, variations in $\dot{V}/\dot{Q}$ ratios produce intermediate effects on arterial blood gas tensions. The full range of $\dot{V}/\dot{Q}$ effects on end-capillary blood gas tensions is illustrated in Figure 65–9. However, the effect of an abnormal $\dot{V}/\dot{Q}$ on the P_{O_2} and P_{CO_2} of expired air and arterial blood can be simplified if we consider a hypothetic lung with three alveolar capillary units characterized by low (0.1), high (10.0), and normal (1.0) $\dot{V}/\dot{Q}$ ratios. If the overall ventilation is 5.25 L/min and pulmonary perfusion is 5.25 L/min, the distribution of ventilation and

perfusion is that illustrated in Figure 65–13. The 5.25 L of expired gas includes 0.25 L from the low $\dot{V}/\dot{Q}$ alveolus, which has a low Pa_{O_2} and high Pa_{CO_2}; 2.5 L from the normal $\dot{V}/\dot{Q}$ alveolus with normal gas tensions; and 2.5 L from the high $\dot{V}/\dot{Q}$ alveolus, which has an increased Pa_{O_2} and low Pa_{CO_2} reflecting the wasted ventilation. Arterial blood, on the other hand, receives 2.5 L of flow from the capillary with a low $\dot{V}/\dot{Q}$ ratio; blood from this alveolar capillary unit has a low O_2 content and arterial hypoxemia is the inevitable consequence.

The Pc_{O_2} and CO_2 content of blood from low $\dot{V}/\dot{Q}$ alveoli are also higher than normal. However, this excess CO_2 can be compensated for if there is sufficient perfusion from alveoli with high $\dot{V}/\dot{Q}$ ratios and a low CO_2 content. Because CO_2 is a potent stimulus to ventilation, a small increase in Pa_{CO_2} stimulates an increase in overall ventilation so that the arterial Pc_{O_2} is maintained at normal levels. In contrast, because of the sigmoidal relationship between P_{O_2} and O_2 content, the O_2 content of arterial blood from alveoli with a high $\dot{V}/\dot{Q}$ ratio does not increase enough to compensate for low $\dot{V}/\dot{Q}$ units (see Fig. 65–11).

This ability to increase the overall level of ventilation to maintain a normal Pa_{CO_2} may be compromised in individuals with an inordinate amount of ventilation to high $\dot{V}/\dot{Q}$ alveoli (high V_{DS}/V_T ratio). In these patients the level of $\dot{V}_E$ required to maintain an adequate level of alveolar ventilation for CO_2 elimination may encroach on or exceed their ventilatory reserve. In this instance, to prevent respiratory muscle fatigue, the patient compromises on a lower $\dot{V}_E$ that can be maintained comfortably, but CO_2 retention is the result. Thus, whereas hypoxemia is an inevitable consequence of $\dot{V}$-$\dot{Q}$ mismatching, hypercapnia may also result if there is a bimodal distribution of $\dot{V}/\dot{Q}$ ratios with an inordinate amount of ventilation to high $\dot{V}/\dot{Q}$ regions that prevents adequate compensatory hyperventilation for the excess CO_2 content of blood from areas with a low $\dot{V}/\dot{Q}$ ratio.

CLINICAL ASSESSMENT OF GAS EXCHANGE

The clinical assessment of gas exchange begins with an analysis of the arterial blood gases. Hypoxemia most commonly is due to $\dot{V}$-$\dot{Q}$ mismatching, but increased shunt flow, diffusion impairment, and hypoventilation are other poten-

Figure 65–13. Mismatching of ventilation and perfusion produces arterial hypoxemia because the large volume of poorly oxygenated blood from the alveolus on the left ($\dot{V}/\dot{Q} = 1/10$) is not compensated by the small amount of well-oxygenated blood derived from the alveolus on the right ($\dot{V}/\dot{Q} = 10/1$). The Pc_{O_2} of expired air falls because alveolar gas from the alveolus on the right contains little CO_2. See text for details.

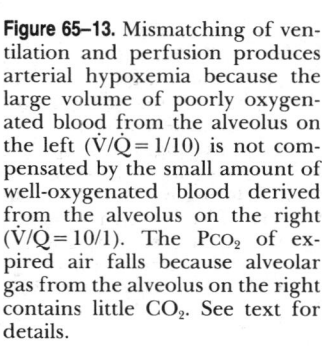
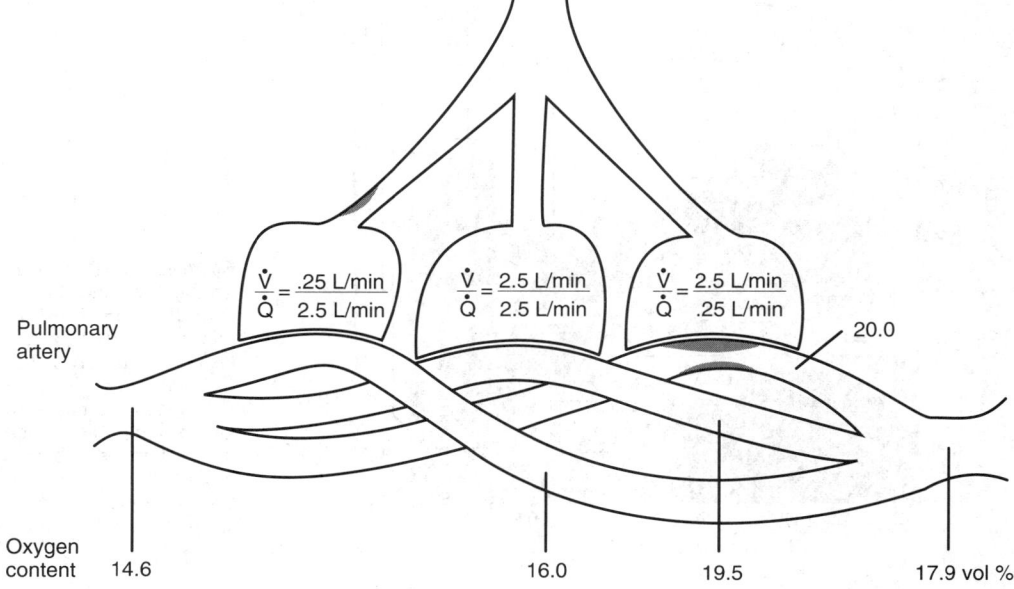

tial causes of arterial desaturation. In contrast, hypercapnia always indicates alveolar hypoventilation. The hypoventilation may be due to a reduction in the overall level of ventilation, as during anesthesia, or may reflect decreased effective alveolar ventilation caused by increased ventilation of high $\dot{V}/\dot{Q}$ alveoli in the patient with chronic obstructive pulmonary disease. In the latter instance the absolute level of minute ventilation typically is increased but, because of the wasted ventilation to high $\dot{V}/\dot{Q}$ alveoli, ventilation to well-perfused gas exchange units is reduced. This wasted ventilation is reflected by an abnormally high V_{DS}/V_T ratio.

Alveolar-Arterial Oxygen Difference

Even in a previously healthy individual without lung disease, alveolar hypoventilation produces hypoxemia and hypercapnia. When alveolar ventilation falls, the Pa_{CO_2} must increase (Equation 8). The alveolar Po_2, which is inversely related to alveolar P_{CO_2}, can be calculated from the alveolar gas equation as

$$P_{AO_2} = P_{IO_2} - P_{ACO_2}\left(F_{IO_2} + \frac{1 - F_{IO_2}}{R}\right) \quad (18)$$

where $P_{IO_2} = (P_B - P_{H_2O}) \times F_{IO_2}$. The partial pressure of water in saturated inspired gas is 47 mm Hg, so, if $P_B = 760$ mm Hg, $P_{IO_2} = (760 - 47) \times 0.209 = 149$ mm Hg in a subject breathing room air. If R is not measured, a value of 0.8 is assumed. For a subject breathing room air ($F_{IO_2} = 0.209$), Equation 18 can be simplified to

$$P_{AO_2} = 149 - P_{ACO_2}/0.8 \quad (19)$$

An alveolar-arterial O_2 difference ($P_{AO_2} - Pa_{O_2}$) develops because of the previously described effects of $\dot{V}$-$\dot{Q}$ mismatching, shunt, and diffusion impairment on gas exchange. Because there is normally some $\dot{V}/\dot{Q}$ heterogeneity and a small physiologic shunt is present, the normal $P_{AO_2} - Pa_{O_2}$

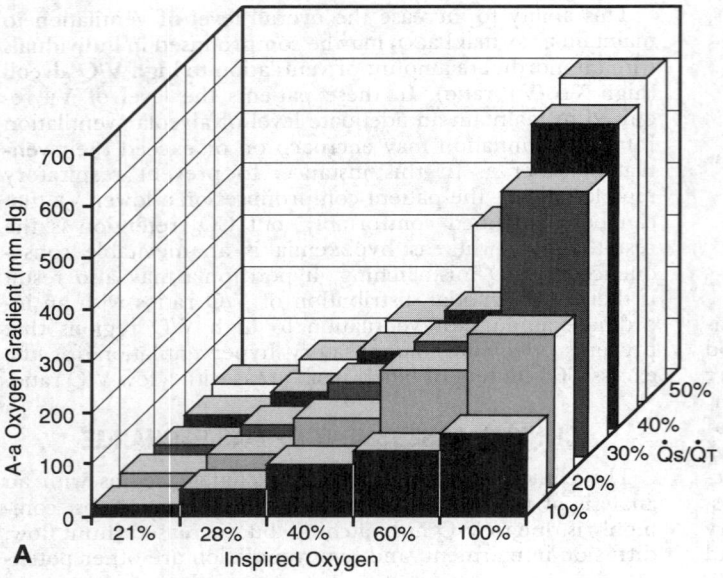

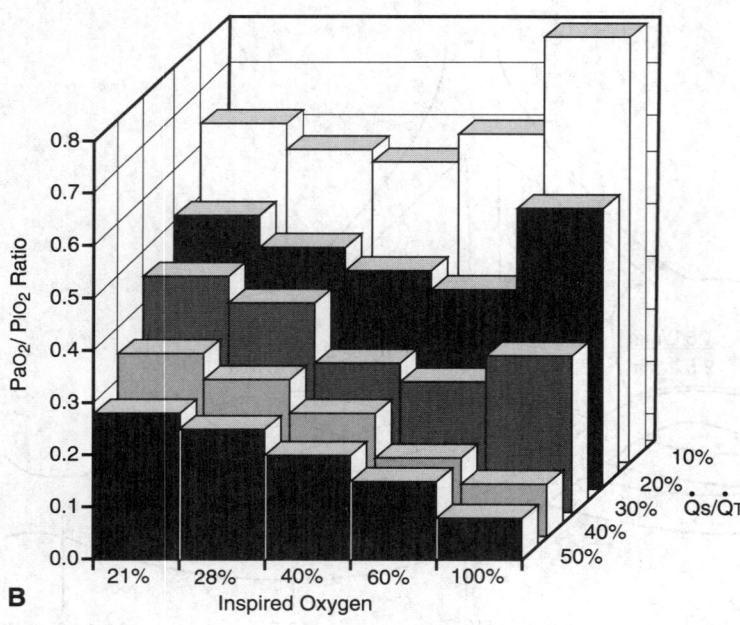

Figure 65–14. Effect of changes in F_{IO_2} on $P_{AO_2} - Pa_{O_2}$ (O_2 gradient, *A*) and the arterial/inspired O_2 ratio (Pa_{O_2}/P_{IO_2}, *B*) with different-size shunts. For each shunt the $P_{AO_2} - Pa_{O_2}$ increases with F_{IO_2} and, although it is greater for larger $\dot{Q}s/\dot{Q}_T$ at any given F_{IO_2}, it is too variable to be useful for characterizing gas exchange during changes in F_{IO_2}. The Pa_{O_2}/P_{IO_2} ratio has been used to characterize the severity of gas exchange abnormalities at differing levels of F_{IO_2}, but it also changes with changes in F_{IO_2}. The direction of change in Pa_{O_2}/P_{IO_2} with increases in F_{IO_2} is different for different $\dot{Q}s/\dot{Q}_T$ values, demonstrating a steady decrease for $\dot{Q}s/\dot{Q}_T$ greater than 30% and biphasic changes for $\dot{Q}s/\dot{Q}_T$ of 30% or less.

may reach 10 mm Hg in a 20-year-old person breathing room air.[51] The $P_{A_{O_2}} - P_{a_{O_2}}$ widens with age because of airway closure and lower $\dot{V}/\dot{Q}$ ratios at the lung bases in older individuals. Values up to 20 mm Hg are normal in a 65-year-old individual breathing room air.

As the $P_{a_{CO_2}}$ rises and the $P_{A_{O_2}}$ falls because of alveolar hypoventilation, even when there is normal gas exchange and complete equilibration of pulmonary capillary blood with alveolar gas at all gas exchange units, arterial hypoxemia is present. However, the $P_{A_{O_2}} - P_{a_{O_2}}$ should be normal. If other abnormalities of gas exchange such as diffusion limitation, shunting, or ventilation-perfusion mismatching are present in addition to alveolar hypoventilation, the difference should be increased. Thus the greatest clinical use of $P_{A_{O_2}} - P_{a_{O_2}}$ should be to distinguish between simple alveolar hypoventilation, such as might occur in patients with neuromuscular disease or depressed respiratory drive (increased $P_{a_{CO_2}}$ and normal $P_{A_{O_2}} - P_{a_{O_2}}$, and hypoventilation complicated by further abnormalities in lung function such as infection, edema, or atelectasis (increased $P_{a_{CO_2}}$ and increased $P_{A_{O_2}} - P_{a_{O_2}}$). Unfortunately, this approach is an oversimplification that ignores the dependence of $P_{A_{O_2}} - P_{a_{O_2}}$ on the $P_{A_{O_2}}$.

$P_{A_{O_2}} - P_{a_{O_2}}$ can be calculated when a patient is receiving supplemental O_2. However, the value increases with increasing inspired O_2 concentration[52] (Fig. 65–14). The magnitude of the increase depends on the relative contributions of $\dot{V}$-$\dot{Q}$ mismatching, shunt, and diffusion impairment to the hypoxemia. It is difficult to predict how $P_{A_{O_2}} - P_{a_{O_2}}$ will vary in an individual patient. Some have advocated normalizing $P_{a_{O_2}}$ for varying O_2 concentrations by calculating the ratio of arterial to inspired O_2. This approach ignores the nonlinear relationship between $P_{A_{O_2}}$ and $P_{a_{O_2}}$ and suffers from the same limitations as does comparison of the $P_{A_{O_2}} - P_{a_{O_2}}$ values obtained at different inspired O_2 concentrations.

$P_{A_{O_2}} - P_{a_{O_2}}$ may also be difficult to interpret in patients with hypercapnia when $P_{A_{O_2}}$ is decreased. The elegant analysis presented by Fahri and Rahn more than 35 years ago indicated that the $P_{A_{O_2}} - P_{a_{O_2}}$ should decrease with decreases in $P_{A_{O_2}}$ unless diffusion limitation is the major source of the $P_{A_{O_2}} - P_{a_{O_2}}$ gradient.[53] This was observed to be the case in a group of hypercapnic patients with advanced obstructive pulmonary disease who were breathing room air; it was found that $P_{A_{O_2}} - P_{a_{O_2}}$ varied inversely with $P_{a_{CO_2}}$.[54] In the patients with the most severely elevated $P_{a_{CO_2}}$ values (range 59 to 81 torr) and therefore the lowest $P_{A_{O_2}}$ values, $P_{A_{O_2}} - P_{a_{O_2}}$ was normal. Furthermore, when patients experienced a change in $P_{a_{CO_2}}$, $P_{A_{O_2}} - P_{a_{O_2}}$ changed in the opposite direction, decreasing with a further increase in $P_{a_{CO_2}}$. All of these patients had distinctly abnormal gas exchange values as reflected by an increased venous admixture, and when $P_{a_{CO_2}}$ changed, the venous admixture tended to change in the same direction. Thus, $P_{A_{O_2}} - P_{a_{O_2}}$ may be misleading when utilized to assess gas exchange in the patient with alveolar hypoventilation and hypercapnia. Normal values for $P_{A_{O_2}} - P_{a_{O_2}}$ do not exclude significant additional abnormalities in gas exchange, and constant or decreasing values with progressive hypoventilation may indicate additional deterioration of intrinsic lung function.

Venous Admixture

Calculation of the venous admixture (Equation 17) provides an alternative means of quantitating the impairment in gas exchange. In this approach all of the abnormalities in gas exchange (including those resulting from $\dot{V}$-$\dot{Q}$ mismatching and diffusion limitation) are treated as if they were due to a hypothetical shunt through unventilated lung. Because

the contributions of $\dot{V}$-$\dot{Q}$ mismatching and diffusion limitation to arterial desaturation decrease as the inspired O_2 concentration increases, the calculated venous admixture generally falls during supplemental O_2 administration. The venous admixture measured while a patient is breathing 100% O_2 represents true right-to-left shunt.

The venous admixture calculation is based on the O_2 content difference between pulmonary capillary blood and arterial blood. The discordant relationship between $P_{A_{O_2}} - P_{a_{O_2}}$ and the venous admixture that has been observed in hypercapnic patients breathing room air may be explained by the change in slope of the oxyhemoglobin curve in the region of the $P_{A_{O_2}}$ that occurs with hypercapnia (Fig. 65–15). For example, patients with $P_{a_{CO_2}}$ greater than 60 torr have a $P_{A_{O_2}}$ of about 60 torr. This value falls near the shoulder of the oxyhemoglobin dissociation curve, below which small decreases in P_{O_2} correspond to large decreases in O_2 saturation. As a result, the $P_{A_{O_2}} - P_{a_{O_2}}$ may be normal despite a substantial saturation difference between pulmonary capillary and arterial blood.

Although the venous admixture is a useful measure of gas exchange, it is difficult to calculate without access to a computer for computation of arterial and pulmonary capillary O_2 contents.[55, 56] Furthermore, in the critically ill patient pulmonary blood flow and mixed venous saturation are frequently abnormal. Widening of the arteriovenous O_2 content difference, which may occur in the patient with congestive heart failure or whenever the cardiac output fails to increase in proportion to metabolic demand, results in a decreased mixed venous P_{O_2} and O_2 content. It is intuitive that for a given venous admixture, lowering the O_2 content of the mixed venous blood that is added to the oxygenated pulmonary capillary blood decreases the O_2 content of arterial blood[57] (Fig. 65–16). However, if one assumes a normal cardiac output and mixed venous O_2 content in calculating the venous admixture, progressive decreases in the mixed

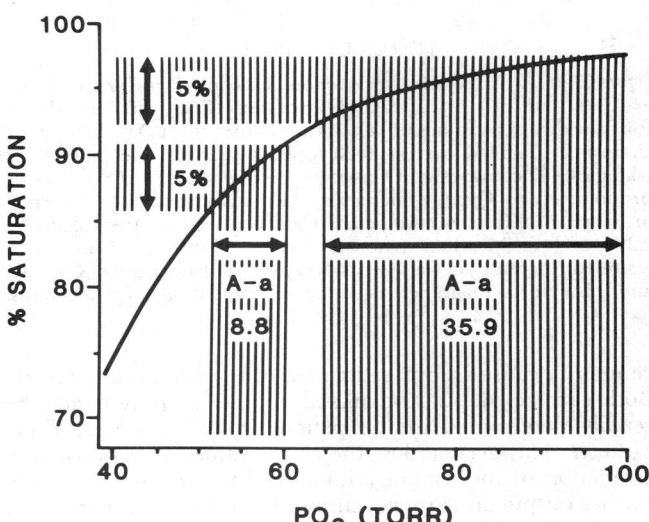

Figure 65–15. Normal oxyhemoglobin dissociation curve, illustrating the different changes in P_{O_2} associated with the same change in saturation at normal alveolar P_{O_2} (100 torr) versus low alveolar P_{O_2} (60 torr). If a given amount of shunt or ventilation-perfusion maldistribution produces a 5% drop in saturation between pulmonary capillary and arterial blood, this creates a 35.9-torr alveolar-arterial gradient if the alveolar P_{O_2} is normal but only an 8.8-torr alveolar-arterial gradient if the alveolar P_{O_2} is 60 torr, as in the patient with a $P_{a_{CO_2}}$ of 60 to 80 torr. (From Gray BA, Blalock JM: Interpretation of the alveolar-arterial oxygen difference in patients with hypercapnia. Am Rev Respir Dis 143:4, 1991.)

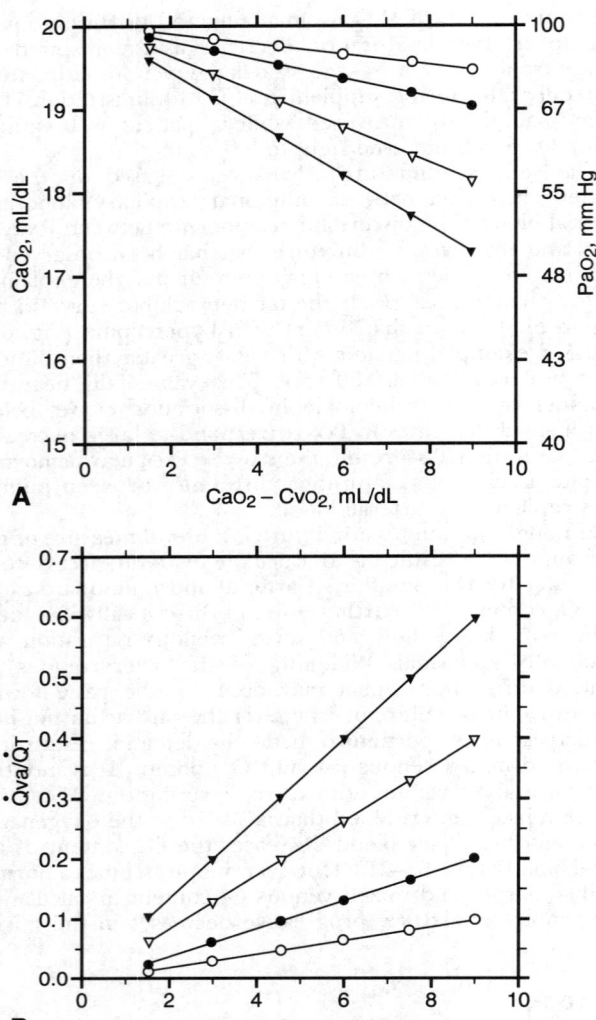

A

B

Indicator gases of different solubilities are infused into a peripheral vein, and their elimination via expired air and retention in arterial blood are measured. Retention of the extremely insoluble gas sulfur hexafluoride reflects blood flow through alveolar capillaries with extremely low $\dot{V}/\dot{Q}$ ratios (<0.001), whereas the appearance of the highly soluble gas acetone in the expired gas indicates perfusion of alveoli with high $\dot{V}/\dot{Q}$ ratios (>100). By infusing six gases of various solubilities, it is possible to reconstruct the $\dot{V}/\dot{Q}$ profile of the entire lung. In a young healthy individual the range of $\dot{V}/\dot{Q}$ ratios is narrow (0.3 to 3.0) and homogeneously distributed around a mean of 1.0.[49]

Clinical studies utilizing this technique have shown that $\dot{V}$-$\dot{Q}$ mismatching is the major cause of hypoxemia in most forms of lung disease.[60–62] Diffusion impairment and right-to-left intrapulmonary shunt may also contribute to the abnormal gas exchange, but blood flow to poorly ventilated areas with low $\dot{V}/\dot{Q}$ ratios accounts for most of the hypoxemia in the critically ill.[63] Even when the expired minute ventilation is normal or increased, maldistribution of ventilation relative to perfusion is reflected by heterogeneity in the distribution of $\dot{V}/\dot{Q}$ ratios (Fig. 65–17). The development of regions with high $\dot{V}/\dot{Q}$ ratios is reflected by an increase in the V_D/V_T ratio, whereas the appearance of low $\dot{V}/\dot{Q}$ areas increases the venous admixture. This technique has provided invaluable insight into the physiologic derangements respon-

Figure 65–16. *A.* Effect of arteriovenous O_2 content difference ($CaO_2 - C\bar{v}O_2$, mL/dL) on arterial O_2 content (CaO_2, mL/dL) shown for four different values of venous admixture ($\dot{Q}va/\dot{Q}T$): 0.05 (open circles), 0.10 (filled circles), 0.20 (open triangles), and 0.30 (filled triangles). The lowering of CaO_2 by a widened $CaO_2 - C\bar{v}O_2$ is more pronounced as $\dot{Q}va/\dot{Q}T$ increases. PaO_2 is indicated on the right ordinate. *B.* Effect of the actual $CaO_2 - C\bar{v}O_2$ on the calculated value of $\dot{Q}va/\dot{Q}T$ when a normal $CaO_2 - C\bar{v}O_2$ of 4.5 mL/dL is assumed. Increases in $CaO_2 - C\bar{v}O_2$ cause overestimation of $\dot{Q}va/\dot{Q}T$, and this error is magnified as the actual value of $\dot{Q}va/\dot{Q}T$ increases.

venous O_2 cause an overestimation of the venous admixture. Both cardiac output and mixed venous saturation may be readily determined in the patient by using a Swan-Ganz catheter. However, unless the actual values are known, any estimation of the venous admixture that assumes a normal cardiac output and arteriovenous O_2 content difference must be viewed with the understanding that an elevated venous admixture may reflect either an abnormality in gas exchange in the patient with normal cardiac function or a lesser abnormality in gas exchange combined with reduced venous O_2 content in the patient with a low cardiac output.

Multiple Inert Gas Elimination Technique

Introduction of the multiple inert gas elimination technique by Wagner and colleagues allowed investigators to characterize the distribution of $\dot{V}/\dot{Q}$ ratios in the lung.[58, 59]

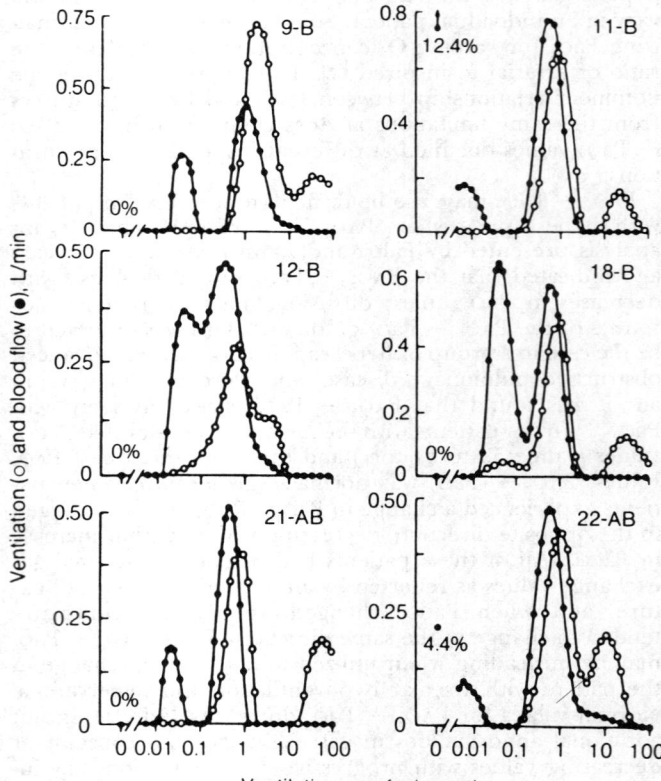

Figure 65–17. Maldistribution of ventilation (open circles) and perfusion (filled circles) observed in patients with chronic obstructive pulmonary disease. Note the increased ventilation to lung units with high $\dot{V}/\dot{Q}$ ratios and increased blood flow to lung units with low $\dot{V}/\dot{Q}$ ratios. This is one of several different patterns observed. (From Wagner PD, Dantzker DR, Dueck R, et al: Ventilation-perfusion inequality in chronic obstructive pulmonary disease. Reproduced from the Journal of Clinical Investigation, 1977, volume 59, pp 203–216 by copyright permission of the American Society of Clinical Investigation.)

sible for the impaired gas exchange in critically ill patients, but unfortunately its complexity precludes its routine use at the bedside.

THERAPEUTIC INTERVENTIONS

Treatment of the critically ill patient with respiratory failure is aimed at maintaining gas exchange while improving the underlying cardiac and pulmonary function. Supplemental O_2, mechanical ventilation, and pharmacologic therapy with bronchodilators, vasodilators, and inotropic agents are commonly employed to support the patient's vital functions and reverse the underlying pathophysiology. It is important to recognize that, in addition to their primary effect, each of these interventions may have secondary effects on cardiac or pulmonary function that reduce their ability to improve gas exchange.

Oxygen

O_2 therapy is the cornerstone of management for the hypoxemic patient. Because most hypoxemia is due to $\dot{V}$-$\dot{Q}$ mismatching, the PaO_2 readily improves with supplemental O_2. A PaO_2 of 60 mm Hg is sufficient to increase the hemoglobin saturation to 90%. O_2 levels greater than this produce little further increase in the arterial O_2 content because of the sigmoid shape of the hemoglobin-O_2 dissociation curve. An inspired O_2 concentration of 40% or less is usually sufficient to increase the PaO_2 to 60 mm Hg in patients with hypoxemia caused by $\dot{V}$-$\dot{Q}$ mismatching. However, individuals with acute lung injury and severe $\dot{V}$-$\dot{Q}$ derangements including increased shunt flow may not be able to achieve this level even while breathing 100% O_2.

Supplemental O_2 increases the local PO_2 in poorly ventilated alveoli. The consequent reduction in alveolar nitrogen content may lead to alveolar collapse and the development of microatelectasis if deep breathing or other measures such as positive airway pressures are not employed to maintain alveolar expansion.[64] To the extent that the reflex adjustment of ventilation to perfusion caused by hypoxic vasoconstriction is attenuated, $\dot{V}/\dot{Q}$ ratios may change throughout the lung. Pulmonary hypertension may be relieved. Because the supplemental O_2 improves the oxygenation of blood from poorly ventilated regions, its overall effect on arterial oxygenation is beneficial.

Drug Therapy

The homeostatic redistribution of perfusion to match ventilation may be seriously impaired by the administration of bronchodilators and vasoactive agents that interfere with hypoxic vasoconstriction. Systemic absorption of inhaled bronchodilators may worsen $\dot{V}$-$\dot{Q}$ relationships and increase arterial hypoxemia even while having a beneficial effect on bronchial smooth muscle tone.[65] The use of nitroprusside and other vasodilators that block hypoxic vasoconstriction can produce significant hypoxemia by increasing perfusion to poorly ventilated alveoli.[66]

The effect of other interventions on hypoxic vasoconstriction may be more subtle. Cardiac output may be increased in the critically ill patient by administration of fluids and/or inotropic agents. Increases in pulmonary blood flow per se may indirectly worsen $\dot{V}$-$\dot{Q}$ mismatching. If O_2 consumption remains constant, increasing cardiac output increases the mixed venous PO_2. Increasing mixed venous PO_2, either directly or indirectly by increasing alveolar O_2, attenuates hypoxic vasoconstriction and increases the venous admixture.[67]

Mechanical Ventilation

The effect of positive pressure ventilation on pulmonary blood flow has already been discussed. The situation becomes even more complex when the multiple effects of positive end-expiratory pressure are considered. The improvement in arterial oxygenation with positive end-expiratory pressure is associated with an increase in functional residual capacity and is thought to be due to the prevention of airway closure and improved ventilation to low $\dot{V}/\dot{Q}$ alveoli. However, increases in lung volume increase pulmonary vascular resistance, and, if the less affected regions of the lung are more compliant than their diseased counterparts, the relative perfusion of the spared areas might be decreased.[68, 69] Positive end-expiratory pressure also increases the intrathoracic pressure, decreasing venous return and cardiac output. The increase in intrathoracic pressure is transmitted to the extra-alveolar vessels, increasing pulmonary arterial pressure. However, the increase in pulmonary arterial pressure is less than the increment in alveolar pressure, so additional regions of zone 1 and zone 2 may be produced. These phenomena account for the increase in $PaCO_2$ that is sometimes observed if excessive positive end-expiratory pressure is employed.

Despite these considerations, the physician should not hesitate to use mechanical ventilation and pharmacologic therapy to maintain gas exchange and reverse the underlying pathophysiology in a critically ill patient. One must recognize that therapeutic interventions may have secondary detrimental effects on gas exchange and provide enough supplemental O_2 to maintain oxygenation until the underlying disease process can be corrected.

References

1. Halmagyi DFJ, Kinney JM: Metabolic rate in acute respiratory failure complicating sepsis. Surgery 77:492, 1975.
2. Blackburn GL, Bistrian BR, Miami BS, et al: Nutrition and metabolic assessment of the hospitalized patient. JPEN 1:11–22, 1977.
3. Browning JA, Linberg SE, Tunney S, et al: The effects of fluctuating FIO_2 on metabolic measurements in mechanically ventilated patients. Crit Care Med 10:82, 1982.
4. Hey EN, Lloyd BB, Cunningham DJC, et al: Effects of various respiratory stimuli on the depth and frequency of breathing in man. Respir Physiol 1:193, 1966.
5. Jones NL, McHardy GJR, Naimark A, et al: Physiological dead space and alveolar-arterial gas pressure differences during exercise. Clin Sci 31:19, 1966.
6. Daly WJ, Bondurant S: Direct measurement of respiratory pleural pressure in man. J Appl Physiol 18:513, 1963.
7. Milic-Emili J, Henderson AM, Dolovich MB, et al: Regional distribution of inspired gas in the lung. J Appl Physiol 21:749, 1966.
8. Begin R, Renzetti AD, Bigler AH, et al: Flow and age dependence of airway closure and dynamic compliance. J Appl Physiol 38:199, 1975.
9. Kaneko K, Milic-Emili J, Dolovich MB, et al: Regional distribution of ventilation and perfusion as a function of body position. J Appl Physiol 21:767, 1966.
10. Otis AB, McKerrow CB, Bartlett RA, et al: Mechanical factors in distribution of pulmonary ventilation. J Appl Physiol 8:427, 1956.
11. Bone RC: Diagnosis of causes for acute respiratory distress by pressure-volume curves. Chest 70:740, 1976.
12. Connors AF, McCaffree DR, Gray BA: Effect of inspiratory flow rate on gas exchange during mechanical ventilation. Am Rev Respir Dis 124:537, 1981.
13. Mead J, Takashima T, Leith D: Mechanical interdependence of distensible units in the lung. Fed Proc 26:551, 1967.
14. Hubmayr RD, Rodarte JR, Walters BJ, et al: Regional ventilation during spontaneous breathing and mechanical ventilation in dogs. J Appl Physiol 63:2467, 1987.
15. Terry PB, Traystman RJ, Newball HH, et al: Collateral ventilation in man. N Engl J Med 298:10, 1978.
16. Buist AS: The single breath nitrogen test. N Engl J Med 293:438, 1975.
17. Meneely GR, Kaltreider NL: The volume of the lung determined by helium dilution: Description of the method and comparison with other procedures. J Clin Invest 28:129, 1949.
18. Darling RC, Cournard A, Richards DW Jr: Studies on the intrapulmonary mixture of gases. III. An open circuit method for measuring residual air. J Clin Invest 19:609, 1940.

19. Brody JS, Stemmler EJ, DuBois AB: Longitudinal distribution of vascular resistance in the pulmonary arteries, capillaries, and veins. J Clin Invest 47:783, 1968.
20. Raj JU, Chen P: Microvascular pressures measured by micropuncture in isolated perfused lamb lungs. J Appl Physiol 61:2194, 1986.
21. Folkow B: The haemodynamic consequences of adaptive structural changes of the resistance vessels in hypertension. Clin Sci 41:1, 1971.
22. Permutt SJ, Howell JBL, Proctor DJ: Effect of lung inflation on static pressure-volume characteristics of pulmonary vessels. J Appl Physiol 16:64, 1961.
23. Roos A, Thomas LJ Jr, Nagel EL, et al: Pulmonary vascular resistance as determined by lung inflation and vascular pressures. J Appl Physiol 16:77, 1961.
24. Howell JBL, Permutt S, Proctor DF, et al: Effect of inflation of the lung on different parts of pulmonary vascular bed. J Appl Physiol 16:71, 1961.
25. Maseri A, Caldini P, Harward P, et al: Determinants of pulmonary vascular volume. Circ Res 31:218, 1972.
26. West JB, Dollery CT, Naimark A: Distribution of blood flow in isolated lung; Relation to vascular and alveolar pressures. J Appl Physiol 19:713, 1964.
27. Permutt S, Bromberger-Barnea B, Bane HN: Alveolar pressure, pulmonary venous pressure and the vascular waterfall. Med Thorac 19:239, 1962.
28. Hughes JMB, Glazier JB, Maloney JE: Effect of lung volume on the distribution of pulmonary blood flow in man. Respir Physiol 4:58, 1968.
29. Nemery B, Wijns W, Piret L, et al: Pulmonary vascular tone is a determinant of basal lung perfusion in normal seated subjects. J Appl Physiol 54:262, 1983.
30. Fishman AP: Hypoxia on the pulmonary circulation: How and where it acts. Circ Res 38:221, 1976.
31. Reid LM: Structure and function in pulmonary hypertension. Chest 89:279, 1986.
32. Enson Y, Thomas HM, Bosken CH, et al: Pulmonary hypertension in interstitial lung disease: Relation of vascular resistance to abnormal lung structure. Trans Assoc Am Physicians 88:248, 1975.
33. Burrows B, Kettel LJ, Hiden AH, et al: Patterns of cardiovascular dysfunction in chronic obstructive lung disease. N Engl J Med 286:912, 1972.
34. Naimark A, Dugard A, Rangno RE: Regional pulmonary blood flow and gas exchange in hemorrhagic shock. J Appl Physiol 25:301, 1968.
35. Hughes JMB, Glazier JB, Rosenzweig DY, et al: Factors determining the distribution of pulmonary blood flow in patients with raised pulmonary venous pressure. Clin Sci 37:847, 1969.
36. Neuhaus A, Bentz RR, Weg JG: Pulmonary embolism in respiratory failure. Chest 73:460, 1978.
37. Moser KM, LeMoine JR, Nachtway FJ, et al: Deep venous thrombosis and pulmonary embolism: Frequency in a respiratory intensive care unit. JAMA 246:1422, 1981.
38. Chastre J, Cornud F, Bouchama A, et al: Thrombosis as a complication of pulmonary-artery catheterization via the internal jugular vein. N Engl J Med 306:278, 1982.
39. Tomashefski JF, Davies P, Boggis C, et al: The pulmonary vascular lesions of the adult respiratory distress syndrome. Am J Pathol 112:112, 1983.
40. Hyman AL, Mathe AA, Leslie CA, et al: Modification of pulmonary vascular responses to arachidonic acid by alterations in physiologic state. J Pharmacol Exp Ther 207:388, 1978.
41. Hales CA, Sonne L, Peterson M, et al: Role of thromboxane and prostacyclin in pulmonary vasomotor changes after endotoxin in dogs. J Clin Invest 68:497, 1981.
42. Parsons PE, Worthen GS, Moore EE, et al: The association of circulating endotoxin with the development of the adult respiratory distress syndrome. Am Rev Respir Dis 140:294, 1989.
43. Okusawa S, Gelfand JA, Ikejima T, et al: Interleukin 1 induces a shock-like state in rabbits. J Clin Invest 81:1162, 1988.
44. Starmes HF Jr, Warren RS, Jeevanandam M, et al: Tumor necrosis factor and the acute metabolic response to tissue injury in man. J Clin Invest 82:1321, 1988.
45. Stephens K, Ishizaka A, Larrick J, et al: Tumor necrosis factor causes increased pulmonary permeability and edema. Am Rev Respir Dis 137:1364, 1988.
46. Wagner PD: Diffusion and chemical reaction in pulmonary gas exchange. Physiol Rev 57:257, 1977.
47. Roughton FJW, Forster RE: Relative importance of diffusion and chemical reaction rates in determining rate of exchange of gases in the human lung, with special reference to true diffusing capacity of pulmonary membrane and volume of blood in lung capillaries. J Appl Physiol 11:290, 1957.
48. Forster RE: Exchange of gases between alveolar air and pulmonary capillary blood: Pulmonary diffusing capacity. Physiol Rev 37:391, 1957.
49. Wagner PD, Laravuso RB, Uhl RR, et al: Continuous distributions of ventilation perfusion ratios in normal subjects breathing air and 100% O_2. J Clin Invest 54:54, 1974.
50. Riley RL, Cournand A: 'Ideal' alveolar air and the analysis of ventilation-perfusion relationships in the lungs. J Appl Physiol 1:825, 1949.
51. Raine JM, Bishop JM: A-a difference in O_2 tension and physiological dead space in normal man. J Appl Physiol 18:284, 1963.
52. Cole RB, Bishop JM: Effect of varying inspired O_2 tension on alveolar-arterial O_2 tension difference in man. J Appl Physiol 18:1043, 1963.
53. Fahri LE, Rahn H: A theoretical analysis of the alveolar-arterial O_2 difference with special reference to the distribution effect. J Appl Physiol 7:699, 1955.
54. Gray BA, Blalock JM: Interpretation of the alveolar-arterial oxygen difference in patients with hypercapnia. Am Rev Respir Dis 143:4, 1991.
55. Severinghaus JW: Simple, accurate equations for human blood O_2 dissociation computations. J Appl Physiol 46:599, 1979.
56. Kelman GR: Digital computer subroutine for the conversion of oxygen tension into saturation. J Appl Physiol 21:1375, 1966.
57. Mithoefer JC, Ramirez C, Cook W: The effect of mixed venous oxygenation on arterial blood in chronic obstructive pulmonary disease. Am Rev Respir Dis 117:259, 1978.
58. Wagner PD, Saltzman HA, West JB: Measurement of continuous distributions of ventilation-perfusion ratios: Theory. J Appl Physiol 36:588, 1974.
59. West JB: State of the Art: Ventilation-perfusion relationships. Am Rev Respir Dis 116:919, 1977.
60. Wagner P, Dantzker D, Dueck D, et al: Ventilation-perfusion inequality in chronic obstructive lung disease. J Clin Invest 59:203, 1977.
61. Wagner PD, Dantzker DR, Iacovoni VE, et al: Ventilation perfusion inequality in asymptomatic asthma. Am Rev Respir Dis 118:511, 1978.
62. Manier G, Castaing Y, Guernard H: Determinants of hypoxemia during the acute phase of pulmonary embolism in humans. Am Rev Respir Dis 132:232, 1985.
63. Dantzker DR, Brook CJ, Dehart P, et al: Ventilation-perfusion distributions in the adult respiratory distress syndrome. Am Rev Respir Dis 120:1039, 1979.
64. Dantzker DR, Wagner PD, West JB: Instability of lung units with low V_A/Q ratios during O_2 breathing. J Appl Physiol 38:886, 1975.
65. Gazioglu K, Condemi JJ, Hyde RW, et al: Effect of isoproterenol on gas exchange during air and oxygen breathing in patients with asthma. Am J Med 50:185, 1971.
66. Colley PS, Cheney FW, Hlastala MP: Ventilation-perfusion and gas exchange effects of sodium nitroprusside in dogs with normal and edematous lungs. Anesthesiology 47:338, 1977.
67. Sandoval J, Long GR, Skoog C, et al: Independent influence of blood flow rate and mixed venous Po$_2$ on shunt fraction. J Appl Physiol 55:1128, 1983.
68. Maunder RJ, Shuman WP, McHugh JW, et al: Preservation of normal lung regions in the adult respiratory distress syndrome. JAMA 255:2463, 1986.
69. Kanarek DJ, Shannon DC: Adverse effect of positive end-expiratory pressure on pulmonary perfusion and arterial oxygenation. Am Rev Respir Dis 112:457, 1975.

CHAPTER 66

Lung Defense

Laurel Wiegand
Herbert Y. Reynolds

A healthy person confronts the environment with a lung surface the size of a tennis court. This surface has delicate barrier characteristics to facilitate rapid and efficient gas exchange. Thousands of liters of ambient air containing a potentially hazardous mixture of gases, particulate matter, and airborne microorganisms flow over this surface daily. Upper airway secretions are also frequently aspirated during sleep, even in normal individuals.[1] Both inhalation and aspiration allow routine contamination of the lower respiratory tract with exogenous and endogenous microbial and particulate debris, yet infection is rare in healthy humans.

This extraordinary resistance to disease is maintained by an intricate system of mechanical and immunologic defenses that span the respiratory tract from nares to alveoli (Fig. 66–1). These defenses function in concert to discourage contamination of the lower respiratory tract and to eliminate trespassing pathogens that do reach this region.

A sufficient inoculum of virulent microorganisms can overwhelm the respiratory defenses and lead to the development of pneumonia. Healthy hosts are not invulnerable. However, pneumonia is more common and carries a more ominous prognosis in hosts with defective or compromised lung defense mechanisms. Critically ill patients who require care in the intensive care unit (ICU) are at particular risk for the development of serious pneumonia and can be considered vulnerable hosts. In this chapter we examine how specific features of critical illness compromise the normally effective respiratory defense network, increasing the risk of serious infectious pneumonia in this population of patients. The discussion begins with a general review of normal respiratory tract defense mechanisms.

NORMAL LUNG DEFENSE MECHANISMS

The lung defense system begins in the upper airways, which participate in many important respiratory functions including the modification of inspired air and the filtration and clearance of the inspired load of pathogens and particulate debris. Upper airway structures provide a series of physical barriers to the inhalation and aspiration of these materials and also assist with mechanical clearance through the gag and cough reflexes and the mucociliary escalator. In addition, upper airway secretions contain various antimicrobial products that participate in host defense.

Nasopharynx and Oropharynx

The nasopharynx and oropharynx present the first in a series of mechanical and immunologic barriers to inspired pathogens (see Fig. 66–1). The nasal septum and turbinates provide a convoluted surface lined with ciliated, mucus-secreting columnar epithelial cells that overlie a submucosa rich in plasma cells and lymphocytes similar to that found in the conducting airways. The oropharyngeal cavity is lined by stratified squamous epithelium that is bathed in salivary and parotid gland secretions rich in immunoglobulin A (IgA) and other protective substances. The convoluted, sticky mucosal surface of the supraglottic airways effectively filters

and entraps inhaled particles more than 10 μm in diameter.[2] Although microbes are smaller than 10 μm, they are often adherent to particles in this size range. Particle-laden upper airway secretions can then be swallowed, expectorated, or forcibly expelled by sneezing or coughing. The nasopharynx, larynx, and large airways are studded with neuronal sensory afferents that are responsible for such clearance-oriented reflexes. The gag reflex closes off the glottis to prevent aspiration of upper airway and gastric secretions, and the cough and sneeze reflexes expel foreign material from both the nasopharynx and the conducting airways. The larynx and vocal cords add to the mechanical barrier confronting particles larger than 10 μm and participate in the protective gag and cough clearance reflexes.

Microbial Ecosystem of Upper Airways

Maintenance of a normal microbial ecosystem on the mucosal surface lining the upper airways may be another important component of the host defense system.[3] Mechanical factors such as chewing, abrasion of the oropharyngeal surfaces by the tongue, expectoration, and swallowing help to prevent bacterial overgrowth by reducing the burden of microorganisms and senescent cells on mucosal surfaces. The normal flora and its mucosal microenvironment inhibit abnormal mucosal colonization with virulent organisms by complex and poorly understood mechanisms. Factors that influence the microflora of the upper respiratory tract may include nutrient supply, growth factors, local pH, and tissue tropism, or the propensity of certain organisms to establish themselves in specific mucosal niches.[4, 5] In addition to competing for binding sites on epithelial cell surfaces, normal oropharyngeal microbial flora may prevent the growth of pathogenic bacteria by interbacterial interference or inhibition.[6, 7]

Particle Size

As illustrated in Figure 66–1, the fate of particles less than 10 μm in size varies.[2] Particles smaller than 0.5 μm tend to remain suspended in air and are exhaled in the next breath. Most particles between 3 and 10 μm in size impact aerodynamically at the branch points of many generations of airways and are subsequently cleared from the conducting airways by the mucociliary escalator and cough. In addition, at such points of impact, mucosal lymphoid structures termed bronchus-associated lymphoid tissue may capture

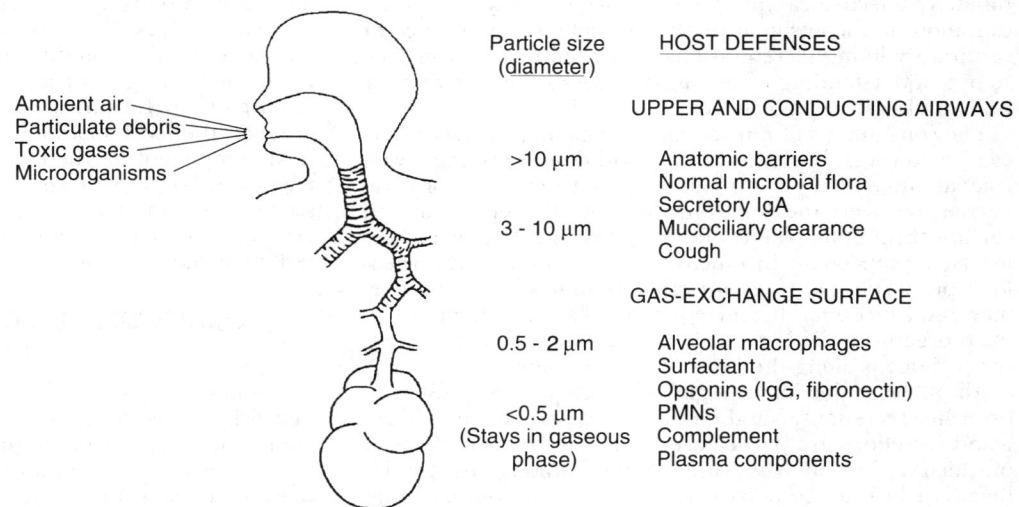

Figure 66–1. Mechanical and immunologic defenses protecting the respiratory tract.

trapped pathogens, although the clinical significance of this mechanism in humans remains to be established.[8-10]

Mucociliary Transport System

The details of the intricate structure and function of the mucociliary transport system are beyond the scope of this chapter but have been reviewed elsewhere.[11, 12] This system functions throughout most of the respiratory tract to sweep trapped debris toward the mouth so it can be removed by coughing, swallowing, or expectoration. This clearance mechanism becomes particularly important in the subglottic conducting airways, which are lined with ciliated epithelial cells down to the level just proximal to the respiratory bronchioles. Mucus is secreted from goblet cells and submucosal glands and facilitates adherence of particles to the airway surface for transport along the mucociliary escalator. Periciliary fluid bathes the bases of the cilia and an overlying layer of mucus interacts with the tips of the cilia.[11] The exact biochemical composition of periciliary fluid and mucus is not known, but precise regulation of fluid and electrolyte gradients across mucosal epithelial cells is required for optimal mucociliary function.[13] Autonomically mediated alterations in blood flow through an intricate nasal vascular network allow the rapid modulation of the temperature and humidity of inspired air necessary for the normal rheologic and biologic function of mucus and other airway secretions.[14] Cilia beat in a complex, dynamic fashion with frequencies ranging from 12 to 15 Hz to maintain a constant flow of mucus and trapped particles toward the mouth. Normal transport rates range from 0.5 to 20 mm/min. Tracer studies have demonstrated that virtually all material deposited on the ciliary epithelium in normal persons is removed in less than 24 hours.[11]

Respiratory Tract Secretions

Respiratory tract secretions also contribute to host defense via a variety of immune and nonimmune mechanisms. These secretions include the constituents of mucus produced by goblet cells and bronchial glands, serous and Clara's cell products, immunoglobulins, iron transport proteins, and many other factors, which have been reviewed in detail elsewhere.[15] The list of putative antimicrobial factors in these secretions continues to grow. For example, the iron transport proteins lactoferrin and transferrin, which are present in airway mucosal secretions and alveolar lining fluid, respectively, may act as nonimmune host factors by regulating the free iron supplies necessary for bacterial growth.[15] Unfortunately, selective sampling techniques to allow precise localization and assessment of the physiologic significance of respiratory lining secretions have not been readily available, so our understanding of the importance of these factors for human disease remains to be established.

The constituents of mucus remain incompletely characterized.[16] However, it is clear that, in addition to playing a vital role in mucociliary transport, mucus provides a physical barrier between the environment and the epithelial cell surface throughout the conducting airways. The macromolecular glycoproteins in mucus that contribute to the rheologic properties necessary for effective mucociliary transport may also function as ligands for the cell surface receptors of microorganisms. This could facilitate the removal of potential pathogens along the mucociliary escalator.

All of the major immunoglobulin isotypes are present in bronchial secretions. Nasal washings and parotid and salivary gland secretions are particularly rich in secretory IgA, most of which is probably synthesized locally. Although the precise details of IgA antibody participation in host defense remain uncertain,[17] secretory IgA antibody can agglutinate or neutralize microorganisms, block the uptake of antigens, and inhibit the adherence of specific pathogens to the mucosal surface.[18] Mucosal secretions from the trachea and conducting airways are the least precisely characterized, but it appears that the ratio of immunoglobulin G (IgG) to IgA increases progressively toward the distal airways.[19] IgG antibody can neutralize certain microbes, activate complement, and agglutinate particulate antigens and is the most effective opsonizing antibody.

Alveolar Defense System

Particles or microbes between 0.5 and 2 μm in size, such as a single bacterium, can elude the trapping mechanisms just described and reach the terminal gas exchange units, which include the alveoli and respiratory bronchioles.[14] These distal units are not cleansed by coughing or the mucociliary transport system.[14] Ciliated epithelium and mucus-secreting cells disappear just proximal to the respiratory bronchioles. The terminal air sacs are lined with a flat epithelial cell layer composed of type I and type II pneumonocytes. Alveolar macrophages may roam freely over the alveolar surface and are postulated to function as the primary phagocytic cell defense system. Alveolar macrophages act as scavengers to ingest and kill trespassing microorganisms through phagocytosis and the production of oxygen radicals and proteases. Animal data have demonstrated that aerosolized bacteria deposited on the alveolar surface are rapidly captured and ingested by alveolar macrophages.[20-22] Inside the macrophage, the fate of the invading pathogen varies with its virulence and the inoculum size.[15] The macrophage may be able to kill or contain the organism. Cell-mediated immune stimulation may be necessary to complete the action. A number of cellular mediators generated from T lymphocytes can energize and activate macrophages to improve their phagocytic and bactericidal properties. Alternatively, the macrophage may recruit additional help through the elaboration of chemotactic factors that attract polymorphonuclear and other inflammatory cells into the alveolus.

The alveolar defense system may be augmented by the diverse actions of other soluble agents in the alveolar space, such as surfactant, fibronectin, immunoglobulins, and certain complement components.[15, 23] Surfactant phospholipids and fragments of fibronectin, a large surface glycoprotein, may act as nonimmune opsonins to facilitate macrophage phagocytosis. IgG is the principal opsonic antibody available in fluid sampled from bronchoalveolar lavage of the distal air spaces. Complement may promote bacterial attachment to macrophages or work with specific IgG antibody to augment receptor binding interactions. In addition, a microbe might trigger the activation of the alternative complement pathway for direct lysis of the organism.

When the local anatomic, mechanical, secretory, and cellular components of the respiratory defense network cannot adequately cope with an infectious challenge, they are assisted by complex systemic responses that include the recruitment of blood-borne phagocytic cells and humoral and cell-mediated immune factors.[15]

COMPROMISED LUNG DEFENSES IN CRITICAL ILLNESS

Pneumonia results when the respiratory host defense network is overwhelmed. Critically ill patients are especially vulnerable, and the development of pneumonia in an ICU patient carries an ominous prognosis despite aggressive therapy. In one study, 50% mortality was reported in ICU patients with pneumonia compared with 4% mortality in those without pneumonia.[24] Pneumonia in the critically ill is also associated with increased cardiopulmonary instability, the development of multiple organ system failure, and an increased length of ICU stay in survivors. As many as 5% of hospitalized patients are estimated to acquire pneumonia during admission,[25, 26] and the risk is highest in patients admitted to the ICU. The reported incidence varies from 12% in a general medical ICU[27] to over 20% in mechanically ventilated patients[28] to as much as 70% in patients with the adult respiratory distress syndrome.[29–31]

Although pneumonia leading to cardiopulmonary decompensation may be the initial cause of illness in the ICU patient, more frequently pneumonia arises as a nosocomial, or hospital-acquired, infection. The responsible pathogens are diverse, particularly in severely immunocompromised hosts, in whom unusual opportunistic pathogens are more frequent. However, the most common etiologic agents remain aerobic gram-negative bacilli.[32] Gram-negative bacillary pneumonias such as those caused by *Pseudomonas aeruginosa* are associated with a uniquely high mortality[24, 26] and are a major contributor to overall hospital mortality.[33, 34] Factors that place the critically ill patient at particular risk for the development of nosocomial pneumonia are the focus of the remainder of this discussion.

Microorganisms can invade the lung via several routes. Although direct inoculation or aerosolization of microbial pathogens into the lung has been reported to occur with contaminated ventilatory equipment, this problem has been largely eliminated by employing rigorous standards for the handling of equipment, utilizing humidifying cascades that do not generate aerosols, and introducing the unit dose medication system.[35–39] Pneumonia also develops infrequently after hematogenous or contiguous spread from other infected sites. However, most nosocomial pneumonias are due to aspiration of endogenous organisms that have colonized the upper respiratory tract.

Airway Colonization

Johanson and coworkers were among the first to demonstrate a close relationship between upper airway colonization with aerobic gram-negative bacilli and the subsequent development of pneumonia.[27] Nosocomial pneumonia occurred in 23% of colonized patients compared with 3% of noncolonized patients, and colonization preceded the development of pneumonia in 85% of cases.[27]

There is a strong relationship between illness severity and risk of abnormal colonization of the upper airways. In a study by Johanson and coworkers,[40] oropharyngeal cultures were collected from hospitalized patients and colonization rates were related to the severity of the underlying illness. Oropharyngeal colonization was reported to occur in 6% of healthy subjects, 35% of moderately ill patients, and 73% of severely ill patients.[40] More than 50% of the critically ill patients were colonized within the first 4 days of hospitalization.[40] The striking difference in the prevalence of colonization between critically ill patients and healthy subjects suggests important differences in host susceptibility. Although some healthy individuals have gram-negative bacillary colonization of the upper respiratory tract, these organisms are usually transient residents and are cultured in small numbers.[41] In fact, healthy persons are relatively resistant to colonization even when aggressively challenged with gram-negative bacteria.[42] Exactly why critically ill patients are so predisposed to colonization by pathogenic organisms is poorly understood. However, multiple insults are probably involved and can be divided into factors that alter bacterial binding or adherence to mucosal cells and factors that enhance exposure to pathogenic organisms.

Bacterial Adherence

Colonization has been strongly associated with enhanced adherence of pathogenic bacteria to the mucosal epithelial cells that line the oropharynx and trachea.[43] Various microbes have specialized appendages, such as pili or fimbriae, that allow binding of the organism to specific receptors on mucosal epithelial cells. These receptors are often simple carbohydrate moieties. Adherence to epithelial cells prevents physical removal of the organism and is a prerequisite for stable colonization with normal commensal flora. However, the ability of bacteria and other pathogens to adhere to host tissues is an important virulence factor. Bacterial adherence may enhance cell surface exposure to bacterial products, allowing overgrowth or invasion by virulent strains. The complexity of bacterial-epithelial adhesive interactions has been reviewed.[44] Although it is clear that adherence is regulated in a highly complicated fashion,[44] our current understanding of the physiologic significance of available data is hampered by the lack of in vivo experiments.

Most of the available data pertain to the binding of pathogenic gram-negative rods, the most common and serious cause of nosocomial pneumonia in ICU patients. Adherence of pathogenic bacteria to oropharyngeal cells can be increased by many factors such as serious illness, surgery, endotracheal intubation, malnutrition, azotemia, and smoking.[42, 45] Enhanced bacterial adherence in systemic illness may be related to salivary and inflammatory cell proteases that modify or expose specific epithelial receptor binding sites. Similar mechanisms may operate in the lower airways, where the binding of bacteria to tracheal cells is reportedly increased by tracheostomy, endotracheal intubation, malnutrition, general surgery, and viral infection.[42, 46] Chronically tracheostomized patients with enhanced bacterial adherence have higher sputum levels of neutrophil-derived elastase than patients with lower levels of adherence.[47] Salivary protease activity has also been observed to increase in critically ill patients.[48] This increase in salivary protease activity was associated with increased adherence of *P. aeruginosa* to buccal epithelial cells and a decrease in cell surface fibronectin.[48] Fibronectin is a large surface glycoprotein that has been shown to facilitate the binding of microorganisms to epithelial cells.[48] During critical illness, an increase in salivary and inflammatory cell protease-mediated cleavage of cell surface fibronectin has been postulated to expose receptor sites for gram-negative bacterial attachment. However, Mason and coworkers[49] reported that fibronectin could not be demonstrated on the buccal surface of healthy humans, suggesting that increased adherence of bacterial pathogens may be mediated by mechanisms other than loss of cell surface fibronectin.

Other Factors

Physical Factors. Other factors have been postulated to influence bacterial adherence in systemic illness. These include alterations of pH and other physical characteristics of the mucosal microenvironment.[50] Poor nutritional status may affect the integrity of mucosal epithelial cells and alter the normal bacterial-epithelial adhesive interactions.[51] Bacterial adherence in both the upper airways and trachea may be influenced by mucosal trauma, commonly caused by endotracheal tubes,[52] nasogastric tubes, and suctioning catheters. Many ICU patients are treated with broad-spectrum antibiotics that eliminate normal flora and may promote pathogenic colonization by compromising normal interbacterial inhibition mechanisms and altering normal adhesive interactions.[7, 53–55] The possible influences of other pharmacologic agents and therapeutic modalities such as oxygen on bacterial adherence have not been well studied.

Intensive Care Unit Environment. Critically ill patients may also be predisposed to bacterial colonization and overgrowth in the upper airways because several aspects of the intensive care environment increase exposure of the patient to potential endogenous and exogenous pathogens. Organisms may be transmitted between patients and staff via poorly washed hands of hospital personnel, which frequently harbor aerobic gram-negative bacilli and *Staphylococcus aureus*.[24, 56, 57] However, the patient's own intestinal flora is likely to be the most important source of organisms. Fecal-oral transmission may lead to upper airway colonization. In addition, various factors promote bacterial overgrowth of the stomach and the subsequent retrograde movement of organisms to the pharynx, a phenomenon that is probably facilitated by nasogastric tubes. Enteral alimentation, antacids, and histamine type 2 blockers allow gastric overgrowth with enteric flora as gastric pH increases.[58–60] These agents have been associated with increased gastric colonization followed by oropharyngeal colonization and may increase the risk of nosocomial pneumonia.[58–61]

Various procedures common in the intensive care setting may also facilitate bacterial colonization of the upper airways. All ICU practitioners are familiar with the extraordinary difficulty of maintaining good nasopharyngeal and oropharyngeal hygiene in intubated patients. The nasal and pharyngeal mucosa invariably becomes eroded and often caked with secretions. The presence of endotracheal and nasogastric tubes can impair swallowing and the other mechanical clearance mechanisms that normally help to reduce the bacterial burden in the nose and pharynx, thus promoting bacterial overgrowth. Nasal mucosal trauma and edema caused by endotracheal and nasogastric tubes also compromise sinus drainage and eustachian tube function and increase the risk of bacterial overgrowth leading to nosocomial sinusitis and otitis.[62, 63]

Aspiration and Direct Inoculation. Upper airway colonization by pathogenic organisms provides a source of huge numbers of virulent organisms that may subsequently contaminate the lung. These organisms may reach the lower respiratory tract by aspiration or by direct inoculation through an endotracheal or tracheostomy tube. Aspiration occurs commonly in hospitalized patients and is facilitated by endotracheal, tracheostomy, and nasogastric tubes.[36, 64, 65] Depressed consciousness related to primary neurologic disease, metabolic encephalopathy, sedatives, narcotics, and anesthesia also increases the risk of aspiration,[1] as do esophageal disorders.[66] In addition, endotracheal and tracheostomy tubes bypass upper airway defense mechanisms and allow direct inoculation of pathogens into the tracheobronchial tree.

Size and Virulence of Inoculum. When the lower respiratory tract becomes contaminated, the risk of colonization and subsequent infection depends on the size and virulence of the inoculum and the integrity of the lower respiratory tract host defense mechanisms. The cough reflex and the mucociliary transport system play vital roles in clearing debris from the airways down to the level of the respiratory bronchioles.[14] Cough and other protective reflexes often function poorly in critically ill patients with upper airway structural abnormalities, depressed consciousness, or motor weakness caused by drugs and various neurologic disorders.[67] Cough may be abolished altogether or compromised to the extent that it simply results in moving secretions from one lung to the other.

Most studies of mucociliary dysfunction are descriptive rather than mechanistic, and the relevance of in vitro and animal data to human susceptibility to colonization and infection is uncertain. Mucociliary function may be impaired by the destruction of ciliated epithelium, exposure to ciliotoxic agents, or alterations in the composition of mucus. Multiple insults are common in critically ill patients. For example, tracheal injury by cuffed endotracheal or tracheostomy tubes has been shown to cause rapid destruction of ciliated epithelium in an animal model.[68] Such injury was associated with arrested mucus transport and distal accumulation of mucus.[68] In addition, tube or cuff damage may stimulate mucus production and alter mucus composition to promote further mucus accumulation and ciliary dysfunction in the lower airways.[11] Procedures such as bronchoscopy and tracheal suctioning also cause mucosal injury and similarly interfere with mucociliary transport.[69, 70] Ciliated epithelium may be directly destroyed by the aspiration of acidic gastric contents.[71] Widespread destruction of ciliated epithelium has been observed after respiratory tract infection with bacteria, viruses, and mycoplasmas.[12, 72]

Specific Organisms and Disease States. Certain microbes (mycoplasmas, viruses, *Bordetella pertussis*) and inflammatory cell products have been shown to be directly ciliotoxic[73–75] by complex and poorly understood mechanisms. For example, ciliary beat frequency decreased after exposure to *P. aeruginosa* proteinases and human neutrophil elastase in vitro.[73] Others have reported ciliary dysfunction in nasal epithelial cells after exposure to the supernatant from a *P. aeruginosa* culture and pyocyanin was isolated as the putative culprit.[74] Chemical mediators from inflammatory cells and serum may impair mucociliary transport by altering mucus, ion, and water transport across epithelial cells.[12]

Considerable data suggest that mucociliary function is chronically impaired in certain disease states such as chronic bronchitis that are commonly found in ICU patients.[11] We know little about the influence of aging and malnutrition on this system. The influences of multiple acute systemic illnesses such as sepsis and renal failure on mucociliary function have also not been well characterized. Drugs such as anticholinergics, antihistamines, aspirin, barbiturates, ethanol, and narcotics have all been reported to depress mucociliary transport in animal and human studies.[11, 76–78] Other therapeutic modalities, such as high oxygen concentrations, have been shown to cause epithelial cell damage and impaired ciliary function,[11] although the significance of these effects for human disease remains speculative.

Alveolar and Systemic Defenses

A microbe that has eluded the defense network in the upper and conducting airways enters the terminal gas exchange units, which are composed of respiratory bronchioles, alveolar ducts, and alveoli. Animal studies using bolus inoculations of bacterial pathogens have shown that the normal lung effectively clears small bacterial loads.[79] However, minute volumes of upper airway secretions in colonized hosts are likely to provide bacterial loads far in excess of those resulting in the predictable development of pneumonia in animal models.[79–82] Thus, the increased prevalence of nosocomial pneumonia in ICU patients may be most importantly related to factors that enhance distal lung unit exposure to large inocula of virulent organisms.

Alveolar and systemic defenses may also be impaired in critical illness. Alveolar defenses such as macrophage function may be compromised by immunosuppressive therapy, oxygen toxicity, uremia, acidosis, pulmonary edema, intercurrent viral infection, and sepsis.[23, 83] For example, significant impairment of alveolar macrophage secretion of chemotactic factors and complement components has been observed during glucocorticoid and cyclophosphamide administration in animals.[84, 85] In addition, many ICU patients have overt defects in systemic immune function caused by bone marrow suppression, immunosuppressive therapy, the acquired immunodeficiency syndrome, or various immunoglobulin deficiency states that place them at specific risk for the development of certain opportunistic infections. In the compromised host who has bone marrow failure and inadequate reserves of inflammatory cells, the back-up inflammatory response may be ineffective. In patients with acquired immunodeficiency syndrome or those receiving immunosuppressive therapy, cell-mediated immunity and granuloma formation are impaired, which may in turn blunt appropriate alveolar macrophage stimulation.[15]

Each compromising factor adds to the disintegration of the normally protective lung defense network. For example, many ICU patients are elderly. The increased risk of pneumonia in the elderly is probably a consequence of increased oropharyngeal colonization with virulent organisms, impaired mechanical clearance mechanisms, and weakened systemic humoral and cellular immunity.[83, 86, 87] These problems are related to the aging process itself and to the increased prevalence of chronic illnesses, malnutrition, and use of multiple medications in the aged.[83, 86, 88] Exposure of the elderly patient to the additive insults of the ICU environment and acute illness further augments the risk. Thus, the impairment in host defense in critically ill patients is usually multifactorial, resulting from various aspects of ICU care, acute and chronic systemic illness, and underlying host factors. Compromise of the lung defense system is a major contributor to pulmonary sepsis and death in these patients.

References

1. Huxley EJ, Viroslav J, Gray WR, et al: Pharyngeal aspiration in normal adults and patients with depressed consciousness. Am J Med 64:564, 1978.
2. Hatch TF: Distribution and deposition of inhaled particles in the respiratory tract: Conference on airborne infection. J Bacteriol Rev 25:237, 1961.
3. Mackowiak PA: The normal microbial flora. N Engl J Med 307:83, 1982.
4. Gibbons RJ, van Houte J: Selective bacterial adherence to oral epithelial surfaces and its role as an ecological determinant. Infect Immun 3:567, 1971.
5. Niederman MS, Ferranti RD, Zeigler A, et al: Respiratory infections complicating long-term tracheostomy. The implication of persistent gram-negative tracheobronchial colonization. Chest 85:39, 1984.
6. Murray PR, Rosenblatt JE: Bacterial interference by oropharyngeal and clinical isolates of anaerobic bacteria. J Infect Dis 134:281, 1976.
7. Sprunt K, Redman W: Evidence suggesting importance of role of interbacterial inhibition in maintaining balance of normal flora. Ann Intern Med 58:579, 1968.
8. Berman JS: Lymphocytes in the lung: Should we continue to exalt only BALT? Am J Respir Cell Biol 3:101, 1990.
9. Mestecky J: The common mucosal immune system and current strategies for induction of immune responses in external secretions. J Clin Immunol 7:265, 1987.
10. Pabst R, Gehrke I: Is the bronchus-associated lymphoid tissue (BALT) an integral structure of the lung in normal mammals, including humans? Am J Respir Cell Mol Biol 3:131, 1990.
11. Wanner A: Clinical aspects of mucociliary transport. Am Rev Respir Dis 116:73, 1977.
12. Wanner A: Mucociliary clearance in the trachea. Clin Chest Med 7:247, 1986.
13. Welsh MG: Electrolyte transport by airway epithelia. Physiol Rev 67:1143, 1987.
14. Proctor DF: The upper airways. I. Nasal physiology and defense of the lung. Am Rev Respir Dis 115:97, 1977.
15. Reynolds HY: Integrated host defense against infections. In: Crystal RG, West JB, Barnes PJ, et al (eds): The Lung: Scientific Foundations. New York, Raven Press, p 1899, 1991.
16. Wu R, Carlson DM: Structure and synthesis of mucins. In: Crystal RG, West JB, Barnes PJ, et al (eds): The Lung: Scientific Foundations. New York, Raven Press, p 183, 1991.
17. Mestecky J, McGhee JR: Immunoglobulin A: Molecular and cellular interactions involved in IgA biosynthesis and immune response. Adv Immunol 40:153, 1987.
18. Kaltreider HB: Normal immune response. In: Crystal RG, West JB, Barnes PJ, et al (eds): The Lung: Scientific Foundations. New York, Raven Press, p 499, 1991.
19. Kaltreider HB, Chan MKL: The class-specific immunoglobulin composition of fluids obtained from various levels of the canine respiratory tract. J Immunol 116:423, 1976.
20. Green G, Kass EH: The role of the alveolar macrophage in the clearance of bacteria from the lung. J Exp Med 119:167, 1964.
21. Jackson S, Southern PM, Pierce AK, et al: Pulmonary clearance of gram negative bacilli. J Lab Clin Med 69:883, 1967.
22. Laurenzi GA, Beman L, First M, et al: A quantitative study of the deposition and clearance of bacteria in the murine lung. J Clin Invest 43:759, 1964.
23. Sibille Y, Reynolds HY: Macrophages and polymorphonuclear neutrophils in lung defense and injury. Am Rev Respir Dis 141:471, 1990.
24. Stevens RM, Teres D, Skillman JJ, et al: Pneumonia in an intensive care unit. Arch Intern Med 134:106, 1974.
25. LaForce FM: Hospital-acquired gram-negative rod pneumonias: An overview. Am J Med 70:664, 1981.
26. Sanford JP, Pierce AK: Lower respiratory tract infections. In: Bennett JV, Brachman PS (eds): Hospital Infections. Boston, Little, Brown, p 255, 1979.
27. Johanson WG, Pierce AK, Sanford JP, et al: Nosocomial respiratory infections with gram-negative bacilli. Ann Intern Med 77:701, 1972.
28. Craven DE, Kunches LM, Kilinsky V, et al: Risk factors for pneumonia and fatality in patients receiving continuous mechanical ventilation. Am Rev Respir Dis 133:792, 1986.
29. Ashbaugh DG, Petty TL: Sepsis complicating the acute respiratory distress syndrome. Surg Gynecol Obstet 135:865, 1972.
30. Seidenfeld JJ, Pohl DF, Bell RC, et al: Incidence, site, and outcome of infections in patients with the adult respiratory distress syndrome. Am Rev Respir Dis 134:12, 1986.
31. Zapol WM, Snider MT, Hill JD, et al: Extracorporeal membrane oxygenation in severe acute respiratory failure: A randomized prospective study. JAMA 242:2193, 1979.
32. Horan TC, White JW, Jarvis WR, et al: Nosocomial infections surveillance, 1984. MMWR CDC Surveill Summ 35(1SS):17SS, 1986.
33. Gross PA, Neu HC, Aswapokee P, et al: Deaths from nosocomial infection: Experience in a university hospital and a community hospital. Am J Med 68:219, 1980.
34. Gross PA, Van Antwerpen C: Nosocomial infections and hospital deaths: A case-control study. Am J Med 75:658, 1983.
35. Craven DE, Connolly MG, Lichtenberg DA, et al: Contamination of medical ventilators with tubing changes every 24 or 48 hours. N Engl J Med 306:1505, 1982.
36. Cross AS, Roup B: Role of respiratory assistance devices in endemic nosocomial pneumonia. Am J Med 70:681, 1981.
37. Pierce AK, Sanford JP: Bacterial contamination of aerosols. Arch Intern Med 131:156, 1973.
38. Reiznarz JA, Pierce AK, Mays BB, et al: The potential role of inhalation therapy equipment in nosocomial pulmonary infection. J Clin Invest 44:831, 1965.
39. Sanders CV, Luby JP, Johanson WG, et al: *Serratia marcescens* infections from inhalation therapy medications: Nosocomial outbreak. Ann Intern Med 73:15, 1970.
40. Johanson WG, Pierce AK, Sanford JP: Changing pharyngeal flora of hospitalized patients. Emergence of gram-negative bacilli. N Engl J Med 281:1138, 1969.
41. Rosenthal S, Tager IB: Prevalence of gram-negative rods in the normal pharyngeal flora. Ann Intern Med 83:355, 1975.
42. Palmer LB: Bacterial colonization: Pathogenesis and clinical significance. Clin Chest Med 8:455, 1987.
43. Niederman MS: Bacterial adherence as a mechanism of airway colonization. Eur J Clin Microbiol Infect Dis 8:15, 1989.
44. Roberts DD: Interactions of respiratory pathogens with host cell surface and extracellular matrix components. Am J Respir Cell Mol Biol 3:181, 1990.
45. Higuchi JH, Johanson WG: The relationship between adherence of *Pseudomonas aeruginosa* to upper respiratory cells in vitro and susceptibility to colonization in vivo. J Lab Clin Med 95:698, 1980.
46. Niederman MS, Merrill WW, Ferranti RD, et al: Nutritional status and bacterial binding in the lower respiratory tract in patients with chronic tracheostomy. Ann Intern Med 100:795, 1984.
47. Niederman MS, Merrill WW, Polomski L, et al: Influence of sputum IgA and elastase on tracheal cell bacterial adherence. Am Rev Respir Dis 133:255, 1986.
48. Woods DE, Straus DC, Johanson WG, et al: Role of salivary protease activity in adherence of gram-negative bacilli to mammalian buccal epithelial cells in vivo. J Clin Invest 68:1435, 1981.
49. Mason CM, Bawdon RE, Pierce AK, et al: Fibronectin is not detectable on the intact buccal epithelial surface of normal rats or humans. Am J Respir Cell Mol Biol 3:563, 1990.
50. Palmer LB, Merrill WW, Niederman MS, et al: Bacterial adherence to respiratory tract cells. Relationships between in vivo and in vitro pH and bacterial attachment. Am Rev Respir Dis 133:384, 1986.
51. Niederman MS, Mantovani R, Schoch P, et al: Patterns and routes of tracheobronchial colonization in mechanically ventilated patients. The

role of nutritional status in colonization by *Pseudomonas* species. Chest 95:155, 1989.

52. Ramphal R, Small PM, Shands JW Jr, et al: Adherence of *Pseudomonas aeruginosa* to tracheal cells injured by influenza infection or by endotracheal intubation. Infect Immun 27:614, 1980.

53. Petersdorf RD, Cortin JA, Hoeprich PD, et al: A study of antibiotic prophylaxis in unconscious patients. N Engl J Med 257:1001, 1957.

54. Sanders WE, Sanders CC: Modification of normal flora by antibiotics: Effects on individuals and the environment. In: Root RK, Sande MA (eds): Contemporary Issues in Infectious Disease, Volume 1, New Dimensions in Antimicrobial Therapy. New York, Churchill Livingstone, p 217, 1984.

55. Tillotson JR, Finland M: Bacterial colonization of the respiratory tract complicating antibiotic therapy of pneumonia. J Infect Dis 119:597, 1969.

56. Albert RK, Condie F: Hand-washing patterns in medical intensive care units. N Engl J Med 304:1465, 1981.

57. Maki DG: Control of colonization and transmission of pathogenic bacteria in the hospital. Ann Intern Med 89:777, 1978.

58. Driks MR, Craven DE, Celli BR, et al: Nosocomial pneumonia in intubated patients given sucralfate as compared with antacids or histamine type 2 blockers. N Engl J Med 317:1376, 1987.

59. Moulin GC, Patterson DG, Hedley-White J, et al: Aspiration of gastric bacteria in antacid-treated patients: A frequent cause of postoperative colonization of the airway. Lancet 1:242, 1982.

60. Pingleton SK, Hinthorn DR, Liu C: Enteral nutrition in patients receiving mechanical ventilation. Multiple sources of tracheal colonization include the stomach. Am J Med 80:827, 1986.

61. Tryba M: Risk of acute stress bleeding and nosocomial pneumonia in ventilated intensive care unit patients: Sucralfate versus antacids. Am J Med 83(suppl 3B):117, 1987.

62. Caplan ES, Hoyt NJ: Nosocomial sinusitis. JAMA 247:639, 1982.

63. Knodel AR, Beekman JF: Unexplained fevers in patients with nasotracheal intubation. JAMA 248:868, 1982.

64. Cameron JL, Reynolds J, Zuidema GD: Aspiration in patients with tracheostomies. Surg Gynecol Obstet 136:68, 1973.

65. Spray SB, Zuidema GD, Cameron JD: Aspiration pneumonia: Incidence of aspiration with endotracheal tubes. Am J Surg 131:701, 1976.

66. Belsey R: The pulmonary complications of oesophageal disease. Br J Dis Chest 54:342, 1960.

67. Irvin RS, Rosen MJ, Braman SS: Cough. A comprehensive review. Arch Intern Med 137:1186, 1977.

68. Alexopolus C, Jansson B, Lindholm CE: Mucus transport and surface damage after endotracheal intubation and tracheostomy. An experimental study in pigs. Acta Anaesthesiol Scand 28:68, 1984.

69. Landa JF, Kwoka MA, Chapman GA, et al: Effects of suctioning on mucociliary transport. Chest 77:202, 1980.

70. Sackner MA, Landa JF, Greeneltch N, et al: Pathogenesis and prevention of tracheobronchial damage with suction procedures. Chest 64:284, 1973.

71. Wynne JW, Ramphal R, Hood CI: Tracheal mucosal damage after aspiration. Am Rev Respir Dis 124:728, 1981.

72. Afzelius BA: Immotile-cilia syndrome and ciliary abnormalities induced by infection and injury. Am Rev Respir Dis 124:107, 1981.

73. Amitani R, Wilson R, Rutman A, et al: Effects of human neutrophil elastase and *Pseudomonas aeruginosa* proteinases on human respiratory epithelium. Am J Respir Cell Mol Biol 4:26, 1991.

74. Wilson R, Cole P: The effect of bacterial products on ciliary function. Am Rev Respir Dis 138(suppl):49, 1988.

75. Wilson R: Secondary ciliary dysfunction. Clin Sci 75:113, 1988.

76. Gerrity TR, Cotromanes E, Garrard CS, et al: The effect of aspirin on the lung mucociliary clearance. N Engl J Med 308:139, 1983.

77. Hermens WAJJ, Merkus FWHM: The influence of drugs on nasal ciliary movement. Pharmacol Res 4:445, 1987.

78. West S, Brandon B, Stolley P, et al: A review of antihistamines and the common cold. Pediatrics 56:100, 1975.

79. Toews GB, Gross GN, Pierce AK: The relationship of inoculum size to lung bacterial clearance and phagocytic response in mice. Am Rev Respir Dis 120:559, 1979.

80. Ansfield MJ, Woods DE, Johanson WG Jr.: Lung bacterial clearance in murine pneumococcal pneumonia. Infect Immun 17:195, 1977.

81. Berendt RF: Relationship of method of administration to respiratory virulence of *Klebsiella pneumoniae* for mice and squirrel monkeys. Infect Immun 20:581, 1978.

82. Toews GB: Nosocomial pneumonia. Clin Chest Med 8:467, 1987.

83. Skerrett SJ, Niederman MS, Fein AM: Respiratory infections and acute lung injury in systemic illness. Clin Chest Med 10:469, 1989.

84. Pennington JE, Harris EA: Influence of immunosuppression on alveolar macrophage chemotactic activities in guinea pigs. Am Rev Respir Dis 123:299, 1981.

85. Pennington JE, Matthews WJ, Marion JE, et al: Cyclophosphamide and cortisone acetate inhibit complement biosynthesis by guinea pig bronchoalveolar macrophages. J Immunol 123:1318, 1979.

86. Esposito AL: The effect of common pharmacologic agents on pulmonary antibacterial defenses: Implications for the geriatric patient. Clin Chest Med 8:373, 1987.

87. Valenti MW, Trudell RG, Bentley DW: Factors predisposing to oropharyngeal colonization with gram-negative bacilli in the aged. N Engl J Med 298:1108, 1978.

88. Martin TR: The relationship between malnutrition and lung infections. Clin Chest Med 8:359, 1987.

CHAPTER 67

Respiratory Failure: An Overview

Paul N. Lanken

Respiratory failure refers to the end result of a host of clinical disorders characterized by severe impairment in pulmonary gas exchange. The clinical disorders associated with respiratory failure can be divided into two basic types: (1) hypercapnic respiratory failure, resulting in elevated $PaCO_2$ (>45 torr) and (2) hypoxemic respiratory failure, resulting in PaO_2 less than 55 torr despite administration of at least 60% supplemental oxygen (Fig. 67–1). Because both types are life threatening if gas exchange abnormalities are severe and because the underlying diseases and therapies may differ significantly, understanding the mechanisms and characteristics of each type of respiratory failure and its differential diagnoses is important not only in caring for patients with overt respiratory failure but also possibly in preventing its development.

COMPONENTS OF THE RESPIRATORY SYSTEM

Pulmonary gas exchange occurs as a result of a sequential interplay of a number of components of the overall respi-

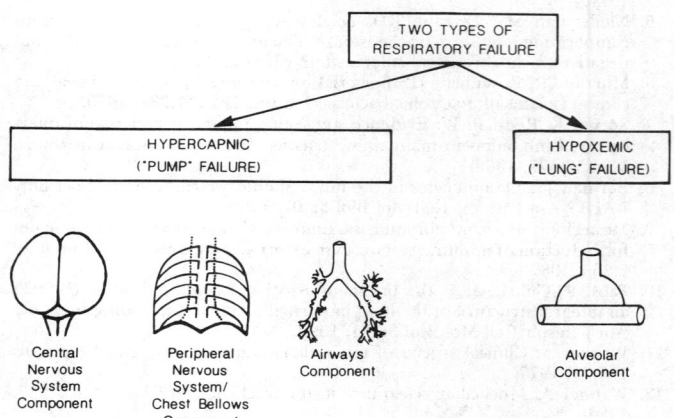

Figure 67–1. Acute respiratory failure can be divided into two types: hypercapnic respiratory failure with $PaCO_2$ greater than 45 torr and hypoxemic respiratory failure with PaO_2 less than 55 torr despite 60% or higher concentrations of inspired O_2. Hypercapnic respiratory failure, also described as respiratory pump failure (pump failure), is due to failure of one or more of three components of the respiratory system: (1) CNS ventilatory drive, (2) peripheral nervous system and chest bellows, including the respiratory muscles, and (3) the conducting airways. Hypoxemic respiratory failure results from impairment of the fourth component of the overall respiratory system, the alveoli.

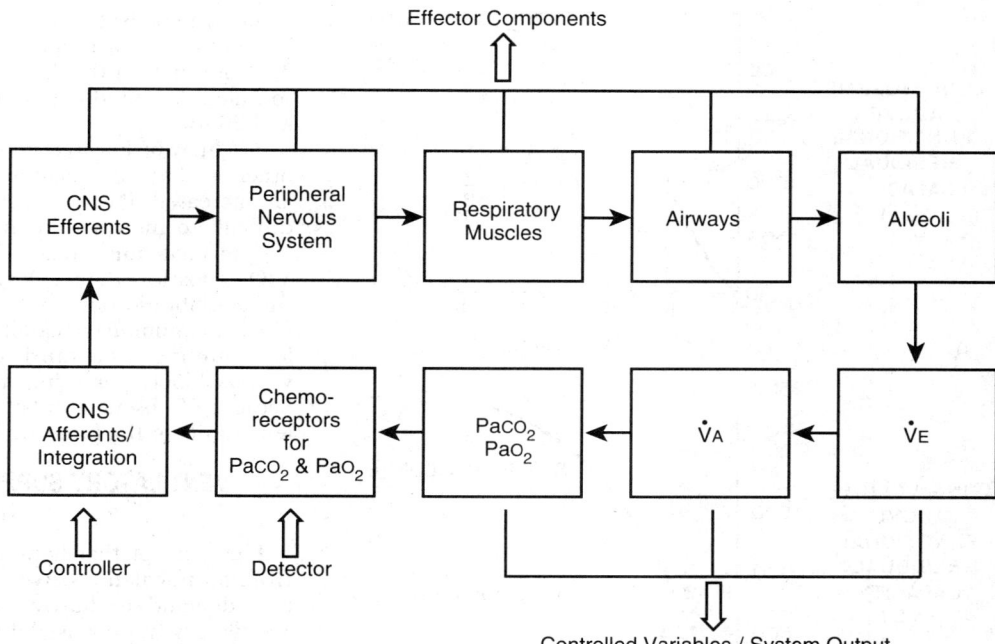

Figure 67–2. The overall respiratory system, described in Figure 67–1, is an integral part of a complex feedback system whose effector components consist of the central neural drive to ventilate, the neural connections to the respiratory muscles, the muscles themselves, the conducting airways, and the alveoli. The controlled variables, or system output, consist of minute ventilation, alveolar ventilation, and $PaCO_2$ and PaO_2. The arterial levels of PO_2 and PCO_2 are detected by peripheral and central chemoreceptors (detector), which then send information back to the CNS controller. The CNS controller, in turn, responds to abnormalities in PaO_2 or $PaCO_2$ by modifying the activity of the effector components.

ratory system. This system has classically been divided into four functional and structural components[1] (see Fig. 67–1): (1) the central neural drive, (2) the peripheral nervous system (the phrenic nerves and other respiratory motor neurons) and the chest bellows (i.e., the respiratory muscles plus the thorax and abdominal structures surrounding the lungs), (3) the airways, and (4) the alveoli. These four components work together as the effector arm of a more complex feedback system (Fig. 67–2) whose role is to maintain homeostasis of $PaCO_2$ and PaO_2 at rest, during exercise, and in diseased states. Because respiratory failure may result from impaired functioning of one, or a combination, of these four components, analysis of each component's functioning should aid in the understanding and management of clinical cases of respiratory failure.

Components of the Respiratory Pump

Inspiration occurs through the actions of the respiratory pump,[2, 3] whose components normally function in the following sequence (see Fig. 67–2): (1) The central neural drive initiates the process by generating rhythmic oscillations under central nervous system (CNS) control in response to changes in $PaCO_2$ and PaO_2 as well as other influences. (2) These neural impulses are conducted from the medulla via the spinal cord to the phrenic and other motor neurons innervating the diaphragm and other respiratory muscles. (3) These muscles inflate the lungs by creating a negative pleural pressure within the thorax by expanding the chest wall and displacing adjacent abdominal contents. (4) The subatmospheric pressure in the alveoli generates the flow of air through the airways by convection. (5) Further movement and mixing of O_2 and CO_2 occur by gaseous diffusion in distal airways and in alveolar spaces.

The respiratory pump produces a certain minute ventilation (expired volume per unit time, $\dot{V}E$) and alveolar ventilation ($\dot{V}A$) by controlling the depth of tidal volumes and the respiratory rate. Changes in alveolar ventilation alter $PaCO_2$ according to the following relationship:[1, 2]

$$\dot{V}A = K \times \dot{V}CO_2/PaCO_2 \qquad (1)$$

where $\dot{V}CO_2$ is the CO_2 production per minute and K is a constant, 863.

The relationship between the pressure generated by the respiratory pump and the resulting tidal volume is shown in Figure 67–3. Figure 67–3*A* schematically illustrates a normal static pressure-volume curve of the respiratory system,[4] that is, the lung and chest wall plus adjacent abdominal contents. The slope of this curve represents the respiratory system's static compliance (Cst), which is defined as

$$Cst = \Delta V/\Delta P \qquad (2)$$

where ΔV is the tidal volume and ΔP is the end-inspiratory static alveolar pressure, the elastic recoil pressure of the respiratory system.

Figure 67–3*B* schematically shows a normal dynamic pressure-volume curve added to the normal static curve shown in Figure 67–3*A*. These demonstrate that, during a spontaneous inspiration, the respiratory muscles must not only generate forces to expand the lungs and chest wall equivalent to the static recoil pressure for a given tidal volume (see Fig. 67–3*A*) but also generate the additional pressure gradient needed to move that tidal volume through the airways. The magnitude of this pressure gradient is determined by inspiratory flow rate and airway resistance. Normally these pressures are relatively modest because of the remarkably efficient mechanical properties of the respiratory apparatus. For a normal individual with a static compliance of the respiratory system of 100 mL/cm H_2O and airway resistance of 4 cm H_2O/L/s breathing at an inspiratory flow rate of 0.5 L/s, the respiratory muscles would need to overcome pressures of only 6 to 7 cm H_2O to produce a tidal volume of about 400 mL.

Alveolar Component

The alveolar component of the respiratory system represents the gas-exchanging units where O_2 and CO_2 diffuse passively across the alveolar capillary membrane; the diffusion is due to differences in PO_2 and PCO_2 across this membrane, that is, between mixed venous and pulmonary capillary blood on the one side and individual alveolar spaces

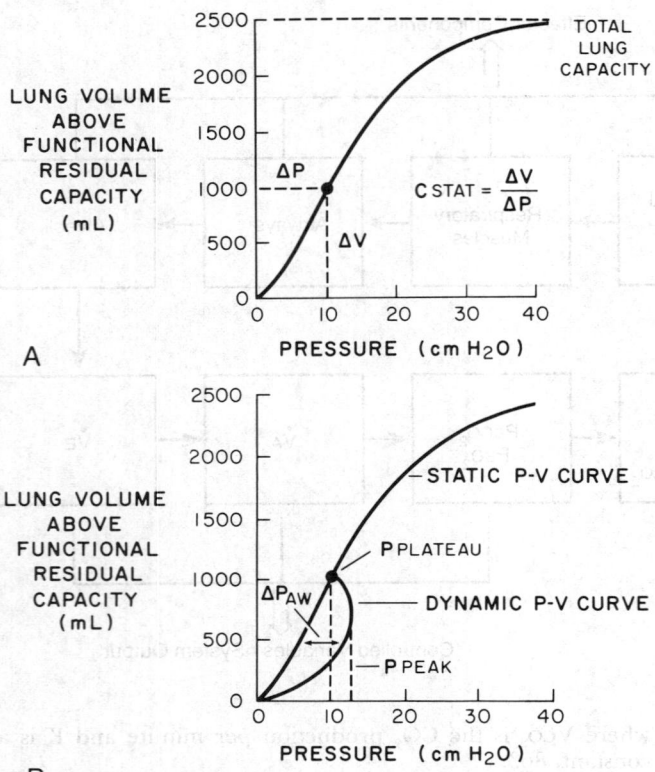

LUNG VOLUME ABOVE FUNCTIONAL RESIDUAL CAPACITY (mL)

$$C \, STAT = \frac{\Delta V}{\Delta P}$$

A

PRESSURE (cm H₂O)

LUNG VOLUME ABOVE FUNCTIONAL RESIDUAL CAPACITY (mL)

B

PRESSURE (cm H₂O)

Figure 67–3. *A.* Schematic static pressure-volume curve of a normal respiratory system (lung plus chest wall and adjacent abdomen) relating end-inspiratory lung volume to the system's recoil pressure. The slope of the curve is the static compliance (C_{st}) of the respiratory system, the ratio of the change in volume (ΔV) to the change in pressure (ΔP). In this example, C_{st} is 100 mL/cm H_2O. *B.* The same static pressure-volume curve (static P-V curve) of the respiratory system as in *A*, with the addition of a dynamic pressure-volume curve (dynamic P-V curve) representing the pressure drop across the conducting airways during normal inspiration. In this example, to inspire a 1.0-L tidal volume, the respiratory muscles not only must overcome the recoil pressure (P plateau) of the respiratory system to expand the lungs and chest wall but also must generate an additional pressure (P peak) to establish the pressure gradient that results in inspiratory flow. (From Lanken PN: Mechanical ventilation. In: Fishman AP [ed]: Pulmonary Diseases and Disorders. 2nd ed. New York, McGraw-Hill, p 2373, 1988. Reproduced with permission of McGraw-Hill, Inc.)

on the other. Although P_{O_2} in an individual alveolus is determined by the fraction of inspired oxygen, F_{IO_2} and the ventilation/perfusion ($\dot{V}/\dot{Q}$) ratio of that alveolus, the mean alveolar partial pressure of oxygen, P_{AO_2}, for the entire lung can be calculated from the alveolar gas equation:

$$P_{AO_2} = P_{IO_2} - P_{ACO_2}/R \qquad (3)$$

where P_{IO_2} is the partial pressure of inspired oxygen, P_{ACO_2} is estimated as equal to P_{ACO_2}, and R is the respiratory ratio, usually assumed to be 0.8 (except when $F_{IO_2} = 1.0$, when its value is 1). The respiratory ratio R is the non–steady-state equivalent of the respiratory quotient RQ, defined as

$$RQ = \dot{V}_{CO_2}/\dot{V}_{O_2} \qquad (4)$$

Compared with its relatively direct control of P_{ACO_2}, the respiratory pump can change levels of P_{AO_2} much less effectively. The respiratory pump can increase P_{AO_2} only modestly through hyperventilation, that is, by lowering P_{ACO_2} and P_{ACO_2} as a consequence of increased $\dot{V}_A$. Conversely, the respiratory pump can decrease P_{AO_2} only

through hypoventilation because the resulting rise in P_{ACO_2} lowers P_{AO_2} according to the alveolar gas equation (Equation 3). Note that, in this latter circumstance, $P_{AO_2} - P_{aO_2}$, the so-called A-a gradient, should remain normal, between 10 and 20 torr.

P_{aO_2} may be lowered in disease states by three mechanisms other than hypoventilation, all of which are characterized by an increased $P_{AO_2} - P_{aO_2}$ (although this value may be difficult to interpret in the presence of hypercapnia[5]): (1) $\dot{V}/\dot{Q}$ mismatching, that is, increased number of alveoli with $\dot{V}/\dot{Q}$ ratios less than 1.0; (2) diffusion defects that prevent full equilibration of P_{O_2} between the alveolar space and the blood in pulmonary capillaries; and (3) increased right-to-left shunting. This third mechanism can occur with mixed venous blood perfusing alveoli with a $\dot{V}/\dot{Q}$ ratio of zero because of absent ventilation or through anatomic right-to-left shunts in the lungs or heart.

VENTILATORY SUPPLY VERSUS VENTILATORY DEMAND

The concept that hypercapnic respiratory failure results from an imbalance between ventilatory supply and ventilatory demand is illustrated schematically in Figure 67–4. Ventilatory supply is defined as the maximal sustainable ventilation (MSV), the highest spontaneous ventilation that an individual can maintain indefinitely without developing respiratory muscle fatigue.[2, 3] Ventilatory demand refers to an individual's spontaneous minute ventilation, which, if sustained, would result in a certain "preset" level of P_{ACO_2} as determined by the central controlling mechanism of the feedback loop (see Fig. 67–2). As illustrated in Figure 67–4A, a normal individual has a great deal of ventilatory reserve at rest with an MSV far exceeding resting minute ventilation. For example, a normal 40-year-old man who weighs 70 kg has an estimated MSV of about 80 L/min, which is estimated as half of his predicted maximal voluntary ventilation of approximately 160 L/min.[6] This may be compared with a resting minute ventilation of about 6 to 7 L/min (~90 mL/kg/min). In disease, ventilatory supply (MSV) may be markedly reduced and ventilatory demand increased so that they approximate each other as shown in Figure 67–4B, with the patient balanced on the edge of respiratory failure. Further reductions in MSV and/or increases in ventilatory demand eventually lead to respiratory muscle fatigue and overt hypercapnic respiratory failure (see Fig. 67–4C).

Ventilatory Supply

The ability to maintain or increase total ventilation ($\dot{V}_E$) to keep P_{ACO_2} levels within the normal range depends, to a large degree, on an intact respiratory pump. Despite extensive clinical and laboratory knowledge related to the respiratory muscles and development of skeletal muscle fatigue,[2, 7] the basic cellular, molecular, and biochemical mechanisms involved in respiratory muscle fatigue in disease states remain poorly defined. As a consequence, empirical observations have been utilized to assess maximal sustainable ventilation as expressed by the following relationships:

$$MSV = \frac{1}{2}MVV \qquad (5)$$

where MVV is the maximal voluntary ventilation,[6] although a greater fraction of MVV may be sustained after endurance training.[8]

$$MSV = \frac{1}{2}(40 \times FEV_1) = 20 \times FEV_1 \qquad (6)$$

where FEV_1 is the forced expired volume in the first second of expiration. This relationship is derived from Equation 5 because normally MVV approximately equals $FEV_1 \times 40$.[1]

NORMAL VENTILATION

Demand < Supply

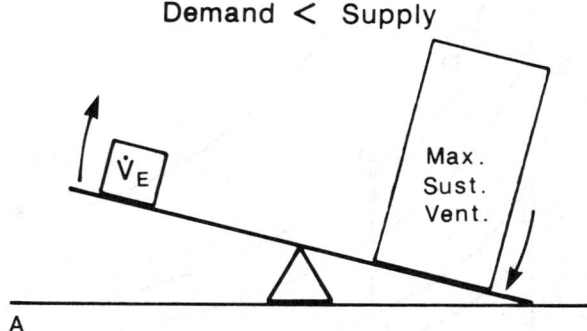

A

BORDERLINE VENTILATORY FAILURE

Demand ≅ Supply

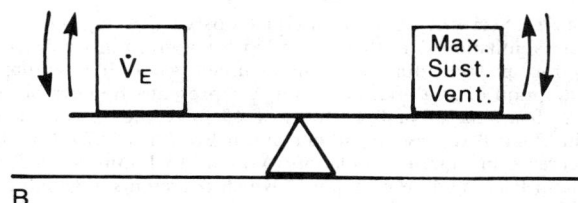

B

OVERT VENTILATORY FAILURE

Demand > Supply

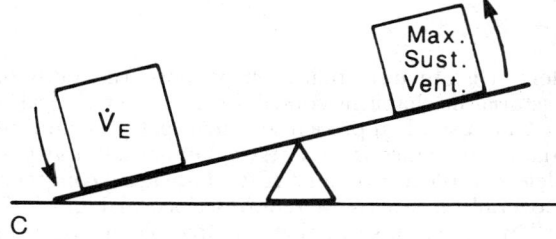

C

Figure 67–4. Schematic representation of the balance between ventilatory demand, defined as an individual's spontaneous minute ventilation, $\dot{V}_E$, needed to achieve a certain Pa_{CO_2}, and ventilatory supply, defined as his or her maximal sustainable ventilation (Max. Sust. Vent.) under different conditions. *A.* The normal situation, in which maximal sustainable ventilation far outweighs resting minute ventilation. *B.* The effects of disease in which increased ventilatory demand approximately equals a decreased ventilatory supply, resulting in a state of borderline ventilatory failure. *C.* A further increase in ventilatory demand has occurred compared to *B;* demand now exceeds maximal sustainable ventilation and will lead to overt hypercapnic respiratory failure when respiratory muscle fatigue occurs. See text for further details.

It would not be valid in the presence of upper airway obstruction or in patients whose respiratory muscles have poor endurance.

$$MSV = 30 \times VC \qquad (7)$$

where VC is the vital capacity. Equation 7 is derived from Equation 6 because normally forced vital capacity (FVC) = VC and $FEV_1/FVC = 0.75$. Note that this relationship would

not be valid in individuals with obstructive airways disease whose FEV_1/FVC is less than 0.75.

Table 67–1 lists a number of different mechanisms involving multiple distinct factors that may compromise the effectiveness of the respiratory pump and thereby limit a patient's MSV. Equations 5 to 7 must be applied to specific clinical situations with caution for several reasons. Patients with certain neuromuscular diseases, such as myasthenia gravis, may be subject to early fatigue and have an MSV considerably less than ½MVV. In addition, bedside MVV measurements involving patients who are sedated or confused may be unreliable and underestimate the true MVV because of poor cooperation or comprehension by the patient during the maneuver.[9]

TABLE 67–1
FACTORS AND EXAMPLES REDUCING VENTILATORY SUPPLY

Category	Examples
Decreased respiratory muscle strength	
Fatigue or borderline fatigue	During recovery period from fatigue,[25, 34] high respiratory rates,[9] increased Pdi/Pdimax,*[3, 9] increased inspiratory time[3]
Disuse atrophy	Prolonged mechanical ventilation; status post–phrenic nerve injury
Malnutrition	Protein-calorie starvation[24, 35]
Electrolyte abnormalities	Low serum phosphate,[14] low potassium
Arterial blood gas abnormalities	Low pH,[2] high P_{CO_2},[36] low Po_2[2]
Fatty infiltration of diaphragm	Obesity
Unfavorable alteration in force-length relationship	Flattened domes of diaphragms caused by hyperinflation[2, 24]
Increased muscular energetics or decreased substrate supply	
High elastic work of breathing[20]	Low lung or chest wall compliance,[19] high respiratory rates
High resistive work of breathing[20]	Expiratory airway obstruction, high flow rates
Low perfusion of diaphragm	Circulatory shock states,[37] anemia, increased time when muscle is actively contracting[2, 3]
Decreased motor neuron function	
Decreased phrenic neural output	Polyneuropathy, Guillain-Barré syndrome, phrenic nerve transection or injury, poliomyelitis
Decreased neuromuscular transmission	Myasthenia gravis, paralyzing agents
Abnormal respiratory mechanics	
Flow limitation (FEV_1, FIV_1)[38, 39]	Bronchospasm, upper airway obstruction, airway secretions
Loss of lung volume	Post–lung resection, large pleural effusions
Other restrictive defects	Incisional or other pain-limiting inspiration; tense abdomen caused by ileus, peritoneal dialysis, or ascites

*Pdi/Pdimax is the ratio of the transdiaphragmatic pressure gradient produced for a given breath to the individual's maximal transdiaphragmatic pressure gradient.

Ventilatory Demand

The level of an individual's spontaneous minute ventilation is determined by the central controller component of the respiratory system, which drives the respiratory pump to maintain a certain level of $Paco_2$ (see Fig. 67–2). The physiological variables that determine a given level of minute ventilation to maintain a certain $Paco_2$ are defined by the following equations:

$$\dot{V}_E = \dot{V}_A + \dot{V}_{DS} \qquad (8)$$

where $\dot{V}_{DS}$ is dead space ventilation and is equal to the product of the respiratory rate and physiologic dead space, V_{DS}, the sum of anatomic dead space and alveolar dead space associated with alveoli with $\dot{V}/\dot{Q}$ ratios greater than 1.0. By substituting $(V_{DS}/V_T) \times \dot{V}_E$, where V_T is tidal volume and V_{DS}/V_T is the dead space/tidal volume ratio, for the term V_{DS} in this equation and rearranging terms, the following equation is derived:

$$\dot{V}_E = \dot{V}_A /(1 - V_{DS}/V_T) \qquad (9)$$

Equation 1 can be modified by substituting $RQ \times \dot{V}_{O_2}$ for $\dot{V}_{CO_2}$ (Equation 2); when this modified Equation 1 is substituted for $\dot{V}_A$ in Equation 8, one can derive the following equation of ventilatory demand:

$$\dot{V}_E = K \times (\dot{V}_{O_2} \times RQ)/[Paco_2 /(1 - V_{DS}/V_T)] \qquad (10)$$

This equation is represented graphically by Figure 67–5, which illustrates how V_{DS}/V_T and $Paco_2$, as independent physiologic variables, together determine $\dot{V}_E$.[10] In Figure 67–5, each curve is an isopleth with a certain value for V_{DS}/V_T whose shape is determined by the hyperbolic relationship between $Paco_2$ and $\dot{V}_E$ that is evident in Equation 10 (when $\dot{V}_{O_2}$ and RQ are constant as in Fig. 67–5). The example in Figure 67–5 illustrates that a first stepwise increase in spontaneous minute ventilation is needed to keep $Paco_2$ at 40 torr if V_{DS}/V_T increases from a normal of 0.3 to 0.75 because of respiratory disease, such as the adult respiratory distress syndrome.[11] A second stepwise increase in minute ventilation is required if $Paco_2$ decreased from 40 to 30 torr, as in hyperventilation stimulated by hypoxemia. Finally, if $\dot{V}_{O_2}$ increases above 200 mL/min (the value assumed as a constant in graphing the isopleths), as in sepsis, a third increase in minute ventilation (not illustrated) would be needed to maintain the same level of $Paco_2$. In the latter circumstance, the increased $\dot{V}_{O_2}$ would in effect shift the V_{DS}/V_T curves vertically.

If these changes in ventilatory demand occurred in a patient with sepsis and adult respiratory distress syndrome, simultaneous decreases in the patient's ventilatory supply would also be expected: decreased lung compliance, restricted tidal volumes, and atelectasis plus possible adverse effects of acidosis, hypoxemia, and limited blood perfusion on respiratory muscle function, as listed in Table 67–1. These changes in demand and supply, if severe, would reverse the normal relationship of supply outweighing demand and result in overt hypercapnic respiratory failure (see Fig. 67–4). Table 67–2 lists changes in the factors on the right-hand side of Equation 10 that would increase ventilatory demand and important clinical examples for each factor. Changes in these factors in the reverse direction would tend to reduce ventilatory demand and possibly prevent respiratory muscle fatigue and hypercapnic respiratory failure.

FAILURE OF INDIVIDUAL RESPIRATORY SYSTEM COMPONENTS

Because respiratory failure in a patient is often a final common pathway manifestation of multiple diseases and

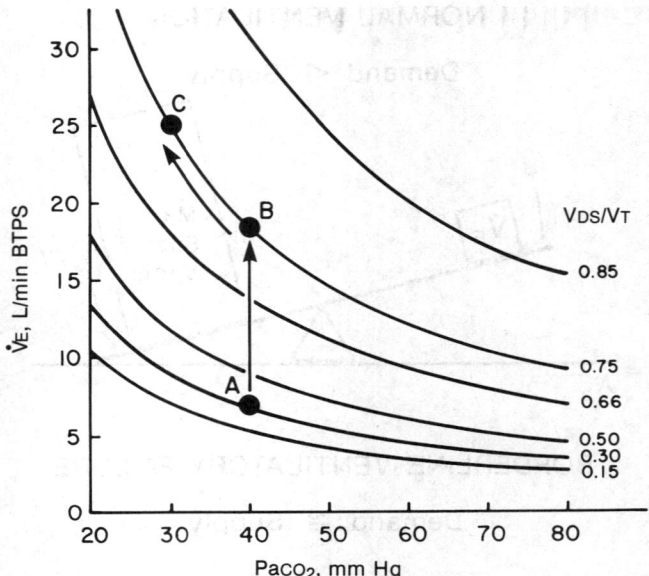

Figure 67–5. Series of isopleths of equal V_{DS}/V_T showing the level of minute ventilation ($\dot{V}_E$) that is needed for a given level of arterial Pco_2 for an individual with an assumed value for minute O_2 consumption of 200 mL/min. Point A represents the normal situation with a V_{DS}/V_T of 0.3, $Paco_2$ of 40 torr, and $\dot{V}_E$ of about 7 L/min. Point B represents an increase in V_{DS}/V_T to 0.75, for which an increase in minute ventilation to about 18 L/min is needed to maintain $Paco_2$ at 40 torr. Point C, which represents moving up the V_{DS}/V_T isopleth of 0.75 to decrease $Paco_2$ from 40 to 30 torr, requires a total ventilation of about 25 L/min or about 3.5 times the original resting $\dot{V}_E$. See text for further comments. (Adapted from Selecky PA, Wasserman K, Klein M, et al: A graphic approach to assessing interrelationships among minute ventilation, arterial carbon dioxide tension and ratio of physiologic dead space to tidal volume in patients on respirators. Am Rev Respir Dis 117:181, 1978.)

disorders, it is apparent that such patients frequently have multifactorial mechanisms contributing to their clinical condition. One useful approach to such patients and their potential complexities is to assess systematically the potentially deleterious contributions of the individual components of the overall respiratory system described in Figure 67–1. The following sections describe the physiologic and clinical characteristics of respiratory failure occurring as a consequence of impairment of one of the four components of the respiratory system.

TABLE 67–2	
FACTORS AND EXAMPLES INCREASING VENTILATORY DEMAND	
Categories	**Clinical Examples**
Increased V_{DS}/V_T	Asthma, emphysema, adult respiratory distress syndrome,[11] pulmonary emboli
Increased O_2 consumption	Fever, sepsis, trauma, shivering, increased work of breathing,[20] massive obesity
Increased respiratory quotient	Excessive carbohydrate feeding[40]
Decreased $Paco_2$	Hypoxemia, metabolic acidosis, central neurogenic hyperventilation, anxiety, sepsis, renal and hepatic failure

TABLE 67-3

TYPICAL CHANGES IN ARTERIAL BLOOD GASES $P_{AO_2} - P_{aO_2}$, AND VENTILATION IN ACUTE RESPIRATORY FAILURE CAUSED BY FAILURE OF INDIVIDUAL COMPONENTS OF THE RESPIRATORY SYSTEM*

Failed Respiratory System Component	pH	Pa_{CO_2}	Pa_{O_2}	$P_{AO_2} - Pa_{O_2}$	Ventilation Total	Alveolar
Central nervous system	↓	↑	↓	NL	↓	↓
Peripheral nervous system or chest bellows	↓	↑	↓	↑	↓	↓
Airways						
In asthma						
Early phase (before respiratory failure)	↑	↓	NL	↑	↑	↑
Crossover point	NL	NL	NL to ↓	↑	↑	NL
Extremely severe obstruction or respiratory muscle fatigue	↓	↑	↓	↑	↑	↓
In flare of COPD						
Non–CO_2 retainer	↓	↑	↓	↑	↑	↓
CO_2 retainer						
Baseline	↓	↑	↓	↑	NL	↓
Flare	↓	↑↑	↓↓	↑	NL or ↑	↓
Alveoli						
Before respiratory muscle fatigue	↑	↓	↓↓	↑↑	↑	↑
After respiratory muscle fatigue	↓	↑	↓↓	↑↑	↑	↓

*Note: ↑ = increased, ↑↑ = very increased, ↓ = decreased, ↓↓ = very decreased, NL = in the normal range.

Impairment of Central Neural Drive Component

Common examples of the acute form of this disorder include overdoses of sedative, narcotic, or other prescription drugs that have sedating properties, such as tricyclic antidepressants, and certain structural disorders of the CNS involving the respiratory center, such as diffuse meningoencephalitis or localized abnormalities affecting the medulla. Chronic forms, such as metabolic alkalosis or methadone maintenance therapy, effectively raise the threshold of the CNS controller to increases in Pa_{CO_2}, the end result being a chronic respiratory acidosis. Acute superimposed on chronic forms of this type of disorder may occur as part of the obesity-hypoventilation syndrome or in severe myxedema. Iatrogenic causes of this disorder include overaggressive use of postoperative narcotics, residual effects of long-acting narcotics used intraoperatively, and metabolic alkalosis.

The initial step in the pathophysiology of this type of component failure is decreased central neural drive, leading to decreased tidal volumes and/or respiratory rates. These result in decreased minute ventilation and decreased alveolar ventilation according to Equations 8 and 9, which in turn result in a rise in Pa_{CO_2} (Equation 1) and hypercapnic respiratory failure (Table 67–3). Although pulmonary function testing may be difficult to perform because of poor cooperation by the patient, the patient may demonstrate a fairly well preserved vital capacity and maximal inspiratory pressure during relatively lucid periods. Arterial blood gas changes typically confirm an acute respiratory acidosis.

Treatment recommended for this form of respiratory failure includes reversal of the impairment by means of a specific pharmacologic agent, if possible, such as intravenous administration of naloxone for narcotic-induced respiratory failure. Nonspecific pharmacologic stimulation of ventilation may be problematic because of the concomitant need for tracheal intubation to protect against aspiration. Even successful reversal of the respiratory depression does not obviate the need for admission to a special care unit to monitor the patient's respiratory status closely. Inadequate airway protection because of loss of the patient's gag reflex is common in drug overdoses and frequently leads to tracheal intubation with mechanical ventilation if hypoventilation occurs.

Peripheral Nervous System–Chest Bellows Component

Clinical causes of neuromuscular weakness of the respiratory muscles are acute demyelinating polyneuropathy (Guillain-Barré syndrome), generalized myasthenia gravis, acute polymyositis, acute respiratory muscle weakness[12, 13] such as those associated with hypokalemia or hypophosphatemia,[14] and acute poliomyelitis and cervical spinal cord injury affecting the phrenic motor neurons (C3-5 nerve roots). Iatrogenic causes include residual effects of paralyzing agents, cholinergic crisis resulting from use of anticholinesterase agents to treat myasthenia gravis, and respiratory muscle fatigue resulting from prior attempts at weaning from mechanical ventilation. The latter may persist for up to 24 hours if observations on other skeletal muscles can be applied to the diaphragm.[15]

In respiratory failure caused by neuromuscular weakness despite adequate central neural drive, transpulmonary pressure gradients cannot produce normal tidal volumes because of (1) disruption of the CNS transmission at various points along the neuromuscular pathway from spinal cord to diaphragms or (2) intrinsic weakness of the respiratory muscles. Increases in respiratory rate via the feedback loop (see Fig. 67–2) initially compensate for the small tidal volumes to maintain minute and alveolar ventilation. Eventually, with further weakness, the patient can no longer compensate for the inadequate tidal volumes or produce spontaneous sighs. Loss of sighs and the low tidal volume breathing result in progressive atelectasis, probably because of loss of surface activity of alveolar surfactant, and eventually lung compliance decreases.[16, 17] This further reduces the patient's tidal volumes because the same transpulmonary pressure, when applied to lungs with a lower compliance, results in a lower tidal volume (Fig. 67–6A). Ventilatory supply is thus limited directly by the decreased respiratory muscle function and indirectly by the decreased lung compliance. In addition, the patient's ventilatory demand is increased because of an increased V_{DS}/V_T caused primarily by the shallow tidal volumes without a corresponding decrease in the patient's dead space as well as by modest increases in the elastic work of breathing (see Fig. 67–6A). As a result of these changes, the patient eventually experiences decreased alveolar venti-

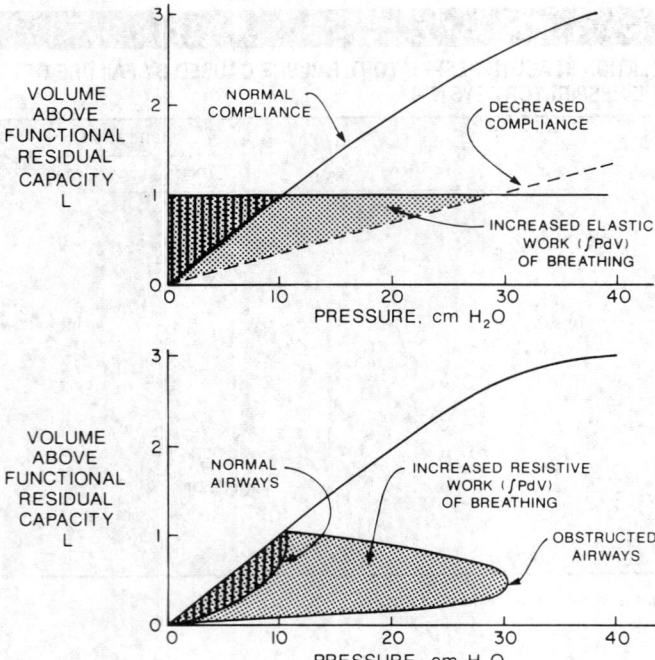

Figure 67–6. *A.* Schematic representation of a normal static pressure-volume curve *(solid curve)* of the respiratory system with its static compliance decreased to approximately one third of its normal value *(dashed line).* With this change in compliance, to inspire the same tidal volume of 1.0 L, the respiratory muscles would need to overcome a threefold increased recoil pressure; in addition, the decreased compliance results in an increased elastic work of breathing *(stippled area),* the product of pressure and volume ($\int P \, dV$), that is also approximately three times greater than the normal elastic work of breathing *(vertically striped area). B.* Dynamic pressure-volume curves representing the increase in pressure that must be generated during inspiration to overcome the effects of increased airway obstruction. In addition, the resistive work of breathing is greatly increased as indicated by the area *(vertical stripes)* enclosed by the normal inspiratory loop (normal airways) compared to the area *(stippled)* in the loop associated with increased airway resistance (obstructed airways). (Adapted from Lanken PN: Weaning from mechanical ventilation. In: Fishman AP [ed]: Pulmonary Diseases and Disorders: Update 1. New York, McGraw-Hill, p 366, 1982. Reproduced with permission of McGraw-Hill, Inc.)

lation and a rise in PacO₂. Patients with neuromuscular weakness may also have poor gag reflexes and lack effective coughs. As a consequence, they have significant areas of atelectasis and commonly suffer from aspiration pneumonias. Both may contribute to clinically significant hypoxemia.

This class of disorders also includes primary problems with the thoracic cage, or chest bellows, which expands the lungs. These include acute injury such as flail chest,[18] post-operative changes such as those after an extensive thoracoplasty, and chronic conditions such as severe kyphoscoliosis.[12, 19] Other mechanical limitations to lung expansion include massive abdominal obesity, large pleural effusions, or distended loops of bowel or ascites. Acute respiratory failure may occur after major thoracic trauma because of a flail chest. In such cases, the negative pleural pressure generated by the respiratory muscles leads to inward displacement of a large proportion of the thorax rather than lung expansion with an adequate tidal volume. If the chest wall injury is substantial in area, it also limits spontaneous sighs, as do narcotic analgesics. In these circumstances, the same mechanisms that limit ventilatory supply in neuromuscular weakness also occur, with the additional detrimental effects of associated atelectasis, possible lung contusion, and

limitation of chest wall motion because of pain. As noted for neuromuscular weakness, shallow tidal volumes increase VDS/VT and the elastic work of breathing (see Fig. 67–6A). The eventual result of the imbalance between ventilatory supply and demand is hypercapnic respiratory failure (see Table 67–3).

In chronic problems with the chest bellows, such as severe kyphoscoliosis, the elastic work of breathing, greatly increased because of the deformed chest wall, increases V̇O₂ (see Fig. 67–6A). Normally the work of breathing represents less than 5% of an individual's total O₂ consumption; however, its contribution may increase up to 25% or more when patients are breathing against high mechanical loads[20, 21] (see Fig. 67–6). When patients with severe kyphoscoliosis develop acute respiratory failure, the greatly increased work of breathing and restriction of lung volumes chronically limit ventilatory supply, which may be acutely compromised by development of a lower respiratory tract infection. Ventilatory demand is increased with an increase in VDS/VT because of shallow tidal volume breathing and an increase in V̇O₂ because of an elevated work of breathing.

Arterial blood gas changes in respiratory failure caused by neuromuscular weakness or severe alterations in function of the chest bellows generally resemble those resulting from impaired central neural drive. An acute or chronic respiratory acidosis is seen with a variable fall in the arterial pH depending on the degree of renal compensation, which starts to increase the serum bicarbonate concentration after 24 hours of hypercapnia (see Table 67–3). PaO₂ may be decreased because of alveolar hypoventilation (according to Equation 3), atelectasis, or aspiration pneumonia. Bedside pulmonary function tests as a rule reveal decreased vital capacity, MVV, and maximal inspiratory and expiratory static pressures.

Therapy for these disorders depends on the specific condition that results in respiratory failure. Otherwise, as a standard approach, tracheal intubation is indicated to protect the airway from aspiration and/or to provide positive pressure mechanical ventilation. If aspiration is not of significant concern, other forms of mechanical ventilation, such as positive pressure volume-cycled ventilation delivered via a continuous positive airway pressure mask[22] or nasal prongs that are specially fitted to the nares of the patient, have been found to be effective in some patients with neuromuscular weakness. Nocturnal mechanical ventilation is especially valuable in patients with diaphragmatic weakness that results in periods of severe hypoventilation and arterial oxygen desaturation during rapid eye movement sleep, because rapid eye movement sleep induces a state-related hypotonia in their accessory muscles of ventilation.

Airways Disease

Acute examples of impairment of the airways component leading to respiratory failure include acute upper airway obstruction as in acute epiglottitis, status asthmaticus,[2, 23] and acute decompensations of chronic obstructive pulmonary disease (COPD). Chronic forms of this disorder include COPD and advanced cystic fibrosis with chronic hypercapnia.

In these disorders, the mechanism of CO₂ retention is complex and commonly multifactorial. For example, in status asthmaticus, lung hyperinflation results in an array of conditions limiting ventilatory supply. Hyperinflation leads to an unfavorable length-tension relationship of the diaphragm. Tidal volumes decrease if the increased functional residual capacity rises into the flattened portion of the pressure-volume curve (see Fig. 67–3). Airway obstruction also severely reduces FEV₁, which causes a marked, direct decrease in MSV (Equation 6). Ventilatory demand increases as the $\dot{V}O_2$ rises in response to a greatly increased resistive work of breathing (see Fig. 67–6B), and VDS/VT may increase strikingly because of V-Q mismatching. Respiratory muscles eventually fatigue if the airway obstruction and high demand for ventilation persist, and this may lead to rapid development of respiratory failure. In patients who have an acute flare of COPD, the mechanism of respiratory failure is similar to that described earlier with the same factors limiting ventilatory supply and raising ventilatory demand.[24]

Bedside pulmonary function testing typically reveals a reduced forced vital capacity, reduced FEV_1, and severely diminished peak flow. Inspiratory maximal pressure may be in the normal range or reduced because of severe hyperinflation or development of respiratory muscle fatigue. In acute or chronic upper airway obstruction, these flow rates are likewise decreased and the flow-volume loop has characteristic plateaus according to the site of obstruction.

With regard to changes in arterial blood gases, patients with status asthmaticus typically go through three distinct phases of clinical importance. First, the patients early in their course with mild-to-moderate obstruction tend to have moderate hypocapnia with $PaCO_2$ of the order of 30 torr, reflecting predominantly nonchemical (i.e., vagal) stimuli from pulmonary receptors to the central respiratory center. In addition, there is mild hypoxemia with an increased PAO_2 − PaO_2 because of V-Q mismatching. Second, as the airway obstruction becomes more severe and the respiratory muscles begin to exhibit fatigue, the $PaCO_2$ appears normal at approximately 40 torr, which is known as the crossover point. This point is notable and ominous because it may represent a $PaCO_2$ rising from previous hypocapnic levels because of acute respiratory muscle fatigue and/or severe airway obstruction. At this point acute hypercapnic respiratory failure may be imminent. The clinical maxim for status asthmaticus is that a "normal" PCO_2 should be considered *not* normal and a possible indication for urgent or emergent intubation and mechanical ventilation. Third, with extreme airway obstruction, with or without respiratory muscle fatigue, patients can develop acute respiratory acidosis with extremely high levels of $PaCO_2$. Hypoxemia also occurs unless the patient is receiving supplemental O_2. Mild decrements in serum bicarbonate levels are commonly present because of renal compensation of the chronic respiratory alkalosis that occurred during the several days when the patient was hyperventilating at home in the early phase of acute asthma. These patterns of arterial blood gas changes are summarized in Table 67–3.

In acute flares of COPD in patients who are not chronic CO_2 retainers, pulmonary function test results and arterial blood gas changes are similar to those described for acute asthma. In contrast, in the COPD patient with chronic hypercapnia, the increased $PaCO_2$ is accompanied by renal compensation for the chronic respiratory acidosis; this results in smaller than normal decrements in arterial pH for a further acute rise in $PaCO_2$ as listed in Table 67–3. Although bedside pulmonary function test results for patients with exacerbations of COPD are similar to those for patients with acute asthma, the best way to assess pulmonary function is by frequent measurements of arterial blood gases. Because patients with acute asthma and flares in COPD frequently sit bolt-upright while in severe respiratory distress, it may be difficult to appreciate paradoxical respirations coinciding with the onset of inspiratory diaphragmatic fatigue.[25] Furthermore, this clinical sign is not specific for respiratory muscle fatigue but may occur in response to high resistive workloads,[26] which is the case in acute airways disease.

Careful monitoring of the patient's clinical condition and arterial blood gas levels is important in the rational management of these disorders. For example, in administering O_2 to patients with COPD it should be kept in mind that hypercapnia may worsen: approximately 30% of patients acutely ill with COPD flares have acute rises in $PaCO_2$ requiring intubation, approximately 60% have modest rises manageable without intubation, and about 10% do not have significant changes in $PaCO_2$.[27] Several mechanisms account for the observed rise of $PaCO_2$ after administration of supplemental O_2: (1) removal of the hypoxic stimulus for central neural drive in patients who presumably have lost the normal response to rises in $PaCO_2$; (2) the Haldane effect, in which CO_2 bound to hemoglobin is released into the plasma because of increased O_2 saturation; and (3) a contribution related to an increase in VDS/VT presumably mediated through release of hypoxic vasoconstriction at the microcirculatory level leading to an increased proportion of alveoli with $\dot{V}/\dot{Q}$ ratios greater than 1.0.[28]

As a rule, tracheal intubation and positive pressure mechanical ventilation are indicated in acute hypercapnic respiratory failure associated with asthma or in acute flares of COPD when the changes in $PaCO_2$, PaO_2 or pH become life threatening—for example, when the arterial pH is less than 7.25.

For patients with COPD with borderline respiratory failure who require only modest inspiratory peak pressures (e.g., less than 25 cm H_2O), supplemental positive pressure ventilation delivered via nasal continuous positive airway pressure mask may allow sufficient time for the airway obstruction to respond to other therapy and to avoid tracheal intubation.[29] This may be an especially attractive therapeutic alternative for patients with severe COPD who have been intubated in the past and may have been difficult to wean. Another modality that might help to avoid tracheal intubation is the application of a continuous positive airway pressure mask at pressure levels less than the patient's intrinsic or occult positive end-expiratory pressure (PEEP), that is, auto-PEEP.[30] This technique has been shown to decrease the work of breathing and respiratory distress during weaning of this type of patient and may serve as a useful preventive measure.[31, 32]

Alveolar Component

Common clinical examples are characterized by diffuse alveolar flooding of different types: adult respiratory distress syndrome, cardiogenic pulmonary edema, extensive pneumonias, diffuse pulmonary hemorrhage, and near-drowning. A massive acute pulmonary embolus with opening of a patent foramen ovale in response to acute pulmonary hypertension and ensuing right-sided heart failure is also in the differential diagnosis.

Flooding of alveoli leads to hypoxemic respiratory failure because it results in a large right-to-left shunt across the lungs caused by continued flow of mixed venous blood through the nonventilated alveoli, that is, those with a $\dot{V}/\dot{Q}$ ratio of zero. Also probably contributing to the profound hypoxemia observed in these types of clinical disorders are V-Q mismatching with perfusion of alveoli with very low $\dot{V}/\dot{Q}$ ratios, that is, extremely low levels of ventilation, and diffusion defects caused by thickening of the air-blood barrier in alveoli partially filled with fluid.

Hypoxemic respiratory failure has a number of important clinical features. First, because of the large right-to-left shunt, these patients show minimal, if any, improvement in PaO_2 with supplemental O_2. Second, hypoxemia with O_2 saturations of 88% or less may become rapidly life threatening with further falls in PaO_2 because this degree of O_2 saturation occurs on the steep, linear portion of the hemoglobin dissociation curve. Third, because O_2 concentrations of 60% or more are potentially toxic to the lungs, therapy with such high concentrations by itself is strong indication for intubation and mechanical ventilation with PEEP to try to maintain adequate arterial oxygenation at a lower FIO_2.

Ventilatory demand in these disorders is usually high because minute ventilation is increased by hypoxemia, high VDS/VT, increased work of breathing because of the stiff lungs, and resetting of the $PaCO_2$ threshold to maintain a lower than normal $PaCO_2$ mediated by stimulation of vagally mediated juxtacapillary receptors by interstitial edema. Conversely, ventilatory supply is decreased by loss of lung volume because of diffuse alveolar flooding, extremely low lung compliance, and degrees of respiratory muscle fatigue induced by high respiratory rates, high elastic loads, hypoxemia, and possibly a decreased blood supply to the diaphragm resulting from coexistent shock. As a consequence, patients with hypoxemic respiratory failure may develop concomitant hypercapnic respiratory failure.

Bedside measurement of pulmonary function, which may be difficult to perform because of severe respiratory distress, confirms a low vital capacity, high respiratory rate, and low MVV; maximal inspiratory pressures may be lowered, reflecting respiratory muscle fatigue or poor cooperation. Changes in arterial blood gases show severe hypoxemia and an elevated $PAO_2 - PaO_2$ even when the patient is breathing 100% O_2. The degree of hypoxemia is also reflected in low PaO_2/PAO_2 or PaO_2/FIO_2 ratios.[33] Alveolar hyperventilation is commonly seen early in this disorder; the patient may then progress to hypercapnic respiratory failure as described earlier (see Table 67–3).

Therapy for this type of disorder includes the following goals: restoration of safe levels of arterial oxygenation at nontoxic concentrations of supplemental O_2 and specific treatment of the etiologic agent and mechanism of injury, if possible. High right-to-left shunt fractions should be treated not with high, potentially toxic concentrations of O_2 but rather with interventions to decrease the elevated shunt fraction. These include lowering pulmonary capillary pressures through diuresis or other methods of intravascular volume contraction, for example, ultrafiltration in patients with renal failure, specific cardiac therapy in cases of congestive heart failure, and judicious application of PEEP via tracheal intubation and mechanical ventilation in cases of diffuse alveolar flooding. However, if hypoxemic respiratory failure occurs in the context of the syndrome of multiple organ system failure, more complex therapeutic tactics must be developed to accomplish these goals of therapy while minimizing their potentially adverse effects on nonpulmonary organ dysfunction.

Conclusion

Acute respiratory failure is a commonly occurring life-threatening condition whose causes are legion and whose pathophysiologic mechanisms are multifactorial. In hypercapnic respiratory failure, ventilatory demand outweighs ventilatory supply, eventually leading to respiratory muscle fatigue and rises in $PaCO_2$. In hypoxemic respiratory failure, the gas-exchanging properties of fluid-filled alveoli are severely impaired, resulting in severe hypoxemia predominantly caused by increases in the degree of right-to-left shunting of mixed venous blood through nonventilated but still perfused alveoli. For hypercapnic respiratory failure, improved understanding of the mechanisms limiting ventilatory capacity and factors leading to increased demand for ventilation can guide effective preventive and supportive therapy. Likewise, for hypoxemic respiratory failure, standard therapeutic approaches address the primary need to ensure safe levels of arterial oxygenation by treating the offending agent and mechanism of disease, if possible, and by decreasing the high shunt fraction while trying to minimize deleterious effects of this therapy on the lungs and other organs.

References

1. Lanken PN: Weaning from mechanical ventilation. In: Fishman AP (ed): Update: Pulmonary Diseases and Disorders. New York, McGraw-Hill, p 366, 1982.
2. Roussos C, Macklem PT: The respiratory muscles. N Engl J Med 307:786, 1982.
3. Roussos C, Macklem PT: Clinical implications of respiratory muscle fatigue. In: Fishman AP (ed): Pulmonary Diseases and Disorders. New York, McGraw-Hill, p 2275, 1988.
4. Lanken PN: Mechanical ventilation. In: Fishman AP (ed): Pulmonary Diseases and Disorders. New York, McGraw-Hill, p 2373, 1988.
5. Gray BA, Blalock JM: Interpretation of the alveolar-arterial oxygen difference in patients with hypercapnia. Am Rev Respir Dis 143:4, 1991.
6. Zoche GP, Fritts HW, Cournand A: Fraction of maximum breathing capacity available for prolonged hyperventilation. J Appl Physiol 14:1073, 1960.
7. NHLBI Workshop summary: Respiratory muscle fatigue. Report of the Respiratory Muscle Fatigue Workshop Group. Am Rev Respir Dis 142:474, 1990.
8. Leith DE, Bradley M: Ventilatory muscle strength and endurance training. J Appl Physiol 41:508, 1976.
9. Yang KL, Tobin MJ: A prospective study of indexes predicting the outcome of trials of weaning from mechanical ventilation. N Engl J Med 324:1145, 1991.
10. Selecky PA, Wasserman K, Klein M, et al: A graphic approach to assessing interrelationships among minute ventilation, arterial carbon dioxide tension and ratio of physiologic dead space to tidal volume in patients on respirators. Am Rev Respir Dis 117:181, 1978.
11. Gattinoni L, Pesenti A, Bombino M, et al: Relationships between lung computed tomographic density, gas exchange and PEEP in acute respiratory failure. Anesthesiology 69:812, 1988.
12. Grippi MA, Fishman AP: Respiratory failure in structural and neuromuscular disorders involving the chest bellows. In: Fishman AP (ed): Pulmonary Diseases and Disorders. 2nd ed. New York, McGraw-Hill, p 2299, 1988.
13. Kelly B, Luce J: The diagnosis and management of neuromuscular diseases causing respiratory failure. Chest 99:1485, 1991.
14. Aubier M, Murciano D, Lecocguic Y, et al: Effect of hypophosphatemia on diaphragmatic contractility in patients with acute respiratory failure. N Engl J Med 313:420, 1985.
15. Edwards RHT, Hill DK, Jones DA, et al: Fatigue of long duration in human skeletal muscle after exercise. J Physiol (Lond) 272:7690, 1977.
16. Bendixen HH, Smith GM, Mead J: Pattern of ventilation in young adults. J Appl Physiol 19:195, 1964.
17. Bendixen HH, Hedley-Whyte J, Chir B, et al: Impaired oxygenation in surgical patients during general anesthesia with controlled ventilation. A concept of atelectasis. N Engl J Med 269:991, 1963.
18. Cullen P, Modell JH, Kirby RR, et al: Treatment of flail chest. Use of intermittent mandatory ventilation and positive end-expiratory pressure. Arch Surg 110:1099, 1975.
19. Bergofsky EH, Turino GM, Fishman AP: Cardio-respiratory failure in kyphoscoliosis. Medicine 38:263, 1959.
20. Otis AB: The work of breathing. In: Fenn WO, Rahn H (eds): Handbook of Physiology, Section 3, Respiration. Washington, DC, American Physiological Society, p 463, 1964.
21. Cournand A, Richards DW Jr, Bader RA, et al: The oxygen cost of breathing. Trans Assoc Am Physicians 67:162, 1954.
22. Ellis ER, Bye PTP, Bruderer JW, et al: Treatment of respiratory failure during sleep in patients with neuromuscular disease: Positive-pressure ventilation through a nose mask. Am Rev Respir Dis 135:148, 1987.
23. Weiner P, Suo J, Fernandez E, et al: The effect of hyperinflation on respiratory muscle strength and the efficiency in healthy subjects and patients with asthma. Am Rev Respir Dis 141:1501, 1990.
24. Derenne J, Fleury B, Pariente R: Acute respiratory failure of chronic obstructive pulmonary disease. Am Rev Respir Dis 138:1006, 1988.
25. Cohen CA, Zagelbaum G, Gross D, et al: Clinical manifestations of inspiratory muscle fatigue. Am J Med 73:308, 1982.
26. Tobin MJ, Perez W, Guenther SM, et al: Does rib cage–abdominal paradox signify respiratory muscle fatigue? J Appl Physiol 63:851, 1987.
27. Campbell EJM: The J. Burns Amberson lecture. The management of acute respiratory failure in chronic bronchitis and emphysema. Am Rev Respir Dis 96:626, 1967.
28. Aubier M, Murciano D, Milic-Emili J, et al: Effects of the administration of O_2 on ventilation and blood gases in patients with chronic obstructive pulmonary disease during acute respiratory failure. Am Rev Respir Dis 122:747, 1980.
29. Marion W: Intermittent volume cycled mechanical ventilation via nasal

mask in patients with respiratory failure due to COPD. Chest 99:681, 1991.

30. Pepe PE, Marini JJ: Occult positive end-expiratory pressure in mechanically ventilated patients with airflow obstruction. The auto-PEEP effect. Am Rev Respir Dis 126:166, 1982.
31. Petrof B, Legaré M, Goldberg P, et al: Continuous positive airway pressure reduces work of breathing and dyspnea during weaning from mechanical ventilation in severe chronic obstructive pulmonary disease. Am Rev Respir Dis 141:281, 1990.
32. Brochard L, Isabey D, Piquet J, et al: Reversal of acute exacerbations of chronic obstructive lung disease by inspiratory assistance with face mask. N Engl J Med 323:1523, 1990.
33. Gilbert R, Keighley JF: The arterial/alveolar oxygen tension ratio. An index of gas exchange applicable to varying inspired oxygen concentrations. Am Rev Respir Dis 109:142, 1974.
34. Roussos C: Respiratory muscle fatigue and ventilatory failure. Chest 97 (suppl):89S, 1991.
35. Donahoe M, Rogers RM, Wilson DO, et al: Oxygen consumption of the respiratory muscles in normal and in malnourished patients with chronic obstructive pulmonary disease. Am Rev Respir Dis 140:385, 1989.
36. Weinberger SE, Schwartzstein RM, Weiss JW: Hypercapnia. N Engl J Med 321:1223, 1989.
37. Hussain S, Simkus G, Roussos C: Respiratory muscle fatigue: A cause of ventilatory failure in septic shock. J Appl Physiol 48:2033, 1985.
38. Lane DJ, Howell JBL, Giblin B: Relation between airway obstruction and CO_2 tension in chronic obstructive airway disease. Br Med J 3:707, 1968.
39. Rebuck AS, Read J: Assessment and management of severe asthma. Am J Med 51:788, 1971.
40. Covelli HD, Black JW, Olsen MS, et al.: Respiratory failure precipitated by high carbohydrate loads. Ann Intern Med 95:579, 1981.

CHAPTER 68

Mechanical Respiratory Failure

Lewis R. Kline
Victor A. Ferrari

DEFINITION OF MECHANICAL RESPIRATORY FAILURE

Acute respiratory failure can be classified into two broad categories on the basis of whether there is hypoxemic lung failure or primary compromise of the respiratory "pump," that is, hypercapnic respiratory failure. The former type of respiratory failure indicates disruption of the lung parenchyma, whereas the latter signifies a failure of gas exchange because of severe hypoventilation. Although the two types often coexist in a patient, it remains useful to conceptualize the pathophysiology of respiratory failure in this fashion. This chapter focuses on mechanical respiratory failure and highlights the functional organization of the neuromuscular and skeletal systems of the respiratory pump. Specific diseases are reviewed that can cause either acute respiratory failure or an acute decompensation superimposed on chronic respiratory insufficiency. Two general disease processes can lead to mechanical respiratory failure: disorders that affect the neuromuscular system and structural disorders of the thorax and upper airway (Table 68–1). The resulting sequelae of ventilatory pump failure are discussed, and general and specific treatment measures are reviewed including newer treatment measures that have an impact on

the outcome of these patients as they improve and leave the intensive care unit.

FUNCTIONAL ANATOMY OF THE RESPIRATORY SYSTEM

Functionally, the chest wall consists of two compartments, the rib cage and the abdomen, separated by the diaphragm. The rib cage is a complex structure made up of the sternum, thoracic vertebrae, ribs, and costal cartilages. Because of their articulations, the ribs can move in three planes: lateral, cephalocaudal, and ventral.[1, 2] The muscles that move the ribs in a cephalad, lateral, and dorsoventral direction promote inspiration; those that decrease chest wall volume are expiratory (Fig. 68–1). Although the motion of the ribs is usually along one axis during normal breathing, during disease states certain deformities of the rib cage can occur that have profound effects on the efficiency of the chest wall pump (see later).

In contrast to the relative rigidity of the rib cage, the abdominal compartment is essentially a flexible fluid-filled container. When the abdominal contents are compressed, equal displacement in the opposite direction must occur. Posterior displacement of these contents is, however, limited because of the dorsal sections of the ribs and the spine and pelvic bones. Accordingly, downward movement of the diaphragm during inspiration initiates an outward ventral displacement of the abdominal wall. During active expiration, the contraction of the abdominal muscles results in inward movement of the liquid contents and upward passive movement of the diaphragm into the chest.

The diaphragm, a dome-shaped structure, is the major muscle of inspiration and assumes an even larger role in the supine position than in the upright position.[3] Two compo-

TABLE 68–1

STRUCTURAL AND NEUROMUSCULAR DISORDERS OF THE CHEST BELLOWS LEADING TO ACUTE AND/OR CHRONIC RESPIRATORY FAILURE

Structural abnormalities
 Kyphoscoliosis*
 Obesity*
 Ankylosing spondylitis*
 Fibrothorax*
 Thoracoplasty*
 Flail chest†
Neuromuscular disorders
 Disorders of the spinal cord and anterior horn cells
  Spinal cord injury or destruction*†
  Amyotrophic lateral sclerosis*
  Poliomyelitis*†
  Encephalomyelitis (e.g., with carcinoma)*
  Multiple sclerosis (rare cause)*
 Disorders of peripheral nerves
  Guillain-Barré syndrome*†
  Isolated disease of the phrenic nerves*†
 Disorders of the neuromuscular junction
  Myasthenia gravis*
  Eaton-Lambert syndrome*
 Myopathic disorders
  Muscular dystrophies*
  Polymyositis*†
  Periodic paralysis†

*Leads to chronic respiratory failure and superimposed acute exacerbations.
†Leads to acute respiratory failure.
From Grippi MA, Fishman AP: Respiratory failure in structural and neuromuscular disorders involving the chest bellows. In: Fishman AP (ed): Pulmonary Diseases and Disorders. 2nd ed. New York, McGraw-Hill, p 2300, 1988. Reproduced with permission of McGraw-Hill, Inc.

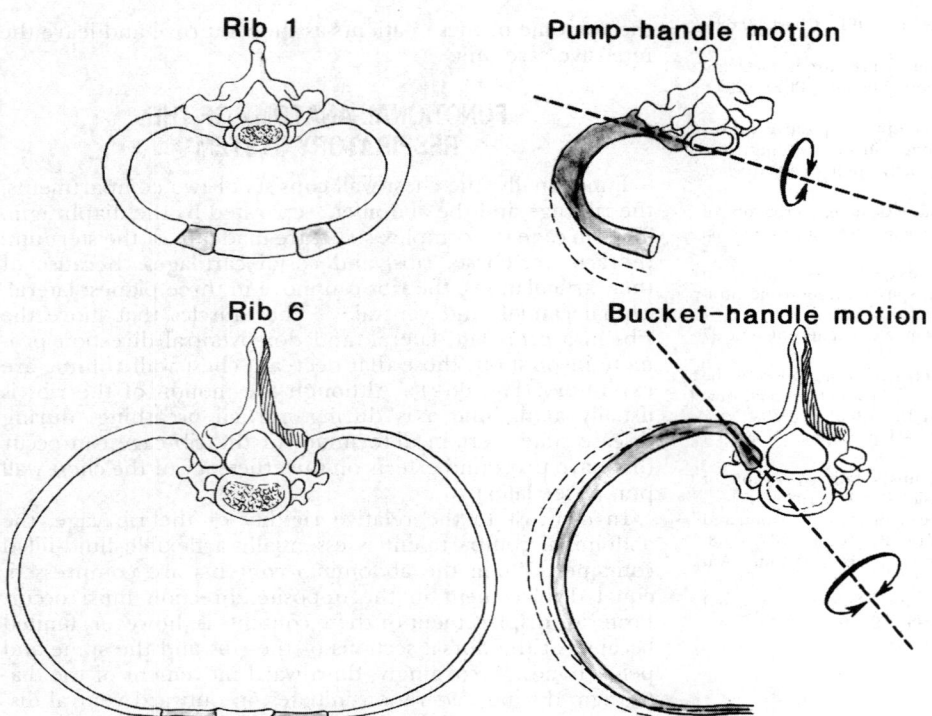

Figure 68–1. Functional anatomy of the human rib cage. In the upper ribs *(top)*, rotation of the rib-neck axis *(broken line)* in an inspiratory direction increases the anteroposterior diameter of the rib cage (pump handle motion), whereas in the lower ribs *(bottom)*, rotation of the rib-neck axis causes an increase in the lateral diameter of the rib cage (bucket handle motion). (From De Troyer A, Estenne M: Functional anatomy of the respiratory muscles. Clin Chest Med 9:175, 1988.)

nents, the costal portion and the crural portion, make up this muscle as it radiates from a central tendon to the peripheral bony structures. There is increasing evidence that each portion has a different function in view of their distinct zones of insertion and levels of innervation. Whereas the crural portion, innervated by the intermediate and lower cervical roots, may play a role as part of the esophageal sphincter, the costal portion, innervated by the upper cervical roots, is principally involved in inspiration.[4, 5] The diaphragm is a cylinder-shaped muscle capped by a tendinous dome; the cylindric portion inserts on the inner aspect of the rib cage (Fig. 68–2) to form what is known as the zone of apposition.[6] As the diaphragm contracts, the apposed muscle fibers shorten, which causes the dome to move caudally, resulting in a significant piston-like movement.[7] In effect, as the diaphragm contracts and moves caudally, the volume displacement creates a negative intrathoracic pressure while forcing the abdominal liquid contents to move outward. (For a more detailed explanation of the complex relationships of the diaphragm, chest wall, and abdomen, see ref 1.) Thus, as the diaphragm descends during inspiration, there is synchronous outward movement of both the chest wall and the abdomen; bedside observation of chest wall and abdominal motions can provide valuable clues about normal diaphragmatic function, as outlined later.

In addition to the diaphragm, the parasternal muscles are always active in inspiration and cause both an elevation of the ribs and a descent of the sternum.[8] Controversy still exists about the relative roles of the internal and external intercostal muscles and whether they are important in respiration.[1] Like the parasternal muscles, the scalene muscles are active during quiet inspiration. Contrary to popular belief, they are more than accessory muscles of respiration and act to lift the rib cage during inspiration. Many other muscles may contribute to inspiration when the respiratory system is stressed. Most important among these are the sternocleidomastoid muscles that both elevate the upper rib cage and cause cranial displacement of the sternum. The muscles of the abdomen (rectus muscle of the abdomen,

external and internal obliques, transverse muscle of the abdomen) serve primarily an expiratory function when the respiratory system is stressed. As these muscles contract during expiration, they drive the diaphragm upward into the chest. When the abdominal muscles relax at end expiration, they can contribute to the ensuing inspiratory effort by allowing passive descent of the diaphragm before the

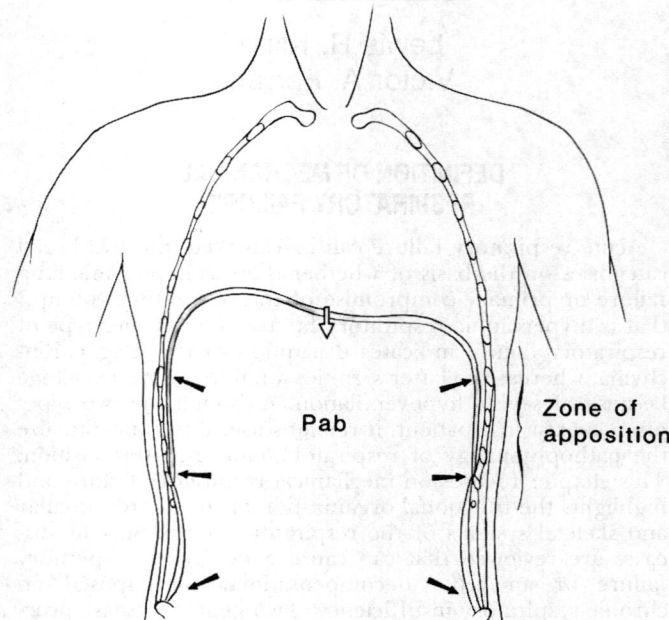

Figure 68–2. Appositional opponent of diaphragmatic action. Descent of the diaphragmatic dome during inspiration *(open arrow)* causes an increase in abdominal pressure (Pab) that is transmitted through the apposed diaphragm to expand the lower rib cage *(black arrows)*. (From De Troyer A, Estenne M: Functional anatomy of the respiratory muscles. Clin Chest Med 9:175, 1988.)

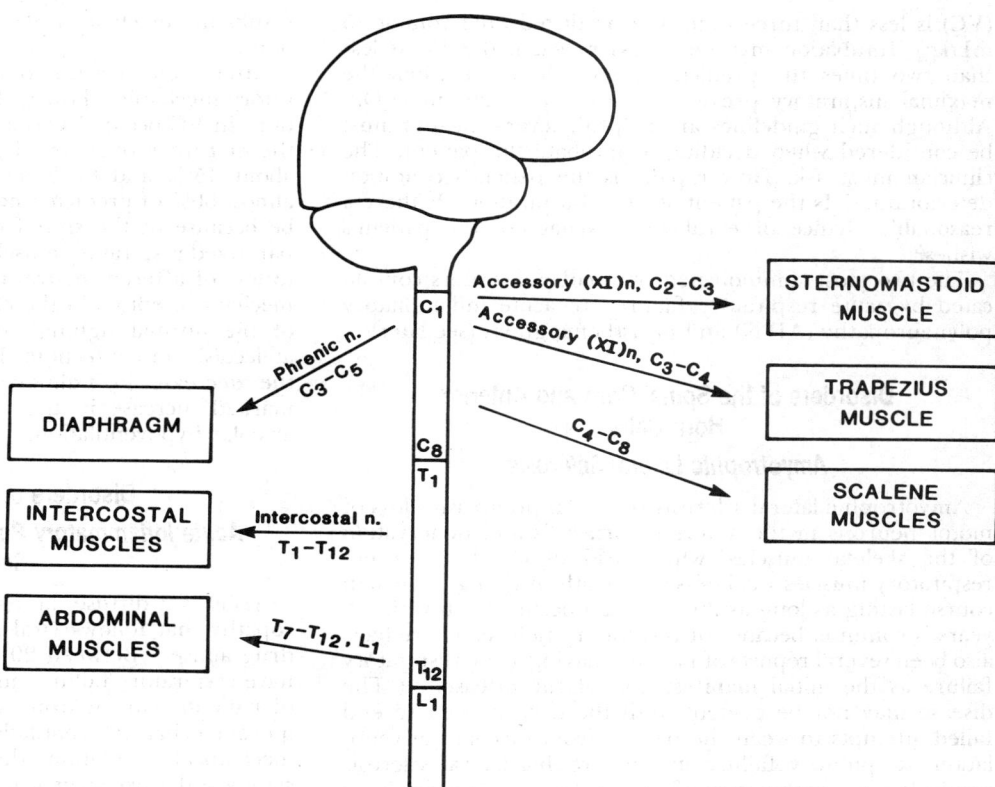

Figure 68–3. The motor innervation of the major respiratory muscle groups. (From Tobin MJ: Respiratory muscles in disease. Clin Chest Med 9:263, 1988.)

onset of the active inspiratory contraction. When mechanical respiratory failure is due to neuromuscular disease, the innervation of the muscles just described becomes an important consideration. Innervation of these muscles that contribute to the respiratory pump extends from the upper cervical cord to the thoracic-lumbar junction (Fig. 68–3).

RESPIRATORY FAILURE RESULTING FROM NEUROMUSCULAR DISEASE

To gain an appreciation of the pathogenesis of various neuromuscular disorders, it is useful to review the functional neuroanatomy of respiration (see Fig. 68–3). The respiratory pattern generator, an ill-defined cellular network with inherent automaticity, is located in the medulla situated near the floor of the fourth ventricle. These cells provide excitatory inputs to both inspiratory and expiratory muscles through projections to anterior horn cells in the contralateral spinal cord. In addition to this automatic system, a voluntary system projects to anterior horn cells from higher centers in the cortex. Diseases such as amyotrophic lateral sclerosis and poliomyelitis destroy anterior horn cells and produce respiratory muscle weakness. Inhibitory modulation in the spinal cord arises in part from glycinergic interneurons, and loss of this inhibition, as can occur in tetanus, creates uncontrollable respiratory muscle spasm leading to respiratory failure. In turn, when an action potential is conducted down the axon, acetylcholine (ACh) is presynaptically released across the synaptic junction. A whole host of diseases can disrupt this axonal transmission by interfering with sodium channels (various toxins) or by causing demyelination (e.g., Guillain-Barré syndrome, diphtheria). When postsynaptic receptors at the neuromuscular junction are stimulated by ACh, contraction of the respiratory muscles ensues. If the release of ACh is hindered by entities such as Eaton-Lambert syn-

drome, botulism, or snake venom, or if ACh receptors are lost as in myasthenia gravis, mechanical failure can occur. Finally, respiratory muscles must be functional to promote ventilation to meet metabolic demands. Inflammatory diseases, such as polymyositis, and metabolic disorders, such as acid maltase deficiency, can impair the normal contraction of respiratory muscles. In short, any disruption of the neuromuscular axis can ultimately produce respiratory pump failure (see Table 68–1).

Clinical Features

Unless a patient with neuromuscular disease manifests acute respiratory failure caused by cor pulmonale or aspiration pneumonia, the underlying disorder may go undetected. This may be because general muscle weakness prevents patients from stressing their limited ventilatory capacity.[9] These patients typically have reduced lung volumes (i.e., restrictive lung disease) related to respiratory muscle weakness,[10] and decreased lung compliance,[11] presumably related to the presence of diffuse microatelectasis. Chest wall compliance is also diminished because of stiffening of the rib cage[12] and possibly because of muscle spasticity.[13] Patients with neuromuscular disease assume a rapid shallow breathing pattern.[14] The reduced lung volumes ultimately lead to decreased oxygen stores, hypoventilation, and oxyhemoglobin desaturation. Nocturnal symptoms are often the earliest manifestation,[15] but as the underlying neuromuscular disease progresses, bulbar weakness may begin to coexist, resulting in hoarseness, dysphagia, apneas, and inability to clear secretions. Although the alveolar-arterial oxygen gradient is usually well maintained,[14] P_{CO_2} levels begin to rise as respiratory muscle strength falls to 30% of the predicted normal value.[16] The ability to cough and clear secretions may be reduced when the vital capacity

(VC) is less than three times the predicted tidal volume (5 mL/kg). Intubation may be necessary when the VC is less than two times the predicted tidal volume or when the maximal inspiratory pressure is less than -20 cm H_2O.[17] Although such guidelines are helpful, several factors must be considered when deciding to intubate the patient. The clinician must ask: How rapidly is the patient's condition deteriorating? Is the patient at risk of aspiration? Is there a reasonable chance of extubation? What are the patient's wishes?

The two most common neuromuscular disorders complicated by acute respiratory failure are acute inflammatory polyneuropathy (AIPN) and myasthenia gravis (see later).

Disorders of the Spinal Cord and Anterior Horn Cells

Amyotrophic Lateral Sclerosis

Amyotrophic lateral sclerosis results in progressive loss of motor neurons in the anterior horn cells and denervation of the skeletal muscles, which lead ultimately to severe respiratory muscles weakness and death. Although a benign course lasting as long as 20 years can occur, death within 3 years is common because of respiratory failure. There have also been several reports of patients' having acute respiratory failure as the initial manifestation of the disease.[18-22] The disease may not be evident until there have been several failed attempts to wean the patient from mechanical ventilation. Respiratory failure in amyotrophic lateral sclerosis results from a combination of factors. Because anterior horn cell loss is most marked in the cervical, lumbosacral, and lower thoracic spine, the function of the inspiratory and expiratory muscles is compromised. Weakness of the diaphragm and external intercostal muscles leads to reduced inspiratory pressures and lung volumes. In addition, abdominal muscle weakness results in an ineffective cough and the retention of secretions. Dysfunction of the pharyngeal and laryngeal muscles predisposes the patient to bulbar symptoms and aspiration pneumonia. A number of studies have shown that there is a reduced survival rate when the bulbar area of the central nervous system is affected first.[22]

In view of the relentless progressive deterioration of these patients, the management of respiratory failure presents not only complicated medical problems, but social and ethical issues as well. The decision to intubate a patient with amyotrophic lateral sclerosis will likely create a situation in which the patient will depend permanently on a ventilator. However, with newer ventilation techniques for use in the home, this decision does not always indicate a hopeless condition (see later). Frank discussions with the patient and family about the impending respiratory problems and available options should occur as soon as the diagnosis is clear.

Injury of the Spinal Cord

The anatomic location of the acute injury determines the extent of the respiratory manifestations. High cervical cord lesions (C1-2) cause paralysis of the diaphragm and the intercostal, scalene, and abdominal muscles.[13, 23] Because the phrenic nerves remain intact, phrenic pacing of the diaphragm is an option.[13, 23, 24] Middle cervical cord lesions (C3-5) destroy the phrenic motorneurons. This type of diaphragmatic paralysis cannot be ameliorated with phrenic pacing. When injuries of the lower cervical and thoracic cord occur, the diaphragm and neck muscles remain functional. As a result, these injuries do not usually result in prolonged mechanical ventilation.[25] Lower cervical and high thoracic cord injuries cause paralysis of the expiratory muscles, which

results in defective cough and clearance of bronchial secretions.

After acute cervical cord injury, measurements of respiratory mechanics show a change over time. Marked reductions in VC occur; VC is about 30% of predicted normal in the first week of injury. By the fifth week, VC increases to about 45%, and by 5 months after injury, it doubles to almost 60% of predicted normal.[26] Much of this change may be because of the shift from flaccidity to spasticity of the paralyzed respiratory muscles. In addition, acute injury leads to loss of afferent neural information from the respiratory mechanoreceptors in the chest wall. This may result in loss of the normal sighing mechanism, with development of atelectasis and infection. The loss of muscle strength and the decrease in pulmonary compliance contribute to a marked increase in the work of breathing with ensuing alveolar hypoventilation.

Disorders of Peripheral Nerves

Acute Inflammatory Polyneuropathy (Guillain-Barré Syndrome)

AIPN is a diffuse, autoimmune, demyelinating polyneuropathy that follows viral illness, surgery, and intravenous drug abuse.[27] Between 20 and 50% of patients with AIPN have respiratory failure, and AIPN accounts for about 50% of patients with neuromuscular disease who ultimately require mechanical ventilation.[17, 27] Because of advances in mechanical ventilation, the prognosis of AIPN has risen significantly; excellent functional recovery can be expected in 85% of cases.[28] Mortality for this disease is less than 5%.

The clinical features of the polyneuritis are similar to those of acute and chronic poliomyelitis. A monophasic course is followed by 95% of patients, with 90% reaching a nadir of muscle weakness by 15 days and a plateau in progression by 4 weeks.[28] In addition to motor weakness, the disease is often accompanied by paresthesias, cranial neuropathies, and general autonomic disturbances. The more rapid the onset of the syndrome, the more likely that the patient will manifest respiratory failure.[17, 29-34] Criteria for intubation have varied among centers, but a reduced VC of 12 to 15 mL/kg coupled with a rapid fall of VC during 4 to 6 hours has been a reliable indicator for intervention.[31] Overall, the duration of ventilatory support required for patients with AIPN is quite variable, ranging from a few weeks to 2 months or more. Pulmonary embolism is a major complication of immobilization in up to one third of AIPN patients.[35]

In addition to the general treatment measures described later for mechanical respiratory failure, plasma exchange has been reported to be beneficial if begun by the seventh day of illness, or in severe patients who require artificial ventilation.[36, 37] There is no proven role for corticosteroids, and such therapy may be harmful in these patients.[38]

Disorders of the Neuromuscular Junction

Myasthenia Gravis

Myasthenia gravis is an autoimmune disease in which the motor end plate has a decrease in ACh receptor sites. Antibodies to the ACh receptor are present, and clinical severity of the disease seems to parallel the extent of ACh receptor loss, but not the titer of ACh antibodies.[39] Patients have a high incidence of thymomas and other autoimmune diseases. Myasthenia gravis accounts for 30% of cases of neuromuscular respiratory failure;[17] approximately 20% of all patients with myasthenia gravis have episodes of acute respiratory failure. Precipitating factors include myasthenic crisis, cholinergic crisis, steroid-induced muscle weakness, and infection. Because of the numerous therapies that exist for this disease, it is essential that the diagnosis be established as soon as possible.

The decision to intubate the patient with myasthenic crisis, as in all cases of neuromuscular failure, must be tailored to the individual. Of the various physiologic parameters, the VC is the most utilized. The decrease in VC is due largely to a decrease in the maximal expiratory pressure secondary to weakness of the expiratory muscles. (The maximal expiratory pressure is actually the most abnormal measure in myasthenia gravis.) A VC of less than 15 mL/kg or less than 1 L indicates the need for intubation.[40, 41] The patient's condition can deteriorate rapidly, necessitating frequent monitoring of respiration. After mechanical ventilation is instituted, the average time to extubation is 14 days.[27]

Anticholinesterases are the mainstay of treatment in myasthenia gravis. These agents enhance transmission at the neuromuscular junction and thereby augment respiratory muscle strength. Unfortunately, these agents also increase bronchial secretions and the work of breathing, and their use is therefore usually reduced or stopped during myasthenic crisis. Hence, high doses of steroids are used in conjunction with plasmapheresis.[42, 43] Plasmapheresis usually promotes improvement by the third plasma exchange; the effects of steroids are not evident for several weeks. With these current approaches, mortality has been reduced from more than 40% to less than 10%

Diseases of the Respiratory Muscles
Diaphragmatic Paralysis

Diaphragmatic paralysis often goes unrecognized until a patient is unable to be weaned from the ventilator. The frequency of occurrence of this disorder has grown at many centers with the increase in cardiac and other thoracic surgeries. In general, patients with unilateral diaphragmatic paralysis have only minor respiratory impairment unless there is coexistent pulmonary disease; those with bilateral paralysis are highly symptomatic. A myriad of causes of bilateral diaphragmatic paralysis have been identified, including spinal cord injury (see earlier), infections, polyneuropathies, motor neuron disease, myopathies, systemic lupus erythematosus, paraneoplastic syndromes, idiopathic disorders, and accidental or surgical trauma.[45] Because the disorder is unrecognized or diagnosis is delayed, these patients can present with chronic hypoventilation, nocturnal oxygen desaturations, cor pulmonale, or acute respiratory failure. During rapid eye movement sleep when skeletal muscles are naturally atonic, profound hypoventilation may occur in these patients as a result of inhibition of the intercostal and accessory muscles.[46]

Patients have a restrictive defect seen during pulmonary function testing secondary to the muscle weakness. Because gravitational effects displace the diaphragm cephalad, there is a 40% or greater reduction in VC in the supine position compared with measurement in the erect position.[13] Classically, paradoxical abdominal motion is observed on inspiration when the patient is supine. Fluoroscopy is the method most commonly used to establish the diagnosis; the patient is asked to sniff, which results in paradoxical motion (upward) of the diaphragm. However, this technique can be misleading for two reasons. First, 6% of healthy subjects will exhibit paradoxical motion during the sniff test.[47] Second, some patients with this disorder do not have paradoxical motion because they learn to contract their abdominal muscles at end expiration, which forces the diaphragm upward. At the onset of inspiration, relaxation of the abdominal

muscles causes diaphragmatic descent.[13] More sophisticated evidence of impairment of the phrenic-diaphragmatic axis requires phrenic nerve stimulation, recording of the diaphragmatic electromyogram, and transdiaphragmatic pressure measurements. Although these techniques are useful, they can be difficult to perform, especially in the mechanically ventilated patient.

As just noted, when bilateral diaphragmatic paralysis is present, it may be extremely difficult to wean patients from mechanical ventilation. After other contributing conditions such as pneumonia have been adequately treated, the patients should be placed in the erect position. Often, a tracheostomy is necessary because of the prolonged illness of these patients. The goal should be to achieve daytime freedom from the ventilator, with the tracheostomy plugged. A form of nocturnal ventilatory support should be chosen either through the tracheostomy or via nasal positive pressure ventilation (see later) to avoid the adverse consequences of chronic hypoventilation and respiratory muscle fatigue. With proper management, good-quality life can be achieved and the prognosis can be excellent. One study reported a minimal need for rehospitalization because of acute respiratory decompensation and cited a median length of survival of 7 years.[13]

Respiratory Muscle Fatigue

Much has been written about the role of respiratory muscle fatigue in mechanical respiratory failure. By definition, respiratory muscle fatigue is a reversible state caused by extreme effort that exceeds the strength and endurance of the respiratory muscles. Three general types of fatigue have been described: central fatigue, transmission fatigue, and contractile fatigue.[48] All are likely to be important in clinical fatigue. Briefly, central fatigue results from a decrement in central neural drive to the respiratory muscles as they become overused. Reversible transmission fatigue results when neural or neuromuscular conduction decreases during high respiratory muscle demand. Contractile fatigue is a reversible process whereby the muscular force developed in response to neural drive begins to fall. This occurs when the length-tension or force-velocity relationship of the muscle has not been altered, and no drug effect is present.[48]

As patients attempt to shift from mechanical ventilation to spontaneous breathing, it is clear that there are high demands on the respiratory muscles relative to their ability to endure a large workload. Nevertheless, few studies unequivocally establish respiratory muscle fatigue during weaning attempts. However, most investigators believe that respiratory muscle fatigue plays an important role in patients who are being weaned from mechanical ventilation.

STRUCTURAL ABNORMALITIES LEADING TO RESPIRATORY FAILURE
Chest Wall Disorders

Like neuromuscular disease, chest wall disorders typically result in a restrictive pattern of pulmonary physiology, with reductions in both total lung capacity and VC. The respiratory pattern is generally one of shallow and more rapid respirations, and decreased ventilation leads to ventilation-perfusion mismatching. In diseases of the chest wall, loss of ventilatory capacity often first manifests as dyspnea on exertion and decreased exercise tolerance. When severe disease is present, the work of breathing may exceed the ventilatory capacity, and hypercapnic respiratory failure results.

TABLE 68–2

CAUSES OF KYPHOSCOLIOSIS

Idiopathic causes
Neuromuscular diseases
  Muscular dystrophy
  Poliomyelitis
  Cerebral palsy
  Friedreich's ataxia
Bone disorders
  Osteoporosis
  Osteomalacia
  Vitamin D–resistant rickets
  Tuberculous spondylitis
  Neurofibromatosis
Connective tissue diseases
  Marfan's syndrome
  Ehlers-Danlos syndrome
  Morquio's syndrome
Thoracic cage structural disorders
  Thoracoplasty
  Empyema
  Trauma

Kyphoscoliosis

Kyphoscoliosis is the most studied chest wall disorder causing respiratory failure. The term refers to an abnormal curvature of the spine in a posterior (kyphosis) or lateral (scoliosis) direction, or combination of the two (kyphoscoliosis). The causes include diseases of the vertebrae, connective tissue, or neuromuscular system of the vertebral column (Table 68–2), and 80% of cases are idiopathic in origin,[49] with an as yet undefined inheritance pattern,[50] and a female sex predominance of 4 to 1. Kyphoscoliosis causes less than 1% of adult chronic respiratory failure and must be severe to do so, assuming the absence of other pulmonary disease.

The physiologic abnormalities and clinical manifestations depend largely on the angle of deformity. In general, the greater the degree of curvature, the more likely the patient will experience respiratory failure. Bergofsky and colleagues demonstrated that the patients with the most severe degree of spinal abnormality had the most advanced respiratory failure.[51] They also demonstrated that the types of spinal curvature are additive in their contribution to respiratory failure: the combination of moderate scoliosis and moderate kyphosis is equivalent to the presence of a severe degree of either. For ventilatory failure to develop with severe scoliosis alone, it is thought that the curvature must exceed 100° (see later description), and until this point is reached, no significant reduction in pulmonary function occurs.[52]

In terms of the physical abnormalities produced by the disease process, the initial lateral displacement of the spine, or primary curve, results in two additional vertebral changes: (1) a secondary curve develops (presumably to counterbalance the primary curve); and (2) the vertebral column rotates on its longitudinal axis such that the ribs on the convex side of the deformity are splayed and displaced posteriorly, forming a gibbus (hump) and compressing the ribs on the concave side.[53] The degree or angle of deformity is known as the Cobb angle and is determined using intersecting lines drawn through the upper and lower limbs of the primary curve (Fig. 68–4). Severe scoliosis is a rare finding, and the incidence in the general population of an angle greater than 70° is 1 in 10,000.[54]

Clinically, most patients younger than 35 years of age, even with a severe deformity, are asymptomatic. As they age, however, changes such as degenerative joint disease and ossification of points of rotation decrease the compliance of the rib cage and lead to symptoms such as dyspnea, decreased exercise capacity, respiratory infections, and acute respiratory failure. Angles of curvature greater than 120° are often associated with overt signs of respiratory failure, including alveolar hypoventilation, pulmonary hypertension, and cor pulmonale. As a general rule, until kyphoscoliosis becomes severe, it has little effect on respiratory function. However, in the setting of concomitant lung disease (e.g., emphysema, acute bronchitis, and pneumonia), even patients with moderate deformities may become symptomatic. No significant abnormality on physical examination or chest x-ray film identifies patients with early respiratory failure until cor pulmonale is detected.

Pathophysiology. One of the key mechanisms of respiratory failure is a decrease in both the static and the dynamic compliances of the chest wall and lungs, with the rib cage having the predominant effect, especially with aging. Compliance in patients with severe disease may be as low as 25% of normal values and correlates well with the angle of deformity.[55] These changes increase the work of breathing as a direct result of the increase in elastic resistance of the chest wall. Thus, a patient with severe kyphoscoliosis could perform four to five times the normal work of breathing at normal tidal volumes and respiratory rates. To minimize this work, patients breathe at smaller tidal volumes and at higher respiratory rates, thus increasing dead space ventilation and causing inefficient carbon dioxide elimination. These changes in mechanics lead to a restrictive pulmonary function pattern; total lung capacity and VC are decreased in patients with scoliosis greater than 90°,[56, 57] and these volumes decrease in proportion to the angle of curvature.[56, 58] There is a severe decrease in the diffusing capacity of the lungs for carbon monoxide in all adults.[52, 56, 57, 59, 60]

Patients with chronic ventilatory failure demonstrate hypercapnia, hypoxemia, and a widened alveolar-arterial gradient.[51, 55] The degree of hypercapnia and hypoxemia seems to correlate more with the patients' age and inspiratory muscle strength than with the severity of spinal abnormality.[61] In certain studies,[61, 62] maximal inspiratory and expiratory pressure were found to be decreased. Although the decrease in maximal expiratory pressure may be due in part to a reduction in total lung capacity, it is likely also due to the distortion of the chest wall. It has been proposed that although respiratory muscle weakness may contribute to respiratory failure, the presence of respiratory failure itself may lead to progressive muscle weakness. In one study,[61] all patients with kyphoscoliosis had low maximal inspiratory pressure, but the patients with respiratory failure had the lowest values. In addition, there was better correlation between maximal inspiratory pressure and both PCO_2 and PO_2 than with the degree of curvature of the spine. The chest cage abnormality also leads to a smaller total pulmonary vascular bed.[62] The lungs of patients with respiratory failure are between 30 and 65% of normal size at post mortem. As many as one third of patients have additional lung disease such as bronchiectasis and emphysema, but the remaining two thirds show only atelectasis.

Reflex respiratory responses to increased inspired carbon dioxide are preserved in patients with kyphoscoliosis. However, with the development of alveolar hypoventilation and hypercapnia, the ventilatory response becomes blunted. The probable mechanisms for this dampened response include the limitation in performance of the chest bellows because of increased work of breathing, and the chronic adaptation of the central chemoreceptors to increased bicarbonate concentration in the cerebrospinal fluid. There have also been reports of abnormalities in central respiratory control caused by sleep apnea and other sleep disorders in these patients, and further investigations are ongoing.[63]

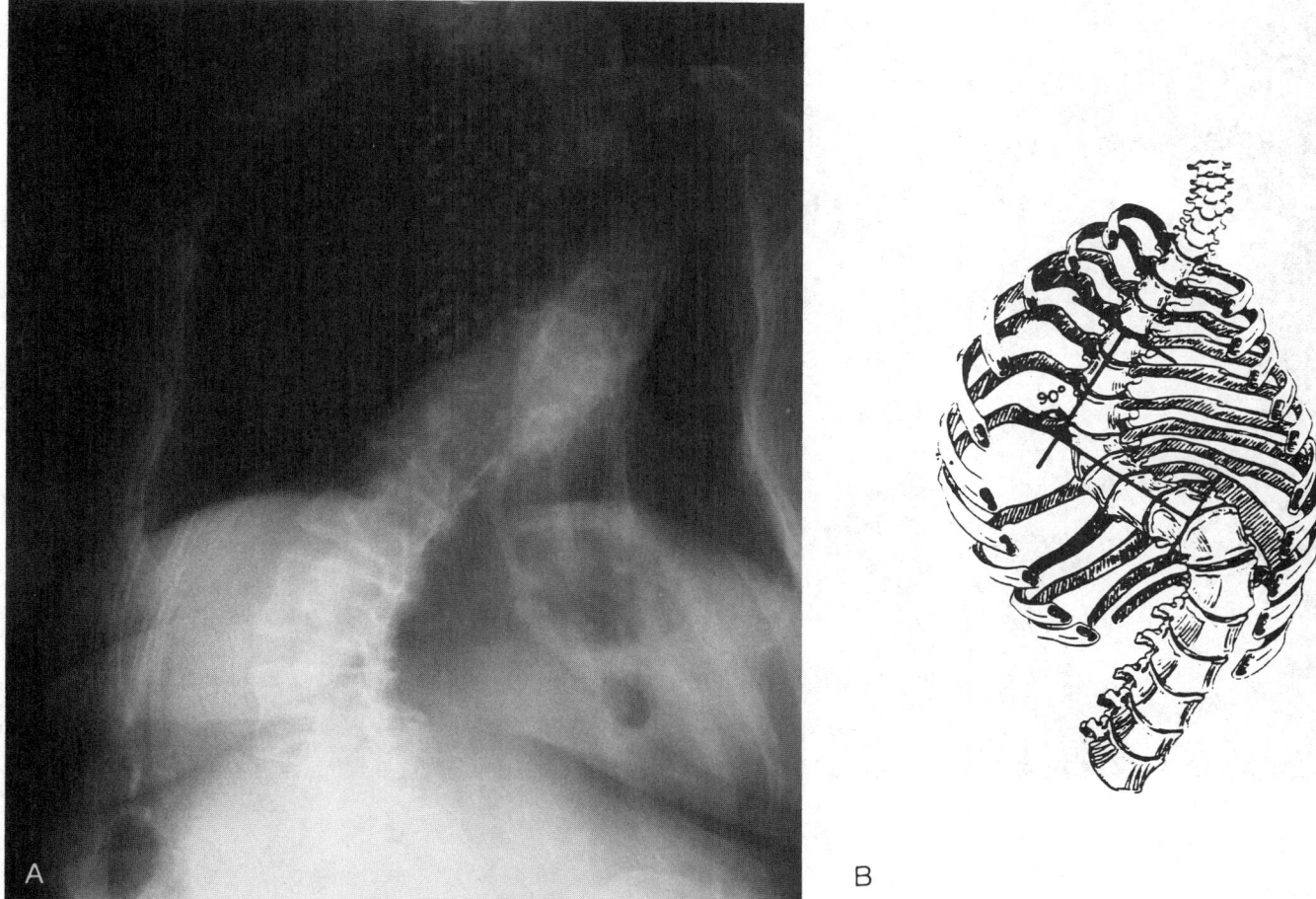

Figure 68–4. Kyphoscoliosis. *A.* Posteroanterior radiographic view of the thoracic abnormality. *B.* Drawing demonstrating the serpiginous course of the vertebral column with primary and compensatory (or secondary) curves. The Cobb angle is measured by identifying the cranial and caudal vertebrae at the locations of change in direction of curvature and drawing perpendicular lines from the upper border of the upper vertebra and lower border of the lower vertebra. The Cobb angle is formed where these perpendicular lines cross. (From Grippi MA, Fishman AP: Respiratory failure in structural and neuromuscular disorders involving the chest bellows. Fishman AP [ed]: Pulmonary Diseases and Disorders. 2nd ed. New York, McGraw-Hill, p 2300, 1988. Reproduced with permission of McGraw-Hill, Inc.)

Ankylosing Spondylitis

Ankylosing spondylitis is a systemic rheumatic disorder that produces synovitis, chondritis, and juxta-articular osteitis, resulting in fibrosis and ossification of the ligamentous structures of the spine and rib cage (Fig. 68–5). The disease is closely associated with the human leukocyte antigen B27 histocompatibility antigen and has a strong familial inheritance pattern. About 20% of white patients with the antigen have manifestations of the disease, and up to 95% of white patients with ankylosing spondylitis have the antigen. The criteria for diagnosis include the following: (1) chronic low-back pain with decreased motion of the spine; (2) x-ray evidence of bilateral sacroiliitis; and (3) less than 2.5 cm of chest wall expansion (measured at the level of the fourth intercostal space). Systemic manifestations develop in 10 to 20% of chronically affected patients and involve the ocular (iritis), cardiac (aortic regurgitation, heart block), and skeletal (peripheral arthritis) systems. The classic bamboo spine (Fig. 68–6) occurs in less than 1% of patients.[64] Respiratory involvement is mild, and ventilatory failure is rare except in the presence of diaphragmatic dysfunction or other lung disease.

Flail Injury of the Chest

Acute respiratory failure caused by traumatic flail injury of the chest has traditionally been ascribed to a mechanical disruption of the chest wall. The mechanism for the respiratory abnormality was believed to be a paradoxical inward movement of the flail segment, inefficient ventilation of the underlying parenchyma, and paradoxical respiration of the other lung segments, or pendelluft. The theory held that during inspiration, the alveoli under the flail segment were actually emptying rather than filling (Fig. 68–7).

An examination of this phenomenon has led to an alternative theory that contusion of the underlying lung parenchyma is the major cause of respiratory failure. By treating the patient with intermittent mandatory ventilation and adequate pain control, internal stabilization of the chest wall was facilitated, and patients improved more rapidly than those who underwent surgical stabilizing procedures.[65, 66]

Obesity and Obesity-Hypoventilation Syndrome

For this discussion, the distinction between obese patients and obese patients with hypoventilation should be kept clearly in mind. There are important physiologic differences

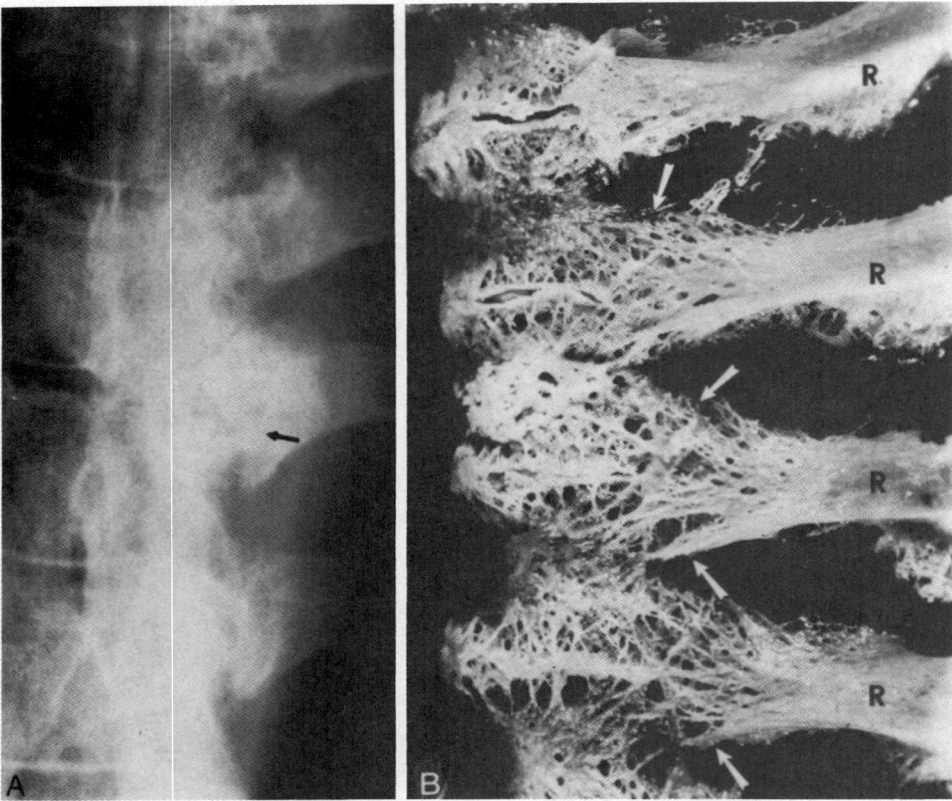

Figure 68–5. Ankylosing spondylitis. Costovertebral joint erosions and costovertebral joint ankylosis in a 60-year-old man with a long history of ankylosing spondylitis. *A.* An oblique frontal radiograph of the thoracic spine demonstrates bone erosions about many costovertebral articulations, especially prominent at one level *(arrow)*. Characteristic "squaring" of the vertebral bodies and narrowing of the intervertebral spaces are evident as well. *B.* A photograph of the lateral aspect of a macerated thoracic spine of a spondylitic cadaver demonstrates extensive bony ankylosis *(arrows)* of the heads of the ribs (R) and vertebral bodies. Ossification of disks is also seen. (Modified from Resnick D, Niwayama G: Diagnosis of Bone and Joint Disorders. 2nd ed. Philadelphia, WB Saunders, p 1132, 1988.)

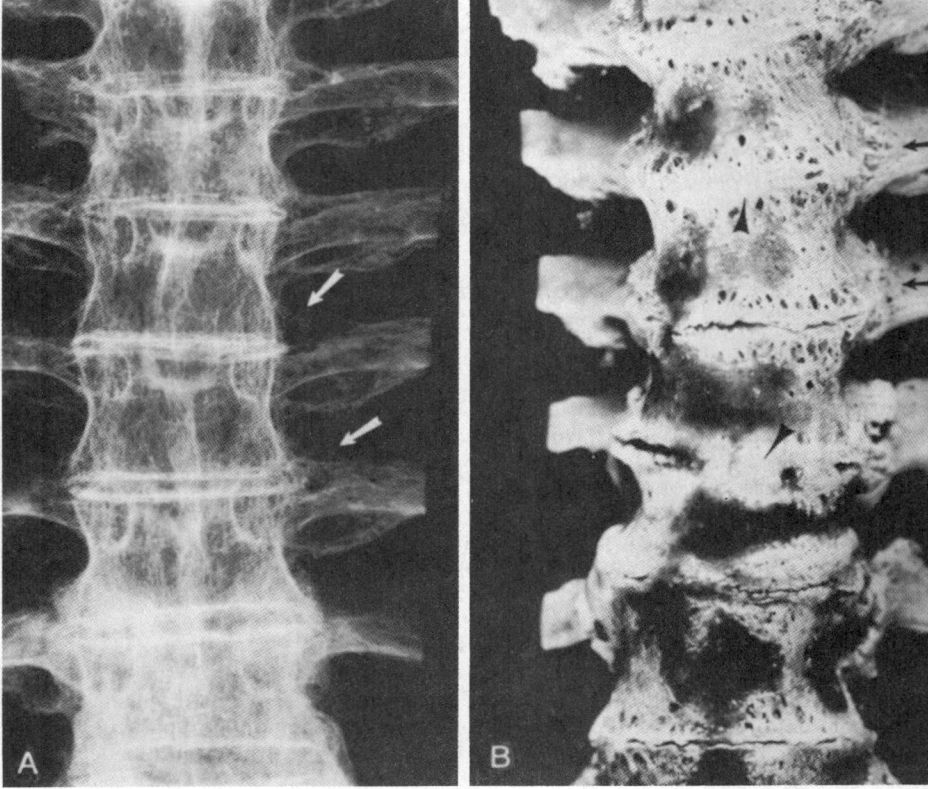

Figure 68–6. Classic bamboo spine of ankylosing spondylitis. An anteroposterior radiograph *(A)* and photograph (anterior view) *(B)* of a macerated whole spine reveal widespread syndesmophytosis, leading to symmetric ossification of multiple intervertebral disks *(arrowheads in B)*. An undulating spinal contour has been produced. Note the costovertebral joint ankylosis *(arrows)*, which contributes to limitation of chest cage expansion. (Modified from Resnick D, Niwayama G: Diagnosis of Bone and Joint Disorders. 2nd ed. Philadelphia, WB Saunders, p 1121, 1988.)

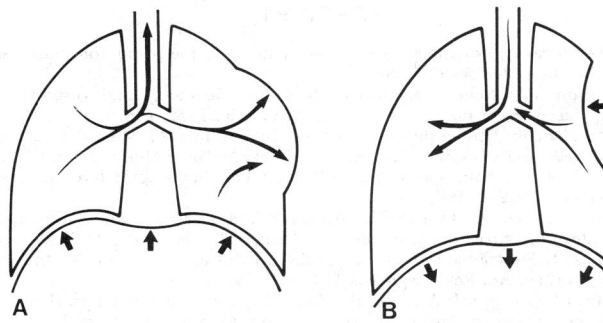

Figure 68–7. The theory of pendelluft. In expiration *(A)*, the flail segment expands and air from the opposite lung fills the lung under the region of paradoxical movement. In inspiration *(B)*, air in the lung beneath the flail segment moves to help expand the opposite lung. (From Trinkle JK, Harman PK, Grover FL: Chest trauma. Fishman AP [ed]: Pulmonary Diseases and Disorders. 2nd ed. New York, McGraw-Hill, p 2450, 1988. Reproduced with permission of McGraw-Hill, Inc.)

between these two groups that have a significant impact on their treatment. Most studies of pulmonary disease in obese patients have defined obesity as having a gross weight of between 150 and 200% of ideal body weight.

Compliance. Obesity has significant effects on the work of breathing and the compliance of the chest bellows system. In morbidly obese patients (weight > 150% of ideal body weight), the chest wall becomes stiff and noncompliant because of the excessive tissue contained in the chest and abdomen,[67–69] and it becomes even less compliant when the patient is supine.[67] The work of breathing is increased by the mass-elastic load that this tissue presents, as well as the flow-resistive load provided by the increased resistance of the nasopharyngeal segment seen in many patients. These mechanical loads increase the respiratory muscle work necessary to maintain eucapnia, even during wakefulness.[70] In obese eucapnic patients, chest wall compliance is close to normal,[71] whereas obese hypercapnic patients may have chest wall compliances of up to one third of normal values. Lung compliance is also decreased in obese patients,[68, 69] which may be due to either increased pulmonary blood volume or increased dependent airway closure.[69]

Pulmonary Function Studies. A restrictive pattern is produced in obesity, with significant reductions in expiratory reserve volume, functional residual capacity and total lung capacity, and a smaller tidal volume. The VC and maximal voluntary ventilation are reduced in proportion to the increase in body weight and the decrease in chest wall compliance,[67–69] with contributions from respiratory muscle dysfunction and decreased lung compliance.

Ventilation. Patients with severe obesity are generally hypoxemic, with a widened alveolar-arterial oxygen gradient caused by ventilation-perfusion mismatching. Alveolar collapse and airway closure at the bases contribute significantly to this phenomenon.[67, 69, 72, 73] The work of breathing is increased in obese patients because of the need to eliminate a higher daily production of carbon dioxide, coupled with the decreased compliance of the respiratory system. The hypoxic ventilatory drive for eucapnic obese patients is normal or even increased,[74, 75] whereas hypercapnic obese patients have decreased responses to hypoxia, hypercapnia, and increases in mechanical loads.[75–77]

Hemodynamics. Because of the large amount of excess working tissue, the cardiac output and blood volume are both increased. Systemic hypertension and subsequently pulmonary hypertension are often present. During sleep, the arterial oxygen saturation repeatedly decreases, with associated elevation in systemic and pulmonary vascular resistance. Alveolar ventilation stimulates increased hypoxic pulmonary vasoconstriction during sleep, which eventually leads to pulmonary hypertension during waking hours. The hypoxia and hypercapnia may predispose the patient to ventricular arrhythmias, especially during long apneic periods. In addition, there is a cyclic variation in cardiac output, with the nadirs occurring after apneic episodes.[78, 79]

GENERAL MANAGEMENT OF MECHANICAL RESPIRATORY FAILURE

Failure of the ventilatory pump to provide an adequate level of alveolar ventilation is the common end point in both neuromuscular and structural disorders. To treat the resulting hypercapnia, the first line of therapy is rest in the form of ventilatory support. A minimum of 12 hours is required to restore respiratory muscle contractility.[80, 81] Another vital aspect in treatment is the reversal of hypoxemia and the use of supplemental oxygen. The importance of hypoxic vasoconstriction in this process cannot be overemphasized, and this simple maneuver may have a major impact on pulmonary hemodynamics and regional ventilation-perfusion relationships. Attention must be paid to the many steps that contribute to respiratory failure from neuromuscular disease or mechanical derangements of the chest wall. As noted, many reversible processes may compound acute mechanical respiratory failure. Therapy should be directed at clearing respiratory secretions and managing pneumonia or heart failure. In addition, chest physiotherapy, incentive spirometry, or when indicated, bronchoscopy should be used to reverse atelectasis. Other metabolic abnormalities, especially hypoxemia, should be treated promptly. Moreover, both hypercapnia and acidosis directly reduce diaphragmatic contractility and endurance.[82] Hypophosphatemia and hypokalemia also have detrimental effects on respiratory muscle function and require rapid correction. If the patient has obstructive airways disease, as evidenced by bronchospasm, appropriate medications should be administered.

In some patients, attempts are made to improve respiratory mechanics. Patients with kyphoscoliosis may benefit from large-volume inflations via intermittent positive pressure breathing; improvement in pulmonary compliance by reversal of microatelectasis may last for several hours after such treatments.[59] Unfortunately, this form of therapy has not been effective in neuromuscular disease. Surgery for correction of severely scoliotic patients can be useful, but little improvement results after age 20, and the complication rate can be as high as 50%.[83]

Traditionally, improvements in respiratory mechanics were achieved in patients with flail chest by surgically stabilizing the thorax. Later experiments with respiratory failure resulting from flail injury have demonstrated that internal fixation by mechanical ventilation alone, as well as treatment of pulmonary contusion, may be a more successful method for weaning patients more rapidly from ventilation and decreasing the duration of hospital stays.[65, 84] The importance of adequate pain control to improve ventilatory function has also received attention, and the use of epidural delivery systems appears to be effective in this group of patients.[66]

Pharmacotherapy for Mechanical Respiratory Muscle Failure

Some drugs have proved to have a positive inotropic effect on respiratory muscles. For example, preliminary data indicate that aminophylline may increase diaphragmatic strength and delay the onset of diaphragmatic fatigue.[85] Although studies have established this effect in experimental settings, clinical efficacy remains controversial, and a full discourse is beyond the scope of this chapter. Other studies are beginning to focus on the sympathomimetic amines and digitalis. All of these agents may have important therapeutic implications, and further studies are needed to explore this promising field.

Nutrition

The use of dietary measures to decrease carbon dioxide production and improve ventilatory performance remains controversial but is under continued study.[86–88] In one report,[86] dietary restriction of carbohydrate intake to 50 g resulted in a mean decrease in Pco_2 of 9 mm Hg and a mean increase in Po_2 of 12 mm Hg. There was no significant change in weight during the study in these hospitalized patients who served as their own controls.

Mechanical Ventilation in the Home Environment

Many patients, after surviving the acute insult that resulted in mechanical respiratory failure, cannot regain sufficient levels of spontaneous ventilation to live independently of the mechanical ventilator. Accordingly, there has been growing interest in ventilatory support devices for use in the home. These devices may take the form of rocking beds, positive pressure ventilators via tracheostomy, or negative pressure ventilators with a poncho or other type of cuirass.[89–92] Although some patients require one of these ventilatory techniques on a continuous basis, many need only nocturnal ventilation. These techniques have been shown to prolong survival and to improve the quality of life for these patients. Intermittent nightly mechanical ventilation under negative pressure[93] or under positive pressure via tracheostomy can alter the natural evolution of mechanical respiratory failure after discharge from the hospital. However, these techniques have certain inherent difficulties and potential complications. Negative pressure ventilatory devices are often uncomfortable and can induce obstructive sleep apnea. There are also many complications with tracheostomy, such as infection, and psychologic factors often prevent tolerance.

Some clinicians have been using an alternative method to replace tracheostomy, in the form of a nasal mask or silicone fittings for the nostrils. These appliances are usually affixed to the head with Velcro straps and have been adapted to positive pressure ventilators from nasal continuous positive pressure devices for the treatment of sleep apnea. Although the method was originally proposed for the treatment of neuromuscular disorders, the technique can be extended to other disorders that result in hypoventilation, particularly at night. The silicone pieces fitted to the nostrils may provide more comfort and less possibility of air leaks.

Like positive pressure ventilation via tracheostomy, nasal ventilation prevents nocturnal oxygen desaturation and provides an improved sense of well-being during the day. Moreover, there are few complications and the technique is less cumbersome than the alternative methods just described. However, leaks through the mouth can result in hypoventilation, and a chin strap to keep the mouth closed may be needed. Nasal ventilation should not be considered for the patient who is entirely dependent on the ventilator, but rather for those for whom nocturnal rest is desired. Thus, the need for tracheostomy can be replaced or postponed by nasal ventilation. All of the methods discussed require a supportive family and home environment. These elements are always crucial to any successful ventilatory program in the home.

References

1. De Troyer A, Estenne M: Functional anatomy of the respiratory muscles. Clin Chest Med 9:175, 1988.
2. Wilson TA, Rehder K, Krayer S, et al: Geometry and respiratory displacement of human ribs. J Appl Physiol 62:1872, 1987.
3. Macklem P: The respiratory muscles. In Fishman AP (ed): Pulmonary Diseases and Disorders. 2nd ed. New York, McGraw-Hill, p 2269, 1988.
4. De Troyer A, Sampson M, Sigrist S, et al: The diaphragm: Two muscles. Science 213:237, 1981.
5. Sant'Anbrogio G, Frazier DT, Wilson MF, et al: Motor innervation and pattern of activity of cat diaphragm. J Appl Physiol 18:43, 1963.
6. Mead J: Functional significance of the area of apposition of diaphragm to rib cage. Am Rev Respir Dis 119:31, 1979.
7. Mead J, Loring SH: Analysis of volume displacement and length changes of the diaphragm during breathing. J Appl Physiol 53:750, 1982.
8. De Troyer A, Sampson MG: Activation of the parasternal intercostals during breathing efforts in human subjects. J Appl Physiol 52:524, 1982.
9. Smith P, Calvery MB, Edwards RHT, et al: Practical problems in the respiratory care of patients with muscular dystrophy. N Engl J Med 316:1197, 1987.
10. Gibson GJ, Pride MB, Newsome-Davis J, et al: Pulmonary mechanics in patients with respiratory muscle weakness. Am Rev Respir Dis 115:389, 1977.
11. De Troyer A, Borenstein S, Cordier R: Analysis of lung volume restriction in patients with respiratory muscle weakness. Thorax 35:603, 1980.
12. Estenne M, De Troyer A: The effects of tetraplegia on chest wall statics. Am Rev Respir Dis 134:121, 1986.
13. Tobin MJ: Respiratory muscles in disease. Clin Chest Med 9:263, 1988.
14. Begin R, Bureau MA, Lupien I, et al. Control of breathing in Duchenne's muscular dystrophy. Am J Med 69:227, 1980.
15. Rochester DF, Arora NS: Respiratory muscle failure. Med Clin North Am 67:573, 1983.
16. Braun NMT, Arora NS, Rochester DF: Respiratory muscle and pulmonary function in polymyositis and other proximal myopathies. Thorax 38:616, 1983.
17. O'Donohue WJ, Baker JP, Bell GM, et al: Respiratory failure in neuromuscular disease: Management in a respiratory care unit. JAMA 235:733, 1976.
18. Fromm GB, Wisdom PJ, Block AJ: Amyotrophic lateral sclerosis presenting with respiratory failure. Chest 71:612, 1977.
19. Hill R, Martin J, Hakin A: Acute respiratory failure in motoneuron disease. Arch Neurol 40:30, 1983.
20. Daros M, Spiro AJ, Severdlow M: Respiratory failure in amyotrophic lateral sclerosis. NY State J Med 84:570, 1984.
21. Meyrignale C, Poirer J, Dagos JD: Amyotrophic lateral sclerosis presenting with respiratory insufficiency as the major complaint. Eur Neurol 24:115, 1985.
22. Braun SR: Respiratory system in amyotrophic lateral sclerosis. Neurol Clin 5:9, 1987.
23. Danon J, Druz WS, Goldberg NB, et al: Function of the isolated paced diaphragm and the cervical accessory muscles in C1 quadriplegics. Am Rev Respir Dis 119:909, 1979.
24. Garrido H, Mazaira J, Gutierrez P, et al: Continuous respiratory support in quadriplegic children by bilateral phrenic nerve stimulation. Thorax 42:573, 1987.
25. Wicks AB, Menter RR: Long-term outlook in quadriplegic patients with initial ventilatory dependency. Chest 90:406, 1986.
26. Ledsome JR, Sharp JM: Pulmonary function in acute cervical cord injury. Am Rev Respir Dis 124:41, 1981.
27. Bennett DA, Bleck TP: Diagnosis and treatment of neuromuscular causes of acute respiratory failure. Clin Neuropharmacol 11:303, 1988.
28. Loffel NB, Rossi LN, Mumenthaler M, et al: The Landry-Guillain-Barré syndrome: Complications, prognosis, and natural history in 123 cases. J Neurosci 33:71, 1977.
29. Moore P, James O: Guillain-Barré syndrome: Incidence, management and outcome of major complications. Crit Care Med 9:549, 1981.
30. Gracey DR, McMichan JC, Divertie MB, et al: Respiratory failure in Guillain-Barré syndrome. A 6-year experience. Mayo Clin Proc 57:742, 1982.
31. Ropper AH, Kehne SM: Guillain-Barré syndrome: Management of respiratory failure. Neurology 35:1662, 1985.
32. Newsum JK, Smith RM, Crocker D: Intubation for acute respiratory failure in Guillain-Barré syndrome. JAMA 242:1650, 1979.
33. Sunderrajan EV, Dasvenport J: The Guillain-Barré syndrome: Pulmonary-neurologic correlations. Medicine 64:333, 1985.
34. Ropper AH: Severe acute Guillain-Barré syndrome. Neurology 36:429, 1986.
35. Raman TK, Blake JA, Harris, TM: Pulmonary embolism in Landry-Guillain-Barré-Strohl syndrome. Chest 60:555, 1971.
36. Dyck PJ, Kurtzke JF: Plasmapheresis in Guillain-Barré syndrome (editorial). Neurology 35:1105, 1985.
37. Guillain-Barré Syndrome Study Group: Plasmapheresis and acute Guillain-Barré syndrome. Neurology 35:1096, 1985.
38. Hughes RAC, Newsom-Davis JM, Perkin GD, et al: Controlled trial of prednisolone in acute polyneuropathy. Lancet 2:750, 1978.

39. Engel AG: Myasthenia gravis and myasthenic syndromes. Ann Neurol 16:519, 1984.
40. Pascuzzi RM, Johns TR: Myasthenia gravis: The patient evaluation. Semin Neurol 2:231, 1982.
41. Gracey DR, Howard FM, Divertie MB: Mechanical ventilation for respiratory failure in myasthenia gravis. Mayo Clin Proc 58:597, 1983.
42. Gracey DR, Howard FM, Divertie MB: Plasmapheresis in the treatment of ventilator-dependent myasthenia gravis patients. Chest 85:739, 1983.
43. Seybold ME: Plasmapheresis in myasthenia gravis. Ann NY Acad Sci 505:584, 1987.
44. Cohen MS, Younger D: Aspects of the natural history of myasthenia gravis: Crisis and death. Ann NY Acad Sci 377:670, 1981.
45. Shim C: Motor disturbances of the diaphragm. Clin Chest Med 1:125, 1980.
46. Skatrud J, Iber C, McHugh W, et al: Determinants of hypoventilation during wakefulness and sleep in diaphragmatic paralysis. Am Rev Respir Dis 121:587, 1980.
47. Alexander C: Diaphragm movements and the diagnosis of diaphragmatic paralysis. Clin Radiol 17:79, 1966.
48. Aldrich TK: Respiratory muscle fatigue. Clin Chest Med 9:225, 1988.
49. James J: Scoliosis. 2nd ed. Edinburgh, Churchill Livingstone, p 1, 1976.
50. Litwin SD: Genetic Determinants of Pulmonary Disease. New York, Marcel Dekker, p 182, 1978.
51. Bergofsky EH, Turino GM, and Fishman AP: Cardiorespiratory failure in kyphoscoliosis. Medicine 38:263, 1959.
52. Jones R, Kennedy J, Hasham F, et al: Mechanical inefficiency of the thoracic cage in scoliosis. Thorax 36:456, 1981.
53. Grippi MA, Fishman AP: Respiratory failure in structural and neuromuscular disorders involving the chest bellows. In: Fishman AP (ed): Pulmonary Diseases and Disorders. 2nd ed. New York, McGraw-Hill, p 2300, 1988.
54. Kane WJ: Prevalence of scoliosis. Clin Orthop 126:43, 1977.
55. Kofer ER: Idiopathic scoliosis—Gas exchange and the age dependence of arterial blood gases. J Clin Invest 58:825, 1976.
56. Weber B, Smith J, Briscoe W, et al: Pulmonary function in asymptomatic adolescents with idiopathic scoliosis. Am Rev Respir Dis 111:389, 1975.
57. Caro C, Dubois A: Pulmonary function in kyphoscoliosis. Thorax 16:282, 1961.
58. Weinstein S, Zavalo D, Ponseti I: Idiopathic scoliosis. J Bone Joint Surg 63:702, 1981.
59. Sinha R, Bergofsky E: Prolonged alteration of lung mechanisms in kyphoscoliosis by positive pressure hyperinflation. Am Rev Respir Dis 106:47, 1972.
60. Cooper D, Rajas T, Mellins R, et al: Respiratory mechanics in adolescents with idiopathic scoliosis. Am Rev Respir Dis 130:16, 1984.
61. Lisboa C, Moreno R, Fava M, et al: Inspiratory muscle function in patients with severe kyphoscoliosis. Am Rev Respir Dis 132:48, 1985.
62. Naeye R: Kyphoscoliosis and cor pulmonale. Am J Pathol 38:561, 1961.
63. Mezon B, West P, Israels J, et al: Sleep breathing abnormalities in kyphoscoliosis. Am Rev Respir Dis 122:617, 1980.
64. Rosenow E, Strimlan C, Muhm J, et al: Pleuropulmonary manifestations of ankylosing spondylitis. Mayo Clin Proc 52:641, 1977.
65. Trinkle JK: Flail chest and pulmonary contusion. In: Trinkle JK, Grover FL (eds): Management of Thoracic Trauma Victims. Philadelphia, JB Lippincott, p 39, 1980.
66. Mackersie RC, Schackford SR, Hoyt DB, et al: Continuous epidural fentanyl analgesia: Ventilatory function improvement with routine use in treatment of blunt chest injury. J Trauma 27:1207, 1987.
67. Naimark A, Cherniak RM: Compliance of the respiratory system and its components in health and obesity. J Appl Physiol 15:377, 1960.
68. Sharp J, Henry J, Sweeny S, et al: The total work of breathing in normal and obese men. J Clin Invest 43:728, 1964.
69. Rochester D, Guson Y: Current concepts in the pathogenesis of the obesity-hypoventilation syndrome. Am J Med 57:402, 1974.
70. Arch AM, Remmers JE, Bunce H III: Supraglottic airway resistance in normal subjects and patients with occlusive sleep apnea. J Appl Physiol 53:1158, 1982.
71. Suratt P, Wilheit S, Hsiao H, et al: Compliance of chest wall in obese subjects. J Appl Physiol 57:403, 1984.
72. Holley H, Milic-Emili J, Becklake M, et al: Regional distribution of pulmonary ventilation and perfusion in obesity. J Clin Invest 46:475, 1967.
73. Hurewitz A, Susskind H, Harold W: Obesity alters regional ventilation in lateral decubitus position. J Appl Physiol 59:774, 1985.
74. Burki N, Baker R: Ventilatory regulation in eucapnic morbid obesity. Am Rev Respir Dis 129:538, 1984.
75. Sampson M, Grassino A: Load compensation in obese patients during quiet tidal breathing. J Appl Physiol 55:1269, 1983.
76. Garay SM, Rapoport D, Sorkin B, et al: Regulation of ventilation in the obstructive sleep apnea syndrome. Am Rev Respir Dis 124:451, 1981.
77. Zwillich C, Suton F, Pierson D, et al: Decreased hypoxic ventilatory drive in the obesity-hypoventilation syndrome. Am J Med 59:343, 1975.
78. Shepard JW Jr: Cardiopulmonary consequences of obstructive sleep apnea. Mayo Clin Proc 65:1250, 1990.
79. Zwillich C, Devlin T, White D, et al: Bradycardia during sleep apnea: Characteristics and mechanisms. J Clin Invest 69:1286, 1982.
80. Roussos C, Macklem PT: The respiratory muscles. N Engl J Med 307:786, 1982.
81. Rochester DF, Arora NS: Respiratory muscle failure. Med Clin North Am 67:573, 1983.
82. Juan G, Calcerley P, Talamo C, et al: Effects of carbon dioxide on diaphragmatic function in human beings. N Engl J Med 310: 874, 1984.
83. Swank S, Lonstein J, Moe J, et al: Surgical treatment of adult scoliosis. J Bone Joint Surg 63:268, 1981.
84. Shackford SR, Virgilio RW, Peters RM: Selective use of ventilatory therapy in flail chest injury. J Thorac Cardiovasc Surg 81:194, 1981.
85. Aubier M: Pharmacotherapy of respiratory muscles. Clin Chest Med 9:311, 1988.
86. Kwan R, Mir MA: Beneficial effects of dietary carbohydrate restriction in chronic cor pumonale. Am J Med 82:751, 1987.
87. Tirlapur VG, Mir MA: Effect of low calorie intake on abnormal pulmonary physiology in patients with chronic hypercapneic respiratory failure. Am J Med 77:987, 1984.
88. Wilson DO, Rogers RM, Hoffman RM: Nutrition and chronic lung disease. Am Rev Respir Dis 132:1347, 1985.
89. Garay S, Turino G, Goldring R: Sustained reversal of chronic hypercapnia in patients with alveolar hypoventilation syndromes. Am J Med 70:269, 1981.
90. Hoeppner V, Cockroft D, Dosman J, et al: Nighttime ventilation improves respiratory failure in secondary kyphoscoliosis. Am Rev Respir Dis 129:240, 1984.
91. Wiers W, LeCultre R, Dellinga O, et al: Cuirass respiratory treatment of chronic respiratory failure in scoliotic patients. Thorax 32:221, 1977.
92. Fulkerson W, Wilkins J, Esbenshade A, et al: Life threatening hypoventilation in kyphoscoliosis: Successful treatment with a molded body brace-ventilator. Am Rev Respir Dis 129:185, 1984.
93. Leger P, Jennequin M, Gerard E, et al: Home positive pressure ventilation via nasal mask for patients with neuromuscular disorders. Eur Respir J 2(suppl 7):640, 1989.

CHAPTER 69

Central Respiratory Failure, Including Sleep Disorders

Richard J. Schwab
Joanne E. Getsy
Allan I. Pack

Respiratory failure can be broadly categorized into hypercapnic respiratory failure ($P_{CO_2} > 45$ torr) and hypoxemic respiratory failure ($P_{O_2} < 50$ torr, on room air).[1] This chapter discusses hypercapnic respiratory failure and sleep disorders. The respiratory system can be subdivided into four components: (1) the central nervous system (CNS) provides the neural drive to ventilation; (2) the peripheral nervous system and respiratory muscles provide information to move the chest wall and diaphragm, which generates airflow; (3) the endobronchial tree (extrathoracic and intrathoracic airways) enables air to reach gas exchange units; (4) the alveoli provide the surface area for oxygen–carbon dioxide exchange between air and blood. If any component of this system fails, respiratory failure can ensue. This chapter focuses on the CNS and sleep disorders as a cause of respiratory failure.

Many diseases that commonly present in the intensive care unit (ICU) can be exacerbated by sleep. Asthma, chronic obstructive pulmonary disease (COPD), cardiovascular diseases including both arrhythmias and coronary artery disease, restrictive lung diseases, and interstitial lung disease

---

TABLE 69-1

EXTRAPULMONARY VENTILATORY FAILURE

I. Central nervous system
   A. Drug overdose (narcotics, barbiturates)
   B. Cerebral vascular accident or hemorrhage
   C. Trauma
   D. Infection
   F. Neoplasm
   F. Postseizure
   G. Primary alveolar hypoventilation
II. Peripheral nervous system and respiratory muscles
   A. Spinal cord lesions
      1. Trauma, neoplasm, hemorrhage, infection
      2. Poliomyelitis
      3. Multiple sclerosis
   B. Peripheral nervous system
      1. Guillain-Barré syndrome
      2. Peripheral neuritis
      3. Anterior horn cell
         a. Amyotrophic lateral sclerosis
      4. Neuromuscular junction
         a. Myasthenia gravis
         b. Eaton-Lambert syndrome
         c. Botulism
         d. Neuromuscular blocking agents
         e. Organophosphate poisoning
         f. Neuromuscular blocking antibiotics
           (aminoglycosides)
   C. Respiratory muscle weakness or myopathies
      1. Polymyositis
      2. Muscular dystrophy
      3. Periodic paralysis
      4. Respiratory muscle fatigue
      5. Metabolic causes
         a. Hypophosphatemia
         b. Hypokalemia
         c. Myxedema
   D. Chest wall disorders
      1. Thoracoplasty
      2. Flail chest
      3. Kyphoscoliosis
      4. Fibrothorax
      5. Ankylosing spondylitis
III. Sleep disorders
   A. Central sleep apnea
   B. Obstructive sleep apnea
   C. Obesity-hypoventilation syndrome

can all worsen during sleep. Alternatively, patients who present with unexplained hypercapnia, cor pulmonale, pulmonary hypertension, or alveolar hypoventilation may have a primary sleep disorder as the underlying cause of these disorders. In this chapter, we first review CNS respiratory failure and then present an overview of sleep and the control of breathing during sleep. We review central and obstructive sleep apnea as well as the treatment of these sleep disorders. We address the use of nasal nocturnal ventilation in the management of hypoventilation. We discuss sleep and sleep deprivation in the ICU. Finally, we focus on the major diseases in the ICU affected by sleep and describe patients who present with respiratory failure in the ICU who are manifesting underlying primary sleep disorders.

CENTRAL NERVOUS SYSTEM RESPIRATORY FAILURE

Table 69–1 gives the causes of extrapulmonary ventilatory failure by site of involvement. Diseases causing acute and chronic respiratory failure are listed.[1-11] Respiratory failure secondary to abnormalities of the peripheral nervous system and the respiratory muscles is discussed fully in Chapter 40.

Briefly, any disorder of the spinal cord, peripheral nervous system, anterior horn cell, neuromuscular junction, or respiratory muscles can result in or precipitate respiratory failure. The most common cause of respiratory failure related to loss of the central drive for respiration involves drug overdoses. Many medications when taken in overdose can lead to respiratory failure. The most common medications include narcotics, benzodiazepines, and barbiturates. Any depressant drug, however, given in sufficient dosage can lead to suppression of ventilatory drive and subsequent respiratory failure. These patients may be unconscious and a diagnosis can usually be made with a toxicology screen. In any comatose or semicomatose patient with hypercapnia, drug overdose should be suspected. Structural abnormalities of the CNS (e.g., cerebrovascular accident, trauma, infection, and neoplasm) usually present with focal neurologic findings. Hypercapnia ensues in these conditions secondary to abnormalities that reduce the premotor drive to phrenic and other respiratory motor neurons.

Metabolic abnormalities including hypothyroidism (myxedema coma) and metabolic alkalosis can also result in hypoventilation and, if severe, respiratory failure.[4, 5] Metabolic alkalosis can easily be diagnosed with an arterial blood gas analysis. Hypothyroidism is often subtle and the diagnosis can be easily missed unless it is considered and a careful history and physical examination are obtained. These disorders rarely cause ventilatory failure by themselves but can be a contributing factor to the development of ventilatory failure.

Chronic hypercapnia and hypoxemia in the absence of known respiratory muscle weakness, neurologic disease, or other cause of mechanical respiratory failure are considered the idiopathic primary alveolar hypoventilation syndrome. Although this disease has an unknown etiology, a decrease in the central respiratory drive appears to result from an abnormality in the respiratory center.[12-14] The most severe episodes of hypoventilation occur during sleep in these patients. This disease can occur in all age groups and presents insidiously with a dearth of pulmonary symptoms. Patients complain of lassitude, abnormal sleep patterns, excessive daytime sleepiness, and morning headaches. The disease may first manifest itself after a patient is sedated with a medication or anesthetic. Pulmonary hypertension and right-sided congestive heart failure may eventually develop secondary to the chronic hypoxia and hypercapnia. The diagnosis is confirmed by finding hypoxia, hypercapnia, and respiratory acidosis in the absence of other causes of extrapulmonary ventilatory failure. Although patients have relatively few pulmonary complaints, the arterial blood gas abnormalities are often severe, with P_{CO_2} values of about 50 to 70 torr and P_{O_2} values of 40 to 50 torr.[12-14] Patients with primary alveolar hypoventilation can hyperventilate voluntarily to normalize their P_{CO_2}, unlike most patients with hypercapnia on the basis of underlying lung disease (COPD). Some patients with primary alveolar hypoventilation syndrome may be able to maintain relatively normal respiration while awake but during sleep, with the loss of their wakefulness drive to breathe, develop significant hypoventilation and periods of apnea.[12-14] There is a continuum between primary alveolar hypoventilation syndrome and central sleep apnea, although patients with central sleep apnea do not generally manifest daytime hypercapnia.

All of these causes of extrapulmonary respiratory failure (CNS, peripheral nervous system, and respiratory muscles, listed in Table 69–1) are worsened during sleep, when significant changes take place in the neural control of ventilation. In addition, there are certain conditions in which the primary events resulting in respiratory failure occur during sleep, and, if severe, may result in daytime hypercapnia. Before considering these sleep disorders (see Table 69–1), we briefly consider the changes in neural control of ventilation that occur during sleep and give a brief overview of sleep states.

PHYSIOLOGY OF SLEEP

Although sleep appears to be a passive state, it is actually a complex process during which various physiologic changes occur. Within sleep there are two distinct states: non–rapid eye movement (NREM) sleep (quiet or slow-wave sleep) and rapid eye movement (REM) sleep (paradoxical or active sleep). These two states are found in virtually all mammals and birds, and each state has its own set of physiologic and electroencephalographic (EEG) hallmarks.[15] NREM sleep can be divided by EEG criteria into four stages (Fig. 69–1). Each stage in NREM sleep represents a deeper sleep stage, with the arousal threshold being the highest in stage 4 (delta sleep) and the lowest in stage 1 sleep. REM sleep is characterized by marked CNS metabolic activity, and it is during

this time that dreaming principally occurs. During REM sleep there are episodic rapid eye movements and characteristic EEG activity that is similar to that in wakefulness (see Fig. 69–1). The rapid eye movements are associated with flurries of central neuronal activity. These flurries of activity do not generally result in peripheral movements because there is active suppression of motor neuron activity in REM sleep (i.e., muscle atonia), although there can be periodic ("phasic") twitching of the extremities. REM sleep and NREM sleep alternate throughout the night in a cyclic fashion. Cycles of REM sleep typically last 10 to 20 minutes and occur approximately every 90 to 110 minutes; as the night progresses the REM cycles lengthen.[16] These sleep processes have several important physiologic consequences that affect breathing, which we now consider.

CONTROL OF VENTILATION DURING SLEEP

We have begun to learn a great deal about the control of ventilation during sleep in normal subjects and in patients

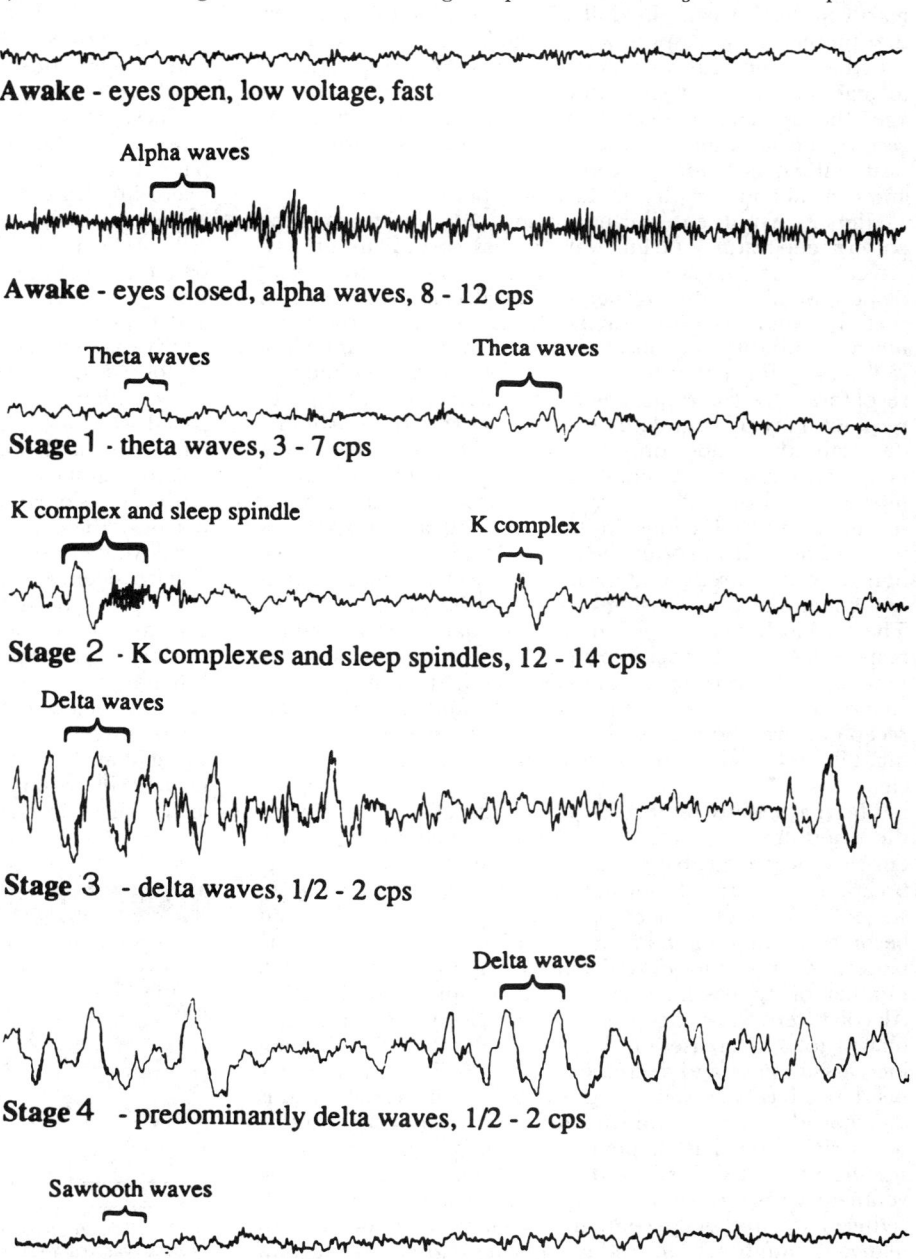

Figure 69–1. Isolated polysomnographic data showing EEG patterns in the awake state, the four different EEG stages of NREM sleep (stages 1 to 4), and the EEG pattern of REM sleep. The characteristic wave patterns for the different sleep stages are noted. (EEGs courtesy of the Penn Center for Sleep Disorders.)

Awake - eyes open, low voltage, fast

Alpha waves

Awake - eyes closed, alpha waves, 8 - 12 cps

Theta waves   Theta waves

Stage 1 - theta waves, 3 - 7 cps

K complex and sleep spindle   K complex

Stage 2 - K complexes and sleep spindles, 12 - 14 cps

Delta waves

Stage 3 - delta waves, 1/2 - 2 cps

Delta waves

Stage 4 - predominantly delta waves, 1/2 - 2 cps

Sawtooth waves

REM Sleep - sawtooth waves, low voltage, fast

TABLE 69–2

EFFECTS OF SLEEP ON VENTILATION IN NORMAL SUBJECTS*

Characteristic	NREM	REM
Breathing pattern	Periodic (stage 1, 2)[20–24] Regular (stage 3, 4)[20–24]	Irregular[20–24] ± apneas
Po_2	↓ 3–10 mm Hg[20, 25–28]	↓ [32–36]
Pco_2	↑ 2–8 mm Hg[20, 25–29]	↑ [37–40]
Alveolar ventilation	↓ [20, 21]	↓ ↓ [33, 38, 39]
Tidal volume	↓ [20, 21]	↓ ↓ [33, 38, 39]
Hypoxic ventilatory response	↓ [18, 38, 41–43, 46]	↓ ↓ [18, 38, 41–43, 46]
Hypercapnic ventilatory response	↓ [18, 39, 43–46]	↓ ↓ [18, 39, 43–46]
Oxygen consumption	↓ ↓ (15–25%)[20, 21, 47, 48]	↓ [20, 48]
Upper airway resistance	↑ [30]	↑ ↑ [31]

*All values compared with those during wakefulness.

with sleep-related respiratory disorders. Breathing is generated by a network oscillator thought to be situated primarily in the pons and medulla. There is evidence, however, that there may be respiratory pacemaker cells.[17] The major function of the central pattern generator for respiration is to maintain homeostasis in the respiratory system, that is, keep the arterial blood gases normal. The respiratory center receives information from three major sources: higher cortical centers, mechanical receptors in the chest wall and lung, and central and peripheral chemoreceptors.

Higher cortical centers can override the respiratory central pattern generator. During wakefulness cortical inputs can affect ventilation; for example, anxiety can cause hyperventilation. Similarly, during sleep, when dreaming occurs, the cortical centers may have a significant impact on the medullary respiratory neurons.[18] Receptors in the lung and chest wall send information to the respiratory center. Pulmonary receptors (stretch, rapidly adapting [irritant], and C fiber receptors) are all stimulated by different varieties of stimuli. Such stimuli include lung inflation, deflation, and inhaling noxious compounds. Stimulation of rapidly adapting and C fiber receptors results in a rapid, shallow breathing pattern secondary to reductions in tidal volume and inspiratory time.[18] The central pattern generator also receives information from the carotid body, which acts as the major peripheral chemoreceptor sensing changes in Po_2, Pco_2, and pH. The carotid body responds quickly to changes in Po_2 and is responsible for the increase in ventilation that occurs with hypoxia. The central chemoreceptors in the medulla respond primarily to changes in Pco_2 and/or pH. These receptors are thought to be situated in the ventrolateral medulla, relatively close to the surface of the fourth ventricle.[19]

There are many important physiologic effects of sleep on the respiratory system. These effects change during different sleep stages (Table 69–2). As noted in Table 69–2, the breathing pattern of normal subjects may be periodic in stage 1 and stage 2 sleep, particularly in the elderly, but becomes regular in stages 3 and 4.[20–24] In REM sleep the pattern of respiration is distinctly irregular and a small number of apneas may occur even in normal subjects.[20–24] Alveolar ventilation decreases during sleep, secondary primarily to a decrease in the tidal volume with resulting increases in Pco_2 and decreases in Po_2.[20, 21, 25–29] Upper airway resistance has been shown to be increased in sleep, which is a major determinant of the decrease in minute ventilation.[30, 31] The resultant hypoxemia and hypercapnia are more significant in REM sleep than in NREM sleep.[32–39] The ventilatory response to both hypercapnia and hypoxia is also reduced during sleep compared with waking levels, with many, although not all, studies showing a greater reduction

in REM sleep than in NREM sleep.[18, 38–46] Oxygen consumption decreases 15 to 25% in normal subjects during sleep.[20, 21, 47] In one study oxygen consumption was greater in REM sleep than in NREM sleep, but other studies have suggested that oxygen consumption is more dependent on circadian rhythms than on sleep stage.[47–49]

These physiologic changes that occur during sleep do not have major clinical significance in normal subjects, but in patients with underlying pulmonary disease they may have major implications.[16] Several studies have demonstrated that hypoxemia and hypercapnia associated with REM and NREM sleep are significant in patients with COPD, idiopathic pulmonary fibrosis, and cystic fibrosis.[32, 34–36] Patients with these diseases also have blunted responses to hypoxia and hypercapnia during sleep compared with wakefulness, which can contribute to the development of respiratory acidosis during sleep.[32, 34–36] In patients with COPD, arterial desaturations during sleep can approach 10 to 35% compared with baseline when they are awake.[34, 36, 40] Therefore, patients with COPD or any type of respiratory failure are at risk for significant hypoxemia and hypercapnia during sleep.

The physiologic changes that occur during sleep affect not only the control of the respiratory system but also the cardiovascular system. The hemodynamic changes that occur during sleep are summarized in Table 69–3. In general, blood pressure decreases during NREM sleep and fluctuates considerably during REM sleep (at times blood pressure during REM sleep may be elevated over levels during wakefulness).[20, 21, 50–55] The heart rate drops 5 to 10% during NREM sleep and has considerable variability during REM sleep. Cardiac output decreases in NREM sleep and is variable in REM sleep.[20, 21, 51, 54] These hemodynamic changes may be important in hypotensive patients and those with low cardiac outputs. It is important for physicians managing

TABLE 69–3

HEMODYNAMIC CHANGES DURING SLEEP IN NORMAL SUBJECTS*

Characteristic†	NREM	REM
BP	↓ 10–15%[20, 50, 51, 55]	Variable, higher than NREM[20, 50, 51, 55]
HR	↓ 5–10%[20, 52, 53]	Variable, resting level[20, 52, 53]
CO	↓ 10%[20, 21, 51, 54]	Variable, ↓ [20, 21, 51, 54]
SVR	↓ [20, 21]	↓ [20, 21]
PAP	↑ [20]	↑ [20]

*Values compared with those during wakefulness.
†BP = blood pressure; HR = heart rate; CO = cardiac output; SVR = systemic vascular resistance; PAP = pulmonary arterial pressure.

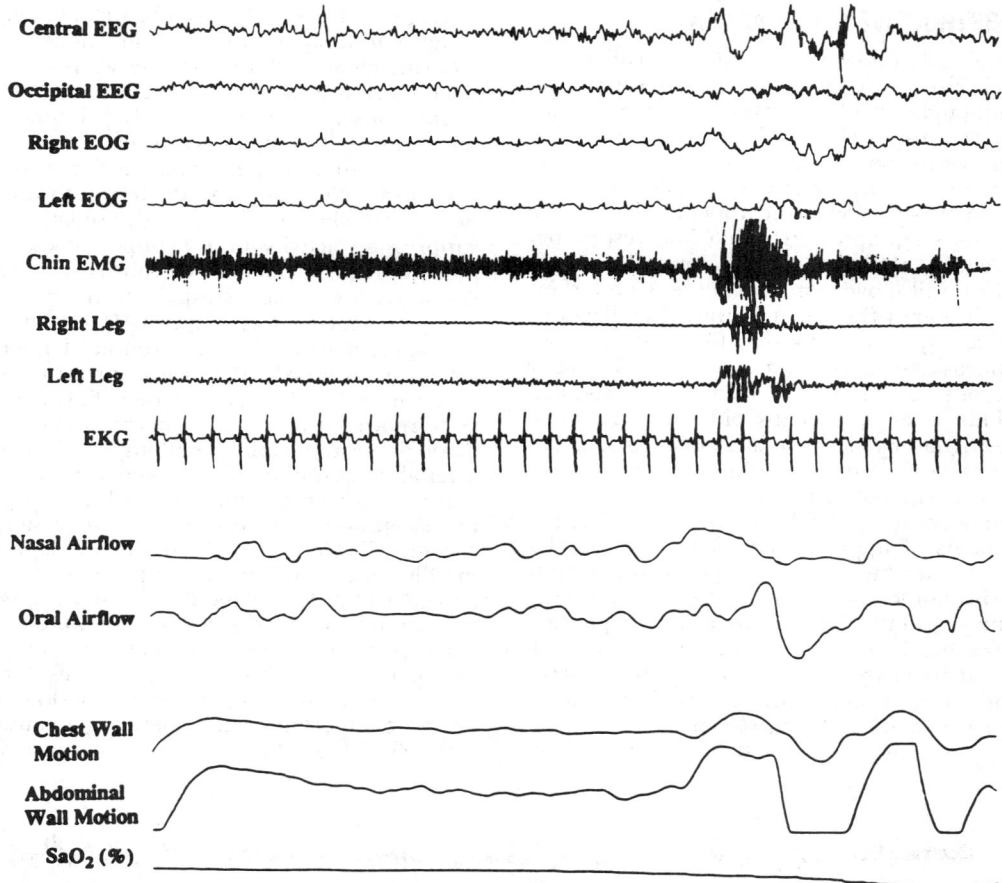

Figure 69–2. Polysomnogram of a patient with central sleep apnea syndrome. Note the lack of nasal and oral airflow in conjunction with the lack of chest wall and abdominal motion during the apnea. The latter indicates absence of respiratory effort. At the end of the central apnea there is an arousal, as shown by the increase in EMG activity. EOG = electro-oculogram; EMG = electromyogram; EKG = electrocardiogram; SaO_2 = arterial oxyhemoglobin saturation. (Polysomnogram courtesy of the Penn Center for Sleep Disorders.)

patients in ICUs or cardiac care units to be aware of the hemodynamic and ventilatory changes that occur in patients during sleep. Certain changes that they observe in these closely monitored situations may be consequences of normal physiologic alterations.

CENTRAL SLEEP APNEA

Central sleep apnea is defined as recurrent episodes of apnea (cessation of airflow for 10 seconds or more) during sleep in the absence of any respiratory muscle effort.[16, 56–58] The pathogenesis of central sleep apnea involves temporary abolition of central drive to the respiratory pump muscles. These apneic episodes result in repeated periods of hypoxia, hypercapnia, and acidemia. Central sleep apnea may be idiopathic or associated with a number of neurologic conditions, including autonomic dysfunction, neuromuscular disease, Shy-Drager syndrome, bulbar poliomyelitis, myasthenia gravis, encephalitis, and brain stem infarct.[16, 56, 58, 59] Any disease affecting the central pattern generator can lead to central sleep apnea. The clinical features of central sleep apnea have a wide spectrum from little physiologic significance to end-stage pulmonary hypertension and right-sided heart failure. Recurrent episodes of respiratory failure and chronic alveolar hypoventilation are found predominantly in patients whose central sleep apnea is a manifestation of a defect in the respiratory center or neuromuscular system.[16, 60]

These patients with hypercapnic central sleep apnea develop hypoxemia, right-sided heart failure, pulmonary hypertension, and polycythemia. On the other hand, patients with nonhypercapnic central sleep apnea, secondary to transient abnormalities in respiratory drive during sleep, do not develop chronic pulmonary or cardiovascular complications but present with insomnia, sleep disruption, daytime sleepiness, and frequent arousals during the night.[16, 56, 60]

The diagnosis of central sleep apnea is made by demonstrating recurrent episodes of apnea without chest wall or abdominal wall movement on a polysomnogram (Fig. 69–2). When central sleep apnea is diagnosed, patents should be studied during the day to determine whether they hypoventilate during wakefulness. This can be determined by assessing their arterial PCO_2. The management of patients with central sleep apnea is dependent on whether they have hypercapnic or nonhypercapnic sleep apnea. In patients with nonhypercapnic central sleep apnea management strategies include acetazolamide, oxygen, and nasal continuous positive airway pressure (CPAP).[61–65] CPAP is reasonable first-line therapy in patients with nonhypercapnic central sleep apnea, but the mechanism of CPAP therapy in this condition is not clear, although it may involve stimulation of upper airway afferents.[64, 65] In patients with hypercapnic central sleep apnea the treatment is the same as that for primary alveolar hypoventilation syndrome and consists of some form of nocturnal ventilation (see under Nasal Nocturnal Ventilation).

OBSTRUCTIVE SLEEP APNEA

Obstructive apneas, secondary to intermittent collapse of the upper airway, are more common during sleep than central apneas, although mixed patterns can occur. Obstructive sleep apnea syndrome (OSAS) is a common clinical problem with a prevalence of at least 1 to 4% in the general population.[66] It is defined as recurrent episodes of apnea during sleep caused by occlusion of the upper airway. Unlike patients with central sleep apnea, who have no respiratory drive, in patients with OSAS there is respiratory effort (chest wall and abdominal wall movement) but there is no airflow because of the occlusion of the upper airway. The diagnosis can be made with a polysomnogram (Fig. 69–3) demonstrating repetitive apneas associated with arousals and usually arterial desaturations. The disorders commonly associated with OSAS include obesity, hypothyroidism, facial bone abnormalities (retrognathia, micrognathia), macroglossia, acromegaly, nasal obstruction, hypertrophy of the uvula, and adenoidal or tonsillar enlargement.[67]

The exact pathogenesis of OSAS is not clear, but the primary determinants of upper airway caliber are intraluminal pressure and the activity of the upper airway dilator muscles. The extrathoracic location of the upper airway exposes it to positive intraluminal pressure during expiration and negative intraluminal pressure during inspiration. In the awake state, activity of the upper airway dilator muscles during inspiration counterbalances the negative intraluminal pressure generated by chest wall contraction.[68, 69] Many patients with sleep apnea have a narrowed upper airway even during wakefulness. This can be well demonstrated by newer imaging techniques, including magnetic resonance imaging and cine computed tomography scans[70] (Fig. 69–4). During sleep there is a decrease in the activity of the upper airway dilator muscles; this is especially prominent in REM sleep, the period when obstructive events are usually most severe.[16, 66, 69, 71, 72] Without upper airway dilator muscle activity, negative intraluminal pressure during inspiration promotes upper airway closure. Accordingly, sedatives and alcohol, by suppressing activity of the upper airway dilator muscles, increase the incidence of obstructive sleep apnea.[73–75] An obstructive apnea is usually terminated by moving from a deeper stage of sleep (e.g., REM) to a lighter stage of sleep (or wakefulness) with an arousal. Upper airway dilator activity is restored by this arousal process and airway patency is regained.[16, 69] The patient then falls back asleep and the cycle repeats itself. This cycle can occur hundreds of times throughout the night, resulting in repetitive episodes of arterial desaturation and markedly fragmented sleep.

It is not surprising that the cardinal symptoms of obstructive sleep apnea are excessive daytime sleepiness and loud snoring (Table 69–4). The disease is most common in middle-aged men but can be present in both sexes and in all age groups.[16] In patients with sleep apnea, loud snoring is followed by quiet periods interrupted by loud "snorts" when breathing is restored. Many patients indicate that their bed partners witness apneas. Patients may fall asleep at inappropriate times, such as in the middle of a conversation or, more important, while operating an automobile. Patients with OSAS have three to seven times as many car accidents

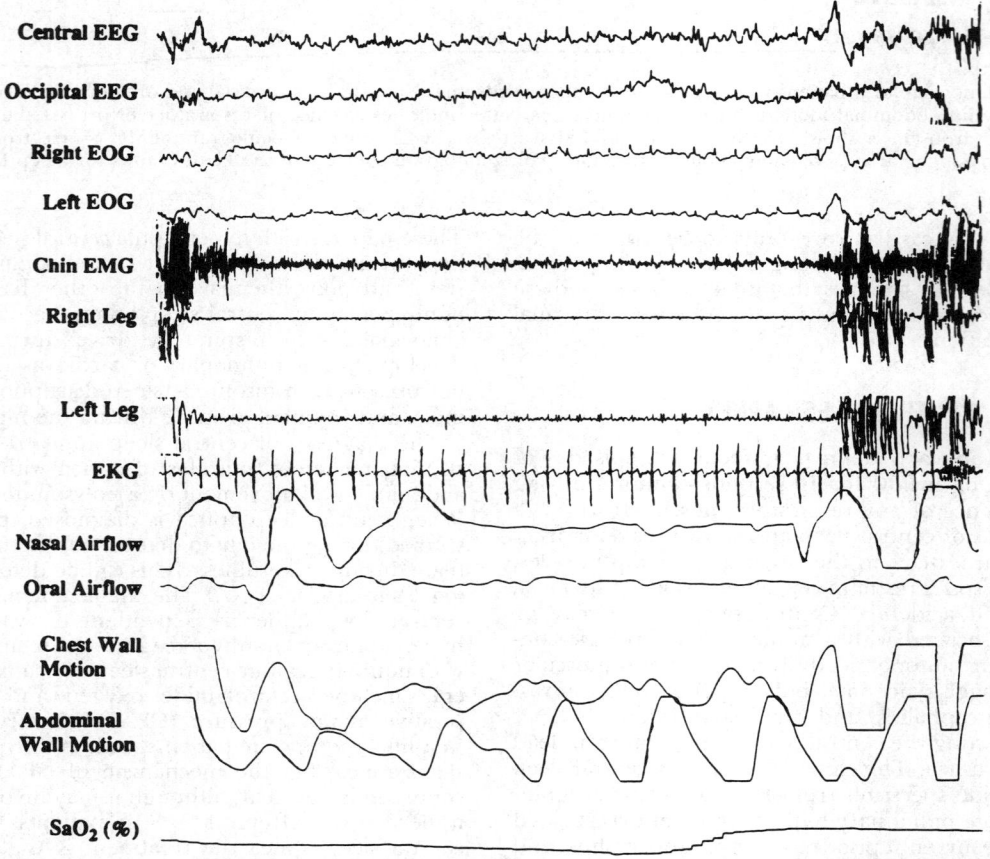

Figure 69–3. Polysomnogram of a patient with obstructive sleep apnea syndrome (OSAS). Note the lack of nasal and oral airflow with persistent chest wall and abdominal motion during the apnea. During the apnea there is a drop in the arterial oxyhemoglobin saturation curve (SaO₂), as well as abdominal and chest wall paradox. At the end of the apnea there is an arousal, as shown by the increase in EMG activity. (Polysomnogram courtesy of the Penn Center for Sleep Disorders.)

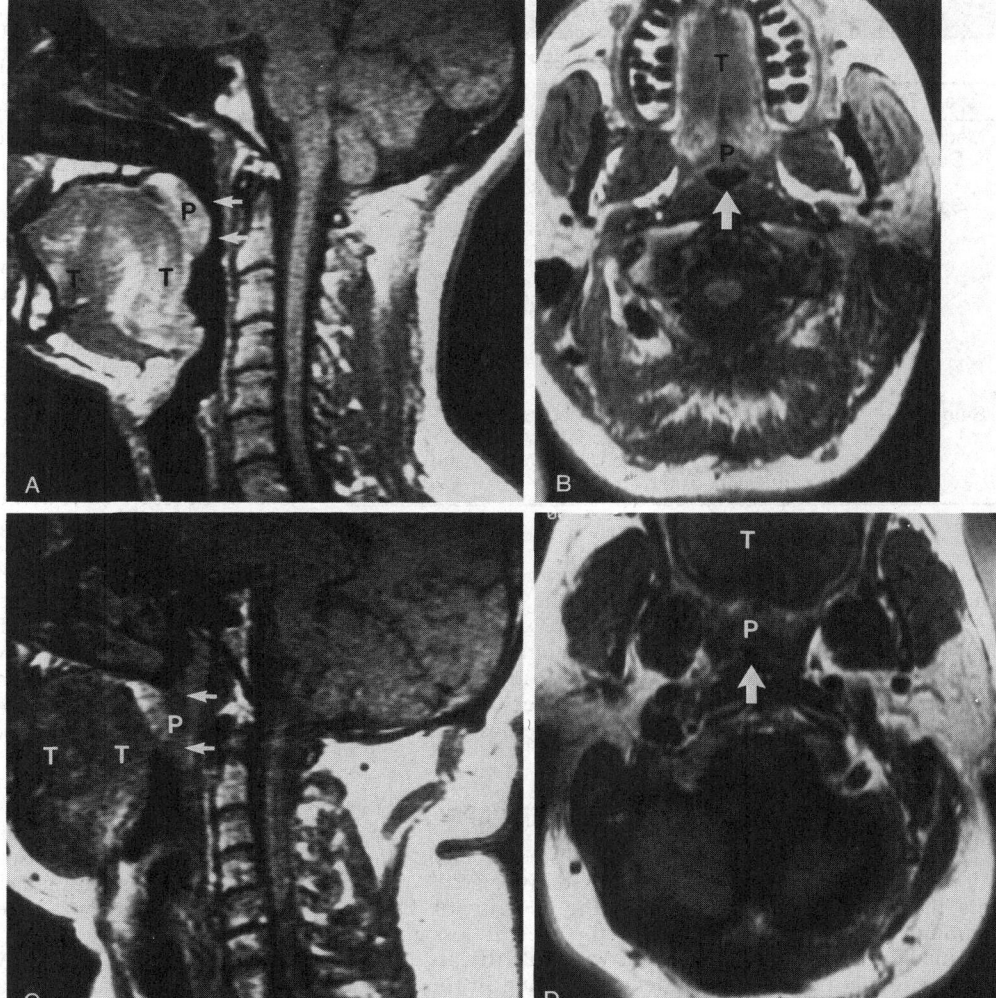

Figure 69–4. *A–D.* Differences in size of the upper airway between a normal subject and a patient with OSAS. *A.* Midline sagittal magnetic resonance image in a normal subject. Note the normal configuration of the retropalatal airway (*arrows*). *B.* Axial magnetic resonance image in the same normal subject at the level of the soft palate. Note the normal size and configuration of the airway at this level (*arrow*). *C.* Midline sagittal magnetic resonance image in a patient with OSAS. Note the virtual obliteration of the retropalatal airway (*arrows*). *D.* Axial magnetic resonance image in the same patient with OSAS at the level of the soft palate. Note the marked narrowing of the airway at this level (*arrow*).

as normal subjects, presumably because of their overwhelming sleepiness.[76, 77] The patients with the most severe sleep apnea (determined by arterial oxyhemoglobin desaturation during apneic episodes) have the highest car accident rates.[76, 78] Patients with milder disease maintain wakefulness in conversation but fall asleep when not engaged in other activities, for example, at meetings or when watching television. Other classic symptoms include personality changes (especially irritability), morning headaches, intellectual impairment, palpitations, and memory loss.[57, 66, 67, 79] The car-

dinal signs of OSAS include obesity, mild hypertension, and in severe cases cardiac arrhythmias, pulmonary hypertension, edema, and polycythemia.[57, 66, 67, 79] Approximately 10 to 15% of patients with severe OSAS develop pulmonary hypertension and right-sided heart failure. In mild cases of OSAS none of these signs may develop. It appears that daytime hypoxemia and hypercapnia in addition to nighttime hypoxemia are necessary for development of pulmonary hypertension and right-sided heart failure.[16, 80]

The "gold standard" for making the diagnosis of obstructive sleep apnea is an overnight polysomnogram (see Fig. 69–3) demonstrating repeated apneic episodes in the presence of respiratory effort, associated with arousals and arterial oxyhemoglobin desaturations. Overnight oximetry, which may detect recurrent oxyhemoglobin desaturations associated with apneic episodes, can be used for screening, although the accuracy of this test has not been fully determined in large studies.[16] Furthermore, overnight polysomnography, in contrast to oximetry, provides enough information to determine whether other conditions causing excessive daytime sleepiness, such as nocturnal myoclonus, are present. The multiple sleep latency test may be performed to determine the severity of daytime sleepiness. In a normal patient the mean latency to sleep during the naps of the latency test is more than 10 minutes, whereas in a patient with sleep apnea the mean latency to sleep is usually less than 5 minutes (pathologic sleepiness) and may be lower.

TABLE 69–4
DIAGNOSIS AND EVALUATION OF OBSTRUCTIVE SLEEP APNEA SYNDROME
Clinical clues to the diagnosis of OSAS
Middle-aged, overweight men
Loud snoring
Excessive daytime sleepiness
Witnessed apneas
Hypertension
Unexplained hypercapnia or pulmonary hypertension
Work-up of OSAS
Screening overnight oximetry (optional)
Overnight polysomnogram (gold standard for the diagnosis)
Multiple sleep latency test to determine degree of sleepiness

TABLE 69–5

TREATMENT OF OBSTRUCTIVE SLEEP APNEA

Type of Therapy	Treatment
Medical	
General measures	Weight loss
	Avoidance of alcohol, sedatives
Specific measures	Positional therapy
	Sleeping primarily in lateral positions (for patients with mild disease)
	Orthodontic devices
	Tongue-retaining devices
	Pharmacologic agents
	Oxygen
	Nasal CPAP
	BiPAP
Surgical	Treatment of nasal obstruction
	Uvulopalatopharyngoplasty
	Hyoid or mandibular advancement
	Tracheostomy

In patients with severe obstructive sleep apnea REM episodes can be demonstrated on naps during the latency test that resemble those in a patient with narcolepsy. This is presumably caused by the severe sleep fragmentation and deprivation. The polysomnogram can be helpful in stratifying the severity of disease and determining whether the apneas are position dependent, occurring in the supine position but not in the lateral decubitus position.[81–83]

TREATMENT OF OBSTRUCTIVE SLEEP APNEA

Treatment modalities for OSAS are listed in Table 69–5. All patients should avoid alcohol and sedatives.[57, 73–75] Weight loss has been shown to decrease the severity of OSAS, although it is difficult to sustain the weight loss in this population of patients.[84] In patients with mild disease apneas may be totally position dependent, occurring in the supine but not in the lateral decubitus position. For patients with position-dependent sleep apnea, sleeping in the lateral decubitus posture often alleviates the apnea.[81, 82] This is accomplished by inserting a tennis ball in a pocket sewn in the back of the patient's night shirt to prevent the patient from lying in the supine position. Tongue-retaining and mandibular-positioning devices have been helpful in some patients, but there are only a few studies showing efficacy and this therapy has not been widely used.[79, 85, 86] Pharmacologic agents that have been used in the past include acetazolamide and medroxyprogesterone, which increase ventilatory drive, and protriptyline, which increases upper airway muscle tone and decreases the amount of REM sleep.[57, 87–90] Each of these medications has significant side effects and none has been shown conclusively to result in substantial improvement in patients with OSAS.[67] Oxygen therapy abolishes apneas in some patients but increases the number of apneas in other patients.[67, 91–94] Oxygen therapy may blunt oxyhemoglobin desaturations but is unlikely to alter the degree of sleep fragmentation caused by the obstructive apneas or the resultant excessive daytime sleepiness. Therefore, oxygen therapy should be considered only for patients who do not respond to conventional therapy.[93]

The treatment of choice at present for patients with OSAS is nasal CPAP therapy. This therapy has been shown convincingly to reduce the incidence of apneic episodes and the daytime sleepiness in patients with both obstructive and central sleep apnea.[64, 65, 95–97] It provides a pneumatic splint for the airway, preventing collapse during sleep when upper airway dilator muscle activity is reduced. The pressure

necessary to abolish apneas varies between patients and should be determined in the sleep laboratory. Nasal CPAP therapy is well tolerated, and several studies have confirmed long-term compliance with this type of therapy.[97–99] Local problems related to the airflow and increased pressure, such as rhinitis and nasal irritation, may occur but usually can be treated with either humidification of the CPAP system or nasal decongestants.

A newer technique for delivering positive airway pressure has been developed that allows independent regulation of the inspiratory positive airway pressure (IPAP) and expiratory positive airway pressure (EPAP). This system, called BiPAP (bilevel positive airway pressure), can decrease the need for high levels of expiratory pressure while maintaining high levels of inspiratory pressure.[100] Because the negative intraluminal pressure during inspiration tends to collapse the airway and the positive intraluminal pressure during expiration tends to widen the airway, the IPAP level of conventional CPAP may be more important than the EPAP level of CPAP.[68, 69, 100] Furthermore, reduction in EPAP levels using the BiPAP system should decrease the high mean airway pressure generated with routine CPAP and improve the comfort of the patient. In one study BiPAP has been shown to be as effective as conventional CPAP in patients with OSAS.[100] However, BiPAP is more expensive than conventional CPAP therapy and has not yet been shown to be more effective than conventional CPAP. BiPAP should be reserved for patients who do not tolerate CPAP, particularly for those who report difficulties with exhalation. Newer CPAP systems are also capable of maintaining relative airway pressure stability during respiration and ramping up to a prescribed CPAP pressure. These CPAP machines use a feedback system with a microprocessor to maintain a stable CPAP pressure during inspiration and expiration. The ramp function enables these machines to increase the CPAP pressure gradually over a selected time interval from a low pressure to the prescribed set pressure. When patients use this ramp system, the CPAP pressure is lowest while they are falling asleep and increases after they have fallen asleep.

In general, surgical therapy for patients with OSAS should be reserved for patients with specific anatomic abnormalities or selected patients who do not respond to CPAP therapy. Nasal surgery can be helpful if there is a discrete nasal obstruction such as a tumor or polyp.[67, 101] Nasal septal deviation may exacerbate apneic episodes but by itself is not usually a cause of significant OSAS.[67] In patients with clear cephalometric abnormalities (i.e., micrognathia, retrognathia), a mandibular advancement procedure may be indicated.[67, 102, 103] Similarly, patients with OSAS who have marked tonsillar or adenoidal hypertrophy usually improve when these tissues are removed.[101]

The most common surgical procedure for OSAS is uvulopalatopharyngoplasty (UPPP).[104] This procedure consists of removal of the tonsils and adenoids, uvula, distal margin of the soft palate, and any excessive pharyngeal tissue. In nonselected patients with OSAS, UPPP decreases the respiratory disturbance index by 50% in 50 to 60% of patients.[104–107] Success rate in patients undergoing a UPPP appears to be related to the site of obstruction; patients with oropharyngeal (retropalatal) obstruction have the best results and those with hypopharyngeal obstruction have the worst results.[104–107] Computed tomographic scans have been used to help determine which category a patient fits into.[107] Unfortunately, in most patients with OSAS the upper airway is narrowed in multiple sites, making it difficult to achieve success solely with a UPPP.[104] Many patients who undergo a UPPP may still require nasal CPAP therapy. UPPP has several significant complications (pain, infection, hemorrhage, nasopharyngeal reflux, and rhinolalia) and at least a

50% failure rate. It should be reserved for selected patients with oropharyngeal obstruction who fail or refuse nasal CPAP therapy.[67, 104]

Tracheostomy is still a viable treatment for patients with OSAS but should be considered only for patients with severe disease resulting in incapacitating hypersomnolence, malignant arrhythmias, and/or cardiac failure who have not responded to medical or surgical therapy.[67, 104] Tracheostomy is usually 100% effective in relieving OSAS but is not easily accepted by patients. Gastric bypass has also been performed in patients with OSAS with favorable results.[108, 109] This type of surgery should be limited to morbidly obese patients with significant sleep apnea in whom other modalities of weight loss have failed. Before surgery, methods for controlling the apneas during sleep are required.

Regardless of the type of therapy chosen, patients with OSAS should be followed closely by a physician familiar with sleep-related breathing disorders. Periodic assessment of the patient's response to therapy is necessary. Patients may need periodic home oximetry or other studies to make sure that they are not developing nocturnal arterial desaturation and that their level of CPAP is still adequate.[67] Although the treatment of OSAS has come a long way, the present treatment modalities still have significant limitations and newer medical and/or surgical treatment regimens need to be developed.

OBESITY-HYPOVENTILATION SYNDROME

Although most patients (75%) with OSAS are obese, only 10 to 15% hypoventilate when they are awake with resulting daytime hypercapnia and hypoxemia.[16, 80] Such patients often experience pulmonary hypertension and right-sided heart failure and are said to have the obesity-hypoventilation, or pickwickian, syndrome. It is not entirely clear why obese patients develop daytime hypercapnia, but it appears to involve a decrease in central respiratory drive in conjunction with a reduction in chest wall compliance secondary to obesity.[110–113] Multiple modalities have been used in the treatment of the obesity-hypoventilation syndrome. Weight loss and correction of any lower airway obstruction (bronchodilator therapy) are reasonable initial therapeutic alternatives.[84, 111] Progesterone has been used with varying results to try to augment central respiratory drive.[114, 115] Tracheostomy and nasal CPAP therapy have been used with reasonable success in these patients.[95, 113, 116] Lastly, nasal ventilation during sleep has been a successful method of correcting hypercapnia in these patients.[117] In patients with obesity-hypoventilation syndrome and obstructive apneas, a reasonable initial approach is to use nasal CPAP at a level that alleviates the obstructive apneas and hypopneas. Supplemental oxygen may be needed to blunt the oxyhemoglobin desaturations that accompany the breathing disorders during sleep. If this fails to relieve the nocturnal hypercapnia, nocturnal ventilation with a nasal mask should be the next line of therapy.

NASAL NOCTURNAL VENTILATION

The management of patients with daytime hypercapnia secondary to central sleep apnea, obesity-hypoventilation syndrome, primary alveolar hypoventilation syndrome, neuromuscular disease, and other causes of extrapulmonary ventilatory failure is similar, with some type of ventilatory assistance being necessary to correct the hypercapnia and respiratory acidosis. In these patients, ventilation limited to nighttime use can often correct the daytime hypercapnia. One of the newer, innovative and noninvasive treatment modalities for extrapulmonary respiratory failure is nocturnal nasal positive pressure ventilation. In nasal ventilation, a CPAP mask or nasal "pillows" (which fit directly into the nostrils) are used with a conventional volume-cycled ventilator. In general, the assist control mode of ventilation is chosen with a tidal volume set at approximately 10 mL/kg. Pressure cycle ventilation can also be used for nasal ventilation. One such system is the BiPAP S/T system. Using this system, a high level of inspiratory pressure (15 to 20 cm H_2O) should be sufficient to ventilate the patient. A back-up respiratory rate can support the patient if the rate falls below a preset value. Regardless of the mode of ventilation, the respiratory rate should be adjusted to maintain an appropriate P_{CO_2}. For patients with severe hypercapnia, the respiratory rate should be increased gradually over several nights to avoid a precipitous drop in P_{CO_2}. A patient being initially prepared for nocturnal ventilation should be admitted to an ICU or step-down unit to familiarize the patient with the ventilator and set up the initial parameters. Table 69–6 provides a protocol for initiation of nasal ventilation. The exhaled volume in patients undergoing nasal ventilation is usually lower than the tidal volume set on the ventilator because of leaks in the mask and system. Therefore, the delivered tidal volume should be increased until the exhaled volume (measured on the ventilator or with a hand-held spirometer) is approximately equal to the desired tidal volume. A chin strap may be necessary to prevent mouth leaks. There have been many studies demonstrating the efficiency of nocturnal nasal ventilation in patients with alveolar hypoventilation syndromes, neuromuscular disease, kyphoscoliosis, and other causes of restrictive lung disease, quadriplegia, and the pickwickian syndrome.[118–124]

SLEEP IN THE INTENSIVE CARE UNIT

Consideration of sleep and sleep physiology is also of general relevance to management of all patients in ICUs. One important aspect is how sleep deprivation affects such patients. ICUs have expanded, with more critically ill patients being treated with sophisticated life-support devices in a high-technology environment. Sleep can become difficult in this setting of frequent diagnostic, therapeutic, and nursing procedures. In this environment, light and sound levels are often well above normal, resulting in sensory overload.[125] Lighting in the ICU is usually on for 24 hours, disturbing sleep patterns and possibly affecting circadian rhythms.[125] Noise is a constant source of stimulation. The average noise level in the ICU can remain high over 24 hours because of the need for constant monitoring. To fall asleep, noise levels of less than 35 to 40 dB are recommended (although the exact level depends on the type of noise and whether it is continuous or episodic).[125] However, in the ICU noise levels ranging from 45 to 80 dB have been recorded.[125–127] Other causes of sleep disturbance in the ICU include crowding, noxious odors, pain, and frequent contact with patients. Pain experienced by recovering patients is an especially common problem leading to sleep disturbances in the ICU.[125]

Sensory overload with resultant sleep deprivation is thought to lead to the so-called ICU syndrome, or ICU psychosis.[128] The clinical manifestations of this syndrome include a spectrum of psychologic reactions including depression, delirium, anxiety, hallucinations, fear, and disorientation.[128] Patients manifesting this syndrome can become combative, confused, and extremely difficult to manage. The ICU syndrome is of significant concern because it can hinder clinical recovery by adding stress to the patient's psychologic and physical status.[129] Although a number of factors (severity of illness, age, medications, metabolic aberrations) can contribute to the ICU syndrome, sleep depri-

TABLE 69–6

NASAL VENTILATION PROTOCOL

I. Set-up
  A. Elective admission to ICU or step-down unit
    1. Mean length of stay 4–5 d to adjust to nocturnal ventilation.
    2. Obtain appropriate fitting CPAP mask or nasal pillows.
      a. Chin strap may be needed to keep the mouth closed.
II. Ventilator parameters
  A. Volume cycled
    1. Tidal volume
      a. For most patients, use 10 mL/kg.
      b. Obese patients (>100 kg), use 5–7 mL/kg.
    2. Respiratory rate
      a. Adjust rate to obtain appropriate Pco_2; start with 12 breaths/min.
    3. Fio_2
      a. In patients with a normal alveolar-arterial gradient, room air (Fio_2 21%) is usually sufficient.
      b. Aim to keep oxygen saturations > 92–94%.
    4. Mode
      a. Assist control mode is preferred for most patients.
  B. Pressure cycled (BiPAP S/T)
    1. Pressure levels
      a. Initial IPAP of 18–20 cm H_2O and EPAP of 2 cm H_2O.
    2. Respiratory rate
      a. Initial timed respiratory rate of 12 breaths/min.
      b. To decrease Pco_2, increase either IPAP or respiratory rate or both.
    3. Fio_2
      a. In patients with a normal alveolar-arterial gradient, room air (Fio_2 21%) is usually sufficient.
      b. Aim to keep oxygen saturations > 92–94%.
    4. Mode
      a. Use spontaneous/timed mode.
III. Monitoring nasal ventilation
  A. Exhaled volume (for volume-cycled ventilator)
    1. Although exhaled volume should theoretically equal the tidal volume, because of leaks in the system the exhaled volume is often less than the tidal volume.
    2. Increase the tidal volume until the average exhaled volume (measure on the ventilator or with a hand-held spirometer) equals the desired tidal volume.
  B. Arterial blood oxygen saturation (Sao_2)
    1. Oximeters are needed to adjust Fio_2, keep $Sao_2 \geq$ 92%.
  C. Pco_2
    1. Arterial blood gases should be checked frequently to determine appropriate Pco_2 and make ventilator adjustments. An indwelling arterial line can be used.
  D. Arterial blood gases
    1. A morning arterial blood gas analysis with the patient awake should be obtained 2–3 d after implementing nocturnal nasal ventilation to evaluate Pco_2 before and after ventilation.

vation is clearly a component.[128, 129] Some of the mental status changes observed in the ICU appear to be reproduced in normal subjects with experimental sleep deprivation.[129, 130] After 2 to 5 days of sleep deprivation, experimental subjects develop slurred speech, irritability, and disorientation.[129, 130] Further sleep deprivation in experimental subjects results in hallucinations and paranoia. When these sleep-deprived subjects were allowed one night of normal sleep, the signs of psychosis resolved; analogously, when patients are transferred out of the ICU the symptoms of this syndrome disappear.[129, 130] The ICU syndrome usually occurs on the third to seventh day after admission to the ICU and can remit within 48 hours of leaving the ICU.[125]

Patients in the ICU manifest signs of both sleep deprivation and sleep fragmentation (inability to progress through the normal sleep stages), both of which can contribute to the ICU syndrome.[131, 132] Polysomnographic studies of patients' sleep patterns in the ICU suggest that multiple abnormalities occur.[133] ICU patients manifest increased stage 1 sleep, increased arousals with awakenings, increased latency to sleep onset with decreased REM sleep, shortened REM periods, and decreased total sleep efficiency.[132–134] It has been demonstrated that patients in the ICU often sleep during the day.[131] Consequently, they are deprived of normal amounts of sleep, continuity of sleep stages, and time for quality sleep.

Research is needed to further investigate sleep patterns in the ICU, and effective means of enhancing sleep in the ICU need to be developed. In the meantime, certain recommendations can be made to enhance the quality of sleep in the ICU: (1) all ICUs should be built with individual rooms for patients so that noise and light can be minimized by closing observation doors; (2) to reduce sensory overload, especially at night, conversation should be minimized and noise control structures and light dimmers should be used (it is important to try to maintain normal light-dark cycles that entrain the circadian rhythm); (3) safe alarm systems must be developed that alert the staff to potential medical problems but do not disturb sleep; (4) the routine practice of obtaining vital signs throughout the night, early morning chest radiographs, or phlebotomy (5:00 to 6:30 AM) should be followed only if absolutely necessary; (5) procedures and interventions (including baths and bed changes) should be planned to maximize uninterrupted sleep time so that patients can attain consolidated sleep and deep sleep stages; (6) sleep should be considered a priority, not a luxury, in the ICU, because sleep deprivation can affect the patient's recovery and contribute to the ICU syndrome.[129, 131] For these initiatives to be implemented, ICU physicians and nurses must be aware of the sleep disturbances occurring in their patients and develop a coordinated plan to enhance the quality of sleep in their ICU.

Unfortunately, many of these initiatives are difficult to achieve in the ICU, and patients often require some type of sedation to sleep. The ideal sedative or hypnotic would be short acting, have minimal drug interactions, have no effects on the cardiovascular or pulmonary systems, and be able to simulate normal sleep patterns while not exerting its sedative effect beyond the routine sleep period.[135–137] Such a medication does not yet exist. At present, the benzodiazepines are the best hypnotics for patients in the ICU. Positive attributes of benzodiazepines include amnesia, anxiolysis, sedation, muscle relaxation, and the availability of short-acting preparations.[135] Unfortunately, benzodiazepines have significant effects on sleep architecture as well as on the control of the respiratory system. Benzodiazepines reduce delta sleep, enhance stage 2 sleep at the expense of other stages of sleep, and often have effects that last into the next day or night.[137, 138] Benzodiazepines have minimal or no effect on REM sleep.[139] Short-acting benzodiazepines (trizolam, midazolam, lorazepam) are the medications of choice for promoting sleep in the ICU without sedation being carried over into the next day or night.[135] Respiratory depressant effects of benzodiazepines are usually not significant in normal hosts but may become a significant problem in patients who tend to have alveolar hypoventilation. Hypercapnia may develop in the COPD patient being weaned from the ventilator if he or she is oversedated with benzodiazepines.[140] The benefits of sedation must be weighed against the side effects in all patients. Sleep is a major concern in the ICU, and physicians who run ICUs should be aware of the effects of sleep deprivation on physiologic function as well as mechanisms for enhancing sleep.

MEDICAL ILLNESSES EXACERBATED BY SLEEP

Several medical conditions may become worse during sleep, and this can have direct implications for the care of patients with these conditions in the ICU. Asthma is worse at night in many patients. Up to two thirds of asthmatics develop nocturnal bronchoconstriction, the cause of which is unclear.[141, 142] These asthmatic patients, who have been called "morning dippers," can have falls in the forced expiratory volume in 1 second and peak flow of 50% during the night.[141, 142] Unstable patients or patients recovering from recent asthmatic attacks commonly manifest nocturnal bronchoconstriction.[143] Studies have demonstrated that asthmatic attacks at night are not related to any specific sleep stage.[141] Asthmatic patients admitted to the ICU should be expected to experience falls in their expiratory flow rates at night. Weaning the asthmatic from the ventilator should be done cautiously at night. Therapeutic agents, including long-acting bronchodilators such as oral theophylline or oral beta-agonists, can be given before sleep to help prevent nocturnal bronchoconstriction.

Patients with COPD can deteriorate at night. As discussed under Control of Ventilation During Sleep, arterial oxyhemoglobin desaturations during sleep in patients with COPD can approach 10 to 35%, compared with a baseline during wakefulness.[34, 36, 40] The hypoxemic episodes are especially significant during REM sleep.[32-36] Similarly, hypercapnia can be exacerbated during sleep in patients with COPD, with the hypercapnic episodes being more significant in REM sleep than NREM sleep.[37-40] Cardiac arrhythmias can become an important problem at night in patients with COPD.[144, 145] Both ventricular and atrial ectopias have been associated with hypoxemic episodes during sleep in patients with COPD. Cardiac ischemia, demonstrated by ST depression on electrocardiograms, has been found in hypoxic patients with COPD.[145] Fortunately, most of the cardiac abnormalities can be reversed with oxygen administration. Patients with COPD exacerbations in the ICU should be monitored carefully for cardiac complications. Other patients with lung disease, including those with interstitial lung disease, cystic fibrosis, and restrictive lung disease (kyphoscoliosis), have been noted to have hypoxemia during sleep.[32, 35, 146-148] As a rule, any patient with significant lung disease residing in the ICU is at risk of developing hypoxemia during sleep.

Little is known about the interaction of sleep and cardiovascular disease, yet ischemic episodes and arrhythmias often occur at night.[149] Nocturnal angina is a common entity in both REM sleep and NREM sleep, although there is no predominance in a specific sleep stage.[150, 151] There appears to be a propensity for myocardial infarction to occur between 6:00 AM and 12:00 noon, but again the relationship to sleep physiology is unclear.[152, 153] More research is needed to determine the frequency of nocturnal angina and myocardial infarction during sleep and whether these disorders are related to dreaming and REM sleep. The incidence of ventricular arrhythmias has been demonstrated to increase, decrease, or remain the same during sleep; similar findings have been reported with ventricular arrhythmias and sleep stage.[149, 154-156] Some patients are predisposed to ventricular arrhythmias at night, but it is not clear what factors precipitate the rhythm disturbance and whether it is sleep related. It is reasonable, however, to monitor via telemetry all patients with coronary artery disease or arrhythmias admitted to the ICU.

PRIMARY SLEEP DISORDERS AND RESPIRATORY FAILURE

Many patients who come to the ICU in respiratory failure actually have an underlying sleep disorder. For example, a typical patient admitted to the ICU with respiratory failure requiring intubation often has obesity, shortness of breath, cough, hypoxemia, hypercapnia, polycythemia, and right-sided heart failure. The working diagnosis is usually COPD. However, many of these patients do not have COPD but have underlying sleep apnea. How can we determine which patients have a sleep disorder? One simple test is voluntary hyperventilation for 30 to 60 seconds; in patients with intrinsic lung disease, hypercapnia is not usually corrected by hyperventilation, but in patients with respiratory control problems (central or obstructive sleep apnea or hypoventilation syndromes) hypercapnia can be corrected.[157] Similarly, alveolar-arterial oxygen gradients should be abnormal in patients with COPD but normal in patients with respiratory control problems. Pulmonary function tests also help to distinguish between COPD and sleep apnea. Patients with underlying sleep apnea often show some degree of restrictive pulmonary function results secondary to obesity rather than obstructive pulmonary function results secondary to lower airway obstruction. However, the simplest way to diagnose unsuspected sleep disorders is by history. Simple questioning of the patient or family about sleep problems (e.g., excessive daytime sleepiness, snoring, witnessed apneas) often suggests a diagnosis of a sleep disorder. If a sleep disorder is suspected, overnight polysomnography to confirm a diagnosis should be performed.

For patients with cor pulmonale, pulmonary hypertension may be a manifestation of OSAS. These patients experience recurrent hypoxemic episodes at night (secondary to the repeated apneas), leading to elevation of pulmonary artery pressures (hypoxic vasoconstriction), which, presumably, leads to chronic pulmonary hypertension. In all patients with unexplained pulmonary hypertension a diagnosis of sleep apnea should be considered. This is especially important because sleep apnea is a treatable condition, whereas most of the other causes of pulmonary hypertension are not treatable. As a general rule, all patients who present with unexplained hypercapnia, polycythemia, pulmonary hypertension, or cor pulmonale should be questioned about sleep apnea or hypoventilation syndromes and evaluated for these disorders if the symptom complex is suggestive.

Sleep apnea syndromes can also masquerade in other scenarios. For example, patients may initially have significant sleep apnea only after receiving sedatives, hypnotics, or narcotics.[158] After the administration of one of these medications, patients may experience significant apnea requiring admission to the ICU and/or mechanical ventilation. Such patients should have a work-up for sleep apnea or hypoventilation syndromes. Likewise, a patient who is difficult to wean after surgery may have an underlying sleep disorder causing persistent hypercapnia.[158] Patients with renal failure are at risk for sleep apnea, so any patient who develops respiratory failure in the presence of renal failure should at least be questioned about the possibility of sleep apnea.[159] Endocrine abnormalities including hypothyroidism can be associated with obstructive sleep apnea. Therefore, it is essential for physicians in the ICU to be familiar with sleep disorders, recognize the presentations, ask the appropriate questions, and be able to proceed with an evaluation of sleep apnea. It is important to remember that sleep-related breathing disorders are treatable conditions, unlike many of the conditions that we see in the ICU.

References

1. Balk R, Bone RC: Classification of acute respiratory failure. Med Clin North Am 67:551, 1983.
2. Pratter MR, Irwin RS: Respiratory failure. VI. Extrapulmonary causes. In: Rippe J, Csete M (eds): Manual of Intensive Care Medicine. Boston, Little, Brown, p 179, 1983.

3. Rogers RM, Gray BA: Recognition of acute and chronic respiratory failure and an algorithm for selecting therapy. In: Baum GL, Wolinsky E (eds): Textbook of Pulmonary Diseases. Boston, Little, Brown, p 949, 1983.
4. Williams MH, Shim CS: Ventilatory failure. Am J Med 48:477, 1970.
5. Demers RR, Irwin RS: Management of hypercapnic respiratory failure: A systematic approach. Respir Care 24:328, 1979.
6. Goldring RM, Cannon PJ, Heinemann HO, et al: Respiratory adjustment to chronic metabolic alkalosis in man. J Clin Invest 47:188, 1968.
7. Hughes JMB: Central respiratory failure reversed by treatment. Brain 90:675, 1967.
8. Garlind T, Linderholm H: Hypoventilation syndrome in a case of chronic epidemic encephalitis. Acta Med Scand 162:343, 1958.
9. Sivak ED, Streib EW: Management of hypoventilation in motor neuron disease presenting with respiratory insufficiency. Ann Neurol 7:188, 1980.
10. Devereaux MW, Keane JR, Davis RL: Automatic respiratory failure. Arch Neurol 29:46, 1973.
11. Colice GL, Bernat JL: Neurologic disorders and respiration. Clin Chest Med 10:521, 1989.
12. Phillipson EA: Hypoventilation syndromes. In: Murray JF, Nadel JA (eds): Textbook of Respiratory Medicine. Philadelphia, WB Saunders, p 1831, 1988.
13. Rhoads GG, Brody JS: Idiopathic alveolar hypoventilation: Clinical spectrum. Ann Intern Med 71:271, 1969.
14. Rodman T, Close HP: The primary hypoventilation syndrome. Am J Med 5:808, 1959.
15. Carskadon MA, Dement WA: Normal human sleep: An overview. In: Kryger MH, Roth T, Dement WC (eds): Principles and Practice of Sleep Medicine. Philadelphia, WB Saunders, p 3, 1989.
16. Phillipson EA: Sleep disorders. In: Murray JF, Nadel JA (eds): Textbook of Respiratory Medicine. Philadelphia, WB Saunders, p 1841, 1988.
17. Feldman JL, Smith JC: Cellular mechanisms underlying modulation of breathing pattern in mammals. Ann NY Acad Sci 563:114, 1989.
18. Douglas NJ: Control of ventilation during sleep. In: Kryger MH, Roth T, Dement WC (eds): Principles and Practice of Sleep Medicine. Philadelphia, WB Saunders, p 249, 1989.
19. Millhorn DE, Eldridge FL: Role of ventrolateral medulla in regulation of respiratory and cardiovascular systems. J Appl Physiol 61:1249, 1986.
20. Shepard JW Jr: Gas exchange and hemodynamics during sleep. Med Clin North Am 69:1243, 1985.
21. Shepard JW Jr: Cardiopulmonary consequences of obstructive sleep apnea. Mayo Clin Proc 65:1250, 1990.
22. Krieger J: Breathing during sleep in normal subjects. Clin Chest Med 6:577, 1985.
23. Shore ET, Millman RP, Silage DA, et al: Ventilatory and arousal patterns during sleep in normal young and elderly subjects. J Appl Physiol 59:1607, 1985.
24. Pack AI, Silage DA, Millman RP, et al: Spectral analysis of ventilation in elderly subjects awake and asleep. J Appl Physiol 64:1257, 1988.
25. Birchfield RI, Sieker HO, Heyman A: Alterations in respiratory function during natural sleep. J Lab Clin Med 54:216, 1959.
26. Birchfield RI, Sieker HO, Heyman A: Alterations in blood gases during natural sleep and narcolepsy: A correlation with the electroencephalographic stages of sleep. Neurology 8:107, 1958.
27. Bulow K: Respiration and wakefulness in man. Acta Physiol Scand 59(suppl 209):1, 1963.
28. Robin ED, Whaley RD, Crump CH, et al: Alveolar gas tensions, pulmonary ventilation and blood pH during physiologic sleep in normal subjects. J Clin Invest 37:981, 1958.
29. Reed DJ, Kellogg RH: Changes in respiratory response to CO_2 during natural sleep at sea level and at altitude. J Appl Physiol 13:325, 1958.
30. Henke KG, Dempsey JA, Kowitz JM, et al: Effects of sleep-induced increases in upper airway resistance on ventilation. J Appl Physiol 69:617, 1990.
31. Orem J, Netick A, Dement WC: Increased upper airway resistance to breathing during sleep in the cat. Electroencephalogr Clin Neurophysiol 43:14, 1977.
32. Muller NL, Francis PW, Gurwitz D, et al: Mechanism of hemoglobin desaturation during rapid-eye-movement sleep in normal subjects and in patients with cystic fibrosis. Am Rev Respir Dis 121:463, 1980.
33. Block AJ, Boysen PG, Wynne JW, et al: Sleep apnea, hypopnea and oxygen desaturation in normal subjects: A strong male predominance. N Engl J Med 300:513, 1979.
34. Fleetham JA, Mezon B, West P, et al: Chemical control of ventilation and sleep arterial oxygen desaturation in patients with COPD. Am Rev Respir Dis 122:583, 1980.
35. Tatsumi K, Kimura H, Kunitomo F, et al: Arterial oxygen desaturation during sleep in interstitial pulmonary disease: Correlation with chemical control of breathing during wakefulness. Chest 95:962, 1989.
36. Douglas NJ, Calverley PMA, Leggett RJE, et al: Transient hypoxaemia during sleep in chronic bronchitis and emphysema. Lancet 1:1, 1979.
37. Naifeh KH, Severinghaus JW, Kamiya J, et al: Effect of aging on estimates of hypercapnic ventilatory response during sleep. J Appl Physiol 66:1956, 1989.
38. Douglas NJ, White DP, Weil JV, et al: Hypoxic ventilatory response decreases during sleep in normal men. Am Rev Respir Dis 125:286, 1982.
39. Douglas NJ, White DP, Weil JV, et al: Hypoxic ventilatory response in sleeping adults. Am Rev Respir Dis 126:758, 1982.
40. Flick MR, Block AJ: Continuous in-vivo monitoring of arterial oxygenation in chronic obstructive lung disease. Ann Intern Med 86:725, 1977.
41. White DP, Douglas NJ, White DP, et al: Hypoxic ventilatory response decreases during sleep in normal premenopausal women. Am Rev Respir Dis 126:530, 1982.
42. Berthon-Jones M, Sullivan CE: Ventilatory and arousal responses to hypoxia in sleeping humans. Am Rev Respir Dis 125:632, 1982.
43. Hedemark LL, Kronenberg RS: Ventilatory and heart rate responses to hypoxia and hypercapnia during sleep in adults. J Appl Physiol 53:307, 1982.
44. Gothe B, Altose MD, Goldman MD, et al: Effect of quiet sleep on resting and CO_2-stimulated breathing in humans. J Appl Physiol 50:724, 1981.
45. Berthon-Jones M, Sullivan CE: Ventilation and arousal responses to hypercapnia in normal sleeping humans. J Appl Physiol 57:59, 1984.
46. Douglas NJ: Control of ventilation during sleep. Clin Chest Med 6:563, 1985.
47. Fraser G, Trinder J, Colrain IM, et al: Effect of sleep and circadian cycle on sleep period energy expenditure. J Appl Physiol 66:830, 1989.
48. Brebbia DR, Altshuler KZ: Oxygen consumption rate and electroencephalographic state of sleep. Science 150:1621, 1965.
49. Webb P, Hiestand M: Sleep metabolism and age. J Appl Physiol 38:257, 1975.
50. Coccagna G, Mantovani M, Brignani F, et al: Arterial pressure changes during spontaneous sleep in man. Electroencephalogr Clin Neurophysiol 31:277, 1971.
51. Khatri IM, Freis ED: Hemodynamic changes during sleep. J Appl Physiol 22:867, 1967.
52. Bristow JD, Honour AJ, Pickering TG, et al: Cardiovascular and respiratory changes during sleep in normal and hypertensive subjects. Cardiovasc Res 3:476, 1969.
53. Snyder F, Hobson JA, Morrison DF, et al: Changes in respiration, heart rate, and systolic blood pressure in human sleep. J Appl Physiol 19:417, 1964.
54. Miller JC, Horvath SM: Cardiac output during human sleep. Aviat Space Environ Med 47:1046, 1976.
55. Lugaresi E, Coccagna G, Farneti P, et al: Snoring. Electroencephalogr Clin Neurophysiol 39:59, 1975.
56. White DP: Central sleep apnea. In: Kryger MH, Roth T, Dement WC (eds): Principles and Practice of Sleep Medicine. Philadelphia, WB Saunders, p 513, 1989.
57. Kales A, Vela-Bueno A, Kales JD: Sleep disorders: Sleep apnea and narcolepsy. Ann Intern Med 106:434, 1987.
58. Tobin MJ, Cohn MA, Sackner MA: Breathing abnormalities during sleep. Arch Intern Med 143:1221, 1983.
59. McNicholas WT, Rutherford R, Grossman R, et al: Abnormal respiratory pattern generation during sleep in patients with autonomic dysfunction. Am Rev Respir Dis 128:429, 1983.
60. Bradley TD, McNicholas WT, Rutherford R, et al: Clinical and physiologic heterogeneity of the central sleep apnea syndrome. Am Rev Respir Dis 134:217, 1986.
61. White DP, Zwillich CW, Pickett CK, et al: Central sleep apnea: Improvement with acetazolamide therapy. Arch Intern Med 142:1816, 1982.
62. McNicholas WT, Carter JL, Rutherford R, et al: Beneficial effect of oxygen in primary alveolar hypoventilation with central sleep apnea. Am Rev Respir Dis 125:773, 1982.
63. Martin RJ, Sanders MH, Gray BA, et al: Acute and long-term ventilatory effects of hyperoxia in the adult sleep apnea syndrome. Am Rev Respir Dis 125:175, 1982.
64. Issa FG, Sullivan CE: Reversal of central sleep apnea using nasal CPAP. Chest 90:165, 1986.
65. Hoffstein V, Slutsky AS: Central sleep apnea reversed by continuous positive airway pressure. Am Rev Respir Dis 135:1210, 1987.
66. Strohl KP, Cherniack NS, Gothe B: Physiologic basis of therapy for sleep apnea. Am Rev Respir Dis 134:791, 1986.
67. Kaplan J, Staats BA: Obstructive sleep apnea. Mayo Clin Proc 65:1087, 1990.
68. Schwab RJ, Gefter WB, Kline LR, et al: Dynamic imaging of the upper airway during a respiratory cycle. Am Rev Respir Dis 143:A793, 1991.
69. Block AJ, Faulkner JA, Hughes RL, et al: Factors influencing upper airway closure. Chest 86:114, 1984.
70. Hoffman EA, Gefter WB: Multimodality imaging of the upper airway, MRI, MR spectroscopy, and ultrafast x-ray CT. In: Suratt P, Remmers JE (eds): Sleep and Respiration. New York, Wiley-Liss, p 291, 1990.
71. Sauerland EK, Orr WC, Hairston LE: EMG patterns of oropharyngeal muscles during respiration in wakefulness and sleep. Electromyogr Clin Neurophysiol 12:307, 1981.
72. Sauerland EK, Harper RM: The human tongue during sleep: Electromyographic activity of the genioglossus muscle. Exp Neurol 51:160, 1976.
73. Taasan VC, Block AJ, Boysen PG, et al: Alcohol increases sleep apnea and oxygen desaturation in asymptomatic men. Am J Med 71:240, 1981.
74. Dolly FR, Block AJ: Effect of flurazepam on sleep-disordered breathing and nocturnal oxygen desaturation in asymptomatic subjects. Am J Med 73:239, 1982.

75. Krol RC, Knuth SL, Bartlett D: Selective reduction of genioglossal muscle activity by alcohol in normal human subjects. Am Rev Respir Dis 129:247, 1984.
76. Findley LJ: Automobile driving in sleep apnea. In: Suratt P, Remmers JE (eds): Sleep and Respiration. New York, Wiley-Liss, p 337, 1990.
77. Findley LJ, Unverzagt ME, Suratt PM: Automobile accidents involving patients with obstructive sleep apnea. Am Rev Respir Dis 138:337, 1988.
78. Findley L, Fabrizio M, Thommi G, et al: Severity of sleep apnea and automobile crashes. N Engl J Med 320:868, 1989.
79. Westbrook PR: Sleep disorders and upper airway obstruction in adults. Otolaryngol Clin North Am 23:727, 1990.
80. Bradley TD, Rutherford R, Grossman RF, et al: Role of daytime hypoxemia in the pathogenesis of right heart failure in the obstructive sleep apnea syndrome. Am Rev Respir Dis 131:835, 1985.
81. Chaudhary BA, Chaudhary TK, Kolbeck RC, et al: Therapeutic effect of posture in sleep apnea. South Med J 79:1061, 1986.
82. Kavey NB, Blitzer A, Gidro-Frank S, et al: Sleeping position and sleep apnea syndrome. Am J Otolaryngol 6:373, 1985.
83. George CF, Millar TW, Kryger MH: Sleep apnea and body position during sleep. Sleep 11:90, 1988.
84. Smith PL, Gold AR, Meyers DA, et al: Weight loss in mildly to moderately obese patients with obstructive sleep apnea. Ann Intern Med 103:850, 1985.
85. Clark GT, Nakano M: Dental appliances for the treatment of obstructive sleep apnea. J Am Dent Assoc 118:611, 1989.
86. Cartwright RD, Samelson CF: The effects of nonsurgical treatment for obstructive sleep apnea. JAMA 248:705, 1982.
87. Strohl KP, Hensley MJ, Saunders NA, et al: Progesterone administration and progressive sleep apneas. JAMA 245:1230, 1981.
88. Orr WC, Imes NK, Martin RJ: Progesterone therapy in obese patients with sleep apnea. Arch Intern Med 139:109, 1979.
89. Brownell LG, West P, Sweatman P, et al: Protriptyline in obstructive sleep apnea. N Engl J Med 307:1037, 1982.
90. Bonora M, St John WM, Bledsoe TA: Differential elevation by protriptyline and depression by diazepam of upper airway respiratory motor activity. Am Rev Respir Dis 131:41, 1985.
91. Smith PL, Haponik EF, Bleecker ER: The effects of oxygen in patients with sleep apnea. Am Rev Respir Dis 130:958, 1984.
92. Gold AR, Bleecker ER, Smith PL: A shift from central and mixed sleep apnea to obstructive sleep apnea resulting from low-flow oxygen. Am Rev Respir Dis 132:220, 1985.
93. Fletcher EC, Munafo DA: Role of nocturnal oxygen therapy in obstructive sleep apnea. Chest 98:1497, 1990.
94. Phillips BA, Schmitt FA, Berry DTR, et al: Treatment of obstructive sleep apnea. Chest 98:325, 1990.
95. Sullivan CE, Issa FG, Berthon-Jones M, et al: Reversal of obstructive sleep apnoea by continuous positive airway pressure applied through the nares. Lancet 1:862, 1981.
96. Sanders MA: Nasal CPAP effect on patterns of sleep apnea. Chest 86:839, 1984.
97. Westbrook PR: Treatment of sleep disordered breathing: Nasal continuous positive airway pressure (CPAP). In: Suratt P, Remmers JE (eds): Sleep and Respiration. New York, Wiley-Liss, p 387, 1990.
98. Sanders MH, Gruendl CA, Rogers RM: Patient compliance with nasal CPAP therapy for sleep apnea. Chest 90:330, 1986.
99. O'Brien CF, Mahowald MW, Schleuter J, et al: Continuous positive airway pressure in obstructive sleep apnea: Initial response and long-term followup. Am Rev Respir Dis 133:A342, 1986.
100. Sanders MH, Kern N: Obstructive sleep apnea treated by independently adjusted inspiratory and expiratory positive airway pressures via nasal mask. Chest 98:317, 1990.
101. Koopmann CF, Moran WB: Surgical management of obstructive sleep apnea. Otolaryngol Clin North Am 23:787, 1990.
102. Guilleminault C, Riley R, Powell N: Obstructive sleep apnea and abnormal cephalometric measurements. Chest 86:793, 1984.
103. Partinen M, Guilleminault C, Quera-Salva M, et al: Obstructive sleep apnea and cephalometric roentgenograms. Chest 93:1199, 1988.
104. Shepard JW, Olsen KD: Uvulopalatopharyngoplasty for treatment of obstructive sleep apnea. Mayo Clin Proc 65:1260, 1990.
105. Weil JV, Cherniack NS, Dempsey JA, et al: Respiratory disorders of sleep. Am Rev Respir Dis 136:755, 1987.
106. Sher AE: Surgery for obstructive sleep apnea. In: Suratt P, Remmers JE (eds): Sleep and Respiration. New York, Wiley-Liss, p 407, 1990.
107. Shepard JW, Thawley SE: Evaluation of the upper airway by computerized tomography in patients undergoing uvulopalatopharyngoplasty for obstructive sleep apnea. Am Rev Respir Dis 140:711, 1989.
108. Sugerman HJ, Fairman RP, Lindeman AK, et al: Gastroplasty for respiratory insufficiency of obesity. Ann Surg 193:677, 1981.
109. Victor DW, Sarimento CF, Yanta M, et al: Obstructive sleep apnea in the morbidly obese. Arch Surg 119:970, 1984.
110. Rochester DF, Enson Y: Current concepts in the pathogenesis of the obesity-hypoventilation syndrome. Am J Med 57:402, 1974.
111. Bradley TD, Rutherford R, Lue F, et al: Role of diffuse airway obstruction in the hypercapnia of obstructive sleep apnea. Am Rev Respir Dis 134:920, 1986.
112. Lopata M, Onal E: Mass loading, sleep apnea, and the pathogenesis of obesity hypoventilation. Am Rev Respir Dis 125:640, 1982.
113. Rapoport DM, Garay SM, Epstein H, et al: Hypercapnia in the obstructive sleep apnea syndrome. Chest 89:627, 1986.
114. Lyons HA, Huang CT: Therapeutic use of progesterone in alveolar hypoventilation associated with obesity. Am J Med 44:881, 1968.
115. Sutton FD, Zwillich CW, Creagh CE, et al: Progesterone for outpatient treatment with pickwickian syndrome. Ann Intern Med 83:476, 1975.
116. Rapoport DM, Sorkin B, Garay SM, et al: Reversal of the "pickwickian syndrome" by long-term use of nocturnal nasal-airway pressure. N Engl J Med 307:931, 1982.
117. Nordberg J, Kline L: Nocturnal ventilation via nasal CPAP mask in pickwickian syndrome. Am Rev Respir Dis 139:A115, 1989.
118. Leger P, Jennequin J, Gerard M, et al: Home positive pressure ventilation via nasal mask for patients with neuromuscular weakness or restrictive lung or chest-wall disease. Respir Care 34:73, 1989.
119. Bach JR, Alba AS: Management of chronic alveolar hypoventilation by nasal ventilation. Chest 97:52, 1990.
120. Carrey Z, Gottfried SB, Levy RD: Ventilatory muscle support in respiratory failure with nasal positive pressure ventilation. Chest 97:150, 1990.
121. Goldberg AI, Cane RD, Childress D, et al: Combined nasal intermittent positive-pressure ventilation and rocking bed in chronic respiratory insufficiency. Chest 99:627, 1991.
122. Bach JR, Alba A, Mosher R, et al: Intermittent positive pressure ventilation via nasal access in the management of respiratory insufficiency. Chest 92:168, 1987.
123. Kerby GR, Mayer LS, Pingleton SK: Nocturnal positive pressure ventilation via nasal mask. Am Rev Respir Dis 135:738, 1987.
124. Ellis ER, Bye PTP, Bruderer JW, et al: Treatment of respiratory failure during sleep in patients with neuromuscular disease. Am Rev Respir Dis 135:148, 1987.
125. Baker CF: Sensory overload and noise in the ICU: Sources of environmental stress. Crit Care Q 6:66, 1984.
126. Falk S, Woods, NF: Hospital noise-levels and potential health hazards. N Engl J Med 289:774, 1973.
127. Snyder-Halpern R: The effect of critical care unit noise on patient sleep cycles. Crit Care Q 7:41, 1985.
128. Weber RJ, Oszko MA, Bolender BJ, et al: The intensive care unit syndrome: Causes, treatment, and prevention. Drug Intell Clin Pharm 19:13, 1985.
129. Helton MC, Gordon SH, Nunnery SL: The correlation between sleep deprivation and the intensive care unit syndrome. Heart Lung 9:464, 1980.
130. Kollar EJ, Pasnau RO, Rubin RT, et al: Psychological, psychophysiological, and biochemical correlates of prolonged sleep deprivation. Am J Psychiatry 126:488, 1969.
131. Richards KC, Bairnsfather L: A description of night sleep patterns in the critical care unit. Heart Lung 17:35, 1988.
132. Hilton AB: Quantity and quality of patient's sleep and sleep-disturbing factors in a respiratory intensive care unit. J Adv Nurs 1:453, 1976.
133. Aurell J, Elmqvist D: Sleep in the surgical intensive care unit: Continuous polygraphic recording of sleep in nine patients receiving postoperative care. Br Med J 190:1029, 1985.
134. Broughton R, Baron R: Sleep patterns in the intensive care unit and on the ward after acute myocardial infarction. Electroencephalogr Clin Neurophysiol 45:348, 1978.
135. Dobb GJ, Murphy DF: Sedation and analgesia during intensive care. Clin Anaesthesiol 3:1055, 1985.
136. Sedation in the intensive care unit (editorial). Lancet 1:1388, 1984.
137. Timsit-Berthier M, de Thier D, Machowsky R, et al: Sleep and wake after benzodiazepine hypnotics: A 20-hour EEG comparison of lormetazepam and flunitrazepam. Curr Med Res Opin 9:552, 1985.
138. Borbély AA, Mattmann P, Loepfe M, et al: Effect of benzodiazepine hypnotics on all-night EEG spectra. Hum Neurobiol 4:189, 1985.
139. Roth T, Roehrs T, Zorick F, et al: Pharmacological effects of sedative-hypnotics, narcotic analgesics, and alcohol during sleep. Med Clin North Am 69:1281, 1985.
140. Robinson RW, Zwillich CW: The effects of drugs on breathing during sleep. In: Kryger MH, Roth T, Dement, WC (eds): Principles and Practice of Sleep Medicine. Philadelphia, WB Saunders, p 501, 1989.
141. Douglas NJ: Asthma. In: Kryger MH, Roth T, Dement, WC (eds): Principles and Practice of Sleep Medicine. Philadelphia, WB Saunders, p 591, 1989.
142. Clark TJH, Hetzel MR: Diurnal variation of asthma. Br J Dis Chest 71:87, 1977.
143. Connolly CK: Diurnal rhythms in airway obstruction. Br J Dis Chest 73:357, 1979.
144. Shepard JW Jr, Garrison MW, Grither DA, et al: Relationship of ventricular ectopy to nocturnal oxygen desaturation in patients with chronic obstructive pulmonary disease. Am J Med 78:28, 1985.
145. Tirlapur VG, Mir MA: Nocturnal hypoxemia and associated electrocardiographic changes in patients with chronic obstructive airways disease. N Engl J Med 305:125, 1982.
146. Mezon BL, West P, Israels J, et al: Sleep breathing abnormalities in kyphoscoliosis. Am Rev Respir Dis 122:617, 1980.
147. Bye PTP, Issa F, Berthon-Jones M, et al: Studies of oxygenation during sleep in patients with interstitial lung disease. Am Rev Respir Dis 129:27, 1984.

148. Perez-Padilla R, West P, Lertzman M, et al: Breathing during sleep in patients with interstitial lung disease. Am Rev Respir Dis 132:224, 1985.
149. George CFP: Cardiovascular diseases. In: Kryger MH, Roth T, Dement, WC (eds): Principles and Practice of Sleep Medicine. Philadelphia, WB Saunders, p 617, 1989.
150. Murao S, Harumi K, Katayama S, et al: All-night polygraphic studies of nocturnal angina pectoris. Jpn Heart J 7:295, 1972.
151. King MJ, Zir LM, Kaltman AJ, et al: Variant angina associated with angiographically demonstrated coronary artery spasm and REM sleep. Am J Med Sci 265:419, 1973.
152. Muller ME, Stone PH, Turi ZG, et al: Circadian variation in the frequency of onset of acute myocardial infarction. N Engl J Med 313:1315, 1985.
153. Mitler MM, Kripke DF: Circadian variation in myocardial infarction. N Engl J Med 314:1187, 1986.
154. Smith R, Johnson L, Rothfeld D, et al: Sleep and circadian arrhythmias. Arch Intern Med 130:751, 1972.
155. Orr WC, Stahl ML, Whitsett T, et al: Physiological sleep patterns and cardiac arrhythmias. Am Heart J 97:128, 1979.
156. Rosenberg MJ, Uretz E, Denes P: Sleep and ventricular arrhythmias. Am Heart J 106:703, 1983.
157. Martin RJ: Respiratory failure during sleep. In: Schwarz MI (ed): Pulmonary Grand Rounds. Philadelphia, BC Decker, p. 206, 1990.
158. Kryger MH: Management of obstructive sleep apnea: Overview. In: Kryger MH, Roth T, Dement, WC (eds): Principles and Practice of Sleep Medicine. Philadelphia, WB Saunders, p. 584, 1989.
159. Kimmel PL, Miller G, Mendelson WB: Sleep apnea syndrome in chronic renal disease. Am J Med 86:308, 1989.

CHAPTER 70

Respiratory Failure in Cardiac Disease

David M. F. Murphy

Pulmonary disorders arising from cardiac disease cause some of the most frequently encountered diagnostic and therapeutic problems in the intensive care unit setting. Interpreting the complex interplay between the cardiac, pulmonary, and circulatory systems in the acutely ill patient requires a clear understanding of cardiopulmonary physiology and the pulmonary consequences of disordered cardiac function.

DEFINITION OF RESPIRATORY FAILURE

Respiratory failure occurs when the respiratory system fails to maintain external gas exchange. Any component of the system may fail, leading to failure of the system as a whole. To the extent that the heart and lungs are closely coordinated in the maintenance of adequate tissue oxygenation, failure of the cardiac system can lead to failure in the respiratory system. Respiratory failure may present acutely or develop more slowly and lead to a chronic condition. Both of these forms also may be divided into hypoxemic and/or hypercapnic categories. The criteria used to define these two situations are derived from arterial blood gas measurements, the hallmark of hypoxemic failure being a PaO_2 of less than 60 mm Hg, whereas a $PaCO_2$ of greater than 50 mm Hg characterizes hypercapnic failure.[1] Hypoxemic failure usually results from disordered function at the alveolar capillary level, whereas hypercapnic failure often results from alveolar hypoventilation. When respiratory failure occurs as a result of cardiac disease, the most common underlying mechanisms are increased shunting, ventilation-perfusion ($\dot{V}$-$\dot{Q}$) inequality, and hypoventilation.

MECHANISMS OF RESPIRATORY FAILURE IN CARDIAC DISEASE

In most circumstances respiratory failure in cardiac disease is of the hypoxemic form. In some situations, such as acute pulmonary edema, PCO_2 may rise rapidly to levels associated with respiratory failure,[2] but hypercapnic respiratory failure usually occurs only in the most advanced stages of hypoxemic respiratory failure.

Shunting

Cardiac disease may cause hypoxemia as a result of anatomic shunting, as occurs in some congenital heart diseases, such as atrial or ventricular septal defects, patent ductus arteriosus, or Fallot's tetralogy.[3] Intrapulmonary right-to-left shunts also can occur with arteriovenous malformations. More frequently, a physiologic shunt develops when lung units are not ventilated because of alveolar flooding or atelectasis while uninterrupted blood flow continues to these units. This is a frequent phenomenon in the intensive care unit setting and occurs in the context of acute pulmonary edema,[4] pneumonia,[5] atelectasis,[6] and acute massive pulmonary embolism.[7]

A physiologic shunt represents the equivalent of a $\dot{V}/\dot{Q}$ ratio of zero. Although $\dot{V}/\dot{Q}$ ratios can extend from zero to infinity, normal values are usually centered about unity with a range from 0.6 to 3.0.

The presence of a shunt is detected at the bedside by having the patient inspire oxygen at a concentration of 100%, as this eliminates the hypoxemia of $\dot{V}$-$\dot{Q}$ inequality, diffusion impairment, and hypoventilation.[8] A one-way valve system can be used to deliver 100% oxygen for 20 minutes, followed by sampling of the PaO_2. Failure to achieve a PaO_2 of at least 600 mm Hg indicates a clinically significant shunt.[9] The shunt fraction can be calculated more precisely from the shunt equation:

$$\frac{\dot{Q}s}{\dot{Q}} = \frac{0.0013(PAO_2 - PaO_2)}{0.0031(PAO_2 - PaO_2) + (CaO_2 - C\bar{v}O_2)}$$

where $\dot{Q}s$ = shunt flow
$\dot{Q}$ = total pulmonary blood flow
PAO_2 = alveolar oxygen pressure
PaO_2 = arterial oxygen pressure
CaO_2 = arterial oxygen content
$C\bar{v}O_2$ = mixed venous oxygen content

and measurements of $C\bar{v}O_2$ are obtained from pulmonary arterial catheterization data.[10]

With each percentage rise in shunt flow there is a marked decrease in PaO_2, which emphasizes the profound effect of venous admixture on PaO_2. In the presence of a low cardiac output, small changes in shunt flow can significantly lower PaO_2.[10]

In the critically ill patient, several factors affect the shunt fraction.[11] For example, shunting is reduced with decreases in total pulmonary blood flow but is increased when hypoxic vasoconstriction is relieved. Mechanical influences such as edema-induced vessel compression reduce the shunt fraction. Pharmacologic agents such as nitroprusside, diltiazem, and prostaglandin E increase shunting, and agents such as aspirin, indomethacin, and almitrine decrease shunting. The diuretic furosemide reduces shunting by redistributing blood

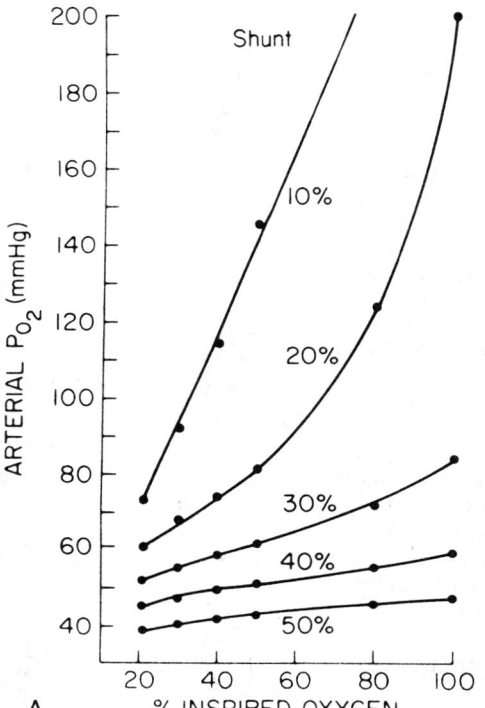

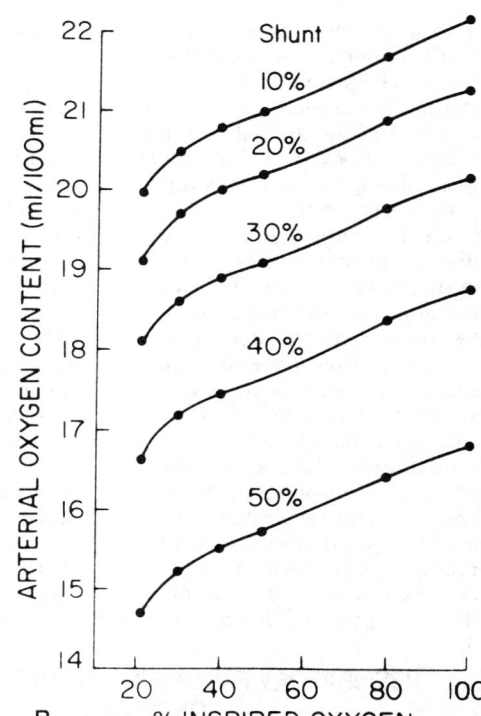

Figure 70–1. *A.* Effect of changing the inspired oxygen concentration on PaO_2 and oxygen content for lung shunts of 10 to 50%. The increase in PaO_2 with increasing inspired oxygen is small for lungs with large shunts. *B.* However, because of the shape of the hemoglobin dissociation curve, the increase in oxygen content is considerable. (From Dantzker DR: Adult respiratory distress syndrome. Clin Chest Med 3:57, 1982.)

flow to areas that are unaffected by edema at the same time that it increases cardiac output. Positive end-expiratory pressure (PEEP) reduces shunt by opening collapsed lung units and increasing functional residual capacity.

Because of the relationship between shunt fraction and total pulmonary blood flow, shunting may increase with increases in cardiac output. This phenomenon is not clearly understood,[12] but it may result from preferential increases in perfusion to flooded alveoli at the intralobar level. Another explanation is that increases in $C\bar{v}O_2$ increase shunt fraction by altered blood flow distribution[13] even though cardiac output remains constant.

Low levels of mixed venous oxygen pressure, $P\bar{v}O_2$, result from an imbalance between oxygen delivery and oxygen needs.[14] A low cardiac output,[15] oxygen content, or hemoglobin concentration or an increase in oxygen consumption ($\dot{V}O_2$) can lead to a low $P\bar{v}O_2$. A single value of $C\bar{v}O_2$ may result from a series of different combinations of PaO_2 and cardiac output over a range of systemic oxygen transport. However, when cardiac output and PaO_2 change in opposite directions, the resultant $P\bar{v}O_2$ may be unpredictable.[16]

In the presence of a large shunt, PaO_2 responds poorly to increases in the fraction of inspired oxygen (FIO_2) because hypoxemia is the result of admixture of blood that traverses unventilated alveoli. At lower levels of shunt, there is a rise in PaO_2 with increasing FIO_2, but at higher degrees of shunt the effect on PaO_2 of increasing FIO_2 even to 100% decreases significantly[17] (Fig. 70–1). Because high concentrations of oxygen are toxic to the lung, mechanical ventilation, sometimes in association with PEEP, should be used to treat this situation. Oxygen itself may produce atelectasis, because as FIO_2 increases, alveolar oxygen is taken up faster by capillary blood than it can be replaced from the alveolar air, leading to local atelectasis and increased shunting.[18]

Ventilation-Perfusion Inequality

This mechanism is less important than physiologic shunting in cardiogenic edema but is of some importance in congestive heart failure, dilated cardiomyopathy, myocardial infarction, and mitral stenosis. When an abnormal distribution of $\dot{V}/\dot{Q}$ ratios develops, the result is hypoxemia and hypercapnia.[19] However, the presence of alveolar hypoxia usually causes vasoconstriction of the arterioles leading to those particular lung units in an effort to regulate the $\dot{V}/\dot{Q}$ ratios back toward normal.[20] Elevation of left atrial pressure[21] and certain drugs (nitroprusside, nitroglycerin, beta-agonists, and calcium channel blockers) can interfere with this regulatory mechanism.[22] Hypercapnia stimulates the respiratory center to increase ventilation and restore the arterial carbon dioxide tension to normal, resulting in the common clinical finding of hypoxemia and normocapnia. If the level of ventilation required is particularly high, respiratory muscle fatigue can result from the excessive work of breathing, causing hypoventilation, uncompensated hypercapnia, and respiratory acidosis.[23]

Hypoventilation and Respiratory Muscle Fatigue

An increased respiratory workload resulting from changes in lung mechanics may cause respiratory muscle fatigue and hypercapnic respiratory failure.[24] Respiratory muscle contraction depends on the use of high-energy compounds, which are easily exhausted and must be constantly regenerated by aerobic and anaerobic pathways.[25] Because these pathways are dependent on muscle blood flow, muscle contractility is also dependent on respiratory muscle blood flow.[26] When an excessive workload is imposed on the respiratory muscles or respiratory muscle blood flow is reduced, the ability to renew high-energy compounds may be exceeded and muscle fatigue results.[27]

In the absence of disease, respiratory muscle blood flow apparently does not limit respiratory muscle function,[28] but in the presence of either cardiogenic[29] or septic shock[30] respiratory muscle blood flow may be of critical importance. In animal studies, cardiogenic shock causes systemic hypoxemia and acidemia leading to increased ventilation. Despite an increase in respiratory muscle blood flow, lactate production increases, respiratory muscle fatigue develops, and finally hypercapnic respiratory failure and respiratory arrest result. However, if cardiogenic shock is produced in mechanically ventilated animals, diaphragmatic fatigue is prevented and the animals survive.[27, 29]

Septic shock produces effects similar to those of cardiogenic shock.[30] In animal studies, endotoxin injection leads to progressive respiratory muscle fatigue and death resulting from respiratory failure.[31] Despite an increase in total blood flow, anaerobic metabolism develops, as shown by increases in diaphragmatic lactate levels. This indicates impairment in the ability of the diaphragm to utilize the oxygen supplied by the increase in blood flow. These changes are probably due to the effects of endotoxin on oxygen extraction. During shock, an increase in respiratory muscle blood flow may affect the blood flow to other vital organs. In situations in which cardiac function is impaired and the respiratory muscle needs for oxygen are high, a significant proportion of cardiac output may be diverted to meet the metabolic needs of the respiratory muscles, reducing the blood flow available to other vital structures. Mechanical ventilation can relieve this problem by allowing the respiratory muscles to rest, thus reducing their blood flow needs and increasing the proportion of blood flow available to other organs.[27, 29]

RESPIRATORY FAILURE IN SELECTED CARDIAC CONDITIONS

Respiratory failure may occur in the context of acute, subacute, or chronic cardiac disease.

Cardiogenic Shock

This condition occurs most frequently with acute myocardial infarction. In the absence of complications such as acute septal or papillary muscle rupture, infarction of at least 40% of the left ventricular muscle is usually necessary to precipitate this condition.[32] Cardiogenic shock is characterized by a blood pressure of less than 80 mm Hg, a pulmonary capillary wedge pressure greater than 18 mm Hg, a cardiac index of less than 1.8 L/min/m², oliguria with a urine output less than 500 mL in 24 hours, and signs of peripheral hypoperfusion.

Because oxygen transport is adversely affected by decreases in cardiac output, hemoglobin concentration, and arterial oxygen saturation, it is important that PaO_2 be maintained at 60 mm Hg (90% saturation) or more to help maintain organ function. This can be achieved initially with cardiopulmonary resuscitation followed by intubation, mechanical ventilation, and supplementary oxygen. If these measures fail to achieve a PaO_2 greater than 60 mm Hg despite FIO_2 values of 60%, careful application of PEEP may raise the PaO_2 without adversely affecting left ventricular function and oxygen transport.[33]

Because the effects of PEEP on cardiac output are not always predictable in the setting of ventricular dysfunction, the objective should be to optimize oxygen transport with acceptable filling pressures by changing the other variables as needed. Maximal improvement in static lung compliance has been shown to correlate with maximal oxygen transport in normovolemic patients.[34]

Validated measurements of mixed venous oxygen saturation are sometimes useful as a guide to assessing the adequacy of the oxygen transport system.[35] Values less than 40% merit increasing oxygen transport by increasing oxygen content and maximizing cardiac output with careful use of inotropes and vasodilators,[36] remembering that some vasodilators such as nitroglycerin[37] and sodium nitroprusside may increase intrapulmonary shunting and decrease PaO_2.[38]

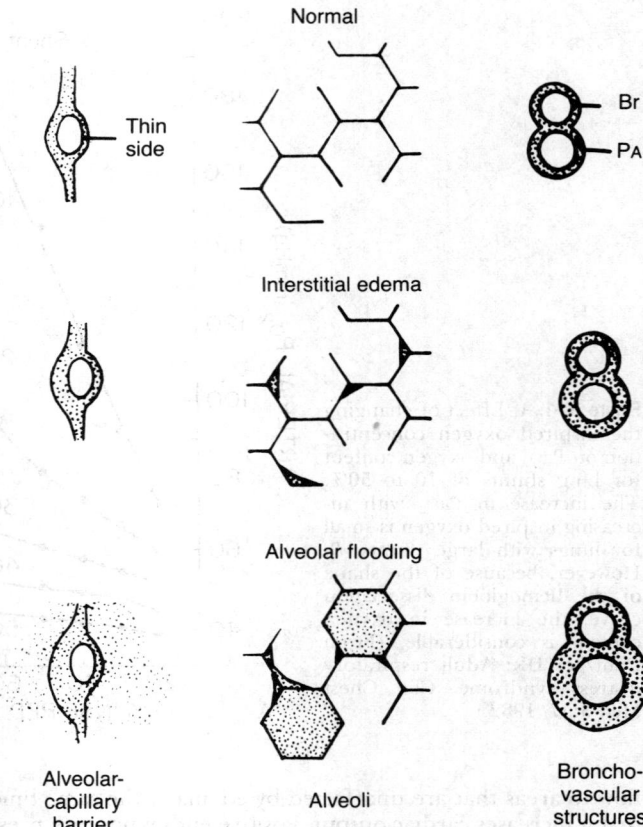

Figure 70–2. Progression from interstitial to alveolar edema associated with peribronchial (and perivascular) cuffing. *(Top)* Normal lung. The alveolar capillary septum incorporates the capillary eccentrically to form a thick and a thin side. The alveoli are free of fluid. The peribronchovascular interstitial space is normal. *(Middle)* Interstitial pulmonary edema. The thick side of the alveolar capillary septum is widened. The peribronchovascular interstitial space is thickened by excess fluid. *(Bottom)* Fluid has escaped from the alveolar interstitium with the alveoli. Alveolar flooding is not uniform. There is marked peribronchovascular edema. (From Murphy DMF, Fishman AP: Pulmonary disorders produced by cardiac disease. In: Fishman AP [ed]: Pulmonary Diseases and Disorders. 2nd ed. New York, McGraw-Hill, p 1103, 1988. Reproduced with permission of McGraw-Hill, Inc.)

Failure to achieve an adequate cardiac output should warrant early consideration of intra-aortic balloon counterpulsation, which increases coronary perfusion while unloading the left ventricle.[39] Because cardiogenic shock is associated with mortality rates as high as 90%, it is important to rule out other treatable causes of decreased cardiac output such as hypoxemia, acidosis, sepsis, hemorrhage, myocardial depressant drugs, or decreases in cardiac output induced by positive pressure ventilation.

Myocardial Infarction

The pulmonary consequences of myocardial infarction in the absence of shock depend on whether pulmonary congestion, interstitial edema, or frank alveolar edema results (Fig. 70–2). After acute myocardial infarction, pulmonary vascular pressures remain elevated for about a week, and in the absence of frank alveolar edema the main functional abnormalities are widening of the alveolar-arterial oxygen difference ($PAO_2 - PaO_2$), hypoxemia, and acute respiratory alkalosis.[40, 41] Hypoxemia usually persists for about 3 weeks,[42] with the level of PaO_2 probably related to airway closure resulting from interstitial fluid collection.[43] The use of pul-

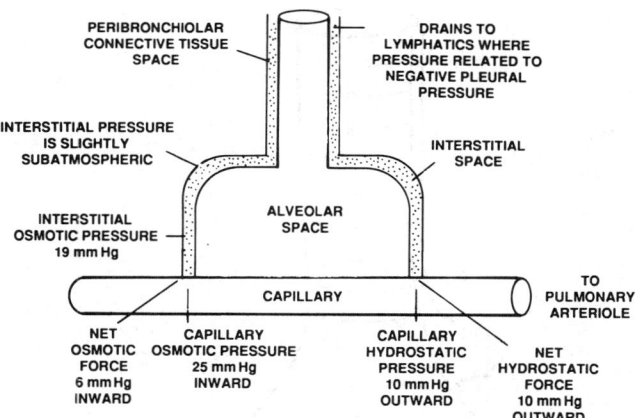

Figure 70–3. Diagrammatic representation of the Starling forces that determine the movement of fluid across the alveolar capillary membrane in the normal lung. Fluid moves out of the capillary because the net hydrostatic force outward (capillary hydrostatic pressure less interstitial hydrostatic pressure) is 4 mm Hg greater than the net osmotic pressure inward (capillary osmotic pressure less interstitial osmotic pressure).

monary arterial catheterization data to manage patients with acute myocardial infarction is common but is not associated with a reduced in-hospital mortality, shortened hospital stay, or improved long-term survival.[44] Two large retrospective studies found no decrease in the fatality rate in patients managed with pulmonary arterial catheters who developed pulmonary edema and cardiogenic shock.[45, 46]

Pulmonary Edema

Although this is covered in chapter 83, certain aspects merit further emphasis. A precise balance between the hydrostatic and osmotic forces of the lung is necessary to maintain the functional integrity of the alveolar space. The interplay between these factors was initially proposed by Ernest Starling in 1896.[47] Further development of this important concept led to an equation that describes the relationship of hydrostatic pressure and osmotic pressures to the net flow of fluid across a semipermeable membrane:

$$F = K_f[(Pcap - Pisf) - \sigma(\pi plasma - \pi isf)]$$

where F = rate of fluid filtration
K_f = filtration coefficient
Pcap = capillary hydrostatic pressure
Pisf = interstitial fluid hydrostatic pressure
πplasma = oncotic pressure of plasma
πisf = oncotic pressure of interstitial fluid
σ = osmotic reflection coefficient of the endothelium

The filtration of fluid across the membrane is governed by the opposing hydrostatic and osmotic pressures in conjunction with the permeability of the endothelium, with the lymphatic system removing any excess fluid that accumulates[48] (Fig. 70–3). When the capacity of the lymphatics to remove fluid is overloaded, filtered fluid accumulates in the interstitial space, initially on the thick side of the alveolar capillary membrane but then extending to the peribronchiolar and perivascular connective tissue spaces (see Fig. 70–2).

Pulmonary edema may be separated into increased permeability edema or hydrostatic pulmonary edema. Because the latter is often due to cardiac disease, the terms cardiogenic and noncardiogenic edema are often used. In hydrostatic pulmonary edema the rate of fluid filtration across the

alveolar capillary membrane initially increases as hydrostatic pressure rises in the microvasculature.[49] This often occurs as a direct result of increases in pulmonary capillary wedge pressures, with pressures greater than 18 mm Hg being associated with increased interstitial fluid, dyspnea, and detectable radiographic changes.[50] A large number of conditions can cause elevation in the hydrostatic pressure of the lungs' microcirculation (Table 70–1).

The true average hydrostatic pressure of the microcirculation in the lung is actually greater than the left atrial pressure and more closely approximates left atrial pressure plus 0.4 times the difference between the pulmonary arterial and left atrial pressure.[51] Also, the hydrostatic pressure of the microcirculation is related to the height in the lung at which it is measured.[52] It has been suggested that the inflection point of the pulmonary artery profile immediately after balloon occlusion is a direct measure of the microcirculation's hydrostatic pressure;[53] however, this does not conform to mathematically derived predictions.[54]

In studies of the mechanisms controlling removal of pulmonary edema fluid in animals, the reabsorbtion of water and protein could not be explained solely on the basis of hydrostatic and osmotic pressures.[55] This observation and the finding that adult rat type II alveolar epithelial cells are probably able to absorb sodium and thus water raise the possibility that active ion transport by the alveolar epithelium is involved in clearance of alveolar fluid.[56] In human experiments, when sequential samples of pulmonary edema fluid were analyzed for albumin and total protein in patients with both cardiogenic and noncardiogenic edema, the patients who improved clinically showed an increased protein con-

TABLE 70–1
CONDITIONS THAT RESULT IN INCREASED MICROVASCULAR HYDROSTATIC PRESSURE

Pressure Effect	Condition
Increased left ventricular end-diastolic pressure	Coronary artery disease Acute myocardial infarction Angina Left ventricular aneurysm Aortic valvular disease Aortic stenosis Aortic regurgitation Dysfunctional prosthetic aortic valve Cardiomyopathy Congestive Restrictive Hypertrophic Arrhythmias Pericarditis Fluid overload High-output states
Increased left atrial pressure	Mitral valve disease Mitral stenosis Mitral regurgitation Dysfunctional prosthetic mitral valve Left atrial myxoma Left atrial thrombus
Increased pulmonary venous pressure	Pulmonary veno-occlusive disease Fibrosing mediastinitis Mediastinal tumor Congenital cardiac anomalies
Neurogenic	Subarachnoid hemorrhage Cerebrovascular accidents High-altitude pulmonary edema

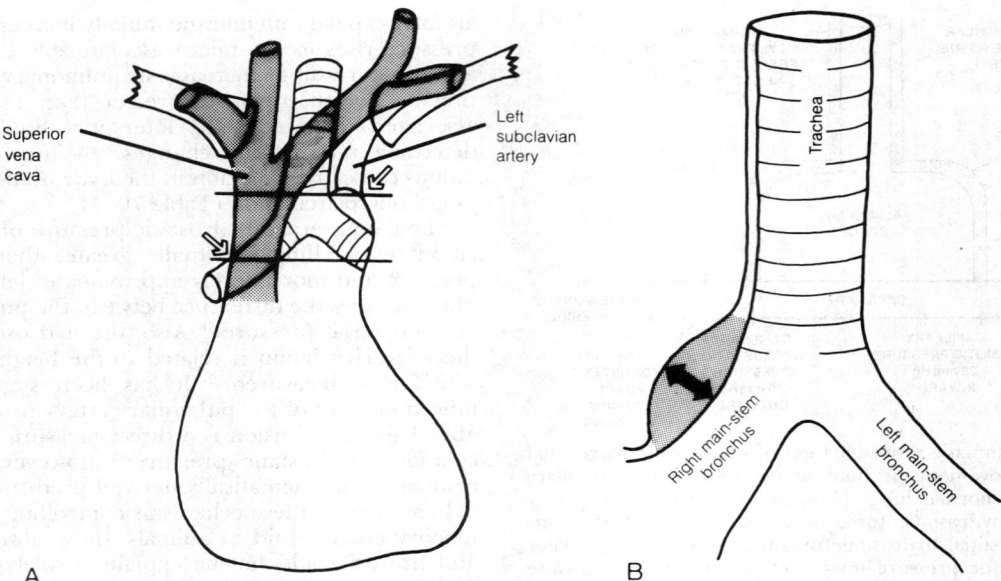

Figure 70–4. Radiographic indices of expanded blood volume and increased central venous pressures. *A.* The width of the vascular pedicle. The left border of the pedicle is formed by the relatively indistensible subclavian artery. The right border of the pedicle is formed by the more compliant right bronchocephalic vein above and the superior vena cava below. The landmarks on which the measurements are made are indicated by the two arrows. The upper limit of normal for the width of the vascular pedicle is 53 mm. *B.* The distended azygos vein. The upper limit of normal diameter in the conventional upright radiograph is 7 mm. (From Murphy DMF, Fishman AP: Pulmonary disorders produced by cardiac disease. In: Fishman AP [ed]: Pulmonary Diseases and Disorders. 2nd ed. New York, McGraw-Hill, p 1103, 1988. Reproduced with permission of McGraw-Hill, Inc.)

centration in the alveolar edema fluid.[57] This supports the concept of active ion transport across the alveolar epithelium as a mechanism for clearance of edema fluid.

In the intensive care setting, measurements of the prevailing hemodynamic conditions are used to assess cardiac function and to determine prognosis.

Radiology

Chest radiography remains the most sensitive technique available for the early detection of pulmonary edema.[58] The chest roentgenogram also permits some degree of objective measurement of the extent of extravascular lung water. Several experimental studies of patients with acute myocardial infarction have shown that the chest radiograph can detect interstitial pulmonary edema even before the development of clinical symptoms.[59] Animal experiments in which radiographic changes were related to gravimetrically measured extravascular lung water revealed that a chest radiologist could recognize hazy shadowing when the amount of lung water was more than 30% above the mean normal value.[60]

When radiographic scoring systems have been used to grade pulmonary edema, most studies have revealed that the sensitivity of the radiologic methods equaled or exceeded that of extravascular lung water measurements. A relationship with extravascular lung water measurements was demonstrated when optimal radiographic techniques were used with upright, cooperative cardiac patients and when precise radiographic criteria were used to describe the presence of interstitial pulmonary edema for the purpose of scoring. However, when portable equipment was used to obtain chest roentgenograms of supine, critically ill patients, less correlation with extravascular lung water measurements was demonstrated and no clear correlation existed between changes in lung water and changes in radiographic score.[61]

Other radiographic measurements that are sometimes clinically useful include the azygos vein width measured with the patient in the upright position, which correlates well with mean right atrial pressure (Fig. 70–4). The normal azygos vein width in a conventional radiograph is 7 mm. Another useful measurement on a radiograph taken with the patient in the upright position is the vascular pedicle width (Figs. 70–4 and 70–5). In cardiac patients the width of the pedicle correlates well with total circulating blood volume.[62]

Pulmonary Function

With the development of alveolar edema, air entry is reduced to flooded air spaces, shunting and V̇-Q̇ mismatch increase, and both lung volumes and static compliance decrease.[63] If hyperventilation is present, there may be a reduction in $PaCO_2$ and a respiratory alkalosis.

Detailed noninvasive measurements of the mechanical properties of the total respiratory system can now be obtained in critically ill patients with ventilators equipped with measuring devices. Using these, measurements of early changes in respiratory mechanics in seriously ill patients have been obtained. Studies of patients with cardiogenic pulmonary edema have revealed the presence of intrinsic PEEP (or auto-PEEP) averaging about 3 cm H_2O. Also, respiratory resistance has been found to be elevated in patients who have no evidence of airway disease. The increase in respiratory resistance may reflect narrowing of bronchial lumens because of vagal reflexes[64] or decrease in lung volume rather than compression of airways by interstitial fluid or congested arteries.[65] Measurements of static compliance, an indication of the amount of fluid in the air spaces, have been significantly correlated with the pulmonary oxygenation index—the PaO_2/PAO_2 ratio.[66] This ratio is a stable index of pulmonary oxygenation frequently used in reference to $PAO_2 - PaO_2$ for critically ill patients.[67]

Treatment of Acute Pulmonary Edema

When pulmonary congestion gives way to frank alveolar edema, urgent therapy is necessary to prevent progressive

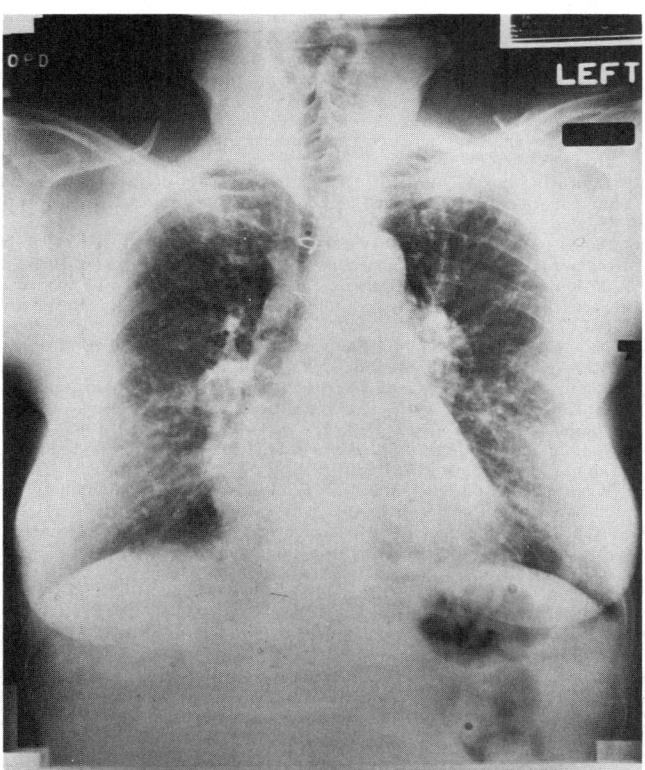

Figure 70–5. Chest radiography of a woman with mitral stenosis showing an enlarged azygos vein and vascular pedicle with upper zonal cephalization.

acute respiratory failure leading to death. If PaO_2 cannot be maintained at 60 mm Hg or higher with a supplementary oxygen concentration of 60%, continuous positive airway pressure should be administered via a high-flow venturi face mask at 10 cm H_2O, because improved gas exchange and reduced respiratory work may offset the need for ventilator treatment.[68] Intubation and continuous positive pressure ventilation with an inspiratory/expiratory time ratio of 1:2 should be commenced if this fails to increase PaO_2 sufficiently. If arterial oxygen levels remain unsatisfactory, PEEP may be added, with careful monitoring of cardiac output, mixed venous O_2 saturation, pulmonary arterial wedge pressure, and arterial blood pressure as necessary. PEEP improves oxygenation by reducing functional residual capacity and decreasing $\dot{V}$-$\dot{Q}$ mismatch and intrapulmonary shunting[69] but may decrease cardiac output and thus reduce oxygen transport by reducing venous return to the right ventricle and altering ventricular geometry.[70] If the condition continues to deteriorate despite a high FIO_2 and PEEP at 15 cm H_2O with peak airway pressure reaching 65 to 70 cm H_2O, inverse ratio ventilation at 1:1 to 3:1 could be considered.[71] Ultrafiltration can be used when acute pulmonary edema is refractory to diuretic therapy.[72]

Congestive Heart Failure

The mortality resulting from this condition remains high, with 50% of patients dying within a year of the onset of symptoms.[73] Traditionally, congestive heart failure means combined left and right ventricular failure with evidence of systemic and pulmonary venous hypertension and a low cardiac output. Any of the causes of left-sided heart failure can cause increased pulmonary arterial pressure and patho-

logic changes in the pulmonary vascular bed leading to right ventricular failure (Table 70–2).

Pathophysiology

Chronic left ventricular failure is associated with increases in pulmonary venous and capillary pressures leading to pulmonary congestion, interstitial edema, or occasionally frank alveolar edema (see Fig. 70–2).

Radiology

The chest roentgenogram in congestive heart failure reveals cardiomegaly, upper zonal cephalization, and evidence of interstitial or frank alveolar edema (see Fig. 70–5). Because estimates of heart size from chest radiographs taken with portable equipment are variable, the size of the pulmonary vessels, not the heart, is the most important criterion in the detection of congestive heart failure. Atypical patterns of edema also may result from positioning of the patient, pulmonary parenchymal abnormalities, or an abnormal pulmonary vascular bed.[74] Right-sided or bilateral pleural effusions are often present. Concealed large right subpulmonic effusions may be suggested by the presence of a shoulder on the contour of the diaphragm.

Pleural Effusion

Transudative pleural effusions occur with congestive heart failure in up to 72% of patients,[75] most of whom have elevated systemic and pulmonary venous pressures,[76] but are uncommon with cor pulmonale or mitral stenosis.[77] Some authors consider that biventricular failure is necessary for the development of pleural effusion. Experiments reveal that pleural effusions occur when right atrial pressure increases in the presence of a reduced osmotic pressure. In a prospective study, the formation of pleural effusions in patients with congestive heart failure was strongly correlated with pulmonary venous hypertension.[78] Transudative pleural effusions occur in heart failure because high left atrial pressure leads to edema fluid traversing the visceral pleural membrane, as the pleural space pressure is lower than visceral interstitial hydrostatic pressure. Another pos-

TABLE 70–2	
CAUSES OF CONGESTIVE HEART FAILURE	
Type of Heart Failure	**Cause**
Right sided	Left-sided heart failure
	Chronic ischemic heart disease
	Mitral regurgitation, acute and chronic
	Hypertensive heart disease
	Severe aortic stenosis
	Aortic regurgitation, chronic
Independent right and left sided	Congestive cardiomyopathy, idiopathic
	Cardiomyopathy caused by infiltration (amyloid, sarcoid, connective tissue disease)
	Cardiomyopathy, inflammatory (viral, parasitic, metals, cytotoxins)
	Right ventricular infarction
	Intracardiac shunts (atrial septal defect, ventricular septal defect, patent ductus arteriosus)

sible cause of increased filtration from the visceral pleura is that visceral pleural venous drainage is toward the pulmonary veins and increasing pulmonary venous back pressure increases the microvascular pressure in the visceral pleura.

Increasing accumulation of pleural fluid causes increasing dyspnea. Smaller effusions tend to displace rather than compress the lung, so that after thoracentesis lung expansion is usually smaller than the volume of fluid removed from the pleural space.[79] Larger effusions have a space-occupying effect, but oxygenation is preserved because perfusion is reflexly reduced to the compressed underventilated lung, moving the $\dot{V}/\dot{Q}$ ratio toward normal.[80] Relief of dyspnea after thoracentesis is not due to improved gas exchange, as blood gas values may even deteriorate, but results from reduction in size of the thoracic cage, allowing the inspiratory muscles to operate on a more advantageous portion of their length-tension curve.

Treatment

Therapy for respiratory failure occurring in concert with congestive heart failure includes fluid restriction, diuretic therapy, and the use of inotropes and vasodilators.[81] Pulmonary edema may lead to respiratory muscle fatigue and hypoxemia with increased work of breathing and metabolic demands. In this situation, continuous positive airway pressure applied via a face mask reduces the work of breathing by decreasing the large negative intrathoracic pressures, reduces shunting by increasing functional residual capacity, and lowers filling pressures without decreasing stroke volume or cardiac output.[68] If continuous positive airway pressure by mask is contraindicated (because of unconsciousness, exhaustion, lack of cooperation of the patient, or technical difficulties), intubation and positive pressure ventilation should be instituted.[82]

Formerly, intra-aortic balloon conterpulsation was restricted to patients with cardiogenic shock, but advances in the percutaneous intra-aortic insertion method have increased its use in a variety of conditions leading to severe left ventricular failure including postcardiotomy shock, acute mitral regurgitation, ventricular septal rupture, refractory unstable angina, and refractory ventricular arrhythmias.[82]

Prognosis

In general, good correlations between mortality resulting from congestive heart failure and severity of disease scores (Acute Physiology and Chronic Health Evaluation [APACHE] II) have been described.[83] However, when APACHE II scores have been used to predict mortality of patients with respiratory failure caused by cardiogenic pulmonary edema, less accurate prognostic information has been obtained.[84]

Dilated Cardiomyopathy

Dilated cardiomyopathy is a disease of cardiac muscle that is associated with a marked reduction in ventricular contractility. Poor contraction of the ventricle leads to mural thrombi, which can be detected in 20% of patients by echocardiography,[85] and may lead to systemic embolism in up to 15% of cases. With atrial fibrillation the incidence of systemic embolism rises to 33%.[86] Atrial and ventricular arrhythmias are common and may lead to sudden death.

References

1. Fishman AP, Hansen-Flaschen J: Acute respiratory failure: Introduction. In: Fishman AP (ed): Pulmonary Diseases and Disorders. 2nd ed. New York, McGraw-Hill, p 3185, 1988.
2. Aberman A, Fulop M: The metabolic and respiratory acidosis of acute pulmonary edema. Ann Intern Med 76:173, 1972.
3. Murphy DMF, Fishman AP: Pulmonary disorders produced by cardiac disease. In: Fishman AP (ed): Pulmonary Diseases and Disorders. 2nd ed. New York, McGraw-Hill, p 1103, 1988.
4. Bongard FS, Matthay MA, Mackensie RC, et al: Morphologic and physiologic correlates of increased extravascular lung water. Surgery 96:395, 1984.
5. Light RB, Mink WN, Wood LDH: Pathophysiology of gas exchange and pulmonary perfusion in pneumococcal lobar pneumonia in dogs. J Appl Physiol 50:524, 1981.
6. Dantzker DR: Pulmonary gas exchange. In: Dantzker DR (ed): Cardiopulmonary Critical Care. Orlando, FL, Grune & Stratton, p 36, 1986.
7. D'Alonzo GE, Bower JS, DeHart P, et al: The mechanism of abnormal gas exchange in acute massive pulmonary embolism. Am Rev Respir Dis 128:170, 1983.
8. West JB: Ventilation/Blood Flow and Gas Exchange. 3rd ed. Oxford, Blackwell Scientific Publications, p 96, 1977.
9. Wagner PD: Mixed venous P_{O_2} ($P\bar{v}_{O_2}$) and arterial P_{O_2}, P_{CO_2} and pH. In: Chusid EL (ed): The Selective and Comprehensive Testing of Adult Pulmonary Function. New York, Futura Publishing, p 183, 1983.
10. Pontoppidan H, Geffin B, Lowenstein E: Acute respiratory failure in the adult. 2. N Engl J Med 287:743, 1972.
11. Wagner PD, Rodriguez-Roisin R: Clinical advances in pulmonary gas exchange. Am Rev Respir Dis 143:883, 1991.
12. Bren PH, Schumacker PT, Hedeinstierna G, et al: How does increased cardiac output increase shunt in pulmonary edema? J Appl Physiol 53:1273, 1982.
13. Fishman AP: Hypoxia on the pulmonary circulation. How and where it acts. Circ Res 38:221, 1976.
14. Dantzker DR (ed): Cardiopulmonary Critical Care. Orlando, FL, Grune & Stratton, p 38, 1986.
15. Shapiro B: Arterial blood gas monitoring. Crit Care Clin 4:483, 1988.
16. Carble PV, Gray BA: Effect of opposite changes in cardiac output arterial pO_2 on relationship between mixed venous pO_2 and oxygen transport. Am Rev Respir Dis 140:891, 1989.
17. Dantzker DR: Adult respiratory distress syndrome. Clin Chest Med 3:37, 1982.
18. Dantzker DR, Wagner PD, West JB: Unstability of lung units with low VA/Q ratios during oxygen breathing. J Appl Physiol 38:886, 1975.
19. West JB: Ventilation-perfusion inequality and overall gas exchange in computer models of the lung. Respir Physiol 7:88, 1969.
20. Grant BJB: Effect of local pulmonary blood flow control on gas exchange. J Appl Physiol 53:1100, 1982.
21. Bergofsky EH: Acute control of the normal pulmonary circulation. In: Moser KM (ed): Pulmonary Vascular Disease. New York, Marcel Dekker, p 223, 1979.
22. Brent BN, Berger HJ, Mathay RA, et al: Contrasting acute effects of vasodilators (nitroglycerin, nitroprusside and hydralazine) on right ventricular performance in patients with chronic obstructive pulmonary disease and pulmonary hypertension. Am J Cardiol 51:1682, 1983.
23. Roussos C: Ventilatory failure and respiratory muscles. In: Roussos C, Macklem PT (eds): The Thorax, Part B. New York, Marcel Dekker, p 1253, 1985.
24. Cohen CA, Zagelbaum G, Gross D, et al: Clinical manifestations of respiratory muscle fatigue. Am J Med 73:308, 1982.
25. Supinski, GS: Respiratory muscle blood flow. Clin Chest Med 9:211, 1988.
26. Supinski GS, DiMarco A, Gonzalez J, et al: Reversibility of diaphragmatic fatigue by mechanical hyperperfusion. Am Rev Respir Dis 133:A337, 1986.
27. Viires N, Sillye G, Aubier M, et al: Regional blood flow: Distribution in dog during induced hypotension and low cardiac output. J Clin Invest 72:935, 1983.
28. Fregosi RF, Dempsey JA: Effects of exercise in normoxia and acute hypoxia on respiratory muscle metabolites. J Appl Physiol 60:1274, 1986.
29. Aubier M, Tuppenbach T, Roussos C: Respiratory muscle fatigue during cardiogenic shock. J Appl Physiol 51:499, 1981.
30. Hussain SN, Simkus G, Roussos C: Respiratory muscle fatigue. A cause of ventilatory failure in septic shock. J Appl Physiol 58:2033, 1985.
31. Hussain SN, Rutledge F, Graham R: Effects of norepinephrine and fluid administration on diaphragmatic O_2 consumption in septic shock. J Appl Physiol 63:1368, 1987.
32. Pasternak RC, Braunwald E, Sobel BE: Acute myocardial infarction. In: Braunwald E (ed): Heart Disease, a Textbook of Cardiovascular Medicine. 3rd ed. Philadelphia, WB Saunders, p 1222, 1988.
33. Calvin JE, Driedger AA, Sibbald WJ: Positive end expiratory pressure (PEEP) does not depress left ventricular function in patients with pulmonary edema. Am Rev Respir Dis 124:121, 1981.
34. Suter PM, Fairley B, Isenberg MD: Optimum end-expiratory airway pressure in patients with acute pulmonary failure. N Engl J Med 292:284, 1975.
35. Kandel G, Aberman A: Mixed venous oxygen saturation. Its role in the assessment of the critically ill patient. Arch Intern Med 143:1400, 1983.
36. Passmore JM: Hemodynamic support of the critically ill patient. In: Dantzker DR (ed): Cardiopulmonary Critical Care. Orlando, FL, Grune & Stratton, p 393, 1988.

37. Berthelsen A, St Haxholdt O, Husum B, et al: PEEP reverses nitroglycerine induced hypoxemia following coronary artery bypass surgery. Acta Anaesthesiol Scand 30:243, 1986.
38. Mookherjee S, Keighley JFH, Warner RA, et al: Hemodynamic ventilatory and blood gas changes during infusion of sodium nitroferrin-cyanide (nitroprusside). Chest 72:273, 1977.
39. Moulopoulos S, Stamatelopoulos S, Petrou P: Intra-aortic balloon assistance in intractable cardiogenic shock. Eur Heart J 7:396, 1986.
40. McNicol MW, Kirby BJ, Bhoola KD, et al: Pulmonary function in acute myocardial infarction. Br Med J 2:1270, 1965.
41. McNicol MW, Kirby BJ, Bhoola KD, et al: Changes in pulmonary function 6–12 months after recovering from myocardial infarction. Lancet 2:1441, 1966.
42. Valentine PA, Fluck DC, Mounsey JPD, et al: Blood gas changes after acute myocardial infarction. Lancet 2:837, 1966.
43. Demedts M, Sniderman A, Utz G, et al: Lung volumes including closing volume, and arterial blood gas measurements in acute ischemic left heart failure. Bull Physiopathol Respir 10:11, 1974.
44. Dalen JE: Does pulmonary artery catheterization benefit patients with acute myocardial infarction? Chest 98:1313, 1990.
45. Zion MM, Balkin J, Rosenmann D, et al: Use of pulmonary artery catheters in patients with acute myocardial infarction. Chest 98:1331, 1990.
46. Gore JM, Goldberg RJ, Spodick DH, et al: A community wide assessment of the use of pulmonary artery catheters in patients with acute myocardial infarction. Chest 92:721, 1987.
47. Starling EH: On the absorption of fluids from the connective tissue space. J Physiol (Lond) 19:312, 1896.
48. Gee MH, Spath JA: The dynamics of the lung fluid filtration system in dogs with edema. Circ Res 46:796, 1980.
49. Erdmann JA, Vaughn TR, Brigham K, et al: Effect of increased vascular pressure on lung fluid balance in unanesthetized sheep. Circ Res 37:271, 1975
50. McHugh TJ, Forrester JS, Adler L, et al: Pulmonary vascular congestion in acute myocardial infarction: Hemodynamic and radiologic correlations. Ann Intern Med 76:29, 1972.
51. Weidemann HP, Matthay MA, Matthay RA: Cardiovascular pulmonary monitoring in the intensive care unit (part 1). Chest 85:537, 1984.
52. Blake LH, Staub NC: Pulmonary vascular transport in sheep. A mathematical model. Microvasc Res 12:197, 1976.
53. Cope DK, Allison KC, Parmentier JL, et al: Measurement of effective pulmonary capillary pressure using the pressure profile after pulmonary artery occlusion. Crit Care Med 14:16, 1986.
54. Seigel LC, Pearl RG: Measurement of the longitudinal distribution of pulmonary vascular resistance from pulmonary artery occlusion pressure profiles. Anaesthesiology 68:305, 1988.
55. Matthay MA, Landolt CC, Staub NC: Differential liquid and protein clearance from the alveoli of anaesthetized sheep. J Appl Physiol 53:96, 1982.
56. Mason RJ, Williams MC, Widdicombe JH, et al: Transepithelial transport by pulmonary alveolar type II cells in primary culture. Proc Natl Acad Sci USA 79:6033, 1982.
57. Matthay MA, Weiner-Kronish JP: Intact epithelial barrier function is critical for the resolution of alveolar edema in humans. Am Rev Respir Dis 142:1250, 1990.
58. Prichard JS: Edema of the Lung. Springfield, IL, Charles C Thomas, 1982.
59. Pistolesi M, Miniati M, Milne ENC, et al: The chest roentgenogram in pulmonary edema. Clin Chest Med 6:316, 1985.
60. Snashall PD, Keyes SJ, Morgan B, et al: Lung volume changes in early pulmonary edema in dogs. Clin Sci 55:23, 1978.
61. Halprin BD, Feeley TW, Mihm FG, et al: Evaluation of portable chest roentgenogram for quantitating extravascular lung water in critically ill adults. Chest 85:649, 1985.
62. Pistolesi M, Milne ENC, Miniati M, et al: The vascular pedicle of the heart and the vena azygous. Part II. Acquired heart disease. Radiology 152:9, 1984.
63. Sharp JT, Burnell IL, Griffith GT, et al: The effects of therapy on pulmonary mechanics in human pulmonary edema. J Clin Invest 40:665, 1961.
64. Chung HG, Keyes SJ, Morgan BM, et al: Mechanisms of airway narrowing in acute pulmonary edema in dogs: Influence of the vagus and lung volume. Clin Sci 65:289, 1983.
65. Michel RP, Zocchi L, Rossi A, et al: Does interstitial edema compress airways and arteries in the lungs? A morphometric study. J Appl Physiol 62:108, 1987.
66. Broseghini C, Brandolese R, Poggi R, et al: Respiratory mechanics during the first day of mechanical ventilation in patients with pulmonary edema and chronic airway obstruction. Am Rev Respir Dis 138:355, 1988.
67. Gilbert R, Auchincloss JH, Kuppinger M, et al: Stability of the arterial/alveolar oxygen partial pressure ratio. Crit Care Med 7:267, 1979.
68. Räsänen J, Heikkla J, Downs J, et al: Continuous positive airway pressure by face mask in acute cardiogenic pulmonary edema. Am J Cardiol 55:296, 1985.
69. Rose MD, Downs JB, Heenan TJ: Temporal responses of functional residual capacity and oxygen tension to changes in positive end expiratory pressure. Crit Care Med 9:79, 1981.
70. Schuster S, Erbel R, Weilermann LS, et al: Hemodynamics during PEEP ventilation in patients with severe left ventricular failure studied by transesophageal echocardiography. Chest 97:1181, 1990.
71. Gurevitch MJ, Van Dyke J, Young E, et al: Improved oxygen and lower peak airway pressure in severe adult respiratory distress syndrome: Treatment with inverse ratio ventilation. Chest 89:211, 1989.
72. Susini G, Zuccketti M, Bortone F, et al: Isolated ultrafiltration in cardiogenic pulmonary edema. Crit Care Med 18:14, 1990.
73. Killip T: Epidemiology of congestive heart failure. Am J Cardiol 56:2A, 1985.
74. Goodman LR, Putman CE: Diagnostic imaging in acute cardiopulmonary disease. Clin Chest Med 5:247, 1984.
75. Leuollen EC, Cain DT: Pleural effusion: A statistical study of 436 patients. N Engl J Med, 252:79, 1955.
76. Mellins RB, Levine OR, Fishman AP: Effect of systemic and pulmonary venous hypertension on pleural and pericardial fluid accumulation. J Appl Physiol 29:564, 1970.
77. Chetty KG: Transudative pleural effusions. Clin Chest Med 6:49, 1985.
78. Wiener-Kronish JP, Matthay MA, Callen PW, et al: Relationship of pleural effusions to pulmonary hemodynamics in patients with congestive heart failure. Am Rev Respir Dis 132:1253, 1985.
79. Brown NE, Zamel N, Aberman A: Changes in pulmonary mechanics and gas exchange following thoracentesis. Chest 74:540, 1978.
80. Anthonisen NR, Martin RR: Regional lung function in pleural effusion. Am Rev Respir Dis 116:201, 1977.
81. Francus G, Archer SL: Diagnosis and management of acute congestive heart failure in the intensive care unit. J Intensive Care Med 4:84, 1989.
82. Perret, CL: Management of severe heart failure. Acta Anaesthesiol Belg 39(suppl 2):103, 1988.
83. Knaus WA, Draper EA, Wagner DP, et al: APACHE II: A severity of disease classification system. Crit Care Med 13:818, 1985.
84. Fedullo AJ, Swinburne AJ, Wahl GW, et al: APACHE II score and mortality in respiratory failure due to cardiogenic pulmonary edema. Crit Care Med 16:1218, 1988.
85. Taliercio C, Seward J, Driscoll D, et al: Idiopathic dilated cardiomyopathy in the young. Clinical profile and natural history. J Am Coll Cardiol 6:1126, 1985.
86. Fuster V, Gersh B, Giullawi E, et al: The natural history of idiopathic dilated cardiomyopathy. Am J Cardiol 47:525, 1981.

CHAPTER 71

Acute Respiratory Failure in Chronic Obstructive Pulmonary Disease

J. Randall Curtis
Leonard D. Hudson

Chronic obstructive pulmonary disease (COPD) is a common disorder, affecting an estimated 10 million individuals in the United States, and in 1988 this disease was the fourth leading cause of death in the United States.[1] COPD refers to chronic bronchitis and/or (usually and) emphysema, which is accompanied by airflow obstruction as measured by spirometry. Chronic bronchitis is a diagnosis made by a history of cough productive of sputum (on most days at least 3 months per year for 2 consecutive years). Emphysema is a pathologic diagnosis, but the diagnosis can be suggested by certain clinical and laboratory findings. Emphysema can be presumed in a chronically dyspneic patient with airflow obstruction but no history of chronic bronchitis; also, the finding of a significant reduction in diffusing capacity in any patient with major airflow obstruction strongly suggests the presence of emphysema. Acute respiratory failure (ARF) in patients with COPD is one of the most frequent causes of admission to the intensive care unit (ICU). In this chapter we address some of the features of ARF that are unique to these patients. Perhaps most relevant to the patient with COPD is the difficulty in defining ARF in the setting of chronic respiratory insufficiency. When ARF has been identified in the COPD patient, one must immediately search for the precipitating event while simultaneously initiating action based on several principles of management. Early in the care of these patients, the physician is often faced with the difficult decision of whether and when to utilize endotracheal intubation and mechanical ventilation. The decision regarding mechanical ventilation should be approached with the knowledge of current survival data for COPD patients with ARF. Finally, there are frequently ethical and societal issues raised by the care of these patients.

The COPD patient with a history of gradually increasing dyspnea and sputum production, and with respiratory distress and diffuse expiratory wheezes, can be diagnosed as having an acute exacerbation of COPD. Although the scenario of dyspnea and increased sputum suggests exacerbation of COPD, these patients may present in more cryptic ways. For instance, patients can present with symptoms of central nervous system dysfunction ranging from irritability to coma attributable to the effects of hypoxia and/or acidosis on the central nervous system. Patients also can present with evidence of the effects of hypoxia or acidosis on the cardiovascular system, such as tachycardia, arrhythmia, or infarction. The possibility of an acute exacerbation of COPD must be in the differential diagnosis in order that appropriate diagnostic and therapeutic measures be taken.

When ARF is suspected, the diagnosis must be confirmed by arterial blood gas analysis. The presence of hypoxemia, hypercapnia, and acidosis can be used to define this disorder, but it is difficult to set specific levels of $Paco_2$ or Pao_2 because patients' baseline values may be markedly abnormal. It is more helpful to define ARF as a functional disturbance of physiologic mechanisms manifested in the arterial blood gas values by two criteria: (1) a significant change from baseline values—a drop in a patient's baseline Pao_2 and/or rise in $Paco_2$—and (2) a level of Pao_2 or pH associated with potential morbidity or mortality. In general, patients with ARF have a Pao_2 less than 55 mm Hg and a $Paco_2$ greater than 50 mm Hg. The pH is helpful in assessing the degree of hypoventilation that is acute versus the degree that is chronic and compensated because renal compensation by retention of bicarbonate takes time (usually several days). In acute respiratory acidosis without renal compensation, the pH drops by 0.08 for each 10-point rise in the $Paco_2$. In chronic respiratory acidosis with normal renal compensation, the pH drops by 0.03 for each 10-point rise in the $Paco_2$. This relationship between $Paco_2$ and pH is particularly helpful in assessing acute exacerbations in COPD patients because they frequently present with acute, superimposed on chronic, respiratory acidosis.

For the COPD patient diagnosed with ARF, there are four principles of management: (1) correct life-threatening hypoxemia, (2) correct life-threatening acidosis, (3) treat the underlying processes, and (4) prevent complications. Measures to correct hypoxemia should be instituted immediately; the timing of measures to correct acidosis varies according to the clinical situation (discussed in detail later). However, at the same time that oxygen therapy is started, the physician should also begin a thorough search for the etiology of the ARF because definitive treatment of the underlying processes depends on accurate diagnosis of the precipitating event.

PRECIPITATING EVENTS

Identification of a precipitating event is a critical feature in caring for the COPD patient with ARF. Without identification and treatment of the precipitating event, treatment of the respiratory failure is suboptimal and may not succeed. Almost any systemic or pulmonary illness can tip the carefully compensated COPD patient toward respiratory failure. Such illnesses can be grouped by their effect on pulmonary mechanics. For instance, an illness could produce ARF by one or more of six mechanisms: (1) decreasing ventilatory drive (oversedation, hypothyroidism, brain stem lesion); (2) decreasing muscle strength or function (malnutrition, shock, myopathy, hypophosphatemia, hypomagnesemia, hypocalcemia, myasthenia gravis, central or peripheral nervous system lesion); (3) decreasing chest wall elasticity (rib fracture, pleural effusion, ileus, ascites); (4) decreasing the lungs' resiliency or capacity for gas exchange (atelectasis, pulmonary edema, pneumonia); (5) increasing the airway resistance (bronchospasm, increased secretions or failure to clear usual secretions, upper airway obstruction, airway edema as in smoke inhalation); or (6) increasing metabolic oxygen requirements (systemic infection, hyperthyroidism). In addition to these six mechanisms, it is important to recognize the role of impaired cough and failure to clear secretions. Many disorders create one or more of the listed mechanisms while simultaneously interfering with the clearance of secretions (e.g., oversedation, myopathy, myasthenia gravis, rib fracture). When secretion clearance is impaired, the secretions can both contribute to the ARF and interfere with efforts to correct the ARF.

Despite the long list of disorders that can precipitate ARF, the most important precipitants of ARF in the COPD patient are airway infection, pulmonary embolus, congestive heart failure, anatomic interference with chest wall function, and medication noncompliance. These are important precipitants because they are relatively common, potentially reversible, and often overlooked. Each is discussed in more detail. Another important precipitant is oversedation. This is often iatrogenic and should be considered when prescribing sedating medication to a patient with COPD.

Airway Infection

Although difficult to study, probably the most common precipitant of ARF in COPD patients is airway infection. Pneumonia is often poorly tolerated by COPD patients and, in one series of COPD patients with ARF, was judged to be the precipitant of ARF in 20%.[2] Pneumonia in patients with COPD differs from pneumonia in normal hosts primarily in the bacteriology. COPD patients are more likely to harbor unusual organisms such as gram-negative enteric bacteria and *Legionella* and are more likely to have antibiotic-resistant organisms. This is presumably due to decreased clearance of organisms (because of impaired cough and impaired host defenses), frequent exposure to hospital environments, and frequent courses of antibiotics.

Acute bronchitis clearly plays a major role in ARF in patients with COPD. Defining this role is difficult; many of the agents thought to cause tracheobronchitis are normal flora of the upper airway and frequently are chronic contaminants of the lower airway in the absence of an acute exacerbation. Consequently, interpretation of sputum culture is difficult at best. *Haemophilus influenzae* and *Streptococcus pneumoniae* have been found in cultures of transtracheal aspirates of 80% of patients with acute exacerbations of chronic bronchitis,[3] but colonization may be difficult to distinguish from invasive infection. Fagon and colleagues[4] performed fiberoptic bronchoscopy in 54 COPD patients with ARF requiring intubation. In each case the clinical impression was that acute bronchitis caused the ARF. Using protected brush specimens, bacteria were recovered from only 50% of patients. *Haemophilus* and *Streptococcus* species represented 74% of all agents recovered, although enteric gram-negative rods made up 18% of the isolates. No clinical, laboratory, or radiologic feature identified the patients with positive cultures.

Viral agents and *Mycoplasma pneumoniae* play a role in ARF in COPD patients, but again the degree of their involvement is unclear. Viral agents, especially influenza viruses and rhinoviruses, can be identified in 20 to 30% of acute respiratory illnesses in patients with COPD.[5, 6] Glezen and colleagues[7] have shown that the peak occurrence of hospitalization of persons with acute respiratory disease coincided with the peak of influenza virus activity each year in Houston from 1978 to 1981. Chronic pulmonary disorders, especially in persons over 65 years of age, were the most common underlying illnesses. Even more intriguing is the potential role of viral and mycoplasmal infection in setting the stage for a secondary bacterial infection. There is evidence that viral respiratory illnesses are associated with increased isolation of *S. pneumoniae* and *H. influenzae* and that invasive *H. influenzae* infection, as determined by seroconversion, may also be the sequela of viral infection.[8] Potential mechanisms by which viral agents may lead to secondary bacterial respiratory infection include decreased mucociliary clearance and impaired phagocyte function.[9]

Although their use is controversial, empirical antibiotics should be used to treat most COPD patients with ARF and no clear noninfectious precipitant. This is not because there is good evidence suggesting an infectious precipitant in these cases but because these patients are critically ill and there is to date no effective way to distinguish the subgroup of patients that would benefit from antibiotics. In addition, some evidence does exist that patients treated with antibiotics do better than those from whom antibiotics are withheld, particularly if the patients present with dyspnea, increased sputum production, and sputum purulence.[10]

Pulmonary Embolus

Pulmonary embolus can clearly precipitate ARF in the COPD patient, and some evidence suggests that patients with COPD are at increased risk for pulmonary emboli. Although incidence reports vary, one series reported a 50% incidence of pulmonary emboli at autopsy in patients with severe COPD.[11] There are several reasons why these patients might be at increased risk for pulmonary emboli, including a high incidence of cor pulmonale with right ventricular mural thrombi.[11] There is also some evidence that COPD patients may be at increased risk because of abnormalities in platelet production[12] and function.[13] Of course, these patients frequently have limited physical activity because of poor pulmonary reserve and may have a high incidence of deep venous thrombosis.

Because the mortality resulting from diagnosed but untreated pulmonary embolus is approximately 30%,[14] the diagnosis of embolus in the COPD patient with ARF is an important issue. Unfortunately, patients with COPD frequently have only nonspecific symptoms and signs to suggest pulmonary embolism. Pleuritic chest pain and hemoptysis occur less frequently in COPD patients,[15] and dyspnea and hypoxemia can usually be attributed to another cause. Interestingly, some COPD patients with respiratory failure caused by pulmonary embolus have a decrease in $Paco_2$ from their usual baseline hypercapnia.[16] This feature, although insensitive, should raise the suspicion of pulmonary embolus. In fact, Chopin and colleagues described the use

of capnography to diagnose pulmonary embolism in COPD patients with ARF on the basis of their relative increase in CO_2 elimination compared with COPD patients with other causes of ARF.[17] This technique needs to be validated before acceptance for wide clinical application. Chest x-ray abnormalities, such as Hampton's hump (a density along the pleural surface with convexity pointing toward the hilum), Westermark's sign (unilateral blanching), and changes in the pulmonary hilum, although not overly sensitive or specific in the patient without COPD, are essentially useless in the patient with severe COPD.

The ventilation-perfusion ($\dot{V}/\dot{Q}$) scan can be a useful diagnostic tool in patients with COPD. Previous studies questioned the utility of $\dot{V}/\dot{Q}$ in COPD patients,[18, 19] especially those with ARF.[20] Data from the national collaborative prospective investigation of pulmonary embolism diagnosis (PIOPED) now indicate that the diagnostic utility of $\dot{V}/\dot{Q}$ scans for acute pulmonary embolism is not impaired by the presence of pre-existing cardiac or pulmonary disease.[21]

A serologic test that could support or rule out the diagnosis of pulmonary embolus would be a major contribution. Measurement of the D dimer, a specific derivative of cross-linked fibrin, in plasma has been proposed as an assay that may be able to rule out pulmonary embolus in 35% of patients with an indeterminate $\dot{V}/\dot{Q}$ scan, thus sparing these patients an angiogram.[22] The test needs further validation, particularly in patients with COPD.

Pulmonary angiography remains the "gold standard" for diagnosing pulmonary embolus. Previous data suggested that patients with cor pulmonale are at a slightly increased risk of complications of pulmonary angiography[23, 24] and that false-negative results could be obtained for patients with ARF[19] and COPD patients with recurrent multiple small emboli.[25] However, data from the prospective investigation of pulmonary embolism diagnosis indicate that pulmonary angiography is both safe and accurate in COPD patients.[26]

The need for angiography can often be eliminated by the finding of a deep venous thrombosis, which in itself is an indication for anticoagulation. Consequently, impedance plethysmography, lower extremity duplex Doppler ultrasonography, or contrast or radionuclide venography should be considered for all patients for whom pulmonary embolus is in the differential diagnosis. A negative study might necessitate further tests, perhaps a pulmonary angiogram, depending on the degree of clinical suspicion, but a positive study may obviate further work-up.

Treatment of pulmonary embolus with anticoagulants is the same in patients with COPD as in those without. The role of thrombolytic agents is not yet clearly defined, but patients with ARF may benefit from thrombolysis, particularly when right-sided heart function and pulmonary circulation are compromised.[27, 28]

Heart Function and Fluid Status

Assessment of heart function and fluid status in the COPD patient with ARF can be difficult. Respiratory distress and poor fluid intake before admission can result in negative fluid balance and decreased cardiac output. Underlying cor pulmonale and signs of right-sided heart failure may coexist with volume depletion, and if diuretic therapy is used in this circumstance the result could be circulatory collapse. Unfortunately, the prevalence of cor pulmonale increases with increasing severity of COPD. Forty percent of patients with a forced expiratory volume in 1 second (FEV_1) of less than 1.0 L and 70% of those with an FEV_1 of less than 0.6 L have cor pulmonale.[29] Hence, COPD patients presenting with ARF are at high risk of coincident cor pulmonale. Assessment of heart function is further complicated by the nonspecific presentation of cor pulmonale in COPD patients. Although Doppler echocardiography can accurately make or exclude this diagnosis in most patients,[30] this technology may be neither available nor appropriate in the initial, often emergent, assessment of the COPD patient with ARF.

The patient with COPD may also have volume overload and left-sided failure that precipitates ARF. These patients frequently have coexisting ischemic heart disease and are at risk for cardiogenic pulmonary edema. Initial evaluation should therefore be approached with a high index of suspicion for both volume depletion with compromised cardiac output and volume overload and pulmonary edema. In general, this issue can be resolved with a careful physical examination and a chest x-ray study. Occasionally, pulmonary arterial catheterization may be necessary to assist in the evaluation.

Anatomic Precipitants

Pleural effusion, rib fracture, pneumothorax, and upper airway obstruction are unusual precipitants of ARF in patients with COPD, but because specific therapy may be corrective, these diagnoses should be considered in each case. The patient with severe COPD may be unable to compensate for a relatively small increase in ventilatory workload caused by any of these abnormalities.

Pleural effusions cause both lung collapse and chest wall expansion and in doing so might be expected to decrease gas exchange and worsen respiratory muscle mechanics. In fact, thoracentesis of large volumes has not been shown to improve gas exchange[31] but has been shown to reduce the size of the thoracic cage and allow respiratory muscles to operate on a more advantageous portion of the length-tension curve.[32] One could speculate that the COPD patient with hyperinflation would have even more to gain from therapeutic thoracentesis.

A painful rib fracture causes splinting of the chest wall and intercostal muscle spasm. Local nerve block or epidural analgesia can reduce the need for potentially dangerous systemic analgesics and could obviate the need for mechanical ventilation.

The elderly COPD patient with spontaneous pneumothorax may present with dyspnea and anxiety but without chest pain.[33] The diagnosis may be difficult to make in the patient with severe and especially bullous emphysema. Although discussed in more detail as a complication of mechanical ventilation, this diagnosis should be entertained in all COPD patients with ARF.

Upper airway obstruction is a rare cause of ARF in COPD, but because intubation or tracheostomy can be lifesaving, this diagnosis should not be missed. COPD patients are frequently at increased risk of oropharyngeal cancers, and patients with prior endotracheal intubations are at increased risk of tracheal stenosis.

Noncompliance

Noncompliance with bronchodilator and anti-inflammatory medications may produce an exacerbation of COPD leading to ARF. Noncompliance is undoubtedly heightened by the relatively complicated medication regimen of many patients with COPD, which involves multiple oral and inhaled agents. One study showed that 54% of COPD patients significantly underused their medications in a 3-month period.[34] Questions about medication use may allow a physician and patient to develop ways to simplify or clarify the patient's regimen and thereby improve compliance.

MANAGEMENT OF ACUTE RESPIRATORY FAILURE IN CHRONIC OBSTRUCTIVE PULMONARY DISEASE

Utilization of Intensive Care

After deciding that hospital admission is necessary for the patient with COPD and acute exacerbation, the physician must decide to which category of nursing unit the patient is to be admitted. In the past, one of us suggested that all COPD patients with ARF initially should be admitted to an ICU, at least overnight. With the changes that have occurred over the last decade in hospital utilization patterns, this suggestion no longer seems either feasible or appropriate. In general, patients admitted to hospitals have a greater acuity of illness now than 10 years ago. Consequently, access to intensive care beds is more limited. At the same time, nurses and respiratory therapists on acute care wards have become more experienced in managing patients with greater acuity of illness, and intermediate care units have become more common. Currently we recommend that the decision about whether to admit a COPD patient with acute exacerbation to the acute care ward, an intermediate care unit, or an ICU be individualized and that both patient-related and institution-related factors be taken into account.

All patients with a diagnosis of ARF by the blood gas criteria given earlier are potentially unstable. However, if the patient's acute precipitating cause has been diagnosed and is potentially responsive to appropriate therapy, if current blood gas abnormalities are not life threatening with appropriate oxygen therapy, if the patient is cooperative with treatment (for example, with bronchodilator administration, oxygen therapy, and secretion clearance), and if appropriate nursing and respiratory care and observation can be provided on an acute care ward, admission to that site might be warranted. An ICU setting is necessary for patients who need closer observation and monitoring than can be provided outside the ICU. Such observation may be necessary because of a greater risk of deterioration or of complications, as well as for those requiring mechanical ventilation. Also, some patients may require a level of respiratory therapy that is not available in the acute care ward setting. An intermediate care unit or a noninvasive monitoring unit might be ideal for delivering the level of monitoring and care that is required for many COPD patients with an exacerbation.

A prior decision by the patient not to receive cardiopulmonary resuscitation should cardiopulmonary arrest occur, or not to have endotracheal intubation and mechanical ventilation, should not be a basis for excluding the patient from an ICU. An ICU is entirely appropriate as a site for delivering aggressive care to the respiratory patient but stopping short of mechanical ventilation or cardiopulmonary resuscitation. An exception would exist if the patient also had made it clear that he or she did not want aggressive treatment and that comfort was the only goal of therapy. The goals of therapy should be clearly identified and communicated to all the caregivers so that the approach to the patient is consistent.

Principles of Management

The diagnosis of ARF allows the practitioner to apply principles of management (Table 71-1) that are appropriate to all patients with ARF. The way these principles are applied to patients with COPD in ARF differs markedly from the way they are applied to patients with other types of ARF such as the adult respiratory distress syndrome. These principles include: correction of life-threatening hypoxemia, correction of life-threatening acidosis, treatment of the un-

---

TABLE 71-1

PRINCIPLES OF MANAGEMENT OF ACUTE RESPIRATORY FAILURE IN PATIENTS WITH CHRONIC OBSTRUCTIVE PULMONARY DISEASE

1. Correct life-threatening hypoxemia
   a. Usually requires only small increases in F_{IO_2} (1–2 L/min by nasal prongs).
   b. Infiltrate or pulmonary edema suggests the presence of a shunt, and a higher F_{IO_2} may be required.
   c. Usually the therapeutic goal is a Pa_{O_2} of 55–65 mm Hg (associated with nearly complete oxygen saturation of hemoglobin).
   d. Observe for signs of CO_2 retention and check arterial blood gases after increments in F_{IO_2}.
2. Correct life-threatening acidosis
   a. Usually is less urgent than correcting hypoxemia.
   b. Usually is accomplished with therapy to improve airflow and remove secretions.
   c. Decision to use mechanical ventilation depends more on clinical status (especially mental status) than level of pH or P_{CO_2}.
   d. Bicarbonate therapy is rarely indicated.
3. Treat underlying disease process
   a. Treatment aimed at increasing airflow:
      First line: use ipratroprium and/or inhaled beta-agonist, systemic corticosteroids.
      Second line: use theophylline.
   b. Treatment aimed at improving secretion removal: use hydration, chest percussion, inhaled heated moisture as indicated.
   c. Precipitating events are treated as indicated.
4. Prevent complications
   a. Cardiac dysrhythmias: maintain oxygenation and normalize electrolyte values; monitor level of theophylline, if used.
   b. Pulmonary thromboembolism: use subcutaneous heparin for prophylaxis if not contraindicated.
   c. Treat gastrointestinal complications.
      Prophylaxis of gastrointestinal bleeding: sucralfate vs. H_2 blocker.
      Nasogastric suctioning: if aerophagia is a problem.
   d. Nosocomial infection: use sucralfate for prophylaxis of gastrointestinal bleeding.
   e. Prevent barotrauma and impaired cardiac output because of intrinsic PEEP on mechanical ventilation.
      Use modest tidal volume (7–8 mL/kg).
      Minimize $\dot{V}_E$, peak and mean airway pressures.
      If intrinsic PEEP develops, attempt to
         Decrease respiratory rate.
         Increase inspiratory flow rate (approximately 5–6 × $\dot{V}_E$).
         Decrease tidal volume.
         Try pressure support.

---

derlying disease process, and prevention and treatment of complications.

Correction of Hypoxemia

Correction of hypoxemia in the COPD patient with ARF usually requires administration of a small increase in the fraction of inspired oxygen (F_{IO_2}), which can be achieved with a low flow of oxygen via nasal prongs. An alternative to nasal prongs is a face mask employing the Venturi principle to entrain air so that a fixed percentage of oxygen can be delivered, ranging from approximately 24 to 35%. A small increment in F_{IO_2} suffices because these patients usually have a combination of hypoventilation and $\dot{V}/\dot{Q}$ mismatching; the hypoxemia with both of these physiologic mechanisms is responsive to changes in inspired oxygen content.

Occasionally, patients with COPD and ARF require ad-

ministration of a higher F_{IO_2}. These patients have some degree of shunting contributing to their hypoxemia in addition to the other physiologic mechanisms of hypoxemia mentioned earlier. The shunting in these patients may be associated with pneumonia or congestive heart failure, both of which result in airless areas of lung to which some degree of blood flow continues.

Initial oxygen therapy can be guided by an assessment of the chest x-ray film together with the clinical symptoms and signs and the initial Pa_{O_2}. If the chest x-ray film does not show pulmonary infiltrates (e.g., the clear chest x-ray film associated with exacerbation of bronchitis) and the Pa_{O_2} is in the 40s to low 50s on room air, oxygen therapy can be started at 1 to 2 L/min by nasal prongs, adjusting this flow rate according to subsequent arterial blood gas determinations. On the other hand, if a significant new pulmonary infiltrate is seen on the chest x-ray film, a greater increase in supplemental oxygen is warranted as initial therapy—either a higher flow rate by nasal prongs or a higher F_{IO_2} by face mask (e.g., 35 to 40%) with repeated arterial blood gas measurements within a short time (15 to 30 minutes) to allow further adjustment.

In either case, the level of supplemental oxygen needed should be evaluated and adjusted according to repeated arterial blood gas measurements while at the initial level of oxygen therapy. The goal of therapy is to provide adequate oxygen saturation (e.g., >90%) without a significant increase in Pa_{CO_2} associated with respiratory acidosis. Usually a Pa_{O_2} between 55 and 65 mm Hg is adequate and a reasonable goal of initial therapy. This level allows nearly complete saturation of the hemoglobin with oxygen but avoids progressive retention of CO_2 in most (but not all) patients.

Oxygen must be delivered to COPD patients in a controlled fashion because some patients clearly have progressive retention of CO_2 with progressive respiratory acidosis when given oxygen in excessive amounts. The use of controlled oxygen therapy was popularized by EJ Moran Campbell, at that time of Hammersmith Postgraduate Medical Centre and Hospital in London, England.[35] Campbell described the rationale and importance for this and popularized a mask using the Venturi principle of entraining air, the so-called Venti-mask, as a means of achieving controlled oxygen therapy. Others have since shown that low flow rates of supplemental oxygen delivered by nasal prongs are also effective as a means of providing controlled oxygen therapy.[36, 37]

A minority of COPD patients with ARF have increases in Pa_{CO_2} with oxygen therapy.[35, 38] Bone and colleagues found that the presence of severe hypoxemia ($Pa_{O_2} < 49$ mm Hg) and acidemia (pH < 7.35) predicted a greater risk of increase in Pa_{CO_2} with oxygen therapy.[39] Warren and coworkers found that severe acidemia was the best prognostic factor but failed to confirm severe hypoxemia as a significant predictor.[40] The risk is clearly minimized if oxygen is given in a controlled and monitored fashion.[35–38]

The reason traditionally given for retention of CO_2 with excessive amounts of oxygen in COPD patients in ARF has been removal of the hypoxic drive to breathe. It was assumed that these patients, particularly those with chronic CO_2 retention, were no longer sensitive to CO_2 ventilatory drive and were dependent on their hypoxic drive to maintain adequate ventilation. When oxygen was administered, it was assumed that the hypoxic drive to breathe was no longer functional and the subsequent rise in CO_2 in some of these patients was related to hypoventilation. This mechanism has been questioned. New data suggest that the CO_2 retention in response to oxygen administration is probably multifactorial and that an increase in $\dot{V}/\dot{Q}$ ratio may be the predominant mechanism rather than hypoventilation resulting from suppression of the hypoxic drive to breathe.[41–43]

Aubier and colleagues found that patients with COPD had a ventilatory drive during ARF that was five times greater than that in their chronic stable state. Although administration of oxygen caused a modest reduction in ventilatory drive, drive was still several times greater than that in stable patients and the small change in minute ventilation ($\dot{V}E$) did not account for the large increase in $PaCO_2$.[41, 42] They concluded that despite a reduction of the hypoxic stimulus of oxygen administration, the respiratory muscle activity remained great enough to maintain $\dot{V}E$ at nearly the same value as when the patient was breathing room air. They further concluded that the changes in $PaCO_2$ after the administration of oxygen were mainly due to increased inhomogeneity of $\dot{V}/\dot{Q}$ distribution within the lungs, resulting in an increase of dead space or wasted ventilation. Stradling subsequently questioned these data and argued that global hypoventilation was the major effect, as originally thought, with an additional contribution by the Haldane effect and a relatively minor contribution by increased $\dot{V}/\dot{Q}$.[44] However, a study by Sassoon and coworkers of stable patients with severe COPD while breathing oxygen supports the idea that the changes in PCO_2 while breathing oxygen are primarily due to changes in $\dot{V}/\dot{Q}$ with an increased ratio of dead space to tidal volume.[43] Regardless of the mechanism, the clinician must recognize that progressive respiratory acidosis is a potential complication of inappropriate oxygen administration in a minority of patients with COPD and ARF. This complication can be minimized by providing oxygen in a dose adequate to improve oxygen saturation and oxygen delivery but not to be associated with progressive increase in $PaCO_2$.

Correction of Life-Threatening Acidosis

The type, urgency, and intensity of therapy to correct acidosis depend on the clinical status and the degree of respiratory acidosis. If the patient is obtunded or comatose and cannot be aroused, immediate intubation and mechanical ventilation are warranted, even without having arterial blood gas analysis available. Severe acidosis (pH < 7.2) might warrant administration of small amounts of bicarbonate intravenously.[45, 46] However, in most patients, some time is available for correcting the acidosis. That is, the acidosis does not have to be corrected immediately, but therapy should begin a trend in the right direction. The main goal of therapy is to improve the pH from potentially life-threatening levels of acidosis. The option of mechanical ventilation is available but usually is not necessary. Most patients have improvement in the acidosis with treatment of the underlying airflow obstruction including administration of bronchodilators, corticosteroids, and secretion clearance measures. The decision regarding endotracheal intubation and mechanical ventilation or use of mechanical ventilation by face mask is discussed later.

The use of respiratory stimulants remains controversial,[47, 48] and no controlled clinical trials have shown undisputed clinical benefit. Doxapram administration is associated with a smaller increase in $PaCO_2$ during oxygen therapy compared with placebo,[49, 50] but the best-designed study found no difference in frequency of intubation and mechanical ventilation between the treatment and control groups.[50]

Treatment of the Underlying Disease Process

Treatment of the underlying process is directed at two aspects: the acute precipitating event and the chronic airflow obstruction. Diagnosis and treatment of the acute precipitating event have been covered. Treatment of the chronic airflow obstruction is aimed at two general goals: an increase in the diameter of airways (through bronchodilation and reduction of edema and inflammation) and enhanced removal of airway secretions.

Treatment Aimed at Improving Airflow. Medications to decrease airway resistance include bronchodilators and corticosteroids. Many COPD patients with acute exacerbation appear to have a component of increased airflow obstruction that is partially responsive to bronchodilator agents. Although the amount of reversibility may be relatively small, gaining this therapeutic advantage can be extremely important in management of these patients. The available bronchodilators include beta-adrenergic agents, anticholinergic agents, and theophylline medications. Of the three types of bronchodilator medications, the beta-adrenergic and anticholinergic agents in their aerosolized form have a greater relative bronchodilator effect than theophylline. Beta-adrenergic and anticholinergic agents are both effective; there is no clear-cut advantage of one drug versus another in most studies of COPD outpatients,[51–55] although results of other studies favor ipratropium over a beta-adrenergic agent.[56, 57] Studies of COPD patients both as stable outpatients[51–53] and during acute exacerbations[53–55] have demonstrated that a maximal bronchodilator response is achieved with one of these agents given in adequate doses and that adding the other agent gives relatively little or no additional effect. Therefore, which drug is used as initial therapy may be decided according to the preference of the individual physician. However, in the patient with ARF, if one agent does not produce the desired effect, the other agent should be added on a trial basis.

Several beta$_2$-selective agents can be administered. These include metaproterenol, albuterol, terbutaline, isoetharine, pirbuterol, and bitolterol. They can be administered either via a metered-dose inhaler (MDI) or as a solution with a nebulizer. The MDI is cheaper, and if the patient is able to use one correctly and cooperate with therapy this is the preferred route of administration.[58, 59] The MDI should be used with a spacer or reservoir for two reasons.[60] First, a spacer traps the large particles, which would otherwise precipitate and deposit in the mouth and be absorbed with subsequent systemic toxic effects. Second, a spacer lessens the need for coordination of the inhalation with activation of the MDI; this may be of particular benefit in a dyspneic patient with a high respiratory rate. The usual dose of medication given to a stable outpatient can be increased in the setting of ARF, with the patient being monitored for tachycardia. Also, more frequent dosing may be required, again determined according to the effect on the individual patient but as frequent as every 2 hours or even hourly in some situations. Initially, 10 to 20 inhalations over a relatively short time may be warranted, as long as the patient is evaluated during the administration for both beneficial effect and possible toxicity. If the patient breathing spontaneously is unable to use an MDI effectively because of the acuity of illness, a nebulizer with a mouthpiece should be employed, at least during the initial acute phase of the illness. In the patient receiving mechanical ventilation, the beta-adrenergic aerosol can be administered by an MDI through an adaptor in the ventilator tubing.[61] Because of possible precipitation of the medication in the ventilator tubing, larger than usual doses are required.

Ipratropium bromide is an anticholinergic agent that is available only in an MDI.[62] Ipratropium is a quaternary ammonium structure, whereas atropine sulfate is a tertiary ammonium agent. The quaternary structure is associated with lipid insolubility; therefore ipratropium, unlike atropine, crosses biologic barriers with difficulty. This difference accounts for the pharmacologic properties that distinguish ipratropium from atropine. Ipratropium is poorly absorbed into the blood stream, has few systemic side effects, has a more selective respiratory effect, and has a longer duration of action. Ipratropium bromide administered via an MDI, therefore, is the preferred anticholinergic agent. Again, doses larger than those conventionally recommended for the stable outpatient may be necessary. Also, the dosing interval may have to be shortened, as with the beta-adrenergic agents. Atropine methonitrate is a quaternary ammonium compound available in solution form in European and other countries but not in the United States. Atropine sulfate in a solution form can be used for patients in North America if nebulized delivery is required. Atropine sulfate should be given every 3 to 4 hours with more frequent dosing if necessary as judged clinically.

Studies of theophylline compared with other bronchodilator agents administered to patients with acute severe asthma have questioned the role of theophylline in this condition. The efficacy of intravenous aminophylline in the treatment of patients hospitalized because of an exacerbation of COPD was studied with a randomized, double-blind, placebo-controlled design.[63] Patients received either intravenous aminophylline or placebo, in addition to inhaled nebulized metaproterenol, intravenous methylprednisolone, antibiotics, and supplemental oxygen. There were no significant differences between the placebo and aminophylline groups in spirometric measurements, dyspneic indices, or arterial blood gas values. Although the difference in overall incidence of side effects between the two groups was not statistically significant, there was a strong trend toward more side effects in the aminophylline group (7 of 15 vs. 1 of 13) and gastrointestinal complaints were greater in the aminophylline group (6 of 15 vs. 0 of 13; $P < .05$). One possible criticism of this study is the relatively small sample size (total n = 28), which increases the chance of a beta or type II error. Also, in interpreting the data one must keep in mind that these patients were receiving large doses of intravenous corticosteroids in addition to an inhaled beta-adrenergic agent. However, it seems fair to conclude that aminophylline adds relatively little benefit in most patients with COPD and ARF who are treated with corticosteroids and beta-adrenergic agents. For the patient not receiving theophylline at the time of hospital admission, we recommend beginning therapy with beta-adrenergic and anticholinergic aerosols and systemic corticosteroids but not starting theophylline initially. However, if by 12 to 24 hours no substantial improvement has occurred, we would add theophylline. If the patient is already receiving theophylline, we recommend that it be continued and the dose be adjusted according to theophylline blood levels. Acutely, it can be given intravenously in the form of aminophylline. However, if the patient is able to take oral agents and gastrointestinal function is thought to be intact, theophylline is well absorbed from the gut and can be administered orally. If there is any question regarding efficacy of the oral route in a given patient, it is prudent to begin with intravenous administration.

If the COPD patient has an acute exacerbation severe enough to warrant admission to the hospital, we recommend administration of corticosteroids initially, unless specific contraindications exist. The recommendation for administration of corticosteroids in patients with both COPD and ARF is based on the only controlled randomized trial of corticosteroid administration in this population of patients.[64] Consecutive patients with COPD admitted to hospital with acute bronchitis as the precipitating condition for ARF were randomized to receive methylprednisolone (0.5 mg/kg every 6 hours for 3 days) versus placebo. Other treatment was standardized. The steroid-treated group demonstrated a greater improvement in FEV$_1$ at any time point after the

first 12 hours for the rest of the 3 days of the study. There was no difference in eventual outcome, although survival was high in both groups. No increase in side effects or complications was attributable to corticosteroids. Another study examined COPD patients presenting to the emergency department with acute exacerbations.[65] The patients were randomized to receive either intravenous methylprednisolone or placebo in addition to other therapy and were followed for 5 hours. There were no differences in the number of patients admitted to the hospital or in pulmonary function at the end of the 4.5-hour mean period. No difference was noted in patients presenting with repeated exacerbations within the next several days, although follow-up after discharge from the emergency department was not rigorous. The apparent conflict in results between these two studies may be explained by the period of follow-up. Taken together, these results suggest that, although benefit is not seen by 5 hours, benefit measured by objective improvement in pulmonary function can be seen by 12 hours after administration. The other impressive finding in the first study, by Albert and colleagues, was that more patients who received corticosteroids had a marked improvement in pulmonary function; 12 of 22 corticosteroid patients showed a greater than 40% increase in FEV$_1$ at the end of 3 days compared with only 3 of 21 patients receiving placebo.[64] Relatively few COPD patients respond to corticosteroids when they are clinically stable,[66] and this study suggests that some COPD patients who do not respond to corticosteroids when clinically stable may respond during acute exacerbations.[67]

In conclusion, we recommend that the COPD patient admitted to the hospital for ARF be treated initially with corticosteroids plus either beta-adrenergic or anticholinergic bronchodilator aerosol in an aggressive fashion (or a combination of both bronchodilators). Theophylline should be added if there is not a significant improvement during the next 12 to 24 hours.

Treatment Aimed at Improving Secretion Removal. Most patients with acute exacerbations of COPD have an increase in airway secretions because of either increased production related to an acute inflammatory or infectious condition or increased retention resulting from impairment of cough and other airway clearance mechanisms. Any therapeutic measures that can be added to help the patient in clearing secretions may be important. There is limited objective information about measures that are clearly effective, especially in patients with ARF. Corticosteroids may play a role in loosening secretions or making them less viscous. Chest percussion might be helpful, although it may be both uncomfortable and physiologically compromising to place the patients in extreme bronchial drainage positions, and usually these must be modified.[68, 69] If chest percussion and postural drainage are used, they should be given as a therapeutic trial and the resulting sputum production should be compared with the sputum production when the patient coughs spontaneously after bronchodilator therapy without chest percussion and postural drainage. Measures that might improve the effectiveness of coughing include instructing the patient in proper cough technique (although most patients have learned this for themselves), having the patient in a sitting position (because coughing in a supine or partially upright position is difficult), and using effective bronchodilation with encouragement of cough immediately afterward. Adequate hydration of the patient makes sense, the hypothesis being that secretions in a well-hydrated patient are less viscous. There are, however, few data to support this.[70] There is also no evidence that administration of fluid directly into the airways is helpful. However, some patients find that inhalation of heated moist aerosol helps them raise secretions, and in such patients this measure should be used empirically.

Prevention and Treatment of Complications

The outcome for critically ill patients is often related to whether complications of the patient's disease or therapy develop. Whenever possible, potential complications should be anticipated and preventive measures taken. Heightened awareness of possible complications can help in early diagnosis and management and may improve outcome. It is beyond the scope of this chapter to review all possible complications.[71] The major complications that can be anticipated in the management of ARF in patients with COPD are briefly reviewed.

Cardiac Dysrhythmias. Cardiac dysrhythmias are frequent in COPD patients with ARF.[72-75] Both supraventricular and ventricular dysrhythmias occur with approximately equal frequencies.[72] Dysrhythmias in these patients often have a multifactorial etiology.[71] Possible etiologic factors include the following:

1. The acute lung disease with its associated hypoxemia and acidosis
2. Underlying heart disease, including ischemic heart disease and right-sided heart failure with right-sided heart dilatation
3. Other metabolic abnormalities commonly found in these patients, including electrolyte abnormalities and increased catecholamine levels
4. Iatrogenic factors such as medications frequently used for these patients, including sympathomimetics and theophylline, and procedures performed, including right-sided heart catheterization

The approach to management of dysrhythmias in these patients often varies from the approach to dysrhythmias caused by a primary cardiac problem such as ischemic heart disease. Frequently, no acute therapy can change the underlying cause of the dysrhythmia in patients with primary cardiac disease, so pharmacologic antiarrhythmic therapy becomes the primary intervention. As with any other patient with life-threatening dysrhythmia (ventricular fibrillation or ventricular tachycardia with hypotension), electrical cardioversion or antiarrhythmic therapy should be employed if the cardiac rhythms are thought to be an acute threat to life in the patient with COPD. However, if the rhythm is not an acute threat to life, the major approach in these patients is to identify and treat the metabolic causes of the dysrhythmia—especially hypoxemia and acidosis or alkalosis—and to treat the underlying lung disease or diseases. Antiarrhythmic pharmacologic therapy is necessary only when correction of the other possible etiologic factors has not been successful.

Pulmonary Thromboembolism. Pulmonary embolism may occur as a complication in the COPD patient with ARF. As discussed earlier, pulmonary embolism as a precipitating cause of ARF in the patient with COPD can be a difficult diagnosis to make.[19, 76] The same caveats apply to diagnosing pulmonary embolism when it develops as a complication. A high degree of suspicion for this complication is probably the most important diagnostic prerequisite.

Gastrointestinal Complications. Gastric distention and intestinal ileus occur in COPD patients with ARF. Aerophagia is a frequent occurrence in these dyspneic patients and many metabolic abnormalities can predispose to ileus. Both gastric dilatation and ileus may further compromise diaphragm function. Also, these complications predispose to aspiration of gastric contents.

A high incidence of gastrointestinal bleeding has been reported in patients with ARF.[77] Possible preventive or therapeutic measures in these patients include enteral feeding[78] and administration of antacids, H_2 blockers, or sucralfate. Enteral feeding and sucralfate are currently preferred means of prevention. Sucralfate has found favor because of reports that its use is associated with a lower frequency of nosocomial pneumonias than use of antacids.[79, 80]

Nosocomial Infections. Nosocomial infections, particularly pneumonias, are perhaps the most severe complications in these patients, especially in terms of their adverse effect on outcome. The factors predisposing to nosocomial infection and the prevention and treatment of infection in these patients are similar to those in other critically ill patients and are covered elsewhere in this text.

Complications Associated with Mechanical Ventilation. These complications include barotrauma, intrinsic positive end-expiratory pressure (or auto-PEEP) with lung hyperinflation and its associated complications, and nosocomial infection. Barotrauma and auto-PEEP are dealt with later. In addition, airway complications can be related to the endotracheal tube or tracheostomy. In most patients with COPD and ARF, maintenance of an endotracheal tube airway is preferred if the period of mechanical ventilator support is expected to be relatively short, because one study found that serious airway complications were probably more frequent with tracheostomy than with prolonged use of an endotracheal tube.[81] Therefore, tracheostomy is not warranted in most patients. However, if the episode of ARF requiring mechanical ventilation is likely to be prolonged and yet ultimately reversible, early tracheostomy may be justified.

Mechanical Ventilation

Most patients with COPD in ARF do not require mechanical ventilation for a successful outcome. However, some patients do not survive without a period of mechanical ventilation. In patients with COPD and ARF receiving mechanical ventilation, data suggest that the likelihood of surviving the acute episode is relatively good.[2, 82] There are no specific values of PaO_2, $PaCO_2$, or pH that provide a basis for deciding whether a patient will benefit from mechanical ventilation. Rather the decision is a clinical one, based on knowledge of the patient's baseline pulmonary and functional states and the reversibility of the precipitating event, as well as current symptoms and physical examination with arterial blood gas values as supporting data.

The primary determinant of the decision in most instances is the patient's mental status. If the patient is alert and able to cooperate with treatment, a period of aggressive therapy but without endotracheal intubation and mechanical ventilation (so-called conservative therapy) is warranted, regardless of the arterial blood gas data. If the patient is somnolent and unable to cooperate with treatment and stimulation and initial therapeutic measures do not improve the mental state, endotracheal intubation and mechanical ventilation should be considered regardless of the severity of the arterial blood gas abnormalities. One study suggests that if the patient fails a trial of conservative therapy and is subsequently intubated and ventilated, the outcome is significantly worse than if the decision for intubation and mechanical ventilation was made on admission.[83] This difference in outcome is more likely dependent on the selection of patients than on any delay in mechanical ventilation therapy.

One reason to avoid mechanical ventilation in COPD patients whenever possible (as opposed to its use in other patients with ARF) is the effect on secretion removal. Effective coughing is the primary means of secretion clearance. Stable patients with severe COPD have impaired coughing, because a high airflow is necessary for optimal coughing. Optimal coughing is also dependent on the ability to close the glottis, which allows intrathoracic pressure to increase with subsequent high velocities of airflow when the glottis is suddenly opened. Placement of an endotracheal tube through the larynx prevents glottic closure and thus further impairs the cough mechanism. Although respiratory care and nursing personnel can suction secretions from central airways in the intubated patient, this is not as effective as coughing in removing secretions from distal airways or preventing nosocomial lower airway infections. Because both secretion clearance and nosocomial infection are major problems in the COPD patient with ARF, the cough mechanism should be protected and encouraged whenever possible. If the patient is unresponsive, she or he cannot cough effectively. Consequently, endotracheal intubation to allow mechanical ventilation does not have the same detrimental effect on secretion clearance in the obtunded patient.

The specifics of mechanical ventilation management are dealt with in other chapters in this text. Only the aspects specifically related to patients with COPD are covered here. These include ventilatory requirements in COPD and complications of mechanical ventilation in the COPD patient.

Ventilatory requirements are usually normal or only modestly increased in the patient with COPD. A normal to slightly increased $\dot{V}E$ is usually adequate for CO_2 removal, depending on the precipitating cause of the ARF (causes associated with an increase in CO_2 production or in dead space result in higher $\dot{V}E$ requirements). Therefore, a modest tidal volume (VT) and $\dot{V}E$ should be used initially to prevent alkalemia from developing especially in patients with compensated respiratory acidosis in their chronic state. Although a VT of 10 mL/kg of body weight is usually suggested, tidal volumes of 7 to 8 mL/kg suffice and potentially are associated with fewer complications, especially with less chance of developing auto-PEEP. Because ventilatory requirements are modest in most patients with COPD and ARF, any ventilator mode is usually adequate to achieve the goals of mechanical ventilation in these patients. However, some of the modes of ventilation are more apt to be associated with development of complications than others, and comfort of the patient is also a factor. These considerations should be taken into account when determining the ventilatory mode.

Auto-PEEP and barotrauma are two major complications of mechanical ventilation in patients with COPD. The two may be related because auto-PEEP and its air trapping with progressively higher lung volumes and elevated pressures probably predispose to the development of barotrauma. Auto-PEEP is a frequent development and should be monitored for in all patients with COPD receiving mechanical ventilation.[84, 85] Risk factors for the development of auto-PEEP include chronic airflow obstruction, older age, and high $\dot{V}E$ requirements.[85] Auto-PEEP is also particularly dangerous in COPD patients because the increased lung compliance in these patients results in more of the alveolar pressure being transmitted to the pleural space. Therefore, there is a greater propensity for impairment in venous return and reduction of cardiac output. If the presence of auto-PEEP is not recognized, the clinician frequently draws faulty conclusions based on the available data. If a pulmonary arterial catheter is in place, the increased alveolar and pleural pressures associated with auto-PEEP result in falsely elevated intrathoracic vascular pressures including pulmonary arterial wedge pressure. With a high wedge pressure and fall in cardiac output, the clinician may decide that the patient is on the descending limb of the Starling curve and may administer a diuretic. This could result in a reduction in the intravascular volume, which would further contribute to the reduction in venous return and impairment of cardiac output.

When it has been determined that a degree of auto-PEEP is present, the treatment focuses on two aspects. First, the ultimate goal of treatment is improvement of airflow and justifies maximal therapeutic measures aimed at reducing airflow obstruction. The second aspect of therapy concerns manipulation of the mechanical ventilation mode and settings. The goal of changing the ventilator settings is to allow a longer period for exhalation and thus allow dissipation of the trapped air that results in auto-PEEP. This can be accomplished by increasing the inspiratory flow rate and shortening the time for inhalation or decreasing the respiratory rate and thus increasing the time for exhalation. One might also try decreasing the VT and thus the amount of air given to a patient with each ventilator breath, making it easier to exhale the lower VT in the time available for exhalation. One would expect reducing VT or the respiratory rate to result in an increase in PCO_2. However, auto-PEEP and its attendant trapped air are usually associated with an increase in dead space. Thus, if a reduction in VT or respiratory rate were effective in decreasing auto-PEEP and dead space, the reduced $\dot{V}E$ might be associated with more efficient gas exchange and relatively little change in alveolar ventilation and $PaCO_2$. Connors and associates studied the effect of varying inspiratory flow rate on gas exchange in patients with ARF.[86] An increased inspiratory rate (and thus a shorter inspiratory time for delivering the same VT) was associated with a decrease in dead space in patients with COPD but not other patients with ARF. They did not measure auto-PEEP, but it is likely that the improved gas exchange was associated with a reduction in this measurement. If auto-PEEP develops while the patient is on the assist-control mode of ventilation, changing to intermittent mandatory ventilation and allowing the patient to take some spontaneous breaths might allow some of the trapped gas to dissipate, with an accompanying reduction in auto-PEEP.

Work of breathing may be an issue in choosing a ventilatory mode. Controlled mechanical ventilation is associated with the lowest work of breathing and the assist-control mode usually with the second lowest. However, Marini and coworkers have shown that with the assist-control mode some patients continue to make an active inspiratory effort when they have triggered the inspiration and continue this effort throughout inspiration despite the fact that the entire breath is delivered by the ventilator.[87] Therefore these patients continue to have muscular work during inspiration. One of the variables that affects this phenomenon is the inspiratory flow rate delivered by the ventilator. Active inspiratory work is more likely to occur with a relatively low inspiratory flow rate. Thus, with the assist-control mode one should employ a high inspiratory flow rate, both to minimize inspiratory work and to allow a longer exhalation. Also, patients should be examined to determine whether they are using their inspiratory muscles during the ventilator-delivered breath. During intermittent mandatory ventilation the patient obviously performs work during the spontaneous breathing portion of the ventilation. In this mode the amount of work can be controlled by varying the respiratory rate. The pressure support mode of ventilation reduces ventilatory work (with the amount of work dependent on the pressure value selected) and allows the patient more control over the ventilatory waveform, so it often provides a more comfortable form of ventilation. Whether having the patient perform some work with intermittent mandatory or pressure support ventilation and gradually reducing the amount of ventilator work and increasing the patient's work of breathing is beneficial in training the inspiratory muscles and hastening weaning is not yet known; a thorough discussion of this topic is beyond the scope of this chapter.

Several reports have recommended relatively early administration of mechanical ventilation or continuous positive airway pressure delivered via face mask or nasal mask, in an attempt to treat respiratory acidosis, reduce work of breathing, and avoid endotracheal intubation.[88–95] These methods may be useful with selected patients. However, most reports have been of uncontrolled studies,[88–94] and the only controlled study in COPD patients with ARF is reported in abstract only at the time of this writing.[95] Another report (also on an uncontrolled study) described several patients with obstructive pulmonary disease who failed to respond to nasal positive pressure ventilation and required endotracheal intubation.[96] This report also documents the marked increase in use of nursing staff resources required with this type of noninvasive ventilation. Therefore, the efficacy of and proper selection of patients for these methods remain in question.

Nutritional Support

Although nutritional support for COPD patients in ARF is fairly well accepted,[97, 98] the best method of support remains unclear. It is clear that COPD patients in ARF are likely to show signs of protein-calorie malnutrition,[99] which can be chronic, acute, or, most likely, acute associated with baseline chronic malnutrition.[100] It is also relatively clear that specific nutritional deficiencies can exacerbate respiratory muscle weakness. Such nutritional deficiencies include hypophosphatemia,[101, 102] hypocalcemia,[103] and hypomagnesemia[104] and should be corrected when present.

Difficulty arises in determining the degree of protein-calorie support. Large carbohydrate loads increase CO_2 production in COPD patients[98] and can result in hypercapnic acidosis with respiratory failure or in unsuccessful weaning from mechanical ventilation. In the ventilated patient this usually can be prevented by increasing the minute ventilation,[105] but this is not feasible before intubation or when extubation is being attempted. Substituting lipid calories for carbohydrate calories decreases the respiratory quotient and CO_2 production[105] and is a feasible maneuver in these patients. In COPD patients requiring longer periods of ventilatory support, this change in feeding regimen should be attempted just before a weaning attempt but not when ventilatory demands are such that weaning is not an option. In patients without COPD, protein supplementation seems to increase oxygen consumption and ventilatory sensitivity to CO_2.[106] The role of protein supplementation in respiratory support of the COPD patients is unclear.

Although further studies are needed to define the optimal form and timing of nutritional support, in general enteral or parenteral nutrition should be considered if a patient requires more than a day of mechanical ventilation. In contrast to previous recommendations of 4000 to 5000 calories per day, these patients probably require only about 2000 calories per day.[97] The patient with moderately high minute ventilation who is not tolerating attempts to be weaned from the ventilator may require a temporary decrease in or discontinuation of nutritional support.

In most situations, the preferred route of nutritional supplementation is through the gastrointestinal tract. However, COPD patients with ARF have delayed colonic transit time and diffuse digestive motor dysfunction[107] and may be at increased risk for bowel pseudo-obstruction and perforation.[108] For this reason, total parenteral nutrition should be considered for critically ill ventilated COPD patients. Nonetheless, even for these patients, a careful trial of enteral feeding is indicated as long as the gastrointestinal tract is functional.

OUTCOME OF ACUTE RESPIRATORY FAILURE IN PATIENTS WITH CHRONIC OBSTRUCTIVE PULMONARY DISEASE

Information about mortality resulting from ARF in a COPD patient is critical for the physician assessing appropriate therapy and also for the patient and family making decisions regarding aggressiveness of treatment. Unfortunately, the available data on mortality suffer from several limitations. First, the reported series do not include all patients with COPD and ARF because some patients elect not to be admitted to an ICU or even to a hospital and hence may not be available to researchers. Second, many studies use different definitions of ARF and most studies do not describe clinical variables that affect mortality in enough detail to allow comparison of the populations of patients. Third, there is a relative lack of recent data. With these limitations in mind, some generalizations can be made from the literature.

The mortality of COPD patients with ARF has generally been defined as either in-hospital mortality or mortality at 30 days. Before 1978, mortality rates in 10 studies reported in the English language [46, 83, 107–116] ranged from 12 to 37% and averaged 28%. From 1978 forward three studies have reported mortalities of 6%,[117] 7%,[39] and 16%.[118] Although the definitions of respiratory failure differ in many of these studies, analysis of each study suggests a general trend toward improved in-hospital survival.[119] This improved survival raises the question of whether improvements in care of patients have had an impact on outcome. In addition, examination of these studies suggests that the severity of the underlying disease and the severity of the acute precipitating illness are both important determinants of overall mortality.

Despite the relatively promising in-hospital survival, the long-term prognosis for COPD patients after ARF is less optimistic. Five-year mortality has been reported as 70%[120] and 84%.[121] It is not clear, however, that the episode of ARF actually changes long-term mortality. In fact, comparison of the data of Martin and colleagues on survival of COPD patients with ARF to survival data for historical controls without ARF suggests that there is little difference.[117] There is clear evidence relating long-term survival to FEV_1,[122] and there is some evidence that if a patient survives an episode of ARF, prior mechanical ventilation does not influence long-term mortality.[83, 123] This implies that the clinician should not use a current episode of ARF in estimating a patient's chance of long-term survival.

Even an accurate measure of the overall mortality of ARF does not help the clinician or patient as much as the ability to use a particular patient's clinical variables to predict his or her chance of surviving an episode of ARF. Several researchers have shown that mortality is markedly increased if the pH is below 7.23 to 7.26,[40, 46] whereas the level of $Paco_2$ is less important. However, the pH does not have the predictive power necessary to aid the clinician in the decision to withhold aggressive treatment. Kaelin and colleagues analyzed the outcome of 39 episodes of ARF in 35 COPD patients and were unable to identify any clinical features predictive of death.[124] Menzies and colleagues retrospectively examined their experience with 95 COPD patients and found that survival was significantly associated with premorbid level of activity, FEV_1, serum albumin level, and severity of dyspnea.[2] No one variable was a powerful enough predictor to aid in clinical decision making. These authors developed a complex mathematic model to estimate survival on the basis of these variables. Prospective validation is necessary to determine the utility of this and other such models.

In summary, estimates of in-hospital mortality resulting from ARF in COPD patients vary from 6 to 40%, presumably primarily because of issues related to selection of patients and perhaps also improvements in clinical management. Long-term prognosis does not seem to be influenced by a resolved episode of ARF. To date, clinical predictors of mortality are inadequate to allow reasonable certainty in predicting the outcome for an individual patient.

ETHICAL AND FINANCIAL ISSUES

The primary ethical question that arises in caring for COPD patients with ARF is that of withholding and withdrawing mechanical ventilation. Over the past half century the rapid technologic advances in life support have led to a series of ethical questions regarding therapy at the end of life. These questions can be complicated by two occasionally competing principles: patients' autonomy in health care decisions and health care workers' right to not offer, begin, or maintain futile treatment. Most of these questions are not unique to the COPD patient with ARF and are discussed in detail elsewhere in this text and in several policy statements.[125–129] However, several aspects of withholding or withdrawing support are different in the COPD patient.

One shortcoming of living wills and advance directives is that they generally cannot specify the exact circumstances under which certain therapies are withheld, because specifics of disease, severity, and potential treatment usually cannot be predicted. However, the patient with end-stage COPD can anticipate ARF and, with his or her physician, describe specific circumstances under which mechanical ventilation should be withheld or withdrawn. This kind of advanced planning can make the end of life much less traumatic for patient, family, and physician.

It is generally accepted that physicians serve patients best, if advance directives are not available, by the presumption in favor of sustaining life and providing aggressive treatment. This is common sense for a young patient without chronic disease, but for an unknown elderly COPD patient there may be some hesitation to provide mechanical ventilation because of fear of mortality, ventilator dependence, or poor quality of life. We consider that these are all misguided arguments for withholding mechanical ventilation from a patient unknown to the physician. Mortality data, as described earlier, do not allow us to predict with any certainty which patients will survive ARF. In addition, there is some evidence that patients who recover from an episode of ARF have survival curves similar to those of comparable patients without an episode of ARF.[117] The fear of ventilator dependence in the patient unknown to a physician is actually a fear of withdrawing support already initiated. There is no ethical difference between withholding and withdrawing support[126, 127] (despite a real emotional difference). In addition, institution of mechanical ventilation can allow time to evaluate the patient's condition or to determine the patient's, family's, and health care team's concerns. In our experience, true failure to wean from mechanical ventilation despite improvement in the precipitating event is rare, even in the patient with severe COPD. Finally, quality of life is subjective and in part dependent on the patient's general sense of well-being and satisfaction with life.[130–133] In general, primary physicians consider their older patients' quality of life to be worse than do the patients.[134] Physicians, especially when unfamiliar with a patient, should not make the mistake of projecting their own values onto the patient.

Economic issues are becoming increasingly important factors in health care policy decisions. ICUs for adults represent 6% of all hospital beds and 15% of all hospital costs.[135] Wagner surveyed 3884 patients admitted to an ICU and found that the 6% of these patients requiring mechanical ventilation for more than 7 days consumed 37% of the total ICU resources.[136] Although these figures are critical in matters of policy, caregivers should not allow the financial cost of treatment to play a significant role in the decision to withhold or withdraw mechanical ventilation from an individual patient.

Currently, end-stage COPD is not a well-accepted indication for lung transplantation. However, young patients (roughly 45 years of age) with obstructive pulmonary disease caused by α_1-antitrypsin deficiency or chemical inhalation have had successful transplantations.[137] These patients have prolonged postoperative courses with frequent complications and require long-term immune suppression. Whether this becomes a feasible option for slightly older patients with COPD depends on technologic advances, economic resources, and organ availability. It seems likely that this treatment will pose some difficult questions for our medical system.

References

1. US Bureau of the Census: Statistical Abstract of the United States: 1991. (111th ed. Washington, DC, US Government Printing Office, 1991.
2. Menzies R, Gibbons W, Goldberg P: Determinants of weaning and survival among patients with COPD who require mechanical ventilation for acute respiratory failure. Chest 95:398, 1989.
3. Schreiner A, Bjerkestrand G, Digranes A, et al: Bacteriologic findings in the transtracheal aspirate from patients with acute exacerbation of chronic bronchitis. Infection 6:54, 1978.
4. Fagon J, Chastre J, Trouillet J, et al: Characterization of distal bronchial microflora during acute exacerbation of chronic bronchitis. Am Rev Respir Dis 142:1004, 1990.
5. Smith CB, Golden CA, Kanner RE, et al: Association of viral and *Mycoplasma pneumoniae* infections with acute respiratory illness in patients with chronic obstructive pulmonary diseases. Am Rev Respir Dis 121:225, 1980.
6. Gump DW, Phillips CA, Forsuth BR, et al: Role of infection in chronic bronchitis. Am Rev Respir Dis 113:465, 1976.
7. Glezen WP, Decker M, Perrolta DM: Survey of underlying conditions in persons hospitalized with acute respiratory disease during influenza epidemics in Houston, 1976–1981. Am Rev Respir Dis 136:550, 1987.
8. Smith CB, Golden CA, Klauber MR, et al: Interactions between viruses and bacteria in patients with chronic bronchitis. J Infect Dis 154:552, 1976.
9. Couch RB: The effects of influenza on host defenses. J Infect Dis 144:284, 1981.
10. Anthonisen NR, Manfreda J, Warren CPW, et al: Antibiotic therapy in exacerbations of chronic obstructive pulmonary disease. Ann Intern Med 106:196, 1987.
11. Baum GL, Fisher FD: The relationship of fatal pulmonary insufficiency with cor pulmonale, right-sided mural thrombi and pulmonary emboli: A preliminary report. Am J Med Sci 240:609, 1960.
12. Martin JF, Slater DN, Trowbridge EA: Abnormal intrapulmonary platelet production: A possible cause of vascular and lung disease. Lancet 1:793, 1983.
13. Cordova C, Musca A, Viola F, et al: Platelet hyperfunction in patients with chronic airways obstruction. Eur J Respir Dis 66:9, 1985.
14. Dalen JE, Alpert JS: Natural history of pulmonary embolism. Prog Cardiovasc Dis 17:259, 1975.
15. Sharma GVRK, Sasahara AA: Diagnosis of pulmonary embolism in patients with chronic obstructive pulmonary disease. J Chronic Dis 28:253, 1975.
16. Lippmann M, Fein A: Pulmonary embolism in the patient with chronic obstructive pulmonary disease. Chest 79:39, 1981.
17. Chopin C, Fesard P, Mangalaboyi J, et al: Use of capnography in diagnosis of pulmonary embolism during acute respiratory failure of chronic obstructive pulmonary disease. Crit Care Med 18:353, 1990.
18. Alderson PO, Biello DR, Sachariah KG, et al: Scintigraphic detection of pulmonary embolism in patients with obstructive pulmonary disease. Radiology 138:661, 1981.
19. Smith R, Ellis K, Alderson PO: Role of chest radiography in predicting the extent of airway disease in patients with suspected pulmonary embolism. Radiology 159:391, 1986.
20. Neuhaus A, Bentz RR, Weg JC: Pulmonary embolism in respiratory failure. Chest 73:460, 1976.
21. Stein PD, Coleman RE, Gottschalk A, et al: Diagnostic utility of ventilation/perfusion lung scans in acute pulmonary embolism is not diminished by pre-existing cardiac or pulmonary disease. Chest 100:604, 1991.
22. Bounameaux H, Cirafici P, de Moerloose P, et al: Measurement of D-dimer in plasma as diagnostic aid in suspected pulmonary embolism. Lancet 337:196, 1991.
23. Mills SR, Jackson DC, Sullivan DC, et al: Angiographic evaluation of chronic pulmonary embolism. Radiology 136:301, 1980.
24. Perlmutt LM, Braun SD, Neuman GE, et al: Pulmonary arteriography in the high risk patient. Radiology 162:187, 1987.
25. Fanta CH, Wright TC, McFadden ER: Differentiation of recurrent pulmonary emboli from chronic obstructive lung disease as a cause of cor pulmonale. Chest 79:92, 1981.
26. The PIOPED Investigators: Value of the ventilation/perfusion scan in

acute pulmonary embolism. Results of the prospective investigation of pulmonary embolism diagnosis (PIOPED). JAMA 263:2753, 1990.

27. Urokinase Pulmonary Embolism Trial Study Group: Urokinase pulmonary embolism trial: Phase 1 results: A cooperative study. JAMA 214:2163, 1970.

28. Hirsh J: Treatment of pulmonary embolism. Annu Rev Med 28:91, 1987.

29. Klinger JR, Hill NS: Right ventricular dysfunction in chronic obstructive pulmonary disease. Chest 99:715, 1991.

30. Marchandise B, DeBruyne B, Delaunoise L, et al: Noninvasive reduction of pulmonary hypertension in chronic obstructive pulmonary disease by Doppler echocardiography. Chest 91:361, 1987.

31. Light RW: Thoracentesis (diagnostic and therapeutic) and pleural biopsy. In: Pleural Diseases. Philadelphia, Lea & Febiger, p 237, 1983.

32. Estenne M, Yernault J, DeTroyer A: Mechanism of relief of dyspnea after thoracentesis in patients with large pleural effusions. Am J Med 74:813, 1983.

33. George RB, Herbert SJ, Shames JM, et al: Pneumothorax complicating pulmonary emphysema. JAMA 234:389, 1975.

34. Campbell EJM: The J Burns Amberson lecture: The management of acute respiratory failure in chronic bronchitis and emphysema. Am Rev Respir Dis 96:626, 1967.

35. Renzetti AD Jr, McClement JH, Litt BD: The Veterans Administration cooperative study of pulmonary function. 3. Mortality in relation to respiratory function in chronic obstructive pulmonary disease. Am J Med 41:115, 1966.

36. Bigelow BD, Petty TL, Levine BE, et al: The effect of oxygen breathing on arterial blood gases in patients with chronic airway obstruction living at 5,200 feet. Am Rev Respir Dis 96:28, 1967.

37. Cherniack RM, Hakimpour K: The rational use of oxygen in respiratory insufficiency. JAMA 71:456, 1967.

38. Pierson DJ: The toxicity of low-flow oxygen therapy. Respir Care 28:889, 1983.

39. Bone RC, Pierce AK, Johnson RL: Controlled oxygen administration in acute respiratory failure in chronic obstructive pulmonary disease: A reappraisal. Am J Med 65:896, 1978.

40. Warren PM, Flenley DC, Millar JS, et al: Respiratory failure revisited: Acute exacerbations of chronic bronchitis between 1961–1968 and 1970–1976. Lancet 1:467, 1980.

41. Aubier M, Murciano D, Fournier M, et al: Central respiratory drive in acute respiratory failure of patients with chronic obstructive pulmonary disease. Am Rev Respir Dis 122:191, 1980.

42. Aubier M, Murciano D, Milic-Emili J, et al: Effects of the administration of O_2 on ventilation and blood gases in patients with chronic obstructive pulmonary disease during acute respiratory failure. Am Rev Respir Dis 122:747, 1980.

43. Sassoon CSH, Hassell KT, Mahutte CK: Hyperoxic-induced hypercapnia in stable chronic obstructive pulmonary disease. Am Rev Respir Dis 135:907, 1987.

44. Stradling JR: Hypercapnia during oxygen therapy in airways obstruction: A reappraisal. Thorax 41:897, 1986.

45. Addis GJ: Bicarbonate buffering in acute exacerbations of chronic respiratory failure. Thorax 20:337, 1965.

46. Kettel LJ, Diener CF, Morse JO, et al: Treatment of acute respiratory acidosis in chronic obstructive lung disease. JAMA 217:1503, 1971.

47. Bickerman HA, Chusid EL: The case against the use of respiratory stimulants. Chest 58:53, 1970.

48. Woolf CR: The use of "respiratory stimulant" drugs. Chest 58:49, 1970.

49. Riordan JF, Sillett RW, McNicol MW: A controlled trial of doxapram in acute respiratory failure. Br J Dis Chest 69:57, 1975.

50. Moser KM, Luchsinger PC, Adamson JS, et al: Respiratory stimulation with intravenous doxapram in respiratory failure. N Engl J Med 288:427, 1973.

51. Easton PA, Jadue C, Dhingra S, et al: A comparison of the bronchodilating effects of a beta-2 adrenergic agent (albuterol) and an anticholinergic agent (ipratropium bromide), given by aerosol alone or in sequence. N Engl J Med 315:735, 1986.

52. LeDoux EJ, Morris JF, Temple WP, et al: Standard and double-dose ipratropium bromide and combined ipratropium bromide and inhaled metaproterenol in COPD. Chest 95:1013, 1989.

53. Karpel JP: Bronchodilator responses to anticholinergic and beta-adrenergic agents in acute and stable COPD. Chest 99:871, 1991.

54. Karpel JP, Pesin J, Greenberg D, et al: A comparison of the effects of ipratropium bromide and metaproterenol sulfate in acute exacerbations of COPD. Chest 98:835, 1990.

55. Rebuck AS, Chapman KR, Abboud R: Nebulized anticholinergic and sympathomimetic treatment of asthma and chronic obstructive airways disease in the emergency room. Am J Med 87:1091, 1987.

56. Gross NJ, Skorodin MS: Role of the parasympathetic system in airway obstruction due to emphysema. N Engl J Med 311:421, 1984.

57. Braun SR, McKenzie WN, Copeland C, et al: A comparison of the effect of ipratropium and albuterol in the treatment of chronic obstructive airway disease. Arch Intern Med 149:544, 1989.

58. Jasper AC, Mohsenifar Z, Kahan S, et al: Cost-benefit comparison of aerosol bronchodilator delivery methods in hospitalized patients. Chest 91:614, 1987.

59. Turner JR, Corkery KJ, Eckman D, et al: Equivalence of continuous flow nebulizer and metered-dose inhaler with reservoir bag for treatment of acute airflow obstruction. Chest 93:476, 1987.

60. Godden DJ, Crompton GK: An objective assessment of the tube spacer in patients unable to use a conventional pressurized aerosol efficiently. Br J Dis Chest 75:165, 1981.

61. Fernandez A, Lazaro A, Garcia A, et al: Bronchodilators in patients with chronic obstructive pulmonary disease on mechanical ventilation. Am Rev Respir Dis 141:164, 1990.

62. Gross NJ: Drug therapy: Ipratropium bromide. N Engl J Med 319:486, 1988.

63. Rice KL, Leatherman JW, Duane PG, et al: Aminophylline for acute exacerbations of chronic obstructive pulmonary disease. Ann Intern Med 107:305, 1987.

64. Albert RK, Martin TR, Lewis SW: Controlled clinical trial of methylprednisolone in patients with chronic bronchitis and acute respiratory insufficiency. Ann Intern Med 92:753, 1980.

65. Emerman, CL, Connors AE, Lukens TW, et al: A randomized controlled trial of methylprednisolone in the emergency treatment of acute exacerbations of COPD. Chest 95:563, 1989.

66. Mendella LA, Manfreda J, Warren CPW, et al: Steroid response in stable chronic obstructive pulmonary disease. Ann Intern Med 96:17, 1982.

67. Hudson LD, Monti CM: Rationale and use of corticosteroids in chronic obstructive pulmonary disease. Med Clin North Am 74:661, 1990.

68. Tyler ML: Complications of positioning and chest physiotherapy. Respir Care 27:458, 1982.

69. Connors AF, Hammon WE, Martin RH, et al: Chest physical therapy: The immediate effect on oxygenation in acutely ill patients. Chest 78:559, 1980.

70. Chopra SK, Taplin GV, Simmons DH: Effects of hydration and physical therapy on tracheal transport velocity. Am Rev Respir Dis 115:1009, 1977.

71. Sherman C, Hudson LD: Complications of acute respiratory failure. In: Bone RC, George RB, Hudson LD (eds): Acute Respiratory Failure. New York, Churchill Livingstone, p 317, 1987.

72. Hudson LD, Kurt TL, Petty TL: Arrhythmias associated with acute respiratory failure in patients with chronic airway obstruction. 63:661, Chest 1973.

73. Holford FD, Mithoefer JC: Cardiac arrhythmias in hospitalized patients with chronic obstructive pulmonary disease. Am Rev Respir Dis 108:879, 1973.

74. Sideris DA, Katsadoros DP, Valianos G, et al: Type of cardiac dysrhythmias in respiratory failure. Am Heart J 81:32, 1975.

75. Khokhar N: Cardiac arrhythmias associated with acute respiratory failure in chronic obstructive pulmonary disease. Milit Med 146:856, 1981.

76. Moser KM, LeMoine JR, Nachtwey FJ, et al: Deep venous thrombosis and pulmonary embolism, frequency in a respiratory intensive care unit. JAMA 246:1422, 1981.

77. Harris SK, Bone RC, Ruth WE: Gastrointestinal hemorrhage in patients in a RICU. Chest 72:301, 1977.

78. Pingleton SK, Hadzima SK: Enteral alimentation and gastrointestinal bleeding in mechanically ventilated patients. Crit Care Med 11:13, 1983.

79. Driks MR, Craven DE, Celli B, et al: Nosocomial pneumonia in intubated patients given sucralfate as compared with antacids or histamine type-2 blockers. N Engl J Med 317:1376, 1987.

80. Tryba M: Risk of acute stress bleeding and nosocomial pneumonia in ventilated intensive care patients: Sucralfate versus antacids. Am J Med 83(suppl 3B):117, 1987.

81. Stauffer JL, Olson DE, Petty TL: Complications and consequences of endotracheal intubation and tracheostomy. Am J Med 70:65, 1981.

82. Petty TL: Intensive and Rehabilitative Respiratory Care. 3rd ed. Philadelphia, Lea & Febiger, p 238, 1982.

83. Sluiter HJ, Blokzijl EJ, Van Dijl W, et al: Conservative and respirator treatment of acute respiratory insufficiency in patients with chronic obstructive lung disease. Am Rev Respir Dis 105:932, 1972.

84. Pepe PE, Marini JJ: Occult positive end-expiratory pressure in mechanically ventilated patients with airflow obstruction; The auto-PEEP effect. Am Rev Respir Dis 126:166, 1982.

85. Brown DG, Pierson DJ: Auto-PEEP is common in mechanically ventilated patients: A study of incidence, severity and detection. Respir Care 31:1069, 1986.

86. Connors AF, McCaffree DR, Gray BA: Effect of inspiratory flow rate on gas exchange during mechanical ventilation. Am Rev Respir Dis 124:537, 1981.

87. Marini JJ, Rodriguez RM, Lamb V: The inspiratory workload of patient-initiated mechanical ventilation. Am Rev Respir Dis 134:902, 1986.

88. Brochard L, Isabey D, Piquet J, et al: Reversal of acute exacerbations of chronic obstructive lung disease by inspiratory assistance with a face mask. N Engl J Med 323:1523, 1990.

89. Carrey Z, Gottfried SB, Levy RD: Ventilatory muscle support in respiratory failure with nasal positive pressure ventilation. Chest 97:150, 1990.

90. Conway J, Carroll M, Brown A, et al: The successful reversal of hypoxia using nasal intermittent positive pressure ventilation plus added oxygen in respiratory failure due to acute exacerbations of chronic airways disease. Am Rev Respir Dis 4(int conf suppl):A74, 1991.

91. Miro AM, Hertig I, Shivaram U: Continuous positive airway pressure (CPAP) in chronic obstructive patients with pulmonary disease (COPD) in acute hypercapneic respiratory failure. Am Rev Respir Dis 4(int conf suppl):A472, 1991.

92. Shivaram U, Cash M: Nasal CPAP in the management of decompensated hypercapnic respiratory failure. Am Rev Respir Dis 4(int conf suppl):A472, 1991.

93. Elliott MW, Steven MH, Phillips GD, et al: Non-invasive mechanical ventilation for acute respiratory failure. Br Med J 300:358, 1990.

94. Meduri GU, Conoscenti CC, Menashe P, et al: Noninvasive face mask ventilation in patients with acute respiratory failure. Chest 95:865, 1989.

95. Bott J, Carroll M, Conway JH, et al: The effect of nasal intermittent positive pressure ventilation on acute exacerbations of chronic obstructive pulmonary disease (COPD). Am Rev Respir Dis 4(int conf suppl):A472, 1991.

96. Chevrolet J-C, Jolliet P, Abajo B, et al: Nasal positive pressure ventilation in patients with acute respiratory failure. Difficult and time-consuming procedure for nurses. Chest 100:775, 1991.

97. Koretz RL: Nutritional support. Chest 88:2, 1985.

98. Derenne J, Fleury B, Pariente R: Acute respiratory failure of chronic obstructive pulmonary disease. Am Rev Respir Dis 138:1006, 1988.

99. Driver AG, McAlvery MT, Smith JL: Nutritional assessment of patients with chronic obstructive pulmonary diseases and acute respiratory failure. Chest 82:568, 1982.

100. Guidet B, Lebricon T, Staikowsky F, et al: Nutritional status of patients with chronic obstructive pulmonary disease in acute respiratory failure (ARF). Am Rev Respir Dis 143(suppl):A451, 1991.

101. Newman JH, Neff TA, Ziporin T: Acute respiratory failure associated with hypophosphatemia. N Engl J Med 296:1101, 1977.

102. Aubier M, Murciano D, LeCoeguic Y, et al: Effect of hypophosphatemia on diaphragmatic contractility in patients with acute respiratory failure. N Engl J Med 313:420, 1985.

103. Aubier M, Viires N, Piquet J, et al: Effects of hypocalcemia on diaphragmatic strength generation. J Appl Physiol 58:2054, 1985.

104. Dhingra S, Solven F, Wilson A, et al: Hypomagnesemia and respiratory muscle power. Am Rev Respir Dis 129:497, 1984.

105. Herve P, Simonneau G, Girad P, et al: Hypercapnic acidosis induced by nutrition in mechanically ventilated patients: Glucose versus fat. Crit Care Med 13:537, 1985.

106. Rodriguez JL, Askanazi J, Weissman C, et al: Ventilatory and metabolic effects of glucose infusions. Chest 88:512, 1985.

107. Bonmarchand G, Denis P, Weber J, et al: Motor abnormalities of digestive and urinary tract in patients on ventilator for acute exacerbation of chronic obstructive pulmonary disease. Dig Dis Sci 34:1231, 1989.

108. Golden G, Chandler JG: Colonic ileus and cecal perforation in patients requiring mechanical ventilatory support. Chest 68:661, 1975.

109. Smith JP, Stone RW, Muschenheim C: Acute respiratory failure in chronic lung disease: Observations on controlled oxygen therapy. Am Rev Respir Dis 97:791, 1968.

110. Asmundson T, Kilburn KH: Survival of acute respiratory failure. Ann Intern Med 70:471, 1969.

111. Burk RH, George RB: Acute respiratory failure in chronic obstructive pulmonary disease. Arch Intern Med 132:865, 1973.

112. Gottlieb LS, Belchum OJ: Course of chronic obstructive lung disease following first onset of respiratory failure. Chest 63:5, 1973.

113. Moser KM, Shibel LJM, Beamon AJ: Acute respiratory failure in obstructive lung disease. JAMA 225:705, 1973.

114. Seriff NS, Khan F, Lazo BJ: Acute respiratory failure. Med Clin North Am 57:1539, 1973.

115. Cullen JH, Kaemmerlen JT: Acute ventilatory failure in chronic obstructive lung disease. Am Rev Respir Dis 98:998, 1968.

116. Vanderbergh E, Van De Woetijne KP, Gyselen A: Conservative treatment of acute respiratory failure in patients with chronic obstructive lung disease. Am Rev Respir Dis 98:60, 1968.

117. Martin TR, Lewis SW, Albert RK: The prognosis of patients with chronic obstructive pulmonary disease after hospitalization for acute respiratory failure. Chest 82:310, 1982.

118. Dardes N, Campo S, Chiappini MG, et al: Prognosis of COPD patients after an episode of events respiratory failure. Eur J Respir Dis 69(suppl 146):377, 1986.

119. Hudson LD: Survival data in patients with acute and chronic lung disease. Am Rev Respir Dis 140:519, 1989.

120. Dolce JJ, Crisp C, Mazella B, et al: Medication adherence patterns in chronic obstructive pulmonary disease. Chest 99:837, 1991.

121. Shachor Y, Liberman D, Tamir A, et al: Long-term survival of patients with chronic obstructive pulmonary disease following mechanical ventilation. Isr J Med 25:617, 1989.

122. Asmundsson T, Kilburn KH: Survival after acute respiratory failure. Ann Intern Med 80:50, 1974.

123. Gillespie DJ, Marsh HMM, Divertie MB, et al: Clinical outcome of respiratory failure in patients requiring prolonged (>24 hours) mechanical ventilation. Chest 90:364, 1986.

124. Kaelin RM, Assimacopoulos A, Chevrolet J: Failure to predict six-month survival of patients with COPD requiring mechanical ventilation by analysis of simple indices. Chest 92:971, 1987.

125. NIH workshop summary: Withholding and withdrawing mechanical ventilation. Am Rev Respir Dis 124:1327, 1986.

126. NIH workshop on withholding and withdrawing mechanical ventilation. Am Rev Respir Dis 140(suppl):S1, 1989.

127. Task Force in Ethics of the Society of Critical Care Medicine: Consensus report on the ethics of foregoing life-sustaining treatments in the critically ill. Crit Care Med 18:1435, 1990.

128. American College of Chest Physicians/Society of Critical Care Medicine Consensus Panel: Ethical and moral guidelines for the initiation, continuation, and withdrawal of intensive care. Chest 97:949, 1990.

129. American Thoracic Society statement. Withholding and withdrawing life-sustaining therapy. Am Rev Respir Dis 115:478, 1991.

130. Dracup K, Raffin T: Withholding and withdrawing mechanical ventilation: Assessing quality of life. Am Rev Respir Dis 140(suppl):S44, 1989.

131. Pearlman RA, Uhlmann RF: Quality of life in elderly, chronically ill outpatients. J Gerontol 46:M31, 1991.

132. McSweeny AJ, Grant I, Heaton RK, et al: Life quality of patients with chronic obstructive pulmonary disease. Arch Intern Med 142:473, 1982.

133. Prigatano GP, Wright EC, Levin D: Quality of life and its predictors in patients with mild hypoxemia and chronic obstructive pulmonary disease. Arch Intern Med 144:1613, 1984.

134. Uhlman RF, Pearlman RA: Perceived quality of life and preferences for life-sustaining treatment in older adults. Arch Intern Med 151:495, 1991.

135. Spivak D: The high cost of acute health care: A review of escalating costs and limitations of such exposure in intensive care units. Am Rev Respir Dis 136:1008, 1987.

136. Wagner DP: Economics of prolonged mechanical ventilation. Am Rev Respir Dis 140(suppl):S14, 1989.

137. Emery RW, Graif JL, Hale K, et al: Treatment of end-stage chronic obstructive pulmonary disease with double lung transplantation. Chest 99:533, 1991.

CHAPTER 72

Acute Severe Asthma

Jonathan E. Gottlieb
James E. Fish

Asthma is a disorder characterized by variable airflow obstruction, bronchial hyper-responsiveness, and associated symptoms of wheezing, chest tightness, cough, and dyspnea. It is a heterogeneous disorder with respect to etiologic factors, pathologic features, and clinical presentation. Because of this heterogeneity, it is uncertain whether asthma represents a truly distinct nosologic entity with unique pathogenesis or multiple disorders with common clinical manifestations.

For the overwhelming majority of asthmatic patients, their disease is usually well controlled with drug therapy or with no medication at all. Despite a high prevalence of disease, asthma-related deaths are fortunately rare. In fact, only a minority of patients ever require emergency medical therapy because of uncontrollable symptoms, and even 80 to 90% of these are successfully treated in the emergency room setting. Thus, only a small fraction of patients fail to respond to outpatient management as well as more aggressive treatment in the emergency room. This small minority nevertheless account for almost 500,000 hospitalizations annually in the United States.[1] Severe and persistent asthma that is resistant to conventional therapy is known as *status asthmaticus*, a life-threatening condition that presents unique challenges to the treating physician. Although much of the following discussion applies to asthma in general, the primary focus is on severe, life-threatening asthma, its pathogenesis and pathophysiology, and strategies for management.

EPIDEMIOLOGY

Estimates of asthma occurrence rates in North America and elsewhere in the world vary considerably, reflecting different standards for identifying asthmatic patients in population surveys. It is nevertheless accepted that there is a worldwide distribution of asthma, with higher prevalence rates in more developed or industrialized societies.[2–5] The highest prevalence rates (11 to 17%) have been reported for children in Australia and New Zealand.[6–8] Prevalence rates in the United States are between 3 and 8.5% in children 5 to 15 years of age and between 3 and 6% in older adolescents and adults.[9–11] Population-based surveys also suggest that there has been a global increase in asthma prevalence since the late 1970s.[12–15]

Prevalence rates in the United States are higher for males during late adolesence and early adulthood and higher for females after age 30 years.[16] The incidence of new cases is estimated at 1.2 to 1.6 cases per 100 subject-years during the first decade of life, with approximately 0.3 new cases per 100 subject-years occurring after age 20 years. New cases in patients older than age 40 years are more likely to occur in women and in individuals with a prior history of respiratory symptoms during childhood.[16] Although there is much to learn about the natural history of asthma, it appears that more than 50% of children having asthma in the first decade of life experience remission of symptoms by age 20 years.[17] Approximately 40 to 50% of subjects who experience such remissions, however, have a recurrence of disease after age 30 years.[18] The natural history of asthma in adult patients is even less predictable, but it is thought that remissions are less likely than in children.

Of great concern is the striking increase in morbidity and mortality from asthma during the past decade in most of the developed world. After a decline from 0.4 death per 100,000 population to approximately 0.2 per 100,000 in the 1970s, mortality in the United States increased by approximately 6.2% per annum during the 1980s in patients between 5 and 34 years of age.[19] Although accurate population-based figures are not available for patients older than the age of 35 years, data from the National Center for Health Statistics suggest that in this age group asthma mortality also increased between 1968 and 1982.[20] The corresponding increase in overall asthma morbidity[21] and the apparent increase in prevalence are of equal concern because they are occurring during a period of declining morbidity and prevalence of many other chronic respiratory diseases.

PATHOGENESIS

Nonspecific airway hyper-responsiveness is a feature common to all types of asthma. Hyper-responsiveness manifests as cough and bronchospasm with exposure to nonspecific (nonallergenic) irritants, and it can be demonstrated in the laboratory as an exaggerated airway response to inhaled methacholine or histamine, exercise, or hyperventilation.[22–27] The underlying cause of airway hyper-responsiveness is not known, although it is believed that cellular effector pathways leading to airway inflammation may be responsible.[28, 29] Airway hyper-responsiveness is almost invariably present in symptomatic asthmatic individuals, but it is not specific for this condition. Approximately 10 to 15% of asymptomatic individuals without a history of airways disease may demonstrate airway hyper-responsiveness in the laboratory,[23] and so too may patients with cystic fibrosis,[30] those

with chronic obstructive pulmonary disease,[31, 32] and patients with recent viral respiratory tract infections.[33, 34]

Although asthma is generally viewed as an acquired disorder, it seems likely that genetic determinants that influence atopy and airway responsiveness interact with environmental factors to create increased risk. The basic pathophysiologic abnormality responsible for the clinical manifestations of asthma is airway obstruction. The major elements of obstruction include constriction of airway smooth muscle, mucus secretion, and edema of the airway wall. These processes may be acute or chronic and each is potentially reversible. Numerous environmental and endogenous factors have been implicated as triggers of asthma, and on the basis of current information, such stimuli appear to act by operating through effector mechanisms involving neural and cellular pathways. Neural effector pathways involve reflex activation of postganglionic parasympathetic fibers that release acetylcholine at end-organ tissues, causing smooth muscle constriction and mucous gland secretion.[35, 36] These reflexes may be initiated by activation of afferent irritant receptors in the airways. Stimulation of nonmyelinated C fiber endings in airway epithelium may also cause an axon reflex with in situ release of neuropeptides in airway tissues. Neuropeptides of particular interest are substance P and neurokinin A, both of which have been histochemically localized in human lung tissue.[37, 38] Although substance P can contract airway smooth muscle,[39] it appears to have more potent effects on microvascular permeability and secretion of mucus.[40, 41] Neurokinin A, on the other hand, has been shown to be more potent than substance P as a bronchoconstrictor.[38, 42] The development of substance P receptor antagonists will aid us in more precisely defining the role of neurokinins in asthma pathogenesis.[43]

The involvement of cellular pathways in asthma has been recognized for some time, primarily in the context of immunoglobulin E–mediated mast cell activation and allergic airway reactions. Binding of allergen to mast cell–bound immunoglobulin E antibody molecules results in changes in cell membrane properties with the de novo generation of biologically active lipid mediators and the release of granules containing other, preformed biologic mediators. The exact sequence of events, the cell species involved, and the role of specific chemical mediators in the inflammatory processes that follow mast cell activation are not known. However, there is evidence that a number of cell species, including eosinophils,[44, 45] neutrophils,[46] macrophages,[47, 48] and lymphocytes,[49, 50] may be involved. These cells are capable of generating and releasing a variety of mediators and cytokines that have direct pathobiologic effects on airways as well as the ability to recruit other inflammatory cells to airway tissues. A partial list of mediators that are of putative importance and their biologic effects is given in Table 72–1. Although inhaled aeroallergens and immunoglobulin E–mediated allergic airway reactions are recognized as important initial steps in inflammatory airway responses, evidence suggests that mast cells may be responsive to nonimmunologic stimuli as well. Histamine-releasing factors have been identified in nasal secretions and in supernatants from mononuclear cells and neutrophils.[51–55]

Histopathologic studies in asthma reveal the presence of lymphocytic and eosinophilic infiltration, thickened basement membranes, epithelial denudation, submucosal edema, and increased smooth muscle mass.[56–58] Bronchoalveolar lavage studies in asthmatics have also revealed the presence of increased numbers of eosinophils and mast cells.[59, 60] Most of these studies have been carried out in selected patients, and although the findings may be valid for patients having chronic, mild-to-moderate disease, it is important to note that they may not be characteristic of the larger asthmatic

TABLE 72–1

CELL-DERIVED CHEMICAL MEDIATORS AND THEIR POTENTIAL BIOLOGIC EFFECTS IN ASTHMA*

Mediator	Cell Source	Bronchospasm	Mucosal Edema	Secretion of Mucus	Cell Infiltration	Tissue Damage
Histamine	MC	+	+	+		
Prostaglandin D_2	MC	+		+		
Leukotrienes C_4, D_4, E_4	MC, EOS	+	+	+		
Thromboxane B_2	AM, PMN	+		+		
Leukotriene B_4	Am, PMN				+	
Platelet-activating factor	MC, AM, PMN, EOS		+	+	+	
EOS chemotaxin	MC				+	
PMN chemotaxin	MC, AM				+	
Superoxide radicals	AM, PMN, EOS					+
Major basic protein	EOS					+
Cationic proteins	EOS					+

*MC = mast cells; EOS = eosinophils; AM = alveolar macrophages; PMN = polymorphonuclear leukocytes; + = effect present.

population. Prior autopsy studies have demonstrated the importance of mucous plugging in patients with severe acute and fatal asthma. Moreover, it has been suggested that patients experiencing sudden asphyxial episodes of asthma may have bronchospasm as the primary pathologic change and airway inflammation may be less of a factor.[61] Autopsy results showing no evidence of mechanical obstruction in fatal asthma support the importance of acute bronchospasm in some patients.[62]

PATHOPHYSIOLOGY

Airway obstruction is the most prominent pathophysiologic abnormality in acute severe asthma, and it accounts for a variety of alterations in gas exchange and cardiopulmonary function (Table 72–2). Hypoxemia is typically mild,[63] even in patients requiring mechanical ventilation; and so too correction of hypoxemia usually requires only modest increases in inspired oxygen tension. Multiple inert gas elimination techniques have been used to determine that hypoxemia is a function of ventilation-perfusion inequalities and unrelated to intrapulmonary shunting. The dispersion of pulmonary blood flow distribution can be severely abnormal, with only moderate dispersion of ventilation; hence, ventilation-perfusion inequalities are characterized by a bimodal distribution, with perfusion directed to populations with either normal or low ventilation/perfusion ratios.[64] A similar pattern of ventilation-perfusion relationships has been reported in less severe asthma.[65] The absence of significant

TABLE 72–2

PHYSIOLOGIC ALTERATIONS IN SEVERE ASTHMA

Increased airway resistance (decreased FEV_1, peak expiratory flow rate)

Increased airway closure at high lung volumes (decreased vital capacity; increased residual volume, functional residual capacity, and often total lung capacity)

Increased pulmonary arterial pressure relative to pleural pressure (electrocardiographic evidence of right ventricular strain or P-pulmonale)

Increased fluctuations in pleural pressure with resulting increased fluctuations in systolic arterial pressure (pulsus paradoxus)

Increased ventilation-perfusion mismatch (decreased Pao_2, increased ratio of dead space volume to tidal volume; increased $Paco_2$ in severe cases)

Increased oxygen consumption, carbon dioxide production, and cardiac output

shunting explains why only modest levels of inspired oxygen tension are needed to correct hypoxemia and suggests that redistribution of pulmonary blood flow, in addition to increased cardiac output and perhaps collateral ventilation, is responsible for the preservation of Pao_2. The extent of ventilation-perfusion mismatching does not always correspond to the severity of obstruction. In fact, improved airway obstruction after bronchodilator treatment is often associated with a paradoxical drop in Pao_2,[66] most likely owing to an exaggeration of ventilation-perfusion mismatching.

Dead space ventilation in asthma is usually increased so that a higher total ventilation is required to maintain adequate alveolar ventilation and normal Pco_2. Despite this increase in dead space ventilation and an increase in carbon dioxide production caused by greater work of breathing, asthmatic patients typically have $Paco_2$ values below or near normal because of hyperventilation.[63] Any increase in the $Paco_2$ is an indication of respiratory failure and a potentially fatal situation.

Airway narrowing and increased resistance to airflow cause air trapping and hyperinflation owing to incomplete emptying of some areas of lung and because of airway closure.[67, 68] Progressive air trapping and hyperinflation lead to an increase in residual volume and functional residual capacity and, in some cases, an elevation of total lung capacity as well.[69] The higher distending pressures that attend hyperinflation may in part be beneficial, because elastic parenchymal elements of the lung exert radial traction on airways, in effect reducing airway resistance and increasing airway caliber.[70] Because breathing at higher lung volumes requires greater inspiratory muscle forces to overcome the higher elastic recoil of the lungs and thorax, the work of breathing is augmented. Moreover, overdistention of the lung causes an increase in the radius of curvature of the diaphragm, establishing a suboptimal length-tension relationship, not only for the diaphragm itself but also for the accessory respiratory muscles.[71] This adds further to the work of breathing in terms of oxygen consumption per liter of ventilation. At times, the oxygen cost of breathing can exceed local oxygen delivery to respiratory muscles and so lead to lactic acidosis, muscle fatigue, and ultimately respiratory failure.[72, 73]

Typical pulmonary function findings in the severe episode include a significant increase in residual volume and a corresponding decrease in vital capacity and 1-second forced expiratory volume (FEV_1). The reduction in vital capacity correlates well with the severity of the episode, and in some cases, the vital capacity may be only slightly larger than the tidal volume. During a severe episode, residual volume can exceed the patient's normal total lung capacity; to maintain ventilation in these extreme circumstances, there is an obligate increase in total lung capacity. Increases in total lung capacity are thought to be related to increased activity of inspiratory intercostal and accessory muscles of breathing.[69, 71, 74, 75]

Lung hyperinflation and the marked pleural pressure changes that occur between inspiration and expiration during breathing at high lung volumes can cause considerable stress on the cardiovascular system. A marked increase in pulmonary arterial pressure relative to pleural pressure has been demonstrated during acute episodes. Because the outer surface of the right ventricle is surrounded by pleural pressure, there is a resultant degree of pulmonary hypertension in proportion to the degree of lung hyperinflation.[76, 77] Moreover, the exaggerated drop in pleural pressure during inspiration at high lung volumes effectively increases left ventricular afterload, because muscle tension of the left ventricle depends on systemic arterial pressures relative to pleural pressures. The negative inspiratory pleural pressures seen in severe asthma therefore lead to a decrease in left ventricular stroke volume and arterial pulse pressure, in part accounting for the pulsus paradoxus of severe asthma.[78]

Severe asthma is usually accompanied by a significant increase in oxygen consumption and a corresponding increase in cardiac output.[79] Although these changes may be related to increased work of breathing, other factors such as anxiety and increased levels of circulating catecholamines may also contribute.

CLINICAL MANIFESTATIONS

Typical symptoms of asthma include wheezing, chest tightness, cough, and dyspnea. One or more of these symptoms can occur on an intermittent basis, with symptom-free intervals intervening, or they may be persistent with episodic worsening. Occasionally, the asthmatic patient may have the sole symptom of cough, either productive or nonproductive. Although some studies have shown that up to 40% of patients with unexplained cough have demonstrable evidence of airway hyperreactivity and therefore a possible underlying asthmatic diathesis,[80] such patients generally have relatively normal lung function and represent the milder end of the disease spectrum.

In acute severe asthma, a specific trigger or precipitating factor is often not identified. Nevertheless, the medical history should attempt to define the potential role of atopy and aeroallergen exposure, antecedent viral respiratory tract infections, chemical or pollutant exposure, drug or food sensitivity, occupational exposure, or use of drugs known to precipitate asthma. Sudden, asphyxial fatal and near-fatal episodes of asthma have been associated with aeroallergen exposure,[81] profound emotional episodes,[60] ingestion of aspirin or other nonsteroidal anti-inflammatory drugs,[82] and the use of beta-blockers.[83] Successful identification of a precipitating factor, although difficult, may help prevent subsequent life-threatening episodes.

Typical physical findings during an acute episode include tachypnea, wheezing, prolonged expiration, and tachycardia. Signs of a particularly severe episode include a respiratory rate greater than 32 breaths/min, use of accessory respiratory muscles, heart rate greater than 120 beats/min, and exaggerated pulsus paradoxus.[84, 85] Cyanosis, diaphoresis, difficulty in maintaining speech, inability to lie supine, and altered consciousness are also signs of severe and potentially fatal asthma.[86] The absence of wheezing is unreliable as an indicator of severity, because it may be observed in both mild and severe episodes when ventilation is poor. In fact, a "silent" chest is a common finding in patients with severe,

TABLE 72–3
CLINICAL SIGNS OF LIFE-THREATENING ASTHMA
Previous or recurrent episodes of status asthmaticus
Inability to lie flat
Quiet chest
Difficulty in talking
Altered consciousness
Cyanosis
Use of accessory muscles
$FEV_1 < 20\%$ of predicted value; peak expiratory flow rate < 150 L/min
Pulsus paradoxus (>18 mm Hg)
Pneumothorax or pneumomediastinum
$Pao_2 < 50$ mm Hg
Any elevation in $Paco_2$

sudden asphyxial episodes.[60] Clinical signs associated with severe, life-threatening asthma are listed in Table 72–3.

INITIAL EVALUATION

Despite a general correlation between asthma symptoms and physiologic impairment, symptom complaints and physical findings may be an imprecise means of predicting severity in a particular episode.[87, 88] Therefore, objective measures of mechanical lung function and gas exchange are required for proper initial evaluation. Measurements of FEV_1 or peak expiratory flow rate and arterial blood gases are the most commonly used tests in this regard. Often, patients may be in such distress that they are unwilling or unable to perform respiratory maneuvers required to obtain FEV_1 or peak expiratory flow rate measurements. In this case, the inability to perform the test speaks to the severity of the episode. Patients demonstrating FEV_1 values less than 20% of predicted normal or peak expiratory flow rate measurements less than 150 L/min are at risk for acute respiratory failure. Lack of significant improvement in these measurements after initial bronchodilator therapy in the emergency room setting portends poor outcome without longer-term aggressive treatment in the hospital, preferably in the intensive care setting.

Severe hypoxemia ($Pao_2 < 50$ mm Hg) is also a sign of life-threatening asthma. Any elevation in $Paco_2$ is indicative of respiratory failure and deserves close observation and aggressive management. It should be noted that severe hypoxemia and elevations in $Paco_2$ are uncommon and occur in less than 10% of patients with acute asthma.[88] A $Paco_2$ value in the range of 38 to 44 mm Hg should be cause for concern, as it may reflect poor ventilatory reserve in a patient who, on the basis of the acute episode, should have a lower $Paco_2$ owing to hyperventilation.

The chest x-ray film is usually unremarkable, except for evidence of hyperinflation and bronchial wall thickening. However, in the acute severe episode, radiographs should be obtained to rule out complications that may alter patient management, such as pneumothorax, pneumomediastinum, heart failure, pneumonia, and lobar atelectasis. Sinus tachycardia is the most common electrocardiographic abnormality in acute asthma, but in severe circumstances, the electrocardiogram may also reveal right axis deviation and transient P-pulmonale caused by right ventricular strain.[89, 90] In the older patient, the electrocardiogram is most useful in excluding ischemic heart disease and arrhythmias. Blood tests and sputum examination are of limited value unless there is suspicion of infection. Elevated peripheral blood eosinophil counts (>500/mm³) are a frequent finding in patients with acute asthma who are not already taking corticosteroids.

Leukocytosis, on the other hand, is usually not a feature of asthma unless patients are taking corticosteroids. Expectorated sputum may have a purulent (yellow-green) discoloration owing to the presence of numerous eosinophils. The presence of eosinophils and eosinophil products, including Charcot-Leyden crystals and Curschmann's spirals, may help distinguish asthma from chronic bronchitis. Serum potassium levels should be measured because inhaled beta-agonists have been known to decrease serum potassium levels.[91] In addition, liver function studies and plasma theophylline levels should be checked to determine safe theophylline dosages.

MANAGEMENT

The first steps taken in the management of severe asthma are determined by the results of initial blood gas measurements and the duration and character of the episode. For example, many patients have gradual deterioration over days or even weeks despite aggressive outpatient treatment with inhaled beta-agonists, corticosteroids, and methylxanthines. This picture of gradual worsening occurs frequently after viral respiratory tract infections, with seasonal aeroallergen exposure, after adjustments in medication regimens, or with poor compliance with therapy. In this setting, intensification of chemotherapy is often all that is needed to halt progression and achieve gradual reversal. If respiratory failure is present and mechanical ventilation is indicated, there is usually sufficient time to prepare the patient for semielective intubation and to give sedation and even paralytic agents if necessary. By contrast, sudden and rapid deterioration during several hours is sometimes noted to occur, especially in young male patients.[61] If they are fortunate enough to be seen in time, these patients must be immediately treated with intubation, assisted ventilation, and correction of acidosis. Although there is no confirming histopathologic evidence, it has been argued that the latter more explosive situation arises from abrupt and intense bronchoconstriction, whereas more gradual deterioration reflects chronic, progressive inflammation.

In all cases, however, the first imperative is to determine whether the patient has respiratory failure ($PaCO_2 > 45$ mm Hg) and, if so, whether ventilatory support is required to maintain adequate oxygenation and control acidemia. In general, hypercapnia per se is not an absolute indication for assisted ventilation. Because the elements of airway obstruction in asthma are reversible, hypercapnia usually is corrected rapidly with initial therapy and does not necessitate intubation or mechanical ventilation. In fact, less than 10% of asthmatics require mechanical ventilation to treat hypercapnia,[92] whereas most patients experience normalization of $PaCO_2$ levels within hours after initiating drug therapy. As a rule, $PaCO_2$ elevations in the range of 50 to 60 mm Hg are well tolerated if the patient remains alert and is able to cooperate with treatment.

Endotracheal Intubation

Intubating the patient with acute severe asthma can be a technical challenge. Patients are often unable to assume the supine position because of anxiety and respiratory distress.[86] They have frequently eaten or taken liquids within hours of presentation, so that the risk of gastric aspiration is high. This risk is further augmented by treatment with methylxanthines, which may promote nausea and vomiting. In addition, manipulation of the upper airway can worsen bronchospasm or induce laryngeal spasm.

Ideally, intubation should be performed by individuals with considerable experience in difficult intubations. If the

TABLE 72–4
INITIAL DRUG TREATMENT OF SEVERE ASTHMA

1. Administer beta-adrenergic agents by inhalation every 20 min for the first hour.
   a. Albuterol, 0.5 mL of 0.5% solution (2.5 mg) in 2.5 mL of normal saline; or
   b. Metaproterenol, 0.3 mL of 5% solution (15 mg) in 2.5 mL of normal saline; or
   c. Isoproterenol,* 0.5 mL of 0.5% solution (2.5 mg) in 2 mL of normal saline
2. Alternatively, if the patient is unable to use a nebulizer, give epinephrine (0.3 mL of 1:1000 dilution) by subcutaneous injection.
3. Begin theophylline IV infusion; adjust dose to achieve serum level of 12–15 μg/mL.
4. Begin parenteral corticosteroids early. Administer methylprednisolone, 60 mg q 6 hr.

*Isoproterenol has the advantage of a more rapid onset of peak therapeutic action than albuterol. However, cardiovascular side effects of tachycardia and arrhythmias are more frequent with isoproterenol.

patient is unable to lie flat, nasotracheal intubation can be performed with the patient in the sitting position. However, this is less desirable than orotracheal intubation, because larger-diameter endotracheal tubes can be passed via the oral route, permitting easier access for suctioning and, if necessary, lavage. Sedation can be effectively achieved with a short-acting benzodiazepine such as midazolam in 1- to 2-mg increments; a total dose of 10 to 15 mg may be necessary. Of the muscle relaxants, vecuronium or pancuronium are preferred because they are less likely to cause histamine release than either succinylcholine or atracurium.[93, 94]

Various agents have been used successfully to sedate patients with status asthmaticus, including short- or intermediate-duration benzodiazepines, such as lorazepam. In general, the patient who requires assisted ventilation for status asthmaticus has been under great emotional and physical stress and has endured many sleepless hours. Accordingly, we use sedatives liberally during the first 24 to 36 hours of ventilator management to reduce anxiety and allow the patient to rest.

Medications

The pharmacologic treatment of acute severe asthma or status asthmaticus differs from the usual treatment of asthma in terms of intensity, particularly with respect to medication dosages and frequency of administration (Table 72–4). Initial treatment in the emergency room usually entails administration of sympathomimetic agents, either by injection or by inhalation, depending on the patient's ability to tolerate use of a nebulizer. Albuterol (2.5 to 5.0 mg, given as 0.5 to 1.0 mL of 0.5% solution in 2.5 mL of normal saline) can be given by inhalation, repeating the dose as often as every 20 to 30 minutes for the first 1 to 2 hours. Isoproterenol can be substituted if more rapid onset of bronchodilatation is needed, although isoproterenol is associated with a higher risk of tachycardia and arrhythmias. For patients unable to cooperate with the use of a nebulizer, epinephrine (0.3 mL of 1:1000 dilution) or terbutaline (0.25 mg) may be given by subcutaneous injection, again as often as every 20 to 30 minutes during the first 1 to 2 hours. Because of potential cardiac side effects of injected sympathomimetics, the inhalational route is preferred for older patients and those with known cardiac disease.

Intravenous beta-agonists have been used in children failing to respond to inhaled aerosol therapy.[95, 96] Several studies, initially with albuterol[97] and more recently with terbutaline,[98] suggested a role for intravenous selective beta₂-agonists in the treatment of adults with severe asthma. However, direct comparisons of inhaled and intravenous selective beta-agonist drugs failed to demonstrate a clear advantage of the intravenous approach in terms of greater improvement in lung function or gas exchange.[99–103] Given their greater potential for cardiac toxicity, intravenous beta-agonists should be reserved as a possible lifesaving measure in those who fail to respond to conventional inhaled therapy.

The optimal frequency of administration of inhaled beta-agonists after the initial hour of therapy is unknown, although experience indicates that an interval of 90 to 120 minutes is safe. Beta-agonists may also be given safely by continuous nebulization during a 2-hour interval.[103] Although this approach offers some advantages with regard to reducing reliance on respiratory therapy or nursing personnel, further studies are needed to determine whether this approach is safe or practical for longer treatment periods.

In our experience, corticosteroids are almost always required for successful resolution of severe asthma. The timing of administration and the corticosteroid dose used are the most important considerations. Because there is a several hours' lag period between time of administration and the onset of appreciable improvement in lung function,[104, 105] steroids should be given as soon as possible. Although the optimal corticosteroid dose has not been established, some studies indicated that higher doses may achieve earlier improvement.[106, 107] The duration of high-dose treatment is usually limited to days; therefore, the risks associated with such therapy are minimal.

Although oral prednisone is rapidly absorbed from the gut[108] and has been shown to give comparable results to intravenous hydrocortisone in severe asthma,[109] we recommend the use of parenteral steroids to ensure adequate blood and tissue levels. One approach is to give methylprednisolone in doses of 60 to 240 mg every 6 hours until there is objective evidence of improvement in lung function. Methylprednisolone is preferred to hydrocortisone because of its smaller mineralocorticoid effect and lower likelihood of causing hypokalemia.[110] If the patient's condition continues to deteriorate while he or she is taking steroids in these prescribed doses, we consider administering even higher doses on the premise that the potential benefits outweigh the risks in this life-threatening situation.

The use of methylxanthines in asthma is becoming increasingly controversial, in part because of the low therapeutic index of these compounds, but also because of questions concerning the benefits of such therapy. As single therapy for the acute episode, theophylline is not as effective as either inhaled or injected sympathomimetic agents, nor does it enhance the benefits achieved by these other agents when used as combined therapy during the initial hours of treatment.[111, 112] Other studies examining the longer-term effects of aminophylline in hospitalized asthmatic patients concluded that it did not add significant benefit to other standard therapies.[113] Although provocative, these studies are not, in our view, sufficiently definitive at this point to recommend eschewing the use of theophylline altogether. It is recognized that methylxanthines are effective bronchodilators and that some asthmatic patients taking theophylline deteriorate if the medication is discontinued. Further, methylxanthines have potential benefits other than improvement in airflow rates, such as improved diaphragmatic contractility and enhanced mucociliary clearance rates.[114, 115]

Until larger studies are carried out to clarify in full detail the risks and benefits of theophylline therapy, a conservative approach, giving theophylline in doses approximating 0.5

mg/kg/h with the goal of achieving a blood level of 10 to 15 mg/L is warranted. The infusion rate is lowered to 0.25 mg/kg/h in patients with congestive heart failure or liver disease and in patients taking medications that might reduce drug elimination and increase serum levels, such as cimetidine, ciprofloxacin, and erythromycin.[116, 117] We generally avoid a loading dose in patients already taking theophylline as a maintenance medication and instead confirm the serum concentration so that proper adjustments in the level can be made safely. For intravenous use, anhydrous theophylline is preferred to aminophylline because it lacks the ethylene diamine moiety that causes hypersensitivity reactions. It is imperative that serum theophylline concentrations be monitored on a daily basis to maintain adequate levels and avoid toxicity.

Anticholinergic agents have been used in the treatment of asthma for many years,[118] and although they are recognized as having bronchodilator activity, their proper role in the treatment of status asthmaticus is not established.[119] In general, anticholinergic agents have a slower onset of bronchodilator action than do beta-agonists and they achieve their peak effect 30 to 90 minutes after administration.[120] Moreover, the peak effect achieved is usually less than that seen with beta-agonists in status asthmaticus.[121, 122] Several studies have furnished support for the use of the quaternary ammonium compound ipratropium bromide in combination therapy with beta-agonists in severe asthma.[123–126] A rational approach is to ascertain whether the patient who responds poorly to beta-agonists has a good response to anticholinergics and, if so, consider alternating inhaled anticholinergics with beta-agonists. Special mention concerning the use of magnesium sulfate in acute severe asthma is made only because of reports of its efficacy in a small number of patients.[127] A single intravenous dose of magnesium sulfate (1.2 g in 50 mL of saline) resulted in improved peak airflow and fewer hospitalizations. Given the modest level of improvement and the lack of any larger experience or more detailed studies, we have no recommendations regarding the use of this smooth muscle relaxant.

A number of other drugs have been used in the management of severe asthma, and although most are of questionable value as conventional therapy, some have merit in specific circumstances. For example, mucolytic agents, such as N-acetylcysteine, are thought to reduce sputum viscosity by breaking down disulfide bonds that link glycoproteins and other constituents of mucus. Their ability to improve the clearance of secretions in asthma is controversial.[128] We do not recommend that N-acetylcysteine be used routinely because of its potential to cause nausea and trigger bronchospasm. When indicated, we administer N-acetylcysteine (10% solution) in a volume of 2 to 5 mL directly through the bronchoscope to remove retained secretions.

Antibiotics were once used routinely in the treatment of asthma but now they are recommended only when there is reasonable clinical evidence of infection. In contrast to viral respiratory pathogens, bacteria rarely cause lower respiratory tract infections that lead to exacerbations of asthma.[129, 130] On the other hand, worsening asthma has been associated with acute bacterial sinusitis, a condition requiring aggressive and often prolonged antibiotic therapy.[131–133]

A number of other drug compounds have been recommended for the treatment of chronic severe asthma, including methotrexate,[134–136] gold,[137, 138] and troleandomycin.[139] In general, these compounds have been promulgated as being potentially useful on the basis of their anti-inflammatory activity and, hence, their potential as steroid-sparing agents. The evidence that any of these agents significantly alters the course of chronic asthma is far from convincing. Likewise, there is no demonstrable role for any of these agents in the emergency treatment of acute severe asthma.

TABLE 72–5

MECHANICAL VENTILATION IN ASTHMA

Standard Approaches

Suppress patient-initiated ventilation (intermittent mandatory ventilation or assist/control mode) by using adequate minute ventilation.

Use a pattern of high-flow ventilation to maximize expiratory time and decrease intrinsic positive end-expiratory pressure (PEEP).

Administer sedation (lorazepam, 1–2 mg q 6–8 h IV) and, if necessary, paralyzing agents (vecuronium, 0.02–0.05 mg/kg, or pancuronium, 0.02–0.05 mg/kg).

Attempt to achieve adequate Pao_2 ($\geq$60 mm Hg), $Paco_2$ ($\leq$50 mm Hg), pH (7.25–7.55) and peak airway pressure ($\leq$60 cm H_2O).

Extraordinary Measures

Use controlled hypoventilation with bicarbonate infusion to maintain artrial pH >7.25.

Administer helium-oxygen (40:60) mixtures as source of ventilatory gas.

Consider prophylactic tube thoracostomy to protect against tension pneumothorax if inflation pressures remain >70 cm H_2O.

Administer low-level (5 cm H_2O) PEEP to decrease work of breathing in the recovering asthmatic patient with high intrinsic PEEP.

Perform segmental bronchial lavage via fiberoptic bronchoscope.

Consider administration of isoflurane or enflurane anesthetics.

Mechanical Ventilation

The major goals of mechanical ventilation are to restore respiratory muscle strength and to maintain adequate arterial blood pH (Table 72–5). Oxygenation is rarely difficult, and typically 0.3 to 0.5 inspired oxygen fraction is sufficient to maintain adequate oxygen saturation. Although carbon dioxide elimination may frequently be abnormal after mechanical ventilation is initiated, if adequate arterial pH is maintained at a level of 7.3 or higher, modestly elevated $Paco_2$ levels can be tolerated.

In severe asthma, the work of breathing may exceed the patient's ability to breathe comfortably or efficiently. Therefore, complete respiratory muscle rest should be achieved promptly with ventilatory assistance. Intermittent mandatory ventilation or assist/control mode ventilation may be used interchangeably, as long as the patient is adequately sedated and the rate and tidal volume output of the ventilator is set to be in synchrony with the patient's own breathing pattern. If neuromuscular paralysis is required, vecuronium has several advantages over other nondepolarizing relaxants, because it undergoes spontaneous deacetylation, and unlike pancuronium, it is not dependent on renal excretion. Further, the brief (62-minute) half-life of vercuronium allows for more rapid recovery of muscle function after discontinuation of drug administration. Atracurium and succinylcholine should not be used in status asthmaticus because of their tendency to release histamine.[93, 94]

Because of the underlying physiology, several unique problems are encountered in ventilating the asthmatic patient. For example, increased airway resistance results in high inspiratory airway pressures, thus raising the risk of barotrauma. Moreover, incomplete emptying of alveoli at end expiration produces intrinsic positive end-expiratory pressure (PEEP), also called auto-PEEP. The limited ability to ventilate adequately because of high pressures and the added dead space attendant with intrinsic PEEP may cause an elevation in $Paco_2$.

Although conventional practice dictates using low inspiratory flow rates to minimize peak inspiratory pressure, evidence suggests that better gas exchange and lower intrinsic PEEP levels may be achieved with a pattern of low tidal volumes and high flow rates.[140] The risk of elevated peak inspiratory pressures from high flow rates appears to be offset by lower intrinsic PEEP levels. The rationale for this approach is based on the thesis that elevated pressures are better tolerated by proximal airways than distal structures in terms of barotrauma, but this has not been proved.

Intrinsic PEEP is measured by occluding the expiratory port of the ventilator at end expiration.[141] This maneuver is analogous to the commonly measured plateau pressure, but it is performed at end expiration instead of end inspiration. With the port occluded, alveolar pressures upstream from newly opened sites of collapse are transmitted downstream to the airway opening. Thus, at end expiration, airway pressure may read at or near zero on the ventilator manometer, but after occluding the ventilator port, the pressure rises to the level of alveolar pressure, or the level of intrinsic PEEP. It is not unusual to find intrinsic PEEP levels between 10 and 20 cm H_2O in severe asthma. In sedated, paralyzed patients, intrinsic PEEP has effects similar to those of extrinsic PEEP: namely, increased intrathoracic pressures, decreased venous return, increased pulmonary vascular resistance with impedance of right ventricular emptying, and ventricular interdependence with diastolic dysfunction of the left ventricle. Drug therapy to reduce airway obstruction and longer expiratory times during the ventilatory cycle using low tidal volumes and high inspiratory flow rates are the most effective measures for reducing intrinsic PEEP. For most asthmatics, optimal ventilation can be achieved by using tidal volumes of 6 to 10 mL/kg, respiratory rates of 20 to 30 breaths/min, and inspiratory flows of 80 to 100 L/min. However, some patients fail to respond to these measures and other approaches are needed.

If peak airway pressures exceed 70 cm H_2O, tidal volume, inspiratory flow, or respiratory rate may be reduced. Of these, a reduction in tidal volume or rate is preferred initially, because this more effectively decreases hyperinflation and intrinsic PEEP. Although a reduction of inspiratory flow may decrease peak pressure, it also reduces emptying time and may lead to increased hyperinflation. Almost any maneuver that brings peak airway pressure into a more reasonable range may also result in further hypoventilation, increased $Paco_2$, and a fall in pH. In this instance, controlled hypoventilation can be used with infusion of bicarbonate to maintain adequate blood pH.[142, 143] The danger of administering bicarbonate, apart from problems associated with volume overload and hypertonicity, is the possibility that life-threatening alkalosis might occur if airway obstruction suddenly reverses and alveolar ventilation is restored. Therefore, bicarbonate should be given in quantities sufficient to produce an adequate pH (7.25 to 7.30) rather than normal blood pH.

Administration of helium-oxygen mixtures in a ratio of 40:60 has been advocated as an effective means of reducing density-dependent resistance, improving gas exchange, and at the same time lowering dynamic pressures.[144] Although this approach may have some application in addressing problems of high peak pressures and high $Paco_2$, further experience is needed to make general recommendations.

The use of extrinsic PEEP in ventilator management in patients with obstructive airways disease has been advocated by some investigators,[145] although other researchers have shown untoward effects.[146] In our view, there is no sound physiologic reason for using extrinsic PEEP in managing intubated asthmatic patients. In fact, PEEP has been shown to be detrimental in the sedated, paralyzed patient in whom ventilation is dictated by ventilator settings.[147]

However, for selected patients who are recovering and actively initiating their own breaths, the judicious application of small amounts of PEEP can be helpful in allowing them to trigger the ventilator with reduced effort. Because most ventilators employ demand valves or stepper motors to adjust inspiratory flow in response to a negative pressure deflection (inspiratory effort), patients with high levels of intrinsic PEEP may be at a special disadvantage. With intrinsic PEEP of 10 cm H_2O, for example, the patient needs to reduce alveolar pressure by 12 cm H_2O to produce the necessary 2 cm H_2O negative deflection to trigger the ventilator. Because of current ventilator design, the application of 5 cm H_2O of PEEP results in subtraction of 5 cm H_2O from the pressure required to trigger; thus, the patient with 10 cm H_2O intrinsic PEEP needs to generate only 7 cm H_2O inspiratory pressure. In the mechanically ventilated asthmatic patient who (1) is not paralyzed, (2) initiates ventilator-delivered breaths, (3) has high levels of intrinsic PEEP, and (4) manifests respiratory distress with suprasternal retractions, use of accessory muscles, or other signs, the judicious use of small levels of PEEP may temporarily facilitate synchrony with the ventilator.

Other Measures

If peak inspiratory pressures remain elevated (>70 cm H_2O) and intrinsic PEEP cannot be lowered below 20 cm H_2O with conventional aggressive measures, consideration should be given to other nonconventional but potentially lifesaving measures. For example, prophylactic tube thoracostomy may protect against sudden death occurring in association with tension pneumothorax. Whether pneumothorax correlates better with peak, mean, or end-expiratory pressures is not known. Nevertheless, the risk of barotrauma in mechanically ventilated asthmatic patients is significant, with a reported incidence as high as 33%.[148–154]

General anesthesia has also been used in life-threatening asthma, and because this form of therapy is viewed as a last resort, most published reports of its use are anecdotal. The goals of general anesthesia are to achieve rapid bronchodilatation and to allow time for other therapeutic measures to take effect. Inhalant anesthetics, including halothane, isoflurane, and enflurane, produce significant bronchodilatation during the induction of anesthesia.[155–158] The mechanism of bronchodilatation has been related to a direct effect on smooth muscle as well as indirect effects mediated by catecholamine release and antagonism of cholinergic and histaminergic effects.[159–161] The halogenated compounds are strongly arrhythmogenic, although isoflurane and enflurane are less potent in this regard.[157–162] Ketamine also has smooth muscle–relaxant effects, and it may be given by continuous intravenous infusion.[163–166] Because the bronchodilator effects of ketamine are thought to be related to adrenergic stimulation, it is uncertain whether ketamine offers any advantages over parenteral beta-agonists.[164] Ketamine is contraindicated in patients with hypertension, preeclampsia, and increased intracranial pressure. As a rule, bronchospasm returns when general anesthesia is terminated, unless other specific therapeutic measures have started to work. The use of these agents is considered extreme and potentially dangerous.

Removal of impacted secretions by fiberoptic bronchoscopy can also be of benefit.[152, 167, 168] Sudden deterioration in gas exchange or increasing resistance to mechanical ventilation as reflected by increasing inflation pressures may be an indication of mucous plugging of airways. Adequate preoxygenation, sedation, and occasionally, general anesthesia are required for satisfactory results. For peripheral secretions, lavage of a bronchopulmonary segment with repeated infusions of warm saline in 50-mL aliquots facilitates removal of plugs and casts of small airways. The amount of lavage fluid returned after suctioning may be a small fraction of the amount infused owing to the intense airway obstruction. If secretions are inordinately viscous, adding N-acetylcysteine (2 to 5 ml of 10% solution) to the saline may be helpful.[168] This application of bronchoscopic segmental lavage has virtually replaced volume-controlled whole lung lavage performed by gravity-dependent fluid exchange.[169–171] The benefits of improved oxygenation and increased compliance after bronchoscopic lavage may be offset by early worsening of these measurements,[167] as well as the possibility of an increased incidence of bronchopulmonary infections.[152]

COMPLICATIONS

Complications of asthma are uncommon, and when they do occur, they are often a consequence of treatment rather than the disease itself. Sinus tachycardia is an expected finding during an acute episode. More serious arrhythmias, however, such as supraventricular tachycardia and ventricular premature contractions, are infrequent and usually subside as airflow obstruction improves.[89, 172, 173] Careful cardiac monitoring is nevertheless important in managing elderly patients, especially those with underlying heart disease, because either methylxanthines or beta-agonist agents in excessive doses may increase the incidence of arrhythmia. Whether the combined use of methylxanthines and beta-agonists poses an added risk of serious arrhythmias is controversial.[174–177] Severe asthma may also be associated with metabolic acidosis resulting from lactic acidosis of unknown cause.[73, 92] Metabolic acidosis is reported to occur in up to 48% of patients hospitalized for asthma.[92] Other metabolic disturbances include hypokalemia caused by beta-agonist therapy[91, 178] and hypophosphatemia resulting from intracellular shifts in phosphorus during correction of respiratory acidosis.[179] The potential clinical consequences of hypophosphatemia include decreased diaphragmatic muscle contractility[180] and altered tissue oxygenation.[181]

Barotrauma with pneumomediastinum and pneumothorax are among the most serious complications of acute asthma. Barotrauma is extremely rare as a spontaneous occurrence. Most often, it occurs as a complication of mechanical ventilation and its prevention has already been considered. Occlusion of a major airway by mucous plugging can cause acute respiratory distress, atelectasis, altered gas exchange, and hypotension. Emergency removal of a major airway plug by endoscopy and suction may be required to restore ventilation.

The complications of acute and chronic asthma are frequently related to drug therapy, especially methylxanthine therapy. Nausea and gastrointestinal disturbances are considered early manifestations of theophylline toxicity, but in our experience, tachycardia, tremor, and anxiety are more reliable signs of toxicity. It is important to remember that toxic symptoms may develop in some patients at blood levels of less than 20 mg/L.[182] At higher levels, generally greater than 35 mg/L, seizures and serious cardiac rhythm disturbances may occur. Serial serum measurements of theophylline are recommended to avoid untoward effects. When signs of toxicity are present or when serum levels exceed 20 mg/L, theophylline administration should be discontinued. If the patient shows signs of serious toxicity or excessive levels and has recently taken oral theophylline, further systemic absorption of drug from the gastrointestinal tract can be decreased with administration of oral activated charcoal (50 to 100 g) and a cathartic, preferably 100 mL of 70% sorbitol.[183] Activated charcoal enhances theophylline clearance,[184, 185] thus making it useful in the treatment of overdose by the intravenous route also. The recommended regimen for this is 20 g every 2 hours.[186] Charcoal hemoperfusion should also be considered in cases of life-threatening theophylline intoxication, especially if normal clearance mechanisms are impaired, as in liver disease.[187, 188] Because seizures associated with theophylline intoxication may result in residual neurologic abnormalities,[183] the use of prophylactic antiepileptic therapy should be considered.

Concern has been raised as to whether inhaled beta$_2$-agonist therapy can have untoward effects on airway responsiveness and symptom control.[189, 190] Notably, such concerns relate to the long-term use of inhaled beta$_2$-agonists for outpatient maintenance therapy, and even in this situation, the issue is controversial and in need of further facts before definitive conclusions can be drawn. With respect to managing acute severe asthma, beta-agonists, in conjunction with corticosteroids, remain the treatment of choice and are central to proper management.

DIFFERENTIAL DIAGNOSIS

Several conditions may mimic acute asthma and should be considered in the differential diagnosis, especially in the patient with new-onset asthma. Obstruction of a major airway caused by laryngeal edema, tracheal stenosis, vocal cord paralysis, neoplasm, foreign body, or tracheomalacia may cause asthma-like symptoms. Obstruction of the upper airway is associated with inspiratory stridor and hoarseness. An unusual cause of upper airway obstruction presenting as asthma is vocal cord dysfunction wherein paradoxical movement (adduction) of the true and false cords occurs during inspiration.[191–193] Patients with this abnormality often have psychiatric disorders and episodic hoarseness in addition to paroxysmal dyspnea and wheezing. Direct visualization of the airway by laryngoscopy and bronchoscopy and maximal expiratory flow volume loops are important tools in the diagnosis of upper airway obstruction.

Bronchospasm and wheezing may also occur with acute pulmonary embolism. The differential diagnosis should take advantage of ventilation-perfusion scanning, especially after bronchodilator administration because improved ventilation may correct perfusion abnormalities in the asthmatic patient. Determination of the carbon monoxide diffusion capacity may also be helpful, because it is usually normal in acute asthma and reduced with pulmonary embolism. So-called cardiac asthma may occur in association with left ventricular dysfunction or mitral valve disease. The signs and symptoms are easily mistaken for those of asthma, especially because of the prominence of nocturnal dyspnea and wheezing. Careful attention to radiographic and electrocardiographic signs of congestive heart failure and ischemic heart disease can usually detect an underlying cardiac disorder.

Chronic or acute aspiration of oropharyngeal or gastric contents may cause cough, chest tightness, and wheezing and may be confused with an acute asthmatic episode. Exclusion of diffuse pulmonary infiltrates by chest radiography helps to rule out massive aspiration. A careful history, imaging studies of swallowing function and gastric emptying, and 24-hour monitoring of lower esophageal pH may be required to document aspiration or gastroesophageal reflux as a cause of symptoms.

The overlap between asthma and other causes of chronic airway obstruction is well recognized. Patients with chronic obstructive pulmonary disease may have acute exacerbation, with symptoms and signs that are virtually indistinguishable from those of asthma. Although the treatment of these patients does not differ significantly from the treatment of the severe asthmatic, there is considerable difference in the expected outcome of treatment and the prognosis for longer-term recovery. A history of cigarette smoking and chronic productive cough suggests chronic obstructive pulmonary disease as the primary underlying disorder.

References

1. Weiss KB: Seasonal trends in US asthma hospitalizations and mortality. JAMA 263:2323, 1990.
2. Cookson JB: Prevalence rates of asthma in developing countries and their comparison with those in Europe and North America. Chest 91:97S, 1987.
3. Van Niekerk CH, Weinberg EG, Shore SC, et al: Prevalence of asthma: A comparative study of urban and rural Xhosa children. Clin Allergy 9:319, 1979.
4. Waite DA, Eyles EF, Tonkin SL, et al: Asthma prevalence in Tokelauan children in two environments. Clin Allergy 10:71, 1980.
5. Smith JM, Harding LK, Cumming G: The changing prevalence of asthma in schoolchildren. Clin Allergy 1:57, 1971.
6. Britton WJ, Woolcock AJ, Peat J, et al: Prevalence of bronchial hyper-responsiveness in children: The relationship between asthma and skin reactivity to allergens in two communities. Int J Epidemiol 15:202, 1986.
7. Williams H, McNicol KN: Prevalence, natural history and relationship of wheezy bronchitis and asthma in children. An epidemiological study. Br Med J 4:321, 1969.
8. Sears MR, Jones DT, Silva PA, et al: Asthma in seven year old children: A report from the Dunedin Multidisciplinary Child Development Study. NZ Med J 95:533, 1982.
9. National Center for Health Statistics: Current Estimates from the National Health Interview Survey: U.S., 1987. Vital and Health Statistics. Public Health Service. Washington, DC, US Government Printing Office, 1987. Department of Health and Human Services publication (PHS)88-1594. Series 10, No. 166.
10. Dodge RR, Burrows B: The prevalence and incidence of asthma and asthma-like symptoms in a general population sample. Am Rev Respir Dis 122:567, 1980.
11. Broder I, Higgins MW, Mathews KP, et al: Epidemiology of asthma and allergic rhinitis in a total community, Tecumseh, Michigan. J Allergy 53:127, 1974.
12. Halfon N, Newacheck PW: Trends in the hospitalization for acute childhood asthma, 1970–84. Am J Public Health 76:1308, 1986.
13. Gergen PJ, Mullally DI, Evans R III: National survey of prevalence of asthma among children in the United States, 1976 to 1980. Pediatrics 81:1, 1988.
14. Smith JM: The prevalence of asthma and wheezing in children. Br J Dis Chest 70:73, 1976.
15. Mitchell EA: Increasing prevalence of asthma in children. NZ Med J 96:463, 1983.
16. Barbee RA, Dodge R, Lebowitz MI, et al: The epidemiology of asthma. Chest 87:21S, 1985.
17. Bronnimann SB, Burrows B: Natural history of asthma. Chest 87:214, 1985.
18. Burrows B: The natural history of asthma. J Allergy Clin Immunol 80:373, 1987.
19. Weiss KB, Wagener DK: Changing patterns of asthma mortality. Identifying target populations at high risk. JAMA 264:1683, 1990.
20. Evans R III, Mullally DI, Wilson RW, et al: National trends in the morbidity and mortality of asthma in the US. Prevalence, hospitalization and death from asthma over two decades: 1965–1984. Chest 91:65S, 1987.
21. Gergen PJ, Weiss KB: Changing patterns of asthma hospitalization among children: 1979 to 1987. JAMA 264:1688, 1990.
22. Fish JE, Menkes HA: Airway reactivity: Role in acute and chronic disease. In: Simmons DH (ed): Current Pulmonology, Volume 5. New York, John Wiley & Sons, p 169, 1984.
23. Fish JE: In vivo methods for study of allergy: Skin and mucosal tests, techniques and interpretation—bronchial challenge testing. In: Middleton E, Reed CE, Ellis EF, et al (eds): Allergy: Principles and Practice. 3rd ed. St Louis, CV Mosby, p 447, 1988.
24. Cockcroft DW, Killian DM, Mellon JA, et al: Bronchial reactivity to inhaled histamine: A method and clinical survey. Clin Allergy 7:235, 1977.
25. Hargreave FE, Ryan G, Thomson N, et al: Bronchial responsiveness to histamine or methacholine in asthma: Measurement and clinical significance. J Allergy Clin Immunol 68:347, 1981.
26. Anderson SD: Current concepts of exercise-induced asthma: A review. Allergy 38:289, 1983.
27. McFadden ER Jr, Ingram RH Jr, Strauss RH, et al: Exercise-induced asthma. Observations on the initiating stimulus. N Engl J Med 301:763, 1979.
28. O'Byrne PM, Dolovich J, Hargreave FE: Late asthmatic responses. Am Rev Respir Dis 136:740, 1987.
29. Djukanovic R, Roche WR, Wilson JW, et al: Mucosal inflammation in asthma. Am Rev Respir Dis 142:434, 1990.

30. Mellis CM, Levison H: Bronchial reactivity in cystic fibrosis. Pediatrics 61:446, 1978.
31. Parker CD, Bilbo RE, Reed CE: Methacholine aerosol as a test for bronchial asthma. Arch Intern Med 115:452, 1965.
32. Simonsson BG: Clinical and physiological studies on chronic bronchitis. III. Bronchial reactivity to inhaled acetylcholine. Acta Allerg 20:325, 1965.
33. Empey DW, Laitinen LA, Gold WM, et al: Mechanisms of bronchial hyperreactivity in normal subjects after upper respiratory tract infection. Am Rev Respir Dis 113:131, 1976.
34. Little JW, Hall WJ, Douglas RG Jr, et al: Airway hyperreactivity and peripheral airway dysfunction in influenza A infection. Am Rev Respir Dis 118:295, 1978.
35. Widdicombe JG, Barnes PJ: Cholinergic mechanisms in bronchial hyperresponsiveness and asthma. In: Kaliner MA, Barnes PJ, Persson CGA (eds): Asthma: Its Pathology and Treatment. New York, Marcel Dekker, p 327, 1991.
36. Barnes PJ: Cholinergic control of airway smooth muscle. Am Rev Respir Dis 136:S42, 1987.
37. Lundberg JM, Hokfelt T, Martling C-R, et al: Substance P–immunoreactive sensory nerves in the lower respiratory tract of various mammals including man. Cell Tissue Res 235:251, 1984.
38. Martling CR, Theodorsson-Norheim E, Lundberg JM: Occurrence and effects of multiple tachykinins: Substance P, neurokinin A, neuropeptide K in human lower airways. Life Sci 40:1633, 1987.
39. Lundberg JM, Martling C-R, Saria A: Substance P and capsaicin-induced contraction of human bronchi. Acta Physiol Scand 119:49, 1983.
40. Rogers DF, Carstairs JR, Alton EWFW, et al: Tachykinins and mucus secretion in human bronchi in vitro. Am Rev Respir Dis 137:12, 1989.
41. Rogers DF, Awvdkij B, Barnes PJ: Effects of tachykinins on mucus secretion in human bronchi in vitro. Eur J Pharmacol 174:2983, 1989.
42. Advenier C, Naline E, Drapean G, et al: Relative potencies of neurokinins in guinea-pig and human bronchus. Eur J Pharmacol 139:133, 1987.
43. Snider RM, Constantine JW, Lowe JA III, et al: A potent nonpeptide antagonist of the substance P (NK$_1$) receptor. Science 251:435, 1991.
44. Filley WV, Holley KE, Kephart GM, et al: Identification by immunofluorescence of eosinophil granule major basic protein in lung tissues of patients with bronchial asthma. Lancet 2:11, 1982.
45. Bousquet J, Chanez P, Lacoste JY, et al: Eosinophilic inflammation in asthma. N Engl J Med 323:1033, 1990.
46. Metzger WJ, Zavala D, Richerson, HB, et al: Local allergen challenge and bronchoalveolar lavage of allergic asthmatic lungs. Description of the model and local airway inflammation. Am Rev Respir Dis 135:433, 1987.
47. Dunnill MS: The pathology of asthma. In: Middleton E, Reed CE (eds): Allergy: Principles and Practice. St Louis, CV Mosby, p 678, 1978.
48. Godard P, Chaintreuil J, Damon M, et al: Functional assessment of alveolar macrophages: Comparison of cells from asthmatics and normal subjects. J Allergy Clin Immunol 70:88, 1982.
49. Corrigan CJ, Kay AB: CD4 T-lymphocyte activation in acute severe asthma. Am Rev Respir Dis 141:970, 1990.
50. Kus J: Lymphocyte activation by house dust allergen in asthma: Analysis with monoclonal antibodies. Clin Exp Allergy 20:165, 1990.
51. Kaplan AP, Haak-Frendscho M, Fauci A, et al: A histamine-releasing factor from activated human mononuclear cells. J Immunol 135:2027, 1985.
52. Thueson DO, Speck LS, Lett-Brown MA, et al: Histamine-releasing activity (HRA). I. Production by mitogen or antigen-stimulated human mononuclear cells. J Immunol 123:626, 1979.
53. Schulman ES, Liu MC, Proud D, et al: Human lung macrophages induce histamine release from basophils and mast cells. Am Rev Respir Dis 131:230, 1985.
54. MacDonald SM, Lichtenstein LM, Proud D, et al: Studies of IgE-dependent histamine releasing factors. Heterogeneity of IgE. J Immunol 139:506, 1987.
55. White MV, Kaliner MA: Neutrophils and mast cells. I. Human neutrophil derived histamine releasing activity. J Immunol 139:1624, 1987.
56. Jeffery PK, Wardlaw AJ, Nelson FC, et al: Bronchial biopsies in asthma. An ultrastructural, quantitative study and correlation with hyperreactivity. Am Rev Respir Dis 140:1745, 1989.
57. Beasley R, Roche WR, Roberts JA, et al: Cellular events in the bronchi in mild asthma and after bronchial provocation. Am Rev Respir Dis 139:806, 1989.
58. Laitinen LA, Heino M, Laitinen A, et al: Damage of the airway epithelium and bronchial reactivity in patients with asthma. Am Rev Respir Dis 131:599, 1985.
59. Kirby JG, Hargerave FE, Gleich GJ, et al: Bronchoalveolar cell profiles of asthmatic and nonasthmatic subjects. Am Rev Respir Dis 136:379, 1987.
60. Wardlaw AJ, Dunnette S, Gleich GJ, et al: Eosinophils and mast cells in bronchoalveolar lavage in subjects with mild asthma. Am Rev Respir Dis 137:62, 1988.
61. Wasserfallen J-B, Schaller M-D, Feihl F, et al: Sudden asphyxic asthma: A distinct entity? Am Rev Respir Dis 142:108, 1990.
62. Reid LM: Mucus as a contributory factor. In: Weiss GB (ed): Status Asthmaticus. Baltimore, University Park Press, p 59, 1978.
63. McFadden ER, Lyons HA: Arterial-blood gas tension in asthma. N Engl J Med 278:1028, 1968.
64. Rodriguez-Roisin R, Ballester, E, Roca, J, et al: Mechanisms of hypoxemia in patients with status asthmaticus requiring mechanical ventilation. Am Rev Respir Dis 139:732, 1989.
65. Wagner PD, Dantzker DR, Iacovoni VE, et al: Distributions of ventilation-perfusion ratios in asthma. Am Rev Respir Dis 118:511, 1978.
66. Palmer KNV: Effect of bronchodilator drugs on arterial blood gas tensions in bronchial asthma. Postgrad Med J 47(suppl):75, 1971.
67. Pepe PE, Marini JP: Occult positive end-expiration pressure in mechanically ventilated patients with airflow obstruction. Am Rev Respir Dis 126:166, 1982.
68. Pride NB, Macklem PT: Lung mechanics in disease. In: Macklem PT, Mead J: Handbook of Physiology, Section 3, The Respiratory System, Volume III, Mechanics of Breathing, Part 2. Bethesda, American Physiological Society, p 659, 1986.
69. Woolcock A, Read J: Lung volumes in exacerbations of asthma. Am J Med 50:75, 1972.
70. Pride NB, Permutt S, Riley RL, et al: Determinants of maximal expiratory flow from the lungs. J Appl Physiol 23:646, 1967.
71. Martin J, Powell E, Shore S, et al: The role of respiratory muscles in the hyperinflation of bronchial asthma. Am Rev Respir Dis 121:441, 1980.
72. Jardim J, Farkas G, Prefant C, et al: The failing inspiratory muscles under normoxic and hypoxic conditions. Am Rev Respir Dis 124:274, 1981.
73. Appel D, Rubenstein R, Schrager K, et al: Lactic acidosis in severe asthma. Am J Med 75:580, 1983.
74. Newball HH, Menkes HA, Permutt S, et al: Lung volumes and compliance in myasthenia gravis and reversible airway obstruction. Am Rev Respir Dis 114:639, 1976.
75. Peress L, Sybrecht G, Macklem PT: The mechanism of increase in total lung capacity during acute asthma. Am J Med 61:165, 1976.
76. Permutt S: Some physiologic aspects of asthma: Bronchomuscular contraction and airways calibre. Ciba Found Study Group 38:63, 1971.
77. Permutt S: Physiologic changes in the acute asthmatic attack. In: Lichtenstein LM, Austen KF (eds): Asthma—Physiology, Immunopharmacology and Treatment. New York, Academic Press, 1973.
78. Fish JE, Summer WR: Acute lower airway obstruction: Asthma. In: Moser KM, Spragg RG (eds): Respiratory Emergencies. 2nd ed. St. Louis, CV Mosby, p 144, 1982.
79. Summer WR: Physiological changes in the acute asthmatic attack. In: Weiss EB (ed): Status Asthmaticus. Baltimore, University Park Press, p 81, 1978.
80. Irwin RS, Corrao WM, Pratter MR: Chronic persistent cough in the adult: The spectrum and frequency of causes and successful outcome of specific therapy. Am Rev Respir Dis 123:413, 1981.
81. O'Hollaren MT, Yuninger JW, Offord KP, et al: Exposure to an aeroallergen as a possible precipitating factor in respiratory arrest in young patients with asthma. N Engl J Med 324:359, 1991.
82. Cohen RD, Bateman ED, Potgieter PD: Near-fatal bronchospasm in an asthmatic patient following ingestion of flurbiprofen. S Afr Med J 61:803, 1982.
83. Benatar SR, Opie LH: Sudden death in asthmatics receiving beta-blockers. S Afr Med J 62:308, 1982.
84. Knowles GK, Clark TJH: Pulsus paradoxus as a valuable sign indicating severity of asthma. Lancet 2:1356, 1973.
85. Rebuck AS, Pengelly.LD: Development of pulsus paradoxus in airway obstruction. N Engl J Med 288:66, 1973.
86. Brenner BE, Abraham E, Simon RR: Position and diaphoresis in acute asthma. Am J Med 74:1005, 1983.
87. Shim CS, Williams MH Jr: Evaluation of the severity of asthma: Patients vs. physician. Am J Med 68:11, 1980.
88. McFadden ER Jr: Asthma: Airway dynamics, cardiac function, and clinical correlates. In: Middleton E, Reed CE, Ellis EF, et al (eds): Allergy: Principles and Practice. 3rd ed. St Louis, CV Mosby, p 1018, 1988.
89. Grossman J: The occurrence of arrhythmias in hospitalized asthmatic patients. J Allergy Clin Immunol 57:310, 1976.
90. Gelb AF, Lyons HA, Fairshter RD, et al: P-pulmonale in status asthmaticus. J Allergy Clin Immunol 64:18, 1979.
91. Haalboom JRE, Deenstra A, Struyvenberg A: Hypokalemia induced by inhalation of fenoterol. Lancet 1:2215, 1985.
92. Mountain RD, Heffner JE, Brackett NC Jr, et al: Acid-base disturbances in acute asthma. Chest 98:651, 1990.
93. Ertama PM: Histamine liberation in surgical patients following administration of neuromuscular blocking drugs. Ann Clin Res 14:27, 1982.
94. Bowman WC: Pre- and postjunctional cholinoreceptors at the neuromuscular junction. Anesth Analg 59:935, 1980.
95. Bohn D, Kalloghlian A, Jenkins J, et al: Intravenous salbutamol in the treatment of status asthmaticus in children. Crit Care Med 12:892, 1984.
96. Herman JJ, Noah ZL, Moody RR: Use of intravenous isoproterenol for status asthmaticus in children. Crit Care Med 11:716, 1983.
97. Williams S, Seaton A: Intravenous or inhaled salbutamol in severe acute asthma. Thorax 32:555, 1979.
98. Van Renterghem D, Lamont H, Elinck W, et al: Intravenous versus nebulized terbutaline in patients with acute severe asthma: A double-blind randomized study. Ann Allergy 59:313, 1987.

99. Lawford P, Jones BJM, Milledge JS: Comparison of intravenous and nebulised salbutamol in initial treatment of severe asthma. Br Med J 276:84, 1978.

100. Bloomfield P, Carmichael J, Petrie GR, et al: Comparison of salbutamol given intravenously and by intermittent positive pressure breathing in life threatening asthma. Br Med J 78:848, 1979.

101. Williams SJ, Winner SJ, Clark TJH: Comparison of inhaled and intravenous terbutaline in acute severe asthma. Thorax 36:639, 1981.

102. O'Connell MB, Iber C: Continuous intravenous terbutaline infusions for adult patients with status asthmaticus. Ann Allergy 64:213, 1990.

103. Colacone A, Wolkove N, Stern E, et al: Continuous nebulization of albuterol (salbutamol) in acute asthma. Chest 97:693, 1990.

104. Ellul-Micallef R, Fenech FF: Intravenous prednisone in chronic bronchial asthma. Thorax 30:312, 1975.

105. Fanta C, Rossing TH, McFadden ER Jr: Glucocorticoids in acute asthma. A clinical controlled trial. Am J Med 74:845, 1983.

106. Haskell RJ, Wong BM, Hansen JE: A double blind randomized clinical trial of methylprednisolone in status asthmaticus. Arch Intern Med 143:1324, 1983.

107. Ratto D, Alfonso C, Sipsey J, et al: Are intravenous corticosteroids required in status asthmaticus? JAMA 260:527, 1988.

108. Morrison PJ, Bradbrook ID, Rogers HJ: Plasma prednisolone levels from enteric and nonenteric coated tablets estimated by an original technique. Br J Clin Pharmacol 4:597, 1977.

109. Harrison BD, Stokes TC, Hart GJ: Need for intravenous hydrocortisone in addition to oral prednisolone in patients admitted to hospital with severe asthma without ventilatory failure. Lancet 1:181, 1986.

110. Collins JV, Harris PWR, Clark TJH, et al: Intravenous corticosteroids in treatment of acute bronchial asthma. Lancet 2:1047, 1970.

111. Rossing TH, Fanta CH, Golstein DH, et al: Emergency therapy of asthma: Comparison of the acute effects of parenteral and inhaled sympathomimetics and infused aminophylline. Am Rev Respir Dis 122:365, 1980.

112. Fanta CH, Rossing TH, McFadden ER: Treatment of acute asthma: Is combination therapy with sympathomimetics and methylxanthines indicated? Am J Med 80:5, 1986.

113. Self TH, Abou-Shala N, Burns R, et al: Inhaled albuterol and oral prednisone therapy in hospitalized adult asthmatics. Does aminophylline add any benefit? Chest 98:1317, 1990.

114. Aubier M, DeTroyer A, Sampson M, et al: Aminophylline improves diaphragmatic contractility. N Engl J Med 305:249, 1981.

115. Sutton PP, Pavia D, Bateman JRM, et al: The effect of oral aminophylline on lung clearance in man. Chest 80:889, 1981.

116. Jonkman JHG: Therapeutic consequences of drug interactions with theophylline pharmacokinetics. J Allergy Clin Immunol 78:736, 1986.

117. Raoof S, Woolschlager CM, Khan F: Ciprofloxacin increases serum theophylline level. Am J Med 82:115, 1987.

118. Gandevia B: Historical review of the parasympatholytic agents in the treatment of respiratory disorders. Postgrad Med J 51:13, 1975.

119. Gross NJ: Ipratropium bromide. N Engl J Med 319:486, 1988.

120. Ruffin RE, Fitzgerald JD, Rebuck AS: A comparison of the bronchodilator activity of Sch 1000 and salbutamol. J Allergy Clin Immunol 59:139, 1977.

121. Ward MJ, Fentem PH, Smith WHR, et al: Ipratropium bromide in acute asthma. Br Med J 282:598:1981.

122. Leahy BC, Gomm SA, Allen SC: Comparison of nebulized salbutamol with nebulized ipratropium bromide in acute asthma. Br J Dis Chest 77:159, 1983.

123. Bryant DH: Nebulized ipratropium bromide in the treatment of acute asthma. Chest 88:24, 1985.

124. Ward MJ, Macfarlane JT, Davies D: A place for ipratropium bromide in the treatment of severe acute asthma. Br J Dis Chest 79:374, 1985.

125. Beck R, Robertson C, Galdes-Sebaldt M, et al: Combined salbutamol and ipratropium bromide by inhalation in the treatment of severe acute asthma. J Pediatr 107:605, 1985.

126. McGivern DV, Fentem PH, Macfarlane JT, et al: Responses to the sequential administration of salbutamol and ipratropium bromide during recovery from acute severe asthma. Thorax 39:227, 1984.

127. Skobeloff EM, Spivey WH, McNamara RM, et al: Intravenous magnesium sulfate for the treatment of acute asthma in the emergency department. JAMA 262:1210, 1989.

128. Franceschinis R, Lualdi P: Mucolytics and oral acetylcysteine. Eur J Respir Dis 111:1980.

129. Berman SZ, Mathison DA, Stevenson DD, et al: Transtracheal aspiration studies in asthmatic patients in relapse with "infective" asthma and in subjects without respiratory disease. J Allergy Clin Immunol 56:206, 1975.

130. Hall WJ, Hall CB: Bacterial and viral infections in etiology and therapy. In: Weiss EB, Segal MS (eds): Bronchial Asthma: Mechanisms and Therapeutics. Boston, Little, Brown, p 435, 1976.

131. Slavin RG, Cannon RE, Friedman WH, et al: Sinusitis and bronchial asthma. J Allergy Clin Immunol 66:250, 1980.

132. Phipatanakul CS, Slavin RG: Bronchial asthma produced by paranasal sinusitis. Arch Otolaryngol 100:109, 1974.

133. Slavin RG: Relationship of nasal disease and sinusitis to bronchial asthma. Ann Allergy 49:76, 1982.

134. Mullarkey MF, Lammert JK, Blumenstein BA: Long-term methotrexate treatment in corticosteroid-dependent asthma. Ann Intern Med 112:577, 1990.

135. Mullarkey MF, Blumenstein BA, Andrade WP, et al: Methotrexate in the treatment of corticosteroid-dependent asthma: A double-blind crossover study. N Engl J Med 318:603, 1988.

136. Erzurum SC, Leff JA, Cochran JE, et al: Lack of benefit of methotrexate in severe, steroid-dependent asthma. A double-blind, placebo-controlled study. Ann Intern Med 114:353, 1991.

137. Muranaka M, Miyamoto T, Shida T, et al: Gold salt in the treatment of bronchial asthma—a double-blind study. Ann Allergy 40:132, 1978.

138. Klaustermeyer WB, Noritake ST, Kwong FK: Chrysotherapy in the treatment of corticosteroid-dependent asthma. J Allergy Clin Immunol 79:720, 1987.

139. Wald JA, Friedman BF, Farr RS: An improved protocol for the use of troleandomycin (TAO) in the treatment of steroid-requiring asthma. J Allergy Clin Immunol 78:36, 1986.

140. Tuxen DV, Lane S: The effects of ventilatory pattern on hyperinflation, airway pressures, and circulation in mechanical ventilation of patients with severe airflow obstruction. Am Rev Respir Dis 136:827, 1987.

141. Pepe PE, Marini JP: Occult positive end-expiration pressure in mechanically ventilated patients with airflow obstruction. Am Rev Respir Dis 126:166, 1982.

142. Darioli W, Perret C: Mechanical controlled hypoventilation in status asthmaticus. Am Rev Respir Dis 129:385, 1984.

143. Menitore SM, Goldring RM: Combined ventilator and bicarbonate strategy in the management of status asthmaticus. Am J Med 74:898, 1983.

144. Gluck EH, Ohorato DJ, Castriotta RD: Helium-oxygen mixtures in intubated patients with status asthmaticus and respiratory acidosis. Chest 98:693, 1990.

145. Smith TC, Marini JP: Impact of PEEP on lung mechanics and work of breathing in severe airflow obstruction. J Appl Physiol 65:1488, 1988.

146. Tuxen DV: Detrimental effects of positive end-expiratory pressure during controlled mechanical ventilation of patients with severe airflow obstruction. Am Rev Respir Dis 140:5, 1989.

147. Marini JP: Should PEEP be used in airflow obstruction? Am Rev Respir Dis 140:1, 1989.

148. Pingleton SK: Complications of acute respiratory failure. Am Rev Respir Dis 137:1463, 1988.

149. Steier M, Chung N, Roberts EB, et al: Pneumothorax complicating continuous ventilatory support. J Thorac Cardiovasc Surg 67:17, 1974.

150. Scoggin CH, Sahn SA, Petty TL: Status asthmaticus. A nine-year experience. JAMA 238:1158, 1977.

151. Braman SS, Koeminerlen JT: Intensive care of status asthmaticus. A 10 year experience. JAMA 264:366, 1990.

152. Luksza AR, Smith P, Coakley J, et al: Acute severe asthma treated by mechanical ventilation: 10 years' experience from a district general hospital. Thorax 41:459, 1986.

153. Cullen OJ, Caldera DL: Pulmonary barotrauma in critically ill patients. Anesthesiology 50:187, 1979.

154. Mansel JK, Stogner SW, Petrini MF, et al: Mechanical ventilation in patients with acute severe asthma. Am J Med 89:42, 1990.

155. Schwartz SH: Treatment of status asthmaticus with halothane. JAMA 251:2688, 1984.

156. Parnass SM, Feld JM, Chamberlin WH, et al: Status asthmaticus treated with isoflurane and enflurane. Anesth Analg 66:193, 1987.

157. Johnston RG, Noseworthy TW, Friesen EG, et al: Isoflurane therapy for status asthmaticus in children and adults. Chest 97:698, 1990.

158. Bierman MI, Brown M, Muren O, et al: Prolonged isoflurane anesthesia in status asthmaticus. Crit Care Med 14:832, 1986.

159. Fletcher SW, Flacke W, Alper MH: The actions of general anesthetic agents on tracheal smooth muscle. Anesthesiology 29:517, 1968.

160. Hickey RF, Graf PD, Nadel JA, et al: The effects of halothane and cyclopropane on total pulmonary resistance in the dog. Anesthesiology 31:334, 1969.

161. Hirshman CA, Edelstein G, Peetz S, et al: Mechanism of action of inhalational anesthesia on airways. Anesthesiology 56:107, 1982.

162. Johnston RR, Eger EI, Wilson C: A comparative interaction of epinephrine with enflurane, isoflurane, and halothane in man. Anesth Analg 55:709, 1976.

163. L'Hommedieu CS, Arens JJ: The use of ketamine for the emergency intubation of patients with status asthmaticus. Ann Emerg Med 16:568, 1987.

164. Betts EK, Parkin CE: Use of ketamine in an asthmatic child. Anesth Analg 50:420, 1971.

165. Corssen G, Gutierrez J, Reeves JG, et al: Ketamine in the anaesthetic managment of asthmatic patients. Anesth Analg 51:588, 1972.

166. Fisher MM: Ketamine for status asthmaticus. Anaesthesia 32:771, 1977.

167. Weinstein HJ, Bone RC, Ruth WE: Pulmonary lavage in patients treated with mechanical ventilation. Chest 72:583, 1977.

168. Millman M, Millman FM, Goldstein IM, et al: Repeated bronchoscopy and lavages in a severely ill elderly patient. Immunol Allerg Prac 12:298, 1990.

169. Ramirez RJ, Obenour WH Jr: Bronchopulmonary lavage in asthma and chronic bronchitis: Clinical and physiologic observations. Chest 59:146, 1971.

170. Kylstra JH, Rausch DC, Hall KD, et al: Volume-controlled lung lavage

in the treatment of asthma, bronchiectasis, and mucoviscidosis. Am Rev Respir Dis 103:651, 1971.

171. Rogers RM, Bruanstein MS, Shuman JF: Role of bronchopulmonary lavage in the treatment of respiratory failure: A review. Chest 62:955, 1972.

172. Rebuck AS, Read J: Assessment and management of severe asthma. Am J Med 51:788, 1971.

173. Molfino NA, Nannini LJ, Martelli AN, et al: Respiratory arrest in near-fatal asthma. N Engl J Med 324:285, 1991.

174. Nicklas RA, Whitehurst VE, Donohoe RF, et al: Combined use of beta-adrenergic agonists and methyl xanthines (letter). N Engl J Med 307:557, 1982.

175. Crane J, Pearce N, Flatt A, et al: Prescribed fenoterol and death from asthma in New Zealand, 1981–1983: Case-control study. Lancet 1:917, 1989.

176. Kemp JP, Chervinsky P, Orgel HA, et al: Concomitant bitolterol mesylate aerosol and theophylline for asthma therapy, with 24 hr electrocardiographic monitoring. J Allergy Clin Immunol 73:32, 1984.

177. Flatt A, Burgess C, Windom H, et al: The cardiovascular effects of inhaled fenoterol alone and during treatment with oral theophylline. Chest 96:1317, 1989.

178. Swenson ER, Aitken ML: Hypokalemia occurs with inhaled albuterol. Am Rev Respir Dis 131:A99, 1985.

179. Laaban J-P, Waked M, Laromiguiere M, et al: Hypophosphatemia complicating management of acute severe asthma. Ann Intern Med 112:68, 1990.

180. Aubier M, Mruciano D, Lecocguie Y, et al: Effect of hypophosphatemia on diaphragmatic contractility in patients with acute respiratory failure. N Engl J Med 313:420, 1985.

181. Knochel JP: Deranged phosphorus metabolism. In: Seldin DW, Giebisch G (eds): The Kidney: Physiology and Pathophysiology. New York, Raven Press, p 1397, 1985.

182. Jacobs MH, Senior RM, Kessler G: Clinical experience with theophylline: Relationship between dosage, serum concentration and toxicity. JAMA 235:1983, 1976.

183. Goldberg MJ, Park GD, Berlinger WG: Treatment of theophylline intoxication. J Allergy Clin Immunol 78:811, 1986.

184. Mahutte CK, True RJ, Michiels TM, et al: Increased serum theophylline clearance with orally administered activated charcoal. Am Rev Respir Dis 128:820, 1983.

185. Sessler CN, Glauser FL, Cooper KR: Treatment of theophylline toxicity with oral activated charcoal. Chest 87:325, 1985.

186. Park G, Radomski L, Goldberg M, et al: Effect of size and frequency of multiple oral charcoal doses on theophylline clearance. Clin Pharmacol Ther 34:663, 1983.

187. Park GD, Spector R, Robert RJ, et al: The use of hemoperfusion for theophylline intoxication. Am J Med 74:961, 1983.

188. Greenberg A, Piraino BH, Kroboth PD, et al: Severe theophylline toxicity. Role of conservative measures, antiarrhythmic agents, and charcoal hemoperfusion. Am J Med 76:854, 1984.

189. Sears M, Taylor DR, Lake DC, et al: Regular inhaled beta-agonist treatment in bronchial asthma. Lancet 336:1391, 1990.

190. β₂ agonists in asthma: Relief, prevention, morbidity. Lancet 336:1411, 1990.

191. Patterson R, Schatz M, Horton M: Munchausen's stridor: Non-organic laryngeal obstruction. Clin Allergy 4:307, 1974.

192. Rogers JH, Stell PM: Paradoxical movement of the vocal cords as a cause of stridor. J Laryngol Otol 92:157, 1978.

193. Christopher KL, Wood RP III, Eckert C, et al: Vocal-cord dysfunction presenting as asthma. N Engl J Med 308:1566, 1983.

CHAPTER 73

Adult Respiratory Distress Syndrome

Clinical Features

John H. Hansen-Flaschen

The adult respiratory distress syndrome (ARDS) is a common disorder. Although the actual incidence is unknown, current estimates suggest that more than 150,000 cases occur each year in the United States alone. ARDS can develop in previously healthy individuals, but more often, this disorder complicates major surgery, trauma, or a serious medical illness. More than 20 years have elapsed since ARDS came into focus as a distinct category of respiratory failure,[1] yet the mortality of this condition remains exceedingly high and no specific treatment is available as yet. However, survival can be improved by meticulous supportive therapy that is based on a thorough understanding of the pathophysiology and clinical course of this disorder.

DEFINITION

The meaning of the term *adult respiratory distress syndrome* has evolved considerably during the past two decades as the spectrum of disorders that cause respiratory failure has gradually come into focus. Today, ARDS is defined as an acute lung injury that results in widespread bilateral pulmonary infiltrates, severe refractory hypoxemia, and a marked reduction in lung compliance. Experienced clinicians recognize typical cases of ARDS with little difficulty; however, several related conditions can be confused with this form of respiratory failure. For that reason, certain aspects of the definition warrant special emphasis.

In ARDS, respiratory failure results from widespread injury to the gas-exchanging components of the lungs. Cardiac pulmonary edema and massive aspiration of blood are examples of disorders that can cause a similar clinical condition in the absence of severe injury to the lungs. Left-sided heart failure, in particular, may be difficult to distinguish from ARDS, especially in cases of severe diastolic dysfunction when the cardiac silhouette appears normal on chest radiograph. Left-sided heart failure can usually be differentiated from ARDS by careful measurement of the pulmonary capillary wedge pressure using a balloon flotation catheter; however, cardiac pulmonary edema and ARDS frequently coexist.[2–4] When ARDS is suspected in a patient with an elevated pulmonary capillary wedge pressure ($>$18 to 20 mm Hg), the diagnosis can be made with confidence only if lung infiltrates fail to improve 24 to 48 hours after the wedge pressure has been restored to normal.

Damage to the lungs must be acute in onset. ARDS typically progresses to respiratory failure within 6 to 48 hours after initial injury to the lungs[5, 6] (Fig. 73–1). Bleomycin toxicity and disseminated tuberculosis are examples of disorders that often progress to respiratory failure during weeks rather than days. Such instances of subacute lung injury should not be included in the category of ARDS.

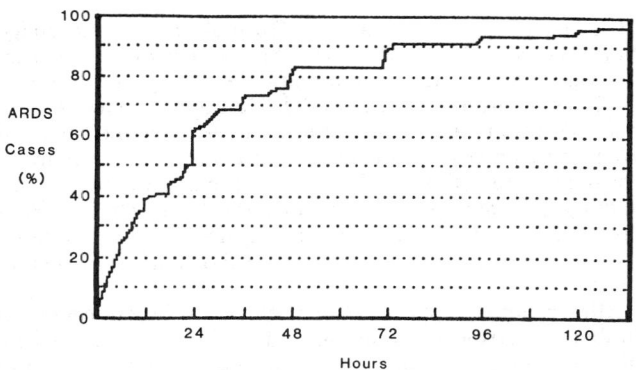

Figure 73–1. Time to onset of ARDS after a predisposition was identified in 83 patients followed prospectively. (Reproduced, with permission, from Fowler AA, Hamman RF, Good JT, et al, Adult respiratory distress syndrome: Risk with common predispositions. Ann Intern Med. 1983; 98:593–597.)

Pulmonary infiltrates are not necessarily diffuse in ARDS; however, they must be extensive and bilateral, or widespread in the remaining lung after pneumonectomy. Excluded by this criterion are focal conditions that can cause respiratory failure, such as lobar pneumonia and unilateral pulmonary edema after evacuation of a pneumothorax.

Disturbances in gas exchange and pulmonary mechanics must be severe. No cutoff criteria have been universally accepted for the severity of the physiologic disturbances in ARDS. However, the term is generally reserved for episodes of acute lung injury that necessitate mechanical ventilation and administration of oxygen at a concentration exceeding 50%. Murray and colleagues proposed an acute lung injury scoring system that may prove useful in estimating the severity of ARDS.[7]

ARDS is not limited to adults. The first published description of the syndrome was titled "Acute respiratory distress in adults" to distinguish this condition from respiratory distress syndrome of premature neonates.[1] However, ARDS is now known to occur in people of all ages, including mature newborns.[8, 9]

In the past, many authors equated the clinical disorder ARDS with the pathologic entity permeability pulmonary edema. These two terms should not be used interchangeably. Although some degree of permeability edema is invariably present at the onset of ARDS, other important structural abnormalities of the lung typically emerge as ARDS evolves. Indeed, the permeability of the pulmonary vascular bed may return to normal in the advanced stages of ARDS as fibrosis and cyst-like spaces progressively dominate the architecture of the lungs.[10] Moreover, many episodes of permeability pulmonary edema never result in the severe physiologic impairment that is required for the designation ARDS.

Although ARDS is frequently accompanied by acute injury to other organs, this condition should not be viewed exclusively as the pulmonary manifestation of the multiple organ system failure syndrome. ARDS occurs without concomitant failure of other organs in such diverse conditions as aspiration of gastric contents, *Pneumocystis carinii* pneumonia, and massive air embolism.

CAUSES AND ASSOCIATED DISORDERS

Like the terms interstitial nephritis and acute hepatitis, the term ARDS designates a category of organ dysfunction that encompasses many distinct disorders. Almost since the first descriptions of the syndrome, some physicians argued against the lumping together of diverse conditions that differ markedly in pathogenesis and prognosis.[11–13] These experts recommended substitution of a specific etiologic diagnosis whenever possible so as not to obscure important differences among the many causes of acute lung injury. However, clinicians have found that identification of a specific cause is impossible in many instances, whereas in other situations, the lung injury appears multifactorial in origin. For this reason, and because the principles of supportive therapy tend to be similar regardless of the cause, the term ARDS continues to be widely used in clinical practice.

Nevertheless, physicians should not be content with a diagnosis of ARDS. Pursuit of a specific cause or predisposition is appropriate in every instance, for many of the conditions that precipitate ARDS can be treated, and other disorders can be prevented from recurring if a specific predisposition is identified. Moreover, the prognosis for recovery from ARDS varies considerably according to the cause.[6]

To date, more than 50 causes of ARDS have been identified.[14, 15] Additional causes continue to emerge as adverse pulmonary reactions to new therapies are discovered. Many of the known causes occur uncommonly and are readily apparent from the history. Dramatic examples include attempted suicide by hanging, imperfect preservation of a transplanted lung, inhalation of chlorine gas, and measles pneumonia. Other causes may be exceedingly difficult to identify with certainty, such as rare drug reactions and occult aspiration.

Epidemiologic studies have shown that most episodes of ARDS encountered in U.S. hospitals are associated with a few common causes or predisposing conditions, singly or in combination[16, 17] (Table 73–1). Septic syndrome appears to be the single most important cause of ARDS in hospitalized patients.[18–21] In fact, sepsis is so commonly implicated in ARDS that this cause should be considered first in any patient with otherwise unexplained ARDS in association with a new fever, hypotension, or a clinical predisposition to serious infection. ARDS is classically attributed to sepsis with gram-negative bacteria;[22] however, infections with gram-positive organisms and fungi can also precipitate the syndrome.[20] In critically ill patients, the source of sepsis is often difficult to identify. Postmortem studies suggest that the origin of sepsis-induced ARDS is likely to be the abdomen if the site of infection escapes detection during life.[2, 23] Experimental observations suggest that severely ill or injured patients can have sepsis-induced ARDS from the gut even in the absence of focal infection.[24, 25] Malnutrition and prolonged catabolism promote translocation of bacteria or endotoxin directly from the lumen of the intestine into the systemic circulation by impairing the barrier function of the gut mucosa and the phagocytic function of hepatic Kupffer's cells.[24]

Infectious pneumonia may be the most common cause of

TABLE 73–1

COMMONLY ASSOCIATED WITH ONSET OF ADULT RESPIRATORY DISTRESS SYNDROME

Septic syndrome
Aspiration of gastric contents
Bilateral pneumonia
Bilateral lung contusion
Near-drowning
Multiple fractures
Extensive surface burns
Massive drug overdose
Massive blood transfusion

TABLE 73–2

IMPORTANT UNUSUAL CAUSES OF ADULT RESPIRATORY DISTRESS SYNDROME IN HOSPITALIZED PATIENTS

> Leukoagglutinin transfusion reaction
> Protamine
> Opiates
> Radiologic contrast media
> Neurogenic pulmonary edema
> Venous air embolism
> Diffuse alveolar hemorrhage
> Relief of upper airway obstruction
> Tracheoesophageal fistula

ARDS in patients with ARDS that develops outside of the hospital.[17] Nosocomial pneumonias frequently cause ARDS as well. Some infecting organisms, such as *Streptococcus pneumoniae, Mycoplasma pneumoniae,* legionella, and influenza virus, can cause ARDS by spreading rapidly throughout both lungs. Other pulmonary infections seem to initiate ARDS while remaining localized by precipitating a diffuse pulmonary inflammatory response that is analogous to the lung injury caused by sepsis originating outside of the thorax.

Aspiration of gastric contents is another common cause of ARDS.[17, 26] Approximately one third of hospitalized patients who experience a clinically recognized episode of gastric aspiration subsequently have the syndrome.[5, 6] In the original description of massive gastric aspiration, Mendelson suggested that a pH of less than 2.5 is necessary to cause severe lung injury.[27] Animal studies have shown that aspiration of nonacidic stomach contents can also cause widespread damage to the lungs, suggesting that gastric enzymes and small food particles also contribute to the lung injury.[28]

Severe trauma and surface burns are frequently associated with the development of ARDS.[29] Several mechanisms can contribute to acute lung injury in this setting. Lung contusion is an important cause of ARDS that develops within 24 hours after blunt injury to the chest. Fat embolism sometimes causes ARDS in patients with long bone fractures.[30] This complication characteristically appears 12 to 48 hours after the injury but may be less common in the United States than it was in the past now that trauma victims are routinely and effectively immobilized before transport to the hospital. Septic syndrome is probably the most common cause of ARDS that develops several days or more after severe trauma or burn. Some investigators suggested that a systemic syndrome closely resembling sepsis can be precipitated by extensive injury to soft tissues after trauma, burn, or prolonged hypotension even in the absence of infection.[29]

Several unusual causes of ARDS deserve attention because they are difficult to identify unless specifically considered (Table 73–2). Leukoagglutinin reactions occasionally cause severe acute lung injury during or immediately after transfusion of a blood product.[31, 32] The blood bank can confirm this diagnosis by testing a sample of the transfused plasma for antibodies directed against white blood cells from the recipient. When ARDS develops immediately after cardiopulmonary bypass or cardiac catheterization, an idiosyncratic reaction to protamine may be the precipitating event.[33, 34] Radiologic contrast media and high therapeutic doses of opiates[35] also occasionally cause ARDS in susceptible individuals.[36]

Neurogenic pulmonary edema is frequently overlooked as a cause of acute respiratory distress in hospitalized patients, especially when the neurologic event is an intracerebral bleed or a seizure.[37] Venous air embolism can occasionally cause full-blown ARDS: outside of the operating room, the most common portal of entry for the air is a central venous catheter left open to the air.[38] Diffuse alveolar hemorrhage should be considered whenever ARDS develops in association with a large, otherwise unexplained drop in the hemoglobin concentration of the blood. Hemoptysis may be minimal or absent before intubation. Alveolar hemorrhage is emerging as a common cause of ARDS after bone marrow transplantation. The mechanism is thought to involve circulating inflammatory cells because the hemorrhage generally occurs during recovery of the marrow and because corticosteroids appear to reduce the mortality of this complication.[39]

After relief of upper airway obstruction by endotracheal intubation or tracheostomy, some individuals have permeability pulmonary edema that is sufficiently severe to require mechanical ventilation. This peculiar reaction appears to be more common in children and young adults.[40] Sometimes, the unexpected development of ARDS is the only indication that an intubated patient has a tracheoesophageal fistula. This dreaded complication of intubation usually necessitates surgical repair.

The cause of ARDS can often be determined by careful review of the events preceding the onset of lung injury. Because ARDS generally appears within 1 or 2 days after the precipitating event, the search can be narrowed considerably. If pneumonia or alveolar hemorrhage is suspected, bronchoalveolar lavage may confirm the diagnosis by identifying the infecting organism or by recovering hemosiderin-laden macrophages that are characteristic of bleeding in the distal air spaces. Lung lavage is sometimes helpful in diagnosing gastric aspiration if vegetable matter or skeletal muscle is found in the fluid. Open lung biopsy can be performed with acceptable morbidity, even on patients who require high concentrations of inspired oxygen and positive end-expiratory pressure (PEEP). However, the findings are usually nonspecific, unless respiratory failure is caused by pneumonia or by widespread malignancy.

ARDS frequently develops in a setting of catastrophic acute illness or injury such that a specific precipitating event for the lung injury cannot be identified with certainty. In such instances, presumptive treatment of sepsis is often justified.

PATHOPHYSIOLOGY

ARDS represents a final common pathway that leads to a form of acute respiratory failure characterized by several distinctive physiologic disturbances. After the lung injury has advanced to the stage necessitating mechanical ventilation, all of these abnormalities are present, to varying degrees of severity, regardless of the precipitating cause. Most of the physiologic disturbances in ARDS are readily identifiable at the bedside as outlined later.

Hypoxemia

Hypoxemia is characteristically severe in ARDS: some patients die of hypoxemia despite optimal supportive therapy. Studies using the multiple inert gas technique have shown that the alveolar-arterial difference in partial pressure of oxygen is widened in ARDS, primarily because blood is shunted from right to left through nonventilated lung units.[41, 42] Shunting is thought to result from perfusion of atelectatic or fluid-filled alveoli and is often most severe in the first several days after onset of ARDS.[43] Lung regions that have low ventilation/perfusion ratios are sometimes present as well, but their contribution to hypoxemia in most patients with ARDS appears to be minimal.[44] In contrast, the hypoxemia observed in most chronic lung disorders is caused primarily by mismatching of ventilation and perfusion.[44]

The fact that hypoxemia is caused primarily by intrapulmonary shunting in ARDS has several important implications for the supportive therapy of patients with this disorder. Arterial hypoxemia associated with a moderate-to-large shunt responds poorly to high concentrations of inspired oxygen but often improves after addition of PEEP. Shunt-associated hypoxemia can also be improved by changing the position of the patient at frequent intervals. This occurs because atelectasis and alveolar edema tend to be worse in the dependent portions of the lung where blood flow is augmented by gravity.[45, 46] Rolling the patient to a new position increases blood flow to aerated portions of the lung and reduces the shunt fraction, at least until atelectasis and edema redistribute to the new dependent regions. Intrapulmonary shunting also gives rise to a complex dependency of PaO_2 on cardiac output and central venous Po_2. Although the effects on shunt fraction and PaO_2 are difficult to predict in individual patients, increases in cardiac output and venous Po_2 generally tend to improve systemic oxygen delivery in ARDS.[44]

Accurate measurement of the shunt fraction requires simultaneous measurement of the arterial and venous Po_2.[47] If a pulmonary arterial catheter is not in place for sampling of central venous blood, shunt can be estimated by measurement of the alveolar-arterial difference while the patient breathes 100% oxygen. Assuming a normal cardiac output, the shunt fraction is approximately equal to alveolar-arterial difference in partial pressure of oxygen divided by 20 at a fraction of inspired oxygen of 1.[48] A PaO_2 of 50 torr while the patient is receiving 100% oxygen corresponds to a shunt of approximately 50% in a patient who has a normal cardiac output. Shunt fractions larger than 50% are usually not compatible with survival for longer than a few minutes.

Increased Physiologic Dead Space

As ARDS evolves, the physiologic dead space often increases while hypoxemia remains stable or becomes less severe.[43] Presumably, the dead space abnormality worsens during the remodeling of acutely injured lung as ventilation is restored to gas-exchanging units that are poorly perfused because of progressive occlusion or obliteration of the pulmonary capillary bed.[10] The dead space–to–tidal volume ratio frequently exceeds 0.6 in ARDS and sometimes approaches 0.9 (the normal dead space fraction is 0.15 to 0.35, depending on the pattern of breathing).

If the rate of production of carbon dioxide remains constant, changes in the physiologic dead space can be followed at the bedside by observing the minute ventilation required to sustain a normal $Paco_2$. Patients with ARDS sometimes require a minute ventilation greater than 30 L/min to maintain a $Paco_2$ of 40 torr (normally, 6 to 8 L/min is required). A large increase in the dead space fraction can cause unavoidable hypercapnia and may delay weaning from mechanical ventilation in patients who are unable to sustain an elevated minute ventilation during spontaneous breathing.

Decreased Pulmonary Compliance

The compliance of the lungs is invariably reduced in ARDS. Decreased compliance is the primary reason that high driving pressures are required to inflate the lungs.[47] The reduction in compliance is usually attributed to an increase in the elastance of lung tissue that is diffusely hypercellular and edematous. An alternative explanation has emerged. Computed tomographic (CT) scans and studies

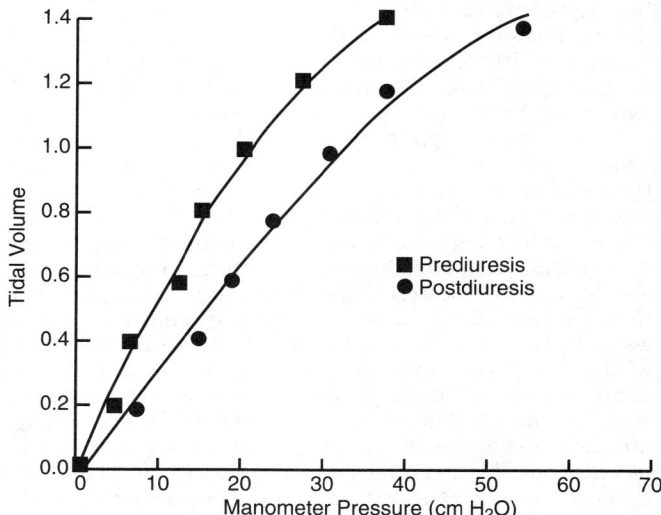

Figure 73–2. Plateau airway pressures, plotted as a function of inspired tidal volume, for a patient with ARDS before and after diuresis. Static compliance of the thorax is the slope of the curve at a given tidal volume (tidal volume/[plateau pressure − PEEP]). The compliance curve moved to the left after diuresis, indicating an improvement in chest compliance.

of gas exchange using multiple inert gases have shown that lung injury is distributed heterogeneously in many patients with ARDS.[41, 45, 46] Areas of dense consolidation or atelectasis are interspersed with regions that remain nearly normal in structure and function. If the consolidated areas do not participate in ventilation, lung expansion during inhalation may result primarily from ventilation of aerated units that retain near-normal elastance. According to this theory, the overall compliance of the lungs is reduced in ARDS, not so much because the injured lung is more elastic, but because the volume of lung available for ventilation is markedly reduced.[49]

If the patient makes no effort to breathe during the respiratory cycle, the static compliance of the thorax (lungs, chest wall, and diaphragm) can be estimated rapidly at the bedside. The ventilator is set to provide an end-inspiratory pause of 0.3 to 0.5 second; then the plateau airway pressure is measured during each inspiratory pause as successive breaths are delivered at increasing tidal volumes in 100- or 200-mL increments (Fig. 73–2). With this information, a static pressure-volume curve can be generated by plotting tidal volume against the corresponding change in airway pressure (end-inspiratory plateau pressure − PEEP).[48, 50] The static compliance of the thorax is the slope of the curve (tidal volume/[plateau pressure − PEEP]) at a designated tidal volume. The static compliance of the healthy thorax generally exceeds 100 mL/cm H_2O of inflating pressure at a tidal volume of 8 mL/kg. Compliance often falls as low as 10 to 20 mL/cm H_2O in severe ARDS. Serial measurements of static thoracic compliance can be helpful in determining the clinical course of ARDS and in assessing response to therapeutic interventions such as diuresis[50] (see Fig. 73–2).

Increased Airway Resistance

Because of difficulties inherent in measuring resistance of the airways during mechanically assisted ventilation, considerably less is known about the effects of ARDS on airway function than on other mechanical properties of the lungs. That is unfortunate because airway resistance may affect the supportive therapy of ARDS in at least three ways: (1) as the inspiratory resistance of the airways is increased, higher driving pressures are needed to inflate the lungs; (2) when expiratory airway resistance is increased, the time required for passive exhalation is prolonged with the effect that end-expiratory air trapping (auto-PEEP, or intrinsic PEEP) can occur at higher respiratory rates; and (3) airway resistance increases the work of breathing and may delay weaning from mechanical ventilation.

Many studies have shown that endotracheal tubes add considerable resistance to airflow in patients who require mechanical ventilation. Several research techniques are available to measure the resistance of the native airways beyond the endotracheal tube during mechanical ventilation.[46] Studies with these techniques generally show that the resistance of the bronchial tree is increased in ARDS.[31, 48] However, interpretation of airway resistance measurements during acute respiratory failure remains problematic. If the lungs are functionally small in ARDS because of widespread, patchy consolidation, the airflow resistance of the entire bronchial tree is expected to increase in proportion to the number of airways that do not contribute to ventilation, even if the caliber of the functioning airways remains unchanged.[49] Whether small or medium-sized airways are significantly narrowed in ARDS remains unknown. Also unknown is the extent to which reversible bronchospasm may be present in this condition.

Although airway resistance is difficult to measure directly in patients undergoing mechanical ventilation, clinicians can obtain a useful index of inspiratory airway resistance by observing the difference between the peak dynamic pressure at end inspiration and the plateau pressure measured during an end-inspiratory pause. Provided that the tidal volume and inspiratory flow rate remain constant between measurements, changes in this pressure difference reflect changes in the total inspiratory resistance of the airways.[48, 50] A rough indication of expiratory airway resistance can be obtained by noting the duration of a passive expiration from a high lung volume.

Pulmonary Hypertension

In patients with ARDS, right-sided heart catheterization often discloses a difference of 5 to 10 cm H_2O or more between the pulmonary arterial diastolic pressure and the pulmonary capillary wedge pressure, indicating the presence of pulmonary hypertension. Early after the onset of lung injury, pulmonary hypertension is thought to be caused by vasoconstriction, platelet thrombosis, and perivascular edema. After several weeks, remodeling of damaged pulmonary arterioles and extensive obliteration of the alveolar capillary bed contribute to the increase in pulmonary vascular resistance as well.[10] Although pulmonary hypertension is usually mild or moderate in severity, right-sided heart failure sometimes occurs in patients with severe ARDS.[51]

Dependence of Oxygen Uptake on Oxygen Supply

In 1973, Powers and coworkers reported that systemic oxygen uptake is dependent on oxygen delivery in patients with ARDS, even at normal or near-normal rates of oxygen delivery.[51a] Their results generated considerable interest because studies using healthy animals have consistently shown that oxygen uptake remains virtually independent of oxygen delivery until the delivery rate falls below a threshold value that is considerably lower than the normal range.[52] The discrepancy between healthy laboratory animals and patients with ARDS raised the possibility that ARDS causes or is associated with a pathologic defect in oxygen extraction throughout the body.

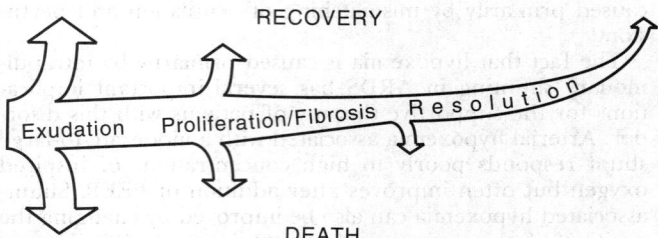

Figure 73–3. ARDS tends to evolve along a similar pathway regardless of cause, although many patients leave this path along the way to recover or to die.

Several subsequent studies also found a linear relationship between oxygen uptake and oxygen delivery in patients with ARDS.[52a, 52b] Other published reports extended this finding to patients with a variety of acute and chronic cardiopulmonary disorders, including sepsis, congestive heart failure, pulmonary hypertension, and chronic obstructive pulmonary disease.[53] Indeed, the possibility has been raised that supply dependency of oxygen uptake may represent normal physiologic behavior in humans and not a manifestation of pathologic oxygen extraction as previously suggested.[52, 53] Other evidence supports a view, long held by some physiologists, that supply dependency of oxygen uptake is an artifact of the techniques usually used to measure oxygen delivery in critically ill patients.[32, 54] This important issue is unlikely to be resolved until methodological differences are reconciled and more data become available on the relationship between oxygen uptake and delivery in healthy humans at rest.

CLINICAL COURSE: RADIOGRAPHIC-PATHOLOGIC CORRELATION

Like most organs, the lung manifests a limited repertoire of responses to acute injury. Regardless of the inciting factors, ARDS tends to evolve, during days or weeks, along a similar pathway that is marked by characteristic changes on chest radiographs and pathologic specimens. Not all patients travel the entire pathway—many deviate along the way to recover or to die; however, the main route is well recognized and stereotypic (Fig. 73–3).

In those patients who have the full-blown syndrome, the radiographic and pathologic features of ARDS typically evolve through three distinct but overlapping phases. The exudative phase lasts for several days and is characterized by accumulation of protein-rich edema fluid and widespread infiltration of inflammatory cells. Survivors of the original insult often enter a second, protracted phase of proliferation and fibrosis, which is distinguished by lung cell replication and formation of new connective tissue. If the functional integrity of the lungs is not destroyed during the second phase, and if the patient does not die of sepsis or some other complication, then ARDS finally resolves during a remarkable third phase of repair and recovery.

Exudative Phase

ARDS invariably begins with a physically or chemically mediated injury to the alveolar capillary membranes of the lungs. This injury gives rise to the increased-permeability pulmonary edema and acute inflammatory changes that characterize the exudative phase of the syndrome. Considering the devastating consequences of the injury, the initial anatomic damage to the lungs is often surprisingly subtle. Indeed, the earliest structural abnormalities can be seen only

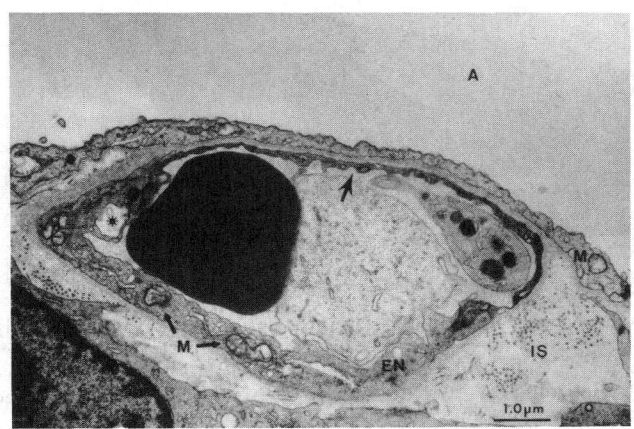

Figure 73–4. Exudative phase of ARDS. Electron micrograph showing a portion of an alveolar wall. The endothelium (EN), although damaged, appears intact. → = necrotic endothelial cell; * = abnormal cytoplasmic vacuole; IS = edematous interstitial space; A = alveolar space; M = mitochondria. (From Fisher AB: Pulmonary oxygen toxicity. In: Fishman AP [ed]: Pulmonary Diseases and Disorders. 2nd ed. New York, McGraw-Hill, p 2334, 1988. Reproduced with permission of McGraw-Hill, Inc.)

with the aid of an electron microscope. At the onset of edema formation, when the alveolar capillary membranes still appear intact by light microscopy, ultrastructural studies show cytologic evidence of widespread injury to endothelial and epithelial cells. Typical changes include focal swelling of the cytoplasm, abnormally large cytoplasmic vacuoles, disrupted mitochondria, and pyknosis of the nuclei.[55–57] Even in severely damaged areas, large discontinuities are rarely seen in the endothelial surface, suggesting that viable endothelial cells spread out quickly to close the gaps left behind when neighboring cells necrose and slough away (Fig. 73–4). In contrast, as the initial injury progresses, the epithelial surface of the alveolar capillary membrane often appears severely disrupted (Fig. 73–5). Fragmentation and sloughing of necrotic type 1 epithelial cells uncover large areas of denuded basement membrane. Gaps in the epithelial surface are closed, only after several days, by proliferation of type 2 epithelial cells.[58]

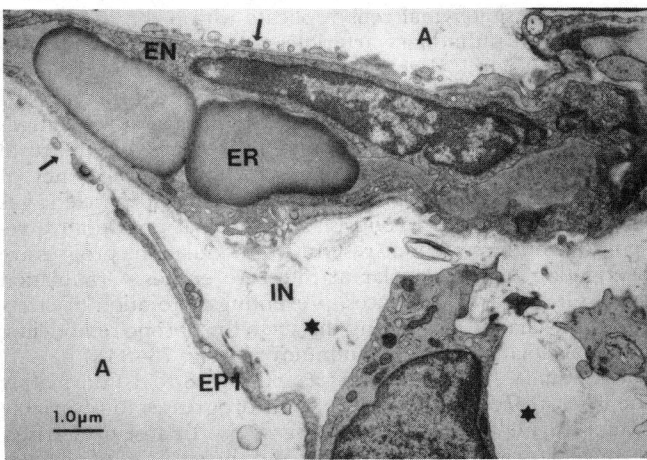

Figure 73–5. Exudative phase of ARDS. Electron micrograph showing fragmentation (→) of epithelial cells (EPI) and accumulation of edema fluid (*) within the interstitial spaces (IN) of an alveolar wall. EN = endothelial cell; ER = erythrocytes within a capillary lumen; A = alveolar space.

Damage to the endothelial and epithelial surfaces of the alveolar walls promotes leakage of protein-rich edema fluid into the extravascular spaces of the lungs.[59] The interstitial spaces of the alveolar walls are widened by edema, fibrin, and extravasated red blood cells. Much more fluid swells the connective tissue spaces surrounding the bronchovascular bundles and along the intralobular septa. Many of the alveoli and some of the alveolar ducts fill with edema fluid, whereas others are collapsed by external compression or by alterations in surface tension (Fig. 73–6).

A characteristic feature of the early injury is the formation of hyaline membranes focally along the surfaces of the distal air spaces. These coarse bands of eosinophilic material are composed of plasma proteins and cellular debris trapped within a fibrin mesh. The presence of hyaline membranes distinguishes the exudative edema of early diffuse alveolar damage from the protein-poor edema fluid of hemodynamic edema.

Within hours after the initial insult, resident macrophages release a host of peptide mediators known as cytokines.[60] Some of these cytokines, notably tumor necrosis factor, act directly on pneumocytes to initiate or amplify the inflammatory response to acute lung injury. Other macrophage-derived cytokines function as powerful chemoattractants for neutrophils and blood-borne mononuclear cells. Partly in response to release of these chemoattractants, circulating leukocytes adhere to the endothelium of the alveolar capillaries and migrate across the damaged endothelium. By 24 to 48 hours after the onset of lung injury, neutrophils are seen histologically throughout the interstitial and alveolar spaces and can be recovered from the distal airways by bronchoalveolar lavage.[38, 61] Neutrophils are thought to play a major role in early progression of acute lung injury by releasing reactive metabolites of oxygen and several potent proteases that damage structural components of the lung directly.[62]

The coagulation system is also activated during the exudative phase of ARDS. Microthrombi form throughout the pulmonary microcirculation, interfering with gas exchange and contributing to the thrombocytopenia that is often observed during this phase. Platelet-fibrin thrombi are most prevalent in the capillaries and the smaller arterioles, whereas laminated fibrin clots tend to form in the preacinar and interacinar arterioles.[63] Still larger arteries are occluded by thrombi that are visible in pathologic specimens without the aid of a microscope. These thrombi can be seen angiographically using a bedside balloon occlusion technique as intraluminal filling defects in segmental and subsegmental arteries.[64] The macrothrombi can cause hemorrhagic infarcts that are most prominent beneath the visceral surface where collateral circulation is normally limited.[65]

At the onset of ARDS, radiographic manifestations of acute lung injury usually lag behind the pathologic changes. Even after the development of respiratory distress and hypoxemia, chest radiographic abnormalities are often absent or easily overlooked.[66] A modest reduction in lung volume may be accompanied by blurring of the bronchovascular margins and by subtle ground-glass infiltrates that are often first seen in retrospect. However, as edema fluid accumulates, alveolar consolidation spreads rapidly throughout both lungs. Air bronchograms are often prominent unless left-sided heart failure or fluid overload accompanies the acute lung injury, in which case edema fluid often fills many of the distal airways.

By 24 to 48 hours, portable chest films typically show dense patchy infiltrates (Fig. 73–7) or homogeneous consolidation throughout both lungs. This latter pattern is some-

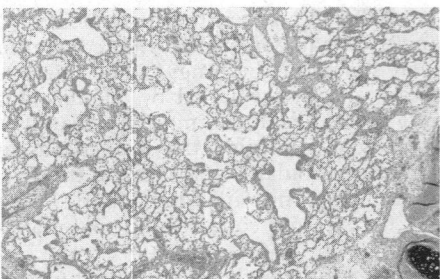 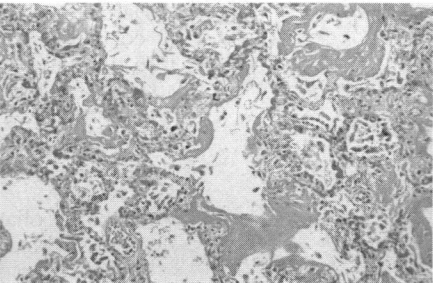 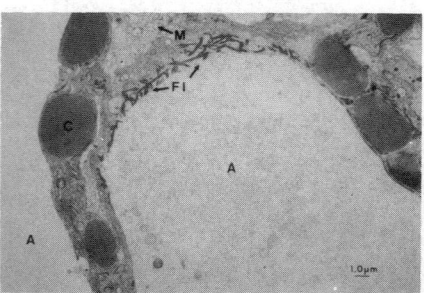

Figure 73–6. Exudative phase of ARDS. *A.* Many alveoli are filled with a protein-rich exudate containing erythrocytes; however, the architecture of the alveolar membranes and the alveolar ducts is preserved. Hyaline membranes line one of the alveolar ducts. *B.* Higher-power view showing increased cellularity of alveolar walls and several hyaline membranes. *C.* Electron micrograph of an alveolar wall separating two alveolar spaces (A). One of the alveolar spaces is flooded with protein-rich edema fluid. Part of the surface of this alveolar space is covered by a hyaline membrane containing strands of fibrin (FI). C = capillary lumen containing sludged erythrocytes; M = injured mitochondria.

times referred to as a bilateral whiteout. Mechanical ventilation with PEEP frequently reduces the density of the radiographic infiltrates at this stage of the injury by re-expanding atelectatic air spaces and by driving some of the edema fluid out of the alveoli into adjacent interstitial spaces.[67, 68] This effect can lead to the false impression that the lung injury has improved.

CT scans of the chest obtained shortly after the development of ARDS show that the early changes are often distributed heterogeneously within the lungs.[45, 46, 49] Patchy areas of consolidation are typically most prominent in the dependent posterobasal segments. The uppermost regions may appear fully aerated on CT cross-sections, even when supine chest films suggest diffuse opacification. The gradient of consolidation often shifts to an inverted pattern within minutes after the patient is rolled from a supine to a prone position, suggesting that gravity plays an important role in determining the distribution of atelectasis and alveolar edema. These findings have helped to explain some of the abnormalities in gas exchange and lung mechanics that characterize the initial phase of ARDS, as described earlier.

Some patients recover quickly and completely after the

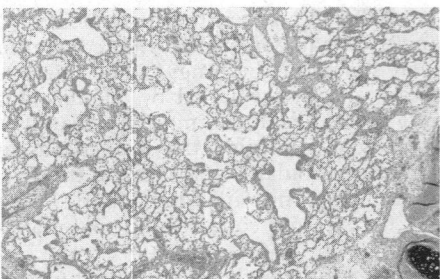

Figure 73–7. Early exudative phase of ARDS. This chest radiograph, obtained immediately before intubation, shows widespread, patchy, bilateral infiltrates.

exudative phase of ARDS. For reasons that remain poorly understood, their lungs never show the progressive inflammatory and proliferative changes that characterize the second phase of the full-blown syndrome. Certain forms of acute lung injury typically cause ARDS with rapid recovery, such as high-altitude pulmonary edema, fat embolism, neurogenic pulmonary edema, and many acute drug reactions. It is possible that these injuries cause minimal necrosis of lung cells compared with other types of injury that are commonly associated with delayed recovery, such as sepsis, aspiration, and certain pneumonias.

Proliferation and Fibrosis

In those patients whose disease progresses to the second phase of ARDS, proliferative changes begin as early as 3 or 4 days after initial injury with spread of type 2 epithelial cells along the alveolar walls. These cuboid cells fill in the gaps along the alveolar epithelial surface left behind by sloughing of necrotic type 1 cells. Subsequent differentiation of the type 2 cells into type 1 cells restores the squamous surface of the damaged alveolar walls. Within the adjacent interstitium, fibroblasts and myofibroblasts proliferate and begin to modify the extracellular connective tissue. Other fibroblasts migrate into the alveolar spaces and proliferate there, forming granulation tissue.[70, 71] The walls of small blood vessels are also involved in the early proliferative changes. Mesenchymal cells replicate within the intima and the media of pulmonary arterioles and deposit new connective tissue there.[72] These proliferative changes narrow the vascular lumina and predispose to intraluminal thrombosis.

If appropriately regulated, the early proliferative changes in ARDS repair the damaged lungs and restore the structural integrity of the alveolar capillary membranes.[73] Patency of airways and alveolar capillaries is restored and efficient gas exchange resumes. In contrast, if the initial proliferative response continues without restorative modulation, progressive obliteration of the alveolar architecture ensues. Granulation tissue fills the alveolar spaces, preventing restoration of effective gas exchange and setting the stage for fibrotic remodeling of the alveolar capillary membranes[71, 74] (Fig. 73–8A).

Pulmonary fibrosis appears as early as 8 to 10 days after the onset of respiratory failure and progresses to a variable extent during the ensuing days or weeks. In advanced cases, the alveolar capillary membranes and the surfaces of alveolar ducts are progressively replaced by dense, irregular bands of fibrous tissue[74] (see Fig. 73–8B). Some alveoli collapse and are obliterated; others join together, forming fewer but larger distal air spaces and dilated alveolar ducts. The intima of small arteries and the walls of some veins and lymphatic

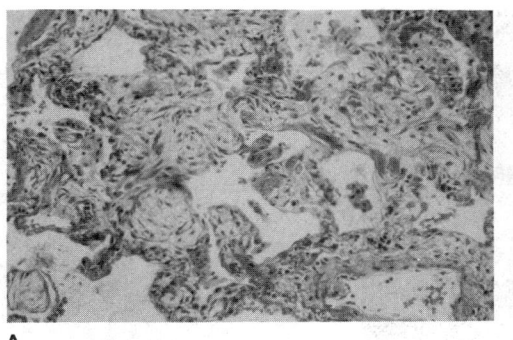 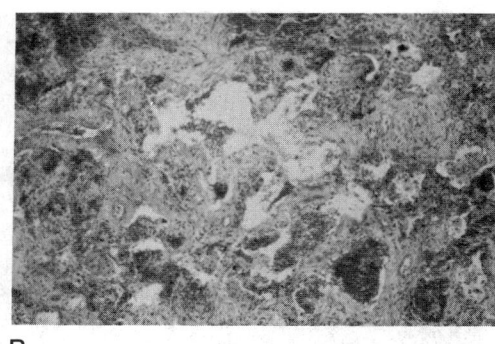

Figure 73–8. Proliferative and fibrotic stage of ARDS. Samples of an open lung biopsy obtained 3 weeks after onset of respiratory failure. *A.* The alveolar architecture is distorted by proliferative changes and fibrosis. Note the whorls of granulation tissue filling some of the air spaces. *B.* Dense bands of fibrous tissue have replaced normal alveolar walls. Some distal air spaces are collapsed; a dilated alveolar duct is also seen.

A   **B**

vessels are also widened and distorted by concentric fibrosis. After 3 or 4 weeks, the most severely damaged areas of the lungs may resemble a sponge: innumerable cystic air spaces and dilated bronchioles are separated by thick walls of hypocellular connective tissue.[10, 72] In other instances, part or all of the lung is consumed by nosocomial bronchopneumonia or infected abscesses that often progress despite the use of appropriate antibiotics.

The radiographic appearance of the lungs changes dramatically during the proliferative and fibrotic phase of ARDS. Confluent alveolar infiltrates become less dense and homogeneous as edema fluid is resorbed and distal air spaces are reopened. Reticular infiltrates emerge in some areas, whereas ground-glass opacities predominate in others.[75] During the second and third weeks, as fibrotic remodeling occurs, the lower lung fields often take on a salt-and-pepper appearance. This stippling effect may represent the radiographic manifestation multiple dilated distal air spaces walled by thickened fibrous lung tissue (Figs. 73–9 and 73–10).

Pulmonary barotrauma is a frequent and important complication of ARDS during the proliferative and fibrotic phase.[66] Driven by positive pressure mechanical ventilation, air leaks from damaged distal airways or ruptured alveoli into the adjacent interstitial spaces. The extra-alveolar air then dissects centrally along bronchovascular sheaths, causing pulmonary interstitial emphysema, or distally to the periphery of the lungs, forming subpleural air cysts. Radiographically, the subpleural air cysts appear as discrete, rounded lucencies that are typically located in the lower lung fields[76] (see Fig. 73–9). Occasionally, a subpleural air cyst grows so big that it can be mistaken for a tension pneumothorax. Pulmonary interstitial emphysema is more difficult to see on chest radiograph: the extra-alveolar air is sometimes recognized as lucent bands surrounding central blood vessels (reverse air bronchograms), or as small, evanescent, rounded lucencies in the perihilar region.[77]

From the bronchovascular sheaths, extra-alveolar air is often driven centrally across the hilum of the lung into the mediastinum.[66] Pneumomediastinum is seen on chest radiographs as a thin radiolucent stripe along the outside edge of the heart and central vessels. Mediastinal air enters the pleural spaces through discontinuities in the parietal pleura, causing pneumothorax. Air can also escape from the chest to the subcutaneous tissues of the neck and trunk or to the retroperitoneal space by dissecting along deep fascial planes. Rarely, air breaks into the peritoneal space and collects under the diaphragm, simulating air from a ruptured abdominal viscus.

Loculated pneumothoraces sometimes occur repeatedly during the advanced phase of proliferation and fibrosis, necessitating two or three chest tubes on each side. Pockets of pleural air often gravitate to anterior or perimediastinal locations, where they are difficult to see on portable chest radiographs—lateral films or CT scans may be required for visualization (Fig. 73–11).

Repair and Recovery

The lung function of many patients who enter the second phase of ARDS never seems to improve beyond a certain plateau. Either these patients are too ill to heal or the gas-exchanging components of their lungs are so extensively destroyed that the healing process cannot restore an adequate blood-gas interface.[73] These patients require mechanical ventilation and high concentrations of inspired oxygen until they die. Other patients do ultimately recover despite extensive fibrosis. The mechanical properties and gas-exchanging function of their lungs return toward normal during a third phase of ARDS that sometimes continues as long as 6 to 12 months after mechanical ventilation is discontinued.[78]

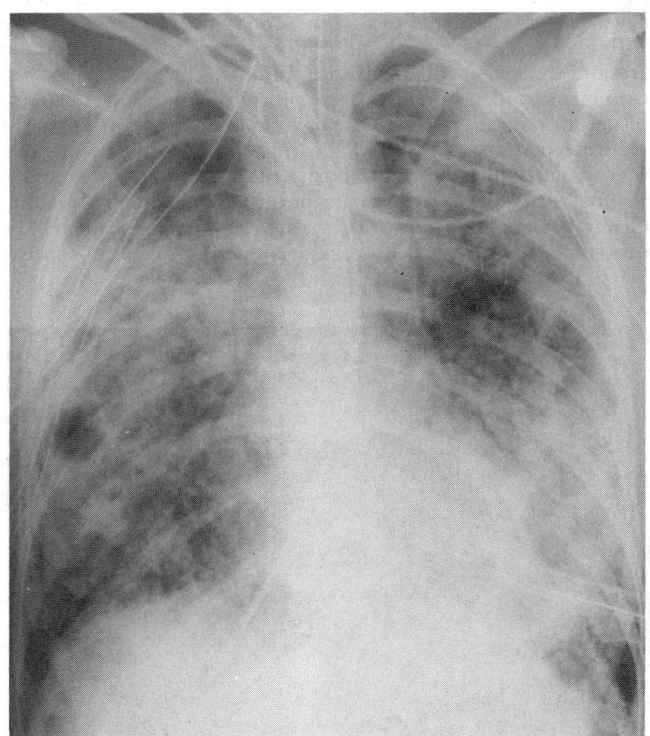

Figure 73–9. Proliferative and fibrotic phase of ARDS. Coarse, reticular infiltrates are seen in some areas; ground-glass opacities predominate in other areas. The right lower lobe contains a salt-and-pepper infiltrate. A small subpleural air cyst is present in the right mid-lung field.

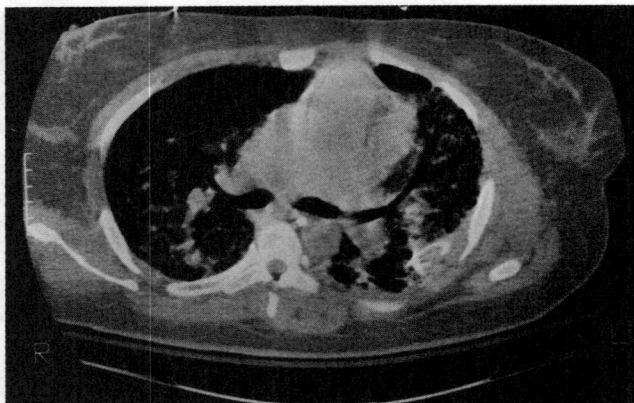

Figure 73–10. Proliferative and fibrotic phase of ARDS. High-resolution CT scan obtained 3 weeks after onset of ARDS, showing cystic air spaces and coarse, reticular infiltrates indicative of fibrosis.

Remarkably little is known about the reparative phase of advanced ARDS because few pathologic specimens are obtained during this time.[58] Serial chest radiographs show progressive clearing of dense reticular infiltrates, suggesting that fibrous tissue is resorbed or rearranged. Months after the onset of ARDS, radiographic residua may be limited to a few linear densities or a shaggy appearance of the heart borders and diaphragm (Fig. 73–12). The radiographic appearance of the lungs may even return to normal.[77]

Up to 75% of patients are left with a mild or moderate impairment in lung function and occasional individuals are permanently disabled by severe chronic lung disease.[78-80] Residual impairment is particularly likely after ARDS associated with viral pneumonia.[78] Pulmonary function studies performed 1 year or longer after recovery from ARDS show a variety of abnormalities in patients who remain dyspneic with exercise. The carbon monoxide diffusing capacity is frequently reduced, primarily because of a decrease in capillary blood volume. In some of these patients, persistence of pulmonary hypertension may be an important cause of residual exercise limitation.[80] Lung volumes are often preserved, although occasional patients retain a moderate-to-severe restrictive pattern on pulmonary function testing. Other patients are left with a surprising degree of airflow obstruction, with or without associated air trapping. Reactiv-

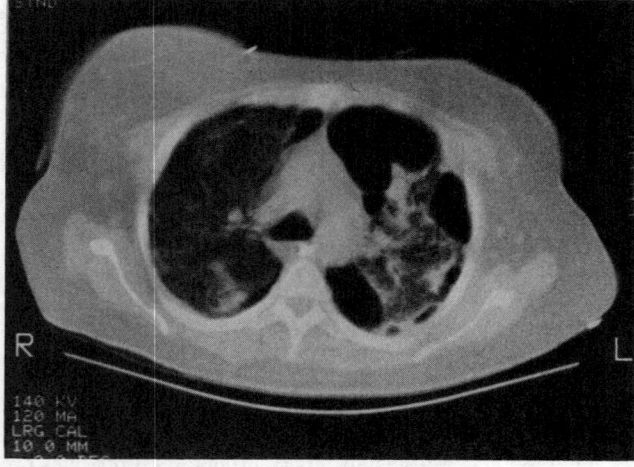

Figure 73–11. Advanced proliferative and fibrotic phase of ARDS. This CT scan shows multiple bilateral loculated pneumothoraces. Portions of the lung tissue appear fibrotic and cystic.

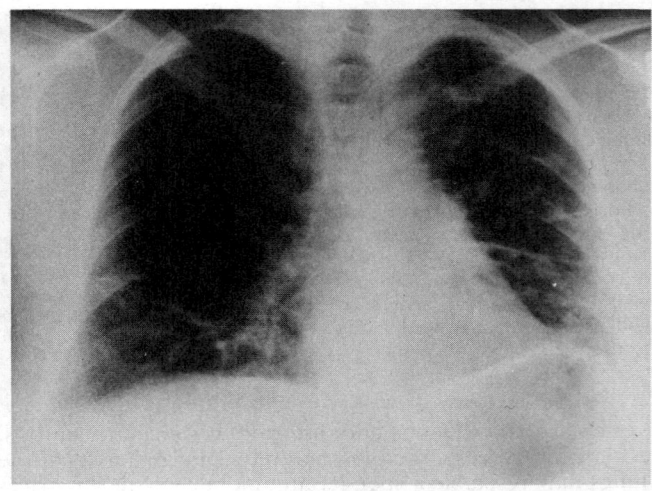

Figure 73–12. Recovery from ARDS. This chest radiograph was obtained 8 months after onset of ARDS. Note the shaggy heart border and the presence of linear densities in both lower lung fields.

ity to methacholine inhalation and reversible bronchospasm are sometimes observed in patients who have no prior history of obstructive airways disease, suggesting that ARDS has triggered or uncovered a form of asthma in these patients.[81]

In contrast to most patients who experience a progressive improvement in exercise tolerance during the first several months of recovery, some individuals become more dyspneic during this time. Failure to improve after ARDS should raise the possibility of tracheal stenosis at the site of the endotracheal tube cuff or the tracheostomy stoma.[78] A flow-volume loop and tracheal tomograms can be useful in screening for this potentially correctable problem; bronchoscopy confirms the diagnosis.

PROGNOSIS

Published survival rates for ARDS vary considerably but average approximately 50%[2, 6, 18, 23, 81-83] (Fig. 73–13). Although useful in emphasizing the devastating impact of ARDS, the overall survival figures for this condition are potentially misleading in other respects. Less than 20% of patients who die with ARDS actually succumb to respiratory failure; most die early as a result of the underlying illness

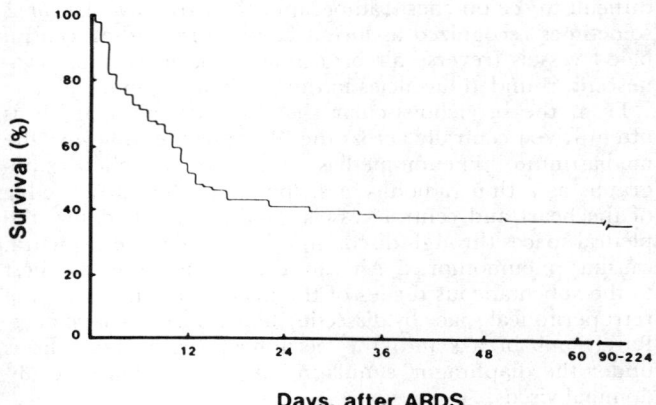

Figure 73–13. Percentage of survival of 88 patients with ARDS followed prospectively for up to 229 days. Sixty-five percent of the patients ultimately died. (From Fowler AA, Hamman RF, Zerbe GO, et al: Adult respiratory distress syndrome: Prognosis after onset. Am Rev Respir Dis 132:472, 1985.)

or injury that precipitated respiratory failure, or later because of sepsis or multiple organ system failure.[2, 84]

Overall survival rates for ARDS are also misleading in that the prognosis for individuals varies dramatically according to precipitating factors and underlying health status. Epidemiologic studies have identified subsets of patients with ARDS who have an excellent prognosis for full recovery on the one hand, or a near-certain likelihood of death on the other. For example, the mortality for conscious patients with ARDS after near-drowning is less than 10%,[85, 86] whereas the mortality for those who have ARDS in association with septic shock generally exceeds 80%.[18, 22] Mortality approaches 100% for individuals who experience ARDS as a complication of severe hepatic dysfunction.[83, 87]

Close examination of subsets that vary in prognosis suggest that the nature and severity of coexisting disorders are more important than the cause of ARDS in determining survival. Analysis of mortality rates in a prospective multicenter trial of methylprednisolone for ARDS[83] illustrates this point. Retrospectively, the authors were able to divide the 99 patients enrolled in this study evenly into two groups according to the presence or absence of four coexisting conditions: liver failure (bilirubin level > 4 mg/dL), renal failure (creatinine level > 4 mg/dL), coma after cardiopulmonary resuscitation, or rapidly fatal malignancy. The mortality for the group of patients who met one or more of those criteria was 95%; mortality for the other group was only 30%. Another study found a strong correlation between the number of organs that fail and the mortality rate for critically ill patients.[84] These observations suggest that a useful estimate of the prognosis for an individual with ARDS can be made only by considering the combined impact of all of the patient's acute and chronic health impairments.

Research under way at the University of Utah suggests that survival may be improved by incorporation of computer-driven treatment protocols in the supportive treatment of patients with severe ARDS. Additional improvements in survival are not likely to be achieved until physicians learn how to prevent multiple-organ injury and systemic infection in patients at risk for critical illness.

References

1. Ashbaugh DG, Bigelow DB, Petty TL, et al: Acute respiratory distress in adults. Lancet 2:319, 1967.
2. Montgomery AB, Stager MA, Carrico J, et al: Causes of mortality in patients with the adult respiratory distress syndrome. Am Rev Respir Dis 132:485, 1985.
3. Goris RJA, Boekhorst TPA, Nuytinck JKS, et al: Multiple organ failure: Generalized autodestructive inflammation? Arch Surg 120:1109, 1985.
4. Zimmerman GA, Morris AH, Cengiz M: Cardiovascular alterations in the acute respiratory distress syndrome. Am J Med 73:25, 1982.
5. Pepe PE, Potkin RT, Reus DH, et al: Clinical predictors of the adult respiratory distress syndrome. Am J Surg 144:124, 1982.
6. Fowler AA, Hamman RF, Good JT, et al: Adult respiratory distress syndrome: Risk with common predispositions. Ann Intern Med 98:593, 1983.
7. Murray JF, Mathay MA, Luce J, et al: An expanded definition of the adult respiratory distress syndrome. Am Rev Respir Dis 138:720, 1988.
8. Faix R, Viscardi RM, DiPietro MA, et al: Adult respiratory distress syndrome in full-term newborns. Pediatrics 83:971, 1989.
9. Royall JA, Levin DL: Adult respiratory distress syndrome in pediatric patients. I. Clinical aspects, pathophysiology, pathology, and mechanisms of lung injury. J Pediatr 112:169, 1988.
10. Tomashefski JF: Pulmonary pathology of the adult respiratory distress syndrome. Clin Chest Med 11:593, 1990.
11. Effros RM, Mason GR: An end to ARDS. Chest 89:162, 1986.
12. Fishman AP: Shock lung: A distinctive nonentity. Circulation 47:921, 1973.
13. Murray JF: The adult respiratory distress syndrome (may it rest in peace). Am Rev Respir Dis 111:716, 1975.
14. Hansen-Flaschen JH, Fishman AP: Adult respiratory distress syndrome: Clinical features and pathogenesis. In: Fishman AP (ed): Pulmonary Diseases and Disorders. 2nd ed. New York, McGraw-Hill, p 2201, 1988.
15. Hudson LD: Causes of the adult respiratory distress syndrome: Clinical recognition. Clin Chest Med 3:195, 1982.
16. Pepe PE, Fowler AA, Hamman RF, et al: Adult respiratory distress syndrome: Risk with common predispositions. Ann Intern Med 99:293, 1983.
17. Baumann WR, Jung RC, Koss M, et al: Incidence and mortality of adult respiratory distress syndrome: A prospective analysis from a large metropolitan hospital. Crit Care Med 14:1, 1986.
18. Fein AM, Lippmann M, Holtzman H, et al: The risk factors, incidence and prognosis of ARDS following septicemia. Chest 83:40, 1983.
19. Weinberg PF, Matthay MA, Webster RO, et al: Biologically active products of complement and acute lung injury in patients with sepsis syndrome. Am Rev Respir Dis 130:791, 1984.
20. Niederman MS, Fein AM: Sepsis syndrome, the adult respiratory distress syndrome and nosocomial pneumonia. Clin Chest Med 11:633, 1990.
21. Bone RC, Fisher CJ, Clemmer TP, et al: A controlled clinical trial of high-dose methylprednisolone in the treatment of severe sepsis and septic shock. N Engl J Med 317:653, 1987.
22. Kaplan RL, Sahn SA, Petty TL: Incidence and outcome of the respiratory distress syndrome in gram-negative sepsis. Arch Intern Med 139:867, 1979.
23. Bell RC, Coalson J, Smith JD, et al: Multiple organ failure and infection in adult respiratory distress syndrome. Ann Intern Med 99:293, 1983.
24. Runcie C, Ramsay G: Intraabdominal infection: Pulmonary failure. World J Surg 14:196, 1990.
25. Deitch EA, Ma WJ, Ma L, et al: Protein malnutrition predisposes to inflammatory-induced gut-origin septic states. Ann Surg 211:560, 1990.
26. Bynum LJ, Pierce AK: Pulmonary aspiration of gastric contents. Am Rev Respir Dis 114:1129, 1976.
27. Mendelson CL: The aspiration of stomach contents into the lungs during obstetric anesthesia. Am J Obstet Gynecol 52:191, 1946.
28. Wynne JW: Aspiration pneumonitis: Correlation of experimental models with clinical disease. Clin Chest Med 3:25, 1982.
29. Demling RH: Current concepts on the adult respiratory distress syndrome. Circ Shock 30:297, 1990.
30. Schonfeld SA, Ploysongsang Y, DiLisio R, et al: Fat embolism prophylaxis with corticosteroids. Ann Intern Med 99:438, 1983.
31. Wright PE, Bernard GR: The role of airflow resistance in patients with the adult respiratory distress syndrome. Am Rev Respir Dis 139:1169, 1989.
32. Vermeij CG, Feenstra BWA, Adrichem WJ, et al: Independent oxygen uptake and oxygen delivery in septic and postoperative patients. Chest 99:1438, 1991.
33. Olinger GN, Becker RM, Bonchek LI: Noncardiogenic pulmonary edema and peripheral vascular collapse following cardiopulmonary bypass: Rare protamine reaction? Ann Thorac Surg 29:20, 1980.
34. Maggart M, Stewart S: The mechanisms and management of noncardiogenic pulmonary edema following cardiopulmonary bypass. Ann Thorac Surg 43:231, 1987.
35. Lusk JA, Maloley PA: Morphine-induced pulmonary edema. Am J Med 84:367, 1988.
36. Borish L, Matloff SM, Findlay SR: Radiologic contrast media–induced noncardiogenic pulmonary edema: Case report and review of the literature. J Allergy Clin Immunol 74:104, 1984.
37. Colice GL, Matthay MA, Bass E, et al: Neurogenic pulmonary edema. Am Rev Respir Dis 130:941, 1984.
38. Clark MC, Flick MR: Permeability pulmonary edema caused by venous air embolism. Am Rev Respir Dis 129:633, 1984.
39. Metcalf J, Armitage J, Arneson M, et al: The effect of glucocorticoids on survival and development of subsequent opportunistic infections in bone marrow transplant patients with diffuse alveolar hemorrhage. Am Rev Respir Dis 143:A474, 1991.
40. Sofer S, Bar-Ziv J, Scharf SM: Pulmonary edema following relief of upper airway obstruction. Chest 86:401, 1984.
41. Dantzger DR, Brook CJ, Dehart P, et al: Ventilation-perfusion distributions in the adult respiratory distress syndrome. Am Rev Respir Dis 120:1039, 1979.
42. Dantzger DR: Gas exchange in the adult respiratory distress syndrome. Clin Chest Med 3:57, 1982.
43. Shimada Y, Yoshiya I, Tanaka K, et al: Evaluation of the progress and prognosis of the adult respiratory distress syndrome. Chest 76:180, 1979.
44. Wagner PD, Rodriguez-Roisin R: Clinical advances in pulmonary gas exchange. Am Rev Respir Dis 143:883, 1991.
45. Gattinoni L, Pesenti A, Bombino M, et al: Relationships between lung computed tomographic density, gas exchange, and PEEP in acute respiratory failure. Anesthesiology 69:812, 1988.
46. Maunder RJ, Shuman WP, McHugh JW, et al: Preservation of normal lung regions in the adult respiratory distress syndrome. JAMA 255:2463, 1986.
47. Shapiro AR, Peters RM: A nomogram for planning respiratory therapy. Chest 72:197, 1977.
48. Marini JJ: Monitoring during mechanical ventilation. Clin Chest Med 9:73, 1988.
49. Marini JJ: Lung mechanics in ARDS. Clin Chest Med 11:673, 1990.
50. Bone RC: Diagnosis of causes for acute respiratory distress by pressure-volume curves. Chest 70:740, 1976.
51. Brunet F, Dhainaut JF, Devaux JY, et al: Right ventricular performance

in patients with acute respiratory failure. Intensive Care Med 14:474, 1988.

51a. Powers SR, Mannal R, Neclerio M, et al: Physiologic consequences of positive end-expiratory pressure (PEEP) ventilation. Ann Surg 178:865, 1973.

52. Schumacker PT, Samsel RW: Oxygen supply and consumption in ARDS. Clin Chest Med 11:715, 1990.

52a. Danek SJ, Lynch JP, Weg JG, et al: The dependence of oxygen uptake on oxygen delivery with adult respiratory distress syndrome. Am Rev Respir Dis 122:387, 1980.

52b. Mohsenifar Z, Goldbach P, Tashkin DP, et al: Relationship between O_2 delivery and O_2 consumption in the adult respiratory distress syndrome. Chest 84:267, 1983.

53. Dantzger DR, Foresman B, Gutierrez G: Oxygen supply and utilization relationships. Am Rev Respir Dis 143:675, 1991.

54. Ronco JJ, Phang T, Wally KR, et al: Oxygen consumption is independent of changes in oxygen delivery in severe adult respiratory distress syndrome. Am Rev Respir Dis 143:1267, 1991.

55. Albertine KH: Ultrastructural abnormalities in increased-permeability pulmonary edema. Clin Chest Med 6:345, 1985.

56. Katzenstein AA, Myers JL, Mazur MT: Acute interstitial pneumonia: A clinicopathologic, ultrastructural, and cell kinetic study. Am J Surg Pathol 10:256, 1986.

57. Bachofen M, Weibel ER: Alterations in the gas exchange apparatus in adult respiratory insufficiency associated with septicemia. Am Rev Respir Dis 115:589, 1977.

58. Bachofen M, Weibel ER: Structural alterations of lung parenchyma in the adult respiratory distress syndrome. Clin Chest Med 3:35, 1982.

59. Pratt PC, Vollmer RT, Shelburne JD, et al: Pulmonary morphology in a multihospital collaborative extracorporeal membrane oxygenation project: I. Light microscopy. Am J Pathol 95:191, 1979.

60. Rinaldo JE, Christman JW: Mechanisms and mediators of ARDS. Clin Chest Med 11:621, 1990.

61. Fowler AA, Hyers TM, Fisher BJ, et al: The adult respiratory distress syndrome: Cell populations and soluble mediators in the airspaces of patients at high risk. Am Rev Respir Dis 136:1225, 1987.

62. Dorinsky PM, Gadek JE: Lung neutrophils in the adult respiratory distress syndrome: Clinical and pathophysiological significance. Am Rev Respir Dis 133:218, 1986.

63. Tomashefski JF, Davies P, Boggis L, et al: The pulmonary vascular lesions of the adult respiratory distress syndrome. Am J Pathol 112:112, 1983.

64. Greene R, Jantsch H, Boggis C, et al: Respiratory distress syndrome with new considerations. Radiol Clin North Am 21:699, 1983.

65. Jones R, Reid LM, Zapol WM, et al: Pulmonary vascular pathology: Human and experimental studies. In: Zapol WM, Falke KJ (eds): Acute Respiratory Failure. New York, Marcel Dekker, p 23, 1985.

66. Aberle DR, Brown K: Radiologic considerations in the adult respiratory distress syndrome. Clin Chest Med 11:737, 1990.

67. Johnson TH, Altman AR, McCaffree RD: Radiologic considerations in the adult respiratory distress syndrome treated with positive end expiratory pressure (PEEP). Clin Chest Med 3:89, 1982.

68. Malo J, Jameel A, Wood LDH: How does positive end-expiratory pressure reduce intrapulmonary shunt in canine pulmonary edema? J Appl Physiol 57:1002, 1984.

69. Stark P, Greene R, Kott MM, et al: CT findings in ARDS. Radiologe 27:367, 1987.

70. Fukuda Y, Ishizaki M, Masuda Y, et al: The role of intra-alveolar fibrosis in the process of pulmonary structural remodeling in patients with diffuse alveolar damage. Am J Pathol 126:171, 1987.

71. Bitterman PB, Henke CA: Fibroproliferative disorders. Chest 99:81S, 1991.

72. Marinelli WA, Henke CA, Harmon KR, et al: Mechanisms of alveolar fibrosis after acute lung injury. Clin Chest Med 11:657, 1990.

73. Clark RA: The commonality of cutaneous wound repair and lung injury. Chest 99:57S, 1991.

74. Kuhn C: Patterns of lung repair: A morphologist's view. Chest 99:11S, 1991.

75. Greene R: Adult respiratory distress syndrome: Acute alveolar damage. Radiology 163:57, 1987.

76. Albelda SM, Gefter WB, Kelley MA, et al: Ventilator-induced subpleural air cysts: Clinical, radiographic and pathologic significance. Am Rev Respir Dis 127:360, 1983.

77. Unger JM, England DM, Bogust GA: Interstitial emphysema in adults: Recognition and prognostic implications. J Thorac Imaging 4:86, 1989.

78. Eliott CG: Pulmonary sequelae in survivors of ARDS. Clin Chest Med 11:789, 1990.

79. Peters JI, Bell RC, Prihoda TJ, et al: Clinical determinants of abnormalities in pulmonary function in survivors of the adult respiratory distress syndrome. Am Rev Respir Dis 139:1163, 1989.

80. Ghio AJ, Elliott CG, Crapo RO, et al: Impairment after adult respiratory distress syndrome. Am Rev Respir Dis 139:1158, 1989.

81. Simpson DL, Goodman M, Spector SL, et al: Long-term follow-up and bronchial reactivity testing in survivors of the adult respiratory distress syndrome. Am Rev Respir Dis 117:449, 1978.

82. Seidenfeld JJ, Pohl DF, Bell RC, et al: Incidence, site and outcome of infections in patients with the adult respiratory distress syndrome. Am Rev Respir Dis 134:12, 1986.

83. Bernard GR, Luce JM, Sprung CL, et al: High dose corticosteroids in patients with the adult respiratory distress syndrome: A randomized double-blinded trial. N Engl J Med 317:1565, 1987.

84. Knaus WA, Wagner DP: Multiple organ failure: Epidemiology and prognosis. Crit Care Clin 5:221, 1989.

85. Modell JH, Graves SA, Ketover A: Clinical course of 91 near-drowning victims. Chest 70:231, 1976.

86. Oakes DD, Sherick JP, Maloney JR, et al: Prognosis and management of victims of near-drowning. J Trauma 22:544, 1982.

87. Matuschak GM, Rinaldo JE, Pinsky MR, et al: Effect of end stage liver failure on the incidence and resolution of the adult respiratory distress syndrome. J Crit Care 2:162, 1987.

88. Schwartz DB, Bone RC, Balk RA, et al: Hepatic dysfunction in the adult respiratory distress syndrome. Chest 95:871, 1989.

89. Dubois M, Lotze MT, Diamond WJ, et al: Pulmonary shunting during leukoagglutinin-induced noncardiogenic pulmonary edema. JAMA 244:2186, 1980.

90. Lewis RW, Rudd N, Pittman JA: Blood transfusion complications: Leukoagglutinin reactions. Obstet Gynecol 65:78S, 1985.

Clinical Management

Paul N. Lanken

OVERVIEW OF THERAPY AND PROGNOSIS

Clinical management of patients with ARDS is, as a rule, based on a combination of both specific and nonspecific treatments. *Specific* therapies are those directed against exogenous agents causing the syndrome or against endogenous mediators that are considered to be the primary causes of ARDS. *Nonspecific* therapies include various types of supportive care not only for the respiratory failure attributable to ARDS itself but also for the commonly accompanying multiple organ system failure (MOSF). Current clinical management of ARDS is derived primarily from prior clinical experience and, by extrapolation, from animal investigations. However, despite numerous clinical reports since the first description of ARDS in 1967[1] and extensive laboratory studies,[2, 3] no prospective, controlled, randomized, multicenter clinical trial has confirmed that any therapeutic intervention is effective in preventing ARDS or in improving the survival rate for patients with established ARDS. Finally, in most reported series, patients who have ARDS in association with sepsis alone[4] or together with a variety of predisposing causes[5–8] have overall mortality rates of 50 to 75%, a range that is virtually unchanged from that reported in the original 1967 series.[1]

Although reported overall survival rates of ARDS patients have not shown improvement during the past two decades, this may be attributable to factors other than genuine lack of progress in treating these patients. For example, later reports may have included ARDS patients with more severe illness and/or otherwise higher risks of death compared with those of earlier series.[9] These considerations illustrate a fundamental problem related to ARDS clinical series: a general lack of identification of prognostic factors that have been validated to predict risk of death at the onset of ARDS. This deficiency has serious implications for designing and interpreting clinical trials. First, without such factors, control and experimental groups in an ARDS clinical trial cannot be stratified prospectively, or analyzed retrospectively, for major factors correlating with risk of death at the start of the trial to ensure initial comparability of the two groups. Lack of these prognostic factors also prevents meaningful comparisons among different controlled clinical trials or between an uncontrolled clinical trial and historical controls. Table 73–3 provides some parameters commonly used to describe patients in ARDS clinical trials together with their status as prognostic factors.

Also making it difficult to compare ARDS clinical studies is the marked variability in the clinical characteristics of ARDS patients. These characteristics include (1) different etiologies or associated causes with probable differences in humoral and cellular mediators of lung injury; (2) differences in patterns and degrees of lung injury and in the evolution and resolution of that injury; (3) variations in the type, degree, and timing of medical interventions; and (4) various degrees and severity of concomitant non–respiratory organ system failure.

THREE PARADIGMS OF ARDS

Because of the highly variable clinical presentation and course of ARDS, clinical management is described here in terms of the following simplified scheme, in which ARDS is viewed as one of three distinct clinicopathologic paradigms: (1) ARDS as failure of a single organ, the lung, in the initial acute exudative phase of lung injury; (2) ARDS, again as failure of the lung alone, but in the subacute (or chronic) proliferative and fibrotic phase, which follows the acute phase after 1 to 2 weeks of respiratory support; and (3) ARDS as failure of the lung as an integral part of the syndrome of acute MOSF. Viewing ARDS as three distinct paradigms may somewhat oversimplify the clinical and pathologic manifestations of ARDS because these manifestations may overlap in many patients and because lung dysfunction and pathologic changes evolve in a continuous

---

TABLE 73–4

THREE PARADIGMS OF ADULT RESPIRATORY DISTRESS SYNDROME WITH ASSOCIATED CAUSES OF DEATH

Paradigm 1: Single-Organ Failure of the Lung in the Initial Acute Exudative Phase
Hypoxemic respiratory failure
Complications of mechanical ventilation (e.g., barotrauma)
Precipitating cause of ARDS

Paradigm 2: Single-Organ Failure of the Lung in the Subacute Proliferative and Fibrotic Phase
Nosocomial infections, especially pneumonia and sepsis
Pulmonary fibrosis after several weeks or more of mechanical ventilation
Complications of mechanical ventilation (e.g., barotrauma)
Hypoxemic respiratory failure

Paradigm 3: ARDS as an Integral Part of MOSF
Circulatory shock
Ischemic injury of other organs (e.g., brain, bowel, or extremities)
Coagulopathy and hemorrhage
Hepatic failure
Nosocomial infections
Respiratory causes listed under paradigm 2

---

rather than a stepwise manner. However, dividing this complex syndrome into three separate entities is justified because of the different clinical manifestations, therapeutic issues, and causes of death (Table 73–4). In addition, the purpose of this three-part model of ARDS is to provide an organizational structure to help in understanding of the vast array of therapeutic interventions with their different rationales and goals (Table 73–5).

PARADIGM 1: ARDS AS ACUTE LUNG FAILURE IN THE ACUTE EXUDATIVE PHASE

Clinical and Pathologic Features

This paradigm, also known as the acute exudative phase of ARDS, reflects the original classic description of ARDS,[1] featuring acute respiratory failure with marked hypoxemia, diffuse alveolar infiltrates, and severely diminished lung compliance in the absence of left-sided congestive heart failure. More recent clinical definitions of ARDS, such as that describing a semiquantitative lung injury score,[10] are still based primarily on this original paradigm of ARDS. Commonly associated causes of this manifestation of ARDS include injurious agents that reach the alveoli via the airways (e.g., as in gastric aspiration, toxic gas inhalation, and viral or other diffuse pneumonias [Fig. 73–14]) or via the blood stream (e.g., as in fat emboli syndrome or massive air embolism). Pathologic change in the lung consists of diffuse pulmonary edema that floods alveoli with protein-rich fluid, variable degrees of intra-alveolar hemorrhage, and infiltration by inflammatory cells. Hyaline membranes, which are evidence of intra-alveolar fibrin formation, may develop during this phase despite only several days of exposure to high concentrations of oxygen. There may also be evidence of intravascular coagulation and/or extensive destruction of alveolar epithelium.[11-15] The pathophysiologic mechanism is related to primary injury of the alveolar capillary membrane that results in its increased permeability.

In this phase, death resulting from hypoxemic respiratory failure or from the clinical condition that precipitated the ARDS is the major threat to the patient. Before treatment with assisted ventilation, hypercapnic respiratory failure may

---

TABLE 73–3

PROGNOSTIC VALUE OF VARIOUS PARAMETERS IN ADULT RESPIRATORY DISTRESS SYNDROME

Parameter	Effect on Mortality
Physiological Factors at Onset of ARDS*	
Indices of hypoxemia	
Pao_2/Fio_2	Not validated
Pao_2/PAo_2	Not validated
Lung injury score[10]	Not validated
MOSF	
APACHE score	Higher score predicts higher mortality[7]
Associated Causes of ARDS	
Pneumocystis pneumonia	Increased mortality† (>90%) in AIDS[55]
Bone marrow transplantation	Increased mortality† (>95%)[56]
End-stage liver disease	Increased mortality† (>95%)[57]
Fat emboli	Decreased mortality† (<10%)[58]
Clinical Course After Onset of ARDS	
Improving oxygenation	Decreased mortality[4]
More positive fluid balance	Increased mortality[41, 43]
Reduced pulmonary arterial occlusion pressure	Decreased mortality[42]
Failure of other organs	Increased mortality[59]
Sepsis	Increased mortality[6]

*Fio_2 = fraction of inspired oxygen; PAo_2 = alveolar partial pressure of oxygen; APACHE = Acute Physiology and Chronic Health Evaluation.
†Compared with mortality rates of 50–70% in large series whose common causes of ARDS were sepsis, multiple trauma, and aspiration.[5-8]

TABLE 73–5

THREE PARADIGMS OF ADULT RESPIRATORY DISTRESS SYNDROME WITH THERAPEUTIC APPROACHES

Paradigm 1: Single-Organ Failure of the Lung (Acute Exudative Phase)
Specific therapy
  None known except for ARDS resulting from specific treatable causes
Supportive therapy
  Oxygen therapy
  Conventional mechanical ventilation with PEEP
  Variations of conventional mechanical ventilation
    Inverse ratio ventilation
    Controlled hypercapnia
    Controlled hypothermia
    Exogenous surfactant administration
  Nonconventional support of gas exchange
    High-frequency ventilation
    Extracorporeal membrane oxygenation (ECMO)
    Extracorporeal carbon dioxide removal (ECCO$_2$R)
  Lowering of pulmonary capillary hydrostatic pressure

Paradigm 2: Single-Organ Failure of the Lung (Subacute Proliferative and Fibrotic Phase)
Specific therapy
  Anti-inflammatory therapy
Supportive therapy
  Prevention of pulmonary oxygen toxicity
  Prevention of pulmonary barotrauma
  Prevention of lung injury resulting from alveolar overdistension
  Prevention and treatment of nosocomial infections

Paradigm, 3: ARDS as an Integral Part of MOSF
Specific therapy
  Treatment of septic syndrome
    Anti-inflammatory therapy
    Monoclonal antibody therapy
Supportive therapy
  Circulatory support
  Supportive therapy for failure of other individual organ systems (e.g., renal, hepatic, bone marrow, and coagulation)
  Nutritional and other general intensive care therapy

also develop because of respiratory muscle fatigue. A variety of parameters have been used to define abnormalities of lung function during this phase (e.g., the ratio of arterial to alveolar partial pressure of oxygen; see Table 73–3). These parameters relate to the degree of alveolar flooding and associated impairment of oxygenation. Although these parameters have been useful as inclusion criteria for ARDS clinical trials, none has been validated as a prognostic indicator for risk of death at the onset of ARDS. This lack of prognostic value suggests that they may not accurately reflect the degree and nature of the initial lung injury and/or the subsequent response of the lung to injury, both of which presumably determine survival. Outcomes from this phase vary markedly among patients: of those who survive, some have rapid and complete recovery, whereas others experience a slow and prolonged recovery phase (i.e., paradigm 2; see later). Nonsurvivors may die swiftly after only hours or several days as a result of overwhelming hypoxemic respiratory failure or after several weeks or even months of continued mechanical ventilation as a result of a nosocomial infection.

Clinical Management: Specific Therapy

Although no known intervention reverses the permeability defect of the alveolar capillary membrane, in certain conditions, specific therapy may be directed against the etiologic agent or condition resulting in the ARDS. Table 73–6 lists examples of underlying conditions associated with ARDS

that have specific therapies. These examples emphasize the importance of attempting to find a potentially treatable cause of ARDS at its onset.

As early as 1971, glucocorticosteroids (or steroids) had been recommended as therapy for ARDS with the aim of decreasing a presumed inflammatory reaction.[16] Although the concept that an inflammatory reaction occurs during the initial injury in lungs in ARDS appears confirmed, the effectiveness of steroid therapy for ARDS has not. After 16 years of using steroids to treat ARDS, a prospective, randomized, placebo-controlled, multicenter clinical trial in 1987 showed that high-dose steroid therapy for ARDS did not decrease mortality of patients with established ARDS.[8] Nor did steroids prevent the occurrence of ARDS or hasten its resolution in patients with sepsis; indeed, steroid therapy in patients with ARDS caused by sepsis significantly increased the mortality from and the duration of ARDS.[17] This history of steroid therapy for ARDS emphasizes the importance of confirming the efficacy of new interventions in ARDS before their widespread use. It also raises questions about the efficacy of other elements of current clinical management of ARDS whose benefit has been assumed from clinical experience rather than confirmed by appropriately designed controlled clinical trials.

Clinical Management: Supportive Therapy

Oxygen Therapy

The main goal of oxygen therapy is to prevent death resulting from severe hypoxemia. Initial therapy for early ARDS is supplemental oxygen to maintain Pao$_2$ above 55 mm Hg (or an arterial oxygen saturation of 88%). As severe ARDS evolves and the patient's minute ventilation increases, oxygen therapy quickly changes from low-flow modalities such as nasal prongs and simple face masks to high-flow systems such as tightly fitting non-rebreathing or rebreathing reservoir bags. These systems may prevent the need for intubation if the ARDS rapidly reverses.

Another temporizing alternative to intubation is use of a continuous positive airway pressure mask that can deliver virtually 100% oxygen (because of the tight seal between the mask and the face) as well as PEEP.[18] The latter is important because the hypoxemia in ARDS is characteristically resistant to supplemental oxygen by itself (Fig. 73–15). This resistance is due to increased right-to-left shunting of mixed venous blood across the lungs because completely fluid-filled or collapsed alveoli continue to be perfused. More appropriate treatment than simply raising the fraction of inspired oxygen (Fio$_2$) is to decrease this high right-to-left shunt. This may

TABLE 73–6

UNDERLYING TREATABLE CAUSES OF ADULT RESPIRATORY DISTRESS SYNDROME

Infectious Causes
Bacterial sepsis
Diffuse pneumonia caused by bacteria (e.g., *Legionella*)
Diffuse pneumonia caused by viruses (e.g., cytomegalovirus)
Diffuse pneumonia caused by *Pneumocystis carinii*
Other diffuse pulmonary infections (e.g., miliary tuberculosis)

Diffuse Pulmonary Hemorrhage
Goodpasture's syndrome
Systemic lupus erythematosus
Wegener's granulomatosis
Autologous bone marrow transplantation

Drug Reactions
Aspirin toxicity

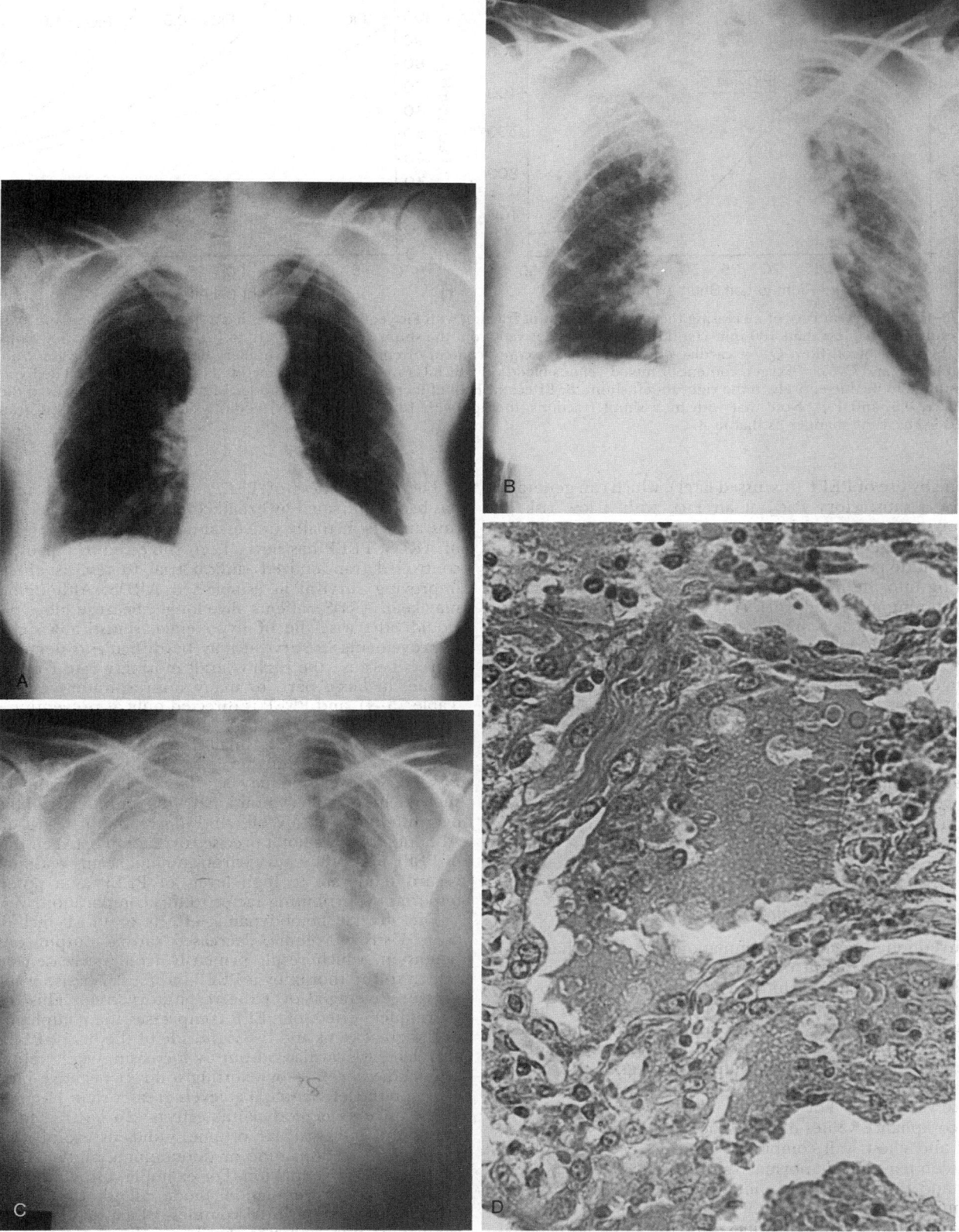

Figure 73–14. Paradigm 1 of ARDS. Patient with multiple myeloma who was receiving high-dose glucocorticosteroid therapy developed ARDS related to *Pneumocystis carinii*. *A.* Baseline chest radiograph. *B.* Chest radiograph on day of admission. *C.* Chest radiograph 1 day later (patient refused intubation and died that night). *D.* Photomicrograph of hematoxylin-eosin–stained section showing alveolar flooding. Sample of patient's lung was taken at postmortem examination.

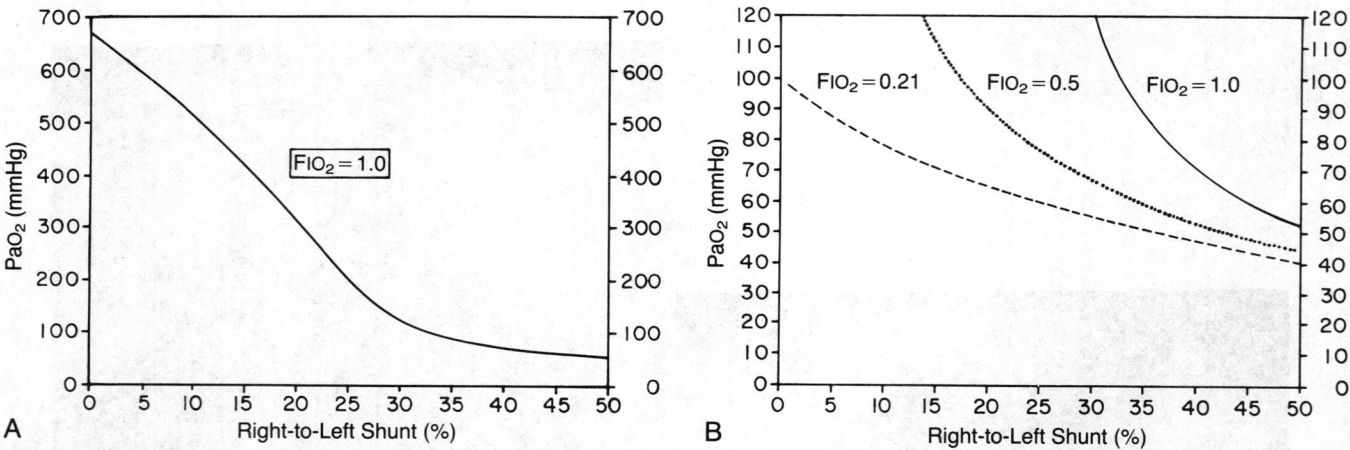

Figure 73–15. *A*. Effect on PaO_2 of increasing the right-to-left shunt fraction with FIO_2 equal to 1.0. Note that a shunt greater than approximately 33% results in PaO_2 less than 100 mm Hg. This graph was derived from the shunt equation ($Qs/QT = [Cc'O_2 - CaO_2]/[Cc'O_2 - C\bar{v}O_2]$, where Qs = the shunt blood flow, QT = cardiac output, $Cc'O_2$ = oxygen content of end-pulmonary capillary blood, CaO_2 = oxygen content of arterial blood, and $C\bar{v}O_2$ = oxygen content of mixed venous blood) in which $CaO_2 - C\bar{v}O_2$ was assumed to be 4.5 mL/100 dL. The hypoxemia was assumed to be due entirely to the right-to-left shunt. *B*. Effect on PaO_2 of increasing the right-to-left shunt with gas mixtures of different FIO_2 (0.21, 0.5, and 1.0). Note that with high shunt fractions, therapy with 100% oxygen only modestly increases PaO_2. This graph was derived in the same manner as that in *A*.

be done by use of PEEP (discussed later), which can generally achieve a satisfactory PaO_2 at an FIO_2 with a low risk of pulmonary oxygen toxicity.

Disadvantages of a continuous positive airway pressure mask include potential leaks or disconnections, danger from vomiting into the mask, respiratory muscle fatigue because of continuing increased work of breathing, and provision of only temporary delays in intubation. There is also a potential risk of pulmonary oxygen toxicity because patients may be exposed to high concentrations of oxygen for several days or longer. Although the exact lower limit of oxygen concentration that is toxic for lungs of ARDS patients is unknown, some evidence suggests that oxygen concentrations higher than 60% for more than 24 hours may result in permanent lung damage in these patients.[19] Breathing 90 to 100% oxygen for more than 48 hours despite diuresis and continuous positive airway pressure would be a strong indication for intubation and initiation of mechanical ventilation with PEEP.

Conventional Mechanical Ventilation with Positive End-Expiratory Pressure

Conventional mechanical ventilation with PEEP has been the standard treatment of ARDS since originally reported in 1967.[1] As a rule, volume- or time-controlled positive pressure ventilators have been used because they can deliver adequate tidal volumes at high peak pressures and at high inspiratory flows. High airway pressures are needed to inflate exceedingly stiff (i.e., poorly compliant) lungs in ARDS, and high flows are needed to supply ARDS patients' increased minute ventilation. For example, ARDS patients commonly have compliance values of the static respiratory system (i.e., lungs and chest wall combined) equal to 10 to 25 mL/cm H_2O, compared with normal values of 50 to 100 mL/cm H_2O, and they may have minute ventilations greater than 25 L/min.[20]

The application of PEEP increases the lung's functional residual capacity, which correlates closely with a decrease in the right-to-left shunt across the lungs.[21, 22] PEEP may also increase the respiratory system's compliance,[22, 23] thereby changing static and dynamic pressure-volume curves of the respiratory system (Fig. 73–16).

The effectiveness of PEEP in improving PaO_2 in ARDS has been confirmed by broad clinical experience. Because of this and its virtually universal acceptance in the treatment of ARDS, PEEP has never been subjected to a prospective, controlled, randomized clinical trial to test its efficacy in improving survival in established ARDS. Although PEEP may keep ARDS patients alive longer because more patients would otherwise die of hypoxemia, statistically significant improvements in survival may be difficult to demonstrate. This is because the high overall mortality rate from ARDS is due, in large part, to many nonrespiratory causes (see Table 73–4), and PEEP is directed only at preventing death from hypoxemic respiratory failure. Hypoxemic respiratory failure accounts for a small fraction of deaths in most reported series.[6, 7] Furthermore, the beneficial effects of PEEP on oxygenation may be offset by its deleterious effects, such as barotrauma, additional lung injury attributable to overdistention of alveoli, and decreased cardiac output. Although there is not a precise correlation between the level of PEEP and pulmonary barotrauma, it seems reasonable to regard moderate to high levels of PEEP as a potentially important contributing factor to this complication.

The adverse hemodynamic effects of PEEP include decreased stroke volume, decreased cardiac output, and hypotension, which result primarily from decreased venous return to the thorax by a PEEP-induced increase in pleural pressure averaged over the respiratory cycle. This "central tourniquet" effect of PEEP compresses the compliant walls of the great veins and the right side of the heart. PEEP may also decrease cardiac output by increasing right ventricular afterload, as well as by exerting a direct negative inotropic effect on the left ventricle at levels greater than 15 cm H_2O.[24] These adverse hemodynamic effects can be treated by expansion of intravascular volume, judicious use of inotropic agents such as dopamine or dobutamine, and/or alteration of the mode of ventilation. For example, use of an intermittent mandatory ventilation mode allows the patient to breathe spontaneous tidal volumes, which in addition to the ventilator's tidal volumes should result in a more negative time-averaged pleural pressure.

To understand the rationale and mechanism of PEEP, it may be helpful to consider the lungs in this stage of ARDS as consisting of three regions (Fig. 73–17): a normal region with essentially fluid-free alveoli; a recruitable region in

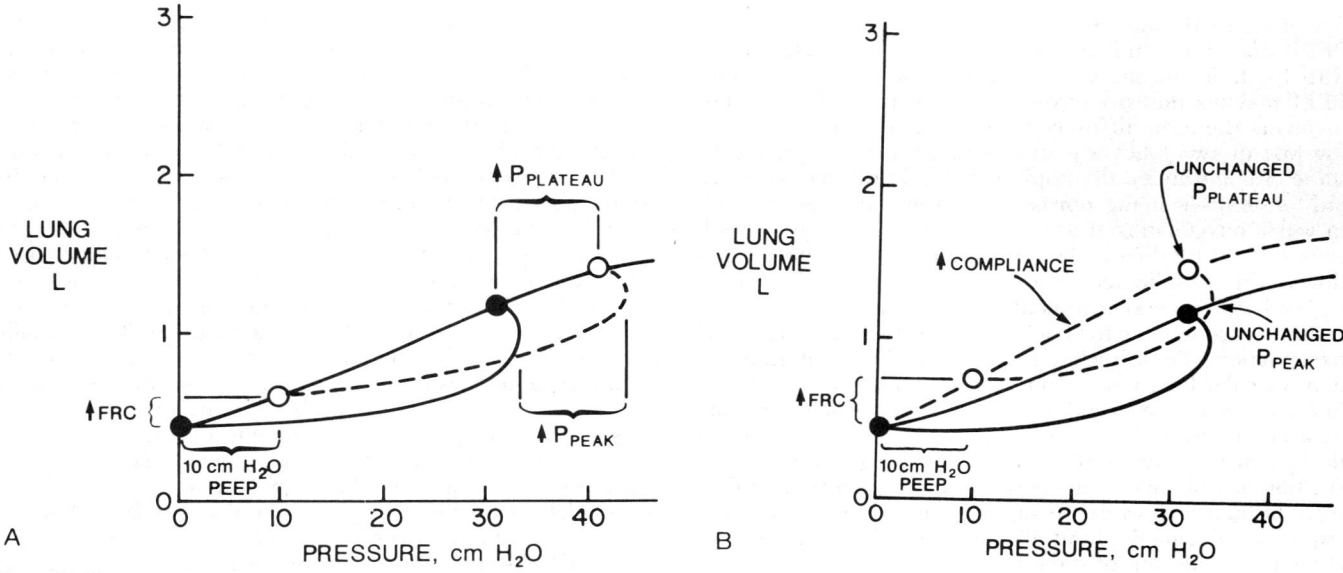

Figure 73-16. *A.* Schematic representation of the effect of addition of 10 cm H$_2$O of PEEP on dynamic inspiratory pressure-volume curves during positive pressure ventilation. In ARDS, the static pressure-volume curve *(solid line connecting the four circles)* of the total respiratory system (lungs and chest wall combined) shows a decreased functional residual capacity (FRC) and a decreased slope caused by low lung compliance. An inspiratory dynamic pressure-volume curve is shown with zero PEEP *(solid line with filled circles)* and after the addition of 10 cm H$_2$O PEEP *(dashed line with open circles).* Note that the addition of PEEP moves the end-expiratory location of the curve, that is, functional residual capacity, along the original static pressure-volume curve and also results in a higher peak pressure (Ppeak) and a higher end-inspiratory pressure (Pplateau) compared with the situation for zero PEEP. *B.* Schematic representation of the effect of PEEP on static and dynamic pressure-volume curves in ARDS. In some patients with ARDS, the addition of PEEP may increase the slope of the static pressure-volume curve of the respiratory system *(dashed line intersecting the ordinate)* compared with zero PEEP *(solid line).* This may result in little or no change in peak and plateau pressures for the same tidal volumes. (Modified from Lanken PN: Mechanical ventilation. In: Fishman AP [ed]: Pulmonary Diseases and Disorders. 2nd ed. New York, McGraw-Hill, p 2373, 1988. Reproduced with permission of McGraw-Hill, Inc.)

which alveoli are atelectatic or partially filled with fluid; and a nonrecruitable region in which alveoli are completely filled with fluid.[25, 26]

First, in the normal region, PEEP raises the end-expiratory pressure and volume of normal alveoli along their individual pressure-volume curves. However, during inspiration, PEEP plus the ventilator's tidal volume may cause high alveolar pressures and result in alveolar overdistention. Normal lungs generally reach full expansion when transpulmonary pressures are 35 to 40 cm H$_2$O. Pressures greater than this may

excessively distend the alveoli, which has been found to cause acute lung injury in experimental studies.[27, 28]

Second, in the recruitable region, PEEP reinflates both the atelectatic alveoli and the partially fluid-filled alveoli, possibly by redistributing the original fluid within their confines. This increases the ventilation/perfusion ratios for these alveoli from zero, or close to zero, and accounts for the decrease in the right-to-left shunt in ARDS and improved oxygenation. However, alveoli in this region may also be overdistended for the same reasons as just discussed.

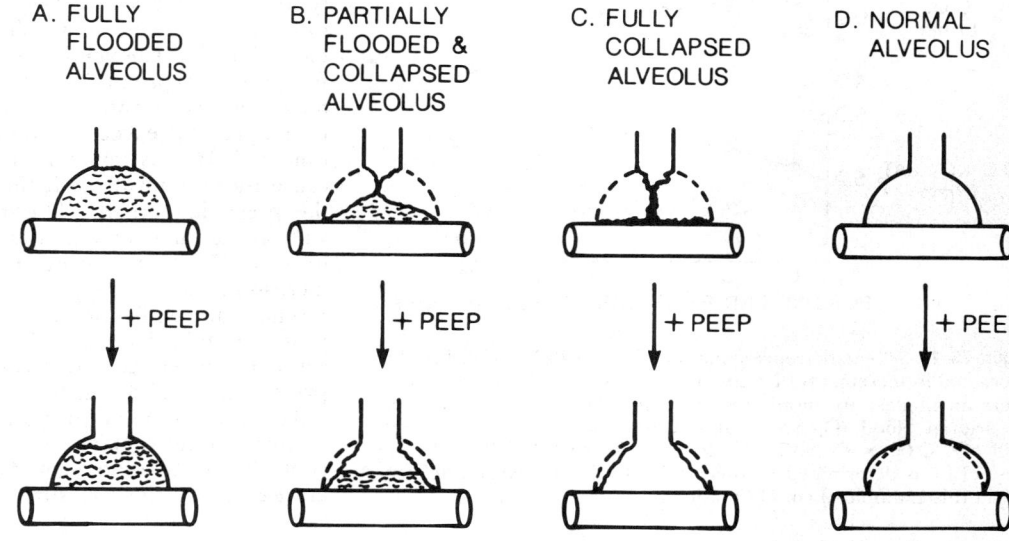

Figure 73-17. Schematic representation of the effect of PEEP on recruitable and nonrecruitable regions of the lung in ARDS. The nonrecruitable region is represented in *A* and the recruitable region in *B* and *C*. *A.* PEEP has no effect on alveoli that are completely filled with fluid. *B.* PEEP redistributes fluid and expands alveoli that are partially filled with fluid and atelectatic. *C.* PEEP expands fully collapsed alveoli. *D.* PEEP may overdistend normal alveoli.

Finally, in the nonrecruitable region, the application of PEEP does not reinflate alveoli that are completely filled with fluid. By means of this model, one can explain why PEEP may not improve oxygenation in certain disorders not involving the lung diffusely, such as pneumonia consolidating one or two lobes with the remaining lobes normal. In these circumstances, the application of PEEP may result in only distention of the normal region and may even result in worse oxygenation if greater pressures in normal alveoli caused by PEEP divert a larger fraction of pulmonary blood flow to the consolidated area.

Besides alveolar recruitment just described, other mechanisms may contribute to beneficial effects of PEEP on arterial oxygenation. These include a redistribution of pulmonary extravascular lung water from the intra-alveolar space to the interstitial space; prevention of small-airway collapse during expiration, thus improving the lung's overall ventilation/perfusion ratio; and decreases in the right-to-left shunt fraction attributable to decreases in cardiac output. In contrast, little, if any, evidence supports the concept that PEEP "squeezes" edema fluid out of alveoli, back into the intravascular space, and out of the lung.

The first therapeutic goal of PEEP during this phase of ARDS is to restore safe levels of Pao_2 as rapidly as possible. This goal can usually be achieved by targeting a Pao_2 between 55 and 65 mm Hg (i.e., an arterial saturation of about 90%), unless a higher Pao_2 is found to be needed for an individual patient (such as for severe arterial oxygen

desaturation with airway suctioning). The second therapeutic goal of PEEP in this phase is to allow stepwise lowering of the patient's inspired oxygen concentrations, initially from toxic concentrations (95 to 100%) to safer concentrations (40 to 60%), while maintaining adequate levels of arterial oxygenation. Both the beneficial effects of PEEP on oxygenation and its adverse hemodynamic effects can be monitored systematically during the performance of a "best-PEEP" trial (Fig. 73–18), whose therapeutic goal is maximizing oxygen delivery (i.e., the product of cardiac output and oxygen saturation of arterial blood).[23] An alternative approach to a best-PEEP trial is simply to apply increments of PEEP until Pao_2 is increased to a satisfactory level or until a clinically significant fall in cardiac output or blood pressure occurs. If hypoxemia and toxic Fio_2 remain the most life-threatening problems, the circulatory problems can be overcome as described earlier and the increments of PEEP continued until satisfactory oxygenation or nontoxic levels of Fio_2 are reached. Levels of PEEP between 10 and 15 cm H_2O are generally adequate to restore arterial oxygenation but, in severe cases, much higher levels may be required. In some cases of critically severe hypoxemia in the acute phase of ARDS (paradigm 1), elevations of PEEP to 25 to 35 cm H_2O may be needed to preserve oxygenation; however, this level of PEEP, plus aggressive attempts to lower pulmonary capillary pressures, may severely compromise cardiac output and lead to MOSF.

In the treatment of this phase of ARDS, after the most effective level of PEEP is determined and if it is tolerated without hemodynamic compromise or signs of barotrauma, many clinicians hold PEEP constant while trying to taper the patient's inspired oxygen concentration stepwise to the 40 to 60% range. After that Fio_2 range is reached, attempts would then be made to lower the PEEP in steps of 2.5 or 3 cm H_2O to as low as permitted by the patient's Pao_2. The stepwise lowering of PEEP is done purposively in small decrements, because arterial oxygenation may fall precipitously with abrupt removal of PEEP and may take several hours to recover fully in some patients.[20, 23] For the same reason, most clinicians minimize routine suctioning of the patient's airways and do not remove PEEP while pulmonary arterial occlusion pressures are measured.

Variations of Conventional Mechanical Ventilation with Positive End-Expiratory Pressure

Inverse Ratio Ventilation. Besides PEEP, another method of increasing end-expiratory pressure, and hence functional residual capacity, is inverse ratio ventilation, in which inverse ratio refers to ratio of inspiratory time to expiratory time more than 1:1. Conventional ratios, 1:3 to 1:1, prolong time for passive expiration to facilitate return of blood to the heart. In inverse ratio ventilation, inspiration is deliberately prolonged to exceed expiratory time by two to four times.[29, 30] In this manner, tidal volumes are "stacked" because there is insufficient time for complete exhalation of the preceding breath. This results in lung hyperinflation with an elevated end-expiratory alveolar pressure, that is, intrinsic PEEP (or auto-PEEP). Inverse ratio ventilation also increases mean airway pressure compared with conventional mechanical ventilation using the same tidal volume and pressure limit. This technique increases Pao_2, probably because of its effects on mean airway and end-expiratory pressures, but also possibly because of an altered pattern of inflation of alveoli in lungs of patients with ARDS.

Inverse ratio ventilation may be performed in a pressure-controlled or a volume-controlled mode.[30] One of the main attractions of the pressure-controlled mode is enhanced

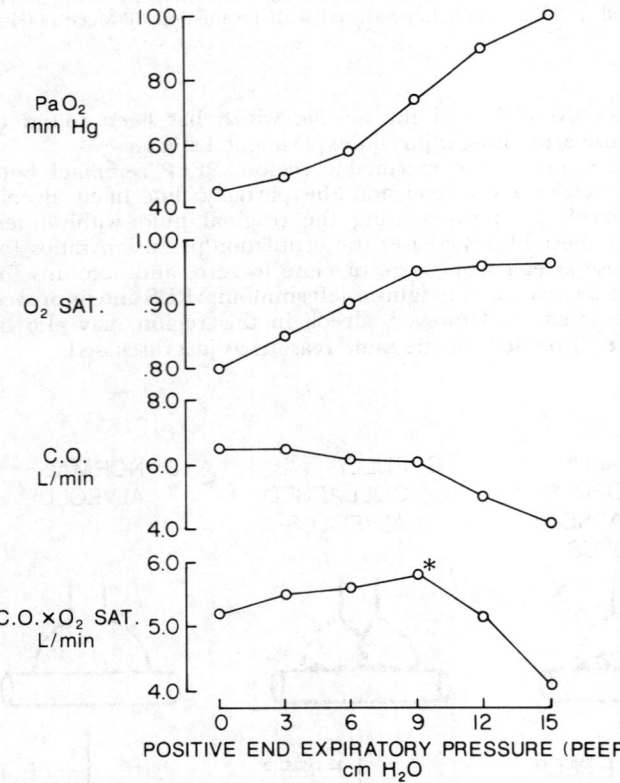

Figure 73–18. Schematic representation of a best-PEEP trial. PEEP is increased in increments of 3 cm H_2O (abscissa), and various parameters (ordinates) are monitored including Pao_2, oxygen saturation of arterial blood (O_2 SAT), and cardiac output (C.O.). Oxygen delivery (C.O. × O_2 SAT) is calculated for each PEEP level. The best PEEP is determined by the maximal value of oxygen delivery or, in this example, 9 cm H_2O (asterisk).[23]

protection against the potentially deleterious effects of high alveolar pressures leading to barotrauma or alveolar overdistension. Adverse effects of inverse ratio ventilation are the same as those for conventional mechanical ventilation, but they include the potential for greater hemodynamic compromise because of higher mean airway pressures as well as a possible greater risk of barotrauma as a result of unrecognized high alveolar pressure. Controlled clinical trials are needed to compare this technique with conventional mechanical ventilation to assess its role in therapy for ARDS.

Controlled Hypercapnia. Controlled hypercapnia has been used successfully as a ventilation strategy for patients with status asthmaticus.[31] In this approach, the ventilator's minute ventilation is deliberately limited to avoid high inspiratory pressures and their adverse sequelae. One result is higher than normal $Paco_2$. This approach can be adapted for treatment of the acute exudative phase of ARDS, which requires high peak inspiratory pressures to keep $Paco_2$ within the normal range. Under these circumstances, controlled hypoventilation would result in lower airway and alveolar pressures, compared with conventional ventilation, because of smaller tidal volumes and lower inspiratory flow rates. These smaller tidal volumes, in turn, would decrease the potential for alveolar overdistension and alveolar injury. However, this technique generally requires that the patient be heavily sedated and paralyzed, with the ventilator in the control mode. Controlled hypercapnia should be considered as investigational in the treatment of ARDS until controlled clinical trials establish its efficacy and safety.

Controlled Hypothermia. Two rationales are proposed for this technique. The first is that total oxygen consumption would be decreased by lowering the core temperature of the patient, and the second is that lower than normal core temperatures would permit vital organs such as the brain to tolerate greater degrees of hypoxemia. The end result would enable tissue oxygenation to be maintained at a lower than normal Pao_2 and hence permit lowering of the Fio_2. This technique is generally used only when hypoxemic respiratory failure is extremely severe (e.g., Pao_2 less than 50 mm Hg with $Fio_2 = 1.0$) and the patient has been exposed to high, potentially toxic concentrations of oxygen for several days or longer. Although these rationales seem to be attractive, experimental evidence to support the usefulness of the technique is equivocal[32] and clinical experience remains anecdotal.[33] Animal experiments suggest that controlled hypothermia reliably decreases total oxygen consumption but does not necessarily allow a decrease in Fio_2 because of a concomitant decrease in oxygen delivery attributable to depression of cardiac function. Furthermore, hypothermia may predispose a patient to a platelet coagulopathy and has unknown effects on the processes involved in lung repair and host defense.

Therapy with Exogenous Surfactant. Studies of lungs of patients with ARDS support the concept that there is a deficiency of functionally active surfactant in ARDS. Although the syndrome was originally so named because of similarities with the respiratory distress syndrome of neonates,[1] neonates manifest hypoxemic respiratory failure primarily because of lack of surfactant as a result of immature lungs. This has been confirmed by studies showing that exogenous surfactant has been successful in both preventing and treating the neonatal syndrome.[34] In contrast, most evidence points to the primary mechanism in the pathogenesis of ARDS as an increase in permeability of an injured alveolar capillary membrane. Nevertheless, lack of functional surfactant could contribute to hypoxemia because alveoli without it would be inherently unstable and tend to collapse (see Fig. 73–17). Surfactant activity in ARDS could be lost by several means: by being washed out by alveolar flooding;

by inactivation after contact with plasma proteins, especially albumin;[35] and by injury to type II alveolar cells, which normally produce surfactant. Prospective controlled clinical trials of surfactant administration in patients with early ARDS without MOSF (corresponding to paradigm 1) are now under way. The hypothesis being tested is that administration of exogenous surfactant to the alveolar space would restore functional surfactant activity. This effect may increase overall survival by improving oxygenation and lung compliance, thus reducing the risks of oxygen toxicity, barotrauma, and lung injury related to alveolar overdistension.

Nonconventional Support of Gas Exchange

High-Frequency Ventilation. High-frequency mechanical ventilation provides relatively small tidal volumes at respiratory rates much greater than normal (e.g., exceeding 100 breaths/min).[36] Although no controlled studies demonstrate that this type of ventilator leads to improved survival of ARDS patients, its potential advantage lies in its capacity to keep tidal volumes and peak airway pressures relatively low while still providing adequate oxygenation. However, carbon dioxide clearance with high-frequency ventilation may be only partially effective and somewhat unpredictable. High-frequency ventilation may have a role in selected patients with ARDS and large bronchopleural fistulas.[37] In such patients, air leaks through the fistula during conventional mechanical ventilation with the normal (8 to 10 mL/kg) tidal volumes may be so great that alveolar hypoventilation results (Fig. 73–19). An alternative to high-frequency ventilation is use of a volume-controlled ventilator at lower tidal volumes (4 to 5 mL/kg) and higher rates (40 to 60 breaths/min) to attempt to lower the pressure gradient across the fistula.

Extracorporeal Membrane Oxygenation (ECMO). During the acute exudative phase of ARDS, some patients do not

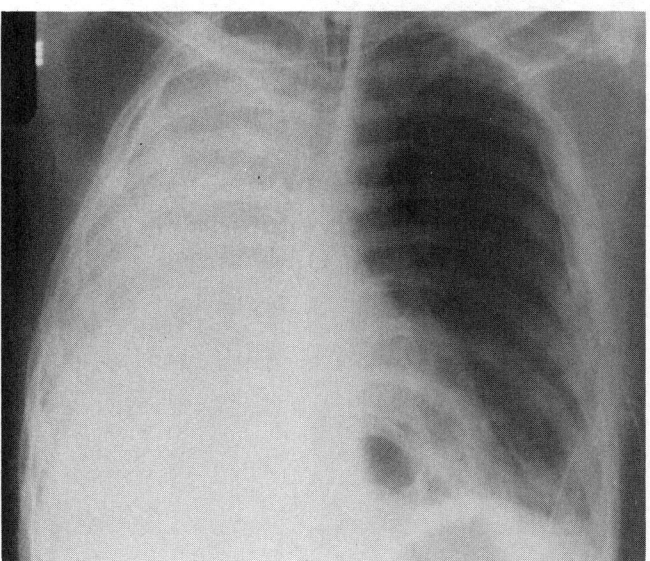

Figure 73–19. Successful use of jet ventilation for bronchopleural fistula. Chest radiograph of a 20-year-old man with ARDS and a large bronchopleural fistula from the left lung. The patient had been in a motorcycle accident and sustained a laceration of the right lung, which had been treated by pneumonectomy. Postoperatively, he had ARDS in the left lung complicated by loculated pneumothoraces and large air leaks via multiple chest tubes (evident in the radiograph). After increasing hypercapnia occurred during conventional mechanical ventilation and PEEP, the patient was treated with high-frequency jet ventilation for more than 1 month. The air leaks eventually stopped and he was discharged from the hospital.

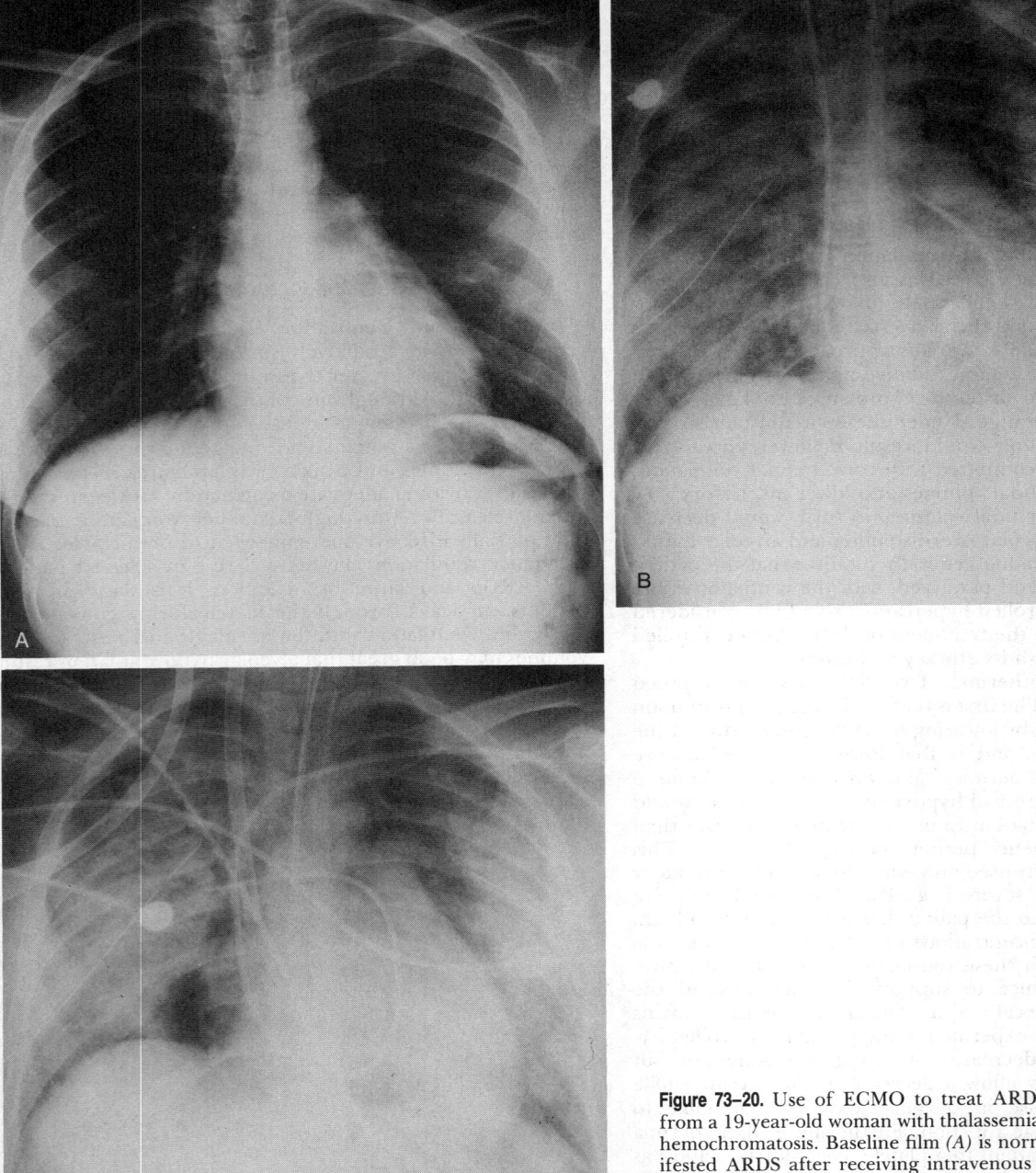

Figure 73–20. Use of ECMO to treat ARDS. Chest radiographs from a 19-year-old woman with thalassemia major and secondary hemochromatosis. Baseline film *(A)* is normal. The patient manifested ARDS after receiving intravenous desferrioxamine. She was treated with conventional mechanical ventilation and PEEP but had bilateral tension pneumothoraces treated by the use of chest tubes *(B)*. Because of persistent, severe hypoxemia (PaO_2 < 50 mm Hg with FIO_2 = 0.8 to 1.0 and 15 cm H_2O PEEP for more than 1 week), she was treated via ECMO, with one catheter located in the superior vena cava and the other in the femoral vein *(C)*. Despite this treatment, her lungs did not improve and she died after 8 days of ECMO.

respond to standard mechanical ventilation with PEEP, even with 100% inspired oxygen and vigorous attempts to lower pulmonary capillary pressures. Such patients may have life-threatening hypoxemia with PaO_2 below 50 mm Hg and may experience significant bradycardias because of hypoxia especially with coughing, suctioning, or turning. Under such circumstances, some clinicians resort to artificial means of gas exchange for oxygenation (Fig. 73–20). ECMO, or oxygenation by means of an artificial membrane lung via a

venoarterial route of perfusion, was the subject of a controlled, prospective multicenter study of ARDS.[38] Although ECMO was found to improve oxygenation, it did not improve survival, with an approximate 90% mortality in both ECMO-treated and control groups. These results suggest that the patients in this study represented a subset of ARDS patients whose lungs had been injured so severely that recovery from respiratory failure was unlikely. Because proliferative and fibrotic changes in the lungs were prominent at autopsy,[13] the ARDS in many of these patients appears to have progressed during the study from paradigm 1, the acute exudative phase, to paradigm 2, the subacute proliferative and fibrotic phase. The overall mortality rate of patients enrolled in the ECMO study, even in the control group, was worse than that observed in other ARDS studies (i.e., 90% mortality vs. 50 to 75% mortality). These differences in mortality have been ascribed to a more severely ill patient population that was selected by the ECMO entry criteria (criterion 1, or "fast entry": $PaO_2 < 50$ mm Hg for more than 2 hours at FIO_2 of 1.0 and PEEP ≥ 5 cm H_2O; or criterion 2, or "slow entry": $PaO_2 < 50$ mm Hg for more than 12 hours after 48 hours of maximal medical therapy at $FIO_2 = 0.6$ and PEEP ≥ 5 cm H_2O *and* right-to-left shunt $\geq 30\%$ at $FIO_2 = 1.0$ and PEEP ≥ 5 cm H_2O). However, these entry criteria have not been validated as predictors of increased mortality. An alternative reason for the markedly higher mortality rate in the ECMO study might have been differences in associated causes: a much higher prevalence (approximately 60%) of viral pneumonias and death resulting from respiratory failure compared with that in other series.

Extracorporeal Carbon Dioxide Removal (ECCO$_2$R). A hiatus followed the disappointing results of the 1979 ECMO study, after which artificial gas exchange was returned to clinical treatment of adults with ARDS, largely because of efforts of Gattinoni and coworkers.[39] In their approach, the artificial membrane was used during venovenous perfusion by means of femoral or saphenous veins; the membrane's main purpose was to remove carbon dioxide. By doing so, the requirements for minute ventilation were reduced with the aim of preventing overdistention of lung alveoli. The potential for oxygen toxicity was also reduced by providing partial oxygenation across the artificial membrane, as well as by providing apneic oxygenation with nontoxic oxygen concentrations. In some centers in Europe, this technique has become standard therapy for severe ARDS, especially for patients who do not respond to PEEP. The basis for this acceptance was that survival results with ECCO$_2$R exceeded those of the 1979 ECMO study despite use of the same entry criteria. Because of the issues (noted earlier) concerning comparisons among different clinical trials and the use of historical controls, a prospective, randomized clinical trial of ECCO$_2$R was begun in the United States. The preliminary results of this controlled trial demonstrate no survival advantage with ECCO$_2$R compared with the control therapy available, and both groups show survival rates much better (40 to 50%) than those of the 1979 ECMO study despite use of the same entry criteria.[40] It remains to be determined for which subset of ARDS patients, if any, is the use of this expensive technology medically justified.

Reduction of Pulmonary Capillary Hydrostatic Pressure

Whether attributable to ARDS or heart failure, pulmonary edema forms as a passive process by the net effect of the Starling forces across the alveolar capillary membrane. Increased permeability of this membrane in ARDS is represented in the Starling equation both as a higher than normal filtration coefficient (i.e., conductance) and as a lower reflection coefficient for proteins. Under these circumstances, capillary hydrostatic pressure is the predominant force that maintains fluid flow from capillary to alveolar space until the alveoli are virtually filled. The net oncotic pressure gradient opposing this flux is also decreased because of increased oncotic pressure in the alveolar fluid resulting from leakage of plasma into alveoli. The important conclusion from this brief consideration of lung fluid balance in

ARDS is that formation of alveolar edema responds with a higher than normal "gain" to increases in pulmonary capillary hydrostatic pressure. The clinical corollary of this conclusion is that keeping the pulmonary capillary hydrostatic pressure as low as possible should minimize formation of edema in ARDS. However, if this pressure is too low, cardiac output can be jeopardized and end-organ perfusion may be sacrificed. Fluid balance in ARDS can be monitored noninvasively by clinical assessments of daily and cumulative fluid input and output, changes in body weight, and changes in oxygenation and compliance in response to decreasing intravascular volume. Alternatively, invasive monitoring can be done by means of a pulmonary arterial flotation catheter with measurement of pulmonary arterial occlusion pressure and cardiac output and the response of such parameters to diuresis or volume challenges.

Some clinicians advocate reducing pulmonary capillary pressures as standard therapy in ARDS because of the effect on decreasing edema formation. However, the exact role of intravascular volume reduction and the optimal level of pulmonary capillary pressure in the management of ARDS in general remain to be established. Although fluid restriction and reduction of pulmonary capillary pressure as therapy for ARDS have support from several clinical studies,[41–43] no prospective controlled studies with ARDS patients have tested these measures directly. The difficulties of studying fluid balance in ARDS are illustrated by considering one study. In this report, clinical variables of survivors and nonsurvivors were examined retrospectively, and nonsurvivors were distinguished by their having significantly greater positive fluid balance during the initial 24 hours of therapy.[41] However, this study was not designed as an experiment in which fluid administration was controlled, so patients with greater net fluid balance may have been given more fluid simply because it was judged to be clinically indicated. Thus, patients with more severe illness could have received more fluid; this would explain the link between positive fluid balance and the observed higher death rate. Pending conclusive data about optimal fluid balance in ARDS, it seems prudent to reduce pulmonary capillary pressure as long as adequate perfusion of vital organs is maintained. However, it remains to be determined how best to monitor adequacy of perfusion for various organs.

PARADIGM 2: ARDS AS SINGLE-ORGAN FAILURE OF THE LUNG IN THE SUBACUTE PROLIFERATIVE AND FIBROTIC PHASE

Clinical and Pathologic Features

Patients can often be successfully managed through the acute exudative phase of ARDS only to remain dependent on mechanical ventilation until death. They cannot be weaned from the ventilator because of high minute ventilations, they have recurrent infections, and they commonly continue to have signs of inflammation such as fever and leukocytosis. Some of these patients die subsequently of progressive or unremitting respiratory failure, as occurred in patients in the 1979 ECMO study.[38] Others die primarily because of nosocomial pneumonias or sepsis and MOSF while still ventilator dependent.[6, 7] Pathologic studies of lungs from nonsurvivors as early as 1 week after onset of ARDS indicated extensive inflammatory cell infiltration, cellular proliferation, and early fibrosis of the interstitial and alveolar spaces.[12, 14, 20] The presence of hyaline membranes lining alveolar walls and the similarity of these pathologic changes to those observed in experimental oxygen toxicity have suggested that oxygen toxicity may be a major contributing mechanism to development of this phase of lung injury in

ARDS.[13, 20] In addition, patients in this phase of ARDS also appear to be much more susceptible than other types of ventilator-dependent patients to nosocomial pneumonias.[7] These pneumonias prolong ventilator dependence and may eventually result in sepsis and death.

Clinical Management: Specific Therapy

No specific therapy prevents cellular proliferation and pulmonary fibrosis from occurring during this phase. Although steroid therapy has been found to be ineffective in preventing or treating ARDS caused by sepsis as noted earlier,[8, 17] steroid therapy in uncontrolled series appeared to speed resolution of inflammation and epithelial cell proliferation during this phase of ARDS.[44, 45] However, these patients represented a select subset of ARDS patients. Their clinical status corresponded to paradigm 2 of ARDS rather than paradigm 1 or 3 for which steroids have been found to be not only ineffective but also deleterious. Each patient had been systematically assessed before starting steroid therapy to rule out the presence of active infection as the cause of signs of inflammation. However, questions regarding definition of subsets of ARDS patients who might benefit from steroids and the appropriate time to begin such therapy must be answered from controlled clinical trials before these agents can be recommended for any phase of ARDS.

Clinical Management: Supportive Therapy

Respiratory support is continued with special attention (as previously discussed) to avoid pulmonary oxygen toxicity and to prevent pulmonary barotrauma and lung injury caused by overdistention of alveoli. General supportive intensive care principles and approaches should be used during this phase. It is not clear why patients in this phase of ARDS have such a high risk of death resulting from nosocomial infections, especially pneumonias and sepsis, and why appropriate administration of antibiotics has not decreased this risk.[6, 7] Further investigation of the nature of defects in lung defenses will be needed before progress in this aspect of ARDS can be anticipated.

PARADIGM 3: ARDS AS AN INTEGRAL PART OF MULTIPLE ORGAN SYSTEM FAILURE
Clinical and Pathologic Features

In paradigm 2, patients with isolated lung injury frequently manifest MOSF later in the clinical course of illness. In paradigm 3, the reverse occurs: ARDS develops concurrently with or shortly after the onset of MOSF. For example, ARDS occurs in a substantial proportion (10 to 25%)[17, 46] of patients with gram-negative sepsis. Septic shock and MOSF are described more fully in other chapters (Chapters 22 through 28). It is generally accepted that ARDS and MOSF in paradigm 3 occur as manifestations of a generalized permeability defect in the systemic and pulmonary vascular beds resulting from a generalized inflammatory process. The prognosis for patients with sepsis appears to be determined predominantly by the extent and degree of organ system failure and the underlying disorders.[47]

Clinical Management: Specific Therapy
Treatment of Systemic Factors by Anti-Inflammatory Agents

Up to recently, specific treatment of ARDS as part of the syndrome of MOSF has consisted of treatment of the underlying infectious process causing the septic syndrome. Although steroid therapy for established ARDS was not beneficial (as noted earlier), another hypothesis had been that earlier administration of high-dose steroids might improve the outcome of sepsis and septic shock as well as decrease the occurrence of sepsis-induced ARDS. However, clinical trials testing this hypothesis also showed the lack of efficacy of steroid therapy for sepsis per se[48, 49] and the occurrence of ARDS in sepsis was not significantly decreased.[17] Prostaglandin E_1, another anti-inflammatory agent that is also a systemic and pulmonary vasodilator, was found to improve outcomes in a single-center, prospective controlled study of patients who had ARDS with sepsis or postoperative respiratory failure.[50] However, in a multicenter study of prostaglandin E_1 used for patients with sepsis and ARDS, no significant improvement in mortality or in duration of ARDS was found.[4] These negative findings occurred despite significant improvement in oxygen delivery in the treated group compared with controls. These results for prostaglandin E_1 illustrate the need to confirm results for a new therapy in a large multicenter trial to avoid potential selection bias or other types of bias caused by enrolling patients from a single institution.

Other agents besides steroids or prostaglandin E_1 have the potential to modulate the generalized inflammatory reaction in sepsis and its adverse effects. These include cyclooxygenase inhibitors such as ibuprofen, which is currently undergoing a multicenter, controlled clinical trial. Effects of these agents in improving outcome from sepsis with or without ARDS or in preventing sepsis-induced ARDS are currently unknown.

Monoclonal Antibody Therapy of Sepsis

Monoclonal antibody therapy against endotoxin (i.e., monoclonal antibodies with epitopes for the lipid A region of endotoxin) has been effective in decreasing mortality in certain categories of patients with sepsis and gram-negative infections.[46, 51] Despite improvement in survival in these subsets of septic patients, no decrease was observed in the occurrence of ARDS after such therapy. However, one study noted improvement in the resolution rate for dysfunction of several organs including the lungs.[51] These results indicate that the major determinant of mortality in sepsis or septic shock is not ARDS but rather MOSF. Conclusions regarding the relationship of endotoxin, antiendotoxin therapy, and ARDS must be deferred until additional information about basic mediators of ARDS in sepsis are better understood and until results from controlled clinical trials of monoclonal antibodies against other possible mediators, such as tumor necrosis factor, become known.

Clinical Management: Supportive Therapy
Hemodynamic Management and Expansion of Intravascular Volume

Sepsis and MOSF result in increased vascular permeability leading to intravascular hypovolemia. This, in turn, decreases cardiac output by decreasing preload. In ARDS, a similar leakage of plasma occurs from pulmonary capillaries into alveoli. Because of the need to restore intravascular volume, replacement fluid therapy is standard treatment of sepsis and septic shock. However, this treatment also tends to raise pulmonary capillary hydrostatic pressure and cause an increased influx of fluid into the lungs. The clinician managing a patient with septic shock, MOSF, and ARDS must balance the goal of restoring adequate blood volume by volume expansion to treat the septic shock and the goal of limiting, or possibly reducing, pulmonary capillary pressure to treat the ARDS. Accurate fluid monitoring is the first step in responding to this clinical dilemma. Next, fluid therapy should be based on a judgment of whether sepsis or ARDS is the most life-threatening condition. These difficult circumstances have led to different clinical approaches. Some clinicians use volume loading, but not producing pulmonary arterial occlusion pressures greater than 15 cm H_2O, because of the relative ineffectiveness of additional preload to increase cardiac output[52, 53] and because of exacerbation of ARDS at higher pressures. Other clinicians keep pulmonary arterial occlusion pressures lower while increasing cardiac output by other means.[53] Still others continue volume loading and other interventions to increase cardiac function until a supernormal oxygen delivery is achieved.[54] As discussed earlier, although ARDS studies have shown that nonsurvivors, as a group, have a more positive fluid balance than survivors,[41–43] limiting fluid therapy has not been shown to improve survival. The final answer to this issue needs to be determined by prospective controlled clinical studies.

CONCLUSIONS

Until more specific therapy is identified and proved of value in decreasing mortality in ARDS, therapy should be guided by following two therapeutic considerations. First, conventional mechanical ventilation with PEEP should be used to prevent hypoxemia and to limit effects of oxygen toxicity, but with attention to avoiding alveolar overdistention. Second, efforts should be made to achieve a negative fluid balance without compromising oxygen delivery or end-organ function. Nosocomial infections and death resulting from sepsis occurring 1 week to many weeks after the onset of ARDS remain serious problems and indicate that interventions to augment lung defense mechanisms are needed as an important part of the supportive care of the ARDS patient.

The key to uniformly successful therapy of ARDS will ultimately lie in its prevention. This, in turn, will depend on accurate identification of the cause of ARDS and its basic mechanisms at the cellular and molecular levels. In addition, improved knowledge of the basic processes that determine how the lung responds to this type of injury will be essential. Better understanding of how to modulate that response is needed to prevent the lung from evolving along the frequently lethal "final common pathway" that currently typifies ARDS.

References

1. Ashbaugh DG, Bigelow DB, Petty TL, et al: Acute respiratory distress in adults. Lancet 2:319, 1967.
2. Rinaldo JE, Christman JW: Mechanisms and mediators of ARDS. Clin Chest Med 11:621, 1990.
3. Tate RM, Repine JE: Neutrophils and the adult respiratory distress syndrome. Am Rev Respir Dis 128:552, 1983.
4. Bone RC, Slotman G, Maunder R, et al: Randomized double-blind, multicenter study of prostaglandin E_1 in patients with the adult respiratory distress syndrome. Chest 96:114, 1989.
5. Fowler AA, Hamman RF, Good JT, et al: Adult respiratory distress syndrome: Risk with common predispositions. Ann Intern Med 98:593, 1983.
6. Bell RC, Coalson J, Smith JD, et al: Multiple organ failure and infection in adult respiratory distress syndrome. Ann Intern Med 99:293, 1983.
7. Montgomery AB, Stager MA, Carrico J, et al: Causes of mortality in patients with the adult respiratory distress syndrome. Am Rev Respir Dis 132:485, 1985.
8. Bernard GR, Luce JM, Sprung CL, et al: High dose corticosteroids in patients with the adult respiratory distress syndrome: A randomized double-blinded trial. N Engl J Med 317:1565, 1987.
9. Rinaldo JE: The prognosis of the adult respiratory distress syndrome. Chest 90:471, 1986.
10. Murray JF, Mathay MA, Luce J, et al: An expanded definition of the adult respiratory distress syndrome. Am Rev Respir Dis 138:720, 1988.
11. Kapanci Y, Weibel ER, Kaplan HP, et al: Pathogenesis and reversibility of the pulmonary lesions of oxygen toxicity in monkeys. Lab Invest 20:101, 1969.
12. Bachofen M, Weibel ER: Alterations in the gas exchange apparatus in adult respiratory insufficiency associated with septicemia. Am Rev Respir Dis 115:589, 1977.
13. Pratt PC, Vollmer RT, Shelburne JD, et al: Pulmonary morphology in a multihospital collaborative extracorporeal membrane oxygenation project: I. Light microscopy. Am J Pathol 95:191, 1979.
14. de los Santos R, Seidenfeld JJ, Anzueto A, et al: One hundred per cent oxygen lung injury in adult baboons. Am Rev Respir Dis 136:657, 1987.
15. Tomashefski JF: Pulmonary pathology of the adult respiratory distress syndrome. Clin Chest Med 11:593, 1990.
16. Petty L, Ashbaugh DG: Adult respiratory distress syndrome. Chest 60:233, 1971.
17. Bone RC, Fisher CJ Jr, Clemmer TP, et al: Early methylprednisolone treatment for septic syndrome and the adult respiratory distress syndrome. Chest 92:1032, 1987.
18. Venus B, Jacobs HK, Lim L: Treatment of the adult respiratory distress syndrome with continuous positive airway pressure. Chest 76:257, 1979.
19. Elliot CG, Rasmusson BY, Crapo RO, et al: Prediction of pulmonary function abnormalities after adult respiratory distress syndrome (ARDS). Am Rev Respir Dis 135:634, 1987.
20. Lamy M, Fallat RJ, Koeniger E, et al: Pathologic features and mechanisms of hypoxemia in adult respiratory distress syndrome. Am Rev Respir Dis 114:267, 1976.
21. Falke K, Pontoppidan H, Kumar A, et al: Ventilation with end-expiratory pressure in acute lung disease. J Clin Invest 51:2315, 1972.
22. Ranieri VM, Eissa NT, Corbeil C, et al: Effects of positive end-expiratory pressure on alveolar recruitment and gas exchange in patients with the adult respiratory distress syndrome. Am Rev Respir Dis 144:544, 1991.
23. Suter PM, Fairley HB, Isenberg MD: Optimum end-expiratory airway pressure in patients with acute pulmonary failure. N Engl J Med 292:284, 1975.
24. Jardin F, Farcot JC, Boisante L, et al: Influence of positive end-expiratory pressure on left ventricular performance. N Engl J Med 304:387, 1981.
25. Gattinoni L, Pesenti A, Bombino M, et al: Relationships between lung computed tomographic density, gas exchange, and PEEP in acute respiratory failure. Anesthesiology 69:812, 1988.
26. Maunder RJ, Shuman WP, McHugh JW, et al: Preservation of normal lung regions in the adult respiratory distress syndrome. JAMA 255:2463, 1986.
27. Kolobow R, Moretti MP, Gumagalli R, et al: Severe impairment in lung function induced by high peak airway pressure during mechanical ventilation. An experimental study. Am Rev Respir Dis 135:312, 1987.
28. Dreyfuss D, Soler P, Basset G, et al: High inflation pressure pulmonary edema: Respective effects of high airway pressure, high tidal volume and positive end-expiratory pressure (PEEP). Am Rev Respir Dis 137:1159, 1988.
29. Tharatt RS, Allen RP, Albertson TE: Pressure controlled inverse ratio ventilation in severe adult respiratory failure. Chest 94:755, 1988.
30. Marcy TW, Marini JJ: Inverse ratio ventilation in ARDS. Chest 100:495, 1991.
31. Darioli R, Perret C: Mechanical controlled hypoventilation in status asthmaticus. Am Rev Respir Dis 129:385, 1984.
32. Johnston WE, Vinten-Johansen J, Strickland RA, et al: Hypothermia with and without end-expiratory pressure in canine oleic pulmonary edema. Am Rev Respir Dis 140:110, 1989.
33. Hurst JM, DeHaven CB, Branson R, et al: Combined use of high-frequency jet ventilation and induced hypothermia in the treatment of refractory respiratory failure. Crit Care Med 13:771, 1985.
34. Merritt TA, Hallman M, Bloom BT, et al: Prophylactic treatment of very premature infants with human surfactant. N Engl J Med 315:785, 1986.
35. Ikegami M, Kaneda M, and Nozaki M: A protein inhibitor of surfactant in the airways of patients with adult respiratory distress syndrome. Am Rev Respir Dis 131:135, 1985.
36. Slutsky AS: Nonconventional methods of ventilation. Am Rev Respir Dis 138:175, 1988.
37. Albelda SM, Hansen-Flaschen JH, Taylor E, et al: Evaluation of high-frequency jet ventilation in patients with bronchopleural fistulas by quantitation of the airleak. Anesthesiology 63:551, 1985.
38. Zapol WM, Snider MT, Hill JD, et al: Extracorporeal membrane oxygenation in severe acute respiratory failure. A randomized prospective study. JAMA 242:2193, 1979.
39. Gattinoni L, Pesenti A, Mascheroni D, et al: Low frequency positive-pressure ventilation with extracorporeal CO_2 removal in severe acute respiratory failure. JAMA 256:881, 1986.
40. Suchyta MR, Clemmer TP, Orme JF, et al: Increased survival of ARDS patients with severe hypoxemia (ECMO criteria). Chest 99:951, 1991.
41. Simmons RS, Berdine GG, Seidenfeld JJ, et al: Fluid balance and the adult respiratory distress syndrome. Am Rev Respir Dis 132:485, 1987.
42. Humphrey HJ, Hall J, Sznajder JI, et al: Improved survival following pulmonary capillary wedge pressure reduction in patients with ARDS. Chest 97:1176, 1990.
43. Schuller D, Mitchell JP, Calandrino FS, et al: Fluid balance during

pulmonary edema; Is fluid gain a marker or a cause of poor outcome? Chest 100:1068, 1991.

44. Hooper RG, Kearl RA: Established ARDS treated with a sustained course of adrenocortical steroids. Chest 97:138, 1990.

45. Meduri GU, Belenchia JM, Estes RJ, et al: Fibroproliferative phase of ARDS; Clinical findings and effects of corticosteroids. Chest 100:943, 1991.

46. Ziegler EJ, Fisher CJ Jr, Sprung CL, et al: Treatment of gram-negative bacteremia and septic shock with HA-1A human monoclonal antibody against endotoxin. N Engl J Med 324:429, 1991.

47. Knaus WA, Wagner DP: Multiple systems organ failure: epidemiology and prognosis. Crit Care Clin 5:221, 1989.

48. Bone RC, Fisher CJ Jr, Clemmer TP, et al: A controlled clinical trial of high-dose methylprednisolone in the treatment of severe sepsis and septic shock. N Engl J Med 317:659, 1987.

49. Veterans Administration Systemic Sepsis Cooperative Study Group: Effect of high-dose glucocorticoid therapy on mortality in patients with clinical signs of systemic sepsis. N Engl J Med 317:659, 1987.

50. Holcroft JW, Vassar MJ, Weber CJ: Prostaglandin E₁ and survival in patients with the adult respiratory distress syndrome: A prospective trial. Ann Surg 203:371, 1986.

51. Greenman RL, Schein RMH, Martin MA, et al: A controlled clinical trial of E5 murine monoclonal IgM antibody to endotoxin in the treatment of gram-negative sepsis. JAMA 266:1097, 1991.

52. Ognibene FP, Parker MM, Natanson C, et al: Depressed left ventricular performance: Response to volume infusion in patients with sepsis and septic shock. Chest 93:903, 1988.

53. Prewitt RM, Matthay MA, Ghignone M: Hemodynamic management in the adult respiratory distress syndrome. Clin Chest Med 4:251, 1983.

54. Shoemaker WC, Appel PL, Kram HB: Prospective trial of supranormal values of survivors as therapeutic goals in high risk surgical patients. Chest 94:1176, 1988.

55. Wachter RM, Luce JM, Turner J, et al: Intensive care of patients with the acquired immunodeficiency syndrome. Outcome and changing patterns of utilization. Am Rev Respir Dis 134:891, 1986.

56. Schuster DP, Marion JM: Precedents for meaningful recovery during treatment in a medical intensive care unit: Outcome in patients with hematologic malignancy. Am J Med 75:402, 1983.

57. Matuschak GM, Rinaldo JE, Pinsky MR, et al: Effect of end stage liver failure on the incidence and resolution of the adult respiratory distress syndrome. J Crit Care 2:162, 1987.

58. Schonfeld SA, Ploysongsang Y, DiLisio R, et al: Fat embolism prophylaxis with corticosteroids. Ann Intern Med 99:438, 1983.

59. Pontoppidan H, Huttemeier PC, Quinn DA: Etiology, demography, and outcome. In: Falke KJ, Zapol WM (eds): Acute Respiratory Failure. New York, Marcel Dekker, p 1, 1985.

CHAPTER 74

Pulmonary Hypertension and Right-Sided Heart Failure

Harold I. Palevsky

Pulmonary hypertension and resulting right-sided heart failure are frequent problems in the critical care setting. Usually occurring as a consequence of exacerbations of an underlying disease processes, these conditions contribute significantly to morbidity and mortality of patients.

Cor pulmonale is a term used to denote enlargement of the right ventricle by hypertrophy and/or dilation as a consequence of processes not primarily involving the heart. Although most often caused by airway processes or parenchymal lung disease, cor pulmonale may also develop as a result of disorders of ventilatory drive (in the setting of normal lungs), abnormalities of the respiratory bellows (e.g., disorders of the thoracic cage, neuromuscular disorders), or processes directly affecting the pulmonary vascular bed. Invariably, in cor pulmonale, pulmonary hypertension develops before right ventricular failure. In chronic conditions, both hypertrophy and dilation contribute to right ventricular enlargement; in acute conditions, dilation predominates because of insufficient time for hypertrophy to occur. In most cases, if the pulmonary hypertension causing an increased right ventricular afterload is not relieved, eventually right ventricular failure results.

This chapter briefly reviews the physiology and pathogenesis of pulmonary hypertension. The most common causes of pulmonary hypertension and cor pulmonale are presented, along with an approach to the evaluation for pulmonary vascular disease. Finally, both standard and newer treatment options for pulmonary hypertension and right-sided heart failure are discussed.

NORMAL PULMONARY CIRCULATION

The pulmonary circulation is normally a high-capacitance, low-resistance circuit. It is unique among the organ vascular beds in that it accommodates the entire cardiac output and is largely passive, lacking elaborate mechanisms for autoregulation of its blood pressure. Through vascular recruitment and distention, the normal pulmonary circulation can accommodate several multiples of resting cardiac output with only slight increments in pulmonary arterial pressure.

Although low, the normal pulsatile pulmonary arterial pressure is sufficient to overcome pulmonary vascular resistance and to keep pulmonary blood flow equal to systemic blood flow. The normal pulmonary blood flow is accomplished with an average pressure drop (in mean pressure) of only 5 to 10 mm Hg between the pulmonary artery and the left atrium (Table 74–1). For normal subjects younger than the age of 40 years, even during exercise, the upper limit of mean pulmonary arterial pressure at sea level is 30 mm Hg. In well-trained athletes achieving cardiac outputs greater than 20 L/min, mean pulmonary arterial pressures may be higher.[1]

Owing to the contribution of hypoxemia to resting pulmonary arterial tone, the criteria for defining pulmonary hypertension depend on altitude; at sea level, a resting mean pulmonary arterial pressure greater than 20 mm Hg is considered abnormal; at an altitude of 15,000 ft, the normal range for mean pulmonary arterial pressure extends to 25 mm Hg. Mild resting pulmonary hypertension at sea level generally signifies a limitation of the pulmonary vascular tree and/or an elevated pulmonary blood flow. In general, the minimally abnormal pulmonary arterial pressures increase significantly when either vascular tone or blood flow increases (e.g., during acute hypoxia or exertion). These pressures are important only in terms of the strain imposed on the right ventricle, and intermittent increases in right ventricular afterload may be of lesser significance than sustained increases. However, over time, even intermittent imposition of strain on the right ventricle results in muscular hypertrophy and possibly eventuates in heart failure.

Often, pulmonary hypertension is not diagnosed until an explanation is sought for right ventricular hypertrophy or right-sided heart failure. The normal right ventricle can generate systolic pressures up to approximately 50 mm Hg in response to an acute increase in afterload. If the afterload has developed gradually so that the right ventricle has had time to hypertrophy, it can generate substantially higher pressures, even up to systemic arterial pressure levels. How-

TABLE 74–1

NORMAL HEMODYNAMIC VALUES AT SEA LEVEL

Parameter	At Rest	During Moderate Exercise
Cardiac output (L/min)	6	16
Heart rate (beats/min)	80	130
Right atrial pressure (mm Hg)	4–6	6–8
Pulmonary arterial pressures (mm Hg)		
Systolic	20–25	30–35
Diastolic	10–12	11–14
Mean	14–18	20–25
Pulmonary wedge pressure (mm Hg)	6–10	10–14
Systemic arterial pressure (mm Hg)	120/80	150/95
Mean	90–100	110–120
Pulmonary vascular resistance (U)	0.7–1	0.6–0.9

ever, if the elevated afterload is maintained, it is likely that the ventricle will ultimately fail.

The pressure drop across the pulmonary vascular bed is frequently related to the pulmonary blood flow (cardiac output) using an equation analogous to Ohm's law:

Pulmonary vascular resistance =

$$\frac{\text{mean pulmonary arterial} - \text{pulmonary arterial wedge}}{\text{pulmonary blood flow (L/min)}}$$
$$\frac{\text{pressure (mm Hg)} \quad \text{pressure (mm Hg)}}{\text{pulmonary blood flow (L/min)}}$$

Expressed this way, the normal pulmonary vascular resistance is approximately 1 U. Resistance may also be expressed in dyne • s/cm[5] by multiplying the numerator of this equation by 80; expressed in this way, normal pulmonary vascular resistance is approximately 50 to 100 dyne • s/cm.[5]

However, this resistance equation, adapted from Poiseuille's law, is based on the laminar flow of a newtonian fluid through rigid tubes and does not readily apply to the pulmonary circulation. The normal pulmonary vascular bed is composed of elastic, distensible vessels, not rigid tubes; they change in diameter with changes in pulmonary blood volume, flow, and pressure.[2] In addition, pulmonary blood flow is pulsatile and turbulent rather than laminar. The pulmonary blood volume is altered by changes in blood flow, transthoracic pressures, and the gravitational effects of posture. Because blood is a non-newtonian fluid, its apparent viscosity changes with different flow velocities. The resistance equation seems to be most applicable to the abnormal pulmonary circulation in which vessel walls are thickened and have become more rigid; it may not accurately describe the highly distensible, normal pulmonary circulation.

Because the relationship between pressure and flow in the normal pulmonary circulation is not linear, resistance is not a constant but varies with the flow through the system, with the pressure drop across the pulmonary circulation, and with the other factors noted earlier. This complicates interpretation of calculated values for pulmonary vascular resistance, especially in evaluating the effect of a therapeutic intervention on the pulmonary circulation. The substitution of mean pulmonary arterial pressure for the pressure drop between the pulmonary artery and the left atrium in the numerator of the resistance equation deprives the calculation of any physiologic meaning.

Comparing changes in the calculated pulmonary vascular resistance can also be problematic; the same degree of change may have different physiologic significance. For example, a decrease in calculated pulmonary vascular resistance caused by an increased cardiac output in association with a decrease in pulmonary arterial pressure and a stable

heart rate is a more desirable clinical state than is an equivalent decrease in pulmonary vascular resistance resulting from a greater increase in cardiac output, an unchanged pulmonary arterial pressure, and tachycardia.

PATHOGENESIS OF PULMONARY HYPERTENSION

Although changes in left-sided heart filling pressure, cardiac output, heart rate, hematocrit, and blood volume may all contribute to the development of pulmonary hypertension, the major contributing factor is an elevation in the pulmonary vascular resistance, localized primarily to the precapillary arteries and arterioles. This increase in vascular resistance may be anatomic or vasoconstrictive in origin; often, both mechanisms are involved. Regardless of cause, when the pulmonary vascular reserve is compromised by a progressive reduction in the extent and/or the distensibility of the pulmonary vascular bed, it is initially observed that increases in cardiac output result in pulmonary hypertension. Over time, lesser and lesser increments in pulmonary blood flow (cardiac output) are required to raise the pulmonary arterial pressures. Eventually, even the resting cardiac output produces elevated pulmonary arterial pressures.

Oxygen Tensions

The most potent stimulus for pulmonary vasoconstriction is alveolar hypoxia, acting on the adjacent small pulmonary arteries and arterioles. The mediators involved in transducing the response are as yet not identified. Systemic arterial hypoxemia augments the local effects of alveolar hypoxia indirectly by way of sympathetic neural reflexes.[3] In chronic hypoxemia, the effects of these pulmonary vasoconstrictive stimuli are often augmented by increased blood viscosity caused by secondary polycythemia. Episodic exacerbations of hypoxemia result in progressive pulmonary vascular impairment and may lead to development of sustained pulmonary hypertension, even though recovery from early episodes is frequently associated with the return of pulmonary arterial pressures to normal levels.[4]

Acid-Base Status

Acidosis (pH < 7.2) also elicits pulmonary vasoconstriction. In humans, acidosis acts synergistically with hypoxia, whereas alkalosis diminishes the vasoconstrictive response to hypoxia.[2] The biologic basis of this is not understood.

Carbon Dioxide

Unlike the situation in hypoxia, carbon dioxide appears to contribute to pulmonary hypertension by way of the acidosis generated by carbon dioxide retention rather than by direct vasoconstriction.[2] Carbon dioxide retention may be self-perpetuating; hypercapnia blunts the responsiveness of respiratory centers to carbon dioxide and promotes retention of bicarbonate by the kidney.[5] Not only the hypercapnia resulting from disorders of the lungs or ventilation, but also that seen in response to metabolic alkalosis, results in ventilatory depression, with consequent progressive hypercapnia, hypoxia, and pulmonary vasoconstriction.

Mediators of Vascular Tone

Investigations into the mechanisms by which vascular smooth muscle tone is regulated have placed renewed emphasis on the role of the pulmonary endothelium in the uptake and metabolism of vasoactive compounds and have led to the description of potent mediators of both vasodilation and vasoconstriction.

Among the compounds described, prostacyclin (prostaglandin I_2), the predominant metabolite of arachidonic acid, appears to play an important role in the local modulation of vascular tone.[6] Endothelium-derived relaxing factor is a product of the intact vascular endothelium and acts on adjacent vascular smooth muscle. After intensive efforts to characterize endothelium-derived relaxing factor, it appears that it may be the short-lived, diffusible, free radical nitroxide (NO•), which acts by stimulating guanylate cyclase in the smooth muscle to increase cyclic guanosine monophosphate levels.[7, 7a]

Endothelins, a family of 21-amino-acid peptides, are circulating hormones with potent smooth muscle constrictive effects.[8] These compounds are produced by both pulmonary vascular endothelial cells and bronchiolar respiratory epithelial cells and, in experimental preparations, can cause both significant pulmonary vasoconstriction and airway smooth muscle constriction. There is speculation that endothelin may be the mediator of hypoxic pulmonary vasoconstriction.[9, 9a]

Although not yet a consideration in management of patients, additional mediators of vascular tone will certainly be identified in the future, and modification of the balance between the mediators of vasodilation and vasoconstriction will be of clinical relevance.

Histologic Changes in Microvasculature

Histologic changes occurring either as an initiating process or as a consequence of increased flow, pressure, or sheer stress within the pulmonary microvasculature contribute to the maintenance and progression of pulmonary vascular disease.[10] Changes can be observed within the media, the intima, the lumen, or any combination of these locations. Up to a point, the microvascular changes are likely to be reversible if the inciting mechanism can be removed; however, eventually a point is reached when the microvascular changes become fixed.[11, 12]

Compounding the contributions of proliferative histologic changes in the pulmonary microvascular bed to increasing the pulmonary vascular resistance is the occurrence of in situ thrombosis. Observed in pulmonary hypertensive states regardless of cause, this is likely a consequence of alterations in endothelial function reducing local fibrinolytic activity and/or release of inhibitors of platelet activation (e.g., prostacyclin), as well as endothelial injury predisposing to platelet deposition and the initiation of thrombosis.[13, 14] The frequency of microvascular thrombosis led to the suggestion that anticoagulation, or the use of inhibitors of platelet activation, may have a role in all patients with pulmonary vascular disease, regardless of the pathogenesis of the process.[14]

CAUSES OF PULMONARY HYPERTENSION AND COR PULMONALE

Pulmonary hypertension occurs far more commonly as a consequence of an identifiable and concurrent disease process than as primary (unexplained or idiopathic) pulmonary hypertension. The mechanisms by which these underlying conditions cause pulmonary hypertension vary considerably (Table 74–2): heart diseases cause increased pulmonary venous pressure, or increased pulmonary blood flow; in contrast, parenchymal lung diseases and thromboembolic disease obliterate or obstruct segments of the pulmonary vascular bed.

TABLE 74–2

CAUSES OF PULMONARY HYPERTENSION

Hyperkinetic
  Intracardiac shunt lesions
    Atrial septal defect, ventricular septal defect, anomalous venous return (total and partial)
  Pulmonary arteriovenous fistulas

Passive
  Elevated left ventricular end-diastolic pressure
    Coronary heart disease, cardiomyopathy, aortic valve disease, constrictive pericarditis
  Mitral valve stenosis or obstruction
  Left atrial obstruction
    Myxoma, neoplasm, thrombus
    Pulmonary venous obstruction
    Neoplasm, adenopathy, fibrosing mediastinitis

Obliterative
  Pulmonary parenchymal disease
    Obstruction (bronchitis, emphysema, bronchiectasis)
    Restrictive physiology (fibrosis of any causes, thoracic cage abnormalities)
  Pulmonary arteritis
    Scleroderma, systemic lupus erythematosus, other collagen-vascular disease and vasculitis, schistosomiasis

Obstructive
  Pulmonary embolism—acute and chronic
    Venous thromboemboli, tumor emboli
  Pulmonary arterial thrombosis
    Sickle cell disease, Eisenmenger's sydrome (e.g., tetralogy of Fallot)

Vasoconstrictive
  Hypoxemia
    Sleep apnea syndromes, neuromuscular disorders, high-altitude disease

Idiopathic
  Primary pulmonary hypertension, including pulmonary veno-occlusive disease (small intrapulmonary veins)
  Diet-related pulmonary hypertension (e.g., aminorex, toxic oil syndrome)
  Coexistent portal and pulmonary hypertension
  Persistent fetal circulation

Congenital Heart Disease

Congenital cardiac defects that result in persistent left-to-right shunting within the heart or between the great vessels often cause pulmonary hypertension.[15, 16] Because acute left-to-right shunts and the intermittent increases in cardiac output seen with exercise do not cause appreciable pulmonary hypertension in normal lungs, factors other than the level of pulmonary blood flow have been invoked to explain the pulmonary hypertension seen in chronic left-to-right shunts. The duration and persistence of the hemodynamic abnormalities, secondary morphologic changes occurring within the pulmonary vasculature, reflex pulmonary vasoconstriction induced by distention of pulmonary veins or the left atrium, and coexisting hypoxemia have all been proposed as contributing factors. Depending on the congenital cardiac defect, and whether increased pulmonary blood pressure or blood flow is the major abnormality, the intima or media of the pulmonary vessels may be primarily affected. With the persistence of the hemodynamic abnormalities, these secondary changes in the pulmonary resistance vessels may become the dominant mechanism for sustaining the pulmonary hypertension and in determining its reversibility.[11]

Acquired Disorders of the Left Side of the Heart

Passive pulmonary hypertension occurs as a consequence of an increase in the outflow pressure required of the pulmonary circulation (e.g., from the increase in left atrial and left ventricular end-diastolic pressure in congestive heart failure, or from the increase in left atrial pressure in mitral stenosis). Over time, a reactive (vasoconstrictive) process augments this passive component, further increasing the pulmonary vascular resistance and the magnitude of the pulmonary hypertension.[17] Histologic changes occurring in the pulmonary vascular bed as a consequence of elevated pressures may cause the pulmonary hypertension to become fixed. These secondary structural changes occur initially in the pulmonary venous microcirculation and then develop in the pulmonary arterial beds. Prominent among the histologic findings are (1) intimal and/or medial hypertrophy that progresses to fibrosis of the pulmonary veins and venules that is followed by similar changes in the muscular pulmonary arteries and arterioles; (2) perivascular interstitial edema exhibiting a gravitational dependence, which not only increases pulmonary vascular resistance but also stimulates perivascular fibrosis; (3) occlusion of small pulmonary vessels by in situ thrombi, occurring as a consequence of slow pulmonary blood flow and damage to the pulmonary microvascular endothelium. Treatment of the cause of pulmonary venous hypertension may reduce pulmonary venous and arterial pressures and allows for regression of the reversible components of the secondary vascular changes.[17]

Left ventricular failure is a common cause of passive pulmonary hypertension and also of right ventricular failure. However, in most cases, the degree of pulmonary hypertension present is not sufficient to account for the development or the severity of the right-sided heart failure. This discrepancy between the apparent afterload of the right ventricle and the development of right-sided heart failure may, in part, be due to involvement of the right ventricle and especially the intraventricular septum by the pathologic process that is affecting the left ventricle.

Pulmonary Venous Disease

Obstruction of the large pulmonary veins as they enter or course through the mediastinum may result from entrapment in a neoplastic or inflammatory process or from compression by enlarged lymph nodes. Causes of this obstruction include primary or metastatic neoplasm (e.g., lymphoma and breast or lung carcinoma), infection (e.g., tuberculosis and histoplasmosis), inflammatory processes that affect lymph nodes or the mediastinum (e.g., sarcoidosis and sequelae of radiation therapy), or uncertain sources (e.g., fibrosing mediastinitis). This obstruction of the central pulmonary veins results in a passive form of pulmonary hypertension, with resultant histologic changes developing in the microvascular beds similar to those described earlier in acquired cardiac disease. Although this form of secondary pulmonary hypertension, with obstruction of the large pulmonary veins resulting from a structural cause is often referred to as pulmonary veno-occlusive disease, it should be distinguished from unexplained (primary or idiopathic) pulmonary veno-occlusive disease. In this latter condition, the small pulmonary veins and venules are directly affected by an inflammatory process of unknown etiology that leads to luminal compromise and fibrosis.

Obstructive Airways Disease

Chronic obstructive airways disease (chronic obstructive pulmonary disease, chronic bronchitis and emphysema) is the leading cause of pulmonary hypertension and cor pulmonale in the United States. The pulmonary hypertension develops primarily as a consequence of the alveolar and arterial hypoxemia resulting from alterations in ventilation-perfusion relationships. Characteristically, the pulmonary hypertension occurs in two different patterns: episodically during an acute respiratory tract infection in the patient with emphysema and chronically in the patient with chronic bronchitis. It is frequent that, in patients first seen during an exacerbation of their respiratory disease, clinical distinction between chronic bronchitis and emphysema may be difficult.

Chronic bronchitis and emphysema often coexist with the component of chronic bronchitis predominantly responsible for the alveolar hypoxia and the low Po_2, high Pco_2, and resultant low pH that produce pulmonary hypertension. Emphysema contributes to the development of pulmonary hypertension through obliteration of segments of the pulmonary vascular bed. However, in most cases, emphysema alone does not result in pulmonary hypertension, even when involvement of the lungs is extensive, because of the distensibility of the remaining portions of the pulmonary vascular bed, because of limitations of the exercise-related increases in cardiac output imposed by the patient's lung disease, and because ventilation-perfusion relationships are not as severely disturbed as in chronic bronchitis.

Interstitial Lung Disease

Interstitial lung disease can result from a wide variety of diffuse processes such as sarcoidosis, asbestosis, radiation pneumonitis, and many of the collagen-vascular diseases, or it can be idiopathic. Common to these disorders is an interstitial cellular inflammation leading to parenchymal fibrosis and a restrictive ventilatory defect, with diminished lung volumes and relatively normal airflow. The inflammatory infiltrate entraps and eventually destroys the microvasculature, decreasing the capacity of the pulmonary vascular bed and limiting the distensibility of the remaining vessels, thus increasing the pulmonary vascular resistance. Over time, these changes, coupled with closure of peripheral airways by the peribronchiolar inflammatory process, result in arterial hypoxemia and accelerate the progression of pulmonary hypertension to right ventricular failure.

Alveolar Hypoventilation in Patients with Normal Lungs

Pulmonary hypertension may develop in individuals who demonstrate alveolar hypoventilation despite normal lungs and gas exchange. As in patients with ventilation-perfusion abnormalities, the important pathogenetic factors appear to be alveolar hypoxia, arterial hypoxemia and hypercapnia, and respiratory acidosis. The alveolar hypoventilation in these patients originates in either an inadequate ventilatory drive or an ineffective respiratory muscle pump (chest bellows). Disorders associated with alveolar hypoventilation include the sleep apnea syndromes, neuromuscular disorders (e.g., myasthenia gravis, Guillain-Barré syndrome, and many of the muscular dystrophies), central respiratory drive impairment (e.g., after a cerebrovascular accident, Ondine's curse), thoracic cage abnormalities (e.g., kyphoscoliosis), and extreme obesity.

The clinical presentation is determined by the cause and pathogenesis of the alveolar hypoventilation. In sleep apnea syndromes, alveolar hypoxia, arterial hypoxemia, and hypercapnia are initially manifested only during sleep. In neuromuscular disorders and thoracic cage abnormalities, alveolar hypoxia and arterial hypoxemia (and hypercapnia) may appear initially only during exertion (or in some instances during sleep), when ventilation fails to keep pace with metabolic demand. In both groups of patients, blood gas tensions may be normal while the patient is awake and at rest; over time, the patient's status deteriorates and resting blood gas tensions remain abnormal. Pulmonary hypertension may initially be present only when hypoxia is present; over time, it becomes persistent.

Treatment is directed toward the pathogenesis of the alveolar hypoventilation. In the neuromuscular disorders and in kyphoscoliosis, some success has been achieved by resting the respiratory muscles at night using negative-pressure (cuirass-type) ventilators or, more recently, ventilation using specialized nasal masks. This prevents chronic fatigue of the respiratory muscles and appears to minimize alveolar hypoventilation, even during daytime. In the obstructive sleep apnea syndromes, preventing obstruction through use of nasal continuous positive airway pressure or a tracheostomy eliminates the arterial hypoxemia and its cardiopulmonary consequences. In other conditions in which specific therapies are not available, the use of supplemental oxygen to prevent hypoxia and arterial hypoxemia is often of benefit.

Collagen-Vascular Diseases

Pulmonary vascular disease is an important clinical component of many collagen-vascular diseases, most frequently being seen in systemic lupus erythematosus and in progressive systemic sclerosis (scleroderma) and its variant syndromes. In these patients, pulmonary hypertension usually develops as a consequence of interstitial inflammation, interstitial fibrosis, or pulmonary vasculitis.[18-21] However, in some patients, the pulmonary interstitium appears to be uninvolved and the histologic lesions in the pulmonary vessels resemble those of primary pulmonary hypertension. This observation led to speculation that some patients with primary pulmonary hypertension represent cases of collagen-vascular disease (particularly scleroderma and its variants) confined to the pulmonary vasculature. This hypothesis is supported by the similarities in pulmonary vascular histologic findings, by similar age and sex distribution of the patients, and by the high frequency of Raynaud's phenomenon and antinuclear antibodies in patients with primary pulmonary hypertension.[22] An alternative hypothesis is that, in some of these patients, the occurrence of pulmonary hypertension and Raynaud's phenomenon represents a generalized vasoconstrictive disorder affecting both the systemic and pulmonary vascular beds. Although it is possible to demonstrate a pulmonary vasoconstrictor response in some patients with Raynaud's phenomenon, the clinical significance of this finding remains uncertain.[23]

Systemic Lupus Erythematosus

Systemic lupus erythematosus is a multisystem disease of unknown cause that is characterized by autoantibodies and circulating immune complexes; inflammatory changes occur in the connective tissues, in the blood vessels, and on serosal surfaces. The lungs and the pleura are involved more frequently in lupus than in other connective tissue diseases; the reported incidence being up to 70%. The high incidence of pulmonary hypertension occurring in systemic lupus erythematosus, as well as its frequent progression to right-sided heart failure, has been noted. A 10:1 female-to-male predominance has been reported in the cases of pulmonary hypertension associated with systemic lupus erythematosus; most of the patients also have been found to exhibit Raynaud's phenomenon.[18]

The histopathologic lesions in patients with lupus usually resemble those of primary pulmonary hypertension; vasculitis and extensive immune complex deposition are rare. This pulmonary hypertension has also been attributed to microthrombi developing as a consequence of the hypercoagulable state that occurs in the presence of circulating anticardiolipin antibodies; however, this is not a universal finding. Unfortunately, as in primary pulmonary hypertension, treatment of pulmonary hypertension associated with systemic lupus erythematosus using either anticoagulants or pulmonary vasodilators has had only modest success.

Progressive Systemic Sclerosis (Scleroderma)

Progressive systemic sclerosis (scleroderma) and its variants (e.g., the CREST [calcinosis cutis, Raynaud's phenomenon, esophageal dysfunction, sclerodactyly, and telangiectasia] syndrome, and associated overlap syndromes) have a high incidence of pulmonary vascular disease with considerable morbidity and mortality from the resultant pulmonary hypertension.[20, 24] The CREST syndrome variant of scleroderma was initially thought to be relatively benign, with little visceral involvement. However, long-term follow-up studies have shown a substantial incidence of pulmonary vascular involvement in these patients. In one prospective study involving cardiac catheterization of patients with progressive systemic sclerosis or the CREST syndrome variant, pulmonary hypertension, either as an isolated finding or in association with pulmonary parenchymal or cardiac disease, was found in up to one third of patients with progressive systemic sclerosis, and in up to one half of patients with the CREST syndrome.[24] The pulmonary vascular disease may be independent of pulmonary parenchymal or other visceral diseases; its occurrence is associated with a marked reduction in survival.[20] As in the case of systemic lupus erythematosus, the pathologic changes of these lesions are often indistinguishable from those of primary pulmonary hypertension.

Pulmonary Thromboembolic Disease

Pulmonary hypertension occurs as a consequence of both acute and chronic (unresolved) pulmonary thromboembolism. Acute pulmonary thromboembolism is reviewed in Chapter 75. Chronic thromboembolic occlusion of the pulmonary vasculature remains misdiagnosed and misunderstood and consists of two distinct syndromes with quite different patterns of vascular involvement, different pathogenetic mechanisms, and different therapeutic options.[25] The first syndrome is in situ thrombotic occlusion of small pulmonary arteries; the second is chronic (unresolved) thromboembolic occlusion of large pulmonary arteries.

Thrombotic Occlusion of Precapillary Pulmonary Microvasculature

Thrombotic and recanalized lesions of the small muscular pulmonary arteries and pulmonary arterioles are found in histologic specimens from patients with pulmonary hypertension of any cause. They have also been classified as one of the histologic subtypes of primary pulmonary hypertension (Table 74–3). These microvascular lesions are found in the absence of a detectable source of embolization and in the absence of emboli in the larger pulmonary vessels. In the past, these thrombotic and recanalized lesions were attributed to one or more showers of microemboli. However, it is more likely that they are the result of in situ thrombosis rather than multiple pulmonary emboli. This in situ thrombosis occurs as a consequence of injury to the pulmonary microvascular endothelium by high intravascular pressures

TABLE 74–3
HISTOLOGIC LESIONS OF PRIMARY PULMONARY HYPERTENSION*

1. Primary pulmonary arteriopathy with
   a. Plexiform lesions (with or without thrombotic lesions)
   b. Thrombotic lesions
   c. Isolated medial hypertrophy
   d. Intimal fibrosis and medial hypertrophy
   e. Isolated arteritis
2. Pulmonary veno-occlusive disease
3. Pulmonary capillary hemangiomatosis

*Classification schema of National Heart, Lung, and Blood Institute Primary Pulmonary Hypertension Registry.[27]

and flows, resulting in alterations in the local balance between coagulation and fibrinolysis, and/or platelet aggregation on the injured microvascular endothelium.

Histologic proof of the presence of microthrombi in the pulmonary vascular bed does not appear to be necessary for management of patients. On lung scan, patients with microthromboemboli demonstrate patchy inhomogeneity in their perfusion pattern without defects that correspond to anatomic segments or subsegments; pulmonary angiography is unnecessary and cannot detect thrombi in vessels of this small caliber. Treatment is often empirical and consists of long-term anticoagulation with warfarin-type agents and/or the administration of antiplatelet agents. Because these lesions are so common, it has been suggested that all patients with pulmonary hypertension be treated for microthrombi. Vasodilators have also been advocated, even though, as in other forms of pulmonary hypertension, appreciable benefit is infrequent.

Chronic Proximal Pulmonary Thromboembolism

This clinical syndrome is a result of occlusion of portions of the proximal pulmonary arterial tree by organized thrombotic material.[25] It is still uncertain whether this obstruction is due to recurrent, unrecognized pulmonary emboli occurring over years, or to a single embolic event that, instead of lysing, propagates and organizes. The latter scenario is more likely. Failure of local fibrinolytic mechanisms apparently allows the clot to propagate (antegrade and retrograde), to obstruct portions of the pulmonary vascular bed, and to decrease the compliance of the central pulmonary vessels. By the time that the diagnosis is made, the obstructing material has become organized and fibrotic and no longer resembles an acute thrombus.

It is important to recognize this cause of pulmonary hypertension because of the availability of specific surgical therapy.[26–28] Ventilation-perfusion lung scanning is the cornerstone of screening for this diagnosis. All patients with pulmonary hypertension of uncertain cause should undergo lung scans. Perfusion defects that are segmental or larger necessitate proceeding with pulmonary angiography. Selective contrast pulmonary angiography is the current standard for diagnosis, because perfusion lung scans underestimate both the number and the extent of thromboembolic lesions. This is particularly true when the organized thromboembolic material is not obstructing a vessel but is adherent to the vessel wall, compromising luminal diameter and vascular compliance. Identification of the precise location and extent of the organized clot is necessary for decisions as to suitability for surgery. Although contrast pulmonary angiography poses some risk in patients with pulmonary hypertension, the use of magnification views with the selective or subselective injections of small contrast volumes minimizes this.[29]

Fiberoptic angioscopy and magnetic resonance imaging are both under active investigation as modalities that may be helpful in defining the lesions of proximal thromboembolic pulmonary hypertension.[30, 31, 31a]

Surgery is considered for patients in whom clot in lobar or more proximal pulmonary arteries is persistent after at least 6 months of anticoagulation. Thromboendarterectomy is done, via a median sternotomy, using deep hypothermic cardiopulmonary bypass with intermittent periods of circulatory arrest.[29] Hemodynamic improvement is usually quite dramatic and the patients improve correspondingly (i.e., by at least two functional classes according to the New York Heart Association classification).[26] Surgical mortality originally reported to exceed 15% has been reduced to approximately 6%.[29] Patients require lifetime anticoagulation and/or placement of an inferior vena cava filter after this procedure.

Primary Pulmonary Hypertension

Primary pulmonary hypertension is a clinical syndrome characterized by pulmonary hypertension in the absence of sufficient underlying cardiac, pulmonary, or systemic disease to account for it; it is unexplained pulmonary hypertension. The diagnosis requires that three criteria be met: (1) clinical, radiographic, and electrocardiographic evidence suggesting pulmonary hypertension; (2) demonstration of elevated pulmonary arterial pressures and pulmonary vascular resistance in association with a normal pulmonary wedge pressure; and (3) inability to find a cause of the pulmonary hypertension in conditions related to the heart, the lungs, or the systemic circulation or in systemic disease.

Primary pulmonary hypertension is an uncommon disorder. Although the onset may occur at any age, symptoms are usually first manifested in early adulthood. The mean age at the time of diagnosis is usually 30 to 36 years, 9% of patients being older than the age of 60 years.[32] The sex incidence is approximately equal in childhood, but females predominate after puberty. In adults, the female-to-male ratio has ranged from 1.7:1 to 5:1 in different studies; the female-to-male predominance is higher among black persons.[32] The time delay from onset of first symptoms, generally fatigue or dyspnea, to the diagnosis of primary pulmonary hypertension, is about 2 years.

The heterogeneity of the patient population and late diagnosis complicate understanding the pathogenesis and the natural history of primary pulmonary hypertension.[32, 33] It has been observed that neither the age at which the disorder is recognized nor the level of pulmonary arterial pressure correlates with survival. In contrast, the level of cardiac output does have prognostic value, a low value correlating with a worsened prognosis.[33, 34, 34a]

The vascular lesions associated with primary pulmonary hypertension are in the precapillary, muscular pulmonary arteries and arterioles, which compose the major site of resistance in the pulmonary circulation. Several different histologic patterns have been identified in patients with primary pulmonary hypertension (Table 74–3); until recently, these lesions were interpreted in terms of pathogenetic mechanisms. However, it now seems clear that there are only a limited number of ways in which the pulmonary microvasculature can respond to injury and that a variety of these histologic patterns can occur in a single patient. The different lesions observed represent different stages in the response to a vascular injury, possibly related to differences in the nature of the initiating process, the rapidity of development of the inciting stimulus and how long it continues, and differences in the severity and duration of the resulting pulmonary hypertension.[12, 35, 36]

Therapeutic options for patients with primary pulmonary

hypertension are few.[37] Anticoagulation has been suggested because of the prevalence of microthrombotic lesions in histologic specimens.[12–14, 35, 36] The value of anticoagulation is uncertain, particularly in patients with syncope (up to 55% of patients with primary pulmonary hypertension) and hemoptysis (up to 15% of patients with primary pulmonary hypertension). Oxygen therapy, to prevent arterial hypoxemia (especially during exercise) and to avoid hypoxic pulmonary vasoconstriction, should be considered in all patients, especially those with a low diffusing capacity (e.g., <60% of predicted value). Vasodilator therapy has been of benefit in selected patients[37, 38] (see later).

Dietary Pulmonary Hypertension

Pulmonary hypertension with the histologic features of primary pulmonary hypertension has occurred in humans after the ingestion of certain substances (e.g., aminorex).[39] This observation, along with the development of pulmonary hypertension in animals fed monocrotaline, a pyrrolizine alkaloid contained in shrubs of the *Crotalaria* species, has raised questions as to the role of ingested materials in the pathogenesis of some instances of idiopathic pulmonary hypertension.

The pulmonary hypertension attributed to aminorex, an appetite suppressant, has generated great interest as a potential model for the pathogenesis and course of unexplained pulmonary hypertension. Introduced in Switzerland, Austria, and Germany in 1965, aminorex was related on epidemiologic grounds to the outbreak of primary pulmonary hypertension that occurred in those countries in 1966. After aminorex was withdrawn from over-the-counter sales in 1968, the epidemic subsided. Attempts to duplicate the histologic changes observed in patients by administering aminorex to animals have been consistently unsuccessful. Nonetheless, several important observations were made concerning the epidemic: (1) pulmonary hypertension developed in only a small fraction of all those who ingested aminorex, suggesting interaction with a genetic predisposition; (2) the development of pulmonary hypertension could not be related to either total dosage or duration of aminorex use (again suggesting the role of an underlying predisposition to develop primary pulmonary hypertension); and (3) in some patients, the pulmonary hypertension regressed after removal of the drug.

Primary Pulmonary Hypertension in Association with Portal Hypertension

A syndrome with clinical and histologic features indistinguishable from those of primary pulmonary hypertension has been observed in conjunction with portal hypertension of multiple different causes.[40, 40a] The incidence of this association appears to be at least five to six times that of primary pulmonary hypertension in the general population.[41, 41a] The liver is suspected of playing a role either by failing to inactivate a vasoconstrictor substance or by producing a metabolic intermediate that damages the pulmonary vascular endothelium. Alternatively, a vasodilator substance normally produced in the liver is no longer made owing to the hepatic injury. At present, the etiology of coexistent pulmonary and portal hypertension remains speculative.

There is little therapeutically to offer these patients. Anticoagulation is contraindicated, vasodilators have generally been ineffective, and the patients are not usually considered to be candidates for transplantation, as treatment would require transplantation of multiple organs.

Pulmonary Vascular Disease in the Toxic Oil Syndrome

In 1981, more than 20,000 people in Spain became ill as a consequence of ingestion of a toxic oil. During the acute illness, pulmonary hypertension was noted to accompany acute lung injury in up to 20% of patients. With recovery from the acute illness, the prevalence of pulmonary hypertension declined so that by 4 years after the acute illness, only 1.5% of involved individuals demonstrated pulmonary hypertension. In a small subgroup of patients, the pulmonary hypertension became progressive, with clinical and pathologic characteristics similar to those of primary pulmonary hypertension. This syndrome appears to have an incidence of approximately 1.6 per 1000 patients and is rapidly progressive, with death occurring in 83% of patients during 6.5-year follow-up. Were it not known that these patients had toxic oil syndrome, these patients would be thought to have primary pulmonary hypertension.[41b]

The recognition of this syndrome is of considerable interest for the insights it provides about the mechanisms of pulmonary vascular injury. The toxic oil syndrome is characterized by damage to vascular endothelium throughout the body.[41c] This damaged endothelium promotes in situ thrombosis, which contributes to pulmonary vascular obstruction. In addition, the initial endothelial insult leads to intimal proliferation and myointimal cell migration, which result in the characteristic medial and intimal hyperplasia and fibrosis characteristic of primary pulmonary hypertension. Plexiform-like lesions have also been observed in this syndrome. Although many details remain to be uncovered, the development of a primary pulmonary hypertension–like syndrome after a single ingestion of a toxic compound is quite thought provoking. The infrequent prevalence of this syndrome suggests that a predisposition to vascular injury must be present in an individual before the toxic substance can initiate the injury, which eventuates in progressive pulmonary vascular disease.[41b]

Pulmonary Hypertension in Association with Human Immunodeficiency Virus Infection

During the past several years, there has been increased recognition of an association between pulmonary hypertension and infection with human immunodeficiency virus type 1. Initially described in hemophiliacs,[41d] this association has been found in patients infected with human immunodeficiency virus type 1 who have not been intravenous drug users and who have never had opportunistic pulmonary infections. Pulmonary hypertension appears to have an incidence of approximately 0.5% in patients infected with this virus.[41e]

Although vascular endothelial cells are often CD4+, initial investigations have not found evidence of direct viral infection of the pulmonary artery endothelial cells.[41f] Evidence suggests that lymphokines and other mediators released by the inflammatory response to viral infection cause changes in the pulmonary vascular endothelium that progress to the obstructing lesions, which eventually result in pulmonary hypertension. Although further investigation of this association is ongoing, this does represent the first identified instance of a viral infection resulting in a clinical and pathologic syndrome similar to primary pulmonary hypertension.

Adult Respiratory Distress Syndrome

Pulmonary hypertension has been observed to occur frequently in the setting of acute lung injury or the adult respiratory distress syndrome. The elevations of pulmonary vascular resistance are generally modest, with average reported pulmonary vascular resistance values ranging from 145 to 700 dyne • s/cm[5], although values as high as 2400 dyne • s/cm[5] have been observed.[42] The level of pulmonary hypertension does not appear to correlate with the shunt fraction observed in adult respiratory distress syndrome.

Explanations proposed for this increased vascular resistance include pulmonary microvascular obstruction caused by interstitial edema or cellular infiltration; injury to endothelial cells resulting in swelling and/or promotion of in situ thrombosis; vasoconstriction as a consequence of neurohumoral mediators, acid-base status, or hypoxia; and hemodynamic alterations attributable to positive pressure ventilation and the imposition of positive end-expiratory pressures. It is likely that different mechanisms are operative at different times in the pathologic process, with vasoconstriction occurring early, and cellular obstruction of the microvasculature and in situ thrombosis occurring later.

The presence or severity of pulmonary hypertension does not correlate with mortality of adult respiratory distress syndrome.[43] However, in animal studies, pulmonary arterial pressures correlate with the development of edema and increases in lung weight and lymph flow; these appear to correlate with the adequacy of gas exchange.[44]

DIAGNOSIS OF PULMONARY VASCULAR DISEASE

Owing to the large reserve capacity of the normal pulmonary circulation, which allows it to accept large increases in pulmonary blood flow without substantial elevations in pulmonary arterial pressures, extensive pulmonary vascular changes must be present before pulmonary hypertension develops.[2] When symptoms do develop, they occur first during exertion, presenting as easy fatigability, dyspnea, chest pain, and/or presyncope or syncope. Right-sided heart failure occurs subsequently and manifests itself as peripheral edema, early satiety, and/or right upper quadrant pain.

Results of physical examination with the patient at rest, particularly before the pulmonary vascular changes have become extensive, are often normal; examination during exertion may be necessary to suggest the presence of disease of the pulmonary circulatory bed. The difficulty in early diagnosis is compounded by the unavailability of noninvasive screening techniques for pulmonary hypertension. As a consequence, consideration of the presence of pulmonary hypertension often waits until severe symptoms or abnormalities in the chest radiograph or electrocardiogram are present.[1]

Symptoms

No symptom is specific for pulmonary hypertension.[45, 46] Because of this, there is often a significant delay between the onset of symptoms and the establishment of the diagnosis of pulmonary hypertension.[32] Only after the pulmonary hypertension results in the development of right ventricular hypertrophy are specific findings likely to be present on physical examination at rest and on noninvasive testing (electrocardiogram, chest radiograph, echocardiogram). If the increased afterload is not reduced, right-sided heart failure, with its characteristic physical findings, develops.

The most frequent initial symptom of pulmonary hypertension is exertional dyspnea. This dyspnea, as is the case with easy fatigability, is often blamed on anxiety or lack of physical fitness. Various explanations for this dyspnea have been proposed, including hypoxic stimulation of peripheral chemoreceptors, stimulation of interstitial irritant receptors, stimulation of stretch receptors in the pulmonary arteries,

and inability of cardiac output to match metabolic need. It is likely that each explanation plays a role in some patients, although none has proved to be universal.

Syncope or presyncope (lightheadedness during exertion) is another symptom commonly seen in pulmonary hypertension. Most frequently, this occurs later in the course of the disease in patients with high resting pulmonary arterial pressures. This symptom is usually attributed either to an inability to adequately increase cardiac output during exertion (in association with exercise-induced systemic vasodilation) or to a bradyarrhythmia. It is often considered an indicator of a poor prognosis.

Chest pains may occur in up to 50% of patients with severe pulmonary hypertension; these often resemble typical angina and are thought to be a consequence of right ventricular ischemia. Hemoptysis has been observed to occur with all causes of pulmonary hypertension. In postcapillary pulmonary vascular disorders, the bleeding may be from dilated submucosal veins in the airways. In precapillary pulmonary hypertension, aneurysms of alveolar capillaries have been identified in some patients; in others, the underlying inflammatory process has involved the microvasculature and has resulted in bleeding.

Hoarseness may be seen in long-standing, severe pulmonary hypertension. It is due to paralysis of the left vocal cord as a result of the compression of the left recurrent laryngeal nerve between the aorta and the left pulmonary artery (Ortner's syndrome). Early satiety, right upper quadrant epigastric pain, or both may develop when hepatic congestion and distention of Glisson's capsule occur as a consequence of right-sided heart failure and elevation of systemic venous pressures.

Signs

The physical signs of pulmonary hypertension are similar regardless of the underlying cause or pathogenetic mechanism. Early on, the jugular venous pulse configuration is dominated by the a wave. As the pulmonary hypertension progresses and right-sided heart failure with tricuspid insufficiency develops, the a wave becomes less prominent, and the v wave becomes proportionally larger. A right ventricular S_4 may be present with the prominent a wave. The right ventricle becomes palpable at the lower left sternal border or in the subxiphoid region, and pulmonary arterial valve closure becomes palpable in the second left intercostal space.

On auscultation, P_2 is accentuated and S_2 is initially narrowly split. Often, a sharp systolic ejection click is heard over the pulmonary artery in the second left intercostal space. A right atrial S_3 gallop is often present. A tricuspid insufficiency murmur is frequently heard at the left sternal border. Owing to the relatively large pressure gradient present across the tricuspid valve in pulmonary hypertension, the murmur present is high pitched and quite different from the low-pitched, blowing insufficiency murmur associated with organic tricuspid disease. This murmur may not evidence significant respiratory variation. A pulmonic insufficiency murmur may also be appreciated.

In addition to exhibiting the signs and symptoms of right ventricular hypertrophy and/or right-sided heart failure, pulmonary hypertension may manifest as unexplained arterial hypoxemia. Frequently, the hypoxemia is relatively unresponsive to the administration of supplemental oxygen. This shunt, which may be transient in nature, may be occurring at an intrapulmonary level, as a consequence of increased flow through vessels in relatively poorly ventilated lung zones or may be at an intracardiac level, through a reopened foramen ovale. An intravenous injection of ^{99m}Tc-

TABLE 74–4

EVALUATION OF SUSPECTED PULMONARY HYPERTENSION

Laboratory studies
  Complete blood count, coagulation profile, liver function tests, collagen-vascular screen
Chest radiograph
Electrocardiogram
Pulmonary function tests
  Spirometry, lung volumes, diffusing capacity, arterial blood gas determination
Ventilation-perfusion lung scan
  Pulmonary angiogram (if lung scan or clinical history suggests proximal pulmonary embolism)
Echocardiogram
Exercise test
Right-sided heart catheterization

labeled macroaggregated albumin may be useful for distinguishing these: a patent foramen ovale shunts particles to the systemic circulation where they are trapped in the brain, the liver, and the kidneys and are seen as uptake in those organs during imaging with a gamma camera. Shunts at the pulmonary microvascular level still trap all of the imaging agent and imaging studies obtained over systemic organs will not demonstrate any uptake of the ^{99m}Tc-labeled macroaggregated albumin.

Diagnostic Studies

Except for cardiac catheterization (with exercise), available diagnostic techniques do not detect early pulmonary hypertension. However, these studies, particularly when used serially, are useful in following the course of pulmonary hypertension in patients in whom right ventricular hypertrophy or enlargement of the pulmonary arteries has already occurred. The unexpected finding of right ventricular hypertrophy on either an electrocardiogram or an echocardiogram, or of right-sided heart enlargement or enlargement of the pulmonary arteries on a chest radiograph, should raise concern as to the presence of pulmonary hypertension and trigger further investigation.

Diagnostic tests may have a role in determining the cause of the pulmonary vascular disorder (Table 74–4). The complete blood count, blood coagulation tests, liver function tests, and serologic studies for collagen-vascular disease may be useful: polycythemia raises the possibility of chronic hypoxia or hemoglobinopathy; hypercoagulable states suggest thrombosis; abnormal liver function study results raise the possibility of concurrent pulmonary hypertension and portal hypertension; abnormal serologic findings can suggest the presence of a systemic connective tissue disorder.

Chest radiographs and pulmonary function tests (spirometry and determination of lung volumes and diffusing capacity) are useful in suggesting disorders of the airways, intrinsic pulmonary parenchymal disease, or abnormalities of the mediastinum. A ventilation-perfusion lung scan is necessary to distinguish thromboembolic pulmonary vascular disease (e.g., large vessel [surgically treatable], unresolved pulmonary embolism) from other causes of pulmonary hypertension.[25, 26] Pulmonary angiography is generally reserved for patients with a clinical history or a lung scan suggestive of proximal pulmonary emboli. An echocardiogram can demonstrate structural cardiac abnormalities, such as valvular disease, septal defects, and myxomas. Right-sided heart catheterization remains necessary for determining the degree of the pulmonary hypertension, for excluding certain cardiac lesions, and for testing vasodilator agents.

TREATMENT OF PULMONARY HYPERTENSION

The treatment of pulmonary hypertension is directed toward any reversible component of the underlying pathogenetic process while relieving any hypoxemia, hypercapnia, or acidosis that might be contributing to right-sided heart strain. In addition to specific measures, several categories of treatment may be helpful in patients with pulmonary hypertension regardless of cause.

Oxygen Supplementation

In patients demonstrating arterial hypoxemia—resting, exertional, or nocturnal—there is a role for careful oxygen supplementation aiming to treat the hypoxic vasoconstriction and to reduce the afterload on the right ventricle, while also reducing any contribution of the hypoxemia to arrhythmogenesis. The performance of a sleep study looking for nocturnal arterial desaturation should be considered in all patients with unexplained pulmonary hypertension. Exertional arterial desaturation should be considered in all patients with a low diffusing capacity (e.g., <60% of predicted value);[47, 48] these patients should be exercised to tolerance while arterial oxygen saturation is monitored with pulse oximetry. Although oxygen administration entails some risk in patients with obstructive pulmonary disease by potentially decreasing respiratory drive and alveolar ventilation and thereby worsening respiratory acidosis,[5] the supplementation of oxygen directed to maintain an arterial oxygen tension of greater than 60 mm Hg, or an arterial oxygen saturation of greater than 90%, reduces the mortality of cor pulmonale and improves cognitive function and quality of life. The guidelines for supplemental oxygen therapy are well detailed in reviews.[49–51]

A new therapy also directed toward improving arterial oxygenation in chronic obstructive airways disease (chronic obstructive pulmonary disease) involves the use of almitrine bismesylate, a carotid body stimulant, which may also augment hypoxic vasoconstriction and improve ventilation-perfusion matching within the lungs without affecting minute ventilation.[52, 53] In a long-term, randomized, double-blind trial of this agent in hypoxemic, hypercapnic patients with chronic obstructive pulmonary disease, the study group had fewer hospitalizations and episodes of right-sided heart failure than did the control group.[54] However, these results await more extensive trials before this investigational drug therapy can be used as a substitute for long-term oxygen supplementation.

Treatment of Heart Failure

Right-sided heart failure in pulmonary hypertension and cor pulmonale may be transient if the exacerbating factors can be controlled. The usual therapies for heart failure are used: low-salt regimen and administration of digitalis and diuretics.[2, 55] Phlebotomy to decrease the circulating blood volume (and hematocrit) may be of benefit in patients with secondary polycythemia;[56] repeated phlebotomies may be needed to maintain the benefit. Diuretics should be given with care, particularly in patients with abnormalities of ventilatory control, because metabolic alkalosis may complicate their use; alkalosis, in turn, contributes to ventilatory insufficiency by depressing the ventilatory response to carbon dioxide. Moreover, diuresis may increase blood viscosity by increasing the hematocrit. In critically ill patients, overdiuresis can result in inadequate filling of the right side of the heart and may compromise cardiac output and arterial oxygenation.

Anticoagulation

As noted earlier, both acute and chronic pulmonary thromboembolism may result in pulmonary hypertension and right-sided heart failure, and pulmonary hypertension of any cause seems to have the potential to initiate in situ thrombosis in the pulmonary microvascular beds.[13, 14, 57] Moreover, after the patient is in right-sided heart failure, venous thrombosis and pulmonary embolism are frequent complications of the resultant venous stasis and decreased physical activity. Because of these observations, it is suggested that anticoagulation (or treatment with antiplatelet agents) be considered for any patient with pulmonary hypertension, without waiting for the development of overt right-sided heart failure. Routine prophylaxis for venous thrombosis, usually with subcutaneous heparin administration, is advisable for all periods of hospitalization or prolonged immobility. This is particularly important in critically ill patients, who often have many factors predisposing to thrombosis and who may not be able to indicate the onset of new symptoms.

Vasodilator Therapy

For more than 30 years, vasodilator therapy has been used to try to dilate the pulmonary resistance vessels and to decrease the right ventricular afterload. Unfortunately, vasodilator administration is potentially hazardous, necessitating that therapy be initiated in a critical care unit setting. Studies of vasodilator therapy have been complicated by uncertainty as to the long-term significance of a favorable acute vasodilator response.[58, 59] It is also not known if the lack of an acute response during a vasodilator trial indicates that there will be no benefit from long-term vasodilator administration.

The optimal response to the administration of a vasodilator agent is an increase in cardiac output accompanied by a reduction in pulmonary arterial pressure with minimal decrease in systemic arterial blood pressure. More frequently, the response has been an increase in cardiac output, in association with relatively unchanged pulmonary arterial pressures. This hemodynamic profile decreases the calculated pulmonary vascular resistance; the increase in cardiac output is generally accompanied by an improved exercise tolerance. However, despite the increase in pulmonary blood flow (cardiac output), the sustained high pulmonary arterial pressure and the improved cardiac output may result in an increase in the right ventricular work, particularly if there is any increase in heart rate. For this reason, clinical improvement may be short-lived unless the pulmonary arterial pressure falls.

Unfortunately, vasodilating agents often affect the systemic vascular bed more than the pulmonary vascular bed. For this reason, vasodilator therapy should be initiated in a critical care unit setting with full hemodynamic monitoring, including measurement of pulmonary arterial pressures and cardiac output, systemic blood pressure, and arterial oxygenation. If administration of a vasodilator results in systemic vasodilation without a compensatory increase in cardiac output, systemic hypotension results. This hypotension may be difficult to manage: vasopressors administered to cause systemic vasoconstriction may worsen the pulmonary hypertension, thereby increasing the right ventricular afterload. Systemic hypotension may also decrease coronary perfusion and contribute to right ventricular failure.

To avoid the untoward consequences of systemic vasodilation, particularly in response to a long-acting, orally administered agent, efforts have been devoted to finding screening agents for pulmonary vascular reactivity. Prostacyclin currently appears to be the best agent for this purpose.[60, 60a] However, after a patient responds to a screening agent, efforts must be undertaken to identify an agent for long-term therapy. Studies to identify an agent for extended vasodilator therapy are complicated by the need to evaluate multiple agents and by the need to assess for vasodilation both at rest and during exercise.[12, 61, 62] Often, a more substantial response is seen in the blunting of the exercise-induced increase in pulmonary arterial pressures (secondary to increased blood flow) than is observed at rest.

Despite the initial enthusiasm for long-term vasodilator therapy, particularly in patients with primary pulmonary hypertension, only about one third of all patients who receive vasodilator therapy experience stabilization or improvement with pharmacologic therapy. In responders, different agents have proved effective in different patients. Calcium channel blockers, notably nifedipine or diltiazem, are the most commonly used oral agents,[63] but occasionally other vasodilators, used singly or in combination, have proved effective. Prolonged intravenous infusions of prostacyclin, or its analogues, may be of benefit in stabilizing patients who have failed to respond to other therapies, and in sustaining them until they can undergo lung or heart-lung transplantation.[64]

Transplantation

Despite the therapies cited earlier, the pulmonary hypertension and right-sided heart failure often pursue a progressive course. For selected patients, transplantation of either a single lung or of two lungs, or of a lung-heart block, may provide dramatic relief of cardiorespiratory failure. Although these types of surgical interventions are still under development and are limited in availability, they can be lifesaving after the medical therapies have been exhausted. Reports have expanded the indications for lung transplantation and have documented improved patient survival with both lung and lung-heart transplantation.[65–73]

References

1. Palevsky HI: Exercise and the pulmonary circulation. In: Leff A (ed): Cardiopulmonary Exercise Testing. Orlando, FL, Grune & Stratton, p 89, 1986.
2. Fishman AP: Pulmonary circulation. In: Fishman AP (ed): Handbook of Physiology, Section 3, The Respiratory System, Volume I, Circulation and Nonrespiratory Functions. Bethesda, American Physiological Society, p 93, 1985.
3. Archer SL, McMurtry IF, Weir EK: Mechanisms of acute hypoxic and hyperoxic changes in pulmonary vascular reactivity. In: Weir EK, Reeves JT (eds): Pulmonary Vascular Physiology and Pathophysiology. New York, Marcel Dekker, p 241, 1989.
4. Unger M, Atkins M, Briscoe WA, et al: Potentiation of pulmonary vasoconstriction with intermittent repeated hypoxia. J Appl Physiol 43:662, 1977.
5. Derenne J-P, Fluery B, Pariente R: Acute respiratory failure of chronic obstructive lung disease. Am Rev Respir Dis 138:1006, 1988.
6. Van Grondelle A, Worthen GS, Ellis D, et al: Altering hydrodynamic variables influences PGI_2 production by isolated lungs and endothelial cells. J Appl Physiol 57:388, 1984.
7. Peach MJ, Johs RA, Rose CE Jr: The potential role of interactions between endothelium and smooth muscle in pulmonary vascular physiology and pathophysiology. In: Wir EK, Reeves JT (eds): Pulmonary Vascular Physiology and Pathophysiology. New York, Marcel Dekker, p 643, 1989.
7a. Cremona G, Dinh-Xuan AT, Higenbottam TW: Endothelium-derived relaxing factor and the pulmonary circulation. Lung 169:185, 1991.
8. Lerman A, Hildebrand FL Jr, Margulies KB, et al: Endothelin: A new cardiovascular regulatory peptide. Mayo Clin Proc 64:1441, 1990.
9. Vanhoutte PG: Endothelium and control of vascular function. State of the art. Hypertension 13:658, 1989.
9a. Stewart DJ, Levy RD, Cernacek P, et al: Increased plasma endothelin-1 in pulmonary hypertension: Marker or mediator of disease? Ann Intern Med 114:464, 1991.
10. Reid LM: Vascular remodeling. In: Fishman AP (ed): The Pulmonary Circulation: Normal and Abnormal Mechanisms, Management, and the National Registry. Philadelphia, University of Pennsylvania Press, p 259, 1990.

11. Rabinovitch M, Keave JF, Norwood WI: et al: Vascular structure in lung tissue obtained at biopsy correlated with pulmonary hemodynamic findings after repair of congenital heart defects. Circulation 69:655, 1984.

12. Palevsky HI, Schloo BL, Pietra GG, et al: Primary pulmonary hypertension: Vascular structure, morphometry and responsiveness to vasodilator agents. Circulation 80:1207, 1989.

13. Weir EK, Archer SL, Edwards JE: Chronic primary and secondary thromboembolic pulmonary hypertension. Chest 93:149S, 1988.

14. Cohen M, Fuster V, Williams WD: Anticoagulation in the treatment of pulmonary hypertension. In: Fishman AP (ed): The Pulmonary Circulation: Normal and Abnormal Mechanisms, Management, and the National Registry. Philadelphia, University of Pennsylvania Press, p 501, 1990.

15. Perloff JK: Congenital heart disease and pulmonary hypertension. In: Moser KM (ed): Pulmonary Vascular Diseases. New York, Marcel Dekker, p 489, 1979.

16. Edwards JE: Congenital pulmonary vascular disorders. In: Moser KM (ed): Pulmonary Vascular Diseases. New York, Marcel Dekker, p 527, 1979.

17. Dexter L: Pulmonary vascular disease in acquired heart disease. In: Moser KM (ed): Pulmonary Vascular Diseases. New York, Marcel Dekker, p 427, 1979.

18. Asherson RA, Oakley CM: Pulmonary hypertension and systemic lupus erythematosus. J Rheumatol 13:1, 1986.

19. Bunch TW, Trancredi RG, Lie JT: Pulmonary hypertension in polymyositis. Chest 79:105, 1981.

20. Stupi AM, Steen VD, Owens GD, et al: Pulmonary hypertension in CREST syndrome variant of systemic sclerosis (scleroderma). Arthritis Rheum 29:515, 1986.

21. Kobayashi H, Sano T, Fi K, et al: Mixed connective tissue disease with fatal pulmonary hypertension. Acta Pathol Jpn 32:1121, 1982.

22. Rich S, Kieras K, Hart K, et al: Antinuclear antibodies in primary pulmonary hypertension. J Am Coll Cardiol 8:1307, 1986.

23. Fahey PJ, Utell MJ, Condemi JJ, et al: Raynaud's phenomenon of the lung. Am J Med 76:263, 1984.

24. Ungerer RG, Tashkin DP, Furst D, et al: Prevalence and clinical correlates of pulmonary arterial hypertension in progressive systemic sclerosis. Am J Med 75:65, 1983.

25. Rich S, Levitsky S, Brundage BH: Pulmonary hypertension from chronic pulmonary thromboembolism. Ann Intern Med 108:425, 1988.

26. Moser KM, Daily PO, Peterson K, et al: Thromboendarterectomy for chronic, major vessel thromboembolic pulmonary hypertension: Immediate and long-term results in 42 patients. Ann Intern Med 107:560, 1987.

27. Daily PO, Dembitsky WP, Iversen S, et al: Risk factors for pulmonary thromboendarterectomy. J Thorac Cardiovasc Surg 99:670, 1990.

28. Moser KM, Auger WR, Fedullo PF: Chronic major-vessel thromboembolic pulmonary hypertension. Circulation 81:1735, 1990.

29. Nicod P, Peterson K, Levine M, et al: Pulmonary angiography in severe chronic pulmonary hypertension. Ann Intern Med 107:565, 1987.

30. Shure D, Gregoratos G, Moser KM: Fiberoptic angioscopy: Role in the diagnosis of chronic pulmonary arterial obstruction. Ann Intern Med 103:844, 1985.

31. Gefter WB, Palevsky HI, Dinsmore BJ, et al: Identification of chronic thromboembolic pulmonary hypertension with MR imaging. Radiology 169:218, 1988.

31a. Hatabu H, Gefter WB, Konishi J, et al: Magnetic resonance approaches to the evaluation of pulmonary vascular anatomy and physiology. Magn Res Q 7:208, 1991.

32. Rich S, Dantzker DR, Ayres SM, et al: Primary pulmonary hypertension: A national study. Ann Intern Med 107:216, 1987.

33. Glanville AR, Burke CM, Theodore J, et al: Primary pulmonary hypertension: Length of survival in patients referred for heart-lung transplantation. Chest 91:675, 1987.

34. Voelkel NF, Reeves JT: Primary pulmonary hypertension. In: Moser K (ed): Pulmonary Vascular Disease. New York, Marcel Dekker, p 574, 1979.

34a. D'Alonzo GE, Barst RJ, Ayres SM, et al: Survival in patients with primary pulmonary hypertension. Results from a national prospective registry. Ann Intern Med 115:343, 1991.

35. Loyd JE, Atkinson JB, Pietra GG, et al: Heterogeneity of pathologic lesions in familial primary pulmonary hypertension. Am Rev Respir Dis 138:952, 1988.

36. Pietra GG, Edwards WD, Kay JM, et al: Histopathology of primary pulmonary hypertension: A qualitative and quantitative study of pulmonary blood vessels from 58 patients in the National Heart, Lung, and Blood Institute Primary Pulmonary Hypertension Registry. Circulation 60:1198, 1989.

37. Palevsky HI, Fishman AP: The management of primary pulmonary hypertension. JAMA 265:1014, 1991.

38. Palevsky HI, Fishman AP: Vasodilator therapy for primary pulmonary hypertension. Annu Rev Med 36:563, 1985.

39. Gurtner HP: Aminorex pulmonary hypertension. In: Fishman AP (ed): The Pulmonary Circulation: Normal and Abnormal Mechanisms, Management, and the National Registry. Philadelphia, University of Pennsylvania Press, p 397, 1990.

40. Edwards BS, Wier EK, Edwards WD, et al: Coexistent pulmonary and portal hypertension: Morphologic and clinical features. J Am Coll Cardiol 10:1233, 1987.

40a. Robalino BD, Moodie DS: Association between primary pulmonary hypertension and portal hypertension: Analysis of its pathophysiology and clinical, laboratory and hemodynamic manifestations. J Am Coll Cardiol 17:492, 1991.

41. McDonnell PJ, Toye PA, Hutchins GM: Primary pulmonary hypertension and cirrhosis: Are they related? Am Rev Respir Dis 127:437, 1983.

41a. Hadengue A, Benhayoun MK, Lebrec D, et al: Pulmonary hypertension complicating portal hypertension: Prevalence and relation to splanchnic hemodynamics. Gastroenterology 100:520, 1991.

41b. Gomez-Sanchez MA, Saenz De La Calzada C, Gomez-Pajuelo C, et al: Clinical and pathologic manifestations of pulmonary vascular disease in the toxic oil syndrome. J Am Coll Cardiol 18:1539, 1991.

41c. Martinez-Tello FJ, Tellez I: Extracardiac vascular and neural lesions in the toxic oil syndrome. J Am Coll Cardiol 18:1043, 1991.

41d. Goldsmith GH, Bally RG, Brettler DB, et al: Primary pulmonary hypertension in patients with classic hemophilia. Ann Intern Med 108:797, 1988.

41e. Speich R, Jenni R, Opravil M, et al: Primary pulmonary hypertension in HIV infection. Chest 100:1268, 1991.

41f. Mette SA, Palevsky HI, Pietra GG, et al: Primary pulmonary hypertension in association with human immunodeficiency virus infection: A possible viral etiology for some forms of hypertensive pulmonary arteriopathy. Am Rev Respir Dis 145:1196, 1992.

42. Rounds SIS: Pulmonary circulatory control in lung injury. In: Weir EK, Reeves JT (eds): Pulmonary Vascular Physiology and Pathophysiology. New York, Marcel Dekker, p 403, 1989.

43. Fowler AA, Hamman RF, Zerbe GO, et al: Adult respiratory distress syndrome: Prognosis after onset. Am Rev Respir Dis 132:472, 1985.

44. Permutt S: The role of pulmonary arterial pressure in experimentally induced acute lung injury. In: Zapol WM, Falke KJ (eds): Acute Respiratory Failure. New York, Marcel Dekker, p 227, 1985.

45. Reeves JT, Groves BM: Approach to the patient with pulmonary hypertension. In: Weir EK, Reeves JT (eds): Pulmonary Hypertension. Mt Kisco, NY, Futura Publishing, p 1, 1984.

46. Rubin LJ: Clinical evaluation. In: Rubin LJ (ed): Pulmonary Heart Disease. Boston, Martinus Nijhoff Publishing, p 107, 1984.

47. Owens GR, Rogers RM, Pennock BE, et al: The diffusing capacity as a predictor of arterial oxygen desaturation during exercise in patients with chronic obstructive pulmonary disease. N Engl J Med 310:1218, 1984.

48. Kelley MA, Panettieri RA Jr, Krupinski AV: Resting single-breath diffusing capacity as a screening test for exercise induced hypoxemia. Am J Med 80:807, 1986.

49. Fulmer JD, Snider GL: ACCP-NHLBI National Conference on Oxygen Toxicity. Chest 86:234, 1987.

50. Flenley DC: Long-term home oxygen therapy. Chest 87:99, 1985.

51. Timms RM, Khaja FU, Williams GW: The nocturnal oxygen therapy trial. Hemodynamic response to oxygen therapy in chronic obstructive pulmonary disease. Ann Intern Med 102:29, 1985.

52. Bell RC, Mullins RC III, West LG, et al: The effect of almitrine bismesylate on hypoxemia in chronic obstructive pulmonary disease. Ann Intern Med 105:342, 1986.

53. Gothe B, Cherniack NS, Bachand RT, Jr, et al: Long-term effects of almitrine bismesylate on oxygenation during wakefulness and sleep in chronic obstructive pulmonary disease. Am J Med 84:436, 1988.

54. Voisin C, Howard P, Ansquer JC: Vectarion international multicentre study. Bull Eur Physiopathol Respir 23:169S, 1987.

55. Rubin LJ, Peter RH: Therapy of pulmonary heart disease. In: Rubin JJ (ed): Pulmonary Heart Disease. Boston, Martinus Nijhoff Publishing, p 325, 1984.

56. McGrath RC, Weil JV: Adverse effects of normovolemic polycythaemia and hypoxia on hemodynamics in the dog. Circ Res 43:793, 1978.

57. Voelkel NF, Weir EK: Etiologic mechanisms in primary pulmonary hypertension. In: Weir EK, Reeves JT (eds): Pulmonary Vascular Physiology and Pathophysiology. New York, Marcel Dekker, p 513, 1989.

58. Reeves JT, Groves BM, Turkevich D: The case for treatment of selected patients with primary pulmonary hypertension. Am Rev Respir Dis 134:343, 1986.

59. Eysmann SB, Palevsky HI, Reichek N, et al: Echo/Doppler and hemodynamic correlates of vasodilator responsiveness in primary pulmonary hypertension. Chest 99:1066, 1991.

60. Palevsky HI, Long W, Crow J, et al: Prostacyclin and acetylcholine as screening agents for pulmonary vasodilator responsiveness in patients with primary pulmonary hypertension. Circulation 82:2018, 1990.

60a. Morgan JM, McCormack DG, Griffiths MJ, et al: Adenosine as a vasodilator in primary pulmonary hypertension. Circulation 84:1145, 1991.

61. Palevsky H, Pietra GG, Fishman AP: Pulmonary veno-occlusive disease and its response to vasodilator agents. Am Rev Respir Dis 142:426, 1990.

62. Gassner A, Sommer G, Fridrich L, et al: Differential therapy with calcium antagonists in pulmonary hypertension secondary to COPD: Hemodynamic effects of nifedipine, diltiazem, and verapamil. Chest 98:829, 1990.

63. Rich S, Brundage BH: High-dose calcium channel blocking therapy for primary pulmonary hypertension: Evidence for long-term reduction in pulmonary arterial pressure and regression of right ventricular hypertrophy. Circulation 76:134, 1987.

64. Rubin LJ, Mendoza J, Hood M, et al: Treatment of primary pulmonary hypertension with continuous intravenous prostacyclin (epoprostenol). Ann Intern Med 112:485, 1990.

65. Montefusco CM, Veith FJ: Lung transplantation. Surg Clin North Am 66:503, 1986.
66. Hutter JA, Despins P, Higenbottam T, et al: Heart-lung transplantation. Better use of resources. Am J Med 85:4, 1988.
67. Grossman RF, Frost A, Zamel N, et al: Results of single-lung transplantation for bilateral pulmonary fibrosis. N Engl J Med 322:727, 1990.
68. Cooper JD, Patterson GA, Grossman R, et al: Double-lung transplantation for advanced chronic obstructive lung disease. Am Rev Respir Dis 139:303, 1989.
69. Trulock EP, Egan TM, Kouchoukos NT, et al: Single lung transplantation for severe chronic obstructive pulmonary disease. Chest 96:738, 1989.
70. Stevens JH, Raffin TA, Baldwin JC: The status of transplantation of the human lung. Surg Gynecol Obstet 169:179, 1989.
71. McCarthy PM, Starnes VA, Theodore J, et al: Improved survival after heart-lung transplantation. J Thorac Cardiovasc Surg 99:54, 1990.
72. Calhoon JH, Grover FL, Gibbons WJ, et al: Single lung transplantation. Alternative indications and technique. J Thorac Cardiovasc Surg 101:816, 1991.
73. Pasque MK, Trulock EP, Kaiser LR, et al: Single-lung transplantation for pulmonary hypertension. Circulation 84:2275, 1991.

CHAPTER 75

Pulmonary Embolism in the Critically Ill Patient

Mark A. Kelley

Pulmonary embolism is a major clinical disorder that affects 0.5 million patients annually in the United States. The mortality of pulmonary embolism, estimated to be as much as 30%, falls to below 10% when this condition is properly diagnosed and treated.[1, 2] Therefore, pulmonary embolism is a significant health hazard for which the outcome is greatly influenced by correct diagnosis and treatment. Although there have been no large published studies of pulmonary embolism in critically ill patients, most reported series of pulmonary embolism have included patients with cardiopulmonary disease, often in the critical care setting. A large body of experience is contained in the multicenter diagnostic study Prospective Investigation of Pulmonary Embolism Diagnosis.[3] In this study, the vast majority of patients suspected of having pulmonary embolism had cardiopulmonary disease and/or malignancy. Because patients with such advanced stages of illness are often seen in the critical care setting, pulmonary embolism is encountered frequently by the critical care physician.

This chapter focuses on the pathogenesis of, physiologic consequences of, and diagnostic approaches to acute pulmonary embolism, with particular emphasis on critical care medicine. Major therapeutic issues, particularly for patients with complicating factors such as bleeding disorders and underlying cardiopulmonary disease, are also addressed.

GENERAL CONCEPTS
Concept of Thromboembolism

Pulmonary emboli result from the formation of a clot in the venous system, which subsequently migrates up the venous circulation to become lodged in the pulmonary vasculature. Carefully performed autopsy studies have shown that serious pulmonary embolism almost always originates from a clot arising in the major capacitance venous vessels above the knee or in the vena cava.[4–6] A venous clot may also form in the pelvic veins in association with pelvic inflammation or malignancy. Thrombi arising in the superior vena cava or its tributary vessels have been increasingly recognized.[7, 8] Such clot formation may result from invasive instrumentation such as central venous catheter placement or from long-term use of indwelling catheters for infusion. In patients with dilated right ventricles, a mural clot may also form within that cardiac chamber and subsequently travel to the pulmonary arteries. Although these examples are more frequently seen in the critical care setting, most pulmonary emboli still arise from the venous vessels between the popliteal fossa and the right side of the heart.

There is a close relationship between deep venous thrombosis and pulmonary embolism, but the two do not usually present simultaneously. Patients with proximal deep venous thrombosis usually have no symptoms of pulmonary emboli, even though the majority of such patients have abnormal lung scans suggesting this diagnosis.[9, 10] Similarly, patients with pulmonary embolism usually have clinically silent deep venous thrombosis. Nonetheless, both disorders can lead to the same outcome, fatal pulmonary embolism. Therefore, the term *thromboembolism* has been used to describe the syndrome of venous thrombosis with its potential for migration to the pulmonary circulation.[11]

Pathogenesis of Venous Thrombosis

The mechanisms for the formation of venous clot are complicated and remain incompletely understood. More than 100 years ago, Virchow suggested a triad that leads to venous clot formation: stasis of blood flow, hypercoagulability of blood, and vessel wall injury.[12] Although the biochemistry of blood clotting is better understood in modern times, Virchow's description is still useful. Injury to major vessels, as might occur with direct trauma, surgical manipulation, or venous catheter insertion, may cause endothelial damage leading to formation of a local clot and its subsequent propagation. Venous stasis, a common condition in immobilized, critically ill patients, results in a sluggish venous blood flow and a propensity for thrombus formation.

Considering the third component of Virchow's triad, hypercoagulability, requires a brief review of the coagulation system.[13, 14] The usual trigger for thrombus formation is endothelial injury, which exposes subendothelial collagen to circulating platelets. These platelets stick to the injury site and form a platelet plug through the cyclooxygenase system. As this platelet plug is forming, the clotting cascade is activated by one of two pathways. Endothelial collagen can activate the intrinsic clotting pathway through activation of factor XII. Alternatively, if tissue thromboplastin is released by injured tissue, the extrinsic pathway is activated through factor VII. In most forms of tissue injury, both mechanisms are probably operative.

This clotting process is balanced by an endogenous thrombolytic system designed to limit the clot and subsequently dissolve it when the vessel injury has resolved. This process is initiated by the release of tissue plasminogen activator (TPA) from injured cells near the fibrin clot. TPA cleaves circulating plasminogen to its active form, plasmin. In turn, the plasmin acts locally within the clot matrix to dissolve fibrin.[14]

Although this relationship between thrombosis and thrombolysis is well known, a biochemical abnormality leading to a hypercoagulable state cannot be demonstrated in most patients with thromboembolism. Uncommonly, some patients with recurrent venous thromboses are found to have a congenital biochemical abnormality that influences clotting. For example, patients with antithrombin III deficiency have excessive production of thrombin, whereas protein C–deficient patients have difficulty inhibiting fibrin formation and promoting fibrinolysis. The hypercoagulable state of malignancy may be the result of the release of a tissue thromboplastin-like substance elaborated from the tumor.[14] There is indirect evidence of a clotting abnormality in patients who have withstood surgery or trauma. Clot formation is detectable through fibrinogen scanning in patients undergoing surgery and has been associated with a decrease in fibrinolytic activity in the immediate postoperative period.[15, 16] However, it is unusual to find clotting abnormalities associated with the other diverse conditions leading to pulmonary embolism, such as congestive heart failure, stroke, and obesity.

Incidence of Thromboembolism

The incidence of thromboembolism has been extensively studied in postoperative patients but less is known about other patient groups. Fatal pulmonary embolism has been documented in approximately 1% of patients after general surgery; in 4 to 7% after emergency hip surgery; and in 0.3 to 1.7% after elective hip surgery.[17, 18] The incidence of nonfatal pulmonary embolism is not well known for surgical patients, but in at least one report, up to 18% of patients had new lung perfusion defects after surgery.[19] Because of these statistics, considerable research has been devoted to the prevention of postoperative venous thrombosis, largely through the use of low-dose heparin.

The incidence of thromboembolism in other types of patients, particularly those with nonsurgical conditions, has not been extensively studied and must be inferred from other types of information. About 3% of patients with myocardial infarction have pulmonary embolism if they are not treated with anticoagulation.[20] Low-dose heparin in such patients reduces the incidence of deep venous thrombosis from 23 to 4%.[21] Patients with neurologic disorders who are immobilized are particularly vulnerable to pulmonary embolism, the incidence of which can likewise be reduced with low-dose heparin.[22, 23] Other conditions such as malignancy and congestive heart failure are well-known predisposing factors to thromboembolism and are commonly encountered in the critical care unit.

Autopsy studies have suggested that pulmonary embolism is a common cause of unexpected death. Although the incidence of undiagnosed, fatal pulmonary embolism may be declining slightly,[24] it remains a common finding among autopsied patients who had been receiving mechanical ventilation.[25] In about 5% of these autopsied patients, the diagnosis of pulmonary embolism was missed, an oversight that probably influenced patient outcome. Similar statistics apply to patients undergoing unsuccessful cardiopulmonary resuscitation, 8% of whom have been found to have pulmonary emboli at autopsy.[26] Therefore, in the critical care setting, pulmonary embolism is a constant threat that can be seen in a variety of patient groups.

Physiologic Consequences of Pulmonary Embolism

Deep venous thrombosis may lead to few clinical consequences until the clot migrates into the pulmonary circulation and triggers several cardiopulmonary events. The first and least understood are the often transient signs of tachypnea and tachycardia. The clinical observation is that most patients with pulmonary embolism manifest these signs with or without major hemodynamic or gas exchange abnormal-

ities. This suggests that some ventilation-perfusion abnormalities and/or reflexes may be stimulated by the embolus or by mediators such as serotonin released from platelets in the clot.

In the critically ill patient, pulmonary embolism often produces the more life-threatening consequences of hypoxemia and reduced right-sided heart performance and cardiac output. Such consequences are usually the result of massive pulmonary emboli. In the normal human, the pulmonary vasculature has considerable redundancy. Therefore, the pulmonary vascular bed must be substantially obliterated before either gas exchange or blood flow is reduced. For example, the normal human can tolerate a pneumonectomy with no change in resting pulmonary artery pressure or resting arterial blood gas values. Similarly, with pulmonary embolism, clot that occludes less than 40% of the pulmonary circulation is usually well tolerated and causes only transient changes in hemodynamics and arterial blood gas values.[27]

The relationship between hypoxemia and the degree of pulmonary embolism is now better understood.[28, 29] Investigations using multiple inert gas techniques have shown that pulmonary emboli direct blood flow away from areas of normal ventilation-perfusion match (Fig. 75–1). This redirected blood must flow through a limited vascular bed with a fixed ventilation, resulting in a lower ventilation/perfusion ratio. In massive pulmonary embolism, this effect is magnified because a relatively small portion of the pulmonary vascular bed must accommodate most of the pulmonary blood flow with only a limited amount of ventilation. This, in effect, results in a shunt through this limited vascular bed. A corollary is that, for a previously normal individual, the presence of arterial hypoxemia from pulmonary embolism implies that substantial clot has obliterated most of the pulmonary vasculature.

In previously healthy individuals, hemodynamic abnormalities from pulmonary embolism are also associated with a massive clot.[27] Because of the redundancy of the pulmonary circulation, small pulmonary emboli are easily tolerated because blood flow is redirected to other available parts of the pulmonary circulation. However, when the clot burden reaches approximately 40 to 50% of the pulmonary circulation, this adaptive capacity is reduced and pulmonary arterial resistance begins to rise. In patients with cardiopulmonary disease and reduced pulmonary vascular reserve, correspondingly smaller degrees of clot are required to produce pulmonary hypertension[30, 31] (Fig. 75–2).

The right ventricle is a volume-dependent organ that, in contrast to the left ventricle, cannot adjust its stroke volume to acute changes in afterload. If the normal right ventricle is subjected to an abrupt afterload stress, such as from pulmonary embolism, the chamber acutely dilates. This right ventricular dilation then produces tricuspid insufficiency and a marked fall in cardiac output. In contrast, when afterload slowly increases from pulmonary hypertension, as may occur with congestive heart failure or chronic lung disease, the right ventricle hypertrophies and begins to resemble the left ventricle in its performance characteristics.

These physiologic observations help to explain the lethal consequences of pulmonary embolism. In patients with a previously normal cardiopulmonary system, a relatively modest amount of clot may produce transient physiologic effects, but usually cardiac output and gas exchange are preserved by redirecting pulmonary blood flow through other pulmonary vessels. However, if a massive clot burden occludes the pulmonary circulation, hypoxemia occurs because of the reduced pulmonary vasculature available for gas exchange. In addition, the right ventricle fails because of the acute rise in pulmonary vascular resistance. This can result in hypotension and death (Fig. 75–3). In patients with

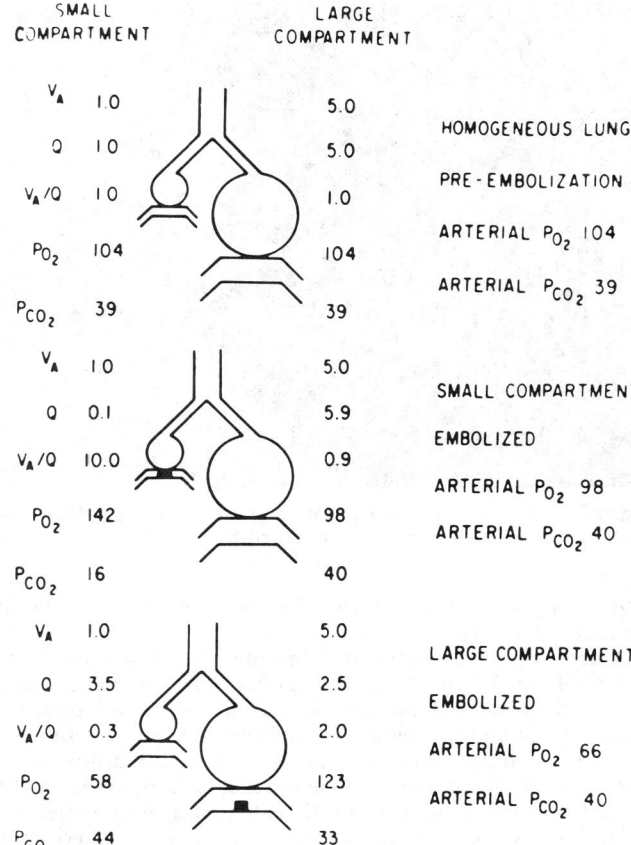

Figure 75–1. Ventilation and perfusion are matched in the two-compartment lung model demonstrated in the top panel. In the middle panel, small-compartment blood flow has been reduced by 90% and diverted to the large compartment, resulting in the development of a high–alveolar ventilation/perfusion ratio ($\dot{V}A/\dot{Q}$) unit but a minimal decrease in the $\dot{V}A/\dot{Q}$ of the larger compartment (1 to 0.9). Thus, no significant hypoxemia develops (104 to 98 mm Hg). In the bottom panel, large-compartment blood flow has been reduced by 50% and diverted to the small compartment. This leads to 58% of the blood flow distributed to a lung unit with a $\dot{V}A/\dot{Q}$ of 0.3 and significant hypoxemia develops (104 to 66 mm Hg). Mixed venous gas tensions remained constant and physiologic. (From D'Alonzo GE, Dantzker DR: Gas exchange alterations following pulmonary thromboembolism. Clin Chest Med 5:415, 1984.)

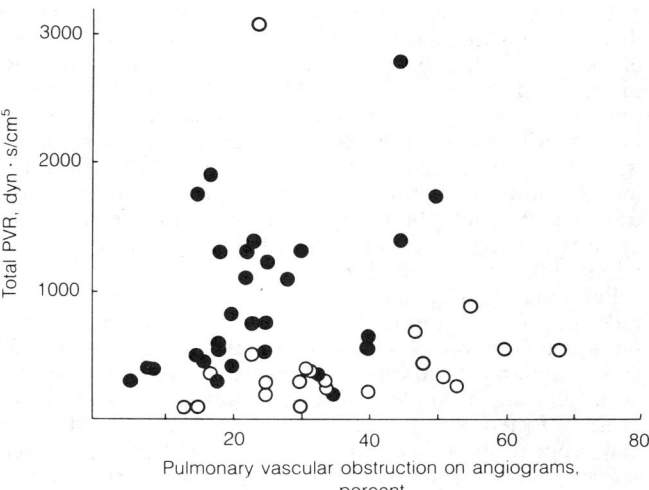

Figure 75–2. The relationship between pulmonary vascular resistance (PVR) and pulmonary vascular occlusion from pulmonary embolism as judged by the pulmonary angiogram. In previously normal patients (open circles), pulmonary vascular resistance becomes elevated only with large clot burdens. In patients with previous cardiopulmonary disease (filled circles), less vascular obstruction is required to elevate pulmonary vascular resistance. (From Sharma GVRK, McIntyre KM, Sharma S, et al: Clinical and hemodynamic correlates in pulmonary embolism. Clin Chest Med 5:428, 1984.)

cardiopulmonary disease, these consequences of pulmonary embolism may occur even with modest clot burdens. As discussed later, such physiologic effects become important when considering the therapeutic strategy of pulmonary embolism.

DIAGNOSIS
Clinical Manifestations

Pulmonary embolism can present in a number of confusing ways, particularly in the patient with underlying cardiopulmonary disease. The classic symptom complex of hemoptysis, dyspnea, and pleuritic chest pain is not usually seen together in any single patient. These symptoms are largely nonspecific because they can also be associated with other common disorders such as pneumonia, myocardial infarction, and congestive heart failure.[11]

In the critical care setting, the situation is particularly complicated because most patients have pre-existing cardiopulmonary disease. Consequently, pulmonary embolism is often suspected in the critically ill patient because of hemodynamic compromise and/or severe gas exchange abnormalities. Even so, the manifestations of pulmonary embolism can be masked by the physiologic abnormalities of other conditions such as pulmonary edema and sepsis. Thus, the physician is often in the unenviable position of considering pulmonary embolism in many situations in the critical care unit.

Because of the nonspecific clinical presentation of pulmonary embolus, the clinician must rely on laboratory studies to arrive at an accurate diagnosis. Routine blood studies are of no diagnostic value in the critically ill patient with pulmonary embolus.[11] Despite some interest in a serum marker for pulmonary embolus,[32] no single blood study has yet been associated with an accurate diagnosis. The use of arterial blood gas determinations may be helpful because a normal P_{O_2} or alveolar-arterial gradient is not common with pulmonary embolus.[33, 34] However, such normal findings are unlikely in a critical care setting.

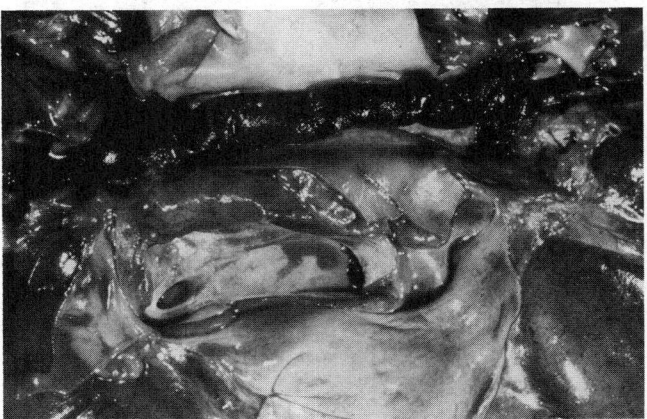

Figure 75–3. Massive, fatal pulmonary embolus occluding the main pulmonary artery.

The electrocardiogram in pulmonary embolism most often demonstrates nonspecific ST-T wave changes. At least one of the electrocardiographic manifestations of acute cor pulmonale ($S_1Q_3T_3$, complete right bundle branch block, P-pulmonale, or right axis deviation) is present in 25% of patients with acute pulmonary embolism. Left axis deviation is as common as right axis deviation in this disorder. The most common arrhythmia consists of premature atrial contractions. Probably the most useful role of the electrocardiogram is to diagnose acute myocardial infarction, which may mimic pulmonary embolism.[35]

Pulmonary embolism may be manifested on the chest radiograph in a number of different ways. Most often, pulmonary embolism is associated with infiltrates, effusions, and/or atelectasis, largely attributable to pulmonary infarction, splinting from pleurisy, or perhaps altered compliance in the affected area.[36] Occasionally, a pulmonary infarction may appear as a Hampton hump—a peripheral wedge-shaped parenchymal lung defect with an accompanying pleural effusion. Of interest is that large pulmonary emboli tend not to produce pulmonary infarction and therefore may be associated with minimal chest radiographic abnormalities. If the clot is massive enough to obliterate the blood flow to one lung, the vasculature to that lung may appear markedly diminished, giving the so-called Westermark sign. Although these radiographic patterns may occasionally be useful, they may not be helpful in critically ill patients, who often have abnormal chest radiographs because of other conditions such as pneumonia and congestive heart failure.

Diagnostic Studies

The most useful tests for diagnosing pulmonary emboli are imaging studies of the pulmonary vasculature and noninvasive studies of the lower extremities. The application of

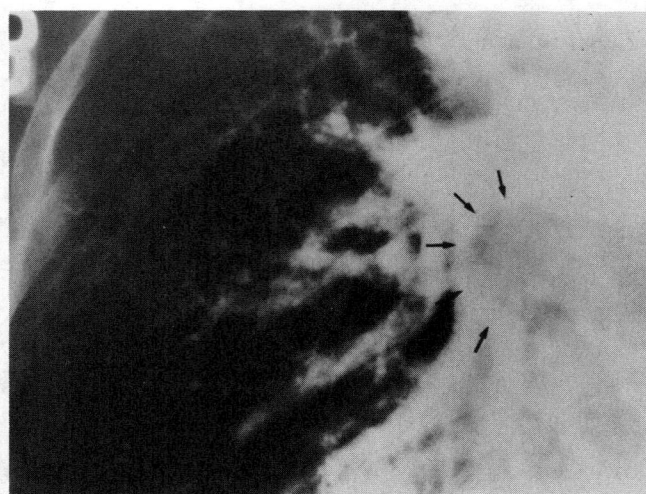

Figure 75–5. Pulmonary arteriogram demonstrating large clot in the right main pulmonary artery, as outlined by arrows.

these diagnostic technologies has been reviewed[37] and is summarized here.

The ventilation-perfusion radionuclide lung scan is an essential diagnostic test for pulmonary embolism and has undergone considerable investigation in the past decade.[3, 38–42] The technology of radionuclide lung scanning is simple and noninvasive but may require some adjustments for the critically ill patient. The perfusion component of the scan, which is the most useful clinically, requires the injection of radioactive technetium tagged to macroaggregated albumin. This radioactive material lodges in well-perfused lung zones so that poorly perfused areas appear as cold spots on the scan. Such defects could be from vascular disorders, as occurs in pulmonary emboli, or from alveolar disease, such as pneumonia, which is associated with both perfusion and ventilation defects. The ventilation scan, in theory, helps to distinguish between these possibilities. Radioactive gases have been utilized for the ventilation scan, including radioactive xenon, and a variety of radioactive aerosols have also been used to image the airways during inhalation.

From a practical viewpoint, the ventilation scan may be undesirable and even impossible in the critically ill patient. Except through sophisticated exhaust systems, radioactive gases cannot be used in mechanically ventilated patients. Other patients with respiratory distress may not tolerate the closed ventilation systems or the work of breathing required for the ventilation scan. Furthermore, although the ventilation scan has received much attention in the literature, it remains unclear how much additional information it adds to the perfusion scan.

The lung scan is an excellent screening test for pulmonary embolism. A normal scan showing minimal or no defects effectively rules out the diagnosis of pulmonary embolism.[43, 44] Abnormal scans have been classified by probability for pulmonary embolus. A high-probability scan, with segmental defects corresponding to anatomic occlusion of the pulmonary vasculature, is associated with at least an 85% likelihood of pulmonary embolus[3, 37] (Fig. 75–4). Other scan interpretations showing less specific findings are not accurate enough alone to be relied on for correct diagnosis. Unfortunately, most patients with pulmonary emboli fall into these uncertain diagnostic categories of either an intermediate- or low-probability lung scan.[37]

The pulmonary angiogram remains the "gold standard" for diagnosing pulmonary embolism. When performed by experienced investigators using selective arterial injections,

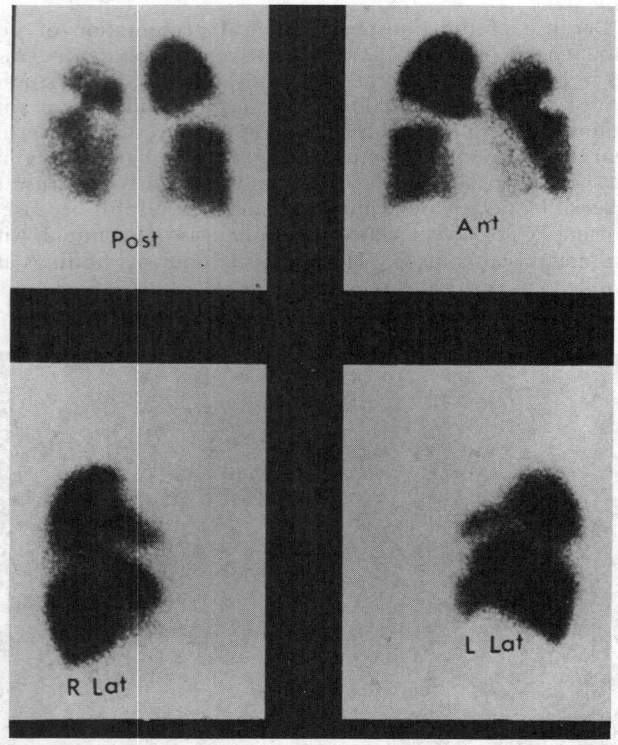

Figure 75–4. High-probability perfusion lung scan that demonstrates wedge-shaped defects corresponding to areas of vascular occlusion from pulmonary emboli. Ventilation scan showed no defects.

this study is extremely accurate in detecting clinically important pulmonary emboli with a negligible false-negative rate[3, 45-47] (Fig. 75–5). In the Prospective Investigation of Pulmonary Embolism Diagnosis study, pulmonary angiography had a mortality of less than 1% in a population of extremely ill patients.[3] However, it is unknown whether the accuracy and safety of the pulmonary angiogram are reproducible outside a tertiary hospital setting.

Another option for diagnosing pulmonary embolism is investigation of the veins of the lower extremities. The logic is that, for most patients, proximal deep venous thrombosis is the source of pulmonary emboli and, if detected, would be treated the same way as pulmonary embolism[37] (Fig. 75–6). Although contrast venography is the standard for diagnosing venous disease, it is invasive and may even promote phlebitis. Alternatively, there are two noninvasive techniques to examine the deep venous system. The most widely studied is impedance plethysmography, which detects venous occlusion from the popliteal fossa to the right atrium. This study has at least a 90% accuracy compared with that of venography, is easy to perform, and requires little operator experience for correct interpretation.[37] Duplex Doppler ultrasonography, a more recent technique, can provide dramatic images of the venous system.[48] This technology has not been

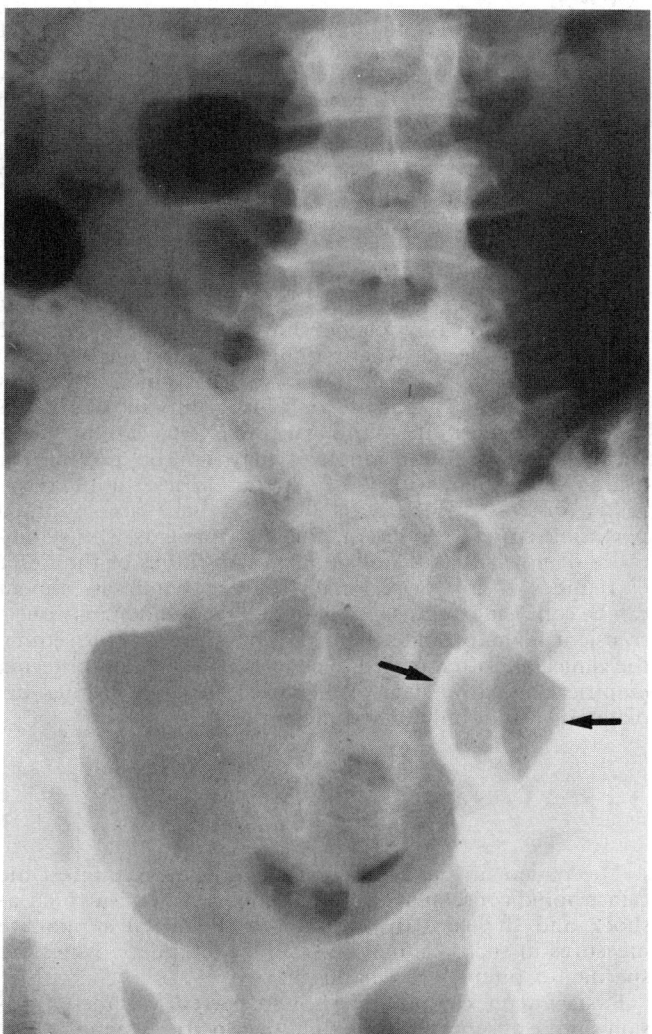

Figure 75–6. Large ileofemoral thrombus outlined by contrast venography in patient with lower-extremity trauma and documented pulmonary emboli.

studied as widely as impedance plethysmography but has been found useful in detecting clots below the knee.

These noninvasive technologies of lung scanning and venous studies have been combined, and a diagnostic approach to pulmonary embolism has been proposed (Fig. 75–7). In this strategy, the lung scan is used to detect patients whose scans are normal or have high-probability defects. The patients with normal scans are extremely unlikely to have pulmonary embolism, whereas patients with high-probability scans can be assumed to have this disorder. Exceptions include patients with previous thromboembolic disease whose perfusion defects could be old findings and patients with extrinsic compression of the pulmonary artery from neoplasm.

Patients with low-probability scans may not require workup or treatment for pulmonary embolism if the clinical suspicion of this disorder is low (<20%). Otherwise, venous studies of the lower extremities can be performed to document proximal deep venous thrombosis. If the results are normal, patients without cardiopulmonary disease can probably be followed with serial venous studies. The significance of these normal venous study results in patients with cardiopulmonary disease is unknown.

Other physiologic measurements used in the critical care setting may help in diagnosing pulmonary embolism. For example, respiratory compliance can be measured in ventilated patients. Pulmonary embolism alone usually does not alter lung compliance, except in the rare occasion when it presents as pulmonary edema.[49] Physiologic dead space may also rise with pulmonary embolism and also can be measured directly or by monitoring expired carbon dioxide in the ventilated patient.[50]

With the use of a pulmonary arterial flotation catheter, hemodynamic assessment may be helpful in diagnosing pulmonary embolism. In massive pulmonary embolism, pulmonary vascular resistance is elevated above baseline and is accompanied by signs of impaired right ventricular performance such as tricuspid regurgitation, elevated right ventricular pressure, and low cardiac output. A common misconception is that massive pulmonary emboli produce major elevations in pulmonary arterial pressure. As described earlier, abrupt increases in pulmonary vascular resistance result in acute right ventricular failure and reduced cardiac output. Because of this fall in cardiac output, only modest elevations of pulmonary arterial pressure are encountered in the previously healthy patient with massive pulmonary emboli (Fig. 75–8). However, because much of the pulmonary vascular space has been obliterated, calculated pulmonary vascular resistance remains markedly elevated.[27, 30, 31]

In many critically ill patients, echocardiography may be employed to examine ventricular wall motion, to determine valve competence, and to detect pericardial effusion. Echocardiographic findings such as tricuspid regurgitation or new right ventricular dilation suggest the diagnosis of pulmonary embolism.[51] In some patients, a free-floating embolus may even be seen in the right atrium or ventricle.[51-53]

Diagnostic Scenarios

Despite the diagnostic complexities, critically ill patients with suspected pulmonary embolism often fall into several common scenarios. In each situation, a few key diagnostic steps are helpful and can be supplemented by other types of physiologic information available in the critical care unit.

In the first and most straightforward scenario, the patient with no previous cardiopulmonary disease has moderate hemodynamic compromise and/or gas exchange abnormalities. Common problems such as pneumonia, pulmonary edema, and myocardial infarction can often be ruled out

DIAGNOSTIC ALGORITHM

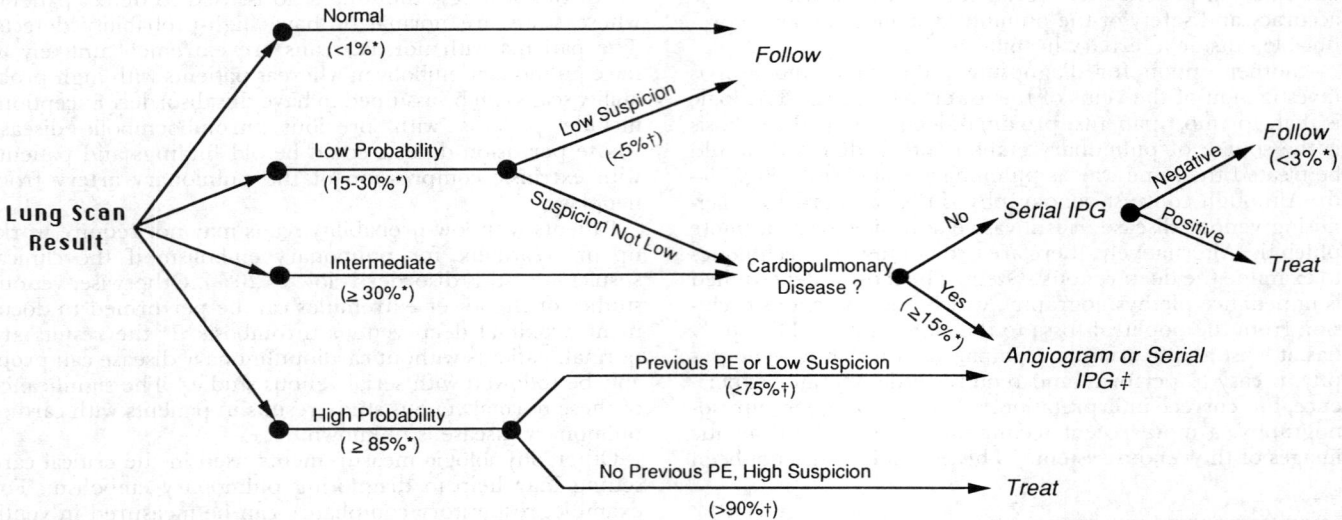

Figure 75–7. Diagnostic algorithm. A normal scan effectively rules out pulmonary embolism (PE). A high-probability scan supports the diagnosis of pulmonary embolism, except in the presence of previous pulmonary embolism or low clinical suspicion. Other scan results were less helpful except the combination of low probability and low clinical suspicion. An abnormal impedance plethysmography (IPG) study supports the diagnosis of thromboembolism. A normal result reliably excludes this disorder only in patients with nondiagnostic scans and no cardiopulmonary disease. Percentages in parentheses indicate likelihood of pulmonary embolism. ★ Strongly supported by clinical studies; † suggested by clinical studies, needs confirmation; ‡ a single normal impedance plethysmographic result may not be sufficient to rule out thromboembolism. (Reproduced, with permission, from Kelley MA, Carson JL, Palevsky HI, et al, Diagnosing pulmonary embolism: New facts and strategies. Ann Intern Med. 1991; 114:300–306.)

clinically. The next immediate step in such a patient is to perform a radionuclide lung scan. If pulmonary emboli are responsible for substantial hemodynamic and gas exchange abnormalities, major clotting should be present and appear on the lung scan as multiple, segmental or lobar perfusion scan defects. A low-probability lung scan is inconsistent with massive pulmonary embolism and suggests that an alternative diagnosis be pursued. An indeterminate lung scan result necessitates other diagnostic tests such as either a pulmonary angiogram or noninvasive studies of the lower extremities. In patients without pre-existing cardiopulmonary disease, the latter have been shown to be accurate in ruling out thromboembolism.[54] However, it is unknown if such a strategy applies to critically ill patients. Therefore, a normal noninvasive venous study result may not rule out thromboembolism in this patient group.

In a second and more dramatic scenario, the patient is admitted with shock and/or hypoxic respiratory failure necessitating mechanical ventilation. The presence of normal pulmonary compliance with severe hypoxemia suggests a pulmonary vascular process. Invasive hemodynamic monitoring with a pulmonary flotation catheter may reveal right-sided heart failure with high pulmonary vascular resistance. Even if these findings are suggestive of pulmonary embolism, further studies are often needed for confirmation. If the patient can be transported out of the critical care unit, a perfusion lung scan could be obtained to demonstrate substantial vascular occlusion. Pulmonary angiography may be preferable because of its high diagnostic accuracy. If the patient cannot be transported out of the critical care unit, other options are bedside pulmonary angiography[55] and noninvasive studies of the lower extremities.

A third scenario often occurring in the critical care setting

features the patient with known cardiopulmonary disease who has a transient setback, such as worsening hemodynamic characteristics or physiologic shunt. In such a case, the clinician must decide whether this deterioration is due to underlying cardiopulmonary disease or to some other event such as pulmonary embolism. This group of patients is probably the most difficult to assess in critical care medicine because noninvasive technology may not be useful. For example, a patient with known pneumonia or adult respiratory distress syndrome is likely to have an abnormal perfusion scan. In addition, for such patients, the significance of normal results of noninvasive studies of the lower extremities is unknown. Finally, hemodynamic assessment can be confusing because small pulmonary emboli may cause transient hemodynamic changes. Therefore, in this setting, the clinician is often forced to choose between administering empirical therapy, such as heparin, and establishing the diagnosis with a pulmonary angiogram.

THERAPY

Immediate Support

The patient in the critical care setting may manifest the catastrophic consequences of pulmonary embolism such as shock and hypoxia. In addition to the usual supportive measures in such a situation, several therapeutic issues are specific for pulmonary embolism.

First, if acute cor pulmonale is suspected, volume expansion (in the absence of overt fluid overload) is essential. The failing right ventricle may also perform better with the use of beta-agonist drugs such as dobutamine or dopamine. If the patient has a cardiac arrest, external compression during

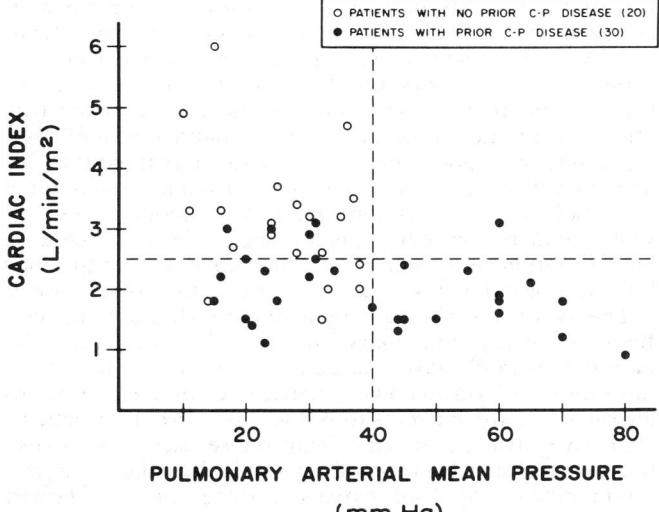

Figure 75–8. Relationship between cardiac index and pulmonary artery pressure in patients with pulmonary emboli. Patients without previous cardiopulmonary (C-P) disease never developed high pulmonary arterial pressure even with severe reductions in cardiac index. Elevations in pulmonary arterial pressure were confined to patients with pre-existent cardiopulmonary disease. (From Sharma GVRK, McIntyre KM, Sharma S, et al: Clinical and hemodynamic correlates in pulmonary embolism. Clin Chest Med 5:428, 1984.)

cardiopulmonary resuscitation may fragment a clot in the main pulmonary artery and relieve proximal vascular obstruction.

Patients with such a massive clot usually have severe hypoxemia attributable to ventilation-perfusion mismatch. This hypoxemia can also be worsened by low cardiac output and/or shunting across a patent foramen ovale. In such cases, it may be difficult to improve arterial blood gas values unless there is an accompanying improvement in cardiac performance. If pulmonary emboli are unilateral, hypoxemia may be positional, as gravity influences the ventilation-perfusion relationship. The effects of positional variation on ventilation-perfusion match in pulmonary embolism may be variable and, in fact, paradoxical. In one report, ventilation-perfusion match was optimized when the lung with the clot was in the dependent position.[56] This observation was contrary to the usual situation in which the ventilation/perfusion ratio is optimized with the unaffected lung in the dependent position. Regardless of the mechanism, positional hypoxemia may be a clue to the presence of pulmonary embolism, and variations in position may help to reduce hypoxemia.

Treatment of Clot

The majority of patients probably survive the initial insult of pulmonary embolism. If given time, the endogenous lytic system can usually dissolve the clot. The danger is that, in the meantime, venous thrombosis progresses, and additional thrombus migrates to the pulmonary circulation. Therefore, the principal therapeutic strategy in pulmonary embolism is to prevent additional clot formation in the venous system by interrupting the thrombotic process with anticoagulation. The exception is a minority of patients for whom the degree of the pulmonary embolism is substantial. These patients often have hemodynamic compromise, and in such a tenuous physiologic state, any additional clot burden could prove fatal. In such cases, it may be desirable to reduce the clot volume by the use of thrombolytic therapy. Finally, in

patients who cannot tolerate anticoagulation or thrombolytic therapy, alternative methods of treating pulmonary emboli include vena cava occlusion and catheter or surgical embolectomy.

Anticoagulation

Unless contraindicated, patients suspected of having pulmonary emboli should undergo rapid anticoagulation with heparin. This drug binds to circulating antithrombin III and produces a conformational change so that antithrombin III becomes 1000 times more effective in inhibiting thrombin. Heparin's effect on antithrombin III also causes it to block activated factor X early in the clotting cascade. Through these two mechanisms, heparin both interrupts and inhibits the clotting process. The antithrombin effect directly blocks the activated clotting cascade as it produces large quantities of thrombin. In addition, heparin's effect on factor X blocks early stages of the clotting cascade before its amplification through succeeding pathways.[14] This effect explains why low-dosage heparin is so successful in preventing venous thrombosis.[57, 58] Heparin's relatively short half-life of 0.5 to 2 hours is unaffected by renal or hepatic failure. Consequently, clotting studies can normalize relatively rapidly when heparin administration is discontinued.

Although there are other options for administering heparin, the continuous intravenous infusion of this drug is probably the most efficacious and most commonly used method. In patients with normal results of clotting studies, a bolus of approximately 5000 U is provided, followed by continuous infusion of approximately 1000 U/h.[57] The activated partial thromboplastin time (PTT) is used to adjust the subsequent heparin dose. Heparin should be administered to prolong the PTT to 15 to 25 seconds longer than the patient's own PTT or a similar interval beyond the middle range of the normal laboratory value for PTT.[57] Although it has been empirically observed that heparin requirement is much higher in the first few days of therapy, the adjustment of heparin is probably not necessary much more frequently than every 24 hours. It has been well shown that therapeutic doses of heparin are necessary to prevent recurrent thromboembolic events.[57, 59, 60]

Bleeding is the major complication of heparin administration, and its incidence has been reported to range from 5 to 20%.[61] The upper limit of this range likely applies to patients with problems such as multiple venous access sites, those with stress ulceration of the gastric mucosa, and patients undergoing invasive surgical procedures. In such patients, platelet-activating agents should be avoided because these drugs increase the likelihood of bleeding complications. Prolongation of the PTT beyond the therapeutic range is also associated with a high bleeding rate. Therefore, in the patient being treated for thromboembolism, strict attention to the PTT should be maintained. When bleeding does occur, it can usually be stopped with interruption of the heparin administration and attention to the bleeding site. If more rapid clotting control is necessary, protamine can be administered to bind heparin to form an inactive complex.

Heparin can also induce thrombocytopenia and even thrombosis. This phenomenon usually occurs 5 to 10 days after the start of heparin therapy and is usually seen in patients who have previously been treated with heparin.[14, 57, 62] Although the exact mechanism is unclear, this disorder may result from an immune reaction against platelets, mediated by the endothelium.[62] Most patients receiving heparin therapy have some slight decline in platelet count; however, a steadily falling platelet level, particularly below 50,000/mm³, strongly suggests heparin-induced thrombocytopenia. In such cases, heparin administration should be stopped and alternative methods of anticoagulation considered. Because of the possibility of this complication, patients receiving heparin should have platelet counts measured every few days.

Warfarin is the most commonly used form of long-term anticoagulation after thromboembolism. This drug acts by inhibiting the action of clotting factors II, VII, IX, and X, thus prolonging the prothrombin time. Warfarin can also reduce levels of protein C, a naturally occurring inhibitor of fibrinolysis. This effect on protein C occurs before the inhibition of the other clotting factors and, in theory, a hypercoagulable state can occur within the first 1 to 2 days of warfarin therapy. Therefore, in the presence of ongoing thrombosis, warfarin should not be given before an antithrombotic effect has been established with heparin.

As a result of considerable clinical investigation, the target of anticoagulation achieved by warfarin has been lowered to a prothrombin time of 1.25 to 1.5 times the patient's own control value.[57] This degree of anticoagulation is highly successful in the prevention of recurrent thrombosis and yet has a much lower complication rate compared with higher target levels of the prothrombin time.

The administration of warfarin is a clinical challenge because of warfarin's many interactions with other medications. Therefore, in a critical care setting, warfarin is not usually employed, except in the most stable of patients whose drug regimen is constant. Instead, most clinicians prefer to use heparin in the critical care unit because it has few drug interactions and its short half-life makes it quite easy to adjust anticoagulation effects.

Thrombolytic Therapy

As described earlier, thrombolytic therapy should be employed when it is necessary to rapidly dissolve clot. Trials comparing streptokinase and urokinase with heparin have not demonstrated that thrombolytic therapy alters survival in patients with pulmonary emboli.[63, 64] However, these studies were not designed to show a difference in mortality but simply to document that thrombolytic therapy dissolves clot more rapidly than does heparin. There are three major drugs available for thrombolysis: streptokinase, urokinase, and TPA. Although the three drugs have somewhat different properties, they all act by triggering the conversion of plasminogen to plasmin. The ideal thrombolytic agent dissolves clots without producing a systemic fibrinolytic effect. In theory, such a drug might reduce bleeding complications. Unfortunately, all fibrinolytic agents, including TPA, must achieve some degree of systemic lytic effect to produce therapeutic results. Therefore, the choice of lytic agents depends on other issues such as cost, ease of administration, and onset of action.

Although the properties of thrombolytic agents have been reviewed,[65, 66] a few highlights are worthy of emphasis. Streptokinase, a commonly employed drug in both the pulmonary and coronary circulations, is a foreign protein derived from bacteria. Streptokinase must form a complex with plasminogen, which then cleaves other circulating plasminogen to its active form of plasmin. In theory, this complexing might result in clinical situations in which there is no more available circulating plasminogen as a source of plasmin. However, practically, this is not a common problem because most patients achieve a lytic effect with this drug.

Urokinase, a human protein, is more expensive than streptokinase but may have somewhat more rapid onset of action. In contrast to streptokinase, urokinase directly cleaves plasminogen to plasmin. Although streptokinase may induce formation of antistreptococcal antibodies, urokinase is nonantigenic and may be used multiple times in the same patient.

TPA has been widely used in the coronary circulation. In contrast to initial theory, this drug seems to be most effective when given in doses sufficient to sustain a systemic lytic affect. As a human protein it is also nonantigenic and has a rapid onset of action. New trials have demonstrated that this drug may be given for brief periods and still have substantial thrombolytic effect.[67] If confirmed by additional trials, this short regimen may reduce hemorrhagic side effects because both duration and intensity of thrombolytic therapy may influence bleeding risk.[67] Like urokinase, TPA is expensive.

The use of thrombolytic agents requires clinical judgment. Because treated pulmonary embolism has less than 10% mortality, it would take a large clinical trial to demonstrate the efficacy of thrombolytic therapy. Until then, it seems logical to use these agents to reduce clot burden in patients who have cardiopulmonary compromise. Aside from cost, there is no clear advantage of any single thrombolytic agent. Streptokinase, the least expensive drug with the largest clinical experience, may be the preference of many clinicians, despite some problems with antigenic side effects. Urokinase and TPA may be better choices if a rapid dissolution of the clot is desired. The pharmacologic action and side effects of these three thrombolytic agents are summarized in Table 75–1.

The complications of thrombolytic therapy can largely be prevented by careful patient selection. Any active bleeding site or recent central nervous system disease (probably within the past 3 to 6 months) is generally considered an absolute contraindication to thrombolytic therapy. Most clinicians avoid thrombolytic therapy if invasive procedures, surgery, or severe trauma has occurred within the previous 7 days. There are other relative contraindications but their risks must be weighed against the clinical need for thrombolytic therapy.

Clinical laboratory studies of coagulation are not useful in predicting hemorrhagic complications of lytic therapy.[68] The use of such studies appears to be limited to documenting that a lytic state has been established. The concomitant use of heparin and antiplatelet agents may also increase the risk of bleeding with thrombolytic agents and thus should be avoided while lytic therapy is being utilized.

Other Therapies

Another variation in the treatment of pulmonary embolism is the infusion of thrombolytic agents through a catheter placed in the pulmonary artery. In theory, this local infusion might be more effective in dissolving clots by delivering drug directly to the thrombus and perhaps even reducing the dose requirement of thrombolytic therapy. However, this approach has not proved any more efficacious than systemic thrombolytic therapy and may even be associated with more side effects resulting from catheter-related complications.[69]

In some critically ill patients, anticoagulation and thrombolytic therapy may be contraindicated because of bleeding complications. Preventing the migration of venous clots into the pulmonary circulation can be achieved by blocking the inferior vena cava through mechanical means. The surgical interruption of the inferior vena cava by ligation, sutures, or external clips has largely been replaced by endovascular filtration devices, which can be placed through percutaneous catheters. A number of such devices have been developed, all employing similar technology. This consists of a stainless steel filter that has low-resistance characteristics and can be inserted through a large-bore catheter. These devices have hooks that engage in the wall of the vena cava to provide a

TABLE 75–1

COMPARISON OF THROMBOLYTIC AGENTS

Drug	Source	Action	Dosage*	Side Effects	Cost
Streptokinase	Cultures of streptococcal bacteria	Combines with circulating plasminogen to form activator complex; cleaves plasminogen to produce plasmin	IV bolus of 250,000 U over 30 min followed by maintenance dose of 100,000 U/h for 12–24 h for PE	Bleeding; antigenic; cannot be used again (?); systemic fibrinolysis	Modest
Urokinase	Human urine or recombinant DNA technology	Cleaves circulating plasminogen directly; more rapid(?)	4000 U/kg IV over 20 min followed by maintenance of 4000 U/kg/h for 12–24 h for PE	Bleeding (nonantigenic)	5–10 times streptokinase
TPA	Recombinant DNA technology	Cleaves plasminogen within clot; requires systemic fibrinolysis; more rapid(?)	IV infusion of 100 mg over 2 h for PE	Bleeding (nonantigenic)	Similar to urokinase

*PE = pulmonary embolism.

permanent placement. The most widely studied device is the Greenfield filter, which does not require long-term anticoagulation and has a good patency record.[70] However, the Greenfield filter has been plagued by such problems as malposition, vena cava perforation, and femoral venous thrombosis at the insertion site.[71, 72] These difficulties led to the development of a mesh filter known as the bird's nest filter. Because of its redundant cluster of wires, this filter does not require precise alignment along the axis of the cava and it has a patency rate similar to that of the Greenfield filter.[73] More recently, attention has been focused on the development of retrievable filters, which can be removed after the patient's potential for thromboembolism recedes. To date, none of these filtration devices have been subjected to controlled trials to compare efficacy and safety.[74]

In selected cases, the clinician may resort to embolectomy to rescue a patient who is dying of hemodynamic shock from pulmonary emboli. Clearly, when possible, such severely compromised patients should be first be considered for thrombolytic therapy. However, if such therapy is ineffective or contraindicated, mechanical removal of clots from the pulmonary circulation may be appropriate. Although there is considerable controversy about the role of surgical embolectomy, it may be helpful in selected patients. Much of the surgical experience in this area antedates the availability of thrombolytic agents and therefore cannot be simply compared with current experience when such medical therapy is available. Nonetheless, important themes in these surgical experiences are useful. The overall mortality of patients undergoing embolectomy for acute massive pulmonary embolism is about 30%. However, this mortality jumps to about 70% for patients taken to surgery in the setting of a cardiac arrest.[75–77] Therefore, if this therapeutic surgical approach is chosen, it should be undertaken with some haste before the patient becomes moribund.

Another option is embolectomy performed through a percutaneous catheter. With this technique, a specially designed suction catheter is used to remove a central clot from the pulmonary artery.[78] Although this procedure can be dramatically effective and avoids surgery, its general success rate is not yet known (Figs. 75–9 and 75–10).

Summary of Therapeutic Approaches

For most patients with pulmonary embolism, anticoagulation is a simple and effective therapy. Such patients usually

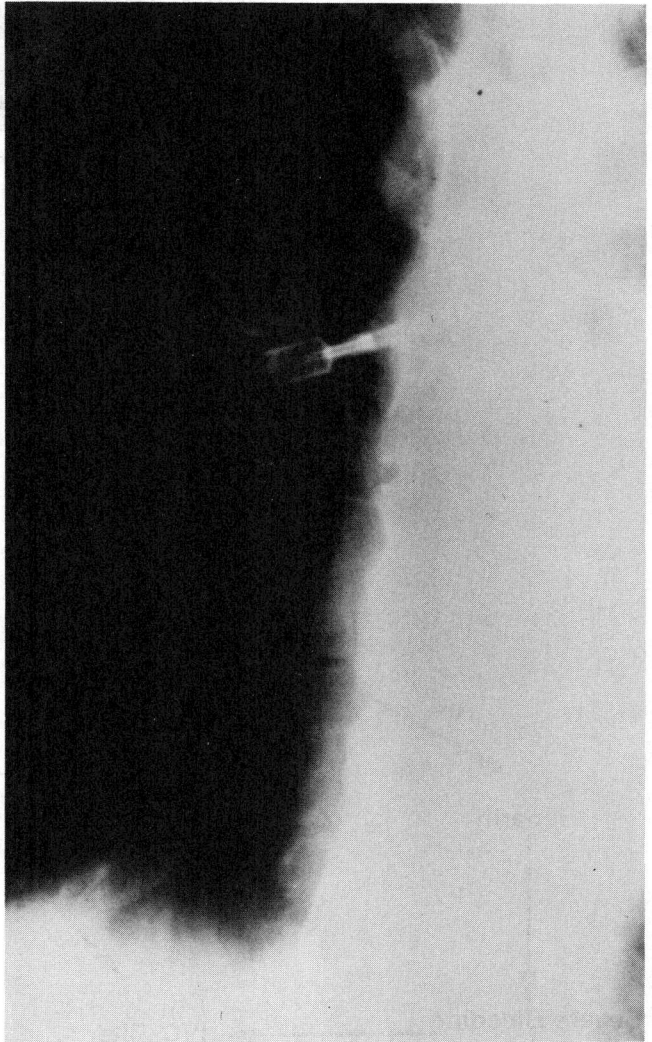

Figure 75–9. Embolectomy suction catheter within the right main pulmonary artery before catheter embolectomy for massive pulmonary embolus.

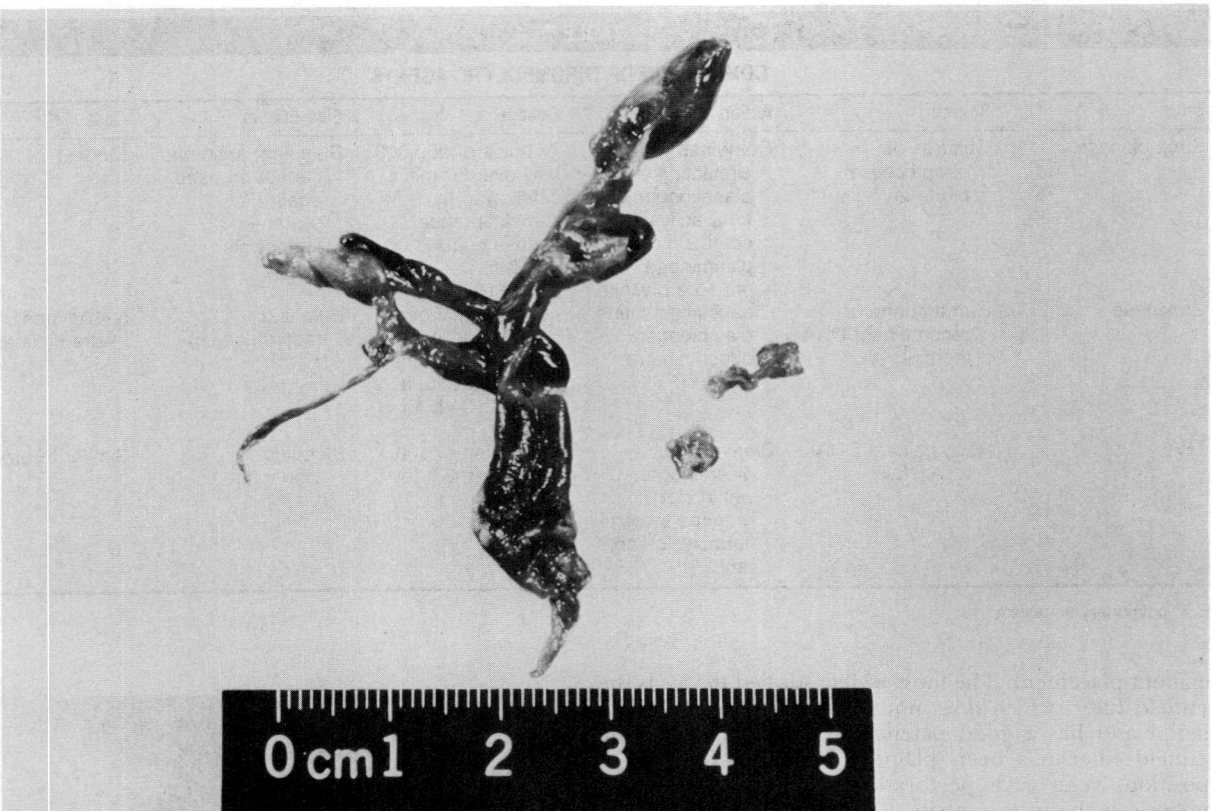

Figure 75–10. Large pulmonary embolus removed by suction catheter embolectomy.

**THERAPEUTIC
STRATEGY**

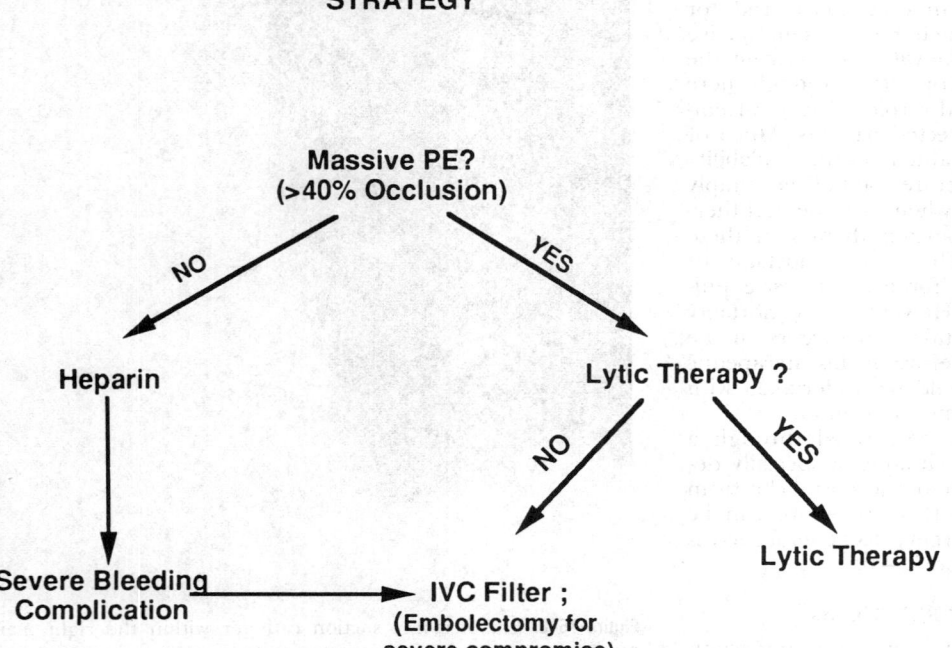

Figure 75–11. Therapeutic algorithm for treating pulmonary embolism. See text for details. PE = pulmonary embolism; IVC = inferior vena cava.

have nonmassive pulmonary emboli (i.e., occluding less than 40% of the pulmonary vasculature) and have nonlethal clinical manifestations such as dyspnea and pleurisy. However, such patients are also unlikely to be admitted to the critical care unit. Critically ill patients with pulmonary embolism usually have massive clot manifested by hemodynamic compromise, hypoxia, or syncope—all symptoms that prompt critical care unit admission. Despite the lack of a randomized trial, there is consensus that massive pulmonary embolism should, when possible, be treated with thrombolytic therapy.[79] This approach reduces the clot burden in the venous system and thereby the potential for more emboli. Lytic therapy also dissolves clots in the pulmonary vasculature, thus reducing vascular resistance and improving right ventricular performance. Therefore, thrombolytic therapy should be strongly considered for patients with hemodynamic compromise, severe hypoxemia, or large clot burdens as judged by lung scan or angiogram.

Unfortunately, thrombolytic therapy may not be possible in some critically ill patients because of potential bleeding complications. In such cases, the strategy should be directed toward ensuring that no additional clot reaches the pulmonary circulation. Therefore, in patients with massive pulmonary embolism who are not candidates for lytic therapy, an inferior vena cava filter offers a high degree of protection from additional emboli. A similar strategy applies to patients who must stop anticoagulant therapy because of bleeding complications.

Finally, embolectomy should be considered when other measures are contraindicated or have failed and the patient continues to have severe cardiopulmonary compromise. The choice of catheter versus surgical embolectomy is a matter of judgment and local experience. Before either maneuver, an inferior vena cava filter should be placed immediately to prevent more emboli. These therapeutic approaches are summarized in Figure 75–11.

References

1. Dalen JE, Alpert JS: Natural history of pulmonary embolism. Prog Cardiovasc Dis 17:257, 1975.
2. National Institutes of Health Consensus Conference: Prevention of venous thrombosis and pulmonary embolism. JAMA 256:744, 1986.
3. The PIOPED Investigators: Value of the ventilation/perfusion scan in acute pulmonary embolism: Results of the Prospective Investigation of Pulmonary Embolism Diagnosis (PIOPED). JAMA 263:2753, 1990.
4. Sevitt S, Gallagher W: Venous thrombosis and pulmonary embolism. Br J Surg 48:475, 1961.
5. McLachlin J, Paterson JC: Some basic observations on venous thrombosis and pulmonary embolism. Surg Gynecol Obstet 93:1, 1951.
6. Havig GO: Source of pulmonary emboli. Acta Chir Scand 478(suppl):42, 1977.
7. Adelstein DJ, Hines JD, Carter SG, et al: Thromboembolic events in patients with malignant superior vena cava syndrome and role of anticoagulation. Cancer 62:2258, 1988.
8. Wanscher B, Frifelt JJ, Smith-Silverstein C, et al: Thrombosis caused by polyurethane double-lumen subclavian superior vena cava catheter and hemodialysis. Crit Care Med 16:624, 1988.
9. Moser KM, LeMoine JR: Is embolic risk conditioned by location of deep venous thrombosis? Ann Intern Med 94:439, 1981.
10. Huisman MV, Buller HR, Ten Cate JW, et al: Unexpected high prevalence of silent pulmonary embolism in patients with deep venous thrombosis. Chest 95:498, 1989.
11. Moser KM: Venous thromboembolism: State of the art. Am Rev Respir Dis 141:235, 1990.
12. Virchow R: Die Verstopfung der Lungenarterie und ihre Folgen. Br Exp Pathol Physiol 2:227, 1846.
13. Colman RW, Rubin RN: Prophylaxis and treatment of thromboembolism based on pathophysiology of clotting mechanisms. In: Fishman AP (ed): Pulmonary Diseases and Disorders. 2nd ed. New York, McGraw-Hill, p 1049, 1988.
14. Kessler CM: Anticoagulation and thrombolytic therapy: Practical considerations. Chest 95:245S, 1989.
15. Flanc C, Kakkar VV, Clarke MB: The detection of venous thrombosis of the legs using 125I-labelled fibrinogen. Br J Surg 55:742, 1968.
16. Kakkar VV: The 125I-labelled fibrinogen test and phlebography in the diagnosis of deep vein thrombosis. Milbank Mem Fund Q 50:206, 1972.
17. International Multi-center Trial: Prevention of fatal postoperative pulmonary embolism by low doses of heparin. Lancet 2:45, 1975.
18. Hirsh J, Hull RO, Raskob GE: Epidemiology and pathogenesis of venous thrombosis. J Am Coll Cardiol 8:104B, 1986.
19. Browse NC, Clemenson G, Croft DN: Fibrinogen detectable thrombosis in the legs and pulmonary embolism. Br Med J 1:603, 1974.
20. Veterans Administration Cooperative Clinical Trial: Anticoagulation in acute myocardial infarction: Results of a cooperative clinical trial. JAMA 225:724, 1973.
21. Kakkar V: Prevention of venous thrombosis and pulmonary embolism. Am J Cardiol 65:50C, 1990.
22. Warlow C, Ogstum D, Douglas AS: Deep venous thrombosis of the legs after strokes. Br Med J 1:1178, 1976.
23. McCarthy ST, Robertson D, Turner JJ, et al: Low dose heparin as prophylaxis against deep vein thrombosis after stroke. Lancet 2:800, 1977.
24. Goldman L, Sayson R, Robbins S: Diagnostic yield of the autopsy in a university hospital and a community hospital. N Engl J Med 308:1000, 1983.
25. Papadakis MA, Mangrone CM, Lee KK, et al: Treatable abdominal pathologic conditions and unsuspected neoplasms at autopsy in veterans who received mechanical ventilation. JAMA 265:885, 1991.
26. Bedall SE, Fulton EJ: Unexpected findings and complications at autopsy after cardiopulmonary resuscitation (CPR). Arch Intern Med 146:1725, 1986.
27. Sharma GVRK, McIntyre KM, Sharma S, et al: Clinical and hemodynamic correlates in pulmonary embolism. Clin Chest Med 5:421, 1984.
28. Dantzker DR, Bower JS: Alterations in gas exchange following pulmonary thromboembolism. Chest 81:495, 1982.
29. D'Alonzo GE, Dantzker DR: Gas exchange alterations following pulmonary thromboembolism. Clin Chest Med 5:411, 1984.
30. McIntyre KM, Sasahara AA: The hemodynamic response to pulmonary embolism in patients without prior cardiopulmonary disease. Am J Cardiol 28:288, 1971.
31. McIntyre KM, Sasahara AA: Determinants of right ventricular function and hemodynamics after pulmonary embolism. Chest 65:534, 1974.
32. Vargo JS, Becker DM, Philbrick JT, et al: Plasma DNA: A simple, rapid test for aiding the diagnosis of pulmonary embolism. Chest 97:63, 1990.
33. Cvitanic O, Marino PL: Improved use of arterial blood gas analysis in suspected pulmonary embolism. Chest 95:48, 1989.
34. Wilson JE, Pierce AK, Johnson RL Jr, et al: Hypoxemia in pulmonary embolism. A clinical study. J Clin Invest 50:481, 1971.
35. Stein PD, Dalen J, McIntyre KM, et al: The electrocardiogram in acute pulmonary embolism. Prog Cardiovasc Dis 17:247, 1975.
36. Bynum LJ, Wilson JE: Radiographic features of pleural effusions in pulmonary embolism. Am Rev Respir Dis 117:829, 1978.
37. Kelley MA, Carson JL, Palevsky HI, et al: Diagnosing pulmonary embolism: New facts and strategies. Ann Intern Med 114:300, 1991.
38. Alderson PO, Biello DR, Gottschalk A, et al: Tc-99m DTPA aerosol and radioactive gases compared as adjuncts to perfusion scintigraphy in patients with suspected pulmonary embolism. Radiology 153:515, 1984.
39. Hull RD, Hirsh J, Carter CJ, et al: Diagnostic value of ventilation-perfusion lung scanning in patients with suspected pulmonary embolism. Chest 88:819, 1985.
40. Biello DR, Mattar AG, McKnight RC, et al: Ventilation-perfusion studies in suspected pulmonary embolism. Am J Roentgenol 133:1033, 1979.
41. Alderson PO, Rujanavech W, Secker-Walker RH, et al: The role of Xe-133 ventilation studies in the scintigraphic detection of pulmonary embolism. Radiology 120:633, 1976.
42. Hull RD, Hirsh J, Carter CJ, et al: Pulmonary angiography, ventilation lung scanning, and venography for clinically suspected pulmonary embolism with abnormal perfusion lung scan. Ann Intern Med 98:891, 1983.
43. Kipper MS, Moser KM, Kortman KE, et al: Long term follow-up of patients with suspected embolism and normal lung scan. Chest 82:411, 1982.
44. Hull RD, Raskob GE, Coates G, et al: Clinical validity of a normal perfusion lung scan in patients with suspected pulmonary embolism. Chest 97:23, 1990.
45. Novelline RA, Blaterwich OH, Athanasoulis CA, et al: The clinical course of patients with suspected pulmonary embolism and a negative pulmonary arteriogram Radiology 176:561, 1976.
46. Cheely R, McCartney WH, Perry JR, et al: The role of non-invasive tests versus pulmonary angiography in the diagnosis of pulmonary embolism. Am J Med 70:17, 1981.
47. Hull RD, Raskob GE, Carter CJ, et al: Pulmonary embolism in outpatients with pleuritic chest pain. Arch Intern Med 148:838, 1988.
48. White RH, McGanan JP, Dashback MM, et al: Diagnosis of deep-vein thrombosis using duplex ultrasound. Ann Intern Med 111:297, 1989.
49. Hyers TM, Fowler AA, Wicks AB: Focal pulmonary edema after massive pulmonary embolism. Am Rev Respir Dis 123:232, 1981.
50. Eriksson L, Wollmer P, Olsson CG, et al: Diagnosis of pulmonary embolism based upon alveolar dead space analysis. Chest 96:357, 1989.
51. Kasper W, Meinertz, Hankel B, et al: Echocardiographic findings in patients with proved pulmonary embolism. Am Heart J 112:1284, 1986.

52. Farfel Z, Schechter M, Vered Z, et al: Review of echocardiographically diagnosed right heart entrapment of pulmonary emboli-in-transit with emphasis on management. Am Heart J 113:171, 1987.
53. Kinney EL, Wright RJ: Efficacy of treatment of patients with echocardiographically detected right-sided heart thrombi: A meta-analysis. Am Heart J 118:569, 1989.
54. Hull RD, Raskob GE, Coates G, et al: A new non-invasive strategy for patients with suspected pulmonary embolism. Arch Intern Med 149:2549, 1989.
55. Rosengarten PL, Tuxen DV, Weeks AM: Whole lung pulmonary angiography in the intensive care unit with two portable chest x-rays. Crit Care Med 17:274, 1989.
56. Badr MS, Grossman JE: Positional changes in gas exchange after unilateral pulmonary embolism. Chest 98:1514, 1990.
57. Hyers TM, Hull RD, Weg JG: Antithrombotic therapy for venous thromboembolic disease. Chest 95:37S, 1989.
58. Watson-Williams E: Antithrombotic and fibrinolytic therapy. Clin Chest Med 7:469, 1986.
59. Wheeler AP, Jaquiss RDB, Newman JH: Physician practices in the treatment of pulmonary embolism and deep venous thrombosis. Arch Intern Med 148:1321, 1988.
60. Doyle DJ, Turpie AGG, Hirsh J, et al: Adjusted subcutaneous heparin or continuous intravenous heparin in patients with acute deep vein thrombosis. Ann Intern Med 107:441, 1987.
61. Levine MN, Raskob G, Hirsh J: Hemorrhagic complications of long-term anticoagulant therapy. Chest 95:26S, 1989.
62. Cines DB, Tomaski A, Tannenbaum S: Immune endothelial cell injury in heparin-associated thrombocytopenia. N Engl J Med 316:581, 1987.
63. Urokinase-streptokinase embolism trial and phase 2 results. A cooperative study. JAMA 229:1606, 1974.
64. Marder VJ, Sherry S: Thrombolytic therapy: Current status. N Engl J Med 318:1512, 1585, 1988.
65. Loscalzo J: An overview of thrombolytic agents. Chest 97:117S, 1990.
66. Kessler CM: The pharmacology of aspirin, heparin, coumarin, and thrombolytic agents: Implications for therapeutic use in cardiopulmonary disease. Chest 99:97S, 1991.
67. Levine M, Hirsh J, Weitz J, et al: A randomized trial of a single bolus dosage regimen of recombinant tissue plasminogen activator in patients with acute pulmonary embolism. Chest 98:1473, 1990.
68. Hirsh DR, Goldhaber SZ: Laboratory parameters to monitor safety and efficacy during thrombolytic therapy. Chest 99:113S, 1991.
69. Leeper KV, Popovich J, Lesser BA, et al: Treatment of massive acute pulmonary embolism. The use of low doses of intrapulmonary arterial streptokinase combined with full doses of systemic heparin. Chest 93:234, 1988.
70. Kanter B, Moser KM: The Greenfield vena cava filter. Chest 93:170, 1988.
71. Greenfield LJ, Cho KJ, Tauscher JR: Limitations of percutaneous insertion of Greenfield filters. Cardiovasc Surg 31:344, 1990.
72. Pais SO, Tobin KD, Austin CB, et al: Percutaneous insertion of the Greenfield inferior vena cava filter: Experience with ninety-six patients. J Vasc Surg 8:460, 1988.
73. Martin B, Martyak TE, Stoughton TL, et al: Experience with the Gianturco-Roehm bird's nest vena cava filter. Am J Cardiol 66:1275, 1990.
74. Yune HY: Inferior vena cava filter: Search for an ideal device. Radiology 172:15, 1989.
75. Clarke DB, Abrams LD: Pulmonary embolectomy: A 25 year experience. J Thorac Cardiovasc Surg 92:442, 1986.
76. Gray HH, Morgan JM, Paneth M, et al: Pulmonary embolectomy for acute massive pulmonary embolism: An analysis of 71 cases. Br Heart J 60:196, 1988.
77. Meyer G, Tamisier D, Sors H, et al: Pulmonary embolectomy: A 20-year experience at one center. Ann Thorac Surg 51:232, 1991.
78. Greenfield LJ: Vena caval interruption and pulmonary embolectomy. Clin Chest Med 5:495, 1984.
79. National Institutes of Health Consensus Development Conference: Thrombolytic therapy in thrombosis. Ann Intern Med 93:141, 1980.

CHAPTER 76

Pleural Disease

Richard G. Wood
Gary T. Kinasewitz

The pleural cavity is the potential space between the visceral pleura, which envelops the lung, and the parietal pleura, which covers the opposing surfaces of the chest wall, the mediastinum, and the diaphragm. In health, these serous membranes are separated by a thin layer of fluid. The accumulation of excess fluid within the pleural space in response to inflammation and/or injury to the pleural membrane is a hallmark of pleural disease. In some patients, the effusion reflects the local response to disease within or adjacent to the pleura itself. In others, particularly in critically ill patients, the effusion is just one manifestation of a complex systemic illness affecting many organs. On rare occasions, the pleural disease per se may be life threatening and necessitate management in the intensive care unit (ICU).

Recognition of the pleural involvement can provide important clues as to the cause of the underlying illness. When pleural disease occurs in the course of an illness, it may signal disease progression, the development of a complication, or inadequacy of therapy. Failure to treat the pleural disease appropriately can increase the morbidity and mortality of disorders in the critically ill patient.

PHYSIOLOGY

If one opens the thoracic cavity and examines the surfaces of the parietal and visceral membranes macroscopically, they appear similar. Each is covered by a single layer of mesothelial cells situated on a layer of connective tissue. However, there are important anatomic differences between the visceral and parietal pleurae. The blood supply of the parietal pleura is derived from the systemic circulation, whereas the visceral pleura has a dual arterial supply from both bronchial and pulmonary vessels; the former is predominant in humans.[1] The capillaries of the visceral pleura drain into the pulmonary veins so that the hydrostatic pressure in the visceral pleural capillaries is lower than that in the parietal pleura.

The lymphatic drainage of the two pleural surfaces also differs. The lymphatics of the parietal pleura are the major avenue by which protein, cells, and particulate matter leave the pleural space.[2] The mesothelial surface of the parietal pleura contains pores (stoma) that connect to the lacunae, dilated lymphatic spaces, in the submesothelial connective tissue layer.[3] Lymphatics within the lung parenchyma beneath the visceral pleura do not have stomas to communicate with the pleural cavity and do not participate in clearance of protein or particulate matter from the pleural cavity.

Fluid Dynamics

The thin layer of fluid that normally separates the two pleural surfaces is formed as an ultrafiltrate of plasma. The movement of fluid between the submesothelial capillaries and the pleural space can be described in terms of Starling's law of transcapillary exchange (Fig. 76–1). Simply stated, filtration or reabsorption of fluid across the semipermeable capillary endothelial-pleural mesothelial membrane is deter-

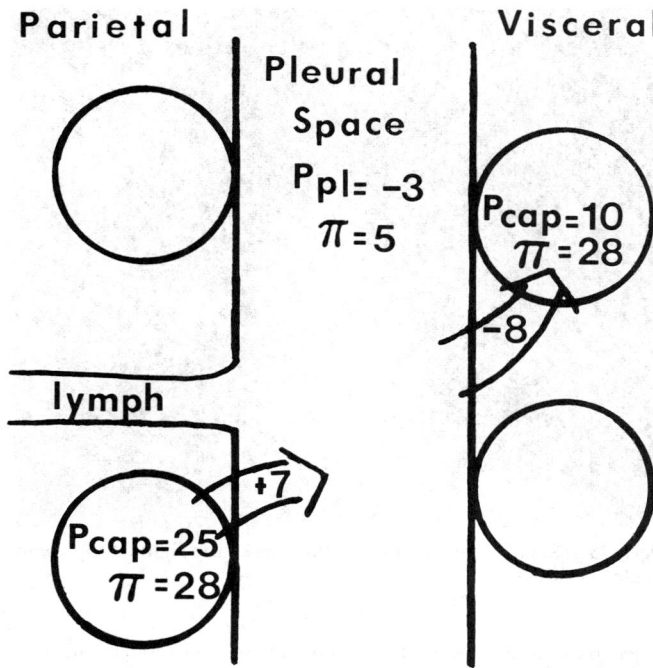

Figure 76–1. Distribution of hydrostatic (P) and oncotic (π) pressures across the parietal and visceral pleura. Fluid movement (F) can be described in terms of the Starling equation as

$$F = K_f[(Pcap - Ppl) - \sigma(\pi cap - \pi pl)]$$

where K_f and σ are the filtration coefficient and the osmotic reflection coefficient for protein, respectively; cap indicates capillary, pl, pleura. (Normally, σ is approximately 0.9.) The numbers in the open arrows indicate the direction and magnitude of the pressure differences that promote filtration and reabsorption across the parietal and visceral pleurae, respectively. (From Kinasewitz GT, Fishman AP: Pleural dynamics and effusion. In: Fishman AP [ed]: Pulmonary Diseases and Disorders. 2nd ed. p 2119, 1988. Reproduced with permission of McGraw-Hill, Inc.)

mined by the balance between the hydrostatic and oncotic pressures across the pleura.[4] Even though the protein concentration in plasma is greater than that in the pleural fluid, the hydrostatic pressure difference across the parietal pleura exceeds the oncotic pressure gradient opposing fluid filtration, and pleural fluid is filtered from the parietal membrane. The hydrostatic pressure in the visceral pleural capillaries is similar to that with the pulmonary circulation. Thus, under normal circumstances, the balance of Starling's forces promotes fluid reabsorption across the visceral pleura.

Pleural Fluid Pressures

The tendency of the chest wall to expand and the lung to collapse produces a slightly subatmospheric pleural fluid pressure at the end of expiration (functional residual capacity).[5] Pleural pressure fluctuates during the respiratory cycle and decreases to even more negative levels during a spontaneous inspiration (Fig. 76–2). Quiet expiration is a passive process in which relaxation of the inspiratory muscles permits the pleural pressure to rise back to end-expiratory levels. However, active expiratory efforts by spontaneously breathing critically ill patients with respiratory failure may generate extremely high intrapleural pressures during the expiratory phase of the respiratory cycle.

During positive pressure ventilation, pleural pressure rises during inspiration and falls back to subatmospheric values during expiration. When positive end-expiratory pressure is

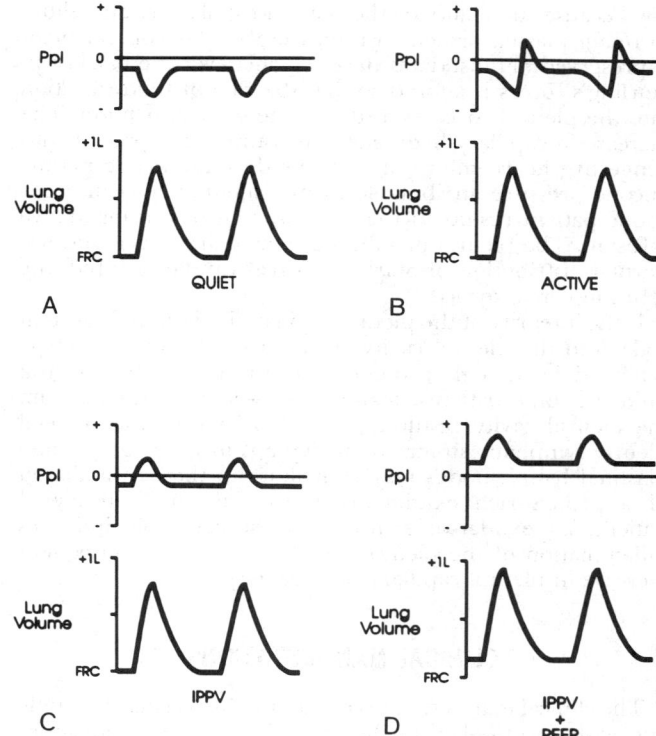

Figure 76–2. Respiratory variations in pleural pressure (Ppl) *A.* During spontaneous respiration pleural pressure is slightly subatmospheric at end expiration (functional residual capacity [FRC]). It decreases during inspiration and then returns to the end-expiratory level during quiet respiration. *B.* Even during spontaneous breathing, active expiratory muscle contraction may produce positive pleural pressures during expiration. *C.* Intermittent positive pressure ventilation (IPPV) reverses the pleural pressure changes during the respiratory cycle. Pleural pressure rises during inspiration and falls back to subatmospheric levels during expiration. *D.* Applying positive end-expiratory pressure (PEEP) during mechanical ventilation (IPPV) may result in a positive intrapleural pressure throughout the entire respiratory cycle.

applied to the ventilator circuit, the intrapleural pressure may be positive throughout the respiratory cycle. This positive intrapleural pressure can have important effects on venous return and intravascular pressures (see Chapter 65).

Pathogenesis of Pleural Effusions

Pleural effusions develop whenever the rate of fluid accumulation exceeds that of fluid removal. Effusions are generally classified as either transudates or exudates on the basis of the protein and lactate dehydrogenase (LDH) concentrations in the fluid (Table 76–1). This classification has important implications regarding the pathogenesis of the effusion. The protein content of a transudative effusion is

TABLE 76–1

DISTINGUISHING TRANSUDATIVE FROM EXUDATIVE EFFUSIONS

Criteria	Critical Value*
Pleural fluid–to–serum protein ratio	>0.5
Pleural fluid LDH level	>200 IU/L
Pleural fluid–to–serum LDH ratio	>0.6

*If any one critical value is exceeded, the effusion is an exudate.

low because the ability of the pleural capillary endothelium to retain plasma proteins within the vascular compartment is preserved. Transudates develop whenever the balance in Starling's forces is altered so that the rate of fluid filtration into the pleural space exceeds its rate of reabsorption. The increase in capillary hydrostatic pressure in the patient with congestive heart failure or with the decrease in the plasma oncotic pressure attributable to hypoalbuminemia in a cirrhotic patient results in the development of a transudative effusion. The pleural membranes per se are intact, and if a normal distribution of Starling's forces can be restored, the effusion is reabsorbed.

If the integrity of the pleural capillary is disrupted, protein leaks into the pleural cavity. Exudative effusions are characterized by a high protein concentration in the pleural fluid. In some patients, inadequate protein clearance from the pleural cavity resulting from blockage of the parietal pleural lymphatic stomas or malignant invasion of the mediastinal lymph nodes may contribute to the accumulation of a protein-rich exudate. However, in the critically ill patient, an exudative effusion almost inevitably indicates inflammation of the pleural membranes with a consequent increase in pleural capillary permeability.

CLINICAL MANIFESTATIONS

The clinical manifestations of pleural disease may be subtle and easily overlooked in the critically ill patient with more obvious and life-threatening abnormalities. Although an occasional effusion may be asymptomatic, most patients with pleural disease complain of chest pain, cough, and dyspnea. Pleuritic chest pain caused by inflammation of the pleural membranes characteristically increases with inspiration and may be localized to a specific area of the chest wall. Pain attributable to involvement of the diaphragmatic portion of the parietal pleura may be referred to the ipsilateral shoulder. A nonproductive cough may arise from reflex stimulation of receptors within the compressed lung. A productive cough suggests the presence of an infiltrate in the underlying lung. Dyspnea is also common and probably is multifactorial in origin. A large effusion acts as a space-occupying lesion and reduces all lung volumes. Ventilation-perfusion mismatching produces hypoxemia. A large effusion also allows the chest wall to expand outward so that the resting length of the inspiratory muscles is shortened. Removing a modest amount of fluid may relieve the patient's dyspnea, even in the absence of any significant improvement in arterial oxygenation or vital capacity. This symptomatic improvement is due to the consequent shift of the chest wall volume-pressure curve, which allows the inspiratory muscles to contract from a more advantageous position on their length-tension curve.[6]

Physical examination is helpful in permitting the physician to detect the presence of a pleural effusion. Although it may be difficult to appreciate the ipsilateral enlargement of the hemithorax produced by a large effusion, chest wall movement during inspiration may be restricted and lag on the affected side. The auscultation of a friction rub produced by the rubbing together of the two pleural surfaces is pathognomonic of pleural involvement. Pleural rubs typically disappear as the effusion enlarges and separates the visceral from the parietal membrane. Tactile fremitus and vocal fremitus are decreased, the percussion note is dull, and breath sounds are diminished or absent on the side of a large pleural effusion. Although atelectasis may produce similar auscultatory findings, the trachea tends to shift toward the atelectatic lung, whereas a large effusion produces tracheal deviation away from the affected hemithorax. Occasionally, a massive effusion may increase intrathoracic

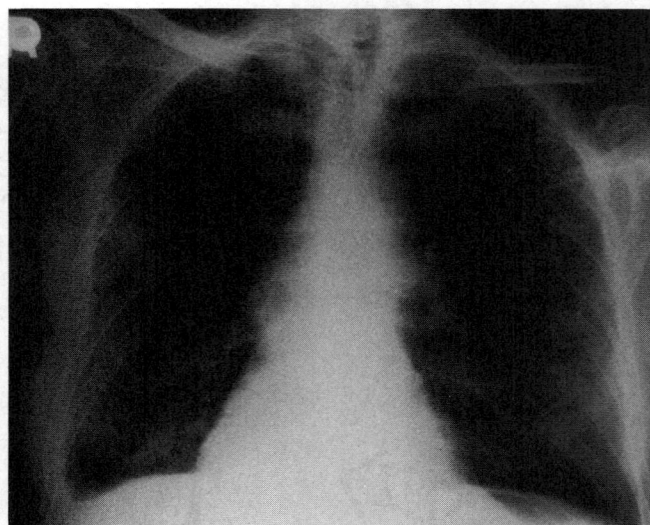

Figure 76–3. Small pleural effusion. Blunting of the right costophrenic angle is evident.

pressures to the point at which venous return is compromised and systemic hypotension ensues.

ASSESSMENT
Radiography and Ultrasonography

The presence of a pleural effusion may be verified (or first recognized) by examination of the chest radiograph.[7] Fluid tends to accumulate in the dependent portions of the thoracic cavity so that the earliest indication of a pleural effusion is a homogeneous density that obliterates the costophrenic angle (Fig. 76–3). Approximately 500 mL of fluid must accumulate before the lateral costophrenic angle appears blunted on an upright radiograph.[8] The presence of a subpulmonic effusion may be suspected when the distance between the stomach bubble and the air-containing left lower

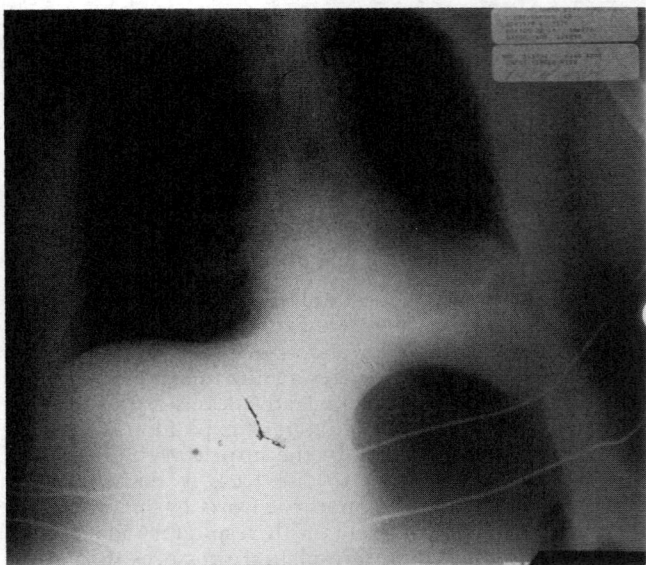

Figure 76–4. Subpulmonic effusions. Increased distance between stomach bubble and air-containing left lower lobe of the lung is due to a left subpulmonic effusion, whereas the homogeneous hepatic shadow is indicative of a right subpulmonic effusion.

lobe of the lung is increased (Fig. 76–4). Recognition of a subpulmonic effusion in the right hemithorax is more difficult. A homogeneous hepatic shadow and an inability to visualize the pulmonary vessels behind the dome of the right hemidiaphragm may be subtle clues to the presence of an effusion beneath the right lung.

It can be difficult or impossible to obtain a true upright radiograph in a critically ill patient. Whenever a semierect or supine film is obtained, free-flowing fluid layers posteriorly and imparts a hazy density to the affected hemithorax. The presence of a posterior effusion should be suspected when one hemithorax is more opaque than its counterpart

but vessels can still be appreciated within the lung parenchyma. Lateral decubitus views obtained in the ICU verify the presence of free-flowing fluid within the pleural space. However, intense pleural inflammation may produce localized obliteration of the pleural space. If this occurs, the effusion may loculate in an atypical location or fail to layer out against the chest wall on the decubitus view (Fig. 76–5).

Ultrasonography can be helpful in confirming the presence of a small pleural effusion and in distinguishing between a loculated effusion and parenchymal disease.[9, 10] Pleural effusions are visualized as an echo-free area beneath the chest wall and can be distinguished from the multiple

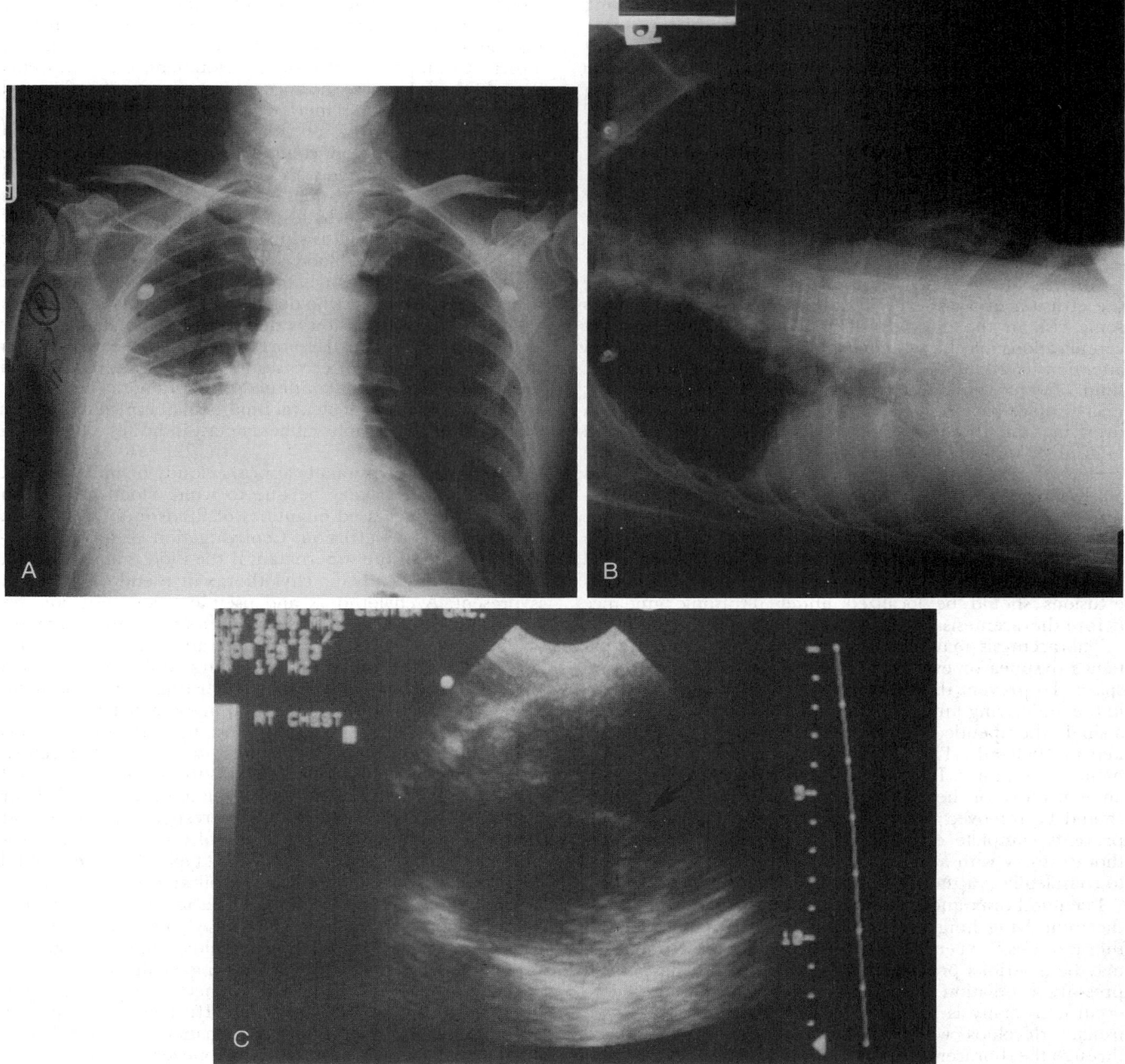

Figure 76–5. Loculated effusion. *A.* Standard anteroposterior radiograph showing opacity at the right base. *B.* Right lateral decubitus film shows a small amount of free-flowing pleural fluid layering against the chest wall. *C.* Ultrasonography of lateral right hemithorax reveals large septations *(arrow)* within an echo-free area, indicating a loculated pleural effusion; 1500 mL of purulent fluid was drained via tube thoracostomy.

echoes reflected by an infiltrate within the parenchyma of the lung (see Fig. 76–5C). The technique is simple, is inexpensive, and can be performed at the bedside in the ICU. It may be invaluable in localizing a loculated effusion for aspiration and can guide the placement of thoracostomy tubes to drain an empyema.

Computed tomography can provide valuable information in the evaluation of a pleural effusion, but transportation of a critically ill patient with multiple tubes and intravascular catheters who requires ventilatory support to the computed tomographic scanner room may impose an unnecessary risk. Computed tomography is extremely helpful in distinguishing between a peripheral lung abscess and an empyema with an air-fluid level.[11] Most empyemas form an obtuse angle at the chest wall and are lenticular. The separated pleural membranes are uniformly thickened and the underlying lung parenchyma is compressed by an empyema. Lung abscesses usually abut the pleura at an acute angle without displacement of the pulmonary vessels and possess irregular cavity walls. In each patient, the potential benefit of obtaining more detailed information to supplement the radiographic and ultrasound findings must be weighed against the risk of transporting an unstable patient to the radiology suite.

Pleural Fluid
Thoracentesis

Analysis of the pleural fluid often indicates the cause of the effusion in a critically ill patient. Thoracentesis entails some risk in the critically ill patient.[12] The incidence of complications may be minimized if the operator pays careful attention to technique and removes only a small amount of fluid. Twenty milliliters provides a sufficient sample for microscopic, bacteriologic, and clinical analysis. The skin overlying the thoracentesis site is sterilely prepared and infiltrated with local anesthetic. The periosteum of the underlying rib and parietal pleura are also infiltrated, and an 18-gauge needle attached to a 20-mL syringe is introduced over the top of the rib to minimize the likelihood of damage to the intercostal vessels, which course in the groove beneath each rib. The needle is advanced until the pleural cavity is entered and fluid is obtained. Small or loculated effusions should be localized under ultrasonic guidance before thoracentesis.

Thoracentesis may also be performed to relieve the patient's dyspnea or evacuate blood or pus from the pleural space. To prevent the development of re-expansion edema in the underlying lung, the amount of fluid removed during a single therapeutic thoracentesis to relieve dyspnea is limited to 1000 mL. This usually produces marked improvement in symptoms. In contrast, if one is attempting to drain an empyema or hemothorax, as much fluid as possible should be removed before the development of loculations prevents complete evacuation of the pleural space. Tube thoracostomy with a large-bore tube frequently is required to completely evacuate the pleural space in these patients.

Pneumothorax and bleeding resulting from laceration of the underlying lung are the most feared complications of thoracentesis.[13, 14] Persistent air leak or bronchopleural fistula may be a serious problem in the patient receiving positive pressure ventilation. Pneumothorax has been reported to occur in as many as 12% of all thoracenteses. Fortunately, it usually develops when air is inadvertently introduced through the thoracentesis needle. In this instance, the patient with a small pneumothorax may be closely monitored with serial chest films. However, unless the operator recognizes that this complication has occurred during the procedure, tube thoracostomy to treat a potential pulmonary air leak is indicated. Bleeding may occur as a consequence of laceration of an intercostal vessel. Splenic and hepatic lacerations are possible if the thoracentesis needle penetrates beneath the diaphragm. Despite these risks, pleural effusions in critically ill patients frequently indicate a complication or new problem that necessitates additional therapy. Unless the cause of the effusion is obvious (e.g., new bilateral effusions in the elderly patient with acute pulmonary edema), a diagnostic thoracentesis should be performed.

Pleural Fluid Analysis

Gross visual inspection of the sample may be sufficient to establish or confirm a clinical diagnosis. The aspiration of blood from the pleural cavity of a patient with multiple traumatic rib fractures confirms the presence of a hemothorax. Similarly, if one obtains pus from the pleural space of a patient with pneumonia, the development of an empyema is established. In these instances, microscopic inspection and chemical analysis serve merely to confirm the diagnosis.

The small amount (less than 15 mL) of pleural fluid normally present is straw colored and odorless. The presence of red blood cells in fluid with a reddish tint can be confirmed by microscopic examination. As few as 5000 red blood cells per cubic millimeter, which is equivalent to adding 1 mL of blood to a liter of fluid, is sufficient to impart a reddish hue to the fluid. If the red blood cell count exceeds $100,000/mm^3$, the fluid appears grossly hemorrhagic. A bloody effusion in the critically ill patient who does not have a bleeding diathesis suggests that the effusion is due to trauma, malignancy, or pulmonary infarction. Hemorrhage as a consequence of a traumatic tap usually decreases as fluid is removed. Unless the fluid clears with continued aspiration, a hematocrit should be obtained. A pleural fluid hematocrit value greater than 25% of the peripheral hematocrit indicates a hemothorax.

Pleural fluid occasionally appears cloudy or milky on first examination. This may be due to white blood cells in an empyema or increased quantities of lipids in a chylothorax or pseudochylous effusion. Centrifugation of this fluid reveals clearing of the supernatant if the fluid is an empyema, but it remains cloudy if a chylothorax or pseudochylothorax is present. A chylothorax and pseudochylous effusion are distinguished by their triglyceride and cholesterol contents.

The total white blood cell count and differential count may suggest the cause of the pleural effusion.[15] Normal pleural fluid contains less than 1000 cells per cubic millimeter, and the majority of these are mesothelial cells, monocytes, and small lymphocytes. Most transudates have less than 1000 cells per cubic millimeter with a similar differential count. Exudates typically have 1000 to 10,000 white blood cells per cubic millimeter. Neutrophils are the major cellular constituent of an acute inflammatory response. Because most effusions in critically ill patients are of recent onset, neutrophils are usually the predominant cell type. If the neutrophil count exceeds $100,000/mm^3$, a complicated parapneumonic effusion or empyema should be suspected. Gram's stain and cultures should always be performed whenever an infectious cause is suspected. In selected patients, samples should be submitted for acid-fast bacilli and fungal culture.

If the effusion is chronic, lymphocytes may be the predominant cell type.[16] Lymphocytic effusions are frequently encountered in patients with malignancy, pleural tuberculosis, and rheumatoid arthritis. Whenever malignancy is a consideration, the pleural fluid should also be sent for cytologic examination. Occasionally, pleural fluid may contain more than 10% eosinophils. Pleural fluid eosinophilia frequently develops when a pneumothorax is present.[17]

However, in some critically ill patients, it may develop during the course of a resolving infection or drug reaction.

Pleural effusions are generally classified as transudative or exudative on the basis of the protein and LDH levels in the pleural fluid[18] (see Table 76–1). Pleural effusions with a pleural fluid–to–serum protein ratio of greater than 0.5, an LDH level greater than 200 IU, or an LDH pleural fluid–to–serum concentration ratio of greater than 0.6 are classified as exudates. If none of these criteria is met, the fluid is a transudative effusion.

Measurements of the pleural fluid glucose concentration and pH are helpful in determining the cause of an exudative effusion.[19–21] Normally, the pleural fluid glucose concentration and pH are similar to those of serum. Whenever a large number of metabolically active cells or bacteria are present in the pleural cavity, glucose is metabolized to lactic acid and carbon dioxide and the pH falls.[22] The glucose and pH measurements provide similar information. Measurement of pH is rapid, whereas the glucose level may not be available for several hours. A pH of less than 7.2 or a glucose concentration of less than 40 mg/dL in a rapidly developing effusion is usually indicative of a complicated parapneumonic effusion. Extremely low glucose levels (<10 mg/dL) and pH values less than 7.0 are characteristically present in the effusions that develop as a complication of esophageal rupture.[23] Low glucose levels and pH may also be found in long-standing effusions caused by rheumatoid arthritis, malignancy, and tuberculosis. The diagnosis of these conditions is usually suspected on the basis of clinical findings and can be confirmed by cytologic examination, culture, and biopsy.

The pleural fluid amylase concentration should always be measured in critically ill patients with abdominal symptoms. Some patients with pancreatitis develop a pleural effusion during the course of their disease. The pleural fluid amylase levels in pancreatic effusions are usually greater than the corresponding serum levels.[24] Extremely high amylase levels should suggest the presence of a pancreatopleural fistula or esophageal rupture.[25] The pleural fluid amylase is of salivary rather than pancreatic origin in the latter condition. Lung cancer and other neoplasms can also produce increased pleural fluid amylase levels.[26]

Additional tests may be performed on the pleural fluid sample to identify unusual causes of pleural effusion. The need for further testing is usually based on clinical suspicion and the interpretation of these specialized tests is discussed in relation to specific disease entities.

APPROACH TO PLEURAL EFFUSION IN CRITICALLY ILL PATIENTS

The pleura may be involved in a wide variety of disorders, some of which are chronic. When an acutely ill patient is admitted to the ICU, the intensivist must always consider the possibility that the effusion is due to a coexistent condition and is unrelated to the patient's life-threatening problem. The recent onset of chest pain or dyspnea increases the probability that the effusion is a manifestation of the patient's underlying illness. When an effusion develops after hospitalization in the ICU, it almost inevitably indicates progression of the underlying disease process or the development of a new complication.

The incidence of different types of pleural effusions varies depending on the population examined. Malignancy and infection are two equally common causes of pleural disease in the general population. However, patients with malignant effusions are usually hospitalized on a general ward. In contrast, profound hypoxemia and sepsis are commonly observed in the patient with an untreated empyema and these individuals often require intensive care. The following

TABLE 76–2
CAUSES OF TRANSUDATIVE EFFUSIONS IN CRITICALLY ILL PATIENTS

Congestive heart failure	Urothorax
Hypoalbuminemia	Iatrogenic
Cirrhosis	Misplaced central line
Nephrosis	Peritoneal dialysis
Malnutrition	

discussion focuses on the evaluation and management of those forms of pleural disease that are likely to be encountered in the critically ill patient.

Transudates

The initial step in determining the cause of a pleural effusion is to decide whether the effusion is a transudate or an exudate on the basis of pleural fluid protein and LDH levels. Transudates develop because the balance in Starling's forces across the pleural capillaries is altered so that fluid filtration exceeds the rate of fluid reabsorption. Because the capillary endothelium per se is intact and retains its normal sieving characteristics, the cell and protein contents in a transudative effusion are low.

Most transudative effusions in critically ill patients are due to congestive heart failure (Table 76–2). Some of these individuals have overt heart disease when they are admitted to the ICU. Others have occult cardiac dysfunction that is not clinically apparent until they are challenged with a large volume of fluid. The increased systemic capillary pressures accelerate the rate of fluid filtration across the parietal pleura, and simultaneously, when pressures within the visceral pleural capillaries increase, fluid is also filtered from the surface of the lung into the pleural cavity. The development of transudative effusions in patients with cardiac disease is best correlated with the development of pulmonary venous hypertension.[27]

Transudative effusions may also develop when the plasma oncotic pressure is reduced.[28] In this instance, hydrostatic pressure within the pleural capillaries may be normal, but the oncotic pressure gradient that retards the filtration of fluid into the pleural cavity is reduced. Albumin is the principal plasma protein responsible for the oncotic pressure difference across the capillary endothelium, and transudative effusions frequently develop in patients with hypoalbuminemia attributable to hepatic cirrhosis or the nephrotic syndrome. Transudative effusions may also develop in the critically ill patient whose serum albumin level falls because of an inadequate calorie intake.

Transudative effusions can also develop when low-protein ascitic fluid leaks across the diaphragm into the pleural space. Some patients with hepatic cirrhosis have microscopic defects in their diaphragm, which allow the free passage of ascitic fluid into the thoracic cavity.[29, 30] The effusions in such patients can reach massive proportions and be particularly difficult to manage. A similar phenomenon has been observed in patients with renal disease undergoing peritoneal dialysis.[31] In the patient with hydronephrosis and a ureteral fistula, urine may track up through the retroperitoneum and produce an effusion with a low protein concentration.[32] If a urothorax is suspected, measurement of the pleural fluid creatinine level may be diagnostic. Whenever a transudative effusion develops shortly after a central catheter is placed, one must exclude the possibility that it is an iatrogenic effusion resulting from an improperly placed catheter in the pleural space. Although perforation of a major vessel

---

TABLE 76–3

CAUSES OF EXUDATIVE EFFUSIONS IN CRITICALLY ILL PATIENTS

Pneumonia	Adult respiratory distress syndrome
Simple	Abdominal diseases
Complicated	Postoperative
Empyema	Pancreatitis
Pulmonary embolism	Subphrenic abscess
Trauma	Esophageal rupture
Hemothorax	Enteropleural fistulas
Chylothorax	Drug reactions

---

frequently produces a hemothorax, if significant bleeding does not occur, the new effusion may be a transudate with a glucose and electrolyte composition similar to that of the fluid that has been administered via the central venous catheter.

Treatment of most transudative effusions is directed at correction of the underlying problem. Occasionally, a therapeutic thoracentesis is indicated for the relief of dyspnea. However, unless the underlying pathophysiology is reversed, the fluid rapidly reaccumulates. Diuretics are the mainstay of therapy. Although albumin infusion may be useful in the malnourished patient with hypoalbuminemia, it rapidly escapes the vascular compartment of patients with cirrhosis and nephrosis and is rarely indicated for the treatment of pleural disease in such patients.

Exudates

Exudative pleural effusions are characterized by an increase in the protein and LDH levels within the pleural fluid. The presence of an exudative effusion implies a disruption of the integrity of the capillary-endothelial barrier to protein entry into the pleural space, interruption of the normal lymphatic pumping mechanism for protein clearance, or both. The acute response to pleural injury is an outpouring of neutrophils into the pleural space. Infiltration of the pleural membranes may produce an intense local reaction, and patients often complain of pleuritic chest pain.

The normal mechanisms regulating pleural fluid filtration and reabsorption are more seriously deranged when an exudative effusion develops, and these effusions may be more difficult to manage than a transudative effusion. In addition to treatment of the underlying disorder, local measures may be required to control the effusion and to preserve the integrity of the pleural membranes. Whenever diagnostic thoracentesis confirms the presence of an exudative effusion in a critically ill patient, its cause should be established so that proper therapy can be instituted. An exudative effusion may be just one manifestation of a life-threatening problem in the critically ill patient. The majority of exudative effusions that occur in critically ill patients are due to the conditions given in Table 76–3.

Pneumonia

An effusion that develops in association with pneumonia is termed a *parapneumonic effusion*. Parapneumonic effusions are extremely common. They have been prospectively observed in 50% of patients with pneumococcal pneumonia and occur with even greater frequency in patients with anaerobic pneumonias.[33, 34] These organisms are responsible for most community-acquired pneumonias. In patients hospitalized in an ICU, oropharyngeal colonization with *Staphylococcus aureus* and enteric gram-negative rods is the rule, and more than 60% of patients with pneumonia caused by these organisms experience a parapneumonic effusion.[34]

Parapneumonic effusions are the initial stage in a process that can, if untreated, develop into an empyema.[35] Parapneumonic effusions accumulate because the underlying parenchymal infection increases the permeability of the adjacent pleural vessels. There is an outpouring of protein-rich fluid in response to the adjacent lung infection. If the pneumonia progresses to involve the pleural surface, bacterial invasion of the pleural cavity may occur. After bacteria are within the pleural fluid, the infection may spread to involve the entire pleural cavity. The neutrophil concentration in the effusion increases, and the fluid becomes frankly purulent. Fibrin deposition on the pleural surfaces may lead to loculation. If the purulent fluid cannot be evacuated, fibroblasts migrate along the fibrinous deposits to produce the thick collagenous peel that may encase the lung. Depending on the virulence of the infectious organism and the host's resistance, the progression from parapneumonic effusion to empyema may occur in hours to days.

Whenever a pleural effusion is present in a patient with pneumonia, a diagnostic thoracentesis should be performed to determine if it is a simple parapneumonic effusion or a complicated one with the potential to progress to a frank empyema. Gram's stain and culture of the aspirated fluid may reveal the organism responsible for the parapneumonic effusion and dictate the choice of antibiotic therapy. However, unless the Gram's stain is positive or frank pus is aspirated, the distinction between a simple and a complicated parapneumonic effusion is based on the pleural fluid glucose, pH, and LDH measurements. Effusions with a glucose level less than 40 mg/dL, pH lower than 7.1, and LDH level greater than 1000 IU/L are complicated and almost inevitably necessitate chest tube drainage.[36] If the glucose level is greater than 60 mg/dL, the pH greater than 7.3, and the LDH level less than 500 IU/L, the effusion is a simple parapneumonic one and can be expected to resolve with antibiotic therapy. Borderline effusions with glucose, pH, and LDH values between these extremes may not require immediate tube thoracostomy. However, after 12 to 24 hours of therapy, a repeated thoracentesis should be performed. If organisms are present or the biochemical indices deteriorate, tube thoracostomy is indicated.

Simple parapneumonic effusions usually respond to antibiotic therapy. Antibiotic penetration across the inflamed pleural membranes is excellent. Adequate levels are achieved with intravenous therapy, and the intrapleural administration of antibiotics is not warranted.[37] If a complicated parapneumonic effusion is identified, tube thoracostomy drainage should be initiated as soon as possible to prevent the development of loculations, which may make it difficult or impossible to completely drain the pleural space. A thrombolytic agent can be instilled via the chest tube in an attempt to lyse the intrapleural adhesions.[38–40] However, the risk of bleeding from the inflamed pleural surfaces is considerable, and many critically ill patients have additional contraindications to the use of thrombolytic therapy.[41] We prefer to drain as much of the effusion as possible via a thoracostomy tube and treat small residual loculations with high-dose antibiotics. If tube thoracostomy is performed early in the course of the disease, surgical drainage or decortication is rarely necessary.

An empyema is a purulent infection within the pleural space, which usually develops as a complication of a pneumonia. However, empyemas can also be a consequence of thoracic surgery, penetrating chest wounds, and esophageal rupture.[42, 43] Transdiaphragmatic extension of abdominal infections and septic emboli from distant locations are other causes of empyema. Most empyemas can be managed as complicated parapneumonic effusions, but because the purulent empyema fluid rapidly loculates within the pleural cavity, open drainage in the operating room may be ultimately required to remove a nidus of infection.

Pulmonary Embolism

Critically ill patients who have undergone operative procedures, experienced massive trauma, or simply are immobilized in bed by invasive monitoring devices are at risk for deep venous thrombosis and pulmonary embolism.[44] Because many critically ill patients may be dyspneic because of their primary disorder or too obtunded to complain of new symptoms, the recognition of a newly developing exudative effusion may be the first clinical clue to the presence of a pulmonary embolus. Pleural effusions develop in 50% of patients with pulmonary emboli.[45] They classically are described as a bloody exudate with neutrophilic predominance, but one or more of these features may be absent.[46] In most patients, the effusion develops as a consequence of local ischemia or infarction, which increases the permeability of the pleural capillaries. The effusions, which usually are small or modest in size, develop within hours of the embolus and resolve spontaneously during the next several days. Recrudescence of the pleural effusion should suggest recurrent embolization. In an occasional patient, the effusion is a transudate attributable to heart failure.

Pulmonary embolism is a common disorder and this diagnosis should be suspected whenever an unexplained exudative effusion is recognized.[47] The evaluation and management of the patient with a pulmonary embolus are discussed in Chapter 75. Pleural effusions caused by pulmonary emboli do not require any specific therapy. Appropriate treatment of the pulmonary embolic disease prevents recurrent emboli, and the associated effusions resolve during several days.

Trauma

Hemothorax. Blunt trauma that fractures ribs and penetrating injuries to the chest are the usual causes of a hemothorax.[48] The penetrating trauma may be iatrogenic. Laceration of a subclavian vein or injury to the intercostal vessels during a thoracentesis may result in a hemothorax. Aortic dissection, pulmonary infarction, and malignancy are uncommon causes of hemothorax.

The presence of a hemothorax, which should be suspected whenever a patient with trauma has a pleural effusion, can be verified by aspirating blood from the pleural cavity. In contrast to the blood that is aspirated during a traumatic tap, blood that has been in the pleural space for a length of time is defibrinated and does not clot when it is aspirated. The hemoglobin concentration of a hemothorax usually exceeds 25% of that in blood, whereas a serosanguineous effusion rarely has a hemoglobin level greater than 1 g/dL. The fluid obtained during a traumatic tap clears after centrifugation, whereas fluid from a hemothorax may retain a reddish tint if it has been present long enough for hemolysis to occur.

The majority of hemothoraces are due to bleeding from the lung.[49] When the hemothorax is due to trauma, it usually is accompanied by a pneumothorax (hemopneumothorax) (Fig. 76–6). Hemorrhage from the low-pressure pulmonary vessels generally stops spontaneously. Massive hemothorax suggests bleeding from a systemic vessel such as an intercostal artery.

Blood is reabsorbed from the pleural space, and it is not mandatory that every hemothorax be evacuated.[49, 50] However, an acute hemothorax is usually managed with a chest tube to oppose the visceral and parietal pleural surfaces and achieve tamponade of the bleeding site. Thoracostomy tube drainage is mandatory if a hemopneumothorax is present.

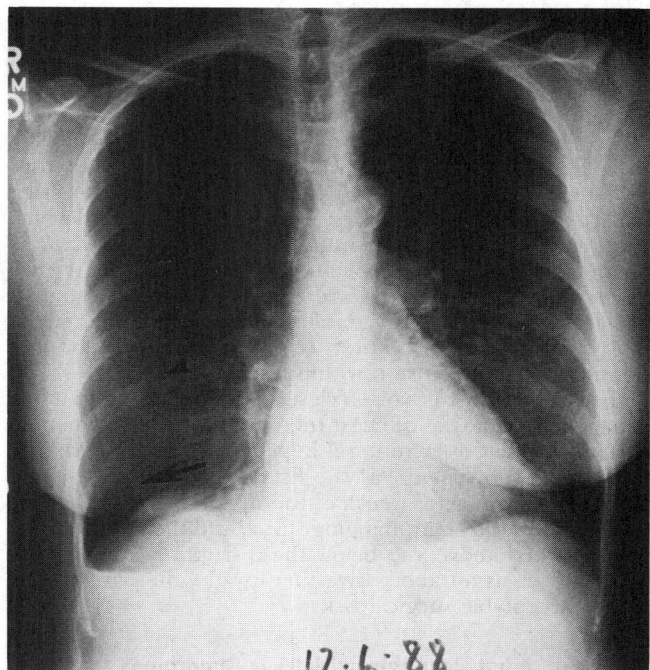

Figure 76–6. Hemopneumothorax. Multiple fractured right posterior ribs are evident *(arrowheads)*. Upright posteroanterior radiograph shows visceral pleura *(arrow)* of the collapsed right lung and an air-fluid interface in the right hemithorax.

Continued chest tube drainage after initial evacuation of the hemothorax indicates persistent bleeding. If the rate of blood loss exceeds several hundred milliliters per hour and is not slowing, thoracotomy may be necessary to repair the bleeding vessels.

An occasional hemothorax caused by penetrating trauma becomes secondarily infected, but chest tube drainage does not reduce the incidence of empyema formation.[51] Less than 10% of patients with a large hemothorax deposit enough fibrin on their pleural surfaces to prevent re-expansion of the underlying lung.[49] Because most hemothoraces resolve spontaneously, decortication to free the trapped lung can be deferred until it is clear that further resolution of the pleural disease is unlikely and the restrictive impairment is severe enough to warrant surgical intervention.

Chylothorax. A chylothorax is due to a disruption of the thoracic duct, which allows the lipid- and lymphocyte-rich chyle to enter the pleural space. The thoracic duct enters the thoracic cavity through the right hemidiaphragm and ascends anterior to the vertebral column before crossing over to the left side at the level of the fifth thoracic vertebra and continuing up to the neck, where it empties into the junction of the left internal jugular and subclavian veins. Depending on the level of the injury, the chyle accumulates in the right or the left pleural cavity.

Although malignant obstruction of the thoracic duct is the most common cause of chylothorax, most chylothoraces diagnosed in the ICU are due to trauma.[52] Traumatic chylothorax can be a consequence of a crush injury to the chest or be caused by penetrating wounds to the neck or the chest. The thoracic duct is close to the aortic arch, the subclavian vessels, and the esophagus and may be disrupted during surgery on these structures. Inadvertent laceration of the thoracic duct during catheterization of the subclavian vein can also produce a chylothorax.

A chylothorax should be suspected whenever milky or opalescent fluid is aspirated from the pleural cavity. Chyle is nonirritating so the fluid contains many lymphocytes rather than the neutrophils that are characteristic of an empyema. A chylous effusion must be differentiated from a pseudochylous effusion, which may have a similar appearance. The fat in a chylous effusion consists of chylomicrons, triglyceride, cholesterol, and phospholipid. The triglyceride level exceeds 110 mg/dL, whereas the concentration of cholesterol is low. Pseudochylous effusions contain high levels of cholesterol (often exceeding 1000 mg/dL), which accumulate owing to the continued breakdown of chronic inflammatory cells in a long-standing effusion. If the triglyceride and cholesterol levels are equivocal, lipoprotein analysis confirms the presence of chylomicrons in a chylothorax.[53] Ingestion of butter colored with lipophilic dye stains the chylous effusion within hours.

Thoracic duct fistulas often close spontaneously, and initial management is a trial of chest tube drainage complemented by a low-fat diet or parenteral hyperalimentation to reduce the formation of chyle.[54] If the fistula does not close spontaneously after several weeks of therapy, the site of the leak can be localized by lymphangiography, and the thoracic duct can be ligated above and below the disruption.[55–57] Tetracycline sclerosis is an alternative therapy for the patient who is an unacceptable surgical risk.

Adult Respiratory Distress Syndrome

The adult respiratory distress syndrome complicates the course of many patients admitted to the ICU. Because many of these patients have pneumonia, generalized sepsis, or abdominal catastrophes or have severe trauma, it is difficult to determine precisely the frequency with which the pleural effusions they develop are solely a consequence of their adult respiratory distress syndrome. Yet there is a considerable body of experimental evidence to suggest that pleural effusions should be a relatively common occurrence in these patients.

Whenever a significant amount of pulmonary edema develops, fluid leaks from the surface of the lung into the pleural cavity. Exudative pleural effusions have been described in experimental models of adult respiratory distress syndrome produced by ethchlorvynol administration and oleic acid infusion (which mimics the fat embolism syndrome).[58–60] It remains to be determined if the exudative effusions are a consequence of increased pleural capillary permeability or are simply due to the leak of the protein-rich pulmonary edema fluid across the visceral pleura.[59, 60]

These experimental observations have clinical relevance. Bilateral exudative pleural effusions have been reported as a complication of ethchlorvynol-induced permeability edema.[61] Radiographically apparent pleural effusions have been observed in more than a third of patients with adult respiratory distress syndrome.[62] Because the pleural effusions presumably develop as a response to the lung injury, it is not unexpected that they resolve without specific therapy as the underlying problem improves.

Abdominal Disease

Pleural effusions frequently develop in response to operative manipulation or inflammation in the abdomen. As many as 50% of patients undergoing abdominal surgery have a small effusion within the first 48 to 72 hours postoperatively.[63, 64] The effusion typically occurs on the side where the surgery was performed. Whenever there is infection or sterile inflammation beneath the diaphragm, the potential exists for extension of the inflammatory process into the pleural cavity. Exudative effusions may occur in response to generalized peritonitis or a subphrenic abscess.[65]

TABLE 76–4

ADDITIONAL CAUSES OF EXUDATIVE EFFUSIONS

Neoplastic diseases
　Metastatic disease
　Mesothelioma
Infections
　Tuberculosis
　Actinomycosis and nocardiosis
　Fungal infections
　Viral infections
　Parasitic infections
Collagen-vascular diseases
　Rheumatoid pleuritis
　Systemic lupus erythematosus
　Drug-induced lupus
　Immunoblastic lymphadenopathy
　Sjögren's syndrome
　Wegener's granulomatosis
Postpericardiectomy or post–myocardial infarction syndrome
Asbestos exposure
Sarcoidosis
Uremia
Meigs' syndrome
Yellow nail syndrome
Trapped lung
Radiation therapy
Electrical burns

Individuals with pancreatitis are particularly prone to have pleural effusions because the leakage of enzyme-rich pancreatic fluid across the diaphragm evokes an exudative pleural response. Pancreatic effusions are recognized in 20% of such patients.[66, 67] Occasionally, an effusion may develop as a consequence of a fistula between the pleural cavity and the pancreas, gallbladder, or bowel.[68–70]

A diagnostic thoracentesis should be performed whenever a pleural effusion develops in a patient with abdominal symptoms. A pleural fluid amylase level that is higher than the corresponding serum level is indicative of a pancreatic effusion. If the thoracentesis excludes pleural infection, the effusion can be managed by treating the underlying disorder.

Other Disorders

An occasional effusion in a critically ill patient is unrelated to the patient's life-threatening illness (Table 76–4). Whenever a lymphocytic effusion is encountered, malignancy should be considered. However, a chronic tuberculous effusion is also characterized by a predominance of lymphocytes, and disseminated tuberculosis can be a life-threatening illness. It is beyond the scope of this chapter to review all the causes of pleural effusions, and the interested reader is referred to comprehensive reviews.[71, 72]

PNEUMOTHORAX*

A pneumothorax is gas within the pleural space. Spontaneous pneumothoraces do occur, typically in a young, otherwise healthy individual. However, most pneumothoraces that develop in critically ill patients are due to either pulmonary disease or trauma. The latter can be accidental or iatrogenic. Regardless of how it develops, a pneumothorax increases the morbidity and complicates the management of the seriously ill patient. Its most dramatic manifestation, tension pneumothorax, is a life-threatening catastrophe,

---

*See also Chapter 78.

which can be rapidly fatal if it is not promptly recognized and decompressed.

Clinical Manifestations

The symptoms and physical findings of a unilateral pneumothorax depend on its size and may be obscured by the underlying pulmonary disease. Chest pain and dyspnea occur in 80 to 90% of patients. Dyspnea is most severe in patients with large pneumothoraces and in those with significant lung disease. Nonproductive cough, unusual chest noises, abnormal chest wall movement, hemoptysis, syncope, and weakness also occur.

Distinctive clinical signs can be elicited when the pneumothorax is large. The percussion note is unduly resonant on the affected side, usually in association with reduced or absent tactile fremitus. Breath sounds are often diminished to absent; occasionally, bronchial breath sounds are heard that are amphoric or metallic in quality. The trachea and the mediastinum may shift away from the side on which the pneumothorax is present. Tapping one coin on the anterior chest wall with another elicits a metallic ringing note that can be heard over the posterior aspect of the same hemithorax; this finding helps to distinguish a pneumothorax from a large bulla. Often, a pleural friction rub is heard. A left pneumothorax, but more often mediastinal emphysema, is sometimes accompanied by a clicking or crunching sound that is synchronous with the heartbeat (Hamman's sign).

The vital capacity and other lung volumes are reduced, as is pulmonary compliance. Arterial hypoxemia is common but tends to ameliorate with time as blood flow in the collapsed lung decreases to match the ipsilateral decrease in ventilation. This reflex adjustment of ventilation to blood flow may be compromised in the patient with pulmonary disease.

Tension Pneumothorax

A tension pneumothorax exists when abnormally high pressure in the pleural space not only produces major lung collapse and displacement of mediastinum but also impedes venous return to the right atrium. This syndrome occurs in 3 to 5% of patients with spontaneous pneumothorax and even more frequently in patients with parenchymal disease.[73] In an uncomplicated pneumothorax, some of the pleural gas escapes during expiration and pleural pressure usually remains subatmospheric. Pleural pressures may exceed 20 cm H_2O in a tension pneumothorax. The positive pressure in the pleural space is sustained by a check valve mechanism. Strong inspiratory efforts promote the entry of air into the pleural space, but the check valve prevents its egress during expiration, so that the intrapleural pressure continues to rise, collapsing the lung and impairing venous return.

On physical examination, the trachea is deviated to the side opposite the pneumothorax, whereas the affected side is tympanic and breath sounds are inaudible. The heart is also displaced to the contralateral side. The decreased venous return produces neck vein distention and systemic hypotension.

Radiographic Manifestations

When a pneumothorax is present, the visceral pleura can be visualized radiographically as a delicate line that is outwardly convex, separated from the parietal pleural surface by a mantle of gas. Pleural adhesions or underlying parenchymal disease may cause the collapse to be asymmetric. Recognition of a pneumothorax can be particularly difficult on a supine chest radiograph because the air accumulates along the anterior aspect of the lung and may not displace the lateral border of the lung from the chest wall. The sudden reappearance of a clearly demarcated diaphragm and cardiac shadow should suggest the presence of an anterior pneumothorax, which can be verified by obtaining a film with the patient in the upright or decubitus position (Fig. 76–7).

An expiratory chest radiograph can be helpful in detecting a small pneumothorax. During maximal expiration, the volume of the lung decreases while the volume of the pneumothorax remains unchanged; therefore, the proportion of the hemithorax occupied by the pneumothorax is increased. Moreover, expiration increases the density of the lung (but not the pneumothorax), increasing the contrast between them. A film obtained with the patient in the lateral decubitus position with the affected side up is sometimes helpful in distinguishing between a pneumothorax and a

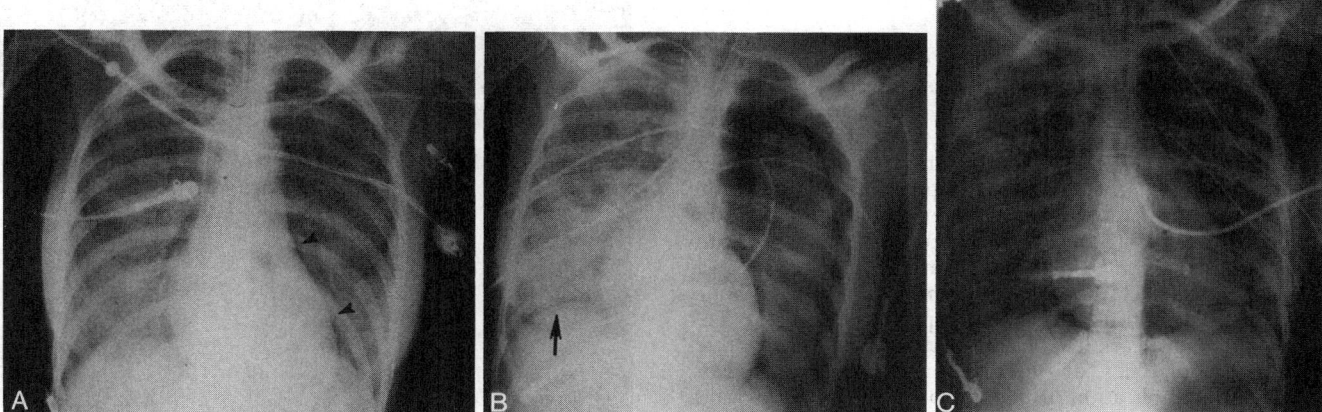

Figure 76–7. *A.* Barotrauma. Portable supine radiograph of young female with adult respiratory distress syndrome mechanically ventilated with positive end-expiratory pressure. Pneumothorax is suggested by lucency along the left border of the heart (*arrowheads*). *B.* Repeated supine radiograph 12 hours later shows large pneumothorax on the left. The appearance of a lucency above the right hemidiaphragm (*arrow*) suggests a pneumothorax on that side. *C.* After tube thoracostomy for treatment of the left-sided pneumothorax, subcutaneous emphysema can be identified in the left side of the chest extending to the neck region. Subpleural air cyst is visible in right lower lung field. Increased lucency along the diaphragm and right-sided heart border are clearly visible, indicating progression of the right-sided pneumothorax.

large cyst or bulla because free air in the pleural cavity accumulates along the uppermost part of the chest wall.

If a tension pneumothorax is present, the chest radiograph may demonstrate a shift of the mediastinum to the contralateral side with depression of the ipsilateral diaphragm. An air-fluid interface occurs in as many as 25% of patients who have a spontaneous pneumothorax. Accumulation of a large quantity of pleural fluid within hours of onset of the pneumothorax strongly suggests either hemopneumothorax or rupture of the esophagus into the pleural space. Thoracentesis should be done promptly to determine whether the fluid is blood or gastric contents.

Pneumothorax in the Critically Ill Patient

Traumatic pneumothorax can be caused by either penetrating or blunt injury to the thorax. Automobile accidents, stab and gunshot wounds, and crush injuries are common causes of pneumothorax. Iatrogenic trauma is not uncommon. Pneumothorax is a well-recognized complication of thoracotomy but can also occur after neck or abdominal surgery. Thoracentesis, pleural biopsy, transbronchial biopsy, and subclavian vein catheterization are among the more common iatrogenic causes of pneumothorax. Pneumothorax has also been observed after the development of a pneumoperitoneum during peritoneal dialysis.

A secondary pneumothorax is a serious complication and may occur in patients with lung disease. Patients with suppurative pulmonary infections may have tissue necrosis and a bronchopleural fistula leading to a pyopneumothorax.[74] This complication most commonly occurs with staphylococcal pneumonias but may also be a complication of infections caused by *Klebsiella, Pseudomonas, Actinomycosis, Nocardia,* and anaerobic mouth organisms.

Pneumothorax can also occur in the decompensated patient with asthma or chronic obstructive pulmonary disease.[75] Air trapping and increased alveolar pressures lead to rupture of alveoli, followed by the dissection of air into the interstitium and then to the visceral pleura or the mediastinum. The presence of a pneumomediastinum or subcutaneous emphysema should alert the physician to the possibility of a pneumothorax in these patients. Pneumothorax is an unusual manifestation of pulmonary infarction. Esophageal perforation is a rare but potential lethal cause of pneumothorax.[76]

Barotrauma

Pneumothorax occurs in 3 to 5% of mechanically ventilated patients.[77] Obstructive airways disease, necrotizing pneumonia, excessive tidal volumes, and high end-expiratory pressures all increase the risk of pneumothorax during positive pressure ventilation. Subcutaneous emphysema and the radiographic appearance of subpleural air cysts in the interstitium are frequent harbingers of an impending pneumothorax.[78, 79] Clinically, the occurrence of a pneumothorax is often signaled by cardiopulmonary distress associated with tachypnea, loss of synchrony with the ventilator, and a precipitous rise in the peak inspiratory pressure. The pathogenesis appears to be the rupture of overinflated emphysematous blebs, or overdistention of infected parenchyma by the application of positive pressure to the airways. In the normal lung, peak inflation pressures greater than 80 cm H_2O are dangerous; considerably lower pressures can cause rupture in the diseased lung. Continuous positive pressure ventilation carries an even higher risk of pneumothorax. About 16% of patients subjected to a positive end-expiratory pressure of 8 to 17 cm H_2O have pneumothorax.[80] The patient who experiences a pneumothorax while being

mechanically ventilated is at high risk to progress to a tension pneumothorax. Therefore, any pneumothorax in a mechanically ventilated patient calls for immediate chest tube placement to decompress the pleural space.

Bronchopleural Fistula

A bronchopleural fistula is a communication between the tracheobronchial tree and the pleural space. In the critically ill patient, most bronchopleural fistulas are a consequence of necrotizing pulmonary infections that cavitate into the pleural space[81] (Fig. 76–8). Bronchopleural fistulas can also develop after penetrating injuries to the chest or as a result of pulmonary barotrauma. Surgical resection of necrotic or infected lung parenchyma entails a particularly high risk of the subsequent development of a bronchopleural fistula. Dehiscence of a bronchial stump after resection of carcinoma is relatively uncommon, and when this occurs, residual tumor is frequently detected in the margin of the resection.[74] This is a particularly feared complication after pulmonary resection because of the frequency with which the pleural space becomes contaminated.

Management

Pneumothorax is a serious and potentially life-threatening complication in a critically ill patient. Therefore, aggressive management is warranted. When the pneumothorax is due to iatrogenic puncture of the lung in a patient who does not have significant pulmonary disease, tube thoracostomy with a small (No. 12 French) pneumothorax catheter applied to continuous suction may suffice to re-expand the lung. However, air leaks through a diseased lung can be considerable, and we favor the insertion of a large (No. 28 French) thoracostomy tube, which also drains any associated effusion (see Chapter 78). A large thoracostomy tube should always be inserted whenever a hemopneumothorax or pyopneu-

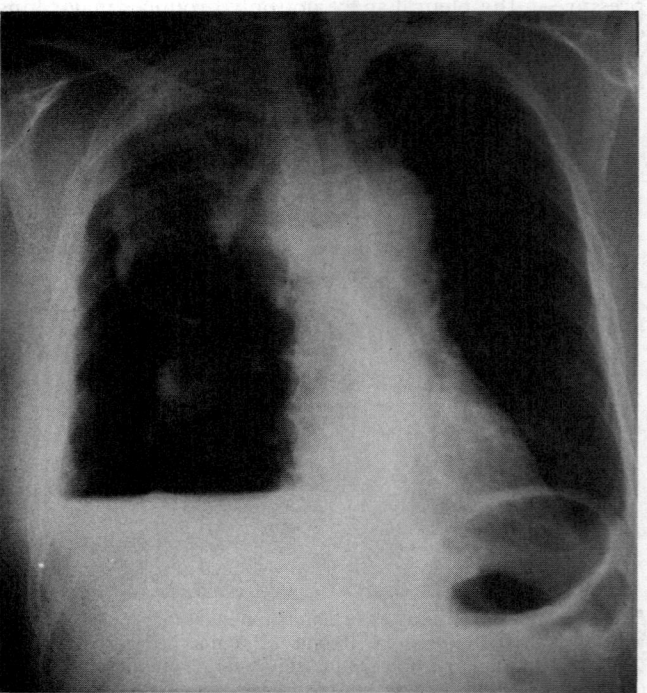

Figure 76–8. Bronchopleural fistula. The collapsed lung can be seen above the air-fluid level, which extends across the entire pleural cavity.

mothorax is present. Additional chest tubes may be required if the initial tube fails to fully re-expand the lung and evacuate the pleural space.

A few days of continuous suction is usually sufficient to appose the pleural surfaces and seal the air leak. Persistent air leak through infected or necrotic tissue can be a particularly difficult problem. In the patient with respiratory insufficiency who requires mechanical ventilation with positive end-expiratory pressure, the bronchopleural fistula may not close until the underlying pulmonary disease improves.[82, 83]

Surgical intervention is required if the bronchopleural fistula fails to close spontaneously. However, because of associated medical problems, surgery may not be feasible until the patient's general status improves. Thoracotomy to close a bronchopleural fistula in a patient with acute respiratory failure should be delayed until the patient can be sustained with minimal ventilatory assistance.

References

1. Von Hayek H: The Human Lung. New York, Hafner, 1960.
2. Broaddus VC, Wiener-Kronish JP, Staub NC: Clearance of lung edema into the pleural space of volume-loaded anesthetized sheep. J Appl Physiol 68:2623, 1990.
3. Wang N: The preformed stomas connecting the pleural cavity and the lymphatics in the parietal pleura. Am Rev Respir Dis 111:12, 1975.
4. Kinasewitz GT, Fishman AP: Influence of alterations in Starling forces on visceral pleural fluid movement. J Appl Physiol 51:671, 1981.
5. Lai-Fook S: Mechanics of the pleural space: Fundamental concepts. Lung 165:249, 1987.
6. Estenne M, Yernault J, de Troyer A: Mechanism of relief of dyspnea after thoracentesis in patients with large pleural effusions. Am J Med 74:813, 1983.
7. Henschke CI, Davis SD, Romano PM, et al: The pathogenesis, radiologic evaluation, and therapy of pleural effusions. Radiol Clin North Am 27:1241, 1989.
8. Collins JD, Burwell D, Furmanski S, et al: Minimal detectable pleural effusions. Radiology 105:51, 1972.
9. Kohan JM, Poe RH, Israel RH, et al: Value of chest ultrasonography versus decubitus roentgenography for thoracentesis. Am Rev Respir Dis 133:1124, 1986.
10. Matalon TA, Neiman HL, Mintzer RA: Noncardiac chest sonography. Chest 83:675, 1983.
11. Stark DD, Federle MP, Goodman PC, et al: Differentiating lung abscess and empyema: Radiography and computed tomography. AJR 141:163, 1983.
12. Godwin JE, Sahn SA: Thoracentesis: A safe procedure in mechanically ventilated patients. Ann Intern Med 113:800, 1990.
13. Seneff MG, Corwin RW, Gold LH, et al: Complications associated with thoracentesis. Chest 90:97, 1986.
14. Collins TR, Sahn SA: Thoracentesis: Clinical value, complications, technical problems, and patient experience. Chest 91:817, 1987.
15. Light RW, Erozan YS, Ball WC Jr: Cells in pleural fluid. Their value in differential diagnosis. Arch Intern Med 132:854, 1973.
16. Yam LT: Diagnostic significance of lymphocytes in pleural effusions. Ann Intern Med 66:972, 1967.
17. Adelman M, Albelda SM, Gottlieb J, et al: Diagnostic utility of pleural fluid eosinophilia. Am J Med 77:915, 1984.
18. Light RW, Macgregor MI, Luchsinger PC, et al: Pleural effusions: The diagnostic separation of transudates and exudates. Ann Intern Med 77:507, 1972.
19. Houston MC: Pleural fluid pH: Diagnostic, therapeutic and prognostic value. Am J Surg 154:333, 1987.
20. Good JT, Taryle DA, Maulitz RM, et al: The diagnostic value of pleural fluid pH. Chest 78:55, 1980.
21. Light RW, MacGregor MI, Ball WC, et al: Diagnostic significance of pleural fluid pH and Pco₂. Chest 64:591, 1973.
22. Sahn SA, Reller LB, Taryle DA, et al: The contribution of leukocytes and bacteria to the low pH of empyema fluid. Am Rev Respir Dis 128:811, 1983.
23. Good JT, Antony VB, Reller LB, et al: The pathogenesis of the low pleural fluid pH in esophageal rupture. Am Rev Respir Dis 127:702, 1983.
24. Light RW, Ball WC: Glucose and amylase in pleural effusions. JAMA 255:257, 1973.
25. Cameron JL, Kieffer RS, Anderson WJ, et al: Internal pancreatic fistulas. Ann Surg 184:587, 1976.
26. Kramer MR, Saldana MJ, Cepero RJ, et al: High amylase levels in neoplasm-related pleural effusions. Ann Intern Med 110:567, 1989.
27. Wiener-Kronish JP, Matthay MA, Callen PW, et al: Relationship of pleural effusions to pulmonary hemodynamics in patients with congestive heart failure. Am Rev Respir Dis 132:1253, 1985.
28. Black LF: The pleural space and pleural fluid. Mayo Clin Proc 47:493, 1972.
29. Lieberman FL, Hidemura R, Peters RL, et al: Pathogenesis and treatment of hydrothorax complicating cirrhosis with ascites. Ann Intern Med 64:341, 1966.
30. Chen A, Ho YS, Tu YC, et al: Diaphragmatic defect as a cause of massive hydrothorax in cirrhosis of liver. J Clin Gastroenterol 10:663, 1988.
31. Rudnick MR, Coyle JF, Beck LH, et al: Acute massive hydrothorax complicating peritoneal dialysis, report of 2 cases and review of the literature. Clin Nephrol 12:38, 1979.
32. Miller KS, Wooten S, Sahn SA: Urinothorax: A cause of low pH transudative pleural effusion. Am J Med 85:448, 1988.
33. Taryle DA, Potts DE, Sahn SA: The incidence and clinical correlates of parapneumonic effusions in pneumococcal pneumonia. Chest 74:170, 1978.
34. Light RW, Girard WM, Jenkinson SG, et al: Parapneumonic effusions. Am J Med 69:507, 1980.
35. Andrews NC, Parker EF, Shaw RR, et al: Management of nontuberculous empyema. Am Rev Respir Dis 85:935, 1962.
36. Light RW, Sahn SA: The sun should never set on a parapneumonic effusion. Chest 95:945, 1989.
37. Taryle DA, Good JT, Morgan EJ, et al: Antibiotic concentrations in human parapneumonic effusions. J Antimicrob Chemother 7:171, 1981.
38. Willsie-Ediger SK, Salzman G, Reisz G, et al: Use of intrapleural streptokinase in the treatment of thoracic empyema. Am J Med 300:296, 1990.
39. Moulton JS, Moore PT, Mencini RA: Treatment of loculated pleural effusions with transcatheter intracavitary urokinase. AJR 153:941, 1989.
40. Bergh NP, Ekroth R, Larsson S, et al: Intrapleural streptokinase in the treatment of haemothorax and empyema. Scand J Thorac Cardiovasc Surg 11:265, 1977.
41. Godley PJ, Bell RC: Major hemorrhage following administration of intrapleural streptokinase. Chest 86:486, 1984.
42. Yeh TJ, Hall DP, Ellison RG: Empyema thoracis: A review of 110 cases. Am Rev Respir Dis 88:785, 1963.
43. Bartlett JG: Bacterial infections of the pleural space. Semin Respir Infect 3:308, 1988.
44. Neuhaus A, Bentz RR, Weg JG: Pulmonary embolism in respiratory failure. Chest 73:460, 1981.
45. Bynum LJ, Wilson JE: Radiographic features of pleural effusions in pulmonary embolism. Am Rev Respir Dis 117:829, 1978.
46. Bynum LJ, Wilson JE: Characteristics of pleural effusions associated with pulmonary embolism. Arch Intern Med 136:159, 1976.
47. Moser KM, LeMoine JR, Nachtway FJ, et al: Deep venous thrombosis and pulmonary embolism: Frequency in a respiratory intensive care unit. JAMA 246:1422, 1981.
48. Griffith GL, Todd EP, McMillin RD, et al: Acute traumatic hemothorax. Ann Thorac Surg 26:204, 1978.
49. Weil PH, Margolis IB: Systematic approach to traumatic hemothorax. Am J Surg 142:692, 1981.
50. Wilson JM, Boren CH, Peterson SR, et al: Traumatic hemothorax: Is decortication necessary? J Thorac Cardiovasc Surg 77:489, 1979.
51. Eddy AC, Luna GK, Copass M: Empyema thoracis in patients undergoing emergent closed tube thoracostomy for thoracic trauma. Am J Surg 157:494, 1989.
52. Bessone LN, Ferguson TB, Burford TH: Chylothorax. Ann Thorac Surg 12:527, 1971.
53. Stouts BA, Ellefson RD, Budahn LL, et al: The lipoprotein profile of chylous and nonchylous pleural effusions. Mayo Clin Proc 55:700, 1980.
54. Robinson CLN: The management of chylothorax. Ann Thorac Surg 39:90, 1985.
55. Milson RW, Kron IL, Rheuban KS, et al: Chylothorax: An assessment of current surgical management. J Thorac Cardiovasc Surg 89:221, 1985.
56. Dulchansky SA, Ledgerwood AM, Lucas CE: Management of chylothorax after blunt chest trauma. J Trauma 28:1400, 1988.
57. Spiro JD, Spiro RH, Strong RW: The management of chyle fistula. Laryngoscope 100:771, 1990.
58. Miller KS, Harley RA, Sahn SA: Pleural effusions associated with ethchlorvynol lung injury result from visceral pleural leak. Am Rev Respir Dis 140:764, 1989.
59. Weiner-Kronish JP, Broaddus VC, Albertine KH, et al: Relationship of pleural effusions to increased permeability pulmonary edema in anesthetized sheep. J Clin Invest 82:1422, 1988.
60. Blomqvist H, Berg B, Frostell C, et al: Net fluid leakage in experimental pulmonary edema in the dog. Acta Anaesthesiol Scand 34:377, 1990.
61. Miller KS, Sahn SA: Bilateral exudative pleural effusions following intravenous ethchlorvynol administration. Chest 95:464, 1989.
62. Weiner-Kronish JP, Matthay MA: Pleural effusions associated with hydrostatic and increased permeability pulmonary edema. Chest 93:852, 1988.
63. Light RW, George RB: Incidence and significance of pleural effusion after abdominal surgery. Chest 69:621, 1976.
64. Nielsen PH, Jepsen SB, Olsen AD: Postoperative pleural effusion following upper abdominal surgery. Chest 96:1133, 1989.
65. Schwartz ID, Olson LC: Left pleural effusion: Masking subphrenic abscess—Caused by *Salmonella enteritidis* serotype Heidelberg. Clin Pediatr 28:266, 1989.

66. Uchiyama T, Yamamoto T, Mizuta E, et al: Pancreatic ascites—A collected review of 37 cases in Japan. Hepatogastroenterology 36:244, 1989.
67. McKenna JM, Craig RM, Chandraseekhar AJ, et al: The pleuropulmonary complication of pancreatitis. Chest 71:197, 1977.
68. Donrej W, Kullins P, Petritech W, et al: Colobronchial fistula: A rare complication of Crohn's disease. Am Rev Respir Dis 142:1225, 1990.
69. Cunningham LW, Grobman M, Poz HL, et al: Cholecystopleural fistula with cholelithiasis presenting as a right pleural effusion. Chest 97:751, 1990.
70. Pisani RJ, Zeller FA: Bilious pleural effusion following liver biopsy. Chest 98:1535, 1990.
71. Sahn SA: The pleura. Am Rev Respir Dis 138:184, 1988.
72. Light RW: Pleural Diseases. 2nd ed. Philadelphia, Lea & Febiger, 1990.
73. Macklin MT, Macklin CC: Malignant interstitial emphysema of the lungs and mediastinum as an important occult complication in many respiratory diseases and other conditions: An interpretation of clinical literature in light of laboratory experiment. Medicine 23:281, 1944.
74. Hankins JR, Miller JE, Attar S, et al: Bronchopleural fistula: Thirteen year experience with 77 cases. J Thorac Cardiovasc Surg 76:755, 1978.
75. George RB, Herbert SJ, Shames JM, et al: Pneumothorax complicating pulmonary emphysema. JAMA 234:389, 1975.
76. Sabanathan S, Eng J, Pradhan GN: Boerhaave's syndrome complicating acute myocardial infarction. Case report. Scand J Thorac Cardiovasc Surg 24:87, 1990.
77. Zwillich CW, Pierson DJ, Creagh CE, et al: Complications of assisted ventilation. Am J Med 57:161, 1974.
78. Woodring JH: Pulmonary interstitial emphysema in the adult respiratory distress syndrome. Crit Care Med 13:786, 1985.
79. Albelda SM, Gefter WB, Kelley MA, et al: Ventilator-induced subpleural air cysts: Clinical, radiographic, and pathologic significance. Am Rev Respir Dis 127:360, 1983.
80. Steier M, Ching N, Roberts EB, et al: Pneumothorax complicating continuous ventilatory support. J Thorac Cardiovasc Surg 67:17, 1974.
81. Barker WL, Faber LP, Ostermiller WE, et al: Management of persistent bronchopleural fistulas. J Thorac Cardiovasc Surg 62:393, 1971.
82. Bishop MJ, Benson MS, Pierson DJ: Carbon dioxide excretion via bronchopleural fistulas in adult respiratory distress syndrome. Chest 91:400, 1987.
83. Blanch PB, Koens JC, Layon AJ: A new device that allows synchronous intermittent inspiratory chest tube occlusion with any mechanical ventilator. Chest 97:1426, 1990.

CHAPTER 77

Aspiration

Gregory R. Owens

Aspiration of either oropharyngeal or gastric contents leads to a wide spectrum of effects, ranging from no clinical sequelae to fulminant respiratory failure. Aspiration occurs much more commonly than is recognized clinically. Studies suggest that as many as 45% of normal individuals and up to 70% of patients with a depressed sensorium aspirate oropharyngeal contents during sleep.[1] Likewise, in studies utilizing dye, evidence of aspiration of gastric contents was found in 7 to 16% of patients undergoing surgery.[2–4] Few sequelae of these minor episodes of aspiration were noted. These facts should not be taken to mean that aspiration does not cause disease. Indeed, aspiration is often cited as the major cause of death associated with anesthesia.[5] This chapter focuses on the two major clinical syndromes associated with aspiration: aspiration pneumonitis and aspiration pneumonia, which have distinct clinical presentations and different treatments. The reader is referred to Chapter 67 for discussion of the diagnosis and management of aspiration pneumonia.

RISK FACTORS

The risk factors for aspiration have been well characterized,[6] and the three major categories are shown in Table 77–1. The most common risk factor for aspiration is an altered level of consciousness, which diminishes the reflex response of the upper airway to aspiration. The two most frequent causes of aspiration in this category are anesthesia, particularly during emergency or obstetric surgery, and the use of alcohol and sedative agents. In addition, patients with a history of a seizure disorder or patients experiencing a cerebrovascular accident are at risk for aspiration.

A second category of risk factors includes diseases that alter the motor function of the esophagus or the hypopharynx. Diseases such as systemic sclerosis and achalasia are associated with dilatation of the esophagus, and these patients often have repetitive bouts of aspiration.

The third category of risk factors includes mechanical disruption of glottic closure or gastroesophageal sphincter function. The use of nasogastric tubes is associated with dysfunction of both the larynx and the lower gastroesophageal sphincter. When nasogastric tubes are utilized to feed patients, the combination of the two defects plus gastric distention often leads to aspiration. The use of tracheotomy tubes is associated with a high frequency of aspiration because of the inhibition of normal laryngeal movement.[7] Even the placement of endotracheal tubes, often used to protect the airway, is associated with a small, but significant, risk of aspiration.[8] In addition to mechanical disruption of the lower esophageal sphincter, pharmacologic alteration of its function also occurs.[9] Both theophylline and beta-agonists have been shown to decrease lower esophageal sphincter pressure and thus predispose to aspiration. Likewise, narcotics such as morphine and sedatives such as the benzodiazepines cause a decrease in lower esophageal sphincter pressure.

CLINICAL ASPECTS OF ASPIRATION PNEUMONITIS AND ASPIRATION PNEUMONIA

The development of aspiration pneumonitis occurs after the aspiration of gastric contents, which are usually sterile. A chemical burn of the tracheobronchial tree and pulmonary parenchyma follows if the volume of the aspirate is sufficiently large or pH of the aspirate is sufficiently low.

The onset of the clinical syndrome is usually well delineated. The patient often is noted to vomit and aspirate while being intubated or during the placement of a nasogastric tube. A latent period of 1 to 12 hours is followed by the

TABLE 77–1

CONDITIONS THAT PREDISPOSE TO ASPIRATION

Altered consciousness
  Alcoholism
  Drug abuse
  Use of sedatives
  Seizures
  General anesthesia
  Central nervous system disorders

Dysphagia
  Esophageal disorder
  Neurologic deficits

Mechanical disruption of defense barriers
  Nasogastric tube
  Endotracheal tube
  Tracheostomy

TABLE 77-2

CLINICAL SIGNS AFTER ASPIRATION OF GASTRIC CONTENTS

Sign	Number of Patients (N-50)	Percentage of Patients with the Finding
Fever, total	47	94
99–102°F	24	48
>102°F	23	46
Tachypnea	39	78
Rales	36	72
Cough	18	36
Cyanosis	16	32
Wheezing	16	32
Apnea	15	30
Shock	12	24

From Bynum L, Pierce A: Pulmonary aspiration of gastric contents. Am Rev Respir Dis 114:1129, 1976.

rapid onset of shortness of breath accompanied by a cough, which may be productive of thin, frothy fluid.[10] Table 77–2 details the clinical features noted in one study of aspiration pneumonitis.[11]

Results of laboratory studies are usually normal, with the exception of an alteration in arterial blood gas values, which usually reveal hypoxemia and a respiratory alkalosis.[11] Chest radiography may be helpful because the location of the pneumonitis tends to be stereotypic owing to the effects of gravity and the propensity for hospitalized patients to lie in the supine position. Areas that are commonly involved with aspiration pneumonitis (and aspiration pneumonia) are dependent areas of the lung. Thus, the superior segments of the lower lobes and the posterior segment of the right upper lobe are commonly involved. Figure 77–1 documents the location of pulmonary damage after aspiration in relationship to the position of the patient during the episode of aspiration. The infiltrates noted are usually alveolar in nature. If the aspiration is massive, the adult respiratory distress syndrome may occur with bilateral alveolar infiltrates.[12]

The clinical course of aspiration pneumonia is quite different from that of aspiration pneumonitis. Aspiration pneumonia develops after the aspiration of oropharyngeal contents alone or a mixture of oropharyngeal and gastric contents. Unlike the case with aspiration pneumonitis, the episode of aspiration is often not witnessed. The clinical course of the disease may be relatively slow paced in contrast to the often fulminant onset of aspiration pneumonitis.[13] The diagnosis is often inferred clinically when a patient with a known risk factor for aspiration, especially an altered level of consciousness, has pneumonia in an area characteristic of aspiration pneumonia. Laboratory evaluation is usually not productive. Although thought to be virtually pathognomonic of aspiration pneumonia, foul-smelling sputum is seen in less than 20% of patients.[14]

The microbiologic characteristics of aspiration pneumonia depend on where the aspiration occurred. The organisms typically seen in aspiration pneumonia occurring outside the hospital are predominantly anaerobic, with *Peptostreptococcus*, *Bacteriodes melaninogenicus*, and *Fusobacterium nucleatum* representing the most common species. The predominance of anaerobic organisms in these pneumonias is due to their prevalence in the saliva of nonhospitalized persons. Normal people harbor approximately 10^8 bacteria per milliliter of

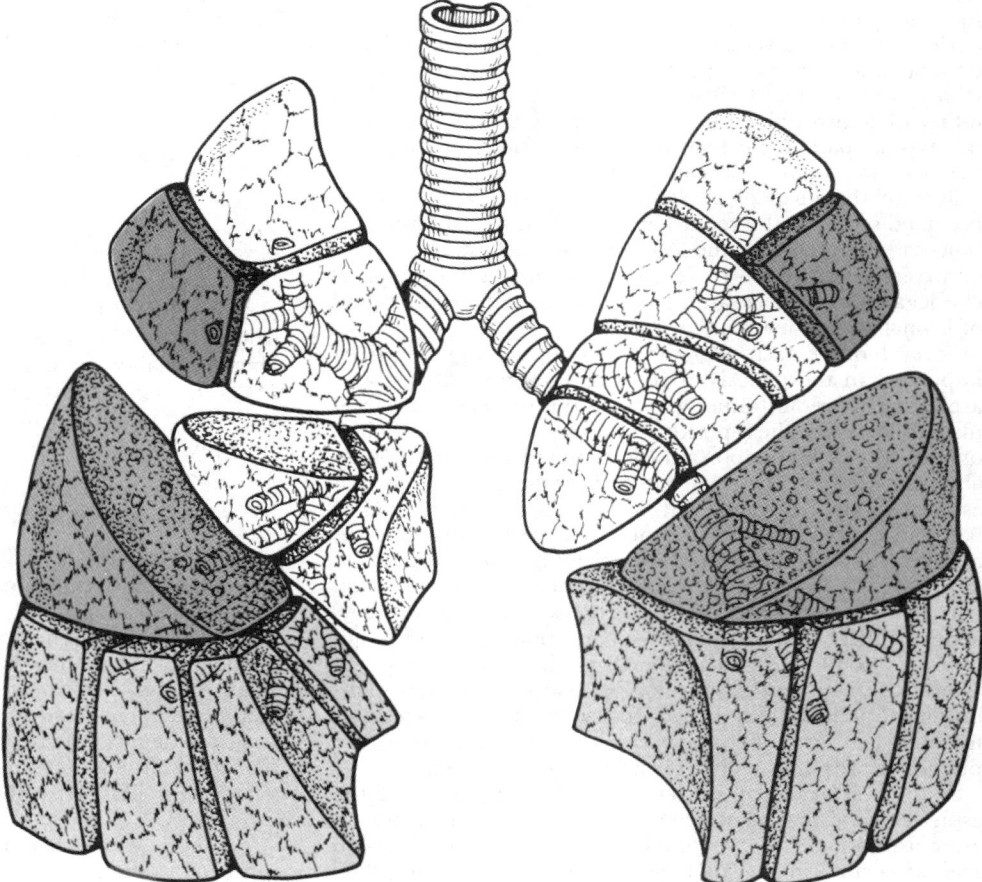

Figure 77-1. The gravity dependence of aspiration (note that the lungs are represented as inwardly rotated so that part of the lateral surface is displayed). In an erect patient, aspiration involves primarily the basal segments of the lower lobes. The superior segments of the lower lobes are primarily affected in a supine patient, and the posterior segments of the upper lobes are primarily affected in patients in the lateral decubitus position. (From Shapiro MS, Matthay RA: Pulmonary aspiration: Keys to effective therapy. J Respir Dis 1989; 10[6]:59–74.)

saliva, whereas persons with poor oral hygiene can have bacterial counts as high as 10^{11}/mL of saliva.[15]

Aspiration of oropharyngeal contents occurring in the hospital may lead to quite different consequences. Within the first 4 days of hospitalization, approximately 40% of patients have colonization of the upper airway.[16] The colonization occurs not with anaerobic organisms, but with aerobic organisms, most typically gram-negative rods such as *Pseudomonas aeruginosa*, *Escherichia coli*, and *Proteus* species.[17] In addition, *Staphylococcus aureus* is commonly found. Interestingly, after the initial period of colonization, few additional patients become colonized, so that the pool of patients at risk for an aerobic aspiration pneumonia does not constantly expand as the duration of hospitalization is prolonged.[18] This implies some yet unexplained difference in susceptibility of patients to upper airway colonization.

ASPIRATION PNEUMONITIS
Pathologic Changes

Since Mendelson's classic description of aspiration pneumonitis in obstetric patients,[19] the pathologic changes and pathophysiology of this syndrome have been well characterized. The majority of experimental studies have shown that the pH and volume of the aspirated material correlate with the extent of lung damage.[20, 21] These studies suggest that a pH less than 2.5 and a volume greater than 25 mL are usually necessary for lung damage to occur.

The information about the pathologic changes in the lung resulting from aspiration comes primarily from animal models. When gastric juice was marked with methylene blue and aspirated into dogs, the dye marker was noted at the surface of the lung in 12 to 18 seconds.[22] Atelectasis was noted immediately, and by 3 minutes it had become extensive. Routine pathologic studies performed during this early period revealed alveolar hemorrhage, pulmonary edema, desquamation of the superficial cell layers of the trachea with complete loss of ciliated and nonciliated cells, and an influx of neutrophils into the alveoli.[23] Figure 77–2 shows the typical pathologic features of aspiration pneumonitis. Electron microscopy revealed necrosis of type I alveolar cells.[24] In the next 24 to 36 hours, alveolar consolidation occurred owing to the remarkable influx of neutrophils, and mucosal sloughing of the trachea and airways sometimes occurred. After 72 hours, resolution of the pathologic process began with a decrease in neutrophils and regeneration of bronchial epithelium.

Several other factors in addition to pH appear to be important in the genesis of pulmonary abnormalities after aspiration. Foremost among these is the presence of particulate foodstuff in the aspirate.[25] In a dog model of aspiration, one of the most important determinants of pulmonary abnormalities was the presence of food particles. Dogs that aspirated gastric contents with food particles, but at a pH of 5.9, had hypoxemia and intrapulmonary shunting that was as severe as those in animals aspirating hydrochloric acid at a pH of 1.8. Aspiration of hydrochloric acid and food particles was associated with the most severe physiologic abnormalities. The pathologic changes noted after the aspiration of food particles differ from those seen with acid aspiration. Foodstuff aspiration is associated with a peribronchial inflammatory reaction, which is followed by a mononuclear granulomatous response in addition to the pulmonary reaction seen after acid-only aspiration.

Additional evidence suggests that the osmolarity of the aspirated fluid may play a role in the genesis of lung disease after aspiration.[26] Hypersomolar solutions (as would been seen after antacid therapy) with concentrations above 2000

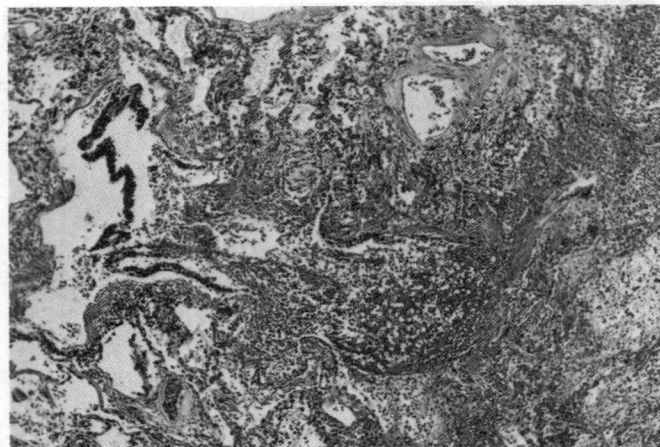

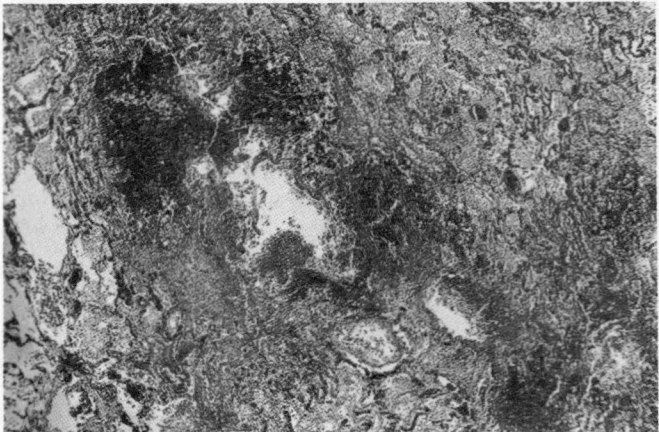

Figure 77–2. Pathologic findings from a patient who died 48 hours after aspiration. (*Top*) Bronchial necrosis (at center, with remaining bronchial epithelium to left of center); fibrinous, hemorrhagic alveolar reaction about bronchus. Hematoxylin-eosin stain; × 50. (*Bottom*) More marked bronchial necrosis with abscess information. Hematoxylin-eosin stain; × 35. (From Dines DE, Titus JL, Sessler AD: Aspiration pneumonitis. Mayo Clin Proc 45:347, 1970.)

mOsm/L were shown to cause severe lung damage, whereas, with solutions of less osmolarity, no damage occurred.

Finally, the typically quoted critical volume of 25 mL may be misleading.[27] In a rat model of aspiration, larger-volume aspiration could be relatively well tolerated with a pH of 1.8, whereas small-volume aspirates with extremely low pH values (1.0) were almost uniformly fatal. This study demonstrated the important interaction of pH and the volume of the aspirate.

Prevention

The prevention of aspiration syndromes begins with an awareness of the causes of aspiration and the gravity of its occurrence. Patients with altered mental status should not be placed in the supine position, but rather in the decubitus position. Likewise, these patients should not have nasogastric tube feedings performed until an endotracheal tube has been placed. The head of the bed should be elevated during these feedings to decrease the likelihood of regurgitation. The residual gastric volume should be monitored. Finally, constant infusion of feedings is preferred over bolus delivery.

It would seem obvious that the most straightforward approach to the prevention of aspiration pneumonitis is the elimination of gastric acid. Because pH is thought to be the primary determinant of the pulmonary effects of aspiration, elimination of that risk factor should lead to a decrease in the likelihood of aspiration. Indeed, multiple studies have shown that it is possible through the use of histamine H_2 receptor antagonists (ranitidine, cimetidine), metoclopramide, or antacids to decrease the gastric volume and to increase the pH into the range that is typically thought not to be associated with aspiration pneumonitis.[28–30] These studies suggested that, because these risk factors had been decreased, the frequency of aspiration should decrease.

Although theoretically plausible, this hypothesis has never been tested clinically, and data suggest that it may not be true. First, aspiration pneumonitis has developed in patients who received prophylaxis with antacids and whose gastric pH was well above the critical value of 2.5.[31] There is a second and more important problem associated with the neutralization or elimination of gastric acid. Several studies have shown that the chronic use of antacids and histamine H_2 receptor antagonists in critically ill patients is associated with an increased risk of the development of nosocomial gram-negative pneumonias.[32, 33] This increased frequency of pneumonia is thought to be due to colonization of the now nonacidic stomach by bacteria, followed by regurgitation and aspiration of the neutral, but colonized, gastric contents.

Thus, at the current time, it is not clear whether pharmacologic prophylaxis for aspiration should be utilized. Certainly, with short-term administration, such as preoperatively, there is virtually no risk to the use of acid-neutralizing agents. However, long-term use of prophylactic agents requires further study.

Treatment

Because the aspirate spreads through the lung widely and extremely rapidly, and because the acid damage to the airways and pulmonary parenchyma is virtually instantaneous, measures aimed at acid neutralization are of no value.[34] Indeed, some information suggests that the extent of the damage may actually be increased by bronchial lavage.[35] Immediate efforts should be made to obtain and maintain airway patency by vigorous endotracheal suctioning. Bronchoscopy should be considered if there is evidence of large food particles in the suctioned material or if the chest radiograph shows evidence of segmental or lobar atelectasis.[36]

There is a growing consensus about the use of corticosteroids in patients with aspiration pneumonitis. Although early studies, usually poorly controlled and with few subjects enrolled, suggested that parenchymal damage was reduced and survival was greater in corticosteroid-treated patients,[37–39] more recent studies cast doubt on these earlier studies. Well-controlled studies have been performed both in patients with aspiration pneumonitis[40] and in those with the adult respiratory distress syndrome[41, 42] and have reached the same conclusions. All three studies had identical outcomes and showed that corticosteroid treatment did not lead to decreased death rates or more rapid improvement. In addition, there was a higher frequency of gram-negative pneumonias noted in patients with either aspiration pneumonitis or adult respiratory distress syndrome. This finding is almost certainly due to adverse effects of corticosteroids on white blood cell function. Laboratory evaluations have shown that corticosteroid-treated animals have an increased susceptibility to infection, and especially to infection with gram-negative bacilli.[43]

Because aspiration pneumonitis is a chemical burn, not an infection, of the lung, it seems obvious that antibiotics are not effective in this clinical syndrome. Interestingly, however, there is no agreement in the literature about the use of antibiotics in aspiration pneumonitis, and some authors strongly support their use.[10, 11, 44] However, the use of broad-spectrum antibiotics may select for more virulent or resistant organisms and may also increase the likelihood of drug toxicity. Perhaps the best approach is to delay the use of antibiotics until definite evidence of bacterial infection is noted.

Ventilatory support measures are critical in the therapy of patients with aspiration pneumonitis. Supplemental oxygen alone may be adequate in patients with evidence of minimal aspiration. However, the use of mechanical ventilation with positive end-expiratory pressure may be necessary in patients with evidence of more significant aspiration.

It was suggested that patients with aspiration pneumonitis may be at increased risk for barotrauma.[45] This study showed a 10-fold increase in the development of pneumothorax and pneumomediastinum in patients with aspiration pneumonitis compared with that in other patient groups requiring mechanical ventilation. The authors suggested that the aspirated acid destroyed lung tissue and increased the susceptibility of the lung to the mechanical forces generated by the ventilator.

Prognosis

The morbidity and mortality associated with aspiration pneumonitis are substantial and different from those noted in Mendelson's description of the disease. Mendelson noted no deaths in his patients.[19] More recent studies showed mortality rates of 35 to 60%.[46, 47] One study actually found mortality rates to be 100% when the pH of the aspirate was less than 1.75.[22]

No recent studies have evaluated the long-term prognosis of patients with aspiration pneumonitis. However, one report suggested that patients may experience pulmonary fibrosis after an episode of aspiration pneumonitis.[48] The frequency of this occurrence is unknown.

SUMMARY

Aspiration of oropharyngeal or gastric contents is a relatively frequent event but often is attended by no clinical sequelae. In patients who aspirate gastric contents with a pH less than 2.5 or a volume greater than 25 mL, a chemical burn of the lung may occur, leading to pneumonitis. The main therapy of this pneumonitis is supportive with oxygen and sometimes mechanical ventilation. There is no evidence that pharmacologic therapy is necessary or important. Likewise, it is not clear that pharmacologic therapy is effective when given prophylactically. The mortality in this clinical syndrome is substantial and related to the pH and volume of the aspirate.

References

1. Huxley E, Viroslav J, Gray W, et al: Pharyngeal aspiration in normal adults and patients with depressed consciousness. Am J Med 64:564, 1978.
2. Culver GA, Makel HP, Beecher HK: Frequency of aspiration of gastric contents by the lungs during anesthesia and surgery. Ann Surg 133:289, 1951.
3. Berson W, Adriani J: "Silent" regurgitation and aspiration of gastric content during anesthesia. Anesthesiology 15:644, 1954.
4. Gardner AMN: Aspiration of food and vomit. Q J Med 27:227, 1958.
5. Edwards G, Morton H, Pask E, et al: Deaths associated with anesthesia. Anesthesia 11:194, 1956.
6. Hughes R, Freilich R, Bytell D, et al: Aspiration and occult esophageal disorders. Chest 80:489, 1981.
7. Cameron J, James R, Zuidema G: Aspiration in patients with tracheostomies. Surg Gynecol Obstet 136:68, 1973.

8. Spray S, Zuidema G, Cameron J: Aspiration pneumonia. Am J Surg 131:701, 1976.
9. Bartlett J: Aspiration pneumonia. Clin Notes Respir Dis 18:3, 1980.
10. Dines D, Baker W, Scantland W: Aspiration pneumonitis—Mendelson's syndrome. JAMA 176:229, 1961.
11. Bynum L, Pierce A: Pulmonary aspiration of gastric contents. Am Rev Respir Dis 114:1129, 1976.
12. Dines DE, Titus JL, Sessler AD: Aspiration pneumonitis. Mayo Clin Proc 45:347, 1970.
13. Bartlett J, Gorbach S, Finegold S: The bacteriology of aspiration pneumonia. Am J Med 56:202, 1974.
14. Bartlett J: Anaerobic bacterial infections of the lung. Chest 91:901, 1987.
15. Rosebury T: Microorganisms Indigenous to Man. New York, McGraw-Hill, 1966.
16. Johanson W, Pierce A, Sanford J, et al: Nosocomial respiratory infections with gram negative bacilli. Ann Intern Med 77:701, 1972.
17. Johanson W, Pierce A, Sanford J: Changing pharyngeal bacterial flora of hospitalized patients. N Engl J Med 281:1137, 1969.
18. Langer M, Mosconi P, Cigada M, et al: Long term respiratory support and risk of pneumonia in critically ill patients. Am Rev Respir Dis 140:302, 1989.
19. Mendelson C: Aspiration of stomach contents into the lungs during obstetric anesthesia. Am J Obstet Gynecol 52:191, 1946.
20. Teabeaut J: Aspiration of gastric contents: Experimental study. Am J Pathol 28:51, 1952.
21. Lewis RT, Burgess JH, Hampson LG: Cardiorespiratory studies in critical illness. Arch Surg 103:335, 1971.
22. Hemelberg W, Bosomworth P: Aspiration pneumonitis: Experimental studies and clinical observations. Anesth Analg 43:669, 1964.
23. Greenfield L, Singleton R, McCaffree D, et al: Pulmonary effects of experimental graded aspiration of hydrochloric acid. Ann Surg 170:74, 1969.
24. Wynne JW, Modell JH: Respiratory aspiration of stomach contents. Ann Intern Med 87:466, 1977.
25. Schwartz D, Wynne J, Gibbs C, et al: The pulmonary consequences of aspiration of gastric contents at pH values greater than 2.5. Am Rev Respir Dis 121:119, 1980.
26. Rogers MA, Toung JK, Gurtner G, et al: The effects of osmolarity on pulmonary damage in aspiration. Anesthesiology 61:A490, 1984.
27. James CF, Modell JH, Gibbs CP, et al: Pulmonary aspiration—Effects of volume and pH in the rat. Anesth Analg 63:665, 1984.
28. Manchikanti L, Colliver JA, Marrero TC, et al: Ranitidine and metoclopramide for prophylaxis of aspiration pneumonitis in elective surgery. Anesth Analg 63:903, 1984.
29. Manchikanti L, Grow JB, Colliver JA, et al: Bicitra (sodium citrate) and metoclopramide in outpatient anesthesia for prophylaxis against aspiration pneumonitis. Anesthesiology 63:378, 1985.
30. Colman RD, Frank M, Loughnan BA, et al: Use of I.M. ranitidine for the prophylaxis of aspiration pneumonitis in obstetrics. Br J Anaesth 61:720, 1988.
31. Brown BR: Pulmonary aspiration syndrome after inhalation of gastric fluid containing antacids. Anesthesiology 51:452, 1979.
32. Craven D, Kunches L, Kilinsky V, et al: Risk factors for pneumonia and fatality in patients receiving mechanical ventilation. Am Rev Respir Dis 133:792, 1986.
33. Driks M, Craven D, Celli B, et al: Nosocomial pneumonia intubated patients given sucralfate as compared with antacids or histamine type 2 blockers. The role of gastric colonization. N Engl J Med 317:1376, 1987.
34. Awe W, Fletcher W, Jacob S: The pathophysiology of aspiration pneumonitis. Surgery 50:232, 1966.
35. Taylor G, Pryse-Davis J: Evaluation of endotracheal steroid therapy in acid pulmonary aspiration syndrome. Anesthesiology 29:17, 1968.
36. Kim I, Brummitt W, Humphrey A, et al: Foreign body in the airway: A review of 202 cases. Laryngoscope 83:347, 1973.
37. Bannister W, Sattilaro A: Vomiting and aspiration during anesthesia. Anesthesiology 23:251, 1962.
38. Lawson D, Defalco A, Phelps J, et al: Corticosteroids as treatment for aspiration of gastric contents: An experimental study. Surgery 59:845, 1966.
39. Tinstman T, Dines D, Arms R: Postoperative aspiration pneumonia. Surg Clin North Am 53:859, 1973.
40. Wolfe J, Bone R, Ruth W: Effects of corticosteroids in the treatment of patients with gastric aspiration. Am J Med 63:719, 1977.
41. Bone R, Fischer C, Clemmer T, et al: Early methylprednisolone treatment for septic syndrome and the adult respiratory distress syndrome. Chest 92:1032, 1987.
42. Weigelt J, Norcross J, Borman M, et al: Early steroid therapy for respiratory failure. Arch Surg 120:536, 1985.
43. Kass E, Finland M: Corticosteroids and infection. Adv Intern Med 9:45, 1958.
44. McCormick P: Immediate care after aspiration of vomit. Anesthesia 30:658, 1975.
45. DeLatorre F, Tomasa A, Klamburg J, et al: Incidence of pneumothorax and pneumomediastinum in patients with aspiration pneumonia requiring ventilatory support. Chest 72:141, 1977.
46. Cameron JL, Mitchell WH, Zuidema GD: Aspiration pneumonia. Arch Surg 106:49, 1973.
47. Cameron JL, Zuidema GD: Aspiration pneumonia—Magnitude and frequency of the problem. JAMA 219:1194, 1972.
48. Sladen A, Zanca P, Hadnott W: Aspiration pneumonia—The sequelae. Chest 59:448, 1971.

CHAPTER 78

Life-Threatening Pulmonary Hemorrhage

Stephen A. Mette
Steven M. Albelda

Life-threatening bleeding from the lungs may occur as either massive hemoptysis or diffuse alveolar (pulmonary) hemorrhage. Both clinical entities are associated with a high mortality when not treated expeditiously and definitively. However, they are distinct in clinical presentation and pathophysiology. Massive hemoptysis is defined as significant (and often dramatic) bleeding from the airways, usually from a bronchial arterial source, and is associated with few or no chest radiographic changes. In contrast, diffuse alveolar hemorrhage can be insidious and is usually associated with hypoxemia, anemia, and diffuse radiographic changes, but little hemoptysis. Bleeding, in this case, originates from pulmonary capillaries. Successful treatment of massive hemoptysis depends on the concerted efforts of the intensive care specialist, the pulmonologist, the anesthesiologist, the thoracic surgeon, and the interventional radiologist to stabilize the patient, localize the bleeding site, protect the airway, and provide temporizing or curative intervention. Management of the alveolar hemorrhage syndromes is oriented toward medical stabilization and nonsurgical intervention and most frequently involves immunosuppressive therapy.

MASSIVE HEMOPTYSIS

Massive hemoptysis has been variably defined as 300 to 600 mL of expectorated blood during a 24-hour period.[1-3] Because aspiration of blood and asphyxiation are the usual causes of death in patients with massive hemoptyses,[4] any amount of blood in the tracheobronchial tree that may compromise the airway should be considered life threatening. The rate of hemorrhage and the general medical condition of the patient appear to predict mortality better than the volume of blood loss.[1]

Massive hemoptysis is almost always due to localized disease such as carcinoma of the lung, tuberculosis, and other infectious or inflammatory processes. Tuberculosis continues to be the major cause of significant hemoptysis worldwide, but is relatively less common in the United States than in Southeast Asia and the underdeveloped parts of the world. Along with tuberculosis, bronchiectasis, lung abscess, necrotizing pneumonia, pulmonary aspergilloma, and cystic fibrosis are the major causes of massive hemoptysis in industrialized countries (Table 78–1). Carcinoma of the lung causes hemoptysis in as many as 50% of patients with this

TABLE 78–1

CAUSES OF LIFE-THREATENING HEMOPTYSIS

Infectious or Inflammatory
  Tuberculosis
  Bronchiectasis
  Lung abscess
  Necrotizing pneumonia
  Aspergilloma
  Cystic fibrosis
  Lung sequestration

Neoplastic
  Bronchogenic carcinoma
  Bronchial adenoma

Cardiovascular
  Mitral stenosis
  Severe, chronic congestive heart failure
  Arteriovenous malformations
  Pulmonary infarction

Iatrogenic or Traumatic
  Bronchoscopic lung biopsy
  Pulmonary arterial rupture (from flow-directed catheter)
  Pulmonary contusion
  Foreign body aspiration

Other
  Alveolar hemorrhage syndromes
  Pneumoconiosis
  Broncholithiasis

disease,[5] but it remains a relatively infrequent cause of life-threatening hemoptysis. Bronchial adenoma, pneumoconiosis, arteriovenous malformations, mitral stenosis, pulmonary emboli, and trauma are rare causes of massive hemoptysis. Iatrogenic hemoptysis from bronchoscopic transbronchial biopsies and pulmonary infarction related to the use of flow-directed pulmonary arterial catheters are unusual but important complications of those procedures.

Of the two distinct blood supplies to the lung (pulmonary and bronchial circulations), the bronchial circulation is most often the source of bleeding in massive hemoptysis. Chronic inflammation frequently produces a rich supply of bronchial arterial collaterals that bleed when they are eroded by the inflammatory process. Other systemic vessels such as the internal mammary, long thoracic, intercostal, and diaphragmatic arteries may also have collateralization with the bronchial circulation or even entirely supply the diseased area. Identification of the source of the vascular supply to the bleeding becomes important when planning angiographic or surgical intervention. The pulmonary circulation may be the source of hemoptysis from pulmonary arterial trauma (e.g., flow-directed catheters), certain arteriovenous malformations, or chest trauma.[6] The vascular supply to some arteriovenous malformations, bronchiectasis, and lung sequestration may also involve fistula formation between the bronchial and pulmonary circulations. Pulmonary venous–bronchial venous plexus may dilate in the face of high pulmonary venous pressures and can be the source of bleeding in severe mitral stenosis.[7]

Assessment

An expeditious assessment utilizes historical features and results of the physical examination, laboratory and radiographic tests, and bronchoscopic evaluation to locate the bleeding site and plan its management.

History and Physical Examination

A well-directed history can quickly help narrow the differential diagnosis of hemoptysis. Previous pneumonia or tuberculosis suggests the possibility of bronchiectasis, whereas a history of cigarette smoking in patients older than 40 years of age makes lung cancer a more likely diagnosis. Patients often have difficulty in quantitating the amount of expectorated blood but can usually say how long they have had hemoptysis. Establishing whether the blood was expectorated, vomited, or cleared from a posterior nasal source is not always easy. Focusing on the quality of the blood may be helpful. Blood mixed with pus suggests lung abscess or necrotizing pneumonia, especially if the patient gives a history of fever. Frothy blood indicates a pulmonary source, and the physician should seek a history of congestive or mitral valvular disease. Chest pain or a lateralizing sensation has not been found to be a good predictor for localizing the site of hemoptysis.[8]

A rapid yet thorough physical examination must be performed in an effort to localize the bleeding source and stabilize the patient's condition. Because asphyxiation with aspirated blood is of major concern, a quick assessment of the airway should be made. Oral endotracheal intubation should be performed in the obtunded patient or in any situation in which the airway is inadequately protected. Although exsanguination is unusual in massive hemoptysis, hypotension from poor oral intake or coexisting sepsis should be addressed with intravenous volume repletion.

Examination of the nose, mouth, and pharynx is vital in the search for an upper airway site of bleeding. Posterior nasopharyngeal epistaxis can be confused with a pulmonary source of bleeding and thus warrants investigation if blood is found in the oropharynx. Telangiectasia on the lips or oral mucosa is suggestive of oral or upper gastrointestinal bleeding attributable to hereditary telangiectasia (Osler-Weber-Rendu disease).

The chest examination may help isolate the source of the disease to one hemithorax or identify a potential cardiac cause of bleeding. Evidence of unilateral consolidation, wheezing, or rales could indicate the bleeding site and help focus bronchoscopic or radiographic examination. However, aspirated blood from a nonpulmonary source or from the contralateral lung may confound efforts at localization by physical examination. Cardiac examination findings consistent with congestive heart failure or the auscultatory findings of mitral stenosis necessitate further investigation if a pulmonary source is not found. Chest trauma leading to rib fracture and pulmonary contusion can also be discerned from careful examination of the thorax.

Other helpful physical examination findings include clubbing (which is associated with bronchiectasis, cystic fibrosis, and lung cancer), cervical or supraclavicular adenopathy (lung cancer), and petechiae, diffuse bleeding, palpable purpura, or hematuria (coagulopathies, vasculitis, renal-pulmonary hemorrhage syndromes).

Laboratory and Radiographic Tests

Emergent laboratory analysis should be undertaken in all patients with massive hemoptysis. These include coagulation studies (prothrombin time, partial thromboplastin time, platelet count, and bleeding time in patients taking aspirin or those with renal failure); hemoglobin determination; white blood cell count; serum electrolyte, serum creatinine, and blood urea nitrogen levels; and an arterial blood gas determination. Blood should be sent for typing and cross-matching in anticipation of thoracotomy and possible transfusion requirements. Sputum should be sent for bacterial, acid-fast bacilli, and fungal cultures as well as analysis with Gram's, acid-fast, and fungal stains. A urinalysis should also be done to look for evidence of blood and glomerulonephritis. Skin and serologic tests for fungal infection are seldom helpful. However, serum precipitating antibodies to aspergillus may be helpful in diagnosing a pulmonary aspergilloma. An intermediate-strength purified protein derivative should be tested on patients whose tuberculin status is not known. If the patient is stable enough, some measurement of pulmonary function is useful to evaluate suitability for surgical resection. A bedside determination of the forced expiratory volume in 1 second, or even the peak flow, can be of value in this situation.

The chest radiograph remains the most important imaging study in determining the site and cause of hemoptysis. Unilateral cavitary disease may indicate a necrotizing infection or lung carcinoma, whereas diffuse bilateral alveolar infiltrates suggest diffuse alveolar hemorrhage. Congenital heart disease and mitral stenosis may also be implicated radiographically. When there is radiographically evident lung disease involving both hemithoraces, such as in bilateral cavitating tuberculosis, localization of the source of bleeding may be difficult. Furthermore, alveolar infiltrates may be due to aspirated blood alone and may not be helpful in diagnosing the cause or the location of bleeding. A high-quality chest radiograph is therefore a vital diagnostic tool but one that usually requires adjunctive measures to localize the source of bleeding.

Other radiographic tests can be used for both diagnosis and management of life-threatening hemoptysis. Computed tomography of the chest may help define the disease process (mycetoma, pleural or chest wall involvement) and aid the thoracic surgeon to plan the appropriate surgical intervention. Radioisotopic ventilation-perfusion and pulmonary arterial angiography are useful in the unusual situation in which pulmonary embolism causes significant hemoptysis. Angiography of the bronchial circulation is helpful in detecting the site of bleeding as well as defining the vascular anatomy of the bleeding lesion. Although visualization of extravasated dye requires active bleeding of at least 2 mL/min, the vascular supply to the bleeding site must often be inferred by the abnormal vascular anatomy. Angiography may also play an important role in treating the nonsurgical candidate by enabling the angiographer to perform therapeutic embolization of the bleeding vessels.

Bronchoscopy has become the most important diagnostic procedure in localizing the site of bleeding.[4, 9, 10] It also serves as an important modality in stabilizing the actively bleeding patient. The choice between rigid and flexible fiberoptic bronchoscopy depends on several factors, including the skills of the bronchoscopist, the facility with which bronchoscopy can be done, and the rate of bleeding.[4] The flexible fiberoptic bronchoscope lends itself to rapid access to the tracheobronchial tree, at the bedside, through an endotracheal tube of at least 8 mm. It has the advantage of directly visualizing the upper lobes and the segmental and subsegmental bronchi, where localization and local control of the bleeding can be attempted. Rigid bronchoscopy requires skills not always quickly available to the intensivist. However, it is far superior to the flexible bronchoscope in the evacuation of large amounts of blood and blood clots. This technique also permits better lavage of the hemorrhagic area followed by tamponade packing of the bleeding airway.

Management

Because rapid and effective treatment of massive hemoptysis is critically important, the patient should be admitted to the intensive care unit where the skills and resources of the intensivist are readily available. Consultation with a pulmonologist, a thoracic surgeon, an interventional radiologist, and an anesthesiologist should be initiated while stabilization is under way.

Medical Management

Initial management should be aimed at protection of the airway and hemodynamic stabilization. If the patient is actively bleeding or if respiratory failure seems imminent, oral endotracheal intubation with an 8-mm or larger single-lumen endotracheal tube should be performed. Nasotracheal intubation should be avoided, as epistaxis may complicate management and fiberoptic bronchoscopy becomes more difficult. In addition, a nasotracheal tube is not long enough to intubate a mainstem bronchus selectively, should this become necessary.

If the bleeding lung has been identified, the normal lung may need to be isolated to prevent fatal aspiration. Selective intubation of the right mainstem bronchus can be accomplished by blindly advancing the endotracheal tube until breath sounds are no longer auscultated in the left side of the chest. Bronchoscopic guidance into the left main bronchus is usually required when attempting to intubate the left lung. The technique also helps avoid right upper lobe obstruction by the endotracheal tube when the right main bronchus requires intubation. The use of double-lumen endotracheal tubes (Carlens' or Robertshaw's) has little advantage over selective main bronchial intubation. Moreover, their use is associated with considerable complications, including the need for frequent checking for positioning and the potential for bronchial mucosal erosion in the mechanically ventilated patient.[11, 12] Because of their small lumen, suctioning of the airways is also compromised.

Supplemental oxygen should be initiated early in the course of treatment, because worsening oxygenation usually occurs as bleeding continues. Mechanical ventilation is often needed because patients frequently have underlying lung disease. Positive end-expiratory pressure has been advocated as a possible therapeutic modality; this is achieved by attempting to accomplish tamponade of the bleeding vessel with positive intrathoracic pressures.[13] However, caution must be exerted not to compromise the patient hemodynamically as well as potentially worsen ventilation-perfusion mismatch in localized lung disease. Positioning the patient with the bleeding lung down (if known) may help minimize aspiration of blood into the contralateral lung.

Hemodynamic stabilization requires two large-bore intravenous catheters for the administration of fluid, blood, and intravenous medications. Four to six units of type-specific and cross-matched blood must be available for the patient who may potentially need thoracotomy.

Further stabilization involves correcting metabolic abnormalities. If there is a coagulopathy, fresh frozen plasma or cryoprecipitate (if the fibrinogen level is less than 100 mg/dL) should be administered. The patient should be kept lying still, and chest percussion should be avoided. Sedation with a benzodiazepine can help with the extreme anxiety these patients often experience. However, suppression of the cough reflex with narcotics is best avoided, especially in the nonintubated patient, to aid with the expectoration of blood in the airways. Initiating appropriate antibiotic administration when a necrotizing pneumonia or tuberculosis is suspected, although prudent, does not alter immediate outcome. Congestive heart failure should be treated if present. If bleeding continues, intravenous administration of vasopressin (0.2 to 0.4 U/min) has anecdotally been associated with hemostasis.[14]

Endobronchial Management

After initial stabilization, bronchoscopic inspection of the airways should be performed. The fiberoptic flexible bronchoscope has greater versatility, although it has limitations, especially in the face of massive bleeding (see earlier). Either the fiberoptic or the rigid bronchoscope can be used for localization of the bleeding airway and may also be used to control hemorrhage until further definitive therapy can be employed. Topical epinephrine (at a 1:20,000 dilution) may be administered if the bleeding site is small and active bleeding is not profuse. Iced isotonic saline lavage was used effectively to curtail hemorrhage in several reported series.[15, 16] Isolation or tamponade of the bleeding segmental or subsegmental bronchus can be attempted with a Fogarty catheter passed through a fiberoptic bronchoscope.[15] This technique is best used to retard the flow of blood into the main bronchi while awaiting surgical or angiographic management of the bleeding source. If the patient is not actively bleeding, the application of fibrin precursors onto the bleeding site may provide sufficient coagulative hemostasis in patients who are otherwise not surgical candidates or in whom definitive therapy may be delayed.[17] The use of laser photocoagulation has no role in the acutely bleeding patient with massive hemoptysis, but the technique may offer palliation in patients with small recurrent focal oozing of blood in the major airways.

Endovascular Treatment

Angiography of the bronchial or other systemic vessels (e.g., internal mammary, intercostal, and long thoracic arteries) that supply the bleeding lesion may be used to help define the vascular anatomy and stabilize the patient in preparation for surgical extirpation.[18–20] Angiographic patterns can help identify the cause of the bleeding by noting the hypervascularity of an inflammatory lesion or the characteristic systemic-to-pulmonary vascular anomalies found in arteriovenous malformations, bronchiectasis, and lung sequestration. Angiographic embolization should generally be reserved for those patients for whom surgery is not an option. Significant success in controlling the hemorrhage has been reported for a variety of bleeding sources, including tuberculosis, bronchogenic carcinoma, and bronchiectasis.[20, 21] This technique must be done with great care by a skilled angiographer to avoid spinal arterial or retrograde embolization. Rebleeding recurs in about 20% of cases depending on the cause, but is most pronounced in aspergillomas.[18] Bleeding from aspergillomas has been successfully palliated with percutaneous intracavitary instillation of amphotericin B.[22]

Surgery

Surgical resection of the bleeding lung tissue is the definitive therapy for massive hemoptysis and should be considered for all patients who are acceptable candidates. Determination of inoperability excludes patients with severe lung disease (postoperative predicted forced expired volume in 1 second is less than 800 mL or carbon dioxide retention is documented by arterial blood gas determination), patients with unresectable carcinomas, and patients whose prognosis from their underlying disease is unreasonably poor. Furthermore, surgery should not be undertaken without localization of the bleeding site to one hemithorax.

Iatrogenic Massive Hemoptysis

Two commonly used diagnostic techniques, fiberoptic bronchoscopy and pulmonary arterial catheterization, are occasionally associated with life-threatening hemoptysis. Bronchoscopic bronchial and transbronchial biopsies have a 1 to 4% risk of significant bleeding in the nonimmunocompromised or uremic patient.[23, 24] These bleeds, if massive,

should be treated in the same manner outlined for other causes of massive hemoptysis.

Pulmonary arterial injury or rupture after inflation of the balloon of a flow-directed catheter has been reported with increasing frequency. More than 40 cases have been documented,[25] with mortality of approximately 40%.[25, 26] The diagnosis is made when hemoptysis occurs during insertion of the catheter or after balloon inflation. If pulmonary arterial injury or rupture is suspected, angiographic contrast can be injected through the distal catheter port. Extravasation of contrast material out of the pulmonary artery into the parenchyma or into the bronchus or identification of a false aneurysm confirms the diagnosis.[27–29] Treatment must be prompt, but the choice of therapy is controversial. The catheter should be kept in place or pulled back proximal to the rupture site. Carefully reinflating the balloon in this position may stop the bleeding, but the results are often not permanent. Reversal of anticoagulation is essential. Embolization with 10 mL of autologous clot injected through the catheter has been reported to stop bleeding.[27] The patient should be intubated, and positive end-expiratory pressure may be initiated in an attempt to achieve tamponade of the pulmonary artery. If bleeding continues, however, segmentectomy or lobectomy may be needed.

DIFFUSE ALVEOLAR HEMORRHAGE

Diffuse alveolar or pulmonary hemorrhage occurs as a consequence of a variety of disorders, including anti–glomerular basement membrane (anti-GBM) antibody disease (Goodpasture's syndrome), vasculitis and immune complex disease (Wegener's granulomatosis, systemic lupus erythematosus), idiopathic rapidly progressive glomerulonephritis, administration of certain medications (D-penicillamine), coagulopathies, and some idiopathic syndromes (Table 78–2). Several classification schemes have been proposed,[30–32] generally based on the presence or absence of (1) renal disease,

TABLE 78–2
CLASSIFICATION OF DIFFUSE ALVEOLAR HEMORRHAGE

Characteristics*	Diseases*
I. AH with GN and anti-GBM antibody	Classic Goodpasture's syndrome
II. AH with renal disease without demonstrable immunologic abnormalities	Uremic lung bleeding, legionnaires' disease, cresentic GN without anti-GBM antibody or immune complexes
III. AH with GN and immune complex disease	SLE, Wegener's granulomatosis, HSP, cryoglobulinemia, MCTD, systemic vasculitis
IV. AH with immune complexes but without renal disease	SLE, Wegener's granulomatosis, systemic vasculitis
V. AH with anti-GBM antibody but without renal disease	Early Goodpasture's syndrome
VI. AH without renal disease or immunologic disorder (idiopathic disorders, bleeding disorders, acute lung injury, miscellaneous)	DIC, thrombocytopenia, leukemia, anticoagulant use, ARDS, toxic inhalation, mitral stenosis, drugs, idiopathic pulmonary hemosiderosis

*AH = alveolar hemorrhage; GN = glomerulonephritis; SLE = systemic lupus erythematosus; HSP = Henoch-Schönlein purpura; MCTD = mixed connective tissue disease; DIC = disseminated intravascular coagulation; ARDS = adult respiratory distress syndrome.
Adapted from Albelda SM, Gefter WB, Epstein DM, et al: Diffuse pulmonary hemorrhage: A review and classification. Radiology 154:289–297, 1985.

CLASSIFICATION OF DIFFUSE PULMONARY HEMORRHAGE

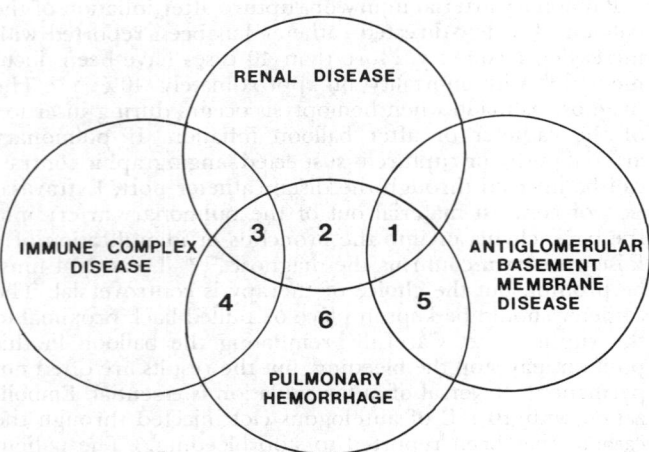

Figure 78–1. Classification of diffuse pulmonary hemorrhage. 1 = pulmonary hemorrhage associated with glomerulonephritis and anti-GBM antibody; 2 = pulmonary hemorrhage associated with renal disease without demonstrable immunologic abnormalities; 3 = pulmonary hemorrhage associated with glomerulonephritis and immune complex disease; 4 = pulmonary hemorrhage and immune complex disease without renal disease; 5 = pulmonary hemorrhage associated with anti-GBM antibodies without renal disease; 6 = pulmonary hemorrhage without demonstrable immunologic associations or renal disease. (From Albelda SM, Gefter WB, Epstein DM, et al: Diffuse pulmonary hemorrhage: A review and classification. Radiology 154:289–297, 1985.)

(2) involvement of immune complexes, (3) anti-GBM antibody, and (4) pulmonary hemorrhage resulting from non-immunologic or renal disease. There is, however, clinical overlapping of the different pathologic entities, which may lead to diagnostic confusion (Fig. 78–1). Regardless of the cause, the alveolar hemorrhage syndromes are characterized by diffuse bleeding from the acinar microvasculature into the pulmonary alveoli.[33] Although these syndromes are unusual, mortality of this group of diseases is high and requires prompt recognition and specialized treatment. Without early treatment of the alveolar hemorrhage syndromes, respiratory failure, pulmonary fibrosis, and irreversible renal failure may occur.

Assessment

Alveolar hemorrhage syndromes are often characterized by the clinical triad of hemoptysis, anemia, and diffuse alveolar infiltrates.[34] Clinical manifestations include dyspnea, cough, and hypoxemia.[32] Alveolar hemorrhage often occurs without frank hemoptysis,[35–38] a presentation that commonly leads to initial misdiagnoses.[34, 39] Alveolar infiltrates are a constant feature of these syndromes, but there is no specific pattern of parenchymal involvement for alveolar hemorrhage. The usual radiographic appearance is that of diffuse alveolar filling (Fig. 78–2), although the pattern may vary from bilateral diffuse to unilateral patchy infiltrates.[31, 40] Lack of associated findings, such as adenopathy, pleural effusions, and cavitation, supports the diagnosis of alveolar hemorrhage. However, alveolar filling processes (e.g., pulmonary edema, diffuse pneumonia, and alveolar proteinosis) may appear radiographically identical.

In the absence of hemoptysis, the diagnosis of alveolar hemorrhage can often be confirmed with the help of additional studies. Fiberoptic bronchoscopy with bronchoalveolar lavage to determine the hemosiderin content of alveolar macrophages has been shown to be useful in diagnosing alveolar bleeding.[41, 42] The pulmonary uptake of carbon monoxide should be increased in patients with alveolar bleeding. Monitoring the pulmonary uptake of carbon dioxide in patients with alveolar hemorrhage may be a sensitive indicator of rebleeding.[43, 44] Other methods to detect acute acinar bleeding include nuclear lung scanning with technetium Tc 99m sulfur colloid[45] or technetium Tc 99m pertechnetate–labeled red blood cells,[46, 47] but their reliability is questionable. The diagnosis of an alveolar hemorrhage syndrome can usually be made from the clinical presentation and radiologic criteria alone.

Diagnosis of specific disease entities requires additional testing. Anti-GBM antibody disease requires the presence of circulating serum anti-GBM antibody[48, 49] or the demonstration of linear anti-GBM immunoglobulin G immunofluorescent staining on a renal biopsy specimen[50] (Fig. 78–3). Although the same antibody binds to the alveolar septal basement membrane, alveolar basement membrane immunofluorescent staining is observed less commonly.[48, 51] Renal biopsy tissue is preferable to lung tissue for diagnostic purposes, and renal biopsy should be considered early in the search for a specific cause. Other serologic tests to rule out systemic lupus erythematosus, systemic vasculitis, and Wegener's granulomatosis should also be performed. These include levels of antinuclear antibody, complement, rheumatoid factor, cryoglobulins, and circulating antineutrophilic cytoplasmic antibodies.[52]

All patients with suspected alveolar hemorrhage should also undergo assessment of renal function with determination of blood urea nitrogen and serum creatinine levels. Urinalysis is essential to check for blood or red blood cell casts. Paranasal sinus films may help in the diagnosis of Wegener's granulomatosis. Coagulation studies, Gram's stains and culture of the sputum, and urine *Legionella* antigen studies must all be considered part of the evaluation for the patient with alveolar hemorrhage.

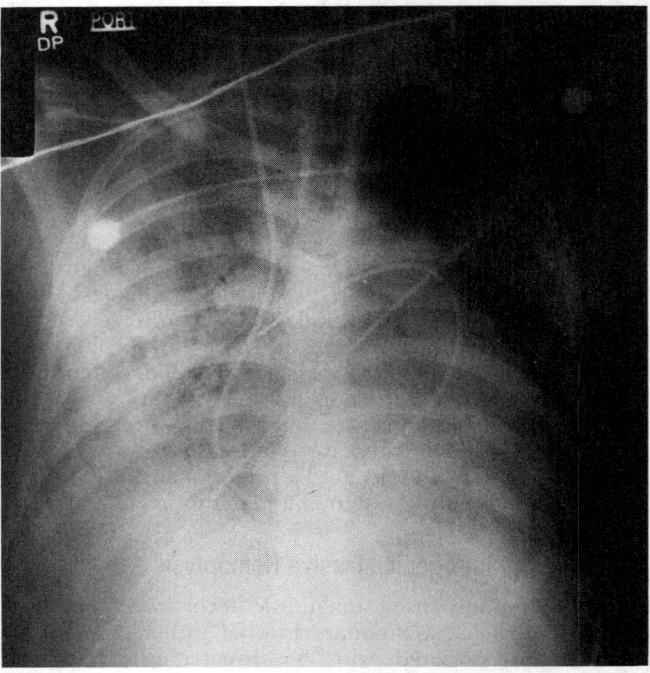

Figure 78–2. Diffuse pulmonary hemorrhage in a 21-year-old man with known systemic lupus erythematosus. The patient had a fever, dyspnea, and hemoptysis.

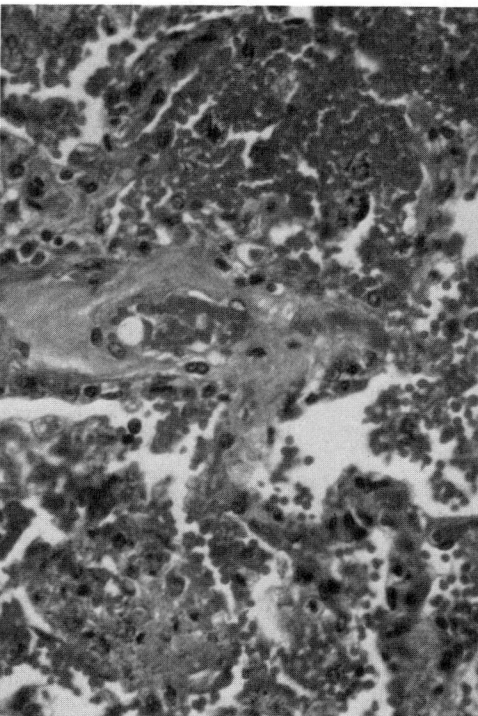 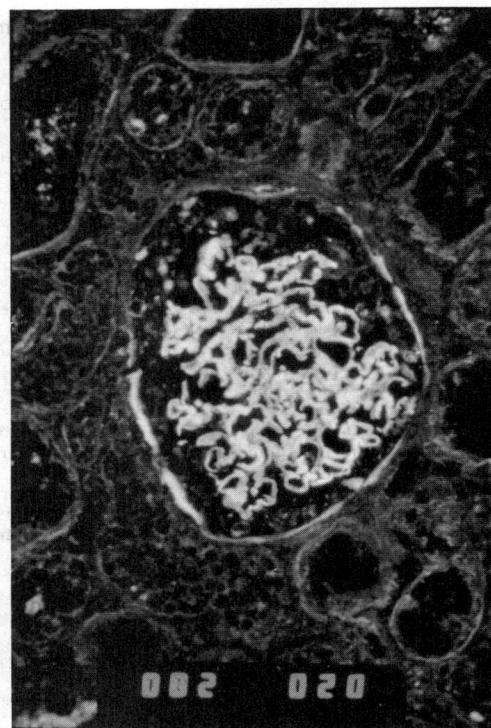

Figure 78–3. Massive hemoptysis in a 59-year-old woman with Good-pasture's syndrome. *(Left)* Lung biopsy specimen showing alveolar hemorrhage. × 250. *(Right)* Anti–immunoglobulin G immunofluorescent staining showing the linear pattern of anti-GBM antibody in a glomerulus from the same patient. × 400.

Management

There are two major goals in treating alveolar hemorrhage syndromes. The first is to control alveolar bleeding. The second is to prevent or halt the progression of renal or other extrapulmonary disease. After significant renal damage in anti-GBM antibody and immune complex disease has occurred, there is little hope of regaining renal function. Although there are several published recommendations for the treatment of the different immunologically mediated syndromes,[30, 34, 53, 54] there have been no controlled clinical trials to document their efficacy.

Specific therapeutic regimens rely on prompt and accurate diagnosis. Treatment of alveolar hemorrhage syndromes caused by immunologic mechanisms (e.g., anti-GBM antibody disease, systemic lupus erythematosus, systemic vasculitis, and Wegener's granulomatosis) is best accomplished with pulsed doses of steroids[30] beginning with methylprednisolone at 1 g/d for 3 to 5 days followed by daily prednisone (1 to 2 mg/kg/d). Plasma exchange therapy performed on a daily basis for a total of 10 to 14 exchanges has been suggested for anti-GBM antibody disease,[30, 53] with the rationale that circulating antibody can be removed, while antibody resynthesis is prevented by high-dose steroids and cytotoxic agents. Plasmapheresis does not appear to be effective in managing alveolar hemorrhage attributable to immune complex disease, but some clinicians continue to advocate its use, citing anecdotal reports that suggest therapeutic success.[55] The use of immunosuppressive cytotoxic agents such as cyclophosphamide and azathioprine is also controversial. Their combined use with steroid administration and plasmapheresis is recommended for anti-GBM antibody disease (cyclophosphamide, 1 to 2 mg/kg/d, or azathioprine, 1 mg/kg/d).[30, 54] Cyclophosphamide treatment of the renal component of necrotizing vasculitis has been shown to be effective if therapy is begun before significant glomerular damage has occurred.[56, 57] However, its efficacy in controlling alveolar hemorrhage is less certain. Bilateral nephrectomy is no longer warranted for these disorders.[34, 58]

Control of alveolar bleeding may also necessitate ancillary measures such as administration of fresh frozen plasma or cryoprecipitate for coagulopathies, antibiotics for diffuse pneumonia, and arginine vasopressin for the platelet dysfunction of uremia. Because the pathologic changes of many alveolar hemorrhage syndromes are thought to be capillaritis and venulitis,[33] monitoring and reducing pulmonary arterial occlusion pressures may help limit any hemodynamic component of bleeding.

Monitoring treatment success can be accomplished by several methods. Cessation of acute alveolar hemorrhage should result in clearing of alveolar infiltrates on radiographs within 2 to 10 days,[40] unless there is underlying lung disease. In mechanically ventilated patients, an improvement in pulmonary compliance may reflect a cessation of bleeding. As mentioned earlier, measurement of the carbon dioxide diffusing capacity may indicate the amount of fresh blood in the alveoli.[44] Finally, in anti-GBM antibody disease as well as in the vasculitides, a halt in the decline of renal function may indicate effectiveness of treatment.

SUMMARY

Life-threatening pulmonary hemorrhage occurs in a variety of diseases and clinical situations. It deserves prompt attention to establish a diagnosis and plan treatment so that the poor survival associated with this group of disorders is lessened. The patient with massive hemoptysis may require endotracheal intubation, mechanical ventilation, volume resuscitation, and correction of coagulopathies and metabolic abnormalities. Bronchoscopy (either rigid or fiberoptic) should be performed early to help establish location and diagnosis. It may also serve to temporize the bleeding until definitive therapy can be undertaken. Surgical resection must be considered early in the appropriate patient. Angiographic embolization may be an alternative modality in the nonsurgical candidate.

For the patient with diffuse alveolar hemorrhage, an expeditious search for the cause is essential to help preserve organ function, especially that of the kidneys. A renal biopsy must be considered early to help differentiate the various disorders.

References

1. Crocco JA, Rooney JJ, Fankhushen DS, et al: Massive hemoptysis. Arch Intern Med 121:495, 1968.
2. Gourin A, Garzon AA: Operative management of massive hemoptysis. Ann Thorac Surg 18:52, 1974.
3. Conlan AA, Hurwitz SS, Krige L, et al: Massive hemoptysis. Review of 123 cases. J Thorac Cardiovasc Surg 85:120, 1983.
4. Bobrowitz ID, Ramakrishna S, Shim YS, et al: Comparison of medical vs surgical treatment of major hemoptysis. Arch Intern Med 143:1343, 1983.
5. Weaver LJ, Solliday N, Cugell DW, et al: Selection of patients with hemoptysis for fiberoptic bronchoscopy. Chest 76:7, 1979.
6. Barth DH, Mertens MA: Interventional radiology. Med Clin North Am 68:1647, 1984.
7. Ferguson FC, Kobilak RE, Deitrick JE: Varices of the bronchial veins as a source of hemoptysis in mitral stenosis. Am Heart J 28:445, 1944.
8. Kinasewitz GT, Long RJ, George RB: Inability of awake patients to correctly locate a cough stimulus. South Med J 78:970, 1985.
9. Smiddy JF, Elliott RC: The evaluation of hemoptysis with fiberoptic bronchoscopy. Chest 64:168, 1973.
10. Garzon AA, Gourin A: Surgical management of massive hemoptysis. A ten-year experience. Ann Surg 187:267, 1978.
11. Wolfe JD, Simmons DH: Hemoptysis: Diagnosis and management. West J Med 127:383, 1977.
12. Gourin A, Garzon AA: Control of hemorrhage in emergency pulmonary resection for massive hemoptysis. Chest 68:120, 1975.
13. Noseworthy TW, Anderson BJ: Massive hemoptysis. Can Med Assoc J 135:1097, 1986.
14. Magee G, Williams MJ Jr: Treatment of massive hemoptysis with intravenous Pitressin. Lung 160:165, 1982.
15. Imgrund SP, Goldberg SK, Walkenstein MD, et al: Clinical diagnosis of massive hemoptysis using the fiberoptic bronchoscope. Crit Care Med 13:438, 1985.
16. Conlan AA, Hurwitz SS: Management of massive hemoptysis with the rigid bronchoscope and cold saline lavage. Thorax 35:901, 1980.
17. Bense L: Intrabronchial selective coagulative treatment of hemoptysis. Report of three cases. Chest 97:990, 1990.
18. Uflacker R, Kaemmerer A, Picon PD, et al: Bronchial artery embolization in the management of hemoptysis: Technical aspects and long term results. Radiology 157:637, 1985.
19. Vujic I, Pyle R, Hungerford GD, et al: Angiography and therapeutic blockade in the control of hemoptysis. The importance of nonbronchial systemic arteries. Radiology 143:19, 1982.
20. Remy J, Arnaud A, Fardou H, et al: Treatment of hemoptysis by embolization of bronchial arteries. Radiology 122:33, 1977.
21. Uflacker R, Kaemmerer A, Neves C, et al: Management of massive hemoptysis by bronchial artery embolization. Radiology 146:627, 1983.
22. Shapiro MJ, Albelda SM, Mayock RL, et al: Severe hemoptysis associated with pulmonary aspergilloma: Percutaneous intracavitary treatment. Chest 94:1225, 1988.
23. Herf SM, Suratt PM, Arora NS: Deaths and complications associated with transbronchial lung biopsy. Am Rev Respir Dis 115:708, 1977.
24. Zavala DC: Pulmonary hemorrhage in fiberoptic transbronchial biopsy. Chest 70:584, 1976.
25. Remy T, Siproudhis L, Laurent JF, et al: Massive hemoptysis from iatrogenic balloon catheter rupture of pulmonary artery: Successful early management by balloon tamponade. Crit Care Med 15:272, 1987.
26. Hannan AT, Brown M, Bigman O, et al: Pulmonary artery catheter induced hemorrhage. Chest 85:128, 1984.
27. Rubin SA, Puckett RP: Pulmonary artery–bronchial fistula: A new complication of Swan-Ganz catheterization. Chest 75:515, 1979.
28. Barash PG, Nardi D, Hammond G, et al: Catheter-induced pulmonary artery perforation. Mechanisms, management and modifications. J Thorac Cardiovasc Surg 82:5, 1981.
29. Kron IL, Piepgrass W, Carebello B, et al: False aneurysm of the pulmo-
nary artery: A complication of pulmonary artery catheterization. Ann Thorac Surg 33:629, 1982.
30. Leatherman JW, Davies SF, Hoidal JR: Alveolar hemorrhage syndromes: Diffuse microvascular lung hemorrhage in immune and idiopathic disorders. Medicine 63:343, 1984.
31. Albelda SM, Gefter WB, Epstein DM, et al: Diffuse pulmonary hemorrhage: A review and classification. Radiology 154:289, 1985.
32. Bradley JD: The pulmonary hemorrhage syndromes. Clin Chest Med 3:593, 1982.
33. Morgan PGM, Turner-Warwick M: Pulmonary hemosiderosis and pulmonary hemorrhage. Br J Dis Chest 75:225, 1981.
34. Briggs WA, Johnson JP, Teichman S, et al: Antiglomerular basement membrane antibody–mediated glomerular nephritis and Goodpasture's syndrome. Medicine 58:348, 1979.
35. Eagen JW, Memoli VA, Roberts JL, et al: Pulmonary hemorrhage in systemic lupus erythematosus. Medicine 57:545, 1978.
36. Palmer PE, Finley TN, Drew WL, et al: Radiographic aspects of occult pulmonary haemorrhage. Clin Radiol 29:139, 1978.
37. Bombardieri S, Paoletti P, Ferri C, et al: Lung involvement in essential mixed cryoglobulinemia. Am J Med 66:748, 1979.
38. Robboy SJ, Minna JD, Colman RW, et al: Pulmonary hemorrhage syndrome as a manifestation of disseminated intravascular coagulation: Analysis of ten cases. Chest 63:718, 1973.
39. Leatherman JW, Sibley RK, Davies SF: Diffuse intrapulmonary hemorrhage and glomerulonephritis unrelated to antiglomerular basement membrane antibody. Am J Med 72:401, 1982.
40. Fraser RG, Paré JAP, Paré PD, et al: Goodpasture's syndrome and idiopathic pulmonary hemosiderosis. In: Fraser RG, Paré JAP, Paré PD, et al (eds): Diagnosis of Diseases of the Chest. 3rd ed. Philadelphia, WB Saunders, p 1181, 1989.
41. Finley TN, Aronow A, Consentino AM, et al: Occult pulmonary hemorrhage in anticoagulated patients. Am Rev Respir Dis 112:23, 1975.
42. Kahn FW, Jones JM, England DM: Diagnosis of pulmonary hemorrhage in the immunocompromised host. Am Rev Respir Dis 136:155, 1987.
43. Ewan PW, Jones HA, Rhodes CG, et al: Detection of intrapulmonary hemorrhage with carbon monoxide uptake. N Engl J Med 295:1391, 1976.
44. Addleman M, Logan AS, Grossman RF: Monitoring intrapulmonary hemorrhage in Goodpasture's syndrome. Chest 87:119, 1985.
45. Winzelberg GG, Wholey MH, Sachs M: Scintigraphic localization of pulmonary bleeding using technetium Tc 99m sulfur colloid: A preliminary report. Radiology 143:757, 1982.
46. Coel MN, Druger G: Radionuclide detection of the site of hemoptysis. Chest 81:242, 1982.
47. Winzelberg GG, Laman D, Sachs M, et al: Detection of pulmonary hemorrhage with technetium-labeled red cells. J Nucl Med 22:884, 1981.
48. Wilson CB, Dixon FJ: Renal injury from immune reactions involving antigens in or of the kidney. In: Brenner BM, Stein J (eds): Contemporary Issues in Nephrology, Volume 3. New York, Churchill Livingstone, p 46, 1979.
49. Weislander J, Bygren P, Heinegard D: Antiglomerular basement membrane antibody: Antibody specificity in different forms of glomerulonephritis. Kidney Int 23:855, 1983.
50. Wilson CB, Dixon FJ: Anti–glomerular basement membrane antibody–induced glomerulonephritis. Kidney Int 3:74, 1973.
51. Beechler CR, Enquist RW, Hunt KK, et al: Immunofluorescence of transbronchial biopsies in Goodpasture's syndrome. Am Rev Respir Dis 121:869, 1980.
52. Nolle B, Specks U, Ludemann J, et al: Anticytoplasmic antibodies: Their immunodiagnostic value in Wegener's granulomatosis. Ann Intern Med 111:28, 1989.
53. Lockwood CM, Boulton Jones JM, Lowenthal RM, et al: Recovery from Goodpasture's syndrome after immunosuppression treatment and plasmapheresis. Br Med J 2:252, 1975.
54. Peters DK, Rees AJ, Lockwood CM: Treatment and prognosis of antiglomerular basement membrane antibody mediated nephritis. Transplant Proc 14:513, 1982.
55. Millman RP, Cohen TB, Levinson AI, et al: Systemic lupus erythematosus complicated by acute pulmonary hemorrhage: Recovery following plasmapheresis and cytotoxic therapy. J Rheumatol 8:1021, 1981.
56. Fauci AS, Haynes BF, Katz P: The spectrum of vasculitis: Clinical, pathologic, immunologic and therapeutic considerations. Ann Intern Med 89:660, 1978.
57. Fauci AS, Haynes BF, Katz P, et al: Wegener's granulomatosis: Prospective clinical and therapeutic experience with 85 patients over 21 years. Ann Intern Med 98:76, 1983.
58. Glassrock RJ: Goodpasture's syndrome. In: Massry SG, Glassrock RJ (eds): Textbook of Nephrology. Baltimore, Williams & Wilkins, p 719, 1983.

CHAPTER 79

Acute Smoke Inhalation

Jacob Loke

Toxic gas inhalation can result in lung injury. Sources include indoor conflagration as in smoke inhalation attributable to fires,[1] occupational exposure,[2–5] industrial accidents (e.g., the toxic gas release in Bhopal, India, in 1985[6]) and military uses[7, 8] (e.g., poison gas). In acute toxic gas inhalation, whether from smoke inhalation or industrial accidents, the effect on the lung depends on the degree of exposure and the toxic gases or chemicals involved. In the most severe case, the victim has acute respiratory distress, severe arterial hypoxemia, pulmonary edema, respiratory failure, and adult respiratory distress syndrome that necessitate endotracheal intubation and mechanical ventilation.

Unless specific toxic gases or chemicals can be documented in an industrial accident, physicians must treat the lung injury without identifying the toxic gases, with supportive measures such as administration of oxygen, bronchodilators, and in certain cases, antibiotics or corticosteroids. Exposure to many toxic gases may occur in the fire environment,[9, 10] but clinically only measurements of carboxyhemoglobin (COHb) can be made in fire victims to assess the amount of carbon monoxide inhaled. In certain research institutes or hospitals, the determination of cyanide in blood samples of fire victims may be possible.

This chapter reviews acute smoke inhalation and the different commonly encountered toxic gases causing lung injuries.

FIRE ENVIRONMENT

It is estimated that there were about 2.1 million fires in the United States in 1989, of which 688,000 were structure fires and 74.6% were residential fires.[11] Four thousand six hundred fifty-five people died as a result of structure fires, and cigarette-ignited fires were the leading cause of house fire deaths.[12] In the home, wood furniture, upholstery, carpets, wood and plastic paneling on walls and ceilings, polyurethane materials, papers, and clothing are all potentially combustible materials and can release different toxic products of combustion.[13, 14] Major toxic chemical products of combustion from polyvinyl chloride material[15] present in wall and floor covering or telephone cable insulation include hydrogen chloride and carbon monoxide. The polyurethane materials in upholstery generate isocyanates and hydrogen cyanide on combustion. In addition to hydrogen cyanide, ammonia and acrolein are produced in the combustion of nylon and Acrilan, respectively. Nylon and Acrilan are used in some carpets and many other items.

The flammability of the products in the home and the thermal decomposition modes of these materials affect the amount of toxic gases that is produced in fires.[16] More toxic gases may be released when substances are decomposed in the pyrolysis state (smoldering or nonflaming condition) than in the combustion state (flaming mode), and the degree of emission of toxic gases from the burning of plastic polymers can be different under flaming and nonflaming conditions. The spread of a fire and smoke production depends on the quantity of combustible material that is available, the presence of the flammable materials, ventilation, the space in which the combustion may spread, and the fire protection system. In addition to the smoke and toxic gases from fires, there is the generation of high temperatures or heat from the flames, which can lead to severe burns and upper airway injury and direct death of the fire victims. If combustion occurs in a poorly ventilated environment, oxygen is depleted in the ambient air, which can cause arterial hypoxemia in individuals breathing an oxygen-deficient atmosphere. Secondary effects of fires include mechanical or structural damage of the home, causing the collapse of walls or roofs onto the fire victims. However, the majority of deaths from fires are due to the acute smoke inhalation, not to the high temperatures or burns or trauma from the falling structural parts of homes.

Smoke and Toxic Gases

Smoke is a suspension of visible small particles in hot air and toxic gases. The burning of carbonaceous material produces black smoke, and this is due to the particles of carbon or soot to which organic acids and aldehydes can adhere.[17] White smoke may result from the combustion of plastic polymers.

Carbon Monoxide

Carbon monoxide is the most dangerous gas that is produced in fires. Carbon-containing material is present in every home, residential building, or office. During the incomplete combustion of carbonaceous material associated with diminished oxygen in the ambient air or ventilation, carbon monoxide is generated. A significant amount of carbon monoxide can be present, especially in poorly ventilated places such as basements or closed spaces. This can lead to significant morbidity and mortality of fire victims and even firefighters, especially when they do not use respirators during inspection of poorly ventilated spaces after the fires have been extinguished.

Carbon monoxide is an odorless, colorless, tasteless, poisonous gas and competes with oxygen for the binding sites on the hemoglobin molecules. The affinity of carbon monoxide for hemoglobin is 210 times greater than that of oxygen. Carbon monoxide causes a shift of the oxygen-hemoglobin dissociation curve to the left and decreases oxygen release at the tissue level.[18, 19] Tissue hypoxia ensues.

The signs and symptoms of tissue hypoxia attributable to carbon monoxide intoxication are reflected in the central nervous system and the cardiovascular system because there is a greater amount of oxygen utilization by these organs. The central nervous system abnormalities depend on the level of carbon monoxide poisoning and include headache, dizziness, impairment in the performance of psychomotor tests,[20] behavioral incapacitation,[21] reduced visual discrimination, and in severe cases, confusion, ataxia, convulsions, and coma. Retinal hemorrhages may occur. A cherry red color of the skin and mucous membranes has been described, but this is an uncommon finding and is not a reliable sign. Direct determination of the blood COHb level[22, 23] is used for the diagnosis of carbon monoxide poisoning.

There is an increase in pulse rate and cardiac output with no significant changes in ventilation with acute carbon monoxide poisoning. Myocardial tissue oxygen tension from coronary sinus measurements has been shown to be decreased. In addition, there is a decrease in exercise tolerance and the presence of myocardial ischemia in patients with coronary arterial disease who are exposed to low levels of carbon monoxide (COHb level of 4.5%). Transmural myocardial infarction and myocardial toxicity have been reported in patients with carbon monoxide poisoning.[24]

Carbon monoxide is supposed to be nontoxic to the lung per se. However, an ultrastructural study of the lungs of rabbits exposed to carbon monoxide showed epithelial and endothelial cell swelling, interstitial edema, and depletion of lamellar bodies in alveolar type II cells.[25] This study postulates that carbon monoxide poisoning may induce noncardiogenic pulmonary edema in humans. However, in a study from the U.S. Army Institute of Surgical Research in Texas, the lungs of carbon monoxide–exposed sheep showed no histologic abnormalities.[26]

Other acute effects of carbon monoxide poisoning include lactic acidosis, diabetes insipidus, disseminated intravascular coagulation, myonecrosis, and hyperglycemia.

Hydrogen Cyanide

In a study of toxic gases produced during building fires in the Dallas area, carbon monoxide, hydrogen cyanide, hydrogen chloride, aldehydes (formaldehyde and acetaldehyde), total hydrocarbons, and free radicals of gases were demonstrated.[27] Carbon monoxide levels exceeded the short-term exposure limit (400 ppm) in an average of 28.5% of the fires; hydrogen cyanide was present in only 12% of the fires, whereas hydrogen chloride was found in only 9%. Dangerous levels of hydrogen cyanide and hydrogen chloride were not detected in this study. Although hydrogen cyanide is not a major toxic gas in fires,[28] fire fatalities have been shown to have significant cyanide levels and lethal cyanide blood levels have been demonstrated in air crash fatalities. The presence of combustible material, such as polyurethane, nylon and Acrilan, wool, and silk, should make one suspect the presence of a significant hydrogen cyanide level in the fire environment. The smoldering and combustion of polyurethane foam used in upholstered furniture produce hydrogen cyanide,[28] whereas the combustion of polyvinyl chloride causes the release of hydrogen chloride.

Hydrogen cyanide is a colorless gas with an odor of bitter almonds, which is probably not detectable in the fire environment.[29] This gas is a histotoxic hypoxic poison, which interferes with the utilization of oxygen at the cellular level by disrupting the cytochrome *c* oxidase in the mitochondria. This effect of cyanide leads to anaerobic metabolism and lactic acidosis. In the initial phase of intoxication, hydrogen cyanide produces central nervous system hypoxia and stimulates respiration until the depressant effects on the central nervous system become evident. The clinical manifestations vary with the blood cyanide levels.[30] A blood cyanide level of 2.5 mg/L or more is considered to reflect severe poisoning, and the affected person has dilated pupils, is comatose, and is hypotensive with slow, gasping respirations. Hydrogen cyanide in combination with carbon monoxide can have an additive or synergistic adverse effect on cerebral metabolism. Consequently, some fire victims may have such central nervous system depression that they are incapable of escape from the scene of a fire even when there is a sublethal concentration of hydrogen cyanide in the fire environment. There is no rapid method for determination of cyanide blood levels in most hospital clinical laboratories.

Hydrogen Chloride

It has become increasingly evident that plastic and its polymers have an important role in morbidity and mortality when these materials are involved in a fire. Mortality has been seen in smoke inhalation fire victims without burns and with severe chemical lung injury and only minimal elevation of the COHb level. Death is due to the toxic effects of gases such as hydrogen chloride, hydrogen cyanide, and other toxic gases.

The burning of polyvinyl chloride,[15] which is present in many plastic polymers, results in the release of hydrogen chloride. Hydrogen chloride is a hydroscopic substance, which in combination with water vapor causes the production of hydrochloric acid in the form of an aerosol. Hydrochloric acid has corrosive properties and produces significant irritation of the mucous membranes of the eyes, the nose, and the respiratory tract. Chlorine gas and phosgene are not produced with the thermal degradation of the polyvinyl chloride.

It has been shown that, in a low-energy controlled fire environment with the presence of wood, paper, clothing, polyvinyl chloride, and other synthetic materials, free radicals were produced with the equivalent oxidative power of chlorine gas. The signs and symptoms of chlorine gas exposure depend on the severity of the chlorine gas inhalation. There is severe irritation of the eyes, the upper airways, and the respiratory tract, which can be lethal when the chlorine concentration exceeds 430 ppm after 30 minutes of exposure. Tremendous heat is also released from the burning of plastic polymer, especially polyurethane. This can lead to the melting of iron and steel in structural supports, causing the structural collapse of homes and buildings.

Aldehydes

In the comparison of smoke produced from the combustion of wood versus smoke from the burning of kerosene, more carbon monoxide and aldehydes were present in wood smoke than in kerosene smoke. Furthermore, in experimental animals exposed to wood smoke, there was increased mortality and pulmonary injury in these animals compared with the kerosene smoke–exposed animals.[17] Aldehydes, including formaldehyde, acetaldehyde, and acrolein, are among the noxious and irritant gases produced in fires. Aldehydes irritate the skin, the eyes, and the mucous membranes, and acrolein has been shown to cause pulmonary edema in experimental animals.

Additional Toxic Gases

Nitrogen dioxide, oxides of nitrogen and sulfur, metallic oxides, ammonia, isocyanates, and organic hydrocarbons can also be present in the fire environment.

Thermal Factors

Although the toxic and irritant gases produced in the fire environment are the leading causes of morbidity and mortality in fire victims, flames and heat are the other major lethal factors. They cause significant burns of the body surface and inflict thermal injury on the upper airways. The pathophysiology and therapy of surface burns are not discussed in this chapter. Instead the focus is on the thermal injury of the airway. Unless steam is produced in the fire environment,[31] thermal injury to the fire victim is confined to the upper airways and does not involve the peripheral airways.

Thermal inhalation injury was present in 2.9% of 2297 burn patients at the Brooke Army Medical Center in Fort Sam Houston, Texas.[32] However, in a review of the records of 1058 consecutive burn patients treated between 1980 and 1984 at the same institute, inhalation injury was present in 35.3% (373 patients); inhalation injury was diagnosed by bronchoscopy and/or ventilation-perfusion lung scan.[33] Fire victims with thermal inhalation injury are those who sustain burns in a closed environment or are close to the fires or ignition source.[34] Thermal inhalation injury patients usually have burns on the face, and there is severe erythema of the oropharyngeal area associated with coughing of carbonaceous material or sputum, shortness of breath, hoarseness, and wheezing.[35] As a result of the oropharyngeal burn, there is upper airway obstruction caused by laryngeal edema and/or laryngospasm, which can be life threatening. In fire victims involved with the same degree of smoke inhalation, as assessed by the COHb level, the respiratory tract damage is more severe in burned individuals compared with non-burned patients.

PATHOPHYSIOLOGY

In the absence of burns and thermal upper airway injury, toxic inhalation in a fire can lead to pulmonary changes:[1, 36, 37] (1) impairment of the mucociliary function; (2) hypersecretion of mucus and an inflammatory response in the tracheobronchial tree; (3) alteration in biochemical factors in the lung, including surfactant; (4) cellular and immunologic changes leading to increased vascular permeability, pulmonary edema, and alveolar hemorrhage; (5) bronchoconstriction; and (6) pulmonary infection.

The mucociliary blanket of the lung transports particulate matter from the lung through the ciliary process, and mucus is expelled by reflexes such as coughing. In animal studies, acute inhalation of wood smoke without thermal injury causes disruption of the mucociliary blanket of the tracheobronchial tree. In addition, the acute irritation of the airways produces an increase in airway secretion of mucus, which, coupled with the impairment of the mucociliary function, results in the clinical picture of tracheobronchitis.

By using the technique of bronchoalveolar lavage in patients with acute smoke inhalation, a spectrum of inflammatory responses with mobilization of inflammatory cells such as alveolar macrophages has been demonstrated.[38] Similar results have been shown in laboratory animals.[39] In addition, there is alteration in the structure and chemotactic function of the pulmonary alveolar macrophage.[38] These effects, combined with alterations of the mucociliary blanket, may explain in part the increased susceptibility to pulmonary infection of patients with smoke inhalation.[40]

The bronchoconstriction seen in patients with smoke inhalation may be due to the direct inhalation of the irritant gases or fumes or inhalation of particles adhering to different aldehydes. Vagus-mediated reflex bronchoconstriction may also play a role. Bronchoconstriction can cause ventilation-perfusion mismatch, and if combined with the carbon monoxide or a low inspired oxygen concentration in the fire environment, may lead to arterial hypoxemia.[41]

CLINICAL EVALUATION

Patients with acute smoke inhalation may have a nonproductive cough, eye irritation, and mild respiratory distress, or they may have acute shortness of breath, cyanosis, hypotension, and loss of consciousness. There may be burns on the face and other parts of the body associated with a smell of smoke and carbonaceous material on the clothes of the fire victims. Initial examination includes determining vital signs, the respiratory status, and arterial oxygenation of the patient, together with obtaining blood samples for routine studies, including a COHb level. Facial burns and thermal inhalation injury may be evident in patients with coughing, sore throat, hoarseness, and stridor.

Physical examination may reveal stridor in the neck region and wheezes in the lung. Fiberoptic bronchoscopy may be indicated to evaluate the upper and lower airways, especially in patients with thermal inhalation injury[34] and burns. If significant stridor or laryngeal edema or upper airway swelling is seen on fiberoptic laryngoscopy and is associated with respiratory distress and significant arterial hypoxemia, endotracheal intubation may be needed to protect the upper airways. In patients who are not intubated, lung function tests, especially flow-volume studies, may demonstrate upper airway obstruction[35] or acute airway obstruction.[1, 42, 43]

The mental status of the patients should be determined because severe arterial hypoxemia, severe carbon monoxide intoxication, drug abuse, and alcohol intoxication can cause an alteration in mental status leading to loss of consciousness and coma. Patients who are lethargic and hypoxemic with underlying chronic obstructive pulmonary disease may need to be intubated. When the patient is intubated and mechanically ventilated, fiberoptic bronchoscopy is not indicated unless there is significant thermal injury with sloughing of the bronchial mucosa or significant carbonaceous material and secretions in the airways associated with significant hypoxemia and/or lobar atelectasis. Sputum should be sent for Gram's stain and cultures.

The chest radiograph is not a sensitive indicator of inhalation lung injury and may be normal initially in patients with cough and respiratory distress and arterial hypoxemia. Focal and patchy pulmonary infiltrates may be seen as late as 24 to 36 hours after exposure.[44] Diffuse pulmonary infiltrates or pulmonary edema is noted in patients with progressive lung injury or initially in patients with severe smoke inhalation. In fire victims who jump from a high building to escape the fire, pneumothorax, hemothorax, pulmonary contusion, and rib and bone fractures may be noted on the chest radiograph.

Acute myocardial ischemia or infarction can occur in fire victims with underlying ischemic heart disease. Fire victims with heart disease, chest pain, and dyspnea should be hospitalized for observation to exclude acute myocardial ischemia, especially if the blood COHb level is elevated (in nonsmokers, the COHb level is less than 2%, whereas in smokers, it ranges from 5 to 10%).

Laboratory studies including COHb level and arterial blood gas determination should be performed for fire victims with significant respiratory distress and underlying cardiac or pulmonary disease. The COHb level is valuable in determining the severity of acute smoke inhalation and indirectly reflects also the amount of other toxic and irritant gases that are inhaled in the fire environment. Patients with abnormal COHb levels may have a normal PaO_2 and a normal calculated oxygen saturation. However, the measured arterial oxygen saturation and arterial oxygen content are both decreased. In the presence of a normal COHb level, other toxic gases such as cyanide should be suspected, especially if there is a severe metabolic acidosis in the arterial blood gases with abnormal PaO_2. Falsely elevated values of blood hemoglobin and COHb levels can be seen in patients with elevated levels of triglycerides and chylomicrons.

Mechanical ventilation and oxygen therapy decrease the half-life of COHb level. Therefore, the COHb level in blood measured initially at the hospital is usually lower than the blood sample at the fire scene.

Patients with altered mental status should also be screened for toxins, including alcohol. In one study, there was an increase in blood alcohol levels in 32% of autopsied fire victims.[45] Drug abuse screening may need to be done in selected fire victims with history of drug abuse and abnormal mental status changes, including coma.

MANAGEMENT

The therapy of fire victims with smoke inhalation[46] depends on the clinical presentation, the severity of the inhalation injury with or without thermal upper airway involvement, arterial oxygenation, COHb level, and the presence of other medical illness such as ischemic heart disease, chronic obstructive airways disease, and asthma. Treatment modalities include oxygen inhalation, administration of inhaled or oral or intravenous bronchodilators, chest physiotherapy, administration of corticosteroids or antibiotics, endotracheal intubation, tracheostomy, and mechanical ventilation.

Maintaining adequate oxygenation is vital in management of patients. The arterial blood gas values and COHb level are necessary to evaluate the need for oxygen therapy. If the patient is awake and alert, 100% oxygen can be delivered by means of a face mask. Patients with chronic obstructive pulmonary disease who require high-concentration oxygen therapy and have carbon dioxide retention may need to be intubated, especially if signs of lethargy are present. The half-life of COHb is decreased to approximately 80 minutes by breathing 100% oxygen, and this can be decreased even faster with hyperbaric oxygen.[47] At 2.5 atm of oxygen, the COHb level decreases to 20% in about 50 minutes.

The prognosis of carbon monoxide poisoning depends on the COHb level and, to a lesser extent, on the blood pH. High COHb levels, greater than 40%, for prolonged periods may produce late neurologic sequelae. In a study of three fire victims with an average COHb level of 51% and an average pH of 6.89, all had full neurologic recovery in spite of the presence of severe metabolic acidosis and severe carbon monoxide intoxication.[48] They had early intubation and mechanical ventilation with 100% oxygen. These procedures are recommended in fire victims with severe carbon monoxide intoxication (COHb level > 40 to 50%), and this mode of oxygen delivery may decrease the morbidity and mortality and may reduce the late neurologic sequelae of carbon monoxide poisoning. When a hyperbaric oxygen chamber is available, the application of hyperbaric oxygen is indicated in severe carbon monoxide poisoning, because this is the most efficacious mode of oxygen administration to decrease the COHb level. In mild-to-moderate carbon monoxide poisoning without severe metabolic acidosis and neurologic dysfunction, 100% oxygen can be given by face mask and the COHb determined serially. The half-life of COHb is 4 to 6 hours.

When wheezing is present or there is evidence or history of chronic obstructive airways disease or asthma, bronchodilator therapy can be given by the oral, inhaled, or intravenous route. Beta$_2$-agonists can be delivered by inhalation or nebulization, and racemic epinephrine aerosol inhalation may benefit patients with upper airway obstruction or stridor who do not need to be intubated. Chest physiotherapy with inhaled bronchodilator therapy may be of value in patients with copious sputum production.

Fever, purulent sputum production, leukocytosis, and infiltrates on the chest radiograph indicate the onset of pulmonary infection and pneumonia. The clinical findings of patients together with the Gram's stain of the sputum and the sputum culture determine the use of specific antibiotic therapy. At the U.S. Brooke Army Medical Center, the medical burn team does not recommend prophylactic aerosol therapy with gentamicin in fire victims with inhalation injury and significant surface burns.[34] It has been estimated that, in burn patients, there was an increased mortality (maximum of 20%) and pneumonia (maximum of 40%) in fire victims with inhalation injury compared with those who had no inhalation injury.[33]

Corticosteroids have been used to treat patients with pulmonary thermal and acrid smoke injury.[49] However, it has been shown that the corticosteroid-treated group of patients with surface burns with inhalation injury has an increased mortality, as well as rate of infections,[50] compared with that of the placebo-treated group. Thus, the use of corticosteroids to treat patients with inhalation injury and surface burns is not recommended.

In smoke inhalation without surface burns, there is an inflammatory response in the lung as evident by the data from bronchoalveolar lavage studies. Although corticosteroids may block this inflammatory response,[51] they may also increase the propensity for infection. The effectiveness of inhaled corticosteroids in ameliorating the inflammatory response in the lungs of patients with inhalation injury remains to be studied. In patients with smoke inhalation, corticosteroids have been recommended to be given early in one large dose.[52] Other investigators have shown no beneficial effect on pulmonary injury–related morbidity and mortality after mild smoke inhalation injury (COHb level of 14%).[53] Although there are no well-controlled studies, some experts recommend a trial of corticosteroids (about 2 mg/kg/d of methylprednisolone equivalent) for 24 to 48 hours in patients without thermal surface burns but with evidence of upper airway obstruction, respiratory insufficiency, and/or severe bronchospasm.

In some inhalation injury occurring in chemical plants in which hydrogen cyanide is suspected, specific antidotes (available as the Cyanide Antidote Package [Lilly]) with inhaled amyl nitrite pearls and 10% sodium nitrite and 25% sodium thiosulfate solutions are indicated.

Finally, in patients with severe arterial hypoxemia and diffuse lung infiltrates associated with clinical findings compatible with the adult respiratory distress syndrome, mechanical ventilation and the use of positive end-expiratory pressure may be indicated. In a report from the U.S. Army Institute of Surgical Research in Texas, high-frequency percussive ventilation may be beneficial in inhalation injury to decrease the incidence of pulmonary infection and iatrogenic barotrauma when compared with conventional ventilation.[54]

The late pulmonary complications of acute smoke inhalation include the development of chronic obstructive airways disease, recurrent chronic bronchitis or pneumonia, bronchiectasis, tracheal stenosis, hyperreactivity of the airways, interstitial fibrosis, and respiratory insufficiency.

References

1. Loke J, Matthay RA, Walker-Smith GJ: The toxic environment and its medical implications with special emphasis on smoke inhalation. In: Loke J (ed): Pathophysiology and Treatment of Inhalation Injuries. New York, Marcel Dekker, p 453, 1988.
2. Rabinovitch S, Greyson ND, Weiser W, et al: Clinical and laboratory features of acute sulfur dioxide inhalation poisoning: Two year follow up. Am Rev Respir Dis 139:556, 1989.
3. Sferlazza SJ, Beckett WS: The respiratory health of welders. Am Rev Respir Dis 143:1134, 1991.
4. Jones RN, Hughes, JM, Glindmeyer H, et al: Lung function after acute chlorine exposure. Am Rev Respir Dis 134:1190, 1986.
5. Rosenthal T, Baum GL, Frand U, et al: Poisoning caused by inhalation of hydrogen chloride, phosphorus oxychloride, phosphorus pentachloride, oxalyl chloride and oxalic acid. Chest 73:623, 1978.
6. Kamat SR, Mahashur AA, Tiwari AKB, et al: Early observation on pulmonary changes and clinical morbidity due to the isocyanate gas leak at Bhopal. J Postgrad Med 31:63, 1985.
7. Sidell FR: What to do in case of an unthinkable chemical warfare attack or accident. Postgrad Med 88:70, 1990.
8. Urbanetti J: Battlefield chemical inhalation injury. In: Loke J (ed): Pathophysiology and Treatment of Inhalation Injuries. New York, Marcel Dekker, p 281, 1988.
9. Lowry WT, Juarez L, Petty CS, et al: Studies of toxic gas production during actual structural fires in the Dallas area. J Forensic Sci 30:59, 1985.
10. Terrill JB, Montgomery RR, Reinhardt CF: Toxic gases from fires. Science 200:1343, 1978.
11. Karter Jr MJ: Fire loss in the United States during 1989. Fire J 84(5):56, 1990.
12. Mierley MC, Baker SP: Fatal house fires in an urban population. JAMA 249:1466, 1983.
13. Alarie Y: The toxicity of smoke from polymeric materials during thermal decomposition. Annu Rev Pharmacol Toxicol 25:325, 1985.
14. Hartzell GE, Packham SC, Switzer WG: Toxic products from fires. Am Ind Hyg Assoc J 44:248, 1983.

15. Dyer RF, Esch VH: Polyvinyl chloride toxicity in fires: Hydrogen chloride toxicity in fire fighters. JAMA 235:393, 1976.
16. Committee on Fire Toxicology: Fire and Smoke: Understanding the Hazards. National Research Council, Board on Environmental Studies and Toxicology. Washington, DC, National Academy Press, 1986.
17. Zikria BA, Ferrer JM, Floch HF: The chemical factors contributing to pulmonary damage in "smoke poisoning." Surgery 71:704, 1972.
18. Ayres SM, Giannelli S Jr, Mueller H: Carboxyhemoglobin and the access to oxygen. Arch Environ Health 26:8, 1973.
19. Winter PM, Miller JN: Carbon monoxide poisoning. JAMA 236:1502, 1976.
20. Beard RR, Grandstaff N: Carbon monoxide exposure and cerebral function. Ann NY Acad Sci 174:385, 1970.
21. Purser DA, Berrill KR: Effects of carbon monoxide on behavior in monkeys in relation to human fire hazard. Arch Environ Health 38:308, 1983.
22. Hirsch CS, Bost RO, Gerber SR, et al: Carboxyhemoglobin concentrations in flash fire victims. Report of six simultaneous fire fatalities without elevated carboxyhemoglobin. Am J Clin Pathol 68:317, 1977.
23. Zikria BA, Budd DC, Floch F, et al: What is clinical smoke poisoning? Ann Surg 181:151, 1975.
24. Anderson RF, Allensworth DC, Degroot WJ: Myocardial toxicity from carbon monoxide poisoning. Ann Intern Med 67:1172, 1967.
25. Fein A, Grossman RF, Jones JG, et al: Carbon monoxide effect on alveolar epithelial permeability. Chest 78:726, 1980.
26. Shimazu T, Ikeuchi H, Hubbard GB, et al: Smoke inhalation injury and the effect of carbon monoxide in the sheep model. J Trauma 30:170, 1990.
27. Lowry WT, Peterson J, Petty CS, et al: Free radical production from controlled low-energy fires: Toxicity considerations. J Forensic Sci 30:73, 1985.
28. Levin BC, Paabo M, Fultz ML, et al: Generation of hydrogen cyanide from flexible polyurethane foam decomposed under different combustion conditions. Fire Mater 9(3):125, 1985.
29. Hall AH, Rumack BH: Clinical toxicology of cyanide. Ann Emerg Med 15:1067, 1986.
30. Clark CJ, Campbell D, Reid WH: Blood carboxyhaemoglobin and cyanide levels in fire survivors. Lancet 1:1332, 1981.
31. Moritz AR, Henriques FC Jr, McLean R: The effects of inhaled heat on the air passages and lungs. Am J Pathol 21:311, 1945.
32. DiVincenti FC, Pruitt BA Jr, Reckler JM: Inhalation injuries. J Trauma 11:109, 1971.
33. Shirani KZ, Pruitt BA, Mason AD Jr: The influence of inhalation injury and pneumonia on burn mortality. Ann Surg 205:82, 1987.
34. Shirani KZ, Moylan JA, Pruitt BA Jr: Diagnosis and treatment of inhalation injury in burn patients. In: Loke J (ed): Pathophysiology and Treatment of Inhalation Injuries. New York, Marcel Dekker, p 239, 1988.
35. Haponik EF, Meyers DA, Munster AM, et al: Acute upper airway injury in burn patients. Serial changes of flow-volume curves and nasopharyngoscopy. Am Rev Respir Dis 135:360, 1987.
36. Cahalane M, Demling RH: Early respiratory abnormalities from smoke inhalation. JAMA 251:771, 1984.
37. Landa J, Avery WG, Sachner MA: Some physiologic observations in smoke inhalation. Chest 61:62, 1972.
38. Demarest GB, Hudson LD, Altman LC: Impaired alveolar macrophage chemotaxis in patients with acute smoke inhalation. Am Rev Respir Dis 119:279, 1979.
39. Loke J, Paul E, Virgulto JA, et al: Rabbit lung after acute smoke inhalation. Cellular responses and scanning electron microscopy. Arch Surg 119:956, 1984.
40. Fick RB Jr, Paul ES, Merrill WW, et al: Alterations in the antibacterial properties of rabbit pulmonary macrophages exposed to wood smoke. Am Rev Respir Dis 129:76, 1984.
41. Genovesi MG, Tashkin DP, Chopra S, et al: Transient hypoxemia in firemen following inhalation of smoke. Chest 71:441, 1977.
42. Sheppard D, Distefano S, Morse L, et al: Acute effects of routine firefighting on lung function. Am J Ind Med 9:333, 1986.
43. Whitener DR, Whitener LM, Robertson KJ, et al: Pulmonary function measurements in patients with thermal injury and smoke inhalation. Am Rev Respir Dis 122:731, 1980.
44. Putman CE, Loke J, Matthay RA, et al: Radiographic manifestations of acute smoke inhalation. Am J Roentgenol 129:865, 1977.
45. Levine MS, Radford EP: Fire victims: Medical outcomes and demographic characteristics. Am J Public Health 67:1077, 1977.
46. Fein A, Leff A, Hopewell PC: Pathophysiology and management of the complications resulting from fire and the inhaled products of combustion: Review of the literature. Crit Care Med 8:94, 1980.
47. Norkool DM, Kirkpatrick JN: Treatment of acute carbon monoxide poisoning with hyperbaric oxygen: A review of 115 cases. Ann Emerg Med 14:1168, 1985.
48. Strohl KP, Feldman NT, Saunders NA, et al: Carbon monoxide poisoning in fire victims: A reappraisal of prognosis. J Trauma 20:78, 1980.
49. Chester EH, Kaimal PJ, Payne CB Jr, et al: Pulmonary injury following exposure to chlorine gas. Possible beneficial effects of steroid treatment. Chest 72:247, 1977.
50. Pruitt BA Jr, McManus AT: Opportunistic infections in severely burned patients. Am J Med 76:146, 1984.
51. Dressler DP, Skornik WA, Kupersmith S: Corticosteroid treatment of experimental smoke inhalation. Ann Surg 183:46, 1976.
52. Mellins RB, Park S: Respiratory complications of smoke inhalation in victims of fires. J Pediatr 87:1, 1975.
53. Robinson NB, Hudson LD, Riem M, et al: Steroid therapy following isolated smoke inhalation injury. J Trauma 22:876, 1982.
54. Cioffi WG, Graves TA, McManus WF, et al: High-frequency percussive ventilation in patients with inhalation injury. J Trauma 29:350, 1989.

CHAPTER 80

Pulmonary Consequences of Trauma

John M. Luce

The pulmonary system may be involved directly or indirectly in single- or multiple-system trauma. Direct involvement occurs most often after thoracic injuries, such as tracheobronchial rupture and pulmonary contusion, that physically damage the airways or the lungs. Indirect involvement results from injuries to extrathoracic structures such as the central nervous system or the abdomen. By themselves, these injuries may compromise pulmonary function to the extent that endotracheal intubation and mechanical ventilation are required. Alternatively, the surgical treatment of trauma may necessitate transient intubation and mechanical ventilation, or these therapies may be used to treat complications in the postoperative period. Finally, a number of injuries, including those mentioned earlier, are associated with a condition once called post-traumatic respiratory failure or insufficiency and more commonly referred to as the adult respiratory distress syndrome (ARDS).

This chapter reviews the three topics of thoracic trauma, extrathoracic trauma, and ARDS primarily from an intensivist's point of view, although some discussion related to surgery is included. Because several aspects of extrathoracic trauma and ARDS are covered elsewhere in this section, thoracic trauma is the major focus of this chapter.

THORACIC TRAUMA

Approximately 25% of civilian trauma deaths in the United States result from thoracic trauma, and in another 25 to 50% of cases, thoracic injury contributes to a fatal outcome. Most thoracic injuries are due to motor vehicle accidents or falls that cause blunt trauma, although an increasing number are caused by penetrating knife or gunshot wounds. Although many patients with such injuries die outside the hospital, a significant fraction reach the hospital and are admitted to the intensive care unit (ICU) either directly or via the operating room. Trunkey noted that only 15% of patients with thoracic trauma require major surgery; the great majority, 85% can be managed with relatively simple procedures, including tube thoracostomy.[1]

Large-bore (No. 32 to 40 French) siliconized tubes generally are used in patients with trauma to drain intrapleural blood or fluid, monitor the rate of further bleeding, and

---

TABLE 80–1

COMMON INTRATHORACIC INJURIES

Injuries of the Thoracic Cage
Rib fractures
Sternal fracture
Flail chest

Aberrant Air
Subcutaneous emphysema
Pneumomediastinum
Pneumothorax
Pneumoperitoneum
Pneumatocele
Systemic air embolism

Other Pleural Abnormalities
Hemothorax
Chylothorax

Respiratory Tract Injuries
Upper airway obstruction
Tracheobronchial rupture

Pulmonary Injuries
Pulmonary contusion
Pulmonary laceration and hematoma

Cardiovascular Injuries
Myocardial contusion
Cardiac rupture and penetration
Cardiac tamponade
Aortic rupture

Other Intrathoracic Injuries
Esophageal perforation
Diaphragmatic rupture

---

evacuate air. Blood may clot in smaller tubes, which also may be inadequate in providing air evacuation. Initially, chest tubes usually are inserted into the fifth intercostal space at the anterior midaxillary line and directed posteriorly and upward to drain blood, fluid, and air.[1] Other chest tubes may be directed anteriorly if air evacuation only is required. Most tubes are placed under negative pressure until evaluation of blood, fluid, and air is complete, after which they may be switched to water seal drainage.

Common Intrathoracic Injuries

Rib fractures are the most common injury sustained after blunt thoracic trauma[2] (Table 80–1). They are particularly frequent among older persons with rigid and brittle thoracic skeletons and may occur either in isolation or as a sign of severe underlying injury. Thoracic ribs five through nine are most commonly broken as a result of trauma, and these injuries may be associated with pneumothorax or hemothorax. Fractures of thoracic ribs one through three, which normally are protected by the clavicle, the scapula, and the shoulder musculature, may be associated with tracheobronchial rupture and rupture of the thoracic aorta, among other severe injuries.[3] Fractures of thoracic ribs 10 through 13 may be associated with injury of the spleen, the liver, or the diaphragm.

In addition to their association with underlying trauma, rib fractures usually cause intense pain that may lead to splinting, diminished respiratory efforts, and an inhibited cough. These conditions in turn may be responsible for atelectasis, pneumonia, and abnormal respiratory gas exchange. The presence of rib fractures is suggested by an altered breathing pattern and by point tenderness and crepitance on physical examination of the chest. Fractures also may be visualized on the routine chest radiograph or on special views. Because such fractures usually can be diagnosed clinically and because they are often associated with severe trauma that requires urgent intervention, there rarely, if ever, is an indication to obtain rib detail views in the trauma setting. Severe pulmonary compromise attributable to rib fractures is reflected by a tidal volume of less than 5 mL/kg, a forced vital capacity of less than 10 mL/kg, or hypoxemia and hypercapnia on arterial blood gas analysis.[2]

The treatment of rib fractures requires attention to the pain they cause. Systemic analgesics and external stabilization with tape or binders should generally be avoided, because both reduce cough and respiratory efforts. Instead, if only one or two ribs are broken, they can be treated with intercostal nerve blocks using 0.5% bipivacaine, single injections of which usually provide basal pain relief for approximately 12 hours. If more prolonged relief is required, and especially if more than a few ribs are broken, patients should receive epidural analgesia with either morphine or fentanyl.[4] After pain has been relieved, patients should be encouraged to deep breathe or perform incentive spirometry.

Rib fractures may be associated with immediate or delayed pneumothorax in some patients with trauma. Simple pneumothorax, which is discussed later, may be converted to tension pneumothorax by positive pressure ventilation (PPV). Such conversion is especially dangerous in the operating room, where the cause of sudden collapse of the patient may not be appreciated. Because of this, many surgeons recommend that all patients with traumatic rib fractures undergo tube thoracostomy if they are to be mechanically ventilated or to undergo general anesthesia.

Sternal fractures result from severe blows to the anterior chest and therefore are associated with underlying trauma even more often than are routine rib fractures. They are frequently accompanied by local hematomas and may also be diagnosed by lateral radiographs if time permits. Extremely painful sternal fractures are best treated with epidural analgesia. Approximately 25% of these injuries necessitate operative reduction and fixation, especially in children.[5]

Flail chest results either from multiple contiguous or segmental rib fractures or from bilateral disruption of rib attachments to the sternum. Such injuries produce a segment of chest wall that moves in response to changes in pleural pressure rather than to the pull of the respiratory muscles.[2] Flail chest is diagnosed by the detection of paradoxical chest wall movement either by visual inspection or on palpation of the chest. Chest radiographs may also be helpful in identifying multiple rib fractures or separation of ribs from the sternum.

The respiratory embarrassment that results from flail chest was previously explained in terms of pendelluft, signifying a to-and-fro movement of end-expired air between the two lungs that increased dead space ventilation during the breathing cycle. Acceptance of this concept of pendelluft led to a series of maneuvers, from taping the fractured ribs to stabilizing them with orthopedic devices, to limit the paradoxical movement of the flail segment.[6] External stabilization of this sort then gave way to internal stabilization using PPV to reduce paradoxical movement. Patients were hyperventilated to induce apnea and were ventilated for several weeks, often through a tracheostomy, to allow their injuries to heal.[7]

Eventually, the idea of impaired ventilation resulting from pendelluft was challenged by animal and human studies.[2] The concept of pendelluft then was discarded in favor of the theory that the pressure gradients developed by the respiratory muscles are dissipated by the paradoxically moving segment of chest wall so that the work of breathing increases. At the same time, pulmonary contusion under the flail segment also may contribute to abnormal gas exchange.[8]

As the pathophysiology of flail chest has been better understood, management has shifted from obligatory internal stabilization with PPV to the use of this modality only in patients who experience significant respiratory failure.[9-11] Because such failure may involve ARDS in patients with severe pulmonary contusion, positive end-expiratory pressure (PEEP) may also be required. Nonventilatory management of flail chest necessitates continued observation of patients in an ICU setting, with frequent sampling of arterial blood gases and perhaps forced vital capacity maneuvers. Pain relief is provided with intercostal nerve blocks or, more commonly, epidural analgesia. When pain is relieved, chest physiotherapy, incentive spirometry, and other techniques to maintain lung volume can be applied.[2]

Aberrant Air

Aberrant air and *extrarespiratory air* are terms used to describe air (or some other gas) that appears where it is not normally seen after a variety of disease processes, including thoracic trauma. Air found under the skin, commonly in areas such as the thorax and the head and neck, is called *subcutaneous emphysema*. Mediastinal emphysema, or *pneumomediastinum*, refers to air in the mediastinum, which envelops the upper trachea and includes the pericardium. *Pneumothorax* describes air in the pleural space; *pneumoperitoneum* is air in the peritoneum; *pneumatocele*, or pulmonary cyst, is air in the lung parenchyma.[12]

Although air may reach these locations from an external source, as might occur when the lung is lacerated by a jagged rib end or a foreign object, aberrant air is usually caused by internal rupture of a bronchus or the alveoli. Such rupture may result either from trauma or from overdistention related to PPV and PEEP. When alveolar rupture occurs, the air may remain localized in the form of a pneumatocele. More commonly, it may enter the distal bronchovascular space and track to the mediastinum, where it may cause pneumomediastinum or decompress into the subcutaneous tissue, into the retroperitoneal space and from there into the peritoneum, or into the pleural space via the mediastinal pleura.[13, 15] Other causes of pneumothorax are tracheobronchial and esophageal rupture (discussed later).

Although subcutaneous emphysema usually does no more than alter patient appearance, it also may prevent eye opening and interfere with respiration. Similarly, pneumomediastinum may rarely compress the trachea, the great vessels, and the heart.[16, 17] Impaired cardiac output resulting from pneumopericardium has been reported,[18] as has intracranial hypertension attributable to impaired central venous return in a patient with pneumomediastinum.[19] Pneumoperitoneum, on the other hand, may prompt unnecessary surgical exploration of the abdomen. Pneumothorax, especially if a large amount of air enters but cannot leave the pleural space and thus is under tension, may cause respiratory failure and cardiovascular collapse.

Whether respiratory failure or cardiovascular collapse is the most important cause of clinical deterioration in patients with tension pneumothorax is unclear. A low cardiac output caused by impaired venous return resulting from continuously high pleural pressures is the traditional explanation for such deterioration. However, as reviewed by Light,[20] animal experiments have demonstrated that worsening arterial blood gas values rather than diminished venous return are responsible. Human data are not available to help determine the exact pathophysiology of this disorder.

Subcutaneous emphysema is easily diagnosed by the disfigurement it causes and by crepitance.[15] Pneumomediastinum may also be reflected in a sound during the cardiac cycle that is called mediastinal crunch.[16] The physical signs of pneumothorax are ipsilateral hyperresonance and diminution of breath sounds, fremitus, and contralateral tracheal deviation. Patients with tension pneumothorax usually appear distressed, with labored respirations, cyanosis, tachycardia, and diaphoresis. Arterial blood gas determinations generally reveal severe hypoxemia and perhaps respiratory and metabolic acidosis. Aberrant air may also be visualized by a variety of radiographic procedures, including the routine chest radiograph.

Aberrant air may resolve spontaneously as the air is dissipated and the ruptured alveoli or airways heal themselves. The resolution is accelerated if patients breathe 100% oxygen, which mixes with the aberrant air and facilitates its reabsorption. However, because the air leak may continue and because it may be associated with severe underlying conditions, tube thoracostomy drainage frequently is required. Tube thoracostomy definitely should be performed in patients with known or suspected tension pneumothorax; this procedure may be preceded by placement of a 16-gauge catheter into the anterior second intercostal spare to evacuate air. In addition, bilateral chest tubes often are placed empirically in trauma patients who have subcutaneous emphysema and are suspected of having tracheobronchial rupture or tension pneumothorax and who are likely to receive PPV and PEEP. Although this approach may not be necessary in many instances, it usually is justified.

Systemic air embolism is another form of an embolism that has been reported after both penetrating and blunt thoracic injury.[21-24] Air embolism results when a traumatic fistula is created between a bronchus and a pulmonary vein. Air enters the vein during either spontaneous or, more likely, mechanical ventilation and then may pass through the left ventricle into the cardiac or cerebral arteries or farther into the systemic circulation. Although air embolism may occur coincident with or shortly after trauma, it also may develop days or weeks later in patients who receive PPV with or without PEEP and thereafter sustain pneumothorax or other forms of aberrant air.[25]

Immediate systemic air embolism should be suspected after thoracic trauma in patients who evidence focal neurologic deficits in the absence of obvious head injury, patients who manifest cardiovascular collapse after the initiation of PPV, and patients in whom air is recovered from the left ventricle or visualized in the coronary arteries. Patients with the delayed form while receiving PPV and PEEP have the combination of aberrant air on the chest radiograph, recurrent episodes of cerebral infarction or myocardial injury, and a characteristic pattern of livedo reticularis of the lower extremities.[25] Therapy includes the administration of 100% oxygen, insertion of intravascular catheters to remove air, and surgery to isolate the injured lung and repair fistulas. Systemic arterial froth attributable to an embolism is an ominous prognostic sign.

Other Pleural Abnormalities

The term *hemothorax* (the presence of blood in the pleural space) is reserved for patients in whom the hematocrit of the pleural fluid is at least 50% of that of the peripheral blood.[26] Hemothorax frequently accompanies pneumothorax in patients with thoracic trauma. Pleural blood accumulation is generally limited when it results from lung laceration or capillary rupture because the pulmonary circulation is a low-pressure system. However, massive hemothorax may occur if intercostal or internal mammary vessels or the great vessels of the chest are torn.

Before or after hemothorax has been confirmed by chest radiography, early placement of chest tubes is indicated in patients who have experienced intrathoracic blood loss on the order of 500 to 1000 mL/h. Autotransfusion should be considered in such circumstances, although mild coagulopathies may occur,[27] and the rate of continued blood loss should be monitored closely. Thoracotomy is usually recommended if the rate of bleeding exceeds 500 mL during the subsequent 6 to 8 hours and is required in approximately 20% of patients with hemothorax.[26] Whether or not surgery is performed, the chest tubes should remain in place until the bleeding falls below approximately 100 mL in 24 hours, or until a concurrent air leak is resolved.

Early thoracotomy was previously recommended to evaluate clotted blood and prevent pleural sequelae in patients with traumatic hemothorax who did not require immediate exploration or in those whose pleural spaces were not drained completely with chest tubes. Subsequent studies showed that residual hemothoraces are usually reabsorbed on their own and rarely cause persistent lung restriction.[28] Indeed, fibrothorax is estimated to occur in less than 1% of patients with hemothorax.[26] Similarly, pleural empyema is not a common consequence of traumatic hemothorax, occurring in from 1 to 4% of patients. It is therefore accepted today that chest tube drainage is sufficient to drain most hemothoraces and that their early decortication is not generally required.

Chylothorax is the presence of chyle in the pleural space resulting from disruption of the thoracic duct or a major lymphatic tributary. Chyle is bacteriostatic and not irritating to the pleura, so it does not cause a pleural reaction that seals the pleural space and prevents additional chyle from accumulating. The thoracic duct normally conveys up to 2500 mL of chyle daily, an amount that increases markedly after fat ingestion. In addition to containing triglycerides, chyle contains electrolytes and protein in concentrations similar to those in serum. The primary cellular component of chyle is the T lymphocyte.[26] Thus, prolonged loss of chyle may result in nutritional depletion, water and electrolyte loss, and T cell depletion.[29]

Chylothorax may not be obvious immediately after thoracic trauma because the flow of chyle through the thoracic duct is depressed when activity and diet are restricted. When they are apparent radiographically, chylous pleural effusions may be diagnosed by the presence of milky fluid rich in lymphocytes and refractile fat droplets under the microscope. Such effusions usually resolve spontaneously or in response to chest tube drainage and a low-fat diet.[30] Surgical ligation of the thoracic duct, chemical pleurodesis, or pleuroperitoneal shunting are indicated if the effusions do not clear, if they interfere with pulmonary function, or if they are associated with extreme nutritional loss or cellular immune depression.[26, 31]

Respiratory Tract Injuries

Upper airway obstruction is most often due to a foreign body or secretions in patients with thoracic trauma. Occasionally, however, it may result from maxillofacial injury or fracture of the larynx. The latter condition is associated with stridor, difficulty in phonation, and crepitance over the site of injury. Oropharyngeal obstructions can usually be removed by a sweep of the finger, although aspirated objects such as teeth or food particles may necessitate laryngoscopy or bronchoscopy for removal. Emergency cricothyrotomy should be performed in patients with maxillofacial injury but not in those with complete laryngeal fracture, whose upper airway cannot be maintained otherwise. Tracheostomy through the second or third tracheal ring may be necessary for airway maintenance in patients with severe maxillofacial injury or laryngeal fracture.

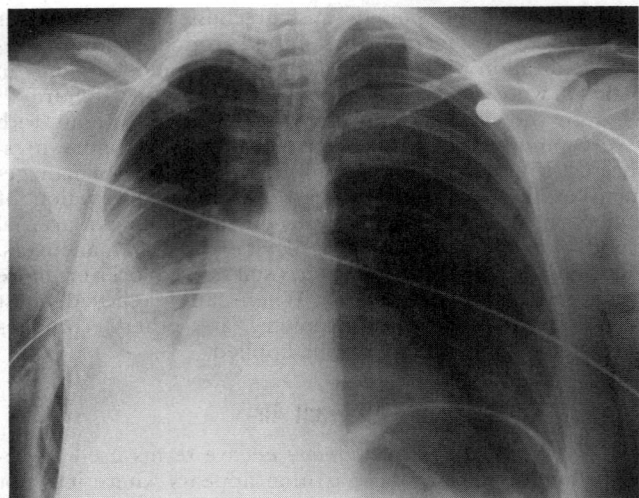

Figure 80–1. Chest radiograph from 52-year-old woman with type 1 tear of right mainstem bronchus. Right lung has failed to re-expand after tube thoracostomy, and it falls away from right hilum owing to gravity.

Tracheobronchial rupture is usually associated with subcutaneous emphysema, fracture of the upper three ribs, and other signs of severe thoracic trauma. Tracheobronchial disruption occurs for the most part within an inch of the carina; circumferential tears of the bronchi are most typical. Injury at this site is thought to occur because the more proximal trachea is relatively fixed within the mediastinum, whereas the distal bronchi are subjected to shear forces during deceleration owing to the pendulum-like effect of the lungs. Bursting forces may also be generated within the large airways, particularly if the glottis is closed.[2, 32]

Two common forms of tracheobronchial rupture have been identified. In the first, the bronchus ruptures into the pleural cavity, causing a pneumothorax that cannot be resolved by tube thoracostomy. Because the lung is not adequately suspended, it may seem to fall away from the hilum on the chest radiograph, rather than collapsing toward it as normally occurs with pneumothorax. This characteristic radiographic finding, called the falling lung sign, is much more specific for tracheobronchial rupture than for a simple pneumothorax[33] (Fig. 80–1). Patients with type 1 acute tracheobronchial rupture usually have respiratory distress and hemoptysis. Bronchoscopy is useful in confirming the diagnosis of tracheobronchial rupture,[34] although it is not warranted in all patients with thoracic trauma and pneumothorax. Patients with type 1 tracheobronchial rupture may be managed with an endotracheal tube passed beyond the point of rupture before thoracotomy.[35–38]

In the second type of tracheobronchial rupture, the disruption usually is incomplete and may not communicate with the pleural space. If pneumothorax is present, it generally resolves with chest tube placement. The bronchial tear then heals with stricture formation, either causing no symptoms or leading to atelectasis or bronchiectasis of the ipsilateral lung. Complicated strictures of the latter type may necessitate surgical repair. In addition, focal bronchiectasis may be amenable to surgery.

Pulmonary Injuries

Pulmonary contusion results from the application of compressive forces to the lung and may or may not be associated with overlying rib fractures. The forces create a bruise

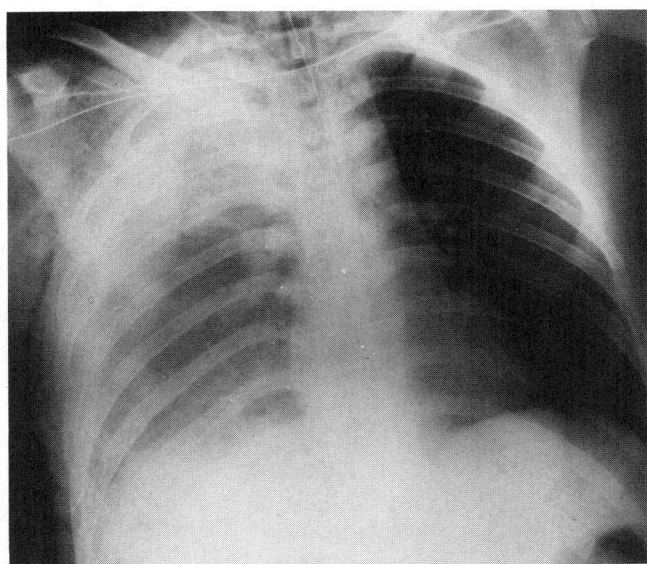

Figure 80–2. Right-sided pulmonary contusion on chest radiograph of 37-year-old man.

characterized by increased capillary permeability, edema formation, hemorrhage, altered surfactant function, and subsequent inflammation.[39, 40] These changes are similar to those produced by blast injury.[2] The physiologic result is decreased compliance of the affected lung, increased work of breathing, and altered gas exchange attributable to edema and atelectasis, which can be complicated by the effects of concurrent flail chest.[41] If the contusion is sufficiently diffuse or is associated with other factors such as fat embolism or sepsis, patients may manifest ARDS.

Pulmonary contusion usually becomes radiographically apparent within 1 hour of injury, although there may be a time lag of 3 to 4 hours.[2] Typically, the chest radiograph shows a poorly defined infiltrate, often but not always in an area of rib trauma (Fig. 80–2). Depending on the severity of injury and its treatment, resolution may occur within days to weeks after parenchymal lung injury.

Treatment of pulmonary contusion is dictated by the severity of injury and associated problems. Patients with small contusions and normal or near-normal gas exchange need only monitoring, whereas those with extensive contusions, flail chest, and other injuries may require intubation and mechanical ventilation. Because both crystalloid and colloid solutions leak into the bruised area of the lung as long as capillary permeability is increased, the type of fluid used during resuscitation is not critical. Empirical antibiotics or corticosteroids are not indicated in this condition. Fortunately, contusion usually is not a progressive disease unless pneumonia or other processes supervene.[42]

Pulmonary laceration attributable to blunt or penetrating trauma may cause bleeding, air leak, or systemic air embolism by the mechanisms mentioned earlier. Lacerations are usually treated by tube thoracostomy alone unless severe complications develop.[43] A conservative approach is also indicated for pulmonary hematoma, which occurs when bleeding from a laceration is contained by the lung parenchyma or the pleura, and for traumatic pneumatocele, in which lung cyst develops. The only indications for surgical treatment of these last two conditions are infection in the cavity that is unresponsive to appropriate antibiotic therapy and lesions that increase in size under observation.[44, 45]

Cardiovascular Injuries

Myocardial contusion results from sudden deceleration on the application of great pressure to the chest and is commonly seen in patients with injuries caused by a steering wheel, including sternal fracture.[46–48] It has been thought to occur in up to 75% of patients with blunt thoracic trauma, although it has been reported in only 15% of patients with fatal thoracic injuries.[2] Although coronary arterial lacerations and thrombosis may occur in this situation, contusion usually represents an intramural hematoma in the myocardial wall with no evidence of myocardial rupture.[49] This either may cause no complications or may lead to supraventricular or ventricular dysrhythmias or to congestive failure related to decreased compliance and dyskinesia of the wall.[50–52]

The true incidence of myocardial contusion is unknown because diagnostic criteria are both insensitive and nonspecific. Patients in whom the diagnosis is most likely to be made have anterior chest pain and electrocardiographic abnormalities such as ST-T wave changes.[50–52] The levels of the MB fraction of creatine kinase are elevated, although the amount of myocardial damage does not correlate with levels of the MB isoenzyme of creatine kinase, and abnormal wall motion or a decreased ejection fraction may be demonstrated on two-dimensional echocardiography.[53–57] Technetium scanning has also been used to evaluate cardiac performance, but this technique is not recommended over echocardiography.[58, 59]

Patients with known contusion who manifest potentially lethal dysrhythmias should be treated with lidocaine, pronestyl, or other agents.[60] Inotropic agents and intra-aortic balloon counterpulsation have been used for severe congestive heart failure.[61] The long-term care of patients who survive these problems is uncertain because myocardial contusion is not usually an ischemic injury. Similarly, the optional management of patients with anterior chest pain but no other symptoms is unclear. Although ICU admission has been recommended for all patients with suspected contusion, those who have no electrocardiographic changes or evidence of impaired cardiac function probably can be monitored outside of the ICU.[62] Follow-up echocardiography and electrocardiography are recommended for patients with confirmed contusions.[2]

Cardiac rupture and penetration are seen infrequently in the ICU because patients with these problems usually die outside of the hospital. However, patients may survive both conditions, especially if their right ventricles are less than fully injured or their atria leak blood slowly. Patients with cardiac rupture or penetration have either shock or signs of pericardial tamponade.[63–66] Evidence of valvular disruption or an intraventricular septal defect also may be present.[67] The treatment is surgical, although temporizing measures such as pericardiocentesis may be used.

Cardiac tamponade in trauma patients usually results from cardiac rupture, penetrating wounds of the heart, or retrograde aortic rupture. These conditions allow a collection of blood in the pericardium sufficient to interfere with diastolic filling of the ventricles and, as blood pressure falls, perfusion of the coronary circulation. The rate of formation of hemopericardium varies among patients; many patients with tamponade resulting from cardiac rupture or penetration die immediately, whereas a few with slow bleeding may not be diagnosed until they have completed surgery for other problems and are in the ICU.[65, 66]

Depending on the rate of bleeding and other factors, the well-known triad of arterial hypotension, central venous hypertension, and distant heart sounds may or may not be present in patients with cardiac tamponade. Nevertheless, the significance of an elevated central venous pressure after chest trauma is such that a central venous pressure catheter probably should be placed in most patients who sustain major thoracic injury. An exaggerated pulsus paradoxus, the fall in blood pressure that is normally seen as cardiac output declines in inspiration, also is an inconsistent finding. A widened cardiac silhouette is rarely present on the chest radiograph because the pericardium has not been stretched sufficiently to accommodate large volumes of blood in acute tamponade. Because of these factors, tamponade must often be diagnosed by two-dimensional echocardiography or empirical pericardiocentesis. When tamponade is known to exist, volume should be infused and pericardiocentesis or creation of a subxiphoid pericardial window should usually be performed to stabilize patients before definitive cardiorrhaphy.[68, 69]

Aortic rupture is the most common cause of immediate death among accident victims who do not survive long enough to reach the hospital. Approximately 15% of patients with traumatic rupture survive temporarily, but 90% of these survivors die within the next 10 weeks if surgery is not provided.[70] In patients who are alive on arrival at the hospital, intrathoracic bleeding is prevented by either the aortic adventitia or the pleura, creating a false aneurysm that usually leaks gradually or massively within the next few days. In survivors and nonsurvivors of motor vehicle accidents, the aorta usually ruptures at its isthmus just distal to the descending origin of the subclavian artery, although the ascending aortic root may also rupture during falls. It is thought that, during deceleration, the heart and the proximal aorta move forward and twist while the descending aorta is held in place, this at a time when intraluminal pressure is greatly elevated.[71, 72]

Patients with aortic rupture classically have shock or signs of cardiac tamponade. Many have concurrent head injury and are unconscious. Paraplegia also may be present as a consequence of compression of the intercostal arteries supplying the spinal cord.[2] If conscious, patients may complain of intense interscapular pain. Hoarseness from recurrent laryngeal nerve compression may occur, as may hypertension in the upper extremities and hypotension below, a sign called acute coarctation. A systolic murmur also may be heard in the mid-scapular area or at the base of the heart.

The chest radiograph of patients with traumatic aortic rupture may or may not reveal fractures of one or more of the upper three ribs.[73] Apical capping attributable to subpleural blood and pleural abnormalities caused by hemothorax may also be present. However, the most sensitive and specific finding on routine chest radiography is mediastinal widening, which should lead to more definitive diagnostic maneuvers in the appropriate clinical setting [74, 75] (Fig. 80–3). Computed tomography may identify aortic rupture.[76, 77] However, aortography is usually needed to confirm the diagnosis and direct surgical repair, which requires left thoracotomy with or without partial left-sided heart bypass.[2] Hypertension should be avoided in the perioperative period.

Other Intrathoracic Injuries

Esophageal perforation is a rare injury that may follow penetrating chest trauma, although the esophagus has been known to rupture after blunt thoracic or abdominal injuries. If the lesion is below the cervical esophagus, patients most often have chest pain and, eventually, fever. The chest radiograph may reveal pneumomediastinum, pneumothorax, or a pleural effusion, which usually is left sided and has a low pH and elevated amylase level. The definitive diagnosis is usually made by esophageal contrast studies

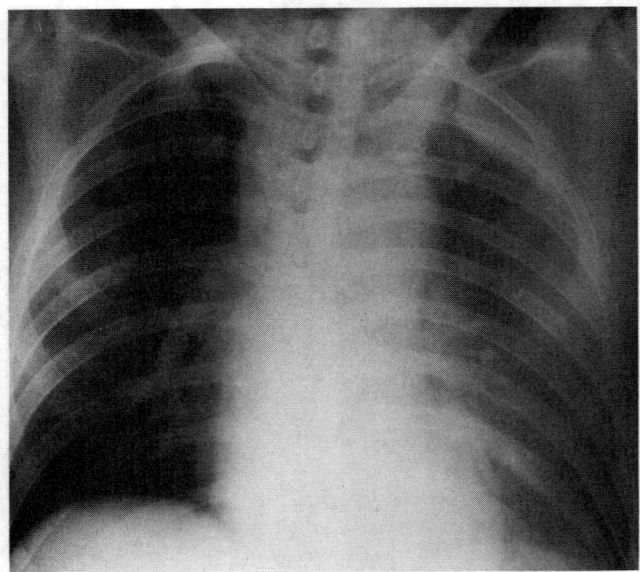

Figure 80–3. Chest radiograph obtained with the patient in the supine position, showing widened mediastinum and left-sided pleural effusion in 47-year-old man with traumatic aortic rupture.

and/or esophagoscopy. Treatment includes chest tube drainage and surgical repair.[78]

Diaphragmatic rupture may follow blunt or penetrating trauma to the chest or, more commonly, the abdomen. Although laceration may occur at any site, herniation of subdiaphragmatic contents after blunt trauma usually involves either the central diaphragmatic tendon or its lateral costal insertion and is generally found on the left side.[79–89] Injury may be suspected if the diaphragm appears high in the chest or visceral herniation is seen on the chest radiograph. Placement of a nasogastric tube and insertion of contrast material usually confirm the diagnosis.[85] As is true of several of the conditions discussed earlier, injury to the diaphragm may be identified late in the hospital course or, much later, when patients may have incarcerated hernias.[86, 87] This injury is treated surgically with a thoracotomy or a laparotomy or a combined procedure.

EXTRATHORACIC TRAUMA

As noted earlier, injury to extrathoracic structures may indirectly compromise pulmonary function or patients may experience complications perioperatively. The closest area to the thorax is the abdomen, and because the abdomen and the thorax function together in series, respiratory problems are as common after intra-abdominal trauma and surgery as they are after trauma and surgery to the chest. In addition, pulmonary embarrassment frequently accompanies trauma to the head, the cervical spinal cord, and the extremities.

Common Extrathoracic Injuries

Abdominal injuries account for approximately 6% of trauma but contribute to at least 25% of the deaths.[88] Like thoracic trauma, abdominal trauma is of two types: blunt and penetrating. Blunt abdominal trauma usually is the more difficult to diagnose but accounts for fewer deaths than does penetrating injury. Any intra-abdominal structure may be damaged by either kind of trauma, but wounds to the spleen, the liver, the pancreas, the large bowel, and the major vessels are the most common.[89, 90] Because abdominal trauma is both common and difficult to diagnose, peritoneal lavage and exploratory laparotomy are frequently performed in trauma patients.[88, 91]

Abdominal trauma and surgery are associated with a high incidence of complications such as atelectasis and pneumonia, especially in patients with pre-existing obesity or chronic obstructive pulmonary disease.[92-94] This high incidence in turn relates to several abnormalities in pulmonary function, including a decrease in functional residual capacity of approximately 25%, a decrease in vital capacity of 60%, and a decline in arterial oxygenation that may persist for several days.[95-97] Radiographic evidence of atelectasis also is common, and clearance of mucus is diminished in the airways.[98]

One explanation for the atelectasis and impaired clearance of secretions observed after abdominal operations is abnormal function of the diaphragm. This possibility was supported by a study of postcholecystectomy patients who demonstrated characteristic declines in vital capacity and functional residual capacity.[99] Furthermore, the patients also manifested a reduction in pleural and intra-abdominal pressures normally generated by contraction of the diaphragm. In four patients studied by magnetometry, this reduction in diaphragmatic strength was associated with a breathing pattern seen in patients with bilateral diaphragmatic paralysis. Whether the diaphragmatic dysfunction was due to inadequate pain control or a neural mechanism is unclear.

Post-traumatic pulmonary complications may be prevented or ameliorated by a variety of techniques to end lung expansion, including continuous positive airway pressure and incentive spirometry.[100, 101] Epidural analgesia offers great advantages over systemic morphine administration in this situation.[102] However, many patients, including those with injuries outside as well as within the abdomen, require intubation and mechanical ventilation, frequently for prolonged periods. The duration of PPV required for such patients presumably relates in part to persistent dysfunction of the diaphragm.

Head injury frequently accompanies injury to other areas of the body and accounts for approximately half of all trauma fatalities.[103] Comatose patients with either diffuse brain damage or intracranial mass lesion such as epidural or subdural hematomas have depressed gag and cough reflexes and therefore are subject to upper airway obstruction, aspiration, and respiratory tract infection. Indeed, bacterial pneumonia is the most common complication of head injury. Pulmonary edema may also occur in such patients as a result of fluid aspiration or ARDS related to neurogenic mechanisms, aspiration, or sepsis.[104]

Because of these common complications, intubation and mechanical ventilation are routine in patients with severe head injury. Mechanical ventilation is also used to hyperventilate such patients and thereby lower intracranial pressure. Because PEEP raises mean intrathoracic pressure and may raise intracranial pressure by impeding cerebral venous pressure, it should be used only when necessary to improve oxygenation in patients with severe head injury. The standard respiratory care practices of inducing cough and deep tracheal suctioning may also increase intracranial pressure and ideally should be performed cautiously and during intracranial pressure monitoring.

Quadriplegia resulting from acute cervical spinal cord trauma, spinal arterial infarction, or compression by tumor is often associated with profound respiratory compromise. Injuries at or above the cord segments C3-5 involve the phrenic nerves and cause partial or complete bilateral hemidiaphragmatic paralysis. In addition, intercostal muscle paralysis caudad to the lesion limits the normal outward expansion of the middle and upper rib cage, further compromising inspiration. Expiration is also greatly reduced because of paralysis of the abdominal and other expiratory muscles. Sternocleidomastoid, scalene, and trapezoid activity persists in high cord injuries, but the efficiency of these muscles is greatly reduced. Because of their extensive respiratory muscle dysfunction, quadriplegics with high cervical cord injury are unable to generate an adequate vital capacity. Hypoxemia is common and results from both hypoventilation and microatelectasis.[106, 107]

Quadriplegic patients with lesions in the lower cervical cord, whose phrenic nerve nuclei are completely or partially intact, can contract their diaphragms to a variable extent. Nevertheless, they lack the intercostal muscle activity necessary to stabilize the rib cage so the hemidiaphragms can function properly; as a result, their inspiratory function is compromised. Like quadriplegics with higher-level defects, these patients also have lost the use of their abdominal and other expiratory muscles. This combination of expiratory and inspiratory weakness prevents them from coughing and clearing secretions, placing them at high risk for respiratory tract infections.[106]

As is evident from the earlier discussion, a large percentage of patients with acute spinal cord injuries require ventilatory support. Vital capacity is commonly between 1.2 and 1.5 L after these injuries and is accompanied by reductions in inspiratory and expiratory pressures.[108] As might be expected, the higher the level of the spinal cord lesion, the more profound the respiratory failure is. Fortunately, however, the need for ventilatory support is often temporary. As the initial phase of spinal shock passes, chest wall flaccidity is replaced with spasticity, and pulmonary function significantly improves as the more rigid chest wall resists collapse. One study reported an increase in the vital capacity of a group of quadriplegics from 1.5 L on admission to 2.7 L 18 weeks later.[109] Overall, approximately 80% of patients with injuries at or below the C-4 level can eventually be safely weaned from mechanical ventilation.

Fat embolism syndrome is a form of pulmonary and other organ system dysfunction that develops after long-bone and pelvic fractures in as many as 10% of trauma patients.[110] The cause is believed to be an interaction of marrow fat embolized to the lungs and other organs with platelets, neutrophils, and free fatty acids.[111] This interaction results in increased capillary permeability and inflammation that may cause pulmonary edema severe enough to constitute ARDS.[112] Confusion and other central nervous system dysfunction may result directly from this interaction or from hypoxemia caused by lung injury. Autopsy studies reveal fat globules, edema, alveolar hemorrhage, and hyaline membrane in the lung, and petechiae and edema of the brain.[113]

Patients with fat embolism syndrome may have a classic triad of confusion, dyspnea, and petechiae from 12 to 72 hours after injury.[113] Other patients may lack petechiae but nevertheless manifest abnormalities in respiratory gas exchange and diffuse radiographic infiltrates[114] (Fig. 80-4). Diagnosis must be based on only clinical presentation because laboratory tests such as detection of lipuria or circulating fat globules are nonspecific for the syndrome. Therapy includes immobilization of fractures and support with PPV and PEEP for respiratory failure. Corticosteroids have been administered after the diagnosis of fat embolism syndrome on the premise that they stabilize lysosomal and capillary membranes, but their effectiveness in this situation has not been demonstrated. However, steroids were shown to prevent the syndrome in patients at risk in one series.[118]

ADULT RESPIRATORY DISTRESS SYNDROME*

The term ARDS is used to describe patients with diffuse chest radiographic infiltrates, reduced lung compliance, ex-

---

*See also Chapter 73.

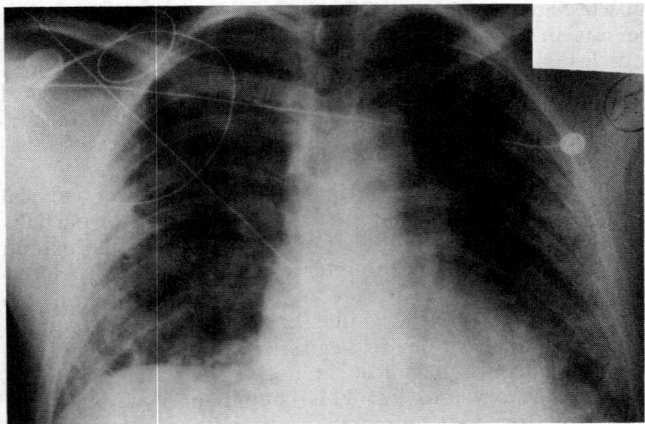

Figure 80–4. Diffuse chest radiographic infiltrates attributed to fat embolism syndrome in 24-year-old man with femoral fracture.

treme dyspnea, and severe arterial blood gas abnormalities who require PPV and PEEP for prolonged periods.[116-118] The characteristic pathologic charges of ARDS include disordered pulmonary capillaries, lung inflammation and edema, hyaline membranes, and fibrosis.[119]

The incidence of ARDS is unclear. Seven of the 12 patients listed by Ashbaugh and coworkers[120] in their first description of ARDS in 1967 had trauma, and this group later estimated that 21 of 500 patients managed by the respiratory care services at the University of Colorado from 1964 to 1968 manifested the clinical criteria of ARDS.[121] Horowitz and coauthors noted that 3 of 49 consecutive patients admitted to the trauma service at Parkland Memorial Hospital in Dallas had shock lung.[116] Fulton and Jones described posttraumatic pulmonary insufficiency in 44 of 399 trauma patients at Louisville General Hospital in 1973. At San Francisco General Hospital, Lewis and associates found that 40 of 6196 admissions to the trauma service for 1972 through 1975 required mechanical ventilation for 15 days or longer.[118]

Reviews from the University of Washington[122] and the University of Colorado[123] indicate that trauma is indeed a major risk factor for ARDS. Traumatic conditions associated with the syndrome include head trauma,[124] pulmonary arterial reperfusion,[125] pancreatitis,[126] lung re-expansion,[127] near-drowning,[128] burns and smoke inhalation,[129] aspiration,[130] lung contusion,[39, 40] fat embolism syndrome,[110-114] massive transfusion,[130] intravascular coagulation,[131] and shock,[116] although hypotension per se is infrequently associated with ARDS.[122, 132] Why these various conditions are associated with ARDS is unclear, but a unifying theory is that they all lead to a generalized inflammatory response in which the lungs are injured in the process.[133]

Although one or more of the conditions noted earlier may account for ARDS shortly after trauma, many patients experience the syndrome after several days. Here, ARDS probably results from the superimposition of pulmonary[134] or systemic infection[135] in patients who are immunosuppressed owing to their injuries. Indeed, sepsis was associated with ARDS in a significant number of the trauma patients described by Horovitz and colleagues[116] and Fulton and Jones,[117] and it also figured prominently in other surgical series.[136, 137] Sepsis was the major risk factor for ARDS in a review from the University of Washington,[122] and it was the leading cause of death in patients who died after 3 days in the ICU at that institution.[138] Prevention of trauma and of the infections that frequently follow it is an obvious approach to preventing ARDS.

References

1. Trunkey DD: Thoracic trauma. In: Trunkey DD, Lewis FR (eds): Current Therapy of Trauma 1983–1984. Philadelphia, BC Decker, p 85, 1984.
2. Shackford SR: Blunt chest trauma: The intensivist's perspective. J Intensive Care Med 1:125, 1986.
3. Richardson JD, McElvein RB, Trinkle JK: First rib fracture: A hallmark of severe trauma. Ann Surg 181:251, 1975.
4. Chayen MS, Rudick V, Borvine A: Pain control with epidural injection of morphine. Anesthesiology 53:338, 1980.
5. Rutherford RB, Campbell DN: Thoracic injuries. In: Zuidema GD, Rutherford RB, Ballinger WB (eds): The Management of Trauma. 4th ed. Philadelphia, WB Saunders, p 391, 1985.
6. Carlisle HB, Sutton JP, Stevenson SE: New technique for stabilization of the flail chest. Am J Surg 112:133, 1966.
7. Ransdell HT: Treatment of flail chest injuries with a piston respirator. J Trauma 5:412, 1968.
8. Clark GC, Schecter WP, Trunkey DD: Variables affecting outcome in blunt chest trauma: Flail chest vs. pulmonary contusion. J Trauma 28:298, 1988.
9. Trinkle JK, Richardson JD, Franz JL, et al: Management of flail chest without mechanical ventilation. Ann Thorac Surg 19:355, 1975.
10. Shackford SR, Smith DE, Zarins CK, et al: The management of flail chest. Am J Surg 132:759, 1976.
11. Richardson JD, Adams L, Flint LM: Selective management of flail chest and pulmonary contusion. Ann Surg 196:481, 1982.
12. Maunder RJ, Pierson DJ, Hudson LD: Subcutaneous and mediastinal emphysema. Arch Intern Med 144:1447, 1984.
13. Macklin MT, Macklin CC: Malignant interstitial emphysema of the lungs and mediastinum as an important occult complication in many respiratory diseases and other conditions: An interpretation of the clinical literature in the light of laboratory experiment. Medicine 23:281, 1944.
14. Robertson HT, Lakshminarayan S, Hudson LD: Lung injury following a 50-metre fall into water. Thorax 33:175, 1978.
15. Pierson DJ: Disorders of the mediastinum. In: Murray JF, Nadel JA (eds): Textbook of Respiratory Medicine. Philadelphia, WB Saunders, p 1781, 1988.
16. Pierson DJ: Pneumomediastinum. In: Murray JF, Nadel JA (eds): Textbook of Respiratory Medicine. Philadelphia, WB Saunders, p 1795, 1988.
17. Van Stiegmann G, Brantigan CO, Hopeman AR: Tension pneumomediastinum. Arch Surg 112:1212, 1977.
18. Cummings RG, Wesly RLR, Adams DH, et al: Pneumopericardium resulting in cardiac tamponade. Ann Thorac Surg 37:511, 1984.
19. Coelho JCU, Tonnesen AS, Allen SJ, et al: Intracranial hypertension secondary to tension subcutaneous emphysema. Crit Care Med 13:512, 1985.
20. Light RW: Pneumothorax. In: Murray JF, Nadel JA (eds): Textbook of Respiratory Medicine. Philadelphia, WB Saunders, p 1745, 1988.
21. Thomas AN, Stephens BG: Air embolism: A cause of morbidity and death after penetrating chest trauma. J Trauma 14:633, 1974.
22. Graham JM, Beall AC, Mattox KL, et al: Systemic air embolism following penetrating trauma to the lung. Chest 72:449, 1977.
23. Ponn RB, Zatarain G, Gerzberg L, et al: Systemic air embolism in experimental penetrating lung injuries. J Thorac Cardiovasc Surg 74:766, 1977.
24. King MW, Aitchison JM, Nel JP: Fatal air embolism following penetrating lung trauma: An autopsy study. J Trauma 24:753, 1984.
25. Marini JJ, Culver BH: Systemic gas embolism complicating mechanical ventilation in the adult respiratory distress syndrome. Ann Intern Med 110:699, 1989.
26. Light RW: Chylothorax, hemothorax, and fibrothorax. In: Murray JF, Nadel JA (eds): Textbook of Respiratory Medicine. Philadelphia, WB Saunders, p 1760, 1988.
27. Napoli VM, Symbas PJ, Vroon DH, et al: Autotransfusion from experimental hemothorax: Levels of coagulation factors. J Trauma 27:296, 1987.
28. Wilson JM, Boren CH, Peterson SR, et al: Traumatic hemothorax: Is decortication necessary? J Thorac Cardiovasc Surg 77:489, 1979.
29. Breaux JR, Marks C: Chylothorax causing reversible T-cell depletion. J Trauma 28:705, 1988.
30. Ramzy AI, Rodriguez A, Cowley RA: Pitfalls in the management of traumatic chylothorax. J Trauma 22:513, 1982.
31. Milsom AW, Kron IL, Rheuban KS, et al: Chylothorax: An assessment of current surgical management. J Thorac Cardiovasc Surg 89:221, 1985.
32. Bertelsen S, Howitz P: Injuries of the trachea and bronchi. Thorax 27:188, 1972.
33. Kumpe DA, Oh KS, Wyman SM: A characteristic pulmonary finding in unilateral complete bronchial transection. Am J Roentgenol 110:704, 1970.
34. Hara KS, Prakash UBS: Fiberoptic bronchoscopy in the evaluation of acute chest and upper airway trauma. Chest 96:627, 1989.
35. Urschel HC, Razzuk MA: Management of acute traumatic injuries of tracheobronchial tree. Surg Gynecol Obstet 136:113, 1973.

36. Collins JP, Ketharanathan V, McConchie I: Rupture of major bronchi resulting from closed chest injuries. Thorax 28:371, 1973.
37. Grover FL, Ellestad C, Arom KV, et al: Diagnosis and management of major tracheobronchial injuries. Ann Thorac Surg 28:384, 1979.
38. Thompson DA, Rowlands BJ, Walker WE: Urgent thoracotomy for pulmonary or tracheobronchial injury. J Trauma 28:276, 1988.
39. Oppenheimer L, Craven KD, Forkert L, et al: Pathophysiology of pulmonary contusion in dogs. J Appl Physiol 47:718, 1979.
40. Pison U, Seeger W, Buchhorn R, et al: Surfactant abnormalities in patients with respiratory failure after multiple trauma. Am Rev Respir Dis 140:1033, 1989.
41. Craven KD, Oppenheimer L, Wood LDH: Effects of contusion and flail chest on pulmonary perfusion and oxygen exchange. J Appl Physiol 47:729, 1979.
42. Bongard FS, Lewis FR: Crystalloid resuscitation of patients with pulmonary contusion. Am J Surg 148:145, 1984.
43. Graham JM, Mattox KL, Beall AC: Penetrating trauma of the lung. J Trauma 19:665, 1979.
44. Ganske JG, Dennis DL, Vanderveer JB: Traumatic lung cyst: Case report and literature review. J Trauma 21:493, 1981.
45. Stulz P, Schmitt HE, Hasse J, et al: Traumatic pulmonary pseudocysts and paramediastinal air cyst: Two rare complications of blunt chest trauma. J Trauma 24:850, 1984.
46. Parmley LF, Manion WC, Mattingly TW: Nonpenetrating traumatic injury of the heart. Circulation 18:371, 1958.
47. Saunders CR, Doty DB: Myocardial contusion. Surg Gynecol Obstet 144:595, 1977.
48. Rothstein RJ: Myocardial contusion. JAMA 250:2189, 1983.
49. Doty DB, Anderson AE, Rose EF, et al: Cardiac trauma: Clinical and experimental correlations of myocardial contusion. Ann Surg 180:452, 1974.
50. Sutherland GR, Calvin JE, Driedger AA, et al: Anatomic and cardiopulmonary responses to trauma with associated blunt chest injury. J Trauma 21:1, 1981.
51. Harley DP, Mena I, Narahara KA, et al: Traumatic myocardial dysfunction. J Thorac Cardiovasc Surg 87:386, 1984.
52. Liedtke AJ, DeMuth WE: Nonpenetrating cardiac injuries: A collective review. Am Heart J 86:687, 1973.
53. Miller FA, Seward JB, Gersh BJ, et al: Two-dimensional echocardiographic findings in cardiac trauma. Am J Cardiol 50:1022, 1982.
54. Kumar SA, Puri VK, Mittal VK, et al: Myocardial contusion following nonfatal blunt chest trauma. J Trauma 23:327, 1983.
55. King RM, Mucha P, Seward JB, et al: Cardiac contusion: A new diagnostic approach utilizing two-dimensional echocardiography. J Trauma 23:610, 1983.
56. Hiatt JR, Yeatman LA, Child JS: The value of echocardiography in blunt chest trauma. J Trauma 28:914, 1988.
57. Helling TS, Duke P, Beggs CW, et al: A prospective evaluation of 68 patients suffering blunt chest trauma for evidence of cardiac injury. J Trauma 29:961, 1989.
58. Brantigan CO, Burdick D, Hopeman AR, et al: Evaluation of technetium scanning for myocardial contusion. J Trauma 18:460, 1978.
59. Potkin RT, Werner JA, Trobaugh GB, et al: Evaluation of noninvasive tests of cardiac damage in suspected cardiac contusion. Circulation 66:627, 1982.
60. Fabian TC, Mangiante EC, Patterson R, et al: Myocardial contusion in blunt trauma: Clinical characteristics, means of diagnosis, and implications for patient management. J Trauma 28:50, 1988.
61. Snow N, Lucas AE, Richardson JD: Intra-aortic balloon counterpulsation for cardiogenic shock from cardiac contusion. J Trauma 22:426, 1982.
62. Healey MA, Brown R, Fleiszer D: Blunt cardiac injury: Is this diagnosis necessary? J Trauma 30:137, 1990.
63. Trinkle JK, Toon RS, Franz JL, et al: Affairs of the wounded heart: Penetrating cardiac wounds. J Trauma 19:467, 1979.
64. Evans J, Gray LA, Rayner A, et al: Principles for the management of penetrating cardiac wounds. Ann Surg 189:777, 1978.
65. Williams JB, Silver DG, Laws HL: Successful management of heart rupture from blunt trauma. J Trauma 21:534, 1981.
66. Martin TD, Flynn TC, Rowlands BJ, et al: Blunt cardiac rupture. J Trauma 24:287, 1984.
67. Sparrow JG, Miller DW: Ventricular septal defect following blunt thoracic and abdominal trauma: Case report. J Trauma 29:690, 1989.
68. Breaux EP, Dupont JB, Albert HM, et al: Cardiac tamponade following penetrating mediastinal injuries: Improved survival with early pericardiocentesis. J Trauma 19:461, 1979.
69. Arom KV, Richardson JD, Webb G, et al: Subxiphoid pericardial window in patients with suspected traumatic pericardial tamponade. Ann Thorac Surg 23:545, 1977.
70. Parmley LF, Mattingly TW, Manion WC, et al: Nonpenetrating traumatic injury of the aorta. Circulation 17:1086, 1958.
71. Symbas PN, Tyras DH, Ware RE, et al: Traumatic rupture of the aorta. Ann Surg 178:6, 1972.
72. Kirsh MM, Behrendt DM, Orringer MB, et al: The treatment of acute traumatic rupture of the aorta: A 10-year experience. Ann Surg 184:308, 1976.
73. Shackford SR, Virgilio RW, Smith DE, et al: The significance of chest wall injury in the diagnosis of traumatic aneurysms of the thoracic aorta. J Trauma 18:493, 1978.
74. Gundry SR, Williams S, Burney RE, et al: Indications for aortography in blunt thoracic trauma: A reassessment. J Trauma 22:664, 1982.
75. Gundry SR, Burney RE, Mackenzie JR, et al: Assessment of mediastinal widening associated with traumatic rupture of the aorta. J Trauma 23:293, 1983.
76. Egan TJ, Neiman HL, Herman RJ, et al: Computed tomography in the diagnosis of aortic aneurysm dissection or traumatic injury. Radiology 136:141, 1980.
77. Heiberg E, Wolverson MK, Sundaram M, et al: CT in aortic trauma. AJR 140:1119, 1983.
78. Beal SL, Pottmeyer EW, Spisso JM: Esophageal perforation following external blunt trauma. J Trauma 28:1425, 1988.
79. Ebert PA, Gaertner RA, Zuidema GD: Traumatic diaphragmatic hernia. Surg Gynecol Obstet 125:59, 1967.
80. Pomerantz M, Rodgers BM, Sabiston DC: Traumatic diaphragmatic hernia. Surgery 64:529, 1968.
81. Estrera AS, Platt MR, Mills LJ: Traumatic injuries of the diaphragm. Chest 75:306, 1979.
82. Ward RE, Flynn TC, Clark WP: Diaphragmatic disruption secondary to blunt abdominal trauma. J Trauma 21:35, 1981.
83. Van Vugt AB, Schoots FJ: Acute diaphragmatic rupture due to blunt trauma: A retrospective analysis. J Trauma 29:683, 1989.
84. Sharma OP: Traumatic diaphragmatic rupture: Not an uncommon entity—Personal experience with collective review of the 1980's. J Trauma 29:678, 1989.
85. Shea L, Graham AD, Fletcher JC, et al: Diaphragmatic injury: A method for early diagnosis. J Trauma 22:539, 1982.
86. Feliciano DV, Cruse PA, Mattox KL, et al: Delayed diagnosis of injuries to the diaphragm after penetrating wounds. J Trauma 28:1135, 1988.
87. Madden MR, Paull DE, Finkelstein JL, et al: Occult diaphragmatic injury from stab wounds to the lower chest and abdomen. J Trauma 29:292, 1989.
88. Trunkey DD: Abdominal trauma. In: Trunkey DD, Lewis FR (eds): Current Therapy of Trauma 1983–1984. Philadelphia, BC Decker, p 93, 1984.
89. Graham JM, Mattox KL, Jordan GL: Traumatic injuries of the pancreas. Am J Surg 136:744, 1978.
90. Kashuk JL, Moore EE, Millikan S, et al: Major abdominal vascular trauma—A unified approach. J Trauma 22:672, 1982.
91. Fischer RP, Beverlin BC, Engrav LH, et al: Diagnostic peritoneal lavage. Am J Surg 136:701, 1978.
92. Wightman JAK: A prospective survey of the incidence of postoperative pulmonary complications. Br J Surg 55:85, 1968.
93. Latimer RG, Dickman M, Day WC, et al: Ventilatory patterns and pulmonary complications after upper abdominal surgery determined by preoperative and postoperative computerized spirometry and blood gas analysis. Am J Surg 122:622, 1971.
94. Pierce AK, Robertson J: Pulmonary complications of general surgery. Annu Rev Med 28:211, 1977.
95. Stein M, Koota GM, Simon M, et al: Pulmonary evaluation of surgical patients. JAMA 181:103, 1962.
96. Zikria BA, Spencer JL, Kinney JM, et al: Alterations in ventilatory function and breathing patterns following surgical trauma. Ann Surg 179:1, 1974.
97. Ali J, Weisel RD, Layug AB, et al: Consequences of postoperative alterations in respiratory mechanics. Am J Surg 128:376, 1974.
98. Gamsu G, Singer MM, Vincent HH, et al: Postoperative impairment of mucous transport in the lung. Am Rev Respir Dis 114:673, 1976.
99. Ford GT, Whitelane WA, Rosenal TW, et al: Diaphragm function after upper abdominal surgery in humans. Am Rev Respir Dis 127:431, 1983.
100. Stock MC, Downs JB, Gauer PK, et al: Prevention of postoperative pulmonary complications with CPAP, incentive spirometry, and conservative therapy. Chest 87:151, 1985.
101. O'Donohue WJ Jr: National survey of the usage of lung expansion modalities for the prevention and treatment of postoperative atelectasis following abdominal and thoracic surgery. Chest 87:76, 1985.
102. Spence AA, Smith G: Postoperative analgesia and lung function: A comparison of morphine with extradural block. Br J Anaesth 43:144, 1971.
103. Bartkowski HM, Pitts LH: Neurologic injury. In: Trunkey DD, Lewis FR (eds): Current Therapy of Trauma 1983–1984. Philadelphia, BC Decker, p 47, 1984.
104. Luce JM: Medical management of head injury. Chest 89:864, 1986.
105. Borel C, Hanley D, Diringer MN, et al: Intensive management of severe head injury. Chest 98:180, 1990.
106. Luce JM: Medical management of spinal cord injury. Crit Care Med 13:126, 1985.
107. Schmidt-Norowa WW, Altman AR: Atelectasis and neuromuscular respiratory failure. Chest 85: 792, 1984.
108. Mansel JK, Norman JR: Respiratory complications and management of spinal cord injuries. Chest 97:1446, 1990.
109. Ledsome JR, Sharp JM: Pulmonary function in acute cervical cord injury. Am Rev Respir Dis 124:41, 1981.
110. Moylan JA, Evenson MA: Diagnosis and treatment of fat embolism. Annu Rev Med 28:85, 1977.
111. Gossling HR, Donohue TA: The fat embolism syndrome. JAMA 241:2740, 1979.

112. Barie PS, Minnear FL, Malik AB: Increased pulmonary vascular permeability after bone marrow injection in sheep. Am Rev Respir Dis 123:648, 1981.

113. Dines DE, Burgher LW, Okazaki H: The clinical and pathologic correlation of fat embolism syndrome. Mayo Clin Proc 50:407, 1975.

114. Fabian TC, Hoots AV, Stanford DS, et al: Fat embolism syndrome: Prospective evaluation in 92 fracture patients. Crit Care Med 18:42, 1990.

115. Schonfeld SA, Ploysongsang Y, DiLisio R, et al: Fat embolism prophylaxis with corticosteroids. Ann Intern Med 99:438, 1983.

116. Horovitz JH, Carrico CJ, Shires GT: Pulmonary response to major injury. Arch Surg 108:349, 1974.

117. Fulton RL, Jones CE: The cause of post-traumatic pulmonary insufficiency in man. Surg Gynecol Obstet 140:179, 1975.

118. Lewis FR, Blaisdell FW, Schlobohm RM: Incidence and outcome of posttraumatic respiratory failure. Arch Surg 112:436, 1977.

119. Blaisdell FW, Schlobohm RM: The respiratory distress syndrome: A review. Surgery 74:251, 1973.

120. Ashbaugh DG, Bigelow DB, Petty TL, et al: Acute respiratory distress in adults. Lancet 2:7511, 1967.

121. Ashbaugh DG, Petty TL, Bigelow DB, et al: Continuous positive-pressure breathing (CPPB) in adult respiratory distress syndrome. J Thorac Cardiovasc Surg 57:31, 1969.

122. Pepe PE, Potkin RT, Reus DH, et al: Clinical predictors of the adult respiratory distress syndrome. Am J Surg 144:124, 1982.

123. Fowler AA, Hamman RF, Good JT, et al: Adult respiratory distress syndrome: Risk with common predispositions. Ann Intern Med 98:593, 1983.

124. Colice GL, Matthay MA, Bass E, et al: Neurogenic pulmonary edema. Am Rev Respir Dis 130:941, 1984.

125. Horgan MJ, Lum H, Malik AB: Pulmonary edema after pulmonary artery occlusion and reperfusion. Am Rev Respir Dis 140:1421, 1989.

126. Nicod L, Leuenberger PH, Seydoux C, et al: Evidence for pancreas injury in adult respiratory distress syndrome. Am Rev Respir Dis 131:696, 1985.

127. Pavlin DJ, Nessly ML, Cheney FW: Increased pulmonary vascular permeability as a cause of re-expansion edema in rabbits. Am Rev Respir Dis 124:422, 1981.

128. Hoff BH: Multisystem failure: A review with special reference to drowning. Crit Care Med 7:310, 1979.

129. Achauer BM, Allyn PA, Furnas DW, et al: Pulmonary complications of burns: The major threat to the burn patient. Ann Surg 177:311, 1973.

130. Hudson LD: Causes of the adult respiratory distress syndrome—Clinical recognition. Clin Chest Med 3:195, 1982.

131. Bone RC, Francis PB, Pierce AK: Intravascular coagulation associated with the adult respiratory distress syndrome. Am J Med 61:585, 1976.

132. Fishman AP: Shock lung. Circulation 47:921, 1973.

133. Rinaldo JE, Rogers RM: Adult respiratory-distress syndrome. N Engl J Med 306:900, 1982.

134. Johanson WG, Holcomb JR, Coalson JJ: Experimental diffuse alveolar damage in baboons. Am Rev Respir Dis 126:142, 1982.

135. Pietra GG, Rüttner JR, Wüst W, et al: The lung after trauma and shock—Fine structure of the alveolar-capillary barrier in 23 autopsies. J Trauma 21:454, 1981.

136. Ashbaugh DG, Petty TL: Sepsis complicating the acute respiratory distress syndrome. Surg Gynecol Obstet 135:865, 1972.

137. Clowes GHA, Hirsch E, Williams L, et al: Septic lung and shock lung in man. Ann Surg 181:681, 1975.

138. Montgomery AB, Stager MA, Carrico CJ, et al: Causes of mortality in patients with the adult respiratory distress syndrome. Am Rev Respir Dis 132:485, 1985.

CHAPTER 81

Acute Drug-Induced Lung Injury

Edward C. Rosenow III
Richard J. Pisani

Many drugs are known to induce lung injury, both acute and chronic, as well as to produce bronchospasm and pleural disease.[1-7] The critical care medicine physician must be aware of the drugs that can produce any adverse pulmonary injury, especially the drugs known to induce an acute or subacute injury that might require admittance of the patient to a critical care unit. Table 81–1 lists the drugs that have a well-documented potential to injure the lung and those (marked with an asterisk) that can produce acute or subacute respiratory insufficiency requiring critical care management. The mechanism of almost all of these is unknown, with a few exceptions that are discussed under the separate drug classifications.

There is no diagnostic test to confirm or refute the possibility of acute lung injury with the following exceptions: (1) elevated salicylate level in acetylsalicylic acid (ASA)–induced noncardiac pulmonary edema, (2) presence of leukoagglutinin-induced antibodies in blood tranfusion–related noncardiac pulmonary edema, and (3) findings of a hemolytic-uremic syndrome characteristic of mitomycin C toxicity.

The three types of drug toxicities that are considered in this chapter in relation to acute to subacute respiratory insufficiency are bronchospasm, adult respiratory distress sydrome (ARDS), and noncardiac pulmonary edema. There is, of course, significant clinical overlap between ARDS and noncardiac pulmonary edema. These can be separated by the observation that noncardiac pulmonary edema is a self-limited process associated with minimal inflammatory cell infiltration of the interstitium, whereas ARDS is associated not only with evidence of capillary leak and intra-alveolar pulmonary fluid but also with a significant element of inflammatory cell infiltration. Presumably, in noncardiac pulmonary edema the main mechanism is increased alveolar capillary leakage of fluid with little stimulation of inflammatory cells to respond, whereas in ARDS the predominant insult may provoke inflammatory cell infiltration with a secondary transudation of fluid.

Interestingly, there is not much detail available about the histology of many of these reactions other than isolated case reports. One supposition is that the more rapid the clearing of the infiltrate, the more likely it is to represent noncardiac pulmonary edema rather than an inflammatory response.

However, almost all of the drugs listed in Table 81–1 can produce disease of sufficient extent to cause respiratory insufficiency eventually, possibly resulting in admission to an intensive care unit. It is important to have an overall picture of the presentations for all of the drugs listed in Table 81–1 to develop a better perspective of the drug reactions that present acutely versus those that are subacute to chronic.

This is an arbitrary breakdown, but it may be of value in discerning the nature of the drug-induced pulmonary disease reactions.

DRUGS INDUCING BRONCHOSPASM

Increased airway reactivity may occur with many acute interstitial lung disease reactions if there is an element of underlying hyperreactivity. Certain reactions, such as acute nitrofurantoin interstitial pneumonitis, may be associated with bronchospasm producing a combined obstructive and restrictive lung disease.[8, 9] In 2 to 5% of patients with asthma, symptoms are aggravated by the ingestion of ASA as well as most of the nonsteroidal anti-inflammatory agents. There is little documentation of obstructive lung disease in patients with ASA-induced noncardiac pulmonary edema, and it is likely that the mechanisms are widely disparate to the point that there is no overlap in this particular reaction.[10, 11]

Bronchospasm to the point of respiratory failure and death may occur with the beta-blockers, particularly those that are not cardioselective. Studies using impedance techniques have shown that most beta-blockers can produce increased airway resistance in normal individuals. Thus beta-blockers should be avoided in patients with an element of obstructive lung disease as well as those with hyperreactive

TABLE 81-1
DRUG-INDUCED PULMONARY DISEASE CLASSIFICATION

Chemotherapeutic	**Analgesics**
Cytotoxic	*Heroin
Azathioprine	*Methadone
*Bleomycin	*Naloxone
Busulfan	*Placidyl
Chlorambucil	*Propoxyphene
Cyclophosphamide	*Salicylates
Etoposide	**Cardiovascular**
Melphalan	*Amiodarone
*Mitomycin	Angiotensin-converting
Nitrosoureas	enzyme inhibitors
Procarbazine	Anticoagulants
Vinblastine	*Beta-blockers
Noncytotoxic	Dipyridamole
*Methotrexate	*Fibrinolytic agents
*Cytosine arabinoside	*Protamine
*Bleomycin	Tocainide
*Procarbazine	**Inhalants**
Antibiotic	Aspirated oil
*Amphotericin B	*Oxygen
Nitrofurantoin	**Intravenous**
*Acute	*Blood
Chronic	Morrhuate sodium
Sulfasalazine	Ethiodized oil
Sulfonamides	(lymphangiogram)
Anti-inflammatory	Talc
*Acetylsalicylic acid	**Miscellaneous†**
Gold	Bromocriptine
Methotrexate	Dantrolene
Nonsteroidal anti-	*Fat emulsion
inflammatory agents	*Hydrochlorothiazide
*Penicillamine	Methysergide
Immunoreactive	Oral contraceptives
Cyclosporine	*Tocolytic agents
*Interleukin-2	*Tricyclic antidepressants
Corticosteroids	*L-Tryptophan
Bronchospasm	Radiation
Nitrofurantoin (acute)	*Systemic lupus
Acetylsalicylic acid	erythrematosus (drug-
Nonsteroidal anti-	induced)
inflammatory agents	*Complement-mediated
Beta-blockers	leukostasis
Dipyridamole	*Interleukin-2

*Patients typically present with acute or subacute respiratory insufficiency.

†Bleomycin plus oxygen is associated with ARDS, mitomycin plus 5-fluorouracil with noncardiac pulmonary edema, and methotrexate (intrathecal) with noncardiac pulmonary edema.

airways disease because both groups are greatly predisposed to worsening with their use. More than two dozen deaths have resulted from the use of timolol ophthalmologic solution, and it should also be avoided in any individual with obstructive lung disease.[12] Typically, the patient does not mention this medication because it is an eye drop and not taken by mouth. Betaxolol, another beta-blocker, is safer and a good alternative medication.

Dipyridamole has been associated with several episodes of acute bronchospasm in patients with underlying chronic obstructive pulmonary disease who were given the drug for radionuclide ventriculography. Intravenous theophylline will rapidly reverse the bronchospasm.[13]

CHEMOTHERAPEUTIC DRUGS

We have divided chemotherapeutic drug–induced lung disease into two categories: cytotoxic and noncytotoxic. Cytotoxic injury to the lung is associated with a typical histologic pattern of atypia in a type II pneumocyte. This cytotoxic reaction is progressive and fatal unless the drug is discontinued and corticosteroids are added or the dose is boosted. In contrast, in noncytotoxic lung disease there is no evidence of cellular atypia and, with the exception of disease caused by cytosine arabinoside, the course is rarely fatal.

The manifestations of a cytotoxic drug reaction may begin weeks to months and sometimes years after drug exposure with the onset of nonproductive cough, dyspnea, and usually fever (although this may not occur daily).[1–3, 5, 7] Laboratory studies are of little value. The chest roentgenogram shows a diffuse interstitial process often with an alveolar component (Fig. 81–1). Initially, the infiltrate can be well localized or asymmetric. As the process continues, a diffuse "whiteout" of both lungs may occur. Pleural effusions are present in a small percentage of patients. Pulmonary function testing shows diminished volumes as well as decreased carbon monoxide diffusing capacity, with reduction in the latter frequently preceding the clinical and roentgenologic changes. Histologic pattern, as stated, is usually that of atypia of the type II pneumocyte. The differential diagnosis of diffuse pulmonary disease in the immunocompromised host should include opportunistic infection, drug-induced lung disease, recurrence of an underlying process such as lymphoma or leukemic infiltrate into the lungs, idiopathic pulmonary fibrosis (this may well be a somewhat atypical pattern for a drug and/or radiation effect), and "unrelated" conditions such as pulmonary emboli, ARDS, sepsis, community-acquired pneumonia, or congestive heart failure.

Toxic pulmonary reactions to bleomycin and mitomycin can lead to an ARDS-like picture but are distinguished by their unique clinical features. Bleomycin therapy within the year combined with supplemental oxygen therapy with a fraction of inspired oxygen greater than 0.25 can produce an ARDS-like picture beginning 1 to 4 days after initiation of oxygen therapy (Fig. 81–2).[14, 15] This may occur even when it has been over a year since bleomycin was given. Therefore, anyone who has received bleomycin at any time in his or her lifetime should be given oxygen very cautiously. The reaction may be fatal unless the mechanism is recognized, the fraction of inspired oxygen is reduced to less than 0.25, and corticosteroids are given.

The second unique reaction to a member of this group of cytotoxic drugs is mitomycin-induced hemolytic-uremic syndrome, which is frequently associated with a noncardiac pulmonary edema.[16, 17] This reaction is usually associated with concomitant use of a leukocyte transfusion or 5-fluorouracil. It is fatal in more than half of the cases.

Of the noncytotoxic drugs (see Table 81–1), cytosine

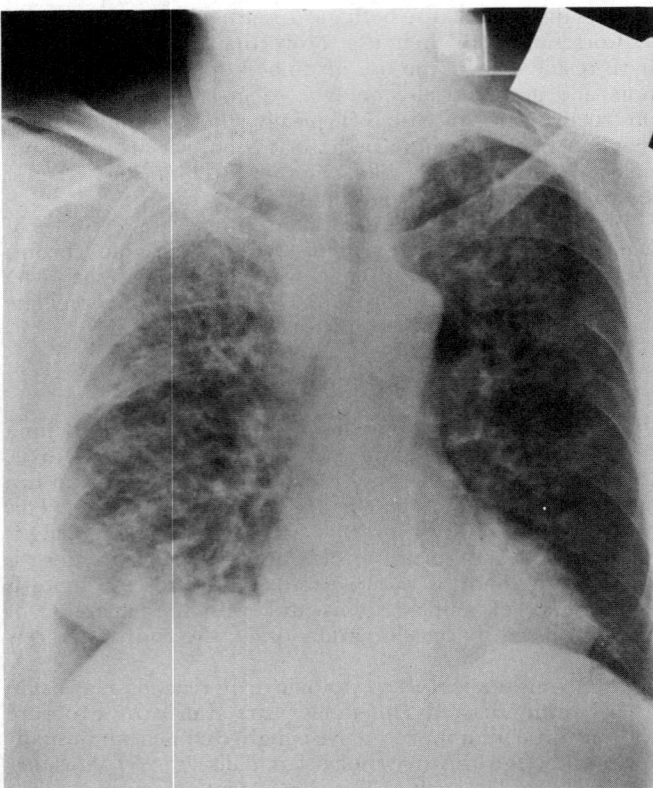

Figure 81–1. Chest roentgenogram of a 75-year-old man who received cyclophosphamide (Cytoxan) for treatment of Wegener's granulomatosis. Dyspnea, cough, and fever developed over several weeks and progressed even though the drug was discontinued and corticosteroids were given.

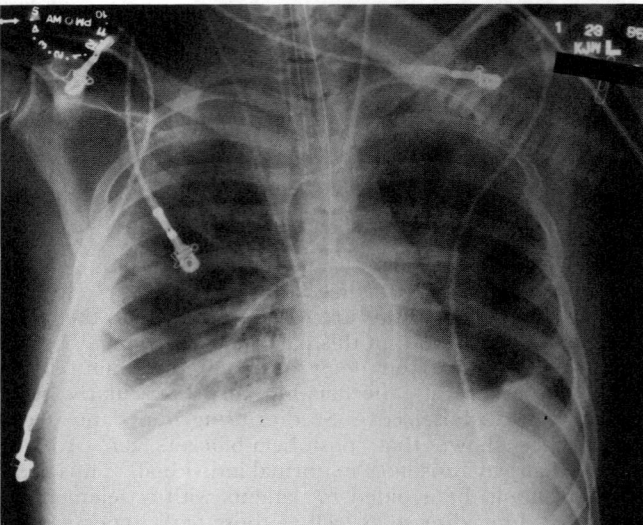

Figure 81–2. Chest roentgenogram of a 46-year-old man who had diffuse infiltrates beginning 1 day after resection of infarcted bowel and who was receiving bleomycin. Open lung biopsy eliminated other causes. He responded to lowering of the fraction of inspired 713oxygen below 0.25 and treatment with corticosteroids.

arabinoside produces a form of noncardiac pulmonary edema unlike that in any other drug-induced pulmonary disease (Fig. 81–3).[18, 19] Progressive dyspnea and fever begin while the patient is receiving the medication or within 4 weeks. The lung histologic specimen shows little infiltration of inflammatory cells into the interstitium; instead, an intense proteinaceous pulmonary edema is present in the intra-alveolar spaces. The mortality is about 50%; corticosteroids are the treatment of choice.

Methotrexate is one of the few drugs known to produce granulomas in the lung. It is associated with the onset of pulmonary disease 10 days to several weeks after initiation of therapy.[2, 3, 5, 7] A hypersensitivity reaction is probably involved, and about half of the cases are associated with peripheral blood eosinophilia. The disease is rarely fatal, and although response to discontinuation of the drug is excellent, corticosteroids may be used to resolve the infiltrate more rapidly. Methotrexate is the only drug known to produce hilar lymphadenopathy, which occurs in about 10% of the cases. Intrathecal methotrexate has been associated with several case reports of a fatal noncardiac pulmonary edema.

Bleomycin and procarbazine can each produce both cytotoxic and noncytotoxic reactions. The noncytotoxic reactions are associated with eosinophilia in about half the cases. They are characterized by rapid onset and resolution of pulmonary infiltrates, especially with the use of corticosteroids.

ANTIBIOTICS

Amphotericin B, given after a transfusion of granulocytes, can produce an ARDS-like picture.[20] In one series, the reaction occurred in about 5% of the patients. The mechanism may involve aggregation of polymorphonuclear leukocytes in the pulmonary capillaries. Although most of the cases reported have occurred with concomitant transfusion of granulocytes, there are several reports of this reaction occurring when amphotericin B is given without any other agent.

Acute nitrofurantoin pneumonitis may begin within a few hours to 10 days after initiation of therapy and manifest as an acute interstitial intra-alveolar process mimicking a noncardiac pulmonary edema (Fig. 81–4).[8, 9] There is little in the literature about the histology of this reaction, although bronchoalveolar lavage has shown polymorphonuclear neutrophils in the few cases in which a histologic study has been

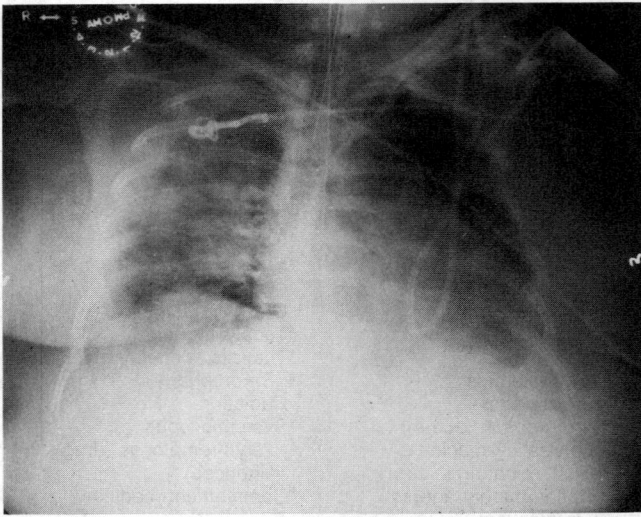

Figure 81–3. Chest roentgenogram of a 58-year-old woman with acute leukemia who was receiving cytosine arabinoside. During 1 week, the patient developed progressive pulmonary infiltrates with fever that was thought to be due to ARDS, but histologic diagnosis confirmed changes typical of cytosine arabinoside–induced noncardiac pulmonary edema.

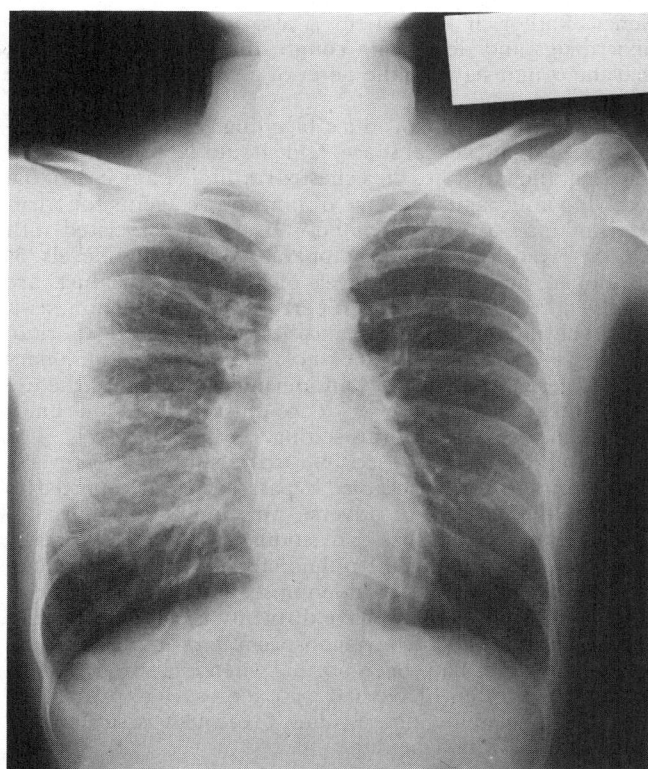

Figure 81–4. Chest roentgenogram of a 26-year-old woman with acute onset of dyspnea and a temperature up to 40°C 1 day after nitrofurantoin treatment was begun for urinary infection. The chest x-ray film cleared within 36 hours after the medication was stopped.

done. Clinically, the process resembles a noncardiac pulmonary edema in its rapid resolution with discontinuation of the medication. Few fatal cases have occurred. There is no overlap in acute and chronic nitrofurantoin pneumonitis. The latter resembles idiopathic interstitial pneumonitis and fibrosis clinically, radiologically, and histologically. Sulfasalazine produces subacute to chronic pulmonary infiltrates frequently associated with eosinophilia.[21] Sulfonamides have also been associated with pulmonary infiltrate with eosinophilia syndrome.

Any of the aminoglycoside antibiotics can produce respiratory insufficiency through the induction of respiratory muscle weakness.[22] This usually occurs after overdosage but can also be seen in patients with pre-existing respiratory muscle weakness or renal insufficiency.

ANTI-INFLAMMATORY AGENTS

ASA aggravates bronchospasm in 2 to 5% of asthmatics, sometimes producing acute respiratory insufficiency.[10] More than 200 proprietary drugs contain ASA, and it is important that the clinician obtain a careful drug history. The most serious pulmonary reaction, noncardiac pulmonary edema, is a prostaglandin-mediated process that occurs in 25% of the patients with a salicylate level greater than 40 mg/dL (Fig. 81–5).[11] Central nervous system stimulation by ASA produces a respiratory alkalosis. $PaCO_2$ is usually below 20 torr and this should indicate the need to obtain a salicylate level. Although most cases result from an intentional overdosage, one third occur as accidental toxicity in patients taking ASA on a long-term basis.

Methotrexate given as an anti-inflammatory agent at low doses of 10 to 15 mg/wk for rheumatoid arthritis produces a granulomatous interstitial process in about 5% of the patients receiving the medication.[23] Several deaths have resulted from respiratory failure. The onset is subacute and the process is reversible if the medication is discontinued and corticosteroids are given.

Penicillamine is used for immune suppression in a number of inflammatory disorders, including various liver diseases and rheumatoid arthritis. It can induce systemic lupus erythematosus and bronchiolitis obliterans. In addition, there have been reports of more than 10 cases of penicillamine-induced Goodpasture's syndrome, which can occur acutely to subacutely.[24] The clinical course mimics that of Goodpasture's syndrome of spontaneous onset.

IMMUNOREACTIVE DRUGS

Treatment with corticosteroids at immunosuppressive levels is well known to result in opportunistic infections. This may occur in diseases that do not normally produce an immunocompromised state, such as temporal arteritis or inflammatory bowel disease. *Pneumocystis carinii* pneumonia, cytomegalovirus pneumonia, invasive aspergillosis, and others disorders must be considered in this setting as well as in the typical immunocompromised host.

Interleukin-2 has been associated with several cases of noncardiac pulmonary edema with respiratory failure. Cardiac toxicity manifested by pulmonary edema, arrhythmias, and impaired cardiac output has also been described.[25] Pulmonary edema resolves spontaneously within several days of termination of therapy. Induction of hyperreactive airways disease with use of interleukin-2 has also been reported. The concomitant use of tumor-infiltrating lymphocytes may contribute to the pulmonary toxicity of interleukin-2.[26]

ANALGESICS

Heroin-induced noncardiac pulmonary edema may be the single most common cause of drug-induced pulmonary disease in the world.[1, 2, 4, 5] The mechanism is unknown, but it may involve a direct effect on the alveolar capillary membrane or may be mediated through the central nervous system. Respiratory rate and depth are depressed, producing an elevated $PaCO_2$. Response to supportive therapy and the

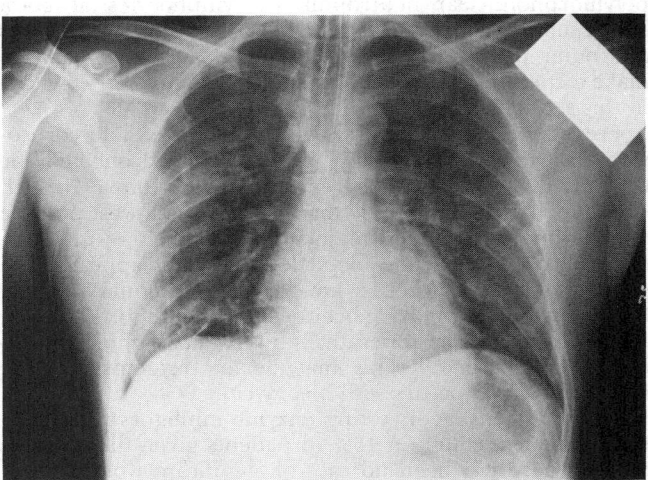

Figure 81–5. Chest roentgenogram of a 42-year-old man with ASA-induced pulmonary edema resulting from intentional overdosage. $PaO_2 = 60$ torr; $PaCO_2 = 13$ torr.

use of naloxone to reverse central nervous system depression is excellent. Unfortunately, aspiration occurs in about half of the patients and may be complicated by bacterial pneumonia. Similar reactions have occurred with oral or intravenous methadone, naloxone, ethchlorvynol, propoxyphene, and other sedative medications. The main clinical clues are depressed respirations and hypercapnia associated with miosis of the pupils.

Noncardiac pulmonary edema has been associated with the synthetic narcotic analgesic naloxone, not necessarily in overdoses.[27-29]

CARDIOVASCULAR DRUGS

Amiodarone produces amiodarone pulmonary toxicity in 6% of the patients receiving the drug. Most of the affected patients have received amiodarone for at least 2 months at an average dose of 400 mg/d, although the reaction has occurred at lower daily dosages.[30] In about one third of the patients the onset is subacute, mimicking that of pneumonia and possibly pulmonary embolism, and in two thirds the onset of interstitial and/or intra-alveolar pneumonitis is more insidious. Fever may or may not be present. Amiodarone pulmonary toxicity is fatal in about 10% of the patients, but it is unpredictable which 10% will progress in respiratory insufficiency and die even when the medication is discontinued and corticosteroids are added.

Amiodarone induces phospholipid deposition in many cells including alveolar macrophages. Although the presence of lipid-filled macrophages is not diagnostic of amiodarone pulmonary toxicity (they are present in many patients who die of nonpulmonary causes), their absence virtually excludes the disorder. The sedimentation rate is elevated in almost all patients with amiodarone pulmonary toxicity, contrary to what would be expected with congestive heart failure or pulmonary embolism, which are two of the major alternatives in the differential diagnosis in these patients with coronary artery disease. When the syndrome of amiodarone pulmonary toxicity presents acutely to subacutely (as it does in one third of the patients), pneumonia is a major consideration and one in which the sedimentation rate may also be elevated.

A ^{67}Ga scan is positive in all patients with amiodarone pulmonary toxicity, as it would be with pneumonia. Bronchoalveolar lavage may show a normal differential (in addition to lipid-filled macrophages) or may show an increase in polymorphonuclear neutrophils or lymphocytes or both. When there is an increase in the neutrophils or lymphocytes and other possible causes are excluded, it is reasonable to make a specific diagnosis of amiodarone pulmonary toxicity in this setting.

Treatment is to discontinue amiodarone and add corticosteroids. However, for many patients amiodarone may be the only drug that controls ventricular arrhythmia. In such cases, an attempt should be made to use the lowest possible amiodarone dose and to maintain such patients with corticosteroids. (Amiodarone blood levels do not appear to be good predictors of whether amiodarone pulmonary toxicity has occurred.) There have been several case reports of acute ARDS occurring postoperatively in patients who have received amiodarone.[31] This may be an oxygen-synergistic reaction, such as occurs with bleomycin.

The angiotensin-converting enzyme inhibitors produce a nonproductive cough in 15% of patients given these drugs. So far, there has been no case of significant worsening of obstructive lung disease such as occurs with the beta-blockers.[32] This group of drugs is mentioned here not because they can produce an acute reaction with respiratory insuffi-

ciency. Rather, if the patient is also receiving some other toxic drugs and develops a cough, the clinician may think that the cough signifies the onset of a reaction to one of the other drugs.

Anticoagulants can produce bleeding into any tissue, including lung or pleural space, and should be considered the source of the infiltrates on a chest x-ray film of any individual receiving anticoagulants. Use of fibrinolytic agents for treatment of intra-arterial thrombosis has been associated with ARDS; typically, thrombocytopenia, diminished levels of fibrinogen, and increased levels of fibrin split products are observed.[33, 34] This is not a reperfusion phenomenon, as it has involved all of the lung and has occurred after fibrinolytic therapy for thrombosis of a coronary artery. Pulmonary emboli were not involved. Considering the extent of the use of fibrinolytic agents, the incidence must be quite low, but it should be considered in this setting.

Protamine sulfate as used by cardiac surgeons to reverse heparinization during cardiac bypass has been reported to produce three types of adverse pulmonary reactions: (1) anaphylactoid generalized reaction, (2) severe bronchospasm, and (3) noncardiac pulmonary edema.[35, 36] All three of these reactions have a sudden onset and progress rapidly. The anesthesiologist may have difficulty in providing ventilation because of the bronchospasm and hyperinflation. Wedge pressures have been normal when measured. Almost half of these patients have had prior exposure to protamine, including protamine zinc insulin. Treatment is supportive, but the reaction may be fatal.

Tocainide is a lidocaine derivative used in treating various dysrhythmias. There are more than 40 known cases of tocainide-induced pneumonitis and fibrosis, almost always of insidious onset.[37] There is a good response to discontinuing the medication and using corticosteroids.

Hydrochlorothiazide can produce a noncardiac pulmonary edema. It occurs only with the hydroxyl radical product of chlorothiazide. Most of those affected have been women and all were receiving intermittent therapy.[38]

INHALANTS

Aspirated oil, such as mineral oil, can produce a focal process mimicking a solitary pulmonary nodule or a segmental pneumonitis. It may, however, insidiously produce a diffuse process, which can progress to respiratory failure.

Oxygen toxicity occurs in any individual receiving a sufficiently high fraction of inspired oxygen for more than 48 hours. In its early phases it is inflammatory and reversible, but after several days it enters a fibrotic irreversible stage with respiratory insufficiency.[39]

INTRAVENOUS

Donor blood from multiparous females who have developed antilymphocytic antibodies to the fetus can transmit these antibodies to the recipient, who has onset of noncardiac pulmonary edema within 1 to 4 hours of initiation of the blood transfusion.[40] The reaction can occur with any blood product, not just red blood cells. In addition to dyspnea and cough resulting from noncardiac pulmonary edema, generalized rash occurs in about half of the cases. Hypotension and fever may also be seen. Treatment is supportive. It is not known whether corticosteroids are of any benefit.

Morrhuate sodium and sodium tetradecyl sulfate are drugs used for sclerosing esophageal varices through the flexible esophagoscope. Its use has been associated with ARDS, beginning within 8 to 24 hours of the initial therapy.[41-43] Experimental animal studies showed a transient increase in pulmonary arterial pressures, and lymph flow returned to baseline in 2 to 8 hours. We have seen 14 cases of respiratory insufficiency secondary to morrhuate sodium administration, and 107 cases of pleural effusion were attributed to this drug at the time of variceal injection.[43a]

MISCELLANEOUS DRUGS

Intralipid or fat emulsion can produce a fat overload syndrome with sudden development of coagulopathy, hepatosplenomegaly, increase in triglyceride levels, and variable end-organ dysfunction including severe hypoxic respiratory failure.[44, 45] Fat emulsion was reported to produce little or no impairment of pulmonary function in normal individuals but to increase the alveolar-arterial oxygen gradient and intrapulmonary shunt in patients with ARDS; therefore it should be given with caution in this group of patients.[46]

A tocolytic agent is a drug used by obstetricians to inhibit uterine contraction during premature labor.[47] The most common tocolytic agents are albuterol (salbutamol) and ritodrine. Physiologically these drugs produce arterial dilatation with an increased intravascular fluid volume. If the drug fails to inhibit uterine contractions, it is discontinued and the mother often receives corticosteroids to accelerate fetal lung maturation. As a result of discontinuing the tocolytic agent, the arterial tone returns to normal in the presence of increased intravascular fluid. The mineralocorticoid effect of the corticosteroids promotes enhanced fluid retention. The outcome may be the development of pulmonary edema, which mimics several entities including aspiration pneumonitis, congestive heart failure, and amniotic fluid embolus. Clues to tocolytic agent–induced pulmonary edema include a drop in the hematocrit caused by hemodilution and a drop in the blood pressure as a result of vasodilation. Treatment is supportive, including the use of oxygen and diuretics.

Overdosage with antidepressant medications is the single most common drug-related reason for emergency room admission.[48] At least 30%, and up to 50%, of patients with tricyclic antidepressant overdosage have abnormal chest roentgenograms, some because of aspiration pneumonia. However, about 10% develop evidence of noncardiac pulmonary edema. Eighty percent have a widened alveolar-arterial oxygen gradient, and most of these patients require mechanical ventilation for some time. The presence of hypotension on admission to the emergency room is highly correlated with the presence of pulmonary edema.

L-Tryptophan is associated with several pleuropulmonary abnormalities: pulmonary hypertension, interstitial pneumonitis, pleural effusion, and a Guillain-Barré type of respiratory muscle weakness with respiratory failure. Most of the deaths in L-tryptophan–induced disease are associated with severe respiratory muscle weakness and respiratory failure.[49-51]

Drug-induced systemic lupus erythematosus can be seen acutely and clinically mimics spontaneous-onset systemic lupus erythematosus with apparent weakness of the diaphragm, interstitial pneumonitis, pericardial effusion, pleural effusion, and increased pulmonary arterial pressure.[52] More than 40 medications are known to induce lupus, but by far the most common drugs or group of drugs are isoniazid, hydralazine, procainamide, the anticonvulsants, and penicillamine. Drug-induced lupus must be considered in any patient receiving these medications who has unexplained pleuropulmonary findings.

Complement-mediated leukostasis with severe noncardiac pulmonary edema can occur with several different medications but particularly with iodinated compounds.[53-56] We think this was the mechanism for the fatal reactions in two patients receiving amiodarone who underwent pulmonary angiograms because of suspected pulmonary emboli. Amiodarone is an iodinated compound and may predispose patients to this reaction; however, many of these patients have had coronary angiograms and other tests using contrast media without this severe reaction. We now use only a nonionic contrast agent in patients receiving amiodarone.

References

1. Treatment-induced respiratory disorders. In: Akoun GM, White JP (eds): Drug-Induced Disorders, Volume 3. Amsterdam, Elsevier, p 377, 1989.
2. Rosenow EC III: Drug-induced lung diseases. In: Kelly WNT (ed): Textbook of Internal Medicine. Philadelphia, JB Lippincott, p 1939, 1989.
3. Cooper JAD Jr, White DA, Matthay RA: Drug-induced pulmonary disease. Part I: Cytotoxic drugs. Am Rev Respir Dis 133:321, 1986.
4. Cooper JAD Jr, White DA, Matthay RA: Drug-induced pulmonary disease. Part II: Noncytotoxic drugs. Am Rev Respir Dis 133:488, 1986.
5. Rosenow EC III: Drug-induced pulmonary disease. In: Murray JF, Nadel JA (eds): The Textbook of Respiratory Medicine. Philadelphia, WB Saunders, p 1681, 1988.
6. Snyder LS, Hertz MI: Cytotoxic drug-induced lung injury. Semin Respir Infect 3:217, 1988.
7. Rice KL: Pulmonary infiltrates associated with noncytotoxic drugs. Semin Respir Infect 3:229, 1988.
8. Holmberg L, Boman G: Pulmonary reactions to nitrofurantoin. 447 cases reported to the Swedish Adverse Drug Reaction Committee 1966–1976. Eur J Respir Dis 62:180, 1981.
9. Sovijarvi ARA, Lemola M, Stenius B, et al: Nitrofurantoin-induced acute, subacute and chronic pulmonary reactions. Scand J Respir Dis 58:41, 1977.
10. Picado C, Castillo JA, Montserrat JM, et al: Aspirin-intolerance as a precipitating factor of life-threatening attacks of asthma requiring mechanical ventilation. Eur Respir J 2:127, 1989.
11. Thisted B, Krantz T, Strom J, et al: Acute salicylate self-poisoning in 177 consecutive patients treated in ICU. Acta Anaesthesiol Scand 31:312, 1987.
12. Dunn TL, Gerber MJ, Shen AS, et al: The effect of topical ophthalmic instillation of timolol and betaxolol on lung function in asthmatic subjects. Am Rev Respir Dis 133:264, 1986.
13. Eagle KA, Boucher CA: Intravenous dipyridamole infusion causes severe bronchospasm in asthmatic patients. Chest 95:258, 1989.
14. Goldiner PL, Carlon GC, Cvitkovic E, et al: Factors influencing postoperative morbidity and mortality in patients treated with bleomycin. Br Med J 1:1664, 1978.
15. Van Barneveld PWC, Sleijfer DT, VanDerMark TW, et al: Natural course of bleomycin-induced pneumonitis. A follow-up study. Am Rev Respir Dis 135:48, 1987.
16. Verweij J, van Zanten T, Souren T, et al: Prospective study on the dose relationship of mitomycin C–induced interstitial pneumonitis. Cancer 60:756, 1987.
17. Sheldon R, Slaughter D: A syndrome of microangiopathic hemolytic anemia, renal impairment, and pulmonary edema in chemotherapy-treated patients with adenocarcinoma. Cancer 58:1428, 1986.
18. Jehn U, Göldel N, Rienmüller R, et al: Non-cardiogenic pulmonary edema complicating intermediate and high-dose ara C treatment for relapsed acute leukemia. Med Oncol Tumor Pharmacother 5:41, 1988.
19. Andersson BS, Luna MA, Yee C, et al: Fatal pulmonary failure complicating high-dose cytosine arabinoside therapy in acute leukemia. Cancer 65:1079, 1990.
20. Dutcher JP, Kendall J, Norris D, et al: Granulocyte transfusion therapy and amphotericin B: Adverse reactions? Am J Hematol 31:102, 1989.
21. Sullivan SN: Sulfasalazine lung. Desensitization to sulfasalazine and treatment with acrylic coated 5-ASA and azodisalicylate. J Clin Gastroenterol 9:461, 1987.
22. Holtzman JL: Gentamicin and neuromuscular blockade (letter). Ann Intern Med 84:55, 1986.
23. Carson CW, Cannon GW, Egger MJ, et al: Pulmonary disease during the treatment of rheumatoid arthritis with low dose pulse methotrexate. Semin Arthritis Rheum 16:186, 1987.
24. Peces R, Riera JR, Arbolea LR, et al: Goodpasture's syndrome in a patient receiving penicillamine and carbimazole. Nephron 45:316, 1987.
25. Conant EF, Fox KR, Miller WT: Pulmonary edema as a complication of interleukin-2 therapy. AJR 152:749, 1989.
26. Lazarus DS, Kurnick JT, Kradin RL: Alterations in pulmonary function in cancer patients receiving adoptive immunotherapy with tumor-infiltrating lymphocytes and interleukin-2. Am Rev Respir Dis 141:193, 1990.
27. Prough DS, Roy R, Bumgarner J, et al: Acute pulmonary edema in healthy teenagers following conservative doses of intravenous naloxone. Anesthesiology 60:485, 1984.

28. Stadnyk A, Grossman RF: Nalbuphine-induced pulmonary edema. Chest 90:773, 1986.
29. Taff RH: Pulmonary edema following naloxone administration in a patient without heart disease. Anesthesiology 59:576, 1983.
30. Martin WJ II, Rosenow EC III: Amiodarone pulmonary toxicity. Recognition and pathogenesis (part 1). Chest 93:1067, 1988.
31. Kay GN, Epstein AE, Kirklin JK, et al: Fatal postoperative amiodarone pulmonary toxicity. Am J Cardiol 62:490, 1988.
32. Gibson GR: Enalapril-induced cough. Arch Intern Med 149:2701, 1989.
33. Kerstein MD, Adinolfi MF: Pulmonary dysfunction associated with streptokinase therapy. Arch Surg 121:852, 1986.
34. Martin TR, Sandblom RL, Johnson RJ: Adult respiratory distress syndrome following thrombolytic therapy for pulmonary embolism. Chest 83:151, 1983.
35. Shapira N, Schaff HV, Piehler JM, et al: Cardiovascular effects of protamine sulfate in man. J Thorac Cardiovasc Surg 84:505, 1982.
36. Culliford AT, Thomas S, Spencer FC: Fulminating noncardiogenic pulmonary edema. A newly recognized hazard during cardiac operations. J Thorac Cardiovasc Surg 80:868, 1980.
37. Feinberg L, Travis WD, Ferrans V, et al: Pulmonary fibrosis associated with tocainide: Report of a case with literature review. Am Rev Respir Dis 141:505, 1990.
38. Grace AA, Morgan AD, Strickland NH: Hydrochlorothiazide causing unexplained pulmonary edema. Br J Clin Pract 43:79, 1989.
39. Jackson RM: Pulmonary oxygen toxicity. Chest 88:900, 1985.
40. Popovsky MA, Abel MD, Moore SB: Transfusion-related acute lung injury associated with passive transfer of antileukocyte antibiodies. Am Rev Respir Dis 128:185, 1983.
41. Korula J, Baydur A, Sassoon C, et al: Effect of esophageal variceal sclerotherapy (EVS) on lung function. A prospective controlled study. Arch Intern Med 146:1517, 1986.
42. Monroe P, Morrow CF Jr, Millen JE, et al: Acute respiratory failure after sodium morrhuate esophageal sclerotherapy. Gastroenterology 85:693, 1983.
43. Saks BJ, Kilby AE, Dietrich PA, et al: Pleural and mediastinal changes following endoscopic injection sclerotherapy of esophageal varices. Radiology 149:639, 1983.
43a. Zeller FA, Cannon CR, Prakash UBS: Thoracic manifestations after esophageal variceal sclerotherapy. Mayo Clin Proc 66:727, 1991.
44. Kollef MH, McCormack MT, Caras WE, et al: The fat overload syndrome: Successful treatment with plasma exchange. Ann Intern Med 112:545, 1990.
45. Bass J Jr, Friedl W, Jeranek W: Intralipid causing adult respiratory distress syndrome. J Natl Med Assoc 76:401, 1984.
46. Hwang TL, Huang SL, Chen MF: Effects of intravenous fat emulsion on respiratory failure. Chest 97:934, 1990.
47. Pisani RJ, Rosenow EC III: Pulmonary edema associated with tocolytic therapy. Ann Intern Med 110:714, 1989.
48. Roy TM, Ossorio MA, Cipolla LM, et al: Pulmonary complications after tricyclic antidepressant overdose. Radiology 170:667, 1989.
49. Travis WD, Kalafer ME, Robin HS, et al: Hypersensitivity pneumonitis and pulmonary vasculitis with eosinophilia in a patient taking an L-tryptophan preparation. Ann Intern Med 112:301, 1990.
50. Kilbourne EM, Swygert LA, Philen RM, et al: Guidance on the eosinophilia-myalgia syndrome (editorial). Ann Intern Med 112:85, 1990.
51. Tazelaar HD, Myers J, Drage CW, et al: Pulmonary disease associated with L-tryptophan-induced eosinophilic myalgia syndrome. Clinical and pathologic features. Chest 97:1032, 1990.
52. Tororitis MC, Rubin RL: Drug-induced lupus. Genetic, clinical, and laboratory features. Postgrad Med 78:149, 1985.
53. Schneiderman H, Hammerschmidt DE, McCall AR, et al: Fatal complement-induced leukostasis after diatrizoate injection. Principles of clinicopathologic diagnosis. JAMA 250:2340, 1983.
54. Solomon DR: Anaphylactoid reaction and non-cardiac pulmonary edema following intravenous contrast injection. Am J Emerg Med 4:146, 1986.
55. Boden WE: Anaphylactoid pulmonary edema ("shock lung") and hypotension after radiologic contrast media injection. Chest 81:759, 1982.
56. Delacour JL, Floriot C, Wagschal G, et al: Non-cardiac pulmonary edema following intravenous contrast injection. Intensive Care Med 15:49, 1988.

CHAPTER 82

Barotrauma, Decompression Sickness, and Air Embolism

Stephen R. Thom

Disorders such as decompression sickness (DCS) and air embolism used to be viewed as within the purview of only a small group of physicians involved in military, naval, or aerospace operations. This is no longer the case. Scuba diving has become a common recreational activity as well as an industrial and scientific tool. It is currently estimated that there are some 2.7 million sport divers in the United States, and nearly 300,000 new divers are trained per year. There are between 500 and 600 diving injuries treated each year and approximately 90 fatalities.[1] Physicians in coastal communities are most likely to be called on to treat these injuries. In addition, iatrogenic air embolism is an increasingly recognized problem in daily medical practice. There are no accurate estimates of the frequency of iatrogenic embolism. Efforts to assess the risk of some procedures have led to the conclusion that many go unreported.[2] Therefore, knowledge of the treatment for this condition is an obligatory element of critical care practice that is independent of geography.

PATHOPHYSIOLOGY OF GAS BUBBLE–RELATED DISORDERS

The physical principles related to bubble-mediated disorders are straightforward. In the ocean the ambient environmental pressure increases by 1 atmosphere (atm) for every 33 ft. Therefore, at a depth of say 66 ft, ambient pressure is that of the atmosphere plus 2.0 atm for the water, equaling 3.0 atmospheres absolute (ata). Compressed air from scuba (self-contained underwater breathing apparatus) equipment is delivered at ambient pressure. Hence, the work of breathing is nominally increased by the resistance of the system and not by the hydrostatic pressure impinging on the chest wall.

Gas is dissolved in the body in proportion to its partial pressure according to Henry's law. However, the rate at which a tissue becomes saturated is virtually always limited by the rate of gas delivery and thus the local blood flow. Gas uptake is unequal throughout the body because blood flow is unequally distributed in the body and also because the solubility of inert gas (e.g., nitrogen, 79% of air) in tissues depends on with the lipid/water ratio. As an average figure, the half-time for body saturation with nitrogen at a given partial pressure is estimated to be 23 minutes.[3]

In like manner, gas must be removed from tissues on decompression. In his now classic approach to assessing decompression risk, Haldane theorized that DCS could be avoided if no tissue nitrogen partial pressure were allowed to exceed twice the absolute pressure.[3] He calculated decompression tables based on the hypothesis that there are five different tissue half-times (i.e., rates of perfusion) in the body. Remarkably little has changed in nearly 100 years, and current decompression tables are largely based on Haldane's theory. The fundamental issue is that on decompression some degree of supersaturation of tissues is tolerated, without bubble formation, as a driving force for removal of nitrogen from tissues to the plasma. Gas is then transported to the lungs, where gas tension in the blood quickly equilibrates with the alveolar gas tension.

Diffusion of gas from one body compartment to another, for example, muscle to fat, does not significantly affect uptake and removal of inert gas under normal circumstances. In the pathologic state when bubbles form, however, diffusion takes on enormous importance. Gas in the bubble is physically isolated from the circulation and gas transport across the phase boundary is required to eradicate the bubble. The result is that the elimination of this gas after decompression is markedly slower than its uptake at depth.[4-6]

A bubble can present a mechanical obstruction if it occurs in a vascular space. Doppler bubble detectors have been used effectively in animals and humans to track bubbles after decompression. Bubbles appear to arise almost exclusively in the venous circulation and hence in an area of lower hydrostatic pressure. Arterial bubbles are seen with extreme decompression stress, and their presence is usually associated with severe DCS.[7, 8] The site of origin of these bubbles is unclear but is probably venous. The mechanisms by which these bubbles may gain arterial entry are discussed in detail later.

Extravascular bubbles have been found in the eye, urine, cerebrospinal fluid, and myelin in animals subjected to severe decompression stress.[3, 9, 10] Gas accumulation in the joints and periarticular tissues of humans has been shown with decompression to altitude.[11] One can speculate on how extravascular bubbles may impede blood flow, particularly in an area bounded by a poorly compliant capsule. However, direct evidence supporting this mechanism in DCS is sparse.

The intracellular environment appears to be remarkably resistant to bubble formation. Explosive decompression of microorganisms from hundreds of atmospheres produces bubbles only when there is a pre-existing gas phase.[12] Erythrocytes and even erythrocyte vesicles are similarly resistant, suggesting that it is not a cytoplasmic characteristic but rather some structuring of water by the cell membrane boundary that prevents gas nucleation.[13]

Inert gas bubbles in the plasma result in a nonpolar environment that can denature globular proteins. On contact with a bubble, the protein can unfold and insert the formerly sequestered hydrophobic domain into the bubble. Lipoproteins denatured in this manner may be one source of the fat emboli that sometimes occur in severe DCS.[14] A similar mechanism has been proposed for bubble introduction during cardiopulmonary bypass.[15]

Bubbles can also precipitate an acute inflammatory reaction. Hageman's factor is directly activated by bubbles, leading to activation of the intrinsic clotting system and kinin.[16, 17] Complement, activated by the alternative pathway, appears to have major importance in the development of symptoms on decompression. It was shown that complement activation in response to bubbles is variable within the population, and those more sensitive to complement activation are also more susceptible to DCS.[18] Animals depleted of complement do not show evidence of DCS when subjected to provocative decompression.[19]

Platelets degranulate in response to interactions with bubbles,[20] causing both platelet depletion and formation of circulating thrombi. Complement-mediated recruitment and activation of polymorphonuclear leukocytes set the stage for further microvascular insults. Pulmonary hypertension seen in association with venous air embolism appears to be due to agents released by activated platelets and polymorphonuclear leukocytes and not local factors such as bubble occlusion of capillary lumen or thromboxane production.[21, 22] There are still other local effects of bubbles that are not well defined. Cerebral arterial microemboli, small enough to pass

through the vasculature without being trapped, provoke an immediate marked arteriolar vasodilatation that lasts approximately 90 minutes. This effect is followed by a progressive decrease in flow, below the normal level, and an associated depression of neural function.[23]

BAROTRAUMA

Pressure-induced injury, barotrauma, arises from two mechanisms. The more common form occurs when exogenous pressure cannot be adequately communicated or equalized with that in an air-filled body space. The more catastrophic second form occurs on decompression when high-pressure gas within the body cannot be vented to the environment at a rate sufficient to prevent overexpansion trauma.

Ear-Sinus Barotrauma

The most common diving problem arises because mucosal congestion fails to allow adequate eustachian tube ventilation to equalize the pressure in the external ear with that in the middle ear. As a diver descends in the water, pressure causes an inward distortion of the tympanic membrane which may then rupture. Pain, vertigo, tinnitus, and hearing loss may occur. Although not life threatening, this injury is extremely uncomfortable and may lead to panic, particularly in the novice diver, that may precipitate more severe injury (e.g., drowning, uncontrolled ascent, and pulmonary overexpansion injury). Often the injury stops short of frank tympanic membrane rupture. The patient complains of ear pain and a sensation of ear blockage or diminished hearing. On examination one finds gradations of hemorrhage within the substance of the eardrum. Treatment includes cessation of diving until signs and symptoms clear and easy autoinflation of the ears is demonstrated. Oral decongestants may also be used. In a case of tympanic membrane perforation, a complete otologic evaluation is indicated, but fortunately most perforations heal spontaneously.

A diver who performs a forceful Valsalva maneuver at depth while trying to equalize pressure in the middle ear may generate sufficient pressure to rupture the round window. The mechanism is usually an explosive rupture caused by the transmission of cerebrospinal fluid pressure that is increased by both ambient hydrostatic pressure and the Valsalva maneuver.[24] At times, implosive rupture occurs when a diver manages to increase the middle-ear pressure in an excessively forceful manner. Tinnitus, vertigo, and hearing loss are the immediate sequelae. Treatment is largely expectant, and otologic evaluation is mandatory. In the acute setting, the greatest concern is differentiation of this disorder from inner-ear DCS, for which recompression treatment should be undertaken. Generally, a history of onset of symptoms during compression rather than on ascent or after leaving the water allows distinction between the two injuries.

Sinus barotrauma related to inadequate pressure equilibration can occur among scuba divers and aviators.[25] Blockages of the sinus ostia are caused by congestion of the nasal mucosa or a mass. With a rapid increase in ambient pressure that is poorly transmitted to a sinus, mucosal engorgement, edema, and inflammation result. Headache, epistaxis, and localized sinus pain are common symptoms. Sinus barotrauma can also result from a sudden decrease in environmental pressure if a one-way valve blockage occurs at a sinus ostium. Pressure within the sinus builds and in the extreme may be sufficient to rupture the sinus. Pneumocephalus, shown in Figure 82–1, occurred with frontal sinus rupture in a diver with an upper respiratory tract infection who had previous sinus surgery. In cases such as these, careful obser-

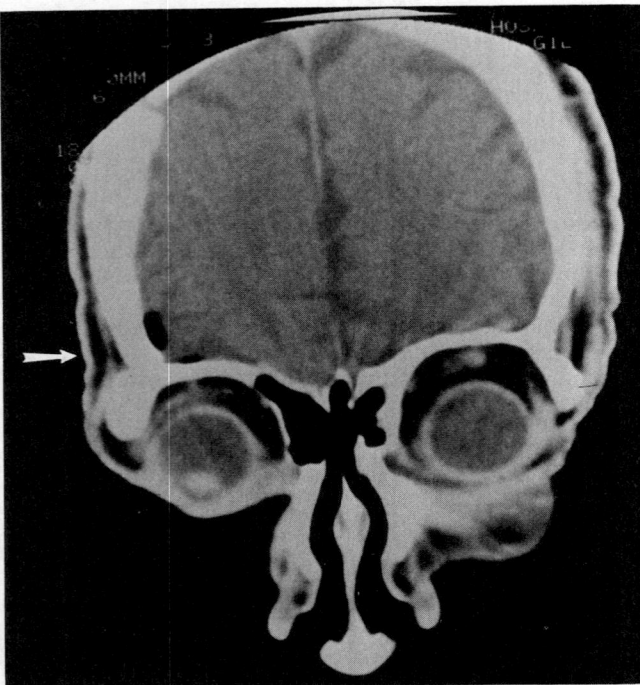

Figure 82–1. Pneumocephalus (*arrow*) after decompresssion in an individual with a history of previous sinus surgery and congestion resulting from an upper respiratory tract infection.

vation and prophylactic antibiotics for meningitis risk are used. The patient in this case had no untoward developments, and a computed tomogram 1 month later was normal.

Pulmonary Barotrauma

Professional breath-hold diving is a common practice in some areas of the world (e.g., women divers of Japan *[ama]* and Korea *[hae-nyo]*). It is also an exceedingly common recreational practice, albeit rarely to the depths visited by professionals. As a diver descends in the water and pressure increases, the gas in the lungs is compressed. The depth at which injury occurs is somewhat variable. In theory, pulmonary edema and alveolar rupture with hemorrhage occur when total lung volume is decreased below residual lung volume. For example, if a diver with a total lung capacity of 6.5 L and a residual volume of 1.5 L dives to 110 ft (4.3 ata), lung volume decreases to residual volume. Remarkably, this is only half as deep as some individuals have gone on a breath-hold dive. It is thought that this may be related to a significant reduction in a diver's residual volume because of immersion. In these situations, intrathoracic blood volume may be increased by as much as 1 L.[26, 27]

Open water scuba diving is commonly undertaken to a depth of 100 ft. This situation is entirely different from breath-hold diving because the demand regulator on a diver's air tank delivers gas at ambient pressure. Hence, there is no loss of lung volume, but the stage is set for overexpansion when pressure is decreased as the diver ascends. Probably the most common source of pulmonary overexpansion injury in daily medical practice is mechanical ventilation. Alveolar rupture has been observed when trans-alveolar pressure ranged from 20 to 80 mm Hg, with the intact chest wall providing an extra measure of resilience.[28, 29] The site of rupture appears to be the common border of the alveolar base and vascular sheath.[30] A pressure differential of 80 mm Hg occurs over only 3.5 ft in the ocean.

Scuba divers who ascend while holding their breath are at risk, as are those with underlying pulmonary disorders such as reduced pulmonary compliance, hyperactive airways (e.g., asthmatics), and any condition that partially obstructs the airway.[31, 32] There are several manifestations of overexpansion injury and they require somewhat different approaches to clinical management.

It is rare for diving-related overexpansion injury to stop short of alveolar rupture and the appearance of air beyond the visceral pleural boundary. On occasion, however, a diver may present with dyspnea, hypoxia, and hemoptysis without manifestations of more typical overexpansion injuries.[33] Treatment is supportive, with maintenance of adequate oxygenation and, perhaps most important, ruling out more severe overexpansion injuries and DCS.

After alveolar rupture, air may dissect the perivascular sheath to the mediastinum and pericardium. This diagnosis of mediastinal emphysema is established by chest x-ray study (Fig. 82–2). Typically, a radiolucent band is found laterally along the cardiac border on the posteroanterior film and almost always is seen retrosternally in the lateral view.[34] The diagnosis is often made incidentally, but on occasion subcutaneous emphysema or chest discomfort is noted. The only other physical finding may be a crackling sound over the heart during systole, Hamman's sign, present in about one half of cases.[35] There is no specific treatment for this disorder, but ventilation with 100% oxygen is recommended to hasten nitrogen elimination. Rarely, cervical mediastinotomy is required if a tension pneumomediastinum occurs.

Overexpansion with a tear of the visceral pleural may cause a pneumothorax to develop. Although a simple pneumothorax may arise initially, a scuba diver at depth may rapidly develop a tension pneumothorax as the volume of gas increases exponentially on ascent (Fig. 82–3). With a simple pneumothorax, patients may present with dyspnea and chest pain and may be found to have a unilateral

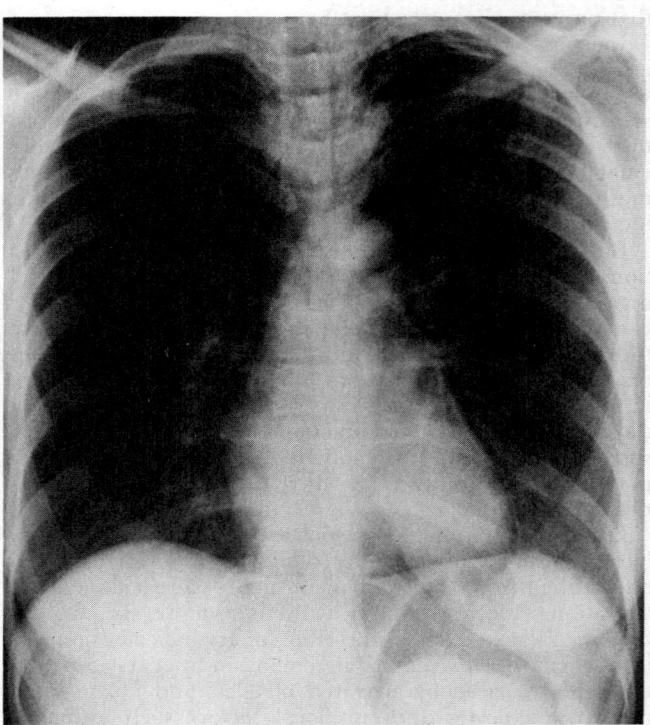

Figure 82–2. Pneumomediastinum in an asymptomatic scuba diver after a rapid ascent from 45 ft in sea water. Note the radiolucent band along the left cardiac border.

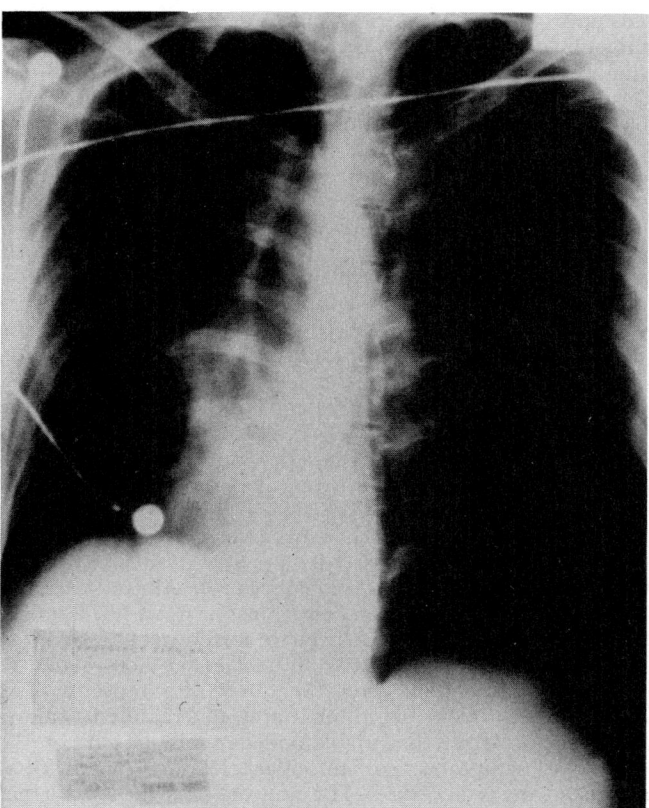

Figure 82–3. Left tension pneumothorax with shift of mediastinal structures.

decrease in breath sounds, hyperresonance to percussion, and, in approximately one fourth of cases, subcutaneous emphysema.[36] With a tension pneumothorax, patients may also exhibit tracheal deviation, distended neck veins, and cyanosis. Compromised venous return associated with this condition is a life-threatening emergency. Immediate chest decompression is typically accomplished by insertion of a large-bore needle into the second intercostal space in the midline of the affected hemithorax. After this a tube thoracostomy can be made, usually in the fourth intercostal space in the midaxillary line.

DECOMPRESSION SICKNESS

DCS is caused by bubbles of inert gas in the blood and body tissues. The variety and severity of symptoms depend on the volume and location of the bubbles. Over time, all body tissues become saturated with inert gas, and the concentration of the gas is proportional to its partial pressure (Henry's law). On decompression, gas must be removed from tissues, and significant rapid lowering of pressure leads to bubble formation. This is true regardless of the pressure at which the body is first saturated. Therefore, DCS is a disorder not only of scuba divers but also of aviators and astronauts.

Clinical Manifestations

In DCS there is a continuum of signs and symptoms ranging from skin itching and vague constitutional symptoms to shock and cardiopulmonary arrest. Inert gas bubbles precipitate DCS, but the disorder is not simply related to the presence of such bubbles. It is now clearly established that a diver may have bubbles form and not develop evidence of DCS. In fact, 5 to 10% of inert gas absorbed by the tissues in a normal dive is released as bubbles after decompression.[5, 37] These observations have led to the view that bubble formation is not widespread but rather limited to discrete nucleation sites. The volume or "load" or bubbles and their location in the body determine whether symptoms occur. Doppler ultrasound detectors have been used to good advantage in studying some aspects of DCS in humans. Relatively low bubble grades are generally good predictors of safe decompression profiles; however, high grades (evidence of a large number of bubbles) are poor predictors of individual risk of DCS.

Regardless of which symptoms a patient may report, the onset of the symptoms is usually relatively prompt. Approximately three fourths of patients experience symptoms within 1 hour of decompression.[1] Ninety percent develop symptoms within 12 hours of decompression. A small number may not present for 24 to 48 or more hours after diving, which makes diagnosis difficult at times. An added source of confusion arises when divers fly soon after diving. Conventional aircraft are not pressurized to 1.0 ata; therefore, flight represents an added decompression risk to a diver who may have a subclinical bubble load. It is now a rather common occurrence to care for patients who have developed DCS while in a jet returning from a diving vacation. To diminish this problem it is generally recommended that divers wait a minimum of 24 hours after diving before they fly.

Patients frequently describe fatigue, malaise, and a sense of foreboding as a prodrome to more severe manifestations of DCS. On rare occasions, these may be their only complaints. It is speculated that these general complaints are related to a bubble load sufficient to precipitate some of the secondary biochemical changes described under Pathophysiology of Gas Bubbles but below a threshold for more serious symptoms. Other hypotheses include bubble involvement in cerebral centers for wakefulness and adrenocortical exhaustion.[38, 39]

Pruritus is relatively common among individuals exposed to high inert gas pressures in a hyperbaric chamber and is thought to be due to formation of small bubbles in the skin. This is not a manifestation of systemic bubble formation or a prodrome to DCS. Among patients who have been diving, cutaneous manifestations evolve from areas of pruritus to localized erythema and then to mottled areas of cyanosis. Presumably, signs and symptoms arise because of vasospasm or obstruction of venous drainage by bubbles in the skin. A rarer cutaneous finding that is frequently associated with musculoskeletal DCS is a raised patch of skin, usually with follicular depressions, a peau d'orange effect. This is thought to reflect lymphatic obstruction by bubbles.[40]

Among the most common manifestation of DCS is an achy limb pain, which occurs in 50 to 70% of cases.[41, 42] Characteristically, the pain is at first vaguely localized and over time increases in intensity and becomes periarticular. More than one site may be affected, but a bilaterally symmetric distribution is rare. Virtually any joint may be involved. Interestingly, the shoulder is most frequently affected in scuba divers, whereas the hip is the most common site among aviators and those who work in compressed air in tunnels. Symptoms are thought to arise because of bubbles in the periarticular tissues.[43] The mechanism by which pain is produced remains unclear but probably involves physical deformation (e.g., stretch) of noncompliant tissues and impaired blood flow. Perhaps the most convincing evidence for this comes from high-altitude research, in which individuals with gas in periarticular, noncompliant tissues all complained of symptoms, whereas those with only intra-articular gas had none.[11] The secondary biochemical effects of bubbles may also be involved.

A general perception for many years has been that approximately one third of patients with DCS have signs and symptoms relatable to impairment of the nervous system. Newer estimates suggest, however, that the incidence may be closer to 60%.[1] Most of these cases involve spinal cord dysfunction, usually in the lower thoracic or upper lumbar region. Weakness and paresthesias of a leg are reported, which may progress to paraplegia. Band-like abdominal pain is sometimes also present. Bowel and bladder dysfunction, most typically urine retention, must be specifically assessed in these cases. Peripheral nerve involvement with patchy hypoesthesia, hyperesthesia, or paresthesia is sometimes reported.[41, 44] Cerebral DCS, protean in its presentation, may be manifest as a vague change in personality, loss of memory, visual disturbance, or acute psychosis.[44, 45] In 90% or more of these cases, symptoms occur within 1 hour of surfacing.[46]

Hypotheses regarding pathogenesis of neurologic DCS are numerous. There is compelling evidence that spinal cord DCS arises largely from venous stasis. Inert gas bubbles liberated from the spinal cord region appear to coalesce and occlude venous outflow.[47, 48] This mechanism does not, however, explain all clinical phenomena, and some aspects of spinal cord DCS as well as other neurologic forms of DCS may be due to bubble formation within the substance of nervous tissue.[49] When neurologic symptoms evolve in a delayed fashion after decompression, microvascular arterial embolization may be involved.[50]

Vestibular DCS is manifested by a sudden onset of vertigo, often with tinnitus, nausea, vomiting, and nystagmus and sometimes with hearing loss. It is referred to as "the staggers" in diving circles. Pathogenesis is thought to involve the presence of bubbles in the eighth cranial nerve neural connections or, more likely, in the inner ear. Animal data suggest that bubbles in the semicircular canals rupture the membranes and damage the cochlea, resulting in hemorrhage.[51]

In perhaps 2 to 8% of DCS cases, the venous bubble load is sufficient to precipitate symptoms of pulmonary embolism. In animals subjected to severe decompression profiles, Doppler detection of bubbles in the pulmonary arteries is associated with elevated pulmonary arterial and right ventricular pressures and decreased cardiac output and arterial oxygenation.[52, 53] The pulmonary insult may be compounded by bubble-mediated activation of polymorphonuclear leukocytes and platelets. In humans, initial manifestations may be only cough and substernal discomfort. Over minutes to hours patients progress to frank dyspnea, cyanosis, and shock. Decompression stress has been demonstrated to alter pulmonary microvascular permeability.[54]

Treatment

In all forms of DCS, attention should be paid to the possibility of intravascular volume depletion caused by the surface activity of bubbles, which triggers secondary inflammation.[55, 56] Specific electrolyte disturbances are not characteristic of DCS, although both hypo- and hyperkalemia have been reported.[57, 58] A chest x-ray film should be obtained when possible to assess whether overexpansion injury has occurred, and arterial oxygenation should be determined.

Definitive treatment of DCS includes hyperbaric oxygen administration in a recompression chamber. Emergent treatment should always include 100% oxygen ventilation. This treatment decreases the plasma nitrogen concentration, increasing the gradient of nitrogen from bubbles to plasma. Impressive early improvement of symptoms can be seen with this approach, which is expected to decrease the volume of the bubbles. This process is then augmented in a hyperbaric chamber. Treatment is most commonly begun at 2.8 ata. Based on Boyle's law, pressurization directly decreases bubble volume, thus decreasing tissue distortion and vascular compromise. The increased pressure also increases the inert gas partial pressure within the bubble, which hastens complete elimination of the bubble as oxygen ventilation maintains a plasma inert gas partial pressure of virtually zero.

Hyperbaric oxygen therapy often takes 4 hours or more, as bubble elimination may be slow in areas of poor flow where platelet- and polymorphonuclear leukocyte–mediated intravascular "sludging" and edema have occurred. Over the course of treatment, stepwise decompression is carried out. The outcome depends on the severity of the initial injury, which is reflected by both the signs and symptoms and the rapidity of onset of symptoms on decompression. In serious forms of DCS involving pulmonary and neurologic insults (called type II DCS), cure or nearly complete resolution of symptoms is seen in 60 to 75% of cases.[42, 44, 45] Delay of treatment is expected to have an adverse effect; indeed, in one study success decreased from 75% to only 57% when treatment was delayed beyond 12 hours.[42] Altitude-induced DCS seems to have an even better prognosis with treatment, and complete recovery has been reported in 97% or more of cases.[59, 60] This improved rate may in part be related to more rapid treatment after the onset of symptoms. The average delay from symptom onset to treatment among injured sport divers is variable and depends in part on the severity of symptoms. For musculoskeletal, or type I, DCS, the mean delay is 6 days. For neurologic symptoms it has been variously reported as 16 to 30 hours.[1, 45] However, even when patients present after delays of days, successful treatment has been reported.[42, 61]

Emergency on-scene treatment with hydration and 100% oxygen may result in improvement or even complete resolution of symptoms before arrival at an emergency department. This should not dissuade the practitioner from proceeding with recompression therapy, however. Although at times there is continued recovery among divers who are not treated with recompression, this is usually seen only with musculoskeletal or extremely mild neurologic cases.[1, 45] Moreover, some patients suffer a relapse, and if treatment is initially withheld there is further delay and thus a diminished chance for successful recompression treatment.

Adverse effects of hyperbaric oxygen therapy are relatively rare. Alterations in pulmonary function in association with standard, repetitive hyperbaric oxygen exposures have not been observed.[62, 63] Symptoms of carinal irritation and dry cough, which precede measurable decrements in pulmonary function, occur on rare occasion in divers who respond slowly and therefore undergo extended recompression therapy.[62] Sinus barotrauma is of more theoretic than practical significance in the context of diving injuries, as these patients have already exhibited an ability to equalize pressure in their sinuses with compression. The most pronounced manifestation of oxygen toxicity associated with clinical use of hyperbaric oxygen involves the central nervous system. Grand mal seizures occur in approximately 1 in 10,000 compressions and fortunately are not associated with pathologic changes.[64–66] Intermittent hyperbaric oxygen can cause myopia, but usually this is seen only in older patients who undergo repetitive treatments. Myopia is thought to be due to an alteration in the lens structure. It is virtually always temporary and reverses within approximately 6 weeks after treatment is terminated.[67] Nuclear cataract formation has been noted among patients who have undergone intermittent treatment over many months and received hyperbaric oxygen for more than 200 hours.[68] This is well in excess of the treatment recommended for DCS.

Additional forms of therapy that have been recommended for DCS include heparin and coumarin anticoagulants, corticosteroids, and various nonsteroidal anti-inflammatory drugs. Anticoagulants are not now recommended for inner-ear DCS, in which hemorrhage is often seen.[69] The value of corticosteroids is debated. In one animal study involving spinal cord DCS, methylprednisolone provided no added benefit with concomitant recompression therapy.[70] Because of the involvement of platelets with intravascular bubbles, there has been some interest in the potential for using aspirin and other antiaggregating agents in decompression stress situations. Prophylactic use of antiplatelet drugs was found to be beneficial in several[71, 72] but not all[73] animal studies. Prophylactic aspirin has failed to prevent the post-decompression fall in platelet survival in humans. Anti-inflammatory drugs appear to have merit in treating residual pain after treatment of musculoskeletal DCS, as symptoms may indeed be due to inflammation.[74]

AIR EMBOLISM

Etiology

Any breach of the vascular wall that allows contact of air with blood can give rise to air embolism. There are situations in which pathologic events are more common, and the severity of symptoms varies with the ultimate location of the bubbles.

Rapid decompression such that the rate of gas efflux from the lungs is lower than the rate of gas volume change precipitates pulmonary overexpansion. Uncontrolled ascent from scuba diving at depths of 3.5 ft or more and sudden loss of cabin pressure in an aircraft are the two events most likely to cause for accidental injury. Rupture of the alveolar capillary wall in these instances provides conditions for development of arterial gas emboli. Trauma to the great vessels can have a similar effect but becomes a concern only after treatment of the primary injury and restoration of intravascular volume.[75] Insufflation of air into the vagina, particularly in a pregnant woman, may also give rise to air embolism. This would be expected to result in a venous embolic picture, but it may also lead to arterial emboli.[76] There are also fatal instances associated with childbirth without purposeful injection of air.[77]

Air embolism is an ever-present danger in medical procedures. The early history of this subject has been reviewed.[78] Brauer, in 1906, was probably the first to recognize fatal iatrogenic embolism, which was in the setting of pneumothorax formation and irrigation of empyema cavities. Essentially any invasive chest procedure can cause air embolism. Reported causes range from a relatively simple thoracentesis[75] to open heart surgery with extracorporeal oxygenation or circulation. Stoney and colleagues[2] suggested that the recorded cases of air embolism with cardiopulmonary bypass may only be a small fraction of the total. In a retrospective survey they identified an incidence of 1 per 1000 procedures. Air embolism associated with cranial surgery, especially with the patient in a sitting or Fowler's position, commonly precipitates venous (pulmonary) air embolism.[79] Air-cooled laser surgery of the uterine cavity has been recognized to cause venous gas embolism, and gas cooling should no longer be done.[80] Starzl and colleagues[81] reported suspected cerebral air embolism in 9 of 48 liver transplantation cases. Air introduced with vascular anastomosis of the graft is hypothesized to gain access to the arterial circulation through a pulmonary arteriovenous fistula in these patients with chronic liver disease. Arterial catheterization, arteriography, and hemodialysis are additional recognized sources.[82] There is also some risk with intravenous lines, especially central venous catheters.[83] With a pressure gradient of only 5 cm H_2O, air can pass through a 14-gauge catheter at the rate of 100 mL/s.[83]

Signs and Symptoms

Bubbles entering the venous circulation usually lodge in the lungs. Symptoms, if they occur at all, are therefore referable to this organ. Animal experiments demonstrate that both the total quantity of air and its rate of entry determine whether serious injuries occur. Injection of 5 to 7.5 mL/kg/min may be rapidly fatal, whereas volumes of air well in excess of 5 mL/kg are tolerated if the rate of entry is less than 1 mL/min.[84, 85] Bubbles precipitate pulmonary hypertension, edema, and eventually right-sided heart failure. The movement of bubbles within the right side of the heart can occasionally be auscultated over the precordium, the sound being vaguely reminiscent of a sponge being squeezed. The sound is heard throughout the cardiac cycle and is historically referred to as a "millwheel" murmur.[86] There are times when there may be no signs or only mild wheezing. Laboratory findings may include hypoxia and evidence of right-sided heart strain on electrocardiography. Rarely, an air-fluid level in the pulmonary artery, a pathognomonic sign, has been reported.[87]

Symptoms and signs of arterial gas embolism depend on the final location of the bubbles. Bubbles typically break up as they reach branch points in the arteriolar network and ultimately lodge in vessels with diameters ranging from 30 to 60 μm.[88] Kidney embolization may be manifest as renal failure, hematuria, or proteinuria. Failure of other visceral organs, gastrointestinal bleeding, and uterine bleeding have been described. Skin involvement may appear as cyanotic "marbling." Perhaps of historical interest are the so-called Liebermeister's sign, a sharply defined area of tongue pallor, and air bleeding—observation of air when a vessel is incised or a needle inserted. In my experience, these signs are typically noted in settings when the diagnosis is patently obvious and the outcome fatal.

The most serious clinical events arise with embolization to the coronary arteries and central nervous system. As little as 0.5 mL of air can precipitate myocardial infarction.[89] Potentially fatal dysrhythmias are also reported.[28] Cerebral gas emboli may be manifest as seizures, discrete cranial nerve dysfunction, hemisensory or motor deficits, or loss of vision. Often, however, bilateral asymmetric defects are noted, as are alterations in the level of consciousness. There are remarks in the literature suggesting that cerebral embolism of up to 1 mL of air is well tolerated.[90] This is now thought to be due to extracranial passage of air through anastomotic channels. Injection of only tenths of a milliliter of air can lead to profound morbidity or death, although individual outcome may vary.[91] The buoyancy of bubbles has some impact on their distribution. In the upright posture head embolization is more likely than trunk embolization.

There are local and systemic cardiovascular responses to cerebral air embolism. Cardiac dysrhythmias mediated by autonomic discharge and catecholamine release, as well as hypertension, may occur. Cerebrovascular responses include immediate vasodilatation with reactive hyperemia of the tissues surrounding the area of infarction. Loss of autoregulation causes passive transfer of systemic pressure to the central nervous system and elevated intracranial pressures.[91, 92]

The diagnosis of cerebral air embolism should be entertained wherever central nervous system deficits arise after a vascular lumen is opened to air. Neurologic findings in a scuba diver diving in less than 30 ft of sea water (a scenario in which DCS in extremely unlikely) should as a rule be presumed to be due to pulmonary overpressurization injury and cerebral air embolism.

Arterial gas embolism in a situation in which only venous emboli should occur is referred to as paradoxical arterial embolism. It is particularly because of the possibility of this occurring that iatrogenic venous air emboli should not be taken lightly. Venous bubbles can enter the arterial circulation across a cardiac septal defect. Perhaps 30% of the population have a patent foramen ovale.[93] The normal pressure differential between the left and right atria and the valve covering over the foramen keeps the septum competent under most circumstances. In a setting of pulmonary embolism with elevated right-sided heart pressures this situation changes. Transient opening may also be associated with something as benign as a Valsalva maneuver.[94] Paradoxical embolism has gained attention as a possible etiology for cerebral deficits among scuba divers with DCS. Several studies have established a high likelihood of atrial septal defects in this group of patients.[95, 96] The possibility of microvascular air emboli triggering DCS has been discussed in relation to several cases with particularly severe neurologic deficits.[97]

There are other possible mechanisms for the passage of air bubbles from the pulmonary to the systemic circulation. The possibility of arteriovenous fistula in patients with chronic liver disease has already been mentioned. Transpulmonic passage of venous bubbles through the capillary network has been hypothesized in cases of massive showering of the lungs with bubbles.[98] In addition, the efficiency of filtration of venous bubbles by the pulmonary circulation can be significantly altered by several general anesthetics, including halothane and nitrous oxide.[99] In settings in which pulmonary overpressurization injuries have occurred, the possibility of air entry into the arterial vasculature because of microscopic barotrauma, without overt pneumothorax, has been suggested.[100]

Treatment

Supportive care with attempts to maintain oxygenation and circulation is a standard, accepted approach to venous gas embolism. The buoyancy of bubbles has some impact on their location. Durant and colleagues,[86] in 1947, demonstrated in animals that massive air embolism to the right ventricle sufficient to block the pulmonary artery can be made to rise away from the outflow tract to the apex, with resumption of blood flow. Placement of patients in the left lateral decubitus position, the Durant maneuver, appears to improve outcome when oxygen and vasopressors are also used.[101] When air has entered the arterial circulation, however, buoyancy forces cannot overcome arterial blood pressure.[102] There has been concern about the potential for elevating intracranial pressure in patients with concomitant cerebral air embolism by performing this maneuver. The current recommendation is to refrain from positioning a patient in this manner or to do so only transiently to dislodge bubbles that have not yet entered the pulmonary artery.

There have been reports of dramatic improvements in cardiopulmonary function in some patients when a catheter was advanced into the right side of the heart and the air evacuated.[103] Experience has been gained in treating pulmonary air embolism with hyperbaric oxygen and recompression almost exclusively in patients with DCS and pulmonary involvement. As one might expect, symptoms usually resolve rapidly with treatment based on principles already discussed.[42] In other situations associated with pulmonary air embolism and severe obstruction of pulmonary blood flow, little experience with recompression has been reported. If patients do not succumb rapidly because of cor

pulmonale, supportive measures often improve clinical status. In this case ventilation with 100% oxygen can be extremely beneficial in reducing bubble volume. Air in the pulmonary arteriolar network is removed principally by diffusion into the alveolar space rather than into plasma.[104] Bronchodilators are also frequently used to combat bronchospasms in these patients.

As with DCS, emergent treatment of arterial air embolism includes hydration and 100% oxygen ventilation. Simple physics provides the basis for expecting therapeutic benefit with recompression therapy. Direct observation of cerebral vessels has verified that gas bubbles are compressed and perfusion is improved when an animal is treated in a hyperbaric chamber.[88] Because changes in bubble volume are directly proportional to pressure, there has been some effort to determine what pressure may be most efficacious. Bubbles disappear from the cerebral circulation with compression to between 3.0 and 4.0 ata. A direct comparison of 2.8- and 6.0-ata compression showed little overall difference.[105] This is attributed largely to the fact that the greatest change in volume of a bubble occurs with early compression, such as going from 1.0 to 2.0 ata (from 100 to 50% of former bubble size) versus 5.0 to 6.0 ata (from 20 to 17% of former bubble size). This observation has considerable practical importance because one-person hyperbaric chambers capable of 3.0-ata compression are relatively common in the United States, whereas only a few centers with larger chambers are capable of administering 6.0 ata (Fig. 82–4).

Prognosis is generally improved with earlier treatment of cerebral air embolism. There appears to be a rather sharp decrease in clinical efficacy after approximately a 4- to 5-hour delay. In one series involving diving-related cerebral air embolism, treatment was successful in 48 of 66 cases (73%) if treatment was begun within 4 hours.[106] Similar observations have been made in a smaller series of cases of iatrogenic cerebral air embolism.[107] Of eight patients treated within 5 hours of onset of symptoms, five (63%) recovered completely and three had partial resolution. Among six patients treated 11 to 25 hours later, complete resolution was seen in only two, partial resolution in two, and no change in two.

Emergent treatment with 100% oxygen and hydration ameliorates some of the acute symptoms of cerebral air embolism. In one series of 42 sport divers, 56% had some improvement in symptoms in transit to a hyperbaric chamber.[108] With a mean delay to treatment of only 3 hours, 78% of divers in this series had complete or nearly complete recovery with recompression therapy. A number of patients may experience complete resolution of symptoms without receiving recompression therapy. In one series of 81 sport divers, 2 had complete resolution.[1] In another series of 34 cases, 8 patients who presented with no initial loss of consciousness and apparently rather mild symptoms spontaneously recovered.[45]

Particularly among severely injured patients, some have neurologic deterioration after seemingly successful recompression treatment. Because of this, there has been an examination of recompression profiles as well as the possible use of adjunctive measures during recompression therapy. The etiology of relapse is unclear. Hypotheses include slow re-expansion of in situ residual gas on decompression, re-embolization from an underlying pulmonary injury, and the so-called postischemic reperfusion phenomenon. Comparison of several recompression profiles in animals suggests that use of more hyperbaric oxygen and lower pressures (e.g., 2.8 ata) rather than an initial high-pressure exposure with air at 6.0 ata may decrease the incidence of relapses.[106] Therapeutic adjuncts that have shown some promise in animal trials include lidocaine[109] and a combination of pros-

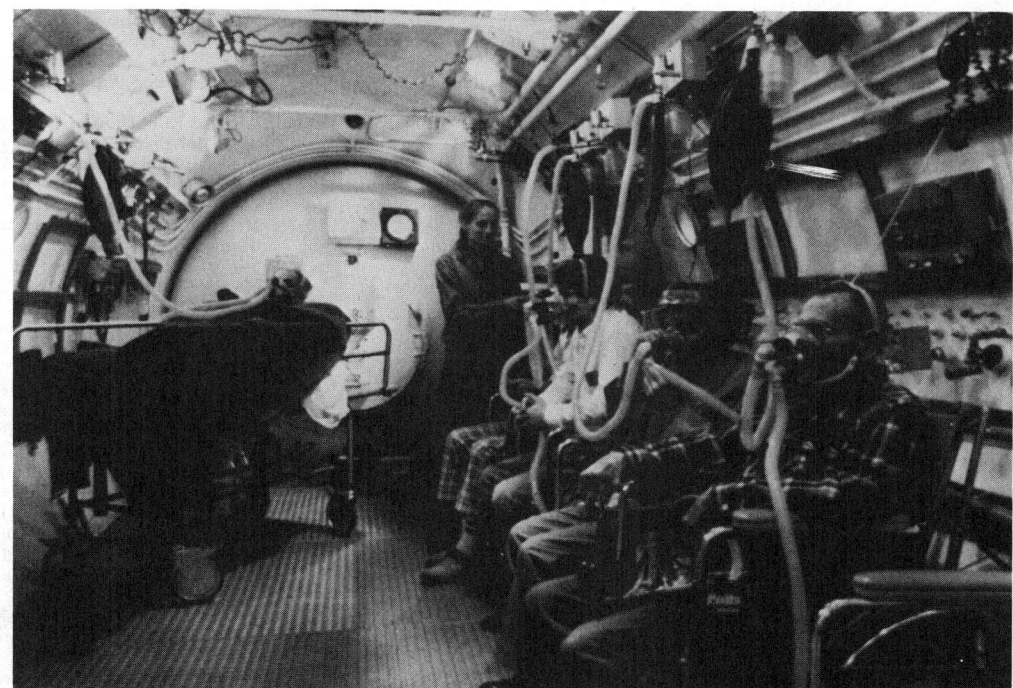

Figure 82–4. Main hyperbaric chamber at the Institute for Environmental Medicine, University of Pennsylvania. The chamber is compressed to as much as 6 ata with air, and patients breathe supplemental oxygen via a tight-fitting (continuous positive airway pressure) face mask, hood, or endotracheal tube. Mechanical ventilation can be carried on in the chamber, as well as intravenous infusions, cardiac and arterial line monitoring, and transvenous cardiac pacing.

taglandin I_2, indomethacin, and heparin.[110] The use of bolus doses of steroids may decrease the frequency of relapse,[106] but evidence for the benefit of this treatment is inconclusive. The standard treatment for patients with residual deficits is repetitive, intermittent hyperbaric oxygen, and stepwise improvements are often seen over several days.[111]

Aeromedical transport has become a common means of conveyance for critically injured patients. Because of the decrease in atmospheric pressure with altitude, however, there is a risk to patients with DCS or air embolism. A patient's condition may worsen acutely because of expansion of bubbles. Because prognosis is closely linked to expeditious recompression therapy, the clinician must make a choice of transport mode based on the severity of a patient's injuries and differences in transport times with ground versus aeromedical evacuation. Ideally, transport in an aircraft pressurized to 1.0 ata should be arranged when distances are great. Several military and civilian aircraft, such as the Cessna Citation and Learjet, can be pressurized to sea level. More commonly, the distances involved in moving patients to a recompression chamber in the continental United States make helicopter transport a consideration. The risk to a patient can be diminished by making certain that the lowest safe altitude is maintained (e.g., 300 to 500 ft, depending on the terrain). The medical crew can help to combat enlargement of bubbles by maintaining ventilation with 100% oxygen and adequate hydration.

There continues to be a misconception in the general medical community that hyperbaric chambers are few and are not equipped to manage critically injured patients. In fact, most chamber systems are capable of maintaining cardiovascular support and mechanical ventilation of patients undergoing hyperbaric treatment. Information on chambers in all geographic regions is outlined in publications by the Undersea and Hyperbaric Medical Society, Bethesda, MD. Emergency information can be obtained through the Divers Alert Network by calling 919–684–8111.

References

1. Divers Alert Network: Report on 1988 Diving Accidents. Durham, NC, Duke University, 1989.
2. Stoney WS, Alford WC, Burrus GR, et al: Air embolism and other accidents using pump oxygenators. Ann Thorac Surg 29:336, 1980.
3. Boycott AE, Damant GCC, Haldane JS: The prevention of compressed air illness. J Hyg 8:342, 1908.
4. D'Aoust BG, Smith KH, Swanson HT: Decompression-induced decrease in nitrogen elimination in awake dogs. J Appl Physiol 41:348, 1976.
5. Hills BA: Effect of decompression per se on nitrogen elimination. J Appl Physiol 45:916, 1978.
6. Kindwall ER, Baz A, Lightfoot EN, et al: Nitrogen elimination in man during decompression. Undersea Biomed Res 2:285, 1975.
7. Gardette B: Correlation between decompression sickness and circulating bubbles in 232 divers. Undersea Biomed Res 6:99, 1979.
8. Spencer MP, Campbell SD, Sealey JL, et al: Experiments on decompression bubbles in the circulation using ultrasonic and electromagnetic flow meters. J Occup Med 11:238, 1969.
9. Cockett ATK, Nakamura RM, Franks JJ: Recent findings in the pathogenesis of decompression sickness (dysbarism). Surgery 58:384, 1965.
10. Gersh I, Hawkinson GE, Rathbun EN: Tissue and vascular bubbles after decompression from high pressure atmospheres—Correlation of specific gravity with morphological changes. J Cell Comp Physiol 24:35, 1944.
11. Ferris EB, Engle GL: The clinical nature of high altitude decompression sickness. In: Fulton JF (ed): Decompression Sickness. Philadelphia, WB Saunders, p 4, 1951.
12. Hemmingsen EA, Hemmingsen BB, Owe JJ, et al: Lack of bubble formation in hypobarically decompressed cells. Aviat Space Environ Med 58:742, 1987.
13. Hemmingsen BB, Steinberg NA, Hemmingsen EA: Intracellular gas supersaturation tolerances of erythrocytes and resealed ghosts. Biophys J 47:491, 1985.
14. Haymaker W: Decompression sickness. In: Lubarsh O, Henke F, Rassle R (eds): Handbuch der speziellen Pathologischen: Anatomie und Histologie, Volume XIII, Part 1. Berlin, Springer-Verlag, p 1600, 1957.
15. Lee WH, Krumhaar D, Fonkalsrud ER, et al: Denaturation of plasma proteins as a cause of morbidity and death after intracardiac operations. Surgery 50:29, 1961.
16. Hallenbeck JM, Bove AA, Moquin RB, et al: Accelerated coagulation of whole blood and cell-free plasma by bubbling in vitro. Aerospace Med 44:712, 1973.
17. Hallenbeck JM, Bove AA, Elliott DH: The bubble as a nonmechanical trigger in decompression sickness. In: Ackles KN (ed): Blood-Bubble Interactions in Decompression Sickness. Downsview, Defense and Civil Institute of Environmental Medicine, p 129, 1973. Publication 73-CP-960.
18. Ward CA, McCullough D, Fraser WD: Relation between complement activation and susceptibility to decompression sickness. J Appl Physiol 62:1160, 1987.
19. Ward CA, McCullough D, Yee D, et al: Complement activation involvement in decompression sickness of rabbits. Undersea Biomed Res 17:51, 1990.
20. Philp RB, Schacham P, Gowdey CW: Involvement of platelets and microthrombi in experimental decompression sickness: Similarities with disseminated intravascular coagulation. Aerospace Med 42:494, 1971.

21. Domb M, Goldstein J, Vincent JL, et al: Hemodynamic, gasometric and hematological effects of air infusion in dogs: Leukotriene inhibition with U 60,257. Bull Eur Physiopathol Respir 22:375, 1986.
22. Fukushima M, Kobayashi T: Effects of thromboxane synthase inhibition on air emboli lung injury in sheep. J Appl Physiol 60:1828, 1986.
23. Helps SC, Parsons DW, Reilly PL, et al: The effect of gas emboli on rabbit cerebral blood flow. Stroke 21:24, 1990.
24. Farmer JC: Otological and paranasal sinus problems in diving. In: Bennett PB, Elliott DH (eds): The Physiology and Medicine of Diving and Compressed Air Work. 3rd ed. London, Bailliere Tindall, p 507, 1982.
25. Neblett LM: Otolaryngology and sport scuba diving: Update and guidelines. Ann Otol Rhinol Laryngol 94(suppl 115):2, 1985.
26. Craig AB: Depth limits of breath hold diving (an example of Fennology). Respir Physiol 5:14, 1968.
27. Schaefer KE, Allison RD, Dougherty JH, et al: Pulmonary and circulatory adjustment determining the limits of depths in breath-hold diving. Science 162:1020, 1968.
28. Rukstinat GJ, LeCount ER: Air in the coronary arteries. JAMA 91:1776, 1928.
29. Malhotra MS, Wright HC: Effects of raised intrapulmonary pressure on the lungs of fresh unchilled cadavers. J Pathol Bacteriol 82:198, 1961.
30. Macklin MT, Macklin CC: Malignant interstitial emphysema of the lungs and mediastinum as an important occult complication in many respiratory diseases and other conditions: An interpretation of the clinical literature in light of laboratory experiments. Medicine 23:281, 1944.
31. Colebatch HJH, Smith MM, Ng CKY: Increased elastic recoil as a determinant of pulmonary barotrauma in divers. Respir Physiol 26:55, 1976.
32. Liebow AA, Stark JE, Vogel J, et al: Intrapulmonary air trapping in submarine escape training casualties. US Armed Forces Med J 10:265, 1959.
33. Balk M, Goldman JM: Alveolar hemorrhage as a manifestation of pulmonary barotrauma after scuba diving. Ann Emerg Med 19:930, 1990.
34. Fraser RG, Pane JAP: Diagnosis of Diseases of the Chest, Volume 3. 2nd ed. Philadelphia, WB Saunders, p 1812, 1977.
35. Wilson R: Thoracic injuries. In: Tintinalli J (ed): A Study Guide in Emergency Medicine, Volume 3. Dallas, American College of Emergency Physicians, p 16.31, 1978.
36. Kirsh MM, Sloan H: Blunt Chest Trauma: General Principles of Management. Boston, Little, Brown, p 919, 1977.
37. Powell MR, Spencer MP, von Ramm OT: Ultrasonic surveillance of decompression. In: Bennett PB, Elliott DH (eds): The Physiology of Diving and Compressed Air Work. 3rd ed. London, Bailliere Tindall, p 404, 1982.
38. Dewey WA: Decompression sickness—An emerging recreational hazard. N Engl J Med 267:759, 1962.
39. Rozsahegyi I, Roth B: Participation of the central nervous system in decompression. Ind Med Surg 35:101, 1966.
40. Edmonds C, Thomas RL: Medical aspects of diving—Part 4. Med J Aust 2:1367, 1972.
41. Rivera JC: Decompression sickness among divers: An analysis of 935 cases. Milit Med 129:316, 1964.
42. Green RD, Leitch DR: Twenty years of treating decompression sickness. Aviat Space Environ Med 58:362, 1987.
43. Daniels S, Davies JM, Paton WDM, et al: Recent experiments using ultrasonic imaging to monitor bubble formation in divers. In: Bachrach AJ, Matzen MM (eds): Underwater Physiology, Volume VIII. Bethesda, Undersea Medical Society, p 249, 1984.
44. Erde E, Edmonds C: Decompression sickness: A clinical series. J Occup Med 17:324, 1975.
45. Dick PK, Massey EW: Neurologic presentation of decompression sickness and air embolism in sports divers. Neurology 35:667, 1985.
46. Francis TJR, Pearson RR, Robertson AG, et al: Central nervous system decompression sickness: Latency of 1070 human cases. Undersea Biomed Res 15:403, 1989.
47. Hallenbeck JM, Bove AA, Elliott DH: Mechanisms underlying spinal cord damage in decompression sickness. Neurology 25:308, 1975.
48. Hallenbeck JM: Cinephotomicrography of dog spinal vessels during cord-damaging decompression sickness. Neurology 26:190, 1976.
49. Francis TJR, Pezeshkpour AH, Dutka AJ, et al: Is there a role for the autochthonous bubble in the pathogenesis of spinal cord decompression sickness? J Neuropathol Exp Neurol 47:475, 1988.
50. Francis TJR, Pezeshkpour AH, Dutka AJ: Arterial gas embolism as a pathophysiologic mechanism for spinal cord decompression sickness. Undersea Biomed Res 16:439, 1989.
51. Money KE, Buckingham IP, Calder IM, et al: Damage to the middle and the inner ear in underwater divers. Undersea Biomed Res 12:77, 1985.
52. Bove AA, Hallenbeck JM, Elliott DH: Circulatory responses of venous air embolism and decompression sickness in dogs. Undersea Biomed Res 1:207, 1974.
53. Neuman TR, Spragg R, Howard R, et al: Cardiopulmonary consequences of decompression stress. Am Rev Respir Dis 177:162, 1978.
54. Chryssanthou C, Springer M, Lipschitz S: Blood-brain and blood-lung barrier alteration by dysbaric exposure. Undersea Biomed Res 4:117, 1977.
55. Bove AA, Hallenbeck JM, Elliott DH: Changes in blood and plasma volumes in dogs during decompression sickness. Aerospace Med 45:49, 1974.
56. Barnard EEP, Hanson JM, Rowton-Lee MA, et al: Post-decompression shock due to extravasation of plasma. Br Med J 2:154, 1966.
57. Kindwall EP, Margolis I: Management of severe decompression sickness with treatment ancillary to recompression: Case report. Aviat Space Environ Med 46:1065, 1975.
58. Melamed Y, Ohry A: The treatment and the neurological aspects of diving accidents in Israel. Paraplegia 18:127, 1980.
59. Wirjosemito SA, Touhey JE, Workman WT: Type II altitude decompression sickness (DCS): U.S. Air Force experience with 133 cases. Aviat Space Environ Med 60:256, 1989.
60. Davis JC, Anderson GK, Douglas G, et al: Altitude decompression sickness: Hyperbaric therapy results in 145 cases. Aviat Space Environ Med 48:722, 1977.
61. Myers RAM, Bray P: Delayed treatment of serious decompression sickness. Ann Emerg Med 14:254, 1985.
62. Clark JM, Lambertsen CJ: Pulmonary oxygen toxicity: A review. Pharmacol Rev 23:37, 1971.
63. Hart GB, Strauss MB, Riker J: Vital capacity of quadriplegic patients treated with hyperbaric oxygen. J Am Paraplegia Soc 7:91, 1984.
64. Clark JM: Oxygen toxicity. In: Bennett PB, Elliott DH (eds): The Physiology and Medicine of Diving and Compressed Air Work. 3rd ed. London, Bailliere Tindall, p 200, 1982.
65. Davis JC: Hyperbaric medicine: Patient selection, treatment procedures, and side effects. In: Davis JC, Hunt TK (eds): Problem Wounds: The Role of Oxygen. New York, Elsevier, p 225, 1988.
66. Hart GB, Struass MB: Central nervous system oxygen toxicity in a clinical setting. In: Bove AA, Bachrack AJ, Greenbaum LJ (eds): Undersea and Hyperbaric Physiology, Volume IX. Bethesda, Undersea and Hyperbaric Medical Society, p 695, 1987.
67. Lyne AJ: Ocular effects of hyperbaric oxygen. Trans Ophthalmol Soc UK 98:66, 1978.
68. Palmquist BM, Philipson B, Barr PO: Nuclear cataract and myopia during hyperbaric oxygen therapy. Br J Ophthalmol 68:113, 1984.
69. Farmer JC, Thomas WG, Youngblood DA, et al: Inner ear decompression sickness. Laryngoscope 86:1315, 1976.
70. Francis TJR, Dutka AJ: Methyl prednisolone in the treatment of acute spinal cord decompression sickness. Undersea Biomed Res 15:165, 1989.
71. Popovic P, Popovic V, Honeycutt C: Levodopa and aspirin pretreatment beneficial in experimental decompression sickness. Fed Proc 40:423, 1981.
72. Inwood MJ: Experimental evidence in support of the hypothesis that intravascular bubbles activate the hemostatic process. In: Ackles KN (ed): Blood-Bubble Interactions in Decompression Sickness. Downsview, Defense and Civil Institute of Environmental Medicine, p 171, 1973. Publication 73-CP-960.
73. Bennett PB, Brock AJ: Action of selected drugs on decompression sickness in rats. Aerospace Med 40:607, 1969.
74. Douglas JD: Intramuscular diclofenac sodium as adjuvant therapy for type I decompression sickness: A case report. Undersea Biomed Res 13:457, 1986.
75. Thomas AN: Air embolism following penetrating lung injuries. J Thorac Cardiovasc Surg 66:533, 1973.
76. Bray P, Myers RAM, Cowley RA: Orogenital sex as a cause of nonfatal air embolism in pregnancy. Obstet Gynecol 61:653, 1983.
77. Mylks GW, Brown AB, Robinson CR: Air embolism during labor. Can Med Assoc J 56:427, 1947.
78. Schlaepfer K: Air embolism following venous diagnostic or therapeutic procedures in diseases of the pleura and lung. Johns Hopkins Med J 33:321, 1922.
79. Hunter AR: Air embolism in the sitting position. Anaesthesia 17:467, 1962.
80. Gas/air embolism associated with intrauterine laser surgery. FDA Drug Bull 20:6, 1990.
81. Starzl TE, Schneck SA, Mazzoni G, et al: Acute neurological complication after liver transplantation with particular reference to intraoperative cerebral air embolus. Ann Surg 187:236, 1978.
82. Baskin SE, Wozniak R: Hyperbaric oxygenation in the treatment of hemodialysis associated air embolism. N Engl J Med 293:184, 1975.
83. Flanagan JP, Gradisar IA, Gross RJ, et al: Air embolus—A lethal complication of subclavian puncture. N Engl J Med 281:488, 1969.
84. Oppenheimer MJ, Durant TM, Lynch P: Body position in relation to venous air embolism and the associated cardiovascular-respiratory changes. Am J Med Sci 225:362, 1953.
85. Richardson HF, Coles BC, Hall GE: Experimental gas embolism. Can Med Assoc J 36:584, 1937.
86. Durant TM, Long J, Oppenheimer MJ: Pulmonary (venous) air embolism. Am Heart J 33:269, 1947.
87. Kinard RE, Williams JE, Orrison WW: Venous air embolism. South Med J 80:96, 1987.
88. Waite C, Mazzone WF, Greenwood ME, et al: Dysbaric cerebral air embolism. In: Lambertsen CJ (ed): Underwater Physiology, Volume III. Washington, DC, National Academy of Sciences, p 205, 1967.

89. Spencer FC, Rossi NP, Yu SC, et al: The significance of air embolism during cardiopulmonary bypass. J Thorac Cardiovasc Surg 49:615, 1965.

90. Van Allen CM, Hrdina LS, Clark J: Air embolism from the pulmonary vein. A clinical and experimental study. Arch Surg 19:567, 1929.

91. De la Torre E, Meredith J, Netsky MG: Cerebral air embolism in the dog. Arch Neurol 6:67, 1962.

92. Evans DE, Kobrine AI, Weathersby PK, et al: Cardiovascular effects of cerebral air embolism. Stroke 12:338, 1981.

93. Thompson T, Evans WP: Paradoxical embolism. Q J Med 23:135, 1930.

94. Lynch JJ, Schuchard GH, Gross CM, et al: Prevalence of right-to-left arterial shunting in a healthy population: Detection by Valsalva maneuver contrast echocardiography. Am J Cardiol 53:1478, 1984.

95. Wilmshurst PT, Byrne JC, Webb-Peploe MM: Relation between interatrial shunts and decompression sickness in divers. Lancet 1:1302, 1989.

96. Moon RE, Camporesi EM, Kisslo JA: Patent foramen ovale and decompression sickness in divers. Lancet 1:513, 1989.

97. Neuman TS, Bove AA: Combined arterial gas embolism and decompression sickness following no-stop dives. Undersea Biomed Res 17:429, 1990.

98. Butler BD, Hills BA: Transpulmonary passage of venous air emboli. J Appl Physiol 59:543, 1985.

99. Butler BD, Leiman BC, Katz J: Arterial air embolism of venous origin in dogs: Effect of nitrous oxide in combination with halothane and pentobarbitone. Can J Anaesth 34:570, 1987.

100. Golding FC, Griffiths P, Hempleman HV, et al: Decompression sickness during construction of the Danforth Tunnel. Br J Ind Med 17:167, 1960.

101. Gottlieb JD, Ericsson JA, Sweet RB: Venous air embolism. Anesth Analg 44:773, 1965.

102. Butler BD, Laine GA, Leiman BC, et al: Effect of the Trendelenburg position on the distribution of arterial air emboli in dogs. Ann Thorac Surg 45:198, 1988.

103. Marshall WK, Bedford RF: Use of a pulmonary artery catheter for detection and treatment of venous air embolism: A prospective study in man. Anesthesiology 52:131, 1980.

104. Pressor RG, Kirk KR, Haselby KA, et al: Fate of air emboli in the pulmonary circulation. J Appl Physiol 67:1898, 1989.

105. Leitch DR, Greenbaum LJ, Hallenbeck JM: Cerebral arterial air embolism: Is there benefit in beginning HBO treatment after 6 bar? Undersea Biomed Res 11:221, 1984.

106. Leitch Dr, Green RD: Pulmonary barotrauma in divers and the treatment of cerebral arterial gas embolism. Aviat Space Environ Med 57:931, 1986.

107. Murphy BP, Harford FJ, Cramer FS: Cerebral air embolism resulting from invasive medical procedures. Ann Surg 201:242, 1985.

108. Kizer KW: Dysbaric cerebral air embolism in Hawaii. Ann Emerg Med 16:535, 1987.

109. Evans DE, Catron DW, McDermott JJ, et al: Effect of lidocaine after experimental cerebral ischemia induced by air embolism. J Neurosurg 70:97, 1989.

110. Hallenbeck JM, Leitch DR, Dutka AJ, et al: Prostaglandin I$_2$, indomethacin and heparin promote postischemic neuronal recovery in dogs. Ann Neurol 12:145, 1982.

111. Leitch DR: Treatment of air decompression illness in the Royal Navy. In: Davis JC (ed): Treatment of Serious Decompression Sickness and Arterial Gas Embolism. Bethesda, Undersea Medical Society, p 11, 1979. Report 34 WS (SDS).

CHAPTER 83

Pulmonary Edema: Lung Water Balance in Relation to Physiologic Monitoring and Clinical Outcome in the Critically Ill

Mark A. Camp
Barry A. Gray

We are born with pulmonary edema and, if we live long enough, we will likely die with pulmonary edema. Pulmonary edema occurs with left ventricular failure, mitral valve dysfunction, intravascular volume overload, and various forms of lung injury. Edema plays a major role in the clinical and physiologic expression of the respiratory aspects of these disorders. The purpose of this chapter is to examine our current understanding of both the pathophysiology of pulmonary edema and, more important, the physiologic mechanisms that keep the lungs dry. We focus on the aspects of these concepts that are related to physiologic monitoring and therapeutic intervention in the critically ill patient. With the wide application of pulmonary arterial catheterization in the intensive care unit, it becomes important to understand the relation of pulmonary capillary pressure to the other factors that determine lung water balance. Similarly, knowledge of the forces that operate in the interstitial space of the lung is necessary to understand the effects of different forms of positive pressure breathing.

FACTORS DETERMINING LUNG WATER BALANCE

The lung has two barriers to the formation of pulmonary edema: the vascular endothelium, which impedes the formation of interstitial pulmonary edema, and the respiratory epithelium, which impedes the formation of alveolar edema. Fluid filtration from the vasculature to the interstitium occurs through the walls of the smaller-caliber vessels of the lung, which consist of a single layer of endothelial cells. The lower respiratory tract is lined by a single layer of respiratory epithelium. These cells are normally impermeable to both fluids and solutes. They represent the barrier to the formation of alveolar edema when excess fluid accumulates in the interstitial space. Lung water balance depends on the balance of forces acting across these barriers.[1]

Vascular Endothelium. Two primary forces must be considered when describing fluid balance across the vascular endothelium of the lung: the hydrostatic pressure gradient and the osmotic pressure gradient. The same two forces act across any semipermeable membrane and are illustrated by the equation first presented by Ernest Starling in 1896:[2]

$$F = K_f[(Pcap - Pisf) - \sigma(\pi plasma - \pi isf)] \quad (1)$$

where F = rate of fluid filtration
K_f = filtration coefficient
Pcap = capillary hydrostatic pressure
Pisf = interstitial fluid hydrostatic pressure
πplasma = oncotic pressure of plasma
πisf = oncotic pressure of interstitial fluid

σ   = osmotic reflection coefficient of the endothelium

Pcap and πplasma are the intravascular components of these forces—the capillary hydrostatic pressure, which acts to filter fluid into the interstitial space, and the oncotic pressure, which exerts an effect in the opposite direction. Pisf and πisf are the extravascular components of these forces, the interstitial hydrostatic pressure serving to oppose fluid filtration from the vascular space (when positive) and the πisf acting in the opposite direction.

The vascular endothelium has two different variables in the Starling equation: K_f and σ. The filtration coefficient K_f represents permeability to water and is the product of vascular surface area (S) and hydraulic conductivity (L_p). The reflection coefficient σ depends on permeability to protein. Its value is 1 if a barrier is totally impermeable to protein and 0 if the barrier is fully permeable.

Classification of Pulmonary Edema. Pulmonary edema is generally classified according to the mechanism that produces the increase in fluid flux across the vascular endothelium. Thus, the terms *high-pressure, hydrostatic,* and *cardiogenic* pulmonary edema refer to conditions associated with elevated Pcap, and the terms *low-pressure, high-permeability,* and *noncardiogenic* pulmonary edema refer to conditions in which K_f is elevated and σ is reduced. Of course, reduced πplasma could also produce a form of pulmonary edema associated with low Pcap and normal permeability.

Two aspects of the Starling equation deserve attention. First, if the hydraulic conductivity of the membrane is increased, fluid filtration is more sensitive to small changes in the hydrostatic pressure gradient, Pcap − Pisf. Second, as the membrane becomes more permeable to protein (σ approaches 0), the entire oncotic portion of the equation approaches 0 and the hydrostatic pressure gradient assumes major importance. Thus, the Starling relationship suggests that the distinction between high-pressure pulmonary edema and low-pressure pulmonary edema may not necessarily decide appropriate therapy. Whether the mechanism of pulmonary edema is increased pressure or increased permeability, the principal vehicle for therapeutic intervention might be a reduction in Pcap.

Alveolar Epithelium. Analogous transmembrane forces act across the alveolar epithelium.[1] There are two principal differences. First, the alveolar barrier is much less permeable to both fluid and solutes of any size. The result is that under normal conditions essentially no fluid or protein is able to enter the alveolar space. During the formation of pulmonary edema the alveolar barrier prevents the formation of alveolar edema until a substantial amount of interstitial edema (35% increase in lung water) has accumulated.[3-5] When alveolar flooding does occur there appears to be a transformation of the alveolar membrane from an impermeable barrier to a barrier that is freely permeable to both water and solute. The nature and site of this transformation are not well understood.[1] The second principal difference is that, unlike the endothelium, the alveolar epithelium exhibits active transport[6] that can promote resorption of fluid against an oncotic pressure gradient.[7]

Quantitative Aspects of the Starling Equation and Pulmonary Edema. Guyton and Lindsey in 1959 performed a classic series of experiments in which they progressively increased left atrial pressure (Pla) in dogs by acutely constricting the thoracic aorta.[8] They found that Pla greater than 24 mm Hg resulted in pulmonary edema formation in animals with a normal protein concentration. In selected animals, they decreased the plasma protein content by performing plasmapheresis. In these animals with reduced πplasma (protein content = 47% of control), Pla greater

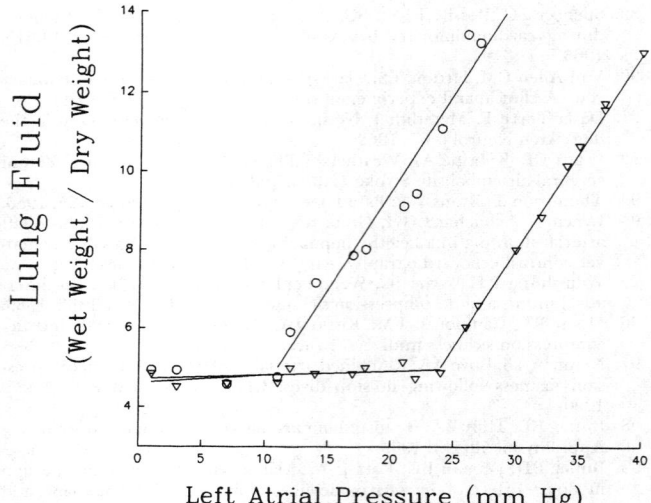

Figure 83–1. Fluid in the lungs of dogs subjected to 0.5 hour of Pla elevation to various values. (▽) Dogs with normal plasma protein concentration. (○) Dogs whose plasma protein concentration had been reduced to an average equal to 47% of the normal value. (This graph illustrates the findings of Guyton and Lindsey.[8])

than 11 mm Hg caused edema formation (Fig. 83–1). It should be noted that the normal colloid osmotic pressure was 24 mm Hg in these experiments. When plasma oncotic pressure was normal there was no tendency for edema formation with increases in pressure if Pla was less than 24 mm Hg. When oncotic pressure was reduced there was no increase in lung water at pressures less than 11 mm Hg. These experiments suggested that there was a threshold Pla for pulmonary edema above which vascular fluid would leak out into the lung. This threshold appeared to occur when the Pla exceeded the πplasma, implying that σ is equal to one and that Pisf and πisf could be ignored. As is often the case, this is an oversimplification of the complex situation in vivo. Subsequent studies from that laboratory and many others have made it clear that lung water balance is more complex for a number of reasons. First, at normal vascular pressures there is continuous transvascular filtration of fluid, which is removed from the interstitial space by the pulmonary lymphatics.[9] This indicates that there is a net unbalanced gradient for fluid filtration under normal conditions; that is, Pcap − σπplasma is greater than Pisf − σπisf. Second, because pulmonary lymph contains plasma proteins, σ is less than 1 and πisf is not 0. Third, Pcap and Pla are not equivalent.[10] Fourth, Pisf is not 0,[4] and in fact both Pisf and πisf play important roles in lung water balance.[10-12] To formulate a rational approach to the interpretation of hemodynamic data and πplasma measurements, it is necessary to examine these concepts in more detail.

Capillary Pressure

The microcirculation of the lungs lacks media and adventitia at diameters of less than 75 μm on the arterial side and less than 200 μm on the venous side.[13, 14] The bulk of fluid and protein exchange occurs through these vessels, which have a single layer of endothelium directly situated on the basement membrane and an assortment of pathways for intra- and extracellular transport of water and solute (Fig. 83–2).[15-19] A clear distinction should be made between Pla or pulmonary capillary wedge pressure (Ppcw), which is an estimate of Pla, and the pressure in these microvessels, which is the hydrostatic force promoting fluid filtration in the lung (Pcap in the Starling equation).[20] The difference between

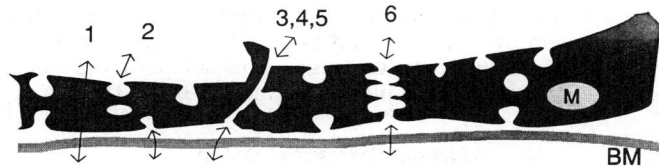

Figure 83–2. Diagram indicating six possible mechanisms for transport of fluid and solute through four pathways across the pulmonary endothelium. The pathways and mechanisms are as follows: (1) Cellular, directly through endothelial cell membranes and cytoplasm (water, small nonpolar solutes, lipid-soluble solutes). (2) Vesicular, small cytoplasmic vesicles thought to shuttle back and forth between opposing cell surfaces and to exchange fluid and solutes by equilibrating contents at each surface. (3 to 5) The intercellular junction, which allows transport by three mechanisms: (3) lateral diffusion in cell membranes through junctional complexes may provide a pathway for water-insoluble solutes; (4) narrow junctions may provide pathways for diffusion and ultrafiltration exchange of water and lipid-insoluble solutes up to the size of small plasma proteins; (5) wide junctions permit exchange of plasma proteins and other large molecules as well. The structure of the junctions appears to vary from arterial to venous regions of the microvascular bed. (6) Transitory open channels formed by the confluence of chains of micropinocytotic vesicles may provide an additional extracellular transport pathway. M = mitochondrion; BM = basement membrane. (Adapted from Renkin EM: Multiple pathways of capillary permeability. Circ Res 41:735–743, 1977, by permission of the American Heart Association, Inc.)

Pcap and Pla depends on the longitudinal distribution of pulmonary vascular resistance. A number of experimental techniques for determining the arterial and venous components of pulmonary vascular resistance and the actual Pcap have been evaluated.[10, 20–24] In general, it appears that 60% of pulmonary vascular resistance is in the upstream precapillary segment and 40% is downstream between the capillaries and the left atrium.[10] Thus Pcap is approximately 40% of the difference between pulmonary arterial pressure (Ppa) and Pla added to Pla.

Holloway and colleagues[21] developed a technique that allows Pcap to be estimated under clinical conditions by examining the pressure tracing as the pulmonary arterial catheter is being wedged (Fig. 83–3). The intersection between the initial rapid pressure fall, caused by run-off from the arterial segment into the more compliant capillary segment, and the later more slowly developing pressure fall, caused by run-off from the capacitance of the capillary bed into the veins and left atrium, is the estimated Pcap. Under normal conditions with Ppa − Pla = 10 mm Hg, Pcap would be 4 mm Hg greater than Pla. With elevated pulmonary vascular resistance the difference between Pcap and Pla increases, but not always in a predictable fashion. The venous fraction of pulmonary vascular resistance may vary from 0.2 to 0.7 in patients with acute respiratory failure, depending on the endogenous release or exogenous administration of vasoactive agents.[25–28]

Vertical Gravitational Effects

Regional Pcap also deviates from Pla because of gravitational effects. For every centimeter below the left atrium, regional Pcap exceeds the Pcap at the left atrial level by 1 cm H_2O (0.73 mm Hg). The opposite is true for regions above the left atrium except for zone 1, where Ppa is 0. The relevance of this gravitational gradient to regional lung water balance depends on the gravitational gradient for Pisf. Although the data are conflicting, depending on the method used to estimate Pisf, it appears that the gravitational gradient for Pisf is between 0.6 and 0.8 cm H_2O/cm vertical distance.[29, 30] This partially explains the well-recognized clin-

ical phenomenon that edema tends to accumulate in the most dependent regions of the lung.

Interstitial Fluid Pressure

The interstitial pressure in the lung is more difficult to determine than the intravascular pressure.[1] Several different techniques have been used to estimate Pisf, including insertion of micropipettes,[31] implantation of cotton wicks,[32] implantation of hollow perforated capsules,[11, 33] and measurement of intra-alveolar fluid resorptive pressures in occluded fluid-filled segments.[29] At the outset it should be recognized that there are three components of interstitial pressure: total tissue pressure, solid tissue pressure, and interstitial fluid pressure.[34] Total tissue pressure is the sum of solid tissue pressure and interstitial fluid pressure.[35] Total tissue pressure, the pressure measured by cannulas, needles, and balloons, is usually atmospheric or slightly positive in peripheral tissues, depending on the relationship between tissue volume and mechanical constraints. In the lung, total tissue pressure is subatmospheric and variable between interstitial compartments (see later). The fluid component of tissue pressure is the force important in water and solute movement (i.e., Pisf). Despite their individual limitations, all of the methods used to estimate Pisf reveal a negative value in the lung and other tissues.[11, 29, 31–33]

The difference between total tissue pressure and interstitial fluid pressure, the solid tissue pressure, is generated by the surface-surface interactions and the deformation of solid

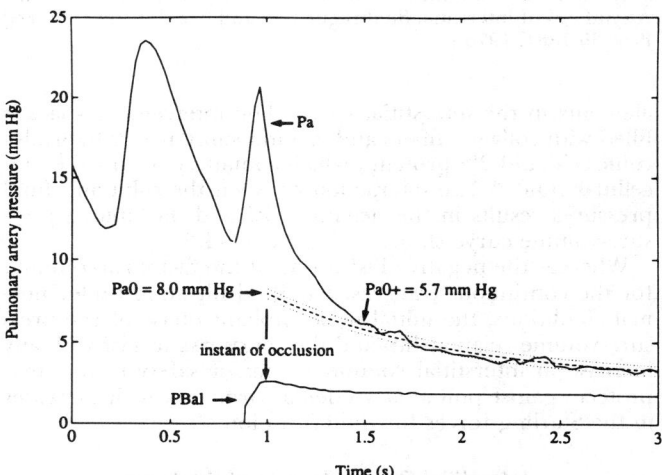

Figure 83–3. Pressures in the pulmonary artery (Pa) and balloon of a Swan-Ganz catheter (PBal) are shown to illustrate the procedure for estimation of pulmonary Pcap. An exponential has been fitted to the pressure data for the 2 seconds after occlusion using the pressure at 10 seconds as the asymptotic value for the wedge pressure. Two estimates of Pcap derived from this procedure are shown. PaO is the value obtained by extrapolation of the exponential back to the instant of occlusion. PaO+ is the value of Pa at the point where the recorded pressure trace deviates from the exponential by the mean standard error of the extrapolation. This corresponds to the value for Pcap that would be selected at the bedside by a trained observer examining the pressure profile for the break point between the initial rapid pressure fall and the later more slowly developing pressure fall. Compared with a more direct estimate of Pcap by the double-occlusion technique, PaO+ tends to provide an underestimate, but both estimates are within 2 mm Hg of Pcap even when the longitudinal distribution of vascular resistance is perturbed by the infusion of histamine or serotonin. (From Hakim TS, Maarek JMI, Chang HK: Estimation of pulmonary capillary pressure in intact dog lungs using the arterial occlusion technique. Am Rev Respir Dis 140:217, 1989.)

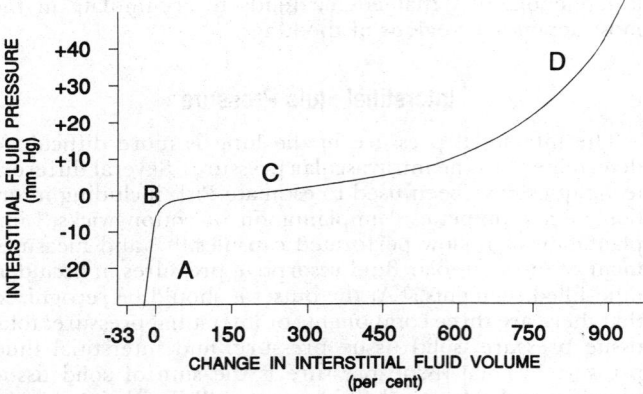

Figure 83–4. Pressure-volume curve of the interstitial space. The interstitial space normally exists in a compacted state with little or no free fluid. The solid structures resist further compaction and deformation, which results in a negative Pisf. With the accumulation of minute quantities of interstitial fluid the solid-solid interaction is released, resulting in a steep rise in fluid pressure. The pressure-volume curve for interstitial fluid exhibits relatively noncompliant behavior; that is, small increases in interstitial fluid volume evoke large increases in Pisf (point A). With the accumulation of more fluid, a point is reached at which the solids are being separated and solid-solid interaction is eliminated (point B). Solid tissue pressure is 0, and the compliance for interstitial fluid is equal to that of the total tissue space. Beyond this point, the interstitial fluid space becomes relatively compliant and large amounts of fluid accumulate with little further increase in Pisf (point C). When the volume limit of the tissue is reached, there is a second stage of reduced compliance (point D). (Modified from Guyton AC, Taylor AE, Brace RA: A synthesis of interstitial fluid regulation and lymph formation. Fed Proc 35:1881, 1976.)

elements in the interstitial space. The intercellular space is filled with collagen fibers and ground substance (98% hyaluronic acid and 2% protein), which contains entrapped extracellular fluid.[36] The interaction between the solid and fluid pressures results in the negative Pisf and the unique pressure-volume curve shown in Figure 83–4.[37]

Whereas the negative Pisf is one of the factors accounting for the continuous transvascular fluid filtration under normal conditions, the initial noncompliant phase of the pressure-volume relationship and the sharp rise in Pisf with any increase in interstitial volume are major safety factors that protect against pulmonary edema formation with increases in the Starling forces for fluid filtration.

Interstitial Compartments of the Lung

The pulmonary microvasculature and interstitium can be divided into two compartments, alveolar and extra-alveolar,[38] based on how the total interstitial pressure changes with changes in alveolar pressure and lung volume (Fig. 83–5).[39] Most of the capillaries are located in the alveolar septa, where the perimicrovascular pressure is directly affected by changes in alveolar pressure (PA).[40, 41] This is called the alveolar interstitial compartment. The other vessels are located in the extra-alveolar compartment. The extra-alveolar compartment includes three anatomically distinct regions: the bronchovascular sheath surrounding the airway, pulmonary artery, and lymphatics; the interstitial space surrounding the pulmonary vein and lymphatics; and the interstitial space surrounding the corner vessels of the alveoli. The perimicrovascular pressure in the extra-alveolar space is less than that surrounding the alveolar vessels and does not experience the direct effect of changes in PA.[42–44] A precise description of the behavior of the pressures in

these two compartments requires careful attention to the intervention by which PA and lung volume are changed as well as a suitable reference pressure, usually either alveolar gas pressure or average pleural surface pressure (Ppl).

Alveolar Interstitial Space

Total tissue pressure in the alveolar interstitial compartment (PxA) is directly affected by PA and by surface tension forces generated at the alveolar air-liquid interface and follows the law of Laplace.[45]

$$\text{PxA} = \text{PA} - (2T/R) \qquad (2)$$

where PxA = total perivascular tissue pressure
  T = surface tension at the air-liquid interface
  R = radius of curvature of the air-liquid interface

Normally PxA is -3 to -4 mm Hg, relative to PA. With an increase in lung volume T and R increase as alveolar surface area increases, but the effect of increased T predominates and PxA decreases relative to PA. At the same time, with an increase in lung volume the transpulmonary pressure (Ptp = PA − Ppl) increases and alveolar vessel perimicrovascular pressure increases relative to Ppl. The difference between PxA and PA is normally minimized by the action of pulmonary surfactant, which is produced by the type II alveolar cells. Any reduction in surfactant activity would then be

PULMONARY EDEMA

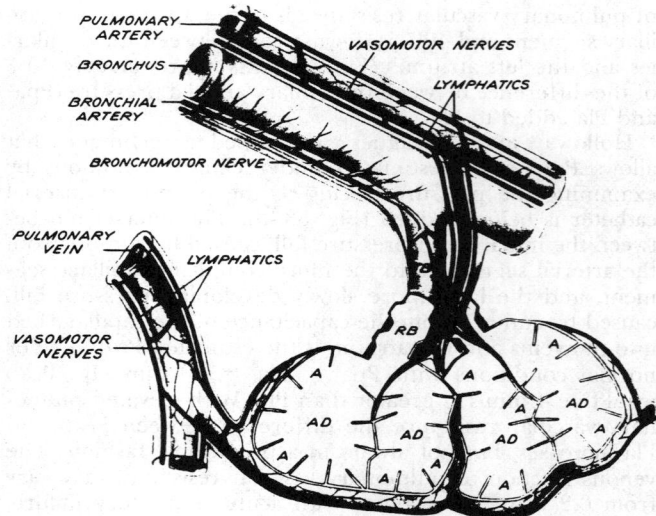

Figure 83–5. Drawing illustrating the interstitial compartments of the lung in relation to lung water balance. In the interstitial space surrounding the alveoli (A) and alveolar ducts (AD) the total tissue pressure is related primarily to PA and surface tension. The interstitial space surrounding the bronchus and pulmonary artery and that surrounding the pulmonary vein constitute one component of the extra-alveolar compartment. The other component of the extra-alveolar compartment is at the corners of the alveoli, where the radial traction of expanding alveoli protects against the direct effect of changes in PA. The total tissue pressure in the extra-alveolar spaces is determined by mechanical interdependence between adjacent structures of different compliances and is generally more negative than either PA or pleural pressure. The pressures in the tissue spaces surrounding the terminal bronchus (TB) and respiratory bronchiole (RB) are probably intermediate between those in the alveolar and extra-alveolar spaces.[4] (From Staub NC: Lung structure and function—1982. Basics Respir Dis 10:1, 1982.)

expected to increase the difference between P_A and P_{XA} and therefore favor pulmonary edema formation by lowering P_{isf}. Indeed, this has been demonstrated in a canine model by Albert and coworkers.[46] The decrease in surfactant activity that occurs during the development of pulmonary edema may also augment the gradient for further fluid filtration.[47]

Extra-Alveolar Interstitial Space

The total perivascular tissue pressure in the extra-alveolar compartment (P_{XE}) depends on mechanical interdependence with surrounding structures. Studies have shown that it is normally more negative than P_{pl}, that is, about -10 cm H_2O when P_{pl} is -5 cm H_2O. With an increase in lung volume the tethering effect of expanding alveoli and radial traction by the surrounding connective tissues causes this pressure to fall even lower.[5, 39, 48–51] Thus, with increases in P_A, P_{pl}, and transpulmonary pressure (P_{tp}) during positive pressure lung inflation the P_{XE} decreases relative to P_A, and when P_{tp} is increased to 25 cm H_2O, $P_A - P_{XE}$ may increase to as much as 40 cm H_2O, that is, 15 cm H_2O below P_{pl}.[39] This concept is relevant to an understanding of the effect of positive end-expiratory pressure (PEEP).

Effect of Positive Airway Pressure

The increase in P_{XA} makes it tempting to speculate that the improvement in gas exchange and compliance seen with PEEP in patients with any kind of pulmonary edema[52, 53] is the result of a decrease in lung water fostered by a decrease in the hydrostatic gradient for fluid filtration. However, studies have failed to demonstrate that PEEP produces a consistent decrease in lung water or the rate of pulmonary edema formation.[41, 54–62] The primary beneficial effect of PEEP on gas exchange and pulmonary compliance stems from the increase in lung volume and the prevention of alveolar atelectasis.[53] At the same time it has been shown that the increase in P_{XA} and decrease in P_{XE} result in a redistribution of edema fluid from the alveolar to extra-alveolar compartment, which would also improve gas exchange and compliance.[62]

Interpretation of Wedge Pressure Measurements During Positive End-Expiratory Pressure

When wedge pressure is used to gauge left ventricular preload in patients receiving PEEP, a consideration of cardiac mechanics makes it clear that the appropriate reference pressure is pleural, or juxtacardiac, rather than atmospheric. Ventricular preload is a concept related to myocardial wall tension during diastole, which is a function of the transmural distending pressure difference, $P_{la} - P_{pl}$ or $P_{pcw} - P_{pl}$. When wedge pressure is used to assess the propensity for pulmonary edema formation in patients receiving PEEP, the appropriate reference pressure is not as clear. The change in the filtration pressure gradient for alveolar microvessels ($P_{cap} - P_{XA}$) could be approximated by using P_A as the reference, that is, looking at the change in $P_{pcw} - P_A$. On the other hand, the change in the filtration pressure gradient for extra-alveolar microvessels ($P_{cap} - P_{XE}$) would probably be even greater than that calculated using P_{pl} as the reference; that is, looking at the change in $P_{pcw} - P_{pl}$ would underestimate the filtration pressure gradient. Because as much as 50% of transvascular fluid filtration in the lung may occur from extra-alveolar vessels,[4] the possibility that the effective filtration pressure gradient may increase with the application of PEEP despite a decrease in $P_{pcw} - P_{pl}$ cannot be discounted.[40, 61, 63] Of course, disparate changes in the longitudinal distributions of pulmonary vascular resistance in the alveolar and extra-alveolar vessels with PEEP could further confound the interpretation of wedge pressure in relation to the true filtration pressure gradient, $P_{cap} - P_{isf}$.[25]

Oncotic Pressures

A great deal of debate has focused on the importance of plasma oncotic pressure in the prevention and resolution of pulmonary edema. Plasma oncotic pressure can be calculated from the measured serum concentrations of albumin (alb) and globulin (glob).[64]

$$\pi alb = 2.8C + 0.18C^2 + 0.012C^3$$

$$\pi glob = 1.6C + 0.15C^2 + 0.006C^3$$

$$\pi tot = 2.1C + 0.16C^2 + 0.0009C^3$$

where C = protein concentration (g/dL)
π = colloid oncotic pressure (mm Hg)
πtot = total oncotic pressure, assuming $C_{alb}/C_{glob} = 1.0$

It can also be measured directly by using a commercially available oncometer pressure transducer system.[65] The oncometer has the advantage of providing the estimate from a single rapid measurement, but caution should be exercised in applying this measurement made with an artificial membrane of a given σ in vitro to the clinical situation, where the σ in vivo may differ significantly.

Those who advocate augmentation of plasma oncotic pressure by infusion of colloids base their conclusion on demonstrable improvements in gas exchange in clinical studies[66] and attenuation of lung water accumulation in laboratory experiments.[67] The key issue in the debate is related to the time course of the increase in the oncotic pressure gradient ($\pi plasma - \pi isf$).[4] Because transvascular filtrate contains plasma protein,[12] it must be realized that any increase in plasma oncotic pressure eventually increases interstitial oncotic pressure, but how rapidly does this occur? An understanding of the physiologic factors that determine the transvascular oncotic pressure gradient should help explain the divergent results, which depend on experimental design and experimental conditions.

The equation for solute flux across the vascular endothelium identifies the factors responsible for maintenance of the concentration gradient ($C_{plasma} - C_{isf}$) for any particular solute.[4]

$$J_s = PS(C_{plasma} - C_{isf}) + (1 - \sigma) \times C_s \times J_v \quad (3)$$

where J_s = net transvascular flux of solute in question
PS = permeability–surface area product for the solute
J_v = net transvascular volume flow
C_s = average concentration of the solute across the barrier, that is, $(C_{plasma} + C_{isf})/2$
σ = reflection coefficient for the solute

The equation states that solute movement is the sum of the diffusive flux (resulting from the transvascular solute concentration difference) and the amount that flows in solution during filtration (solvent drag). The diffusive flux tends to bring solute concentrations into equilibrium ($C_{isf} = C_{plasma}$). The solvent drag component tends to dilute interstitial solute concentration (J_s/J_v) toward a limit determined by σ, $(1 - \sigma)C_s$.[4] Solutes are restricted in proportion to their molecular size. The smaller molecules (molecular weight less than 1000) have equal concentrations on both sides of the endothelium because σ is small and PS is relatively large. The larger molecules (molecular weight greater than 60,000), which include the plasma proteins with a high σ and relatively lower PS, do not pass freely across the barrier.[1] As a result, the concentration of protein in the interstitium is different from that in the plasma, which allows an oncotic gradient to exist, but the gradient is subject to change with changes in PS, σ, and Jv. Recall that Jv is the same as F in the Starling equation and therefore a function of K_f and (Pcap − Pisf). The studies of Vaughan and associates showed that interstitial fluid contains albumin at a concentration equal to 60 to 80% of that in plasma under normal conditions and that labeled albumin infused into the vascular space equilibrates with interstitial albumin with a half-time of 1.5 to 4.0 hours.[68] The rate of equilibration is increased if Pcap is elevated (increased Jv) or endothelial permeability is increased (increased Jv and PS, decreased σ).[4, 68]

Interstitial Oncotic Pressure

With our current technology it is not possible to measure πisf directly. Part of the problem is that colloids are not distributed evenly throughout the extracellular compartment of the interstitial space[69] and the excluded volume depends on the state of tissue hydration among other factors.[4] Investigators have used the efferent lung lymph from the right lymph duct in the dog and from the caudal mediastinal lymph node in the sheep to estimate transvascular filtrate composition and πisf.[65, 68, 70–72] Normally πisf is 60 to 80% of πplasma,[9, 12, 73] not because σ is low but because the transvascular filtration rate is low. In other words, the diffusive flux component of Equation 3 predominates under normal conditions because of low Jv.[1] If Jv becomes zero, Cisf equilibrates with Cplasma. Thus lymph flow is necessary to maintain the oncotic gradient, πplasma − πisf.

Interstitial Protein Wash-Down Phenomenon

With increases in Pcap under conditions of normal endothelial permeability, the fluid filtered is an ultrafiltrate of plasma with a low protein concentration (because the solvent drag component becomes more important with increases in Jv). This leads to a reduction in interstitial protein concentration. This is most easily demonstrated by the progressive decrease in lung lymph protein oncotic pressure with elevation of Pcap, as shown in Figure 83–6. Consequently, the oncotic gradient opposing fluid filtration (πplasma − πisf) increases.[12] This increase is approximately 50% of the increase in Pcap. Thus, although the relatively high πisf tends to promote fluid filtration under normal conditions, this protein wash-down phenomenon becomes an important safety factor that protects against the development of pulmonary edema under conditions of increased Pcap. Clearly, the value of πplasma is important in the effectiveness of this safety factor because πplasma − πisf cannot exceed πplasma. In fact, because Cisf cannot fall below (1 − σ)Cplasma,[4] the limiting value is somewhat less than πplasma.[12, 72]

With increases in transvascular filtration resulting from increases in endothelial permeability, this protein wash-down safety factor would not be operative because of the decrease in σ and increase in PS. Thus the importance of πplasma is diminished in the low-pressure, high-permeability type of edema that occurs in adult respiratory distress syndrome (ARDS).

Significance of Plasma Oncotic Pressure

From the foregoing considerations it should be apparent that the importance of πplasma is different under different

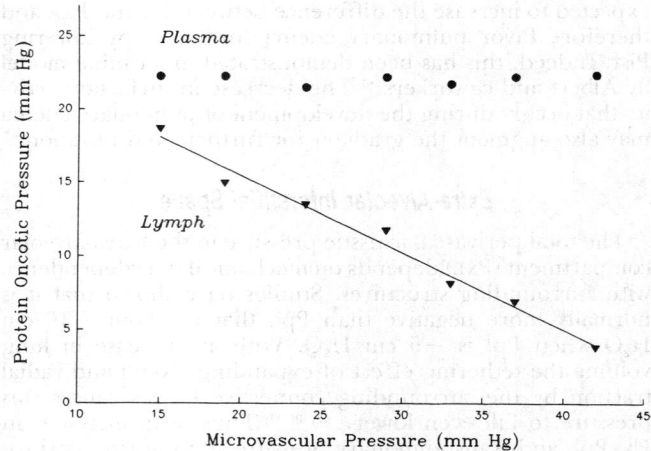

Figure 83–6. Protein oncotic pressure in plasma and lung lymph from a sheep with a chronic lymph fistula and a balloon in the left atrium. Microvascular pressure has been calculated from pressures in the left atrium (Pla) and pulmonary artery (Ppa) as 0.6Pla + 0.4 Ppa. With various elevations of Pla produced by inflation of the left atrial balloon, lymph flow increases and lymph oncotic pressure decreases. Assuming that πlymph = πisf, this interstitial protein wash-down phenomenon would increase πplasma − πisf and offset the increase in Pcap. Estimates from different laboratories indicate that the increase in the πplasma − πisf is equal to 50% of the increase in Pcap. (Modified using mm Hg in place of cm H_2O to illustrate the findings of Erdmann AJ III, Vaughan TR Jr, Brigham KL, et al: Effect of increased vascular pressure on lung fluid balance in unanesthetized sheep. Circ Res 37:271–284, 1975, by permission of the American Heart Association, Inc.)

conditions. Under conditions of chronic hypoproteinemia, πisf is also reduced and the Starling forces may be normally balanced despite a high value for Pcap − πplasma. With acute hypoproteinemia the tendency for the decrease in πisf to lag behind the fall in πplasma leaves the Starling forces temporarily unbalanced, possibly leading to acute pulmonary edema at nearly normal values for Pcap, as in the classic experiment of Guyton and Lindsey.[8] The importance of πplasma stems not only from the steady-state value for Pcap − πplasma but also from the protective effect of the protein wash-down phenomenon with increases in Pcap. For example, Zarins and coworkers[70] found no increase in lung water with an acute 75% reduction in πplasma at constant Ppcw (5 mm Hg) in baboons, and Rackow and colleagues[67] demonstrated a beneficial effect of augmenting πplasma when they compared the effects of crystalloid and colloid infusion to increase Ppcw from 5 to 15 mm Hg in dogs with the same degree of acute hypoproteinemia. The animals receiving crystalloid solution experienced a significant increase in lung water.

In any case, the beneficial effects of plasma colloid pressure augmentation are short-lived because of the equilibration of exogenous vascular colloid with interstitial fluid. When Pcap is high, the increased turnover of colloid causes equilibration to proceed within 12 hours to the new steady-state difference in π between plasma and interstitial fluid.[4] The benefits are further limited when capillary injury leads to reduced values for σ and increased values for PS, as occurs in ARDS. This is due not only to increased turnover with increased PS and Jv but also to the reduced effectiveness of the oncotic pressure gradient (πplasma − πisf) when σ is reduced.

Lymphatic Drainage

Net lung water balance depends not only on the rate of transvascular fluid filtration but also on the rate at which

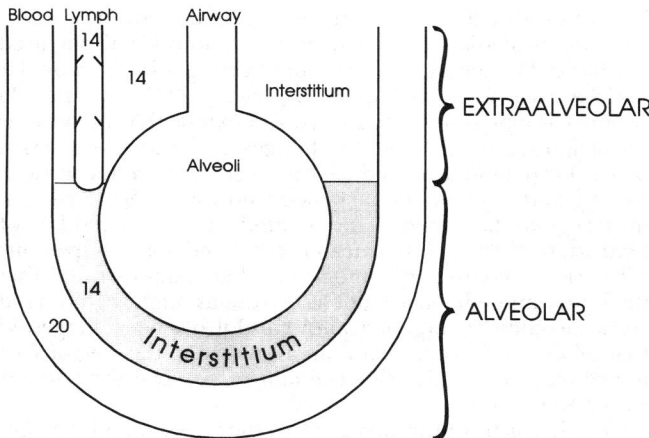

Figure 83–7. Schematic model of the terminal respiratory unit indicating the liquid and solute exchange compartments. The two interstitial compartments are the alveolar interstitium and the extra-alveolar interstitium. The initial lymphatics are at the junction of the two interstitial compartments and are situated to receive lymph flow from the alveolar interstitium. The lymphatics themselves, however, are situated in the extra-alveolar compartment. The numbers indicate protein osmotic pressure (in millimeters of mercury). It is thought that under normal conditions the osmotic pressure in the two interstitial compartments is the same. Filtration occurs throughout the length of the microcirculation and can occur in either the alveolar or extra-alveolar compartment. (Modified from Matthay MA, Landolt CC, Staub NC: Differential liquid and protein clearance from the alveoli of anesthetized sheep. J Appl Physiol 53:96, 1982.)

this fluid is removed by the pulmonary lymphatics. The lymphatic vessels of the lung begin at the edge of the alveolar compartment but are for the most part located in the extra-alveolar compartment[74–77] (Fig. 83–7). Extrapolation of animal data to estimate lymph flow in a normal 70-kg person yields a value of approximately 20 mL/h.[78] The lymphatics have the capability of increasing fluid transport approximately 10-fold when required by increased Starling forces[78] or even more under the influence of increased capillary permeability.[4] This capability is more pronounced under chronic conditions of increased capillary pressure, which results in hypertrophy of existing lymphatic vessels.[79–82] The flow of lymph is down a pressure gradient that extends from the alveolar regions of the lung to more central regions near the hilum. Because lymphatics have valves, lymph flow may be facilitated by respiratory movements, which produce intermittent compression and dilatation of the lymph vessels located in the extra-alveolar space. Lymphatics also contain smooth muscle, and the pumping action of its contractions can generate considerable pressure gradients.[83]

Lymphatic Outflow Back Pressure

Pulmonary lymphatics empty into systemic veins in the thorax, and questions have been repeatedly asked about the importance of central venous pressure in the transport function of the pulmonary lymphatics. According to one school of thought, the lymphatic pumps can generate up to 25 cm H_2O[84] and there is no evidence that venous pressures in the range compatible with life can interfere with lymph flow from the lungs.[4, 77] On the other hand, Allen and colleagues have cited experiments from their laboratory supporting the concept that central venous pressure elevations impair the lymphatic clearance of fluid from the lungs under conditions of increased transvascular filtration produced by either elevated Pcap or increased permeability.[85]

This group noted a continuous relationship between central venous pressure and impairment of lymphatic function and cautioned that values for right atrial pressure frequently encountered in the intensive care unit may influence lung water balance through this mechanism.

Lymphatic Obstruction or Disruption

Obstruction or disruption of pulmonary lymphatics can occur in the clinical setting of malignancy or lung transplantation. How important is this to lung water balance? Although clinical observations may be difficult to interpret in view of other complicating features of the disease process, there are some germane observations in laboratory animals. Ligation of the lymphatics produces transient interstitial edema and a tendency for enhanced lung water accumulation with elevations in capillary pressure.[86] Autologous lung transplantation in dogs also produces transient elevations of lung water, without alveolar edema, which is maximal at 3 days and back to normal by 6 weeks.[87] The mild and transient nature of the response to lymphatic ligation or transection probably reflects the fact that lymphatics regenerate quite rapidly.[88]

FORMATION OF PULMONARY EDEMA

When the transvascular filtration rate exceeds the capacity of the lymphatics, pulmonary edema results. The sequence of edema formation appears to be the same whether the increase in transvascular filtration is the result of elevated Pcap or of increased permeability.[13] Accumulation of fluid occurs initially in the interstitium of the bronchovascular sheath. This is followed by thickening of the interstitial space of the alveolar septa. If the edema becomes severe, flooding of the alveoli occurs.[13] Whether the initial fluid cuffs in the bronchovascular sheath result from fluid filtered from septal capillaries or extra-alveolar vessels is not clear.

Alveolar Edema

Although interstitial edema can produce measurable changes in lung mechanics and gas exchange,[89] the clinical and radiologic manifestations of pulmonary edema are largely the result of alveolar edema. Alveolar flooding is apparently an all-or-none process. Individual alveoli are either completely flooded or dry with only minimal accumulations of fluid at the corners. Partially fluid-filled alveoli are not found.[13] The edema fluid interferes with surfactant activity, which may cause alveolar atelectasis.[47] The site of fluid entry into the alveoli during the alveolar flooding stage has been the subject of much investigation and heated debate.[90–96] Some favor fluid entry across the normally impermeable alveolar membrane. Others have favored entry "upstream" in the terminal airways with subsequent alveolar flooding. Current opinion seems to favor the latter explanation.[1, 96–99]

It seems clear that alveolar edema begins to develop when interstitial volume or pressure reaches some critical level, but the mechanism is not clear. The importance of surface tension at the air-liquid interface is agreed on by most authorities.[1, 4] The critical point may be reached when total alveolar interstitial pressure approaches alveolar gas pressure simply because the structural strength of the alveolar epithelium does not allow it to restrain positive tissue pressure.[34] With some forms of capillary injury there may be direct disruption of the alveolar epithelium, which hastens the process of alveolar flooding, even when the offending agent is carried by the blood.[100]

Protein Concentration of Interstitial and Alveolar Fluid

The protein concentration of interstitial fluid and lymph reflects the mechanism of increased fluid filtration. When filtration is increased by elevated Pcap with normal endothelial permeability, interstitial protein wash-down reduces the interstitial fluid protein concentration.[12] The same is true for increased filtration produced by reduced πplasma.[70] When filtration is caused by increased permeability, that is, increased K_f and PS for protein with reduced σ, interstitial protein concentration is increased.[68, 101] In contrast, the protein concentration of alveolar edema fluid is the same as that of interstitial fluid, regardless of the cause of the pulmonary edema.[102] This indicates disruption of some component of the epithelial barrier in both types of pulmonary edema. The clinical correlate of this is that the mechanism of pulmonary edema can sometimes be established by a measurement of the protein concentration in alveolar edema fluid.

Fein and colleagues[103] compared measurements of alveolar edema fluid protein concentrations, Ppcw, and clinical diagnoses in 24 patients with florid pulmonary edema. They reported that in patients with low-pressure pulmonary edema the edema fluid/plasma total protein concentration ratio was always 0.6 or more (average 0.94 ± 0.45 SEM), whereas in patients with high-pressure cardiogenic pulmonary edema it was always 0.56 or less (average 0.46). In subsequent studies, more overlap in the total protein concentration ratio has been found, suggesting that there may be a spectrum for the pathogenesis of pulmonary edema that ranges from the pure cardiogenic type with high Pcap and normal permeability to the noncardiogenic type with low Pcap and elevated permeability.[104, 105] The intermediate type has some degree of both elevated Pcap and increased permeability, which combine to create a transvascular filtration rate sufficient to produce alveolar edema. It has also been noted that the albumin/globulin ratios of edema fluid relative to plasma differ depending on the mechanism of edema. This would be predicted from Equation 3 if cardiogenic edema represented a normal distribution of decreasing PS and increasing σ for protein of increasing molecular radius and noncardiogenic edema represented a relative increase in PS and decrease in σ for larger protein molecules.[105] Thus, whereas the edema fluid sampled from patients with cardiogenic pulmonary edema tends to have relatively more albumin and less globulin, that sampled from patients with high-permeability edema tends to have an albumin/globulin ratio similar to that of plasma.[104] However, as we shall see, the process of edema resolution may cloud the interpretation of alveolar fluid protein measurements in terms of the difference between high-pressure edema and edema resulting from increased permeability.

PULMONARY BLOOD FLOW DISTRIBUTION IN PULMONARY EDEMA

Pulmonary blood flow redistribution with the development of pulmonary edema requires discussion because of its importance for certain clinical aspects of the problem. The hypoxemia associated with pulmonary edema is largely a manifestation of the flow of mixed venous blood through the capillaries of flooded alveoli, where no oxygenation can occur. Hence, blood flow redistribution away from edematous regions serves to minimize hypoxemia. Blood flow distribution is also important in the pathophysiology of edema formation. When there is increased capillary pressure or capillary injury, the important determinants of transvascular filtration rate are K_f and Pcap. Both are influenced by

blood flow distribution. To the extent that blood flow redistribution is mediated by changes in the number of perfused capillaries,[106] there are proportional changes in the vascular surface area S, as well as K_f ($K_f = L_p \times S$) and the PS product for plasma proteins. To the extent that blood flow redistribution is mediated by changes in the upstream resistance, Pcap should be reduced in regions of reduced flow. Redistribution of pulmonary blood flow away from edematous regions has been demonstrated in animal models of hydrostatic[106–109] and permeability[110–113] edema. In patients with ARDS, computed tomography has demonstrated that the injury and edema are not as diffuse as might be inferred from the chest roentgenogram,[114] and it has been suggested that blood flow redistribution away from the regions of injury may be a major determinant of survival for patients with ARDS.[115]

Certain forms of therapy can produce subsequent changes in flow distribution after edema has formed. A number of studies have demonstrated changes in gas exchange with the administration of vasoactive drugs in laboratory animals with pulmonary edema[110, 116, 117] and in patients with ARDS.[27, 28] This suggests that vasoconstriction is involved in the initial redistribution of flow, but other mechanisms such as vascular compression caused by increased interstitial pressure[106–108] or the loss of tethering forces with reduced alveolar volume[106, 109] may be involved as well. The increase in flow to edematous regions with the application of PEEP may reflect both redistribution of flow away from more normal regions because of vascular compression[110, 118] and a decrease in the resistance of edematous regions associated with alveolar expansion.[108] With PEEP the net effect on oxygenation depends on the relative improvement in regional ventilation compared with the increase in flow to edematous regions.[117, 118] It remains to be seen whether the change in flow distribution with vasodilator therapy has an adverse effect on lung fluid balance.

RESOLUTION OF PULMONARY EDEMA

When pulmonary edema has formed and the underlying cause has been reversed, what processes are involved in the resolution of the pulmonary edema? Interest in the clearance of pulmonary edema fluid is relatively new compared with that in the area of edema pathogenesis, which has fascinated physiologists for more than a century.[2] Most of the new insights into the problem have resulted from the application of new and innovative techniques in the past decade.

Interstitial Fluid Clearance

Interstitial pulmonary edema is apparent on the chest radiograph when approximately 500 mL (70-kg person) of edema fluid is present.[119] Theoretically possible routes of interstitial edema removal include the lymphatics, the pulmonary circulation, the bronchial circulation, and the pleural space.[119, 120] Studies in dogs and sheep have shown that the lymphatics are responsible for approximately one third of pulmonary edema clearance.[120–123] The lymphatic flow rate does not change simultaneously with changes in Pcap but demonstrates a marked hysteresis; for a given Pcap lymph flow is greater if Pcap is decreasing from a higher level than if it is increasing from a lower level, suggesting that the accumulated interstitial fluid rather than Pcap "drives" lymph flow.[122] A study in sheep has demonstrated that the pleural space accounts for 23 to 29% of the total edema fluid cleared from the lung, suggesting that this may be an important route of edema clearance and that obliteration of the pleural space (e.g., pleurodesis) might increase the tendency of the lungs to develop pulmonary edema.[120] The

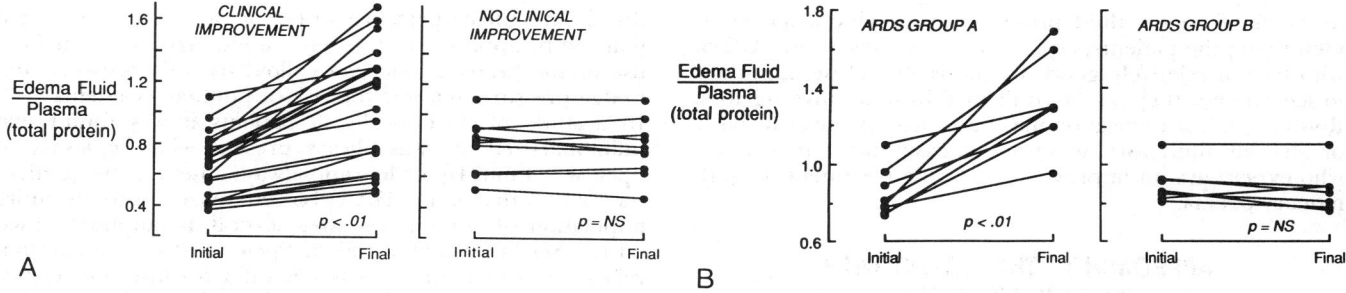

Figure 83–8. Edema fluid/plasma total protein concentration ratios for intubated patients with pulmonary edema. Individual data points indicating the initial value and the final value obtained 1 to 12 hours later are connected by lines. *A.* Data for all 34 patients are displayed as two groups: clinical improvement, the 24 patients who experienced an improvement as judged by improved oxygenation, and no clinical improvement, the 10 patients who experienced no improvement as judged by stable or worsening oxygenation. *B.* Data for the 16 patients judged to have increased capillary permeability, based on a wedge pressure less than 16 mm Hg, have been divided into two groups: ARDS group A, the 9 patients who experienced an improvement in oxygenation (22% mortality), and ARDS group B, the 7 patients who experienced no improvement in oxygenation (71% mortality). Note that the initial concentration ratio was greater than 0.6 in all patients in both ARDS groups. In the hydrostatic edema group the average concentration ratio was 0.54 ± 0.11. (From Matthay MA, Weiner-Kronish JP: Intact epithelial barrier function is critical for the resolution of alveolar edema in humans. Am Rev Respir Dis 142:1250, 1990.)

relative contribution of the pulmonary versus the bronchial circulation to edema clearance remains unclear. Interstitial pulmonary edema resolves rather rapidly. Studies in dogs and sheep have shown that crystalloids infused into the lungs rapidly enter the interstitium and then are removed with a half-life of approximately 3 hours.[42, 124] This is further supported by clinical studies demonstrating resolution of isolated interstitial pulmonary edema within 12 to 24 hours.[125]

Alveolar Fluid Clearance

As previously noted, the alveolar epithelium is quite "tight," with a reflection coefficient approaching 1 (perfectly impermeable).[18, 42, 126, 127] This means that the membrane, if intact, is a substantial barrier to overcome in the resolution of alveolar edema. During the formation of pulmonary edema, the concentration of protein in the alveolar fluid equals that in the interstitium, indicating that the previously impermeable epithelium has become permeable.[102] During the reparative phases of pulmonary edema, however, the membrane may return to its previously impermeable state. The rate of clearance of alveolar liquid is inversely proportional to the protein concentration in the alveolar liquid.[7, 42, 128] For example, Staub[128] instilled Ringer's lactate, serum, and a 14 g/dL albumin solution into the lungs of sheep and measured the rate of clearance. The half-life for clearance of Ringer's lactate was 3 hours, the half-life for clearance of serum was 6 hours, and in the 4-hour study period only 10% of the albumin solution was cleared. The concentration of protein in the instilled serum increased over a 4-hour period from 6.0 to 8.5 g/dL, confirming that liquid was being cleared faster than protein. In other studies it was found that the protein oncotic pressure had increased to 40 to 50 cm H_2O after 4 hours.[119] It has also been demonstrated that the clearance of liquid from the alveoli slows down with progressive increases in protein concentration,[7] which is not unexpected if one examines the Starling forces. The movement of liquid against this substantial gradient suggests an active transport process.

Studies have confirmed that the alveolar epithelium actively transports sodium from alveolar to interstitial fluid (and water follows passively).[6, 129–139] The studies have been done in dogs, sheep, and cultured human cells and can be summarized as follows: The Na^+ channel blocker amiloride and the Na^+,K^+-ATPase blocker ouabain inhibit fluid transport, and furosemide (which blocks Na^+-Cl^- cotransport)

has no effect. Both terbutaline and epinephrine stimulate fluid transport; propranolol does not alter baseline clearance but blocks terbutaline-induced stimulation of fluid transport. The clinical implications of these findings are still unclear. The protein in the alveolus is removed at a much lower rate (i.e., 1% per hour) than the fluid.[7, 42] Despite numerous studies,[7, 42, 140–148] the exact mechanisms of protein removal remain undetermined but may include diffusion, mucociliary clearance, transcellular vesicular transport, and engulfment by macrophages.[119]

Clinical Measurement of Pulmonary Edema Clearance

Matthay and Weiner-Kronish[149] obtained sequential samples of airway fluid and serum from 34 intubated patients with pulmonary edema who were classified as having edema on the basis of either altered hydrostatic forces or increased permeability, as seen in ARDS. They noted that 24 patients experienced an improvement in gas exchange and most of these also had radiographic evidence of improvement. The other 10 experienced no change or deterioration. Although 83% of the patients who had hydrostatic edema showed improvement, 56% of the patients with ARDS also improved. Comparing protein measurements obtained at the time of intubation with those obtained over the next 1 to 12 hours, they found that those who experienced improvement all demonstrated increases in edema fluid total protein concentration (3.8 ± 3.9 to 5.6 ± 1.6 g/dL) and in the edema fluid/plasma total protein concentration ratio as shown in Fig. 83–8. The group who failed to improve showed no change (4.2 ± 1.0 to 4.1 ± 1.1 g/dL). They also noted a striking difference in mortality among the patients with increased permeability. The nine ARDS patients with an increase in edema fluid protein (Fig. 83–8B) experienced 22% mortality, compared with 71% in the other seven patients with ARDS. The authors concluded that the integrity of the alveolar epithelium is critical to recovery from pulmonary edema.

These results make it necessary to interpret edema fluid protein measurements with caution in terms of establishing the etiologic importance of hydrostatic and permeability factors. A low edema fluid protein concentration (50% or less of that in plasma) indicates hydrostatic edema, but a high value (60% or more of that in plasma) may be due to either increased permeability or resolution of hydrostatic edema. These observations also suggest that sequential measurement of edema fluid protein may provide a means of identifying the patients, especially in the subset with ARDS, who have a relatively good prognosis. It will be important to see whether they can be confirmed by other investigators. Routine clinical application may be limited by the availability of alveolar fluid for the second measurement in patients who experience an improvement during treatment for pulmonary edema.

APPROACH TO THE PATIENT WITH PULMONARY EDEMA
Cardiogenic Pulmonary Edema

When pulmonary edema is associated with acute elevation of Pla, the mechanism is obvious and the clinical outcome depends on the ability of therapy to reduce Pla and Pcap without producing an unacceptable decrease in cardiac output. Often this can be accomplished without resort to hemodynamic measurements, but in the more difficult cases it may be necessary to use measurements of cardiac output and Ppcw as a guide to therapy. The target range for Ppcw to ensure the resolution of pulmonary edema is not readily identified. In the setting of acute myocardial infarction relatively minor alterations in pulmonary hemodynamics can produce progressive decrements in gas exchange and lung mechanics.[150] On the other hand, the clinical observation that patients with gradually acquired increases in Pla can tolerate pressures as high as 30 mm Hg without developing clinical or radiologic evidence of pulmonary edema has fascinated clinicians and physiologists for years. There is no consensus on or satisfactory animal model for this phenomenon.

The factors that protect the lung when Pcap increases include the sharp increase in Pisf with small increases in interstitial fluid volume, the increase in the oncotic pressure gradient (πplasma − πisf) resulting from interstitial fluid protein wash-down, and the clearance of filtered fluid and protein by the pulmonary lymphatics. Although the relative importance of these different safety factors is debated, it appears that protein wash-down accounts for approximately 50% and increased Pisf and lymphatic clearance each account for approximately 25% of the lung's ability to withstand an increase in Pcap without developing pulmonary edema.[4] The protein wash-down effect,[1] lymphatic hypertrophy,[81] and perhaps altered compliance of the interstitial space[4] are all thought to contribute to the compensation for a chronic increase in Pcap. It is also possible that small amounts of alveolar edema are present and that an augmented alveolar epithelial resorptive capacity prevents the development of clinically detectable edema.

The most important safety factor, interstitial protein wash-down, depends on the integrity of the endothelial barrier. Even mild capillary injury diminishes the capacity of this mechanism. It is possible that edema in the setting of acute myocardial infarction is different from other forms of cardiogenic edema because of the release of substances that produce an increase in the permeability of pulmonary capillaries,[151] but there is not general agreement on this.[152]

The individual with a wedge pressure greater than 18 mm Hg and clinical evidence of pulmonary edema is ordinarily excluded from clinical studies to examine pathogenesis or therapeutic interventions in ARDS. However, it must be appreciated that an individual patient could have come to this condition as the result of capillary injury superimposed on chronic left atrial hypertension. A Ppcw of 20 mm Hg may be low compared with the patient's baseline compensated condition.

In any case, it should be recognized that there can be no threshold capillary pressure for pulmonary edema formation that can be applied to all patients. Some have advocated the use of the gradient between colloid osmotic pressure and wedge pressure to assess the risk of pulmonary edema.[153, 154] In a study of 36 critically ill patients it was found that pulmonary edema was always present when πplasma − Ppcw was 4 mm Hg or less and always absent if the gradient was greater than 4 mm Hg.[153] To generalize this to the entire population of patients requires several assumptions based on the Starling equation. First, Ppcw must bear a constant relationship to Pcap. This is not valid because the relative size of postcapillary resistance in the pulmonary circulation varies widely in many clinical conditions.[25, 26, 155] Second, there must be in vivo equivalence between Ppcw and the effective oncotic pressure corresponding to πplasma, which is $\sigma \times \pi$plasma. Because σ is not 1, nor is it the same in all patients, this assumption cannot be supported. Third, it must be assumed that the balance of extravascular forces, Pisf and πisf, is the same in all patients. Clearly, conditions associated with chronic elevation of Pla or chronic hypoproteinemia produce alterations in the interstitial forces. Further clinical investigation is needed to establish the prognostic value of the πplasma − Ppcw gradient in view of the obvious theoretic problems. This should not be taken to discount the importance of πplasma. It is clearly an important factor not only in the Starling equation for the steady state but also in establishing the effectiveness of interstitial fluid protein wash-down with elevations in Pcap. To the extent that πplasma reflects serum protein concentration and the general metabolic state of the patient, it is also an important prognosticator for survival in any type of critical illness.

Noncardiogenic Pulmonary Edema and the Adult Respiratory Distress Syndrome

The importance of therapy directed at reducing edema formation by altering the Starling forces in patients with ARDS is highly controversial. Some authorities argue that ARDS is primarily a problem of inflammation and that alteration of the Starling forces would be expected to have no effect on outcome.[156] The fact that mortality in ARDS is more closely related to infection and multiple organ system failure than to hypoxemic respiratory failure[157] lends credence to the assertion that treatment of pulmonary edema to improve lung function has no effect on outcome. Others have provided evidence that neither gas exchange nor survival is correlated with lung water accumulation.[115]

However, there are two sides to this issue. The Starling equation implies that reduction in Pcap could assume major importance in the treatment of pulmonary edema even in the presence of pulmonary capillary injury. Using an animal model of ARDS, Prewitt and coworkers[158] demonstrated that wedge pressure reduction was the most effective means of reducing lung water accumulation. Clinical studies suggesting that these factors may be important to clinical outcome are beginning to appear.

Negative fluid balance and weight loss are significantly correlated with decreased requirements for mechanical ventilation and improved survival in patients with ARDS,[159] and increased lung water is associated with increased mortality.[160] Of course, there are many ways in which a large positive fluid balance could be a marker for poor survival, as in gastrointestinal hemorrhage, sepsis, or pump failure. Attempts to compare groups of patients randomized to routine treatment with those randomized to protocols designed to restrict fluid and decrease lung water suggest improved survival,[160] but the needs of individual patients often result in a considerable discrepancy between the treatment intended and the treatment actually received. As might be

TABLE 83-1

CLINICAL LUNG WATER MEASUREMENTS: COMPARISON OF METHODS*

Criterion	CXR	SGI	TDI	CT	MRI	PET
Accuracy	3.0	2.2	2.9	2.8	2.0	3.1
Sensitivity	2.5	2.6	2.7	2.9	2.2	3.0
Reproducibility	3.2	3.0	3.1	3.5	2.8	3.0
Noninvasiveness	4.0	3.3	1.9	3.5	4.0	2.1
Practicality	4.0	2.4	3.2	1.2	0.6	0.6
Economy	4.0	2.8	3.0	1.1	1.0	1.0
Average	3.5	2.7	2.8	.2.5	2.1	2.1

*Clinical suitability of six methods for lung water measurement. In 1984 the National Institutes of Health conducted a workshop on the clinical application of lung water measurements. After the conference the participants were asked to grade each method on a scale of 0 to 4 with respect to six criteria. The six methods are CXR, chest radiograph; SGI, soluble gas inhalation; TDI, thermal dye indicator dilution; CT, computed tomography; MRI, magnetic resonance imaging; and PET, positron emission tomography. The grade assigned for cost has been inverted and expressed as economy.
Adapted from Staub NC: Clinical use of lung water measurements: Report of a workshop. Chest 90:588, 1986.

expected, the patients with less fluid gain have lower indices of severity of illness, but even after accounting for severity of illness by statistical means net fluid balance appears to be a significant independent predictor of survival.[161] When vigorous therapy, including diuretics, phlebotomy, dialysis, and/or ultrafiltration, is applied to all patients with ARDS, there appears to be a subset who experience a decrease in Ppcw and have a marked improvement in survival.[162]

Thus, as in cardiogenic pulmonary edema, survival in noncardiogenic pulmonary edema may depend on the ability of the patient to achieve a reduction in Pcap without an unacceptable decrement in cardiac output and systemic oxygen transport. In the former, because capillary permeability is normal, Ppcw must be reduced from the abnormal to the normal range. In the latter, because permeability is increased, filling pressure must be reduced from normal to low normal. The improved survival that has been demonstrated does not necessarily refute the assertion that mortality is related to infection and multiple organ system failure rather than respiratory failure. These observations suggest that reducing pulmonary edema in patients with ARDS may reduce the requirement for ventilatory support and thus reduce the risk of these complications. It may be that mortality resulting from infection and multiple organ system failure in patients with ARDS is the result of treatment rather than the natural history of the syndrome.

If the most effective therapy in both types of pulmonary edema is that which reduces Pcap, the distinction between edema resulting from alteration in hydrostatic forces and that resulting from increased permeability may not be of fundamental importance. Of course, it is always important to identify cardiac dysfunction to establish prognosis and develop a treatment plan specific to the type of hemodynamic derangement. Similarly, if the etiology of increased permeability can be identified, it may be possible to direct specific therapy at the underlying condition.

CLINICAL MEASUREMENT OF PULMONARY EDEMA

Allen and colleagues[85] concluded their review of advances in pulmonary edema by noting that clinical research is impaired by the lack of a reliable technique for lung water measurement. In 1984 the National Institutes of Health conducted a workshop on the clinical application of lung water measurements.[163] The participants used a scale of 0 to 4 to rate methods of lung water measurement on the basis of six criteria: accuracy, sensitivity, reproducibility, noninvasiveness, practicality, and cost. For the purpose of this comparison we restrict our comments to six methods: portable chest roentgenogram, soluble gas inhalation, thermal dye indicator dilution, computed tomography, magnetic

resonance imaging, and positron emission tomography. The ratings are shown in Table 83-1. With respect to accuracy, positron emission tomography received the highest rating, followed by portable chest roentgenogram and thermal dye indicator dilution. The relatively high ratings received by the chest roentgenogram for accuracy, sensitivity, and reproducibility may reflect the high quality of the radiographs presented. The caliber of radiographs of critically ill patients routinely obtained with portable equipment under the conditions encountered in the emergency room or intensive care unit is highly variable and usually somewhat less than publication quality. Changes in lung gas volume clearly influence our perception of the quantity of lung water, leading to the clinical impression that PEEP improves lung water balance, and should be avoided when using sequential films to estimate clinical progress. With respect to noninvasiveness, thermal dye indicator dilution received the lowest rating, but in the patient who already requires right-sided heart and arterial catheterization for hemodynamic monitoring there is minimal additional risk. With respect to practicality, computed tomography, magnetic resonance imaging, and positron emission tomography received the lowest ratings because of the logistics of transfer of the critically ill patient to the imaging facility, especially for sequential studies on successive days.

Indicator Dilution Methods

Because first-pass indicator dilution is the method that has been most widely used to quantify lung water in clinical studies, it deserves special comment. The original method of Chinard used the mean transit time difference for radiolabeled water and albumin to compute the extravascular volume of distribution for water.[164, 165] Brigham and coworkers[115] used a modification of this method in a clinical study of patients with ARDS and concluded that mortality did not correlate with lung water. The next major steps toward clinical applicability came with the use of heat as the diffusible indicator,[166] the substitution of indocyanine green dye–labeled albumin as the intravascular indicator,[167] and the development of a dedicated microprocessor for bedside use.[168] Utilizing these newer methods, Schuster's group[160, 161] concluded that fluid balance and lung water are important determinants of mortality in ARDS.

The theoretic and practical limitations of the first-pass mean transit approach in general[169] and specifically the thermal dye method[170] have been reviewed. The greatest limitation of the molecular tracer methods is related to their dependence on the extent of pulmonary vascular recruitment. Thus they measure a greater fraction of the actual lung water when cardiac output or pulmonary arterial pressure is increased[171] and when edema is produced by hydrostatic forces rather than capillary injury.[172] In contrast, the thermal dye method detects pulmonary edema equally well in the presence of high pressure or diffuse capillary injury and has good sensitivity and specificity.[173] The major limitation of the thermal dye method occurs when injury is not homogeneous, as in hydrochloric acid aspiration.[170] Under these conditions the fraction of lung water detected depends on the distribution of pulmonary blood flow relative to the regions of injury, and interventions such as PEEP or vasodilators, which redistribute blood flow back to the region of injury, cause a greater fraction of lung water to be detected.[118] The problem is not that the thermal indicator does not "see" the poorly perfused edematous regions but rather that the method used to extrapolate indicator dilution curves to exclude recirculating indicator also excludes indicator slowly emerging from these regions. With the development of better methods for analyzing the curves[174] the thermal dye method could provide an accurate estimate of lung water in all types of injury uninfluenced by changes in blood flow distribution.

At present we must conclude that there is no method for quantitative monitoring of pulmonary edema that would be satisfactory for routine clinical application. It is anticipated that improved technology will provide a method that might be satisfactory for application to clinical investigation, but it will probably be cumbersome and costly in terms of both capital expenditure and the personnel needed to obtain reliable results. The return, of course, would be a better understanding of the factors that determine the course of pulmonary edema in various clinical situations and the importance of therapy directed at edema resolution in terms of clinical outcome.

References

1. Staub NC: The pathogenesis of pulmonary edema. Prog Cardiovasc Dis 23:53, 1980.
2. Starling EH: On the absorption of fluids from the connective tissue spaces. J Physiol (Lond) 19:312, 1896.
3. Snashall PD, Weidner WJ, Staub NC: Extravascular lung water after extracellular fluid expansion in dogs. J Appl Physiol 42:624, 1977.
4. Taylor AE, Parker JC: Pulmonary interstitial spaces and lymphatics. In: Fishman AP, Fisher AB (eds): Handbook of Physiology, Section 3, Respiration, Volume I. Bethesda, American Physiological Society, p 167, 1985.
5. Lai-Fook SJ: Perivascular interstitial fluid pressure measured by micropipettes in isolated dog lungs. J Appl Physiol 52:9, 1982.
6. Goodman BE, Fleischer RS, Crandall RD: Evidence for active Na⁺ transport by cultured monolayers of pulmonary alveolar epithelial cells. Am J Physiol 245:C78, 1983.
7. Matthay MA, Berthiaume Y, Staub NC: Long-term clearance of liquid and protein from the lungs of unanesthetized sheep. J Appl Physiol 59:928, 1985.
8. Guyton AC, Lindsey AW: Effect of elevated left atrial pressure and decreased plasma protein concentration on the development of pulmonary edema. Circ Res 7:649, 1959.
9. Staub NC: Steady state pulmonary transvascular water filtration in unanesthetized sheep. Circ Res 28/29(suppl 1):135, 1971.
10. Gaar KA, Taylor AE, Owens LJ, et al: Pulmonary capillary pressure and filtration coefficient in the isolated perfused lung. Am J Physiol 213:910, 1967.
11. Meyer BJ, Meyer A, Guyton AC: Interstitial fluid pressure. V. Negative pressure in the lung. Circ Res 22:263, 1968.
12. Erdmann AJ III, Vaughan TR Jr, Brigham KL, et al: Effect of increased vascular pressure on lung fluid balance in unanesthetized sheep. Circ Res 37:271, 1975.
13. Staub NC, Nagano H, Pearce ML: Pulmonary edema in dogs, especially the sequence of fluid accumulation in the lungs. J Appl Physiol 22:227, 1967.
14. Staub NC: The pathophysiology of pulmonary edema. Hum Pathol 1:419, 1970.
15. Renkin EM: Multiple pathways of capillary permeability. Circ Res 41:735, 1977.
16. Staub NC: Pulmonary edema due to increased micro-vascular permeability to fluid and proteins. Circ Res 43:143, 1978.
17. Simionescu M, Simionescu N, Palade GE: Permeability of muscle capillaries to small heme peptides. Evidence for the existence of patent transendothelial channels. J Cell Biol 64:586, 1975.
18. Schneeberger EE, Karnovsky MJ: Substructure of intercellular junctions in freeze-fractured alveolar-capillary membranes of mouse lung. Circ Res 38:404, 1976.
19. Inoue S, Michel RP, Hogg JC: Zonulae occludens in alveolar epithelium and capillary endothelium of dog lungs studied with the freeze-fracture technique. J Ultrastruct Res 56:215, 1976.
20. Gaar KA, Taylor AE, Owens LJ, et al: Effect of capillary pressure and plasma proteins on the development of pulmonary edema. Am J Physiol 213:79, 1967.
21. Holloway H, Perry M, Downey J, et al: Estimation of effective pulmonary capillary pressure in intact lungs. J Appl Physiol 54:846, 1983.
22. Battacharya J, Staub NC: Direct measurement of microvascular pressure in the isolated perfused dog lung. Science 210:327, 1980.
23. Gabel JC, Drake RE: Pulmonary capillary pressure in intact dog lungs. Am J Physiol 235:H569, 1978.
24. Hakim TS, Maarek JMI, Chang HK: Estimation of pulmonary capillary pressure in intact dog lungs using the arterial occlusion technique. Am Rev Respir Dis 140:217, 1989.
25. Collee GG, Lynch HE, Hill RD, et al: Bedside measurement of pulmonary capillary pressure in patients with acute respiratory failure. Anesthesiology 66:614, 1987.
26. Cope DK, Allison RC, Parmentier JL, et al: Measurement of effective pulmonary capillary pressure using the pressure profile after pulmonary artery occlusion. Crit Care Med 14:16, 1986.
27. Radermacher P, Santak B, Becker H, et al: Prostaglandin E₁ and nitroglycerin reduce pulmonary capillary pressure but worsen ventilation-perfusion distributions in patients with adult respiratory distress syndrome. Anesthesiology 70:601, 1989.
28. Radermacher P, Santak B, Wüst HJ, et al: Prostacyclin for the treatment of pulmonary hypertension in the adult respiratory distress syndrome: Effects on pulmonary capillary pressure and ventilation-perfusion distributions. Anesthesiology 72:238, 1990.
29. Parker JC, Guyton AC, Taylor AE: Pulmonary interstitial and capillary pressures estimated from intra-alveolar fluid pressures. J Appl Physiol 44:267, 1978.
30. Levine OR, Mellins RB: Effect of gravity on the interstitial pressure of the lung in intact dogs. J Appl Physiol 33:357, 1972.
31. Wiederhielm CA, Weston BV: Microvascular, lymphatic, and tissue pressures in the unanesthetized mammal. Am J Physiol 225:992, 1973.
32. Scholander PF, Hargens AR, Miller SL: Negative pressure in the interstitial fluid of animals. Science 161:321, 1968.
33. Guyton AC: A concept of negative interstitial fluid pressure based on pressures in implanted perforated capsules. Circ Res 12:399, 1963.
34. Guyton AC, Taylor AE, Granger HJ: Analysis of types of pressure in the pulmonary spaces: Interstitial fluid pressure, solid tissue pressure, and total tissue pressure. In: Giuntini C (ed): Central Hemodynamics and Gas Exchange. Torino, Italy, Minerva Medica, p 41, 1971.
35. Guyton AC, Taylor AE, Brace RA: A synthesis of interstitial fluid regulation and lymph formation. Fed Proc 35:1881, 1976.
36. Schubert M: Intercellular macromolecules containing polysaccharides. Biophys J 4(suppl):119, 1965.
37. Guyton AC: Interstitial fluid pressure, II. Pressure-volume curves of interstitial space. Circ Res 16:452, 1965.
38. Staub NC: Lung structure and function—1982. Basics Respir Dis 10:1, 1982.
39. Howell JBL, Permutt S, Proctor DF, et al: Effect of inflation of the lung on different parts of pulmonary vascular bed. J Appl Physiol 16:71, 1961.
40. Bφ G, Hauge A, Nicolaysen G: Alveolar pressure and lung volume as determinants of net transvascular fluid filtration. J Appl Physiol 42:476, 1977.
41. Woolverton NC, Brigham KL, Staub NC: Effect of positive pressure breathing on lung lymph flow and water content in sheep. Circ Res 42:550, 1978.
42. Matthay MA, Landolt CC, Staub NC: Differential liquid and protein clearance from the alveoli of anesthetized sheep. J Appl Physiol 53:96, 1982.
43. Staub NC: Effects of alveolar surface tension on the pulmonary vascular bed. Jpn Heart J 7:386, 1966.
44. Nicolaysen G, Hauge A: Determinants of transvascular fluid shifts in zone-I isolated rabbit lungs. Microvasc Res 17(part 2):S113, 1979.
45. West JB: Respiratory Physiology—The Essentials. 2nd ed. Baltimore, Williams & Wilkins, 1979.
46. Albert RK, Lakshminarayan S, Hildebrandt J, et al: Increased surface tension favors pulmonary edema formation in anesthetized dogs' lungs. J Clin Invest 63:1015, 1979.
47. Said SI, Avery ME, Davis RK, et al: Pulmonary surface activity in induced pulmonary edema. J Clin Invest 44:458, 1965.
48. Blake LH, Staub NC: Pulmonary vascular transport in sheep. A mathematical model. Microvasc Res 12:197, 1976.
49. Lai-Fook SJ, Toporoff B: Pressure-volume behavior of perivascular interstitium measured in isolated dog lung. J Appl Physiol 48:939, 1980.
50. Hauge A, Nicholaysen G: Studies on transvascular fluid balance and capillary permeability in isolated lungs. Bull Physiopathol Respir 7:1197, 1971.

51. Canada E, Benumof JL, Tousdale FR: Pulmonary vascular resistance correlated in intact normal and abnormal canine lungs. Crit Care Med 10:719, 1982.
52. Ashbaugh DC, Petty TL, Bigelow DB: Continuous positive pressure breathing (CPPB) in adult respiratory distress syndrome. J Thorac Cardiovasc Surg 57:31, 1969.
53. Kumar A, Falke KJ, Feffin B: Continuous positive pressure ventilation in acute respiratory failure. N Engl J Med 283:1430, 1970.
54. Caldini P, Leith JD, Brenan MJ: Effect of continuous positive pressure ventilation (CPPV) on edema formation in dog lung. J Appl Physiol 39:672, 1975.
55. Toung TJ, Saharia P, Mitzner WA: The beneficial and harmful effects of positive end-expiratory pressure. Surg Gynecol Obstet 147:518, 1978.
56. Pang LM, Rodriguez F, Stalcup SA: Effects of hyperinflation and atelectasis on fluid accumulation in the puppy lung. J Appl Physiol 45:284, 1978.
57. Demling RH, Staub NC, Edmonds LH: Effect of end expiratory airway pressure on accumulation of extravascular lung water. J Appl Physiol 38:907, 1975.
58. Hopewell PC: Failure of positive end-expiratory pressure to decrease lung water content in alloxan-induced pulmonary edema. Am Rev Respir Dis 120:813, 1979.
59. Hopewell PC, Murray JF: Effects of continuous positive-pressure ventilation in experimental pulmonary edema. J Appl Physiol 40:568, 1976.
60. Miller WC, Rice DL, Linger KM: Effect of PEEP on lung water content in experimental noncardiogenic pulmonary edema. Crit Care Med 9:7, 1981.
61. Goldberg HS, Mitzner W, Batra G: Effect of transpulmonary and vascular pressures on rate of pulmonary edema formation. J Appl Physiol 43:14, 1977.
62. Pare PD, Warriner B, Baile EM, et al: Redistribution of pulmonary extravascular water with positive end-expiratory pressure in canine pulmonary edema. Am Rev Respir Dis 127:590, 1983.
63. Albert RK, Lakshminarayan S, Kirk W, et al: Lung inflation can cause pulmonary edema in zone I of in situ dog lungs. J Appl Physiol 59:815, 1980.
64. Landis EM, Pappenheimer JR: Exchange of substances through the capillary walls. In: Hamilton WF (ed): Handbook of Physiology, Section 2, Circulation, Volume II. Washington, DC, American Physiological Society, p 961, 1963.
65. Weil MH, Morissette M, Michaels S, et al: Routine plasma colloid oncotic pressure measurements. Crit Care Med 3:229, 1974.
66. Skillman JJ, Parikh BM, Tanenbaum BJ: Pulmonary venous admixture—Improvement with albumin and diuresis. Am J Surg 119:440, 1970.
67. Rackow EC, Weil MH, Macneil AR, et al: Effects of crystalloid and colloid fluids on extravascular lung water in hypoproteinemic dogs. J Appl Physiol 62:2421, 1987.
68. Vaughan TR, Erdmann AJ, Brigham KL, et al: Equilibration of intravascular albumin with lung lymph in unanesthetized sheep. Lymphology 12:217, 1979.
69. Sellinger SL, Bland RD, Demling RH, et al: Distribution volumes of [^{131}I]albumin, [^{14}C]sucrose, and ^{36}Cl in sheep lung. J Appl Physiol 39:773, 1975.
70. Zarins CK, Rice CL, Peters KM, et al: Lymph and pulmonary response to isobaric reduction in plasma oncotic pressure in baboons. Circ Res 43:925, 1978.
71. Staub NC: Extravascular forces in lung affecting fluid and protein exchange. Am Rev Respir Dis 115(6 part 2):159, 1977.
72. Staub NC: Pulmonary edema. Physiol Rev 54:678, 1974.
73. Warren MF, Drinker CK: The flow of lymph from the lungs of the dog. Am J Physiol 136:207, 1942.
74. Hayck H von: The Human Lung. New York, Hafner Press, 1960.
75. Miller WS: The Lung. 2nd ed. Springfield, IL, Charles C Thomas, 1947.
76. Nagaishi C: Functional Anatomy and Histology of the Lung. Baltimore, University Park Press, 1972.
77. Rusznyàk J, Földi M, Szabó G: Lymphatics and Lymph Circulation: Physiology and Pathology. 2nd ed. Oxford, Pergamon Press, 1967.
78. Staub NC: "State of the art" review. Pathogenesis of pulmonary edema. Am Rev Respir Dis 109:358, 1974.
79. Sampson JJ, Leeds SE, Uhley HN, et al: Studies of lymph flow and changes in pulmonary structures as indexes of circulatory changes in experimental pulmonary edema. Isr J Med Sci 5:826, 1969.
80. Uhley HN, Leeds SE, Sampson JJ, et al: Some observations on the role of the lymphatics in experimental acute pulmonary edema. Circ Res 9:688, 1961.
81. Uhley HN, Leeds SE, Sampson JJ, et al: Role of pulmonary lymphatics in chronic pulmonary edema. Circ Res 11:966, 1962.
82. Leeds SE, Uhley HN, Sampson JJ, et al: Significance of changes in the pulmonary lymph flow in acute and chronic experimental pulmonary edema. Am J Surg 114:254, 1967.
83. Hall JG, Morris B, Woolley G: Intrinsic rhythmic propulsion of lymph in the unanesthetized sheep. J Physiol (Lond) 180:336, 1965.
84. Pang LM, Mellins RL, Rodriguez-Martinez F: Effect of acute lymphatic obstruction on fluid accumulation in the chest in dogs. J Appl Physiol 39:985, 1975.
85. Allen SJ, Drake RE, Williams JP, et al: Recent advances in pulmonary edema. Crit Care Med 15:963, 1987.

86. Magno M, Szidon JP: Hemodynamic pulmonary edema in dogs with acute and chronic lymphatic ligation. Am J Physiol 231:1777, 1976.
87. Cowan GSM Jr, Staub NC, Edmunds LH Jr: Changes in the fluid compartments and dry weights of reimplanted dog lungs. J Appl Physiol 40:962, 1976.
88. Eraslan S, Turner MD, Hardy JD: Lymphatic regeneration following lung reimplantation in dogs. Surgery 56:970, 1964.
89. Iliff LD, Greene RE, Hughes JMB: Effect of interstitial edema on the distribution of ventilation and perfusion. J Appl Physiol 33:462, 1972.
90. Schulz H: The Submicroscopic Anatomy and Pathology of the Lung. Berlin, Springer-Verlag, 1959.
91. Cottrell TS, Levine OR, Senior RM, et al: Electron microscopic alterations at the alveolar level in pulmonary edema. Circ Res 21:783, 1967.
92. Finegold MJ: Interstitial pulmonary edema. Lab Invest 16:912, 1967.
93. Cunningham AL, Hurley JV: Alpha-naphthyl-thiourea–induced pulmonary oedema in the rat: A topographical and electron-microscopic study. J Pathol 106:25, 1972.
94. Whayne TF Jr, Severinghaus JW: Experimental hypoxic pulmonary edema in the rat. J Appl Physiol 25:729, 1968.
95. Iliff LD: Extra-alveolar vessels and edema development in excised dog lungs. Circ Res 28:524, 1971.
96. Staub NC: Pathways for fluid and solute fluxes in pulmonary edema. In: Fishman AP, Renkin EM (eds): Pulmonary Edema. Bethesda, American Physiological Society, p 113, 1979.
97. Goshy M, Lai-Fook SJ, Hyatt RE: Perivascular pressure measurements by wick-catheter technique in isolated dog lobes. J Appl Physiol 46:950, 1979.
98. Gee MH, Williams DO: Effect of lung inflation on perivascular cuff fluid volume in isolated dog lung lobes. Microvasc Res 17:192, 1979.
99. Gee MH, Staub NC: Role of bulk fluid flow in protein permeability of the dog lung alveolar membrane. J Appl Physiol 42:144, 1977.
100. Montaner JSG, Tsang J, Evans KG, et al: Alveolar epithelial damage. J Clin Invest 77:1786, 1986.
101. Brigham KL, Woolverton WC, Blake LH, et al: Increased sheep lung vascular permeability caused by pseudomonas bacteremia. J Clin Invest 54:792, 1974.
102. Vreim CE, Snashall PD, Staub NC: Protein composition of lung fluids in anesthetized dogs with acute cardiogenic edema. Am J Physiol 231:1466, 1976.
103. Fein A, Grossman RF, Jones JG, et al: The value of edema fluid protein measurement in patients with pulmonary edema. Am J Med 67:32, 1979.
104. Sprung CL, Rackow EC, Fein A, et al: The spectrum of pulmonary edema: Differentiation of cardiogenic, intermediate, and noncardiogenic forms of pulmonary edema. Am Rev Respir Dis 124:718, 1981.
105. Sprung CL, Long WM, Marcial EH, et al: Distribution of proteins in pulmonary edema. The value of fractional concentrations. Am Rev Respir Dis 136:957, 1987.
106. Muir AL, Hogg JC, Naimark A, et al: Effect of alveolar liquid on distribution of blood flow in dog lungs. J Appl Physiol 39:885, 1975.
107. Hughes JMB, Glazier JB, Maloney JE, et al: Effect of extra-alveolar vessels on distribution of blood flow in the dog lung. J Appl Physiol 25:701, 1968.
108. Muir AL, Hall DL, Despas P, et al: Distribution of blood flow in the lung in acute pulmonary edema in dogs. J Appl Physiol 33:763, 1972.
109. Ritchie BC, Schauberger G, Staub NC: Inadequacy of peri-vascular edema hypothesis to account for distribution of pulmonary blood flow in lung edema. Circ Res 24:807, 1969.
110. Ali J, Wood LDH: Factors affecting perfusion distribution in canine oleic acid pulmonary edema. J Appl Physiol 60:1498, 1986.
111. Malik AB, Van der Zee H, Neumann PH, et al: Effects of pulmonary edema on regional pulmonary perfusion in the intact dog lung. J Appl Physiol 49:834, 1980.
112. Tsang JY, Baile EM, Hogg JC: Relationship between regional pulmonary edema and blood flow. J Appl Physiol 60:449, 1986.
113. Velazquez M, Schuster DP: Pulmonary blood flow distribution after lobar oleic acid injury: A PET study. J Appl Physiol 65:2228, 1988.
114. Maunder, RJ, Shuman WP, McHugh JW, et al: Preservation of normal lung regions in the adult respiratory distress syndrome. JAMA 255:2463, 1986.
115. Brigham KL, Kariman K, Harris TR, et al: Correlation of oxygenation with vascular permeability–surface area but not with lung water in humans with acute respiratory failure and pulmonary edema. J Clin Invest 72:339, 1983.
116. Bishop MJ, Huang T, Cheney FW: Effect of vasodilator treatment on the resolution of oleic acid injury in dogs. Am Rev Respir Dis 131:421, 1985.
117. Mink SN, Light RB, Cooligan T, et al: Effect of PEEP on gas exchange and pulmonary perfusion in canine lobar pneumonia. J Appl Physiol 50:517, 1981.
118. Carlile PV, Hagan SF, Gray BA: Perfusion distribution and lung thermal volume in canine hydrochloric acid aspiration. J Appl Physiol 65:750, 1988.
119. Matthay MA: Resolution of pulmonary edema: Mechanisms of liquid, protein, and cellular clearance from the lung. Clin Chest Med 6:521, 1985.
120. Broaddis VC, Weiner-Kronish JP, Staub NC: Clearance of pulmonary

edema into the pleural space of volume loaded anesthetized sheep. J Appl Physiol 68:2623, 1990.

121. Bland RD, Hansen TR, Haberkem CM: Lung fluid balance in lambs before and after birth. J Appl Physiol 53:992, 1982.

122. Gee MH, Spath JA Jr: The dynamics of the lung fluid filtration system in dogs with edema. Circ Res 46:796, 1980.

123. Raj U, Bland RD: Elevated pulmonary microvascular pressure retards lung liquid clearance in lambs. Am Rev Respir Dis 131:A397, 1985.

124. Courtice FC, Phipps PJ: The absorption of fluid from the lungs. J Physiol (Lond) 105:186, 1949.

125. Pistolesi M, Guintini C: Assessment of extravascular lung water. Radiol Clin North Am 16:551, 1978.

126. Gorin AB, Stewart PA: Differential permeability of the endothelial and epithelial barrier to albumin flux. J Appl Physiol 47:1315, 1979.

127. Taylor AE, Guyton AC, Bishop VS: Permeability of the alveolar membrane to solutes. Circ Res 16:353, 1965.

128. Staub NC: Alveolar flooding and clearance. Am Rev Respir Dis 127:S44, 1983.

129. Bachofen M, Weibel ER: Alterations of the gas exchange apparatus in adult respiratory insufficiency associated with septicemia. Am Rev Respir Dis 116:589, 1977.

130. Berthiaume Y, Staub NC, Matthay MA: Terbutaline and epinephrine increase the rate of alveolar liquid clearance in anesthetized sheep. Fed Proc 44:1910A, 1985.

131. Boucher RC, Stutts MJ, Gatzy JT: Regional differences in bioelectric properties and ion flow in excised canine airways. J Appl Physiol 51:706, 1981.

132. Goodman BE, Brown JEJ, Crandall ED: Regulation of transport across pulmonary alveolar epithelial cell monolayers. J Appl Physiol 57:703, 1984.

133. Goodman BE, Crandall ED: Dome formation in primary cultured monolayers of alveolar epithelial cells. Am J Physiol 243:C96, 1982.

134. Crandall ED Palombo RL, Goodman BE: Effects of terbutaline on sodium flux from alveolar to vascular fluid in isolated perfused rat lung. Am Rev Respir Dis 129:A345, 1984.

135. Mason RJ, William MC, Widdicombe JH, et al: Transepithelial transport by pulmonary alveolar type II cells in primary culture. Proc Natl Acad Sci USA 79:6033, 1982.

136. Olver RE: Fluid balance across the fetal alveolar epithelium. Am Rev Respir Dis 127:S33, 1983.

137. Olver RE, Davis B, Morris MG, et al: Active transport of Na$^+$ and Cl$^-$ across the canine tracheal epithelium in vitro. Am Rev Respir Dis 112:811, 1975.

138. Sugahara K, Caldwell JH, Mason RJ: Electric currents flow out of domes formed by cultured epithelial cells. J Cell Biol 99:1541, 1984.

139. Wright EM: Solute and water transport across epithelia. Am Rev Respir Dis 127:S3, 1983.

140. Conhaim RL, Gropper MA, Staub NC: Effect of lung inflation on alveolar-airway barrier protein permeability in dog lung. J Appl Physiol 55:1249, 1983.

141. Courtice FC, Simmonds WJ: Absorption from the lungs. J Physiol (Lond) 109:103, 1949.

142. Dominguez EAM, Leibow AA, Bensch KG: Studies on the pulmonary air-tissue barrier: Absorption of albumin by the alveolar wall. Lab Invest 16:905, 1967.

143. Drinker CR, Hardenbergh E: Absorption from the pulmonary alveoli. J Exp Med 86:7, 1947.

144. Egan EA, Nelson RM, Olver RE: Lung inflation and alveolar permeability to non-electrolytes in the adult sheep in vivo. J Physiol (Lond) 260:409, 1976.

145. Freedman FB, Johnson JA: Equilibrium and kinetic properties of the Evans blue albumin system. Am J Physiol 216:675, 1969.

146. Meyer EC, Ottaviano R, Higgins JJ: Albumin clearance from alveoli: Tissue permeation vs. airway displacement. J Appl Physiol 43:487, 1977.

147. Schultz AB, Grisner JT, Grande F: Absorption of radioactive albumin from the lungs of normal dogs. J Lab Clin Med 61:494, 1963.

148. Zumsteg TA, Havill AM, Gee MH: Relationships among lung extravascular fluid compartments with alveolar flooding. J Appl Physiol 53:267, 1982.

149. Matthay MA, Weiner-Kronish JP: Intact epithelial barrier function is critical for the resolution of alveolar edema in humans. Am Rev Respir Dis 142:1250, 1990.

150. Gray BA, Hyde RW, Hodges M, et al: Alterations in lung volumes and pulmonary function in relation to hemodynamic changes in acute myocardial infarction. Circulation 59:551, 1979.

151. Gee MH, Gwirtz PA, Spath JA: Extravascular water content of heart and lungs after acute myocardial ischemia. J Appl Physiol 45:102, 1978.

152. Parker JC, Campbell L, Gilchrist S, et al: Failure of myocardial ischemia to increase pulmonary microvascular permeability in dogs. J Appl Physiol 56:691, 1984.

153. Rackow EC, Fein IA, Leppo J: Colloid osmotic pressure as a prognostic indicator of pulmonary edema and mortality in the critically ill. Chest 72:709, 1977.

154. Weil MH, Carlson RW: Colloid osmotic pressure and pulmonary edema (editorial). Chest 72:692, 1977.

155. Taylor AE, Cope DK, Allison RC, et al: Capillary pressure measurement in human lungs. In: Zapol WM, Lemaire F (eds): Adult Respiratory Distress Syndrome. New York, Marcel Dekker, p 353, 1991.

156. Rinaldo JE, Rogers RM: Adult respiratory-distress syndrome. N Engl J Med 306:900, 1982.

157. Bell RC, Coalson JJ, Smith JD, et al: Multiple organ system failure and infection in adult respiratory distress syndrome. Ann Intern Med 99:293, 1983.

158. Prewitt RM, McCarthy J, Wood LDH: Treatment of acute low pressure pulmonary edema in dogs. J Clin Invest 67:409, 1981.

159. Simmons RS, Berdine GG, Seidenfield JJ, et al: Fluid balance and the adult respiratory distress syndrome. Am Rev Respir Dis 135:924, 1987.

160. Eisenberg PR, Hansbrough JR, Anderson D, et al: A prospective study of lung water measurements during patient management in an intensive care unit. Am Rev Respir Dis 136:662, 1987.

161. Schuller D, Mitchell JP, Calandrino FS, et al: Fluid balance during pulmonary edema: Is fluid gain a marker or a cause of poor outcome? Chest 100:1068, 1991.

162. Humphrey H, Hall J, Sznajder I, et al: Improved survival in ARDS patients associated with a reduction in pulmonary capillary wedge pressure. Chest 97:1176, 1990.

163. Staub NC: Clinical use of lung water measurements: Report of a workshop. Chest 90:588, 1986.

164. Chinard FP, Enns T, Nolan MF: Pulmonary extravascular water volumes from transit time and slope data. J Appl Physiol 17:179, 1962.

165. Chinard FP: Estimation of extravascular lung water by indicator-dilution techniques. Circ Res 37:137, 1975.

166. Noble WH, Obdrzalek J, Kay JC:. A new technique for measuring pulmonary edema. J Appl Physiol 34:508, 1973.

167. Gee MH, Miller PD, Stage AF, et al: Estimation of pulmonary extravascular fluid volume by use of thermodilution (abstract). Fed Proc 30:379, 1971.

168. Lewis FR, Elings VB, Sturm JA: Bedside measurement of lung water. J Surg Res 27:250, 1979.

169. Effros RM: Lung water measurements with the mean transit time approach. J Appl Physiol 59:673, 1985.

170. Allison RC, Carlile PV, Gray BA: Thermodilution measurement of lung water. Clin Chest Med 6:439, 1985.

171. Turino GM, Pine MB, Shubrooks SJ Jr, et al: The volume of extravascular water of the lung in normal man and in disease. Bull Physiopathol Respir 7:1161, 1971.

172. Pearce ML, Yamashita J, Beazell J: Measurement of pulmonary edema. Circ Res 16:482, 1965.

173. Gray BA, Beckett RC, Allison RC, et al: Effect of edema and hemodynamic changes on extravascular thermal volume of the lung. J Appl Physiol 56:878, 1984.

174. Bock J, Deuflhard P, Hoeft A, et al: Thermal recovery after passage of the pulmonary circulation assessed by deconvolution. J Appl Physiol 64:1210, 1987.

Mechanical Ventilation and Weaning

Robert C. Hyzy
John Popovich, Jr.

Mechanical ventilation is one of the most frequently applied interventions in modern critical care units. Techniques for providing artificial ventilation have been considered for centuries. The poliomyelitis epidemics of the 1950s led to the development of techniques of application and organized care units that currently form the basis of respiratory intensive care.

INDICATIONS FOR MECHANICAL VENTILATION

The decision to initiate mechanical ventilation of a patient entails a major commitment of hospital resources and a set

TABLE 84-1

ABNORMALITIES SUGGESTIVE OF THE NEED FOR MECHANICAL VENTILATION

Parameter	Value
Loss of ventilatory reserve	
Respiratory rate	>35 breaths/min
Tidal volume	<5 mL/kg
Vital capacity	<10 mL/kg
Negative inspiratory force	>−25 cm H_2O
Minute ventilation	>10 L/min
Rise in P_{CO_2}	>10 mm Hg
Refractory hypoxemia	
Alveolar-arterial gradient (F_{IO_2} = 1.0)	>450 mm Hg
Pa_{O_2}/PA_{O_2}	<0.15
Pa_{O_2} with supplemental O_2	<55 mg Hg

of unique and serious complications. Traditional parameters often used to evaluate the need for mechanical ventilation are listed in Table 84-1. The main indications for institution of mechanical ventilation are inability to oxygenate the arterial blood adequately and loss of the capacity to sustain adequate alveolar ventilation. The indications for initiating mechanical ventilation are often not clear-cut, and specific clinical factors must be taken into account. In general, it is important to consider mechanical ventilation early in a patient's course of illness, but this depends on the disease process. For example, a patient with severe chronic obstructive pulmonary disease (COPD) and CO_2 retention may be in a chronic state of ventilatory failure and respiratory muscle fatigue.[1] An attempt to reverse the factors, such as worsening bronchospasm or congestive heart failure, that may have led to worsening of the patient's status may avoid the necessity of instituting mechanical ventilation. In contrast, an asthmatic patient with normal arterial blood gas values may require mechanical ventilation early if signs of fatigue persist or progress despite therapy.[2]

Common disorders in which mechanical ventilation may be indicated are listed in Table 84-2 and include acute pulmonary parenchymal diseases, such as severe pneumonia or the adult respiratory distress syndrome (ARDS). Mechanical ventilation is usually indicated in these disorders because of hypoxemia refractory to other measures or excessive work of breathing. Cardiogenic pulmonary edema can produce

TABLE 84-2

CONDITIONS OFTEN REQUIRING MECHANICAL VENTILATION

Acute pulmonary parenchymal disease
  Pneumonitis: infective, aspiration, and others
  Adult respiratory distress syndrome
Cardiogenic pulmonary edema
  Acute myocardial infarction
  Cardiomyopathy
Primary ventilatory failure
  Guillain-Barré syndrome
  Myasthenia gravis
  Drug overdose
Airways disease
  Exacerbations of chronic obstructive pulmonary disease
  Asthma
Systemic illnesses
  Shock
  Sepsis
Miscellaneous
  Intraoperative: general anesthesia
  Chest trauma

similar physiologic derangements but may respond to therapy before mechanical ventilation is necessary. In addition, cardiac disease may contribute to ventilatory failure if respiratory muscle fatigue occurs because of inadequate perfusion of the respiratory muscles.[3]

Primary ventilatory failure can occur for several reasons but is a less common indication for mechanical ventilation. Etiologies are generally neurologic and include myasthenia gravis, Guillain-Barré syndrome, poliomyelitis, spinal cord or head trauma, and drug overdose. Obesity-related hypoventilation and idiopathic hypoventilation are less commonly encountered. Disorders of the chest wall, such as kyphoscoliosis, can also manifest with ventilatory failure. The presence of primary ventilatory failure may be suggested by CO_2 retention in the presence of a normal or nearly normal alveolar-arterial O_2 gradient. However, the concomitant presence of atelectasis or parenchymal fibrosis in this setting may result in a widened alveolar-arterial O_2 gradient.

The exacerbation of underlying obstructive airways disease is a frequent indication for the initiation of mechanical ventilation. Depending on the clinical circumstances, refractory hypoxemia or ventilatory failure or both may serve as an indication for mechanical ventilation.[1, 4]

Systemic illnesses leading to respiratory failure include sepsis and shock. In some circumstances, mechanical ventilation is indicated in these disorders despite the preservation of relatively normal arterial blood gas levels. For example, a patient in shock may develop a progressive metabolic acidosis. The extent to which the lungs compensate adequately for metabolic acidosis may be determined by calculating what the appropriate P_{CO_2} would be for a given acidosis: expected $P_{CO_2} = 1.5[HCO_3^-] + 8 \pm 2$. If the P_{CO_2} rises out of the range of appropriate compensation, mechanical ventilation should be strongly considered even if the pH is relatively well maintained. In this setting, the increased demand on the respiratory system to compensate for the metabolic acidosis by hyperventilation, combined with the propensity to develop respiratory muscle fatigue secondary to hypoperfusion, may lead to a respiratory arrest if intervention is withheld.[5] In general, early institution of mechanical ventilation is indicated in shock states.

In most settings in which mechanical ventilation is indicated, alterations in lung mechanics, such as increased airway resistance and decreased lung compliance, result in increased work of breathing by the ventilatory muscles, especially the diaphragm. The initiation of mechanical ventilation (other than controlled mechanical ventilation with paralysis) ameliorates the patient's work to a considerable although incomplete extent.[6] The ventilatory muscles continue to perform some work, although the magnitude of this work tends not to be fatiguing when at least 80% of the minute ventilation is delivered from the machine.[7] Used appropriately, support with mechanical ventilation creates an opportunity for reversal of the underlying condition and alleviates the patient's ventilatory work to an extent that permits the diaphragm to rest and recover from circumstances that have produced or might produce diaphragmatic fatigue and life-threatening hypercapnia.[8]

Mechanical ventilation may be performed by either positive pressure or negative pressure mechanical ventilators. Both types of ventilators create the development of a pressure gradient between the mouth and alveoli such that air flows into the lungs.

NEGATIVE PRESSURE VENTILATION

Historically, the most important negative pressure ventilator is the iron lung.[9] The patient is placed into an airtight cylindrical tank that encompasses the body below the neck.

When the tank is cyclically evacuated of gas, negative pressure is generated around the chest and abdomen. A negative alveolar-mouth pressure gradient is thereby created, and gas flows into the lungs. Exhalation is passive and occurs when the tank pressure is allowed to return to atmospheric pressure. The iron lung is large and difficult to work with because it restricts access to a significant portion of the patient's body by nursing personnel. This mode of ventilation works best in patients with neuromuscular diseases such as poliomyelitis, whose lungs, thoracic cage, and airways are relatively normal. The airway remains unprotected from aspiration. Also, discoordination between inspiratory movement of the thorax and opening of the glottis can occur, hampering effective ventilation by producing upper airway obstruction. Finally, the negative pressure applied to the abdomen leads to pooling of venous blood in the splanchnic vasculature and impaired venous return. This phenomenon, referred to as tank shock, may be responsible for the development of systemic hypotension often observed in patients ventilated with the iron lung.

The cuirass ventilator, a modification of the tank ventilator, consists of a shell that is fastened only to the thorax and upper abdomen. Airflow occurs into the lungs again by the generation of a negative pressure around the thorax and abdomen. Because this device covers less of the body than the iron lung, nursing care is easier. However, the cuirass is less effective as a mode of mechanical ventilation for the same reason.[10] Reports of the use of intermittent cuirass negative pressure ventilation for patients with chronic hypercapnia resulting from neuromuscular disease[11, 12] and COPD[13, 14] have suggested a potential role for these ventilators in relieving the chronically fatigued diaphragm. Nocturnal or even weekly use of these ventilators may allow the patient to reset his or her P_{CO_2} at a lower point during the day when the cuirass ventilator is not being used. The development of a lower P_{CO_2} may in turn help to alleviate symptoms of arterial hypoxemia by increasing the alveolar oxygen tension as dictated by the alveolar air equation. Whether this form of intervention significantly affects morbidity and mortality in these groups of patients awaits further study.

The rocking (oscillating) bed is also frequently classified as a negative pressure ventilator, but it really functions as a diaphragmatic assist device. As the patient is alternately rocked in the Trendelenburg and the reverse Trendelenburg positions, diaphragmatic excursions occur because the abdomen alternately compresses and decompresses the diaphragm. Rocking bed ventilation has been used successfully in patients with diaphragmatic paralysis after coronary artery bypass surgery as a means of partial ventilatory support.[15]

POSITIVE PRESSURE VENTILATION: PHYSIOLOGY AND ITS CONSEQUENCES

Although full[16] and partial[17] ventilatory support may be provided via nasal mask to patients with acute respiratory failure with some success, positive pressure ventilation generally requires the presence of an endotracheal tube. When airway pressure is elevated above atmospheric pressure, the airway pressure gradient between the central airway and the alveoli leads to an inflow of air into the alveoli. Exhalation takes place passively when the mouth pressure is returned to atmospheric, and the gradient is reversed.

Positive pressure ventilation has effects on both the gas transfer function of the lung and its mechanical function. The distribution of ventilation makes gas exchange less efficient in the positive pressure–ventilated lung. Because of the regional inhomogeneities of diseased lung, the distribution of ventilation is never uniform throughout the lungs.

Different lung units receive different proportions of the delivered volume, which depend on the compliance of the alveolus and the resistance of associated airways. A noncompliant lung unit may receive significantly less volume while a compliant unit is simultaneously overventilated. As a result, positive pressure ventilation increases ventilation of the more compliant, nondependent upper lung zones. This results in an increase in the physiologic dead space as nondependent lung areas become underperfused in relation to ventilation and fail to participate in gas exchange. In addition, because the diaphragm is no longer pulling open the dependent lung regions that already have a low ventilation/perfusion ratio, increased shunting of blood through the lung can occur.[18] However, positive pressure ventilation may enhance the ability of the lung to undertake its respiratory function of oxygenating the blood by elevating mean airway pressure and functional residual capacity (FRC). This tends to decrease shunting by maintaining airway and alveolar patency in areas of alveolar collapse. This is also one proposed explanation for the ability of positive end-expiratory pressure (PEEP) to improve oxygenation. The adverse physiologic effects of positive pressure ventilation are a consequence of both the inhomogeneities of gas distribution (e.g., barotrauma; intrinsic PEEP, or auto-PEEP) and the global increase in intrathoracic pressure with inspiration (hemodynamic effects).

Pulmonary Barotrauma

In the mechanically ventilated patient, barotrauma is the development of extra-alveolar air as a result of alveolar rupture. Clinically, barotrauma may be manifested by the development of pneumothorax, bronchopleural fistula, pulmonary interstitial emphysema, pneumomediastinum, pneumoperitoneum, or subcutaneous emphysema. The location of the abnormal air collection developed depends on the location of the rupturing alveolus and its adjacent structures. Alveolar rupture into the pleural space produces pneumothorax, whereas rupture elsewhere is manifested clinically according to the further dissection of air along contiguous fascial planes.[19]

Patients with diseases affecting lung compliance are predisposed to the development of pulmonary barotrauma. Patients with emphysema have elevated lung compliance and may experience barotrauma more readily because of areas of anatomic weakness in the lung parenchyma. Patients with ARDS have decreased lung compliance and have elevated airway pressures when mechanically ventilated with volume-cycled ventilators. Elevations in airway pressure are transmitted, albeit imperfectly, to the alveolar space and serve as a distending pressure that predisposes the alveolus to rupture. Diseased lung units are inhomogeneously ventilated by positive pressure ventilation and empty at different rates. As a consequence, changes in peak airway pressure reflect the common airway resistive forces mutually overcome by the ventilator rather than changes at the alveolar level.[20] Transepithelial pressure (alveolar minus interstitial pressure) is more indicative of the distending stress at the alveolar level producing barotrauma,[18] but this cannot be routinely measured. Nevertheless, elevations in peak airway pressure during volume-cycled mechanical ventilation are correlated with the development of barotrauma. In one report,[21] 43% of patients in acute respiratory failure with low lung compliance having peak airway pressures greater than 70 cm H_2O developed barotrauma, compared with 8% of patients with peak pressures ranging from 50 to 70 cm H_2O. There were no episodes of barotrauma in patients whose peak airway pressures were less than 50 cm H_2O. This study suggests that mechanical ventilation that results in the de-

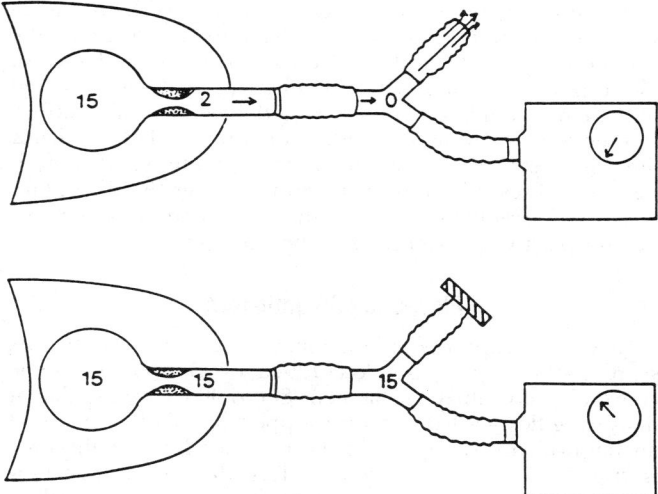

Figure 84–1. Measurement of auto-PEEP. (*Top*) Just before the next ventilator inflation cycle, alveolar pressure remains positive (15 cm H₂O) as flow continues through critically narrowed airways. (*Bottom*) When the expiratory port is occluded at end expiration, pressures equilibrate across the area of narrowing and the ventilator manometer deflection approximates the driving pressure outward (auto-PEEP). (From O'Quin R, Marini JJ: Pulmonary artery occlusion pressure: Clinical physiology, measurement and interpretation. Am Rev Respir Dis 128:319, 1983.)

velopment of peak airway pressures less than 50 cm H₂O is unlikely to produce barotrauma, and this serves as a useful therapeutic goal when achievable.

Volutrauma

There is solid experimental evidence that alveolar overdistention can result in lung injury pathophysiologically similar to that in ARDS.[22] Strategies of ventilatory support in patients with ARDS utilizing tidal volumes in excess of 10 mL/kg may result in the overdistention of more compliant alveoli that receive the tidal volume delivered by the machine.[23] Theoretically, this worsens the acute lung injury, although the extent to which this is clinically important is unknown at this time. As a result of these predominantly laboratory studies, some authors advocate the use of smaller tidal volumes in conjunction with higher levels of PEEP to provide ventilatory support to patients with ARDS,[24] even at the expense of significant degrees of hypercapnia.[25]

Auto–Positive End-Expiratory Pressure

Just as with spontaneous respiration, exhalation during mechanical ventilation is largely a passive event and continues until FRC is achieved, that is, until the elastic recoils of the opposing lungs and chest wall reach equilibrium. Differences in emptying between diseased lung units and more normal lung units mean that, under circumstances of respiratory failure, a positive pressure breath initiated by the patient or ventilator may be delivered before exhalatory airflow from the preceding breath has ceased. This phenomenon is termed *intrinsic PEEP* or *auto-PEEP*[26] and represents the remaining positive airway pressure present at the time of breath initiation.

Mechanical ventilators are vented to ambient atmospheric pressure. The presence of auto-PEEP cannot be detected unless the exhalatory port venting to the atmosphere is occluded at end expiration (Fig. 84–1). Patients who are mechanically ventilated because of obstructive airways dis-

ease have a large degree of inhomogeneity in the emptying of lung units and can experience auto-PEEP even at a relatively low minute ventilation. Auto-PEEP is common in mechanically ventilated patients. In one series,[27] auto-PEEP was found in 39% of patients whose minute ventilation exceeded 10 L/min and in 100% of patients whose minute ventilation exceeded 20 L/min. Patients with diffuse lung disease, such as ARDS, may develop auto-PEEP at high minute ventilations because the distribution of ventilation is markedly inhomogeneous and airway resistance may be elevated in this setting. The importance of the development of auto-PEEP in a patient who is being fully supported by mechanical ventilation lies in its ability to increase alveolar and intrathoracic pressure and thereby exacerbate the hemodynamic and other effects of positive pressure ventilation.

Hemodynamic Effects

In the thorax, vascular filling is determined by transmural pressure, the difference between intravascular and intrathoracic pressure (Fig. 84–2). With positive pressure ventilation, intrathoracic pressure is positive during inspiration. Consequently, transmural right atrial pressure increases and, as a result, the gradient for systemic venous return of blood to the heart decreases. In addition, large lung volumes compress the pulmonary vascular bed and thereby increase pulmonary vascular resistance and decrease right ventricular output. Increased pulmonary vascular resistance also causes

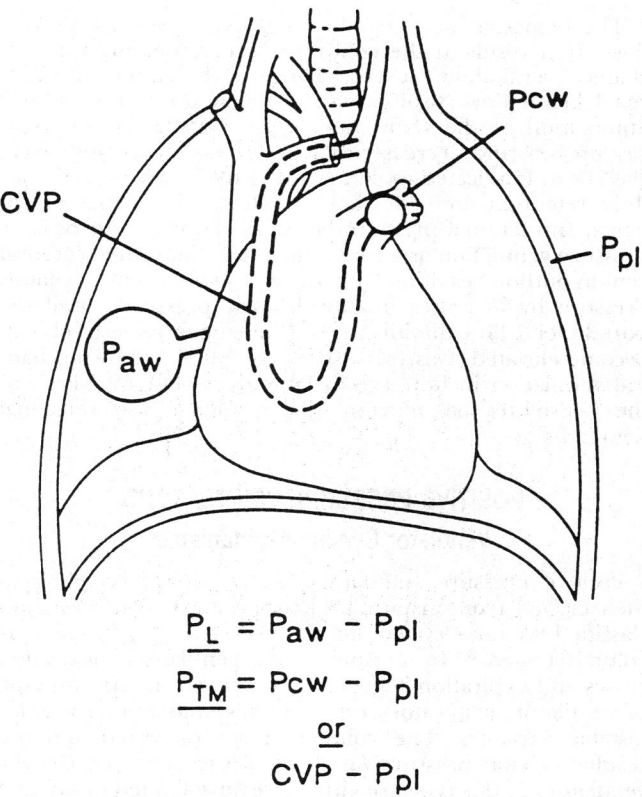

$$P_L = P_{aw} - P_{pl}$$

$$P_{TM} = P_{cw} - P_{pl}$$

or

$$CVP - P_{pl}$$

Figure 84–2. Relationship among transpulmonary pressure (PL [P_L in figure]), airway pressure (Paw [P_{aw}]), and pleural pressure (Ppl [P_{pl}]). Note that the effective cardiac filling pressure, or transmural pressure (Ptm [P_{TM}]) is also influenced by Ppl. Therefore, Paw or measured cardiac filling pressures (wedge pressure [Pcw] or central venous pressure [CVP]) are more accurate if referenced to Ppl. (From Boysen PG, McGough PG: Pressure-control and pressure support ventilation: Flow patterns, inspiratory time, and gas distribution. Respir Care 33:126, 1988.)

a shift of the interventricular septum of the heart to the left and impairs diastolic filling of the left ventricle (ventricular interdependence). As a consequence of these effects, cardiac output may fall and systemic hypotension may result with positive pressure ventilation, especially if hypovolemia is present.[28] The presence of auto-PEEP or exogenously applied PEEP increases intrathoracic pressure further and accentuates these hemodynamic effects.[29] In patients with left ventricular failure, increases in intrathoracic pressure with positive pressure ventilation may serve to improve left ventricular performance by decreasing transmural filling pressure and decreasing effective left ventricular afterload.[30]

The pulmonary capillary wedge pressure (Ppcw) measured by a Swan-Ganz catheter is referenced to atmospheric pressure and hence does not take intrathoracic pressure into account. During positive pressure mechanical ventilation with PEEP, the development of significant elevations in intrathoracic pressure may result in elevations of Ppcw that are not reflective of the true transmural filling pressure and falsely suggest the presence of adequate left ventricular filling pressure when this is not the case. An estimate of transmural pressure in this setting may be made by subtracting one half of the PEEP level from the Ppcw if the lung compliance is normal or one fourth of the PEEP applied if lung compliance is reduced.[31] Please refer to Chapter 85 for an in-depth discussion of the hemodynamic effects of positive pressure ventilation.

Other Effects

The hemodynamic sequelae of positive pressure ventilation often result in the compromise of other organs. Mechanical ventilation causes a change in the pattern of intrarenal blood flow, promoting salt retention in the kidney. Stimulation of the renin-angiotensin system, elevations of vasopressin, and decreases in atrial natriuretic peptide have each been implicated as contributing to the development of fluid retention and edema in mechanically ventilated patients. Intracranial pressure becomes elevated with positive pressure ventilation as a consequence of diminished cerebral venous outflow resulting from the elevation of central venous pressure by increases in intrathoracic pressure. Similarly, portal blood flow diminishes and hepatic enzyme levels can become elevated. Gastrointestinal complications of mechanical ventilation include the development of stress ulcers of the gastrointestinal mucosa with resultant gastrointestinal hemorrhage.

POSITIVE PRESSURE VENTILATORS
Ventilator Cycling Mechanisms

Positive pressure ventilators are classified according to their cycling from inspiration to expiration. Ventilators are classified as time cycled, pressure cycled, flow cycled, or volume cycled.[32] In a time-cycled ventilator, inspiration ceases and expiration begins after a preset time. In this type of ventilator, inspiratory time and respiratory rate are adjustable variables. The volume of gas delivered and the resultant airway pressure vary from breath to breath. Usually ventilators of this type are either pressure limited or volume limited. Time-cycled ventilators have little use in adults but are still used for neonates (Babybird-2, Bear Cub BP-200).

Pressure-Cycled Ventilators

In a pressure-cycled ventilator, inspiration ceases when a preset maximal pressure is reached. The maximal pressure delivered is controlled directly, and the lung volume developed varies. Increased airway resistance caused by bronchospasm or mucous plugging can lead to a change in the volume of gas delivered. A decrease in the compliance of the lung or chest wall, such as might occur with increased pulmonary interstitial edema, would have a similar effect. Consequently, ventilation with a pressure-cycled ventilator does not ensure that an adequate minute ventilation is delivered. Pressure preset ventilators such as the Bird Mark series were frequently used in the past to administer intermittent positive pressure breathing therapy.

Flow-Cycled Ventilators

Newer microprocessor-controlled mechanical ventilators such as the Puritan-Bennett 7200a or Bear-5 and some conventional ventilators (Siemens Servo 900c) are capable of delivering flow-cycled pressure support ventilation. A preset airway pressure is applied to the patient when the machine is triggered and is cycled off after the inspiratory flow decreases to a predetermined percentage of its peak values (Fig. 84–3).[33] This modality differs from pressure-cycled ventilators in that the preset pressure is sustained until flow tapers. As a result, pressure support ventilation (PSV) tends to be more comfortable for the patient, who has a greater degree of control over ventilator cycling.

Volume-Cycled Ventilators

Volume-cycled ventilators are the mainstay of conventional ventilatory support in the adult critical care unit. Here, the controlled variables, tidal volume and inspiratory flow, determine airway pressure and inspiratory time. At a constant respiratory frequency, a consistent minute ventilation is delivered. Variations in airway resistance or lung compliance lead to alterations in airway pressures but do not affect minute ventilation. Figure 84–4 shows how variations in airway resistance, lung compliance, inspiratory flow rate, and tidal volume affect airway pressure and inspiratory time. If the peak airway pressure exceeds the high-pressure limit set by the operator, the remainder of the tidal volume is vented to the atmosphere and is not received by the patient. In addition, when high airway pressures are generated, a certain amount of the tidal volume is lost in the ventilator tubing because of the compliance of the tubing. Therefore, even in a volume-cycled ventilator the delivered tidal volume can vary somewhat.

Volume-cycled ventilators that can achieve an inspiratory flow of 100 L/min at a pressure of 100 cm H_2O are sufficient to support most patients in acute respiratory failure. These ventilators, such as the Bourns Bear-1 and Puritan-Bennett MA-1, have a constant gas flow pattern (square wave). Newer microprocessor-controlled mechanical ventilators, such as the Puritan-Bennett 7200, Bear-5, and Engstrom Erica, allow various flow patterns, such as constant, decelerating, and sinusoidal patterns (Fig. 84–5). In choosing the inspiratory flow pattern and rate, an attempt is made to optimize gas exchange while minimizing high peak inspiratory pressures, which may be associated with barotrauma. In many instances the flow pattern makes little difference. However, the ramp wave pattern, which provides decelerating inspiratory flow, may distribute ventilation more evenly than other types of waveforms.[34] As a result, peak inspiratory pressure, dead space, and the alveolar-arterial gradient may be found to be lower in certain patients, such as those with obstructive airways disease, when ventilated with this waveform. Nonetheless, mean airway pressure may still rise, increasing intrathoracic pressure and resulting in adverse hemodynamic consequences. Newer microprocessor-controlled ventilators also have the ability to apply an inspiratory hold that inhibits

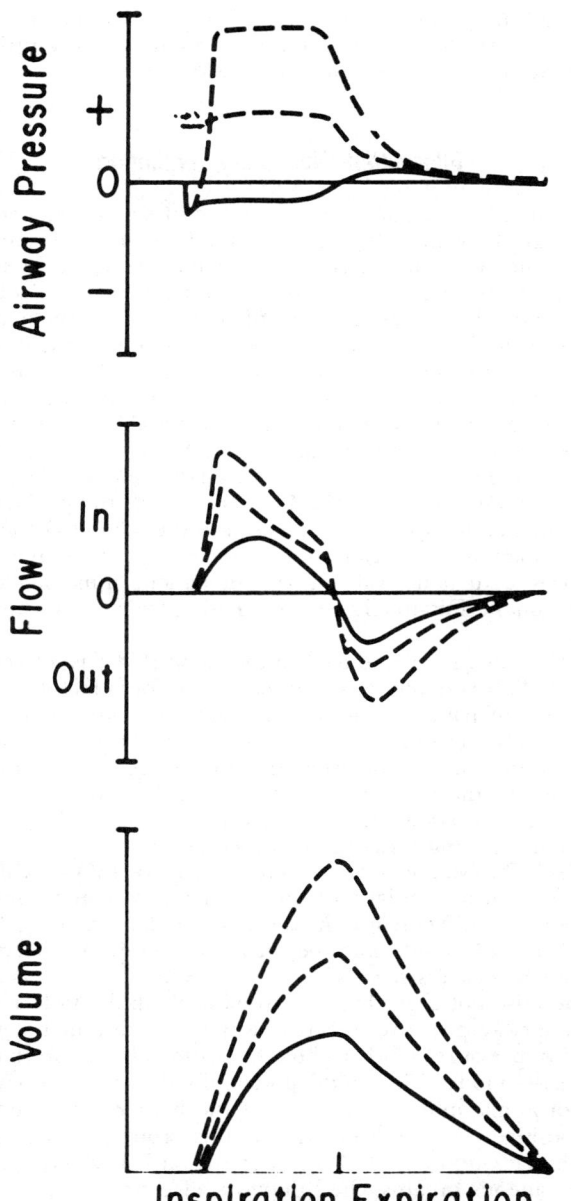

Figure 84–3. Pressure support ventilation. Pressure, flow, and volume as measured in the distal endotracheal tube during unsupported and pressure-supported spontaneous breaths in intubated patients. Note that the unsupported patient (*solid lines*) must first generate an initial negative pressure "spike" to open ventilator demand valves and then must maintain a small amount of negative pressure to produce flow through the ventilator circuitry. The addition of increasing levels of pressure support (*dashed lines*), however, provides plateaus of positive pressure that augment the spontaneous tidal volume in accordance with the patient's spontaneous inspiratory flow demand and inspiratory time pattern. (From MacIntyre NR: Pressure support ventilation: Effects on ventilatory reflexes and ventilatory muscle workloads. Respir Care 32:447, 1987.)

the exhalation of an inspired volume until after a preset pause (end-inspiratory pause). This can lead to an improved distribution of gas in the lung through collateral ventilation (pendelluft flow) but also results in elevations of mean airway pressure.

There are three modes of triggering the inspiratory phase in volume-cycled mechanical ventilators: controlled, assist-control (A-C) and intermittent mandatory ventilation (IMV)

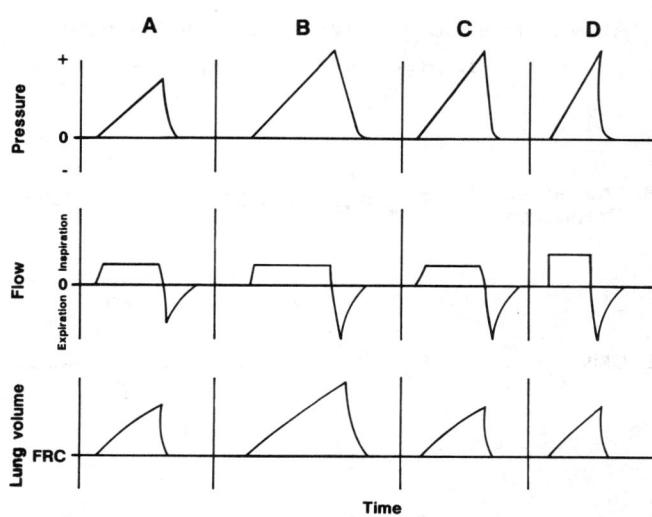

Figure 84–4. Pressure, flow, and volume waveforms for a volume-cycled ventilator using a constant flow generator (square wave). *A.* Baseline. *B.* Increased delivered tidal volume. *C.* Decreased lung compliance. *D.* Increased inspiratory flow rate. An increase in peak airway pressure occurs as a result of conditions *B, C,* and *D.* (Adapted from Spearman CB, Sheldon RL, Egan DF: Egan's Fundamentals of Respiratory Therapy. 4th ed. St Louis, CV Mosby, p 524, 1982.)

(Fig. 84–6). Modern volume-cycled ventilators can function in any of the three inspiratory modes with only a few modifications.

Controlled Mechanical Ventilation

In controlled ventilation, minute ventilation is completely dependent on the rate and tidal volume set on the ventilator. The patient cannot routinely move air through the closed ventilator circuit. Any respiratory efforts made by the patient therefore do not contribute to minute ventilation. Controlled ventilation is the required ventilatory mode in patients who are making no respiratory effort (i.e., patients with spinal cord injury or drug overdose) and those who have been subjected to pharmacologic paralysis. In certain patients, intentional paralysis and controlled ventilation are used to achieve better oxygenation or ventilation. Neuromuscular paralysis decreases O_2 consumption, in part because of a decrease in respiratory muscle work.[35] For this reason neuromuscular paralysis can be an effective therapeutic adjunct in patients with refractory hypoxemia or refractory hyper-

VENTILATOR FLOW AND PRESSURE WAVEFORMS

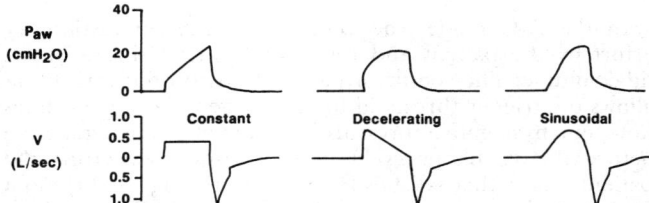

Figure 84–5. Airway pressure (Paw) and flow rate (V) shown for constant, decelerating, and sinusoidal inspiratory flow waveforms. Inspiratory time and tidal volume were held constant. Peak inspiratory airway pressure is lowest but mean airway pressure is highest with the decelerating inspiratory flow waveform. (From Banner MJ, Lampotang S: Clinical use of inspiratory and expiratory flow waveforms. In: Kacmarek RM, Stoller JK [eds]: Current Respiratory Care. Philadelphia, BC Decker, p 138, 1988.)

Airway Pressure Waveform During Various Modes of Ventilation

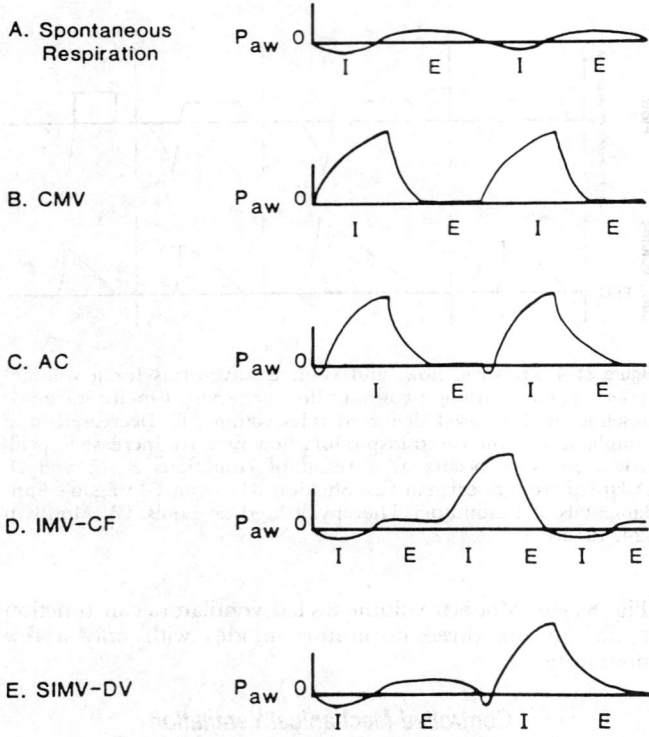

Figure 84-6. Airway pressure during various modes of ventilation. CMV = controlled mechanical ventilation; AC = assist-control; IMV-CF = intermittent mandatory ventilation delivered by a continuous flow circuit; SIMV-DV = synchronized intermittent mandatory ventilation delivered by a demand valve circuit; P_{aw} = airway pressure; I = inspiration; E = expiration. (From Tobin MJ, Dantzker DR: Mechanical ventilation and weaning. In: Dantzker DR [ed]: Cardiopulmonary Critical Care. Orlando, FL, Grune & Stratton, p 216, 1986.)

capnia. Neuromuscular paralysis and controlled mechanical ventilation are also sometimes used for the asthmatic who is difficult to ventilate.[36, 37] In this setting, controlled mechanical ventilation is performed to ensure adequate oxygenation. Hypercapnia is allowed to occur, and respiratory acidosis is corrected with bicarbonate administered intravenously.

Assist-Control Mechanical Ventilation

In the A-C mode, the ventilator senses an inspiratory effort by the patient and responds by delivering a preset tidal volume. The ventilator has a sensitivity adjustment that allows the trigger threshold to be changed. This determines how much negative pressure the patient must generate before the ventilator cycles. Every inspiratory effort the patient makes that satisfies the ventilator's trigger threshold leads to delivery of the preset tidal volume. The presence of auto-PEEP increases the effective trigger threshold. Thus the amount of negative pressure that must be generated by the patient to trigger the ventilator increases by the amount of auto-PEEP present.[38] Work by the patient is required to trigger the ventilator and continues to be performed during inspiration.[39] To ensure against the possibility of hypoventilation, a control mode back-up rate is set on the ventilator.

If the time between two spontaneous inspiratory efforts is greater than the interval corresponding to the back-up rate, a breath of the same tidal volume is delivered.

Intermittent Mandatory Ventilation

With IMV, the patient is allowed to breath spontaneously through the ventilator circuit at a tidal volume and rate that he or she determines according to need. At regular intervals the ventilator delivers breaths based on a preset tidal volume and rate. The degree of ventilatory support the patient receives is based on the IMV rate selected. Originally IMV was delivered with continuous gas flow through the circuitry and was not synchronized with the patient's respiratory efforts. Most newer systems have the capability to synchronize the intermittent ventilator breath with an inspiratory effort by the patient, a modality termed *synchronized intermittent mandatory ventilation* (SIMV). This avoids the problem of a ventilated breath being delivered to the patient at the end of a spontaneous inspiration. However, this modification utilizes a demand valve that the patient must make an additional effort to trigger,[40] increasing the work of breathing.

IMV was first introduced in the early 1970s as a weaning tool.[41] Subsequently, its use has been broadened to full support of patients who are in acute respiratory failure. A national survey of more than 1200 hospital-based respiratory care departments showed IMV to be the most common mode of full ventilatory support (71.6%) and the most frequently used weaning technique (90.2%).[42] The use of IMV in weaning is discussed subsequently.

Several advantages have been claimed for IMV as a mode of mechanical ventilation.[43] In patients who cannot synchronize with the ventilator in the A-C mode, switching from A-C to IMV mode may be advantageous if the need for sedation is excessive.

Because not every breath involves the application of positive airway pressure, mean airway pressure (but not peak airway pressure) tends to be less in the IMV mode than in the A-C mode. This could potentially decrease the risk of barotrauma and obviate some of the hemodynamic effects of positive pressure ventilation in this group of patients. At lower back-up rates of IMV, when the patient is taking more spontaneous breaths, the inhibitory effect of positive pressure on venous return and cardiac output is lessened. IMV may be particularly advantageous for a patient receiving PEEP who may have even greater cardiovascular compromise secondary to mechanical ventilation. Some proponents of IMV have suggested that the IMV mode confers an advantage over the A-C mode in the setting of respiratory alkalosis.[44, 45] It is thought that hyperventilation in the IMV mode is avoided by the patient's determining the tidal volume. More recent evidence suggests that differences in P_{CO_2} and pH between the A-C and IMV modes, if present at all, are small and not clinically significant.[46, 47] IMV has been said to be useful in maintaining and improving respiratory muscle strength because patients spontaneously breathe during a portion of the minute ventilation. Beneficial effects on hemodynamics realized at low levels of IMV back-up require increased diaphragmatic work and blood flow to meet the patients' minute volume demand. Whether patients with cardiac dysfunction who are ventilated with low rates of SIMV to realize potential hemodynamic benefits can meet the increased metabolic demands of a harder-working diaphragm makes the use of SIMV in the setting of cardiac compromise problematic.

Full Ventilatory Support: Choice of Mode in Conventional Mechanical Ventilation

Generally speaking, patients with acute respiratory failure should receive full ventilatory support. To the extent that it is possible, the patient should be relieved of the work of breathing by the machine to rest the diaphragm and permit time for the underlying pulmonary derangement to be reversed. It is now clear that, short of neuromuscular paralysis, the diaphragm and other respiratory muscles continue to perform work when fully supported by assisted mechanical ventilation.[7] Assisted ventilation, whether provided by the A-C or SIMV mode, requires that the patient generate sufficient negative pressure by inspiratory muscle contraction to trigger the machine. Marini and colleagues[7] have shown that when a patient is fully supported and the A-C mode is changed gradually over to decreasing amounts of mechanical support in the SIMV mode, the amount of inspiratory work per liter of ventilation increases progressively. At levels of SIMV support less than 80% of the assist minute ventilation, a potential fatiguing inspiratory load is created. Consequently, offering the acutely ill patient less than 80% of minute ventilation through SIMV back-up may be insufficient to rest the fatigued diaphragm and, in fact, may be fatiguing to the diaphragm on an ongoing basis. When the patient receives more than 50% of minute ventilation from the machine in the SIMV mode, the possible hemodynamic benefits of spontaneously breathing through the ventilator circuitry by negative pressure in SIMV may be lost. In one study,[48] only when patients received less than half of their minute ventilation from the machine in the SIMV mode were there increases in cardiac output, mean blood pressure, and wedge pressure compared with the values when the patients were supported in the A-C mode. However, increases in O_2 consumption above values seen in the A-C mode resulted. This suggests that the hemodynamic benefits gained at low SIMV back-up rates were offset by increases in work of breathing. Hence, patients receiving full ventilatory support by SIMV should probably receive at least 80% of their minute ventilation from the machine. At this level of support there is no particular advantage of one modality over the other, and the choice may be more a function of the clinician's familiarity with the method than the patient's benefit.

Full Ventilatory Support: Settings, Alarms, and Adjustments

A summary of suggested initial ventilation settings for providing full ventilatory support is presented in Table 84–3. The rationale for these and other ventilator settings is discussed later.

TABLE 84–3
SUGGESTED INITIAL VENTILATOR SETTINGS

Parameter	Type or Value
Mode	Assist control
Tidal volume	10–12 mL/kg
Flow rate	40 L/min
Flow waveform	Constant (square wave)
I/E ratio	1:3
Rate	10–20 breaths/min
O_2 concentration	100%
Trigger sensitivity	−1 to −3 cm H_2O

Respiratory Rate and Tidal Volume

The respiratory rate is generally set between 10 and 20 breaths/min when a patient is first given ventilation. This rate frequently must be adjusted based on observation of the patient and arterial blood gas analysis. The initial rate that is set may be somewhat dependent on the mode selected for use, in that patients receiving controlled mechanical ventilation and IMV are totally or largely dependent on the set rate to obtain a sufficient minute volume. The initial respiratory rate selected for these modalities should therefore err somewhat on the higher side when compared with the A-C mode.

Conventionally, the recommended tidal volume is about 12 mL/kg ideal body weight. This recommendation was based on the ability of these supraphysiologic tidal volumes to prevent atelectasis-induced hypoxemia in anesthetized patients with relatively normal lungs who were mechanically ventilated.[49] The use of 10 to 15 mL/kg tidal volumes made the former practice of episodic hyperinflation "sigh" breaths unnecessary.[50] Experimental evidence[51, 52] has suggested that large tidal volumes may induce lung injury, a phenomenon called "volutrauma." This may be most likely to occur in the setting of ARDS, where the tidal volume is delivered exclusively to only a portion of the lung.[23] On the basis of currently available information, no final recommendation can be made. However, it is reasonable to utilize tidal volumes no greater than 12 mL/kg for patients with diffuse lung disease to reduce the possibility of inducing significant volutrauma.

Other settings in which reductions in tidal volume are below the conventionally applied amount of 10 to 15 mL/kg include obstructive airways disease, in the presence of fibrotic lung disease, or after lung resection. Here the goal is to minimize airway pressure and thereby reduce the risk of barotrauma.

Flow Rate, Pattern, and Inspiratory/Expiratory Ratio

The peak flow rate determines the maximal inspiratory flow delivered by the ventilator in the inspiratory phase. An initial flow rate of 40 L/min is usually appropriate; however, higher rates of inspiratory flow are frequently necessary to produce adequate gas exchange, especially in patients with obstructive airways disease. Increasing the inspiratory flow rate shortens inspiratory time and thus decreases the inspiratory/expiratory (I/E) ratio. Because decreases in respiratory rate and tidal volume are often not possible in that alveolar ventilation needs to be maintained, improvements in the I/E ratio may be achieved by increasing the inspiratory flow. Conventionally, an I/E ratio of at least 1:2 is required and a ratio of 1:3 or more is preferable. Inspiratory time is determined by the tidal volume and the inspiratory flow rate. Expiratory time is determined by the inspiratory flow rate and the respiratory rate. Adjusting the I/E ratio so that inspiratory time is shorter and expiratory time is longer results in lower intrathoracic pressure and also lessens auto-PEEP. This can help avoid or ameliorate the hemodynamic consequences of positive pressure ventilation.

However, increasing the inspiratory flow rate increases the risk of barotrauma because peak airway pressures increase. As discussed earlier, newer microprocessor-controlled ventilators often allow the use of different inspiratory flow patterns. Altering the waveform may allow the patient to be ventilated at a higher inspiratory flow rate, yet at lower peak and mean airway pressures. The ramp wave pattern may be especially useful in this regard. The optimal values of flow rate and flow pattern must be determined empirically at the bedside.

Fraction of Inspired Oxygen

The fraction of inspired O_2 (FIO_2) is easily adjusted on most volume-cycled ventilators by a simple O_2 blender. In pressure-cycled ventilators, FIO_2 may vary in relation to airway resistance and lung compliance. When initiating mechanical ventilation, it is best initially to utilize higher FIO_2 settings. Attempts should always be made, however, to utilize the lowest possible FIO_2 that maintains adequate arterial O_2 saturation. An arterial O_2 saturation greater than 90% may generally be achieved by attaining a PaO_2 above 60 mm Hg. However, when acidemia and hypercapnia shift the O_2 dissociation curve to the right, a higher FIO_2 may be required to achieve the higher PaO_2 that is necessary to saturate hemoglobin above the 90% level. In addition, in patients with large shunts, such as those with ARDS, changes in FIO_2 affect PaO_2 to relatively minor degrees, and significant reductions in FIO_2 may be permitted with only a minimal decrease in PaO_2. Ideally, to decrease the risk of O_2 toxicity, an FIO_2 below 50% is suggested if possible.

Trigger Sensitivity

Ventilators set in the A-C mode have a sensitivity dial that determines how much negative inspiratory pressure or flow the patient must develop in the ventilator tubing to trigger the ventilator to deliver a preset tidal volume by positive pressure. Sensitivity should be selected to allow the patient to trigger the ventilator easily and avoid a prolonged period between the initial effort and the machine breath. Auto-PEEP increases the effective trigger sensitivity of the mechanical ventilator. When auto-PEEP is present, the patient must generate enough negative pressure in the ventilator tubing to overcome not only the trigger sensitivity set on the ventilator but also the auto-PEEP. This may lead to dyspnea and anxiety. Conversely, if the machine is set to be too sensitive, it "auto-cycles." That is, the machine triggers a breath immediately after the preceding one is delivered, regardless of the patient's effort. Usually a trigger sensitivity of -1 to -3 cm H_2O is used.

Temperature and Humidity

Humidification of the ventilated gas is important to prevent desiccation of the tracheal mucosa. Most ventilators have a cascade humidifier with a temperature monitor to ensure that gas temperature is appropriate. Delivered gas should be kept at a relative humidity of 80 to 100% and a temperature of 32 to 37°C.

Alarms

The most important alarms on a volume-cycled ventilator are the high-pressure alarm, the low-exhaled-volume alarm, and the apnea (low-pressure) alarm. The high-pressure alarm is routinely set at a level 10 to 15 cm H_2O above the peak inspiratory pressure. If this level is exceeded during the delivery of the machine breath, the alarm sounds and the remainder of the tidal volume is vented to the atmosphere and not delivered to the patient. High-pressure alarms are often triggered by the asynchrony of the patient with the ventilator. Although this is frequently related to coughing, other more serious problems may have developed. These include development of a kink in the endotracheal tube, displacement of the endotracheal tube into a mainstem (usually right) bronchus, development of a worsening bronchospasm or mucous plugging, pneumothorax (especially tension pneumothorax), and decreased lung compliance.

Volume-cycled ventilators measure the exhaled tidal volume and signal a decrease in this volume. The low-exhaled-volume alarm may signify that the patient has become disconnected from the ventilator or that an air leak from the patient or from the ventilator circuitry has developed, such as may occur in the setting of bronchopleural fistula or an endotracheal tube cuff leak. In this setting, the low-airway-pressure alarm may also signal. The low-airway-pressure alarm also signals if the inspiratory flow rate is set below the needs of the patient and the patient is actively drawing air into the lungs by generating negative pressure while the machine is attempting to deliver a positive pressure tidal volume.

Adjustments: Alveolar Ventilation and Arterial Oxygenation

The patient must be examined on an ongoing basis to be certain that the ventilatory pattern is smooth and that airway or hemodynamic compromise has not taken place. In addition, ensuring adequate ventilation requires evaluation of arterial blood gases and adjustment of ventilator settings to correct the abnormalities detected. Arterial blood gas assays are used to determine whether an appropriate minute ventilation is being delivered and whether oxygenation is adequate. Alveolar ventilation in liters per minute is determined by the tidal volume minus the dead space measured in liters multiplied by the number of breaths per minute. Because the $PaCO_2$ is inversely proportional to the alveolar ventilation, changes in tidal volume and respiratory rate may alter the $PaCO_2$. If tidal volume and dead space are kept constant, the respiratory rate needed in the A-C mode to obtain a desired $PaCO_2$ can be determined by using the following formula:

$$\frac{\text{Required respiratory rate}}{\text{Current respiratory rate}} = \frac{\text{current } PaCO_2}{\text{desired } PaCO_2}$$

Solving for the required respiratory rate gives the ventilator rate that should be set to achieve the desired $PaCO_2$. The actual $PaCO_2$ attained, however, may be slightly different from the desired value because of alterations in dead space that may result when respiratory rate is changed. Occasionally, the amount of dead space present may become clinically significant. For example, a patient with severe obstructive airways disease may have so much dead space ventilation that a decrease in the respiratory rate may lead to a decrease in $PaCO_2$ because of prolongation of the expiratory time and greater airway emptying. Dead space ventilation can be estimated by using the following formula for the ratio of dead space to tidal volume:

$$\frac{V_{DS}}{V_T} = \frac{PaCO_2 - P\overline{E}CO_2}{PaCO_2}$$

where $PaCO_2$ = arterial PCO_2
$P\overline{E}CO_2$ = exhaled gas PCO_2 (mixed)
V_{DS} = dead space volume
V_T = tidal volume

The exhaled gas PCO_2 may be measured by capnography. V_{DS}/V_T improves as pulmonary parenchymal disease resolves but may be useful in other clinical circumstances. For example, an increase in V_{DS}/V_T without a clear explanation may signal development of pulmonary embolic disease. In addition, the measurement of V_{DS}/V_T may be useful in managing patients with obstructive airways disease who have air trapping, as mentioned earlier.

Patients mechanically ventilated in the A-C or IMV mode set their own $PaCO_2$ according to their respiratory drive. This alone or combined with psychogenic hyperventilation can result in significant alkalemia, which may have serious consequences when the pH exceeds 7.56. In this setting, the alkalemia cannot be corrected simply by altering the ventilator rate. Changing to the IMV mode from the A-C mode does not help because the patient's own respiratory drive still permits significant respiratory alkalosis to take place. Administering sedatives to blunt the respiratory drive or adding dead space to the ventilator circuitry may prove useful. Occasionally, the patient must be paralyzed and ventilated in the controlled mode if the problem is severe enough and refractory to other manipulations. A pH in excess of 7.70 generally results in cardiac arrhythmias and could prove fatal.

The adequacy of oxygenation is assessed by evaluating the PaO_2. To determine the adjustment in FIO_2 necessary to achieve a desired PaO_2, the arterial/alveolar ratio (PaO_2/PAO_2) may be used. Unlike the alveolar-arterial gradient ($PAO_2 - PaO_2$), the arterial/alveolar ratio stays relatively constant if the patient remains clinically stable. To determine the FIO_2 needed to achieve the desired PaO_2, the following formula may be utilized:

$$\frac{Current\ PaO_2}{Current\ PAO_2} = \frac{desired\ PaO_2}{required\ PAO_2}$$

The alveolar O_2 concentration is calculated by using the alveolar gas equation:

$$PAO_2 = PIO_2 - PaCO_2/R$$

where R is the respiratory quotient (generally equal to 0.8) and PIO_2 is the PO_2 of the inspired gas:

$$PIO_2 = (atmospheric\ pressure - water\ vapor\ pressure) \times FIO_2$$
$$= (760 - 47) \times FIO_2$$

Values of 760 mm Hg for atmospheric pressure and 47 mm Hg for water vapor pressure are valid at sea level and are altered at increasing elevations. Once the required PAO_2 is known, the required FIO_2 may be calculated from PIO_2 and $PaCO_2$. If arterial hypoxemia persists despite high levels of FIO_2, the institution of PEEP may be indicated.

POSITIVE END-EXPIRATORY PRESSURE

PEEP is the result of impeding the normally passive expiratory phase of respiration so that a constant positive airway pressure is maintained. PEEP is useful in improving oxygenation, particularly in patients, such as those with cardiogenic pulmonary edema or diffuse lung injury, who have small lung volumes and decreased lung compliance. In these clinical settings the pressure-volume inflation curve of the lungs is shifted to the right, meaning that end-expiratory volume (FRC) is reduced and higher airway pressures result from delivery of the same tidal volume. In this setting the addition of PEEP is thought to redistribute lung water and recruit atelectatic alveoli. This increases FRC and shifts the pressure-volume curve back toward its normal position. With the addition of PEEP formerly collapsed alveoli become ventilated, thus decreasing intrapulmonary shunting and improving arterial oxygenation.[53]

As higher levels of PEEP are applied, additional increases in FRC cause lung volume to reach the flattened upper portins of the pressure-volume curve. When the same tidal volume is applied by volume-cycled mechanical ventilation, the resultant airway pressures rise sharply under these conditions. Pleural and intrathoracic pressures rise correspondingly, and the risks of barotrauma and hemodynamic embarrassment increase as a result. Thus compliance increases as PEEP is applied initially to patients with a decreased FRC but decreases when the level of PEEP becomes too great, as compliance is the slope of the pressure-volume curve. At high levels of PEEP alveolar overdistention may compress adjacent blood vessels and increase dead space.

According to these principles of lung mechanics, optimal PEEP may be obtained by determining the PEEP level at which compliance is maximized and VDS/VT is minimized.[54] However, pressure-volume curves obtained with large-volume syringes are often impractical for routine use at the bedside, and end-tidal CO_2 measurements required to calculate dead space may be unreliable in this setting.[55]

The cardiovascular effects of PEEP are an accentuation of the cardiovascular effects of positive pressure ventilation. PEEP may cause a precipitous fall in cardiac output. As with positive pressure ventilation, much of this effect is due to increased thoracic pressure leading to increased transmural right atrial pressure and a decreased gradient for venous return to the right side of the heart. Increased resistance of the pulmonary vasculature caused by positive airway pressure and PEEP leads to impaired emptying of the right ventricle and a shift in the interventricular septum into the left ventricle, impairing diastolic filling of the left ventricle and resuting in a depression in cardiac output.

The addition of PEEP leads to problems in interpretation of the Ppcw. The Ppcw is assumed to reflect the left ventricular end-diastolic pressure and thereby assess end-diastolic volume. Depending on the location of the pulmonary arterial catheter tip, Ppcw readings in patients receiving positive pressure ventilation, and especially in those receiving PEEP, may reflect alveolar pressure rather than capillary pressure. The lung can be divided into three zones, called West zones. In the supine patient in a critical care unit, perfusion goes preferentially to the posterior (dependent) lung zones because of the influence of gravity. Ventilation goes preferentially to the anterior lung zones, which are not collapsed at end expiration. In the anteriormost lung zone, West zone 1, alveolar pressure exceeds both pulmonary arterial and pulmonary venous pressures. If the catheter is wedged in this zone, the Ppcw tracing reflects alveolar pressure rather than capillary pressure. In zone 2 alveolar pressure still exceeds pulmonary venous pressure, but in zone 3 alveolar pressure is exceeded by both pulmonary arterial and pulmonary venous pressures. Only if the pulmonary arterial catheter wedges in West zone 3, the most dependent and hence posterior portion of the lung in the supine patient in the critical care unit, is the Ppcw likely to be an accurate reflection of left ventricular end-diastolic pressure. Fortunately, because Swan-Ganz catheters are flotation guided by the inflated balloon, they are preferentially located in West zone 3, where the flow is greatest. A cross-table lateral chest x-ray film may be obtained to help assess the anterior-posterior placement of the Swan-Ganz catheter if the question arises. Momentarily disconnecting the patient from the ventilator is not recommended. West zones are physiologically dynamic and not anatomic in nature. In the presence of severe hypovolemia, mechanical ventilation with high PEEP, or large tidal volumes, the amount of lung that is in zone 3 is lessened because of alveolar overdistention and there is an increased possibility that the catheter is in zone 1 or zone 2. In these settings, Ppcw is overestimated if transmitted alveolar pressure is mistakenly interpreted as Ppcw.

Even if the catheter wedges in a zone 3 location, elevations in intrathoracic pressure with positive pressure ventilation and PEEP can result in overestimation of Ppcw, as discussed earlier. This is because the filling of the heart is determined by the transmural pressure, not merely the intravascular pressure measured by the Swan-Ganz catheter. In patients with low lung compliance, such as those with ARDS, approximately 25% of the PEEP value may be subtracted from the measured Ppcw to obtain a more accurate estimate of the transmural wedge pressure.[31]

Renal, gastrointestinal, and central nervous system effects of PEEP are similar to the effects of positive pressure ventilation discussed earlier. In addition, the risk of barotrauma is increased by the addition of PEEP.

Some investigators have demonstrated a humorally mediated depression in left ventricular contractility in animals ventilated with PEEP.[56] Alterations in coronary artery perfusion have been demonstrated and used to explain alterations in contractility of the heart that may be found with PEEP.

Please refer to Chapter 85 for further discussion of the hemodynamic effects of mechanical ventilation.

Indications for Positive End-Expiratory Pressure

The use of PEEP for patients with diffuse lung injury and severe hypoxemia, such as diffuse pneumonia and ARDS, has gained widespread acceptance. The use of PEEP can result in adequate arterial oxygenation and hemoglobin saturation, which are essential for the delivery of sufficient amounts of O_2 to the peripheral tissues. Even ARDS patients who have acceptance levels of arterial oxygenation may benefit by the addition of PEEP, as it may allow adequate oxygenation to be maintained at a lower inspired O_2 concentration, thus decreasing the risk of O_2 toxicity. Although it is not known what level of FIO_2 is safe in avoiding O_2 toxicity, a goal of an FIO_2 of 0.5 or less is generally desirable but not always possible.

In ARDS, PEEP is entirely supportive and acts merely to improve arterial oxygenation by increasing FRC. The use of prophylactic PEEP in patients at risk for ARDS has been shown to have no impact on the incidence or subsequent course of ARDS.[57] High levels of PEEP during the clinical course of patients with ARDs were shown to have a beneficial effect on outcome,[58] but this has not been confirmed in prospective controlled studies. Therefore, the possibility that the application of PEEP may benefit patients with ARDS remains controversial. Hickling and colleagues have proposed that the use of PEEP in conjunction with a small tidal volume (5 mL/kg) may improve survival in patients with ARDS by avoiding the injury caused by alveolar distention (volutrauma).[25]

PEEP has been used in other clinical settings with mixed results. In patients after cardiac surgery, PEEP has not been shown to prevent atelectasis.[59] Patients with localized lung diseases such as pneumonia often have worsening hypoxemia with the addition of PEEP. Here ventilation-perfusion mismatch is increased by ventilating areas of infiltrate where compensatory vasoconstriction has occurred. Nonetheless, an empirical trial of PEEP in this setting may be considered if the patient has hypoxemia that is refractory to 100% inspired O_2 and body positioning. PEEP has also been used for patients with chest wall disorders, such as flail chest, to stabilize the chest wall and has been used in disorders characterized by instability of the tracheobronchial tree, such as bronchomalacia, in an attempt to maintain the patency of the airways. Some authors consider the application of small amounts of PEEP (i.e., 3 to 5 cm H_2O) to be "physiologic," overcoming the decrease in FRC seen with endotracheal intubation when the glottic apparatus is bypassed.[60]

Small amounts of PEEP applied via the ventilator have been employed to counteract the effects of auto-PEEP in patients with COPD receiving full ventilatory support. This can serve to decrease the effective trigger sensitivity of the machine and unload the inspiratory muscles of respiration.[61] Great care must be taken to use an amount of applied PEEP less than the amount of auto-PEEP so that patients do not have worsening dynamic hyperinflation, increasing the risk of hemodynamic embarrassment and barotrauma.[62] Although using PEEP to oppose auto-PEEP in patients receiving full ventilatory support has some theoretic advantages, it has not been shown to be beneficial to the patient in a clinically meaningful way. Prolonging the expiratory phase of respiration remains the preferred ventilatory intervention for managing patients with significant amounts of auto-PEEP.

There are no absolute contraindications to the use of PEEP. Some relative contraindications include unilateral lung disease, obstructive lung disease, elevated peak and mean airway pressures, bronchopleural fistula, hypovolemia, elevated intracranial pressure, and pulmonary embolism. As mentioned previously, utilization of PEEP for patients with unilateral lung disease, although generaly not helpful, may occasionally be warranted. In patients with pulmonary emboli, PEEP may worsen hypoxemia by compressing pulmonary vessels that had been unobstructed by emboli through overdistention of alveoli. Thus, PEEP should be avoided in the setting of hypoxemia resulting from pulmonary embolic disease.

Optimization of Positive End-Expiratory Pressure

Various strategies have been employed to determine the optimal or "best" PEEP for patients with ARDS. Albert,[63] wary of the detrimental effects of PEEP, advocates the lowest PEEP that results in an adequate PaO_2 at an FIO_2 less than 0.6 or 0.7 rather than seeking to achieve other specific end points that have not been shown to affect survival in this condition.

Nevertheless, alternative strategies deserve mention. The lung compliance approach involves the determination of pressure-volume curves by using a large-volume (2-L) syringe to inflate the chest passively. Bedside measurements of lung compliance (tidal volume/end-inspiratory airway pressure − PEEP) are inappropriate for this use because chest wall compliance is incorporated in this calculation and is inconstant in critical care unit patients. There has been renewed interest in determining pressure-volume curves in ARDS patients since the finding of Gattinoni and colleagues[23] that the recruited portions of the lungs of patients with ARDS have relatively normal compliance values and receive most of the tidal volume delivered from the mechanical ventilator. As a means of achieving maximal recruitment without alveolar overdistention, which might produce volutrauma, they advocated that PEEP be applied to recruit additional lung units and increase FRC until the slope (compliance) abruptly increases. These concepts remain to be tested clinically, as the authors acknowledged, and cannot be recommended for clinical use at present.

Applying increasing amounts of PEEP to minimize the amount of blood shunted through the lungs to values at or approaching 15% has been advocated by some authors provided that cardiac output has not diminished.[64]

PEEP can dramatically improve oxygenation, but the beneficial effects can be negated by impairment of cardiac function. Perhaps the best way to reconcile these opposing effects is to optimize the delivery of O_2 to the tissues. O_2 delivery ($\dot{D}O_2$) is the product of O_2 content of the arterial blood and cardiac output:

$$\dot{D}O_2 = O_2 \text{ content} \times \text{cardiac output} \times 10$$
$$= (Hb \times 1.39 \times SaO_2) + (0.003 \times PaO_2) \times CO \times 10$$

where Hb = hemoglobin concentration (g/dL)
SaO_2 = arterial O_2 saturation
CO = cardiac output (L/min)

This equation shows that if cardiac output decreases to a greater extent than arterial O_2 content increases, O_2 delivery decreases. When instituting a therapeutic trial of PEEP in adults, an initial level of about 4 to 5 cm H_2O is selected. Arterial blood gas analysis is performed and, if adequate arterial oxygenation (i.e., saturation greater than 90%) can be achieved at an FIO_2 of 0.5 or less, PEEP is not increased further. If arterial oxygenation is still inadequate, PEEP is increased in increments of approximately 3 to 5 cm H_2O. At these levels of PEEP, an indwelling pulmonary arterial catheter must be placed to determine cardiac output. With refractory hypoxemia, PEEP is increased and repeated blood gas and cardiac output analyses are performed. When a sufficient amount of PEEP has been added, cardiac output begins to drop and consequently O_2 delivery may drop as well. At that point, it is usually necessary to decrease PEEP to the previous level and thereby optimize cardiac output and O_2 delivery. If a patient is thought to have a decreased circulating blood volume, a judicious infusion of fluid may be attempted at the higher level of PEEP to increase cardiac output. In the appropriate clinical setting, attempts may be made to increase cardiac output through the use of inotropic drugs or afterload reduction. Regardless of additional therapeutic maneuvers such as volume infusion, inotropes, or afterload reduction, the best PEEP in this case is the value that results in the maximal O_2 delivery.

With an indwelling pulmonary arterial catheter, the mixed venous O_2 pressure ($P\bar{v}O_2$) can also be obtained. Even in patients who have ARDS or sepsis, a low $P\bar{v}O_2$ (less than 28 mm Hg) means that more O_2 is being extracted at the tissue level, as the result of either increased tissue demand or decreased O_2 delivery. If $P\bar{v}O_2$ increases with therapeutic manipulations, tissue perfusion is improved and, therefore, tissue O_2 extraction is less. Thus, $P\bar{v}O_2$ indirectly reflects the cardiac output and tissue O_2 consumption. These variables are related by the Fick equation as follows:

$$CO = \dot{V}O_2/(CaO_2 - C\bar{v}O_2)$$

where $\dot{V}O_2$ = O_2 consumption
  CaO_2 = O_2 concentration of arterial blood
  $C\bar{v}O_2$ = O_2 concentration of mixed venous blood

Often, $P\bar{v}O_2$ does not accurately reflect tissue perfusion in patients with sepsis or ARDS because of altered vasoregulatory mechanisms and peripheral physiologic shunting in these disorders. As a result, $P\bar{v}O_2$ may be spuriously elevated in patients with ARDS or septicemia. Here, it may be helpful to look at the trends in serum lactate levels to better assess tissue perfusion. A rising serum lactate level and an elevated $P\bar{v}O_2$ suggest both serious tissue hypoperfusion and peripheral shunting. In addition, it has been shown that O_2 consumption may be dependent on O_2 delivery in patients with ARDS. This means that $\dot{V}O_2$ in the foregoing equation is not constant. Thus, an alternative to optimizing arterial O_2 delivery in patients with ARDS is maximization of O_2 consumption. In summary, optimizing the level of PEEP in patients with diffuse lung disease by maximizing O_2 delivery and consumption, although not perfect, probably offers the best opportunity to influence relevant variables positively.

ALTERNATIVES TO CONVENTIONAL MECHANICAL VENTILATION

Conventional mechanical ventilation with volume-cycled positive pressure mechanical ventilators is sufficient to provide full ventilatory support under most clinical circumstances. In the adult critical care unit, institution of one of the alternative modalities discussed in this section may be contemplated in an attempt to provide support to patients with complex ventilatory needs or high-mortality conditions, such as ARDS. However, no prospective controlled studies

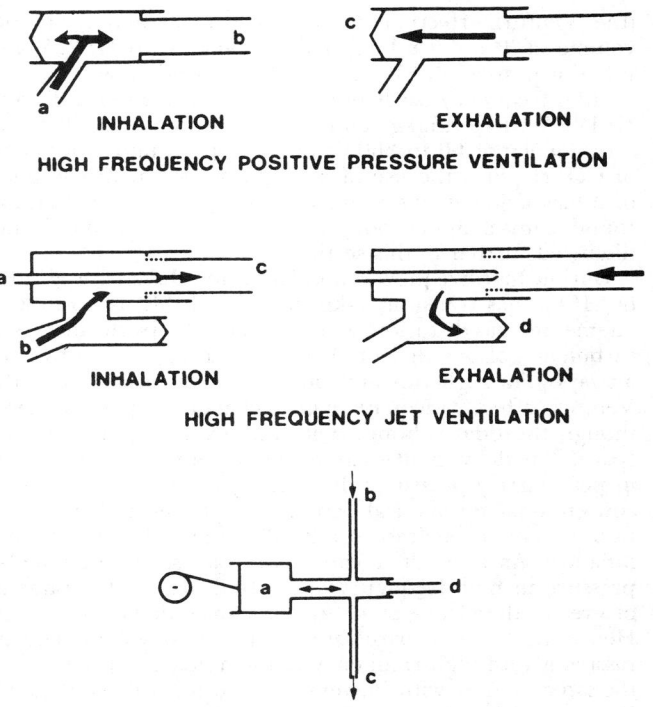

Figure 84–7. Modes of high-frequency ventilation. (*Top*) High-frequency positive pressure ventilation. High-pressure conditioned gas (a) is delivered during inhalation and flows predominantly through an endotracheal tube (b) to the patient with partial escape to the atmosphere. During exhalation the gas exits through an optional one-way valve (c). (*Middle*) High-frequency jet ventilation. Conditioned high-pressure gas enters from a cannula (a) at a selected level along the endotracheal tube or trachea (c). This gas entrains additional conditioned gas (b) (the Venturi effect). During exhalation the gas exits passively through an optional one-way valve (d). (*Bottom*) High-frequency oscillation. The piston or diaphragm (a) oscillates while fresh conditioned gas (bias flow) enters (b) and exhaust gas exits (c) at a balanced constant rate. The bias flow ports can be positioned anywhere along the path from the external tip of the endotracheal tube to within the trachea itself. (From Saari A, Rossing T, Drazen JM: Physiological basis for new approaches to mechanical ventilation. Reproduced, with permission, from the Annual Review of Medicine, Vol. 35, © 1984 by Annual Reviews Inc.)

have been published that suggest an improvement in morbidity or mortality with the use of any of these techniques.

High-Frequency Ventilation

High-frequency ventilation utilizes extremely high respiratory rates to deliver tidal volumes below the volume of the anatomic dead space to achieve adequate pulmonary gas exchange.[65] There are three basic types of high-frequency ventilation: high-frequency positive pressure ventilation (HFPPV), high-frequency jet ventilation (HFJV), and high-frequency oscillation (Fig. 84–7). HFPPV utilizes respiratory rates between 60 and 100 breaths/min with tidal volumes between 3 and 6 mL/kg. With a responsive exhalation valve, inspiration and expiration can take place through the same endotracheal tube. Inspiratory time should be no greater than one third of the entire cycle. HFJV utilizes respiratory rates of approximately 100 to 200 and occasionally up to 400 breaths/min. Tidal volumes similar to those in HFPPV are delivered through a small (14 to 16 gauge) catheter placed in the lumen of the endotracheal tube. The addition of an associated continuous high-flow system allows entrainment of additional gas of an adjustable O_2 concentration (the Venturi effect) and an approximate delivered tidal volume of 3 to 4.5 mL/kg. Exhalation in both HFPPV and HFJV is passive. PEEP may be added in either setting.

High-frequency oscillation is different from HFPPV and HFJV. A 1 to 3 mL/kg column of gas is rapidly oscillated at a frequency of 60 to 3000 vibrations per minute. Removal of CO_2 requires the use of a CO_2 absorber or the addition of a biased gas flow system. High-frequency oscillation has found clinical application mainly in neonates and is not discussed further in this section.

During high-frequency ventilation in adults with HFPPV or HFJV, gas transport takes place probably as a result of augmented gas diffusion, which is facilitated by the increased turbulence of gas delivered by convection to the proximal airways. Through this and other mechanisms, such as the Venturi effect, adequate gas exchange is possible even though the tidal volumes delivered are less than the dead space. The delivery of such low-tidal-volume breaths results in peak airway pressures that usually are less than those in conventional mechanical ventilation. However, high respiratory frequencies lead to auto-PEEP and dynamic hyperinflation. As a result, mean airway pressure and alveolar pressure in high-frequency ventilation may be the same as or greater than those attained with conventional techniques. Hence, the risks of barotrauma and hemodynamic embarrassment with high-frequency ventilation are approximately the same as those with conventional mechanical ventilation.[66] During high-frequency ventilation, the respiratory excursion of the chest wall may be lessened by stimulation of airway mechanoreceptors and subsequent vagal inhibition of phrenic nerve activity.[67] Thus high-frequency ventilation

(especially HFPPV) has proved useful in upper airway and thoracic surgery procedures, where a motionless thorax or the ability to ventilate through a small catheter may be beneficial.

Patients with ARDS may be successfully ventilated by high-frequency ventilation.[68, 69] In the largest randomized study published to date, no improvement in survival was associated with the use of high-frequency ventilation compared with conventional mechanical ventilation.[66] HFJV may be useful in ventilating patients in whom large persistent bronchopleural fistulas have developed, and it has been approved by the Food and Drug Administration for this purpose.[70] The magnitude of the bronchopleural air leak seen after the institution of HFJV may be less than, the same as, or even greater than that seen beforehand during conventional mechanical ventilation because of increases in alveolar pressure resulting from the institution of HFJV. It is impossible to predict whether HFJV will be of benefit in a particular patient with a large bronchopleural fistula. The clinical response to this modality must be determined empirically. Worsening oxygenation and hypercapnia may result from the institution of HFJV in patients with acute lung injury and persistent bronchopleural fistula.[71] The use of HFJV may be associated with the development of necrotizing tracheobronchitis; however, this is seldom a clinically significant problem. Obstructive lung disease is a relative contraindication to the institution of HFJV. Patients in whom this therapeutic modality is instituted should receive a low driving pressure, an inspiratory time less than 40%, and frequencies between 100 and 150 breaths/min. An approach to the institution of HFJV is shown in Figure 84–8.

- Driving pressure (DP) of 35 psi†
- Inspiratory time (IT) of 30 percent
- Frequency (F) of 150 breaths per min
- FIo_2 of 1.0
- PEEP of 0 cm H_2O or equal to that used during conventional ventilation

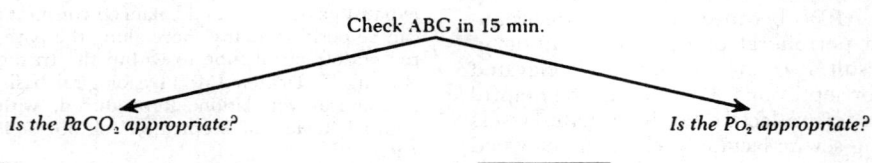

Check ABG in 15 min.

Is the $PaCO_2$ appropriate?

Is the Po_2 appropriate?

If hypercapnic:*
1. Increase DP by 5-psi increments up to maximum of 50 psi.
2. Increase IT in 5-percent increments up to maximum of 40 percent.
3. Increase F in 10-breaths/min increments up to maximum of 250.‡
4. Can add conventional tidal volume breaths or pressure support.

If hypoxic:*
1. Add PEEP in 3-cm H_2O to 5-cm H_2O increments.
2. Increase DP by 5-psi increments up to maximum of 50 psi.
3. Increase IT in 5-percent increments up to maximum of 40 percent.

If hypocapnic:*
1. Decrease DP by 5-psi decrements.
2. Decrease IT by 5-percent decrements to minimum of 20 percent.
3. Decrease F in 10-breaths/min decrements to minimum of 100.‡

If hyperoxic:*
1. Decrease FIo_2.
2. Decrease PEEP if present.

Figure 84–8. Initial jet ventilator settings. *Careful monitoring of peak, mean, and end-expiratory airway pressures and minute ventilation and oximetry should be performed when any change is made in ventilatory parameters. Only experienced personnel should use HFJV. †If the patient was hypoxic with controlled mechanical ventilation, driving pressure should be adjusted as necessary to achieve a mean airway pressure equal to that present during controlled mechanical ventilation. If minute ventilation under those conditions is not at least equal to that present during controlled mechanical ventilation, driving pressure should be further increased until this condition is met before obtaining arterial blood gas levels. If the patient was hypercapnic with controlled mechanical ventilation, driving pressure should be adjusted as necessary to achieve a minute ventilation two times that present during controlled mechanical ventilation. If mean airway pressure exceeds 110% of that present during controlled mechanical ventilation before obtaining that minute ventilation, arterial blood gas levels should be obtained at that point before further increasing driving pressure. ‡In individual patients, changes in rate may have opposite effects. ABG = arterial blood gas. (From Standiford TJ, Morganroth ML: High frequency ventilation. Chest 96:1383, 1989.)

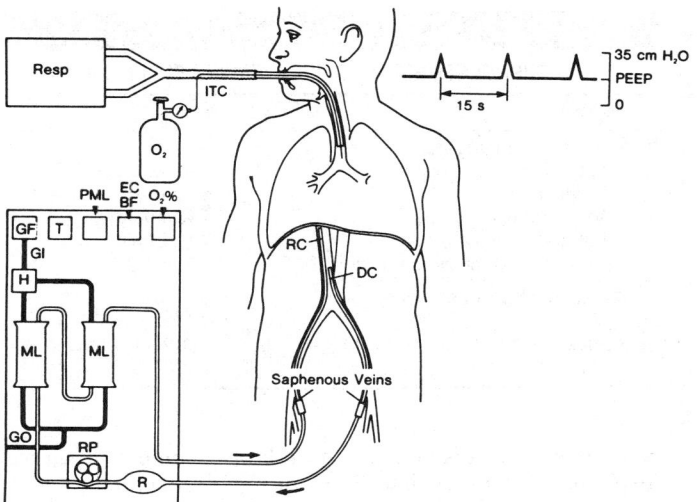

Figure 84–9. Cannulation and perfusion circuit for extracorporeal CO_2 removal. DC = blood drainage catheter; ECBF = extracorporeal blood flow; GF = gas flow monitor; GI = gas inlet; GO = gas outlet; H = humidifier; ITC = intratracheal catheter; ML = membrane lung; $O_2\%$ = venous drainage blood O_2 monitor; PML = membrane lung pressure, in-out; R = venous reservoir; RC = blood return catheter; Resp = respirator; RP = roller pump; T = ambient temperature control. (From Gattinoni L, Pesenti A, Mascheroni D, et al: Low-frequency positive pressure ventilation with extracorporeal CO_2 removal in severe acute respiratory failure. JAMA 256:881–886, 1986. Copyright 1986, American Medical Association.)

Pressure-Controlled Inverse Ratio Ventilation

Pressure-controlled inverse ratio ventilation is a form of controlled mechanical ventilation that has been used in patients with diffuse airways disease with refractory hypoxemia. By utilizing either heavy sedation or neuromuscular paralysis, the inspiratory/expiratory ratio is altered such that an I/E of 2:1 to 4:1 is employed. Significant reductions in peak airway pressure may result, although mean airway pressure increases. Although pressure-controlled inverse ratio ventilation may be administered in a fashion that is well tolerated hemodynamically,[72] the risk of hemodynamic compromise is significant because of the induction of significant amounts of auto-PEEP.[73] Complications including pneumothorax, hypotension, and bradysystolic arrest have been described. In the small, uncontrolled series published to date, patients with refractory hypoxemia have been oxygenated by this means, although survival has not been improved.[74, 75] This modality remains experimental and has as yet not been studied in a prospective controlled fashion. Its use is best restricted to centers where experimental, controlled protocols are being used.

Low-Frequency Ventilation with Extracorporeal CO_2 Removal

In the 1970s a large National Institutes of Health–sponsored multicenter trial evaluated the role of extracorporeal membrane oxygenation in patients with severe ARDS and found no improvement in survival from the 90% mortality rate seen in the control group.[76] However, interest in vascular bypass of the lungs has continued as injured lung units may potentially benefit by not undergoing conventional positive pressure ventilatory support in this setting. Gattinoni and colleagues[77] have evaluated extracorporeal CO_2 removal utilizing venovenous bypass as a means of minimizing posi-

tive pressure breaths to just 3 to 5 per minute, enough to ensure adequate oxygenation (Fig. 84–9). Nearly 45% survival was seen among patients treated by this method, patients whose gas exchange was as severely compromised as those studied in the extracorporeal membrane oxygenation trial. This study was retrospective and nonrandomized. Improved survival may have been merely the result of more fastidious care, as a study at the University of Utah has shown.[78] Final recommendations regarding the clinical utility of this experimental modality cannot be made at present.

Airway Pressure Release Ventilation

Airway pressure release ventilation is an alternative means of ventilatory support with putative advantages for use in patients with severe acute lung injury.[79, 80] With this modality, continuous positive airway pressure is supplied to inflate the lungs. The pressure is released cyclically, allowing the airway pressure to drop, the lungs to empty of gas, and CO_2 to be removed (Fig. 84–10). This modality remains experimental and has not been adequately studied in clinical trials.

WEANING AND PARTIAL VENTILATORY SUPPORT

Weaning is the process of transferring the work of breathing back to the patient so that independence from the mechanical ventilator is regained. The difficulty in achieving this goal is dependent on the severity of the patient's underlying illness and the extent to which the patient's respiratory muscles have been deconditioned by mechanical support. Most patients are easily weaned from short periods of mechanical ventilation.[81] Indeed, patients who are mechanically ventilated intraoperatively or while sedated by a drug overdose usually do not require anything more elaborate than a brief period of nonaugmented spontaneous breathing through the endotracheal tube (T piece weaning) before extubation. On the other hand, patients who are surviving courses of mechanical ventilation as the result of ARDS, pneumonia, exacerbations of COPD, septicemia, pulmonary edema, or other complicated medical conditions often require prolonged periods to be successfully weaned.

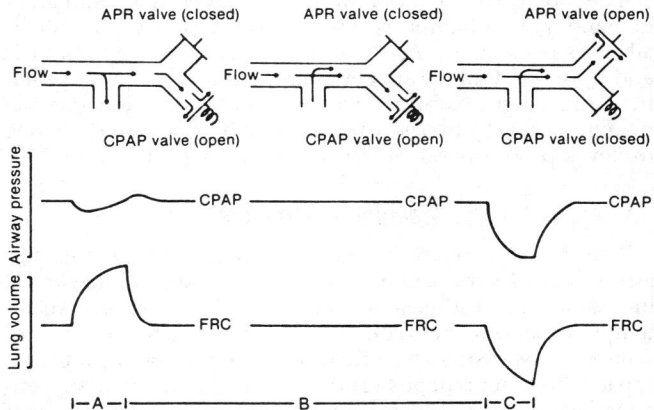

Figure 84–10. Concept of airway pressure release (APR) ventilation. *A.* Continuous flow CPAP. *B.* During exhalation with CPAP, the CPAP valve opens and the APR valve closes. *C.* During airway pressure release from the preset CPAP level to ambient pressure, the CPAP valve closes and the APR valve opens. After closure of the APR valve, FRC is established. (From JB Downs, MC Stock, Airway pressure release ventilation: A new concept in ventilatory support, Crit Care Med, 15, 459–461, © by Williams & Wilkins, 1987.)

Clinical Considerations
Optimizing the Patient for Weaning

Respiratory muscle endurance is required to sustain independence from the mechanical ventilator and should be considered from the standpoint of neuromuscular capacity and mechanical work demand. The need for continued mechanical ventilation is influenced by factors contributing to both sides of this equation. The weanable patient must be clinically stable with a ventilatory requirement that can be met by the patient.

Infection can prolong the course of respiratory failure by elevating the central drive to breathe in order to meet increases in both O_2 consumption and CO_2 production. Similarly, the ability of the lungs to compensate for metabolic acidosis with a respiratory alkalosis may increase the ventilatory requirement beyond that which the patient can meet. Hyperalimentation with a large carbohydrate load can increase CO_2 production and impede weaning.[82]

The demands placed on the respiratory system by derangements such as pneumonia, obstructive lung disease, ARDS, or cardiogenic pulmonary edema decrease as these disorders improve. Effective alveolar ventilation is enhanced and hypoxemia improves as dead space decreases. Ventilatory requirement, manifested as minute ventilation, decreases as a result, making weaning feasible.

The ability to meet the ventilatory requirement in a sustained fashion can be hampered by factors such as hypophosphatemia,[83, 84] hypomagnesemia,[85] anemia, and a low cardiac output. In the presence of left ventricular dysfunction the inability to meet increased blood flow requirements of the diaphragm in the setting of recovery from acute respiratory failure may be sufficient to prevent weaning. A study be Lemaire and colleagues[86] demonstrated the development of left ventricular dysfunction in difficult to wean patients with COPD and ischemic cardiac disease in whom spontaneous ventilation had been initiated through an endotracheal tube. When the patients were restudied 1 week later after diuresis and successful weaning, hemodynamic profiles similar to the values seen a week earlier before the trial of spontaneous breathing were found. Hence the inability of the cardiac system to meet the blood supply and energy requirement of the diaphragm may be clinically occult before weaning is initiated.

The ability of the diaphragm to meet the ventilatory demand may be hampered by other means as well. Metabolic alkalosis or sedation may blunt respiratory drive. Thoracic and upper abdominal surgery may lead to postoperative left hemidiaphragm paralysis. Patients undergoing left internal mammary artery bypass surgery may be particularly prone to develop postoperative left hemidiaphragm paralysis.[15]

Weaning Parameters

The decision to begin weaning is aided by the objective assessment of various measures that corroborate the clinical impression of readiness for weaning (Table 84–4). An attempt is made to evaluate recovery from acute respiratory failure by assessing the efficiency of oxygenation and the capacity for spontaneous ventilation. The efficacy of oxygenation may be assessed without removing the patient from the ventilator. However, the standard weaning parameters listed in Table 84–4 are obtained by briefly removing the patient from the ventilator.

A tidal volume in excess of 5 mL/kg and a vital capacity in excess of 10 mL/kg are generally considered acceptable for initiation of weaning. The negative inspiratory force is thought to be an important indicator of respiratory muscle strength.[87] It is also less effort dependent than other parameters. However, it is dependent on lung volume. A negative inspiratory force less than -20 cm H_2O is acceptable if this value is obtained at FRC, but a value less than -30 cm H_2O is acceptable if the patient is permitted to exhale down to residual volume by occluding the inspiratory port. A decrease in resting minute ventilation to less than 10 L/min occurs in conjunction with improvements in pulmonary parenchymal disease or a decrease in the central drive to breathe as with the resolution of infection. The maximal voluntary ventilation is the most effort dependent of the standard weaning parameters and as such is often difficult to obtain. However, the relative proportion of minute ventilation to maximal voluntary ventilation is a good indicator of ventilatory reserve.[88] The ability to double minute ventilation with the maximal voluntary ventilation maneuver has been found to be a specific but not sensitive indicator of weaning ability.[89]

The standard weaning parameters are most useful in the population of mechanically ventilated patients with readily reversible disease and those who require only short-term mechanical ventilation intraoperatively. Fortunately, this population appears to constitute the majority of patients. The standard weaning parameters are less useful in patients who have had a more prolonged course of mechanical ventilation. Here the attainment of most or all of these parameters can precede successful weaning by days or weeks[90, 91] or may not be achieved by the time successful weaning has taken place.[89] A study by Morganroth and colleagues[90] found no additional improvement in weaning parameters when successful weaning was accomplished in COPD patients who had been difficult to wean. Other factors such as psychologic well-being are involved in facilitating weaning.[92] However, physiologic limitations to weaning may be present that are not assessed because of lack of specificity and sensitivity of the standard weaning parameters. This has led investigators to look for other, more reliable methods of predicting the likelihood of weaning success. The central neurologic drive to breathe[93] and the inspiratory work of breathing[94, 95] are two potentially useful weaning parameters undergoing clinical scrutiny.

The inspiratory work of breathing required to oxygenate and ventilate the patient adequately is determined by integrating the area enclosed by the pressure-volume curve generated by an esophageal balloon, an estimate of pleural pressure. Fiastro and colleagues[91] showed that patients such as those mentioned earlier who have satisfied the traditional weaning parameters remained unweanable until the inspiratory work of breathing per liter and per minute decreased below certain threshold values. This experimental and somewhat invasive means of assessing ability to wean has potential for widespread clinical applicability but requires additional study because of the limited number of patients evaluated.

TABLE 84–4
MEASUREMENTS ESTABLISHING WEANING POTENTIAL

Parameter	Value
Standard weaning parameters	
Negative inspiratory force	< -20 cm H_2O
Tidal volume	>5 mL/kg
Vital capacity	>10 mL/kg
Minute ventilation ($\dot{V}E$)	<10 L/min
Maximal voluntary ventilation	$>2 \times \dot{V}E$
Assessment of gas exchange	
V_{DS}/V_T	<0.60
Alveolar-arterial gradient ($F_{IO_2} = 1.0$)	$<300–350$ mmHg
Pa_{O_2}/F_{IO_2} ratio	>200

A less invasive measurement, the airway occlusion pressure ($P_{0.1}$), has also been used as a weaning parameter. The airway occlusion pressure is the amount of negative pressure generated during the first 0.1 second of inspiration. The measurement of $P_{0.1}$ is independent of effort by the patient and is thought to reflect the neurologic drive to breathe. Patients with acute respiratory failure resulting from COPD have increased values of $P_{0.1}$ in an attempt to compensate for an overburdening mechanical load.[96] A study by Sassoon and coworkers[97] suggested that $P_{0.1}$ may be useful when measured before extubation, although Montgomery and colleagues[98] found pre-extubation measurements of $P_{0.1}$ to be useful only for assessing ventilatory reserve. Only increases in $P_{0.1}$ before extubation with CO_2 rebreathing, suggesting the presence of significant ventilatory reserve, were found to discriminate weanable patients from those who were not weanable. Absolute measurements of $P_{0.1}$ without CO_2 rebreathing were not useful in this regard. In addition, persistently elevated $P_{0.1}$ values correspond to fatigue-indicative changes in the diaphragmatic electromyogram of patients who are not ready to be weaned and undergo weaning trials.[99] These studies suggest that the central neurologic drive to breathe, as measured by $P_{0.1}$, correlates with the ability of the respiratory muscles to perform the work needed to sustain a patient without the mechanical ventilator. Further study is needed to delineate the role of this noninvasive, effort-independent weaning tool.

Respiratory Muscles

The institution of mechanical ventilation is thought to rest the respiratory muscles, allowing recovery from diaphragmatic fatigue, even though the diaphragm is not completely at rest and significant work of breathing is performed during mechanical ventilation.[6] During this time, deconditioning of the respiratory muscles may occur, resulting in decreased diaphragmatic strength. The institution of a weaning trial results in the imposition of an elastic and resistive load on the respiratory muscles. Meeting this requirement without reinduction of fatigue constitutes a successful weaning episode. Weaning trials may be conceptualized from the standpoint of respiratory muscle training. Spontaneous breathing through an endotracheal tube imposes a resistive load that increases the inspiratory work of breathing but can also serve to increase respiratory muscle strength. Hyperventilation during the weaning trial may improve respiratory muscle endurance. Aldrich and colleagues[100, 101] suggested that significant respiratory muscle training is unlikely to occur with routine weaning approaches and have reported success in weaning difficult patients by using inspiratory resistive loading devices. Although different approaches to weaning have theoretic implications for respiratory muscle training, a successful period of weaning by any means enhances the likelihood of future success.

Regardless of the approach selected, the development of respiratory muscle fatigue indicates a failed weaning attempt and the need for continued mechanical support. As fatigue ensues, the diaphragm contracts more maximally[102] but continues to act as a pressure generator.[103] Hypercapnia occurs, preceded by the onset of rapid, shallow breathing.[104] Abdominal paradox may provide a valuable clue to the development of diaphragmatic fatigue[105] but, when present in lesser amounts, may simply indicate an increased respiratory workload such as that seen when breathing through an endotracheal tube.[106] Clinical guides to the development of a failed weaning attempt are included in Table 84–5.

Approaches to Weaning

Weaning is best instituted early in the day at a time when sufficient personnel are available for close observation. The

---

TABLE 84–5

CLINICAL INDICATORS SUGGESTIVE OF A FAILED WEANING ATTEMPT

Parameter	Value
Respiratory rate	Increase >10 breaths/min
Pulse	Increase >20 breaths/min
Blood pressure	Increase or decrease >20 mm Hg systolic
PaO_2	Decrease to <60 mm Hg with supplemental O_2
$PaCO_2$	Increase >10 mm Hg
pH	Decrease >0.10 unit

---

patient should be rested, alert, and cooperative and positioned as upright as possible to minimize the effect of the abdominal contents in compressing the diaphragm. There are several methods of progressive weaning, including the conventional T piece approach, IMV, and methods incorporating weaning adjuncts such as PSV and continuous positive airway pressure (CPAP).

Conventional (T Piece) Weaning

Conventional weaning is undertaken by removing the patient from the ventilator for progressively longer trials of spontaneous breathing. The patient breathes humidified O_2 through a T-shaped adapter that is connected to the endotracheal or tracheostomy tube. An O_2 source and humidifier provide inspired gas flow at least twice the patient's resting minute ventilation.[107] FIO_2 should be increased to approximately 10% more than had been delivered by the ventilator to compensate for acute oxygenation reductions. A reservoir tube that holds approximately 120 cm^3 of gas constitutes the remainder of the T adapter and serves to prevent CO_2 rebreathing and entrainment of room air.

Conventional T piece weaning requires careful observation of the patient because breaths are spontaneously generated and apnea-triggered alarms or machine breaths are not provided by the ventilator circuitry. Some degree of dyspnea and anxiety is common when mechanical ventilation is discontinued and the patient is allowed to breathe spontaneously. However, a significant increase in respiratory rate and a decrease in tidal volume often reflect the need for reinstitution of mechanical support.[104] The development of uncompensated hypercapnia during the weaning trial suggests not only a failed weaning trial but probably also sufficient diaphragmatic fatigue to mandate mechanical support for 12 to 24 hours before additional weaning is contemplated.

The initial weaning trial often consists of breathing through the T tube for approximately 15 to 30 minutes. Repeated measurements of weaning parameters and/or arterial blood gases should be performed at the end of the trial to ensure that the patient has successfully completed the weaning trial without the induction of fatigue. After a successful initial weaning trial, additional weaning trials of a longer duration are instituted. Protocols must be individualized according to the patient's abilities. Easily weaned postoperative patients may be extubated after an initial 30-minute trial. The difficult to wean patient can require several days of gradually increasing periods without ventilation during the day, with periods of rest with ventilation in between. This may help to recondition the respiratory muscles.

When a patient is capable of tolerating extended periods of breathing through the T tube with little or no rest in between, extubation is considered provided that continued artificial airway access is not needed for other reasons, such as tracheobronchial toilet or airway protection.

Intermittent Mandatory Ventilation

IMV has been discussed in the section on positive pressure ventilation. IMV was first developed in the 1970s as a weaning technique. Patients are progressively weaned from the ventilator by a stepwise decrease in the IMV rate of usually 1 to 3 breaths/min at each step. This requires spontaneous respiration to account for a larger and larger portion of the patient's minute ventilation. The IMV rate of patients with good underlying mechanics and ventilation parameters can be decreased quickly over the course of a few hours. If weaning fails at a given IMV rate, an increase in the back-up IMV rate may be reinstituted or the patient may be rested more completely in the A-C mode. When patients have achieved an IMV rate of 0, they may either be converted to a T piece apparatus or be maintained on the ventilator at the 0 IMV rate. Extubation can take place soon thereafter.

For weaning in the SIMV mode, the patient remains connected to the ventilator and triggers a demand valve in the inspiratory limb before receiving a spontaneously generated breath. Breathing spontaneously through the ventilator circuitry during IMV increases the resistive breathing load beyond that imposed by the presence of an endotracheal tube. Additional work is required to trigger the demand valve, which may be especially important if auto-PEEP is present. A study by Marini and coworkers[7] suggested that the inspiratory work of breathing at low levels of IMV back-up is potentially fatiguing when the patient's lung mechanics have not improved to the point where the additional respiratory load imposed by spontaneous breaths is tolerated. Just as with conventional weaning, patients who become fatigued with IMV weaning and have significant amounts of hypercapnia should be rested for 12 to 24 hours by the reinstitution of total ventilatory support. IMV weaning is most likely to be successful in patients with less deranged pulmonary mechanics in whom weaning can take place over several hours rather than several days. This includes postoperative patients and patients recovering from readily reversible insults such as drug overdoses.

There is no convincing evidence that IMV weaning takes less time than conventional T tube weaning. In the majority of patients who receive mechanical ventilation, weaning is easily accomplished by either means. Hence, for this group the choice between weaning modes is probably not of great consequence. Patients with underlying cardiac disease may have less difficulty moving from mechanical ventilation to spontaneous ventilation when less than 50% of their minute ventilation comes from the mechanical ventilator.[48] However, the additional imposed respiratory muscle workload and the concomitant need for greater diaphragmatic blood flow may potentially negate this benefit.[86] Patients with abnormal lung mechanics who require several days for successful weaning probably are best weaned by progressive T tube trials because of the imposed workload of weaning spontaneously through the ventilator circuitry with SIMV. Consideration may be given to using partial ventilatory assist methods such as PSV to overcome this handicap.

Pressure Support Ventilation

PSV is not a weaning modality but rather a form of mechanical ventilation that is used to provide partial ventilatory support to patient-initiated breaths. In the pressure support mode, a preset amount of positive pressure is delivered during inspiration when the machine has been triggered via a demand valve.[33]

Pressure support is flow cycled in that the amount of positive airway pressure applied is halted after the patient's inspiratory flow has tapered off to a predetermined percentage of the peak inspiratory flow (see Fig. 84–3). As a result, synchrony with the ventilator is assured and pressure support is a comfortable, well-tolerated means of ventilatory support.

The goals for using pressure support as a weaning adjunct are twofold. Lower levels of pressure support may be applied to overcome the resistance of the endotracheal tube. At higher (greater than 10 cm H_2O) levels of pressure support, tidal volume is augmented. In each instance, some amount of the work of breathing ordinarily performed by the patient is shifted to the machine.

No clear guidelines have been established for determining the level of pressure support at which the patient should be started to achieve either of the two objectives. A study by Fiastro and coworkers[108] showed that the amount of pressure support required to overcome the resistance of the endotracheal tube varies as a function of tube diameter and inspiratory flow. Pressure support of as much as 20 cm H_2O may be required to overcome the resistance of a 7-mm endotracheal tube at an inspiratory flow of 0.8 L/s. In general, pressure support of 5 to 10 cm H_2O is usually sufficient to overcome, at least in part, the resistance of the endotracheal tube.

Several formulas have been advanced for determining a starting pressure support level to augment tidal volume.[109] These include

$$\text{Pressure support (cm } H_2O) = \text{maximal inspiratory pressure}/3$$
$$= \text{peak inspiratory pressure} - \text{static pressure}$$
$$= [(\text{peak inspiratory pressure} - \text{static pressure})/\text{flow rate}] \times \text{peak spontaneous flow}$$

When support has been instituted the tidal volume should be determined and compared with the patient's spontaneous tidal volume. PSV is thought to contribute to ventilatory muscle training by improving respiratory muscle endurance. As decreasing levels of pressure support are used, an increase in respiratory rate and a decrease in tidal volume are usually noted, effectively shifting the work of breathing over to the machine. However, just as successful weaning episodes permit longer T piece trials and lower IMV rates, lower pressure support levels become better tolerated as the patient's lung mechanics improve and ventilatory muscle training takes place.

In the setting of IMV weaning, PSV may be added to overcome endotracheal tube and ventilator circuitry resistance encountered during spontaneous breaths. Initially, an IMV support rate that delivers approximately 80% of the patient's minute ventilation is used and the other breaths are spontaneously generated with the help of pressure support. Subsequently, the patient's IMV back-up rate is decreased, as before, until finally the patient is breathing spontaneously with the help of pressure support through the ventilator circuitry at an IMV of 0. The pressure support level is then decreased and the patient is extubated at a low level of PSV or after a successful T piece trial.

Pressure support is also used as a weaning adjunct alone without an SIMV back-up. If PSV is used to overcome the resistance of the endotracheal tube and ventilator circuitry, progressive trials of PSV are employed in place of T piece trials with the patient rested by returning to ventilator use in between trials. When the patient is capable of tolerating long periods without the ventilator at a low level of pressure support, a T piece trial and/or extubation is undertaken. Alternatively, the patient may be given a higher level of PSV around the clock and gradually weaned to a low level of PSV before extubation. If there is significant airway obstruction, PSV applied in this manner may be unable to provide sufficient minute ventilation.[110] Pressure support must be used with caution when employed without an SIMV back-up rate in patients with airway obstruction and significant bronchospasm. Brochard and colleagues[111] found that different threshold levels with PSV were required to prevent diaphragmatic electromyographic changes suggestive of fatigue in patients being weaned from mechanical ventilation who had previously failed a T piece trial. Presumably, the threshold level of PSV decreases as weaning progresses. Thus, pressure support seems well suited as a weaning adjunct for the patient who is thought to be ready for weaning but is unable to tolerate an initial 30-minute T piece trial, at least in part because of the resistive load of the endotracheal tube.

No clinical trials have been performed showing a decrease in overall weaning time through the use of PSV. Clinically, the initiation of pressure support weaning trials in patients unable to tolerate conventional T piece trials potentially introduces a lead time bias. That is, patients able to tolerate PSV trials before tolerating T piece trials may ultimately be extubated at the same time as patients who have only T piece trials. The number of patients needed to confirm the presence of at least a 1-day difference in the time to extubation while avoiding a type II error is prohibitively great, and this has thus far prevented such a study from taking place.

PSV has been supplied by mask to provide partial ventilatory support to patients with exacerbations of COPD in an attempt to obviate the need for endotracheal intubation and conventional mechanical ventilation. In the only published study to date,[17] only 1 of 13 patients required intubation when treated with a flow-by triggered mask PSV device, compared with 11 of 13 patients who required intubation and mechanical ventilation and a historical, matched control group. This prospective study could not be observer "blinded." Because the study was not randomized, further confirmation of these results is required before widespread implementation can be recommended.

Continuous Positive Airway Pressure

CPAP is delivered throughout the respiratory cycle and may be utilized both in patients who are intubated and in those who are not. CPAP may be a useful adjunct to the weaning process in patients who have high O_2 requirements. In this setting, CPAP acts similarly to PEEP in decreasing shunting and improving arterial hypoxemia. Similarly, CPAP may be used in a patient who requires a high FIO_2 before the institution of mechanical ventilation. Finally, CPAP can be used as an adjunct in weaning patients with obstructive airways disease who have significant amounts of auto-PEEP.

A study by Petrof and colleagues[112] showed significant decreases in auto-PEEP and the inspiratory work of breathing when CPAP was applied to weaning COPD patients. The effects of CPAP on weaning duration were not addressed in this study. Decreases in the respiratory muscle workload would potentially be of benefit, although this remains unproved. Despite significant increases in end-expiratory lung volume at high levels of CPAP (e.g., 10 to 15 cm H_2O), decreases in the elastic work of breathing were found and worsening dynamic hyperinflation was not thought to have occurred. Nonetheless, the use of levels of CPAP in excess of the amount of auto-PEEP present is essential to prevent this from occurring.[38] As a result, no more than approximately 5 cm H_2O CPAP can be recommended on an empirical basis if it is to be used for this purpose.

Traditionally, CPAP can be delivered either by continuous flow or by demand flow. Demand flow is commonly used when providing CPAP via a mechanical ventilator to avoid the high gas flow required in the continuous flow mode. Demand flow CPAP involves the opening of a demand valve by patient-generated work in order to trigger the flow of gas. This imposed workload may be especially important to patients with obstructive airways disease and auto-PEEP (the study by Petrof and associates used continuous flow CPAP). Flow-by CPAP is a newer mode of administration. Flow-by CPAP is triggered by a decrease in the flow of a small amount of gas that is sent past the patient in the ventilator circuit. Less inspiratory work by the patient is required because a demand valve is not present.[113, 114] Clinical experiences are limited at this time, although a flow-by CPAP approach appears promising.

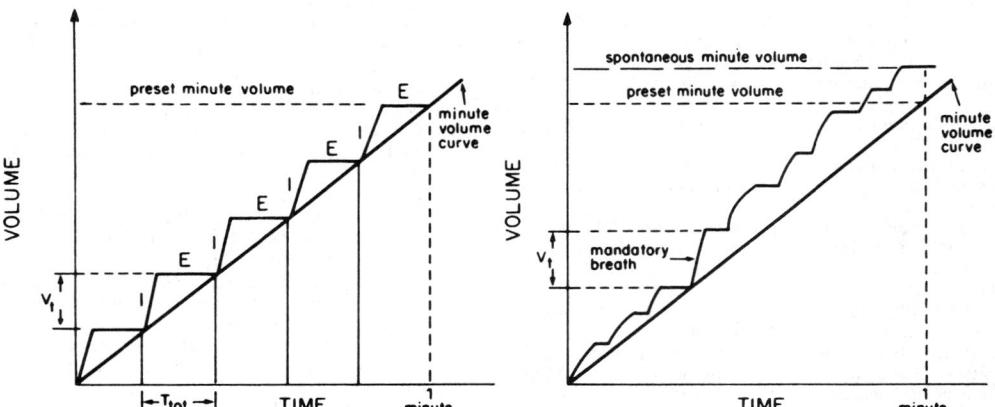

Figure 84–11. Mandatory minute volume ventilation. The adequacy of ventilation is judged against the volume cumulation rate (minute volume curve) predicted from the guaranteed minute volume (preset minute volume). When no cycles are called for by the patient within a certain period (T_{tot}), a tidal breath (V_t) is delivered by the machine (*left*). As long as the volume moved during spontaneous breathing exceeds the expected values, mandatory breaths are withheld. However, if the spontaneous rate slows sufficiently that the spontaneous and minute volume curves intersect, a mandatory breath is delivered (*right*). I = inspiration; E = expiration. (From Marini JJ: Mechanical ventilation. Curr Pulmonol 9:164, 1988.)

Mandatory Minute Volume

Mandatory minute volume is a means of partial ventilatory support whereby machine breaths are applied episodically when the patient's spontaneous breathing through the ventilator circuitry drops below a predetermined minute ventilation.[115] This ensures adequate minute ventilation. If the predetermined minute ventilation is exceeded by the patient's spontaneous respirations, no machine breaths are delivered (Fig. 84–11). This means of support was originally available only with the Hamilton-Veolar ventilator and clinical experience with it is limited at this time.

Extubation

When the patient is capable of performing the work of breathing and the patient is weaned from the mechanical ventilator, extubation may then be performed. Occasionally after weaning, the endotracheal tube is left in place for a few days to provide access for suctioning of tracheobronchial secretions or to protect the airway.

For extubation, the patient should be awake and alert. The stomach should be emptied of its contents to avoid the ill effects of an aspiration at the time of extubation. The patient should be situated upright and the trachea and oral cavity should be thoroughly suctioned. Air is removed from the cuff of the endotracheal tube, and the endotracheal tube is withdrawn after the patient has taken a deep inspiration. When the tube has been removed, the patient is encouraged to cough and oral secretions are again suctioned.

Acknowledgment. The authors gratefully acknowledge the contribution of Ms. Charisse Lukaszek in the preparation of this manuscript.

References

1. Schmidt GA, Hall JB: Acute on chronic respiratory failure: Assessment and management of patients with COPD in the emergent setting. JAMA 261:3444, 1989.
2. Scoggin CH, Sahn SH, Petty TL: Status asthmaticus: A nine year experience. JAMA 238:1158, 1977.
3. Aubier M, Trippenbach T, Roussos C: Respiratory muscle fatigue during cardiogenic shock. J Appl Physiol 51:499, 1981.
4. Derenne JP, Fleury B, Pariente R: Acute respiratory failure of chronic obstructive pulmonary disease. Am Rev Respir Dis 138:1006, 1988.
5. Viires N, Sillye G, Aubier M, et al: Regional blood flow: Distribution in dog during hypotension and low cardiac output. J Clin Invest 72:935, 1983.
6. Marini JJ, Rodriguez M, Lamb V: The inspiratory workload of patient-initiated mechanical ventilation. Am Rev Respir Dis 134:902, 1986.
7. Marini JJ, Smith TC, Lamb V: External work output and force generation during synchronized intermittent mechanical ventilation: Effect of machine assistance on breathing effort. Am Rev Respir Dis 136:1169, 1988.
8. Weinberger SE, Schwartztein RM, Weiss JW: Hypercapnia. N Engl J Med 321:1223, 1989.
9. Drinker P, Shaw LA: An apparatus for the prolonged administration of artificial respiration. I. Design for adults and children. J Clin Invest 7:229, 1927.
10. Hill NS: Clinical applications of body ventilators. Chest 90:897, 1986.
11. Garay SM, Turino GM, Goldring RM: Sustained reversal of chronic hypercapnia in patients with alveolar hypoventilation syndrome. Am J Med 70:269, 1981.
12. Driver AG, Blackburn BB, Marcuard SP, et al: Bilateral diaphragm paralysis treated with cuirass ventilation. Chest 92:683, 1987.
13. Cropp A, Dimarco AF: Effects of intermittent negative pressure ventilation on respiratory muscle function in patients with severe chronic obstructive pulmonary disease. Am Rev Respir Dis 135:1056, 1987.
14. Guitierrez M, Bertoza T, Contreras G, et al: Weekly cuirass ventilation improves blood gases and inspiratory muscle strength in patients with chronic airflow limitation and hypercarbia. Am Rev Respir Dis 136:617, 1988.
15. Abd AG, Braun NMT, Baskin MI, et al: Diaphragmatic dysfunction after open heart surgery: Treatment with a rocking bed. Ann Intern Med 111:881, 1989.
16. Meduri GU, Conoscenti CG, Menashe P, et al: Non-invasive face mask ventilation in patients with acute respiratory failure. Chest 95:865, 1989.
17. Brochard L, Isabey D, Piquet J, et al: Reversal of acute exacerbations of chronic obstructive lung disease by inspiratory assistance with a face mask. N Engl J Med 323:1523, 1990.
18. Snyder JV, Carroll GC, Shuster DP, et al: Mechanical ventilation: Physiology and application. Curr Probl Surg 21:1, 1984.
19. Maunder RJ, Pierson DJ, Hudson LD: Subcutaneous and mediastinal emphysema: Pathophysiology, diagnosis and management. Arch Intern Med 144:1447, 1984.
20. Hubmayr RD, Abel MD, Rehder K: Physiologic approach to mechanical ventilation. Crit Care Med 18:103, 1990.
21. Petersen GW, Baier H: Incidence of pulmonary barotrauma in a medical ICU. Crit Care Med 11:67, 1983.
22. Hickling KG: Ventilatory management of ARDS: Can it affect outcome? Intensive Care Med 16:219, 1990.
23. Gattinoni L, Pesenti A, Aralli L, et al: Pressure-volume curve of total respiratory system in acute respiratory failure: Computed tomographic scan study. Am Rev Respir Dis 136:730, 1987.
24. Corbridge TC, Wood LDH, Crawford GP, et al: Adverse effects of large tidal volume and low PEEP in canine acid aspiration. Am Rev Respir Dis 142:311, 1990.
25. Hickling KG, Henderson SJ, Jackson R, et al: Low mortality associated with low volume pressure limited ventilation with permissive hypercapnia in severe adult respiratory distress syndrome. Intensive Care Med 16:372, 1990.
26. Pepe PE, Marini JJ: Occult positive end-expiratory pressure in mechanically ventilated patients with airflow obstruction: The auto-PEEP effect. Am Rev Respir Dis 126:166, 1982.
27. Brown DG, Pierson DJ: Auto-PEEP is common in mechanically ventilated patients: A study of incidence, severity and detection. Respir Care 31:1069, 1986.
28. Pinsky MR: Cardiopulmonary interaction: The effects of negative and positive pleural pressure changes on cardiac output. In: Dantzker DR (ed): Cardiopulmonary Critical Care. Orlando, FL, Grune & Stratton, p 109, 1986.
29. Quist J, Pontoppidan H, Wilson RS, et al: Hemodynamic responses to mechanical ventilation with PEEP. Anesthesiology 42:45, 1971.
30. Rasanen J, Nikki P, Heikkila J: Acute myocardial infarction complicated by respiratory failure: The effects of mechanical ventilation. Chest 85:21, 1984.
31. Marini JJ, O'Quin R, Culver BH, et al: Estimation of transmural cardiac pressures during ventilation with PEEP. J Appl Physiol 53:384, 1982.
32. Banner MJ, Blanch P, Desautels: Mechanical ventilators. In: Kirby RB, Banner MJ, Downs JB (eds): Clinical Applications of Ventilatory Support. New York, Churchill Livingstone, p 401, 1990.
33. MacIntyre NR: Respiratory function during pressure support ventilation. Chest 89:677, 1986.
34. Al-Saady N, Bennett D: Decelerating inspiratory flow wave form improves lung mechanics and gas exchange in patients on intermittent positive pressure ventilation. Intensive Care Med 11:68, 1985.
35. Field S, Kelley SM, Macklem PT: The oxygen cost of breathing in patients with cardiorespiratory disease. Am Rev Respir Dis 126:7, 1982.
36. Daroli R, Perret C: Mechanical hypoventilation in status asthmaticus. Am Rev Respir Dis 129:385, 1984.
37. Menitove R, Goldring R: Combined ventilation and bicarbonate strategy in the management of status asthmaticus. Am J Med 74:898, 1983.
38. Tobin MJ, Lodato RF: PEEP, auto-PEEP and waterfalls. Chest 96:449, 1989.
39. Marini JJ, Capps JS, Culver BH: The inspiratory work of breathing during assisted mechanical ventilation. Chest 87:612, 1985.
40. Christopher KL, Neff TA, Bowman JL, et al: Intermittent mandatory ventilation systems. Chest 87:625, 1985.
41. Downs JB, Klein EF, Desautels D, et al: IMV: A new approach to weaning patients from mechanical ventilation. Chest 64:331, 1973.
42. Venus B, Smith RA, Mathru M: National survey of methods and criteria used for weaning from mechanical ventilation. Crit Care Med 15:530, 1987.
43. Weisman IM, Rinaldo JE, Rogers RM, et al: Intermittent mandatory ventilation. Am Rev Respir Dis 127:641, 1983.
44. Downs JB, Perkins HM, Medell JH: Intermittent mandatory ventilation. Arch Surg 109:519, 1974.
45. Cullen P, Modell JH, Kirby RR, et al: Treatment of flail chest: Use of intermittent mandatory ventilation and positive end-expiratory pressure. Arch Surg 110:1099, 1975.
46. Culpepper JA, Rinaldo JE, Rogers RM: Effects of mechanical ventilator mode on tendency towards respiratory alkalosis. Am Rev Respir Dis 132:1075, 1985.
47. Hudson LD, Hurlow RS, Craig KC, et al: Does intermittent mandatory ventilation correct respiratory alkalosis in patients receiving assisted mechanical ventilation? Am Rev Respir Dis 132:1071, 1985.
48. Groeger JS, Levinson MR, Carlon GC: Assist control versus synchronized intermittent mandatory ventilation during acute respiratory failure. Crit Care Med 17:607, 1989.
49. Pontoppidan H, Geffin B, Lowenstein E: Acute respiratory failure in the adult. N Engl J Med 287:799, 1972.
50. Farley HB: Sigh as a dodo: An editorial. Respir Care 25:5, 1976.

51. Dreyfuss D, Soler P, Basset G, et al: High inflation pressure pulmonary edema: Respective effects of high airway pressure, high tidal volume and positive end-expiratory pressure. Am Rev Respir Dis 137:1159, 1988.
52. Hernandez LA, Peevy KJ, Moise AA, et al: Chest wall restriction limits high airway pressure induced lung injury in young rabbits. J Appl Physiol 66:2364, 1989.
53. Shapiro BA, Cane RD, Harrison RA: Positive end-expiratory pressure therapy in adults with special reference to acute lung injury: A review of the literature and suggested clinical correlations. Crit Care Med 12:127, 1984.
54. Suter PM, Fairley HB, Isenberg MD: Optimum end-expiratory airway pressure in patients with acute pulmonary failure. N Engl J Med 292:284, 1975.
55. Hoffman RA, Krieger BP, Kramer MR, et al: End-tidal carbon dioxide in critically ill patients during changes in mechanical ventilation. Am Rev Respir Dis 140:1265, 1989.
56. Grindlinger GA, Manny J, Justic R, et al: Presence of negative inotropic agents in canine plasma during positive end-expiratory pressure. Circ Res 45:460, 1979.
57. Pepe PE, Hudson LE, Carrico HJ: Early application of positive end-expiratory pressure in patients at risk for the adult respiratory distress syndrome. N Engl J Med 311:281, 1984.
58. Kirby RR, Downs JB, Civetta JM, et al: High level positive end-expiratory pressure (PEEP) in acute respiratory insufficiency. Chest 67:156, 1975.
59. Good JT, Wolz JF, Anderson JT, et al: The routine use of positive end-expiratory pressure after open heart surgery. Chest 76:387, 1979.
60. Smith RA: Physiologic PEEP. Respir Care 33:620, 1988.
61. Smith TC, Marini JJ: Impact of PEEP on lung mechanics and work of breathing in severe airflow obstruction. J Appl Physiol 65:1488, 1989.
62. Tuxen DV: Detrimental effects of positive end-expiratory pressure during controlled mechanical ventilation of patients with severe airflow obstruction. Am Rev Respir Dis 140:5, 1989.
63. Albert RK: Least PEEP: Primum non-nocere. Chest 87:2, 1985.
64. Gallagher JJ, Civetta JM, Kirby RR: Terminology update: Optimal PEEP. Crit Care Med 6:323, 1978.
65. Standiford TJ, Morganroth ML: High-frequency ventilation. Chest 96:1380, 1989.
66. Carlon GC, Howland WS, Ray C, et al: High-frequency jet ventilation: A prospective randomized evaluation. Chest 84:551, 1983.
67. Thompson WK, Marchak BE, Bryan AC: Vagotomy reverses apnea induced by high frequency oscillatory ventilation. J Appl Physiol 51:1484, 1981.
68. Shuster DP, Klain M, Snyder J: Comparison of high frequency jet ventilation to conventional mechanical ventilation during severe acute respiratory failure in humans. Crit Care Med 10:625, 1982.
69. Holzapel L, Perrin RF, Gaussorgues P, et al: Comparison of high-frequency jet ventilation in adults with respiratory distress syndrome. Intensive Care Med 13:100, 1987.
70. Carlon GC, Ray C Jr, Klain M, et al: High-frequency positive-pressure ventilation in management of a patient with bronchopleural fistula. Anesthesiology 52:160, 1980.
71. Bishop MJ, Benson MS, Sato P, et al: Comparison of high frequency ventilation with conventional mechanical ventilation for bronchopleural fistula. Anesth Analg 66:833, 1987.
72. Abraham E, Yoshihara G: Cardiopulmonary effects of pressure controlled inverse ratio ventilation in severe respiratory failure. Chest 96:1356, 1989.
73. Duncan SR, Rizk NW, Raffin TA: Inverse ratio ventilation: PEEP in disguise? Chest 92:390, 1987.
74. Gurevitch MJ, Van Dyke J, Young ES, et al: Improved oxygenation and lower peak airway pressure in severe adult respiratory distress syndrome. Treatment with inverse ratio ventilation. Chest 89:211, 1986.
75. Tharratt RS, Allen RP, Albertson TE: Pressure controlled inverse ratio ventilation in severe adult respiratory failure. Chest 94:755, 1988.
76. Zapol WM, Snider MT, Hill JD, et al: Extracorporeal membrane oxygenation in severe acute respiratory failure. JAMA 242:2193, 1979.
77. Gattinoni L, Pesenti A, Mascheroni D, et al: Low-frequency positive-pressure ventilation with extracorporeal CO_2 removal in severe acute respiratory failure. JAMA 256:881, 1986.
78. Suchyta MR, Elliott CG, Clemmer TP, et al: The adult respiratory distress syndrome: A report of survival and modifying factors. Am Rev Respir Dis 143:A677, 1991.
79. Downs JB, Stock MC: Airway pressure release ventilation: A new concept in ventilatory support. Crit Care Med 15:459, 1987.
80. Stock MC, Downs JB, Frolicher DA: Airway pressure release ventilation. Crit Care Med 15:462, 1987.
81. Sporn PHS, Morganroth ML: Discontinuation of mechanical ventilation. Clin Chest Med 9:113, 1988.
82. Dark DS, Pingleton SK, Kerby GR: Hypercapnia during weaning: A complication of nutritional support. Chest 88:141, 1985.
83. Agusti AGN, Torres A, Estopa R, et al: Hypophosphatemia as a cause of failed weaning: The importance of metabolic factors. Crit Care Med 12:142, 1984.
84. Aubier M, Murciano D, Lecocgnuic Y, et al: Effect of hypophosphatemia on diaphragmatic contractility in patients with acute respiratory failure. N Engl J Med 313:420, 1985.
85. Mollow DW, Dhinga S, Solven F, et al: Hypomagnesemia and respiratory muscle power. Am Rev Respir Dis 129:497, 1984.
86. Lemaire F, Teboul JL, Cinotti L, et al: Acute left ventricular dysfunction during unsuccessful weaning from mechanical ventilation. Anesthesiology 69:171, 1988.
87. Sahn SA, Lakshminarayan S, Petty TL: Weaning from mechanical ventilation. JAMA 235:2208, 1976.
88. Sahn SA, Lakshminarayan S: Bedside criteria for discontinuation of mechanical ventilation. Chest 63:1002, 1973.
89. Tahvanainen J, Salenpera M, Nikki P: Extubation criteria after weaning from intermittent mandatory ventilaty and continuous positive airway pressure. Crit Care Med 11:702, 1983.
90. Morganroth ML, Morganroth SL, Nett LM, et al: Criteria for weaning from prolonged mechanical ventilation. Arch Intern Med 144:1012, 1984.
91. Fiastro JF, Habib MP, Shon BY, et al: Comparison of standard weaning parameters and work of breathing in mechanically ventilated patients. Chest 94:232, 1988.
92. Holliday JE, Hyers TM: The reduction of weaning time from mechanical ventilation using tidal volume and relaxation biofeedback. Am Rev Respir Dis 141:1214, 1990.
93. Herrara M, Blasco J, Venegas J, et al: Mouth occlusion pressure ($P_{0.1}$) in acute respiratory failure. Intensive Care Med 11:134, 1985.
94. Peters RM, Hilberman M, Hogan JS, et al: Objective indications for respiratory therapy in post-trauma and postoperative patients. Am J Surg 124:262, 1972.
95. Proctor HJ, Woolson R: Prediction of respiratory muscle fatigue by measurements of the work of breathing. Surg Gynecol Obstet 136:367, 1973.
96. Aubier M, Murciano D, Fournier M, et al: Central respiratory drive in acute respiratory failure of patients with chronic obstructive pulmonary disease. Am Rev Respir Dis 122:191, 1980.
97. Sassoon C, Te TT, Mahutte CK, et al: Airway occlusion pressure: An important indicator for successful weaning in patients with chronic obstructive pulmonary disease. Am Rev Respir Dis 135:107, 1987.
98. Montgomery AB, Holle RHO, Neagley SR, et al: Prediction of successful ventilator weaning using airway occlusion pressure and hypercapnic challenge. Chest 91:496, 1987.
99. Murciano D, Boczkowski J, Lecocguic Y, et al: Tracheal occlusion pressure: A simple index to monitor respiratory muscle fatigue during acute respiratory failure in patients with chronic obstructive pulmonary disease. Ann Intern Med 108:800, 1988.
100. Aldrich TK, Karpel JP: Inspiratory muscle resistive training in respiratory failure. Am Rev Respir Dis 138:461, 1985.
101. Aldrich TK, Karpel JP, Uhrlass RM, et al: Weaning from mechanical ventilation: Adjunctive use of inspiratory muscle resistive training. Crit Care Med 17:143, 1989.
102. Pourriat JL, Lamberto CH, Hoang PH, et al: Diaphragmatic fatigue and breathing pattern during weaning from mechanical ventilation in COPD patients. Chest 90:703, 1986.
103. Swartz MA, Marino PL: Diaphragmatic strength during weaning from mechanical ventilation. Chest 88:736, 1985.
104. Tobin MJ, Perez W, Guenther SM, et al: The pattern of breathing during successful and unsuccessful trials of weaning from mechanical ventilation. Am Rev Respir Dis 134:1111, 1986.
105. Cohen C, Zagelbaum G, Gross D, et al: Clinical manifestations of respiratory muscle fatigue. Am J Med 73:308, 1982.
106. Tobin MJ, Guenther SM, Perez W, et al: Konno-Mead analysis of ribcage-abdominal motion during successful and unsuccessful trials of weaning from mechanical ventilation. Am Rev Respir Dis 135:1320, 1987.
107. Dean SE, Keenan RL: Spontaneous breathing with a T-piece circuit: Minimum fresh gas/minute volume ratio which prevents rebreathing. Anesthesiology 56:449, 1982.
108. Fiastro JF, Habib MP, Quan SF: Pressure support compensation for inspiratory work due to endotracheal tubes and demand continuous positive airway pressure. Chest 93:499, 1988.
109. Hughes CW, Popovich J: Uses and abuses of pressure support ventilation. J Crit Illness 4:25, 1989.
110. Marini JJ, Crooke PS, Truwit JD: Determinants of pressure-preset ventilation: A mathematical model of pressure control. J Appl Physiol 67:1081, 1989.
111. Brochard L, Hauf A, Lorino H, et al: Inspiratory pressure support prevents diaphragmatic fatigue during weaning from mechanical ventilation. Am Rev Respir Dis 139:513, 1989.
112. Petrof BJ, Legare M, Goldberg P, et al: Continuous positive airway pressure reduces work of breathing and dyspnea during weaning from mechanical ventilation in severe chronic obstructive pulmonary disease. Am Rev Respir Dis 141:281, 1990.
113. Sassoon CSH, Giron AE, Ely EA, et al: Inspiratory work of breathing on flow-by and demand flow CPAP. Crit Care Med 17:1108, 1989.
114. Saito S, Tokioka H, Kosaka F: Efficacy of flow-by during continuous positive airway pressure and ventilation. Crit Care Med 18:654, 1990.
115. Hewlett AM, Platt AS, Terry VG: Mandatory minute volume: A new concept in weaning from mechanical ventilation. Anaesthesia 32:163, 1977.

CHAPTER 85

Hemodynamic Effects of Mechanical Ventilation

William J. Fulkerson, Jr.
Claude A. Piantadosi

Positive intrathoracic pressures created by mechanical ventilators produce significant changes in cardiovascular and extrapulmonary organ system function. Soon after positive pressure ventilation was introduced as a therapeutic modality, investigators noted marked changes in hemodynamic function in animals and humans with various modes of support. In 1935, Moore and associates reported a marked decrease in cardiac output during both intermittent positive pressure ventilation (IPPV) and continuous positive pressure ventilation (CPPV) in dogs.[1] This finding was confirmed later in humans by other investigators.[2, 3] Work by Cournand and colleagues in 1948 clarified the importance of the applied waveform on cardiovascular effects of IPPV.[4] Changes in cardiac output were shown to be minimized during positive pressure breathing with relatively rapid inflation, rapid deflation, and an inspiratory/expiratory time ratio on the order of 1:2. The inspiratory/expiratory ratio proved to be the most important of these factors.

The application of high intrathoracic pressures was found to produce dramatic cardiovascular effects in most patients. However, marked reductions in cardiac output and systemic arterial pressure were less common during clinical use of IPPV than during CPPV. These findings originally led to the virtual elimination of CPPV from clinical practice. Interest in CPPV returned when Ashbaugh and colleagues reported the practice of mechanical ventilation with positive end-expiratory pressure (PEEP) for treatment of refractory hypoxemia in patients with diffuse lung injury and respiratory failure.[5] This report led to the widespread use of PEEP in treatment of the adult respiratory distress syndrome (ARDS), despite the adverse cardiovascular effects of the modality.

Since 1967, the effects of PEEP on the cardiovascular system have been studied in detail, and a wealth of complex and sometimes contradictory data has been generated about the hemodynamic effects of IPPV and PEEP. A broad range of experimental and clinical studies have shown that the most important hemodynamic consequence of positive pressure ventilation is a fall in cardiac output, which may impair systemic oxygen transport to tissues. This chapter reviews the basic hemodynamic effects of positive pressure ventilation and PEEP in the context of clinical practice in the intensive care unit. Understanding and avoiding the potential negative effects of this life-supportive therapy can be essential to the survival of the critically ill patient.

MECHANICAL EFFECTS OF POSITIVE PRESSURE VENTILATION ON CARDIAC FUNCTION

Cardiac output is the product of ventricular stroke volume and heart rate. Heart rate is influenced by sympathetic and parasympathetic nervous system activity. Stroke volume is determined predominantly by three factors: (1) preload, the length of cardiac muscle fibers at the start of contraction, proportional to ventricular end-diastolic volume and esti-

mated by end-diastolic pressure; (2) afterload, the tension the muscle develops during systole, usually equated with blood pressure; and (3) contractility. Preload and afterload are presumed to correlate clinically with specific intravascular pressures. Intravascular pressure within the chest fluctuates with airway pressure, however, and absolute intravascular values may not reflect the pressure actually responsible for distention of the cardiac ventricles. This distending, or transmural, pressure is the difference between the pressure inside and outside a vascular structure and represents the actual pressure reflective of ventricular filling. Positive pressure ventilation produces alterations in airway pressure, pleural pressure, and therefore transmural pressure, affecting the right and left ventricles differently (Table 85–1).

Right Ventricle

Positive pressure ventilation and PEEP may have a significant effect on right ventricular preload and subsequently cardiac output. Pressure within the intrathoracic venae cavae rises as airway pressure is increased by positive pressure ventilation, resulting in reduced venous return from the periphery to the right atrium.[4, 6–8] During CPPV, pressure within the right ventricle increases, but subtracting intrapleural pressure from intracardiac pressure reveals that transmural right ventricular end-diastolic pressure actually declines when either IPPV or CPPV with 12 cm H_2O of PEEP is applied.[4, 8] This led to the assumption that right ventricular end-diastolic volume decreased along with the decrease in transmural filling pressure and that right ventricular stroke output responded as expected according to Starling's law of the heart. Other investigators suggested that transmural right ventricular pressure may not reflect right ventricular preload because of uneven transmission of intrathoracic pressures to juxtacardiac regions related to the mechanics of lung distention and compression of the mediastinum.[9] Other studies confirmed reductions in right ventricular end-diastolic volume by assessing volume changes directly. Fewel and colleagues determined that right ventricular end-diastolic volume decreased significantly in dogs receiving CPPV.[10] These data suggested that IPPV with PEEP caused a reduction in right and then left ventricular stroke volume, primarily by impeding venous return.

Right ventricular afterload may vary considerably with positive airway pressure because lung volume is a primary determinant of pulmonary vascular resistance. Pulmonary vascular resistance is increased at low lung volumes owing to hypoxic vasoconstriction of larger pulmonary arterioles. Pulmonary vascular resistance decreases with lung inflation

TABLE 85–1
ADVERSE CARDIAC EFFECTS OF POSITIVE PRESSURE VENTILATION AND POSITIVE END-EXPIRATORY PRESSURE

Right Ventricle
Reduced systemic venous return or right ventricular preload
Increased right ventricular afterload
Possible decreased contractility in ischemic myocardium

Left Ventricle
Decreased left ventricular preload related to
  Decrease in right ventricular preload
  Increase in pulmonary vascular resistance
Decreased contractility related to
  Myocardial ischemia
  Possible circulating negative inotropic agents
  Left ventricle–dependent decrease in volume secondary to right ventricular dilation and ventricular interdependence

to functional residual capacity and then rises with further increases in lung volume.[11] Some investigators demonstrated that mechanical lung inflation can increase the impedance to right ventricular outflow significantly.[12, 13] Most studies suggest that right ventricular outflow is affected minimally by small tidal volumes and that IPPV causes little change in afterload.[14] With addition of PEEP, however, pulmonary vascular resistance increases as lung volume increases. In patients requiring PEEP, pulmonary vascular resistance may already be increased owing to reduced cross-sectional area of the pulmonary circulation by disease. Thus, patients with pulmonary microcirculation disruption or thrombosis, such as those with ARDS, may be most susceptible to increases in right ventricular afterload while receiving high levels of PEEP.

Decreased right ventricular contractility during positive pressure ventilation has been postulated by some investigators. Scharf and coworkers demonstrated in dogs that an increase in pulmonary arterial pressure led to increases in right ventricular volume and right ventricular end-diastolic pressure and a decline in stroke volume and right ventricular ejection fraction.[15] Other work, however, indicates good preservation of right ventricular contractility until systolic pulmonary arterial pressures exceed 50 mm Hg.[16] Other studies reported that right ventricular function is generally normal in animals receiving IPPV and up to 20 cm H_2O of PEEP. In a report of patients undergoing coronary bypass surgery, a reduction in right ventricular ejection fraction was observed owing to PEEP in a small minority of patients, whereas most patients exhibited decreases in preload with PEEP.[17] The currently available experimental data and clinical experience suggest that right ventricular contractility is not impaired by IPPV and PEEP in most instances. A decline in right ventricular contractility attributable to PEEP, however, could occur in the presence of coronary arterial disease and reduced myocardial blood flow.

Left Ventricle

The effect of positive pressure ventilation on left ventricular hemodynamics is complex, and conflicting data exist about the mechanisms. Left ventricular preload is coupled directly to right ventricular outflow. As right ventricular outflow decreases with increasing intrathoracic pressure from PEEP, left ventricular preload should decrease. Studies monitoring left ventricular volume suggested that a decline in preload is a major physiologic factor in the fall in cardiac output during PEEP.[4, 7, 18, 19] Other researchers suggested that decreases in cardiac output from the addition of PEEP to IPPV are greater than would be predicted solely on the basis of decreases in venous return.[20] Animal and human experiments demonstrated significant decreases in the left ventricular stroke volume with increasing PEEP even with elevated right and left ventricular filling pressures. In these investigations, it was concluded that the observed reductions in cardiac output during PEEP were not due to a mechanical decrease in right ventricular filling but might represent depression of left ventricular function.[21, 22] The reasons for disparate conclusions about the effects of IPPV and CPPV on left ventricular function probably reside within the diverse experimental models and the techniques used to estimate filling pressures.

During changes in intrathoracic pressure, estimates of intravascular pressure must account for alterations in the measurements attributable to pressure changes outside the vascular structures, as noted earlier. The actual transmural distending pressure is difficult to assess during positive pressure ventilation. The problem has been approached by measuring esophageal, pleural, and anterior pericardial

pressures and adjusting measured intravascular pressures for the apparent extracardiac pressures. Using thin pressure transducers placed in juxtacardiac positions, Marini and associates demonstrated that most measurements of transmural pressure are erroneous.[9] Furthermore, measurement of esophageal pressure is position dependent and may underestimate juxtacardiac pressures and lead to overestimation of transmural pressures.[23] A practical and accurate bedside method of estimating transmural distending pressures while patients receive positive pressure ventilation is elusive. It seems safe to conclude, however, that declines in cardiac output at a PEEP of 15 cm H_2O and above are due primarily to decreased venous return, and secondary effects may be mediated through changes in left ventricular afterload and contractility.

In contrast to the negative effects of PEEP on left ventricular preload, it has been suggested that IPPV actually may be advantageous in some instances by decreasing afterload. Positive intrathoracic pressure should result in a decrease in left ventricular transmural pressure and decrease the wall tension necessary for the left ventricle to maintain a given volume. This mechanism should lead to decreased left ventricular afterload. Animal models in which left ventricular ejection fraction is maintained during initiation of PEEP tend to confirm this.[10] Augmentation of cardiac function by IPPV with large tidal volumes was also observed in an animal model of congestive heart failure.[14] Other studies demonstrated improved cardiac output with positive pressure breathing in patients with shock.[24] Despite the possible decrease in afterload attributable to positive pressure, it is unlikely that IPPV with PEEP (i.e., positive intrathoracic pressure throughout the respiratory cycle) would be clinically advantageous.

Evaluation of contractility during IPPV with PEEP is hampered clinically by difficulties in assessing contractility adequately at specific times during the ventilatory cycle. Several possible ways for PEEP to alter contractility have been suggested, including myocardial ischemia attributable to altered coronary blood flow.[25] Changes in myocardial blood flow during PEEP, however, are correlated with a decrease in cardiac output and easily reversed by volume infusion.[7, 26] Thus, the evidence of altered contractility caused by myocardial ischemia during CPPV has not been convincing. Other ways that PEEP might alter left ventricular contractility include activation of vagal reflexes leading to negative chronotropic, inotropic, and vasodilatory effects.[27] Other studies suggested decreased contractility during PEEP ventilation secondary to circulating humoral factors.[28, 29] Negative inotropic effects of ventricular interdependence may also contribute to a decrease in left ventricular function.[30]

Ventricular Interdependence

Changes in the volume of either ventricle may affect the distensibility or volume of the opposite ventricle, because the heart is confined by the pericardium. Postmortem heart studies demonstrated that the filling pressure for each ventricle is influenced by the volume status of the opposing ventricle.[31] Bemis and others showed that, for a given left ventricular end-diastolic pressure, the left ventricular volume depends on filling of the right ventricle.[32] Therefore, if right ventricular volume increases with increasing PEEP owing to increasing pulmonary vascular resistance, a decrease in left ventricular volume might be anticipated. This effect has been demonstrated by echocardiographic assessment of ventricular volume in patients with ARDS treated with high levels of PEEP.[33] These studies showed that transmural right and left ventricular end-diastolic pressures decreased in these patients, but the left ventricular filling

TABLE 85–2

NEUROHUMORAL RESPONSES TO POSITIVE PRESSURE VENTILATION

Hormone or Peptide	Response	Reference
Plasma renin and aldosterone	Increased	40
Vasopressin (antidiuretic hormone)	Increased	52
Atrial natriuretic peptide	Decreased	54
Prostaglandins	Increased	29

volume was more affected than the right because the interventricular septum bulged into the left ventricle and limited filling. This is consistent with other studies of acute right ventricular volume overload using more precise measurements of right and left ventricular geometry.[34, 35]

Studies of ventricular function in open and closed chest animals revealed, however, that decreased cardiac function in closed chest animals ventilated with PEEP did not occur in open chest animals when the heart was free from interaction with lung. Pericardiectomy also did not alter the cardiovascular responses to increase expiratory pressure.[7] These and similar studies led to the conclusion that an increased ventricular interdependence mechanism is not a major factor in PEEP-induced decreases in cardiac output. Thus, the primary mechanisms of reduction of cardiac output from IPPV and PEEP appear to be decreased venous return and heart-lung interactions.[36–38]

Neurohumoral Factors Associated with Positive Pressure Ventilation

Cardiac output may be altered by excitation of the autonomic nervous system via activation of cardiopulmonary receptors during IPPV and CPPV.[39] Reflex cardiac depression during pulmonary overdistention with PEEP was observed after stimulation of lung C fiber receptors.[21] Stimulation of these receptors induces vagally mediated hypotension, bradycardia, and decreases in stroke volume. Depression of cardiac output by humorally active compounds released into the circulation after lung inflation has been hypothesized on the basis of animal studies.[40] Endogenous release of a negative inotrope (e.g., a prostanoid metabolite) may contribute to depression of cardiac output during positive pressure ventilation.[29] Furthermore, other humoral and hormonal responses attributable to the hemodynamic effects of IPPV and CPPV may affect regulation of cardiac output and the regional distribution of blood flow.[28, 40] Some of these humoral responses to positive pressure ventilation are summarized in Table 85–2. Thus, changes in cardiovascular hemodynamics under the influence of IPPV and CPPV may not result only from mechanical mechanisms. These humoral effects all appear to be modest, however, and none have been shown unequivocally to be clinically significant in patients receiving IPPV and PEEP.[41]

EFFECTS OF POSITIVE PRESSURE VENTILATION ON TISSUE OXYGENATION

Adequate oxygen delivery (Do_2) to the tissues and avoidance of hypoxia at the cellular level are fundamental therapeutic goals in critically ill patients. At the present time, systemic measurements of oxygen transport are used to infer the status of oxygen availability for oxidative metabolism by the tissues. Assessment of oxygen delivery to the tissues requires measurement of cardiac output ($\dot{Q}$) and arterial oxygen content (Cao_2). Calculation of oxygen delivery is based upon the Fick principle:

$$\dot{V}o_2 = \dot{Q} \times (Cao_2 - C\bar{v}o_2)$$

where $\dot{V}o_2$ is oxygen consumption of the body and $C\bar{v}o_2$ is mixed venous oxygen content.

$$Do_2 = \dot{Q} \times Cao_2$$

Such systemic measurements are useful when the total oxygen delivery to the body tissues becomes limited and oxygen consumption declines. Systemic measurements are difficult to interpret, however, when regional inequities in oxygen delivery and oxygen consumption develop during diffuse disease processes such as sepsis and ARDS, which often necessitate ventilatory support.[42]

Regional Blood Flow and Oxygenation

Several experimental studies indicate that IPPV and PEEP selectively alter the distribution of cardiac output, although there is little evidence that they decrease regional oxygen consumption.[26, 43, 50] Experimentally, moderate levels of PEEP, whether applied to normal or injured lungs, reduce cardiac output and systemic oxygen delivery. This reduction is accompanied by differences in the distribution of perfusion to various regional vascular beds. Relative to IPPV, PEEP reduces blood flow to the splanchnic, bronchial, and adrenal circulations but has little effect on total renal blood flow.[48] Significant reductions in total coronary and subendocardial flow also occur in proportion to the decline in cardiac output. A more recent study also reported similar effects of PEEP on coronary blood flow and on the distribution of cardiac output.[26] These and other studies[51] showed no evidence of anaerobic metabolism in normal tissues with blood flow reduction after administration of PEEP. Thus, there is insufficient evidence to conclude that changes in organ blood flow produced by PEEP definitely contribute to multiple organ system failure in ARDS and sepsis. Some of the effects of IPPV and PEEP on specific regional circulatory beds are summarized later.

During IPPV, increases in intrathoracic pressure produce transient increases in intra-abdominal pressure. These abdominal pressure changes are associated with increases in portal venous pressure and decreases in portal venous blood flow to liver. Portal venous blood flow can be reduced by more than 25% by IPPV with high tidal volumes and by more than 50% with the application of 5 to 7 cm H_2O of PEEP.[45] CPPV also decreases portal blood flow and increases portal pressure significantly after acute experimental lung injury induced by oleic acid infusion.[46] These CPPV-related changes in portal pressure and blood flow suggest an increase in portal vascular resistance presumably by the mechanical influence of CPPV on portal vessels and perhaps by direct compression of hepatic parenchyma.[47] Decreases in portal and hepatic blood flow accompanying PEEP also correlate directly with reduced cardiac output and can be largely reversed by maintaining cardiac output with volume infusion.[43] Hence, the portal venous effects of CPPV are normally of little consequence. However, the liver could be more vulnerable to ischemia if systemic blood pressure and arterial perfusion were simultaneously decreased.

The renal response to IPPV and CPPV has been well studied, but there is not yet a consensus on the precise mechanisms of sodium and water retention and decreased urine output observed in patients on PEEP. The renal responses to CPPV are somewhat variable and probably depend on the magnitude and duration of PEEP.[49] Some experimental evidence points to changes in the intrarenal distribution of blood flow and the release of vasopressin during CPPV.[46, 47, 52] CPPV decreases fractional blood flow to the outer renal cortex and enhances sodium reabsorption.[49]

The effects of CPPV on glomerular filtration rate and the renin-angiotensin axis are uncertain because the results of the measurements have been variable. In one study, CPPV and continuous positive airway pressure were found to produce similar depression of glomerular filtration rate and urine output. However, continuous positive airway pressure stimulated vasopressin levels and urinary sodium retention less than CPPV.[53] Of note, CPPV and its associated decrease in atrial filling pressure reduce the secretion of atrial natriuretic peptide.[54] Atrial natriuretic peptide has potent natriuretic and diuretic effects, and it inhibits secretion of aldosterone and renin. Thus, reduced atrial natriuretic peptide secretion may contribute to the sodium and water retention accompanying CPPV. The antidiuretic effect of CPPV on renal function may be ameliorated by treatment with low-dose dopamine [55] and by lower body positive pressure.[54]

The effects of IPPV and CPPV on cerebrovascular hemodynamics are potentially important in several clinical settings. Clinical studies of the effects of CPPV on the brain have reported variable effects of PEEP on cerebrovascular hemodynamics.[56–60] CPPV decreases venous return to the thorax and increases extrathoracic venous pressure as discussed earlier. In the brain, the increase in cerebral venous pressure may increase intracranial pressure (ICP).[56–59] An elevated ICP may decrease the cerebral perfusion pressure, the difference between mean arterial pressure and ICP, which is critical for maintaining cerebral blood flow. ICP in many patients, including some with pre-existing high ICP, is unaffected by CPPV, however, owing to cerebrovascular autoregulation.[58] The transmission of positive airway pressure to the extrathoracic vessels and subsequently the brain may also be reduced by low lung compliance.[61]

Nevertheless, CPPV may compromise cerebrovascular hemodynamic function in certain patients with brain injury.[56–59] Patients with brain edema are at special risk from decreased brain perfusion during CPPV for the reasons cited earlier and because of further compromise of cerebral perfusion pressure when cardiac output is depressed by CPPV. Severe brain injury may impair cerebrovascular autoregulation, and reduced cerebral oxygen delivery in these patients may compound the clinical problem. The importance of small changes in cerebral perfusion pressure caused by CPPV is difficult to assess in the absence of deterioration of the patient's neurologic status.[60] In situations involving comatose patients, such as after prolonged postcardiopulmonary arrest, CPPV should be used cautiously to avoid a critical decrease in cerebral perfusion pressure by worsening an elevation in ICP and decreasing cardiac output. If significant levels of PEEP are necessary to maintain pulmonary gas exchange in a comatose patient and aggressive therapy is indicated, monitoring ICP invasively should be considered. For patients with brain injury who require CPPV, the infusion of large volumes of crystalloid to restore venous return after instituting PEEP should be avoided because this practice may also increase the ICP.[62]

ASSESSMENT OF TISSUE OXYGEN DELIVERY DURING MECHANICAL VENTILATION

The preceding discussion emphasized that the interaction of positive pressure ventilation and PEEP with the hemodynamic status of individual patients is complex and may vary significantly depending on underlying disease processes. In general, most studies suggest that PEEP levels less than or equal to 10 cm H_2O are associated with minimal cardiovascular effects. Routine intensive care monitoring, including blood pressure, heart rate, respiratory rate, neurologic status, and urine output, may be adequate in these patients. Intrinsic PEEP, or auto-PEEP, however, can develop in the lungs of ventilated patients as a result of air trapping owing to inadequate expiratory time or dynamic airway collapse, especially in patients with pre-existing obstructive pulmonary disease. Therefore, this complication must be suspected when inordinate cardiovascular responses occur in predisposed ventilated patients.

In patients who begin with compromised cardiovascular function, alterations in hemodynamic status and oxygen delivery are possible even at low levels of PEEP. As levels of PEEP reach 15 cm H_2O and above, the risk of decreased cardiac output, hypotension, and the development of inadequate tissue oxygenation increases. At higher levels of PEEP, invasive hemodynamic monitoring may be necessary for more sensitive and accurate assessment of systemic oxygen transport. An indwelling arterial catheter should be placed for continuous monitoring of blood pressure and for assessing arterial oxygenation. Pulmonary arterial catheterization with a balloon-tipped catheter should be used to estimate pulmonary capillary wedge pressure (PCWP), measure cardiac output by thermodilution, and obtain mixed venous blood samples for oxygen content analysis.

Proper interpretation of complex oxygen transport variables entails understanding the confounding effects of IPPV and CPPV on cardiovascular hemodynamics. Using the pulmonary arterial catheter to measure PCWP for estimation of left ventricular end-diastolic pressure may be particularly troublesome at high levels of PEEP, and some correction for juxtacardiac pressure must be made if assessment of transmural pressure is desired. The best clinical estimate of transmural pressure may be the esophageal pressure with the patient in the lateral decubitus position,[9] but this is far from perfect and may be difficult clinically. In some models of diffuse lung injury, approximately one half of PEEP levels in excess of 10 cm H_2O are transmitted to the juxtacardiac area. Routinely subtracting this value from the measured PCWP after conversion of centimeters of water to millimeters of mercury is a rough estimate of the distending pressure. As noted earlier, it is this distending pressure and not the absolute measured wedge pressure that correlates with ventricular volume. However, even when left ventricular end-diastolic pressure can be measured directly, it may not correlate well with left ventricular end-diastolic volume when external forces, including lung volume and pleural, pericardial, or right ventricular pressure, interact with the left ventricle or when left ventricular compliance is impaired.[32]

Absolute values of PCWP generally cannot be interpreted in patients receiving IPPV and PEEP but must be viewed in relation to cardiac output at several different PCWP values. The PCWP is also an important concern when discontinuing patients from PEEP. If PEEP is suddenly reduced or removed in patients who are euvolemic or have volume overload, the redistribution of intravascular volume to the thorax may promote sudden pulmonary edema, shunting, and critical hypoxemia.[8, 59, 63, 64] For this reason, we do not advocate discontinuation of PEEP suddenly or transient removal of patients from the mechanical ventilator while they are receiving moderate-to-high levels of PEEP. In addition, reinitiation of the PEEP effect of redistributing extravascular lung water to the conducting or nonrespiratory areas of the lung may be delayed, and the patient could have significant interval morbidity.

The additional data obtained from an indwelling pulmonary arterial catheter, including mixed venous oxygen content, cardiac output, and arterial oxygen content measurements, allow assessment of systemic oxygen delivery and oxygen consumption during positive pressure ventilation. These calculations are useful to assess overall oxygen delivery and utilization by the body, but both are averages resulting from the requirements of all the tissues of the body. Therefore, these systemic measures do not reflect the metabolic activity or oxygenation of specific organs or tissue beds. Some clinicians have also advocated the use of mixed venous oxygen saturation to monitor cardiac output, but this approach is inappropriate in disease states with disturbed relationships between oxygen delivery and extraction at the tissue level such as sepsis and ARDS.[42] Adequate methods for assessing regional oxygen delivery and extraction are not yet available, but the development of several research techniques offers future clinical promise.[65] Until regional methods are available, tissue oxygenation should be managed during mechanical ventilation by optimizing oxygen delivery to support oxygen consumption as much as possible while monitoring clinical and laboratory signs of end-organ function. Critically ill patients with delivery-dependent tissue oxygen extraction may benefit from pharmacologic support of supranormal cardiac output.[66]

It seems advisable to recommend the least PEEP rule when trying to avoid the hemodynamic complications of mechanical ventilation. Optimal PEEP becomes the lowest level of PEEP that provides an acceptable arterial oxygen saturation at a fraction of inspired oxygen of 0.5 or less without damaging oxygen delivery.[66] Alternative methods of mechanical ventilation, including pressure-controlled ventilation with reversal of the inspiratory/expiratory ratio and airway pressure-release ventilation, may result in decreased airway pressures in some patients without worsening hypoxemia. Hemodynamic and respiratory responses to these modes of ventilation have not been adequately studied, however, and routine clinical use cannot be recommended.

In some cases, high levels of PEEP must be used despite falling cardiac output, and additional therapy may be necessary to counteract the deleterious hemodynamic response. Many studies demonstrated that volume replacement improves the reduction in cardiac output attributable to PEEP,[8, 26] but volume infusion in patients that need PEEP the most (e.g., patients with ARDS) may worsen the underlying pulmonary process. The increased permeability of the pulmonary microcirculation in ARDS may predispose to alveolar flooding with only slight increases in the PCWP or pulmonary venous pressure. Indeed, two studies suggested that ARDS patients with a negative fluid balance and lower PCWP have an improved survival.[68, 69] Additional therapeutic measures such as transfusion to hemoglobin levels greater than 10 mg/dL, suppression of fever, adjustment of ventilator flow rates and tidal volumes, and judicious administration of sedatives and paralytic agents should be used if appropriate to improve oxygen delivery, decrease noncritical oxygen consumption, and lower airway pressure. Inotropic agents such as dobutamine and dopamine should be used to support depressed or insufficient cardiac output by enhancing contractility without requiring higher preload, but these agents increase myocardial oxygen demand and may be harmful to ischemic myocardium.

CONCLUSION

Many physiologic factors are involved in the hemodynamic responses to positive pressure ventilation and PEEP under various cardiovascular stresses. Assessment of the individual patient must take into account changes in pleural pressure, mode of ventilation, underlying pulmonary and cardiac disease, systemic oxygen requirements, and intravascular volume status. An understanding of the impact of these variables allows the physician to evaluate hemodynamic alterations intelligently during therapy with mechanical ventilation. Therapeutic goals should be directed at limiting cardiovascular compromise by using the least PEEP clinically acceptable and optimizing systemic oxygen delivery to sustain the oxygen consumption of the body.

References

1. Moore RL, Humphreys GH, Wreggit WR: Studies on the volume output of blood from the heart in anaesthetized dogs before thoracotomy and after thoracotomy and intermittent or continuous inflation of the lungs. J Thorac Surg 5:159, 1935.
2. Motley, HL, Cournand A, Eckman M, et al: Physiolgical studies on man with the pneumatic balance resuscitator, "Burns model." J Aviation Med 17:431, 1946.
3. Werkö L: The influence of positive pressure breathing on the circulation in man. Acta Med Scand Suppl 193:1, 1947.
4. Cournand A, Motley HL, Werkö L, et al: Physiological studies of the effects of intermittent positive pressure breathing on cardiac output in man. Am J Physiol 152:162, 1948.
5. Ashbaugh DG, Bigelow DB, Petty TL, et al: Acute respiratory distress in adults. Lancet 2:319, 1967.
6. Braunwald E, Binion JT, Morgan WL Jr, et al: Alterations in central blood volume and cardiac output induced by positive pressure breathing and counteracted by metaraminol (Aramine). Circ Res 5:670, 1957.
7. Fewell JE, Abendschein DR, Carlson CJ, et al: Mechanism of decreased right and left ventricular end-diastolic volumes during continuous positive-pressure ventilation in dogs. Circ Res 47:467, 1980.
8. Qvist J, Pontoppidan H, Wilson RS, et al: Hemodynamic responses to mechanical ventilation with PEEP: The effect of hypervolemia. Anesthesiology 42:45, 1975.
9. Marini JJ, Culver BH, Butler J: Mechanical effect of lung inflation with positive pressure on cardiac function. Am Rev Respir Dis 124:382, 1979.
10. Fewell JE, Abendschein DR, Carlson CJ, et al: Continuous positive pressure ventilation decreases right and left ventricular end-diastolic volumes in dog. Circ Res 46:125, 1980.
11. Simmons PH, Linde CM, Miller JH, et al: Relation between lung volume and pulmonary vascular resistance. Circ Res 9:465, 1961.
12. Henning RJ, Heyman V, Aclover I, et al: Cardiopulmonary effects of oleic acid–induced pulmonary edema and mechanical ventilation. Anesth Analg 65:925, 1986.
13. Scharf SM, Caldini P, Ingram RH Jr: Cardiovascular effects of increasing airway pressure in the dog. Am J Physiol 232:H35, 1977.
14. Pinsky MR, Summer WR, Wise RA, et al: Augmentation of cardiac function by elevation of intrathoracic pressure. J Appl Physiol 54:950, 1983.
15. Scharf SM, Brown R: Influence of the right ventricle on canine left ventricular function with PEEP. J Appl Physiol 52:254, 1982.
16. Vlahakes GJ, Turley K, Hoffman JIE, et al: The pathophysiology of failure in acute right ventricular hypertension: Hemodynamic and biochemical correlations. Circulation 63:87, 1986.
17. Neidhart PP, Suter PM: Changes of right ventricular function with positive end-expiratory pressure (PEEP) in man. Intensive Care Med 14(suppl 2):471, 1988.
18. Brown DR, Bazaral MG, Nath PH, et al: Canine left ventricular volume response to mechanical ventilation with PEEP. Anesthesiology 54:409, 1981.
19. Viquerat CE, Righetti A, Suter PM: Biventricular volumes and function in patients with adult respiratory distress syndrome ventilated with PEEP. Chest 83: 509, 1983.
20. Prewitt RM, Wood LDH: Effect of positive end-expiratory pressure on ventricular function in dogs. Am J Physiol 236:H534, 1979.
21. Cassidy SS, Roberson CH, Pierce AK: Cardiovascular effects of positive end-expiratory pressure in dogs. J Appl Physiol 44:743, 1978.
22. Cassidy SS, Eschenbacher WL, Robertson CH Jr, et al: Cardiovascular effects of positive-pressure ventilation in normal subjects. J Appl Physiol 47:453, 1979.
23. Marini JJ, O'Quin R, Culver BH, et al: Estimation of transmural cardiac pressures during ventilation with PEEP. J Appl Physiol 53:384, 1982.
24. Pinsky MR, Summer WR: Cardiac augmentation by phasic high intrathoracic pressure support in man. Chest 84:370, 1983.
25. Tucker HJ, Murray JF: Effects of end-expiratory pressure on organ blood flow in normal and diseased dogs. J Appl Physiol 34:573, 1973.
26. Dorinsky PM, Hamlin RL, Gadek JE: Alterations in regional blood flow during positive end-expiratory pressure ventilation. Crit Care Med 15:106, 1987.
27. Biondi JW, Schulman DS, Matthay RA: Effects of mechanical ventilation on right and left ventricular function. Clin Chest Med 9:55, 1988.
28. Patten MT, Liebman PR, Manny J, et al: Humorally mediated alterations in cardiac performance as a consequence of positive end-expiratory pressure. Surgery 84:201, 1975.
29. Dunham B, Grindlinger G, Utsunomiya T, et al: Role of prostaglandins in positive end-expiratory pressure–induced negative inotropism. Am J Physiol 241:H783, 1981.
30. Weber KT, Janicki JS, Shroff S, et al: Contractile mechanics and interaction of the right and left ventricles. Am J Cardiol 47:686, 1981.
31. Taylor RR, Covell JW, Sonnenblick EH, Ross J Jr: Dependence of

ventricular distensibility on filling of the opposite ventricle. Am J Physiol 213:711, 1967.

32. Bemis CE, Serur JR, Borkenhagen D, et al: Influence of right ventricular filling pressure on left ventricular pressure and dimension. Circ Res 34:498, 1974.

33. Jardin F, Farcot JC, Boisante L, et al: Influence of positive end-expiratory pressure on left ventricular performance. N Engl J Med 304:387, 1981.

34. Badke FR: Left ventricular dimensions and function during right ventricular pressure overload. Am J Physiol 242:H611, 1982.

35. Moulopoulos SD, Sarcas A, Stamatellopoulos S, et al: Left ventricular performance during by-pass or distension of the right ventricle. Circ Res 17:484, 1965.

36. Culver BH, Marini JJ, Butler J: Lung volume and pleural pressure effects on ventricular function. J Appl Physiol 50:630, 1981.

37. Wise R, Robotham J, Bromberger-Barnea B, et al: The effect of PEEP on left ventricular function in right heart bypassed dogs. J Appl Physiol 51:541, 1981.

38. Wise R, Robotham J, Bromberger-Barnea B, et al: Elevation of left ventricular diastolic pressure by PEEP in the isolated in-situ heart. Physiologist 22:134, 1979.

39. Sellden H, Delle M, Sjovall H, et al: Reflex changes in sympathetic nerve activity during mechanical ventilation with PEEP in sino-aortic denervated rats. Acta Physiol Scand 130:15, 1987.

40. Payen DM, Brun-Buisson CJL, Carli PA, et al: Hemodynamic, gas exchange, and hormonal consequences of LBPP during PEEP ventilation. J Appl Physiol 62:61, 1987.

41. Robotham JL, Scharf SM: Effects of positive and negative pressure ventilation on cardiac performance. Clin Chest Med 4:161, 1983.

42. Danek SJ, Lynch JP, Weg JG, et al: The dependence of oxygen uptake on oxygen delivery in the adult respiratory distress syndrome. Am Rev Respir Dis 122:387, 1980.

43. Bredenberg CE, Paskanik AM: Relation of portal hemodynamics to cardiac output during mechanical ventilation with PEEP. Ann Surg 198:218, 1983.

44. Lutch JS, Murray JF: Continuous positive-pressure ventilation: Effects on systemic oxygen transport and tissue oxygenation. Ann Intern Med 76:193, 1972.

45. Johnson EE: Splanchnic hemodynamic response to passive hyperventilation. J Appl Physiol 38:156, 1975.

46. Johnson EE, Hedley-Whyte J: Continuous positive pressure ventilation and portal flow in dogs with pulmonary edema. J Appl Physiol 33:385, 1972.

47. Johnson EE, Hedley-Whyte J: Continuous positive pressure ventilation and choledochoduodenal flow resistance. J Appl Physiol 39:937, 1975.

48. Manny J, Justice R, Hechtman HB: Abnormalities in organ blood flow and its distribution during positive end-expiratory pressure. Surgery 85:425, 1979.

49. Hall SV, Johnson EE, Hedley-Whyte J: Renal hemodynamics and function with continuous positive pressure ventilation in dogs. Anesthesiology 41:452, 1974.

50. Berry AJ, Geer RT, Marshall C, et al: The effect of long-term controlled mechanical ventilation with positive end-expiratory pressure on renal function in dogs. Anesthesiology 61:406, 1984.

51. Sugimoto H, Ohashi N, Sarnada Y, et al: Effects of positive end-expiratory pressure on tissue gas tensions and oxygen transport. Crit Care Med 12:661, 1984.

52. Baratz RA, Philbin DM, Patterson RW: Plasma antidiuretic hormone and urinary output during continuous positive pressure breathing in dogs. Anesthesiology 34:510, 1971.

53. Chin WDN, Cheung HW, Driedger AA, et al: Assisted ventilation in patients with pre-existing cardiopulmonary disease. Chest 4:503, 1988.

54. Andrivet P, Adnot S, Brun-Brisson C, et al: Involvement of ANF in the acute antidiuresis during PEEP ventilation. J Appl Physiol 65:1967, 1988.

55. Hemmer M, Suter PM: Treatment of cardiac and renal effects of PEEP with dopamine in patients with acute respiratory failure. Anesthesiology 50:399, 1979.

56. Cooper KR, Boswell PA, Chio SC: Safe use of PEEP in patients with severe head injury. J Neurosurg 63:552, 1985.

57. Shapiro HM, Marshall CF: ICP responses to PEEP in head injured patients. J Trauma 18:254, 1978.

58. Aidinis SJ, Lafferty J, Shapiro HM: Intracranial responses to PEEP. Anesthesiology 45:275, 1976.

59. Apuzzo MLJ, Weiss MH, Peterson V, et al: Effect of positive end expiratory ventilation on intracranial pressure in man. J Neurosurg 46:227, 1977.

60. Frost EAM: Effects of PEEP on intracranial pressure and compliance in brain-injured patients. J Neurosurg 47:195, 1977.

61. Huseby JS, Pavlin EG, Butler J: Effect of positive end-expiratory pressure on intracranial pressure in dogs. J Appl Physiol 44:25, 1978.

62. Doblar DD, Santiago TV, Kahn AU, et al: The effect of positive end-expiratory pressure ventilation (PEEP) on cerebral blood flow and cerebrospinal fluid pressure in goats. Anesthesiology 55:244, 1981.

63. Lemaire F, Jean-Louis T, Cinotti L, et al: Acute left ventricular dysfunction during unsuccessful weaning from mechanical ventilation. Anesthesiology 69:171, 1988.

64. Beach T, Millen E, Grenvik A: Hemodynamic response to discontinuance of mechanical ventilation. Crit Care Med 1:85, 1973.

65. Collaborative Group on Intracellular Monitoring: Intracellular monitoring in experimental respiratory failure. Am Rev Respir Dis 138:484, 1988.

66. Shoemaker WC, Appel PL, Kram HB, et al: Prospective trial of supranormal values of survivors as therapeutic goals in high-risk surgical patients. Chest 94:1176, 1988.

67. Weisman IM, Ricaldo JE, Rogers RM: Positive end-expiratory pressure in adult respiratory failure. N Engl J Med 307:1381, 1982.

68. Simmons RS, Berdine GG, Seidenfeld JJ, et al: Fluid balance and the adult respiratory distress syndrome. Am Rev Respir Dis 135:924, 1987.

69. Humphrey H, Hall J, Sznajder I, et al: Improved survival in ARDS patients associated with a reduction in pulmonary capillary wedge pressure. Chest 97:1176, 1990. (Comment in: Chest 97:1025, 1990.)

CHAPTER 86

Oxygen Toxicity

Michael F. Beers
Aron B. Fisher

Since the discovery of oxygen more than 200 years ago by Joseph Priestley,[1] the therapeutic value of supplemental oxygen breathing in the treatment of hypoxemia caused by respiratory or cardiac insufficiency has become widely recognized. Concomitant with its first description, toxicity from oxygen exposure was recognized by Priestley,[1] Lavoisier,[2] and others.[3] With the advent of improved oxygen delivery systems, mechanical ventilation, and the modern intensive care unit, oxygen therapy and its complications have spurred a renewed interest in its relevance to care of patients.[4–10]

In every sense, oxygen must be thought of as a drug with a therapeutic window associated with the level and duration of its administration. The potential adverse effects of exposing patients to high oxygen tensions can be divided into two categories: (1) alterations of normal physiologic functions and (2) oxygen-induced tissue damage.[4] The physiologic changes involve perturbations of both pulmonary and extrapulmonary homeostasis and are easily correctable if recognized promptly. Extrapulmonary physiologic effects of hyperoxia include suppression of erythropoiesis, systemic vasoconstriction, and depression of cardiac output. Pulmonary physiologic effects of hyperoxia include depression of hypoxic ventilatory drive, pulmonary vasodilation, and absorption atelectasis.

In addition to its adverse physiologic effects, oxygen in high concentrations is cytotoxic. All respiring cells are potentially susceptible to the toxic effects of elevated partial pressure of oxygen; however, the major toxic effects seen clinically are related to damage to the lungs. The pulmonary pathologic alteration associated with excessive oxygen exposure was described by Lorrain-Smith nearly 100 years ago.[3] Today, lung damage from high concentrations of inspired oxygen is thought to be a major contributing comorbid process in the management of patients in the intensive care unit with respiratory failure. In addition, outpatient oxygen administration and hyperbaric oxygen therapy (oxygen delivered at pressures > 1 ata*) place larger

---

* ata = atmosphere absolute. Pressure at sea level = 1 ata.

segments of the population at risk for oxygen-associated injury.[5]

The toxic (and therapeutic) manifestations of oxygen administration are a function of the partial pressure of oxygen rather than the percentage of oxygen in inspired gases. Hyperoxia is defined as any inspired oxygen concentration greater than normal atmospheric (0.21 ata). Normobaric hyperoxia is defined as an elevated oxygen concentration (0.21 to 1.0 ata) delivered at a total pressure equal to 1 ata (i.e., sea level). Hyperbaric hyperoxia denotes an oxygen concentration greater than 0.21 ata delivered at a total pressure greater than 1 ata. As we examine subsequently, the molecular and cellular basis of tissue injury is thought to be mediated by biochemically reactive free radicals whose formation is directly dependent on oxygen concentration. Because oxygen concentration is directly proportional to partial pressure, breathing 100% oxygen at 0.8 ata (an altitude of 5000 ft [e.g., in Denver]), 80% oxygen at 1 ata (sea level), or 40% oxygen at 2 ata (in a hyperbaric chamber) for the same duration produces similar toxicity.

In the intensive care setting, oxygen toxicity is most often manifest under normobaric hyperoxic conditions. The pathophysiologic effects of hyperbaric hyperoxia have been extensively reviewed by others.[14-16] Therefore, this chapter describes molecular mechanisms, pathophysiology, clinical manifestations, diagnosis, and approaches to management in those conditions associated with excessive free radical production during normobaric hyperoxic exposure in patients with acute respiratory failure.

MOLECULAR AND CELLULAR MECHANISMS

Free Radical Theory

It is now generally accepted that the toxic effects of oxygen in the lung are the direct result of increased concentrations of highly reactive oxygen-derived free radicals.[17-20] In 1954, Gerschman and associates published a report in which they demonstrated in mice that the pathophysiologic changes of oxygen toxicity and x-irradiation were similar, involving at least one common mechanism, the production of oxidizing free radicals.[20]

All aerobic cells, including those of the lung, utilize oxygen as a metabolic substrate for the generation of ATP via oxidative phosphorylation and in a variety of oxygenation and hydroxylation reactions.[18, 19] The oxygen molecule per se appears to be relatively nonreactive and nontoxic. The sequential addition of electrons (e^-) to oxygen can form highly reactive free radicals, as follows:

$$O_2 \xrightarrow{e^-} O_2^- \xrightarrow{e^- + 2H} H_2O_2 \xrightarrow{e^-} OH\cdot \xrightarrow{e^- + H} H_2O$$

Superoxide anion (O_2^-), hydrogen peroxide (H_2O_2), and hydroxyl radical ($OH\cdot$) represent one-, two-, and three-electron reduction products of oxygen, respectively. Singlet oxygen (O_2^*), a potent electrophile, is also generated as a by-product of oxygen-dependent metabolism.

During normal cellular metabolism, almost all of molecular oxygen is completely converted to water, and the enzymes responsible for the reduction reactions (e.g., cytochrome oxidase) release little or none of the partially reduced oxygen intermediates owing to their high affinity for such compounds. However, these reactions, as well as others, including auto-oxidation of tissue enzymes and metabolites, can serve as incomplete electron donors (i.e., less than four electrons) to molecular oxygen, generating and releasing reactive oxygen intermediates.[11]

Figure 86–1 depicts the general mechanisms responsible for the generation of these toxic species of oxygen reduction.

$$(1)\quad O_2 + A^{2+} \longrightarrow O_2^- + A^{3+}$$

$$(2)\quad O_2 + H_2A \longrightarrow H_2O_2 + A$$

$$(3)\quad O_2^- + H_2O_2 \xrightarrow{Fe^{3+}} OH\cdot + OH^- + O_2$$

Figure 86–1. General mechanisms for the generation of toxic species of oxygen reduction. (1) Superoxide anion (O_2^-) is generated by the one-electron reduction of molecular oxygen (O_2) through a variety of electron donors (represented by A^{2+}). (2) Hydrogen peroxide (H_2O_2) is generated by the two-electron reduction of molecular oxygen, usually via enzymatic catalysis. (3) The interaction of superoxide and hydrogen peroxide in the presence of metals can generate hydroxyl radical. (Adapted from Fisher AB: Molecular mechanisms of oxygen toxicity. Appl Cardiopulmonary Pathophysiol 3:121, 1989.)

O_2^- (Reaction 1) and hydrogen peroxide (Reaction 2) are each generated via both enzymatic and nonenzymatic processes. Although both molecular species can have direct toxic effects, their interaction via the Haber-Weiss cycle in the presence of metallic ions (typically Fe^{3+}) can generate hydroxyl radical (Reaction 3), which represents the most dangerous of the oxygen-derived products.

Free Radical Production in Lung

It is likely that most of these generalized mechanisms and metabolic intermediates occur in the lung. Hyperoxia has been shown to stimulate increases in oxygen radical production in whole rat lungs, lung mitochondria, lung microsomes, and lung nuclear membranes, providing important support for the free radical hypothesis.[21-25] Toxic oxygen radicals (specifically O_2^-) have been directly measured inside pulmonary endothelial cells in culture by electron spin paramagnetic resonance during hyperoxic exposure.[26]

Within the lung, all subcellular compartments are sources of free radical production. The reactions responsible involve both the direct reduction of oxygen and the auto-oxidation of partially reduced tissue components to generate O_2^-, hydrogen peroxide, and $OH\cdot$. Mitochondria appear to be the major subcellular source of O_2^-, which is produced by the oxidation of ubisemiquinone during normal functioning of the mitochondrial electron transport chain and by auto-oxidation of NADH dehydrogenase.[19] Additional O_2^- is generated by (1) the endoplasmic reticulum through the auto-oxidation of flavins (e.g., cytochrome P-450)[18] or other components; (2) microsomes during turnover of NADPH–cytochrome c reductase;[18] and (3) plasma membranes by auto-oxidation of cytochromes[17] and during prostaglandin synthesis.[27] Hydrogen peroxide is produced at most of the aforementioned sites by the dismutation of O_2^- and via oxidase activity (e.g., urate oxidase) in peroxisomes.[25] As mentioned earlier, $OH\cdot$ is generated presumably where concentrations of O_2^- and hydrogen peroxide are greatest, near their production sites.

Mechanisms of Cellular Toxicity

The cytotoxic effects of hyperoxia derive from the interaction of superoxide anion and other oxygen radicals with key cellular components. The biochemical alterations produced by the oxidation of cellular components are depicted in Table 86–1. Although all cellular components can react with oxygen radicals, lipid peroxidation and protein oxidation are thought to represent important mechanisms of oxygen toxicity.[27, 28] Lipids containing unsaturated fatty acids are particularly susceptible. Lipid hydroperoxides produced as intermediates are extremely toxic and can propagate the

TABLE 86–1

BIOCHEMICAL ALTERATIONS AND CELLULAR DYSFUNCTION FROM OXYGEN FREE RADICAL DAMAGE

Oxidized Cell Component	Cellular Manifestation
Lipids	
Lipid peroxidation	Damage to cell and organelle membranes
Surfactant	Altered lung mechanics
Eicosanoids	Changes in cellular metabolism and intracellular signaling
Proteins	Inactivation of enzymes and transport proteins
	Altered cellular and intercellular permeability
Nucleic acids	Inhibition of cell growth and division
Pyridine nucleotides	Altered intermediary metabolism
Complex carbohydrates	Altered recognition of macromolecules

Adapted from Fisher AB: Pulmonary oxygen toxicity. In: Fishman AP (ed): Pulmonary Diseases and Disorders. 2nd ed. New York, McGraw-Hill, p 2332, 1988. Reproduced with permission of McGraw-Hill, Inc.

peroxidation process in an autocatalytic manner.[12] Proteins are inactivated by reaction of radicals with sulfhydryl groups,[12] cross-linkage of proteins,[28] or oxidation of constituent amino acids. Destruction of lipid and protein results in damage to cellular and organellar membranes, inactivation of key enzymes, and disruption of cellular transport. In addition, DNA, pyridine nucleotides, and complex carbohydrates are also susceptible to oxidative processes leading to mutagenesis, growth inhibition, and alteration of intermediary metabolism.

Cellular Antioxidant Strategies

The half-life and tissue levels of most reactive oxygen species are low, in part owing to an elaborate network of cellular antioxidant defenses. Antioxidant mechanisms include any cellular process that (1) prevents formation of free radicals, (2) converts oxidants to less reactive species, (3) compartmentalizes reactive species away from important cellular structures, or (4) initiates repair of molecular injury by free radicals.[29]

The biochemical defenses available to the cell for detoxification of oxygen radicals are listed in Table 86–2. It is convenient to divide cellular oxygen radical defenses into three basic categories: (1) enzymatic scavenging systems that directly catalyze removal of free radicals, (2) enzyme-cofactor systems that utilize a recyclable (renewable) intermediate to remove or prevent oxygen radicals, and (3) nonenzymatic free radical scavengers that rereduce oxygen radicals or quench radical-producing reactions.

The major enzymatic oxygen radical scavenger in the lungs is superoxide dismutase.[30] Superoxide dismutase is a metalloprotein present in three distinct forms characterized by metallic cofactors. Copper-zinc superoxide dismutase is a dimeric protein, which is predominantly cytosolic;[31, 32] manganese superoxide dismutase is found mainly in mitochondria.[32, 33] In addition, copper superoxide dismutase, a tetrameric peptide, has been isolated from plasma. All forms of superoxide dismutase catalyze the dismutation of O_2^- to hydrogen peroxide at high rates. Hydrogen peroxide is then removed enzymatically either by the glutathione redox cycle (see later) or by catalase.

The glutathione redox cycle is the most important cellular scavenger of hydrogen peroxide and represents a unique system utilizing multiple enzymes and a renewable low-

molecular-weight scavenger.[34] Glutathione peroxidase, a metalloprotein containing selenium, removes both hydrogen peroxide and lipid peroxides at the expense of reduced glutathione oxidation. Reduced glutathione is regenerated by glutathione reductase, utilizing NADPH derived from the pentose monophosphate shunt pathway. The ability to recycle reduced glutathione makes the glutathione redox cycle a pivotal antioxidant defense system.

Low-molecular-weight, nonenzymatic free radical scavengers include ascorbic acid (vitamin C), α-tocopherol (vitamin E), and β-carotene (vitamin A).[29] These nonrecyclable compounds are essentially derived from extrinsic (dietary) sources. High-molecular-weight antioxidants in the lung include albumin, which binds extracellular iron, thus helping to limit Haber-Weiss–type reactions, and mucus, which binds inhaled oxidants.

Modification of Oxygen Toxicity

In addition to intrinsic cellular antioxidant mechanisms, the susceptibility of cells or organisms to oxygen toxicity can be modified by certain factors.

Many drugs used therapeutically act synergistically with hyperoxia, accelerating free radical production and worsening oxygen toxicity. Bleomycin has been shown to increase lung injury and fibrosis through enhanced production of O_2^-.[35] Potentiation of oxygen toxicity by disulfiram has been shown to occur via the inhibition of cytosolic superoxide dismutase by diethyldithiocarbamate produced in vivo from the conversion (reduction) of disulfiram.[36] The metabolism of nitrofurantoin[37] and paraquat[38] results in production of superoxide or hydroxyl radicals, and oxygen has been shown to increase their cytotoxicity.

Modification of dietary intake can also modify oxygen tolerance. Protein malnutrition as well as dietary deficiency of any of the antioxidant quenchers (see Table 86–2) can alter the response to hyperoxia. The adverse effects of vitamin A and vitamin E deficiency are especially well described.[39, 40] Protein deficiency is thought to potentiate toxicity from hyperoxia owing to a lack of sulfur-containing amino acids, which are crucial for glutathione synthesis.[41, 42]

Oxygen tolerance has been increased in experimental animal models by exposure to sublethal oxygen concentrations[43] or by injection of endotoxin[44, 45] or oleic acid. Induced tolerance correlated with an increased concentration of antioxidant enzymes in the lung; however, it should be noted that each compound can also independently produce lung damage in animal models. Conversely, fever, hyperthyroidism, and glucocorticoid excess all decrease oxygen tolerance in animal models, which is attributable to increased free radical generation. Thus, modulation of oxygen toxicity via methods of antioxidant enzyme induction or increased production of oxygen free radicals is in accordance with the oxidant-antioxidant balance theory and may become important clinically.

PATHOPHYSIOLOGY

The toxic effects of oxygen in the lung occur when free radical production during hyperoxic exposure overwhelms intrinsic antioxidant defenses; excess free radicals interact with cellular components, resulting in cytotoxic events, which produce a characteristic cascade of events to produce biochemical, cellular, morphologic, and physiologic changes.

The biochemical changes were described in detail earlier. The sequence of cellular and morphologic changes has been extensively reviewed.[9, 46] Most data have come from animal models, but limited amounts of human data also exist. The changes that occur in the lung in response to oxygen

TABLE 86–2

CELLULAR ANTIOXIDANT STRATEGIES*

Antioxidant	Function	Comment
Enzymes		
Superoxide dismutase—mitochondria	Dismutates O_2^- to H_2O_2	Contains Mn^{2+}
Superoxide dismutase—cytosol	Dismutates O_2^- to H_2O_2	Contains Cu^{2+}, Zn^{2+}
Catalase	Dismutates H_2O_2 to H_2O	Peroxisomal
Enzyme-Cofactor Systems		
GSH	Cofactor for antioxidant enzymes (listed below)	Synthesized in cells from amino acids
	Quenches oxygen-derived radicals directly	glutamic acid, glycine, and cysteine
Glutathione peroxidase†	Removes H_2O_2 and lipid peroxides	Uses GSH → GSSG
Glutathione S-transferase	Restores sulfhydryl groups	Uses GSH → GSSG
Glutathione reductase	Resynthesizes GSH from GSSG	NADPH as cofactor
Free Radical Scavengers		
α-Tocopherol (vitamin E)	Quenches lipid peroxidation chain reaction	Dietary source
Ascorbic acid (vitamin C)	Quenches oxygen-derived radicals	Dietary source
β-Carotene (vitamin A)	Quenches singlet oxygen	Dietary source

*GSH = glutathione (reduced form); GSSG = glutathione (oxidized form); O_2^- = superoxide anion; H_2O_2 = hydrogen peroxide; NADPH = nicotine adenine dinucleotide phosphate, reduced.
†Contains selenium.

exposure are similar among different species,[9, 47–49] although the duration and severity of individual stages vary.

Primary Morphologic and Cellular Changes

There appear to be four basic phases in the development of oxygen toxicity in lung tissue.[46] The first three phases (initiation, inflammation, and destruction) occur during exposure to both lethal (e.g., 100% oxygen at 1 ata) and sublethal doses of hyperoxia. The fourth phase, proliferation and/or fibrosis, occurs if there is return to sublethal oxygen levels. If lethal exposures persist, ongoing destruction leads to death.

Initiation Phase. The initial phase of oxygen toxicity takes place in the first few hours after exposure to lethal doses of oxygen and during longer periods with sublethal hyperoxia and continues throughout the duration of the exposure. Although no significant evidence of morphologic injury is apparent, several important events are occurring. Enhanced rates of oxygen radical formation have been noted in mitochondria,[21] microsomes,[23] and nuclear membranes[24] by pathways described earlier. Decreased rates of protein synthesis, alterations in tracheobronchial clearance of particulates, and changes in endothelial cell function are also observed before the onset of morphologic changes.

Inflammatory Phase. The earliest morphologic changes in the lung in response to hyperoxia occur as a consequence of primary cellular damage and involve subtle changes in endothelial cell structure resulting in pericapillary accumulation of fluid.[47–49] Lymph fluid collected from sheep exposed to 100% oxygen for 72 hours and injected intravenously with ³H-labeled dextran demonstrated an increased concentration of labeled dextran compared with plasma, indicating leakage from the pulmonary microcirculation via disruptions in the endothelial lining.[50] The proteinaceous fluid that accumulates often forms hyaline membranes, and the pathologic picture is one of noncardiogenic pulmonary edema with morphologic characteristics of diffuse alveolar damage associated with the adult respiratory distress syndrome and other forms of lung injury (Figs. 86–2 and 86–3).

This fluid exudate is rapidly followed by accumulation of inflammatory blood cell elements and release of mediators.[51–54] A rapid influx of platelets within the pulmonary capillary bed after 48 hours of exposure to 100% oxygen has been described.[51] Neutrophil recruitment soon follows

and has been associated with an amplification of the morphologic injury. However, the role of the neutrophil remains controversial, as other studies have shown that induced neutropenia does not prevent development of pulmonary edema or lung microvascular injury during hyperoxic exposure in rabbits or lambs.[55] This suggests that the neutrophil may contribute to, but is not essential for, the development of the inflammatory phase of pulmonary oxygen toxicity.

Destruction Phase. Overt cellular destruction begins shortly after the inflammatory phase. The earliest evidence of impending cellular destruction appears at the ultrastructural level. Observed changes in lung epithelial and endothelial cells include membrane damage, vacuolation of cytoplasm, mitochondrial swelling, and nuclear degeneration.[47, 48] Soon after, frank cell death is seen and exposure of the basement membrane occurs.

The differential sensitivity of various lung cells to oxygen toxicity is species specific. In the sheep and the rat, capillary endothelial cells are the most oxygen sensitive and manifest the earliest ultrastructural alterations. In the primate, type I epithelial cells often show greater sensitivity.[48] The granular pneumonocyte (type II cell) is relatively resistant to oxidant injury and, during recovery (see later), these cells appear to proliferate and repopulate denuded alveolar membranes.

Proliferation and/or Fibrosis. If exposure to toxic levels of oxygen is terminated, a subacute and chronic stage, the proliferative phase, develops. The cell proliferative response blunts the destructive phase and may partially account for survival of the animal. As noted earlier, proliferation of type II pneumonocytes occurs as an attempt to restructure the alveolus.[48, 56] In addition, there is an influx and proliferation of interstitial cells[47, 49, 57] (fibroblasts, monocytes, and macrophages), which appears to be mediated by both cytokine[58, 59] and autocrine factors[60] with deposition of collagen.[61] In baboons, lung histologic characteristics and function have been shown to return to normal within 6 months of recovery from severe oxygen toxicity,[62] but in other settings, the end result may instead be varying degrees of fibrosis or emphysema. The controlling factors remain ill defined.

Taken in toto, the pathophysiologic and morphologic changes associated with hyperoxic stress are similar to other forms of diffuse alveolar damage. There is an initial inflammatory response (exudative phase) followed by fibrosis and repair (proliferative phase), which is not essentially different

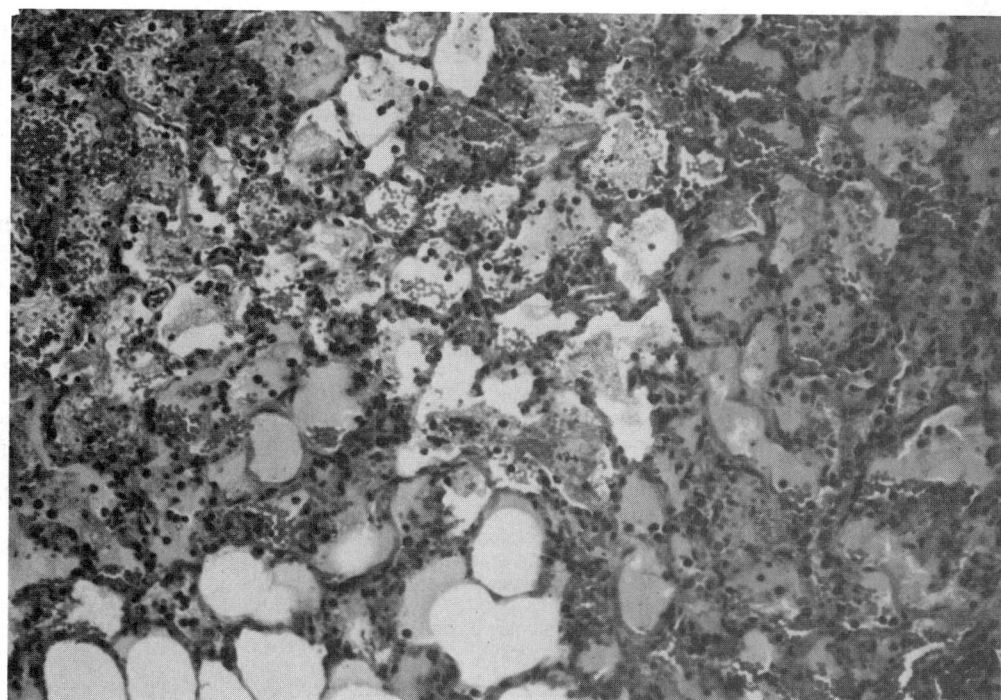

Figure 86–2. Morphologic changes in oxygen toxicity. Light micrograph of the lungs of sheep after 84 hours of 100% oxygen breathing. The alveolar walls are diffusely thickened and alveolar edema is present. Intense inflammatory changes are highlighted by the presence of neutrophil infiltration of the interstitium. (Courtesy of JH Hansen-Flaschen.)

from that in other forms of adult respiratory distress syndrome.

Secondary Changes

The cellular changes that occur in response to toxic oxygen exposure also produce secondary, contributory changes in lung physiology and function. The increased capillary permeability that occurs because of cellular damage results in decreased lung compliance, an increased alveolar-arterial oxygen gradient, and a decreased carbon monoxide diffusing capacity.

Hyperoxia has also been reported to alter the pulmonary surfactant system. It appears reasonably well established that there is a decrease in surface activity of alveolar surfactant material recovered from animals exposed to hyperoxic conditions.[63–66] Although alterations in surfactant phospholipid content,[65, 66] surfactant protein synthesis,[67, 68] and levels of surfactant protein messenger RNA have been reported[67, 68] after hyperoxic exposure, the exact mechanism remains unclear. One potential explanation appears to be inactivation of the biophysical activity of surfactant by serum proteins that leak into the alveolar space. Pathophysiologically, reduced surfactant function contributes to the changes in

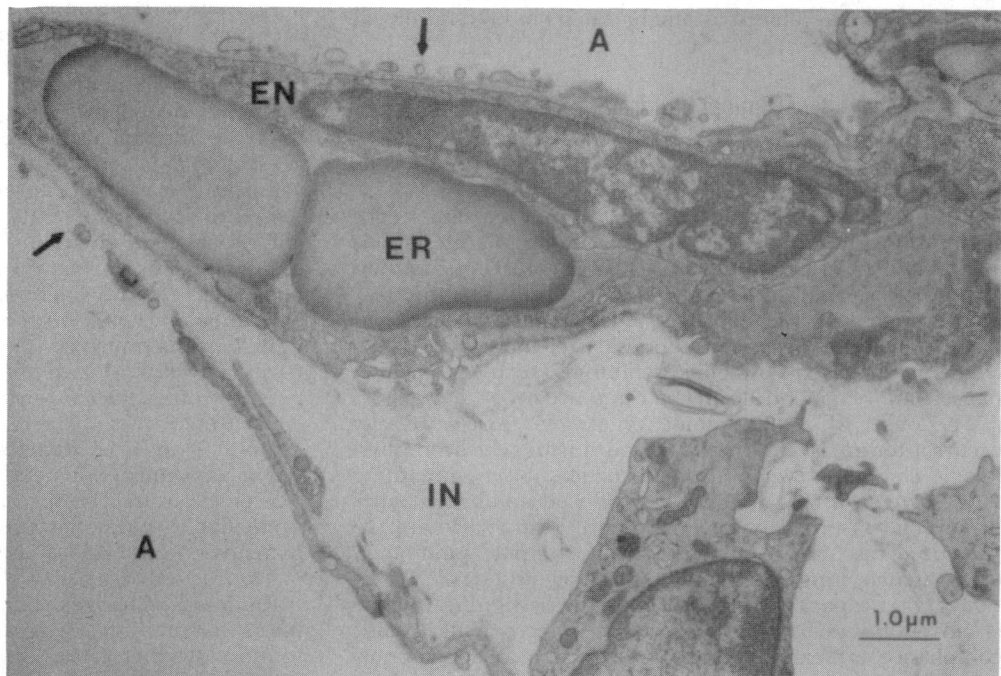

Figure 86–3. Electron microscopic changes in the lungs of sheep breathing 100% oxygen for 70 hours. There is marked interstitial edema (IN). Type I epithelial cells (arrows) show fragmentation and swelling of intracellular organelles. EN = endothelial cell; A = alveolus; ER = erythrocyte. (Courtesy of JH Hansen-Flaschen and GG Pietra.)

TABLE 86-3

SEQUENCE OF PULMONARY CHANGES DURING HYPEROXIC EXPOSURE IN HUMANS

[O_2] at 1 atm	Exposure Duration	Manifestation
100%*†	>12 h	Decreased tracheobronchial clearance; decreased forced vital capacity; cough; chest pain
	>24 h	Altered endothelial function
	>36 h	Increased alveolar-arterial oxygen gradient; decreased carbon monoxide diffusing capacity
	>48 h	Increasing alveolar permeability; pulmonary edema; surfactant inactivation
	>60 h	Adult respiratory distress syndrome
60%*	≥7 d	Mild chest discomfort without changes in lung mechanics; possible changes in morphometry
24-28%	Months	Subclinical pathologic changes; no clinical toxicity documented

*Data from normal volunteers.[69-73, 77]
†Data from patients with irreversible brain damage.[74]

lung function found during the terminal stages of oxygen intoxication through alteration in normal alveolar surface tension.

CLINICAL MANIFESTATIONS AND DIAGNOSIS

The precise concentration of oxygen that is toxic to humans has been difficult to establish. Table 86-3 summarizes the sequence of clinical and physiologic changes observed in humans after various hyperoxic exposures. Most of the data have come from normal, healthy subjects, and the effects of other factors such as age, nutritional status, and concomitant illness as might be seen in critically ill patients is unknown.

Clinical Syndromes
Acute Toxicity: Tracheobronchitis and Adult Respiratory Distress Syndrome

Normal volunteers exposed to 100% oxygen experience symptoms within 12 to 24 hours. The earliest manifestations are related to effects on the tracheobronchial mucosa and include substernal chest pain and nonproductive cough.[69] Measurements of tracheobronchial function show decreased particle clearance as early as 6 hours after the start of 100% oxygen exposure.[70] Systemic symptoms such as malaise, nausea, anorexia, and headache often occur.

The onset of acute pulmonary oxygen toxicity usually occurs after an asymptomatic period during which no physiologic changes develop. In nine male subjects, breathing 100% oxygen for 6 to 12 hours produced no abnormalities in alveolar-arterial oxygen gradient, pulmonary arterial pressure, vascular resistance, cardiac output, pulmonary extravascular lung water, or chest x-ray findings.[71] By 24 hours, vital capacity was shown to decrease significantly.[9, 69, 72, 73] By 48 hours, 98% oxygen produced decrements in static compliance and carbon monoxide diffusing capacity in normal volunteers,[72] and in patients with irreversible brain dam-

age given 100% oxygen, the alveolar-arterial oxygen gradient increased precipitously after 40 to 60 hours of exposure.[74] The longest voluntary exposure to 100% oxygen reported is 110 hours. This patient experienced severe dyspnea, a marked decrease in pulmonary function, and acute respiratory failure.[75]

Chronic Pulmonary Syndromes

Although not well understood in humans, the subacute and chronic phases of oxygen poisoning are well documented in animals and appear to be related to dose and duration of the exposure. The best known clinical syndrome of chronic pulmonary oxygen toxicity in humans occurs in the newborn receiving oxygen for treatment of neonatal respiratory distress syndrome. Persistent morphologic changes with healing may produce the chronic disorder of pulmonary development referred to as bronchopulmonary dysplasia.[5] The effects of long-term exposure of adults to inspired oxygen concentrations of 60 to 100% is less clear, although morphometric changes after 13 days of such exposures in brain-dead patients have been described.[76] Data for longer exposures at even lower levels of inspired oxygen are unavailable.

Diagnosis

The studies described earlier indicate that, although early (reversible) physiologic, anatomic, and biochemical changes can be detected after short exposure to hyperoxia, humans can tolerate 100% oxygen at sea level for 24 hours without serious pulmonary injury. It should also be apparent that pulmonary oxygen toxicity develops insidiously after a variable lag period during which the biochemical and cellular changes described earlier are beginning to occur. Thus, early clinical detection of oxygen toxicity during the lag phase is currently impossible, and diagnostic tests directed toward identification of biochemical changes such as lipid peroxidation improve accuracy but are as yet unavailable for clinical use. Currently, diagnosis of oxygen poisoning depends on nonspecific symptom complexes or abnormal pulmonary function in the proper clinical setting.

Symptoms. Development of chest pain followed by tachypnea and cough in a patient breathing elevated concentrations of oxygen should alert the clinician to the possibility of oxygen toxicity. The study by Montgomery and colleagues suggested that there is no better index of oxygen toxicity than the individual's subjective symptoms of retrosternal chest pain.[77] In critically ill patients requiring mechanical ventilation or with an altered mental status, the detection of these subjective complaints becomes difficult to impossible.

Physical Examination. The presence of rales suggestive of interstitial or alveolar edema may be noted but is certainly nonspecific for the diagnosis.

Pulmonary Function Tests. Decreases in vital capacity, pulmonary compliance, or carbon monoxide diffusing capacity as well as a widening of the alveolar-arterial partial pressure of oxygen have been observed during hyperoxic exposures.[72, 73]

Monitoring serial changes in vital capacity has been proposed as a means of detecting and following injury from oxygen exposure;[9] however, in the intensive care unit, measurements of pulmonary function (especially vital capacity maneuvers) are often limited by cooperation of the patient or by practicality.

Radiologic Changes. The chest x-ray findings of increased interstitial markings or an alveolar filling process are similar to those of other causes of diffuse alveolar damage and are nonspecific.

Biochemical Tests. The early appearance of pentane and ethane in expired respiratory gases (by-products of lipid peroxidation),[78, 79] the presence of by-products of collagen breakdown in lung lavage,[80] and decreases in clearance of serotonin[81] or other biogenic amines by the lung[82] have been demonstrated in animals, but the diagnostic utility of these tests in detecting oxygen poisoning in clinical practice is still unproved.

PREVENTION AND THERAPY

As with any drug, oxygen should be administered judiciously in doses to achieve therapeutic efficacy but to limit toxicity. Because the early detection of oxygen toxicity has remained elusive and specific therapy is lacking, avoidance of pulmonary oxygen toxicity remains the cornerstone of management. The best approach is adherence to guidelines for doses that have been found to be without major side effects.[5]

Guidelines for Oxygen Administration

100% Oxygen. Oxygen in concentrations up to 100% can be administered during cardiopulmonary resuscitation and in the transport and initial management of critically ill patients. Patients not receiving mechanical ventilation should be monitored for evidence of respiratory depression. If needed, inspired 100% oxygen can be used for up to 24 hours without producing significant lung injury. During this period, management should be directed toward improving pulmonary gas exchange, optimizing oxygen delivery, and limiting tissue metabolic demands so that inspired oxygen can be lowered to nontoxic (<50%) levels.

Oxygen Less Than 100%. A fraction of inspired oxygen of 0.5 or less can be administered safely to most patients for up to weeks, although idiosyncrasies of individual patients (e.g., prior bleomycin use) may dictate less tolerance. The maximal safe duration for oxygen exposures between 0.5 and 1.0 is less certain, although it is expected that these concentrations can be tolerated longer than 24 hours.

Therapy of Oxygen Toxicity

After clinical pulmonary oxygen toxicity is recognized, efforts should be directed at limiting further production of oxidizing free radicals. This involves four major maneuvers:

○ TABLE 86–4

AGENTS WITH POTENTIAL ANTIOXIDANT EFFICACY

Compound	Species	Route of Administration	Reference
N-Acetylcysteine	Rat	IV	85
	Human	IV	90
Vitamin E*	Rat	IV	40
	Human	Enteral	89,90
Vitamin A*†	Rat	—	39
Ascorbic acid*	Human	IV	90
Superoxide	Rat	IV	87
dismutase*	Rabbit	IV	88
	Rat	Intratracheal	91
Catalase*	Rat	IV	87
	Rabbit	IV	88
Surfactant	Rat	Intratracheal	63,64
Deferoxamine	Rat	IV	86
Selenium*	Human	IV	90

*Complete toxic and therapeutic profiles not fully established in humans.
†Not tested as replacement therapy; seen in deficient animal model.

---

1. Reduction of inspired oxygen concentration to less than 0.5 ata (50% at sea level). If unacceptable arterial hypoxemia develops (PaO_2 < 60 mm Hg), other therapeutic measures must be instituted. Positive end-expiratory pressure[83] or newer ventilator modalities such as inverse inspiratory/expiratory ventilation[84] can be attempted to decrease intrapulmonary shunting, thus reducing inspired oxygen levels.

2. Optimization of oxygen delivery. Both optimizing cardiac output (potentially with the use of invasive pulmonary arterial catheter monitoring) and correcting anemia improve tissue delivery of oxygen, allowing a lower fraction of inspired oxygen.

3. Limiting oxygen consumption. Control of fever, treatment of pyrogenic infection, sedation, muscle paralysis, and use of active cooling have all been used to decrease oxygen demand.

4. Use of antioxidants. On the basis of accumulating evidence that oxidant mechanisms and free radical formation underlie oxygen toxicity, an alternative approach currently under investigation is the administration of oxyradical scavengers that could limit the damage from elevated levels of inspired oxygen.[29] Agents such as those described in Table 86–4 have shown promise in reducing or limiting oxygen toxicity in several animal models.

Continuous infusion of N-acetylcysteine in rats exposed to 100% oxygen results in decreased mortality and less lung edema.[85] Deferoxamine, an iron-chelating agent, provides partial protection against hyperoxic lung damage in rats, presumably by limiting Haber-Weiss–type reactions.[86] Improvements in the plasma half-life of intravenously administered superoxide dismutase and catalase through conjugation to polyethylene glycol has been shown to limit oxygen damage in rats and rabbits.[87, 88] Vitamin A–deficient rats have shown an increased susceptibility to oxygen poisoning.[39] A single uncontrolled trial of vitamin E (α-tocopherol) administration in humans with adult respiratory distress syndrome has shown a beneficial effect.[89] The most intriguing pharmacologic agent for increasing oxygen tolerance is bacterial endotoxin. The mechanism is unknown and is species specific to rats and lambs,[40, 45] but primates have not been tested.

To date, no controlled trial using antioxidant compounds in humans at risk for hyperoxic exposure has been published; however, intriguing preliminary results have been obtained in a small, randomized series of critically ill patients receiving mechanical ventilation in which administration of vitamin E, ascorbic acid, N-acetylcysteine, and selenium substantially reduced intensive care unit mortality.[90] Although these data are encouraging, the potential toxicities of such a regimen are unknown and further studies with larger series are clearly warranted before formal recommendations can be made.

SUMMARY

Management of patients in the intensive care unit with elevated fractions of inspired oxygen alters normal respiratory physiology and damages lung tissue. Pulmonary oxygen toxicity begins at the subcellular level when the production of highly reactive oxygen free radicals exceeds local cellular defenses. This in turn triggers a cascade of events starting with cellular damage and progressing through alterations in lung mechanics and pulmonary gas exchange, significantly increasing patient morbidity and mortality. The mainstay of therapy is prevention, and oxygen should be administered at the lowest possible concentration to ensure adequate tissue oxygenation. Currently, no specific therapy is available for the treatment of oxygen toxicity, although several agents that act as oxyradical scavengers have shown promise in animal models and preliminary clinical studies.

References

1. Priestley J: Experiments and Observations on Different Kinds of Air, Volume 2. London, J. Johnson (printer), 1775.
2. Duveen DI: Lavoisier. In: Readings from Scientific American. Scientific Genius and Creativity. New York, WH Freeman, p 35, 1982.
3. Lorrain-Smith J: The pathological effects due to increase of oxygen tension in the air breathed. J Physiol (Lond) 24:19, 1899.
4. Fisher AB: Oxygen therapy. Side effects and toxicity. Am Rev Respir Dis 122:61, 1980.
5. Fisher AB: Pulmonary oxygen toxicity. In: Fishman AP (ed): Pulmonary Diseases and Disorders. 2nd ed. New York, McGraw-Hill, p 2331, 1988.
6. Bryan CL, Jenkinson SG: Oxygen toxicity. Clin Chest Med 9:141, 1988.
7. Deneke SM, Fanburg BL: Normobaric oxygen toxicity of the lung. N Engl J Med 302:76, 1980.
8. Klein J: Normobaric pulmonary oxygen toxicity. Anesth Analg 70:195, 1990.
9. Clark JM, Lambertsen CJ: Pulmonary oxygen toxicity: A review. Pharmacol Rev 23:37, 1970.
10. Frank L, Massaro DM: Oxygen toxicity. Am J Med 69:117, 1980.
11. Fisher AB: Molecular mechanisms of pulmonary oxygen toxicity. Appl Cardiovasc Pathophysiol 3:121, 1989.
12. Wispe JR, Roberts RJ: Molecular basis of pulmonary oxygen toxicity. Clin Perinatol 14:651, 1988.
13. Lodato RF: Oxygen toxicity. Crit Care Clin 6:749, 1990.
14. Lambertsen CJ: Effects of hyperoxia on organs and tissues. In: Robin ED (ed): Extrapulmonary Manifestations of Respiratory Disease. New York, Marcel Dekker, p 239, 1978.
15. Schaefer KE: Hyperbaria—O_2 toxicity. In: Loeppky JA, Riedesel ML (eds): Oxygen Transport to Human Tissues. Amsterdam, Elsevier/North Holland Biomedical Press, p 291, 1982.
16. Bert P; Hitchcock MA, Hitchcock FA, trans: Barometric Pressure; Researches in Experimental Physiology. Columbus, OH, College Book, 1943.
17. Freeman BA, Crapo JD: Biology of disease: Free radicals and tissue injury. Lab Invest 47: 412, 1982.
18. Fisher AB, Forman HJ: Oxygen utilization and toxicity in the lungs. In: Fishman AP, Fisher AB (eds): Handbook of Physiology, Section 3, The Respiratory System, Volume I, Circulation and Nonrespiratory Functions. Bethesda, American Physiological Society, p 231, 1985.
19. Fisher AB: Intracellular production of oxygen-derived free radicals. In: Halliwell B (ed): Oxygen Radicals and Tissue Injury. Bethesda, Federation of American Societies for Experimental Biology, p 34, 1987.
20. Gerschman R, Gilbert DL, Nye SW, et al: Oxygen poisoning and x-irradiation: A mechanism in common. Science 119:623, 1954.
21. Freeman BA, Crapo JD: Hyperoxia increases oxygen radical production in rat lungs and lung mitochondria. J Biol Chem 256:10986, 1981.
22. Turrens JF, Freeman BA, Crapo JD: Hyperoxia increases H_2O_2 release by lung mitochondria and microsomes. Arch Biochem Biophys 217:411, 1982.
23. Yusa T, Crapo JD, Freeman BA: Hyperoxia enhances lung and liver nuclear superoxide generation. Biochim Biophys Acta 798:167, 1984.
24. Boveris A, Chance B: The mitochondrial generation of hydrogen peroxide: General properties and effect of hyperbaric oxygen. Biochem J 134: 707, 1973.
25. Boveris A, Oshino N, Chance B: The cellular production of hydrogen peroxide. Biochem J 128:617, 1972.
26. Zweir JL, Duke SS, Kuppusamy P, et al: Electron paramagnetic evidence that cellular oxygen toxicity is caused by the generation of superoxide and hydroxyl free radicals. FEBS Lett 252:12, 1989.
27. Logan MR, Davies RE: Lipid oxidation: Biological effects and antioxidants—A review. Lipids 15:485, 1980.
28. Freeman BA, Sharman MC, Mudd JB: Reaction of ozone with phospholipid vesicles and human erythrocyte ghosts. Arch Biochem Biophys 197:264, 1979.
29. Heffner JE, Repine JE: Pulmonary strategies of anti-oxidant defense. Am Rev Respir Dis 140:531, 1989.
30. Fridovich IA : Superoxide dismutases. Annu Rev Biochem 44:147, 1975.
31. Fridovich IA: Superoxide radical: An endogenous toxicant. Annu Rev Pharmacol Toxicol 23:239, 1983.
32. Slot JW, Genze HJ, Freeman BA, et al: Intracellular localization of copper-zinc and manganese superoxide dismutase in rat liver parenchyma. Lab Invest 55:363, 1986.
33. Smith P, Heath D: Paraquat. CRC Crit Rev Toxicol 4:411, 1976.
34. Ross D, Norbeck K, Moldeus P: The generation and subsequent fate of glutathionyl radicals in biological systems. J Biol Chem 260:15028, 1985.
35. Martin WJ II, Kachel DL: Bleomycin-induced pulmonary endothelial injury: Evidence for the role of iron catalyzed toxic oxygen-derived species. J Lab Clin Med 110:153, 1987.
36. Forman HJ, York JL, Fisher AB: Mechanism for the potentiation of oxygen toxicity by disulfiram.J Pharmacol Exp Ther 212:452, 1980.
37. Martin WJ II, Powis GW, Kachel DL: Nitrofurantoin-stimulated oxidant production in pulmonary endothelial cells. J Lab Clin Med 105:271, 1985.
38. Smith LL: Mechanism of paraquat toxicity in lung and its relevance to treatment. Hum Toxicol 6:31, 1987.
39. Cohen-Addad N, Bollinger R, Chou J, et al: Vitamin A deficiency and pulmonary oxygen toxicity: Morphometric studies in the murine lung. Pediatr Res 23:76, 1988.
40. Frank L, Neriishi K: Endotoxin treatment protects vitamin-E deficient rats from pulmonary oxygen toxicity. Am J Physiol 247:R520, 1984.
41. Fanburg BL, Deneke SM: Protein deficiency potentiates oxygen toxicity. Exp Lung Res 14:911, 1988.
42. Deneke SM, Lynch BA, Fanburg BL: Effects of low protein diets or feed restriction on rat lung glutathione and oxygen toxicity. J Nutr 115:726, 1985.
43. Sjostrom K, Crapo JD: Structural and biochemical adaptive changes in rat lungs after exposure to hyperoxia. Lab Invest 48:68, 1983.
44. Frank L, Summerville J, Massaro D: Protection from oxygen toxicity with endotoxin. Role of endogenous antioxidant enzymes of the lung. J Clin Invest 65:1104, 1980.
45. Frank L, Roberts RJ: Endotoxin protection against oxygen-induced acute and chronic lung injury. J Appl Physiol 45:577, 1979.
46. Crapo JD: Morphological changes in pulmonary oxygen toxicity. Annu Rev Physiol 48:721, 1986.
47. Crapo JD, Barry B, Foscue HA, et al: Structural and biochemical changes in rat lungs occurring during exposures to lethal and sublethal doses of oxygen. Am Rev Respir Dis 122:123, 1980.
48. Kapanci Y, Weibel ER, Kaplan HP, et al: Pathogenesis and reversibility of oxygen toxicity in monkeys, II. Ultrastructural and morphometric studies. Lab Invest 20:101, 1969.
49. Kapanci Y, Tosco R, Eggermann J, et al: Oxygen pneumonitis in man: Light- and electron-microscopic morphometric studies. Chest 62:162, 1972.
50. Hansen-Flaschen JH, Lanken PN, Pietra GG, et al: Effect of 100% O_2 on passage of uncharged dextrans from blood to lung lymph. Am J Physiol 60:1797, 1986.
51. Barry B, Crapo JD: Patterns of accumulation of platelets and neutrophils in rat lungs during exposure to 100% and 85% oxygen. Am Rev Respir Dis 132:548, 1985.
52. Fox RB, Hoidal JR, Brown DM, et al: Pulmonary inflammation due to oxygen toxicity: Involvement of chemotactic factors and polymorphonuclear leukocytes. Am Rev Respir Dis 123:521, 1981.
53. Fox RB, Shasby M, Harada RN, et al: A novel mechanism for pulmonary oxygen toxicity: Phagocyte mediated lung injury. Chest 80:3S, 1985.
54. Rinaldo JE, English D, Levine J, et al: Increased retention of radiolabeled neutrophils in early oxygen toxicity. Am Rev Respir Dis 137:345, 1988.
55. Raj JU, Hazinski TA, Bland RD: Oxygen induced lung microvascular injury in neutropenic rabbits and lambs. J Appl Physiol 58:921, 1985.
56. De los Santos R, Seidenfeld JJ, Anzueto A: One hundred percent oxygen lung injury in adult baboons. Am Rev Respir Dis 136:657, 1987.
57. Harrison GA: Ultrastructural changes in rat lung during long term exposure to oxygen. Exp Med Surg 29:96, 1971.
58. Tanswell AK: Cellular interactions in pulmonary oxygen toxicity in vitro: Hyperoxic induction of fibroblast factors which alter growth and lipid metabolism of pulmonary epithelial cells. Exp Lung Res 5:23, 1983.
59. Freeman BA, Tanswell AK: Biochemical and cellular aspects of pulmonary oxygen toxicity. Adv Free Radical Biol Med 1:133, 1985.
60. Tzaki MG, Byrne PJ, Tanswell AK: Cellular interactions in pulmonary oxygen toxicity in vitro: II. Hyperoxia causes adult rat lung fibroblast cultures to produce apparently autocrine growth factors. Exp Lung Res 14:403, 1988.
61. Valiimaki M, Juva K, Rantanen J, et al: Collagen metabolism in rat lungs during chronic intermittent exposure to oxygen. Aviat Space Environ Med 46:684, 1975.
62. Wolfe WG, Robinson LA, Moran JF, et al: Reversible pulmonary oxygen toxicity in the primate. Ann Surg 188:530, 1978.
63. Armbruster S, Klein J, Stouten EM, et al: Surfactant in pulmonary oxygen toxicity. Adv Exp Med Biol 215:345, 1987.
64. Holm BA, Notter RH, Matalon S: Pulmonary physiological and surfactant changes during injury and recovery from hyperoxia. J Appl Physiol 59:1402, 1985.
65. Gross NJ, Smith DM: Impaired surfactant phospholipid metabolism in hyperoxic mouse lungs. J Appl Physiol 51:1198, 1981.
66. Abe M, Tierney DF: Lung phospholipids during recovery from oxygen toxicity are altered by hydrocortisone. Exp Lung Res 12:119, 1987.
67. Nogee LM, Wispe JR: Effects of pulmonary oxygen injury on airway content of surfactant protein A. Pediatr Res 24:568, 1988.
68. Nogee LM, Wispe JR, Clark JC, et al: Increased expression of pulmonary surfactant proteins in oxygen exposed rats. Am J Respir Cell Mol Biol 4:102, 1991.
69. Comroe JH, Dripps RD, Dumke PR, et al: Oxygen toxicity. The effects of inhalation of high concentrations of oxygen on normal men at sea level and at a simulated altitude of 18,000 feet. JAMA 128:710, 1945.
70. Sackner MA, Landa J, Hirsch J, et al: Pulmonary effects of oxygen breathing: 6 hour study in normal men. Ann Intern Med 82:40, 1975.
71. Van de Water JN, Kagey KS, Miller IT, et al: Response of the lung to 6 to 12 hours of 100 percent oxygen inhalation in normal man. N Engl J Med 283:621, 1970.

72. Caldwell PRB, Lee WL, Schildkraut HS, et al: Changes in lung volume, diffusing capacity, and blood gases in men breathing oxygen. J Appl Physiol 21:1477, 1966.
73. Harabin AL, Homer LD, Weathersby PK, et al: An analysis of decrements in vital capacity as an index of pulmonary oxygen toxicity. J Appl Physiol 63:1130, 1987.
74. Barber RE, Lee J, Hamilton WK: Oxygen toxicity in man: A prospective study in patients with irreversible brain damage. N Engl J Med 283:1478, 1970.
75. Dolezal V: The effect of long lasting oxygen inhalation upon respiratory parameters in man. Physiol Bohemoslov 11:149, 1962.
76. Kapanci Y, Tosco R, Eggermann J, et al: Oxygen pneumonitis in man. Chest 62:162, 1972.
77. Montgomery AB, Luce JM, Murray JF: Retrosternal pain is an early indicator of oxygen toxicity. Am Rev Respir Dis 139:1548, 1989.
78. Reily CA, Cohen G, Lieberman M: Ethane evolution: A new index of lipid peroxidation. Science 183:208, 1974.
79. Morita S, Snider MT, Inada Y: Increased N-pentane excretion in humans: A consequence of pulmonary oxygen exposure. Anesthesiology 64:730, 1986.
80. Adamson IY, King GM, Bowden DH: Collagen breakdown during acute lung injury. Thorax 43:562, 1989.
81. Block ER, Fisher AB: Depression of serotonin clearance by rat lungs during oxygen exposure. J Appl Physiol 42:33, 1977.
82. Dobuler KJ, Catravas JD, Gillis CN: Early detection of oxygen induced lung injury in conscious rabbits. Reduced in vivo activity of angiotensin-converting enzyme and removal of 5-hydroxytryptamine. Am Rev Respir Dis 126:534, 1982.
83. Shapiro BA, Cane RD, Harrison RA: Positive end-expiratory pressure therapy in adults with reference to acute lung injury: A review of the literature and suggested clinical correlations. Crit Care Med 12:127, 1984.
84. MacIntyre, N: New forms of mechanical ventilation. Clin Chest Med 9:47, 1988.
85. Patterson CE, Butler JA, Byrne FD, et al: Oxidant lung injury: Intervention with sulfhydryl reagents. Lung 163:23, 1985.
86. Boyce NW, Campbell D, Holdsworth SR: Modulation of normobaric pulmonary oxygen toxicity by hydroxyl radical inhibition. Clin Invest Med 10:316, 1987.
87. White CW, Jackson JH, Abuchowski A, et al: Polyethylene glycol–attached antioxidant enzymes decrease pulmonary oxygen toxicity in rats. J Appl Physiol 66:584, 1989.
88. Jacobson JM, Michael JR, Jafri MH, et al: Antioxidants and antioxidant enzymes protect against pulmonary oxygen toxicity in the rabbit. J Appl Physiol 68:1252, 1990.
89. Wolf HRD, Seeger HW: Experimental and clinical results in shock lung treatment with vitamin E. Ann NY Acad Sci 393:392, 1982.
90. Sawyer MAJ, Novick W, Marino PL: Antioxidant therapy and survival in ARDS: A clinical study (abstract). Crit Care Med 17:S153, 1989.
91. Padmanabhan RV, Gudapaty R, Leiner IE, et al: Protection against pulmonary toxicity in rats by the intratracheal administration of liposome-encapsulated superoxide dismutase or liposomes. Am Rev Respir Dis 132:164, 1985.
92. Matalon S, Holm BA, Notter RH: Mitigation of pulmonary hyperoxic injury by administration of exogenous surfactant. J Appl Physiol 62:756, 1987.

CHAPTER 87

Adjunct Methods of Respiratory Therapy

Gregory Tino
Michael A. Grippi

During the past several decades, significant advances have been made in the management of the critically ill patient. Some have had far-reaching clinical, ethical, and socioeconomic implications (e.g., the use of mechanical ventilation[1]). In the United States, critical care accounts for 2 to 3% of many hospital budgets;[2] the average daily charges for a patient in a critical care unit exceed $3,000.[3] Respiratory care, including adjunct measures such as chest physiotherapy and nebulization of inhaled medications, has become an integral part of the management of critically ill patients; the annual cost is calculated in *billions* of dollars. In fact, respiratory care accounts for about 3% of hospital expenditures in the United States.[2] Despite this huge investment, controversy abounds about the efficacy of a number of respiratory therapy modalities.[4] Therefore, a logical and selective application of these techniques, based on data available in the medical literature, is important from both patient care and financial perspectives.

This chapter focuses on three adjunct methods of respiratory care in the critical care unit: (1) chest physiotherapy, including incentive spirometry; (2) inhaled therapeutic agents; and (3) use of supplemental oxygen.

CHEST PHYSIOTHERAPY

Chest physiotherapy refers to techniques designed to maintain lung expansion, assist mucociliary clearance, relieve airway obstruction, and improve ventilatory function[5,6] (Table 87–1). Included are chest percussion and postural drainage, incentive spirometry, deep breathing exercises, coughing, forced expiratory maneuvers, and mechanical aids such as intermittent positive pressure breathing and continuous positive airway pressure. Currently, chest percussion with postural drainage and incentive spirometry are the physiotherapy techniques most widely utilized in the United States.[7]

Methods
Chest Percussion and Postural Drainage

Chest percussion may be delivered by respiratory therapists, nurses, or other appropriately trained medical personnel. The technique consists of striking discrete areas of the chest wall with both hands alternating in rapid succession; the hands are held in a slightly cupped position with the fingers closed, resulting in the trapping of air between the hands and the chest wall. Treatment may be targeted to specific anatomic locations or may be applied systematically to both hemithoraces. Mechanical vibration devices are also used; however, they offer no clear advantages over manual techniques.[8,9] Percussion is often combined with postural drainage, through which the patient's position is periodically changed to promote gravity-dependent movement of secretions from individual lobes toward the trachea.[10] Subsequently, the secretions are expelled by suctioning or having the patient cough. The rationale for use of chest percussion and postural drainage is based on several physiologic principles: (1) airway obstruction from any cause may result in loss of lung volume and increased resistance in central and peripheral airways;[6,11] (2) airway obstruction produces altered ventilation-perfusion relationships and impaired gas exchange;[5,6] and (3) inadequate mucus clearance leads to

TABLE 87–1

GOALS OF CHEST PHYSIOTHERAPY

Maintenance of adequate lung expansion
Enhancement of mucociliary clearance
Relief of airway obstruction and decrease in work of breathing
Improvement of ventilatory function and gas exchange

pooling of secretions and delayed removal of potentially infected material from the respiratory tract.[12]

Incentive Spirometry

The incentive spirometer was developed by Bartlett and associates more than two decades ago.[13] The device measures the volume of a breath when the patient, with his or her glottis open, performs a sustained, maximal inspiration to total lung capacity. The spirometer can be used with or without supervision after appropriate instruction of patients.

A key element in the use of the incentive spirometer is provision of visual feedback to the patient of his or her progress. The patient must be alert and should be encouraged to use the device as frequently as several times per hour.[14] The goal is to prevent microatelectasis and macroatelectasis, which result in diminished lung compliance, increased work of breathing, and hypoxemia.[14-16] The sustained inspiratory efforts help prevent collapse of alveolar units and decrease physiologic dead space.[17, 18]

Indications

Chest physiotherapy is widely prescribed in the United States (Fig. 87–1). According to a national survey conducted in 1985 to evaluate the use of chest physiotherapy in the prevention of postoperative pulmonary complications, incentive spirometry and chest percussion were ordered in 81 and 95% of hospitals, respectively.[7] In the majority of institutions surveyed, other modalities were also used in various combinations. Despite this popularity, the efficacy of chest physiotherapy in a broad range of clinical conditions has been disputed.[4, 19]

The lack of information addressing the utility of chest physiotherapy in the critical care setting is striking. Although significant increases in oxygenation have been reported after mechanical vibration, position change, and suctioning of mechanically ventilated patients,[20] these results have not been demonstrated consistently.[21, 22] Hence, recommenda-

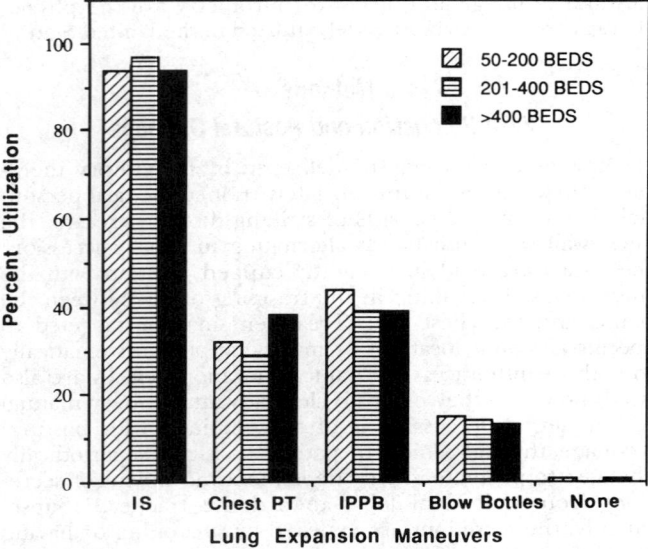

Figure 87–1. Lung expansion maneuvers prescribed prophylactically in the United States—utilization by hospital size. IS = incentive spirometry; IPPB = intermittent positive pressure breathing; PT = physiotherapy. (Adapted from O'Donohue WJ: National survey of the usage of lung expansion modalities for the prevention and treatment of postoperative atelectasis following abdominal and thoracic surgery. Chest 87:77, 1982.)

TABLE 87–2
INDICATIONS FOR CHEST PHYSIOTHERAPY

Accepted Indications
Treatment of lobar atelectasis
Prevention of postoperative pulmonary complications in high-risk situations (e.g., COPD) after thoracic or upper abdominal surgery
Respiratory failure complicated by copious airway secretions
Maintenance or improvement of pulmonary function in cystic fibrosis
Exacerbation of bronchiectasis

Questionable Indications
Chronic bronchitis with scant airway secretions
Status asthmaticus
Pneumonia
Respiratory compromise attributable to neuromuscular and skeletal disorders associated with reduced compliance (e.g., kyphoscoliosis)

tions on the use of chest physiotherapy techniques in critically ill patients have been based on extrapolation of data documenting their benefit in patients with a variety of medical conditions encountered outside the critical care unit. In general, the indications for chest physiotherapy include (1) prevention and treatment of atelectasis and (2) improvement of pulmonary function in patients with cystic fibrosis and other disorders characterized by copious sputum production (Table 87–2).

Treatment of Atelectasis

The value of chest physiotherapy, particularly incentive spirometry, in the prevention of atelectasis in surgical patients has been debated extensively. Atelectasis remains the most common postoperative pulmonary complication.[23] It may be evident as segmental, lobar, or whole lung collapse; hypoxemia may be seen despite a normal chest x-ray film, so-called microatelectasis.[24] Disruption of the normal sigh and cough mechanisms, coupled with transient decrements in lung volume and respiratory drive commonly seen postoperatively, contributes to its development.[25-27] The result is often clinically significant hypoxemia, arising primarily from ventilation-perfusion mismatch.[27, 28]

In an early controlled trial of chest physiotherapy (including postural drainage) for patients undergoing cholecystectomy,[29] the incidence of atelectasis and other pulmonary complications was reduced substantially in the treated group (42% vs. 27%). The incidence was even lower (12%) in patients taught the techniques before surgery. In another large, prospective study, patients were randomly assigned preoperatively to four groups, each receiving one of the following treatment regimens: intermittent positive pressure breathing, incentive spirometry, deep breathing exercises, or no prophylactic management.[30] The incidence of postoperative pulmonary complications, including atelectasis, was reduced by more than half in each of the treated groups (48% vs. 21 to 22%). No significant side effects of treatment were noted, and hospital stay was shortened in those patients receiving incentive spirometry. These studies, as well as others, support the use of chest physiotherapy in preventing postoperative atelectasis in high-risk patients, especially when the measures are initiated before surgery.[27, 31, 32]

In addition to controversy over the use of chest physiotherapy in the prophylaxis of atelectasis, disputes about its use in the active treatment of this problem also occur. Although some experts believe that, in most cases, atelectasis does not require treatment,[23] other investigators advocate rather aggressive management with fiberoptic bronchoscopy[33] or nasal continuous positive airway pressure[34] when the atelectasis is significant (i.e., lobar or greater). However, in one study comparing fiberoptic bronchoscopy with chest physiotherapy, no advantage was demonstrated for bronchoscopy combined with chest physiotherapy over chest physiotherapy alone.[35] Given the potential adverse effects of bronchoscopy and positive airway pressure ventilation in the intubated patient,[36] chest physiotherapy should be considered an effective and safe option in the management of acute atelectasis in this patient population.[19, 37]

Management of Cystic Fibrosis and Other Pulmonary Disorders

Cystic fibrosis remains the most common lethal genetic disorder of white persons. Its pulmonary manifestations include hypersecretion of mucus and chronic bacterial infections. Complications of advancing disease are airway obstruction, bronchiectasis, atelectasis, pneumothorax, cor pulmonale, and respiratory failure, often leading to admission to the critical care unit.[38] Although there are no specific data on which to evaluate chest physiotherapy in the critically ill patient with cystic fibrosis, it is used widely and has been found effective in improving mucus clearance and pulmonary function.[5, 19] One study reported a twofold increase in sputum volume in patients with cystic fibrosis who were treated with percussion and postural drainage compared with coughing maneuvers alone.[39] This beneficial effect on bronchial clearance was substantiated in other reports as well.[19, 40, 41] Objective measures of pulmonary function in patients with cystic fibrosis are also favorably influenced; increases in peak expiratory flow rate,[42] specific conductance,[43] vital capacity, and forced expiratory volume in 1 second[44] have been demonstrated.

Chest physiotherapy may be beneficial in other acute or chronic pulmonary conditions (e.g., bronchiectasis).[19, 20, 45] In addition, there may be a role for chest physiotherapy in disorders characterized by impaired lung inflation and inability to mobilize secretions (e.g., neuromuscular diseases, kyphoscoliosis, and severe obesity).[14]

Adverse Effects

Incentive spirometry is generally well tolerated.[30] However, chest percussion and postural drainage may be associated with adverse effects, particularly in critically ill patients. For example, acute bronchoconstriction, wheezing, and decrements in expiratory flow rate have been reported.[44, 46] In addition, children treated with percussion and postural drainage after cardiac surgery for congenital heart disease have been reported to have more severe and refractory atelectasis than those not receiving chest physiotherapy.[47]

Adverse effects on gas exchange have also been described. A significant decline in mean arterial oxygen tension immediately after percussion and postural drainage, presumably owing to ventilation-perfusion inequality, has been reported. Similarly, transient drops in mean arterial oxygenation have been noted in other studies of critically ill patients,[48] although long-term sequelae, if any, have not been described. However, such reductions were not observed in patients producing moderate or large amounts of mucopurulent sputum.[49] These findings do not preclude the use of chest physiotherapy in such patients; rather, they suggest that patients in a critical care unit should be monitored carefully during treatment, and supplemental oxygen should be administered, as indicated.

Finally, a number of adverse hemodynamic and metabolic changes have been described during chest physiotherapy in

TABLE 87–3
GOALS OF AEROSOL THERAPY
Bronchodilation
Airway humidification
Mucolysis and enhanced mucokinesis
Direct antimicrobial action
Adjunctive treatment of upper airway obstruction
? Adjunctive treatment of ARDS

mechanically ventilated patients, including increases in heart rate, systolic and mean arterial blood pressure, cardiac output, oxygen consumption, and carbon dioxide production.[50] Decreases in arterial pH and minute ventilation and increases in $PaCO_2$ have also been noted, although the clinical significance of these changes is unclear.

In summary, chest physiotherapy, as adjunctive respiratory therapy in selected critical care situations, is clearly beneficial. Proper monitoring of vital signs and oxygen saturation is important. Routine use, particularly of chest percussion and postural drainage, in asthma or exacerbations of chronic bronchitis without excessive secretions cannot be supported by the current literature. Similarly, it is clear that these modalities do not have a routine role in the treatment of pneumonia or the prevention of its complications. Further studies are necessary to more precisely define the role of chest physiotherapy in the critical care unit.

USE OF AEROSOLS AND INHALED MEDICATIONS

A variety of aerosols are used commonly in the modern critical care unit to treat a broad range of acute and chronic respiratory disorders. The goals of aerosol therapy (Table 87–3) include bronchodilation, enhanced mucokinesis and mucolysis, humidification, and direct pulmonary deposition of antimicrobial agents. Useful techniques of producing and delivering aerosols have been developed in the past three decades, and much has been written on the validity of the clinical and scientific bases supporting their use.[4, 51] Before addressing the efficacy of specific inhalation medications, a brief review of the basic principles of aerosol generation and deposition is warranted.

Principles of Aerosol Generation and Deposition

An aerosol is defined as an airborne suspension of fine solid or liquid particles, ranging in size from 10^{-4} to 10^2 μm.[52, 53] Natural aerosols may include dust, bacteria, yeast, molds, and products of combustion. The challenge inherent in medical aerosol technology is the manufacture of particles with the stability and size necessary for deposition in desired sites, including the lower respiratory tract.

The behavior of aerosols depends on a number of factors (Table 87–4): particle size, concentration, electrical charge, surface tension, and humidity.[53–56] Most therapeutic aerosols are composed primarily of spheric molecules of heterogeneous sizes; they are referred to as polydisperse.[53] Particle size distribution is expressed by a measure known as the mass median diameter. In a given aerosol, half of the mass is in particle sizes above, and half below, the mass median diameter.[55, 56] Another useful designation of an aerosol particle's dimension is based on its aerodynamic properties and is known as the aerodynamic equivalent diameter.[52, 53, 55, 56] In general, the larger the particle, the more proximal is its deposition in the respiratory tract.

Deposition of aerosols in the lung is also influenced by other physical properties of the particles.[52–56] For example,

TABLE 87–4
FACTORS AFFECTING AEROSOL BEHAVIOR AND STABILITY
Particle size and concentration
Gravitational settling (sedimentation)
Inertial impaction
Route of administration (oral or nasal)
Presence of underlying obstructive pulmonary disease
Others
Particle electrical charge
Particle surface tension
Ambient humidity
? Ventilatory pattern

the gravitational settling, or sedimentation, of a particle denotes its depositional velocity onto a surface, as influenced by gravitational forces. The settling speed is also affected by particle density and diameter. Simply stated, larger, more dense particles are deposited more quickly. Another important variable is inertial impaction, a term that reflects the oppositional forces determining deposition (namely, gravity and the resistance offered to flow by the medium through which the particle is moving). The latter increases as airstream direction shifts. In the respiratory tract, this is analogous to the movement of aerosols across airway bifurcations; as the course of flow changes, smaller, more central particles deposit less readily and are carried more distally.

Clearance of deposited material is usually accomplished by the mucociliary elevator, via cough, via phagocytosis by alveolar macrophages, and for some soluble elements, by systemic absorption and metabolism.[54–57]

Clinical Applications

From a clinical standpoint, several issues are of particular importance in providing effective inhalation therapy. The preferred route of administration is the mouth, because increased resistance in the nasal passages augments inertial impaction there.

As alluded to earlier, particle size is also crucial (Table 87–5); about 65% of particles with an aerodynamic equivalent diameter of 10 μm or greater are trapped in the oropharynx.[53] For particles of less than 5 μm, especially those less than 2 μm, alveolar deposition predominates.[53, 54]

The role of ventilatory pattern in aerosol deposition is controversial.[58] For example, some studies suggest that slow inhalation to moderately large lung volumes, followed by breath holding, optimizes delivery to the lower respiratory tract.[59, 60] The significance of this factor in patients in the critical care unit, where ventilatory patterns may not be stable, is largely unknown.

TABLE 87–5	
AEROSOL PARTICLE SIZE AND SITE OF RESPIRATORY TRACT DEPOSITION	
Particle Size (μm)	**Deposition in Respiratory Tract**
>100	Do not enter tract
5–100	Trapped in nose
2–5	Deposited proximal to alveoli
1–2	Can enter alveoli, with 95–100% retention
0.25–1	Minimal settling in airways
<0.25	Predominantly alveolar deposition

From Spearman CB, Sheldon RL, Egan DF: Humidity and aerosol therapy. In: Spearman CB, Sheldon RL, Egan DF (eds): Egan's Fundamentals of Respiratory Therapy. 4th ed. St Louis, CV Mosby, p 353, 1982.

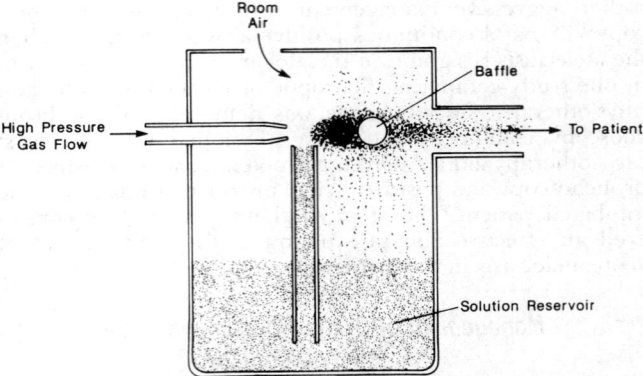

Figure 87–2. The jet nebulizer. See text for details. (From Fishman AP [ed]: Pulmonary Diseases and Disorders: Update 1. New York, McGraw-Hill, p 370, 1982.)

In addition, underlying lung pathologic change dramatically affects aerosol distribution. Although uniform parenchymal deposition is the rule in normal patients, asymmetric uptake with a significant perihilar distribution is characteristic of chronic obstructive pulmonary disease (COPD).[61, 62]

Finally, the importance of proper humidification cannot be overstated; care must be taken to provide enough moisture to mimic room air conditions and to prevent overdrying and thermal airway damage. At the same time, overhumidification can change particulate properties and affect deposition.[52–54, 56, 63]

The generation of aerosols is accomplished by the comminution of liquid or solid materials into smaller particles. This is an energy-requiring, two-step process, which begins with mechanical disruption of the material, followed by its dispersion.[53, 55, 56] Although condensation of vaporized materials is an alternative process, it is not clinically practical, given the thermal instability of most substances used in inhalation therapy. The generation of therapeutic aerosols is accomplished by using nebulizers that produce stable particles, usually less than 20 to 30 μm in diameter. Two principal types of nebulizers are routinely employed in the critical care unit: jet and ultrasonic. In addition, a third type of delivery device, the metered-dose inhaler, is being used more commonly in the critical care setting.

Jet Nebulizer

The jet nebulizer (Fig. 87–2), also known as the pneumatic atomizer, is the most widely used apparatus for aerosolizing liquids.[53–56, 64] In addition, it is the most commonly used device for delivering bronchodilators in intubated patients.[65] The jet nebulizer has no moving parts; the liquid to be nebulized is stored in a reservoir and is entrained by Venturi's action into a feeding tube by a high-pressure stream of air or oxygen. The liquid is comminuted by a baffle and then dispersed by turbulent flow. Larger droplets hit the nebulizer wall owing to inertial impaction and, subsequently, return to the reservoir. Although contaminated aerosol reservoirs have been reported in several outbreaks of nosocomial pneumonia,[66–68] the availability of disposable respiratory equipment has markedly reduced the incidence of this source of infection.[68]

Ultrasonic Nebulizer

The ultrasonic nebulizer (Fig. 87–3) is more complicated than the jet device. Energy for aerosol production is derived from a piezoelectric transducer.[53–56, 69] The apparatus is

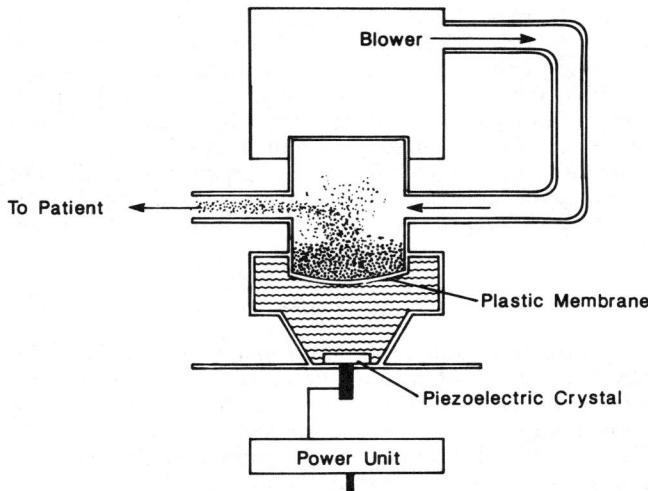

Figure 87–3. The ultrasonic nebulizer. See text for details. (From Fishman AP [ed]: Pulmonary Diseases and Disorders: Update 1. New York, McGraw-Hill, p 370, 1982.)

divided into two compartments: (1) the power chamber, which contains the transducer, and (2) the nebulizer chamber, which contains the solution to be nebulized. High-frequency vibrations produced by a piezoelectric crystal are transmitted to the nebulizer chamber through a coupling fluid via a flexible plastic membrane. The aerosolized liquid is delivered to the patient by either a carrier gas or by spontaneous ventilatory effort. A major advantage of the ultrasonic nebulizer is its ability to generate large aerosol volumes.[64] Consequently, it has been used widely to aerosolize saline and water for maximal humidification of inspired air.[54, 69] It is also an important tool for induction of respiratory secretions for cytologic and bacteriologic studies.[56, 70] Mucolytic agents and some antibiotics have been delivered by this method, but widespread applicability has been hampered by concerns about drug viscosity and a theoretic concern about chemical disruption of pharmacologic agents by ultrasonication.[54]

Metered-Dose Inhaler

The metered-dose inhaler is a portable device used to generate aerosols from either liquids or solids.[53] It is the most frequently prescribed outpatient bronchodilator delivery system.[71, 72] Its components include a small vial, which houses the specific medication, and an inert gas propellant. When activated, the propellant nebulizes the agent and delivers it in a predetermined dosage. Most metered-dose inhalers provide bronchodilator particles with a mass median diameter ranging from 2.8 to 4.3 μm.[53] Although side effects have been reported, including cardiac dysrhythmias thought to be related to the propellant,[56, 65] the use of metered-dose inhalers is safe and effective, even in critically ill patients. A study comparing the delivery of albuterol from a metered-dose inhaler with that from a jet nebulizer in mechanically ventilated patients with airway obstruction showed the methods to be equally efficacious. The cost savings with the metered-dose inhaler were substantial.[65]

Pharmacologic Agents Delivered as Aerosols

With the basic tenets of aerosol generation and deposition as a background, this discussion focuses on classes of nebulized pharmacologic agents commonly used in the critical care unit. The most important of these include bronchodilators, antimicrobial agents, mucolytics, and helium-oxygen mixtures. Because of its potential role in the treatment of patients with the adult respiratory distress syndrome (ARDS), a brief description of aerosolized surfactant is also provided.

Bronchodilators

The use of nebulized bronchodilators for the treatment of reversible airway obstruction dates to 1935 when inhaled epinephrine was first introduced.[73] Since then, a number of other agents have been developed. These drugs demonstrate varying degrees of receptor selectivity and duration of action (Table 87–6). In general, sympathomimetic drugs that produce bronchial smooth muscle relaxation are the most commonly prescribed and widely studied.[74-77] Their efficacy in providing rapid bronchodilation with few adverse effects after inhalation in patients with acute and chronic airflow obstruction is well documented.[75, 76, 78] In the critical care unit, inhaled beta-agonists are a key component of the therapy of patients with respiratory failure attributable to airway obstruction, including severe asthma.[79] However, these agents have no proven benefit in other disorders, such as acute pulmonary edema. Accordingly, their routine use in the critically ill, ventilator-dependent patient with other forms of pulmonary or cardiac disease cannot be justified.[80] Even when the drugs are indicated, the choice of specific agent and the mode of delivery remain topics for debate.

The most frequently reported and worrisome side effects of sympathomimetic bronchodilators, especially in patients with underlying cardiovascular disease, are cardiac dysrhythmias.[72, 74, 81] In general, the preferred agents are those that selectively stimulate airway beta-receptors. Examples include isoetharine, terbutaline, metaproterenol, and albuterol. These agents are all efficacious, and a general endorsement for the preferential use of any one of them cannot be made. Albuterol appears to have a longer duration of action[82] and increased beta$_2$-receptor selectivity.[83] Terbutaline is most often used orally.[74] Isoetharine has a shorter duration of action.[77, 80] With any of these drugs, interaction with skeletal muscle and central nervous system beta-receptors may produce tremor, anxiety, and nausea.[77] Upper airway deposition of aerosols may be substantial in cases of severe airway obstruction.[61, 62, 76] The ideal safe and effective dosage range of these agents has not been determined in critically ill patients.

	Type*			Duration of
Agent	**Alpha**	**Beta₁**	**Beta₂**	**Action**
Epinephrine	3+	4+	3+	Short
Racemic epinephrine	2+	3+	2+	Short
Ephedrine	2+	3+	3+	Long
Isoproterenol		4+	4+	Short
Isoetharine		1+	3+	Medium
Metaproterenol		2+	2+	Long
Terbutaline		1+	3+	Long
Albuterol		1+	4+	Long
Fenoterol		1+	4+	Long

TABLE 87–6

RECEPTOR SITE STIMULATION, RELATIVE STRENGTH, AND DURATION OF ACTION OF SOME ADRENERGIC DRUGS

*1 + = minor effect; 4 + = strong effect.
†Short, 0.5–2 h; medium, 2–4 h; long, 4–6 h.
From Peters JA: Pharmacology for respiratory therapy. In: Spearman CB, Sheldon RL, Egan DF (eds): Egan's Fundamentals of Respiratory Therapy. 4th ed. St Louis, CV Mosby, p 396, 1982.

In many institutions, the delivery of inhaled bronchodilators in the critical care unit is provided almost exclusively by pressurized nebulizers. However, evidence is now mounting that these agents can be equally effectively delivered using a metered-dose inhaler in selected intubated patients.[65, 85] The efficacy and safety of the metered-dose inhaler have been demonstrated in the treatment of both ambulatory and non–critically ill hospitalized patients with bronchospasm, at substantially less cost.[76, 84-86] Dosage adjustments must be made to account for endotracheal tube deposition and for changes in inspiratory flow rate, which can alter drug delivery.[65, 85] Further investigation is required to determine the optimal use of aerosol-generating devices in the critically ill patient.

Anticholinergic agents such as ipratropium bromide, as well as corticosteroids and cromolyn sodium, are all effective for treating airflow obstruction.[76] However, their utility in patients in the critical care unit is unknown.

Antimicrobial Agents

The development and use of aerosolized antimicrobials in the treatment of pulmonary infections have been undertaken with several goals in mind: (1) avoidance of the toxicities of systemically administered agents, (2) direct deposition of active drugs in the lungs, (3) enhanced drug penetration of infected lung tissue, and (4) improvement in results of treatment of gram-negative respiratory infections.

A variety of antibacterial and antifungal inhalation drugs is available. Neomycin, penicillin derivatives, aminoglycosides, and amphotericin B are examples. Their use as prophylactic or therapeutic agents in the critical care unit remains highly controversial. In a large study of surgical patients in a critical care unit who were treated prophylactically with inhaled polymyxin B, the incidence of colonization with *Pseudomonas aeruginosa* declined.[87] However, some patients had pneumonia with drug-resistant gram-negative bacilli. The resultant mortality rate was 64%, higher than that reported previously, without prophylactic administration.[87] Other investigations also failed to demonstrate a decrease in mortality or elimination of the need for systemic therapy in patients in a critical care unit treated with prophylactic inhaled antibiotics.[88, 89] Furthermore, these medications are not devoid of toxicity; refractory bronchospasm in patients with obstructive pulmonary disease has been documented.[90]

Treatment of most established pulmonary infections with inhalation antimicrobials alone cannot be supported by available data. Legitimate ethical considerations have precluded randomized investigations. Aerosolized agents may have a role when combined with intravenous therapy in recalcitrant respiratory tract infections, but additional research is required to substantiate the role of this form of treatment.

Although the routine use of antimicrobial agents delivered through inhalation is not well defined, the administration of aerosolized pentamidine in the prophylaxis of *Pneumocystis carinii* pneumonia in patients with the acquired immunodeficiency syndrome has become widely accepted[91, 92] (see Chapter 50). In addition, reports suggest that aerosolized pentamidine is also effective as the sole agent in the treatment of mild disease.[93, 94] Drug delivery to the alveolar spaces, with minimal upper respiratory tract deposition and few side effects, is accomplished by using a nebulizer, the Respirgard II.[95] Hence, in patients with mild *P. carinii* pneumonia, aerosolized pentamidine may be considered a viable therapeutic option, especially in patients with a contraindication to other drugs such as trimethoprim-sulfamethoxazole. However, the drug should not be used alone in severe infections. Untoward effects include cough, bronchospasm,[94] and rarely, hypoglycemia,[96] maculopapular rash,[97] and pancreatitis.[98] Disseminated pneumocytosis and atypical clinical and radiographic presentations of *P. carinii* pneumonia have also been noted in patients receiving aerosolized pentamidine prophylaxis.[99] Interestingly, there is evidence that when the aerosol form is used in conjunction with intravenous pentamidine in severe infections, plasma concentrations of the drug are higher in ventilated patients than in patients breathing spontaneously.[100] The basis of this finding is unknown.

Mucolytics

Retained secretions represent a major problem for critically ill patients with asthma, lower respiratory tract infections, and cystic fibrosis. In addition to the methods of chest physiotherapy described earlier, mucolytic agents have been widely used in this setting. These drugs alter the rheologic properties of sputum. Examples include detergents and wetting agents such as tyloxapol, which lower mucous surface tension.[74, 90] Aerosolized proteolytic enzymes (e.g., trypsin and pancreatic dornase) were used extensively in the past; however, adverse effects, including fever, hoarseness, and bronchospasm, as well as questionable in vivo efficacy, have limited their use at present.[74, 90] Perhaps the best known agent is *N*-acetylcysteine. *N*-Acetylcysteine disrupts glycoprotein bonds, thereby reducing sputum viscosity and consistency.[80, 90, 101] It is available in 10 and 20% solutions that can be aerosolized or instilled directly into the airways through a bronchoscope. The in vitro effects of *N*-acetylcysteine are clear,[102] and some clinical studies suggest favorable changes in sputum viscosity after use in patients with asthma and chronic bronchitis.[103, 104] Nevertheless, no controlled studies clearly justify the use of *N*-acetylcysteine in the critical care unit; it may be a useful adjunctive measure for clearing secretions that have been refractory to other treatment modalities. Bronchospasm, particularly in patients with known reactive airways disease, is the most commonly reported side effect.[80, 90, 105] Inhaled bronchodilators should be administered concurrently in high-risk, and perhaps all, patients.

Helium-Oxygen (Heliox) Mixtures

Helium is an inert, virtually insoluble, low-density gas, which, when mixed with oxygen, has important clinical applications. The lower density of the gas mixture, compared with that of air or oxygen alone, increases its diffusibility and promotes laminar flow in obstructed airways.[106] Inspiratory and expiratory flow rates are increased, and airway resistance and the work of breathing are decreased.[106-108] Typical gas mixtures range from 60 to 80% helium, combined with 20 to 40% oxygen. The mixtures are relatively expensive; they are free from significant adverse reactions. Although helium-oxygen mixture had widespread application in past decades for the treatment of bronchospasm,[109] newer treatment modalities have limited its role largely to the management of upper airway obstruction.[110, 111] Nonetheless, helium-oxygen mixture may be of value in the management of critically ill patients with status asthmaticus and refractory hypercapnia. Data demonstrate that the use of helium-oxygen, in conjunction with other modalities, including inhaled beta-agonists, subcutaneous epinephrine, and steroids, results in significant reductions in $PaCO_2$ and airway pressure in mechanically ventilated asthmatics.[107] A re-evaluation of helium-oxygen therapy in other conditions encountered in the critical care unit may be warranted; at present, its use should be considered in selected clinical circumstances.

Surfactant

Surfactant is a complex detergent produced by type II pneumonocytes that line the alveolar spaces.[112] It is composed of phospholipids, neutral lipids, and protein; its primary constituent is dipalmitoyl phosphatidylcholine, which accounts for 50% of the complex. Because of its ability to reduce surface tension in alveoli, even at low expiratory lung volumes, surfactant fulfills several important physiologic functions: (1) maintenance of lung compliance, (2) prevention of alveolar edema, and (3) preservation of lung inflation.[112-115] It has long been recognized that surfactant deficiency is the etiologic factor in respiratory distress syndrome of preterm infants.[116] This disorder is characterized by diminished lung compliance, atelectasis, and intrapulmonary shunting.[112] Within the past decade, a number of artificial surfactants that can be delivered by aerosol or through direct intratracheal instillation have been introduced. Several randomized, controlled trials have addressed their use in the treatment of respiratory distress syndrome.[113, 114, 117, 118] Although the studies differ in the length of therapy and in the surfactant preparations used, most have demonstrated a fall in airway pressure and enhanced gas exchange in treated infants.[114, 119, 120] Reduced mortality and a lower incidence of complications of respiratory distress syndrome, including intraventricular hemorrhage and bronchopulmonary dysplasia, have also been reported.[121] Other studies dispute these results.[119] Adverse effects appear to be minimal, although an early report indicated an apparent increased incidence of patent ductus arteriosus in treated infants.[118]

Alterations in surfactant synthesis and secretion have been implicated in patients with diffuse lung injury secondary to ARDS. These abnormalities have been shown in both animal models[122] and clinical studies.[123] Because intrapulmonary shunting and a reduction in lung compliance are the physiologic hallmarks of ARDS, there is growing interest in the use of artificial surfactant in its management. Beneficial effects have been noted in a number of animal models.[124, 125] In one preliminary report in humans, transient improvement in oxygenation was seen in patients with severe ARDS after the administration of a single dose of exogenous surfactant.[126] At present, large multicenter, randomized, controlled trials to assess the efficacy of aerosolized surfactant in ARDS resulting from sepsis and trauma are under way. It is hoped that the initial enthusiasm for the use of this agent will be corroborated.

OXYGEN THERAPY

Since its discovery in the late 18th century, oxygen has been employed extensively in medical practice. Despite this long-standing history, its use in many clinical circumstances remains controversial. Critically ill patients routinely receive supplemental oxygen—perhaps not surprisingly, given the spectrum of cardiopulmonary disorders that prompt admission to the critical care unit. It has been only recently, however, that the pharmacology of oxygen has been delineated. This discussion provides an overview of the indications for oxygen therapy and a brief description of the systems available for oxygen delivery.

Indications

Simply stated, the goals of oxygen therapy are (1) treatment of hypoxemia and (2) prevention of the consequences of insufficient oxygen delivery to peripheral tissues. The pathophysiologic mechanisms of hypoxemia and tissue hypoxia and the role of oxygen supplementation are, however, not straightforward. Hypoxemia may arise through a variety

TABLE 87–7
INDICATIONS FOR OXYGEN THERAPY

Accepted Indications
Acute arterial hypoxemia of any cause (Po_2 < 60 mm Hg or oxygen saturation < 90%)
Chronic hypoxemic states (e.g., COPD)
Normoxemic hypoxia
   Carbon monoxide poisoning
   Anemia
   Diminished tissue perfusion attributable to cardiac failure
   Methemoglobinemia

Questionable Indications
Acute myocardial infarction without hypoxemia
Angina
Dyspnea without hypoxemia
Nocturnal oxygen desaturation (e.g., COPD and sleep apnea)
Sickle cell crisis

of mechanisms, including alveolar hypoventilation (as seen in neuromuscular disorders), diffusion abnormalities, ventilation-perfusion mismatching, right-to-left shunting, and the breathing of hypoxic gas mixtures.[127] The response to supplemental oxygen depends on the mechanism(s) of hypoxemia operative in an individual patient. Increases in the fraction of inspired oxygen (FIO_2) may produce dramatic improvements in PaO_2 in conditions characterized by mild or moderate ventilation-perfusion mismatching, such as pneumonia.[128] However, increasing the FIO_2 is often of little benefit in ARDS, in which there is substantial intrapulmonary shunting.[129]

Tissue hypoxia generally occurs when oxygen consumption exceeds oxygen delivery. Oxygen delivery is the product of cardiac output and the oxygen content of arterial blood; the latter is a function of hemoglobin concentration, PaO_2, and the oxyhemoglobin dissociation curve.[130]

There is no single, easily measured variable that reliably identifies tissue hypoxia. Rather, inadequate peripheral oxygenation is suggested by altered end-organ function, the presence of lactic acidosis, a decreased cardiac output, and a reduced PO_2 in mixed venous blood. Supplemental oxygen administration can certainly increase the dissolved oxygen concentration in the absence of improved pulmonary gas exchange; however, it may have a less beneficial effect on tissue oxygen delivery if severe anemia or reduced cardiac output is present. In such situations, supplemental oxygen constitutes a small part of a larger management scheme. Knowledge of the underlying pathophysiology governs the proper use of oxygen in conjunction with other therapeutic modalities.

Given the many clinical settings in which oxygen therapy is employed, guidelines concerning its appropriate use are important. Concerns about the cost and safety of oxygen administration are paramount. Despite the growing body of knowledge regarding oxygen therapy, its utility in some situations is controversial and often unsupported. Table 87–7 summarizes accepted and questionable indications for oxygen therapy. In general, the major indications for oxygen therapy include acute hypoxemia, chronic hypoxemia, and normoxemic hypoxia.

Acute Hypoxemia

The most common and universally accepted indication for the use of supplemental oxygen is a PaO_2 value below 60 mm Hg or an arterial oxygen saturation of less than 90%.[131, 132] Initiation of therapy is usually based on appropriate laboratory documentation, but careful, empirical oxygen therapy is defensible in the short-term when hypoxemia or tissue hypoxia are clinically likely. The goal of treatment is reversal of the hypoxemia using the lowest concentration of supplemental oxygen possible. Periodic reassessment is mandatory. Although data from controlled trials supporting the efficacy of supplemental oxygen under these circumstances are scarce, the potential effects of untreated hypoxia on various organ systems justifies its use. In patients with intercurrent hypercapnia, such as those with advanced COPD, care must be taken to avoid exacerbating the hypercapnia by overzealous oxygen therapy.

Chronic Hypoxemia

Long-standing hypoxemia induces a number of compensatory physiologic responses aimed at maximizing oxygen delivery. Examples include the development of secondary polycythemia and a rightward shift of the oxyhemoglobin dissociation curve.[132] COPD is the most frequent pulmonary cause of chronic hypoxemia. A number of studies have addressed long-term oxygen therapy in this population of patients. Early reports suggested beneficial effects of supplemental oxygen,[133, 134] and two large studies from the early 1980s firmly established its efficacy.[135, 136] Both reported lower mortality rates for chronically hypoxic patients receiving continuous oxygen therapy than for those treated with oxygen intermittently or with no oxygen at all. In addition, patients with hypercapnia, pulmonary hypertension, and polycythemia tended to benefit more.[135] Similar studies of patients with chronic hypoxemia caused by severe interstitial lung disease do not exist. Prompt identification of patients with chronic hypoxemia and institution of therapy in the critical care unit, after the patient is clinically stable, are important.

Normoxemic Hypoxia

A number of clinical conditions fall under the heading of normoxemic hypoxia (i.e., tissue hypoxia in the absence of hypoxemia). A classic example is carbon monoxide poisoning. Carbon monoxide has a great affinity for hemoglobin and reduces oxygen binding and transport. Impaired oxygen unloading at the tissue level is the result. The PaO_2 is invariably normal, especially early in the course of carbon monoxide poisoning; the measured oxygen content is reduced. Treatment with supplemental oxygen at high concentrations (e.g., 100%) significantly diminishes the half-life of carboxyhemoglobin and may increase tissue oxygen delivery.[137]

Other examples of normoxemic hypoxia include severe anemia, cardiogenic shock, and disorders characterized by alterations in hemoglobin-oxygen interactions (e.g., methemoglobinemia). Although no large controlled trials have specifically addressed the value of supplemental oxygen in these settings, the pathophysiology of tissue hypoxia supports its use in situations in which inadequate tissue oxygen delivery is clinically likely.[130, 131]

The value of supplemental oxygen in a number of settings in which it has been used traditionally remains unproved. The best example is uncomplicated acute myocardial infarction, without accompanying hypoxemia. Although supplemental oxygen has been reported to limit infarct size in animal models[138] and to diminish myocardial ischemia in humans,[139] even when the baseline PaO_2 is normal, these findings have been disputed.[140] Furthermore, routine use of oxygen for treatment of angina pectoris,[130] dyspnea without hypoxemia,[131] nocturnal desaturation,[132, 141] and sickle cell crisis,[127] although common practice, has not been clearly proved beneficial.

Like other drugs, oxygen can produce adverse effects.

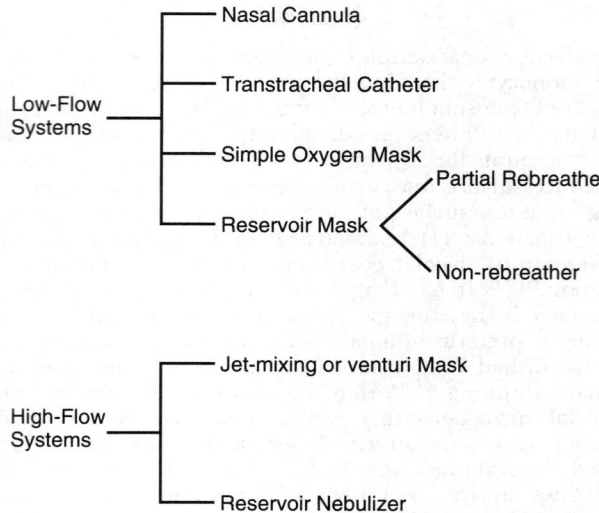

Figure 87–4. Oxygen delivery systems. See text for details.

The most devastating complication of high-flow oxygen therapy is pulmonary cytotoxicity and parenchymal fibrosis. Another well-known adverse effect is oxygen-induced hypoventilation in patients with hypercapnic respiratory failure.[132, 141] In addition, alveolar nitrogen washout and interference with surfactant function produce structural alveolar changes and intrapulmonary shunting.[106, 127] The potential hazards of supplemental oxygen should encourage its rational use.

Oxygen Delivery Systems

A variety of oxygen delivery systems are available for clinical use (Fig. 87–4). They may be divided into two groups: low-flow and high-flow systems.

Low-Flow Systems

In general, low-flow systems provide a fraction of the patient's minute ventilatory requirement as pure oxygen, rather than fulfill the total ventilatory demand (because the patient breathes some room air with each inspiration). Because the flow rates are low (4 to 6 L/min), the actual inspired oxygen concentration varies according to the minute ventilation.[142] Hence, these devices are also known as variable performance systems.[106] A variety of low-flow devices are available.

Nasal Cannulas. Nasal cannulas are the most commonly used low-flow devices.[127] One hundred percent oxygen is provided at rates up to 6 L/min; at low levels of minute ventilation, the FIO_2 may be as high as 50%.[131] Flow rates higher than 6 L/min are usually poorly tolerated by patients. Conservation devices have been developed to allow lower mean flow rates.[143] Nasal catheters are also available, but they are used uncommonly. Because the FIO_2 cannot be easily predicted, the use of nasal cannulas is not advisable in patients with unstable hypercapnic respiratory failure.

Simple Oxygen Masks. Simple masks are usually made of plastic and fit over the patient's nose and mouth; exhalation ports are built-in. Oxygen flow rates of 5 to 6 L/min generate an FIO_2 of 30 to 60%. Although simple masks are not equipped with a reservoir bag, their design creates the potential for carbon dioxide retention, especially at flow rates below 5 L/min. Therefore, lower flow settings are discouraged to prevent carbon dioxide rebreathing. As for other variable performance devices, the FIO_2 depends on the ventilatory pattern.

Reservoir Masks. Reservoir masks are essentially simple masks fitted with a bag into which source oxygen flows and from which the patient inhales. Reservoir masks provide FiO_2 of greater than 50% at flow rates between 4 and 10 L/min. The flow rates used preclude significant carbon dioxide rebreathing by maintaining partial bag inflation during the ventilatory cycle. Reservoir masks are of two types: non-rebreathing and partial rebreathing. With the former, a one-way valve between the mask and the reservoir bag ensures that only source oxygen enters the bag during exhalation, thereby preventing rebreathing of exhaled gas. In contrast, the partial rebreathing apparatus lacks this valve, allowing the patient to inspire exhaled gas. Ideally, this gas represents dead space volume and is composed primarily of oxygen, thus conserving the source gas. Although reservoir masks generally provide high FiO_2, 90 to 100% is rarely achieved in practice, for a variety of technical reasons, including a poor mask fit.

Transtracheal Catheters. During the past several years, a number of systems have been developed through which oxygen is delivered directly into the trachea via a catheter placed percutaneously. These transtracheal oxygen delivery systems are designed specifically for long-term oxygen therapy in patients whose oxygen requirements are generally stable. Advantages of their use include elimination of the need for nasal cannulas and lower required oxygen flow rates. Of course, catheter placement is an invasive procedure, and the technique necessitates careful local care and periodic catheter changes to prevent infection.

High-Flow Systems

High-flow, or fixed performance, systems are designed to provide an inspired gas flow that exceeds the minute ventilatory requirement of the patient. Unlike the case with low-flow systems, the FiO_2 is unaffected by the minute ventilation, so that specific FiO_2 values are reliably delivered.[130, 131] The prototype high-flow system is the jet-mixing, or venturi, mask, introduced by Campbell in 1960.[144] Oxygen flows at high velocity into the mask through a narrow orifice, where creation of a lower pressure allows mixing with room air in a constant air/oxygen ratio. This occurs, at least in part, in accordance with the Venturi modification of the Bernoulli principle, which describes the restoration of pressure distal to obstruction of gas flow by dilation of the passage. With the venturi mask, higher flow rates translate into higher oxygen concentrations because of a lower level of air entrainment. Alternatively, increases in the size of mask side ports through which air is entrained result in lower FiO_2 because of higher air/oxygen ratios. The range of FiO_2 levels for which these masks are most reliable is 24 to 40%.[145-147] Oxygen requirements of 50% or greater are best provided by other modalities (e.g., reservoir masks or mechanical ventilation). Venturi masks are most useful in clinical situations in which the administration of supplemental oxygen needs to be monitored carefully to avoid alveolar hypoventilation (e.g., in patients with hypercapnic COPD).[147]

Other examples of high-flow oxygen systems include reservoir nebulizers, T tubes, tracheostomy collars, continuous positive airway pressure masks, and oxygen tents.

References

1. Swinburne AJ, Fedullo AJ, Shayne D: Mechanical ventilation: Analysis of increased use and patient survival. J Intensive Care Med 3:315, 1988.
2. Ayres SM: Magnitude of use and costs of in-hospital respiratory therapy. Am Rev Respir Dis 122(suppl):11, 1980.
3. Elpern EH, Silver MR, Rosen RL, et al: The non-invasive respiratory care unit: Patterns of use and financial implications. Chest 99:205, 1991.
4. Pierce AK: Scientific basis of in-hospital respiratory therapy. Am Rev Respir Dis 122(suppl):1, 1980.
5. Rochester DF, Goldberg SK: Techniques of respiratory physical therapy. Am Rev Respir Dis 122(suppl):133, 1980.
6. Menkes H, Britt J: Physical therapy: Rationale for physical therapy. Am Rev Respir Dis 122(suppl):127, 1980.
7. O'Donohue WJ: National survey of the usage of lung expansion modalities for the prevention and treatment of postoperative atelectasis following abdominal and thoracic surgery. Chest 87:76, 1985.
8. Darrow G, Anthonisen NR: Physiotherapy in hospitalized medical patients. Am Rev Respir Dis 122(suppl):155, 1980.
9. Maxwell M, Redmond A: Comparative trial of manual and mechanical percussion technique with gravity-assisted bronchial drainage techniques in patients with cystic fibrosis. Arch Dis Child 54:542, 1979.
10. Gaskell DV, Webber BA: The Brompton Hospital Guide to Chest Physiotherapy. Oxford, Blackwell Scientific Publications, 1977.
11. Macklem PT, Mead J: Resistance of central and peripheral airways as measured by a retrograde catheter. J Appl Physiol 22:395, 1967.
12. Newhouse M, Sanchin J, Brenenstock J: Lung defense mechanisms. N Engl J Med 295:990, 1976.
13. Bartlett RH, Gazzaniga AB, Geraghty TR: The yawn maneuver: Prevention and treatment of postoperative pulmonary complications. Surg Forum 22:196, 1971.
14. Murray JF: Indications for mechanical aids to assist lung inflation in medical patients. Am Rev Respir Dis 122(suppl):121, 1980.
15. Martin RT, Rogers RM, Gray BA: Mechanical aids to lung expansion: The physiologic basis for use of mechanical aids to lung expansion. Am Rev Respir Dis 122(suppl):105, 1980.
16. Fletcher R, Larsson A: Gas exchange in the partially atelectatic lung. Anaesthesia 40:1186, 1985.
17. Ferris BG, Pollard DS: Effect of deep and quiet breathing on pulmonary compliance in man. J Clin Invest 39:143, 1960.
18. Knelson JH, Howatt WF, Demuth GR: Effect of respiratory pattern on alveolar gas exchange. J Appl Physiol 29:328, 1970.
19. Kiriloff LH, Owens GR, Rogers RM, et al: Does chest physical therapy work? Chest 88:436, 1985.
20. Holody B, Goldberg H: The effect of mechanical vibration physiotherapy on arterial oxygenation in acutely ill patients with atelectasis or pneumonia. Am Rev Respir Dis 124:372, 1981.
21. Laws A, McIntyre R: Chest physiotherapy: A physiologic assessment during intermittent positive pressure ventilation in respiratory failure. Anaesth Soc J 16:487, 1969.
22. MacKenzie C, Shin B, McAslan T: Chest physiotherapy: The effect on arterial oxygenation. Anesth Analg 57:28, 1978.
23. O'Donohue WJ: Prevention and treatment of post-operative atelectasis. Can it and will it be adequately studied? Chest 87:1, 1985.
24. Prys-Roberts E, Nunn JF, Dobson RH, et al: Radiographically undetectable pulmonary collapse in the supine position. Lancet 2:399, 1967.
25. Jackson CV: Preoperative pulmonary evaluation. Arch Intern Med 148:2120, 1988.
26. Meyers JR, Lembeck L, O'Kane H, et al: Changes in functional residual capacity of the lung after operation. Arch Surg 110:576, 1975.
27. Tisi GM: Preoperative evaluation of pulmonary function: Validity, indications and benefits. Am Rev Respir Dis 119:293, 1979.
28. Benumof JL: Mechanism of decreased blood flow to atelectatic lung. J Appl Physiol 46:1047, 1979.
29. Thoren L: Postoperative pulmonary complications: Observations on their prevention by means of physiotherapy. Acta Chir Scand 107:194, 1954.
30. Celli BR, Rodriquez KS, Snider GL: A controlled trial of intermittent positive-pressure breathing, incentive spirometry and deep breathing exercises in preventing pulmonary complications after abdominal surgery. Am Rev Respir Dis 130:12, 1984.
31. Roukema JA, Carol EJ, Prins JG: The prevention of pulmonary complications after upper abdominal surgery in patients with non-compromised pulmonary status. Arch Surg 123:30, 1988.
32. Oikkonen M, Karjalainen K, Kahara V, et al: Comparison of incentive spirometry and intermittent positive pressure breathing after coronary artery bypass graft. Chest 99:60, 1991.
33. Mahajan VK, Catron PW, Huber GL: The value of fiberoptic bronchoscopy in the management of pulmonary collapse. Chest 73:817, 1978.
34. Duncan SR, Negrin S, Mihm FG, et al: Nasal continuous positive airway pressure in atelectasis. Chest 92:621, 1987.
35. Marini JJ, Pierson DJ, Hudson L: Acute lobar atelectasis: A prospective comparison of fiberoptic bronchoscopy and respiratory therapy. Am Rev Respir Dis 119:971, 1979.
36. Lindholm CE, Ollman B, Snyder JV, et al: Cardiorespiratory effect of fiberoptic bronchoscopy in critically ill patients. Chest 74:362, 1978.
37. Marini JJ: Management of lobar atelectasis. Respir Care 28:204, 1983.
38. Scanlin TF: Cystic fibrosis. In: Fishman, AP (ed): Pulmonary Diseases and Disorders. 2nd ed. New York, McGraw-Hill, p 1273, 1988.
39. Loring M, Penning C: Evaluation of postural drainage by measurement of sputum volume and consistency. Am J Phys Med 50:215, 1971.
40. Wong J, Keens T, Wannamaker E, et al: Effects of gravity in tracheal transport rates in normal subjects and in patients with cystic fibrosis. Pediatrics 60:146, 1977.
41. Rossman CM, Waldes R, Sampson D, et al: Effect of chest physiotherapy on the removal of mucus in patients with cystic fibrosis. Am Rev Respir Dis 126:131, 1982.
42. Tecklin J, Holsclaw D: Evaluation of bronchial drainage in patients with cystic fibrosis. Phys Ther 55:1081, 1975.

43. Cochrane GM, Webber BA, Clarke SW: Effects of sputum on pulmonary function. Br Med J 2:1181, 1977.
44. Feldman J, Traver GA, Taussig LM: Maximal expiratory flows after postural drainage. Am Rev Respir Dis 119:239, 1979.
45. Mazzocco M, Kiriloff L, Owens G, et al: Physiologic effects of chest percussion and postural drainage in patients with bronchiectasis. Am Rev Respir Dis 129:A-52, 1984.
46. Campbell AH, O'Connell JM, Wilson F: The effect of chest physiotherapy upon the FEV$_1$ in chronic bronchitis. Med J Aust 1:33, 1975.
47. Reines, HD, Sade RM, Bradford BF, et al: Chest physiotherapy fails to prevent postoperative atelectasis in children after cardiac surgery. Ann Surg 195:451, 1982.
48. Tyler ML, Hudson LD, Grose BL, et al: Prediction of oxygenation during chest physiotherapy in critically ill patients. Am Rev Respir Dis 121(suppl):218, 1980.
49. Connors AF, Hammon WE, Martin RJ, et al: Chest physical therapy: The immediate effect on oxygenation in acutely ill patients. Chest 78:559, 1980.
50. Klein P, Kemper M, Weissman C, et al: Attenuation of the hemodynamic responses to chest physical therapy. Chest 93:38, 1988.
51. Pierce AK, Saltzman HA: Conference on the scientific basis of respiratory therapy. Am Rev Respir Dis 110:1, 1974.
52. Morrow PE: Aerosol characterization and deposition. Am Rev Respir Dis 110:88, 1974.
53. Swift DL: Aerosols and humidity therapy: Generation and respiratory deposition of therapeutic aerosols. Am Rev Respir Dis 122:71, 1980.
54. Spearman CB, Sheldon RL, Egan DF: Humidity and aerosol therapy. In: Spearman CB, Sheldon RL, Egan DF (eds): Egan's Fundamentals of Respiratory Therapy. 4th ed. St Louis, CV Mosby, p 335, 1982.
55. Swift DL, Litt M: Physical and physiological principles of aerosol deposition and mucociliary clearance. In: Burton GG, Hodgkin JE (eds): Respiratory Care: A Guide to Clinical Practice. 2nd ed. Philadelphia, JB Lippincott, p 358, 1984.
56. Helmholz HF, Burton GG: Applied humidity and aerosol therapy. In: Burton GG, Hodgkin JE (eds): Respiratory Care: A Guide to Clinical Practice. 2nd ed. Philadelphia, JB Lippincott, p 379, 1984.
57. Camner P: Clearance of particles from the human tracheobronchial tree. Clin Sci 59:79, 1980.
58. Brain JD, Valberg PA: Deposition of aerosol in the respiratory tract: State of the art. Am Rev Respir Dis 120:1325, 1979.
59. Newman SP, Pavia D, Clarke SW: Improving the bronchial deposition of pressurized aerosols. Chest 80(suppl):909, 1981.
60. Dolovich M, Ruffin RE, Roberts R, et al: Optimal delivery of aerosols from metered dose inhalers. Chest 80(suppl):911, 1981.
61. Lin MS, Goodwin DA: Pulmonary distribution of an inhaled radioaerosol in obstructive pulmonary disease. Radiology 118:645, 1976.
62. Taplin GV, Poe ND, Isawa T, et al: Radioaerosol and xenon gas inhalation and lung perfusion scintigraphy. Scand J Respir Dis 85(suppl):144, 1974.
63. Wells RE, Perera RD, Kinney JM: Humidification of oxygen during inhalational therapy. N Engl J Med 268:644, 1963.
64. Mercer TT: Production of therapeutic aerosols: Principles and techniques. Chest 80(suppl):813, 1981.
65. Gay PC, Patel HG, Nelson SB, et al: Metered dose inhalers for bronchodilator delivery in intubated mechanically ventilated patients. Chest 99:66, 1991.
66. Reinarz JA, Pierce AK, Mays BB: The potential role of inhalational therapy equipment in nosocomial pulmonary infections. J Clin Invest 44:831, 1965.
67. Phillips I: *Pseudomonas aeruginosa* respiratory tract infection in patients receiving mechanical ventilation. J Hyg 65:229, 1967.
68. Pierce AK, Sanford JP, Thomas GD: Long term evaluation of decontamination of inhalational therapy equipment and the occurrence of necrotizing pneumonia. N Engl J Med 282:528, 1970.
69. Boucher RMG, Kreuter J: The fundamentals of the ultrasonic atomization of medicated solutions. Ann Allergy 26:591, 1968.
70. Hensler NM, Spivey CG, Dees TM: The use of hypertonic aerosol in production of sputum for diagnosis of tuberculosis. Chest 40:639, 1961.
71. Clarke SW, Newman SP: Differences between pressurized aerosol and stable drug particles. Chest 80(suppl):907, 1981.
72. Clarke SW: Inhaler therapy. Q J Med 67:355, 1988.
73. Graeser JB, Rowe AH: Inhalation of epinephrine for the relief of asthmatic symptoms. J Allergy 6:415, 1935.
74. Peters JA: Pharmacology for respiratory therapy. In: Spearman CB, Sheldon RL, Egan DF (eds): Egan's Fundamentals of Respiratory Therapy. 4th ed. St Louis, CV Mosby, p 380, 1982.
75. Miller WF: Aerosol therapy in acute and chronic respiratory disease. Arch Intern Med 131:148, 1973.
76. Newhouse MT, Dolovich MB: Current concepts: Control of asthma by aerosols. N Engl J Med 315:870, 1986.
77. Popa V: Beta-adrenergic drugs. Clin Chest Med 7:313, 1986.
78. Detroyer A, Yernault JC, Rodenstein D: Influence of beta-2 agonist aerosols on pressure-volume characteristics of the lungs. Am Rev Respir Dis 118:987, 1978.
79. Summer WR: Status asthmaticus. Chest 1(suppl):875, 1985.
80. Marino PL: The pharmacotherapy of respiratory failure. In: Marino PL: The ICU Book. Philadelphia, Lea & Febiger, p 328, 1991.

81. Neville E, Corris PA, Vivian J, et al: Nebulized salbutamol and angina. Br Med J 285:796, 1982.
82. Snider GL, Laguanda R: Albuterol and isoproterenol aerosols: A controlled study of duration of effect in asthmatic patients. JAMA 221:682, 1972.
83. Hendeles L: Asthma therapy: State of the art. Am Rev Respir Dis 9:82, 1988.
84. Summer W, Elston R, Tharpe L, et al: Aerosol bronchodilator delivery methods: Relative impact on pulmonary function and cost of respiratory care. Arch Intern Med 149:618, 1989.
85. Berenberg MJ, Baigelman W, Cupples LA, et al: Comparison of metered dose inhaler attached to an aero-chamber with an updraft nebulizer for the administration of metaproterenol in hospitalized patients. J Asthma 22:87, 1985.
86. Crogan SJ, Bishop MJ: Laboratory reports: Delivery efficiency of metered dose aerosols given via endotracheal tubes. Anesthesiology 70:1008, 1989.
87. Feeley TW, Du Moulin GC, Hedley-Whyte J, et al: Aerosol polymyxin and pneumonia in seriously ill patients. N Engl J Med 293:471, 1975.
88. Greenfield S, Teres D, Bushnell LS, et al: Prevention of gram negative bacillary pneumonia using aerosol polymyxin as prophylaxis. I. Effect on the colonization pattern of the upper respiratory tract of seriously ill patients. J Clin Invest 52:2935, 1973.
89. Levine BA, Petroff PA, Slade L, et al: Prospective trials of dexamethasone and aerosolized gentamicin in the treatment of inhalational injury in the burned patient. J Trauma 18:188, 1978.
90. Wanner A, Rao A: Clinical indications for and effects of bland, mucolytic and anti-microbial aerosols. Am Rev Respir Dis 122:79, 1980.
91. Centers for Disease Control: Guidelines for prophylaxis against *Pneumocystis carinii* pneumonia for persons infected with human immunodeficiency virus. JAMA 262:335, 1989.
92. The San Francisco Community Prophylaxis Trial: Aerosolized pentamidine for prophylaxis against *Pneumocystis carinii* pneumonia. N Engl J Med 323:769, 1990.
93. Montgomery AB, Debs RJ, Luce JM, et al: Aerosolized pentamidine as sole therapy for *Pneumocystis carinii* pneumonia in patients with acquired immunodeficiency syndrome. Lancet 2:480, 1987.
94. SooHoo GW, Mohsenifar Z, Meyer RD: Inhaled or intravenous pentamidine therapy for *Pneumocystis carinii* pneumonia in AIDS: A randomized trial. Ann Intern Med 113:195, 1990.
95. Simonds AK, Newman SP, Johnson MA, et al: Alveolar targeting of aerosol pentamidine: Toward a rational delivery system. Am Rev Respir Dir 141:827, 1990.
96. Karboski JA, Godley PJ: Inhaled pentamidine and hypoglycemia. Am J Med 108:490, 1988.
97. Berger T, Tappero JW, Leoung GS, et al: Aerosolized pentamidine and cutaneous eruptions. Ann Intern Med 110:1035, 1989.
98. Murphy RL, Noskin GA, Ehrenpreis ED: Acute pancreatitis associated with aerosolized pentamidine. Am J Med 88:53N, 1990.
99. Jules-Elysee KM, Stover DE, Zaman MB, et al: Aerosolized pentamidine: Effect on diagnosis and presentation of *Pneumocystis carinii* pneumonia. Ann Intern Med 112:750, 1990.
100. Girard DM, Clair B, Certain A, et al: Comparison of plasma concentrations of aerosolized pentamidine in non-ventilated and ventilated patients with pneumocystosis. Am Rev Respir Dis 140:1607, 1989.
101. Dorow P: Mucolytics: When dispensable, when necessary? Lung 168(suppl):622, 1990.
102. Hirsch SR, Zastrow JE, Kory RC: Sputum liquefying agents: A comparative in vitro evaluation. J Lab Clin Med 74:346, 1969.
103. Kory RC, Hirsch SR, Giraldo J: Nebulization of N-acetylcysteine combined with a bronchodilator in patients with chronic bronchitis: A controlled study. Dis Chest 54:504, 1968.
104. Grater WC, Cato A: Double-blind study of acetylcysteine-isoproterenol and saline-isoproterenol in non-hospitalized patients with asthma. Curr Ther Res 15:660, 1973.
105. Rao S, Wilson DB, Brooks RC, et al: Acute effects of nebulization of N-acetylcysteine on pulmonary mechanics and gas exchange. Am Rev Respir Dis 102:17, 1970.
106. Spearman CB, Sheldon RL, Egan DF: Gas therapy. In: Spearman CB, Sheldon RL, Egan DF: Egan's Fundamentals of Respiratory Therapy. 4th ed. St Louis, CV Mosby, p 422, 1982.
107. Gluck EH, Onorato DJ, Castriotta R: Helium-oxygen mixtures in intubated patients with status asthmaticus and respiratory acidosis. Chest 98:693, 1990.
108. Ishikawa S, Segal MS: Reappraisal of helium-oxygen therapy in patients with chronic lung disease. Ann Allergy 31:536, 1973.
109. Barach AL: The use of helium in the treatment of asthma and obstructive lesions of the larynx and trachea. Ann Intern Med 9:739, 1935.
110. Skrinskas GJ, Hyland RH, Hutcheon MA: Using helium-oxygen mixtures in the management of acute upper airway obstruction. Can Med Assoc J 128:555, 1983.
111. Lu TS, Ohmura A, Wong KC, et al: Helium-oxygen in the treatment of upper airway obstruction. Anesthesiology 45:678, 1976.
112. Jobe A, Machiko I: Surfactant for the treatment of respiratory distress syndrome. Am Rev Respir Dis 136:1256, 1987.
113. Vidyasagar D, Shimada S: Pulmonary surfactant replacement in respiratory distress syndrome. Clin Perinatol 14:991, 1987.

114. Merritt TA, Hallman M, Spragg R, et al: Exogenous surfactant treatments for neonatal respiratory distress syndrome and their potential role in the adult respiratory distress syndrome. Drugs 38:591, 1988.
115. Clements JA: Dependence of pressure-volume characteristics of lungs on intrinsic surface active material. Am J Physiol 187:592, 1956.
116. Avery EM, Mead J: Surface properties in relation to atelectasis and hyaline membrane disease. Am J Dis Child 97:517, 1959.
117. Enhoring G, Hill D, Sherwood G, et al: Improved ventilation of prematurely delivered primates following tracheal deposition of surfactant. Am J Obstet Gynecol 132:529, 1978.
118. Fujiwara T, Maeta H, Chida S, et al: Artificial surfactant therapy in hyaline membrane disease. Lancet 1:55, 1980.
119. Horbar JD, Soll RF, Sutherland JM, et al: A multicenter randomized placebo-controlled trial of surfactant therapy for RDS. N Engl J Med 320:959, 1989.
120. Robertson B: Neonatal respiratory distress syndrome and surfactant therapy: A brief review. Eur Respir J 3(suppl):735, 1989.
121. Hallman M, Merritt TA, Jarvenpa AL, et al: Exogenous human surfactant for therapy of severe RDS: A randomized prospective clinical trial. J Pediatr 106:963, 1985.
122. Berry D, Ikegami M, Jobe A: Respiratory distress and surfactant inhibition following vagotomy in rabbits. J Appl Physiol 61:1741, 1986.
123. Petty TL, Silvers GW, Paul GW, et al: Abnormalities in lung elastic properties and surfactant function in ARDS. Chest 75:571, 1979.
124. Matalow S, Holm BA, Notler RH: Mitigation of pulmonary hyperoxic injury by administration of exogenous surfactant. J Appl Physiol 62:756, 1987.
125. Berggren P, Lachmann B, Curstedt T, et al: Gas exchange and lung morphology after surfactant replacement in experimental adult respiratory distress syndrome induced by repeated lung lavage. Acta Anaesthesiol Scand 30:321, 1986.
126. Richman PS, Spragg RG, Merritt TA, et al: Administration of porcine-lung surfactant to humans with ARDS: Initial experience. Am Rev Respir Dis 135:A5, 1987.
127. Snider GL, Rinaldo JE: Oxygen therapy in medical patients hospitalized outside of the intensive care unit. Am Rev Respir Dis 122:29, 1980.
128. Meakins J: Observations on the gases in human arterial blood in certain pathological pulmonary conditions and their treatment with oxygen. J Pathol Bacteriol 24:79, 1921.
129. Bone RC: Treatment of severe hypoxemia due to the adult respiratory distress syndrome. Arch Intern Med 140:85, 1980.
130. Block ER: Oxygen therapy. In: Fishman AP (ed): Pulmonary Diseases and Disorders. 2nd ed. New York, McGraw-Hill, p 2317, 1988.
131. Fulmer JD, Snider GL: ACCP-NHLBI National Conference on oxygen therapy. Chest 86:234, 1984.
132. Anthonisen NR: Hypoxemia and oxygen therapy. Am Rev Respir Dis 126:729, 1982.
133. Stark RD, Finnegan P, Bishop JM: Long-term domiciliary oxygen therapy in chronic bronchitis with pulmonary hypertension. Br J Med 1:467, 1973.
134. Levine BE, Bigelow B, Hamstra RD, et al: The role of long-term continuous oxygen administration in patients with chronic airway obstruction with hypoxemia. Ann Intern Med 66:639, 1967.
135. Nocturnal Oxygen Therapy Trial Group: Continuous or nocturnal oxygen therapy in hypoxemic chronic obstructive lung disease. Ann Intern Med 93:391, 1980.
136. Medical Research Council Working Party: Long-term domiciliary oxygen therapy in chronic hypoxic cor pulmonale complicating chronic bronchitis and emphysema. Lancet 1:681, 1981.
137. Turino GM: Effect of carbon monoxide on the cardiorespiratory system—carbon monoxide toxicity: Physiology and biochemistry. Circulation 63:253A, 1981.
138. Maroko PR, Radvany P, Braunwald E, et al: Reduction of infarct size by oxygen inhalation following acute coronary occlusion. Circulation 52:366, 1975.
139. Madias JE, Madias NE, Wood WB: Precordial ST-segment mapping: Effects of oxygen inhalation on ischemic injury in patients with acute myocardial infarction. Circulation 53:411, 1976.
140. Rawles JM, Kenmura ACF: Controlled trial of oxygen in uncomplicated myocardial infarction. Br Med J 1:1121, 1976.
141. Rudolph M, Banks RA, Semple SJC: Hypercapnia during oxygen therapy in acute exacerbations of chronic respiratory failure. Lancet 2:483, 1977.
142. Goldstein RS, Young J, Rebuck AS: Effect of breathing pattern on oxygen concentration received from standard face masks. Lancet 2:1118, 1982.
143. Claiborne RA, Paynter DE, Dutt AK, et al: Evaluation of the use of an oxygen conservation device in long-term oxygen therapy. Am Rev Respir Dis 136:1095, 1987.
144. Campbell EJM: A method of controlled oxygen administration which reduces the risk of carbon dioxide retention. Lancet 2:12, 1960.
145. Friedman SA, Weber B, Briscoe WA, et al: Oxygen therapy: Evaluation of various air-entraining masks. JAMA 228:474, 1974.
146. Mithoefer JC, Karetzky MS, Mead GD: Oxygen therapy in respiratory failure. N Engl J Med 277:947, 1967.
147. Shiff MM, Massaro DM: Effect of oxygen administration by a venturi apparatus on arterial blood gas values in patients with respiratory failure. N Engl J Med 277:950, 1967.

CHAPTER 88

Long-Term Airway Management

Bradford K. Grassmick
Joseph Bander

Artificial airways have had a long history in medicine. The Egyptians may have performed airway access procedures as long as 5500 years ago. Hippocrates (500 BC) used an artificial airway in patients with peritonsillar abscess to maintain an open breathing passage. Artificial airways were relatively rare until the early 19th century when diphtheria was epidemic, which resulted in the development of tracheotomy by Brehomean and Trosseau.

Intubation in the modern era progressed with the work of MacEwen in Scotland who developed a series of tubes for the delivery of anesthesia, and O'Dwyer in New York who used tubes to maintain patent airways in diphtheria patients.

After the poliomyelitis epidemics of the 1950s, mechanical ventilatory support became common practice.[1] Injuries to the trachea were caused by the relatively stiff red rubber tubes with their small low-compliance cuffs and led to the evolution of the modern endotracheal tube. Although the design of endotracheal tubes has improved, airway injury with intubation is still a significant problem.

FUNCTIONS OF ARTIFICIAL AIRWAY

Patients undergo endotracheal intubation for a variety of reasons: (1) delivery of anesthesia during operative procedures, (2) maintenance of oxygenation and ventilation during respiratory failure, (3) provision of a patent airway in patients with an upper airway obstruction, (4) access for suctioning, (5) protection of the airway from the aspiration of secretions, and (6) a means for hyperventilation in patients with increased intracranial pressure.

In pursuing these goals, an endotracheal tube must fulfill four contradictory functions:

1. The tube should provide as *large* a diameter as possible for ventilation, especially spontaneous ventilation, and for access to the lower airways for suctioning and bronchoscopy.
2. The diameter of the tube should be as *small* as possible to avoid damage to the fragile structures of the glottis.
3. The tube should provide a *tight* seal in the trachea to prevent the loss of delivered tidal volume and to decrease the risk of aspiration.
4. The endotracheal cuff should exert *minimal* pressure to avoid injury to the mucosa and the tracheal cartilages.

ANATOMY

The prominent structures in the supraglottic region include the epiglottis, valleculae, and piriform sinuses (Fig. 88–1). Separating the epiglottis from the base of the tongue are the valleculae. The epiglottis merges laterally with the arytenoepiglottic folds and the piriform sinuses. The epiglottis, the valleculae, and the piriform sinuses are often injured during intubation attempts. Within the glottic opening (Fig. 88–2) are the true vocal cords, which lie under the false vocal cords. The vocal cords attach anteriorly to the

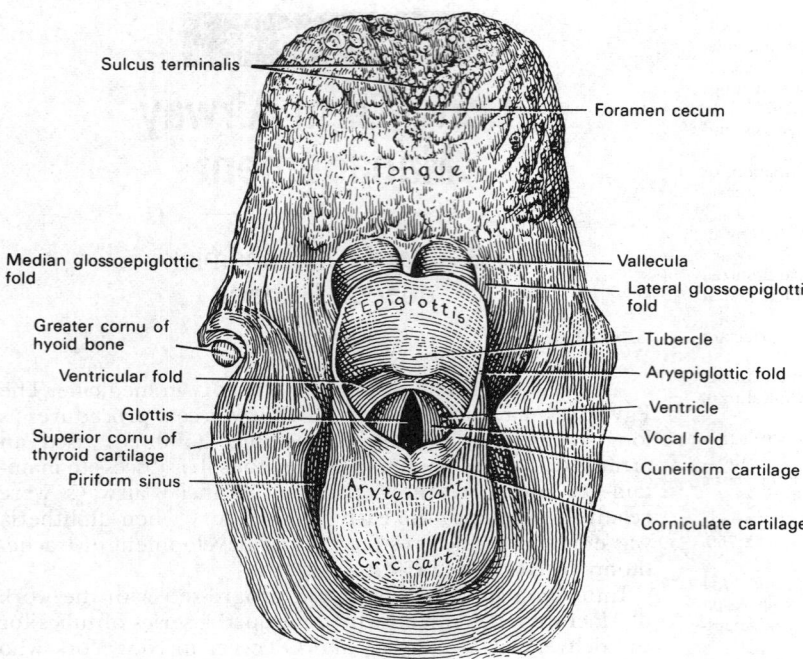

Figure 88–1. Supraglottic anatomy showing epiglottis, the valleculae, and the piriform sinus. (From Clemente C [ed]: Gray's Anatomy. 30th ed. Philadelphia, Lea & Febiger, 1985.)

thyroid cartilage and posteriorly to the arytenoid cartilages, which give them mobility. The area between the arytenoid cartilages is the posterior commissure. The arytenoid cartilages and the posterior commissure are frequently injured by endotracheal tubes. The narrowest portion of the airway is the subglottic region, consisting of the cricoarytenoid muscles, which lie just under the vocal cords.

The trachea extends from the 6th cervical vertebra to the 11th thoracic vertebra, a distance of approximately 11 cm, to the carina. The average distance from the incisors to the carina is 27 cm in men and 23 cm in women. An oral endotracheal tube is in appropriate position when it is between 18 and 22 cm at the incisors.[2] The trachea is composed of 16 to 20 cartilaginous rings, which are open posteriorly but joined by the tracheal muscle. The rings are joined to one another by fibroelastic tissue.[2] Tracheas vary significantly in the cross-sectional anatomy, with the most

common being C-, U-, and D-shaped cartilaginous rings in both males and females[3, 4] (Fig. 88–3). The anteroposterior diameter of the trachea in males varies from 15 to 19 mm and may increase with age.[2] In females, the diameter is 13 to 17 mm.[1] There is no correlation between tracheal size and habitus (i.e., height, weight, or body surface area).[5] There is, however, a correlation with gender, with females having smaller airways than males.

AIRWAY INJURY

Injuries resulting from artificial airways occur primarily in the larynx and in the trachea. Injuries to the supraglottic area consist of hematomas, edema, and lacerations of the epiglottis and the piriform sinuses. False passages have been produced in the piriform sinus by overzealous intubation attempts. Edema and abrasions of the vocal cords may result in chronic fibrosis and granuloma formation. Paralysis of the vocal cords may occur from nerve injury,[6, 7] but more commonly, vocal cord impairment is the result of damage to the arytenoid cartilages or stenosis of the posterior commissure. Injury to the cricoarytenoid muscles may result in subglottic stenosis. Injury to the tracheal mucosa and/or cartilage may occur at the level of the endotracheal or tracheostomy tube cuff or anywhere along the length of the tube. Tracheomalacia or dilatation of the trachea occurs at the level of the endotracheal or tracheostomy tube cuff. Tracheal stenosis occurs with healing of mucosal injury and may occur anywhere along the length of mucosal contact by an endotracheal tube or tracheostomy tube. The various types of airway injury are discussed later.

Injury to Larynx
Supraglottic Injury

Supraglottic laryngeal injuries include lacerations of the epiglottis, piriform sinuses, and vocal cords. Edema of the pharynx or epiglottis may occur in as many as 33% of intubated patients, and supraglottic injuries can be seen in 44% of such patients.[8, 9] As many as 86% of patients note

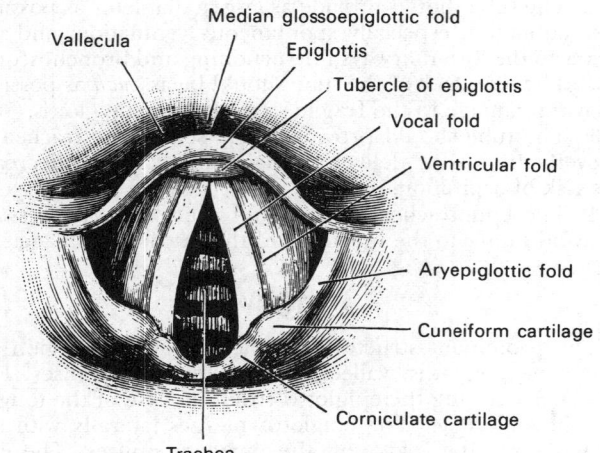

Figure 88–2. Glottic anatomy showing true and false vocal cords, the arytenoid cartilages, and the posterior commissure. (From Clemente C [ed]: Gray's Anatomy. 30th ed. Philadelphia, Lea & Febiger, 1985.)

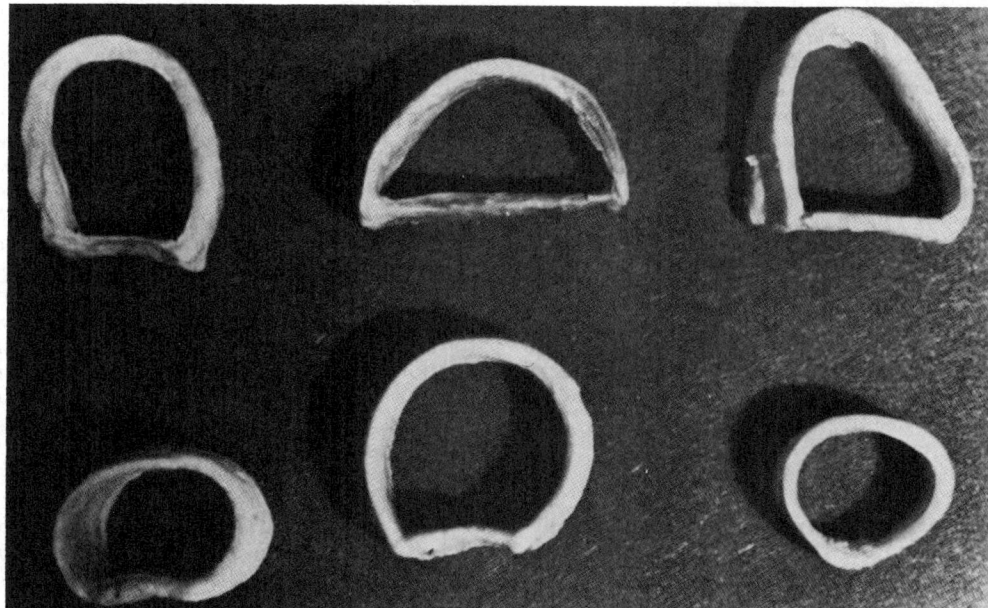

Figure 88–3. Tracheal cross-sectional shapes showing variation in anatomy. (Adapted from Mackenzie CF: Compromises in the choice of endotracheal or nasotracheal intubation and tracheostomy. Heart Lung 12:485, 1983.)

hoarseness even without visible injury. In atraumatic intubations, about 6% of patients may have evidence of laryngeal injury.[8] The most frequent findings were hematomas and lacerations of the vocal cords, especially the left cord, the epiglottis, the false vocal cords, and the piriform sinuses. Paralysis of the vocal cords is rare.

The vast majority of injuries resolve within weeks and usually without sequelae. The major factors contributing to laryngeal injury include the proficiency of the operator, individual anatomic variation of the patient, the degree of relaxation of the patient, and the urgency with which the intubation is performed.[8, 10, 11]

Glottic and Subglottic Injury

Injury to the vocal cords, the arytenoid cartilages, and the posterior commissure are the most serious sequelae of en-

dotracheal intubation. Vocal cord injury most commonly takes the form of erythema or ulceration on the posteriomedial portions of the vocal cords, where the endotracheal tube makes contact with the cords (Fig. 88–4). The most common symptom is hoarseness, but swelling of the cords and stridor may develop after extubation, necessitating reintubation or tracheostomy. The chronic sequelae may include granuloma formation on the cords and fibrosis resulting in impaired vocal cord function and loss of airway patency. True paralysis of the vocal cords because of compression and injury to the recurrent laryngeal nerve has also been reported.[6, 12] Although paralysis is uncommon and usually unilateral, there are reports of bilateral vocal cord paralysis from intubation.[7]

Injury to the arytenoid cartilages, which provide mobility to the vocal cords, and to the posterior commissure may occur acutely with erythema and ulceration at the points of contact with the endotracheal tube (Fig. 88–5). The most serious complication is the development of stenosis of the

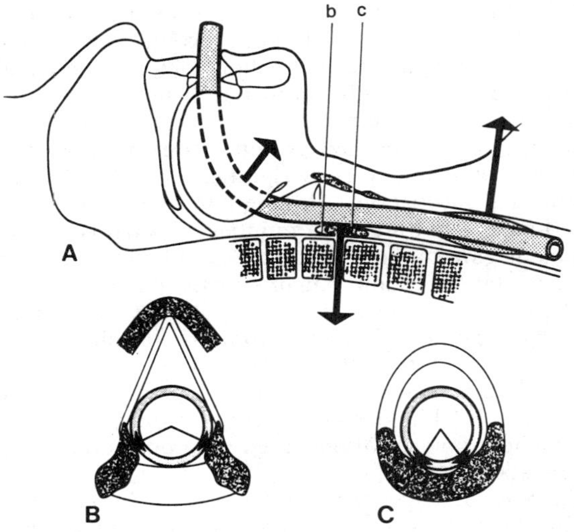

Figure 88–4. Contact points of the endotracheal tube with the arytenoid cartilages and the posterior commissure. (From Lindholm CE: Prolonged endotracheal intubation. Acta Anesthesiol Scand Suppl 33:62, 1969.)

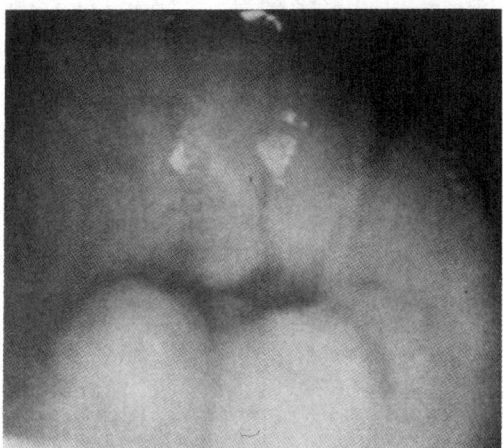

Figure 88–5. Acute inflammation of vocal cords and arytenoid cartilages. (From Whited RE: A prospective study of laryngotracheal sequelae in long-term intubation. Laryngoscope 94:367, 1984.)

posterior commissure, which may result in permanent airway impairment (Fig. 88–6).

Injury to the subglottic area acutely may produce ulceration and edema in the airway and cause stridor on extubation. Chronic stenosis from subglottic injury may result in upper airway obstruction. Often, chronic stenosis is slowly progressive and may not become evident for months or even a year after discharge of the patient from the hospital.[13] The overall incidence of acute laryngeal injury has been reported to be as high as 94%.[14] The incidence of permanent sequelae of laryngeal injury that necessitates surgical intervention such as tracheostomy or repair of stenosis has been reported to be as low as 0% and as high as 10%.[13, 15]

Many factors have been evaluated in the pathogenesis of glottic injury, but three factors (duration of intubation, tube diameter, and head motion) appear to have significant roles. Other factors, including previous smoking, history of steroid use, airway infections, high inspiratory oxygen concentrations, chronic diseases, and race, have been implicated, but not confirmed, in the pathogenesis of airway injury.[16–18]

Duration of Intubation. Since the advent of mechanical ventilation in the 1950s, there has been an ongoing debate as to how long patients may safely be endotracheally intubated and at what point an intubated patient should receive a tracheostomy. In the 1960s, it was common practice to routinely perform a tracheostomy after 48 to 72 hours of intubation. With the development of more compliant tube material (polyvinyl chloride, silicone, Silastic) and high-volume, low-pressure cuffs, endotracheal intubation times have increased to more than 2 to 3 weeks and considerations other than duration of intubation affect the timing of a tracheostomy.[19]

In a prospective study of 52 patients who required ventilatory support for up to 11 days, there was airway injury correlated with the duration of the intubation. Other contributing factors were larger tube size, female sex, and the use of steroids.[17] There was also a higher incidence of airway injury in the patients who underwent early tracheostomy.[17] The most serious complications of tracheostomy included tracheal stenosis and tracheoesophageal fistula. The most serious complications of endotracheal intubation, subglottic stenosis, occurred less frequently than the complications of tracheostomy. The conclusion of the authors was that endotracheal intubation for periods of up to 11 days would have spared 80% of patients a tracheostomy and its complications.

In another study, there was no statistical correlation between the duration of endotracheal intubation and glottic injury, although patients who underwent early tracheostomy were less likely to have glottic injury and more likely to have tracheal injuries.[9] These investigators concluded that the complications of tracheostomy were more serious than those of endotracheal intubation for up to 3 weeks.[9]

Other studies have demonstrated a relationship between duration of intubation and laryngotracheal injury. Whited found that patients intubated for 5 days had only a 2% incidence of chronic laryngeal problems.[20] This figure rose to 4% for patients intubated from 6 to 10 days, whereas 14% of patients intubated for 11 days or longer had chronic laryngeal problems.

Nowak and colleagues demonstrated that glottic injury occurred in 9% of patients who were intubated for up to 6 days, increased to 18.7% for patients intubated for up to 13 days, and was 38% in patients intubated for more than 14 days.[21]

Colice and associates examined patients intubated for an average of 10 days.[14] Although laryngeal edema and vocal cord ulcerations were common, these injuries usually resolved. However, intubation for longer than 10 days was associated with moderate-to-severe laryngeal pathologic changes.

Several studies were unable to find a correlation between laryngotracheal injury and the duration of intubation. Dunham and LaMonica found no significant difference in the incidence of complications in patients who were endotracheally intubated between 7 and 21 days compared with those who underwent early tracheostomy and were ventilated for the same period.[22] The study found that there was a tendency for patients who underwent early tracheostomy to have a higher incidence of airway injury than those who underwent tracheostomy later.[22] Case reports have shown that patients may tolerate prolonged endotracheal intubation without significant airway injury at extubation.[15] Elliott and colleagues reviewed 30 survivors of adult respiratory distress syndrome intubated for an average of 16 days and found that 3 patients had subsequent laryngeal or tracheal injury necessitating repair. There was no significant difference in the duration in intubation, positive end-expiratory pressure, or age of the patients with injury compared with those without.[13] Via-Reque and Rattenborg described six patients who were endotracheally intubated from 55 to 155 days without airway impairment.[23]

The weight of published evidence suggests that the incidence of glottic injury rises significantly after 10 days of endotracheal intubation. Although most of the injury resolves during 4 to 8 weeks, a number of patients experience permanent glottic injury resulting in functional airway impairment. The question remains unsettled, however, as to how long endotracheal intubation should be maintained before conversion to a tracheostomy is considered. Several studies suggested that the complications of tracheostomy may be more serious than the complication of endotracheal intubation.[9, 22, 24] The decision to convert the patient's airway to a tracheostomy is often based on considerations other than duration alone.[19]

Tube Size. Experimentally, the size of the endotracheal tube has been shown to influence airway injury.[25] Patients nasally intubated have significantly less injury to the arytenoid and corniculate cartilages.[26] Differences in injury with oral and nasal endotracheal tubes may be more a function of tube size, position in the posterior pharynx, or inherent

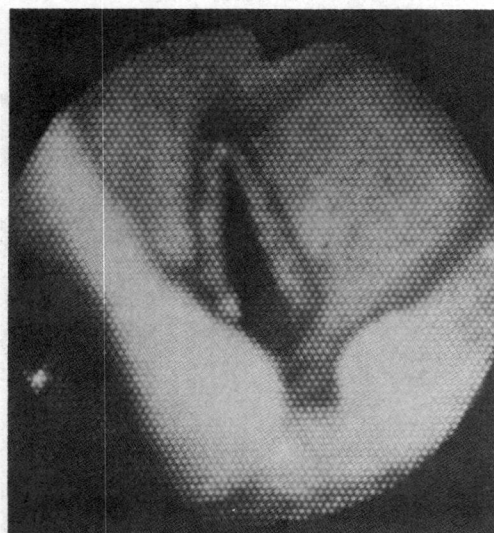

Figure 88–6. Chronic posterior commissure stenosis. (From Whited RE: A prospective study of laryngotracheal sequelae in long-term intubation. Laryngoscope 94:367, 1984.)

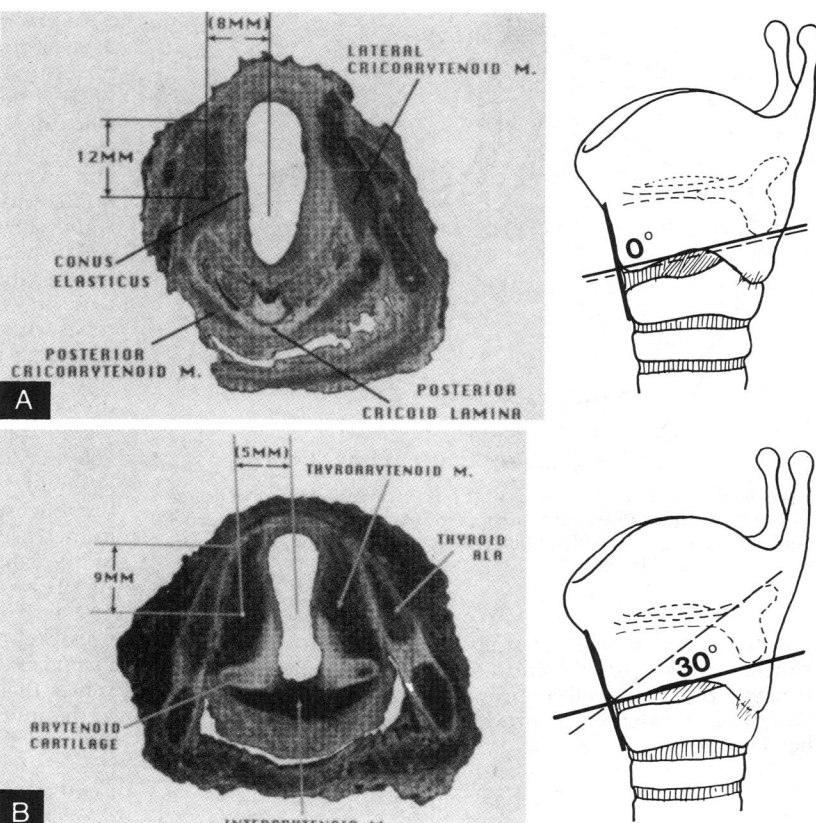

Figure 88–7. Male *(A)* and female *(B)* subglottic anatomy showing limited transverse diameters. (Adapted from Lipton RJ, McCaffrey TV, Cahill DR: Sectional anatomy of the larynx: Implications for the transcutaneous approach to endolaryngeal structures. Ann Otol Rhinol Laryngol 98:141, 1989.)

stability of the nasal tubes.[27] The subglottic portion of the airway has a significantly smaller transverse diameter than anterioposterior diameter[1] (Fig. 88–7). Glottic size is related only to sex rather than to height, weight, or body size. Endotracheal tubes have an external diameter approximately 2 mm larger than the internal diameter.[28] Placement of a 9-mm internal diameter tube in most male patients causes overdistention of the subglottis, and an 8-mm internal diameter tube overdistends the subglottis in most females patients.[6] Several studies found female patients to be more susceptible to airway injury because of their smaller airway.[16, 17]

Intralaryngeal pressure increases with tube size, and mucosal perfusion pressure is exceeded by forces from even the smallest tube (Table 88–1). Patients intubated with tubes larger than 8-mm internal diameter have greater damage

after relatively short periods (<70 hours) of intubation than patients with smaller tubes.[29]

To reduce the risk of glottic injury, tubes that approximate the patient's subglottic dimensions should be used. The appropriate size of endotracheal tube for most men is 8.0- to 8.5-mm internal diameter, and for most women, 7.0- to 7.5-mm internal diameter.

Head Motion. The endotracheal tube lies on the posterior glottis, and because the glottis acts as a fulcrum, the pressures exerted with motion of the tube may be much greater than those at rest (Fig. 88–8). There is increased incidence of laryngeal injury in patients who have severe agitation.[14, 20, 21, 22, 30] By comparison, patients with flaccid paralysis appear to have less laryngotracheal injury than other patients. Motion of the head causes the tube to rock back and forth over the arytenoid cartilages and posterior commissure, greatly increasing the forces on those fragile structures.

The endotracheal tube can move as much as 2 cm cephalad with head extension and 2 cm caudally with neck flexion[27] (Fig. 88–9). If the endotracheal tube is too close to the carina or enters the right mainstem bronchus, the patient may cough or struggle on the ventilator, increasing the likelihood of laryngeal injury. Inadvertent right mainstem intubation may occur in as many as 9.6% of intubations,[9, 31–33] may not be detectable by auscultation, and has been associated with increased mortality.[25]

Agitation may result in self-extubation. The reported incidence of self-extubation ranges from 13 to 33%,[9, 34] with a resultant increase in complications.[9, 22, 32, 34, 35] The use of nasal tubes has been advocated as a means to decrease spontaneous dislocation of the endotracheal tube[34] but may result in sinusitis or nasal necrosis.[35, 36] Several mask appliances have been developed that decreased the incidence of

TABLE 88–1
PRESSURE RECORDINGS FROM SIDE PORT INFUSION CATHETER IN DOG

PVC Endotracheal Tube Inside Diameter (mm)*	Peak Parietal Pressure (to nearest 25 mm Hg)
6.0	75
7.0	95
8.0	180
9.0	375

*PVC = polyvinyl chloride.
From Waymuller EA, Bishop MS, Hibbard AW, et al: Quantification of intralaryngeal pressure exerted by endotracheal tubes. Ann Otol Rhinol Laryngol 92:444, 1983.

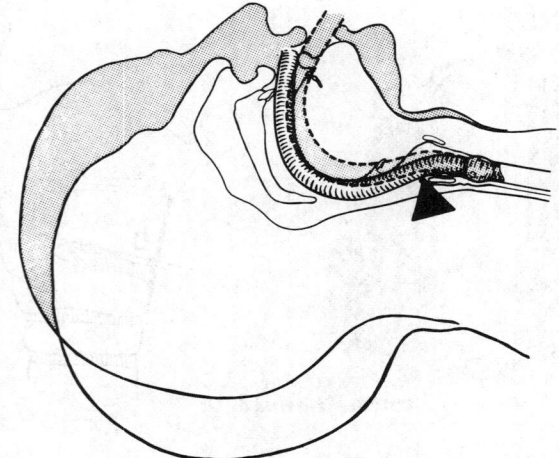

Figure 88–8. Arytenoid cartilages and posterior commissure acting as fulcrum for the endotracheal tube. (From Whited RE: A prospective study of laryngotracheal sequelae in long-term intubation. Laryngoscope 94:367, 1984.)

self-extubation in clinical trials.[37] Vigilance in monitoring, restraining the patient, and adequately securing the endotracheal tubes, as well as providing adequate sedation and analgesia, is essential to prevent complications in the intubated patient.

Tracheal Injury

Injury to the trachea from endotracheal intubation occurs in two areas: where the endotracheal tube cuff comes into contact with the tracheal mucosa and underlying cartilage and where the tip of the endotracheal tube contacts the tracheal wall.

Injury to the tracheal mucosa occurs in all patients who are endotracheally intubated for prolonged periods.[9, 20] The majority of injuries resolve spontaneously, but tracheal stenosis at the cuff site develops in as many as 11% of patients who undergo long-term intubation.[9] Tracheomalacia may develop from overdistention of the endotracheal tube cuff, and over time, tracheal stenosis may develop as fibrosis occurs with healing. The true incidence of tracheal dilatation is unknown.

Tracheal injury at the level of the cuff is the result of two factors, intracuff pressures and mechanical motion of the cuff on the mucosa. The early red rubber endotracheal tubes with small noncompliant cuffs required high intracuff pressures to provide an adequate seal of the airway.[38, 39] A significant portion of the intracuff pressure was transmitted directly to the mucosa of the trachea, resulting in damage to the tracheal mucosa[18] (Fig. 88–10). Although the high-volume, low-pressure cuffs currently in use seal at much lower pressures, all the intracuff pressure is transmitted to the mucosa. Overdistention of the low-pressure cuffs results in increased intracuff pressures, which then resemble those of the small-volume, high-pressure cuffs[38, 39] (Fig. 88–11). As pressure on the mucosa increases, blood flow decreases in a nearly linear fashion (Fig. 88–12). Even low intracuff pressures of 20 mm Hg or less result in a significant decrease in mucosal blood flow.[40] As intracuff pressures increase to values that approach systemic arterial pressure, blood flow in the mucosa approaches zero.[41]

Blood flow to the tracheal mucosa is reduced with cuff pressures exceeding 30 mm Hg.[41, 42] As pressures increase to 40 to 50 mm Hg, mucosal blood flow ceases and ischemic damage becomes widespread. Therefore, intracuff pressures should be kept as low as possible to prevent injury to the tracheal mucosa.[38–43] Several investigators suggested using the minimal leak technique to determine intracuff pressure. In a study by Off and coworkers, 54% of the patients had acceptable intracuff pressures of 25 mm Hg or less, and

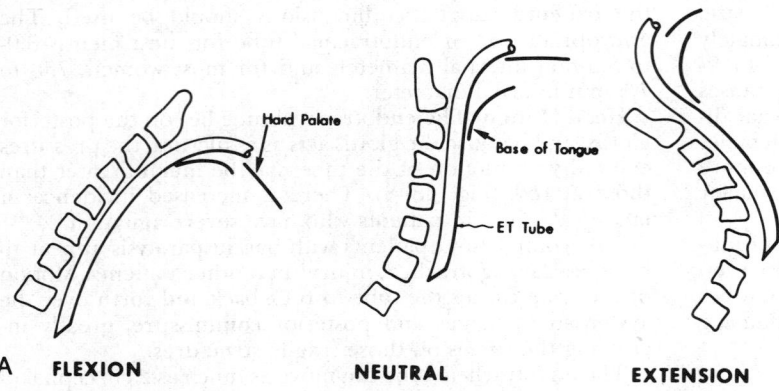

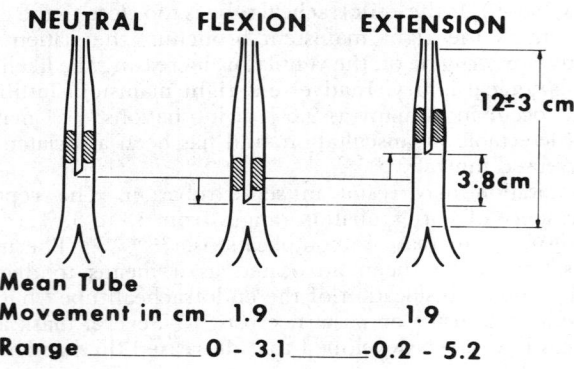

Figure 88–9. Movement of the tip of endotracheal tube with head flexion and extension. (Adapted from PA Conrardy, LR Goodman, F Lainge, et al, Alteration of endotracheal tube position, Crit Care Med, 4, 8–12, © by Williams & Wilkins, 1976.)

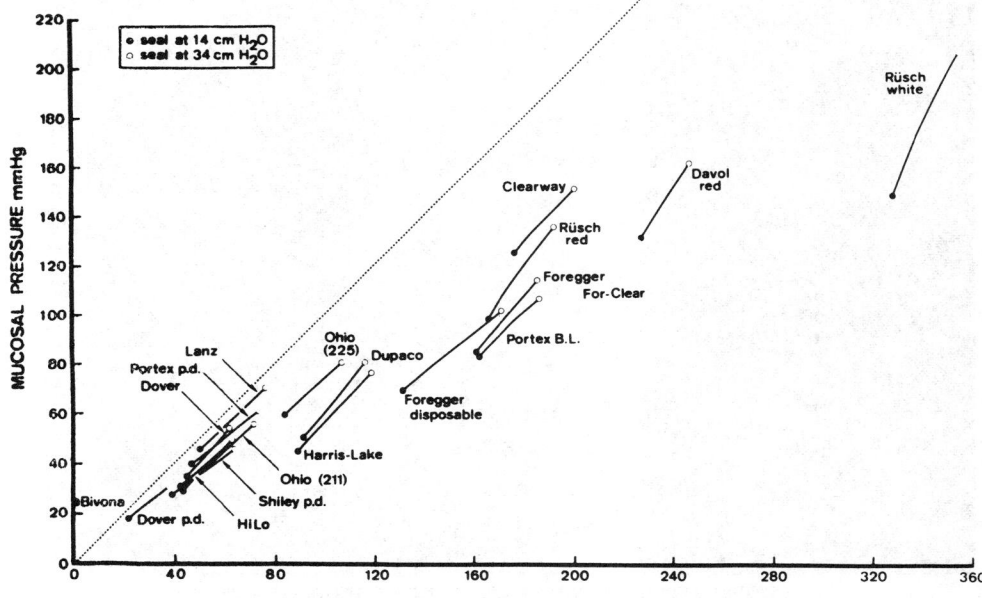

Figure 88–10. Relationship of intracuff pressure and pressure on the tracheal mucosa. (From Dobrin P, Canfield T: Cuffed endotracheal tubes: Mucosal pressures and tracheal wall blood flow. Am J Surg 133:562, 1977.)

intracuff pressures could be reduced to acceptable levels in another 24% by allowing a small leak at end inspiration. In the remaining 22%, intracuff pressures were not correctable, and as a group, those patients had higher peak and static airway pressures.[44]

Balancing the concern for minimizing intracuff pressures is the need to maintain an adequate airway seal to prevent the loss of tidal volume, to prevent aspiration, and to prevent the loss of positive end-expiratory pressure during mechanical ventilation. Anatomic variations may not allow an adequate seal at reasonable cuff pressures.[45, 46] Most airways are U, C, or D shaped.[4, 5] Placement of a round cuff in a nonround trachea causes portions of the airway not to be sealed (Fig. 88–13) unless the circumference of the cuff approximates that of the airway. Studies in anatomic models of circular and noncircular airways revealed that many brands of tubes would seal only at excessively high intracuff pressures, which in turn generate high lateral wall pressures. This was particularly true of small tubes in noncircular airways.[47]

Chandler and Crawley evaluated the size of the cuff necessary to provide an adequate seal to avoid excessive intracuff pressures.[48] Using a single brand of endotracheal tube, they found that most male patients obtained an adequate seal with an 8.5-mm internal diameter tube with a cuff diameter of 26 mm. In female patients, the majority of airways were sealed with a 7.5-mm internal diameter tube with a cuff diameter of 20.5 mm. Intracuff pressures were less than 17 mm Hg.[48]

Unfortunately, cuff diameters are not uniform among all brands of endotracheal tubes. Using a tube with too small a

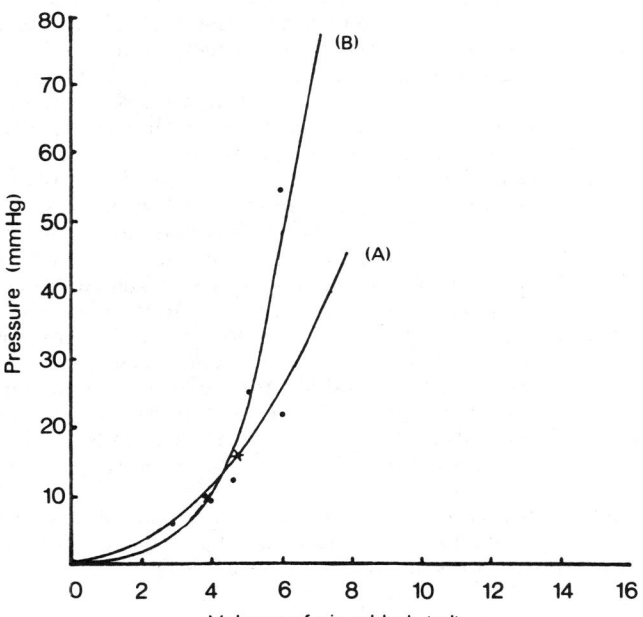

Figure 88–11. Change in intracuff pressure with overinflation. Curve A obtained in vivo; curve B, in rigid tube of same nominal tracheal diameter (20.2 mm). (From Chandler M, Crawley BE: Rationalization of the selection of endotracheal tubes. Br J Anaesth 58:111, 1986.)

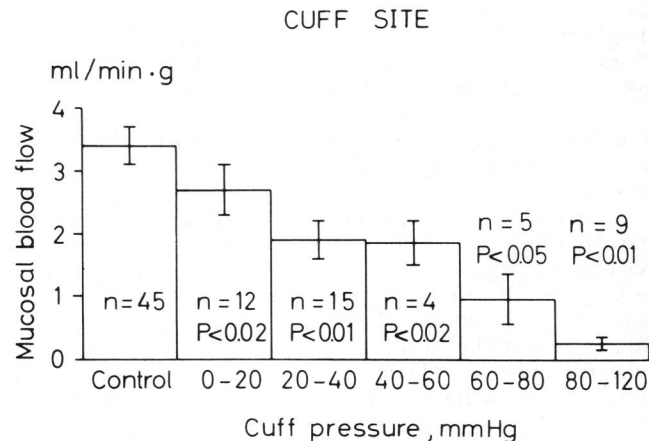

Figure 88–12. Decrease in mucosal perfusion with increasing intracuff pressure. (From Nordin U, Lindholm CE, Wolgast M: Blood flow in the rabbit tracheal mucosa under normal conditions and under the influence of tracheal intubation. Acta Otolaryngol Suppl 345:23, 1977.)

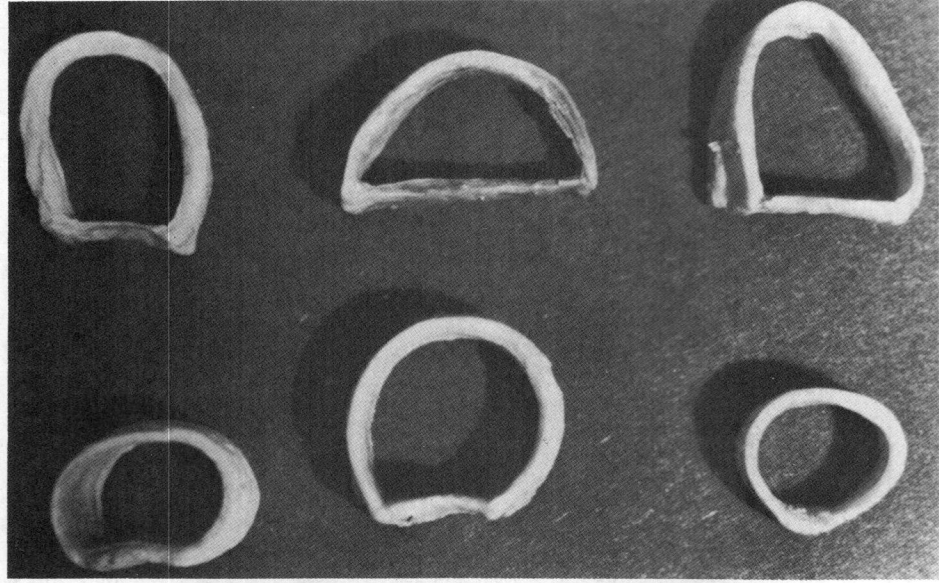

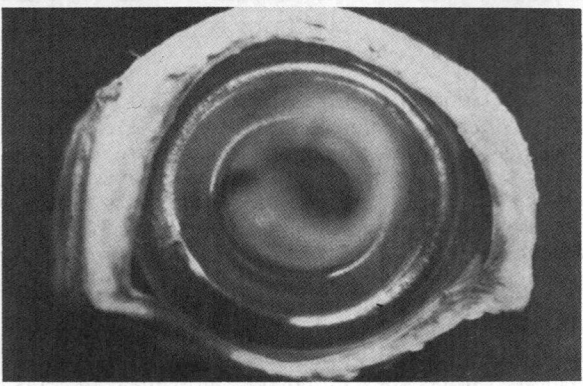

Figure 88–13. Failure of a round endotracheal cuff to seal a nonround trachea. (Adapted from Mackenzie CF: Compromises in the choice of endotracheal or nasotracheal intubation and tracheostomy. Heart Lung 12:485, 1983.)

cuff results in an inadequate seal at reasonable intracuff pressures or requires overdistention of the cuff, producing high intracuff pressures to seal the airway. Using a tube with too large a cuff results in the airway's being sealed before the cuff is fully inflated. Partial inflation of large-volume, low-pressure cuffs allows small folds to form in the wall of the cuff, which in turn allows aspiration of secretions to occur. Clinically, it is recognized that endotracheal tubes do not completely protect the airway from aspiration and that larger tubes may provide less protection than smaller tubes.[49] There is a significant decrease in the incidence of aspiration with the use of positive end-expiratory pressure.[50]

Because the tracheal mucosa is fragile enough to be injured by a weighted cotton swab, part of the injury induced by cuffs may be the result of shear force on the mucosa generated by the tube cuff with movement.[51] Nordin and others found that the mechanical shear forces developed by the contact of even an uninflated cuff on the tracheal mucosa result in damage.[25, 26, 52, 53] These findings reinforce the need to keep head motion to a minimum.

Overly large endotracheal tube cuffs may not be fully inflated when the airway is sealed, and the endotracheal tube may not be held in the center of the trachea. As a result, the tip of the tube may come in contact with the wall of the trachea and cause injury to the tracheal mucosa[25] (Fig. 88–14). The conclusion is that the cuff of the endotracheal tube should closely match the circumference of the trachea to avoid both underinflation and overdistention. However, movements of the endotracheal tube from patient activity may still result in injury to the mucosa.

The pulsatile increases in intracuff pressure with mechanical ventilation may also contribute to the tracheal dilatation occasionally seen in patients receiving mechanical ventilatory support, even when cuff pressures are acceptable. Tracheal dilatation has been found to be much more pronounced in animals that received positive pressure mechanical ventilation than spontaneously breathing animals.[54]

Acute tracheal injury may result in tracheal stenosis as fibrosis occurs with healing. Symptoms usually develop weeks to months after extubation.[53, 56] Patients may not be symptomatic until there has been a 75% reduction in the tracheal lumen.[57] The most common complaint is exertional dyspnea. Flow-volume loops and radiographs are used to evaluate upper airway obstruction but are not especially sensitive unless obstruction is severe. Other techniques such as computed tomographic scans and acoustic reflection techniques show promise in diagnosing tracheal stenosis. Stenoses at the cuff site are usually about 4 to 5 cm in length.[58] Surgical repair of tracheal lesions at the level of the cuff generally produces good results compared with that of glottic and subglottic injury.[56, 59–61] Overall, the incidence of tracheal injury from endotracheal intubation that requires surgical repair appears to be about 3%.[13]

Other Complications of Endotracheal Tubes

There is a high incidence of paranasal sinusitis related to the use of nasotracheal tubes.[36, 62–66] In patients intubated for longer than 5 days, up to 26% may have sinusitis necessitating antibiotics and removal of the tube.[63]

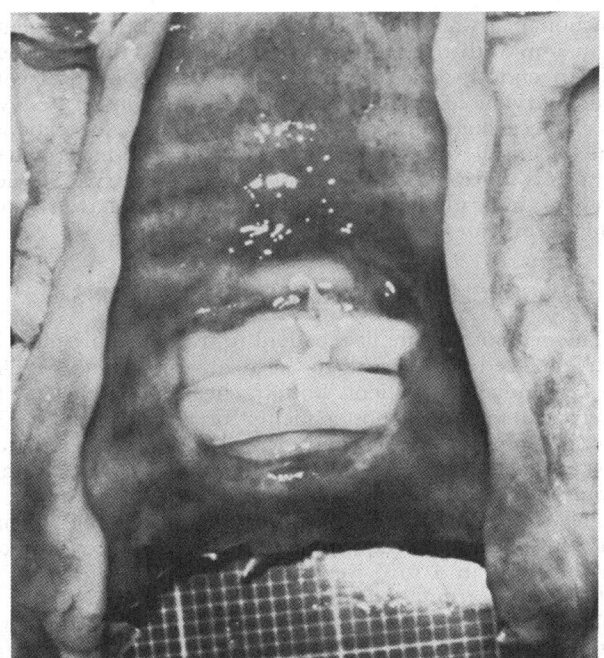

Figure 88–14. Cuff and tube tip injury to the tracheal wall. (From Whited RE: A study of endotracheal tube injury to the subglottis. Laryngoscope 95:1216, 1985.)

Sinusitis may not always be clinically apparent with purulent drainage and may be demonstrated only by computed tomographic scans.[64] Patients intubated by blind nasotracheal intubation as an emergency procedure experienced sinusitis more quickly than patients electively intubated in the operating room.[66] Sinusitis can lead to the development of septic retrograde thrombophlebitis in the intracranial sagittal sinus and life-threatening subdural empyema. The incidence of intracranial complications of sinusitis may be as high as 10%, with up to 30% mortality.[67] Other complications of nasal intubation include bleeding and nasal necrosis from prolonged intubation.[36] Given the frequent and potentially severe complications, nasal intubations should be avoided except under unusual circumstances.[64–66]

Tracheostomy

To determine the optimal timing of a tracheostomy entails balancing the relative risks and benefits of tracheostomies. The purported benefits of tracheostomies are comfort of the patient, including for speech and swallowing; more effective suctioning and oral hygiene; ease of replacement if accidental extubation occurs; and avoidance of injury to the glottis by by-passing the vocal cords.[35, 68, 69] The relative risks of tracheostomy include the risks associated with transport of critically ill patients to the operating room;[70, 71] intraoperative problems, such as bleeding and loss of airway control;[57, 72, 73] and postoperative problems, including infection, hemorrhage, tracheal stenosis and erosion into the innominate artery, and death.[46, 52, 74]

Stauffer and colleagues found a relatively high incidence of early complications with tracheostomy, including infection (36%), hemorrhage (36%), and cardiac arrest (4%).[9] The overall early complication rate was 66% for tracheostomies, with an average of 1.6 complications for each tracheostomy. Intraoperative technical problems were encountered in 10% of all the tracheostomies performed. The early complication rate for endotracheal intubation was 66% and included excessive cuff pressures (19%), self-extubation (13%), aspi-

ration (8%), and right mainstem intubation (2%). The conclusion was that the early complications of tracheostomy were more serious than those of endotracheal intubation.[9]

Other researchers found similarly high rates of both fatal and nonfatal complications of tracheostomy. Mortality rates from 0 to 7.9% were described.[75, 76] Fatal complications related to tracheostomy include infection, airway obstruction, hemorrhage, intraoperative cardiac arrest, and tension pneumothoraces.[77–79] Acute nonfatal complication rates range from 10 to 65%[57, 75] and include tracheitis and stomal infection, hemorrhage, pneumothorax, and tube obstruction or dislocation.[57, 75, 77–81] Emergency tracheostomies appear to have a higher complication rate compared with that for elective procedures.

Ulceration at the cuff site occurs in most patients with a tracheostomy. Healing of the stoma occurs by approximation of the incised cartilaginous rings, which can result in tracheal stenosis.[57] Asymptomatic tracheal stenosis can occur in up to 16% of such patients. Symptomatic stenosis causing airway impairment necessitated surgical correction in as many as 8% of the patients.

Patients with stenosis after tracheostomy usually have dyspnea, stridor, wheezing, or cough. Respiratory distress, difficulty with secretions, or cyanosis may also occur. Tracheoesophageal fistulas are relatively rare. The onset of symptoms may occur anytime from immediately after extubation to as long as 6 years after extubation.[55]

Large series of patients with tracheostomy showed that narrowing of the tracheal lumen of more than 50% occurred at rates between 5 and 25%. The rates of functional impairment ranged from 1.5 to 10%.[75] Functional impairment of the airway is thought to occur when the tracheal lumen approaches 5 mm in diameter[55] or when the lumen is reduced by 75% or more.[57]

A particularly catastrophic complication of tracheostomy is trachea–innominate artery erosion. The incidence of this complication has been reported to be between 0.02 and 1.3%.[82, 83] Trachea–innominate artery fistulas appear to be associated with operating under less than optimal conditions and placing a low tracheostomy stoma.[83] The mortality associated with erosion into the artery is approximately 50%, ranging from 23 to 94%. Erosion usually occurs within 4 weeks after the tracheostomy and may be heralded by minor tracheal bleeding and pulsation of the tracheal cannula. These findings are not present in the majority of cases, however, and the usual presentation is of massive bright red bleeding necessitating urgent surgical intervention.[26]

Persistent tracheal stomas and tracheomalacia occur in a small percentage of patients.[57] Persistent stomas were thought to be related to infection and steroid use that interferred with healing. Tracheomalacia usually occurred between the stoma and cuff sites from the loss of cartilaginous support. Injury to the cartilage may be the result of infection and/or pressure necrosis.[57]

Overall, it appears that the complications of tracheostomy, both acute and chronic, are more severe than those of endotracheal intubation.

Infectious Complications of Endotracheal and Tracheostomy Tubes

Colonization occurs in endotracheal tubes within 24 hours. Oropharyngeal secretions collect around the cuff of the endotracheal tube with resultant aspiration. With exhalation, secretions are blown into the endotracheal tube, where microorganisms adhere to the polyvinyl chloride tube material.[84] Colonization of the endotracheal tube presents an increased risk of nosocomial infection.[85] By comparison, colonization of tracheostomies occurs primarily at the stoma. The majority of organisms are aerobic gram-negative bacilli, although anaerobic organisms are found in 35% of cultures. These organisms are distinct from those found in the upper and lower airways.[86]

In burn patients, infections related to tracheostomies can be devastating. In a study from Shriner's Burn Institute, the incidence of pulmonary infections in patients with tracheostomies was 78% compared with 12.5% in patients who did not receive a tracheostomy.[87] In the patients with a tracheostomy and pulmonary sepsis, cultures of these areas and the burn wound had a 100% correlation. The majority of the organisms were gram-negative organisms.[86, 87] Mortality was 100% in the patients with pulmonary infection and a tracheostomy, whereas mortality was only 25% in patients with pulmonary sepsis but without a tracheostomy.[87]

Overall, intubation is associated with approximately a 1.5% incidence of nosocomial infection.[88] This represents a fourfold increase in risk of infection compared with that in patients who are not intubated and may account for 11% of hospital-associated pneumonia. Tracheostomies alone are associated with a 25% incidence of infection, which increased to 66% when patients received ventilation. This risk is minimal for patients undergoing ventilation for less than 24 hours but increases significantly after the fifth day of intubation.

Tracheostomy Versus Prolonged Endotracheal Intubation

Given the complications of tracheostomy, it has been suggested that prolonged endotracheal intubation for as long as 4 to 6 weeks may be less traumatic than tracheostomy.[59] However, there are some groups for whom early tracheostomy is beneficial. In patients with head injury with compromised neurologic function, aspiration from glottic dysfunction is common.[47] Patients with the poorest cognitive function can have a mortality rate of 24% from aspiration pneumonia when decannulated.[21] Therefore, even with the significant airway injuries that tracheostomies can cause, there is greater risk with an unprotected airway in patients with head injury with severe cognitive defects.[21, 47] These patients may be candidates for early tracheostomy. In contrast, burn patients, whose mortality is far greater with tracheostomy than with endotracheal intubation, would be better served by prolonged intubation.

With the exception of these two groups of patients, the question remains open as to when to consider tracheostomy for endotracheally intubated patients. The advantages of a tracheostomy (i.e., patient's comfort, ease of suctioning, and avoidance of laryngeal injury) have not been confirmed but continue to be proposed as justification for the procedure.

More than 90% of intensive care unit nurses in one survey believed that tracheostomies were superior to endotracheal intubation for the patient's comfort, the ease of handling secretion and suctioning, facilitation of communication, and the ease of mouth care.[81] The majority of nurses thought that tracheostomies were better tolerated psychologically.[81] The majority of the positive responses were from neurosurgical nurses, which may represent a bias with a select population of patients. The results of Stauffer and colleagues suggest that difficulty in suctioning with oral or nasal endotracheal tubes is uncommon, as was discomfort caused by endotracheal tubes.[9] Improved ability to communicate and the ability to swallow may warrant the consideration of a tracheostomy. A study indicates that nearly half of patients undergoing ventilation experienced anxiety or fear. The primary reason was the inability to communicate.[89]

Although a tracheostomy may decrease laryngeal injury by by-passing the vocal cords, airway injury can still occur. Cuff site injury is noted with both endotracheal tubes and tracheostomy tubes, but stomal lesions, which may result in functional airway impairment in about 10% of patients, occur only with tracheostomies.[75] Laryngeal injury attributable to endotracheal intubation may result in vocal cord injury, arytenoid cartilage damage, or subglottic stenosis, which necessitate surgical repair in 5 to 10% of patients. The technical difficulty of repair suggests that tracheal stenosis is more remediable than laryngeal injury.[68] Studies, however, indicate that laryngeal injury repairs have reasonable success rates.[52, 61, 90–92]

CONCLUSIONS AND RECOMMENDATIONS

The decision to submit a patient to tracheostomy must be individualized with regard to the relative risks and benefits for that individual patient. Endotracheal intubation may be safely maintained in most patients for up to 10 days. The development of acute laryngotracheal injury at this juncture does not correlate with permanent injury[14] and therefore should not be used as the sole justification for conversion to tracheostomy. Tracheostomy may be indicated for patients who are expected to require mechanical ventilatory support for longer than 4 to 6 weeks. Certain other categories of patients who are at risk may also be considered for early tracheostomy. Patients who experience stridor after extubation may require a tracheostomy until resolution of the laryngeal injury. Patients with severe neurologic injuries at risk for aspiration or those who require frequent pulmonary toilet may benefit from a tracheostomy.

Major benefits of tracheostomy for the long-term ventilator-bound patient are the ease with which the patient may be recannulated if an extubation occurs, the ease of clearing secretions from the inner cannula of the tracheostomy tube, and the facilitation of eating or communication in those patients who find oral intubation intolerable. Careful attention to utilization of appropriately sized tubes, 8.0- to 8.5-mm internal diameter in male patients and 7.0- to 7.5-mm internal diameter in females, minimizes the risk of injury as a result of tube size. In addition, preventing excessive head motion should reduce injury. If the risk of injury has been lessened (i.e., utilizing appropriate tube size and minimizing agitation and head movement) and the patient is making progress in weaning, it is reasonable to maintain the patient with an endotracheal tube for indefinite periods rather than subject the patient to a tracheostomy with its risk of complications.

References

1. Mackenzie CF, Hallesey MD, Clark D, et al: Adult tracheal and laryngeal dimensions as an indicator for correct tracheal tube use (abstract). Anesthesiology 57:A500, 1982.
2. Morris IR: Functional anatomy of the upper airway in airway management and anesthesia in the emergency department. Emerg Med Clin North Am 6:639, 1988.
3. Mehta S, Myat HM: The cross-sectional shape and circumference of the human trachea. Ann R Coll Surg Engl 66:356, 1984.
4. Mackenzie CF, McAslan TC, Shin B, et al: The shape of the human adult trachea. Anesthesiology 49:48, 1978.
5. Mackenzie CF, Shin B, Whitley N, et al: The relationship of human tracheal size to body habitus (abstract). Anesthesiology 51:S378, 1978.
6. Minuck M: Unilateral vocal-cord paralysis following endotracheal intubation. Anesthesiology 45:448, 1976.
7. Brandwein M, Abramson AL, Shikowitz MJ: Bilateral vocal cord paralysis following endotracheal intubation. Arch Otolaryngol Head Neck Surg 112:877, 1986.
8. Peppard SB, Dickens JH: Laryngeal injury following short term intubation. Ann Otol Rhinol Laryngol 92:327, 1983.
9. Stauffer JL, Olson DE, Petty TL: Complications and consequences of endotracheal intubation and tracheotomy. Am J Med 70:60, 1981.
10. Donnelly WA, Grossman AA, Grem FM: Local sequelae of endotracheal anesthesia. Anesthesiology 9:490, 1948.
11. Kambicm V, Radsel Z: Intubation lesions of the larynx. Br J Anaesth 50:587, 1978.
12. Snider GL: Historical perspective on mechanical ventilation: From simple life support system to ethical dilemma. Am Rev Respir Dis 140:S2, 1989.

13. Elliot CG, Rasmusson BY, Crapo RO: Upper airway obstruction following adult respiratory distress syndrome. Chest 94:526, 1988.
14. Colice GL, Stukel TA, Dain B: Laryngeal complications of prolonged intubation. Chest 96:877, 1989.
15. Pecora DV: Prolonged endotracheal intubation. Chest 82:130, 1982.
16. Gaynor EB, Greenberg SB: Untoward sequelae of prolonged intubation. Laryngoscope 95:1461, 1985.
17. El-Naggar M, Sadagopan S, Levine H, et al: Factors influencing choice between tracheostomy and prolonged translaryngeal intubation in acute respiratory failure: A prospective study. Anaesth Analg 55:195, 1976.
18. Kastanos N, Estopa Miró R, Agastí-Vidal A: Laryngotracheal injury due to endotracheal intubation. Incidence, evolution and predisposing factors. A prospective long-term study. Crit Care Med 11:362, 1983.
19. Watson CB: A survey of intubation practices in critical care medicine. Ear Nose Throat J 62:474, 1983.
20. Whited RE: A prospective study of laryngotracheal sequelae in long-term intubation. Laryngoscope 94:369, 1984.
21. Nowak P, Cohn AM, Guidice MA: Airway complications in patients with closed-head injuries. Am J Otolaryngol 8:91, 1987.
22. Dunham CM, LaMonica C: Prolonged tracheal intubation in the trauma patient. J Trauma 24:120, 1984.
23. Via-Reque E, Rattenborg C: Prolonged nasotracheal intubation. Crit Care Med 9:637, 1989.
24. Finfer SR, MacKenzie SIP, Saddler JM, et al: Cardiovascular responses to tracheal intubation: A comparison of direct laryngoscopy and fibreoptic intubation. Anaesth Intensive Care 17:44, 1989.
25. Whited RA: A study of endotracheal tube injury to the subglottis. Laryngoscope 95:1216, 1985.
26. Dubeck MN, Wright BD: Comparison of laryngeal pathology following long-term oral and nasal endotracheal intubations. Anesth Analg 75:663, 1978.
27. Conrardy PA, Goodman LR, Lainge F, et al: Alterations of endotracheal tube position. Crit Care Med 4:8, 1976.
28. Bernhard WN, Yost L, Joynes D, et al: Intracuff pressures in endotracheal and tracheostomy tubes. Chest 87:720, 1985.
29. Mathias DB, Wedley JR: The effects of cuffed endotracheal tubes on the tracheal wall. Br J Anesth 46:849, 1974.
30. Woo P, Kelly G, Kirshner P: Airway complications in the head injured. Laryngoscope 99:725, 1989.
31. Faryle DA, Good JT, Sahn SA: Emergency room intubation—Complications and survival. Chest 75:541, 1979.
32. Rashkin MC, Davis T: Acute complications of endotracheal intubation. Chest 89:165, 1986.
33. Zwillich CW, Presson DJ, Aeagh CE, et al: Complications of assisted ventilation. Am J Med 57:161, 1974.
34. Ripoli I, Lindholm CE, Carrol R, et al: Spontaneous dislocation of endotracheal tube position. Anesthesiology 49:50, 1978.
35. Mackenzie CF: Compromises in the choice of endotracheal or nasotracheal intubation and tracheostomy. Heart Lung 12:485, 1978.
36. Zwillich C, Pierson DJ: Nasal necrosis: A complication of nasotracheal intubation. Chest 64:376, 1973.
37. Fasota FJ, Hoffman LA, Zullo TG, et al: Evaluating two methods used to stabilize oral endotracheal tubes. Heart Lung 16:140, 1987.
38. Dobrin P, Canfield T: Cuffed endotracheal tubes: Mucosal pressures and tracheal wall blood flow. Am J Surg 133:562, 1977.
39. Leigh JM, Maynard JP: Pressure on the tracheal mucosa from cuffed tubes. Br Med J 1:1173, 1979.
40. Nordin U, Lindholm CE, Wolgast M: Blood flow in the rabbit tracheal mucosa under normal conditions and under the influence of tracheal intubation. Acta Otolaryngol Suppl 345:23, 1977.
41. Nordin U, Engstrom B, Lindholm CE: Surface structures of the tracheal wall after different durations of intubation. Acta Otolaryngol 215(suppl 345):59, 1977.
42. Seegobin RD, van Hasselt GL: Endotracheal cuff pressure and tracheal mucosal blood flow: Endoscopic study effects of four large volume cuffs. Br Med J 288:965, 1984.
43. Cooper JD, Grillo HC: The evolution of tracheal injury due to ventilatory assistance through cuffed tubes. Ann Surg 169:334, 1969.
44. Off D, Braun SR, Thompkins B, et al: Efficacy of the minimal leak technique of cuff inflation in maintaining proper intracuff pressures for patients with cuffed artificial airways. Respir Care 28:1115, 1983.
45. Bernhard WN, Cottrell JE, Suchumarar C, et al: Adjustment of intracuff pressure to prevent aspiration. Anesthesiology 50:363, 1979.
46. Seegobin RD, van Hasselt GL: Aspiration beyond endotracheal cuffs. Can Anaesth Soc J 33:273, 1986.
47. Plunkett PF, Ashavas-Penault S: The effect of tracheal shape on the pressure dynamics of severe commercially available endotracheal tube cuffs: An in vivo study. Respir Care 26:45, 1981.
48. Chandler M, Crawley BE: Rationalization of the selection of tracheal tubes. Br J Anaesth 58:111, 1986.
49. Pavlin EG, VanNimwegan D, Hornbein TF: Failure of a high-compliance low-pressure cuff to prevent aspiration. Anesthesiology 42:216, 1975.
50. Janson BA, Poulton TJ: Does PEEP reduce the incidence of aspiration around endotracheal tubes? Can Anaesth Soc J 33:157, 1986.
51. Holding AC: Laryngotracheal damage during intratracheal anesthesia. Ann Otol 80:565, 1971.
52. Nordin U, Engstrom B, Fansson B, et al: Surface structure and vascular anatomy of the tracheal wall under normal conditions and after intubation. Acta Otolaryngol 215(suppl 345):35, 1977.
53. Schmidt WA, Schaap RN, Mortensen JD: Immediate mucosal effects of short-term short-cuff, endotracheal intubation. Arch Pathol Lab Med 103:516, 1979.
54. King K, Mandava B, Kamen JM: Tracheal tube cuffs and tracheal dilatation. Chest 67:458, 1975.
55. Weber AL, Grillo HC: Tracheal stenosis: An analysis of 151 cases. Radiol Clin North Am 16:291, 1978.
56. Geffin B, Grillo HC, Cooper JD, et al: Stenosis following tracheostomy for respiratory care. JAMA 216:1984, 1971.
57. Dane TEB, King EG: A prospective study of complications after tracheostomy for assisted ventilation. Chest 67:398, 1975.
58. Hoffstein V, Zaml N: Tracheal stenosis measured by the acoustic reflection technique. Am Rev Respir Dis 130:472, 1984.
59. Brooks R, Bartlett RH, Gazzaniga AB: Management of acute and chronic disorders of the trachea and subglottis. Am J Surg 150:24, 1985.
60. Andrews MJ, Poarm FG: An analysis of 59 cases of tracheal lesions following tracheostomy with cuffed assisted ventilation with special reference to diagnosis and treatment. Br J Surg 60:208, 1973.
61. Hawkins DB: Glottic and subglottic stenosis from endotracheal intubation. Laryngoscope 86:329, 1976.
62. Grindlinger GA, Niehoff J, Hughes SL, et al: Acute paranasal sinusitis related to nasotracheal intubation of head injured patients. Crit Care Med 15:214, 1987.
63. O'Reilly MJ, Reddick E, Black W, et al: Sepsis from sinusitis in nasotracheally intubated patients. Am J Surg 147:601, 1984.
64. Kronberg FG, Goodwin WJ: Sinusitis and intensive care unit patients. Laryngoscope 95:936, 1985.
65. Meyer P, Guérin JM: Acute paranasal sinusitis and nasotracheal intubation. Crit Care Med 16:205, 1988.
66. Deutschman CS, Wilton P, Senia J, et al: Paranasal sinusitis associated with nasotracheal intubation: A frequently unrecognized and treatable source of sepsis. Crit Care Med 14:111, 1986.
67. Remmler D, Boles R: Intracranial complications of frontal sinusitis. Laryngoscope 90:1814, 1980.
68. Heffner JE: Medical indications for tracheostomy. Chest 96:186, 1989.
69. Marsh HM, Gillespie DJ, Baumgartner AE: Timing of tracheostomy in the critically ill patient. Chest 96:190, 1989.
70. Braman SS, Dunn SM, Armico CA, et al: Complications of intrahospital transport in critically ill patients. Ann Intern Med 197:469, 1987.
71. Gervais HW, Eberle B, Konietzke D, et al: Comparison of blood gases of ventilated patients during transport. Crit Care Med 15:761, 1987.
72. Duyal VS, El-Masri W: Tracheostomy in intensive care setting. Laryngoscope 96:58, 1986.
73. Freman L, Hedenstierna G, Schuldt B: Stenosis following tracheostomy. Anaesthesia 31:479, 1976.
74. Mackenzie CF, Shin B, Whitley IV, et al: Human tracheal circumference as an indication of correct cuff size. Anesthesiology 53:S414, 1980.
75. Lindholm CE: Survey of the literature concerning intubation and tracheostomy. Acta Anesth Scand 13:10, 1969.
76. Skaggs JA, Cogbill CL: Tracheostomy: Management, mortality, complications. Am Surg 35:393, 1969.
77. Rogers LA: Complications of tracheotomy. South Med J 62:1496, 1969.
78. Paloschi G, Lynn RB: Observation upon elective and emergency tracheostomy. Surg Gynecol Obstet 138:356, 1965.
79. Stemmer EA, Oliver C, Carey JP, et al: Fatal complications of tracheotomy. Am J Surg 131:288, 1976.
80. Toye FJ, Weinstein JD: Clinical experience with percutaneous tracheostomy and cricothyroidostomy in 100 patients. J Trauma 26:1034, 1986.
81. Astrachan DI, Kirchner JC, Goodwin WJ: Prolonged intubation vs tracheotomy: Complications, practical and psychological considerations. Laryngoscope 98:1165, 1988.
82. Aass AS: Complications of tracheostomy and long-term intubation: A follow-up study. Acta Anaesth Scand 19:127, 1975.
83. Jones JW, Reynolds M, Hewitt RL, et al: Tracheo-innominate artery erosion. Ann Surg 184:194, 1976.
84. Scottile FD, Marrie TJ, Prough DS, et al: Nosocomial pulmonary infection: Possible etiologic significance of bacterial adherence to endotracheal tubes. Crit Care Med 14:265, 1986.
85. Kerver AJH, Rommos JH, Mevissen-Verhage EAE, et al: Prevention of colonization and infection in critically ill patients: A prospective randomized study. Crit Care Med 16:1087, 1988.
86. Bartlett JG, Faling LJ, Willey S: Quantitative tracheal bacteriologic and cytologic studies in patients with long-term tracheostomies. Chest 74:635, 1978.
87. Eckhauser FE, Billote J, Burke JF, et al: Tracheostomy complicating massive burn injury. Am J Surg 127:418, 1974.
88. Cross AS, Roup B: Role of respiratory assistance devices in endemic nosocomial pneumonia. Am J Med 70:681, 1981.
89. Bergbon-Engberg I, Haljamae H: Assessment of patient's experience of discomforts during respiratory therapy. Crit Care Med 17:1068, 1989.
90. Grillo HC: Primary reconstructive of airway after resection of subglottic laryngeal and upper tracheal stenosis. Ann Thorac Surg 33:3, 1982.
91. Stell PM, Maron AGD, Stanley RE, et al: Chronic laryngeal stenosis. Ann Otol Rhinol Laryngol 94:108, 1985.
92. Smith RJH: Laryngotracheal Stenosis. Head Neck Surg 10:38, 1987.

The Cardiovascular System

Section Editor

Joshua Wynne

CHAPTER 89

Circulatory Shock

Mark E. Astiz
Eric C. Rackow
Max Harry Weil

Circulatory shock results from derangements of the cardiovascular system such that perfusion of systemic tissues is critically reduced. Eight principal components of the circulatory system that regulate systemic perfusion can be identified (Fig. 89–1). Derangements of any of these components can result in hemodynamic deterioration and circulatory failure. The first component is intravascular volume, which serves to modulate mean circulatory pressure and thereby venous return and ventricular filling.[1] Decreases in intravascular volume because of loss of red blood cells, plasma, or water decrease mean circulatory pressure and venous return. The heart is the second component. Cardiac output is determined by contractility, heart rate, and loading conditions.[2] Inotropic and chronotropic incompetence can result from structural abnormalities and circulating depressant substances. The third component is the resistance circuit defined primarily by the metarterioles, where 80% of the resistance drop across the systemic circuit occurs.[3] Changes in arteriolar tone determine ventricular loading conditions and the distribution of systemic blood flow. Excessive increases in arteriolar resistance increase impedance to left ventricular ejection and decrease microcirculatory flow. Other alterations in regional resistance may result in distributive abnormalities of systemic blood flow and mismatching of tissue blood supply with tissue metabolic requirements.[4, 5] The capillary exchange network is the fourth component. This circuit includes the largest fractional cross-sectional area of the vascular tree and is the site of nutrient exchange and fluid flux between the intravascular and extravascular compartments. Increases in capillary hydrostatic pressures or capillary permeability contribute to loss of intravascular

volume and edema formation, and increases in non-nutrient capillary flow compromise tissue nutrient exchange.[6, 7] The venular resistance vessels are the fifth component of the cardiovascular system. These vessels are responsible for 10 to 15% of the systemic resistance gradient. Excessive venular resistance increases capillary hydrostatic pressures, thereby increasing microvascular fluid flux and exacerbating intravascular fluid loss. Arteriovenous connections are the sixth component. These vascular pathways connect arterioles and venules. Opening of these channels can result in systemic and tissue hypoxia by bypassing the normal capillary exchange system.[8, 9] The venous capacitance is the seventh component and is made up of the medium-sized and large veins. In these vessels, 80% of the intravascular volume normally resides.[10] Increases in venous capacitance decrease effective circulating blood volume by decreasing venous return, and decreases in venous capacitance mobilize volume toward the central compartment, thereby increasing venous return.[11, 12] Finally, mainstream patency is the eighth component. Obstruction of mainstream blood flow in the pulmonary and systemic arterial beds can impede right and left ventricular ejection, and obstruction in the venous circuit limits venous return.

HEMODYNAMIC PARAMETERS

The hemodynamic parameters used to assess the integrity of the circulatory system include heart rate, arterial pressure, central venous pressure, pulmonary arterial wedge pressure, and cardiac output. Decreases in heart rate are indicative of chronotropic incompetence, which may be related to structural abnormalities or reflex-mediated responses as seen in severe, acute hypotension and acute inferior myocardial infarction.[13] Increases in heart rate may be indicative of underlying cardiac disease or, in the case of supraventricular tachycardia, may reflect compensatory mechanisms to maintain cardiac output and systemic perfusion.

Arterial hypotension is commonly used to identify the development of circulatory shock. Blood pressure is optimally monitored with proximal intra-arterial pressures. Vasoconstrictive influences, accentuated in hypodynamic circulatory failure, reduce the accuracy of noninvasive and peripheral measurements, resulting in falsely low values recorded for blood pressure.[14] The importance of arterial pressure is based on the relationship of mean arterial pres-

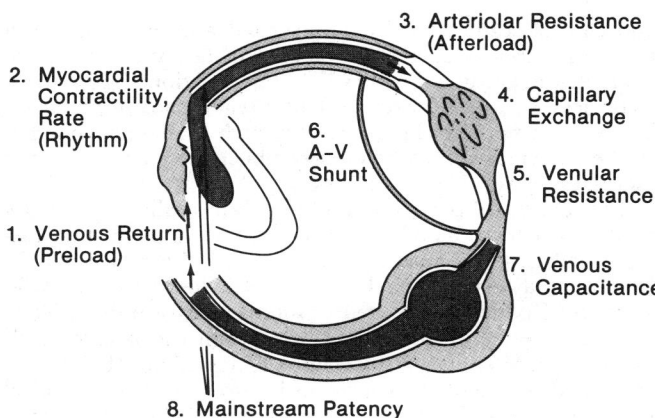

Figure 89–1. Functional components of the circulatory system of import in the regulation of systemic perfusion. (From Weil MH, von Planta M, Rackow EC: Acute circulatory failure [shock]. In: Braunwald E [ed]: Heart Disease: A Textbook of Cardiovascular Medicine. 4th ed. Philadelphia, WB Saunders, p 569, 1992.)

sure to organ perfusion.[15] Normally, organ blood flow is autoregulated within a range of mean arterial pressures between 60 and 120 mm Hg. As the mean arterial pressure decreases below the autoregulated range, blood flow becomes pressure dependent and tissue hypoperfusion ensues.[16]

Marked decreases in cardiac output and tissue blood flow may occur even within the normal range of arterial blood pressure. Potent vasoconstriction, mediated by sympathoadrenal reflexes, is activated in low-flow states to increase peripheral vascular resistance and maintain arterial pressure. These mechanisms redistribute systemic blood flow to more vital organs, creating critical regional hypoperfusion that may exist despite apparently normal levels of arterial pressure.[17, 18] Conversely, depending on regional vasodilatory mechanisms and cardiac output, organ perfusion may be maintained despite lower levels of arterial pressure. Thus, blood pressure is not a consistently good indicator of the adequacy of tissue perfusion.[19–22]

Central venous and pulmonary arterial wedge pressures are monitored as indirect indices of intravascular volume and ventricular preload. The correlation with blood volume is generally poor except at either extreme of the measurement.[23] The relationship between filling pressure and preload may be difficult to assess because of the influence of changes in ventricular compliance related to either underlying illness or therapeutic interventions such as positive end-expiratory pressure.[24] In ventricles with decreased compliance, elevated filling pressures may give a false impression of the adequacy of ventricular filling.

The relationship of cardiac output to loading conditions corrected for the influence of heart rate is used to assess ventricular ionotropic competence. The response of stroke volume to fluid infusion is extremely useful in separating the effects of inadequate preload from decreases in myocardial contractility.[25, 26] Noninvasive measurements of ejection fraction and calculation of systolic and diastolic volumes help better define loading conditions and ventricular contractility.[2] Although extremely low levels of cardiac output are associated with a poor prognosis in virtually all forms of shock, increased levels do not necessarily indicate an improved outcome, particularly in septic shock.[27] As with other flow measurements, cardiac output must ultimately be interpreted with regard to metabolic demands to assess adequacy of blood flow in meeting tissue metabolic requirements.

Systemic and pulmonary vascular resistance can be calculated from the ratio of arterial pressure to cardiac output. Excessive vasodilation is suggested by hypotension and decreased systemic vascular resistance. Increased levels indicate either compensatory mechanisms to maintain arterial pressure or pathologic increases in vascular tone. Venous tone cannot be specifically monitored. However, in the absence of ongoing volume loss, the administration of large amounts of fluid with only small changes in central venous or pulmonary wedge pressures suggests decreased venous tone and increased venous capacitance.[28]

PATHOPHYSIOLOGY OF SHOCK

Patients with circulatory shock usually present with acute hypoperfusion of tissues associated with a hypodynamic systemic circulation. Hypoperfusion is manifested by evidence of end-organ hypoperfusion, including changes in mental status; decreased urine output; cool, clammy extremities; and decreased peripheral pulses. In patients with shock associated with a hyperdynamic circulation, such as septic shock, the extremities may be warm because of peripheral vasodilation.

The development of circulatory shock is most often related to decreases in cardiac output. The hypodynamic form of shock initiates several physiologic responses directed at preserving cardiac output and arterial pressure. Heart rate increases in an attempt to maintain cardiac output. Neurohumorally mediated increases in arteriolar resistance maintain arterial pressure and redistribute blood flow away from less vital areas such as the skin and splanchnic bed to more vital tissues such as the brain and the heart.[17, 18] The same reflexes increase venous tone, thereby initially augmenting central blood volume and venous return.[11] Activation of the renin-angiotensin system and increased vasopressin release enhance renal conservation of salt and water and augment arteriolar tone.

With progressive shock these mechanisms ultimately fail. Prolonged venular and arteriolar vasoconstriction promotes the egress and loss of intravascular volume. Ongoing hypotension may produce myocardial ischemia and dysfunction. Further increases in peripheral resistance compromise cardiac output by increasing ventricular afterload.[29] Progressive ischemia and acidosis decrease arteriolar tone, producing terminal arteriolar vasodilation, further compromising microvascular integrity, and increasing intravascular fluid loss.[30] In experimental hemorrhagic shock, an irreversible stage is reached at which resuscitation cannot be achieved.[31] The clinical applicability of this concept and the mechanisms responsible for irreversibility are unclear.

In some patients, primarily those with septic shock, the development of shock is characterized by systemic vasodilation and increases in cardiac output. The progression of shock is associated with profound vasodilation refractory to endogenous or exogenous vasopressors.[20, 32] These patients are characterized by a hyperdynamic circulatory state in which, despite marked increases in cardiac output, there is maldistribution of blood flow and arterial pressure falls because of progressive loss of vascular tone. The development of a hypodynamic circulation occurs as a terminal process in these patients.

OXYGEN METABOLISM

Oxygen is the most important substrate transported by the circulatory system. Circulatory shock represents an imbalance between tissue oxygen requirements for metabolic activity and tissue oxygen delivery. A fundamental feature of fatal progression of circulatory shock is a decline in

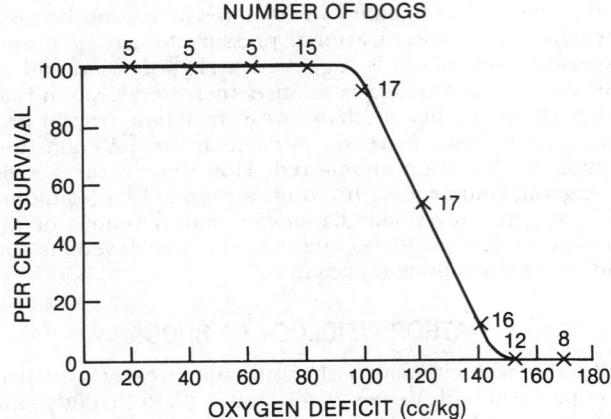

Figure 89–2. The relationship between oxygen deficit and survival during experimental shock produced by hemorrhage. (From Crowell JW, Smith EE: Oxygen deficit and irreversible hemorrhagic shock. Am J Physiol 206:313, 1964.)

systemic oxygen consumption. Experimentally, the severity of the shock is directly related to the severity of the oxygen debt. Irreversibility of shock and mortality are determined by cumulative systemic oxygen debt (Fig. 89–2).[33] In most cases, the primary deficit is inadequate oxygen delivery as a result of decreases in cardiac output and/or oxygen saturation and hemoglobin. A primary hypermetabolic syndrome with markedly increased oxygen requirements complicates some forms of shock, as in patients with trauma, sepsis, and burns.[34] Under normal conditions, systemic oxygen consumption is maintained independently of oxygen delivery through changes in oxygen extraction.[35] The normal oxygen extraction ratio is 25%, and this can increase up to 75 to 80% under conditions of marked decreases in tissue blood flow. As critical levels of oxygen delivery are reached, oxygen extraction is maximized and levels of capillary oxygen tension are reached below which there is an inadequate gradient for the diffusion of oxygen from the capillaries to the tissues. At this point, oxygen consumption falls and a linear relationship between oxygen delivery and oxygen consumption is observed.[35, 36] Anaerobic metabolism ensues, and pyruvic acid is diverted away from the citric acid cycle and lactic acid is produced.[37] Anaerobic glycolysis results in a decrease in high-energy phosphates.[38, 39] Only 2 mol of ATP is produced per mole of glucose metabolized anaerobically, compared with 38 mol of ATP when glucose is metabolized aerobically. Thus, lactic acidosis and the development of a linear relationship between oxygen consumption and oxygen delivery serve as markers of critical hypoperfusion and tissue energy deficit.[40]

Lactic acidosis may also be observed clinically despite less than maximal oxygen extraction. This pattern is characteristic of septic shock, but it may be observed in other clinical settings as well.[41] Several mechanisms have been postulated to account for these observations, including primary metabolic injury, shifts in the oxygen dissociation curve, and distributive abnormalities of systemic or microcirculatory blood flow leading to regional imbalances in oxygen supply and demand.[42] The observation that flow-dependent oxygen consumption characterizes these patients is most consistent with primarily distributive abnormalities of blood flow that do not preclude oxygen utilization.[40, 43, 44]

Assessment of blood lactate concentration is a useful method of assessing systemic perfusion.[45, 46] Addition of pyruvate and determination of the lactate/pyruvate ratio do not enhance the value of this measurement.[45] Experimental

and clinical studies have demonstrated a clear relationship between increases in arterial blood lactate level and critical decreases in oxygen delivery.[37, 47] The relationship between lactic acidosis and flow-dependent oxygen consumption has been confirmed in clinical studies.[40, 43, 44] In experimental studies, decreases in high-energy phosphates coincide with increases in tissue lactic acid levels.[38, 39]

The severity of perfusion failure and mortality are directly related to arterial blood lactate levels, with mortality increasing as lactate concentration exceeds 2 mM/L[45, 46] (Fig. 89–3). When the arterial blood lactate level is less than 2 mM/L, survival of patients admitted to intensive care units is likely to be greater than 90%. However, when the lactate levels exceed 8 mM/L, survival declines to less than 10%.[46] The rate of clearance of lactic acidosis is also a marker of clinical improvement and response to therapy. Failure of arterial lactate levels to decrease after a therapeutic intervention or further increases are ominous and prognosticate a poor outcome.[48] Under conditions of normal perfusion, such as after a seizure or exercise, lactic acid is rapidly cleared with a half-life of approximately 60 minutes.[49] During recovery from circulatory shock, clearance is frequently prolonged and the half-life is approximately 24 hours.[48] Hepatic failure, although increasing clearance time, does not appear to affect the clinical correlation between lactic acidosis and hypoperfusion.[50]

METABOLIC CHANGES

The onset of circulatory shock is associated with a myriad of hormonal changes that are directed at the preservation of organ perfusion and metabolic function.[51] The sympathoadrenal system is activated and there are marked increases in catecholamine levels, which have several effects including augmentation of cardiac function, vasoconstriction, increase in metabolic rate, and stimulation of glycogenolysis and lipolysis.[52, 53] Vasopressin release is increased and the renin-angiotensin system is also activated.[54, 55] These hormonal changes augment vascular tone and stimulate salt and water retention, thereby protecting plasma volume. Peripheral conversion of thyroxine to triiodothyronine is significantly impaired, resulting in decreased triiodothyro-

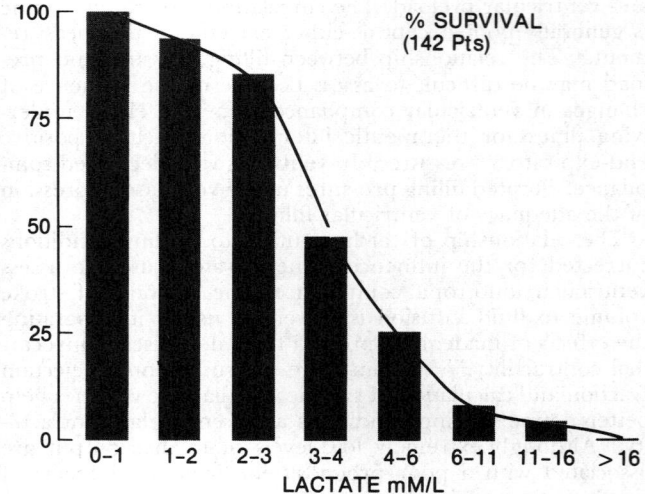

Figure 89–3. Relationship between concentrations of arterial blood lactate and survival in clinical shock states. (From Weil MH, Shubin H: Metabolic consequences of cardiogenic shock. In: Meltzer LE, Dunning AJ [eds]: Textbook of Coronary Care. Amsterdam, Excerpta Medica, p 634, 1972.)

nine levels and the formation of an inactive metabolite (reverse triiodothyronine).[56, 57] Glucagon and cortisol secretions are also increased significantly. Coupled with the influence of different cytokines, they stimulate peripheral protein breakdown and promote hepatic gluconeogenesis.[58–60] Insulin levels are usually decreased, reflecting the suppression of pancreatic insulin release by catecholamines.[58, 61]

Hyperglycemia is frequently observed because of enhanced gluconeogenesis, glycogenolysis, and insulin resistance.[58, 61] Fatty acid and total serum lipid levels are usually decreased despite elevated catecholamine levels that predispose to lipolysis.[62] This is presumably due to the decreased perfusion of adipose tissues. Glucose becomes the major metabolite as anaerobic metabolism begins. Fatty acid oxidation decreases and protein is increasingly used as an energy source. Proteolysis results in increases in total serum amino acids and urea concentration. Ongoing shock produces depletion of tissue high phosphate levels with eventual release of breakdown products of purine metabolism.[63, 64]

MEDIATORS

Various substances are released that mediate the circulatory and metabolic changes seen during shock. Activation of some of these mediators occurs as part of the stress response, and other substances are released when tissue hypoxia occurs. Exogenous factors such as allergens and infectious agents activate cellular, hormonal, and plasma cascades, which in turn activate multiple mediator systems. Factors such as traumatic injury and inflammatory lesions such as pancreatitis and burns are capable of activating the same mediator pathways. Among the important mediators activated during circulatory shock are the neuroendocrine system, complement, the clotting cascade, and arachidonic acid metabolites. Activation of macrophages, neutrophils, and platelets with the release of cytokines, enzymes, and other vasoactive substances is also important.

Derivatives of membrane phospholipids are important mediators of shock.[65, 66] Activation of phospholipase A_2 releases arachidonic acid from membrane phospholipids. Prostaglandins and thromboxane are produced through the cyclooxygenase pathway and leukotrienes and lipoxins through the lipoxygenase pathways. Platelet-activating factor, another phospholipid derivative, may have a regulatory role in eicosanoid synthesis.[67] These substances variably affect smooth muscle tone, are capable of activating platelets and leukocytes, and can increase microvascular permeability. Inhibitors of platelet-activating factor, prostaglandins, leukotrienes, and thromboxane have been demonstrated to increase survival in experimental models of anaphylactic, septic, and hemorrhagic shock.[65, 66]

Increases in β-endorphins, endogenous opiates, have been reported in hemorrhagic and septic shock.[68] These substances may contribute to hypotension through their vasodilatory activity. Naloxone, an opiate antagonist, increases cardiac output and arterial pressure in hemorrhagic and septic shock.[69] This activity appears to be mediated through a sympathomimetic effect because both sympathectomy and adrenal medullectomy abolish the pressor response to naloxone.[68]

Bacterial toxins are major mediators of septic shock.[70, 71] Their biologic activity is manifested through the activation of a variety of cellular, plasma, and humoral mediator systems. Endotoxin, a lipopolysaccharide component of the outer membrane of gram-negative bacterial cell walls, is postulated to be a major mediator of gram-negative septic shock.[71] Other virulence factors produced by gram-negative organisms include exotoxins and proteases.[72] Gram-positive organisms contain peptidoglycans, exotoxins, polysaccha-

rides, and other substances that mediate systemic and local responses to the organisms.[70, 73, 74]

Cytokines derived from macrophages and other cells are the principal mediators released by the action of bacterial toxins.[71, 75–77] Tumor necrosis factor, interleukin-6, and interleukin-1 have been implicated in the pathogenesis of septic shock. They appear to modulate the hemodynamic, metabolic, and neurohormonal changes that are observed during sepsis. Increased levels of tumor necrosis factor and interleukins have been correlated with mortality resulting from septic shock.[78, 79] The activity of these substances appears in part to be mediated through prostaglandins and the subsequent activation of a wide range of mediator systems.[80] Cytokines may also directly affect organ function, as evidenced by the myocardial depression associated with tumor necrosis factor.[81]

Immune mechanisms are also important in anaphylactic shock. During anaphylaxis, antigen combines with receptor-bound immunoglobulin E, leading to activation of mast cells and basophils, which in turn release a wide range of primary mediators.[82–84] Histamine, leukotrienes, platelet-activating factor, and prostaglandins are all among the mediators that produce the increased microvascular permeability, bronchoconstriction, and hypotension that occur during anaphylactic shock.[84]

Several other plasma cascades are activated during shock and may contribute to organ injury. Activation of the complement system releases C3a and C5a, which cause hypotension, increase microvascular permeability, and activate neutrophils with the subsequent release of oxygen radicals and proteolytic enzymes.[66, 85–87] Disseminated intravascular coagulation may result from activation of the clotting system through either the intrinsic or the extrinsic pathway.[88, 89] Deposition of fibrin and development of microthrombosis can result in organ injury. Kinins are also generated from precursor molecules, by plasma and tissue kallikreins.[90, 91] Bradykinin is the predominant vasoactive peptide, and it produces vasodilation and increased microvascular permeability.

Substances released from endothelial cells may also modulate vascular tone during circulatory shock. Endothelin, a potent vasoconstrictor, is synthesized and secreted by endothelial cells.[92] Increased levels have been reported during cardiogenic shock and in response to endotoxin.[92, 93] Endothelium-derived relaxing factor, nitric oxide, is a potent vasodilator and may have a role in cytokine-induced hypotension.[94, 95]

CELLULAR FUNCTION

Hypoperfusion and ischemia initiate a sequence of events resulting in cellular dysfunction and death.[96, 97] The initial insult occurs at the cell membrane, where the transmembrane potential decreases because of failure of the proton pump.[98, 99] As a result, cell swelling occurs and water and sodium are accumulated intracellularly with loss of intracellular potassium and magnesium. Activation of Na^+,K^+-ATPase depletes ATP, stimulating the mitochondria. Cyclic AMP levels decrease as anaerobic conditions limit high-energy phosphate production. Calcium regulation is impaired and intracellular accumulation occurs.[93] Cells begin to swell with initial enlargement of the endoplasmic reticulum. Blebs appear at the cell surfaces because of changes in microfilament and microtubule function. As cellular injury worsens, mitochondrial dysfunction and uncoupling occur, further depressing electron transport.[100] The mitochondria condense with increased separation between the inner and outer membranes. Swelling of the mitochondria marks the transition to irreversible cellular injury. Dense aggregates representing denatured proteins appear in the mitochondria and cytoplasm, and dissolution of chromatin is observed. Lysosomal breakdown and calcium precipitation occur. Terminal fracture of the plasma membrane, mitochondria, endoplasmic reticulum, and nuclear envelope is observed.

ORGAN FUNCTION

Cardiac dysfunction is commonly observed in all forms of shock. In the setting of acute myocardial infarction, coronary hypoperfusion, cardiac ischemia, and myocardial injury are primary determinants of cardiac dysfunction.[101] The extent of total myocardial injury correlates directly with the development of shock during acute myocardial infarction, with the loss of 40% or more of myocardial mass producing cardiogenic shock.[102]

The role of coronary hypoperfusion in mediating cardiac dysfunction is less secure in other forms of shock.[103] Myocardial depressant substances appear to be important factors contributing to cardiac function in septic shock and possibly hemorrhagic shock.[104-106] Several different substances that can adversely affect cardiac function have been isolated in clinical and experimental studies. A direct correlation between the concentration of some of these substances and clinical myocardial depression has been observed in septic shock.[101] Other mediators, including tumor necrosis factor and endorphins, have potential myocardial depressant effects.[81] Decreased cardiac responsiveness to exogenous and endogenous catecholamines may also contribute to cardiac systolic dysfunction during circulatory shock. Markedly elevated levels of circulating catecholamines can produce adrenergic receptor down-regulation. Indeed, in congestive heart failure and septic shock the ionotropic effect of beta-adrenergic stimulation is depressed in parallel with decreased catecholamine-responsive adenylate cyclase activity and reduced beta-adrenergic receptor density.[107, 108] Diastolic function is also altered in septic and cardiogenic shock.[109-111] Decreased compliance and ventricular relaxation are observed early, with eventual evolution to a dilated cardiomyopathy.[112] In cardiogenic shock, these changes result from ischemia and tissue injury. The factors contributing to decreased compliance in septic shock are unclear.

Increases in minute ventilation with associated increased work of breathing and the development of respiratory muscle fatigue frequently complicate circulatory shock.[113] A significant metabolic burden may be placed on the patient as the oxygen demands of the respiratory muscles increase.[114] Hypoperfusion of the respiratory muscles may exacerbate this problem and contribute to respiratory muscle dysfunction and ventilatory failure. Respiratory muscle dysfunction related to disease states such as sepsis may further compromise ventilatory function.[115]

Noncardiogenic and cardiogenic pulmonary edema may compromise tissue oxygenation during circulatory shock by producing intrapulmonary shunting and arterial hypoxemia. The development of these complications significantly increases mortality resulting from shock.[116, 117] Hydrostatic pulmonary edema is observed primarily with cardiac failure and after excessive fluid infusion. Decreases in colloid osmotic pressure during crystalloid resuscitation may also contribute to pulmonary edema.[118] The lung injury of adult respiratory distress syndrome is produced by activated mediator systems affecting the alveolar capillary membrane and pulmonary vascular response. Adult respiratory distress syndrome is a frequent complication of traumatic and septic shock; it is usually observed within 24 hours after resuscitation, and virtually all cases occur within 72 hours.[117, 119]

Decreases in glomerular filtration result primarily from renal hypoperfusion during shock.[120] As cardiac output falls, the renal fraction of cardiac output falls and renal blood flow decreases. Increases in tone of efferent arterioles initially maintain glomerular filtration. Ultimately, this mechanism fails and renal insufficiency occurs.[121] Increases in renal vascular resistance during vasopressor infusion may exacerbate the decrease in renal blood flow, further compromising renal function.[120] Elevated left atrial pressures during cardiogenic shock may protect renal blood flow through increased release of atrial natriuretic hormone and activation of vasodilatory reflexes.[122] During septic shock, intrarenal shunting may also contribute to decreases in renal function.[123] Intraluminal tubular obstruction, alterations in the filtration coefficient, vasoconstriction, and tubular back leak are mechanisms that contribute to the development of acute tubular necrosis during circulatory shock.[121] Other factors, such as rhabdomyolysis, nephrotoxic drug administration, and contrast infusion, further increase the risk of renal failure in critically ill patients. Decreases in free water clearance are a useful marker of incipient renal insufficiency during circulatory shock.[124, 125]

The liver is the major metabolic organ of the body and is the site of nearly 90% of the body's reticuloendothelial cell mass. During circulatory shock, hepatic hypoperfusion and congestion impair hepatic metabolic activity and phagocytic clearance by the hepatic reticuloendothelial system.[126, 127] Activation of Kupffer's cells with subsequent cytokine release may also contribute to hepatic injury.[128] Modest increases in levels of transaminases, bilirubin, and alkaline phosphatase characterize ischemic injury, and more dramatic increases in transaminase levels occur in severe cases of hypoxic liver injury (i.e., shock liver).[129, 130] These changes are usually transient and not clinically significant if perfusion is restored to normal levels. Pathologically, centrilobular necrosis, central venous and sinusoidal congestion, cholestasis, and edema are features of ischemic liver injury.[130]

Gastrointestinal hypoperfusion during circulatory shock can be the source of significant complications. Intestinal ischemia compromises the integrity of the intestinal mucosal barrier, promoting translocation of bacteria and endotoxin across the mucosa wall into the systemic circulation.[131, 132] In cases of severe ischemia, hemorrhagic ulcerations and necrotic bowel may be observed.[133] Hypoperfusion of the gastrointestinal tract and mediator release predispose to stress ulceration of the stomach and hemorrhage.[134, 135] Biliary ischemia is postulated to be a factor in the development of acalculous cholecystitis.[136] Pancreatitis associated with hypoperfusion is relatively uncommon but may be seen in cases of prolonged ischemia and circulatory failure.[137] The pancreas may also be a source of myocardial depressant factor, which impairs cardiac performance during circulatory shock.[138]

Microcirculatory and rheologic abnormalities contribute to hypoperfusion during circulatory shock. The normal hyperemic response to ischemia is attenuated, suggesting impaired microvascular reserve.[139, 140] Reduced microvascular flow results from decreased cardiac output and vasoconstrictive influences. Decreased capillary flow and changes in red blood cell deformability predispose to red blood cell aggregation and increased blood viscosity.[141] Aggregation of activated white blood cells and platelets produces intravascular clumping and further compromises capillary blood flow. Impaired reticuloendothelial clearance of particulate matter potentiates these processes.[142] Tissue edema may also impede tissue oxygenation by increasing intercapillary distances and thereby limiting the diffusion of oxygen into cells.[143, 144]

Coagulation abnormalities are frequently observed during circulatory shock. They may reflect underlying illnesses, the effect of medications, and hemodilution. The development of disseminated intravascular coagulation is a serious complication of shock.[145, 146] The coagulation process can be activated by tissue factors, endothelial cell injury, and external factors such as endotoxin. The resulting microthrombosis and fibrin deposition may impair organ blood flow and potentiate organ injury, although this issue is controversial.[146] Typical laboratory findings include a microangiopathic hemolytic anemia, prolongation of the prothrombin time and partial thromboplastin time, decreased platelet count and fibrinogen concentration, and increased concentration of fibrin monomers and split products. Therapy is directed at reversing the underlying process.

Changes in mental status are frequently observed in patients with circulatory shock and have been correlated with poor outcome in some forms of shock.[147] Blood flow is preferentially redirected to the brain and heart in low-flow states. However, as the mean systemic arterial pressure decreases below 60 mm Hg, cerebral hypoperfusion ensues, with ischemic injury developing in arterial border zones of the cerebral cortex.[148, 149] The development of respiratory alkalosis with associated hypercapnia and cerebral vasoconstriction may exacerbate this process.[149] Coexistent metabolic alterations such as hypoxemia, acidosis, and electrolyte abnormalities may also impair cerebral function. Other metabolic disturbances, such as the abnormalities of amino acid metabolism that are observed in patients with septic shock, may also contribute to the development of an encephalopathy.[150]

CLINICAL CLASSIFICATION OF SHOCK

Clinical shock can be categorized into four primary circulatory defects (Table 89–1).[151] The first three categories, which are characterized by decreased cardiac output and tissue blood flow, represent hypodynamic forms of shock. Hypovolemia is the most common cause of circulatory failure and results from a critical reduction in intravascular blood volume. This may be clinically apparent as in hemorrhage or excessive gastrointestinal losses or may be more occult with third spacing of intravascular volume as in acute pulmonary edema or intra-abdominal sepsis. Cardiogenic shock is produced by cardiac inotropic and/or chronotropic incompetence and can represent the initial and sole abnormality as in acute myocardial infarction or an evolutionary process as in septic shock. Obstructive shock is produced by obstruction of one of the critical conduits of the circulatory bed. Pulmonary embolism, vena caval obstruction, aortic aneurysm, and cardiac tamponade are all examples of obstructive shock.

The distributive form of circulatory shock is the fourth category and is characterized by maldistribution of blood flow and/or blood volume. This type of shock is best exemplified by patients with sepsis. Cardiac output is usually increased early in the course of sepsis and septic shock, but maldistribution of blood flow with vasodilation of systemic vascular beds leads to inadequate tissue perfusion despite the hyperdynamic circulatory state. Alterations in vascular tone may decrease effective circulating blood volume in this form of shock, resulting in venous pooling and decreased venous return. Under these circumstances, cardiac output is decreased and the patient has a hypodynamic circulatory state. Arteriovenous shunting and systemic or microcirculatory disturbances in the distribution of blood flow reduce tissue nutrient flow. Septic shock, spinal shock, and narcotic overdose are examples of clinical syndromes involving distributive forms of circulatory shock.

INITIAL THERAPY

In approaching the patient with circulatory shock, the most immediate priority is establishing cardiopulmonary stability. Simultaneously, possible etiologies for the development of shock are assessed. The ventilation-infusion-pump (VIP) approach is one which we have found to be useful in initially stabilizing the patient.[152] The "V" refers to ventilation and oxygenation. Patients with shock should all be initially treated with high-flow oxygen systems at high fractions of inspired oxygen (i.e., 50% or greater) to optimize arterial oxygen saturation and therefore oxygen delivery. This requires the use of a mask system with a flow rate in excess of the patient's minute ventilation. Because minute ventilation is frequently increased in shock, gas flow rates in the range of 20 to 40 L/min should be utilized.[153] Nasal prongs or low-flow systems do not provide adequate rates of gas flow to ensure that a high fraction of inspired oxygen is being delivered.

The decision to use endotracheal intubation involves several issues. In obtunded patients, independent of gas exchange abnormalities, endotracheal intubation should be rapidly completed to ensure airway control. The degree of respiratory work and the anticipated likelihood of rapid reversal of the patient's clinical status are the next concern. Increased respiratory rates, greater than 30 breaths/min, when coupled with evidence of accessory muscle use and paradoxical abdominal movements, are indicative of markedly increased respiratory work and impending ventilatory failure.[154] When associated with clinical conditions that are not promptly reversible, they indicate the need for endotracheal intubation. From a physiologic perspective, these clinical signs are evidence of increased respiratory muscle metabolic and oxygen requirements. Accordingly, a possible benefit of intubation in this setting is a decrease in respiratory work and overall systemic oxygen consumption with subsequent redistribution of systemic blood flow away from respiratory muscles to other hypoperfused areas of the body.[155] Persistent respiratory acidosis is also indicative of ventilatory failure and the need for ventilatory support. Finally, the development of severe hypoxia with a PaO$_2$ less than 50 to 60 mm Hg and a fraction of inspired oxygen greater than 50 to 60% should be an indication for intubation.

The potential complications of intubation in the patient with shock should be anticipated.[156] If sedation is required, hypotension may be profoundly worsened by both the direct vasodilatory effect of the agents utilized and the decrease in endogenous catecholamines that occurs with sedation.[157] Therefore, if possible, intubation should be done with the use of minimal sedation or, if necessary, with short-acting reversible agents in patients with circulatory shock.

The second important complication of ventilatory support

TABLE 89–1

CLASSIFICATION OF SHOCK

Type	Defect	Examples
Hypovolemic	Decreased intravascular volume	Hemorrhage Dehydration
Cardiogenic	Decreased cardiac function	Acute myocardial infarction Cardiomyopathy
Obstructive	Intravascular obstruction	Pulmonary embolism Superior vena cava syndrome
Distributive	Maldistribution of blood flow and/or blood volume	Septic shock Spinal shock

is the effect of increased intrathoracic pressure on venous return. This is especially an issue in hypovolemic patients with circulatory shock, who are sensitive to increases in intrathoracic pressure and further decreases in venous return.[158, 159] The placement of large-bore intravascular catheters for fluid administration and prior infusion of fluid can mitigate this complication. The early use of positive end-expiratory pressure exacerbates this tendency.[160] Accordingly, positive end-expiratory pressure should be introduced judiciously after restoring intravascular volume and achieving a degree of circulatory stability.

The "I" refers to infusion. Overwhelmingly, patients with circulatory shock have evidence of significant volume deficits. This is even true of approximately one third of the patients with myocardial infarction complicated by hypoperfusion.[161] Fluid infusion is optimally guided by measurement of ventricular filling. Because of the high incidence of impaired cardiac performance and pulmonary pathology in patients with shock, pulmonary arterial occlusive (wedge) pressure should be utilized to guide fluid infusion.[162, 163]

During a fluid challenge for volume repletion during shock, significant aliquots should be infused. We have found a standardized fluid challenge protocol to be helpful (Table 89–2).[164] An aliquot of 200 mL of 5% colloid solution or 600 mL of physiologic salt solution is infused for a period of 10 minutes. The pulmonary arterial diastolic pressure or pulmonary arterial wedge pressure is monitored, and if the change is less than 3 mm Hg the fluid infusion is continued. If wedge pressure increases by more than 7 mm Hg, the fluid challenge is discontinued because significant left ventricular dysfunction, either systolic or diastolic, is present and other pharmacologic or mechanical interventions are necessary to improve cardiac performance. If the increment in wedge pressure is between 3 and 7 mm Hg, the fluid infusion should be stopped for 10 minutes and restarted if the pressure recedes to within 3 mm Hg of the previous measurement. When measurement of filling pressure of the left side of the heart is not immediately available, the fluid challenges can be guided by central venous pressure assessment using end points of 2 and 5 mm Hg. Alternatively, clinical end points of arterial pressure, heart rate, and urine output may also be used, while taking care to assess the patient for possible fluid overload.

Fluid infusion is optimized when a level of filling pressure is reached that is associated with the maximal increase in cardiac output. This level varies between patients, depending on the underlying pathologic alteration that affects myocardial performance. In patients with marked decreases in ventricular compliance, as after acute myocardial infarction, the optimal level of wedge pressure ranges between 15 and 20 mm Hg, whereas in patients with septic shock levels of 10 to 15 mm Hg are reported.[162, 165] In either case, the delineation of optimal filling pressure should be individualized by judging the changes in wedge pressure and cardiac output during fluid infusion. Excessive fluid administration beyond optimal fluid pressures accrues no benefit in cardiac output and may compromise oxygen delivery by producing pulmonary edema and arterial oxygen desaturation. In addition, some reports suggest that excessive increases in filling pressure may significantly increase ventricular wall tension, producing myocardial ischemia and ventricular dysfunction.[166]

Most fluid resuscitation is initiated with asanguineous fluids. Either isotonic crystalloid or iso-oncotic colloid solutions should be utilized for expansion of the intravascular volume.[167] The volume of distribution of iso-oncotic fluids is primarily limited to the intravascular space. The volume of distribution of isotonic crystalloids includes the interstitial space; thus, the volume of crystalloids required may be three to four times that of colloids. Hyperoncotic fluids are dependent on mobilization of extravascular fluid for their optimal effect and therefore should not be utilized for fluid resuscitation. Hypertonic fluids have been used in selected clinical settings and their role is still being defined. The choice of crystalloid or colloid remains controversial. Colloid solutions are associated with a reduction in total fluid requirements and may be associated with less pulmonary and systemic edema.[118]

The use of asanguineous fluid is dependent on the ability of most patients to tolerate euvolemic hemodilution. Decreases in hematocrit decrease blood viscosity and impedance to ventricular ejection, resulting in increased stroke volume and cardiac output. For most patients there is little benefit to increasing the hematocrit above 30%.[168, 169] However, in patients with impaired cardiac function, cardiac output may not increase sufficiently and higher levels of hemoglobin are usually required to maintain systemic oxygen delivery.[170] In patients with initial hematocrits less than 30%, the need for red blood cells should be considered early. In general, decreases of 1 to 3 g/dL of hemoglobin can be expected with large-volume resuscitation of patients with shock.[118]

The "P" refers to pump. There are three major considerations in evaluating cardiac performance in patients with circulatory shock. The first is whether the patient has a viable rhythm. Ventricular and supraventricular tachycardias must be treated promptly, and in the hypotensive patient cardioversion is the treatment of choice. Pacing may be needed to sustain heart rate in patients with bradycardias, and in some cases, such as right ventricular infarction, there are hemodynamic benefits of sequential atrioventricular pacing.[171] The second important consideration is obstructive shock that is immediately life threatening and reversible, that is, pericardial tamponade or tension pneumothorax. These diagnoses should always be considered and may warrant empirical interventions, depending on the clinical setting. The third consideration is the need for pharmacologic support of cardiovascular function. After ensuring adequate volume repletion, catecholamines may be used to achieve hemodynamic stability. Inotropic agents are used to increase cardiac output and oxygen delivery to systemic tissues, thereby reversing perfusion failure. Dobutamine, which has predominantly beta-adrenergic activity, can be used as an inotropic agent in patients with low cardiac output but adequate arterial pressure.

If vasopressor drugs are utilized, they should be titrated to maintain the minimal acceptable arterial pressures (60 to 70 mm Hg, mean pressure) to avoid worsening systemic hypoperfusion through excessive vasoconstriction. Dopamine, which has combined alpha- and beta-adrenergic and

---

TABLE 89–2

STANDARDIZED FLUID CHALLENGE*

Fluid infusion of 200 mL colloid or 600 mL crystalloid for 10 min

PAWP-Related Changes
If increase in PAWP ≤ 3 mm Hg, continue infusion
If increase in PAWP > 3 mm Hg and ≤ 7 mm Hg, hold infusion
   until increase in PAWP ≤ 3 mm Hg and then restart infusion
If increase in PAWP > 7 mm Hg, discontinue infusion

CVP-Related Changes
If increase in CVP ≤ 2 mm Hg, continue infusion
If increase in CVP > 2 mm Hg and ≤ 5 mm Hg, hold infusion
   until increase in CVP ≤ 2 mm Hg and then restart infusion
If increase in CVP > 5 mm Hg, discontinue infusion

*PAWP = pulmonary arterial wedge pressure; CVP = central venous pressure.

dopaminergic activity, is preferred for patients who are hypotensive. Levarterenol is a more potent alpha-adrenergic agent and may be used in patients who remain hypotensive or respond to dopamine with excessive tachycardia. In these patients, low doses of dopamine, 1 to 3 μg/kg/min may be used to preserve renal blood flow by taking advantage of renal dopaminergic effects.[172] Although these vasopressor agents are often utilized, there are few data to indicate that their use improves outcome.[173] Indeed, they have potentially severe adverse effects, including increasing myocardial oxygen requirements and, in the case of vasopressors, worsening systemic hypoperfusion.

The use of vasodilators is limited primarily to patients with predominantly cardiac failure but adequate blood pressure. Nitroprusside is a preferred agent because of its balanced arterial and venous activity, which allows for decreasing preload and afterload.[174] When ongoing ischemia is a concern, nitroglycerin, which is predominantly a venodilator, may be utilized.[175] To avoid exacerbating hypotension, these drugs should be slowly titrated to a desired dose and left-sided heart filling pressure should be maintained between 15 to 18 mm Hg.[171] Worsening arterial hypoxemia may be observed with these agents because of increases in intrapulmonary shunting and can be an issue for patients with borderline oxygenation.[176]

The use of alkali therapy in patients with shock and lactic acidemia is controversial.[177] Tissue hypoperfusion produces tissue hypoxia and diminished washout of tissue carbon dioxide. Decreased pulmonary excretion because of decreased pulmonary blood flow contributes to the tissue accumulation of carbon dioxide.[178] Substantial decreases in cardiac output are often associated with significant increases in venous and tissue carbon dioxide.[179–181] Titration of lactic acid with sodium bicarbonate generates additional carbon dioxide through the activity of carbonic anhydrase. Thus, there is a potential for exacerbating tissue acidosis and potentially adversely affecting tissue and cellular function with alkalization.[182, 183] Studies to date have not demonstrated that alkali therapy enhances survival, effectively reduces tissue acidosis, or improves cardiovascular function during circulatory shock.[183, 184] Accordingly, we do not currently recommend alkali therapy for lactic acidosis resulting from circulatory shock.

Depending on the etiology of circulatory shock, specific therapeutic interventions warrant consideration. In patients with cardiogenic shock, thrombolytic therapy and early angioplasty may be of benefit.[185] When mechanical defects exist, such as a ventricular septal defect or mitral valve incompetence, placement of an intra-aortic balloon and early surgical intervention should be considered.[186, 187] Identification of the site of infection, surgical drainage if necessary, and appropriate antibiotic therapy are crucial in the treatment of patients with septic shock.[188, 189] The use of epinephrine in addition to fluids is critical in patients with anaphylactic shock to stabilize mast cell and basophil cell membranes.[190] Histamine antagonists and corticosteroids are adjunctive therapies.[191] In patients with hemorrhagic shock, the site of bleeding must be promptly identified and addressed with appropriate surgical or nonsurgical therapies. Coagulation abnormalities exacerbating the bleeding must also be corrected. Traumatic shock requires a similar approach, with identification of the site of injury and the necessary surgical interventions.

NEWER THERAPIES

There has been increasing interest in the role of different mediators in the development of circulatory shock. The use of specific inhibitors of mediator activity can be expected in the near future. Immunotherapies directed at endotoxin and tumor necrosis factor are undergoing clinical trials in patients with septic shock.[192–195] Inhibitors of lipid mediators, such as platelet-activating factor, thromboxane, and leukotrienes, are being studied as possible interventions in septic, burn, and anaphylactic shock.[65, 196] The administration of prostaglandins with cytoprotective features is also being investigated.[197, 198] Naloxone, a competitive inhibitor of β-endorphins, may have a role in septic and hemorrhagic shock, although additional studies are necessary.[199]

Attention is also focused on the development of organ insufficiency after circulatory shock. In patients who are initially successfully resuscitated, a major cause of mortality is subsequent onset of multiple organ system failure.[200, 201] Accordingly, ischemic and reperfusion injuries are being investigated. Calcium channel blockers, oxygen radical scavengers, and inhibitors of lipid mediators may all have a role in attenuating organ injury during the ischemic period and after reperfusion.[202, 203]

Immunoincompetence and a hypercatabolic stress response are also features of the postresuscitation phase of many of these clinical forms of shock.[204, 205] These factors increase susceptibility to subsequent infection and organ failure. Immunomodulatory therapy with biologic response modifiers, more optimal forms of metabolic support, and therapies aimed at modulating the stress response are areas of clinical investigation in which advances can be expected.[142, 206, 207]

SUMMARY

Circulatory shock results from derangement of the cardiovascular system such that perfusion of systemic tissues is critically reduced, producing tissue oxygen and energy deficits. Many substances mediate the circulatory and metabolic changes seen during shock. In treating the patient with circulatory shock, the immediate priority is establishing cardiopulmonary stability. Depending on the etiology of the shock syndrome, specific therapeutic interventions warrant subsequent consideration. Newer therapies focused on modulating mediator activity hold promise for the future.

References

1. Guyton AC, Jones CE, Coleman TG: Graphical analysis of cardiac output regulation. In: Circulatory Physiology: Cardiac Output and Regulation. 2nd ed. Philadelphia, WB Saunders, p 237, 1973.
2. Braunwald E, Sonnenblick EH, Ross J Jr: Mechanisms of cardiac contraction and relaxation. In: Braunwald E (ed): Heart Disease. A Textbook of Cardiovascular Medicine. 4th ed. Philadelphia, WB Saunders, p 351, 1992.
3. Zweifach BW: Quantitative studies in microcirculatory structure and function. I. Analysis of pressure distribution in the terminal vascular bed of the cat mesentery. Circ Res 34:848, 1974.
4. Cain SM: Review: Supply dependency of oxygen uptake in ARDS—Myth or reality? Am J Med Sci 228:119, 1984.
5. Dahn M, Lange P, Libdell K, et al: Splanchnic and total body oxygen consumption differences in septic and injured patients. Surgery 101:69, 1987.
6. Schmid-Schönbein H: Microrheology of erythrocytes, blood viscosity and the distribution of blood flow in the microcirculation. In: Guyton AC (ed): Cardiovascular Physiology II. Baltimore, University Park Press, p 1, 1976.
7. Brigham KL, Woolverton WC, Blake LH, et al: Increased sheep lung vascular permeability caused by pseudomonas bacteremia. J Clin Invest 54:792, 1974.
8. Castaing Y, Munier G: Hemodynamic disturbances and VA/Q matching in hypoxemic cirrhotic patients. Chest 96:1064, 1989.
9. Archie JP: Anatomic arterial-venous shunting in endotoxic and septic shock in dogs. Ann Surg 186:171, 1972.
10. Weidman MP: Dimensions of blood vessels from distributing artery to collecting vein. Circ Res 12:556, 1963.
11. Rothe CF: Reflex control of the veins and vascular capacitance. Physiol Rev 63:1281, 1983.

12. Rothe CF: Physiology of venous return. Arch Intern Med 146:977, 1986.
13. Secher N, Sander-Jensen K, Werner C, et al: Bradycardia during severe but reversible hypovolemic shock in man. Circ Shock 14:267, 1984.
14. Cohn JN: Blood pressure measurements in shock: Mechanism of inaccuracy in auscultatory and palpatory methods. JAMA 199:118, 1967.
15. Johnson PC: Review of previous studies and current theories of autoregulation. Circ Res 15(suppl):2, 1964.
16. Bond R, Green H: Peripheral circulation. In: Altura B (ed): Handbook of Shock and Trauma. New York, Raven Press, p 29, 1983.
17. Abboud FM, Heistud D, Mark A, et al: Reflex control of the peripheral circulation. Prog Cardiovasc Dis 18:371, 1976.
18. Rutherford RB, Balis JS, Trow RS, et al: Comparison of hemodynamic and regional blood flow changes at equivalent stages of hemorrhagic and endotoxin shock. J Trauma 16:886, 1976.
19. Nishijma H, Weil MH, Shubin H, et al: Hemodynamic and metabolic studies on shock associated with gram-negative bacteremia. Medicine 52:287, 1973.
20. Parker M, Shelhamer J, Natanson C, et al: Serial cardiovascular variables in survivors and nonsurvivors of human septic shock: Heart rate as an early predictor of prognosis. Crit Care Med 15:923, 1987.
21. Shoemaker W, Czer L: Evaluation of the biologic importance of various hemodynamic and oxygen transport variables. Crit Care Med 7:424, 1979.
22. Henning R, Weil MH, Weiner F: Blood lactate as a prognostic indicator of survival in patients with acute myocardial infarction. Circ Shock 9:307, 1982.
23. Baek S, Makabali CG, Byran-Brown C, et al: Plasma expansion in surgical patients with high central venous pressure: The relationship of blood volume to hematocrit, CVP, pulmonary wedge pressure and cardiorespiratory changes. Surgery 78:304, 1975.
24. Raper R, Sibbald W: Misled by the wedge? Chest 89:427, 1986.
25. Rackow EC, Kaufman BS, Falk JL, et al: Hemodynamic response to fluid repletion in patients with septic shock: Evidence for early depression of cardiac performance. Circ Shock 22:11, 1987.
26. Mohr P, Monson D, Owczarski C, et al: Sequential cardiorespiratory events during and after dextran-40 infusion in normal and shock patients. Circulation 39:379, 1969.
27. Parker MM, Shelhamer JH, Bacharach SL, et al: Profound but reversible myocardial depression in patients with septic shock. Ann Intern Med 100:483, 1984.
28. Echt M, Duweling J, Guer U, et al: Effective compliance of the total vascular bed and the intrathoracic compartment derived from changes in central venous pressure induced by volume changes in man. Circ Res 64:61, 1974.
29. Mueller H, Ayers S, Grace W: Principal defects which account for shock following acute myocardial infarction in man: Implications for treatment. Crit Care Med 1:27, 1973.
30. Flint LM, Cryer HM, Simpson CJ, et al: Microcirculatory norepinephrine constriction response in hemorrhagic shock. Surgery 96:240, 1984.
31. Wiggers CJ: The present status of the shock problem. Physiol Rev 22:74, 1942.
32. Groeneveld J, Bronsveld W, Thijs L: Hemodynamic determinants of mortality in human septic shock. Surgery 99:140, 1986.
33. Crowel JW, Smith EE: Oxygen deficit and irreversible hemorrhagic shock. Am J Physiol 206:313, 1964.
34. Siegel JH, Cerra FB, Coleman B, et al: Physiologic and metabolic correlations in human sepsis. Surgery 86:163, 1979.
35. Schwartz S, Frantz RA, Shoemaker WC: Sequential hemodynamic and O₂ transport response to hypovolemia, anemia and hypoxia. Am J Physiol 241:864, 1981.
36. Adams RP, Dietman LA, Cain SM: A critical value for O₂ transport in the rat. J Appl Physiol 53:660, 1982.
37. Cain SM: Appearance of excess lactate in anesthetized dogs during anemic and hypoxic hypoxia. Am J Physiol 209:604, 1965.
38. Chaudry I, Wichterman K, Baue A: Effect of sepsis on tissue adenine nucleotide levels. Surgery 85:205, 1979.
39. Chaudry IH, Sayeed M, Baue A: Effect of hemorrhagic shock on tissue adenine nucleotides in conscious rats. Can J Physiol Pharmacol 52:181, 1976.
40. Haupt M, Gilbert E, Carlson R: Fluid loading increases oxygen consumption in septic patients with lactic acidosis. Am Rev Respir Dis 131:912, 1985.
41. Astiz ME, Rackow EC, Kaufman BS, et al: Relationship of oxygen delivery and mixed venous oxygenation to lactic acidosis in patients with sepsis and acute myocardial infarction. Crit Care Med 16:655, 1988.
42. Rackow EC, Astiz ME, Weil MH: Cellular oxygen metabolism during sepsis and shock: The relationship of oxygen consumption to oxygen delivery. JAMA 259:1989, 1988.
43. Kaufman BS, Rackow EC, Falk JL: The relationship between oxygen delivery and consumption during fluid resuscitation of hypovolemic and septic shock. Chest 85:336, 1984.
44. Annat G, Viale JP, Percival C, et al: Oxygen delivery and uptake in the adult respiratory distress syndrome. Am Rev Respir Dis 133:999, 1986.
45. Weil MH, Afifi AA: Experimental and clinical studies on lactate and pyruvate as indicators of the severity of acute circulatory failure (shock). Circulation 41:989, 1970.
46. Cady L, Weil MH, Afifi A, et al: Quantification of critical illness with special reference to blood lactate. Crit Care Med 1:75, 1973.
47. Rashkin M, Bosken C, Baughman R: Oxygen delivery in critically ill patients. Relationship to lactate and survival. Chest 87:580, 1985.
48. Falk JL, Rackow EC, Leavy J, et al: Delayed lactate clearance in patients surviving circulatory shock. Acute Care 11:212, 1985.
49. Orringer CE, Eustace JC, Wunsch CD, et al: Natural history of lactic acidosis after grand mal seizures. N Engl J Med 297:796, 1977.
50. Kruse J, Zaidi S, Carlson R: Significance of blood lactate in critically ill patients with liver disease. Am J Med 83:77, 1987.
51. Waters J, Wilmore D: The metabolic response to trauma and sepsis. In: DeGroot L (ed): Endocrinology. 2nd ed. Philadelphia, WB Saunders, p 2367, 1989.
52. Benedict CR, Grahame-Smith DG: Plasma noradrenaline and adrenaline concentration and dopamine-β-hydroxylase activity in patients with shock due to septicemia, trauma and hemorrhage. Q J Med 47:1, 1979.
53. Davies CL, Newman RJ, Molyneux SG, et al: The relationship between plasma catecholamine and the severity of injury in man. J Trauma 24:99, 1984.
54. Claybaugh JR, Share L: Vasopressin, renin and cardiovascular response to continuous slow hemorrhage. Am J Physiol 224:519, 1973.
55. Beaty O, Sloup CH, Schmid HE Jr, et al: Renin response and angiotensinogen control during graded hemorrhage and shock in the dog. Am J Physiol 231:1300, 1976.
56. Phillips R, Vallente W, Caplan E, et al: Circulating thyroid hormone changes in acute trauma. Prognostic implications for clinical outcome. J Trauma 24:116, 1984.
57. Kaptein E, Weiner J, Robinson W, et al: Relationship of altered thyroid hormone indices to survival in nonthyroidal illness. Clin Endocrinol 16:565, 1982.
58. Marchuk JB, Finley RJ, Groves AC, et al: Catabolic hormones and substrate patterns in septic patients. J Surg Res 23:177, 1977.
59. Melby JC, Spink WW: Comparative studies on adrenal cortical function and cortisol metabolism in patients with shock due to infections. J Clin Invest 37:1791, 1958.
60. Mack E, Egdhal RH: Cortisol secretion in hemorrhagic shock. Surg Forum 18:48, 1967.
61. Heibert JM, Sveldner JS, Egdhal RH: Altered insulin and glucose metabolism produced by epinephrine during hemorrhagic shock in the adrenalectomized primate. Surgery 74:223, 1973.
62. Daniel A, Pierce C, Shizgal H, et al: Protein and fat utilization in shock. Surgery 84:588, 1978.
63. Crum C, Simon R, Dantzker D, et al: Evidence for adenosine triphosphate degradation in critically ill patients. Chest 88:763, 1985.
64. Woolliseroft J, Calfer H, Fox I: Hyperuricemia in acute illness: A poor prognostic sign. Am J Med 72:58, 1982.
65. Lefer A: Significance of lipid mediators in shock states. Circ Shock 27:3, 1989.
66. Slotman GJ, Burchard KW, Williams JJ, et al: Interaction of prostaglandins, activated complement, and granulocytes in clinical sepsis and hypotension. Surgery 99:744, 1986.
67. Fletcher JR, DiSimone AG, Earnest MA: Platelet activating factor receptor antagonist improves survival and attenuates eicosanoid release in severe endotoxemia. Ann Surg 211:312, 1990.
68. Bernton EW, Long JB, Holaday JW: Opioids and neuropeptides: Mechanisms in circulatory shock. Fed Proc 44:290, 1985.
69. Faden AJ, Holaday JW: Opiate antagonists: A role in the treatment of hypovolemic shock. Science 205:317, 1979.
70. Danner R, Suffredini A, Natanson C, et al: Microbial toxins: Role in the pathogenesis of septic shock and multiple organ failure. In: Bihari D, Cerra F (eds): New Horizons. Multiple Organ Failure. Fullerton, CA, Society of Critical Care Medicine, p 151, 1989.
71. Morrison DC, Ryan JL: Endotoxins and disease mechanisms. Annu Rev Med 38:417, 1987.
72. Pollack M: The role of exotoxin A in pseudomonas disease and immunity. Rev Infect Dis 5(suppl 5):S979, 1983.
73. Sheagren J: Staphylococcus aureus. N Engl J Med 310:1368, 1984.
74. Styrt B, Gorbach S: Recent development in understanding of the pathogenesis and treatment of anaerobic infection. N Engl J Med 321:240, 1989.
75. Beutler B, Cerami A: Cachectin. More than a tumor necrosis factor. N Engl J Med 316:379, 1987.
76. Dinarello CA: Interleukin A. Rev Infect Dis 61:51, 1984.
77. Jacobs R, Traber D: Immune cellular interactions during sepsis and septic injury. Crit Care Clin 5:9, 1989.
78. Calandra T, Baumgartner JD, Grau GE, et al: Prognostic values of tumor necrosis factor/cachectin, interleukin-1, interferon-α, and interferon-γ in the serum of patients with septic shock. J Infect Dis 161:982, 1990.
79. Hack CE, De Groot ER, Felt-Bersma RJ, et al: Increased plasma levels of interleukin-6 in sepsis. Blood 74:1704, 1989. (Comment in: Blood 75:1897, 1990.)
80. Revhaug A, Michie HR, Manson JM, et al: Inhibition of cyclo-oxygenase

attenuates the metabolic response to endotoxin in humans. Arch Surg 123:162, 1988.

81. Natanson C, Eichenholz PW, Danner RL, et al: Endotoxin and tumor necrosis factor challenges in dogs simulate the cardiovascular profile of human septic shock. J Exp Med 169:823, 1989.

82. Ishizaka T: Analysis of triggering events in mast cells for immunoglobin E–mediated histamine release. J Allergy Clin Immunol 67:90, 1981.

83. Kagey-Sobotka A, MacGlashan DW, Lichtenstein LM: Role of receptor aggregation in triggering IgE mediated reactions. Fed Proc 41:12, 1982.

84. MacGlashan D, Lichtenstein L: Mast cell and basophil derived mediators of allergic diseases. In: Lessoff M, Lec T, Kemeny D (eds): Allergy. Baltimore, Williams & Wilkins, p 201, 1987.

85. Vogt W: Anaphylatoxins: Possible roles in disease. Complement 3:177, 1986.

86. McCabe WR: Serum complement levels in bacteremia due to gram-negative organisms. N Engl J Med 288:21, 1973.

87. Hack C, Nijjens J, Bersma F, et al: Elevated plasma levels of the anaphylatoxins C3a and C5a are associated with fatal outcome in sepsis. Am J Med 86:20, 1989.

88. Suffredini AF, Harpel PC, Parrillo J: Promotion and subsequent inhibition of plasminogen activation after administration of intravenous endotoxin to normal subjects. N Engl J Med 320:1165, 1989.

89. Siegel T, Seligsohn U, Aghai E, et al: Clinical and laboratory aspects of disseminated intravascular coagulation (DIC). A study of 188 cases. Thromb Haemost 39:122, 1978.

90. Nies AS, Forsyth R, Williams H, et al: Contribution of kinins to endotoxin shock in unanesthetized rhesus monkeys. Circ Res 22:155, 1969.

91. Alving B, Hojima Y, Pisano J, et al: Hypotension associated with prekallikrein activator (Hageman-factor fragments) in plasma protein fraction. N Engl J Med 299:66, 1978.

92. Lerman A, Hildebrand F, Margulies K: Endothelin: A new cardiovascular regulatory peptide. Mayo Clin Proc 65:1441, 1990.

93. Cernace KP, Stewart DJ: Immunoreactive endothelin in human plasma: Marked elevations in patients in cardiogenic shock. Biochem Biophys Res Commun 161:562, 1989.

94. Furchgott RF, Zawadzki JV: The obligatory role of endothelial cells in the relaxation of arterial smooth muscle by acetylcholine. Nature 288:373, 1980.

95. Kilbourn RG, Belloni P: Endothelial cell production of nitrogen oxides in response to interferon-gamma in combination with tumor necrosis factor, interleukin-1 or endotoxin. J Natl Cancer Inst 82:772, 1990.

96. Chaudry IH: Cellular mechanisms in shock and ischemia and their correlation. Am J Physiol 245:R117, 1983.

97. Trump B, Berezesk I, Cowley R: The cellular and subcellular characteristics of acute and chronic injury with emphasis on the role of calcium. In: Cowley R, Trump B (eds): Pathophysiology of Shock, Anoxia and Ischemia. Baltimore, Williams & Wilkins, p 301, 1982.

98. Shires GT, Cunningham JN, Backer CR, et al: Alterations in cellular membrane function during hemorrhagic shock in primates. Ann Surg 176:288, 1972.

99. Sayeed MM: Membrane sodium-potassium transport and ancillary phenomenon in circulatory shock. In: Cowley R, Trump B (eds): Pathophysiology of Shock, Anoxia and Ischemia. Baltimore, Williams & Wilkins, p 112, 1982.

100. Mela L, Bacalzo LV Jr, Miller ID: Defective oxidative metabolism of rat mitochondria in hemorrhagic and endotoxin shock. Am J Physiol 220:571, 1971.

101. Wakers FJ, Lie K, Becker AE, et al: Coronary artery disease in patients dying from cardiogenic shock or congestive heart failure in the setting of acute myocardial infarction. Br Heart J 38:906, 1976.

102. Page DL, Caulfield JB, Kastor JA, et al: Myocardial changes associated with cardiogenic shock. N Engl J Med 285:133, 1971.

103. Cunnion RE, Shaer GL, Parker MM, et al: The coronary circulation in human septic shock. Circulation 73:637, 1986.

104. Greene LJ, Shapanka R, Glen TM, et al: Isolation of a myocardial depressant factor from plasma of dogs in hemorrhagic shock. Biochim Biophys Acta 491:275, 1977.

105. Parrillo JE, Burche C, Shelhamer JH, et al: A circulating myocardial depressant substance in humans with septic shock. J Clin Invest 76:1539, 1985.

106. Benussayag C, Christeff N, Auclair M, et al: Early released lipid soluble cardiodepressant factor and elevated estrogenic substances in human septic shock. Eur J Clin Invest 14:288, 1984.

107. Bristow MR, Ginsburg R, Minobe W, et al: Decreased cathecholamine sensitivity and beta-adrenergic receptor density in failing human hearts. N Engl J Med 307:205, 1982.

108. Romano FD, Jones SB: Characteristics of myocardial beta-adrenergic receptors during endotoxicosis in the rat. Am J Physiol 251:R359, 1986.

109. Diamond G, Forrester JS: Effect of coronary artery disease and acute myocardial infarction on left ventricular compliance in man. Circulation 45:11, 1972.

110. Jafri SM, Lavine S, Field BE, et al: Left ventricular diastolic function in sepsis. Crit Care Med 18:709, 1990.

111. Alyono D, Reng WS, Chau RY, et al: Characteristics of ventricular function in severe hemorrhagic shock. Surgery 94:250, 1983.

112. Parker M, Shelhamer J, Bacharach S, et al: Profound but reversible myocardial depression in patients with septic shock. Ann Intern Med 100:483, 1984.

113. Aubier M, Trippenbach T, Roussos C: Respiratory muscle fatigue during cardiogenic shock. J Appl Physiol 5:499, 1981.

114. Field S, Kelly S, Macklem P: The oxygen cost of breathing in patients with cardiorespiratory disease. Am Rev Respir Dis 126:9, 1982.

115. Buckzowski J, Dureuil B, Bronger C, et al: Effects of sepsis on diaphragmatic function in rats. Am Rev Respir Dis 138:260, 1988.

116. Rackow EC, Fein A, Siegel J: The relationship of the colloid osmotic pulmonary artery wedge pressure gradient to pulmonary edema and mortality in critically ill patients. Chest 82:433, 1982.

117. Fein AM, Lippmann M, Holtzman H, et al: The risk factors: Incidence and prognosis of ARDS following septicemia. Chest 83:40, 1983.

118. Rackow EC, Falk JL, Fein IA, et al: Fluid resuscitation in circulatory shock: A comparison of the cardiorespiratory effect of albumin, heta-starch and saline solutions in patients with hypovolemic and septic shock. Crit Care Med 11:839, 1983.

119. Pepe PE, Potkin RT, Reus DH, et al: Clinical predictors of the adult respiratory distress syndrome. Am J Surg 144:124, 1982.

120. Tristani F, Cohn J: Studies in clinical shock and hypotension. Circulation 62:839, 1970.

121. Myer B, Moran S: Hemodynamically mediated acute renal failure. N Engl J Med 314:97, 1986.

122. Kahl F, Flint J, Szidon J: Influence of left atrial distention on renal vasomotor tone. Am J Physiol 226:240, 1974.

123. Rector R, Goyal S, Rosenberg I, et al: Sepsis: A mechanism for vasodilation in the kidney. Ann Surg 178:222, 1972.

124. Jones L, Weil MH: Changes in urinary output and free water clearance in patients with acute circulatory shock. J Urol 102:121, 1969.

125. Baek S, Makabali G, Brown R, et al: Free water clearance patterns as predictors and therapeutic guides in acute renal failure. Surgery 77:632, 1975.

126. Cowley RA, Mansberger AR, Rudo F, et al: A comparison of levels of blood ammonia and other metabolites in portal and systemic circulation during shock. Surg Forum 10:450, 1960.

127. Grun M, Brolsch CE, Walter J: Influence of portal hepatic blood flow on RES function. In: Liehr H, Grun M (eds): Reticuloendothelial System and Pathogenesis of Liver Disease. New York, Elsevier/North Holland Biomedical Press, p 149, 1980.

128. Keller G, West M, Cerra F, et al: Macrophage-mediated modulation of hepatic function in multiple-system failure. J Surg Res 37:555, 1985.

129. Brohult J, Gillquest J: Serum enzyme levels as a measure of liver reaction after hypovolemic shock and operations in man. Acta Chir Scand 134:353, 1968.

130. Birgens H, Henrickson J, Matzen P, et al: The shock liver: Clinical and biochemical finding in patients with centrilobular liver necrosis following cardiogenic shock. Acta Med Scand 204:417, 1978.

131. Lillihei RC: The intestinal factor in irreversible shock. Surgery 42:1043, 1957.

132. Fink MP: Gastrointestinal mucosal injury in experimental models of shock, trauma, and sepsis. Crit Care Med 19:627, 1991.

133. Bhagwat AG, Hawk WA: Terminal hemorrhagic necrotizing enteropathy. Am J Gastroenterol 45:163, 1966.

134. Skillman JJ, Britinelli LS, Goldman H, et al: Respiratory failure, hypotension sepsis and jaundice. A clinical syndrome associated with lethal hemorrhage from acute stress ulceration of the stomach. Am J Surg 123:25, 1971.

135. Robert A, Kaufman GL Jr: Stress ulcers, erosions, and gastric mucosal injury. In: Sleisenger MH, Fordtran JS (eds): Gastrointestinal Disease. Pathophysiology, Diagnosis, Management. 4th ed. Philadelphia, WB Saunders, p 772, 1989.

136. Orlando R, Gleason E, Drezner A: Acute acalculous cholecystitis in the critically ill patient. Am J Surg 45:472, 1983.

137. Ellison E: The pancreas in shock. In: Hardaway RM (ed): Shock: The Reversible Stage of Dying. Littleton, MA, PSG Publishing, p 403, 1988.

138. Lefer AM: Role of a myocardial factor in the pathogenesis of shock. Am J Physiol 222:450, 1972.

139. Astiz ME, Tilly E, Rackow EC, et al: Peripheral vascular tone in sepsis. Chest 99:1072, 1991.

140. Thoren O: Blood flow patterns of the forearm of critically ill post-traumatic patients. Acta Chir Scand 443(suppl):11, 1974.

141. Voerman HJ, Groeneveld AB: Blood viscosity and circulatory shock. Intensive Care Med 15:72, 1989.

142. Saba TM, Jaffe E: Plasma fibronectin (opsonic glycoprotein): Its synthesis by vascular endothelial cells and role in cardiopulmonary integrity after trauma as related to reticuloendothelial function. Am J Med 68:577, 1980.

143. Heughan C, Ninikoski J, Hunt TK: Effect of excessive infusion of saline solution on tissue oxygen transport. Surg Gynecol Obstet 135:257, 1972.

144. Rhodes G, Taylor M, Newell JC, et al: Effect of dopamine, ethanol and mannitol on cardiopulmonary function in adults with respiratory distress syndrome. J Thorac Cardiovasc Surg 82:203, 1981.

145. Feinstein D: Treatment of disseminated intravascular coagulation. Semin Thromb Hemost 14:351, 1988.

146. Mant M, King E: Severe, acute disseminated intravascular coagulation. Am J Med 67:557, 1979.
147. Sprung CL, Peduzzi PN, Shatney CH, et al: Impact of encephalopathy on mortality in the sepsis syndrome. Crit Care Med 18:801, 1990.
148. Brierley J: Ischemic necrosis along brain arterial boundary zones: Some aspects of its etiology. Adv Neurol 26:155, 1979.
149. Lindenberg R: Patterns of CNS vulnerability in acute hypoxemia including anesthesia accidents. In: Schade JP, McMeneny WH (eds): Selective Vulnerability of the Brain in Hypoxemia: A Symposium. Philadelphia, FA Davis, p 189, 1963.
150. Takezeka J, Taenuka N, Nishigima M: Amino acids and thiobarbituric reactive substances in cerebrospinal fluid and plasma of patients with septic encephalopathy. Crit Care Med 11:876, 1983.
151. Hinshaw LB, Cox BG: The Fundamental Mechanism of Shock. New York, Plenum Publishing, p 13, 1972.
152. Weil MH, Shubin H: The "VIP" approach to the bedside management of shock. JAMA 207:337, 1969.
153. American College of Chest Physicians National Heart, Lung and Blood Institute Conference on Oxygen Therapy. Arch Intern Med 144:1645, 1984.
154. Cohen C, Zagelbaum G, Gross G, et al: Clinical manifestations of inspiratory muscle fatigue. Am J Med 73:308, 1982.
155. Viires N, Sillye G, Aubier M, et al: Regional blood flow distribution in dogs during induced hypotension and low cardiac output: Spontaneous breathing versus artificial ventilation. J Clin Invest 74:935, 1983.
156. Natanson C, Shelhamer J, Parrillo J: Intubation of the trachea in the critical care setting. JAMA 253:1160, 1985.
157. Hoar P, Nelson N, Mangano D, et al: Adrenergic response to morphine-diazepam anesthesia for myocardial revascularization. Anesth Analg 60:406, 1981.
158. Cournand A, Moteley HL, Werko L, et al: Physiological effects of intermittent positive pressure breathing on cardiac output in man. Am J Physiol 152:162, 1978.
159. Rankin J, Olsen C, Arentzen C, et al: The effects of airway pressure on cardiac function in intact dogs and man. Circulation 66:108, 1982.
160. Harken A, Brennan M, Smith B, et al: The hemodynamic response to positive end-expiratory ventilation in hypovolemic patients. Surgery 76:786, 1974.
161. Forrester JS, Diamond G, Swan JH: Correlative classification of clinical and hemodynamic function after acute myocardial infarction. Am J Cardiol 31:137, 1977.
162. Packman M, Rackow EC: Optimum filling pressures during fluid resuscitation of patients with hypovolemic and septic shock. Crit Care Med 11:165, 1983.
163. Forrester JS, Diamond G, McHugh TJ, et al: Filling pressures in the right and left sides of the heart in acute myocardial infarction. N Engl J Med 285:190, 1971.
164. Weil MH, Henning RJ. New concepts in the diagnosis and fluid treatment of circulatory shock. Anesth Analg 58:124, 1979.
165. Crexells C, Chatterjee K, Forrester J, et al: Optimal level of filling pressure in the left side of the heart in acute myocardial infarction. N Engl J Med 289:1263, 1973.
166. Mangano D, VanDyke D, Ellis R: The effect of increasing preload on ventricular output and ejection in man. Circulation 62:535, 1980.
167. Falk JL, Rackow EC, Weil MH: Colloid and crystalloid fluid resuscitation. In: Shoemaker WC, Ayres S, Grenvick A, et al (eds): Textbook of Critical Care. 2nd ed. Philadelphia, WB Saunders, p 1055, 1989.
168. Fortune J, Feustel P, Saifi J, et al: Influence of hematocrit on cardiopulmonary function after acute hemorrhage. J Trauma 27:243, 1987.
169. Czer LS, Shoemaker WC: Optimal hematocrit value in critically ill postoperative patients. Surg Gynecol Obstet 147:363, 1978.
170. Roseberg B, Wulff K: Hemodynamics following normovolemic hemodilution in elderly patients. Acta Anaesthesiol Scand 25:402, 1981.
171. Topol E, Goldschlager W, Ports W, et al: Hemodynamic benefit of atrial pacing in right ventricular myocardial infarction. Ann Intern Med 96:594, 1982.
172. Schaaer G, Fink M, Parrillo J: Norepinephrine alone versus norepinephrine plus low dose dopamine: Enhanced renal blood flow with combination pressor therapy. Crit Care Med 13:492, 1985.
173. Ruiz C, Weil MH, Carlson R: Treatment of circulatory shock with dopamine. JAMA 242:165, 1979.
174. Chatterjee K, Parmley W, Ganz W, et al: Hemodynamic and metabolic responses to vasodilator therapy in acute myocardial infarction. Circulation 48:1183, 1973.
175. Flaherty J, Reid P, Kelley D, et al: Intravenous nitroglycerin in acute myocardial infarction. Circulation 51:132, 1975.
176. Mookherjee S, Keighley JF, Warner RA, et al: Hemodynamic, ventilating and blood gas changes during infusion of sodium nitroferricyanide (nitroprusside). Chest 72:273, 1977.

177. Narins RG, Cohen JJ: Bicarbonate therapy for organic acidosis. The case for its continued use. Ann Intern Med 106:615, 1987.
178. Falk JL, Rackow EC, Weil MH: End-tidal carbon dioxide concentration during cardiopulmonary resuscitation. N Engl J Med 18:607, 1988.
179. Brantigan JW, Ziegler EC, Hynes KM, et al: Tissue gases during hypovolemic shock. J Appl Physiol 37:117, 1974.
180. Weil MH, Rackow EC, Trevino R, et al: Differences in acid-base state between venous and arterial blood during cardiopulmonary resuscitation. N Engl J Med 315:153, 1986.
181. Halmagyi D, Kennedy M, Varga D: Hidden hypercapnia in hemorrhagic hypotension. Anesthesiology 33:594, 1970.
182. Graf H, Arieff H, Leach W: Evidence for a detrimental effect of bicarbonate therapy in hypoxic lactic acidosis. Science 227:754, 1985.
183. Kette F, Weil MH, von Planta M, et al: Buffer agents do not reverse intramyocardial acidosis during cardiac resuscitation. Circulation 81:1660, 1990.
184. Cooper D, Walley K, Wiggs B, et al: Bicarbonate does not improve hemodynamics in critically ill patients who have lactic acidosis. Ann Intern Med 112:492, 1990.
185. Lee L, Bates E, Pitt B, et al: Percutaneous transluminal coronary angioplasty improves survival in acute myocardial infarction complicated by cardiogenic shock. Circulation 78:1345, 1988.
186. Resnekov L: Cardiogenic shock. Chest 83:893, 1983.
187. Goldberger M, Tabak S, Shah P: Clinical experience with intra-aortic balloon counterpulsation in 112 consecutive patients. Am Heart J 111:497, 1986.
188. Bryan CS, Reynolds KL, Brenner ER: Analysis of 1,186 episodes of gram-negative bacteremia in non-university hospitals: The effects of antimicrobial therapy. Rev Infect Dis 5:629, 1983.
189. Kreger BE, Craven DE, McCabe WR: Gram-negative bacteremia. IV. Re-evaluation of clinical features and treatment of 612 patients. Am J Med 68:344, 1980.
190. Barach EM, Nowak RM, Lee TG, et al: Epinephrine for the treatment of anaphylactic shock. JAMA 251:2118, 1984.
191. Church MK, Holgate ST: The development of drug therapy. In: Lessof MH, Lee TH, Kemeny DM (eds): Allergy: An International Textbook. Baltimore, Williams & Wilkins, p 599, 1987.
192. Ziegler EJ, McCutchan JA, Fierer J, et al: Treatment of gram-negative bacteremia and shock with human antiserum to a mutant *Escherichia coli*. N Engl J Med 307:1225, 1982.
193. Greenman RL, Schein RM, Martin MA, et al: A controlled clinical trial of E5 murine monoclonal IgM antibody to endotoxin in the treatment of gram-negative sepsis. The XOMA Sepsis Study Group. JAMA 266:1097, 1991. (Comment in: JAMA 266:1125, 1991.)
194. Ziegler E, Fischer C, Staube R, et al: Prevention of death from gram-negative bacteremia and sepsis by HA-IA, a human monoclonal antibody specific for lipid A of endotoxin. N Engl J Med 324:429, 1991.
195. Tracy KJ, Beutler B, Lowry SF, et al: Shock and tissue injury induced by recombinant human cachectin. Science 234:470, 1986.
196. Rockwell W, Ehrlich H: Ibuprofen in acute care. Ann Surg 211:78, 1990.
197. Bihari D, Smithies M, Grimson A, et al: The effects of vasodilation with prostacyclin on oxygen delivery and uptake in critically ill patients. N Engl J Med 317:497, 1987.
198. Hartl W, Herndon D, Wolfe R: Kinin/prostaglandin system: Its therapeutic value in surgical stress. Crit Care Med 18:1167, 1990.
199. Faden A: Opiate antagonists and thyrotropin-releasing hormone. Potential role in the treatment of shock. JAMA 252:1177, 1984.
200. Fry DE, Pearlstein L, Fulton RL, et al: Multiple system organ failure. The role of uncontrolled infection. Arch Surg 115:136, 1980.
201. Kraus W, Draper E, Wagner D, et al: Prognosis in acute organ system failure. Ann Surg 202:685, 1985.
202. McCord J: Oxygen-derived free radicals in postischemic tissue injury. N Engl J Med 312:159, 1985.
203. Cheung J, Bonventre J, Mulis C, et al: Calcium and ischemic injury. N Engl J Med 314:1670, 1986.
204. Christou N: Host-defense mechanisms in surgical patients: A correlative study of the delayed hypersensitivity skin-test response, granulocyte function and sepsis. Can J Surg 28:39, 1985.
205. Abraham E: Host defense abnormalities after hemorrhagic trauma and burns. Crit Care Med 17:934, 1989.
206. McArdle AH, Palmason C, Brown R, et al: Early arterial feeding of patients with major burns: Prevention of catabolism. Ann Plast Surg 13:396, 1984.
207. Moore E, Jones T: Benefits of immediate jejunostomy feedings after major abdominal trauma. A prospective randomized trial. J Trauma 26:874, 1986.

CHAPTER 90

Acute Myocardial Ischemia*

Joshua Wynne

Although mortality has been halved during the last 25 years, coronary artery disease (CAD) is still a leading cause of death in the United States. It causes about 500,000 deaths each year and more than 2 million hospitalizations for unstable angina pectoris (UAP) and acute myocardial infarction (AMI).[1–3]

The fall in mortality in CAD is likely multifactorial in origin: risk factor modification (e.g., control of hypertension, cessation of cigarette smoking, lowering cholesterol, sensible exercise), improved medical treatment strategies, improved mechanical revascularization by angioplasty and bypass surgery, and treatment of arrhythmias and other complications of acute myocardial ischemia through the use of cardiac and intensive care units.

DEFINITIONS

There is a wide spectrum of clinical presentations in ischemic heart disease, ranging from silent CAD to AMI. Silent CAD and exertional angina pectoris are chronic forms of CAD and are usually due to enhanced myocardial demand for nutrients that exceeds the ability of a coronary artery narrowed by an atherosclerotic plaque to increase flow appropriately. The acute ischemic syndromes (UAP and AMI) are caused most commonly by a primary reduction in coronary blood flow, often occur at rest, and may lead to myocardial damage.

UAP—also called preinfarction angina, crescendo angina, acute coronary insufficiency, and intermediate coronary syndrome—is characterized by severe but transient myocardial ischemia.[3] Although its presentation, including clinical and electrocardiographic features, may be indistinguishable from that of a myocardial infarction, no necrosis occurs. Recurrent episodes of ischemia are common and, in some cases, are premonitory of the development of an infarct.

AMI occurs when ischemia persists for a sufficient length of time to produce myocardial necrosis; perhaps half of the patients presenting with AMI experience a prodrome of UAP.[3] AMI may be associated with Q waves on the electrocardiogram (ECG) or only ST segment and T wave abnormalities (so-called non–Q wave infarction).

HISTORICAL PERSPECTIVE

The modern era in the treatment of AMI dates to the 1950s and 1960s with the development of cardiac care units, the introduction of lidocaine for treating ventricular arrhythmias, the development of external defibrillators, the technique of cardiopulmonary resuscitation, and the use of hemodynamic monitoring.[2] In the 1960s and 1970s there were increasing attempts to limit the size of myocardial infarctions by pharmacologic and other means, aimed prin-

cipally at reducing the demand for oxygen and nutrients by the myocardium. The past decade has witnessed a crusade aimed at improving myocardial perfusion in the acutely ischemic patient by pharmacologic, catheter-based, and surgical means.

MECHANISMS

Acute myocardial ischemia results when there is an imbalance between nutrient supply and demand. In most cases, the basic cause is narrowing of one or more of the large epicardial coronary arteries by an atherosclerotic plaque, but various nonatherosclerotic mechanisms may be involved on occasion (Table 90–1). Of particular importance in younger patients is cocaine abuse, which may cause myocardial ischemia in several different ways; coronary artery spasm,[4] often with associated thrombosis, appears to be the most frequent cause of myocardial ischemia in this setting.

Atherosclerotic narrowing of the coronary arteries accounts for the vast majority of acute ischemic episodes. In most cases the luminal diameter of a coronary artery must be narrowed by at least 70% before there is sufficient reduction in coronary flow to exceed the metabolic needs of the myocardium. Such an imbalance occurs most commonly when there is a fixed stenosis in the coronary artery that allows adequate blood flow at rest but becomes limiting when an increase in coronary blood flow is needed to match the increase in myocardial oxygen demand that occurs during physical or other activities. This inability of coronary flow to increase appropriately leads to a supply-demand imbalance, and typical angina pectoris occurs (although there is increasing evidence that three fourths of such ischemic episodes may be clinically silent[5]). Management of such patients involves strategies to reduce the heightened myocardial oxygen demand during exercise by limiting the attendant increase in heart rate, blood pressure, and/or contractility (e.g., with beta-adrenergic blockers or calcium channel blockers) or by

TABLE 90–1
NONATHEROSCLEROTIC CAUSES OF MYOCARDIAL ISCHEMIA

Intrinsically normal coronary artery
  Embolus
    Infective endocarditis
    Left atrial myxoma
    Mitral valve prolapse
    Paradoxical embolus
    Atrial or ventricular thrombus
  Spasm
    Cocaine abuse
    Nitroglycerin withdrawal
  Hematologic abnormalities
    Hypercoagulable state
    Sickle cell disease
Abnormal coronary artery
  Spasm
    Variant (Prinzmetal's) angina
  Vasculitis
    Syphilis
    Kawasaki's disease
    Takayasu's disease
    Polyarteritis nodosa
    Systemic lupus erythematosus
  Congenital disorder
    Anomalous origin
  Acquired disorders
    Aortic or coronary dissection
    Trauma (including surgical)
    Cardiac catheterization mishaps

---

*Because of extraordinary lay and professional interest in this field, a large number of clinical trials are under way, the results of which may temper or change the recommendations contained within this chapter. The reader is urged to supplement the overview presented here with the latest information contained within journals. To aid in this task, the titles and acronyms of ongoing major trials are given wherever possible.

improving perfusion down the coronary artery itself (with percutaneous transluminal coronary angioplasty [PTCA] or coronary artery bypass graft [CABG] surgery) or its collateral supply (with nitrates).

The factors responsible for transforming a previously stable patient with exertional angina pectoris (or a patient with previously silent CAD) into a patient with acute myocardial ischemia have evoked intense speculation since the turn of the century. It is becoming increasingly clear that such a transition usually results from a primary reduction in coronary perfusion (with a lesser contribution from increased demand), usually caused by an abrupt change in the architecture of the atherosclerotic plaque that triggers platelet deposition, thrombus formation, coronary vasoconstriction, and a resultant reduction in flow down the artery.

Plaque Disruption

The initiating event in most cases of acute myocardial ischemia appears to be ulceration, fissuring, or rupture of an atherosclerotic plaque with resulting interruption of the covering endothelium, leading in some cases to deep injury to the wall of the vessel because of hemorrhage within the plaque[6] (Fig. 90–1). The precise factors that precipitate plaque disruption are not known, although soft plaques with a high lipid content appear to be at particular risk,[7] especially if subjected to increased turbulence and hemodynamic shear forces[8] (Fig. 90–2). A fibrous cap overlies the lipid pool contained within the atherosclerotic plaque, and deep tears seem to occur at the junction of the cap with the normal vessel wall (Fig. 90–3). Attendant hemorrhage and thrombosis extend into the lipid pool, distorting and increasing the size of the plaque itself.[6] Perhaps surprisingly, the protuberant plaques that produce the most severe coronary artery stenoses appear to be less prone to disruption than moderately stenotic plaques (<60 to 70% stenosis).[9] Although severe stenoses seem to progress to complete occlusion more commonly than less severe stenoses, this transition often is clinically silent and not invariably associated with acute infarction. It is speculated that this occurs because the initial tight stenosis recruits collateral blood flow that maintains myocardial perfusion when the vessel closes.[8]

Thrombus Formation

Disruption of the plaque exposes collagen, atheromatous material, and other constituents that lead to platelet activa-

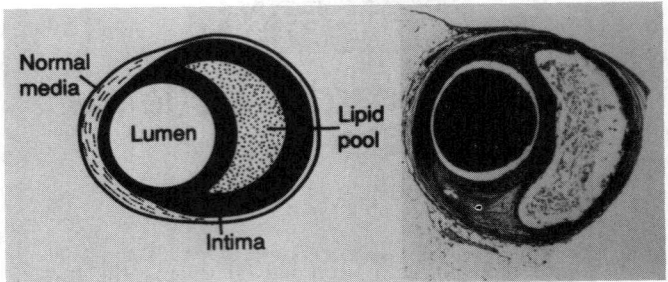

Figure 90–2. Diagrammatic representation *(left)* and photomicrograph *(right)* of a histologic transverse section of a coronary artery with an eccentric stenosis. The lumen of the histologic specimen contains a mass of gelatin and barium used in postmortem angiography. The lipid pool is separated from the lumen by the plaque cap. Elastic-hematoxylin stain, × 20. (From Davies MJ: A macro and micro view of coronary vascular insult in ischemic heart disease. Circulation 82[suppl II]:38–46, 1990, by permission of the American Heart Association, Inc.)

tion and adherence and subsequent thrombus formation[8] (Fig. 90–4). The thrombus may be partially or totally occlusive, with resulting acute reduction in coronary blood flow (Figs. 90–5 and 90–6). If a totally occluding thrombus forms and remains in situ, a Q wave myocardial infarction typically results. It has been speculated that a partially occlusive clot (or one that is lysed by the body's natural thrombolytic mechanisms) may cause the other acute ischemic syndrome (UAP, non–Q wave myocardial infarction). Fuster and colleagues have suggested that mild plaque injury is associated with a mild thrombogenic stimulus, producing partial or transient thrombosis with attendant transient ischemia as is seen in UAP.[8] More extensive vessel wall injury may produce more occlusive or persistent thrombosis and result in prolonged episodes of ischemia or non–Q wave infarction. Deep injury may lead to persistent thrombotic occlusion of the vessel and the clinical syndrome of Q wave infarction.[10] It seems that mild degrees of endothelial injury (e.g., with mere fissuring of the plaque) produce thrombi with a high

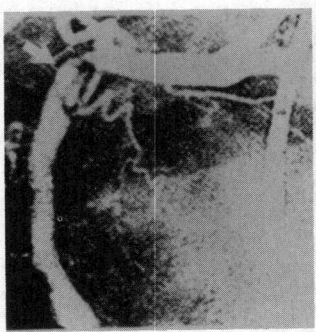 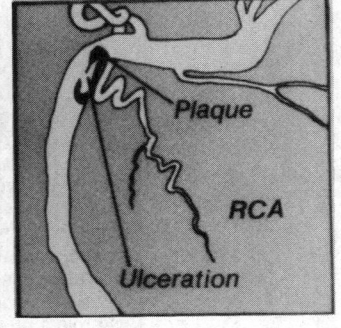

Figure 90–1. Digital subtraction coronary angiogram *(left)* and corresponding sketch *(right)* of a right coronary artery (RCA), showing a severe proximal stenosis with plaque fissuring *(arrow at left)* in a patient with UAP. (From Myler RK, Shaw RE, Stertzer SH, et al: Unstable angina and coronary angioplasty. Circulation 82[suppl II]:88–95, 1990, by permission of the American Heart Association, Inc.)

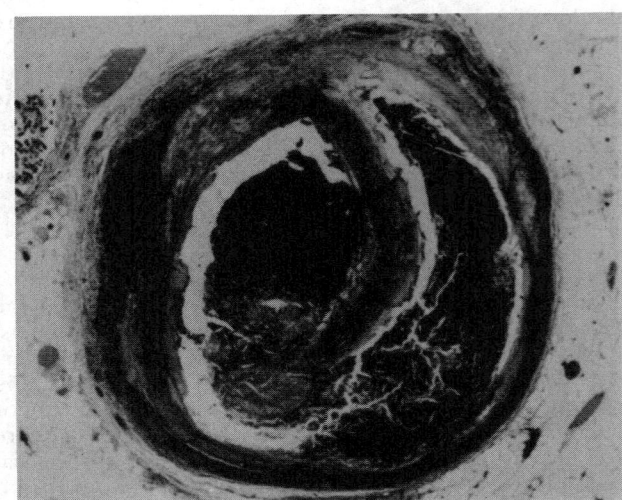

Figure 90–3. Photomicrograph of a histologic transverse section of a coronary artery with a fissured plaque. The fissure in the cap is at the lower left. The lipid pool contains a dark mass of thrombus that projects into the lumen but is not totally occlusive. Trichrome stain, × 20. (From Davies MJ: A macro and micro view of coronary vascular insult in ischemic heart disease. Circulation 82[suppl II]:38–46, 1990, by permission of the American Heart Association, Inc.)

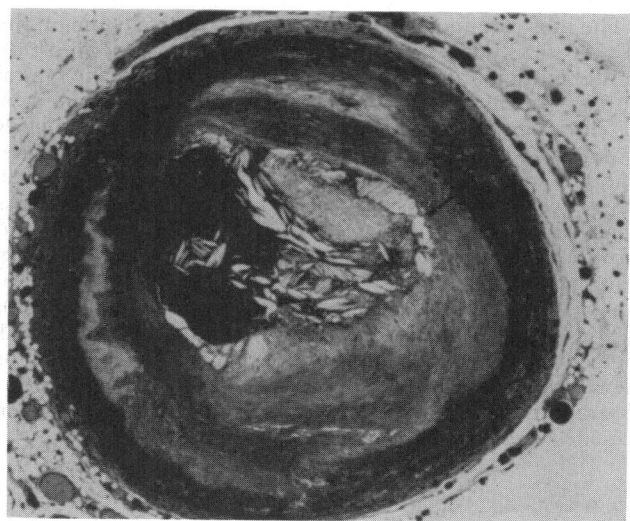

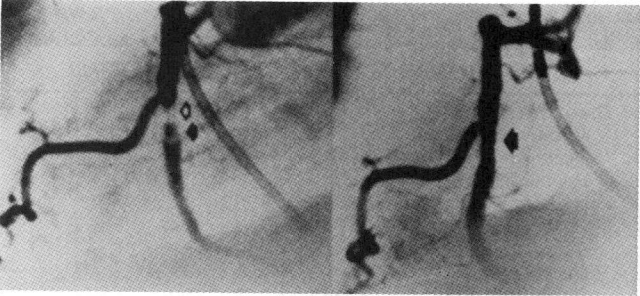

Figure 90–6. Coronary angiogram *(left)* of a right coronary stenosis *(open arrow)* and intraluminal thrombus (filling defect, *filled arrow*). After angioplasty and thrombolysis *(right)*, the stenosis is markedly improved and the clot has disappeared. (From Myler RK, Shaw RE, Stertzer SH, et al: Unstable angina and coronary angioplasty. Circulation 82[suppl II]:88–95, 1990, by permission of the American Heart Association, Inc.)

Figure 90–4. Photomicrograph of a histologic transverse section of a coronary artery with an occlusive thrombus overlying a fissured plaque. The thrombus (stained dark) within the lumen contains cholesterol crystals extruded from the plaque. Trichrome stain, × 20. (From Davies MJ: A macro and micro view of coronary vascular insult in ischemic heart disease. Circulation 82[suppl II]:38–46, 1990, by permission of the American Heart Association, Inc.)

erythrocyte-fibrin composition, and such clots are particularly sensitive to lysis by the intrinsic fibrinolytic system or exogenously administered agents.[11] Deeper injury (as would occur with plaque rupture, with extrusion of collagen and cholesterol esters) would attract more platelet deposition, with formation of more platelet-rich clots that may be more resistant to thrombolysis by intrinsic or exogenously administered agents.

Vasoconstriction

Diseased coronary arteries often have associated functional smooth muscle and are capable of vasoconstriction. It ap-

pears that platelet aggregation at the site of plaque disruption leads to the release of vasoactive compounds (serotonin, thromboxane A_2) that may narrow the vessel further and produce additional reduction in coronary flow.[12] The normal and intact endothelium protects against vasoconstriction by releasing a variety of vasodilating agents (e.g., prostacyclin and endothelium-derived relaxing factor). Coronary vessels that are even mildly atherosclerotic appear to lose their ability to resist vasoconstriction,[13] perhaps because of impaired production or release of endothelium-derived relaxing factor[14] and related compounds.

DIAGNOSIS OF UNSTABLE ANGINA PECTORIS AND ACUTE MYOCARDIAL INFARCTION

History

Certain characteristics of the chest discomfort of acute ischemia may permit differentiation from noncardiac causes of chest pain, but symptoms are often atypical and in some cases (perhaps 20%) silent.[15] Useful features that suggest acute ischemic pain include radiation of pain to the left shoulder or arm and pain of similar quality to that of the patient's usual exertional angina pectoris or a prior AMI. Features that suggest nonischemic pain include radiation to the back, abdomen, or legs; pain reproduced by palpation; or a "stabbing" quality of the discomfort.[16]

A wide variety of conditions (Table 90–2) may mimic the discomfort of acute myocardial ischemia; misdiagnosis may have catastrophic results (such as if anticoagulants and thrombolytic agents are given to a patient with a pericardial effusion or a dissecting aortic aneurysm). Algorithms have been developed for determining the likelihood of AMI in patients who present to the emergency room with chest pain. The most useful factors in distinguishing ischemic from nonischemic pain are the quality, location, and radiation of the chest pain; accompanying electrocardiographic features of ischemia; and abnormal cardiac enzyme levels during a 12-hour period of observation.[16] Additional diagnostic studies (such as transesophageal echocardiography or computed tomographic scanning for aortic dissection) are required in some patients to arrive at a firm diagnosis (Table 90–3).

Electrocardiogram

Acute myocardial ischemia usually but not invariably is associated with electrocardiographic changes, and a normal ECG may be found even with a documented myocardial infarction. Diagnostic changes on the ECG are most common

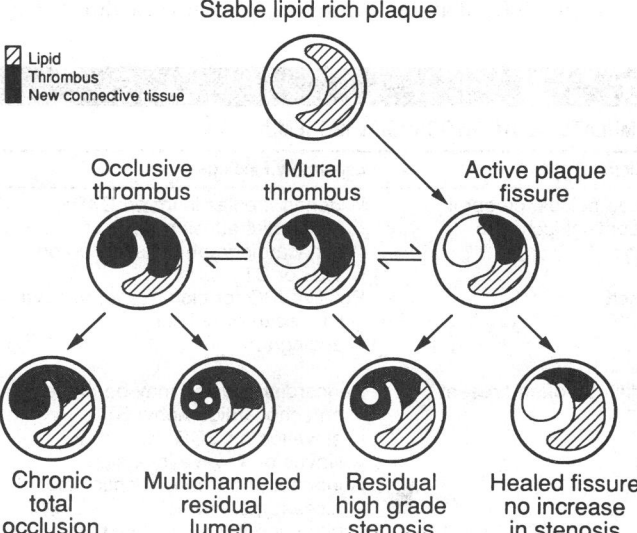

Stable lipid rich plaque

☑ Lipid
■ Thrombus
■ New connective tissue

Occlusive thrombus   Mural thrombus   Active plaque fissure

Chronic total occlusion   Multichanneled residual lumen   Residual high grade stenosis   Healed fissure no increase in stenosis

Figure 90–5. Diagrammatic representation of the progression, healing, and possible outcomes of an episode of plaque fissuring. (From Davies MJ: A macro and micro view of coronary vascular insult in ischemic heart disease. Circulation 82[suppl II]:38–46, 1990, by permission of the American Heart Association, Inc.)

TABLE 90-2

IMPORTANT NONCORONARY CAUSES OF CHEST PAIN

Cardiovascular
  Mitral valve prolapse
  Dissecting aortic aneurysm
  Pericarditis
  Hypertrophic cardiomyopathy
  Pulmonary arterial hypertension
  Aortic stenosis
Pulmonary
  Pulmonary embolus or infarction
  Pneumothorax or mediastinal emphysema
  Pleuritis
Neuromuscular
  Costochondritis and chest wall disorders
  Herpes zoster
  Nerve entrapment (radicular and thoracic outlet syndromes)
Psychologic
  Hyperventilation
  Neurosis or anxiety disorder
Gastrointestinal
  Esophageal reflex
  Gastritis
  Pancreatitis
  Gallbladder disease

with disease of the left anterior descending coronary artery (90%), followed by the disease of the right anterior descending coronary artery (70 to 80%) and left circumflex disease (50%).[17] Comparison with a prior ECG or one obtained when chest pain is absent is often useful in identifying ischemia as the cause of chest pain.

As a rule, ST elevation on the ECG implies transmural ischemia, usually caused by a reduction in flow in a large epicardial coronary artery as would be seen with vasospasm (variant angina) or acute thrombosis. ST depression usually indicates subendocardial ischemia, often produced by heightened myocardial oxygen demand in the setting of a fixed supply. Q waves usually indicate myocardial necrosis, although transient Q waves may be seen with severe but reversible ischemia.[18] The term Q wave infarct is now preferred to transmural infarct because some anatomic transmural infarcts do not produce Q waves and many nontransmural infarcts are associated with Q waves.[19]

The most common manifestation of acute ischemia on the ECG is an ST segment shift (either elevation or depression). In the setting of an occlusive coronary thrombus, the typical pattern on the ECG is initial T wave peaking, followed by ST elevation in the leads over the ischemic site and then R wave loss and the development of Q waves as necrosis occurs. The ST segment elevation then begins to recede, and T wave inversion follows (Fig. 90–7). Mirror image changes occur with posterior Q wave infarction (ST depression and growth in the size of R waves in leads V_1 and V_2). Right ventricular infarction is indicated on the ECG by ST elevation in leads applied to the right precordium (V_{3R} and V_{4R}).

Non–Q wave infarction usually is associated with ST segment and T wave abnormalities. Similar changes may be seen during pain in patients with UAP but the electrocardiographic pattern typically returns to baseline between episodes of pain.

Enzymes

When myocardial cells die, their cell membranes lose their integrity and intracellular enzymes diffuse out of the cell and enter the circulation. The attendant rise in serum levels of myocardial enzymes is the definitive determinant of whether or not infarction has occurred.[2] Although serum enzyme levels do not have perfect sensitivity or specificity (particularly a single determination of one enzyme), they are the mainstay of the diagnosis of AMI (Table 90–4).

Creatine kinase (CK) is found in abundance in brain and cardiac and skeletal muscle, with lesser amounts in the liver, kidney, spleen, lung, and gastrointestinal tract. Serum levels of CK are detectable 4 to 8 hours after AMI, peak at 12 to 24 hours, and return to normal in 3 to 4 days.[20] Peak levels do not correlate well with the size of an infarct because reperfusion can lead to more washout into the serum despite a smaller infarct. Muscle trauma of various types (intramuscular injection, cardioversion or defibrillation, rhabdomyolysis) may lead to CK release, as may a cerebrovascular accident or hypothyroidism.

The MB isoenzyme of CK is found only in trace amounts in skeletal muscle and other tissues, and its rise usually indicates myocardial necrosis. On occasion, elevated CK-MB levels are seen after strenuous exercise, in hypothyroidism, with the cardiomyopathies, and after cardiac trauma resulting from defibrillation, contusion, and myocarditis.[20] CK-

TABLE 90-3

CHARACTERISTICS OF CONDITIONS THAT MAY SIMULATE ACUTE MYOCARDIAL ISCHEMIA

Disease	History	Examination	Laboratory Findings*
Aortic dissection	Tearing, severe pain, often radiation to back	Diminished pulses, cerebral or abdominal ischemic damage	Widened mediastinum on CXR; pericardial effusion on echocardiography; dissection on TEE or CT
Pulmonary embolism	Risk factor for venous stasis (bed rest, cast, malignancy); dyspnea prominent	Tachypnea	Positive IPG for clot in legs; positive lung scan or pulmonary angiogram
Pericarditis	Positional and pleuritic pain	Pericardial rub often present	Pericardial effusion may be present on echocardiography; ST elevation on ECG without Q waves or T wave inversion
Gastrointestinal disorders	Discomfort related to meals or position (reflux)		Abnormal endoscopy (peptic ulcer disease); abnormal ultrasonography (gallbladder)
Pneumothorax	Abrupt onset of pleuritic chest pain and dyspnea	Unilateral diminished breath sounds	CXR confirmation

*CT = computed tomographic imaging; CXR = chest x-ray film; IPG = impedance plethysmography; TEE = transesophageal echocardiography.

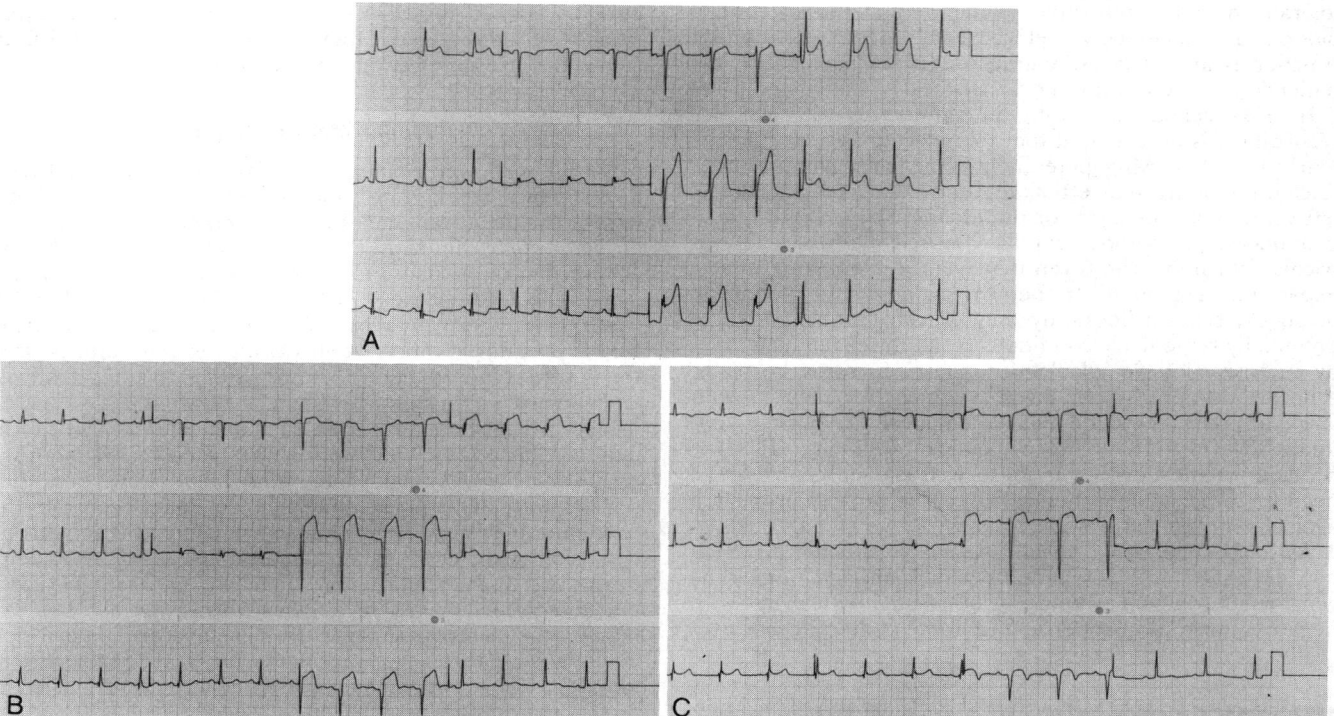

Figure 90–7. Evolutionary electrocardiographic changes in a patient with an acute anterior myocardial infarction. *A.* Hyperacute changes, with ST segment elevation and peaking of T waves. *B.* Twelve hours later. Development of Q waves. *C.* Ten days later. Development of T wave inversion with continued ST segment elevation. (Courtesy of Electrocardiographic Laboratory, Harper Hospital, Detroit, MI.)

MB is released into and cleared from the serum slightly faster than total CK. In less than 20% of patients with myocardial infarction, CK-MB levels are elevated but total CK levels do not exceed the normal range (although they may rise and fall). This so-called intranormal bump usually probably indicates a small but real degree of myocardial necrosis.[20]

Lactate dehydrogenase (LDH) and its five isoenzymes are found in most tissues as well as the heart. Isoenzyme LDH1 (and to a lesser extent LDH2) predominates in heart tissue, and skeletal muscle and liver have predominately LDH5. LDH1 is also found in erythrocytes, kidney, brain, stomach, and pancreas.[21] LDH appears in the serum 8 to 12 hours after myocardial infarction, peaks at 3 to 6 days, and returns to normal in 8 to 14 days. Determination of LDH levels is most useful if it is suspected that AMI occurred more than 24 hours previously and CK and CK-MB determinations are not diagnostic[20] (see Table 90–4). Because of the widespread occurrence of LDH in the body, greater reliability in diagnosing an infarct is achieved by looking at the LDH1/LDH2 ratio. A ratio greater than 1.0 is relatively sensitive and specific for myocardial necrosis.

Other serum enzymes (myoglobin, aspartate aminotransferase) appear in the serum after infarction, but they have limited clinical utility and should not be assessed routinely. It is important to emphasize that it takes time for any enzyme to appear in the serum, and it is typical for the serum enzyme levels to be normal in the early phases of a myocardial infarction; thus, at present a single normal enzyme value by no means excludes the possibility of AMI. It is hoped that in the future there will be such a laboratory test, perhaps assaying for the presence of the isoforms of enzymes.[22]

Echocardiography

Although two-dimensional echocardiography may detect a regional wall motion abnormality in the majority of patients with acute infarction (as well as demonstrate a transient regional abnormality during ischemia in patients with UAP), assessment of left ventricular function is not necessary in every patient with an acute ischemic syndrome. It is wasteful to obtain a multiplicity of ventricular function studies (e.g., echocardiography, radionuclide ventriculography, computed tomography, nuclear magnetic resonance imaging, and/or cardiac catheterization), because they all provide similar functional information.

In UAP, echocardiography is perhaps most useful for assessing ventricular performance in patients who appear clinically to have marginal function and who might not

---

TABLE 90–4

RECOMMENDATIONS FOR USE OF SERUM ENZYME DETERMINATIONS IN DIAGNOSIS OF PRESUMED ACUTE MYOCARDIAL INFARCTION

CK and CK-MB values should be obtained on admission and at 12 and 24 h later.

If AMI may have occurred more than 24 h before admission and if CK and CK-MB values are not diagnostic, total lactate dehydrogenase (LDH) value should be obtained.

If total LDH value is elevated, LDH isoenzyme values should be obtained; an LDH1/LDH2 ratio > 1.0 is indicative of AMI.

If chest pain recurs after admission, CK and CK-MB values should be obtained at 0, 12, and 24 h.

Routine use of enzyme determinations other than CK, CK-MB, and LDH is not recommended at present.

Adapted, with permission, from Lee TH, Goldman L, Serum enzyme assays in the diagnosis of acute myocardial infarction. Recommendations based on a quantitative analysis. Ann Intern Med 1986; 105:221–233.

tolerate negative inotropic agents (e.g., beta-adrenergic blockers and calcium channel blockers). Assessing ventricular function is an aid in estimating prognosis, particularly for patients who are to undergo CABG.

In AMI, echocardiography (in conjunction with Doppler recordings) is an essential tool for selected patients, particularly for identifying potentially remediable complications (including pericardial effusion, ventricular septal rupture, left ventricular aneurysm or pseudoaneurysm, mitral regurgitation with or without papillary muscle rupture, left ventricular thrombi, right ventricular infarction, and infarct expansion) (Fig. 90–8). In the AMI patient with hypotension or shock, echocardiography may quickly distinguish these potentially remediable conditions from power failure caused by extensive left ventricular infarction. In some hospitals, echocardiography is employed routinely for patients with large infarcts (based on eletrocardiographic findings and total CK level > 1000 IU/L or CK-MB level > 150 IU/L) to provide prognostic information as well as data regarding the need for anticoagulant therapy to treat or provide protection against ventricular thrombi.[2]

As in UAP patients, assessment of ventricular function may be useful in AMI patients with suspected borderline ventricular function who are to be treated with drugs with negative inotropic properties. In some centers, echocardi-

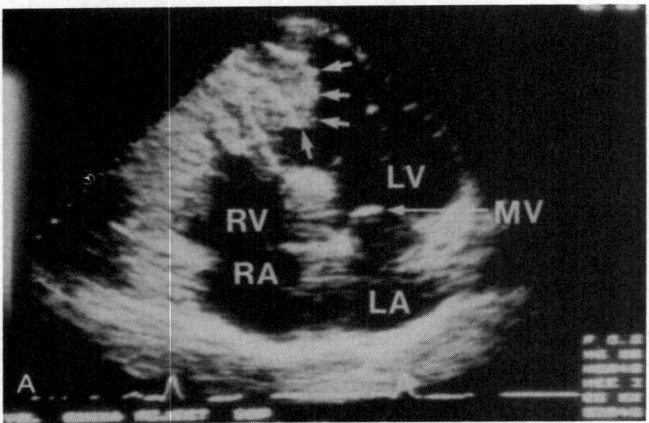

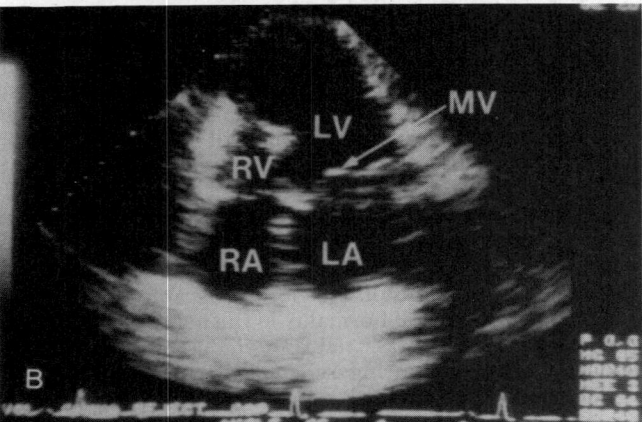

Figure 90–8. Apical four-chamber views of two-dimensional echocardiograms in patients with (arrows, A) and without (B) left ventricular mural thrombosis. LA = left atrium; LV = left ventricle; MV = mitral valve; RA = right atrium; RV = right ventricle. (From Turpie AG, Robinson JG, Doyle DJ, et al: Comparison of high-dose with low-dose subcutaneous heparin to prevent left ventricular mural thrombosis in patients with acute anterior myocardial infarction. Reprinted, by permission of the New England Journal of Medicine, 320; 352–357, 1989.)

ography is used for all AMI patients to help in estimating prognosis, although its superiority over other clinical indicators and exercise testing is not established.

Radionuclide Techniques

Radionuclide ventriculography, like echocardiography, allows assessment of global and regional biventricular function. It has the advantage of providing quantitative estimates of ventricular function in virtually all patients, whereas echocardiography may yield inadequate images in 10 to 15% of patients (e.g., because of body habitus or lung disease). Coupled with use of a bicycle ergometer, it may provide useful prognostic information during exercise and is used for postinfarction patients.[23] It has the disadvantages of cost and radiation exposure.

Myocardial perfusion agents such as thallium-201 or technetium-99m isonitrile derivatives are taken up by the myocardium in proportion to regional blood flow, and thus regions with ischemia or infarction do not concentrate the compounds. Differentiation of ischemic from necrotic tissue is possible with serial resting thallium-201 imaging by demonstrating "redistribution" or "filling in" of an initial defect in subsequent images in regions with ischemia but not infarction. For the most part, however, myocardial perfusion imaging is performed during and after dynamic exercise to look for regions with reversible ischemia (particularly in the postinfarction patient).[24]

Infarct-avid agents such as technetium-99m pyrophosphate or antimyosin antibody fragments can detect, localize, and quantitate necrotic tissue.[25] Disadvantages include lack of significant accumulation before 24 hours after infarction, relative insensitivity in non–Q wave infarction, and inability to distinguish new from old large infarcts. This technique usually is reserved for uncommon situations in which the diagnosis of possible AMI remains unclear 1 to 3 days after the suspected infarct.

MANAGEMENT: GENERAL MEASURES
Monitoring

After initial evaluation and stabilization in the emergency department, patients with acute ischemia should be transferred expeditiously to the cardiac or intensive care unit. In some cases it may be appropriate to admit the patient to a unit with a lower intensity of care (observation or step-down unit) if the initial symptoms are atypical or the clinical presentation suggests a stable course. In either case, continuous electrocardiographic monitoring is mandatory for the early detection and treatment of arrhythmias. A modified lead V_1 is employed routinely, coupled to a visual monitor and often a computerized, automated arrhythmia detection unit. In other cases, particularly when the patient is unstable or hypotensive, the patient may be transferred directly to the cardiac catheterization laboratory and only later to the cardiac care unit.

Electrocardiographic monitoring is discontinued after 12 to 24 hours in patients who have not had an AMI and after 48 to 72 hours in those who have, unless they manifest hemodynamic instability, persistent ischemia, or arrhythmia.[2, 16]

Activity

Patients with acute ischemia are placed at bed rest, usually with permission for either a bedside commode or bathroom privileges. Activity is advanced as tolerated; with the more aggressive management strategies currently employed, AMI patients are often ambulant within several days after admission to the hospital. This is in marked contrast to management policies of only a few decades ago, when patients were put at bed rest for an extended length of time.

The duration of total hospitalization for AMI has fallen progressively during the last few decades. Typical length of stay may be as short as 5 to 6 days for an uncomplicated infarct. Selected patients undergoing successful reperfusion therapy have been discharged in as few as 3 days, although this is not yet the established standard of care in the United States.[26]

Diet

Patients usually are given a clear or full liquid diet for the first 24 hours, except for patients who may need to go urgently to the cardiac catheterization laboratory or those who are nauseated from their infarct or analgesic agents, who are given nothing by mouth. The diet is advanced on the second day to a low-cholesterol diet with no added salt. Dietary instruction by the dietitian or nurse (for both the patient and family) at the time of hospitalization for acute ischemia is extremely valuable because the patient and family usually are highly motivated to prevent future problems.

MANAGEMENT: SPECIFIC MEASURES
Hemodynamic Monitoring

A balloon flotation right-sided heart catheter is required in a minority of patients with UAP or AMI, usually in the setting of low cardiac output, hypotension, cardiogenic shock, and/or pulmonary edema (Table 90–5). It is particularly useful in clarifying the etiology of circulatory insufficiency and distinguishing among hypovolemia, left ventricular contractile dysfunction, right ventricular infarction, ventricular septal rupture, mitral regurgitation, and cardiac tamponade. Adjunctive noninvasive evaluation (including two-dimensional echocardiography and the radionuclide techniques) may complement the clinical and hemodynamic assessment.

Intra-arterial pressure monitoring is employed principally in the setting of severe hypotension (Table 90–6). Although the radial artery is often cannulated for pressure measurement, this pressure may be falsely low in cardiogenic shock because of peripheral vasoconstriction. If such a situation is

---

TABLE 90–5

INDICATIONS FOR BALLOON FLOTATION CATHETER IN ACUTE MYOCARDIAL ISCHEMIA

Definite
   Severe or progressive congestive heart failure
   Cardiogenic shock or progressive hypotension
   Mechanical complications of AMI
      Ventricular septal defect
      Mitral regurgitation
Possible
   Hypotension not responding to fluid administration
   Before giving fluids to a patient with suspected pulmonary
      congestion
   Stable AMI patients with mild pulmonary congestion
   Monitoring intravenous vasodilator or inotropic therapy

Adapted from Gunnar RM, Passamani ER, Bourdillon PD, et al: Guidelines for the early management of patients with acute myocardial infarction. A report of the American College of Cardiology/American Heart Association Task Force on Assessment of Diagnostic and Therapeutic Cardiovascular Procedures (Subcommittee to Develop Guidelines for the Early Management of Patients with Acute Myocardial Infarction). Reprinted with permission from the American College of Cardiology (Journal of the American College of Cardiology, 1990, Vol 16, pp 249–292).

TABLE 90–6

INDICATIONS FOR ARTERIAL PRESSURE MONITORING IN ACUTE MYOCARDIAL ISCHEMIA

Definite
   Patients with severe hypotension (<80 mm Hg) or cardiogenic
      shock
   Patients receiving vasopressor agents
Possible
   Patients receiving intravenous vasodilators
   Patients receiving intravenous inotropic agents
   Patients with life-threatening arrhythmias
   Patients requiring frequent arterial blood gas determinations
      (e.g., for management of a respirator)

Adapted from Gunnar RM, Passamani ER, Bourdillon PD, et al: Guidelines for the early management of patients with acute myocardial infarction. A report of the American College of Cardiology/American Heart Association Task Force on Assessment of Diagnostic and Therapeutic Cardiovascular Procedures (Subcommittee to Develop Guidelines for the Early Management of Patients with Acute Myocardial Infarction). Reprinted with permission from the American College of Cardiology (Journal of the American College of Cardiology, 1990, Vol 16, pp 249–292).

---

suspected, a central artery (e.g., femoral) should be employed. Central intra-arterial pressure monitoring often is used in patients receiving vasopressor agents for a similar reason.

More controversial is whether direct arterial pressure monitoring is required for patients receiving intravenous vasodilators and inotropic agents. Although some patients require such direct monitoring, many can be treated without incident with indirect blood pressure determinations, particularly when an automated blood pressure device is used.

Oxygen

Supplemental oxygen is administered routinely for the acute ischemic syndromes because patients who have otherwise uncomplicated courses may be modestly hypoxemic initially, presumably on the basis of pulmonary ventilation-perfusion mismatches. More intensive management (endotracheal intubation and mechanical ventilation) is required for only a minority of patients (such as those in fulminant pulmonary edema or cardiogenic shock).

Nitrates

Nitroglycerin has long been a mainstay of the treatment of acute myocardial ischemia. Its principal action is as a venodilator; it acts as an arteriolar dilator only in high doses. Nitroglycerin's beneficial effects are due to dilatation of epicardial coronary arteries, reduction of venous return (preload), and enhancement of collateral flow into the ischemic region. Nitroglycerin is used most commonly to relieve ischemic pain; it has a lesser role in limiting infarct size. The major serious side effect of nitrates is hypotension; the principal minor side effect is headache. Because of the deleterious effects of hypotension during acute ischemia, nitroglycerin is relatively contraindicated in patients with systolic blood pressure less than 90 mm Hg, in the setting of marked bradycardia or tachycardia, and in patients with suspected right ventricular infarction (who are highly dependent on an adequate venous return to maintain an acceptable cardiac output).[2]

Only preparations with rapid onset and offset of activity (sublingual, topical, and intravenous) should be used in the acute setting; long-acting nitrates are reserved for the convalescent and outpatient phases of management. For the initial management of ischemic pain, one or more sublingual nitroglycerin tablets are often employed, but for the pro-

TABLE 90–7

TYPICAL DOSES OF NITRATES FOR ACUTE MYOCARDIAL ISCHEMIA

Agent	Dose
Intravenous nitroglycerin	10–300 μg/min
2% nitroglycerin ointment	0.5–2 inches q 4–8 h
Transdermal nitroglycerin	0.1–0.6 mg/h (5–30 cm² q 24 h)
Isosorbide dinitrate (oral)	10–40 mg q 6 h
Sublingual nitroglycerin	0.3–0.4 mg q 5 min × 3

phylaxis or treatment of recurrent ischemia, intravenous nitroglycerin is preferred (Table 90–7). Invasive monitoring of blood and filling pressures is not required unless the patient has complicating factors (e.g., hypotension, possible right ventricular infarction). An infusion pump is mandatory, and initial doses of 10 to 20 μg/min can be increased as necessary to achieve pain relief or until incipient hypotension or tachycardia appears. There is no absolute upper dose limit, but additional pharmacologic or other intervention usually is indicated if good pain relief is not achieved with 200 to 300 μg/min. Simultaneous administration of acetaminophen usually helps to reduce headache. Once an adequate response has been achieved and before the patient is transferred out of the unit, intravenous nitroglycerin should be changed to a topical (e.g., ointment) or long-acting oral form. Tolerance of the effects of nitrates occurs with continued use, and an intermittent dosing schedule with oral forms should be instituted as soon as the patient's condition is sufficiently stable.

Although there have been relatively few randomized studies of the efficacy of nitrates in UAP, clinical experience confirms their benefits. Best effects are achieved with intravenous therapy, often with concomitant beta-adrenergic blocker therapy.[27]

Nitroglycerin is used routinely in patients with suspected or documented AMI, but the rationale for doing so is somewhat controversial. Although there is no doubt about the efficacy of nitrates in relieving ischemic pain, their routine use is usually prompted by a desire to reduce infarct size and mortality. The available data do not support the common practice of giving intravenous nitroglycerin to all patients with acute myocardial infarction, although intravenous nitroglycerin may reduce infarct size and mortality in some patients. We find it to be of greatest benefit when it is given to patients with moderate or large AMIs (especially anterior in location) who present soon after the onset of pain.[2, 28, 29] There are relatively sparse data regarding the use of nitrates after thrombolytic therapy. Although limited data suggest some beneficial effect on left ventricular function,[30] nitroglycerin has been implicated as a cause of heparin resistance.[31] If nitroglycerin is used in this setting, it is important to ensure an adequate anticoagulation effect.

Lidocaine

Lidocaine is the drug of choice for treating serious arrhythmias in the setting of acute ischemia. Ventricular tachycardia and other complex ventricular arrhythmias often respond to lidocaine administration. Although the risk of ventricular fibrillation is reduced by about one third by the routine use of lidocaine in the AMI setting, overall mortality is not, perhaps because of an increased risk of asystole.[2, 32] Therapy with lidocaine usually is initiated with a loading dose of 1 mg/kg (not to exceed 100 mg), followed 20 to 30 minutes later by a second bolus of 0.5 mg/kg, although on rare occasions cadditional boluses are required at 10-minute

intervals until a total dose of 4 mg/kg is given.[2] To maintain adequate plasma levels, an infusion of 20 to 50 μg/kg/min (usually around 2 to 4 mg/min) is started. Lidocaine is metabolized by the liver, and elimination is prolonged in patients with liver disease; the half-life of elimination is also prolonged in patients with AMI, in the elderly, in patients in congestive heart failure, and in patients in shock, and an appropriate dose reduction is required. Lidocaine levels usually begin to increase after 24 hours or so, and a reduction in infusion rate of 1 mg/min or more at 12 hours after initiating therapy is desirable. Side effects usually are neurologic, and common manifestations include confusion, paresthesias, dizziness, tremor, slurred speech, and seizure activity.

Asymptomatic ventricular arrhythmias of one form or another are common in stable CAD, and although their presence usually indicates an increased risk of mortality, treatment of the arrhythmia may actually decrease survival, presumably by a proarrhythmic side effect.[33] Thus, ventricular arrhythmias usually are treated in the chronic setting only if symptomatic.

In the setting of acute ischemia, the threshold for precipitating ventricular fibrillation is lower and there is more rationale for treating asymptomatic arrhythmias. Because the available data do not support routine prophylactic use of lidocaine, it should be used only in certain settings in which its benefits outweigh its potential or actual risks (Table 90–8). We usually discontinue lidocaine after 24 to 48 hours, and often no further antiarrhythmic therapy is required.

If treatment of ventricular arrhythmias is necessary but lidocaine is not effective, procainamide is the next agent usually employed. A loading dose of 10 to 15 mg/kg (not to exceed 1000 mg total, or an infusion rate of 50 mg/min) followed by a maintenance dose of 20 to 80 μg/kg/min often is effective. However, the likelihood of other side effects (proarrhythmia, conduction defects, hypotension) is somewhat higher than with lidocaine.

Analgesia

The pain associated with acute ischemia is important therapeutically for several reasons. It usually is a manifestation of ongoing ischemia and can be used as a barometer of the efficacy of therapy unless it is due to another process (pericarditis, pulmonary embolism, reflex esophagitis). Continuing pain should ordinarily lead to intensification of the anti-ischemic program, with additional pharmacologic (e.g., beta-adrenergic blockers and calcium channel blockers), mechanical (intra-aortic balloon pump, angioplasty), or surgical (CABG) therapy. In addition, pain leads to an increase in

TABLE 90–8

INDICATIONS FOR INTRAVENOUS LIDOCAINE IN ACUTE MYOCARDIAL ISCHEMIA

Sustained ventricular tachycardia or fibrillation
Ventricular premature depolarizations that are
   Frequent (>6/min)
   Closely coupled (R on T)
   Multiform in configuration or occurring in bursts of three or
   more in succession

Adapted from Gunnar RM, Passamani ER, Bourdillon PD, et al: Guidelines for the early management of patients with acute myocardial infarction. A report of the American College of Cardiology/American Heart Association Task Force on Assessment of Diagnostic and Therapeutic Cardiovascular Procedures (Subcommittee to Develop Guidelines for the Early Management of Patients with Acute Myocardial Infarction). Reprinted with permission from the American College of Cardiology (Journal of the American College of Cardiology, 1990, Vol 16, pp 249–292).

myocardial oxygen demand through sympathetic stimulation (tachycardia, hypertension, increased contractility) and thus can worsen the supply-demand imbalance.

Intravenous morphine sulfate in 2- to 5-mg doses is the drug of choice and should be given in sufficient quantities to relieve pain and anxiety (along with specific anti-ischemic therapy). Additional benefits include venous and arterial vasodilatation, with an attendant fall in preload and afterload.

Calcium Channel Blockers

Calcium channel blocking agents act to dilate coronary and systemic arteries, often resulting in enhanced myocardial perfusion and peripheral vasodilation. Their beneficial effects in acute ischemia result from both an improvement in myocardial blood flow and a reduction in demand by reducing wall tension (and, to a lesser extent, heart rate and contractility). There is speculation that their use may favorably influence the cellular calcium overload that occurs during infarction and that they may ameliorate the resulting myocyte necrosis. Although the drugs are negative inotropic agents, in most cases the contractile depression is compensated for by reflex sympathetic stimulation as a consequence of vasodilation. Patients with obvious or incipient congestive heart failure ordinarily should be treated with other agents, and even patients without manifest failure but with ventricular depression should be treated with calcium channel blockers with caution.

There are important differences among the various agents. The dihydropyridines (nifedipine, nicardipine) are potent vasodilators, whereas verapamil has more effect on atrioventricular conduction, explaining its efficacy in supraventricular arrhythmias. Combining a dihydropyridine agent with a beta-adrenergic blocker may limit the potentially deleterious increase in heart rate that occurs with monotherapy.

These agents are often successful in reducing or eliminating recurrent episodes of rest pain in UAP, particularly in the setting of coronary spasm without underlying CAD (Prinzmetal's angina). The use of nifedipine alone (without a concomitant beta-adrenergic blocker) is not recommended except in Prinzmetal's angina, because it appears to be ineffective and possibly detrimental in routine UAP.[34, 35]

Assessing the overall benefit of calcium channel blockers in UAP has been hindered by the relatively small number of well-designed randomized trials. What is noteworthy is the contrast between the apparent acute clinical benefit of verapamil, diltiazem, and nifedipine plus a beta-adrenergic blocker and the lack of a long-term beneficial effect in preventing subsequent infarction or death.[36–38] Thus, although calcium channel blockers may help to stabilize a patient with UAP, more definitive therapy is eventually required in many patients. This often requires revascularization with either PTCA or CABG.

As in UAP, there have been surprisingly few adequate controlled clinical trials of the routine use of calcium channel blockers in the AMI setting.[38, 39] The largest reported experience has been with nifedipine, usually as monotherapy without a concomitant beta-adrenergic blocker. Over a dozen studies involving almost 10,000 patients with threatened or confirmed AMI have demonstrated no benefit of nifedipine in preventing progression to AMI; limiting infarct size; or reducing mortality, reinfarction rates, or the frequency of postinfarction angina.[38–40] Four of the trials are large, so it is unlikely that the negative results are due to a type II error. Several trials have even suggested higher mortality in patients receiving nifedipine. Nifedipine also had no obvious

beneficial effect on ventricular function or recurrent ischemia when given with thrombolytic therapy.[41]

About a half-dozen clinical trials are available to assess the benefit of verapamil in AMI and a minority are of adequate sample size.[36, 38, 39] Only one study (the second Danish Trial, DAVIT-II) suggested a beneficial effect of verapamil and only in preventing reinfarction in patients without heart failure.[42] Taken together, the available data do not support the routine use of verapamil in the AMI setting because early outcome (including mortality) is not unequivocally improved and infarct size is not reduced.[38, 39] The early use of verapamil (especially when given intravenously) may be harmful, because one study found an increased risk of sinoatrial arrest and atrioventricular block.[38]

Only a few adequate studies of diltiazem in AMI are available. Overall, diltiazem has not been demonstrated to have a major beneficial effect in AMI, and it may be associated with an increased risk of sinoatrial arrest and atrioventricular conduction block.[2] It is only in the subgroup of patients with non–Q wave AMI that diltiazem may be of some benefit.[40] In patients with non–Q wave AMI who do not have large infarcts, depressed left ventricular function, and especially pulmonary congestion, diltiazem appears to reduce the incidence of early reinfarction and recurrent severe angina pectoris.[43–46] Diltiazem has been found to have a deleterious effect in patients with non–Q wave AMI and depressed left ventricular function.[46]

The lack of convincing evidence to support the routine use of calcium channel blockers in AMI (except for non–Q wave AMI patients without left ventricular contractile dysfunction) should not negate their short-term benefits in treating postinfarction angina. Although adequate data from controlled clinical trials are not available, calcium channel blockers (especially diltiazem) seem to be useful clinically in treating AMI patients with postinfarction angina, particularly if coronary arteriography and acute interventional therapy are unavailable or contraindicated. Monotherapy with nifedipine probably should not be used in this setting under almost any circumstances. There are insufficient data to know whether any of the calcium channel blockers are of particular benefit or hazard when given after thrombolytic therapy.[47]

Virtually all of the reported experience has been obtained with the regular dosage forms of the calcium channel blockers; the sustained-release forms usually are not used in the acute setting. In the case of nifedipine, the use of a sustained-release form theoretically might be beneficial if it avoided an acute drug effect with hypotension, but the potential risks of a sustained drug effect if a complication develops usually militate against using such long-acting forms.

Nifedipine (almost always with a beta-adrenergic blocker) is given in divided doses of 40 to 120 mg/d. Verapamil is not used frequently in the cardiac or intensive care unit setting (except intravenously for supraventricular arrhythmias), but when employed it usually is given in divided oral doses of 360 mg/d. Diltiazem usually is used in doses of 60 to 90 mg four times a day (240 to 360 mg/d) (Table 90–9).

Beta-Adrenergic Blockers

Beta-adrenergic blockers have multiple actions that are of variable benefit during acute ischemia, including the following:

1. Reducing myocardial oxygen demand by lowering heart rate, blood pressure, and contractility
2. Blocking adverse effects of catecholamines
3. Reducing platelet aggregation

TABLE 90–9

TYPICAL DOSES OF CALCIUM CHANNEL BLOCKERS FOR ACUTE MYOCARDIAL ISCHEMIA

Agent	Dose
Verapamil	80–120 mg t.i.d. or q.i.d.
Diltiazem	60–90 mg t.i.d. or q.i.d.
Nifedipine	10–30 mg t.i.d. or q.i.d.
Nicardipine	20–40 mg t.i.d.

4. Improving myocardial blood flow (at least by prolonging diastole by reducing heart rate)
5. Antiarrhythmic properties

Because of these actions, these agents can ameliorate the deleterious effects of ischemia by reducing nutrient demand and improving coronary blood flow. They decrease mortality by reducing arrhythmias, myocardial damage, and complications such as myocardial rupture.[2, 38]

The initial use of beta-adrenergic blockers in UAP antedated current understanding of the syndrome and the importance of a primary reduction in perfusion in its pathogenesis; it was previously held that UAP was merely a more severe form of demand-type angina pectoris, and thus it seemed logical to use a drug clearly efficacious in reducing the determinants of myocardial oxygen demand. Because UAP is now thought to be due to a primary reduction in perfusion (resulting from plaque fissuring, coronary vasospasm, and/or labile thrombus formation), the rationale for using a beta-adrenergic blocker is more equivocal (although reducing demand would seem to be beneficial even if the primary problem is a reduction in myocardial nutrient supply).

Although clinical experience indicates that beta-adrenergic blockers are of some value in the management of UAP, there have been relatively few adequate clinical trials with sufficiently large populations of patients to form firm conclusions.[37] The pooled results of the available studies suggest that beta-adrenergic blockers in UAP have no more than a modest effect in preventing subsequent AMI (about a 13% reduction) and no definite effect on reducing mortality.[37] Furthermore, most of the trials are confounded by the simultaneous administration of long-acting nitrates. On the other hand, UAP caused by coronary spasm (Prinzmetal's angina) is invariably worsened by the use of these agents; an increase in ischemia after the use of beta-adrenergic blockers should suggest the possibility of coronary vasospasm.

In the AMI setting, on the other hand, the benefits of beta-adrenergic blockers are clear. Beneficial effects occur with both early and late treatment in the following periods:

1. An early treatment period (within the first few hours of infarction), with therapy designed to limit infarct size as well as reduce the risk of complications and reduce mortality.
2. A late treatment period (commencing days to weeks after completed infarction), designed to reduce the risk of reinfarction as well as complications and mortality.

In more than two dozen trials an intravenous beta-adrenergic blocker has been used within 12 hours of onset of AMI.[38, 39] Pooled data from these trials suggest that treatment can reduce early mortality by 13%, nonfatal infarction by 19%, and nonfatal cardiac arrest by 16%. Mortality appears to be reduced most when treatment is given early, and it appears that the principal reason for lowered mortality is the prevention of cardiac rupture.[38] The benefits of beta-adrenergic blockers extend to patients receiving thrombolytic therapy, in whom fewer nonfatal reinfarctions and recurrent ischemic events are seen with therapy.[48]

Assessing the degree of infarct limitation is difficult in the clinical setting (in contrast to an experimental animal model), because the best method for measuring infarct size (histologic) cannot be used with patients. Furthermore, the available studies differ in study design and methodology. Nevertheless, early beta-adrenergic blocker therapy appears to have a modest effect in limiting infarct size.[38]

Beneficial effects of a variety of beta-adrenergic blockers (both cardioselective and noncardioselective) have been reported, with no clear advantage of one agent over another.[2] An ultra–short-acting agent has some theoretic appeal, although no firm data are available.[49] Because there are theoretic reasons for questioning the use of agents with intrinsic sympathomimetic activity, their use ordinarily is proscribed.

Because of the modest benefit of beta-adrenergic blockers and their potential for serious side effects, they are given most commonly when there is evidence of excess sympathetic stimulation (manifested by tachycardia or systolic hypertension) and no evidence of incipient or actual left ventricular decompensation and heart failure. The numerous absolute and relative contraindications to beta-adrenergic blockers (Table 90–10) should be borne in mind. Because of these contraindications, less than half of the patients receiving thrombolytic therapy are eligible for a beta-adrenergic blocker.[50]

Oral beta-adrenergic blocker therapy started after the acute phase (so-called secondary prevention) has been studied in several placebo-controlled trials involving over 35,000 patients. Long-term therapy begun within the first few days after an infarction and continued for at least 2 years results in about a one fourth reduction in reinfarction and mortality.[38] The benefit appears to be the same regardless of infarct location, size, and type (Q wave or non–Q wave) and age of the patient.[39] Both sudden mortality and nonsudden mortality are reduced, suggesting a beneficial effect in reducing both ischemia and arrhythmias. Even patients with mild and compensated congestive heart failure seem to derive benefit.[51] Low-risk patients appear to derive benefits as well as high-risk patients,[52] but side effects (fatigue, sexual dysfunction) may be problematic enough to outweigh the benefits in very low risk patients.[2]

Most studies of beta-adrenergic blockers have used relatively large doses. Intravenous regimens include metoprolol,

TABLE 90–10

CONTRAINDICATIONS TO BETA-ADRENERGIC BLOCKER THERAPY

Definite
 Heart rate < 60 beats/min, especially if there is evidence of sinus node dysfunction
 Systolic blood pressure < 100 mm Hg
 Moderate or severe left ventricular failure
 Signs of peripheral hypoperfusion
 Severe chronic obstructive pulmonary disease
 Atrioventricular conduction abnormalities
Possible
 History of asthma
 Severe peripheral vascular disease
 Insulin-dependent diabetes mellitus
 Concurrent use of verapamil or diltiazem

Adapted from Gunnar RM, Passamani ER, Bourdillon PD, et al: Guidelines for the early management of patients with acute myocardial infarction. A report of the American College of Cardiology/American Heart Association Task Force on Assessment of Diagnostic and Therapeutic Cardiovascular Procedures (Subcommittee to Develop Guidelines for the Early Management of Patients with Acute Myocardial Infarction). Reprinted with permission from the American College of Cardiology (Journal of the American College of Cardiology, 1990, Vol 16, pp 249–292).

TABLE 90-11

TYPICAL DOSES OF BETA-ADRENERGIC BLOCKERS FOR MYOCARDIAL ISCHEMIA

Agent	Oral	Intravenous
Propranolol	40–80 mg q.i.d.	
Metoprolol	50–100 mg b.i.d.	5 mg q 5 min × 3
Timolol	10–20 mg b.i.d.	
Nadolol	40–80 mg q.d.	
Atenolol	50–100 mg q.d.	5 mg × 1 or 2

5 mg every 2 to 5 minutes for a total of up to 15 mg, atenolol, 5 mg once or twice, and propranolol, 5 to 8 mg given during 10 to 15 minutes (although this use of intravenous propranolol is not approved by the Food and Drug Administration) (Table 90–11). Esmolol offers the theoretic advantages of a short duration of action, but there are insufficient data for a firm conclusion regarding its use.[49]

Thrombolytic Therapy

Because of the likely role of thrombus in the pathogenesis of UAP and its central role in AMI, there has been great interest in treatment strategies for lysing intracoronary thrombi. Although the body's intrinsic fibrinolytic system usually partially or completely dissolves clots that cause infarcts, it often takes 1 to 2 days to weeks for this to occur. Work with animal models suggests that lysis must occur within as little as 1 to 2 hours for reperfusion of an occluded coronary bed to be effective in salvaging myocardium otherwise destined for necrosis.[53] These data cannot be extrapolated directly to humans, but they suggest the conceptual approach of "speeding up" the body's natural thrombolytic system by administering exogenous agents.

Three such agents currently are available for use in the United States, and additional thrombolytic agents are on the horizon.[54] Each agent activates the fibrinolytic system at a different point. Recombinant single-chain tissue plasminogen activator (TPA), like the compound produced normally by the body, cleaves plasminogen into the active enzyme plasmin, which degrades the fibrin in clots into degradation products and produces clot dissolution. Naturally occurring TPA (and commercially produced recombinant TPA for that matter) is largely inactive unless complexed with fibrin-bound plasminogen; this keeps the natural fibrinolytic system in check and prevents activation of unbound circulating plasminogen, which would produce continuous fibrinogen-olysis and a systemic lytic state. Although recombinant TPA is relatively "clot specific" and leads to less fibrinogenolysis than other lytic agents, it is not specific for the thrombi in coronary arteries; it dissolves any clot (including hemostatic plugs at puncture sites or in the cerebral circulation), and serious bleeding is no less common than with the other agents.[55]

Streptokinase, a bacterial protease, combines with bound and unbound (circulating) plasminogen and thus degrades the fibrin in clots as well as circulating fibrinogen, producing a systemic lytic state. Anisoylated plasminogen–streptokinase activator complex (APSAC) is activated only after binding to fibrin, but once activated it produces a systemic lytic state similar to that with streptokinase (in the doses ordinarily employed). Urokinase and the related compounds prourokinase and single-chain urokinase–plasminogen activator directly activate plasminogen, although these agents currently are not approved for use as intravenous thrombolytic agents for coronary thrombosis.

The initial method of administration of thrombolytics was intracoronary. Reperfusion may be achieved in about three fourths of AMI patients, but there has been no clear beneficial impact on mortality; pooled data from several trials reveal a nonsignificant 18% lower mortality in patients so treated.[38, 56] Additional disadvantages include expense, logistic problems related to the availability of cardiac catheterization laboratories and trained staff, and the need to transport seriously ill patients.[2] For all of these reasons, intracoronary thrombolysis currently is used only as adjunctive therapy during PTCA and rarely as the primary intervention.

Currently, the preferred method of administration of thrombolytic therapy is intravenous. Several well-designed, large, prospective controlled trials have shown that early administration of intravenous thrombolytic therapy reduces mortality by one fourth to one third after acute Q wave AMI associated with ST elevation.[57–63] Whether a similar benefit occurs in patients with non–Q wave AMI or UAP is not yet established, and trials are under way.

Selection of Patients

Whether all patients with AMI should receive thrombolytic therapy is controversial.[57] The benefit of therapy has been conclusively established in the subset of patients less than 75 years of age who present within 6 hours of symptom onset with electrocardiographic evidence of at least a moderate-sized anterior infarct (and who lack other specific contraindications). Although a 25 to 30% reduction in mortality can be expected in this subgroup, it constitutes a minority of patients hospitalized with AMI. Only about one third of hospitalized AMI patients are considered to be eligible for thrombolysis and only half of them actually receive therapy (Fig. 90–9). The remaining two thirds are considered to be ineligible because of age (>75 years), late presentation (>4 to 6 hours), nondiagnostic ECG, or other contraindication (Table 90–12).[57] Yet mortality overall is lowest in the group of patients without contraindications to lytic therapy and highest in those who are thought to have contraindications, particularly advanced age or late presentation. In these groups the mortality rate approaches 25%[64] (Fig. 90–10).

Age has long been considered a relative but strong contraindication to lytic therapy, and many of the larger trials excluded elderly patients because they are at increased risk of bleeding (especially intracranial). In the trials in which elderly patients were included, there appeared to be a

Total Population=675,000

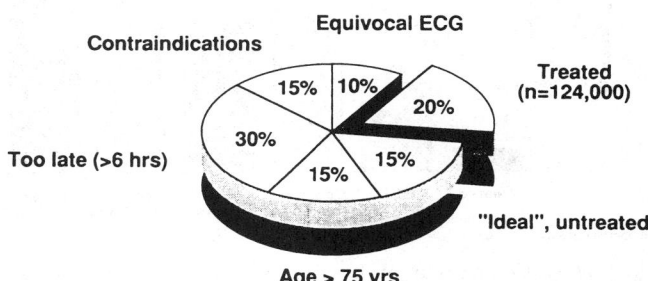

Figure 90–9. Approximate proportions of patients eligible and ineligible for thrombolysis according to traditional recommendations and practices. (Reproduced, with permission, from Muller DWM, Topol EJ, Selection of patients with acute myocardial infarction for thrombolytic therapy. Ann Intern Med 1990; 113:949–960.)

TABLE 90-12

CONTRAINDICATIONS TO THROMBOLYTIC THERAPY

Active internal bleeding
Suspected aortic dissection
Prolonged or traumatic cardiopulmonary resuscitation
Recent head trauma or known intracranial neoplasm
Diabetic hemorrhagic retinopathy or other hemorrhagic
　ophthalmologic condition
Pregnancy
History of hemorrhagic cerebrovascular accident

Adapted from Gunnar RM, Passamani ER, Bourdillon PD, et al: Guidelines for the early management of patients with acute myocardial infarction. A report of the American College of Cardiology/American Heart Association Task Force on Assessment of Diagnostic and Therapeutic Cardiovascular Procedures (Subcommittee to Develop Guidelines for the Early Management of Patients with Acute Myocardial Infarction). Reprinted with permission from the American College of Cardiology (Journal of the American College of Cardiology, 1990, Vol 16, pp 249–292).

greater lowering of mortality in the elderly patients than in the younger patients.[50, 58] Until further data become available, age should not be considered a contraindication to lytic therapy in an otherwise healthy patient with significant myocardium at risk and without other specific contraindications.

Late presentation (after 4 to 6 hours) often has been used to disqualify patients for lytic therapy, because clinical and experimental data have not demonstrated any significant myocardial salvage when ischemic myocardium is reperfused after more than 4 hours.[53, 57] Despite this, several studies (most notably the ISIS-2 trial) have shown a decrease in early mortality in patients treated 7 to 24 hours after symptom onset.[58] A meta-analysis using pooled data from almost three dozen thrombolytic trials similarly suggests a reduction in mortality for patients treated late.[56] The ongoing LATE (Late Assessment of Thrombolytic Efficacy) study is designed to address this issue definitively. Until definitive information is available, it seems reasonable to treat patients presenting between 6 and 12 hours after symptom onset, particularly if there is evidence of ongoing ischemia (manifested by chest pain) and findings of a moderate or larger infarct on the ECG.[57]

Why mortality should be reduced in such patients despite lack of infarct limitation or improvement in ventricular function is unknown. According to the "open artery hypoth-

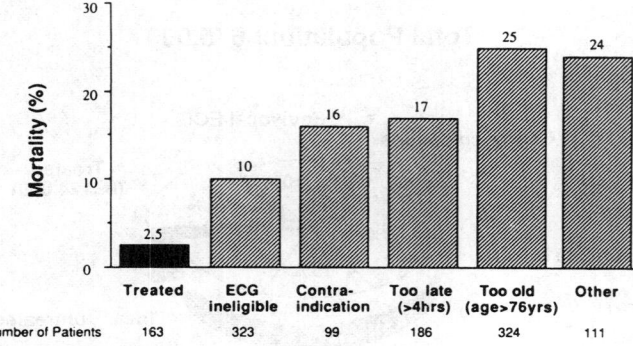

Figure 90–10. Comparison of hospital mortality rates of patients treated with thrombolysis by TPA with that of patients considered to be ineligible for thrombolytic therapy. The extremely low mortality for the treated group contrasts with the substantial mortality in the untreated groups, particularly the elderly and late-presenting groups. Data adapted from Cragg and colleagues.[64] (Reproduced, with permission, from Muller DWM, Topol EJ, Selection of patients with acute myocardial infarction for thrombolytic therapy. Ann Intern Med 1990; 113:949–960.)

esis,"[55] effects other than myocardial salvage result from early reperfusion, including a reduction in aneurysm formation,[65, 66] a reduction in ventricular arrhythmias,[67, 68] a reduction in left ventricular thrombus formation,[69] and the provision of a conduit for collateral blood flow into other jeopardized vessels.[57]

The location and extent of infarcts are related to the efficacy of lytic therapy. The mortality reduction with anterior infarcts (which are associated with at least a twofold higher mortality with conventional therapy than inferior infarcts[57]) is substantial and in some patients may be more than 50%. The benefit with inferior infarcts is more modest. It appears that the benefit of thrombolytic therapy is related more to the size of an infarct than its location; anterior infarcts tend to be about twice the size of inferior infarcts and thus derive the greater benefit. The larger the infarct, the greater the overall mortality but also, it seems, the greater the benefit from lytic therapy.[57, 70]

Previous infarct patients may benefit from thrombolytic therapy, but the available data are mixed. One large study (the GISSI trial)[59] showed no benefit of lytic therapy in patients with prior infarcts, another study showed higher mortality, and several others suggested a lowering of mortality similar to that in patients suffering their first myocardial infarction.[57, 58, 63] Until the issue is clarified, it seems reasonable to use lytic agents to treat patients with prior infarcts as long as the indications for doing so are clear and there are no strong contraindications.

Hypertension is considered a relative contraindication to thrombolytic therapy because of the risk of precipitating intracranial hemorrhage, which occurs in about 0.5% of patients treated with standard doses. Clear risk factors for bleeding include increased age and large doses of thrombolytic agent. Some studies have suggested a correlation between the risk of intracranial bleeding and blood pressure,[48] but other studies have not confirmed this association.[57–59] It seems appropriate to consider the use of lytic agents for hypertensive patients, provided that the blood pressure is reduced to 180/120 or less and kept at these levels or less for the duration of lytic therapy.[57]

A prior cerebral ischemic event has been treated as a strong contraindication to thrombolytic therapy. Because patients who had a stroke or a transient cerebral ischemic episode within the preceding 3 to 6 months have been routinely excluded from trials of thrombolytic therapy, there are inadequate data for firm guidelines. Although it is reassuring that there does not appear to be an excess of hemorrhagic strokes in AMI patients given lytic therapy who had prior nonhemorrhagic strokes within 6 months, the safety of lytic therapy in this setting is not established.[57]

Cardiopulmonary resuscitation has been a relative contraindication to lytic therapy because severe intrathoracic hemorrhage may follow the chest compression associated with it. The available data suggest, however, that the risk of bleeding is low, particularly if the duration of cardiopulmonary resuscitation is less than 10 minutes.[57]

Recent surgery has been a strong contraindication to lytic therapy because patients who have had recent major surgical procedures (including noncompressible vascular punctures, childbirth, and needle biopsy of organs) are at increased risk of bleeding. Although definitive data are unavailable, thrombolytic agents have been utilized with acceptable morbidity 14 days or more after a surgical operation or procedure and even earlier in a few cases.[71]

Selection of Thrombolytic Agent

Three agents are commercially available in the United States: streptokinase; TPA, also called alteplase and duteplase; and APSAC, also called anistreplase.

Streptokinase is the oldest of the thrombolytic agents and costs about one tenth as much as TPA and APSAC. On the other hand, TPA produces greater initial vessel patency (70 to 75%) than APSAC (60 to 70%) or streptokinase (50 to 60%) (Fig. 90–11). It seems that TPA and streptokinase produce similar patency by 1 to 2 days (Fig. 90–12). However, greater vessel patency has not translated into more myocardial salvage or lower mortality. Left ventricular function improves after thrombolytic therapy (usually to a small degree), with equivalent efficacy of streptokinase and TPA.[72] The ISIS-3 trial has provided mortality data, although the results of the study have been questioned because of the dose, route of administration, and timing of the concomitant heparin therapy. Nevertheless, this comparison of the agents showed no difference in mortality in patients treated with streptokinase, TPA, or APSAC.[73] Whether combining thrombolytic agents offers any advantage is under study.

A disadvantage of streptokinase and APSAC is that they are antigenic. Occasional allergic reactions and hypotension may accompany their use, but the reactions are usually mild and pretreatment with corticosteroids and/or antihistamines is not required. In 1 to 2%, reactions are severe enough to require cessation of the infusion. Because antibodies may

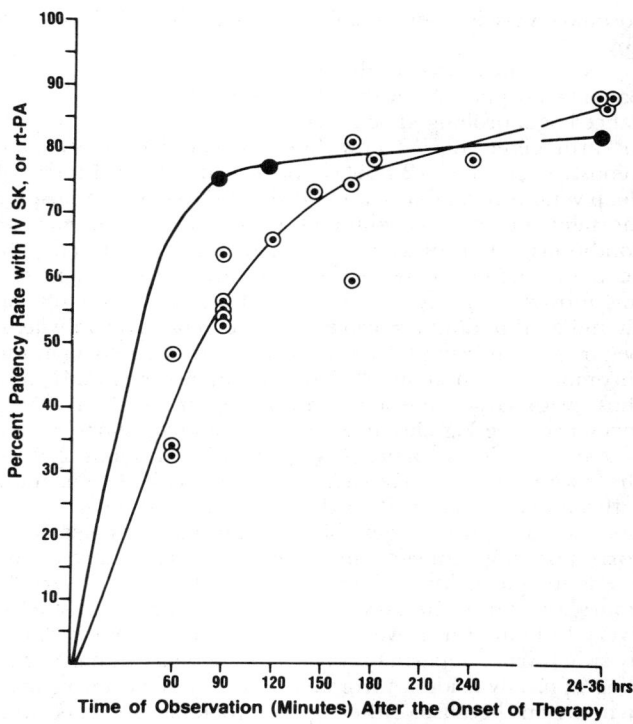

Figure 90–12. Frequency of reperfusion after thrombolytic therapy with intravenous streptokinase (IV SK, ☉) or recombinant TPA (rt-PA, ●) as a function of elapsed time after initiation of therapy. Although recombinant TPA achieves earlier thrombolysis, both agents show equivalent patency rates at 24 hours. (Reproduced, with permission, from Sherry S, Marder VJ, Streptokinase and recombinant tissue plasminogen activator [rt-PA] are equally effective in treating acute myocardial infarction. Ann Intern Med 1991; 114:417–423.)

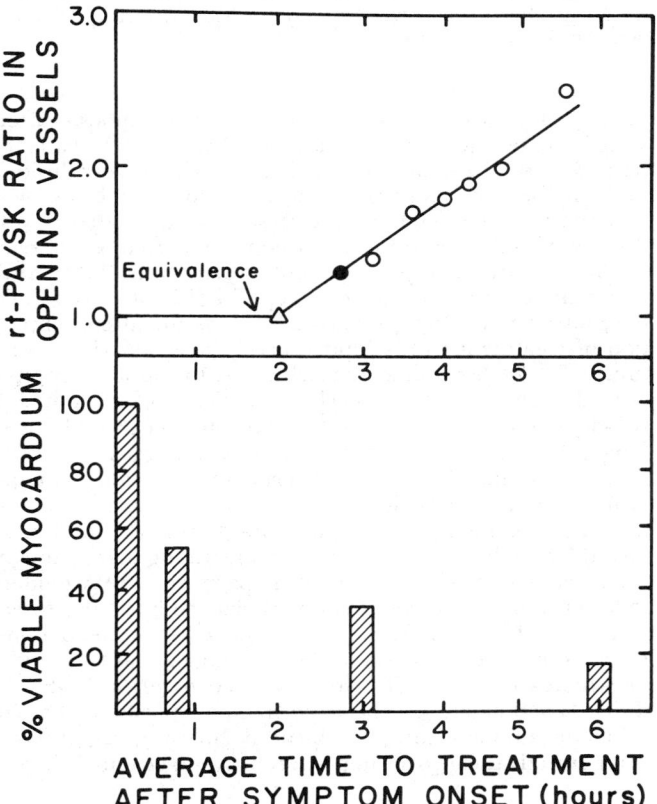

Figure 90–11. Data from three studies (△, ○, ●) demonstrating the relative efficacy of recombinant TPA and streptokinase (rt-PA/SK ratio) in achieving vessel patency in patients with myocardial infarction (*top*) and the percentage of viable myocardium in dogs with coronary occlusion (*bottom*) as a function of time after onset. The greater the time delay after symptom onset, the more likely recombinant TPA is than SK to achieve thrombolysis, but there is likely to be less viable myocardium that potentially can be salvaged. (Reproduced, with permission, from Sherry S, Marder VJ, Streptokinase and recombinant tissue plasminogen activator [rt-PA] are equally effective in treating acute myocardial infarction. Ann Intern Med 1991; 114:417–423.)

develop after initial treatment with streptokinase or APSAC, retreatment with either agent within 6 to 12 months may lead to a severe allergic reaction or neutralization of the effect of the agent. For these reasons, we ordinarily switch to TPA in this setting.

Although TPA is relatively clot specific and produces less of a systemic lytic state than either streptokinase or APSAC, this has not translated into fewer bleeding complications. In the ISIS-3 trial, the risk of stroke (especially hemorrhagic) was highest with TPA. It has been speculated that the production of a systemic lytic state by streptokinase and APSAC reduces the risk of rethrombosis of the infarct-related coronary artery; TPA produces the least fibrinogenolysis but has the highest reocclusion rate. Of the three agents, APSAC had the least desirable profile in the ISIS-3 trial. It had no advantage in reduced mortality overall, and allergic reactions, minor bleeding, and cerebral hemorrhage were all more common than with streptokinase.[73]

Heparin

Anticoagulants have been used for years for patients with acute myocardial ischemia, but firm data supporting their use have become available only in recent years. Efforts to limit the formation, propagation, and embolization of thrombi in UAP and AMI have been directed at multiple sites of potential clot formation: (1) deep venous thrombosis and resulting pulmonary embolism in patients at bed rest, (2) left ventricular mural thrombi after AMI, (3) re-formation of coronary thrombi in UAP, and (4) reocclusion of coronary vessels after initially successful thrombolytic therapy.

Deep venous thrombi develop in more than one third of patients hospitalized with AMI, especially those with advanced age, prolonged bed rest, and congestive heart failure or cardiogenic shock.[74] Low-dose heparin (5000 U subcutaneously every 8 or 12 hours) appears to reduce the risk of deep venous thrombosis after AMI[75] and to lower in-hospital mortality of patients admitted with a variety of medical conditions.[76] For these reasons, patients hospitalized with acute ischemia who are neither fully ambulatory nor receiving intravenous heparin or oral warfarin anticoagulation should at a minimum receive low-dose heparin prophylaxis, begun on admission to the hospital.[2] Left ventricular mural thrombi occur in about 20% of all patients with AMI, and those with large anterior infarcts have more than a 50% incidence[2] (see Fig. 90–8). The risk of systemic embolization is about 2% in all patients with AMI[77] and about 10% in those with thrombi.[78] Heparin reduces the risk of developing a thrombus by one half to three fourths,[79] although it has not been unequivocally established that this translates into a corresponding reduction in the risk of embolic stroke and attendant mortality. A higher dose of 12,500 U every 12 hours for at least 10 days appears to be superior to 5000 U every 12 hours for preventing mural thrombi.[79] We ordinarily switch from heparin to warfarin in patients with echocardiographically evident thrombi or large akinetic left ventricular regions because of the logistic problems associated with prolonged subcutaneous drug administration.

Heparin in full intravenous doses is effective in relieving recurrent ischemia in UAP[80, 81] and in reducing the likelihood of progression to AMI. In one study the combination of aspirin and heparin was no more beneficial than heparin alone, and bleeding complications were more common.[80] Whether mortality and progression to AMI are reduced to a similar degree as with aspirin is not clear. Thus, the relative merits of heparin, aspirin, and their combination in UAP are still uncertain.[82] In view of this (and until a properly designed randomized trial is performed), we routinely administer both heparin and aspirin to patients presenting with UAP, particularly because frequently it is not clear on presentation whether a patient merely has unstable angina or has suffered an infarction.

Despite the large number of trials of anticoagulant therapy in AMI during the past three decades, the evidence for a beneficial effect (at least on mortality) has been equivocal. Pooled data from the available trials suggest that mortality is reduced, perhaps by about one fifth.[38, 39] Whether these data are still relevant is questionable, however, because patients today are ambulatory earlier, are treated with other ancillary agents, often receive thrombolytic therapy, and so forth.

The use of anticoagulants after thrombolytic therapy is controversial; results appear to differ depending on the thrombolytic agent and the dose of heparin employed. In three of four studies of vessel patency in AMI patients treated with TPA, full-dose intravenous heparin started during or at the end of TPA infusion resulted in a significant improvement in early vessel patency[83–85] (Fig. 90–13). There are inadequate data regarding vessel patency after treatment with streptokinase or APSAC, but mortality data are available. In the SCATI trial, mortality after thrombolytic therapy was lower in the patients who also received heparin (2000 U intravenously followed by 12,500 U subcutaneously every 12 hours).[86] Mortality was also lower in the GISSI-2 trial in patients treated with streptokinase but not TPA.[50, 87] These results may be explained by the greater systemic anticoagulant state produced by streptokinase compared with TPA. Less heparin appears to be necessary to maintain a sufficient

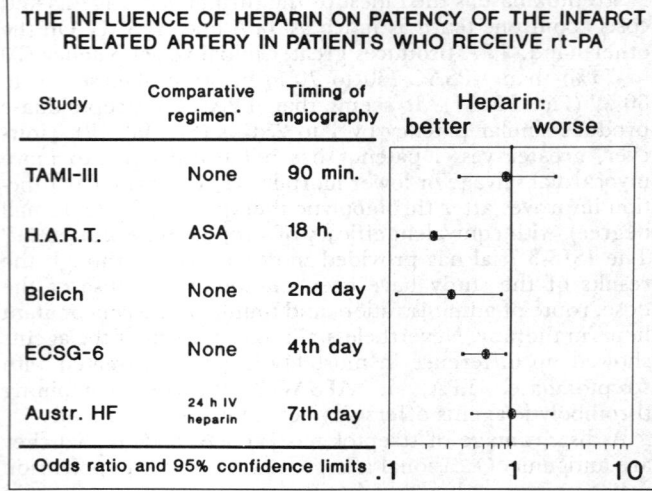

Study	Comparative regimen*	Timing of angiography	Heparin: better ⟷ worse
TAMI-III	None	90 min.	
H.A.R.T.	ASA	18 h.	
Bleich	None	2nd day	
ECSG-6	None	4th day	
Austr. HF	24 h IV heparin	7th day	

Odds ratio and 95% confidence limits: .1   1   10

Figure 90–13. Influence of heparin on patency of the infarct-related artery in patients who received recombinant TPA (rt-PA). ASA = aspirin; Austr HF = Australian Heart Foundation Study; Bleich = ref 83; ECSG-6 = Sixth European Cooperative Study Group Trial; H.A.R.T. = Heparin-Aspirin Reperfusion Trial; IV = intravenous; TAMI-III = Third Thrombolysis and Angioplasty in Myocardial Infarction Trial. (From Prins MH, Hirsh J: Heparin as an adjunctive treatment after thrombolytic therapy for acute myocardial infarction. Am J Cardiol 67:3A, 1991.)

degree of anticoagulation to prevent rethrombosis after streptokinase therapy than after TPA therapy. Patients treated with TPA are at particular risk of reocclusion, probably because there is less fibrinogenolysis and less systemic anticoagulation. For these reasons, we and others favor the use of full-dose intravenous heparin started at the end of thrombolytic therapy in patients treated with TPA[47] and either high-dose subcutaneous heparin (12,500 U) or full-dose intravenous therapy started 3 to 4 hours after completion of treatment with streptokinase.[88] The heparin is continued for 24 hours and then changed to the low prophylactic dosage unless there is a clinical indication for continued full-dose anticoagulant (e.g., cardiogenic shock with prolonged bed rest). There are some data to suggest that full-dose intravenous heparin is superior to subcutaneous heparin after treatment with streptokinase[88] but at the risk of increased hemorrhagic complications.[50, 87] The ISIS-3 trial has added to the controversy by demonstrating that although the combination of subcutaneous heparin with TPA tended to lower mortality, this was counterbalanced by an increased risk of cerebral hemorrhage.[73] Definitive recommendations must await the completion of the ongoing Global Utilization of Streptokinase and TPA for Occluded Arteries (GUSTO) Trial. Whether any of the experimental specific thrombin inhibitors under study (e.g., hirudin, hirugen, argatroban) offer any advantage over heparin remains to be established.[47]

Warfarin

Because the risk of embolization from a left ventricular thrombus is highest in the first 2 to 3 months after infarction (especially in the first 10 days), chronic warfarin anticoagulation has been suggested for patients with echocardiographically visible thrombi or large akinetic ventricular regions.[2, 89, 90] One small study has suggested that aspirin may be as efficacious as long-term anticoagulation for treating left ventricular mural thrombi, but the use of aspirin instead of warfarin should be considered unestablished at present.[91] The risk of embolism diminishes after 3 months after in-

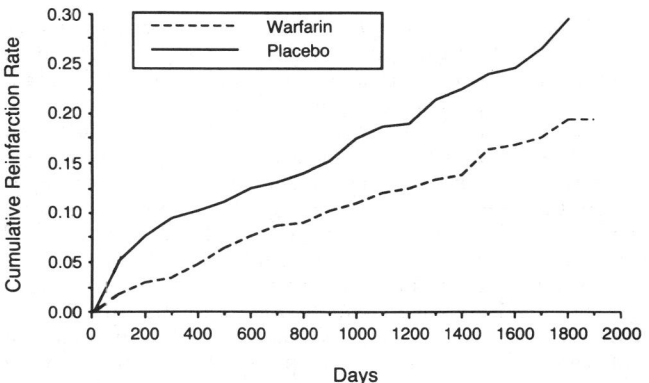

Figure 90–14. Cumulative reinfarction rate in patients with myocardial infarction given warfarin or placebo. (From Smith P, Arnesen H, Holme I: The effect of warfarin on mortality and reinfarction after myocardial infarction. Reprinted, by permission of the New England Journal of Medicine, 323; 147–152, 1990.)

farction, and it may be possible to discontinue warfarin at that time, particularly if echocardiography or radionuclide ventriculography shows that the noninfarcted ventricular regions contract well. On the other hand, it is advisable to continue warfarin therapy indefinitely (to prolong the prothrombin time to 1.3 to 1.5 times the control value) in patients with an enlarged and diffusely hypocontractile ventricle.[2] Warfarin appears to reduce mortality for at least 3 years after infarction,[92] perhaps by preventing occlusion or reocclusion of stenotic coronary arteries (Fig. 90–14). Mortality is reduced by about one fourth and cerebrovascular accidents by more than one half, with serious bleeding occurring only in 0.6% of patients each year.[92] It remains unestablished whether aspirin alone or in combination with warfarin offers any advantage.

Aspirin

Three large randomized trials have established a role for aspirin in the treatment of UAP.[80, 93, 94] Pooled data from the studies (which involved more than 2000 patients) demonstrated about a 40% reduction in both progression to AMI and mortality.[37]

Substantial benefit is also conferred by aspirin in the AMI setting. The large ISIS-2 study demonstrated that mortality could be reduced by almost one fourth by aspirin, with similar additional benefit occurring with the addition of streptokinase.[58] The risk of reinfarction was cut in half, and the benefits of aspirin occurred even though it was started as long as 24 hours after infarction. Because substantial benefit was found even in the absence of concomitant thrombolytic therapy, aspirin in a dose of approximately 160 mg/d should be used routinely in AMI, with the first dose given immediately on presentation.[2] We ordinarily continue aspirin indefinitely after AMI.

The optimal dose of aspirin remains unestablished. Various dosing schedules have been used in various clinical trials, making comparison difficult. A dose of 80 mg of aspirin appears to be sufficient in most patients to inhibit platelet aggregation by blocking platelet cyclooxygenase, and a dose greater than 325 mg may lead to undesirable gastrointestinal side effects including bleeding. Although larger doses of aspirin theoretically might lead to coronary vasoconstriction, the true upper dose limit has not been established. Accordingly, a dose of 160 to 325 mg/d can be recommended,[38] although a lower dose (80 to 160 mg/d) has been suggested for patients receiving concomitant heparin and/or warfarin therapy.[78] There appears to be no advantage to adding dipyridamole to aspirin. Various new platelet antagonists are under study, including a monoclonal antibody directed against the platelet glycoprotein IIb/IIIa receptor.[47] What roles these agents may play is uncertain pending the completion of experimental and clinical trials of their safety, efficacy, and relative merits.

Surgical Revascularization

Emergency surgical revascularization is rarely required because of intractable recurrent ischemia in UAP. Current intensive medical therapy with intravenous nitrates, calcium channel blockers, heparin with or without aspirin, beta-adrenergic blockers, and intra-aortic balloon pumping or PTCA can control recurrent ischemia at rest in almost all patients. The more typical timing of CABG in the setting of UAP is after an initial period of stabilization. In some patients CABG is advisable after such a period of stabilization but before hospital discharge because of angina pectoris that is precipitated by ambulation despite an optimal medical program; if a patient cannot be rendered pain free on ambulation in the hospital, it is unlikely the patient will be able to manage at home without even more recurrent ischemia. Other patients require early surgical revascularization because of the angiographic severity of their CAD (such as those with significant left main coronary arterial stenosis, in which revascularization is associated with improved long-term survival).

More controversial is whether all patients with UAP should be considered for cardiac catheterization and CABG if the coronary anatomy is favorable. CABG has been shown to reduce the frequency and severity of anginal episodes in chronic stable angina pectoris,[95] and the same appears to be true in UAP as well.[96] The largest prospective trial is the Veterans Affairs Cooperative Study, which randomized about 500 UAP patients to medical or medical plus surgical therapy.[96] In the surgery group, CABG was performed on average a little more than a week after presentation. Five-year follow-up revealed no mortality difference in the group overall, although those with triple-vessel disease or a depressed left ventricular ejection fraction fared better with CABG.[97, 98] After a 5-year period, almost half the medically treated patients required surgical revascularization because of unacceptable symptoms. The surgical patients experienced greater improvement in their quality of life, as manifested by improved treadmill exercise performance, reduced need for medications, fewer symptoms, and fewer subsequent hospitalizations. Balancing these beneficial effects was the lack of difference between medically and surgically treated patients in the frequency of recurrent UAP and myocardial infarction, with reduced mortality only in certain surgical subgroups (those with triple-vessel disease and/or left ventricular dysfunction).

In the AMI setting, a few groups advocate emergency CABG for patients presenting within 6 hours of onset, because CABG is the most definitive way to achieve coronary revascularization, particularly in patients with multivessel CAD.[99–101] Although these nonrandomized studies have suggested improved survival and/or myocardial salvage, the logistics of proceeding with emergency cardiac catheterization and CABG in a sufficiently timely fashion to be beneficial are daunting enough to be impractical at present for most hospitals.

Most cases of surgical revascularization early in the course of AMI are to treat mechanical complications of the infarction (Table 90–13).

Papillary muscle rupture may produce profound mitral regurgitation and low cardiac output, and although treat-

TABLE 90–13
INDICATIONS FOR EARLY CARDIAC SURGERY IN ACUTE MYOCARDIAL INFARCTION
Severe recurrent ischemia
Mechanical complication
Mitral regurgitation or papillary muscle rupture
Ventricular septal defect
Pseudoaneurysm
Left ventricular aneurysm
High-risk characteristics
Strongly positive exercise test
Left main coronary artery stenosis
Selected patients with multivessel CAD

ment with vasodilators and the intra-aortic balloon pump (IABP) may stabilize the patient, urgent mitral valve replacement and CABG are usually indicated.

Ventricular septal defects are managed in a similar fashion, with initial stabilization followed by urgent cardiac catheterization and insertion of an IABP and then early surgery to close the ventricular septal defect and revascularize the coronary arteries.

Free wall rupture is a catastrophic complication of AMI that almost invariably leads to death; in a few cases surgery has saved patients who otherwise surely would have died. In most cases, cardiac tamponade and electrical-mechanical dissociation occur so rapidly that nothing short of heroic measures is likely to be beneficial. In some patients, free wall rupture is self-contained, leading to left ventricular pseudoaneurysm. In such a situation, the myocardial rupture temporarily becomes sealed off by clot and adhesions between the epicardium and pericardium. Unlike a true aneurysm, pseudoaneurysms are prone to rupture with invariably fatal outcome. Accordingly, early surgical revascularization is indicated in virtually all cases.

Percutaneous Transluminal Coronary Angioplasty

Coronary angioplasty is a major advancement in the treatment of acute myocardial ischemia. In UAP, several uncontrolled studies have demonstrated that PTCA can achieve mechanical revascularization of stenotic or occluded coronary arteries with results generally comparable to the experience in stable angina pectoris[102–108] (see Fig. 90–6). Success rate and complications do not differ substantially from those in elective PTCA, and early results appear to be similar to those achieved with CABG.[104] Long-term results are affected by the restenosis problem; at least one third of PTCA sites become restenotic, usually within a 6-month period. Nevertheless, PTCA in UAP may at least allow hospital discharge and a period of stabilization.

Various innovative adaptations of balloon angioplasty have appeared, including atherectomy, laser, and stent delivery devices.[109] All have a limited role at present, and restenosis continues to be a major problem. Atherectomy offers the potential advantage of removing the potentially thrombogenic plaque, and laser balloon angioplasty has found a niche in resealing PTCA-induced coronary dissections and sparing the patient the need for an emergency CABG operation.[110] Nevertheless, these new techniques have not lived up to initial expectations and balloon angioplasty remains the standard against which all new techniques are compared.

The role of standard PTCA in AMI continues to evolve. Three separate roles have been identified: (1) primary angioplasty, as an alternative to thrombolytic or surgical therapy; (2) adjunctive angioplasty, as a routine procedure after thrombolytic therapy; and (3) deferred or delayed angioplasty, with PTCA performed only for specific indications, usually recurrent myocardial ischemia.

Primary angioplasty consists of immediate cardiac catheterization and angioplasty of the infarct-related vessel alone, without thrombolytic or other specific concomitant reperfusion therapy. Its use is restricted to centers with the requisite facilities, support services, and expertise. In such centers, the available data, although limited, suggest that it may be an acceptable alternative to thrombolytic therapy.[111–116] It offers the advantage of immediately demonstrating the coronary anatomy. Because of the logistic problems associated with primary angioplasty, it has not enjoyed widespread application. It is used most commonly for patients who have strong contraindications to thrombolytic therapy, such as those who have had recent surgery.

Adjunctive angioplasty, performed after intravenous thrombolytic therapy, is attractive from a theoretic standpoint because most patients are left with a residual significant coronary stenosis despite successful lysis of the clot and about one fourth of patients do not achieve coronary reperfusion with standard thrombolytic therapy. Three major clinical trials involving more than 1000 patients have addressed this issue and have come to remarkably similar conclusions.[48, 117, 118] Despite a procedural success rate of 90% or greater, routine immediate PTCA after TPA lytic therapy did not improve global or regional left ventricular function compared with that achieved with delayed or elective PTCA or TPA alone. Complications and mortality were higher in the immediate PTCA groups, and emergency CABG was required about three times more frequently (Fig. 90–15). Although subsequent recurrent ischemic events are less common after immediate PTCA,[117] the associated risks do not favor such an approach at present.

No definitive data are yet available for so-called rescue angioplasty, in which immediate PTCA is performed only in patients with a persistently occluded artery despite thrombolytic therapy. The Thrombolysis and Angioplasty in Myocardial Infarction (TAMI) study subjected such patients to routine PTCA in a nonrandomized fashion and found a high mortality and reocclusion rate and considerable clinical instability.[117] Although more encouraging data have been reported as well, immediate or rescue PTCA cannot be recommended at present, pending the results of larger prospective randomized trials.

Deferred or delayed angioplasty has been advocated to reduce the coronary stenosis that persists even after successful thrombolytic therapy. Although about 15% of patients receiving thrombolytic agents have no stenosis greater than

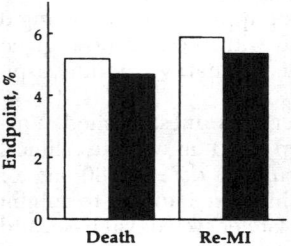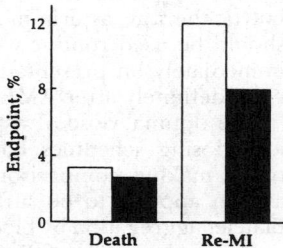

Figure 90–15. Results of two trials *(left and right)* comparing routine (open bars) with selective (filled bars) strategies for cardiac catheterization and angioplasty after AMI. Prophylactic angioplasty offered no advantage in terms of the risk of death or reinfarction (Re-MI). (Reproduced, with permission, from Topol EJ, Holmes DR, Rogers WJ, Coronary angiography after thrombolytic therapy for acute myocardial infarction. Ann Intern Med 1991; 114:877–885.)

50% when studied after their infarct, the majority have at least one significant residual stenosis. The stenosis typically is the result of both ulcerated atheromatous material and some degree of residual clot.[2]

The most definitive data available comparing an invasive strategy with a "watchful waiting" strategy after AMI have come from the Thrombolysis in Myocardial Infarction Phase II Trial (TIMI-II).[48] More than 3000 patients treated with TPA were randomized to either an invasive strategy of cardiac catheterization within a day or two after their AMI, followed by PTCA if appropriate, or a conservative strategy of angiography and PTCA only if postinfarction angina or ischemia on predischarge exercise testing developed. No differences between the two groups were found in mortality, rest or exercise ventricular function, or reinfarction rate. Thus, the results of this large study suggest that PTCA should be performed after AMI only for specific clinical indications such as resting or inducible ischemia, severe left ventricular dysfunction, or serious ventricular arrhythmias that are convincingly related to ischemia.[2]

Intra-Aortic Balloon Pump

The IABP, typically inserted via the femoral artery, is of value in three principal settings: cardiogenic shock (with or without right ventricular infarction), refractory UAP or postinfarction angina, and mechanical complications of AMI such as papillary muscle rupture with severe mitral regurgitation and ventricular septal rupture. Most IABPs are inserted using a percutaneous approach, although a surgical cutdown is required on occasion. An IABP cannot be inserted in some patients with iliofemoral disease because of tortuosity and narrowing of the vessel and/or attendant limb ischemia. Although the percutaneous approach utilizing a central guidewire has simplified insertion, complications occur in more than one third of patients.[119, 120] Vascular complications are most common but infection also is of concern, particularly if the device is left in place for more than a few days. The IABP is ineffective or contraindicated in patients with aortic aneurysms, aortic regurgitation, severe arrhythmias, tachycardia, and severe peripheral vascular disease.

Benefits of the IABP stem from deflation of the balloon just before systole (causing a reduction in afterload) and inflation of the balloon in diastole (augmenting diastolic flow and attendant coronary perfusion). In patients with UAP or AMI with recurrent episodes of pain despite maximal medical therapy, the IABP typically relieves the pain. The next step usually involves catheterization and mechanical revascularization with either PTCA or CABG. In cardiogenic shock the IABP may afford temporary stabilization, but it has not altered the otherwise dismal prognosis in this condition unless coupled with mechanical revascularization.

Similar benefits are seen with severe mitral regurgitation and ventricular septal rupture after AMI. These often desperately ill patients usually can be stabilized quite effectively with afterload reduction therapy and balloon counterpulsation. However, the IABP by itself has not changed appreciably the poor prognosis for these patients unless surgical correction of the defect is performed concomitantly.

Standard Care
Unstable Angina Pectoris

Most patients with UAP (in the absence of left ventricular failure) can be stabilized with an aggressive medical program, which usually includes intravenous nitroglycerin and intravenous heparin (Table 90–14). We usually prefer to add

---

TABLE 90–14
INITIAL MANAGEMENT OF UNSTABLE ANGINA PECTORIS

Hospitalization in cardiac or intensive care unit or step-down unit
Intravenous heparin to prolong partial thromboplastin time to 1.5–2 times control
Consider adding aspirin
Begin diltiazem or verapamil (if not already given); consider nifedipine or nicardipine if patient is already receiving a beta-adrenergic blocker
Intravenous nitroglycerin titrated to pain relief and side effects
Consider adding a beta-adrenergic blocker if not already given
Cardiac catheterization if pain recurs despite maximal medical program; consider IABP, PTCA, CABG

---

aspirin in the absence of contraindications or an enhanced clinical risk of bleeding complications, because it may be difficult to decide prospectively whether a patient has just UAP or has had some degree of myocardial necrosis. If a patient has been taking a beta-adrenergic blocker or a calcium channel blocker, we usually continue the medication. The only exception to this is a patient who is receiving monotherapy with a dihydropyridine calcium channel blocker, in which case we either switch to another agent (usually diltiazem) or add a beta-adrenergic blocker. For patients who previously were not receiving antianginal medications, diltiazem (or verapamil) is started; a beta-adrenergic blocker may be added as needed.

In the uncommon patient with true coronary artery spasm and no fixed coronary artery stenosis, treatment is with nitroglycerin and a calcium channel blocker. Beta-adrenergic blockers are proscribed, and heparin and aspirin probably are unnecessary. Until cardiac catheterization is performed, however, it often is difficult to make a definitive diagnosis of coronary artery spasm. The diagnosis becomes more likely if there is a worsening of angina pectoris when a beta-adrenergic blocker is used, because the drug may lead to unopposed alpha-adrenergic stimulation with an attendant increase in coronary vascular tone.

It usually takes a few days for the dosages of medications to be optimized. Intravenous medications should be converted to oral or topical forms or discontinued. Strong consideration is given to cardiac catheterization as an aid to subsequent decisions regarding management. In some patients it may be appropriate to forgo catheterization if an exercise test demonstrates good exercise capacity without evidence of high-grade ischemia.

In patients who have continued ischemia at rest or with minimal exertion despite an optimal medical program, cardiac catheterization is mandatory. Depending on the demonstrated coronary anatomy, a decision can be made to insert an IABP, perform PTCA, or proceed with CABG surgery.

Acute Myocardial Infarction

The initial management of a patient with AMI is centered on relief of pain, re-establishment of coronary blood flow to the ischemic region if possible, limitation of infarct size, and surveillance for arrhythmia and other complications (Table 90–15). All patients with suspected or confirmed infarction need to be closely monitored and treated as soon as feasible with aspirin (in the absence of a contraindication). Pain relief should be a priority, and strong consideration should be given to thrombolytic therapy. Many patients who qualify for lytic therapy do not receive it, especially the patients who might profit most from it.[57, 64] Intravenous beta-adrenergic blockers and nitroglycerin may be efficacious in selected

TABLE 90–15

INITIAL MANAGEMENT OF ACUTE MYOCARDIAL INFARCTION

Hospitalization in cardiac or intensive care unit setting
Oxygen by nasal prongs
Aspirin
Analgesia for pain
Consider thrombolytic therapy
Consider intravenous beta-adrenergic blocker, especially in
    setting of reflex tachycardia, hypertension, or recurrent pain
Consider intravenous nitroglycerin, especially for recurrent pain
At least low-dose subcutaneous heparin; consider high-dose
    subcutaneous or intravenous full-dose heparin after
    thrombolytic therapy, in patients with large anterior infarcts,
    ventricular thrombi, and congestive heart failure

patients, and all patients should receive at least low-dose subcutaneous heparin prophylaxis. In the absence of complications, patients with AMI should be ready for transfer out of the cardiac or intensive care unit to a step-down unit with telemetry within 1 to 3 days. A phase I rehabilitation program should be initiated early in the patient's hospitalization, and planning for discharge should be begun soon after admission.

If patients are able to tolerate a progressive ambulation protocol without recurrent angina pectoris or other problems, a submaximal predischarge exercise tolerance test often is performed. Patients demonstrating inducible or spontaneous postinfarction angina pectoris should undergo cardiac catheterization. Further management decisions hinge on the results of the catheterization.

Risk factor modification is an important issue for all patients with acute ischemia, whether they have had an infarction or not. Lifestyle changes (e.g., cessation of cigarette smoking, consumption of a sensible diet, reliability in taking medications) are best initiated in the hospital. Appropriate evaluation and initial management of hypercholesterolemia, hypertension, diabetes mellitus, and obesity are begun in the hospital and continued on an outpatient basis.

MANAGEMENT: COMPLICATIONS

Various complications may occur in the acute ischemic syndromes. Some (especially arrhythmias) may be found in both UAP and AMI, but most occur solely in the setting of AMI.

Supraventricular Arrhythmias

Various supraventricular brady- and tachyarrhythmias may occur in the setting of acute myocardial ischemia. In most cases the arrhythmia is the result (direct or indirect) of the underlying ischemia, but in some cases a rapid supraventricular arrhythmia may precipitate acute myocardial ischemia; successful termination of the arrhythmia typically results in resolution of the ischemia. Because tachycardia increases myocardial oxygen demand and thereby may precipitate ischemia, an arrhythmia that might ordinarily be well tolerated may cause significant problems if it occurs in the acute setting. For this reason, prompt therapy of supraventricular arrhythmias in the setting of acute ischemia usually is indicated, even though there is seldom anything unique about the arrhythmia or its treatment.

One treatment caveat concerns the use of digitalis glycosides in the acutely ischemic patient. These agents may increase myocardial oxygen demands, and some data suggest that the use of digitalis during and after AMI is associated

with increased mortality.[121] Although these data are disputed, we ordinarily prefer to use other agents (e.g., beta-adrenergic blockers, verapamil) in the acutely ischemic patient unless left ventricular function is sufficiently compromised that alternative agents are undesirable.

Sinus tachycardia is one of the more ominous arrhythmias in the setting of AMI. Although often related to pain, anxiety, hypovolemia, atrial infarction, or pericarditis, its appearance in the absence of one of these factors suggests significant incipient depression of ventricular performance, with sympathetic nervous system stimulation recruited to help maintain perfusion. Such patients typically have little cardiac reserve and are often on the verge of frank pulmonary edema or cardiogenic shock. Treatment of sinus tachycardia usually is directed at the underlying process. In patients in whom the sinus tachycardia is not due to incipient or actual pump failure, administration of beta-adrenergic blockers is beneficial. However, because of the deleterious effects of beta-adrenergic blockers in pump failure, noninvasive assessment of ventricular function and even invasive assessment of hemodynamics should be done before beta-adrenergic blockers are used if there is any doubt about the cause of sinus tachycardia.

Ventricular Arrhythmias

Ventricular arrhythmias occur in virtually all forms of heart disease as well as in normal subjects. Even repetitive ventricular arrhythmias may be found in apparently normal subjects. Yet despite their ubiquity, an increase in the number and complexity of ventricular arrhythmias in the setting of CAD is a marker of patients at increased risk of mortality. For this reason, treatment of such arrhythmias is often considered. Yet the treatment of asymptomatic ventricular arrhythmias paradoxically may lead to *increased* mortality, presumably because of a proarrhythmic effect of the antiarrhythmic agent itself.[33]

In trying to decide which patient with ventricular arrhythmia to treat, four major variables should be considered:

1. Is the patient acutely ischemic? If so, consideration should be given to treatment because the threshold for precipitating repetitive ventricular arrhythmias and ventricular fibrillation is lower.

2. Is there left ventricular contractile dysfunction? The presence of ventricular dysfunction puts the patient in a higher risk category and strengthens the argument for treatment.

3. Is the arrhythmia symptomatic or does it produce hemodynamic compromise? There is little argument that recurrent sustained ventricular tachycardia producing hemodynamic compromise requires antiarrhythmic therapy. On the other hand, treating ventricular bigeminy that is well tolerated may be overly aggressive.

4. Have all potentially remediable causes of arrhythmia been corrected (such as hypokalemia, hypoxemia, or acid-base disturbance)?

If the answer to all four of these questions is "yes," treatment with an antiarrhythmic agent is indicated. Decisions are more difficult in other situations; nevertheless, it usually is appropriate to use specific antiarrhythmic therapy in equivocal cases, at least until additional information is available (for example, until AMI is ruled out, at which point antiarrhythmic agents might be discontinued).

Antiarrhythmic agents are often used during the period of thrombolytic drug administration, because reperfusion of a previously occluded coronary artery may lead to the abrupt appearance of a variety of brady- and tachyarrhythmias, including ventricular tachycardia and even ventricular fibrillation. Yet it is now known that such early arrhythmias (termed reperfusion arrhythmias) often occur in the absence of reperfusion, and in any event true reperfusion arrhythmias may not respond to lidocaine and other first-line antiarrhythmic agents.

Arrhythmias occurring during the course of an AMI may be grouped as early (within the first 12 to 24 hours) and late (after the first day or two). Early arrhythmias, including ventricular fibrillation, that do not occur in the setting of severe pump failure are not associated with a poor long-term prognosis, and the in-hospital mortality is similar to[122] or only mildly increased over[123] that of patients without ventricular fibrillation. Ventricular arrhythmias that persist or appear later are more ominous. Whereas persistence of ventricular arrhythmias at the time of hospital discharge is a marker of increased posthospitalization mortality,[124] treatment of asymptomatic arrhythmia may actually increase mortality.[33] How to manage such patients is a controversial and difficult issue and is best referred to an electrophysiologist or cardiologist with a special interest in arrhythmias.

Symptomatic ventricular arrhythmias, including sustained ventricular tachycardia and ventricular fibrillation, that occur late in the post-AMI course are associated with a high risk of recurrent arrhythmia and death. Aggressive management is indicated in all cases and the advice of a consultant familiar with the management issues is imperative.

Conduction Abnormalities

Episodes of myocardial ischemia (particularly those caused by coronary vasospasm) may be associated with transient abnormalities of sinus node function and of atrioventricular conduction. Treatment of the ischemia usually resolves the conduction abnormality, and pacing is rarely required. Conduction abnormalities occurring during AMI are more worrisome because they are associated with double the in-hospital mortality[125] and reduced long-term survival. Particularly in the setting of an anterior infarct, they often are associated with extensive necrosis in the upper portion of the septum. With inferior infarcts, conduction defects are more likely to be transient, because they are often due to atrioventricular node ischemia rather than necrosis of the conduction tissue.

How much benefit accrues from temporary pacing in the setting of AMI is controversial. Although data are not available to show that temporary pacing lowers mortality, it is thought that some patients are saved (Table 90–16). Furthermore, the presence of a temporary pacemaker in a patient at high risk of developing complete heart block reduces the stress on the patient, the family, and the nursing and medical staff when sudden heart block does occur.

External pacemakers are available and may obviate the need for the prophylactic insertion of a temporary pacing wire in a patient at high risk of complete heart block.

Pump Failure in Acute Myocardial Infarction

There are three principal hemodynamic categories of pump failure in AMI; each requires a different therapeutic approach. The categories are left ventricular pump failure without hypotension, cardiogenic shock, and right ventricular pump failure caused by right ventricular infarction.[2] In all cases of pump failure (whether manifested by elevated filling pressures or diminished cardiac output), it is important to exclude a variety of conditions that may have similar presentations, including volume depletion, cardiac tamponade, pulmonary embolism, and pre-existing conditions such as chronic pulmonary disease with cor pulmonale.

TABLE 90–16
INDICATIONS FOR TEMPORARY PACING IN ACUTE MYOCARDIAL INFARCTION

Definite
  Asystole
  Complete heart block
  Right bundle branch block with left anterior or posterior hemiblock developing during AMI
  Left bundle branch block developing during AMI
  Type II second-degree atrioventricular block
  Symptomatic bradycardia not responding to atropine
Possible
  Type I second-degree atrioventricular block with hypotension not responding to atropine
  Sinus bradycardia with hypotension not responding to atropine
  Recurrent sinus pauses not responding to atropine
  Atrial or ventricular overdrive pacing for incessant ventricular tachycardia
  Left bundle branch block with first-degree heart block of unknown duration
  Bifascicular block of unknown duration

Adapted from Gunnar RM, Passamani ER, Bourdillon PD, et al: Guidelines for the early management of patients with acute myocardial infarction. A report of the American College of Cardiology/American Heart Association Task Force on Assessment of Diagnostic and Therapeutic Cardiovascular Procedures (Subcommittee to Develop Guidelines for the Early Management of Patients with Acute Myocardial Infarction). Reprinted with permission from the American College of Cardiology (Journal of the American College of Cardiology, 1990, Vol 16, pp 249–292).

Assessment of hemodynamic classification is possible with bedside hemodynamic determinations, often supplemented by noninvasive cardiac functional imaging. However, unlike the patient with noncardiogenic shock, the patient with hemodynamic embarrassment caused by AMI often is better served by hemodynamic assessment in the cardiac catheterization laboratory as part of a formal cardiac catheterization than by a bedside procedure. This permits simultaneous determination of coronary anatomy, coronary angioplasty if appropriate, and insertion of an IABP catheter under controlled conditions. For such patients the cardiac catheterization laboratory is the ideal intensive care unit, permitting both diagnostic and sophisticated therapeutic interventions.

Pump failure without hypotension is manifested by a left ventricular filling pressure greater than 15 mm Hg, a systolic arterial pressure greater than 100 mm Hg, and a cardiac index less than 2.5 L/min/m²; there are variable degrees of tissue hypoperfusion and pulmonary congestion.[2] The primary therapy is with vasodilators, typically either intravenous nitroglycerin (particularly if there is active ischemia and/or prominent pulmonary congestion) or nitroprusside (particularly if hypertension is present and/or tissue hypoperfusion is prominent) (Table 90–17). Intravenous dobutamine or amrinone is added if the response to vasodilators is inadequate. If blood pressure is inadequately maintained, dopamine rather than dobutamine often is used. Insertion of an IABP or mechanical coronary artery revascularization may be required as well.

For the patient with pulmonary congestion and preserved cardiac output, treatment often is initiated with an intravenous diuretic (e.g., furosemide in a 10- to 40-mg initial dose). An inadequate diuretic response is treated with larger doses and/or the addition of another agent such as metolazone. Excessive diuresis with attendant volume depletion, prerenal azotemia, and hypokalemia must be avoided. If the response to a diuretic still is inadequate, a vasodilator can be added, with careful attention to volume status. Positive inotropic agents (digitalis and sympathomimetic agents) are best avoided in this setting if possible.

Cardiogenic shock is manifested by an arterial systolic

TABLE 90–17

GUIDELINES FOR USE OF INTRAVENOUS CATECHOLAMINES AND VASODILATORS IN PUMP FAILURE AFTER MYOCARDIAL INFARCTION

Catecholamines
A. Begin with a low dose and titrate every 10–15 min to a therapeutic end point without provoking unacceptable adverse effects.
   1. Dopamine: Begin with 1–3 µg/kg/min and increase by 50- to 75-µg increments.
   2. Dobutamine: Begin with 2–5 µg/kg/min and increase by 50- to 75-µg increments.
   3. Norepinephrine: Begin with 1–3 µg/min and increase by 0.5- to 2-µg increments. Preferably use in combination with alpha-blocker (e.g., phentolamine).
B. Use acidic solutions as diluents.
C. Observe for adverse effects.
   1. Sinus tachycardia (rarely bradycardia may occur with norepinephrine-induced hypertension).
   2. Accelerated atrioventricular conduction and increased ventricular response in supraventricular arrhythmias.
   3. Atrial and ventricular premature beats and tachyarrhythmias.
   4. Worsening or provocation of ischemia or ventricular dysfunction.
   5. Tissue hypoperfusion because of excessive vasoconstriction and necrosis (from extravascular extravasation) may result from use of dopamine or norepinephrine.
   6. Nausea and vomiting.

Vasodilators
A. Begin with low doses and titrate every 10–15 min to a therapeutic end point without provoking adverse effects.
   1. Sodium nitroprusside: Begin with 10–20 µg and increase by 10 to 20 µg/min increments.
   2. Intravenous nitroglycerin: Begin with 10–20 µg and increase by 10 to 20 µg/min increments.
   3. Intravenous phentolamine: Begin with 0.5 mg/min and increase by 0.25 mg/min increments.
   4. Use freshly prepared solutions of nitroprusside (<6–8 h old), and shield the reservoir from light.
B. Preferably use nonabsorbent plastic tubing when using intravenous nitroglycerin to avoid adherence of nitroglycerin to plastic tubing.
C. Observe for adverse effects.
   1. Flushing, headaches, and hypotension.
   2. Reflex tachycardia; rarely reflex bradycardia occurs with nitroglycerin.
   3. Worsening or precipitation of ischemia because of excessive hypotension and tachycardia and, possibly, maldistribution of coronary nutrient flow (nitroprusside).
   4. Arterial desaturation resulting from intrapulmonary shunting.
   5. Methemoglobinemia (nitroglycerin and nitroprusside).
   6. Thiocyanate and cyanide intoxication (nitroprusside).
   7. Precipitation of increased intracranial and intraocular pressure (nitrates).
   8. Ethanol intoxication during prolonged high-dose infusions of intravenous nitroglycerin containing ethanol as a vehicle.

Miscellaneous
A. Infuse these potent drugs through free-flowing non–posture-dependent, large-bore, intravenous, preferably central, lines using well-calibrated constant-infusion pumps.
B. Avoid abrupt cessation of infusion (unless serious adverse effects occur) and preferably wean gradually.
C. Avoid flushing infusion lines through which catecholamines or vasodilators are infusing.
D. If cardiac outputs are being determined using a pulmonary arterial catheter, avoid infusing drugs through right atrial port of pulmonary arterial catheter.

Adapted from Shah PK, Swan HJC: Complications of acute myocardial infarction. In: Parmley WW, Chatterjee K (eds): Cardiology. Philadelphia, JB Lippincott, p 17, 1990.

pressure less than 90 mm Hg, left ventricular filling pressure greater than 15 mm Hg, and cardiac output less than 2.5 L/min/m².[2] Because of the exceedingly high mortality in this subset (80 to 100% with conventional therapy), the patient ordinarily should be stabilized as well as possible and brought to the cardiac catheterization laboratory. After instrumentation and assessment of hemodynamic status, an IABP is inserted and coronary arteriography performed. If the infarct-related artery can be opened with PTCA, the outlook improves substantially, with mortality reduced by half to about 40%.[126]

Right ventricular infarction is manifested by elevated right atrial and right ventricular diastolic pressures (>10 mm Hg), cardiac index less than 2.5 L/min/m², systolic pressure less than 100 mm Hg, and normal or elevated left ventricular filling pressure.[2] Such hemodynamics are seen in about 10% of inferior infarctions, even though some degree of right ventricular infarction can be demonstrated in one third to one half of patients with inferior infarcts (and only occasionally in anterior infarction). These patients are quite volume sensitive and may require large amounts of fluids to maintain cardiac output. Vasodilators (especially nitrates) and diuretics are best avoided. If volume infusion results in inadequate improvement, dobutamine infusion and insertion of an

IABP may be of benefit. Angioplasty of an occluded right coronary artery may be necessary and can be lifesaving. Because the long-term prognosis in these patients is typically excellent (there is often only a limited degree of concomitant left ventricular damage), management should be extremely aggressive, even in the presence of profound shock.

It is important to differentiate right ventricular infarction from cardiac tamponade, which it can resemble. In right ventricular infarction the interventricular septum shifts toward the left ventricle; this impairs left ventricular filling and can lead to elevation of both right and left ventricular filling pressures. Differentiation is by echocardiography, which demonstrates right ventricular dysfunction and little or no pericardial fluid. The diagnosis of right ventricular infarction is supported by ST segment elevation in the right precordial electrocardiographic leads, although often this is a transient finding.[127]

Mechanical Complications in Acute Myocardial Infarction

The mechanical complications that may follow infarction include mitral regurgitation caused by ischemia or necrosis of the papillary muscles and adjacent ventricular wall; myocardial rupture, including free wall rupture, pseudoaneurysm formation, and ventricular septal rupture; and left ventricular expansion and aneurysm formation. They all involve disruption of necrotic myocardium, have important short-term and long-term consequences, and are potentially treatable.

Infarct Expansion

This is the most common of the mechanical complications, occurring in almost one third of AMIs, especially anterior in location. It consists of thinning and lengthening of the necrotic segment in the absence of additional necrosis and results in regional dilatation.[128] Much of the acute dilatation appears to occur within the first several days after an AMI, when the infarct has the least tensile strength.[129] Expansion sets the stage for subsequent cardiac rupture in some patients but also the progressive dilatation, distortion of ventricular shape, and aneurysm formation that are associated with a particularly poor prognosis.[130, 131] Preliminary data suggest that the process can be attenuated to some degree by using beta-adrenergic blockers and converting enzyme inhibitors to reduce afterload[132, 133] (Fig. 90–16). Definitive recommendations must await the results of the Survival and Ventricular Enlargement Trial (SAVE), a double-blind placebo-controlled trial of captopril in post-AMI patients with ejection fraction of 40% or less.

It is likely that ventricular aneurysms are the end result of infarct expansion. Aneurysms form as fibrous tissue replaces necrotic myocardium and occur after the period of healing after infarction. Long-term sequelae associated with ventricular aneurysm include pump failure with congestive heart failure, mural thromboembolism, angina pectoris, and ventricular arrhythmias. Surgical resection of a localized aneurysm with otherwise well-preserved ventricular function often is effective in improving heart failure symptoms; coupled with electrophysiologic mapping or additional procedures such as endocardial resection, it may be effective as well for malignant ventricular arrhythmias. Anticoagulation ordinarily is adequate to prevent embolism, and surgical resection rarely is required simply to reduce the risk of thromboembolic phenomena.

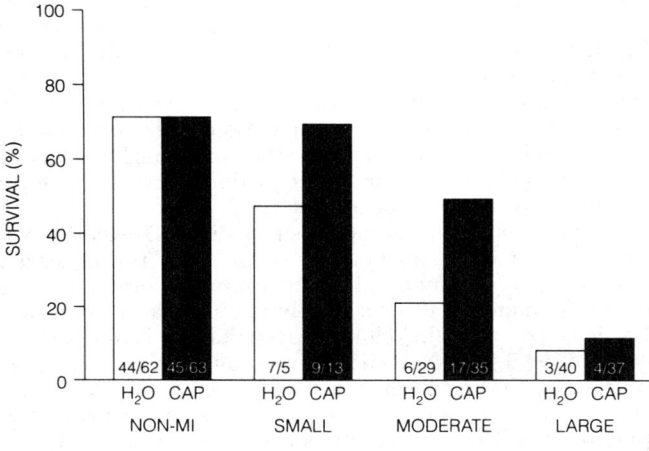

Figure 90–16. One-year survival after experimental myocardial infarction (MI) in a rat model. Captopril (CAP) improved long-term survival compared with saline placebo (H_2O), especially for animals with moderate-sized infarcts. (From Pfeffer MA, Pfeffer JM: Ventricular enlargement and reduced survival after myocardial infarction. Circulation 75[suppl IV]:93–97, 1987, by permission of the American Heart Association, Inc.)

Myocardial Rupture

Rupture is the most dramatic consequence of infarct expansion and may occur in three principal forms: ventricular septal rupture, free wall rupture, and left ventricular pseudoaneurysm formation. All three tend to occur during the first week after AMI and all are associated with high mortality.

Rupture of the interventricular septum occurs in 1 to 2% of infarctions and may be associated with chest pain, congestive heart failure, hypotension, and hypoperfusion. The attendant left-to-right shunt produces right-sided volume overload with elevated pulmonary blood flow and reduced systemic cardiac output. A new systolic murmur usually appears, accompanied by a palpable thrill in about half of the cases. The diagnosis often can be established using bedside two-dimensional echocardiography and color flow Doppler recordings, which can demonstrate the location of the defect. Confirmation is provided by right-sided heart catheterization that demonstrates a step-up in oxygen saturation from right atrium to pulmonary artery.

Management is through the use of vasodilators, diuretics, and inotropic agents as appropriate. After initial stabilization, the patient should be brought rapidly to the cardiac catheterization laboratory for insertion of an IABP, confirmation of the site and size of the defect, and definition of the coronary artery anatomy. The patient should then undergo surgery without delay with closure of the defect, resection of infarcted tissue as necessary, and CABG as appropriate. Such an aggressive approach can achieve a 50 to 75% survival rate, whereas without operation the survival is about 50% at 1 week and under 10% at 1 year.[134]

Free wall rupture is a catastrophic complication of AMI and may account for as much as one fourth of the acute peri-infarction mortality.[135] It occurs more commonly after a first infarction, in women older than 70 years of age, and in patients with systemic hypertension.[135] The clinical presentation typically is one of sudden chest pain followed by hypotension, distended neck veins, electrical-mechanical dissociation, and death. In a few cases the attendant pericardial tamponade is walled off for a variable time, resulting in a more subacute presentation. Even then, it is a rare patient who survives free wall rupture; immediate surgery is the only hope for survival.

Pseudoaneurysm formation occurs when sufficient adhesions develop between the epicardium and pericardium to contain (at least temporarily) a free wall rupture. A pseudoaneurysm is unlike a true left ventricular aneurysm because no myocardial tissue is present in the wall of the aneurysm and all that prevents rupture of the aneurysmal wall is clot and pericardial adhesions. Because breakdown of the adhesions and clot results in fatal cardiac tamponade, surgical repair is indicated on an emergency basis.

The diagnosis usually is established by two-dimensional echocardiography, which demonstrates distortion of the normal myocardial architecture, mural and often intracavitary thrombus, absent or expansile (dyskinetic) regional wall motion, and often some degree of localized or free pericardial fluid. Cardiac catheterization is performed to define the coronary artery anatomy, but left ventriculography is not required routinely and may be harmful. Surgical correction consists of excising necrotic myocardium and associated thrombus and sewing together the left ventricular walls surrounding the rupture; concomitant coronary revascularization is performed as necessary.

Mitral Regurgitation

Mitral regurgitation post infarction is due to ischemia or infarction of the papillary muscles and adjacent ventricular wall. The regurgitation may be mild with ischemia or fulminant when associated with rupture of the body of the papillary muscle. Although commonly thought to cause mitral regurgitation in the AMI setting, rupture of the avascular chordae tendineae is an infrequent occurrence. The papillary muscles are particularly vulnerable to ischemia as a consequence of their endocardial location distant from the coronary arteries. In the case of the posteromedial papillary, a single blood supply from the posterior descending coronary artery (usually a branch of the right) is an additional risk factor. The severity of the resulting mitral regurgitation is a function of the degree of papillary muscle ischemia. Pronounced papillary muscle ischemia or infarction may be associated with a surprisingly limited degree of ischemia or infarction of the adjacent ventricular wall despite profound mitral regurgitation.

The appearance of a new systolic murmur during the course of an AMI suggests mitral regurgitation caused by papillary muscle ischemia or infarction (or, less commonly, rupture of the interventricular septum), but the quality, intensity, and timing of the murmur may bear little relationship to the severity of the regurgitant leak. In some cases, the appearance of acute mitral regurgitation is heralded by pulmonary edema and hypotension with little or no murmur. More ominous is rupture of one or more of the heads of the papillary muscle or even of the body of the muscle itself, an occurrence that leads to intractable pulmonary edema and shock if not managed with aggressive medical stabilization and surgical repair.

The diagnosis of papillary muscle rupture is suggested by the appearance of a new systolic murmur or the sudden onset of pulmonary edema, usually despite an electrocardiographically small infarct (usually inferior or posterior in location). Differentiation from ventricular septal rupture (which may also produce a new murmur) may be achieved by two-dimensional echocardiography with color flow Doppler recording, which may demonstrate the disrupted leaflets and flail chordae tendineae with attached papillary muscle remnants (Table 90–18). Right-sided heart catheterization with a balloon flow-directed catheter demonstrates reduced pulmonary arterial oxygen saturation, the absence of an oxygen step-up of a left-to-right shunt, and often large regurgitant ("CV") waves. Definitive diagnosis is provided by cardiac catheterization, which should be performed after initial stabilization with vasodilators, diuretics, and inotropes as necessary. In the cardiac catheterization laboratory an IABP is inserted, the coronary anatomy defined, and the mitral regurgitation documented. Once mitral regurgitation has been confirmed, surgery should proceed expeditiously because the mortality of medically treated patients is 50% within 24 hours and more than 90% by 2 months.[136, 137] Mitral valve replacement and coronary revascularization can save more than half of these patients.[136]

Pericarditis

Pericarditis not associated with self-limited ventricular rupture occurs in two principal time periods, one early (within the first several days after AMI) and the other (presumably of autoimmune origin) later (weeks to months after infarction).

Early pericarditis occurs within the first few days after infarction in about 10% of AMI patients, although it appears to be occurring less commonly as thrombolytic therapy becomes more widespread. It occurs more frequently in larger and more complicated (particularly Q wave) infarcts and is related to epicardial or pericardial inflammation in the region of infarction.[138] Although anticoagulation therapy may lead to the development of a hemorrhagic pericardial effusion (rarely with tamponade) in an occasional patient, thrombolytic, antiplatelet, and anticoagulant therapy has been surprisingly well tolerated overall.

Differentiation from anginal pain is important because recurrent angina usually indicates ongoing ischemia or new necrosis that needs to be addressed with specific anti-ischemia strategies. Pain also causes sympathetic stimulation, with a resultant increase in myocardial oxygen demand. The factors that suggest pericarditis include a positional and pleuritic component and a type of pain different from that reported by the patient at the onset of the infarct. The ECG is usually not helpful in the distinction, because of the existing ST segment and T wave abnormalities.[139] An echocardiogram similarly may not be helpful in diagnosis, because pericarditis often occurs with little or no pericardial fluid, and fluid may be present without clinical pericarditis. The presence of a one-, two-, or three-component pericardial function rub is confirmatory, but the rub may be evanescent. Treatment is with aspirin in anti-inflammatory doses; steroidal and nonsteroidal agents are effective as well but are more problematic because of their potentially serious side effects, including the demonstration in animal models of impaired healing of the infarcted region[140] and increases in coronary vascular resistance.[141]

Delayed or postinfarction pericarditis (Dressler's syndrome) now is an uncommon occurrence, for uncertain reasons. It is presumed to be autoimmune in origin because of the frequency with which antimyocardial antibodies may be detected, and the clinical presentation is marked by constitutional symptoms suggestive of immune complex phenomena, including fever, malaise, anorexia, serositis (especially pericardial and pleural), arthralgias or arthritis, and pulmonary infiltrates. Treatment is with nonsteroidal anti-inflammatory agents, often for a prolonged course, because Dressler's syndrome has a protracted course usually of several weeks duration and tends to recur. Doses of medication must be tapered slowly and corticosteroids are required on occasion. Other sequelae of pericardial inflammation (such as tamponade and chronic constrictive pericarditis) are uncommon.

TABLE 90–18

DIFFERENTIATION OF PAPILLARY MUSCLE RUPTURE AND VENTRICULAR SEPTAL RUPTURE

Features	Papillary Muscle Rupture with Severe Mitral Regurgitation	Ventricular Septal Rupture
Clinical		
Frequency	1% of infarcts	1–2% of infarcts
Timing	Day 3–5	Day 3–5
Infarct location	Inferoposterior	Anterior equals inferior
Murmur	May be soft or absent	Loud
Precordial thrill	Rare	Present in 50%
Diagnostic		
Two-dimensional echocardiogram	Flail mitral apparatus	Septal defect visualized
Doppler recording	Mitral regurgitation	Left-to-right shunt
Pulmonary arterial catheterization	Large regurgitant ("CV") waves in "wedge" tracing	Oxygen step-up in pulmonary artery; CV waves may be present

TABLE 90–19
PRINCIPAL CARDIOPULMONARY CAUSES OF RECURRENT POSTINFARCTION CHEST PAIN
Myocardial ischemia Infarction extension Infarction expansion Myocardial rupture or pseudoaneurysm Pericarditis Pulmonary embolism

Recurrent Chest Pain

Ischemic chest pain in the immediate postinfarction period is of concern because it suggests the vulnerability of still viable myocardium to progression to infarction. Rapid differentiation from other causes of chest pain is important (Table 90–19). Careful attention to the history, physical examination, ECG, and serially determined serum enzymes usually allow at least a presumptive differential diagnosis.

Infarct extension may cause chest pain as a consequence of reocclusion of a subtotally narrowed coronary artery. Infarct extension occurs in 5 to 10% of AMI patients and should be diagnosed only if there is re-elevation of the serum enzymes.[142] In some patients it may occur without chest pain.[143] Because it is associated with increased mortality and may further damage an already impaired ventricle, aggressive pharmacologic management is indicated. Cardiac catheterization often is appropriate so that the cause of the ischemia can be ascertained; in some cases PTCA is appropriate to try to reopen a reoccluded coronary artery.[48]

Infarction expansion (see earlier) may also cause chest pain, although no additional necrosis is involved and serum enzyme levels are not altered. A form of cardiac rupture, it is presumed to result from slippage of the damaged myocytes, particularly if subjected to high left ventricular wall stresses (afterload).[128] Prevention is the only therapy available; it appears that beta-adrenergic blockers and particularly converting enzyme inhibitors may offer some protection against expansion.

Recurrent ischemia is distinguished from infarct extension only by the subsequent course; the serum enzyme levels are not re-elevated with postinfarction angina as they are with infarct extension. Ischemia may be due to impaired perfusion of the peri-infarct zone or increased demand resulting from regional dyskinesia or may be "ischemia at a distance" because of supply-demand imbalance in a ventricular region distant from the infarction.[144] Distant ischemia is of particular concern as it may represent additional myocardium at risk, often a region distal to an additional coronary stenosis that becomes evident after an AMI because of attendant hypotension, hypoxemia, reduced collateral blood flow, or increased myocardial oxygen demand caused by ventricular dilatation and increased levels of circulating catecholamines. It is no wonder that distant ischemia may be associated with a less favorable prognosis than ischemia in the peri-infarction region.[144] Cardiac catheterization may be of considerable value in clarifying the etiology of recurrent ischemia by defining the status of the culprit coronary artery causing the infarction, as well as establishing the presence and severity of the additional coronary artery stenoses that form the substrate for distant ischemia.

Non–Q Wave Infarction

Non–Q wave infarcts tend to be smaller than Q wave infarcts and are typically subendocardial in location. The incidence of non–Q wave infarcts appears to be increasing, perhaps as a consequence of the effectiveness of pharmacologic therapy that aborts a threatened Q wave infarct and transforms it into a smaller and less confluent infarct by quickly re-establishing coronary perfusion. The concern with non–Q wave infarcts is that the unstable plaque that led to the initial infarction maintains its instability and potential for rethrombosis, re-exposing myocardium to the risk of infarction. In support of this concern are data showing a higher rate of reinfarction, postinfarction angina, and late mortality than in Q wave infarcts[40] (Fig. 90–17).

Although non–Q wave infarcts are associated with less myocardial damage and hence lower early (hospital) mortality than Q wave infarcts (Fig. 90–18), this advantage is lost in the subsequent months and years. For this reason, a non–Q wave infarct often is managed in a manner akin to that for UAP, with a low threshold for cardiac catheterization and mechanical revascularization, particularly in patients demonstrating spontaneous or exercise-induced myocardial ischemia. Pharmacologic therapy has been employed with some success in an attempt to reduce the late morbidity and mortality in non–Q wave infarction.

MANAGEMENT: PREDISCHARGE
Unstable Angina Pectoris

The majority of patients with UAP may be stabilized in the hospital on a pharmacologic antianginal regimen that renders the patient pain free (see Table 90–14). Only a minority remain so unstable that urgent or emergency mechanical revascularization with either PTCA or CABG is required. The patients who cannot be rendered pain free despite an optimal medical program should undergo expeditious cardiac catheterization, with consideration given to insertion of an IABP. Depending on the coronary anatomy, further plans can be made to achieve coronary revascularization.

Patients who are rendered pain free by medical therapy should be considered potentially unstable, however, because the diseased plaque that initiated the episode of UAP retains its ability to compromise coronary blood flow. The available data indicate that although CABG relieves subsequent ischemic symptoms better than medical therapy, mortality is improved only in patients with left main coronary artery stenosis or a reduced ejection fraction.[96–98] Echocardiography

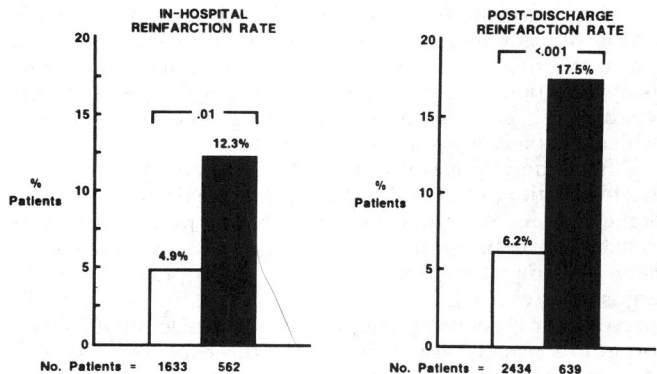

Figure 90–17. Incidence of reinfarction rates during (*left*) and after (*right*) hospitalization for Q wave (open bars) and non–Q wave (filled bars) myocardial infarction. (From Gibson RS: Current status of calcium channel–blocking drugs after Q wave and non–Q wave myocardial infarction. Circulation 80[suppl IV]:107–109, 1989, by permission of the American Heart Association, Inc.)

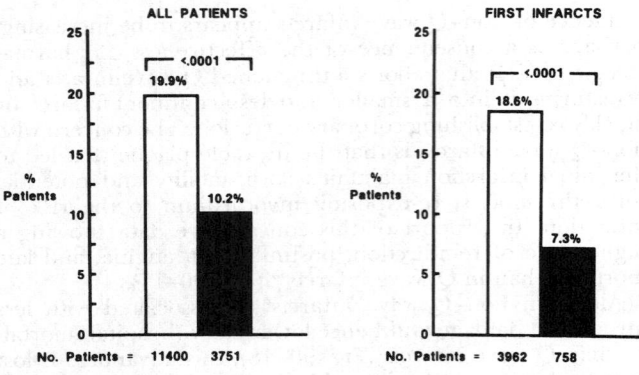

Figure 90–18. Short-term mortality rates for *(left)* all patients and *(right)* those sustaining their first Q wave (open bars) or non–Q wave (filled bars) myocardial infarction. (From Gibson RS: Current status of calcium channel–blocking drugs after Q wave and non–Q wave myocardial infarction. Circulation 80[suppl IV]:107–109, 1989, by permission of the American Heart Association, Inc.)

and radionuclide ventriculography can identify high-risk patients with ventricular dysfunction, but defining coronary anatomy is possible only with coronary arteriography. For these reasons we usually have a low threshold for performing cardiac catheterization after hospitalization for UAP. For patients not proceeding directly to catheterization, an exercise tolerance test with thallium imaging may provide useful information, including exercise capacity and evidence of silent or inducible myocardial ischemia. If a patient demonstrates angina at a low level of effort, significant ischemia on the ECG or thallium scan, or other worrisome findings suggestive of global left ventricular ischemia such as exertional hypotension, prompt diagnostic cardiac catheterization is indicated. Exercise testing should not be performed if the patient continues to exhibit spontaneous pain or ischemia on minimal exertion. In such patients, expeditious cardiac catheterization should be undertaken. Exercise testing is appropriate only if the patient has been rendered totally asymptomatic and stable by pharmacologic management.

Acute Myocardial Infarction

Whereas the initial phase of management of an AMI is directed at restoring coronary perfusion, limiting infarct size, and treating arrhythmias and other complications (see Table 90–15), later in-hospital management is directed at risk factor modification, cardiac rehabilitation, and identification of patients at increased risk of subsequent ischemic or arrhythmic events. There is no better time than during hospitalization to begin discussing the lifestyle, diet, exercise, medication, and other posthospitalization changes with which the patient will need to comply.

After a period of bed rest and limited activity early in the hospitalization, most AMI patients become deconditioned to some degree. A graded exercise plan as part of a cardiac rehabilitation program has been shown to be remarkably safe, although the precise exercise prescription should be adjusted according to the severity of the infarct and the presence or absence of complications. Cardiac rehabilitation programs usually are divided into three phases: phase I, during the acute hospitalization; phase II, during outpatient convalescence; and phase III, during long-term recovery.

Identifying patients at increased risk of recurrent ischemia is of critical importance before or in the weeks after hospital discharge, because mechanical revascularization of such high-risk patients may be efficacious in preventing serious sequelae. Patients sustaining a complicated infarct, manifested by congestive heart failure, hypotension, ongoing ischemia, serious arrhythmias, or a mechanical defect, should undergo early cardiac catheterization because the 1-year postinfarction mortality for such patients may be as high as 20 to 50%.[145]

Identifying patients with an apparently uncomplicated infarct who are at increased risk of posthospitalization morbidity and mortality is a formidable problem, because these complications often are a function of the stability or instability of the disrupted plaque; we currently have no completely reliable tool for assessing this risk. In the prethrombolytic era, exercise testing (often with use of a radionuclide such as thallium) was able to separate a low-risk group with an annual mortality rate of a few percent from a moderate-risk group with 10% mortality in the first year after AMI.[145] In the current thrombolytic era, exercise testing has not been as reliable in identifying moderate-risk patients.[146–148] In the study with the most definitive follow-up, more than 500 patients were followed for 5 years after reperfusion therapy and the predischarge exercise test was not predictive of reinfarction or death in the follow-up period.[63]

While acknowledging these data, we still recommend performing an exercise test in the early post-AMI period to establish exercise capacity and to identify patients with inducible ischemia. Patients with an abnormal stress test should then undergo cardiac catheterization so that appropriate management decisions may be made. Exercise testing may be performed during the hospitalization, in which case the test is arbitrarily halted at a set point (submaximal). Alternatively, it may be performed in the weeks after discharge, in which case a symptom-limited test is performed. Those with "negative" tests may still be at some risk if the plaque remains unstable; we have no established technique for assessing the potential for rethrombosis of a given lesion. It is hoped that a new technique such as intravascular ultrasonography may provide this prognostic information.

Assessment of ventricular function also provides important prognostic information. Resting radionuclide ventriculography or echocardiography may identify patients with depressed ventricular function who may benefit from mechanical revascularization. One approach is to couple exercise testing with either technique to provide both resting and exercise functional information.

Although ambulatory electrocardiographic monitoring provides important prognostic information by identifying patients at increased risk, there is no persuasive evidence that treating asymptomatic ventricular arrhythmias reduces the risk of subsequent mortality.[33] Even as few as 10 ventricular premature depolarizations per hour in a post-AMI patient are associated with an increased mortality rate over the subsequent 2 years.[124, 149] Unless the arrhythmias can be correlated with periods of active myocardial ischemia, antiarrhythmic therapy has not been shown to be efficacious in reducing mortality. Whether formal electrophysiologic testing or newer techniques such as the signal-averaged ECG provide any further useful information is controversial;[68, 150–154] even if they could provide additional risk stratification data, how to treat the high-risk patient remains enigmatic.

Attention to coronary risk factors is important in all patients admitted to the hospital with acute myocardial ischemia. In addition to counseling on diet, stress management, cigarette smoking, and exercise, screening and treatment should be performed for hyperlipidemia, hypertension, and diabetes mellitus. Discharge medications should be reviewed with the patient and family, and as simplified a program as possible should be adopted to maximize compliance. Arrangements for follow-up care are vital, as are precise instructions regarding what to do if symptoms recur.

Please refer to the other chapters in this section for additional information.

References

1. National Center for Health Statistics: Monthly Vital Statistics Report 36:13, 1988.
2. Gunnar RM, Passamani ER, Bourdillon PD, et al: Guidelines for the early management of patients with acute myocardial infarction. A report of the American College of Cardiology/American Heart Association Task Force on Assessment of Diagnostic and Therapeutic Cardiovascular Procedures (subcommittee to develop guidelines for the early management of patients with acute myocardial infarction). J Am Coll Cardiol 16:249, 1990.
3. Braunwald E: Unstable angina. A classification. Circulation 80:410, 1989.
4. Lange RA, Cigarroa RG, Flores ED, et al: Potentiation of cocaine-induced coronary vasoconstriction by beta-adrenergic blockade. Ann Intern Med 112:897, 1990.
5. Rozanski A, Berman DS: Silent myocardial ischemia. I. Pathophysiology, frequency of occurrence, and approaches toward detection. Am Heart J 114:615, 1987.
6. Davies MJ: A macro and micro view of coronary vascular insult in ischemic heart disease. Circulation 82(suppl II):38, 1990.
7. Falk E: Plaque rupture with severe pre-existing stenosis precipitating coronary thrombosis. Characteristics of coronary atherosclerotic plaques underlying fatal occlusive thrombi. Br Heart J 50:127, 1983.
8. Fuster V, Stein B, Ambrose JA, et al: Atherosclerotic plaque rupture and thrombosis. Evolving concepts. Circulation 82(suppl II):47, 1990.
9. Ambrose JA, Tannenbaum MA, Alexopoulos D, et al: Angiographic progression of coronary artery disease and the development of myocardial infarction. J Am Coll Cardiol 12:56, 1988.
10. Fuster V, Badimon L, Cohen M, et al: Insights into the pathogenesis of acute ischemic syndromes. Circulation 77:1213, 1988.
11. Richardson SG, Allen DC, Morton P, et al: Pathological changes after intravenous streptokinase treatment in eight patients with acute myocardial infarction. Br Heart J 61:390, 1989.
12. Golino P, Buja LM, Ashton JH, et al: Effects of thromboxane and serotonin receptor antagonists on intracoronary platelet deposition in dogs with experimentally stenosed coronary arteries. Circulation 78:701, 1988.
13. Ludmer PL, Selwyn AP, Shook TL, et al: Paradoxical vasoconstriction induced by acetylcholine in atherosclerotic coronary arteries. N Engl J Med 315:1046, 1986.
14. Griffith TM, Lewis MJ, Newby AC, et al: Endothelium-derived relaxing factor. J Am Coll Cardiol 12:797, 1988.
15. Kannel WB, Abbott RD: Incidence and prognosis of unrecognized myocardial infarction. An update from the Framingham study. N Engl J Med 311:1144, 1984.
16. Lee TH, Juarez G, Cook EF, et al: Ruling out acute myocardial infarction. A prospective multicenter validation of a 12-hour strategy for patients at low risk. N Engl J Med 324:1239, 1991.
17. Schweitzer P: The electrocardiographic diagnosis of acute myocardial infarction in the thrombolytic era. Am Heart J 119:642, 1990.
18. Bateman TM, Czer LSC, Gray RJ, et al: Transient pathologic Q waves during acute ischemic events: An electrocardiographic correlate of stunned but viable myocardium. Am Heart J 106:1421, 1983.
19. Raunio H, Rissanen V, Romppanen T, et al: Changes in the QRS complex and ST segment in transmural and subendocardial myocardial infarctions. A clinicopathologic study. Am Heart J 98:176, 1979.
20. Lee TH, Goldman L: Serum enzyme assays in the diagnosis of acute myocardial infarction. Recommendations based on a quantitative analysis. Ann Intern Med 105:221, 1986.
21. Sobel BE, Shell WE: Serum enzyme determinations in the diagnosis and assessment of myocardial infarction. Circulation 45:471, 1972.
22. Seacord LM, Abendschein DR, Nohara R, et al: Detection of reperfusion within one hour after coronary recanalization by analysis of isoforms of the MM creatine kinase isoenzyme in plasma. Fibrinolysis 2:151, 1988.
23. Ahnve S, Gilpin E, Henning H, et al: Limitations and advantages of the ejection fraction for defining high risk after acute myocardial infarction. Am J Cardiol 58:872, 1986.
24. Hakki A, Nestico PF, Heo J, et al: Relative prognostic value of rest thallium-201 imaging, radionuclide ventriculography and 24-hour ambulatory electrocardiographic monitoring after myocardial infarction. J Am Coll Cardiol 10:25, 1987.
25. Volpini M, Guibbini R, Gei P, et al: Diagnosis of acute myocardial infarction by indium-lll antimyosin antibodies and correlation with the traditional techniques for the evaluation of extent and localization. Am J Cardiol 63:7, 1989.
26. Topol EJ, Burek K, O'Neill WW, et al: A randomized controlled trial of hospital discharge three days after myocardial infarction in the era of reperfusion. N Engl J Med 318:1083, 1988.
27. Curfman GD, Heinsimer JA, Lozner EC, et al: Intravenous nitroglycerin in the treatment of spontaneous angina pectoris: A prospective, randomized trial. Circulation 67:276, 1983.
28. Jugdutt BI, Warnica JW: Intravenous nitroglycerin therapy to limit myocardial infarct size, expansion, and complications. Effect of timing, dosage and infarct location. Circulation 78:906, 1988.
29. Yusuf S, MacMahon S, Collins R, et al: Effect of intravenous nitrates on mortality in acute myocardial infarction: An overview of the randomised trials. Lancet 1:1088, 1988.
30. Rentrop KP, Feit F, Sherman W, et al: Late thrombolytic therapy preserves left ventricular function in patients with collateralized total coronary occlusion: Primary end point findings of the Second Mount Sinai–New York University Reperfusion Trial. J Am Coll Cardiol 14:58, 1989.
31. Becker RC, Corrao JM, Bovill EG, et al: Intravenous nitroglycerin-induced heparin resistance: A qualitative antithrombin III abnormality. Am Heart J 119:1254, 1990.
32. MacMahon S, Collins R, Peto R, et al: Effects of prophylactic lidocaine in suspected acute myocardial infarction. An overview of results from the randomized controlled trials. JAMA 260:1910, 1988.
33. The Cardiac Arrhythmia Suppression Trial (CAST) Investigators: Preliminary report: Effect of encainide and flecainide on mortality in a randomized trial of arrhythmia suppression after myocardial infarction. N Engl J Med 321:406, 1989.
34. Holland Interuniversity Nifedipine/Metoprolol Trial (HINT) Research Group: Early treatment of unstable angina in the coronary care unit: A randomised, double-blind, placebo controlled comparison of recurrent ischaemia in patients treated with nifedipine or metoprolol or both. Br Heart J 56:400, 1986.
35. Muller JE, Turi ZG, Pearle DL, et al: Nifedipine and conventional therapy for unstable angina pectoris. A randomized, double-blind comparison. Circulation 69:728, 1984.
36. Lubsen J: Medical management of unstable angina. What have we learned from the randomized trials? Circulation 82(suppl II):82, 1990.
37. Yusuf S, Wittes J, Friedman L: Overview of results of randomized clinical trials in heart disease. II. Unstable angina, heart failure, primary prevention with aspirin, and risk factor modification. JAMA 260:2259, 1988.
38. Yusuf S, Sleight P, Held P, et al: Routine medical management of acute myocardial infarction. Lessons from overviews of recent randomized controlled trials. Circulation 82(suppl II):117, 1990.
39. Yusuf S, Wittes J, Friedman L: Overview of results of randomized clinical trials in heart disease. I. Treatments following myocardial infarction. JAMA 260:2088, 1988.
40. Gibson RS: Current status of calcium channel blocking drugs after Q wave and non–Q wave myocardial infarction. Circulation 80(suppl IV):107, 1989.
41. Erbel R, Pop T, Meinertz T, et al: Combination of calcium channel blocker and thrombolytic therapy in acute myocardial infarction. Am Heart J 115:529, 1988.
42. The Danish Study Group on Verapamil in Myocardial Infarction: Effect of verapamil on mortality and major events after acute myocardial infarction (the Danish Verapamil Infarction Trial II—DAVIT II). Am J Cardiol 66:779, 1990.
43. Gibson RS, Boden WE, Theroux P, et al: Diltiazem and reinfarction in patients with non–Q-wave myocardial infarction. Results of a double-blind, randomized, multicenter trial. N Engl J Med 315:423, 1986.
44. Gibson RS, Young PM, Boden WE, et al: Prognostic significance and beneficial effect of diltiazem on the incidence of early recurrent ischemia after non–Q wave myocardial infarction: Results from the Multicenter Diltiazem Reinfarction Study. Am J Cardiol 60:203, 1987.
45. Boden WE, Krone RJ, Kleiger RE, et al: Diltiazem reduces long-term cardiac event rate after non–Q wave infarction: Multicenter Diltiazem Post-Infarction Trial (MDPIT). Circulation 78(suppl IV):579, 1988.
46. The Multicenter Diltiazem Postinfarction Trial Research Group: The effect of diltiazem on mortality and reinfarction after myocardial infarction. N Engl J Med 319:385, 1988.
47. Popma JJ, Topol EJ: Adjuncts to thrombolysis for myocardial reperfusion. Ann Intern Med 115:34, 1991.
48. The TIMI Study Group: Comparison of invasive and conservative strategies after treatment with intravenous tissue plasminogen activator in acute myocardial infarction. Results of the Thrombolysis in Myocardial Infarction (TIMI) Phase II Trial. N Engl J Med 320:618, 1989.
49. Kirshenbaum JM, Kloner RA, Antman EA, et al: Use of an ultra short-acting β-blocker in patients with acute myocardial ischemia. Circulation 72:873, 1985.
50. The International Study Group: In-hospital mortality and clinical course of 20891 patients with suspected acute myocardial infarction randomised between alteplase and streptokinase with or without heparin. Lancet 336:71, 1990.
51. The MIAMI Trial Research Group: Metoprolol in acute myocardial infarction (MIAMI): A randomised placebo-controlled international trial. Eur Heart J 6:199, 1985.
52. Goldman L, Sia STB, Cook EF, et al: Costs and effectiveness of routine therapy with long-term beta-adrenergic antagonists after acute myocardial infarction. N Engl J Med 319:152, 1988.
53. Reimer KA, Jennings RB: The wavefront phenomenon of myocardial ischemic cell death. II. Transmural progression of necrosis within the framework of ischemic bed size (myocardium at risk) and collateral flow. Lab Invest 40:633, 1979.
54. Verstraete M: Thrombolytic treatment in acute myocardial infarction. Circulation 82(suppl II):96, 1990.

55. Sherry S, Marder VJ: Streptokinase and recombinant tissue plasminogen activator (rt-PA) are equally effective in treating acute myocardial infarction. Ann Intern Med 114:417, 1991.

56. Yusuf S, Collins R, Peto R, et al: Intravenous and intracoronary fibrinolytic therapy in acute myocardial infarction: Overview of results on mortality, reinfarction and side-effects from 33 randomized controlled trials. Eur Heart J 6:556, 1985.

57. Muller DWM, Topol EJ: Selection of patients with acute myocardial infarction for thrombolytic therapy. Ann Intern Med 113:949, 1990.

58. ISIS-2 Collaborative Group: Randomised trial of intravenous streptokinase, oral aspirin, both, or neither among 17187 cases of suspected acute myocardial infarction: ISIS-2. Lancet 2:349, 1988.

59. Gruppo Italiano per lo Studio della Streptochinasi nell 'Infarto Miocardico (GISSI): Effectiveness of intravenous thrombolytic treatment in acute myocardial infarction. Lancet 1:397, 1986.

60. Wilcox RG, von der Lippe G, Olsson CG, et al: Trial of tissue plasminogen activator for mortality reduction in acute myocardial infarction. Anglo-Scandinavian Study of Early Thrombolysis (ASSET). Lancet 2:525, 1988.

61. AIMS Trial Study Group: Effect of intravenous APSAC on mortality after acute myocardial infarction: Preliminary report of a placebo-controlled clinical trial. Lancet 1:545, 1988.

62. Gruppo Italiano per lo Studio della Streptochinasi nell 'Infarto Miocardico (GISSI): Long-term effects of intravenous thrombolysis in acute myocardial infarction: Final report of the GISSI study. Lancet 2:871, 1987.

63. Simoons ML, Vos J, Tijssen JGP, et al: Long-term benefit of early thrombolytic therapy in patients with acute myocardial infarction: 5-year follow-up of a trial conducted by the Interuniversity Cardiology Institute of the Netherlands. J Am Coll Cardiol 14:1609, 1989.

64. Cragg DR, Friedman HZ, Bonema JD, et al: Outcome of patients with acute myocardial infarction who are ineligible for thrombolytic therapy. Ann Intern Med 115:173, 1991.

65. Hockman JS, Choo H: Limitation of myocardial infarct expansion by reperfusion independent of myocardial salvage. Circulation 75:299, 1987.

66. Hale SL, Kloner RA: Left ventricular topographic alterations in the completely healed rat infarct caused by early and late coronary artery reperfusion. Am Heart J 116:1508, 1988.

67. Kersschot IE, Brugada P, Ramentol M, et al: Effects of early reperfusion in acute myocardial infarction on arrhythmias induced by programmed stimulation: A prospective, randomized study. J Am Coll Cardiol 7:1234, 1986.

68. Sager PT, Perlmutter RA, Rosenfeld LE, et al: Electrophysiologic effects of thrombolytic therapy in patients with a transmural anterior myocardial infarction complicated by left ventricular aneurysm formation. J Am Coll Cardiol 12:19, 1988.

69. Eigler N, Maurer G, Shah PK: Effect of early systemic thrombolytic therapy on left ventricular mural thrombus formation in acute anterior myocardial infarction. Am J Cardiol 54:261, 1984.

70. Mauri F, Gasparini M, Barbonaglia L, et al: Prognostic significance of the extent of myocardial injury in acute myocardial infarction treated by streptokinase (the GISSI trial). Am J Cardiol 63:1291, 1989.

71. Verstraete M, Miller GAH, Bounameaux H, et al: Intravenous and intrapulmonary recombinant tissue-type plasminogen activator in the treatment of acute massive pulmonary embolism. Circulation 77:353, 1988.

72. White HD, Rivers JT, Maslowski AH, et al: Effect of intravenous streptokinase as compared with that of tissue plasminogen activator on left ventricular function after first myocardial infarction. N Engl J Med 320:817, 1989.

73. ISIS-3 (Third International Study of Infarct Survival) Collaborative Group: ISIS-3: A randomised comparison of streptokinase vs tissue plasminogen activator vs antistreplase and of aspirin plus heparin vs aspirin alone among 41 299 cases of suspected acute myocardial infarction. Lancet 339:753, 1992.

74. Chesboro JH, Fuster V: Antithrombotic therapy for acute myocardial infarction: Mechanisms and prevention of deep venous, left ventricular and coronary artery thromboembolism. Circulation 74(suppl III):1, 1986.

75. Gallus AS: Overview of the management of thrombotic disorders. Semin Thromb Hemost 15:99, 1989.

76. Halkin H, Goldberg J, Modan M, et al: Reduction of mortality in general medical in-patients by low-dose heparin prophylaxis. Ann Intern Med 96:561, 1982.

77. Meltzer RS, Visser CA, Fuster V: Intracardiac thrombi and systemic embolization. Ann Intern Med 104:689, 1986.

78. Fuster V, Stein B, Halperin JL, et al: Antithrombotic therapy in cardiac disease: An approach based on pathogenesis and risk stratification. Am J Cardiol 65:38C, 1990.

79. Turpie AGG, Robinson JG, Doyle DJ, et al: Comparison of high-dose with low-dose subcutaneous heparin to prevent left ventricular mural thrombosis in patients with acute transmural anterior myocardial infarction. N Engl J Med 320:352, 1989.

80. Theroux P, Ouimet H, McCans J, et al: Aspirin, heparin or both to treat acute unstable angina. N Engl J Med 319:1105, 1988.

81. Neri Serneri GG, Gensini GF, Poggesi L, et al: Effect of heparin, aspirin, or alteplase in reduction of myocardial ischaemia in refractory unstable angina. Lancet 335:615, 1990.

82. Hirsh J: Heparin. N Engl J Med 324:1565, 1991.

83. Bleich SD, Nicholas TC, Schumacher RR, et al: Effect of heparin on coronary arterial patency after thrombolysis with tissue plasminogen activator in acute myocardial infarction. Am J Cardiol 66:1412, 1990.

84. Hsia J, Hamilton WP, Kleiman N, et al: A comparison between heparin and low-dose aspirin as adjunctive therapy with tissue plasminogen activator for acute myocardial infarction. N Engl J Med 323:1433, 1990.

85. de Bono DP, Simoons ML, Tijssen J, et al: Effect of early intravenous heparin on coronary patency, infarct size, and bleeding complications after alteplase thrombolysis: Results of a randomised double blind European Cooperative Study Group trial. Br Heart J 67:122, 1992.

86. The SCATI (Studio sulla Calciparina nell'Angina e nella Trombosi Ventricolare nell'Infarto) Group: Randomised controlled trial of subcutaneous calcium-heparin in acute myocardial infarction. Lancet 2:182, 1989.

87. Gruppo Italiano per lo Studio della Sopravvivenza nell'Infarto Miocardico. GISSI-2: A factorial randomised trial of alteplase versus streptokinase and heparin versus no heparin among 12,490 patients with acute myocardial infarction. Lancet 336:65, 1990.

88. Prins MH, Hirsh J: Heparin as an adjunctive treatment after thrombolytic therapy for acute myocardial infarction. Am J Cardiol 67:3A, 1991.

89. Resnekov L, Chediak J, Hirsh J, et al: Antithrombotic agents in coronary artery disease. Chest 95(suppl):52S, 1989.

90. Hirsh J, Poller L, Deykin D: Optimal therapeutic range for oral anticoagulants. Chest 95(suppl):5S, 1989.

91. Kouvaras G, Chronopoulos G, Soufras G, et al: The effects of long-term antithrombotic treatment on left ventricular thrombi in patients after an acute myocardial infarction. Am Heart J 119:73, 1990.

92. Smith P, Arnesen H, Holme I: The effect of warfarin on mortality and reinfarction after myocardial infarction. N Engl J Med 323:147, 1990.

93. Lewis HD, Davis JW, Archibald DG, et al: Protective effects of aspirin against acute myocardial infarction and death in men with unstable angina. Results of a Veterans Administration Cooperative Study. N Engl J Med 309:396, 1983.

94. Cairns JA, Gent M, Singer J, et al: Aspirin, sulfinpyrazone or both in unstable angina. Results of a Canadian multicenter trial. N Engl J Med 313:1369, 1985.

95. Peduzzi P, Hultgren H, Thomsen J, et al: Ten-year effect of medical and surgical therapy on quality of life: Veterans Administration Cooperative Study of Coronary Artery Surgery. Am J Cardiol 59:1017, 1987.

96. Booth DC, Deupree RH, Hultgren HN, et al: Quality of life after bypass surgery for unstable angina. 5-year follow-up results of a Veterans Affairs Cooperative Study. Circulation 83:87, 1991.

97. Scott SM, Luchi RJ, Deupree RH, et al: Veterans Administration Cooperative Study for Treatment of Patients with Unstable Angina. Results in patients with abnormal ventricular function. Circulation 78(suppl I):113, 1988.

98. Parisi AF, Khuri S, Deupree RH, et al: Medical compared with surgical management of unstable angina. Five year mortality and morbidity in the Veterans Administration Study. Circulation 80:1176, 1989.

99. Phillips SJ, Zeff RH, Skinner JR, et al: Reperfusion protocol and results in 738 patients with evolving myocardial infarction. Ann Thorac Surg 41:119, 1986.

100. DeWood MA, Spores J, Notske RN, et al: Medical and surgical management of myocardial infarction. Am J Cardiol 44:1356, 1979.

101. Flameng W, Sergeant P, Vanhaecke J, et al: Emergency coronary bypass grafting for evolving myocardial infarction. Effects on infarct size and left ventricular function. J Thorac Cardiovasc Surg 94:124, 1987.

102. Meyer J, Schmitz H, Erbel B, et al: Transluminal angioplasty in patients with unstable angina pectoris. In: Kaltenbach M (ed): Transluminal Coronary Angioplasty and Intracoronary Thrombolysis. Berlin, Springer-Verlag, p 367, 1982.

103. Williams DO, Riley RS, Singh AK, et al: Evaluation of the role of coronary angioplasty in patients with unstable angina pectoris. Am Heart J 102:1, 1981.

104. Faxon DP, Detre KM, McCabe CH, et al: Role of percutaneous transluminal coronary angioplasty in the treatment of unstable angina. Report from the National Heart, Lung, and Blood Institute Percutaneous Transluminal Coronary Angioplasty and Coronary Artery Surgery Study Registries. Am J Cardiol 53:131C, 1983.

105. DeFeyter P, Serruys PW, vanden Brand M, et al: Emergency coronary angioplasty in refractory unstable angina. N Engl J Med 313:342, 1985.

106. Plokker HW, Ernst SM, Bal ET, et al: Percutaneous transluminal coronary angioplasty in patients with unstable angina pectoris refractory to medical therapy: Long-term clinical and angiographic results. Cathet Cardiovasc Diagn 14:15, 1988.

107. Wohlgelernter D, Cleman M, Highman HA, et al: Percutaneous transluminal coronary angioplasty of the "culprit lesion" for management of unstable angina pectoris in patients with multivessel coronary artery disease. Am J Cardiol 58:460, 1986.

108. Sharma B, Wyeth RP, Kolath GS, et al: Percutaneous transluminal coronary angioplasty of one vessel for refractory unstable angina pectoris: Efficacy in single and multivessel disease. Br Heart J 59:280, 1988.

109. Cook SL, Eigler NL, Shefer A, et al: Percutaneous excimer laser coronary angioplasty of lesions not ideal for balloon angioplasty. Circulation 84:632, 1991.
110. Jenkins RD, Safian RD, Dean WE, et al: Laser balloon angioplasty for unstable ischemic syndromes (abstract). J Am Coll Cardiol 15(suppl A):245A, 1991.
111. Hartzler GO, Rutherford BD, McConahay DR, et al: Percutaneous transluminal coronary angioplasty with and without thrombolytic therapy for treatment of acute myocardial infarction. Am Heart J 106:965, 1983.
112. Pepine CJ, Prida X, Hill JA, et al: Percutaneous transluminal coronary angioplasty in acute myocardial infarction. Am Heart J 107:820, 1985.
113. Hartzler GO, Rutherford BD, McConahay DR: Percutaneous transluminal coronary angioplasty: Application for acute myocardial infarction. Am J Cardiol 53:117C, 1984.
114. Sriram R, Mullen GM, Foschi A, et al: Percutaneous transluminal coronary angioplasty in acute myocardial infarction without prior thrombolytic therapy. Am J Cardiol 55:842, 1985.
115. O'Neill W, Timmis GC, Bourdillon PD, et al: A prospective randomized clinical trial of intracoronary streptokinase versus coronary angioplasty for acute myocardial infarction. N Engl J Med 314:812, 1986.
116. Rothbaum DA, Linnemeier TJ, Landin RJ, et al: Emergency percutaneous transluminal coronary angioplasty in acute myocardial infarction: A 3 year experience. J Am Coll Cardiol 10:264, 1987.
117. Topol EJ, Califf RM, George BS, et al: A randomized trial of immediate versus delayed elective angioplasty after intravenous tissue plasminogen activator in acute myocardial infarction. N Engl J Med 317:581, 1987.
118. Simoons ML, Arnold AER, Betriu A, et al: Thrombolysis with tissue plasminogen activator in acute myocardial infarction: No additional benefit from immediate percutaneous coronary angioplasty. Lancet 1:197, 1988.
119. Goldberger M, Tabak SW, Shah PK: Clinical experience with intra-aortic balloon counterpulsation in 112 consecutive patients. Am Heart J 111:497, 1986.
120. Isner JM, Cohen SR, Virmani R, et al: Complications of the intraaortic balloon counterpulsation device: Clinical and morphologic observations in 45 necropsy patients. Am J Cardiol 45:260, 1980.
121. Muller JE, Turi ZG, Stone PH, et al: Digoxin therapy and mortality after myocardial infarction. N Engl J Med 314:265, 1986.
122. Tofler GH, Stone PH, Muller JE, et al: Prognosis after cardiac arrest due to ventricular tachycardia or ventricular fibrillation associated with acute myocardial infarction (the MILIS study). Am J Cardiol 60:755, 1987.
123. Volpi A, Maggioni A, Franzosi MG, et al: In-hospital prognosis of patients with acute myocardial infarction complicated by primary ventricular fibrillation. N Engl J Med 317:257, 1987.
124. Bigger JT Jr, Fleiss JL, Kleiger R, et al: The relationships among ventricular arrhythmias, left ventricular dysfunction, and mortality in the 2 years after myocardial infarction. Circulation 69:250, 1984.
125. De Guzman M, Rahimtoola SH: What is the role of pacemakers in patients with coronary artery disease and conduction abnormalities? Cardiovasc Clin 13:191, 1983.
126. Lee L, Bates ER, Pitt B, et al: Percutaneous transluminal coronary angioplasty improves survival in acute myocardial infarction complicated by cardiogenic shock. Circulation 78:1345, 1988.
127. Bellamy GR, Rasmussen HH, Nasser RN, et al: Value of two-dimensional echocardiography, electrocardiography, and clinical signs in detecting right ventricular infarction. Am Heart J 112:304, 1986.
128. Lamas GA, Pfeffer MA: Left ventricular remodeling after acute myocardial infarction: Clinical course and beneficial effects of angiotensin-converting enzyme inhibition. Am Heart J 121:1194, 1991.
129. Erlebacher JA, Weiss JL, Weisfeldt ML, et al: Early dilation of the infarcted segment in acute transmural myocardial infarction: Role of infarct expansion in acute left ventricular enlargement. J Am Coll Cardiol 4:201, 1984.
130. Meizlish JL, Berger HJ, Plankey M, et al: Functional left ventricular aneurysm formation after acute anterior transmural myocardial infarction. Incidence, natural history, and prognostic implications. N Engl J Med 311:1001, 1984.
131. Lamas GA, Vaughan DE, Parisi AF, et al: Effects of left ventricular shape and captopril therapy on exercise capacity after anterior wall acute myocardial infarction. Am J Cardiol 63:1167, 1989.
132. Sharpe N, Murphy J, Smith H, et al: Treatment of patients with symptomless left ventricular dysfunction after myocardial infarction. Lancet 1:255, 1988.
133. Nabel EG, Topol EJ, Galeana A, et al: A randomized, double-blind, placebo-controlled pilot trial of combined early intravenous captopril and tPA therapy in acute myocardial infarction (abstract). Circulation 80(suppl II):112, 1989.
134. Gray RJ, Sethna D, Matloff JM: The role of cardiac surgery in acute myocardial infarction. I. With mechanical complications. Am Heart J 106:723, 1983.
135. Bates RJ, Beutler S, Resnekov L, et al: Cardiac rupture—Challenge in diagnosis and management. Am J Cardiol 40:429, 1977.
136. Nishimura RA, Schaff HV, Shub C, et al: Papillary muscle rupture complicating acute myocardial infarction: Analysis of 17 patients. Am J Cardiol 51:373, 1983.

137. Clements SG, Story WE, Hurst JW, et al: Ruptured papillary muscle, a complication of myocardial infarction: Clinical presentation, diagnosis and treatment. Clin Cardiol 8:93, 1985.
138. Tofler GH, Muller JE, Stone PH, et al: Pericarditis in acute myocardial infarction: Characterization and clinical significance. Am Heart J 117:86, 1989.
139. Krainin FM, Flessas AP, Spodick DH: Infarction-associated pericarditis. Rarity of diagnostic electrocardiogram. N Engl J Med 311:1211, 1984.
140. Silverman HW, Pfeifer MP: Relation between use of anti-inflammatory agents and left ventricular free wall rupture during acute myocardial infarction. Am J Cardiol 59:363, 1987.
141. Friedman PL, Brown EJ Jr, Gunther S, et al: Coronary vasoconstrictor effect of indomethacin in patients with coronary-artery disease. N Engl J Med 305:1171, 1981.
142. Maisel AM, Ahnve S, Gilpin E, et al: Prognosis after extension of myocardial infarct: The role of Q wave or non–Q wave infarction. Circulation 71:211, 1985.
143. Muller JE, Rude RE, Braunwald E, et al: Myocardial infarct extension: Occurrence, outcome, and risk factors in the Multicenter Investigation of Limitation of Infarct Size. Ann Intern Med 108:1, 1988.
144. Schuster EH, Bulkley BH: Early post-infarction angina. Ischemia at a distance and ischemia in the infarct zone. N Engl J Med 305:1101, 1981.
145. Fioretti P, Brower RW, Simoons ML, et al: Prediction of mortality in hospital survivors of myocardial infarction. Comparison of predischarge exercise testing and radionuclide ventriculography at rest. Br Heart J 52:292, 1984.
146. Topol EJ, Holmes DR, Rogers WJ: Coronary angiography after thrombolytic therapy for acute myocardial infarction. Ann Intern Med 114:877, 1991.
147. Weiss AT, Maddahi J, Shah PK, et al: Exercise-induced ischemia in the streptokinase-reperfused myocardium: Relationship to extent of salvaged myocardium and degree of residual coronary stenosis. Am Heart J 118:9, 1989.
148. Touchstone DA, Beller GA, Nygaard TW, et al: Functional significance of predischarge exercise thallium-201 findings following intravenous streptokinase therapy during acute myocardial infarction. Am Heart J 116:1500, 1988.
149. The Multicenter Postinfarction Research Group: Risk stratification and survival after myocardial infarction. N Engl J Med 309:331, 1983.
150. Lewis SJ, Lander PT, Taylor PA, et al: Evolution of late potential activity in the first six weeks after acute myocardial infarction. Am J Cardiol 63:647, 1989.
151. Turitto G, Caref EB, Macina G, et al: Time course of ventricular arrhythmias and the signal averaged electrocardiogram in the post-infarction period: A prospective study of correlation. Br Heart J 60:17, 1988.
152. Cripps T, Bennett D, Camm J, et al: Prospective evaluation of clinical assessment, exercise testing and signal-averaged electrocardiogram in predicting outcome after acute myocardial infarction. Am J Cardiol 62:995, 1988.
153. Kuchar DL, Thorburn CW, Sammel NL: Late potentials detected after myocardial infarction: Natural history and prognostic significance. Circulation 74:1280, 1986.
154. Gomes JA, Winters SL, Martinson M, et al: The prognostic significance of quantitative signal-averaged variables relative to clinical variables, site of myocardial infarction, ejection fraction and ventricular premature beats: A prospective study. J Am Coll Cardiol 13:377, 1989.

CHAPTER 91

Left-Sided Heart Failure

Richard P. Lewis
Carl V. Leier

SPECTRUM OF LEFT-SIDED HEART FAILURE

Left-sided heart failure is a common problem in the intensive care setting. Its most extreme manifestation is cardiogenic shock, for which the prognosis is dire. Acute pulmonary edema, another dramatic form, also requires urgent therapy and has a significant mortality. At the other extreme is transient and often reversible left ventricular dysfunction associated with sepsis and other toxic states.[1] The most common form of left-sided heart failure is low-output chronic congestive heart failure (CHF), which may be seen as the initial presentation or as an exacerbation.

Left-sided heart failure can be due to systolic dysfunction of the left ventricle, aortic or mitral valvular disease, or predominant diastolic dysfunction of the left ventricle. There are more than 400,000 new cases annually in the United States. Therapy for the various manifestations of left-sided heart failure varies with the severity and nature of the presentation. This chapter deals with the more acute forms of left-sided heart failure, although general principles of chronic therapy are also discussed. The most common causes of left-sided heart failure are listed in Table 91–1.

Left-sided heart failure is usually accompanied by fluid retention and is therefore termed *congestive heart failure*. However, the extent of fluid retention does not correlate with the severity of left-sided heart failure, in part because of modern diuretic therapy. Furthermore, the severity of left ventricular dysfunction does not correlate closely with symptomatic limitation. Patients with chronic left-sided heart failure may experience successful peripheral vascular adaptations and tolerate remarkable degrees of left ventricular dysfunction with minimal symptoms.

Patients with chronic left-sided heart failure are grouped into three broad categories, mild, moderate, and severe CHF, with the mild category corresponding to New York Heart Association functional class I–II, the moderate category to class III, and the severe category to class IV. The 2-year mortality for mild heart failure is 5 to 10%; for moderate heart failure, 20 to 25%; and for severe heart failure, 70 to 80%.

MYOCARDIAL RESPONSES IN LEFT-SIDED HEART FAILURE

Left ventricular myocardial failure is best defined as a state wherein there is insufficient myocardial mass to meet the demands of systolic contraction. This state can be the result of an excessive mechanical load or intrinsic myocardial disease. The myocardial response in either case is hypertrophy.[2-7] Hypertrophy involves addition of new contractile units (sarcomeres). The stimulus for hypertrophy is still unclear but is related to myocardial wall stress.

According to the formulation of Laplace, myocardial wall stress is given approximately by the formula

$$S = Pr/2h$$

where S = wall stress
P = ventricular pressure
r = ventricular radius
h = ventricular wall thickness

Thus, wall stress is directly related to systolic pressure and volume and inversely related to wall thickness.

Cardiac hypertrophy is present in all types of chronic left ventricular disease and has two major forms. In pressure loads, as in aortic stenosis or arterial hypertension, sarcomeres are added in parallel so that the wall thickness increases without increased cavitary dimensions. In volume loads (aortic or mitral regurgitation or "remodeling" after myocardial infarction) sarcomeres are added in series as well as in parallel and the cavity volume increases. Although hypertrophied muscle is less efficient than normal muscle, the cardiac hypertrophic response to a pressure or volume load may be successful enough to allow normalization of wall stress for each individual contractile unit.[8, 9] Thus, the

TABLE 91–1

COMMON CAUSES OF LEFT-SIDED HEART FAILURE

Acute Left-Sided Heart Failure
  Acute myocardial infarction
    Massive anterior infarction
    Right ventricular infarction syndrome (inferior infarction)
    Papillary muscle rupture or dysfunction
    Ruptured interventricular septum
  Aortic stenosis
  Uncontrolled hypertension
  Ruptured chordae tendineae (myxomatous valve disease)
  Subacute bacterial endocarditis of aortic and/or mitral valve
  Sepsis
  Chronic obstructive pulmonary disease
  Myocarditis
  Complications in patients with chronic heart disease
    Atrial fibrillation
    Pregnancy
    Renal failure
  End-stage chronic left-sided heart failure

Chronic Left-Sided Heart Failure
  Cardiomyopathy
    Dilated
    Ischemic
    Hypertensive
    Other (obstructive, restrictive)
  Valvular heart disease
    Aortic regurgitation
    Mitral regurgitation
    Mitral stenosis

ejection fraction remains normal. This is referred to as compensated left ventricular disease (Fig. 91–1).

Eventually the hemodynamic load worsens or intrinsic myocardial dysfunction progresses, and hypertrophy is no longer adequate for the total wall stress of the ventricle. At this point, myocardial energy is diverted from fiber-shortening work to maintain wall stress and the ejection fraction falls. This condition is referred to as decompensated left ventricular disease, and there ensues progressive left ventricular dilatation ("pathologic" dilatation) that initiates an irreversible heart failure cycle.

The mechanism of pathologic dilatation remains unclear. It does not involve overstretched sarcomeres, as has long been believed. It probably involves slippage of myocardial fiber layers caused by excessive wall stress.[4] As the ventricle becomes dilated it assumes a more spheric shape, which in

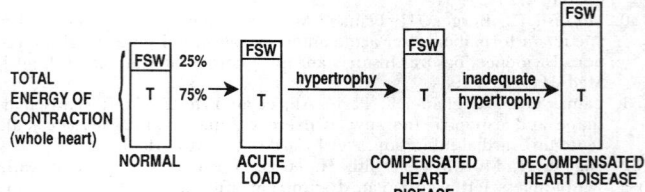

Figure 91–1. Schematic illustration of the effects of an acute load on the total energy of contraction for the whole heart. An acute load causes a fall in fiber-shortening work (FSW) as energy is directed to maintaining wall tension (T). As compensatory hypertrophy develops, the relative proportion of energy for FSW is restored and the ejection fraction returns to normal. Eventually, the amount of hypertrophy becomes inadequate because of either progressive increase in load (e.g., aortic stenosis) or ischemic death of myocardium. At this point, the FSW again drops and the ejection fraction falls. The total energy of contraction, however, is further increased.

itself mitigates the advantage of the helical inner and outer fiber layers, which enable nearly complete systolic emptying when the ventricle has the normal ellipsoidal shape. There is evidence that increased sphericity is more common in the myopathic ventricle than in a ventricle that has dilated in response to a volume load.[10]

Although pathologic dilatation enables a stroke volume of normal size to be maintained in spite of a low ejection fraction, it has many disadvantages. Pathologic dilatation increases left ventricular dimensions and therefore wall stress. In addition, the dilated heart with a low ejection fraction cannot reduce wall stress during the last half of systole because of the less than normal decrease in left ventricular volume during systole. Evidence is accumulating that therapeutic measures that reduce wall stress in chronic left ventricular disease may mitigate the process of pathologic dilatation (discussed later).[11]

Myocardial systolic wall stress is the primary determinant of myocardial oxygen consumption. Other determinants are fiber-shortening work, tachycardia, and positive inotropic stimulation. Myocardial oxygen consumption in turn determines coronary blood flow requirements. When left ventricular mass increases as a result of hypertrophy, the myocardial oxygen consumption increases and resting coronary blood flow must increase in a parallel fashion because the myocardium normally extracts the maximal amount of oxygen from the arterial blood. This requires growth in both the microcirculation and epicardial coronary arteries, and the latter is often limited by atherosclerosis. When pathologic dilatation develops, the situation is aggravated because the oxygen consumption per gram of myocardium is also increased over normal as a result of excessive wall stress. Thus, the heart in most patients with left-sided heart failure requires substantially more oxygen delivery than normal.[12-14]

Coronary blood flow can be compromised by increased left ventricular end-diastolic pressure, which is usually present in patients with CHF. Because arterial diastolic pressure is usually normal or low, the high left ventricular end-diastolic pressure reduces the coronary perfusion gradient. Sinus tachycardia, atrial flutter, and fibrillation also reduce coronary blood flow by reducing diastolic coronary perfusion time (Fig. 91–2). Left ventricular coronary perfusion is virtually all diastolic. Thus, hypertrophied hearts are easily rendered ischemic even in the absence of coronary artery disease. Ischemic dysfunction is present in many patients with left-sided heart failure and is potentially remediable.[12] If unrecognized, however, chronic ischemia, especially in the subendocardium, can lead to cell death and fibrosis.[14] Many forms of treatment of left ventricular dysfunction undoubtedly produce clinical improvement by improving subendocardial blood flow and reversing ischemic dysfunction (see later).[15]

Hypertrophy with or without subendocardial fibrosis and ischemia reduces ventricular diastolic compliance.[16] In some disorders, notably chronic arterial hypertension, and in old age, left ventricular diastolic dysfunction is an early manifestation of left-sided heart failure. Such patients have high filling pressures and relatively intact systolic function but may nonetheless develop a clinical picture resembling that of CHF. It is important to recognize this subset of patients because chronic therapy differs significantly from the therapy employed when systolic dysfunction is the major problem.

Chronic left ventricular diastolic dysfunction results in hypertrophy of the left atrium to meet the increased pressure load for ventricular filling. The hypertrophied left atrium can produce as much pressure with atrial systole as is normally produced by the right ventricle. Atrial systole may account for nearly half of ventricular diastolic filling.

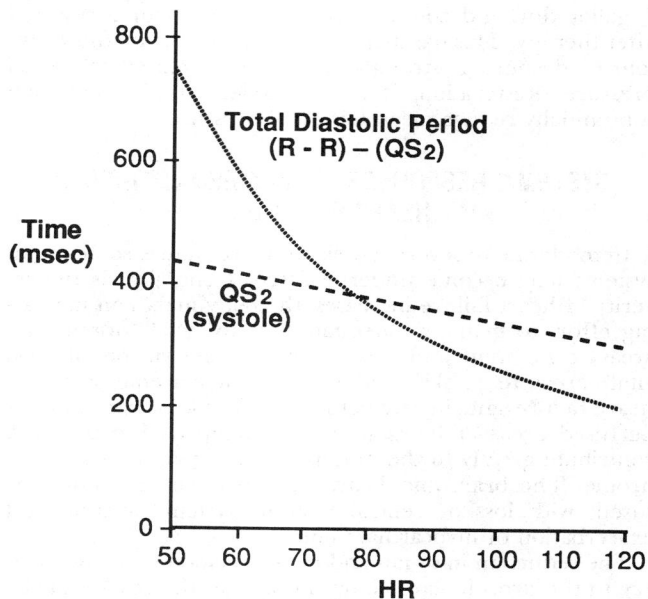

Figure 91–2. The total diastolic period (RR–QS$_2$) is not linearly related to heart rate as is the systolic period measured from systolic time intervals (QS$_2$). (From Boudoulas H, Rittgers SE, Lewis RP, et al: Changes in diastolic time with various pharmacologic agents. Implication for myocardial perfusion. Circulation 60:164–169, 1979. Reproduced with permission. Copyright 1979 American Heart Association.)

Eventually, however, left atrial wall stress exceeds the compensatory hypertrophic response and atrial dilatation and failure occur. At this point, the magnitude of the left atrial systolic pressure wave (the a wave) drops and mean left atrial pressure increases. This results in the appearance of a predominant S$_3$ instead of an S$_4$ gallop (Fig. 91–3). The presence of an S$_3$ gallop, which is in reality the result of atrial failure, is a useful clinical indicator of advanced left-sided heart failure.

Left atrial dysfunction is more rapidly reversible than ventricular dysfunction and occurs as a result of either therapy with inotropic agents or reduction of preload and afterload to the left atrium. Thus, patients may exhibit an

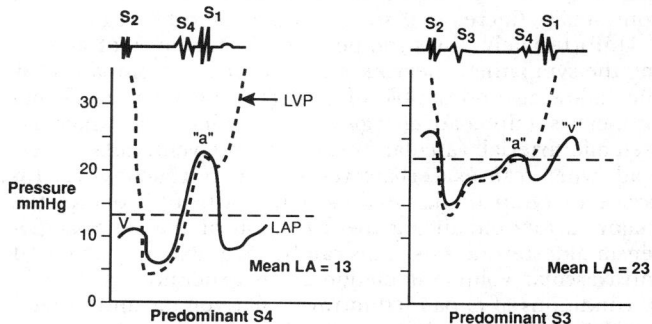

Figure 91–3. Schematic illustration of the left atrial (LAP) and left ventricular (LVP) diastolic pressures and phonocardiogram in chronic heart disease associated with a predominant S$_3$ or S$_4$ gallop. When there is a predominant S$_4$, there is a large atrial contraction (a wave) producing a loud S$_4$ gallop and low mean left atrial pressure. When the atrium fails, the mean left atrial pressure rises. The v wave height increases, resulting in a high filling pressure in early diastole producing a loud S$_3$ gallop. (Reprinted from Lewis RP: Digitalis. In: Leier CV [ed]: Cardiotonic Drugs: A Clinical Survey. New York, Marcel Dekker, p 85, 1987 by courtesy of Marcel Dekker, Inc.)

S₃ gallop during decompensation but an S₄ gallop is restored after therapy. This has major implications because the symptom of dyspnea is strongly related to increased left atrial pressure. Restoration of a normal left atrial systole can substantially reduce mean left atrial pressure.

SYSTEMIC RESPONSES TO IMPAIRED LEFT-SIDED HEART FUNCTION

In moderate to severe left-sided heart failure, some organ systems may become underperfused. Generally, as the severity of heart failure increases, the body makes an increasing effort to maintain adequate flow to "vital" organs and areas (e.g., brain and heart) via vasoconstriction of "less vital" areas (e.g., skin and viscera). In extreme stages of heart failure and in circulatory shock, the various underperfused areas and organs may develop dysfunction and contribute greatly to the multiple organ system failure syndrome. The brain and heart may also become underperfused, with loss of central nervous system function and exacerbation of myocardial failure.

The reduction in organ and regional blood flow is secondary to the drop in cardiac output and to the release of the vasoconstricting neurohumoral substances norepinephrine, angiotensin II, and vasopressin. Vasodilating substances (e.g., atrial natriuretic factor, local bradykinin, local prostaglandin, and various vascular endothelium-relaxing factors) are also released in advanced left-sided heart failure, but in most situations the vasodilating effects of these substances are overwhelmed by the effects of the vasoconstricting compounds.

Activation of the Sympathetic Nervous System

The mechanisms causing enhanced activity of the sympathetic nervous system in heart failure are not fully understood or known.[17–19] It may in fact represent inappropriate activation of the bodily defense mechanisms against hypovolemia. It is generally thought that reduced blood pressure, pulse pressure, and flow in the region of arterial high-pressure baroreceptors play a major role in activating the sympathetic nervous system. Hypoperfusion of various organs and regions probably contributes to the activation of the sympathetic nervous system as well. The activation of the sympathetic nervous system represents an effort to augment cardiac output via enhancement of ventricular contractility (increase of stroke volume) and heart rate.

Unfortunately, this "compensatory" maneuver of activating the sympathetic nervous system is often accompanied by the following undesirable effects: (1) The vasoconstricting properties (alpha-adrenergic) of norepinephrine increase systemic arterial vascular resistance and ventricular afterload, which can exacerbate ventricular dysfunction. (2) Increase of sympathetic nervous system activity is one of the major factors enhancing the activation of the renin-angiotensin-aldosterone axis. This can be favorable in a setting of intravascular volume depletion but is generally detrimental in conditions of expanded intravascular volume and congestive left-sided heart failure. (3) The activation of the sympathetic nervous system can effect venoconstriction to reduce relative venous capacitance and contribute to an inordinate increase in central blood volume and excessive preload. (4) Heightened sympathetic nervous system activity increases myocardial oxygen consumption; this is extremely important in patients with hypoperfused myocardium (e.g., patients with coronary artery obstruction), who cannot increase myocardial blood flow to match the increase in oxygen demands. (5) When the sympathetic nervous system activity is present

for prolonged periods, down-regulation of some myocardial inotropic receptors occurs, thereby blunting the inotropic response.[20]

The heightened sympathetic nervous system tone accounts for many of the clinical manifestations of left-sided heart failure including tachycardia, increased anxiety, restlessness, altered rest and sleep patterns, central pallor, cool moist palms and feet, and cardiac arrhythmias (particularly when it is combined with underlying structural heart disease, electrolyte abnormalities, or other disorder).

Activation of the Renin-Angiotensin-Aldosterone Axis

The activation of this axis sets up a number of pathophysiologic events in heart failure, most related to elevated angiotensin II and aldosterone levels. In heart failure, elevated angiotensin II greatly enhances vasoconstriction, increasing systemic vascular resistance and afterload with resultant depression of cardiac systolic function; augments sympathetic nervous system tone by increasing the release of, blocking the reuptake of, and increasing the sensitivity to norepinephrine at the nerve ending; stimulates the thirst center; releases arginine vasopressin, enhancing water retention at the kidney level; and increases aldosterone release. Elevated aldosterone in heart failure causes salt and water retention by the kidney, increasing total body salt and water content, intravascular volume, and preload, and increases salt and water content of arterioles, impairing their ability to dilate and thus further augmenting systemic vascular resistance and ventricular afterload. Aldosterone causes hypokalemia via sodium-potassium exchange at the distal tubule and may lead to hypomagnesemia as well.

Increased Vascular Resistances and Ventricular Afterload

It is important not to confuse blood pressure with systemic vascular resistance. Basically, systemic vascular resistance = mean blood pressure/cardiac output. In heart failure, mean blood pressure may be in the normal range or even low, but systemic vascular resistance and ventricular afterload can be high because, at that particular level of blood pressure, the cardiac output is markedly depressed. Stated another way, systemic vascular resistance is markedly increased in conditions of marked reduction in cardiac output such that mean blood pressure is maintained at a normal level or is slightly reduced. This is an important consideration with respect to therapeutics because in many phases of left-sided heart failure, therapies are directed at primarily reducing systemic vascular resistance with a resultant increase in stroke volume and cardiac output so that systemic blood pressure is maintained (pulse pressure is even augmented) in the presence of drug-reduced vascular resistance. Alternatively, allowing an additional increase in systemic vascular resistance in these patients results in further reduction in cardiac output and further deterioration of overall cardiovascular function.

As noted earlier, ventricular afterload represents the overall workload on the ventricle during systole and is defined as wall stress. Therefore, anything that increases ventricular systolic pressure (via increases in aortic impedance or systemic vascular resistance) or ventricular systolic volume increases afterload. Because of the detrimental relationship between ventricular afterload and ventricular function in patients with impaired cardiac function, therapeutics are often directed at reducing the determinants of ventricular afterload, particularly in those with adequate blood pressure.

For the normal ventricle, an increase in ventricular after-

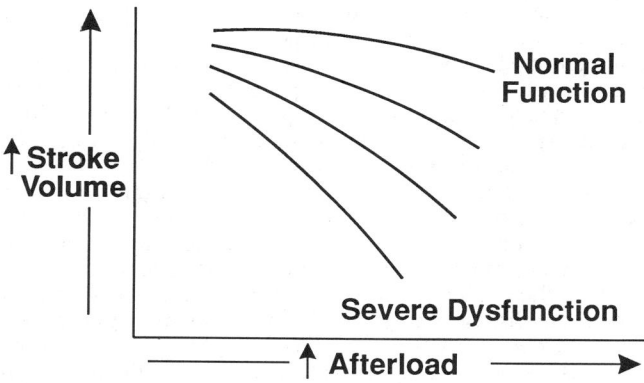

Figure 91–4. Schematic illustration of the effect of increasing afterload on left ventricular stroke volume. When left ventricular dysfunction is present there is an augmented effect.

load is generally well tolerated without much overall change in ventricular function, but this is not the case for the failing ventricle (Fig. 91–4). The magnitude of the detrimental effect varies directly with the severity of ventricular dysfunction and with the amount of afterload or wall stress imposed on the failing ventricle. Basically, in the evolution of left-sided heart failure, the hearts with the most dysfunction are generally those that experience the greatest wall stress and afterload and thus the greatest deterioration in ventricular function for any increase in wall stress or afterload.

Elevation of Ventricular Preload

Preload, at the most basic level, is the amount of diastolic stretch placed across the actin-myosin filament before muscle contraction. With respect to the intact ventricle, the precontraction stretch across the actin-myosin filaments is directly related to the amount of cellular stretch, which in turn is directly related to ventricular diastolic volume. The ventricular diastolic volume is directly (but not linearly) related to ventricular diastolic pressure and ventricular compliance. Therefore, in the setting of heart failure, preload increases with increased intravascular volume (salt and water retention) and with enhanced venoconstriction (shifts blood volume centrally). In ventricles with poor compliance, the increased intravascular volume and venoconstriction are reflected primarily in large increases in left ventricular end-diastolic pressure (and pulmonary capillary pressure) with little increase in the actin-myosin stretch.

The importance of preload or actin-myosin stretch is related to the close association of ventricular preload and systolic function; this association is represented by the Frank-Starling ventricular function curves (Fig. 91–5). The Frank-Starling curves or preload–systolic function curves indicate that ventricular systolic function increases with an increase in stretch across the actin-myosin filament. The increase in preload is generally considered a favorable ventricular compensatory mechanism. Often, the increase in central blood volume and ventricular volume leads to an adequate increase in systolic function so that the patient remains "compensated."

"Noncompensated" patients are those who continue to have symptomatic reduction in stroke volume and cardiac output despite the increase in ventricular preload. These patients have signs and symptoms of increased intravascular volume and high ventricular filling pressures with the various clinical manifestations of congestion, including high

pulmonary capillary wedge pressures, high pulmonary arterial pressures, pulmonary edema, elevated right-sided heart pressures, hepatomegaly, pedal edema, and so forth.

The pathophysiology of left-sided heart failure has a wide spectrum of severity, from mild to marked, and duration of presentation, from chronic to acute. Patients who present with the symptoms over time are generally regarded as having chronic heart failure and are generally managed by correcting the underlying cardiac lesion with digitalis, diuretics, vasodilators, and converting enzyme inhibitors in varying combinations. Patients whose symptoms occur rather abruptly require more dramatic forms of intervention, generally with parenterally administered inotropic drugs, diuretics, and/or vasodilators.

PULMONARY CONGESTION AND EDEMA

Increases in pulmonary blood volume and interstitial fluid volume are uniformly present in CHF.[21] The increased pulmonary fluid volume decreases lung compliance, compresses the small airways, and impairs oxygen diffusion. Normally, the low intravascular pressure in the pulmonary circulation ensures that the lungs are nearly the last organ to sequester fluid in fluid-overloaded states. However, when left atrial pressure rises as a result of chronic left-sided heart disease, the lungs may become one of the first organs to accumulate fluid.

Increased left atrial pressure required by diminished ventricular diastolic compliance requires an increase in pulmonary blood volume. This is manifest on the chest x-ray film by prominence of the upper lobe pulmonary veins. As the pressure further increases, edema forms in the interstitial spaces when the lymphatic system is overwhelmed. This interstitial edema compresses small airways and capillaries, and perivascular edema effaces the sharp delineation of vascular structures from surrounding tissues. The chest x-ray film therefore shows engorged lymphatics and loss of definition of the lower lobe vasculature (where intravascular pressure is normally highest because of gravity). The final stage is frank alveolar edema, which tends to be most prominent centrally (butterfly pattern), but this pattern may be altered when structural pulmonary disease is present. Pulmonary edema is favored when the serum albumin level is low.

The most common causes of acute pulmonary edema are hypertensive heart disease, aortic and mitral valve disease, and occlusive coronary artery disease, particularly acute myocardial infarction. It is of interest that the classic picture

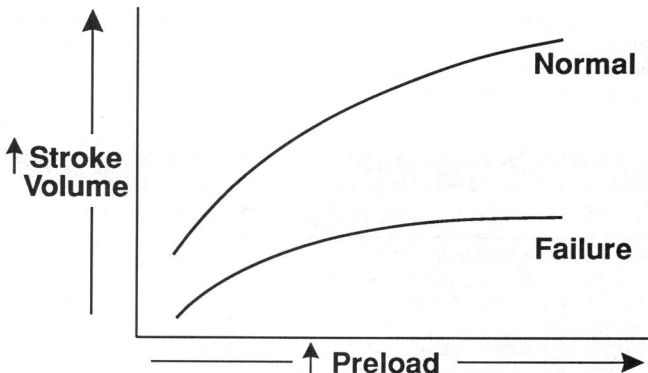

Figure 91–5. Schematic illustration of the Frank-Starling relationship. As preload increases, stroke volume increases. In left-sided heart failure, the stroke volume for any preload is smaller and increases less with increases in preload.

of pulmonary edema is virtually confined to isolated left-sided heart disease. When the right ventricle decompensates in patients with left ventricular disease, or when tricuspid valve disease or pericardial disease is present, the usual pattern is that of pulmonary congestion and pleural effusions but not pulmonary edema.

Acute pulmonary edema is nearly always associated with a massive sympathetic nervous system discharge. This causes redistribution of the peripheral blood volume centrally, and the cardiac output may actually be increased in the early stage of pulmonary edema. There may be a marked increase in systemic arterial blood pressure.

CLINICAL EVALUATION OF LEFT-SIDED HEART FAILURE

The routine history and physical examination provide important information for evaluation and management of left-sided heart failure. The etiology is frequently established from the history. It is essential to search for precipitating factors in patients who present initially with left-sided heart failure or in whom there has been an exacerbation. Identification of such precipitating factors may be important for determining optimal therapy (Table 91–2). The most common precipitating factors are inadequate dietary sodium restriction, development of atrial flutter or fibrillation, and discontinuation of previously effective therapy. Acute pulmonary edema is commonly related to physical or emotional stress.

The physical examination provides data on the extent of fluid overload in the lungs (rales, wheezing, effusions). Patients with pulmonary edema are severely dyspneic and in the early stages there may be minimal rales. The jugular venous pressure is always increased with right-sided heart failure, and the waveforms may give a clue to tricuspid valve disease or pericardial disease. When peripheral edema is present, there is generally at least 10 to 15 lb of fluid retention.

When biventricular failure is present there is often a parasternal lift similar to that seen with mitral valve disease. The left-sided heart impulse is nearly always displaced laterally and is usually diffuse. There is often a visible or palpable S_3 or S_4 gallop. Perhaps the most important physical sign in patients with left-sided heart failure is an S_3 gallop, which identifies a group with advanced left ventricular dysfunction (see later). This often subtle finding is frequently missed unless the patient is auscultated in the lateral decubitus position in a quiet setting using the bell piece of the stethoscope. Murmurs of mitral and tricuspid regurgitation are frequently present in left-sided heart failure. Also, the physical examination suggests whether primary aortic or mitral valve disease is the cause of a left-sided heart failure, but it should be remembered that in end-stage aortic valve stenosis the systolic murmur may be unimpressive.

TABLE 91–2

PRECIPITATING FACTORS FOR LEFT-SIDED HEART FAILURE

Reduction or termination of therapy
Inadequate dietary sodium restriction
Uncontrolled hypertension
Arrhythmia
Negative inotropic agents (class I antiarrhythmics, calcium channel blocking agents, beta-adrenergic blocking agents)
Nonsteroidal anti-inflammatory agents
Excess ethanol
Pulmonary emboli
Physical, emotional, and environmental stress

The routine electrocardiogram indicates the presence of acute or old myocardial infarction. The presence of left bundle branch block indicates that significant myocardial disease is present. Cardiac enlargement and changes related to pulmonary congestion are important radiographic findings. Absence of cardiac enlargement in a patient with left-sided heart failure suggests ischemic disease.

All patients presenting with left-sided heart failure should have an echocardiogram. Echocardiographic studies can define left ventricular anatomy and function, left atrial size, and valvular function. In addition, echocardiography can establish the diagnosis of hypertrophic cardiomyopathy and pericardial disease. Echocardiography also gives an estimate of right-sided heart function. (When right-sided heart dilatation is present, the clinical course is usually more advanced.) Patients with predominant diastolic dysfunction are identified by an echocardiographic study that shows relatively intact systolic function and Doppler findings of impaired diastolic filling.

Cardiac catheterization to establish the status of the coronary arteries may be indicated when active ischemia or acute myocardial infarction is the suspected cause of left-sided heart failure. Occasionally, it may be difficult to distinguish between cardiogenic and noncardiogenic pulmonary edema, and measurement of the pulmonary capillary wedge pressure can provide the critical differentiation. The pulmonary capillary wedge pressure is generally above 25 mm Hg in cardiogenic pulmonary edema, but it must be remembered that successful therapy of pulmonary edema can rapidly restore the wedge pressure to nearly normal levels at a time when the radiographic findings may still be present.

THERAPY OF ACUTE AND/OR SEVERELY DECOMPENSATED LEFT-SIDED HEART FAILURE

As soon as the condition of acute left-sided heart failure is recognized, pharmacologic intervention is promptly instituted.[22–27] This pharmacologic intervention should be regarded not as a curative or final form of therapy but rather as stabilization therapy to allow the performance of diagnostic procedures including echocardiography and cardiac catheterization. The purpose of performing these diagnostic procedures early in the course of the patient's illness is to arrive at a diagnosis of a condition that can then be surgically cured or greatly ameliorated; examples include acute valvular insufficiency, ruptured interventricular septum, and severe aortic or mitral stenosis. Invasive hemodynamic monitoring is often required to help guide therapy in severely ill patients (see later). In general, the prognosis of the patient is greatly compromised if there is undue or inappropriate delay in diagnosis and therapy or if the acute cardiac condition is caused by lesions that cannot be repaired surgically or by other means.[28, 29]

Criteria and Application of Acute Pharmacologic Intervention

The clinical signs of left-sided heart failure include those related to low cardiac output (e.g., tachycardia, hypotension, reduced pulse pressure, reduced peripheral perfusion, altered sensorium, reduced renal function and urine flow) and/or elevated left ventricular diastolic pressure (e.g., base-to-apex vascular redistribution on chest x-ray film, ventricular gallop sounds, pulmonary edema).

If the patient has the signs and symptoms of low cardiac output without evidence for elevated ventricular diastolic pressure and/or with signs of volume depletion, fluid volume is administered as a primary intervention. This form of intervention can be safely carried out simply by following clinical symptoms and signs including normalization of blood pressure, peripheral perfusion, heart rate, improved renal function, and increased urine flow.

Virtually all other conditions of acute left-sided heart failure require additional pharmacologic support, initiated and adjusted using clinical and hemodynamic guidelines. Although one can safely initiate pharmacologic intervention in most of these patients without hemodynamic data, the optimal selection of drugs, doses, concomitant volume administration, and so forth requires the insertion and use of flow-directed thermodilution pulmonary arterial catheters. The ability to estimate left ventricular filling pressures via a clinical criterion is poor at best. If systemic blood pressure cannot be reliably determined by cuff sphygmomanometer, an arterial line should also be placed. These catheters enable frequent clinical assessment, and the data obtained allow the clinician to make the best pharmacologic choices (drugs and doses) and alter them at a moment's notice during the tenuous course of many of these patients.

The selection and adjustment of pharmacologic support of patients with acute left-sided heart failure are guided by (1) the status of left ventricular filling pressure, (2) the clinical and hemodynamic status of left ventricular function and output, and (3) systemic blood pressure and systemic perfusion. Because most patients with acute left-sided heart failure have clinical and hemodynamic evidence of reduced ventricular function and cardiac output and of impaired systemic perfusion, the most fundamental guidelines for pharmacologic selection and adjustments are related to ventricular filling pressures and systemic blood pressure (Fig. 91–6).

Patients with left ventricular filling pressures (as estimated by the pulmonary artery occlusive pressure or pulmonary capillary wedge pressure) of less than 15 to 18 mm Hg at any level of systemic blood pressure may benefit greatly from the cautious and hemodynamically guided administration of fluid volume. Pharmacologic supplementation is required for virtually all patients with acute or decompensated left-sided heart failure whose left ventricular filling pressures are greater than 18 mm Hg or who arrive at that

level with fluid administration but fail to demonstrate an improvement of their compromised left-sided heart function.

At this particular point, we are dealing with patients with elevated left ventricular filling pressures, reduced cardiac output, and varying levels of systemic blood pressure. Drug selection is generally based on the level of systemic blood pressure. At systolic blood pressures of 100 mm Hg or more, vasodilating agents are selected with the expectation that the reduction in systemic vascular resistance and aortic impedance will improve ventricular function; increase stroke volume and cardiac output; enhance systemic perfusion, renal function, and urine output; and reduce the elevated ventricular filling pressures.[30-32] The primary drugs are nitroglycerin and nitroprusside, both administered intravenously. The selection of one drug over the other is based on several factors, including personal preference. Generally, more aggressive afterload reduction, as may be required for the management of acute mitral regurgitation or acute aortic valvular insufficiency, is best achieved with nitroprusside. Most situations requiring afterload reduction, particularly in the setting of acute left-sided heart failure secondary to myocardial ischemia syndromes, are best managed with intravenous nitroglycerin.[33]

At the other end of the spectrum, the patient with elevated filling pressures; marked reduction in ventricular function, stroke volume, and cardiac output; and a marked reduction in systemic perfusion and systemic blood pressure (≤70 mm Hg) requires drugs with vasopressor activity. The therapeutic goal here is to increase systemic blood pressure to a level guaranteeing maintenance flow to brain, kidney, and myocardium. Dopamine is the drug of choice in this setting. Norepinephrine is occasionally added if dopamine fails to bring systemic blood pressure into the acceptable range. When systemic blood pressure has been brought to a systolic level of at least 80 mm Hg and a diastolic level of at least 60 mm Hg, dobutamine can be added to further augment hemodynamics. Because of its more favorable effects on the myocardial oxygen supply/demand ratio and overall hemodynamics, dobutamine is often added to dopamine administration when the fundamental problem of severe systemic

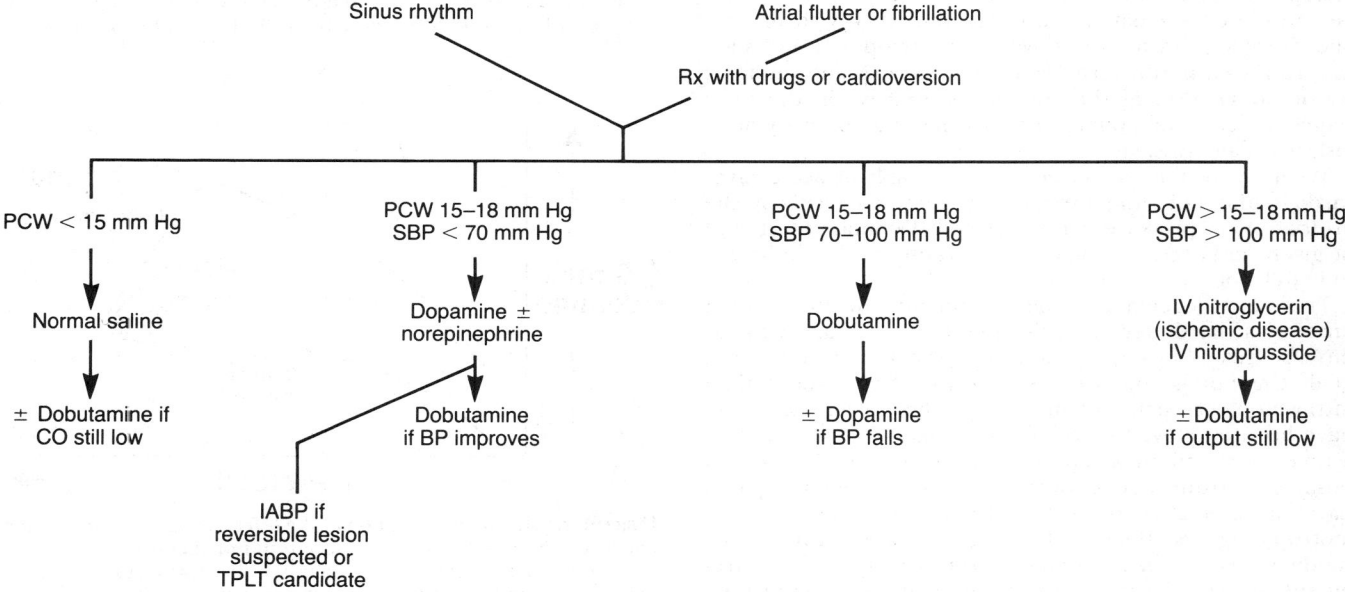

Figure 91–6. Therapy of severe acute left ventricular failure. PCW = pulmonary capillary wedge; SBP = systemic blood pressure; CO = cardiac output; TPLT = transplantation.

hypotension has been addressed with the vasopressor (dopamine or norepinephrine).

Dobutamine is the drug indicated for most patients whose systemic blood pressure is between the previous two extremes.[23, 34, 35] Administration of dobutamine in this setting generally increases ventricular function, stroke volume, and cardiac output; improves systemic perfusion; normalizes systemic blood pressure; increases pulse pressure; and brings ventricular filling pressures down to an acceptable range. If the administration of dobutamine is accompanied by a substantial augmentation of systemic blood pressure (to systolic pressures of 110 to 120 mm Hg or more), vasodilator therapy can be added to further improve central hemodynamics and reduce ventricular filling pressures. If the administration of dobutamine is accompanied by some reduction in systemic blood pressure, dopamine can be added to avert the development of threatening hypotension.

When administering parenteral therapy to severely ill patients with left-sided heart failure, careful monitoring of fluid intake and output and body weight is required. Parenteral diuretics must usually be employed to compensate for the intravenous fluid load. This is especially difficult when renal failure is present and the response to diuretics is altered.

THERAPY OF ACUTE PULMONARY EDEMA

Acute pulmonary edema is a medical emergency and the patient should be in a monitored intensive care setting.[36] However, treatment should begin promptly when the patient is seen (often by emergency medical service paramedics or in the emergency room). An arterial blood gas determination should be done as quickly as possible, especially in more advanced cases in which respiratory (and often metabolic) acidosis may be present.[37] In such patients, intubation is usually required and morphine sulfate should be avoided. Such patients are a high-risk group.

Patients should be placed in the sitting position and oxygen administered by face mask. Furosemide should be given intravenously (40 to 60 mg). This potent agent produces immediate venodilatation and subsequent diuresis.[38] To further enhance venodilatation, nitrates may be added, as a sublingual tablet, a nitrate paste, or intravenously if the arterial pressure is markedly elevated. Nitroprusside should be considered for patients who respond poorly to nitrates and diuretics and for those with a catastrophic event such as a ruptured mitral valve. Intravenous morphine sulfate is a traditional form of therapy and is effective in the early stages of acute pulmonary edema when a respiratory alkalosis is usually present.

When acute pulmonary edema is a result of acute myocardial infarction, the prognosis is dire, especially if the arterial blood pressure is not elevated. Dobutamine should be given, and urgent coronary angiography is often indicated to search for a correctable lesion.

Pulmonary edema may be precipitated by the sudden onset of atrial flutter or fibrillation, and these arrhythmias must be treated promptly. Slowing the ventricular rate is the goal. Digoxin is somewhat slower for this purpose than intravenous verapamil or intravenous beta-blockers, but all have been employed successfully. Digoxin has an onset of action of 30 minutes but has the advantage that it is a positive inotropic agent. Both beta-blockers and verapamil have an onset of action of 2 to 3 minutes but are negative inotropic agents. Beta-blocking agents have a physiologic rationale because excessive adrenergic activity, which is frequently present, facilitates atrioventricular node conduction. In severely ill patients, urgent cardioversion is the preferred initial treatment, especially for atrial flutter, which is often more difficult to control and easier to cardiovert.

In the past, theophylline has been employed when it is not clear whether acute respiratory distress is due to pulmonary edema or bronchospasm. Although this agent is useful for bronchospasm, it can produce serious ventricular arrhythmias and should not be used unless pulmonary disease is strongly suspected as the etiology.

INTRA-AORTIC BALLOON COUNTERPULSATION

Insertion of a percutaneous intra-aortic balloon pump (IABP) is an appropriate approach for certain subsets of patients with left-sided heart failure.[39–41] This device is indicated when there is reason to suspect a surgically remediable cause in a patient with severe left-sided heart failure poorly responsive to pharmacologic therapy. If the decision is made to insert an IABP, it should be inserted before irreversible deterioration of bodily organs occurs. Often the IABP must be inserted to allow a diagnostic cardiac catheterization to be performed. The IABP is indicated for patients with refractory left-sided heart failure who are considered to be possible candidates for cardiac transplantation or those already on the cardiac transplantation list.

Insertion of an IABP is less clearly indicated for a patient (usually after an acute myocardial infarction) who has severe left ventricular failure without obvious remediable cause. In some of these patients, an urgent angioplasty or coronary bypass can be performed if it appears that there is viable myocardium. Often, however, there is end-stage myocardial damage and no surgical or other intervention is possible. Some of these patients can eventually be weaned from the balloon pump, but most have persistent severe left ventricular dysfunction. Thus, insertion of an IABP in this setting requires considerable clinical judgment.

THERAPY OF CHRONIC CONGESTIVE HEART FAILURE

Therapy for chronic CHF is not dealt with here in detail because it is beyond the scope of this text.[42, 43] However, many patients are already receiving such therapy or require initiation of therapy. Therefore, the intensivist must have a basic familiarity with the major classes of drugs used for therapy of chronic left-sided heart failure. The physiologic

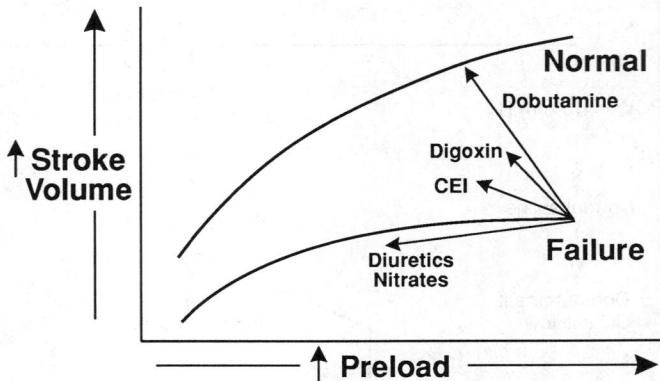

Figure 91–7. Schematic illustration of the effects of various therapeutic agents on the Frank-Starling relationship in patients with left-sided heart failure. Inotropic agents have the greatest effect on stroke volume, and preload-reducing agents (diuretics, nitrates, converting enzyme inhibitors [CEI]) have the least effect.

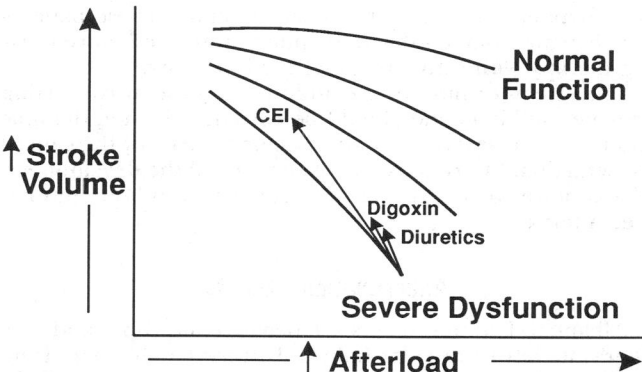

Figure 91–8. Schematic illustration of the effects of various therapeutic agents that reduce afterload. Converting enzyme inhibitors (CEI) have the greatest effect.

effects of agents employed for therapy of chronic left-sided heart failure are summarized in Figures 91–7 and 91–8.

Digitalis

Until the 1960s digitalis was the mainstay of therapy of left-sided heart failure.[22, 44] Its use was characterized by a high incidence of toxicity (25% in hospitalized patients), in large part because of the high doses employed. The introduction of serum digoxin measurement in 1970 and subsequent understanding of the complex pharmacokinetics of digitalis have led to a dramatic reduction in toxicity. The positive inotropic effect of digitalis results from an increase in intracellular calcium induced by inhibition of the enzyme Na^+,K^+-ATPase (sodium pump). The response is finite, and nearly maximal effects are achieved at the empirically derived recommended steady-state serum levels (Fig. 91–9).

Many of the actions of digitalis are related to its autonomic nervous system effects.[45] Therapeutic levels increase parasympathetic tone, and toxic levels increase adrenergic tone. The electrophysiologic effect of digitalis at therapeutic levels is to slow the sinus rate and atrioventricular nodal conduc-

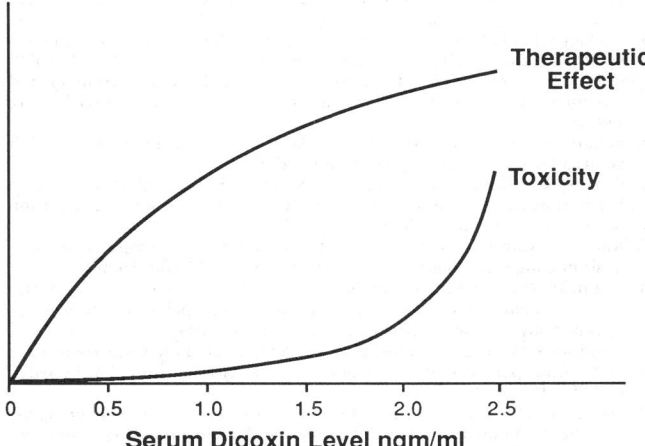

Figure 91–9. Schematic illustration of the relationship between therapeutic effect and toxicity of digoxin in relation to the steady-state serum digoxin level. At a level of 1.5 to 2.0 ng/mL, the maximal therapeutic effect with minimal toxicity is achieved. (Reprinted from Lewis RP: Digitalis. In: Leier CV [ed]: Cardiotonic Drugs: A Clinical Survey. New York, Marcel Dekker, p 85, 1987 by courtesy of Marcel Dekker, Inc.)

tion. Toxic levels may induce a variety of arrhythmias. Typical toxic arrhythmias are automatic tachycardias such as paroxysmal atrial tachycardia with block, junctional tachycardia, and ventricular tachycardia. These toxic tachyarrhythmias typically respond to the administration of potassium. In patients with conduction disease, digitalis may produce high-grade sinoatrial or atrioventricular nodal block that does not respond to potassium (and in fact may be aggravated by potassium). Digoxin-specific antibody fragments have been introduced that have provided prompt reversal of life-threatening digitalis toxic arrhythmias.[46]

Numerous randomized clinical trials have established the efficacy of digitalis in patients with CHF associated with sinus rhythm.[47–49] In fact, digitalis benefits are additive to those of both diuretics and converting enzyme inhibitors.[50] These three agents have now been termed triple therapy.

The beneficial effects of digitalis in the failing circulation are complex and comprehensive (Table 91–3). The inotropic effect of digitalis is more striking in the failing heart. In this setting, digitalis is about 50% as potent an inotrope as isoproterenol. A major beneficial effect of digitalis is to restore normal baroreceptor function. The arterial baroreceptors are depressed in chronic CHF, which helps perpetuate the excessive neurohumoral response. Restoration of baroreceptor function "turns off" the sympathetic nervous system and the renin-angiotensin system, resulting in net arterial and venous dilatation (reduced preload and afterload).

Digitalis has beneficial effects on myocardial energetics in most patients. Digitalis generally slows the heart rate, which allows greater diastolic coronary perfusion time. The overall efficiency of the heart as a pump is increased by elimination of nonconducted beats in patients with atrial fibrillation and high ventricular rate. Digitalis also improves left atrial function by restoring the atrium's ability to generate an effective systolic contraction, thereby reducing mean left atrial pressure. Finally, digitalis is a diuretic agent both by its direct effect on the renal tubules and by its indirect effect of increasing renal blood flow by inhibition of the sympathetic nervous system.

Digitalis should be used for all patients with moderately severe heart failure and patients with class IV heart failure if there are no contraindications. Generally, a loading dose of 1 mg of digoxin is divided over 24 hours (given parenterally in severely ill patients). In patients with cardiogenic shock, acute myocardial infarction, or acute pulmonary edema, all of which are associated with maximal adrenergic nervous system output, benefit of the inotropic effect of

TABLE 91–3
CIRCULATORY RESPONSE TO DIGITALIS IN LEFT-SIDED HEART FAILURE

Digitalis Effect	Circulatory Response
Inotropic stimulation	Enhanced if myocardial beta-receptors down-regulated
Restoration of baroreceptor responsiveness	Reduction in neurohumoral response
	Arterial and venous dilatation
Improvement of myocardial energetics	Increased myocardial blood flow by slowing heart rate
	Elimination of ineffectual beats (atrial fibrillation)
Improvement of atrial contractile function	Lowered mean left atrial pressure
Promotion of diuresis	Direct tubular inhibition of sodium reabsorption
	Reflex increase in renal blood flow

digitalis is difficult to demonstrate. Therefore, the drug should be reserved for those with atrial fibrillation. The only contraindications to digitalis are significant ventricular arrhythmias not responsive to restoration of electrolyte abnormalities or high-grade atrioventricular block in the absence of a pacemaker.

Diuretics

Diuretics are the cornerstone of pharmacotherapy of fluid retention in patients with left ventricular failure.[51] Diuretics are not without hazard. Three common major complications include overdiuresis, potassium and magnesium depletion, and metabolic alkalosis. Overdiuresis may be subtle because the symptoms (dyspnea and fatigue) are identical with those of left-sided heart failure. It is essential to maintain an accurate weight history for proper management of patients receiving diuretics.

Diuretic-induced hypokalemia and hypomagnesemia have been implicated in the predisposition to arrhythmic sudden death. Careful monitoring of serum potassium and magnesium levels to maintain these values in the high-normal range can produce remarkable improvement in ventricular ectopy, especially if the patient is receiving digitalis. Most patients tolerate oral potassium poorly, so potassium-sparing diuretics (spironolactone, amiloride, or triamterene) are preferred. When metabolic alkalosis results from vigorous diuresis, acetazolamide should be added until the serum bicarbonate level is restored to normal.

It is not widely appreciated that the bioavailability of oral furosemide is poor in patients with CHF. This can be suspected when excessive doses are required without apparent benefit. In the intensive care setting, furosemide should generally be given intravenously. It should be recognized that nonsteroidal anti-inflammatory agents inhibit the effect of furosemide.

Thiazide agents act more distally than furosemide in the renal tubule and are therefore additive. Metolazone is particularly effective even when glomerular filtration rate is low and should be combined with furosemide in refractory cases.

Vasodilators

Of the numerous direct- and indirect-acting vasodilators that have been introduced for the therapy of CHF in the past 20 years, most have not survived the test of randomized clinical trials, because of either drug tolerance or patients' intolerance.[43, 52] Converting enzyme inhibitors have emerged as the most efficacious vasodilators. These agents not only improve symptoms but also prolong life.[53] This is probably because converting enzyme inhibitors are the most physiologic vasodilators, as they inhibit the renin-angiotensin system. These agents produce both arterial and venous dilatation. It may take several weeks to achieve the full clinical benefit of these agents. Long-term studies show improvement in functional classification, less rehospitalization and fewer emergency room visits, improved exercise capacity, less ventricular ectopy, and improved survival. A study of patients after large anterior myocardial infarctions indicated that postinfarction left ventricular dilatation (remodeling) was mitigated, suggesting one mechanism for improved survival.[54]

There is as yet no consensus about which converting enzyme inhibitor is preferable, although captopril has the advantage that low doses can be used when initiating therapy. Often the initial dose must be substantially lower than the eventual maintenance dose. Converting enzyme inhibitors should be tried in all patients with overt CHF, but caution is advised in treating patients with severe hypoten-

sion, hyponatremia, and prerenal azotemia. These patients may benefit from a 3-day dobutamine infusion before starting therapy with converting enzyme inhibitors.[55]

The effects of nitrates are additive to those of converting enzyme inhibitors and should be considered when diastolic dysfunction is severe or angina pectoris is part of the clinical presentation.[56] Care must be taken to avoid the development of tolerance to the nitrates by providing a 6-hour nitrate-free interval.

Antiarrhythmic Agents

All antiarrhythmic agents are negative inotropes and may aggravate left ventricular failure. Unfortunately, there is no evidence that therapy of asymptomatic ventricular arrhythmia, which is nearly universally present in patients with left ventricular dysfunction, can prolong life. In fact, the Cardiac Arrhythmia Suppression Trial involving patients after myocardial infarction suggests that the opposite may be true.[57]

Ventricular ectopy in patients with left-sided heart failure should be treated initially by careful maintenance of normal serum electrolyte levels and avoidance of hypoxemia. This is successful in a high percentage of cases. In other patients, a low dose of a selective beta-adrenergic blocking agent should be considered because adrenergic hyperactivity commonly precipitates arrhythmias in these patients. Such therapy may have other benefits as well in patients with left-sided heart failure.[58]

It appears that nearly half of the deaths of patients with left ventricular failure are sudden and probably related to arrhythmia. This has produced a therapeutic dilemma. Generally, if the ventricular arrhythmia is symptomatic (i.e., sustained ventricular tachycardia) after optimal therapy, an electrophysiologic study should be performed to guide therapy. If empirical drug therapy is to be tried, amiodarone appears to be the most efficacious agent, although it does have a potential for pulmonary toxicity.[59] In other patients, the automatic implantable defibrillator has proved successful.[60]

References

1. Parker MM, Shelhammer JM, Bachrach SL, et al: Profound but reversible myocardial depression in patients with septic shock. Ann Intern Med 100:483, 1984.
2. Linzback AJ: Heart failure from the point of view of quantitative anatomy. Am J Cardiol 5:370, 1960.
3. Rackley CE, Dalldorf FG, Hood WP Jr, et al: Sarcomere length and left ventricular function in chronic heart disease. Am J Med Sci 259:90, 1970.
4. Ross J Jr, Sonnenblick EH, Taylor RR, et al: Diastolic geometry and sarcomere lengths in the chronically dilated canine left ventricle. Circ Res 38:49, 1971.
5. Panidis IP, Kotler MN, Ren JF, et al: Development and regression of left ventricular hypertrophy. J Am Coll Cardiol 3:1309, 1984.
6. Ginzton LE, Conant R, Rodrigues DM, et al: Functional significance of hypertrophy of the noninfarcted myocardium after myocardial infarction on humans. Circulation 80:816, 1989.
7. Katz AM: Cardiomyopathy of overload—A major determinant of prognosis in congestive heart failure. N Engl J Med 322:100, 1990.
8. Spann JF, Buccino RA, Sonnenblick EM, et al: Contractile state of cardiac muscle obtained from cats with experimentally produced ventricular hypertrophy and heart failure. Circ Res 21:341, 1967.
9. Boudoulas H, Mantzouratos D, Sohn YH, et al: Left ventricular mass and systolic performance in chronic systemic hypertension. Am J Cardiol 57:232, 1986.
10. D'Cruz IA, Shroff SG, Janicki JS, et al: Differences in the shape of the normal, cardiomyopathic, and volume overloaded human left ventricle. J Am Soc Echocardiogr 2:408, 1989.
11. Unverferth DV, Mahegan JP, Magorien RD, et al: Regression of myocardial cellular hypertrophy with vasodilator therapy in chronic congestive heart failure associated with idiopathic dilated cardiomyopathy. Am J Cardiol 51:1392, 1983.
12. Unverferth DV, Magorien RD, Lewis RP: The role of subendocardial ischemia in perpetuating myocardial failure in patients with nonischemic congestive cardiomyopathy. Am Heart J 105:176, 1983.

13. Laskey WK, Reichek N, Sutton MSJ, et al: Matching of myocardial oxygen consumption to mechanical load in human left ventricular hypertrophy and dysfunction. J Am Coll Cardiol 3:291, 1984.

14. Unverferth DV, Baker PB, Surft SE, et al: Matching of myocardial oxygen consumption to mechanical load in human left ventricular hypertrophy and dysfunction. J Am Coll Cardiol 3:291, 1984.

15. Unverferth DV, Magorien RD, Altshield R, et al: The hemodynamic and metabolic advantages gained by a five-day infusion of dobutamine in patients with congestive cardiomyopathy. Am Heart J 106:29, 1983.

16. Gaasch WH, Bing OHL, Mirsky I: Chamber compliance and myocardial stiffness in left ventricular hypertrophy. Eur Heart J 3:139, 1982.

17. Braunwald E: Pathophysiology of heart failure. In: Braunwald E (ed): Heart Disease: A Textbook of Cardiovascular Medicine. Philadelphia, WB Saunders, p 426, 1988.

18. Levine TB, Frances GS, Goldsmith SR, et al: Activity of the sympathetic nervous system and renin-angiotensin system assessed by plasma hormone levels and their relation to hemodynamic abnormalities in congestive heart failure. Am J Cardiol 49:1659, 1982.

19. Kluger J, Cody RJ, Laragh JM: The contributions of sympathetic tone and the renin-angiotensin system to severe chronic congestive heart failure: Response to specific inhibitors (prazosin and captopril). Am J Cardiol 49:1667, 1982.

20. Bristow MR, Ginsberg R, Minobe W, et al: Decreased catecholamine sensitivity and beta-adrenergic receptor density in failing human hearts N Engl J Med 307:205, 1982.

21. Ingram RH, Braunwald E: Pulmonary edema: Cardiogenic and noncardiogenic. In: Braunwald E (ed): Heart Disease: A Textbook of Cardiovascular Medicine. Philadelphia, WB Saunders, p 544, 1988.

22. Leier CV (ed): Cardiotonic Drugs: A Clinical Survey. New York, Marcel Dekker, 1986.

23. Leier CV, Unverferth DV: Medical therapy of end-stage congestive and ischemic cardiomyopathy. Cardiovasc Clin 19:243, 1988.

24. Leier CV: Approach to the patient with hypotension and shock. In: Kelley WN (ed): Textbook of Internal Medicine. Philadelphia, JB Lippincott, p 393, 1989.

25. Gunnar RM, Loeb HS: Shock in acute myocardial infarction: Evolution of physiological therapy. J Am Coll Cardiol 1:154, 1983.

26. Hands ME, Rutherford JD, Muller JE, et al: The in-hospital development of cardiogenic shock: Incidence, predictors of occurrence, outcome and prognostic factors. J Am Coll Cardiol 14:40, 1989.

27. Schreiber TL, Miller DH, Zola B: Management of myocardial infarction shock: Current status. Am Heart J 117:435, 1989.

28. Pifarre R, Spinazzola A, Nemickas R, et al: Emergency aortocoronary bypass for acute myocardial infarction. Arch Surg 103:525, 1971.

29. Lee L, Bates ER, Pitt B, et al: Percutaneous transluminal coronary angioplasty improves survival in cardiogenic shock complicating acute myocardial infarction. Circulation 78:1345, 1988.

30. Franciosa JA, Limas CH, Gutha NH, et al: Improved left ventricular function during nitroprusside infusion in acute myocardial infarction. Lancet 1:650, 1972.

31. Chatterjee K, Swan HJC, Kaushik VS, et al: Effects of vasodilator therapy for severe pump failure in acute myocardial infarction on short-term and late prognosis. Circulation 53:797, 1976.

32. Leier CV, Bambach D, Thompson MJ, et al: Central and regional hemodynamic effects of intravenous isosorbide dinitrate, nitroglycerin and nitroprusside in patients with congestive heart failure. Am J Cardiol 48:1115, 1981.

33. Gold HK, Chiariello M, Leinbach RC, et al: Deleterious effects of nitroprusside on myocardial injury during acute myocardial infarction. N Engl J Med 293:1003, 1975.

34. Leier CV, Heban P, Huss P, et al: Comparative systemic and regional hemodynamic effects of dopamine and dobutamine in patients with cardiac failure. Circulation 58:466, 1978.

35. Gillespie TA, Ambos HD, Sobei BE, et al: Effects of dobutamine in patients with acute myocardial infarction. Am J Cardiol 39:588, 1977.

36. Sprung CL, Rackow EC, Fein IA, et al: The spectrum of pulmonary edema: Differentiation of cardiogenic, intermediate, and noncardiogenic forms of pulmonary edema. Annu Rev Respir Dis 124:718, 1981.

37. Aberman A, Fulop M: The metabolic and respiratory acidosis of acute pulmonary edema. Ann Intern Med 76:173, 1972.

38. Dikshit K, Vyden JK, Forrister JS, et al: Renal and extrarenal hemodynamic effects of furosemide in congestive heart failure after myocardial infarction. N Engl J Med 288:1087, 1973.

39. Scheidt S, Wilner G, Mueller H, et al: Intra-aortic balloon counterpulsation in cardiogenic shock: Report of a cooperative clinical trial. N Engl J Med 288:979, 1973.

40. DeWood MA, Notske RN, Hensley GR, et al: Intra-aortic balloon counterpulsation with or without reperfusion for myocardial infarction shock. Circulation 61:1105, 1980.

41. Hill JD, Farrar DJ, Hershon JJ, et al: Use of a prosthetic ventricle as a bridge to cardiac transplantation for postinfarction cardiogenic shock. N Engl J Med 314:626, 1986.

42. Packer M (ed): Symposium on the therapeutic challenges in the management of congestive heart failure. J Am Coll Cardiol 12:262, 547, 1988.

43. Packer M: Vasodilator and inotropic drugs for the treatment of chronic heart failure: Distinguishing hype from hope. J Am Coll Cardiol 12:1299, 1988.

44. Lewis RP: Digitalis: A drug that refuses to die. Crit Care Med 18:(S1)5, 1990.

45. Ribner HS, Plucinski DA, Hsieh AM, et al: Acute effects of digoxin on total systemic vascular resistance in congestive heart failure due to dilated cardiomyopathy: A hemodynamic hormonal study. Am J Cardiol 56:896, 1985.

46. Antman EM, Wenger TL, Butler VP Jr, et al: Treatment of 150 cases of life-threatening digitalis intoxication with digoxin-specific Fab antibody fragments. Circulation 81:1744, 1990.

47. Yusef S, Wittes J, Bailey K, et al: Digitalis—A new controversy regarding an old drug. The pitfalls of inappropriate methods. Circulation 73:14, 1986.

48. The Captopril-Digoxin Multicenter Research Group: Comparative effects of therapy with captopril and digoxin in patients with mild to moderate heart failure. JAMA 259:539, 1988.

49. DiBianco R, Shabetai R, Kostuk W, et al: A comparison of oral milrinone, digoxin, and their combination in the treatment of patients with chronic heart failure. N Engl J Med 320:677, 1989.

50. Gheorghiade M, Hall V, Lakier JB, et al: Comparative hemodynamic and neurohormonal effects of intravenous captopril and digoxin and their combinations in patients with severe heart failure. J Am Coll Cardiol 13:134, 1989.

51. Smith TW, Braunwald E, Kelly RA: Management of heart failure. In: Braunwald E (ed): Heart Disease: A Textbook of Cardiovascular Medicine. Philadelphia, WB Saunders, p 485, 1988.

52. Mulrow CD, Mulrow JP, Linn WD, et al: Relative efficacy of vasodilator therapy in chronic congestive heart failure. Implications of randomized trials. JAMA 259:3422, 1988.

53. The CONSENSUS Trial Study Group: Effects of enalapril on mortality in severe congestive heart failure. Results of the Cooperative North Scandinavian Enalapril Survival Study (CONSENSUS). N Engl J Med 316:1429, 1987.

54. Pfeffer MA, Lamas GA, Vaughn DE, et al: Effect of captopril on progressive ventricular dilatation after anterior myocardial infarction. N Engl J Med 319:80, 1988.

55. Unverferth DV, Magorien RD, Lewis RP, et al: Long-term benefit of dobutamine in patients with congestive cardiomyopathy. Am Heart J 100:622, 1980.

56. Leier CV, Huss P, Magorien RD, et al: Improved exercise capacity and differing arterial and venous tolerance during chronic isosorbide dinitrate therapy for congestive heart failure. Circulation 67:817, 1983.

57. The Cardiac Arrhythmia Suppression Trial (CAST) Investigators: Preliminary report: Effect of encainide and flecainide on mortality in a randomized trial of arrhythmia suppression after myocardial infarction. N Engl J Med 321:406, 1989.

58. Waagstern F, Caidahl K, Wallentin I, et al: Long-term β-blockade in dilated cardiomyopathy effects of short- and long-term metoprolol treatment followed by withdrawal and readministration of metoprolol. Circulation 80:551, 1989.

59. Cleland JGF, Dargie HJ, Findlay IN, et al: Clinical, haemodynamic, and antiarrhythmic effects of long term treatment with amiodarone of patients in heart failure. Br Heart J 57:436, 1987.

60. Marchlinski FG, Flores BT, Buxton AE, et al: The automatic implantable cardioverter-defibrillator. Efficacy, complications, and device failures. Ann Intern Med 104:481, 1986.

CHAPTER 92

Right-Sided Heart and Pericardial Disease

Steven J. Lavine

RIGHT VENTRICLE

Determinants of Right Ventricular Function

The right ventricle and left ventricle are arranged in series connected by the pulmonary circulation and eject the same stroke volume. To accomplish this, both ventricles must operate with similar ventricular function curves and utilize

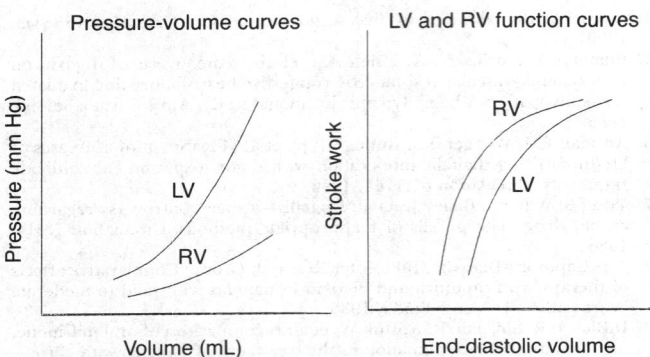

Figure 92–1. Diastolic ventricular pressure-volume curves (graphic) for the left and right ventricles with normal function are shown on the left. Ventricular function curves are shown on the right. The right ventricle is more distensible, as demonstrated by the rightward shift of the diastolic pressure-volume curve and leftward shift of the ventricular function curves.

the Frank-Starling mechanism to adjust stroke volume to changing loading conditions such as alterations in posture.[1] However, the left ventricle is stiffer than the right ventricle and has a smoother internal topography. Consequently, the right ventricle is thinner and more distensible and operates at lower filling pressures. The resting ejection fraction is lower, and it ejects against a lower afterload (exerted in part by the pulmonary circulation). Figure 92–1 shows the pressure-volume and ventricular function curves for both right and left ventricles and illustrates the lower distensibility of the left ventricle.[2] The left ventricular function curve is positioned rightward, demonstrating a higher end-diastolic volume (and probably end-diastolic pressure) for the same stroke volume.

The determinants of right ventricular systolic performance are identical with those that govern left ventricular systolic performance and include contractility, preload, and afterload.[3, 4] Right ventricular contractility may be impaired by diseases that affect both ventricles, such as various forms of cardiomyopathy. More commonly, right ventricular systolic performance is affected by alterations in afterload produced by pulmonary hypertension. The response to acute changes produced by increases in afterload or decreases in contractility or preload involves compensations whose purpose is to maintain right ventricular stroke volume. These compensations include increased sympathetic output and increased heart rate to increase contractility.[3] The Frank-Starling mechanism is recruited in response to increased afterload or decreased contractility and results in right ventricular dilatation.[1] Right ventricular dilatation does increase right ventricular afterload according to the Laplace principle: $S = Pr/2h$, where S = stress, P = right ventricular pressure, r = radius, and $2h$ = wall thickness. Consequently, wall stress increases further, depressing right ventricular performance because of the inverse relation between ventricular systolic performance and afterload.[5] More long-term compensations result in hypertrophy of the right ventricle to reduce wall stress and maintain right ventricular performance.

Both the left ventricle and the right ventricle are encased in a pericardial shell that has limited elasticity. Consequently, acute increases in the volume of one or more intracardiac chambers may result in the pericardium restraining its intracardiac contents.[6, 7] Therefore, the diastolic pressure-volume relation of the left and right ventricles is in part determined by the pericardium.[8, 9] The influence of the pericardium appears more important with acute chamber

dilatation and less important with chronic dilatation, as the pericardium has time to stretch and remodel.[10] The ventricular septum is a shared wall between the left and right ventricles that permits both a systolic and a diastolic interaction between ventricles. This interaction is further facilitated by the pericardium during both systole and diastole.[11] Clinically, the diastolic ventricular interaction is of considerable importance. Right ventricular dilatation and congestive heart failure resulting from chronic cor pulmonale flatten the ventricular septum and alter left ventricular shape. Consequently, the left ventricular pressure-volume curve is shifted leftward and upward so that smaller left ventricular diastolic volumes result in similar left ventricular filling pressures (Fig. 92–2).[12] If left ventricular dysfunction and left ventricular end-diastolic pressure elevation accompany pre-existing right ventricular dysfunction, right ventricular filling pressures may be further accentuated because of the straightening of the ventricular septum. Elevated left ventricular end-diastolic pressures may lead to further elevations in the pulmonary arterial pressure, resulting in further right ventricular dysfunction because of increases in afterload.

Causes of Right Ventricular Dysfunction Seen in the Critical Care Setting

An exhaustive listing of causes of right ventricular dysfunction is beyond the scope of this discussion. The reader, if interested, may wish to examine a textbook on cardiovascular disease or pulmonary medicine.

Cor Pulmonale

Cor pulmonale can be operationally defined as right ventricular hypertrophy, dysfunction, or congestive heart failure caused by pulmonary disease in the absence of

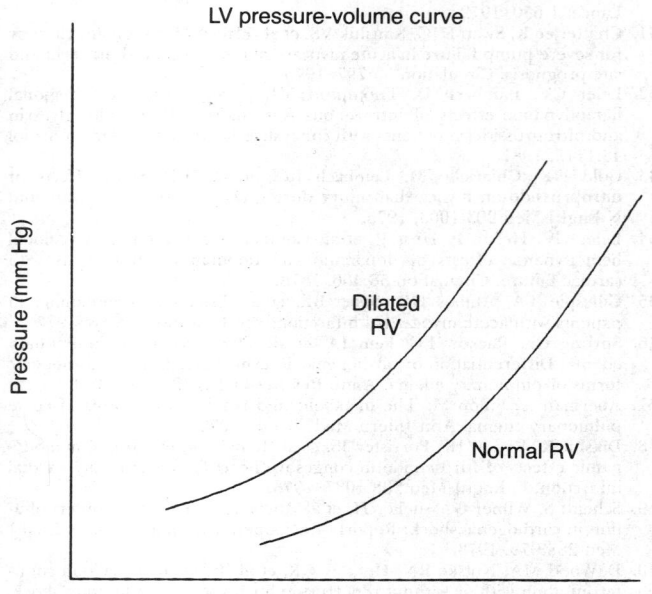

Figure 92–2. Diastolic pressure-volume curves (graphic) are shown for the left ventricle with and without right ventricular dilatation. Right ventricular dilatation, especially if associated with right ventricular filling pressure elevation, shifts the left ventricular pressure-volume curve to the left.

TABLE 92–1
CAUSES OF COR PULMONALE

Chronic obstructive pulmonary disease
  Emphysema
  Chronic bronchitis
  Cystic fibrosis
Restrictive lung disease
  Sarcoidosis
  Pulmonary fibrosis
  Scleroderma
Pulmonary vascular disease
  Recurrent pulmonary embolism
  Primary pulmonary hypertension
Chest wall deformity and neuromuscular disorders
  Kyphoscoliosis
  Sleep apnea
  Myasthenia gravis

clinically important left-sided heart disease or congenital heart disease. Cor pulmonale is a not infrequent finding in autopsy series, in which incidences as high as 40% have been noted.[13, 14] The causes of cor pulmonale are many and are best considered in broad categories, which are listed in Table 92–1. Cor pulmonale may be chronic, as in any of the diseases listed in Table 92–1, or acute, as in massive or repeated pulmonary embolism. Chronic cor pulmonale is a result of either vasoconstriction or anatomic restriction of the vascular bed.

Signs and Symptoms. Signs and symptoms depend on both the etiology of cor pulmonale and the extent of right ventricular failure. Symptoms associated with right ventricular failure include fatigue, dizziness, chest pain, and dyspnea, although dyspnea may also be related to the underlying cause of cor pulmonale. Gastrointestinal symptoms may be caused by gut edema. Signs of right ventricular failure include tachycardia, hypotension, and systemic venous hypertension manifested by jugular venous distention, hepatomegaly, leg edema, and ascites. A left parasternal lift, a palpable pulmonary artery segment, a loud P_2, a right ventricular S_4, and the murmurs of tricuspid and pulmonary regurgitation may also be present.

Laboratory and Diagnostic Testing. *Chest Roentgenography.* Enlargement of the right ventricle is best seen as filling in of the retrosternal air space on the lateral chest x-ray film. From the posteroanterior or anteroposterior projection, the border of the left side of the heart appears to be lifted off the diaphragm. The pulmonary outflow tract may also be enlarged. The pulmonary vasculature may appear pruned in the distal lung fields in vascular etiologies of cor pulmonale. Other x-ray findings vary depending on the etiology of cor pulmonale.

Electrocardiography. The electrocardiogram (ECG) is nonspecific in cor pulmonale. There are some specific but insensitive findings for acute pulmonary emboli (i.e., $S_1Q_3T_3$ or incomplete right bundle branch block), but these findings reflect right ventricular hypertrophy or enlargement. With cor pulmonale, an S_1Q_3 pattern, a right axis deviation, an R/S ratio less than 1 in V_6, an R/S ratio greater than 1 in V_1, incomplete right bundle branch block, right atrial enlargement, or low voltage may be seen.[13] The incidence of these findings on the ECG depends on the etiology of cor pulmonale.

Assessment of Left Ventricular and Right Ventricular Function and Size. Left ventricular and right ventricular size can be assessed by using either radionuclide angiography or two-dimensional and Doppler echocardiography. Radionuclide angiography, first pass or equilibrium, can assess left and right end-diastolic volume and determine ejection fraction. The normal right ventricular ejection fraction is greater than 45%.[15] Echocardiography can also assess left and right ventricular size, wall thickness, and function (Fig. 92–3). Doppler (pulsed, continuous, and color flow mapping) echocardiography can assess the presence of accompanying mitral regurgitation, which may further increase the pulmonary arterial pressure. Also, the extent of tricuspid regurgitation, often afterload dependent (based on the pulmonary arterial pressure), can be assessed with color flow mapping. An assessment of the peak tricuspid regurgitation velocity can estimate accurately pulmonary arterial systolic pressure in the absence of pulmonic stenosis using the simplified Bernoulli equation:[16]

$$PG = 4V^2$$

where PG = pressure gradient between the right ventricle and right atrium
V = peak continuous wave velocity from the tricuspid regurgitation spectrum

Adding the mean right atrial pressure estimated from the central venous pressure to this gradient yields the pulmonary arterial systolic pressure. Pulmonary arterial diastolic pressure can be estimated from the end-diastolic pulmonary regurgitation velocity by using continuous-wave Doppler echocardiography. Tricuspid regurgitation velocity greater than 3 m/s and pulmonic regurgitation end-diastolic velocity

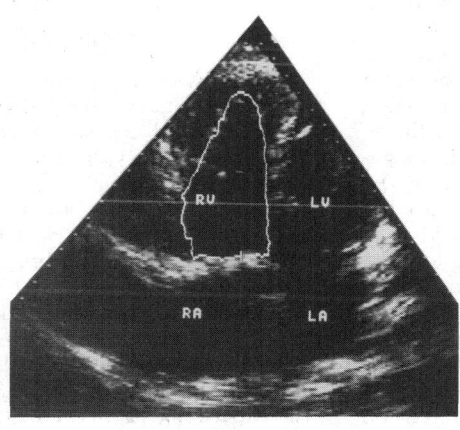

Figure 92–3. End-diastolic (ED) and end-systolic (ES) frames from the four chamber view are shown in a representative patient with right ventricular infarction. The endocardial borders have been outlined and show right ventricular systolic dysfunction. The right atrium (RA) is also dilated. LA = left atrium; LV = left ventricle; RV = right ventricle.

greater than 2 m/s suggest a pulmonary arterial systolic pressure of 40 mm Hg and pulmonary arterial diastolic pressure of 20 mm Hg.

Right-Sided Heart Catheterization. Right-sided heart catheterization is useful in assessing the presence of pulmonary hypertension, right ventricular pressures, right atrial pressures, and cardiac output. Right ventricular contrast ventriculography can be performed for the assessment of right ventricular function, although noninvasive techniques are more than adequate substitutes. Vasoactive maneuvers (i.e., 100% oxygen or vasodilators) can be utilized to determine whether the pulmonary circulation is reactive. In addition, left-sided heart catheterization can determine whether left ventricular end-diastolic pressures are increased and whether pulmonary hypertension is in part contributed to by elevated left ventricular filling pressures.

Differential Diagnosis. Differential diagnosis includes the many etiologies of cor pulmonale. From the standpoint of right ventricular congestive heart failure, signs of systemic venous congestion may be seen with (1) right ventricular congestive heart failure caused by congenital heart disease, (2) pulmonary vascular disease, (3) passive congestion secondary to left ventricular congestive heart failure or mitral stenosis, (4) obstruction of right ventricular inflow, as in superior vena cava syndrome or tricuspid stenosis, and (5) pericardial diseases including cardiac tamponade with slow compression or constrictive pericarditis.

Therapeutic Options. Because the causes of cor pulmonale are diverse, therapeutic options have some diversity. Paramount in therapy is lowering the pulmonary arterial pressure to improve right ventricular function. This can be accomplished by improved oxygenation, reduction of passive congestion by diuresis, heparin therapy or thrombolysis in pulmonary embolism,[17] vasodilators (in some patients) with primary pulmonary hypertension, and tracheostomy to improve ventilation in sleep apnea.[18] The use of digoxin has always been controversial.[19, 20] Its use is best limited to patients with accompanying left ventricular dysfunction or atrial fibrillation. Phlebotomy to reduce the hematocrit to less than 55% decreases viscosity and both the pulmonary and systemic vascular resistances.[21] Finally, theophylline may have a number of beneficial effects, including a reduction in bronchospasm, improvement in biventricular function, and a diuretic effect.[22, 23]

Right Ventricular Dysfunction Secondary to Congenital Heart Disease

Table 92–2 lists a number of congenital anomalies associated with right-sided heart failure. The list is by no means exhaustive and is applicable to the patient who survives to adulthood. In a broad characterization of these lesions, causes can be divided into right ventricular volume overload, right ventricular outflow tract obstruction, intrinsic right ventricular dysfunction, and severe pulmonary hypertension (Eisenmenger's reaction).[24] In lesions associated with Eisenmenger's reaction or with congenital anomalies with obligatory venous admixture (systemic vein emptying into the arterial circulation), right-to-left shunting occurs with hypoxemia resulting in further pulmonary vasoconstriction.

Various laboratory and other diagnostic testing can be helpful in assessing the nature of the congenital anomaly; the degree of right ventricular dysfunction; and the oxygenation, hemodynamic, and acid-base status of the patient. Although cyanosis may always be present in a particular patient, increasing degrees of cyanosis associated with worsening hypoxemia may be seen during periods of hypotension resulting in decreased pulmonary blood flow, as may be seen

TABLE 92-2
CONGENITAL LESIONS ASSOCIATED WITH RIGHT VENTRICULAR DYSFUNCTION IN ADULTS
Right ventricular volume overload
Atrial septal defect
Ebstein's anomaly
Right ventricular pressure overload
Pulmonic stenosis
Tetralogy of Fallot
Intrinsic right ventricular dysfunction
Right ventricular dysplasia
Pulmonary arterial hypertension; Eisenmenger's reaction
Aortic shunts (patent ductus arteriosus, aortopulmonary window)
Ventricular shunts (ventricular septal defect)
Atrial shunts (atrial septal defect, total anomalous pulmonary venous return)

with sepsis. The ECG is usually nonspecific but demonstrates right ventricular hypertrophy and enlargement often associated with right ventricular strain. Incomplete right bundle branch block, right axis deviation, and precordial ST segment and T wave abnormalities may be seen. Chest roentgenography demonstrates right ventricular enlargement, which is best seen in the lateral projection. Suffused pulmonary vasculature in the case of an atrial septal defect associated with right ventricular volume overload or pruning associated with severe pulmonary hypertension may be seen. Two-dimensional echocardiography and Doppler echocardiography have been extremely useful diagnostic tools. The anatomic nature of the defect, the direction and size of a shunt, or an obstruction across a valve can often be demonstrated by echocardiography.

Management of right ventricular dysfunction in these patients should be directed toward finding the cause of the decompensation. Sepsis, nausea, vomiting, diarrhea, electrolyte disturbance, unexplained hypotension, and arrhythmias may contribute to decompensation. Intensification of hypoxemia and cyanosis may occur with hypotension, leading to further right-to-left shunting and acidosis. Correction of hypotension, bicarbonate administration to reduce acidosis, appropriate fluid replacement, and the use of alpha-adrenergic agents improve the hypoxemia and increased pulmonary arterial pressures that hypoxia can aggravate. The use of digoxin to improve right ventricular function has been controversial at best. Vasodilators with greater selectivity for the pulmonary circulation have not always proved to be useful and often dilate the systemic circulation, which may lead to greater right-to-left shunting.[25]

Right Ventricular Infarction

Pathophysiology. The inferior wall of the right ventricle receives coronary blood flow from the left anterior descending artery and conus branch of the right coronary artery. This dual supply tends to protect the right ventricular anterior wall. However, the posterior wall of the right ventricle receives its blood supply from the right coronary artery (and occasionally from the left circumflex artery), which supplies the inferoposterior left ventricular wall. Right ventricular infarction most commonly occurs with inferoposterior myocardial infarction involving the posterior septum.[26] The right ventricle is generally thought to be protected even with severe right coronary stenosis because of its thin wall, rich collaterals, and ability to receive nutrients via diffusion. Right ventricular hypertrophy may afford some disadvantage because it may increase myocardial oxygen demand and impede collateral flow, although this has not been uniformly noted.[26, 27]

Infarction of the posterior right ventricular wall and posterior septum may result in varying degrees of right ventricular dysfunction. The full-blown clinical spectrum of right ventricular infarction characterized by clear lungs, jugular venous distention, atrioventricular block, and hypotension occurs in less than 10% of patients with acute right ventricular infarction.[28] Approximately 15 to 30% of all myocardial infarctions have associated right ventricular infarction,[28, 29] and this increases to 40 to 70% when only inferoposterior infarctions are considered.[30, 31] In the full-blown clinical picture, the right ventricle is reduced to a passive conduit between the right atrium and left atrium. Consequently, preload to the left atrium is markedly reduced, resulting in hypotension.[28] The right ventricle dilates in an attempt to recruit the Frank-Starling mechanism. This compensation results in marked increases in right ventricular and right atrial filling pressures. If a pressure gradient exists between the right atrium and left ventricle, forward flow to the left atrium ensues. Coexistence of left ventricular infarction in the inferoposterior and posterior septal walls is common. Significant left ventricular dysfunction accompanying right ventricular infarction is a further impedance to maintaining left ventricular preload. Consequently, maintaining a gradient from the right atrium to the left atrium becomes more difficult.[28, 32] If the right ventricle must dilate significantly to maintain stroke volume, increased pericardial restraining forces may limit increases in left ventricular preload, increase left and right ventricular filling pressures, and contribute to hypotension.[33]

Clinical Presentation. The patient may manifest, in the course of an acute inferoposterior myocardial infarction, restlessness, anxiety, and reduced perfusion suggesting reduced cardiac output. On physical examination, the patient may have bradycardia (and atrioventricular block), signs of reduced perfusion, and hypotension. Neck vein distention with an increased y descent, pulsus paradoxus, positive Kussmaul's sign, and right ventricular third and fourth heart sounds may be present.[26, 28, 32]

Laboratory and Other Diagnostic Modalities. Levels of creatine kinase and isoenzymes are often higher than might be expected for the amount of ST segment elevation and Q waves seen on the ECG.[34] The ECG demonstrates an inferior myocardial infarction, ST segment depression in the precordial leads, and ST segment elevation in the right-sided precordial leads.[35] Chest x-ray study reveals cardiomegaly without pulmonary vascular congestion. Echocardiography reveals regional left ventricular hypokinesia with akinesia in the inferoposterior walls. The right ventricle (see Fig. 92–3) is often dilated, with hypokinesia of the septum and posterior right ventricular wall, abnormal septal motion, and tricuspid regurgitation.[36] Radionuclide angiography reveals similar findings although they may resolve in time. Technetium pyrophosphate scanning in the left anterior oblique projection reveals left ventricular uptake as well as right ventricular posterior wall uptake that denotes the areas of infarction.[37] Cardiac catheterization often reveals total occlusion of the right coronary artery and occasionally of the left circumflex artery if a left dominant system is present. Circumferential right ventricular infarction may occur with left anterior descending occlusions or conus branch occlusions of the right coronary artery. Right-sided pressures are high with low pulmonary arterial pressures. Pressure tracings may look identical for the right atrium, right ventricle, and pulmonary artery with severe infarction (Fig. 92–4). The right ventricular tracing shows a square root sign with low right ventricular pulse pressures. Pulsus alternans may be seen in the pulmonary arterial pressure tracing. Right-sided pressure (mean right atrial pressure) may be greater than or equal to the left ventricular end-diastolic pressure.[26, 28, 32]

Differential Diagnosis. Differential diagnosis includes cardiac tamponade, constrictive pericarditis, restrictive cardiomyopathy, and massive pulmonary embolism.[38] Several of the clinical findings are suggestive of cardiac tamponade (neck vein distention, hypotension, pulsus paradoxus, equalization of right-sided pressures) and constrictive pericarditis or restrictive cardiomyopathy (jugular venous distention, equilibration of right-sided pressures, and square root sign). However, echocardiography can quickly exclude or include cardiac tamponade or restrictive cardiomyopathy caused by amyloid and may give clues to effusive constrictive pericarditis. Other modalities, such as computed tomographic scanning or magnetic resonance imaging, can assess pericardial thickness. Angiography or lung scan is critical in the diagnosis of pulmonary embolism.

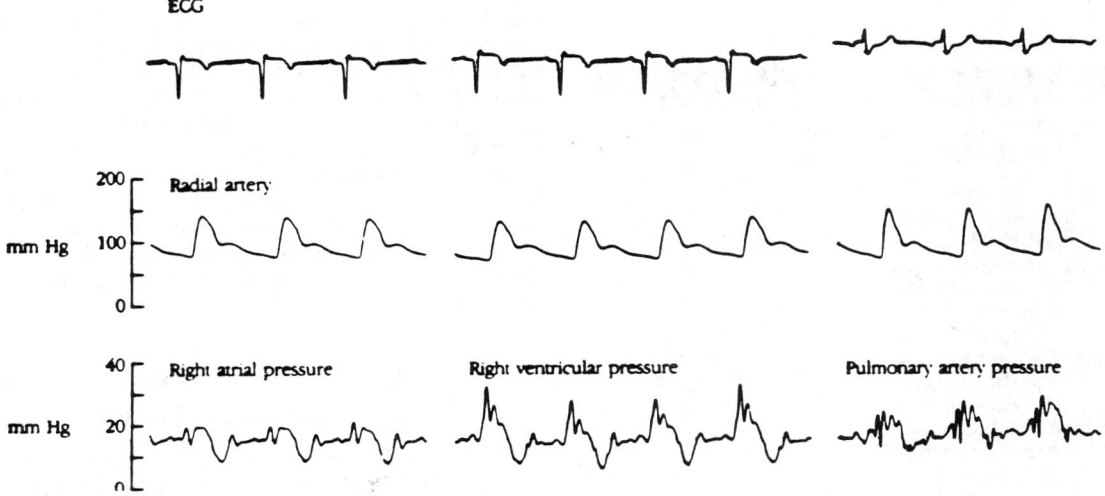

Figure 92–4. Sequential right atrial, right ventricular, and pulmonary arterial tracings for a patient with right ventricular infarction. The pressure tracings for each chamber are similar. The right ventricular tracings show a low pulse pressure and a dip and plateau configuration. (From Lorell B, Leinbach RC, Pohost GM, et al: Right ventricular infarction: Clinical diagnosis and differentiation from cardiac tamponade and pericardial constriction. Am J Cardiol 43:465, 1979.)

Therapy. A pressure gradient from the right atrium to the left atrium is needed for flow, and because the right ventricle is poorly compliant, volume loading may quickly accomplish this goal. The presence of left ventricular dysfunction may lead to severe pulmonary congestion and impede effective preload delivery to the left side of the heart. To maintain an effective gradient across the pulmonary circulation, left ventricular filling pressures can be lowered with nitroprusside. Inotropic stimulation of both right and left sides may be useful. Oxygen may be used as an adjunct to therapy to reduce pulmonary resistance and right ventricular afterload. If the patient has bradycardia or atrioventricular block, restoration of atrial-ventricular synchrony may increase blood pressure significantly because 50% of stroke volume may be derived from an effectively timed atrial contraction.[39, 40]

Right Ventricular Dysfunction Secondary to Left Ventricular Dysfunction

The most common cause of right ventricular dysfunction is left ventricular dysfunction or obstruction of inflow to the left ventricle. The causes of left ventricular dysfunction or inflow obstruction are numerous and can be classified into several broad categories (Table 92–3), including cardiomyopathy, valvular heart disease, coronary artery disease, obstruction to left ventricular inflow (mitral stenosis), and congenital heart disease. Presenting symptoms include dyspnea on exertion progressing to orthopnea and paroxysmal nocturnal dyspnea, chest pain, fatigue, palpitations, and syncope. The incidence of individual symptoms depends on the etiology. For example, angina is more likely to occur in coronary disease or valvular heart disease with left ventricular outflow obstruction and hypertrophy. Physical findings include jugular venous distention, abnormal carotid contours, rales, evidence of systemic venous hypertension, left parasternal lift, third and fourth heart sound gallops, mitral and tricuspid regurgitation, and increased pulmonic component of the second heart sound. Other murmurs may also be present with coexisting valvular heart disease. Mitral regurgitation and tricuspid regurgitation may also be present because of biventricular dilatation resulting in altered left ventricular geometry and tricuspid annular dilatation.

Cardiomegaly with pulmonary vascular congestion may be seen on the chest x-ray film. The ECG often demonstrates conduction disease, left ventricular hypertrophy, and non-

TABLE 92–3
CAUSES OF LEFT VENTRICULAR DYSFUNCTION LEADING TO RIGHT VENTRICULAR DYSFUNCTION
Cardiomyopathy
Congestive (dilated)
Restrictive (e.g., amyloid, idiopathic)
Coronary artery disease
After myocardial infarction
Ischemic cardiomyopathy
Ischemic mitral regurgitation
Valvular heart disease
Mitral regurgitation
Aortic valve disease
Congenital heart disease
Ventricular septal defect
Patent ductus arteriosus
Left ventricular inflow obstruction
Mitral stenosis
Cor triatriatum
Pulmonary venous obstruction

specific ST segment and T wave abnormalities. A previous myocardial infarction may also be noted. Echocardiography is especially revealing for valvular heart disease and cardiomyopathy of various causes. Previous myocardial infarction may be manifested by hypokinesia and scarring of the affected wall as seen by echocardiography. Doppler echocardiography and color flow mapping can often reveal the extent and severity of valvular heart disease. Pulmonary arterial systolic pressure can be estimated from the peak tricuspid regurgitation velocity by use of the modified Bernoulli's equation.[16] Finally, cardiac catheterization and left ventriculography can demonstrate the extent and severity of coronary disease or valvular heart disease. In the critical care unit, right-sided heart catheterization using pulmonary arterial flotation catheters may be useful for pulmonary arterial and pulmonary arterial wedge pressure monitoring. Right ventricular and pulmonary arterial pressures are likely to be elevated and cardiac output depressed.

Therapeutic options primarily address the cause of left ventricular dysfunction or left ventricular inflow obstruction. Diuretics to reduce left ventricular and subsequently right ventricular filling pressures are important therapeutic options. Biventricular dilatation is likely to lead to accentuation of filling pressures on both sides. As filling pressures continue to rise, they may begin to equilibrate. This finding indicates the importance of not only ventricular interdependence but also pericardial restraint in biventricular congestive heart failure.[11, 41–43] Diuretics reduce venous return and reduce total intracardiac size, resulting in a reduction of intrapericardial contact stress.[44] Vasodilators such as nitroprusside, a balanced venous and arteriolar dilator, not only reduce filling pressures on the left and right sides but also increase cardiac output via arterial vasodilatation. Because intracardiac pressure is a function of transmural pressure plus pericardial pressure, changing pericardial pressure by reducing intracardiac size has important and dramatic effects on the right and left ventricular filling pressures.[45] Both Smiseth and colleagues[42] experimentally and Smith[43] clinically have noted marked downward displacement of the left ventricular pressure-volume curve with nitroprusside therapy in congestive heart failure. When transmural pressures are substituted for intracardiac pressures, the downward displacement is eliminated and the plot moves up and down a single curve. A graphic example of this finding is demonstrated in Figure 92–5. Angiotensin-converting enzyme inhibitors may be given orally and may also have, via different mechanisms, venodilation and arteriolar dilatation effects. Inotropic therapy with dobutamine or amrinone (a type III phosphodiesterase inhibitor) leads to clinical improvement as both ventricles may demonstrate inotropic influence. Amrinone has the additional advantage of being an arteriolar vasodilator. Atrial fibrillation may accompany biventricular dysfunction, and digitalization may be useful for both controlling the rate and adding inotropic support. Digoxin and angiotensin-converting enzyme inhibitors when used together have a synergistic effect on left ventricular performance in patients with congestive heart failure.[46]

PERICARDIUM

Anatomy and Function

The cardiac chambers are enveloped by a serosal sac that is one cell thick on the surface of the heart (visceral pericardium), and the parietal pericardium (the outer portion of the sac) is composed of a single cell layer with a fibrous coat. The pericardium envelops the cardiac chambers and reflects around the hila, great vessels, and left atrium. There is a

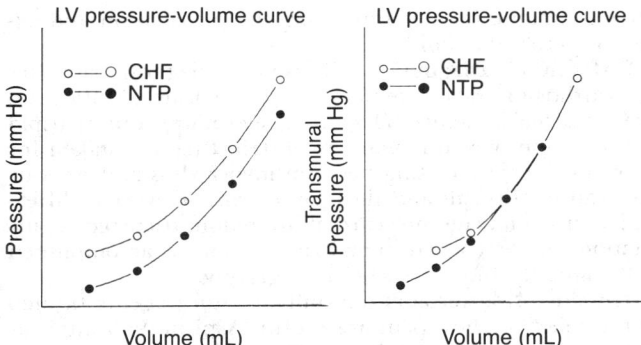

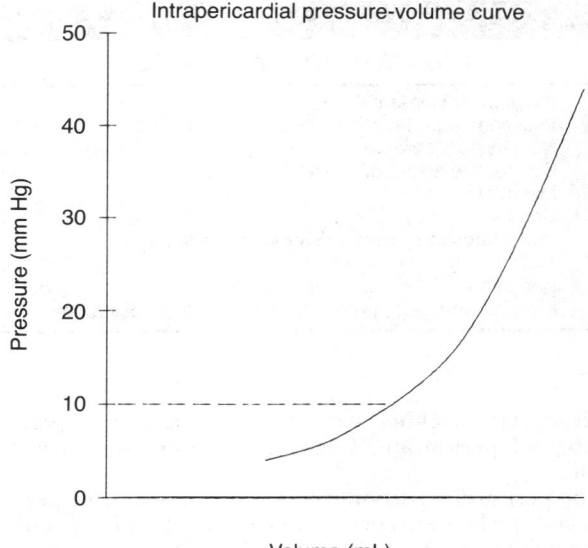

Figure 92-5. Left ventricular diastolic pressure-volume curves (graphic) for an idealized patient with left-sided congestive heart failure (CHF) and after therapy with nitroprusside (NTP) are shown on the left. There is a downward displacement of the left diastolic pressure-volume curve with nitroprusside. The influence of pericardial restraint is shown on the right. Transmural pressure (intracavitary pressure − pericardial pressure) is substituted for intracavitary pressure. Transmural pressure-volume curves for a patient with left-sided heart failure (congestive heart failure) and after nitroprusside therapy are shown on the right. The curves are nearly superimposable.

Figure 92-6. Graphic representation of the intrapericardial pressure-volume curve. The curve is depicted as an exponential function with a rapid rise in pressure for small volume increments beginning at 10 mm Hg.

potential space between the parietal pericardium and visceral pericardium in which fluid may accumulate. The pericardium has multiple functions, several of which are listed in Table 92-4.[6, 7] From a clinical standpoint, restraint of chamber dilation, retardation of infectious processes, and ventricular coupling are the most important functions. Breakdown or overuse of any of these functions can contribute to hemodynamic embarrassment. For example, purulent pericarditis producing cardiac tamponade is a life-threatening illness. Cardiac dilation, although chronic, can lead to increased pericardial restraining forces that further increase intracardiac pressures.[43]

Although the pericardium has some degree of elasticity, it becomes essentially inelastic with any significant cardiac dilation. Figure 92-6 is a graphic example of pressure-volume characteristics of the pericardium. At lower volumes, the pericardium can increase its volume with minimal fluid pressure incrementation. However, with larger increases in volume, pericardial pressure begins to rise exponentially. This exponential rise begins at pressures of 10 to 12 mm Hg.[6, 7] Not surprisingly, the left[47] and the right ventricles have similar pressure-volume curves with exponential rises in pressure for small volume increments at 10 to 12 mm Hg.

In the normal left ventricle, intrapericardial pressures are assumed to be negligible. This conclusion is based on fluid catheter measurements. However, fluid catheter measure-

ments assess only hydrostatic pressure. Smiseth and colleagues[44] have offered a different approach to this issue. They hypothesized that the underlying left and right ventricles exert a constant force on the pericardium. Several investigators have attempted to measure this force with the use of air-filled or fluid-filled flat Silastic balloons. Their data indicate that in a normal left ventricle, pericardial pressure as surface contact pressure is between 40 and 80% of the mean right atrial pressure. This percentage of mean right atrial pressure increases with increases in the left and right ventricular filling pressures.[48-50] Smiseth and colleagues[44, 51] demonstrated excellent correlation of fluid-filled intrapericardial Silastic balloon catheter measurements with hydrostatic pressure measurements in the presence of a pericardial effusion. Furthermore, they demonstrated that the difference between intracardiac pressures before and after pericardiectomy was similar to the intrapericardial pressure measured with the flat Silastic balloon in the normal left ventricle without a pericardial effusion.

If the pericardium thickens, becomes scarred, or becomes involved by other pathologic processes, the restraining properties may increase, resulting in a greater degree of coupling.

Diseases of Pericardium
Acute Pericarditis

Acute pericarditis is the result of many causes, as listed in Table 92-5. The inflammatory process may result in an effusion, and if the effusion develops rapidly enough cardiac tamponade may ensue. Almost all causes of acute pericarditis may result in pericardial effusion. Some causes (neoplastic) are more likely to result in cardiac tamponade or constrictive pericarditis (tuberculosis).[6, 7]

Symptoms and Signs. Although acute pericarditis may be asymptomatic, there is often chest pain. Three varieties of chest pain have been described. First is the classic description of central discomfort made worse by recumbence and improved by sitting erect; this chest pain may also radiate to the trapezius ridge. Second is the description of a pleural-like pain, and third is the description of a pain that resembles

TABLE 92-4
FUNCTIONS OF THE PERICARDIUM
Lubrication
Fixes the heart in position
Isolates the heart from other structures (retards infectious processes)
Limits the extent of acute cardiac dilation
Facilitates atrial filling
Limits atrioventricular valve regurgitation under conditions of increased left ventricular size and pressure
Facilitates systolic and diastolic ventricular interdependence

TABLE 92–5
ETIOLOGY OF ACUTE PERICARDITIS
Idiopathic disorders Infection: viral, tuberculosis, fungal, bacterial Neoplastic disorders Connective tissue diseases Myxedema Uremia Postinfarction or postpericardiotomy disorders Trauma Radiation Drug related (e.g., procainamide, minoxidil) disorders

angina pectoris. Other symptoms may be based upon the etiology of pericarditis. Constitutional symptoms may also occur.

The pericardial friction rub is pathognomonic of pericarditis and can be heard even with a pericardial effusion. Rubs may be faint or loud or may completely disappear. Pericardial friction rubs usually have three components (systolic, early filling, and later filling) but can have two components with atrial fibrillation and with rapid heart rates.

Laboratory and Diagnostic Studies. Cardiac enzyme levels are expected to be normal unless underlying myocarditis is present. Elevations of the white blood cell count, erythrocyte sedimentation rate, and acute-phase reactants can be seen. The ECG (Fig. 92–7) is extremely helpful in diagnosing pericarditis. Four stages have been described.[52, 53] In the first stage, there is concave ST segment elevation in most leads. During stage II the ST segments return to baseline and T waves flatten in these leads. PR depression may also be seen. In stage III, T wave inversion occurs diffusely. Stage IV represents normalization of the ECG. Stages I through III may occur in rapid progression. Progression of stage III to stage IV may take several weeks to months. The chest x-ray film may show enlargement of the cardiac silhouette with effusions greater than 250 mL. Echocardiography is a sensitive technique for demonstrating the distribution and extent of pericardial fluid.

Differential Diagnosis. Differential diagnosis includes myocarditis (T wave inversion), acute myocardial infarction or myocardial ischemia (ST segment elevation), and tricuspid regurgitation or ventricular septal defect (rub mistaken for murmur). Differentiating between myocarditis and pericarditis can be difficult and they can coexist. However, differentiation from acute myocardial infarction, tricuspid regurgitation, or ventricular septal defect can be accomplished both clinically and with echocardiography.

Therapy. Nonsteroidal anti-inflammatory agents titrated to the relief of chest pain are useful. Aspirin (900 mg four times a day) and indomethacin (25 mg four times a day) can be used. However, nonaspirin agents should not be used with pericarditis associated with acute myocardial infarction as they may thin the myocardial scar.[54] Corticosteroids should be avoided if possible but can be used if all other measures fail. Treatment of known etiologic agents should be immediately addressed.

Post–Myocardial Infarction Pericarditis

Post–myocardial infarction pericarditis occurs in approximately 20% of patients on the second to fifth day after myocardial infarction.[55, 56] Infarction is uniformly transmural and tends to be larger in patients with rubs. Chest pain is not always present but when present is clearly different from ischemic pain. The pain tends to be pleuritic and associated with fever and other systemic symptoms. ST segment deviations may be seen diffusely and may normalize the ST segment depression seen in reciprocal leads from the ST segment elevation seen with the acute infarction. T waves that were previously inverted may become upright. However, electrocardiographic changes may be subtle. A pericardial rub is often present.[57, 58] The pericarditis tends to have a course of 1 to 3 days and can be successfully managed with aspirin. Ibuprofen and steroids are contraindicated as they may influence infarct healing.[54, 59]

Pericardial effusion after myocardial infarction may be

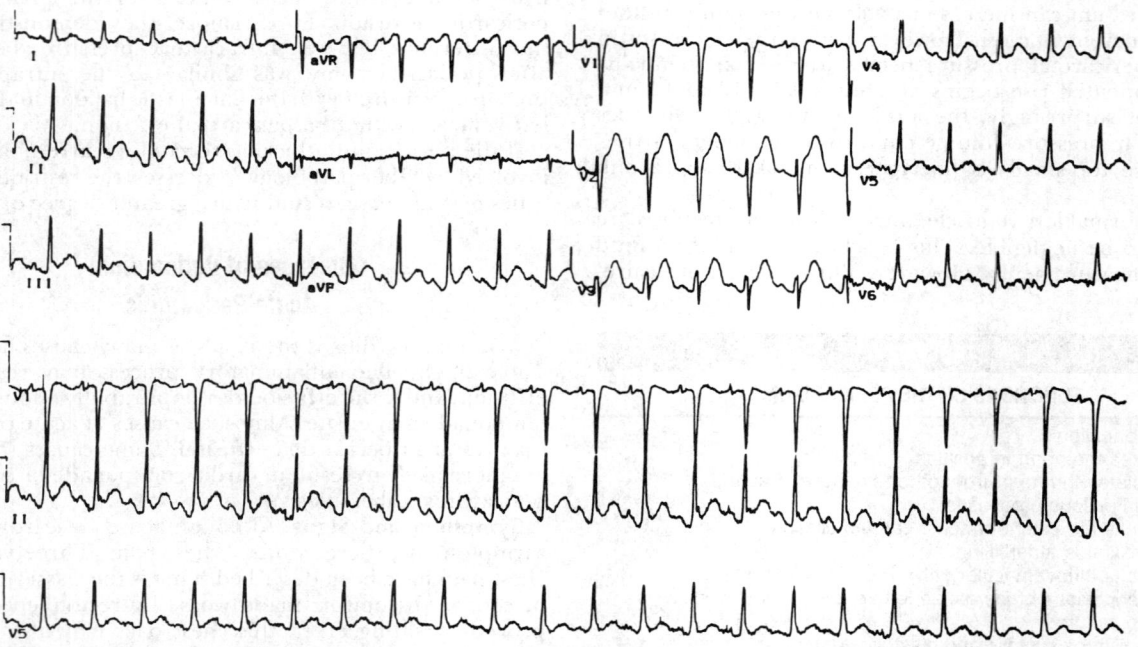

Figure 92–7. Twelve-lead ECG of a patient with acute viral pericarditis. ST segment elevation is seen diffusely. PR interval depression is noted in leads II, III, and aV$_F$.

the only presentation of pericarditis as a rub may be absent in half the patients.[60] Anticoagulation is not strictly contraindicated. However, cardiac tamponade occurs with a low incidence and when present tends to be seen with acute anterior myocardial infarction. With thrombolysis, approximately 1% of patients develop hemorrhagic effusions leading to cardiac tamponade. In each case, heparin and aspirin were also used.[61]

Pericardial Effusion

Any etiology of acute pericarditis can lead to the accumulation of pericardial fluid. Approximately 250 mL of fluid is needed for the effusion to become clinically obvious by physical examination or chest x-ray study. Larger amounts of fluid can accumulate if the accumulation is slow enough to allow the pericardium to stretch and remodel.

Signs and Symptoms. The effusion per se may produce few if any symptoms. The underlying pericarditis or associated illness may produce varied symptoms. Larger effusions may compress adjacent structures, producing hoarseness, dysphagia, and dyspnea. Physical examination may reveal a rub in more than 50% of patients and may reveal distant heart sounds. The effusion may compress the left lower bronchus, producing bronchial breath sounds; this has been termed Ewart's sign. Pulsus paradoxus should not be present unless the pericardial effusion is compressive.

Laboratory and Diagnostic Studies. Chest radiography reveals a dilated cardiac silhouette with a smooth contour and a water bottle appearance. Lung fields are clear and a pleural effusion may be present. The ECG may reveal low voltage. Echocardiography is the preferred diagnostic procedure and demonstrates an echo-free space both posteriorly and anteriorly (Fig. 92–8). Two-dimensional echocardiography can be invaluable in demonstrating the size and distribution of pericardial fluid. An echo-free space seen only anteriorly may or may not represent fluid. Usually, posterior or apical deposition of fluid occurs first in the gravity-dependent sites. However, if the right ventricular free wall is hypermobile, an anterior free space is more likely to be fluid than adipose. Right atrial angiography has demonstrated an effusion as an increased space between the edge of the dye and the edge of the cardiac silhouette on fluoroscopy. Finally, computed tomographic scanning or

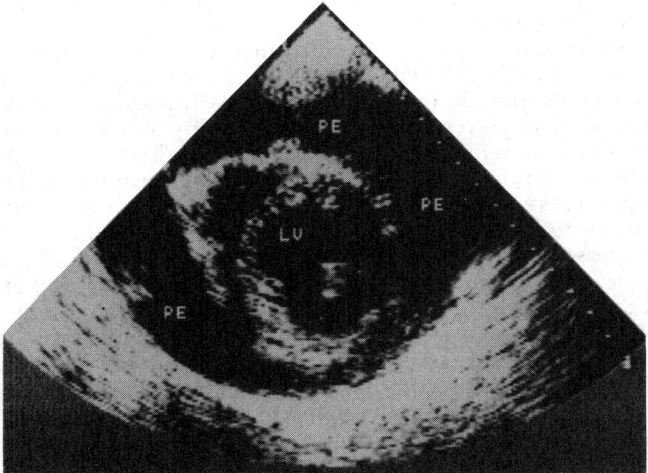

Figure 92–8. Stop frame from a two-dimensional echocardiogram taken in the parasternal short-axis view demonstrating a large circumferential pericardial effusion (PE). LV = left ventricle.

magnetic resonance imaging can be useful and sensitive in the demonstration of a pericardial effusion.

Diagnostic and Therapeutic. If the effusion does not produce hemodynamic embarrassment and there is no infection, no specific therapy is needed. However, its cause may still be in question. The presence of an associated systemic illness may point to its cause, but a pericardiocentesis is often required to obtain fluid for chemistry assays; glucose, protein, rheumatoid factor, antinuclear antibody, and complement determination; culture; and cytologic tests. If metastatic disease is suspected, a subxiphoid resection or window would be useful for obtaining fluid, cytologic, and histologic samples. There is some evidence that a window results in apposition of the visceral pericardium and parietal pericardium and obliteration of the intrapericardial space.[62] Pericardiocentesis can also be performed electively either in the catheterization laboratory with full hemodynamic monitoring and intrapericardial measurement or in the critical care setting with electrocardiographic guidance by connecting an exploring electrode to the pericardiocentesis needle. If the needle touches the wall of the heart, ST segment elevation is seen. Finally, ultrasound guidance may also provide information about the needle's placement, the location of fluid, and the amount of fluid still to be drained. It may be specifically helpful in the case of a loculated effusion.[63]

Cardiac Tamponade

Cardiac tamponade is an emergent situation in which pericardial fluid is accumulating with such rapidity and under such pressure that cardiac filling and cardiac output are compromised.[64] Because the pericardium is nonelastic, the pressure begins to rise in an exponential fashion with increasing volume after a certain amount of fluid has accumulated[6, 7] (see Fig. 92–6). Alterations in the pericardium because of pathologic processes may make it even less compliant. As the intrapericardial pressure rises with increasing intrapericardial volume, cardiac filling is restricted. A series of compensatory mechanisms comes into play. As the filling volume and stroke volume fall, adrenergic stimulation ensues, resulting in increased heart rate, increased contractility, and increased systemic venous adrenergic tone, which increases venous return and the systemic venous pressure. Cardiac tamponade is not an all-or-none phenomenon but a spectrum of compressive physiology. Reddy and coworkers[65] described three hemodynamic phases of cardiac tamponade. In phase I, the pericardial, left ventricular, and right ventricular pressures are increased but not equilibrated. Cardiac output is not compromised. In phase II, right ventricular and pericardial pressures are equilibrated with each other but not with left ventricular pressure. Cardiac output is depressed and pulsus paradoxus is present. During phase III, all pressures are equilibrated, cardiac output is markedly depressed, and pulsus paradoxus is present in all patients.

Etiology. Cardiac tamponade can occur with any of the causes of acute pericarditis that lead to effusion. It is more common with malignancy, uremia, and penetrating trauma and after cardiac surgery. Anticoagulation used during active pericarditis may increase the chance of cardiac tamponade.

Signs and Symptoms. The symptoms of cardiac tamponade are not specific to this entity. They may be related to hypotension or the underlying acute pericarditis or to chronic illness associated with the acute pericarditis. Cardiac tamponade, when compressive and more chronic, is likely to produce symptoms of weakness, fatigue, and some degree of breathlessness. Physical examination reveals systemic venous hypertension with distended neck veins, prominent x descent of the neck veins with decreased y descent, leg edema, and ascites if chronic. Heart sounds may be distant and the patient may be hypotensive, especially if hemopericardium is present.[66] Pulsus paradoxus is present in nearly all patients and is defined as a decrease in blood pressure of more than 10 mm Hg with inspiration. Normally, in the absence of a pericardial effusion, inspiration increases venous return to the right side of the heart and increases the pulmonary vascular capacitance, resulting in decreased return to the left side of the heart. In the presence of a hemodynamically significant pericardial effusion resulting in limited intrapericardial space, inspiration increases the volume of the right side of the heart, which results in decreased left ventricular volume and stroke volume because of leftward shifting of the ventricular septum.[67] A pericardial friction rub may also be present. Pulsus paradoxus may be absent with an atrial septal defect, severe aortic regurgitation, left ventricular congestive heart failure (left-sided pressure stays greater than right-sided pressure), severe tamponade with hypotension, and low-pressure tamponade because of intravascular volume depletion.

Diagnostic Studies. *Electrocardiography.* The ECG is nonspecific and may suggest pericarditis (ST segment elevation or PR depression) or pericardial effusion (low voltage). Electrical alternation involving the P, QRS, and T waves is suggestive of tamponade and more specifically of malignant etiologies of tamponade.[68]

Echocardiography. Echocardiography reveals a large pericardial effusion, although the effusion may be loculated. Signs of compression such as right atrial or right ventricular collapse may be present. Right atrial collapse occurs during ventricular systole when the pressure and volume are lowest and the intrapericardial pressure is high.[69] Right atrial collapse (Fig. 92–9) can be seen on the apical four-chamber or parasternal short-axis echocardiogram as invagination of the right atrial free wall. Right atrial collapse is quite sensitive but can be seen in the absence of cardiac tamponade, with pericardial effusion alone. Right ventricular collapse in early diastole is a more specific sign[70] (Fig. 92–10). Right atrial or right ventricular collapse may not occur when right-sided pressures are elevated. In this circumstance, intrapericardial pressures may not exceed either right atrial or right ventric-

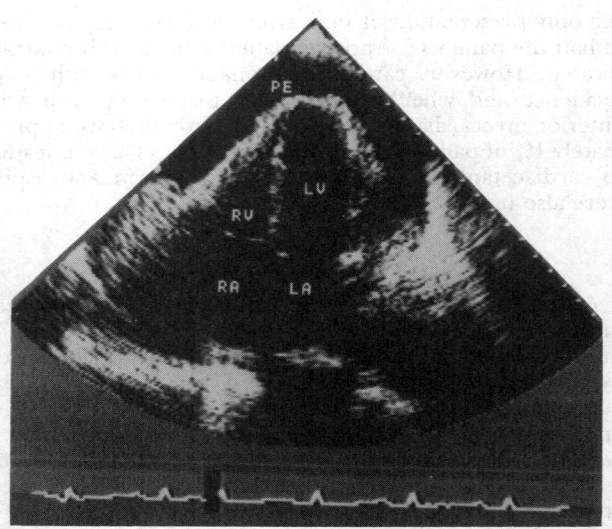

Figure 92–10. Stop frame in diastole from a two-dimensional echocardiogram taken in the apical four-chamber view in a patient with cardiac tamponade. The left ventricle (LV) is expanding while the right ventricle (RV) remains collapsed in early diastole. RA = right atrium; LA = left atrium; PE = pericardial effusion.

ular filling pressures. Right atrial and right ventricular collapse may also be attenuated with right ventricular hypertrophy, because a thicker right ventricular wall is less likely to collapse. There are other echocardiographic signs, including alteration of left ventricular and right ventricular size with inspiration on M mode, alteration in the mitral echogram EF slope, and alterations in the transmitral and tricuspid flow velocities with inspiration.[71] However, these signs are more reflective of the mechanisms governing pulsus paradoxus.

Right-Sided Heart Catheterization and Pericardiocentesis. Right-sided heart catheterization can be performed either in the hemodynamic laboratory or at the bedside with a thermodilution pulmonary arterial catheter. Right atrial, right ventricular, pulmonary arterial diastolic, and intrapericardial pressures are nearly identical and cardiac output is variably depressed (Fig. 92–11). Often, right-sided heart catheterization is performed as a prelude to pericardiocentesis for both therapeutic and diagnostic purposes. Intrapericardial hydrostatic pressures are equilibrated with right-sided pressures.

Pericardiocentesis can be performed using an anterior or subcostal approach. Fluoroscopic, electrocardiographic, or echocardiographic guidance is helpful. Echocardiographic guidance is preferred because it can pinpoint the needle entrance, location, and extent of fluid.[63] Withdrawal of as little as 50 mL can result in considerable reduction in right-sided pressures, especially intrapericardial hydrostatic pressure, which may fall to low levels and be associated with an increase in cardiac output (Fig. 92–12). Examination of the pericardial pressure-volume curve (see Fig. 92–6) reveals an exponential rise of pressure for a small increment in volume. Tamponade occurs on the upslope of this curve. However, clinical experience often indicates that greater volumes must be removed before the baseline hemodynamic state is restored. The process that produces the fluid may also alter the pericardium and the characteristics of the intrapericardial pressure-volume curve.

If pericardiocentesis cannot be performed immediately, the patient can be stabilized by optimizing his or her volume status, enhancing contractility, and reducing afterload.[72]

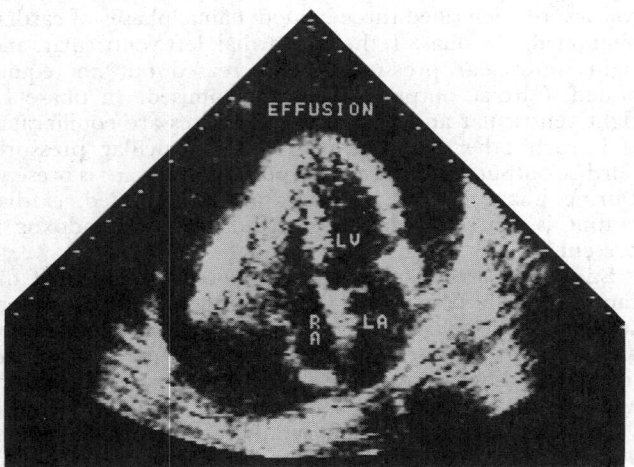

Figure 92–9. Stop frame from a two-dimensional echocardiogram taken in the apical four-chamber view in a patient with cardiac tamponade. A large pericardial effusion is present. Right atrial (RA) invagination or collapse is seen during ventricular systole. LV = left ventricle; LA = left atrium.

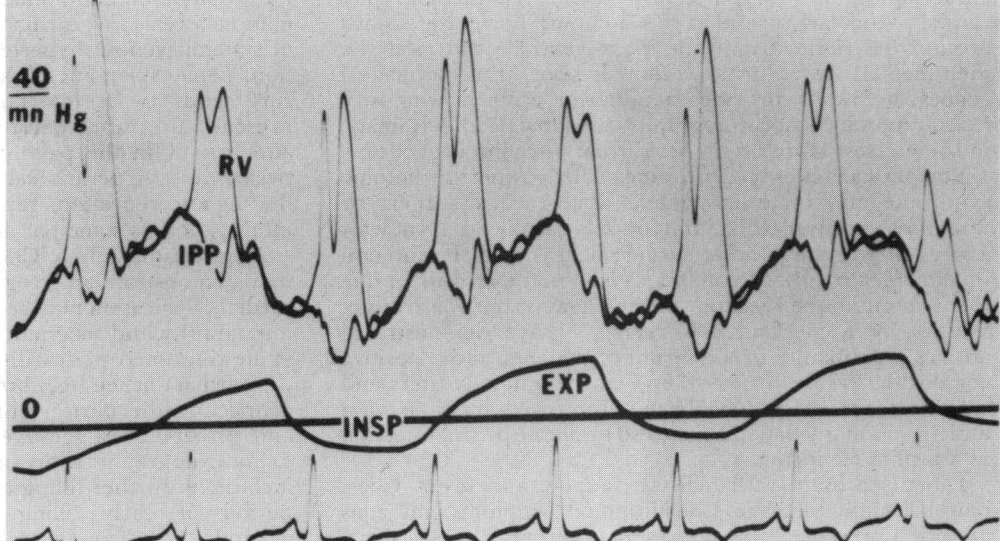

Figure 92–11. Right ventricular (RV) pressure and intrapericardial pressure (IPP) in a patient with cardiac tamponade. Equalization of diastolic pressure is seen with inspiration (INSP) and expiration (EXP). (From Reddy PS: Hemodynamics of cardiac tamponade. In: Reddy PS, Leon DF, Shaver JA [eds]: Pericardial Disease. New York, Raven Press, p 167, 1982.)

However, these treatment strategies provide only stabilization. Ultimately, pericardiocentesis must be performed.

Although observation for reaccumulation may suffice for idiopathic or viral etiologies, other etiologies such as malignancy may require more definitive procedures, including a pericardial window, subcutaneous resection, or installation of a sclerosing or chemotherapeutic agent.[73] The choice depends on the patient, the presence of malignancy, and the long-term response of the patient to the treatment of carcinoma.

Pericardial Involvement After Cardiac Surgery

Cardiac Compression. Cardiac compression may occur after cardiac surgery as the drains are removed or when they fail to drain properly. In the presence of bleeding, a considerable amount of fluid may accumulate with a locular distribution. Significant accumulation may result in isolated right-sided or left-sided heart compression. The patient may have hypotension, neck vein distention, and a rub but may not demonstrate pulsus paradoxus. Electrocardiography and

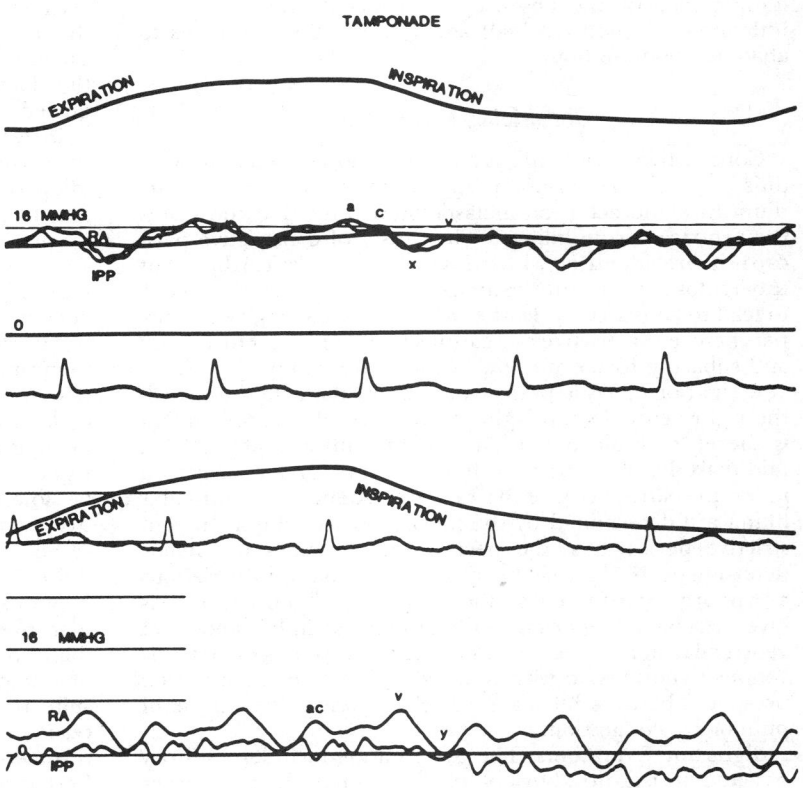

Figure 92–12. *(Top)* Equalization of right atrial (RA) pressure and intrapericardial pressure (IPP) in a patient with cardiac tamponade. *(Bottom)* After pericardiocentesis; the right atrial and intrapericardial pressures are markedly reduced. The intrapericardial pressure is now near 0 (a, c, x, and y are the right atrial venous waves). (From Reddy PS: Hemodynamics of cardiac tamponade. In: Reddy PS, Leon DF, Shaver JA [eds]: Pericardial Disease. New York, Raven Press, p 163, 1982.)

chest radiography may not be helpful. Echocardiography can be particularly useful in this situation. Locular effusions around the right atrium and right ventricle can easily be identified. If the acoustic window is poor, transesophageal echocardiography provides a posterior acoustic window.[74] Localization by echocardiography can allow needle drainage in some cases. More often, pericardial resection is needed.

Postpericardiotomy Syndrome. The postpericardiotomy syndrome may occur in patients after cardiac surgery or after a recent myocardial infarction. It usually occurs at least 1 week after either cardiac surgery or myocardial infarction in about 10 to 40% of patients. It is hypothesized to be due to an autoimmune reaction directed against the epicardium. Studies by Engle and coworkers[57, 58] have demonstrated antiheart antibodies in the serum of patients, and a positive correlation has been noted between the antibody titers and the incidence of this syndrome. Increased titers to viral antigens in many patients may also implicate a viral infection as a facilitative factor.

Patients present with malaise, fatigue, and fever. Chest pain is usually pleuritic. Constitutional symptoms and signs are often present. Physical examination reveals a pericardial friction rub. Chest radiography may reveal pleural effusion in two thirds of patients, pulmonary infiltrates occasionally, and enlargement of the cardiac silhouette in half. Electrocardiographic findings usually include nonspecific ST segment and T wave alterations, which may be difficult to discern because of existing ST segment and T wave abnormalities. Echocardiography may reveal a pericardial effusion, which may have been present previously. This syndrome is usually recognized clinically. However, the pericardial effusion may be quite large and cardiac tamponade can occur especially with the use of anticoagulants. Cardiac tamponade should be managed by pericardiocentesis followed by treatment with anti-inflammatory agents. Pericardiectomy should be reserved for recurring cardiac tamponade. In the absence of cardiac tamponade, anti-inflammatory (nonsteroidal) agents cause the symptoms to abate in about 48 hours.

Constrictive Pericarditis

Constrictive pericarditis is a complication of acute pericarditis in which the parietal pericardium and visceral pericardium fuse and act as an inelastic membrane that constrains the ventricles from filling.[75] The causes of constrictive pericarditis are identical with those of acute pericarditis, but tuberculosis, radiation, trauma, and uremia are more likely to lead to constriction. In the case of tuberculosis, years may pass before constrictive pericarditis is recognized. More acute and subacute forms are now being encountered.

A rigid or inelastic pericardium limits the extent to which the right ventricle and right atrium can fill. Diastolic filling is therefore rapid and early and discontinues abruptly in mid-diastole. Biventricular filling occurs under increased filling pressures because the rate and extent of biventricular filling are determined by the inelastic pericardium. In constrictive pericarditis, the pericardium becomes the major determinant of diastolic behavior and respiratory variations are poorly transmitted to the right side of the heart.[76] As biventricular filling occurs with an increase in left and right ventricular filling pressures, signs and symptoms of systemic venous hypertension with reduced cardiac output are often present. These findings are more prominent than those of pulmonary congestion.

Signs and Symptoms. The presentation includes a history of acute pericarditis, but not all patients have had an earlier episode. Patients complain of dyspnea on exertion, easy fatigability, and abdominal and leg swelling. Physical examination reveals low cardiac output and signs and symptoms of systemic venous hypertension including neck vein distention, hepatosplenomegaly, edema, and ascites. Blood pressure tends to be low normal, atrial fibrillation is often present, and pulsus paradoxus is usually seen in only 20% and usually in the patients who have effusive constrictive pericarditis. A pericardial knock[77] is the hallmark physical finding and represents rapid deceleration of left ventricular inflow; there is some parallel with the S_3 sound.

Diagnostic Studies. Chest radiography and fluoroscopy may demonstrate an irregular cardiac silhouette, and pericardial calcification may be shown by fluoroscopy. Computed tomography and magnetic resonance imaging may demonstrate thickened pericardium. Echocardiography may show pericardial thickening, fibrous strands in the pericardial fluid connecting the pericardium with the left ventricular wall, and physiology suggestive of restricted cardiac filling.[78–80] Echocardiographic signs suggesting restricted cardiac filling include no further filling of the posterior free wall after the period of early filling, ventricular expansion ending abruptly,[80] and an increase in the extent of rapid filling shown by transmitral Doppler echocardiography.[81] The pericardium may bind down the left ventricular free wall, limiting its motion. The ventricular septum may demonstrate a notching motion on M mode. However, the diagnosis is most reliably secured by cardiac catheterization. Right- and left-sided heart catheterization reveals equalization of diastolic right- and left-sided heart pressures.[82] Right ventricular systolic pressure is usually less than 50 mm Hg. Respiratory variations are not transmitted to the heart, as demonstrated by Kussmaul's sign. A square root sign on the right or left ventricular pressure tracing (Fig. 92–13) and prominent x and y descents of the right atrial pressure can also be seen. Catheterization findings that represent restriction and enhanced early diastolic filling, when combined with anatomic evidence for a thickened pericardium, make the diagnosis of constrictive pericarditis secure. Despite cardiac catheterization and various noninvasive techniques, the diagnosis may still be elusive and surgery may be required.

Differential Diagnosis. Constrictive pericarditis must be distinguished from restrictive cardiomyopathy, including idiopathic, amyloid, and other infiltrative cardiomyopathies. Amyloid is easy to differentiate on the basis of echocardiographic appearance and biopsy examination. Idiopathic restrictive cardiomyopathy can best be differentiated on the basis of catheterization findings and the absence of a thickened pericardium. With restrictive cardiomyopathy, left ventricular filling pressures are greater than right ventricular filling pressures, the pulmonary arterial pressure is greater than 50 mm Hg, and the pericardium is normal. If pericardial knock is absent, an S_3 sound may be present. Fluid loading may increase left ventricular pressures more than right ventricular pressures.[82] Early diastolic filling tends to be slower with restrictive cardiomyopathy than with constrictive pericarditis.[81, 83] However, significant overlap of these catheterization and diastolic filling findings may make it difficult to be able to differentiate the two entities. If there is pre-existing left ventricular dysfunction, the left ventricular pressures may be greater than the right ventricular filling pressures even with constriction. The demonstration of a thickened pericardium therefore becomes critical. Despite the findings from computed tomography, magnetic resonance imaging, and Doppler echocardiography, surgery is sometimes needed for diagnostic and therapeutic reasons. Restrictive cardiomyopathy is not curable; however, constrictive pericarditis is curable and should be treated aggressively.

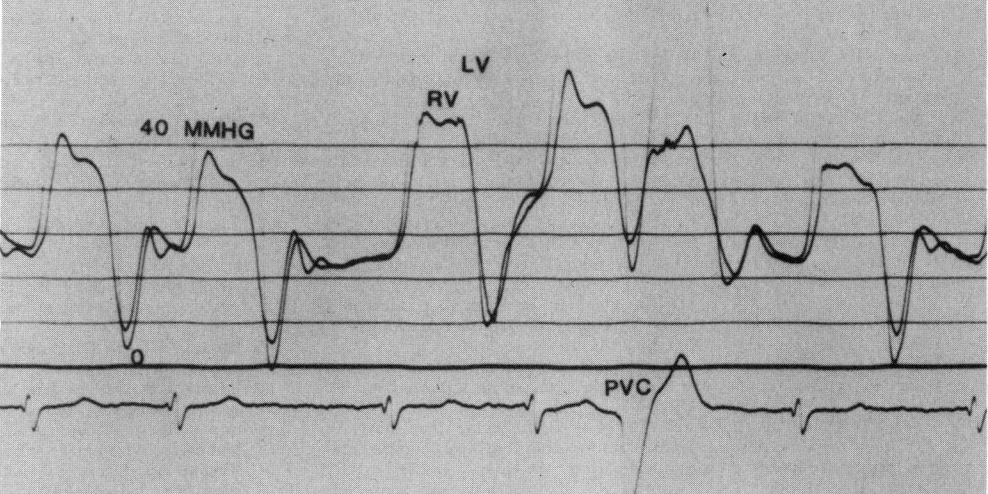

Figure 92–13. Simultaneous left ventricular (LV) and right ventricular (RV) pressure tracings for a patient with constrictive pericarditis and atrial fibrillation. Both right and left ventricular pressures are equalized in diastole and show the characteristic dip and plateau (square root sign). (From Reddy PS: Constrictive pericarditis. In: Reddy PS, Leon DF, Shaver JA [eds]: Pericardial Disease. New York, Raven Press, p 282, 1982.)

Therapy. Pericardiectomy is the only definitive therapy presently available. Careful and complete resection is often needed. Surgery is time consuming and results in significant loss of blood and fluids. Medical therapy consists of efforts to reduce systemic venous hypertension, primarily by administration of diuretics before surgery.

Effusive Constrictive Pericarditis

The presentation of patients with effusive constrictive pericarditis may be variable. Symptoms and signs may suggest either constriction or tamponade. The difference in presentation often has to do with the degree of pericardial effusion present. This entity was originally described with the presentation of cardiac tamponade. After pericardiocentesis, the hemodynamics resembled those seen with constrictive pericarditis.[84, 85] The etiologies of effusive constrictive pericarditis are similar to those of cardiac tamponade and constrictive pericarditis. The diagnostic and therapeutic approaches to effusive constrictive pericarditis are similar to the approaches to pericardial effusion, cardiac tamponade, or constrictive pericarditis. Echocardiography, right-sided heart catheterization, computed tomography or magnetic resonance imaging, and pericardial resection may be utilized.

References

1. Sarnoff SJ, Berglund E: Ventricular function: I. Starling's law of the heart studied by means of simultaneous right and left ventricular function curves in the dog. Circulation 9:706, 1954.
2. Weber, KT, Janicki JS, Shroff SG, et al: The right ventricle: Physiologic and pathophysiologic considerations. Crit Care Med 11:323, 1983.
3. Braunwald E: Regulation of the circulation. I. N Engl J Med 290:1124, 1974.
4. Sibbald WJ, Driedger AA: Right ventricular function in acute disease states: Pathophysiologic considerations. Crit Care Med 11:339, 1983.
5. Grossman W, Braunwald E, Mann T, et al: Contractile state of the left ventricle in man as evaluated for the end systolic pressure–volume relation. Circulation 56:845, 1977.
6. Spodick DH: The normal and diseased pericardium: Current concepts of pericardial physiology, diagnosis and treatment. J Am Coll Cardiol 1:240, 1983.
7. Spodick DH: The pericardium: Structure, function and disease spectrum. In: Spodick DH (ed): Pericardial Diseases. Philadelphia, FA Davis, p 1, 1976.
8. Ross J: Acute displacement of the diastolic pressure volume curve of the left ventricle. Circulation 59:32, 1979.
9. Ludbrook PA, Byrne JD, McKnight RC: Influence of right ventricular hemodynamics on left ventricular diastolic pressure–volume relation in man. Circulation 59:21, 1979.
10. Freeman GL, Lewinter MM: Pericardial adaptations during chronic cardiac dilatation in dogs. Circ Res 54:294, 1984.
11. Bove A, Santamore W: Ventricular interdependence. Prog Cardiovasc Dis 23:365, 1981.
12. Krayenbuehl HP, Turina J, Hess O: Left ventricular function in chronic pulmonary hypertension. Am J Cardiol 41:1150, 1978.
13. Robin ED, Gaudia R: Cor pulmonale. Including a short note on pulmo cordis (cardiac lung disease). DM May:3; 1970.
14. Fishman AP: Chronic cor pulmonale. Am Rev Respir Dis 114:775, 1976.
15. Berger HJ, Matthay RA, Pytlik LM, et al: First pass radionuclide assessment of right and left ventricular performance in patients with cardiac and pulmonary disease. Semin Nucl Med 9:275, 1975.
16. Berger M, Haimowitz A, VanTosh A, et al: Quantitative assessment of pulmonary hypertension in patients with tricuspid regurgitation using continuous wave Doppler. J Am Coll Cardiol 6:359, 1985.
17. Dalen JE, Bana JS Jr, Brooks HL, et al: Resolution rate of acute pulmonary embolism in man. N Engl J Med 280:1194, 1969.
18. Motta J, Guilleminault C, Schroeder JS, et al: Tracheostomy and hemodynamic changes in sleep-induced apnea. Ann Intern Med 89:454, 1978.
19. Green LH, Smith TW: The use of digitalis in patients with pulmonary disease. Ann Intern Med 87:459, 1977.
20. Mathur PN, Powles P, Pugsley SO, et al: Effect of digoxin on right ventricular function in severe chronic airflow obstruction: A controlled clinical trial. Ann Intern Med 95:283, 1981.
21. Weisse AB, Moschos CB, Frank MJ, et al: Hemodynamic effects of staged hematocrit reduction in patients with stable cor pulmonale and severely elevated hematocrit levels. Am J Med 58:92, 1975.
22. Matthay RA, Berger HJ, Loke J, et al: Effect of aminophylline upon right and left ventricular performance in chronic obstructive pulmonary disease. Noninvasive assessment by radionuclide angiocardiography. Am J Med 58:92, 1975.
23. Matthay RA, Berger HJ, Davies R, et al: Improvement in cardiac performance by oral long-acting theophylline in chronic obstructive pulmonary disease. Am Heart J 104:1022, 1982.
24. Perloff JK: Post-pediatric congenital heart disease in adults. In: Roberts WC (ed): Congenital Heart Disease in Adults. Philadelphia, FA Davis, 1979.
25. Friedman WF: Congenital heart disease in infancy and childhood. In: Braunwald E (ed): Heart Disease: A Textbook of Cardiovascular Medicine. 3rd ed. Philadelphia, WB Saunders, p 896, 1988.
26. Isner JM, Roberts WC: Right ventricular infarction complicating left ventricular infarction secondary to coronary heart disease. Am J Cardiol 42:885, 1978.
27. Erhardt LR: Clinical and pathological observations in different type of acute myocardial infarction: A study of 84 patients deceased after treatment in coronary care unit. Acta Med Scand 26:7, 1974.
28. Cohn JN, Giuka NH, Brodeur MI, et al: Right ventricular infarction. Am J Cardiol 33:209, 1974.
29. Ratliffe NB, Hackel DB: Combined right and left ventricular infarction: Pathogenesis and clinicopathological correlation. Am J Cardiol 45:217, 1980.
30. Reduto LA, Berger HJ, Cohen LS: Sequential radionuclide assessment of left and right ventricular performance after transmural myocardial infarction. Ann Intern Med 89:441, 1978.
31. Tobinick E, Schelbert HR, Henning H: Right ventricular ejection fraction in patients with acute anterior and inferior myocardial infarction assessed by radionuclide angiography. Circulation 57:1078, 1978.
32. Baigrie RS, Haa A, Morgan CD, et al: Spectrum of right ventricular involvement in inferior wall myocardial infarction: A clinical, hemodynamic, and noninvasive study. J Am Coll Cardiol 1:1396, 1983.
33. Goldstein JA, Vlahakes GJ, Verrier ED: The role of right ventricular

systolic dysfunction and elevated intrapericardial pressure in the genesis of low output in experimental right ventricular infarction. Circulation 65:513, 1982.

34. Strauss HD, Sobel BE, Roberts W: The influence of occult right ventricular infarction on enzymatic estimated infarct size, hemodynamics and prognosis. Circulation 62:503, 1980.
35. Chou T, Van Der Belkahn J, Allen J, et al: Electrocardiographic diagnosis of right ventricular infarction. Am J Med 70:1175, 1981.
36. Lopez-Sendon J, Garcia-Fernandez MA, Coma-Canella F, et al: Segmental right ventricular function after acute myocardial infarction: Two-dimensional echocardiographic study in 63 patients. Am J Cardiol 51:390, 1983.
37. Wackers FJ, Lie KI, Sokole EB: Prevalence of right ventricular involvement in inferior wall infarction assessed with myocardial imaging with thallium-201 and technetium-99m pyrophosphate. Am J Cardiol 42:358, 1978.
38. Lorell B, Leinbach RC, Pohost GM, et al: Right ventricular infarction: Clinical diagnosis and differentiation from cardiac tamponade and pericardial constriction. Am J Cardiol 43:465, 1979.
39. Topol EJ, Goldschlager N, Ports TA: Hemodynamic benefit of atrial pacing in right ventricular myocardial infarction. Ann Intern Med 96:594, 1982.
40. Isner JM, Fisher GP, DelNegro AA, et al: Right ventricular infarction with hemodynamic decompensation due to transient loss of augmentation: Successful treatment with atrial pacing. Am Heart J 102:792, 1981.
41. Lavine SJ, Campbell CA, Gunther SJ: Diastolic filling in acute left ventricular dysfunction: Role of the pericardium. J Am Coll Cardiol 12:1326, 1988.
42. Smiseth OA, Refsum H, Junemann M, et al: Ventricular diastolic pressure-volume shifts during acute ischemic left ventricular failure in dogs. J Am Coll Cardiol 3:966, 1984.
43. Smith ER, Smiseth OA, Kingma I, et al: Mechanism of action of nitrates. Role of changes in venous capacitance and in the left ventricular diastolic pressure-volume relation. Am J Med 76:14, 1984.
44. Smiseth OA, Kingma I, Refsum H, et al: The pericardial hypothesis: Mechanism of acute shifts of the left ventricular diastolic pressure-volume relation. Clin Physiol 5:403, 1985.
45. Smiseth OA, Refsum H, Tyberg JV: Pericardial pressure assessed by right atrial pressure: A basis for calculation of left ventricular transmural pressure. Am Heart J 108:603, 1984.
46. Captopril-Digoxin Multicenter Research Group: Comparative effects of captopril and digoxin in patients with mild to moderate heart failure. JAMA 259:539, 1988.
47. Gaasch WH, Levine HJ, Quinones MA, et al: Left ventricular compliance: Mechanism and clinical implications. Am J Cardiol 38:645, 1976.
48. Mann DL, Lew W, Bon-Hayaski E, et al: In vivo mechanical behavior of canine pericardium. Am J Physiol 251:H349, 1986.
49. Assanelli D, Lew WY, Shabetai R, et al: Influence of the pericardium on right and left ventricular filling in the dog. J Appl Physiol 63:1025, 1987.
50. Slinker BK, Dutchey RV, Bill SP, et al: Right heart pressure does not equal pericardial pressure in the potassium chloride arrested canine heart in situ. Circulation 76:359, 1987.
51. Smiseth OA, Frais MA, Kingma I, et al: Assessment of pericardial constraint in dogs. Circulation 71:158, 1985.
52. Spodick DH: Diagnostic electrocardiographic sequences in acute pericarditis: Significance of PR segment and PR vector changes. Circulation 48:575, 1973.
53. Spodick DH: The electrocardiogram in acute pericarditis: Distributions of morphologic and axial changes by stages. Am J Cardiol 33:470, 1974.
54. Brown EJ, Kloner RA, Schoener FJ, et al: Scar thinning due to ibuprofen administration following experimental myocardial infarction. Am J Cardiol 51:877, 1983.
55. Toffler GH, Muller JE, Stone PH, et al: Pericarditis in acute myocardial infarction: Characterization and clinical significance. Am Heart J 117:86, 1989.
56. Gregoratos G: Pericardial involvement in acute myocardial infarction. Cardiol Clin 8:601, 1990.
57. Engle MA, Ito T: The post-pericardiotomy syndrome. Am J Cardiol 7:73, 1961.
58. Engle MA, McCabe JC, Ebert PA: The post-pericardiotomy syndrome and antiheart antibodies. Circulation 49:401, 1974.
59. Hammerman H, Kloner RA, Hole S, et al: Dose dependent effects of short term methyl prednisolone on myocardial infarct extent, scar formation, and ventricular function. Circulation 68:446, 1983.
60. Sugiura T, Iwasaka T, Takayama Y, et al: Factors associated with pericardial effusion in acute Q wave myocardial infarction. Circulation 8:477, 1990.
61. Rankin J, deBruyne B, Benit E, et al: Cardiac tamponade early after thrombolysis for acute myocardial infarction: A rare but not reported hemorrhagic complication. J Am Coll Cardiol 17:280, 1991.
62. Sugimoto JT, Little AG, Ferguson MK, et al: Pericardial window: Mechanisms of efficacy. Ann Thorac Surg 50:442, 1990.
63. Hanaki Y, Kamiya H, Todoraki H, et al: New two dimensional echocardiographically directed pericardiocentesis in cardiac tamponade. Am J Cardiol 66:1487, 1990.
64. Fowler NO: Physiology of cardiac tamponade and pulsus paradoxus. II.

65. Reddy PS, Curtis EI, Uretsky SF: Spectrum of hemodynamic changes in cardiac tamponade. Am J Cardiol 66:1487, 1990.
66. Spodick DH: Acute pericardial disease. Pericarditis, effusion, and tamponade. JCE Cardiol 14:9, 1979.
67. Shabetai R, Fowler NO, Fenton JC, et al: Pulsus paradoxus. J Clin Invest 44:1882, 1965.
68. Spodick DH: Electric alternation of the heart. Its relation to the kinetics and physiology of the heart during cardiac tamponade. Am J Cardiol 10:155, 1962.
69. Kronzon I, Cohen ML, Winer HE: Diastolic atrial compression. A sensitive echocardiographic sign of cardiac tamponade. J Am Coll Cardiol 2:770, 1983.
70. Armstrong WF, Schilt BF, Helper DJ, et al: Diastolic collapse of the right ventricle with cardiac tamponade: An echocardiographic study. Circulation 65:1491, 1982.
71. Burstow DJ, Oh JK, Bailey KR, et al: Cardiac tamponade: Characteristic Doppler observations. Mayo Clin Proc 64:312, 1989.
72. Kerber RE, Gascho JA, Litchfield R, et al: Hemodynamic effects of volume expansion and nitroprusside compared with pericardiocentesis in patients with acute cardiac tamponade. N Engl J Med 307:929, 1982.
73. Hancock EW: Neoplastic pericardial disease. Cardiol Clin 8:673, 1990.
74. Kochar GS, Jacobs LE, Kotler MN: Right atrial compression in post operative cardiac patients: Detection by transesophageal echocardiography. J Am Coll Cardiol 16:511, 1990.
75. Shabetai R: Constrictive pericarditis. In: Shabetai R (ed): The Pericardium. New York, Grune & Stratton, p 154, 1981.
76. Shabetai R, Fowler NO, Guntheroth WG: The hemodynamics of cardiac tamponade and constrictive pericarditis. Am J Cardiol 26:480, 1970.
77. Spodick DH: Acoustic phenomena in pericardial disease. Am Heart J 81:114, 1971.
78. Schnittger I, Bowden RE, Abrams J, et al: Echocardiography: Pericardial thickening and constrictive pericarditis. Am J Cardiol 42:388, 1978.
79. Martin RP, Bowden R, Filly K, et al: Echocardiography: Pericardial thickening and constrictive pericarditis. Am J Cardiol 42:388, 1978.
80. Voeklel AG, Pietro DA, Folland ED, et al: Echocardiographic features of constrictive pericarditis. Circulation 58:871, 178.
81. Appleton CP, Hatle LK, Popp RL: Demonstration of restrictive physiology by Doppler echocardiography. J Am Coll Cardiol 11:757, 1988.
82. Lorell BH, Grossman W: Profile in constrictive pericarditis, restrictive cardiomyopathy, and cardiac tamponade. In: Grossman W (ed): Cardiac Catheterization and Angiography. 3rd ed. Philadelphia, Lea & Febiger, p 427, 1986.
83. Tyberg TL, Goodyear AVN, Hurst VW, et al: Left ventricular filling in differentiating restrictive amyloid cardiomyopathy and constrictive pericarditis. Am J Cardiol 47:791, 1981.
84. Spodick DH, Kumar S: Subacute constrictive pericarditis with cardiac tamponade. Dis Chest 54:62, 1968.
85. Hancock EW: Subacute effusive constrictive pericarditis. Circulation 43:183, 1971.

Metabolic and Toxic Effects on the Cardiovascular System

Prabodh M. Mehta
Robert A. Kloner

Acid-base disturbances are extremely common in critically ill patients. These patients often have mixed respiratory alkalosis and metabolic acidosis.[1] Respiratory alkalosis caused by hyperventilation is most often multifactorial in these patients and can be due to anxiety, hypoxemia, congestive heart failure (CHF), fever, sepsis, liver disease, central nervous system disease, drugs, and mechanical ventilation. Respiratory alkalosis was found in 45% of all arterial blood gas measurements in a medical intensive care unit.[2] A combination of mixed respiratory alkalosis and metabolic acidosis in patients in intensive care units has been associated with a high mortality. The effects of acid-base disturbances on cardiovascular function are a result of their direct action on myocardial contractility and peripheral vasculature and their indirect effects related to stimulation of the sympathoadrenal system (Fig. 93–1).

ACIDOSIS AND CARDIOVASCULAR SYSTEM

The negative inotropic effect of acidosis was first recognized by Klug in 1879[3] and subsequently reported by Smith in a detailed study in 1926.[4] Initial work showing a cardiodepressant effect of systemic acidosis[5] was followed by reports that suggested no significant effect of severe acidosis on myocardial contractility.[6, 7] This conflict was resolved after it was recognized that the effects of systemic acidosis in vitro are quite different from those seen in the intact animal. Acidosis is a strong stimulant of the sympathoadrenal system. It causes release of norepinephrine from nerve endings and both epinephrine and norepinephrine from the adrenal gland.[8] The positive inotropic influence of the released catecholamines tends to negate the direct cardiodepressant influence of systemic acidosis. The extent of the overall change in the intracellular concentration of hydrogen ions related to acid-base abnormalities is determined in part by the composition of the intracellular buffers. Although the predominant influence of acidosis on intracellular pH is related to changes in PCO_2, an additional mechanism involves a process by which an intracellular hydrogen ion is exchanged with an extracellular cation. Animal experiments suggest that a net transmembrane flux of hydrogen and bicarbonate ions occurs across skeletal and cardiac muscle in response to acid-base disturbances.[9] Work by Clancy and colleagues suggested that catecholamines attenuate the expected decrease in intracellular pH owing to acidosis by causing an alteration of the transmembrane flux of acid-base radicals.[10] The overall influence of acidosis on the cardiovascular system is dependent on not only its direct

· TABLE 93–1
FACTORS THAT INFLUENCE THE EFFECTS OF ACIDOSIS ON MYOCARDIAL FUNCTION

Stimulation of sympathoadrenal system
  Release of catecholamines
  Alteration of transmembrane ionic fluxes
 	
Direct negative inotropic effect of acidosis
  Changes in intracellular pH
  Duration of acidosis
  Metabolic vs. respiratory acidosis

effects on the myocardium but also its indirect effects on the sympathoadrenal system as well as the status of the left ventricle before the onset of acidosis (Table 93–1).

In a canine study, Steinhart and colleagues studied the effects of beta-adrenergic activity and the cardiovascular response to severe respiratory acidosis.[11] In control animals, severe hypercapnic acidosis (pH 6.48 ± 0.02) led to a decrease in the cardiac output, depression of left ventricular function, and subsequent death. In a second group of animals, administration of isoproterenol during hypercapnic acidosis did not result in depression of myocardial function. Furthermore, death did not occur even with higher degrees of respiratory acidosis than in the control group. The third group of animals received propranolol, which resulted in a much more rapid and severe depression of myocardial function compared with that in the control animals, and the occurrence of death with less severe degrees of respiratory acidosis. These results indicate that beta-adrenergic receptor stimulation prevents hypercapnic heart failure and beta-adrenergic receptor blockade worsens the effects of respiratory acidosis. Rose and colleagues studied the effects of pulmonary hypertension and hypercapnic acidosis on right ventricular performance in conscious dogs[12] (Fig. 93–2). They demonstrated that beta-adrenergic blockade in the setting of increased right ventricular afterload and hypercapnic acidosis resulted in a more rapid decline of right ventricular function.

Patients with chronic CHF have high levels of circulating catecholamines[13] and reduced myocardial norepinephrine receptor concentrations.[14] Systemic acidosis in this population of patients may produce a more profound negative inotropic effect, and this may be seen with a lesser degree of acidosis because the compensatory sympathoadrenal mechanism may be blunted. Patients already receiving beta-adrenergic receptor–blocking agents are also expected to have more pronounced deleterious effects of systemic acidosis.[11, 12]

Pathophysiology

The decrease in contractility seen from an increase in PCO_2 (respiratory acidosis)[15] is greater than that from a decrease in bicarbonate (metabolic acidosis). Carbon dioxide rapidly enters the cell, reducing the intracellular pH, whereas both hydrogen and bicarbonate ions enter and exit the myocyte slowly, causing a smaller reduction in intracellular pH.[15, 16] Techniques for measurement of intracellular pH have confirmed the hypothesis that intracellular pH changes more rapidly in response to an extracellular respiratory acidosis than to metabolic acidosis.[17] Steenbergen and associates demonstrated that, in the rat heart, a 0.5-unit decline in extracellular pH and no change in intracellular pH resulted in only a 25% decrease in the developed left ventricular pressure. In contrast, when the same change in extracellular pH was accompanied by a 0.25-unit decline in

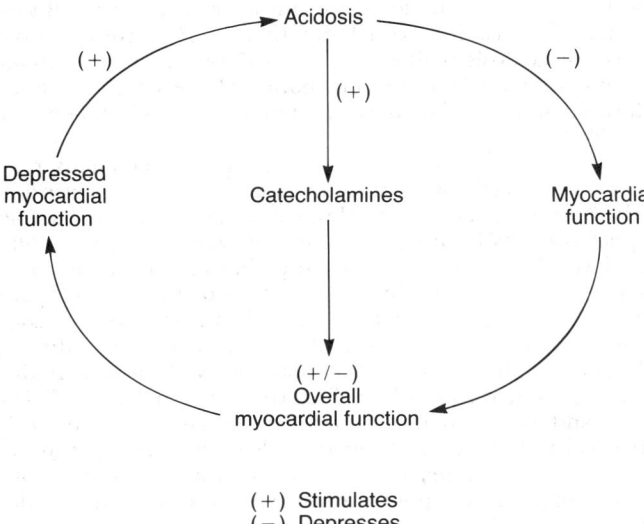

Figure 93–1. Effects of acid-base disturbances on cardiovascular function.

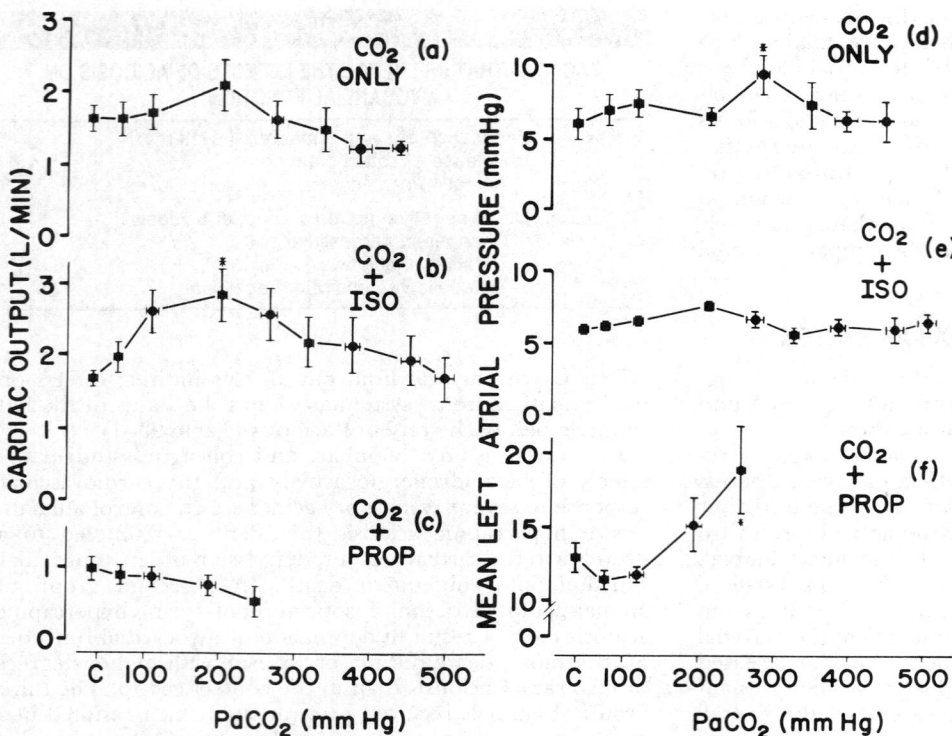

Figure 93–2. Influence of beta-adrenergic activity on the myocardial response to severe respiratory acidosis in 18 dogs. Effect of increased $PaCO_2$ on cardiac output and mean left atrial pressure. Groups a and d: only carbon dioxide administered. Groups b and e: carbon dioxide and isoproterenol (ISO). Group c and f: carbon dioxide and propranolol (PROP). Point C = value obtained before intervention, with animals breathing 100% oxygen. (From Steinhart CR, Purmutt S, Gurtner GH, et al: Beta-adrenergic activity and cardiovascular response to severe respiratory acidosis. Am J Physiol 244:H46, 1983.)

intracellular pH, there was an 80% decline in left ventricular pressure. The major determinant of intracellular pH is PCO_2. Changes in extracellular pH resulting from metabolic effects cause small changes in intracellular pH owing to the small flux of hydrogen ions that occurs across the plasma membrane.[18, 19]

Mechanisms of Negative Inotropic Effect

Several mechanisms have been suggested to explain the effect of acidosis on myocardial contractility, and the data are mainly based on in vitro and in vivo animal experimentation (Table 93–2). Study of energy production during systemic acidosis has shown that the decreased energy utilization during depressed contractility is not related to decreased energy production.[18] Experimentally, lack of available energy can be inferred if it is demonstrated that the ratio of adenosine triphosphate to adenosine diphosphate or of creatine phosphate to creatine is lower than normal. The initial decrease in left ventricular pressure seen with respiratory acidosis is associated with increased levels of creatine phosphate and increased ratio of adenosine triphosphate to adenine diphosphate.[20] In artificial buffer acidosis, there is a slight increase in the ratio of creatine phosphate to creatine.[18] These data suggest that acidosis does not primarily cause reduced energy production, and therefore lack of substrate cannot account for the negative inotropic effect of acidosis.

TABLE 93–2
MECHANISMS OF NEGATIVE INOTROPIC EFFECT OF SYSTEMIC ACIDOSIS
Inhibition of slow Ca^{2+} current
Decreased Ca^{2+} pool and Ca^{2+} release
Altered binding and uptake of intracellular Ca^{2+}
Diminished tension generated by myofibrils in response to Ca^{2+}

At the cellular level, the effects of acidosis have been investigated extensively and are quite complex. Acidosis decreases the tension developed by isolated myofibrils at any given extracellular calcium concentration.[21, 22] However, the intracellular transport of calcium and the binding of calcium to the sarcolemma are affected by acidosis. An intracellular competition between hydrogen and calcium ions for binding sites on troponin has been demonstrated.[20, 23] Thus, acidosis decreases the binding of calcium to troponin. Ricciardi and coworkers performed experiments with rat cardiac muscle.[24] They studied the relation between generated force and sarcomere length in an isolated preparation under control conditions and with varying degrees of respiratory acidosis and different calcium concentrations. They found that the negative inotropic effect of respiratory acidosis was most pronounced with the least calcium concentration at all sarcomere lengths. They concluded that the negative inotropic effect of acidosis is due to a competition of hydrogen and calcium ions for binding to troponin. However, others have shown that the binding of calcium to troponin is independent of pH.[25]

Safer and coworkers proposed that hydrogen ions may interfere directly with calcium entry into the myocardial cells.[26] An inhibition of the slow calcium current attributable to acidosis has been demonstrated in various experimental models.[27–29] Metabolic acidosis in embryonic chick ventricles depresses the amplitude and duration of the slow calcium current.[30] About one half of the calcium involved in contraction comes from calcium influx into the myocytes during the plateau phase of the action potential, with the remainder coming from release of calcium from internal stores.[31] Fabiato and Fabiato demonstrated the presence of an intracellular calcium-dependent calcium release.[32] A decrease in the calcium influx caused by acidosis decreases the contraction-producing calcium pool directly and also secondarily decreases the release of calcium from internal stores. Use of calcium-sensitive fluorescein ionophores has greatly helped in elucidating the cellular mechanism underlying the effects of acidosis. Studies performed in cultured chick embryonic and adult guinea pig ventricular myocytes have shown that intracellular acidosis markedly decreases the sensitivity of the contractile elements to calcium ions.[33] In addition, there is probably an impairment of calcium extrusion via sodium-calcium exchange, impairment of calcium uptake by sarcoplasmic reticulum, and competition between hydrogen and calcium ions for intracellular calcium-binding sites.

Acidosis also has important electrophysiologic effects on the ventricular myocardium. Studies with guinea pig papillary muscles showed that extracellular respiratory as well as metabolic acidosis causes a reduction in conduction velocity, resting potential, and maximal rate of rise of the action potential upstroke (maximal velocity).[34] The effects of respiratory acidosis were of greater magnitude and occurred more rapidly than the effects of metabolic acidosis, and acidosis altered the relationship between resting membrane potential and maximal velocity. The inhomogeneities in conduction may be important in the creation of re-entry circuits and in the development of re-entrant ventricular arrhythmia, particularly in association with acute ischemia.

Effect of Acid-Base Disturbances on Vascular System

Systemic acidosis induces vasodilatation of most arterial vessels, leading to a decrease in peripheral vascular resistance.[35, 36] Catecholamines released owing to the acidosis counteract this direct effect.[36, 37] However, the response of the peripheral vasculature to both alpha- and beta-adrenergic stimulation is decreased in the presence of low pH. On the other hand, the effects of metabolic or respiratory alkalosis on the peripheral vasculature have not been well elucidated. Some data suggest that alkalosis also causes arterial vasodilatation in the peripheral vascular system. The net effect of either acidosis or alkalosis on the peripheral vascular system depends on the degree of acid-base disturbance, the rapidity with which it develops, and the state of the individual before the onset of acidosis or alkalosis.

Acidosis causes constriction of the venous system.[38] This may lead to decreased venous capacitance, resulting in a shift of blood into the central circulation, causing elevated pulmonary vascular volume and pressure with clinical manifestations of cardiac volume overload. Underlying left ventricular dysfunction or depressed left ventricular contractility attributable to systemic acidosis could exacerbate this effect.

In contrast to their effects on the peripheral vascular system where both may cause vasodilatation, acidosis and alkalosis have different effects on the coronary vasculature.[39, 40] Acidosis causes coronary vasodilatation and alkalosis augments vascular tone.[41] Experiments performed on isolated canine coronary arteries revealed that metabolic as well as respiratory changes in acid-base disturbances produced a similar degree of change in the coronary vasomotor tone. This suggests that the extracellular ionic changes mediate the effects of acidosis and alkalosis on coronary vascular tone. Furthermore, extracellular hydrogen ion changes induce variations in the contractile activity of coronary vascular smooth muscle by modulating calcium efflux.[41]

In contrast to these in vitro experiments, studies performed in the intact rabbit heart by using the radioactive microsphere technique by Eliades and Weiss[42] showed that hypercapnic acidosis caused a significant increase in regional myocardial blood flow but metabolic acidosis did not have this effect. The effects of hypercapnic acidosis were blocked in the animals that had carotid denervation or in those that were pretreated with propranolol. This study suggested that carbon dioxide mediates its changes on the coronary vasculature not only by direct action but also via the sympathoad-

renal system. The vasoconstrictor effect of respiratory alkalosis on the coronary vascular tone is clinically utilized as a diagnostic tool for inducing vasospasm in patients with Prinzmetal's angina.

Treatment of Metabolic Acidosis

Metabolic acidosis caused by excessive lactic acid production is commonly seen after cardiopulmonary arrest and other conditions characterized by decreased cardiac performance and reduced tissue perfusion. In these conditions, the combination of circulatory insufficiency and hypoxemia reduces tissue oxygen availability, leading to anaerobic metabolism and lactic acidosis. Lactic acidosis per se has a direct negative inotropic effect on myocardial function, and therefore its treatment constitutes an important part of interrupting the downward spiral in cardiovascular function that is seen in these patients. Lactic acidosis has traditionally been treated with intravenous sodium bicarbonate. This has not been shown to improve outcome for patients and, in addition, causes a significant solute and volume overload. In a model of hypoxic lactic acidosis, the administration of sodium bicarbonate was accompanied by depression of cardiac function, acceleration of lactate production, and a paradoxical lowering of the blood pH and bicarbonate concentrations[43] (Figs. 93–3 and 93–4).

Arieff and colleagues studied the effects of intravenous sodium bicarbonate in dogs with phenformin-induced lactic acidosis.[44] They compared the effects of sodium bicarbonate with those of equimolar amounts of sodium chloride or no therapy in 47 dogs with lactic acidosis. They found that treatment of experimental lactic acidosis with sodium chloride, sodium bicarbonate, or no therapy resulted in no change of blood pH and bicarbonate and a similar mortality. In addition, sodium bicarbonate administration resulted in a significant decline of liver and erythrocyte intracellular pH, significant reductions in cardiac output and hepatic portal vein blood flow, and an increase in the gut lactic acid production. These changes were not seen with sodium chloride infusion. Thus, sodium bicarbonate was not useful in decreasing mortality and may indeed have deleterious effects in this model.

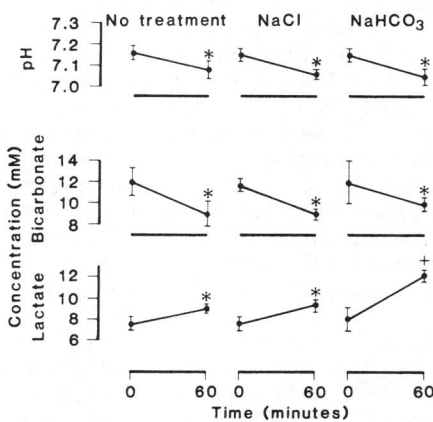

Figure 93–3. Detrimental effect of bicarbonate therapy in hypoxic lactic acidosis. Blood pH and bicarbonate and lactate concentrations in dogs during 60 minutes of therapy of hypoxic lactic acidosis. $*$ = $P < .05$ compared with control at 0 minutes. $+$ = $P < .01$ compared with animals receiving sodium chloride as well as animals receiving no treatment. (From Graf H, Leach W, Arieff AI: Evidence for a detrimental effect of bicarbonate therapy in hypoxic lactic acidosis. Science 227:754, 1985. Copyright 1985 by AAAS.)

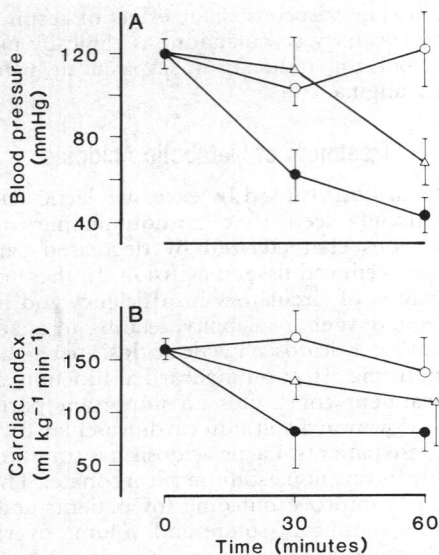

Figure 93–4. Hemodynamic changes in dogs demonstrating a detrimental effect of bicarbonate therapy in hypoxic lactic acidosis. Sodium chloride (open circles), sodium bicarbonate (filled circles), or no therapy (open triangles). Treatment with sodium bicarbonate resulted in significant decreases in both mean arterial blood pressure (A) and cardiac index (B). (From Graf H, Leach W, Arieff AI: Evidence for a detrimental effect of bicarbonate therapy in hypoxic lactic acidosis. Science 227:754, 1985. Copyright 1985 by AAAS.)

The deleterious effects of exogenous bicarbonate administration in lactic acidosis may be related to (1) generation of carbon dioxide as a result of administration of bicarbonate, which crosses the intracellular membrane and leads to worsening of intracellular acidosis; (2) enhanced glycolysis, which accelerates lactic acid production as the pH increases; and (3) an increase in the binding of oxygen and hemoglobin, which then impairs tissue oxygen availability.

Administration of an experimental agent, a mixture of sodium carbonate and sodium bicarbonate (Carbicarb), in an animal model of hypoxic lactic acidosis has been shown to have beneficial effects. Bersin and Arieff induced hypoxic lactic acidosis in 28 dogs[45] (Figs. 93–5 and 93–6). Thirteen received sodium bicarbonate and 15 received Carbicarb after development of lactic acidosis. After therapy, the arterial pH rose with Carbicarb administration from 7.22 to 7.27 ($P < .01$) and fell with sodium bicarbonate from 7.18 to 7.13 ($P < .01$). Mixed venous P_{CO_2} did not change with Carbicarb but increased with sodium bicarbonate; arterial lactate stabilized with Carbicarb but rose with sodium bicarbonate administration. Cardiac output was unchanged with Carbicarb but decreased with sodium bicarbonate. Carbicarb thus appears to be superior to sodium bicarbonate for the treatment of experimental hypoxic lactic acidosis.

Dichloroacetate has been under investigation as an alternative mode of therapy for lactic acidosis. It stimulates pyruvate dehydrogenase to catalyze the oxidation of lactate and pyruvate. Experiments in dogs with nonhypoxic lactic acidosis induced by either phenformin infusion or hepatectomy showed that dichloroacetate lowered blood lactic acid levels, improved systemic pH and bicarbonate concentration, and normalized the cardiac output.[46] In a rat model of hypoxic lactic acidosis, dichloroacetate significantly attenuated the rise in blood lactate levels and maintained a higher blood pH and bicarbonate level compared with those in control animals[47] (Fig. 93–7). In a canine model of asphyxia-induced cardiac arrest, dichloroacetate-treated animals had a significantly faster rate of decline in lactic acid levels that continued to the final sampling period.[48]

In a nonblinded study, Stacpoole and colleagues gave dichloroacetate to 29 patients with lactic acidosis of various causes[49] (Fig. 93–8). In 23 patients, dichloroacetate improved or resolved the metabolic acidosis. Among patients who responded with at least a 20% reduction in blood lactic acid levels, mean survival time was 60 hours compared with 26 hours among the nonresponders. In addition, there was no evidence of toxicity to dichloroacetate. Although this was an open, nonblinded, nonrandomized study, it indicated that the use of dichloroacetate clearly improves the acid-base status in patients with lactic acidosis. This improvement may reduce the chance of early death and provide an opportunity to reverse other life-threatening complications associated with lactic acidosis. A prospective randomized multicenter study of sodium dichloroacetate for treatment of lactic acidosis is in progress.

Use of Sodium Bicarbonate During Cardiopulmonary Resuscitation

In the past, it was believed that metabolic acidosis was ubiquitous during cardiopulmonary resuscitation (CPR), and in view of the known negative effects of acidosis on cellular metabolism and cardiovascular function, treatment with large amounts of sodium bicarbonate was recommended during CPR. Subsequently, it was recognized that acidosis is far less severe when adequate basic life support is initiated within a reasonable time.[50] Because of this understanding, in 1980, it was recommended that arterial blood gas measurement be relied on to determine the dose of bicarbonate infusion. However, it was subsequently shown that bicarbonate administration induced hyperosmolarity, hypernatremia,

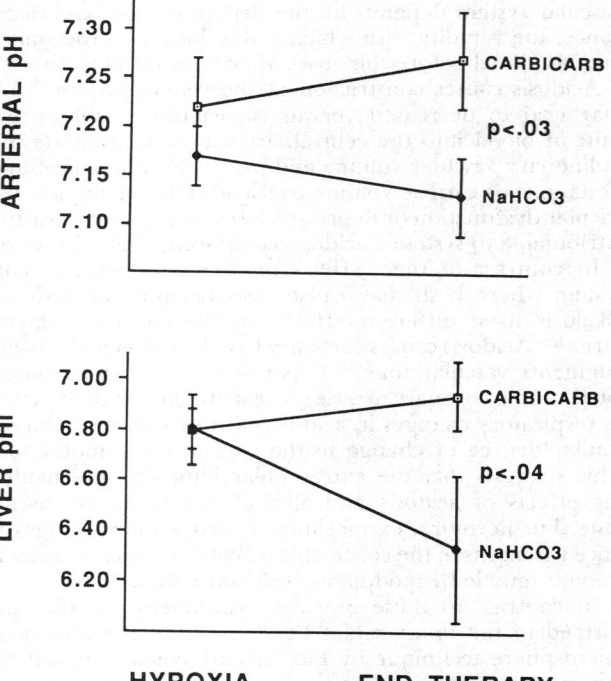

Figure 93–5. Effects of Carbicarb and sodium bicarbonate on arterial pH and liver intracellular pH during hypoxia in an animal model of hypoxic lactic acidosis. (From Bersin RM, Arieff AI: Improved hemodynamic function during hypoxia with Carbicarb, a new agent for the management of acidosis. Circulation 77:227, 1988. By permission of the American Heart Association, Inc.)

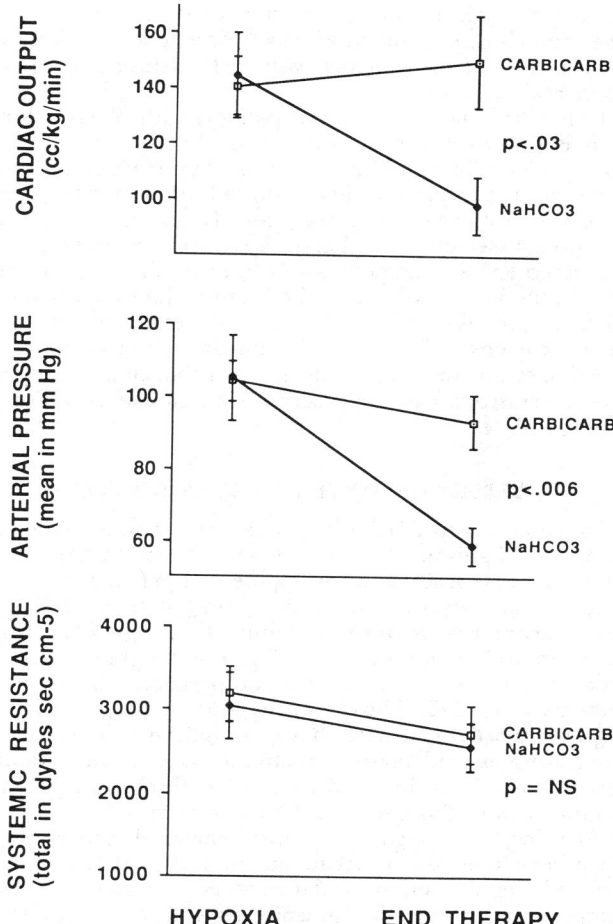

Figure 93–6. Improved hemodynamics attributable to Carbicarb administration in contrast to sodium bicarbonate administration during hypoxic lactic acidosis in dogs. (From Bersin RM, Arieff AI: Improved hemodynamic function during hypoxia with Carbicarb, a new agent for the management of acidosis. Circulation 77:227, 1988, by permission of the American Heart Association, Inc.)

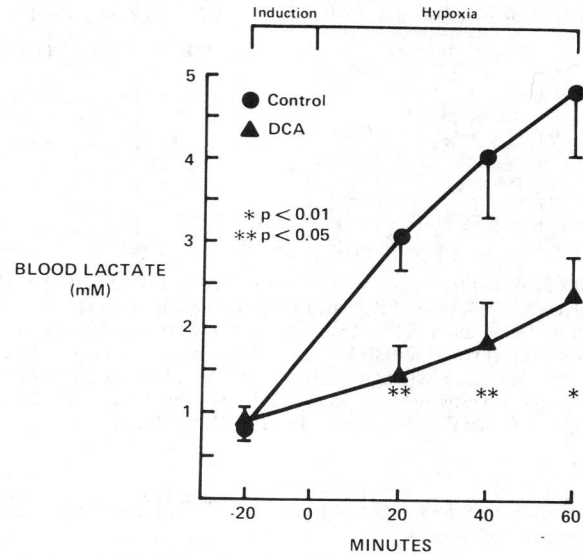

Figure 93–7. Beneficial effect of dichloroacetate (DCA) in a model of hypoxic lactic acidosis. (From Romeh SA, Tannen RL: Therapeutic benefit of dichloroacetate (DCA) in experimentally induced hypoxic lactic acidosis. J Lab Clin Med 107:378, 1986.)

and transient alkalosis with associated arrhythmias.[51, 52] It was recognized that the ability to defibrillate animals was independent of the pH,[53] and therefore the use of bicarbonate before defibrillation is not justified. Use of bicarbonate creates a paradoxical effect on the acid-base status. Sodium bicarbonate does counteract acidemia, but while doing so it induces the production of large amounts of carbon dioxide, which easily crosses the cellular membrane. Therefore, there is a paradoxical increase in acidosis, both intracellularly and in the venous circulation. Thus, bicarbonate can contribute to cellular dysfunction because of increased levels of carbon dioxide in the myocardium and venous blood.

The cause of acidemia during cardiac arrest has been extensively investigated. In a porcine model of CPR, increases in the arteriovenous carbon dioxide and pH gradients were found during cardiac arrest.[54] Weil and colleagues noted that, during CPR, patients exhibited a mild acidosis in the arterial blood but severe acidosis in the mixed venous blood[55] (Fig. 93–9). In a subset of 13 patients, the bicarbonate level before and during CPR was not altered, suggesting that the gradient between arterial and mixed venous blood pH was due solely to carbon dioxide.[55]

Von Planta and colleagues documented the presence of an arteriovenous gradient for hydrogen ions and carbon dioxide across the coronary circulation in an animal model

of cardiac arrest and CPR.[56] Cardiac arrest was electrically induced in anesthetized, mechanically ventilated pigs. During CPR, there was rapid onset of profound myocardial acidosis with an increase in intramyocardial hydrogen ion concentration. Great cardiac vein P_{CO_2} increased also, and there was myocardial lactic acid production. These investigations concluded that buffers like bicarbonate that increase bicarbonate concentration reduce arterial acidosis caused by CPR but may exacerbate venous and likely tissue acidosis.

Bishop and Weisfeldt showed deleterious effects of sodium bicarbonate administration during CPR in dogs as well as in patients.[50] During CPR in dogs, bicarbonate administration led to significant increase in arterial P_{CO_2} and serum osmolality. In humans, they found a significant increase in serum osmolality with the use of sodium bicarbonate. In one patient

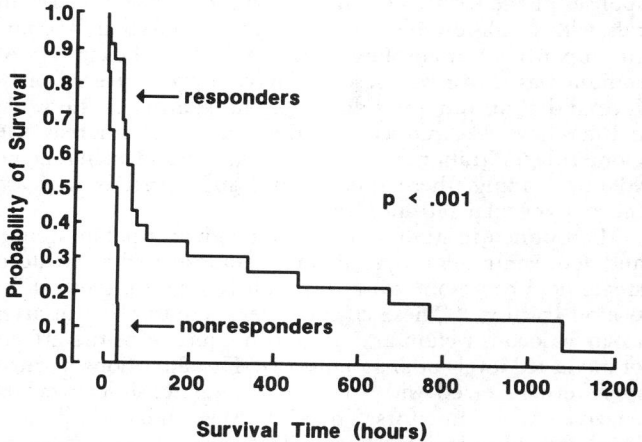

Figure 93–8. Effects of dichloroacetate in patients with lactic acidosis. Survival time curves among patients who responded with at least a 20% reduction in blood lactic acid concentration (responders) versus nonresponders. (Reproduced, with permission, from Stacpoole PW, Lorenz AC, Thomas RG, et al. Dichloroacetate in the treatment of lactic acidosis. Ann Intern Med. 1988; 108:58–63.)

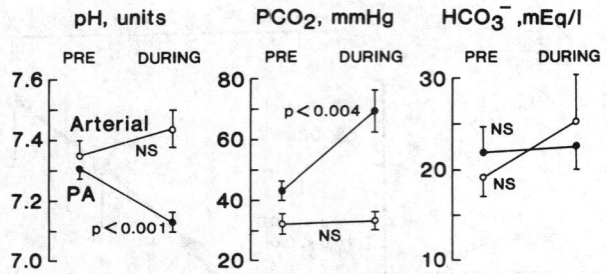

Figure 93–9. Arterial and mixed venous (PA) pH, P_{CO_2}, and bicarbonate (HCO_3^-) before (PRE) and during cardiopulmonary resuscitation in 13 patients. The means ± SEM are shown. NS denotes not significant. (From Weil MH, Rackow EC, Trevino R, et al: Difference in acid-base state between venous and arterial blood during cardiopulmonary resuscitation. Reprinted, by permission of the New England Journal of Medicine, 315;153–156, 1986.)

with inadequate ventilation during CPR, bicarbonate caused a marked rise in P_{CO_2} and a fall in arterial pH.

It therefore appears that repeated use of intravenous bicarbonate is not indicated during CPR. The optimal method of resuscitating patients with cardiac arrest lies in avoiding the problems of acidosis and low perfusion pressure by early definitive care, which in most instances is defibrillation. Sodium bicarbonate is not recommended for routine management, even for unwitnessed cardiac arrests. Its use is reserved until other measures, namely defibrillation, cardiac compression, and drugs such as epinephrine and antiarrhythmic agents, have already been used. In patients with pre-existing metabolic acidosis with or without hyperkalemia and in the emergency treatment of severe hypercalcemia, bicarbonate should be used. The initial dose is 1 mEq/kg intravenously, and subsequently 0.5 mEq/kg should be given but only after 10 minutes and with careful monitoring of blood acid-base balance.

CONGESTIVE HEART FAILURE
Metabolic Disturbances

Chronic CHF elicits several compensatory mechanisms that involve the vascular system and various hormones. Decreased renal plasma blood flow leads to stimulation of the renin-angiotensin-aldosterone system. The adaptive responses of the kidneys occur early in the course of CHF. In rats with small-to-moderate myocardial infarction, a clear-cut impairment of absolute as well as fractional excretion of sodium was shown.[57] These rats have normal arterial pressure and peak pumping ability of the ventricle. The renal plasma flow was reduced in these animals, whereas the glomerular filtration rate was not altered. During acute volume loading, these rats did not appropriately increase their glomerular filtration rate.

Micropuncture studies in rats with a myocardial infarction and left ventricular dysfunction demonstrated a reduced single-nephron glomerular filtration rate and increased filtration fraction.[58] These changes were due to efferent arteriolar vasoconstriction and are a consequence of the effects of increased levels of angiotensin II. The alterations in these rats were reversed with the use of angiotensin-converting enzyme (ACE) inhibitors. The reduced renal blood flow and increased filtration fraction led to avid reabsorption of sodium and water in the proximal convoluted tubule. The augmented renin and angiotensin II levels resulted in increased secretion of aldosterone, which causes increased distal tubular reabsorption of sodium and water. In addition, the increased sympathetic nerve activity and the elevated

circulating catecholamines contributed to the renal sodium retention via direct tubular effects.[59] Plasma vasopressin level is also elevated in patients with CHF, causing increased water reabsorption.

Hyponatremia is common in patients with severe CHF.[60] This is due to a number of factors. The decreased renal plasma blood flow and increased filtration fraction lead to a decrease in the distal delivery of sodium and filtrate and impairment of free water excretion. In addition, increased vasopressin secretion further reduces free water excretion. Increased levels of angiotensin II induce thirst and increase free water intake, which further causes dilutional hyponatremia. The use of diuretics without restriction of water intake worsens the problem of hyponatremia. In fact, excessive diuresis further augments the neurohormonal and renal mechanisms that cause low serum sodium concentration in the first place.

Angiotensin-Converting Enzyme Inhibition

In patients with CHF, renal vasoconstriction is a compensatory mechanism. With progressive heart failure, renal perfusion falls, leading to development of prerenal azotemia. The activation of the renin-angiotensin system in CHF plays a significant role in the development of high blood urea nitrogen and creatinine levels. There is a significant correlation between serum creatinine and plasma renin activity in patients with CHF. Those with hyponatremia (a marker of high renin activity in CHF) have a significantly higher blood urea nitrogen and plasma creatinine concentrations and a lower renal blood flow and glomerular filtration rate when compared with those without hyponatremia.[61]

ACE inhibitors such as captopril, enalapril, and lisinopril have been used in the treatment of CHF. ACE inhibitors are both venous and arteriolar dilators. The acute hemodynamic improvement with these agents is sustained, and long-

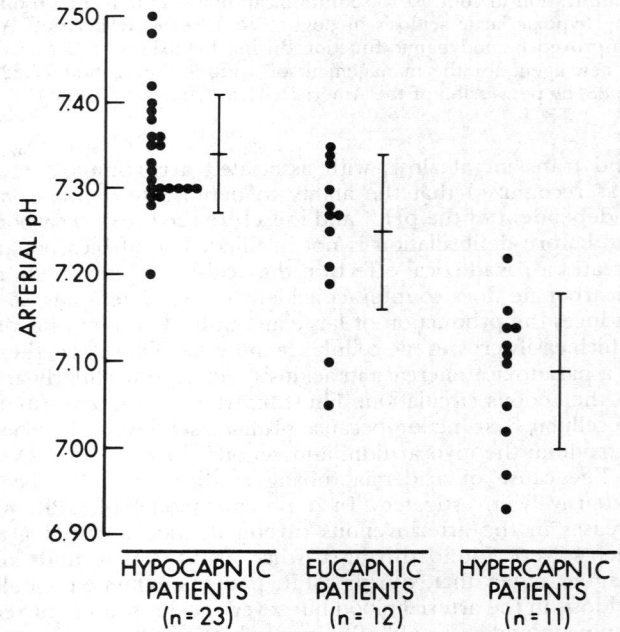

Figure 93–10. Arterial pH in 46 patients with acute pulmonary edema before treatment. Hypocapnia is arterial P_{CO_2} less than 35 mm Hg; eucapnia is P_{CO_2} between 35 and 45 mm Hg; hypercapnia is P_{CO_2} greater than 45 mm Hg. The mean values are significantly different ($P < .005$). (Reproduced, with permission, from Aberman A, Fulop M. The metabolic and respiratory acidosis of acute pulmonary edema. Ann Intern Med. 1972; 76:173–184.)

term improvement in exercise tolerance has been shown. In a randomized double-blind study, enalapril was shown to reduce mortality in patients with severe CHF.[62] Similar results have been shown with the use of captopril.[63]

When initiating therapy with these agents, one should start with low doses (6.25 mg three times daily for captopril or 2.5 mg once or twice a day for enalapril) to avoid hypotension and worsening of renal failure, especially in those with hyponatremia. Increase in the dosages should be gradual and slow, as peak improvement in exercise capacity may not occur for several weeks. Deterioration in renal function with the use of ACE inhibitors can be prevented by avoiding hypotension and overdiuresis. The use of ACE inhibitors improves renal function in patients with severe cardiac failure and reduces the requirement for diuretic agents. Serum sodium concentrations have also been shown to normalize in hyponatremic patients with the addition of captopril to their medical regimen.[64]

PULMONARY EDEMA: ACID-BASE DISTURBANCES

Patients with pulmonary edema attributable to acute left ventricular failure often have acid-base disturbances. These patients are commonly acidemic, which is most often due to a combination of metabolic and respiratory acidosis.[65] The respiratory acidosis is due to carbon dioxide retention because of increased work of breathing, muscle exhaustion, diminished responsiveness of the respiratory center, and imbalance of pulmonary ventilation and perfusion.

Aberman and Fulop reported on arterial blood gas measurements in 50 consecutive patients with acute pulmonary edema caused by left ventricular failure[65] (Figs. 93–10 and 93–11). They found acidemia (pH < 7.36) in 38 of the 46 patients studied before therapy. Eleven patients had arterial P_{CO_2} greater than 45 mm Hg and 12 had normal P_{CO_2}. The hypercapnia did not correlate with the severity of the pul-

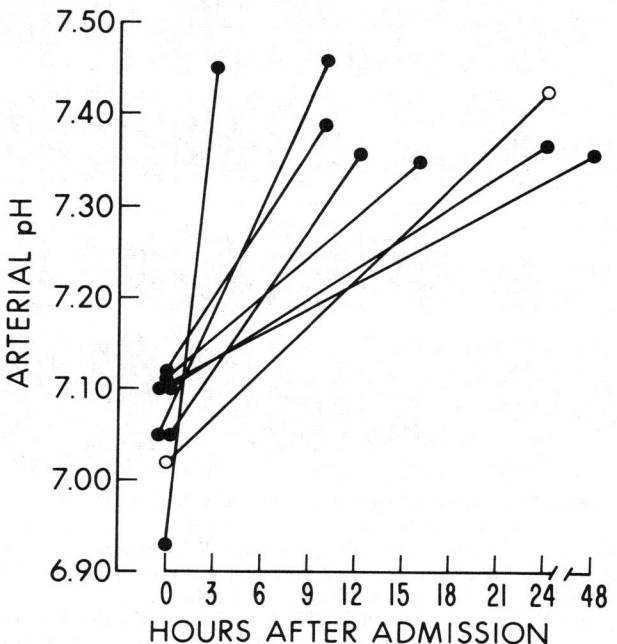

Figure 93–11. Arterial pH before and after treatment of pulmonary edema in eight severely acidemic patients (pH < 7.13). Open circles refer to the sole patient given assisted ventilation. (Reproduced, with permission, from Aberman A, Fulop M. The metabolic and respiratory acidosis of acute pulmonary edema. Ann Intern Med. 1972; 76:173–184.)

monary edema. In another study of 18 patients with acute pulmonary edema, 14 had a blood pH of less than 7.36, and blood lactate concentrations were elevated in 15 of the 18 patients (>2 mmol/L).[66] The ratio of plasma lactate to pyruvate was elevated, suggesting that the increased lactate concentration was caused by tissue hypoxemia and hypoperfusion.

Metabolic acidosis rapidly resolves with therapy of pulmonary edema and so does the respiratory acidosis. Rarely, respiratory acidosis may require intubation with assisted ventilation. Even in patients with severe metabolic acidosis, bicarbonate therapy was not required. Clinical improvement was accompanied by decreased lactic acidosis, regneration of bicarbonate level, and return of pH to normal. Hence, the mainstay of therapy for acid-base abnormalities in patients with pulmonary edema remains the treatment of the pulmonary edema itself.

ELECTROLYTE ABNORMALITIES AND CARDIOVASCULAR FUNCTION
Calcium

Calcium plays an important role in triggering and modulating the contractile function of the heart muscle. It also plays an important role in secretory and permeability events at the cellular level.[67] Intracellular calcium in the heart muscle is readily exchangeable and in rapid equilibrium with plasma ionized calcium. Hypocalcemia causes electrocardiographic changes and, in its severe form, can lead to cardiovascular collapse and cardiac arrest.[68–70] In addition, hypocalcemia has been implicated as a cause of decreased left ventricular contractility.

Although hypocalcemia is common in the critically ill patient, infusion of calcium chloride and correction of ionized calcium in this group of patients produces only a transient improvement in cardiovascular function[71] (Desai T, Geheb M, unpublished data). The improvement is not sustained even with continuous calcium infusion and maintenance of the serum ionized calcium levels within the normal range. Auffant and colleagues showed that hypocalcemia was common after cardiopulmonary bypass; however, correction of plasma calcium did not significantly change the measures of myocardial pump function.[72]

Long-standing chronic hypocalcemia may lead to chronic abnormalities in cardiovascular function. Patients with chronic renal failure have chronic hypocalcemia. Henrich and associates evaluated left ventricular function after hemodialysis in patients with hypocalcemia.[73] Half of the patients underwent hemodialysis, wherein the ionized calcium level was corrected, whereas in the other half, the ionized calcium level was left uncorrected. There was significant improvement in indices of left ventricular function in those who had their ionized calcium level corrected. This effect did not result from a change in plasma norepinephrine concentration, nor was it related to an increase in plasma bicarbonate or a decrease in blood urea nitrogen, creatinine, or magnesium levels. A change in serum ionized calcium level was the only difference among the variables tested. Hypocalcemia in patients with chronic renal failure is accompanied by secondary hyperparathyroidism. Henrich and colleagues did not measure whether there was a significant change in the serum parathyroid levels.[73] Drueke and colleagues demonstrated that, in severely hyperparathyroid uremic patients, left ventricular dysfunction improved after parathyroidectomy.[74]

Hypocalcemia leads to increased ventricular irritability and electrocardiographic changes are related to prolongation of phase 2 of the action potential. This is manifested by a

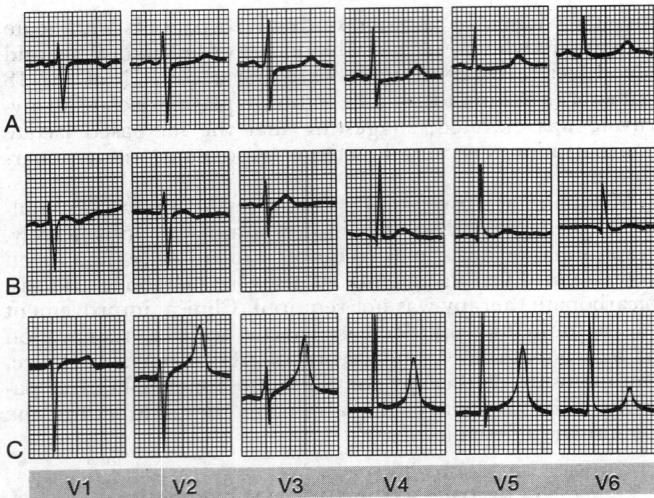

Figure 93–12. Electrocardiographic changes in hypocalcemia, hypercalcemia, and hypocalcemia with hyperkalemia. *A.* At a Ca^{2+} level of 5.7 mg/dL, the QT interval is prolonged, characteristic of hypocalcemia. *B.* Tracing recorded at a Ca^{2+} level of 16.0 mg/dL shows the short ST segment of hypercalcemia. *C.* Tracing was recorded at a K^+ level of 6.0 mEq/L, Ca^{2+} of 5.5 mg/dL, and phosphorus level of 12.0 mg/dL. The prolonged QT interval and the tented T wave reflect hypocalcemia and hyperkalemia, which are often present in chronic renal disease. (From Fisch C: Electrocardiography and Vectorcardiography. In: Braunwald E [ed]: Heart Disease: A Textbook of Cardiovascular Medicine. 4th ed. Philadelphia, WB Saunders, p 116, 1992.)

prolongation of the ST segment and the QT interval[75] (Fig. 93–12). The QTa (Q to the apex of the T wave) and QT intervals are prolonged, but the QT_c interval rarely is greater than 140% of normal. If there is accompanying hypokalemia, then in addition to the prolongation of the ST segment, there is the presence of a U wave. If the T wave is flattened, the U wave gives an impression of a markedly prolonged QT interval, which actually is the QU interval. In contrast, hypercalcemia shortens phase 2 of the action potential and the ST segment. The QT interval is shortened, and the ST segment may be depressed with inversion of T waves. The QT and the QT_c intervals do not correlate well with serum calcium levels; however, the QTa interval correlates best with the calcium level.

Phosphorus

There are many causes of hypophosphatemia,[76] and it is especially common in hospitalized alcoholic patients. The serum phosphorus level may be normal when patients are admitted to the hospital but then declines to low values within 1 to 3 days after the patients are treated with intravenous glucose.[77, 78] Respiratory alkalosis is also common in the critically ill patient and, if sustained, leads to hypophosphatemia. Myocardial dysfunction resulting from phosphate deficiency has been shown in both animals and humans.[79, 80] Fuller and associates studied the effects of chronic hypophosphatemia in dogs.[79] Phosphate deficiency was accompanied by a significant decline in the stroke volume, peak blood flow velocity, and maximal left ventricular rate of change of pressure. Dietary repletion of phosphate in these animals corrected the hemodynamic abnormalities.[79] In critically ill patients with hypophosphatemia (<2 mg/dL), decreased cardiac output was seen and improved significantly after phosphate repletion.[80] Intravenous phosphate should be used with caution, as rapid administration can lead to marked abnormalities in the electrocardiogram and the

development of atrial arrhythmias. It can also lead to peripheral vasodilatation and marked hypotension, along with severe depression of left ventricular function.

Potassium

Hypokalemia is quite common in patients with CHF who are being treated with diuretics. This can lead to serious arrhythmias, especially in patients who are receiving digitalis preparations. Potassium replacement in these patients should be in the form of potassium chloride because there is accompanying hypochloremic metabolic alkalosis (Fig. 93–13). On the electrocardiogram, hypokalemia is accompanied by flattening of the T waves and appearance of U waves. The depressed T waves and the presence of U waves give a false impression of an increased QT interval. Hypokalemia causes ventricular ectopic beats and could lead to ventricular tachycardia, especially in patients with underlying heart disease.

Hyperkalemia is also accompanied by serious cardiovascular side effects. Electrocardiographically, hyperkalemia leads to peaking of symmetric T waves, and with further increase in potassium levels, there is broadening of the QRS complex and prolongation of the PR interval. These changes are seen with a potassium level of greater than 6.5 mEq/L. With further increases in the serum potassium level to approximately 8 mEq/L, the atrial excitability is suppressed, and there is complete atrioventricular dissociation with a sine wave pattern followed by ventricular fibrillation or asystole. Serious hyperkalemia is often seen in patients with chronic renal failure and should be treated emergently.

In the short term, 10 to 20 mL of 10% calcium chloride given intravenously can promptly antagonize the effects of hyperkalemia. This effect, however, is short-lived. Specific measures to lower serum potassium levels include intrave-

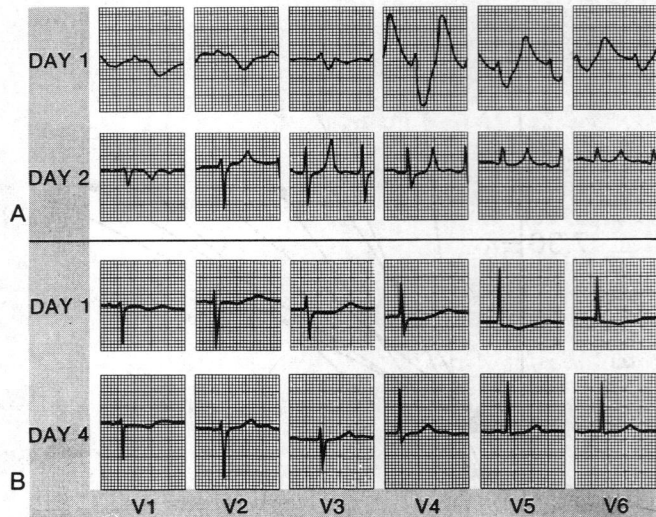

Figure 93–13. Electrocardiographic changes in hyperkalemia *(A)* and hypokalemia *(B)*. *A.* On day 1, at a K^+ level of 8.6 mEq/L, the P wave is no longer recognizable and the QRS complex is diffusely prolonged. Initial and terminal QRS delay is characteristic of K^+-induced intraventricular conduction and is best illustrated in leads V_2 and V_6. On day 2, at a K^+ level of 5.8 mEq/L, the P wave is recognizable with a PR interval of 0.24 sec and, the duration of the QRS complex is approximately 0.10 sec and, the T waves are characteristically tented. *B.* On day 1, at a K^+ level of 1.5 mEq/L, the T and U waves are merged. The U wave is prominent and the QU interval prolonged. On day 4, at a K^+ level of 3.7 mEq/L, the tracing is normal. (From Fisch C: Electrocardiography and Vectorcardiography. In: Braunwald E [ed]: Heart Disease: A Textbook of Cardiovascular Medicine. 4th ed. Philadelphia, WB Saunders, p 116, 1992.)

nous administration of sodium bicarbonate (one to two ampules, 44 to 88 mEq). Metabolic alkalosis transiently shifts potassium intracellularly, thereby lowering the serum potassium levels. In addition, intravenous glucose with insulin (50 mL of 50% dextrose in water and 10 U of regular insulin) should be given; this initiates a potassium level–lowering effect within 15 minutes, and the effect lasts for 4 to 6 hours. Definitive treatment of the hyperkalemia consists of oral or rectal administration of cation-exchange resin (sodium polystyrene sulfonate [Kayexalate], 25 to 50 g) and emergent dialysis in patients with severe renal dysfunction.

Magnesium

Causes of hypomagnesemia are multiple, but it is most commonly seen in association with the use of diuretics and in patients who abuse alcohol.[81] Tissue magnesium deficiency can occur without reduced serum levels; however, hypomagnesemia appears to be the most expeditious clinical method of identifying magnesium depletion.[82] Magnesium depletion has been implicated in aggravating potassium depletion and interferes with potassium repletion.[83] Ventricular arrhythmias, especially in those with underlying heart disease, are commonly seen in relation to hypokalemia. In these patients, uncorrected hypomagnesemia prevents normalization of potassium levels despite large doses of potassium supplements. It is therefore important to diagnose and correct hypomagnesemia in patients with ventricular arrhythmias. On the surface electrocardiogram, changes in relation to hypomagnesemia are predominantly those related to associated hypokalemia. Intravenous magnesium administration has been shown to be effective in treating some patients with serious ventricular arrhythmias.[84]

In a group of patients with torsades de pointes, intravenous magnesium was shown to be effective in treating the arrhythmia.[85] The mechanism behind the action of intravenous magnesium in these patients remains unclear, as not all had hypomagnesemia.

Magnesium deficiency has also been implicated as a factor contributing to the development of serious ventricular arrhythmias in patients with severe CHF. However, a study of patients with heart failure by Ralston and colleagues did not show a significant difference between serum and tissue magnesium concentrations in patients with heart failure and serious ventricular arrhythmias when compared with those in patients with heart failure without serious ventricular arrhythmias.[86] In vivo and in vitro, magnesium has been demonstrated to have antiarrhythmic properties,[87, 88] and the effectiveness of intravenous magnesium administration in patients with serious ventricular arrhythmias may result not because of the correction of magnesium depletion but from its direct electrophysiologic effects. The precise role of magnesium therapy in ventricular arrhythmias remains investigational.

EFFECTS OF COCAINE ON CARDIOVASCULAR FUNCTION

Cocaine-related cardiovascular complications are being increasingly recognized. Myocardial ischemia or infarction related to the use and abuse of cocaine has been well documented. Nademanee and colleagues performed 24-hour ambulatory electrocardiographic monitoring and exercise stress testing in 21 long-term cocaine users during the first few weeks of drug withdrawal.[89] Eight of the 21 individuals had frequent episodes of ST segment elevation recorded during ambulatory electrocardiographic monitoring, and 1 patient had an abnormal treadmill test result. Many of these episodes of ST segment elevation were not associated with

chest pain (silent). Thirty-eight percent of this group gave a history of chest pain suggestive of angina. This indicates that the incidence of ischemia in this group of young patients (mean age, 34 years) is high, and in some patients, ischemia may be silent.

There are more than 63 documented cases of myocardial ischemia or infarction in association with cocaine use.[90] The actual incidence is probably much higher than this. In these patients, coronary thrombosis appears to be an important pathophysiologic factor for myocardial infarction; however, underlying coronary arterial stenosis was seen in only 43% of these patients. The possible effects of cocaine on the coronary circulation include coronary arterial spasm, intimal proliferation, and accelerated arteriosclerosis. Generalized coronary vasospasm has been documented in both animals and humans with an acute dose of cocaine.[91–93]

Dressler and colleagues performed an autopsy series on 17 long-term cocaine users with a mean age of 32 years.[94] Coronary arterial narrowings of 25% or more were seen in 76% of patients and narrowings of 75% or more were seen in 47%. This high incidence of coronary stenosis in a young population of patients suggests that cocaine may cause or accelerate coronary arteriosclerosis.

Thrombolytic therapy has been found to be successful in treating patients who develop Q wave myocardial infarction in association with cocaine use; however, contraindications such as cocaine-related cerebrovascular accident, severe hypertension, seizures, and bleeding disorders must not be present.[90] If patients have an overdose of cocaine, beta-blockers may be indicated for a hyperadrenergic state with hypertension but should be used with caution, as they may worsen coronary arterial vasospasm. Calcium channel blockers have been shown to be valuable in the therapy of experimental cocaine-induced heart disease.[95] Cocaine-induced vasoconstriction has been shown to be calcium dependent, and in vitro experiments documented that vasoconstriction with cocaine hydrochloride could be attenuated by diltiazem.[96] Transient severe myocardial dysfunction has been reported in association with cocaine overuse, and this is probably a reversible process, which may require inotropic support.

Electrophysiologic Effects

Sudden cardiac death and a wide variety of ventricular arrhythmias have been reported in cocaine users. Myocardial ischemia and cocaine-induced myocarditis may create the substrate that leads to malignant arrhythmias. In addition, cocaine has direct electrophysiologic effects, namely, prolongation of intraventricular conduction time and QT interval.[97] These changes have been observed in vitro as well as in animals and humans. In patients who have ventricular arrhythmias resulting from cocaine overdose, the initial therapy consists of reversal of metabolic and respiratory acidosis attributable to seizures and hypoventilation. Although beta-blockers have been useful to counteract the hyperadrenergic state and hypertension, they may worsen coronary arterial vasospasm. Conventional type I-A antiarrhythmic agents should be used with caution in patients who have prolongation of the QT interval.

Other Cardiovascular Complications

Myocarditis and dilated cardiomyopathy with acute CHF have occurred with cocaine abuse. In a study reported by Isner and colleagues, one patient at autopsy demonstrated scattered foci of myocardial fibrosis.[98] In another patient, endomyocardial biopsy revealed myocyte necrosis and diffuse inflammatory cell infiltrates, including eosinophils. In an autopsy study of 40 patients with a history of significant cocaine use, Virmani and colleagues found myocarditis in 20%, with cellular infiltrates consisting of lymphocytes, macrophages, and occasional eosinophils.[99] Experimental studies suggest a direct myocardial depressant action of cocaine.[95]

Aortic dissection and rupture have been reported after cocaine use. This is most likely due to the elevated blood pressure resulting from the effects of cocaine on blocking the reuptake of catecholamines. Hypertensive emergencies in patients with cocaine use should be treated initially with beta-blockers and intravenous sodium nitroprusside.

References

1. Wilson RF, Gibson D, Percinel AK, et al: Severe alkalosis in critically ill surgical patients. Arch Surg 105:197, 1972.
2. Mazzara JT, Ayres SM, Grace WJ: Extreme hypocapnia in the critically ill patient. Am J Med 56:450, 1974.
3. Klug F: Ueber den Einfluss gasartiger Korper auf die Function des Froschherzens. Arch Anat Physiol 435, 1879.
4. Smith HW: The action of acids on turtle heart muscle with reference to the penetration of anions. Am J Physiol 76:411, 1926.
5. Gremels H, Stalling EH: On the influence of hydrogen ion concentration and of anoxaemia upon the heart volume. J Physiol (Lond) 61:297, 1926.
6. Downing SE, Talner NS, Gardner TH: Cardiovascular responses to metabolic acidosis. Am J Physiol 208:237, 1965.
7. Smith NT, Corbarcia AN: Myocardial resistance to metabolic acidosis. Arch Surg 92:892, 1966.
8. Rocamora JM, Downing SE: Preservation of ventricular function by adrenergic influences during metabolic acidosis in the cat. Circ Res 24:373, 1969.
9. Gonzalez NC, Clancy RL: Inotropic and intracellular acid-base changes during metabolic acidosis. Am J Physiol 228:1060, 1975.
10. Clancy RL, Gonzalez NC, Fenton RC: Effect of beta-adrenoreceptor blockade on rat cardiac and skeletal muscle pH. Am J Physiol 230:959, 1976.
11. Steinhart CR, Purmutt S, Gurtner GH, et al: Beta-adrenergic activity and cardiovascular response to severe respiratory acidosis. Am J Physiol 244:H46, 1983.
12. Rose CE, Benthuysen KV, Jackson JT, et al: Right ventricular performance during increased afterload impaired by hypercapneic acidosis in conscious dogs. Circ Res 52:76, 1983.
13. Thomas JA, Marks BH: Plasma norepinephrine in congestive heart failure. Am J Cardiol 41:233, 1978.
14. Bristow MR, Ginsburg R, Minobe W, et al: Decreased catecholamine sensitivity and beta-adrenergic receptor density in failing human hearts. N Engl J Med 307:205, 1982.
15. Cingolani HE, Mattiazi AR, Blesa ES, et al: Contractility in isolated mammalian heart muscle after acid base changes. Circ Res 26:269, 1970.
16. Cingolani HE, Blesa ES, Gonzalez NC, et al: Extracellular vs intracellular pH as a determinant of myocardial contractility. Life Sci 8:775, 1969.
17. Poole-Wilson PA, Cameron IR: A comparison of the control of intracellular pH in cardiac and skeletal muscle. Clin Sci 44:15P, 1973.
18. Steenbergen C, Deleeuw G, Rich T, et al: Effects of acidosis and ischemia on contractility and intracellular pH of rat heart. Circ Res 41:849, 1977.
19. Woodbury JW: Fluxes of H^+ and HCO_3^- across frog skeletal muscle cell membranes. In: Siesjo BK, Sorensen SC (eds): Ion Homeostasis of the Brain. New York, Academic Press, p 270, 1971.
20. Williamson JR, Safer B, Rich T, et al: Effects of acidosis on myocardial contractility and metabolism. Acta Med Scand Suppl 87:95, 1975.
21. Donaldson SKB, Heamansen L, Bolles L: Differential effects of H^+ on Ca^{++} activated force from skinned fibres from soleus cardiac and adductor magnus muscles of rabbits. Pfluegers Arch 376:55, 1978.
22. Rupp H: Modulation of tension generation at the myofibrillar level: An analysis of the effect of magnesium, pH, sarcomere length and state of phosphorylation. Basic Res Cardiol 75:295, 1980.
23. Katz AM, Hecht HH: The early pump failure of the ischemic heart. Am J Med 47:497, 1969.
24. Ricciardi L, Bucx JJJ, Ter Keurs HEDJ: Effects of acidosis on forced-sarcomere length and force-velocity relations of rat cardiac muscle. Cardiovasc Res 20:117, 1986.
25. Stull JD, Buss JE: Calcium binding properties of beef cardiac troponin. J Biol Chem 253:5932, 1978.
26. Safer B, Morad M, Williamson JR: Effects of H^+ on myocardial contractility. Circulation 48(suppl IV):212, 1973.
27. Wada Y, Goto M: Effects of pH on the processes of excitation-contraction coupling of bull frog atrium. Jpn J Physiol 25:605, 1975.
28. Kohlhardt TM, Haap K, Figulla HR: Influence of low extracellular pH upon the calcium inward current and isometric contractile force in mammalian ventricular myocardium. Pfluegers Arch 366:31, 1976.
29. Fry CH, Poole-Wilson PA: Effects of acid base changes on excitation

contraction coupling in guinea pig and rabbit cardiac ventricular muscle. J Physiol (Lond) 313:141, 1981.
30. Vogel S, Sperelakis N: Blockade of myocardial slow cation channels at low pH. Am J Physiol 233:C99, 1977.
31. Morad M, Goldman Y: Excitation-contraction coupling in heart muscle: Membrane control of development of tension. Prog Biophys Mol Biol 27:257, 1973.
32. Fabiato A, Fabiato F: Contractions induced by a calcium-triggered release of calcium from the sarcoplasmic reticulum of single skinned cardiac cells. J Physiol (Lond) 249:469, 1975.
33. Kohmoto O, Spitzer KW, Movsesian MA, et al: Effects of intracellular acidosis on $[Ca^{2+}]i$ transients, transsarcolemmal Ca^{2+} fluxes, and contraction in ventricular myocytes. Circ Res 66:622, 1990.
34. Kagiyama Y, Hill JL, Gettes LS: Interaction of acidosis and increased extracellular potassium on action potential characteristics and conduction in guinea pig ventricular muscle. Circ Res 51:614, 1982.
35. Wildenthal K, Mierzviak DS, Myers RW, et al: Effects of acute lactic acidosis on left ventricular performance. Am J Physiol 214:1352, 1968.
36. Kontos HA, Richardson DW, Patterson JL: Vasodilator effect of hypercapneic acidosis on human forearm vessels. Am J Physiol 215:1403, 1968.
37. Wendling MG, Eckstein JW, Abboud FM, et al: Cardiovascular responses to carbon dioxide before and after beta-adrenergic blockade. J Appl Physiol 22:223, 1967.
38. Sharpey-Schafer EP, Semple SJG, Halls RW, et al: Venous constriction after exercise: Its relation to acid base changes in venous blood. Clin Sci 29:397, 1965.
39. Scheuer J: The effect of respiratory and metabolic alkalosis on coronary flow, hemodynamics, and myocardial carbohydrate metabolism. Cardiologia 52:275, 1968.
40. Rooke DT, Sparks HV Jr: Effect of metabolic vs. respiratory acid base changes in isolated coronary arteries. Experientia 37:982, 1981.
41. Rinaldi GJ, Amado Cattaneo E, Cingolani HE: Interaction between calcium and hydrogen ions in canine coronary arteries. Mol Cell Cardiol 19:773, 1987.
42. Eliades D, Weiss HR: Effect of hypercapnea on coronary circulation. Cardiovasc Res 20:127, 1986.
43. Graf H, Leach W, Arieff AI: Evidence for a detrimental effect of bicarbonate therapy in hypoxic lactic acidosis. Science 227:754, 1985.
44. Arieff AI, Leach W, Park R, et al: Systemic effects of $NaHCO_3$ in experimental lactic acidosis in dogs. Am J Physiol 242:F586, 1982.
45. Bersin RM, Arieff AI: Improved hemodynamic function during hypoxia with Carbicarb, a new agent for the management of acidosis. Circulation 77:227, 1988.
46. Park R, Arieff AI: Treatment of lactic acidosis with dichloroacetate in dogs. J Clin Invest 70:853, 1982.
47. Romeh SA, Tannen RL: Therapeutic benefit of bichloroacetate in experimentally-induced hypoxic lactic acidosis. J Lab Clin Med 107:378, 1986.
48. Gin-Shaw SL, Barsan WG, Eymer V, et al: Effects of dichloroacetate following canine asphyxial arrest. Ann Emerg Med 17:473, 1988.
49. Stacpoole PW, Lorenz AC, Thomas RG, et al: Dichloroacetate in the treatment of lactic acidosis. Ann Intern Med 108:58, 1988.
50. Bishop RL, Weisfeldt ML: Sodium bicarbonate administration during cardiac arrest: Effect on arterial pH, PCO_2, and osmolality. JAMA 235:506, 1976.
51. Mattar JA, Weil MH, Shubin H, et al: Cardiac arrest in the critically ill: II. Hyperosmolal states following cardiac arrest. Am J Med 56:162, 1974.
52. Lawson NW, Butler GH, Ray CT: Alkalosis and cardiac arrhythmias. Anesth Analg 52:951, 1973.
53. Kerber RE, Pandian NG, Hoyt R, et al: Effect of ischemia, hypertrophy, hypoxia, acidosis, and alkalosis on canine defibrillation. Am J Physiol 244:H825, 1983.
54. Grundler WG, Weil MH, Rackow EC: Arteriovenous carbon dioxide and pH gradients during cardiac arrest. Circulation 74:1071, 1986.
55. Weil MH, Rackow EC, Trevino R, et al: Difference in acid-base state between venous and arterial blood during cardiopulmonary resuscitation. N Engl J Med 315:153, 1986.
56. von Planta M, Weil MH, Gazmuri RJ, et al: Myocardial acidosis associated with CO_2 production during cardiac arrest and resuscitation. Circulation 80:684, 1989.
57. Hostetter TH, Pfeffer JM, Pfeffer MA, et al: Cardiorenal hemodynamics and sodium excretion in rats with myocardial infarction. Am J Physiol 245:98, 1983.
58. Ichikawa I, Pfeffer JM, Pfeffer MA, et al: Role of angiotensin II in altered renal function of congestive heart failure. Circ Res 55:669, 1984.
59. Dzau VJ, Creager MA: Neurohormonal systems in heart failure. Heart Failure 2:3, 1986.
60. Packer M: Adaptive and maladaptive actions of angiotensin II in patients with severe congestive heart failure. Am J Kidney Dis 10(1 suppl 1):66, 1987.
61. Dzau VJ: Renal effects of angiotensin-converting enzyme inhibition in cardiac failure. Am J Kidney Dis 10(1 suppl 1):74, 1987.
62. The Consensus Trial Study Group: Effects of enalapril on mortality in severe congestive heart failure: The results of the cooperative north Scandanavian enalapril survival study. N Engl J Med 316:1429, 1987.

63. Newman TJ, Maskin CS, Dennick LG, et al: Effects of captopril on survival in patients with heart failure. Am J Med 84(suppl 3A):140, 1988.
64. Packer M, Medina N, Yushak M: Correction of dilutional hyponatremia in severe chronic heart failure by converting enzyme inhibition. Ann Intern Med 100:782, 1984.
65. Aberman A, Fulop M: The metabolic and respiratory acidosis of acute pulmonary edema. Ann Intern Med 76:173, 1972.
66. Fulop M, Horovitz M, Aberman A, et al: Lactic acidosis in pulmonary edema due to left ventricular failure. Ann Intern Med 79:180, 1973.
67. Bihler I: Role of calcium in heart metabolism. Can J Physiol Pharmacol 62:884, 1984.
68. Bristow MR, Schwartz D, Binetti G, et al: Ionized calcium and the heart. Elucidation of in vivo concentration-response relationships in the open-chest dog. Circ Res 41:565, 1977.
69. Bunker JP, Bendixen HH, Murphy AJ: Hemodynamic effects of intravenously administered sodium citrate. N Engl J Med 266:372, 1962.
70. Gain EA: The problem of cardiac collapse associated with the massive transfusion of citrated blood. Can Anaesth Soc J 9:207, 1962.
71. Porter DL, Ledgerwood AM, Lucas CE, et al: Effect of calcium infusion on heart function. Am Surg 49:369, 1983.
72. Auffant RA, Downs JB, Amick R: Ionized calcium concentration and cardiovascular function after cardiopulmonary bypass. Arch Surg 116:1072, 1981.
73. Henrich WL, Hunt JM, Nixon JV: Increased ionized calcium and left ventricular contractility during hemodialysis. N Engl J Med 310:19, 1984.
74. Drueke T, Fauchet M, Fleury J, et al: Effect of parathyroidectomy on left ventricular function in hemodialysis patients. Lancet 1:112, 1980.
75. Scheidegger D, Drop LJ: The relationship between duration of QT interval and plasma ionized calcium concentration: Experiments with acute, steady-state (Ca++) changes in the dog. Anesthesiology 51:143, 1979.
76. Knochel JP: Hypophosphatemia. West J Med 134:15, 1981.
77. Knochel JP: Hypophosphatemia in the alcoholic. Arch Intern Med 140:613, 1980.
78. Ryback RS, Eckardt MJ, Pautler CP: Clinical relationships between serum phosphorus and other blood chemistry values in alcoholics. Arch Intern Med 140:673, 1980.
79. Fuller TJ, Nichols WW, Brenner BJ, et al: Reversible depression in myocardial performance in dogs with experimental phosphorus deficiency. J Clin Invest 62:1194, 1978.
80. Connor LR, Wheeler WS, Bethune JE: Effect of hypophosphatemia on myocardial performance in man. N Engl J Med 297:901, 1977.
81. Whang R: Magnesium deficiency: Pathogenesis, prevalence, and clinical implications. Am J Med 82(suppl 3A):24, 1987.
82. Whang R: Routine serum magnesium determination—A continuing unrecognized need. Magnesium 6:1, 1987.
83. Whang R, Flink EB, Dyckner T, et al: Magnesium depletion as a cause of refractory potassium repletion. Arch Intern Med 145:1686, 1985.
84. Altura BM, Altura BT: New perspectives on the role of magnesium in the pathophysiology of the cardiovascular system: Clinical aspects. Magnesium 4:226, 1985.
85. Tzivoni D, Banai S, Schuger C, et al: Treatment of torsade de pointes with magnesium sulfate. Circulation 77:392, 1988.
86. Ralston MA, Murnane MR, Unverferth DV, et al: Serum and tissue magnesium concentrations in patients with heart failure and serious ventricular arrhythmias. Ann Intern Med 113:841, 1990.
87. Roden DM, Iansmith BH: Effects of low potassium or magnesium concentrations on isolated cardiac tissue. Am J Med 82(suppl 3A):18, 1987.
88. Kulick DL, Hong R, Ryzen E, et al: Electrophysiologic effects of intravenous magnesium in patients with normal conduction systems and no clinical evidence of significant cardiac disease. Am Heart J 115:367, 1988.
89. Nademanee K, Gorelick DA, Josepheson MA, et al: Myocardial ischemia during cocaine withdrawal. Ann Intern Med 111:876, 1989.
90. Rezkalla SH, Hale S, Kloner RA: Cocaine-induced heart diseases. Am Heart J 120:1403, 1990.
91. Isner JM, Chokshi SK: Cocaine and vasospasm. N Engl J Med 321:1604, 1989.
92. Hale SL, Alker KJ, Rezkalla SH, et al: Adverse effects of cocaine on cardiovascular dynamics, myocardial blood flow, and coronary artery diameter in an experimental model. Am Heart J 118:927, 1989.
93. Lange RA, Cigarroa RG, Yancey CW, et al: Cocaine induced coronary artery vasoconstriction. N Engl J Med 321:1557, 1989.
94. Dressler FA, Malebejadeh S, Roberts WC: Quantitative analysis of amounts of coronary arterial narrowing in cocaine addicts. Am J Cardiol 65:303, 1990.
95. Hale SL, Alker KJ, Rezkalla SH, et al: Nifedipine protects the heart from the acute deleterious effects of cocaine if administered before but not after cocaine. Circulation 83:1437, 1991.
96. Rongione AJ, Isner JV: Cocaine-induced contraction of vascular smooth muscle is inhibited by calcium channel blockade. J Am Coll Cardiol 13:78A, 1989.
97. Hale SL, Lehmann MH, Kloner RA: Electrocardiographic abnormalities after acute administration of cocaine in the rat. Am J Cardiol 63:1529, 1989.
98. Isner JV, Mark Estes NA III, Thompson PD, et al: Acute cardiac events temporally related to cocaine abuse. N Engl J Med 315:1438, 1986.
99. Virmani R, Robinowitz M, Smialek JE, et al: Cardiovascular effects of cocaine: An autopsy study of 40 patients. Am Heart J 115:1068, 1988.
100. Edwards J, Rubin RN: Aortic dissection and cocaine abuse. Ann Intern Med 107:779, 1987.

CHAPTER 94

Disorders of Cardiac Rhythm and Conduction in the Medical Intensive Care Unit

Alfred E. Buxton
Jodie L. Hurwitz

Cardiac arrhythmias frequently complicate the course of critically ill patients. Intensive care physicians must be prepared to deal with two types of arrhythmias. The first are those due to pre-existing primary rhythm disturbances. Examples of these are supraventricular tachycardia caused by atrioventricular (AV) nodal re-entry and recurrent sustained ventricular tachycardia (VT) in patients who had a prior myocardial infarction. Patients with primary rhythm disorders often enter the medical intensive care unit already receiving antiarrhythmic therapy. When such patients develop illnesses that require intensive care, the resulting metabolic derangements often necessitate a change in the dose or even temporary discontinuation of antiarrhythmic agents, thus exposing the patient to the possibility of arrhythmia exacerbations. Alterations in the metabolism of certain antiarrhythmic agents in acute medical illnesses may result in arrhythmic and nonarrhythmic drug toxicity. Furthermore, metabolic disturbances such as electrolyte abnormalities resulting from the patient's acute illness may alter the effects of pre-existing antiarrhythmic therapy, provoking drug toxic arrhythmias or other adverse reactions such as alteration in pacing thresholds.

The second category comprises arrhythmias arising as a result of the acute and chronic noncardiac medical disorders responsible for the patient's being in the medical intensive care unit. Examples of these are multifocal atrial tachycardia and atrial fibrillation in patients with acute pulmonary decompensation and the arrhythmias that result from severe electrolyte abnormalities. Many of these arrhythmias do not cause symptoms and would pass unnoticed if the patient were not undergoing electrocardiographic monitoring. Usually this type of arrhythmia is best treated by correcting the underlying medical or metabolic abnormality, rather than treating the arrhythmia primarily, because patients in these situations are at significantly increased risk for adverse drug reactions. Thus, it is incumbent on the physician caring for the critically ill to treat the whole patient rather than the electrocardiogram (ECG). Most patients with rhythm disorders in the first category are likely to be cared for in the coronary care unit. Therefore, most of the patients in the medical intensive care unit are likely to have cardiac rhythm disturbances in the second category.

CELLULAR ELECTROPHYSIOLOGY

For adequate diagnosis of rhythm and conduction disturbances, some basic properties of cardiac cells must be understood. Furthermore, the effects of antiarrhythmic agents on cardiac cells must be understood if pharmacologic antiarrhythmic therapy is to be administered effectively and safely.

CARDIAC ACTION POTENTIAL

Under normal resting conditions, the inside of cardiac cells is negatively charged with respect to the exterior. The potential maintained across the cell membrane is dependent on the concentration of ions (Na^+, K^+, Cl^-, Ca^{2+}) on the two sides. The movement of ions across the cell membrane is dependent on both electrical and chemical gradients. An electrical stimulus alters membrane conductivity to these ions, which begins a series of events that result in an action potential. The action potential itself is made up of five different phases defined by movement of the specific ions (Fig. 94–1).[1, 2]

During phase 0, Na^+ moves quickly into the cell, causing the transmembrane potential to increase to positive values. The maximal rate of rise of the Na^+ conductance or phase 0 upstroke is also termed V_{max} or dV/dt. Phase 1 is the early rapid repolarization phase (transient outward current mediated by K^+ ions). Phase 2, the plateau phase, is due to a slow inward current carried largely by calcium and is an important determinant of the action potential duration. Phase 3 constitutes rapid repolarization to a more negative resting potential. It is due to both a decrease in the slow inward current and an increase in the outward flow of K^+ ions. During phase 4, the resting membrane potential returns to its most negative values. If spontaneous diastolic depolarization is present, it occurs during this phase. Potassium efflux via K^+ channels, as well as an Na^+-K^+ pump moving Na^+ out of the cell and K^+ into the cell, is primarily responsible for this phase.

Cardiac cells that display spontaneous (phase 4) diastolic depolarization are said to display automaticity; normally, the only cells that have this property are sinoatrial (SA), certain AV nodal cells, and His-Purkinje cells.[1] In normal hearts the SA node discharges most rapidly and thus acts as the primary pacemaker.

The speed with which an action potential propagates is called conduction velocity. Conduction velocity is dependent on the resting membrane potential of the cell, the rate of rise of phase 0 or V_{max}, and cell-to-cell coupling.[3, 4] Cells of the sinus node and AV node normally have a less negative resting membrane potential than other cardiac cells and have a gradual upstroke during phase 0 that is carried by Ca^{2+} ions; thus, they display slow conduction. Slow conduction can also be seen in diseased tissue. Purkinje's and myocardial cells are depolarized rapidly (with rapid conduction), and this initial fast current is carried by an inward sodium current. The ions themselves move across the membrane through channels, which are fairly specific for their own ion (i.e., Na^+ channel, Ca^+ channel, K^+ channel, and Cl^- channel). The channels have gating mechanisms that operate at different membrane potentials, so at certain membrane potentials one ion channel is inactive (cannot be opened) while another is open, allowing its specific ions to pass freely.[5] The gates respond to changes in the transmembrane potential in a time-dependent manner, controlling ion flow and acting to define the different phases of the action potential.

CARDIAC ACTION POTENTIAL

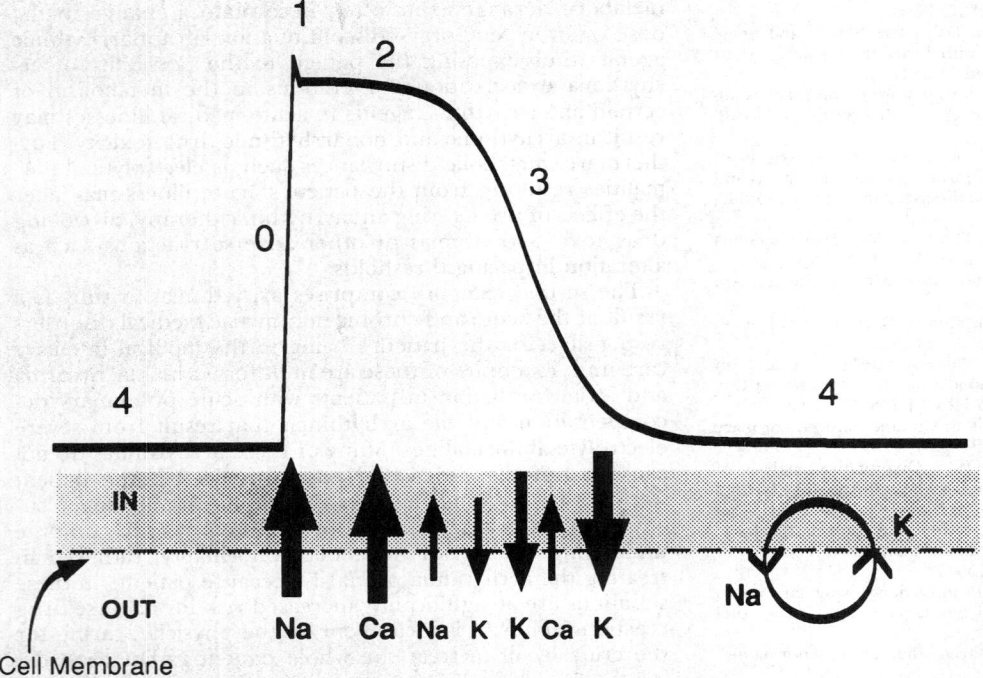

Figure 94–1. The cardiac action potential with phases 0, 1, 2, 3, and 4. The upward arrows represent ion movement into the cell, and downward arrows represent ion movement out of the cell. The width of each arrow represents the magnitude of current contribution during a specific phase. During phase 4 the Na^+-K^+ pump maintains resting membrane potential. See text for more details.

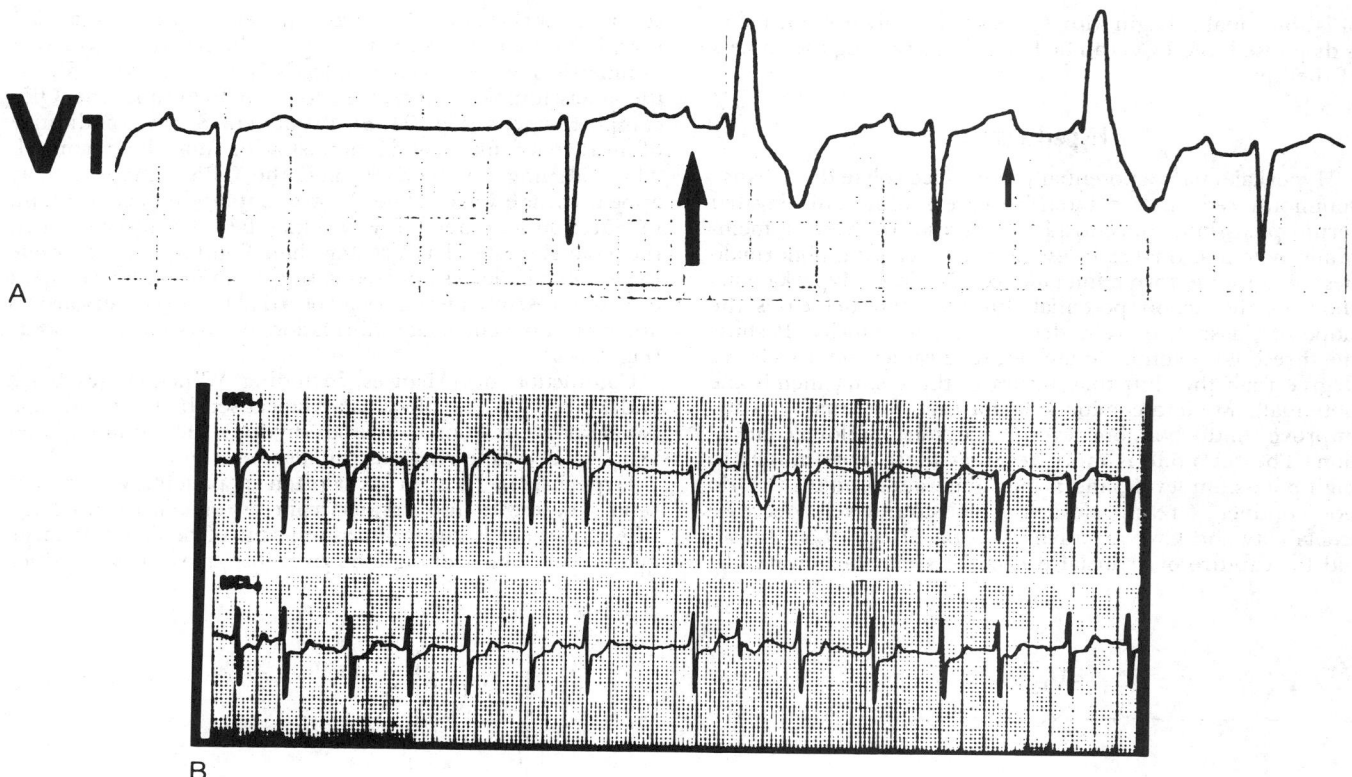

Figure 94–2. Examples of aberrant intraventricular conduction caused by functional right bundle branch block. *A.* Two complexes followed by a run of atrial tachycardia. The first premature atrial complex (*large arrow*) is followed by a QRS complex having right bundle branch aberration. The short RR interval caused by the premature atrial complex follows a much longer RR interval during normal sinus rhythm. The third P wave in the atrial tachycardia (*small arrow*) also causes a relatively short RR interval after a longer RR interval. Note that the third P wave of the tachycardia also conducts with a longer PR interval because of delay in AV nodal conduction. *B.* The Ashman phenomenon. In the middle of the simultaneous rhythm strips, a relatively long pause during atrial fibrillation is followed by a shorter conduction interval that results in a right bundle branch block aberration.

Another property of cardiac cells important in understanding mechanisms of arrhythmias and drug effects is refractoriness. The refractory period is the period of inexcitability that follows the action potential. It is determined in the electrophysiology laboratory by the introduction of premature stimuli over a range of coupling intervals after an action potential. The action potential that is generated by a late premature stimulus (i.e., late in diastole) is normal. As the premature stimulus occurs earlier in diastole it encounters phase 3 of the previous action potential. The resulting premature action potential has a lower than normal V_{max} because it began at a membrane potential that was less negative than normal. Ultimately, with progressively earlier stimuli, there comes a point where no response occurs. The time from the beginning of the first action potential to the point at which no subsequent action potential can be generated is called the effective refractory period. The effective refractory period is a function of the duration of the first action potential and the state of the Na$^+$ channels after the first action potential. After Na$^+$ channels are activated, they enter an inactivated state from which they cannot be opened before returning to the resting state.

AV nodal cells have unique properties that distinguish them from cardiac muscle cells and cells of the His-Purkinje system.[6] The AV nodal cells remain refractory for a significant time after the termination of the action potential. This translates into frequency-dependent changes in AV nodal conduction such that if the atrial rate increases (assuming that the autonomic nervous system tone remains constant)

or a premature atrial impulse occurs, conduction through the AV node slows. On the ECG, this is manifest as a prolonged PR interval. This decremental conduction is a normal physiologic response of the AV node.[7, 8]

His-Purkinje and myocardial cells respond differently to increases in stimulation rate or premature stimuli: as heart rate increases, the refractory period of the cells shortens. Likewise, if the heart rate decreases, the refractory period lengthens. The refractory period of the bundle branches is determined by the previous RR interval: a long RR interval lengthens refractoriness of the bundle branches on the subsequent beat. If a long RR interval is followed by a significantly shorter RR interval (long-short response), one of the bundle branches may be refractory and the resulting QRS complex appears aberrant with a bundle branch block morphology (Fig. 94–2A). This can occur with premature atrial beats, supraventricular tachycardias, and some ventricular complexes during atrial fibrillation. In the latter rhythm, the irregular RR intervals cause long-short responses at the bundle branches, yielding an aberrant or wide QRS complex (Ashman's phenomenon) (see Fig. 94–2B).[6]

ELECTROLYTE ABNORMALITIES

Knowledge of the ionic basis of the action potential makes it obvious that electrolyte abnormalities may result in cardiac arrhythmias and alter the ECG.[9] The ECG can be useful in diagnosing and estimating electrolyte imbalances but can be confusing if it reflects abnormalities of several electrolytes or is abnormal to begin with. Once an electrolyte abnormality is diagnosed, the ECG can be helpful in assessing the success of therapy.

Hyperkalemia

Hyperkalemia is a potentially lethal electrolyte disturbance commonly seen in the intensive care setting. An elevated serum potassium concentration decreases the resting membrane potential (makes it less negative), causing abnormalities of impulse formation and conduction. Hyperkalemia shortens the action potential duration and decreases the slope of phase 4, thereby decreasing automaticity. It shifts the threshold potential to less negative values (but to a lesser degree than the shift that occurs in the resting membrane potential). Moderate hyperkalemia therefore may actually improve conduction, but severe hyperkalemia slows conduction. The SA node is more resistant than atrial muscle to high potassium levels, and it may generate impulses that do not conduct. Greatly elevated potassium levels decrease excitability and have negative inotropic effects. The threshold for capture of artificial pacemakers may be elevated by

severe hyperkalemia. At potassium levels greater than 5.5 mEq/L the first electrocardiographic abnormality is peaked, symmetric T waves, usually in leads II, III, and V_2 to V_4. As the potassium level increases to 8 to 9 mEq/L, the QRS complex widens (Fig. 94–3). Prominent S waves indicative of intraventricular conduction slowing may be recorded. The widening can progress and the QRS complexes may appear as sine waves. The P wave amplitude decreases and its duration lengthens. P waves may become invisible when the potassium level is greater than 9 mEq/L. In extreme hyperkalemia (levels approximating 12 mEq/L), ST segment elevation resembling that in myocardial injury or pericarditis appears and ventricular fibrillation or asystole may occur (Fig. 94–4).

Conduction disturbances, including Wenckebach's block and Mobitz's II AV block, may be caused by hyperkalemia. Accelerated junctional escape rhythms are common and ventricular escape rhythms can also be seen.

Hyperkalemia is seen most often in patients with severe renal failure. It also results from iatrogenic causes (e.g., when a patient is given potassium salts of penicillin in large quantities). Massive digitalis overdose may also produce

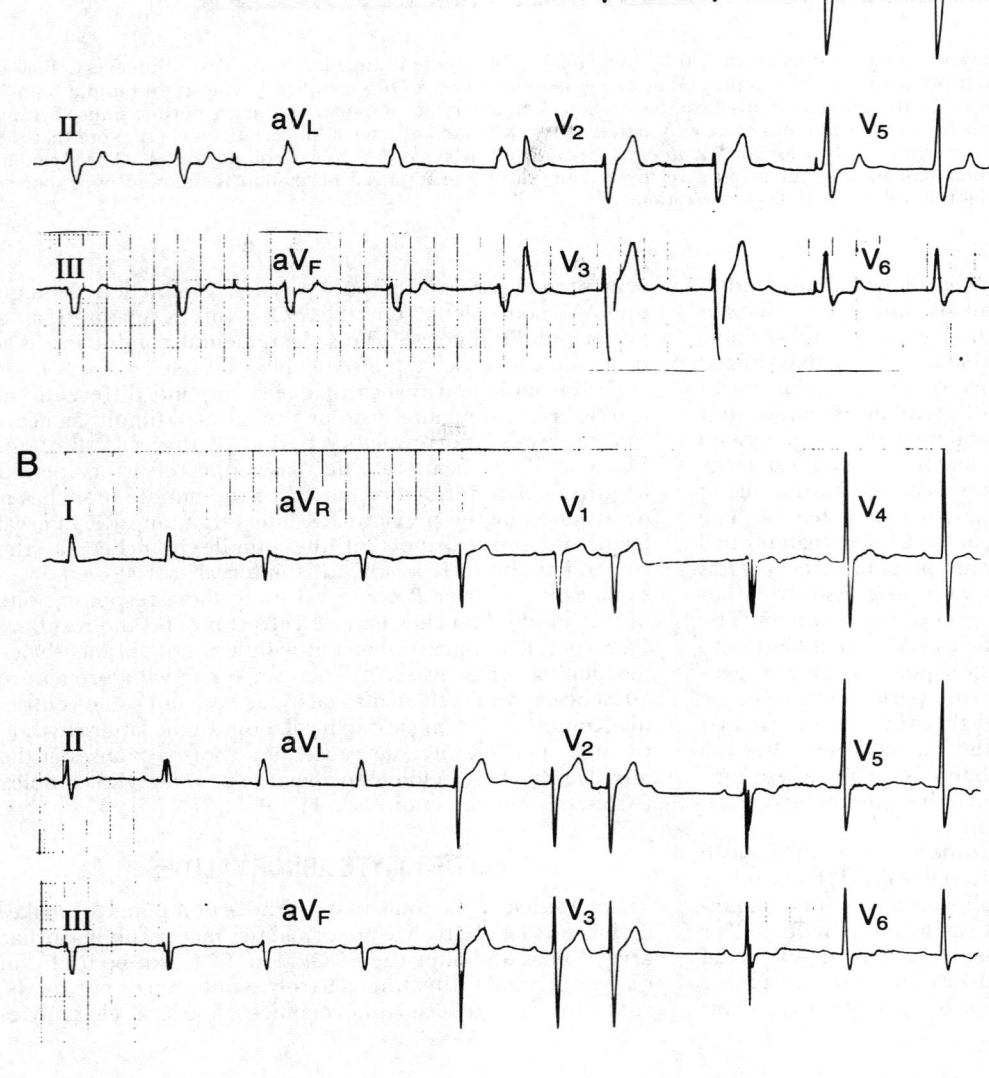

Figure 94–3. Example of mild hyperkalemia. *A.* A 12-lead ECG for a patient with a potassium level of 8.4 mEq/L shows sinus rhythm with markedly prolonged PR interval, widening of the terminal component of the QRS complex, and slurring of the junction between the QRS complex and the ST segment. The T waves are peaked symmetrically. *B.* ECG recorded after hyperkalemia resolved (potassium 5.5 mEq/L). Notice the narrowing of the QRS complex, abbreviation of the PR interval, and return to baseline of the ST segments.

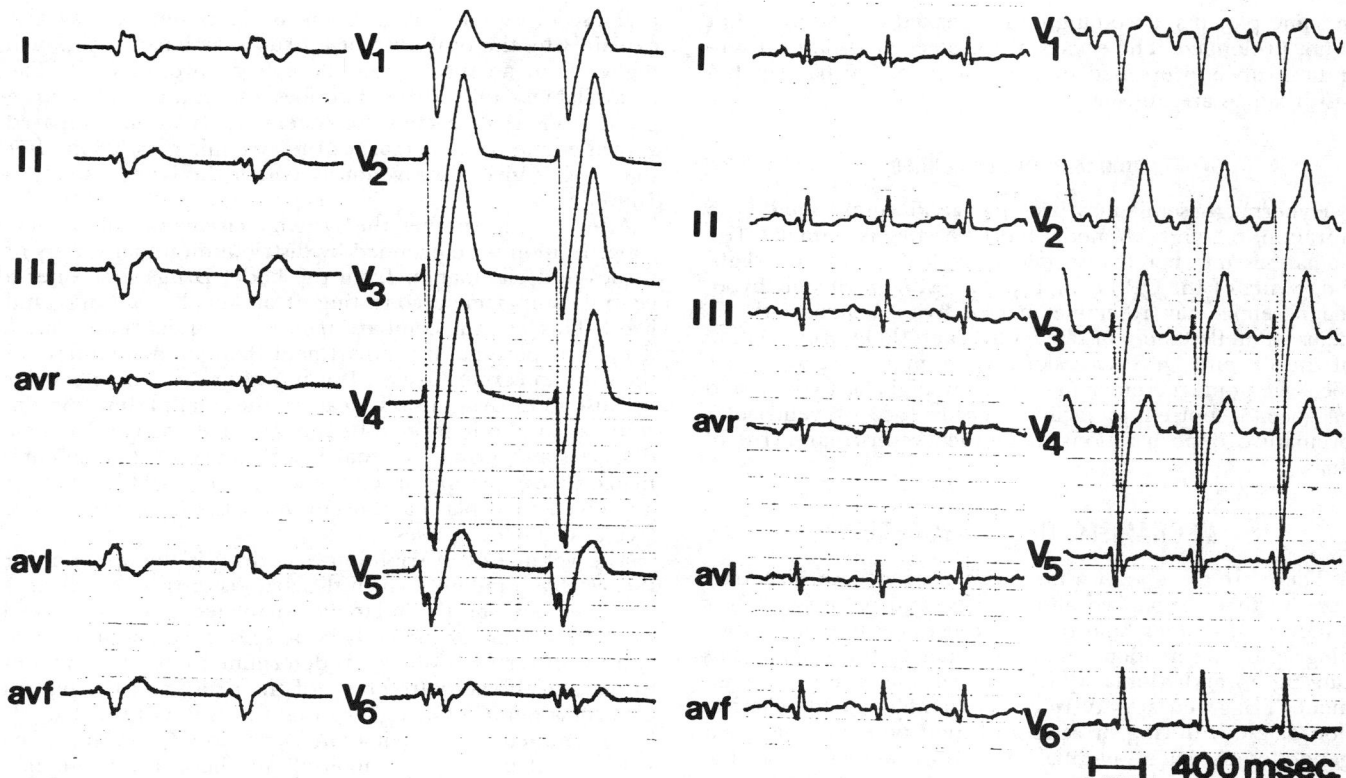

Figure 94–4. Example of advanced hyperkalemia. Atrial activity is not apparent in the ECG at the left. The QRS complex is markedly widened and the ST segment is absent. The QRS complex joins the T wave. The ECG at the right is for the same patient after treatment. (From Josephson ME, Wellens HJJ: How to Approach Complex Arrhythmias. Minneapolis, Medtronic, 1990. Used by permission of Medtronic, Inc.)

hyperkalemia. Acidosis prevents potassium from entering cells and results in elevated levels. Hyperkalemia can exacerbate the toxic (non–long QT) effects of quinidine-like drugs with resultant increases in QRS duration.

Minimal elevation of potassium can be treated with diuretics. Moderately severe elevations of potassium can be treated with 50 mL of 10% glucose solution intravenously and 10 U of regular insulin subcutaneously. This reduces the potassium level by 1 to 2 mEq/L and its effects can last for hours. Sodium bicarbonate intravenously (one or two ampules) can shift potassium into the cells. This effect occurs within 1 hour and also lasts for several hours, and it is particularly beneficial in patients with a metabolic acidosis. The most rapid way to reverse the effects of life-threatening hyperkalemia is to administer 10 to 30 mL of 10% calcium gluconate intravenously during a 1- to 5-minute period. However, none of these procedures removes potassium from the body. To accomplish this, cation-exchange resins can be given orally or as a retention enema. Hemodialysis and peritoneal dialysis can also be used to treat hyperkalemia and acidosis.

Hypokalemia

Hypokalemia increases the resting membrane potential (makes it more negative), hyperpolarizing the cell. This may result in spontaneous automatic activity and slowing of intracardiac conduction. Delayed repolarization (prolongation of the QT interval), ST segment depression, and decreased T wave amplitude may be seen on the surface ECG. Because these are nonspecific alterations in the ECG, it is usually prominent U waves that first signal hypokalemia. The etiology of the U wave is still not well understood. U waves are best seen in the midprecordial leads and are considered abnormal when they are either 1 mm in amplitude or taller than the T wave in the same lead. They are usually seen when the potassium level is less than 2.7 mEq/L. In advanced hypokalemia, the amplitude and duration of the P wave may be increased and the QRS duration may be prolonged, but these findings are rare.

Severe hypokalemia may cause paroxysmal atrial tachycardia with block, AV block (both first and second degree), AV dissociation, and ventricular fibrillation, as well as torsades de pointes. Hypokalemia increases the chance of digitalis toxic arrhythmias and may predispose to the drug-induced long QT syndrome (see later).

Hypercalcemia

Hypercalcemia decreases the QT interval by shortening the ST segment. When the calcium level reaches 16 mg/dL, T wave prolongation occurs and the QT interval actually becomes more normal; however, the ST segment is still short. The QRS complex rarely changes, although severe hypercalcemia may prolong the QRS duration slightly. With markedly elevated calcium levels, the U wave may increase. Arrhythmias are not commonly seen in patients with elevated calcium levels. AV block may occur, but arrhythmias such as sinus arrest, paroxysmal VT, and sudden death are usually the result of a sudden increase in serum calcium level, such as after an intravenous bolus.

Hypocalcemia

In hypocalcemia the QT interval is prolonged as a result of an increase in the ST segment. The T wave may change in some patients, becoming either peaked or flattened, but is not prolonged. The effects of elevated potassium concentration can be worsened by hypocalcemia. Cardiac rhythm disturbances are unusual.

Magnesium Abnormalities

Hypermagnesemia may prolong the PR interval and QRS duration. SA and AV nodal blocks occur occasionally. Hypomagnesemia may cause tall peaked T waves and slight narrowing of the QRS complex. The ECG in chronic hypomagnesemia may resemble that of hypokalemia, with ST depression, flattening of the T wave, and slight prolongation of the PR and QRS. Occasionally, prominent U waves are seen. Hypomagnesemia may worsen digitalis toxicity and has been reported to facilitate occurrence of ventricular premature depolarizations and other ventricular arrhythmias.

MECHANISMS OF TACHYCARDIAS

There are three known mechanisms of tachycardias; triggered activity, enhanced automaticity, and re-entry.[5, 10] It is important to understand the differences because electrocardiographic observations may give clues to the mechanisms causing an arrhythmia, which in turn may influence treatment. Triggered activity refers to spontaneous depolarization of a cell during or after an action potential that itself generates an action potential. It is always dependent on the presence of a previous action potential. It is thought to be secondary to abnormal calcium fluctuations across the cell membrane. At present, the only clinical arrhythmias for which there is evidence of triggered activity are some digitalis toxic arrhythmias and some types of ventricular tachycardia. Enhanced or abnormal automaticity refers to spontaneous depolarization occurring in partially depolarized cells that are not usually automatic, and it is not dependent on the membrane changes of the previous action potential. Both of these mechanisms are thought to occur as a result of abnormal ion fluxes across the cell membrane. Re-entry refers to a tachycardia in which a continuously circulating wave front of electrical activity occurs. Initiation of re-entry requires an area of unidirectional block and an area of slow conduction. The area of unidirectional block allows conduction to occur in one direction only, and the conduction slowing allows recovery of excitability in the area of the unidirectional block so that the impulse can conduct retrogradely, completing the "circuit." Re-entry may arise in cells with abnormalities of function or in tissue with normal electrophysiologic properties in which conduction is slowed because of abnormal intercellular coupling. This mechanism is commonly seen in patients with coronary artery disease and is the type of tachycardia most easily inducible in the electrophysiology laboratory.

PHARMACOKINETICS

The pharmacokinetics of a drug describe its disposition in the body over time.[3, 11] These properties include the processes of absorption, distribution, metabolism, and excretion. After a drug is given orally, its absorption depends on its physical characteristics as well as the characteristics of the gastrointestinal tract. Other drugs and disease states can also alter absorption time by such mechanisms as change in gastric pH and decrease in gastrointestinal motility as seen with diabetes.

Once a drug is absorbed, it may be metabolized before reaching the systemic circulation, either in the gut wall or the liver. This is called first-pass metabolism and limits the oral use of certain drugs (such as lidocaine). It may also explain why the oral dose of a drug may have to be much higher than an intravenous dose (e.g., propranolol). The bioavailability of a drug describes the amount of a drug given orally that reaches the systemic circulation compared with the amount that reaches the systemic circulation after the drug is given intravenously (when the bioavailability is 100%).

After a drug reaches the systemic circulation, its plasma concentration is determined by distribution into a variety of tissues and elimination from the body. Drugs first enter a central compartment consisting of plasma, heart, lungs, and liver. This central compartment is in equilibrium with a deeper or peripheral compartment that involves binding of the drug in certain tissues. It is important to remember this because most drug assays measure the total plasma concentration (i.e., both protein-bound and free drug). In some disease states (such as renal insufficiency or hypoalbuminemic states), plasma protein binding is lowered, so that for any given total plasma concentration the concentration of free available drug rises.

The volume of distribution of a drug is the apparent or theoretic volume into which the drug is distributed. It does not have any specific anatomic correlates and may exceed the total volume of the body because of tissue binding. The volume of distribution (V_d) is determined from the amount of drug in the body (the dose of the drug) and the plasma concentration (C_p) during a constant infusion of the drug. It is determined by the equation $V_d = dose/C_p$. Most antiarrhythmic drugs are metabolized in the liver. Some metabolites have active antiarrhythmic properties (such as 3-methoxy-O-desmethylencainide and O-desmethylencainide, metabolites of encainide), whereas others have detrimental and additive effects (such as the metabolites of lidocaine). For most antiarrhythmic drugs, elimination occurs by a first-order process in which a constant proportion of drug is removed per unit time. Some antiarrhythmic drugs, such as phenytoin and propafenone, have saturable clearance and elimination is described as a zero-order process; that is, a certain amount (instead of proportion) of drug is removed per unit time. Elimination is described by the elimination half-life ($t_{1/2}$), or the time it takes for the plasma concentration to decrease to half of its initial value. After four to five elimination half-lives about 90% of a drug is eliminated from the body. Because drug accumulation mirrors elimination, it also takes four to five elimination half-lives for a drug concentration to reach steady-state values. The elimination half-life is a function of both the volume of distribution and the clearance (Cl) and is described by the equation $t_{1/2} = 0.693 \times V_d/Cl$. Conditions that lower both the volume of distribution and clearance usually do not change the elimination half-life of a drug (e.g., lidocaine in the setting of heart failure). Diseases that decrease clearance alone increase elimination half-life (e.g., lidocaine in the setting of hepatic disease). When a drug is given intravenously the plasma concentration at steady state (C_{pss}) depends on the clearance and the infusion rate (I): $C_{pss} = I/Cl$. If the infusion rate is increased, the final plasma concentration is increased but the time required to reach steady state does not change. If a therapeutic plasma concentration is desired quickly, it is often necessary to give a loading dose followed by a constant infusion. The volume of distribution determines the plasma concentration achieved after a loading dose is given.

ANTIARRHYTHMIC AGENTS

Antiarrhythmic drugs have historically been separated according to the Vaughan Williams classification.[12, 13] This classification separates drugs according to their effects on cell membrane ionic channels and receptors. The antiarrhythmic drugs available today often overlap several classes, but this general classification remains helpful.

Class I drugs act by blocking the Na^+ or fast channel and depressing conduction. Class I drugs are further separated on the basis of their effects on repolarization and the kinetics of their interaction with the Na^+ channel. Class IA drugs (quinidine, procainamide, and disopyramide) prolong conduction and repolarization. As a result, they widen the QRS complex and prolong the QT interval. They dissociate from the Na^+ channel with an intermediate time course (5 to 10 seconds). Class IB drugs (lidocaine and its oral congeners, mexiletine and tocainide) shorten the action potential duration and rapidly dissociate from the Na^+ channel (less than 1 second). They have minimal effects on the ECG. Class IC drugs (encainide, flecainide, and propafenone) significantly affect depolarization by prolonging the QRS and slowly dissociate from the Na^+ channel (about 30 to 60 seconds). Their effects on the Na^+ channel are manifest on the ECG as prolongation of the QRS interval, usually with minimal effect on repolarization. These drugs also depress AV nodal function, prolonging the PR interval.

Class II drugs are the beta-blockers, of which propranolol is the prototype. Class III drugs primarily prolong repolarization and therefore prolong the QT interval. This class of drugs includes amiodarone; bretylium; an active metabolite of procainamide (N-acetylprocainamide); and sotalol. Many of these drugs also have other actions, such as the sodium channel–blocking effects of amiodarone and the beta-blocking effects of sotalol. Class IV drugs are the calcium channel blockers. They can also depress automaticity, in addition to depressing AV nodal function. They appear to have minimal electrophysiologic effects on atrial and ventricular muscle cells.

As stated earlier, this is a general classification of antiarrhythmic drugs. Although it is useful in describing the effects of drugs on cardiac cells, it does not necessarily describe the mechanisms responsible for the drug effects on clinical arrhythmias. Drug effects on the autonomic nervous system also influence the response to arrhythmias. Regardless of the mechanisms of drug action, therapy of the individual patient often remains empirical. Nonetheless, we can gain general information about antiarrhythmic agents from this classification and make an educated decision concerning which drugs are likely to be useful for the treatment of specific arrhythmias (Table 94–1).

NORMAL SINUS RHYTHM

The sinus node, located at the junction of the superior vena cava and the right atrium, is the primary pacemaker of the heart because its discharge rate exceeds that of other automatic tissue. It is sensitive to changes in autonomic nervous system tone; it increases the heart rate in response to sympathetic stimulation, as in fever, pain, or hypotension, and decreases the heart rate in response to increases in vagal tone, which predominates during sleep. Normal sinus rhythm is characterized by P waves that are usually upright in all limb leads except aV_R. The rate is by convention between 60 and 100 beats/min.

RHYTHM DISTURBANCES: BRADYARRHYTHMIAS AND CONDUCTION ABNORMALITIES

Sinus Node Dysfunction[14]

Sinus Bradycardia

Sinus bradycardia is diagnosed when the sinus rate slows to less than 60 beats/min. Patients with sinus bradycardia are usually asymptomatic, but inappropriate sinus bradycardia can cause fatigue, presyncope, and, rarely, syncope. Sinus bradycardia can be a normal and expected response in young adults, especially resting athletes. It is also a normal response during sleep, when heart rates of 35 to 40 beats/min can be observed. Sinus bradycardia can be a response to beta-blockers. When it occurs in response to calcium channel blockers, digitalis, or antiarrhythmic drugs such as sotalol, amiodarone, propafenone, or quinidine, it may indicate underlying sinus node dysfunction. It is a response to acute ventricular ischemia, acute hypertension, acidemia, hypercapnia, and hypothermia in critically ill patients. It can be seen in 10 to 15% of patients after myocardial infarction, especially after inferior infarction. Other less common causes include senile amyloidosis, hypothyroidism, advanced liver disease, typhoid fever, and brucellosis. It occurs during vasovagal syncope and is an isolated finding in the elderly. No treatment is needed unless a patient is symptomatic. When seen in the setting of acute myocardial infarction, unless associated with hemodynamic compromise, no therapy is needed. If cardiac output is inadequate, atropine (1.0 to 2.0 mg) can be given intravenously. Occasionally, symptomatic patients may need implantation of a permanent pacemaker or, in the acute setting, a temporary pacemaker.

Sinoatrial Exit Block

Intermittent failure of conduction of sinus impulses to the surrounding atrial tissue is called second-degree SA exit block or sinus exit block. It is caused by block at the junction of the SA node and atrium and is not due to a change in the sinus discharge rate. The surface ECG shows intermittent absence of P waves with a pause that is a multiple of the sinus or PP interval. Most instances of SA exit block are not associated with symptoms. Rarely a patient feels fatigue, dizziness, or presyncope, depending on the length of the pause. It occurs most often in elderly patients and is usually a chronic problem, not one that is seen in critically ill patients. It can be caused by acute myocarditis, acute myocardial infarction, excessive vagal stimulation, or fibrosis involving the atrium. Quinidine, procainamide, and digitalis have been reported to cause sinus exit block. If there are no associated symptoms, no treatment is necessary. If it is symptomatic, a pacemaker should be placed.

Sinus Arrest

Failure of spontaneous sinus impulse formation is called sinus arrest. There may be no atrial escape or ectopic atrial pacemaker rhythm, resulting in periods of ventricular asystole if an adequate lower escape pacemaker is not present. The electrocardiographic manifestation is a pause that is not a multiple of the PP interval. The presence of symptoms depends on the duration of the pause. Patients may have fatigue, presyncope, and syncope. Digitalis, beta-blockers, and calcium channel blockers can cause sinus arrest. Ischemia and intrinsic conduction system disease are also causes. If the patient continues to be symptomatic after reversible causes are treated, pacemaker placement should be considered.

Sick Sinus Syndrome

Sick sinus syndrome (also known as tachycardia-bradycardia syndrome) is a rhythm that consists of periods of bradycardia alternating with periods of tachycardia. These periods are often interspersed with normal sinus rhythm. The tachycardia is usually an atrial tachycardia, often paroxysmal atrial fibrillation or flutter. The bradycardia can be a symptomatic

TABLE 94–1

CHARACTERISTICS OF CLASSES OF ANTIARRHYTHMIC AGENTS*

Classification	Effects on ECG	Elimination Half-Life	Route of Excretion	Initial Dose	Usual Therapeutic Level	Disease States Requiring Reduction	Drug Interactions	Miscellaneous
I. Sodium channel blockers								
I-A. Quinidine	↑ QT ↑ QRS	4–17 h	Hepatic	Quinidine sulfate 200 mg q 6 h PO	2–5 µg/mL	Hepatic disease	Digoxin; cimetidine; amiodarone; may alter warfarin requirements	Contraindicated with long QT, ↓K+, ↓Mg2+, myasthenia gravis
I-A. Procainamide	↑ QT ↑ QRS	2–5 h	Hepatic and renal (60%)	Regular: 500–1200 mg q 4 h PO	4–10 µg/mL	Renal disease	Amiodarone	Contraindicated with long QT, ↓Mg2+, myasthenia gravis
I-A. Disopyramide	↑ QT ↑ QRS	6–15 h	Hepatic and renal (varied)	150 q 6–8 h PO	2–5 µg/mL	Renal disease, hepatic disease	May ↑ warfarin, beta-blockers; verapamil	Contraindicated with long QT, ↓Mg2+, prostatism, glaucoma, LV dysfunction
I-B. Lidocaine	Slight ↓ QT	1–2 h	Hepatic	Load with 75/50/50/50 mg q 5 min, then 1–4 mg/min IV	1.5–5 µg/mL	LV dysfunction, hepatic disease	Beta-blockers, norepinephrine ↓ clearance; additive CNS toxicity with tocanide and mexiletine	
I-B. Tocanide		9–18 h	Hepatic and renal (40%)	200–400 mg q 8 h PO	3–10 µg/mL	Renal disease	Care with lidocaine	Agranulocytosis and pulmonary fibrosis in <5%; rashes
I-B. Mexiletine		8–15 h	Hepatic	150 mg t.i.d. PO		Hepatic disease	Care with lidocaine; amiodarone will ↓ clearance	CNS toxicity
I-C. Flecainide	↑ PR ↑ QRS	7–23 h	Hepatic and renal (35%)	50–100 q 12 h PO	0.2–1.0 µg/mL	Renal disease	Beta-blockers and calcium channel blockers ↑ digoxin by 25%	LV dysfunction, conduction system disturbance, NSVT in CAD
I-C. Encainide	↑ PR ↑ QRS	2–3 h extensive metabolizers; 8–12 h poor metabolizers	Hepatic	25 mg q 8 h PO		Renal disease (secondary to metabolites)		NSVT in CAD, LV dysfunction
I-C. Propafenone	↑ PR ↑ QRS	Extensive metabolizers 1–9 h; poor metabolizers 10–32 h	Hepatic	150 mg q 8 h PO		Hepatic disease	Beta-blockers and calcium channel blockers; digoxin ↑ by 30–85%; ↑ warfarin; cimetidine ↓ metabolism	LV dysfunction; bronchospasm
Beta-blockers:								
II. Propranolol	± ↑ PR	3–4 h	Hepatic	20 mg q 6 h PO				Not cardioselective, membrane stabilizing activity
II. Esmolol		9 min	RBC esterase	500 µg/kg, then 50 µg/kg/min IV				Cardioselective; extremely short half-life
II. Metoprolol		3–7 h	Hepatic	100 mg b.i.d. PO, 5 mg IV				Cardioselective; membrane stabilizing activity
III. Amiodarone	↑ QT ± ↑ PR ↑ QRS ↓ sinus rate	8–107 d	Hepatic	Load—10 g in first week, then 200–600 mg/d PO	?1–2.5 mg/ml	Hepatic disease	↑ Digoxin; ↑ warfarin; antiarrhythmic agents	Pre-existing pulmonary disease; conduction system disease; neurotoxcity; hepatic, thyroid toxicity

TABLE 94–1

CHARACTERISTICS OF CLASSES OF ANTIARRHYTHMIC AGENTS* Continued

Classification	Effects on ECG	Elimination Half-Life	Route of Excretion	Initial Dose	Usual Therapeutic Level	Disease States Requiring Reduction	Drug Interactions	Miscellaneous
III. Sotalol	↑ QT	6–8 h	Renal	80 mg b.i.d. PO		Renal disease	Potentiate beta-blockers	Contraindicated with long QT; asthma, LV dysfunction
IV. Calcium channel blockers: verapamil, diltiazem	± ↑ PR	3–7 h	Hepatic	80 mg PO q 8 h or 2.5–15 mg IV (verapamil); 30 mg q 8 h PO (diltiazem)		Hepatic disease	Digoxin will ↑ levels	Increase risk in WPW with atrial fibrillation or LV dysfunction
Digoxin	Varies	1–2 d	Renal	Load 0.25 mg × 4 in 24 h PO	0.5–2.0 µg/mL	Renal disease	↑ with quinidine or amiodarone	Increases risk in WPW with atrial fibrillation; ↑ Ca²⁺, ↓ Mg²⁺
Adenosine	—	<10 s	Taken up by RBCs and vascular endothelial cells	6–12 mg IV	—	—	Decreased effect with theophylline and carbamazepine; effect potentiated by dipyridamole	Transient hypotension, transient heart block

*CNS = central nervous system; LV = left ventricle; NSVT = nonsustained ventricular tachycardia; CAD = coronary artery disease; RBC = red blood cell; WPW = Wolff-Parkinson-White syndrome; ↑ = increases, ↓ = decreases.

sinus pause at the end of the tachycardia, sinus bradycardia, SA block, or sinus arrest. This rhythm disturbance results from overdrive suppression of the sinus node. The atrial tachycardia suppresses the sinus node and frequently the AV node in an exaggeration of the normal response. Symptoms are usually related to hemodynamic compromise, which depends on the rapidity of the ventricular response to the tachycardia, the duration of pauses, and the degree of myocardial dysfunction. Symptoms include dizziness, confusion, fatigue, presyncope, congestive heart failure, and syncope. It is often necessary to treat the tachycardia with digitalis to slow the ventricular response. This medication may exacerbate the bradycardia, and a permanent pacemaker may be needed.

Evaluation of Suspected Sinus Node Dysfunction

It is critical to correlate symptoms with electrocardiographic evidence of sinus node dysfunction. Most patients with intermittent dropped (or absent) P waves have no associated symptoms. To be sure that a treatment (such as pacemaker placement) will benefit the patient, it is important that symptoms of dizziness, presyncope, or even syncope correlate temporally with the periods of bradycardia, dropped P waves, and asystole. Even electrophysiologic studies are not exceptionally helpful for evaluation of sinus node dysfunction. Asymptomatic patients may have an abnormal electrophysiologic study, and symptomatic patients may not have electrophysiologic evidence of sinus node dysfunction. Therefore, documentation of symptoms associated with electrocardiographic abnormalities becomes imperative for good care of the patient. In selected patients, invasive electrophysiologic study may be useful to determine whether sinus node dysfunction exists.

ATRIOVENTRICULAR CONDUCTION BLOCK

With a patient having AV conduction block, it is important to be able to determine the site of conduction disturbance because this determines (1) the probability that a subsidiary

pacemaker (escape rhythm) distal to the site of block will result in a hemodynamically stable rhythm and (2) the risk of progression to complete heart block. Block may occur at any level in the specialized conduction system, from the AV node to the His bundle and bundle branches. Examination of the standard ECG often gives clues to the site of block.

The AV node lies just beneath the right atrial endocardium, superior to the coronary sinus ostium. It is highly sensitive to variations in autonomic tone: sympathetic stimulation accelerates conduction and abbreviates refractoriness, and vagal stimulation has opposite effects. Other factors that may alter AV nodal function include myocardial ischemia, chronic hypertension, digitalis intoxication, beta-blockers and calcium channel blockers, viral myocarditis, infectious mononucleosis, Lyme disease, acute rheumatic fever, sarcoidosis, amyloidosis, neoplasms (cardiac mesotheliomas), aortic stenosis, and mitral stenosis. AV nodal block may also be congenital.

The bundle of His connects to the distal part of the AV node, forming the nonbranching portion as it penetrates the membranous septum. The bundle branches begin at the superior margin of the muscular interventricular septum. The cells of the left bundle branch continue downward as a continuous sheet into the septum beneath the noncoronary aortic cusp, and the right bundle branch continues intramyocardially as an unbranched extension down the right side of the intraventricular septum to the apex of the right ventricle. The Purkinje fibers connect at the ends of the bundle branches, form an interweaving network on the endocardial surface of both ventricles, and transmit the cardiac impulse almost simultaneously to the right and left ventricular endocardium. The most frequent causes of block in the His bundle and the distal Purkinje network are coronary artery disease and idiopathic degenerative processes.

First-Degree Atrioventricular Block

First-degree AV block (prolonged AV conduction) is really a misnomer, because AV conduction time is slowed but not

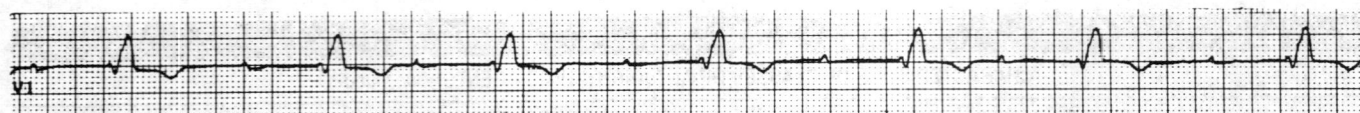

Figure 94–5. Marked sinus bradycardia in association with severe prolongation of the PR interval.

blocked. It is diagnosed when the PR interval is greater than 200 ms (Fig. 94–5). This most often reflects conduction delay in the AV node. In these cases, the QRS duration is usually normal. Less commonly, a long PR interval reflects conduction delay in the His-Purkinje system, and in this case the QRS duration is usually prolonged. Drugs such as digitalis, beta-blockers, and calcium channel blockers may prolong the PR interval, but more frequently this is secondary to intrinsic conduction system disease or hypertension or is seen with increased age. Prolongation of the PR interval is almost never associated with symptoms and, when it occurs in isolation, does not warrant further investigation or therapy. Patients with active endocarditis involving the aortic or mitral valves may develop prolongation of the PR interval as a result of abscess formation in the interventricular system. In these patients, it may antedate progression to higher grades of AV block.

Second-Degree Atrioventricular Block

Second-degree AV block is diagnosed when atrial impulses are blocked when the conduction system should not be refractory. Two kinds are defined: type I (Mobitz's I or Wenckebach's block) and type II (Mobitz's II). Type I block is recognized by progressive prolongation of the PR interval with subsequent shortening of the RR interval until a P wave is not conducted (Fig. 94–6). The hallmark on the ECG is that the conducted beat after the nonconducted P wave has a shorter PR interval than the one conducted before the pause. This pause is not fully compensatory, less than two normal sinus intervals. Any number of conducted impulses may precede the blocked impulse, and often not every PR interval increases before the block. Type I AV block may occur anywhere in the conduction system but usually reflects conduction system disease in the AV node. Therefore, even if this disease progresses to complete conduction block, it is likely to be associated with an escape pacemaker in the His bundle having a rate adequate to support the circulation. It is rare to have significant symptoms associated with this rhythm. Digitalis, beta-blockers, and calcium channel blockers can be a cause of type I AV nodal block. It is seen in ischemic heart disease, especially inferior myocardial infarction. This block can also be caused by heightened vagal tone, such as that seen in resting athletes, and it can be idiopathic in origin. Usually no treatment is necessary.

Type II AV block is most often a reflection of block in the His bundle or lower in the conduction system. This rhythm is more likely to progress to complete heart block, and if this occurs it is associated with a much less stable escape pacemaker having a rate inadequate to support the circulation. The ECG shows a sudden nonconducted P wave not associated with prior prolongation of the PR interval or any alteration in RR intervals (Fig. 94–7). This rhythm is often asymptomatic but is a harbinger of severe conduction system disease. Patients may have intermittent fatigue and lightheadedness. Type II AV block can be caused by ischemia, especially anteroseptal myocardial infarction. Type II block is rarely due to a reversible cause, such as drugs (digitalis, beta-blockers, and calcium channel blockers). Because of the high incidence of progression to complete heart block, this type of AV block is an indication for pacemaker placement. If 2:1 AV block is present on the ECG it is not possible to tell whether it is due to type I or II, and an invasive His bundle catheter evaluation may be needed to determine the site of block.

Complete Heart Block

The terms complete heart block and AV dissociation have been used interchangeably, but the rhythms are different. Complete, or third-degree, heart block indicates that there is no relationship between the atria and the ventricles. When block occurs distal to the His bundle or in the Purkinje system, it is associated with a wide QRS escape complex (Fig. 94–8), whereas block in the AV node or at the level of the His bundle is usually associated with a narrow QRS complex. AV dissociation (see Fig. 94–15) refers to a rhythm in which there is no apparent interaction between the atrium and the ventricle, but complete AV block in some cases may not be determined either because the atrial and ventricular rates are similar or because there is an accelerated subsidiary pacemaker rhythm (e.g., AV junctional rhythm) with a rate higher than that of the sinus. The condition in which the atrial and ventricular rates are almost identical but are not related to each other is called isorhythmic dissociation. Patients with this spectrum of rhythm disturbances are often symptomatic with dizziness, fatigue, presyncope, or syncope. Complete AV block at the AV node level may be caused by digitalis, beta-blockers, antiarrhythmic drugs, and calcium channel blockers. It can also occur during acute inferior or anterior myocardial infarction. Infiltrative (amyloid, sarcoid, scleroderma) conduction system diseases can also cause complete or advanced heart block, as can surgery, electrolyte disturbances, endocarditis, tumors, Chagas' disease, rheumatoid nodules, calcific aortic stenosis, and myxedema. If a patient is symptomatic, pacemaker placement is indicated after correction of reversible causes.

Complete AV block can also be a congenital anomaly. In

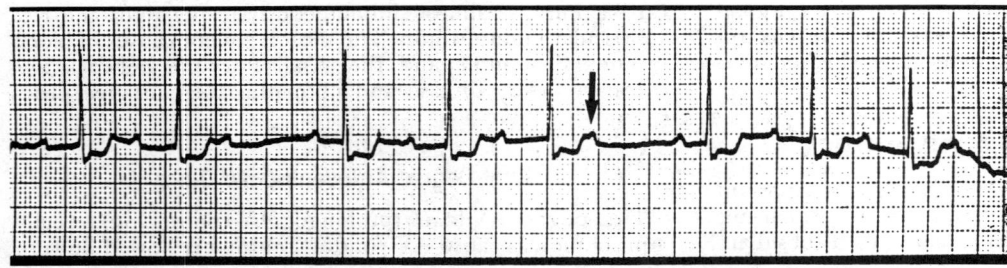

Figure 94–6. Type I (Wenckebach's) second-degree AV block. Notice gradual prolongation of the PR interval followed by a nonconducted P wave (*arrow*). The QRS complex is of normal duration. The block is at the AV nodal level.

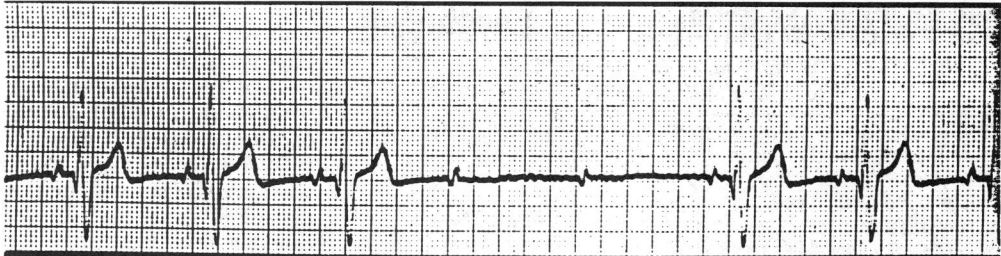

Figure 94-7. Type II second-degree heart block. The fourth and fifth P waves failed to conduct to the ventricles. The conducted PR intervals are constant and normal. Note that the QRS complex is abnormally wide.

these patients, block occurs at the level of the AV node and is associated with a narrow complex junctional rhythm. It is often found fortuitously on the ECG, and asymptomatic patients require no treatment.

PACEMAKERS

Temporary Pacemakers

There are times in the intensive care unit setting when acute severe symptomatic bradyarrhythmias arise and an emergent pacemaker is needed but takes time to place.[15–17] A Zoll external transthoracic cardiac pacing system can be positioned on the chest wall in emergency situations before insertion of a temporary pacing lead. This can be lifesaving but, because of the high output needed for adequate pacing, can also be uncomfortable if skeletal muscle stimulation occurs. It is also possible under these circumstances to use atropine, 1.0 to 2.0 mg intravenously, to increase the heart rate transiently. Low-dose atropine (less than 0.5 mg) is vagomimetic and can significantly slow the heart rate. Isoproterenol at 0.5 to 4 μg/mL intravenously can also be helpful but it is not recommended for patients with coronary artery disease. Both agents increase the heart rate in patients with sinus bradycardia or block at the AV nodal level.

Temporary pacemakers can be used either before permanent pacemaker placement or until reversible problems such as acute ischemia or drug toxicity are treated (see Table 94–2 for specific indications during acute myocardial infarction). The pacing lead is inserted transvenously, usually positioned at the right ventricular apex, and attached to an external generator.

Permanent Pacing

Potential pacemaker patients are divided into three groups according to the necessity for pacemaker placement.[18] Class I includes those who have indications for which there is general agreement that a pacemaker should be placed; class II includes those who have indications for which under certain circumstances placement might be appropriate; class III includes those whose situations are not thought to warrant a pacemaker (Table 94–3). Permanent pacemakers are placed under sterile conditions by a cardiologist or surgeon.

Leads are inserted transvenously (via the subclavian or cephalic vein), positioned in either the right ventricular apex alone (for single-chamber devices) or in the right ventricular apex and right atrial appendage (for dual-chamber devices). The leads are connected to a pulse generator, which is placed in a subcutaneous pocket below the clavicle. Epicardial leads are used when the transvenous approach cannot be used or when the chest is already open, such as during cardiac surgery.

Each patient who has had a permanent pacemaker placed should carry a card with the brand name of the pacemaker, the kind of generator (single or dual chamber), the magnet rate of the pacemaker, and an 800 telephone number with which to call the company with any questions. Each pacemaker company has its own interrogation devices and most hospitals should have several different companies' interrogators.

An Intersociety Commission for Heart Disease code describes the type of pacemaker and its function. The first letter of the code indicates the chamber that is paced: V for ventricular pacing, A for atrial pacing, and D for both chambers. The second letter represents the chamber sensed; it may be V, A, or D, as well as O for none. The third letter indicates whether the pacemaker is inhibited (I), triggered (T), or both (D) when an electrical event occurs; O means that it is asynchronous. The fourth and fifth letters refer to the pacemaker's ability to be programmed (e.g., with rate responsiveness) and whether it has antitachycardia pacing capabilities. For example, VVI means that a pacemaker is capable of ventricular pacing and ventricular sensing and is inhibited when the pacemaker senses an intrinsic QRS. DDDR mode means both atrial and ventricular pacing; both atrial and ventricular sensing; that the appropriate chamber will be inhibited when the P or QRS, respectively, is sensed; and that the pacemaker has rate-responsive capabilities.

A magnet placed over a pacemaker generator turns the pacemaker into asynchronous mode, VOO or DOO. The pacemaker paces the chamber(s) it is programmed to pace but does not sense intrinsic activity. If the patient does not remember what brand of pacemaker he or she has, an overpenetrated x-ray film of the generator almost always shows a visible code that designates the manufacturer.

A frequent problem with dual-chamber pacemakers is pacemaker-mediated tachycardia in patients who have intact

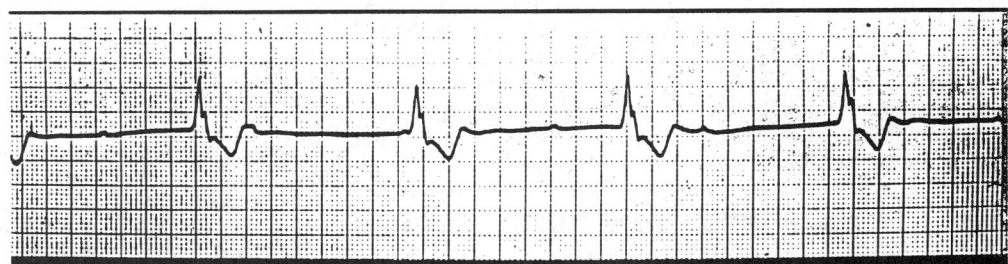

Figure 94–8. Complete heart block. The QRS complex is abnormally wide, suggesting that the level of block is below the AV node.

TABLE 94-2

INDICATIONS FOR TEMPORARY PACING IN THE SETTING OF ACUTE MYOCARDIAL INFARCTION

Class I: Conditions for which there is general agreement that pacemakers should be used
 Asystole
 Complete heart block
 New right bundle branch block + new left anterior or new left posterior fascicular block
 Left bundle branch block
 Type II second-degree AV block
 Symptomatic bradycardia not responsive to atropine

Consider in
 Type I second-degree AV block with associated hypotension not responsive to atropine
 Sinus bradycardia with hypotension not responsive to atropine
 Recurrent sinus pauses not responsive to atropine
 Left bundle branch block with first-degree AV block of unknown duration
 Bifascicular block of unknown duration

ventriculoatrial conduction. When VA conduction is present, retrograde atrial activation occurs after ventricular pacing, and this atrial depolarization may be sensed by the pacemaker. This leads to triggering of ventricular pacing and retrograde conduction to the atria, resulting in an endless loop configuration tachycardia. This tachycardia occurs at the upper rate limit at which the pacemaker is set. It can be terminated by placing a magnet over the pacemaker and treated by reprogramming (increasing) the atrial refractory period so that it exceeds the retrograde ventriculoatrial conduction time.

Alterations in electrolytes that are seen in the intensive care setting, such as hyperkalemia, can cause significant problems with pacemakers. The stimulation threshold can be increased so that the pacemaker no longer paces adequately, or malsensing can occur so that T waves are inappropriately sensed (inhibiting the pacemaker). Inappropriate pacing can trigger VT or ventricular fibrillation, especially during acute myocardial ischemia.

If external cardioversion or defibrillation is necessary in a patient with a permanent pacemaker, positioning of the defibrillation paddles should be perpendicular to the pacemaker generator-lead axis to minimize current flow through the pacemaker generator.

SUPRAVENTRICULAR TACHYARRHYTHMIAS
Sinus Tachycardia

Sinus tachycardia is diagnosed when the sinus rate exceeds 100 beats/min. Sinus tachycardia is characterized by a gradual (as opposed to abrupt) onset and termination. Carotid sinus massage during sinus tachycardia causes slight slowing but not termination. Often the only symptom is palpitations, but more commonly this rhythm is asymptomatic. Sinus tachycardia is usually a physiologic response to such things as dehydration, fever, hyperthyroidism, pain, anxiety, exercise, caffeine, hypotension, congestive heart failure, and hypoxemia. The treatment consists of alleviating underlying causes. It should not be treated primarily, except perhaps to lower myocardial oxygen demand during myocardial infarction or unstable angina.

Atrial Premature Depolarizations

Atrial premature depolarizations (APDs) are early P waves, usually with conducted QRS complexes, that have a mor-

phology that can be similar to that seen during sinus rhythm. The P waves are often visible as a distortion in the T wave. Late diastolic APDs are conducted to the ventricle with a normal PR interval and QRS. Earlier ones are blocked or conducted with a prolonged PR interval (Fig. 94-9) or occasionally with a wide QRS (see Fig. 94-2A). APDs are followed by a pause before returning to normal sinus rhythm. The sum of the pre- and postsystolic PP intervals is usually less than the sum of two sinus PP intervals. This is called a less than fully compensatory pause. This can be helpful in differentiating wide complex beats from ventricular premature depolarizations, in which the pause is usually equal to the sum of two PP intervals (a compensatory pause)

TABLE 94-3

INDICATIONS FOR PERMANENT PACEMAKER PLACEMENT

Class I: Conditions for which there is general agreement that permanent pacemakers should be implanted
 Complete heart block, permanent or intermittent with
  Symptomatic bradycardia
  Congestive heart failure
  Asystole for 3.0 s or longer
 Confusion states that clear with pacing
 Second-degree AV block with symptomatic bradycardia
 Atrial fibrillation, atrial flutter with complete heart block, bradycardia
 After myocardial infarction: persistent advanced second-degree AV block or complete heart block
 Bifascicular block with
  Intermittent complete heart block with symptomatic bradycardia
  Intermittent type II second-degree AV block with symptoms
 Sinus node dysfunction with symptomatic bradycardia
 Recurrent syncope associated with clear events provoked by carotid sinus stimulation and when carotid sinus massage produces at least 3 s of asystole

Class II: Conditions for which permanent pacemakers are frequently used but there is divergence of opinion about the need for their insertion
 Asymptomatic complete heart block with ventricular rates ≥ 40 beats/min
 Asymptomatic type II second-degree AV block
 Asymptomatic type I second-degree AV block at intra-His or infra-His level
 After myocardial infarction:
  First-degree AV block in presence of bundle branch block not documented previously
  Transient advanced AV block and associated bundle branch block
 Bifascicular or trifascicular block with
  Intermittent type II second-degree AV block without symptoms
  Syncope that is not proved to be due to complete heart block
  Pacing-induced infra-His block
 Sinus node dysfunction occurring spontaneously or secondary to drugs with resulting heart rates less than 40 beats/min associated with symptoms
 Recurrent syncope without clear, provocative events and with a hypersensitive cardioinhibitory response

Class III: Conditions for which there is general agreement that a pacemaker would be unnecessary
 First-degree AV block
 Asymptomatic type I second-degree AV block at the AV nodal level
 Transient AV conduction disturbances in the absence of intraventricular conduction defects
 Fascicular blocks with
  No AV block or symptoms
  First-degree AV block with symptoms
 Sinus node dysfunction with no symptoms

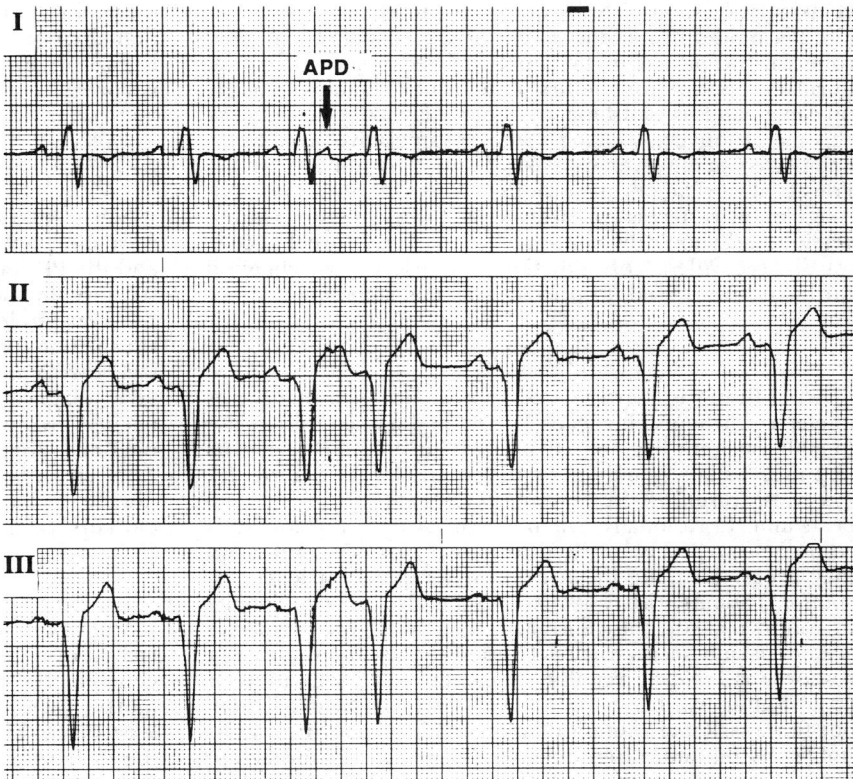

Figure 94–9. Example of atrial premature depolarization (APD). Simultaneous tracings of electrocardiographic leads I, II, III. The fourth P wave is premature (APD). Note that the PR interval of the premature complex is markedly prolonged compared with the PR intervals after the sinus P waves.

unless retrograde conduction to the atria occurs. Symptoms are rare but when they occur are usually palpitations. APDs can be idiopathic, but occasionally caffeine, alcohol, tobacco, and adrenergic stimulants can cause them. Acute decompensation secondary to pulmonary disease is a cause frequently seen in the intensive care unit. Rarely is treatment necessary.

Atrial Fibrillation

Atrial fibrillation occurs frequently in critically ill patients. Atrial fibrillation is characterized by an irregularly irregular ventricular response as a result of disorganized atrial activity. No P waves are visible on the ECG; rarely atrial deflections are visible, varying between 350 and 600 beats/min. The ventricular response can be rapid, although concealed conduction into the AV node usually slows the ventricular response to 100 to 160 beats/min. It can be paroxysmal or persistent. Normally on the ECG there is a wavy baseline with irregular narrow QRS complexes, but aberrant wide complex beats may be present (see Fig. 94–2B). This aberrance results from Ashman's phenomenon, or long-short QRS intervals (discussed earlier). The causes of atrial fibrillation are varied and often treatable. They include acute myocardial infarction, hyperthyroidism, pulmonary embolism, chronic obstructive pulmonary disease, hypertension, atrial septal defect, rheumatic heart disease, mitral valve disease, alcohol binges, cardiomyopathy, metabolic derangements, hemodynamic changes, exercise, acute pericarditis, and the early period after heart surgery. Lone atrial fibrillation is a term used to describe the occurrence of the arrhythmia in patients without recognizable structural heart disease. Atrial fibrillation can be uncomfortable when it occurs suddenly, causing dizziness, presyncope, palpitations, and syncope. If it occurs in the setting of poor left ventricular function, the loss of atrial systole in combination with a high rate can cause significant hemodynamic compromise. The

sudden onset of the arrhythmia and the rapid ventricular response can cause hemodynamic collapse. Hemodynamic collapse can occur for the same reason in patients with diastolic dysfunction resulting from hypertensive heart disease, aortic stenosis, or hypertrophic cardiomyopathy. Patients with Wolff-Parkinson-White (WPW) syndrome frequently develop atrial fibrillation. The presence of an AV bypass tract, which ordinarily lacks decremental conduction properties, allows the development of extremely rapid ventricular responses that can degenerate into ventricular fibrillation.[19] Occasionally, after a paroxysm of atrial fibrillation, a pause occurs that can be symptomatic. Systemic emboli can result from this rhythm; this is more commonly seen in patients with rheumatic mitral valve disease.

If a patient with atrial fibrillation of new onset is hemodynamically unstable, cardioversion using at least 100 J should be performed after adequate sedation or anesthesia. Verapamil and beta-blockers can slow the ventricular response acutely but do not restore sinus rhythm. The onset of action of digoxin is too slow for it to be used in patients who require immediate control of the ventricular response. However, digoxin therapy may be instituted early to help with chronic control of the ventricular response. Digoxin does not convert atrial fibrillation to sinus rhythm, nor does it prevent recurrences. Digoxin or verapamil should not be administered if there is any possibility of WPW syndrome. Both medications may decrease refractoriness of accessory pathways, precipitating ventricular fibrillation. After administration of AV nodal blocking agents, intravenous procainamide can safely convert atrial fibrillation to sinus rhythm in the intensive care setting (12 to 15 mg/kg as a loading dose at 25 to 50 mg/min, watching carefully for hypotension). It is important to rule out reversible causes of atrial fibrillation such as acute pulmonary diseases or heart failure. For long-term treatment, digitalis, beta-adrenergic blocking agents, verapamil, or diltiazem should be given to control ventricular response. Subsequently, quinidine, procainamide, flecainide, propafenone, encainide, sotalol, or amiodarone can be added to help prevent recurrences. If atrial fibrillation occurs for the first time, is not hemodynamically unstable, and is self-limited, there may be no need for chronic prophylaxis. Patients with postoperative atrial fibrillation are usually given 6 weeks of antiarrhythmic therapy.[20] For atrial fibrillation of more than 2 weeks' duration, anticoagulation is necessary for at least 2 weeks before cardioversion and should be continued for at least 2 weeks afterward, regardless of whether electrical or chemical cardioversion is used, to prevent systemic emboli.

Atrial Flutter

Atrial flutter is characterized by sawtooth or flutter waves in electrocardiographic leads II, III, and aV$_F$ at a rate close to 300 beats/min (Fig. 94–10; also see Fig. 94–28). The atrial impulses usually conduct to the ventricles at 2:1 or 4:1 intervals, resulting in a ventricular rate of 75 or 150 beats/min. Occasionally, when the atrial rate has slowed in response to type I antiarrhythmic drugs, 1:1 AV conduction may occur, resulting in an extremely rapid ventricular response. Patients with WPW syndrome also have the ability to conduct 1:1 to the ventricles. Aberrant QRS complexes are not usually seen with atrial flutter because the ventricular response is typically regular. The causes and symptoms of atrial flutter can be the same as those of atrial fibrillation, but flutter is less common than atrial fibrillation. It is a less stable rhythm and often degenerates into atrial fibrillation. Underlying heart disease is more common in patients with atrial flutter than in patients with atrial fibrillation. Because the contribution of the atrial systole is still present to some degree, hemodynamic compromise does not occur as readily. Symptoms are usually related to the ventricular rate. It is often difficult to decrease the ventricular rate below 150 beats/min (2:1 AV block) in patients with atrial flutter, and persistent administration of AV nodal blocking agents may result in drug toxicity before the ventricular rate slows significantly. Thus, the preferred therapy for atrial flutter is cardioversion, and success is often obtained with only 10 to 50 J. Atrial flutter can also be converted to sinus rhythm by overdrive atrial pacing at 115 to 130% of the atrial flutter rate (see Fig. 94–28). Carotid sinus massage may transiently slow the ventricular response but does not terminate the arrhythmia. Antiarrhythmic drugs such as quinidine, procainamide, and disopyramide can be used after adequate digitalization. This latter is extremely important because it is possible for AV conduction to improve as the atrial rate is slowed by antiarrhythmic agents, resulting in a paradoxical increase in ventricular rate.

Sinus Node Re-Entrant Tachycardia

Sinus node re-entry is characterized by a normal sinus P wave morphology. The rate is between 80 and 200 beats/min and the PR interval is related to the rate of the tachycardia. Because the mechanism of this tachycardia is re-entry within the sinus node, it has a sudden onset and termination and is usually initiated by APDs. Vagal stimulation can slow the tachycardia and then cause abrupt termination. For a definitive diagnosis, an invasive electrophysiologic study is needed. Symptoms associated with this tachycardia are palpitations, angina, shortness of breath, and rarely syncope. This rhythm is often associated with underlying cardiac disease and can be treated when symptomatic with beta-blockers, calcium channel blockers, or digitalis.

Multifocal Atrial Tachycardia

Multifocal atrial tachycardia, also known as chaotic atrial tachycardia, is a supraventricular arrhythmia with rates between 100 and 130 beats/min that has varied P wave morphology and PR intervals.[21] By definition there are at least three different P waves and PR intervals. Because of the different PR intervals, the ventricular rhythm appears irregular or chaotic (Fig. 94–11). This rhythm is a supraventricular arrhythmia frequently seen in intensive care settings. This rhythm disturbance is most commonly caused by hypoxia and theophylline therapy, usually in patients with pulmonary disease. It is also seen in older patients with chronic illnesses and can degenerate into atrial fibrillation. A rare cause of this arrhythmia is digitalis toxicity. Primary treatment should be addressed toward the underlying causes, although calcium channel blockers may suppress the arrhythmia. Antiarrhythmic agents are usually ineffective.

Atrial Tachycardias

Atrial tachycardia is a supraventricular arrhythmia with a P wave that precedes each QRS, a definable PR interval, but a P wave morphology different from the sinus P wave

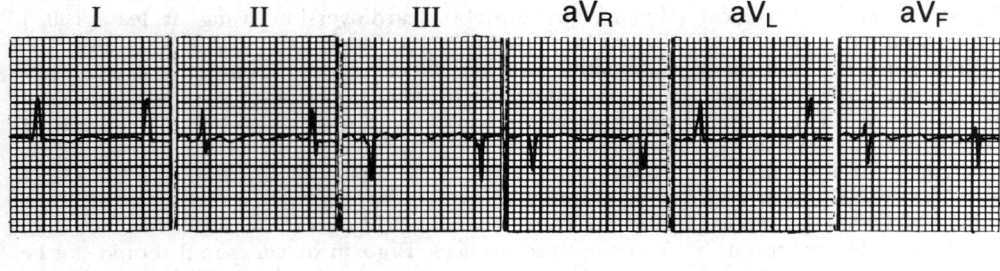

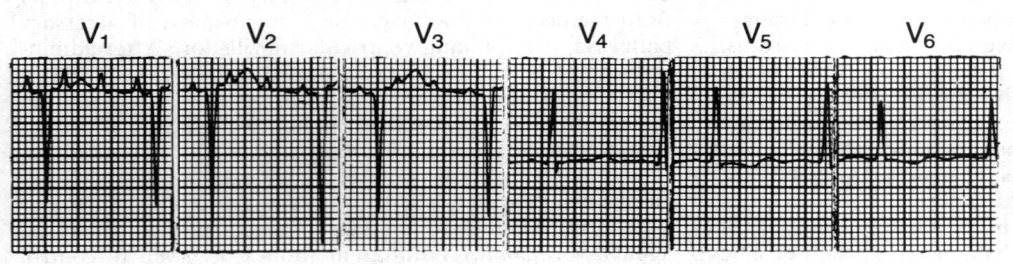

Figure 94–10. Classic atrial flutter. The atrial rate is approximately 300 beats/min. Note that the classic sawtooth appearance is present only in leads II, III, and aV$_F$; atrial activity is upright in leads V$_1$ through V$_3$. This is an unusual example because 3:1 AV block is present, resulting in a ventricular rate slightly less than 100 beats/min.

LEAD I

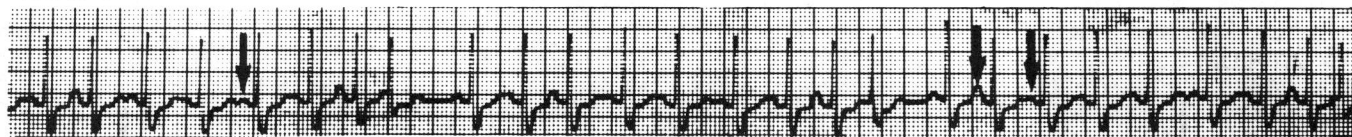

Figure 94–11. Multifocal atrial tachycardia. The arrows point to three different P wave morphologies. Because of the irregular atrial rate the PR intervals after the different P waves vary, depending on the morphology and degree of prematurity of the P wave.

morphology.[22] The mechanism of this tachycardia may be abnormal automaticity or re-entry within the atrium. An atrial focus other than the sinus node becomes the fastest "pacemaker" of the heart and sets the rate for the rest of the heart. The onset of automatic atrial tachycardia is characterized by gradual acceleration over the first few complexes (Fig. 94–12). The first P wave of the tachycardia is identical with the ensuing P waves and different from those in sinus rhythm. In contrast, intra-atrial re-entry is initiated by a premature atrial complex with a morphology different from that of subsequent P waves. Patients may be symptomatic because of the sudden onset and termination of the tachycardia. Digoxin toxicity, chronic obstructive pulmonary disease, coronary artery disease, hypokalemia, theophylline, and adrenergic drugs are known causes of atrial tachycardias. Treatment usually consists of administration of a class IA or IC agent to attempt to suppress the arrhythmia and/or AV nodal blocking agents to control ventricular rate.

Atrioventricular Nodal Re-Entrant Tachycardia

AV nodal re-entrant tachycardia is the most common cause of supraventricular tachycardia. It is a re-entrant rhythm with rates usually between 120 and 250 beats/min that is caused by the presence of dual AV nodal pathways with a slow (alpha) and a fast (beta) conducting pathway.

In typical AV nodal re-entrant tachycardia, the fast pathway has a longer effective refractory period than the slower one; that is, block in the fast pathway occurs at lower rates or in response to APDs of less prematurity. When an early APD encounters the AV node, the fast pathway is refractory and anterograde conduction occurs down the slow pathway (Figs. 94–13 and 94–14A), with subsequent retrograde conduction along the fast pathway. Because both pathways are within the AV node, conduction and subsequent depolarization of both the atria and ventricles occur almost simultaneously. On the surface ECG, the VA interval is quite short (<100 ms). The diagnosis can be suspected on the basis of the 12-lead ECG during tachycardia when either no P waves are visible (because they are within and obscured by the QRS

complex) or the VA interval is extremely short (see Fig. 94–14).

During sinus rhythm, conduction occurs over the fast pathway, resulting in a normal PR interval. Initiation of the tachycardia is usually with an APD and a long PR interval (indicating conduction down the slow pathway). Occasionally, retrograde P waves are seen during the tachycardia. The diagnosis can be made with an esophageal lead tracing that shows a VA interval (onset of earliest ventricular electrogram on the surface ECG leads to onset of earliest atrial spike in esophageal recording lead) of less than 100 ms.[23, 24]

Rarely, the pathways are reversed: during tachycardia, anterograde conduction occurs along the fast pathway and retrograde conduction over the slow pathway. This is termed atypical AV nodal re-entrant tachycardia. Because of the pathway reversal, the ventricles and atria are no longer activated simultaneously. This is manifest on the ECG by retrograde P waves preceding the QRS complex with a relatively short PR interval.

The onset of AV nodal re-entrant tachycardia is sudden, usually without obvious precipitating factors. This tachycardia is not in itself life threatening, but patients with poor left ventricular function may develop hemodynamic compromise. Palpitations, syncope, heart failure, and hypotension are common. If a patient is hemodynamically unstable, cardioversion using 100 to 200 J should be performed after appropriate sedation or anesthesia.

Patients who are hemodynamically stable often respond to vagal maneuvers such as carotid sinus massage. This terminates the tachycardia after slowing in about 80% of patients who are not hypotensive. Carotid sinus massage is performed by applying continuous pressure over the carotid artery pulse at the angle of the jaw (one side at a time) for up to 5 seconds. Carotid sinus massage should not be performed if carotid bruits are present. The initial pharmacologic agent of choice in patients who fail to respond to vagal maneuvers is adenosine (6- to 12-mg intravenous bolus).[25, 26] After termination of tachycardia by adenosine, brief periods of asystole are common. Adenosine is highly effective in terminating tachycardias involving the AV node.

Figure 94–12. Automatic atrial tachycardia. Simultaneous tracings of electrocardiographic leads II and V$_5$. The arrow indicates a late premature atrial complex that begins the automatic tachycardia. Note the gradual acceleration in rate. Note also that the initiating P wave has the same morphology as the subsequent P waves during the tachycardia. (Courtesy of Dennis Cassidy.)

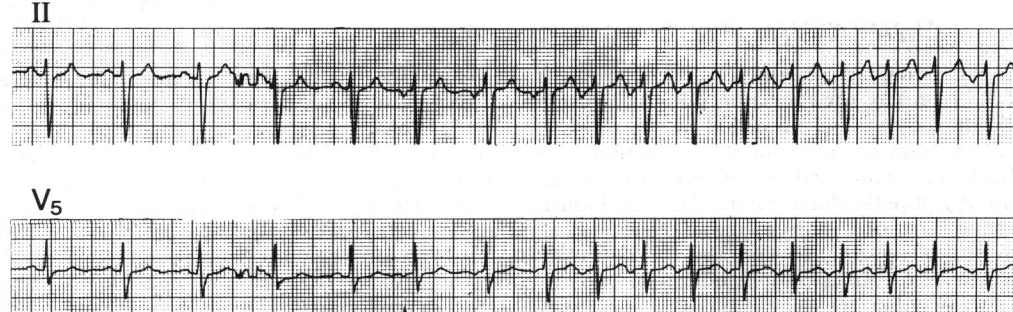

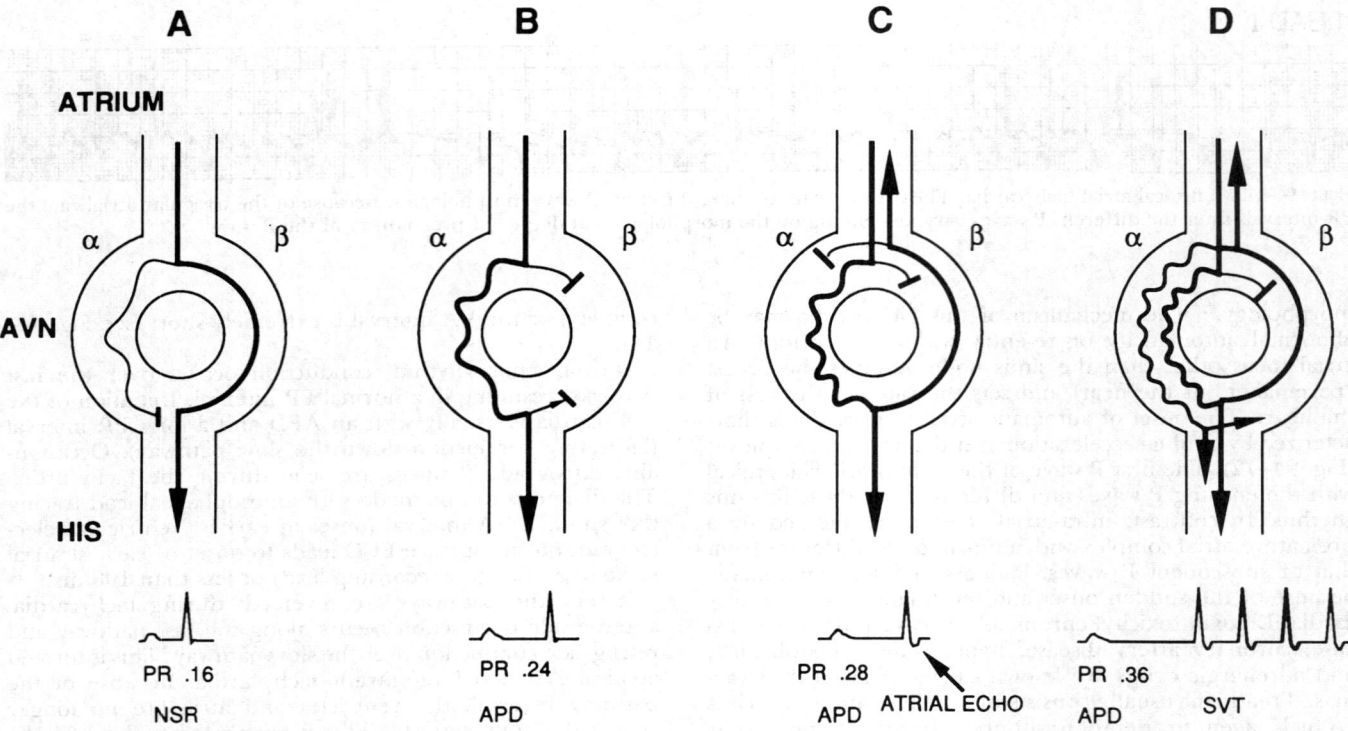

Figure 94–13. Mechanism of AV nodal re-entry. The atrium, AV node (AVN), and His bundle are shown schematically. The AV node is longitudinally dissociated into two pathways with different functional properties. The alpha pathway conducts relatively slowly, and the beta pathway conducts rapidly. In each panel, heavy lines denote excitation in the AV node that is manifest on the surface ECG and light lines denote conduction that is concealed and not apparent on the surface ECG. A. During normal sinus rhythm (NSR) the impulse from the atrium is conducted down both pathways. However, only conduction over the fast (beta) pathway is manifest on the surface ECG, producing a normal PR interval of 0.16 second. B. An APD is blocked in the beta pathway. The impulse is conducted over the alpha pathway to the His bundle and ventricles, producing a PR interval of 0.24 second. Because the impulse is premature, conduction over the alpha pathway occurs more slowly than it would during sinus rhythm. C. A more premature atrial impulse is blocked in the beta pathway but conducted with increased delay in the alpha pathway, producing a PR interval of 0.28 second. The impulse is conducted retrogradely up the beta pathway and then blocked anterogradely in the alpha pathway. D. A still more premature atrial impulse is blocked initially in the beta pathway and conducted over the alpha pathway with increasing delay, producing a PR interval of 0.36 second. Retrograde conduction occurs over the beta pathway and re-entry occurs, producing a sustained supraventricular tachycardia (SVT). (From Josephson ME, Buxton AE, Marchlinski FE: The tachyarrhythmias. In: Wilson JD, Braunwald E, Isselbacher KJ, et al [eds]: Harrison's Principles of Internal Medicine. 12th ed. New York, McGraw-Hill, p 916, 1991. Copyright © 1991 by McGraw-Hill, Inc. Used by permission of McGraw-Hill Book Company.)

Verapamil given intravenously (2.5 to 5.0 mg within 30 seconds to a total dose of 15 mg) can also be successful in terminating the tachycardia. If atrial or ventricular pacing wires are present (e.g., after cardiothoracic surgery), pacing via the wires may be able to stop the tachycardia. Drugs, such as digoxin and beta-blockers, affect the slow pathway and can be used for chronic treatment of tachycardia. Drugs such as procainamide, quinidine, encainide, flecainide, and propafenone that affect the fast pathway may also be given for chronic therapy.

NONPAROXYSMAL JUNCTIONAL TACHYCARDIA

Junctional tachycardia is usually characterized by a narrow QRS complex (or the same QRS as is present during sinus rhythm) that is not preceded by P waves (Fig. 94–15). Atrial activity may result from the sinus node and be dissociated from ventricular activity, or retrograde atrial activation from the AV junction may occur. The mechanism for nonparoxysmal junctional tachycardia is either enhanced automaticity or triggered activity with the QRS similar to that seen in sinus. The rate is influenced by autonomic tone, increased by catecholamines, vagolytic agents, or exercise and slowed with carotid sinus massage. There is usually an acceleration

period on the ECG before stabilization of the rate, which varies from 70 to 150 beats/min. The causes of this tachycardia include digitalis toxicity, inferior myocardial infarction, myocarditis, endogenous or exogenous catecholamines, acute rheumatic fever, and recent open heart surgery. Treatment of the underlying problem is often adequate. These arrhythmias should not be cardioverted (especially if the tachycardia is secondary to digitalis intoxication). Atrial pacing can be used to override and maintain AV conduction.

WOLFF-PARKINSON-WHITE SYNDROME

WPW syndrome is due to one or more extra connections between the atria and ventricles in addition to the normal conduction pathway.[27, 28] These connections are called accessory, or bypass, tracts and can be located anywhere around the AV rings, except the area of aortomitral continuity. In contrast to the decremental conduction properties of the AV node (discussed earlier), the properties of these pathways are typically like those of cardiac muscle without decremental conduction. That is, in response to increased stimulation rates, conduction velocity remains constant. During sinus rhythm, part of the ventricles is activated early (i.e., pre-excited) via this accessory pathway. On the surface ECG a

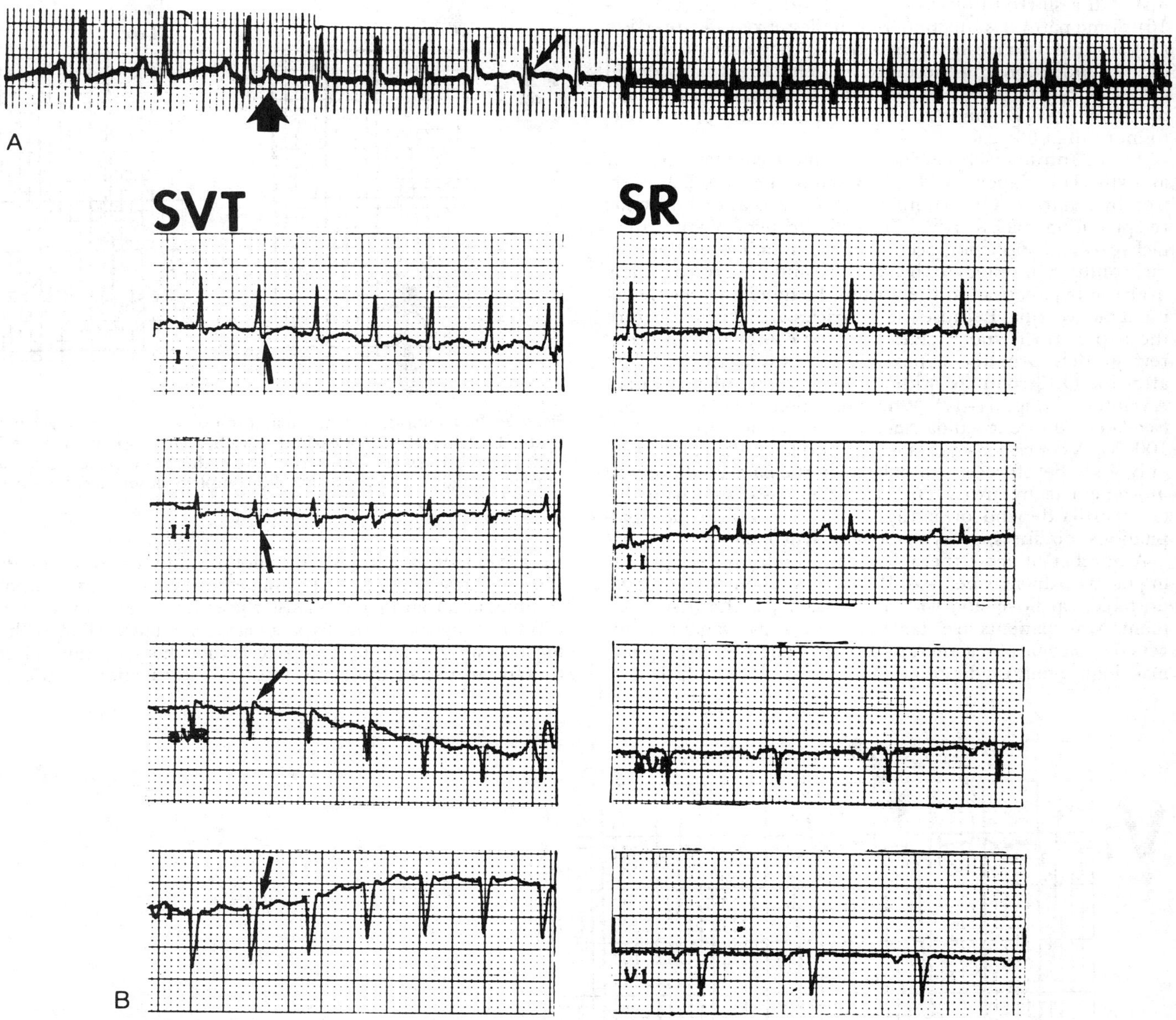

A

SVT   **SR**

B

Figure 94–14. *A.* AV nodal re-entry. The initiating P wave *(thick arrow)* is conducted with a markedly prolonged PR interval, signifying conduction through the "slow" AV nodal pathway. The thin arrow points to the atrial echo superimposed on the end of the QRS. *B.* Tracings from electrocardiographic leads I, II, aV$_R$, and V$_1$ during AV nodal re-entry *(left)* and sinus rhythm *(right)*. During AV nodal re-entry, a terminal negative deflection is visible superimposed on the end of the QRS complex in leads I and II and a terminal positive deflection is superimposed on the end of the QRS complex in leads aV$_R$ and V$_1$ *(arrows)*. These terminal defections are absent during sinus rhythm and represent retrograde atrial activity during the tachycardia.

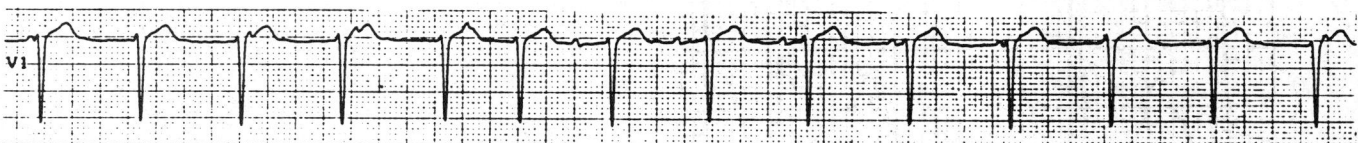

Figure 94–15. Accelerated junctional rhythm at a rate slightly greater than that of sinus rhythm. After the fifth QRS complex the next two P waves are conducted with prolonged PR intervals. The junctional tachycardia then takes over again. The sinus "captures" prove that complete heart block is not present. However, AV dissociation is present at the beginning and the end of the tracing.

short PR interval (<120 ms) and a wide QRS complex (>120 ms) with a slurred upstroke (delta wave) are seen (Fig. 94–16). Some pathways function only in the retrograde direction and are called concealed bypass tracts; they have no antero-grade conduction and therefore no delta waves are seen on the ECG. Bypass tracts are congenital and can cause a variety of arrhythmias beginning at any age, from less than 1 year to more than 60 years.

AV re-entrant tachycardia is the most common type of arrhythmia in patients with WPW syndrome. It is character-ized by a narrow QRS complex referred to as orthodromic reciprocating tachycardia. In orthodromic reciprocating tachycardia, conduction occurs anterogradely over the nor-mal conduction system to the ventricle and then retrogradely over the bypass tract to the atrium, forming a circus move-ment tachycardia. Because the ventricles are activated before the bypass tract, and it takes time for conduction to occur retrogradely over the bypass tract, P waves are inscribed after the QRS complex, with a shorter ventriculoatrial than AV interval (Fig. 94–17). When an esophageal lead is used (see later), the ventriculoatrial interval is always greater than 100 ms. A concealed bypass tract has retrograde conduction only and therefore is still able to participate in the circus movement tachycardia. The symptoms associated with this tachycardia depend primarily on the rate and include pal-pitations, dizziness, presyncope, and syncope.

A number of acute therapies for orthodromic reciprocat-ing tachycardia may be used. If a patient is hemodynamically unstable, cardioversion with 100 to 200 J is the best treat-ment. Most patients are stable enough to use vagal maneu-vers or pharmacologic therapy initially. The preferred phar-macologic agent is adenosine (6 to 12 mg intravenously).[25, 26]

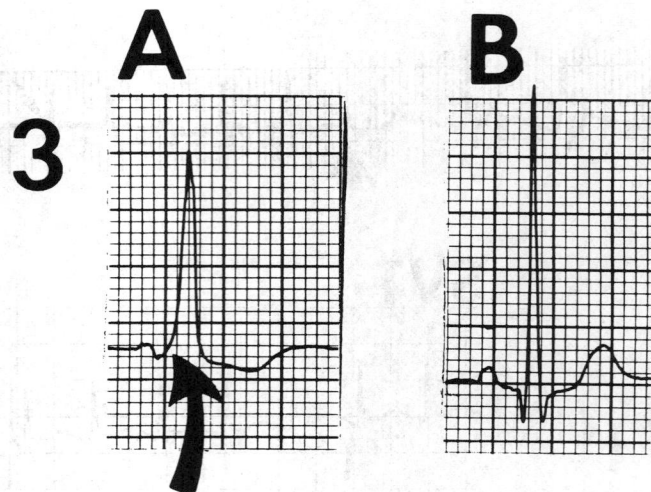

Figure 94–16. Example of ventricular pre-excitation. A tracing from lead III is shown. *A.* Pre-excitation with a short PR interval and delta wave *(arrow).* *B.* Sinus rhythm in the same patient with a normal PR interval and normal QRS complex without a delta wave.

Verapamil or digoxin should not be administered unless there is absolute certainty that the bypass tract cannot conduct anterogradely, because these drugs can shorten the refractory period of the bypass tract, as noted earlier. If the mechanism of the tachycardia is not known, the safest therapy to use in the acute setting is intravenous procain-

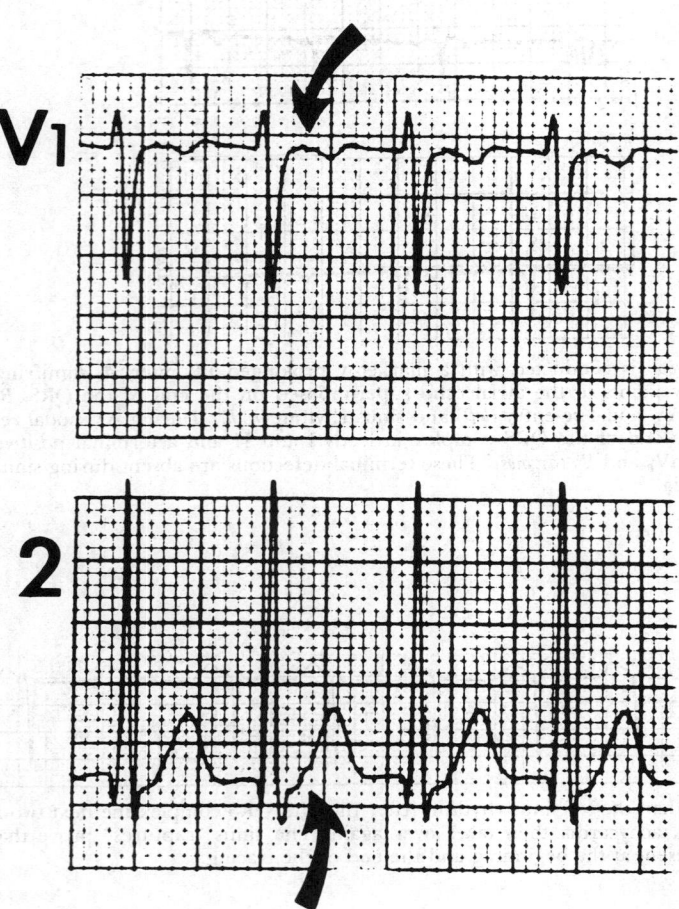

Figure 94–17. Orthodromic AV re-entrant tachycardia. A narrow QRS complex tachycardia at a rate of 140 beats/min is present. Atrial activity follows the QRS complex *(arrows).* Compare the relationship between QRS complex and P waves during this tachycardia with that during AV nodal re-entry depicted in Figure 94–14.

amide. Chronic therapy includes a wide variety of antiarrhythmic agents, catheter ablation, or surgical division.

REGULAR SUPRAVENTRICULAR ARRHYTHMIAS WITH WIDE QRS COMPLEXES IN WOLFF-PARKINSON-WHITE SYNDROME

Antidromic reciprocating tachycardia occurs in about 5% of patients with WPW syndrome.[27] This is a tachycardia with anterograde conduction along the bypass tract and retrograde conduction via the AV node or a second bypass tract. The ventricles are pre-excited by the bypass tract, resulting in a wide QRS complex (>120 ms) with a delta wave and a short PR interval (<120 ms). This can be mistaken for ventricular tachycardia because of the wide QRS interval. The P wave may not be visible on the 12-lead ECG during tachycardia if the rate is high because it may be buried in the T wave. The symptoms depend on the rate. The treatment is the same as that for orthodromic reciprocating tachycardia. Avoid digoxin and verapamil as noted earlier.

Any atrial tachycardia in the presence of a bypass tract may result in a regular wide QRS rhythm. The slurring or the upstroke of the QRS or delta wave should be apparent, however, and the initial QRS forces should be similar to those seen in sinus rhythm. Symptoms and treatment are as described for atrial tachycardias with the exception that digitalis and verapamil should be avoided.

WOLFF-PARKINSON-WHITE SYNDROME: ATRIAL FIBRILLATION

When patients with WPW develop atrial fibrillation, conduction to the ventricles may occur over the accessory tract (Fig. 94–18). This results in a wide QRS complex with a delta wave and an irregularly irregular rhythm. The QRS complex width and morphology may vary depending on the degree to which the ventricles are activated via the bypass tract versus the normal AV conduction system. Atrial fibrillation occurs in approximately 15% of patients with WPW, even if there is no underlying heart disease. Pre-excited atrial fibrillation can be a serious rhythm, as it can degenerate into ventricular fibrillation. This is more likely if the RR intervals are quite short (<260 ms). Digoxin and verapamil are contraindicated in this rhythm because they can decrease refractoriness of the bypass tract, thereby accelerating the ventricular response. For hemodynamically stable rhythms, intravenous procainamide is the best treatment. Procainamide frequently terminates the arrhythmia. Even when type IA agents fail to restore sinus rhythm, they almost always slow the ventricular response by increasing refractoriness of the bypass tract (Fig. 94–19). If the patient is hemodynamically unstable, cardioversion using 100 to 200 J should be performed. Chronic therapy consists of antiarrhythmic agents as outlined under Atrial Fibrillation. Therapy directed at the underlying bypass tract, such as surgery and catheter ablation, is another alternative.[28]

VENTRICULAR ARRHYTHMIAS

Accelerated Idioventricular Rhythm ("Slow Ventricular Tachycardia")

Accelerated idioventricular rhythm is characterized by a wide QRS complex and regular ventricular rate, usually 60 to 110 beats/min. These rhythms are usually asymptomatic and occur in a wide variety of circumstances, including acute myocardial infarction, the early period after open heart surgery, idiopathic cardiomyopathy, acute rheumatic fever, and digitalis toxicity. Because this arrhythmia is usually not associated with symptoms and is not associated with more serious symptomatic arrhythmias, it does not require therapy. It often occurs in the setting of sinus bradycardia and may be suppressed by accelerating the sinus rate with atropine.

Ventricular Premature Complexes

Ventricular premature complexes (VPCs) are recognized by a wide QRS complex (>120 ms) with a bizarre configuration. When VPCs occur in patients without heart disease, the QRS tends to be less wide than when they occur in patients with underlying heart disease. VPCs occur commonly in patients with and without underlying heart disease. As many as 60% of apparently healthy middle-aged men exhibit one or more VPCs during 24 hours of electrocardiographic monitoring, and approximately 70% of patients with chronic coronary disease or cardiomyopathies exhibit VPCs during 24 hours of Holter's monitoring.[29, 30] The mechanism of VPCs varies; in some patients they have been attributed to re-entry, whereas in others protected automatic foci have been implicated. The frequency and number of different morphologies of VPCs often increase during acute medical illnesses, notably acute severe ischemia, especially in the setting of an acute myocardial infarction. Hypokalemia and other electrolyte abnormalities may also provoke VPCs, and they are one of the most common manifestations of digitalis toxicity. Because VPCs rarely cause symptoms, they do not

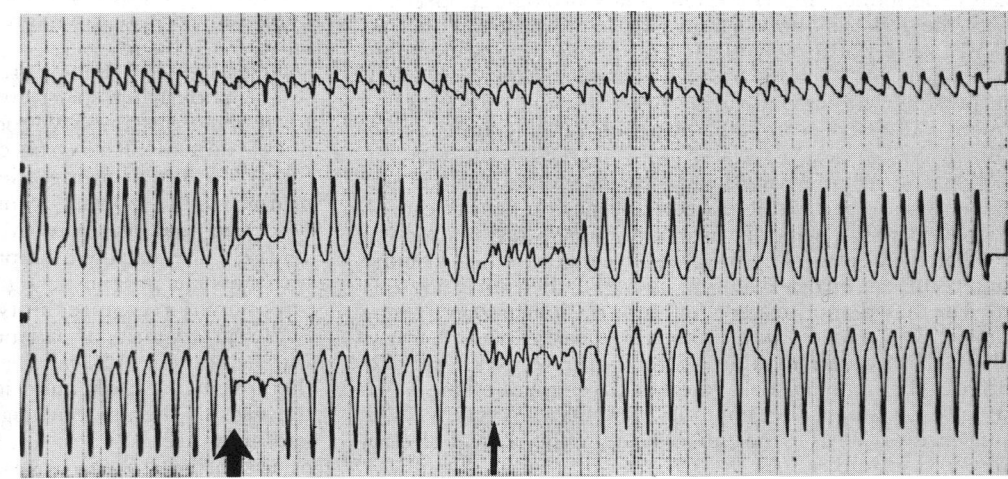

Figure 94–18. Atrial fibrillation in a patient with pre-excitation. Tracings from electrocardiographic leads I, II, and III are shown. The ventricular response to atrial fibrillation is extremely rapid with almost constant variation in QRS intervals. Occasional complexes activate the ventricles predominantly over the normal conduction system, resulting in a narrow QRS complex *(thick arrow)*. The thin arrow points out a second pre-excited QRS complex present during some conducted beats, suggesting the presence of at least two AV bypass tracts.

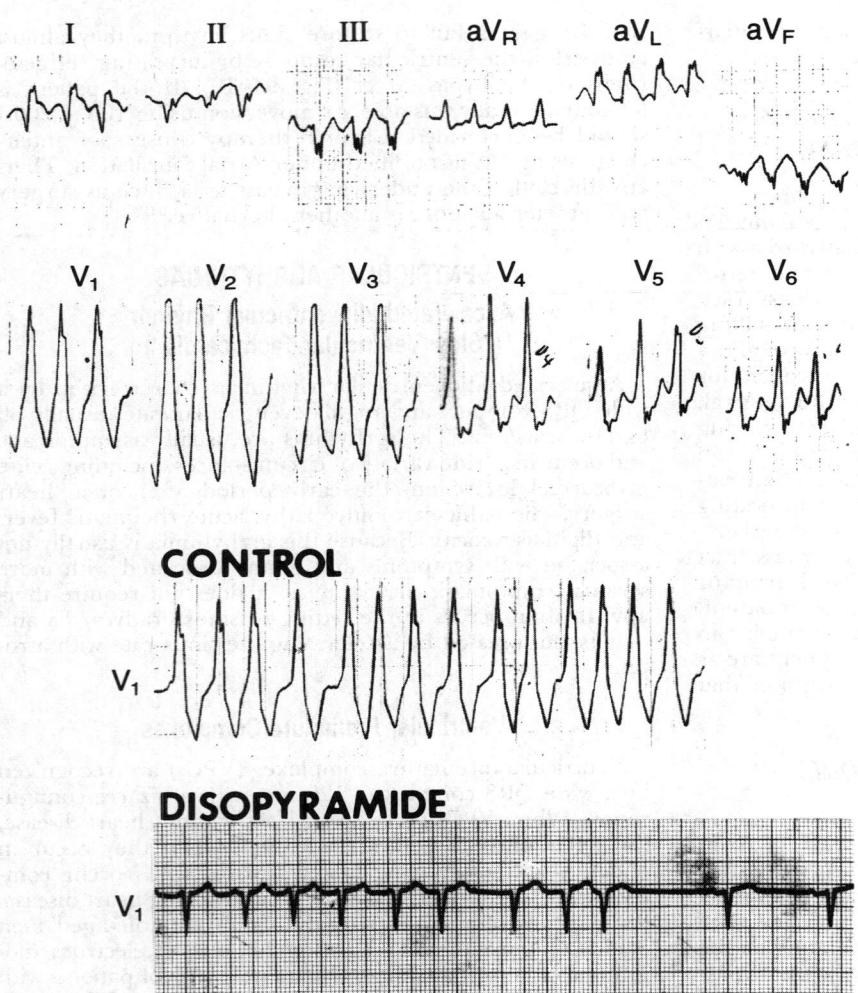

CONTROL

DISOPYRAMIDE

Figure 94–19. Atrial fibrillation in a patient with pre-excitation. *(Top)* The standard 12-lead ECG and a rhythm strip of lead V_1 in the absence of antiarrhythmic drugs. *(Bottom)* After administration of disopyramide, the patient remained in atrial fibrillation, which then terminated spontaneously. Note that the ventricular response during atrial fibrillation after disopyramide is much slower than in the controlled state as a result of loss of pre-excitation. Disopyramide has blocked conduction over the bypass tract. Similar effects occur in response to procainamide and quinidine.

usually require treatment. In the intensive care unit, a sudden increase in frequency of VPCs may be an indication of an acute metabolic abnormality (such as hypoxia) or drug toxicity. In these cases, diagnostic evaluation and therapy should be aimed at the condition underlying the VPCs rather than the VPCs themselves. Occasionally, the cardiac output may be decreased when VPCs occur frequently (as in a bigeminal pattern), effectively halving the heart rate. If this occurs and no primary abnormality (such as digitalis toxicity) can be identified and corrected, pharmacologic suppression with the antiarrhythmic agents may be warranted.

VPCs are not usually treated in the asymptomatic ambulatory patient. VPCs have no adverse prognostic significance in persons without underlying heart disease. Although frequent VPCs and "complex" forms of VPCs (couplets, multiform VPCs) are associated with increased mortality in patients with underlying heart disease such as chronic coronary disease and cardiomyopathies, they do not indicate an increased risk specifically for sudden death (vs. nonsudden cardiac death caused by progressive congestive heart failure or a recurrent myocardial infarction). Furthermore, no study to date has demonstrated that suppression of VPCs alters mortality in patients with underlying heart disease. Because all available antiarrhythmic agents can have significant side effects, the potential risks attending treatment of the VPCs usually outweigh the potential benefits of therapy. The presence of VPCs is not an indication for clinical electrophysiologic studies.

Nonsustained Ventricular Tachycardia

Nonsustained VT ranges from three consecutive VPCs up to 30 seconds at a rate of 100 beats/min or higher. Nonsustained VT may be classified by its morphology (uniform, with each QRS complex having the same morphology, or polymorphic, with constantly varying QRS morphology). Most recorded episodes of nonsustained VT are brief, lasting less than six beats. As such, most episodes of nonsustained VT are not associated with symptoms. Longer episodes of nonsustained VT, especially if rapid, may cause lightheadedness or syncope.

Nonsustained VT most often is discovered in patients with severe underlying structural heart disease. However, one form of nonsustained VT occurs frequently in the absence of heart disease. Paroxysms of repetitive monomorphic (uniform) VT, often having a left bundle branch block configuration with a normal frontal plane QRS axis, have been described that originate in the outflow tract of the right ventricle, are usually asymptomatic, and are not associated with adverse prognostic significance (Fig. 94–20).[31, 32] It is important to recognize this type of nonsustained VT because in the vast majority of patients it is benign and not associated with symptoms. All available pharmacologic antiarrhythmic therapy involves risk, and with this type of nonsustained VT the risks of therapy outweigh the benefits in most patients and they are best left untreated. When this arrhythmia occurs in the absence of structural heart disease, it is often

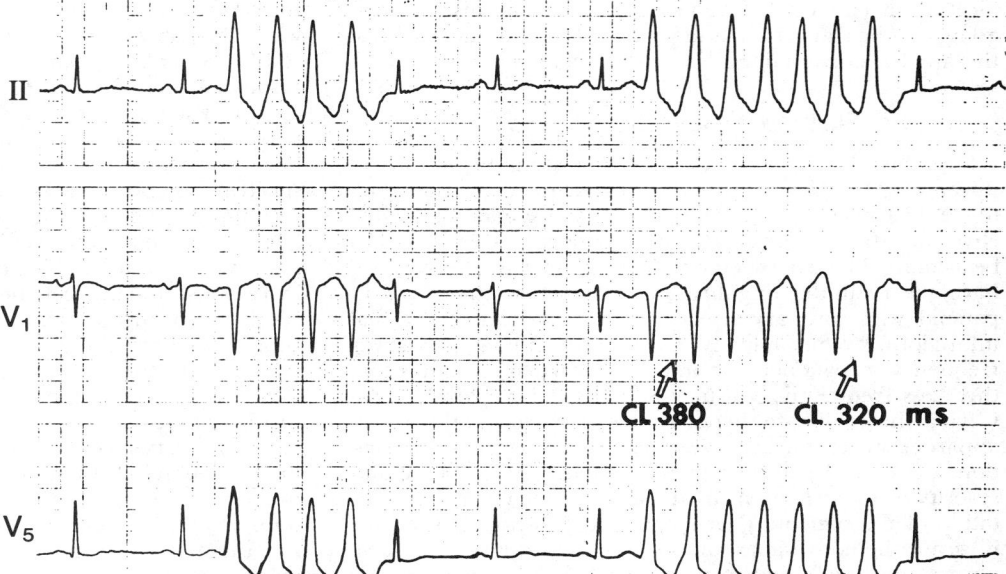

Figure 94–20. Simultaneous tracings from three electrocardiographic leads showing a typical example of repetitive monomorphic ventricular tachycardia in a patient without obvious structural heart disease. The morphology is that of a left bundle branch block with an inferior (normal) frontal plane QRS axis. The cycle length during these episodes is variable, ranging from 320 to 380 ms (rates of approximately 170 beats/min). This patient was asymptomatic during the episodes of VT.

readily suppressed by a variety of antiarrhythmic agents, including beta-adrenergic blocking agents. However, cases have been described in which the antiarrhythmic agents facilitated development of the arrhythmia, converting it from a nonsustained to a sustained and symptomatic form. This type of nonsustained VT is commonly provoked by exercise or catecholamine infusion.

Nonsustained VT is found commonly in patients with hypertrophic and dilated cardiomyopathies (in 20 and 50%, respectively, of patients with these diseases undergoing 24 hours of ambulatory ECG monitoring). Approximately 15% of patients undergoing electrocardiographic monitoring 2 to 4 weeks after myocardial infarction display one or more runs of nonsustained VT, and approximately 5% of patients with chronic coronary artery disease have runs of nonsustained VT during 24 hours of ambulatory ECG monitoring. Nonsustained VT is far more likely to be found in patients with markedly abnormal left ventricular function, regardless of the type of underlying heart disease.[30-33] The mechanism of nonsustained VT appears to vary, depending on the type of associated heart disease. Programmed stimulation is capable of inducing VT in approximately 40% of patients with nonsustained VT and chronic coronary disease, suggesting that the arrhythmia in some of these patients may be due to re-entry. However, nonsustained VT arising in the setting of acute myocardial ischemia or infarction is likely to be due to different mechanisms, possibly abnormal automaticity or re-entry within small areas of the myocardium resulting from functional disparities of refractoriness and conduction. The mechanisms of nonsustained VT in patients with other types of heart disease are unclear at this time, and most patients with nonsustained VT and noncoronary disease do not have the tachycardia induced by programmed stimulation.

Nonsustained VT is associated with increased mortality in patients with all types of underlying heart disease, but it does not appear to predict specifically an increased risk for sudden (vs. nonsudden) cardiac death. It is not clear whether chronic suppression of nonsustained VT would reduce the incidence of sudden death. In the intensive care unit, one should always search for metabolic or other transient abnormalities potentially responsible for precipitating runs of nonsustained VT. The sudden appearance of this arrhythmia may signify the presence of acute myocardial ischemia, severe hypoxia, hypokalemia, or drug toxicity (see later). In these cases, treatment should be directed at the primary abnormality. In the setting of acute ischemia or infarction, increasingly frequent, progressively longer runs of nonsustained (usually polymorphic) VT may herald the onset of ventricular fibrillation, and they should be suppressed (Fig. 94–21). In most other situations, the benefits of suppressing brief (usually asymptomatic) runs of nonsustained VT are unclear. In the occasional patient with severe underlying structural heart disease, frequent runs of nonsustained VT may compromise the cardiac output and warrant suppression. However, this is the exception rather than the rule. Furthermore, patients with severe underlying structural heart disease and brief runs of nonsustained VT may be at increased risk for developing proarrhythmic drug effects or for exacerbation of the underlying ventricular tachyarrhythmia in response to antiarrhythmic drug administration. Here again, the risks of pharmacologic antiarrhythmic therapy may often exceed the benefits of such suppressive therapy, particularly in the asymptomatic patient. Cardiac electrophysiologic studies are useful in identifying patients with nonsustained VT and chronic coronary artery disease who are at high versus low risk for sudden cardiac death. Electrophysiologic studies have not proved useful for risk strat-

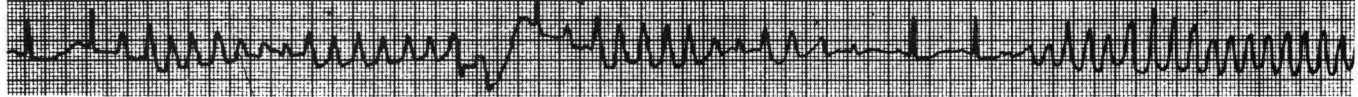

Figure 94–21. Recurrent paroxysms of polymorphic ventricular tachycardia in a patient with ongoing myocardial ischemia. This arrhythmia caused multiple cardiac arrests and was treated by coronary artery bypass grafting. The arrhythmia ceased after revascularization without administration of antiarrhythmic agents.

ification in patients with other types of heart disease. Ongoing studies are evaluating the role of antiarrhythmic therapy for nonsustained VT in these patients.

Sustained Ventricular Tachycardia

Sustained VT is defined as VT exceeding 30 seconds in duration. The minimal rate for diagnosis is generally taken to be 110 beats/min (although in the presence of antiarrhythmic drug therapy the rate may be as low as 100 beats/min). The overwhelming majority of patients with VT have severe underlying heart disease (more than 75% in patients with coronary artery disease and prior myocardial infarction).[34–37] Sustained VT also occurs with much lower frequency in patients with idiopathic dilated cardiomyopathy. Less frequently, VT may be observed in patients with valvular heart disease, hypertrophic cardiomyopathy, or no apparent structural heart disease. The prognostic implications of the tachycardia depend primarily on the type and severity of underlying heart disease and the clinical presentation of the patient. That is, patients in whom VT results in severe hemodynamic compromise or cardiac arrest have a worse prognosis than patients in whom the tachycardia is well tolerated, as recurrences of the arrhythmia are also likely to cause cardiac arrest. Sustained VT may be classified in a number of ways, but it is often useful to assess the QRS morphology. Sustained tachycardias having a constant, uniform morphology occur most frequently in patients with chronic coronary artery disease with a recent or remote myocardial infarction (Fig. 94–22). It is not unusual in this setting for a patient to walk into an emergency room complaining of sudden onset of palpitations that last several hours (sometimes even a day or two). The onset of VT is

sudden and is usually initiated by one or more VPCs. Even when the tachycardia is well tolerated hemodynamically, the sudden onset is associated with transient hypotension, which resolves within several seconds. This hypotension frequently causes syncope at the onset of the episode, which then resolves spontaneously even though the patient continues to have the sustained tachycardia. At the other end of the spectrum, some patients who develop rapid sustained VT with uniform morphology do not tolerate the arrhythmia at all, and it results in immediate hemodynamic collapse manifest as cardiac arrest. The cardiac arrest may develop solely in response to the sustained, usually rapid VT, or it may result from the sustained tachycardia degenerating into ventricular fibrillation.

The acute treatment of patients with uniform, sustained VT is governed by the hemodynamic effects of the tachycardia. The patient who is conscious without severe symptoms may be treated with elective synchronized cardioversion under general anesthesia or by parenteral pharmacologic therapy. Two agents are used primarily for acute intravenous pharmacologic therapy: lidocaine and procainamide. Lidocaine has the advantage that it can be administered quickly as a bolus not requiring dilution (total dose 5 mg/kg given as 75 mg intravenously followed by 50 mg every 5 minutes) with a rapid onset of action. Its major disadvantage is its lack of efficacy in most patients with sustained VT (it is effective in approximately 10%). We prefer to use intravenous procainamide because it is more often effective in terminating VT. Even when procainamide does not terminate an acute episode, it almost always slows the tachycardia significantly (in contrast to minimal effects of lidocaine on the rate of tachycardia). The rate-slowing effect usually produces a more hemodynamically stable state, from which

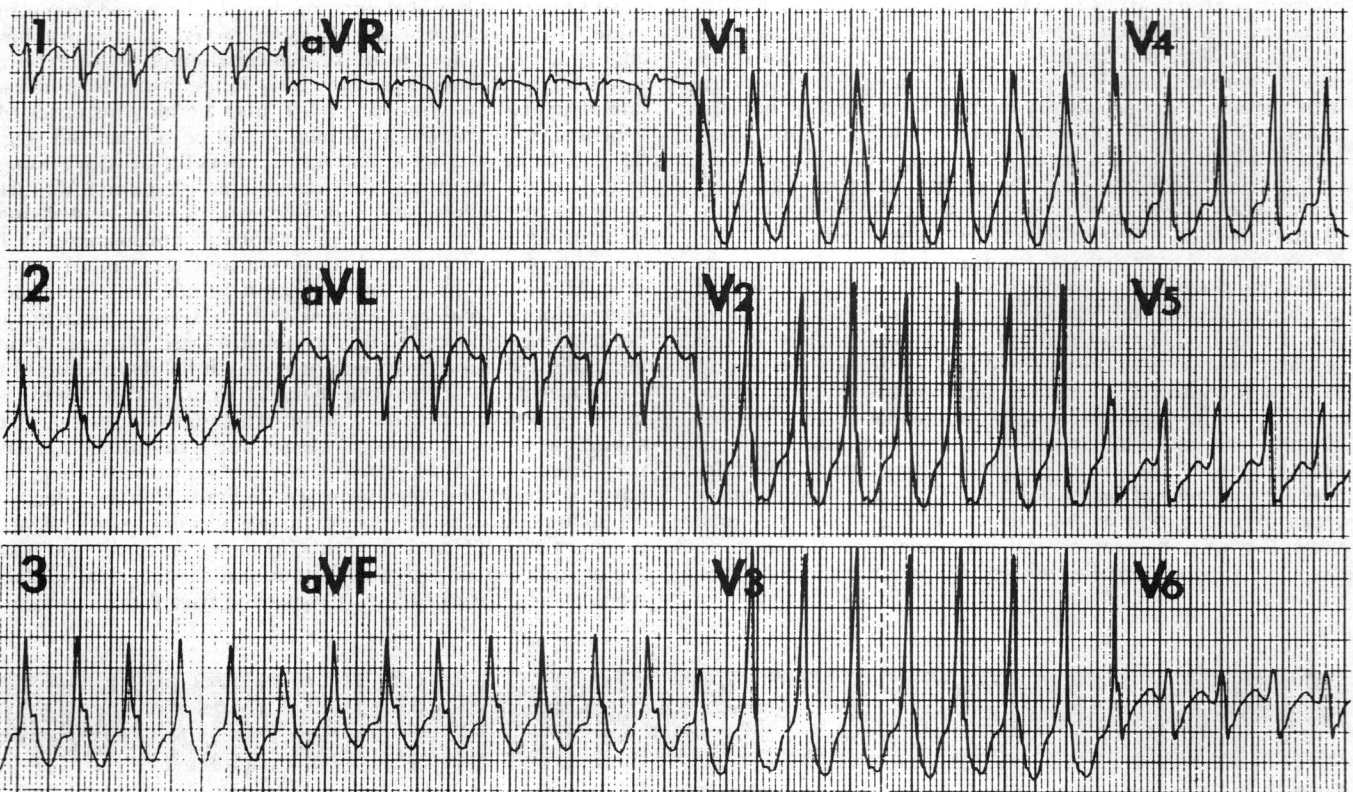

Figure 94–22. Sustained uniform ventricular tachycardia. Note the monophasic R wave in lead V_1 and the R/S ratio less than 1 in lead V_6. AV dissociation is not visible in this tracing.

the patient may then be cardioverted. We administer procainamide acutely as a loading dose of 15 mg/kg given at a rate of 25 to 50 mg/min. The principal side effect is hypotension, and the blood pressure must be checked every 5 minutes when administrating the agent in this manner. For an isolated episode of sustained VT, we do not continue maintenance therapy with lidocaine or procainamide if the arrhythmia terminates during the infusion. However, if the patient has frequent recurrences, the acute loading dose may be followed by oral procainamide or continuation of the intravenous infusion at a rate sufficient to maintain a steady state (0.11 mg/kg/min). These dosages usually result in serum procainamide levels of 8 to 10 μg/mL. We monitor the serum level of procainamide alone and not the combination of procainamide plus N-acetylprocainamide, because no data suggest that the sum of the two levels has any clinical relevance.

As noted earlier, the patient with VT that is poorly tolerated, causing severe hypotension, angina, heart failure, or loss of consciousness, is cardioverted rather than treated pharmacologically. If the patient is conscious, he or she is given an anesthetic or sedative before direct-current synchronized cardioversion.

Most uniform sustained VTs result from re-entry in the myocardium.[34] This mechanism enables many of these tachycardias to be terminated by underdrive or overdrive ventricular pacing. Patients with frequent recurrences may be stabilized by inserting a temporary transvenous right ventricular pacing catheter to terminate episodes rapidly without need for pharmacologic therapy or repeated cardioversions. Pacing should be performed only under continuous electrocardiographic monitoring by an experienced operator with a defibrillator at the bedside, because pacing techniques not infrequently accelerate the tachycardia, converting a stable arrhythmia into a hemodynamically unstable state requiring emergent cardioversion.

Chronic therapeutic options for patients with sustained, uniform VT include oral antiarrhythmic agents and permanent, implanted antitachycardia devices capable of automatically recognizing and terminating the arrhythmia by overdrive pacing or countershock.[38-47] The disadvantage of these therapeutic modalities is that they are palliative and do not cure the patient. However, careful assessment of these therapies by experienced electrophysiologists shows that they involve relatively low short-term morbidity and mortality. Curative therapy for recurrent, sustained uniform VT is now available in the form of guided surgical resection and ablation utilizing endocardial catheters. All chronic therapy is best designed by an experienced electrophysiologic team. Programmed stimulation currently is the best modality for assessing efficacy of pharmacologic and non-pharmacologic therapy for sustained uniform VT.[43, 44] Other techniques such as ambulatory electrocardiographic monitoring are limited by a number of factors. Most patients with recurrent sustained VT have relatively infrequent episodes that are unpredictable. Therefore, ambulatory electrocardiographic monitoring techniques are forced to rely on suppression of VPCs. The effect of the various therapies on VPCs frequently differs from the therapeutic effect on the sustained tachycardia because the mechanism of the VPCs may differ from that of the sustained tachycardia. Approximately one third of patients with sustained VT have only rare isolated VPCs, and monitoring techniques may be inaccurate in determining whether pharmacologic therapy is responsible for suppression of ectopy or disappearance of ectopy is due to random variation of frequency. Finally, individual patients may show a great deal of spontaneous variation in the frequency of ectopy, even in the absence of antiarrhythmic therapy. This spontaneous variation in frequency may mimic antiarrhythmic drug effects.

Polymorphic Ventricular Tachycardia

The hallmark of polymorphic VT is a QRS morphology that changes constantly, in some forms from beat to beat. Multiple electrocardiographic leads may be necessary to detect the morphologic variation because some episodes of polymorphic VT may appear uniform if only one lead is examined. Polymorphic VT is usually divided into episodes associated with a normal QT interval and others associated with prolongation of the QT interval. Polymorphic VT associated with a normal QT interval may be idiopathic without apparent underlying heart disease in rare cases but is most frequently associated with advanced structural heart disease.[37] Polymorphic VT occurs frequently in the setting of acute, severe myocardial ischemia and in patients with cardiomyopathies, both hypertrophic and dilated. Polymorphic tachycardia resulting from acute myocardial ischemia often fails to respond to conventional antiarrhythmic agents, although in some cases it is suppressed by lidocaine or bretylium. Frequently, the only therapy that suppresses this arrhythmia is myocardial revascularization, and in these cases, once revascularization is effected, no further therapy is necessary. Occasionally, polymorphic tachycardias associated with chronic coronary artery disease may be suppressed by conventional antiarrhythmic drugs when acute ischemia is not the precipitating event. The decision to institute pharmacologic therapy must follow careful evaluation of the QT interval on the standard ECG. If the QT interval is markedly prolonged, standard antiarrhythmic agents of the type I class should not be administered. When sustained polymorphic VT causing cardiac arrest occurs in the setting of noncoronary disease, pharmacologic therapy may be difficult to evaluate and is often ineffective. Such patients are best treated with implanted automatic cardioverter-defibrillator devices.[44-46] Although these devices do not prevent episodes of tachycardia, in most cases they are effective in preventing cardiac arrest and sudden death resulting from the tachycardia.

Polymorphic tachycardia with prolongation of the QT interval may occur as a congenital abnormality or be acquired. Patients with the congenital long-QT syndrome usually present with a stereotypic sequence of events. Episodes of syncope usually precede overt cardiac arrest. Episodes of syncope and cardiac arrest caused by the polymorphic VT characteristically follow episodes of extreme sympathetic stimulation, such as startling or sudden awakening in response to aural stimuli.[48-53] The electrocardiographic appearance of polymorphic VT associated with prolongation of the QT interval or torsades de pointes is distinctive. Patients with a congenital long-QT syndrome and torsades de pointes are often effectively treated with beta-adrenergic blocking agents.[48-52] Phenytoin is a second choice for treatment of this arrhythmia. Patients who do not respond to this therapy have undergone left stellate ganglionectomy, but the efficacy of this approach is not clear. In many cases, implanted automatic defibrillators may be the most appropriate therapy if pharmacologic therapy fails.

Torsades de pointes occurring in acquired long-QT syndrome may be idiopathic but most often has clearly recognizable precipitating factors. Episodes of tachycardia usually occur in the setting of bradycardia and are often initiated by VPCs producing a short-long-short series of coupling intervals (Fig. 94–23). This entity was originally recognized in patients with marked bradycardia resulting from complete heart block, but many metabolites and pharmacologic agents

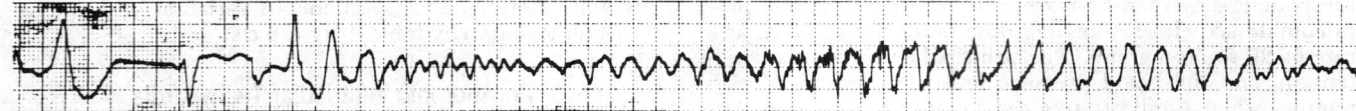

Figure 94–23. Torsades de pointes. Polymorphic ventricular tachycardia began with a long-short sequence in the setting of a prolonged QT interval. Note the continually changing axis during the tachycardia.

are now recognized as frequent precipitating factors (Table 94–4). Hypokalemia and/or hypomagnesemia may trigger this arrhythmia. Virtually all antiarrhythmic drugs, but most commonly type IA drugs such as quinidine or procainamide, especially if accompanied by hypokalemia, are frequent causes. In the case of pharmacologic agents, episodes of torsades de pointes usually occur within several days of initiation of therapy. The incidence of drug-induced torsades de pointes may be increased in patients with atrial fibrillation because of the irregular ventricular response facilitating the short-long-short activation sequence. The occurrence of torsades de pointes in association with type I antiarrhythmic agents does not correlate with serum drug levels.

Therapy of the acquired long-QT syndrome is based on the precipitating abnormality. In the case of marked bradycardia, acute therapy with isoproterenol in a dose sufficient to elevate the heart rate to 100 to 120 beats/min may be effective. Temporary pacing is also effective with either an atrial or ventricular temporary pacemaker sufficient to raise the ventricular rate to 100 to 120 beats/min. If the syndrome is associated with complete heart block, the obvious therapeutic choice is implantation of a permanent pacemaker. Administration of magnesium intravenously may suppress the tachycardia even in the presence of normal serum magnesium levels. When torsades de pointes is precipitated by a pharmacologic agent, the agent must be withdrawn and not readministered. If the arrhythmia occurs during therapy with a type IA antiarrhythmic agent, no other type IA agent should be given. In such cases, amiodarone appears to be a

safe alternative.[54] Electrolyte abnormalities such as hypokalemia or hypomagnesemia must be corrected rapidly. If the offending cause can be identified and corrected, the prognosis in these cases is excellent.

VENTRICULAR FIBRILLATION

Ventricular fibrillation is precipitated by a wide variety of conditions. Severe metabolic abnormalities such as hypokalemia, hyperkalemia, severe hypoxia, and myocardial ischemia frequently precipitate this arrhythmia. Polymorphic VT, in association both with the long-QT syndrome and with a normal QT interval, frequently degenerates into ventricular fibrillation. Rarely, patients with WPW syndrome who develop atrial fibrillation with an extremely rapid ventricular response may develop ventricular fibrillation (see earlier). Electrical accidents involving contact with high-voltage alternating current cause cardiac arrest through ventricular fibrillation. Victims of sudden unexpected cardiac arrest are most often found in ventricular fibrillation. This frequently occurs in a patient with coronary artery disease in response to acute myocardial ischemia and occurs most often within the first 6 hours of the onset of symptoms of acute myocardial infarction. Ventricular fibrillation may also be a primary abnormality in patients with cardiomyopathies, both hypertrophic and dilated. Ventricular fibrillation is frequently initiated by VT, especially in patients with chronic coronary artery disease. After resuscitation, most of these patients do not evolve enzymatic or electrocardiographic evidence of acute myocardial infarction. Such patients are at high risk of recurrent cardiac arrest: approximately 30% over 18 months when no therapy or empirical antiarrhythmic therapy is employed.[55–57] In contrast, patients who develop ventricular fibrillation in the acute phase (first 24 hours) of myocardial infarction appear to be at significantly lower risk for recurrent ventricular fibrillation. Studies of these two groups of patients suggest that most patients who develop ventricular fibrillation in the acute phase of myocardial infarction do so because of the severe myocardial ischemia. After the acute event, most patients are no longer exposed to this risk. In contrast, patients who develop ventricular fibrillation not associated with acute infarction most often have the arrhythmia initiated by VT and appear to have a chronic substrate predisposing to recurrent episodes of cardiac arrest.

The acute management of the patient with ventricular fibrillation consists of unsynchronized defibrillation utilizing high energies ($\geq$200 J). If the arrhythmia is rapidly reversed, intubation is often unnecessary and the patient may stabilize rapidly. However, if the resulting cardiac arrest was prolonged, several days may be required for stabilization. After the initial stabilization, several steps should be taken: a standard 12-lead ECG should be obtained as soon as possible to look for potential precipitating causes (e.g., prolongation of the QT interval) or evidence of acute myocardial infarction. If the patient was undergoing electrocardiographic monitoring at the time of onset of ventricular fibrillation, the preceding rhythm should be carefully examined for potential precipitating events. It should be determined whether the ventricular fibrillation was "primary"

TABLE 94–4

DRUGS ASSOCIATED WITH LONG-QT SYNDROME AND TORSADES DE POINTES

Antiarrhythmic agents (in decreasing order of frequency)
  Quinidine
  Procainamide (especially in patients with high
    N-acetylprocainamide levels)
  Sotalol
  Amiodarone
  Aprindine
  Flecainide
  Encainide
Psychotropic agents
  Phenothiazines
  Neuroleptic agents
Antibiotics
  Ampicillin
  Erythromycin
  Pentamidine
  Trimethoprim-sulfamethoxazole
Other drugs
  Anthracyclines (doxorubicin)
  Chloral hydrate
  Liquid protein diets
  Organophosphorous insecticide poisoning
  Prenylamine
  Probucol
  Terfenadine

or developed after VT. Evidence of bradyarrhythmias preceding the event should be sought. Subsequently, serial ECGs and cardiac enzyme determinations should be obtained to seek evidence of acute myocardial infarction as a precipitating event. It is usual for the serum creatine kinase level to rise to about 300 to 400 IU/mL after one or two direct-current shocks. However, the myocardial fraction of creatine kinase does not rise after rapid defibrillation. When the patient has stabilized, evidence should be sought for the presence and type of underlying structural heart disease. Cardiac catheterization should be performed in all patients to define the coronary artery anatomy. If acute myocardial infarction can be ruled out as a precipitating cause, cardiac electrophysiologic studies should be performed to seek evidence for substrates predisposing to recurrent ventricular fibrillation.

DIGITALIS TOXIC ARRHYTHMIAS

Digitalis affects all cardiac tissues and has been reported to cause virtually all types of cardiac rhythm disturbances. Arrhythmias arising from digitalis toxicity are related to several of its cellular electrophysiologic effects, including depression of normal pacemaker function, slowing of conduction, and development of ectopic rhythms.[58, 59] Depression of pacemaker function may be manifest as sinus node arrest. Depression of conduction may be manifest by sinus node exit block and AV nodal blockade. Ectopic arrhythmias may be due to re-entry, enhanced automaticity, or triggered rhythms associated with delayed afterdepolarizations. Certain ectopic rhythms are characteristic of digitalis toxicity, including atrial tachycardia (Fig. 94–24), nonparoxysmal junctional tachycardia, VPCs, VT, and ventricular fibrillation. Probably the most common manifestation of digitalis effect and toxicity is related to the AV node. All degrees of AV nodal block may result from digitalis, including prolongation of the PR interval, second-degree AV block (usually of the Wenckebach type), and complete AV block (see Fig. 94–24). Complete, or third-degree, AV block is most commonly recognized in patients who receive digitalis for atrial fibrillation or atrial flutter. In these cases, digitalis toxicity is recognized by regularization of the ventricular response to atrial fibrillation. Atrial flutter with varying conduction block to the ventricles or regularization of the ventricular response (i.e., complete heart block with an accelerated junctional rhythm) should raise the suspicion of digitalis toxicity. Production of third-degree AV nodal blockade is often associated with simultaneous development of nonparoxysmal junctional tachycardia caused by enhanced automaticity or triggered activity in the AV junction. The rate of this rhythm may range from 100 to 150 beats/min. However, just as digitalis may provoke exit block at the level of the sinus node, nonparoxysmal junctional tachycardias secondary to digitalis toxicity may be associated with exit block, resulting in irregular ventricular rates.

Another arrhythmia characteristic of digitalis toxicity is bidirectional tachycardia. This arrhythmia, which arises in the fascicles of the specialized conduction system, is usually characterized by a right bundle branch block type of pattern in the precordial leads with alternation of the frontal plane QRS axis (Fig. 94–25). Severe degrees of digitalis toxicity may be manifest by recurrent refractory ventricular fibrillation. Patients with digitalis toxicity are reported to develop refractory ventricular fibrillation in response to cardioversion. All arrhythmias resulting from digitalis toxicity appear to be facilitated in the presence of hypokalemia.

Digitalis toxicity must be suspected in any patient receiving this agent who develops new arrhythmias. Toxicity often is precipitated by the development of renal failure in patients receiving digoxin therapy resulting in elevation of serum drug levels. Toxicity may also be precipitated by the addition of one of the several agents known to elevate serum digoxin levels, such as quinidine, amiodarone, and verapamil. Suicide attempts with digitalis may also produce life-threatening arrhythmias. Children and young adults develop high-grade AV nodal block much more frequently than the elderly as a manifestation of digitalis toxicity. Massive overdose of digitalis may be associated with severe hyperkalemia, presumably as a result of the drug poisoning the Na^+-K^+ exchange pump.

Treatment of digitalis intoxication depends on the type and severity of arrhythmia. Hypokalemia must be corrected rapidly. Minor degrees of intoxication, such as SA block, lesser degrees of AV nodal blockade, and VPCs, may be managed expectantly while the drug is withheld. Severe bradyarrhythmias may respond to intravenous atropine, but if the patient fails to respond temporary pacemaking may be required. Atrial tachycardia with block resulting from digitalis toxicity characteristically responds readily to phenytoin. VT and fibrillation caused by digitalis intoxication may respond to lidocaine, phenytoin, or other type I antiarrhythmic agents. Any high-grade AV block or life-threatening tachyarrhythmias resulting from digitalis toxicity should be treated rapidly with digoxin-specific antibody fragments.[60] Digoxin antibodies rapidly and safely reverse virtually all toxic effects of digoxin and are now widely available. Although these antibodies are prepared from serum proteins, allergic reactions are rare.

WIDE QRS COMPLEX TACHYCARDIA: DIFFERENTIATION OF SUPRAVENTRICULAR FROM VENTRICULAR ORIGINS

The differential diagnosis of a wide QRS complex tachycardia is a frequently encountered clinical problem. Wide QRS complex tachycardia is defined by a QRS duration exceeding 120 ms. Four diagnostic entities must be considered when confronted with such an arrhythmia. First, if the patient exhibits a bundle branch block or intraventricular conduction delay during normal sinus rhythm, any supraventricular tachycardia is likely to result in a wide QRS complex having a morphology similar to that in sinus rhythm. Second, patients with bypass tracts (AV, nodoventricular, nodofascicular) may develop pre-excited supraventricular tachycardias in which the QRS complex is widened

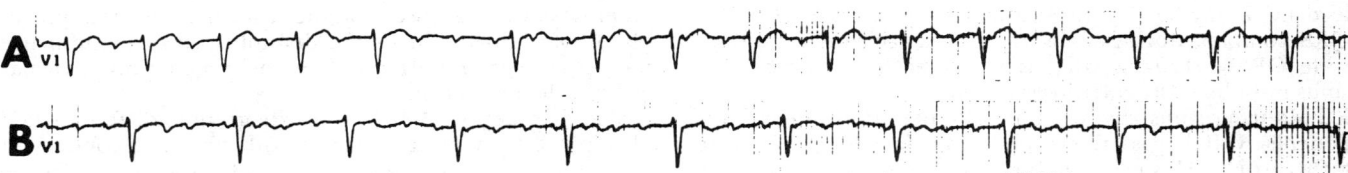

Figure 94–24. Digitalis toxic atrial tachycardia. *A.* Atrial tachycardia with varying degrees of AV conduction block. Note the irregular ventricular rate. *B.* The same atrial tachycardia, now with complete heart block. Notice that the ventricular rate is regular and the P waves no longer bear a relationship to the QRS complex.

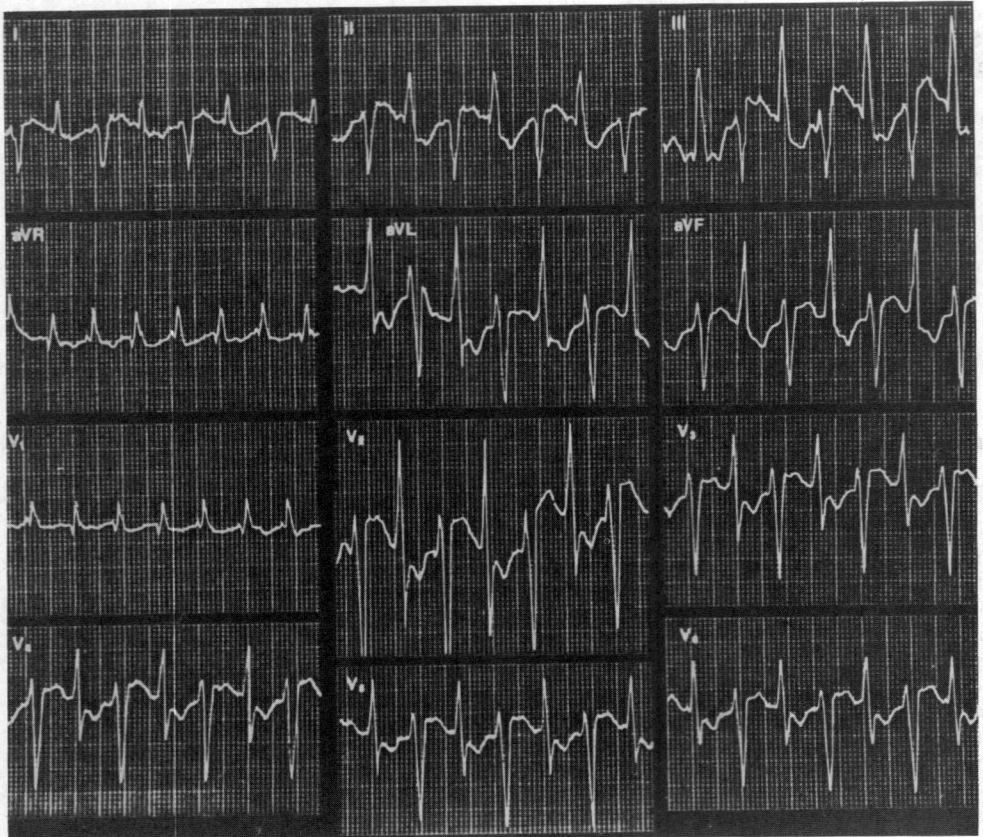

Figure 94–25. Bidirectional ventricular tachycardia in a case of digitalis toxicity. Note the alternating frontal plane axis in the setting of a right bundle branch block, present in V_1. (From Wharton M, Goldschlager N: Interpreting Cardiac Dysrhythmias. Oradell, NJ, Medical Economics Books, p 186, 1987. Reprinted by permission of Blackwell Scientific Publications, Inc.)

because of activation of the ventricles partly or entirely via the bypass tract rather than the normal AV conduction system. Third, supraventricular tachycardia (re-entrant and non–re-entrant) may be conducted to the ventricles over the normal AV conduction system with an aberrant pattern because of functional bundle branch block. Fourth, VT usually has a wide QRS complex. The first factor to consider in differentiating among wide QRS complex tachycardias is whether the rhythm is regular or irregular. Irregularly irregular wide QRS tachycardias occur almost exclusively in the presence of atrial fibrillation. If the QRS complex of an irregularly irregular wide QRS tachycardia is bizarre (not a typical left or right bundle branch pattern), especially if the ventricular rate is over 200 beats/min, atrial fibrillation with conduction over an AV bypass tract should be strongly considered (see Figs. 94–18 and 94–19). Most VTs with uniform morphology vary in cycle length from beat to beat by less than 40 ms (irregular rhythms during VT occur more often in the presence of antiarrhythmic drugs). When atrial fibrillation has been eliminated, the next step is to compare the tachycardia QRS morphology with that during sinus rhythm. If the QRS complex during the tachycardia matches that during the sinus, it is likely to be supraventricular in origin. In such cases, detailed examination of the 12-lead ECG may be helpful. If a patient has a wide, aberrant QRS complex during sinus rhythm, a tachycardia with a wide QRS (>120 ms) that is narrower than that during sinus must be ventricular in origin. Close examination of the ECG during sinus rhythm is usually helpful in identifying patients with bypass tracts who may develop pre-excited tachycardias. However, absence of pre-excitation during sinus rhythm does not exclude the presence of an AV or other type of bypass tract.

Patients who have narrow QRS complexes during sinus rhythm constitute the majority of patients who develop wide QRS complex tachycardias. These are the patients who most often pose difficulties in the differential diagnosis of such tachycardias. This issue has been addressed in a number of studies, and electrocardiographic criteria have been developed that are useful in differentiating supraventricular tachycardias with aberrant intraventricular conduction from tachycardias of ventricular origin.[61–65] However, before even considering the ECG in the differential diagnosis of the tachycardia, the physician would be well advised to consider general characteristics of the patient. More than 80% of sustained VTs having a uniform morphology occur in patients with coronary artery disease and a previous myocardial infarction. Less often, VT occurs in patients with dilated cardiomyopathies, and far less often it occurs in patients with no apparent structural heart disease. Thus, when a patient has a wide QRS tachycardia and a history of myocardial infarction, the odds favor the tachycardia's being ventricular in origin. Conversely, a wide QRS tachycardia in a relatively young, previously healthy patient without evidence of structural heart disease is most likely supraventricular in origin. Obviously, patients with supraventricular tachycardias are not immune to developing coronary or other types of heart disease as they age, and the development of coronary disease or myocardial infarction may influence the occurrence and effects of pre-existing supraventricular tachycardia mechanisms.

The first step in the electrocardiographic differentiation of supraventricular tachycardia with aberrant conduction from VT is to search for evidence of atrial activity in the ECG. The presence of P waves dissociated from the QRS complexes greatly favors a ventricular origin of tachycardia

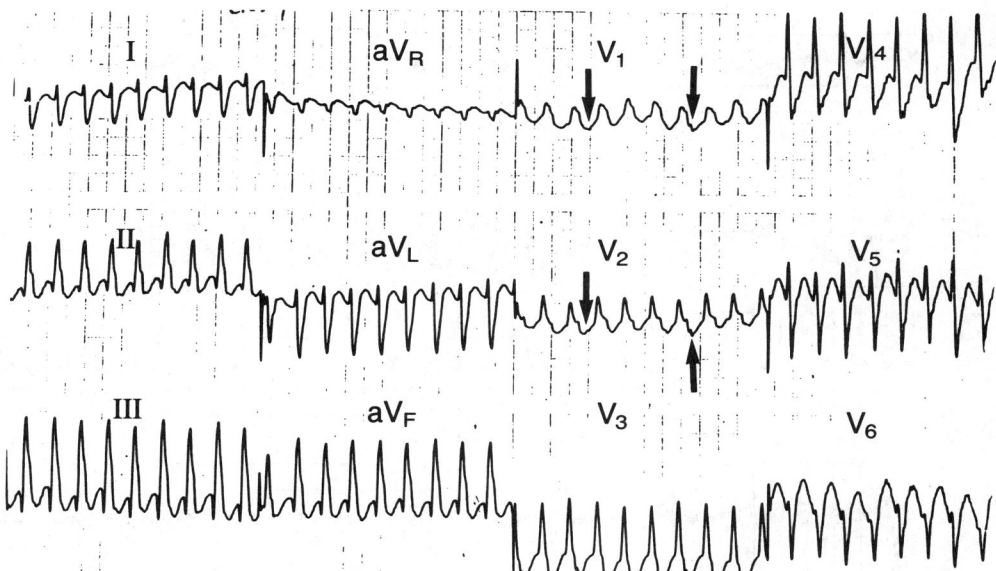

Figure 94–26. Twelve-lead ECG of sustained uniform ventricular tachycardia with a right bundle branch block morphology. AV dissociation is present with P waves marching through the QRS complexes *(arrows)*.

(Fig. 94–26). Accompanying AV dissociation during the tachycardia may be intermittent sinus capture beats having a narrow QRS complex or fusion complexes having an intermittent QRS duration. The presence of these complexes is proof of a ventricular origin of tachycardia. However, failure to identify dissociated atrial activity is not proof of a supraventricular origin of tachycardia, because VT not infrequently is associated with retrograde conduction to the atria in a 1:1 pattern or in a pattern of regular block such as 2:1 or 3:1 (Fig. 94–27). It is useful to remember that examination of the jugular venous pulse may be helpful in this aspect of the differential diagnosis: the presence of intermittent cannon "a" waves results from AV dissociation. On occasion, in spite of careful examination of all 12 standard electrocardiographic leads, evidence of atrial activity cannot be discerned. In such cases, it may be useful to record atrial activity directly via an esophageal electrogram or temporary pacing catheters inserted percutaneously and advanced to the right atrium (Fig. 94–28). The esophageal electrogram is recorded by advancing a temporary pacing catheter into the esophagus just as a nasogastric tube is placed. While the soft catheter is advanced, an electrogram

recording from the leads is continuously monitored to recognize left atrial activity. Patients who have recently undergone open heart surgery usually have temporary atrial pacing leads placed on the epicardium. These leads may be used to record atrial activity directly.

If the patient has a normal QRS duration in sinus rhythm, a number of other criteria may help define the tachycardia mechanism. A QRS duration greater than 140 ms favors a ventricular origin in most cases. Examination of the type of bundle branch block pattern yields other useful criteria. In patients with a right bundle branch block type of QRS, marked left axis deviation (more negative than −30°) strongly favors a ventricular origin of tachycardia (see Fig. 94–27). Right bundle branch block patterns having a monophasic R wave or qR, QR, and RS complexes favor ventricular origin (see Figs. 94–22 and 94–27). A right bundle branch block pattern with a triphasic (rSR') complex in V_1 with the R' having a greater amplitude than the initial R wave favors supraventricular origin (Fig. 94–29). Finally, a predominantly negative QRS complex in V_6 favors ventricular origin of the tachycardia (see Figs. 94–22 and 94–27).

Electrocardiograms having a left bundle branch block QRS

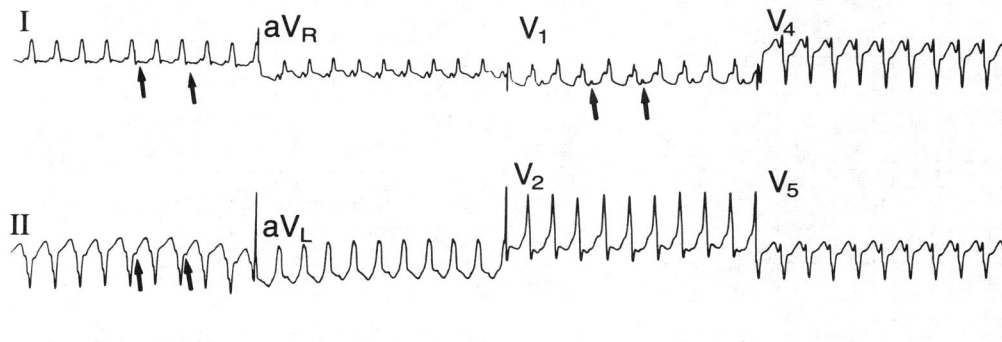

Figure 94–27. Sustained uniform ventricular tachycardia with a right bundle branch block configuration. The arrows indicate atrial activity. VA conduction is present in a 2:1 pattern. Note the marked left axis deviation and the R:S ratio less than 1 in V_6.

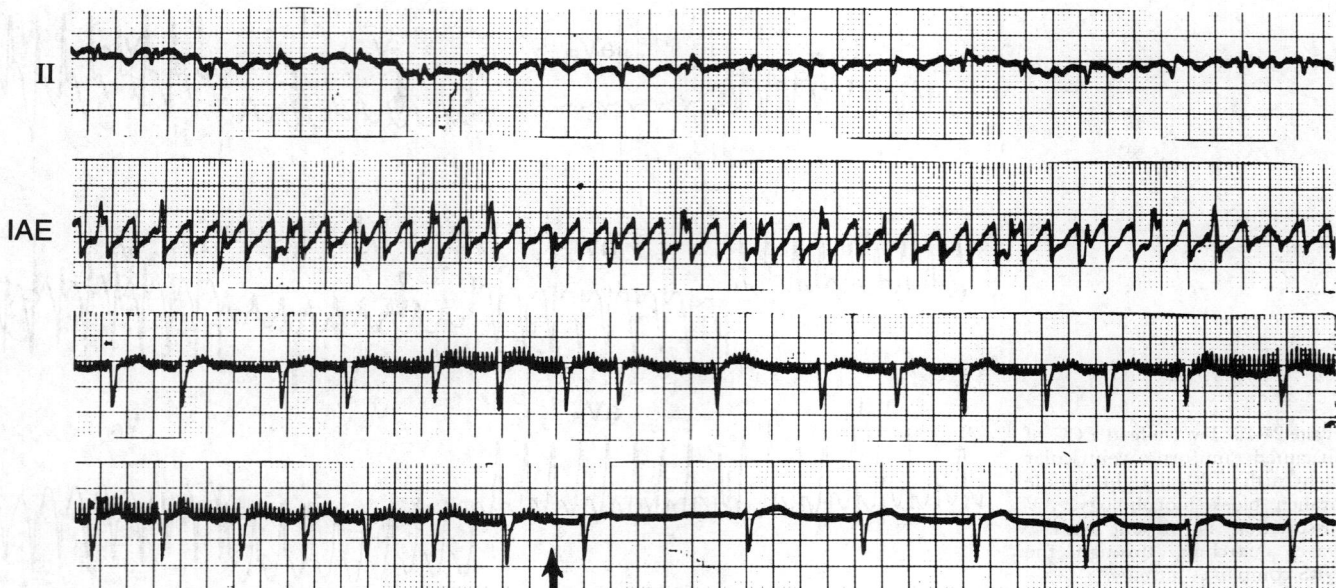

Figure 94–28. Atrial flutter. The top panel shows a tracing from electrocardiographic lead II during atrial flutter. An intra-atrial electrogram (IAE) depicts more clearly regular atrial activity at a rate of 300 beats/min. The bottom two panels show termination of the atrial flutter by overdrive atrial pacing. Stimulus artifact during rapid atrial pacing is superimposed in the tracing from the surface electrocardiographic monitor lead. After termination of rapid atrial pacing *(arrow)*, atrial flutter stops and sinus rhythm is restored.

pattern also have features helpful in differentiating the tachycardia mechanism. It should be noted that left axis deviation in the presence of left bundle branch block is not helpful in differentiating supraventricular from ventricular origin. However, an initial R wave in V_1 or V_2 having a duration greater than 30 ms or an interval from the onset of the initial R to the nadir of the subsequent S wave in V_1 or V_2 greater than 60 ms strongly favors ventricular origin (Fig. 94–30). Notching on the downstroke of the S wave in V_1 or V_2 also favors a ventricular origin of the tachycardia. A Q wave in V_6 with a left bundle branch block pattern also strongly favors ventricular origin.

Two final caveats regarding the differential diagnosis of wide QRS complex tachycardias are in order. First, the tachycardia rate is not helpful in determining the site of origin. Second, the hemodynamic consequences of a tachycardia are not helpful in differentiating between the foregoing mechanisms. It is not unusual, even in patients with prior myocardial infarction, for uniform VT to be well tolerated and not associated with severe hypotension. Conversely, a supraventricular tachycardia in a patient with severe underlying heart disease may cause rapid hemodynamic decompensation. Careful, detailed examination of the 12-lead ECG permits an accurate diagnosis in the majority of wide QRS complex tachycardias when considered in the appropriate context.

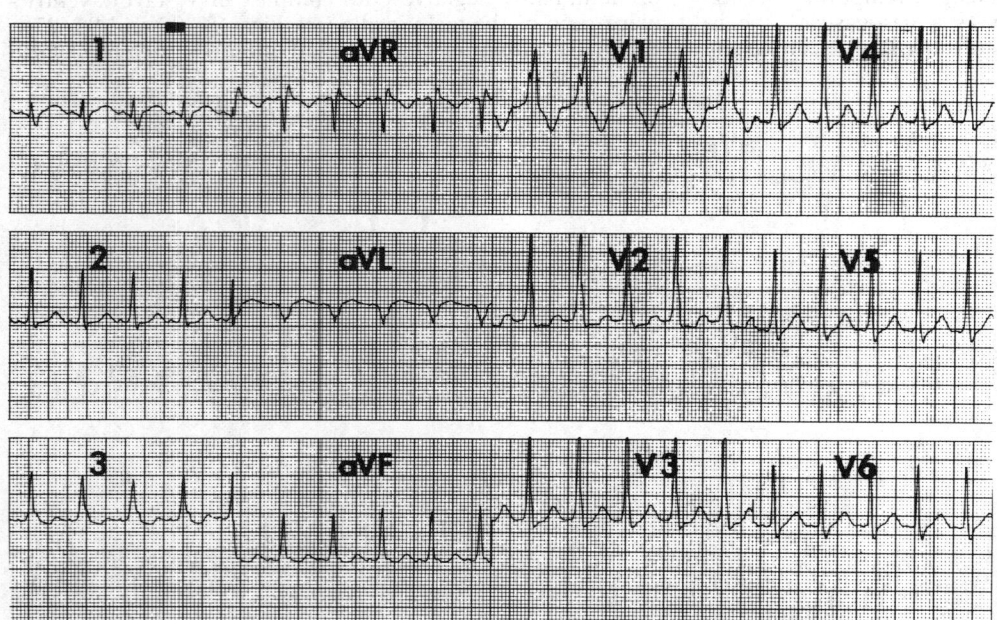

Figure 94–29. Atrial tachycardia in a patient with functional right bundle branch block. Note the rsR′ configuration in V_1 and the R:S ratio greater than 1 in lead V_6. The frontal plane QRS axis is normal.

SVT   VT

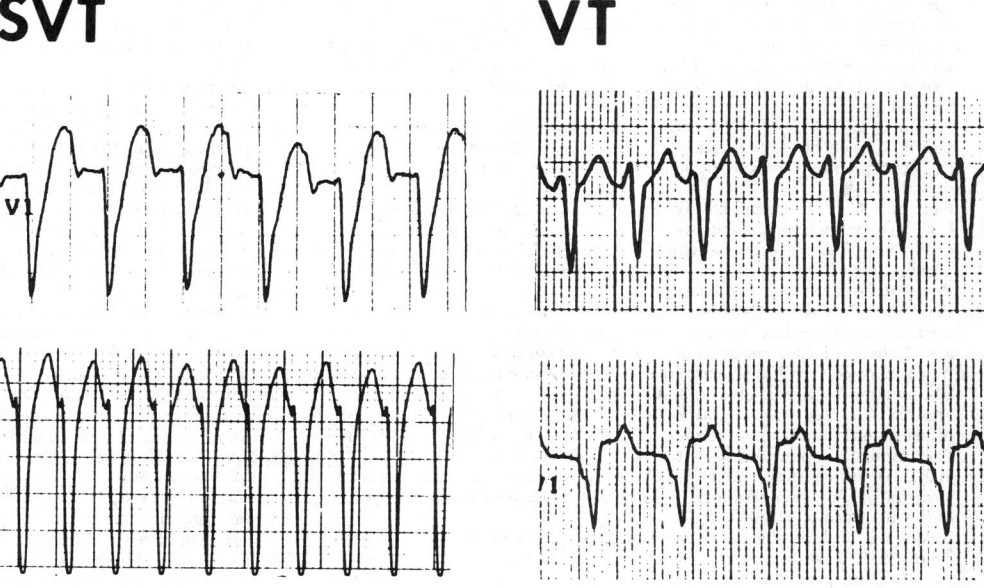

Figure 94–30. Comparison of left bundle branch block aberration during supraventricular tachycardia (SVT) *(left)* in two patients with sustained ventricular tachycardia having a left bundle branch block configuration *(right)*. Each tracing is from ECG lead V₁. *(Left)* During the two examples of SVT, the initial R wave is narrow with a rapid downstroke to the S wave. *(Right)* During VT, note that in the example at the top a broad initial R wave is present. The time from onset of R wave to nadir of the S wave is 80 ms. In the bottom panel, during ventricular tachycardia, there is no initial R wave. The time from onset of QRS to nadir of the S wave is greater than 80 ms, and there is a notch on the downstroke of the S wave.

TACHYCARDIAS: ACUTE TREATMENT

The acute management of any patient with a tachyarrhythmia is determined more by the hemodynamic effects of the arrhythmia than by the specific arrhythmia. That is, if a tachycardia results in such severe hypotension that the patient has lost consciousness, the acute treatment is the same regardless of the arrhythmia: cardioversion or defibrillation to restore sinus rhythm. Thus, a patient with a hypertrophic left ventricle who develops acute atrial fibrillation with a rapid ventricular response causing severe hypotension and a loss of consciousness should be treated by cardioversion, not by AV nodal blocking agents. However, if an acute arrhythmia has precipitated severe symptoms such as unremitting angina, pulmonary edema, and/or severe lightheadedness, one must make a judgment whether to pursue appropriate pharmacologic therapy or administer a short-acting sedative or anesthetic and then perform cardioversion.

At the other extreme, tachyarrhythmias of both supraventricular and ventricular origin may result in a drop in the patient's blood pressure from his or her baseline but no severe symptoms. In this case, several steps should be taken before performing definitive therapy. First, an ECG with multiple standard electrocardiographic leads, preferably a full 12-lead ECG on a multichannel recorder, should be obtained. This is often necessary to establish a precise diagnosis that may influence subsequent diagnostic and therapeutic steps. Even in the case of an apparently uniform VT, a 12-lead ECG should be obtained. In addition, for patients having recurrent episodes of tachycardia, a full 12-lead ECG should be obtained during each of several episodes. Patients with supraventricular tachycardia frequently have multiple mechanisms. Patients with VT may have multiple morphologies of uniform VT, and the number and type may be important in evaluating the efficacy of subsequent therapies. We feel strongly that no matter what the arrhythmia (no matter how bizarre the ECG may appear), no patient should ever be cardioverted or defibrillated while conscious and awake. If the patient is awake, no matter what the diagnosis, there is always time to administer some form of anesthesia or sedation. Thus, the physician must treat the patient, not the ECG or arrhythmia in isolation.

The acute pharmacologic treatment of specific arrhythmias has been covered in previous sections of this chapter. However, in this general discussion, one point is worth emphasizing. In some patients who develop wide QRS complex tachycardias, it may be difficult to differentiate supraventricular tachycardia with aberrant intraventricular conduction from VT. Some physicians use intravenous verapamil as a diagnostic test, reasoning that any tachycardia that terminates in response is supraventricular. However, verapamil is contraindicated as acute therapy for patients with wide QRS complex tachycardias unless the mechanism of the tachycardia is known with certainty or the patient is known to have verapamil-responsive VT. The reason is that administration of verapamil intravenously to patients with hemodynamically stable VT frequently results in acute decompensation.[66, 67]

References

1. Hoffman BF, Cranefield PA: Electrophysiology of the Heart. New York, McGraw-Hill, 1960.
2. Fozzard HA, Arnsdorf MF: Cardiac electrophysiology. In: Fozzard HA, Jennings RB, Haber E, et al (eds): The Heart and Cardiovascular System. New York, Raven Press, pp 1–30, 1986.
3. Thompson KA, Hurwitz JL: Clinical pharmacology and use of antiarrhythmic drugs. In: Waugh R, Ramo B, Wagner G, et al (eds): Cardiac Arrhythmias. Philadelphia, FA Davis. In press.
4. Cranefield PA: The Conduction of the Cardiac Impulse. Mt. Kisco, NY, Futura Publishing, 1975.
5. Hodgkin AL, Huxley AF: A quantitative description of membrane current and its application to conduction and excitation in nerve. J Physiol (Lond) 117:424, 1952.
6. Marriott HJL, Conover MH: Advanced Concepts in Arrhythmias. St Louis, CV Mosby, 1983.
7. Merideth J, Mendez C, Mueller W, et al: Electrical excitability of atrioventricular nodal cells. Circ Res 23:69, 1968.
8. Meijler FL, Janse MJ: Morphology and electrophysiology of the mammalian atrioventricular node. Physiol Rev 68:608, 1988.
9. Commerford PJ, Lloyd EA: Arrhythmias in patients with drug toxicity, electrolyte and endocrine disturbances. Med Clin North Am 65:1051, 1984.
10. Cranefield PF, Wit AL, Hoffman BF: Genesis of cardiac arrhythmias, Circulation 47:190, 1973.
11. Woosley RL, Shand DG: Pharmacokinetics of antiarrhythmic drugs. Am J Cardiol 41:986, 1978.
12. Vaughn-Williams EM: Antiarrhythmic Action. London, Academic Press, 1980.
13. Fenster PE: Clinical pharmacology: Clinical uses of pharmacokinetic principles in prescribing cardiac drugs. Med Clin North Am 68:1281, 1984.

14. Dreifus LS, Michelson EL, Kaplinsky E: Bradyarrhythmias: Clinical significance and management. J Am Coll Cardiol 4:1118, 1984.
15. Hindman MC, Wagner GS, JaRo M, et al: The clinical significance of bundle branch block complicating acute myocardial infarction. 1. Classical characteristics, hospital mortality, and one-year follow-up. Circulation 58:679, 1978.
16. Hindman MC, Wagner GS, JaRo M, et al: The clinical significance of bundle branch block complicating acute myocardial infarction. 2. Indications for temporary and permanent pacemaker insertion. Circulation 58:689, 1978.
17. Gunnar RM, Passamarni ER, Bourdillon PD, et al: Guidelines for the early management of patients with acute myocardial infarction: A report of the American College of Cardiology/American Heart Association Task Force on Assessment of Diagnostic and Therapeutic Cardiovascular Procedures. J Am Coll Cardiol 16:249, 1990.
18. Frye RL, Collins JJ, DeSanctis RW, et al: Guidelines for permanent cardiac pacemaker implantation, May 1984. A report of the Joint American College of Cardiology/American Heart Association Task Force on Assessment of Cardiovascular Procedures (Subcommittee on Pacemaker Implantation). Circulation 70:331A, 1984.
19. Sharma AD, Yee R, Guiraudon G, et al: Sensitivity and specificity of invasive and noninvasive testing for risk of sudden death in Wolff-Parkinson-White syndrome. J Am Coll Cardiol 10:373, 1987.
20. Wu D, Denes P, Amat-y-Leon F, et al: Clinical, electrocardiographic and electrophysiologic observations in paroxysmal supraventricular tachycardia. Am J Cardiol 41:1045, 1978.
21. Kastor JA: Multifocal atrial tachycardia. N Engl J Med 322:1713, 1990.
22. Miles WM, Prystowsky EN: Supraventricular tachycardia in patients without overt preexcitation. Cardiol Clin 4:429, 1986.
23. Gallagher JJ, Smith WM, Kasell J, et al: Use of the esophageal lead in the diagnosis of mechanisms of reciprocating supraventricular tachycardia. PACE 3:440, 1980.
24. Benditt DG, Prichett ELC, Smith WM, et al: Ventriculoatrial intervals: Diagnostic use in paroxysmal supraventricular tachycardia. Ann Intern Med 91:161, 1979.
25. DiMarco JP, Sellers TD, Lerman BB, et al: Diagnostic and therapeutic use of adenosine in patients with supraventricular tachyarrhythmias. J Am Coll Cardiol 6:417, 1985.
26. DiMarco PJ, Miles W, Akhtar M, et al: Adenosine for paroxysmal supraventricular tachycardia: Dose ranging and comparison with verapamil. Ann Intern Med 113:104, 1990.
27. Prystowsky EN: Diagnosis and management of the preexcitation syndromes. Curr Prob Cardiol 13:225, 1988.
28. Gallagher JJ, Gilbert M, Swenson RH, et al: Wolff-Parkinson-White syndrome: The problem, evaluation and surgical correction. Circulation 51:767, 1975.
29. Hinkle LE, Carver ST, Stevens M: The frequency of asymptomatic disturbances of cardiac rhythm and conduction in middle-aged men. Am J Cardiol 24:629, 1969.
30. Califf RM, McKinnis RA, Burks J, et al: Prognostic implications of ventricular arrhythmias during 24 hour ambulatory monitoring in patients undergoing cardiac catheterization for coronary artery disease. Am J Cardiol 50:23, 1982.
31. Buxton AE, Waxman HL, Marchlinski FE, et al: Right ventricular tachycardia: Clinical and electrophysiologic characteristics. Circulation 68:917, 1983.
32. Rahilly GT, Prystowsky EN, Zipes DP, et al: Clinical and electrophysiologic findings in patients with repetitive monomorphic ventricular tachycardia and otherwise normal electrocardiogram. Am J Cardiol 50:459, 1982.
33. Suyama A, Anan T, Araki H, et al: Prevalence of ventricular tachycardia in patients with different underlying heart disease: A study by Holter ECG monitoring. Am Heart J 112:44, 1986.
34. Josephson ME, Horowitz LN, Farshidi A, et al: Recurrent sustained ventricular tachycardia. Circulation 57:431, 1978.
35. McGovern B, Schoenfeld MH, Ruskin JN, et al: Ventricular tachycardia: Historical perspective. PACE 9:449, 1986.
36. Kastor JA: Electrophysiology, pacing and arrhythmia: Ventricular tachycardia. Clin Cardiol 12:586, 1989.
37. Akhtar M: Clinical spectrum of ventricular tachycardia. Circulation 82:1561, 1990.
38. Swerdlow CD, Winkle RA, Mason JW: Determinants of survival in patients with ventricular tachyarrhythmias. N Engl J Med 308:1436, 1983.
39. Wilber DJ, Garan H, Finkelstein D, et al: Out-of-hospital cardiac arrest: Use of electrophysiologic testing in the prediction of long-term outcome. N Engl J Med 318:29, 1988.
40. Josephson ME, Miller JM, Marchlinski FE, et al: Nonpharmacologic therapy of ventricular tachycardia. Clin Cardiol 11:II–17, 1988.
41. Buxton AE, Josephson ME: Ventricular tachycardia—1983. PACE 7:96, 1984.
42. Marchlinski FE: Ventricular tachycardia associated with coronary artery disease. Prog Cardiol 1:231, 1988.
43. Horowitz LN, Josephson ME, Kastor JA: Intracardiac electrophysiologic studies as a method for the optimization of drug therapy in chronic ventricular arrhythmia. Prog Cardiovasc Dis 23:81, 1980.
44. Swerdlow CD, Peterson J: Prospective comparison of Holter monitoring and electrophysiologic study in patients with coronary artery disease and sustained ventricular tachyarrhythmias. Am J Cardiol 56:577, 1985.
45. Mirowski M: The automatic implantable cardioverter-defibrillator: An overview. J Am Coll Cardiol 6:461, 1985.
46. Kelly PA, Cannom DS, Garan H, et al: The automatic implantable cardioverter-defibrillator: Efficacy, complications and survival in patients with malignant ventricular arrhythmias. J Am Coll Cardiol 11:1278, 1988.
47. Lehmann MH, Steinman RT, Schuger CD, et al: The automatic implantable cardioverter defibrillator as antiarrhythmic treatment modality of choice for survivors of cardiac arrest unrelated to acute myocardial infarction. Am J Cardiol 62:803, 1988.
48. Moss AJ, Schwartz PJ, Crampton RS, et al: The long QT syndrome: A prospective international study. Circulation 71:17, 1985.
49. Roden DM, Woosley RL, Primm RK: Incidence and clinical features of the quinidine-associated long QT syndrome: Implications for patient care. Am Heart J 111:1088, 1986.
50. Roden DM, Thompson KA, Hoffman BF, et al: Clinical features and basic mechanisms of quinidine-induced arrhythmias. J Am Coll Cardiol 8:73A, 1986.
51. Jackman WM, Friday KJ, Anderson JL, et al: The long QT syndromes: A critical review, new clinical observations and a unifying hypothesis. Prog Cardiovasc Dis 31:115, 1988.
52. Schwartz PJ: Idiopathic long QT syndrome: Progress and questions. Am Heart J 109:399, 1985.
53. Cranefield PF, Aronson RS: Torsade de pointes and other pause-induced ventricular tachycardias: The short-long-short sequence and early after-depolarizations. PACE 11:670, 1988.
54. Mattioni TA, Zheutlin TA, Sarmiento JJ, et al: Amiodarone in patients with previous drug-mediated torsades de pointes: Long-term safety and efficacy. Ann Intern Med 111:574, 1989.
55. Myerburg RJ, Kessler KM, Estes D, et al: Long-term survival after prehospital cardiac arrest: Analysis of outcome during an 8 year study. Circulation 70:538, 1984.
56. Cobb LA, Baum RS, Alvarez H, et al: Resuscitation from out-of-hospital ventricular fibrillation: 4 years follow-up. Circulation 52(suppl III):223, 1975.
57. Schaffer WA, Cobb LA: Recurrent ventricular fibrillation and modes of death in survivors of out-of-hospital ventricular fibrillation. N Engl J Med 293:259, 1975.
58. Antman EM, Smith TW: Digitalis toxicity. Mod Concepts Cardiovasc Dis 55:26, 1986.
59. Smith TW: Digitalis: Mechanisms of action and clinical use. N Eng J Med 318:358, 1988.
60. Antman EM, Wenger TL, Butler VP, et al: Treatment of 150 cases of life-threatening digitalis intoxication with digoxin-specific Fab antibody fragments: Final report of a multicenter study. Circulation 81:1744, 1990.
61. Wellens HJJ, Bar FWH, Lie KI: The value of the electrocardiogram in the differential diagnosis of a tachycardia with a widened QRS complex. Am J Med 64:27, 1978.
62. Akhtar M: Electrophysiologic bases for wide QRS complex tachycardia. PACE 6:81, 1983.
63. Akhtar M, Shenasa M, Jazayeri M, et al: Wide QRS complex tachycardia: Reappraisal of a common clinical problem. Ann Intern Med 109:905, 1988.
64. Wellens HJJ: The wide QRS tachycardia. Ann Intern Med 104:879, 1986.
65. Kindwall KE, Brown J, Josephson ME: Electrocardiographic criteria for ventricular tachycardia in wide complex left bundle branch block morphology tachycardias. Am J Cardiol 61:1279, 1988.
66. Stewart RB, Bardy GH, Greene HL: Wide complex tachycardia: Misdiagnosis and outcome after emergent therapy. Ann Intern Med 104:766, 1986.
67. Buxton AE, Marchlinski FE, Doherty JU, et al: Hazards of intravenous verapamil for sustained ventricular tachycardia. Am J Cardiol 59:1107, 1975.

CHAPTER 95

Hemodynamic Monitoring

James A. Kruse
Eugenio Armendariz

Pulmonary arterial (PA) catheterization using the balloon flotation catheter was first reported by Lategola and Rahn in the early 1950s and later introduced to clinical practice in the early 1970s by Swan, Ganz, and colleagues.[1-4] Since then, this technique has gained wide usage in the bedside management of patients in the intensive care unit (ICU) setting. A number of options related to the catheter itself have evolved, such as the incorporation of fiberoptic technology for continuous mixed venous oximetry monitoring; rapid-response thermistors that allow measurement of right ventricular (RV) volume and ejection fraction; and extra ports for infusing fluids or drugs, simultaneously monitoring pressures in multiple chambers, or introducing ventricular pacing electrodes. PA catheterization is indicated in many clinical situations (see also Chapter 15) but is particularly useful in evaluating intravascular volume status in patients with hypotension or acute renal failure; in assessing the level of myocardial performance in patients with myocardial infarction, severe heart failure, severe sepsis, circulatory shock, and cardiogenic and noncardiogenic pulmonary edema; and in the perioperative management of high-risk surgical patients.[5-32] The information obtained from invasive right-sided heart catheterization can be useful in titrating therapeutic interventions such as fluid loading, inotropic and afterload-reducing therapy, and positive end-expiratory pressure (PEEP).[15, 20, 22, 25, 30-34] However, because use of this device is not free from complications, it should be used only for specific indications, when the potential benefits surpass the risks, and when the information obtained will probably help in initiating, altering, or monitoring the effects of therapy. Multiple independent clinical investigations have demonstrated that inferring hemodynamic conditions from physical and radiographic findings is inferior to invasive monitoring and that the information resulting from PA catheterization frequently leads to rational changes in therapy.[10, 35-41] The more important question is whether the use of hemodynamic monitoring has a positive effect on the outcome for the patient. This has been difficult to answer from retrospective, uncontrolled studies,[42, 43] but results of prospective, controlled trials suggest that optimizing physiologic variables on the basis of information from invasive monitoring may reduce mortality.[44, 45]

A multicenter trial examining physicians' knowledge of use of the PA catheter concluded that the level of competence is highly variable, and nearly half of those surveyed were unable to derive basic information from PA catheterization findings.[46] The intensivist must be skilled not only in the techniques of catheter insertion and maintenance but also in interpreting the hemodynamic information so obtained. This requires an in-depth understanding of normal and abnormal cardiac physiology, knowledge of the principles underlying the measurement techniques employed for pressure and flow determinations, and knowledge of the derivation of calculated hemodynamic parameters based on these measurements. Awareness of the limitations of these measurement techniques and their application is also important.

ANALYSIS OF PRESSURE WAVEFORMS

The ability to recognize normal and pathologic pressure waveforms is essential to those involved in the use of PA catheters. Normal right atrial and central venous pressure (CVP) waveforms consist of three distinct positive deflections that occur during the cardiac cycle (Fig. 95–1A). The a wave occurs at the end of ventricular diastole, just after the P wave appears on the electrocardiogram, and is due to the increase in pressure resulting from atrial contraction. The decrease in chamber pressure that occurs with subsequent atrial relaxation is known as the systolic dip or x descent. The c wave appears during this period of decreasing pressure, just after the QRS complex, and is thought to result from the force of closure of the tricuspid valve.[47, 48] Continuation of the x descent after this c wave is sometimes referred to as x'. The x' descent ends as venous blood subsequently accumulates in the atrium and exerts increased tension on the chamber walls, thus elevating intra-atrial pressure. This rise in atrial pressure is responsible for the v wave. A diastolic dip, or y descent, follows the opening of the tricuspid valve as the atrium empties into the ventricle. The h wave, mentioned for completeness, is a subtle deflection sometimes seen after the y descent and signals the completion of passive

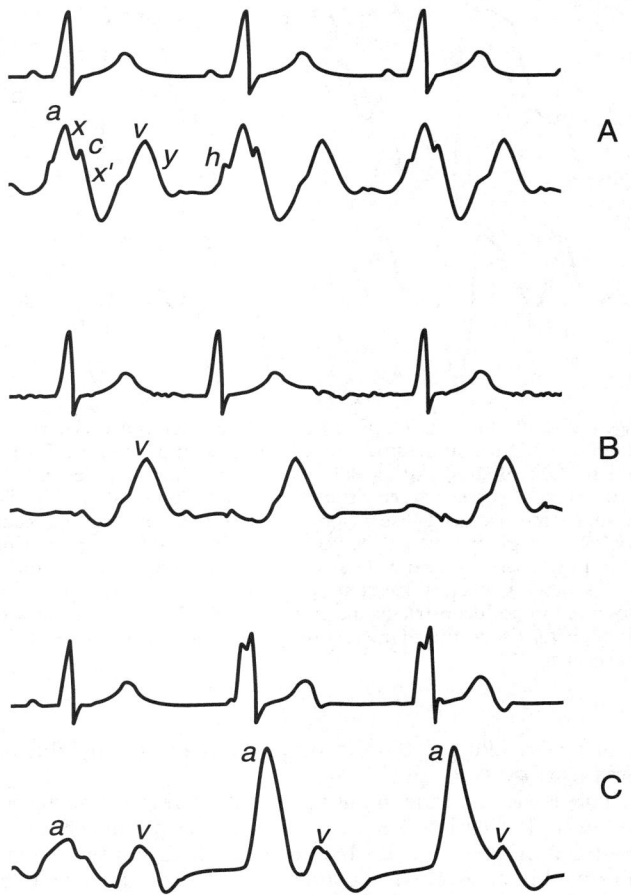

Figure 95–1. Right atrial (or central venous pressure) tracings. *A.* Normal pressure waveform (see text) and simultaneous electrocardiogram. *B.* Reference electrocardiogram and P_{RA} tracing in atrial fibrillation showing absence of a waves. *C.* Reference electrocardiogram and P_{RA} tracing in atrioventricular dissociation. First cycle shows normal a and v waves because atrial systole happens to precede ventricular systole. Giant a waves are seen with next two cycles because right atrium contracts against closed tricuspid valve.

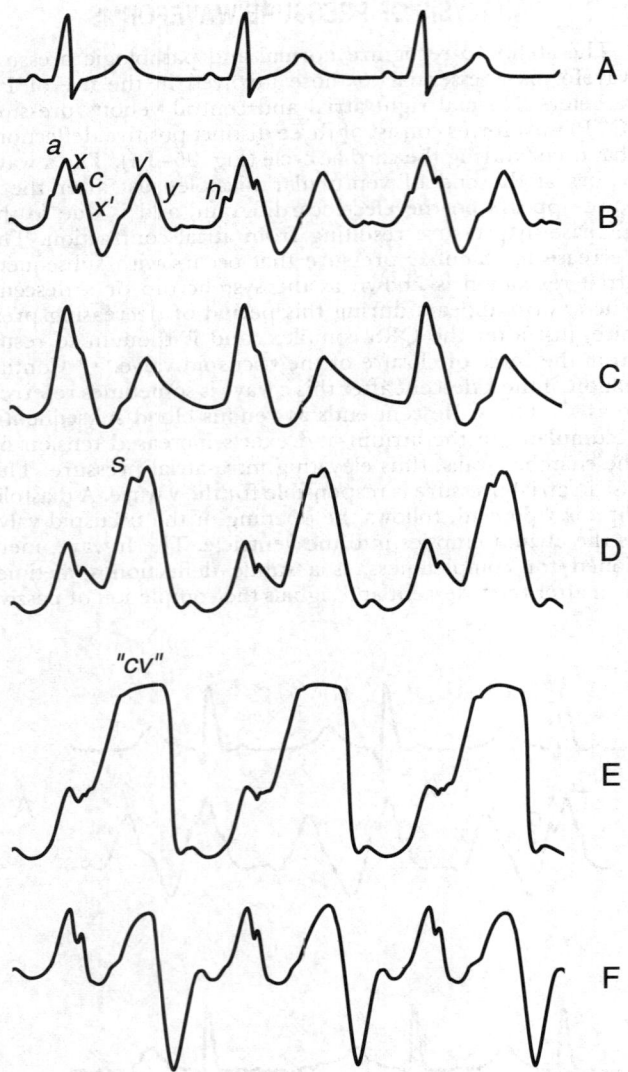

Figure 95–2. Right atrial (or CVP) tracings. *A.* Reference electrocardiogram. *B.* Normal pressure waveform for comparison. *C.* Tricuspid stenosis, demonstrating tall a waves and shallow y descent. *D.* Prominent v waves characteristic of tricuspid regurgitation. In mild to moderate tricuspid insufficiency, a distinct s wave may precede the physiologic v wave. *E.* Severe tricuspid insufficiency showing blunting of the x descent, loss of s wave, melding of the c and v waves, and a steep y descent. *F.* Prominent x and y descents, observed in both constrictive pericarditis and RV myocardial infarction, giving rise to the characteristic M- or W-like appearance of the waveform.

ventricular filling.[49, 50] It is usually apparent only during bradycardia.

The a wave and the initial part of the x descent are absent in atrial fibrillation because there is no organized atrial contraction (see Fig. 95–1*B*). However, giant a waves are observed in atrioventricular dissociation when the atria happen to contract against a closed tricuspid valve (see Fig. 95–1*C*). These large increases in right atrial pressure correspond to the so-called cannon a waves seen on physical examination of the jugular venous pulse and are due to retrograde transmission of the atrial pressure wave to the neck veins. Other causes of prominent a waves include obstruction of RV inflow (e.g., tricuspid stenosis [Fig. 95–2*C*]), decreased RV compliance (e.g., RV hypertrophy), and arrhythmias

(e.g., junctional rhythm with retrograde conduction). Occasionally, atrial flutter with 2:1 atrioventricular block is not apparent from the surface electrocardiogram but may be detected from the right atrial pressure (P_{RA}) tracing by noting two a waves per cardiac cycle.[28] This is most noticeable when the P_{RA} is recorded along with a simultaneous electrocardiographic tracing. A prominent x descent may be observed in pericardial tamponade but the y descent is reduced or absent.[28, 51, 52] Prominent x and y descents can be seen with isolated RV myocardial infarction.[28, 53] Although a steep y descent is typically not apparent in mild RV myocardial infarction, it is commonly observed with more severe degrees of involvement and signifies poor RV compliance.[54] Similar waveform patterns may also be seen in other disease states associated with decreased RV compliance, such as restrictive cardiomyopathy, constrictive pericarditis, and pericardial tamponade. In constrictive pericarditis and RV myocardial infarction both the x and y descents may be quite steep, giving the appearance of an M or W contour to the waveform (see Fig. 95–2*F*).[51, 54, 55] Tricuspid insufficiency is characterized by a prominent systolic pressure wave caused by retrograde regurgitation during ventricular systole. This wave is commonly referred to as a pathologic or giant v wave, and it occurs earlier in systole than the normal or physiologic v wave. With mild to moderate degrees of tricuspid insufficiency a separate positive deflection may be seen, distinct from the physiologic v wave, and has been termed the *s wave* (see Fig. 95–2*D*).[56] With more severe regurgitation, the s and v waves meld into a single wave. With increasingly severe degrees of tricuspid insufficiency, the enlarging v wave encroaches further on the x' descent and may result in melding with the c wave to form a "cv" wave (see Fig. 95–2*E*). This has been referred to as a "ventricularized" right atrial waveform. In tricuspid stenosis, the rate of RV filling is slowed, resulting in a shallow y descent (see Fig. 95–2*C*).

Under normal conditions the jugular venous and right atrial pressures fall during spontaneous inspiration. The inspiratory decline in intrathoracic pressure is transmitted to the central veins and right atrium (Fig. 95–3*B*), and this decrease in back pressure enhances the gradient for venous return. An inspiratory increase in right atrial pressure (see Fig. 95–3*C*) is observed in patients with chronic constrictive pericarditis and occasionally in congestive heart failure, tricuspid stenosis, and restrictive cardiomyopathy. This corresponds to the physical finding known as Kussmaul's sign, the paradoxical inspiratory increase in neck vein distention. Perhaps the most common cause of this phenomenon is right-sided heart failure, and its appearance may be helpful in the bedside diagnosis of RV myocardial infarction and

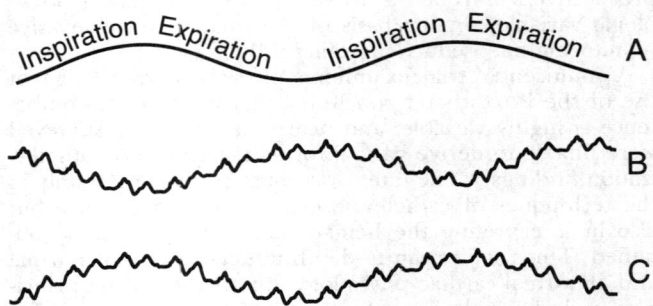

Figure 95–3. Respiratory variation of right atrial or CVP tracings. *A.* Reference respiratory waveform. *B.* CVP tracing for a normal subject breathing spontaneously, showing physiologic inspiratory decrease in CVP. *C.* CVP tracing for a patient with constrictive pericarditis, demonstrating the paradoxical increase in pressure during spontaneous inspiration.

pulmonary embolism.[55, 57, 58] Kussmaul's sign is not characteristic of pericardial tamponade.[59]

The RV pressure waveform is recognized by its marked systolic deflection and a characteristic upsloping during diastole (Fig. 95–4A). Both peak RV systolic and end-diastolic pressure should be noted during bedside catheterization. A significant pressure gradient between right atrial pressure and RV end-diastolic pressure is diagnostic of tricuspid valve stenosis. The "square root sign" (see Fig. 95–4B) refers to an initially rapid rise in RV diastolic pressure followed by a diastolic plateau and is characteristically seen with pericardial constriction.[60] This sign may also be seen in RV myocardial infarction and with restrictive cardiomyopathies but is not typical of pericardial tamponade.[52, 55, 61]

After the catheter tip crosses the pulmonic valve, the PA pressure tracing is observed. This waveform is characterized by a higher diastolic pressure than the RV end-diastolic pressure and by a down-sloping diastolic phase with a prominent dicrotic notch similar to a systemic arterial pressure tracing (Fig. 95–5B, *left*). A marked pressure gradient across the pulmonic valve is indicative of pulmonic stenosis. The PA occlusion pressure (PAOP) tracing is obtained after advancing the catheter farther into the pulmonary artery until the balloon tip lodges in a distal, small-caliber branch of the PA tree and the pressure-monitoring orifice is isolated from pulsatile PA blood flow (see Fig. 95–5B, *right*). The term *pulmonary arterial wedge pressure* is derived from a cardiac catheterization technique that predates the balloon-tipped catheter, in which a non–balloon-equipped catheter is simply advanced into a distal arterial branch until the tip lodges (wedges) in a small-caliber vessel.[62] The balloon-tipped catheter offers several advantages over the older method. First, it allows the catheter to be flow directed. As the catheter is advanced through the central veins, the balloon tip tends to be swept along by the flow of blood and to follow the desired course through the right atrium, right ventricle, and pulmonary artery. This, along with the fact that the observed pressure tracings indicate the position of the catheter tip, allows bedside catheterization without the necessity of fluoroscopic guidance. Second, the balloon minimizes the risk of provoking ventricular arrhythmias while traversing the right ventricle. The endothelium of this chamber is sensitive to physical contact with the tip of the catheter. With the balloon inflated, the catheter tip tends to remain in a central

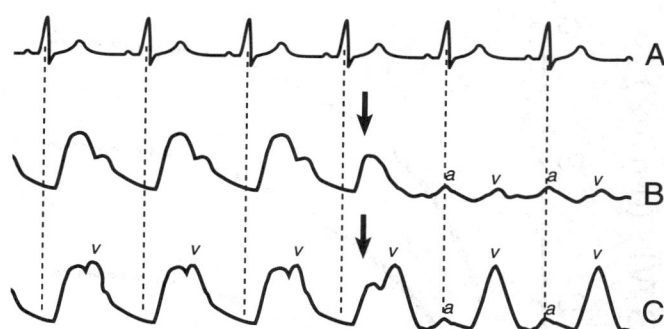

Figure 95–5. PA pressure tracings. Arrows indicate balloon inflation, resulting in conversion to PA occlusion pressure waveforms. *A.* Reference electrocardiogram. *B.* Normal PA waveform showing characteristic dicrotic notch followed by downsloping pressure in diastole *(left)* and normal PAOP tracing *(right)*. *C.* PA *(left)* and PAOP *(right)* tracing observed in severe mitral insufficiency demonstrating pathologic v waves clearly visible after balloon occlusion. Simultaneous electrocardiogram allows differentiation of PA systolic deflections (before balloon inflation) from pathologic v waves (after inflation) by comparing timing of pressure peaks to electrocardiographic cycle.

portion of the blood pool and be less inclined to touch the ventricular wall. Also, the balloon is designed to extend beyond the tip of the catheter when fully inflated, providing a broad, soft, air-cushioned leading surface that protects against focal irritation or trauma to the endothelium. Third, after the initial catheter placement procedure, periodic balloon inflation allows the catheter tip to advance spontaneously to a slightly more distal, occlusive position, allowing measurement of PAOP without a need for manually advancing the catheter. Balloon deflation should then result in the catheter's spontaneously reassuming a slightly more proximal position, with a return of the pulsatile PA waveform. If pulsatile flow is not restored, the catheter tip is too distal and should be withdrawn and the position reassessed. Balloon inflation is done only for brief periods during advancement of the catheter and to obtain periodic PAOP measurements. Continuous balloon inflation should never be allowed to occur because it can result in pulmonary infarction. For the same reason, the PA waveform must be monitored continuously to ensure that the deflated catheter tip has not spontaneously migrated to wedge position. If this occurs, the catheter must be promptly repositioned to a more proximal location. The catheter should never be withdrawn with the balloon inflated because this can potentially snare portions of the tricuspid valve apparatus or damage the vascular intima.

Frank and Starling first delineated the now well-known relationship between ventricular preload and the contractile force generated by the myocardium.[63–66] In the intact heart, preload of the left side of the heart is best defined by left ventricular end-diastolic volume (LVEDV). At a constant level of afterload, heart rate, and intrinsic contractility, increasing LVEDV results in augmentation of stroke volume and cardiac output (Fig. 95–6, curve b). At extremely high levels of LVEDV, further increases in preload result in little or no change in cardiac output, corresponding to the plateau portion of the Starling curve. Cardiac pump performance can be augmented by physiologic or therapeutically mediated decreases in afterload, which shift the Starling curve upward and to the left. Increasing the intrinsic contractility of the heart, such as by stimulation with β-adrenergic catecholamines, has a similar effect (see Fig. 95–6, curve a). On the other hand, increasing afterload or decreasing intrinsic con-

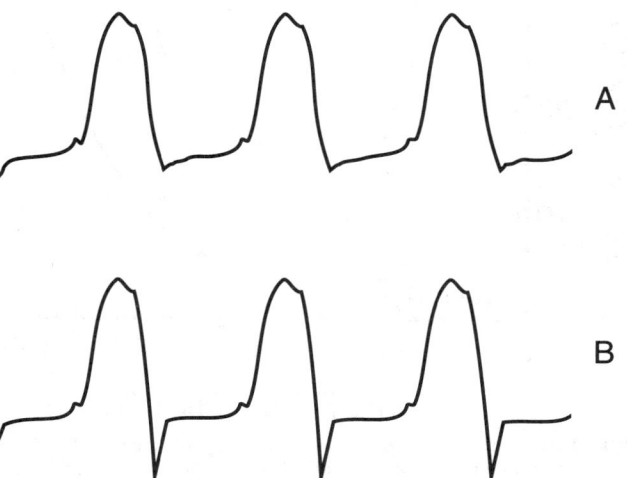

Figure 95–4. Right ventricular pressure tracings. *A.* Normal waveform. *B.* Diastolic dip and plateau, also known as the square root sign, observed in pericardial constriction, right ventricular myocardial infarction, and restrictive cardiomyopathy.

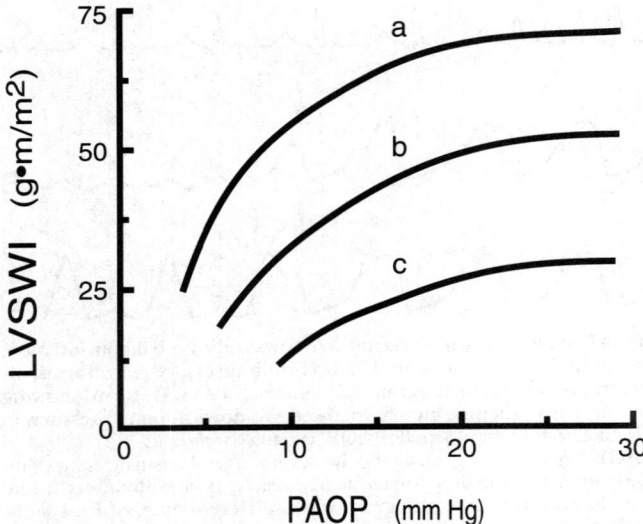

Figure 95–6. Clinical adaptation of the Starling myocardial function curves. Left ventricular stroke work index (LVSWI) is used as a measure of overall left ventricular performance; PAOP is used as an indicator of left ventricular preload. Three function curves are depicted, representing (a) hyperdynamic, (b) normal, and (c) hypodynamic circulatory states. If afterload is considered constant, shifting of the curve is due to a change in the inotropic state of the heart. If intrinsic myocardial contractility is considered constant, shifting is due to a change in left ventricular afterload.

tractility shifts the curve downward and to the right (see Fig. 95–6, curve c), reflecting depression of overall cardiac function.

LVEDV is a function of chamber compliance and distending pressure. Ventricular compliance is defined as the change in diastolic chamber volume that occurs as the result of a change in chamber pressure (dV/dP) and is the reciprocal of ventricular stiffness (dP/dV). Compliance and stiffness vary over the spectrum of end-diastolic volume (Fig. 95–7). Over a narrow range of LVEDV, left ventricular end-diastolic pressure (LVEDP) is approximately proportional to LVEDV, and LVEDP can therefore be used as a measure of left ventricular (LV) preload. Direct determination of LVEDP, however, is impractical outside the cardiac catheterization laboratory. In the absence of mitral valve disease, left atrial pressure (P_{LA}) equilibrates with LVEDP. Direct P_{LA} monitoring is sometimes used to assess LV preload, but the requirement for direct surgical placement of the catheter obviously limits the application of this technique to early postoperative cardiac surgery patients. PA pressure cannot be used to assess P_{LA} or LVEDP because the pulmonary arterioles, capillaries, and venules represent a resistance that creates a pressure drop across the pulmonary vasculature. Viewed another way, it is this pressure gradient that drives blood flow across the pulmonary vasculature. Monitoring left-sided diastolic chamber pressures using the balloon-tipped PA catheter is based on the principle that the effects of resistance on pressure cease to exist if flow is zero. When the balloon is used to occlude a segment of the pulmonary artery, flow distal to the balloon is zero, resistance has no effect on pressure, and pressure at the catheter tip rapidly equilibrates with P_{LA}. In practice, PAOP has generally been shown to correlate well with P_{LA}.[67–71] Thus, PAOP is commonly utilized as a bedside measure of LV preload for the assessment of LV function (see Fig. 95–6). Although P_{RA} or CVP is similarly employed to assess preload, it provides a reflection of the functional state of the right ventricle rather than the left. In conditions in which intrinsic cardiac function

is preserved, changes in preload (e.g., resulting from hypovolemia or fluid overload) are manifest hemodynamically as directionally similar changes in both CVP and PAOP.[12, 20, 72–76] Thus, CVP monitoring is still widely used to assess relative intravascular volume status. However, in the presence of underlying cardiac disease, CVP and PAOP may be markedly disparate. For example, with LV failure LV preload may increase substantially and result in raised LVEDP and increased PA pressure, but if the right side of the heart is able to overcome this imposed increase in RV afterload, RV end-diastolic pressure (and hence CVP) can remain normal. Marked degrees of LV failure are more likely to affect RV function adversely and be manifest as increased CVP. The correlation between CVP and PAOP tends to be low in patients with acute myocardial infarction, other forms of heart disease, or severe sepsis; in patients during the perioperative period; and in patients who are critically ill in general.[20, 22, 72, 75, 77–79] Still, in one study low CVP values (≤5 mm Hg) were highly specific for predicting low or normal PAOP levels (≤12 mm Hg) in critically ill patients with sepsis.[80] When made in conjunction with a complete hemodynamic evaluation including cardiac output determination, CVP measurements allow assessment of RV function. In patients with pericardial effusion, serial CVP values may have the advantage of being a more sensitive indicator of progression to tamponade compared with PAOP alone.[81] CVP determinations have traditionally been made using a water-filled manometer. This technique is less than optimal and should be employed only where transducer monitoring systems are unavailable. Movement of the catheter orifice into the right ventricle results in falsely elevated CVP readings. Transducer-based monitoring systems allow direct visualization of the pressure waveform and alert the clinician to this condition. Because of a meniscus effect, respiratory pressure fluctuations, and other factors, manometer-based measurements have been associated with clinically significant discrepancies compared with electronic methods.[82, 83] Using the PA catheter, P_{RA} and P_{PA} may be simultaneously and continuously monitored by employing two transducers, one connected to the proximal (RA) port and the other to the distal (PA) port. Alternatively, a single transducer allows continuous P_{PA} monitoring and intermittent P_{RA} monitoring (Fig. 95–8).[84]

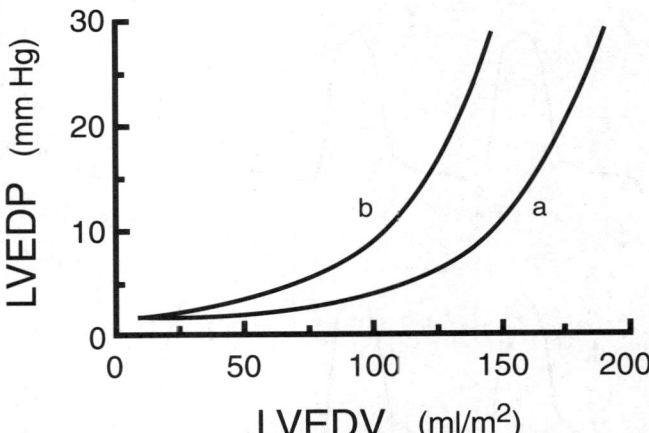

Figure 95–7. Left ventricular end-diastolic pressure (LVEDP) (or PAOP) versus left ventricular end-diastolic volume (LVEDV) (preload). The instantaneous slope of the curve (dP/dV) is defined as ventricular stiffness; its reciprocal (dV/dP) is ventricular compliance. Curve a indicates a normal relationship; curve b, decreased compliance. Note that the relationship between LVEDP (or PAOP) and LV preload varies if compliance changes.

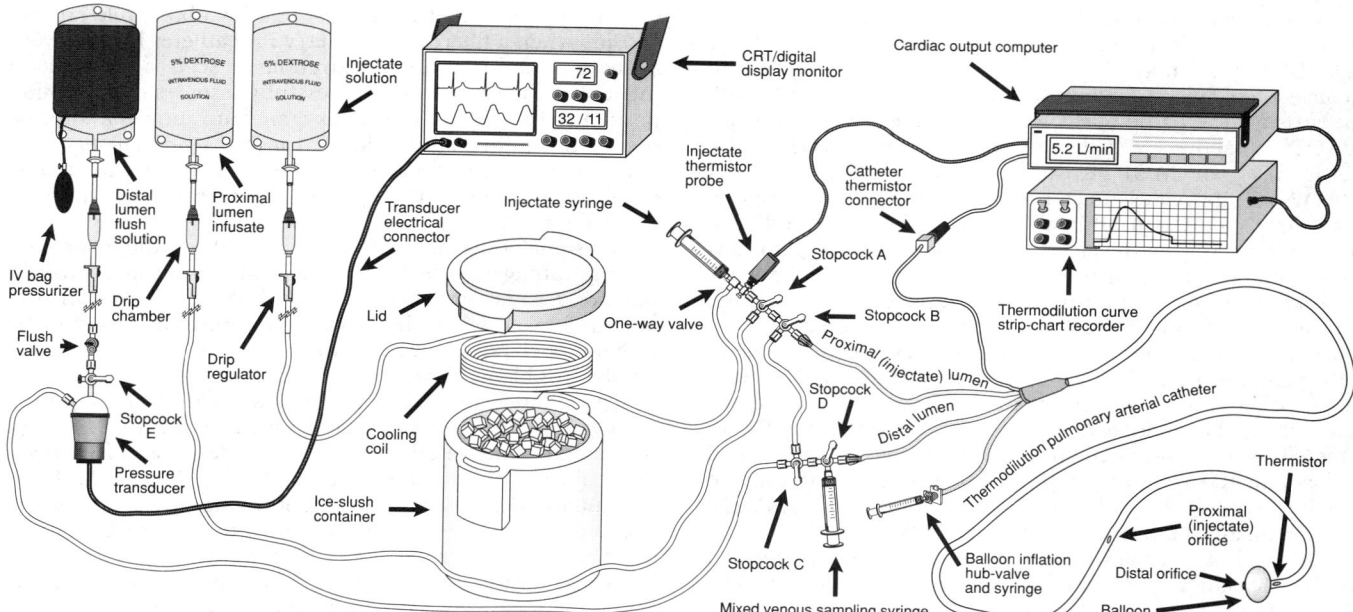

Figure 95–8. Schematic of PA catheter showing representative connections to flush apparatus, injectate source, display monitor, cardiac output computer, and so forth. Adjustment of stopcocks A, B, and C allows thermodilution injection through proximal lumen, right atrial pressure monitoring, or PA pressure monitoring. Alternatively, two pressure transducers may be used for continuous monitoring of both right atrial and PA pressures. Stopcock D allows mixed venous blood sampling from distal catheter orifice. Stopcock E is used to zero transducer system to atmospheric pressure.

Whereas CVP measurements may be made continuously, monitoring of PAOP is necessarily intermittent. This is because the catheter's balloon should not remain inflated for more than a brief period lest pulmonary infarction occur. Normally, PA diastolic pressure closely approximates P_{LA} and PAOP; hence, it is commonly used for continuous monitoring of PAOP, particularly when technical problems preclude direct measurement of PAOP.[69] Although this correlation is generally good, it is not valid when there is pulmonary hypertension associated with pulmonary vascular disease, in which case diastolic P_{PA} may substantially exceed PAOP (Fig. 95–9B). Initial hemodynamic measurements identify the relationship between PAOP and PA diastolic pressure and dictate whether or not left-sided diastolic pressures can subsequently be assessed via PA diastolic pressure monitoring.[85]

Several factors make PAOP less than an ideal reflection of LV preload. Accurate LV volume measurements would be ideal measures of LV preload but are generally unavailable during bedside monitoring. Although PAOP is an indirect measure of LVEDP, even the latter reflects LVEDV only to the extent that LV compliance is constant. Hypertrophic and restrictive cardiac diseases, for example, can lead to significant alterations in LV compliance and hence in the relationship between LVEDP and LVEDV. These are chronic conditions that alter compliance gradually over time, so compliance in these situations should at least remain constant in the acute setting. But because the ventricular diastolic pressure-volume relationship is curvilinear (see Fig. 95–7), chronic changes in compliance alter the degree of change in LVEDP for a given change in LVEDV. In addition, compliance can change acutely for a variety of reasons, most notably from ischemia and administration of certain drugs such as beta-adrenergic agonists and antagonists.[86, 87] Thus, compliance alterations can result in changes in PAOP while LVEDV is constant or even changing in the opposite direction.

Ideally, when monitoring PAOP or P_{LA} for the purpose

of estimating LVEDP and hence LV preload, the pressure should be measured at the peak of the a wave. Ventricular systole normally begins immediately after peak atrial contraction, so the a wave peak corresponds to end diastole. Usually there is only a small difference between peak a wave PAOP and mean PAOP. Although the latter pressure is

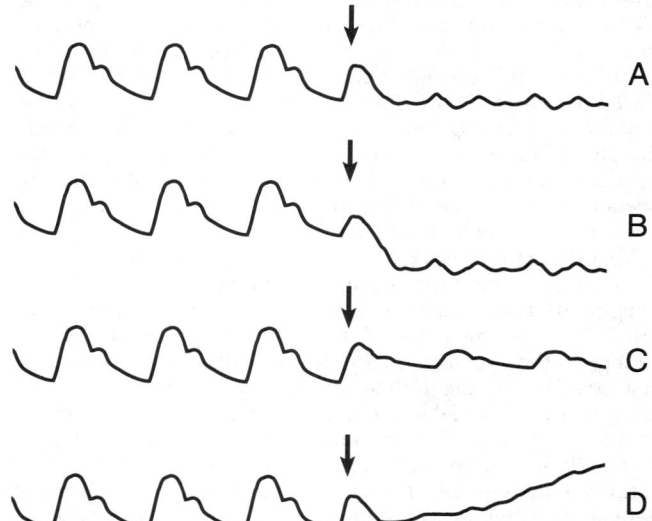

Figure 95–9. PA pressure tracings. Arrows indicate balloon inflation. A. Normal tracing showing expected conversion to PAOP waveform after balloon inflation. B. Tracing observed in pulmonary hypertension showing gradient between diastolic P_{PA} and PAOP. C. Partial occlusion caused by insufficient balloon inflation or excessively proximal catheter tip position, resulting in damped PA pressure tracing rather than true PAOP tracing. Note that damped PA tracing has lower systolic pressure, higher diastolic pressure, and identical mean pressure, compared with preinflation tracing. D. Spurious occlusion waveform caused by "overwedge" condition (see text).

most often used in practice, measurement at the peak of the PAOP a wave is a somewhat more accurate reflection of LVEDP.[16, 88] In mitral insufficiency this difference can be marked and result in falsely high estimation of LVEDP, because a large pathologic v wave raises mean P_{LA} and mean PAOP well above LVEDP. This does not totally preclude the utility of P_{LA} or PAOP measurements in this situation. Mean PAOP still provides an estimate of pulmonary capillary pressure.[89] This is useful for assessing the likelihood of a patient's having or developing pulmonary edema, for differentiating cardiogenic from noncardiogenic pulmonary edema, and for monitoring the effects of fluid loading, diuretics, and other therapies in which the goal may be either to lower pulmonary capillary pressure or to avoid adversely raising it. It may also be possible to use PAOP to assess LVEDP even in the presence of severe mitral regurgitation. If the a and v waves can be identified on the PAOP tracing, peak a wave pressure can be measured and should still adequately reflect LVEDP. The objective is to circumvent the influence of the pathologic v wave on mean P_{LA} or PAOP by measuring the pressure at end diastole.

Although it is usually easy to discern a and v waves in P_{LA} or CVP tracings, it is often difficult in PAOP tracings. The P_{LA} contour undergoes phase shifting and attenuation as the pressure impulse traverses back across the pulmonary vasculature. Manually wedging the catheter (i.e., advancing the catheter through the PA branch with the balloon deflated until impaction of the tip occurs and an atrial pressure tracing is noted) may result in a and v waves clearer than those on PAOP tracings achieved by balloon occlusion.[62] Mean PAOP (rather than peak a wave PAOP) should still be used to assess pulmonary capillary pressure in mitral insufficiency and in general. In mitral stenosis, the pressure gradient across the mitral valve precludes the use of either P_{LA} or PAOP for estimating LVEDP. Pulmonary veno-occlusive disease similarly causes PAOP (but not P_{LA}) to be higher than LVEDP. PAOP and PA diastolic pressure may underestimate LVEDP if there is severe aortic insufficiency.[90] In such patients LV diastolic pressure may continue to rise after mitral valve closure, because of regurgitant LV filling. LVEDP is not reflected by PAOP in this situation because there is no hydraulic continuity between the pulmonary vasculature and the left ventricle while the mitral valve is closed. PA diastolic pressure may also underestimate LVEDP in patients with right bundle branch block. In this situation, the initiation of RV systole lags behind that of the left ventricle. This delay in RV contraction allows PA diastolic pressure to continue to fall in parallel with the left atrial x descent to a level less than LVEDP.

Various criteria have been suggested for confirming that the inflated balloon tip of the PA catheter is truely occluding a segment of pulmonary artery, that is, is in wedge position.[16, 21, 24, 79, 91, 92] The first way to confirm occlusion is to note the change in the pressure tracing from a pulsatile configuration characteristic of the pulmonary artery to a pattern resembling that of an atrial tracing. This left atrial–type waveform should be consistently reproducible with successive inflation and deflation of the catheter balloon. Usually these observations alone suffice, but occasionally it may be difficult to determine whether the change in configuration is due to proper occlusion or to artifactual pressure changes—for example, caused by contact of the catheter tip with the vessel wall or incomplete occlusion (see Fig. 95–9C).

If a blood specimen is drawn from the distal port of the catheter while the balloon is inflated, the specimen represents pulmonary capillary blood rather than mixed venous blood if the catheter is actually in occlusive position.[93–97] Analysis of pulmonary capillary blood gases should demonstrate oxygen tension and saturation levels that equal or exceed arterial levels. This is readily observable at the bedside when a fiberoptic oximetry PA catheter is employed: a sharp rise in oxygen saturation is seen after balloon inflation if the catheter tip successfully assumes the occlusion position. However, a rise in oxygen saturation may not be seen if the catheter tip is located in a PA branch serving a poorly functioning area of lung (e.g., in lobar pneumonia or atelectasis), even though the catheter tip is otherwise optimally positioned.[16, 24]

Occasionally the external portion of the catheter or connecting tubing may become kinked and result in a damped waveform. The internal portion of the catheter can also become kinked when the subclavian approach is used if the catheter becomes pinched between the clavicle and first rib.[98] Similar problems develop if the catheter lumen or tip becomes occluded by thrombus formation. Flushing the distal lumen and observing free flow of intravenous fluid through the catheter and an adequate dynamic response after flushing is abruptly terminated (see Fig. 22–3, Chapter 22) helps in evaluating catheter patency, identifying orifice or luminal occlusion, and ensuring that the waveform is neither overdamped nor hyperresonant.[92, 99] An overdamped waveform is most commonly due to air bubbles in the transducer or tubing or to use of compliant tubing rather than noncompliant pressure tubing. Hyperresonance, ringing, and systolic overshoot can occur when overly long tubing is used to connect the transducer to the catheter hub. It must also be ensured that all tubing connections are tight, stopcocks are properly positioned, the transducer and monitoring system have been properly zeroed and calibrated, and the transducer has been correctly leveled.[85] The level of the midatrium is the reference position for physiologic pressure measurements and corresponds to mid-chest height of the supine patient. This point should be level with the height of the air-fluid interface of the stopcock used to zero the transducer to atmospheric pressure.[100–102]

It is sometimes difficult or impossible to traverse the right side of the heart with the PA catheter in patients with extreme RV dilation, severe pulmonary hypertension, severe tricuspid insufficiency, or profoundly decreased cardiac output. In other situations, the chamber may be traversed normally but the waveforms are less than characteristic. Atrial fibrillation or frequent extrasystoles can cause beat-to-beat fluctuations in pressure measurements that may lead to confusion between RV and PA waveforms. In patients with hyperdynamic states or severe tachycardia it is sometimes difficult to discriminate the RV, PA, and PAOP waveforms.[28] Segmentally occlusive pulmonary embolism can result in complete inability to obtain PAOP.[103–105] Occasionally, balloon inflation results in a steadily increasing pressure that ultimately exceeds the full-scale limit of the monitor screen (see Fig. 95–9D). This is commonly referred to as "overwedging" and is due to impaction of the catheter tip against the vessel wall; wedging into a PA branch that is occluded by thrombus; occlusion of the catheter tip by a defective, overinflated, or asymmetrically inflated balloon; occlusion of the monitoring orifice with clot; or other occlusion or kinking of the catheter.[85] The steadily rising pressure observed on the monitor is due to the slow continuous infusion of pressurized flush solution through the catheter. This slow flush is normally dissipated at the distal catheter orifice and does not affect pressure determinations unless there is an occlusion that prevents normal escape of the flush solution. Repositioning the catheter usually overcomes this problem.

Mean PAOP should always be <u>less</u> than mean PA pressure ($\overline{P_{PA}}$); for mean PAOP to exceed $\overline{P_{PA}}$ would require net blood flow from left atrium to right ventricle. Except perhaps in severe mitral insufficiency, mean PAOP should not exceed PA diastolic pressure.

Use of PAOP to estimate ventricular preload is subject to the limitations of the ventricular pressure-volume relationship. In addition, it is critical to note that the tension developed in the walls of blood vessels or cardiac chambers during passive filling is not determined solely by the intramural pressure. The distending pressure, also known as filling pressure or transmural pressure (P_{tm}), is instead determined by the pressure gradient across the vessel or chamber wall. This can be calculated from intracavitary or intraluminal pressure (P_{il}) and extraluminal pressure (P_{el}) as

$$P_{tm} = P_{il} - P_{el}$$

Although there is conflicting experimental evidence,[16, 106, 107] extraluminal pressure (juxtacardiac pressure) is often equated to pleural or esophageal pressure. That debate notwithstanding, diastolic transmural pressure for the left ventricle should therefore be equal to LVEDP (or PAOP) minus pleural pressure. Correspondingly, for the right ventricle (or right atrium) transmural pressure is equal to RV end-diastolic pressure (or P_{RA}) minus pleural pressure.

Clinical hemodynamic monitoring determines intracavitary or intravascular pressure at the orifice of the indwelling catheter relative to atmospheric pressure; extraluminal pressure is usually unavailable. If pleural pressure (extraluminal pressure) were zero, intraluminal pressure would equal transmural pressure. However, changes in pleural pressure alter the relationship between intraluminal pressure (e.g., CVP or PAOP) and true filling pressure. Any factor that influences intrathoracic pressure can alter pleural and juxtacardiac pressure and thus potentially affect the relationship between intraluminal pressure and filling pressure. Normally, end-tidal pleural pressure is slightly negative and becomes more negative during spontaneous inspiration. Pleural pressure can become markedly negative in patients exerting strenuous inspiratory efforts or performing Müller's maneuver.[108] This commonly occurs in patients with respiratory distress or bronchospasm. On the other hand, pleural pressure is markedly positive during a spontaneous forced expiratory effort, during Valsalva's maneuver, and during inspiration in patients receiving positive pressure ventilation.[109, 110] Breath holding at end expiration has been recommended as a means of obviating these respiratory influences on intravascular pressure during hemodynamic monitoring.[16, 111] Although this is a simple maneuver for normal individuals, it may be impossible for critically ill patients. Even less severely ill patients may have difficulty holding their breath without unconsciously performing Valsalva's maneuver and thereby increasing intrathoracic pressure and altering their hemodynamics. A preferable alternative for estimating filling pressure is to measure intravascular pressures without breath holding, at the end of passive expiration when pleural pressure is closest to zero, and this applies to both the spontaneously breathing patient and the patient receiving positive pressure ventilation.[24, 79, 85, 87, 99, 111-115] Esophageal balloons have been used to estimate extraluminal pressure and allow calculation of transmural pressures; however, their clinical use is not widespread.

For patients exhibiting large respiratory swings in their pressure waveforms, it is critical to ensure that all vascular pressure measurements are made at end expiration. For patients breathing spontaneously, end-expiratory pressure is generally represented by the high point of their CVP and PAOP tracings (Fig. 95–10*B* and *C*). For patients receiving positive pressure ventilation, end expiration is represented by the nadir of the pressure wave tracing (see Fig. 95–10*D* and *F*). This may not hold true for patients who are receiving positive pressure ventilation in an assist-type mode. In this situation inspiration begins when the patient generates a negative inspiratory effort that triggers the ventilator to

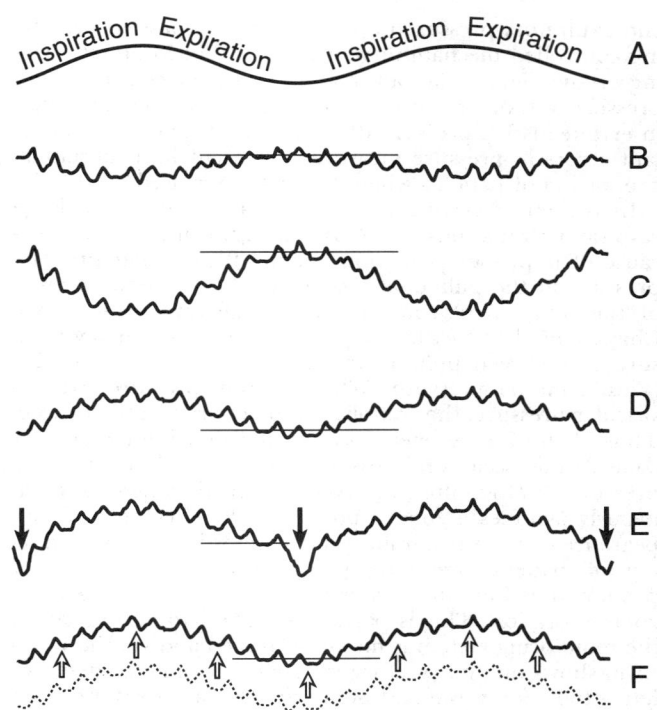

Figure 95–10. Effect of respiration-induced changes in intrathoracic pressure on PAOP tracing. Horizontal line segments indicate level of mean PAOP at end expiration. *A.* Respiratory reference tracing. *B.* Minimal respiratory variation in PAOP waveform, typical of quiet spontaneous breathing in subject with normal lung compliance. *C.* PAOP tracing during deep spontaneous breathing as may be seen in patients with respiratory distress caused by bronchospasm or decreased lung compliance. *D.* PAOP tracing during control mode mechanical ventilation in a patient therapeutically paralyzed or otherwise not making any active respiratory efforts. *E.* PAOP tracing during mechanical ventilation in an assist mode with patient making active inspiratory efforts (*filled arrows*). *F.* Same conditions as *D*, before (*dotted line*) and after (*solid line*) the addition of PEEP. Degree of displacement (*open arrows*) depends on level of PEEP, lung compliance, and tidal volume.

deliver a positive pressure breath. The patient's triggering inspiratory effort may be reflected as an initial negative deflection in the CVP and PAOP tracings (see Fig. 95–10*E*). In this case, even though the patient is receiving positive pressure ventilation, the nadir of the pressure wave tracing may not represent end expiration. Similar discrepancies can occur in patients receiving controlled mechanical ventilation but making inspiratory or expiratory efforts that are not synchronous with the ventilator. Sedation with or without temporary neuromuscular blockade has been employed to circumvent this effect.[116] It is sometimes possible simply to increase the rate of mechanical ventilation and "overdrive" the patient's efforts. In some cases, however, the patient may continue to generate spontaneous inspiratory efforts that make it difficult to determine the point of end expiration. A simultaneous airway pressure waveform is helpful in defining end expiration but usually is not mandatory.[97] Unless the electronic monitor screen has provisions for freezing the tracing and digitally indicating the pressure at the desired point on the waveform by use of a movable cursor, these determinations are best made from a hard copy tracing. If neither of these methods is possible, the digitally indicated "systolic" pressure generally corresponds to the expiratory pressure in spontaneously breathing patients and the "diastolic" pressure reading corresponds to end-expiratory pressure in patients who are passively receiving controlled mechanical ventilation.[79, 99, 117] Routinely relying on the digital read-out that displays the electronic mean pressure without regard to phase of respiration can result in erroneous PA pressure determinations. Clinically important errors in pressure measurement occur in a substantial proportion of patients when this method is used.[21, 85, 114, 115]

In patients receiving positive pressure ventilation, large respiratory variations in PAOP tracings can also occur because of improper positioning of the PA catheter tip. The pressure in the pulmonary vasculature in dependent areas of the lung (West zone 3) exceeds airway pressure (see Chapter 65).[118, 119] At less dependent locations, airway pressure may exceed pulmonary venous (West zone 2) or PA (West zone 1) pressure. Where airway pressure exceeds vascular pressure, the compliant pulmonary vessels collapse. Thus, if the PA catheter tip is located in a West zone 1 or zone 2, the occlusion pressure does not reflect left atrial pressure.[120] Most often the balloon-tipped catheter spontaneously assumes a zone 3 position.[121, 122] However, the appearance of wide respiratory fluctuations in the PAOP tracing of patients receiving mechanical ventilation should prompt the clinician to consider the possibility of a non–zone 3 location. This is particularly likely to be the case if the monitoring system is not overdamped and yet the waveform shows only respiratory variability, with no evidence of left atrial a or v waves.[24] Some degree of airway pressure transmission may occur even when the catheter tip is directed into a zone 3 area. Zone 3 placement is suggested if the degree of respiratory variation observed in the PAOP waveform is also seen in the nonoccluded PA pressure waveform. This can be evaluated by determining the difference between peak inspiratory (pi) PA systolic pressure and end-expiratory (ee) PA systolic pressure, and comparing this to the difference between $PAOP_{pi}$ and $PAOP_{ee}$. It has been stated that a non–zone 3 position is likely when[122, 123]

$$(PAOP_{pi} - PAOP_{ee}) > 1.5 \times (P_{PA,pi} - P_{PA,ee})$$

A zone 3 location can, in most cases, be ensured by obtaining a lateral chest radiograph to demonstrate that the tip of the catheter is below the level of the left atrium.[122, 124] Withdrawing the catheter a short distance and then readvancing it often correct a non–zone 3 location, and it is expedient to attempt such repositioning if there is any question of a non–zone 3 condition. Experimental evidence suggests that placing the patient in the lateral decubitus position, so that the catheter tip is located on the dependent side of the body, is another means of ensuring a zone 3 location.[125] Chest radiography in conjunction with injection of radiocontrast material through the distal pulmonary catheter orifice has been done during balloon occlusion to confirm proper positioning.[126, 127] Although this procedure may allow direct visual confirmation of hydraulic continuity between the catheter tip and the left atrium, it is unsuitable for routine clinical use.

The use of PEEP or continuous positive airway pressure and the development of air trapping (so-called occult PEEP, or auto-PEEP) elevate intrathoracic pressure and can result in further discrepancies between intravascular pressure measurements and transmural pressure.[87, 112, 128, 129] Increasing levels of PEEP generally result in increased central pressures, such as CVP and PAOP, when measured in the usual manner relative to atmospheric pressure (see Fig. 95–10F). However, when intrathoracic pressure is subtracted from the intraluminal CVP or PAOP measurements, the transmural filling pressures, and hence end-diastolic volumes, usually decrease as PEEP is applied.[130–132] Thus, even though PEEP usually raises the measured (intraluminal) pressures, transmural pressures usually fall, reflecting a PEEP-induced decrease in ventricular preload. This is largely due to decreased RV and LV filling caused by the increased intracavitary back pressure that opposes venous return. With much higher levels of PEEP, pulmonary vascular resistance may increase sufficiently to impose a substantial increment in RV afterload. This increase in RV afterload may in some cases be sufficient to result in RV dilation. Thus, the directional change in RV preload depends on the level of PEEP and its combined influence on both venous return and RV afterload. In circumstances that result in RV dilation, the interventricular septum may shift toward the left ventricle so as to encroach on LVEDV and further decrease LV preload.[131] The fraction of airway pressure transmitted to the intrathoracic vasculature varies with pulmonary compliance, making it difficult to evaluate the extent of this discrepancy between intraluminal and transmural pressures.[87, 133]

Various methods have been promulgated to circumvent this source of potential inaccuracy. Although end-expiratory measurements minimize the effects of respiratory excursions, they do not correct for the effects of a constant elevation in intrathoracic pressure as a result of PEEP. Taking steady-state PAOP measurements during temporary discontinuation of PEEP has been advocated.[16] Either PEEP is turned off or the patient is disconnected from the mechanical ventilator circuit and ventilated with a resuscitation bag. Discontinuing PEEP for a short interval allows the effects of raised intrathoracic pressure to abate; however, this technique has serious potential disadvantages. First, discontinuing PEEP may result in severe hypoxemia and atelectasis, which are not always completely reversed when PEEP is reinstituted. Although this technique has been safely implemented in some patients by preoxygenating at an increased fraction of inspired oxygen (FIO_2),[134] severe pulmonary consequences can occur in more severly ill patients.[135–139] Patients requiring high levels of PEEP who are already receiving 100% oxygen are at particular risk. Second, discontinuance of PEEP causes changes in venous return, pulmonary vascular resistance, and ventricular wall tension that can result in a hemodynamic state substantially different from that which exists while the patient is receiving PEEP.[87, 112, 131, 135, 140–145] To mitigate these problems, the nadir PAOP or "pop-off" method has been advocated.[146–148] Pop-off pressure is obtained by abruptly disconnecting the endotracheal tube from the ventilator circuit and immediately measuring PAOP. The interval between disconnection and pressure determination is intentionally short (within 2 seconds) to avoid attaining an equilibrium hemodynamic state while the patient is not receiving PEEP. The abrupt decrease in intrathoracic pressure during pop-off causes a drop in PAOP that occurs before significant alterations in gas exchange, venous return, and afterload are manifest. This technique may not be valid when LV filling pressure is high. Subtracting intrathoracic pressure from PAOP would yield transmural pressure and would obviate the problem altogether. However, as noted earlier, intrathoracic pressure cannot be easily measured in clinical practice. Balloon-equipped esophageal catheters have been used successfully to estimate juxtacardiac pressure,[106] but this technique is not routinely used in practice. The fraction of end-expiratory airway pressure that is transmitted across the alveoli to the pulmonary vasculature averages between one fourth and one half of the applied pressure according to some studies of acute lung injury. Routinely subtracting some fraction of the applied level of PEEP from the measured PAOP has therefore been advocated as yet another method of estimating transmural filling pressure.[87, 112] However, the actual fraction of pressure transmitted depends on the degree to which pulmonary compliance has been affected, which is highly variable from patient to patient. Because of the limitations of these techniques and their potential for adverse effects, PAOP is more commonly measured without discontinuation of PEEP and, in practice, this method is the most satisfactory.[87, 113, 135, 136] In general, the patients receiving high levels of PEEP are those with the least compliant lungs, and hence a smaller fraction of their airway pressure is transmitted to the heart and central vessels.[133] This tends to counter the effect of PEEP on intraluminal pressure determinations.

Pulmonary capillary pressure (P_{cap}) is a major determinant of net fluid flux across the pulmonary capillary endothelium. In general, the higher the pulmonary capillary pressure, the greater the propensity for developing pulmonary edema. In addition to being used to assess LV preload, PAOP is also commonly used to estimate capillary pressure. Thus, PAOP serves as a means of assessing a patient's likelihood of having or developing pulmonary congestion and of differentiating cardiogenic from noncardiogenic pulmonary edema. However, PAOP is not necessarily equal to capillary pressure. In normal lungs, hydrostatic pressure at the level of the pulmonary capillaries is approximately equal to the average of pulmonary venous and pulmonary arterial pressures. This relationship is represented more precisely by the Garr equation:[149]

$$P_{cap} = PAOP + 0.4 \times (\overline{P_{PA}} - PAOP)$$

The coefficient 0.4 is derived from the fact that approximately 40% of total pulmonary vascular resistance occurs on the venous side of the pulmonary capillaries.[150, 151] However, when pulmonary vascular resistance is increased, capillary pressure may differ from this average pressure and from PAOP as well. Although equating mean PAOP with capillary pressure is acceptable in the clinical setting,[24] a more accurate determination of capillary pressure may be made by observing the rate of pressure change during balloon occlusion with the PA catheter.[152] As the pressure declines, two phases are seen: an initial phase of rapid decline followed by a slower, curvilinear fall in pressure, which subsequently equilibrates with P_{LA}.[153] The existence of these two slopes is due to differences between PA and venous resistance. The inflection point of the two slopes should correspond closely to capillary pressure (Fig. 95–11). This method can be employed at the bedside by using a calibrated strip chart recording of the pressure tracing obtained while the balloon

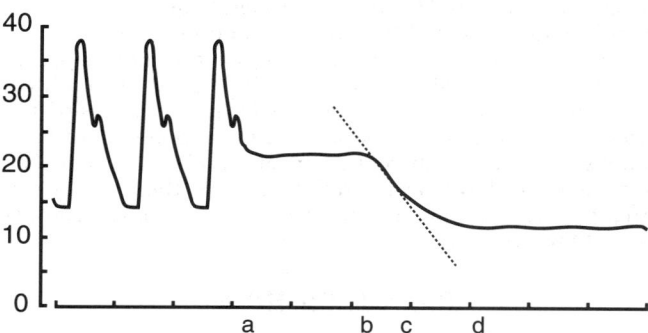

Figure 95–11. Tracing of PA pressure (millimeters of mercury) versus time (seconds), demonstrating method of accurately determining pulmonary capillary pressure by noting the inflection point of the mean P_{PA} tracing immediately after balloon occlusion. At time a, P_{PA} recording is electronically meaned; at time b, balloon is inflated to effect occlusion. Dotted line drawn through initial portion of down-slope aids in locating inflection point (shown at time c), indicative of capillary pressure. Mean PAOP is reached by time d. In this example mean P_{PA} is 22 mm Hg, capillary pressure is 16 mm Hg, and PAOP is 12 mm Hg.

is being inflated; however, optimal determinations require instrumentation capable of displaying a mean pressure tracing. Although not perfectly accurate, the Gaar equation provides a much simpler estimate of capillary pressure that is easily derived without special instrumentation or analysis techniques.[152, 154, 155] Furthermore, although both techniques provide a theoretically more sound estimate of pulmonary capillary pressure, neither has been shown to have a definite practical advantage when applied to critically ill patients.[154]

MEASURING CARDIAC OUTPUT

Balloon-tipped PA catheters are available that do not have thermal sensors and are thus designed for pressure measurements and blood sampling but not for thermodilution measurements. However, all PA catheters used in adult patients in the ICU should have a thermistor near the tip of the catheter to allow complete hemodynamic assessment, including determination of cardiac output by the thermodilution method. Although thermodilution is currently used to the near exclusion of other clinical methods of determining cardiac output, two older methods, the Fick technique and the indocyanine green dye dilution method, have proven validity and are occasionally still used in certain situations at some centers. Both dye and thermal techniques are based on the same principle, namely that an indicator substance injected into the circulation undergoes dilution as it traverses the vasculature and the profile of this dilution in the time domain is related to the rate of blood flow. A working knowledge of the principles involved in the dye dilution method is helpful in understanding the more common thermodilution method.

Indicator Dye Dilution Method

In this technique, sterile indocyanine green dye is used as the indicator substance. After rapid bolus injection into the venous circulation, right side of the heart, or pulmonary artery, the dye rapidly binds to plasma proteins and alters the spectral absorption pattern of the blood. During and immediately after the injection, blood is continuously aspirated at a point downstream from the injection site, usually from a peripheral artery, using an automated syringe pump. A flow-through cuvette, containing a light source, optical filter, and photodetector, is positioned between the syringe pump and the arterial catheter. The output of the photodetector is connected to an instrument that quantitates optical density at the appropriate wavelength, and this may be connected to a strip chart recorder. Representative dye dilution tracings of optical density versus time are shown in Figure 95–12. The ordinate of this plot represents optical density of the blood–green dye mixture, and this is directly proportional to the concentration of green dye according to the Lambert-Beer principle (see Chapters 17 and 19). The delay between injection and the initial appearance of dye at the sampling site represents the appearance time. If complete mixing of dye particles and blood is assumed, the amplitude, duration, and shape of the first-pass dye curve are influenced by the amount of dye injected and the rate of blood flow through the heart (i.e., cardiac output) according to the Stewart-Hamilton equation:[156, 157]

$$\text{Blood flow} = \frac{A \times 60}{k \times \int_0^\tau \Delta C(t)\, dt}$$

where A is the amount of dye (mg) injected, 60 is a constant (s/min) to convert time units from seconds to minutes, the integral term in the denominator represents the area under the indicator dilution curve (mm·s), τ is the data acquisition

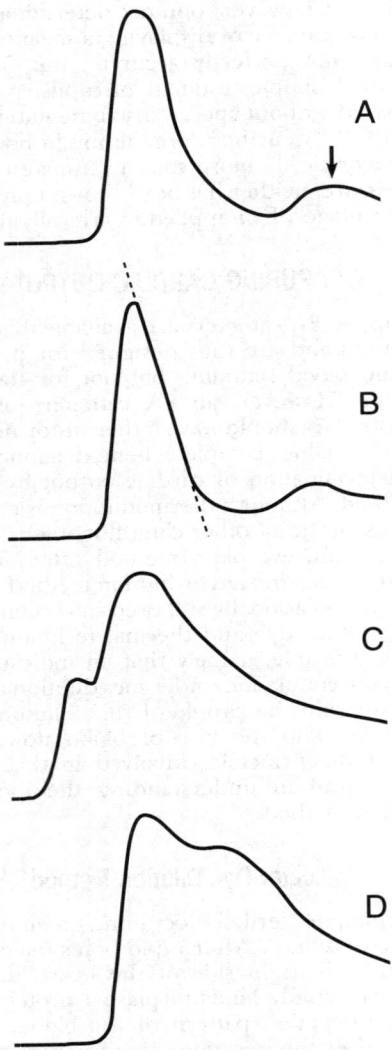

Figure 95–12. Normal dye dilution curve tracings obtained by injection of dye into right atrium with sampling from distal aorta. Vertical dimension is optical density calibrated to dye concentration. *A.* Normal cardiac output curve using linear vertical deflection scale. Arrow indicates normal recirculation peak. *B.* Transformation of normal curve *A* to logarithmic vertical deflection scale yielding linear down-slope. Dotted line demonstrates extrapolation method for circumventing recirculation error. *C.* Effect of right-to-left intracardiac shunting on curve profile. *D.* Effect of left-to-right intracardiac shunting on curve profile.

end point, and *k* is a calibration constant (mg/L/mm) to convert vertical deflection to concentration units. This calibration constant is determined by introducing several blood samples, each prepared to an accurately known concentration of indocyanine green dye, into the cuvette. The resulting deflections in optical density are plotted against the known concentrations, and the calibration factor is derived from the slope of a regression line through these calibration points. The amount of dye injected, *A*, is equal to the concentration of dye in the injectate (mg/mL) times the injectate volume (mL). The integral term is necessary because the dye concentration changes over time. However, if the average concentration of dye represented under the curve is considered, the foregoing equation can be simplified to

$$\text{Cardiac output} = \frac{A \times 60}{C_m \times t \times k}$$

where C_m stands for the mean concentration of dye from the curve and *t* is the duration (seconds) of the indicator curve. The product of C_m and *t* in this equation represents the area under the indicator dilution curve. The area under the indicator dilution curve can be determined graphically by replotting the curve on semilogarithmic graph paper, which should yield an approximately straight line for the down-sloping portion of the curve and allow estimation of the subtended area by calculating the area of the resulting near-triangular waveform. Alternatively, and more accurately, the curve can be traced with a mechanical or electronic planimeter to derive the area. The second peak of optical density (see Fig. 95–12*A*) is due to dye that has traversed the systemic circulation and passed through the monitoring cuvette a second time. This recirculation peak represents the equivalent of additional indicator, which adds to *A* in the preceding equations and interferes with accurate estimation. The recirculation portion of the curve therefore must not be included in calculating the dilution curve area. Using the logarithmic transformation of optical density allows extrapolation of the linear down-slope to baseline, effectively eliminating error caused by this recirculation peak (see Fig. 95–12*B*). Dedicated electronic systems have been developed to perform all these steps automatically and directly display the resultant cardiac output. After first-pass and initial recirculation, indocyanine green is gradually taken up by the liver and excreted in the bile. By monitoring the decay of dye concentration in the blood over a longer period, the indocyanine green method has been used as a means of assessing hepatic blood flow and hepatocellular function.[158, 159]

Pitfalls of the technique include use of outdated dye solutions, inaccurate calibration samples, nonlinearity in the calibration curve, erratic or prolonged injection times, leakage of dye, insufficient mixing in the circulation, blood withdrawal flow rates that are too slow or erratic, the presence of air bubbles or interfering substances in the blood passing through the cuvette, and faulty or uncalibrated instrumentation. Like the thermodilution method, the dye dilution technique generally requires central venous catheterization, although the catheter need not be positioned in the pulmonary artery. It is possible to inject the indicator into a large peripheral vein and sample from a peripheral artery. To obtain cardiac output, it is imperative only that the indicator traverse a point in the circulation where blood flow equals cardiac output before measurement of the indicator concentration. However, peripheral injection and sampling reduce the signal-to-noise ratio and increase the error caused by recirculation, thereby reducing accuracy, particularly at low levels of cardiac output.[160, 161] Further disadvantages of dye dilution methods include the necessity for arterial cannulation and blood wastage or potential complications associated with reinfusion of withdrawn blood. Ear densitometers have been used to obviate these problems. Anaphylactic reactions to indocyanine green have been reported but are rare.[162]

Thermodilution Method

The thermodilution method of measuring cardiac output was introduced by Fegler in 1953.[163] Whereas the dye dilution method employs indocyanine green as the indicator undergoing dilution and measures the change in its concentration over time, the thermodilution method uses thermal energy (heat) as the indicator and measures the change in blood temperature over time. Instead of an extracorporeal densitometer, an intravascular temperature probe is used to quantitate the dilution process. Although the terms heat and temperature are commonly used interchangably, they are technically different. Understanding the relationship between these two physical phenomena is critical to understanding the concept of thermal indicator dilution.

Consider a 1-ton stone that has been heated to 40°C and placed in a small, cool, enclosed, well-insulated room to provide the occupants with heat. The room temperature rises as the mass of stone cools. On the other hand, a single pebble heated to 100°C and placed in the same room would have a negligible effect on the room's temperature, even though the pebble's temperature is much higher than that of the large mass of stone. Thus, the pebble has a higher temperature, but much less heat, than the ton of stone. Heat is therefore the amount of thermal energy possessed by an object and is determined by the temperature of the object as well as its mass. The temperature of a substance, on the other hand, is not dependent on its mass. The relationship between temperature and heat varies from substance to substance and is quantified as the specific heat of the substance. Specific heat (C) is defined by

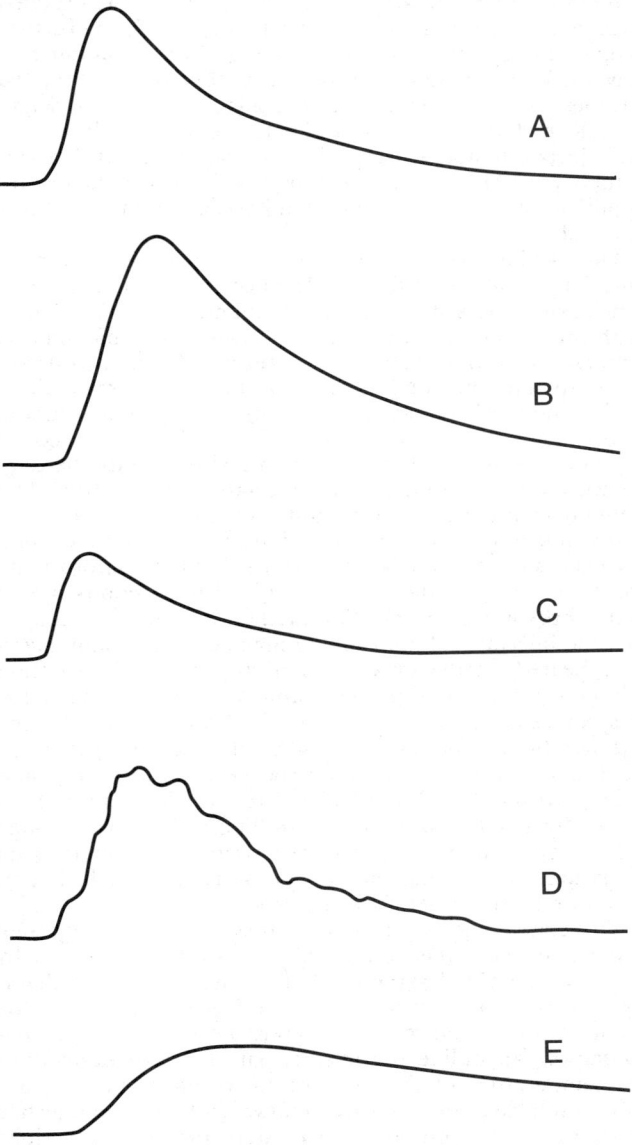

Figure 95–13. Representative thermodilution curve tracings. Note that reversed temperature scale is used for vertical dimension. *A.* Normal cardiac output. *B.* Low cardiac output. *C.* High cardiac output. *D.* "Noisy" tracing caused by erratic injection technique. *E.* Tracing from patient with tricuspid insufficiency.

$$C = \frac{\Delta E}{m \times \Delta T}$$

where ΔE = change in thermal energy of the substance (cal)
   m = mass of the substance (g)
   ΔT = temperature change (°C) of the substance

If the mass and specific heat of a given substance are known, the amount of heat corresponding to a certain temperature change can be calculated from this relationship.

The thermal indicator dilution, or thermodilution, process involves the injection of a known mass of fluid (the injectate) at a known temperature (injectate temperature) into the circulation, while observing its effect on the temperature of blood at some point downstream.[163, 164] Theoretically, the injectate could be any fluid that has either a greater or lesser quantity of heat per unit mass compared to blood. In simpler terms, the injectate could be warmer or cooler than blood. If the injectate were warmer than the body's core temperature, a plot of blood temperature versus time would yield a tracing similar to a dye dilution curve: blood temperature would first rise and then fall as the injected fluid passed the temperature probe. In practice, the injectate temperature is lower than blood temperature and the resulting curve of temperature versus time resembles an inverted dye dilution curve. For consistency with dye dilution curves, thermodilution profiles are often depicted with a reverse temperature axis (Fig. 95–13).

The injectate fluid, usually 5% dextrose in water, is injected into the proximal lumen of the thermodilution PA catheter. The orifice of this lumen is usually positioned within the right atrium. The injectate fluid then mixes with blood in the right atrium and ventricle and passes the distal portion of the catheter, which is typically located in a main branch of the pulmonary artery. The thermal transducer located close to the tip of the catheter converts temperature to an electrical signal that is measured by a microprocessor-based bedside instrument. This computer uses a modification of the Stewart-Hamilton equation to calculate cardiac output as[3]

$$\text{Blood flow} = \frac{(T_b - T_i) \times V_i \times C_i \times S_i \times K_{cal} \times K_{cor} \times 60}{C_b \times S_b \times \int_0^\tau \Delta T_b(t)\, dt}$$

where T_b = baseline blood temperature (°C)
   T_i = injectate temperature
   V_i = injectate volume (mL)
   C_i and C_b = specific heat of injectate and blood (cal/g/°C), respectively
   S_i and S_b = specific gravity of injectate and blood, respectively
   K_{cal} = calibration constant
   60   = time dimension conversion factor (s/min)

and the integral of temperature with respect to time represents the area under the thermodilution curve. Although the specific heat and specific gravity of blood vary with hematocrit, this has a negligible impact on the result, even over a wide range of hematocrit values.[165] The specific gravity terms are needed to convert volume units (for blood and injectate) into mass units. Density terms may be substituted for specific gravity. The specific heat and specific gravity constants together allow calculation of heat from units of temperature and volume. K_{cor} is a correction factor to account for the rise in temperature of the injectate as it traverses the catheter lumen and is warmed somewhat by the catheter and surrounding blood and to account for residual warm fluid in the catheter dead space. Injectate temperature may increase by as much as 8°C because of this phenomenon.[166] K_{cor} has been calculated as[167]

$$K_{cor} = \frac{T_b - T_i'}{T_b - T_i}$$

where T_i is the temperature of the injectate measured just before it is injected into the catheter and T_i' (corrected injectate temperature) is the temperature of the indicator fluid as it exits the right atrial port of the thermodilution catheter. T_i' can be determined empirically and depends chiefly on catheter dimensions and construction. Thermodilution catheter systems have been developed that have two thermistors: one in the usual location at the distal catheter tip and one at the right atrial injectate orifice. With such a system, the output of the proximal thermistor is used to signify injectate temperature and K_{cor} is deleted from the equation.[3, 168, 169]

When a specific catheter design is selected and the specific type and volume of sterile indicator are chosen as the injectate (usually either 5 or 10 mL of 5% dextrose in water), constants can be substituted for the terms K_{cor}, V_i, C_i, and S_i. These constants, as well as C_b and S_b, the calibration constant K_{cal}, and the term 60 s/min can then be combined into a single computation constant, K_{comp}. The equation can be further simplified by solving the integral, or otherwise obtaining the area under the thermodilution curve, and substituting this area as A in place of the integral term in the denominator:

$$\text{Blood flow} = \frac{(T_b - T_i) \times K_{comp}}{A}$$

The solution to this equation yields PA blood flow in liters per minute. Total pulmonary blood flow can be considered right-sided cardiac output, which, except for transient minor differences, is normally equal to left-sided cardiac output (i.e., blood flow from the left ventricle into the systemic circulation). As cardiac output decreases, the degree of deflection in the temperature curve may become more pronounced and the duration of the deflection longer, resulting in a larger area under the curve (see Fig. 95–13B). It is useful to inspect the thermodilution curve routinely. A curve that is atypical may indicate poor injection technique or the presence of a physiologic abnormality that could interfere with the accuracy of the results. For example, the tracing in Figure 95–13D shows a thermodilution curve obtained during an erratic injection. In the presence of a left-to-right shunt, as may occur with ventricular septal defect, patent ductus arteriosus, or partial anomalous pulmonary venous return, pulmonary blood flow exceeds systemic cardiac output. In these conditions, systemic cardiac output as determined by the PA thermodilution catheter may therefore be artifactually high.[170] In addition, a recirculation peak may be apparent on the thermodilution curve because of diversion of the still cool injectate fluid through the shunt and past the catheter tip for a second time. Tricuspid insufficiency causes regurgitation of the injectate fluid from the right ventricle to the right atrium. This has the effect of decreasing the amplitude of maximal temperature deflection and extending the duration of the thermodilution curve (see Fig. 95–13E).[171, 172]

The procedure for performing a thermodilution cardiac output measurement is relatively simple with modern equipment but must be carried out correctly and consistently to ensure accurate and reproducible results. When the catheter has been inserted and proper positioning within the pulmonary artery has been verified, the electrical connector of the catheter's thermistor is connected to the cardiac output computer. A second, external temperature probe is often used to monitor the temperature of the injectate solution (see Fig. 95–8). If used, this probe is also connected to the computer. The computation constant to be used in the cardiac output equation must be entered into the computer. As noted previously, the constant to be employed depends on the model of catheter being used, the temperature of the injectate solution, and the quantity of solution to be injected. Accordingly, the operator must ensure that the computer has been programmed with the proper computation constant. This information is provided in the package insert that accompanies the catheter as well as in the printed documentation for the instrument.

Several types of injection methods are in common use, including the use of prefilled syringes, the two-bag system, and the closed injectate system. Standard 5- or 10-mL syringes can be prefilled and cooled by ICU personnel, but careful technique is required to minimize the risk of bacterial contamination.[173] In one study, the incidence of contamination with this procedure was 16% after storage for 24 hours at room temperature and 45% after 72 hours.[174] If prefilled syringes are placed in an ice-water bath, there is the further danger that syringe leakage or syringe hub contamination may increase the risk of nosocomial bacteremia. Prefilled syringes are also commercially available. These packages typically include a carrier in which the prefilled syringes and the injectate temperature probe are placed, and the carrier is then positioned in an ice water bath. The syringes are tightly sealed; thus the risk of microbial contamination is minimal.

The two-bag system consists of two separate intravenous fluid bags containing the sterile injectate solution, both of which are immersed in the same or identical ice water baths. With this system, fluid in both bags can be maintained at a temperature within 0.5°C of one another.[175] Precautions are taken so that the fluid in one of the bags is maintained sterile, and this bag is used as the source of injectate solution. The external thermistor probe is inserted into the second bag, and the temperature of this fluid represents the temperature of the fluid in the injectate solution bag. The solution in the second bag should be considered contaminated and is not to be used as a source of injectate fluid. Injectate solution can be withdrawn from the appropriate bag by using a needle tap or standard intravenous tubing and a three-way stopcock. This method has the disadvantage that the injectate solution source may become contaminated by repeated needle taps or, if a stopcock and extension tubing are used, by repeated connection and disconnection of syringes at the stopcock. There is also a potential for the injectate fluid to be warmed slightly during transit through the tubing connecting the fluid source and the syringe and during syringe handling.[169] The latter problem can be minimized by avoiding prolonged handling of the filled syringe before injection. Special insulated syringes that contain an air jacket surrounding the syringe barrel are available and minimize such temperature changes.

The closed injectate system consists of a single injectate bag connected to the right atrial port of the PA catheter by way of a specially designed coil of intravenous tubing that is submerged in an ice water bath (see Fig. 95–8).[176–178] At the point of connection to the catheter, there is an attachment containing an in-line thermistor that allows monitoring of the temperature of the injectate as it enters the catheter, thus minimizing temperature errors resulting from injectate warming as the solution is aspirated and during syringe handling. A special valve connects the syringe to both the injectate source tubing and the proximal injectate hub of the PA catheter. This valve allows the injectate solution to be aspirated into the syringe, but during injection the valve automatically closes and directs the fluid into the injectate port of the catheter. This system also has the advantage of minimizing external manipulations, thus decreasing the risk of microbial contamination.[179]

Controls on the cardiac output computer allow the operator to display injectate temperature and blood temperature. Observing these temperatures confirms that the respective temperature sensors are functioning and that their electrical connections are satisfactory. When the computer indicates that the system is ready for measurement, the injectate syringe can be filled to the specified volume, which is usually either 5 or 10 mL for adults. Either 5% dextrose or normal saline solution can be used for thermodilution measurements. Although their specific heats and specific gravities are different, the product of the these two constants yields a nearly identical factor in each case.[167] The injectate fluid is then rapidly injected into the right atrium, and the cardiac output computer displays the result in a matter of seconds.

Small cyclic fluctuations in PA blood temperature occur normally. Typical baseline temperature variations ranging from 0.01 to 0.09°C occur synchronously with respiration and are caused by intrathoracic cooling by inspired air and changes in venous return.[180–184] These fluctuations are nearly absent during apnea and during high rates of mechanical ventilation but can be significant during deep spontaneous respiratory efforts. Because blood temperature is a variable in the computation formula for thermodilution cardiac output, these cyclic changes in PA blood temperature affect the accuracy of the result. Thus, depending on the timing of the injection with respect to the respiratory cycle, slight differences in calculated blood flow result. In addition to this artifactual effect related to injection timing, actual changes in cardiac output occur throughout the respiratory cycle and may have an even more important influence on the resulting measurement. Changes in venous return, pulmonary vascular resistance, ventricular volumes, and LV afterload occur with respiration and influence stroke volume.[110, 185] These changes may be exaggerated in some patients, including those undergoing positive pressure ventilation, spontaneously breathing patients with marked respiratory efforts, and patients with cardiac tamponade, pulmonary embolism, or certain other pathologic states.[52, 55, 58, 108–110, 186, 187] The added variability imposed by these effects can be mitigated by timing the injection with the respiratory cycle, for example, by consistently initiating injection at end expiration. This technique has been shown to improve reproducibility significantly compared with randomly timed injections.[188–190]

Both room temperature and iced injectate solutions are employed clinically. An improved signal-to-noise ratio can be obtained by using a lower injectate temperature and/or a larger injectate volume. If extremely small injectate volumes are used, if the injectate temperature is only slightly lower than blood temperature, or if the patient's cardiac output is quite high, then physiologic variations in PA blood temperature result in a poor signal-to-noise ratio potentially leading to inaccurate flow measurements.[191] Other factors remaining constant, the use of iced injectate results in smaller random and systematic errors than the use of ambient temperature injectate.[192–194] Nevertheless, other investigations have demonstrated empirically that comparable accuracy and reproducibility may be attained by using 10-mL volumes of ambient temperature injectate or iced injectate.[191, 195, 196] However, when 5-mL injectate volumes are employed, greater reproducibility is obtained with injectate at ice water temperature than at room temperature. With 3-mL volumes, iced injectate has been shown to have comparable accuracy but markedly impaired reproducibility. The injectate volume should be measured as accurately as the syringe markings allow. If the actual injectate volume is smaller than indicated

by the computation constant, the cardiac output is overestimated.[197] This is because the induced drop in blood temperature is less, resulting in a higher calculated blood flow. The opposite occurs if the actual injectate volume is greater than that indicated by the computation constant. Routine use of ambient temperature injectate simplifies the procedure by avoiding the need to prepare and wait for the injectate to be cooled and the error caused by warming of the injectate syringe as it is removed from the ice bath.[169, 198] On the other hand, systems with in-line coolers (see Fig. 95–8) allow the use of iced injectate with negligible inconvenience and risk of contamination and may provide slightly more accurate results, particularly when smaller injectate volumes are employed.[176–178, 192]

If injectate temperature were equal to blood temperature, no thermodilution curve would be generated. This situation could theoretically be approached in hypothermic patients undergoing thermodilution measurements with room temperature injectate. Thus, it has specifically been recommended that iced injectate solution should be used in the setting of hypothermia.[199] Shellock and colleagues, however, demonstrated that accurate thermodilution measurements can be obtained using 10-mL volumes of room temperature injectate in patients with moderate degrees of hypothermia (30 to 35°C).[200] Because of increased ventricular arrhythmogenicity, PA catheterization is, in practice, not usually undertaken in ICU patients with more severe degrees of hypothermia. Thus, although the signal-to-noise ratio is decreased in this setting, room temperature injectate is still generally satisfactory for ICU patients with hypothermia.

It is important that the injection be consistently performed in a smooth, rapid fashion, using a steady, even pressure to ensure a constant injection rate. The injection should be as rapid as possible and preferably completed within 2 to 4 seconds when a volume of 5 to 10 mL is used.[192, 199, 201] To this end, hand-held injector devices operating on compressed gas have been developed to automate the injection process and thereby ensure consistent injection rates. Comparing automatic to manual injections, Nelson and Houtchens found a significant difference in resulting cardiac output determinations, but such differences occurred with only a minority of personnel performing the injections.[202] Most of the tested personnel obtained adequate results with manual injections, and overall there was no significant difference between the two techniques.

Various other factors may affect thermodilution results. Thrombus formation over the thermistor has been reported to result in erroneous flow measurements.[203] Infusion of cool intravenous fluids through another central venous access site during thermodilution measurement increases the amount of thermal indicator delivered. Because this added indicator volume is not taken into account by the computation constant, accuracy is adversely affected.[204] This can occur when high flow rates of such fluids are administered through an adjacent central venous catheter, through the side port of an indwelling introducer sheath, or through the extra proximal infusion port available on some thermodilution catheters. The opposite problem may occur if the injectate orifice of the PA catheter is located within the introducer sheath. In this situation part of the injectate volume may flow retrogradely up the sheath and out the side arm, resulting in a delivered injectate volume less than that indicated by the computation constant and a falsely elevated cardiac output value.[205, 206] On the other hand, in situations in which the proximal injection lumen of a PA catheter becomes obstructed, satisfactory results have been obtained by injecting thermal indicator through an introducer sheath, through a secondary right atrial infusion port, through a specialized RV port, or through a separate central venous catheter.[207-209] If the catheter is in wedge position or located so far distally that less than 1 mL of balloon inflation results in complete occlusion, the quantity of thermal indicator reaching the thermistor may be insufficient for an adequate dilution curve.[171] Similarly, erroneous values may be obtained if the catheter tip is lodged in a branch of the pulmonary artery containing an occlusive embolus.[103] Spurious cardiac output values may also be obtained if the catheter is looped within the heart such that the distance between the injectate port and the thermistor is reduced.[210, 211]

The thermodilution curve shown in Figure 95–13A appears smooth. If a fast-response thermistor is employed, the washout phase of the tracing is seen to consist of small deflections synchronous with each cardiac cycle (Fig. 95–14B). These are due to the pronounced change in PA blood temperature during each systole (as warm blood enters the vessel), whereas during diastole there is little change in PA temperature. PA catheters equipped with such thermistors can be used to determine RV volume and ejection fraction. The methodology is based on the law of conservation of energy. The amount of heat energy (E) contained in the right ventricle can be quantitated as

$$E = T \times V \times C \times \rho$$

where V = RV volume (mL)
T = temperature of the RV blood volume (°C)
C = specific heat of blood (cal/g/°C)
ρ = density of blood (g/mL)

The total thermal energy contained in the right ventricle at end diastole is equal to the heat energy remaining from end systole of the previous cycle plus the heat energy that entered the right ventricle during diastole. This can be quantitatively expressed as[212, 213]

$$T_{ed} \times V_{ed} \times C \times \rho = (T_{es} \times V_{es} \times C \times \rho) + [T_B \times (V_{ed} - V_{es}) \times C \times \rho]$$

where T_{ed} = RV blood temperature at end diastole
V_{ed} = RV end-diastolic volume
T_{es} = RV end-systolic blood temperature (from the systole immediately preceding T_{ed})
V_{es} = RV end-systolic volume
T_B = baseline blood temperature

Successive diastolic PA temperatures (T_1 and T_2) may be substituted for the RV temperatures in this formula, and the equation can be algebraically simplified and rearranged to

$$\frac{V_{ed} - V_{es}}{V_{ed}} = 1 - \frac{T_2 - T_B}{T_1 - T_B}$$

The left side of this equation is equivalent to RV ejection fraction (EF_{RV}). The temperature terms on the right side of the equation can be determined graphically from the thermodilution tracing (see Fig. 95–14B). Dedicated cardiac output computers perform the calculations automatically and report EF_{RV} and RV end-systolic and end-diastolic volume, as well as the usual thermodilution cardiac output. In addition to the special thermistor, these PA catheters contain electrodes for sensing the intracavitary electrogram, for accurately timing each systole in relation to the thermodilution curve, and for determining heart rate. The computer also calculates cardiac output by the usual thermodilution method and calculates stroke volume (SV) from cardiac output and heart rate. RV end-diastolic volume is determined from

$$V_{ed} = \frac{SV}{EF_{RV}}$$

and RV end-systolic volume from

$$V_{es} = V_{ed} \times (1 - EF_{RV})$$

EF_{RV} determined by this method compares favorably with ejection fraction measurements made by first-pass and gated nuclear techniques and by biplane ventriculography.[214, 215] The potential clinical role of RV ejection fraction monitoring is under evaluation.[212, 216-220]

The dye dilution method has been used in conjunction with the thermodilution technique to measure extravascular lung water, and some centers have successfully used this procedure clinically. Because the technique depends on both dye and thermodilution principles, it is briefly described here. Iced indocyanine green dye is injected in the usual manner, and both temperature and optical density are monitored at a distal site, typically the femoral artery, by using a special catheter equipped with a thermistor and by using a withdrawl pump and densitometer as with the standard dye dilution method.[221-224] Mean transit times for both the dye and thermal indicators can be calculated from the respective dilution curves. The product of mean transit time and flow is equal to the blood volume between the injection site and the sampling site plus the blood volume of all temporally equidistant sites in other branches of the vasculature.[225] In the case of indocyanine green, the indicator is constrained to the intravascular compartment and gives a true measure of intravascular volume. However, in the case of the thermal indicator some of the indicator (negative heat energy) diffuses out of the pulmonary vasculature, yielding a volume measurement proportional to the combined intravascular and extravascular volume. Extravascular lung water (EVLW) can therefore be calculated from cardiac output (CO) and the thermal (MTT_t) and dye (MTT_d) mean transit times as

$$EVLW = CO \times (MTT_t - MTT_d)$$

Although the methodology has been applied successfully in many clinical and experimental investigations, the requirement for using indocyanine green and arterial sampling makes it cumbersome for routine clinical use. In addition,

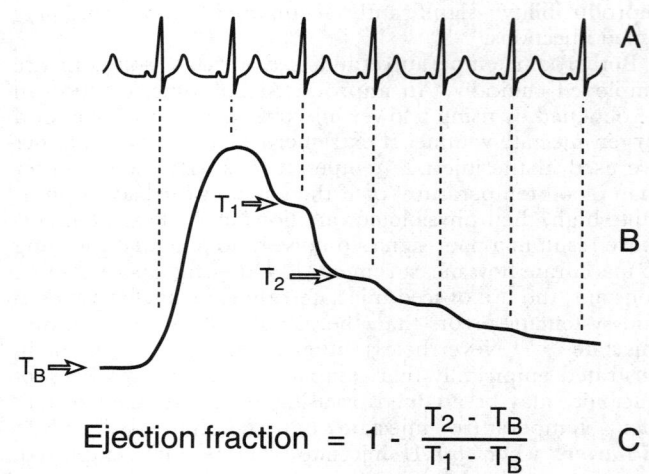

Ejection fraction = $1 - \dfrac{T_2 - T_B}{T_1 - T_B}$

Figure 95–14. Thermodilution measurement of RV ejection fraction using PA catheter equipped with a rapid-response thermistor. *A.* Reference electrocardiogram. *B.* Thermodilution curve (see text). Vertical deflection represents inverse temperature change; T_B is baseline PA blood temperature; T_1 and T_2 are successive PA plateau temperatures. *C.* Formula for calculating RV ejection fraction.

the accuracy of the technique may be limited depending on the type and severity of the pulmonary edema.[221, 224] Finally, the specific role that EVLW measurements might play in the clinical management of critically ill patients has not been well defined.

The Fick Oxygen Method

In the ICU setting, cardiac output is currently measured almost exclusively by the thermodilution method. Before the development of this technique, both the Fick oxygen method and the indocyanine green dye dilution method were commonly employed in the cardiac catheterization laboratory. Although the three techniques have similar accuracy, thermodilution is technically simpler to perform. The Fick oxygen method is based on principles first described by Adolph Fick in 1870, specifically that the quantity of any substance absorbed or released by an organ is the product of blood flow through the organ and the arteriovenous concentration difference of that substance across the organ's vascular bed.[226] In this application, blood flow across the pulmonary vasculature is determined by using oxygen as the marker substance. The arteriovenous oxygen content difference $(CaO_2 - C\bar{v}O_2)$ is obtained from arterial (CaO_2) and mixed venous $(C\bar{v}O_2)$ blood oxygen contents as

$$CaO_2 = (1.39 \times Hb \times SaO_2) + (PaO_2 \times 0.0031)$$
$$C\bar{v}O_2 = (1.39 \times Hb \times S\bar{v}O_2) + (P\bar{v}O_2 \times 0.0031)$$

where 1.39 mL/g = maximal volume of oxygen that can be bound to 1 g of hemoglobin
Hb = hemoglobin concentration (g/dL)
PaO_2 = arterial oxygen tension
SaO_2 = oxyhemoglobin saturation
0.0031 mL/dL/torr = solubility coefficient for oxygen in plasma
$P\bar{v}O_2$ and $S\bar{v}O_2$ = equivalent terms for mixed venous blood

Cardiac output (L/min) is directly proportional to the amount of oxygen (mL) consumed by the body each minute $(\dot{V}O_2)$ and inversely proportional to $CaO_2 - C\bar{v}O_2$ (mL/dL) according to the Fick equation:

$$CO = \frac{\dot{V}O_2}{(CaO_2 - C\bar{v}O_2) \times 10}$$

Oxygen consumption can be determined by analysis of expired gas. A timed collection of expired gas is made using a collapsed Douglas bag, and an aliquot is analyzed for expired oxygen fraction (FEO_2). By knowing FIO_2 and FEO_2, oxygen uptake by the lungs (equivalent to oxygen consumption) can be calculated from

$$\dot{V}O_2 = \frac{(VI \times FIO_2) - (VE \times FEO_2)}{t}$$

where VI and VE = inspired and expired gas volumes (mL)
t = time interval (min) over which volumes are sampled

VI may be measured directly or calculated from the Haldane equation:

$$VI = \frac{VE \times FEN_2}{FIN_2}$$

where

$$FEN_2 = 1 - FEO_2 - FECO_2$$

and

$$FIN_2 = 1 - FIO_2 - FICO_2$$

and the denoted terms refer to the inspired and expired fractional concentrations of the respective gases.[227] $\dot{V}O_2$ measured at ambient conditions depends on ambient temperature and barometric pressure. To standardize gas volume and $\dot{V}O_2$ results, the following conversion factor is often employed to express these measurements as dry gas volume units at standard temperature (273 K) and pressure (1 atm or 760 torr):

$$\frac{PB - PH_2O}{PB} \times \frac{273}{273 + T} \times \frac{PB}{760}$$

where PB = ambient barometric pressure (torr)
PH_2O = water vapor pressure of saturated gas at ambient temperature (torr)
T = ambient temperature (°C)[228]

Bedside instruments are commercially available that connect to the patient's mechanical ventilator circuit and automatically measure oxygen consumption on the basis of the foregoing principles.[229] These devices generally yield acceptable results, but inaccuracies typically become pronounced at high levels of FIO_2.

In animal studies, the Fick method result is highly correlated with pulmonary blood flow determined by direct optical rotameter measurements.[230] Any errors in assaying blood oxygen content, gas volumes or flows, or gas concentrations translate to a corresponding error in $\dot{V}O_2$. Leakage of gas from the circuit is a particularly common source of error. The blood gas measurements reflect instantaneous conditions, but the gas collection occurs over an interval of up to several minutes. Thus, any changes in arterial or mixed venous oxygenation that occur during the procedure also result in error. The bronchial circulation introduces an obligatory, albeit small, degree of error.[228]

Because the foregoing methods of directly determining oxygen consumption are employed at some centers, the Fick oxygen method could be used to measure cardiac output at these institutions. However, the Fick method requires mixed venous blood sampling, which necessitates invasive catheterization, which usually can be done only with a PA catheter. This requirement, technical complexities with the Fick technique, and the wide availability of thermodilution catheters are the chief reasons why the Fick method is seldom used today to measure cardiac output in the ICU. Nevertheless, there are circumstances in which this method can be of practical utility. For example, in the occasional situation in which thermodilution cardiac output results are suspected of being spurious, direct $\dot{V}O_2$ measurements may be used in conjunction with arterial and mixed venous blood gas results to calculate cardiac output and provide an independent check on the thermodilution method.

Comparison of Cardiac Output Measurement Methods

Numerous investigations performed under a wide variety of circumstances have shown good overall correlation between the dye dilution, the thermodilution, and the Fick oxygen methods for determining cardiac output.[3, 168, 192, 198, 231–237] Stetz and associates examined the findings of 14 reports comparing cardiac output measurements by the thermodilution method to measurements by the Fick and dye dilution methods.[231] They concluded that the three methods are equally reliable. Their analysis further demonstrated that because of the inherent variability in thermodilution measurements, successive individual cardiac output determinations that are within 20 to 26% of one another cannot be considered significantly different.[231] To reduce this margin of error, thermodilution measurements are routinely performed at least in triplicate and the results averaged. With this procedure, the threshold for discriminating clinically significant differences decreases to 12 to 15%.

In patients with valvular insufficiency the Fick oxygen method should theoretically be more accurate than indicator dilution techniques.[168, 171, 238–241] In tricuspid insufficiency, regurgitation of indicator from the right ventricle to the right atrium delays complete delivery of indicator to the distal monitoring site, thus increasing transit time and extending the duration of the indicator dilution curve (see Fig. 95–13E). This also results in a decrease in amplitude of the curve, reflecting a decrease in peak dye concentration or thermal change. For both the dye method and the thermodilution method this prolongation decreases signal strength and may thereby adversely affect accuracy. For the dye method the decrease in signal strength (dye concentration), coupled with the transit time delay, has the effect of melding the dilution curve and the recirculation peak, confounding accurate integration under the curve. In the case of thermodilution, there is loss of thermal indicator as a portion of the injectate undergoes additional warming in the right atrium during each successive regurgitation. This loss is unaccounted for in the Stewart-Hamilton equation if the injected negative heat absorbed by right atrial tissue is not released back to the blood during the measurement interval. Such loss of indicator results in a spuriously higher estimate of forward blood flow from the thermodilution curve. The Fick method should be unaffected by valvular regurgitation. Some investigators have demonstrated that cardiac output determined by thermodilution measurements is indeed significantly different from that determined simultaneously by the Fick method in the setting of moderate to severe tricuspid insufficiency but not in the absence of valvular disease.[28, 238, 240, 241] However, other investigators have shown that there is little if any difference between the two techniques in practice, even with severe regurgitation.[172, 242] The discrepancies in these findings are unexplained.

It has also been proposed that the Fick oxygen method should theoretically be more accurate than indicator dilution techniques for patients with states of extremely low cardiac output.[192, 201, 239] As noted, thermal signal loss results in overestimation of cardiac output by the thermodilution method. The lower the flow rate, the greater the degree of warming that occurs as heat is conducted from cardiac tissues into the cooled blood. Thus, thermal signal loss at low flow rates should result in overestimation of cardiac output by the thermodilution method. This has been demonstrated empirically by comparing paired thermodilution determinations and cardiac output measurements by the Fick oxygen method.[237] Subsequent release of thermal indicator from cardiac tissue back into the blood could theoretically result in underestimation of flow at low levels of cardiac output.[201] Recirculation is problematic at low cardiac output when using the dye dilution method.[236] Because thermal dissipation occurs across the systemic circulation, there is little or no recirculation error with the thermodilution technique, unless a left-to-right shunt is present.

Noninvasive and Continuous Cardiac Output Measurement

Various noninvasive methods of determining cardiac output have been investigated. One early method, ballistocardiography, attempted to derive stroke volume and cardiac output by examining the recoil of the body to the physical impulse generated by mechanical systole. Other methods have attempted to derive stroke volume from formulas based on the pulse pressure or by analysis of the central arterial pulse waveform. The pulse pressure (the difference between systolic and diastolic blood pressure) and the pulse waveform

contour have several determinants, including stroke volume, arterial compliance, and systemic vascular resistance (SVR). Assuming that the other factors are constant, pulse pressure should therefore correlate with stroke volume, and cardiac output could be calculated as estimated stroke volume times heart rate. One such formula relating blood pressure to cardiac output is[243]

$$CO = K \times HR \times [163 + HR - (0.48 \times MAP)] \times \int [P_{AO}(t) - P_d] \, dt$$

where HR = heart rate
MAP = mean arterial pressure
P_{AO} = instantaneous aortic pressure
P_d = diastolic aortic pressure

The integral term thus represents the area under the pulse pressure waveform. When continuous blood pressure monitoring is coupled with a computer to perform the calculations, such formulas allow continuous, beat-by-beat stroke volume and cardiac output determinations. Although some studies have shown reasonable agreement between pulse contour methods and thermodilution, others have found severe limitations in accuracy.[243–245] The inclusion of a calibration constant (K) may improve accuracy to a clinically acceptable level; however, this constant must be determined individually using, for example, simultaneous thermodilution measurements.

The Fick method can be applied to carbon dioxide as well as oxygen. Arterial and mixed venous P_{CO_2} values are determined by blood gas analysis, and $\dot{V}_{CO_2}$ is obtained by expired gas analysis, analogous to that described for the Fick oxygen method. This method still requires both arterial and mixed venous blood sampling. However, various methods have been reported for noninvasively estimating mixed venous P_{CO_2} by analyzing expired carbon dioxide during breath-holding or rebreathing maneuvers.[235, 246–249] These techniques appear to have validity but are cumbersome and have not been widely applied, even though they were initially described more than three decades ago. Inhalation of other indicator gases (such as nitrous oxide, acetylene, or inert gases) has also been used.[161] A method combining $\dot{V}_{CO_2}$ measurements with arterial and mixed venous oximetry determinations to estimate cardiac output has been proposed.[250]

Doppler ultrasonography has been employed as a noninvasive means of estimating cardiac output. An ultrasonic transducer is used to direct high-frequency sound waves transcutaneously to the aorta and to detect the reflected waves. Contact of the ultrasound waves with flowing blood within the aorta results in a change in frequency of the reflected waves. According to the Doppler effect, this frequency shift is proportional to the velocity of blood flow (v):

$$v = \frac{f_\Delta \times c}{2 \times f_t \times \cos \theta}$$

where f_t = frequency of the transmitted waves (e.g., 2.5 MHz)
f_Δ = Doppler shift frequency
c = velocity of sound in blood (1570 cm/s)
θ = angle of incidence between the ultrasound beam and the blood flow vector (often 0°)[251, 252]

This provides a reliable measure of aortic blood velocity, but velocity is not the same as flow. Cardiac output is related to ejectate velocity, as well as to heart rate and the cross-sectional area of the aorta, according to

$$CO = HR \times \pi \times r^2 \times \int v(t) \, dt$$

where r is aortic radius, v is aortic blood velocity, and the integral term represents the area under the systolic velocity-time curve.[252] Aortic radius is obtained by one- or two-dimensional echocardiographic imaging or from nomograms based on the subject's age, sex, weight, and height. The ultrasonic probe is usually positioned in the suprasternal notch; the transesophageal approach has also been utilized.[253] Although some investigators have obtained results that correlate closely with thermodilution cardiac output measurements, others have found an unacceptable degree of random variability. Even with refinements, there remain inherent limitations in estimating both aortic cross-sectional area and blood velocity.[254–257] With further developments this method may ultimately find routine application in the ICU.[258]

Another noninvasive method for estimating cardiac output that has received wide attention is electrical impedance cardiography. In this technique a harmless high-frequency alternating current is passed through the thorax while electrical impedance is monitored with surface electrodes. This impedance varies with instantaneous thoracic blood volume and is thereby related to stroke volume. Both empirical and theoretic considerations have been used to developed formulas to transform the impedance waveform into an estimate of stroke volume or cardiac output. One such formula is

$$CO = K_h \times \frac{(0.17 \times H)^3}{4.25} \times \frac{(dZ/dt)_{max}}{Z_0} \times HR \times LVET$$

where K_h = body habitus correction factor
H = body height (cm)
$(dZ/dt)_{max}$ = maximal time rate of change of thoracic impedance during systole (Ω/s)
Z_0 = baseline thoracic impedance (Ω)
HR = heart rate (min^{-1})
$LVET$ = left ventricular ejection time[259, 260]

With commercially available equipment, reasonable correlations with thermodilution cardiac output have been found by some observers,[261–264] but other investigators have had less than satisfactory results.[259, 265–273] The technique is attractive not only because it is noninvasive but also because it allows continuous monitoring. However, it remains to be seen whether the potential of bioimpedance cardiography is realized for routine monitoring in the ICU.

The search for reliable methods of continuous or near-continuous cardiac output monitoring has also included several invasive techniques. In a novel application of thermodilution principles, a catheter-mounted resistive heating element supplies the thermal energy in lieu of a fluid injection.[274–276] An electrical current passes through wires embedded in the catheter, heating the filament in the right atrium and thereby raising the temperature of blood flowing past the heater coil. In this case, positive heat energy is added to the circulation as opposed to the negative heat energy (i.e., cold) supplied by conventional injections of iced or room temperature fluid. The process can be readily automated by using a computer to activate the heating element periodically and calculate cardiac output from the resulting thermodilution curve. Accuracy and reproducibility approach those of conventional bolus thermodilution methods.[275]

The Fick principle has also been applied to continuous cardiac output monitoring. This technique simply integrates three currently used continuous monitoring technologies: digital pulse oximetry, fiberoptic mixed venous oximetry, and breath-by-breath oxygen consumption measurement.[277–279] Arterial oxygen content is estimated from pulse oximetry–derived arterial saturation (SpO$_2$), mixed venous oxygen content is estmiated from PA saturation, and $\dot{V}O_2$ is determined by automated inspired and exhaled gas analysis as described previously. The output of each instrument is interfaced to a computer that calculates cardiac output by the Fick equation. The equations for blood oxygen content also require hemoglobin concentration and arterial and mixed venous oxygen tensions. The former is obtained from periodic routine hematologic assays and entered manually into the computer, and the latter are estimated mathematically by assuming a normal P$_{50}$ and calculating tensions from the respective oxyhemoglobin saturations. If the minor contribution of oxygen tension to oxygen content is ignored, the Fick equation simplifies to

$$CO = \frac{\dot{V}O_2}{k \times Hb \times (SpO_2 - S\bar{v}O_2)}$$

Cardiac output is typically updated approximately once per minute. Fair correlation with simultaneous thermodilution measurements has been demonstrated.[277, 279] Overall accuracy is limited primarily by the inherent inaccuracies of the three component technologies.

DERIVED HEMODYNAMIC VARIABLES

In addition to directly measured hemodynamic parameters, such as CVP, PA pressures, heart rate, and cardiac output, a number of parameters can be derived from the measurements described earlier. These calculated variables can be useful in the overall hemodynamic evaluation of the critically ill patient, for suggesting or corroborating the physiologic disturbance or diagnosis, for assessing severity of illness and outcome, and as quantitative indices for guiding therapy.[6–10, 44, 45, 280, 281]

Mean Arterial Pressure

Systemic arterial blood pressure is constantly changing throughout the cardiac cycle. MAP is the average arterial pressure during one complete cardiac cycle and provides a single numerical value to represent this changing pressure. Arterial catheterization allows the arterial pressure tracing to be displayed using conventional transducer-based monitoring systems. These instruments can accurately determine MAP by integrating the area subtended by the pressure-time waveform. When direct monitoring is not being employed, MAP can be estimated by adding one third of the pulse pressure to the diastolic pressure:

$$MAP = \frac{P_s - P_d}{3} + P_d$$

where P_s and P_d represent systolic and diastolic arterial blood pressure, respectively. Algebraic rearrangement of this equation shows that it is based on the assumptions that the arterial waveform is approximated by a square wave and that systole occupies about one third and diastole two thirds of each cycle:

$$MAP = \left(\frac{1}{3} P_s \right) + \left(\frac{2}{3} P_d \right)$$

Because these formulas can only provide estimates, MAP should be read directly from the electronic monitor whenever arterial catheterization is employed. The same formula can be used to calculate mean PA pressure by substituting the PA systolic and diastolic pressures in place of systemic arterial pressures.

MAP measurement is useful clinically because it provides a more accurate assessment of blood pressure than direct or indirect determinations of systolic and diastolic pressures. As discussed in Chapter 20, systolic and diastolic pressure measurements with fluid-filled transducer-based monitoring systems are subject to artifactual over- or underestimation because of hyperresonance or damping of the waveform that can occur when the resonant frequency and damping coefficient of the system are suboptimal. MAP is much less subject to these dynamic reponse characteristics. In addition, systolic and diastolic pressures vary over the respiratory cycle and during certain arrhythmias. During ventricular bigeminy, for example, systolic pressure can vary significantly with every other heartbeat. Because electronic monitors obtain MAP by averaging the instantaneous pressure over several seconds, the resulting MAP is more representative than systolic and diastolic pressures from a given beat or from peak and nadir pressures over several beats. MAP also provides a rational single parameter for titrating vasoactive pharmacotherapy against blood pressure. Finally, MAP is used in the calculation of certain other derived parameters. Normal MAP is typically in the range of 85 to 100 mm Hg.

Whereas MAP is the average pressure during the entire cardiac cycle, mean systolic pressure (MSP) is the average pressure during systole. Like MAP, this value can be determined by electronic integration, or estimated from[92, 243]

$$MSP = P_d + \frac{2 \times (P_s - P_d)}{3}$$

This variable represents the pressure that the left ventricle works against during systolic ejection and can be used as a simple measure of LV systolic wall tension or afterload.

Body Surface Area

Because the normal range of many physiologic parameters varies with body size, it is frequently useful to index these variables to body surface area (BSA). Body surface area can be calculated using the Dubois formula:[282]

$$BSA = 0.007184 \times W^{0.425} \times H^{0.725}$$

where W is body weight (kg), H is height (cm), and BSA is in square meters. Nomograms based on this formula are also commonly available.

Cardiac Index

The cardiac index (CI) is obtained by dividing the cardiac output by body surface area:

$$CI = \frac{CO}{BSA}$$

This calculation in effect normalizes the patient's cardiac output for body size. Consider two healthy, resting subjects, one 5 ft tall and weighing 55 kg with a cardiac output of 4.7 L/min and the other 6 ft tall and weighing 90 kg with a cardiac output of 5.3 L/min. Although the larger individual has a substantially greater cardiac output than the smaller subject, the shorter person has a greater cardiac index (3.1 L/min/m²) than the taller subject (2.5 L/min/m²). Cardiac index thus allows more accurate comparisons between patients, obviates the need to consider body size during interpretation, and narrows the normal variability associated with cardiac output. Normal cardiac index is approximately 2.6 to 4.0 L/min/m².

Stroke Index

Stroke volume is the quotient of cardiac output and heart rate, expressed in milliliters, and represents the average volume of blood ejected by the heart during systole. Stroke volume is frequently indexed to body surface area, in which

case it is referred to as stroke index (SI). It can be calculated from cardiac index and heart rate as

$$SI = \frac{CI}{HR \times 1000}$$

and is expressed in units of milliliters per square meter. The constant 1000 allows conversion from units of liters to milliliters. As with cardiac index, stroke index represents a physiologic variable (stroke volume) that has been normalized to body size. The resting normal range for stroke index is approximately 35 to 50 mL/m².

Left Ventricular Stroke Work Index

Work is the amount of force required to move a quantity of matter over a certain distance and can be expressed mathematically as the product of force and distance. In hydraulic terms this is equivalent to pressure times volume. The net work performed by the left ventricle is thus equal to the volume of blood ejected times the pressure developed by the contracting myocardium. It can be calculated from

$$LVSWI = 0.0136 \times SI \times (MSP - PAOP)$$

where LVSWI is the LV stroke work index. The constant 0.0136 is derived from the density of mercury (13.6 g/mL) and converts the result to conventional metric units (grammeter per square meter). In the absence of aortic stenosis, mean systolic pressure approximates the average pressure developed by the left ventricle during systole. Although technically less correct,[227, 283] MAP is frequently used in place of mean systolic pressure. LVEDP (approximated in the foregoing formula by PAOP) represents the presystolic baseline pressure and is therefore subtracted from mean systolic pressure. Because the ejected volume is expressed as stroke index in this equation, the result is indexed to body surface area.

It should be noted that the operating level of LV volume can influence myocardial energetics independently of LVSWI. A patient with a dilated left ventricle may have the same LVSWI as a patient with normal or smaller LV dimensions. However, myocardial oxygen consumption is higher in the former patient because, at equal pressures, greater wall tension is needed to develop a given level of pressure in the dilated ventricle, and LV wall tension is a major determinant of mechanical efficiency and myocardial oxygen demand. LVSWI is a complex function of preload, afterload, contractility, and heart rate but is nevertheless a useful bedside indicator of overall pump performance.[227, 283] It takes into account body size (because it is indexed to body surface area) and heart rate and incorporates a crude measure of afterload (mean systolic pressure or MAP). Clinical Starling curves are often constructed by plotting LVSWI against some measure of LV preload, such as LVEDV, LVEDP, or PAOP (see Fig. 95–6). LVSWI has been shown to predict survival in the setting of acute myocardial infarction.[6] The normal range of resting LVSWI is approximately 40 to 60 g·m/m². Increased levels are characteristically observed in systemic hypertension and hypervolemia and decreased levels in circulatory shock and in conditions associated with impaired LV systolic function. Various other indices of ventricular function have been described, including LV dP/dt, peak circumferential fiber-shortening velocity, and ventricular power, but these variables require measurements that are not commonly available in the ICU setting.

Stroke work index for the right vetricle (RVSWI) may be calculated analogously as

$$RVSWI = 0.0136 \times SI \times (\overline{P_{PA}} - P_{RA})$$

RVSWI represents net work performed by the right ventricle against the resistance of the pulmonary circulation. The normal range is approximately 4 to 8 g·m/m². RVSWI is increased in pulmonary embolism and other forms of pulmonary hypertension, and it may be decreased in right-sided heart failure, particularly in forms that are not associated with pulmonary hypertension, such as RV infarction.

Systemic Vascular Resistance

Resistance to flow can be thought of in qualitative terms as the sum of effects that impede fluid flow. If flow is constant and laminar (i.e., nonturbulent) and occurs through straight, rigid tubes, these effects include the frictional forces between the fluid particles (viscosity) and the frictional forces between the fluid particles and the walls of the tube. The latter vary with the inside surface area of the tube, a function of its length and diameter. A quantitative description of these factors can be derived from Poiseuille's law and represented as

$$\text{Resistance} = \frac{8 \times \eta \times l}{\pi \times r^4}$$

where η = viscosity of the fluid
l = length of the tube
r = radius of the tube

Resistance can also be defined as the ratio of pressure to flow and readily calculated if the pressure gradient and flow rate can be measured. The average pressure gradient across the systemic circulation is the difference between MAP (the driving pressure) and mean right atrial pressure or CVP (the back pressure), and total flow through the systemic circulation is equal to cardiac output. Thus, SVR is calculated at the bedside as

$$\text{SVR} = \frac{(\text{MAP} - \text{CVP}) \times 80}{\text{CO}}$$

The factor 80 is employed to convert the result to metric units (dyne·s/cm⁵). Without this factor the resulting dimensions are mm Hg·min/L, also referred to as hybrid resistance units or Wood's units, but these terms are used less frequently today. SVR is often calculated using cardiac index rather than cardiac output in the denominator, thus indexing the variable to body surface area. As noted previously, it is generally preferable to index cardiac output to body surface area. For the same reason it is also preferable to substitute cardiac index for cardiac output in the equation for SVR, which is then referred to as the SVR index. Because cardiac output varies substantially with body surface area but blood pressure does not, it is physiologically sound to index SVR in this way. Note that the SVR index is calculated by substituting cardiac index for cardiac output, and therefore it is equivalent not to SVR divided by body surface area but to SVR multiplied by body surface area. In contrast, the other variables discussed here are all indexed by dividing by body surface area.

Technically, the foregoing formulas for resistance can be applied only to fluids flowing at a constant rate. The total impediment to pulsatile flow is called hydraulic impedance.[284-286] Like resistance, impedance can be defined as the ratio of pressure to flow. However, arterial pressure and flow change continuously during the cardiac cycle, so impedance cannot be calculated from a single pressure and a single flow value. In addition, there is a variable phasic relationship between flow and pressure. Impedance **(Z)** is defined mathematically as the vector sum of fluid resistance (R) and hydraulic reactance (X):

$$\mathbf{Z} = \sqrt{R^2 + X^2}$$

Although resistance is always a positive number, reactance may be positive or negative. It can be broken down into

$$X = X_i - X_c$$

where X_i is inertial reactance and X_c is capacitive reactance. Inertial hydraulic reactance occurs because the mass of blood being propelled through the circulation must be accelerated to a certain peak velocity with each systole. The left ventricle must therefore develop a certain force to effect this acceleration, and this force is independent of that required to overcome the frictional resistance presented by the vascular tree and blood viscosity.[243] The density of blood (and therefore hematocrit), the stroke volume, and the systolic velocity profile are primary determinants of X_i. Note that inertial reactance is not a consideration in systems in which blood flow is unidirectional and constant, because no acceleration or deceleration occurs in a nonpulsatile, linear system. Capacitive reactance occurs because the walls of the arterial vasculature are distensible. With each systole these elastic vessels expand slightly, with the result that the total volume of the arterial tree is increased during systole. Thus, arterial compliance has the effect of causing part of the kinetic energy of each ejected stroke volume to be stored in the arterial tree. A certain amount of this kinetic energy is required to expand these vessels during systole. That potential energy is returned during diastole as the vessels contract passively, propelling the stored blood volume downstream. This phenomenon helps to maintain blood pressure and flow during diastole and is therefore subtractive from inertial reactance. It is also a major factor in defining the shape of the arterial pressure waveform.[287] If the vasculature were made from rigid pipes, arterial pressure would rapidly approach mean capillary pressure after aortic valve closure, capacitive reactance would not be applicable, and impedance would be increased.[288] Because impedance is the vector sum of resistance and reactance, the frequency of flow rate change (i.e., heart rate) is a factor in determining the resulting value for impedance.[285] Thus, heart rate, stroke volume, the degree of compliance of the arterial tree, and hematocrit have effects on impedance that are not taken into account when impedance is simplistically represented by SVR. Nevertheless, SVR is the best available bedside approximation of total impedance and remains a useful clinical tool, primarily as a means of quantitating LV afterload and the degree of systemic vasoconstriction or vasodilation. Normal SVR is approximately 900 to 1400 dyne·s/cm⁵, and normal SVR index is 1600 to 2400 dyne·s·m²/cm⁵. SVR is increased in patients with hypovolemia, those with LV failure, and those receiving vasoconstrictive drugs. SVR is characteristically decreased in patients with sepsis, cirrhosis, aortic insufficiency, arteriovenous fistula, and some types of central nervous system injury and in those receiving vasodilating drugs including certain anesthetic agents.

Pulmonary Vascular Resistance

The pulmonary vascular resistance (PVR) can be calculated analogously to SVR by substituting the pressure gradient across the pulmonary circulation in the numerator of the formula

$$\text{PVR} = \frac{(\overline{P_{PA}} - \text{PAOP}) \times 80}{\text{CO}}$$

(see also Chapters 65 and 74). In addition to the factors discussed under Systemic Vascular Resistance, the presence of critical opening pressures in the pulmonary circulation limits the validity of pulmonary vascular resistance as a true index of impedance.[289] Nevertheless, this variable is useful for quantitatively expressing the level of pulmonary hypertension relative to pulmonary blood flow, for examining the degree of pulmonary vasoconstriction or vasodilation, and for estimating RV afterload. As with SVR, pulmonary vascular resistance is frequently indexed to body surface area, either by substituting cardiac index for cardiac output in the preceding formula or by multiplying pulmonary vascular resistance by body surface area. Normal pulmonary vascular resistance is approximately 100 to 250 dyne · s/cm⁵, and the normal pulmonary vascular resistance index is 200 to 400 dyne · s · m²/cm⁵. Pulmonary vascular resistance is increased in all forms of pulmonary hypertension, including primary pulmonary hypertension and that resulting from LV failure, mitral stenosis, pulmonary embolism, hypoxemia, and acute lung injury. Pulmonary vascular resistance may decrease after correction of hypoxemia and administration of vasodilating drugs.

HEMODYNAMIC PROFILING

A hemodynamic profile is a listing of simultaneously obtained hemodynamic variables representing the patient's cardiovascular status at the time of measurement. It consists of both measured hemodynamic variables (e.g., heart rate, MAP, CVP, PAOP, and cardiac output) and derived hemodynamic variables (e.g., cardiac index, stroke index, LVSWI, SVR index). Invasive hemodynamic monitoring in the ICU frequently involves both systemic arterial catheterization and PA catheterization. In addition to allowing monitoring of vascular and cardiac pressures and cardiac output, these techniques allow convenient access to both arterial and mixed venous blood. Therefore, it is routine to obtain near-simultaneous measurements of not only the hemodynamic information but also arterial and mixed venous blood gases so that primary and derived lung gas exchange variables (e.g., PaO_2, mixed venous oxygen saturation, alveolar-arterial oxygen difference, pulmonary venous admixture) and oxygen transport parameters (e.g., $\dot{V}O_2$, $CaO_2 - C\bar{v}O_2$, oxygen delivery, and oxygen extraction ratio) can be integrated with the hemodynamic data to form a complete physiologic profile. Such profiles provide the clinician with data that, taken together, can be of considerable value in determining the patient's overall physiologic status and in clinical decision making regarding selection and titration of therapy. Table 95–1 lists hemodynamic patterns that are typically observed in several specific pathologic conditions and illustrates the clinical utility of examining hemodynamic measurements as a complete profile rather than simply as individual results. Certain patterns of hemodynamic variables may corroborate

a working diagnosis or suggest a previously unsuspected condition. Finding diastolic equalization of P_{RA}, P_{RV}, P_{PA}, and PAOP, for example, should lead one to consider pericardial tamponade (Fig. 95–15B). In the setting of myocardial infarction, examining the relationship between PAOP and cardiac index enables the clinician to assess severity and mortality risk and to select rationally among various therapeutic options.[15] The synthesis of hemodynamic findings, gas exchange data, indices of oxygen transport, physical findings, and other clinical information provides the maximal opportunity for delineating the patient's underlying disease and severity of illness. Valuable additional information can be obtained by following serial hemodynamic measurements and examining the response to a therapeutic challenge such as fluid loading (see Chapter 89).

Physiologic profiles should be made immediately after initiation of invasive monitoring and periodically thereafter (e.g., every 12 hours) for the duration of catheterization. If necessary, measurements may be made more frequently to assess the effects of therapeutic maneuvers designed to improve perfusion or otherwise favorably influence hemodynamic function. Typically, profiles are obtained before and after a fluid challenge or after initiation of a vasoactive drug infusion. It is also useful to examine the hemodynamic response to withdrawal of ongoing therapy, such as discontinuation of intra-aortic balloon counterpulsation or downward titration of inotropic drug infusions. Because of the volume of information contained in hemodynamic and physiologic profiles, it is important to have a systematic means of collecting and compiling the data. Flow sheets are helpful in this regard. Because a large number of calculations are required to obtain the derived parameters, computer systems are invaluable for generating, displaying, and storing such profiles.

The technical nature of the measurements and the large number of individual values generated from even a single profile guarantee that erroneous results for both primary and derived variables inevitably occur on occasion. The practitioner must be able to identify obviously invalid results. For example, a negative value for pulmonary vascular resistance is physically not possible but may be obtained if PAOP is erroneously reported to be a value greater than the P_{PA}. Certain patterns may suggest that one or more measurements might be erroneous. For example, a normal or elevated mixed venous oxygen saturation would be unusual in the presence of an extremely low cardiac output and should lead the interpreter to question or repeat the measurements. For correct interpretation, knowledge of the physiologic basis of each parameter is only the first step. In addition, one must have a firm grasp of the physiologic relationships

TABLE 95–1								
TYPICAL HEMODYNAMIC PROFILES IN VARIOUS FORMS OF CRITICAL ILLNESS*								
Illness	**CI**	**MAP**	**CVP**	$P_{RV, d}$	$P_{PA, d}$	**PAOP**	**SVRI**	**PVRI**
Cardiogenic shock	↓	↓	↑	↑	↑	↑	↑	N – ↑
Severe LV failure	↓	↓ – N	N	N	↑	↑	↑	N
Acute ventricular septal rupture	↓	↓	↑	↑	↑	↑	↑	N – ↑
RV myocardial infarction	↓	↓	↑ =	↑ =	↓ – N	↓ – N	↑	N
Cardiac tamponade	↓	↓	↑ =	↑ =	↑ =	↑	↑	N – ↑
Critical mitral stenosis	↓	↓ – N	N – ↑	N – ↑	↑	↑	↑	N – ↑
Massive pulmonary embolism	↓	↓	↑	↑	↑	↓ – N	↑	↑
End-stage cor pulmonale	↓	↓ – N	↑	↑	↑	N	↑	↑
Septic shock	↑	↓	↓ – ↑	↓ – ↑	↓ – ↑	↓ – ↑	↓	↑
Hemorrhagic shock	↓	↓	↓	↓	↓	↓	↑	N – ↑

*CI = cardiac index; $P_{RV, d}$ = RV diastolic pressure; $P_{PA, d}$ = PA diastolic pressure; SVRI = systemic vascular resistance index; PVRI = pulmonary vascular resistance index; ↓ = decreased; ↑ = increased; N = normal.

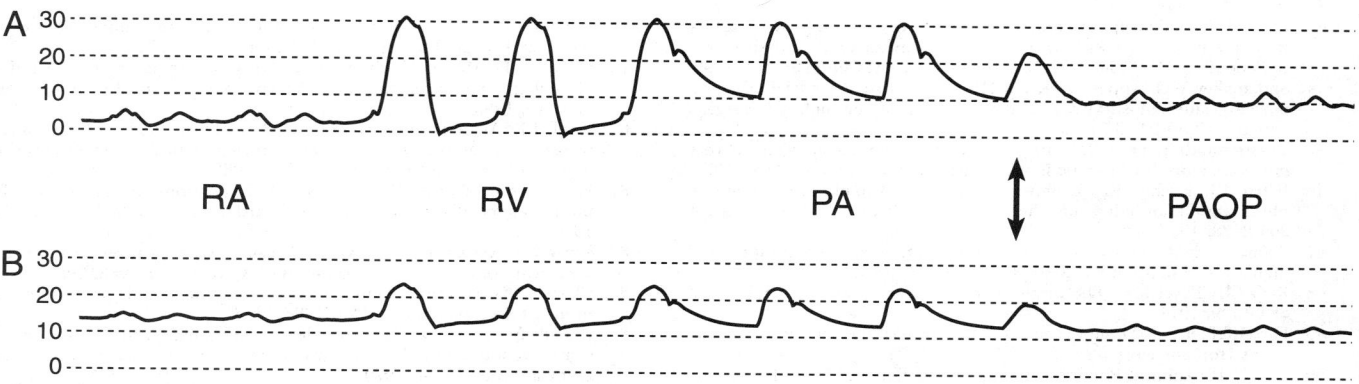

Figure 95–15. Pressure waveform sweep obtained as PA catheter is advanced from right atrial to RV, PA, and finally PAOP position. Arrow indicates transition from P_{PA} to PAOP. *A.* Normal. *B.* Patient with pericardial tamponade. Note increased pressures and diastolic equalization.

between variables and the expected effects of common therapeutic interventions. As an example, one must understand the effects of positive pressure ventilation and PEEP on hemodynamic pressure tracings to interpret such measurements. Along the same lines, the effect of an intracardiac shunt on the accuracy of thermodilution cardiac output determinations must be appreciated lest the clinician be mislead by the resulting measurements.

References

1. Lategola M, Rahn H: A self-guiding catheter for cardiac and pulmonary arterial catheterization and occlusion. Proc Soc Exp Biol Med 84:667, 1953.
2. Swan HJC, Ganz W, Forrester J, et al: Catheterization of the heart in man with use of a flow-directed balloon-tipped catheter. N Engl J Med 283:447, 1970.
3. Ganz W, Donoso R, Marcus HS, et al: A new technique for measurement of cardiac output by thermodilution in man. Am J Cardiol 27:392, 1971.
4. Forrester JS, Ganz W, Diamond G, et al: Thermodilution cardiac output determination with a single flow-directed catheter. Am Heart J 83:306, 1972.
5. Meister SG, Helfant RH: Rapid bedside differentiation of ruptured interventricular septum from acute mitral insufficiency. N Engl J Med 287:1024, 1972.
6. Scheidt S, Wilner G, Fillmore S, et al: Objective haemodynamic assessment after acute myocardial infarction. Br Heart J 35:908, 1973.
7. Shoemaker WC, Chang P, Czer L, et al: Cardiorespiratory monitoring in postoperative patients. I. Prediction of outcome and severity of illness. Crit Care Med 7:237, 1979.
8. Shoemaker WC, Chang P, Bland R, et al: Cardiorespiratory monitoring in postoperative patients. II. Quantitative therapeutic indices as guides to therapy. Crit Care Med 7:243, 1979.
9. Groeneveld ABJ, Nauta JJP, Thijs LG: Peripheral vascular resistance in septic shock: Its relation to outcome. Intensive Care Med 14:141, 1988.
10. Weber KT, Janicki JS, Russel RO, et al: Identification of high risk subsets of acute myocardial infarction. Derived from the Myocardial Infarction Research Units Cooperative Study Data Bank. Am J Cardiol 41:197, 1978.
11. Crexells C, Chatterjee K, Forrester JS, et al: Optimal level of filling pressure in the left side of the heart in acute myocardial infarction. N Engl J Med 289:1263, 1973.
12. Civetta JM, Gabel JC: Flow directed-pulmonary artery catheterization in surgical patients: Indications and modifications of technic. Ann Surg 176:753, 1972.
13. Unger KM, Shibel EM, Moser KM: Detection of left ventricular failure in patients with adult respiratory distress syndrome. Chest 67:8, 1975.
14. Civetta JM, Gabel JC: "Pseudocardiogenic" pulmonary edema. J Trauma 15:143, 1975.
15. Forrester JS, Diamond G, Chatterjee K, et al: Medical therapy of acute myocardial infarction by application of hemodynamic subsets. N Engl J Med 295:1356, 1404, 1976.
16. Pace NL: A critique of flow-directed pulmonary arterial catheterizaton. Anesthesiology 47:455, 1977.
17. Moore CH, Lombardo TR, Allums JA, et al: Left main coronary artery stenosis: Hemodynamic monitoring to reduce mortality. Ann Thorac Surg 26:445, 1978.
18. Sorensen MB, Bille-Brahe NE, Engell HC: Hemodynamic observation

in relation to extensive surgical treatment of patients with increased operative risk. Acta Anaesthesiol Scand 22:287, 1978.
19. Rice CL, Hobelman CF, John DA, et al: Central venous pressure or pulmonary capillary wedge pressure as the determinant of fluid replacement in aortic surgery. Surgery 84:437, 1978.
20. Weil MH, Henning RJ: New concepts in the diagnosis and fluid treatment of circulatory shock. Anesth Analg 58:124, 1979.
21. Pierson DJ, Hudson LD: Monitoring hemodynamics in the critically ill. Med Clin North Am 67:1343, 1983.
22. Packman MI, Rackow EC: Optimum left heart filling pressure during fluid resuscitation of patients with hypovolemic and septic shock. Crit Care Med 11:165, 1983.
23. Shaver JA: Hemodynamic monitoring in the critically ill patient. N Engl J Med 308:277, 1983.
24. Wiedemann HP, Matthay MA, Matthay RA: Cardiovascular-pulmonary monitoring in the intensive care unit. Chest 85:537, 656, 1984.
25. Houston MC, Thompson WL, Robertson D: Shock. Diagnosis and management. Arch Intern Med 144:1433, 1984.
26. Goldenheim PD, Kazemi H: Cardiopulmonary monitoring of critically ill patients. N Engl J Med 311:776, 1984.
27. Amin DK, Shah PK, Swan HJC: The Swan-Ganz catheter: Indications for insertion. J Crit Illness 1:54, 1986.
28. Sharkey SW: Beyond the wedge: Clinical physiology and the Swan-Ganz catheter. Am J Med 83:111, 1987.
29. Broaddus VC, Berthiaume Y, Biondi JW, et al: Hemodynamic management of the adult respiratory distress syndrome. J Intensive Care 2:190, 1987.
30. Natanson C, Hoffman WD, Parrillo JE: Septic shock: The cardiovascular abnormality and therapy. J Cardiothorac Anesth 3:215, 1989.
31. Shoemaker WC, Kram HB, Appel PL: Therapy of shock based on pathophysiology, monitoring, and outcome prediction. Crit Care Med 18:S19, 1990.
32. Rackow EC, Astiz ME: Pathophysiology and treatment of septic shock. JAMA 266:548, 1991.
33. Suter PM, Fairley HB, Isenberg MD: Optimum end-expiratory airway pressure in patients with acute pulmonary failure. N Engl J Med 292:284, 1975.
34. Jardin F, Gurdjian F, Fouilladieu JL, et al: Pulmonary and systemic haemodynamic disorders in the adult respiratory distress syndrome. Intensive Care Med 5:127, 1979.
35. Shell WW, DeWood MA, Peter T, et al: Comparison of clinical signs and hemodynamic state in the early hours of transmural myocardial infarction. Am Heart J 104:521, 1982.
36. Connors AF, McCaffree DR, Gray BA: Evaluation of right-heart catheterization in the critically ill patient without myocardial infarction. N Engl J Med 308:263, 1983.
37. Eisenberg PR, Jaffe AS, Schuster DP: Clinical evaluation compared to pulmonary artery catheterization in the hemodynamic assessment of critically ill patients. Crit Care Med 12:549, 1984.
38. Fein AM, Goldberg SK, Walkenstein MD, et al: Is pulmonary artery catheterization necessary for the diagnosis of pulmonary edema? Am Rev Respir Dis 129:1006, 1984.
39. Tuchschmidt J, Sharma OP: Impact of hemodynamic monitoring in a medical intensive care unit. Crit Care Med 15:840, 1987.
40. Celoria G, Steingrub JS, Vickers-Lahti M, et al: Clinical assessment of hemodynamic values in two surgical intensive care units. Arch Surg 125:1036, 1990.
41. Steingrub JS, Celoria G, Vickers-Lahti M, et al: Therapeutic impact of pulmonary artery catheterization in a medical/surgical ICU. Chest 99:1451, 1991.
42. Gore JM, Goldberg RJ, Spodick DH, et al: A community-wide assessment of the use of pulmonary artery catheters in patients with acute myocardial infarction. Chest 92:721, 1987.

43. Zion MM, Balkin J, Rosenmann D, et al: Use of pulmonary artery catheters in patients with acute myocardial infarction. Analysis of experience in 5,841 patients in the SPRINT Registry. Chest 98:1331, 1990.

44. Shoemaker WC, Appel PL, Kram HB, et al: Prospective trial of supranormal values of survivors as therapeutc goals in high-risk surgical patients. Chest 94:1176, 1988.

45. Tuchschmidt J, Fried J, Astiz M, et al: Supranormal oxygen delivery improves mortality in septic shock patients. Crit Care Med 19:S66, 1991.

46. Iberti TJ, Fischer EP, Leibowitz AB, et al: A multicenter study of physicians' knowledge of the pulmonary artery catheter. JAMA 264:2928, 1990.

47. Potain PCE: Des mouvements et des bruits qui se passent dans les veines jugulaires. Bull Mem Soc Med Hop Paris 4:3, 1967.

48. Rich LL, Tavel ME: The origin of the jugular c wave. N Engl J Med 284:1309, 1971.

49. Hirschfelder AD: Some variations in the form of the venous pulse. Bull Johns Hopkins Hosp 18:265, 1907.

50. Tavel ME: Clinical Phonocardiography and External Pulse Recording. 4th ed. Chicago, Year Book Medical Publishers, pp 64 and 263, 1985.

51. Shabetai R, Fowler NO, Guntheroth WG: The hemodynamics of cardiac tamponade and constrictive pericarditis. Am J Cardiol 26:480, 1970.

52. Hancock EW: Cardiac tamponade. Med Clin North Am 63:223, 1979.

53. Nixon JV: Right ventricular myocardial infarction. Arch Intern Med 142:945, 1982.

54. Coma-Canella I, Lopez-Sendon J: Ventricular compliance in ischemic right ventricular (RV) dysfunction. Am J Cardiol 45:555, 1980.

55. Lorell BH, Leinbach RC, Pohost GM, et al: Right ventricular infarction: Clinical diagnosis and differentiation from cardiac tamponade and pericardial constriction. Am J Cardiol 43:467, 1979.

56. Grossman W (ed): Cardiac Catheterization and Angiography. 2nd ed. Philadelphia, Lea & Febiger, p 322, 1980.

57. Dell'Italia LJ, Starling MR, O'Rourke RA: Physical examination for exclusion of hemodynamically important right ventricular infarction. Ann Intern Med 99:608, 1983.

58. Cohen SI, Kupersmith J, Aroesty J, et al: Pulsus paradoxus and Kussmaul's sign in acute pulmonary embolism. Am J Cardiol 32:271, 1973.

59. Hancock EW: Constrictive pericarditis. Clinical clues to diagnosis. JAMA 232:176, 1975.

60. Jensen DP, Goolsby JP Jr, Oliva PB: Hemodynamic pattern resembling pericardial constriction after acute inferior myocardial infarction with right ventricular infarction. Am J Cardiol 42:858, 1978.

61. Benotti JR, Grossman W, Cohn PF: Clinical profile of restrictive cardiomyopathy. Circulation 61:1206, 1980.

62. Royster RL, Johnson JC, Prough DS, et al: Differences in pulmonary artery wedge pressures obtained by balloon inflation versus impaction techniques. Anesthesiology 61:339, 1984.

63. Frank O: Zur Dynamik des Hertzmuskels. Z Biol 32:370, 1895.

64. Starling EH: Some points in the pathology of heart disease. Effects of heart failure on the circulation. Lancet 1:652, 1896.

65. Patterson SW, Piper H, Starling EH: The regulation of the heartbeat. J Physiol (Lond) 48:465, 1914.

66. Starling EH: The Linacre Lecture on the Law of the Heat. London, Longmans Green, 1918.

67. Batson GA, Chandrasekhar KP, Payas Y, et al: Measurement of pulmonary wedge pressure by the flow-directed Swan-Ganz catheter. Cardiovasc Res 6:748, 1972.

68. Fitzpatrick GF, Hampson LG, Burgess JH: Bedside determination of left atrial pressure. Can Med Assoc J 106:1293, 1972.

69. Lappas D, Lell WA, Gabel JC, et al: Indirect measurement of left-atrial pressure in surgical patients—Pulmonary capillary wedge and pulmonary-artery diastolic pressures compared with left-atrial pressure. Anesthesiology 38:394, 1973.

70. Walston A, Kendall ME: Comparison of pulmonary wedge and left atrial pressure in man. Am Heart J 86:159, 1973.

71. Humphrey CB, Oury JH, Virgilio RW, et al: An analysis of direct and indirect measurements of left atrial filling pressure. J Thorac Cardiovasc Surg 71:643, 1976.

72. Civetta JM, Gabel JC, Laver MB: Disparate ventricular function in surgical patients. Surg Forum 22:136, 1971.

73. Toussaint GPM, Burgess JH, Hampson LG: Central venous pressure and pulmonary wedge pressure in critical surgical illness. Arch Surg 109:265, 1974.

74. Risk C, Rudo N, Falltrick R, et al: Comparison of right atrial and pulmonary capillary wedge pressure. Crit Care Med 6:172, 1978.

75. Mangano DT: Monitoring pulmonary arterial pressure in coronary-artery disease. Anesthesiology 53:364, 1980.

76. Rajacich N, Burchard KW, Hasan FM, et al: Central venous pressure and pulmonary capillary wedge pressure as estimates of left atrial pressure: Effects of positive end-expiratory pressure and catheter tip malposition. Crit Care Med 17:7, 1989.

77. Forrester JS, Diamond G, McHugh TJ, et al: Filling pressures in the right and left sides of the heart in acute myocardial infarction. A reappraisal of central-venous-pressure monitoring. N Engl J Med 285:190, 1971.

78. De Laurentis DA, Hayes M, Matsumsto T, et al: Does central venous pressure accurately reflect hemodynamic and fluid volume patterns in the critical surgical patient? Am J Surg 126:415, 1973.

79. O'Quinn R, Marini JJ: Pulmonary artery occlusion pressure: Clinical physiology, measurement, and interpretation. Am Rev Respir Dis 128:319, 1983.

80. Knobel E, Akamine N, Fernandes CJ Jr, et al: Reliability of right atrial pressure monitoring to assess left ventricular preload in critically ill septic patients. Crit Care Med 17:1344, 1989.

81. Field J, Shiroff RA, Zelis RF, et al: Limitations in the use of the pulmonary capillary wedge pressure. Cardiac tamponade. Chest 70:451, 1976.

82. Verweij J, Kester A, Stroes W, et al: Comparison of three methods for measuring central venous pressure. Crit Care Med 14:288, 1986.

83. Clayton DG: Inaccuracies in manometric central venous pressure measurement. Resuscitation 16:221, 1988.

84. Rhoads MK, Kariman K: A simple and safe method for monitoring of central venous and pulmonary artery pressures with a single transducer. Crit Care Med 7:174, 1979.

85. Quinn K, Quebbeman EJ: Pulmonary artery pressure monitoring in the surgical intensive care unit. Benefits vs difficulties. Arch Surg 116:872, 1981.

86. Visner MS, Arentzen CE, Parrish DG, et al: Effects of global ischemia on the diastolic properties of the left ventricle in the conscious dog. Circulation 71:610, 1985.

87. Eaton RJ, Tazman RM, Avioli LV: Cardiovascular evaluation of patients treated with PEEP. Arch Intern Med 143:1958, 1983.

88. Fisher ML, DeFelice CE, Parisi AF: Assessing left ventricular filling pressure with flow-directed (Swan-Ganz) catheters. Detection of sudden changes in patients with left ventricular dysfunction. Chest 68:542, 1975.

89. Rahimtoola SH, Loeb HS, Ehsani A, et al: Relationship of pulmonary artery to left ventricular diastolic pressure in acute myocardial infarction. Circulation 46:283, 1972.

90. Herbert WH: Limitations of pulmonary artery end-diastolic pressure as the reflection of left ventricular end-diastolic pressure. NY State J Med 72:229, 1972.

91. Morris AH, Chapman RH, Gardner RM: Frequency of technical problems encountered in the measurement of pulmonary artery wedge pressure. Crit Care Med 12:164, 1984.

92. Gardner RM: Hemodynamic monitoring: From catheter to display. Acute Care 12:3, 1986.

93. Brewster H, McIlroy MB: Blood gas tensions and pH of pulmonary "wedge" samples in patients with heart disease. J Appl Physiol 34:413, 1973.

94. Shapiro HM, Smith G, Pribble AH, et al: Errors in sampling pulmonary arterial blood with a Swan-Ganz catheter. Anesthesiology 40:291, 1974.

95. Chlup J, Serf A, Ourednik A, et al: Partial pressures of oxygen and carbon dioxide and pH of blood sampled from wedged pulmonary artery. Clin Sci Mol Med 48:47, 1975.

96. Williams WH, Olsen GN, Allen G, et al: Use of blood gas values to estimate the source of blood withdrawn from a wedged flow-directed catheter in critically ill patients. Crit Care Med 10:636, 1982.

97. Komadina KH, Schenk DA, La Veau P, et al: Interobserver variability in the interpretation of pulmonary artery catheter pressure tracings. Chest 100:1647, 1991.

98. Aitken DR, Minton JP: The "pinch-off sign": A warning of impending problems with permanent subclavian catheters. Am J Surg 148:633, 1984.

99. Tobin MJ: Pulmonary artery catheter problems. Appl Cardiopulm Pathophysiol 3:279, 1990.

100. Pennington LA, Smith C: Leveling when monitoring central blood pressures: An alternative method. Heart Lung 9:1053, 1980.

101. Ross RM: Bedside calibration of pulmonary artery catheters. Chest 84:506, 1983.

102. Gardner RM, Hollingsworth KW: Optimizing the electrocardiogram and pressure monitoring. Crit Care Med 14:651, 1986.

103. Lewis JF, Anderson TW, Fennell WH, et al: A clue to pulmonary embolism obtained during Swan-Ganz catheterization. Chest 81:527, 1982.

104. Quintana E, Sanchez JM, Serra C, et al: Erroneous interpretation of pulmonary capillary wedge pressure in massive pulmonary embolism. Crit Care Med 11:933, 1983.

105. Traeger SM: "Failure to wedge" and pulmonary hypertension during pulmonary artery catheterization: A sign of totally occlusive pulmonary embolism. Crit Care Med 13:544, 1985.

106. Craven KD, Wood LDH: Extrapericardial and esophageal pressures with positive end-expiratory pressure in dogs. J Appl Physiol 51:798, 1981.

107. Marini JJ, O'Quin R, Culver BH, et al: Estimation of transmural cardiac pressures during ventilation with PEEP. J Appl Physiol 53:384, 1982.

108. Buda AJ, Pinsky MR, Ingels NB Jr, et al: Effect of intrathroacic pressure on left ventricular performance. N Engl J Med 301:453, 1979.

109. Pinsky MR, Matuschak GM, Itzkoff JM: Respiratory augmentation of left ventricular function during spontaneous ventilation in severe left ventricular failure by grunting. An auto-EPAP effect. Chest 86:267, 1984.

110. Robotham JL, Scharf SM: Effect of positive and negative pressure ventilation on cardiac performance. Clin Chest Med 4:161, 1983.
111. Riedinger MS, Shellock FG, Swan HJC: Reading pulmonary artery and pulmonary capillary wedge pressure waveforms with respiratory variations. Heart Lung 10:675, 1981.
112. Luce JM: The cardiovascular effects of mechanical ventilation and positive end-expiratory pressure. JAMA 252:807, 1984.
113. Davison R, Parker M, Harrison RA: The validity of determinations of pulmonary wedge pressure during mechanical ventilation. Chest 73:352, 1973.
114. Maran AG: Variations in pulmonary capillary wedge pressure: Variation with intrathoracic pressure, graphic and digital recorders. Crit Care Med 8:102, 1980.
115. Cengiz M, Crapo RO, Gardner RM: The effect of ventilation on the accuracy of pulmonary artery and wedge pressure measurements. Crit Care Med 11:502, 1983.
116. Shuster DP, Seeman MD: Temporary muscle paralysis for accurate measurement of pulmonary artery occlusion pressure. Chest 84:553, 1983.
117. Marini JJ: Respiratory Medicine and Intensive Care for the House Officer. Baltimore, Williams & Wilkins, 1981.
118. West JB, Dollery CT, Naimark A: Distribution of blood flow in isolated lung; relation to vascular and alveolar pressures. J Appl Physiol 19:713, 1964.
119. Green JF: The pulmonary circulation. In: Zelis R (ed): The Peripheral Circulations. New York, Grune & Stratton, p 193, 1975.
120. Tooker J, Huseby J, Butler J: The effect of Swan-Ganz catheter height on the wedge pressure–left atrial pressure relationship during positive-pressure ventilation. Am Rev Respir Dis 117:721, 1978.
121. Kronberg GM, Quan SF, Schlobohm RM, et al: Anatomic locations of the tips of pulmonary artery catheters in supine patients. Anesthesiology 51:467, 1979.
122. Teboul JL, Besbes M, Axler O, et al: Relationship between pulmonary artery occlusive pressure (PAOP) and left ventricular end diastolic pressure: Role of catheter tips location and of PEEP. Intensive Care Med 14(suppl 1):281, 1988.
123. Fretschner R, Kloss T, Guggenberger H, et al: Pulmonary artery occlusion–left atrial pressure gradient: An important factor in determining pulmonary venous vascular resistance in acute pulmonary failure. Crit Care Med 19:399, 1991.
124. Shasby DM, Dauber IM, Pfister S, et al: Swan-Ganz catheter location and left atrial pressure determine the accuracy of the wedge pressure when positive end-expiratory pressure is used. Chest 80:666, 1981.
125. Hasan FM, Malanga AL, Braman SS, et al: Lateral position improves wedge–left atrial pressure correlation during positive-pressure ventilation. Crit Care Med 12:960, 1984.
126. Lefcoe MS, Sibbald WJ, Holliday RL: Wedge balloon catheter angiography in the critical care unit. Crit Care Med 7:449, 1979.
127. Williams WH, Olsen GN, Yergin BM, et al: Opacification of pulmonary veins during wedge angiography. Crit Care Med 9:126, 1981.
128. Pepe PE, Marini JJ: Occult positive end-expiratory pressure in mechanically ventilated patients with airflow obstruction. Am Rev Respir Dis 126:166, 1982.
129. Rice DL, Awe RJ, Gaasch WH, et al: Wedge pressure measurement in obstructive pulmonary disease. Chest 66:628, 1974.
130. Qvist J, Pontoppidan H, Wilson RS, et al: Hemodynamic responses to mechanical ventilation with PEEP: The effect of hypervolemia. Anesthesiology 42:45, 1975.
131. Jardin F, Farcot J-C, Boisante L, et al: Influence of positive end-expiratory pressure on left ventricular performance. N Engl J Med 304:387, 1981.
132. Dhainaut JF, Devaux JY, Monsallier JF, et al: Mechanisms of decreased left ventricular preload during continuous positive pressure ventilation in ARDS. Chest 90:74, 1986.
133. Jardin F, Genevray B, Brun-Ney D, et al: Influence of lung and chest wall compliances on transmission of airway pressure to the pleural space in critically ill patients. Chest 88:653, 1985.
134. de Campo T, Civetta JM: The effect of short-term discontinuation of high-level PEEP in patients with acute respiratory failure. Crit Care Med 7:47, 1979.
135. Downs JB, Douglas ME: Assessment of cardiac filling pressure during continuous positive-pressure ventilation. Crit Care Med 8:285, 1980.
136. Weisman IM, Rinaldo JE, Rogers RM: Positive end-expiratory pressure in adult respiratory failure. N Engl J Med 307:1381, 1982.
137. Luterman A, Horovitz JH, Carrico CJ, et al: Withdrawl from positive end-expiratory pressure. Surgery 83:328, 1978.
138. Beach T, Millen E, Grenvik A: Hemodynamic response to discontinuance of mechanical ventilation. Crit Care Med 1:85, 1973.
139. Rose DM, Downs JB, Heenan TJ: Temporal responses of functional residual capacity and oxygen tension to changes in positive end-expiratory pressure. Crit Care Med 9:79, 1981.
140. Fessler HE, Brower RG, Wise RA, et al: Effects on positive end-expiratory pressure on the gradient for venous return. Am Rev Respir Dis 143:19, 1991.
141. Pick RA, Handler JB, Friedman AS: The cardiovascular effects of positive end-expiratory pressure. Chest 82:345, 1982.
142. Dorinsky PM, Whitcomb ME: The effect of PEEP on cardiac output. Chest 84:210, 1983.
143. Smith PK, Tyson GS Jr, Hammon JW Jr, et al: Cardiovascular effects of ventilation with positive expiratory airway pressure. Ann Surg 195:121, 1982.
144. Tittley JG, Fremes SE, Weisel RD, et al: Hemodynamic and myocardial metabolic consequences of PEEP. Chest 88:496, 1985.
145. Grace MP, Greenbaum DM: Cardiac performance in response to PEEP in patients with cardiac dysfunction. Crit Care Med 10:358, 1982.
146. Carter RS, Snyder JV, Pinsky MR: LV filling pressure during PEEP measured by nadir wedge pressure after airway disconnection. Am J Physiol 249:H770, 1985.
147. Nelson LD, Snyder JV: Technical problems in data acquisition. In: Snyder JV, Pinsky MR (eds): Oxygen Transport in the Critically Ill. Chicago, Year Book Medical Publishers, p 205, 1987.
148. Pinsky M, Vincent J-L, De Smit J-M: Estimating left ventricular filling pressure during positive end-expiratory pressure in humans. Am Rev Respir Dis 143:25, 1991.
149. Garr KA, Taylor AE, Owens LJ, et al: Pulmonary capillary pressure and filtration coefficient in the isolated perfused lung. Am J Physiol 213:910, 1967.
150. Dawson CA, Linehan JH, Rickaby DA: Pulmonary microcirculatory hemodynamics. Ann NY Acad Sci 384:90, 1982.
151. Holloway H, Perry M, Downey J, et al: Estimation of effective pulmonary capillary pressure in intact lungs. J Appl Physiol 54:846, 1983.
152. Isago T, Fujioka K, Traber L, et al: Derived pulmonary capillary pressure changes after smoke inhalation in sheep. Crit Care Med 19:1407, 1991.
153. Cope DK, Allison RC, Parmentier JL, et al: Measurement of effective pulmonary capillary pressure using the pressure profile after pulmonary artery occlusion. Crit Care Med 14:16, 1986.
154. Glauser FL: Derived pulmonary capillary hydrostatic pressure: Time for clinical application? Crit Care Med 19:1335, 1991.
155. Cope DK, Parker JC, Taylor MD, et al: Pulmonary capillary pressures during hypoxia and hypoxemia: Experimental and clinical studies. Crit Care Med 17:853, 1989.
156. Stewart GN: Researches on the circulation time and on the influences which affect it. IV. The output of the heart. J Physiol (Lond) 22:159, 1897.
157. Hamilton WF, Moore JW, Kinsman JM, et al: Studies on the circulation. IV. Further analysis of the injection method, and of changes in hemodynamics under physiological and pathological conditions. Am J Physiol 99:534, 1932.
158. Nxumalo JL, Teranaka M, Schenk WG Jr: Hepatic blood flow measurement. III. Total hepatic blood flow measured by ICG clearance and electromagnetic flowmeters in a canine septic shock model. Ann Surg 187:299, 1978.
159. Kholoussy AM, Pollack D, Matsumoto T: Prognostic significance of indocyanine green clearance in critically ill surgical patients. Crit Care Med 12:115, 1984.
160. Carey JS, Hughes RK: Cardiac output. clinical monitoring and management. Ann Thorac Surg 7:150, 1969.
161. Chamberlain JH: Cardiac output measurement by indicator dilution. Biomed Eng 10:92, 1975.
162. Lund-Johansen P: The dye dilution method for measurement of cardiac output. Eur Heart J 11(suppl I):6, 1990.
163. Fegler G: Measurement of cardiac output in anaesthetized animals by a thermo-dilution method. Q J Exp Physiol 39:153, 1954.
164. Hosie KF: Thermal-dilution technics. Circ Res 10:491, 1962.
165. Andreen M: Computerized measurement of cardiac output by thermo-dilution: Methodologic aspects. Acta Anaesthesiol Scand 18:297, 1974.
166. Meisner H, Glanert S, Steckmeier B, et al: Indicator loss during injection in the thermodilution system. Res Exp Med 159:183, 1973.
167. Ganz W, Swan HJC: Measurement of blood flow by thermodilution. Am J Cardiol 29:241, 1972.
168. Olsson B, Pool J, Vandermoten P, et al: Validity and reproducibility of determination of cardiac output by thermodilution in man. Cardiology 55:136, 1970.
169. Wong M, Skulsky A, Moon E: Loss of indicator in the thermodilution technique. Cathet Cardiovasc Diagn 4:103, 1978.
170. Pearl RG, Siegel LC: Thermodilution cardiac output measurement with a large left-to-right shunt. J Clin Monit 7:146, 1991.
171. Fischer AP, Benis AM, Jurado RA, et al: Analysis of errors in measurement of cardiac output by simultaneous dye and thermal dilution in cardiothoracic surgical patients. Cardiovasc Res 12:190, 1978.
172. Kashtan HI, Maitland A, Salerno TA, et al: Effects of tricuspid regurgitation on thermodilution cardiac output: Studies in an animal model. Can J Anaesth 34:246, 1987.
173. Riedinger MS, Shellock FG, Shah PK, et al: Sterility of prefilled thermodilution cardiac output syringes maintained at room and ice temperature. Heart Lung 14:8, 1985.
174. Burke KG, Larsson E, Maciorowski L, et al: Evaluation of the sterility of thermodilution room-temperature injectate preparations. Crit Care Med 14:503, 1986.
175. Ray C, Carlon GC, Campfield PB, et al: Multiple determinations of cardiac output using a two-bottle technique. Crit Care Med 7:33, 1979.

176. Stawicki JJ, Holford FD, Michelson EL, et al: Multiple cardiac output measurements in man—Evaluation of a new closed-system thermodilution method. Chest 76:193, 1979.

177. Plachetka JR, Larson DF, Salomon NW, et al: Comparison of two closed systems for thermodilution cardiac outputs. Crit Care Med 9:487, 1981.

178. Hammermeister KE, Van Damme J: A simple, new system for maintaining quantities of saline cold and sterile for thermodilution cardiac output measurement. Cathet Cardiovasc Diagn 5:95, 1979.

179. Nelson LD, Martinez OV, Anderson HB: Incidence of microbial colonization in open versus closed delivery systems for thermodilution injectate. Crit Care Med 14:291, 1986.

180. Wessel HU, James GW, Paul MH: Effects of respiration and circulation on central blood temperature of the dog. Am J Physiol 211:1403, 1966.

181. Woods M, Scott RN, Harken AH: Practical considerations for the use of a pulmonary artery thermister catheter. Surgery 79:469, 1976.

182. Afonso S, Herrick JF, Youmans WB, et al: Temperature variations in the venous systems in dogs. Am J Physiol 203:278, 1962.

183. Fegler G: The reliability of the thermodilution method for determination of the cardiac output and the blood flow in central veins. Q J Exp Physiol 42:254, 1957.

184. Okamoto K, Komatsu T, Kumar V, et al: Effects of intermediate positive pressure ventilation on cardiac output measurements by thermodilution in man. Crit Care Med 13:320, 1985.

185. Hoffman JIE, Guz A, Charlier AA, et al: Stroke volume in conscious dogs: Effect of respiration, posture and vascular occlusion. J Appl Physiol 20:865, 1965.

186. Pinsky MR: Hemodynamic effects of mechanical ventilation. Appl Cardiopulm Pathophysiol 3:219, 1990.

187. Reddy PS, Curtiss EI, O'Toole JD, et al: Cardiac tamponade: Hemodynamic observations in man. Circulation 58:265, 1978.

188. Stevens JH, Raffin TA, Mihm FG, et al: Thermodilution cardiac output measurement. Effects of the respiratory cycle on its reproducibility. JAMA 253:2240, 1985.

189. Armengol J, Man GCW, Balsys AJ, et al: Effects of the respiratory cycle on cardiac output measurements: Reproducibility of data enhanced by timing the thermodilution injection in dogs. Crit Care Med 9:852, 1981.

190. Woods M, Scott RN, Harken AH: Practical considerations for the use of a pulmonary artery thermister catheter. Surgery 79:469, 1976.

191. Nelson LD, Anderson HB: Patient selection for iced versus room temperature injectate for thermodilution cardiac output determinations. Crit Care Med 13:182, 1985.

192. Runciman WB, Isley AH, Roberts JG: An evaluation of thermodilution cardiac output using the Swan-Ganz catheter. Anaesth Intensive Care 9:208, 1981.

193. Killpack AK, Davidson LJ, Woods SL, et al: Effect of injectate volume and temperature on measurement of thermodilution cardiac output in acutely ill patients. Circulation 64(suppl IV):165, 1981.

194. Kint PP, van Domburg R, Meij SH: Reproducibility of thermodilution cardiac output measurements. Circulation 64(suppl IV):165, 1981.

195. Riedinger MS, Shellock F: Reproducibility and accuracy of using room temperature vs ice temperature injectate for thermodilution cardiac output determination. Circulation 64(suppl IV):165, 1981.

196. Elkayman U, Berkley R, Azen S, et al: Cardiac output by thermodilution technique. Effect of injectate's volume and temperature on accuracy and reproducibility in the critically ill patient. Chest 84:418, 1983.

197. Reininger EJ, Troy BL: Error in thermodilution cardiac output measurement caused by variation in syringe volume. Cathet Cardiovasc Diagn 2:415, 1976.

198. Riedinger MS, Shellock FG: Technical aspects of the thermodilution method for measuring cardiac output. Heart Lung 13:215, 1984.

199. Raffin TA: The technique of thermodilution cardiac output measurements. J Crit Illness 2:73, 1987.

200. Shellock FG, Riedinger MS, Bateman TM, et al: Thermodilution cardiac output determination in hypothermic postcardiac surgery patients: Room vs ice temperature injectate. Crit Care Med 11:668, 1983.

201. Conway J, Lund-Johansen P: Thermodilution method for measuring cardiac output. Eur Heart J 11(suppl I):17, 1990.

202. Nelson LD, Houtchens BA: Automatic vs manual injections for thermodilution cardiac output determinations. Crit Care Med 10:190, 1982.

203. Bjoraker DG, Ketcham TR: Catheter thrombus lowers cardiac output determinations by thermal dilution. Anesthesiology 57:A155, 1982.

204. Shellock FG, Riedinger MS: Hemodynamic measurement errors caused by catheter introducers. Cathet Cardiovasc Diagn 8:319, 1982.

205. Bearss MG, Yonutas DN, Allen WT: A complication with thermodilution cardiac outputs in centrally-placed pulmonary artery catheters. Chest 81:527, 1982.

206. Stoller JK, Herbst TJ, Hurford W, et al: Spuriously high cardiac output from injecting thermal indicator through an ensheathed port. Crit Care Med 14:1064, 1986.

207. Gibney RTN, Ryan H: Thermodilution cardiac output measurements. Crit Care Med 12:614, 1984.

208. Lee DW, Stevens GH: Comparison of thermodilution cardiac output measurements by injection of the proximal lumen versus side port of the Swan-Ganz catheter. Heart Lung 14:126, 1985.

209. Pesola GR, Carlon GC: Thermodilution cardiac output: Proximal lumen versus right ventricular port. Crit Care Med 19:563, 1991.

210. Iberti TJ, Jayagopal SG: Knotting of a Swan-Ganz catheter in the pulmonary artery. Chest 83:711, 1983.

211. Sciammarella JC Jr: Low cardiac output values due to malposition of a pulmonary artery catheter. Crit Care Med 16:1258, 1988.

212. Vincent J-L: The measurement of right ventricular ejection fraction. Intensive Care World 7:133, 1990.

213. Kettunen R: The thermodilution method in on-line computation of the left ventricular volumes in dogs. Cathet Cardiovasc Diag 11:25, 1985.

214. Dhainaut J-F, Brunet F, Monsallier JF, et al: Bedside evaluation of right ventricular performance using a rapid computerized thermodilution method. Crit Care Med 15:148, 1987.

215. Spinale FG, Smith AC, Carabello BA, et al: Right ventricular function computed by thermodilution and ventriculography. J Thorac Cardiovasc Surg 99:141, 1990.

216. Martin C, Saux P, Albanese J, et al: Right ventricular function during positive end-expiratory pressure. Thermodilution evaluation and clinical application. Chest 92:999, 1987.

217. Dhainaut JF, Lanore JJ, de Gournay JM, et al: Right ventricular dysfunction in patients with septic shock. Intensive Care Med 14:488, 1988.

218. Brunet F, Dhainaut JF, Devaux JY, et al: Right ventricular performance in patients with acute respiratory failure. Intensive Care Med 14:474, 1988.

219. Kimchi A, Ellrodt AG, Berman DS, et al: Right ventricular performance in septic shock: A combined radionuclide and hemodynamic study. J Am Coll Cardiol 4:945, 1984.

220. Biondi JW, Schulman DS, Soufer R, et al: The effect of incremental positive end-expiratory pressure on right ventricular hemodynamics and ejection fraction. Anesth Analg 67:144, 1988.

221. Staub NC: Clinical use of lung water measurements. Report of a workshop. Chest 90:588, 1986.

222. Lewis FR, Elings VB, Sturm JA: Bedside measurement of lung water. J Surg Res 27:250, 1979.

223. Oppenheimer L, Elings VB, Lewis FR: Thermal-dye lung water measurements: Effects of edema and embolization. J Surg Res 26:504, 1979.

224. Pistolesi M, Miniati M, Milne ENC, et al: Measurement of extravascular lung water. Intensive Care World 8:16, 1991.

225. Milnor WR: The heart as a pump. In: Mountcastle VA (ed): Medical Physiology. 13th ed. St Louis, CV Mosby, p 908, 1974.

226. Fick A: Über die Messung des Blutquantums in den Herzventrikeln. Sitzungsber Phys Med Ges Würzburg, p 16, 1870.

227. Yang SS, Bentivoglio LG, Maranhao V, et al: From Cardiac Catheterization Data to Hemodynamic Parameters. 3rd ed. Philadelphia, FA Davis, pp 201 and 373, 1988.

228. Fagard R, Conway J: Measurement of cardiac output: Fick principle using catheterization. Eur Heart J 11(suppl I):1, 1990.

229. Makita K, Nunn JF, Royston B: Evaluation of metabolic measuring instruments for use in critically ill patients. Crit Care Med 18:638, 1990.

230. Seely RD, Nerlich WE, Gregg DE: A comparison of cardiac output determined by the Fick procedure and a direct method using the rotameter. Circulation 1:1261, 1950.

231. Stetz CW, Miller RG, Kelly GE, et al: Reliability of the thermodilution method in the determination of cardiac output in clinical practice. Am Rev Respir Dis 126:1001, 1982.

232. Levett JM, Replogle RL: Thermodilution cardiac output: A critical analysis and review of the literature. J Surg Res 27:392, 1979.

233. Weisel RD, Berger RL, Hechtman HB: Measurement of cardiac output by thermodilution. N Engl J Med 292:682, 1975.

234. Iparraguirre HP, Giniger R, Garber VA, et al: Comparison between measured and Fick-derived values of hemodynamic and oxymetric variables in patients with acute myocardial infarction. Am J Med 85:349, 1988.

235. Blanch L, Fernandez R, Benito S, et al: Accuracy of an indirect carbon dioxide Fick method in determination of the cardiac output in critically ill mechanically ventilated patients. Intensive Care Med 14:131, 1988.

236. Ellis RJ, Gold J, Rees JR, et al: Computerized monitoring of cardiac output by thermal dilution. JAMA 220:507, 1972.

237. van Grondelle A, Ditchey RV, Groves BM, et al: Thermodilution method overestimates low cardiac output in humans. Am J Physiol 245:H690, 1983.

238. Ohteki H, Nagara H, Wada J, et al: Measurement of cardiac output by thermodilution and Fick methods in man—Problems in case of tricuspid regurgitation. Kokyu To Junkan 29:433, 1981.

239. Headley JM: Invasive Hemodynamic Monitoring: Physiological Principles and Clinical Applications. Irvine, CA, Baxter Healthcare Corporation, p 38, 1989.

240. Lipkin DP, Poole-Wilson PA: Measurement of cardiac output during exercise by the thermodilution and direct Fick techniques in patients with chronic congestive heart failure. Am J Cardiol 56:321, 1985.

241. Goldenberg IF, Ochi RP, Emery RW, et al: Overestimation of Fick cardiac output by thermodilution method in patients with severe tricuspid regurgitation. Crit Care Med 16:428, 1988.

242. Hamilton MA, Stevenson LW, Woo M, et al: Effect of tricuspid regurgitation on the reliability of the thermodilution cardiac output technique in congestive heart failure. Am J Cardiol 64:945, 1989.

243. Wesseling KH, de Wit B, Weber JAP, et al: A simple device for the

continuous measurement of cardiac output. Adv Cardiovasc Phys 5:16, 1983.

244. Specht M, Wichmann C, Artenburg C, et al: The influence of vasoactive drugs on continuous cardiac output measurement by the pulse contour method. Crit Care Med 19:S24, 1991.

245. Verdouw PD, Beaune J, Roelandt J, et al: Stroke volume from central aortic pressure? A critical analysis of the various formulae as to their clinical value. Basic Res Cardiol 70:377, 1975.

246. Campbell EJM, Howell JBL: Rebreathing method for measurement of mixed venous P_{CO_2}. Br Med J 2:630, 1962.

247. Franciosa JA: Evaluation of the CO_2 rebreathing cardiac output method in seriously ill patients. Circulation 55:449, 1977.

248. Frankel DZN, Mahutte CK, Rebuck AS: A noninvasive method for measuring the P_{CO_2} of mixed venous blood. Am Rev Respir Dis 117:63, 1978.

249. Hoffstein V, Rebuck AS: Determination of cardiac output based on breath-holding. Crit Care Med 8:671, 1980.

250. Mahutte CK, Jaffe MB, Sassoon CH, et al: Cardiac output from carbon dioxide production and arterial and mixed venous oximetry. Crit Care Med 19:1270, 1991.

251. Valdes-Cruz LM, Horowitz S, Mesel E, et al: A pulsed Doppler echo-cardiographic method for calculation of pulmonary and systemic flow: Accuracy in a canine model with ventricular septal defect. Circulation 68:597, 1983.

252. Huntsman LL, Stewart DK, Barnes SR, et al: Noninvasive Doppler determination of cardiac output in man. Clinical validation. Circulation 67:593, 1983.

253. Singer M, Clarke J, Bennett FED: Continuous hemodynamic monitoring by esophageal Doppler. Crit Care Med 17:447, 1989.

254. Niclou R, Teague SM, Lee R: Clinical evaluation of a diameter sensing Doppler cardiac output meter. Crit Care Med 18:428, 1990.

255. Wong DH, Mahutte CK: Two-beam pulsed Doppler cardiac output measurement: Reproducibility and agreement with thermodilution. Crit Care Med 18:433, 1990.

256. Perrino AC Jr, Barash PG: Concentric beam Doppler: Should we be going in circles? Crit Care Med 18:456, 1990.

257. Donovan KD, Dobb GJ, Newman MA, et al: Comparison of pulsed Doppler and thermodilution methods for measuring cardiac output in critically ill patients. Crit Care Med 15:853, 1987.

258. Wong DH, Onishi R, Tremper KK, et al: Thoracic bioimpedance and Doppler cardiac output measurement: Learning curve and interobserver reproducibility. Crit Care Med 17:1194, 1989.

259. Gotshall RW, Wood VC, Miles DS: Comparison of two impedance cardiographic techniques for measuring cardiac output in critically ill patients. Crit Care Med 17:806, 1989.

260. Huang KC, Stoddard M, Tsueda K, et al: Stroke volume measurements by electrical bioimpedance and echocardiography in healthy volunteers. Crit Care Med 18:1274, 1990.

261. Introna RPS, Pruett JK, Crumrine RC, et al: Use of transthoracic bioimpedance to determine cardiac output in pediatric patients. Crit Care Med 16:1101, 1988.

262. Gotshall RW, Miles DS: Noninvasive assessment of cardiac output by impedance cardiography in the newborn canine. Crit Care Med 17:63, 1989.

263. Jivegard L, Frid I, Haljamae H, et al: Cardiac output determinations in the pig—Thoracic electrical bioimpedance versus thermodilution. Crit Care Med 18:995, 1990.

264. Castor G, Molter G, Helms J, et al: Determination of cardiac output during positive end-expiratory pressure—Noninvasive electrical bioimpedance compared with standard thermodilution. Crit Care Med 18:544, 1990.

265. Miles DS, Gotshall RW, Quinones JD, et al: Impedance cardiography fails to measure accurately left ventricular ejection fraction. Crit Care Med 18:221, 1990.

266. Kalkat GS, Jeyakumar P, Puri VK, et al: Reliability of bioimpedance cardiac output determinations in low and high flow states. Crit Care Med 16:430, 1988.

267. DeMey C, Enterling D: Noninvasive assessment of cardiac output by impedance cardiography: Disagreement between two equations to estimate stroke volume. Aviat Space Environ Med 59:57, 1988.

268. Smith SA, Russell AE, West MJ, et al: Automated non-invasive measurement of cardiac output: Comparison of electrical bioimpedance and carbon dioxide rebreathing techniques. Br Heart J 59:292, 1988.

269. Donovan KD, Dobb GJ, Woods WPD, et al: Comparison of transthoracic electrical impedance and thermodilution for measuring cardiac output. Crit Care Med 14:1038, 1986.

270. Weber J, Heidelmeyer CF, Kubatz E, et al: Die Bestimmung des Herzzeitvolumens unter PEEP-Beatmung mit dem nichtinvasiven Bioimpedanzgerat "NCCOM3" im Vergleich zur Thermodilutionsmethode. Eine Untersuchung an narkotisierten Hunden. Anaesthesist 35:744, 1986.

271. Woo MA, Hamilton M, Stevenson LW, et al: Comparison of thermodilution and transthoracic electrical bioimpedance cardiac output. Heart Lung 20:357, 1991.

272. Preiser JC, Daper A, Parquier J-N, et al: Transthoracic electrical bioimpedance versus thermodilution technique for cardiac output measurement during mechanical ventilation. Intensive Care Med 15:221, 1989.

273. Easterling TR, Benedetti TJ, Carlson KL, et al: Measurement of cardiac output in pregnancy by thermodilution and impedance techniques. Br J Obstet Gynaecol 96:67, 1989.

274. Katayama M, Sekii S, Miyasaka K: Continuous cardiac output measurement by modified thermodilution catheter. Crit Care Med 14:364, 1986.

275. Normann RA, Johnson RW, Messinger JE, et al: A continuous cardiac output computer based on thermodilution principles. Ann Biomed Eng 17:61, 1989.

276. Yelderman M: Continuous measurement of cardiac output with the use of stochastic system identification techniques. J Clin Monit 6:322, 1990.

277. Davies GG, Jebson PJR, Glasgow BM, et al: Continuous Fick cardiac output compared to thermodilution cardiac output. Crit Care Med 14:881, 1986.

278. Tacchino RM, Giovannini I, Castagneto M: Continuous on line cardiac output by Fick method for use in ICU patients. Crit Care Med 14:400, 1986.

279. Doi M, Morita K, Ikeda K: Frequently repeated Fick cardiac output measurements during anesthesia. J Clin Monit 6:107, 1990.

280. Shoemaker WC, Czer LC: Evaluation of the biologic importance of various hemodynamic and oxygen transport variables: Which variables should be monitored in postoperative shock? Crit Care Med 7:424, 1979.

281. Hankeln KB, Senker R, Schwarten JU, et al: Evaluation of prognostic indices based on hemodynamic and oxygen transport variables in shock patients with adult respiratory distress syndrome. Crit Care Med 15:1, 1987.

282. Dubois EF: Basal Metabolism in Health and Disease. Philadelphia, Lea & Febiger, 1936.

283. Parmley WW, Tomoda H, Diamond G, et al: Dissociation between indices of pump performance and contractility in patients with coronary artery disease and acute myocardial infarction. Chest 67:141, 1975.

284. Milnor WR: Arterial impedance as ventricular afterload. Circ Res 36:565, 1975.

285. Milnor WR: Pulsatile blood flow. N Engl J Med 287:27, 1972.

286. Mills CJ, Gabe IT, Gault JH, et al: Pressure-flow relationships and vascular impedance in man. Cardiovasc Res 4:405, 1970.

287. O'Rourke MF, Yaginuma T: Wave reflections and the arterial pulse. Arch Intern Med 144:366, 1984.

288. Urschel CW, Covell JW, Sonnenblick EH, et al: Effects of decreased aortic compliance on performance of the left ventricle. Am J Physiol 214:298, 1968.

289. Gorback MS: Problems associated with the determination of pulmonary vascular resistance. J Clin Monit 6:118, 1990.

Noninvasive Techniques

Steven J. Lavine

Technologic advances in the past 10 to 15 years have led to the expanded use of noninvasive cardiac studies to evaluate chamber size and systolic and diastolic function, characterize hemodynamics, assess myocardial perfusion (using thallium), assess valvular disease, and determine the presence of pericardial disease. The use of both cardiac ultrasonography and nuclear scintigraphy has allowed the physician to correlate pressure and cardiac output information derived via the pulmonary artery and arterial catheter with measures of cardiac volume and function. This has proved to be a powerful clinical addition. Table 96–1 lists the available cardiac ultrasound and nuclear cardiology techniques.

TABLE 96–1

NONINVASIVE CARDIAC IMAGING MODALITIES

Cardiac Ultrasonography
  M mode
  Two-dimensional echocardiography
  Doppler echocardiography
    Pulsed and continuous wave
    Color flow mapping

Nuclear Cardiology
  Perfusion imaging
    Thallium (planar, single-photon emission computed
      tomography)
    Newer technetium agents
  Radionuclide angiography
    First pass
    Equilibrium
      Planar
      Single-photon emission computed tomography

PHYSICS AND INSTRUMENTATION
Cardiac Ultrasonography
Echocardiography

High-frequency ultrasound (2 to 5 mHz in adults) is able to interrogate cardiac structures and distinguish between structures less than 1 mm apart owing to its small wavelength. Ultrasound is emitted via a piezoelectric crystal, which both sends and receives ultrasonic energy, converting the ultrasonic energy to electrical energy and vice versa. Ultrasound is reflected by interfaces between media that have different acoustic impedances or, simply stated, different densities. The amount of reflected energy depends on the difference between the two media. The difference between a solid and a liquid is far greater than that between two solids. A dense object reflects all the energy and there is no transmission beyond the object. In most cases, ultrasound energy is both reflected and transmitted through a given medium. Far-field interrogation of ultrasound is weaker, although ultrasonographs have compensated for this. Moving objects can be interrogated by ultrasound with high resolution. The amplitude of returning signal depends on the density of the interrogated object and the angle of interrogation. Denser and more perpendicular objects have greater amplitude signals.

If amplitude is converted to brightness energy (the B mode) and is displayed over time (1000 samples per second), this produces M-mode echocardiography (the first ultrasound technique introduced). Unfortunately, it provides an "ice pick" (one sector) interrogation, which has a limited field of view but provides high sampling rates (1000 per second). Two-dimensional echocardiography represents interrogation of the heart with a pie shaped beam varying from 30 to 90°. This can be accomplished by oscillating a single transducer through a 30 to 90° sector or by electronically firing a series of transducers (phased array). The increased field of view occurs at the expense of frame rate (30 per second). Images are constructed by using a television format. The relationship between M-mode and two-dimensional echocardiography is depicted in Figure 96–1.

Doppler Echocardiography

Doppler echocardiography utilizes ultrasound energy to record the velocity of moving red blood cells. If a target is moving toward the ultrasound emitter, the frequency returning to the emitter is greater than the emitted frequency. The reverse is expected if the object is moving away from the ultrasound emitter. The difference between the emitted frequency and the returning frequency has been termed the *frequency shift*. This can be expressed as red blood cell velocity using the Doppler equation:

$$V = F_d * C/2F_t(\cos \theta)$$

where V is velocity, C is the velocity of sound in blood (1560 m/s), $\cos \theta$ is the cosine of angle between the Doppler beam and the target, F_d is emitted frequency, and F_t represents reflected frequency.

Unlike the case with amplitude imaging, the best signals are obtained from red blood cells moving parallel to the transducer. Clinically, Doppler ultrasonography can be utilized in a continuous or a pulsed mode. In continuous wave Doppler, one transducer emits and the other receives, allowing a continuous train of signals emitted or received. High velocities can be detected along the path of an interrogating beam. However, localization is not possible other than along the path. Pulsed wave Doppler uses one transducer both to send and to receive the signal. Because one transducer is being used, there is a built-in time delay between the sending and receiving of ultrasound pulses.

This can be varied to sample any given depth:

$$V = d/t$$

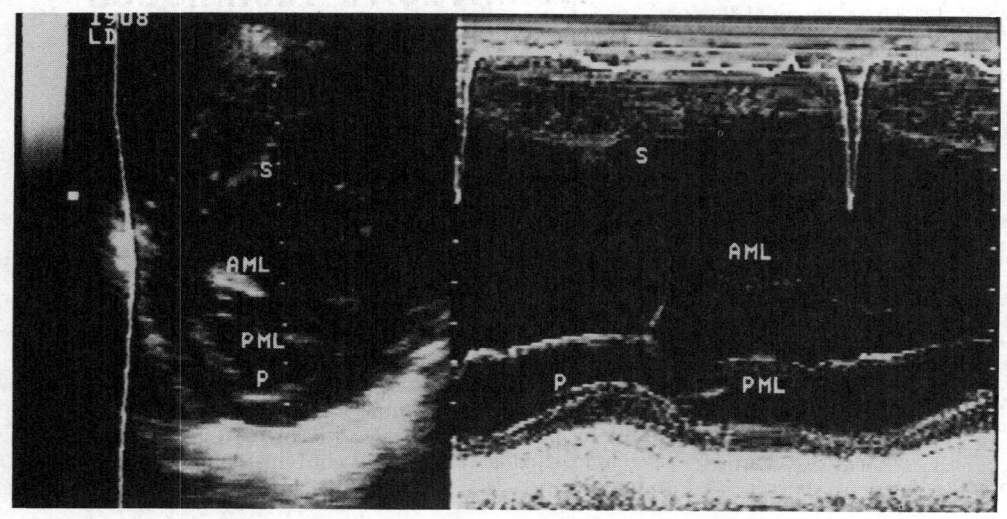

Figure 96–1. Parasternal short-axis view at the mitral leaflet level (*left*) with an M mode of the mitral leaflets (*right*) obtained by cursor (vertical line on short-axis view). AML = anterior mitral leaflet; PML = posterior mitral leaflet; P = posterior wall; S = septum.

where *V* is velocity, *d* denotes distance, and *t* represents time. However, the maximal velocity recordable is limited by the pulsed repetition rate. Velocities higher than this velocity alias (electronically wrap around the zero baseline).

Doppler flow information is processed by using a fast Fourier transform and shown as velocity above or below the baseline, depending on whether flow is moving toward or away from the transducer. Laminar flow is depicted as red blood cell velocities that are uniform and moving in the same direction, whereas turbulent flow is recorded as multiple red blood cell velocities moving in multiple directions owing to oblique signals of lower velocities. Figure 96–2 depicts laminar and turbulent flow. The Doppler beam is usually superimposed on a two-dimensional image for orientation and the velocity recordings are shown on a separate screen (Fig. 96–3).

Doppler information can be superimposed on a two-dimensional image if multiple sample volumes are used along with multiple imaging lines. Blood flow velocity can be depicted by color bars indicating blood flow moving toward the transducer and blood flow moving away from the transducer. Two-dimensional and color flow imaging sequence can be constructed at a rate of less than 30 frames per second and can be used to detect regurgitant lesions, shunts, and other abnormal flow patterns. This form of imaging has been termed *color flow mapping*.

Transducer Locations

Two-dimensional echocardiographic images are obtained as a series of tomographic images from multiple chest wall image locations (Table 96–2; Figs. 96–4 to 96–7). Three orthogonal views are used: long-axis view, short-axis view, and four-chamber view. More recently, a posterior approach has been utilized via transesophageal echocardiography. Transesophageal echocardiography is simply a phased-array transducer mounted on the end of a gastroscope. The instrument is introduced via light sedation through the mouth to multiple levels of the esophagus and the gastroesophageal region. As this is an invasive technique, specific indications exist (Table 96–3), and the imaging planes that can be seen are shown in Figure 96–8. Although transthoracic echocardiography has wide applicability and use in many patients, limited acoustic windows, limited visualization

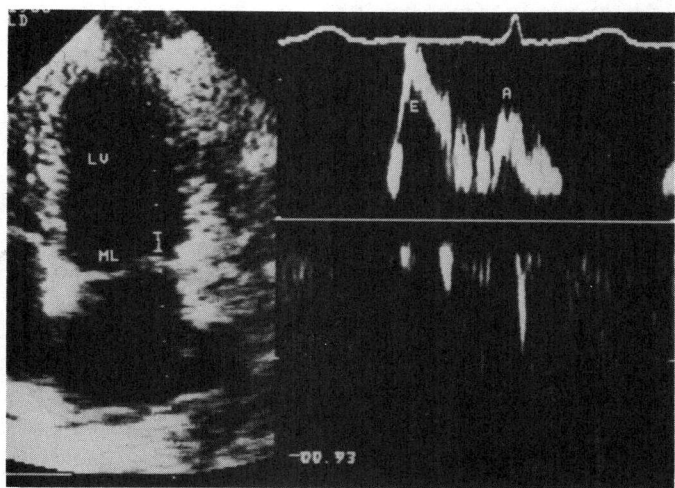

Figure 96–3. Apical chamber view (*left*) of the left ventricle (LV) with the sample volume (*square*) placed in the left ventricle just beyond the mitral leaflet tips (ML). The pulsed Doppler transmitral spectrum is shown on the right with a rapid filling component (E) and atrial filling component (A).

of the aorta, chest wall configuration differences, lung interference, and acoustic shadowing by prosthetic valves limit the diagnostic capability of transthoracic imaging in many patients, especially in those with mechanical mitral prosthetic valves. Imaging posteriorly through the esophagus allows a high-resolution, unimpeded view of the atria, mitral valve prosthesis, aortic root, and ascending and descending aorta.

Radionuclide Imaging

Two major forms of radionuclide imaging are presently available: radionuclide angiography and myocardial perfusion imaging (with thallium). Within the critical care setting, myocardial perfusion imaging (using thallium and other technetium-based agents) has an extremely limited application. The detection of resting or exercise ischemia or infarction either can be accomplished by other techniques (wall

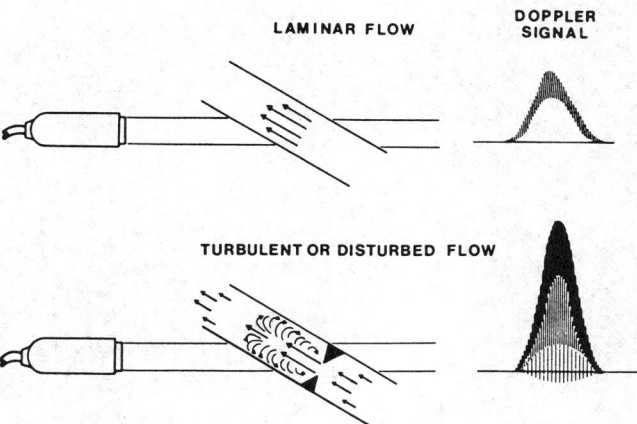

Figure 96–2. Doppler signals recorded from laminar and turbulent flow. With laminar flow, Doppler signals are of similar velocities. Turbulent or disturbed flow occurs across a partial obstruction, resulting in multiple velocities in multiple directions. The Doppler signal shows multiple velocities. (From H Feigenbaum: Echocardiography, 4e. Philadelphia, Lea & Febiger, p 35, 1986. Reprinted with permission.)

TABLE 96–2
TWO-DIMENSIONAL ECHOCARDIOGRAPHIC IMAGING LOCATIONS

1. Parasternal views
  a. Long axis
  b. Short axis
    i. Aortic valve
    ii. Mitral valve
    iii. Papillary muscle
    iv. Infrapapillary muscle
  c. Right ventricular inflow
  d. Four chamber
2. Apical views
  a. Four chamber
  b. Five chamber
  c. Apical two chamber
  d. Apical long axis
3. Subcostal views
  a. Four chamber
  b. Short axis
    i. Aortic
    ii. Mitral
    iii. Left ventricle
4. Suprasternal view

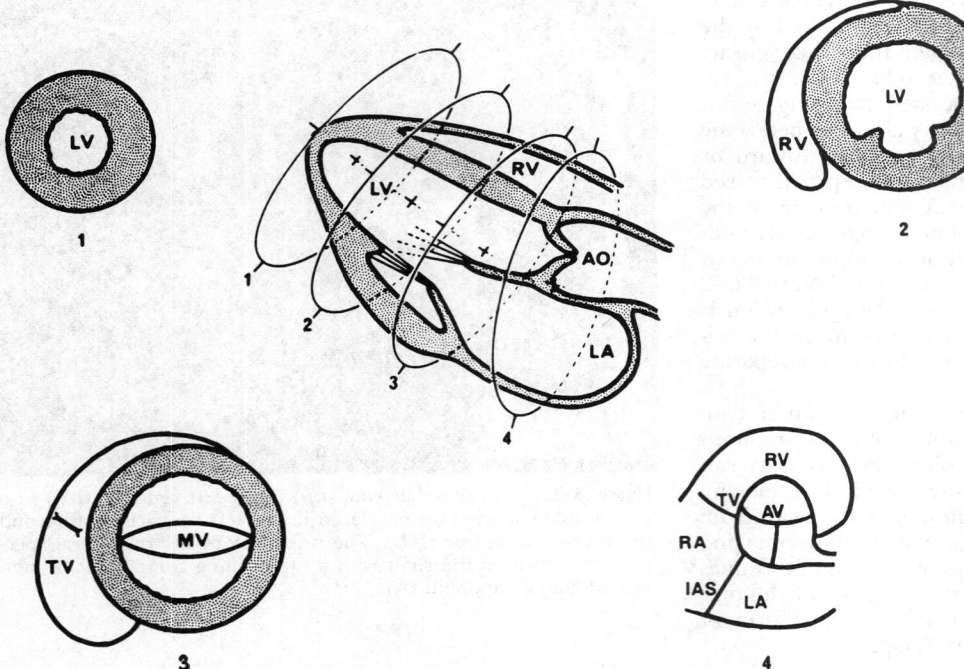

Figure 96–4. Multiple orthogonal short-axis views are depicted on the parasternal long-axis view, (*center*). View 1 is through the apex. View 2 is through the papillary muscles. View 3 is through the mitral leaflets. View 4 is at the base of the heart. LV = left ventricle; RV = right ventricle; AO = aorta; LA = left atrium; MV = mitral valve; TV = tricuspid valve; AV = aortic valve; RA = right atrium; IAS = interatrial septum. (From Braunwald E [ed]: Heart Disease: A Textbook of Cardiovascular Medicine. 4th ed. Philadelphia, WB Saunders, 1992.)

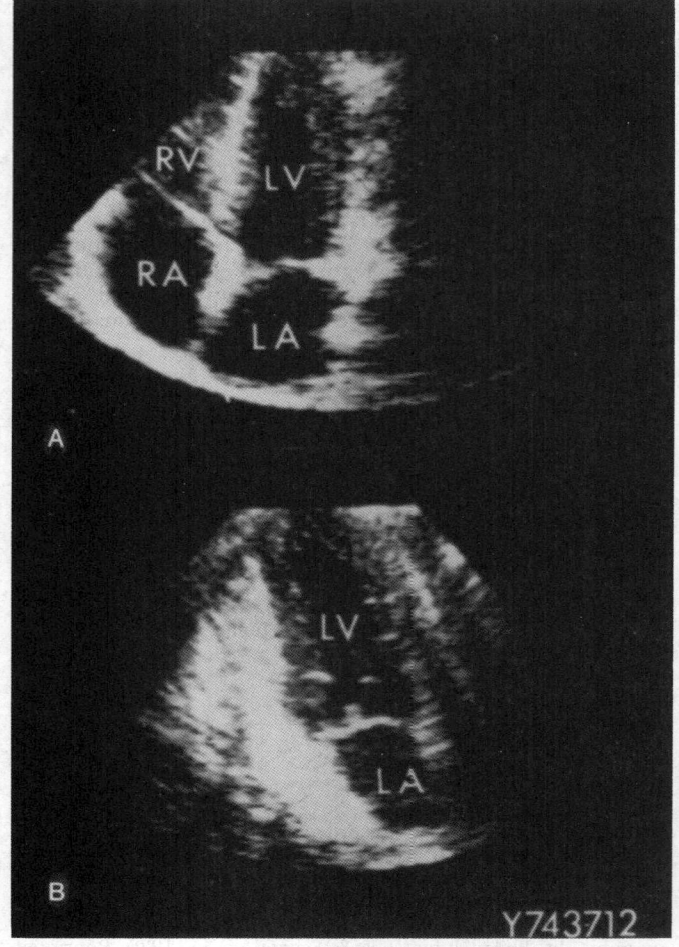

Figure 96–5. Apical four-chamber (*A*) and two-chamber (*B*) views are shown. RV = right ventricle; RA = right atrium; LV = left ventricle; LA = left atrium. (From H Feigenbaum: Echocardiography, 4e. Philadelphia, Lea & Febiger, p 94, 1986. Reprinted with permission.)

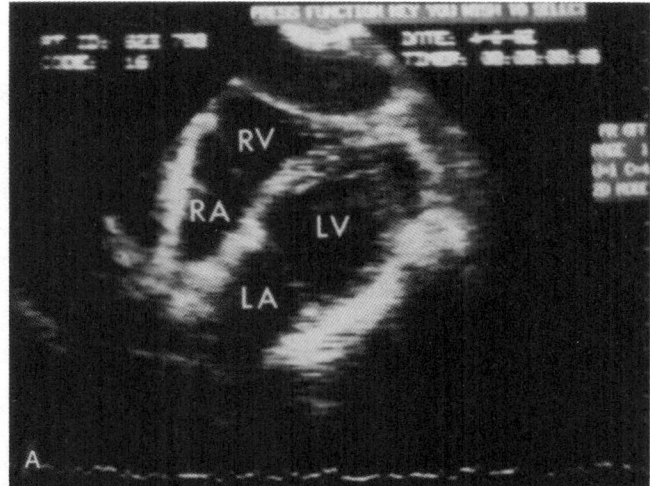

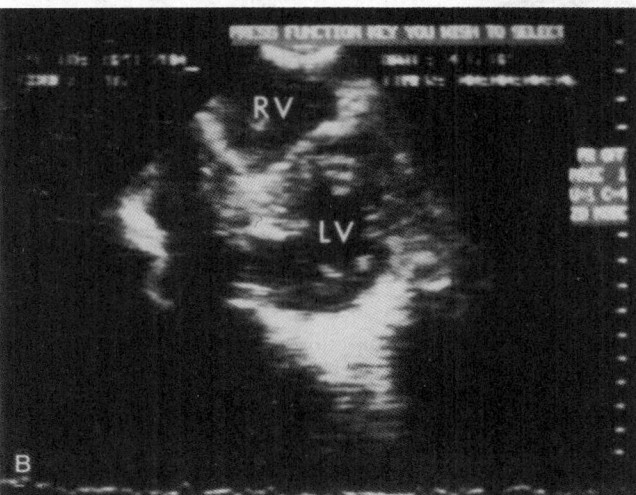

Figure 96–6. Subcostal four-chamber (*A*) and short-axis (*B*) views (left ventricular) are shown. RV = right ventricle; LV = left ventricle; RA = right atrium; LA = left atrium. (From H Feigenbaum: Echocardiography, 4e. Philadelphia, Lea & Febiger, p 96, 1986. Reprinted with permission.)

motion analysis) or is not applicable clinically to the critical care setting (exercise testing). However, radionuclide angiography has considerable applicability, in that chamber size, function, and intracardiac shunts can be evaluated.

Radiopharmaceuticals. The required characteristic of any radiopharmaceutical for radionuclide angiography is that it moves as a bolus through the cardiac chambers and is capable of distributing throughout the blood pool. These two re-

TABLE 96–3
INDICATIONS FOR TRANSESOPHAGEAL ECHOCARDIOGRAPHY
Mitral valve prosthetic dysfunction
Aortic dissection
Atrial masses (tumor or thrombi)
Infective endocarditis
Mitral regurgitation
Atrial septal defect
Limited transthoracic study
Left ventricular function (in critical care unit postoperatively and intraoperatively)
Cardiac surgery (mitral valve repair)

quirements represent the two different techniques: first pass and equilibrium.[1] The agent most commonly used is ^{99m}Tc. ^{99m}Tc attaches to the red blood cell after its first-path transit. Stannous chloride is generally given as a reducing agent to prepare the blood cell for the attachment of the ^{99m}Tc. ^{99m}Tc has a 140-kEv energy and a half-life of 6 hours. It is capable of producing high-quality images and repeated studies.

Image Presentation. In the first-pass type of angiography (Fig. 96–9), a bolus injection is given and imaging commences in the right anterior oblique view tracing the radiopharmaceuticals sequentially through the venae cavae, right-sided heart chambers, the pulmonary circulation, and left-sided heart chambers. A second injection can be given for an intervention study. In the equilibrium type, the red blood cells are reduced with stannous chloride and then the ^{99m}Tc is administered. After the bolus injections, the ^{99m}Tc attaches

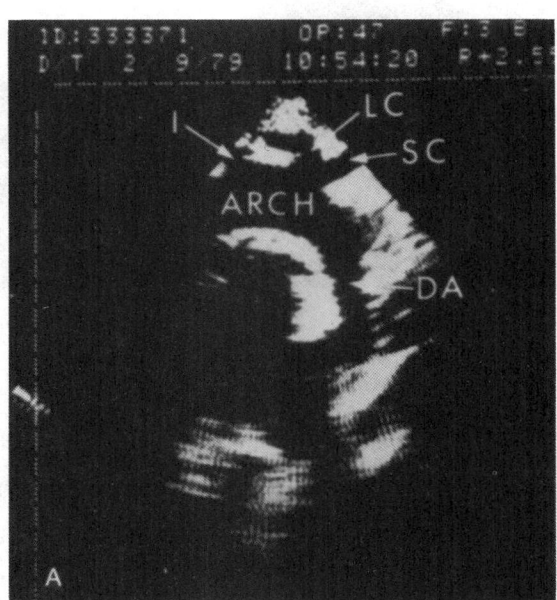

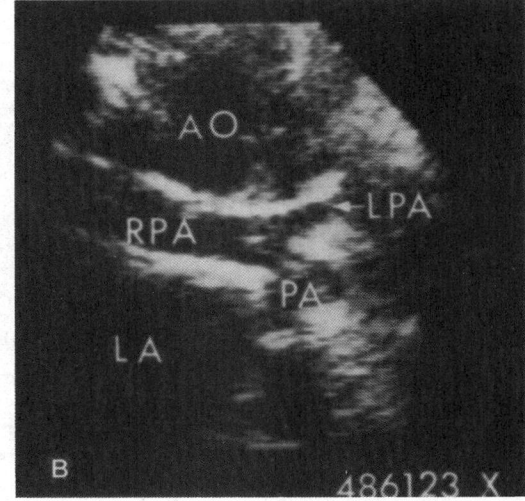

Figure 96–7. Suprasternal views parallel (*top*) and perpendicular (*bottom*) to the arch of the aorta are shown. AO = aorta; I = innominate artery; LC = left common carotid; SC = left subclavian artery; RPA = right pulmonary artery; LPA = left pulmonary artery; PA = pulmonary artery; LA = left atrium; DA = descending aorta. (From H Feigenbaum: Echocardiography, 4e. Philadelphia, Lea & Febiger, p 97, 1986. Reprinted with permission.)

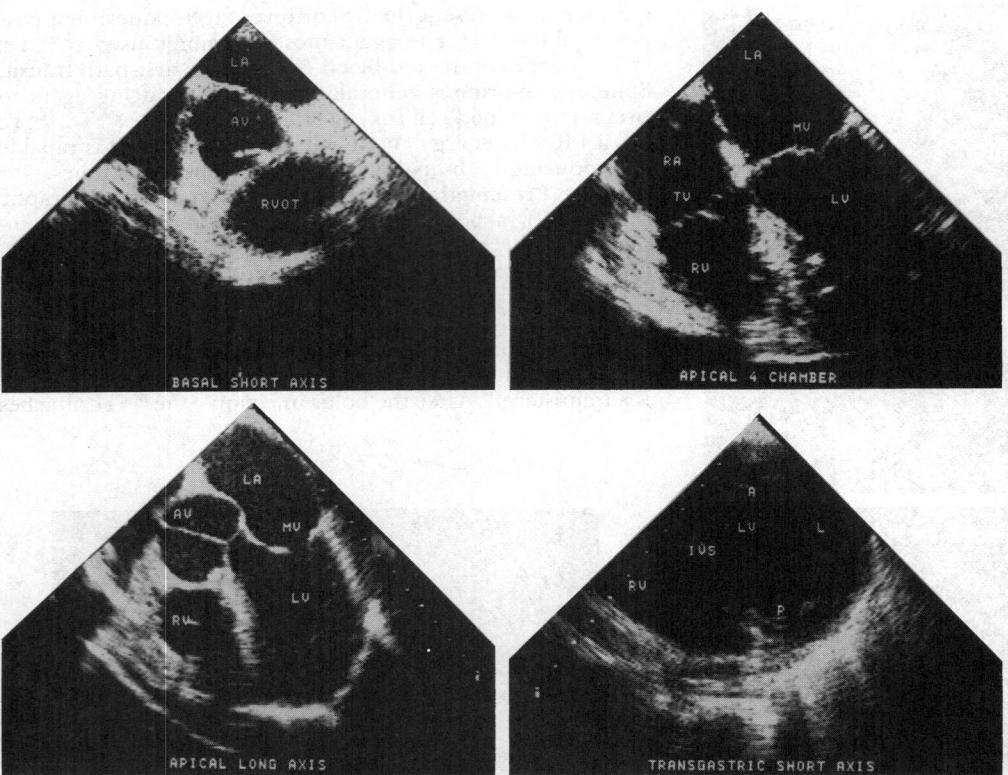

Figure 96–8. Stop frames from a basal short-axis view, apical four-chamber and long axis views, and transgastric view are shown. A = anterior wall; AV = aortic valve; IVS = interventricular septum; L = lateral wall; LA = left atrium; LV = left ventricle; MV = mitral valve; OT = outflow tract; P = posterior wall; PV = pulmonary vein; RA = right atrium; RV = right ventricle; TV = tricuspid valve.

to the red blood cell, producing a blood pool scan that simultaneously depicts the venae cavae, the cardiac chambers, the pulmonary artery, and the aorta. Equilibrium studies can be imaged (Fig. 96–10) in a planar fashion using an anterior or right anterior oblique view and multiple left anterior oblique views. More recently, tomographic imaging has been utilized.

Instrumentation. Detection of photons requires a scintillation camera fitted with a collimator.[2] The collimator (Fig. 96–11) is analogous to lens made up of lead that absorbs photons. Usually, a parallel hole collimator is used. Photons of lesser energy have usually undergone collisions (lost energy) and had their direction altered and are ultimately absorbed by the collimator. Unimpeded photons are able to reach the camera face and depict the structure from which they have emanated.

The camera can be of two types. The Anger type consists of a large sodium iodide crystal with 37 to 91 photomultiplier tubes. The photomultiplier tubes take the photons and their light energy and convert them to electrical energy. The effect of a given photon may be reflected by more than one tube, which allows for greater resolution. However, the photomultiplier tubes can be saturated by repeated photons reaching it and can underestimate the actual radionuclide activity within a given area of the heart. Second, the time delay between the registration of a scintillation event and the next scintillation event is relatively long and photons can go undetected. The second type of camera is the multicrystal camera. Each crystal is capable of registering multiple scintillation events and absorbing multiple photons. The time delay between the registration of events is short. However, the multicrystal camera is like an insect's eye in which there is limited resolution. It has excellent sensitivity and is ideal for first-pass studies. The Anger camera is preferred for equilibrium studies, although first-pass studies can be performed.

Computer. The computer is an integral portion of the instrumentation. An on-board computer exists with a multicrystal camera and is further connected with a computer system capable of image construction, display, and analysis. Equilibrium studies necessitate the use of electrocardiographic gating. Figure 96–12 shows a pictorial example of gating. Essentially, the full cardiac cycle is divided into 20 frames or more. Counts for each $\frac{1}{20}$ of the cardiac cycle are stored in the respective frame. As many as 400 to 500 cycles may be needed for the production of an endless loop cine format for viewing and analysis. Alternatively, the process can be performed by collecting a series of x and y coordinates

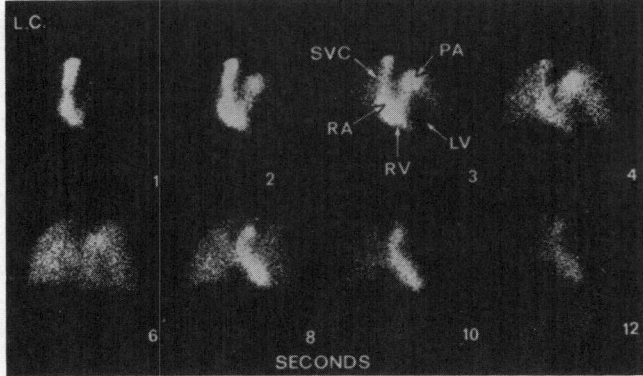

Figure 96–9. First-pass radionuclide angiogram. Tracer is initially in the superior vena cava and right atrium. By 3 seconds, the tracer has entered the pulmonary circulation, and by 8 seconds it has entered the left side of the heart. SVC = superior vena cava; PA = pulmonary artery; LV = left ventricle; RA = right atrium; RV = right ventricle. (From Braunwald E [ed]: Heart Disease: A Textbook of Cardiovascular Medicine. 3rd ed. Philadelphia, WB Saunders, p 317, 1988.)

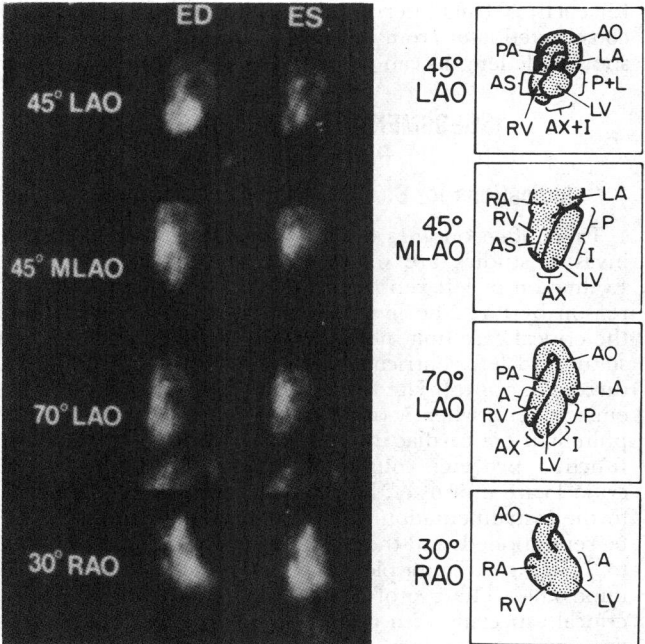

Figure 96–10. Multiview equilibrium radionuclide angiogram. LAO = left anterior oblique; MLAO = modified left anterior oblique; RAO = right anterior oblique; ED = end diastole; ES = end systole; AO = aorta; LA = left atrium; PA = pulmonary artery; LV = left ventricle; AS = anteroseptum; AX = apical; I = inferior; P = posterior; L = lateral; RV = right ventricle; RA = right atrium; A = anterior. (From Braunwald E [ed]: Heart Disease: A Textbook of Cardiovascular Medicine. 3rd ed. Philadelphia WB Saunders, p 319, 1988.)

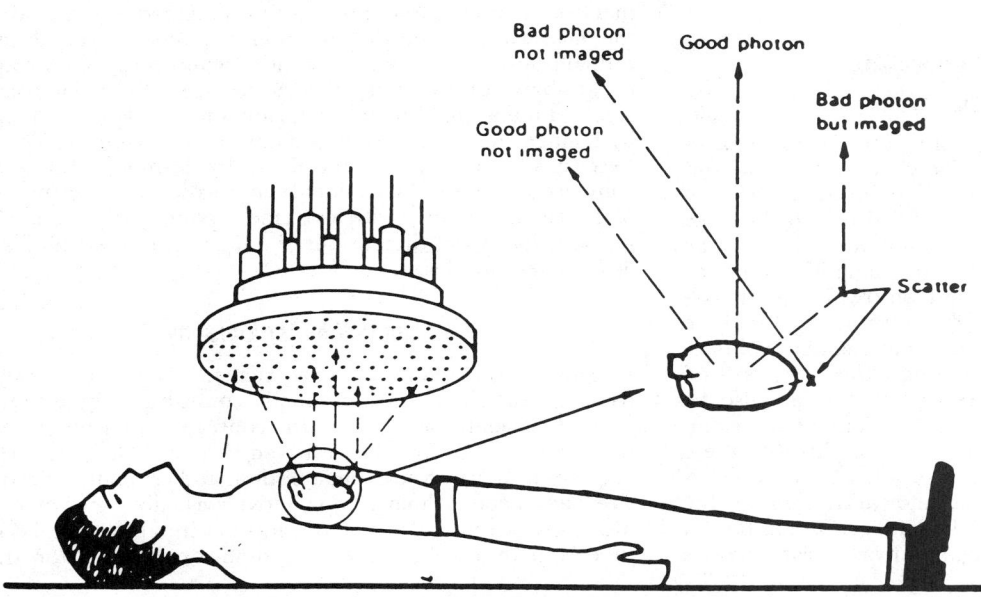

MULTI-CHANNEL COLLIMATOR

Figure 96–11. Multichannel collimator. (From Budinger TF, Rollo FD: Physics and instrumentation. Progr Cardiovasc Dis 20:19, 1977.)

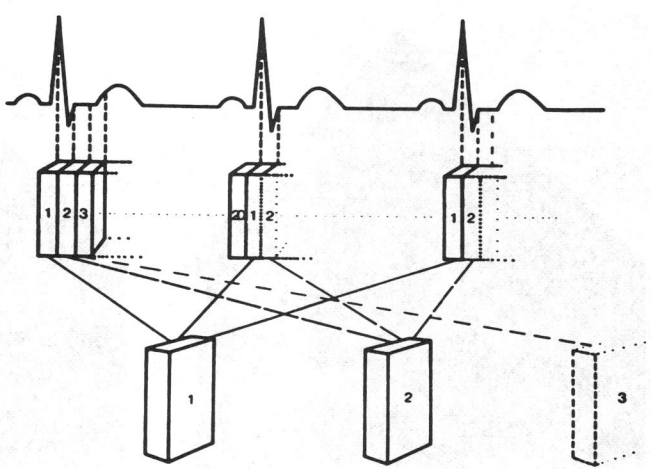

Figure 96–12. Acquisition of scintigraphic data is gated to the patient's electrocardiogram. Counts are stored in frames where frame 1 represents counts from multiple cardiac cycles, occurring during the first portion of the cardiac cycle. (From Braunwald E [ed]: Heart Disease: A Textbook of Cardiovascular Medicine. 3rd ed. Philadelphia, WB Saunders, p 318, 1988.)

for each 0.01-ms interval and storing them. Images can be constructed later from these data, and abnormally long and short cycle lengths can be excluded.

ASSESSMENT OF CARDIOVASCULAR PERFORMANCE
Indications for Studies in the Critical Care Setting

Table 96–4 outlines the more common reasons that noninvasive studies are ordered in the critical care setting. Evaluation of left ventricular function is the most common reason by far. The hypotensive patient, often admitted to the critical care unit, needs evaluation of his or her volume status and left ventricular function to assess the cause and direct the appropriate therapy. Furthermore, in the hypoxemic patient, when it is not clear whether the hypoxemia is pulmonary or cardiac in cause, assessment of left ventricular function provides considerable guidance. Patients in the critical care unit often have limited acoustic windows owing to the instrumentation of their care, their limited ability to be repositioned, and their disease state. Meticulous attention to imaging in multiple planes is important but may be impossible. The use of a transesophageal imaging plane is critical especially with regard to evaluation of aortic dissection, infective endocarditis, murmurs, and left ventricular function (at times).

Assessment of Chamber Size
Echocardiography

Two-dimensional echocardiography can provide images in multiple planes of all the cardiac chambers. Atrial and ventricular volumes can be calculated by outlining the endocardial edge of the chamber (Fig. 96–13) in orthogonal views (views 90° from each other). These area data can be transformed into volume using the area-length formula or Simpson's rule. Correlations with left ventriculographic volume determinations have been 0.80 to 0.85 at end diastole and end systole.[3–5] Correlations with other chamber volumes have had similar correlations, although this has received only limited attention.[6] Estimates of volume can also be determined from single-plane imaging. Commercial echocardiographs contain off-line analysis capability for these calculations. The reader is referred to a textbook on echocardiography for a complete list and derivation of the formulas. Qualitative assessment of chamber size has been a more common practice in many noninvasive laboratories

TABLE 96–4
COMMON INDICATIONS FOR NONINVASIVE STUDIES IN THE CRITICAL CARE SETTING

Evaluation of left ventricular function
Acute myocardial infarction
    Evaluation of left ventricular function
    Mitral regurgitation
    Ventricular septal defect
Pericardial effusion or tamponade
Endocarditis
Evaluation of murmurs
Aortic dissection
Pulmonary hypertension

with surprisingly accurate assessments when compared with those achieved with contrast angiography. Qualitative assessment may include denotations as mild, moderate, or severe, with additional gradations possible.

M-mode echocardiography has been used in the past to characterize left ventricular, right ventricular, and left atrial size. However, these determinations were made with single minor axis dimensions. In the case of the left ventricle, the end-diastolic dimension can be accurate in the absence of a tangential imaging or coexisting regional wall motion abnormalities.[7] However, the minor axis is obtained at the base of the heart. Right ventricular volume estimates are always difficult and have limited accuracy owing to the solid trapezoid shape of the right ventricle, especially when using single dimensions. Finally, determination of left atrial size by a single dimension shares many of the same problems. Left atrial dimension determined by M-mode has been compared with two-dimensional echocardiographic estimates of left atrial volume with extremely poor correlations. At present, left atrial dimensions should not be used to characterize left atrial size.

Radionuclide Angiography

Estimates of right and left ventricular volume are possible using geometric but preferentially count-based determinations. Excellent correlation with contrast ventriculography has been noted for the left ventricle (>0.90).[8–10] Atrial volumes have received little attention, and estimates of atrial size have been primarily qualitative (visually determined). Moving a gamma camera and computer into the critical care unit is both cumbersome and time-consuming. For this

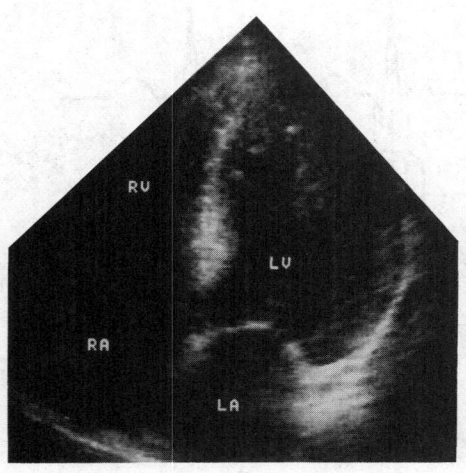
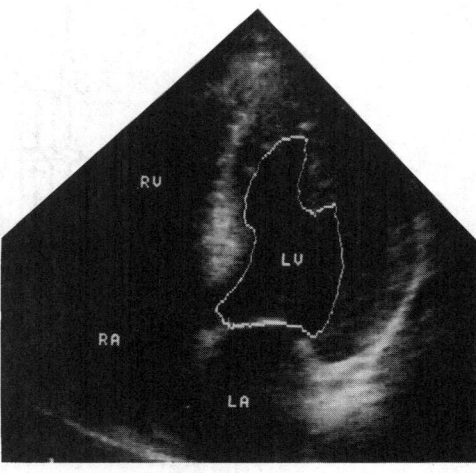

Figure 96–13. Endocardial outline (*right*) of the left ventricle (four-chamber view) at end systole. Stop frame without the endocardial outline (*left*). LV = left ventricle; LA = left atrium; RV = right ventricle; RA = right atrium.

reason, radionuclide angiography has limited use in this setting.

Assessment of Left Ventricular and Right Ventricular Systolic Function

Echocardiography

Two-Dimensional Echocardiography. Left ventricular and right ventricular systolic function can be assessed by using multiple tomographic two-dimensional echocardiographic views. Systolic function is commonly assessed as ejection fraction (EF):

$$EF = (EDV - ESV)/EDV$$

where EDV is end-diastolic volume and ESV represents end-systolic volume. Other indices of left ventricular systolic function are available, including mean and instantaneous systolic ejection rates, end-systolic pressure/volume ratio, and the velocity of circumferential fiber shortening. Good correlations with these indices of left ventricular performance can be found with left ventricular angiographic ejection fraction in the literature.[3-5] Data supporting two-dimensional echocardiographic determination of right ventricular ejection fraction[6] are scanty, primarily because of a limited clinical applicability of determining a specific number and a difficult angiographic assessment. Endocardial outlines of end diastole and systole are traced using an off-line analysis system or the quantitative package of the commercial echocardiograph. Volumes are calculated for end diastole and systole, and an ejection fraction can then be determined. This is applicable for both left and right ventricles.

The tomographic imaging of two-dimensional echocardiography lends itself to the analysis of regional wall motion in multiple tomographic views. Regional wall motion analysis can be be semiquantitative (qualitative) or quantitative. The semiquantitative approach has gained great popularity and is used for wall motion analysis with stress echocardiography.[11] Wall motion for each segment is scored on a 1 to 4 basis, with 1 representing normal and 4 indicating dyskinesis. A wall motion score can be determined for each patient. An alternative method involves quantitative evaluation of end-diastolic and end-systolic images and regional wall motion determination. The left ventricle is divided into multiple segments, and after adjustments for translation and rotation, the regional wall motion can be characterized by radial shortening or area reduction. Multiple computer algorithms exist for this.

M-Mode Echocardiography. Right ventricular systolic function cannot be evaluated by using M-mode echocardiography owing to the ice pick, or 1° sector, view. The left ventricle is interrogated at the base just below the tips of the mitral leaflets. The left ventricular minor axis shortening (fractional shortening) or ejection fraction can be calculated from this single dimension. However, diseases that affect the left ventricle in a focal manner cannot be evaluated by using M-mode echocardiographic measurements.[7] The best example of this is coronary artery disease with a regional wall motion abnormality at the apex. Cardiomyopathy with diffuse left ventricular involvement can be evaluated with M-mode minor axis dimensional changes. Ejection fraction can be calculated but assumes a certain geometry (the major axis is two times the minor axis) that is not true in the spheric ventricle.[7] For this reason, minor axis dimensional change (fractional shortening) is used to characterize left ventricular function. The ventricular septum and posterior wall can be digitized throughout the cardiac cycle. A resulting plot of left ventricular internal dimension versus time can be generated (Fig. 96–14). The peak instantaneous and mean ejection rates can be calculated as well as the velocity of circumferential fiber shortening.[12]

Radionuclide Angiography

First-pass or equilibrium radionuclide angiography can evaluate left ventricular ejection fraction. The first-pass technique either can utilize geometric assumption or can operate on a count-based method for determining left ventricular ejection fraction.[1, 2]

$$\text{Count-based EF} = (EDC - ESC)/(EDC - BK)$$

where EF is ejection fraction, EDC is end-diastolic counts, ESC refers to end-systolic counts, and BK is background counts.

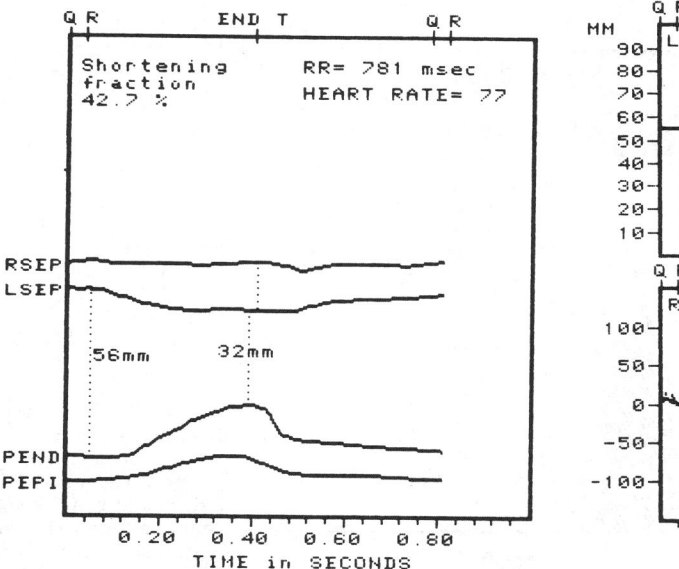
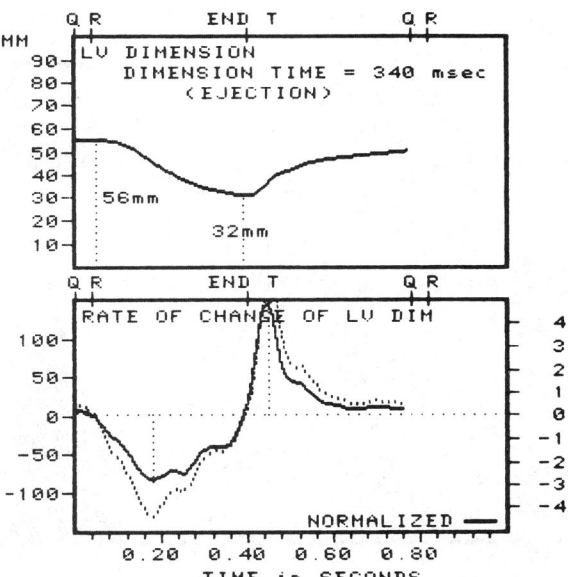

Figure 96–14. Digitized output derived from M mode of the left ventricle is shown on the left. A dimension versus time plot (*upper*) and derivative plot (*lower*) are shown on the right. RSEP = right side of septum; LSEP = left side of septum; PEND = posterior wall of endocardium; PEPI = posterior wall of epicardium; LV = left ventricle.

Similarly, equilibrium acquisition technique lends itself best to the count-based method of left ventricular ejection fraction determination. Correlations with contrast ventriculography are greater than 0.95.[13] Assessment of left ventricular systolic function[1, 2] using mean systolic ejection rate, velocity of circumferential fiber shortening, and peak ejection rate can be performed by analysis of the time-activity curve (Fig. 96–15).

Right ventricular ejection fraction can best be determined by using the first-pass method of acquisition, which both spatially and temporally separates the left ventricle and the right ventricle.[14] Good correlations have been noted with contrast right ventriculography. Assessment of regional wall motion can be qualitative or quantitative. Because the intrinsic resolution may be lower than that of two-dimensional echocardiography, visual assessment of regional wall motion is more difficult. However, semiquantitative visual analysis can be used in an analogous fashion to two-dimensional echocardiography for wall motion analysis. Quantitative methods are also available that divide the left ventricle into multiple segments.[15] However, this analysis is limited to the best septal left anterior oblique view. This represents a serious limitation, as the anterior wall is poorly represented in this view and the apex is foreshortened.

Assessment of Left Ventricular Diastolic Function
Echocardiography

Transmitral Pulsed Doppler Echocardiography. A great deal of attention has been focused on left ventricular diastolic filling, especially in the dyspneic patient and in the patient in whom symptoms of dyspnea are far greater than expected on the basis of the left ventricular systolic function. There is a subset of patients with congestive heart failure with normal systolic function who are believed to have diastolic dysfunction as the cause of their pulmonary congestion.[16] Many of the these patients have congestive heart failure associated with hypertension, left ventricular hypertrophy, and advanced age. Assessment of left ventricular diastolic function has been difficult and has been invasive either with

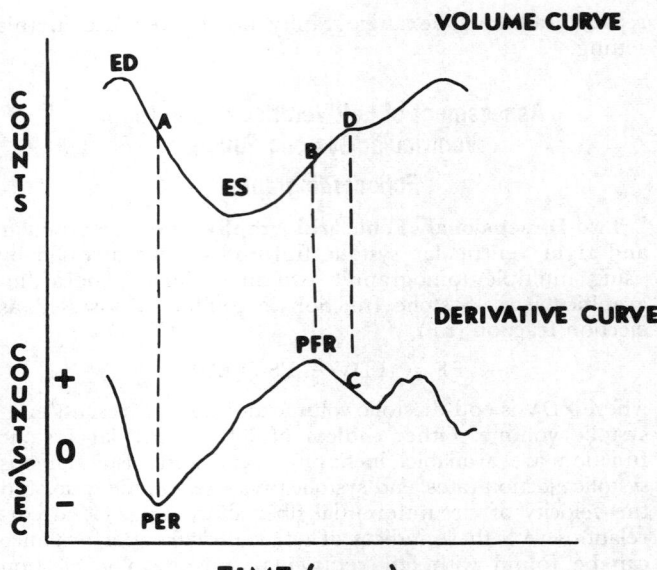

Figure 96–15. A representative time-activity curve for a normal patient is shown along with its derivative curve below. The peak ejection rate (PER) is the maximal negative derivative. Point A is the corresponding point in time on the time-activity curve. The peak filling rate (PFR) is the peak positive derivative after end systole (ES). Point B is the point on the time-activity curve corresponding to the peak filling rate. Point C represents 20% of the peak filling rate and defines the end of the rapid filling period. Point D is the corresponding point on the time-activity curve. ED = end diastole.

construction of left ventricular pressure-volume plots or by digitized M-mode echocardiography.[17] Evaluation of pulsed Doppler transmitral flow has provided a rapid and reproducible method to examine instantaneous transmitral flow or diastolic filling and is often used as a noninvasive means of estimating diastolic function.[18] Figure 96–16 is an example of transmitral flow and the method of evaluation.

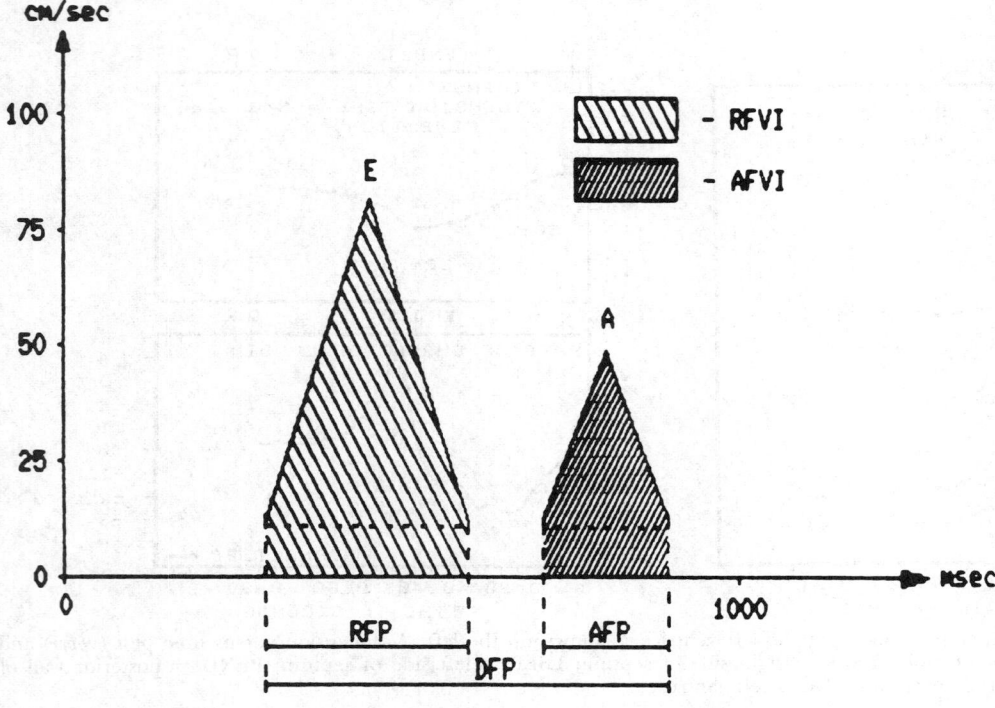

Figure 96–16. A representative transmitral pulsed Doppler spectrum for a normal patient is shown. The rapid filling period (RFP) and its peak (E), the atrial filling period (AFP) and its peak (A), and the corresponding areas beneath the rapid filling (RFVI) and atrial filling (AFVF) spectral curves are shown. DFP = diastolic filling period.

An increased rate and extent of atrial contribution to diastolic filling are commonly seen with hypertension,[19] with coronary artery disease,[20] and in patients with hypertrophied left ventricles.[21] Hypernormalization or normalization of diastolic filling measures can be seen with patients with mitral regurgitation,[19] congestive heart failure,[22] restrictive cardiomyopathy,[23] and constrictive pericarditis.[24] There is a spectrum of diastolic filling alterations that are load dependent or dependent on extrinsic factors (Fig. 96–17). The transmitral flow pattern seen is primarily dependent on the transmitral pressure gradient.[25] Hypernormalization would then imply that there are an increased rate and extent of early diastolic filling, that the transmitral pressure gradient is increased, and that the left atrial pressure at the time of mitral valve opening is increased, as may be seen with mitral regurgitation with or without congestive heart failure.[26] Alternatively, the lack of late diastolic filling may result from increased pericardial restraining properties, as may be seen in patients with dilated left ventricles and elevated left ventricular filling pressures[27] or in patients with constrictive pericarditis.[24] Such restraining influences may make it difficult to generate a gradient, or if a gradient exists,[26] pulmonary venous regurgitation may occur. Some data suggest that the transmitral pressure gradient may be greater than expected to overcome the increased afterload exerted on it by increased left ventricular chamber stiffness.[26] In addition, heart rate can alter diastolic filling by increasing the rate and extent of atrial filling with increasing heart rates.[28] Clearly, diastolic indices can be useful but are dependent on multiple factors.

M-Mode Echocardiography. Digitalization of the ventricular septum and free wall throughout the cardiac cycle can generate a dimension versus time plot (see Fig. 96–14). Differentiation of the diastolic filling portion of this curve and analysis of the dimension versus time curve yield the peak filling rate, its timing, and the percentage of filling volume at various different intervals.[12] These indices can be used to characterize diastolic filling but are dependent on systolic function,[29] heart rate,[28] loading conditions,[29-31] and external constraint.[27]

Clearly, the role of diastolic filling assessment by noninvasive techniques in clinical practices is limited. Perhaps rather than characterizing a disease state, the diastolic filling pattern is best used to assess the loading conditions of the left ventricle. For example, in a dysfunctional left ventricle, a normal diastolic filling pattern suggests significant mitral regurgitation and/or elevated left ventricular end-diastolic pressures.

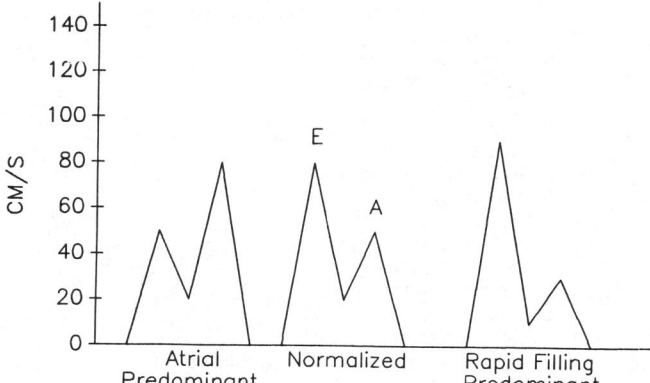

Figure 96–17. Diastolic filling patterns (from transmitral pulsed Doppler spectra) commonly encountered clinically are shown. E = peak rapid filling velocity; A = peak atrial filling velocity.

Radionuclide Angiography

Equilibrium and radionuclide angiography generates a time-activity curve that is analogous to the volume-time curve (see Fig. 96–15). Differentiation of the time-activity curve generates an ejection rate and filling rate analogous to transmitral flow. Peak filling rate and the time to the peak filling rate are measures that have been used to characterize diastolic filling. The percentage of filling volume occurring during one third of diastole and one half of diastole, and at the end of the rapid filling period, has also been used.[32, 33] In patients with coronary artery disease,[32] hypertension,[34] and aortic valve disease,[33] and in some with cardiomyopathy,[22] the peak filling rate and the percentage of filling volume at one third of diastole, at one half of diastole, and at the end of the rapid filling period are reduced, while the time to the peak filling rate is prolonged. However, these indices are load dependent as in patients with coronary artery disease and cardiomyopathy with increased end-diastolic pressures in whom these indices are normalized or even supernormalized.[22] The use of these indices requires knowledge of the influence of loading conditions. Perhaps the best use of these indices may be to characterize the left ventricular hemodynamic state.

Isovolumic Relaxation

Isovolumic relaxation (Fig. 96–18) refers to the time interval between aortic valve closure and mitral valve opening. During this interval, left ventricular pressure declines, left ventricular relaxation commences, and left ventricular endocardium thins, and this period is terminated by the opening of the mitral valve. At the time of mitral valve opening, the left ventricle may not have achieved full relaxation and left ventricular pressure may still continue to decline. Abnormally prolonged relaxation can be characterized by prolongation of this interval. This interval may be prolonged in patients with hypertrophic myocardium,[35] coronary artery disease, and aortic valve disease.[36]

Aortic valve closure can be assessed by the time interval between the R wave and any of the following equivalents of aortic valve closure: M-mode echocardiographic closure of the aortic valve, phonocardiographic A_2, incisura of the carotid pulse tracing, or the end of flow of the transaortic pulsed Doppler spectrum. Mitral valve opening can be assessed by the time interval between the R wave and either of the following equivalents of mitral valve opening: opening of the mitral leaflets on M-mode echogram or the onset of transmitral flow. The isovolumic relaxation period is therefore defined as the R wave–to–mitral valve opening interval minus the R wave–to–aortic valve opening interval. This interval is 60 ± 10 ms in a normal population. However, this interval and its components are influenced by multiple factors (preload, afterload, contractility, and heart rate).[37] For this reason, its clinical utility is limited. Abnormally short isovolumic relaxation periods in the presence of left ventricular dysfunction suggest significant mitral regurgitation (large V wave opens mitral valve early) or elevated left ventricular end-diastolic pressure (increased V wave opens mitral valve earlier).[37]

Analysis of Valvular Function

Analysis of valvular function requires anatomic information of the involved valve, demonstration of obstruction or regurgitation, and identification of the impact on the affected chamber. First-pass or equilibrium radionuclide angiography is useful only for characterizing the impact on the affected chamber. For example, in aortic regurgitation,

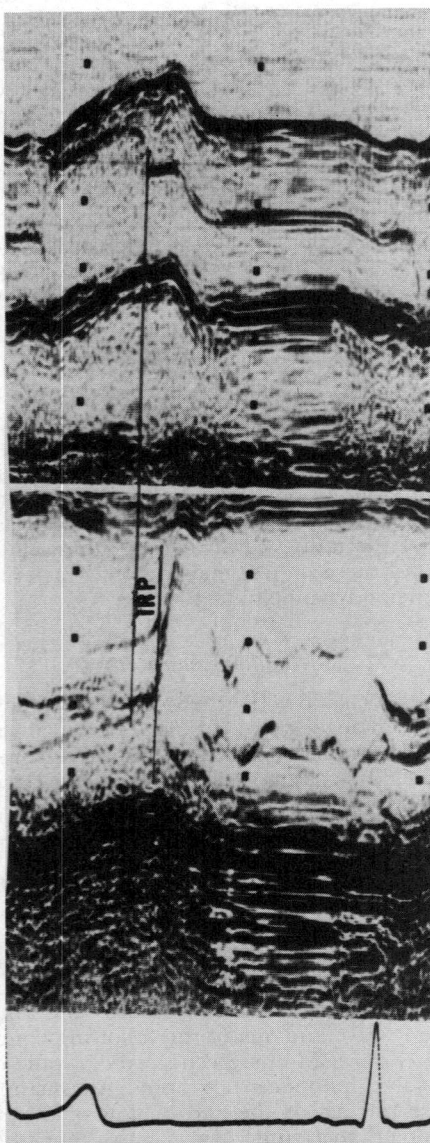

Figure 96–18. An example of one of the multiple methods of determining the isovolumic relaxation period. A simultaneous aortic valve echogram (upper M mode) and mitral valve echogram (bottom M mode) are shown. Aortic valve closure and mitral valve opening are marked by lines drawn perpendicular to these events. The isovolumic relaxation period (IRP) is the time interval between these two events.

left ventricular volume overload is expected with preservation of left ventricular systolic function. If left ventricular systolic function is reduced, and left ventricular size is increasing, potential intervention may be indicated. However, two-dimensional echocardiography and pulsed Doppler echocardiography are more useful, as these studies provide anatomic information, demonstration of the extent of valve involvement, and indication of the impact on the affected cardiac chamber.

M-Mode Echocardiography. M-mode echocardiography provides a high-resolution anatomic evaluation of the affected valve with a small field of view. Visualization of tricuspid and pulmonic valves may be difficult. Interrogation of the affected valve in multiple planes, however, is not possible, which limits the spatial information available. M-

mode echocardiography can provide single (and minor axis) dimensional assessment of left ventricular chamber size and systolic function. This assessment is spatially limited and, in the case of coexisting coronary artery disease, may misrepresent left ventricular function.

Two-Dimensional Echocardiography. Anatomic information regarding valvular function can best be assessed by two-dimensional echocardiography. Table 96–5 summarizes the most common abnormalities of valvular function that can be assessed. This list is lengthy but is not exhaustive. The amount of anatomic information obtainable is considerable (for a full discussion, the reader is referred to a textbook on echocardiography).

Abnormality of valve function can be classified anatomically into stenosis, regurgitation, and abnormal motion characterizing hemodynamic states. Valvular stenosis is seen as thickening of the leaflets with marked reduction in excursion. However, this does not necessarily indicate a significant pressure gradient across the valve, as this may occur with the aortic valve. Regurgitation cannot be assessed by two-dimensional echocardiography directly except by establishing its cause or by demonstrating a flail leaflet. Leaflet motion characterizing a hemodynamic state is an example of how valve motion may parallel transvalvular flow, as in a low cardiac output state (see ref 38, p 188). In addition, early aortic valve closure may be seen with hypertrophic obstructive cardiomyopathy as indicative of early and complete chamber emptying. On the other hand, systolic anterior motion of the mitral valve is another type of abnormal valve motion that does not characterize transvalvular flow but is secondary to a mechanism in which the anterior mitral leaflet

TABLE 96–5
COMMON ABNORMALITIES OF CARDIAC VALVES SEEN ON TWO-DIMENSIONAL ECHOCARDIOGRAPHY

1. Mitral valve
   a. Rheumatic mitral valve disease
   b. Myxomatous degeneration
   c. Calcification of the mitral annulus or leaflets
   d. Infective endocarditis
   e. Flail mitral leaflet
   f. Systolic anterior motion of the mitral leaflets (hypertrophic cardiomyopathy)
2. Aortic valve
   a. Aortic stenosis
   b. Bicuspid valve
   c. Infective endocarditis
   d. Flail leaflet
   e. Aortic valve prolapse
   f. Hypertrophic obstructive cardiomyopathy
3. Tricuspid valve
   a. Tricuspid stenosis
   b. Tricuspid prolapse
   c. Flail leaflet
   d. Infective endocarditis
   e. Dilated annulus
   f. Pulmonary hypertension
   g. Surgically absent valve
4. Pulmonic valve
   a. Pulmonic stenosis
   b. Infundibular stenosis
   c. Infective endocarditis
   d. Flail leaflet
5. Prosthetic valves
   a. Bioprosthetic stenosis or calcification
   b. Ring abscess
   c. Rocking prosthesis
   d. Decreased disk or poppet excursion
   e. Thrombus

is purported to participate in subaortic obstruction in hypertrophic obstructive cardiomyopathy (see ref 38, p 457).

Two-dimensional echocardiography can also assess the impact of valvular disease on chamber size and architecture (Table 96–6). In general, valvular regurgitation dilates both the ventricle and the atrium, depending on the location of the valve. With valvular stenosis, the ventricular chamber preceding the valve hypertrophies with dilation of the affected atrium. Dilation of the hypertrophied ventricular chamber does not occur unless end-stage congestive failure supervenes. In the case of tricuspid regurgitation, both organic factors and pulmonary hypertension are causative. With pulmonary hypertension, it is not uncommon to see four-chamber enlargement. In the case of organic pathologic changes, evidence of right ventricular volume overload with dilation of both the right atrium and the right ventricle is likely. Associated right ventricular hypertrophy may also occur. Alteration in the shape of the ventricular septum may occur with tricuspid regurgitation of organic causes, although this usually is due to volume overload alone.[39]

Doppler Echocardiography. The demonstration of regurgitation and its direction and extent is best accomplished by

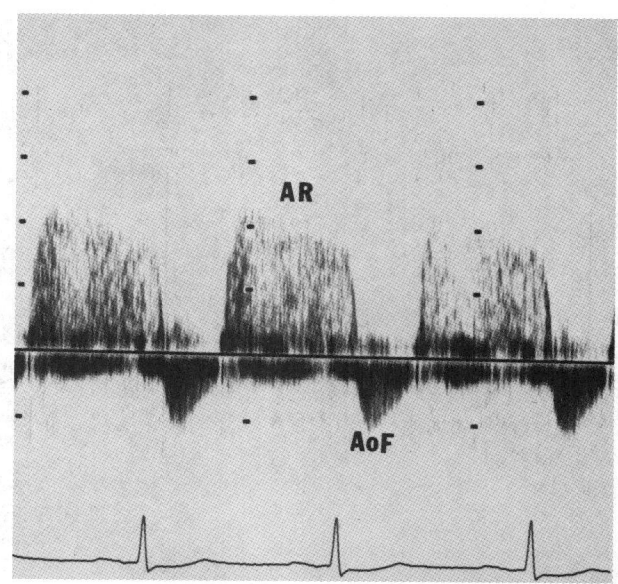

Figure 96–19. Continuous wave Doppler spectral tracing taken through the aortic valve in a patient with chronic moderate aortic regurgitation (AR). Forward aortic flow (AoF) is negatively directed and usually less than 1.7 m/s. In this patient, it is increased owing to the aortic regurgitation. Aortic regurgitation is seen as high velocity (>4 m/s), occurring during diastole, and directed positively (toward the transducer). Calibration: each vertical dot represents 2 m/s.

TABLE 96–6

ALTERATIONS IN CHAMBER SIZE AS ASSESSED BY TWO-DIMENSIONAL ECHOCARDIOGRAPHY IN VALVULAR HEART DISEASE

1. Aortic regurgitation
   a. Dilated left ventricle
   b. Left ventricular hypertrophy
   c. Left atrial dilatation
2. Aortic stenosis
   a. Left ventricular hypertrophy
   b. Left atrial dilatation
3. Mitral stenosis
   a. Left atrial dilatation
   b. Right ventricular dilatation
   c. Right atrial dilatation
   d. Right ventricular hypertrophy
4. Mitral regurgitation
   a. Left atrial dilatation
   b. Left ventricular dilatation
   c. Left ventricular hypertrophy
   d. Dilated right-sided heart chambers
   e. Right ventricular hypertrophy
5. Tricuspid stenosis
   a. Dilated right atrium
   b. Small right ventricle
6. Tricuspid regurgitation
   a. Organic causes
      i. Right atrial dilatation
      ii. Right ventricular dilatation
      iii. Right ventricular hypertrophy
      iv. Flattened ventricular septum (diastole only)
   b. Pulmonary hypertension as cause
      i. Left-sided chamber dilatation
      ii. Right-sided chamber dilatation
      iii. Four-chamber enlargement common
      iv. Right, left, or biventricular hypertrophy
      v. Flattened ventricular septum (systole and diastole)
7. Pulmonic stenosis
   a. Right ventricular hypertrophy
   b. Dilated right atrium
8. Pulmonic regurgitation
   a. Right atrial dilatation
   b. Right ventricular dilatation
   c. Right ventricular hypertrophy
   d. Flattened ventricular septum
   e. If attributable to pulmonary hypertension, same as for tricuspid regurgitation

Doppler imaging. Pulsed and continuous wave Doppler studies across the valve demonstrate the existence of regurgitation by flow being recorded in the direction opposite to forward transvalvular flow and at the appropriate time in the cardiac cycle (Fig. 96–19). Continuous wave Doppler examination is limited in its utility, as it assesses only the peak velocity across the valve. This is of limited hemodynamic utility with the left side of the heart. However, on the right side of the heart, it is useful as it can be utilized to estimate pulmonary arterial pressures[39] (see later). Pulsed wave Doppler studies can be used to map the chamber receiving the regurgitant blood flow to assess the extent of regurgitant flow.

Perhaps the use of color flow mapping is better for this as a 30 to 60° depiction of regurgitant flow by the use of the opposite color as opposed to forward flow and in the appropriate time (systole or diastole) of the cardiac cycle can be depicted (Fig. 96–20). The use of color flow mapping disturbance in the left atrium divided by left atrium area has been used as an estimate of the degree of mitral regurgitation with good to strong correlations with contrast ventriculography.[40] For aortic regurgitation, the width of the regurgitant jet divided by the left ventricular outflow track width or the extent of color flow mapping disturbance into the left ventricle has been used to assess the severity of aortic regurgitation.[41]

Both pulmonic regurgitation and tricuspid regurgitation are often secondary to pulmonary hypertension (afterload), as they are afterload dependent with intact valvular structures, their extent being less important than the estimates of pulmonary arterial pressures. However, in the case of organic pathologic changes, tricuspid regurgitation can be assessed in a similar fashion to mitral regurgitation. Assessing the extent of pulmonic regurgitation by color flow mapping or pulsed or continuous wave Doppler examination has received little attention.

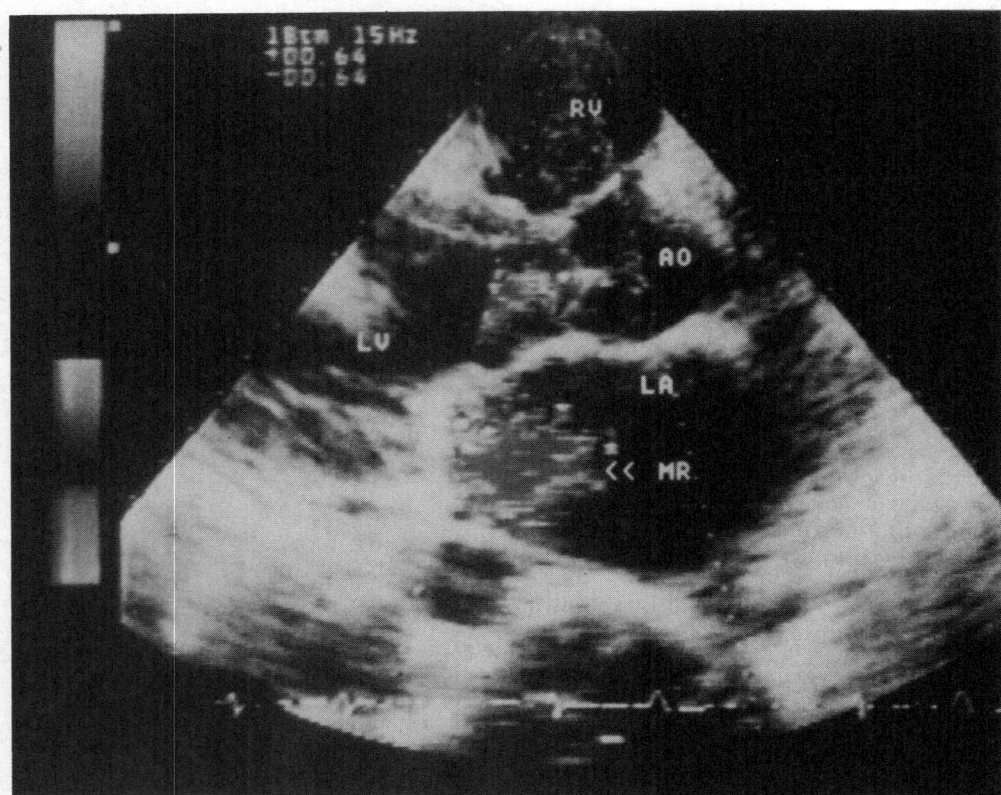

Figure 96–20. Stop frame of parasternal long-axis view of a patient with moderate mitral regurgitation (MR). The mitral regurgitation jet is seen in the left atrium (LA) in systole. LV = left ventricle; AO = aorta; RV = right ventricle.

Valvular stenosis can be assessed by the demonstration of the transvalvular pressure gradient and is characterized by an increased continuous wave velocity across the valve. The modified Bernoulli equation characterizes the relationship between pressure gradient (PG) and velocity (V):

$$PG = 4V^2$$

A pressure gradient determination can be obtained for all four valves (see ref 42, p 23). For the aortic and pulmonic valves, the instantaneous transvalvular pressure grading can be used to characterize the pressure gradient.[43] However, in the case of the aortic valve, the mean pressure gradient may be a more useful measure (see ref 42, pp 127–128). The mean pressure gradient is easily obtainable by outlining the Doppler spectrum utilizing the built-in software of the ultrasonograph, which then determines the mean pressure gradient. Excellent correlations with hemodynamic pressure measurements have been noted for the aortic valve.[44, 45]

An alternative method of evaluation of valvular stenosis uses the continuity equation:

Stenotic valve area × peak velocity across valve =
　　　　prevalve area × peak velocity prevalve

Use of the continuity equation to estimate valve area has been well validated for the aortic valve.[46] The prevalve area represents the area of the left ventricular outflow tract in the case of the aortic valve. These calculations can be performed for pulmonic, mitral, and tricuspid valves, although these are less well validated. The determination of the peak pressure gradient is of less utility for tricuspid and mitral stenosis, although the mean pressure gradient may be useful. The valve area for the tricuspid and mitral valves can be calculated by assessing the rate of transtricuspid or transmitral exponential pressure gradient decline using the formula: valve area = 220/pressure half-time.[17] The pressure half-time is the time interval required for the transmitral or transtricuspid pressure gradient to decline by one half of its original value. If the transmitral velocity is being used, the time required for the velocity to decline by a factor of $1/\sqrt{2}$, or to 70% of its initial velocity. Most ultrasonographs have the software that allows for this rapid calculation. This equation is widely used clinically, although it is an oversimplification. For example, the left atrial–left ventricular compliance (inversely related) and the initial pressure gradient (directly related) are ignored: these two factors influence pressure half-time but in opposite directions.[48]

Transesophageal Echocardiographic Imaging. Transesophageal echocardiography has markedly expanded the capability of Doppler echocardiography (color flow mapping) specifically in the area of valvular regurgitation. As the esophagus is a much closer acoustic interface than the chest wall, greater resolution, sensitivity, and the use of high-frequency transducers have increased the sensitivity for detecting the presence and extent of regurgitation. Specifically, both atria are in near-apposition to the esophagus. The assessment of mitral and tricuspid regurgitation is made much easier, and a high-resolution assessment of valvular anatomy and regurgitation is possible. This has been of great utility in the assessment of prosthetic valve function and regurgitation. In the case of the prosthetic mitral or tricuspid valve, the prosthesis incompletely (bioprosthesis) or completely (mechanical prosthesis) shadows the left and right atria, making assessment of regurgitant flow impossible from the transthoracic imaging plane. Forward mitral and tricuspid flow can be seen with transthoracic imaging but not with transesophageal imaging. With transesophageal imaging, the prosthesis can be seen clearly and with high resolution. Rocking of the valve, valvular thrombus, and other abnormalities can be identified by transesophageal echocardigraphy that often cannot be seen from the chest wall (Fig. 96–21).

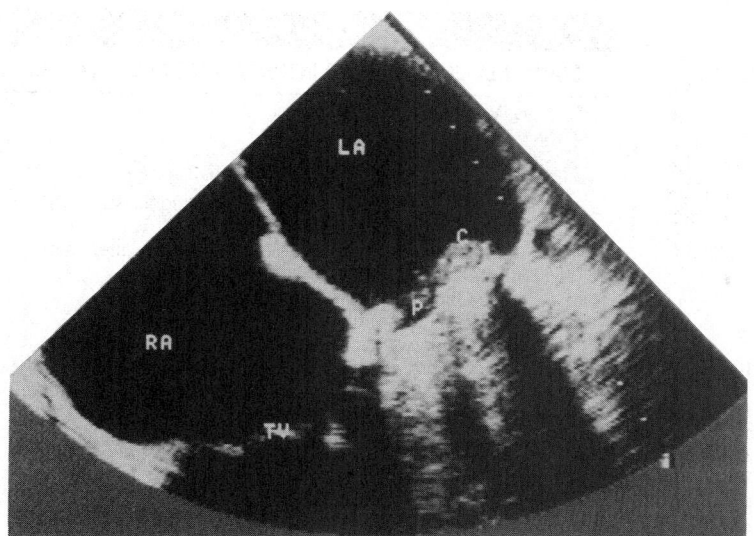
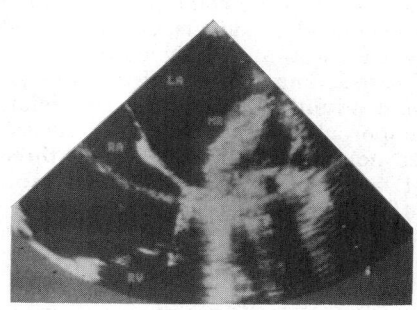

Figure 96–21. Stop frame (*left*) from a transesophageal echocardiogram of a patient with a prosthetic mitral valve (P) with a thrombus (C) attached. Color flow mapping (on the right) revealed moderate to severe mitral regurgitation (MR). LA = left atrium; RA = right atrium; RV = right ventricle; TV = tricuspid valve.

Assessment of Hemodynamics

Estimation of Pulmonary Arterial Pressure

From the tricuspid valve continuous wave velocity, systolic pulmonary arterial pressure can be estimated from the simplified Bernoulli equation (PG = $4V^2$).[42] The pressure gradient calculated represents the pressure difference between the right atrium and the right ventricle in systole. Assuming the absence of pulmonic stenosis and adding an estimate of the mean right atrial pressure from the jugular venous pressure, the pulmonary arterial systolic pressure can be estimated.[39] Similarly, the diastolic pulmonary arterial pressure can be estimated from the pulmonic regurgitation velocity in an analogous fashion.

Estimation of Mean Pulmonary Capillary Pressure

There are presently three methods to estimate the mean pulmonary capillary pressure. No method has gained wide acceptance or applicability.

Echophonocardiographic Method. The ratio of the Q wave to mitral valve closure interval divided by the aortic valve closure–to–E wave of the mitral echogram interval has been used to estimate the mean pulmonary capillary pressure.[49] The rationale behind this ratio is that prolongation of the Q wave to mitral valve closure interval occurs with increased left atrial pressures and the A_2-to-E point of the mitral valve interval decreases in patients with elevated left end-diastolic pressures. Good correlations have been found in patients with mitral stenosis and without mitral stenosis. However, animal studies explored the use of this interval using ischemia and changes in loading conditions to alter the mean pulmonary capillary pressure and found that this method was unable to predict the mean pulmonary capillary pressures. However, ischemia may alter these intervals independent of changes in the mean pulmonary capillary pressure.[50]

Estimates of Aortic Regurgitation Velocity. The left ventricular end-diastolic pressure can be estimated with moderate or greater aortic regurgitation by applying the Bernoulli equation to the end-diastolic aortic regurgitation velocity. The aortic diastolic pressure obtained via blood pressure cuff minus the end-diastolic pressure gradient (estimated from the aortic regurgitant Doppler spectrum) estimates the left ventricular end-diastolic pressure. This evaluation has clearly limited clinical applicability. Milder degrees of aortic regurgitation may not adequately estimate left ventricular end-diastolic pressure, because the velocity is lower owing to the influence of friction from a small regurgitant orifice.

Transmitral Doppler Spectrum or Diastolic Filling Pattern. Certain patterns of diastolic filling[51] are suggestive of elevated left ventricular end-diastolic pressure, although mitral regurgitation can also mimic or accentuate this pattern.[19] Increased left ventricular end-diastolic pressure and increased left atrial pressure at the time of mitral valve opening increase the V wave and increase the early transmitral pressure gradient. This may normalize or even supernormalize the rate and extent of rapid filling and the rapid filling–to–atrial filling ratio. This has been demonstrated both by pulsed Doppler echocardiography and by radionuclide angiography.[22, 52] For example, in patients with congestive cardiomyopathy or coronary artery disease with elevated pulmonary capillary pressures, early redistribution of diastolic filling characterized by an increased rate and extent of rapid filling as compared with that in similar patients with lower pulmonary capillary pressures has been noted.[22] Patients with third heart sounds also had an increase in the rate and extent of rapid filling, a group most likely to have elevated left ventricular end-diastolic pressures.[53] The relationship between the rate and extent of rapid filling divided by the rate and extent of atrial filling and the left ventricular end-diastolic pressure or the mean pulmonary capillary pressure have had only moderate correlations at best.[22] Diastolic filling patterns have multiple determinants that do not permit a stronger correlation and wide clinical applicability to the use of diastolic filling measures to predict the pulmonary capillary pressure. However, normalization or supernormalization of the diastolic filling pattern is strongly suggestive of elevated mean pulmonary capillary pressures in the dilated left ventricle with abnormal systolic function.[51–53]

Identification of Intracardiac Shunts

Table 96–7 lists the commonly encountered intracardiac shunts seen in adult patients. Ostium secundum atrial septal defects are most commonly encountered by far. In the critical care setting, rupture of the sinus of Valsalva aneurysm and postinfarction ventricular septal defects are the most important to recognize. Intracardiac shunts can be assessed noninvasively with regard to three important factors: (1) anatomy, (2) direction and size of shunts, and (3) impact on other cardiac chambers.

Radionuclide Angiography

First-pass techniques are capable of assessing the direction and size of the shunt and the impact on other cardiac chambers. The site of the shunt can be detected if it is a right-to-left shunt by assessing left-sided heart counts during the passage of the radionuclide bolus through the right side of the heart. The ratio of pulmonary to systemic flow can be calculated from analysis of time activity curves over the lungs and left side of the heart.[54] Finally, the size and function of each cardiac chamber can be assessed.

Echocardiography

Lateral beam width may not permit visualization of an atrial or ventricular septal defect by M-mode echocardiography; however, in tetralogy of Fallot, the ventricular septal defect attributable to the overriding aorta is obvious. M-

TABLE 96–7
COMMONLY ENCOUNTERED INTRACARDIAC SHUNTS IN ADULTS

1. Ventricular septal defect
   a. Muscular
   b. Membranous
   c. After myocardial infarction
2. Ventricular septal defect with pulmonic stenosis
   a. Tetralogy of Fallot
   b. Ventricular septal defect with valvar stenosis
3. Atrial septal defect
   a. Ostium primum
   b. Ostium secundum
   c. Sinus venosus
4. Endocardial cushion defects
5. Anomalous pulmonary venous return
   a. With atrial septal defect
   b. Without atrial septal defect
6. Patent ductus arteriosus
7. Ruptured sinus of Valsalva's aneurysm

mode echocardiography cannot demonstrate the shunt or size, but indirect clues can be provided by chamber size (although this is only a single dimension). Abnormal septal motion may indicate an atrial septal defect of a 1.5-to-1 left-to-right shunt.

Two-Dimensional Echocardiography. Two-dimensional echocardiography has the appropriate size of the field of view that allows visualization of the size of the defect as well

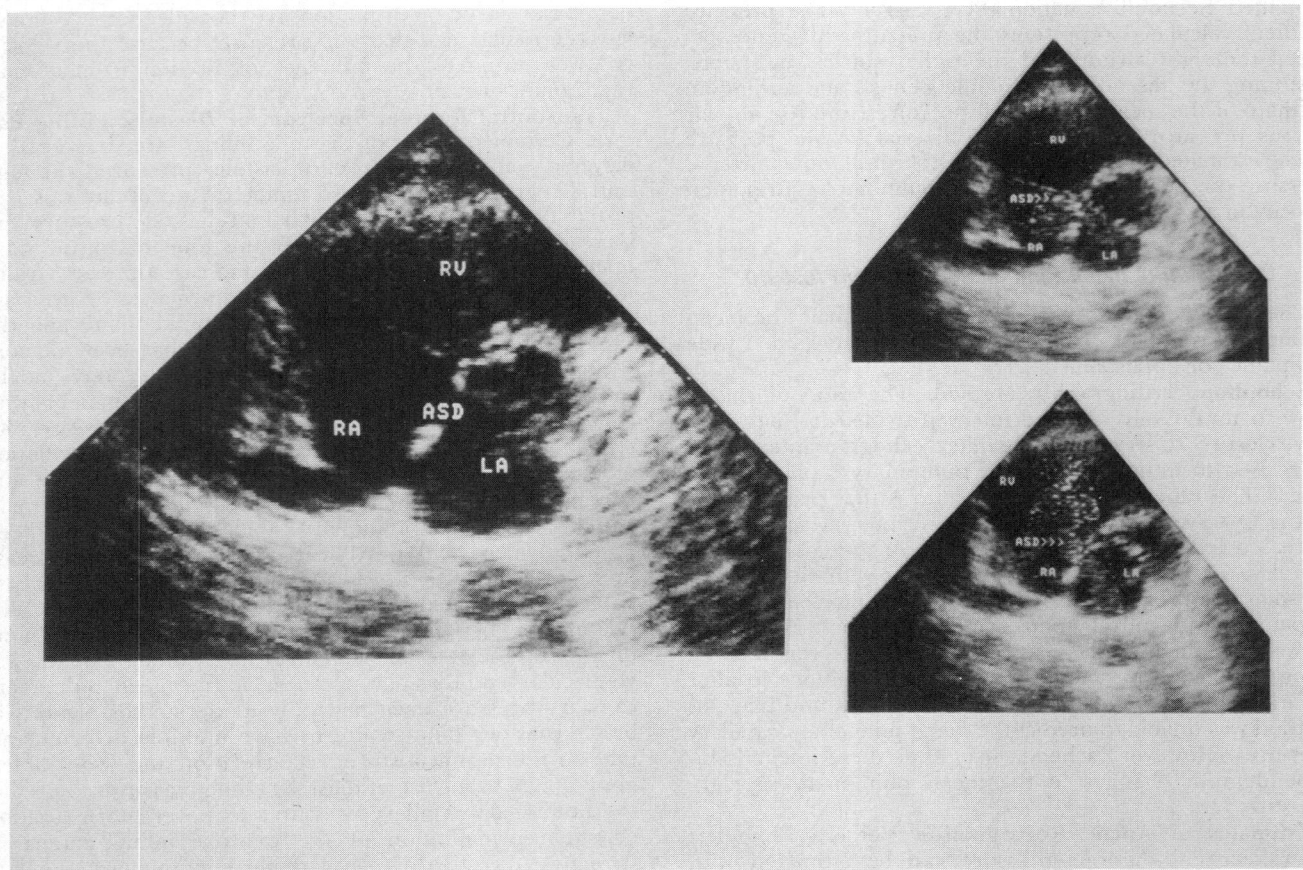

Figure 96–22. Atrial septal defect (ASD) is shown in stop frame on the left. On the upper right atrial septal defect flow is occurring through the defect. Minor manipulation of the transducer demonstrated the full extent of the atrial septal defect flow. RA = right atrium; RV = right ventricle; LA = left atrium.

as potentially the impact on various chambers. For example, a secundum atrial septal defect can be visualized in a subcostal view, along with right atrial and right ventricular dilatation and abnormal ventricular septal motion. However, shunt flow and size of the shunt can only be inferred and estimated. Contrast echocardiography (antecubital vein injection of agitated saline) can demonstrate an atrial septal defect flow either by a negative contrast effect in the atrium (a left-to-right shunt) or by appearance of echo contrast in the left atrium (a right-to-left shunt). Associated lesions can be identified, such as pulmonic or aortic stenosis, coarctation of the aorta, and other abnormalities.

Doppler Echocardiography. The size and direction of the shunt can more easily be demonstrated by Doppler echocardiography. Shunts may be detected with either pulsed wave, continuous wave, or color flow mapping in a variety of views. The direction of flow can also be detected by any of these modalities based on whether flow is toward or away from the transducer (Fig. 96–22). Furthermore, flow is turbulent, which can be demonstrated by multiple velocities recorded with pulsed wave or by increased variance demonstrated by color flow mapping.

Shunt size can be assessed by two basic methods. First, is the classic ratio of pulmonary to systemic flow.[55] This is accomplished by multiplying the area beneath the pulsed wave or continuous wave Doppler integral by the valve area. This yields a good estimate of either pulmonic or systemic flow. However, regurgitation across a valve invalidates the calculation of forward flow across the valve by this technique. Pulmonary flow is usually assessed by flow across the pulmonic or less often the tricuspid valve. Systemic flow is usually assessed by flow across the mitral or aortic valve. Flow assessment across the semilunar valve is probably more accurate, as the mitral or tricuspid valve annulus may change significantly during the cardiac cycle.[56] The second method is by measuring the width of the shunt by color flow mapping.[57] This is really more of semiquantitative method and has much less validation.

Other information available from the Doppler studies includes the velocity of shunt flow. For example, in a restrictive ventricular septal defect with a small shunt flow, one expects the velocity to be higher than with a larger ventricular septal defect. A large shunt might lead to equalization of pressures across the connecting chambers and low velocities. Velocity assessment is less useful for an atrial septal defect.

Detection of Aortic Dissection of Thoracic Aorta

Aortic dissection of thoracic aorta is an emergent situation necessitating prompt therapy. The detection of the aortic dissection and its extent, origin, and exit points are important for therapy and prognosis. The demonstration of intimal tear, false lumen, and blood supply of the major arteries emanating from the aorta is critical. Traditionally, aortography has been the "gold standard." Computed tomographic imaging can act as a screen for detecting aortic dissection. Echocardiography has been used to demonstrate the presence, extent, origin, exit site, and false lumen.[58, 59] Transthoracic imaging can be useful at the valvular level and around the arch, although the resolution is limited.

Transesophageal echocardiography is rapidly emerging as an important imaging procedure. The aorta sits posterior to the esophagus and is easily imageable with high resolution from the upper portion of the descending aorta to the subdiaphragmatic aorta. The area from the valve origin to several centimeters above the valve can also be imaged. As the trachea sits between the esophagus and aorta at the level of the arch, this area is poorly imaged. Biplanar transesoph-

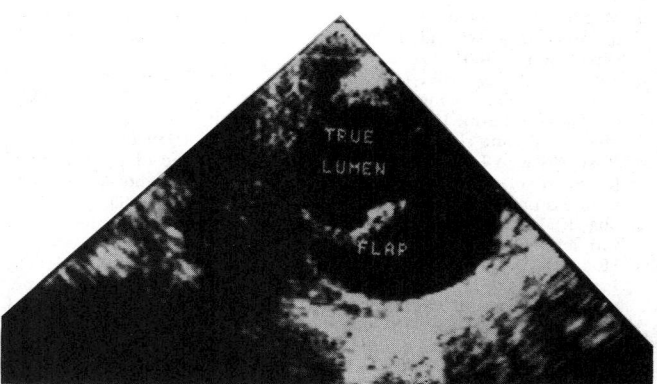

Figure 96–23. Stop frame from a transesophageal echocardiogram of the descending aorta in which aortic dissection is demonstrated. An intimal flap is well visualized. A smaller true lumen is well outlined.

ageal assessment may be useful in this regard. Transesophageal echocardiography demonstrates quite vividly the dissection flap (Fig. 96–23) with a high sensitivity and specificity. Communication between the true and false lumina can be seen with color flow. The origin and exit site of dissection can also be demonstrated. Accompanying aortic regurgitation (in type 1 dissection) can be demonstrated with high resolution. Transesophageal echocardiography can be performed with intravenous sedation in minutes in the critically ill patient, allowing immediate antihypertensive therapy to commence. Aortic angiography can then be performed to determine which vessels are being supplied by the true lumen and which vessels are supplied by the false lumen.

References

1. Letl GP, Buchannan JW, Wagner HN: Monitoring cardiac function with nuclear techniques. Am J Cardiol 46:1125, 1980.
2. Strauss HW, McKusick KA, Bingham JB: Cardiac nuclear imaging: Principles, instrumentation, and pitfalls. Am J Cardiol 46:1109, 1980.
3. Eaton LW, Maughan WL, Shoukas AA, et al: Accurate volume determination in the isolated ejected canine left ventricle by two-dimensional echocardiography. Circulation 60:320, 1979.
4. Folland ED, Parisi AF, Moynihan PF, et al: Assessment of left ventricular ejection fraction and volumes by real-time, two-dimensional echocardiography. A comparison of cineangiographic and radionuclide techniques. Circulation 60:760, 1979.
5. Schiller NB, Acquatella H, Ports TA, et al: Left ventricular volume from paired biplane two-dimensional echocardiography. Circulation 60:547, 1979.
6. Levine RA, Gibson TC, Aretz T, et al: Echocardiographic measurement of right ventricular volume. Circulation 69:497, 1984.
7. Teichholz LE, Kreulen T, Herman MV, et al: Problems in echocardiographic volume determinations: Echocardiographic-angiographic correlations in the presence or absence of asynergy. Am J Cardiol 37:7, 1976.
8. Dehmer GJ, Lewis SE, Hillis LD, et al: Nongeometric determinations of left ventricular volume from equilibrium blood pool scans. Am J Cardiol 34:293, 1980.
9. Massie BM, Kramer BL, Gertz EW, et al: Radionuclide measurement of left ventricular volume: Comparisons of geometric and count-based methods. Circulation 65:725, 1982.
10. Links JM, Becker LC, Schindlebecker G, et al: Measurement of absolute left ventricular volume from gated blood pool studies. Circulation 65:82, 1982.
11. Broderick T, Sawader S, Armstrong WF, et al: Improvement in rest and exercise induced wall motion abnormalities after coronary angioplasty: An exercise-echocardiographic study. J Am Coll Cardiol 15:591, 1990.
12. Gibson DG, Brown D: Measurement of instantaneous left ventricular dimensions and filling rates using echocardiography. Br Heart J 35:1141, 1973.
13. Burrow RD, Strauss HW, Singleton R, et al: Analysis of left ventricular function from multiple gated acquisition cardiac blood pool imaging. Circulation 56:1024, 1977.
14. Berger HJ, Matthay RA, Pytlik LM, et al: First-pass radionuclide assessment of right and left ventricular performance in patients with cardiac and pulmonary disease. Semin Nucl Med 9:275, 1979.

15. Maddox DE, Wynne J, Uren R, et al: Regional ejection fraction: A quantitative radionuclide index of regional left ventricular performance. Circulation 59:1001, 1979.

16. Soufer R, Wohlgelenter D, Vita NA, et al: Intact systolic left ventricular function in clinical congestive heart failure. Am J Cardiol 55:1032, 1985.

17. Gaasch WH, Levine HJ, Quinones MA, et al: Left ventricular compliance: Mechanisms and clinical implications. Am J Cardiol 38:645, 1976.

18. Rokey R, Kuo LC, Zoghbi WA, et al: Determination of parameters of left ventricular diastolic filling with pulsed Doppler echocardiography: Comparison with cineangiography. Circulation 71:543, 1985.

19. Shaikh MA, Lavine SJ: Effect of mitral regurgitation on diastolic filling with left ventricular hypertrophy. Am J Cardiol 61:590, 1988.

20. Stoddard MF, Pearson AC, Kern MJ, et al: Left ventricular diastolic function: Comparison of pulsed Doppler echocardiographic and hemodynamic indexes in subjects with and without coronary artery disease. J Am Coll Cardiol 13:327, 1989.

21. Takenaka K, Dabestani A, Gardin JM, et al: Pulsed Doppler echocardiographic study of left ventricular filling in dilated cardiomyopathy. Am J Cardiol 58:143, 1986.

22. Lavine SJ, Krishnaswami V, Schreiner DP: Diastolic filling in left ventricular dysfunction. Int J Cardiol 8:423, 1985.

23. Appleton CP, Hatke LK, Popp RL: Demonstration of restrictive physiology by Doppler echocardiography. J Am Coll Cardiol 11:757, 1988.

24. Tyberg TL, Goodyear AVN, Hurst VW, et al: Left ventricular filling in differentiating restrictive amyloid cardiomyopathy and constrictive pericarditis. Am J Cardiol 47:791, 1981.

25. Yellin EL, Sonnenblick EH, Frater RWM: Dynamic determinants of left ventricular filling: An overview in cardiac dynamics. In: Baan J, Arntzenius AC, Yellin EL (eds): Cardiac Dynamics. Dordrecht, Netherlands, Martinus Nijhoff, p 145, 1980.

26. Lavine SJ, Held AC, Johnson V: Altered relation between diastolic pressure and flow in left ventricular dysfunction (abstract). Circulation 78(suppl II):115, 1988.

27. Lavine SJ, Campbell CA, Gunther SJ: Diastolic filling in acute left ventricular dysfunction: Role of the pericardium. J Am Coll Cardiol 12:1326, 1988.

28. Gillam LD, Homma S, Novick SS, et al: The influence of heart rate on Doppler mitral inflow patterns (abstract). Circulation 76(suppl IV):123, 1987.

29. Nishimura RA, Abel MD, Hatle LK, et al: Significance of Doppler indices of diastolic filling of the left ventricle: Comparison with invasive hemodynamics in a canine model. Am Heart J 118:1248, 1989.

30. Choong CY, Herrmann HC, Weyman AE, et al: Preload dependence of Doppler derived indexes of left ventricular diastolic function in humans. J Am Coll Cardiol 10:800, 1987.

31. Choong CY, Abascal VM, Thomas JD, et al; Combined influence of ventricular loading and relaxation on the transmitral flow velocity profile in dogs measured by Doppler echocardiography. Circulation 78:672, 1988.

32. Bonow RO, Bacharach SL, Green V, et al: Impaired left ventricular diastolic filling in patients with coronary artery disease; Assessment with radionuclide angiography. Circulation 64:315, 1981.

33. Lavine SJ, Follansbee WP, Shreiner DP, et al: Left ventricular diastolic filling in aortic stenosis. Am J Cardiol 57:1349, 1986.

34. Inouye I, Massie B, Loge D, et al: Abnormal left ventricular filling: An early finding in mild to moderate systemic hypertension. Am J Cardiol 53:120, 1984.

35. Hanrath P, Mathey DG, Siegert R, et al: Left ventricular relaxation and filling patterns in different forms of left ventricular hypertrophy: An echocardiographic study. Am J Cardiol 45:15, 1980.

36. Stewart S, Mason DT, Braunwald E: Impaired rate of left ventricular filling in idiopathic subaortic stenosis and valvular aortic stenosis. Circulation 37:8, 1968.

37. Rahko PS, Shaver JA, Salerni R, et al: Noninvasive evaluation of systolic and diastolic function in severe congestive heart failure secondary to coronary artery disease or idiopathic cardiomyopathy. Am J Cardiol 57:1315, 1986.

38. Feigenbaum H: Echocardiography. 3rd ed. Philadelphia, Lea & Febiger, 1981.

39. Lavine S, Tami L, Jawad I: Pattern of left ventricular diastolic filling associated with right ventricular enlargement. Am J Cardiol 62:444, 1988.

40. Helmcke F, Nanda NC, Hsiung MC, et al: Color Doppler assessment of mitral regurgitation with orthogonal planes. Circulation 75:175, 1987.

41. Baumgartner H, Kratzer H, Helmreich G, et al: Evaluation of aortic regurgitation by color coded two dimensional Doppler echocardiography. Usefulness of different jet parameters for quantification. Am J Noninvasive Cardiol 3:185, 1989.

42. Hatle L, Angelsen B: Doppler Ultrasound in cardiology. Physical principles and Clinical Applications. 2nd ed. Philadephia, Lea & Febiger, 1985.

43. Stamm BR, Martin RP: Quantification of pressure gradients across stenotic valves by Doppler ultrasound. J Am Coll Cardiol 2:707, 1984.

44. Berger M, Berdoff RL, Gallerstein PE, et al: Evaluation of aortic stenosis by continuous wave ultrasound. J Am Coll Cardiol 3:150, 1984.

45. Lima CO, Sahn DJ, Valdes-Cruz, et al: Prediction of the severity of left ventricular outflow tract obstruction by quantitative two-dimensional echocardiographic Doppler studies. Circulation 68:348, 1983.

46. Skjaerpe T, Hegrenaes L, Hatle L: Noninvasive estimation of valve area in patients with aortic stenosis by Doppler ultrasound and two dimensional echocardiography. Circulation 72:810, 1985.

47. Hatle L, Angelsen B, Tromsdal A: Noninvasive assessment of atrioventricular pressure half-time by Doppler ultrasound. Circulation 60:1096, 1979.

48. Thomas JD, Weyman AE: Fluid dynamics model of mitral valve flow: Description with in vitro validation. J Am Coll Cardiol 13:221, 1989.

49. Askenazi J, Koenigsberg DI, Ziegler JH, et al: Echocardiographic estimates of pulmonary artery wedge pressure. N Engl J Med 305:1566, 1981.

50. Lavine SJ, Held AC, Campbell CA, et al: The utility of echophocardiographic timing intervals for the prediction of left ventricular filling pressures. Am J Noninvasive Cardiol 3:249, 1989.

51. Lavine SJ: Left ventricular diastolic function in idiopathic cardiomyopathy: Doppler hemodynamic correlations. Echocardiography 8:151, 1991.

52. Lavine SJ, Arends D: Importance of left ventricular filling pressure on diastolic filling in idiopathic dilated cardiomyopathy. Am J Cardiol 64:61, 1989.

53. Lavine SJ, Arends D: Diastolic filling correlation of the third heart sounds. Am J Noninvasive Cardiol 14:233, 1989.

54. Ashkenazi J, Ahnberg DS, Korngold E, et al: Quantitative radionuclide angionuclide: Detection of and quantitation of left to right shunts. Am J Cardiol 37:382, 1976.

55. Valdez Cruz LM, Horowitz S, Mesel E, et al: A pulsed Doppler echocardiographic method for calculation of pulmonary and systemic flow: Accuracy in a canine model with ventricular septal defect. Circulation 68:597, 1983.

56. Stewart WJ, Jang L, Mich R, et al: Variable effect of change of flow rate through the aortic, pulmonary, and mitral valves on valve area and flow velocity; Impact on quantitative Doppler flow calculations. J Am Coll Cardiol 6:653, 1985.

57. Pollick C, Sullivan H, Cuzee B, et al: Doppler color flow imaging of shunt size in atrial septal defect. Circulation 78:522, 1988.

58. Adachi H, Kyo S, Takamoto S, et al: Early diagnosis and surgical intervention of acute aortic dissection by transesophageal color flow mapping. Circulation 82(suppl IV): 19, 1990.

59. Erbel R, Ensberding R, Daniel W, et al: Echocardiography in the diagnosis of aortic dissection. Lancet 1:457, 1989.

CHAPTER 97

Cardiac Assist Devices and Transplantation

Frank A. Baciewicz, Jr.
Timothy L. Hooper
Larry W. Stephenson

Acute myocardial failure with cardiogenic shock, not responsive to conventional medical therapy, is associated with a mortality approaching 100%.[1, 2] Certain subgroups of patients with cardiogenic shock can now benefit from short-term circulatory support, with the realistic prospect that myocardial recovery, corrective surgery, or transplantation will permit long-term survival. Severe chronic myocardial dysfunction (New York Heart Association class IV) is associated with 50% mortality at 1 year.[3] For this group of patients, although long-term mechanical assistance is a future goal, cardiac transplantation is currently the only accepted form of treatment.

CARDIAC ASSIST DEVICES
General Indications for Use
Cardiac Failure After Open Heart Surgery

Various factors contribute to the development of low cardiac output after open heart surgery, including poor myocardial preservation, intraoperative myocardial infarction, pre-existing myocardial dysfunction, and technical problems during the procedure. Inability to wean the patient from cardiopulmonary bypass despite inotropic therapy has been reported after 4 to 5% of all cardiac operations. The intra-aortic balloon pump (IABP) restores adequate cardiac output in 75 to 80% of cases,[4, 5] but if remaining patients are to be saved, more complete forms of cardiac assistance are needed to reverse the low-output state.

Graft Failure After Heart Transplantation

Postoperative graft dysfunction is the leading cause of early death after cardiac transplantation.[6] Causes of graft dysfunction include pre-existing cardiac dysfunction in the donor, poor graft preservation, high pulmonary vascular resistance in the recipient, and refractory acute or hyperacute rejection. Intra-aortic balloon pumping, often in conjunction with other forms of mechanical assistance, may allow functional recovery of the graft or time for an alternative organ to be sought.[7-9]

Bridge to Transplantation

Approximately 25% of patients awaiting transplantation die before a donor heart becomes available.[10] Clinical deterioration is often precipitous, and in these circumstances cardiac assist devices are increasingly being used to enable an appropriate organ to be found. More than half of such patients have successful transplantation with a survival rate approaching that of the elective procedure.[11]

Acute Myocardial Ischemia and Infarction

The role of assist devices in patients with acute myocardial ischemic complications is unclear. Although the IABP is sometimes useful in the short term for patients with unstable angina or infarction, aggressive medical and surgical interventions are usually more appropriate.[12-14] Use of the IABP has, however, been advocated in patients with postinfarction ventricular septal defects or acute mitral regurgitation to provide hemodynamic improvement before cardiac catheterization and surgical repair.[15]

Other mechanical assist devices may have a role in cardiogenic shock caused by myocardial infarction, but clinical experience in this area is limited. Percutaneous cannulation techniques currently enable rapid institution of circulatory support and thereby play a resuscitative role, for example, after failed angioplasty or massive pulmonary embolism.[16]

Patient Criteria

The decision to undertake circulatory assistance is guided by results of invasive hemodynamic measurements and the response to manipulation of such factors as preload, afterload, and inotropic therapy. Correction of clinical abnormalities that might prejudice myocardial function, such as hypoxia, acidosis, cardiac arrhythmias, and hypo- or hyperthermia, is important.[17-20]

Patients who already have severe liver failure, blood coagulopathy, or renal failure or have had neurologic damage as a result of cardiogenic shock would generally not be considered suitable candidates for mechanical assistance. Further contraindications include systemic disorders such as severe peripheral vascular disease, cerebrovascular disease, metastasis from carcinoma, and sepsis.[17, 21-25]

The precise hemodynamic indications for cardiac assistance are well defined and are outlined in Table 97–1.

TABLE 97–1

CRITERIA FOR INSERTION OF CARDIAC ASSIST DEVICES

Cardiac index < 2 L/min/m²
Systolic blood pressure < 90 mm Hg
Left and/or right atrial pressure > 20 mm Hg
Urine output < 20 mL/h (adults)
Systemic vascular resistance > 2100 dyne · s/cm⁵
Maximal pharmacologic and IABP support

Types of Devices Available
The Intra-Aortic Balloon Pump

The IABP is currently the most widely used form of circulatory assistance. The original concept of arterial counterpulsation has been credited to Clauss and coworkers,[26] although the use of an intra-aortic balloon to generate it was suggested by Moulopoulos and colleagues in 1962.[27] The IABP was first applied clinically by Kantrowitz and associates in 1968 to treat cardiogenic shock.[27a]

The IABP device consists of a balloon catheter and a pump console. The catheter has a polyurethane inflating segment that is positioned in the descending thoracic aorta, and the lumen of the catheter serves as a conduit for helium to be moved back and forth from the balloon to the drive console. The lumen may be a central lumen that permits angiography and aortic pressure monitoring, and it also enables a guidewire to be passed during insertion. The console is designed to deliver a specific volume of gas (carbon dioxide or helium) over a specified time interval, followed by rapid retrieval. The resulting balloon inflation and deflation are synchronized with the electrocardiogram (ECG) and can be adjusted to ensure that inflation occurs after aortic valve closure and deflation immediately before valve opening. In this way, diastolic pressure augmentation is achieved, thus increasing systemic and coronary perfusion and providing systolic unloading of the left ventricle (Fig. 97–1). As a result, both peak left ventricular pressure and myocardial oxygen consumption are decreased and cardiac output is increased.[28]

Contraindications for Use of the Intra-Aortic Balloon Pump. These depend to some extent on the situations in which the IABP is used, but the main contraindications are as follows:

1. The presence of severe occlusive iliac or femoral vascular disease resulting in lack of a vascular insertion site (unless the ascending aorta is being used)
2. Dissecting thoracic aortic aneurysm
3. Abdominal aortic aneurysm
4. Moderate-to-severe aortic regurgitation
5. Inability to use heparin anticoagulation
6. Uncontrolled tachyarrhythmias (inadequate time for effective inflation and deflation of the balloon)
7. Systemic sepsis
8. Severe coagulopathies

A further limitation to the use of the IABP is the presence of severely impaired cardiac function. A cardiac index greater than 1.2 L/min/m² is considered necessary to enable effective diastolic counterpulsation to be generated.

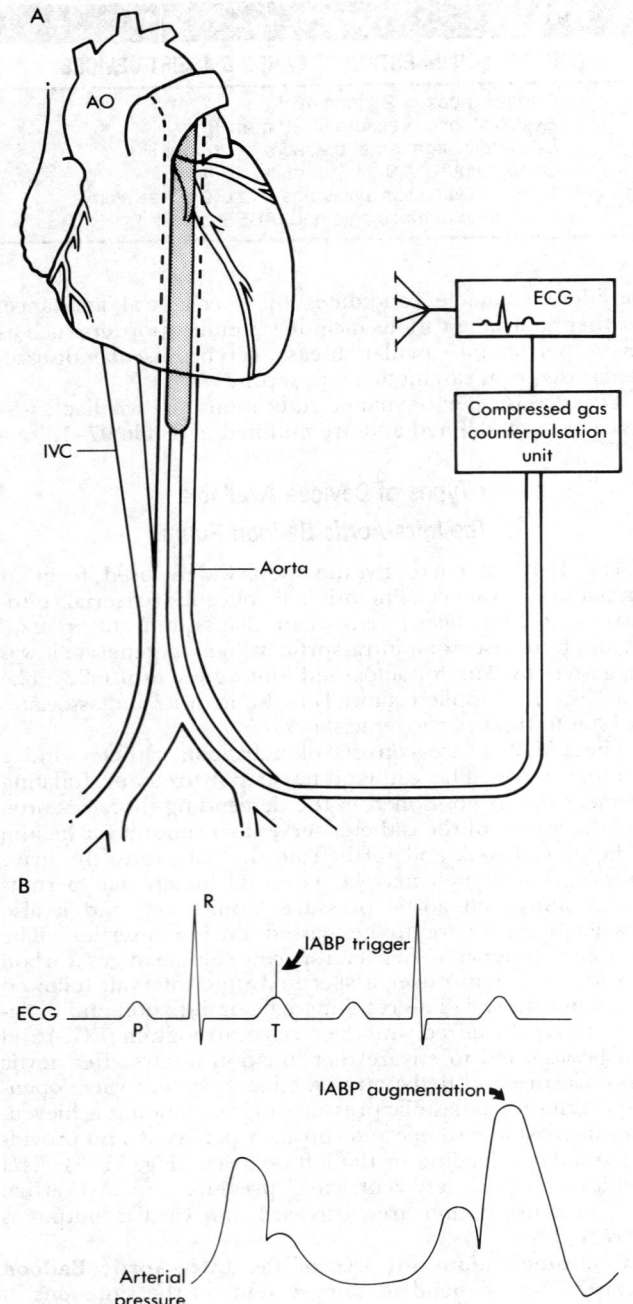

Figure 97–1. *A.* The usual position of an IABP in the descending thoracic aorta below the left subclavian artery. *B.* The IABP triggering from the T wave of the ECG and the resulting increase in diastolic pressure on the arterial pressure tracing. (From Mundth ED: Assisted circulation. In: Sabiston DC, Spencer FC [eds]: Surgery of the Chest, Volume II. 5th ed. Philadelphia, WB Saunders, p 1778, 1990.)

Methods of Insertion. The development and refinement of a relatively safe and effective percutaneous method for IABP catheter insertion, with or without a directing guidewire, have greatly expanded clinical use. Previously, surgical exposure of the femoral artery was required for insertion, and this remains the preferred approach in some institutions. The easier insertion with the percutaneous technique may, however, be associated with a greater incidence of vascular complications.[29]

The balloon is positioned in the proximal descending thoracic aorta, with the catheter tip lying just distal to the left subclavian origin. Satisfactory positioning is confirmed by chest x-ray study. The most commonly used site of insertion of the IABP catheter is the femoral artery. However, in approximately 5 to 10% of patients this approach is unsuccessful, because of tortuosity or occlusive disease of the iliac vessels.[5] In these circumstances, either the ascending aorta can be cannulated directly (during an open cardiac procedure) or alternative sites such as the iliac or axillary arteries may be used.[28]

Complications. Major complications resulting from use of the IABP occur in 4 to 17% of patients and are mostly vascular in nature.[5, 30] Thromboembolism may result in lower limb ischemia, and in up to 1% of cases this may be severe enough to necessitate fasciotomy or amputation. Occasionally, a femorofemoral crossover graft may preserve viability of an ischemic limb in a balloon-dependent patient. Other less common embolic sites include the spinal cord, kidney, and gut. To reduce the likelihood of thromboembolic complications, prophylactic administration of heparin is recommended. Major aortic dissection or aortoiliac perforation is a catastrophic complication, usually resulting in exsanguinating retroperitoneal hemorrhage.

Minor complications include superficial wound infections, bleeding at the site of insertion, and lymphoceles and seromas. They occur in up to 40% of patients.[5, 30] A significant late complication is false aneurysm formation, usually related to previous wound infection.

Overall Results. Failure to wean from cardiopulmonary bypass remains the major indication for the use of the IABP. Successful reversal of the cardiac impairment depends on the nature of the injury and the promptness of IABP intervention.

Reports suggest that patients with left ventricular hypertrophy and an identifiable intraoperative ischemic event are most likely to have a successful outcome with IABP support alone.[5] Patients undergoing isolated coronary procedures fare better than those with pure valvular disease or those with combined coronary and valvular disease.[31]

Approximately 75 to 80% of patients are successfully weaned from bypass with the aid of the IABP and have an overall survival rate of about 50%.[4, 5] Late follow-up of survivors has revealed excellent symptomatic relief and functional status.[32]

Use of balloon counterpulsation in relation to the pulmonary artery has been shown to improve right ventricular ejection, but in the context of postoperative right ventricular failure the device has not proved to be as beneficial as in left-sided heart dysfunction[33] and alternative forms of mechanical assistance are preferred.

Use of the IABP in cardiogenic shock resulting from myocardial infarction may achieve temporary reversal in 75% of patients, but survival is not improved.[28] However, such an intervention may permit time for evaluation of patients with a complicating septal perforation or acute mitral regurgitation before urgent surgery.

The Hemopump

One of the newest forms of cardiac assist is the Hemopump. This device consists of an intra-arterial catheter with a terminal rotating impeller that is placed across the aortic valve.[34] The pump impeller spins at 15,000 to 27,000 rpm and withdraws blood from the left ventricular cavity and propels it into the aorta at flow rates up to 4.0 L/min (Fig. 97–2).

The Hemopump is undergoing clinical trials, and preliminary findings are encouraging. One advantage of the device

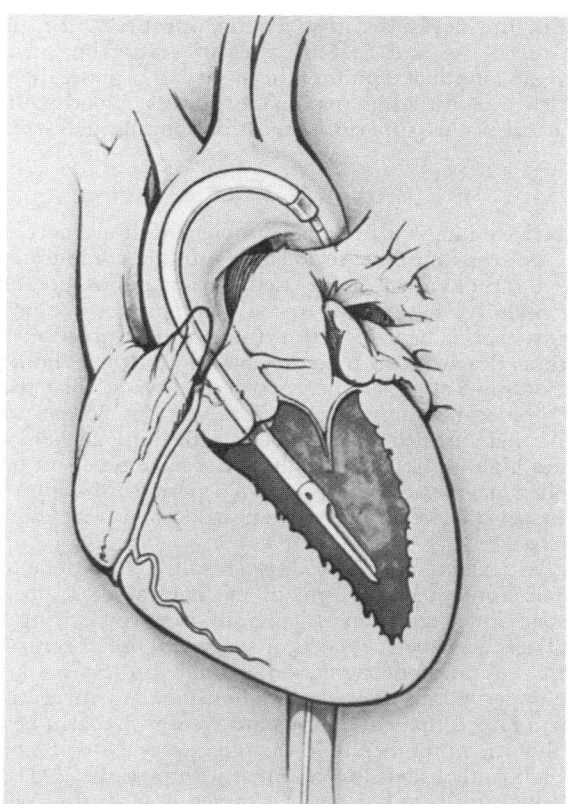

Figure 97–2. Position of the Hemopump within the left ventricular cavity. (From Frazier OH, Wampler RK, Duncan JM, et al: First human use of the Hemopump, a catheter-mounted ventricular assist device. Reprinted with permission from the Society of Thoracic Surgeons [The Annals of Thoracic Surgery, 1990, Vol 49, pages 299–304].)

is that, like the IABP, it can be introduced via a femoral artery cutdown. However, unlike the IABP, the Hemopump does not require a degree of residual ventricular function to provide effective circulatory assistance. Indications for use have included failure to wean from cardiopulmonary bypass, myocardial infarction, severe cardiac allograft rejection, and donor heart failure.

Complications. In the limited clinical experience so far, complications related to use of the Hemopump have been minimal.[35] There have been no evidence of valvular or vascular injury and no thromboembolic problems. Hemolysis related to high pump speeds is of potential concern, particularly if the device is used for prolonged periods, but has not been an important consideration to date.

Results. The initial clinical experience with a group of seven patients with cardiogenic shock, four of whom had not responded to IABP counterpulsation, has been reported.[35] Consistent and effective circulatory support has been achieved for up to 113 hours, and preliminary results indicate an outcome comparable to that with other forms of cardiac assistance. The precise indications and device-related complications will be refined with expanding use.

Ventricular Assist Devices

These devices are usually classified according to the characteristics of the flow they provide—pulsatile or nonpulsatile. They may be used individually to provide left or right ventricular support or in combination to accomplish biventricular assist.

Nonpulsatile Ventricular Assist Devices. Ventricular as-

sist devices (VADs) direct at least part of the intracardiac flow through the device itself. Nonpulsatile systems include roller pumps and centrifugal pumps and necessarily involve extracorporeal circulation.

Roller Pumps Versus Centrifugal Pumps. Roller pumps are the simplest and least expensive forms of cardiac assist devices and are commonly used for cardiopulmonary bypass during conventional open heart surgery. The pump heads are occlusive, with the result that dangerously high afterload pressures and line disruption are potential hazards.[36] The additional risk of gaseous embolization at low preloads necessitates the use of a blood reservoir. Blood trauma may be considerable with these devices, and this tends to restrict their use to the provision of short periods (24 to 48 hours) of support.

Centrifugal pumps have a cone-shaped head that is rotated magnetically and use centrifugal force to move blood through a vortex pump head (Fig. 97–3). Because it is nonocclusive, the pump does not cause major line pressure changes, and it is associated with significantly fewer gaseous emboli than the roller pump.[36] Better blood-handling characteristics allow longer periods of circulatory support (up to 1 week).[37, 38]

For left-sided heart assist, usually the left atrium is cannulated to provide inflow to the pump, with return to the aorta or femoral artery. For right-sided heart support, the right atrium and pulmonary artery are used. By cannulating a major artery and vein and using a membrane oxygenator, a degree of biventricular support is achieved (extracorporeal membrane oxygenation).

Pulsatile Ventricular Assist Devices. Nonpulsatile flow, being nonphysiologic, may contribute to the deterioration in end-organ function seen with prolonged use. Several types of pulsatile VADs have been developed, and they are broadly classified into pneumatically and electrically driven systems.

Pneumatically Driven Ventricular Assist Devices. The most commonly used device of this type is the Pierce-Donachy pump (Fig. 97–4). Typically these devices consist of a flexible polyurethane blood sac enclosed in a rigid chamber. More recent models have a sac with a textured inner surface designed to promote the formation of a pseudointimal lining, which is thought to enhance thromboresistance. Inlet and outlet ports are valved, using either mechanical tilting-disk valves or porcine valves. Pulsatile flow is generated by

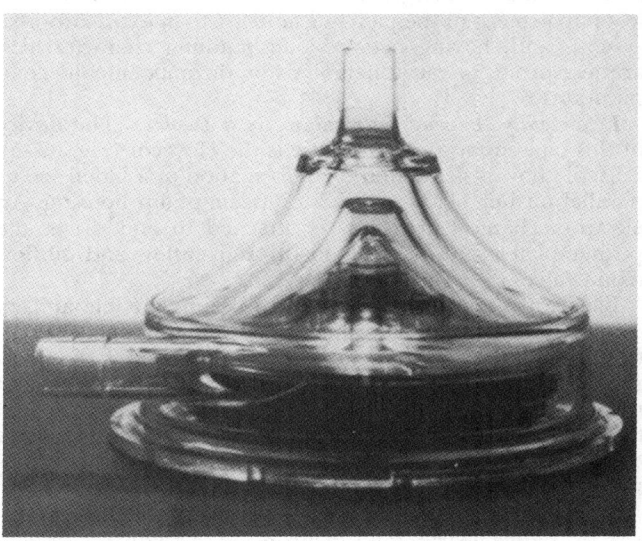

Figure 97–3. Example of a centrifugal pump. (Courtesy of Biomedicus, Inc., Minnetonka, MN.)

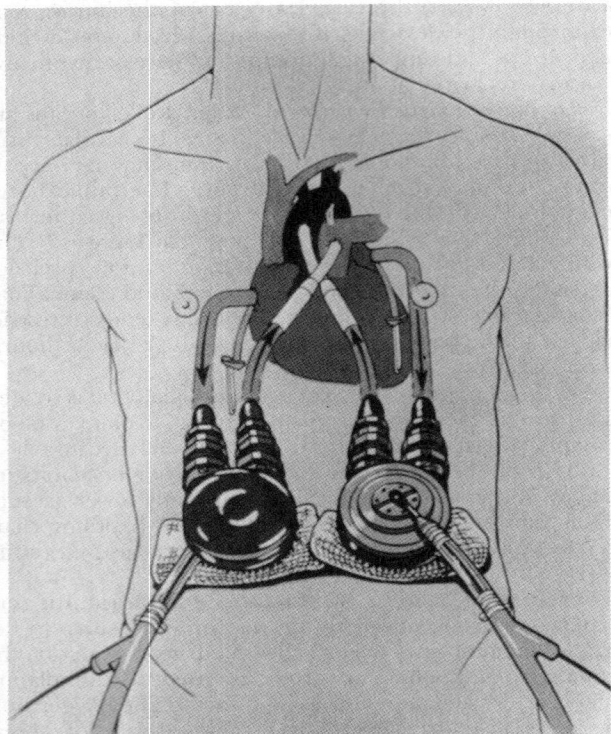

Figure 97–4. Example of the Pierce-Donachy pump. (From Pennington OG, McBride LR, Swartz MT, et al: Use of the Pierce-Donachy ventricular assist device in patients with cardiogenic shock. Reprinted with permission from the Society of Thoracic Surgeons [The Annals of Thoracic Surgery, 1989, Vol 47, pages 130–135].)

compression of the blood sac by gas pulses directed by a hose into the rigid case. Transcutaneous tubing is necessary for connection to the device, which is usually placed on the anterior abdominal wall.

Cannulation techniques used are generally similar to those for nonpulsatile devices, but the left ventricular apex has also been used for left-sided heart assist.

Additional advantages of these devices are that they cause less impairment of the patient's mobility than extracorporeal systems and, having better blood-handling characteristics, are less prone to cause hemolysis or thromboembolic complications.[23]

Electrically Driven Ventricular Assist Devices. The device of this type in most common use is the Novacor (Fig. 97–5). Pulsatile flow is generated by deformation of a blood sac by parallel pusher plates within a cylindric pump housing. An electromechanical armature is attached to and drives the pusher plates, pumping blood through inflow and outflow tissue valves.

Electrical pumps are designed to be implantable and, in conjunction with an experimental power source, are prototypes for future permanent nontethered systems. For current temporary use, an external power line is brought out through the skin. Inflow and outflow cannulas are sutured to the ventricular apex and the thoracic aorta and traverse the diaphragm to reach the pump, which is usually implanted preperitoneally in the abdomen.

Unlike other VADs, this device does not pump in parallel with the native heart but is synchronized to fill during systole, thus directly reducing left ventricular afterload. Disadvan-

tages of the device are that it is inappropriate for left or right atrial use and that in cases of severe biventricular failure an alternative pump is necessary to support the right ventricle. As with the pneumatic devices, blood-handling characteristics are superior to those of nonpulsatile systems.[39]

Complications

Blood trauma is a potential problem with all mechanical assist devices, and the seriousness of this complication is related to the type of device used. Roller pumps, because of their occlusive nature, are particularly prone to cause hemolysis, especially at high flow rates, and in practice this is a serious drawback to their use beyond 24 to 48 hours. In contrast, clinical experience has demonstrated that the superior blood-handling characteristics of centrifugal pumps enable their use for up to a week with minimal hemolysis, even at high flows.[37, 38] Pulsatile VADs have excellent blood-handling properties, and prolonged periods of support for up to several weeks have been associated with minimal hemolysis.[23, 39]

Blood-surface interactions may result in thromboembolic complications with all forms of mechanical assistance, and systemic anticoagulation is generally required during their use. There have been reports of successful use of centrifugal pumps without anticoagulation,[36, 38] but thrombus is known to be deposited inside the pump housing, and currently it is recommended that continuous intravenous heparin be used and that the pump heads be changed every 24 to 48 hours.[40] Thromboembolism is less common with pulsatile VADs, and currently anticoagulation is necessary only during periods of low flow (less than 3 L/min) or for periods of support exceeding 1 week.[23, 41]

Bleeding is an important cause of morbidity whatever the indication and regardless of the type of VAD used. It may be related to defective coagulation caused by prolonged cardiopulmonary bypass or to adverse effects on platelets and coagulation factors associated with any prolonged extracorporeal circulation.[42, 43] The hemorrhagic tendency is aggravated by the requirement for systemic anticoagulation during use of these devices.

Sepsis is a potentially serious complication because patients supported by a VAD have transcutaneous pump cannulas, providing portals of entry for deep tissue or systemic infec-

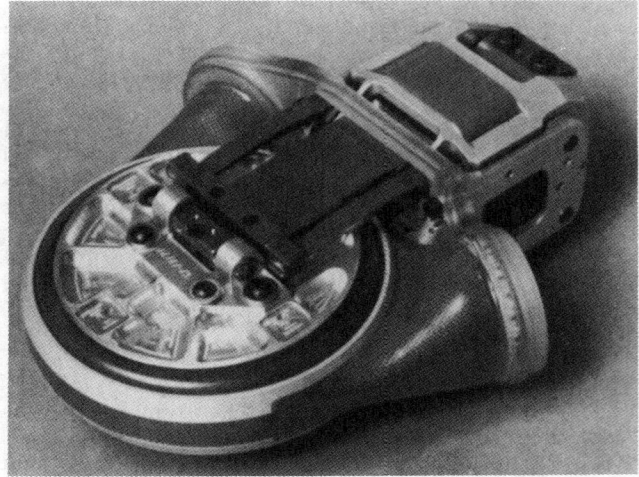

Figure 97–5. Example of an electrically driven ventricular assist device, the Novacor. (Courtesy of Biomedicus, Inc., Minnetonka, MN.)

tion. Transplant patients are at particular risk because their normal immune mechanisms are suppressed.[44] Protracted intensive care, invasive monitoring, and mechanical ventilation all tend to increase the risk of infection.

Multiple organ system failure is the major cause of death in nonsurvivors and is usually attributed to a prolonged period of low cardiac output before institution of mechanical support.[40, 44] Rapid recognition of candidates for cardiac assistance is important in minimizing end-organ damage.

Results

Resuscitation. The use of femorofemoral extracorporeal membrane oxygenation has permitted rapid resuscitation of patients with cardiogenic shock. Both percutaneous[16] and cutdown methods[45] have been described for femoral cannulation, and both roller and centrifugal pumps have been used. Extracorporeal membrane oxygenation systems have generally proved ineffective for periods of support exceeding 48 hours but may allow time for further evaluation of the patient.

Failure to Wean from Cardiopulmonary Bypass. Successful left ventricular assist has been achieved with the roller pump for periods up to 96 hours, with 40% of patients being weaned from support and 30% ultimately discharged.[46] Severe coagulopathy, sepsis, and multiple organ system failure have been major complications in nonsurvivors.

Similar results have been reported with the centrifugal pumps[24, 36, 37] and the pulsatile assist devices,[23, 40] with approximately one third of patients being saved. The long-term outlook for hospital survivors is favorable, with one half to two thirds of patients being in New York Heart Association functional class I or II.[40, 47, 48]

Donor Graft Failure After Heart Transplantation. This eventuality is associated with high mortality, but experience with the use of various types of VADs has increased and there have been isolated reports of successful recovery of graft dysfunction.[7-9]

Bridge to Transplantation. Centrifugal pumps have been used successfully to support candidates for transplantation, generally for short periods (less than 1 week),[49] although support for up to 30 days has been reported.[50] Pulsatile devices have consistently allowed support for longer periods (up to 3 months).[51, 52] More than half of the patients have successful transplantation and two thirds of these are ultimately discharged from the hospital. Long-term survival after transplantation is not quite as good if preoperative support was necessary, but those requiring only univentricular support fare better. The type of VAD used does not appear to influence outcome.[11]

Total Artificial Heart

An orthotopic biventricular replacement prosthesis, the so-called artificial heart, is generally used only as a bridge to transplantation because it requires removal of both native ventricles. Continuous anticoagulation and antiplatelet drugs are required, but prolonged use is still associated with an appreciable incidence of thromboembolic complications.[53] There is also a significant risk of mediastinitis, which contributes to results after transplantation that are inferior to those achieved with other assist devices.[11]

CARDIAC TRANSPLANTATION
Indications for Cardiac Transplantation

Patients with severe myocardial dysfunction, in New York Heart Association functional classes III and IV, despite maximal medical therapy, are potential candidates for transplantation.[10, 54, 55] Patients with acute cardiogenic shock who cannot be weaned from mechanical assist devices may also be considered candidates for transplantation.[56-59] Severe, intractable ventricular arrhythmias are a less common indication, particularly with the advent of the automatic internal cardioverter-defibrillator.

Contraindications to transplantation are relative and continue to be modified with increasing experience. In general, the patient should be 65 years of age or younger and should not have severe renal dysfunction, liver failure, coagulation abnormalities, or central nervous system damage. Severe cerebrovascular or peripheral vascular disease, active infections, or malignancy would preclude transplantation. The patient should have negative results on the tuberculin (purified protein derivative) test, should be seronegative for human immunodeficiency virus, and should not be obese (weighing 20% more than estimated ideal body weight).

Diabetes mellitus, even insulin dependent, is no longer considered an absolute contraindication, but there should not be evidence of severe end-organ damage, such as retinal, renal, peripheral vascular, or neuropathic changes. Severe chronic obstructive pulmonary disease, recent pulmonary infarction, active peptic ulcer disease, or other systemic diseases such as amyloidosis or systemic lupus erythematosus are generally accepted contraindications. The patient should have no recent history of alcohol, smoking, or drug abuse and should be judged to be someone who will comply with the strict medical regimen and follow-up required after transplantation.[54, 60]

If these criteria are satisfied, the patient must have an evaluation of pulmonary vascular resistance. This is the most important factor in determining suitability for orthotopic cardiac transplantation. The pulmonary arterial pressures and pulmonary vascular resistance are commonly elevated in end-stage heart failure because of passive back-up of blood from the failing myocardium.

Pulmonary vascular resistance may be determined by use of an indwelling pulmonary arterial catheter (Swan-Ganz) by subtracting the pulmonary capillary wedge pressure from the mean pulmonary arterial pressure and dividing the result by the cardiac output. This provides pulmonary vascular resistance in Wood units, the normal value being 1 to 2 Wood units. If the pulmonary vascular resistance is significantly elevated, the transplanted heart's right ventricle, which is not accustomed to pumping blood against a high pulmonary resistance, may fail acutely.

If the pulmonary vascular resistance is greater than 3 to 4 Wood units preoperatively, attempts are made to determine whether the elevated pulmonary vascular resistance is reversible by using a vasodilator such as intravenous dobutamine, prostaglandin E_1 or I_2, nitroglycerin, or amrinone. Successful reversal to below 3 Wood units indicates suitability for orthotopic transplantation.

In the acute situation, the pulmonary vascular resistance is usually reactive, responds to pulmonary vasodilators preoperatively and in the operating room, and reverts to normal in the months after transplantation. Hence, a well-preserved donor heart can overcome the elevation of pulmonary vascular resistance. A patient in end-stage heart failure over a protracted period may manifest a fixed, elevated pulmonary vascular resistance that is not responsive to these interventions. It is important that potential recipients awaiting heart transplantation receive repeated right-sided heart catheterization, perhaps twice a year, to ensure that pulmonary vascular resistance has not increased above 3 to 4 Wood units. Irreversible elevation of resistance above this level has been considered an indication for combined heart-lung or heart–single lung transplantation.[54, 60-64]

A more recent option is an orthotopic transplantation

using the heart from a heart-lung recipient (the so-called domino procedure), in whom the presence of pre-existing pulmonary hypertension has resulted in a degree of right ventricular hypertrophy. Such a heart is adapted to an elevated pulmonary vascular resistance.

Donor Selection

Patients with brain death because of trauma, intracranial hemorrhage, or drowning are potential cardiac donors. Criteria for establishment of brain death vary from state to state, and the criteria that apply in one's hospital should be known.

For the determination of brain death, five criteria are usually required: (1) absence of responsiveness to stimulation, with neither spontaneous nor involuntary movement, (2) apnea, (3) absence of brain stem reflexes, (4) exclusion of reversible causes of coma such as hypothermia and drug overdose, and (5) no change in the findings over 12 hours.[65] The usual supporting tests are two electroencephalograms done 12 hours apart and showing no brain activity. Another corroborative test is a brain scan with no evidence of blood flow. Interpretation of the electroencephalogram or brain scan requires two qualified physicians who are not directly associated with the heart transplantation team.[65-68]

In addition to satisfaction of brain death criteria, consent for donation must be obtained from the potential donor's family. In several states, holders of motor vehicle licenses can declare on the license that in the event of brain death they wish to donate their organs and/or tissue. To avoid legal difficulties, if the brain-dead patient had expressed a wish to donate his or her organs (via motor vehicle license or will) and the family opposed it, states have required family consent for donation. Several states have instituted a required request law, according to which the physician declaring death must request or discuss potential donation with the family. These laws have not increased the number of donors.

When the donor is declared brain dead and the family has agreed to donation, several criteria must be satisfied. It is desirable for the donor's age to be less than 40 years for males and less than 45 years for females. Previously, only young donors were used to minimize the possibility of pre-existing coronary artery disease. As the number of candidates awaiting heart transplantation and the number of cardiac transplant centers have increased, the age restriction has been eased, and donors less than 50 years old are considered. However, close attention is given to a donor's history of hypertension, diabetes, smoking, family history of heart disease, and abnormalities of cholesterol and triglyceride blood values if available. It is important to avoid using a graft with significant coronary artery disease because this may aggravate accelerated graft atherosclerosis, the most significant factor limiting long-term survival. Accelerated graft atherosclerosis has been reported to occur in more than 30% of transplant recipients after the first 3 years.[69] Studies have shown a significant increase in the development of coronary atherosclerosis with grafts from donors more than 35 years of age,[55] and screening before selection of a donor heart is important. Our practice is to use older grafts for older recipients or for recipients in desperate need of an organ.

It would be ideal to evaluate the donor heart by coronary angiography to rule out the presence of coronary disease, but this is not possible at all donor hospitals and transport of a donor to an institution with catheterization facilities is not feasible.[68, 70] The logistic constraints of coordinating donor and recipient procedures at distant hospitals make scheduling of angiography impossible.

In addition to the age requirement and the absence of a history of pre-existing cardiac disease, the donor should not have had a prolonged cardiac arrest. A brief cardiac arrest (several minutes) associated with good cardiopulmonary resuscitation and a stable circulation afterward may not exclude the heart for donation. The potential donor should have no history of either blunt (as this may cause a myocardial contusion) or penetrating chest trauma. There should be no history of intracardiac injections, and no evidence of sepsis or lengthy resuscitation with high-dose inotropic support.[68, 70, 71]

The usual evaluation of the donor starts with a brief clinical history including the mechanism of death. Physical examination includes cardiac auscultation to ensure that there are no murmurs. The patient's height and weight are recorded, as are the vital signs. The presence of chest tubes, rib or sternal fractures secondary to trauma, and current inotropic doses are also recorded.

An ECG is necessary to rule out ischemic damage or previous myocardial infarction. This ECG may show nonspecific ST or T wave changes that may be related to brain injury, such as intracranial hemorrhage.[72] An echocardiogram may be needed to assess left ventricular wall function and identify segmental wall dyskinesia if the ECG is abnormal. The echocardiogram is also helpful in checking for a myocardial contusion after chest trauma. It is advantageous to have a cardiologist at the donor's hospital inspect the echocardiogram and report to the transplant surgeon as to the suitability of the organ. Determination of cardiac enzyme levels may also be useful in ruling out myocardial injury.

Arterial blood gases should be analyzed to ensure that the heart is well oxygenated, and a chest x-ray study may be helpful in determining underlying reasons for hypoxia, including pneumothorax or infection. Serum tests, which are necessary within 6 hours of cardiac harvesting, include human immunodeficiency virus status, cytomegalovirus titers, hepatitis B and C screen, and an antibody test for syphilis.

The patient must be examined thoroughly for evidence of sepsis before obtaining the donor heart. An elevated white blood cell count may be related to central nervous system injuries and does not rule the patient out as a potential donor. However, an elevated white blood cell count must be investigated and a potential source of infection identified. Blood cultures, urine, and sputum cultures are obtained routinely. A series from the Texas Heart Institute showed similar short-term outcome for donor hearts obtained from infected donors who were carefully selected and treated with antibiotics before use of the heart in a recipient. These hearts were often used in patients who were rapidly deteriorating and could not wait for an "optimal" organ.[73]

If all these criteria are met, the brain-dead patient is an acceptable donor for a patient with an ABO compatible blood type whose weight is within 20% of the donor's weight. In addition, if the recipient's serum reacts with more than 15% of the serum from a randomly selected panel of donors, a prospective lymphocytotoxic cross-match of recipient serum and donor lymphocytes must be performed to exclude the presence of preformed antibodies. Preformed antibodies might generate hyperacute rejection of the transplanted heart. For the lymphocytotoxic cross-match, serum from the recipient must be kept in a central bank to which a sample of donor blood can be sent for testing to minimize delays. The cross-match is usually performed only for patients within a state's boundaries by that state's organ procurement center. When hearts are procured across state lines or in different areas of the country, this facility may not be available, in which case the transplant team must balance the decision to perform the transplantation with the status of the potential recipient.

The matching of a donor to a potential recipient is usually done by a state or regional organ procurement agency. The recipients are listed by blood type and weight range, and the donor is matched to potential recipients by blood type and weight. The severity of the hemodynamic condition and time on the waiting list are the most important factors in allocating the heart to a specific recipient.

Donor Management

After the donor has met the stringent criteria for donation, the heart must be carefully managed to ensure good function after transplantation. The management of the donor is shared by the organ procurement team in consultation with the intensive care unit staff at the donor hospital. With impending brain death, there are usually several effects on the autonomic nervous system. The initial systemic response to increased intracranial pressure, cerebral injury, hemorrhage, or herniation is an increase in sympathetic discharge, an increase in systemic vascular resistance, and hypertension. Hypertension can be controlled with nitroprusside.[74–76]

When brain death occurs, systemic blood pressure usually falls because of the loss of sympathetic tone and the dilatation of both arteriolar and venous capacitance vessels. Volume replacement is the treatment of choice to restore appropriate filling pressures. During this period of fluid resuscitation, a central venous catheter is a good adjunct, as it enables trends to be followed. Overhydration can cause pulmonary edema and hypoxia, which leads to cardiac dysfunction. The fluid used in resuscitation is usually lactated Ringer's solution, although colloids such as albumin may also be used to restore adequate filling pressures. After adequate fluid resuscitation, systolic blood pressure should be maintained between 90 and 140 mm Hg, which is usually indicated by a central venous pressure between 12 and 18 cm H_2O. If the patient is still hypotensive after volume resuscitation, infusion of 500 mg of dopamine in 500 mL of 5% dextrose should be started to increase the systemic vascular resistance, heart rate, and contractility and to increase the systolic blood pressure to at least 90 mm Hg. Efforts are usually made to maintain the dopamine at less than 10 μg/kg/min because higher dosages may result in graft dysfunction after transplantation.

It is also important to keep the urine output equal to or greater than 1 mL/kg/h. A Foley catheter should be inserted in all potential donors to manage the urine output.

Metabolic acidosis should be treated with intravenous bicarbonate, and the fraction of inspired oxygen, tidal volume, and ventilatory rate should be adjusted to maintain PaO_2 greater than 80 mm Hg and $PaCO_2$ between 30 and 40 mm Hg. Most patients who are on a neurosurgical or neurologic service have $PaCO_2$ maintained below 30 mm Hg to decrease cerebral edema. The hematocrit should be kept greater than 30% and the hemoglobin greater than 10 g/dL, and the donor should be kept at a core temperature of 35°C or higher with a warming blanket.

Donors usually have decreased production of arginine vasopressin, which causes an increase in serum sodium concentration and inappropriately high urine output. This state of diabetes insipidus can be corrected by fluid replacement with 5% dextrose and the use of vasopressin (Pitressin). Twenty units of vasopressin in 1 L of 5% dextrose is titrated to maintain a urine output of about 100 mL/h. The suggested initial dose is 0.8 to 1.0 U/h. Potassium levels must be checked frequently, in view of the excessive urine output and large volumes of fluid being infused.

Thyroid hormone replacement has been proposed for management of the donor. In animal models of brain death, thyroid hormone levels have been reported to fall to 50% of control values within 1 hour while the level of thyroid-stimulating hormone remained unchanged. Novitsky and colleagues suggested that supplementation of thyroid hormone levels may prevent hemodynamic deterioration in the donors and improve graft function after transplantation.[76–78] This view is controversial. Studies by Gifford and coworkers[79] and Macoviak and coworkers[80] have not demonstrated that donor hearts with low thyroxine and triiodothyronine levels at the time of transplantation exhibited worse cardiac function or required more inotropic support postoperatively.

Technique of Cardiac Harvesting

The goal of cardiac harvesting is to remove a hemodynamically stable heart, preserve the heart well, and then implant it less than 4 hours after it is harvested. Ischemic times in excess of 4 hours have been shown to result in worse cardiac function and an increased 30-day mortality.[81]

The procurement takes place in the operating room. The hemodynamics are managed by an anesthesiologist, and there should be a team including operating room and circulating nurses. The procurement team usually comprises one or two surgeons and nurse or organ procurement personnel to infuse the cardioplegic solution.

After the patient has been prepared and draped in a sterile fashion, the sternum is opened using an electric saw if available. If not, a Leischke knife can be used to divide the sternum. The pericardium is then opened, and the superior vena cava, aorta, and inferior cava are dissected from their pericardial attachments. The function of the myocardium is observed to ensure that it agrees with the ECG and echocardiographic data. The aorta and left atrium can be palpated for thrills, indicative of valvular disease, and the coronary arteries examined to ensure that there is no obvious atherosclerotic vascular disease. The myocardium is also observed for hematoma or contusion, which may be a result of blunt chest trauma or periods of cardiopulmonary resuscitation.

If the heart appears to be a suitable organ for harvesting, the teams harvesting the liver, kidney, and lungs are consulted and the method and sequence for excision of the organs are coordinated.

When the time arrives for cardiac harvesting, a cardioplegic catheter is placed in the ascending aorta and attached to the cardioplegic solution. Our institution uses 1 L of 5% dextrose to which 12.5 g of mannitol, 25 mEq of bicarbonate, and 15 mEq of potassium chloride have been added. The patient is then given heparin 300 U/kg, and any central venous catheters that may enter the superior vena cava are withdrawn into the jugular vein. After time is allowed for the heparin to circulate, the superior vena cava is interrupted with a stapling device and the inferior vena cava is transected usually 1 cm above the diaphragm to allow the team harvesting the liver a cuff for the vena caval anastomosis. This inflow occlusion permits the heart to empty after several beats, after which the aortic cross-clamp is placed and infusion of the cardioplegic solution commenced. Simultaneously, the right superior pulmonary vein is transected to decompress the left side of the heart, thus minimizing the risk of myocardial distention. If the lungs are also being harvested, the left side of the heart is alternatively vented by transecting the left atrial appendage rather than the right superior pulmonary vein. While the cardioplegic solution is being infused, the heart is topically cooled with iced saline slush. The aortic root is palpated to make sure that the cardioplegic solution is distending the aortic root and the aortic valve has not been rendered incompetent. Shortly after beginning infusion of the cardioplegic solution and immersion of the heart in iced slush, the ECG should become isoelectric and ventilation can be discontinued.

After the cardioplegic solution has been instilled, the pericardium should be aspirated until dry and the heart removed from the pericardium. This is done by transecting the four pulmonary veins, the pulmonary artery at the bifurcation, and the aorta proximal to the innominate artery (Fig. 97–6).

The excised heart is moved to an adjacent sterile table, and the right atrium is opened to the left of the atrial appendage to allow visualization of the atrial septum and ensure that there is no atrial septal defect. Care should be taken not to touch the area of the sinus node to prevent post-transplantation arrhythmias. The tricuspid and mitral valves are also inspected. The soft tissue between the aorta and pulmonary artery is divided, and the tissue between the four pulmonary veins is transected to ready the heart for transplantation (Fig. 97–7).

The heart is then placed in cold lactated Ringer's solution in a sterile plastic bag. This is placed in a second and a third sterile plastic bag and finally placed in a sealed ice chest. The heart is then transferred to the home institution, where the recipient is being readied for transplantation.[82–84]

Technique for Cardiac Transplantation

Recipients are given antibiotic prophylaxis with a cephalosporin and preoperative immunosuppression including azathioprine at 4 mg/kg intravenously and, if their renal status is stable, cyclosporine at 5 mg/kg orally. In addition, they have 10 U of cross-matched packed red blood cells, 8 U of platelet concentrate, and 4 U of fresh frozen plasma. If the patient has received warfarin (Coumadin) therapy preoperatively, fresh frozen plasma is administered preoperatively, together with 20 mg of vitamin K to restore coagulation.

When the donor heart has been deemed acceptable for cardiac transplantation, the recipient's operation at the home institution is begun. Frequently, the patient has had previous open heart operations and is in precarious hemodynamic balance. Consequently, the reopening of the sternum and further dissection must be done carefully.

Before general anesthesia, the patient has an internal jugular catheter placed, usually through the right internal jugular vein, with subsequent pulmonary arterial (Swan-Ganz) catheter placement. A radial arterial catheter is also introduced to monitor blood pressure. By continually monitoring mixed venous oxygen saturation and cardiac output by using the thermodilution catheter, the hemodynamic management of the recipient is simplified.

A midline sternotomy incision is used. If the procedure is a reoperation, the heart is then dissected carefully out from adhesions. If it is an initial cardiac procedure, the pericardium can be opened without the difficulty of taking down adhesions between the heart, sternum, and pericardium. When the aorta and superior and inferior venae cavae have been dissected free, intravenous heparin can be given and the aortic and vena caval cannulas placed.

If the patient has been hemodynamically unstable, cardiopulmonary bypass can be started at this juncture. This may also simplify division of adhesions if they have proved difficult to deal with. Ideally, however, attempts should be made to delay cardiopulmonary bypass until the donor heart has arrived at the home institution because prolonged cardiopulmonary bypass may result in serious postoperative bleeding (especially in patients who have received preoperative warfarin) and pulmonary and renal dysfunction.

The heart is then excised, beginning at the right atrioventricular junction. This incision is carried down into the coronary sinus and anteriorly to the level of the right atrial appendage. The pulmonary artery and aorta are transected above the valves. The left atrium is entered just posterior to the aortic valve (Fig. 97–8). The left atrium is then excised just posterior to the atrial appendage laterally and medially to the level of the atrial septum. The right and left ventricles are then excised, leaving generous atrial cuffs. In brief, a biventriculectomy is performed. The accompanying diagram

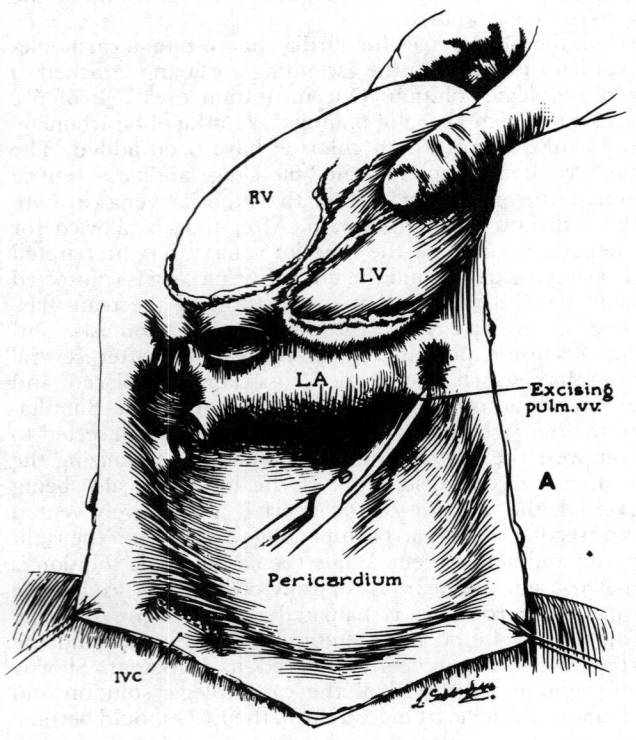
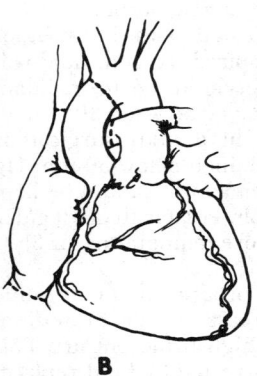

Figure 97–6. *A.* Division of the pulmonary veins at the pericardial reflection. *B.* Lines of division of the pulmonary artery and aorta. (From Baumgartner WA: Operative techniques utilized in heart transplantation. In: Baumgartner WA, Reitz BA, Achuff SC [eds]: Heart and Heart-Lung Transplantation. Philadelphia, WB Saunders, p 113, 1990.)

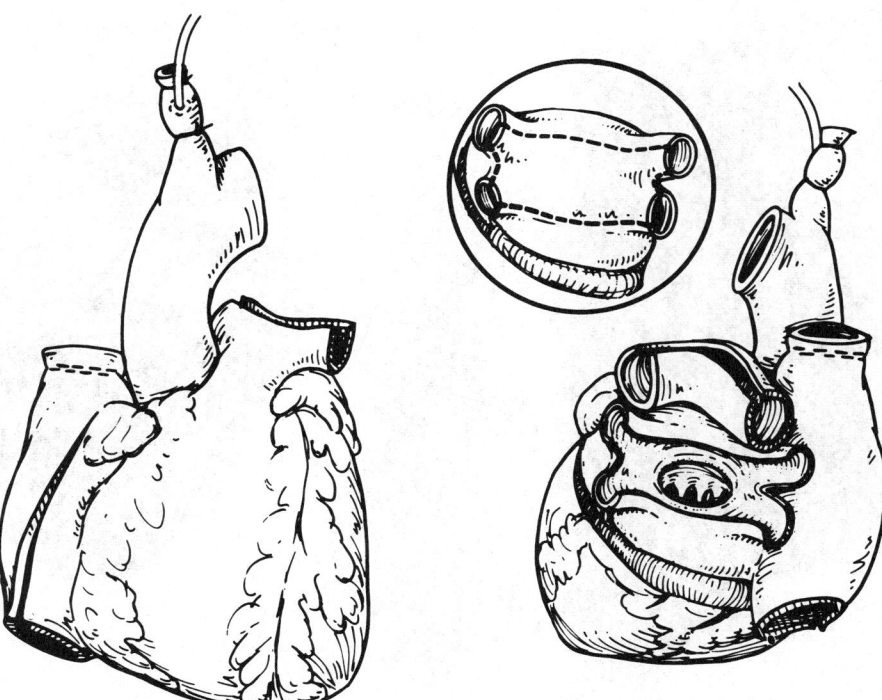

Figure 97–7. Opening of the atria in preparation for reimplantation. (From Fragomeni LS, Rogers G, Kaye MP: Donor identification and organ procurement for cardiac transplantation. Cardiovasc Clin 20:121, 1990.)

shows what remains in the pericardium after excision of the recipient's heart (Fig. 97–9).

The donor heart is then removed from its sterile container. The donor and recipient atria, pulmonary arteries, and aortas are trimmed to appropriate lengths and sizes. The left atrial anastomosis is performed first, using a running 3-0 polypropylene (Prolene) suture, beginning at the base of the left atrial appendage and finishing on the interatrial septum. Before completing the atrial anastomosis, the left ventricular vent is placed across the mitral valve into the donor heart's left ventricular apex to keep it decompressed. After the left atrial anastomosis, a dose of blood cardioplegic solution

containing 10 mEq of potassium chloride is infused through the aortic root using the cardioplegic cannula, which is still in place. The right atrial anastomosis is then fashioned using running 3-0 Prolene sutures. A small opening is left in this atrial anastomosis so that coronary flow can be reinstituted during total cardiopulmonary bypass without distending the right side of the heart. A second dose of blood cardioplegic solution is given through the cardioplegic cannula, which is then removed. The aortic anastomosis is then performed with running 4-0 Prolene sutures. The pulmonary anastomosis is completed with running 4-0 Prolene sutures (Fig. 97–10).

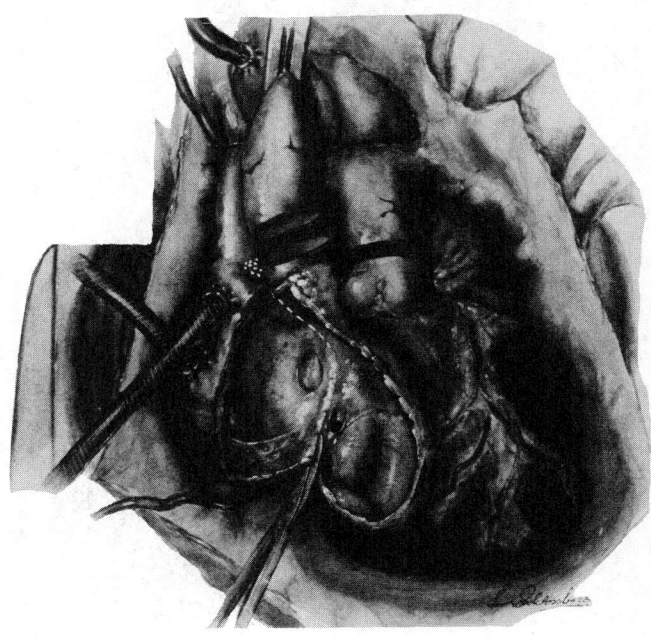

Figure 97–8. Recipient cardiectomy. (From Baumgartner WA: Operative techniques utilized in heart transplantation. In: Baumgartner WA, Reitz BA, Achuff SC [eds]: Heart and Heart-Lung Transplantation. Philadelphia, WB Saunders, p 113, 1990.)

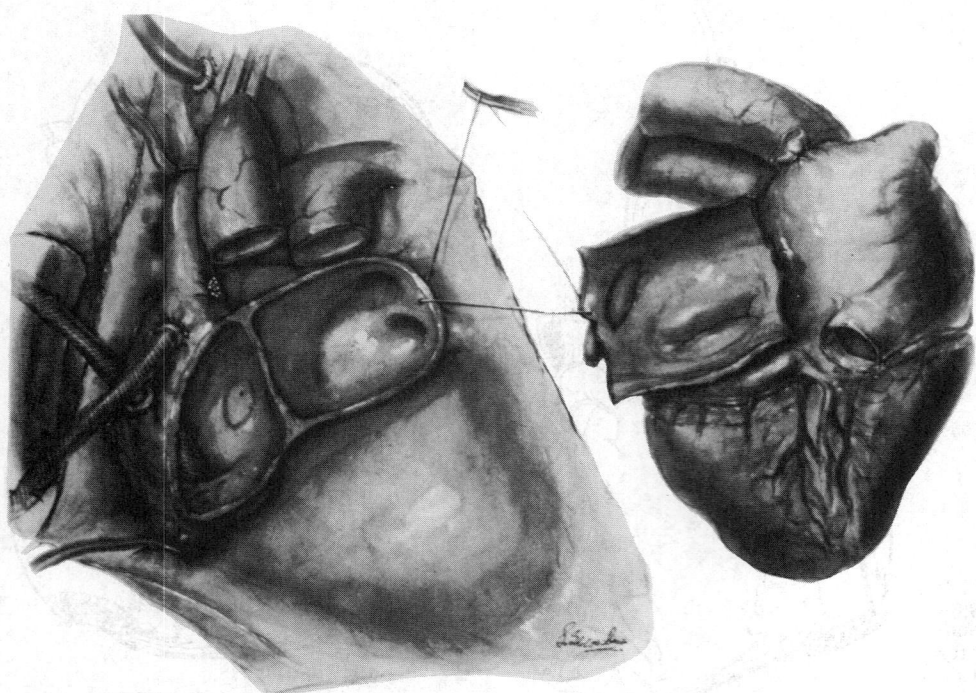

Figure 97–9. The implantation procedure is begun with the left atrial anastomosis. (From Baumgartner WA: Operative techniques utilized in heart transplantation. In: Baumgartner WA, Reitz BA, Achuff SC [eds]: Heart and Heart-Lung Transplantation. Philadelphia, WB Saunders, p 113, 1990.)

The patient, who has been cooled to 28°C throughout the procedure, is then rewarmed. A 19-gauge needle is placed in the ascending aorta to allow egress of air. The aortic cross-clamp is removed with the patient in the head-down position to minimize the risk of cerebral air embolism. As the aortic cross-clamp is removed, 500 mg of methylprednisolone 21-succinate sodium (Solu-Medrol) is given intravenously. The heart usually fibrillates at this point, and,

after ensuring that the left ventricle is decompressed with the left ventricular vent, the heart is defibrillated by direct-current shock. When the heart is beating in a spontaneous rhythm, the right atrial anastomosis is completed. Our policy is then to rewarm, during cardiopulmonary bypass, for half of the total ischemic time, up to 1.5 hours. During this period, the anastomoses are checked for hemostasis. The vena caval tapes are then removed, and a significant portion

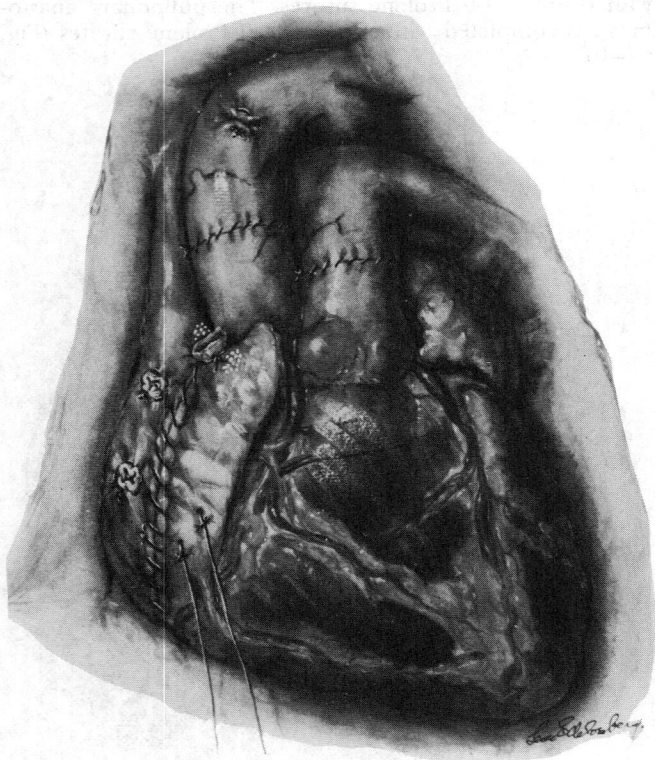

Figure 97–10. Completion of the transplantation procedure with atrial pacer wires in place. (From Baumgartner WA: Operative techniques utilized in heart transplantation. In: Baumgartner WA, Reitz BA, Achuff SC [eds]: Heart and Heart-Lung Transplantation. Philadelphia, WB Saunders, p 113, 1990.)

of the venous return now passes through the transplanted heart. Ventilation is then begun, and the left ventricle is carefully deaired by using a 19-gauge needle and the ventricular vent. After ensuring that the left ventricle is carefully deaired, the vent is removed from the across the mitral valve and the heart is allowed to eject.

When the patient is normothermic, isoproterenol is instituted at 0.5 to 1 µg/min, which usually causes a sinus tachycardia of 100 to 120 beats/min. The patient is then separated from cardiopulmonary bypass, protamine is given to reverse heparin, and the anastomoses are again checked for hemostasis.

Postoperative Management of the Patient with a Transplanted Heart

After the transplantation, the patient is moved to the surgical intensive care unit and placed in a modified isolation room. Our procedure is to allow access to the patient only to those directly involved in his or her care and the immediate family after the patient is stable. On entering the room, one must put on mask, gloves, and a gown. Although strict isolation procedures have not been shown to decrease postoperative infection rates, we have continued these practices in our unit.[85, 86] When the patient moves to the floor, isolation is limited to mask and gloves if contact is made with the patient.

Most patients require cardiotonic agents postoperatively, indicating a degree of graft dysfunction that may be a result of ischemia, inadequate preservation, or changes in the myocardium secondary to increased intracranial pressure, central nervous system herniation, or hemorrhage.

If the patient has an elevated pulmonary vascular resistance before transplantation, the right ventricle of the donor heart may be unable to overcome this resistance. Combinations of nitroglycerin and dobutamine, isoproterenol, amrinone, or prostaglandin E_1 may promote pulmonary vasodilation and thereby improve right ventricular function. The elevated pulmonary vascular resistance usually decreases over the several weeks after transplantation because the elevated pulmonary pressures result from prior left ventricular dysfunction.

The heart usually requires low-dose isoproterenol at 0.4 to 1.0 µg/min to maintain a heart rate about 100 beats/min. The sinus node may be dysfunctional because of trauma, ischemia, or stretch. Isoproterenol or another chronotropic agent may be used to override this sinus node dysfunction. In addition, atrioventricular sequential pacemaking may be used in the presence of sinus node dysfunction. Approximately 5% of transplant patients continue to be bradycardiac or show sinus node dysfunction in the postoperative period and require a permanent transvenous pacemaker. In this situation, we wait approximately 4 weeks before inserting a permanent pacemaker.

Our protocol is to have a pulmonary arterial thermodilution catheter inserted in the operating room before induction of anesthesia, for monitoring of cardiac output by the thermodilution technique, pulmonary arterial pressures, and mixed venous oxygen saturation. Patients can usually have their cardiotonic drugs discontinued by the fourth postoperative day. If the patient is hypertensive, nitroprusside can be used immediately postoperatively to control blood pressure.[86–88]

After transplantation, all efforts are made to wean the patient from the ventilator as soon as possible. This minimizes the risk of pulmonary sepsis, a major cause of morbidity and mortality.

All chest tubes that drain the mediastinum, central monitoring catheters, indwelling urinary catheters, and arterial lines are discontinued as soon as the patient is hemodynamically stable to avoid the risk of postoperative infection.

In the intensive care unit, titers of cytomegalovirus, herpes simplex virus, Epstein-Barr virus, *Toxoplasma, Legionella,* and *Mycoplasma* are routinely obtained postoperatively. These determinations can be repeated later if there is evidence of a clinical infection. Daily blood specimens are sent for a complete blood count including differential, electrolytes, blood urea nitrogen, and creatinine. Liver function tests including aspartate aminotransferase, alanine aminotransferase, alkaline phosphatase, and bilirubin; chest x-ray films; and ECGs are also obtained daily. As the patient becomes more stable, the frequency of these tests can be decreased.[89]

Patients are also usually scheduled for their first endomyocardial biopsy 1 week after transplantation. Usually this biopsy is negative, and our policy has been to transfer the patient to the floor after a negative biopsy.[89]

Immunosuppression and Rejection

To prevent rejection of the transplanted heart, the recipient is given several immunosuppressive drugs before the operation. Our preoperative protocol includes azathioprine at 4 mg/kg intravenously and, if renal status is normal, cyclosporine at 2 mg/kg orally. If renal function is impaired preoperatively, a decreased preoperative dose of cyclosporine is given. In the operating room, as soon as the aortic cross-clamp is removed, 500 mg of Solu-Medrol is given intravenously.

Postoperative immunosuppression includes Solu-Medrol at 100 mg every 8 hours for 24 hours and an antilymphocyte globulin at 10 to 15 mL for 4 to 7 days. Cardiac instability and respiratory instability are reasons for withholding the antilymphocyte globulin. Ranitidine (Zantac), acetaminophen (Tylenol 3), diphenhydramine (Benadryl), and hydrocortisone 21-sodium succinate (Solu-Cortef) are given at the time of antilymphocyte globulin administration. Ranitidine is administered to prevent peptic ulceration. In addition, the azathioprine is continued postoperatively at a dose of 2.0 to 2.5 mg/kg to maintain a white blood cell count of 5000/mm³ or greater. After 24 hours of Solu-Medrol administration, prednisone is begun at 1 mg/kg/d and is tapered by 5 mg/d until a dose of 0.2 mg/kg is achieved. The cyclosporine is given postoperatively when the urine output is greater than 50 mL/h and the blood urea nitrogen and creatinine levels are stable. It can usually be initiated within 24 hours after transplantation. Our policy is to start the cyclosporine at a low dose on a 12-hourly basis and increase the dose to 2 mg/kg every 12 hours. The blood urea nitrogen, creatinine levels, and urine output are followed carefully as the cyclosporine dose is increased. Lasix is usually added when the cyclosporine is initiated to maintain a good urine output. Measurements of cyclosporine levels in the serum help to determine the amount of cyclosporine to be given, although the dose is also guided by urine output, blood urea nitrogen, and creatinine levels and signs of clinical cyclosporine toxicity (Robinson K, Baciewicz FA Jr, unpublished).

The diagnosis of rejection is made from the histologic evaluation of the endomyocardial biopsy specimen. The first biopsy specimen is usually obtained 7 days postoperatively, with the biopsy forceps being introduced through the right internal jugular vein under fluoroscopy. Biopsy specimens are obtained from the right ventricular septal wall. They are usually obtained weekly for the first month, every 2 weeks for the next 2 months, every month for the next 3 months, and then at 2-month intervals for the next 6 months.

Rejection may also be suspected if the patient has unexplained malaise or atrial or ventricular arrhythmias.

Acute rejection is usually treated with 1 g of Solu-Medrol for 3 days and repeated biopsy in 5 to 7 days. Recalcitrant rejection that does not respond to intravenous Solu-Medrol can be treated with a 5- to 7-day course of antilymphocyte globulin or 7 to 10 days of Ortho-Novum monoclonal T3 antibody (OKT3).

Results of Cardiac Transplantation

The 30-day survival rate for orthotopic cardiac transplant recipients is about 90%. The mortality rate is similar for patients from 20 to 65 years of age. Patients in the pediatric age group have higher mortality. The 1-year survival rate is approximately 80% and the 5-year rate about 65%.[6, 89–91]

Patients requiring inotropes, IABP, or left VADs have survival rates approaching those of patients undergoing elective procedures. However, the need for biventricular support or the use of a total artificial heart before transplantation results in a higher mortality.[11, 92]

Within 30 days postoperatively, the leading cause of death is myocardial dysfunction (50%), followed by infection and rejection. After 30 days, the two most frequent causes of death are infection (40%) and rejection (40%) followed by myocardial dysfunction.[6, 89] The 30% incidence of graft coronary atherosclerosis 3 years postoperatively makes it a major contributor to long-term myocardial failure.[69, 93]

References

1. Haddy FJ: Pathophysiology and therapy of the shock of myocardial infarction. Ann Intern Med 73:809, 1970.
2. Scheidt S, Aschiem R, Killup T: Shock after acute myocardial infarction. Am J Cardiol 26:556, 1970.
3. Consensus Trial Study Group: Effects of enalapril on mortality in severe congestive heart failure. N Engl J Med 316:1429, 1987.
4. Pennington DG, Swartz MT, Codd JE: Intra-aortic balloon pumping in cardiac surgical patients: A nine-year experience. Ann Thorac Surg 36:125, 1983.
5. McEnany NT, Kay HR, Buckley MJ: Clinical experience with intra-aortic balloon pump support in 728 patients. Circulation 58(suppl I):124, 1978.
6. Kriett JM, Kaye MP: The Registry of the International Society for Heart Transplantation: Seventh official report—1990. J Heart Transplant 9:323, 1990.
7. Kanter KR, Pennington DG, McBride LR: Mechanical circulatory assistance after heart transplantation. J Heart Transplant 6:150, 1987.
8. Emery RW, Eales F, Joyce LD: Mechanical circulatory assistance after heart transplantation. Ann Thorac Surg 51:43, 1991.
9. Hooper TL, Odom NJ, Fetherston GJ, et al: Successful use of a left ventricular assist device for primary graft failure after heart transplantation. J Heart Transplant 7:385, 1988.
10. Copeland JG, Emery RW, Levinson MM: Selection of patients for cardiac transplantation. Circulation 75:57, 1987.
11. Miller CA, Pae WE Jr, Pierce WS: Combined registry for the clinical use of mechanical ventricular assist pumps and the total artificial heart in conjunction with heart transplantation: Fourth official report—1989. J Heart Transplant 9:453, 1990.
12. Boden WE, Bough EW, Benham I, et al: Unstable angina with episodic ST segment elevation and minimal creatine kinase release culminating in extensive, recurrent infarction. J Am Coll Cardiol 2:11, 1983.
13. Muller KD, Braunwald E: Can infarct size be limited in patients with acute myocardial infarction? Cardiovasc Clin 13:147, 1983.
14. Selden R, Neill WA, Ritzmann LW: Medical versus surgical therapy for acute coronary insufficiency: A randomized study. N Engl J Med 293:1329, 1975.
15. Buckley MJ, Mundth ED, Daggett WM: Surgical management of ventricular septal defects and mitral regurgitation complicating acute myocardial infarction. Ann Thorac Surg 16:598, 1973.
16. Phillips SJ, Zeff RH, Kongtahworn C: Percutaneous cardiopulmonary bypass: Application and indications for use. Ann Thorac Surg 47:121, 1989.
17. Pennington DG, Termuhlen DF: Mechanical circulatory support: Device selection. In: Emery RW, Pritzker MR, Eales F (eds): Cardiac Surgery: State of the Art Reviews, Volume 3, Number 3. Philadelphia, Hanley & Belfus, p 507, 1989.
18. Golding LR, Groves LK, Peter M: Initial clinical experience with a new temporary left ventricular assist device. Ann Thorac Surg 29:66, 1980.
19. Hill JD, Farrar DJ, Hershon JJ: Use of prosthetic ventricle as a bridge to cardiac transplantation for postinfarction cardiogenic shock. N Engl J Med 314:626, 1986.
20. Joyce LD, Johnson KE, Cabrol C: Nine year experience with the clinical use of total artificial hearts as cardiac support devices. Trans Am Soc Artif Intern Organs 34:703, 1988.
21. Litwak RS, Koffsky RM, Jurado RA: Use of a left heart assist device after intracardiac surgery: Technique and clinical experience. Ann Thorac Surg 21:191, 1976.
22. Pennington DG, Codd JE, Merjavy JP: The expanded use of ventricular bypass systems for severe cardiac failure and as a bridge to cardiac transplantation. J Heart Transplant 3:170, 1984.
23. Pennington DG, McBride LR, Swartz MT: Use of Pierce-Donachy ventricular assist device in patients with cardiogenic shock after cardiac operation. Ann Thorac Surg 47:130, 1989.
24. Pennington DG, Merjavy JP, Swartz MT, et al: Clinical experience with a centrifugal pump ventricular assist device. Trans Am Soc Artif Intern Organs 28:93, 1982.
25. Termuhlen DF, Swartz MT, Pennington DG: Predictors for weaning patients from ventricular assist devices. Trans Am Soc Artif Intern Organs 34:131, 1988.
26. Clauss RH, Birtwell WC, Albertal G: Assisted circulation: I. The arterial counterpulsator. J Thorac Cardiovasc Surg 41:447, 1961.
27. Moulopoulos SD, Topaz S, Kolff WJ: Diastolic balloon pumping (with carbon dioxide) in the aorta: A mechanical assistance to the failing circulation. Am Heart J 63:669, 1962.
27a. Kantrowitz A, Tjonneland S, Freed PS, et al: Initial clinical experience with intraaortic balloon pumping in cardiogenic shock. JAMA 203:113, 1968.
28. Bolooki H: Physiology of balloon pumping. In: Bolooki H (ed): Clinical Application of the Intra-Aortic Balloon Pump. 2nd ed. Mount Kisco, NY, Futura Publishing, p 57, 1984.
29. Hauser AM, Gordon S, Ganadharon V: Percutaneous intra-aortic balloon counterpulsation: Clinical effectiveness and hazards. Chest 82:422, 1982.
30. Kantrowitz A, Wasfie T, Freed PS: Intra-aortic balloon pumping 1967 through 1982: Analysis of complications in 733 patients. Am J Cardiol 57:976, 1986.
31. Sturm JT, Fuhrman TN, Sterling R: Combined use of dopamine and nitroprusside therapy in conjunction with intra-aortic balloon pumping for the treatment of post-cardiotomy low output syndrome. J Thorac Cardiovasc Surg 82:13, 1981.
32. Golding LR, Loop FD, Mohan P: Late survival following use of intra-aortic balloon pump in revascularization operations. Ann Thorac Surg 30:48, 1980.
33. Moran JM, Opravil M, Gorman A: Pulmonary artery balloon counterpulsation for right ventricular failure: Clinical experience. Ann Thorac Surg 38:254, 1984.
34. Wampler RK, Moise JC, Frazier OH, et al: In vivo evaluation of a peripheral access axial flow blood pump. Trans Am Soc Artif Intern Organs 34:450, 1988.
35. Frazier OH, Wampler RK, Duncan JM: First human use of the Hemo-pump, a catheter-mounted ventricular assist device. Ann Thorac Surg 49:299, 1990.
36. Campbell CD, Tolitano DJ, Weber KT: Mechanical support for post-cardiotomy heart failure. J Cardiac Surg 3:181, 1988.
37. Hoerr HR, Kraemer MF, Williams JL: In vitro comparison of the blood handling by the constrained vortex and twin roller blood pumps. J Extracorporeal Tech 19:316, 1987.
38. Magovern GJ, Park SB, Maher TD: Use of a centrifugal pump without anticoagulants for postoperative left ventricular assist. World J Surg 9:25, 1985.
39. Starnes VA, Oyer PE, Portner PM: Isolated left ventricular assist as a bridge to cardiac transplantation. J Thorac Cardiovasc Surg 96:62, 1988.
40. Park SB, Liebler GA, Burkholder JA: Mechanical support of the failing heart. Ann Thorac Surg 42:627, 1986.
41. Pennington DG, Kanter KR, McBride LR: Seven years experience with the Pierce-Donachy ventricular assist device. J Thorac Cardiovasc Surg 96:901, 1988.
42. Mohr R, Golan M, Martinowitz U: Effect of cardiac operation on platelets. J Thorac Cardiovasc Surg 92:434, 1986.
43. Esposito RA, Culliford AT, Colvin SV: The role of the activated clotting time in heparin administration and neutralization for cardiopulmonary bypass. J Thorac Cardiovasc Surg 85:174, 1983.
44. Zumbro GL, Kitchens WR, Shearer G: Mechanical assistance for cardiogenic shock following cardiac surgery, myocardial infarction and cardiac transplantation. Ann Thorac Surg 44:11, 1987.
45. Pennington DG, Merjavy JP, Codd JE, et al: Extracorporeal membrane oxygenation for patients with cardiogenic shock. Circulation 70(suppl I):130, 1984.
46. Rose DM, Connolly M, Cunningham JS, et al: Technique and results with a roller pump left and right heart assist device. Ann Thorac Surg 47:124, 1989.
47. Kanter KR, Ruzevich SA, Pennington DG, et al: Follow-up of survivors of mechanical circulatory support. J Thorac Cardiovasc Surg 96:72, 1988.
48. Adamson RM, Demblitsky WP, Reichman RT, et al: Mechanical support: Assist or nemesis? J Thorac Cardiovasc Surg 98:915, 1989.
49. Bolman RM, Cox JL, Marshall W: Circulatory support with a centrifugal pump as a bridge to cardiac transplantation. Ann Thorac Surg 47:108, 1989.

50. Golding LAR, Stewart RW, Sinkewich M: Non-pulsatile ventricular assist bridging to transplantation. Trans Am Soc Artif Intern Organs 34:476, 1988.
51. Hill JD: Bridging to cardiac transplantation. Ann Thorac Surg 47:167, 1989.
52. Portner PM, Oyer PE, Pennington DG: Implantable electric left ventricular assist system: Bridge to transplantation and the future. Ann Thorac Surg 47:142, 1989.
53. Joyce LD, Johnson KE, Toninato CJ, et al: Results of the first 100 patients who received Symbion total artificial hearts as a bridge to cardiac transplantation. Circulation 80(suppl III):192, 1989.
54. Eales F, Emery RW, Joyce LW, et al: Selection of heart transplant recipients and surgical techniques. In: Emery RW, Pritzker MR (eds): Cardiac Surgery: State of the Art Reviews, Volume 4, Number 2. Philadelphia, Hanley & Belfus, p 565, 1988.
55. Pennock JL, Oyer PE, Reitz BA: Cardiac transplantation in perspective for the future: Survival, complications, rehabilitation, and cost. J Thorac Cardiovasc Surg 83:168, 1982.
56. Hardesty RL, Griffith BP, Trento A: Mortally ill patients and excellent survival following cardiac transplantation. Ann Thorac Surg 41:126, 1986.
57. Bolman RM, III, Spray TL, Cox JL: Heart transplantation in patients requiring preoperative mechanical support. J Heart Transplant 6:273, 1987.
58. Shumway SJ, Gardner TJ, Cameron DE: Heart transplantation in patients requiring preoperative inotropic and mechanical support (abstract). J Am Coll Cardiol 11:44A, 1988.
59. Joyce LD: Use of the mini Jarvik-7 total artificial heart as a bridge to transplantation. Heart Transplant 5:203, 1986.
60. Hastillo A, Hess ML: Selection of patients for cardiac transplantation. In: Thompson ME (ed): Cardiac Transplantation. Philadelphia, FA Davis, p 107, 1990.
61. Addonizio LJ, Gersony WM, Robbins RC: Elevated pulmonary vascular resistance and cardiac transplantation. Circulation 76(suppl V):78, 1987.
62. Dreyfus G, Guillemain R, Amrein C: The inability of pulmonary vascular resistance measurements to predict posttransplant right ventricular failure. J Heart Transplant 55:378, 1986.
63. Kormos RL, Thompson M, Hardesty RL: Utility of preoperative right heart catheterization data as a predictor of survival after heart transplantation. J Heart Transplant 5:391, 1986.
64. Kirklin JK, Naftel DC, Kirklin JW: Pulmonary vascular resistance and the risk of cardiac transplantation. J Heart Transplant 7:125, 1988.
65. Medical Consultants on the Diagnosis of Death: Guidelines for the determination of death. JAMA 246:2184, 1981.
66. Fragomeni LS, Rogers G, Kaye MP: Donor identification and organ procurement for cardiac transplantation. In: Thompson ME (ed): Cardiac Transplantation. Philadelphia, FA Davis, p 125, 1990.
67. Cabrol C, Gandjbakhch I, Pavie A: Heart transplantation in Paris, a "La Pitie" Hospital. J Heart Transplant 4:476, 1985.
68. Baumgartner WA: Evaluation and management of the heart donor. In: Baumgartner WA, Reitz BA, Achuff SC (eds): Heart and Heart-Lung Transplantation. Philadelphia, WB Saunders, p 91, 1990.
69. Sarris EG, Mitchell RS, Billingham ME, et al: Inhibition of accelerated cardiac allograft arteriosclerosis by fish oil. J Thorac Cardiovasc Surg 97:841, 1989.
70. Emery RW, Eales F, Von Rueden TJ, et al: The cardiothoracic donor. In: Emery RW, Pritzker MR (eds): Cardiac Surgery: State of the Art Reviews, Volume 2, Number 4. Philadelphia, Hanley & Belfus, p 547, 1988.
71. Baumgartner WA: Evaluation and management of the heart donor. In: Baumgartner WA, Reitz BA, Achuff SC (eds): Heart and Heart-Lung Transplantation. Philadelphia, WB Saunders, p 86, 1990.
72. Fentz V, Gormsen J: Electrocardiographic patterns in patients with cerebrovascular accidents. Circulation 25:22, 1962.
73. Lammermeier DE, Sweeney MS, Haupt HE, et al: Use of potentially infected donor hearts for cardiac transplantation. Ann Thorac Surg 50:222, 1990.
74. Okereke OUJ, Frazier OH, Reese JJ: Cause and importance of donor neurogenic myocardial injury in cardiac transplantation. Transplant Proc 19:1034, 1987.
75. Cushing H: Concerning a definite regulatory mechanism of the vasomotor centre which controls blood pressure during cerebral compression. Johns Hopkins Hosp Bull 12:290, 1901.
76. Novitzky D, Wicomb WN, Cooper DKC: Electrocardiographic, hemodynamic and endocrine changes occurring during experimental brain death in the chacma baboon. J Heart Transplant 4:63, 1984.
77. Wahlers T, Fieguth HD, Jurmann M: Does hormone depletion of organ donors impair myocardial function after cardiac transplantation? Transplant Proc 20:792, 1988.
78. Novitzky D, Cooper DKC, Zuhdi N: The physiological management of cardiac transplant donors and recipients using triiodothyronine. Transplant Proc 20:803, 1988.
79. Gifford RPM, Weaver AS, Burg JE: Thyroid hormone levels in heart and kidney cadaver donors. J Heart Transplant 5:249, 1986.
80. Macoviak JA, McDougall IR, Bayer MF: Significance of thyroid dysfunction in human cardiac allograft procurement. Transplantation 43:824, 1987.
81. Keyne MP: The Registry of the International Society for Heart Transplantation: Fourth official report—1987. J Heart Transplant 6:63, 1988.
82. Lower RR, Shumway NE: Studies on orthotopic transplantation of the canine heart. Surg Forum 11:18, 1960.
83. Watson DC, Reitz BA, Baumgartner WA: Distant heart procurement for transplantation. Surgery 86:56, 1979.
84. Mendez-Picon GJ, Goldman MA, Wolfgang TC: Long distance procurement and transportation of human hearts for transplantation. J Heart Transplant 1:63, 1982.
85. Hess N, Brooks-Brunn JA, Clark D Jr, et al: Complete isolation: Is it necessary? J Heart Transplant 4:458, 1985.
86. Borkon AM, Augustine SM: Immediate postoperative management for the heart transplant recipient. In: Baumgartner WA, Reitz BA, Achuff SC (eds): Heart and Heart-Lung Transplantation. Philadelphia, WB Saunders, p 134, 1990.
87. Stinson EB, Caves PK, Griepp RB: Hemodynamic observations in the early period after human heart transplantation. J Thorac Cardiovasc Surg 69:264, 1975.
88. Stinson EV, Caves PK, Griepp RB: The transplanted heart in the postoperative period. Surg Forum 24:189, 1983.
89. Heck CF, Shumway SJ, Kaye MP: The Registry of the International Society for Heart Transplantation: Sixth official report—1989. J Heart Transplant 8:271, 1989.
90. Baumgartner WA, Augustine S, Borkon AM, et al: Present expectations in cardiac transplantation. Ann Thorac Surg 43:585, 1987.
91. Griffith BP, Hardesty RL, Trento A, et al: Cardiac transplantation: Emerging from an experiment to a service. Ann Surg 47:650, 1986.
92. Hardesty RL, Griffith BP, Trento A, et al: Mortally ill patients and excellent survival following cardiac transplantation. Ann Thorac Surg 41:126, 1986.
93. Billingham ME: Cardiac transplant atherosclerosis. Transplant Proc 19:19, 1987.

CHAPTER 98

Emergency Vascular Surgery in Patients in the Intensive Care Unit

Robert F. Wilson
Lawrence M. Diebel

The main indication for emergency vascular surgery in patients in an intensive care unit (ICU) is occlusion of a critical artery causing severe ischemia of vital organs or an extremity. Occasionally, emergency surgery is required to control hemorrhage from an injured or diseased major vessel or to resect an aneurysm that is leaking or dissecting. A pseudoaneurysm may necessitate resection, especially if it is thought to be infected. Surgical repair of the superior vena cava may be necessary if it has an iatrogenic injury causing a large hematoma or continued bleeding or if it has a severely symptomatic occlusion caused by a benign lesion. An arteriovenous fistula constructed for hemodialysis may have to be narrowed, occluded, or removed if it has become large enough to cause heart failure.

THORAX

Some of the more frequent thoracic problems that may necessitate emergency vascular surgery include aneurysms (arteriosclerotic, dissecting, or traumatic) and infected or leaking vascular anastomoses or grafts.

Aortic Aneurysms
Types of Aneurysms

Arteriosclerotic Aneurysms. Arteriosclerotic aneurysms of the thoracic aorta usually involve the descending aorta or the arch. Most of these, even if rather large, do not require emergency surgery unless there is evidence that they are leaking, expanding rapidly, or occluding an important adjacent structure, such as the superior vena cava or a major bronchus.

Dissecting Aneurysms. Dissecting aneurysms, according to the Stanford classification, are divided into type A (also called DeBakey's types 1 and 2) (involving the ascending aorta) and type B (DeBakey's type 3) (not involving the ascending aorta) (Fig. 98–1). The dissection is considered to be acute if it is less than 14 days old.[1] Patients with type A dissections tend to be younger and usually have inherited defects in the elastic tissue of the medial layer of their aorta. Patients with type B dissections tend to be older, are more frequently hypertensive, and have more age-related degeneration of aortic smooth muscle.

Untreated type A dissections are highly lethal and result in death at a rate of 1 to 2% per hour (30 to 40% by 24 hours and 40 to 60% by 48 hours).[1, 2] The in-hospital mortality rate for untreated dissecting aortic aneurysms usually exceeds 90%. Most patients with type A dissections die of intrapericardial rupture with tamponade. Other causes of death include massive aortic regurgitation with acute left ventricular failure or compromised coronary or cerebral blood flow. Patients with type B dissections usually die of rupture into a pleural cavity.

Aortic dissections generally begin as transverse tears in the ascending aorta 2 to 3 cm above the aortic valve or in the descending aorta within 2 to 3 cm of the left subclavian artery. The dissection usually involves a tear extending from the intima into the media at the junction of its outer third and medial two thirds.

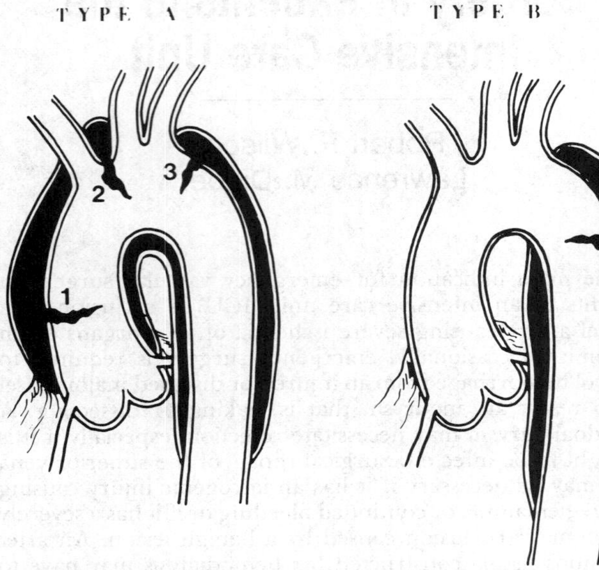

Traumatic Aneurysms. Acute blunt trauma to the thoracic great arteries usually involves, in order of frequency (1) the isthmus (the descending aorta between the left subclavian artery and the ligamentum arteriosum) (75 to 95%), (2) the innominate artery, (3) a subclavian artery, and (4) the ascending aorta.[3] In patients who reach the hospital alive, the injury usually involves only the intima and the media, and the tough adventitial layer is all that prevents a sudden massive exsanguination.

Syphilitic Aneurysms. Because syphilitic aneurysms are associated with a panaortitis, they do not cause dissections. However, these aneurysms, usually arising in the ascending aorta, can grow to a large size, even eroding through the sternum. Fortunately, they are rare now.

Pseudoaneurysms. Pseudoaneurysms may develop in any vessel, usually because of sepsis or technical errors at sites of injury or at suture lines. Infection of prosthetic grafts in the chest is unusual, and if the pseudoaneurysm is not infected or leaking, it can be watched and carefully followed to be sure that it is not increasing in size.

Diagnosis

Although most thoracic aortic aneurysms are discovered incidentally on chest x-ray film, occasionally, they are suspected because of certain clinical findings, such as chest or back pain, loss of pulses in one upper extremity or both lower extremities, and compression of a vital structure. In some instances, their presence was noted during a prior admission.

History. Arteriosclerotic aneurysms are often asymptomatic until relatively late when they erode into or compress adjacent structures or begin to leak. However, dissecting aneurysms are often characterized by a sudden onset of severe tearing pain, which tends to radiate down the back.

A history of a high-speed deceleration injury should make one suspicious of the possibility of a traumatic rupture of the aorta. Symptoms, such as severe back pain or a voice change, may also be suggestive of this diagnosis, but some patients with traumatic rupture of the aorta have relatively little evidence of severe chest trauma.

Physical Examination. Arteriosclerotic aneurysms may occasionally compress the superior vena cava, the trachea, or the esophagus, causing neck vein distention, a pulsating trachea, or dysphagia. A sympathetic effusion, leakage of blood, or compression of a bronchus may cause decreased breath sounds at the lung bases.

Dissecting aneurysms may also cause compression of vital structures or a pleural effusion, but they should be particularly suspected if there are pulse deficits in the radial or femoral arteries. Dissecting aneurysms of the ascending aorta may also cause increasing aortic insufficiency, and the initial phases of rupture through the ascending aorta may cause pericardial tamponade.

Upper extremity hypertension is common with aortic injuries to the proximal descending aorta. Absent or reduced femoral pulses, as with a pseudocoarctation syndrome, are much less frequent, but virtually diagnostic.[4] An absent radial pulse on one side or a bruit over the upper back or supraclavicular areas can be a valuable clinical sign.

Chest Radiography. The great majority of thoracic aneurysms are diagnosed on chest x-ray film as a smooth mass that seems to arise in the mediastinum. In cases of decelerating truncal trauma, the initial chest x-ray film may be normal in 10 to 30% of patients,[5] especially in patients older than 65 years of age. As a consequence, this problem may not become apparent until hours, days, or even years later.

TYPE A   TYPE B

Figure 98–1. The Stanford classification system of aortic dissections. In type A, the ascending aorta is involved, with the intimal tear being located in the ascending aorta (1), 2 to 4 cm above the aortic valve. The aortic arch (2 and 3) is much less apt to be the site of the intimal tear. In type B dissections, the dissection begins in the descending thoracic aorta. (From Miller DC, Stinson EB, Oyer PE, et al: Operative treatment of aortic dissections. Experience with 125 patients over a sixteen-year period. J Thorac Cardiovasc Surg 78:365, 1979.)

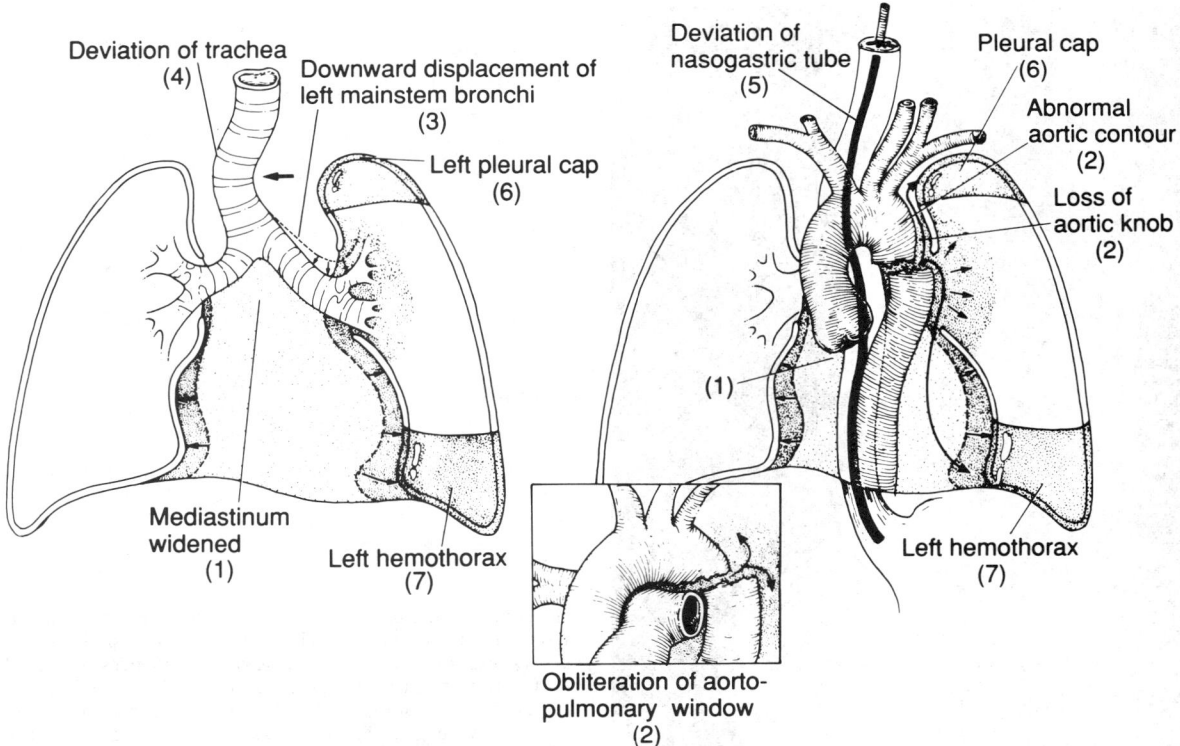

Figure 98–2. Characteristic roentgenographic signs of a traumatic rupture of the descending thoracic aorta include (1) widened mediastinum, (2) obliteration of aorta pulmonary window and loss of normal contour of aortic knob, (3) downward displacement of the left mainstem bronchus, (4) deviation of the trachea to the right, (5) deviation of the nasogastric tube to the right, (6) left-sided pleural cap, and (7) left-sided hemothorax. (From Maggisano R, Cina C: Traumatic rupture of the thoracic aorta. In: McMurty RY, McLellan BA [eds]: Management of Blunt Trauma. Baltimore, Williams & Wilkins, p 213, 1990. © 1990, the Williams & Wilkins Co., Baltimore.)

A number of changes can be seen on plain chest x-ray films that should make one suspicious of traumatic rupture of the aorta (Fig. 98–2). The most accurate radiographic signs of traumatic rupture of the aorta are widening of the superior mediastinum (Fig. 98–3), obscuration or blurring

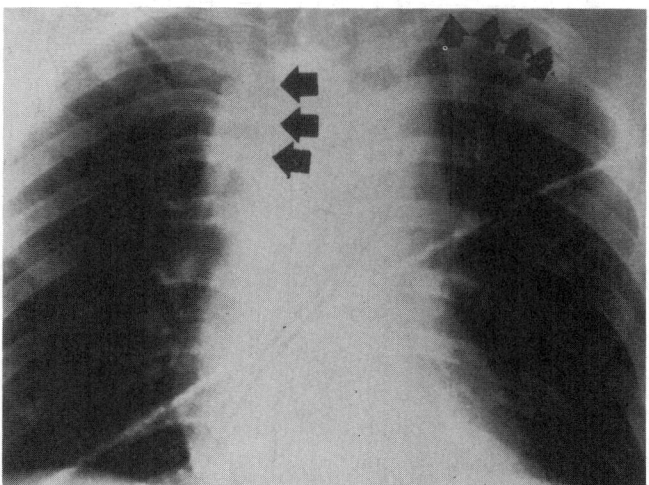

Figure 98–3. Chest x-ray film showing widening of the superior mediastinum, deviation of the trachea to the right (*three arrows*), and a left-sided pleural cap (*four arrows*). (From Maggisano R, Cina C: Traumatic rupture of the thoracic aorta. In: McMurty RY, McLellan BA [eds]: Management of Blunt Trauma. Baltimore, Williams & Wilkins, p 213, 1990. © 1990, the Williams & Wilkins Co., Baltimore.)

of the aortic knob (Fig. 98–4), deviation of the esophagus (nasogastric tube) or trachea more than 1 to 2 cm to the right (Fig. 98–5), and depression of the left mainstem bronchus. Although widening of the superior mediastinum is occasionally due to the pseudoaneurysm itself (Fig. 98–6), it is much more likely to be caused by associated injury to small mediastinal veins.[6–8] Other signs thought to suggest a traumatic rupture of the aorta include left apical cap, loss of the normal clear space between the aortic knob and the left hilum, and displacement or widening of the paratracheal or paravertebral stripes or lines (Fig. 98–7).

In many instances, a technically poor chest x-ray film can make the mediastinum appear widened when it actually is normal. Some of the factors that make a normal mediastinum appear wide include (1) a supine anteroposterior film (rather than a posteroanterior film in an erect patient who is leaning forward 10 to 15°), (2) poor inspiration, and (3) a short distance between the x-ray tube and the patient. The x-ray tube should be at least 100 cm, preferably 150 cm, away from the patient.

Computed Tomography. A computed tomographic (CT) scan, preferably with intravenous contrast materials, can be extremely helpful in defining the position and extent of aortic aneurysms and dissections. It may also be used as a screening test in patients with trauma to determine if there is a mediastinal hematoma.[9, 10] Absence of a mediastinal hematoma on a properly performed CT scan with intravenous contrast is virtually 100% accurate in ruling out a traumatic rupture of the aorta. In aortic dissections, the CT scan may show the false lumen (Fig. 98–8) or even a well-defined intimal flap (Fig. 98–9). The newer generation of CT scanners in the hands of an experienced radiologist may

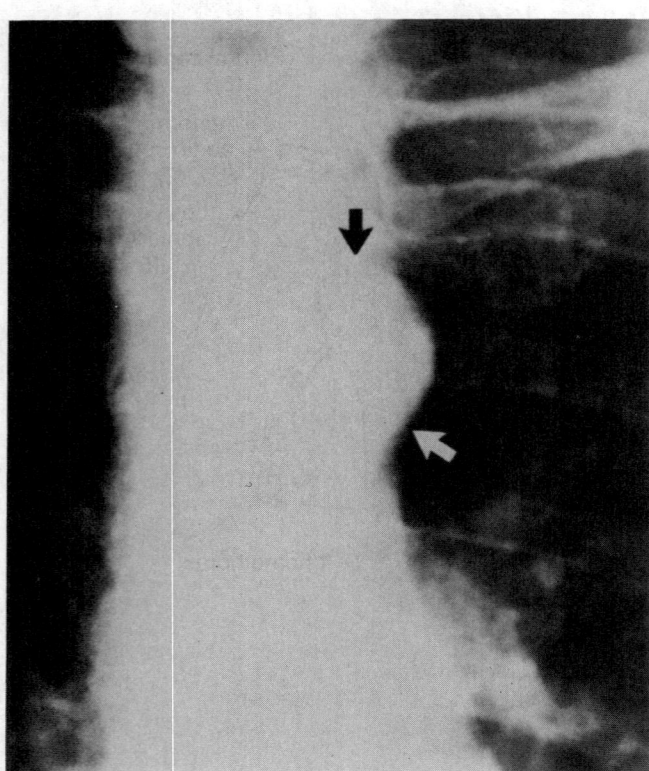

Figure 98–4. Normal aortic outline. The normal aortic knob can be visualized from the 12 o'clock (*black arrow*) to the 4 o'clock (*white arrow*) positions. A normal aortic outline reduces the likelihood of an aortic transection at the isthmus. (From Kerlan RK: Diagnostic arteriography. In: Bongard FS, Wilson SE, Perry MO [eds]: Vascular Injuries in Surgical Practice. East Norwalk, CT, Appleton & Lange, p 62, 1991.)

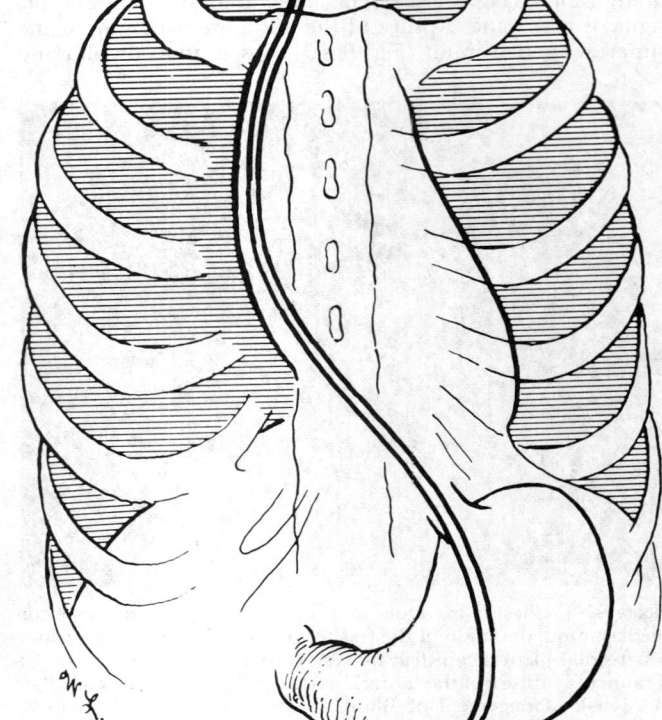

Figure 98–5. Deviation of the esophagus (nasogastric tube) to the right is generally an accurate sign of traumatic rupture of the aorta. If the distance from the nasogastric tube to the spinous process of the fourth thoracic vertebra is greater than 2 cm, it is almost 100% indicative of traumatic rupture of the aorta. (From Wilson RF: Thoracic vascular trauma. In: Bongard FS, Wilson SE, Perry MO [eds]: Vascular Injuries in Surgical Practice. East Norwalk, CT, Appleton & Lange, p 119, 1991.)

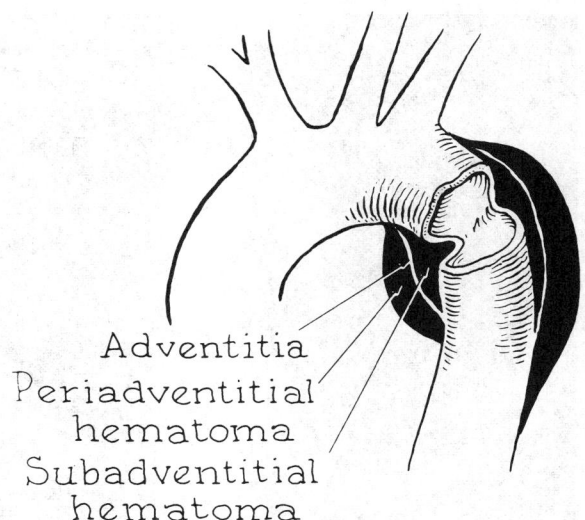

Figure 98–6. The widening of the mediastinum around a traumatic rupture of the aorta usually results from hematoma in the subadventitial and adjacent periadventitial (mediastinal) tissue. The mediastinal hematoma may be large and is due primarily to bleeding from small mediastinal vessels. (From Wilson RF: Thoracic vascular trauma. In: Bongard FS, Wilson SE, Perry MO [eds]: Vascular Injuries in Surgical Practice. East Norwalk, CT, Appleton & Lange, p 119, 1991.)

also provide adequate definition of the anatomy of the dissection to guide surgery; however, the accuracy of the CT scan has been questioned.[11]

Aortography. Angiography is the "gold standard" for establishing the diagnosis and determining the extent of an aortic aneurysm or dissection. However, one of the authors (Wilson RF) knows of at least four traumatic ruptures of the aorta that have had false-negative aortograms. If an aneurysm or dissection is suspected and if there is a possibility that the ICU patient's therapy will be altered because of the findings, an aortogram is indicated. However, if the patient is too ill to have aortic surgery, the risk of transporting the patient to the radiology department and obtaining an aortogram is not warranted. In each case, the likelihood of finding a correctable lesion in a patient who is likely to survive the surgery must be balanced against the risk of movement of the patient to the aortography suite and the effect of 100 to 150 mL of 60% contrast solutions on kidneys, which may have already been damaged by hypotension and pigments, such as myoglobin or free hemoglobin.

During a thoracic aortogram in trauma patients, all areas in question must be visualized clearly. It is important to see the entire aorta and its major branches in the chest as well as the abdomen. A small, smooth eccentric dilatation of the medial portion of the aortic isthmus is a normal variant and has been referred to as the ductus bump (Fig. 98–10). Increased bulging in this area can indicate a traumatic rupture of the aorta (Fig. 98–11). However, the diagnosis is

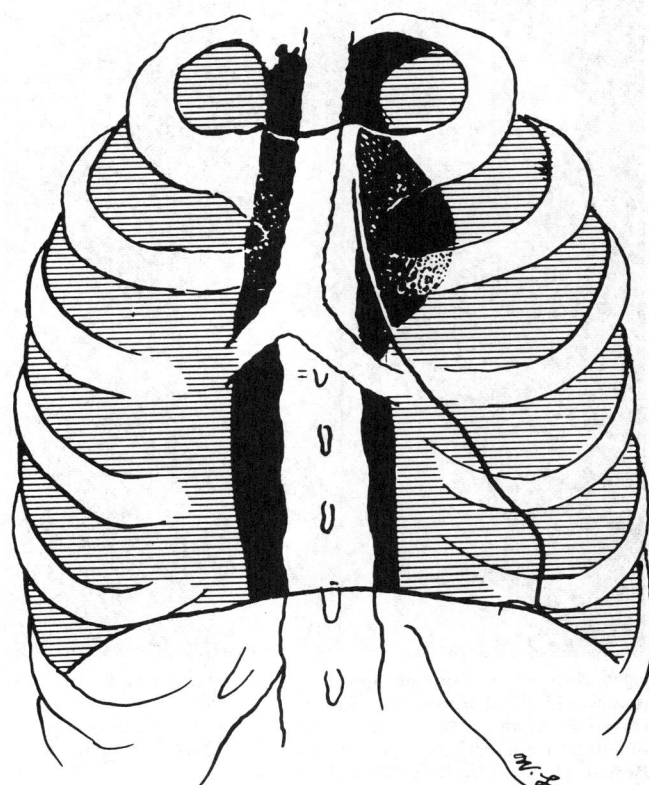

Figure 98–7. Mediastinal hematomas, indicated by the blackened areas, may widen and displace the paratracheal stripe separating the right side of the tracheal air column from the medial border of the right lung by more than 5 mm. Mediastinal hematomas may also displace the right and left paraspinal lines in the lower thorax rather widely from the lateral edges of the thoracic spine. The paraspinal lines are not readily seen on most x-ray films because of overlying structures. (From Wilson RF: Thoracic vascular trauma. In: Bongard FS, Wilson SE, Perry MO [eds]: Vascular Injuries in Surgical Practice. East Norwalk, CT, Appleton & Lange, p 120, 1991.)

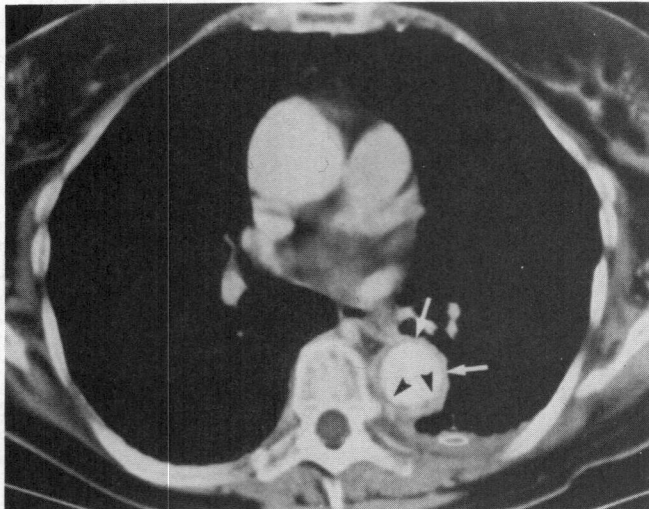

Figure 98–8. CT scan of the chest showing a dissecting aneurysm of the proximal descending aorta. The lumen is opacified and a thin rim of surrounding false lumen can be seen (*white arrows*). There is also central displacement of intimal calcifications (*black arrowheads*) and a small left pleural hematoma. (From Vogelzang RL, Fisher MR: Computed tomography and magnetic resonance imaging in vascular surgical emergencies. In: Bergan JJ, Yao JST [eds]: Vascular Surgical Emergencies. Orlando, FL, Grune & Stratton, p 77, 1987.)

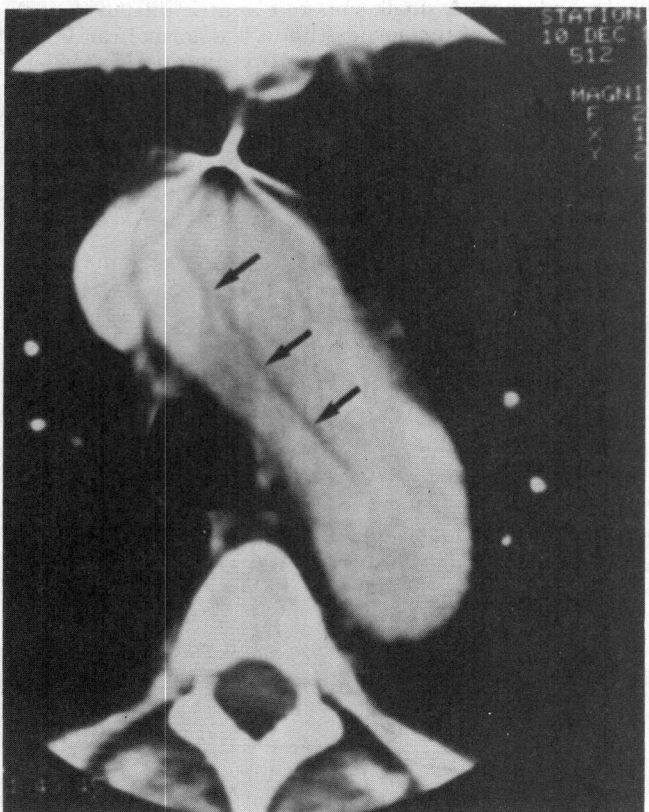

Figure 98–9. Aortogram showing dissection of the aortic arch. There is a well-defined intimal flap (*arrows*) separating the two lumina. (From Vogelzang RL, Fisher MR: Computed tomography and magnetic resonance imaging in vascular surgical emergencies. In: Bergan JJ, Yao JST [eds]: Vascular Surgical Emergencies. Orlando, FL, Grune & Stratton, p 77, 1987.)

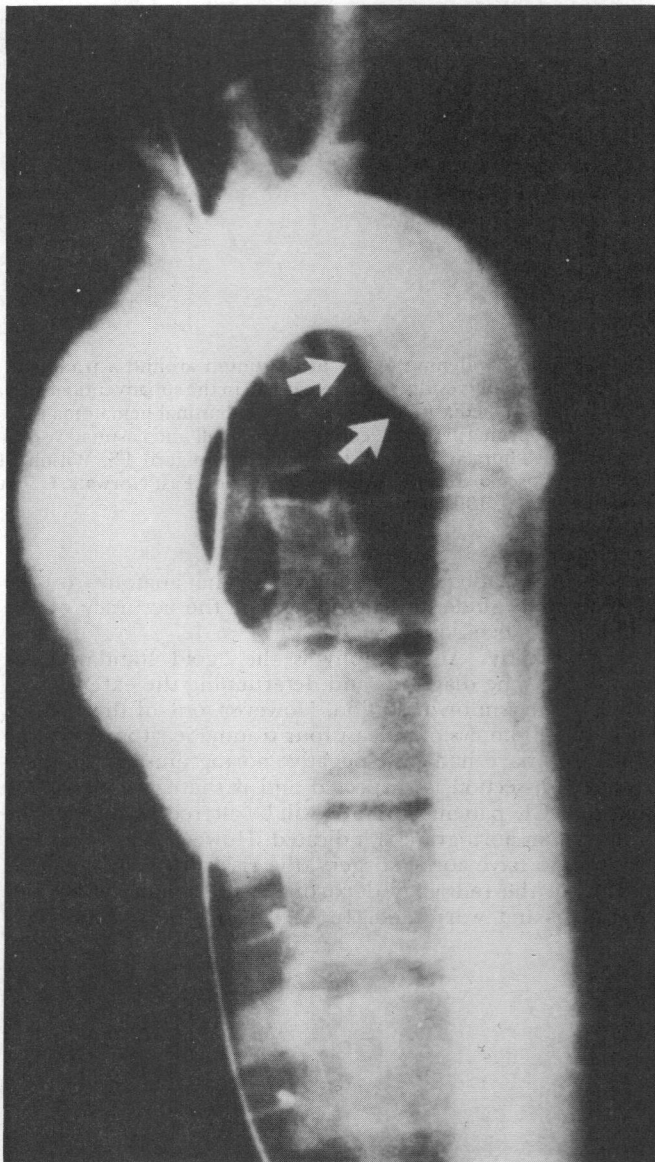

Figure 98–10. Ductus bump. This right posterior oblique arch aortogram shows a smooth, eccentric dilatation (*arrows*) of the medial portion of the aortic isthmus extending toward the insertion of the ligamentum arteriosum. This normal variant should not be confused with an aortic transection. (From Kerlan RK: Diagnostic arteriography. In: Bongard FS, Wilson SE, Perry MO [eds]: Vascular Injuries in Surgical Practice. East Norwalk, CT, Appleton & Lange, p 65, 1991.)

much clearer if an intimal flap can be seen (Fig. 98–12). In many cases, especially if the diagnosis is delayed, the main finding may be a lateral bulge of the aortic wall that indicates the presence of a pseudoaneurysm (Fig. 98–13).

Treatment

Medical Management. Medical therapy of aortic aneurysms includes alleviation of pain and reduction of blood pressure to the lowest level that allows adequate organ perfusion. With most aneurysms or dissections of the aorta, surgery can be delayed, often indefinitely, as long as the systolic blood pressure is maintained below 110 to 120 mm be managed medically. However, surgery is advised for type B dissections if a vital vessel becomes occluded, if there is evidence of bleeding, or if the blood pressure and pain cannot be adequately controlled medically.

With traumatic rupture of the aorta, there is a strong tendency by many surgeons to operate immediately, even if there are severe multiple injuries greatly increasing the risk of surgery. However, if the blood pressure and dp/dt are properly controlled, the traumatic tear of the intima and media can often be handled like a dissection of the descending thoracic aorta, and surgery can be delayed safely for several days or longer.[13–16]

A stable, noninfected pseudoaneurysm at the site of previous vascular surgery can often be managed similarly to a dissection until the patient's condition allows the needed repair.

Surgery. Surgery is recommended for aneurysms that are leaking or expanding rapidly. Urgent surgical repair is recommended for all dissections involving the ascending aorta. Surgery is required for distal dissections only if the dissection is leaking, occludes vital vessels, cannot be managed medically, or shows evidence of progression despite intensive medical therapy.[1]

With surgery involving the proximal aorta total cardiopulmonary bypass is needed. With surgery involving the aortic arch, total cardiopulmonary bypass is needed and one

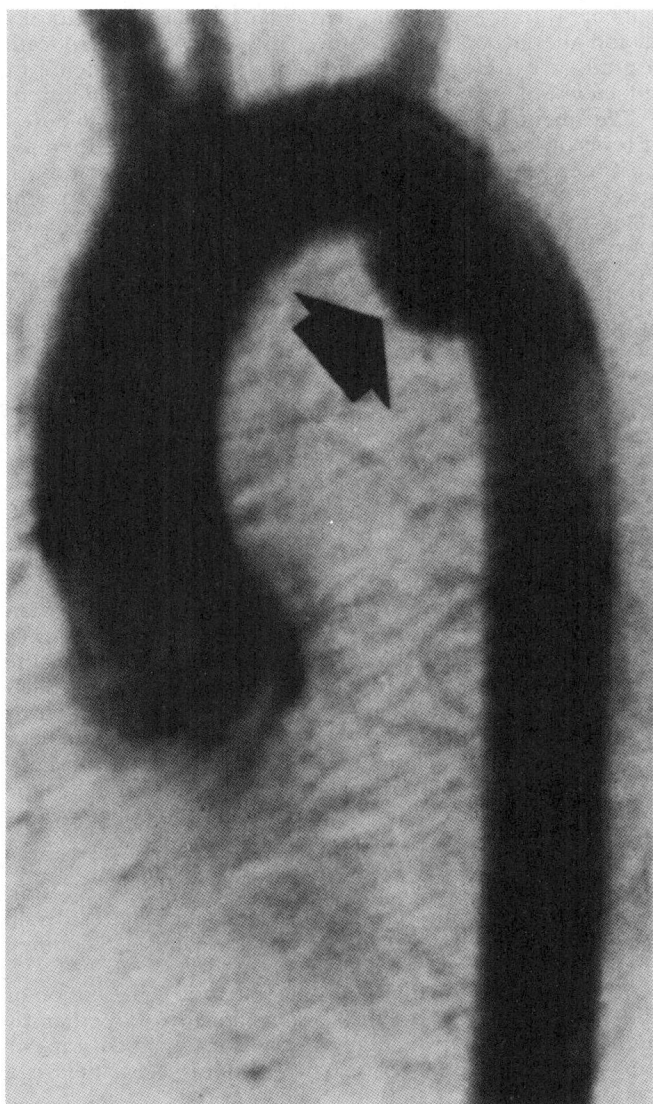

Figure 98–11. Intra-arterial digital subtraction angiogram of a patient involved in a motor vehicle accident who had chest pain and a widened mediastinum (8.5 cm). The pseudoaneurysm formation is seen in projection. This smooth eccentric dilatation coming off the medial side of the isthmus of the aorta (arrow) is much larger than the slight bulging that may normally be seen in this area, referred to as a congenital ductus bump, which is a normal variant. (From Kaebnick HW, Lipchik EO, Towne JB: The role of angiography in emergency vascular surgery. In: Bergan JJ, Yao JST [eds]: Vascular Surgical Emergencies. Orlando, FL, Grune & Stratton, p 57, 1987.)

Hg with an alpha₁-adrenergic blocker and/or vasodilator (such as nitroprusside). At the same time, the dp/dt of the aortic pulse and the reflex tachycardia (caused by the vasodilators) should be reduced by administration of a beta-adrenergic blocker, such as propranolol.[12, 13] However, if the aneurysm is enlarging rapidly or may be leaking, one should operate as soon as there is a reasonable chance that the patient can survive the surgery.

The management of dissecting aneurysms depends largely on the site of the initial opening between the vascular lumen and the dissection.[1] Dissections beginning in the ascending aorta usually require urgent or emergency surgery. In contrast, dissections beginning in the descending aorta can often

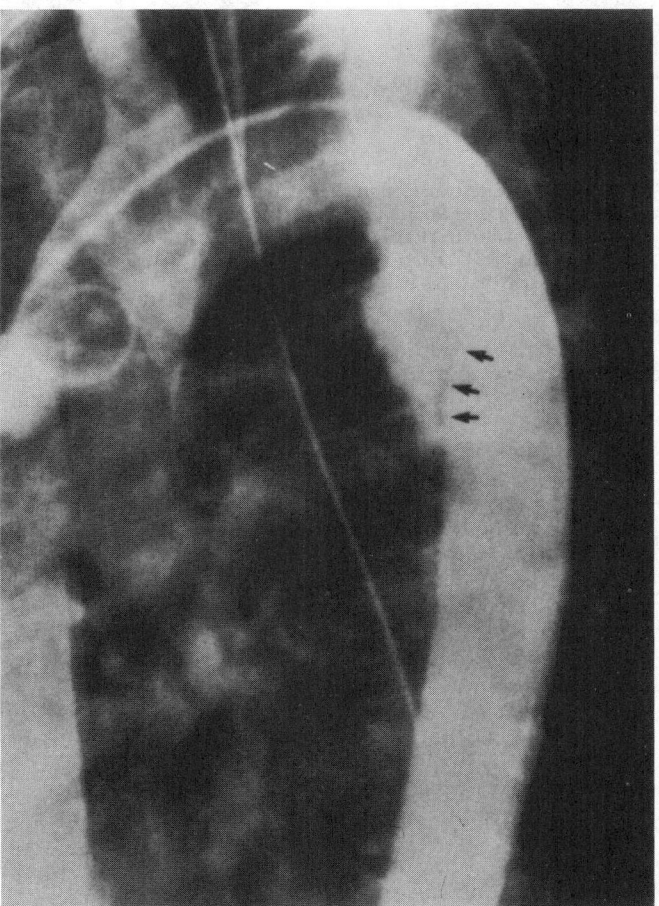

Figure 98–12. Thoracic aortogram shows the pseudoaneurysm and intimal flap (arrows) typical of traumatic rupture of the aorta. (From Maggisano R, Cina C: Traumatic rupture of the thoracic aorta. In: McMurty RY, McLellan BA [eds]: Management of Blunt Trauma. Baltimore, Williams & Wilkins, p 217, 1990. © 1990, the Williams & Wilkins Co., Baltimore.)

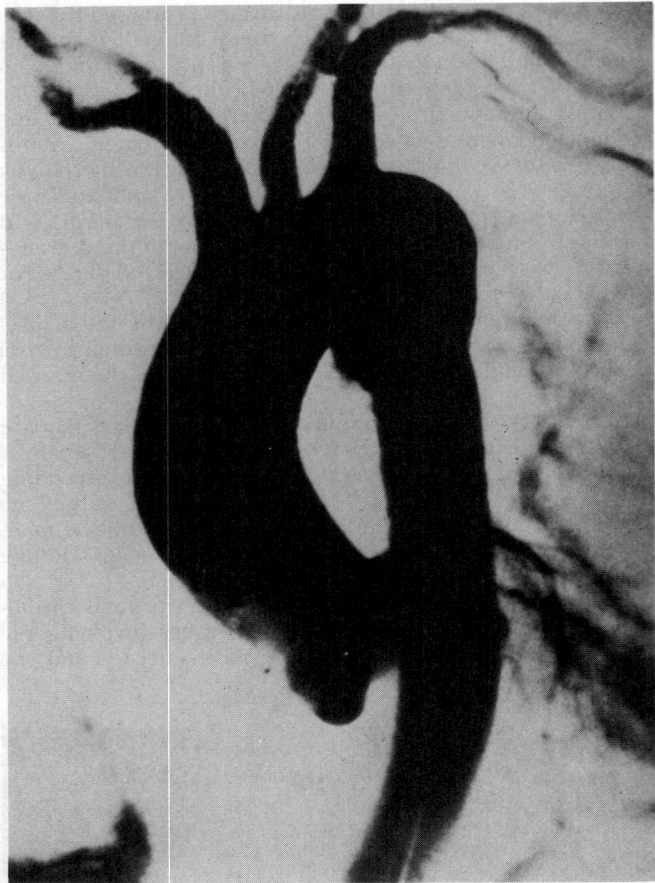

Figure 98–13. Aortic transection. Right posterior oblique subtraction view shows the pseudoaneurysm of the proximal descending thoracic aorta. (From Kerlan RK: Diagnostic arteriography. In: Bongard FS, Wilson SE, Perry MO [eds]: Vascular Injuries in Surgical Practice. East Norwalk, CT, Appleton & Lange, p 66, 1991.)

also has to protect the circulation to the head with separate vascular circuits or severe hypothermia. With surgery involving the descending thoracic aorta, a shunt or partial cardiopulmonary bypass (rather than a simple clamp-and-sew technique) may help to prevent complications, such as proximal hypertension causing left ventricular failure or intracerebral hemorrhage and distal ischemia to the spinal cord and abdominal viscera.

The involved aorta is usually opened, and a prosthetic graft is inserted. If the aneurysm involves the distal thoracic aorta, attaching an island of aorta with the origins of the intercostal arteries from T-8 to T-10 to the graft may reduce the incidence and severity of lower spinal cord ischemia.

Infected Vascular Anastomoses or Grafts

Etiology. Any vascular anastomosis may become infected, but thoracic vascular surgery performed in the presence of an accidental or iatrogenic injury to the esophagus has a greatly increased risk of contamination.

Diagnosis. An elevated white blood cell count and fever in the presence of a pseudoaneurysm or an increasing fluid collection at the site of a prior vascular anastomosis should be considered a vascular infection until proved otherwise. Persistently positive blood cultures for *Staphylococcus epidermidis* in a patient with prior vascular surgery should also make one suspect a vascular infection. However, many

patients with this problem, particularly if they are critically ill and anergic, do not have fever or a leukocytosis. Indeed, a graft or pseudoaneurysm may not show any evidence of infection unless the involved tissue is resected and cultured.

Treatment. With infected grafts or vascular anastomoses, if fever or leukocytosis persists in spite of antibiotic therapy, or if there appears to be evidence of an impending rupture, surgery should be performed as soon as there is any reasonable chance that the patient can survive the procedure. During such surgery, the involved vessel should be resected and an extra-anatomic bypass constructed. Ideally, high blood levels of antibiotics should be present at the time of surgery. In addition, the infected material or tissue should be resected before the new graft is sutured into place.

Occluded Superior Vena Cava

Etiology. Occlusions of the superior vena cava are usually caused by malignancies, such as carcinoma of the lung or lymphomas.[17, 18] However, occasionally, long-term intravenous therapy or total parenteral nutrition through central catheters causes thrombosis of the subclavian and innominate veins and the superior vena cava.

Diagnosis. Acute occlusion of the superior vena cava can cause severe swelling of the head, the neck, and the arms. The skin may become blue or dusky, and the veins of the neck and the arms are often greatly distended. Large collateral veins may also be seen under the skin of the anterior chest and neck. Swelling of the arms, the neck, and the face may be severe, and the patient may become extremely uncomfortable from the tissue swelling. Occasionally, the swelling may involve tissues in and around the upper airway, producing stridor and/or dyspnea.

Extrinsic lesions compressing the superior vena cava can often be seen on the plain chest x-ray film, but a CT scan with contrast medium usually provides much better detail. In many instances, a venacavogram is required to outline the area of occlusion.[18]

Treatment. Malignancies causing extrinsic compression of the superior vena cava are best treated by radiotherapy and/or chemotherapy.[18] Benign occlusions by aneurysms or hematomas should be corrected as soon as the patient is a reasonable surgical risk.

Intraluminal thromboses can often be treated successfully with local thrombolytic therapy. If a catheter is already present, this can be used to infuse the thrombolytic agent. Jeejeebhoy recommended that 7500 IU of urokinase (or an equivalent amount of streptokinase or tissue plasminogen activator) be placed in 3 mL of normal saline solution and injected into the catheter.[19] The catheter is then capped for 3 hours and flushed with 10 mL of saline containing 1000 U of heparin.

Iatrogenic Hemorrhage

In general, mechanical complications of total parenteral nutrition catheters can be divided into vascular injury (resulting in hematomas, bleeding into the chest, brachiocephalic false aneurysms, or arteriovenous fistulas), pleural injury (pneumothorax or hemothorax), hemomediastinum, venous cannulation injury (air embolism or retained catheter fragment), thoracic duct injury, and neurologic injury (phrenic nerve, brachial plexus, recurrent laryngeal nerve, or cervical sympathetic injury).

Hemothorax attributable to insertion of a subclavian vein catheter is not uncommon, and serious complications have been reported in 0.19% of patients for both the subclavian and internal jugular routes.[20–22] If massive hemorrhage occurs, it is usually due to arterial perforation. This complication has occurred in only 1% of patients with the internal jugular approach, but with subclavian vein catheterization, it may occur in 6 to 10%.[23] With perforation of the subclavian or internal mammary artery, concomitant laceration of the pleura may lead to persistent hemorrhage and/or a large hemothorax necessitating surgery. Thoracentesis or insertion of a chest tube can confirm the presence of blood.

Emergency repair or ligation of the involved vessel is recommended if chest tube drainage of blood exceeds 200 to 300 mL/h for more than 3 to 4 hours, if the chest shows increasing hemothorax in spite of well-placed chest tubes, or if there is difficulty stabilizing the patient's vital signs. Occasionally, the bleeding vessel can be occluded by an interventional radiologist.

Catheter Fragments

If an intravenous catheter has been sheared off into a major intrathoracic vein by its needle and cannot be retrieved through a local incision, one should attempt to remove it under fluoroscopic guidance with a flexible forceps inserted via the internal jugular vein. If this is unsuccessful, the catheter can be left in place unless there is evidence that it is a source of sepsis. If it appears to be infected, it should be removed surgically as soon as possible.

Air Embolism

Pathophysiology. Air can enter the vascular system in a variety of ways.[24, 25] Venous air embolism acts primarily by causing an air lock in the outflow tract of the right ventricle and thereby reducing or stopping the flow of blood out of the right side of the heart into the lungs. The amount of venous air that is fatal to adults is estimated to be between 200 and 300 mL, but the rate of air entry is also an important factor.[25]

The mechanisms whereby arterial air emboli cause shock, death, or neurologic abnormalities are different. Air entering the left side of the heart passes quickly into the aorta. Then, depending on the position of the patient, the air may move into the coronary and/or the cerebral arteries. Air entering these vessels can completely obstruct the flow of blood, causing a myocardial infarction or stroke. In dogs, small amounts of air (in the range of 0.5 to 1.0 mL) injected into the coronary circulation have been fatal.[25]

Etiology. In one series, air embolism through central venous catheters caused death in 4 patients and severe neurologic and cardiorespiratory complications in 14 others.[26] Air embolism tends to occur when a central venous catheter is open to air and the central venous pressure is less than atmospheric pressure because of hypovolemia and/or elevation of the head and chest. Sitting or ambulating patients are especially endangered by central venous catheter disconnections.[27] There also may be insidious leaks of air through the hemostasis valves in the introducers used to insert pulmonary arterial catheters.[28]

Systemic air embolism is also a recognized complication of forced positive pressure ventilation, particularly with a penetrating lung injury.[29] The risk of air embolism is increased when ventilatory pressures exceed 60 to 80 cm H_2O.[29]

Clinical symptoms of systemic air emboli include syncope, coma, seizures, cardiac dysrhythmias, and cardiac arrest.[27] A sudden change in cardiovascular or neurologic function shortly after a patient is intubated and ventilated or after a central venous catheter has been inserted or disconnected should be considered to result from air emboli until proved otherwise. During open cardiac massage, the presence of air in the coronary arteries is diagnostic of air embolism, but this is seen in only about 30 to 40% of proven air emboli.[30]

Treatment. Air embolism from intravenous catheters is best prevented by using continuous flush systems[31] and carefully securing all intravenous connections, especially in patients who have subclavian or internal jugular venous catheters and are ambulatory.

The patient with a suspected air embolus should be turned immediately onto her or his left side and her or his legs and pelvis should be elevated so that the intracardiac air tends to move from the outflow tract of the right ventricle to the apex or even back into the right atrium.

If the patient has had a cardiac arrest attributable to air emboli, one should begin closed chest cardiac massage and the intravenous catheter should be aspirated to remove any air that may still be in the catheter or the vein. If this is not rapidly successful, the only chance for resuscitation probably is an immediate thoracotomy with clamping of the involved lung or veins, aspiration of the air from the cardiac chambers and the aorta, and open chest cardiac massage. If cardiopulmonary bypass is available, it can be helpful for maintaining cardiac or cerebral blood flow and possibly also pushing air out of the coronary arteries.

Pulmonary Arterial Rupture

The reported incidence of pulmonary arterial rupture caused by indwelling catheters is about 0.2%.[32] The risk of pulmonary arterial perforation is increased with distal placement of the pulmonary arterial catheter and excessive balloon inflation or vigorous flushing.[33] The risk is also increased in patients with pulmonary hypertension, in patients with mitral valve disease, and in those receiving anticoagulant therapy. Hypothermia during cardiopulmonary bypass, possibly by causing the catheter to stiffen, tends to increase the risk of perforation.[33]

Several other factors also predispose to catheter rupture of the pulmonary artery. If balloon inflation is eccentric, it can force the protruding catheter tip into the wall of the artery. An overwedged pattern suggests that eccentric balloon inflation, overdistention, or both are occurring.[34, 35] If this pattern appears, the balloon should be deflated immediately and the catheter withdrawn until a normal pulmonary arterial tracing returns. If the catheter is advanced too far distally with the balloon deflated, it can also perforate the pulmonary artery.

Hemoptysis in a patient with a pulmonary arterial wedge pressure catheter should suggest the diagnosis of perforation or rupture of the pulmonary artery. Hemoptysis with pulmonary arterial rupture is common, but the severity varies from scant, frothy, pink sputum (which can be mistaken for pulmonary edema) to massive, exsanguinating hemorrhage. Up to 90% of the blood leaking into the tracheobronchial tree may remain in alveoli and small bronchi and not be expectorated.[36] Consequently, a relatively mild hemoptysis may be deceptive and can be associated with extensive bronchial bleeding, causing alveolar flooding and rapid development of hypoxemia.[36, 37] A chest radiograph often reveals a new infiltrate around the tip of the catheter if pulmonary arterial rupture has occurred.[32] However, the initial chest x-ray film is frequently essentially normal.

If the amount of apparent hemoptysis is small and the patient is hemodynamically stable, observation may be all that is needed; however, the pulmonary arterial catheter must not be wedged or flushed vigorously again. Tracheal suctioning and coughing should be minimized, and coagulation abnormalities, if present, must be corrected.

Large amounts of hemoptysis require placement of an occluding balloon (Fogarty's) catheter into the bleeding bronchus or insertion of a double-lumen endotracheal tube. If this does not control the bleeding, an emergency lobectomy or pneumonectomy may be required. However, hemoptysis from pulmonary arterial rupture can be so massive that exsanguination can occur within a few minutes.

Chest Tube Damage to Intercostal Artery

Rarely, insertion of a chest tube can injure an intercostal artery, causing severe continuing bleeding. The easiest way to manage this is to replace the chest tube with a No. 20 to 24 French, 30-mL bag Foley's catheter. After the tip of the Foley catheter is well within the chest, the 30-mL bag is filled with saline and the inflated balloon is then pulled up tightly against the chest wall to compress the intercostal vessels. However, if the blood loss continues to exceed 200 mL/h for more than 2 to 3 hours or if the vital signs become unstable, a thoracotomy is required.

Iatrogenic Injury to Heart

Catheter or Pacemaker Perforation. It has been estimated that the incidence of perforation of the heart by a central venous catheter is about 0.2%.[38] In that report by Burri and Anhefeld, 41 cases with a mortality rate of 83% were cited from the literature. One third of the perforations occurred after 2 days. Elderly patients, apparently because of lipomatosis or thinning of the heart, were more likely to have this complication. Fatal cardiac tamponade may also occur when the intrapericardial catheter, which is plugging the hole in the myocardium, is drawn back into the cardiac chamber. Pacemaker leads can cause similar injuries. Most cardiac penetrations by catheters are apparently asymptomatic. However, if signs and symptoms of tamponade develop, a pericardiocentesis or an epigastric pericardial window may be required. If there is continued bleeding or if shock develops, an emergency thoracotomy is required.

Cardiac Injury During Cardiopulmonary Resuscitation. The incidence of pericardial tamponade with cardiopulmonary resuscitation varies from about 8% with out-of-hospital resuscitations to 2% in the hospital.[39, 40] The injury may be due to direct trauma from the external massage or from attempts at intracardiac injection of drugs.[41, 42] Such attempts were responsible for a hemopericardium found in a third of autopsies done on patients who had cardiopulmonary resuscitation. Consequently, intracardiac injections during cardiopulmonary resuscitation are discouraged.[39]

Lymphatic Duct Injuries

Injury to the major lymphatic ducts in the thoracic inlet by various venipuncture techniques occurs in 0.2 to 4.2% of attempts at catheter placement.[43] These ducts are more likely to be injured with attempted cannulation of an internal jugular vein, especially on the left. Aspiration of serosanguineous fluid indicates the presence of such an injury. The resultant chylothorax occasionally requires surgical intervention, especially if the amount of chylous drainage exceeds 1500 mL/d for more than 10 to 14 days in spite of the patient's taking nothing by mouth or receiving a diet in which all of the fat is medium chain triglycerides.[20]

ABDOMEN

The main problems that may require emergency abdominal vascular surgery in an ICU patient include (1) bleeding from an abdominal aortic aneurysm, (2) occlusion of the aorta or one of its main branches causing critical ischemia, (3) problems (usually occlusion or bleeding) related to previous vascular surgery, (4) delayed manifestations of abdominal vascular trauma, and (5) iatrogenic injury to an intraabdominal vessel.

Abdominal Aortic Aneurysm

A small percentage of older patients in an ICU have an abdominal aortic aneurysm. Such aneurysms can usually be detected by physical examination but may sometimes be difficult to differentiate clinically from a tortuous aorta, especially in obese patients. In an occasional patient, the aneurysm may not be apparent clinically, but it should be suspected if the patient complains of new or increasingly severe lower back pain. Standard x-ray films may detect calcium in the wall of the aneurysm.[44] An ultrasound or CT scan can usually outline the aneurysm, its size, and any blood within its wall (Fig. 98–14) or in the retroperitoneum, indicating dissection or leakage. Occasionally, an aortogram is required to outline the aorta and its major branches.

A large or expanding abdominal aortic aneurysm should be resected or bypassed as soon as the risk of surgery is reasonable. If the aneurysm is leaking, emergency surgery is recommended, almost regardless of the risk.

Occlusion of Branches of Abdominal Aorta

Occlusion of the abdominal aorta or its major branches may be found in patients with severe arteriosclerotic vascular disease and superimposed low-flow states or emboli from the heart. Low cardiac output or emboli may occur after an acute myocardial infarction or with atrial fibrillation. Emboli are especially likely after cardioversion of a chronic atrial fibrillation.

Intestinal Ischemia

Etiology and Incidence. It is essential that acute mesenteric ischemia be diagnosed and treated early. After bowel infarction has occurred, the mortality rate may exceed 70 to 90%. Nonocclusive ischemia without peritoneal signs has a much more favorable outcome.

There are numerous causes of acute intestinal ischemia, which include embolus (20 to 30%) or thrombus (5 to 10%) in the superior mesenteric artery, nonmesenteric artery thrombosis (40 to 60%), and acute mesenteric venous occlusion (5 to 20%).[45] Distal colonic and rectal ischemia is not

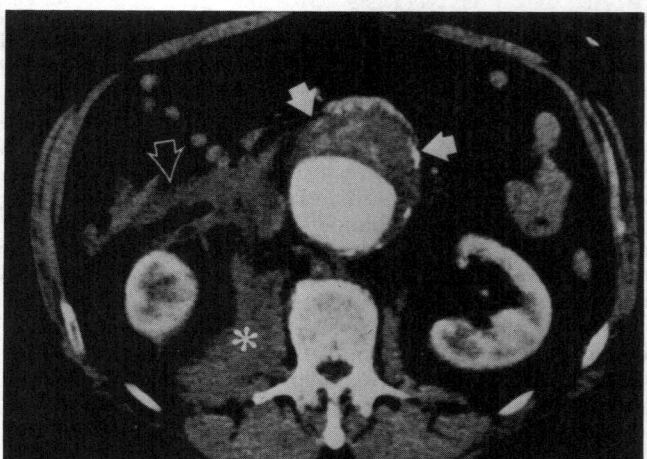

Figure 98–14. CT scan of the abdomen showing a leaking abdominal aortic aneurysm. The aortic aneurysm (*white arrows*) is surrounded by spreading retroperitoneal collections in the anterior perirenal space (*open arrow*), as well as in the right psoas muscle (*). (From Vogelzang RL, Fisher MR: Computed tomography and magnetic resonance imaging in vascular surgical emergencies. In: Bergan JJ, Yao JST [eds]: Vascular Surgical Emergencies. Orlando, FL, Grune & Stratton, p 77, 1987.)

unusual after abdominal aortic aneurysmectomy, especially if a patent inferior mesenteric artery was ligated at the time of surgery.[46] In patients with abdominal aortic aneurysms, the inferior mesenteric artery is usually occluded, unless it was vital for maintaining perfusion to the left side of the colon because of superior mesenteric arterial disease.

If routine colonoscopy is performed after abdominal aortic aneurysm surgery, ischemic colon is found in about 6%.[47, 48] However, clinical evidence of such ischemia is present in only about 2% of patients. With ruptured abdominal aortic aneurysms, colonic ischemia may occur in 60% of cases; however, most of these are not clinically apparent.[49] Small-bowel ischemia is much less common, and it occurs in only 0.15% of patients undergoing abdominal aortic reconstruction.[50]

The small bowel and large bowel usually remain viable if there is gradual arteriosclerotic narrowing of the celiac, superior mesenteric, or inferior mesenteric arteries.[48] As long as one of these vessels remains open, it may provide adequate collateral blood flow to the bowel normally perfused by the other two vessels.

Diagnosis. Diagnosis of intestinal ischemia can be extremely difficult in ICU patients, but early suspicion of mesenteric ischemia followed by rapid diagnostic work-up and treatment appears to be the only method for improving mortality rates. Patients at greatest risk for bowel ischemia are those who undergo repair of a ruptured abdominal aortic aneurysm, particularly if they have no mesenteric Doppler signals after the aortic reconstruction.[48] Other patients at increased risk are those older than 60 years of age with either valvular or atherosclerotic heart disease, especially if heart failure is present and is poorly controlled with digitalis and diuretics.[48] Hypovolemia or hypotension of any cause, recent myocardial infarction, cardiogenic shock, or arrhythmias also increase the risk of intestinal ischemia.

Increasingly severe, constant abdominal pain making the patient restless but with a relatively soft, nontender abdomen on physical examination should make one suspicious of bowel strangulation or ischemia.[51–53] A prior history of abdominal pain, especially after meals, with progressive weight loss is often present in patients with advanced atherosclerosis involving the superior mesenteric artery. Patients with embolic disease often have a history of a prior heart attack or atrial fibrillation. With acute intestinal ischemia, abdominal pain is present in 75 to 90% of patients, and nausea and vomiting are present in about 50 to 60%.[53] Upper gastrointestinal bleeding is uncommon, but guaiac-positive stools are quite frequent.

After abdominal aneurysm surgery, the most common symptom of acute intestinal ischemia is diarrhea, which occurs in about 75% of patients.[45] This may be bloody or nonbloody and usually occurs 24 to 48 hours postoperatively; however, the diarrhea may be delayed for up to 14 days postoperatively. Bloody diarrhea is more ominous and necessitates immediate investigation.[46] An increasing lactic acidosis also necessitates emergency investigation.

Absence of bowel sounds and slight-to-moderate abdominal distention favors the diagnosis of bowel ischemia, but there are many false-positive and false-negative findings. An increasing ileus and a leukocytosis with a shift to the left may also indicate sepsis or nonviable bowel. Abdominal distention is present in 50 to 80%, some peritoneal signs in 60%, ileus in 50%, and shock and fever in about 30% of patients.[45, 51, 52] A severe leukocytosis (white blood cell count ≥20,000/mm³) is seen in less than 50% of patients. A mild elevation in amylase level is common. Other clinical findings include tachycardia (>120 beats/min), hypotension, increased fluid requirements (≥3 L/d above measured losses) to maintain an adequate urine output, and thrombocytopenia.

The presence of physical signs indicating peritoneal irritation is ominous because it usually indicates impending or progressive gangrene. Signs of advancing intestinal ischemia include leukocytosis out of proportion to the physical findings, elevated hematocrit, unexplained metabolic acidosis, and blood-tinged fluid on peritoneal lavage. Any patient who has either bloody diarrhea or persistent nonbloody diarrhea after abdominal aortic surgery should undergo early flexible colonoscopic examination.[48] Adequate examination should include visualization up to the splenic flexure (40 to 50 cm from the anus). If superficial mucosal lesions are discovered on the initial endoscopy, repeated examination should be performed every 12 to 24 hours until it is certain that they are not progressing.

Studies such as arteriography or barium enema examination are usually not helpful in diagnosing colonic ischemia after surgery on abdominal aortic aneurysms. However, with other clinical situations, ischemic colon may sometimes be indicated on barium enema by what looks like thumbprinting of the mucosa of the transverse colon.

Emergency selective arteriography is the keystone of the diagnostic approach to most types of acute mesenteric ischemia of the small bowel.[45, 52] Such arteriography can usually differentiate occlusive from nonocclusive disease. In addition, it can often differentiate embolism, which has a relatively good prognosis, from thrombosis, which has a poor prognosis. With thrombosis, total blockage of the contrast material in the superior mesenteric artery usually occurs about 1 cm from its origin, and both the celiac axis and the superior mesenteric artery generally show significant vascular disease.[57] With an embolus, the first portion of the superior mesenteric artery usually appears to be normal, and the occlusion is usually at the takeoff of the middle colic artery. Consequently, some jejunal branches are still perfused.[53] Venous thrombi in the superior mesenteric vein can sometimes be seen on a CT scan of the abdomen done with intravenous contrast material.

Nonmesenteric intestinal ischemia is diagnosed when mesenteric arterial vasoconstriction is seen on the arteriogram and the clinical picture suggests intestinal ischemia. Shock or the use of vasopressors can make interpretation of the arteriogram difficult.

Treatment. After the diagnosis of acute intestinal ischemia is suspected, vigorous fluid resuscitation is necessary to maintain an adequate blood flow and pressure head in the mesenteric vessels. Pulmonary arterial wedge pressure and cardiac output monitoring may be extremely helpful in attempting to provide optimal blood flow without overloading the heart. Occasionally, low-molecular-weight dextran has been used successfully to expand plasma volume and to decrease intravascular slugging. Because of its vasodilator effect on splanchnic vessels, dopamine is probably the catecholamine of choice if pressure support is necessary. However, no clinical data exist to show its benefit in intestinal ischemia. Rapid administration of digitalis can cause splanchnic vasoconstriction, and therefore, this drug should be used cautiously, especially in elderly patients who may have underlying mesenteric vascular disease.

Systemic antibiotic administration is indicated because of the high incidence of positive blood cultures associated with ischemic bowel. Because excessive dilatation of the bowel can interfere with capillary blood flow, bowel decompression by means of a nasogastric tube can be helpful.

Acute arterial occlusion is best treated by immediate surgical restoration of circulation by embolectomy or aorta–superior mesenteric artery bypass. However, if the colon appears nonviable on direct examination or if the mucosa appears friable, necrotic, and hemorrhagic, emergency colectomy with an end colostomy and a Hartmann pouch is required.[45]

Treatment of nonmesenteric intestinal ischemia can be begun radiologically by administering papaverine (30 to 60 mg/h) through a catheter placed selectively in the superior mesenteric artery.[45] When papaverine is used to treat non-occlusive ischemia, it is continued for 24 hours and then the arteriogram is repeated. Heparin is usually not given concomitantly.

If peritoneal signs are present and abdominal exploration is necessary to determine the viability of the bowel in nonmesenteric ischemia, the surgeon can inject vasodilators and local anesthetics directly into the base of the mesentery in an attempt to improve mesenteric blood flow.[45]

Renal Ischemia

Arterial Disease. Renal vascular occlusive disease may be present with increasing azotemia and a low fractional excretion of sodium.[54] Sudden arterial plugging of major portions of the renal arterial tree may cause flank pain, hematuria, proteinuria, and decreased urine output. Occlusion of smaller renal vessels may be caused by cholesterol, fat, and marrow emboli.[55, 56] Occlusion of only one of the renal arteries may not be apparent unless the patient experiences flank pain. Urine output is usually maintained fairly well as long as one of the kidneys is adequately perfused.

Patients with an acute myocardial infarction, atrial fibrillation, or a ventricular aneurysm have an increased incidence of large arterial emboli. Elderly patients with recent abdominal trauma or aortic surgery can also have cholesterol emboli, sometimes heralded by cutaneous necrotic lesions in the toes (blue toe syndrome) or other tissues below the level of the umbilicus.[57]

The decision for operative intervention is dependent on the amount of renal dysfunction, the site of the thrombi or emboli, and the overall status of the patient. Nonoperative therapy is recommended with distal emboli, for poor-risk patients, and with reasonable function in the other kidney. If the vascular occlusion involves both kidneys or the only functional kidney and the occlusion is in a proximal portion of a renal artery, surgery is generally indicated.[58]

Venous Disease. Venous occlusive disease is relatively uncommon as a cause of acute renal failure. Clues to this entity include proteinuria, lower extremity swelling, and renal function that waxes and wanes without apparent explanation.[56]

Renal venous thrombosis may occur when there is pressure on the inferior vena cava from a malignancy or if a hypercoagulable condition is present. It also tends to occur in glomerulopathies, especially membranous glomerulonephritis.[54] A pulmonary embolus associated with these symptoms and signs indicates the need for venography to exclude clot in the renal veins and the inferior vena cava.[54]

External Iliac Arteries

Hypotension or a low cardiac output greatly increases the likelihood of occlusion of chronically stenosed vessels by thrombi or emboli. The Leriche syndrome of absent femoral pulses, hip or buttock claudication, and impotence attributable to occlusion of the distal aorta is not likely to be detected in critically ill, bedridden patients; however, sudden loss of both pulses at the groin should make one suspect occlusion of the distal aorta. If only one femoral pulse is lost, the occlusion usually involves the common iliac or common femoral artery on that side.

Complications of Major Abdominal Vascular Procedures

The main complications seen after recent vascular surgery are bleeding and occlusion at suture lines. For days, weeks, or even months after vascular surgery in the abdomen, infection may develop or become clinically apparent, especially if a prosthetic graft has been utilized.[44]

Patients undergoing abdominal aortic reconstruction for occlusive disease or an aneurysm require careful postoperative ICU management. These patients often have significant cardiac and respiratory risk factors. The most common cause of death in these patients is an acute myocardial infarction, and careful intraoperative and postoperative hemodynamic monitoring, including pulmonary arterial wedge pressure, cardiac output, and oxygen consumption monitoring, is important to reduce cardiac and peripheral vascular complications.

Postoperative Bleeding

Immediately after resection of an abdominal aortic aneurysm, it is not unusual to have some bleeding into the retroperitoneum. Abdominal distention may not develop until quite late if the bleeding is confined to that area, and aggressive fluid replacement can maintain arterial blood pressure and urine output rather well. Consequently, several hours may pass before the extent of the bleeding is clinically apparent.

Increasing abdominal distention after abdominal vascular surgery is cause for some concern. Such swelling is usually only partly due to ileus. In general, an increase of 1 inch in the circumference of the abdomen is associated with at least 500 to 1000 mL of intra-abdominal fluid (blood) accumulation. Diebel (unpublished data) and others[59] have shown that increasing intra-abdominal pressure can drastically reduce blood flow to the kidneys, the intestines, and the liver. If intra-abdominal pressure as measured with a Foley catheter or nasogastric tube indicates an intra-abdominal pressure exceeding 20 to 30 mm Hg, the abdominal incision should be opened. This can even be done in the ICU if the patient is too unstable to go to the operating room.[59] Other indications for opening the abdominal incision include severe oliguria and increasing metabolic acidosis.

If at all possible, all bleeding and coagulation abnormalities should be corrected before the repeated surgery for postoperative bleeding. This is usually accomplished by administration of platelets, fresh frozen plasma, or cryoprecipitate.

The most common cause of postoperative bleeding is a technical error, but occasionally no specific bleeding site is found. Under such circumstances, the hemorrhage tends to be attributed to prolonged heparin activity or an undiagnosed coagulopathy, such as excessive fibrinolysis.

Graft Infections

The incidences of graft infections after various types of vascular reconstructions are axillofemoral, 15%; femorofemoral, 5%; infrainguinal, 2%; and aortic, less than 1%.[52] More than 75% of aortic graft infections occur in the groin.[60] Early graft infections are often first recognized when swelling, increasing pain, or redness develops in one of the groin incisions.

An abscess or cellulitis in the groin is usually associated with a deeper infection involving whatever graft or suture line has been placed in that area. A CT scan of the abdomen and pelvis can be helpful in diagnosing infection of an aortic prosthetic graft. Findings suggestive of a graft infection include fluid or air around the graft. However, these may be normal findings for up to 4 to 6 weeks after surgery.[61] Indium-labeled leukocyte scans have an overall accuracy of 84% for detecting late graft infections, but the false-positive rate may be as high as 36%.[62]

Aortic-Enteric Fistulas

Any gastrointestinal bleeding in a patient with prior abdominal aortic surgery, even if a graft was inserted years previously, should make one suspicious of an aortic-enteric fistula.[44, 63-65] This usually involves the duodenum at the proximal aortic anastomosis (Fig. 98–15), but it may occasionally involve the distal small bowel at an iliac arterial anastomosis. In some instances, a history of an operation on the aorta is not available, but a long (xiphoid to pubis) midline abdominal scar, particularly when accompanied by bilateral groin incisions, should make one suspect prior aortic surgery. A CT scan showing fluid and gas around the aortic graft is virtually diagnostic of this problem (Fig. 98–16). An aortogram frequently does not show a pseudoaneurysm or fistulous tract in patients with an aortic-enteric fistula.

Abdominal Trauma

Most patients with significant abdominal vascular trauma have hypotension or signs and symptoms associated with local extravasation of blood. However, in some instances, especially with large veins, the initial blood loss may not be obvious enough to warrant re-exploration.[66, 67] Nevertheless, hours or days later, a sudden severe Valsalva's maneuver, which can raise venous and arterial pressures to well over 200 and 300 mm Hg, respectively, may blow out a clot or remove the tamponading effect of a retroperitoneal hematoma. If the patient has a coagulopathy (because of hypotension, liver failure, tissue necrosis, or sepsis), the risk of delayed bleeding is increased further.

Certainly, if a patient with trauma has hypotension that is not clearly due to other causes, one must consider the possibility of intra-abdominal bleeding. Although a diagnostic peritoneal lavage can be extremely helpful for discovering intraperitoneal bleeding, it may not detect blood loss confined to the retroperitoneum. If the patient is stable, a CT scan of the abdomen and pelvis with intravenous and oral contrast media may demonstrate injury to solid organs and intraperitoneal blood. Occasionally, an aortogram may be helpful for detecting injury to a major vessel.

Iatrogenic Injuries

Up to 20% of all intra-aortic balloon pump insertions cause a vascular complication, and the majority of these are

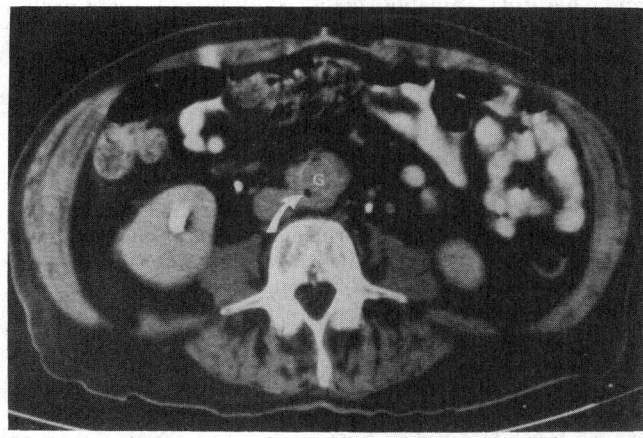

Figure 98–16. Abdominal CT scan showing findings strongly suggestive of the presence of graft-enteral fistula. Aortic graft (G) is surrounded by fluid and gas (*curved arrow*). (From Vogelzang RL, Fisher MR: Computed tomography and magnetic resonance imaging in vascular surgical emergencies. In: Bergan JJ, Yao JST [eds]: Vascular Surgical Emergencies. Orlando, FL, Grune & Stratton, p 77, 1987.)

ischemic in nature.[68] The complication rate is increased if the intra-aortic balloon pump is inserted percutaneously.[69] Most of these injuries or problems involve the femoral artery, but occasionally, an iliac artery or the aorta is damaged.

Occasionally, insertion of femoral arterial catheters to monitor blood pressure or obtain blood samples can also cause injury to the external iliac artery with excessive bleeding into the retroperitoneal space. Such bleeding is usually self-limited, but on rare occasions, it is massive and necessitates emergency surgery.

Any Seldinger's technique using a femoral arterial approach has the potential to occlude or perforate an iliac or femoral artery, causing ischemia in the lower extremities. It can also produce excessive bleeding or a false aneurysm at the groin or in the retroperitoneal pelvis. Patients should be followed closely after such studies to identify these problems before shock or irreversible ischemia develops.

NECK

Some of the vascular problems in the neck that are likely to require emergency surgery in ICU patients include (1) occlusion or bleeding after vascular surgery, (2) injuries caused by insertion of venous catheters, (3) emboli from the heart, (4) bleeding from vessels resulting from erosions caused by infection or by irradiation of head and neck malignancies, and (5) delayed manifestations of trauma.

Complications of Vascular Surgery

After vascular surgery in the neck, there is a 2 to 5% chance of complications related to occlusion, emboli, or bleeding.[70, 71] Although most of these complications occur within 24 hours of surgery, they may occasionally be delayed, and prompt recognition of the problem may be required to prevent death or severe neurologic disability.

Vascular Occlusion or Emboli

The most frequent causes of occlusion of a carotid endarterectomy include technical errors, hypotension, and local hematomas.[71, 72] With any sudden change in neurologic status, an arteriogram or Doppler study of the involved vessels

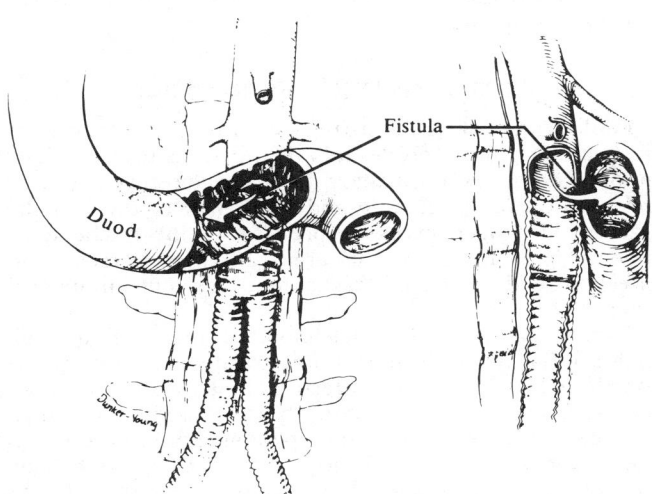

Figure 98–15. Aortoduodenal fistula resulting from abdominal aortic aneurysm. (From Ernst CB: Aortoenteric fistulas. In: Haimovici H [ed]: Vascular Emergencies. East Norwalk, CT, Appleton-Century-Crofts, p 366, 1982.)

can be helpful. If an abnormality is found, or if these studies are not rapidly available, immediate exploration of the operative site should be performed.

Bleeding

Most postoperative bleeding problems occur soon after surgery. However, they are occasionally delayed and may be precipitated by periods of hypertension or unusual agitation, particularly in individuals with abnormal coagulation or platelet function. The bleeding may be manifested as swelling in the neck, airway obstruction from extrinsic pressure, or bleeding through the incision with resultant hypotension.

Airway Obstruction

Airway obstruction with noisy breathing or stridor may occur after almost any type of neck surgery. At times, postoperative bleeding is confined to the deeper spaces of the neck and may be difficult to recognize until rather late. If an airway problem develops rapidly, emergency intubation may not be possible, and the operative incision may have to be opened rapidly to relieve extrinsic compression on the trachea. In rare cases, one may have to provide an emergency airway with a cricothyrotomy, tracheostomy, or large tracheal needle.

In patients with relatively mild symptoms, ultrasonography may be used to detect deeper collections of blood or other fluid in the neck.

Central Venous Catheters

During attempts to insert a catheter into the internal jugular vein, the common carotid or vertebral artery can be injured. This may cause fatal complications from hemorrhage or neurologic damage, especially if the injury is caused by a large-caliber device.[21] If an injury to one of these vessels is suspected of causing excessive bleeding, the device should be left in place until the vessel can be properly controlled and repaired in the operating room.[22] Traumatic arteriovenous fistulas are more frequently associated with internal jugular than with subclavian vein catheters.[73, 74] Rarely, arteriovenous fistulas are created in the vertebral artery during angiographic procedures.[21] Although excessive bleeding may necessitate emergency surgery, most false aneurysms and arteriovenous fistulas can be corrected surgically on a less urgent basis.

Thrombosis of veins occurs regularly when indwelling catheters are left in place for prolonged periods, but clinical symptoms are usually found in only 2 to 6% of patients.[75] Thrombosis of the internal jugular vein in patients who already have neurologic disorders may cause dramatic compromise of cerebral perfusion.[76] Infection of such thrombi can be life threatening, and the device, whether it be a catheter or a transvenous pacemaker lead, should be removed as soon as possible. If the vein remains infected after removal of the device, surgical resection of the infected tissue is usually necessary,[77] especially if the patient remains septic in spite of antibiotics and local drainage.

Emboli

Emboli to the internal carotid artery can occur with atrial fibrillation, acute myocardial infarction, or fungal endocarditis. If the patient's signs and symptoms suggest sudden central nervous system ischemia, and if there is any underlying cardiac disease, a duplex scan or carotid arteriogram should be performed on an emergency basis.

Acute occlusion of a common or internal carotid artery is best treated surgically, and this can often be done under local anesthesia in poor-risk patients. In some high-risk patients with mild deficits, anticoagulation with heparin may be the preferred treatment.[78]

Progressing Strokes and Crescendo Transient Ischemic Attacks

Carotid endarterectomy in patients with an acute complete stroke and altered consciousness has been associated with mortality rates exceeding 40%, whereas medical therapy of such patients has had a mortality rate of only about 20%. However, in about 10 to 15% of patients who have acute symptoms attributable to carotid artery arteriosclerotic disease, the clinical picture is one of either mild but progressing stroke (5 to 10%) or crescendo transient ischemic attacks (2 to 5%).[79] In such patients, medical therapy results in moderate-to-severe deficits or death in about 70 to 80%. In contrast, early surgical correction of the narrowed internal carotid artery reduces the incidence of death or major disability in these patients to about 10 to 30%.

Vascular Erosions
After Radical Neck Dissection

In an occasional ICU patient, a common carotid artery may rupture and bleed massively because of infection or necrosis of an invading carcinoma. This is particularly likely to occur in individuals who have had poor wound healing after a radical neck dissection and irradiation for a cancer of the head and neck.[80] In most instances, there is mild initial (sentinel) bleeding. However, if this is ignored, sudden massive hemorrhage with rapid exsanguination may occur minutes, hours, or days later. Any bleeding from an open wound after a radical neck dissection is an indication for emergency exploration of the wound in the operating room.

Because the leaking vessel is almost invariably infected, separate clean incisions must be used to expose and ligate the uninvolved portion of the vessel proximal and distal to the bleeding site. The involved portion of the vessel can then be excised.

Although there is some risk of stroke after ligation of a common carotid artery, it is relatively low in these patients. The incidence of stroke is particularly low if the common carotid bifurcation is spared. This allows the external carotid artery to provide collateral blood flow to its associated internal carotid artery.

Tracheal–Innominate Arterial Fistulas

Etiology. Occasionally, a tracheotomy tube, either at its tip or at the balloon, erodes into the innominate artery. The innominate artery normally crosses the lower airway near the junction of the middle and lower (distal) third of the trachea. Prolonged excessive pressure of the tracheotomy tube or balloon against this area can cause necrosis and infection of the involved trachea and adjacent innominate artery.[81, 82]

Factors that increase the likelihood of a tracheal–innominate arterial fistula include a low tracheotomy (below the fourth or fifth ring), local infection, high balloon pressure, and pulsation of the tracheotomy tube. Consequently, whenever possible, the tracheotomy opening should be through the second and third tracheal cartilages. Excessive balloon pressure (>30 mm Hg) should also be avoided. If the tracheostomy is pulsating, the tracheotomy dressings should be arranged so that the distal tip of the tube is displaced posteriorly, away from the anterior tracheal wall.

Diagnosis. The first evidence of a tracheal–innominate arterial fistula is generally mild sentinel bleeding from the tracheotomy, usually at least 7 to 14 days after it has been constructed. Bleeding within 24 to 48 hours soon after a tracheotomy is performed is usually due to a technical error, such as failure to secure adequately the isthmus of the thyroid gland or failure to apply an adequate ligature to one of the anterior jugular or anterior thyroid veins. Later bleeding, however, is usually due to suction catheter trauma to an inflamed trachea. Nevertheless, all bleeding from a tracheotomy should be investigated carefully.

The best way to examine the trachea for bleeding is with a flexible bronchoscope. Initially, the bronchoscope is used to examine the distal trachea and tracheobronchial tree. If there is no distal bleeding, the tracheotomy tube is gradually withdrawn while the bronchoscope is used to examine the more proximal portions of the trachea. If the only or main bleeding lesion found is in the anterior trachea where the balloon or tube impinges, there is a strong likelihood that a tracheal–innominate arterial fistula is present.

Management. If a tracheal–innominate arterial fistula is present but the bleeding is not excessive, an endotracheal tube can be inserted beyond the area in question and inflated. This may prevent any sudden bleeding from flooding the lungs while the patient is being taken to the operating room.

If the patient is bleeding significantly, one can try to inflate the balloon further to control the bleeding while the patient is moved to the operating room. If the bleeding is massive or is not controlled by inflating the balloon, one can attempt to control it internally by digital pressure from within the tracheal lumen. One can also try to dissect bluntly along the anterior trachea and then apply digital pressure to the innominate artery at the trachea. During all these steps, arrangements should be made to bring the patient to the operating room for definitive surgery as rapidly as possible.

At surgery, a tracheal–innominate arterial fistula is usually characterized by dense adhesions to the trachea with severe bleeding when the unoccluded artery is dissected off or lifted from the trachea. If the innominate artery is easily dissected off the trachea, appears normal, and does not bleed, a tracheal–innominate arterial fistula was not present; however, a flap of viable muscle should still be inserted between these two structures.

If a tracheal–innominate arterial fistula is found, the normal portions of innominate artery are cut and ligated above and below the fistula, which is then resected without reanastomosis. The involved area of trachea should also be resected. After this, a flap of tissue, usually an adjacent strap muscle, should be inserted between the tracheal repair and the ligated ends of the innominate artery.

Trauma

Penetrating Trauma

Most penetrating injuries to large neck vessels cause enough bleeding to warrant early exploration and repair or ligation. Occasionally, however, a lesion is missed and manifests later as external bleeding, a hematoma, a pseudoaneurysm, or an arteriovenous fistula.

Any later development of bleeding, neck mass, palpable thrill, or audible bruit should alert one to a probable delayed complication of vascular trauma. Whenever possible, an arteriogram should be performed to confirm the diagnosis and to define the lesion before operative correction.

Blunt Trauma and Dissections

Dissection of the layers of the wall of a carotid artery is an uncommon cause of cerebrovascular insufficiency, and most are not diagnosed clinically. However, it may cause severe cerebrovascular accidents or hemorrhage with exsanguination, making this an important vascular surgical problem. The two main types of carotid dissections are traumatic and spontaneous.[83] Traumatic carotid dissection is usually caused by a severe deceleration or hyperextension injury. The internal carotid artery is involved much more frequently that the common carotid artery. Spontaneous dissections may involve any part of the internal carotid artery, but traumatic dissection usually involves the distal artery, often right up to the skull. A spontaneous dissection may result in a jelly roll–like appearance of the artery in cross-section because of curling of the dissected intima and inner media, with the jelly-like thrombus in the false lumen (Fig. 98–17).

Spontaneous carotid dissection usually causes transient ischemic attacks (56%) or completed stroke (30%). An associated sudden onset of ipsilateral headache and neck pain may be helpful in making the diagnosis. With traumatic dissection, there is often delay of 2 to 7 days before localizing neurologic findings develop. This lesion should be suspected in patients with severe head trauma and localized neurologic changes, but no lesion on CT scan of the brain to explain the clinical picture.

The diagnosis is usually made by an arteriogram, which typically shows an extensive narrowing of the internal carotid lumen, often extending up to the skull (Fig. 98–18). This carotid string sign represents elevation and folding of the intima in the dissected segment. In some instances, the carotid arteriogram shows a tapered area of narrowing (referred to as a dunce cap deformity) with distal occlusion (Fig. 98–19).

The treatment of choice is anticoagulation with heparin, and this can produce excellent results.[83] However, if anticoagulation is contraindicated because of associated injuries, if the carotid artery is not totally occluded, and if it is technically feasible, the artery should be explored and repaired. If the carotid stump pressure is greater than 70 mm Hg,

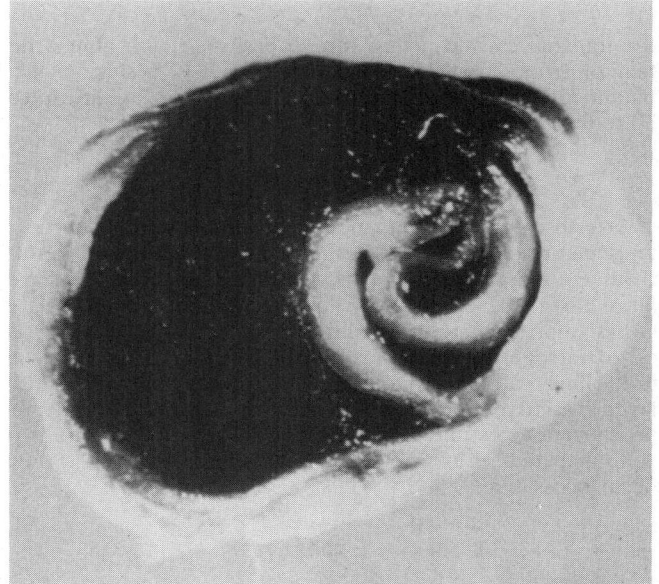

Figure 98–17. Proximal cross-section of a resected carotid artery, showing the dissection within the deep layers of the arterial media with thrombus in the false lumen ("jelly roll–like" appearance) compressing the inner media and intima. (From Krupski WC, Effeney DJ, Ehrenfeld WK: Fibromuscular dysplasia, aneurysms, and spontaneous dissection of the carotid artery. In: Bergan JJ, Yao JST [eds]: Cerebrovascular Insufficiency. Orlando, FL, Grune & Stratton, p 369, 1983.)

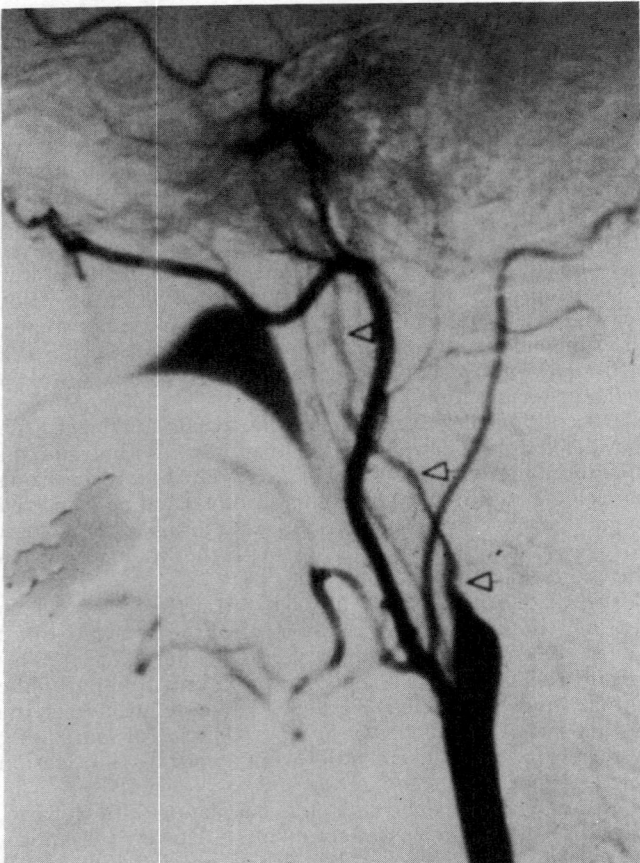

Figure 98–18. The string sign (*arrowheads*) seen on the carotid arteriogram is characteristic of a spontaneous dissection of the internal carotid artery. (From Okuhn SP, Stoney RJ: Carotid artery dissection. In: Bergan JJ, Yao JST [eds]: Vascular Surgical Emergencies, Orlando, FL, Grune & Stratton, p 125, 1987.)

the internal carotid artery can be occluded with almost no fear of stroke. With lower stump pressures, occlusion of a patent internal carotid artery may result in stroke in up to 50 to 60% of cases.

UPPER EXTREMITIES

Arteriosclerosis of the upper extremities seldom necessitates emergency vascular surgery, but ischemia can result from emboli from the heart, especially if the emboli are large and recurrent. More frequent problems usually relate either to arteriovenous fistulas constructed for hemodialysis or to iatrogenic injuries resulting from arteriography or indwelling catheters. Occasionally, trauma may cause delayed vascular problems, particular pseudoaneurysms or arteriovenous fistulas. Although mycotic aneurysms in intravenous drug abusers are less common than in the past, they occur occasionally.

Emboli

Emboli to the upper extremity may arise from the left ventricle after an acute myocardial infarction of the left atrium in patients with chronic atrial fibrillation.[84] Occasionally, endocarditis releases infected emboli that can cause a mycotic aneurysm. Emboli from fungal endocarditis, in contrast to bacterial endocarditis, may be large enough to occlude major vessels.

Any evidence of sudden ischemic changes in an arm or a hand should make one search for a source of emboli, obtain an arteriogram to outline the vascular problem, and begin full-dose heparin administration. Treatment varies with the vessel involved, but emboli causing ischemia can often be removed under local anesthesia in the operating room.

Trauma
Iatrogenic Injuries

Thrombosis. Iatrogenic injuries to vessels in the upper extremity are not uncommon and most frequently involve the radial artery at the wrist attributable to indwelling catheters or the brachial or axillary artery during attempts to perform nerve block.

Thrombosis of the radial artery occurs 5 to 8% of the time that it is cannulated,[85] but surgical intervention is rarely required.[86] Occlusion of the brachial artery occurs with angiography or the use of monitoring catheters in 5 to 41% of cases.[87] However, less than 1 to 2% require surgical intervention to correct ischemia.

The risk of thrombosis increases with the length of time that a radial artery catheter is in place. Radial artery catheters left in place longer than 48 to 72 hours are associated with an increasing risk of thrombosis.[85–87] The size of the cannula also plays a role, and the larger the cannula relative to the diameter of the vessel, the greater is the risk of thrombosis. The risk of thrombosis also increases with tapered catheters and differs depending on the catheter material used (Teflon

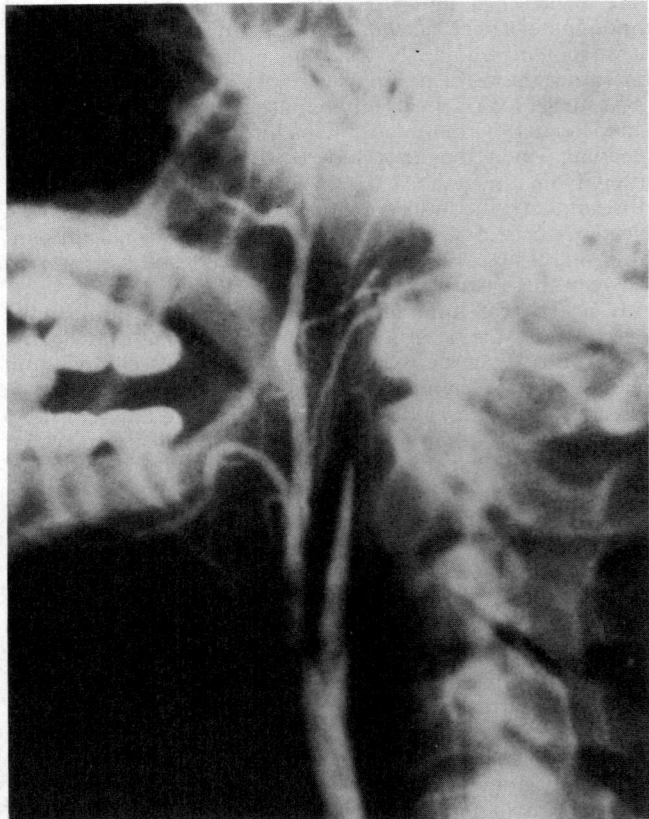

Figure 98–19. Angiogram showing tapered segment of narrowing (dunce cap) with occlusion of the internal carotid artery in a case of spontaneous dissection. (From Okuhn SP, Stoney RJ: Carotid artery dissection. In: Bergan JJ, Yao JST [eds]: Vascular Surgical Emergencies, Orlando, FL, Grune & Stratton, p 125, 1987.)

is less thrombogenic than polyethylene). Intermittent flushing increases the risk of thrombosis, and a continuous dilute heparin flush with a pressurized system is recommended.[31]

Infection. The other major complication that occurs with arterial catheters is infection, particularly if the catheter remains in place longer than 72 to 96 hours in a patient with sepsis elsewhere.[88] Percutaneously inserted catheters have a decreased incidence of infection as compared with those placed by surgical cutdown.

Indwelling vascular lines may be responsible for as much as 10 to 30% of nosocomial bacteremia and may also serve as sites for secondary infection.[88] In Band and Maki's study of 37 catheters exposed to bacteremia, five catheter tips had positive cultures for the same organism.[89] In our ICUs, arterial and venous catheters are usually removed after 72 hours. The tip and the intracutaneous portion are sent for culture if the patient is febrile or has any local signs of inflammation.

Persisting sepsis is occasionally due to a vein that has become occluded and filled with pus. Although suppurative thrombophlebitis usually shows local signs of infection, with redness, swelling, and pain, such evidence may be virtually absent in some patients, especially those who are immunosuppressed. In many instances, the diagnosis can be made or excluded with certainty only by aspirating or cutting down on the vein in question.

Other Complications. Other complications noted with arterial catheters include embolism, skin necrosis, and excessive bleeding from a disconnected line.

Accidental Trauma

Delayed presentation of vascular injuries after accidental trauma may take the form of bleeding, pseudoaneurysms, or occlusion. Management of each of these problems is similar to that noted elsewhere. Because collateral blood flow around the shoulder and the elbow is usually good, emergency surgery for ischemia attributable to vascular problems in these areas is relatively uncommon. However, if the patient is hypotensive, has a low cardiac output, or is receiving large doses of vasopressors, the limb may be threatened.

Occasionally, with blunt trauma to the distal humerus, there may be so much swelling at the elbow that the brachial artery is occluded or the patient may develop a compartment syndrome with later Volkmann's ischemic contracture.

Arteriovenous Fistulas for Hemodialysis

A rather large number of patients with end-stage renal disease have hemodialysis performed via arteriovenous fistulas constructed in the upper extremity. If the patient becomes hypotensive or septic, there is an increased incidence of these grafts' occluding or developing a pseudoaneurysm.[90, 91] If hemodialysis cannot be adequately performed via a double-lumen (Quintin-type) venous catheter and if peritoneal dialysis is not possible, emergency construction of a new arteriovenous fistula may be required.

Occasionally, an arteriovenous fistula gets so large that it can contribute to the development of a high-output cardiac failure. In such circumstances, the fistula should be narrowed with a few sutures. If this is not technically feasible, a new arteriovenous fistula may have to be constructed.

LOWER EXTREMITIES

As with the upper extremities, the lower extremities of ICU patients may require emergency vascular surgery for iatrogenic or accidental trauma.[92, 93] However, the main indication for emergency vascular surgery is acute arterial thromboembolism causing critical ischemia and complications.

Trauma
Penetrating Trauma

Penetrating trauma usually causes early evidence of bleeding or distal ischemia, but sometimes the effects are delayed. Femoral arterial catheters for monitoring blood pressure or for intra-aortic balloon pumping can cause severe distal ischemia, especially in patients with smaller vessels and local arteriosclerotic disease. The ischemia may start with occlusion by an intimal flap (Fig. 98–20). Injuries to the main vessels just above or behind the knee may cause occlusion in a delayed fashion with or without development of a compartmental syndrome.

Arteriovenous fistulas and false aneurysms (Fig. 98–21) in the legs most commonly occur after a penetrating injury. These complications may develop days to years after trauma and can be missed during the initial work-up and operative exploration.[94] This is especially true if the involved vessels are only branches of the main arteries or veins. Therefore, the physician should examine the patient carefully on a regular basis for signs of a late arteriovenous fistula or false aneurysm. An arteriogram demonstrating rapid filling of a vein adjacent to an injured artery is diagnostic of an arteriovenous fistula (Fig. 98–22).

Clinical findings of an arterial injury can include the presence of a bruit or thrill over the injured area. A pulsatile mass may also be present. With large arteriovenous fistulas, high-output cardiac failure may result. Sometimes a large arteriovenous fistula can be diagnosed if local compression slows the heart rate (positive Nicoladani-Branham sign).

When any of these problems are suspected, the best test to confirm the diagnosis is arteriography. Generally, false aneurysms and arteriovenous fistulas should be repaired surgically as soon as they are detected, provided the patient is stable enough to undergo the operation. When needed, such procedures can often be performed under local anesthesia.

Blunt Trauma

Fractures of the femur may injure the adjacent femoral artery. The ischemic effects are usually seen immediately, but in a few patients, they are delayed. The incidence of arterial injuries associated with extremity fractures ranges from about 10% in the civilian population to nearly 30% in military personnel.[95]

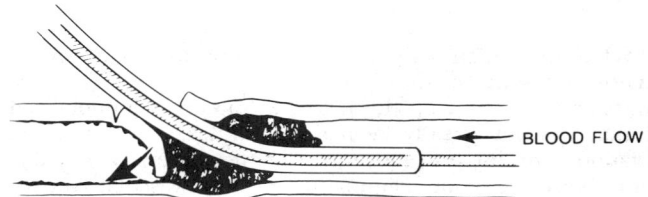

Figure 98–20. Femoral arterial thrombosis occurring after percutaneous insertion of an intra-aortic balloon pump catheter often begins with displacement of the anterior arterial wall into the lumen. Distal arterial run-off is then compromised or completely occluded and eventually total arterial occlusion occurs. (From DeLaria GA: Emergency vascular complications following intraaortic balloon pumping. In: Bergan JJ, Yao JST [eds]: Vascular Surgical Emergencies. Orlando, FL, Grune & Stratton, p 431, 1987.)

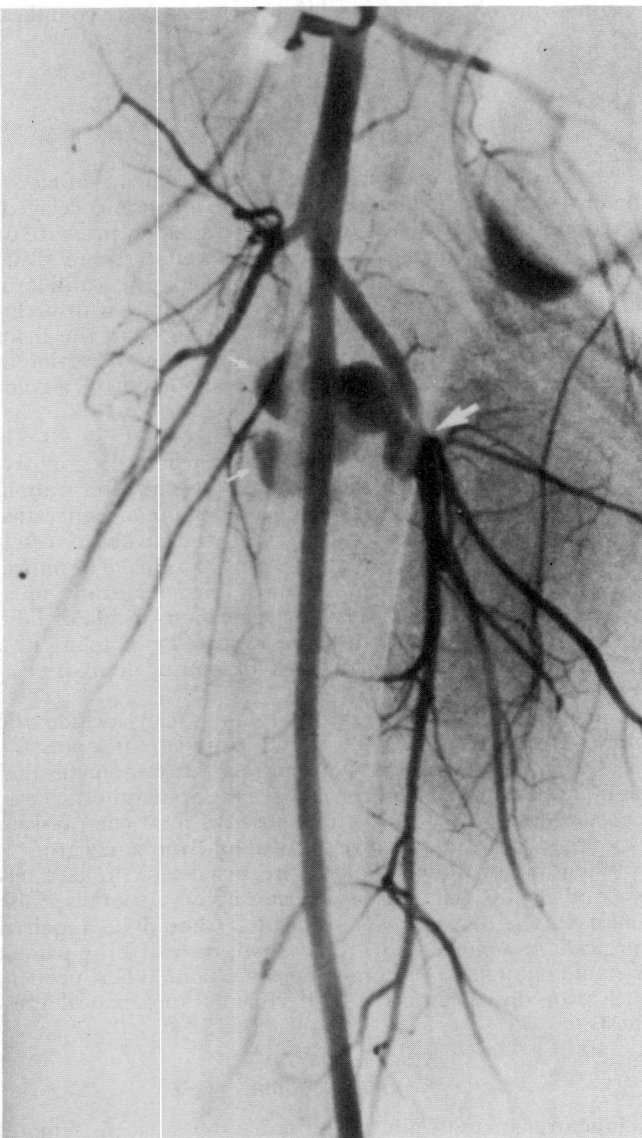

Figure 98–21. Femoral arteriogram showing a false aneurysm of the profunda femoris artery. A knife wound of the thigh of this patient was not believed to have caused a serious injury, but the arteriogram showed a wound of the profunda femoris (*large arrow*) and extravasation of contrast medium into an acute false aneurysm (*small arrows*). (From Perry MO: Penetrating trauma to the extremities. In: Bergan JJ, Yao JST [eds]: Vascular Surgical Emergencies. Orlando, FL, Grune & Stratton, p 165, 1987.)

When the patient with an arterial injury associated with a major extremity fracture is admitted to the ICU, great care must be taken to keep the fracture fragments immobilized if that has not already been done surgically with internal fixation. Any forceful movement of the extremity may disrupt both the bone alignment and the vascular repair, resulting in arterial thrombosis or severe hemorrhage.

The circulation must be assessed frequently, at least hourly, in anyone with a major extremity vascular injury, preferably by palpating the pulses or evaluating distal flow with a Doppler examination. Any change in the circulation necessitates investigation.

With a dislocation of the knee, the popliteal artery is damaged at least 60% of the time. If the vascular injury is not corrected, up to two thirds of these patients may have severe ischemia necessitating an amputation. However, small intimal flaps can probably be followed closely, with or without anticoagulation. Although the popliteal artery may undergo thrombosis acutely, an intimal flap with delayed thrombosis is a more frequent cause of later popliteal arterial occlusion. Fractures of the proximal tibia can produce lesions in the popliteal artery similar to those seen with knee dislocations (Fig. 98–23).

With injuries to the lower leg, especially with combined tibial and fibular fractures, the associated bleeding and muscle swelling may contribute to the formation of a compartmental syndrome. Compartmental syndrome also often occurs when a limb is subjected to an acute ischemic event and then reperfused. After arterial flow is restored, tissue permeability increases and there is local release of toxic oxygen radicals. This results in increased pressure within the fascia-lined muscle compartments of the extremity. This complication occurs after a variety of conditions, including arterial injuries (32%), massive soft tissue injury (19%), venous injuries (14%), and arterial emboli (2%).[96]

Compartment pressure greater than 30 mm Hg can result in progressive nerve and muscle damage, especially if the patient is hypotensive. If this pressure is not promptly relieved surgically, nerve damage can occur within minutes

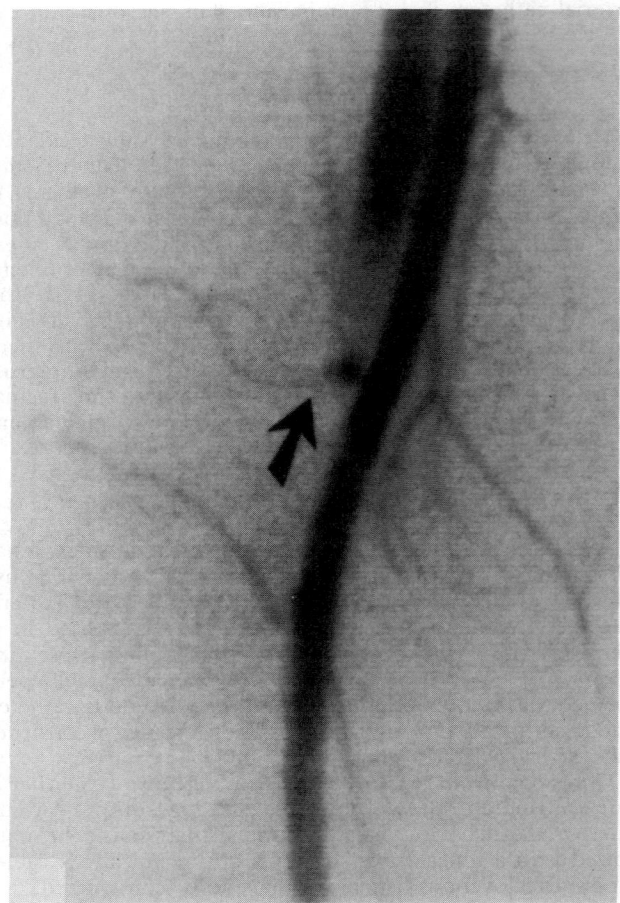

Figure 98–22. Intravenous digital subtraction angiogram. The arrow points to a small false aneurysm; however, the main finding is early opacification of the proximal vein indicating the presence of an arteriovenous fistula. (From Kaebnick HW, Lipchik EO, Towne JB: The role of angiography in emergency vascular surgery. In: Bergan JJ, Yao JST [eds]: Vascular Surgical Emergencies. Orlando, FL, Grune & Stratton, p 57, 1987.)

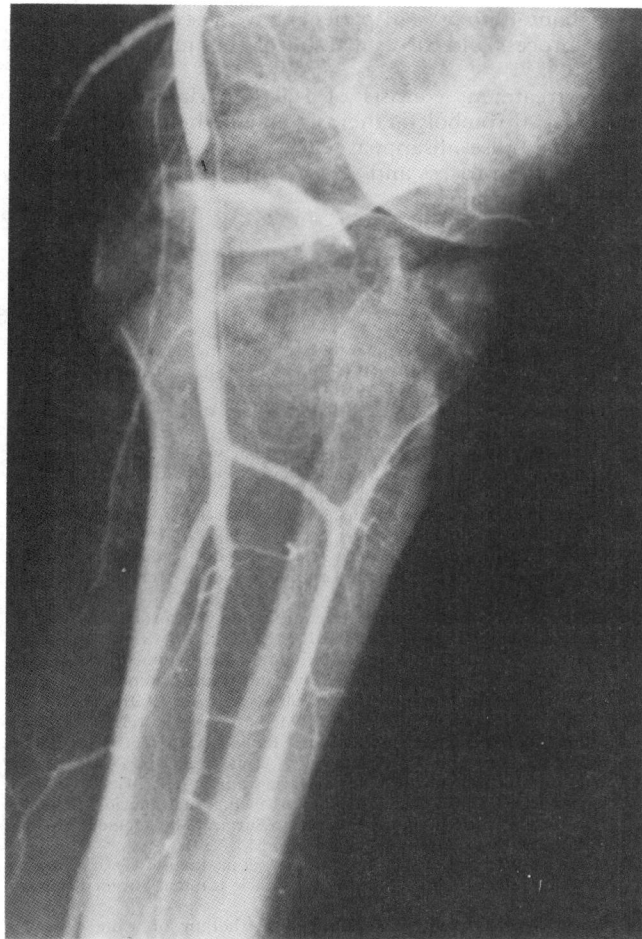

Figure 98–23. Popliteal arteriogram demonstrating an intimal flap with almost complete occlusion of the vessel. This patient had a tibial plateau fracture, but this is also the site of trauma to the popliteal artery during anterior or posterior knee dislocation. (From Bergan JJ: Ligation after acute vascular emergencies. In: Bergan JJ, Yao JST [eds]: Vascular Surgical Emergencies, Orlando, FL, Grune & Stratton, p 43, 1987.)

and can become permanent within 8 to 12 hours. Muscle death often begins within 4 to 6 hours.

Signs of a developing compartmental syndrome are fullness or swelling of an extremity with pain at rest or on palpation, paresthesias in the distribution of the deep peroneal nerve (first dorsal interosseous space), and weakness of the involved muscles, especially the extensor hallucis longus. Even with occlusion of the main vessel, distal pulses may be present in 5 to 15% of cases. Paralysis and loss of sensation tend to be relatively late findings, which often are coincidental with irreversible muscle necrosis.[97]

If a compartmental syndrome is suspected but not obvious, compartment pressures should be measured. This can be done with a variety of devices but generally involves inserting a catheter connected to a pressure transducer into the involved muscle compartment. In the calf, there are four muscle compartments, but the anterior compartment is most likely to be involved.

It has been recommended that fasciotomy be considered for extremity trauma with (1) combined arterial and venous injuries, (2) massive soft tissue damage, (3) delay of more than 4 to 6 hours between wounding and definitive repair, (4) prolonged hypotension, and (5) swelling of the extremity.

Matsen thinks that fasciotomy should be performed when compartment pressures exceed 45 mm Hg;[98] however, we believe that the critical pressure is 30 mm Hg.

If the compartment pressure is greater than 40 mm Hg or if the pressure remains between 30 and 40 mm Hg for longer than 4 hours, a fasciotomy should be performed.[99] Because no absolute critical pressure exists for every patient, fasciotomy should also be considered in patients with pressures less than 30 mm Hg who exhibit clinical signs of compartmental syndrome.[100]

Thromboembolic Occlusions

Acute myocardial infarction or chronic atrial fibrillation may release emboli that are particularly likely to cause leg ischemia by occlusion of the common femoral artery at its bifurcation. Acute hypotension may also cause thrombosis of diseased vessels at the same area or more distally. Severely diseased vessels are particularly prone to thrombosis in patients with a low cardiac output or hypotension.

Although a preoperative arteriogram to define the exact site of occlusion can be of great help to the surgeon, it is not absolutely necessary if the patient has severe renal disease (increasing the risk of contrast studies) or if the viability of the leg is threatened. For example, if one femoral pulse is present and the other has just disappeared, it is clear that the occlusion is in the iliac or common femoral artery. These vessels can often be opened via an incision in the involved groin under local anesthesia in the operating room.

If the foot becomes cold and blue, one can use a Doppler study to help determine the location of the occlusion. The status of the distal vessels on arteriogram is especially helpful in making a decision concerning the possibility of performing a successful infrapopliteal bypass.

After aortic surgery, atherosclerotic plaques may undergo embolization and occlude multiple small vessels distally, producing what is sometimes called trash foot or blue toe syndrome. Treatment involves increasing cardiac output, using vasodilators, and achieving anticoagulation. Occasionally, the emboli may be so extensive that distal surgery is warranted; however, this is seldom successful.

Complications of Vascular Surgery
Graft Thrombosis

Incidence. The incidences of early postoperative graft thrombosis after various arterial reconstructive procedures are axillofemoral, 2 to 25%; femorofemoral, 0 to 13%; femoropopliteal, 5 to 15%; and femorotibial, 15 to 30%.[101, 102]

Etiology. The most common cause of early graft thrombosis is a technical error, such as anastomotic stenosis, intimal flap, and twisting or kinking of the graft. Other causes include stenosis or occlusion of distal outflow vessels, low cardiac output, hypotension, graft compression, and a small-diameter vein graft. A rare cause of early graft failure is a hypercoagulable state attributable to antithrombin III deficiency or abnormal platelet aggregation. For most vascular reconstructions, prosthetic grafts are much more prone to early thrombosis than are vein grafts.

Diagnosis. Graft thrombosis should be suspected if a palpable distal pulse or audible Doppler signal disappears or changes from a biphasic to a monophasic signal (Fig. 98–24). An ankle brachial index that falls by 0.15 or more is also evidence of graft occlusion. Clinical signs, such as the presence of pallor, mottled skin, and coolness of the extremity, tend to be unreliable in the initial postoperative period.

If reoperation for graft thrombosis is performed and no

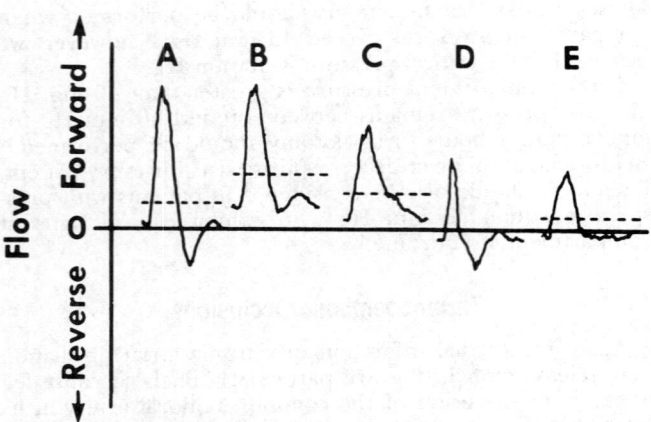

Figure 98–24. Contour of flow pulses in a vein graft. The dotted lines indicate the mean flow. *A.* Unobstructed graft with peripheral vasoconstriction. *B.* Unobstructed graft with peripheral vasodilatation. *C.* Stenosis proximal to the site of the flow probe. *D.* Complete obstruction several centimeters distal to site of flow probe. The pulse contour is nearly normal, but mean flow is zero. *E.* Stenosis just below the flow probe. (From Sumner DS: Noninvasive assessment of peripheral arterial occlusive disease. In: Rutherford RB [ed]: Vascular Surgery. Philadelphia, WB Saunders, p 61, 1989.)

cause of the occlusion is discovered, work-up for a coagulation abnormality should be performed and should include determination of bleeding time, platelet count, prothrombin time, partial thromboplastin time, and fibrinogen levels; antithrombin III assay; platelet aggregation study; and a plasminogen assay.[103]

Therapy. After the diagnosis of graft occlusion is made, 5000 U of heparin should be given intravenously. Thrombectomy and correction of any technical error should then be performed. Additional procedures, such as a proximal aortoiliac surgery or a more distal bypass, may be required to provide adequate inflow or outflow.

Early Complications. Bleeding and early graft occlusion can generally be corrected with local anesthesia, unless there is a problem with inflow from above the groin. In critically ill patients in whom abdominal surgery is contraindicated, a bypass from the femoral artery in the other groin or the axillary artery can usually be performed with local anesthesia.

Late Complications. Late infections of vascular anastomoses or prosthetic grafts cause pseudoaneurysms that progressively enlarge and eventually bleed if not corrected surgically. If an autologous vein graft becomes infected, it often just dissolves and causes severe bleeding if the proximal vessel is still patent. Any of these problems can also cause critical distal ischemia, which may necessitate an extra-anatomic bypass away from the infected area.

False Aneurysms. False aneurysms at vascular suture lines or needle puncture sites are not unusual. These can be treated on an elective basis unless the aneurysm is bleeding, expanding rapidly, or compressing the native vessel, with resultant distal ischemia.

Venous Gangrene

Between 1 and 5% of deep venous thromboses in the lower extremity result in severe swelling and cyanosis of the leg, producing the entity known as phlegmasia cerulea dolens.[104] This is usually associated with some degree of impairment of arterial inflow, and about 30 to 40% of patients have associated frank gangrene or tissue loss. Of

these, about 40 to 50% of patients have a severe generalized disease process and die as a result of the underlying conditions.

Early treatment consists of full heparinization, and in some cases, thrombolytic therapy may be helpful. However, if the pedal pulses disappear, early operative thrombectomy to reverse the process and salvage threatened tissue should be strongly considered.

References

1. Sarris GE, Miller DC: Peripheral vascular manifestations in acute aortic dissection. In: Rutherford RB (ed): Vascular Surgery. 3rd ed. Philadelphia, WB Saunders, p 942, 1989.
2. Miller DC: When to suspect aortic dissection: What treatment? Cardiovasc Med 9:11, 1984.
3. Wilson RF: Injury to the heart and great vessels. In: Henning RJ, Grenvik A (eds): Critical Care Cardiology. New York, Churchill Livingstone, p 411, 1989.
4. Laforte EG: Acute hypertension as a diagnostic clue in traumatic rupture of the thoracic aorta. Am J Surg 110:948, 1965.
5. Wilson RF, Arbulu A, Bassett J, et al: Acute mediastinal widening following blunt chest trauma: Critical decisions. Arch Surg 104:551, 1972.
6. Seltzer SE, D'orsi C, Kirshner R, et al: Traumatic aortic rupture: Plain radiographic findings. AJR 137:1011, 1981.
7. Fisher RG, Hadlock F, Ben-Menachem Y: Laceration of the thoracic aorta and brachiocephalic arteries by blunt trauma. Report of 54 cases and review of the literature. Radiol Clin North Am 19:91, 1981.
8. Woodring JH, Lott FK, Kryscio RJ: Mediastinal hemorrhage: An evaluation of radiographic manifestations. Radiology 151:15, 1984.
9. Mirvis SE, Kostrubiak T, Whitley AO, et al: Role of CT in excluding major arterial injury after blunt thoracic trauma. AJR 147:601, 1987.
10. Varma DGK, Eberly SM: Radiology of mediastinal injuries. In: Webb WR, Besson A (eds): Thoracic Surgery: Surgical Management of Chest Injuries. St Louis, Mosby–Year Book, p 353, 1991.
11. Miller FB, Richardson JD, Thomas HA, et al: Role of CT in diagnosis of major arterial injury after blunt thoracic trauma. Surgery 106:596, 1989.
12. Wheat MW: Current status of medical therapy of acute dissecting aneurysms of the aorta. World J Surg 4:563, 1980.
13. Akins CW, Buckley MJ, Daggett W, et al: Acute traumatic disruption of the thoracic aorta: A ten year experience. Ann Thorac Surg 31:305, 1980.
14. Borman KR, Aurbakken CM, Weigelt JA: Treatment priorities in combined blunt and abdominal aortic trauma. Am J Surg 144:728, 1982.
15. Stiles AR, Cohlmia GS, Smith JH, et al: Management of injuries of the thoracic and abdominal aorta. Am J Surg 150:132, 1985.
16. Maggisano R, Cina C: Traumatic rupture of the thoracic aorta. In: McMurty RY, McLellan BA (eds): Management of Blunt Trauma. Baltimore, Williams & Wilkins, p 206, 1990.
17. Stanford W, Doty DB: The role of venography and surgery in the management of patients with superior vena cava syndrome. Ann Thorac Surg 41:158, 1986.
18. Doty DB, Jones KW: Superior vena cava syndrome. In: Baue AE (ed): Glenn's Thoracic and Cardiovascular Surgery. 5th ed. East Norwalk, CT, Appleton & Lange, p 595, 1991.
19. Jeejeebhoy KN: Enteral and parenteral nutrition. In: Civetta JM, Taylor RW, Kirby RR (eds): Critical Care. Philadelphia, JB Lippincott, p 529, 1988.
20. Wiedemann K, Tuengerthal SJ: Iatrogenic chest injuries. In: Webb WR, Besson A (eds): Thoracic Surgery: Surgical Management of Chest Injuries. St Louis, Mosby–Year Book, p 480, 1991.
21. Morgan RNW, Morrell DF: Internal jugular catheterization: A review of a potentially lethal hazard. Anesthesia 36:512, 1981.
22. Schwartz AJ, Jobes DR, Greenhow DE: Carotid artery puncture with internal jugular cannulation. Anesthesiology 51:160, 1979.
23. Kaiser CW, Koornik AR, Smith N: Choice of route for central venous cannulation: Subclavian or internal jugular vein: A prospective randomized trial. Surgery 17:345, 1981.
24. Flanagan JP, Fradisar A, Gross RJ, et al: Air embolus—A lethal complication of subclavian venipuncture. N Engl J Med 281:488, 1969.
25. Toll MO: Direct blood pressure measurements: Risks, technology evolution and some current problems. Med Biol Eng Comput 22:2, 1984.
26. Coppa GF, Gouge TH, Hofstetter SR: Air embolism: A lethal but preventable complication of subclavian vein catheterization. JPEN 5:166, 1981.
27. Peters JL, Armstrong R, Bradford R, et al: Air embolism: A serious hazard of central venous catheter systems. Intensive Care Med 10:261, 1984.

28. Kondo K, O'Reilly LP, Chiota J: Air embolism associated with an introducer for pulmonary artery catheter. Anesth Analg 63:281, 1984.
29. Graham JM, Beall AD Jr, Mattox KL, et al: Systemic air embolism following penetrating trauma to the lung. Chest 72:449, 1977.
30. Yee ES, Verrier ED, Thomas AN: Management of air embolism in blunt and penetrating thoracic trauma. J Thorac Cardiovasc Surg 85:661, 1983.
31. Gardner RM, Bond EL, Clark JS: Safety and efficacy of continuous flush systems for arterial and pulmonary artery catheters. Ann Thorac Surg 23:534, 1977.
32. McDaniel D, Stone J, Faltas A, et al: Catheter-induced pulmonary artery hemorrhage. J Thorac Cardiovasc Surg 82:1, 1981.
33. Clark CA, Harmon EM: Hemodynamic monitoring: Pulmonary artery catheters. In: Civetta JM, Taylor RW, Kirby RR (eds): Critical Care. Philadelphia, JB Lippincott, p 293, 1988.
34. Page D, Teples D, Hartshoan J: Fatal hemorrhage from Swan-Ganz catheter. N Engl J Med 291:260, 1974.
35. Quinn K, Quebbeman E: Pulmonary artery pressure monitoring in the surgical intensive care unit. Arch Surg 116:872, 1981.
36. Wilson RF, Soullier GW, Wiencek RG Jr: Hemoptysis in trauma. J Trauma 27:1123, 1987.
37. Wiencek RG Jr, Wilson RF: Central lung injuries: A need for early vascular control. J Trauma 28:1418, 1988.
38. Burri C, Anhefeld FW: The Caval Catheter. New York, Springer-Verlag, 1978. Cited in: Weidemann K, Tuengerthal SJ: Iatrogenic chest injuries. In: Webb WR, Besson A (eds): Thoracic Surgery: Surgical Management of Chest Injuries. St Louis, Mosby–Year Book, p 493, 1991.
39. Powner DJ, Holcombe A, Mellow LA: Cardiopulmonary resuscitation–related injuries. Crit Care Med 12:54, 1984.
40. Nagel EL, Fine EG, Krischer JP, et al: Complications of CPR. Crit Care Med 9:424, 1981.
41. Schecter DC: Transthoracic epinephrine injection in heart resuscitation is dangerous. JAMA 234:1184, 1975.
42. Davison R, Barres V, Parker M, et al: Intracardiac injection during cardiopulmonary resuscitation: A low risk procedure. JAMA 244:110, 1980.
43. Teba L, Dedhia HV, Bowen R, et al: Chylothorax review. Crit Care Med 13:49, 1985.
44. Hollier LH, Rutherford RB: Infrarenal aortic aneurysms. In: Rutherford RB (ed): Vascular Surgery. 3rd ed. Philadelphia, WB Saunders, p 909, 1989.
45. Reines HD: Evaluating the acute abdomen in an ICU patient. In: Civetta JM, Taylor RW, Kirby RR (eds): Critical Care. Philadelphia, JB Lippincott, p 574, 1988.
46. Birnbaum W, Rudy L, Wylie EJ: Colonic and rectal ischemia following abdominal aneurysmectomy. Dis Colon Rectum 7:293, 1964.
47. Ernst CB, Hagihara PF, Daugherty ME, et al: Ischemic colitis incidence following abdominal aortic reconstruction. A prospective study. Surgery 80:417, 1976.
48. Ernst CB: Intestinal ischemia following abdominal aortic reconstruction. In: Bernhard VM, Towne JB (eds): Complications in Vascular Surgery. 2nd ed. Orlando, FL, Grune & Stratton, p 325, 1985.
49. Hagihara PF, Ernst CB, Griffin WO Jr: Incidence of ischemic colitis following abdominal aortic reconstruction. Surg Gynecol Obstet 80:417, 1976.
50. Johnson WC, Nabseth DC: Visceral infarction following aortic surgery. Ann Surg 180:312, 1974.
51. Pearce WH, Bergan JJ: Acute intestinal ischemia. In: Rutherford RB (ed): Vascular Surgery. 3rd ed. Philadelphia, WB Saunders, p 1086, 1989.
52. Hurst JM, Fowl RJ: Vascular surgery and trauma. In: Civetta JM, Taylor RW, Kirby RR (eds): Critical Care. Philadelphia, JB Lippincott, p 613, 1988.
53. Bergan JJ, Flinn WR, McCarthy WJ III, et al: Acute mesenteric ischemia. In: Bergan JJ, Yao JST (eds): Vascular Surgical Emergencies. Orlando, FL, Grune & Stratton, p 401, 1987.
54. Beck C: Disordered renal function: Diagnosis. In: Civetta JM, Taylor RW, Kirby RR (eds): Critical Care. Philadelphia, JB Lippincott, p 1319, 1988.
55. Nicholas GG, Demuth WE Jr: Treatment of renal artery embolism. Arch Surg 119:278, 1984.
56. Dean RH: Acute occlusive events involving the renal vessels. In: Rutherford RB (ed): Vascular Surgery. 3rd ed. Philadelphia, WB Saunders, p 1287, 1989.
57. Kempczinski RT: Atheroembolism. In: Kempczinski RF (ed): The Ischemic Leg. Chicago, Year Book Medical Publishers, p 81, 1985.
58. Weaver FA, Meacham PW, Dean RH: Acute renal artery occlusion. In: Bergan JJ, Yao JST (eds): Vascular Surgical Emergencies. Orlando, FL, Grune & Stratton, p 379, 1981.
59. Fietsam R Jr, Villalba M, Glover JL, et al: Intra-abdominal compartment syndrome as a complication of ruptured abdominal aortic aneurysm repair. Ann Surg 55:396, 1989.
60. Goldstone J, Moore WS: Infection in vascular prosthesis: Clinical manifestations and surgical management. Am J Surg 128:225, 1974.
61. O'Hara PJ, Borkowski GP, Hertzer NR, et al: Natural history of periprosthetic air on computerized axial tomographic examination of the abdomen following abdominal aortic aneurysm repair. J Vasc Surg 1:429, 1984.
62. Brunner MC, Mitchell RS, Baldwin JC, et al: Prosthetic graft infection: Limitations of white blood cell scanning. J Vasc Surg 3:42, 1986.
63. Bunt TJ: Synthetic vascular graft infections—II graft-enteric erosions and graft-enteric fistulas. Surgery 94:1, 1983.
64. Reilly LM, Ehrenfeld WK, Goldstone J, et al: Gastrointestinal tract involvement by prosthetic graft infection. The significance of gastrointestinal hemorrhage. Ann Surg 202:342, 1985.
65. Bernhard VM: Aortoenteric fistulas. In: Rutherford RB (ed): Vascular Surgery. 3rd ed. Philadelphia, WB Saunders, p 528, 1989.
66. Wiencek RG, Wilson RF: Abdominal venous injuries. J Trauma 26:777, 1986.
67. Wiencek RG, Wilson RF: Inferior vena cava injuries—The challenge continues. Am Surg 54:423, 1988.
68. DeLaria GA: Emergency vascular complications following intraaortic balloon pumping. In: Bergan JJ, Yao JST (eds): Vascular Surgical Emergencies. Orlando, FL, Grune & Stratton, p 431, 1987.
69. Balooki H: Current status of circulatory support with an intra-aortic balloon pump. Cardiol Clin 3:123, 1985.
70. Kempczinski RF, Brutt TG, Labutta RJ: The influence of surgical specialty and caseload on the results of carotid endarterectomy. J Vasc Surg 3:911, 1986.
71. Hertzer NR: Postoperative management and complications following carotid endarterectomy. In: Rutherford RB (ed): Vascular Surgery. 3rd ed. Philadelphia, WB Saunders, p 1451, 1989.
72. Painter TA, Hertzer NR, O'Hara PJ, et al: Symptomatic internal carotid thrombosis after carotid endarterectomy. J Vasc Surg 5:495, 1987.
73. Dodson T, Quindler E, Crorell R, et al: Vertebral arteriovenous fistula following insertion of central monitoring catheters. Surgery 87:343, 1980.
74. Hansbrough JF, Narrod JA, Rutherford R: Arteriovenous fistula following central venous catheterization. Intensive Care Med 9:287, 1983.
75. Schulier JP, Brion RP, Lustman F: Superior vena cava syndrome following permanent transvenous endocardial pacing. Acta Cardiol 37:39, 1982.
76. Perkins NAK, Cail WS, Bedford RF, et al: Internal jugular vein function after Swan-Ganz catheterization. Anesthesiology 61:456, 1984.
77. Peters JL: Current problems in central venous catheter systems. Intensive Care Med 8:205, 1982.
78. Moore WS: Indications and surgical technique for repair of extracranial occlusive lesions. In: Rutherford RB (ed): Vascular Surgery. 3rd ed. Philadelphia, WB Saunders, p 1373, 1989.
79. Greenhalgh RM, McCollum CN, Bourke BM, et al: Emergency carotid endarterectomy. In: Bergan JJ, Yao JST (eds): Vascular Surgical Emergencies. Orlando, FL, Grune & Stratton, p 139, 1987.
80. Smith LL, Field FI: Management of uncommon lesions affecting the extracranial vessels. In: Rutherford RB (ed): Vascular Surgery. 3rd ed. Philadelphia, WB Saunders, p 1441, 1989.
81. Golz A, Goldsher M, Eliachar I, et al: Fatal hemorrhage following a misplaced tracheotomy. J Laryngol Otol 95:529, 1981.
82. Astrachan DI, Sasaki CT: Tracheotomy. In: Baue AE, (ed): Glenn's Thoracic and Cardiovascular Surgery. 5th ed. East Norwalk, CT, Appleton & Lange, p 611, 1991.
83. Okuhn SP, Stoney RJ: Carotid artery dissection. In: Bergan JJ, Yao JST (eds): Vascular Surgical Emergencies. Orlando, FL, Grune & Stratton, p 125, 1987.
84. Perry MO: Acute limb ischemia. In: Rutherford RB (ed): Vascular Surgery. 3rd ed. Philadelphia, WB Saunders, p 541, 1989.
85. Jones RM, Hill AB, Nahrwold MC, et al: The effect of method of radial artery cannulation on post-cannulation blood flow and thrombus formation. Anesthesiology 55:76, 1981.
86. Bartlett RH, Munster AM: An improved technique for prolonged arterial cannulation. N Engl J Med 279:92, 1968.
87. Barnes R, Foster E, Jannsen A, et al: Safety of brachial artery catheters as monitors in the intensive care unit—Prospective evaluation with the Doppler ultrasonic velocity detector. Anesthesiology 44:260, 1976.
88. Maki DG: Nosocomial bacteremia, an epidemiologic overview. Am J Med 70:719, 1981.
89. Band JD, Maki DG: Infections caused by arterial catheters used for neurodynamic monitoring. Am J Med 67:735, 1979.
90. Haimov M: Circulatory access for hemodialysis. In: Rutherford RB (ed): Vascular Surgery. 3rd ed. Philadelphia, WB Saunders, p 1073, 1989.
91. Sumner DS, Rutherford RB: Diagnostic evaluation of arteriovenous fistulas. In: Rutherford RB (ed): Vascular Surgery. 3rd ed. Philadelphia, WB Saunders, p 1033, 1989.
92. Johnson G Jr: Superficial venous thrombosis. In: Rutherford RB (ed): Vascular Surgery. 3rd ed. Philadelphia, WB Saunders, p 1518, 1989.
93. Yao JST, Flinn WR: Emergency management of superficial venous problems. In: Bergan JJ, Yao JST (eds): Vascular Surgical Emergencies. Orlando, FL, Grune & Stratton, p 461, 1987.
94. Rich NM, Hobson RW, Collins GJ Jr: Traumatic arteriovenous fistulas and false aneurysms. A review of 558 lesions. Surgery 78:817, 1975.

95. Rich NM, Baugh JH, Hughes CW: Acute arterial injuries in Viet Nam—1000 cases. J Trauma 10:359, 1970.

96. Patman RO: Fasciotomy: Indications and technique. In: Rutherford RB (ed): Vascular Surgery. 2nd ed. Philadelphia, WB Saunders, p 513, 1984.

97. Perry MO: Penetrating trauma to the extremities. In: Bergan JJ, Yao JST (eds): Vascular Surgical Emergencies. Orlando, FL, Grune & Stratton, p 165, 1987.

98. Matsen F: Compartmental syndromes. Hosp Pract 15:113, 1980.

99. Russell WL, Burns RP: Acute upper and lower extremity compartment syndromes. In: Bergan JJ, Yao JST (eds): Vascular Surgical Emergencies. Orlando, FL, Grune & Stratton, p 203, 1986.

100. Porter JM, Taylor LM, Baur GM: Non-atherosclerotic vascular disease. In: Moore WS (ed): Vascular Surgery: A Comprehensive Review. New York, Grune & Stratton, p 55, 1983.

101. Szilagyi DE, Elliott JP, Smith RF, et al: A thirty-year survey of the reconstructive surgical treatment of aortoiliac occlusive disease. J Vasc Surg 3:421, 1986.

102. Brewster DC: Early complications of vascular repair below the inguinal ligament. In: Bernhard VM, Towne JB (eds): Complications in Vascular Surgery. 2nd ed. Orlando, FL, Grune & Stratton, p 37, 1985.

103. Towne JB: Hypercoagulable states and unexplained vascular thrombosis. In: Bernhard VM, Towne JB (eds): Complications in Vascular Surgery. 2nd ed. Orlando, FL, Grune & Stratton, p 381, 1985.

104. Dale WA: Venous gangrene. In: Bergan JJ, Yao JST (eds): Vascular Surgical Emergencies, Orlando, FL, Grune & Stratton, p 443, 1987.

SECTION EIGHT

The Renal System and Metabolic Function

Section Editor

Malcolm Cox

CHAPTER 99

Sodium and Volume Homeostasis

Harold M. Szerlip

Numerous homeostatic mechanisms exist to optimize extracellular fluid (ECF) volume and provide adequate perfusion to vital organs. In healthy individuals, despite large fluctuations in salt intake, ECF volume is maintained within narrow limits. In critically ill patients, however, multiple organ system failure and iatrogenic interventions often impair this ability. If not quickly recognized and appropriately treated, excessive ECF volume contraction or expansion may increase morbidity and mortality. An understanding of the factors that regular ECF volume in health and disease is therefore central to the care of the critically ill patient.

MECHANISMS OF SODIUM HOMEOSTASIS
Extracellular Fluid Space

The ECF space contains one third of total body water and is partitioned by vascular endothelium into an intravascular compartment (containing circulating plasma) and an interstitial compartment (bathing all the cells and tissues of the body). A dynamic equilibrium exists between these two compartments, with constant flux of fluid across the capillary bed from the intravascular to the interstitial space and an equal flux of fluid from the interstitial space back into the intravascular space through the lymphatic system.

As initially established by Starling in 1896,[1] the movement of fluid across the capillary bed is determined by the capillary membrane permeability, the hydrostatic pressure gradient (driving fluid out of the intravascular space), and the oncotic pressure gradient (holding fluid within the intravascular space). At the arterial end of the capillary, the sum of these forces shifts fluid across the endothelium into the interstitium. Toward the venous end of the capillary, as capillary

hydrostatic pressure decreases and capillary oncotic pressure increases, interstitial fluid moves back into the capillary (Fig. 99–1). The balance of forces favors net movement of protein-poor plasma from the intravascular to the interstitial space at a rate of approximately 2 mL/min.[2] Lymphatic peristalsis and extrinsic lymphatic compression transport excess interstitial fluid back into the vasculature.[2, 3] If lymphatic return is less than the net transudation of fluid out of the vasculature, the volume of the interstitial space increases, resulting in the formation of edema or the accumulation of fluid in the peritoneal cavity, pleural space, or bowel lumen.

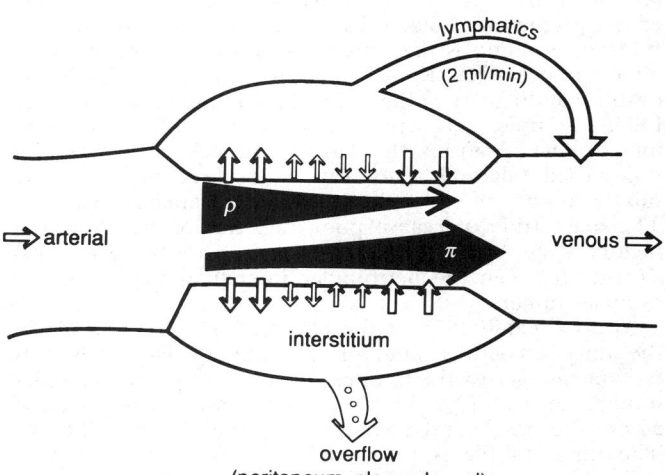

Figure 99–1. Fluid flux across the capillary. At the arterial end of the capillary, the net effect of the Starling forces (hydrostatic, p, and oncotic, π, pressures within the capillary lumen and interstitium) favors the movement of an ultrafiltrate of plasma from the capillary to the interstitium. Toward the venous end of the capillary, as capillary hydrostatic pressure decreases and capillary oncotic pressure increases, fluid moves from the interstitium back into the capillary. Overall, approximately 2 mL/min enters the interstitial space and is returned by the lymphatics into the venous system. If lymphatic return is less than the net transudation of fluid out of the vasculature, expansion of the interstitial space and overflow of fluid into the various body cavities occur.

Because body fluid osmolality is controlled within a narrow range by external water balance, the volume of the ECF space is determined by its solute content. Na^+ is the predominant extracellular solute and because it is essentially excluded from the intracellular space by the action of Na^+,K^+-ATPase, total body Na^+ content determines the volume of the ECF space. However, there is not a single absolute Na^+ content around which ECF volume is defended but rather a series of Na^+ contents depending on Na^+ intake;[4] at high levels of Na^+ intake ECF volume is defended around a value some 10% greater than that at extremely low levels of Na^+ intake. Thus, "normal" ECF volume (total body Na^+ content) varies by approximately 10%, depending on dietary Na^+ intake.

Sodium Balance

Under steady-state conditions, Na^+ intake equals Na^+ excretion. If intake exceeds excretion (positive Na^+ balance), body weight and ECF volume increase. If intake is less than excretion (negative Na^+ balance), body weight and ECF volume decrease. The average American diet contains between 150 and 250 mEq of Na^+ per day. However, critically ill patients rarely have control of their Na^+ intake, which can fluctuate widely depending not only on dietary intake (or lack thereof) but also on the administration of Na^+-containing intravenous fluids and medications.

Na^+ is eliminated from the body through the skin, gastrointestinal tract, and kidney. Although cutaneous and gastrointestinal losses can be extensive in certain disease states, under normal conditions such losses are negligible and the kidney is the major regulator of Na^+ excretion.

Renal Sodium Excretion

Na^+ is freely filtered across the glomerular capillaries, and the filtered load of Na^+ is determined by the product of the glomerular filtration rate (GFR) and the plasma Na^+ concentration. Approximately 99% of the filtered load is reabsorbed as it traverses the nephron; thus, the fractional excretion of Na^+ is usually 1% or less. Between 55 and 65% of the filtered Na^+ is reabsorbed in the proximal tubule. Luminal Na^+ enters proximal tubular cells through a variety of coupled transporters[5] and is then pumped into the lateral intercellular space by Na^+,K^+-ATPase. Because of the high hydraulic conductivity of the luminal membrane, water quickly follows, so fluid reabsorption occurs isotonically in the proximal tubule.[6, 7] From the lateral intercellular space, the reabsorbed salt and water can either leak back into the tubule lumen or enter the peritubular capillary network. The magnitude of reabsorption depends on the "physical factors" (the hydrostatic and oncotic pressure gradients) existing between the peritubular interstitial space and the capillary lumen.

Approximately 25% of the filtered Na^+ is reabsorbed in the thick ascending limb of the loop of Henle. Na^+ is transported across the luminal membrane by a furosemide-inhibitable Na^+-K^+-$2Cl^-$ cotransporter and then extruded across the basolateral membrane by the Na^+,K^+-ATPase.[8] The distal tubule is responsible for the reabsorption of approximately 10% of the filtered Na^+. The Na^+ enters the cell either through a thiazide-inhibitable, neutral NaCl transporter[9, 10] or via an aldosterone-sensitive, amiloride-inhibitable Na^+ channel.[11] As in other parts of the nephron, the energy for Na^+ transport is provided by the Na^+,K^+-ATPase located in the basolateral membrane.

Regulation of Extracellular Fluid Volume
Effective Arterial Blood Volume

The delivery of oxygen and metabolic substrates to tissues and the removal of metabolic waste products depend on absolute intravascular volume, cardiac output, and vascular capacitance or tone. The interplay among these three parameters determines the adequacy (functional integrity) of the vascular space or, as it is commonly called, the effective arterial blood volume (EABV) (Fig. 99–2). A labyrinthine array of homeostatic controls monitors EABV, regulating its individual components in an integrated fashion. Under normal circumstances, cardiac output and vascular capacitance are relatively fixed and intravascular volume is the primary determinant of EABV. In disease states and especially in the critically ill patient, however, it is common for each of these determinants of EABV to be deranged. In patients with multiple organ system failure, for example, it is not unusual for changes in cardiac output or vascular capacitance to produce an ineffective arterial blood volume despite absolute intravascular volume overload; under these circumstances, renal Na^+ retention continues despite excess total body Na^+.

Like any homeostatic system, the system that regulates intravascular and ECF volume consists of an afferent (sensory) limb, which monitors the functional integrity of the circulation, and an efferent (effector) limb, which controls renal Na^+ secretion (Fig. 99–3). The existence of multiple sensors coupled directly or indirectly to numerous effectors minimizes oscillations around the set-point, thereby maintaining total body Na^+ within a narrow range despite large variations in Na^+ intake.

Afferent Limb

Considering that the goal of the volume-regulating system is to optimize intravascular volume, arterial pressure, and tissue perfusion, it is not surprising that monitors are located at points ideally suited for sensing volume, pressure, and tissue perfusion. Some of these sensors have been clearly identified, whereas the existence of others remains presumptive. Roughly 75% of the intravascular volume is contained within the venous side of the circulation, mainly the pulmonary vasculature and cardiac atria; this high-volume, low-pressure system is thus an ideal location for volume sensors. Maneuvers that redistribute interstitial fluid from the lower extremities back into the intravascular space and engorge the central venous circulation (such as head-out water immersion,[12] head-down tilt,[13] and weightlessness[14]) activate these sensors and lead to increased renal Na^+ secretion.

The atria contain richly innervated mechanoreceptors that are activated by atrial distention.[15] Vagal afferents carry the signal to the hypothalamus, where it is integrated with other volume-regulating stimuli. Atrial distention results in decreased sympathetic outflow to the kidneys (increased renal blood flow and Na^+ excretion), increased systemic postcapillary resistance, and decreased arginine vasopressin (decreased Na^+ and water reabsorption), the net result of which is a decrease in intravascular volume. Besides these neurally mediated events, atrial distention also causes the release of a well-characterized natriuretic hormone, atrial natriuretic peptide (ANP).

Whereas intravascular volume is best monitored on the venous side of the circulation, pressure monitoring must occur on the arterial side of the circulation. Baroreceptors in the aortic arch and carotid sinus monitor blood pressure.[16] The importance of these high-pressure monitors in Na^+ homeostasis was initially established in studies of patients with traumatic arteriovenous fistulas.[17] Compression of such fistulas, despite decreasing central venous blood volume, produced prompt natriuresis. Reopening the fistulas, despite causing central venous distention, was antinatriuretic. These baroceptors also operate through vagal afferents.

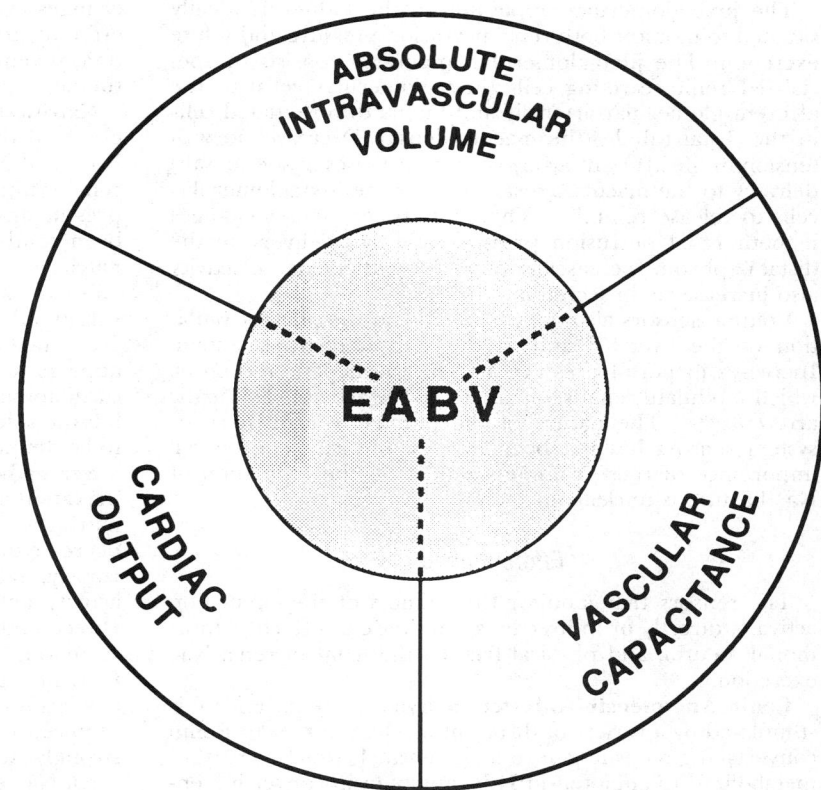

Figure 99–2. Effective arterial blood volume. EABV is a theoretic concept and consists of absolute intravascular volume, cardiac output, and vascular capacitance. Changes in any of these parameters affect EABV.

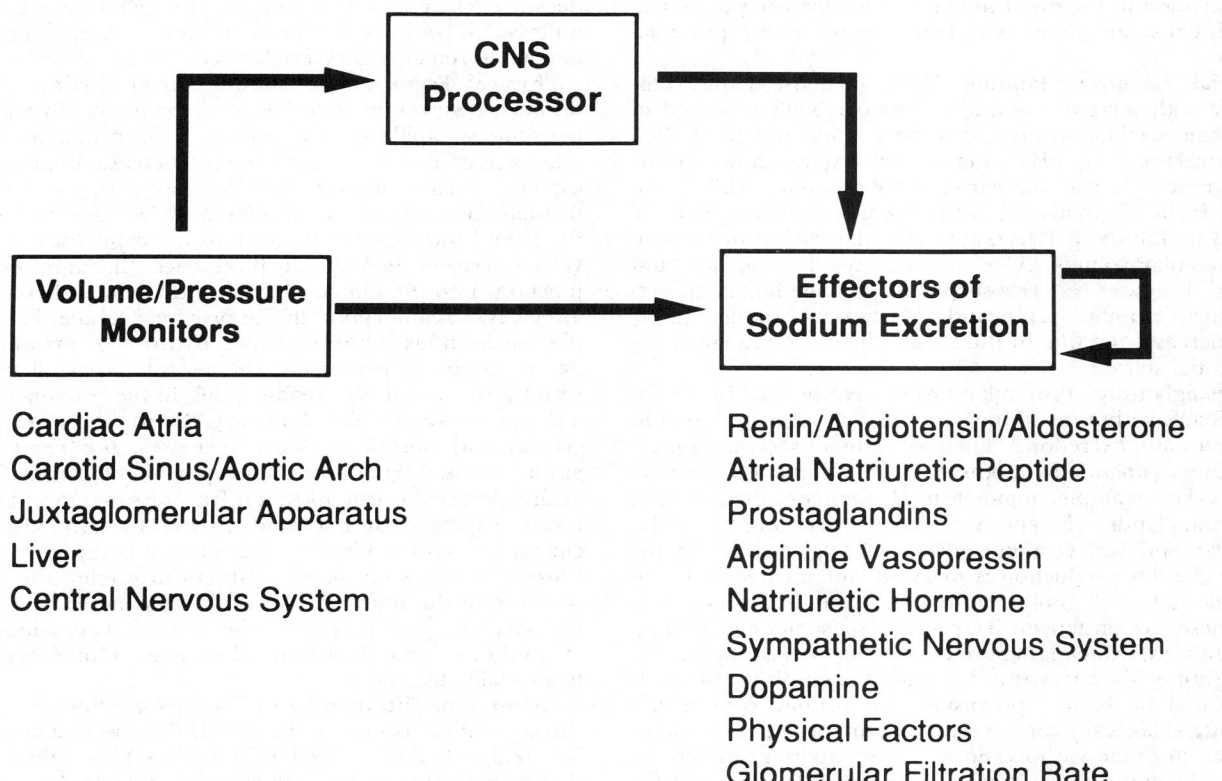

Figure 99–3. Sodium homeostasis. "Sensors" throughout the body monitor blood volume and pressure and directly or indirectly (via a central nervous system processor) regulate "effectors" of sodium excretion. There are feedback loops between the effectors themselves.

The juxtaglomerular apparatus in the kidney is ideally situated to monitor both renal perfusion pressure and solute excretion. The juxtaglomerular apparatus consists of specialized renin-secreting cells (juxtaglomerular cells) in the afferent glomerular arteriole and highly differentiated cells in the distal tubule (the macula densa). Decreases in wall tension in the afferent arteriole and decreases in solute (salt) delivery to the macula densa stimulate the juxtaglomerular cells to release renin.[18, 19] Thus, this system senses changes in both renal perfusion pressure and salt delivery to the distal nephron. Increases in renal sympathetic nerve activity also increase renin secretion.

Volume sensors also appear to exist in the portal circulation of the liver[20, 21] and in the central nervous system. Increases in portal pressure activate the hepatic receptors, which modulate renal sympathetic nerve activity via hepatic afferents.[20, 22] The nature of the putative central nervous system sensors has not been well established. The overall importance of these volume monitors in the regulation of Na+ balance is unclear.

Efferent Limb

The sensors that monitor the fullness of the circulation activate, directly or indirectly, a multitude of effectors (hormonal, neural, and physical factors) that control renal Na+ excretion.

Renin-Angiotensin-Aldosterone System. Renin release is stimulated by a variety of different mechanisms.[18, 19, 23] Renin converts angiotensinogen to angiotensin I, which is further metabolized to angiotensin II by angiotensin-converting enzyme. Besides being a potent vasoconstrictor, angiotensin II directly enhances Na+ reabsorption in the proximal tubule,[24] stimulates aldosterone secretion,[25] and increases the fraction of plasma filtered at the glomerulus by preferentially constricting the efferent arteriole.[26] Aldosterone increases Na+ reabsorption in the distal tubule,[27] and increasing the filtration fraction augments Na+ reabsorption in the proximal tubule.

Atrial Natriuretic Peptide. Although dense bodies compatible with secretory granules were originally observed in histologic sections of atria in 1956,[28] it was not until 1981 that injections of atrial homogenates were shown to be natriuretic.[29] Shortly thereafter, ANP was purified.[30, 31] The active form of circulating ANP is a 28-amino-acid peptide with a multitude of effects that are all aimed at decreasing intravascular volume. ANP increases renal blood flow and GFR,[32] decreases Na+ reabsorption in the medullary collecting duct,[33] inhibits renin and aldosterone production,[34, 35] and increases the flux of fluid from the intravascular to the interstitial space.[36]

Prostaglandins. Prostaglandins are synthesized by a variety of cells within the kidney and play an important role in salt and water excretion.[37] These eicosanoids serve a counterregulatory function by modulating the effects of other hormones. For example, angiotensin II stimulates the synthesis of prostaglandins E_2 and I, which in turn counteract the vascular and Na+-retaining effects of angiotensin.[38] Renal prostaglandin production is markedly augmented in hypovolemic states.[39–42] Inhibition of prostaglandin synthesis under these circumstances decreases GFR (sometimes leading to significant azotemia) and increases Na+ reabsorption.[39–42]

Arginine Vasopressin. Arginine vasopressin release is stimulated by both hypotension and volume contraction. Although classically considered more important in osmoregulation, arginine vasopressin also has important effects on Na+ and volume homeostasis. It is a powerful vasoconstrictor that redistributes cardiac output away from the skin and musculature,[43] increases plasma volume independently of changes in Na+ balance, and, by causing constriction of the efferent arteriole, increases the glomerular filtration fraction, potentiating sodium reabsorption within the proximal tubule.

Natriuretic Hormone. Since De Wardener and colleagues observed that animals maintained a natriuretic response to Na+ loading despite a reduction in GFR, interruption of renal sympathetic efferents, and infusion of arginine vasopressin and mineralocorticoids,[44] an extensive search has been conducted for the purpose of identifying circulating natriuretic hormones. Inhibitors of Na+,K+-ATPase (digitalis-like factors) have been found in the circulation in a variety of volume-expanded states.[45, 46] Digitalis-like factors are a heterogeneous group of compounds, one of which appears to be ouabain itself.[47] High concentrations of this cardiotonic steroid have been identified in the adrenal gland, but the role of these substances in Na+ homeostasis remains to be defined.

Sympathetic Nervous System. Extensive adrenergic innervation exists throughout the length of the nephron. The natriuresis induced by salt loading is associated with a decrease in renal sympathetic efferent nerve activity.[48] Conversely, salt depletion is associated with increased nerve activity and renal denervation blunts Na+ conservation.[48] Direct stimulation of renal sympathetic nerves alters renin secretion, Na+ and water reabsorption, renal blood flow, and GFR in a graded fashion.[49] Renin secretion is increased at low levels of stimulation, whereas more rapid stimulation is required to decrease GFR and renal blood flow. Such data strongly suggest that renal sympathetic nerves modulate renal Na+ excretion.

Dopamine. Both dopamine receptors and dopamine-containing neuronal elements are abundantly present throughout the kidney. Saline loading increases renal dopamine excretion,[50] dopamine antagonists are natriuretic, and dopamine agonists are antinatriuretic.[51] Dopamine appears to decrease Na+ reabsorption in the proximal tubule by inhibiting Na+,K+-ATPase.[52] The signal for release of intrarenal dopamine remains to be established.

Physical Factors. The Starling forces (hydrostatic and oncotic pressure) that exist between the interstitium and the peritubular capillaries are important determinants of Na+ reabsorption in the proximal tubule. Increases in peritubular capillary oncotic pressure and decreases in peritubular hydrostatic pressure favor movement of Na+ and water from the lateral intercellular spaces into the capillaries; the converse increases leakage of fluid back through the tight junctions into the lumen. Anything that alters these factors affects Na+ reabsorption in the proximal tubule. For example, intravenous saline increases hydrostatic pressure and decreases oncotic pressure in the peritubular capillaries; the result is decreased Na+ reabsorption in the proximal tubule and natriuresis. In Na+ depletion, hydrostatic pressure decreases and oncotic pressure increases, the result being antinatriuresis. Whenever the proportion of plasma filtered at the glomerulus (the filtration fraction) changes, the peritoneal capillary oncotic and hydrostatic pressures also change. When the filtration fraction increases (typically because of constriction of the efferent arteriole), the oncotic pressure in the postglomerular capillary increases and Na+ reabsorption also increases. The fraction is commonly increased in volume depletion, whereas in volume expansion it is usually decreased.

Glomerular Filtration Rate. The GFR can fluctuate greatly throughout the course of the day. If the absolute amount of Na+ reabsorbed were fixed, changes in GFR would result in disastrous swings in Na+ excretion. For example, at a GFR of 160 L/d and a serum Na+ concentration of 140 mEq/L, 22,400 mEq of Na+ is filtered, 22,300 mEq is reabsorbed, and only 100 mEq is excreted. A 10% increase in GFR would result in the filtration of an extra 2240 mEq of Na^+. If Na^+ reabsorption were fixed at 22,300 mEq, this increment in filtered load would cause Na^+ depletion and death. Fortunately, changes in GFR are typically accompanied by parallel changes in Na^+ reabsorption so that a fixed proportion (e.g., 99%) of the filtered load is reabsorbed. This linkage between filtration and reabsorption is known as glomerulotubular balance.[53, 54] When filtration is increased by 10%, reabsorption is increased proportionally so that the amount of Na^+ excreted increases from 100 to only 110 mEq. The mechanisms underlying glomerulotubular balance include the physical factors discussed earlier and a variety of luminal factors. For example, variations in GFR change the delivery of organic solutes to the proximal tubule, and increases or decreases in organic solutes such as amino acids are associated with parallel changes in Na^+ reabsorption.[54]

DISORDERS OF EXTRACELLULAR FLUID VOLUME REGULATION

Disorders of ECF volume homeostasis can be divided into two broad categories: states of Na^+ excess and states of Na^+ depletion. Such a classification system is a helpful diagnostic heuristic, but it is overly simplistic and does not always adequately reflect the physiologic basis for the homeostatic response. Because tissue perfusion is the critical element in any consideration of volume homeostasis, it is best to categorize disorders of volume homeostasis by using a tripartite classification system that includes assessments of total body Na^+, absolute intravascular volume, and EABV. In Na^+ depletion, these three parameters always change in parallel. In Na^+-overloaded states, however, they do not always change concordantly.

Extracellular Fluid Volume Depletion

Volume depletion may result from relatively selective loss of fluid from the intravascular space or from proportional loss of intravascular and interstitial fluid (Table 99–1). Chronic Na^+ depletion is generally well tolerated, with pulse, blood pressure, and cardiac output remaining close to normal values despite losses of up to 30% of total body Na^+.[55] In these cases, ECF volume is maintained by increases in total body water at the expense of hyponatremia.

More rapid losses of intravascular volume are less well tolerated. The patient may complain of easy fatigability or of lightheadedness, especially when rapidly assuming the upright position, and may even have a craving for salt and increased thirst. Physical examination, although not an overly sensitive guide to volume status, does provide a rough estimate of ECF volume depletion, the findings reflecting intravascular volume depletion. Acute decreases in intravascular volume of 10 to 15% are associated with supine tachycardia. Losses of 15 to 20% produce orthostatic tachycardia and hypotension. As losses approach 25%, a decline in cardiac output becomes evident and hypotension occurs even in the supine position. When losses reach 40%, tissue perfusion becomes increasingly compromised and vascular collapse (shock) ensues. The value of these hemodynamic changes in assessing the magnitude of intravascular volume depletion may be compromised in patients who are elderly,[56] have autonomic insufficiency, are taking a variety of antihypertensive medications, or have been at prolonged bed rest. Other findings, such as dry mouth or axilla or decreased skin turgor, are less specific and not reliable clues to ECF volume depletion.

TABLE 99-1

CAUSES OF VOLUME DEPLETION

Intravascular depletion
  Hemorrhage
    External
    Internal
  Third spacing of fluid
    Surgical trauma
    Bowel infarction or obstruction
    Pancreatitis
    Burns
Intravascular or interstitial depletion (Na^+ depletion)
  Renal losses (urinary $Na^+ > 20$ mEq/L)
    Diuretics
    Osmotic diuresis
      Hyperglycemia (glucose)
      High protein intake (urea)
      Mannitol
      Radiocontrast dyes
    Abrupt decrease in Na^+ intake in the elderly and in patients
      with chronic renal failure
    Addison's disease
    Postobstructive diuresis
    Polyuric phase of acute renal failure
  Cutaneous losses (urinary $Na^+ < 10$ mEq/L)
    Burns
    Toxic epidermal necrolysis
    Sensible perspiration (sweat)
  Gastrointestinal losses (urinary $Na^+ < 10$ mEq/L)
    Nasogastric suction or vomiting (urinary Na^+ concentration
      may be elevated)
    Diarrhea
    Biliary or pancreatic fistulas

Isolated Intravascular Volume Depletion

Acute hemorrhage selectively depletes the intravascular space and activates neurohumoral mechanisms for preserving tissue perfusion. Rapid external blood loss is usually obvious, but large quantities of blood can also be lost into the thorax, abdomen, retroperitoneum, or large muscles. Although brisk hemorrhage can be viewed as a selective depletion of intravascular volume, changes in blood pressure and pre- and postcapillary resistances soon redistribute ECF volume from the interstitial to the intravascular space, leading to a concurrent decrease in interstitial fluid volume. A similar sequence of events takes place in patients with more chronic blood loss.

Hemorrhage should be considered in any critically ill patient with unexplained hypotension. Internal bleeding may occur after blunt trauma, after open or closed invasive procedures, secondary to a ruptured aneurysm or spleen or an ectopic pregnancy, in hemorrhagic pancreatitis, or spontaneously in patients with bleeding diatheses. Besides suggestive history and signs of volume depletion, the patient may complain of pain in the abdomen, back, flank, groin, or thigh. Occasionally, a bluish yellow discoloration is evident on the flanks and abdomen (Grey Turner's sign) or umbilicus (Cullen's sign). Computed tomography is often helpful in diagnosing internal bleeding. It is important to recognize that before the redistribution of fluid from the interstitial space, the hemoglobin level and hematocrit may be normal.

Relatively selective depletion of intravascular fluid may also occur when fluid is sequestered in so-called third spaces. Large quantities of protein- and sodium-rich fluid may be secluded in the bowel or peritoneum as a result of surgical trauma, bowel infarction or obstruction, or pancreatitis and in the skin after extensive burns. The fluid is not in equilibrium with the ECF and is effectively lost from the circulation.

Because the sequestered fluid is a filtrate of whole blood, hemoconcentration is typically present.

Intravascular and Interstitial Depletion

Depletion of Na+ occurs when excessive amounts of Na+ are lost by the kidneys, gastrointestinal tract, or skin. Such losses are associated with proportional depletion of the intravascular and interstitial fluid compartments. The history and urinary Na+ concentration usually distinguish renal from extrarenal Na+ losses. Because the normal homeostatic response to volume depletion is renal Na+ retention, in the presence of intravascular depletion, a urinary Na+ concentration greater than 20 mEq/L suggests renal Na+ wasting.

Renal Sodium Losses. The most common cause of renal Na+ wasting is the use of diuretics. Diuretics are routinely prescribed for the treatment of edematous disorders or simply to maintain urine output. Because critically ill patients usually have limited access to salt, overzealous use of diuretics frequently results in volume depletion. In addition to an elevated urinary Na+ concentration, volume depletion secondary to overdiuresis is typically associated with hypokalemia and metabolic alkalosis.

Renal Na+ wasting can also arise when the kidney is confronted with an excessive solute load. By decreasing Na+ and water reabsorption in the proximal tubule and loop of Henle, excessive solute loads (osmotic diuresis) can lead to profound ECF volume depletion.[57] Both endogenous and exogenous solutes assault the volume-regulating mechanisms of the critically ill patient. Persistent hyperglycemia, a common problem in the critically ill patient, can increase urine volume by as much as 1500 mL and urinary Na+ excretion by as much as 50 mEq/d.[57] The generation of large quantities of urea as a result of high-protein enteral or parenteral feedings can also cause marked diuresis.[58] Use of mannitol in the treatment of cerebral edema may lead to serious volume depletion. Natriuresis also follows infusions of hypertonic radiographic contrast agents and may convert a negligible degree of Na+ depletion into a clinically significant condition. Because water is lost in excess of Na+, volume depletion caused by osmotic diuresis is often associated with hypernatremia.

Elderly patients and patients with chronic renal failure, both overly represented in the critical care unit, may become Na+ depleted if abruptly given a restricted Na+ diet.[59, 60] Such patients take longer to adapt to a low intake of Na+ than younger individuals or individuals with normal renal function and may lose large amounts of Na+ during the period of adjustment. A more gradual reduction in Na+ intake is far better tolerated.

Another cause of renal salt wasting that must always be considered in the critically ill patient is adrenal insufficiency,[61] especially if hyponatremia and hyperkalemia coexist with volume depletion. The diagnosis can be made with a corticotropin stimulation test. Prompt treatment with both glucocorticoids and mineralocorticoids reverses the salt wasting.

After relief of urinary obstruction or during the recovery phase of acute tubular necrosis, increased urine volume is frequently noted. For the most part, this polyuria results from normal excretion of retained solutes (Na+ and urea) and rarely leads to volume depletion. Occasionally, however, significant Na+ wasting may occur.[62]

Extrarenal Sodium Losses. In certain circumstances, large quantities of hypotonic fluid can be lost from the skin and gastrointestinal tract. The hallmark of extrarenal Na+ depletion is renal Na+ conservation, as reflected by a urinary Na+ concentration less than 10 mEq/L. Because the skin protects the ECF from the external environment, any disruption of this barrier (e.g., burns or toxic epidermal necrolysis) can result in large losses of Na+ and water from the ECF space.[63] In addition, during strenuous exercise (especially in hot, humid climates) large quantities of Na+ can be lost in sweat.[64]

Volume depletion is a common concomitant of gastrointestinal disorders. Protracted vomiting and prolonged nasogastric suction are frequently associated with Na+ depletion. Because the concurrent loss of H+ produces metabolic alkalosis, urinary HCO_3^- excretion is increased and is usually accompanied by obligatory losses of both Na+ and K+. Thus, despite volume contraction, urinary Na+ concentration may be deceptively elevated.[65] However, because of concomitant Cl- depletion, Cl- reabsorption remains high and the urinary Cl- concentration is low.[66]

Normally, stool volume is less than 200 mL/d and accounts for little Na+ excretion. In patients with diarrhea, however, fecal volume can approach 20 L/d with an Na+ concentration similar to that of plasma. In the critical care unit, antibiotic-associated colitis and osmotic diarrhea related to tube feedings are frequent causes of Na+ depletion. Simultaneous losses of $KHCO_3$ in the stool usually produce a hypokalemic metabolic acidosis.

Treatment of Volume Depletion

Treatment of the volume-depleted patient should be aimed at estimating the magnitude of the deficit and replacing it appropriately, replacing ongoing losses, and identifying and correcting the cause(s) of the volume depletion. If signs and symptoms of volume depletion are minimal and the patient can eat, therapy can be as simple as liberalizing Na+ intake. However, if there is any evidence of hemodynamic compromise, parenteral therapy is indicated.

Intravascular volume can be restored with blood, blood products, colloids, or crystalloids. Packed red blood cells are the therapy of choice if there is ongoing blood loss or severe anemia. Fresh frozen plasma should be reserved for volume-depleted patients who also require coagulation factor replacement. Whether to use isotonic crystalloid or one of a variety of available colloids is controversial. Because colloids such as dextran, hydroxyethyl starch (hetastarch), and albumin remain within the intravascular space, they appear to be ideal for rapid intravascular volume expansion. However, most studies comparing colloids and crystalloids have not revealed clear benefits of one over the other.[67] In the elderly, volume repletion with colloid may be associated with a lower incidence of pulmonary edema than repletion with isotonic saline.[68] However, before recommending the use of colloids in the aged, further controlled studies are required. Because of its ease of use and relatively low cost, intravenous isotonic saline (0.9% NaCl) is the best choice for intravascular volume expansion.

Commercially available isotonic saline solutions containing physiologic concentrations of other electrolytes (e.g., Ringer's lactate) should be avoided. If it is necessary to use other electrolytes for repletion, therapy should be tailored to the specific clinical situation. For example, in an acidemic patient, volume expansion can be accomplished by using a solution of half-isotonic (0.45%) saline to which one or two ampules of $NaHCO_3$ (44.8 mEq per ampule) have been added. However, because non–chloride-containing Na+ salts are less well reabsorbed by the kidney[69] and appear to have a greater intracellular distribution than NaCl,[70] such solutions are less efficacious in volume expansion. Hypotonic saline should be used only for hypernatremic, volume-depleted patients and only when the hypovolemia is not life threatening; therapy of the more than mildly volume-depleted, hypernatremic patient should be initiated with isotonic saline.

TABLE 99–2

ELECTROLYTE COMPOSITION OF GASTROINTESTINAL "DRAINAGE FLUIDS"

Type	Concentration			
	Na^+	K^+	HCO_3^-	H^+
Gastric	40–80	5–15	–	80–100
Pancreatic	140–150	0–10	80–100	—
Bile	140–150	0–10	40–50	—
Ileostomy	120–140	5–20	30–60	—
Diarrhea	40–140	20–50	30–50	—

By the time orthostatic tachycardia and hypotension are present, ECF deficits are usually at least 30 mL/kg. However, the exact volume of fluid necessary to replenish the ECF is often difficult to establish. If daily weights or accurate records of the patient's intake and output are available, a more reliable estimate of fluid replacement may be possible. In any event, isotonic saline should be infused until the signs of hemodynamic compromise are no longer present, as demonstrated by a mean arterial blood pressure of at least 70 mm Hg and a urine output of at least 20 to 30 mL/h. The precise rate of fluid administration should be determined by the severity of the hemodynamic compromise and the patient's underlying cardiac and renal status. In a young, otherwise healthy patient whose only problem is intravascular volume depletion, isotonic saline can be infused as rapidly as possible until blood pressure is stabilized. In most critically ill patients, however, cardiac dysfunction and renal insufficiency preclude such vigorous resuscitation. For these patients resuscitation should be initiated with a 250- to 500-mL bolus of isotonic saline, after which additional therapy should be based on careful reassessment of cardiovascular and hemodynamic parameters. Measurement of pulmonary capillary wedge pressure is recommended in patients with poor cardiac function.

After deficits have been replenished, therapy should be directed at replacing ongoing fluid losses. The composition of the maintenance solution depends on the source (composition) of the fluid lost. Although the approximate electrolyte composition of various body fluids is known, direct measurement always provides a much more accurate guide to replacement. The electrolyte composition of the common gastrointestinal "drainage fluids" is provided in Table 99–2.

Extracellular Fluid Volume Overload

Because of the dynamic equilibrium that exists between the intravascular and interstitial spaces, ECF volume overload is typically associated with expansion of both of these compartments. In certain conditions, however, maldistribution of fluid across the capillary membrane results in expansion of the interstitial fluid space at the expense of the intravascular volume.

Despite many pitfalls, the physical examination provides important clues to the presence of ECF volume (total body Na^+) overload. Excess intravascular volume is indicated by distention of the jugular veins and hepatic vascular congestion (usually detected by the presence of so-called hepatojugular reflux). An S_3 gallop and hypertension may also be present but do not reliably correlate with intravascular volume status.

The hallmark of ECF volume expansion is the presence of peripheral edema (expansion of the interstitial space) or ascites. Peripheral edema has been classically divided into so-called pitting edema (associated with congestive heart failure, nephrotic syndrome, cirrhosis, and venous occlusion); the rubbery, nonpitting edema of lymphatic obstruction; and the brawny, unyielding edema of hypothyroidism (myxedema).[71] The more chronic the edema, the greater the likelihood of associated fibrosis and therefore the less the tissues can be pitted. Whether pitting or nonpitting, generalized edema represents expansion of the interstitial space and ECF volume (total body Na^+) overload.

Peripheral edema typically accumulates in dependent areas of the body (e.g., the lower extremities when the patient is sitting or standing, the sacrum and buttocks when the patient is supine) or areas of the body where the subcutaneous tissues are loosely bound by overlying skin (e.g., the periorbital region). By the time peripheral edema becomes discernible at physical examination, the volume of the interstitial space has usually increased by at least 3 to 5 L.

Because of the porous structure of the hepatic sinusoids, increased hepatic venous pressure accelerates the formation of hepatic interstitial fluid and easily overwhelms the hepatic lymphatic drainage system. The peritoneal cavity serves as an escape valve for this fluid, which "sweats" through the liver capsule, forming ascites. Physical examination reveals abdominal distention, shifting dullness, or a fluid wave. The existence of peritoneal fluid is easily confirmed by ultrasonography. Ascites is common in hepatic cirrhosis but is unusual in other edematous disorders.

Interstitial fluid can also accumulate in the lungs (pulmonary edema) and impair gas exchange. Pulmonary edema is characteristic of congestive heart failure but is an unusual manifestation of other Na^+-overloaded conditions unless there is concurrent cardiac disease. Pulmonary edema can also occur in primary pulmonary disorders (e.g., adult respiratory distress syndrome) and is therefore not a reliable sign of ECF volume overload.

Extracellular Fluid Volume Overload with Intravascular Fluid Volume Expansion

Under most circumstances, ECF volume overload is associated with expansion of both the interstitial and intravascular fluid spaces. ECF volume overload may result from primary inability of the kidney to excrete Na^+ (e.g., renal failure) or may be secondary to effective arterial hypovolemia (e.g., congestive heart failure, hepatic cirrhosis, and nephrotic syndrome). In either case, inadequate renal Na^+ excretion leads to positive Na^+ balance and peripheral edema. Although all of these disorders manifest with signs and symptoms of ECF volume overload, it is generally easy to differentiate among them (Table 99–3).

Congestive Heart Failure. As cardiac output declines, blood pressure and tissue perfusion decrease and neurohumoral mechanisms designed to restore blood pressure and renal perfusion are stimulated. Activation of the renin-angiotensin-aldosterone system leads to renal Na^+ retention. Angiotensin II increases systemic vascular tone, thereby supporting blood pressure. In addition, by constricting the efferent arteriole to a greater extent than the afferent arteriole, angiotensin II maintains the GFR even in the presence of diminished renal perfusion. The resulting increase in filtration fraction favors increased proximal tubular Na^+ reabsorption. Angiotensin II also directly stimulates Na^+ reabsorption in the proximal tubule, and aldosterone enhances Na^+ reabsorption in the distal nephron. The fall in cardiac output also leads to an increase in sympathetic tone; this, too, serves to support blood pressure and enhance renal Na^+ reabsorption.

These adjustments increase ECF volume and cardiac preload, thereby restoring cardiac output and renal perfusion

TABLE 99–3

DIFFERENTIAL DIAGNOSIS OF EDEMATOUS DISORDERS*

Disorder	Pulmonary Edema	JVD	Ascites	Peripheral Edema	Proteinuria	U_{Na} (mEq/L)
CHF	Frequent	Normal or elevated	Occasional	Frequent	−/+	<10
Cirrhosis	Rare	Normal	Frequent	Frequent	−	<10
Nephrotic syndrome	Rare	Normal	Rare	Frequent	++++	<10
Renal failure	Occasional	Normal or elevated	Rare	Frequent	−/++	>20

*CHF = congestive heart failure; JVD = jugular venous distention; U_{Na} = urinary Na^+ concentration (mEq/L).

pressure. Simultaneously, counter-regulatory systems, which tend to reduce the systemic vasoconstriction and renal Na^+ retention, are activated.[39, 40] Angiotensin II stimulates the intrarenal synthesis of vasodilatory prostaglandins, and atrial stretch decreases sympathetic outflow to the kidney and leads to release of ANP into the circulation. ANP causes systemic vasodilatation, alters renal hemodynamics, decreases distal tubular Na^+ reabsorption, and inhibits the release of renin and aldosterone. The net effect is a general damping of the systemic vasoconstriction and renal Na^+ retention. Thus, a new steady state is reached in which cardiac output is maintained at the expense of a modest increase in ECF volume.

If cardiac output declines further, additional adjustments in these neurohormonal homeostatic mechanisms are required. A new steady state is again achieved but at the expense of an even greater increase in ECF volume. Eventually, with more advanced heart failure, these mechanisms become maladaptive.[72] Markedly elevated catecholamine levels produce intense vasoconstriction and increase cardiac afterload, leading to a further decline in cardiac output and initiating a downward spiral in cardiac function and a progressive increase in ECF volume. Hyponatremia, oliguria, and prerenal azotemia are common concomitants of severe congestive heart failure.

Treatment. Therapy should be aimed at decreasing cardiac afterload and enhancing intrinsic myocardial function. Although improving cardiac output produces natriuresis, addition of diuretics to further enhance renal Na^+ excretion is an important adjunct to therapy. However, because the failing heart depends on increased preload to maintain cardiac output, aggressive diuresis should be avoided. The treatment of congestive heart failure is discussed in detail in the section on the cardiovascular system.

Cirrhosis. Hepatic cirrhosis is associated with intense renal Na^+ retention, whose pathogenesis has not been clearly elucidated. The long-held idea that portal hypertension results in transudation of fluid from the portal circulation into the peritoneal cavity with subsequent "underfilling" of the vasculature and *secondary* renal Na^+ retention has not been supported by experimental evidence. For example, measurements of intravascular volume in cirrhotic patients during periods of Na^+ retention have revealed expansion rather than contraction of the intravascular space.[73, 74] Furthermore, in animal models of cirrhosis, renal Na^+ retention actually precedes the formation of ascites.[74]

Because of these and other inconsistencies in the underfilling hypothesis, it was proposed that *primary* renal Na^+ retention is the cause of the ECF volume overload in cirrhosis.[73–75] According to the overflow hypothesis, intrahepatic hypertension leads to renal Na^+ retention by activating an incompletely identified hepatorenal reflex. For example, in experimentally induced cirrhosis, prevention of intrahepatic hypertension (by side-to-side portacaval shunting) forestalls Na^+ retention.[76] Interestingly, hepatic denervation (but not renal denervation) alters the early phase of Na^+ retention

in these experimental models,[77] which suggests that the putative hepatic baroreceptors modulate renal Na^+ reabsorption by means unrelated to alterations in renal sympathetic tone.

In an attempt to bring these two hypotheses together, a third hypothesis has been formulated: arterial vasodilation, especially within the splanchnic bed, increases vascular capacitance (decreases "filling" of the arterial system) with subsequent renal Na^+ retention.[78] The arterial vasodilation is presumed to be related to portal hypertension, but the precise mechanism has not been established. Although differing in the presumed cause of renal Na^+ retention during the early or compensated phase of hepatic cirrhosis, all of these hypotheses agree that EABV is inadequate during the decompensated phase of the disease. Decompensated cirrhosis is therefore characterized by a progressive increase in ECF volume (peripheral edema and ascites), oliguria, relative hypotension, and elevated levels of the circulating neurohumoral mediators of renal Na^+ reabsorption (e.g., angiotensin II and catecholamines). Hyponatremia and prerenal azotemia are also common.

Treatment. Ideally, treatment of the ECF volume overload associated with cirrhosis should be based on the pathogenesis of the Na^+ retention. If primary renal Na^+ retention is to blame, increasing Na^+ excretion with diuretics is the ideal therapeutic modality. However, if the Na^+ retention is secondary to either absolute or effective hypovolemia, diuretics could exacerbate the condition by causing a further decline in intravascular volume. Until the underlying pathophysiology is completely understood, the following principles should guide fluid management.

In patients with early, compensated cirrhosis (who have only mild ascites and minimal peripheral edema), therapy should be conservative and consist of dietary Na^+ restriction only. However, because of the severity of salt retention, Na^+ intake should be limited to 10 mEq (250 mg) per day. Such rigorous Na^+ restriction requires the help of a dietitian and considerable diligence on the part of the patient. More aggressive therapy should be instituted only if Na^+ restriction fails and the edema and ascites progress beyond mere cosmetic inconvenience. In that case, the patient should be placed at bed rest, Na^+ restriction continued, and diuretic therapy begun. Cirrhotic patients often have greater natriuresis when treated with the aldosterone antagonist spironolactone than when treated with the usually more potent loop diuretics;[79] this K^+-spacing diuretic is therefore the agent of choice for the cirrhotic patient. Because mobilization of fluid from the interstitial and peritoneal spaces occurs at a limited rate, diuresis should not exceed 1 L/d when edema is present or 500 mL/d when there is no edema.[80]

In late, decompensated cirrhosis, treatment is more problematic. Overly aggressive treatment should be avoided if possible, being initiated only if the edema and ascites threaten to compromise respiratory or cardiovascular function. Although the combination of a loop or thiazide diuretic with spironolactone is frequently efficacious, such therapy often increases morbidity. Large-volume paracentesis (with or without supplemental intravenous albumin administration) has been advocated in the management of ascites.[81, 82] This treatment is a rapid and efficient means of removing excess salt and water and appears to have minimal effects on intravascular volume.[83] It may also improve cardiac preload and increase cardiac output, renal perfusion, and urine volume.[84]

Although sometimes required to support blood pressure in end-stage cirrhosis, intravascular volume expansion with isotonic saline or albumin aggravates volume overload. If necessary, such therapy should be guided by measurements of pulmonary capillary wedge pressure and cardiac output. Intravascular reinfusion of ascites is of limited usefulness, and its routine use is not advocated. Although peritoneovenous shunts are effective in the treatment of refractory ascites, there are many complications associated with their use.[85] Implantation of such devices should be reserved for patients with truly refractory ascites who have maintained reasonably good hepatic synthetic function.

Nephrotic Syndrome. Nephrotic edema has been classically attributed to hypoalbuminemia, with decreased plasma oncotic pressure resulting in intravascular volume depletion as fluid moves out of the vasculature into the interstitium. Intravascular volume depletion then activates renal Na$^+$ retention and ECF volume progressively expands. However, neither clinical observations nor experimental models of nephrosis support this concept.

Clinicians have long been aware that there is little correlation between the degree of hypoalbuminemia and the magnitude of edema. Moreover, individuals with congenital analbuminemia (who have drastically reduced plasma oncotic pressures) do not routinely develop edema. Furthermore, most adults with nephrotic syndrome have no signs or symptoms of intravascular volume depletion; in fact, hypertension is frequently noted. In addition, if the plasma protein concentration is reduced by plasmapheresis, intravascular volume is well maintained until the albumin concentration is less than 2 g/100 mL.[86]

Further evidence against the importance of diminished oncotic pressure in the Na$^+$ retention of nephrotic syndrome comes from studies of experimentally induced minimal change disease. Infusion of puromycin selectively into one kidney produced proteinuria in that kidney only. Despite hypoalbuminemia, only the proteinuric kidney retained Na$^+$.[87] These results imply that the renal Na$^+$ avidity in at least certain types of nephrotic syndrome may be primary and not secondary to either absolute or effective hypovolemia. It should be stressed, however, that this does not exclude the possibility that some patients with nephrotic syndrome are intravascularly depleted[88] or that hypoalbuminemia does not sensitize patients with nephrotic syndrome to what would otherwise be considered relatively trivial hypovolemia-inducing events. The latter consideration is especially important in the critical care setting.

Treatment. A low-Na$^+$ diet and diuretics are the treatments of choice for the edema of nephrotic syndrome. However, aggressive diuresis should be avoided, and patients should be monitored for signs, symptoms, and laboratory evidence of intravascular volume depletion. Although infusion of salt-poor albumin may be natriuretic in some patients with nephrotic syndrome,[89] it is of no long-term benefit and its routine use is not recommended.

Renal Failure. Acute, oliguric renal failure is a common cause of Na$^+$ overload in critically ill patients. Unlike other causes of ECF volume expansion, the Na$^+$ overload associated with renal failure is not a result of enhanced Na$^+$ avidity but rather of the damaged kidneys' inability to match excretion with intake. In chronic renal failure, renal adaptation

usually allows the patient to handle all but extremely excessive dietary Na$^+$ loads, at least until the GFR falls below 10 mL/min.

Treatment. Intake of Na$^+$ should be limited to what can be excreted. Diuretics may increase Na$^+$ excretion but, because they frequently cannot reach their site of action within the nephron, unless extremely high (toxic) doses are given, their usefulness is often limited. A bolus injection of a loop diuretic (e.g., furosemide at 40 mg or bumetanide at 1.0 mg) followed by a continuous infusion (e.g., furosemide at 0.5 mg/kg/h or bumetanide at 1.0 mg/h) may induce natriuresis, while avoiding the toxicity associated with more traditional bolus infusions.[90] In patients who are resistant to diuretics, excess volume can be removed by hemofiltration (see Chapter 109).

Extracellular Fluid Volume Overload with Intravascular Fluid Volume Depletion

Although alterations in the Starling forces (e.g., decreased oncotic pressure and increased capillary permeability) increase the flux of fluid from the intravascular fluid space into the interstitial fluid space, normal homeostatic mechanisms usually prevent changes in these parameters from producing enough maldistribution of fluid to result in intravascular volume depletion. In seriously ill patients, however, the disruption of normal homeostasis, combined with the magnitude of the changes in the Starling forces, may result in symptomatic intravascular volume depletion despite ECF volume overload. Furthermore, because the edematous patient is not immune to hemorrhage or sequestration (third spacing) of intravascular fluid, these causes of intravascular volume depletion must also be considered in the differential diagnosis of the edematous patient with hypotension.

Hypoalbuminemia. Because of increased protein catabolism and poor nutrition, the critically ill patient usually has a decreased serum albumin concentration.[91] Whether hypoalbuminemia alone can cause intravascular volume depletion, renal Na$^+$ retention, and progressive ECF volume expansion is controversial. As previously noted, for otherwise healthy individuals or patients with nephrotic syndrome there are few data supporting this concept. Indeed, expansion of the interstitial space secondary to decreased oncotic pressure is prevented by a variety of countermanding factors, the most important of which is the ability of the lymphatic system to prevent interstitial fluid accumulation by returning fluid to the vasculature.[92] Increased lymph flow also washes out interstitial proteins, thereby decreasing interstitial oncotic pressure and decreasing the flux of fluid across the capillary bed.[93] Finally, the capacitance of the interstitial space is such that any expansion rapidly increases interstitial hydrostatic pressure and hinders further fluid accumulation.[94]

Thus, under otherwise normal conditions it is unlikely that hypoalbuminemia, unless severe, would result in a significant enough maldistribution of ECF to produce intravascular volume depletion and edema. In the bedridden, critically ill patient, however, volume homeostasis is often significantly impaired and the distribution of fluid between the intravascular and interstitial spaces may be adversely affected by hypoalbuminemia. For example, bed rest, malnutrition, changes in pre- and postcapillary sphincter tone, and changes in capillary permeability may all accentuate the role of hypoalbuminemia in the transudation of fluid out of the intravascular space. Furthermore, alterations in the neurohumoral factors that regulate renal Na$^+$ reabsorption, as well as changes in renal function per se, may sensitize the kidneys to the salt-retaining effects of intravascular volume depletion.

Treatment. In hypoalbuminemic, edematous patients with signs and symptoms of intravascular volume depletion, therapy should be directed at enhancing nutrition, improving lymphatic flow with physical therapy, and increasing interstitial hydrostatic pressure in the lower extremities by use of stockings. If, despite such measures, evidence of decreased tissue perfusion (e.g., hypotension and worsening prerenal azotemia) persists, intravascular volume expansion should be initiated. Because isotonic saline only worsens the edema in this situation, colloid solutions are the volume expanders of choice.

Capillary Leak Syndromes. Several well-defined syndromes characterized by hypotension and rapidly developing edema are associated with increased permeability of the capillary endothelium and "leaking" of protein-rich fluid into the interstitium. A diffuse capillary leak has been described after snake bites,[95] after infusion of interleukin-2,[96] and in patients with sepsis.[97, 98] More localized capillary leaks also occur. For example, unilateral pulmonary edema and hypotension have been reported to follow rapid re-expansion of the lung after drainage of air or fluid from the thoracic cavity.[99]

Sepsis is the classic example of a diffuse capillary leak syndrome. Bacterial toxins associated with the cell wall of gram-negative aerobic bacteria (endotoxins) or secreted by gram-positive bacteria (exotoxins) produce a syndrome that is typified in its early phase by increased vascular capacitance, cardiac output, and oxygen consumption and in its later phase by falling cardiac output and increased capillary permeability.[97, 98] The early vasodilation appears to be mediated by histamine and bradykinin. Despite the increased cardiac output, inadequate filling of the circulation and renal Na^+ retention occur. In the later phase, because of the diffuse capillary leak, plasma volume is sequestered in the interstitium.[100, 101] Several factors, including bradykinin, tumor necrosis factor, interleukins, and oxygen free radicals, have been postulated as mediators of the increased capillary permeability.[97]

Treatment. At present, the only effective treatment of the capillary leak syndrome associated with sepsis is early administration of appropriate antibiotics. Whether antibodies against endotoxin would reverse the hemodynamic effects of gram-negative sepsis remains unanswered.[102] Meticulous attention to fluid management is also important. The pulmonary capillary wedge pressure should be maintained in the low-normal range with isotonic saline. Whether colloids should be used is controversial. Because of the presence of the capillary leak, intravenous colloids are unlikely to remain within the intravascular space. Moreover, by increasing interstitial oncotic pressure, they may be detrimental. If intravascular volume repletion alone does not stabilize the patient, blood pressure should be supported by the judicious use of pressors and inotropic agents.

Other Factors Affecting Sodium Excretion in the Critically Ill Patient

Besides the Na^+-retaining conditions already discussed, the precarious state of ECF volume homeostasis in the critically ill patient may be further compromised by medical interventions or concurrent disorders not typically associated with abnormalities in Na^+ balance. Respiratory failure and hypokalemia, both common in critical care units, further diminish the kidneys' ability to excrete Na^+ adequately. So do a variety of commonly employed drugs.

Respiratory Failure. Positive pressure ventilation is associated with a decline in urine output, weight gain, and edema.[103, 104] Increased intrathoracic pressure decreases central venous volume (cardiac preload), thereby activating various mechanisms that result in decreased salt and water excretion by the kidney. Positive end-expiratory airway pressure further compromises renal Na^+ excretion by decreasing cardiac output. In patients with chronic obstructive pulmonary disease, hypercapnia and hypoxemia, independently of any changes in cardiac output, also produce positive Na^+ balance.[105, 106]

Hypokalemia. Even relatively mild hypokalemia (potassium level < 3.0 mEq/L) causes Na^+ retention[107–109] and may lead to edema formation if Na^+ intake is high. The underlying mechanism is not known. However, it does not appear to be related to changes in circulating levels of renin, aldosterone, or catecholamines.[109] Whether intrarenal angiotensin II or prostaglandins have a role deserves further investigation. Whatever the cause, hypokalemia should always be corrected in the critically ill patient both to forestall renal Na^+ retention and to facilitate the therapy of ECF volume overload.

Drugs. Commonly used medications can often disrupt volume homeostasis in the critically ill patient. The Na^+-retaining properties of nonsteroidal anti-inflammatory drugs, for example, are not always appreciated. The inhibition of prostaglandin synthesis acutely reduces Na^+ excretion in normal subjects, but after a few days of positive Na^+ balance a new steady state is achieved. In Na^+-avid states such as congestive heart failure or cirrhosis, however, nonsteroidal anti-inflammatory drugs may produce progressive and striking Na^+ retention.[39–42] They also attenuate the natriuretic effects of loop diuretics.

Calcium channel blockers have been associated with the development of dependent edema. This has been attributed to precapillary vasodilation without concomitant changes in postcapillary tone, resulting in increased transudation of intravascular fluid into the interstitium.[110] The effects of calcium channel blockers on long-term Na^+ balance in individuals with underlying edematous conditions have yet to be studied.

DIURETICS

Diuretics are the mainstay of therapy for ECF volume overload. Although diuretics are usually categorized according to their primary site of action within the nephron, secondary effects in other nephron segments may also be important for their natriuretic action. The major classes of diuretics have predominant sites of action in the proximal tubule (carbonic anhydrase inhibitors), the thick ascending limb of the loop of Henle (loop diuretics), the distal convoluted tubule (thiazides and related diuretics), or the cortical collecting tubules (K^+-sparing diuretics) (Table 99–4). Besides these major diuretics, another agent that is being used with increasing frequency in the critical care unit is dopamine. Osmotic agents and drugs that primarily affect renal blood flow are of limited usefulness and are not discussed.

Carbonic Anhydrase Inhibitors

The natriuretic effects of carbonic anhydrase inhibitors (e.g., acetazolamide) are limited to the proximal tubule. By inhibiting both intracellular and luminal carbonic anhydrase, acetazolamide suppresses Na^+-H^+ exchange, the transport process responsible for most of the Na^+ reabsorption in the proximal tubule. Although inhibition of Na^+ reabsorption in the proximal tubule would be expected to induce significant natriuresis, carbonic anhydrase inhibitors are, in fact, weak diuretics. Because Na^+ reabsorption in more distal nephron sites is delivery dependent, increased reabsorption in these segments of the nephron compensates for the increased delivery out of the proximal tubule. The metabolic

TABLE 99–4

DIURETICS: IMPORTANT ASPECTS OF USE

Diuretic	Site or Mechanism of Action	Dose (mg)	Duration of Action (h)	Fractional Excretion of Sodium (%)	Complications
Carbonic anhydrase inhibitors Acetazolamide	Proximal tubule Inhibits carbonic anhydrase, blocking Na^+-H^+ exchange	250–500 PO or IV b.i.d.	8–12	3	Hypokalemia Metabolic acidosis
Loop diuretics Furosemide Bumetanide Ethacrynic acid	Thick ascending limb of Henle's loop Blocks Na^+-K^+-$2Cl^-$ cotransporter	20–240 PO or IV b.i.d. 0.25–0.5 mg/kg/h IV 0.5–10 PO or IV b.i.d. 1 mg/h IV 25–250 PO b.i.d. 50–100 IV b.i.d.	6 6 6	25	Hypokalemia Hyperuricemia Hypomagnesemia Hyponatremia Metabolic alkalosis Ototoxicity (ethacrynic acid, high-dose furosemide)
Thiazides (and related diuretics) Hydrochlorothiazide Chlorthalidone Chlorothiazide Metolazone	Distal tubule Blocks neutral NaCl transporter	25–100 PO q.d. 25–100 PO q.d. 250–500 IV b.i.d. 2.5–20 PO q.d.	8–12 24–72 2–4 24–48	5	Hypokalemia Hyperuricemia Hyponatremia Metabolic alkalosis
Potassium-sparing diuretics Amiloride Triamterene Spironolactone	Cortical collecting tubule Blocks Na^+ channel Aldosterone antagonist	5–20 PO q.d. 50–150 PO b.i.d. 50–200 PO b.i.d.	12–24 8–12 24–72	2	Hyperkalemia Metabolic acidosis Gynecomastia (spironolactone)

acidosis that results from the associated bicarbonaturia further diminishes the effectiveness of carbonic anhydrase inhibitors.[111] Complications of acetazolamide administration include metabolic acidosis and hypokalemia. Because of its poor natriuretic effect and metabolic side effects, acetazolamide, used alone, has limited usefulness as a diuretic.

Loop Diuretics

Furosemide, bumetanide, and ethacrynic acid are the three loop diuretics presently available in the United States. These drugs are the most potent natriuretic compounds available, the fractional excretion of Na^+ increasing some 25-fold. Furosemide, bumetanide, and, possibly, ethacrynic acid act by inhibiting the Na^+-K^+-$2Cl^-$ cotransporter. Because of their potency, loop diuretics are the agents of choice for treating most Na^+-overloaded patients. Furosemide is the best characterized. In healthy individuals, oral dosing and parenteral dosing are bioequivalent. In most Na^+-avid patients, however, an intravenous dose is approximately twice as effective as an oral dose, even in the absence of gut edema.[112] Thus, when converting from an intravenous to an oral preparation, the dose should be doubled. When bowel edema is present, gastrointestinal absorption is hindered and oral administration is frequently ineffective.[113] Complications include hypokalemia, hyperuricemia, hypomagnesemia, hyponatremia, and metabolic alkalosis. Because of their potency, significant volume contraction may also occur. Ototoxicity may occur with ethacrynic acid and high doses of furosemide.

Thiazides (and Related Diuretics)

The thiazide diuretics (and their relatives such as chlorthalidone) include a broad range of medications that block neutral NaCl transport in the early distal convoluted tubule.[9, 10] These agents are only modestly natriuretic and are usually ineffective when used alone in severely volume-overloaded patients. However, they potentiate the natriuretic action loop of diuretics and are useful in overcoming diuretic resistance. Complications include hypokalemia, hyperuricemia, hyponatremia, and metabolic alkalosis.

Potassium-Sparing Diuretics

Potassium-sparing diuretics act in the cortical collecting tubule. Amiloride and triamterene block the apical membrane Na^+ channel, whereas spironolactone is an aldosterone antagonist. Because K^+ secretion in this nephron segment is indirectly linked to Na^+ reabsorption, these diuretics decrease K^+ secretion. Except for spironolactone, which is useful in the treatment of cirrhotic ascites and edema, these agents are only mildly natriuretic. They are best used for their K^+-sparing effects in combination with more potent diuretics. Complications include hyperkalemia (which can be severe) and metabolic acidosis (which is usually mild). In patients prone to hyperkalemia, K^+-sparing diuretics should be avoided. Spironolactone may also cause gynecomastia.

Dopamine

The kidney is richly endowed with dopaminergic receptors. At low doses (0.5 to 2.0 μg/kg/min), dopamine increases renal blood flow and inhibits proximal tubular Na^+ reabsorption. This combination of effects results in increased Na^+ excretion when dopamine is infused in euvolemic subjects with normal renal function.[114] Dopamine, at doses that activate both dopaminergic and beta-adrenergic receptors (2 to 5 μg/kg/min), is also natriuretic in patients with congestive heart failure.[115] Whether dopamine is a valuable natriuretic agent in other critically ill patients is unclear. By increasing renal blood flow, dopamine increases the delivery of loop

TABLE 99–5

CAUSES OF DIURETIC RESISTANCE

Pseudoresistance
  Dose inadequate
  Dosing interval inappropriate
  Excessive Na⁺ intake
True resistance
  Decreased renal secretion
    Decreased renal blood flow
    Hypoalbuminemia
    Competition for secretion
  Albuminuria
  Increased Na⁺ reabsorption at other nephron segments

diuretics to their site of action in the nephron and may be helpful in overcoming diuretic resistance.[116] However, routine use of dopamine as a diuretic in the intensive care unit is unwarranted.[117] Dopamine should be reserved for volume-overloaded patients who are resistant to other diuretics, and if natriuresis does not occur within 24 hours the dopamine should be discontinued.

Diuretic Resistance

Na⁺-avid patients often appear to be resistant to the natriuretic effects of even the potent loop diuretics. Frequently, the inability to achieve natriuresis with these diuretics is due not to true resistance but rather to inadequate dosing or excessive Na⁺ intake (pseudoresistance) (Table 99–5). However, if a single dose of a loop diuretic does not produce natriuresis, administering the same dose twice or three times a day is also not natriuretic. Because the natriuretic effect of the loop diuretics persists for only 6 hours, if Na⁺ intake is not appropriately restricted the intense Na⁺ reabsorption that occurs during the drug-free interval may negate any beneficial diuretic effects. Even with appropriate Na⁺ restriction, the natriuresis achieved with a single daily dose may not be adequate. Giving the diuretic two or even three times a day then frequently results in satisfactory diuresis. If, despite appropriate dosing and Na⁺ restriction, natriuresis is still not achieved, true diuretic resistance is present. Diuretic resistance is often multifactorial in etiology (see Table 99–5).

Except for spironolactone, all diuretics act from the luminal side of the nephron and depend on proximal tubular secretion for access to the tubular fluid. Their rate of secretion depends on renal blood flow, which is often decreased in Na⁺-retentive patients. To ensure adequate delivery of diuretics to their site of action it is frequently necessary to use large intravenous doses. With severely limited blood flow (e.g., in patients with renal insufficiency) up to 400 mg of furosemide or 10 mg of bumetanide may be necessary to achieve diuresis.

Other causes of inadequate delivery of the diuretic to its site of action include hypoalbuminemia, albuminuria, and competition for secretion in the proximal tubule. Binding of loop diuretics to albumin appears to be necessary for proper secretion of the drug into the renal tubule.[118] In addition, in patients with nephrotic syndrome, binding of the drug by albumin within the tubule may prevent its interaction with the Na⁺-K⁺-2Cl⁻ transporter.[119] In patients with severe renal failure, secretion of loop diuretics may be so impaired by decreased renal blood flow and competition for secretion from uremic toxins that only toxic serum levels would achieve adequate secretion. In these patients, a continuous infusion (rather than a bolus) of the diuretic may induce natriuresis while avoiding toxic side effects.[90] If

constant infusion is unsuccessful, increasing renal blood flow with dopamine may increase delivery of the diuretic to its site of action.[116]

In cases in which reabsorption of Na⁺ at other nephron sites produces resistance, addition of a thiazide often potentiates the effects of a loop diuretic.[120] Although rarely necessary, almost complete nephron blockade can be achieved by further addition of a carbonic anhydrase inhibitor. Because total nephron blockade may result in significant volume contraction, it is recommended only under closely monitored conditions.

References

1. Starling EH: On the absorption of fluid from the connective tissue spaces. J Physiol (Lond) 19:312, 1896.
2. Guyton AC: Textbook of Medical Physiology. 8th ed. Philadelphia, WB Saunders, 1991.
3. Taylor EA: Capillary fluid filtration, Starling forces and lymph flow. Circ Res 49:557, 1981.
4. Bonventre JV, Leaf A: Sodium homeostasis: Steady states without a set point. Kidney Int 21:88, 1982.
5. Jacobson HR, Seldin DW: Proximal tubular reabsorption and its regulation. Annu Rev Pharmacol Toxicol 17:623, 1977.
6. Liu FY, Cogan MG, Rector FC Jr: Axial heterogeneity in the rat proximal convoluted tubule. II. Osmolality and osmotic water permeability. Am J Physiol 247:F822, 1984.
7. Schafer JA, Patlak CS, Andreoli TE: A mechanism of isotonic fluid reabsorption linked to active and passive ion flows in the mammalian superficial pars recta. Am J Physiol 233:F154, 1977.
8. Hebert SC, Andreoli TE: Control of NaCl transport in the thick ascending limb. Am J Physiol 246:F745, 1984.
9. Stokes JB: Sodium chloride absorption by the urinary bladder of the winter flounder: A thiazide sensitive, electrically neutral transport system. J Clin Invest 74:7, 1984.
10. Ellison DH, Velazquez H, Wright FS: Thiazide-sensitive sodium chloride cotransport in the early distal tubule. Am J Physiol 253:F546, 1987.
11. Garty H, Benos DJ: Characteristics and regulatory mechanisms of the amiloride-blockable Na⁺ channel. Physiol Rev 68:309, 1988.
12. Epstein M: Cardiovascular and renal effects of head-out water immersion in man. Circ Res 39:619, 1976.
13. Karnad DR, Tembulkar P, Abraham P, et al: Head-down tilt as a physiological diuretic in normal controls and in patients with fluid retaining states. Lancet 2:525, 1987.
14. Adey WR, Cockett AK, Mack PB, et al: Biosatellite III: Preliminary findings. Science 166:492, 1969.
15. Paintal AS: Vagal sensory receptors and their reflex effects. Physiol Rev 53:159, 1973.
16. Kinchlerm HR: Systemic arterial baroreceptor reflexes. Physiol Rev 56:100, 1976.
17. Epstein FH, Post RS, McDowell M: The effect of an arteriovenous fistula on renal hemodynamics and electrolyte excretion. J Clin Invest 32:233, 1991.
18. Blaine EH, Davis JO, Prewitt RL: Evidence for renal vascular receptor in control of renin secretion. Am J Physiol 220:1591, 1971.
19. Skott O, Briggs JP: Direct demonstration of macula densa–mediated renin secretion. Science 237:1618, 1987.
20. Kostreva DR, Castaner A, Kampine JP: Reflex effects of hepatic baroreceptors on renal and cardiac sympathetic nerve activity. Am J Physiol 238:R390, 1980.
21. Satta A, Contu B, Branca GF, et al: Importance of liver interstitial pressure on sodium retention. Nephron 49:190, 1988.
22. Levy M, Wexler MS: Sodium excretion in dogs with low grade caval constriction: Role of hepatic nerves. Am J Physiol 253:F672, 1987.
23. Davis JO, Freeman RH: Mechanisms regulating renin release. Physiol Rev 56:1, 1976.
24. Cogan MG: Angiotensin II: A powerful controller of sodium transport in the early proximal tubule. Hypertension 5:451, 1990.
25. Brown JJ, Casala-Stenzel J, Cumming AMM, et al: Angiotensin II, aldosterone, and arterial pressure: A quantitative approach. Hypertension 1:159, 1979.
26. Edwards RM: Segmental effects of norepinephrine and angiotensin II on isolated renal microvessels. Am J Physiol 244:F526, 1983.
27. Minuth WW, Steckelings U, Gross P: Complex physiological and biochemical action of aldosterone in toad urinary bladder and mammalian renal collecting duct cells. Renal Physiol 10:297, 1987.
28. Kisch B: Electron microscopy of the atrium of the heart. I. Guinea pig. Exp Med Surg 14:99, 1956.
29. Debold AJ, Borenstein HB, Verers AT, et al: A rapid and potent natriuretic response to intravenous injection of atrial myocardial extract in rats. Life Sci 28:89, 1981.
30. Currie MG, Geller DM, Cole BR, et al: Purification and sequence analysis of bioactive atrial peptides (atriopeptins). Science 223:67, 1984.

31. Atlas SA, Kleinert HD, Camargo MJ, et al: Purification, sequence, and synthesis of natriuretic and vasoactive rat atrial peptide. Nature 309:719, 1984.
32. Huang CL, Lewicki J, Johnson LK, et al: Renal mechanism of action of rat natriuretic factor. J Clin Invest 75:769, 1985.
33. Sonnenberg H, Honrath U, Chong CK, et al: Atrial natriuretic factor inhibits sodium transport in medullary collecting duct. Am J Physiol 250:F963, 1986.
34. Atarashi K, Mulrow PJ, Roberto FS, et al: Effect of atrial peptides on aldosterone production. J Clin Invest 76:1807, 1985.
35. Itoh S, Keishi A, Nushiro N, et al: Effect of atrial natriuretic factor on renin release in isolated afferent arterioles. Kidney Int 32:493, 1987.
36. Almeida FA, Suzuki M, Maack T, et al: Atrical natriuretic factor increases hematocrit and decreases plasma volume in nephrectomized rats. Life Sci 39:1193, 1986.
37. Garrick RE: The renal eicosanoids. In: Goldfarb S, Ziyadeh FN (eds): Contemporary Issues in Nephrology, Volume 23, Hormones, Autocoids, and the Kidney. New York, Churchill Livingstone, p 231, 1991.
38. Schlondorff D, Decandido S, Satriano J: Angiotensin II stimulates phospholipase C and A_2 in cultured rat mesangial cells. Am J Physiol 253:C113, 1987.
39. Dzau VJ: Vascular and renal prostaglandins as counter-regulatory systems in heart failure. Eur Heart J 9(suppl H):15, 1988.
40. Packer M: Interaction of prostaglandins and angiotensin II in the modulation of renal function in congestive heart failure. Circulation 77:I64, 1988.
41. Epstein M: Renal prostaglandins and the control of renal function in liver disease. Am J Med 80(suppl 1A):46, 1986.
42. Stork JE, Dunn MS: Hemodynamic role of thromboxane A_2 and prostaglandin E_2 in glomerulonephritis. J Pharmacol Exp Ther 233:672, 1985.
43. Schmid PG, Abboud FM, Wendling MG, et al: Regional vascular effects of vasopressin: Plasma levels and circulatory response. Am J Physiol 227:998, 1974.
44. De Wardener HE, Mills IH, Clapham WF, et al: Studies on the efferent mechanism of the sodium diuresis which follows the administration of intravenous saline in the dog. Clin Sci 21:249, 1961.
45. De Wardener HE, Clarkson EM: Concept of natriuretic hormone. Physiol Rev 65:659, 1985.
46. Graves SW, Williams GH: Endogenous digitalis-like natriuretic factors. Annu Rev Med 38:433, 1987.
47. Hamlyn JM, Blaustein MP, Bova S, et al: Identification and characterization of a ouabain-like compound from human plasma. Proc Natl Acad Sci USA 88:6259, 1991.
48. DiBona GF: Neural mechanisms in body fluid homeostasis. Fed Proc 45:2871, 1986.
49. DiBona GF: Neural control of renal function: Cardiovascular implications. Hypertension 13:539, 1989.
50. Alexander RW, Gill JR, Yamabe H, et al: Effects of dietary sodium and acute saline infusion on the interrelationship between dopamine excretion and adrenergic activity in man. J Clin Invest 54:194, 1974.
51. Seri I: Dopamine and natriuresis. Mechanism of action and developmental aspects. Am J Hypertens 3:825, 1990.
52. Bertorello A, Hökfelt T, Goldstein M, et al: Proximal tubule Na^+-K^+-ATPase activity is inhibited during high-salt diet: Evidence for DA-mediated effect. Am J Physiol 254:F795, 1988.
53. Gertz KH, Boylan JW: Glomerular-tubular balance. In: Orloff J, Berliner RW (eds): Handbook of Physiology, Section 8, Renal Physiology. Washington, DC, American Physiological Society, p 763, 1973.
54. Haberle DA, von Boyer H: Characteristics of glomerulotubular balance. Am J Physiol 244:F355, 1983.
55. McCance RA: Experimental sodium chloride deficiency in man. Proc R Soc Lond 119:245, 1936.
56. Lipsitz LA: Orthostatic hypotension in the elderly. N Engl J Med 321:952, 1989.
57. Gennari FJ, Kassirer JP: Osmotic diseases. N Engl J Med 291:714, 1974.
58. Gault HM, Dixon ME, Doyle M, et al: Hypernatremia, azotemia, and dehydration due to high-protein tube feeding. Ann Intern Med 68:778, 1968.
59. Epstein M, Hollenberg NK: Age as a determinant of renal sodium conservation in normal man. J Lab Clin Med 87:411, 1976.
60. Dannovitch GM, Bourgoignie J, Bricker NA: Reversibility of the salt losing tendency of chronic renal failure. N Engl J Med 296:14, 1977.
61. Lipsitt MB, Pearson OH: Sodium depletion in adrenalectomized humans. J Clin Invest 37:1395, 1958.
62. Anderson RJ, Linas SL, Berns AS, et al: Nonoliguric acute renal failure. N Engl J Med 296:1134, 1977.
63. Demling RH. Burns. Fluid and electrolyte management. Crit Care Clin 1:27, 1985.
64. Conn JW: The mechanism of acclimatization to heat. Adv Intern Med 3:373, 1949.
65. Kassirer JP, Schwartz WB: The response of normal man to selective depletion of hydrochloric acid. Am J Med 40:10, 1966.
66. Ziyadeh FH, Badr KF: Fractional excretion of chloride in prerenal azotemia. Arch Intern Med 145:1929, 1985.
67. Erstad BL, Gales BJ, Rappaport WD: The use of albumin in clinical practice. Arch Intern Med 151:901, 1991.
68. Rackow EC, Falk JL, Fein IA, et al: Fluid resuscitation in circulatory shock: A comparison of the cardiorespiratory effects of albumin, heta-starch, and saline solutions in patients with hypovolemic and septic shock. Crit Care Med 11:839, 1983.
69. Husted FC, Nolph KD, Maher JF: $NaHCO_3$ and NaCl tolerance in chronic renal failure. J Clin Invest 56:414, 1975.
70. Kurtz TW, Al-Bander HA, Morris RC: "Salt sensitive" essential hypertension in men: Is the sodium ion alone important? N Engl J Med 317:1043, 1987.
71. Katz MA: Interstitial space—The forgotten organ. Med Hypotheses 6:1885, 1980.
72. Dzau VJ: Renal and circulatory mechanisms in congestive heart failure. Kidney Int 31:1402, 1987.
73. Lieberman FL, Ito S, Reynolds TB: Effective plasma volume in cirrhosis with ascites. Evidence that a decreased value does not account for renal sodium retention, a spontaneous reduction in glomerular filtration rate (GFR), and a fall in GFR during drug-induced diuresis. J Clin Invest 48:975, 1969.
74. Levy M: Sodium retention and ascites formation in dogs with experimental portal cirrhosis. Am J Physiol 233:F572, 1977.
75. Lieberman FL, Denison EK, Reynolds TB: The relationship of plasma volume, portal hypertension, ascites, and renal sodium retention in cirrhosis: The overflow theory of ascites formation. Ann NY Acad Sci 170:202, 1970.
76. Unikowsky B, Wexler MJ, Levy M: Dogs with experimental cirrhosis of the liver but without intrahepatic hypertension do not retain sodium or form ascites. J Clin Invest 72:1594, 1983.
77. Levy M, Wexler MJ: Hepatic denervation alters first-phase urinary sodium excretion in dogs with cirrhosis. Am J Physiol 253:F664, 1987.
78. Schrier RW, Arroyo V, Bernardi M, et al: Peripheral arterial vasodilation hypothesis: A proposal for the initiation of renal sodium and water retention in cirrhosis. Hepatology 8:1151, 1988.
79. Perez-Ayuso RM, Arroyo V, Planas R, et al: Random comparative study of efficacy of furosemide versus spironolactone in nonazotemic cirrhosis with ascites: Relationship between diuretic response and the activity of the renin-aldosterone system. Gastroenterology 84:961, 1983.
80. Shear L, Ching S, Gabuzda GJ: Compartmentalization of ascites and edema in patients with hepatic cirrhosis. N Engl J Med 282:1391, 1979.
81. Pinto PC, Amerian J, Reynolds TB: Large-volume paracentesis in nonedematous patients with tense ascites: Its effect on intravascular volume. Hepatology 8:207, 1988.
82. Gines P, Tito L, Arroyo V, et al: Randomized comparative study of therapeutic paracentesis with and without intravenous albumin in cirrhosis. Gastroenterology 94:1493, 1988.
83. Gines P, Arroyo V, Quintero E, et al: Comparison of paracentesis and diuretics in the treatment of cirrhotic with tense ascites. Gastroenterology 93:234, 1987.
84. Guazzi M, Polese A, Magrini F, et al: Negative influences of ascites on the cardiac function of cirrhotic patients. Am J Med 59:165, 1975.
85. Blendis LM, Grieg PD, Langer B: The renal and hemodynamic effects of the peritoneovenous shunt for intractable hepatic ascites. Gastroenterology 77:250, 1979.
86. Joles JA, Koomans HA, Kortlandt W, et al: Hypoproteinemia and recovery from edema in dogs. Am J Physiol 254:F887, 1988.
87. Ichikawa I, Rennke HG, Hoyer JR: Role for intrarenal mechanisms in the impaired salt excretion of experimental nephrotic syndrome. J Clin Invest 71:91, 1983.
88. Meltzer JI, Keim JH, Laragh JH, et al: Nephrotic syndrome: Vasoconstriction and hypervolemic types indicated by renin-sodium profiling. Ann Intern Med 91:688, 1979.
89. Davison AX, Lambie AT, Verth AH, et al: Salt-poor human albumin in management of nephrotic syndrome. Br Med J 1:481, 1974.
90. Rudy DW, Voelker JR, Greene PK, et al: Loop diuretics for chronic renal insufficiency: A continuous infusion is more efficacious than bolus therapy. Ann Intern Med 115:360, 1991.
91. Murray MJ, Marsh, HM, Wochos DN, et al: Nutritional assessment of intensive-care unit patients. Mayo Clin Proc 63:1106, 1988.
92. Zweifach BW: Capillary filtration and mechanisms of edema formation. Pfluegers Arch Suppl:81, 1972.
93. Erdmann AJ, Vaughn TR, Brigham K, et al: Effect of increased vascular pressure on lung fluid balance in unanesthetized sheep. Circ Res 37:271, 1975.
94. Guyton AC: Interstitial fluid pressure. II. Pressure-volume curves of the interstitial space. Circ Res 16:452, 1965.
95. Nelson BK. Snake envenomation. Incidence, clinical presentation and management. Med Toxicol Adverse Drug Exp 4:17, 1989.
96. Chang AE, Rosenberg SA. Overview of interleukin-2 as an immuno-therapeutic agent. Semin Surg Oncol 5:385, 1989.
97. Luce JM: Pathogenesis and management of septic shock. Chest 91:883, 1987.
98. Parrillo JE, Parker MM, Natanson C, et al: Septic shock in humans: Advances in the understanding of pathogenesis, cardiovascular dysfunction, and therapy. Ann Intern Med 113:227, 1990.
99. Mahfood S, Hix WR, Aaron BL: Reexpansion pulmonary edema. Ann Thorac Surg 45:340, 1988.
100. Ellman H: Capillary permeability in septic patients. Crit Care Med 12:629, 1984.

101. Groeneveld ABJ, van Lambalgen TA, Thijs LG: Microvascular permeability in endotoxin and bacterial shock. Acute Care 12:195, 1986.
102. Ziegler EJ, Fisher CJ, Sprung CL, et al: Treatment of gram-negative bacteremia and septic shock with HA-IA human monoclonal antibody against endotoxin. N Engl J Med 324:429, 1991.
103. Murdaugh HV, Sieker HO, Manfredi F: Effect of altered intrathoracic pressure on renal hemodynamics, electrolyte excretion and water clearance. J Clin Invest 38:834, 1959.
104. Sladen A, Laver MB, Pontoppidan H: Pulmonary complications and water retention in prolonged mechanical ventilation. N Engl J Med 279:448, 1968.
105. Kilburn KH, Dowell AR: Renal function in respiratory failure. Arch Intern Med 127:754, 1971.
106. Reihman DH, Farber MO, Weinberger MH, et al: Effect of hypoxemia on sodium and water excretion in chronic obstructive lung disease. Am J Med 78:87, 1985.
107. Fourman P, Hervey GR: An experimental study of edema in potassium deficiency. Clin Sci 14:75, 1954.
108. Lennon EJ, Lemann J: The effect of a potassium-deficient diet on the pattern of recovery from experimental metabolic acidosis. Clin Sci 34:365, 1968.
109. Krishna GG, Chusid P, Hoeldtke RD: Mild potassium depletion provokes renal sodium retention. J Lab Clin Med 109:724, 1987.
110. Williams SA, Rayman G, Tooke JE: Dependent oedema and attenuation of postural vasoconstriction associated with nifedipine therapy for hypertension in diabetic patients. Eur J Clin Pharmacol 37:333, 1989.
111. Presig PA, Toto RD, Alpern RJ: Carbonic anhydrase inhibitors. Renal Physiol 10:136, 1987.
112. Rose BD: Diuretics. Kidney Int 39:337, 1991.
113. Vasko MR, Brown-Cartwright D, Knochel JP, et al: Furosemide absorption is altered in decompensated congestive heart failure. Ann Intern Med 102:314, 1985.
114. McDonald RH Jr, Goldberg LI, McNay JL, et al: Effect of dopamine in man: Augmentation of sodium excretion, glomerular filtration rate, and renal plasma flow. J Clin Invest 43:1116, 1964.
115. Beregovich J, Bianchi C, Rubler S, et al: Dose-related hemodynamic and renal effects of dopamine in congestive heart failure. Am Heart J 87:550, 1974.
116. Linder A.: Synergism of dopamine and furosemide in diuretic resistant oliguric acute renal failure. Nephron 33:121, 1983.
117. Szerlip HM: Renal-dose dopamine: Fact and fiction. Ann Intern Med 115:153, 1991.
118. Inoue M, Okajima K, Itoh K, et al: Mechanism of furosemide resistance in analbuminemic rats and hypoalbuminemic patients. Kidney Int 32:198, 1987.
119. Kirchner KA, Voelker JR, Brater DC: Intratubular albumin blunts the response to furosemide—A mechanism for diuretic resistance in nephrotic syndrome. J Pharmacol Exp Ther 252:1097, 1990.
120. Oster JR, Epstein M, Smoller S: Combination therapy with thiazide-type and loop diuretic agents for resistant sodium retention. Ann Intern Med 99:405, 1983.

CHAPTER 100

Water and Tonicity Homeostasis

Paul M. Palevsky

Disordered water homeostasis, usually manifested as hyponatremia or hypernatremia, is common in the critically ill patient. Volume depletion, cardiac and hepatic dysfunction, renal insufficiency, endocrine disorders, and central nervous system disease may all impair osmoregulation. Thus, the critically ill patient with multiple organ system disease is at increased risk for the development of hypotonicity or hypertonicity in response to osmotic stress.

BODY FLUID OSMOLALITY AND TONICITY

Osmolality and tonicity are closely related but conceptually distinct properties of biologic fluids. Osmolality is a measure of the number of solute particles in an aqueous solution in terms of the number of moles of solute (osmoles) per kilogram of water and is inversely related to the concentration of water in the solution. If two solutions of different osmolalities are separated by an artificial membrane permeable only to water, water diffuses across the membrane down its concentration gradient (from the solution of lesser to the solution of greater osmolality) until osmotic equilibrium is achieved.

Cell membranes are not only freely permeable to water but also selectively permeable to certain solutes. Although all solutes contribute to osmolality, only the solutes whose movement is relatively restricted by cell membranes affect the distribution of water between the extracellular fluid (ECF) and intracellular fluid (ICF) compartments. The concentration of these relatively impermeant ("effective") solutes constitutes the effective osmolality or tonicity of a fluid. Sodium and its associated anions, which are excluded from cells, and glucose are the major determinants of ECF tonicity. Urea, which freely permeates cell membranes and therefore does not alter the distribution of water between the ECF and ICF, does not contribute to tonicity.

Because all body fluids are in osmotic equilibrium, measurements of plasma osmolality (P_{Osm}) reflect the osmolality of both the ECF and the ICF. P_{Osm} may be measured directly or may be estimated from the molar concentrations of the predominant ECF solutes: sodium (and its associated anions), glucose, and urea. Thus

$$P_{Osm} = 2 \times [Na^+] + [BUN] + [glucose]$$

where all concentrations are expressed in millimoles per liter. When blood urea nitrogen (BUN) and glucose are measured in milligrams per deciliter, conversion to millimoles per liter is achieved by using the following equation:

$$P_{Osm} = 2 \times [Na^+] + \frac{[BUN]}{2.8} + \frac{[glucose]}{18}$$

Estimates of P_{Osm} using these formulas are usually within 5 to 10 mOsm/kg of the measured value. An osmole gap, arising from discrepancies between the measured and calculated osmolalities, may result from the presence of routinely unmeasured solute (e.g., ethanol, methanol, and mannitol) in the blood. Under these circumstances, the measured P_{Osm} is appropriately elevated while the calculated value remains within the normal range.

Because tonicity cannot be measured, it must be estimated from the concentration of effective solutes in the plasma. Normally, these solutes are sodium (with its associated anions) and glucose. Thus, plasma tonicity (P_{Ton}) is calculated as

$$P_{Ton} = 2 \times [Na^+] + [glucose]$$

when all values are measured as millimoles per liter or

$$P_{Ton} = 2 \times [Na^+] + \frac{[glucose]}{18}$$

when glucose is measured as milligrams per deciliter. If other osmotically effective solutes, such as mannitol, are present, their concentrations must also be included in the calculation of P_{Ton}.

Under normal circumstances, P_{Osm} and P_{Ton} are virtually identical, differing primarily by the concentration of urea (approximately 5 mOsm/kg). However, during azotemia or when another osmotically ineffective solute (e.g., ethanol) is present, the two values diverge. In the absence of hyperglycemia or elevated levels of other effective solutes (e.g., mannitol), P_{Ton} correlates with the ECF sodium concentration, being approximately twice the plasma sodium concentration (P_{Na}). Thus, hypotonicity is always associated with hyponatremia. Likewise, hypernatremia always implies the presence of hypertonicity. However, hypertonicity cannot always be equated with hypernatremia: In the presence of hyperglycemia or elevated levels of other osmotically effective solutes, hypertonicity may exist with a normal or depressed P_{Na}.

Regulation of P_{Ton} underlies the maintenance of ICF volume. Because the solute content of the ICF is relatively constant over time and the ECF and ICF are in osmotic equilibrium, hypotonicity is associated with fluid shifts into the ICF and intracellular swelling. Conversely, in hypertonic states intracellular dehydration occurs. The clinical manifestations of hypotonicity and hypertonicity are largely attributable to these alterations in cell volume, particularly as they occur within the central nervous system.

MECHANISMS OF WATER AND TONICITY HOMEOSTASIS

The maintenance of a constant body fluid tonicity depends on water balance. Because body fluid tonicity can be viewed as the ratio of total body (osmotically) effective solute (TBES) to total body water (TBW), alterations in TBW produce reciprocal changes in tonicity if TBES remains constant. Thus, increases in TBW produce hypotonicity and deficits result in hypertonicity. Abnormalities in P_{Ton} can also result from disproportionate changes in both TBES and TBW.

Body fluid tonicity is tightly regulated; normal values for P_{Osm} range from 280 to 295 mOsm/kg but do not vary by more than 1 to 2% over time in any individual. Constant tonicity is maintained through appropriate alterations in TBW; at steady state, water balance is achieved through the regulation of both water intake and water excretion.

Water Balance

In healthy individuals, water intake is derived entirely from dietary sources. In addition to the ingestion of liquids, approximately 750 mL of water is ingested daily as preformed water in solid foods and an additional 350 mL is generated through oxidative metabolism.[1] Approximately 0.4 mL of water is produced during metabolism for each gram of amino acids, 0.6 mL for each gram of carbohydrate, and 1.0 mL for each gram of fat.[2]

In patients in the intensive care unit (ICU), water intake is frequently in the form of parenteral fluids given intravenously, diluents for medications, and parenteral nutrition. Parenteral fluid may also be absorbed from intraperitoneal or intravesicular irrigation. In addition, in some circumstances, patients receiving dialysis may have a net gain of water during treatments.

Water excretion can be divided into insensible and sensible losses. Insensible losses occur via the skin and respiratory tract and under basal conditions total approximately 0.6 mL/kg/h (1 L/d for a 70-kg individual).[3] Several factors may increase these losses in the ICU patient. Most important of these is fever, which increases insensible losses by approximately 20% for each 1°C increase in body temperature. Cutaneous water losses are increased in patients with extensive burns, and inadequately humidified supplemental oxygen augments respiratory water losses.

Sensible, or perceived, water losses are primarily gastrointestinal and renal in origin. Gastrointestinal water loss is minimal in healthy individuals, usually totaling less than 100 to 150 mL/d.[4] These losses may increase substantially, exceeding several liters per day, as the result of emesis, diarrhea, and nasogastric, biliary, or enterocutaneous fistula drainage. Additional losses may result from the drainage of ascites and pleural fluid.

Renal losses are the only component of water excretion subject to physiologic regulation, varying in response to alterations in both body fluid tonicity and ECF volume. Hypertonicity and volume depletion stimulate the secretion of arginine vasopressin (AVP) by the neurohypophysis, enhancing water reabsorption and resulting in the excretion of a concentrated urine. In response to hypotonicity, AVP secretion is suppressed, water reabsorption is minimized, and a dilute urine is excreted.

In evaluating changes in water balance it is helpful to divide the urine output into two conceptual components: (1) the volume necessary to excrete urinary solute isosmotically with plasma and (2) the remaining volume, which represents the solute-free water excreted (or reabsorbed) by the kidney. Mathematically, this can be expressed as

$$C_{H_2O} = V \times \left(1 - \frac{U_{Osm}}{P_{Osm}}\right)$$

where C_{H_2O} = solute-free water clearance
V = urine volume
U_{Osm} = urine osmolality
P_{Osm} = plasma osmolality

When the urine is isosmotic, solute-free water clearance is zero. When the urine is dilute ($U_{Osm} < P_{Osm}$), C_{H_2O} has a positive value and represents the rate of solute-free water excretion. When the urine is concentrated ($U_{Osm} > P_{Osm}$), C_{H_2O} assumes a negative value, indicating solute-free water reabsorption by the kidney. (By convention, this is called $T^c_{H_2O}$, the tubular reabsorption of water, where $T^c_{H_2O} = -C_{H_2O}$.)

A more useful assessment of renal water handling is made by evaluating electrolyte excretion rather than total solute excretion. The predominant urinary solutes are sodium and potassium (with their associated anions) and urea; because urea is not an osmotically effective solute, it has no effect on body fluid tonicity. Thus, it is more useful to evaluate renal water handling in terms of electrolyte-free water excretion:[5, 6]

$$C^e_{H_2O} = V \times \left(1 - \frac{U_{Na} + U_K}{P_{Na}}\right)$$

where $C^e_{H_2O}$ = electrolyte-free water clearance
V = urine volume
U_{Na} = urinary sodium concentration
U_K = urinary potassium concentration
P_{Na} = plasma sodium concentration

The importance of the distinction between solute-free and electrolyte-free water clearance is illustrated in the following example. In a patient with a P_{Na} of 150 mmol/L, P_{Osm} of 300 mOsm/kg, U_{Osm} of 300 mOsm/kg, U_{Na} and U_K of 45 and 30 mmol/L, respectively, and a urine volume of 2 L/d, solute-free water clearance is zero {$C_{H_2O} = 2[1 - (300/300)] = 0$} but electrolyte-free water clearance is $C^e_{H_2O} = 2\{1 - [(45 + 30)/150]\} = 1$ L/d. Thus, the patient has a considerable renal electrolyte-free water loss contributing to the hypernatremic state.

Regulation of Water Balance

The maintenance of water balance is dependent on the integrated regulation of water intake and excretion. Renal water excretion provides the major defense against water intoxication and hypotonicity. In contrast, renal water conservation can serve only as an initial defense against dehydration and cannot correct water deficits; augmentation of water intake is necessary for the prevention of progressive hypertonicity.

Regulation of Water Intake

Most water intake is independent of osmoregulatory factors. Approximately 1 L is ingested as preformed or metabolic water in solid foods. An additional 500 to 1500 mL is ingested through social or habitual drinking and is not subject to physiologic regulation. Under normal circumstances, this daily intake of 1.5 to 2.5 L of water is usually more than sufficient to replace obligatory water losses and to maintain normal body fluid tonicity.

Thirst, defined as an intense craving for water, is stimulated by increases in plasma tonicity. The osmotic threshold for thirst is approximately 290 to 295 mOsm/kg, approximately 5 to 10 mOsm/kg higher than that for AVP secretion.[7] Thus, maximal renal water conservation occurs before any significant augmentation of water intake in response to thirst. Not all solutes are equipotent in their stimulation of thirst: Hypertonic saline and mannitol are potent dipsogens, whereas equimolar infusions of glucose and urea have little effect on thirst.[8]

Intravascular volume depletion and hypotension serve as secondary stimuli to thirst through activation of low-pressure vascular stretch receptors and arterial baroreceptors.[9] Hypervolemia-mediated elevation of peripheral and central angiotensin II levels also contributes to the nonosmotic stimulation of thirst.[9, 10]

When individuals with intact thirst sensation have unrestricted access to fluids, water ingestion is a potent defense against hypertonicity; when fully stimulated, thirst-induced water ingestion is sufficient to replace virtually any magnitude of water loss. For example, patients with complete diabetes insipidus (DI) may have urine volumes in excess of 20 L/d; however, if thirst is intact and water intake unrestricted, they are able to match these massive losses with oral water intake, thereby avoiding progressive water depletion and hypertonicity.

As the result of fatigue, obtundation, and multiple organ system illness, critically ill patients are usually unable to control their water intake. They are therefore dependent on prescribed enteral and parenteral fluids for prevention of dehydration and progressive hypertonicity.

Regulation of Water Excretion

Although water losses occur via the skin, respiratory tract, gastrointestinal tract, and kidney, only renal water excretion is subject to extensive physiologic regulation. Renal water excretion can be operationally divided into three interrelated processes: (1) delivery of electrolyte-containing fluid to the "diluting" segments of the nephron (the ascending limb of the loop of Henle and the early distal convoluted tubule), (2) separation of solute and water through the selective reabsorption of electrolyte at these water-impermeable sites, and (3) recombination of solute and water through the selective reabsorption of water from the collecting duct.

The first two of these processes, delivery of fluid to the diluting sites and selective reabsorption of solute, are independent of the prevailing P_{Ton}. The delivery of fluid to the diluting sites determines the maximal rate of electrolyte-free water generation; limitations to fluid delivery restrict electrolyte-free water excretion, even if maximal urine dilution is achieved. The reabsorption of solute at these sites is responsible for the generation of electrolyte-free water and

determines the minimal achievable urinary osmolality. In addition, transport of solute from the tubular lumen into the medullary interstitium is required for establishment of the corticomedullary osmotic gradient. Interference with any of these processes (by intravascular volume depletion, effective arterial hypovolemia, diuretics, or renal disease, for example) impairs renal water handling.

The final urine composition is determined by variable reabsorption of water from the collecting duct, the hydraulic permeability of which is modulated by AVP. When AVP secretion is suppressed, hydraulic permeability is low and a maximally dilute urine ($U_{Osm} < 100$ mOsm/kg) is excreted. As AVP levels rise, water reabsorption increases and a progressively concentrated urine is excreted.

Secretion of AVP varies in proportion to P_{Ton}. In normal individuals, AVP secretion is minimal when P_{Osm} falls below 280 mOsm/kg. As P_{Osm} rises above this threshold, AVP secretion increases linearly, with maximal urine concentration (U_{Osm} of 800 to 1200 mOsm/kg) being achieved when P_{Osm} exceeds 295 mOsm/kg and AVP levels are greater than 5 pg/mL.[11, 12]

The secretion of AVP is solute specific. Hypertonic infusions of saline or mannitol stimulate AVP release, whereas equimolar infusions of urea have a minimal effect.[8, 13] The response to glucose is more complex. Hypertonic glucose infusions decrease circulating AVP levels in normal individuals but stimulate AVP secretion in insulinopenic patients, suggesting that the response to glucose is insulin dependent.[14] Acute hypoglycemia also stimulates AVP release.[12]

AVP release is also physiologically modulated by hemodynamic factors. Changes in intravascular filling are detected by vascular stretch receptors in the intrathoracic veins, pulmonary bed, and left atrium. Changes in arterial pressure are detected by baroreceptors in the aortic arch and carotid sinus. Alterations in ECF volume and blood pressure modulate the osmotic release of AVP; hypovolemia and hypotension augment, and hypervolemia and hypertension inhibit, AVP release at any given level of plasma tonicity.[15] However, the response of AVP secretion to hemodynamic changes is less sensitive than the response to changes in osmolality.[16] Failure to suppress AVP secretion as a result of hemodynamic stimuli commonly contributes to hypotonicity in the ICU patient.

In addition to osmotic and hemodynamic stimuli, various other factors affect AVP secretion. Many of these are of particular significance in the ICU patient: nausea, pain, anxiety, hypoxia, hypercapnia, positive pressure ventilation, pulmonary and central nervous system diseases, certain pharmacologic agents (e.g., opiates), and glucocorticoid and thyroid hormone deficiency all enhance AVP secretion regardless of prevailing body fluid tonicity and ECF volume.

Maximal renal conservation of electrolyte-free water requires generation, maintenance, and appropriate utilization of the corticomedullary osmotic gradient. Gradient generation requires adequate delivery to, and reabsorption of, sodium in, the ascending limb of the loop of Henle and the adequate delivery to, and reabsorption of urea in, the medullary collecting duct. Maintenance of the medullary concentration gradient requires normal medullary blood flow. Interstitial renal disease, loop diuretics (e.g., furosemide and bumetanide), osmotic diuresis, polyuria, and protein malnutrition all impair gradient generation and maintenance and are frequently encountered in critically ill patients. Gradient utilization is strictly AVP dependent; defects in the secretion of AVP or the responsiveness of the collecting duct to AVP produce DI and are also not uncommon in the ICU patient.

DISORDERS OF WATER AND TONICITY HOMEOSTASIS

The symptoms of hypotonicity and hypertonicity are nonspecific. As a result, disturbances of water (tonicity) homeostasis are usually detected through alterations in P_{Na}. Hyponatremia suggests the presence of hypotonicity but may also occur in the setting of normal or elevated P_{Ton}. In contrast, hypernatremia is always indicative of hypertonicity.

Hyponatremia

Isotonic hyponatremia (pseudohyponatremia) is a laboratory artifact arising from alterations in plasma water content associated with severe hyperlipidemia or hyperproteinemia. Because sodium is distributed only in the aqueous phase of plasma (which normally constitutes 93% of the plasma volume), displacement of plasma water by paraproteins or hyperlipidemia decreases the sodium content of plasma despite a constant plasma water sodium concentration. Thus, measurements of plasma (or serum) sodium concentration that depend on total plasma sodium content (e.g., flame photometry) may underestimate the actual plasma water sodium concentration.[17] Pseudohyponatremia should be suspected when the serum is grossly lipemic or viscous. The diagnosis may be confirmed by the presence of a normal measured P_{Osm}. This artifact is obviated if plasma water sodium concentration is measured in undiluted plasma using ion-specific electrodes (direct potentiometry).[17]

Hypertonic hyponatremia occurs when the ECF contains increased concentrations of osmotically effective nonelectrolyte solutes (e.g., glucose and mannitol). The resulting increase in ECF tonicity causes water to shift from the ICF into the ECF, thereby diluting the ECF sodium concentration.

Hypotonic hyponatremia develops when water intake exceeds the sum of insensible, gastrointestinal, and renal electrolyte-free water losses. Because maximal renal electrolyte-free water excretion is 15 to 20 L/d, the development of hypotonicity in the critically ill patient usually reflects the combination of impaired renal electrolyte-free water clearance with either normal or increased water intake.

Hyponatremia (P_{Na} < 135 mmol/L) is common in the critically ill patient. Although the incidence of hyponatremia in the ICU is not well defined, it is much greater than 1%, the rate for patients on general medical-surgical wards,[18] and is associated with a 7- to 60-fold increase in mortality.[18, 19] Although the bulk of this mortality may not result from hypotonicity per se and reflects the severity of underlying disease,[20] severe hyponatremia itself can be life threatening.[21]

Many of the pathogenetic mechanisms resulting in hypotonic hyponatremia are related to changes in ECF volume. Thus, when evaluating a patient with hypotonic hyponatremia, it is useful to construct a differential diagnosis based on ECF volume status (Table 100-1).

Hypovolemic Hypotonicity

When hypotonicity occurs in combination with volume depletion, both TBW and TBES are decreased, but there is a proportionately greater solute than water deficit. The reduction in ECF volume results in enhanced fluid reabsorption in the proximal nephron, decreasing fluid delivery to the renal diluting sites and limiting electrolyte-free water generation. In addition, when volume depletion is of sufficient magnitude, AVP secretion is stimulated, increasing water reabsorption from the collecting duct. This combination of impaired electrolyte-free water generation and increased water reabsorption limits the capacity of the kidneys to excrete a water load. Consequently, when water intake exceeds the diminished electrolyte-free water excretory capacity, hypotonicity ensues.

Any process that produces ECF volume depletion can, if combined with sufficient water intake, result in hypotonicity. Thus, negative sodium balance resulting from excessive renal, gastrointestinal, or cutaneous sodium losses may contribute to the development of hypovolemic hyponatremia. In the critically ill patient, excessive nasogastric or biliary drainage, hemorrhage, sequestration of fluid, cutaneous losses from burns, renal sodium wasting, and under-replacement of intraoperative losses are of special importance in the development of hypovolemic hypotonicity.

Hypervolemic Hypotonicity

In edematous patients, hypotonicity occurs when TBW is disproportionately increased with respect to TBES. The development of positive sodium balance and ECF volume overload is indicative of impaired renal sodium handling as the result of diminished glomerular filtration or enhanced renal tubular sodium reabsorption.

ECF volume expansion in the pathologic edema-forming states (congestive heart failure, hepatic cirrhosis, and nephrotic syndrome) and the capillary leak syndrome (seen, for example, in some patients with endotoxic shock) is associated with diminished effective arterial blood volume (EABV). The pathophysiologic processes contributing to the development of hypotonicity in these states are the same as those underlying hypovolemic hypotonicity. Decreased EABV increases proximal tubular sodium reabsorption, thereby decreasing distal delivery and restricting electrolyte-free water generation, and increases AVP secretion, thereby increasing collecting duct water reabsorption and further reducing electrolyte-free water clearance.

The propensity to manifest hyponatremia under these circumstances is a function of the underlying disorder's hemodynamic impact. For example, early in the course of congestive heart failure, the decrement in EABV is minimal. Consequently, fluid delivery to the distal nephron and AVP secretion are relatively normal and hypotonicity is unusual. As cardiac function worsens, EABV declines and renal electrolyte-free water clearance is progressively restricted. When electrolyte-free water excretion falls below the level of water intake, hypotonicity ensues.

Renal insufficiency may also be associated with hypervolemic hypotonicity. Unlike the edematous disorders, however, renal failure is generally associated with increased absolute intravascular volume and EABV. In chronic renal insufficiency, electrolyte-free water generation is relatively preserved; the decrement in electrolyte-free water excretion results primarily from decreased glomerular filtration.[22] When the glomerular filtration rate falls to 10 mL/min, maximal electrolyte-free water excretion declines from 15 to 20 L/d to less than 2 L/d, markedly reducing the capacity to defend against hypotonicity.

In oliguric acute renal failure, electrolyte-free water excretion is limited by the scant urine output. In nonoliguric acute renal failure, tubular dysfunction may directly impair electrolyte-free water generation, combining with the decreased glomerular filtration rate to restrict significantly electrolyte-free water excretion.

Thus, in renal failure, hypotonicity develops when water intake exceeds the limited electrolyte-free water excretory capacity provided by insensible and renal losses. Fluid management of the patient with renal insufficiency requires careful attention to both sodium and electrolyte-free water

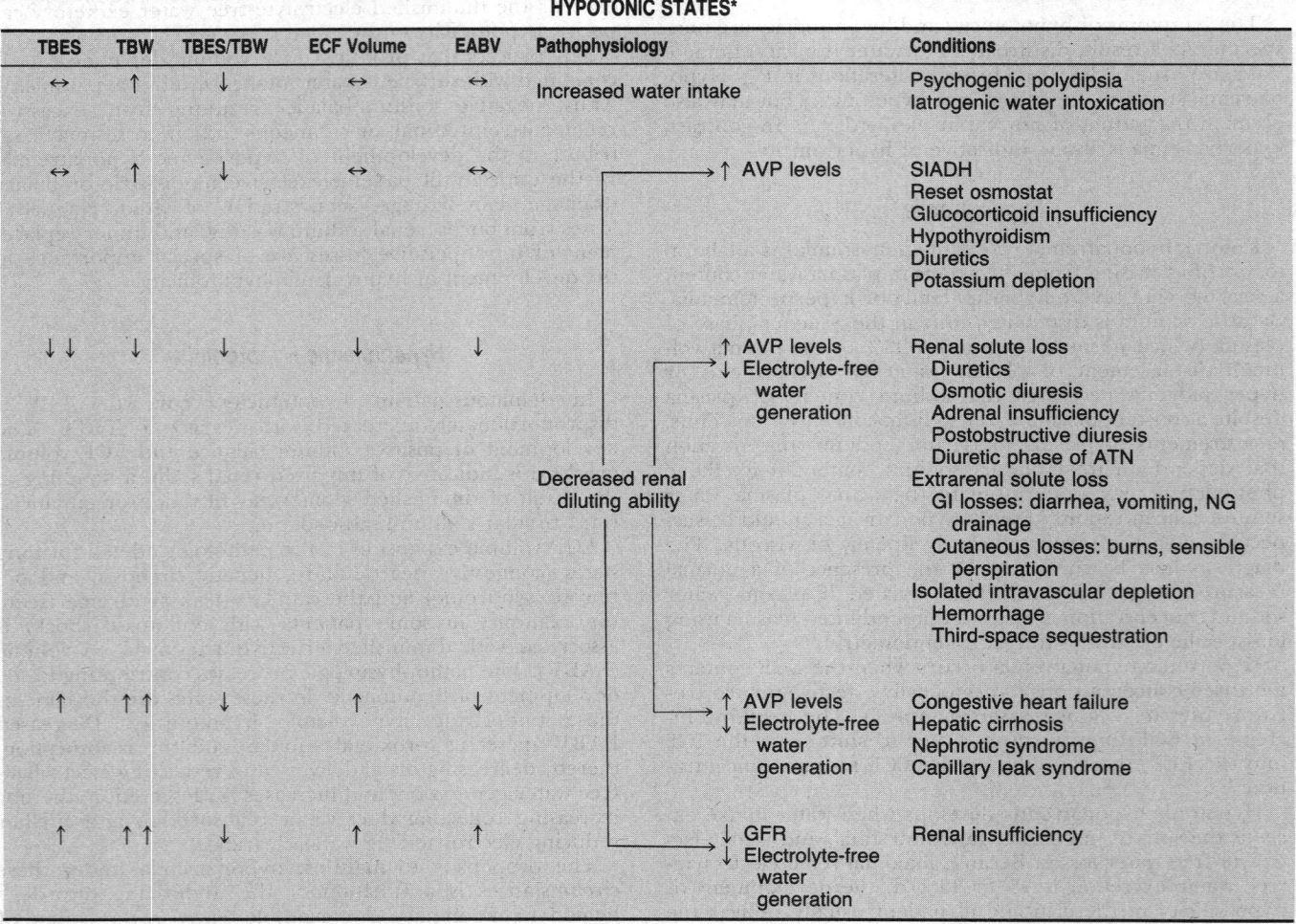

TABLE 100–1

HYPOTONIC STATES*

TBES	TBW	TBES/TBW	ECF Volume	EABV	Pathophysiology		Conditions
↔	↑	↓	↔	↔	Increased water intake		Psychogenic polydipsia Iatrogenic water intoxication
↔	↑	↓	↔	↔		↑ AVP levels	SIADH Reset osmostat Glucocorticoid insufficiency Hypothyroidism Diuretics Potassium depletion
↓↓	↓	↓	↓	↓	Decreased renal diluting ability	↑ AVP levels ↓ Electrolyte-free water generation	Renal solute loss Diuretics Osmotic diuresis Adrenal insufficiency Postobstructive diuresis Diuretic phase of ATN Extrarenal solute loss GI losses: diarrhea, vomiting, NG drainage Cutaneous losses: burns, sensible perspiration Isolated intravascular depletion Hemorrhage Third-space sequestration
↑	↑↑	↓	↑	↓		↑ AVP levels ↓ Electrolyte-free water generation	Congestive heart failure Hepatic cirrhosis Nephrotic syndrome Capillary leak syndrome
↑	↑↑	↓	↑	↑		↓ GFR ↓ Electrolyte-free water generation	Renal insufficiency

*TBES = total body (osmotically) effective solute; TBW = total body water; ECF = extracellular fluid; EABV = effective arterial blood volume; ATN = acute tubular necrosis; GI = gastrointestinal; NG = nasogastric; SIADH = syndrome of inappropriate antidiuretic hormone; GFR = glomerular filtration rate; AVP = arginine vasopressin; ↔ = no change; ↑ = increase; ↓ = decrease.

contents to minimize the risks of both volume overload and hypotonicity.

Euvolemic Hypotonicity

When hypotonicity occurs in the absence of clinical evidence of either volume depletion or volume overload, euvolemic hypotonicity is judged to be present. In these patients, hypotonicity results predominantly from an increase in TBW with little or no change in TBES.

Both excessive water intake and impaired electrolyte-free water excretion may contribute to the development of euvolemic hypotonicity. However, because electrolyte-free water clearance can approach 1 L/h in response to water loading, a patient with normal renal function needs to sustain a heroic water intake to develop hypotonicity on this basis alone. Despite the magnitude of the water ingestion required, profound hyponatremia resulting from primary (psychogenic) polydipsia has occasionally been described in the setting of chronic psychiatric disease.[23, 24] However, careful evaluation of patients with psychogenic polydipsia has usually revealed coexisting defects in AVP secretion and electrolyte-free water generation.[25]

Acute, iatrogenic water intoxication is uncommon. How-ever, large volumes of hypotonic bladder irrigation solution may be absorbed during urologic surgery, producing severe hyponatremia and alterations in mental status (the "post-TURP" [transurethral resection of the prostate] syndrome).[26] Iatrogenic water intoxication may also result from inadvertent intravenous administration of large volumes of hypotonic solutions.

More commonly, disordered AVP secretion underlies the development of euvolemic hypotonicity. Abnormalities in AVP secretion may result from endocrine disorders (glucocorticoid insufficiency and severe hypothyroidism) or be manifest as the syndrome of inappropriate antidiuretic hormone (SIADH). Diuretics and severe potassium depletion may also cause euvolemic hypotonicity. In the ICU, the propensity to develop hypotonicity is frequently exacerbated by the administration of large volumes of hypotonic fluids.

In glucocorticoid deficiency, hypotonicity fails to suppress AVP secretion.[27, 28] The underlying mechanisms are controversial: glucocorticoid deficiency may directly alter AVP secretion; hemodynamic factors resulting from diminished cardiac output and relative hypotension may provide a stimulus for AVP release; and AVP-independent intrarenal factors, in particular, alterations in renal hemodynamics and collecting duct hydraulic permeability, may restrict water excretion.[29, 30] Treatment with physiologic doses of glucocorticoid yields prompt water diuresis and corrects the hypotonicity.[27]

Similarly, in profound hypothyroidism renal water excretion is also often impaired, with elevated circulating AVP levels despite prevailing hypotonicity.[28] The cause of the inappropriate AVP secretion is not known, but it may be related to a fall in cardiac output. AVP-independent impairment of water excretion may result from hemodynamic alterations that diminish glomerular filtration rate and reduce fluid delivery to the diluting sites.

Syndrome of Inappropriate Antidiuretic Hormone. SIADH is the most common cause of hyponatremia in hospitalized patients.[20, 31] The syndrome may result from persistent secretion of AVP in the absence of physiologic osmotic or hemodynamic stimuli, ectopic production of AVP (or other peptides with antidiuretic activity), or increased sensitivity of the collecting duct to AVP.[32] As a result, renal electrolyte-free water excretion is limited, allowing even moderate water intake to lead to progressive hypotonicity. The diagnosis is suggested by an inappropriately concentrated urine ($U_{Osm} > 100$ mOsm/kg) in a euvolemic patient with hypotonic hyponatremia ($P_{Osm} < 280$ mOsm/kg).

The diagnosis of SIADH can be made only if volumetric stimuli for AVP secretion are rigorously excluded. The clinical findings of volume depletion (e.g., tachycardia and orthostatic hypotension) must be absent. The pathologic edema-forming states (congestive heart failure, hepatic cirrhosis, and nephrotic syndrome) are associated with decreased EABV and must also be excluded. In nonedematous patients, clinical assessment based on history and physical findings identifies volume status correctly only about 50% of the time.[33] In the absence of a restricted sodium intake, the urinary sodium concentration provides a better indicator, suggesting intravascular volume depletion if it is less than 30 mmol/L.[33] The diagnosis of SIADH also requires that adrenal and thyroid function be normal.

SIADH is associated with many of the clinical disorders encountered in the critically ill patient (Table 100–2). These disorders may be broadly divided into three categories: neoplasms, pulmonary diseases, and central nervous system disorders. AVP secretion and collecting duct responsiveness are altered by a wide variety of pharmacologic agents, including opiates, barbiturates, antipsychotic agents, carbamazepine, clofibrate, chlorpropamide, several antineoplastic agents, and general anesthetics. Positive pressure ventilation, pain, nausea, and stress are other factors that contribute to the development of SIADH in the critical care setting.

The syndrome of the "reset osmostat" is an important variant of SIADH.[34] Patients with this syndrome regulate P_{Osm} around a depressed set-point. However, because they are able to excrete dilute urine in response to water loading, they do not manifest progressive hypotonicity and generally maintain P_{Na} above 125 mmol/L. It is important to differentiate this disorder from classic SIADH because patients with a reset osmostat are usually asymptomatic and require no specific therapy.

Diuretic-Induced Hypotonicity

Hypotonicity associated with diuretic use merits special mention. Insofar as diuretics produce volume depletion, they contribute to the development of hyponatremia through diminished delivery of fluid to the diluting sites and hemodynamically mediated AVP release. In addition, thiazides and loop diuretics (e.g., furosemide and bumetanide) inhibit sodium reabsorption in the diluting segments of the nephron, further diminishing electrolyte-free water generation.

TABLE 100–2

CAUSES OF SYNDROME OF INAPPROPRIATE ANTIDIURETIC HORMONE

Neoplasms
  Bronchogenic carcinoma
  Carcinoma of the duodenum
  Carcinoma of the pancreas
  Thymoma
  Lymphoma
  Carcinoma of the prostate
Pulmonary diseases
  Tuberculosis
  Pneumonia
  Bronchiectasis
  Pulmonary abscess
  Aspergillosis
  Asthma
  Cystic fibrosis
Central nervous system disorders
  Head trauma
  Subdural hematoma
  Subarachnoid hemorrhage
  Cerebrovascular accident
  Encephalitis
  Meningitis
  Brain tumors
  Guillain-Barré syndrome
  Multiple sclerosis
  Acute intermittent porphyria
Drugs
  Opiates
  Barbiturates
  Tricyclic antidepressants
  Phenothiazines
  Chlorpropamide
  Carbamazepine
  Clofibrate
  Vincristine
  Cyclophosphamide
  General anesthetics
Miscellaneous
  Positive pressure ventilation
  Pain
  Nausea
  Stress

However, thiazide diuretics (and less frequently loop diuretics) have also been associated with severe hyponatremia in the absence of clinical signs of volume depletion.[35] The pathophysiology of this syndrome is uncertain, but direct inhibition of electrolyte-free water generation, hemodynamically mediated AVP release (on the basis of subclinical volume contraction), SIADH, and potassium depletion have all been proposed as mechanisms.[36, 37] In severe potassium depletion, intracellular solute content is diminished, causing water to shift from the ICF to the ECF. In addition, water retention is favored as a result of nonosmotic stimulation of both AVP secretion and thirst.[38–40]

Clinical Manifestations of Hypotonicity

The clinical manifestations of hypotonicity depend on its cause, duration, and magnitude. The primary manifestations of acute hypotonicity result from cerebral edema caused by the osmotic shift of water into the brain.[41] The degree of brain swelling depends on both the rate of development and the magnitude of the hypotonicity and may be sufficient to result in brain stem herniation.[21] In chronic hypotonicity, cerebral swelling is minimized by the loss of intracellular electrolytes and organic solutes.[42–44] These adaptive processes may militate against the development of symptoms, but they may also predispose to complications during treatment.

The signs and symptoms of hypotonicity are nonspecific and are easily obscured in the critically ill patient. Mild hyponatremia ($P_{Na} > 125$ mmol/L) is usually asymptomatic. When hypotonicity develops acutely, nausea, headache, agitation, and confusion may occur when P_{Na} falls below 125 mmol/L. Grand mal seizures, coma, and respiratory arrest ensue in a high percentage of patients with severe acute hypotonicity.[21, 45] Focal neurologic effects are unusual but may occur. The mortality associated with acute hypotonicity is disputed: although some investigators cite mortality rates of approximately 50%,[46, 47] others report rates closer to 5%.[45] Although symptoms generally resolve with treatment, there may be permanent neurologic deficits, possibly as the result of postanoxic encephalopathy after seizures or respiratory arrest.[21]

In chronic hypotonicity (duration greater than 48 hours) manifestations are more vague and nonspecific. Symptoms may range from lethargy and confusion to stupor and coma and there may be a poor correlation between the severity of symptoms and the magnitude of the hypotonicity. Seizures, although less common than in acute hypotonicity, may occur. The mortality rate associated with chronic hypotonicity has been reported to be between 10 and 20%.[18, 19] However, these high mortality rates are probably more indicative of the severity of underlying disease than the result of hypotonicity per se.

Treatment of Hypotonicity

Although severe hypotonicity may have catastrophic consequences, equally catastrophic outcomes may ensue from its treatment. An initial improvement in neurologic symptoms may be followed by the insidious onset of flaccid tetraparesis, pseudobulbar palsy, and alterations in mental status.[41, 48] The pathologic correlate of these findings is demyelination in the central pons (central pontine myelinolysis) and in extrapontine sites where gray matter and white matter are in proximity.[45, 48, 49]

At least three variables have been implicated in the development of this osmotic demyelination syndrome: the duration of the hypotonicity, the rate of correction of the hypotonicity, and the magnitude of correction of the hypotonicity. In acute (<24 hours) hypotonicity, the adaptive mechanisms for extruding solute to maintain brain volume are incomplete. The treatment of acute hypotonicity is therefore associated with less cerebral dehydration than is the correction of chronic hypotonicity. Because cerebral dehydration is postulated to trigger the demyelination (although the mechanism for this has not been elucidated), the osmotic demyelination syndrome rarely follows the correction of acute hypotonicity and is predominantly associated with the treatment of more chronic hypotonicity.[45, 50]

Both the rate and magnitude of the increase in P_{Na} are important in the pathogenesis of the osmotic demyelination syndrome.[41, 45, 51–54] Overly rapid correction of hypotonicity is associated with neurologic deterioration. There is a consensus that the initial therapy of the symptomatic patient should raise the serum sodium level by no more than 1 to 2 mmol/L/h, at least for the first few hours.[55–57] Recommendations regarding the magnitude of the increase in P_{Na} are more divergent, ranging between an increase of no more than 10%[41, 58] and an absolute increase of no more than 25 mmol/L (over 48 hours).[55] Consensus has also yet to be achieved in defining a safe rate of correction of chronic hyponatremia, with recommendations for the increase in P_{Na} ranging between 12 and 20 mmol/L/d.[56, 57]

In summary, the asymptomatic or only minimally symp-

tomatic patient with chronic hypotonicity should be managed conservatively, correcting P_{Na} slowly (≤ 0.5 mmol/L/h). In contrast, symptomatic chronic hypotonicity requires prompt therapy to increase P_{Na} by 1 to 2 mmol/L/h for 2 to 3 hours. As soon as clinical improvement is observed, the rate of correction should be reduced, limiting the total increase in P_{Na} to approximately 10 to 12 mmol/L over the first 24 hours. Similar measures should be instituted in severe acute hyponatremia, even if only minor symptoms (e.g., headache, nausea, and confusion) are present, because more severe symptoms may emerge suddenly. At no point should the initial treatment (within 24 hours) raise P_{Na} beyond about 120 to 125 mmol/L. Normalization of the P_{Ton} can be accomplished gradually thereafter. Throughout the treatment, P_{Na} must be monitored closely to ensure that overcorrection does not occur.

Hypovolemic hypotonicity is best treated with isotonic volume repletion. Correction of volume deficits results in a prompt, and frequently brisk, water diuresis. Occasionally, supplemental electrolyte-free water must be administered to avoid overly rapid correction of the hypotonicity.[58]

In patients with edematous disorders, water restriction is the cornerstone of therapy. The addition of a loop-active diuretic (e.g., furosemide and bumetanide) to increase electrolyte-free water excretion is frequently beneficial, as is the use of an angiotensin-converting enzyme inhibitor in patients with congestive heart failure. Ultimately, however, the correction of hypervolemic hypotonicity depends on treatment of the underlying disease process.

In SIADH also, water restriction is the most important component of therapy. Isotonic saline, although hypertonic relative to the patient's plasma, should be avoided. In euvolemic individuals, the additional sodium is rapidly excreted in the urine, often at extremely high concentrations, causing a net retention of electrolyte-free water and worsening of the hyponatremia. Loop-active diuretics augment renal electrolyte-free water excretion and, when combined with replacement of sodium losses (either orally or with hypertonic saline), are useful in achieving a controlled increase in P_{Na}. Careful monitoring of both P_{Na} and urinary solute losses is mandatory, however.

In patients with SIADH requiring more aggressive therapy, intravenous infusion of 3% saline at 1 to 2 mL/kg/h usually increases P_{Na} by approximately 1 to 2 mmol/L/h.[58] Because hypertonic saline can produce rapid intravascular volume expansion and precipitate acute pulmonary edema, close monitoring is required. Early signs of volume overload should be promptly treated by discontinuing the infusion and administering a loop diuretic.

In addition, in the treatment of SIADH, any potentially offending drugs should be discontinued and specific therapy to correct any underlying disorders instituted. In patients with persistent SIADH, water restriction is usually sufficient. If water restriction is poorly tolerated, treatment with demeclocycline, which blocks AVP-mediated water reabsorption in the collecting duct, may be of benefit.[59]

Hypernatremia

Hypernatremia ($P_{Na} > 145$ mmol/L) is usually attributable to inadequate water intake relative to net electrolyte-free water loss. Less commonly, it may result from the administration of hypertonic sodium-containing solutions or the ingestion of salt. Even relatively mild degrees of hypernatremia normally provoke intense thirst, leading to increased water ingestion that averts progressive hypertonicity.[8, 9] However, in the critically ill patient thirst is frequently impaired by the underlying illness, medications, or impaired mentation. Even when thirst is intact, access to water is usually

TABLE 100–3

HYPERTONIC STATES*

TBES	TBW	TBES/ TBW	ECF Volume	EABV	Pathophysiology	Conditions
↔	↓	↑	↔	↔	Decreased water intake	Primary hypodipsia Essential hypernatremia

↔	↓	↑	↔	↔	Increased water loss
					Inadequate water intake
						Insensible water loss
						    Hyperthermia
						    Hyperventilation
						Renal water loss
						    Hypothalamic DI
						    Nephrogenic DI

↓	↓↓	↑	↓	↓	Hypotonic fluid loss
					Inadequate water intake
						Extrarenal fluid loss
						    Cutaneous losses: burns, sensible
						        perspiration
						    GI losses: diarrhea, vomiting, NG
						        drainage, enterocutaneous fistulas
						        Third-space sequestration: ileus, bowel
						        obstruction, peritonitis, pancreatitis
						Renal fluid loss
						    Diuretics
						    Osmotic diuresis
						    Adrenal insufficiency
						    Postobstructive diuresis
						    Diuretic phase of ATN
						    Chronic renal failure
						    Medullary cystic disease

↑	↔	↑	↑	↑	Pure solute gain	Salt ingestion

↑↑	↑	↑	↑	↑	Hypertonic fluid gain	Hypertonic fluid administration
						    Hypertonic saline
						    Sodium bicarbonate

*TBES = total body (osmotically) effective solute; TBW = total body water; ECF = extracellular fluid; EABV = effective arterial blood volume; ATN = acute tubular necrosis; GI = gastrointestinal; NG = nasogastric; DI = diabetes insipidus; ↔ = no change; ↑ = increase; ↓ = decrease.

limited. Thus, ICU patients are critically dependent on prescribed enteral and parenteral electrolyte-free water to forestall progressive hypernatremia.

As with hypotonicity, hypernatremic disorders can occur in association with normal, increased, or decreased ECF volume (Table 100–3). Thus, the clinical evaluation of hypernatremia should begin with a careful assessment of the patient's volume status.

Euvolemic Hypernatremia

Isolated decreases in TBW are not usually associated with clinical evidence of intravascular or ECF volume depletion. Only one third of a pure water deficit is derived from the ECF and one twelfth from the intravascular compartment. Thus, in a 70-kg individual, a 3% decrease in TBW (which increases P_{Na} by approximately 5 mmol/L) reduces ECF volume by approximately 1 L and blood volume by less than 350 mL. This modest degree of volume depletion is generally not detectable on physical examination but may be manifest through elevations in the blood urea and uric acid concentrations. With extreme degrees of dehydration, however, hemodynamically significant intravascular volume contraction may develop.

Euvolemic hypernatremia may be divided into primary abnormalities of water intake and primary abnormalities of water loss (occurring in association with inadequate water intake). Primary hypodipsia, resulting from malfunction of the hypothalamic osmoreceptors that regulate thirst, is associated with a wide range of intracranial pathology including primary and metastatic tumors of the hypothalamus, granulomatous diseases, vascular abnormalities (most commonly involving the anterior communicating artery), trauma, and hydrocephalus.[11] Hypodipsia has also been described in elderly patients (geriatric hypodipsia) in whom overt hypothalamic pathology is absent.[60] More commonly, hypodipsia in the critically ill patient is attributable to underlying diseases that secondarily decrease thirst or prohibit ad libitum water ingestion.

An important variant of primary hypodipsia is the syndrome of essential hypernatremia, in which there is an upward resetting of the osmotic thresholds for thirst and AVP secretion; the responses to hemodynamic stimuli are normal. Essential hypernatremia therefore represents the hypertonic counterpart of the reset osmostat syndrome.

Excessive electrolyte-free water losses may occur via the insensible route (associated with fever or hyperventilation) or be the result of renal water wasting (DI). When water replacement is insufficient to keep up with ongoing losses, negative water balance and hypernatremia ensue. Hypernatremia caused by increased insensible losses is characterized by oliguria and a high urinary osmolality ($U_{Osm} > 700$ mOsm/kg). In contrast, DI is characterized by polyuria and a less than maximally concentrated urine.

Diabetes Insipidus. DI is produced by deficient AVP secretion (hypothalamic DI) or renal hyporesponsiveness to the hormone (nephrogenic DI). DI is not usually associated with clinically significant hypernatremia because thirst allows water balance to be maintained despite the ongoing polyuria. However, severe hypernatremia may develop if water intake is impaired by intercurrent illness.

Severe or complete forms of DI (either hypothalamic or nephrogenic in origin) classically present with polyuria and a dilute urine ($U_{Osm} < 150$ mOsm/kg). However, in the setting of intravascular volume depletion, U_{Osm} may reach 300 to 400 mOsm/kg as the result of decreased distal tubular flow and AVP-independent water reabsorption. In incomplete or partial forms of DI (either hypothalamic or nephrogenic in origin), polyuria is less pronounced, although water conservation remains submaximal in response to water deprivation or hypertonicity.[61]

The polyuria associated with DI must be differentiated from other polyuric states. The initial step in the evaluation of polyuria is the measurement of total urinary solute content. In the absence of volume contraction, a U_{Osm} greater than 250 mOsm/kg suggests that a solute (e.g., saline, urea, or glucose) diuresis is present and that the diagnosis of DI is unlikely. On the other hand, a dilute urine ($U_{Osm} < 150$ mOsm/kg) indicates a water diuresis, resulting from either primary polydipsia (with secondary polyuria) or DI. Differentiation among hypothalamic DI, nephrogenic DI, and primary polydipsia can be achieved by dehydration testing in combination with measurements of circulating AVP levels.[61, 62]

Hypothalamic DI may result from any process that impairs hypothalamic or neurohypophysial function, including hypophysectomy, head trauma, primary and metastatic tumors, intracranial infections, cerebrovascular diseases, granulomatous diseases, and idiopathic forms[63] (Table 100–4). Nephrogenic DI may result from any process that impairs the responsiveness of the collecting duct to AVP, including a variety of drugs, obstructive uropathy, chronic tubulointerstitial diseases, hypercalcemia, or congenital defects[64] (Table

TABLE 100–4
CAUSES OF HYPOTHALAMIC DIABETES INSIPIDUS

Hypophysectomy
Head trauma
Tumors
  Craniopharyngioma
  Pinealoma
  Cerebral tumors
  Benign cysts
  Leukemia and lymphoma
  Metastatic tumors (especially
    carcinoma of the breast)
Infections
  Encephalitis
  Meningitis
  Tuberculosis
  Syphilis
Cerebrovascular disease
  Cerebrovascular accident
  Aneurysms
  Cavernous sinus thrombosis
  Postpartum pituitary infarction
Granulomatous disease
  Sarcoidosis
  Eosinophilic granuloma
Idiopathic causes
  Sporadic
  Familial

TABLE 100–5
CAUSES OF NEPHROGENIC DIABETES INSIPIDUS

Drugs
  Lithium
  Demeclocycline
  Methoxyflurane
  Amphotericin B
Obstructive uropathy
Chronic tubulointerstitial disease
  Analgesic abuse nephropathy
  Multiple myeloma
  Amyloidosis
  Sarcoidosis
  Sjögren's syndrome
  Sickle cell nephropathy
  Nephrocalcinosis
  Hypokalemic nephropathy
  Polycystic kidney disease
  Medullary cystic disease
Hypercalcemia
Congenital disorders

100–5). Loss of the corticomedullary osmotic gradient because of intrinsic renal disease, protein malnutrition, diuretic therapy, or osmotic diuresis may also limit renal concentrating ability.

Hypothalamic DI is readily treated with hormone replacement. Aqueous AVP may be administered intramuscularly at a dose of 5 to 10 U every 2 to 6 hours. Alternatively, desmopressin (1-desamino-8-D-arginine vasopressin), a synthetic analogue of AVP with a longer half-life and fewer vasoconstrictive effects, can be administered subcutaneously or intravenously at a dose of 1 to 2 µg every 12 to 24 hours or by intranasal insufflation of 5 to 20 µg every 12 hours.[65] In nephrogenic DI, hormone replacement therapy is generally ineffective. Restriction of dietary protein and sodium may attenuate the polyuria by reducing obligate urinary solute excretion. Thiazide diuretics are also of benefit. By inducing mild ECF volume depletion and thereby increasing proximal fluid reabsorption, thiazides decrease distal fluid delivery and enhance AVP-independent water reabsorption in the collecting duct. Amiloride or inhibitors of prostaglandin synthesis have also been efficacious in certain instances.[66, 67]

Hypovolemic Hypernatremia

Patients with excessive hypotonic fluid losses manifest both hypernatremia and ECF volume depletion. In these patients, unlike those with pure water deficits, physical findings of intravascular volume depletion (tachycardia, hypotension, and decreased central venous pressure) are common, as are prerenal azotemia and hyperuricemia.

Hypotonic fluid losses may occur via the skin, gastrointestinal tract, or kidney. Cutaneous fluid losses in patients with extensive burns may be large and contain substantial quantities of electrolytes. Sensible (as opposed to insensible) perspiration also contains significant amounts of electrolyte. Because most gastrointestinal secretions, with the exception of pancreatic and biliary juices, are hypotonic, prolonged nasogastric drainage or diarrhea frequently contributes to the development of hypernatremia in the ICU patient. In patients with ileus, bowel obstruction, peritonitis, or pancreatitis, intravascular volume depletion may occur as the result of sequestration of fluid. These "third-space" losses may contribute to the development of hypovolemic hypernatremia when combined with a water intake that is inadequate to compensate for ongoing electrolyte-free water losses.

Diuretics and osmotic diureses are responsible for most renal hypotonic fluid losses. Hyperglycemia and mannitol administration are common causes of osmotic diuresis in ICU patients. A urea diuresis may follow the relief of urinary tract obstruction and may also contribute to the polyuria of resolving acute renal failure. Parenteral hyperalimentation is also a frequent cause of urea diuresis in the critically ill patient. Hypotonic losses associated with adrenal insufficiency, postobstructive diuresis, polyuric acute renal failure, and some forms of chronic renal insufficiency may also result in hypernatremia.

Urinary indices may be helpful in determining the source of hypotonic fluid losses. Cutaneous, gastrointestinal, and third-space losses are associated with maximal renal sodium and water conservation ($U_{Na} < 10$ mmol/L and $U_{Osm} > 700$ mOsm/kg). In contrast, when the losses are renal in origin, the urinary sodium concentration is elevated ($U_{Na} > 20$ mmol/L) and the osmolality is inappropriately low.

Hypervolemic Hypernatremia

In ICU patients, hypervolemic hypernatremia is primarily an iatrogenic complication, arising from the intravenous administration of hypertonic electrolyte solutions. Most frequently, it occurs after the administration of hypertonic sodium bicarbonate in the treatment of severe metabolic acidosis or during cardiopulmonary resuscitation. Each 50-mL ampule of sodium bicarbonate (containing 44.6 or 50 mmol of sodium) increases P_{Na} in a 70-kg patient by approximately 1 mmol/L. Overcorrection of hypotonicity with 3% saline or inadvertent intravenous administration of hypertonic saline during therapeutic abortions may also produce hypervolemic hypernatremia. Less commonly, hypernatremia may result from accidental ingestion of large quantities of sodium salts.

In the presence of normal renal function and thirst, hypervolemic hypernatremia is transient, being corrected through rapid excretion of solute and ingestion of water. However, persistent hypernatremia results if water intake is restricted or renal function is impaired.

Clinical Manifestations of Hypernatremia

As with hypotonicity, the major clinical manifestations of hypernatremia result from alterations in brain water content.[42, 68] In response to hypertonicity, fluid moves from the ICF into the ECF, maintaining osmotic equilibrium and decreasing cell volume. In the brain, acute hypernatremia is associated with a rapid decrease in water content and an increase in electrolyte concentration. In contrast, in chronic hypernatremia, brain volume is normalized by the accumulation of intracellular solutes, both through the uptake of electrolytes from the ECF and through the generation of organic metabolites including amino acids, polyols, and methylamines.[42, 69, 70] These accumulated intracellular solutes ("idiogenic osmoles") have important therapeutic implications; although they minimize cerebral dehydration during hypertonicity, they increase the risk of cerebral edema during correction of the hypertonic state.

As with hypotonicity, the clinical manifestations of hypernatremia reflect the rapidity of onset, duration, and magnitude of the osmotic stress. In severe acute hypernatremia, brain shrinkage may be substantial, placing traction on intracerebral veins and causing them to rupture.[71] The resulting intracerebral and subarachnoid hemorrhage may produce irreversible neurologic deficits. The manifestations of less profound hypernatremia are nonspecific and include nausea, muscle weakness and fasciculations, and alterations in the sensorium ranging from lethargy to coma. Seizures are uncommon in chronic hypernatremia but may develop after initiation of therapy in as many as 40% of patients.[42] The mortality rate associated with hypernatremia has been reported to range from 40% to more than 70%, depending on its magnitude and rapidity of onset.[72, 73] This mortality, however, probably reflects the severity of predisposing conditions rather than that of the hypernatremia per se.

Treatment of Hypernatremia

Treatment of euvolemic or hypovolemic hypernatremia can be divided into three components: correction of any intravascular volume deficits, repletion of water deficits, and elimination of excessive electrolyte-free water losses. Circulatory compromise must always be treated promptly with isotonic (0.9%) saline or colloid. When adequate volume replacement has been achieved, the electrolyte-free water deficit should be estimated and water replacement initiated. The water deficit may be estimated from body weight and the P_{Na}. Thus

Free water deficit =

$$0.6 \times [\text{body weight (kg)}] \times \left(\frac{[\text{Na}^+]}{140} - 1 \right)$$

Despite the inaccuracies inherent in this formula, the calculation provides a useful first approximation for initiating water replacement therapy.

In acute hypernatremia, the initial phase of water repletion should proceed relatively rapidly: approximately half of the calculated water deficit should be replaced during the first 12 to 24 hours. However, because of the risk of precipitating cerebral edema, P_{Na} should not be lowered more rapidly than 2 mmol/L/h. The remainder of the deficit can then be corrected over the ensuing several days. In chronic hypernatremia, water repletion can be more gradual. In symptomatic patients, P_{Na} should initially be lowered at a rate of no more than 1 to 2 mmol/L/h. When symptoms have resolved, more gradual correction is appropriate.[68] Throughout treatment, neurologic status must be monitored carefully; deterioration after initial improvement in symptoms suggests the development of cerebral edema and mandates temporary discontinuation of water replacement.

No individual fluid regimen is of documented superiority. Water repletion may be accomplished enterally, either orally or by nasogastric tube, or intravenously. Intravenous repletion can be accomplished with hypotonic saline or 5% dextrose in water. Distilled water cannot be administered intravenously because it may cause intravascular hemolysis. When using glucose-containing solutions, the serum glucose concentration should be monitored frequently and, if necessary, insulin therapy initiated to forestall hyperglycemia.

In addition to replacement of the calculated water deficit, ongoing fluid and electrolyte losses must be considered. Urinary, gastrointestinal, and any other losses should be measured and replaced on the basis of their electrolyte content. Insensible losses can be estimated as 0.6 mL/kg/h and increased by 20% for each 1°C elevation in body temperature above normal.

Prompt attention to reducing excessive electrolyte-free water losses is also important. Insensible losses may be reduced by normalizing body temperature with cooling blankets and antipyretics. Hyperglycemia should be controlled and protein loading decreased to limit osmotic diuresis. Nasogastric drainage can be reduced with histamine H_2 receptor blockers (e.g., cimetidine or ranitidine) or proton pump inhibitors (e.g., omeprazole). Diarrhea can be reduced by altering enteral feeding, treating infectious causes, and administering antidiarrheal agents. Specific therapy for DI should be initiated, as appropriate.

Treatment of hypervolemic hypernatremia requires both water repletion and solute removal. Because hypernatremia generally develops rapidly in these patients, the compensatory mechanisms preserving cerebral volume are ineffective and neurologic symptoms may be accentuated. In addition, the concomitant ECF volume expansion may result in pulmonary edema and exacerbate respiratory failure. Treatment must therefore be instituted promptly to forestall neurologic and cardiopulmonary complications. Because water repletion further exacerbates ECF volume overload, a loop diuretic should be simultaneously administered to facilitate solute excretion. In patients with massive volume overload or renal failure, hemodialysis or hemofiltration may be necessary.

Hyperglycemic Hypertonicity

Hyperglycemia is a common cause of hypertonicity. In the critically ill patient with diabetes mellitus, glucose control is frequently poor and hyperglycemia may contribute to morbidity and mortality. Stress, pressor agents, infusions of intravenous glucose, and parenteral hyperalimentation may cause hyperglycemia in patients with no prior history of glucose intolerance.[74]

Hyperglycemia produces hypertonicity both directly, by virtue of the presence of large amounts of glucose in the ECF, and indirectly, through the production of an osmotic diuresis that increases hypotonic fluid losses. The osmotic diuresis results in significant sodium and potassium depletion. However, the effects of these sodium losses on ECF volume are frequently masked by the hyperglycemia, which causes fluid to shift from the ICF to the ECF, thereby maintaining ECF volume despite sodium depletion.

Hyperglycemia may coexist with hyponatremia, hypernatremia, or eunatremia, depending on the magnitude of the osmotic diuresis (which by itself would cause hypernatremia), concomitant water intake (which, if large, would contribute to hyponatremia in a volume-depleted patient and, if small, would exacerbate hypernatremia), and the magnitude of the glucose-related water shift from ICF to ECF (which by itself would cause hyponatremia). The latter relationship is dependent on both the magnitude of the hyperglycemia and the degree of the associated volume depletion.[75] In euvolemic patients, P_{Na} falls by approximately 1.5 mmol/L for each 5 mmol/L increase in the serum glucose concentration. As volume depletion increases, the increment in P_{Na} increases, approaching 2 mmol/L in patients with significant volume depletion. Thus, a "normal" P_{Na} of 140 mmol/L in a severely hyperglycemic patient is indicative of a substantial water deficit.

The therapy of hyperglycemic hypertonicity should begin with the correction of ECF volume deficits using isotonic saline. Volume repletion increases renal glucose clearance and begins to correct the hyperglycemia. Failure to correct volume deficits before initiation of insulin therapy may lead to circulatory collapse as glucose and water move rapidly into cells. Prompt attention must also be given to replacing total body potassium deficits; aggressive insulin therapy before potassium repletion may cause severe hypokalemia. When volume resuscitation has been achieved, treatment with low-dose intravenous insulin should be initiated, with the aim of normalizing the serum glucose concentration over a period of approximately 24 to 48 hours. During this time, hypotonic fluids can be substituted for isotonic saline to correct any coexisting water deficit.

References

1. Teitlebaum I, Berl T, Kleeman CR: The physiology of the renal concentrating and diluting mechanisms. In: Maxwell MH, Kleeman CR, Narins RG (eds): Clinical Disorders of Fluid and Electrolyte Metabolism. 4th ed. New York, McGraw-Hill, p 79, 1987.
2. Inadomi DW, Kopple JD: Fluid and electrolyte disorders in total parenteral nutrition. In: Maxwell MH, Kleeman CR, Narins RG (eds): Clinical Disorders of Fluid and Electrolyte Metabolism. 4th ed. New York, McGraw-Hill, p 945, 1987.
3. Baumber CD, Clark RG: Insensible water loss in surgical patients. Br J Surg 61:53, 1974.
4. Binder HJ, Sandle GI: Electrolyte absorption and secretion in the mammalian colon. In: Johnson LR (ed): Physiology of the Gastrointestinal Tract. 2nd ed. New York, Raven Press, p 1389, 1981.
5. Goldberg M: Hyponatremia. Med Clin North Am 65:251, 1981.
6. Rose BD: New approach to disturbances in the plasma sodium concentration. Am J Med 81:1033, 1986.
7. Zerbe RL, Robertson GL: Osmotic and nonosmotic regulation of thirst and vasopressin secretion. In: Maxwell MH, Kleeman CR, Narins RG (eds): Clinical Disorders of Fluid and Electrolyte Metabolism. 4th ed. New York, McGraw-Hill, p 61, 1987.
8. Zerbe RL, Robertson GL: Osmoregulation of thirst and vasopressin secretion in man: The effects of various solutes. Am J Physiol 244:E607, 1983.
9. Fitzsimons JT: The physiological basis of thirst. Kidney Int 10:3, 1976.
10. Malvin RL, Mouw D, Vander AJ: Angiotensin: Physiologic role in water-deprivation-induced thirst of rats. Science 197:171, 1977.
11. Robertson GL, Aycinena P, Zerbe RL: Neurogenic disorders of osmoregulation. Am J Med 72:339, 1982.
12. Baylis PH: Osmoregulation and control of vasopressin secretion in healthy humans. Am J Physiol 253:R671, 1987.
13. Robertson GL, Shelton RL, Athar S: The osmoregulation of vasopressin. Kidney Int 10:25, 1976.
14. Vokes T, Robertson GL: Effect of insulin on the osmoregulation of thirst and vasopressin. In: Schrier RW (ed): Vasopressin. New York, Raven Press, p 271, 1985.
15. Robertson GL, Althar S: The interaction of blood osmolality and blood volume in regulating plasma vasopressin in man. J Clin Endocrinol Metab 42:613, 1976.
16. Dunn FL, Brennan TJ, Nelson AE, et al: The role of blood osmolality and volume in regulating vasopressin secretion in the rat. J Clin Invest 52:3212, 1973.
17. Weisberg LS: Pseudohyponatremia: A reappraisal. Am J Med 86:315, 1989.
18. Anderson RJ, Chung H-M, Kluge R, et al: Hyponatremia: A prospective analysis of its epidemiology and the pathogenetic role of vasopressin. Ann Intern Med 102:164, 1985.
19. Tierney WM, Martin DK, Greenlee MC, et al: The prognosis of hyponatremia at hospital admission. J Gen Intern Med 1:380, 1986.
20. Anderson RJ: Hospital-associated hyponatremia. Kidney Int 29:1237, 1986.
21. Arieff AI: Hyponatremia, convulsions, respiratory arrest and brain damage after elective surgery in healthy women. N Engl J Med 314:1529, 1986.
22. Bricker NS, Fine LG: The renal response to progressive nephron loss. In: Brenner BM, Rector FC (eds): The Kidney. 2nd ed. Philadelphia, WB Saunders, p 1056, 1981.
23. Jose CJ, Perez-Cruet J: Incidence and morbidity of self-induced water intoxication in state mental hospital patients. Am J Psychiatry 136:221, 1979.
24. Vieweg VWR, David JJ, Rowe WT, et al: Death from self-induced water intoxication among patients with schizophrenic disorders. J Nerv Ment Dis 173:161, 1985.
25. Goldman MB, Luchins DJ, Robertson GL: Mechanisms of altered water metabolism in psychotic patients with polydipsia and hyponatremia. N Engl J Med 318:397, 1988.
26. Rhymer JC, Bell TJ, Perry RC, et al: Hyponatraemia following transurethral resection of the prostate. Br J Urol 57:450, 1985.
27. Agus ZS, Goldberg M: Role of antidiuretic hormone in the abnormal water diuresis of anterior hypopituitarism in man. J Clin Invest 50:1478, 1971.
28. DeRubertis FR, Michelis M, Bloom ME, et al: Impaired water excretion in myxedema. Am J Med 51:41, 1971.
29. Linas SL, Berl T, Robertson GL, et al: Role of plasma arginine vasopressin in the impaired water diuresis of glucocorticoid deficiency. Kidney Int 18:58, 1980.
30. Schwartz MJ, Kokko JP: Urinary concentrating defect of adrenal insufficiency. J Clin Invest 66:234, 1980.
31. Bartter FC, Schwartz WB: The syndrome of inappropriate secretion of antidiuretic hormone. Am J Med 42:790, 1967.
32. Zerbe R, Stropes L, Robertson G: Vasopressin function in the syndrome of inappropriate antidiuresis. Annu Rev Med 31:315, 1980.
33. Chung H-M, Kluge R, Schrier RW, et al: Clinical assessment of extracellular fluid volume in hyponatremia. Am J Med 83:905, 1987.
34. DeFronzo RA, Goldberg M, Agus ZS: Normal diluting capacity in hypo-

natremic patients: Reset osmostat or a variant of the syndrome of inappropriate antidiuretic hormone secretion. Ann Intern Med 84:538, 1976.

35. Ashraf N, Locksley R, Arieff AI: Thiazide-induced hyponatremia associated with death or neurologic damage in outpatients. Am J Med 70:1163, 1981.

36. Kennedy RM, Earley LE: Profound hyponatremia resulting from thiazide induced decrease in urinary diluting capacity in a patient with primary polydipsia. N Engl J Med 282:1185, 1970.

37. Horowitz J, Keynan A, Ben-Ishay D: A syndrome of inappropriate ADH secretion induced by cyclothiazide. J Clin Pharmacol 12:337, 1972.

38. Fichman MP, Vorherr H, Kleman CR: Diuretic-induced hyponatremia. Ann Intern Med 75:853, 1971.

39. Laragh JH: Effect of potassium chloride on hyponatremia. J Clin Invest 33:807, 1954.

40. Berl T, Linas SL, Aisenbrey GA, et al: On the mechanism of polyuria in potassium depletion. The role of polydipsia. J Clin Invest 60:620, 1977.

41. Berl T: Treating hyponatremia: Damned if we do and damned if we don't. Kidney Int 37:1006, 1990.

42. Arieff AI, Guisado R: Effects on the central nervous system of hypernatremic and hyponatremic states. Kidney Int 10:104, 1976.

43. Thurston JH, Hauhart RE, Nelson JS: Adaptive decreases in amino acids (taurine in particular), creatine, and electrolytes prevent cerebral edema in chronically hyponatremic mice: Rapid correction causes dehydration and shrinkage of brain. Metab Brain Dis 2:223, 1987.

44. Verbalis JG, Drutarosky MD: Adaptation to chronic hypoosmolality in rats. Kidney Int 34:351, 1988.

45. Sterns RH: Severe symptomatic hyponatremia: Treatment and outcomes. A study of 64 cases. Ann Intern Med 107:656, 1987.

46. Arieff AI: Central nervous system manifestation of disordered sodium metabolism. Clin Endocrinol Metab 13:269, 1984.

47. Ayus JC, Krothapalli RK, Arieff AI: Changing concepts in treatment of severe symptomatic hyponatremia. Am J Med 78:897, 1985.

48. Sterns RH, Riggs JE, Schochet SS: Osmotic demyelination syndrome following correction of hyponatremia. N Engl J Med 314:1535, 1986.

49. Sterns RH, Thomas DJ, Herndon RM: Brain dehydration and neurologic deterioration after rapid correction of hyponatremia. Kidney Int 35:69, 1989.

50. Norenberg MD, Papendick RE: Chronicity of hyponatremia as a factor in experimental myelinolysis. Ann Neurol 15:544, 1984.

51. Ayus JC, Krothapalli RK, Arieff AI: Treatment of symptomatic hyponatremia and its relation to brain damage. N Engl J Med 317:1190, 1987.

52. Ayus JC, Krothapalli RJ, Armstrong DK: Rapid correction of severe hyponatremia in the rat: Histopathologic changes in the brain. Am J Physiol 248:F711, 1985.

53. Ayus JC, Krothapalli RJ, Armstrong DK, et al: Symptomatic hyponatremia in rats: Effect of treatment on mortality and brain lesions. Am J Physiol 257:F18, 1989.

54. Verbalis JG, Martinez AJ: Osmotic demyelination is dependent on both rate and magnitude of correction of chronic hyponatremia in rats (abstract). Clin Res 37:586A, 1989.

55. Ayus JC, Arieff AI: Symptomatic hyponatremia: Correcting sodium deficits safely. J Crit Illness 5:905, 1990.

56. Sterns RH: The treatment of hyponatremia: First do no harm. Am J Med 88:557, 1990.

57. Berl T: Treating hyponatremia: What is all the controversy about? Ann Intern Med 113:417, 1990.

58. Sterns RH: The management of symptomatic hyponatremia. Semin Nephrol 10:503, 1990.

59. Forrest JN, Cox M, Hong C, et al: Superiority of demeclocycline over lithium in the treatment of chronic syndrome of inappropriate antidiuretic hormone. N Engl J Med 298:173, 1978.

60. Miller PD, Krebs RA, Neal BJ, et al: Hypodipsia in geriatric patients. Am J Med 73:354, 1982.

61. Miller M, Dalakos T, Moses AM, et al: Recognition of partial defects in antidiuretic hormone secretion. Ann Intern Med 73:721, 1970.

62. Zerbe RL, Robertson GL: A comparison of plasma vasopressin measurements with a standard indirect test in the differential diagnosis of polyuria. N Engl J Med 305:1539, 1981.

63. Robinson AG: Disorders of antidiuretic hormone secretion. Clin Endocrinol Metab 14:55, 1985.

64. Singer I: Differential diagnosis of polyuria and diabetes insipidus. Med Clin North Am 65:303, 1981.

65. Richardson DW, Robinson AG: Desmopressin. Ann Intern Med 103:228, 1985.

66. Allen HM, Jackson RL, Winchester MD, et al: Indomethacin in the treatment of lithium-induced nephrogenic diabetes insipidus. Arch Intern Med 149:1123, 1989.

67. Batlle DC, Von Riotte AB, Gaviria M, et al: Amelioration of polyuria in patients receiving long-term lithium therapy. N Engl J Med 312:408, 1985.

68. Brennan S, Ayus JC: Acute versus chronic hypernatremia: How fast to correct ECF volume? J Crit Illness 5:330, 1990.

69. Feig PU, McCurdy DK: The hypertonic state. N Engl J Med 297:1444, 1977.

70. Helig CW, Steomski ME, Blumenfeld JD, et al: Characterization of the major brain osmolytes that accumulate in salt loaded rats. Am J Physiol 257:F1108, 1989.

71. Finberg L, Luttrell C, Redd H: Pathogenesis of lesions in the nervous system in hypernatremic states: Experimental studies of gross anatomic changes and alterations of chemical composition of tissues. Pediatrics 23:46, 1959.

72. Snyder NA, Feigel DW, Arieff AI: Hypernatremia in elderly patients. A heterogeneous, morbid, and iatrogenic entity. Ann Intern Med 107:309, 1987.

73. Mahowald J, Himmelstein D: Hypernatremia in the elderly: Relation to infection and mortality. J Am Geriatr Soc 29:177, 1981.

74. Chung H-M, Kluge R, Schrier RW, et al: Postoperative hyponatremia. Arch Intern Med 146:333, 1986.

75. Moran SM, Jamison RL: The variable hyponatremic response to hyperglycemia. West J Med 142:49, 1985.

CHAPTER 101

Potassium Homeostasis

Lawrence S. Weisberg

The total body potassium (K^+) content of a 70-kg adult is about 3400 mmol, of which only 2% (about 70 mmol) is extracellular.[1] This uneven distribution reflects the large K^+ concentration gradient between the intracellular ($K_i = 150$ mmol/L) and the extracellular ($K_e = 4.5$ mmol/L) fluid compartments. The K_i/K_e ratio is the major determinant of the resting membrane potential, the maintenance of which is crucial for proper functioning of excitable tissues (muscle and nerve).[2] Because even relatively small changes in K_e perturb this ratio, disturbances of K_e (usually measured as changes in the serum K^+ concentration [S_K]) may have serious, even lethal, consequences.

MECHANISMS OF POTASSIUM HOMEOSTASIS

Given the importance of K_i/K_e, it is not surprising that it is tightly regulated. Two separate but cooperative systems participate in K^+ homeostasis. One regulates internal K^+ balance—the distribution of K^+ across cell membranes. The second regulates external K^+ balance—the parity of K^+ excretion with K^+ intake.

Regulation of Internal Potassium Balance

Internal K^+ balance serves to buffer changes in K_e: K^+ moves out of cells during K^+ depletion and into cells after K^+ intake, thereby mitigating drastic alterations of K_i/K_e.[3-5] Factors influencing K^+ distribution include hormones, acid-base balance, body fluid tonicity, exercise, and cell integrity (Table 101–1).

Hormones

The most important hormone modulating internal K^+ balance is insulin, which increases K^+ uptake by muscle, liver, and adipose tissues.[3-5] Raising S_K by 1 to 1.5 mmol/L stimulates pancreatic insulin secretion, implicating insulin in the physiologic modulation of internal K^+ balance. However, whether smaller increments (within the range of normal daily variation) affect insulin secretion remains a matter of

TABLE 101–1

FACTORS AFFECTING INTERNAL POTASSIUM BALANCE

| Factor | Direction of Net Potassium Movement | |
	Into Cells	Out of Cells
Hormones	Insulin Beta$_2$-adrenergic agonists Aldosterone	Alpha-adrenergic agonists
Acid-base balance	Metabolic alkalosis Respiratory alkalosis	Hyperchloremic metabolic acidosis Respiratory acidosis
Body fluid tonicity		Hypertonicity

Miscellaneous		Exercise
		Cell lysis
		   Acute tumor lysis
		   Rhabdomyolysis
		   Hemolysis

debate.[3, 5, 6] Catecholamines also affect internal K$^+$ balance. Epinephrine causes a transient increase in S$_K$ (mediated by activation of alpha-adrenergic receptors) followed by a sustained decrease (mediated by activation of beta$_2$-adrenergic receptors).[6–9] Beta-adrenergic blockers such as propranolol impair potassium tolerance. Beta$_2$-adrenergic agonists enhance cellular K$^+$ uptake, whereas alpha-adrenergic agonists increase K$^+$ efflux. Mineralocorticoids have also been shown to enhance cellular K$^+$ uptake.[10, 11] This shift of K$^+$ into cells may partially offset aldosterone's well-known kaliuretic effects, thereby mitigating body K$^+$ depletion. Glucagon,[3, 4] glucocorticoids, thyroid hormone,[3, 12, 13] and growth hormone[14] may modulate internal K$^+$ balance as well, but their physiologic roles are unknown.

Acid-Base Balance

Our understanding of the effects of acid-base balance on K$^+$ distribution has undergone considerable revision in recent years.[15–17] It is now clear that the direction and magnitude of an acid-base–related change in S$_K$ depend on the specific nature and the duration of the disturbance (Table 101–2). Moreover, a variety of coincidental factors such as renal function, plasma osmolality, circulating hormone levels, and cell integrity may influence the response.

The most consistent and pronounced relationship between changes in pH and S$_K$ occurs in acute mineral acidosis where there is a strong inverse relationship between these two variables: increases by about 0.8 mmol/L for each decline of 0.1 pH units.[15–17] In contrast, in chronic mineral acidosis (of several days' duration), S$_K$ is usually decreased because of associated renal K$^+$ losses. Thus, when hyperkalemia accom-

TABLE 101–2

EFFECTS OF ACID-BASE DISORDERS ON SERUM POTASSIUM CONCENTRATION

Disorder	Change in Serum Potassium Level
Metabolic acidosis	
Hyperchloremic	
Acute	↑ ↑ ↑
Chronic	↑ or ↓
Organic	No change
Metabolic alkalosis	
Acute	↓
Chronic	↓ ↓ ↓
Respiratory alkalosis	↓ ↓
Respiratory acidosis	↑

panies chronic hyperchloremic metabolic acidosis, a defect in renal K$^+$ excretion should always be sought.[15] Unlike acute mineral acidoses, even severe organic (high-anion-gap) acidoses are not usually associated with hyperkalemia,[15–20] and it is now generally accepted that organic acidoses do not directly affect internal K$^+$ balance. However, factors coincident with the acidosis may alter S$_K$. For example, ischemia may result in lactic acidosis and hyperkalemia (because of leaking of K$^+$ from cells). Even the hyperkalemia so commonly seen in patients with diabetic ketoacidosis does not result from the acidemia; rather, it appears to be a consequence of insulin deficiency and hyperglycemia.[20]

Acute metabolic alkalosis (e.g., from sodium bicarbonate administration) results in a consistent but modest decrease in S$_K$,[16, 21] which is greater than can be explained by urinary losses alone and must therefore reflect K$^+$ redistribution. Chronic metabolic alkalosis, however, is associated with large cumulative urinary losses and often results in profound hypokalemia and K$^+$ depletion.[22] Acute respiratory alkalosis is associated with a somewhat greater decrease in S$_K$ but, unlike the case with metabolic alkalosis, the kidney-associated kaliuresis rapidly attenuates and chronic respiratory alkalosis is not associated with hypokalemia.[25] Respiratory acidosis is associated with a predictable but small rise in S$_K$.[16]

Body Fluid Tonicity

K$^+$ shifts out of cells during the infusion of any hypertonic solution, and K$^+$ efflux accompanies endogenously generated hypertonic states as well.[24–26] Hypertonicity-related hyperkalemia assumes particular importance in patients with other defects in K$^+$ homeostasis, such as diabetes mellitus, hypoaldosteronism, and renal insufficiency. Hypotonicity does not affect K$^+$ distribution.

Exercise

Exercise causes a transient shift of K$^+$ out of cells. Clinically significant hyperkalemia may be caused by exercise[27] (and clinically misleading local venous hyperkalemia results from repeated fist clenching during phlebotomy[28]). Physical training attenuates exercise-induced hyperkalemia.[3, 12]

Cell Integrity

Because K$^+$ is present in high concentration inside cells, lysis of cells may results in significant hyperkalemia.

Regulation of External Potassium Balance

The constancy of total body K$^+$ content depends on the balance between K$^+$ intake and K$^+$ excretion (external K$^+$ balance). Although moment-to-moment correlations between S$_K$ and total body K$^+$ are imperfect because of transitory changes in internal K$^+$ balance, sustained perturbations in S$_K$ generally imply disorders of external K$^+$ balance.

Potassium Intake

A typical American diet has a daily K$^+$ content of 50 to 150 mmol. Because the kidney has a prodigious capacity to increase K$^+$ excretion to match intake, normal individuals can gradually increase K$^+$ intake to as much as 600 to 1000 mmol/d without significantly perturbing S$_K$.[29, 30] In contrast, the renal capacity to conserve K$^+$ during K$^+$ deprivation is imperfect, and thus hypokalemia and K$^+$ depletion can result from dietary K$^+$ deficiency alone.[31, 32]

Gastrointestinal Potassium Excretion

Normally, only about 10 to 20 mmol of dietary K^+ is excreted in the stool. Gastrointestinal K^+ losses are increased, but only modestly, by high circulating aldosterone levels and during periods of high K^+ ingestion. Gastrointestinal K^+ losses also account for a significant proportion of total body K^+ elimination in advanced renal insufficiency, when the stool may contain up to 80% of the daily K^+ intake,[14] and in patients with diarrhea. Under most circumstances, however, the kidney is responsible for matching K^+ output to K^+ intake to maintain total body K^+ at a constant level.[6]

Renal Potassium Excretion

K^+ is freely filtered by the glomerulus, and nearly all the filtered K^+ is reabsorbed before the fluid reaches the distal portions of the nephron. The majority of excreted K^+ derives from K^+ secretion in the connecting tubule and cortical collecting duct.[33] Virtually all physiologic regulation of K^+ excretion takes place at these distal sites. Other than K^+ balance itself, two principal factors (distal tubular flow and composition and aldosterone) regulate renal K^+ secretion. In addition, magnesium (Mg^{2+}) is essential for normal renal K^+ conservation.

Hyperkalemia and even increases in dietary K^+ intake without detectable changes in S_K augment renal K^+ secretion.[10] Similarly, hypokalemia and K^+ depletion limit K^+ secretion. These effects are at least partially independent of the associated changes in circulating aldosterone levels.

Distal Tubular Flow and Composition. K^+ secretion is directly proportional to distal tubular flow. Thus, during diuresis, K^+ secretion is enhanced, and during antidiuresis, it is decreased. K^+ secretion is largely independent of sodium (Na^+) delivery to the distal nephron and the distal tubular Na^+ concentration rarely becomes limiting for K^+ secretion. Bicarbonate (HCO_3^-) delivery to the distal nephron stimulates kaliuresis by increasing the electrochemical driving force for K^+ secretion.[33] Other anions, which, like HCO_3^-, are poorly reabsorbed in the distal nephron, have similar effects.

Aldosterone. It is well established that K^+ and aldosterone participate in a homeostatic feedback loop such that hyperkalemia stimulates adrenal aldosterone secretion, which in turn reduces S_K by enhancing renal K^+ excretion. Hypokalemia has the opposite effect. Aldosterone is a potent stimulus to cortical collecting tubule K^+ excretion, especially when distal fluid delivery is maintained. Thus, hypokalemia is a prominent feature of primary aldosteronism (Conn's syndrome) because mineralocorticoid "escape" increases distal delivery.[34] In contrast, when circulating aldosterone levels are high owing to volume depletion or one of the pathologic edema-forming states (secondary aldosteronism), the expected increase in K^+ secretion is mitigated by a decrease in flow. Indeed, it is only when patients with secondary hyperaldosteronism attributable to congestive heart failure or hepatic cirrhosis are treated with diuretics (and distal flow is increased) that hypokalemia commonly ensues.

The effect of dexamethasone (a pure glucocorticoid) on enhancing renal K^+ excretion appears to result entirely from hemodynamic changes (increased glomerular filtration rate and distal flow).[35] Other glucocorticoids may further stimulate K^+ secretion in proportion to their intrinsic mineralocorticoid activity.

Magnesium. Normal Mg^{2+} stores are necessary to maintain the physiologic transmembrane K^+ gradient. Mg^{2+} deficiency is associated with renal K^+ wasting and may result in severe K^+ depletion.[36, 37] Because Mg^{2+}, like calcium (Ca^{2+}), acts to stabilize excitable membranes, the deleterious

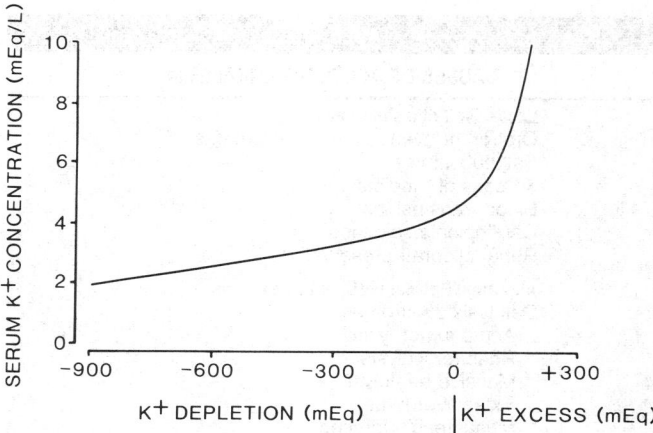

Figure 101–1. Relationship between total body K^+ and the S_K. Note that hypokalemia is not evident until total body K^+ is decreased by approximately 200 mEq. This graph also emphasizes that S_K rises steeply with increases in total body K^+ above normal. (From Weisberg LS, Szerlip HM, Cox M: Disorders of potassium homeostasis in critically ill patients. Crit Care Clin 3:835, 1987.)

myocardial effects of hypokalemia are magnified by concurrent hypomagnesemia.[38]

Acid-Base Balance. Acid-base balance also modulates renal K^+ handling.[23, 33] Whether metabolic or respiratory in origin, acute alkalosis stimulates, and acute acidosis inhibits, renal K^+ secretion. The kaliuresis persists, indeed is enhanced, during the transition from acute to more chronic metabolic alkalosis, and hypokalemia and K^+ depletion are common. In contrast, the kaliuresis of acute respiratory alkalosis attenuates as the disorder becomes more chronic, and significant alterations in total body K^+ are unusual in chronic respiratory alkalosis. During the transition from acute to chronic metabolic acidosis, the initial antikaliuresis is reversed and a prominent kaliuresis may supervene; thus, chronic metabolic acidoses (e.g., classic renal tubular acidosis) are typically associated with hypokalemia and K^+ depletion. Chronic respiratory acidosis has little, if any, effect on body K^+ stores.

In summary, S_K is tightly regulated by two independent but cooperative systems. Internal K^+ balance defends against acute changes in S_K, with cells (mainly muscle and liver) serving as a reservoir for disposal or donation of K^+. External K^+ balance maintains total body K^+ content over the long term. Unfortunately, although the relationship between steady-state S_K and total body K^+ is broadly predictable (Fig. 101–1), minute-to-minute changes in internal K^+ balance make accurate prediction of total body K^+ from a single S_K measurement virtually impossible.

DISORDERS OF POTASSIUM HOMEOSTASIS

Disorders of K^+ homeostasis may be conveniently divided according to the duration of the disturbance: acute if they have been present for less than 48 hours, and chronic if they have been present for days to weeks. Such a distinction is particularly applicable to the intensive care setting where blood chemistry values are sampled frequently and a patient's condition and therapy may change drastically in a short time. Treatment is generally determined by the acuity of the disturbance: the treatment of acute disturbances is largely independent of their cause, whereas the rational treatment of chronic disturbances depends on their pathogenesis. Acute disturbances most often arise from disorders of internal K^+ balance, but chronic disturbances generally imply abnormal external K^+ balance.

TABLE 101–3

CAUSES OF ACUTE HYPERKALEMIA

Excessive Potassium Intake
Oral or intravenous K^+ supplements
Salt substitutes
K^+ salts of medications
Blood transfusions
Cardioplegic solutions
Renal allograft preservatives

Abnormal Potassium Distribution
Cell lysis syndromes
   Acute tumor lysis
   Rhabdomyolysis
   Massive hemolysis
   Extensive burns
   Mesenteric infarction
Pharmacologic agents
   Digitalis intoxication
   Succinylcholine
   Arginine hydrochloride
Hypertonicity
   Glucose
   Sodium chloride
   Mannitol
Acid-base disorders
   Acute hyperchloremic metabolic acidosis
Hyperkalemic periodic paralysis

Acute Oliguric Renal Failure

Acute Hyperkalemia (Table 101–3)

Excessive Potassium Intake

The capacity to tolerate gradual increases in K^+ intake is prodigious. In contrast, the defense against abrupt increases in K^+ intake, although formidable, is limited. Normally, about 50% of an acute K^+ load is excreted in the urine during 4 to 6 hours, and about 90% of the remainder is translocated into cells.[39] These adaptive mechanisms are overwhelmed if large amounts of K^+ are taken in too quickly.[40] Such hyperkalemia is almost always iatrogenic (i.e., caused by overly aggressive K^+ replacement therapy) or the result of a suicide attempt.[41–43] Incomplete mixing of potassium chloride added to intravenous solutions has also caused lethal hyperkalemia.[44] The ability to tolerate K^+ loads declines with disordered internal K^+ balance and impaired renal K^+ excretory capacity.[43] In such circumstances, an otherwise tolerable increase in K^+ intake can cause clinically significant hyperkalemia. Even oral K^+ supplements as small as 30 to 45 mmol daily have resulted in severe hyperkalemia in patients with impaired K^+ homeostasis.[45]

Supplemental K^+ is commonly implicated in acute hyperkalemia.[41–43] Because patients with coronary artery disease may be particularly susceptible to the adverse cardiac electrophysiologic effects of hyperkalemia,[46, 47] K^+ supplements, whether oral or parenteral, should be administered with special care to patients with heart disease. So-called salt substitutes, which contain 40 to 70 mmol of K^+ per teaspoon, may also constitute a significant K^+ load, particularly in patients with impaired K^+ tolerance.[48] Drugs formulated as the K^+ salt (e.g., penicillin), when used in high dosage, also provide relatively large amounts of K^+.[49] Other unusual sources of exogenous K^+ include banked blood,[50, 51] cardioplegic solutions (containing KCl at 20 to 40 mmol/L) used in open heart surgery,[52, 53] and electrolyte solutions used to preserve cadaveric renal allografts (containing concentrations of K^+ approaching intracellular levels).[54]

Abnormal Potassium Distribution

Redistribution of intracellular K^+ to the extracellular space is a common cause of acute hyperkalemia. If only 2% of intracellular K^+ leaks unopposed from cells (and assuming none was excreted in the urine), S_K doubles. Apart from cell lysis syndromes, such dramatic events are rarely encountered. However, impaired internal K^+ balance frequently contributes to the development of hyperkalemia in the face of what for a normal individual would be considered a modest K^+ intake, especially if renal excretory capacity is also compromised.

Cell Lysis Syndromes. The tumor lysis syndrome results from treatment of chemosensitive bulky tumors (usually Burkitt's lymphoma or lymphoblastic lymphoma), with release of intracellular contents, including K^+, into the extracellular fluid.[55] Extreme hyperkalemia,[56, 57] even causing sudden death,[58] has featured prominently in some series. Most of the mortalities were in patients with acute uric acid nephropathy, which impaired their ability to excrete the endogenous K^+ load.[58]

Rhabdomyolysis is associated with a sudden influx of K^+ into the extracellular space.[59] Hyperkalemia is evident in about 40% of patients on presentation and is more common in those whose course is complicated by oliguric acute renal failure.[60–63] A variety of drugs have been associated with rhabdomyolysis.[62] An association with particular relevance to the intensive care setting is cocaine use.[64–67] One third to one half of patients admitted to the hospital with cocaine-associated rhabdomyolysis have acute renal failure, and severe hyperkalemia has been reported in this setting.[64, 65, 67] Lovastatin has also been implicated in rhabdomyolysis-associated severe hyperkalemia in a patient with diabetes mellitus taking an angiotensin-converting enzyme (ACE) inhibitor.[68]

Redistributive hyperkalemia has also been reported in patients with extensive burns, massive hemolytic transfusion reactions,[69] and mesenteric infarction.

Pharmacologic Agents. Massive digitalis overdose has been associated with extreme hyperkalemia,[70] presumably attributable to inhibition of Na^+,K^+-ATPase with unopposed K^+ leak from cells. Succinylcholine depolarizes the motor end plate and, in normal individuals, causes only a trivial K^+ leak from muscle. However, in patients with neuromuscular disorders, the entire muscle may depolarize, causing lethal hyperkalemia. Preoperative hyperreflexia may predict such a response.[71] Arginine hydrochloride, used in the treatment of metabolic alkalosis or for the evaluation of pituitary function, has been reported to cause life-threatening hyperkalemia in patients with renal insufficiency.[72, 73] The hyperkalemia is independent of changes in plasma pH and is thought to relate to displacement of intracellular K^+ by the arginine cation.

Other drugs may cause acute hyperkalemia by causing cell lysis (see earlier) or by interfering with the action of hormones that regulate K^+ homeostasis (see later). Drugs with the latter action do not of themselves cause clinically significant hyperkalemia; rather, they create an environment of impaired K^+ tolerance. For example, a patient receiving supplemental K^+ may develop hyperkalemia only after being started on a regimen of an ACE inhibitor or a beta-adrenergic blocker.

Hypertonicity. The clinical significance of the phenomenon of hypertonicity-related K^+ redistribution is emphasized by the observation that either endogenous hyperglycemia or hypertonic glucose infusions in patients with diabetes mellitus and selective hypoaldosteronism can produce severe, life-threatening hyperkalemia.[24] Hyperglycemia-associated hyperkalemia can be ameliorated by insulin or mineralocorticoid replacement. Glucose-induced hyperkalemia also occurs in diabetic patients with normal circulating aldosterone levels[74] and in insulin-dependent diabetics receiving K^+-sparing diuretics.[75, 76] Hypertonic saline infusions have been associated with hyperkalemia in patients with chronic renal failure.[25] Mannitol-induced hyperkalemia has been described in normal subjects[77] and in patients who, in preparation for neurosurgery, were given hypertonic mannitol to reduce intracranial pressure.[78]

Acid-Base Disorders. The only acid-base disturbance that causes acute hyperkalemia is a mineral or hyperchloremic metabolic acidosis of recent onset, something rarely encountered in clinical practice. Thus, acute hyperkalemia is almost never solely attributable to an acid-base disorder. Although organic acidoses have little or no effect on internal K^+ balance,[16] hyperkalemia and acute organic acidosis may be associated to the extent that they derive from a common cause (e.g., hyperkalemia and lactic acidosis attributable to mesenteric infarction).

Hyperkalemic Periodic Paralysis. Hyperkalemic periodic paralysis is a rare syndrome of episodic hyperkalemia and paralysis and is usually inherited in an autosomal dominant pattern.[79, 80] Attacks may be precipitated by exercise, fasting, exposure to cold, and K^+ administration and prevented by frequent carbohydrate snacks.

Pseudohyperkalemia. Pseudohyperkalemia is discussed later.

Renal Failure

Acute renal failure is often accompanied by acute hyperkalemia.[81] Acute renal failure is a catabolic state associated with release of K^+ from cells; this endogenous K^+ load predisposes to hyperkalemia. Acute tubular necrosis and acute interstitial nephritis may damage the distal nephron, the primary site of K^+ secretion; any limitation in intrinsic K^+ secretory capacity reduces K^+ tolerance. The reduction in glomerular filtration rate of itself may be severe enough to produce oliguria and thereby impair K^+ excretion. Hyperkalemia is more frequent and more severe and develops more rapidly in cases of acute renal failure in which these factors are exaggerated or combined (e.g., severely oliguric or anuric renal failure, or rhabdomyolysis-associated acute tubular necrosis).

Acute Hypokalemia (Table 101–4)

Hypokalemia that develops abruptly in only a few hours is virtually always the result of redistribution of K^+ from the extracellular to the intracellular fluid.

Diabetic Ketoacidosis. A dramatic and life-threatening setting for redistribution hypokalemia is diabetic ketoacidosis (DKA). Although stable patients with insulin-dependent diabetes mellitus usually have normal total body K^+ content,[82] patients with DKA are invariably K^+ depleted because of the glucose-driven osmotic diuresis, poor nutrition, and vomiting.[83] Nonetheless, most patients are normokalemic (or hyperkalemic) on presentation: in one large series, only 4% of patients with DKA had S_K less than 3.5 mmol/L.[84] Insulin deficiency and hyperglycemia account for the preservation of a normal S_K despite severe total body K^+ depletion.[83]

After therapy is instituted, however, S_K typically plummets as K^+ is rapidly translocated into cells. K^+ requirements of up to 120 mmol/h have been reported,[85] with total K^+ supplementation reaching 600 to 800 mmol within the first 24 hours of treatment.[86–88] Both insulin and HCO_3^- have important roles in this transmembrane K^+ shift, K^+ requirements being about one third higher in patients who also receive HCO_3^- replacement than in those receiving insulin alone.[86] Severe hypokalemia during therapy may lead to respiratory arrest[89] and death. In fact, hypokalemia may be the most common single cause of death resulting from DKA uncomplicated by other major illness.[90] Clearly, both K^+ repletion and the judicious (sufficient but not excessive) use of insulin and HCO_3^- are the keystones of therapy.

Refeeding Syndrome. A situation analogous to that encountered during the treatment of DKA arises during aggressive refeeding after prolonged starvation (e.g., anorexia nervosa) or with aggressive hyperalimentation of chronically ill patients. Glucose-stimulated hyperinsulinemia shifts K^+ into cells, rapidly depleting extracellular K^+.[91] Rapid cellular uptake of other ions (e.g., phosphorus ion and Mg^{2+}) occurs as well and may contribute to the high incidence of cardiac electrophysiologic disturbances.[92]

Rapid Blood Cell Production. Treatment of megaloblastic anemias with vitamin B_{12} or folate may result in hypokalemia owing to incorporation of extracellular K^+ into the rapidly expanding red blood cell mass. Similarly, granulocyte-macrophage colony-stimulating factor has been associated with severe redistributive hypokalemia.[93]

Pharmacologic Agents. Insulin and sodium bicarbonate were discussed earlier. Beta-adrenergic agonists may also cause redistribution hypokalemia. For example, the specific $beta_2$-agonist albuterol has been described to cause electrophysiologically significant hypokalemia, especially in patients who are already K^+ depleted.[94] Beta-adrenergic agonist–related K^+ redistribution has been exploited in the treatment of episodes of acute hyperkalemia in patients undergoing maintenance dialysis[95] and may have been responsible for sudden death among patients with chronic lung disease taking beta-agonists by nebulizer.[96]

Postresuscitation Hypokalemia. For the reasons discussed earlier, pharmacologic doses of epinephrine are expected to cause hypokalemia. Postresuscitation hypokalemia may be but one example of this phenomenon. Much lower doses of epinephrine may also be associated with hypokalemia, however. For example, epinephrine, given intravenously in doses about 5% of those recommended for cardiac resuscitation, causes a fall in S_K of about 1 mmol/L.[97] Such doses achieve serum levels of epinephrine comparable with those seen after acute myocardial infarction, and endogenous epinephrine release may explain the transient hypokalemia that has been observed after myocardial infarction or resuscitation from cardiac arrest when exogenous epinephrine has not been employed.[98]

Barium Poisoning. A rare cause of severe redistribution hypokalemia is poisoning with soluble barium salts, which are used in pesticides and depilatories. Barium blocks the channels through which K^+ passively leaves cells, thereby permitting unopposed cellular K^+ uptake by way of Na^+,K^+-ATPase. Manifestations of barium poisoning include pro-

---

TABLE 101–4

CAUSES OF ACUTE HYPOKALEMIA

Treatment of diabetic ketoacidosis
Refeeding syndrome
Rapid blood cell production
   Treatment of megaloblastic anemias
   Granulocyte-macrophage colony-stimulating factor treatment
Pharmacologic agents
   Insulin
   Sodium bicarbonate
   Beta-adrenergic agonists
After resuscitation
After myocardial infarction
Barium poisoning
Hypokalemic periodic paralysis

TABLE 101–5

CAUSES OF CHRONIC HYPERKALEMIA

End-Stage Renal Disease

Mineralocorticoid Deficiency
Addison's disease
Selective hypoaldosteronism
  Hyporeninemic hypoaldosteronism
    Idiopathic
      Diabetes mellitus
      Acquired immunodeficiency syndrome
      Systemic lupus erythematosus
      Obstructive uropathy
      Chronic lead nephropathy
    Pharmacologic agents
      Beta-adrenergic blockers
      Nonsteroidal anti-inflammatory drugs
  Hyperreninemic hypoaldosteronism
    Idiopathic
    Pharmacologic agents
      ACE inhibitors
      Heparin
    Pseudohypoaldosteronism

Intrinsic Potassium Secretory Deficit
Sickle cell disease
Systemic lupus erythematosus
Renal transplantation
  Obstructive uropathy
  Pharmacologic agents: amiloride, triamterene,
    spironolactone

found hypokalemia, hypertension, abdominal pain, vomiting, diarrhea, paralysis, ventilatory failure, and sometimes lethal ventricular arrhythmias.[99–101]

Hypokalemic Periodic Paralysis. Three forms of the rare syndrome hypokalemic periodic paralysis have been described: familial, sporadic, and thyrotoxic.[80] All have in common transient episodes of muscle weakness accompanied by acute hypokalemia caused by cellular K+ uptake. Death resulting from ventilatory failure or cardiac dysrhythmias may occur.

The familial variety is inherited in an autosomal dominant pattern, and symptoms typically begin in the second decade of life. Attacks may be precipitated by carbohydrate or salt ingestion or exercise. Each episode lasts from 1 to 24 hours and persistent weakness between episodes is characteristic. Administration of K+ aborts an acute attack but is ineffective in prevention. Acetazolamide, on the other hand, is remarkably effective in decreasing the frequency of attacks.[102] The sporadic variety is identical with the familial form, except for the absence of a hereditary pattern.

Thyrotoxic periodic paralysis occurs mainly in Asians (usually Japanese). The usual onset of symptoms is in the third decade of life. Severe hypophosphatemia may accompany the hypokalemia.[103] Management consists of treating the hyperthyroidism. Acetazolamide usually worsens the manifestations of thyrotoxic periodic paralysis.[104]

Chronic Hyperkalemia (Table 101–5)
Renal Failure

Although oliguric acute renal failure is commonly associated with hyperkalemia, patients with chronic renal failure usually maintain normal K+ homeostasis until renal function declines to about 10% of normal.[105, 106] Adaptations in both external and internal K+ balance occur.[107, 108] Renal tubular adaptation (increased Na+,K+-ATPase activity) increases the single-nephron K+ secretory rate, and increased flow per nephron further augments K+ secretion. Extrarenal disposition of K+ is likewise enhanced: both aldosterone and insulin appear to have roles in the augmented cellular K+ uptake that occurs in chronic renal failure. Thus, patients with end-stage renal disease who are also mineralocorticoid and/or insulin deficient have a particular predisposition to hyperkalemia.[109]

These adaptive mechanisms allow patients with advanced renal disease to maintain K+ balance, but often only at the extremes of compensation and certainly at the expense of homeostatic flexibility. Any perturbation may rapidly precipitate severe hyperkalemia. Sudden increases in K+ intake may overload the system. Acute reductions in glomerular filtration rate (for example, by hemorrhage, diarrhea, vomiting, or sepsis) impair K+ secretion. Drugs may also disrupt this delicate balance by reducing glomerular filtration rate, inhibiting secretion, or impairing cellular uptake.

Mineralocorticoid Deficiency

Mineralocorticoid deficiency may result from generalized adrenal insufficiency (Addison's disease), hypoaldosteronism, or pseudohypoaldosteronism.

Because of the elaborate nature of K+ homeostasis, mineralocorticoid deficiency alone is unlikely to cause clinically significant hyperkalemia. However, when associated with other defects in renal or extrarenal K+ homeostasis, mineralocorticoid deficiency may precipitate severe hyperkalemia.

Addison's Disease. Up to 50% of patients with Addison's disease have hyperkalemia.[110] Hyperkalemia in the setting of unexplained circulatory collapse should immediately raise the suspicion of addisonian crisis, and glucocorticoid therapy should not be delayed pending confirmation of the diagnosis.

Selective Hypoaldosteronism. A more common setting of mineralocorticoid deficiency is the syndrome of hyporeninemic hypoaldosteronism,[109] generally idiopathic in nature but most often seen in elderly patients with diabetes mellitus and mild-to-moderate renal insufficiency (usually from chronic tubulointerstitial disease). Seventy-five per cent of such patients have asymptomatic hyperkalemia, the remainder having muscle weakness or cardiac arrhythmias. An associated hyperchloremic metabolic acidosis is characteristic. In addition to diabetes mellitus, two other systemic diseases have been associated with this syndrome: the acquired immunodeficiency syndrome[111] and systemic lupus erythematosus.[112] Interestingly, acquired immunodeficiency syndrome is also increasingly recognized as an important cause of generalized adrenal insufficiency.[113, 114] Hyporeninemic hypoaldosteronism has also been associated with obstructive uropathy and chronic lead nephropathy.[115]

Aldosterone deficiency may be induced by a variety of drugs, acting at different sites in the renin-angiotensin-aldosterone axis. Beta-adrenergic receptor blockers predispose patients to hyperkalemia by suppressing renin release. Although symptomatic hyperkalemia from beta-adrenergic blockers alone is rare,[116] serious hyperkalemia may develop in susceptible patients (e.g., those with diabetes mellitus and renal insufficiency).[117] Impaired cellular K+ uptake undoubtedly contributes significantly to the hyperkalemia in such patients as well.[118] Calcium channel blockers may worsen the hyperkalemia associated with beta-adrenergic receptor blockade.[119] Interestingly, calcium channel blockers alone may improve K+ tolerance.[120] Certain calcium channel blockers may also exacerbate the cardiac electrophysiologic complications of hyperkalemia.[121]

Nonsteroidal anti-inflammatory drugs (NSAIDs) have a number of renal effects, several of which may lead to hyperkalemia.[122, 123] By blocking prostaglandin synthesis, NSAIDs decrease glomerular filtration rate and renin secretion.[122, 124] They may also inhibit aldosterone biosynthesis independently of their effects on renin production.[124] Thus, NSAIDs impair renal K$^+$ excretion both directly (reduced aldosterone-dependent K$^+$ secretion) and indirectly (reduced distal tubular flow). NSAID-related hyperkalemia has been reported in patients with both normal[125] and abnormal[126] renal function. Sulindac may cause less hyperkalemia than other NSAIDs.[127] When possible, administration of NSAIDs should be avoided in patients with renal insufficiency or patients who are prone to hyperkalemia because of defects in internal K$^+$ balance.

ACE inhibitors decrease angiotensin II–stimulated aldosterone biosynthesis and have been associated with hyperkalemia, particularly in patients with pre-existing renal insufficiency.[41, 128] Like NSAIDs, ACE inhibitors should be avoided in patients with renal insufficiency, especially those with known or suspected defects in K$^+$ homeostasis.

Heparin directly and selectively inhibits aldosterone biosynthesis.[129, 130] However, clinically significant hyperkalemia is rare, probably because of the influence of other renal and extrarenal homeostatic mechanisms. It is not surprising, therefore, that those cases of severe hyperkalemia in which heparin was implicated occurred in the setting of diabetes mellitus, renal insufficiency,[129, 130] or ACE inhibition.[131]

Pseudohypoaldosteronism. By blocking the renal action of aldosterone, spironolactone inhibits aldosterone-mediated K$^+$ secretion. About 10% of patients treated with spironolactone have clinically significant hyperkalemia, and the incidence rises in patients receiving supplemental K$^+$.[41]

Intrinsic Potassium Secretory Defects

Intrinsic defects in renal K$^+$ secretion occur in a number of different disorders, including sickle cell disease or trait,[132] systemic lupus erythematosus,[133] after renal transplantation,[134] and obstructive uropathy.[135]

Although spironolactone blocks the tubular effects of aldosterone, the two other common K$^+$-sparing diuretics, amiloride and triamterene, inhibit aldosterone-independent K$^+$ secretion. Hyperkalemia is most common in patients with pre-existing renal insufficiency, diabetes mellitus, concurrent use of NSAIDs or ACE inhibitors, and K$^+$ supplementation.[41, 136] The risk of hyperkalemia also increases with age.[137]

Pentamidine has been reported to cause hyperkalemia out of proportion to concomitant acute renal insufficiency in patients with acquired immunodeficiency syndrome.[138] Cyclosporine-induced hyperkalemia has been described in renal transplant recipients.[139]

Chronic Hypokalemia (Table 101–6)

Chronic hypokalemia is virtually always the result of abnormalities in external balance: insufficient K$^+$ intake and/or excessive K$^+$ losses (gastrointestinal or renal). There is a linear relationship between total body K$^+$ depletion and hypokalemia (see Fig. 101–1); provided that there are no gross alterations in internal K$^+$ balance, rough estimates of the magnitude of K$^+$ depletion can be derived from S_K.

Inadequate Potassium Intake

Severe dietary K$^+$ restriction causes hypokalemia in 3 to 7 days in normal humans.[31, 140] In one series of hospitalized patients, inadequate K$^+$ supplementation during intravenous therapy contributed to the development of hypokalemia in 45% of cases and was the sole cause in 6%.[141] Inadequate K$^+$ replacement also contributes to the hypokalemia that frequently complicates diuretic therapy. Other disorders associated with nutritional hypokalemia include anorexia nervosa,[142] the so-called tea-and-toast syndrome, geophagia, and chronic alcoholism.

TABLE 101–6
CAUSES OF CHRONIC HYPOKALEMIA

Inadequate Potassium Intake
Starvation
Anorexia nervosa
Tea-and-toast syndrome
Chronic alcoholism
Inadequate K$^+$ supplementation

Excessive Potassium Losses
Gastrointestinal losses
  Diarrhea
  Villous adenoma
  Long-term laxative abuse
Renal losses
  Gastric fluid loss
    Vomiting
    Nasogastric suction
  Pharmacologic agents
    Diuretics
    Antibiotics
      Amphotericin B
      Carbenicillin, ticarcillin
  Mineralocorticoid excess
    Primary hyperaldosteronism (Conn's syndrome)
      Adrenal adenoma
      Bilateral adrenal hyperplasia
    Secondary hyperaldosteronism
      Hypovolemia
      Renal artery stenosis
      Malignant hypertension
      Renin-secreting tumors
    Miscellaneous causes of mineralocorticoid excess
      Congenital adrenal hyperplasia (11- or 17-hydroxylase deficiency)
      Ectopic ACTH syndrome
      Licorice (glycyrrhetinic acid) ingestion
      Glucocorticoid therapy
Mg^{2+} deficiency
Hypercalcemia
Bartter's syndrome
Liddle's syndrome

Excessive Potassium Losses

Gastrointestinal Potassium Losses. Hypokalemia may develop from both upper and lower gastrointestinal tract fluid losses, but the pathogenesis is quite different in the two situations. With diarrhea, the K$^+$ is lost in the stool, whereas with gastric fluid losses, the K$^+$ is largely lost in the urine. As stool volume rises, the stool K$^+$ concentration usually falls to some extent, thereby attenuating K$^+$ losses.[143] Nonetheless, hypokalemia may occur with diarrhea of any cause. Because alkali is lost in the stool as well, the hypokalemia is usually accompanied by a hyperchloremic metabolic acidosis. In the absence of confounding factors (e.g., concomitant diuretic use), renal K$^+$ conservation generally limits urinary K$^+$ losses to less than 20 mmol/d.[144, 145] Other disorders associated with excessive stool K$^+$ losses include villous adenomas[145] and long-term laxative abuse.[146, 147]

Renal Potassium Losses: Gastric Fluid Loss. Gastric fluid losses (e.g., via vomiting and gastric suction) are a common cause of hypokalemia. Interestingly, most of the K$^+$ losses are renal, not gastric, in origin. The gastric fluid K$^+$ concentration is only 5 to 10 mmol/L, and only massive fluid losses are expected to significantly deplete body K$^+$ stores. However, the associated metabolic alkalosis, increased HCO_3^- delivery to the distal nephron, and secondary hyperaldosteronism all stimulate K^+ secretion.[33] In this situation, the urinary K^+ concentration is typically high, whereas the urinary chloride ion (Cl^-) concentration is low owing to volume contraction.

Pharmacologic Agents. Diuretics are the single most common cause of drug-induced hypokalemia and K^+ depletion. The magnitude of the kaliuresis depends on the site of the action of the diuretic and the prevailing hormonal milieu (especially the circulating aldosterone level).[148, 149] By inhibiting Na^+ and Cl^- reabsorption at sites proximal to the K^+ secretory site, diuretics promote kaliuresis by increasing the distal delivery of fluid. K^+ secretion is further stimulated by secondary aldosteronism to the extent that the patient becomes volume depleted. Thus, hypokalemia frequently accompanies the use of the two most common classes of diuretics: thiazides and loop diuretics ($S_K < 3.5$ mmol/L in 20 and 10% of patients, respectively).[149] Carbonic anhydrase inhibitors, which block sodium bicarbonate reabsorption in the proximal tubule, exert an additional kaliuretic effect by shunting HCO_3^--rich, Cl^--poor fluid to the distal nephron.[148] Combining two K^+-wasting diuretics for added diuretic effect (e.g., furosemide plus metolazone) can result in severe hypokalemia. In such cases, S_K has been found to fall below 3.5 mmol/L in more than 80% of patients and below 3.0 mmol/L in more than half.[149]

Certain antibiotics may also cause renal K^+ wasting and hypokalemia. Ninety percent of patients receiving amphotericin B require K^+ supplementation, the average amount being about 70 mmol/d.[150] The hypokalemia is due, at least in part, to the accompanying renal tubular acidosis[151] and Mg^{2+} depletion.[152] In addition, amphotericin B nonspecifically increases cell membrane permeability, increasing K^+ efflux from renal tubular cells into the tubular fluid.

Penicillin antibiotics, particularly polyanionic derivatives such as carbenicillin and ticarcillin, have been associated with hypokalemia in up to 9% of patients receiving high doses of these drugs.[153] Limited reabsorption of these anionic drugs in the distal nephron creates a favorable electrochemical gradient for K^+ secretion.

Mineralocorticoid Excess. Mineralocorticoids predispose to hypokalemia by stimulating renal K^+ excretion and enhancing cellular K^+ uptake. Mineralocorticoid excess may be primary (e.g., Conn's syndrome); result from absolute or effective hypovolemia (e.g., salt depletion and edematous disorders); or be associated with renal artery stenosis, malignant hypertension, or rarely, renin-secreting tumors. Congenital adrenal hyperplasia, ectopic ACTH syndrome and the ingestion of certain forms of licorice are other causes of mineralocorticoid excess. Hypokalemia is seen in 90% of patients with primary aldosteronism, its severity being directly proportional to Na^+ intake (distal flow).[34] In edematous patients with secondary aldosteronism (e.g., congestive heart failure and hepatic cirrhosis), hypokalemia commonly ensues when diuretic therapy enhances distal flow. Diuretic-induced hypokalemia in congestive heart failure is particularly dangerous because it increases the risk of ventricular arrhythmias.[154] Because almost all glucocorticoids possess some mineralocorticoid activity, prolonged administration of these agents can cause severe hypokalemia, especially in patients who are poorly nourished (and thus already in negative K^+ balance) and in patients receiving diuretics.

Magnesium Deficiency. Mg^{2+} deficiency is a frequently unrecognized cause of renal K^+ wasting and may result in severe K^+ depletion.[155, 156] Because Mg^{2+}, like Ca^{2+}, acts to stabilize excitable membranes, the deleterious effects of hypokalemia on the myocardium are magnified by concurrent hypomagnesemia.[35, 36] Because Mg^{2+} deficiency is associated with marked renal K^+ wasting, the resulting hypokalemia is refractory to K^+ supplementation. This is especially important in patients receiving digoxin, because hypokalemia and hypomagnesemia both potentiate digitalis cardiotoxicity.[37, 157] Thus, hypokalemia that is refractory to aggressive K^+ supplementation should always trigger an evaluation of Mg^{2+} balance. If hypomagnesemia is discovered, repletion of body Mg^{2+} stores reverses the K^+ wasting and allows the repletion of body K^+ stores.

The intensive care setting is fraught with potential causes of hypomagnesemia. Among them are a variety of factors that favor a shift of Mg^{2+} into cells; for example, in malnourished patients (many of whom are already Mg^{2+} deficient), enteral or parenteral feeding can cause profound hypomagnesemia. Mg^{2+} redistribution is also seen during the treatment of patients with anorexia nervosa, DKA, and alcohol withdrawal. In delirium tremens, Mg^{2+} movement into cells is further enhanced by high circulating levels of catecholamines. Finally, alkalosis, especially respiratory alkalosis, favors a shift of Mg^{2+} into cells.

More significant than these internal shifts, however, are those situations favoring increased gastrointestinal or renal Mg^{2+} losses. With malabsorption syndromes or enteral drainage (nasogastric or biliary), Mg^{2+} losses can exceed intake by up to 100 mg/d.[36] Renal Mg^{2+} wasting occurs in osmotic diuresis, in phosphate depletion, and with the use of drugs such as alcohol, diuretics, aminoglycosides, amphotericin B,[150] and cisplatin.[158]

Hypercalcemia. When hypercalcemia causes a salt and water diuresis, it is commonly associated with renal K^+ wasting. In one series, one third of hypercalcemic patients were hypokalemic; the prevalence was 52% in patients with the hypercalcemia of malignancy.[159] Severe hypercalcemia may compound the arrhythmogenic effects of hypokalemia, and forced diuresis, a common treatment of hypercalcemia, may exacerbate hypokalemia.

Bartter's and Liddle's Syndromes. Two rare entities that are characterized by renal K^+ wasting and metabolic alkalosis are Bartter's syndrome, in which patients are typically hypomagnesemic and normotensive,[160] and Liddle's syndrome, in which patients are typically hypertensive.[161] The former is treated with prostaglandin inhibitors and Mg^{2+} and K^+ supplementation, whereas the latter responds to triamterene or amiloride.

Pseudohyperkalemia

A falsely elevated blood K^+ concentration may be seen for a variety of reasons. Normally S_K exceeds the plasma K^+ concentration (P_K) by about 0.4 mmol/L,[162] owing to cell and platelet lysis during clotting. Pseudohyperkalemia is defined as an abnormally large discrepancy between S_K and P_K and is usually seen in patients with severe thrombocytosis,[163, 164] the degree of pseudohyperkalemia being proportional to the platelet count.[164] The same phenomenon has been reported in patients with severe leukocytosis.[165] In both cases, the P_K accurately reflects blood K^+ concentration.[163-165]

Cells left in prolonged contact with plasma at 4°C can lose K^+ and cause pseudohyperkalemia. Hemolysis during specimen collection falsely raises both S_K and P_K.[166] Rapid fist clenching by the patient while the tourniquet is in place before venipuncture is associated with local venous hyperkalemia as muscles release intracellular K^+.[28]

Thus, blood samples for measurement of K^+ concentration should be collected carefully. If a tourniquet is needed for venipuncture, the patient's fist should not be clenched repeatedly. A small-caliber needle and high vacuum in the collection tube may cause hemolysis. An anticoagulated plasma specimen should be used in patients with marked thrombocytosis or leukocytosis. The sample should remain at room temperature, and the plasma should separated from the cells within an hour of venipuncture. Because clinical realities often preclude such ideal practice, clinicians should bear in mind these laboratory artifacts when presented with an abnormal blood K^+ concentration.

Pseudohypokalemia

Severe leukocytosis may cause a spuriously low P_K (pseudohypokalemia) if blood cells are left in contact with the plasma for extended periods at room temperature or higher. This phenomenon results from ongoing cell metabolism in vitro with glucose and K^+ uptake.[166] Unexpected hypokalemia and hypoglycemia in the setting of leukocytosis should alert the clinician to this phenomenon.

CLINICAL MANIFESTATIONS OF POTASSIUM IMBALANCE

Alterations in S_K have a variety of adverse clinical consequences (Table 101–7), the expression of which may be magnified in the critically ill patient. Because K_i/K_e is the major determinant of the resting membrane potential, the most serious of these manifestations are those involving excitable tissues. Small changes in K_e (i.e., S_K) have profound effects on K_i/K_e and thereby on the resting membrane potential. Increases in S_K depolarize the cell, taking the resting membrane potential closer to the threshold for activation, whereas decreases in S_K hyperpolarize the cell.[2]

The relatively long duration of the cardiac action potential depends on a postexcitation decrease in K^+ permeability, which delays recovery to the basal (pre-excitation) state. Increases in S_K blunt this decrease in K^+ permeability and thereby decrease the duration of the action potential. Conversely, decreases in S_K prolong the duration of the action potential.[167]

TABLE 101–7
CLINICAL MANIFESTATIONS OF POTASSIUM IMBALANCE

Hyperkalemia
Cardiac
  Electrocardiographic (ECG) abnormalities
    Conduction defects
    Arrhythmias
Neuromuscular
  Paresthesias
  Weakness or paralysis
Renal
  Decreased ammonia production (hyperchloremic metabolic acidosis)

Hypokalemia
Cardiac
  ECG abnormalities
    Arrhythmias
Neuromuscular
  Weakness or paralysis
  Ileus or gastroparesis
  Rhabdomyolysis
Metabolism
  Glucose intolerance
  Negative nitrogen balance
Renal
  Polyuria or polydipsia
  Increased ammonia production
    Exacerbation of hepatic encephalopathy
    Metabolic alkalosis

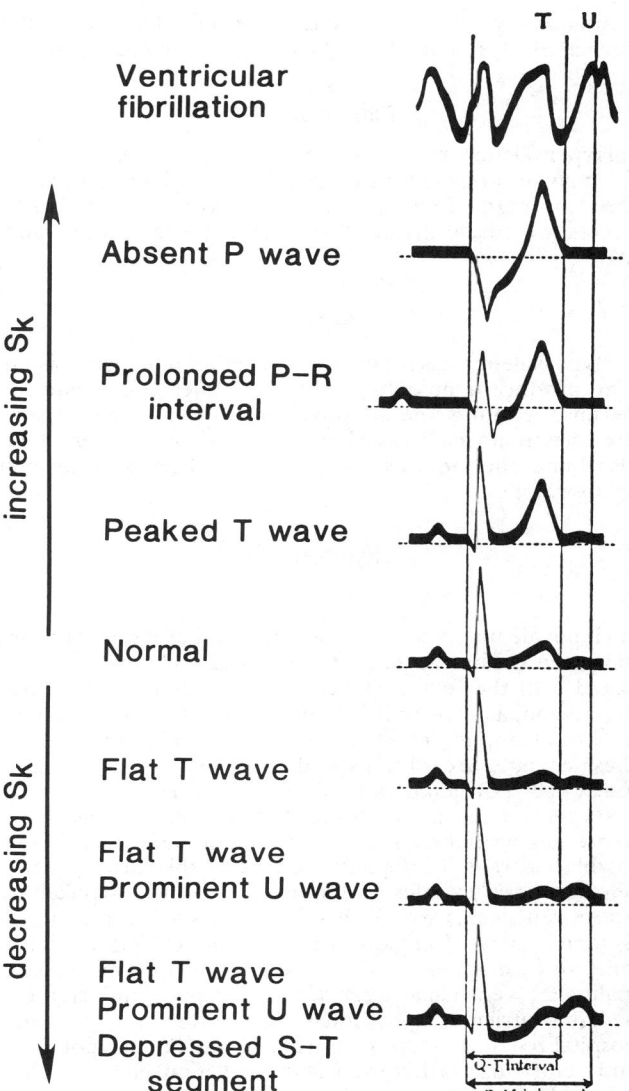

Figure 101–2. ECG manifestations of variations in S_K. (From Weisberg LS, Szerlip HM, Cox M: Disorders of potassium homeostasis in critically ill patients. Crit Care Clin 3:835, 1987.)

Hyperkalemia
Cardiac

Hyperkalemia depolarizes the cell membrane, slows ventricular conduction, and decreases the duration of the action potential. These changes produce the classic electrocardiographic (ECG) manifestations of hyperkalemia, including (in order of their usual appearance) peaking of the T wave, widening of the QRS complex, loss of the P wave, ventricular fibrillation, and asystole[167, 168] (Fig. 101–2). These changes may be modified by a multitude of other factors, such as the extracellular fluid pH, Ca^{2+} concentration and Na^+ concentration, and the rate of rise of S_K.[167]

In the seriously ill patient, in whom there are often numerous confounding variables, typical ECG changes may not accompany changes in S_K. If present, these changes are certainly highly suggestive of hyperkalemia. However, even in their absence, the clinician should be wary when evaluating a hyperkalemic patient. Normal ECGs occur despite extreme hyperkalemia,[169] and the first cardiac manifestation of hyperkalemia may be ventricular fibrillation or asystole.[48]

Consequently, an S_K greater than 6.5 mmol/L, even with a normal ECG, should always be treated as an emergency.

Neuromuscular

Hyperkalemia may result in paresthesias and weakness that may progress to a flaccid paralysis, which typically spares the diaphragm. Reflexes are depressed or absent. Cranial nerves are rarely involved and sensory changes are minimal.[170]

Metabolic

Hyperkalemia decreases basal renal ammoniagenesis and may produce a mild hyperchloremic metabolic acidosis.[171] Because it blunts the adaptive increase in renal ammonia production normally associated with acidemia, hyperkalemia also limits the kidney's ability to defend against metabolic acidosis.[172]

Hypokalemia
Cardiac

Hypokalemia hyperpolarizes the cell membrane and prolongs the cardiac action potential. These changes are associated with the following ECG manifestations: ST segment depression, a decrease in T wave amplitude, and an increase in U wave amplitude[167, 168] (see Fig. 101–2). However, because these changes are all nonspecific, the ECG is a less reliable index of hypokalemia than of hyperkalemia.

Hypokalemia may be associated with an increased incidence of arrhythmias and conduction defects. It is well established that K^+ depletion increases the cardiac toxicity of digitalis glycosides.[173] However, whether hypokalemia causes ventricular arrhythmias in patients not taking digitalis is controversial. Individuals without underlying cardiovascular disease appear not to have an increased incidence of malignant ventricular arrhythmias despite an increase in benign ventricular arrhythmias.[174, 175] However, in individuals hospitalized with acute myocardial infarction, hypokalemia and ventricular tachycardia and fibrillation have been correlated.[176] The hypokalemia seen in this setting may result from increased cellular K^+ uptake owing to high circulating catecholamine levels. However, because K^+ repletion does not reduce the occurrence of these arrhythmias, it is unlikely that hypokalemia is the sole arrhythmogenic factor involved. Nevertheless, because the majority of critically ill patients have underlying cardiovascular disease and, therefore, an increased incidence of sudden death, K^+ deficits should always be judiciously corrected.

Neuromuscular

Modest hypokalemia generally presents as weakness, myalgias, muscle fatigue, and restless legs. With more severe hypokalemia (<2 mmol/L), paralysis may supervene. This usually involves the extremities but may progress to include the trunk and ventilatory muscles.[89, 100, 170] As with hyperkalemia, cranial nerves are spared and sensory function usually remains intact.[170] Smooth muscle dysfunction (ileus, gastroparesis) is more common in hypokalemia than in hyperkalemia. These manifestations may be masked by concomitant hypocalcemia and may appear only when Ca^{2+} stores are repleted. Similarly, in patients with both hypokalemia and hypocalcemia, tetany may occur only after K^+ replacement.[170] Profound hypokalemia may result in rhabdomyolysis.[177] This is believed to be due to a decreased capacity of K^+-deficient muscle to synthesize glycogen and to appropriately

increase blood flow during exercise.[177] Thus, oxygen and metabolic substrate delivery is compromised, especially during exertion. However, rhabdomyolysis has also been reported in hypokalemic hospitalized patients at rest.[178] Even in the absence of frank rhabdomyolysis, elevations of creatine kinase levels may occur with severe hypokalemia and may be misinterpreted as representing myocardial damage (or by decreasing the percentage of the CK_2 [MB] isoenzyme, may obscure the diagnosis of acute myocardial infarction).

Metabolic

Hypokalemia and K^+ depletion cause glucose intolerance because of decreased insulin secretion.[170, 179] Glucose intolerance is more likely to develop in hypokalemic patients who have a genetic predisposition to diabetes.[179]

Hypokalemia and K^+ depletion may also lead to negative nitrogen balance. It is particularly difficult to replace protein stores in malnourished K^+-depleted patients. Nitrogen loss is secondary to increased renal ammonia and urea excretion.[180]

Renal

Hypokalemia and K^+ depletion are associated with polydipsia, polyuria, and nocturia, which appear to result both from decreased renal concentrating ability and from primary polydipsia.[181, 182] K^+ depletion is also commonly associated with metabolic alkalosis owing to increased proximal tubular HCO_3^- reabsorption and increased ammonia excretion.[183] Increased ammoniagenesis in the K^+-depleted patient may exacerbate hepatic encephalopathy in patients with acute or chronic liver failure.[184] Finally, hypokalemia is associated with renal Na^+ retention.[185]

EVALUATION OF DISORDERS OF POTASSIUM HOMEOSTASIS

The diagnostic approach to disorders of K^+ homeostasis is simplified by classifying these disorders according to their duration: acute (or unknown duration) versus chronic.

Acute Hyperkalemia

When S_K rises abruptly, or if S_K is dangerously high (>6.5 mmol/L) on initial presentation, the first step is to obtain an ECG. If there is electrophysiologic evidence of hyperkalemia, treatment should be initiated immediately. Serum electrolytes, glucose, blood urea nitrogen, creatinine and arterial blood gas determinations should be obtained. The urine should be tested for heme pigments to exclude acute rhabdomyolysis or hemolysis. The patient's medications and diet should be reviewed promptly, looking for exogenous sources of K^+ and drugs that are known to impair K^+ tolerance (Table 101–8). Pseudohyperkalemia can be excluded by measuring the P_K; a complete blood count is also helpful in this regard.

Chronic Hyperkalemia

Figure 101–3 provides an approach to the patient with chronic hyperkalemia. A blood urea nitrogen or serum creatinine determination indicates the presence of renal insufficiency, and estimating the glomerular filtration rate provides useful information as well; if the glomerular filtration rate is greater than 10 mL/min, the hyperkalemia is unlikely to be due to solely renal insufficiency. Failure to

TABLE 101–8

PHARMACOLOGIC AGENTS IMPAIRING POTASSIUM TOLERANCE

Agents mainly affecting external K⁺ balance
  K⁺-sparing diuretics
    Amiloride
    Triamterene
    Spironolactone
  ACE inhibitors
  NSAIDs
  Heparin
Agents mainly affecting internal K⁺ balance
  Beta-adrenergic blockers
  Hypertonic solutions
  Digitalis

release cortisol in response to cosyntropin stimulation supports the diagnosis of generalized adrenal insufficiency (Addison's disease). A normal response implies selective hypoaldosteronism, renal unresponsiveness to aldosterone (pseudohypoaldosteronism), or an intrinsic defect in renal K⁺ secretion, and one should then proceed to an assessment of the renin-angiotensin-aldosterone axis. Specifically, one measures plasma renin activity and plasma aldosterone levels before the patient arises from bed in the morning, and again after an intravenous injection of 40 mg of furosemide followed by 2 hours of upright posture. An increase of less than threefold to fivefold in plasma renin activity and plasma aldosterone concentration is diagnostic of hyporeninemic hypoaldosteronism; normal or elevated plasma renin activity

in the face of aldosterone deficiency implies hyperreninemic hypoaldosteronism; and elevated plasma renin activity and plasma aldosterone levels imply pseudohypoaldosteronism or an intrinsic defect in K⁺ secretion.

After mineralocorticoid deficiency is discovered (or suspected), it is of interest to determine whether it alone is responsible for the impairment in K⁺ secretion, to predict response to treatment (hormone replacement). An index that is purported to represent the gradient for renal tubular K⁺ secretion (and that is largely a function of mineralocorticoid effect) is the transtubular K⁺ gradient.[186] It is calculated as follows:

$$(U_K/S_K) \div (U_{OSM}/P_{OSM})$$

where U_{OSM} and P_{OSM} = urine and plasma osmolalities, respectively, and U_K = urine K⁺ concentration. That mineralocorticoid deficiency is responsible for the hyperkalemia is confirmed by measuring the transtubular K⁺ gradient before and 2 hours after an oral dose (0.05 mg) of 9α-fludrocortisone (Florinef). A stimulated value greater than 7 is evidence of normal tubular responsiveness to mineralocorticoid,[186] whereas a value less than 6 implies unresponsiveness. However, some patients require more prolonged exposure to higher doses of 9α-fludrocortisone before responding normally. A transtubular K⁺ gradient of less than 6 after several days of high-dose 9α-fludrocortisone administration is good evidence of tubular unresponsiveness to mineralocorticoid.[187] One may further characterize the defect by attempting to stimulate K⁺ secretion with sodium bicarbonate or sodium sulfate infusions, both of which are markedly kaliuretic in normal individuals. If transtubular

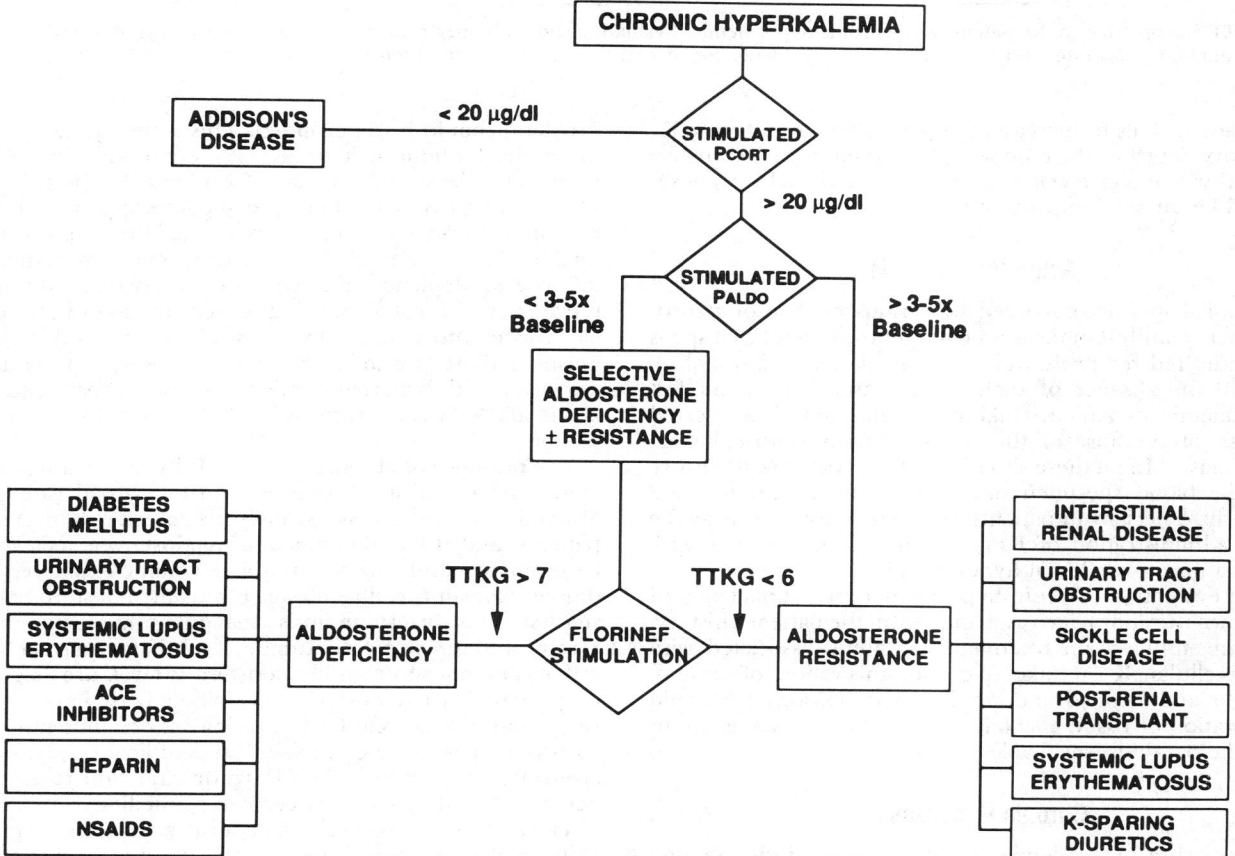

Figure 101–3. Approach to the patient with chronic hyperkalemia. Pᴄᴏʀᴛ = plasma cortisol concentration; Pᴀʟᴅᴏ = plasma aldosterone concentration; TTKG = transtubular K⁺ gradient.

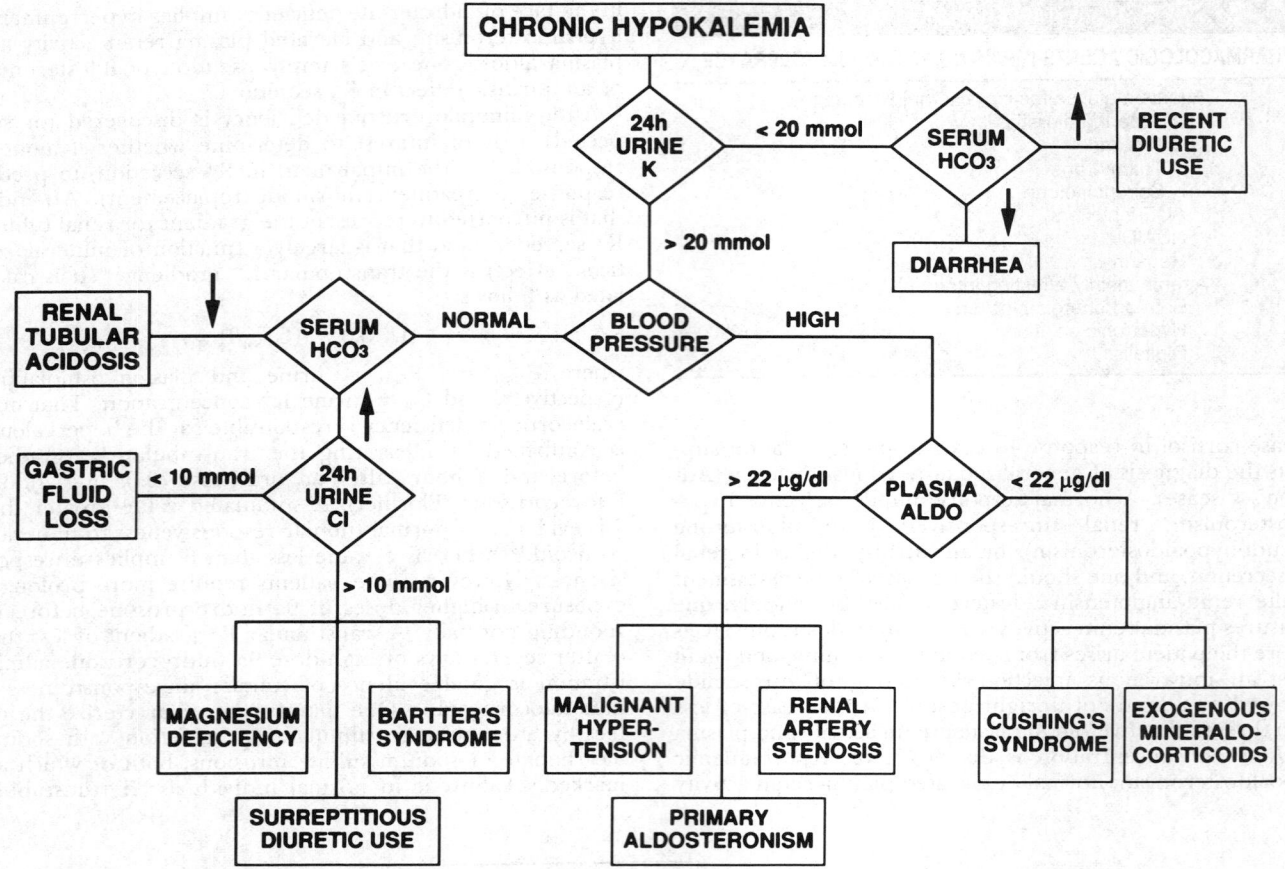

Figure 101–4. Approach to the patient with chronic hypokalemia. Evaluation should be performed with the patient taking at least 100 mEq/d of sodium and potassium, and not receiving diuretic drugs for several days. ALDO = aldosterone.

K^+ gradient fails to increase, the patient has an intrinsic K^+ secretory defect of the type seen, for example, in obstructive uropathy[135] or sickle cell neuropathy,[132] and such diagnoses should be pursued appropriately.

Acute Hypokalemia

Hypokalemia accompanied by serious cardiac or neuromuscular manifestations is an emergency. Urgent therapy is also indicated for profound hypokalemia (S_K of 2 mmol/L), even in the absence of such manifestations. Even modest hypokalemia in patients taking digitalis should be treated aggressively because of the risk of serious ventricular arrhythmias.[173] In all these situations, it is imperative to ensure that the blood specimen has been obtained and handled properly, especially in patients with leukocytosis, because the rapid administration of K^+ in a patient with pseudohypokalemia may cause lethal hyperkalemia.

The evaluation of acute hypokalemia (or hypokalemia of unknown duration) derives mainly from the patient's history, with an emphasis on treatment modalities associated with rapid cellular K^+ uptake (e.g., administration of insulin, HCO_3^-, and beta-adrenergic agonists), reasons for rapid acceleration of tissue anabolism, and a history suggestive of periodic paralysis (see Table 101–4).

Chronic Hypokalemia

After acute hypokalemia and transient K^+ redistribution have been excluded, whether the kidney is responding appropriately to the K^+ deficit (or is the cause of the

problem) should be determined. This is best done by measuring the 24-hour urinary K^+ excretion with the patient receiving at least 100 mmol/d of Na^+ and K^+ (Fig. 101–4). Excretion of less than 20 mmol/d suggests appropriate renal K^+ conservation and points to extrarenal (lower gastrointestinal tract or cutaneous) K^+ losses, or recovery from diuretic-induced K^+ depletion. Excretion of greater than 20 mmol/d is evidence of renal K^+ wasting. Determination of the serum electrolytes and arterial blood gases is also helpful in distinguishing these possibilities: stool K^+ losses are frequently associated with hyperchloremic metabolic acidosis, and metabolic alkalosis is characteristic of diuretic-induced K^+ depletion.

The presence or absence of systemic hypertension conveniently divides renal K^+ wasting into two broad categories. Mineralocorticoid excess is usually the culprit in hypertensive patients, and the renin-angiotensin-aldosterone axis should be evaluated under both basal and volume-expanded conditions. Nonsuppressible plasma renin and aldosterone levels suggest renal artery stenosis, malignant hypertension, or rarely, a renin-secreting tumor. Low basal plasma renin activity and nonsuppressible aldosterone levels are diagnostic of primary hyperaldosteronism. When both basal plasma renin and aldosterone levels are low, exogenous mineralocorticoid ingestion (e.g., certain forms of licorice), Cushing's syndrome (e.g., ectopic ACTH syndrome), and rarely, congenital adrenal hyperplasia become possibilities.

The first step in the evaluation of the normotensive patient with renal K^+ wasting is to look for an accompanying acid-base disorder. Hyperchloremic metabolic acidosis suggests proximal or (classic) distal renal tubular acidosis. On the

TABLE 101-9

EMERGENCY TREATMENT OF HYPERKALEMIA

Therapy	Dose	Onset	Duration	Complications
Membrane Stabilization				
Calcium gluconate (10%)	10-mL IV bolus	Immediate	30–60 min	Digitalis-associated arrhythmias Hypercalcemia
Hypertonic sodium chloride (5%)	50-mL IV bolus	Immediate	Unknown	Volume overload Hypertonicity
Redistribution				
Insulin (short acting)	50 U in 500 mL of 20% dextrose IV at 100 mL/h	20 min	During infusion and 4–6 h thereafter	Hyperglycemia Hypoglycemia
Albuterol	20 mg in 4 mL of normal saline nebulized over 10 min	15 min	>60 min	No response in some patients
Sodium bicarbonate (8.4%)	50-mL bolus IV, then 20 mL/h × 2–3 h	Unknown	Unknown	Volume overload Metabolic alkalosis Hypertonicity
Elimination				
Loop diuretics				
Furosemide	40–80 mg IV	15 min	2–3 h	Volume depletion
Bumetanide	1–2 mg IV			
Sodium polystyrene sulfonate (Kayexalate)	25–50 g (in 15–30 mL of 70% sorbitol) PO or 50 g (in saline) p.r.	1–2 h	Hours	Diarrhea
Dialysis				
Hemodialysis	2–3 h against zero-K$^+$ bath	Immediate	Throughout dialysis	Complications of hemodialysis Cardiac arrhythmias
Peritoneal dialysis	Hourly exchanges with zero-K$^+$ dialysate	Hours	Throughout dialysis	Complications of peritoneal dialysis

other hand, if metabolic alkalosis is present, measuring the 24-hour urinary Cl$^-$ excretion distinguishes between gastric fluid loss (urinary Cl$^-$ excretion < 10 mmol/d), diuretic use or abuse, and Mg^{2+} depletion (urinary Cl$^-$ excretion > 10 mmol/d). Bartter's syndrome also falls into this latter category. Surreptitious diuretic abuse, a common cause of hypokalemia and metabolic alkalosis, particularly in young women concerned about their weight, can be confirmed by sending a urine sample for diuretic drug analysis.

TREATMENT OF POTASSIUM IMBALANCE

Disorders of K$^+$ homeostasis can be conveniently divided according to duration and severity for purposes of treatment as well as for pathogenic categorization. In general, the initial treatment of acute severe hyperkalemia or hypokalemia is independent of the cause of the disturbance, whereas the rational therapy of chronic disorders of K$^+$ homeostasis depends on a thorough understanding of their pathogenesis.

Acute Hyperkalemia

The recommended threshold for instituting emergency therapy for hyperkalemia varies considerably.[188–190] In identifying when hyperkalemia constitutes an emergency, several points should be kept in mind. First, the electrophysiologic effects of hyperkalemia relate to both the absolute S$_K$ and its rate of rise.[167] Second, concurrent metabolic disturbances may ameliorate (e.g., hypernatremia, hypercalcemia, and alkalemia) or exacerbate (e.g., hyponatremia, hypocalcemia, and acidemia) these electrophysiologic effects.[168, 169] Third, although the ECG manifestations of hyperkalemia are generally progressive and proportional to the S$_K$, ventricular fibrillation or asystole may be the first ECG disturbance of hyperkalemia;[46] conversely, a normal ECG may be seen even with severe hyperkalemia.[169]

Thus, it is apparent that neither the ECG nor the S$_K$ alone is an adequate index of the urgency with which hyperkalemia

should be corrected and that the clinical context must always be carefully considered. Any pronouncement of an absolute S$_K$ constituting an emergency must be seen as somewhat arbitrary. Nonetheless, because the treatment of hyperkalemia is safe (if applied properly) and because hyperkalemia is unpredictably lethal, it is prudent to maintain a low threshold for instituting emergency therapy. Most patients manifest ECG changes at S$_K$ greater than 6.7 mmol/L;[168] consequently, the following general guidelines for instituting emergency therapy appear reasonable: (1) S$_K$ greater than 6.5 mmol/L or (2) ECG manifestations of hyperkalemia regardless of the S$_K$.

Treatment is directed at preventing or ameliorating the untoward myocardial electrophysiologic effects of hyperkalemia. Although what constitutes optimal treatment is somewhat controversial,[191–193] the overall therapeutic strategy is not. In chronologic order, the goals of therapy are to (1) antagonize the effect of K$^+$ on excitable cell membranes, (2) redistribute extracellular K$^+$ into cells, and (3) eliminate K$^+$ from the body (Table 101–9).

Membrane Antagonism

Ca^{2+} directly antagonizes the myocardial effects of hyperkalemia.[168, 190] It does not lower S$_K$. Ca^{2+} is beneficial even in patients who are normocalcemic. The preferred agent is calcium gluconate because the Cl$^-$ salt may cause tissue necrosis on extravasation. The dose may be repeated in 5 minutes if no improvement is noted in the ECG or if the ECG deteriorates after initial improvement.

There are several case reports of sudden death in patients given intravenous Ca^{2+} while also receiving digitalis glycosides.[194, 195] Dogs given a large intravenous dose of Ca^{2+} immediately after an intravenous dose of digitalis experienced ventricular asystole; if the Ca^{2+} was infused slowly, however, tolerance increased dramatically.[194] Thus, when severe hyperkalemia has to be treated in patients taking digitalis preparations, it may be wise to administer the Ca^{2+}

as a slow intravenous infusion (10 mL of 10% calcium gluconate in 100 mL of 5% dextrose in water during 20 minutes). In patients who have toxic levels of digitalis, it may be best to avoid Ca^{2+} altogether.

When hyperkalemia develops in a setting of hyponatremia, hypertonic saline can be used to reverse the adverse myocardial and neurologic abnormalities.[196, 197] Whether hypertonic saline is also effective in eunatremic patients is less clear. Like hypertonic saline, hypertonic sodium bicarbonate may exert its greatest beneficial effect in the treatment of severe hyperkalemia by virtue of membrane stabilization (hypernatremia, alkalemia) rather than by K^+ redistribution (see later).

Redistribution

Insulin stimulates K^+ uptake by muscle and liver,[4, 6] leading to a rapid decrease in S_K in both normal subjects and patients with end-stage renal disease.[198] Consequently, it is now accepted as standard therapy for severe hyperkalemia. Frequent monitoring of the blood glucose concentration is important to avoid hyperglycemia or hypoglycemia.

The beta$_2$-adrenergic agonist albuterol has been used to treat hyperkalemia in patients with end-stage renal disease:[199] Nebulized albuterol inhalation causes an abrupt decrease in S_K in about half of the patients studied and had no adverse cardiac effects. The effects of albuterol and insulin were additive.[199] Because half the patients failed to respond to albuterol alone, albuterol should not be used by itself in the treatment of severe hyperkalemia.

Sodium bicarbonate, when given as a slow intravenous infusion (20 to 30 mmol/h during 4 to 6 hours), has been reported to redistribute K^+ into cells; this effect on S_K was independent of changes in pH but correlates with the increase in the serum HCO_3^- concentration.[21] In contrast, shorter-duration infusions of either isotonic or hypertonic (8.4%) sodium bicarbonate (at rates of 2 and 4 mmol/min, respectively, for 1 h) had no effect on S_K. Whether a K^+-lowering effect would have appeared with more prolonged infusion is unknown. Until further studies are performed, however, the effectiveness of sodium bicarbonate in the treatment of severe hyperkalemia must be questioned. For the present, it is perhaps best to reserve hypertonic sodium bicarbonate for the hyperkalemic patient with concurrent hyponatremia and metabolic acidosis.

Elimination

Hyperkalemia often occurs in patients with renal insufficiency. However, even in patients with moderate renal failure, renal K^+ excretion can be enhanced by increasing distal nephron flow. This may be accomplished by volume expansion with saline or sodium bicarbonate and further enhanced by the use of loop diuretics. Bumetanide may have a somewhat greater kaliuretic effect than an equally natriuretic dose of furosemide.[200] Diuretic-induced volume contraction must be avoided, as this decreases distal flow and reduces K^+ excretion.

If advanced renal failure limits renal K^+ excretion, alternative routes of K^+ elimination must be considered. Intestinal K^+ excretion can be enhanced by the oral or rectal administration of sodium polystyrene sulfonate (Kayexalate), a cation-exchange resin. Each gram of resin binds 0.5 to 1.0 mmol of K^+ during about 4 hours. A reduction in S_K is usually seen after 1 to 2 hours. S_K can be expected to decrease by about 0.5 mmol/L after a single dose, but this is highly variable. To avoid the constipating effect of the resin, it is usually given with sorbitol. Patients who cannot tolerate oral medication may receive a retention enema of the resin

in saline. Sorbitol should not be used rectally; it is useful as a cathartic only when taken orally, and there is evidence that sorbitol, when given as an enema, may cause colonic necrosis, particularly in the setting of uremia.[201]

Dialysis is the therapy of last resort in the patient who cannot tolerate, or does not respond to, other K^+ elimination modalities. Hemodialysis lowers S_K more rapidly than peritoneal dialysis. The rate of K^+ removal is directly proportional to the initial S_K, such that by the end of a 3-hour dialysis against a zero-K^+ dialysate, S_K declines by about 40%; a rebound occurs during the next several hours, which negates about half of this reduction, however.[202] Little additional benefit is gained by dialyzing for longer than 3 hours. Hemodialysis using a zero-K^+ bath is safe in most patients but is occasionally associated with ventricular ectopy.[203] Thus, severely hyperkalemic patients undergoing hemodialysis should have continuous ECG monitoring.

Peritoneal dialysis also reduces S_K but the K^+-lowering effect does not correlate well with the amount of K^+ removed, suggesting that the peritoneal glucose and alkali load may enhance cellular K^+ uptake.[204] Because the fall in S_K is considerably slower with peritoneal dialysis than with hemodialysis, peritoneal dialysis is not the preferred modality in the treatment of life-threatening hyperkalemia.

Chronic Hyperkalemia

Chronic hyperkalemia always implies deficient renal K^+ excretion. It follows that the therapy of chronic hyperkalemia should be directed toward stimulating renal K^+ excretion, while at the same time limiting K^+ intake. K^+ intake in adults with chronic hyperkalemia should be restricted to 60 mmol/d. Note that a low-Na^+ diet is almost always a high-K^+ diet. Salt substitutes, which are low in Na^+ but relatively high in K^+, should also be avoided. Also recall that certain drugs (e.g., penicillins) are often formulated as the K^+ salt and when used in high doses may contribute substantially to daily K^+ intake. It is important to search for, and discontinue if possible, all drugs known to impair internal or external K^+ balance (see Table 101–6). Finally, occult urinary tract obstruction should be suspected in all patients with chronic hyperkalemia and a renal ultrasound scan should be obtained.

Thereafter, if the patient remains hyperkalemic and a cause of the hyperkalemia is not found, specific defects in renal K^+ handling should be sought by following the algorithm in Figure 101–3. Therapy for Addison's disease is discussed elsewhere in this section. Specific therapy for selective hypoaldosteronism consists of the oral administration of 9α-fludrocortisone (Florinef). Usual replacement doses are in the range of 0.05 to 0.2 mg daily. However, patients with selective hypoaldosteronism may require higher doses of the hormone, and even so, only about 80% respond with a decrease in S_K.[109] This suggests the presence of partial renal unresponsiveness as well as decreased aldosterone biosynthesis. Unfortunately, the sodium retentive effects of mineralocorticoids appear to be preserved, and a prominent side effect of therapy is fluid overload, often with congestive heart failure.[109]

In cases of apparent mineralocorticoid unresponsiveness, or when mineralocorticoid treatment is complicated by fluid overload, a thiazide or loop diuretic should be added to the regimen. This helps to restore normal volume status and also enhances renal tubular K^+ secretion in many mineralocorticoid-resistant patients. It is crucial to avoid diuretic-induced volume depletion, however, as this exacerbates the underlying K^+ secretory defect.

Patients who fail to respond to the above-mentioned measures may be given an alkalizing agent (e.g., sodium citrate and citric acid [Shohl's solution]), which, by increasing HCO_3^- delivery to the distal nephron, may enhance K^+ secretion. This is especially appropriate for patients whose chronic hyperkalemia is accompanied by so-called type IV renal tubular acidosis, as is commonly the case. The usual dose is 1 to 2 mmol of HCO_3^- equivalent (1 to 2 mL of Shohl's solution) per kilogram of body weight per day in three or four divided doses.

Most patients with chronic hyperkalemia respond to some combination of mineralocorticoid, diuretic, and alkali therapy. For those who do not, and whose S_K remains below 6 mmol/L, it may be best simply to monitor S_K regularly and take care not to perturb K^+ balance in any way. Patients whose S_K exceeds 6 mmol/L should be placed on a regular maintenance regimen of sodium polystyrene sulfonate (Kayexalate).

Acute Hypokalemia

In considering the treatment of hypokalemia, several concepts should be recalled. First, total body K^+ must fall by at least 200 mmol before hypokalemia is even detectable (see Fig. 101–1). In fact, when hypokalemia is uncomplicated by any factors that acutely affect internal K^+ balance, S_K decreases by approximately 0.3 mmol/L for each decrement of 100 mmol of total body K^+.[4] Thus, a low S_K almost always indicates a large total body K^+ deficit. Second, intravenous, and even oral, K^+ loads rapidly enter the extracellular fluid space, within which only about 2% (or 70 mmol) of total body K^+ normally resides. Even though homeostatic mechanisms that defend against hyperkalemia (redistribution of K^+ into cells, enhanced renal K^+ excretion) come into play promptly,[39, 205] if a large amount of K^+ is given too quickly, they are overwhelmed and S_K rises abruptly. Third, alterations in internal K^+ balance may have dramatic effects on the distribution of K^+ loads. For example, during the treatment of DKA, rapid cellular uptake of K^+ may obligate extensive K^+ repletion. Conversely, insulin deficiency so impairs K^+ tolerance that in anephric diabetic patients, virtually the entire load is restricted to the extracellular fluid space.[205] Thus, a K^+ load of only 60 to 70 mmol could be expected to double S_K.

When accompanied by serious cardiac or neuromuscular manifestations, hypokalemia should be treated as an emergency. In addition, urgent therapy is indicated for profound hypokalemia ($S_K < 2$ mmol/L), even in the absence of any overt clinical manifestations, and for moderate hypokalemia ($S_K < 3$ mmol/L) in patients taking digitalis. In these situations, potassium chloride should be administered intravenously.

There is only limited information on which to base a rational prescription of potassium chloride in an emergency.[39, 205–207] In normal individuals, the S_K increases by about 1 mmol/L after a 3-hour intravenous K^+ infusion of 0.6 mmol/kg/h.[39] In anuric patients, a similar rise in S_K follows the 3-hour K^+ infusion of only 0.3 mmol/kg/h.[205] In a diverse intensive care patient population, the mean increase in S_K after a 1-hour infusion of 20 mmol of K^+ (about 0.3 mmol/kg) was 0.25 mmol/L; mild hyperkalemia occurred in about 2% of these treatments.[206] Finally, in patients studied 24 hours after cardiac bypass surgery, a 3-hour K^+ infusion of about 0.2 mmol/kg/h resulted in a mean increase in S_K of 0.4 mmol/L without any complications.[207]

An approach to the treatment of severe hypokalemia is summarized in Table 101–10. Nondiabetic patients with normal renal function should easily tolerate a 1- to 2-hour infusion of potassium chloride at 0.6 mmol/kg/h. In patients with renal insufficiency (of any degree), the infusion rate should be halved (0.3 mmol/kg/h). Patients with uncompli-

TABLE 101–10

EMERGENCY TREATMENT OF HYPOKALEMIA

Patient	Intravenous Potassium Chloride Infusion Rate (mmol/kg/h)
Nondiabetic	
Normal renal function	0.6
Renal insufficiency	0.3
Diabetic	
Normal renal function	0.2
Renal insufficiency	0.1

Protocol
1. Mix potassium chloride in 0.9% saline.
2. Infuse for 1–2 h.
3. Monitor ECG continuously.
4. Recheck S_K at end of infusion.

cated diabetes mellitus should receive no more than 0.2 mmol/kg/h, or no more than 0.1 mmol/kg/h in the setting of renal insufficiency. If the patient is taking drugs that are known to impair internal or external K^+ balance (see Table 101–8), the dose of K^+ should be reduced accordingly. K^+ repletion during the treatment of diabetic ketoacidosis presents particular problems and must be carefully individualized. Whenever K^+ is administered intravenously, the ECG should be monitored continuously and the infusion stopped immediately if signs of hyperkalemia develop.

Using this protocol, the maximal increase in S_K is usually seen at the end of the infusion, and about 50% of the increase is lost during the next 2 to 3 hours at which time a new steady state is achieved. Thus, S_K should be measured at the end of the infusion. If the patient is still dangerously hypokalemic, additional K^+ may be given, recognizing that the rate of rise in S_K is directly proportional to the S_K at the start of the infusion[205] (see Fig. 101–1). If the S_K is in an acceptable range, the measurement should be repeated 2 to 3 hours later, when disposal of K^+ load is complete, to determine the need for further treatment.

Hypokalemia that is not life threatening is best treated with oral K^+ replacement. Because the gastrointestinal absorption of potassium chloride is essentially complete, dangerous hyperkalemia can occur in entirely normal individuals given large doses of potassium chloride elixir, or similar preparations.[208] The maximal increase in S_K is usually seen 1.5 to 2 hours after an oral K^+ load in patients with either normal[40] or impaired[208] renal function. Thus, a single oral dose of potassium chloride should probably not exceed the hourly intravenous dose: 0.6 mmol/kg for a patient with normal renal function, 0.3 mmol/kg for patients with renal insufficiency, and 0.1 to 0.2 mmol/kg for patients with diabetes mellitus, depending on their renal function. S_K should be measured 2 hours after the oral dose to guide further therapy.

Chronic Hypokalemia

The treatment of chronic hypokalemia depends entirely on identifying and, if possible, correcting the cause (see Fig. 101–4). When the cause of the excessive K^+ loss cannot be treated directly, K^+ supplementation or K^+-sparing diuretics should be considered.

References

1. Edelman IS, Leibman J: Anatomy of body water and electrolytes. Am J Med 27:256, 1959.
2. Knochel JP: Potassium gradients and neuromuscular excitability. In:

Seldin DW, Giebisch G (eds): The Kidney: Physiology and Pathophysiology, Volume 2. New York, Raven Press, p 1207, 1985.
3. Sterns RH, Spital A: Disorders of internal potassium balance. Semin Nephrol 7:399, 1987.
4. Sterns RH, Cox M, Feig PU, et al: Internal potassium balance and the control of the plasma potassium concentration. Medicine 60:339, 1981.
5. Cox M, Sterns RH, Singer I: The defense against hyperkalemia: The roles of insulin and aldosterone. N Engl J Med 299:525, 1978.
6. Bia MJ, DeFronzo RA: Extrarenal potassium homeostasis. Am J Physiol 240:F257, 1981.
7. DeFronzo RA, Bia M, Birkhead G: Epinephrine and potassium homeostasis. Kidney Int 20:83, 1981.
8. Brown RS: Extrarenal potassium homeostasis. Kidney Int 30:116, 1986.
9. Williams ME, Gervino EV, Rosa RM, et al: Catecholamine modulation of rapid potassium shifts during exercise. N Engl J Med 312:823, 1985.
10. Young DB: Quantitative analysis of aldosterone's role in potassium regulation. Am J Physiol 255:F811, 1988.
11. Sugarman A, Brown RS: The role of aldosterone in potassium tolerance: Studies in anephric humans. Kidney Int 34:397, 1988.
12. Clausen T, Everts ME: Regulation of the Na,K-pump in skeletal muscle. Kidney Int 35:1, 1989.
13. Kelley DE, Gharib H, Kennedy FP, et al: Thyrotoxic periodic paralysis: Report of 10 cases and review of electromyographic findings. Arch Intern Med 149:2597, 1989.
14. Alexander EA, Perrone RD: Regulation of extrarenal potassium metabolism. In: Maxwell MH, Kleeman CR, Narins RG (eds): Clinical Disorders of Fluid and Electrolyte Metabolism. 4th ed. New York, McGraw-Hill, 109, 1987.
15. Magner PO, Robinson L, Halperin RM, et al: The plasma potassium concentration in metabolic acidosis: A re-evaluation. Am J Kidney Dis 11:220, 1988.
16. Adrogue HJ, Madias NE: Changes in plasma potassium concentration during acute acid-base disturbances. Am J Med 71:456, 1981.
17. Oster JR, Perez GO, Castro A, et al: Plasma potassium response to acute metabolic acidosis induced by mineral and nonmineral acids. Miner Electrolyte Metab 4:28, 1980.
18. Orringer CE, Eustace JC, Wunsch CD, et al: Natural history of lactic acidosis after grand mal seizure: A model for the study of an anion-gap acidosis not associated with hyperkalemia. N Engl J Med 297:796, 1977.
19. Fulop M: Serum potassium in lactic acidosis and ketoacidosis. N Engl J Med 300:1087, 1979.
20. Adrogue HJ, Lederer ED, Suki WN, et al: Determinants of plasma potassium levels in diabetic ketoacidosis. Medicine 65:163, 1986.
21. Fraley DS, Adler S: Correction of hyperkalemia by bicarbonate despite constant blood pH. Kidney Int 12:354, 1977.
22. Kassirer JP, Schwartz WB: The response of normal man to selective depletion of hydrochloric acid: Factors in the genesis of persistent gastric alkalosis. Am J Med 40:10, 1966.
23. Gennari FJ, Cohen JJ: Role of the kidney in potassium homeostasis: Lessons from acid-base disturbances. Kidney Int 8:1, 1975.
24. Goldfarb S, Cox M, Singer I, et al: Acute hyperkalemia induced by hyperglycemia: Hormonal mechanisms. Ann Intern Med 84:426, 1976.
25. Conte G, Del Canton A, Imperatore P, et al: Acute increase in plasma osmolality as a cause of hyperkalemia in patients with renal failure. Kidney Int 38:301, 1990.
26. Makoff DL, DaSilva JA, Rosenbaum BJ: On the mechanism of hyperkalemia due to hyperosmotic expansion with saline or mannitol. Clin Sci 41:383, 1971.
27. Band DM, Lim M, Linton RAF, et al: Changes in arterial plasma potassium during exercise. J Physiol (Lond) 321:74P, 1982.
28. Don BR, Sebastian A, Cheitlin M, et al: Pseudohyperkalemia caused by fist clenching during phlebotomy. N Engl J Med 322:1290, 1990.
29. Sebastian A, Schambelan M: Renal hyperkalemia. Semin Nephrol 7:223, 1987.
30. Schwartz WB: Potassium and the kidney. N Engl J Med 253:601, 1955.
31. Squires RD, Huth EJ: Experimental potassium depletion in normal humans: I. Relation of ionic intakes to the renal conservation of potassium. J Clin Invest 38:1134, 1959.
32. Eaton SB, Konner M: Paleolithic nutrition: A consideration of its nature and current implications. N Engl J Med 312:283, 1985.
33. Wright FS, Giebisch G: Regulation of potassium excretion. In: Seldin DW, Giebisch G (eds): The Kidney: Physiology and Pathophysiology, Volume 2. New York, Raven Press, p 1223, 1985.
34. Melby JC: Primary aldosteronism. Kidney Int 26:769, 1984.
35. Field MJ, Giebisch GJ: Hormonal control of renal potassium excretion. Kidney Int 276:379, 1985.
36. Whang R, Oei TO, Aikawa JK, et al: Magnesium and potassium interrelationships: Experimental and clinical. Acta Med Scand Suppl 647:125, 1981.
37. Wacker WEC, Parisi AF: Magnesium metabolism. N Engl J Med 278:712, 1968.
38. Dyckner T: Relation of cardiovascular disease to potassium and magnesium deficiencies. Am J Cardiol 65:44K, 1990.
39. Sterns RH, Guzzo J, Feig PU: The disposition of intravenous potassium in normal man: The role of insulin. Clin Sci 61:23, 1981.
40. Keith NM, Osterberg AE, Burchell HB: Some effects of potassium salts in man. Ann Intern Med 16:879, 1942.
41. Ponce SP, Jennings AE, Madias NE, et al: Drug-induced hyperkalemia. Medicine 64:357, 1985.
42. Lawson DH: Adverse reactions to potassium chloride. Q J Med 43:433, 1974.
43. Rimmer JM, Horn JF, Gennari FJ: Hyperkalemia as a complication of drug therapy. Arch Intern Med 147:867, 1987.
44. Lankton JW, Siler JN, Neigh JL: Hyperkalemia after administration of potassium from non-rigid parenteral fluid containers. Anesthesiology 39:660, 1973.
45. Perez GO, Oster JR, Pelleya R, et al: Hyperkalemia from single small oral doses of potassium. Nephron 36:270, 1984.
46. Dodge HT, Grant RP, Seavey PW: The effect of induced hyperkalemia on the normal and abnormal electrocardiogram. Am Heart J 45:725, 1953.
47. Hultgren HN, Swenson R, Wettach G: Cardiac arrest due to oral potassium administration. Am J Med 58:139, 1975.
48. Hoyt RE: Hyperkalemia due to salt substitutes. JAMA 256:1726, 1986.
49. Mercer CW, Logic JR: Cardiac arrest due to hyperkalemia following intravenous penicillin administration. Chest 64:358, 1973.
50. Michael JM, Dorner I, Burns D et al: Potassium load in CPD-preserved whole blood and two types of packed red cells. Transfusion 15:144, 1975.
51. Jameson LC, Popic PM, Harms BA: Hyperkalemic death during use of a high-capacity fluid warmer for massive transfusion. Anesthesiology 73:1050, 1990.
52. Friedman BC, Bekes CE: Hyperkalemia post cardiac bypass: Etiology and management. Clin Intensive Care 2:174, 1991.
53. Weber DO, Yarnoz MO: Hyperkalemia complicating cardiopulmonary bypass: Analysis of risk factors. Ann Thorac Surg 34:439, 1982.
54. Soulillou JP, Fillaudeau F, Keribier JP, et al: Acute hyperkalemia risks in recipients of kidney graft cooled with Collins' solution. Nephron 19:301, 1977.
55. Cadman EC, Lundberg WB, Bertino JR: Hyperphosphatemia and hypocalcemia accompanying rapid cell lysis with Burkitt's lymphoma and Burkitt cell leukemia. Am J Med 62:283, 1977.
56. Fennelly JJ, Smyth H, Muldowney FP: Extreme hyperkalemia due to rapid lysis of leukemic cells. Lancet 1:27, 1974.
57. Muggia FM: Hyperkalemia and chemotherapy. Lancet 1:602, 1973.
58. Arseneau JC, Bagler CM, Anderson T, et al: Hyperkalemia, a sequel to chemotherapy of Burkitt's lymphoma. Lancet 1:10, 1973.
59. Better OS: Traumatic rhabdomyolysis ("crush syndrome")—Updated 1989. Isr J Med Sci 25:69, 1989.
60. Gabow PA, Kaehny WD, Kelleher SP: The spectrum of rhabdomyolysis. Medicine 61:141, 1982.
61. Cadnapaphornachai P, Taher S, McDonald FD: Acute drug-associated rhabdomyolysis: An examination of its diverse renal manifestations and complications. Am J Med Sci 280:66, 1980.
62. Curry SC, Chang D, Connor D: Drug- and toxin-induced rhabdomyolysis. Ann Emerg Med 18:1068, 1989.
63. Knochel JP: Rhabdomyolysis and myoglobinuria. Semin Nephrol 1:75, 1981.
64. Rubin RB, Neugarten J: Cocaine-induced rhabdomyolysis masquerading as myocardial ischemia. Am J Med 86:551, 1989.
65. Roth D, Alarcon FJ, Fernandez JA, et al: Acute rhabdomyolysis associated with cocaine intoxication. N Engl J Med 319:673, 1988.
66. Herzlich BC, Arsura EL, Pagala M, et al: Rhabdomyolysis related to cocaine abuse. Ann Intern Med 109:335, 1988.
67. Singhal PC, Faulkner M: Myonecrosis and cocaine abuse. Ann Intern Med 109:843, 1988.
68. Edelman S, Witztum JL: Hyperkalemia during treatment with HMG-CoA reductase inhibitor. N Engl J Med 320:1219, 1989.
69. Schorn TF, Knopse WH: Fatal delayed hemolytic transfusion reaction without previous blood transfusion. Ann Intern Med 110:241, 1989.
70. Smith TW, Butler VP, Haber E, et al: Treatment of life-threatening digitalis intoxication with digoxin-specific Fab antibody fragments: Experience in 26 cases. N Engl J Med 307:1357, 1982.
71. Gronert GR, Theye RA: Pathophysiology of hyperkalemia induced by succinylcholine. Anesthesiology 43:89, 1975.
72. Bushinski DA, Gennari FJ: Life-threatening hyperkalemia induced by arginine. Ann Intern Med 89:632, 1978.
73. Hertz P, Richardson JA: Arginine-induced hyperkalemia in renal failure patients. Arch Intern Med 130:778, 1972.
74. Ammon RA, May WS, Nightingale SD: Glucose-induced hyperkalemia with normal aldosterone levels: Studies in a patient with diabetes mellitus. Ann Intern Med 89:349, 1978.
75. Walker BR, Capuzzi DM, Alexander F, et al: Hyperkalemia after triamterene in diabetic patients. Clin Pharmacol Ther 13:643, 1972.
76. McNay JL, Oran E: Possible predisposition of diabetic patients to hyperkalemia following administration of potassium-retaining diuretic, amiloride (MK 870). Metabolism 19:58, 1970.
77. Morena M, Murphy C, Goldsmith C: Increase in serum potassium resulting from the administration of hypertonic mannitol and other solutions. J Lab Clin Med 73:291, 1969.
78. Buckell M: Blood changes on intravenous administration of mannitol or urea for reduction of intracranial pressure in neurosurgical patients. Clin Sci 27:223, 1964.
79. Gamstrop I: Adynamia episodica heriditaria: A disease clinically resem-

bling familial periodic paralysis but characterized by increasing serum potassium during the paralytic attacks. Am J Med 23:385, 1957.

80. Riggs JE: Periodic paralysis. Clin Neuropharmacol 12:249, 1989.
81. Knochel JP: Biochemical, electrolyte and acid-base disturbances in acute renal failure. In: Brenner BM, Lazarus JM (eds): Acute Renal Failure. 2nd ed. New York, Churchill Livingstone, p 683, 1988.
82. Goodship THJ, Butler PC, Rodham D, et al: Total-body potassium in insulin-dependent diabetes mellitus. Clin Sci 78:377, 1990.
83. Adrogue HJ, Lederer ED, Suki WN, et al: Determinants of plasma potassium levels in diabetic ketoacidosis. Medicine 65:163, 1986.
84. Beigelman PM: Severe diabetic ketoacidosis (diabetic "coma"): 482 episodes in 257 patients; Experience of three years. Diabetes 20:490, 1971.
85. Ionescu-Tirgoviste C, Mincu I: Danger of inadequate administration of potassium. Med J Aust 2:305, 1974.
86. Soler NG, Bennett MA, Dixon K, et al: Potassium balance during treatment of diabetic ketoacidosis: With special reference to the use of bicarbonate. Lancet 2:665, 1972.
87. Pullen H, Doig A, Lambie AT: Intensive intravenous potassium replacement therapy. Lancet 2:809, 1967.
88. Beigelman PM: Potassium in severe diabetic ketoacidosis. Am J Med 54:419, 1973.
89. Dorin RI, Crapo LM: Hypokalemic respiratory arrest in diabetic ketoacidosis. JAMA 257:1517, 1987.
90. Soler NG, Bennett MA, FitzGerald MG, et al: Intensive care in the management of diabetic ketoacidosis. Lancet 1:951, 1973.
91. Solomon MS, Kirby DF: The refeeding syndrome: A review. JPEN 14:90, 1990.
92. Weinsier RL, Krundieck CL: Death resulting from overzealous total parenteral nutrition: The refeeding syndrome revisited. Am J Clin Nutr 34:393, 1981.
93. Viens P, Thyss A, Garnier G, et al: GM-CSF treatment and hypokalemia. Ann Intern Med 111:263, 1989.
94. Lipworth BJ, McDevitt DG, Struthers AD: Prior treatment with diuretic augments the hypokalemic and electrocardiographic effects of inhaled albuterol. Am J Med 86:653, 1989.
95. Allon M, Dunlay R, Copkney C: Nebulized albuterol for acute hyperkalemia in patients on hemodialysis. Ann Intern Med 110:426, 1989.
96. Higgins RM, Cookson WOCM, Lane DG, et al: Cardiac arrhythmias caused by nebulized beta-agonist therapy. Lancet 2:863, 1985.
97. Brown MS, Brown DC, Murphy MB: Hypokalemia from beta$_2$-receptor stimulation by circulating epinephrine. N Engl J Med 309:1414, 1983.
98. Salerno D: Postresuscitation hypokalemia in a patient with a normal prearrest serum potassium level. Ann Intern Med 108:836, 1988.
99. Peach MJ: Cations: Calcium, magnesium, barium, lithium and ammonium. In: Goodman LS, Gilman A (eds): The Pharmacologic Basis of Therapeutics. 5th ed. New York, Macmillan, p 791, 1975.
100. Lewi Z, Bar-Khayim Y: Food-poisoning from barium carbonate. Lancet 2:342, 1964.
101. Diengott D, Rozsa O, Levy N: Hypokalemia in barium poisoning. Lancet 2:343, 1964.
102. Griggs RC, Engel WK, Resnick JS: Acetazolamide treatment of hypokalemic periodic paralysis: Prevention of attacks and improvement of persistent weakness. Ann Intern Med 73:39, 1970.
103. Nora NA, Berns AS: Hypokalemic, hypophosphatemic thyrotoxic periodic paralysis. Am J Kidney Dis 13:247, 1989.
104. Kelley DE, Gharib H, Kennedy FP, et al: Thyrotoxic periodic paralysis: Report of 10 cases and review of electromyographic findings. Arch Intern Med 149:2597, 1989.
105. Van Ypersele de Strihou C: Potassium homeostasis in renal failure. Kidney Int 11:491, 1977.
106. Mitch WE, Wilcox CS: Disorders of body fluids, sodium and potassium in chronic renal failure. Am J Med 72:536, 1982.
107. Gonick HC, Kleeman CR, Rubini ME, et al: Functional impairment in chronic renal disease. III: Studies of potassium excretion. Am J Med Sci 261:281, 1971.
108. Tuck ML, Davidson MB, Asp N, et al: Augmented aldosterone and insulin responses to potassium infusion in dogs with renal failure. Kidney Int 30:883, 1986.
109. DeFronzo RA: Hyperkalemia and hyporeninemic hypoaldosteronism. Kidney Int 17:118, 1980.
110. Burke CW: Adrenocortical insufficiency. Clin Endocrinol Metab 14:947, 1985.
111. Kalin MF, Poretsky L, Seres DS, et al: Hyporeninemic hypoaldosteronism associated with acquired immune deficiency syndrome. Am J Med 82:1035, 1987.
112. Lee FO, Quismorio FP, Troum OM, et al: Mechanisms of hyperkalemia in systemic lupus erythematosus. Arch Intern Med 148:397, 1988.
113. Glasgow BJ, Steinsapir KD, Anders K, et al: Adrenal pathology in the acquired immune deficiency syndrome. Am J Clin Pathol 84:595, 1985.
114. Membreno L, Irony I, Dere W, et al: Adrenocortical function in acquired immunodeficiency syndrome. J Clin Endocrinol Metab 65:482, 1987.
115. Gonzalez JJ, Werk EE Jr, Thrasher K, et al: Renin aldosterone system and potassium levels in chronic lead intoxication. South Med J 72:433, 1979.
116. Bethune DW, McKay R: Paradoxical changes in serum-potassium during cardiopulmonary bypass in association with noncardioselective beta-blockade. Lancet 2:380, 1978.
117. Lundborg P: The effect of adrenergic blockade on potassium concentrations in different conditions. Acta Med Scand Suppl 672:121, 1983.
118. Traub YM, Robinov M, Rosenfeld JB, et al: Elevation of serum potassium during beta blockade: Absence of relationship to the renin-aldosterone system. Clin Pharmacol Ther 28:765, 1980.
119. Kelleher S, Gillum D: Increased serum potassium due to combined calcium channel and beta adrenergic blockade. Kidney Int 27:142A, 1985.
120. Sugarman A, Kahn T: Calcium channel blockers enhance extrarenal potassium disposal in the rat. Am J Physiol 250:F695, 1986.
121. Lee TH, Salomon DR, Rayment CM, et al: Hypotension and sinus arrest with exercise-induced hyperkalemia and combined verapamil/propranolol therapy. Am J Med 80:1203, 1986.
122. Dunn MJ: Nonsteroidal anti-inflammatory drugs and renal function. Annu Rev Med 35:411, 1984.
123. Garella S, Matarese RA: Renal effects of prostaglandins and clinical adverse effects of nonsteroidal anti-inflammatory agents. Medicine 63:165, 1984.
124. Romero JC, Dunlap CL, Strong CG: The effect of indomethacin and other anti-inflammatory drugs on the renin-angiotensin system in man. J Clin Invest 58:282, 1976.
125. Goldzer RC, Coodlley EL, Rosner MJ, et al: Hyperkalemia associated with indomethacin. Arch Intern Med 141:802, 1980.
126. Tan SY, Shapiro R, Franco R, et al: Indomethacin-induced prostaglandin inhibition with hyperkalemia: A reversible cause of hyporeninemic hypoaldosteronism. Ann Intern Med 90:783, 1979.
127. Nesher G, Zimran A, Hershko C: Reduced incidence of hyperkalemia and azotemia in patients receiving sulindac compared with indomethacin. Nephron 48:291, 1988.
128. Textor SC, Bravo EL, Fouad FM, et al: Hyperkalemia in azotemic patients during angiotensin-converting enzyme inhibition and aldosterone reduction with captopril. Am J Med 73:719, 1982.
129. Edes TE, Sunderrajan EV: Heparin-induced hyperkalemia. Arch Intern Med 145:1070, 1985.
130. O'Kelly R, Maga F, McKenna TJ: Routine heparin therapy inhibits adrenal aldosterone production. J Clin Endocrinol Metab 56:108, 1983.
131. Durand D, Ader J-L, Rey J-P, et al: Inducing hyperkalemia by converting enzyme inhibitors and heparin. Kidney Int 34(suppl 25):S196, 1988.
132. Batlle D, Itsarayounguen K, Arruda JAL, et al: Hyperkalemic, hyperchloremic metabolic acidosis in sickle cell hemoglobinopathies. Am J Med 72:188, 1982.
133. DeFronzo RA, Cooke CR, Goldberg M, et al: Impaired renal tubular potassium secretion in systemic lupus erythematosus. Ann Intern Med 86:268, 1977.
134. DeFronzo RA, Goldberg M, Cooke CR, et al: Investigations into the mechanisms of hyperkalemia following renal transplantation. Kidney Int 11:357, 1977.
135. Batlle DC, Arruda JAL, Kurtzman NA: Hyperkalemic distal renal tubular acidosis associated with obstructive uropathy. N Engl J Med 304:373, 1981.
136. Krishna GG, Shulman MD, Narins RG: Clinical use of the potassium-sparing diuretics. Semin Nephrol 8:354, 1988.
137. Hollenberg NK, Mickiewicz C: Hyperkalemia in diabetes mellitus: Effect of a triamterene-hydrochlorothiazide combination. Arch Intern Med 149:1327, 1989.
138. Lachall M, Venuto RC: Nephrotoxicity and hyperkalemia in patients with acquired immunodeficiency syndrome treated with pentamidine. Am J Med 87:260, 1989.
139. Adu D, Turney J, Michael J, et al: Hyperkalemia in cyclosporin-treated renal allograft recipients. Lancet 2:370, 1983.
140. Womersley RA, Darragh JH: Potassium and sodium restriction in the normal human. J Clin Invest 34:456, 1955.
141. Halevy J, Gunsherowitz M, Rosenfeld JB: Life-threatening hypokalemia in hospitalized patients. Miner Electrolyte Metab 14:163, 1988.
142. Elkinton JR, Huth EJ: Body fluid abnormalities in anorexia nervosa and undernutrition. Metabolism 8:376, 1959.
143. Fordtran JS, Dietschy JM: Water and electrolyte movement in the intestine. Gastroenterology 50:263, 1966.
144. Rabinowitz P, Farber M, Friedman IS: A depletion syndrome in villous adenoma of the rectum. Arch Intern Med 109:265, 1962.
145. Shields R: Absorption and secretion of electrolytes and water by the human colon with particular reference to benign adenoma and papilloma. Br J Surg 53:893, 1966.
146. Fleischer N, Brown H, Graham DY, et al: Chronic laxative-induced hyperaldosteronism and hypokalemia simulating Bartter's syndrome. Ann Intern Med 70:791, 1969.
147. Walmsley RN, White GH: Occult causes of hypokalemia. Clin Chem 30:1406, 1984.
148. Velazquez H, Giebisch G: Effect of diuretics on specific transport systems: Potassium. Semin Nephrol 8:295, 1988.
149. Nader PC, Thompson JR, Alpern RJ: Complications of diuretic use. Semin Nephrol 8:365, 1988.
150. Clements JS, Peacock JE: Amphotericin B revisited: Reassessment of toxicity. Am J Med 88:5–22N, 1990.
151. Douglas JB, Healy JK: Nephrotoxic effects of amphotericin B, including renal tubular acidosis. Am J Med 46:154, 1969.
152. Barton CH, Pahl M, Vaziri ND, et al: Renal magnesium wasting associated with amphotericin B therapy. Am J Med 77:471, 1984.

153. Klatersky J, Vanderkelen B, Daneua D, et al: Carbenicillin and hypokalemia. Ann Intern Med 78:774, 1973.
154. Hura CE, Junau RT, Stein JH: Use of diuretics in salt-retaining states. Semin Nephrol 8:318, 1988.
155. Shils ME: Experimental production of magnesium deficiency in man. Ann NY Acad Sci 162:847, 1969.
156. Whang R: Magnesium deficiency: Pathogenesis, prevalence and clinical implications. Am J Med 82(suppl 3A):24, 1987.
157. Brautbar N, Massry SG: Disorders of magnesium metabolism. In: Maxwell MH, Kleeman CR, Narins RG (eds): Clinical Disorders of Fluid and Electrolyte Metabolism. 4th ed. New York, McGraw-Hill, p 831, 1987.
158. Blachley JD, Hill JB: Renal and electrolyte disturbances associated with cisplatin. Ann Intern Med 95:628, 1981.
159. Aldinger KA, Samaan NA: Hypokalemia with hypercalcemia: Prevalence and significance in treatment. Ann Intern Med 87:571, 1977.
160. Bartter FC, Pronove P, Gill JR Jr, et al: Hyperplasia of the juxtaglomerular complex with hyperaldosteronism and hypokalemic alkalosis. Am J Med 33:811, 1962.
161. Liddle GW, Bledsoe T, Coppage WS Jr: A familial renal disorder simulating primary aldosteronism but with negligible aldosterone secretion. Trans Assoc Am Physicians 76:199, 1963.
162. Ladenson JH, Tsai LB, Michael JM, et al: Serum versus heparinized plasma for eighteen common chemistry tests. Am J Clin Pathol 62:545, 1974.
163. Hartmann RC, Auditore JV, Jackson SP, et al: Studies on thrombocytosis: I. Hyperkalemia due to release of potassium from platelets during coagulation. J Clin Invest 37:699, 1958.
164. Graber M, Subramani K, Corish D, et al: Thrombocytosis and serum potassium. Am J Kidney Dis 12:116, 1988.
165. Bronson WR, DeVita VT, Carbone PP, et al: Pseudohyperkalemia due to release of potassium from white blood cells during clotting. N Engl J Med 274:369, 1966.
166. Ladenson JH: Nonanalytical sources of variation in clinical chemistry results. In: Sonnenwirth AC, Jarett L (eds): Gradwohl's Clinical Laboratory Methods and Diagnosis. St Louis, CV Mosby, p 176, 1980.
167. Fisch C: Relation of electrolyte disturbances to cardiac arrhythmias. Circulation 47:408, 1973.
168. Surawicz B: Relationship between electrocardiogram and electrolytes. Am Heart J 73:814, 1967.
169. Szerlip HM, Weiss J, Singer I: Profound hyperkalemia without electrocardiographic manifestations. Am J Kidney Dis 7:461, 1986.
170. Weiner M, Epstein FH: Signs and symptoms of electrolyte disorders. Yale J Biol Med 43:76, 1970.
171. Tannen RL: Relationship of renal ammonia production and potassium homeostasis. Kidney Int 11:453, 1977.
172. Szylman P, Better OS, Chaimowitz C, et al: Role of hyperkalemia in the metabolic acidosis of isolated hypoaldosteronism. N Engl J Med 294:362, 1976.
173. Steiness E: Diuretics, digitalis and arrhythmias. Acta Med Scand Suppl 647:75, 1981.
174. Peters RW, Hamilton J, Hamilton BP: Incidence of cardiac arrhythmias associated with mild hypokalemia induced by low-dose diuretic therapy for hypertension. South Med J 82:966, 1989.
175. Holland QB, Nixon JV, Kuhnert L: Diuretic-induced ventricular ectopic activity. Am J Cardiol 52:1017, 1983.
176. Nordrehaug JE, Von Der Lippe G: Hypokalemia and ventricular fibrillation in acute myocardial infarction. Br Heart J 50:525, 1983.
177. Knochel JP, Schlein EM: On the mechanism of rhabdomyolysis in potassium depletion. J Clin Invest 51:1750, 1972.
178. Drotz DJ, Fan JH, Tai TY, et al: Hypokalemic rhabdomyolysis and myoglobinuria following amphotericin B therapy. JAMA 211:824, 1970.
179. Grunfeld C, Chappell DA: Hypokalemia and diabetes mellitus. Am J Med 75:553, 1983.
180. Walker WG, Sapir DG, Turin M, et al: Potassium homeostasis and diuretic therapy. In: Lant AF, Wilson GM (eds): Modern Diuretic Therapy in the Treatment of Cardiovascular and Renal Disease. Amsterdam, Excerpta Medica, p 331, 1973.
181. Berl T, Linas SL, Aisenbrey GA, et al: On the mechanism of polyuria in potassium depletion: The role of polydipsia. J Clin Invest 60:620, 1977.
182. Mannitius A, Levitin H, Beck D, et al: On the mechanism of renal concentrating ability in potassium deficiencies. J Clin Invest 39:684, 1960.
183. Jones JW, Sebastian A, Hurter HN, et al: Systemic and renal acid-base effects of chronic dietary potassium depletion in humans. Kidney Int 21:402, 1982.
184. Gabuzda GS, Hall PW: Relation of potassium depletion to renal ammonium metabolism and hepatic coma. Medicine 45:481, 1966.
185. Welt AG, Hollander W, Blythe WB: The consequences of potassium depletion. J Chronic Dis 11:213, 1960.
186. Kamel KS, Ethier JH, Richardson RMA, et al: Urine electrolytes and osmolality: When and how to use them. Am J Nephrol 10:89, 1990.
187. Zettle RM, West ML, Josee RG, et al: Renal potassium handling during states of low aldosterone bio-activity: A method to differentiate renal and non-renal causes. Am J Nephrol 7:360, 1987.
188. Rose BD: Hyperkalemia. In: Rose BD (ed): Clinical Physiology of Acid-Base and Electrolyte Disorders. 3rd ed. New York, McGraw-Hill, p 633, 1990.
189. DeFronzo RA: Hyperkalemic states. In: Maxwell MH, Kleeman CR, Narins RG (eds): Clinical Disorders of Fluid and Electrolyte Metabolism. 4th ed. New York, McGraw-Hill, p 572, 1987.
190. Chamberlain MJ: Emergency treatment of hyperkalemia. Lancet 1:464, 1964.
191. Iqbal Z, Friedman EA: Preferred therapy of hyperkalemia in renal insufficiency: Survey of nephrology training-program directors (letter). N Engl J Med 320:60, 1989.
192. Batlle DC, Salem M, Levin ML, et al: More on therapy for hyperkalemia in renal insufficiency (letter). N Engl J Med 320:1496, 1989.
193. Spital A: More on therapy for hyperkalemia in renal insufficiency (letter). N Engl J Med 320:1497, 1989.
194. Bower JO, Mengle HAK: The additive effect of calcium and digitalis: A warning with a report of two deaths. JAMA 106:1151, 1936.
195. Shrager MW: Digitalis intoxication. Arch Intern Med 100:881, 1957.
196. Garcia-Palmieri MR: Reversal of hyperkalemic cardiotoxicity with hypertonic saline. Am Heart J 64:483, 1962.
197. Ballantyne F, Davis LD, Reynolds EW Jr: Cellular basis for reversal of hyperkalemic electrocardiographic changes by sodium. Am J Physiol 229:935, 1975.
198. Blumberg A, Weidmann P, Shaw S, et al: Effect of various therapeutic approaches on plasma potassium and major regulating factors in terminal renal failure. Am J Med 85:507, 1988.
199. Allon M, Copkney C: Albuterol and insulin for treatment of hyperkalemia in hemodialysis patients. Kidney Int 38:869, 1990.
200. Davies DL, Lant AF, Millard NR, et al: Renal action, therapeutic use, and pharmacokinetics of the diuretic bumetanide. Clin Pharmacol Ther 15:141, 1974.
201. Wooton FT, Rhodes DF, Lee WM, et al: Colonic necrosis with Kayexalate-sorbitol enemas after renal transplantation. Ann Intern Med 111:947, 1989.
202. Feig PU, Shook A, Sterns RA: Effects of potassium removal during hemodialysis on the plasma potassium concentration. Nephron 27:25, 1981.
203. Hou S, McElroy PA, Nootens J, et al: Safety and efficacy of low-potassium dialysate. Am J Kidney Dis 13:137, 1989.
204. Brown ST, Ahearn DJ, Nolph KD: Potassium removal with peritoneal dialysis. Kidney Int 4:67, 1973.
205. Sterns RH, Feig PU, Pring M, et al: Disposition of intravenous potassium in anuric man: A kinetic analysis. Kidney Int 15:651, 1979.
206. Kruse JA, Carlson RW: Rapid correction of hypokalemia using concentrated intravenous potassium chloride infusions. Arch Intern Med 150:613, 1990.
207. Manning SH, Angaran DM, Arom KV, et al: Intermittent intravenous potassium therapy in cardiopulmonary bypass patients. Clin Pharm 1:234, 1982.
208. Keith NM, Osterberg AE: The tolerance for potassium in severe renal insufficiency: A study of ten cases. J Clin Invest 26:773, 1947.

CHAPTER 102

Clinical Disorders of Calcium and Magnesium Metabolism in Critically Ill Patients

Michael A. Geheb
Tusar K. Desai

CALCIUM HOMEOSTASIS IN CRITICALLY ILL PATIENTS

With the advent of an economic ion-selective electrode that can rapidly and accurately measure ionized calcium in plasma, there has been a renewal of interest in monitoring plasma calcium in clinical settings.[1] In view of the central role of calcium in the regulation of multiple cellular events (including important aspects of vascular, neurologic, and renal electrolyte biology), disorders of calcium regulation can potentially lead to disorders of substantial clinical significance.[2, 3]

Internal Calcium Distribution

Calcium biology has been extensively reviewed elsewhere and is only briefly summarized here.[4, 5] Under normal circumstances (Fig. 102–1), there is approximately 1200 g (30,000 mmol) of calcium in a 70-kg adult and more than 99% of it is contained in bone. Only 1% of total body calcium or 5.6 g (139 mmol) is distributed between the intracellular (4.3 g, 107 mmol) and the extracellular (1.3 g, 33 mmol) compartments.

External Calcium Balance (Fig. 102–2)

Although ingestion of calcium may vary greatly, a calcium intake of approximately 1000 mg/d (250 mmol/d) is required in a young adult to maintain normal balance. Of this 1000 mg ingested, approximately 800 mg (200 mmol) is excreted in the stool and 200 mg (50 mmol) is absorbed, primarily in the jejunum. Of the calcium filtered through the glomerulus (approximately 10,000 mg/d, 2500 mmol/d), 98% (9800 mg/d, 2450 mmol/d) is reabsorbed and 2% (200 mg/d, 50 mmol/d) is excreted in the urine. Thus, approximately 200 mg (50 mmol) of calcium is absorbed and excreted each day to maintain normal daily balance. Approximately 600 mg (150 mmol) of calcium is exchanged daily between the bone and the extracellular fluid. Daily requirements to maintain calcium balance change radically with age: growing children and young adults require more calcium during active bone formation stages, whereas daily requirements and the ability to absorb calcium decline in the elderly.[4–6]

Extracellular Calcium

Circulating extracellular calcium exists in three forms: protein-bound calcium (approximately 40%); diffusible, nonionized chelates (phosphates, sulfates, citrates, and bicarbonates) of calcium (approximately 15%); and free ionized calcium (approximately 45%), which is the physiologically active fraction (Fig. 102–3).[4, 5, 7, 8] Protein-bound calcium is bound primarily to albumin (70 to 90%); the rest (10 to 30%) is bound to alpha- and beta-globulins. Thus, decreases in serum albumin (which occur frequently in acutely ill patients) cause large declines in extracellular total calcium concentrations. Hypoalbuminemia is also directly associated with decreased concentrations of ionized calcium (Fig. 102–4).[9, 10] Changes in pH alter the binding of calcium to circulating proteins, so that ionized calcium may vary actively without a change in total measured calcium. Acidosis decreases protein binding (increases ionized calcium), whereas alkalosis increases protein binding (decreases ionized calcium).[8, 11] Elevations in free fatty acid levels (which can occur in critically ill patients) increase binding of albumin to calcium and further complicate the ability to estimate ionized calcium from measurements of total calcium and protein.[12] Considering the complexity of these relationships, direct measurement of ionized calcium is needed to evaluate the physiologically active fraction.[10, 12, 13] This is now readily accomplished using ion-selective membrane electrodes. By convention, the ionized calcium value is corrected to a standard pH (usually 7.4), although correction to the patient's arterial pH may have more physiologic significance. At this time, tissue pH is not available as a clinical measurement, although it probably would be the most relevant value. Proper handling of blood specimens under anaerobic conditions (similar to those for blood gas analysis), with minimal delay before measurement, is imperative for accurate determinations.

Maintenance of a constant extracellular concentration of ionized calcium is carefully modulated. The mean ionized calcium value in normal individuals is 1.24 ± 0.03 mmol/L (5.0 ± 0.12 mg; mean ± SD).[6, 10] Thus, extracellular ionized

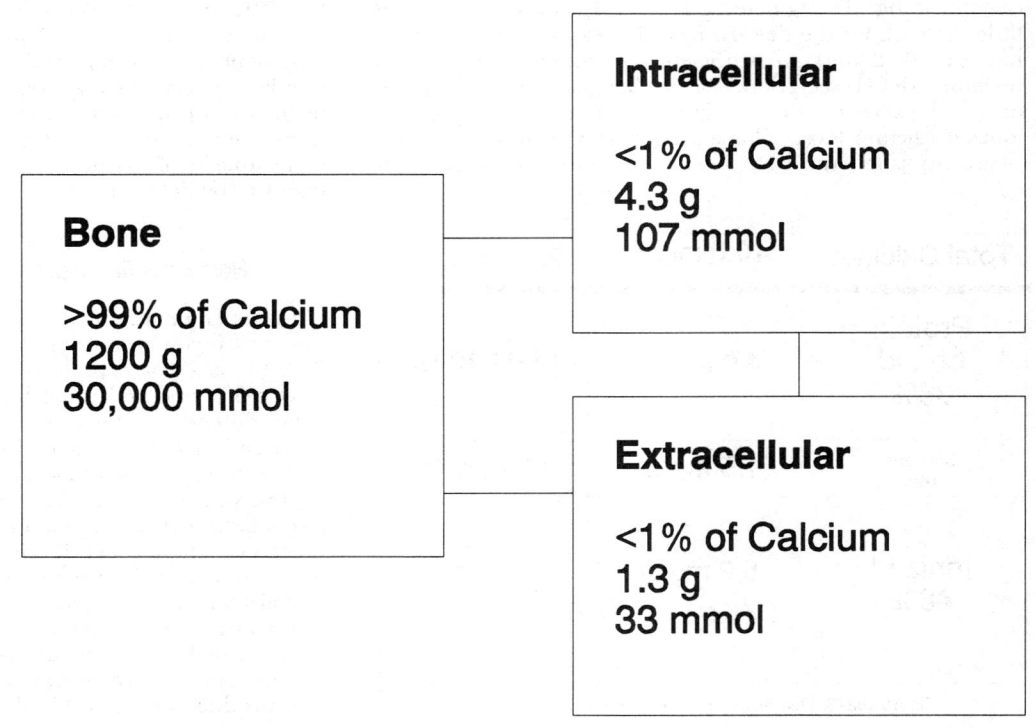

Figure 102–1. Distribution of total body calcium.

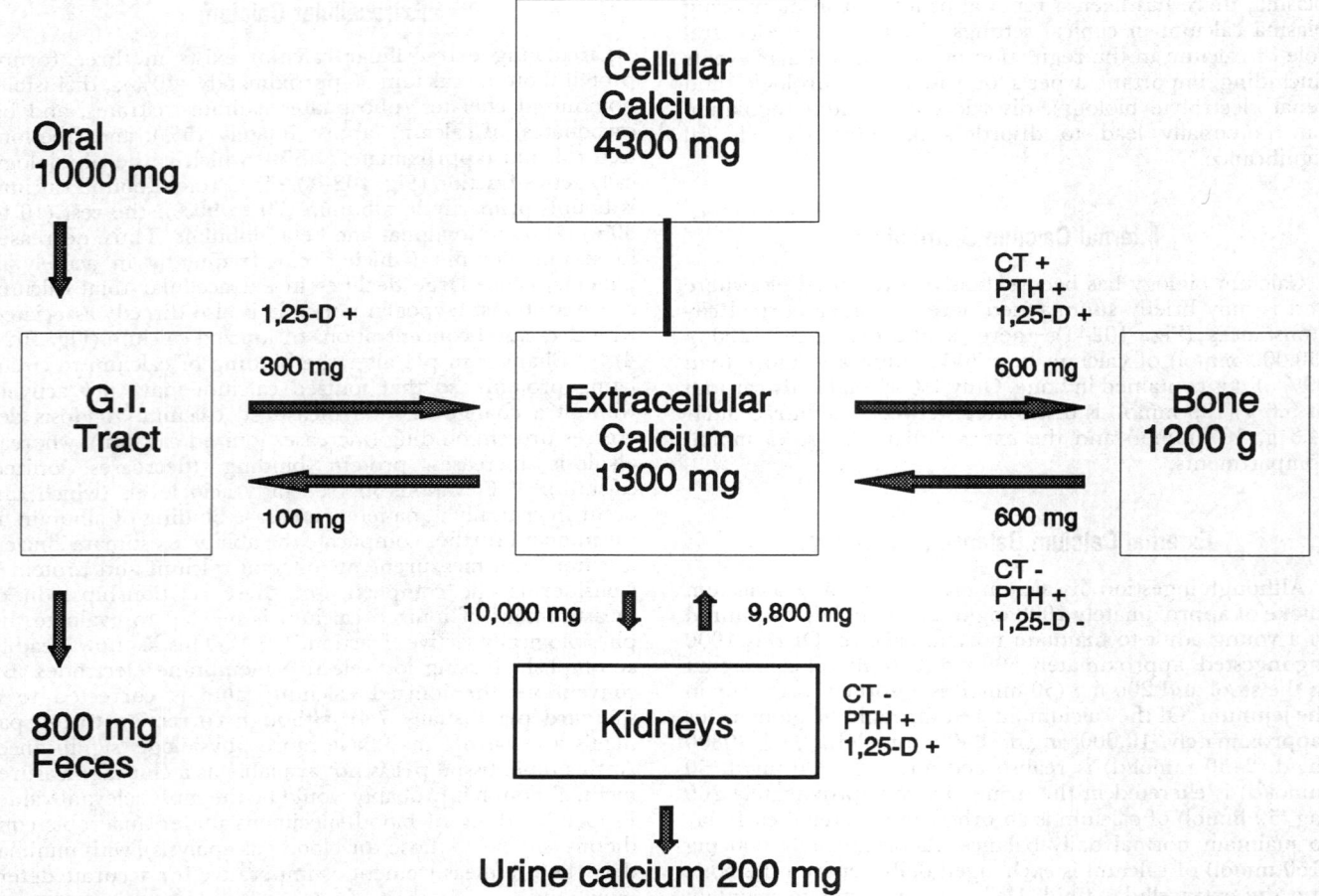

Figure 102–2. Calcium physiology. The distribution of body calcium is shown. On a daily basis, 200 mg of calcium is absorbed in net from the gut and 200 mg is excreted in the urine, thus maintaining balance. 1,25-D = calcitriol; CT = calcitonin; PTH = parathyroid hormone. The + and − signs indicate the effect of the hormone on the fluxes of calcium. Although PTH promotes both bone uptake and resorption, at high levels bone resorption predominates.

calcium is tightly regulated within a 5% range and varies little throughout the day. In fact, decreases as small as 0.03 mmol/L (0.12 mg) are sufficient to stimulate parathyroid hormone (PTH) secretion.[6] Large changes in gut absorption or renal excretion do not lead to substantial changes in ionized calcium level. This extraordinary degree of control is accomplished through the interaction of three calcium-regulating hormones (parathyroid-stimulating hormone, calcitonin, and the vitamin D sterols) and three organ systems (gut, bone, and kidney).[4–6] The existence of another calcium-regulating hormone (gastrocalcin) has been suggested.[14] This hormone is produced in the stomach in response to gastrin stimulation and can lead to hypocalcemia by stimulating bone uptake of calcium. Its role in human physiology remains to be determined.

Hormonal Regulation of Extracellular Calcium

The hormonal regulation of extracellular calcium is intricate and involves multiple feedback loops[4–6] (see Fig. 102–2). PTH is a polypeptide hormone that has many complex effects on bone and renal function, but in general it is the major defender of the organism against hypocalcemia. Small decreases in circulating ionized calcium (<2.5%) stimulate PTH release and elevated concentrations of ionized calcium suppress it.[6] PTH activates bone remodeling by stimulating osteoblastic activity and increasing the number of osteoclasts; however, when PTH levels are elevated and sustained, osteoclastic activity predominates, leading to net calcium mobilization and an increase in circulating calcium. PTH stimulates renal conservation of calcium by promoting reabsorption of filtered calcium from renal tubular fluid. PTH also increases the renal excretion of phosphate and activates the production of 1,25-dihydroxyvitamin D_3 (calcitriol).

Total Calcium	10.5 mg/dL	2.61 mmol/L
Protein bound 38%	4.0 mg/dL	1.00 mmol/L
Chelates 14%	1.5 mg/dL	.37 mmol/L
Ionized 48%	5.0 mg/dL	1.24 mmol/L

Figure 102–3. Distribution of extracellular calcium.

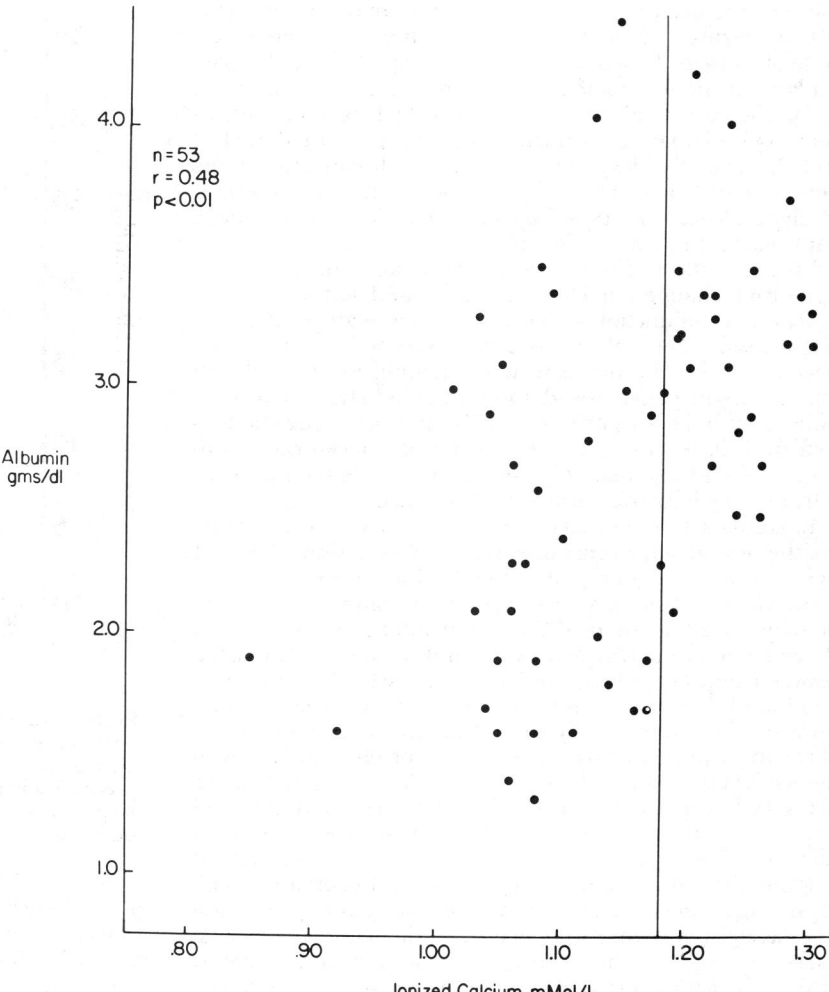

Ionized Calcium vs. Albumin
Patients with No Clinically Identifiable Disorders
of Calcium Metabolism

n = 53
r = 0.48
p < 0.01

Albumin
gms/dl

Ionized Calcium mMol/L

Figure 102–4. Relationship between ionized calcium and serum albumin. (From Desai TK, Carlson RW, Geheb MA: Prevalence and clinical implications of hypocalcemia in acutely ill patients in a medical intensive care unit. Am J Med 84:209, 1988.)

Thus, the concerted actions of PTH converge to preserve or elevate the extracellular calcium concentration.

Calcitonin is a polypeptide hormone that counterbalances many of the effects of PTH.[4–6] It inhibits osteoclastic activity and stimulates osteoblastic activity. It leads to renal calcium retention and induces the production of calcitriol. Its role in adults remains questionable because many of its effects are easily overridden. Calcitonin is probably most important in the growing animal, in which it diverts absorbed calcium to bone.

Calcitriol is the most potent of the vitamin D steroid hormones.[4–6] Its production in proximal tubules of the renal cortex is stimulated by PTH, hypophosphatemia, and calcitonin. Its major delineated action is to stimulate increased absorption of calcium from the small bowel (jejunum). Calcitriol also has many complicated effects at the bone level that facilitate bone remodeling.

Acting in concert, these calcitrophic hormones regulate calcium balance and maintain extracellular calcium at a remarkably constant level (see Fig. 102–2).

DISORDERS OF CALCIUM REGULATION: HYPOCALCEMIA

The most common problem in calcium homeostasis encountered in the critically ill patient is hypocalcemia.[10, 15, 16]

In physiologic terms, hypocalcemia may be considered secondary to the failure of the PTH and vitamin D feedback systems. It may result from an inadequate PTH response to hypocalcemia, vitamin D deficiency, or skeletal resistance to either hormone. In unusual circumstances, it can also result from an excess calcitonin effect. However, the influence of severe acute systemic illness on these homeostatic processes has not been well studied.

Clinical Manifestations
Cardiovascular Disorders

The cardiovascular effects of hypocalcemia are of the greatest concern in the acute care setting. Experimental animal studies have demonstrated a direct correlation between the concentration of calcium in the extracellular fluid and cardiac contractility[17] as well as vascular smooth muscle tension.[18] Ultrastructural studies of various muscle types show differences in the extent of sarcoplasmic reticulum present, with skeletal muscle having the most extensive network, cardiac muscle having an intermediate network, and vascular smooth muscle having the sparsest network.[19] Calcium ions needed to initiate contraction in skeletal muscle are derived almost entirely from its extensive intrinsic network of sarcoplasmic reticulum, whereas cardiac muscle is more dependent upon extracellular calcium as a source. Vascular smooth muscle depends almost entirely on extracellular calcium to initiate contraction.[20] Therefore, it is not surprising that acute drops in extracellular calcium concentration have been reported to precipitate hypotension[21] and left ventricular dysfunction[22-24] with little or no effect on skeletal muscle. Patients with cardiomyopathy may be particularly prone to hypotension or congestive heart failure in the presence of ionized hypocalcemia.[25] Chronic congestive heart failure may be refractory to therapy with digitalis[26] and diuretics or even parenteral sympathomimetic agents (dobutamine) in the presence of hypocalcemia.[25] Correction of hypocalcemia in these patients may lead to dramatic improvement in cardiac function.[27]

Patients with end-stage renal disease also show clinically significant changes in blood pressure and left ventricular function in conjunction with changes in circulatory calcium.[23] Hypotension and left ventricular dysfunction have been associated with the decrease in circulating ionized calcium that occurs in patients undergoing hemodialysis[28] and continuous ambulatory peritoneal dialysis;[29] increasing the ionized calcium level by using either a high-concentration calcium bath during hemodialysis or intravenous infusion of calcium may improve cardiac performance.

In contrast to the observations in patients with cardiomyopathy or end-stage renal disease, the clinical significance of hypocalcemia in acutely ill patients with otherwise normal cardiovascular function remains to be established. In a series of patients admitted to the medical intensive care unit of Detroit Receiving Hospital, we found a direct relationship between ionized calcium and blood pressure.[30] This study also found that the patients with low levels of ionized calcium were not only more likely to be hypotensive but also more likely to require pressor agents. Conversely, patients with higher levels of ionized calcium were less likely to require pressors to support blood pressure. Hypertension occurred only in patients with greater than normal levels of ionized calcium. These patients were admitted with a variety of diagnoses. In all categories, hypocalcemia, hypotension, and sepsis were associated and normocalcemia and hypertension were associated. Other studies have evaluated the cardiovascular effects of calcium infusion: in addition to the pressor effect of calcium, left ventricular performance is improved. The increase in circulating calcium after calcium infusion is temporary, as are the vasopressor and other hemodynamic effects. We have also found that the pressor response to calcium infusion varies inversely with the serum potassium concentration (Fig. 102–5).

Changes of ionized calcium can also affect the electrocardiogram. These effects include prolongation of the QT interval; however, these findings are not specific enough to be of great use for acutely ill patients, who may have multiple other metabolic abnormalities that confound the electrocardiographic interpretation.[4, 7] A single case of torsades de pointes that resolved with correction of hypocalcemia has been described.[31] In our experience, the typical electrocardiographic findings seen in hypocalcemia do not appear to predict which patients will develop cardiovascular compromise. Consequently, although these findings may be of interest to the cardiac electrophysiologist, they are of little practical value to the intensivist.

Neuromuscular Disorders

Neuromuscular irritability, manifested in its most severe forms as seizures and tetany, can also occur in hypocalcemia.[32] Ionized calcium should always be evaluated in the critically ill patient who has neuromuscular instability. Although there are no direct data of which we are aware, in

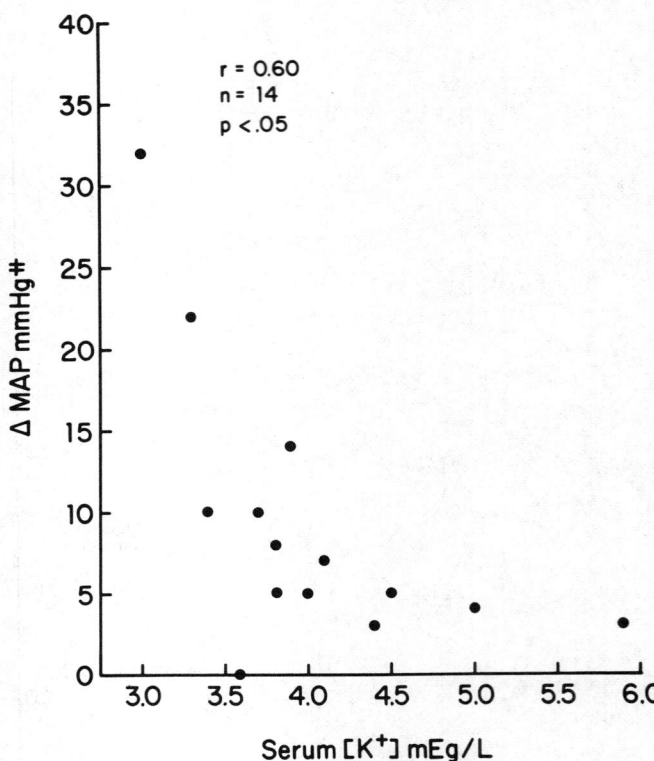

Figure 102–5. Change in mean arterial pressure (MAP) versus pre-infusion serum potassium. Calcium chloride (5 mg/kg) was infused during 20 minutes into patients. The increase in mean arterial pressure was inversely related to the preinfusion concentration of serum potassium. (From Desai TK, Carlson RW, Geheb MA: unpublished observation.)

our experience severe signs of neuromuscular instability are unusual even in patients with severe ionized hypocalcemia. Virtually all of these patients have mental status changes, and it has been difficult to define their relationship to hypocalcemia. In the absence of overt signs of neuromuscular irritability, calcium therapy is not required.

Incidence of Ionized Hypocalcemia in the Medical Intensive Care Unit

The common conditions associated with hypocalcemia in critically ill patients are listed in Table 102–1. In addition, many patients who are severely ill may, with no clear cause, present with hypocalcemia.[10] Several reports have alerted intensive care practitioners to the high prevalence of ionized hypocalcemia in acutely ill patients. However, the reported incidence of this phenomenon ranges widely.[8, 10, 16, 30] The variation in the reported prevalence appears to be related to the severity of illness of the population reported: in populations of patients who are more severely ill, the incidence of ionized hypocalcemia appears to be higher. Chernow and colleagues studied patients in a naval hospital intensive care unit and found an approximately 10% incidence of ionized hypocalcemia.[16] Our experience suggests that in other intensive care populations, ionized hypocalcemia is more common.[10, 30] In the Detroit Receiving Hospital intensive care unit, approximately two thirds of the patients are admitted with ionized hypocalcemia (Fig. 102–6). As the major trauma and critical care center for a large metropolitan area, this hospital primarily serves patients drawn from

TABLE 102–1

CAUSES OF HYPOCALCEMIA

Infection and septic shock
Circulatory shock and cardiac arrest
Renal failure
Acid-base disorders
Chelation
Pancreatitis
Burns
Miscellaneous
    Primary hypoparathyroidism
    Pseudohypoparathyroidism
    Anticonvulsant drugs
    Plicamycin (mithramycin)
    Colchicine

a medically indigent inner city population, in which malnutrition and other chronic health problems are common. This was corroborated when we evaluated patients at Harper Hospital, a tertiary care university hospital with a large cancer center. At this institution, the incidence of ionized hypocalcemia still approached 40% and the condition was seen predominantly in the extremely ill oncologic patients admitted to the intensive care unit. Ionized hypocalcemia is associated with poor outcomes in acutely ill patients.[15] In our series,[10] the mortality rate was four times greater in the hypocalcemic patients (Fig. 102–7). The presence of ionized hypocalcemia seems to correlate with the severity of illness (although direct correlations with severity of illness indices have not been performed). Although multiple causes can be identified (see Table 102–1) in a number of cases, no underlying pathophysiologic cause can be found.

Infection and Septic Shock

The hypocalcemia associated with various forms of infection and septic shock has been difficult to evaluate. Experimental septic shock in the baboon is associated with ionized hypocalcemia.[33] Hypocalcemia in conjunction with the toxic shock syndrome induced by certain strains of *Staphylococcus aureus* is well described.[34] The association of hypocalcemia and sepsis, especially gram-negative sepsis, in humans has been established.[30, 35, 36] The underlying biologic basis for hypocalcemia in these patients remains unclear. However, it is postulated that calcium moves from the extracellular compartment into cells and that the hormonal response to defend against hypocalcemia is inadequate. Zaloga and Chernow reported several different hormonal responses to the hypocalcemia in gram-negative sepsis, including acquired PTH insufficiency, renal 1α-hydroxylase deficiency, vitamin D deficiency, and acquired calcitriol resistance.[35] In experimental studies, endotoxin appears to lead to impaired calcium mobilization from bone.[37] Other studies from our institution suggest that hypoalbuminemic patients (in whom sepsis is more common) have inadequate PTH responses. Our data also demonstrate a direct relationship between 25-hydroxyvitamin D_3 levels and the ionized calcium level.[38] Both hypoalbuminemia and 25-hydroxyvitamin D_3 levels are probably indicative of underlying malnutrition, which is seen commonly in medically indigent patients. Thus, the hypocalcemia of sepsis appears to be marked by a confused hormonal response.

The mechanisms that define the associations between various infectious states (whether toxic shock or gram-negative sepsis) and calcium metabolism are now being delineated. In toxic shock syndrome, although PTH levels increase, high levels of calcitonin have also been described.[34] The

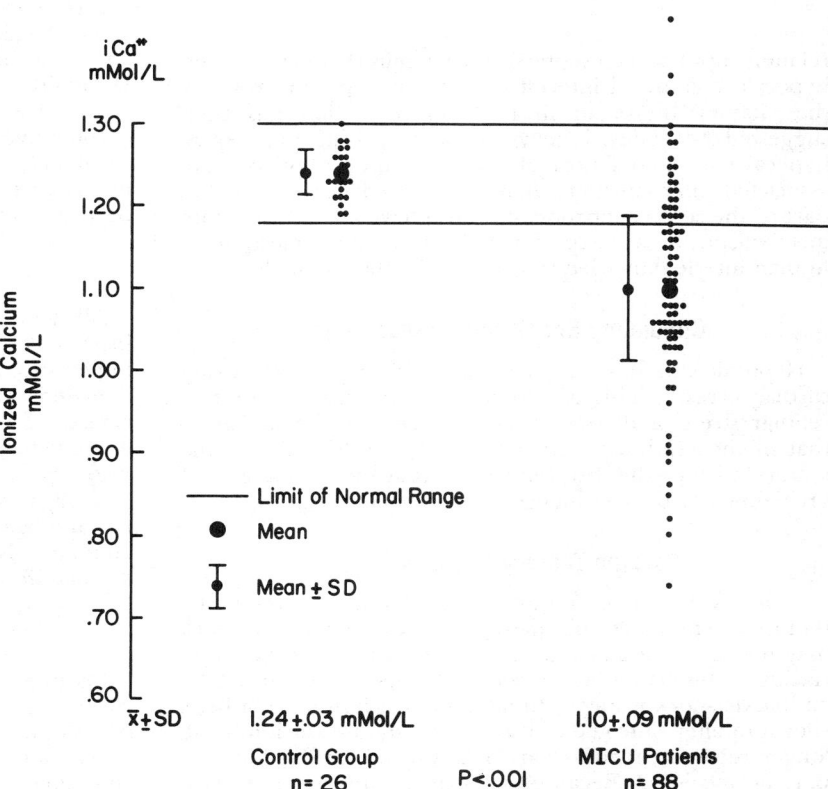

Ionized Calcium

Figure 102–6. Distribution of ionized calcium in patients admitted to the intensive care unit. This graph demonstrates the distribution of ionized calcium in 88 sequential admissions to the intensive care unit of the Detroit Receiving Hospital. Controls were normal nonhospitalized ambulatory individuals. (From Desai TK, Carlson RW, Geheb MA: Prevalence and clinical implications of hypocalcemia in acutely ill patients in a medical intensive care unit. Am J Med 84:209, 1988.)

HOSPITAL MORTALITY RATES

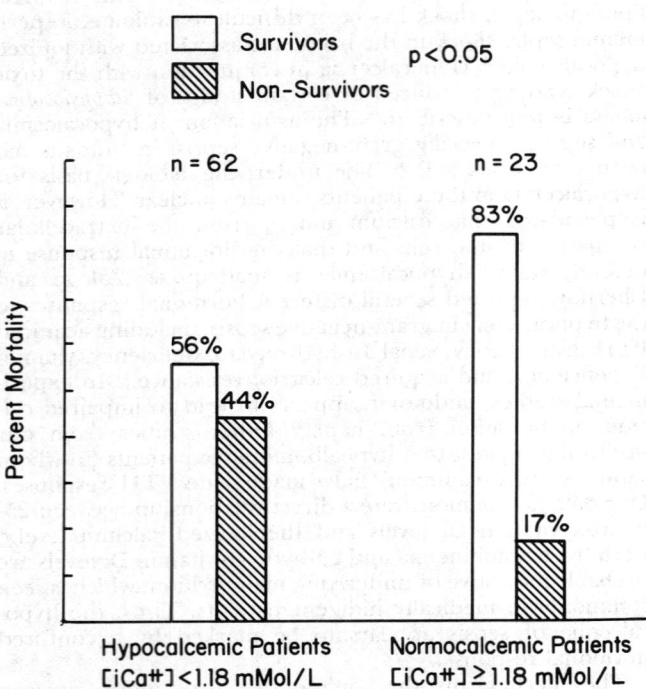

Figure 102–7. Hospital mortality of patients with ionized hypocalcemia. Hospital mortalities were compared according to admitted values for ionized calcium. A value of 1.18 mmol/L was chosen as the lower level of normal based on the values from a control group (see Fig. 102–6). Hospital mortality was four times greater in patients with ionized hypocalcemia. (From Desai TK, Carlson RW, Geheb MA: Prevalence and clinical implications of hypocalcemia in acutely ill patients in a medical intensive care unit. Am J Med 84:209, 1988.)

relationships between septic states, vitamin D deficiency, and hypocalcemia are of interest because an important role for the vitamin D system in immune regulation has been suggested.[39, 40] Thus, it may not be surprising that sepsis, hypocalcemia, and abnormalities in vitamin D regulation are associated. Immune and inflammatory mediators released as part of the septic syndrome may also have a role in calcium metabolism; in an experimental rat model, injection of human interleukin-1 led to transient hypocalcemia.[41]

Circulatory Shock and Cardiac Arrest

Hypocalcemia has also been reported in patients during cardiac arrest.[42] This is another circumstance of extreme cellular stress, and the pathophysiology may be similar to that in the septic patient: movement of calcium from the extracellular to the intracellular compartment as a sign of breakdown of basic cellular control mechanisms.

Calcium Therapy in Shock States

If hypocalcemia is a sign of cellular compromise, the therapy of hypocalcemia in sepsis or cardiovascular shock may not improve outcome. In fact, it has been shown that calcium administration increases the mortality caused by endotoxic shock in rats.[43] In addition, calcium has not been shown to alter outcome in cardiac arrest, and calcium is no longer recommended as part of advanced cardiac life support protocols.[44, 45] Because of the many unanswered ques-

tions about the appropriate approach to the therapy of hypocalcemia associated with circulatory or septic shock,[46] we recommend administration of intravenous calcium only in patients with cardiovascular compromise (hypotension and heart failure) refractory to other therapies. In general, severely depressed levels of hypocalcemia (<0.8 mmol/L, 3.2 mg/dl) are well tolerated and do not require therapy. When calcium is used, we suggest administration of an intravenous bolus of 5 mg/kg elemental calcium during 20 minutes followed by an infusion of 1 to 2 mg/kg/h for several hours until ionized calcium level increases. Response to blood pressure and left ventricular work indices should be monitored. In our experience, ionized calcium levels increase in an unpredictable fashion and the improvements in cardiovascular parameters are short-lived (1 or 2 minutes to several minutes).

Renal Failure

Several mechanisms contribute to the hypocalcemia of renal insufficiency, including 1α-hydroxylase insufficiency (with consequent calcitriol deficiency) and skeletal resistance to PTH.[4, 5, 47] The hyperphosphatemia of renal insufficiency further inhibits 1α-hydroxylase activity.[48] With elevated levels of phosphate, there is also a risk of precipitation of calcium phosphate salts, with further depression of circulating calcium.[49] Generally, these derangements do not occur until renal failure is severe with a glomerular filtration rate (GFR) of less than 25 mL/min.[49] Even then, only 40% of patients with a GFR of less than 20 mL/min exhibit hypocalcemia. Severe hypocalcemia can occur in some patients with oliguric renal failure secondary to rhabdomyolysis.[50] These patients can have marked hyperphosphatemia, hyperuricemia, and elevated creatine kinase levels. Although renal failure is common in the intensive care unit, hypocalcemia should not be assumed to be the result of renal insufficiency unless renal compromise is severe. This generally occurs at serum creatinine levels greater than 4 mg/dL. Efforts to correct hypocalcemia in patients with renal failure should be directed toward reducing serum phosphorus levels and correcting the underlying vitamin D deficiency. Vitamin D should be supplemented only when elevated phosphorus levels have been controlled and only in the setting of the chronic hypocalcemia associated with chronic renal failure. As already noted, cardiovascular performance can improve in patients with renal failure in whom hypocalcemia has been corrected.

Acid-Base Disorders

Alkalemia can lead to a fall in ionized calcium level by increasing protein binding to calcium. This assumes clinical importance in the case of an acidemic patient with a borderline depressed ionized calcium level. Ionized calcium decreases by approximately 0.05 mmol/L (0.2 mg/dL) for each increase in pH by 0.10 unit; however, this effect is blunted in the presence of hypoalbuminemia, which is common in critically ill patients.[12, 51] An increase in circulating lactic acid has also been reported to increase the binding of calcium to albumin.[52] No direct therapy is required unless clinical signs are manifest.

Chelation

Because calcium exists in plasma at a concentration that is close to its limit of solubility, small changes that affect the overall physical chemistry of the plasma solution can lead to precipitation of a variety of calcium salts. Several common clinical circumstances, including blood transfusions and administration of radiographic dye, can also lead to calcium salt precipitation.

Transfusions of blood (preserved with citrate) can lead to hypocalcemia because of the chelation of calcium with citrate.[53] Falls in ionized calcium concentration can be directly related to the rapidity of transfusion and the plasma levels of citrate.[54] Citrate metabolism is compromised in patients with hepatic or renal failure and when hypoperfusion is present.[13] These patients may be particularly susceptible to hypocalcemia after blood transfusions. Plasmapheresis with the infusion of massive amounts of calcium-poor albumin has also been reported to cause hypocalcemia.[55] Although hemodynamic parameters remain stable in the majority of patients with hypocalcemia after transfusion, patients with underlying cardiac compromise may be at risk for hypotension or heart failure.[13, 53, 54, 56] In this group of patients, calcium therapy might be required.

Other less widely appreciated chelating agents include radiographic contrast media and lipid emulsion solutions used with total parenteral nutrition.[12, 13] Radiocontrast agents contain calcium chelators, and the amount of agent used for a routine computed tomographic scan of the head can lower the ionized calcium level by 0.1 to 0.2 mmol/L (0.4 to 0.8 mg/dL) for up to 30 minutes.[57, 58] This may be of clinical significance in the critically ill patient in whom cardiovascular instability may already be problematic.

Pancreatitis

Acute pancreatitis with formation of calcium soaps in peripancreatic areas has been associated with profound hypocalcemia. Alcoholic patients with extremely high triglyceride levels are particularly at risk.[59, 60] Experimental studies suggest that extreme elevations of plasma free fatty acids may have a central role in inducing hypocalcemia.[61] Decreases in serum calcium levels should stimulate PTH secretion in an attempt to correct the serum ionized calcium level toward normal. However, studies evaluating the function of the PTH and vitamin D axis have reported conflicting results[62–64]; although some investigators have reported normal PTH and vitamin D responses to hypocalcemia during acute pancreatitis, others have found an inadequate hormonal response to hypocalcemia. Low intracellular magnesium levels have been associated with the hypocalcemia of pancreatitis.[65] Unless the patient is symptomatic, treatment of hypocalcemia in pancreatitis is not warranted. Hypocalcemia is associated with a poor prognosis.[66] In our experience,[10] the lowest levels of ionized hypocalcemia encountered in the intensive care unit were seen in patients with pancreatitis.

Burns

The ionized calcium concentration can decrease and remain substantially below normal during the course of healing of burns. Therapy is required only if neuromuscular or cardiac signs occur.[67]

Miscellaneous

Other causes of hypocalcemia are distinctly uncommon in the intensive care population. These include primary hypoparathyroidism and pseudohypoparathyroidism. Hypoparathyroidism may result after parathyroid, thyroid, or radical neck surgery.[4, 5] It has also been reported (rarely) after radioiodine therapy[68] and after infiltration of the parathyroid glands with malignancy.[69] Pseudohypoparathyroidism is a syndrome characterized by end-organ resistance to PTH.[4, 5] Both hypoparathyroidism and pseudohypoparathy-

roidism are marked by signs of PTH deficiency, which include hypocalcemia and hyperphosphatemia. These patients are rarely admitted to the intensive care unit unless severe intercurrent illness intervenes. In the presence of severe cardiovascular or neurologic findings, therapy is aimed at correcting circulating calcium levels acutely with calcium infusions (see earlier). In refractory cases vitamin D therapy with dihydrotachysterol (0.25 to 1.0 mg/d) or calcitriol (0.5 to 2.0 μg/d) may be required to correct hypocalcemia.

Anticonvulsant drugs have been reported to induce hypocalcemia (and osteomalacia) in up to 20% of patients receiving long-term anticonvulsant therapy.[70–72] Many mechanisms have been proposed, including induction of microsomal enzymes that increase the degradation of various forms of vitamin D. These drugs may also interfere with gut absorption of calcium[73] and mobilization of calcium from bone.[74] Treatment includes replacement of vitamin D to correct the hypocalcemia.

Inhibition of bone resorption can also occur with other agents that act similarly to calcitonin. These include plicamycin (mithramycin; see discussion later) and colchicine.[75, 76] Both plicamycin and calcitonin are used therapeutically in hypercalcemia. Colchicine poisoning can be marked by hypocalcemia.

Conclusions

In summary, hypocalcemia is exceedingly common in critically ill patients. There are many possible causes of hypocalcemia, but in a substantial number of patients no clear cause can be identified. Therapy for hypocalcemia should be directed to the underlying cause, such as hypomagnesemia. Calcium infusion should be considered cautiously and should be initiated only for patients with cardiovascular or neurologic signs and symptoms. In septic patients, calcium infusion may adversely affect outcome. Specific groups of acutely ill patients in which vitamin D or calcium infusion may prove of benefit have not yet been delineated. At this juncture, hypocalcemia, and especially ionized hypocalcemia, should be viewed as a marker of severity of illness that is associated with a poor prognosis.

DISORDERS OF CALCIUM REGULATION: HYPERCALCEMIA

Hypercalcemia in the general population is most commonly caused by hyperparathyroidism.[77, 78] In hospitalized patients, however, malignancy accounts for approximately 50% of hypercalcemic patients. Patients with hyperparathyroidism and those with renal failure receiving dialysis constitute another 25%. Other causes or unidentified causes account for the rest.[79] In our experience, management of hypercalcemia usually does not require hospitalization in the intensive care unit.[10] When it does, it is the acute complications of malignancy-associated hypercalcemia that require this level of support. Consequently, this chapter emphasizes the complications and therapy of acute hypercalcemia. For other discussions of hypercalcemia the reader is referred to other excellent reviews.[4, 5] Causes of hypercalcemia encountered in the intensive care unit are listed in Table 102–2.

Clinical Manifestations

Depending on the degree of hypercalcemia, patients present with typical signs relative to the neurologic, renal, cardiovascular, and gastrointestinal systems.[80] There are various complications of chronic hypercalcemia, including renal stones,[4, 5] but the intensive care specialist is asked to address

TABLE 102–2

CAUSES OF HYPERCALCEMIA

Malignancy-associated hypercalcemia
    Solid tumors with bone metastases
    Solid tumors without bone metastases
    Hematologic malignancies
Primary hyperparathyroidism
Miscellaneous
    Thyrotoxicosis
    Vitamin D intoxification
    Hypervitaminosis A
    Sarcoidosis (and other granulomatous diseases)
    Adrenal insufficiency
    Milk-alkali syndrome
    Thiazides
    Acute renal failure (rhabdomyolysis)

the acute manifestations. The acutely hypercalcemic patient typically presents with confusion and obtundation, constipation, renal insufficiency, volume depletion, and dehydration.[80] The severity of these signs and symptoms is related to the severity of the hypercalcemia.

Renal Disorders

Renal insufficiency tends to parallel the degree of hypercalcemia[81] and is secondary to a variety of acute changes. These include volume depletion,[4, 82, 83] renal vasoconstriction,[4] and a decrease in glomerular ultrafiltration.[84] Calcium deposition causing tubular obstruction and interstitial nephritis can also occur.[4] In addition, hypercalcemia can lead to a defect in urine-concentrating ability, resulting in polyuria and thus aggravating water and volume losses. Correction of hypercalcemia and volume resuscitation can lead to improvement in renal function as measured by an improvement in the GFR and a decrease in the serum creatinine level.

Cardiovascular Disorders

Hypercalcemia has a positive inotropic effect on the heart, as indicated by shortened systolic time intervals,[85] and the effects of cardiac glycosides are potentiated.[4] The most consistent effect on the electrocardiogram is shortening of the QT interval.[86] There is a direct correlation between blood pressure and ionized calcium in acutely ill patients.[30] Hypertension can also occur after calcium infusion[87] and is common in hypercalcemia caused by hyperparathyroidism[88, 89] and vitamin D intoxication.[90] Hypertension reverses with control of the hypercalcemia. Because blood pressure is supported by hypercalcemia, the degree of volume depletion encountered in these patients is usually underestimated.

Neurologic Disorders

Central nervous system manifestations correlate with the elevation of the serum calcium level and range from lethargy and stupor to coma. Neuromuscular weakness, which is neurogenic (and not myogenic), has been described in hypercalcemia associated with both primary and secondary hyperparathyroidism and reverses with parathyroidectomy.[91–93] In addition to changes in mental status, depression, paranoia, and other neuropsychiatric signs have been described in hypercalcemia.[5] These manifestations improve with correction of the serum calcium level.[80]

Gastrointestinal Disorders

One of the early signs of hypercalcemia is constipation, whereas anorexia, nausea, and vomiting tend to occur later when delays in gastric emptying occur.[4, 5, 80] Gastric ulcers occur in 10 to 15% of patients with primary hyperparathyroidism.[94, 95] There is a complex relationship between stomach hormones and calcium metabolism: calcium infusion stimulates gastrin release, and release of gastrocalcin stimulates calcium uptake in the bone.[4, 5, 14] The exact physiologic roles of these feedback systems in overall calcium homeostasis remain to be defined. Pancreatitis (acute or chronic) is associated with hypercalcemia of any etiology[95–98] and may transiently lower serum calcium.

Miscellaneous Manifestations

Various other signs and symptoms may accompany hypercalcemia, including articular manifestations (pseudogout), metastatic calcification, and pruritus. Many of these are related to chronic hyperparathyroidism (either primary or secondary) and are not usually of concern in the acute setting of the intensive care unit.[4, 5]

Malignancy-Associated Hypercalcemia. Various tumors have been associated with hypercalcemia, including solid tumors (breast, lung, and genitourinary tumors; adenocarcinoma of unknown etiology; head and neck tumors; primary hepatoma; and pancreatic tumors) and hematologic cancers (lymphoma and myeloma).[80] Hypercalcemia can occur with and without bone metastases and can be subdivided into the following categories: solid tumors with bone metastases, solid tumors without bone metastases (humoral hypercalcemia of malignancy), and hematologic malignancies.[99] With current therapies, hypercalcemia can be controlled in the majority of cancer patients. However, it is a grave prognostic factor; in a series of cancer patients, 75% of the patients died within 3 months of the recognition of hypercalcemia.[80] In these patients, when specific cancer therapy was available, survival was longer. Although control of hypercalcemia does little to affect survival, it has major impact on the improvement in symptoms.[80]

Several mechanisms have been described for the induction of hypercalcemia in malignancy, but increased bone resorption is the final common pathway. Although production of PTH is unusual in cancer patients, the production of PTH-related peptide, which mimics the physiologic effects of PTH, is common. Other osteoclast-activating factors produced by tumors include lymphotoxin and tumor necrosis factor. Calcitriol has also been reported to be produced by some lymphomas. On rare occasions, production of prostaglandins (especially the E series, which can be potent simulators of bone resorption) has been reported to cause hypercalcemia. Although prostaglandins may rarely produce hypercalcemia in malignant states, indomethacin and other nonsteroidal antiinflammatory drugs should not be used as first-line therapy.

Malignancy with Bone Metastases. Breast cancer is almost always associated with bone metastases when hypercalcemia is present. Unfortunately, hormonal therapy with estrogens, androgens, or antiestrogens (such as tamoxifen) can precipitate hypercalcemia.[100, 101] Breast cancer cells can induce bone resorption directly, without activation of osteoclasts. The mechanism by which breast cancer induces bone resorption is not clear.[102]

Malignancy Without Bone Metastases. Many cancers (e.g., hypernephroma; pancreatic carcinoma; squamous carcinomas of the lung, cervix, and esophagus; and head and neck tumors) are associated with hypercalcemia without evidence of bone metastases. In most of these cases, humoral hyper-

TABLE 102–3

THERAPY OF HYPERCALCEMIA

Volume expansion
Volume expansion and forced saline diuresis
Plicamycin (mithramycin)
Diphosphonates
Calcitonin
Phosphates
Prostaglandin synthase inhibitors
Glucocorticoids
Miscellaneous
    Gallium nitrate
    WR-2721
    Chloroquine, hydroxychloroquine

calcemia of malignancy is the cause and PTH-related peptide is produced.[103]

Hematologic Malignancies. Multiple myeloma, lymphoma, and leukemia all can involve bone to different extents. In myeloma, osteoclast-activating factor has been cited as the cause of the hypercalcemia.[104] This factor may turn out to be one of several leukocyte cytokines, including lymphotoxin.[105] In lymphomas that may have a component of granulomatous disease (Hodgkin's lymphoma), hypercalcemia can be produced by unregulated production of calcitriol.[106, 107] Patients with cutaneous T cell lymphomas and leukemia induced by infection with human T cell lymphotropic virus type I can also have hypercalcemia.[108] The mechanism is unclear. In general, glucocorticoids are effective in controlling hypercalcemia in myeloma, leukemia, and lymphoma. This is probably secondary to the tumoricidal effect of glucocorticoids in these specific tumors and the ability of glucocorticoid to inhibit osteoclast-activating factor activity. In tumors that produce calcitriol, glucocorticoids can directly inhibit calcitriol-mediated uptake of calcium from the gut.

Other Causes of Hypercalcemia

In addition to hyperparathyroidism there are several other causes of hypercalcemia (see Table 102–2). They are uncommonly encountered, especially in the intensive care unit, and are reviewed elsewhere.[4, 5] It is important to recognize primary hyperparathyroidism because it can be cured through surgery. The measurement of "intact" PTH that is elevated in the presence of hypercalcemia is virtually diagnostic, except when severe renal failure (GFR < 30 mL/min) is present. Because PTH is excreted by the kidneys, PTH levels (depending on the assay utilized) are increased in renal failure.[47]

Therapy

The therapies for hypercalcemia are listed in Table 102–3. Levels of circulating calcium can be lowered by increasing renal calcium excretion, inhibiting gut calcium absorption, or inhibiting bone calcium mobilization. Because bone calcium mobilization is the usual cause of hypercalcemia, therapies directed at inhibiting bone calcium mobilization are usually the most effective after initial therapy.

Volume Expansion and Forced Saline Diuresis. The goal of this therapeutic approach is to dilute circulating calcium and increase renal calcium excretion. In hypercalcemic states, natriuresis, inability to concentrate urine, and decreased intake (sometimes complicated by vomiting) all combine to cause volume depletion, which can be severe. With volume depletion, the GFR decreases, leading to a decline

in calcium excretion that aggravates hypercalcemia. In addition, in hypercalcemic states blood pressure may be relatively maintained, leading to clinical underestimates of volume status. Therefore, rapid replacement of volume deficits is the first step in the therapy of hypercalcemia. Addition of furosemide after volume repletion leads to an increase in sodium chloride, and thus calcium, excretion. Suki and colleagues reported infusion of isotonic saline at 10 to 20 L/d followed by large doses of furosemide.[83] It is important to note that circulating calcium level fell substantially with volume expansion alone before the addition of furosemide. Addition of furosemide allows the clinician to maintain aggressive diuresis and decreases the likelihood of pulmonary edema as a complication. A less aggressive regimen with infusion of isotonic saline at 200 to 300 mL/h and furosemide doses between 40 and 200 mg/d leads to control of hypercalcemia in most cases. With this regimen, the circulating calcium level can be expected to fall by 2 to 3 mg/dL (0.5 to 0.75 mmol/L) during 24 to 48 hours.[4] Magnesium and potassium levels should be monitored and appropriate replacement given as necessary.

Plicamycin (Mithramycin). This cytotoxic agent is an effective inhibitor of osteoclastic activity. It acts relatively rapidly, with an onset of activity within 12 hours and a peak effect within 24 to 48 hours. It is quite effective in treating the hypercalcemia of malignancy.[109] The major side effects of the drug are thrombocytopenia, renal failure, and hepatic failure when given at higher dosages, and it should be avoided in patients with disorders of these systems. The dosage used in the treatment of hypercalcemia is up to 25 μg/kg intravenously, at which the drug appears to be safe. Doses can be repeated every 2 to 3 days as necessary, but toxicity generally limits its use to 2 to 3 weeks. Few studies have compared the relative value of different therapeutic agents in controlling the hypercalcemia of malignancy; however, mithramycin appears to be a particularly effective agent.[110]

Diphosphonates. The diphosphonate (biphosphonate) drugs are analogues of pyrophosphate and are potent inhibitors of bone resorption. The three agents that have been tested clinically are ethane-1-hydroxy-1,1-diphosphonate (etidronate), amino-1-hydroxypropane diphosphonate (ADP), and dichloromethylene diphosphonate (Cl_2MDP). Of these, only etidronate is available in North America. Both ADP and Cl_2MDP are effective in lowering circulating calcium when given either orally or parentally,[111–113] with a slower onset of action by the oral route. ADP is a particularly safe and effective drug; when it was given at a daily dose of 15 mg intravenously (with appropriate volume repletion), virtually all patients with hypercalcemia of malignancy in a large European trial became normocalcemic within 6 days.[114] Cl_2MDP has been removed from use because of a possible association with leukemia.[4] Although etidronate is used orally to control the hypercalcemia of Paget's disease, it is necessary to use the parenteral route in the hypercalcemia of malignancy.[115] The dosage of 7.5 mg/kg/d infused during 2 hours for 2 to 4 days has been used to control hypercalcemia in malignancy.[116]

Calcitonin. Calcitonin directly inhibits osteoclastic activity and is a safe agent. Salmon calcitonin, when given at 4 medical research units/kg subcutaneously every 12 hours, may lower circulating calcium by 2 to 3 mg/dL (0.5 to 0.75 mmol/L). However, the action is short-lived (2 to 3 days).[117] Glucocorticoids may delay the onset of resistance.[118] In general, calcitonin is useful in patients for whom plicamycin is contraindicated.

Phosphates. Phosphate directly inhibits bone resorption in vivo, which may partially explain its calcium-lowering effect. In addition, it complexes directly with calcium.[5] Oral phosphate given at doses of 500 to 1500 mg of elemental phosphorus daily can be effective in lowering the circulating calcium level, especially in hypophosphatemic patients. However, intravenous phosphate can be dangerous and should be reserved for those in whom hypercalcemia is life threatening, hypophosphatemia is present, and other modes of therapy are contraindicated.[119] Under these circumstances, intravenous phosphate can be given as 400 to 800 mg of elemental phosphorus during 12 to 24 hours.[4]

Prostaglandin Synthase Inhibitors. Although prostaglandins have been reported to have some role in the hypercalcemia of malignancy, in general, the prostaglandin synthase inhibitors have been disappointing agents for the control of hypercalcemia.[120]

Glucocorticoids. Glucocorticoids are effective only in specific circumstances. They can be useful in myeloma (in which they inhibit the activity of various osteoclast-activating factors) and in leukemia and lymphomas (in which they have tumor lysis effects). They are also effective in granulomatous diseases such as sarcoidosis and Hodgkin's lymphoma (in which they inhibit vitamin D action in the gut). They are generally ineffective in hyperparathyroid states and in malignancy-associated hypercalcemia other than the tumors just discussed. Dosages of 40 to 100 mg/d have been used. Because of the side effects of glucocorticoids, steroids should be discontinued if the therapy is ineffective.

Other Agents. Gallium nitrate has been used to treat PTH-mediated hypercalcemia and humoral hypercalcemia of malignancy.[121-123] Another agent, WR-2721, inhibits PTH release and possibly bone resorption.[124] Chloroquine and hydroxychloroquine have also been shown to be effective in lowering the calcitriol level in sarcoidosis.[125, 126] The precise role of these agents in the therapy of hypercalcemia awaits further investigation.

Summary

The first step in the treatment of acute symptomatic hypercalcemia of any cause is volume repletion followed by diuretic-induced forced saline diuresis. Especially in malignancy-associated hypercalcemia, plicamycin or intravenous etidronate is the next therapy to be initiated. Calcitonin therapy gives erratic control and glucocorticoids are only specifically indicated. Phosphate therapy (especially intravenous) should be viewed as potentially dangerous and should be reserved for settings in which other therapies cannot be employed.

MAGNESIUM HOMEOSTASIS IN CRITICALLY ILL PATIENTS

Disorders of magnesium metabolism, especially hypomagnesemia, are common in acutely ill patients. Magnesium is involved in the control of many metabolic processes, including oxidative phosphorylation; a variety of enzymatic reactions involving RNA, DNA, and ATP metabolism; and fat and protein metabolism. Magnesium is also essential for neurochemical transmission, skeletal muscle contraction, and cardiac contraction. It is a major regulator of Na^+, K^+-ATPase and plays a major role in the regulation of other intracellular cations. Magnesium counterbalances the effects of calcium in vascular smooth muscle and has a modulating effect on vascular tone.[127-130]

Unlike calcium, ionized magnesium (the physiologically active fraction) is not readily measurable in the clinical situation. Ultrafilterable magnesium may correlate better with ionized magnesium but is not measured routinely in the clinical laboratory.[130, 131]

Internal Magnesium Distribution

Under normal circumstances, there is approximately 24 to 26 g (984 to 1066 mmol) of magnesium in the normal 70-kg adult. A little more than half (14 g, 574 mmol) is distributed in bone and the other half is distributed between cells (12 g, 492 mmol) and the extracellular space (0.3 g, 12.3 mmol).[4] This means that less than 1% of total body magnesium is contained in the extracellular space. Consequently, measured extracellular magnesium is a poor reflection of total body magnesium stores.

External Magnesium Balance

Ingestion of magnesium at 300 to 460 mg/d (12 to 15 mmol/d) is required to maintain normal magnesium balance. Of this, 25 to 60% is absorbed daily, primarily in the jejunum and proximal ileum. Magnesium is excreted through the kidneys; approximately 75% of magnesium is filtered at the glomerulus. The major site of magnesium reabsorption is in the ascending limb of the loop of Henle. Both gut absorption and renal handling of magnesium respond to changes in magnesium intake; especially when magnesium deficiency exists, both gut absorption and renal reabsorption increase. The renal capacity to excrete magnesium is large; thus, hypermagnesemia is unusual in the absence of some degree of renal dysfunction.[132]

Extracellular Magnesium

Extracellular magnesium exists in three forms: protein-bound magnesium (30%), nonionized chelates (bicarbonate, phosphate, and citrate) of magnesium (10%), and free ionized magnesium (60%), which is the physiologically active fraction.[4] Total concentrations of extracellular magnesium vary from 1.7 to 2.3 mg/dL (0.7 to 0.95 mmol/L). As with calcium, the major protein binder of magnesium is albumin (70 to 90% of protein binding) with minor binding to globulin.[4, 132] Protein-bound fractions of magnesium vary directly with pH, protein concentration, and ionized calcium concentration, because to some degree magnesium, hydrogen, and calcium ions all compete for the same binding sites. There is a suggestion that acidemia itself may lead to a shift of magnesium from the intracellular to the extracellular compartments and thus mask underlying magnesium depletion.[133, 134]

Magnesium is usually measured for clinical purposes by spectrophotometric techniques. Unfortunately, hyperbilirubinemia and red blood cell hemolysis interfere with accurate estimation of magnesium because they absorb light at a similar wavelength.[130, 135] Consequently, overestimation of circulating magnesium may occur in these circumstances, which are common in critically ill patients.

A better way to assess the physiologically active fraction of magnesium may be to measure magnesium in protein-free ultrafiltrates of serum.[131, 136] Zaloga and colleagues measured ultrafilterable concentrations of both calcium and magnesium in 64 critically ill patients and found a close correlation between the ultrafilterable and the ionized concentrations of calcium. Based on the relationships between ultrafilterable and ionized calcium, ultrafilterable magnesium was suggested as a better reflector of the physiologically active (ionized) fraction of magnesium.[131] Until better technology (ion-selective electrodes) is clinically available, ultrafilterable magnesium may provide better insights into alterations of magnesium metabolism.

Hormonal Regulation of Magnesium

Although calcitropic and other hormones can affect magnesium handling in both the gut and the kidney,[4, 5, 132] they have little overall effect on magnesium homeostasis. Unlike the intricate mechanisms that exist to regulate calcium homeostasis, there is little recognized similar regulation of magnesium homeostasis. In spite of this, magnesium levels remain remarkably constant.

DISORDERS OF MAGNESIUM REGULATION: HYPOMAGNESEMIA

The most common clinical problem encountered in magnesium metabolism is hypomagnesemia, which is generally equated with total body magnesium depletion. However, the relationship between total body magnesium and blood magnesium varies and is not well understood.[4, 5, 132] Hypomagnesemia is greatly underestimated in the general population of patients; Whang reported hypomagnesemia in 12.5% of routine electrolyte determinations in a Veterans Administration hospital.[129] The estimated incidence of hypomagnesemia in patients admitted to the intensive care unit varies greatly but may be as high as 65%.[137]

Clinical Manifestations of Hypomagnesemia

Electrolyte Disorders

Hypomagnesemia is the most common correctable association with hypocalcemia in acutely ill patients.[7, 10] The association of hypocalcemia and hypomagnesemia is well described.[138–140] However, hypomagnesemia must be severe before inhibition of PTH secretion occurs.[141, 142] Somewhat paradoxically, mild hypomagnesemia stimulates secretion of PTH. Consequently, hypocalcemia should not be attributed to hypomagnesemia unless magnesium levels are less than 1.0 mg/dL (0.4 mmol/L). Hypomagnesemia can also lead to end-organ resistance to the action of PTH.[4, 5] Hypocalcemia cannot generally be corrected without the correction of severe hypomagnesemia.[4, 137, 141–143] Only after magnesium levels are normalized can assessment of other potential causes of hypocalcemia be made.

Magnesium deficiency is commonly associated with hypokalemia. In fact, more than a third of hospitalized patients with hypokalemia have coexistent hypomagnesemia.[144] Hypokalemia has also been described in pure human magnesium deficiency.[129, 144] Loss of intracellular potassium continues in magnesium deficiency in spite of dietary potassium repletion.[145, 146] This loss is presumably due to decreased Na^+,K^+-ATPase activity, which may account for the increased sensitivity to digitalis.[147, 148] In view of the close association of hypomagnesemia and hypokalemia, it is not surprising that the electrocardiographic abnormalities and dysrhythmias encountered in hypomagnesemic patients are similar to those seen in patients with hypokalemia.[4, 147]

Cardiovascular Disorders

Electrocardiographic abnormalities are common but not specific in patients with hypomagnesemia.[147, 149] Cardiac arrhythmias that are refractory to anything other than magnesium repletion also occur in hypomagnesemic patients.[150] These include ventricular tachycardia, fibrillation, and cardiac arrest in both digitalized[148, 151] and nondigitalized[152] patients. Magnesium deficiency is associated with increased myocardial binding to digoxin,[4] and magnesium is effective therapy in digoxin-induced arrhythmias.[148, 153] Both supraventricular and ventricular arrhythmias appear to be more common in hypomagnesemic patients,[154] and magnesium is a treatment of choice for refractory torsades de pointes, a variant of ventricular tachycardia. Magnesium has been reported to be effective therapy for a variety of ventricular

TABLE 102–4
CAUSES OF HYPOMAGNESEMIA
Starvation and refeeding
Alcoholism
Diabetic ketoacidosis
Pancreatitis
Intestinal loss
Renal loss
Diuretics
Osmotic diuresis
Aminoglycosides
Amphotericin B
Cisplatin
Cyclosporine

and supraventricular arrhythmias with and without evidence of magnesium depletion.[147, 155, 156] Routine antiarrhythmic therapy can be unsuccessful in hypomagnesemic patients.[152] Because of the common association of hypomagnesemia and hypokalemia and the difficulty of separating their respective roles in arrhythmogenesis, it is advisable to replace both of these cations in patients who have arrhythmias.

There is evidence for a role of magnesium in the modulation of vascular tone; depletion of magnesium is associated with hypertension.[157] The relation of magnesium depletion to modulation of vascular responses in acutely ill patients requires further delineation.

Neuromuscular Disorders

Neuromuscular irritability has been well described in magnesium deficiency. Signs include tetany, tremors, asterixis, myoclonus, and seizures. Psychiatric manifestations including apathy and depression are also reported.[4, 5] Because of the common association of hypomagnesemia with hypocalcemia, it can be difficult to separate the effects of the respective abnormalities.

Of particular importance in the intensive care unit is the association of skeletal and respiratory muscle weakness in hypomagnesemic patients.[158] Patients with demonstrated magnesium depletion had longer stays in the intensive care unit.[159] Hypomagnesemic patients have shown improvements in respiratory muscle function with repletion of magnesium.[158]

Causes of Hypomagnesemia

Hypomagnesemia can be caused by an abnormality in external magnesium balance that includes inadequate magnesium intake, gastrointestinal malabsorption of magnesium, renal magnesium wasting, or combinations of these. Table 102–4 shows commonly encountered causes of hypomagnesemia in critically ill patients.

Starvation and Refeeding

Prolonged starvation is required to induce hypomagnesemia,[160] and rapid refeeding of a magnesium-deficient patient can lead to hypomagnesemia. Magnesium is required for normal cell synthesis; 0.25 mmol of magnesium is required for each gram of nitrogen incorporated into cells. Consequently, appropriate magnesium repletion is required when initiating nutritional therapy.[161]

Alcoholism

Hypomagnesemia and magnesium deficiency are commonly encountered in acute and chronic alcoholic patients.

The causes of hypomagnesemia are multifactorial and include starvation and diarrhea. Acute alcohol intake can lead to urinary magnesium losses,[162] but the effect is not long-lasting.[163] Coincident phosphate depletion may aggravate renal magnesium losses.[164] Magnesium levels can fall rapidly in alcoholics, perhaps as a result of the provision of magnesium-free calories and the concomitant presence of respiratory alkalosis.[165] Because of the many factors that can be associated with hypomagnesemia in alcoholic patients, it is imperative that magnesium levels be monitored.

Diabetic Ketoacidosis

Magnesium deficiency is commonly encountered in diabetic ketoacidosis and is probably secondary to tissue catabolism and ongoing renal losses.[166]

Pancreatitis

Hypomagnesemia has been reported in pancreatitis, including alcohol-associated pancreatitis. It is multifactorial in etiology and may be related to the effects of alcohol on magnesium metabolism. In addition, magnesium may be deposited in the necrotic tissue around the pancreas.[167]

Intestinal Loss

Malabsorption is a common cause of magnesium deficiency and hypomagnesemia. Chronic diarrhea,[168] short-bowel syndrome (including bypass surgery for obesity[169, 170]) and steatorrhea[171, 172] all lead to fecal magnesium losses. Stool fat binds to magnesium and reduction of stool fat can correct magnesium losses.[172] Prolonged nasogastric suction has also been reported to cause hypomagnesemia.[173]

Renal Loss

The use of several diuretics, including hydrochlorothiazide and furosemide,[4, 83, 174] has been associated with hypomagnesemia. Hypomagnesemia is a particular complication in the treatment of hypercalcemia with aggressive saline diuresis induced with furosemide.[83] Hypercalcemia itself is natriuretic and directly increases urinary magnesium excretion.[175]

Hypomagnesemia has also been reported in experimental postobstructive diuresis,[176] in the diuretic phase of acute renal failure, after renal transplantation, and after the osmotic diuresis associated with uncontrolled diabetes mellitus.[4, 132]

Several drugs encountered in the intensive care unit can also induce renal magnesium wasting. High-dose aminoglycoside therapy (including amikacin, gentamicin, and tobramycin) has been associated with severe hypomagnesemia, hypocalcemia, and hypokalemia.[177–180] Amphotericin B nephrotoxicity has been associated with magnesuria.[181] Tumor therapy with cisplatin has been associated with both acute[182] and chronic[183] magnesuria and hypomagnesemia. Cyclosporine has been reported to cause renal magnesium wasting in both renal[184] and bone marrow transplant[185, 186] patients.

Evaluation

Hypomagnesemia is usually assumed to be associated with total body magnesium deficiency. The underlying cause may be obvious on reviewing the usual associations. In some cases, however, it may be necessary to distinguish renal losses from other causes of hypomagnesemia. Under normal circumstances, renal magnesium excretion of less than 12 to 24 mg/d (0.5 to 1 mmol/d) is assumed to be associated with either nutritional deficiency, gastrointestinal losses, or internal shifts of magnesium. If excretion of magnesium exceeds 36 mg/d (1.5 mmol/d), then renal losses of magnesium for any of the causes cited are assumed to be responsible.[4, 5]

Therapy

Patients with magnesium levels less than 1.0 mg/dL (0.4 mmol/L) should be assumed to be magnesium deficient with a total body magnesium deficit of 1 to 2 mmol/kg body weight.[160] Therapy should be initiated with 1 mEq/kg administered parenterally during the first 24 hours. One gram of magnesium sulfate ($MgSO_4$) contains 4 mmol (92 mg) of elemental magnesium, and a 70-kg individual might require 9 g of $MgSO_4$ in the first day. If tetany or convulsions are present, 2 to 3 g (8 to 12 mmol) of $MgSO_4$ can be given rapidly (in 5 minutes) in a small volume (30 mL) of dextrose in water and an additional 4 to 6 g (16 to 24 mmol) given in the next 2 to 3 hours. Other electrolyte disorders such as hypokalemia commonly coexist and should be addressed at the same time. The hypocalcemia associated with hypomagnesemia may be rapidly corrected as magnesium is repleted. In the presence of renal failure, magnesium dosages must be adjusted downward.

DISORDERS OF MAGNESIUM REGULATION: HYPERMAGNESEMIA

Because renal magnesium excretion is quite efficient, hypermagnesemia occurs only with massive delivery of magnesium to the extracellular fluid space or with more modest magnesium loading in the presence of some degree of renal dysfunction.[4, 5, 187]

Clinical Manifestations

Magnesium produces its effects primarily through its ability to antagonize the effects of calcium at excitable membranes.[188] In general, levels greater than 4.8 mg/dL (2 mmol/L), must be present before clinical effects are evident.[189, 190]

Cardiovascular manifestations include electrocardiographic changes, which vary depending on the degree of elevation of the serum magnesium. Intraventricular conduction delay occurs initially and is followed by first-degree heart block and a prolonged QT interval. At levels greater than 12 mg/dL (5 mmol/L), heart block worsens, until asystole and complete heart block occur at levels greater than 30 mg/dL (12 mmol/L)). Hypermagnesemia is also associated with variable degrees of hypotension.[190]

Hypermagnesemia results in variable degrees of neuromuscular blockade caused by inhibition of acetylcholine release.[187, 190, 195, 196] Diminution of deep tendon reflexes is a useful sign of hypermagnesemia and begins at levels greater than 4.8 mg/dL (2 mmol/L). This diminution generally precedes other signs of hypermagnesemia.[187] Of particular importance is the effect of hypermagnesemia on respiratory muscle function: at levels greater than 16 mg/dL (6.5 mmol/L), hypoventilation secondary to respiratory muscle paralysis can occur.[187, 197–199]

Causes of Hypermagnesemia

Renal Failure. Hypermagnesemia can occur in patients with renal failure (GFR < 30 mL/min),[190] including those receiving dialysis therapy.[197, 200] It generally occurs only when there is excessive intake of magnesium from magnesium-based antacids and purgatives.[190]

Magnesium Overload. Although unusual, elevated levels

of magnesium have been reported in individuals with normal renal function who have received excessive oral or rectal loads of magnesium.[4, 187, 199]

Parenteral Magnesium. Parenteral magnesium is deliberately given to raise levels (2 to 17 mg/dL, 1.2 to 7.0 mmol/L) in the treatment of pregnant eclamptic patients. In this group diminution of tendon reflexes and levels of magnesium are monitored.[94, 187]

Miscellaneous Causes. Acute acidosis,[190] pheochromocytoma,[201] Addison's disease,[190] and hyperparathyroidism[202] have all been associated with mild hypermagnesemia.

Therapy

In a patient with mild symptoms of hypermagnesemia, establishing vigorous diuresis with saline and loop diuretics enhances magnesium excretion.[132, 187]

Calcium directly antagonizes the effects of hypermagnesemia, and hypocalcemia can aggravate the symptoms of hypermagnesemia. In patients with severe signs, intravenous calcium therapy and ventilatory support may be required. In these patients, 1 g of calcium chloride should be administered during 3 minutes and improvements monitored.[187] If necessary, calcium (15 mg/kg) can be infused during 4 hours. In addition to its direct antagonistic effects on magnesium, calcium infusions enhance renal magnesium excretion.[132] In patients in whom renal failure prevents the induction of diuresis, dialysis with magnesium-free dialysate can be lifesaving.[198, 203]

References

1. Fogh-Anderson N, Christiansen TF, Komarny L, et al: Measurement of free calcium ion in capillary blood and serum. Clin Chem 24:1545, 1978.
2. Rassmussen H: The calcium messenger system (part 1). N Engl J Med 314:1094, 1986.
3. Rassmussen H: The calcium messenger system (part 2). N Engl J Med 314:1164, 1986.
4. Sutton RL, Dirks JH: Disturbances of calcium and magnesium metabolism. In: Brenner BM, Rector FC (eds): The Kidney. 4th ed. Philadelphia, WB Saunders, p 841, 1991.
5. Aurbach GD, Marx SJ, Spiegel AM: Parathyroid hormone, calcitonin, and the calciferols. In: Wilson JD, Foster DW (eds): Williams Textbook of Endocrinology. 8th ed. Philadelphia, WB Saunders, p 1397, 1992.
6. Mallette LE: Regulation of blood calcium in humans. Endocrinol Metab Clin North Am 18:601, 1989.
7. Desai TK, Carlson RW, Geheb MA: Hypocalcemia and hypophosphatemia in acutely ill patients. Crit Care Clin 3:927, 1987.
8. Zaloga GP: Hypocalcemia in critically ill patients. Crit Care Med 20:251, 1992.
9. Butler S, Payne R, Gunn I, et al: Correlation between serum ionized calcium and serum albumin in two hospital populations. Br Med J 289:948, 1984.
10. Desai TK, Carlson RW, Geheb MA: Prevalence and clinical implications of hypocalcemia in acutely ill patients in a medical intensive care unit. Am J Med 84:209, 1988.
11. Wybenga DR, Ibbot FA, Cannon DC: Determination of ionized calcium in serum that has been exposed to air. Clin Chem 22:1009, 1976.
12. Zaloga GP, Willey S, Tomasic P, et al: Free fatty acids alter calcium binding: A cause for misinterpretation of serum calcium values and hypocalcemia in critical illness. J Clin Endocrinol Metab 64:1010, 1987.
13. Zaloga GP, Chernow B, Cook D, et al: Assessment of calcium homeostasis in the critically ill surgical patient. Ann Surg 202:587, 1985.
14. Persson P, Hakanson R, Axelson J, et al: Gastrin releases a blood calcium–lowering peptide from the acid-producing part of the rat stomach. Proc Natl Acad Sci USA 86:2834, 1989.
15. Broner CWS, Stidham GL, Westenhircher DF, et al: Hypermagnesemia and hypocalcemia as predictors of high mortality in critically ill pediatric patients. Crit Care Med 18:921, 1990.
16. Chernow B, Zaloga G, McFadden E, et al: Hypocalcemia in critically ill patients. Crit Care Med 10:848, 1982.
17. Bristow MR, Schwartz HD, Binetti G, et al: Ionized calcium and the heart. Circ Res 41:565, 1977.
18. Dillon PF, Murphy RA: Tonic force maintenance with reduced shortening velocity in arterial smooth muscle. Am J Physiol 242:102, 1982.
19. Franzini-Armstrong C: Fine structure of sarcoplasmic reticulum and transverse tubular system in muscle fibers. Fed Proc 23:887, 1964.
20. Bohr DF: Vascular smooth muscle: Dual effect of calcium. Science 139:597, 1963.
21. Chaimowitz C, Abinader E, Benderly A, et al: Hypocalcemic hypotension. JAMA 222:86, 1972.
22. Connor TB, Rosen BL, Blaustein MP, et al: Hypocalcemia precipitating congestive heart failure. N Engl J Med 307:869, 1982.
23. Wong CK, Pun KK, Cheng CH, et al: Hypocalcemic heart failure in end-stage renal disease. Am J Nephrol 10:167, 1990.
24. Wong CK, Lau CP, Cheng CH, et al: Hypocalcemic myocardial dysfunction: Short- and long-term improvement with calcium replacement. Am Heart J 120:381, 1990.
25. Ginsburg R, Esserman LJ, Bristow MR: Myocardial performance and extracellular ionized calcium in a severely failing heart. Ann Intern Med 98:603, 1983.
26. Chopra D, Janson P, Sawin CT: Insensitivity to digoxin associated with hypocalcemia. N Engl J Med 296:971, 1977.
27. Auffant RA, Downs JB, Amick R: Ionized calcium concentration and cardiovascular function after cardiopulmonary bypass. Arch Surg 116:1072, 1981.
28. Maynard JC, Cruz C, Kleerekoper M, et al: Blood pressure response to changes in serum ionized calcium during hemodialysis. Ann Intern Med 104:358, 1986.
29. Feldman AM, Fivush B, Zahka KG, et al: Congestive cardiomyopathy in patients on continuous ambulatory peritoneal dialysis. Am J Kidney Dis 11:76, 1988.
30. Desai TK, Carlson RW, Geheb MA: A direct relationship between ionized calcium and arterial pressure among patients in an intensive care unit. Crit Care Med 16:578, 1988.
31. Akiyama T, Batchelder J, Worsman J, et al: Hypocalcemic torsades de pointes. J Electrocardiol 22:89, 1989.
32. Dubois GD, Arieff AI: Clinical manifestations of electrolyte disorders. In: Arieff AI, DeFronzo RA (eds): Fluid, Electrolytes and Acid-Base Disorders. New York, Churchill Livingstone, p 1087, 1985.
33. Trunkey D, Carpenter MA, Holcroft J: Ionized calcium and magnesium. The effect of septic shock in the baboon. J Trauma 18:166, 1978.
34. Sperber SJ, Blevins DD, Francis JB: Hypercalcitonemia, hypocalcemia, and toxic shock syndrome. Rev Infect Dis 12:736, 1990.
35. Zaloga GP, Chernow B: The multifactorial basis for hypocalcemia during sepsis. Studies of the parathyroid hormone–vitamin D axis. Ann Intern Med 107:36, 1987.
36. Aderka D, Schwartz D, Dan M, et al: Bacteremic hypocalcemia: A comparison between the calcium levels of bacteremic and nonbacteremic patients with infection. Arch Intern Med 147:232, 1987.
37. Zaloga GP, Malcolm D, Chernow B, et al: Endotoxin-induced hypocalcemia results in defective calcium mobilization in rats. Circ Shock 24:143, 1988.
38. Desai TK, Carlson RW, Geheb MA: Parathyroid–vitamin D axis in critically ill patients with unexplained hypocalcemia. Kidney Int 32:S225, 1987.
39. Cohen MS, Mesler DE, Snipes RG, et al: 1,25(OH)$_2$D$_3$ activates H$_2$O$_2$ secretion by human monocyte derived macrophages. Clin Res 33:397A, 1985.
40. Manolagas SC, Deftos LJ: The vitamin D endocrine system and the hematolymphopoietic tissue. Ann Intern Med 100:144, 1984.
41. Boyce BF, Yates AJP, Mundy GR: Bolus injections of recombinant human interleukin-1 cause transient hypocalcemia in normal mice. Endocrinology 125:2780, 1989.
42. Urban P, Scheidegger D, Buchmann B, et al: Cardiac arrest and blood ionized calcium levels. Ann Intern Med 109:110, 1988.
43. Malcolm DS, Zaloga GP, Holaday JW: Calcium administration increases the mortality of endotoxic shock in rats. Crit Care Med. 17:900, 1989.
44. Standards and guidelines for cardiopulmonary resuscitation (CPR) and emergency cardiac care (ECC). JAMA 256:1924, 1986.
45. Zaloga GP, Chernow B: Hypocalcemia and hypophosphatemia in critical illness. JAMA 256:1924, 1986.
46. Chernow B: Calcium: Does it have a therapeutic role in sepsis? Crit Care Med 18:895, 1990.
47. Morrison G, Geheb MA, Earley LE: Chronic renal failure in the kidney. In: Seldin DW, Giebisch G (eds): The Kidney: Physiology and Pathophysiology. New York, Raven Press, p 1901, 1985.
48. Tanaka Y, DeLuca HF: The control of a 25-hydroxy vitamin D metabolism by inorganic phosphorus. Arch Biochem Biophys 154:566, 1973.
49. Coburn JW, Popovtzer M, Massry SG, et al: The physicochemical state and renal handling of divalent ions in chronic renal failure. Arch Intern Med 124:302, 1969.
50. Grossman, RA, Hamilton RW, Morse BM, et al: Nontraumatic rhabdomyolysis and acute renal failure. N Engl J Med 291:807, 1974.
51. Moore E: Ionized calcium in normal serum, ultrafiltrates and whole blood determined by ion-exchange electrode. Clin Invest 49:318, 1970.
52. Schaer H, Bachmann U: Ionized calcium in acidosis: Differential effect of hypercapnic and lactic acidosis. Br J Anaesth 46:842, 1974.
53. Olinger GN, Hottenrot C, Mulder DG, et al: Acute clinical hypocalcemic myocardial depression during rapid blood transfusion and post-operative hemodialysis. J Thorac Cardiovasc Surg 72:503, 1976.
54. Denlinger JK, Nahrwold ML, Gibbs PS, et al: Hypocalcaemia during rapid blood transfusion in anaesthetized man. Br J Anaesth 48:995, 1976.

55. Buskard NA, Varghese Z, Wills MR: Correction of hypocalcaemic symptoms during plasma exchange. Lancet 2:344, 1976.
56. Howland WS, Schweizer O, Jascott D, et al: Factors influencing the ionization of calcium during major surgical procedures. Surg Gynecol Obstet 58:274, 1976.
57. Berger RE, Gomez LS, Mallette LE: Acute hypocalcemic effects of clinical contrast media injections. AJR 138:283, 1982.
58. Caulfield JB, Zir L, Harthorne JW: Blood calcium levels in the presence of arteriographic contrast material. Circulation 52:119, 1975.
59. Cameron JL, Crisler C, Margolis S, et al: Acute pancreatitis with hyperlipemia. Surgery 70:53, 1971.
60. Decaux G, Hallemans R, Mockel J, et al: Chronic alcoholism: A predisposing factor for hypocalcemia in acute pancreatitis. Digestion 20:175, 1980.
61. Warshaw AL, Lee KH, Napier TW, et al: Depression of serum calcium by increased plasma free fatty acids in the rat: A mechanism for hypocalcemia in acute pancreatitis. Gastroenterology 89:814, 1985.
62. Hauser CJ, Kamrath RO, Sparks J, et al: Calcium homeostasis in patients with acute pancreatitis. Surgery 94:830, 1983.
63. Robertson GM, Moore EW, Swift DM, et al: Inadequate parathyroid response in acute pancreatitis. N Engl J Med 294:512, 1976.
64. Weir GC, Lesser PB, Drop LJ, et al: The hypocalcemia of acute pancreatitis. Ann Intern Med 83:185, 1975.
65. Ryzen E, Rude RK: Low intracellular magnesium in patients with acute pancreatitis and hypocalcemia. West J Med 152:145, 1990.
66. Ranson JHC, Rifkind KM, Turner JW: Prognostic signs and non-operative peritoneal lavage in acute pancreatitis. Surg Gynecol Obstet 143:209, 1976.
67. Szyfelbein SK, Drop L, Martyn J: Persistent ionized hypocalcemia in patients during resuscitation and recovery phases of body burns. Crit Care Med 9:454, 1981.
68. Orme MC, Connolly ME: Hypoparathyroidism after iodine-131 treatment of thyrotoxicosis. Ann Intern Med 75:136, 1971.
69. Horwitz CA, Myers WP, Foote FW: Secondary malignant tumors of the parathyroid glands: Report of two cases with associated hypoparathyroidism. Am J Med 52:797, 1972.
70. Hunter J, Maxwell JD, Stewart DA, et al: Altered calcium metabolism in epileptic children on anticonvulsants. Br Med J 4:202, 1971.
71. Tolman, KG, Jubiz W, Sannella JJ, et al: Osteomalacia associated with anticonvulsant drug therapy in mentally ill retarded children. Pediatrics 56:45, 1975.
72. Stamp TC, Round JM, Rowe DJ, et al: Plasma levels and therapeutic effect of 25-hydroxycholecalciferol in epileptic patients taking anticonvulsant drugs. Br Med J 4:9, 1972.
73. Harrison HC, Harrison HE: Inhibition of vitamin D–stimulated active transport of calcium of rat intestine by diphenylhydantoin-phenobarbital treatment. Proc Soc Exp Biol Med 153:220, 1976.
74. Hahn TJ, Scharp CR, Richardson CA, et al: Interaction of diphenyl-hydantoin (phenytoin) and phenobarbital with hormonal mediation of fetal rat bone resorption in vitro. J Clin Invest 62:406, 1978.
75. Ellwood MG, Robb GH: Self-poisoning with colchicine. Postgrad Med J 47:129, 1971.
76. Heath DA, Palmer JS, Aurbach GD: The hypocalcemic action of colchicine. Endocrinology 90:1589, 1972.
77. Mundy GR, Cove DH, Fisken R: Primary hyperparathyroidism: Changes in the pattern of clinical presentation. Lancet 1:1317, 1980.
78. Heath H III, Hodgson SF, Kennedy MA: Primary hyperparathyroidism: Incidence, morbidity, and potential economic impact in a community. N Engl J Med 302:189, 1980.
79. Fisken RA, Heath DA, Bold AM: Hypercalcemia—A hospital survey. Q J Med 196:405, 1980.
80. Ralston SH, Gallacher SJ, Patel U, et al: Cancer-associated hypercalcemia: Morbidity and mortality. Clinical experience in 126 treated patients. Ann Intern Med 112:499, 1990.
81. Lins LE: Reversible renal failure caused by hypercalcemia: A retrospective study. Acta Med Scand 203:309, 1978.
82. Transbol I, Hornum I, Dawids S: Hypercalcemia and sodium-losing renal disease. Scand J Urol Nephrol 4:125, 1970.
83. Suki WN, Yium JM, Von Minden M, et al: Acute treatment of hypercalcemia with furosemide. N Engl J Med 283:836, 1970.
84. Humes HD, Ichikawa I, Troy JL, et al: Evidence for a parathyroid hormone–dependent influence of calcium on the glomerular filtration. J Clin Invest 61:32, 1978.
85. Shiner PT, Harris WS, Weissler AM: Effects of acute changes in serum calcium levels on the systolic time intervals in man. Am J Cardiol 24:42, 1969.
86. Bronsky D, Dubin A, Waldstein SS, et al: Calcium and the electrocardiographic manifestations of hyperparathyroidism and marked hypercalcemia from various etiologies. Am J Cardiol 7:833, 1961.
87. Marone C, Beretta-Piccoli C, Wiedmann P: Acute hypercalcemic hypertension in man: Role of hemodynamics, catecholamines and renin. Kidney Int 20:92, 1981.
88. Daniels J, Goodman AD: Hypertension and hyperparathyroidism: Inverse relation of serum phosphate level and blood pressure. Am J Med 75:17, 1983.
89. Singal AK, Beevers DG: Parathyroid hypertension. Br Med J 286:498, 1983.
90. Earll JM, Kurtzman NA, Moser RH: Hypercalcemia and hypertension. Ann Intern Med 64:378, 1966.
91. Patten BM, Bilezikian JP, Mallette LE, et al: Neuromuscular disease in primary hyperparathyroidism. Ann Intern Med 80:182, 1974.
92. Mallette LE: Review: Primary hyperparathyroidism: An update: Incidence, etiology, diagnosis, and treatment. Am J Med Sci 293:239, 1987.
93. Mallette LE, Patten BM, Engel WK: Neuromuscular disease in secondary hyperparathyroidism. Ann Intern Med 82:474, 1975.
94. Mallette LE, Bilezikian JP, Heath DA, et al: Primary hyperparathyroidism: Clinical and biochemical features. Medicine 53:127, 1974.
95. Christiansen J: Primary hyperparathyroidism and peptic ulcer disease. Scand J Gastroenterol 9:111, 1974.
95. Mixter CA, Keynes M, Cope O: Further experience with pancreatitis as a diagnostic clue to hyperparathyroidism. N Engl J Med 266:265, 1962.
96. Goebell H: The role of calcium in pancreatic secretion and disease. Acta Hepato-Gastroenterol 23:151, 1976.
97. Leeson PM, Fourman P: Acute pancreatitis from vitamin D poisoning in a patient with parathyroid deficiency. Lancet 1:1185, 1966.
98. Meltzer LE, Palmon FR, Paik YK, et al: Acute pancreatitis secondary to hypercalcemia of multiple myeloma. Ann Intern Med 57:1008, 1962.
99. Mundy GR: The hypercalcemia of malignancy. Kidney Int 31:142, 1987.
100. Valentin-Opran A, Eilon G, Saez S, et al: Estrogens and antiestrogens stimulate release of bone resorbing activity of cultured human breast cancer cells. J Clin Invest 75:726, 1985.
101. Legha SS, Powell K, Buzdar AU, et al: Tamoxifen-induced hypercalcemia in breast cancer. Cancer 47:2803, 1981.
102. Eilon G, Mundy GR: Direct resorption of bone by human breast cancer cells in vitro. Nature 276:726, 1978.
103. Broadus AE, Mangin M, Ikeda K, et al: Humoral hypercalcemia of cancer: Identification of a novel parathyroid hormone–like peptide. N Engl J Med 319:556, 1988.
104. Mundy GR, Raisz LG, Cooper RA, et al: Evidence for the secretion of an osteoclast stimulating factor in myeloma. N Engl J Med 291:1041, 1974.
105. Garrett IR, Durie BGM, Nedwin GE, et al: Production of lymphotoxin, a bone-resorbing cytokine, by cultured myeloma cells. N Engl J Med 317:526, 1987.
106. Breslau NA, Mcguire JL, Zerwekh JE, et al: Hypercalcemia associated with increased serum calcitriol levels in three patients with lymphoma. Ann Intern Med 100:1, 1984.
107. Jacobson JO, Bringhurst FR, Harris NL, et al: Humoral hypercalcemia in Hodgkin's disease. Cancer 63:917, 1989.
108. Blayney DW, Jaffe ES, Fisher RI, et al: The human T-cell leukemia/lymphoma virus, lymphoma, lytic bone lesions, and hypercalcemia. Ann Intern Med 98:144, 1983.
109. Perlia CP, Gubisch NJ, Wolter J, et al: Mithramycin treatment of hypercalcemia. Cancer 25:389, 1970.
110. Mundy GR, Wilkinson R, Heath DA: Comparative of available medical therapy for hypercalcemia of malignancy. Am J Med 74:421, 1983.
111. Ralston SH, Gardner MD, Dryburgh FJ, et al: Comparison of amino-hydroxypropylidene diphosphonate, mithramycin, and corticosteroids/calcitonin in treatment of cancer related hypercalcemia. Lancet 2:907, 1985.
112. Jacobs TP, Siris ES, Bilezikian JP, et al: Hypercalcemia of malignancy: Treatment with intravenous dichloromethylene diphosphonate. Ann Intern Med 94:312, 1981.
113. van Breukelen FJM, Bijvoet OLM, Frijlink WB, et al: Efficacy of aminohydroxypropylidene biphosphonate in hypercalcemia: Observations on regulation of serum calcium. Calcif Tissue Int 34:321, 1982.
114. Harinck HJ, Bijvoet OM, Plantingh AT, et al: Role of bone and kidney in tumor induced hypercalcemia and its treatment with biphosphonate and sodium chloride. Am J Med 82:1133, 1987.
115. Jung A: Comparison of two parenteral diphosphonates in hypercalcemia of malignancy. Am J Med 72:221, 1982.
116. Ryzen E, Martodam RR, Troxell M, et al: Intravenous etidronate in the management of hypercalcemia. Arch Intern Med 145:449, 1985.
117. Hosking DJ: Treatment of severe hypercalcemia with calcitonin. Metab Bone Dis Relat Res 2:207, 1980.
118. Binstock ML, Mundy GR: Effect of calcitonin and glucocorticoids in combination on the hypercalcemia of malignancy. Ann Intern Med 93:269, 1980.
119. Heath DA: The use of inorganic phosphate in the management of hypercalcemia. Metab Bone Dis Relat Res 2:213, 1982.
120. Brenner, DE, Harvey HA, Lipton A, et al: A study of prostaglandin E₂, parathormone, and response to indomethacin in patients with hypercalcemia of malignancy. Cancer 44:556, 1982.
121. Warrell RP, Israel R, Frisone M, et al: Gallium nitrate for acute treatment of cancer-related hypercalcemia. Ann Intern Med 108:669, 1988.
122. Warrell RP, Issacs M, Alcock NW, et al: Gallium nitrate for treatment of refractory hypercalcemia from parathyroid carcinoma. Ann Intern Med 107:683, 1987.
123. Warrell RP, Bockman RS, Coonley CJ, et al: Gallium nitrate inhibits calcium resorption from bone and is effective treatment for cancer-related hypercalcemia. J Clin Invest 73:1487, 1984.
124. Glover DJ, Shaw L, Glick JH, et al: Treatment of hypercalcemia in

parathyroid cancer with WR-2721, S-2-(3-aminopropylamino) ethyl-phosphorothioic acid. Ann Intern Med 103:55, 1985.

125. O'Leary TJ, Jones G, Yip A, et al: The effects of chloroquine on serum 1,25-dihydroxyvitamin D and calcium metabolism in sarcoidosis. N Engl J Med 315:727, 1986.

126. Barre PE, Gascon-Barre M, Meakins JL, et al: Hydroxychloroquine treatment of hypercalcemia in a patient with sarcoidosis undergoing hemodialysis. Am J Med 82:1259, 1987.

127. Shils ME: Magnesium in health and disease. Annu Rev Nutr 8:429, 1988.

128. Sjogren A, Edvinsson L, Fallgren B: Magnesium deficiency in coronary artery disease and cardiac arrhythmias. J Intern Med 226:213, 1989.

129. Whang R: Magnesium deficiency: Pathogenesis, prevalence, and clinical implications. Am J Med 82(suppl 3a):24, 1987.

130. Salem M, Munoz R, Chernow B: Hypomagnesemia in critical illness. 7:225, 1991.

131. Zaloga GP, Wilkens R, Tourville J, et al: A simple method for determining physiologically active calcium and Mg concentrations in critically ill patients. Crit Care Med 15:813, 1987.

132. Lau K: Magnesium metabolism: Normal and abnormal. In: Arieff AI, DeFronzo RA (eds): Fluid, Electrolyte, and Acid-Base Disorders. New York, Churchill Livingston, p 575, 1985.

133. Caddell JL, Reed GF: Unreliability of plasma Mg values in asphyxiated neonates. Magnesium 8:11, 1989.

134. Kristiansen VB, Larsen J, Neilsen TC, et al: Correction of respiratory acidosis and transient hypomagnesemia. Acta Med Scand 218:133, 1985.

135. Rehak NN, Chiang BT: Modified magnesium method in the aca III: Elimination of interference by bilirubin. Clin Chem 35:1031, 1989.

136. Chernow B, Roa J, Eguiguren L, et al: Ultrafilterable Mg concentrations in critically ill patients. Circ Shock 27:323, 1989.

137. Ryzen E, Park WW, Singer FR, et al: Magnesium deficiency in a medical ICU population. Crit Care Med 13:19, 1985.

138. Friedman M, Hatcher G, Watson L: Primary hypomagnesemia with secondary hypocalcemia in an infant. Lancet 1:703, 1967.

139. Khilnani P, Munoz R, Salem M, et al: Hypomagnesemia and ionized hypocalcemia are prevalent findings in critically ill neonates. Chest 98:42s, 1990.

140. Rasmussen HS, Cintin C, Aurup P, et al: The effect of intravenous Mg therapy on serum and urine levels of potassium, calcium, and sodium in patients with ischemic heart disease, with and without myocardial infarction. Arch Intern Med 148:1801, 1988.

141. Buckle RM, Care AD, Cooper CW, et al: The influence of plasma magnesium concentration on parathyroid hormone secretion. J Endocrinol 42:529, 1986.

142. Anast CS, Winnacker JL, Forte LR, et al: Impaired release of parathyroid hormone in magnesium deficiency. J Clin Endocrin Metab 42:707, 1976.

143. Fuss M, Cogan C, Gillet R, et al: Magnesium administration reverses the hypocalcemia secondary to hypomagnesemia despite low circulating levels of 25-hydroxyvitamin D and 1,25-dihydroxy vitamin D. Clin Endocrinol 22:807, 1985.

144. Boyd JC, Bruns DE, Wills MR: Frequency of hypomagnesemia in hypokalemic states. Clin Chem 29:178, 1983.

145. Whang R, Morosi H, Rodgers D, et al: The influence of continuing magnesium deficiency on muscle K repletion. J Lab Clin Med 79:895, 1967.

146. Whang R, Flink EB, Dyckner T, et al: Mg depletion as a cause of refractory potassium depletion. Arch Intern Med 145:1686, 1985.

147. Iseri LT, Freed J, Bures AR: Magnesium deficiency and cardiac disorders. Am J Med 58:837, 1975.

148. Seller RH, Cangiano J, Kim KE, et al: Digitalis toxicity and hypomagnesemia. Am Heart J 79:57, 1970.

149. Burch GE, Giles TD: The importance of magnesium deficiency in cardiovascular disease. Am Heart J 94:649, 1977.

150. Iseri LT, Chung P, Tobis J: Magnesium therapy for intractable ventricular tachyarrhythmias in normomagnesemia patients. Am J Med 138:823, 1983.

151. McMullen JK: Asystole and hypomagnesaemia during recovery from diabetic ketoacidosis. Br Med J 1:690, 1977.

152. Chadda KD, Lichstein E, Gupta P: Hypomagnesemia and refractory cardiac arrhythmia in a nondigitalized patient. Am J Cardiol 31:98, 1973.

153. Specter MJ, Schweizer E, Goldman R: Studies on Mg mechanism of action in digitalis-induced arrhythmias. Circulation 52:1001, 1975.

154. Dyckner T: Serum magnesium in acute myocardial infarction. Acta Med Scand 207:59, 1980.

155. Cohen L, Kitzes R: Magnesium sulfate and digitalis—toxic arrhythmias. JAMA 249:2808, 1983.

156. Iseri LT, Chung P, Tobis: Magnesium therapy for intractable ventricular tachyarrhythmias in normomagnesemic patients. West J Med 138:823, 1983.

157. Resnick LM, Gupta RK, Laragh JH: Intracellular free Mg in erythrocytes in essential hypertension: Relation to blood pressure and serum divalent cations. Proc Natl Acad Sci 81:6511, 1984.

158. Molloy DW, Dhingra S, Sloven F, et al: Hypomagnesemia and respiratory muscle power. Am Rev Respir Dis 129:497, 1984.

159. Fiaccodori E, del Canale S, Coffrini E, et al: Muscle and serum Mg in pulmonary intensive care unit patients. Crit Care Med 16:751, 1988.

160. Shils ME: Experimental human magnesium depletion. Medicine 48:61, 1969.

161. Ang SD, Daly JM: Potential complications and monitoring of patients receiving total parenteral nutrition. In: Rombeau JL, Caldwell MD (eds): Clinical Nutrition, Volume 2, Parenteral Nutrition. Philadelphia, WB Saunders, pp 331–343, 1986.

162. McCollister RJ, Flink EB, Lewis, MD: Urinary excretion of magnesium in man following the ingestion of ethanol. Am J Clin Nutr 12:415, 1963.

163. Dick M, Evans RA, Watson L: Effect of ethanol on magnesium excretion. J Clin Pathol 22:152, 1969.

164. Dominguez JH, Gray RW, Lemann J Jr: Dietary phosphate deprivation in women and men: Effects on mineral and acid balances: Parathyroid hormone and the metabolism of 25-OH-vitamin D. J Clin Endocrinol Metab 43:1056, 1976.

165. Wolfe SM, Victor M: The relationship of hypomagnesemia and alkalosis to alcohol withdrawal symptoms. Ann NY Acad Sci 162:973, 1969.

166. Martin HE, Smith K, Wilson ML: The fluid and electrolyte therapy of severe diabetic acidosis and ketosis. Am J Med 24:376, 1958.

167. Hersch T, Siddiqui DA: Magnesium and the pancreas. Am J Clin Nutr 26:362, 1973.

168. Lim P, Jacob E: Tissue magnesium level in chronic diarrhea. J Lab Clin Med 80:313, 1972.

169. Lipner A: Symptomatic magnesium deficiency after small-intestinal surgery bypass for obesity. Br Med J 1:148, 1977.

170. Parfitt AM, Miller MJ, Thomson DL, et al: Metabolic bone disease after intestinal bypass for treatment of obesity. Ann Intern Med 89:193, 1978.

171. Lim P, Jacob E: Tissue magnesium level in chronic diarrhea. J Lab Clin Med 80:313, 1972.

172. Booth CC, Barbouris N, Hanna S, et al: Incidence of hypomagnesaemia in intestinal malabsorption. Br Med J 2:141, 1963.

173. Kellaway G, Ewen K: Magnesium deficiency complicating prolonged gastric suction. NZ Med J 61:137, 1962.

174. Kuller L, Farrier N, Caggiula A, et al: Relationship of diuretic therapy and serum magnesium levels among participants in the multiple risk intervention trial. Am J Epidemiol 122:1045, 1985.

175. Eliel LP, Smith WO, Chanes R, et al: Magnesium metabolism in hyperparathyroidism and osteolytic disease. Ann NY Acad Sci 162:810, 1969.

176. Purkerson ML, Slatopolsky E, Klahr S: Urinary excretion of magnesium, calcium, and phosphate after release of unilateral ureteral obstruction in the rat. Miner Electrolyte Metab 6:182, 1981.

177. Keating MJ, Sethi MR, Bodey GP, et al: Hypocalcemia with hypoparathyroidism and renal tubular dysfunction associated with aminoglycoside therapy. Cancer 39:1410, 1977.

178. Kelnar CJ, Taor WS, Reynolds DJ, et al: Hypomagnesaemic hypocalcemia with hypokalemia caused by treatment with high dose gentamycin. Arch Dis Child 53:817, 1978.

179. Bar RS, Wilson HE, Mazzaferri EL: Hypomagnesemic hypocalcemia secondary to renal magnesium wasting. Ann Intern Med 82:646, 1975.

180. Patel R, Savage A: Symptomatic hypomagnesemia associated with gentamicin therapy. Nephron 23:50, 1979.

181. Burgess JL, Birchall R: Nephrotoxicity of amphotericin B with emphasis on changes in tubular function. Am J Med 53:77, 1972.

182. Schilsky RL, Anderson T: Hypomagnesemia and renal magnesium wasting in patients receiving cisplatin. Ann Intern Med 90:929, 1979.

183. Mavichak V, Coppin CM, Wong NL, et al: Renal magnesium wasting and hypocalciuria in chronic cis-platinum nephropathy in man. Clin Sci 75:203, 1988.

184. Barton CH, Vaziri, ND, Martin DC, et al: Hypomagnesemia and renal magnesium wasting in renal transplant recipients receiving cyclosporine. Am J Med 83:693, 1987.

185. June CH, Thompson CB, Kennedy MS, et al: Profound hypomagnesemia and renal magnesium wasting associated with the use of cyclosporine for marrow transplantation. Transplantation 39:620, 1985.

186. June CH, Thompson CB, Kennedy MS, et al: Correlation of hypomagnesemia with the onset of cyclosporine-associated hypertension in marrow transplant patients. Transplantation 41:47, 1986.

187. Van Hook JW: Hypermagnesemia. Crit Care Clin 7:215, 1991.

188. Iseri LT, French JH: Magnesium: Nature's physiologic calcium blocker. Am Heart J 108:188, 1984.

189. Fishman RA: Neurological aspects of magnesium metabolism. Arch Neurol 12:562, 1965.

190. Mordes JP, Wacker WE: Excess magnesium. Pharmacol Rev 29:273, 1978.

191. Elin RJ: Magnesium metabolism in health and disease. Dis Mon 34:161, 1988.

192. McCubbin JH, Sibai BM, Andella TN, et al: Cardiopulmonary arrest due to acute maternal hypermagnesaemia (letter). Lancet 1:1058, 1981.

193. Olinger ML: Disorders of calcium and magnesium metabolism. Emerg Med Clin North Am 7:796, 1989.

194. Reinhart RA: Magnesium metabolism: A review with special reference to the relationship between intracellular content and serum levels. Arch Intern Med 148:2415, 1988.

195. Wacker WE, Parisi AF: Magnesium metabolism. N Engl J Med 278:658, 712, 772, 1968.

196. Rude RK, Singer FR: Magnesium deficiency and excess. Annu Rev Med 32:245, 1981.

197. Randall RE, Cohen MD, Spray CC, et al: Hypermagnesemia in renal failure: Etiology and toxic manifestations. Ann Intern Med 61:73, 1964.

198. Alfrey AC, Terman DS, Barettschneider L, et al: Hypermagnesemia after renal transplantation. Ann Intern Med 73:367, 1970.
199. Ditzler JW: Epsom-salts poisoning and a review of magnesium-ion physiology. Anesthesiology 32:378, 1970.
200. Coburn JW, Popovtzer MM, Massry SG, et al: The physico-chemical state and renal handling of divalent ions in chronic renal failure. Arch Intern Med 124:302, 1969.
201. Cohen L, Kitzes R: Pheochromocytoma: A rare cause of hypermagnesemia. Magnesium 4:165, 1985.
202. Sutton RA: Plasma magnesium concentration in primary hyperparathyroidism. Br Med J 1:529, 1970.
203. Oren S, Rapoport J, Zlotnik M, et al: Extreme hypermagnesemia due to ingestion of Dead Sea water. Nephron 47:199, 1987.

CHAPTER 103

Phosphorus Homeostasis

Sidney M. Kobrin
Stanley Goldfarb

Phosphorus is among the most abundant constituents of all tissues and a major mineral component of bone. This element plays a fundamental role in cellular integrity and metabolism, particularly the provision of cellular energy in the form of ATP, and the phosphorylation of various enzymes (such as protein kinases) and other proteins that express hormone action. Its concentration influences several metabolic pathways such as glycolysis, gluconeogenesis, ammoniagenesis, and the formation of 1,25-dihydroxy + cholecalciferol (1,25-DHCC). Changes in serum phosphate levels also influence the oxygen-carrying capacity of hemoglobin through regulation of 2,3-diphosphoglycerate (2,3-DPG) synthesis. Phosphorus is also an important constituent of membrane phospholipids that have essential roles in cell integrity and cell signal transduction pathways (through their action as components of the phosphoinositide system).

PHYSIOLOGIC PRINCIPLES

The total body content of phosphorus is about 1000 g, of which approximately 85% is in bone and most of the remainder is intracellular. Less than 1% is located in the plasma, of which 10% is protein bound, 5% is complexed, and the balance is in the form of orthophosphates. It has been customary to express concentrations in terms of elemental phosphorus (referred to as phosphate). The normal fasting serum phosphate level in adults is 3.0 to 4.5 mg/dL (1 mg/dL is equal to 0.32 mmol/L or 0.58 mEq/L). There is a diurnal variation of serum phosphate levels with a morning nadir. Ingestion of carbohydrate lowers the serum phosphate concentration by enhancing cellular uptake and ingestion of phosphate-rich food results in elevation of the serum phosphate level. Therefore, samples for the determination of serum and urinary phosphate concentrations should ideally be obtained with the patient in the fasting state.

The average daily intake of phosphorus in the United States is approximately 1000 mg, mostly provided by dairy products, meats, and eggs and, to a lesser extent, by vegetables and grains. The mechanism of absorption in the small intestine is complex, but most phosphorus is absorbed by passive diffusion. A smaller, but significant, amount is absorbed actively under the influence of 1,25-DHCC.[1] The percentage of dietary phosphorus absorbed by the intestine remains remarkably constant (60 to 65%) for a wide range of phosphorus intake (4 to 30 mg/d). Thus, the dietary intake of phosphorus is an important determinant of the amount of phosphorus absorbed. The gastrointestinal tract also secretes a relatively fixed amount of phosphorus (about 200 mg/d). At a steady state, adults must excrete in the urine an amount of phosphorus equal to the net daily intestinal absorption to maintain normal external balance. This underscores the role of the kidney as the most important regulator of the serum phosphate concentration and total body phosphorus content.

Phosphate is freely filtered at the glomerulus. Approximately 80% of the filtered load is reabsorbed in the proximal convoluted tubule, 10% is reabsorbed beyond the proximal convoluted tubule, and the remainder is excreted in the urine. Tubular phosphate transport occurs by way of a membrane carrier which is activated by cell sodium uptake (sodium-phosphate cotransport), as well as being the result of cellular utilization of phosphate in metabolic pathways. Parathyroid hormone (PTH) and dietary phosphate intake are the two most important regulators of urinary phosphate excretion.[2] A rise in serum PTH levels depresses tubular reabsorption of phosphate (by a process involving stimulation of proximal tubular adenosine 3',5'-cyclic monophosphate production) and leads to phosphaturia.[3] Renal phosphate transport is also directly influenced by dietary phosphate intake.[4] If the diet is deficient in phosphate, there is an immediate and profound reduction in urinary phosphate excretion.[5] The mechanism of this renal phosphate retention is unclear; although suppression of PTH secretion occurs, it is not the primary factor. Urinary phosphate excretion is also markedly influenced by the filtered load of phosphate (the product of serum phosphate concentration and the glomerular filtration rate). As the filtered load increases, the capacity to reabsorb phosphate increases until a maximal rate of transport for phosphate is reached. If the filtered load exceeds the maximal rate of phosphate transport, urinary phosphate excretion is augmented; conversely, if the filtered load is less than the maximal rate of transport, virtually no phosphate appears in the urine.

HYPOPHOSPHATEMIA

Whether hypophosphatemia results in symptomatic cellular phosphate depletion is a complex function of the level of cellular phosphate stores and tissue metabolic activity. Hypophosphatemia may occur with or without a reduction in total body phosphate content (i.e., with or without phosphate depletion). Hypophosphatemia usually results from one or more of the following: decreased intestinal absorption of phosphorus, increased excretion of phosphate in the urine, and translocation of phosphorus from the extracellular to the intracellular fluid compartments (i.e., a change in internal balance) (Table 103–1).

Causes

Gastrointestinal Factors

Because phosphate is ubiquitous in foods, phosphate depletion is rarely due to a selective decrease in phosphate intake. Furthermore, the kidney rapidly responds to dietary phosphate restriction by enhancing tubular phosphate reabsorption, thereby preventing negative phosphate balance. However, because of obligate intestinal phosphate secretion,

TABLE 103–1

CAUSES OF HYPOPHOSPHATEMIA

Predominant Mechanism	Associated Mechanisms		
	Renal Losses	Transcellular Shift	Decreased Intestinal Absorption
Decreased Intestinal Absorption			
Malnutrition or starvation			
Phosphate binders			
Abnormal vitamin D metabolism	+		
Renal Losses			
Primary hyperparathyroidism			
Secondary hyperparathyroidism			
Renal tubular transport defects			
Oncogenic osteomalacia			+
Diuretic phase of acute tubular necrosis			
Postobstructive diuresis			
Renal transplantation		+	+
Acute volume expansion			
Glycosuria			
Idiopathic hypercalciuria			
Transcellular Shifts			
Glucose infusions and refeeding			
Respiratory alkalosis			
Septicemia			
Chronic liver disease			
Hyperadrenergic states			
Hungry bone syndrome			
Metabolic acidosis	+		
Multifactorial Causes			
Alcoholism	+	+	+
Burns		+	+
Diabetic ketoacidosis	+	+	+

prolonged starvation ultimately leads to phosphate depletion and negative phosphate balance. Because protein-calorie malnutrition results in cell breakdown and the release of large amounts of intracellular phosphate, hypophosphatemia may not accompany even severe phosphate depletion.

One situation in which a selective decrease in phosphate intake occurs is worth emphasizing. Critically ill patients in the intensive care setting usually receive total parenteral nutrition if enteral feeding is not possible. Regimens that do not include phosphate may lead to profound hypophosphatemia. Even in this situation, however, the predominant cause of the hypophosphatemia is the rapid cellular uptake of phosphate during refeeding rather than the absence of phosphate supplementation.[6]

An important cause of hypophosphatemia is the ingestion of large amounts of aluminum- or magnesium-containing antacids and calcium salts.[7] In the intestinal lumen, these agents bind both dietary and secreted phosphates, rendering them poorly absorbable. This mechanism is particularly relevant in the intensive care setting where antacids, including the aluminum-containing compound sucralfate, are commonly used to prevent stress ulcers.

Most syndromes of fat malabsorption are also associated with hypophosphatemia. Although increased fecal excretion of phosphate contributes to the negative phosphate balance, the predominant mechanism is the marked phosphaturia resulting from secondary hyperparathyroidism (caused by concomitant calcium and vitamin D malabsorption). Defects in gastrointestinal absorption of phosphate are also noted in patients with familial hypophosphatemic rickets and in some patients undergoing maintenance hemodialysis, presumably because of abnormalities in vitamin D metabolism.

Renal Factors

Decreased renal tubular phosphate reabsorption can be due to intrinsic defects in tubular transport or, more com-monly, to extrinsic factors that inhibit phosphate reabsorption. In both situations, the urine contains significant amounts of phosphate despite hypophosphatemia. The most common causes of renal phosphate wasting are primary or secondary hyperparathyroidism. Hypophosphatemia is a characteristic feature of primary hyperparathyroidism, provided renal function is normal or only modestly impaired. Although secondary hyperparathyroidism is present in most patients with chronic renal disease, hyperphosphatemia (rather than hypophosphatemia) occurs in such patients owing to decreased urinary phosphorus excretion as a consequence of the fall in glomerular filtration rate. Fat malabsorption leads to malabsorption of calcium, hypocalcemia, and secondary hyperparathyroidism. The elevated levels of PTH acting, in this case, on a normal kidney lead to phosphate wasting and hypophosphatemia.

An intrinsic tubular defect of phosphate transport may be a component of Fanconi's syndrome (glycosuria, generalized aminoaciduria, bicarbonaturia, uricosuria, and phosphaturia). Decreased renal tubular phosphate reabsorption is also responsible for hypophosphatemia in familial hypophosphatemic rickets and oncogenic osteomalacia.[8] The latter syndrome was initially described in association with mesenchymal tumors and, more recently, in association with malignant tumors. Reduced 1,25-DHCC levels have been documented in hypophosphatemia, but it is unclear whether this alteration in vitamin D metabolism is an epiphenomenon or a causative factor in the hypophosphatemia.

The diuretic phase of acute tubular necrosis, postobstructive diuresis, and renal transplantation may all be associated with hypophosphatemia. The hypophosphatemia in these situations is multifactorial in cause; the often profound diuresis, the resolving secondary hyperparathyroidism in the face of improving renal function, and continued use of phosphate binders all have roles. In addition, a minority of patients, particularly after renal transplantation, may have an intrinsic defect in tubular phosphate reabsorption.[9]

Hyperglycemia with glycosuria may promote renal phosphate excretion and contribute to phosphate depletion in uncontrolled diabetes.[10] This effect may result from competition between glucose and phosphate for transport across the brush border of the proximal tubule. Acute volume expansion with saline, administration of high-dose glucocorticoids, use of acetazolamide, and chronic metabolic acidosis also promote urinary phosphate excretion.

Transcellular Shifts

Increased cellular phosphate uptake may lead to hypophosphatemia. In the intensive care setting, glucose infusions are a common cause of hypophosphatemia. Glucose-induced insulin release promotes cellular phosphate uptake, and the use of exogenous insulin to treat diabetes mellitus is also associated with hypophosphatemia.[11, 12]

The so-called nutritional recovery syndrome may occur as a consequence of refeeding starved individuals.[13] Initially reported in severely malnourished prisoners of war and concentration camp survivors, this syndrome is now seen most frequently during intravenous feeding of patients with anorexia nervosa or other severe debilitating illnesses. Hypophosphatemia in this setting may be partly due to inadequate phosphate supplementation, but the major cause is cellular uptake of phosphate during refeeding.

Acute respiratory alkalosis is also often associated with marked hypophosphatemia and hypophosphaturia.[14] This phenomenon has been attributed to the associated increase in intracellular pH, which in turn activates glycolysis and increases the formation of phosphate-containing sugars at the expense of serum phosphate levels. However, a marked fall in the serum phosphate concentration generally occurs only when hyperventilation is accompanied by glucose infusions; mild hypophosphatemia is the rule in the absence of concomitant glucose infusion. The hypophosphatemia that develops in gram-negative septicemia and chronic liver disease is presumably due in part to respiratory alkalosis, but other factors may also be operative. Catecholamines have been shown to be important mediators of redistribution hypophosphatemia and may explain, in part, the hypophosphatemia of acute myocardial infarction, sepsis, and burns. The frequent use of catecholamine infusions in the intensive care setting may also have a role in the development of hypophosphatemia in critically ill patients.

Hypophosphatemia may result from therapy that produces rapid new bone formation in a severely demineralized skeleton, a situation often termed the hungry bone syndrome.[10] This syndrome may follow parathyroidectomy for primary hyperparathyroidism, treatment of renal osteodystrophy by parathyroidectomy, renal transplantation, and the medical treatment of severe rickets or osteomalacia. Osteoblastic metastases, particularly in patients with prostatic cancer, may produce similar effects. Patients with rapidly growing tumors such as acute leukemia, lymphomas, and Burkitt's lymphoma sometimes have hypophosphatemia and hypophosphaturia.[15] The underlying mechanism is thought to be rapid tumor growth leading to increased cellular demand for phosphate.

Hypophosphatemia has been reported during the treatment (rewarming) of a profoundly hypothermic patient.[16] Studies also suggest that clinically significant hypophosphatemia may occur in hyperthermic states, in part because of increased renal excretion. The hypophosphatemia of untreated gout has been attributed to respiratory alkalosis produced by pain-induced hyperventilation as well as a reduction in renal phosphate reabsorption caused by tubular damage. Acidosis has also been associated with hypophosphatemia. Before therapy, acidosis promotes the breakdown of intracellular organic compounds, with release of inorganic phosphate, which is excreted in the urine. During the treatment of acidosis, resynthesis of these organic compounds occurs, resulting in an intracellular shift of phosphate and hypophosphatemia.

Multifactorial Causes

Several of the aforementioned mechanisms may be present in an individual patient with hypophosphatemia and phosphate depletion. Indeed, hypophosphatemia is commonly multifactorial in cause. This is perhaps best exemplified by patients with chronic alcoholism, severe burns, and diabetic ketoacidosis. Serum phosphate concentrations may be normal when alcoholic patients are first admitted to the hospital but commonly decline precipitously when therapy is initiated. As many as 30% of male alcoholic patients have hypophosphatemia between the second and fifth days after admission to the hospital.[17] Phosphorus intake is poor in such patients, and intestinal losses from malabsorption (attributable to pancreatic insufficiency), diarrhea and vomiting, and the administration of antacids contribute as well. Renal losses result from the general catabolic state and the phosphaturic effect of ethanol.[10, 14, 18] Intracellular shifts of phosphate are also important: intravenous glucose infusions, and the respiratory alkalosis and hyperadrenergic state that frequently accompany alcohol withdrawal, contribute.[19]

Patients with extensive burns often have hypophosphatemia, with the lowest levels being reported on the fifth hospital day. Multiple causes have been identified, including respiratory alkalosis, catecholamine release, the use of total parenteral nutrition, and the administration of large doses of antacids.[20]

Diabetic patients have normal or low serum phosphate levels, depending on the level of control of the diabetes. Patients with well-controlled, stable diabetes are generally normophosphatemic and have normal total body phosphate stores. Before therapy, patients with diabetic ketoacidosis often have marked negative phosphate balance because of glycosuria, metabolic acidosis, poor phosphate intake, and hypercalciuria. Hypercalciuria, which appears to be related to the severe glycosuria, may lead to secondary hyperparathyroidism, which in turn causes phosphaturia. Despite depleted phosphate stores, the serum phosphate concentration is often normal in patients with diabetic ketoacidosis, presumably because of the enhanced catabolic rate.[11] However, on administration of insulin, the serum phosphate level may fall rapidly, reaching between 1 and 2 mg/dL during the first 24 to 48 hours of therapy.[12] Urinary phosphate excretion is markedly reduced during this period, reflecting enhanced anabolism and insulin-stimulated transcellular shifts of phosphate, and perhaps insulin-induced renal tubular reabsorption of phosphate as well.

Clinical Manifestations

Hypophosphatemia is commonly encountered in clinical practice. Approximately 2% of all patients admitted to a general hospital have serum phosphate levels less than 2 mg/dL.[10] The incidence of hypophosphatemia rises sharply in patients with chronic debilitating diseases or the acute illnesses discussed earlier. Hypophosphatemia may or may not be associated with phosphate depletion. Clinical manifestations may be totally absent in mild hypophosphatemia but may be life-threatening in prolonged severe hypophosphatemia (serum phosphate concentration < 1 mg/dL).

Two fundamental biochemical abnormalities underlie the manifestations of hypophosphatemia: depletion of intracellular ATP and decreased levels of 2,3-DPG.[10, 21] These abnormalities lead to cellular dysfunction (or frank tissue necrosis) and decreased oxygen delivery to vital organs. Typically, acute hypophosphatemia in a previously normal individual is not associated with symptoms because cellular stores are adequate to prevent critically low concentrations from developing. However, in patients with phosphate depletion in whom glycolysis and glycogen formation are then stimulated (e.g., by insulin), ATP levels fall in the face of increased demand and 2,3-DPG production falls.

Hypophosphatemia can cause muscle weakness and even frank rhabdomyolysis,[22] a syndrome recognized by elevation of serum creatine kinase and aldolase levels and myoglobinuria. Alcoholics are most vulnerable, especially during the first few days of hospitalization, when acute hypophosphatemia is superimposed on underlying chronic phosphate deficits.[23] Occasionally, profound weakness, muscle pain, and myoglobinuric acute renal failure may develop.[24] Acute respiratory failure is a serious complication of severe hypophosphatemia.

Phosphate depletion also causes abnormalities in myocardial function[18, 25] and may also affect smooth muscle. Phosphate-depleted animals exhibit decreased vascular reactivity to angiotensin II and norepinephrine. Congestive heart failure is uncommon, however, unless hypophosphatemia is superimposed on significant myocardial disease.

The neuroencephalopathy associated with phosphate deficiency has protean manifestations. Mild phosphate deficiency may cause paresthesias. More extreme hypophosphatemia (serum phosphate levels < 0.5 mg/dL) has been associated with irritability, nervousness, dysarthria, confusion, stupor, and coma.[26] In the alcoholic, these manifesta-

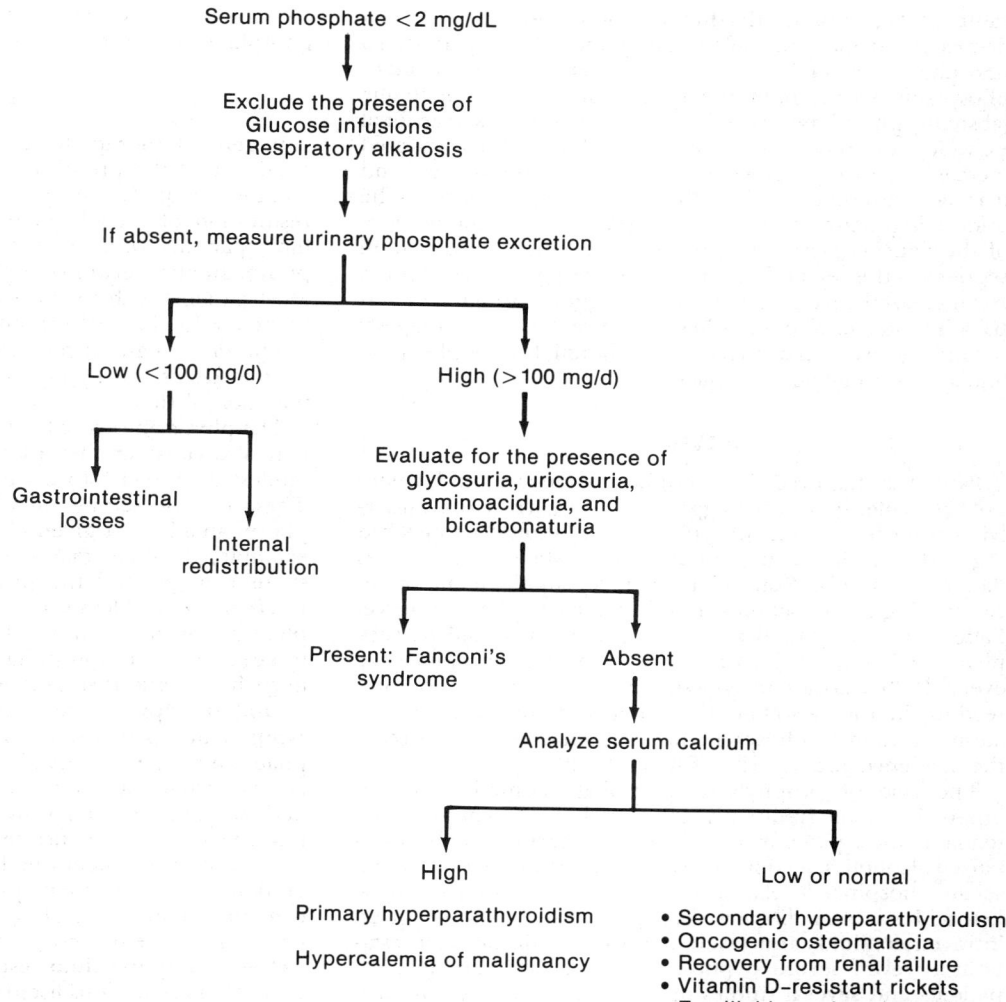

Figure 103–1. Diagnostic work-up of hypophosphatemia.

tions may mimic those of delirium tremens. However, hallucinations are not a feature of hypophosphatemia.

Because of the reduction in red blood cell 2,3-DPG levels, hypophosphatemia shifts the oxyhemoglobin dissociation curve to the left[27] and decreases tissue oxygen delivery. Another important hematologic consequence of hypophosphatemia is a fall in erythrocyte ATP levels.[28] This enhances membrane fragility and decreases erythrocyte elasticity, resulting in decreased red blood cell survival. Hemolysis is rare, except with profound degrees of hypophosphatemia (serum phosphate levels < 0.2 mg/dL). Depressed leukocyte phagocytic activity and migration have also been observed in severe hypophosphatemia[29] and have been implicated in the increased susceptibility to infection in critically ill patients. Thrombocytopenia, decreased platelet survival, and impaired clot retraction have been demonstrated in hypophosphatemic animals.[30] However, it is unclear whether specific bleeding abnormalities occur in hypophosphatemic humans.

Hypercalciuria of sufficient magnitude to cause negative calcium balance and urolithiasis may be seen in hypophosphatemic patients. The major cause of hypercalciuria is a specific defect in calcium reabsorption in the distal nephron.[10, 21] In addition, hypophosphatemia directly stimulates bone resorption and increases 1,25-DHCC levels, which in turn increases intestinal calcium absorption and bone resorption.[10, 21] All of these effects tend to elevate the serum calcium concentration and promote urinary losses of calcium. Hypermagnesiuria commonly complicates phosphate depletion. A tubular defect in magnesium transport and increased mobilization of bone magnesium are responsible.[31]

Metabolic acidosis may result from severe hypophosphatemia because of renal bicarbonate wasting, decreased excretion of titratable acid, and impaired ammoniagenesis.[10] However, the acidemia is usually mild because it is counterbalanced by the mobilization of alkali from bone. Chronic hypophosphatemia is associated with abnormal bone mineralization, which can ultimately lead to rickets and osteomalacia. Bone pain, pathologic fractures, and rheumatic complaints are common in adults with hypophosphatemic osteomalacia. Finally, hypophosphatemia has been associated with insulin resistance and impaired gluconeogenesis.[32]

Diagnostic Approach

In the majority of patients with hypophosphatemia, the underlying cause is usually apparent from the history or from the clinical setting in which the hypophosphatemia occurs. The most common causes of acute hypophosphatemia in patients in intensive care units are glucose infusions and respiratory alkalosis. In cryptic cases, measurement of urinary phosphate excretion may be helpful (Fig. 103–1). Hypophosphatemia attributable to transcellular shifts, deficient intake, or antacid administration leads to a marked decrease in urinary phosphate excretion (<100 mg/d). Renal phosphate wasting is suggested by inappropriate urinary phosphate excretion in the setting of hypophosphatemia (absolute phosphate excretion > 100 mg/d or a fractional excretion of phosphate in excess of 20%). An associated increase in urinary glucose, bicarbonate, amino acid, and uric acid excretion points to Fanconi's syndrome as the underlying cause of the hypophosphatemia. In the absence of the Fanconi syndrome, the serum calcium concentration segregates the remaining causes of renal phosphate wasting. An increased serum calcium level suggests primary hyperparathyroidism, whereas a low serum calcium level suggests secondary hyperparathyroidism, familial hypophosphatemia, or oncogenic osteomalacia.

Prevention

Patients at high risk for hypophosphatemia should, whenever possible, be treated aggressively to correct the underlying disorder. Serum phosphate levels should be checked regularly to detect hypophosphatemia before it reaches dangerous levels. Routine phosphate supplementation in certain high-risk patients has become standard practice. Patients receiving total parenteral nutrition should be supplemented with 10 to 15 mmol of potassium phosphate for every 1000 calories provided.[33] Early resumption of oral feeding in the hospitalized patient and the avoidance of administration of phosphate-binding antacids may decrease the incidence and severity of hypophosphatemia.

The role of prophylactic phosphate administration in other situations frequently associated with hypophosphatemia, namely patients with diabetic ketoacidosis and hospitalized alcoholics, is controversial. Despite normal or elevated serum phosphate levels before therapy, patients with diabetic ketoacidosis often become hypophosphatemic when given intravenous fluids and insulin. However, clinical manifestations of even severe hypophosphatemia are rare in such patients and several studies of prophylactic phosphate supplementations note salutary effects.[34, 35] Nonetheless, phosphate administration may be prudent in two specific situations during the treatment of diabetic ketoacidosis: (1) the small proportion of patients with significant hypophosphatemia (serum phosphate concentration < 1.0 to 1.5 mg/dL) before treatment; and (2) patients who have symptomatic hypophosphatemia during therapy. The prophylactic use of parenteral phosphate when diabetic ketoacidosis is precipitated by some other severe systemic illness (e.g., sepsis, bowel infarction, and myocardial infarction) may also be reasonable.[18] Under these circumstances, even modest hemodynamic, phagocytic, and muscular impairment from phosphate depletion could impair survival, and maintenance of serum phosphate levels in the 2 to 3 mg/dL range is desirable.

Patients with chronic alcoholism can be hypophosphatemic at the time of hospital admission but, more commonly, manifest hypophosphatemia within the first few days of hospitalization. Frequent monitoring of serum phosphate levels is indicated and phosphate supplementation should be begun in the face of progressive hypophosphatemia. However, particular attention must be paid to serum magnesium and calcium levels when phosphate is given to alcoholic patients. Magnesium depletion is common in this population and impairs both PTH secretion and the calcemic response of bone to PTH, sometimes leading to frank hypocalcemia.[36] If serum calcium levels decrease further, because of complexing with the infused phosphate, and the expected calcemic effect of PTH remains limited, severe hypocalcemia may result. Therefore, serum magnesium levels should be checked, and corrected if necessary, before phosphate administration in the alcoholic patient.

Treatment

In general, therapy for hypophosphatemia depends on its severity and the presence or absence of significant clinical manifestations. Correction of the underlying disorder and restoration of an adequate diet are usually sufficient for most patients with asymptomatic mild-to-moderate hypophosphatemia (serum phosphate level of 1.5 to 2.5 mg/dL). Most patients with severe hypophosphatemia (serum phosphate level < 1 mg/dL) should be treated.[18] The presence of symptoms or signs of phosphate depletion, regardless of the magnitude of the hypophosphatemia, always warrants the initiation of therapy.

The physician caring for patients in the intensive care unit may also consider therapy for hypophosphatemia of more modest degree (1.5 to 2.0 mg/dL) in certain circumstances. These include settings in which the contribution of hypophosphatemia to a given clinical finding is ambiguous. For example, a patient may have muscle weakness and mental status changes and the physician may be uncertain as to whether the problem is due entirely or in part to hypophosphatemia or to an unrelated medical condition. It is prudent to keep the serum phosphate concentration above 2 mg/dL in such ambiguous situations.

Oral therapy is preferred for asymptomatic or mildly symptomatic patients. Intravenous administration of phosphate salts is best reserved for patients with severe manifestations of hypophosphatemia or for patients unable to take oral preparations. Therapy is usually initiated with 1 g of phosphate daily and titrated to maintain the serum phosphate concentration at the desired level. The available preparations differ in their pH and sodium and potassium contents. Skim milk (1 g of phosphate per liter) is an excellent source of phosphate. If the patient cannot tolerate lactose or requires fluid restriction, one of the commercially available preparations listed in Table 103–2 may be selected. However, the physician must be aware of the wide range of cation content that accompanies the phosphate in the different preparations: one can provide 1 g of phosphate with 7 to 57 mEq of potassium and 28 to 65 mEq of sodium, depending on the preparation chosen. The preparation that best suits a given patient's metabolic profile should be selected.

Similar to the case with oral preparations, the major differences among intravenous preparations relate to their sodium and potassium contents. In the presence of severe symptoms, intravenous administration of phosphate salts at a dose of 0.08 to 0.16 mmol/kg during 6 hours is an effective and safe regimen. Frequent monitoring of serum phosphate and calcium levels is necessary to prevent hyperphosphatemia and hypocalcemia (levels should be checked after 3 and 6 hours). The infusion should be discontinued after the serum phosphate concentration rises above 1.5 mg/dL. In the presence of renal insufficiency, parenteral phosphate therapy should be used with extreme caution and with frequent monitoring of serum phosphate levels to avoid hyperphosphatemia. If the patient does not soon resume a normal diet, most hypophosphatemic patients require 1 to 2 g of phosphate daily. If renal or gastrointestinal phosphate wasting persists, daily losses should be measured and the daily dose of phosphate adjusted to compensate.

The precipitation of calcium in muscle and soft tissues, which tends to occur if the product of the serum phosphate and calcium concentrations (in milligrams per deciliter) exceeds 70, accounts for the hypocalcemia sometimes associated with phosphate administration. Magnesium supple-

TABLE 103–2

ORAL AND PARENTERAL PHOSPHATE PREPARATIONS

Preparations	Manufacturers	Phosphate Content	Sodium Content	Potassium Content
Oral				
Skim milk		1 mg/mL	0.02 mEq/mL	0.04 mEq/mL
Fleet Phospho-Soda	C.B. Fleet Co., Inc.	150 mg/mL	6 mEq/mL	
K-Phos	Beach Pharmaceuticals	115 mg/tablet		3.7 mEq/tablet
K-Phos Neutral	Beach Pharmaceuticals	250 mg/tablet	12 mEq/tablet	2 mEq/tablet
Neutra-Phos-K	Willen Drug Co.	250 mg/capsule		14 mEq/capsule
Neutra-Phos	Willen Drug Co.	250 mg/capsule	7 mEq/capsule	7 mEq/capsule
Parenteral				
Hyper-Phos K	Hoyt	67 mg/mL		3.3 mEq/mL
Sodium phosphate	Abbott Laboratories	93 mg/mL	4 mEq/mL	
In-Phos	Hoyt	25 mg/mL	1.6 mEq/mL	0.2 mEq/mL
Potassium phosphate	Abbott Laboratories	95 mg/mL		4 mEq/mL

ments, particularly in alcoholic patients, can help to forestall hypocalcemia during phosphate administration. Hypocalcemia prolongs the QT interval, and baseline and follow-up electrocardiograms may be useful when treating high-risk patients. Frequent assessment of serum calcium and phosphate levels indicates whether the rate of phosphate administration should be changed and whether calcium supplementation is necessary.

Oral phosphate has a dose-dependent cathartic effect, a problem usually encountered only when doses exceed 1 g/d. If diarrhea and cramping develop, the dose should be reduced.

HYPERPHOSPHATEMIA

Hyperphosphatemia is defined as a serum phosphate level in excess of 5 mg/dL in adults and greater than 6 mg/dL in children and adolescents. Three general mechanisms are responsible: increased intestinal absorption of phosphate, impaired renal excretion of phosphate, and translocation of phosphate from the intracellular to the extracellular fluid compartment (Table 103–3). In addition, iatrogenic hyperphosphatemia occurs if intravenous phosphate is administered too rapidly.

Causes

Gastrointestinal Factors

Excessive phosphate intake may cause hyperphosphatemia, but this is usually transient. Rapid increases in urinary phosphate excretion defend against hyperphosphatemia unless significant renal impairment is present or massive intake overwhelms the kidney's excretory capacity. Phosphate-containing laxatives or enemas may produce acute elevation in serum phosphate levels in otherwise normal individuals, but this is more common, and of greater magnitude, in patients with an atonic colon, ulcerative colitis, or impaired renal phosphate excretion.[37] Hyperphosphatemia may also develop in newborn infants fed cow's milk, which has a higher phosphate content than human milk, and in states of vitamin D excess.

Renal Factors

Decreased renal excretion of phosphate can be due to renal failure or enhanced renal tubular reabsorption of phosphate. Renal failure is the most common cause of hyperphosphatemia in patients in intensive care units. Despite marked degrees of secondary hyperparathyroidism, phosphate excretion is impaired when the glomerular filtration rate is less than 30 mL/min. The degree of hyperphosphatemia in patients with acute renal failure is variable, with the highest levels occurring in patients in whom the renal failure is due to, or associated with, trauma and rhabdomyolysis.[38] Conditions associated with enhanced tubular reabsorption of phosphate include acromegaly, thyrotoxicosis, sickle cell anemia, and tumoral calcinosis. Certain diphosphonates may also enhance renal phosphate reabsorption.

Finally, impaired renal excretion of phosphate is uniformly seen in hypoparathyroidism and pseudohypoparathyroidism.

Transcellular Shifts

States of increased catabolism or tissue destruction are associated with hyperphosphatemia. Rhabdomyolysis and the tumor lysis syndrome are typical examples. The tumor lysis syndrome is associated with the use of radiotherapy or cytotoxic drugs in patients with leukemia or lymphomas and can cause hyperphosphatemia, hyperkalemia, hypocalcemia, and hyperuricemia.[39] Rhabdomyolysis follows a variety of insults, including narcotic overdose, trauma, and heat stroke and can cause marked hyperphosphatemia and hyperkalemia as potassium and phosphate are released from muscle; hypocalcemia and hyperuricemia may also occur. Both rhabdomyolysis and the tumor lysis syndrome can cause acute

TABLE 103–3

CAUSES OF HYPERPHOSPHATEMIA

Increased Intestinal Absorption
  Excessive intake
  Phosphate-containing laxatives or enemas (iatrogenic or surreptitious)
  Vitamin D excess: endogenous or exogenous

Decreased Renal Excretion
  Acute or chronic renal failure
  Enhanced reabsorption of phosphate (e.g., acromegaly, thyrotoxicosis, sickle cell anemia, tumoral calcinosis, and diphosphonate therapy)
  Hypoparathyroidism
  Pseudohypoparathyroidism

Transcellular Shifts
  Tumor lysis syndrome
  Rhabdomyolysis
  Respiratory acidosis
  Increased catabolism

Intravenous Phosphate Therapy

renal failure. Acute urate nephropathy and the tissue deposition of calcium phosphate contribute to the acute renal failure in both of these conditions. In addition, myoglobinuric acute renal failure frequently complicates rhabdomyolysis. The impaired renal function results in decreased renal phosphate excretion, further aggravating the hyperphosphatemia.

Acute respiratory acidosis can also lead to increases in the serum phosphate concentration, presumably owing to a shift of phosphate into the extracellular fluid.[40]

Clinical Manifestations

The clinical effects of hyperphosphatemia are related to secondary changes in calcium metabolism. Hyperphosphatemia produces hypocalcemia by several mechanisms, including precipitation of calcium phosphate salts, suppression of renal 1-hydroxylase and decreased production of 1,25-DHCC, and decreased absorption of calcium from the gastrointestinal tract, caused by direct effects of phosphate on calcium absorption and reduced 1,25-DHCC levels.[39, 41, 42]

Ectopic calcification is a major complication of hyperphosphatemia. Factors favoring the precipitation of calcium are a calcium-phosphate product greater than 70 and alkalosis. Common sites of soft tissue calcification include blood vessels, periarticular tissue, cornea, lung, and skin. Severe calcification is sometimes referred to as calciphylaxis, and high circulating PTH levels may play a role in its development.

Diagnostic Approach

The cause of hyperphosphatemia is usually obvious from the history and the clinical setting. A reduction in glomerular filtration rate (<30 mL/min) is the most common cause. The serum level of phosphate rarely exceeds 12 mg/dL, even if severe renal failure supervenes, unless large amounts of

phosphate are being added to the circulation. In other hyperphosphatemic conditions, measurement of the urinary excretion of phosphate is helpful in making the diagnosis (Fig. 103–2). Exogenous and endogenous phosphate loads are associated with increased phosphate excretion (>1000 mg/d). In contrast, phosphate excretion is often depressed in patients with increased renal tubular reabsorption. However, because excretion equals intake if the individual is in balance, situations characterized by enhanced renal tubular reabsorption may be associated with high urinary phosphate excretion if phosphate intake is also high. Determination of serum calcium and PTH levels also offers helpful clues to the underlying process. Serum PTH level is low in idiopathic or postsurgical hypoparathyroidism but is elevated in pseudohypoparathyroidism or in secondary hyperparathyroidism (e.g., renal insufficiency).

Treatment

Acute severe hyperphosphatemia with symptomatic hypocalcemia necessitates prompt treatment. If renal failure is not present, urinary phosphate excretion can be increased with the use of isotonic saline or sodium bicarbonate, 1 to 2 liters over 2 hours, and acetazolamide, 500 mg every 6 hours. When renal failure is present, institution of hemodialysis can promptly remove substantial amounts of phosphate and correct both the hyperphosphatemia and the hypocalcemia. When even more rapid control is required, glucose and insulin infusions promote cell phosphate uptake and may ameliorate hyperphosphatemia until dialysis is begun. The chronic hyperphosphatemia seen in chronic renal failure, hypoparathyroidism, or tumoral calcinosis is treated primarily by a low-phosphate diet and aluminum-, magnesium-, or calcium-containing antacids. These preparations bind ingested phosphorus and decrease intestinal absorption.

Acknowledgment. The authors gratefully acknowledge

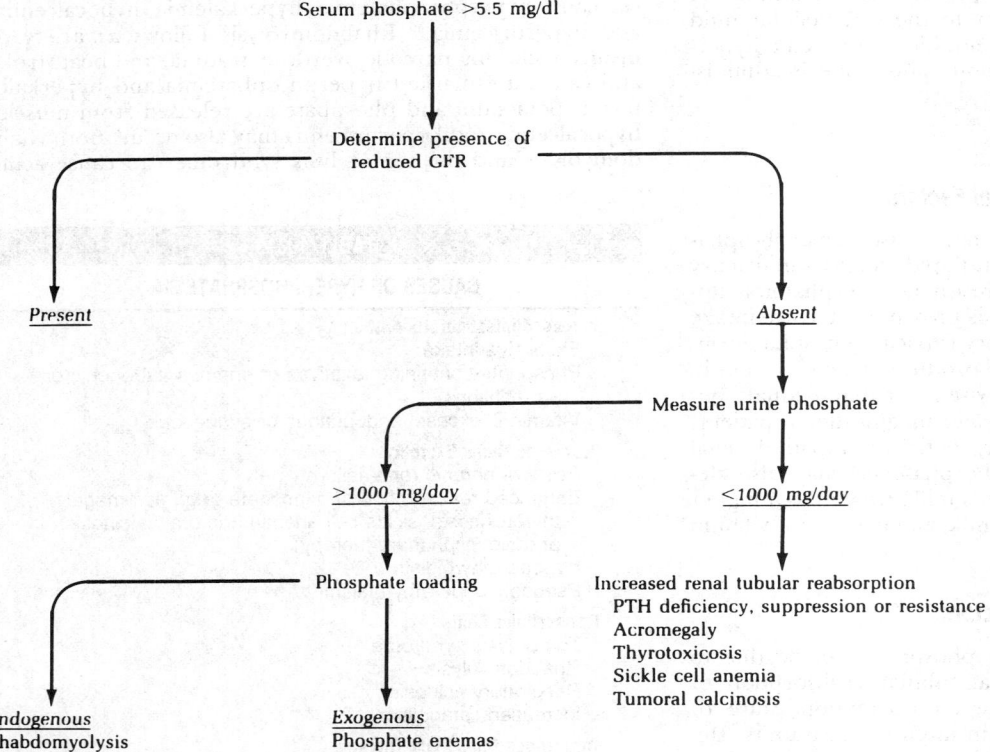

Serum phosphate >5.5 mg/dl

Determine presence of reduced GFR

Present

Absent

Measure urine phosphate

>1000 mg/day

<1000 mg/day

Phosphate loading

Increased renal tubular reabsorption
PTH deficiency, suppression or resistance
Acromegaly
Thyrotoxicosis
Sickle cell anemia
Tumoral calcinosis

Endogenous
Rhabdomyolysis
Tumor lysis

Exogenous
Phosphate enemas
Laxative abuse

Figure 103–2. Diagnostic work-up of hyperphosphatemia. GFR = glomerular filtration rate. (Reprinted with permission from Ziyadeh FN, Goldfarb S: Disorders of phosphate homeostasis. In: Stein JH [ed]: Internal Medicine. 3rd ed. Boston, Little, Brown, p 2339, 1990.)

the expert assistance of Etta Mitchell in preparing the manuscript.

References

1. Kabakoff B, Kendrick NC, DeLuca HF: 1,25-Dihydroxyvitamin D_3 stimulated active uptake of phosphate by rat jejunum. Am J Physiol 243:E470, 1982.
2. Lang F, Greger R, Knox FG, et al: Factors modulating the renal handling of phosphate. Renal Physiol 4:1, 1981.
3. Steele TH: Renal response to phosphorous deprivation: Effects of the parathyroid and bicarbonate. Kidney Int 11:327, 1977.
4. Haramati A, Haas JA, Knox FG, et al: Adaptation of deep and superficial nephrons to changes in dietary phosphate intake. Am J Physiol 244:F265, 1983.
5. Levine BS, Karokawa K, Coburn JW: Early renal adaptation to dietary phosphorus restriction. Adv Exp Med Biol 178:93, 1984.
6. Mashima Y, Ogawa M, Aoki Y, et al: Changes in phosphorus distribution during total parenteral nutrition. JPEN 5:189, 1981.
7. Spencer H, Kramer L, Norris C, et al: Effect of small doses of aluminum containing antacids on calcium and phosphorus metabolism. Am J Clin Nutr 36:32, 1982.
8. Agus ZS: Oncogenic hypophosphatemic osteomalacia. Kidney Int 24:113, 1983.
9. Rosenbaum RW: Decreased phosphate reabsorption after renal transplantation: Evidence for a mechanism independent of calcium and parathyroid hormone. Kidney Int 19:568, 1981.
10. Ziyadeh FN, Goldfarb S: Disorders of phosphate homeostasis. In: Stein JH (ed): Internal Medicine. 3rd ed. Boston, Little, Brown, p 2339, 1990.
11. Keller U, Berger W: Prevention of hypophosphatemia by phosphate infusion during treatment of diabetic ketoacidosis and hyperosmolar coma. Diabetes 29:87, 1980.
12. Forsham PH, Thorn GW: Changes in inorganic serum phosphorus during the intravenous glucose tolerance test as an adjunct to the diagnosis of early diabetes mellitus. Proc Am Diabetes Assoc 9:101, 1949.
13. Silvis SE, Dibartolomeo AG, Aaker HM: Hypophosphatemia and neurologic changes secondary to oral caloric intake: A variant of hyperalimentation syndrome. Am J Gastroenterol 73:215, 1980.
14. Mostellar ME, Tuttle EP: Effects of alkalosis on plasma concentration and urinary excretion of urinary phosphate in man. J Clin Invest 43:138, 1964.
15. Matzner Y, Prococimer M, Polliack A, et al: Hypophosphatemia in a patient with lymphoma in the leukemic phase. Arch Intern Med 141:805, 1981.
16. Levy LA: Severe hypophosphatemia as a complication of the treatment of hypothermia. Arch Intern Med 140:128, 1980.
17. Ryback RS, Eckardt MH, Paulter CP: Clinical relationships between serum phosphorus and other blood chemistry values in alcoholics. Arch Intern Med 140:673, 1980.
18. Rubin MF, Narins RG: Hypophosphatemia: Physiological and practical aspects of its therapy. Semin Nephrol 10:536, 1990.
19. Blachley J, Knochel JP: Alcoholic-induced disturbances in electrolyte and acid-base homeostasis. In Kokko JP, Tannen RL (eds): Fluids and Electrolytes. Philadelphia, WB Saunders, p 513, 1986.
20. Lennquist S, Lindell B, Nordstrom H, et al: Hypophosphatemia in severe burns. Acta Chir Scand 145:1, 1979.
21. Yu GC, Lee DBN: Hypophosphatemia and phosphate depletion. In: Glassock RJ (ed): Current Therapy in Nephrology and Hypertension, Volume 2. Philadelphia, BC Decker, p 26, 1987.
22. Knochel JP: Hypophosphatemia in the alcoholic. Arch Intern Med 140:613, 1980.
23. Knochel JP, Barcenas C, Cotton JR, et al: Hypophosphatemia and rhabdomyolysis. J Clin Invest 62:1240, 1978.
24. Newman JH, Neff TA, Ziporin P: Acute respiratory failure associated with hypophosphatemia. N Engl J Med 296:1101, 1977.
25. Davis SV, Olichwier KK, Chakko SC: Reversible depression of myocardial performance in hypophosphatemia. Am J Med Sci 295:183, 1988.
26. Knochel JP: The pathophysiology and clinical characteristics of severe hypophosphatemia. Arch Intern Med 137:203, 1977.
27. Lichtman MA, Miller DR, Cohen J: Reduced red cell glycolysis, 1,3-diphosphoglycerate and adenosine triphosphate concentration and increased oxygen affinity caused by hypophosphatemia. Ann Intern Med 74:562, 1971.
28. Jacob HS, Amsden T: Acute hemolytic anemia with rigid cells in hypophosphatemia. N Engl J Med 385:1446, 1971.
29. Craddock PR, Yawata Y, Van Santen L, et al: Acquired phagocyte dysfunction: A complication of the hypophosphatemia of parenteral hyperalimentation. N Engl J Med 290:1403, 1974.
30. Yawata Y, Hebbel RP, Silvis S, et al: Blood cell abnormalities complicating the hypophosphatemia of hyperalimentation: Erythrocyte and platelet ATP deficiency associated with hemolytic anemia in hyperalimented dogs. J Lab Clin Med 84:643, 1974.
31. Brautbar N, Lee DB, Coburn WJ, et al: Influence of dietary magnesium in experimental phosphate depletion: Bone and soft tissue mineral changes. Am J Physiol 237:E152, 1979.
32. DeFronzo RA, Lang R: Hypophosphatemia and glucose intolerance: Evidence for tissue insensitivity to insulin. N Engl J Med 303:1259, 1980.
33. Sheldon GF, Grzyb S: Phosphate depletion and repletion: Relation to parenteral nutrition and oxygen transport. Ann Surg 182:683, 1975.
34. Keller U, Berger W: Prevention of hypophosphatemia by phosphate infusion during treatment of diabetic ketoacidosis and hyperosmolar coma. Diabetes 29:87, 1980.
35. Wardrop CAJ: Oxygen availability from the blood and the effect of phosphate replacement on erythrocyte 2,3-DPG and hemoglobin-oxygen affinity in diabetic ketoacidosis. Diabetologia 15:381, 1978.
36. Kobrin SM, Goldfarb S: Magnesium deficiency. Semin Nephrol 10:525, 1990.
37. McConnell TH: Fatal hypocalcemia from phosphate absorption from laxative preparations. JAMA 216:147, 1971.
38. Koffler A, Friedler RM, Massry SG: Acute renal failure due to non-traumatic rhabdomyolysis. Ann Intern Med 85:23, 1978.
39. Tsokos GC, Balow JE, Spiegel RJ, et al: Renal and metabolic complications of undifferentiated lymphoblastic lymphomas. Medicine 60:218, 1981.
40. Giebisch C, Berger L, Pitts R: The extrarenal response to acute acid-base disturbances of respiratory origin. J Clin Invest 34:321, 1955.
41. Gray RW, Wilz DR, Caldas AE, et al: The importance of phosphate in regulating plasma $1,25(OH)_2$ vitamin D levels in humans. J Clin Endocrinol Metab 45:299, 1977.
42. Morgan DB: Calcium and phosphorus transport across the intestine. In Girdwood RM, Smith AW (eds): Malabsorption. Baltimore, Williams & Wilkins, 1969.

CHAPTER 104

Acid-Base Homeostasis

George M. Feldman
Elizabeth B. D. Ripley

Maintenance of acid-base balance is essential to life and is assessed by measuring the H^+ concentration in arterial blood. Alterations of the H^+ concentration, whether in excess or in deficit, are deleterious to cell function, and extremes of acid-base imbalance are rapidly fatal. An elevated H^+ concentration (acidemia) reduces cardiac output and pulmonary blood flow, decreases the affinity of hemoglobin for O_2, and may cause hyperkalemia. A depressed H^+ concentration (alkalemia) reduces cardiac output, increases the affinity of hemoglobin for O_2, reduces the concentration of Ca^{2+} in plasma (thus lowering the seizure threshold), and may cause hypokalemia.

ACID-BASE BALANCE

Understanding acid-base balance (and imbalance) is central to the treatment of patients in the intensive care setting.[1] Two concepts are fundamental in this regard. First, changes in H^+ concentration are reciprocal to changes in OH^- concentration. This means that if H^+ is in excess there is a deficit of OH^- and vice versa. The H^+ concentration is conventionally measured in units of pH (pH $= -\log [H^+]$, where $[H^+]$ is the concentration of H^+ and is expressed in gram equivalents per liter). Second, acid-base balance (as implied by the term balance) is the result of multiple processes that add and remove H^+ and OH^-; each of these separate but sometimes coexisting processes affects blood pH. Dietary intake, cellular metabolism, and the pulmonary, renal, and gastrointestinal systems all modulate acid-base balance. The term *acidosis* is used to describe processes that cause accumulation of H^+ (or deficit of OH^-) in the body, whereas the term *alkalosis* is used to describe processes that cause a deficit of H^+ (or excess of OH^-).

H^+ and OH^- Production

The diet is a major source of both acids and bases.[2, 3] Oxidation of sulfur-containing amino acids (e.g., methionine) produces H^+ (i.e., H_2SO_4), and complete oxidation of carbon compounds yields carbonic acid (i.e., H_2CO_3 or CO_2 + H_2O). H_2SO_4 is an example of a fixed or nonvolatile acid; fixed acids are excreted by the kidneys. H_2CO_3 is volatile and is eliminated by respiration. Incomplete oxidation yields other nonvolatile acids, such as lactic, β-hydroxybutyric, and acetoacetic acids. Base is also generated metabolically; for example, the oxidation of acetate, citrate, and linolate yields OH^-, which in the presence of CO_2 exists principally as HCO_3^-. With a typical American diet, CO_2 production is approximately 220 mmol/kg body weight per day, and nonvolatile H^+ production exceeds OH^- production by approximately 1 mmol/kg/d.

Distribution and Buffering of H^+

Acids and bases are not evenly distributed throughout the body. The cells of some organs selectively transport H^+ and HCO_3^-. At various sites along the gastrointestinal tract and the nephron, for example, certain cells secrete H^+ or HCO_3^-, allowing HCO_3^- or H^+ to accumulate on their antiluminal borders. Thus, as part of the normal digestive process, the stomach secretes H^+, with gastric fluid attaining a pH less than 2 and HCO_3^- accumulating in the blood (thereby generating the so-called postprandial alkaline tide). Acidic gastric juice then enters the small intestine, where it is neutralized by HCO_3^--rich hepatic, pancreatic, and duodenal secretions. In the kidney, 4500 mEq of HCO_3^- is filtered and reabsorbed daily (filtered load of HCO_3^- = plasma HCO_3^- × glomerular filtration rate or 25 mEq/L × 125 mL/min = 4500 mEq/d). The proximal nephron reabsorbs the bulk of the filtered HCO_3^-, thereby forestalling massive HCO_3^- depletion. The distal nephron secretes H^+ at a rate of approximately 1 mEq/kg/d, compensating for net metabolic production of nonvolatile H^+.

By minimizing pH changes (as H^+ and/or HCO_3^- move into and out of organs and cells), buffers contribute to the maintenance of pH within an extremely narrow range. The CO_2-HCO_3^- buffer system is the most important:

$$H_2O + CO_2 \rightleftharpoons H_2CO_3 \rightleftharpoons H^+ + HCO_3^-$$

Because [H_2CO_3] is directly dependent on [CO_2], this equilibrium can be rewritten as

$$H_2O + CO_2 \rightleftharpoons H^+ + HCO_3^-$$

In the more traditional Henderson-Hasselbalch format this becomes

$$pH = pK + \log \frac{[HCO_3^-]}{[CO_2]}$$

where pK is the equilibrium constant (6.1). In this format, it is obvious that pH varies directly with the ratio of base (HCO_3^-) to acid (CO_2). Clinically, [CO_2] in millimoles per liter is determined by measuring the partial pressure of CO_2 in millimeters of mercury or torr (PCO_2) and multiplying by the CO_2 aqueous solubility coefficient (0.03). The normal PCO_2 is 40 torr, yielding a [CO_2] of 1.2 mmol/L (i.e., 40 × 0.03). For the normal [HCO_3^-] of 24 mmol/L, the normal

ratio of base to acid is 24/1.2 = 20, corresponding to a pH of 7.40.

The importance of the CO_2 - HCO_3^- buffer system is due to its abundance and the relationships between the buffer components (CO_2 and HCO_3^-) and the organs that independently regulate their blood concentrations. The kidneys regulate [HCO_3^-] and the lungs regulate PCO_2. Independent homeostatic regulation implies that alterations in systemic pH are minimized as one system compensates for any abnormalities in the other system. For example, in metabolic acidosis the primary abnormality is a decrease in the HCO_3^- concentration, which would reduce the pH. However, because of a compensatory increase in ventilation, PCO_2 decreases, blunting the effect of the HCO_3^- deficit on pH.

As part of homeostatic regulation, in response to acid-base disorders the lungs and kidneys adjust the rate of acid (base) excretion. Although other organs (e.g., the gastrointestinal tract), also handle large quantities of H^+ and HCO_3^-, these acid-base fluxes usually neutralize one another and therefore do not result in net gain of H^+ or HCO_3^- by the body. The respiratory system maintains the arterial blood PCO_2 under strict control. Primary disorders of this system (respiratory acid-base disorders) are discussed in The Pulmonary System section. As noted, the respiratory system also has an essential role in the compensation of metabolic acid-base disorders. To minimize the pH decrement caused by metabolic acidosis, ventilation (and therefore CO_2 excretion) increases, causing PCO_2 to fall. An analogous defense of body fluid pH occurs in metabolic alkalosis: as ventilation is depressed, PCO_2 rises and the increase in pH (alkalemia) is blunted.

Renal Regulation of Acid-Base Balance

To regulate the metabolic component of acid-base balance (i.e., the HCO_3^- concentration), the kidneys must perform two distinct functions: in the proximal tubule, sufficient H^+ to reclaim the filtered load of HCO_3^- must be secreted, and in the distal nephron, sufficient H^+ to neutralize the fixed acid load must be secreted.

HCO_3^- Reclamation

In the proximal nephron (Fig. 104–1), HCO_3^- reclamation occurs via H^+ secretion and titration of luminal HCO_3^- to H_2CO_3. Carbonic anhydrase, an enzyme located in the brush border on the luminal surface of proximal tubular cells, accelerates the dehydration of H_2CO_3 to CO_2 + H_2O, allowing CO_2 to diffuse rapidly out of the lumen into the cell. In the cell, CO_2 + H_2O generates H_2CO_3, which in turn provides H^+ and HCO_3^-. The H^+ is secreted into the lumen while the HCO_3^- exits the basolateral surface of the cell, returning to the blood.

Central to this scheme is the vectorial transport of H^+ (across the luminal membrane) and HCO_3^- (across the basolateral membrane).[4, 5] For the most part, apical (luminal) H^+ secretion depends on Na^+-H^+ exchange, but an H^+-ATPase pump may also be involved. At the basolateral surface, HCO_3^- exits the cell in conjunction with Na^+. Angiotensin II stimulates both apical Na^+-H^+ exchange and basolateral Na^+-HCO_3^- cotransport and may provide the regulatory link between hypovolemia and the increase in proximal tubular HCO_3^- reabsorption that is characteristic of volume-depleted states.[6] The adaptations to metabolic acidosis, respiratory acidosis, and K^+ depletion also involve increasing the effectiveness of proximal tubular HCO_3^- reabsorption by enhancing apical Na^+-H^+ exchange and basolateral Na^+-HCO_3^- cotransport. Parathyroid hormone and acetazolamide inhibit HCO_3^- reabsorption and can in-

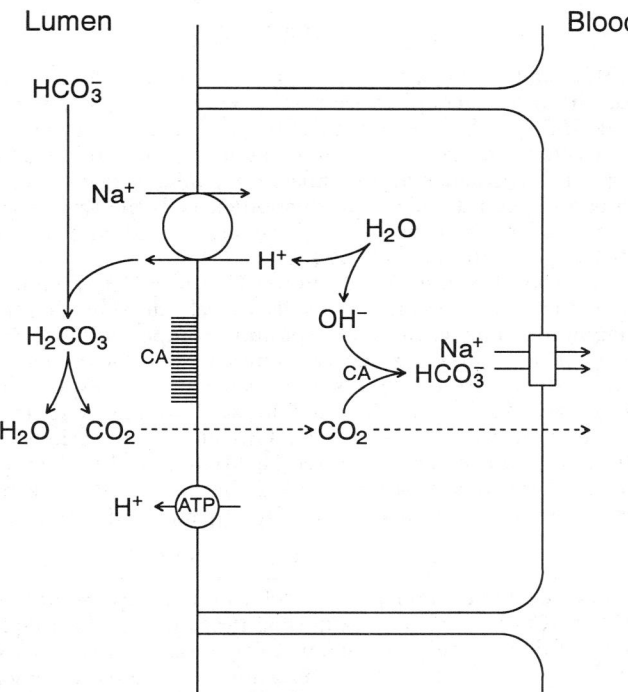

Figure 104–1. Model of HCO_3^- reabsorption in the proximal tubule. The predominant component of H^+ secretion occurs by Na^+-H^+ exchange; a smaller component may occur via an H^+-ATPase pump. Carbonic anhydrase (CA) is located on the luminal brush border and intracellularly. HCO_3^- exits the cell via an Na^+-coupled cotransporter.

duce mild metabolic acidosis. Acetazolamide inhibits brush border carbonic anhydrase activity, thereby slowing H_2CO_3 dehydration.

Fixed Acid Excretion

Metabolically produced, nonvolatile (fixed) acid excretion is a function of the distal portions of the nephron, where H^+ secretion is driven by ATP-dependent H^+ pumps capable of attaining urinary pH values as low as 4.5.[5] In cortical and medullary collecting tubules, H^+ is pumped into the urine by an H^+-ATPase located in the apical cell membrane of alpha intercalated cells (Fig. 104–2). H^+ secretion also depends on H_2CO_3 availability, intracellular carbonic anhydrase activity, and the ability of HCO_3^- to exit the cell across the basolateral membrane in exchange for Cl^-. The H^+-ATPase found in alpha intercalated cells is different from the enzyme found in stomach. A gastric-like H^+, K^+-ATPase, located on the luminal surface of cortical collecting tubule principal cells, may also have a role in renal H^+ secretion (see Fig. 104–2).[7]

Various factors influence distal H^+ secretion.[5] Aldosterone stimulates H^+ secretion both directly (by increasing H^+-ATPase activity) and indirectly (by increasing Na^+ reabsorption). Na^+ reabsorption increases luminal electronegativity (voltage), thereby facilitating the transport of H^+ from neighboring alpha intercalated cells into the lumen. Hypoaldosteronism or resistance to aldosterone (e.g., spironolactone administration) reduces H^+ secretion. Furosemide stimulates H^+ secretion by increasing Na^+ delivery, which also increases principal cell Na^+ reabsorption, luminal electronegativity, and voltage-dependent H^+ secretion. Similar voltage effects are seen after administration of relatively impermeant (in comparison to Cl^-) anions such as sulfate, phosphate, and some penicillin derivatives (e.g., carbenicil-

lin). Reduced Na^+ delivery decreases H^+ secretion, and amiloride, by blocking principal cell Na^+ reabsorption, reduces luminal voltage and voltage-dependent H^+ excretion.

In addition to the ability to acidify the urine, urinary buffers (e.g., ammonia and phosphate) are needed to excrete nonvolatile H^+. To illustrate the critical importance of urinary buffers, consider that a 70-kg person in acid-base balance must excrete about 70 mEq of metabolically produced nonvolatile H^+ in the urine daily. If the urine were buffer free, even at the lowest pH achievable (4.5), more than 2200 L of urine would have to be excreted each day to maintain acid-base balance. In contrast, with normal urinary buffers, the daily fixed acid production is easily excreted in 1 to 2 L. Phosphate and ammonia are the principal urinary buffers. Urinary phosphate depends largely on dietary intake (~1 g/d), whereas ammonia is produced locally by deamination of glutamine in the renal cortex. The ammonia then enters the tubular fluid by nonionic diffusion. Urinary ammonia excretion depends on the rate of ammonia production, urine flow, and distal nephron H^+ secretion (i.e., urinary pH).[8] Secreted H^+ titrates, and thereby traps, diffusible ammonia (NH_3) in its ionic, nondiffusible form (NH_4^+). Ammonia synthesis is influenced by acid-base balance, potassium balance, and circulating glucocorticoid levels. Metabolic acidosis, hypokalemia, and glucocorticoid excess stimulate ammonia production, whereas metabolic alkalosis, hyperkalemia, and glucocorticoid deficiency depress ammonia synthesis.

Disorders of Acid-Base Balance and Compensation

Disorders of acid-base balance—that is, accumulation of excess H^+ (or HCO_3^-) in the body—result from altered H^+

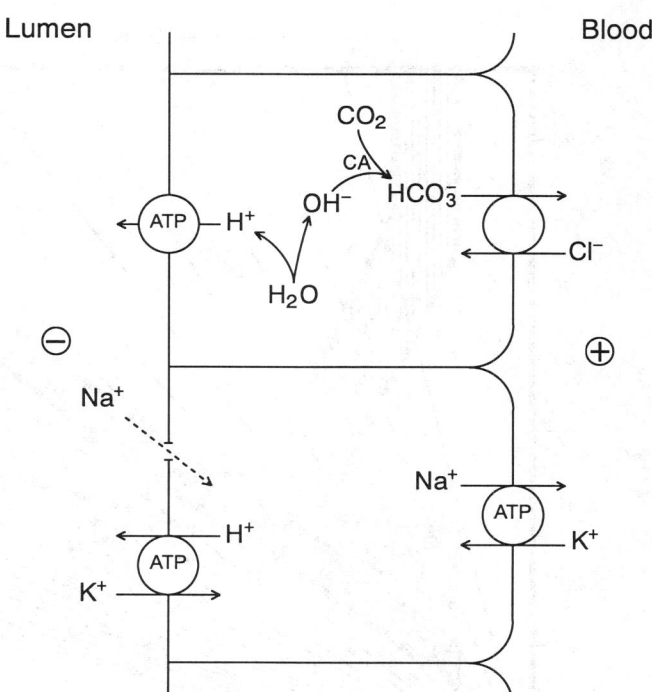

Figure 104–2. Model of acid secretion in the collecting tubule. In the alpha intercalated cell (top cell), H^+ secretion is pumped via an H^+-ATPase pump and HCO_3^- exits the cell by Cl^--HCO_3^- exchange. In neighboring principal cells (bottom cell), Na^+ reabsorption generates a negative voltage in the lumen, aiding H^+ secretion by the alpha intercalated cells. In some cells, H^+ secretion may also involve a gastric-like H^+, K^+-ATPase pump.

(or HCO_3^-) excretion and/or altered H^+ (or HCO_3^-) input. In other words, acidosis occurs when the rate of H^+ intake exceeds the rate of H^+ output or when the rate of base loss exceeds the rate of base intake. Likewise, alkalosis occurs when the rate of base intake exceeds the rate of base loss or when the rate of H^+ excretion exceeds the rate of H^+ input. The type of disorder, metabolic or respiratory, depends on whether the primary abnormality is one of altered HCO_3^- concentration (metabolic) or Pco_2 (respiratory).

After the primary acid-base abnormality, a secondary or compensatory response ensues that has the effect of returning pH toward normal. In response to primary metabolic abnormalities, the compensatory process is respiratory, whereas renal compensation occurs in response to respiratory disorders. Thus, acidemia caused by a metabolic abnormality induces hyperventilation, alkalemia caused by a metabolic abnormality induces hypoventilation, hypercapnia increases renal HCO_3^- generation (H^+ excretion), and hypocapnia decreases net urinary acid excretion. In terms of the Henderson-Hasselbalch equation, the compensatory response alters the $[HCO_3^-]/[CO_2]$ ratio, tending to return the ratio to its initial value of 20. However, because the magnitude of the compensatory response is not as great as that of the primary disturbance, the pH is not completely normalized. Moreover, compensation is not instantaneous; it can take hours or days to be fully expressed.[9] Whereas the renal response to hypercapnia takes several days to be completed, the renal response to hypercapnia is completed in 12 to 24 hours and the respiratory response to metabolic abnormalities (acidemia or alkalemia) is maximal within only a few hours. The pH, Pco_2, and $[HCO_3^-]$ patterns for the lone primary acid-base disorders, including the ensuing compensation, are depicted in Figure 104–3.[10]

METABOLIC ACIDOSIS

Metabolic acidosis, the most common abnormality of acid-base balance, is characterized by a decrease in systemic pH and $[HCO_3^-]$. Severe acidemia (pH < 7.2) reduces cardiac contractility, decreases systemic vascular tone, and predisposes to ventricular arrhythmias. Metabolic acidosis occurs whenever the rate of H^+ production exceeds the rate of H^+ excretion or when the rate of base loss exceeds the rate of HCO_3^- generation (Table 104–1).

In response to the decrement in pH and $[HCO_3^-]$, minute ventilation increases and Pco_2 falls, thereby ameliorating the magnitude of acidification. Respiratory compensation begins immediately but takes several hours to become maximal. The pattern of respiration, known as Kussmaul's respiration, is characterized by an increase in tidal volume and, to a lesser extent, an increase in rate. The fall in Pco_2 varies with the severity of the acidemia (see Fig. 104–3) and is given by Winters' formula,[11] which predicts the arterial Pco_2 (compensation) for a low arterial $[HCO_3^-]$ (primary disturbance):

$$Pco_2 = 1.5 \times HCO_3^- + 8 \, (\pm 2)$$

The so-called anion gap or delta (anion gap = Na^+ − $[Cl^- + tCO_2]$),* which has a normal range of 8 to 16 mEq/L, is helpful in classifying metabolic acidosis.[12] Based on the principle that the cation concentration must equal the anion concentration, an increased difference between measured

---

*Total CO_2 (tCO_2) is often loosely referred to as HCO_3^- but actually encompasses both $[HCO_3^-]$ and dissolved CO_2. Moreover, tCO_2 is typically determined in serum (or plasma) obtained from the venous circulation. Consequently, the venous tCO_2 should be higher than arterial $[HCO_3^-]$ by 2 to 5 mmol/L. Traditionally, tCO_2 is used to calculate the anion gap and the arterial $[HCO_3^-]$ is used with Winters' formula and the acid-base nomogram.

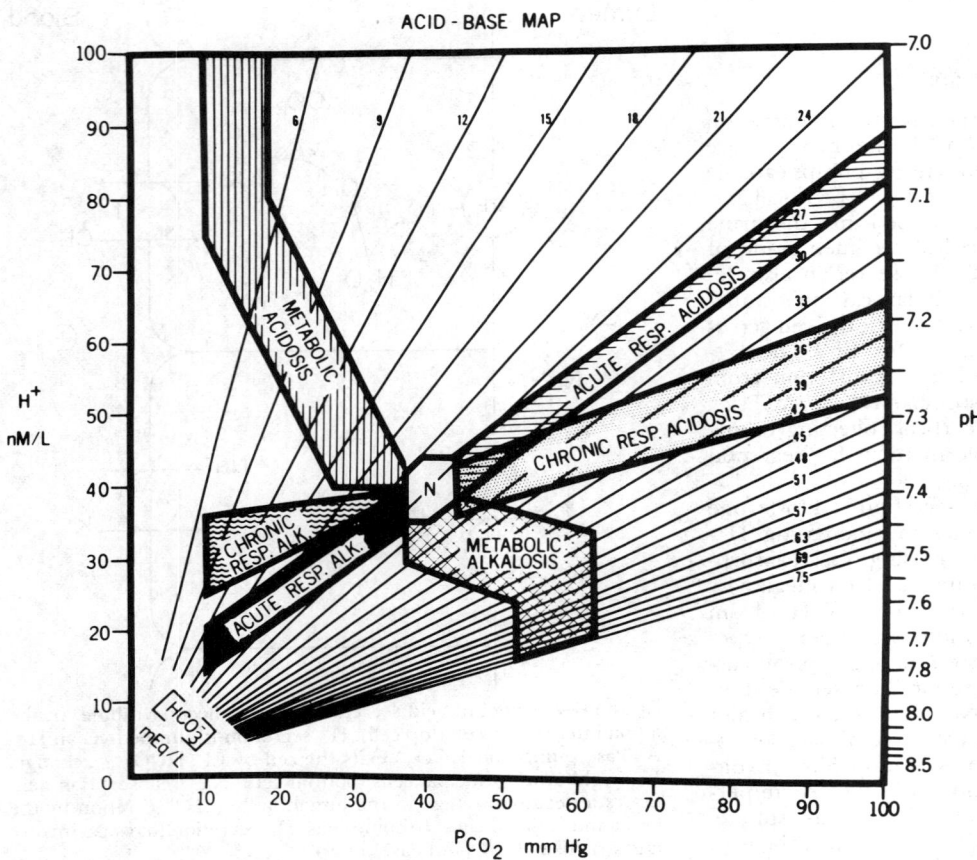

Figure 104–3. Acid-base nomogram showing the 95% confidence limits of compensation for primary acid-base disturbances. N = normal range; RESP = respiratory; ALK = alkalosis. (From Goldberg M, Green SB, Moss ML, et al: Computer-based instruction and diagnosis of acid-base disorders: A systematic approach. JAMA 233:269–275, 1973. Copyright 1973, American Medical Association.)

TABLE 104–1

CAUSES OF METABOLIC ACIDOSIS

Increased H⁺ production
  Metabolic abnormalities (e.g., lactic acidosis, diabetic ketoacidosis)
  Toxins (e.g., methanol, ethylene glycol, salicylate)
  Ingestion of acid (e.g., HCl, NH₄Cl)
Decreased H⁺ excretion (i.e., decreased HCO₃⁻ generation)
  Renal failure
  Renal tubular acidosis (distal renal tubular acidosis, deficient ammonia synthesis)
HCO₃⁻ loss
  Gastrointestinal (e.g., diarrhea)
  Renal (proximal renal tubular acidosis)

cations and anions represents an increase in the unmeasured anions of nonvolatile acids. These anions accumulate either because of increased acid production (e.g., lactate in lactic acidosis, acetoacetate and β-hydroxybutyrate in diabetic ketoacidosis) or because of their retention in renal failure (e.g., phosphate, sulfate). In the absence of a widened anion gap, metabolic acidosis is referred to as hyperchloremic metabolic acidosis (Table 104–2). In contrast to the metabolic source of H⁺ in anion gap acidoses, hyperchloremic acidoses result from excess exogenous H⁺, H⁺ retention caused by renal tubular defects, or base loss via the gastrointestinal tract or kidneys.

Because the anion gap is calculated from three independent laboratory determinations and is influenced by factors unrelated to acid-base balance, there are important limitations to its use. For example, because albumin is the predominant unmeasured anion, the anion gap varies directly with the serum albumin concentration. Because the net negative charge of albumin varies as a function of pH, the contribution of albumin to the anion gap also varies with blood pH: acidemia decreases the anion gap, and alkalemia increases it.[13, 14] Other proteins also have significant charge (either cationic or anionic) and, if present in abnormally high concentration (e.g., gamma globulins in multiple myeloma), affect the anion gap.[15, 16] Some antibiotics (e.g., penicillin derivatives) are administered as salts and can contribute to the anion gap if given in large doses, especially in renal failure, when their excretion is decreased. Abnormal elevations of the other important serum cations, such as Li⁺, Mg²⁺, and Ca²⁺, and the presence of bromide in plasma (which causes a falsely elevated chloride concentration) reduce the size of the anion gap.[17, 18] The normal range for the anion gap has also changed as newer analytic techniques have been introduced; in some instruments the Cl⁻ determination tends to be higher than it was in the past and thus the normal range for the anion gap is reduced.[19] Errors in the determination of tCO₂ can also influence the anion gap. Thus, although the anion gap can provide an important clue to the presence of organic acidosis, it should not replace the direct determination of the organic acid concentrations. This is particularly true in the intensive care unit setting, where hypoalbuminemia and acidemia may obscure the expected widening of the anion gap in patients with lactic acidosis.

Severe hyperkalemia, resulting from a shift of intracellular K⁺ into the extracellular fluid, can occur in acute metabolic acidosis. This alteration in internal K⁺ balance depends on the type of metabolic acidosis rather than on the severity of acidemia. Hyperkalemia occurs in acute hyperchloremic acidosis[20] but not in acute metabolic acidosis caused by excess production of organic acids such as lactic acid.[21, 22] The serum [K⁺] in these circumstances is also influenced by a variety of other factors, including the patient's volume status, plasma insulin and aldosterone concentrations, and renal K⁺ excretory ability. Chronic metabolic acidosis is not associated with hyperkalemia unless there is a concomitant defect in renal K⁺ excretion.

Metabolic Acidosis of Nonrenal Origin
Anion Gap Acidosis

Lactic acidosis and diabetic ketoacidosis, the most common anion gap metabolic acidoses, are discussed in Chapters 105 and 106. Other forms of ketoacidosis are alcoholic ketoacidosis and starvation ketosis.[23] Alcoholic ketoacidosis typically occurs after a drinking binge, during which there is inadequate caloric intake and often vomiting as well. It is marked by elevated β-hydroxybutyrate and free fatty acid concentrations but not by severely elevated glucose or acetoacetate concentrations. Treatment consists of intravenous glucose and electrolytes to replenish deficits. Starvation can produce excess ketoacids as well, but the acidosis is mild, with the [HCO₃⁻] usually remaining above 20 mEq/L.

The metabolic products of methanol (wood alcohol) and ethylene glycol (antifreeze) are toxic organic acids. Methanol is metabolized by alcohol dehydrogenase to formaldehyde and then to formic acid.[24] Formic acid dissociates to H⁺ and formate, causing acidosis and widening the anion gap. Formate is extremely toxic to the optic nerve, causing optic neuritis, papilledema, and blindness. Ethylene glycol is metabolized by alcohol dehydrogenase to glycolaldehyde and then to glycolic, oxalic, and formic acids, all of which dissociate, producing acidosis and widening anion gap. Calcium oxalate crystals, which are usually readily evident in the urine, deposit in renal tubules and other organs, including the brain, heart, and lungs.[25] The treatment of methanol and ethylene glycol toxicity is similar, involving steps to reduce the continued generation of toxic organic acids and steps to diminish their toxicity: (1) remove any residual alcohol in the stomach with activated charcoal, (2) inhibit metabolism of the more toxic alcohol by administering the less toxic alcohol ethanol, (3) maintain a normal systemic pH with HCO₃⁻ administration, and (4) remove both the alcohol and its toxic metabolites with hemodialysis.[26]

Salicylate intoxication can cause anion gap acidosis, inducing both lactic acidosis and ketoacidosis.[27] At lower toxic concentrations, respiratory alkalosis is more common, but at higher doses (and especially in children) salicylate produces

TABLE 104–2

CAUSES OF HYPERCHLOREMIC METABOLIC ACIDOSIS

Nonrenal
  Acid ingestion
    HCl
    NH₄Cl
    Amino acids (arginine hydrochloride, lysine hydrochloride)
  Base loss (gastrointestinal tract)
    Diarrhea and small-bowel losses
    Anion-exchange resins (cholestyramine)
    Ingestion of CaCl₂ or MgCl₂
    Ureterosigmoidostomy
    Ileal loop conduit
Renal
  Acid retention
    Distal renal tubular acidosis (dRTA)
    Deficient ammonia synthesis
  HCO₃⁻ loss
    Proximal renal tubular acidosis (pRTA)

metabolic acidosis. Treatment with HCO_3^- is helpful: raising the pH minimizes the cellular uptake of salicylate and enhances the renal excretion of this organic anion. However, extreme alkalemia may complicate HCO_3^- therapy if aggressive treatment eliminates the metabolic acidosis in a patient with salicylate-induced respiratory alkalosis as well. Careful monitoring of arterial pH and Pco_2 and judicious use of HCO_3^- are mandatory.

Hyperchloremic Acidosis

Administration or ingestion of HCl is an obvious cause of hyperchloremic metabolic acidosis (see Table 104–2). Because they are metabolized to HCl, administered NH_4Cl, arginine hydrochloride, and lysine hydrochloride also cause hyperchloremic acidosis. In contrast to the chloride salts, the acetate salts of these substances do not cause acidosis because acetate is metabolized to HCO_3^-, neutralizing the metabolically produced H^+. Acids other than HCl can also cause normal anion gap acidosis if renal excretion of the accompanying anion is rapid. For example, during the recovery phase of ketoacidosis a normal anion gap acidosis occurs because administered chloride replaces excreted ketoacid anions.[28, 29] Intravenous infusion of saline can dilute the plasma $[HCO_3^-]$ and cause metabolic acidosis if large volumes are administered rapidly. However, the severity of "dilutional" acidosis is effectively blunted by the buffering effects of nonbicarbonate buffers.[30]

Gastrointestinal base loss also leads to hyperchloremic metabolic acidosis (see Table 104–2). Because the ileum and colon normally secrete HCO_3^-,[31] diarrhea typically results in base loss; if this loss is of sufficient magnitude, metabolic acidosis follows. Ingestion of large quantities of cholestyramine (a Cl^--rich, anion-exchange resin) can cause exchange of secreted HCO_3^- for bound Cl^-, resulting in base loss. Similarly, ingestion of calcium or magnesium chloride salts (but not carbonate, acetate, or gluconate salts) results in precipitation of relatively insoluble $CaCO_3$ and $MgCO_3$ and increased fecal base excretion. Finally, because intestinal HCO_3^- secretion occurs by Cl^--HCO_3^- exchange, patients

TABLE 104–3
CAUSES OF PROXIMAL RENAL TUBULAR ACIDOSIS

Primary
  Idiopathic
  Inherited
Secondary to inherited disease
  Cystinosis
  Hereditary fructose intolerance
  Lowe's syndrome
  Wilson's disease
  Carbonic anhydrase deficiency or dysfunction
  Pyruvate carboxylase deficiency
Drugs and toxic agents
  Heavy metals (lead, cadmium, copper, mercury)
  Carbonic anhydrase inhibitors
  Outdated tetracycline
  Arginine and lysine
Miscellaneous
  Hyperparathyroidism
  Multiple myeloma
  Sjögren's syndrome
  Amyloidosis
  Nephrotic syndrome
  Renal transplantation
  Hypervitaminosis D
  Deficiency of vitamin D
  Chronic active hepatitis

TABLE 104–4
CAUSES OF DISTAL RENAL TUBULAR ACIDOSIS

Primary
  Idiopathic
  Inherited
Secondary to inherited disease
  Osteoporosis
  Nerve deafness
  Carbonic anhydrase deficiency or dysfunction
  Hereditary fructose intolerance
Drugs and toxic agents
  Amphotericin B
  Lithium
  Toluene
  Amiloride
Disorders of calcium metabolism
  Nephrocalcinosis
  Idiopathic hypercalciuria
  Hypervitaminosis D
  Hyperparathyroidism
Systemic diseases
  Idiopathic hypergammaglobulinemia
  Multiple myeloma
  Systemic lupus erythematosus
  Sjögren's syndrome
  Hepatic cirrhosis
  Primary biliary cirrhosis
  Chronic active hepatitis
  Interstitial renal disease
  Obstructive uropathy
  Rejection of renal transplant
  Sickle cell disease
  Medullary sponge kidney
  Analgesic nephropathy

with ureterosigmoidostomies and obstructed ileal loop conduits are at risk for enhanced HCO_3^- secretion and excretion; the severity of the resulting acidosis depends on the intestinal surface area exposed to Cl^--rich urine and the duration of the exposure.[32]

Metabolic Acidosis of Renal Origin

Renal insufficiency can be associated with an anion gap metabolic acidosis or a hyperchloremic metabolic acidosis. Reduced filtration of unmeasured anions (e.g., sulfate, phosphate, and organic anions) accounts for the widened anion gap. However, when the filtration of these anions is adequate but renal H^+ or HCO_3^- handling is impaired, hyperchloremic acidosis results. Acidosis resulting from defective HCO_3^- reabsorption in the proximal tubule (and consequently urinary HCO_3^- loss) is called proximal renal tubular acidosis (pRTA) (Table 104–3). Distal renal tubular acidosis (dRTA) is a term that encompasses a variety of defects in distal urinary acidification that limit the excretion of metabolically produced, nonvolatile or fixed H^+ (Table 104–4). In addition to these two broad categories, the failure to synthesize or excrete sufficient quantities of the major urinary buffer (ammonia) diminishes net H^+ excretion and is a common cause of hyperchloremic metabolic acidosis (Table 104–5).

Proximal Renal Tubular Acidosis

Defects in proximal tubular HCO_3^- reabsorption usually occur with other abnormalities in proximal tubule function, including defects in glucose, phosphate, uric acid, and amino acid transport (Fanconi's syndrome). The reduction in serum $[HCO_3^-]$ means that the filtered load of HCO_3^- is diminished in patients with pRTA and that at a steady state proximal

TABLE 104-5

CAUSES OF IMPAIRED NET ACID EXCRETION

Primary aldosterone deficiency
  Adrenal steroid deficiency
    Addison's disease
    Bilateral adrenalectomy
    Bilateral adrenal destruction (hemorrhage, carcinoma)
    Adrenal enzyme defects (21-hydroxylase deficiency, 3β-ol-
      dehydrogenase deficiency, desmolase deficiency,
      acquired immunodeficiency syndrome)
  Isolated aldosterone deficiency
    Familial hypoaldosteronism
    Primary zona glomerulosa defect
    Transient hypoaldosteronism of infancy
    Chronic hypoaldosteronism
    Heparin
    Persistent hypotension
  Inhibition of angiotensin I–converting enzyme
    Primary
    Drugs (e.g., captopril, enalapril)
  Hyporeninemic hypoaldosteronism
    Diabetic nephropathy
    Tubulointerstitial nephropathies
    Nephrosclerosis
    Nonsteroidal anti-inflammatory drugs
    Acquired immunodeficiency syndrome
Resistance to aldosterone
  With salt wasting
    In children
    In adults (methicillin, obstructive nephropathy,
      transplantation, cyclosporine, sickle cell disease)
    Drugs (spironoloactone, amiloride, triamterene)
  Without salt wasting
Chronic renal insufficiency

tubular HCO_3^- reabsorptive capacity is no longer exceeded by the filtered HCO_3^- load and therefore HCO_3^- reclamation is complete. In pRTA, this steady state generally occurs at an HCO_3^- concentration between 14 and 18 mEq/L (compared with ~24 mEq/L in subjects with normal renal function). If the serum $[HCO_3^-]$ exceeds this threshold, HCO_3^- excretion occurs and the urine is alkaline. If the serum $[HCO_3^-]$ is below this threshold, proximal tubular HCO_3^- reabsorption is complete and the urine can be acidified if distal tubule function is intact. Attempts to treat the usually mild acidosis in patients with pRTA are usually unsuccessful because the bicarbonate threshold is exceeded and the administered HCO_3^- is rapidly excreted. However, thiazide-induced contraction of extracellular fluid volume reduces HCO_3^- wasting.[33] K^+ excretion (caused by delivery of relatively impermeant HCO_3^- past the sites of K^+ secretion) is exaggerated by HCO_3^- therapy,[34] but kaliuresis can be reduced with K^+-sparing diuretics.

The diagnosis of pRTA relies on the lowered threshold for HCO_3^- reabsorption and the usually intact distal tubule function. Provided that the plasma $[HCO_3^-]$ is below the threshold, urinary pH is 5.5 or less; to ensure that the plasma $[HCO_3^-]$ is below the HCO_3^- reabsorption threshold, it may be necessary first to administer an acidifying agent, NH_4Cl (0.1 g/kg body weight). Administration of HCO_3^- leads to urinary HCO_3^- excretion and a frankly alkaline urinary pH. Formal evaluation involves quantitation of $[HCO_3^-]$ in plasma and urine to determine the fraction of filtered HCO_3^- that is excreted in the urine ($FE_{HCO_3^-}$):

$$FE_{HCO_3^-} = \frac{[HCO_3^-]_u \times [\text{creatinine}]_p}{[HCO_3^-]_p \times [\text{creatinine}]_u} \times 100$$

where u and p refer to urine and plasma, respectively.[35] For plasma $[HCO_3^-]$ below the reabsorption threshold, FE_{HCO_3}-

is 5% or less; when the plasma $[HCO_3^-]$ is above the threshold, this fraction is 15% or more.

Classic Distal Renal Tubular Acidosis

Classic dRTA arises from a defect in collecting duct H^+ secretion. Studies in animals have shown that gradient-limited defects in H^+ secretion are possible, and the suggested pathogenic mechanisms include reduced H^+ secretion because of diminished lumen voltage or increased H^+ back leak.[36, 37] However, studies in patients with classic dRTA indicate that the H^+ secretory defect is most likely rate limited; that is, there is a quantitative depression of H^+ secretion.[9, 38, 39] Because the medullary collecting duct is responsible for lowering tubule fluid pH below 5.5, a rate-limiting acidification defect is likely to occur in this nephron segment.[9] Hyperaldosteronism resulting from acidosis-induced volume contraction causes K^+ wasting. Hypercalciuria, nephrocalcinosis, and nephrolithiasis often occur in patients with dRTA; children with dRTA fail to grow normally. Acidemia, kaliuresis, and growth retardation are corrected with alkali therapy.

Urinary pH is greater than 5.5 no matter what the severity of the acidemia. Formal diagnosis may require administration of NH_4Cl to ensure the adequacy of the acid stress. An alternative diagnostic procedure utilizes an HCO_3^- challenge.[39] Because of the absence of luminal carbonic anhydrase in the distal nephron, H^+ secretion into HCO_3^--rich distal tubular fluid generates H_2CO_3, which slowly dehydrates to CO_2. This reaction is sufficiently slow that CO_2 is not reabsorbed but rather is excreted in the urine; after the HCO_3^- challenge the urinary P_{CO_2} is normally more than 40 mm Hg higher than the arterial blood P_{CO_2}. In patients with dRTA, however, the urine-to-blood P_{CO_2} gradient is not elevated. In patients with pRTA, distal H^+ secretion is normal and the urine-to-blood P_{CO_2} gradient is normal.

Impaired Net Acid Excretion (Deficient Ammonia Excretion)

Lack of urinary buffer, especially ammonia, limits net H^+ excretion and leads to hyperchloremic metabolic acidosis. An acidic urinary pH (pH < 5.5) is frequently observed because the defect is one of buffer production and excretion rather than cellular H^+ secretion. Also indicating intact distal H^+ secretion, patients with deficient ammonia synthesis have an elevated urine-to-blood P_{CO_2} gradient (normal) after an HCO_3^- challenge. Measurement of the urinary ammonia excretion establishes the diagnosis. Urinary ammonia levels can also be estimated from the urinary anion gap (urinary anion gap = $Na^+ + K^+ - Cl^-$).[40] Patients with normal ammonia synthetic activity who develop hyperchloremic metabolic acidosis (for other reasons) have a negative anion gap because the urinary NH_4^+ concentration is high, whereas patients with ammonia deficiency have a positive urinary anion gap.

Because hyperkalemia inhibits ammonia synthesis, patients with aldosterone deficiency frequently have hyperchloremic metabolic acidosis. Aldosterone deficiency also reduces the rate of H^+ secretion, but it does not affect the maximal lumen-to-blood H^+ gradient that can be achieved (i.e., the urinary pH can be below 5.5).[41–43] In patients with primary hypoaldosteronism, salt wasting and extracellular volume depletion occur and mineralocorticoid replacement (usually with fludrocortisone) repairs K^+ retention, salt wasting, and metabolic acidosis.

In patients with hyporeninemic hypoaldosteronism, salt wasting is not usually apparent until severe salt restriction is imposed.[44] Because a third of the patients with hyporeninemic hypoaldosteronism are hypertensive, it has been suggested that they retain salt and that their expanded extracellular fluid volume suppresses plasma renin activity.[45] Alternatively, reduced plasma renin activity has been explained by a variety of proposed mechanisms, including destruction of the juxtaglomerular apparatus, autonomic insufficiency, prostaglandin deficiency, and alterations in other neurohumoral pathways.[46-49] Compared with patients with primary hypoaldosteronism, patients with hyporeninemic hypoaldosteronism may require higher doses of fludrocortisone because of tubular unresponsiveness. Restriction of dietary K^+ and K^+ removal with a cation-exchange resin are also effective.[50, 51] In patients with hypertension, diuretic therapy may be of benefit[52] but Na^+ depletion should be avoided because hyperkalemia, deficient ammonia synthesis, and hyperchloremic metabolic acidosis commonly supervene.

Hyperkalemia, hyperchloremic metabolic acidosis, and salt wasting also occur in patients with acquired renal diseases involving resistance to exogenous aldosterone[53-55] and those receiving antagonists of aldosterone action. This generalized distal tubular abnormality has also been referred to as a "voltage-dependent" defect.[36, 37, 56-58] If the medullary collecting duct is damaged, abnormalities associated with dRTA are present (i.e., minimal urinary pH > 5.5 and reduced urine-to-blood PCO_2 gradient after an HCO_3^- challenge). Because mineralocorticoids are ineffective, these patients require salt supplements to maintain extracellular fluid volume and to provide adequate Na^+ delivery to the distal nephron for maximal H^+ and K^+ secretion. Additional therapy with $NaHCO_3$ supplementation, K^+ restriction, and a cation-exchange resin may be necessary.

A few patients without salt wasting and renal disease exhibit hyperkalemia, hyperchloremic metabolic acidosis, hypertension, undetectable plasma renin activity, and low plasma aldosterone concentration.[59-63] Because these patients have an increase in distal tubule permeability to Cl^-, salt reabsorption increases and lumen voltage decreases. Consequently, extracellular fluid volume expands, suppressing plasma renin activity and aldosterone production. K^+ secretion is reduced by both low aldosterone levels and diminished lumen voltage, and the resulting hyperkalemia suppresses ammonia synthesis. Treatment with diuretics is effective.

The metabolic acidosis in chronic renal insufficiency is due to deficient ammonia excretion, too. Because ammonia synthesis parallels renal mass, patients with small kidneys have reduced ammonia synthesis as well as altered tubular handling of ammonia.[64-67] There is a clinical impression that deficient ammonia excretion develops at a higher glomerular filtration rate (>30 mL/min) in patients with tubulointerstitial disease than in patients with glomerular disease (20 to 30 mL/min).[68] When the glomerular filtration rate is reduced sufficiently (<15 to 20 mL/min), unmeasured anions are retained and the anion gap increases.[69] Alkali therapy corrects the metabolic acidosis in patients with chronic renal insufficiency and may stop metabolic acidosis–associated bone dissolution.[65]

Treatment

The general therapy of metabolic acidosis should always be geared to correcting the underlying disorder. However, correction of the acidemia is warranted when the pH is less than 7.1. Under these circumstances sufficient $NaHCO_3$ should be infused intravenously to raise the pH above 7.2 and the $[HCO_3^-]$ above 10 mEq/L. The amount of $NaHCO_3$ required varies with the severity of acidosis and the rate of H^+ production (or HCO_3^- loss). The appropriate dose of $NaHCO_3$ can be calculated from the following relationship because the HCO_3^- distribution space is a function of the plasma $[HCO_3^-]$, not the pH:

$$\text{Dose} = \left(0.4 + \frac{2.4}{[HCO_3^-]_{current}} \right) \times \text{body weight} \times ([HCO_3^-]_{desired} - [HCO_3^-]_{current})$$

where body weight is in kg, $[HCO_3^-]$ in mEq/L, and the dose in mEq and the factor $0.4 + 2.4/[HCO_3^-]_{current}$ is the volume of distribution of the administered HCO_3^-.[70] In utilizing this formula, the dose of $NaHCO_3$ should be calculated to raise the $[HCO_3^-]$ above 10 mEq/L; there is no need to correct the $[HCO_3^-]$ completely, and the HCO_3^- should be administered relatively slowly over several hours. Because the rate of H^+ production or HCO_3^- loss is not included in this calculation, it is imperative that arterial blood gases be monitored frequently to assess the adequacy of $NaHCO_3$ therapy.

HCO_3^- therapy is ultimately limited by the concomitant administration of Na^+ and consequent expansion of extracellular fluid volume. It is also well to recall that ampules of $NaHCO_3$ are extremely hypertonic (~1800 mOsm/kg). Because hemodialysis corrects acidosis but avoids the expansion of extracellular fluid volume that accompanies $NaHCO_3$ therapy, it is useful in patients who have increased extracellular fluid volume and/or renal failure. HCO_3^- therapy can also be limited by the titration of H^+ in blood and consequent generation of CO_2 gas, increasing blood PCO_2. If CO_2 is not exhaled, the elevated PCO_2 blunts the anticipated rise in pH, compromising the benefits of base administration. Patients exhibiting this form of CO_2 generation are those with poor or fixed ventilation (i.e., CO_2 retention or ventilator therapy), especially if $NaHCO_3$ is infused rapidly. During metabolic acidosis, rapid HCO_3^- administration can also lead to a paradoxical decrease in cerebrospinal fluid pH.[71] Because CO_2 diffuses rapidly from blood to cerebrospinal fluid (HCO_3^- transport is slow), the cerebrospinal fluid pH becomes more acidic as administered HCO_3^- increases blood pH and ventilation is reduced (PCO_2 increases). The benefits and problems of HCO_3^- therapy in the treatment of lactic acidosis and diabetic ketoacidosis are discussed in Chapters 105 and 106.

METABOLIC ALKALOSIS

In metabolic alkalosis, base accumulation elevates blood pH and $[HCO_3^-]$ (Table 104-6). The accumulated base can be derived from exogenous sources, namely oral or parenteral administration. Alternatively, the base can be generated endogenously by excessive H^+ excretion by the kidneys or gastrointestinal tract. Whatever the mode of generating base, the maintenance of excess total body base depends on reduced renal HCO_3^- excretion. Whereas normal kidneys rapidly excrete excess HCO_3^-, in metabolic alkalosis this capacity is impaired. Identification of the factor(s) responsible for this reduction in renal HCO_3^- excretion is central to the analysis and treatment of metabolic alkalosis.

A significant reduction in glomerular filtration rate reduces HCO_3^- filtration and excretion. Thus, in patients with advanced renal failure, excessive alkali administration coupled with the inability to excrete base leads predictably to metabolic alkalosis.[72, 73] In the absence of renal failure, an elevated plasma $[HCO_3^-]$ increases the filtered HCO_3^- load, and maintenance of metabolic alkalosis is explained by enhanced proximal tubular HCO_3^- reabsorption and/or distal tubular H^+ secretion. For example, extracellular fluid volume contraction increases proximal tubular HCO_3^- reabsorption, at least in part because of activation of the renin-angiotensin-aldosterone system. Angiotensin II enhances proximal tubular HCO_3^- reabsorption directly.[6] Aldosterone

TABLE 104-6

CAUSES OF METABOLIC ALKALOSIS

Exogenous HCO_3^- load with renal failure (including milk-alkali syndrome)
Contraction of extracellular fluid volume
  Gastrointestinal
    Vomiting and gastric aspiration
    Cl^--rich diarrhea (congenital or acquired)
    Villous adenoma
  Renal
    Diuretics
    K^+ depletion
    Posthypercapnic metabolic alkalosis
    Recovery from organic acidosis
    Nonreabsorbable anion
    Refeeding after starvation
    Bartter's syndrome
Expansion of extracellular fluid volume
  High renin
    Renal artery stenosis
    Accelerated hypertension
    Renin-secreting tumors
    Estrogen treatment
  Low renin
    Primary aldosteronism (adenoma, hyperplasia, carcinoma, glucocorticoid suppressible)
    Adrenal enzyme defects (11β-hydroxylase, 17α-hydroxylase)
    Cushing's syndrome (ectopic corticotropin, adrenal carcinoma, adrenal adenoma, pituitary adenoma)
    Other mineralocorticoids (licorice, carbenoxolone, chewing tobacco)

enhances urinary H^+ excretion, both by stimulating distal tubular H^+ secretion and by K^+ depletion, secondarily increasing ammonia generation. Thus, mineralocorticoids can both generate HCO_3^- and maintain the elevated plasma $[HCO_3^-]$.

Metabolic alkalosis impairs central nervous system function and increases neuromuscular irritability. By reducing $[Ca^{2+}]$, severe alkalemia can cause confusion, lethargy, coma, and seizures as well as muscle twitching, spasm, and tetany. Positive Chvostek's and Trousseau's signs are harbingers of more serious neuromuscular dysfunction. Metabolic alkalosis also suppresses ventilation, and frank hypoxemia can occur in severe metabolic alkalosis. For the same reason, metabolic alkalosis may make it more difficult to wean patients from respirators.

Contraction of Extracellular Fluid Volume

Gastrointestinal Causes

HCl loss by vomiting or gastric aspiration is a common cause of metabolic alkalosis.[74] Parietal cells secrete H^+ into the gastric juice at the same time as they release an equal quantity of HCO_3^- into blood. Normally, this process does not provide either an acid or base burden for the body, because the secreted H^+ is neutralized by HCO_3^--rich secretions in the upper small intestine. However, loss of H^+ by vomiting or gastric aspiration interrupts this cycle and results in accumulation of base in the body (base generation). At the same time, extracellular fluid volume depletion occurs because of the loss of Cl^--rich fluid (gastric juice) and because Na^+ and K^+ are lost in the urine after an episode of vomiting when the threshold for HCO_3^- reabsorption is transiently exceeded. Extracellular fluid volume depletion stimulates aldosterone secretion and exacerbates urinary K^+

losses. K^+ depletion enhances proximal tubular HCO_3^- reabsorption and urinary H^+ excretion. After an episode of vomiting the urine is HCO_3^- free (pH < 6), and at all times it is virtually Cl^- free. Expansion of extracellular fluid volume (with NaCl) and repletion of K^+ deficits (with KCl) permit rapid excretion of retained HCO_3^- and correction of the metabolic alkalosis.

More unusual gastrointestinal causes of metabolic alkalosis include congenital and acquired forms of chloridorrhea (Cl^--rich diarrhea) and villous adenomas.[75-78] The acquired form of chloridorrhea has been reported as a transient occurrence in certain viral infections.[78] Chloridorrhea results from lack of normal Cl^--HCO_3^- exchange activity in the ileum and colon, leading to loss of Cl^- and NH_4^+ in HCO_3^--poor diarrhea. Thus, there is simultaneous loss of H^+ (i.e., NH_4^+) and depletion of extracellular fluid volume, generating and maintaining the metabolic alkalosis, respectively. Treatment requires repletion of extracellular fluid volume with NaCl.

Renal Causes

Chloruretic diuretics (e.g., thiazides and furosemide) produce metabolic alkalosis by several mechanisms, including extracellular fluid volume depletion, hyperaldosteronism, and K^+ depletion. Natriuresis and chloriuresis, without concomitant bicarbonaturia, contracts extracellular fluid volume and increases the plasma $[HCO_3^-]$. However, the magnitude of the increase in $[HCO_3^-]$ that can be ascribed to contraction alone is small; the degree of extracellular fluid volume contraction is modest at best, and buffering by nonbicarbonate buffers minimizes the increment in $[HCO_3^-]$.[30] Of more importance is the fact that volume depletion activates the renin-angiotensin-aldosterone system. This enhances proximal tubular HCO_3^- reabsorption and distal tubular H^+ secretion and K^+ excretion. The resulting K^+ deficiency facilitates net acid excretion (bicarbonate generation) by enhancing ammonia generation.[79-82] Increased distal delivery of Na^+-rich fluid also increases H^+ and K^+ excretion.

The renal compensation for chronic hypercapnia involves increased net acid excretion, which elevates the plasma $[HCO_3^-]$. Correction of hypercapnia permits excretion of the excess base but only if the patient receives sufficient dietary Na^+ and Cl^-.[83, 84] So-called posthypercapnic metabolic alkalosis occurs when pre-existing hypovolemia (resulting from dietary salt restriction and/or diuretic administration) is not corrected concomitantly with correction of the hypercapnia. By blunting the respiratory drive, the resulting alkalemia may make weaning from mechanical ventilation difficult. The bicarbonaturic diuretic acetazolamide is sometimes helpful in this situation, especially in patients with underlying heart disease, for whom aggressive Na^+ repletion may be hazardous. If acetazolamide is used for this purpose, special attention must be paid both to repletion of pre-existing K^+ deficits and to replacement of acetazolamide-induced urinary K^+ losses.

Metabolic alkalosis develops occasionally during the recovery from organic acidosis as retained organic anions are converted to HCO_3^-.[85] The patients at risk are those who have retained large quantities of organic anions (i.e., those with severe organic acidosis) and have received vigorous HCO_3^- therapy. Anything that impairs renal HCO_3^- excretion, including severe renal failure, volume depletion, and hypokalemia, increases the risk. Judicious use of HCO_3^- generally forestalls the subsequent development of significant metabolic alkalosis. When little or no HCO_3^- is administered, renal function is normal, Na^+ and K^+ balances are normal, and the recovery from organic acidosis is more commonly associated with the development of hyperchloremic acidosis; the urinary excretion of organic anions during the acidosis represents loss of potential base.

Administration of large amounts of relatively nonreabsorbable anions can induce metabolic alkalosis. For example, carbenicillin and other penicillins are freely filtered, but poorly reabsorbed, by the nephron.[86] When given in large doses, these negatively charged substances obligate the urinary loss of cations, including Na^+, K^+, H^+, and NH_4^+. The resulting volume depletion and hypokalemia augment renal H^+ excretion (base generation). Repletion of Na^+ and K^+ deficits correct the metabolic alkalosis.

The metabolic alkalosis that develops during carbohydrate refeeding after starvation is transient in nature. During starvation, ketoacid production is accelerated and volume depletion is not uncommon. With carbohydrate refeeding (not fats or protein), retained ketoacid anions are converted to HCO_3^- and the renal restoration of extracellular fluid volume limits HCO_3^- excretion.[87-89] Refeeding metabolic alkalosis usually resolves spontaneously within a few days.

Bartter's syndrome is a rare entity that is characterized by metabolic alkalosis, hypokalemia, hypomagnesemia, hyperreninemia, hyperaldosteronism, vascular resistance to the pressor activity of angiotensin II, normal blood pressure, and hyperplasia of the renal juxtaglomerular apparatus.[90] Because inhibition of prostaglandin production restores vascular pressor sensitivity, an abnormality in prostaglandin synthesis may be an important component of this disorder. However, the primary abnormality is thought to be an alteration in NaCl transport in the thick ascending limb of Henle's loop. Bartter's syndrome is seen most often in children and young adults, but the pattern of heredity is not obvious. A similar (acquired) syndrome has been observed after gentamicin treatment. The clinical importance of this syndrome is that it must be distinguished from surreptitious vomiting and laxative or diuretic abuse. To do so may require drug screening. Patients who abuse laxatives have urine that is virtually Cl^- free, whereas patients with Bartter's syndrome have Cl^- in urine. The urinary Cl^- level in patients with diuretic abuse is variable (Fig. 104–4). Therapy is supportive and geared to replenishing extracellular fluid volume and deficiencies of K^+ and Mg^{2+}.

Expansion of Extracellular Fluid Volume

Metabolic alkalosis and extracellular fluid volume expansion coexist in states characterized by mineralocorticoid excess. Excess mineralocorticoid production can be primary (low renin) or secondary (high renin), or mineralocorticoid activity can be increased if degradation is reduced (see Table 104–6).[91-95] Mineralocorticoids stimulate H^+ secretion (by alpha intercalated cells) and K^+ secretion (by principal cells) in the distal nephron. Increased H^+ secretion in conjunction with hypokalemia-induced ammoniagenesis enhances urinary net acid excretion (base generation), causing metabolic alkalosis. Therapy should be directed at the underlying abnormality. Blockade of renal aldosterone receptors with spironolactone can be helpful in situations in which this is not possible. Angiotensin-converting enzyme inhibitors may be of benefit in patients with secondary hyperaldosteronism.

Differential Diagnosis

The pathophysiologic mechanisms underlying the maintenance phase of metabolic alkalosis provide a conceptual framework for classifying and treating acid-base disorders. Renal retention of HCO_3^- depends on either volume contraction or a primary increase in H^+ excretion. Accordingly, metabolic alkalosis can be categorized as saline responsive or saline unresponsive. The patient's history, the physical examination (with particular reference to volume status and blood pressure), and the urinary [Cl^-] are the most important elements in the differential diagnosis (see Fig. 104–4).

Treatment

Treatment of metabolic alkalosis should be directed at correcting or removing the processes that generated the base load and the factors that are maintaining the alkalosis. For example, in diuretic-related metabolic alkalosis diuretics should be discontinued, volume contraction corrected, and K^+ deficits repleted; similar considerations apply to the patient with gastric fluid loss; patients with adrenal adenomas should be treated surgically; and so on. Occasionally,

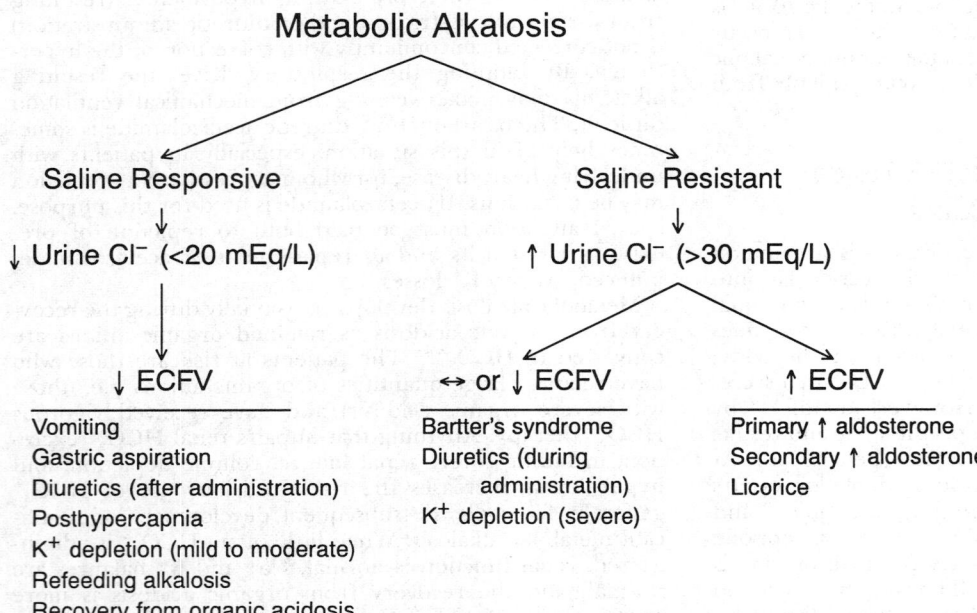

Figure 104–4. Diagnostic schema for metabolic alkalosis. ECFV = extracellular fluid volume.

complications of severe alkalemia, such as seizures, coma, and tetany, require rapid correction of metabolic alkalosis. In these situations, HCl (0.1 to 0.2 mol/L) can be infused into a large vein, with close monitoring of arterial blood gases. The amount of HCl required can be estimated with the same formula used to calculate the HCO_3^- dose to correct metabolic acidosis. Alternative acidifying agents are NH_4Cl and arginine HCl, but the former can be dangerous in patients with liver disease and the latter can cause hyperkalemia.

DIAGNOSTIC APPROACH TO DISORDERS OF ACID-BASE BALANCE

The diagnosis of simple (single) acid-base disturbances is relatively easy because there is only one primary disorder with an appropriate compensatory response. Indeed, many nomograms (e.g., see Fig. 104–3), computer algorithms, and formulas (e.g., Winters' formula) accurately describe the characteristic patterns of single acid-base disturbances.[9–11] Unfortunately, this seemingly simple approach can yield misleading information because patients often present with disorders of short duration and incomplete compensation and because there may be more than one primary disorder (each of unknown severity and duration). Consequently, the acid-base nomogram should never be used as the sole diagnostic tool. Instead, a systematic approach (such as that outlined in Table 104–7) is more likely to yield the correct diagnosis, which, in turn, will lead to appropriate treatment.[96] The strength of this sequential approach is that it

---

TABLE 104–7

DIAGNOSTIC APPROACH TO DISORDERS OF ACID-BASE BALANCE

Identify the medical problems
  History
    Symptoms (e.g., vomiting, diarrhea, polyuria)
    Diseases (e.g., diabetes mellitus, congestive heart failure, chronic obstructive pulmonary disease)
    Medications (e.g., diuretics, laxatives, sedatives)
    Treatment (e.g., ventilation, nasogastric suction, intravenous fluids)
  Physical examination
    Clues (e.g., tetany, jaundice, cyanosis, respiratory rate, blood pressure, fever)
Consider how the medical problems could influence acid-base balance
Examine the laboratory data for evidence of acid-base disorders (confirm or refute your predictions)
  Routine laboratory data (e.g., liver disease, sepsis, renal disease)
  Electrolytes
    Total CO_2 (tCO_2)
      If abnormal, there must be at least a single disturbance
      If normal, there may be multiple disturbances
    Anion gap ($Na^+ - [Cl^- + tCO_2]$)
      Widened gap suggests (anion gap) metabolic acidosis
      Normal gap suggests hyperchloremic acidosis or respiratory alkalosis
      Hypoalbuminemia may obscure widened anion gap
    Potassium
      Altered $[K^+]$ may predict the pH abnormality (decreased K^+ in alkalemia, increased K^+ in acidemia)
  Arterial blood gas
    Are the blood gas values consistent with the previous information?
    Is there a simple or mixed acid-base disturbance?
  Integrate laboratory data with patient's medical problem(s) (Is the entire picture consistent?)

---

greatly simplifies the diagnosis of complex (mixed) acid-base disturbances.

References

1. Davenport HW: The ABC's of Acid-Base Chemistry. 6th ed. Chicago, University of Chicago Press, 1974.
2. Lemann J Jr, Lennon EJ: Role of diet, gastrointestinal tract and bone in acid-base homeostasis. Kidney Int 1:275, 1972.
3. Hills AG: Acid-Base Balance: Chemistry, Physiology, Pathophysiology. Baltimore, Williams & Wilkins, 1973.
4. Moe OW, Preisig PA, Alpern RJ: Cellular model of proximal tubule NaCl and $NaHCO_3$ absorption. Kidney Int 38:605, 1990.
5. Alpern RJ, Stone DK, Rector FC, Jr: Renal acidification mechanisms. In: Brenner BM, Rector FC Jr (eds): The Kidney. 4th ed. Philadelphia, WB Saunders, p 318, 1991.
6. Geibel J, Giebisch G, Boron WF: Angiotensin II stimulates both $Na^+ - H^+$ exchange and Na^+/HCO_3^- contransport in the rabbit proximal tubule. Proc Natl Acad Sci USA 87:7917, 1990.
7. Wingo CS: Active proton secretion and potassium absorption in the rabbit outer medullary collecting duct. J Clin Invest 84:361, 1989.
8. Schoolwerth AC: Regulation of renal ammoniagenesis in metabolic acidosis. Kidney Int 40:961, 1991.
9. Cogan MG, Rector FC Jr: Acid-base disorders. In: Brenner BM, Rector FC Jr (eds): The Kidney. 4th ed. Philadelphia, WB Saunders, p 737, 1991.
10. Goldberg M, Green SB, Moss ML, et al: Computer-based instruction and diagnosis of acid-base disorders: A systematic approach. JAMA 233:269, 1973.
11. Albert MS, Dell RB, Winters RW: Quantitative displacement of acid-base equilibrium in metabolic acidosis. Ann Intern Med 66:313, 1967.
12. Emmett M, Narins RG: Clinical use of the anion gap. Medicine 56:38, 1977.
13. Madias NE, Ayus JC, Adrogue HJ: Increased anion gap in metabolic alkalosis. The role of plasma-protein equivalency. N Engl J Med 300:1421, 1979.
14. Adrogue HJ, Brensilver J, Madias NE: Changes in plasma anion gap during chronic metabolic acid-base disturbances. Am J Physiol 235:F291, 1978.
15. Murray T, Long W, Narins RG: Multiple myeloma and the anion gap. N Engl J Med 292:574, 1975.
16. DeTroyer A, Stolarczyk A, DeBeyl DZ, et al: Value of anion-gap determination in metabolic alkalosis. N Engl J Med 296:858, 1977.
17. Kelleher SP, Raciti A, Arbeit LA: Reduced or absent serum anion gap as a marker of severe lithium intoxication. Arch Intern Med 146:1839, 1986.
18. Blume RS, MacLowry JD, Wolff SM: Limitations of chloride determination in the diagnosis of bromism. N Engl J Med 279:593, 1968.
19. Winter SD, Pearson JR, Gabow PA, et al: The fall of the serum anion gap. Arch Intern Med 150:311, 1990.
20. Burnell JM, Villamil MF, Uyeno BT, et al: The effect in humans of extracellular pH change on the relationship between serum potassium concentration and intracellular potassium. J Clin Invest 35:935, 1956.
21. Fulop M: Serum potassium in lactic and ketoacidosis. N Engl J Med 300:1087, 1979.
22. Brown RS: Extrarenal potassium homeostasis. Kidney Int 30:116, 1986.
23. Halperin ML, Hammeke M, Jose RG, et al: Metabolic acidosis in the alcoholic: A pathophysiologic approach. Metabolism 32:308, 1983.
24. Pamisano J, Gruver C, Adams ND: Absence of anion gap metabolic acidosis in severe methanol poisoning: A case report and review of the literature. Am J Kidney Dis 9:441, 1987.
25. Gabow PA, Clay K, Sullivan JB, et al: Organic acids in ethylene glycol intoxication. Ann Intern Med 105:16, 1986.
26. Pappas SC, Silverman M: Treatment of methanol poisoning with ethanol and hemodialysis. Can Med Assoc J 126:1361, 1982.
27. Temple AR: Acute and chronic effects of aspirin toxicity and their treatment. Arch Intern Med 141:364, 1981.
28. Paulson WD: Anion gap–bicarbonate relation in diabetic ketoacidosis. Am J Med 81:995, 1986.
29. Adrogue HJ, Eknoyan G, Suki WK: Diabetic ketoacidosis: Role of the kidney in acid-base homeostasis re-evaluated. Kidney Int 25:591, 1984.
30. Garella S, Chang BS, Kahn SI: Dilutional acidosis and contraction alkalosis: Review of a concept. Kidney Int 8:279, 1975.
31. Charney AN, Feldman GM: Internal exchange of hydrogen ions: Gastrointestinal tract. In: Seldin DW, Geibisch G (eds): The Regulation of Acid-Base Balance. New York, Raven Press, p 89, 1989.
32. Koch MO, McDougal WS: The pathophysiology of hyperchloremic metabolic acidosis after urinary diversion through intestinal segments. Surgery 98:561, 1985.
33. Arant BS, Greifer IR, Edelmann CM Jr, et al: Effects of chronic salt and water loading in the tubular defects of a child with Fanconi syndrome (cystinosis). Pediatrics 58:370, 1976.
34. Sebastian A, McSherry E, Morris RC Jr: On the mechanism of renal potassium wasting in renal tubular acidosis associated with the Fanconi syndrome (type 2 RTA). J Clin Invest 50:231, 1971.

35. Pitts RF, Lostspeich WD: Bicarbonate and the renal regulation of acid base balance. Am J Physiol 147:138, 1964.
36. Kurtzman NA: Acquired distal renal tubular acidosis. Kidney Int 24:807, 1983.
37. Kurtzman NA: Disorders of distal acidification. Kidney Int 38:720, 1990.
38. Halperin ML, Goldstein MB, Richardson RMA, et al: distal renal tubular acidosis syndromes: A pathophysiological approach. Am J Nephrol 5:1, 1985.
39. Halperin ML, Goldstein MB, Haig M, et al: Studies on the pathogenesis of type I (distal) renal tubular acidosis as revealed by the urinary pCO$_2$ tensions. J Clin Invest 53:669, 1974.
40. Batlle DC, Hizon M, Cohen E, et al: The use of the urinary anion gap in the diagnosis of hyperchloremic metabolic acidosis. N Engl J Med 318:594, 1988.
41. DuBose TD Jr, Caflisch CR: Effect of selective aldosterone deficiency on acidification in nephron segments of the rat renal medulla. J Clin Invest 82:1624, 1988.
42. Chiodi H: Respiratory adaptations to chronic high altitude hypoxia. J Appl Physiol 10:81, 1957.
43. Hulter HN, Ilnicki LP, Harbottle JA, et al: Impaired renal H$^+$ secretion and NH$_3$ production in mineralocorticoid-deficient glucocorticoid-replete dogs. Am J Physiol 232:F136, 1977.
44. Perez GO, Oster JR, Vaamonde CA: Renal acidosis and renal potassium handling in selective hypoaldosteronism. Am J Med 57:809, 1974.
45. Oh MS, Carol HJ, Clemmons JE, et al: A mechanism for hyporeninemic hypoaldosteronism in chronic renal disease. Metabolism 23:1157, 1974.
46. Sparagna M: Hyporeninemic hypoaldosteronism associated with diabetic glomerulosclerosis. J Steroid Biochem 5:369, 1974.
47. Schambelan M, Sebastian A, Biglieri EG: Prevalence, pathogenesis, and functional significance of aldosterone deficiency in hyperkalemic patients with chronic renal insufficiency. Kidney Int 17:89, 1980.
48. DeFronzo RA: Hyperkalemia and hyporeninemic hypoaldosteronism hypoaldosteronism. Kidney Int 17:118, 1980.
49. Nadler JL, Lee FO, Hsueh W, et al: Evidence of prostacyclin deficiency in the syndrome of hyporeninemic hypoaldosteronism. N Engl J Med 314:1015, 1986.
50. Szylman P, Better OS, Chaimowitz C, et al: Role of hyperkalemia in the metabolic acidosis of isolated hypoaldosteronism. N Engl J Med 294:361, 1976.
51. Matsuda D, Nonoguchi H, Tomita K, et al: Primary role of hyperkalemia in the acidosis of hyporeninemic hypoaldosteronism. Nephron 49:203, 1988.
52. Sebastian A, Schambelan M, Sutton JM: Amelioration of hyperchloremic acidosis with furosemide therapy in patients with chronic renal insufficiency and type 4 renal tubular acidosis. Am J Nephrol 4:287, 1984.
53. Rosler A: The natural history of salt-wasting disorders of adrenal and renal origin. J Clin Endocrinol Metab 59:689, 1984.
54. Armanini D, Kuhnle U, Strasser T, et al: Aldosterone-receptor deficiency in pseudohypoaldosteronism. N Engl J Med 313:1178, 1985.
55. Corvol P, Claire M, Oblin ME, et al: Mechanism of the antimineralocorticoid effects of spirolactones. Kidney Int 20:1, 1981.
56. Batlle DC, Sehy JT, Roseman MK, et al: Clinical and pathophysiologic spectrum of acquired distal renal tubular acidosis. Kidney Int 20:389, 1981.
57. Arruda JAL, Kurtzman NA: Mechanisms and classification of deranged distal urinary acidification. Am J Physiol 239:F515, 1980.
58. Batlle DC, Kurtzman NA: Distal renal tubular acidosis: pathogenesis and classification. Am J Kidney Dis 1:328, 1982.
59. Schambelan M, Sebastian A, Rector FC Jr: Mineralocortocoid-resistant renal hyperkalemia without salt wasting (type II pseudohypoaldosteronism): Role of increased renal chloride reabsorption. Kidney Int 19:716, 1981.
60. Licht JH, Amundson D, Hsueh WA, et al: Familial hyperkalaemic acidosis. Q J Med 54:161, 1985.
61. Margolis BL, Lifschitz MD: The Spitzer-Weinstein syndrome: One form of type IV renal tubular acidosis and its response to hydrochlorothiazide. Am J Kidney Dis 7:241, 1986.
62. Travis PS: Case report: Mineralo-corticoid–induced kaliuresis in type II pseudohypoaldosteronism. Am J Med Sci 52:235, 1986.
63. Take C, Ikeda K, Kurwasawa T, et al: Increased chloride reabsorption as an inherited renal tubular defect in familial type II pseudohypoaldosteronism. N Engl J Med 324:488, 1991.
64. Van Slyke DD, Linder GC, Hiller A, et al: The excretion of ammonia and titratable acid in nephritis. J Clin Invest 2:255, 1926.
65. Goodman AD, Lemann J Jr, Lennon EJ, et al: Production, excretion, and net balance of fixed acid in patients with renal acidosis. J Clin Invest 44:495, 1965.
66. Wrong O, Davies HEF: The excretion of acid in renal disease. Q J Med 28:259, 1958.
67. Buerkett J, Martin D, Trigg D, et al: Effect of reduced renal mass on ammonium handling and net acid formation by the superficial and juxtamedullary nephron of the rat. Evidence for impaired reentrapment rather than decreased production of ammonium in the acidosis of uremia. J Clin Invest 71:1661, 1983.
68. Gonick HC, Kleeman CR, Rubini ME, et al: Functional impairment in chronic renal disease. II. Studies of acid excretion. Nephron 6:28, 1969.
69. Widmer B, Gerhardt RE, Harrington JT, et al: Serum electrolyte and acid-base composition. The influence of graded degrees of chronic renal failure. Arch Intern Med 139:1099, 1979.
70. Fernandez PC, Cohen RM, Feldman GM: The concept of the bicarbonate distribution space: The crucial role of body buffers. Kidney Int 36:747, 1989.
71. Posner JB, Plum F: Spinal-fluid pH and neurologic symptoms in systemic acidosis. N Engl J Med 277:605, 1967.
72. Seldin DW, Rector FC Jr: The generation and maintenance of metabolic alkalosis. Kidney Int 1:306, 1972.
73. Orwoll ES: The milk-alkali syndrome: Current concepts. Ann Intern Med 97:242, 1982.
74. Kassirer JP, Schwartz WB: Correction of metabolic alkalosis in man without repair of potassium deficiency. Am J Med 40:19, 1966.
75. Evanson JM, Congenital chloridorrhea or so-called congenital alkalosis with diarrhoea. Gut 6:29, 1965.
76. Pearson A, Sladen GE, Edmonds CJ Jr: The pathophysiology of congenital chloridorrhea. Q J Med 42:453, 1973.
77. Babior BM: Villous adenoma of the colon. Am J Med 41:615, 1966.
78. Kaplan BS, Vitullo B: Acquired chloride diarrhea. J Pediatr 99:211, 1981.
79. Schwartz WB, Relman AS: Metabolic and renal studies in chronic potassium depletion resulting from overuse of laxatives. J Clin Invest 32:258, 1953.
80. Jones JW, Sebastian A, Hulter HN, et al: Systemic and renal acid-base effects of chronic dietary potassium depletion in humans. Kidney Int 21:402, 1982.
81. Hernandez R, Schambelan M, Cogan MG, et al: Dietary NaCl determines severity of potassium depletion–induced metabolic alkalosis. Kidney Int 31:1356, 1987.
82. Garella S, Chazan JA, Cohen JJ: Saline-resistant metabolic alkalosis or "chloride-wasting nephropathy." Ann Intern Med 73:31, 1970.
83. Turino GM, Goldring RM, Heinemann HO: Renal response to mechanical ventilation in patients with chronic hypercapnia. Am J Med 56:151, 1974.
84. Schwartz WB, Hays RM, Polak A, et al: Effects of chronic hypercapnia on electrolyte and acid-base equilibrium. II. Recovery with special reference to the influence of chloride intake. J Clin Invest 40:1238, 1961.
85. Robin ED: Dynamic aspects of metabolic acid base disturbances: phenformin lactic acidosis with alkaline overshoot. Trans Assoc Am Physicians 85:317, 1972.
86. Klastersky J, Vanderkelen B, Daneau D, et al: Carbenicillin and hypokalemia. Ann Intern Med 78:774, 1973.
87. Rapoport A, From GLA, Husdan H: Metabolic studies in prolonged fasting. I. Inorganic metabolism and kidney function. Metabolism 14:31, 1965.
88. Rapoport A, From GLA, Husdan H: Metabolic studies in prolonged fasting. II. Organic metabolism. Metabolism 14:47, 1965.
89. Veverbrants E, Ark RA: Effects of fasting and refeeding. I. Studies on sodium, potassium and water excretion on a constant electrolyte and fluid intake. J Clin Endocrinol 29:55, 1969.
90. Stein JH: The pathogenetic spectrum of Bartter's syndrome. Kidney Int 28:85, 1985.
91. Conn JW, Rovner DW, Cohen EL: Licorice-induced pseudoaldosteronism. hypertension, hypokalemia, aldosteronopenia and suppressed plasma renin activity. JAMA 205:80, 1968.
92. Royston A, Prout BJ: Carbenoxolone-induced hypokalaemia simulating Guillain-Barré syndrome. Br Med J 2:150, 1976.
93. Blacheley JD, Knochel JP: tobacco chewer's hypokalemia: Licorice revisited. N Engl J Med 302:784, 1980.
94. Melby JC: Primary aldosteronism. Kidney Int 26:769, 1984.
95. Laragh JH, Ulick S, Januszewicz V, et al: Aldosterone secretion and primary and malignant hypertension. J Clin Invest 39:1091, 1960.
96. McCurdy DK: Mixed metabolic and respiratory acid-base disturbances: Diagnosis and treatment. Chest 62:35S, 1972.

CHAPTER 105

Lactic Acidosis

James A. Kruse

Lactic acidosis arises chiefly from pathologic conditions that interfere with tissue perfusion and oxygenation.[1-3] Increased concentrations of blood lactate therefore serve as a clinical marker for circulatory shock or more subtle degrees of perfusion impairment. Much less commonly, lactic acidosis is observed in association with certain systemic disorders and a variety of intoxications but without evidence of tissue hypoxia. This chapter reviews the metabolism of lactate, the causes of lactic acidosis, measurement of blood lactate concentration and its clinical utility, and treatment of lactic acidosis.

METABOLISM

Glucose serves as a major substrate for the production of ATP and other high-energy chemical bonds that are used to drive synthetic reactions and other intracellular processes. Most tissues of the body contain the enzymes necessary to carry out the complete oxidation of glucose to carbon dioxide and water. This process can be viewed as three consecutive metabolic pathways, each of which consists of a series of enzyme-facilitated reactions (Fig. 105-1). The first phase begins in the cytosol with the anaerobic conversion of one molecule of glucose to two molecules of pyruvate. A small amount of lactate is normally present in the cell and is in equilibrium with the prevailing pyruvate concentration. Under aerobic conditions, pyruvate then diffuses into the mitochondria, where it is oxidized to acetyl coenzyme A and then to carbon dioxide by way of the tricarboxylic acid, or the Krebs, cycle, completing the second phase. Although some of the cytosolic and mitochondrial reactions involved in the conversion of glucose to carbon dioxide result in the direct phosphorylation of adenosine diphosphate (ADP) to ATP, most ATP is derived from the reduced forms of the flavin and NADH cofactors produced by these pathways. In the final phase of glucose metabolism, these reduced cofactors are oxidized by a series of iron-containing cytochrome proteins located on the inner membrane of the mitochondria, which operate as an electron transport cascade that ends with the reduction of molecular oxygen to water. The oxidative phosphorylation of ADP to form ATP is tightly coupled to this electron transport chain (see Fig. 105-1). Each molecule of NADH that enters the electron transport chain normally results in the formation of three molecules of ATP. Because the flavin cofactors enter further down the chain, only two molecules of ATP are produced per molecule of reduced flavin cofactor.

The complete aerobic oxidation of glucose can thus be summarized by the following net reaction:

$$C_6H_{12}O_6 + 6O_2 + 36ADP + 36P_i \rightarrow$$
$$6CO_2 + 36ATP + 42H_2O$$

where P_i represents inorganic phosphate.

Because oxygen is an absolute requirement for the operation of the electron transport chain and oxidative phosphorylation, tissue hypoxia results in the intracellular accumulation of NADH and reduced flavin cofactors, such as reduced flavin-adenine dinucleotide. In addition, the tricarboxylic acid cycle stops and intracellular pyruvate concentra-

tion increases. Thus, under anaerobic conditions, the accumulation of pyruvate and NADH results in the formation of lactate simply by chemical mass action. This single-step reaction is catalyzed by the enzyme lactate dehydrogenase (LDH):

$$\text{Pyruvate}^- + \text{NADH} + \text{H}^+ \xrightarrow{\text{LDH}} \text{lactate}^- + \text{NAD}^+$$

Because the oxidized form of the nicotinamide cofactor (NAD$^+$) is needed for the conversion of glucose to pyruvate, this cytoplasmic regeneration of NAD$^+$ allows for continuance of the anaerobic metabolism of glucose to pyruvate (Fig. 105-2). The anaerobic conversion of glucose to lactate is called glycolysis, and can be summarized by the net reaction:

$$\text{Glucose} + 2\text{ADP} + 2P_i \rightarrow 2\text{ lactate}^- + 2\text{ATP} + 2H_2O$$

Two moles of lactate are thus produced from each mole of glucose, and the lactate diffuses out of the cell and into the extracellular milieux. Note that the product of this reaction is the lactate anion, not lactic acid. There is no net production of hydrogen ions in this pathway.[4-10] However, hydrogen ions are formed during the subsequent utilization of the ATP produced by glycolysis:

$$\text{ATP} + H_2O \rightarrow \text{ADP} + P_i + \text{H}^+$$

ATP is present in small concentration within the cell and does not accumulate above normal basal concentrations[4, 6, 7, 11] (i.e., ATP does not serve as a reservoir for high-energy chemical storage). Skeletal muscle tissue contains the enzyme creatine kinase (CK) and can synthesize phosphocreatine from ATP; and phosphocreatine serves as a limited storage pool of high-energy phosphate bonds. However, as with other ATP-driven reactions, this process also results in the production of hydrogen ions:

$$\text{Creatine} + \text{ATP} \xrightarrow{\text{CK}} \text{phosphocreatine} + \text{ADP} + \text{H}^+$$

Glycolysis therefore results in the indirect but obligatory generation of hydrogen ions, after the utilization of ATP is taken into consideration. Combining the overall equation for glycolysis and the equation for the hydrolysis of ATP yields

$$\text{Glucose} \rightarrow 2\text{ lactate}^- + 2\text{H}^+$$

Glycolysis can thus be considered to result in acidosis as well as the accumulation of lactate. This stoichiometric relationship considers only the effects of glycolysis on acid-base balance. The organism as a whole may, of course, have independent pathophysiologic processes that result in other acid-base disturbances that alter the overall relationship between systemic acid-base balance and lactate accumulation. Concomitant metabolic or respiratory alkalosis, for example, mitigates the expected effect of increased lactate production on systemic pH. Such mixed acid-base disturbances are common among critically ill patients,[12, 13] and this explains the poor correlation between systemic pH and lactate concentration that is sometimes observed in clinical practice.[14]

At the cellular level, the regulation of these metabolic pathways is by way of feedback control via several key enzymes, notably phosphofructokinase (PFK) in the cytosol and citrate synthase in the mitochondria. These enzymes are allosteric (i.e., their activity is affected by the presence and concentration of certain metabolites). For example, PFK is stimulated by adenosine monophosphate (AMP), by ADP, and by fructose 6-phosphate, whereas ATP, citrate, and hydrogen ions inhibit its activity. These mechanisms regulate the rate of intracellular glucose metabolism and ensure that this rate is matched to the prevailing ATP requirements. The amount of ATP produced by the cell is thereby tightly

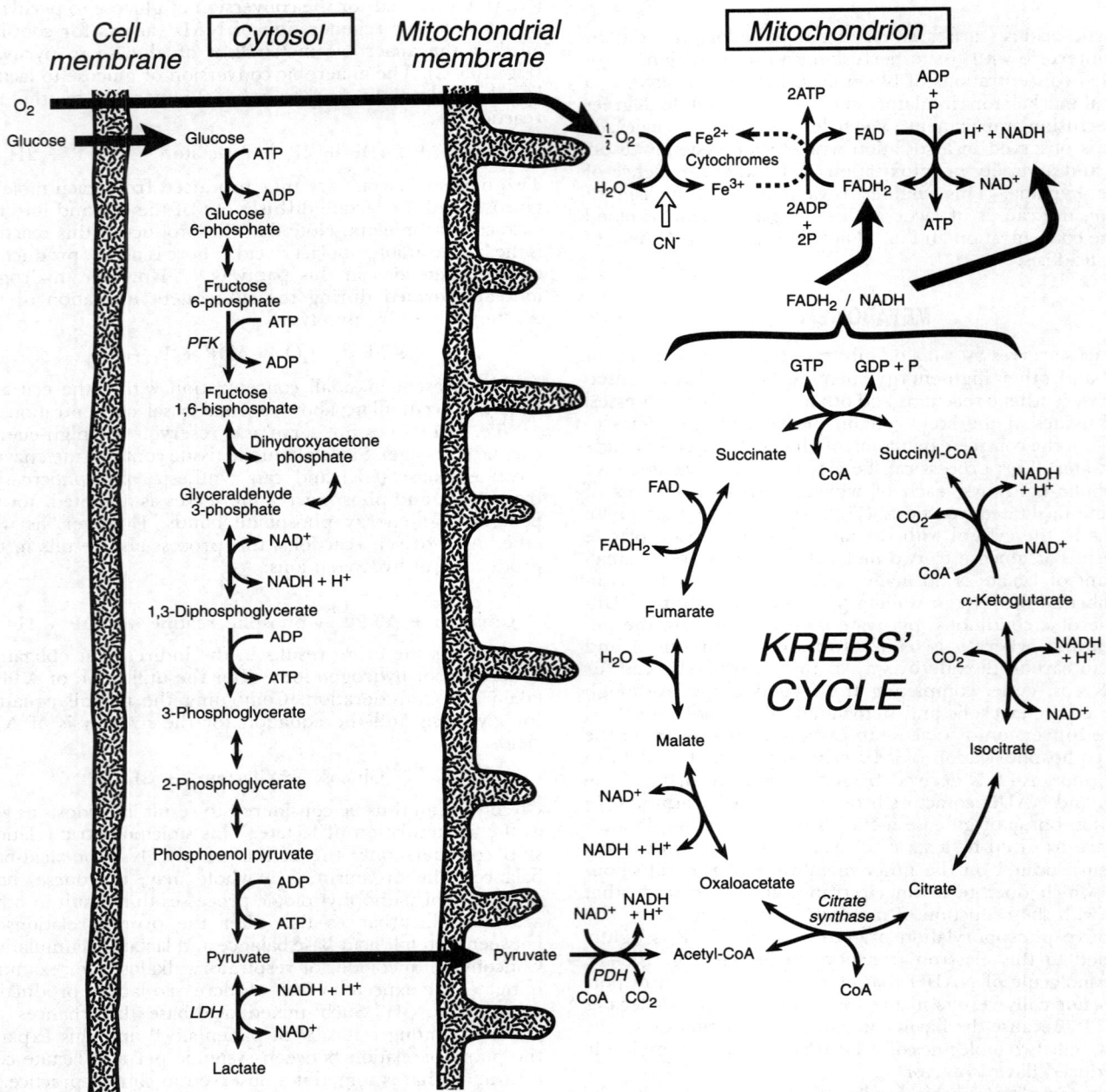

Figure 105–1. Aerobic metabolism of glucose to carbon dioxide and water. PFK = phosphofructokinase; LDH = lactate dehydrogenase; PDH = pyruvate dehydrogenase; P = inorganic phosphate; FAD and FADH$_2$ = oxidized and reduced flavin cofactor, respectively; CoA = coenzyme A.

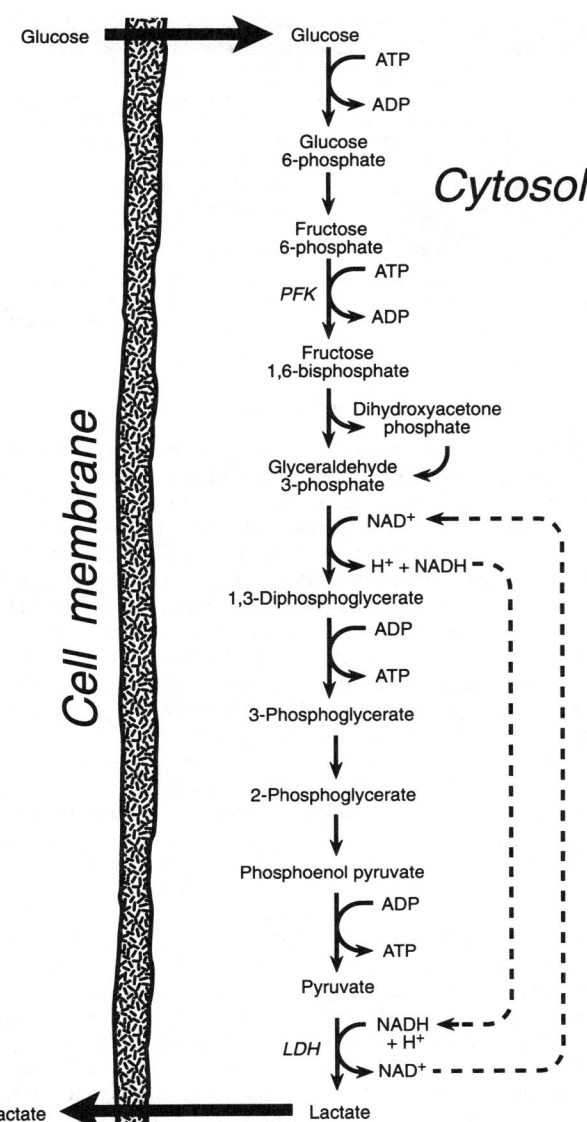

Figure 105–2. Anaerobic metabolism of glucose to lactate.

also be converted back into glucose by the process of gluconeogenesis. However, only two tissues, hepatic and renal cortex, are capable of carrying out this metabolic conversion. The production of lactate by one or more organs, coupled with the reprocessing of this lactate back into glucose, is called the Cori cycle.

Prolonged periods of severe tissue hypoxia, whether caused by increased oxygen demands, severe hypoxemia, inadequate perfusion, or a combination of these factors, result in progressively severe systemic acidosis and oxygen debt. A rough indicator of the extent of this oxygen debt is provided by the severity of the acidosis and, more reliably, the concentration of lactate in extracellular fluids (Fig. 105–3). If the hypoxia is corrected, this oxygen debt can be repaid by generating the needed ATP by way of oxidative metabolism. If uncorrected, the acidosis eventually reaches a degree that adversely affects myocardial function,[15–20] resulting in a decline in cardiac output, worsening organ hypoperfusion, and deeper levels of tissue hypoxia. Both the hypoxia and ultimately the acidosis itself have deleterious effects on cellular functioning that lead to organ system failure and death.

CAUSES

Type A Lactic Acidosis

The classification system formulated by Cohen and Woods divides lactic acidosis into two broad groups, type A and

linked to the amount needed to carry out the metabolic processes necessary for maintaining cellular homeostasis and function.

The net amount of ATP produced by glycolysis is only 2 mol/mol of glucose utilized. From an energetics standpoint, this is inefficient compared with the complete aerobic oxidation of glucose, which yields 36 mol of ATP. The inability of glycolysis to keep pace with ATP requirements and the resulting progressive acidosis limit the utility of this anaerobic pathway except for brief periods of anoxia. Thus, although glycolysis provides a means to compensate for imbalances between cellular oxygen supply and demand, it is only a temporizing measure. Partial reliance on glycolysis may continue for more prolonged periods if the hypoxia is local rather than global. This can occur if one tissue is ischemic and producing lactate, while another tissue that is adequately oxygenated is capable of utilizing this lactate. Many tissues can oxidize lactate, first by converting it to pyruvate, and then by oxidizing pyruvate by way of the tricarboxylic acid cycle. Myocardial tissue utilizes lactate as a preferred substrate under normal conditions.[4] Lactate can

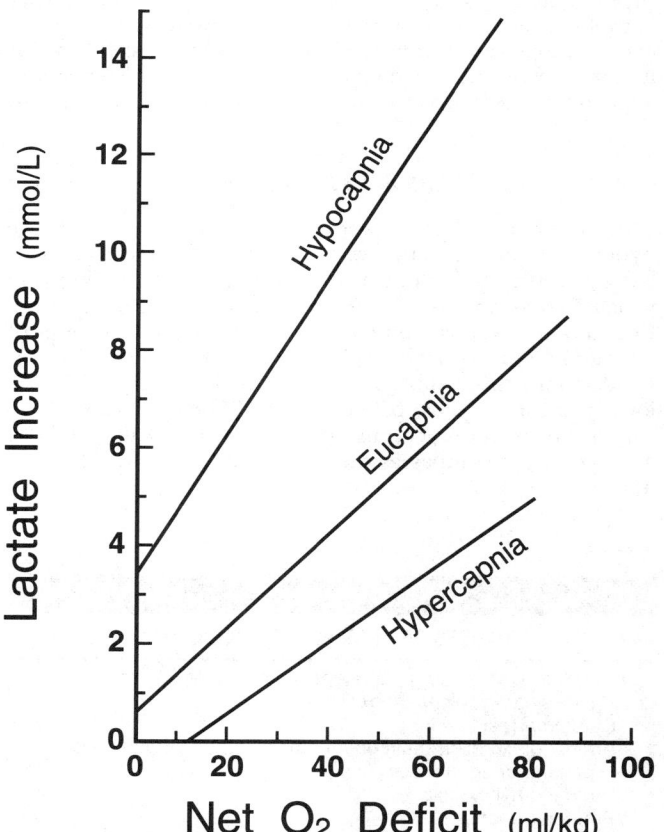

Figure 105–3. Peak lactate increase compared with net oxygen deficit incurred during hypercapnia (PCO_2, 77 torr), eucapnia (PCO_2, 40 torr), and hypocapnia (PCO_2, 18 torr) in anesthetized dogs. (From Cain SM: Effect of PCO_2 on the relation of lactate and excess lactate to O_2 deficit. Am J Physiol 214:1322, 1968.)

type B.[1] In type A lactic acidosis, decreased or inadequate systemic or regional oxygen availability is the underlying mechanism leading to increased lactate production and accumulation (Table 105–1). Circulatory shock is the most common pathologic cause. The same mechanism (i.e., an imbalance between oxygen supply and demand) is also operative physiologically during severe exertion.

With maximal exercise, the energy requirements of skeletal muscle tissue can outstrip the capacity of the respiratory and cardiovascular systems to provide oxygen to the periphery. Lactate production therefore increases, and blood lactate levels can rise markedly. With heavy exercise, lactate levels in the range of 2 to 15 mmol/L are typically observed.[21, 22] With extreme degrees of anaerobic exercise, trained individuals may achieve blood lactate concentrations of 35 mmol/L or greater, with proportionately severe decreases in arterial pH.[23, 24] Increases in blood lactate concentrations attributable to exercise should perhaps not be termed *lactic acidosis* because they represent lactate accumulation that is due to a purely physiologic imbalance in oxygen supply and demand.

A grand mal seizure, although mechanistically similar to strenuous exercise, is a pathologic process that can result in increased blood lactate and metabolic acidosis.[25] In addition to the increase in oxygen demand that occurs with motor seizures, there may also be a compromise in the supply of systemic oxygen. This can occur if the uncontrolled muscle contractions and loss of consciousness interfere with airway patency, ventilation, and/or venous return. Seizures thus represent a prototypic example of type A lactic acidosis, which results from a pathologic imbalance in tissue oxygen supply and demand.[1, 26] Severe asthma represents another pathologic situation in which markedly increased muscular exertion may result in lactate accumulation.[27] As with major motor convulsions, extreme bronchospasm can also result in arterial hypoxemia, as well as hemodynamic embarrassment.

Type B₁ Lactic Acidosis

Although circulatory shock and other forms of tissue hypoxia account for the vast majority of clinical cases of lactic acidosis, there appear to be a number of conditions in which lactate can accumulate without evidence of hypoxia. Cohen and Woods named this heterogeneous group of conditions type B lactic acidosis. Type B has been further divided into three subtypes: type B_1 is associated with various, and for the most part common, disorders (Table 105–2); type B_2 is due to certain drugs or toxins (Table 105–3); and type B_3 encompasses the congenital forms (Table 105–4).

TABLE 105–1

CAUSES OF TYPE A LACTIC ACIDOSIS*

Circulatory shock (e.g., cardiogenic, hypovolemic, and
    septic) or incipient shock
Cardiac arrest
Arterial obstruction (pulmonary embolism, aortic dissection,
    peripheral arterial occlusion)
Profound hypoxemia
Profound anemia
Carbon monoxide poisoning
Motor seizures
Status asthmaticus

*Lactic acidosis associated with inadequate tissue oxygenation.

TABLE 105–2

CAUSES OF TYPE B₁ LACTIC ACIDOSIS*

Hepatic disease	Short bowel syndrome
Diabetes mellitus	Alcoholic ketoacidosis
Sepsis	Thiamine deficiency
Malignancies	Iron deficiency
Renal failure	Alkalemia
Pheochromocytoma	

*Lactic acidosis associated with certain acquired predisposing conditions. A cause-and-effect relationship has not been established with all of the listed disease states and some may actually represent forms of type A lactic acidosis.

Liver Disease

Lactic acidosis has been described in patients with severe liver disease and attributed to decreased hepatic uptake of lactate. Although the liver is an important lactate consumer, other tissues such as the heart, the brain, the kidney, and skeletal muscle are also capable of utilizing lactate.[28–32] On the basis of theoretic calculations, it has been postulated that lactic acidosis would not occur even if hepatic uptake fell to zero, unless there were a concomitant increase in lactate production.[33] Clinically significant increases in blood lactate are seldom observed in patients with advanced liver disease unless there is evidence of circulatory shock.[34, 35] Administration of vasodilators to increase oxygen delivery to patients with hepatic failure has been shown to result in increased oxygen consumption and decreased blood lactate levels.[36, 37] These findings suggest that the increased lactate level sometimes observed in severe liver disease is due to concomitant tissue hypoxia rather than simply decreased hepatic utilization.[38]

Inadequate tissue oxygenation should be a prime consideration in patients with hepatic failure who have lactic acidosis. As with patients with type A lactic acidosis, mortality in patients with severe hepatic disease is correlated with the degree of lactic acidosis.[34, 38] When patients with hepatic impairment have increased blood lactate levels (e.g., after cardiac arrest), their rate of lactate clearance is expected to be impaired compared with that of patients with normal hepatic function.[39, 40] There may be specific biochemical defects that lead to lactic acidosis in patients with Reye's syndrome, a form of severe hepatic disease limited almost exclusively to the pediatric population. Interference with mitochondrial function and deficiencies of hepatic pyruvate

---

TABLE 105–3

CAUSES OF TYPE B₂ LACTIC ACIDOSIS*

Biguanide hypoglycemic agents	Salicylates
Streptozocin	Acetaminophen
Sodium bicarbonate	Ethanol
Fructose	Methanol
Epinephrine	Ethylene glycol
Norepinephrine	Propylene glycol
Ritodrine	Sorbitol
Terbutaline	Xylitol
Papaverine	Halothane
Carbon monoxide	Iron
Sodium nitroprusside	Strychnine
Cyanide	Methyl ethyl ketone
Isoniazid	Amoxapine
Dithiazanine iodide	Nalidixic acid

*Lactic acidosis associated with certain drugs and toxins.

TABLE 105–4

PARTIAL LISTING OF CAUSES OF TYPE B₃ LACTIC ACIDOSIS*

Glucose-6-phosphatase deficiency (glycogen storage disease type I)
Fructose-1,6-bisphosphatase deficiency
Pyruvate carboxylase deficiency
Pyruvate dehydrogenase deficiency
Fructose-1-phosphate aldolase deficiency (hereditary fructose intolerance)
Oxidative phosphorylation defects
MELAS (mitochondrial encephalomyopathy with lactic acidosis and stroke) syndrome

*Lactic acidosis associated with certain inborn errors of metabolism and other apparent congenital forms.

dehydrongenase and pyruvate carboxylase activity have been described in this syndrome.[41, 42]

Cancer

The course of most advanced neoplastic disorders commonly culminates in a critical illness associated with cardiorespiratory dysfunction. Lactic acidosis in this setting is attributable to the underlying systemic hypoperfusion and tissue hypoxia. However, there are reports of cases in which the patient appeared to be quite stable and yet had lactic acidosis, which was sometimes severe and prolonged.[43–53] Lymphoma, leukemia, and breast and lung cancer are among the most frequently reported neoplastic disorders associated with lactic acidosis, but considering the prevalence of these malignancies, this situation is quite rare.

Multiple mechanisms are potentially involved. Large solid tumors may outgrow their blood supply and become ischemic. Extensive neoplastic involvement of the bone marrow may similarly result in local ischemia attributable to compression of the marrow that limits its own blood supply. Evidence of altered intermediary metabolism has been de-

scribed in some malignant tissues. In normal aerobic metabolism, NADH produced in the cytosol is transported into the mitochondria by way of the glycerol phosphate shuttle, which allows for regeneration of cytoplasmic NAD⁺ without producing lactate. Certain neoplastic cells lack the enzyme glycerol-3-phosphate dehydrogenase, which is necessary for this shuttle to operate.[54] Without glycerol-3-phosphate dehydrogenase, NADH accumulates in the cytosol and forces the conversion of pyruvate to lactate (Fig. 105–4). Although this allows for the regeneration of cytoplasmic NAD⁺, it may obligate lactate production even under aerobic conditions.

Diabetes

There are reports of critically ill diabetics having elevated lactate levels, ostensibly without tissue hypoxia.[1, 55] However, since the removal of phenformin from the U.S. market, lactic acidosis occurring in connection with diabetes has become sufficiently uncommon as to question the existence of a true relationship.[35, 56–58] Blood lactate concentrations are not substantially elevated in patients with well-controlled diabetes[59–63] nor is lactic acidosis characteristic of either uncontrolled diabetes or diabetic ketoacidosis.[58, 64, 65] Diabetic ketoacidosis is commonly associated with dehydration, and this can sometimes be severe enough to lead to hypovolemic shock. Sepsis is a frequent precipitant of metabolic decompensation in diabetics, and some patients progress to septic shock. Type A lactic acidosis can therefore occur in severely ill diabetics, and this is likely the mechanism involved in most or perhaps even all cases.[10, 66] It has been postulated that more subtle degrees of hypoperfusion, perhaps attributable in part to diabetes-related vascular disease, may also lead to type A lactate accumulation in some acutely ill diabetics.[30, 67]

Short Bowel Syndrome

In 1979, Oh and colleagues reported a case of high anion gap metabolic acidosis in a patient with a history of bowel resection for mesenteric infarction.[68] The cause of the aci-

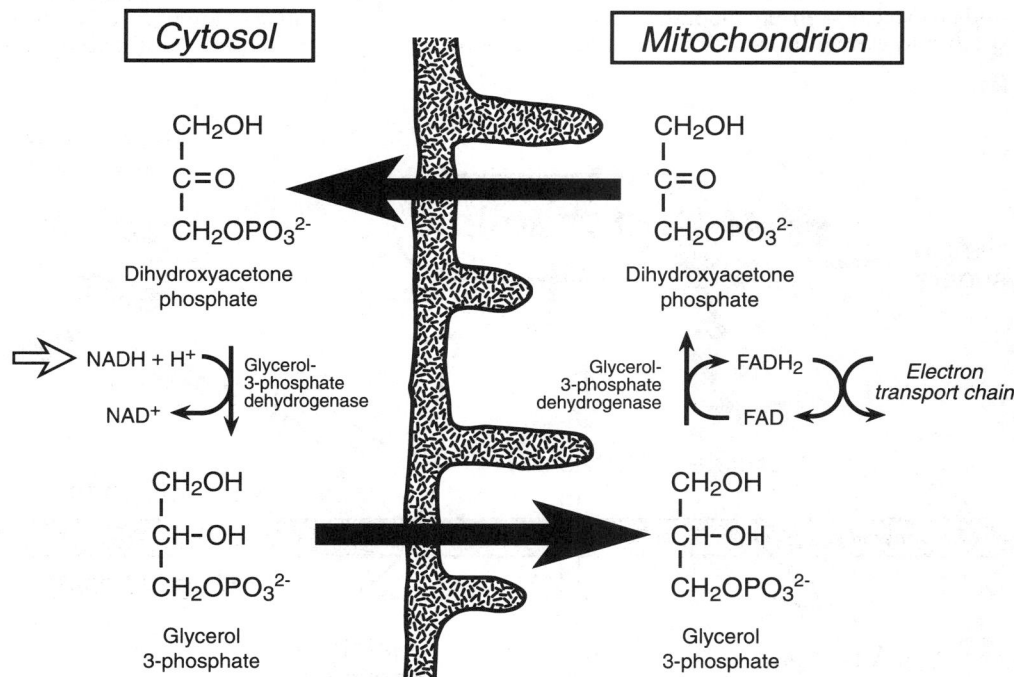

Figure 105–4. The glycerol phosphate shuttle allows for the regeneration of cytoplasmic NAD⁺ from NADH, without producing lactate. In the absense of functional glycerol-3-phosphate dehydrogenase, as may occur in certain neoplastic tissues, NADH accumulation in the cytosol results in increased formation of lactate from pyruvate (see Fig. 105–1).

dosis and the anion gap was not immediately apparent; blood and urine testing for ketones, lactate, and numerous drugs and toxins were negative. Gas chromatography, however, revealed high concentrations of lactate. This assay technique does not distinguish between L-lactate and its stereoisomer D-lactate. Lactate produced by higher animals is the L form, and clinical laboratories therefore commonly employ enzyme-coupled reactions that use L-lactate dehydrogenase or L-lactate oxidase to quantitate blood lactate. Thus, routine lactate assays do not react with D-lactate. The D form, however, is produced by certain bacteria, including certain species that may colonize the lower intestinal tract under certain conditions. Additional sporadic cases of D-lactic acidosis have been documented since this initial report. All have occurred in patients with prior bowel resection or intestinal bypass surgery and have been associated with neurologic manifestations, including stupor, coma, ataxia, slurred speech, nystagmus, asterixis, and behavioral changes[69]

D-Lactic acid is produced by an overgrowth of certain gut flora, notably *Lactobacillus*, *Eubacterium*, and *Bifidobacterium*, accompanied by a concomitant decrease in the usually prevalent *Bacteroides* species[70] (Fig. 105–5). The D-lactic acid is then absorbed from the bowel, resulting in acidosis and accumulation of D-lactate in plasma. The mechanism of the neurologic abnormalities is not known, but they may be due to D-lactate itself or some other bacterial by-product.

A similar syndrome, long recognized by veterinarians, occurs in cattle overfed with grain. The syndrome is characterized by alterations in gut flora, decreased stool pH, lethargy, and ataxia and is sometimes fatal.[71] Definitive diagnosis of D-lactic acidosis hinges on quantitative D-lactate serum levels. This can be accomplished by substituting an enzyme that is specific for the D-lactate isomer (e.g., D-lactate dehydrogenase) in a conventional assay and using a prepared solution of D-lactate as a standard.[72] Alternatively, gas chromatography or nuclear magnetic resonance spectroscopy may be used.[73] This disorder has been successfully treated with oral antibiotics such as vancomycin and neomycin.

Thiamine Deficiency

Deficiency of thiamine (vitamin B₁) can result in beriberi and Wernicke's encephalopathy. Lactic acidosis may also occur and can be severe.[74] Thiamine serves as an obligatory cofactor to several important enzymes, including the pyruvate dehydrogenase system. The ability to oxidize pyruvate to acetate is impaired in thiamine deficiency, and the resulting accumulation of pyruvate leads to increased formation of lactate (see Fig. 105–1).

Alcoholics are particularly at risk for thiamine deficiency. In addition to nutritional deficiency common in alcoholism, ethanol also interferes with thiamine absorption and storage and inhibits the hepatic enzyme pyrophosphokinase, which is needed to activate thiamine.[75] Patients receiving total parenteral nutrition are also at high risk and must receive thiamine supplementation. Several fatal cases of iatrogenic thiamine deficiency associated with lactic acidosis have resulted from the administration of parenteral nutrition formula without thiamine supplementation.[76]

Hyperventilation

Systemic alkalemia results in a small but demonstrable increase in blood lactate concentration. This occurs not only with respiratory alkalemia caused by hyperventilation, but also from metabolic alkalemia (e.g., by administration of sodium bicarbonate). This effect can be demonstrated under otherwise normal conditions (i.e., without evidence of hypoxia). In addition, systemic pH influences the degree of hyperlactatemia resulting from lactic acidosis attributable to exercise or hypoxia (see Fig. 105–3).[77–79] The mechanism may be multifactorial but appears to be predominantly due to the influence of cytosolic pH on the activity of PFK (Fig. 105–6). As pH rises, the catalytic activity of this enzyme increases, resulting in more rapid phosphorylation of fructose 6-phosphate.[80] The remaining steps in the glycolytic sequence follow in an unregulated fashion, leading to the rapid formation of pyruvate. If cellular energy reserves are adequate, the high prevailing ATP concentration inhibits citrate synthase, thus shutting down the tricarboxylic acid cycle and forcing the accumulation of pyruvate. The concentration of NADH also increases owing to the conversion of glyceraldehyde 3-phosphate to 1,3-diphosphoglycerate. By simple chemical mass action, the accumulated NADH and pyruvate are converted to NAD⁺ and lactate. It should be emphasized that the increments in blood lactate level observed in hyperventilated animals and human subjects are mild. Although some early investigations involving hyperventilated anesthetized animals demonstrated high levels of

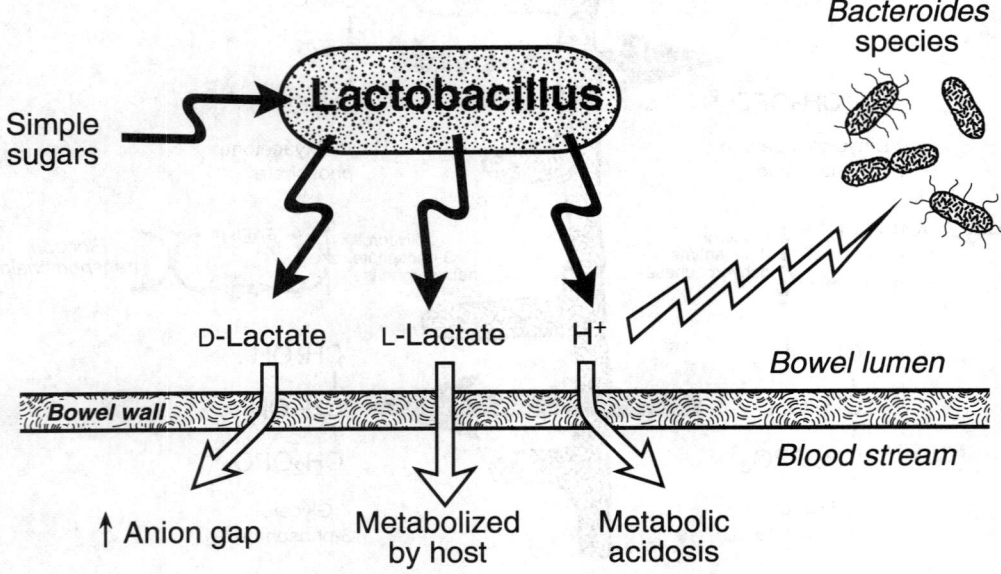

Figure 105–5. Pathophysiology of D-lactic acidosis. Bacterial overgrowth with *Lactobacillus*, *Eubacterium*, or *Bifidobacterium* species may occur after bowel resection or intestinal bypass surgery. These bacteria consume simple sugars available in the bowel lumen and produce acid (hydrogen ions) plus L-lactate and/or D-lactate. Intraluminal pH becomes acidic and inhibits growth of more typical bowel flora, such as *Bacteroides* species. Systemic absorption of D-lactic acid results in a high-anion-gap metabolic acidosis; however, blood lactate concentration is normal if the assay is specific for the L stereoisomer.

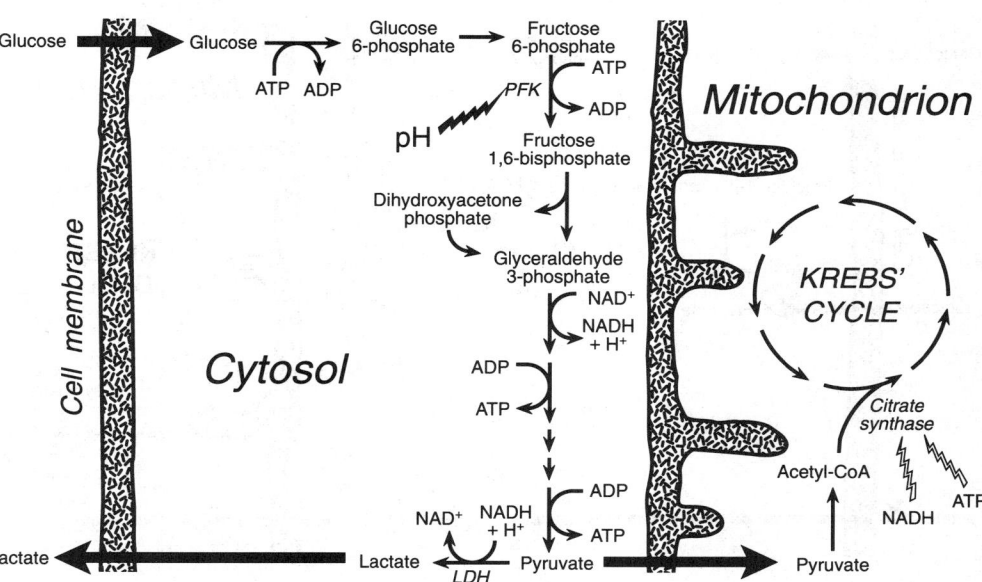

Figure 105–6. Effects of elevated intracellular pH on glucose metabolism. Filled jagged line represents enzyme stimulation; open jagged lines represent enzyme inhibition. Stimulation of PFK, the enzyme controlling the rate-limiting step in the conversion of glucose to pyruvate, results in increased formation of pyruvate. In the presence of adequate cellular energy reserves, citrate sythase is inhibited, preventing oxidation of pyruvate by the tricarboxylic acid cycle. Accumulation of cytosolic pyruvate and NADH leads to increased lactate production. Acetyl-CoA = acetyl coenzyme A.

hyperlactatemia, it is likely that these experimental preparations were complicated by hemodynamic embarrassment.[81]

In one study in which hemodynamic monitoring was employed, hyperventilated dogs had arterial lactate levels in the range of 10 mmol/L; however, marked changes in blood pressure were observed and cardiac output fell by about one third.[82] Other studies showed slight or even no change in lactate levels during hyperventilation.[83] Voluntary hyperventilation by normal subjects to Pco_2 levels in the range of 20 torr, corresponding to an average arterial pH in excess of 7.6, resulted in a mean increase in blood lactate concentration of less than 1 mmol/L.[84] Thus, although common in mechanically ventilated and critically ill patients,[12, 13] alkalemia does not have a clinically significant effect on blood lactate levels.

Other Causes

A variety of other disease states are associated with lactic acidosis and have been labeled as type B_1 causes. These include myocardial infarction, pancreatitis, pulmonary embolism, and use of mechanical ventilation.[1] Critical illness is frequently associated with each of these disorders, and cardiopulmonary dysfunction, including frank circulatory shock, occurs in the most severe cases. Unless evidence is uncovered to suggest otherwise, these illnesses should be considered potential causes of type A lactic acidosis. Elevations in blood lactate level that are observed in severe sepsis can similarly be due to hypoperfusion or to the maldistribution of perfusion that has been well described in this disorder.[85–87] This is supported by studies in which increasing systemic oxygen delivery has frequently been shown to improve oxygen consumption and result in decreases in blood lactate level in patients with sepsis.[88–93] It has also been postulated that lactate levels may be elevated in sepsis, even in the absence of tissue hypoxia caused by changes in the activity of pyruvate dehydrogenase or impairment of oxidative phosphorylation.[10, 94, 95]

Type B_2 Lactic Acidosis
Biguanides

The biguanide hypoglycemic drugs might be considered archetypic causes of type B_2 lactic acidosis. Hundreds of

cases of lactic acidosis have been reported in patients treated with phenformin and, to a much lesser extent, the related biguanides buformin and metformin.[1, 96–99] In many cases, profound degrees of lactate elevation and acidemia have occurred. In the United States, this cause is of only historical interest since this association led to the removal of phenformin from the U.S. market in 1977. At that time, it was estimated that up to 4 of 1000 patients receiving phenformin had lactic acidosis each year, with an overall mortality rate of 50%.[30] Despite intensive investigation, the exact cause of the lactic acidosis has proved elusive. Patients with high blood concentrations of the drug and those with renal and hepatic impairment are known to be at increased risk. The biguanides have been shown to interfere with gluconeogenesis, electron transport, and oxidative phosphorylation and to increase lactate production as well as decrease its utilization.[100–103]

Fructose

Intravenous infusions of fructose have been employed therapeutically for diabetes mellitus and acute ethanol intoxication and in parenteral alimentation formulas. Many cases of severe lactic acidosis have been reported with its use.[1, 104] Unlike glucose, fructose can enter cells in the absence of insulin. High blood levels of fructose are therefore expected to result in diffusion into cells down a concentration gradient. Like glucose, fructose then enters the glycolytic pathway. However, fructose is not phosphorylated by the same enzymes as glucose (Fig. 105–7). Instead, it is able to enter the glycolysis pathway just below the rate-limiting step (i.e., below the level of phosphorylation of fructose 6-phosphate by PFK).[105, 106] By sidestepping this important control point, fructose may be rapidly converted to pyruvate regardless of the ATP requirements of the cell. The accumulation of pyruvate and NADH results in lactate formation. Other mechanisms may also be involved.[100, 107] The sugar alcohols sorbitol and xylitol, both used outside the United States in parenteral nutrition formulas, may cause lactic acidosis by similar mechanisms.[1, 100, 106, 108]

Cyanide

Salts of hydrogen cyanide are widely used in the metal processing and electroplating industries. They are also found

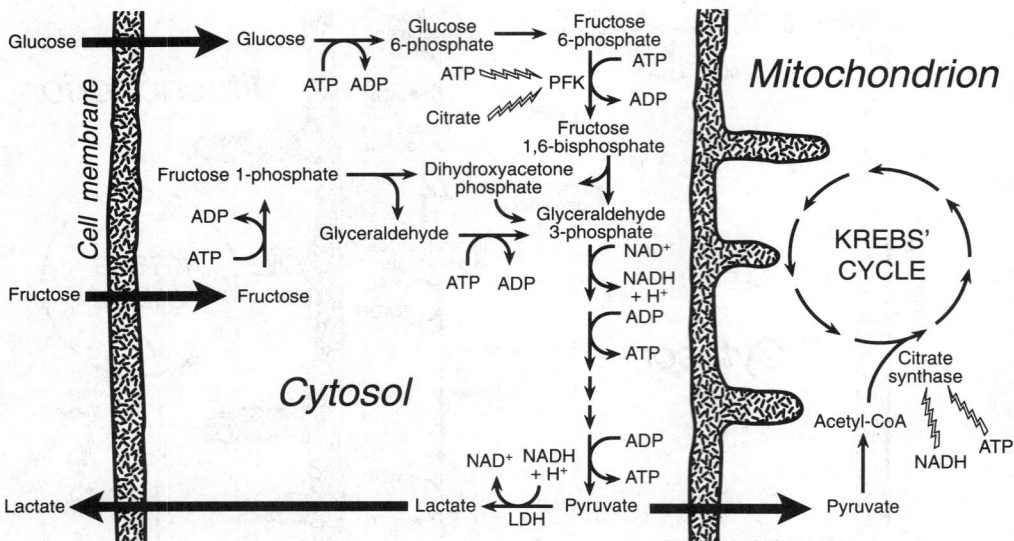

Figure 105–7. Metabolism of fructose. PFK controls the conversion of fructose 6-phosphate to fructose 1,6-bisphosphate, the rate-limiting step in the normal conversion of glucose to pyruvate. Open jagged lines represent enzyme inhibition of PFK and citrate synthase under conditions of adequate cellular energy reserve. Fructose enters the glycolytic pathway below the level of PFK and is thus rapidly converted to pyruvate. Accumulation of cytosolic pyruvate and NADH leads to increased lactate production. Acetyl-CoA = acetyl coenzyme A.

in certain botanicals, such as apricot pits, bitter almonds, and a variety of plant extracts containing amygdalin. The latter substance is the main ingredient in Laetrile, a purportedly antineoplastic agent of dubious efficacy that has caused fatal cyanide poisoning.[109] The antihypertensive agent sodium nitroprusside is metabolized to thiocyanate and cyanide. Clinical use has resulted in lactic acidosis from cyanide poisoning when nitroprusside has been employed at high doses and/or for prolonged periods, particularly in patients with renal insufficiency.[110–112] There have been a few reports of cyanide toxicity from nitroprusside after infusions as short as 35 minutes.[113] Cyanide combines with cytochrome oxidase and blocks the terminal reaction of the intramitochondrial electron transport process[105, 114] (see Fig. 105–1). Production of ATP by oxidative phosphorylation is stopped and anaerobic metabolism is utilized for ATP production, leading to lactic acidosis. The problem is not hypoxia; in fact, tissue and mixed venous oxygen tensions may increase because cellular oxygen utilization is impaired. Nevertheless, the consequences are essentially tantamount to those of tissue hypoxia.

Carbon Monoxide

Lactic acidosis has been observed in cases of severe carbon monoxide poisoning.[115] The decreased oxygen content and the leftward shift in the oxyhemoglobin dissociation curve imposed by formation of carboxyhemoglobin obviously qualifies this as a type A form of lactic acidosis. An additional mechanism may be involved because carbon monoxide can also bind to the cytochromes involved in intramitochondrial electron transport. Interference with this process impedes oxidative phosphorylation in a manner similar to that of cyanide intoxication. Thus, the increased lactate formation seen in severe carbon monoxide poisoning can be classified as both type A and type B lactic acidosis.

Catecholamines

Catecholamine administration may increase blood lactate concentrations by stimulating glycogenolysis. In addition, catecholamines are calorigenic (i.e., they accelerate metabolic demands and therefore increase oxygen requirements). This could result in augmented lactate production in tissues with limited oxygen reserve. Typical pharmacologic doses usually cause only slight elevations of blood lactate levels. Greene, for example, administered epinephrine intravenously to healthy volunteers at a rate of 0.15 μg/kg/min and found that arterial lactate levels increased by 1.3 mmol/L after a 20-minute infusion.[116] A massive overdose of epinephrine, on the other hand, was associated with marked increases.[117]

There are also rare reports that other sympathomimetic agents, including ritodrine, terbutaline, and metaproterenol, cause lactate elevations.[118–120] Other mechanisms may be involved in patients receiving these agents for treatment of severe bronchospasm, including increased oxygen demand resulting from the work of breathing and decreased oxygen delivery caused by hypoxemia or impaired venous return related to changes in intrathoracic pressure.

Regional decreases in oxygen delivery may be due to catecholamine-induced vasoconstriction that results in peripheral tissue ischemia. In patients with borderline cardiac reserve, catecholamine-mediated increases in left ventricular afterload may lead to critical impairment of cardiac output. Large doses of adrenergic agents may therefore cause severe vasoconstriction, leading to lactate production on the basis of both ischemia and myocardial dysfunction. This may be a mechanism involved in the lactic acidosis described in association with rare cases of pheochromocytoma.[121–123] Some of these patients with pheochromocytoma were in extremis and died shortly after their blood lactate level was discovered to be elevated.

Theophylline

Lactic acidosis has been reported in association with severe theophylline intoxication. Generalized seizures as well as probable hypoxemia and/or hemodynamic embarrassment have been reported in these cases.[124, 125] However, because epinephrine and norepinephrine levels have been shown to be increased by theophylline toxicity, catecholamine-induced increases in lactate production could also be a factor.[126–128]

Salicylates and Acetaminophen

Salicylate poisoning has been cited as a cause of lactic acidosis.[35, 100, 129] Although salicylates can potentially interfere with aerobic ATP production by inhibiting enzymes involved in the tricarboxylic acid cycle and by uncoupling oxidative phosphorylation,[130] significant lactate elevation is not characteristic of this drug overdose.[67, 131] A stronger case can be made for the association between lactic acidosis and acetaminophen poisoning. This occurs in about half of severely poisoned patients, can be seen both early and late in the course, and is proportional to the severity of the overdose.[132, 133] There is some evidence that acetaminophen toxicity may stimulate glycolysis and interfere with gluconeogenesis and ATP production.[134] On the other hand, occult hypoperfusion has been uncovered in some cases.[10]

Alcohols and Glycols

Hyperlactatemia occurs in some individuals after ethanol consumption. In one investigation, ethanol was administered orally to healthy volunteers to achieve blood alcohol levels in the range of 390 to 480 mg/dL.[135] Mean blood lactate level rose to 1.3 mmol/L, a change that was statistically significant but of no clinical significance. Fulop and colleagues studied patients presenting to an emergency department with acute ethanol intoxication and discovered that the majority had normal blood lactate concentrations, although a few had mild-to-moderate elevations.[136] Metabolism of ethanol results in increased formation of NADH, thus favoring conversion of pyruvate to lactate. In some subjects, other factors such as thiamine deficiency, alcoholic ketoacidosis, withdrawl seizures, and toxin exposure, are likely to be operative as well.[137]

Methanol and ethylene glycol poisoning may similarly result in lactate elevations by affecting the redox state. Both agents usually cause severe metabolic acidosis and an elevated anion gap without lactic acidosis, however. Methanol is metabolized to formic acid and ethylene glycol to glycolic and other acid intermediates. Poisoning with these toxins can also cause cardiorespiratory impairment, which is severe enough in some cases to produce lactic acidosis from frank circulatory shock. Propylene glycol, considered safe by the U.S. Food and Drug Administration for both oral and parenteral use, is widely used as a solvent in pharmaceuticals and cosmetics. It is a principal vehicle in many drugs commonly employed in critically ill patients, including preparations of phenytoin, digoxin, diazepam, trimethoprim-sulfamethoxazole, nitroglycerin, and others. Multiple dosing with large volumes of such preparations has been associated with lactic acidosis.[138] Serial blood lactate measurements have been highly correlated with both the total dose of administered propylene glycol and the resulting serum levels.[139] Intentional abuse of propylene glycol is rare but has also resulted in lactic acidosis.[140] Long-term administration of the agent has reportedly been associated with seizures,[141] and this could represent one mechanism for increased lactate production. However, seizures have not been universally observed, and lactic acidosis can be explained by conversion of propylene glycol to lactate in the liver[142–144] (Fig. 105–8).

Paraldehyde

Also included in the differential diagnosis of increased anion gap metabolic acidosis is paraldehyde intoxication. This cyclic polymer of acetaldehyde has been reported to cause lactic acidosis, but concomitant seizures or shock provides alternative explanations for the increases in lactate that have been observed.[145] Although the cause of the acidosis in paraldehyde intoxication has not been elucidated, lactic acidosis does not appear to be involved except as a secondary phenomenon.[67]

Iron

Severe iron poisoning, usually by accidental or intentional ingestion of medicinal iron preparations, has been associated with lactic acidosis. Whereas release of protons during the oxidation of ferrous ions may be partially responsible for the acidosis, it does not explain the hyperlactatemia. Although mitochondrial dysfunction may be implicated in the mechanism of the latter,[146] it seems likely that the predominant mechanism is tissue hypoxia. Circulatory shock is a common concomitant of severe iron intoxication.[146, 147] Intractable seizures have also been reported and further exacerbate the imbalance between systemic oxygen supply and demand.

Miscellaneous Agents

There are rare reports of lactic acidosis occurring in patients intoxicated with a variety of other drugs and toxic agents. As with paraldehyde intoxication and iron poisoning, many of these cases were associated with seizures and/or hypotension to an extent that could explain the lactic acidosis on the basis of imbalanced tissue oxygen supply and demand. Alternative causes, such as malignancy or some other factor known to be associated with lactic acidosis, have been present in other cases. Among other agents in this category are strychnine,[148] amoxapine,[149] methyl ethyl ketone,[150] and the antibiotic nalidixic acid.[151, 152] For other agents, a type A cause can be invoked in some but not all of the reported cases. For example, intoxication with the antituberculous agent isoniazid has been reported to cause lactic acidosis. In both animal models and some of the human cases, the mechanism can be explained by the associated persistent generalized seizures that were observed.[100, 153–155] However, there have been a few cases without apparent seizures or other explanations for the lactic acidosis.

From the earlier discussion, it should be appreciated that the lactic acidosis observed in association with some or possibly most of the drugs and toxins described as type B_2 agents may actually represent instances of type A lactic acidosis. This exemplifies an inherent limitation of the classification scheme formulated by Cohen and Woods.[1] It is the

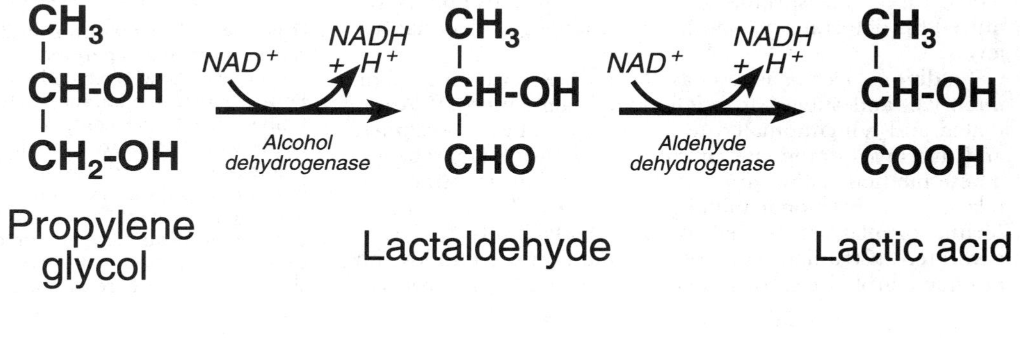

Figure 105–8. Metabolism of propylene glycol by hepatic alcohol dehydrogenase and aldehyde dehydrogenase.

mechanism of the lactic acidosis that underlies this classification: type A are causes ascribed to tissue hypoxia; type B are those that are not due to tissue hypoxia. However, because specific mechanisms are often unknown, particularly when an association is first recognized, de facto categorization under the rubrics of types B_1 and B_2 has for the most part been by simple association. As more cases are reported in greater clinical detail and as more is understood about the mechanisms involved, some or even most of the type B factors may become recognized as actually representing instances of tissue hypoxia. Although frank circulatory shock is readily recognized at the bedside, early or more subtle forms of tissue hypoperfusion may not be. Hypoperfusion and tissue hypoxia are common concomitants of critical illness and the possibility of coexisting hypoxia is sometimes difficult to exclude.

Type B_3 Lactic Acidosis

A variety of congenital forms of lactic acidosis have been described[1, 30, 156–160] (see Table 105–4). Some of these are known to be due to inborn errors of metabolism that have been pinpointed to the deficiency of a single enzyme. All are uncommon. Von Gierke's disease, also known as type I glycogen storage disease, is among the least uncommon and is due to an inherited deficiency of glucose 6-phosphatase. Most of the congenital forms of lactic acidosis manifest in infancy, but some, such as hereditary fructose intolerance, frequently go unrecognized and the diagnosis may first be made in adulthood.[30, 156, 160]

MEASUREMENT AND CLINICAL UTILITY OF LACTATE

Lactic acidosis is a common and expected complication of critical illness that has progressed to the point of severe and global tissue hypoxia. In clinical situations in which there is frank circulatory shock manifest by hypotension and obvious evidence of organ dysfunction, the presence and severity of lactic acidosis underscore the severity of the hypoperfusion state. However, the detection of milder degrees of lactic acidosis, or hyperlactatemia without acidemia, may alert the clinician to more subtle degrees of hypoperfusion. This allows early institution of therapeutic interventions that may improve tissue oxygen delivery, halt or reverse vital organ ischemia, and avert progression to frank or irreversible circulatory shock. Therefore, even relatively mild degrees of lactate elevation may be of clinical importance. This is supported by observations from multiple clinical investigations that blood lactate concentrations in excess of 2.5 to 3.0 mmol/L are associated with increased mortality.[14, 26, 161–166] Changes in arterial pH, carbon dioxide content, and the anion gap are relatively insensitive to these levels of lactate elevation.[14, 167, 168] This is in part due to the normal degree of variability in electrolyte and acid-base values and also occurs because concomitant respiratory and/or metabolic alkalosis are not uncommon in this patient population.[12, 13] Thus, direct measurement of lactate concentration is required for detecting and monitoring changes in blood lactate levels.

Traditional lactate assays have been time consuming, labor intensive, and subject to methodologic limitations.[169] Automated and semiautomated techniques have been developed and are in common use in clinical chemistry laboratories. These methods allow accurate and precise measurement of L-lactate on fractional milliliter quantities of whole blood, serum, or plasma, as well as other body fluids.[169–173] One dedicated instrument currently in common use employs an enzyme-coupled electrochemical lactate sensor that consists

of a lactate oxidase–containing membrane that reacts with lactate to form hydrogen peroxide[174] (Fig. 105–9). The hydrogen peroxide is converted to oxygen at a platinum electrode, resulting in formation of an electric current proportional to the concentration of lactate in the sample.

Pathologic increases in blood lactate concentration occur chiefly in association with either frank circulatory shock or more subtle degrees of tissue hypoperfusion. Although lactic acidosis can occur in a number of conditions other than shock, many of these other conditions are infrequently encountered or result in only minor degrees of elevation in blood lactate level. Therefore, inadequate tissue oxygenation should be the first consideration when a patient with lactic acidosis is encountered. In addition to serving as a marker for detecting inadequate perfusion, serial blood lactate levels can be helpful in monitoring the response to therapeutic interventions designed to improve systemic oxygen delivery. For patients with systemic hypoperfusion and elevated lactate concentrations, the impact of augmenting cardiac output by way of fluid infusions, inotropic agents, or intra-aortic balloon counterpulsation, for example, can be assessed by following sequential changes in blood lactate level. In conjunction with other clinical indicators of organ perfusion (such as urine output and changes in sensorium) and, in

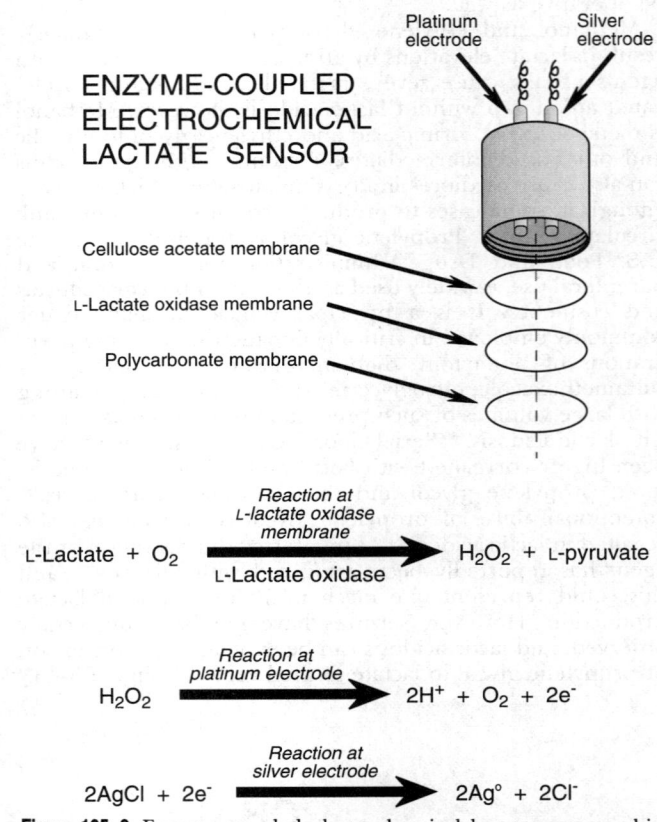

Figure 105–9. Enzyme-coupled electrochemical lactate sensor, which can be used for rapid assay of lactate in microliter quantities of serum, plasma, whole blood, or other lactate-containing body fluids. Polycarbonate membrane excludes large molecules and enzymes. Center membrane contains immobilized L-lactate oxidase, which reacts with lactate to form hydrogen peroxide. Cellulose acetate membrane allows diffusion of hydrogen peroxide but excludes interfering substances from reaching electrodes. Conversion of hydrogen peroxide to oxygen at the platinum anode results in generation of an electron current that is proportional to the concentration of lactate. Conversion of silver chloride to elemental silver at the reference cathode completes the circuit.

selected cases, with invasive hemodynamic measurements, this simple blood test provides a physiologically sound end point for titrating such therapies.

TREATMENT

The treatment of lactic acidosis is directed toward alleviating the underlying cause. Because the most common cause is circulatory shock, the primary aim of treatment in most cases is to restore adequate systemic perfusion and oxygenation. This is frequently accomplished by using supplemental oxygen, intravenous fluids, vasoactive drugs, blood transfusions, and other measures that improve oxygen delivery and mitigate tissue hypoxia. More specific therapy depends on the underlying cause. For example, antibiotic administration and abscess drainage may be indicated in septic shock.

In general, all forms of type A lactic acidosis may be approached in this way; however, there are exceptions. Consider a hemodynamically stable patient with an acute arterial embolism involving an extremity. This is a form of (regional) type A lactic acidosis, but the acidosis is not likely to respond to interventions that simply increase systemic oxygen delivery. The lactic acidosis attributable to generalized seizures requires no treatment per se, because the acidosis ceases when the seizures are halted, assuming that adequate cardiorespiratory function is present. In both cases, treatment of the primary problem alleviates the imbalance in oxygen supply and demand and the lactic acidosis. For cases of true type B lactic acidosis (i.e., cases in which the mechanism is not tissue hypoxia), treatment is limited to that directed against the underlying cause (e.g., thiamine replacement for patients with deficiency of the vitamin, chemotherapy for lactic acidosis associated with malignancy, and appropriate oral antibiotic therapy for patients with D-lactic acidosis).

Sodium bicarbonate has conventionally been used as an adjunct to treat lactic acidosis associated with significant acidemia that is not otherwise immediately reversible. The rationale for its use in this situation is based chiefly on the observation that acidemia itself impairs cardiac function and potentially worsens hypoperfusion.[15-20] This cardiac depression further decreases peripheral oxygen delivery and increases the severity of the lactic acidosis, setting up a descending spiral that culminates in circulatory arrest and death. Correcting the acidemia may break this cycle by improving cardiac function. Acidemia is also arrhythmogenic and diminishes the hemodynamic response to catecholamines.

Arguments against the use of bicarbonate include its potential for causing hyperosmolality and hypervolemia, unfavorably affecting the affinity of hemoglobin for oxygen, and increasing carbon dioxide production and causing mixed venous hypercapnia. In addition, both clinical and experimental reports have demonstrated that administration of sodium bicarbonate may actually stimulate increased lactate production, resulting in further elevation of blood lactate concentration.[47, 175-177] In animal models of lactic acidosis, sodium bicarbonate administration has been demonstrated to depress cardiac output compared with that in controls receiving saline.[175, 177] On the other hand, Cooper and associates infused sodium bicarbonate and sodium chloride into patients with lactic acidosis and were unable to show any difference in hemodynamic effects (Fig. 105–10), although bicarbonate administration did cause ionized hypocalcemia.[178] Their findings have been corroborated by other clinical investigations.[179] The role of bicarbonate in the treatment of lactic acidosis continues to be studied but currently remains controversial.[180-190]

The experimental compound sodium dichloroacetate (DCA) has been shown to lower blood lactate levels in both normal and diabetic animals.[191-195] Blood lactate concentrations are also significantly decreased by DCA in experimental models of lactic acidosis induced by hypoxemia,[196, 197] hypo-

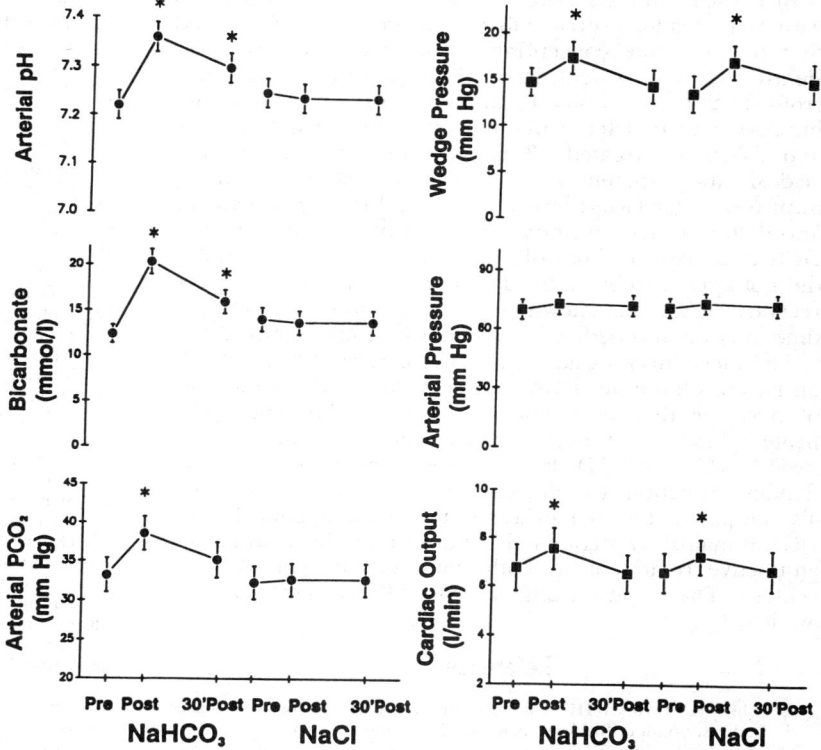

Figure 105–10. Acid-base (*left*) and hemodynamic (*right*) measurements before (Pre) and after (Post) sodium bicarbonate and sodium chloride infusions were administered to critically ill patients with severe lactic acidosis (arterial pH < 7.2). Changes in cardiac output and pulmonary wedge pressure are not attributable to pH correction by sodium bicarbonate because identical changes were observed after sodium chloride administration. All values are mean ± SE. Asterisk indicates *P* < .05 compared with Pre. (Reproduced, with permission, from Cooper DJ, Walley KR, Wiggs BR, et al, Bicarbonate does not improve hemodynamics in critically ill patients who have lactic acidosis. Ann Intern Med 1990; 112:492–498.)

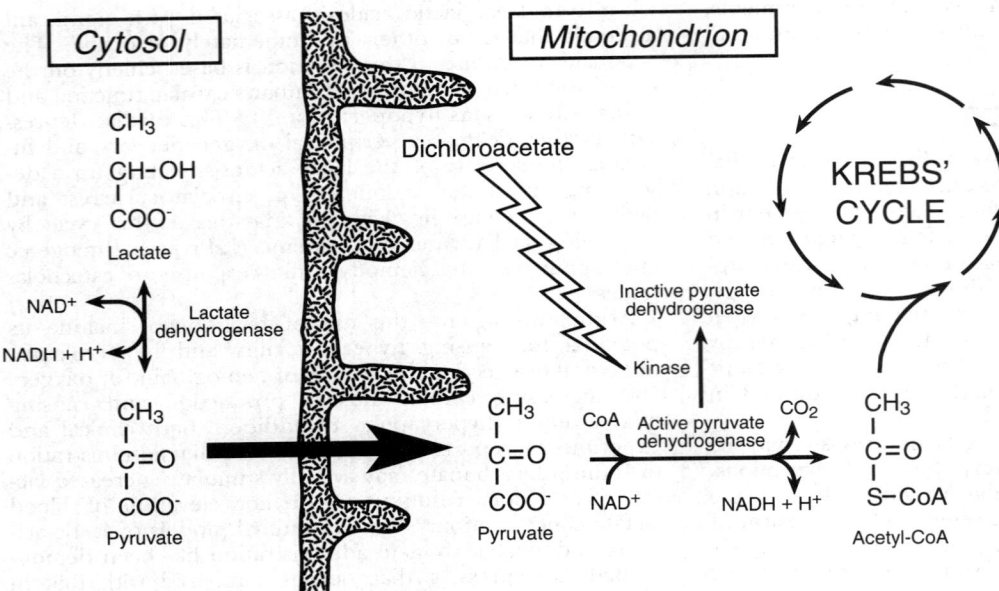

Figure 105–11. Proposed mechanism of action of DCA on lactate metabolism. DCA indirectly augments the activity of pyruvate dehydrogenase by inhibiting a protein kinase that converts pyruvate dehydrogenase to an inactive form. Acetyl-CoA = acetyl coenzyme A.

tension,[198] hepatectomy,[199] phenformin administration,[199] endotoxemia,[200] and sepsis.[201] In addition to favorable effects of DCA on blood lactate levels, several investigations have noted improvement in hemodynamic variables after DCA administration, both in isolated heart preparations and in intact animal models.[196, 199, 202] Blood lactate concentration decreases by 70 to 75% below baseline in healthy volunteers receiving DCA.[203, 204] Although DCA does not appear to decrease peak lactate levels in humans during exhaustive exercise, it does lower the blood lactate level throughout the recovery phase.[205] In patients with coronary artery disease undergoing cardiac catheterization, DCA infusions were shown to improve stroke volume and enhance myocardial efficiency.[206]

Blackshear and associates administered DCA to patients with lactic acidosis attributable to septic shock and found that blood lactate concentration improved, at least transiently.[207] In one patient, lactate levels decreased markedly, from 11.2 to 0.8 mmol/L, and this was associated with improvement in arterial pH and blood pressure. Stacpoole and colleagues treated 13 patients with refractory lactic acidosis and hypotension with DCA and noted significant improvement in lactate level and pH.[208] Most of their patients also demonstrated an improvement in blood pressure after DCA treatment. In both of these series, however, mortality did not appear to be affected by DCA administration. More recently, DCA was shown to favorably influence survival time in adult and pediatric patients with lactic acidosis.[209]

The mechanism of action of DCA is related to its effects on lactate utilization. DCA indirectly stimulates the activity of pyruvate dehydrogenase by inhibiting the action of a protein kinase that normally inactivates the enzyme[195, 201, 205, 210–212] (Fig. 105–11). Because the agent improves hemodynamic function, the decrease in blood lactate level may also be partly due to alleviation of systemic hypoperfusion. DCA remains investigational but appears to be a promising adjunctive treatment in both type A and type B lactic acidosis. The results of ongoing controlled clinical trials are awaited.[213]

References

1. Cohen RD, Woods HF: Clinical and Biochemical Aspects of Lactic Acidosis. London, Blackwell Scientific Publications, 1976.
2. Kruse JA, Carlson RW: Lactate metabolism. Crit Care Clin 5:725, 1987.
3. Buchalter SE, Crain MR, Kreisberg R: Regulation of lactate metabolism in vivo. Diabetes Metab Rev 5:379, 1989.
4. Camici P, Ferrannini E, Opie LH: Myocardial metabolism in ischemic heart disease: Basic principles and application to imaging by positron emission tomography. Prog Cardiovasc Dis 32:217, 1989.
5. Zilva JF: The origin of the acidosis in hyperlactatemia. Ann Clin Biochem 15:40, 1978.
6. Gevers W: Generation of protons by metabolic processes in heart cells. J Mol Cell Cardiol 9:867, 1977.
7. Wilkie DR: Generation of protons by metabolic processes other than glycolysis in muscle cells: A critical review. J Mol Cell Cardiol 11:325, 1979.
8. Gevers W: Generation of protons by metabolic processes other than glycolysis in muscle cells. J Mol Cell Cardiol 11:328, 1979.
9. Mizock BA: Controversies in lactic acidosis. Implications in critically ill patients. JAMA 258:497, 1987.
10. Mizock BA: Lactic acidosis. Dis Mon 35:233, 1989.
11. Johnston DG, Alberti KGMM: Acid-base balance in metabolic acidosis. Clin Endocrinol Metab 12:267, 1983.
12. Wilson RF, Gibson D, Percinel AK, et al: Severe alkalosis in critically ill surgical patients. Arch Surg 105:197, 1972.
13. Mazzara JT, Ayres SM, Grace WJ: Extreme hypocapnia in the critically ill patient. Am J Med 56:450, 1974.
14. Kruse JA, Mehta KC, Carlson RW: Definition of clinically significant lactic acidosis. Chest 100:100S, 1987.
15. McElroy WT Jr, Gerdes AJ, Brown EB Jr: Effects of CO_2, bicarbonate and pH on the performance of isolated perfused guinea pig hearts. Am J Physiol 195:412, 1958.
16. Opie LH, Kadas T, Geevers W: Effect of pH on the function and glucose metabolism of the heart. Lancet 2:551, 1963.
17. Mitchell JH, Wildenthal K, Johnson RL Jr: The effects of acid-base disturbances on cardiovascular and pulmonary function. Kidney Int 1:375, 1972.
18. Yudkin J, Cohen RD, Slack B: The haemodynamic effects of metabolic acidosis in the rat. Clin Sci Mol Med 50:177, 1976.
19. Williamson JR, Safer B, Rich T, et al: Effects of acidosis on myocardial contractility and metabolism. Acta Med Scand [Suppl] 587:95, 1976.
20. Mehta PM, Kloner RA: Effects of acid base disturbance, septic shock, and calcium and phosphorus abnormalities on cardiovascular function. Crit Care Clin 5:747, 1987.
21. Wasserman K, Van Kessel AL, Burton GG: Interaction of physiological mechanisms during exercise. Am J Physiol 22:71, 1976.
22. Stamford BA, Moffatt RJ, Weltman A, et al: Blood lactate disappearance after supramaximal one-legged exercise. J Appl Physiol 45:244, 1978.
23. Osnes J-B, Hermansen L: Acid-base balance after maximum exercise of short duration. J Appl Physiol 32:59, 1972.
24. Schardt FW, Wiegand MK: Continuous blood gas and lactate monitoring during exercise. Fed Proc 45:2930, 1986.
25. Orringer CE, Eustace JC, Wunsch CD, et al: Natural history of lactic acidosis after grand-mal seizures. N Engl J Med 297:796, 1977.
26. Kruse JA: Blood lactate and oxygen transport. Intensive Care World 4:121, 1987.
27. Appel D, Rubenstein R, Schrager K, et al: Lactic acidosis in severe asthma. Am J Med 75:580, 1983.
28. Ritz E, Heidland A: Lactic acidosis. Clin Nephrol 7:231, 1977.

29. Gladden LB: Net lactate uptake during progressive steady-level contractions in canine skeletal muscle. J Appl Physiol 71:514, 1991.
30. Relman AS: Lactic acidosis. In: Brenner BM, Stein JH (eds): Acid-Base and Potassium Homeostasis. London, Churchill Livingstone, p 65, 1978.
31. Yudin J, Cohen RD: The contribution of the kidney to the removal of lactic acid load under normal and acidotic conditions in the conscious rat. Clin Sci 48:121, 1975.
32. Alleyne GAO: Renal metabolic response to acid-base changes. II. The early effects of metabolic acidosis on renal metabolism in the rat. J Clin Invest 49:943, 1970.
33. Woods HF, Connor H, Tucker GT: The role of altered lactate kinetics in the pathogenesis of type B lactic acidosis. In: Porter R, Lawrenson G (eds): Metabolic Acidosis. London, Pitman Publishing, p 307, 1982.
34. Kruse JA, Zaidi SAJ, Carlson RW: Significance of blood lactate in critically ill patients with liver disease. Am J Med 83:77, 1987.
35. Alberti KGMM, Nattrass M: Lactic acidosis. Lancet 2:25, 1977.
36. Gimson A, Bihari D, Wilson C, et al: Delivery dependent oxygen consumption during acute liver failure. Clin Sci 66:12P, 1984.
37. Harrison PM, Wendon JA, Gimson AES, et al: Improvement by acetylcysteine of hemodynamics and oxygen transport in fulminant hepatic failure. N Engl J Med 324:1852, 1991.
38. Bihari D, Gimson AES, Lindridge J, et al: Lactic acidosis in fulminant hepatic failure. Some aspects of pathogenesis and prognosis. J Hepatol 1:405, 1985.
39. Woll PJ, Record CO: Lactate elimination in man: Effects of lactate concentration and hepatic dysfunction. Eur J Clin Invest 9:397, 1979.
40. Almenoff PL, Leavy J, Weil MH, et al: Prolongation of the half-life of lactate after maximal exercise in patients with hepatic dysfunction. Crit Care Med 17:870, 1989.
41. Robinson BH, Gall DG, Cutz E: Deficient activity of hepatic pyruvate dehydrogenase and pyruvate carboxylase in Reye's syndrome. Pediatr Res 11:279, 1977.
42. Tonsgard JH, Getz GS: Effect of Reye's syndrome serum on isolated chinchilla liver mitochondria. J Clin Invest 76:816, 1985.
43. Varanasi UR, Carr B, Simpson DP: Lactic acidosis associated with metastatic breast carcinoma. Cancer Treat Rep 64:1283, 1980.
44. Ellis RW: Breast cancer and lactic acidosis. An unusual metabolic complication. Minn Med 68:441, 1985.
45. Rice K, Schwartz SH: Lactic acidosis with small cell carcinoma. Rapid response to chemotherapy. Am J Med 79:501, 1985.
46. Field M, Block JB, Levin R, et al: Significance of blood lactate elevations among patients with acute leukemia and other neoplastic proliferative disorders. Am J Med 40:528, 1966.
47. Fraley DS, Adler S, Bruns FJ, et al: Stimulation of lactate production by administration of bicarbonate in a patient with a solid neoplasm and lactic acidosis. N Engl J Med 303:1100, 1980.
48. Spechler SJ, Esposito AL, Koff RS, et al: Lactic acidosis in oat cell carcinoma with extensive hepatic metastases. Arch Intern Med 138:1663, 1978.
49. Wesbey G: Lactic acidosis in oat cell carcinoma with extensive hepatic metastases. Arch Intern Med 141:816, 1981.
50. Raju RN, Kardinal CG: Lactic acidosis in lung cancer. South Med J 76:397, 1983.
51. Fields ALA, Wolman SL, Halperin ML: Chronic lactic acidosis in a patient with cancer: Therapy and metabolic consequences. Cancer 47:2026, 1981.
52. Johnson DA, Whelan TV: Lactic acidosis—a review of the association with neoplastic disorder. Milit Med 150:206, 1985.
53. Mintz U, Sweet DL Jr, Bitran JD, et al: Lactic acidosis and diffuse histiocytic lymphoma. Am J Hematol 4:359, 1978.
54. Lehninger AL: Biochemistry. New York, Worth Publishers, p 49, 1970.
55. Daughaday WH, Kipicky RJ, Rasinski DC: Lactic acidosis as a cause of nonketotic acidosis in diabetic patients. N Engl J Med 267:1010, 1962.
56. Fulop M: Lactic acidosis. NY State J Med 82:712, 1982.
57. Kreisberg RA: Lactic acidosis: An update. J Intensive Care Med 2:76, 1987.
58. Kreisberg RA: Lactic acidosis in the patient with diabetes mellitus. Prac Cardiol 6:110, 1980.
59. Anderson J, Mazza R: Pyruvate and lactate excretion in patients with diabetes mellitus and benign glycosuria. Lancet 2:270, 1963.
60. Jervell O: Investigation of the concentration of lactic acid in blood and urine under physiologic and pathologic conditions. Acta Med Scand 24:1, 1928.
61. Tranquada RE, Grant WJ, Peterson CR: Lactic acidosis. Arch Intern Med 117:192, 1966.
62. Huckabee WE: Abnormal resting blood lactate. I. The significance of hyperlactatemia in hospitalized patients. Am J Med 30:833, 1961.
63. Alberti KGMM, Dornhorst A, Rowe AS: Metabolic rhythms in normal and diabetic man. Isr J Med Sci 11:571, 1975.
64. Strandgaard S, Nielsen PE, Bitsch V, et al: Blood lactate and ketone bodies in diabetic ketoacidosis. Acta Med Scand 190:17, 1971.
65. Fulop M, Hoberman HD, Rascoff JH, et al: Lactic acidosis in diabetic patients. Arch Intern Med 136:987, 1976.
66. Frommer JP: Lactic acidosis. Med Clin North Am 67:815, 1983.
67. Harrington JT, Cohen JJ: Metabolic acidosis. In: Cohen JJ, Kassirer JP: Acid-Base. Boston, Little, Brown, p 121, 1982.
68. Oh MS, Phelps KR, Traube M, et al: D-Lactic acidosis in a man with the short-bowel syndrome. N Engl J Med 301:249, 1979.
69. Cross SA, Callaway CW: D-Lactic acidosis and selected cerebellar ataxias. Mayo Clin Proc 59:202, 1984.
70. Stolberg L, Rolfe R, Gitlin N, et al: D-Lactic acidosis due to abnormal gut flora. N Engl J Med 306:1344, 1982.
71. Stowe CM, Werdin RE, Barnes DM, et al: Acute lactacidosis in cattle associated with apiculture. J Am Vet Med Assoc 182:415, 1983.
72. Dahlquist NR, Perrault J, Callaway CW, et al: D-Lactic acidosis and encephalopathy after jejunoileostomy: Response to overfeeding and to fasting in humans. Mayo Clin Proc 59:141, 1984.
73. Traube M, Bock JL, Boyer JL: D-Lactic acidosis after jejunoileal bypass: Identification of organic anions by nuclear magnetic resonance spectroscopy. Ann Intern Med 98:171, 1983.
74. Campbell CH: The severe lactic acidosis of thiamine deficiency: Acute pernicious or fulminating beriberi. Lancet 2:446, 1984.
75. Shorey J, Bhardwaj N, Loscalzo J: Acute Wernicke's encephalopathy after intravenous infusion of high-dose nitroglycerin. Ann Intern Med 101:500, 1984.
76. Centers for Disease Control: Deaths associated with thiamine-deficient total parenteral nutrition. MMWR 38:43, 1989.
77. Takano N: Role of hypocapnia in the blood lactate accumulation during acute hypoxia. Respir Physiol 4:32, 1968.
78. Cain SM: Effect of PCO_2 on the relation of lactate and excess lactate to O_2 deficit. Am J Physiol 214:1322, 1968.
79. Davies SF, Iber C, Keene SA, et al: Effect of respiratory alkalosis during exercise on blood lactate. J Appl Physiol 61:948, 1986.
80. Relman AS: Metabolic consequences of acid-base disorders. Kidney Int 1:347, 1972.
81. Eichenholz A, Mulhausen RO, Anderson WE, et al: Primary hypocapnia: A cause of metabolic acidosis. J Appl Physiol 17:283, 1963.
82. Zborowska-Sluis DT, Dossetor JB: Hyperlactatemia of hyperventilation. J Appl Physiol 22:746, 1967.
83. Sykes MK, Cooke PM: The effect of hyperventilation on "excess lactate" production during anaesthesia. Br J Anaesth 37:372, 1965.
84. Eldridge F, Salzer J: Effect of respiratory alkalosis on blood lactate and pyruvate in humans. J Appl Physiol 22:461, 1967.
85. Parrillo JE, Parker MM, Natanson C, et al: Septic shock in humans. Advances in the understanding of pathogenesis, cardiovascular dysfunction, and therapy. Ann Intern Med 113:227, 1990.
86. Rackow EC, Astiz ME, Weil MH: Cellular oxygen metabolism during sepsis and shock. The relationship of oxygen consumption to oxygen delivery. JAMA 259:1989, 1988.
87. Astiz ME, Rackow EC, Kaufman B, et al: Relationship of oxygen delivery and mixed venous oxygenation to lactic acidosis in patients with sepsis and acute myocardial infarction. Crit Care Med 16:655, 1988.
88. Kaufman BS, Rackow EC, Falk JL: The relationship between oxygen delivery and consumption during fluid resuscitation of hypovolemic and septic shock. Chest 85:336, 1984.
89. Vincent J-L, Roman A, De Backer D, et al: Oxygen uptake/supply dependency. Am Rev Respir Dis 142:2, 1990.
90. Wolf YG, Cotev S, Perel A, et al: Dependence of oxygen consumption on cardiac output in sepsis. Crit Care Med 15:198, 1987.
91. Haupt MT, Gilbert EM, Carlson RW: Fluid loading increases oxygen consumption in septic patients with lactic acidosis. Am Rev Respir Dis 131:912, 1985.
92. Gilbert EM, Haupt MT, Mandanas RY, et al: The effect of fluid loading, blood transfusion, and catecholamine infusion on oxygen delivery and consumption in patients with sepsis. Am Rev Respir Dis 134:873, 1986.
93. Astiz ME, Rackow EC, Falk JL, et al: Oxygen delivery and consumption in patients with hyperdynamic septic shock. Crit Care Med 15:26, 1987.
94. Siegel JH, Cerra FB, Coleman B, et al: Physiological and metabolic correlations in human sepsis. Surgery 86:163, 1979.
95. Harken AH, Lillo RS, Hufnagel HV: The influence of endotoxin on cellular respiration. Surg Gynecol Obstet 140:858, 1975.
96. Misbin RI: Phenformin-associated lactic acidosis: Pathogenesis and treatment. Ann Intern Med 87:591, 1977.
97. Conlay LA, Loewenstein JE: Phenformin and lactic acidosis. JAMA 235:1575, 1976.
98. Wise PH, Chapman M, Thomas DW, et al: Phenformin and lactic acidosis. Br Med J 1:70, 1976.
99. Searle GL, Siperstein MD: Lactic acidosis associated with phenformin therapy. Diabetes 24:741, 1975.
100. Kreisberg RA, Wood BC: Drug and chemical-induced metabolic acidosis. Clin Endocrinol Metab 12:391, 1983.
101. Dietze G, Wicklmayr M, Mehnert H, et al: Effect of phenformin on hepatic balances of gluconeogenesis substrates in man. Diabetologia 14:243, 1978.
102. Arieff AI, Park R, Leach WJ, et al: Pathophysiology of experimental lactic acidosis in dogs. Am J Physiol 239:F135, 1980.
103. Schafer G: Some new aspects of the interaction of hypoglycemia-producing biguanides with biological membranes. Biochem Pharmacol 25:2015, 1976.
104. Craig GM, Crane CW: Lactic acidosis complicating liver failure after intravenous fructose. Br Med J 4:211, 1971.

105. McGilvery RW: Biochemistry. A Functional Approach. Philadelphia, WB Saunders, 1970.

106. Georgieff M, Moldawer LL, Bistrian BR, et al: Xylitol, an energy source for intravenous nutrition after trauma. JPEN 9:199, 1985.

107. Cohen RD, Woods HF: Lactic acidosis revisited. Diabetes 32:181, 1983.

108. Batstone GF, Alberti KGMM, Dewar AK: Reversible lactic acidosis associated with repeated intravenous infusions of sorbitol and ethanol. Postgrad Med J 53:567, 1977.

109. Beamer WC, Shealy RM, Prough DS: Acute cyanide poisoning from laetrile ingestion. Ann Emerg Med 12:449, 1983.

110. Aitken D, West D, Smith F, et al: Cyanide toxicity following nitroprusside induced hypotension. Can Anaesth Soc J 24:651, 1977.

111. Humphrey SH, Nash DA: Lactic acidosis complicating sodium nitroprusside therapy. Ann Intern Med 88:58, 1978.

112. Mellino M, Phillips D: Severe lactic acidosis in a case of nitroprusside resistance. Cleve Clin Q 47:119, 1980.

113. Nightingale SL: New labeling for sodium nitroprusside emphasizes risk of cyanide toxicity. JAMA 265:847, 1991.

114. Hall AH, Rumack BH: Clinical toxicology of cyanide. Ann Emerg Med 15:1067, 1986.

115. Buehler JH, Berns AS, Webster JR, et al: Lactic acidosis from carboxyhemoglobinemia after smoke inhalation. Ann Intern Med 82:803, 1975.

116. Greene NM: Effect of epinephrine on lactate, pyruvate, and excess lactate production in normal human subjects. J Lab Clin Med 58:682, 1961.

117. Kolendorf K, Moller BB: Lactic acidosis in epinephrine poisoning. Acta Med Scand 196:465, 1974.

118. Richards SR, Chang FE, Stempel LE: Hyperlactatemia associated with acute ritodrine infusion. Am J Obstet Gynecol 146:1, 1983.

119. Braden G, Von Oeyen P, Smith M, et al: Mechanisms of ritodrine and terbutaline-induced hypokalemia and pulmonary edema. Kidney Int 27:304, 1985.

120. Braden GL, Johnston SS, Germain MJ, et al: Lactic acidosis associated with the therapy of acute bronchospasm. N Engl J Med 313:890, 1985.

121. Keller U, Mall Th, Walter M, et al: Phaeochromocytoma with lactic acidosis. Br Med J 2:606, 1978.

122. Bornemann M, Hill SC, Kidd GS II: Lactic acidosis in pheochromocytoma. Ann Intern Med 105:880, 1986.

123. Madias NE, Goorno WE, Herson S: Severe lactic acidosis as a presenting feature of pheochromocytoma. Am J Kidney Dis 10:250, 1987.

124. Bernard S: Severe lactic acidosis following theophylline overdose. Ann Emerg Med 20:1135, 1991.

125. Leventhal LJ, Kochar G, Feldman NH, et al: Lactic acidosis in theophylline overdose. Am J Emerg Med 7:417, 1989.

126. Kearney TE, Manoguerra AS, Curtis GP, et al: Theophylline toxicity and the beta-adrenergic system. Ann Intern Med 102:766, 1985.

127. Higbee MD, Kumar M, Galant SP: Stimulation of endogenous catecholamine release by theophylline. A proposed additional mechanism of action for theophylline effects. J Allergy Clin Immunol 70:377, 1982.

128. Vestal RE, Eriksson CE Jr, Musser B, et al: Effect of intravenous aminophylline on plasma levels of catecholamines and related cardiovascular and metabolic responses in man. Circulation 67:162, 1983.

129. Madias NE: Lactic acidosis. Kidney Int 29:752, 1986.

130. Temple AR: Acute and chronic effects of aspirin toxicity and their treatment. Arch Intern Med 141:364, 1981.

131. Bartels PD, Lund-Jacobsen H: Blood lactate and ketone body concentrations in salicylate intoxication. Hum Toxicol 5:363, 1986.

132. Gray TA, Buckley BM, Vale JA: Hyperlactatemia and metabolic acidosis following paracetamol overdose. Q J Med 65:811, 1987.

133. Zabrodski RM, Schnurr LP: Anion gap acidosis with hypoglycemia in acetaminophen toxicity. Ann Emerg Med 13:956, 1984.

134. Caldwell J, Woods HF: Metabolic consequences of the short term exposure of the liver to paracetamol. Clin Sci Mol Med 55:10P, 1978.

135. Kreisberg RA, Owen WC, Siegal AM: Ethanol-induced hyperlactacidemia: Inhibition of lactate utilization. J Clin Invest 50:166, 1971.

136. Fulop M, Bock J, Ben-Ezra J, et al: Plasma lactate and 3-hydroxybutyrate levels in patients with acute ethanol intoxication. Am J Med 80:191, 1986.

137. Halperin ML, Hammeke M, Josse RG, et al: Metabolic acidosis in the alcoholic: A pathophysiologic approach. Metabolism 32:308, 1983.

138. Demey H, Daelemans R, De Broe ME, et al: Propylene glycol intoxication due to intravenous nitroglycerin. Lancet 1:1360, 1984.

139. Keiner MJ, Bailey DN: Propylene glycol as a cause of lactic acidosis. J Anal Toxicol 9:40, 1985.

140. Cate JC, Hedrick R: Propylene glycol intoxication and lactic acidosis. N Engl J Med 303:1237, 1980.

141. Arulanantham K, Genel M: Central nervous system toxicity associated with ingestion of propylene glycol. J Pediatr 93:515, 1978.

142. Rudney H: Propanediol phosphate as a possible intermediate in the metabolism of acetone. J Biol Chem 210:361, 1954.

143. Huff E: The metabolism of 1,2-propanediol. Biochim Biophys Acta 48:506, 1961.

144. Miller ON, Bazzano G: Propanediol metabolism and its relation to lactic acid metabolism. Ann NY Acad Sci 119:957, 1965.

145. Linter SPK: Severe lactic acidosis following paraldehyde administration. Br J Psychiatry 149:650, 1986.

146. Robotham JL, Lietman PS: Acute iron poisoning. Am J Dis Child 134:875, 1980.

147. Henretig RM, Karl SR, Weintraub WH: Severe iron poisoning treated with enteral and intravenous deferoxamine. Ann Emerg Med 12:306, 1983.

148. Boyd RE, Brennan PT, Deng J-F, et al: Strychnine poisoning. Recovery from profound lactic acidosis, hyperthermia, and rhabdomyolysis. Am J Med 74:507, 1983.

149. Cooper GJS, Kletchko S, Tebbutt K, et al: Amoxapine overdosage and primary lactic acidosis. NZ Med J 98:608, 1985.

150. Kopelman PG, Kalfayan PY: Severe metabolic acidosis after ingestion of butanone. Br Med J 286:21, 1983.

151. Gustafson PR: Profound lactic acidosis in a young woman treated with nalidixic acid. Tex Med 81:53, 1985.

152. Leslie PJA, Cregeen RJ, Proudfoot AT: Lactic acidosis, hyperglycaemia and convulsions following nalidixic acid overdosage. Hum Toxicol 3:239, 1984.

153. Neff TA: Isoniazid toxicity: Reports of lactic acidosis and keratitis. Chest 59:245, 1971.

154. Coyer JR, Nicholson DP: Isoniazid-induced convulsions: Part 1. Clinical. South Med J 69:294, 1976.

155. Chin L, Sievers ML, Herrier RN, et al: convulsions as the etiology of lactic acidosis in acute isoniazid toxicity in dogs. Toxicol Appl Pharmacol 49:377, 1979.

156. Burmeister LA, Valdivia T, Nuttall FQ: Adult hereditary fructose intolerance. Arch Intern Med 151:773, 1991.

157. Pagliara AS, Karl IE, Keating JP, et al: Hepatic fructose-1,6-diphosphatase deficiency. A cause of lactic acidosis and hypoglycemia in infancy. J Clin Invest 51:2115, 1972.

158. Driscoll PF, Larsen PD, Gruber AB: MELAS syndrome involving a mother and two children. Arch Neurol 44:971, 1987.

159. Pavlakis SG, Phillips PC, DiMauro S, et al: Mitochondrial myopathy, encephalopathy, lactic acidosis, and strokelike episodes: A distinctive clinical syndrome. Ann Neurol 16:481, 1984.

160. Barela TD, Johnson JD, Hayek A: Metabolic acidosis in the newborn period. Clin Endocrinol Metabol 12:429, 1983.

161. Weil MH, Afifi AA: Experimental and clinical studies on lactate and pyruvate as indicators of the severity of acute circulatory failure (shock). Circulation 41:989, 1970.

162. Broder G, Weil MH: Excess lactate: An index of reversibility of shock in human patients. Science 143:1457, 1964.

163. Cady LD Jr, Weil MH, Afifi AA, et al: Quantitation of severity of critical illness with special reference to blood lactate. Crit Care Med 1:75, 1973.

164. Henning RJ, Weil MH, Weiner F: Blood lactate as a prognostic indicator of survival in patients with acute myocardial infarction. Circ Shock 9:307, 1982.

165. Peretz DI, McGregor M, Dossetor JB: Lacticacidosis: A clinically significant aspect of shock. Can Med Assoc J 90: 673, 1964.

166. Vitek V, Cowley RA: Blood lactate in the prognosis of various forms of shock. Ann Surg 173:308, 1971.

167. Mehta K, Kruse JA, Carlson RW: The relationship between anion gap and elevated lactate. Crit Care Med 14:405, 1986.

168. Iberti TJ, Leibowitz AB, Papadakos PJ, et al: Low sensitivity of the anion gap as a screen to detect hyperlactatemia in critically ill patients. Crit Care Med 18:275, 1990.

169. Harrower JR, Brown CH: Blood lactic acid—A micromethod adapted to field collection of microliter samples. J Appl Physiol 32:709, 1972.

170. Kruse JA, Carlson RW: Lactate measurement: Plasma or blood? Intensive Care Med 16:1, 1990.

171. Westgard JO, Lahmeyer BL, Birnbaum ML: Use of the Du Pont "Automated Clinical Analyzer" in direct determination of lactic acid in plasma stabilized with sodium fluoride. Clin Chem 18:1334, 1972.

172. Boycks E, Michaels S, Weil MH, et al: Continuous-flow measurement of lactate in blood: A technique adapted for use in the emergency laboratory. Clin Chem 21:113, 1975.

173. Piquard F, Schaefer A, Dellenbach P, et al: Rapid bedside estimation of plasma and whole blood lactic acid. Intensive Care Med 7:35, 1980.

174. Weil MH, Leavy JA, Rackow EC, et al: Validation of a semi-automated technique for measuring lactate in whole blood. Clin Chem 32:2175, 1986.

175. Arieff AI, Leach W, Park R, et al: Systemic effects of NaHCO$_3$ in experimental lactic acidosis in dogs. Am J Physiol 242:F586, 1982.

176. Graf H, Leach W, Arieff AI: Metabolic effects of sodium bicarbonate in hypoxic lactic acidosis in dogs. Am J Physiol 249:F630, 1985.

177. Graf H, Leach W, Arieff AI: Evidence of a detrimental effect of bicarbonate therapy in hypoxic lactic acidosis. Science 227:754, 1985.

178. Cooper DJ, Walley KR, Wiggs BR, et al: Bicarbonate does not improve hemodynamics in critically ill patients who have lactic acidosis. Ann Intern Med 112:492, 1990.

179. Mathieu D, Neviere R, Billard V, et al: Effects of bicarbonate therapy on hemodynamics and tissue oxygenation in patients with lactic acidosis: A prospective, controlled clinical study. Crit Care Med 19:1352, 1991.

180. Narins RG, Cohen JJ: Bicarbonate therapy for oganic acidosis. The case for its continued use. Ann Intern Med 106:615, 1987.

181. Stackpoole PW: Lactic acidosis: The case against bicarbonate therapy. Ann Intern Med 105:276, 1986.

182. Cooper DJ, Worthley LIG: Buffer therapies for patients who have lactic acidosis? Intensive Crit Care Dig 9:30, 1990.
183. Graf H, Arieff AI: The use of sodium bicarbonate in the therapy of organic acidosis. Intensive Care Med 12:285, 1986.
184. Ryder REJ: Lactic acidosis: High-dose or low-dose bicarbonate therapy? Diabetes Care 7:99, 1984.
185. Cohen RD, Iles RA: Bicarbonate therapy and lactic acidosis. Diabetes Care 7:509, 1984.
186. Ryder REJ: Bicarbonate therapy and lactic acidosis: A reply. Diabetes Care 7:510, 1984.
187. Weil MH, Trevino RP, Rackow EC: Sodium bicarbonate during CPR. Does it help or hinder? Chest 88:487, 1985.
188. Rumbak MJ: Lactic acidosis. Ann Intern Med 113:254, 1990.
189. Donnelly SM: Lactic acidosis. Ann Intern Med 113:255, 1990.
190. Warren J: Lactic acidosis. Ann Intern Med 113:255, 1990.
191. Weingand KW, Fettman MJ, Phillips RW, et al: Effects of sodium dichloroacetate in awake, healthy, Yucatan miniature swine. Am J Vet Res 47:441, 1986.
192. Ribes G, Valette G, Loubatieres-Mariani M-M: Metabolic effects of sodium dichloroacetate in normal and diabetic dogs. Diabetes 28:852, 1979.
193. Hulter HN, Glynn RD, Sebastian A, et al: Renal and systemic acid-base effects of chronic dichloroacetate administration in dogs. Metabolism 29:997, 1980.
194. Ward RA, Wathen RL, Harding GB, et al: Comparative metabolic effects of acetate and dichloroacetate infusion in the anesthetized dog. Metabolism 34:680, 1985.
195. Evans OB, Stacpoole PW: Prolonged hypolactatemia and increased total pyruvate dehydrogenase activity by dichloroacetate. Biochem Pharmacol 31:1295, 1982.
196. Romeh SA, Tannen RL: Therapeutic benefit of dichloroacetate in experimentally induced hypoxic lactic acidosis. J Lab Clin Med 107:378, 1986.
197. Graf H, Leach W, Arieff AI: Effects of dichloroacetate in the treatment of hypoxic lactic acidosis in dogs. J Clin Invest 76:919, 1985.
198. Dimlich RVW, Biros MH, Widman DW, et al: Comparison of sodium bicarbonate with dichloroacetate treatment of hyperlactatemia and lactic acidosis in the ischemic rat. Resuscitation 16:13, 1988.
199. Park R, Arieff AI: Treatment of lactic acidosis with dichloroacetate in dogs. J Clin Invest 70:853, 1982.
200. Preiser J-C, Moulart D, Vincent J-L: Dichloroacetate administration in the treatment of endotoxin shock. Circ Shock 30:221, 1990.
201. Vary TC, Siegel JH, Tall BD, et al: Metabolic effects of partial reversal of pyruvate dehydrogenase activity by dichloroacetate in sepsis. Circ Shock 24:3, 1988.
202. Burns AH, Giaimo ME, Summer WR: Dichloroacetic acid improves in vitro myocardial function following in vivo endotoxin administration. J Crit Care 1:11, 1986.
203. Wells PG, Moore GW, Rabin D, et al: Metabolic effects and pharmacokinetics of intravenously administered dichloroacetate in humans. Diabetologia 19:109, 1980.
204. Curry SH, Chu P-I, Baumgartner TG, et al: Plasma concentrations and metabolic effects of intravenous sodium dichloroacetate. Clin Pharmacol Ther 37:89, 1985.
205. Carraro F, Klein S, Rosenblatt JI, et al: Effect of dichloroacetate on lactate concentration in exercising humans. J Appl Physiol 66:591, 1989.
206. Wargovich TJ, MacDonald RG, Hill JA, et al: Myocardial metabolic and hemodynamic effects of dichloroacetate in coronary artery disease. Am J Cardiol 61:65, 1988.
207. Blackshear PJ, Fang LS-T, Axelrod L: Treatment of severe lactic acidosis with dichloroacetate. Diabetes Care 5:391, 1982.
208. Stacpoole PW, Harman EM, Curry SH, et al: Treatment of lactic acidosis with dichloroacetate. N Engl J Med 309:390, 1983.
209. Stacpoole PW, Lorenz AC, Thomas RG, et al: Dichloroacetate in the treatment of lactic acidosis. Ann Intern Med 108:58, 1988.
210. Evans OB: Dichloroacetate tissue concentrations and its relationship to hypolactatemia and pyruvate dehydrogenase activation. Biochem Pharmacol 31:3124, 1982.
211. Whitehouse S, Cooper RH, Randle PJ: Mechanism of activation of pyruvate dehydrogenase by dichloroacetate and other halogenated carboxylic acids. Biochem J 141:761, 1974.
212. Crabb DW, Yount EA, Harris RA: The metabolic effects of dichloroacetate. Metabolism 30:1024, 1981.
213. The DCA–Lactic Acidosis Collaborative Study Group: The design of a randomized, multicenter study of sodium dichloroacetate (DCA) as a treatment for lactic acidosis. Controlled Clin Trials 8:291, 1987.

CHAPTER 106

Diabetic Ketoacidosis and Hypoglycemia

Robert A. Kreisberg
Alan M. Siegal

DIABETIC KETOACIDOSIS
Epidemiology

Diabetic ketoacidosis (DKA) continues to be an important and often life-threatening complication of diabetes.[1-4] Approximately 80% of episodes of DKA occur in individuals who already have diabetes mellitus,[1] highlighting the failure of our educational programs and preventive measures. Only 20% of DKA episodes occur in newly diagnosed diabetics, and approximately 90% of those with pre-existing diabetes were receiving insulin. Some patients are repeatedly hospitalized with DKA and are at high risk for complications and death.[5,6] Deaths resulting from DKA and its complications account for about 30 to 50% of the mortality in young patients with type I diabetes mellitus, indicating the seriousness of this complication.[2] Furthermore, the misconception that DKA occurs primarily in patients with type I diabetes mellitus is refuted by the observations that the mean age of patients with DKA is approximately 43 years and that 20% may be obese.[1] Women outnumber men by 1.5:1, and the incidence of DKA per 10,000 diabetics is about twice as high in women as in men. The age distribution of DKA and the rate per 10,000 diabetics emphasize the importance of DKA in individuals older than 45 years of age (45% of total). Previous epidemiologic data suggest that approximately 75% of DKA episodes occur in older diabetics, based on the hospitalization rates for diabetes and the distribution of hospitalization by the old classification system (juvenile and maturity onset).[7] Patients with maturity-onset diabetes constituted 97% of all admissions and 3% of such admissions were for DKA; patients with juvenile-onset diabetes were responsible for 3% of all admissions but 30% were due to DKA; the ratio was 3:1 or 75% in favor of the maturity-onset group.

Although much of our experience with DKA, particularly in recidivistic patients, comes from county institutions or institutions for the indigent,[5,6] which biases our impressions, DKA occurs as frequently in patients from the middle and upper socioeconomic strata as from the low socioeconomic and poverty levels.

DKA occurs with a frequency of about 3 to 8 cases per 1000 diabetes patients per year.[1,4] If diabetes occurs in approximately 6% of the U.S. population, the predicted number of episodes of DKA annually ranges from 45,000 to 120,000.

Precipitating Factors

In approximately 50 to 60% of DKA episodes, an underlying medical illness is the precipitating factor.[4] Discontinuation of insulin is far less frequently a factor than most would believe, accounting for no more than 15 to 25% of all episodes of DKA. In 25 to 30% of episodes, no obvious precipitating factor can be identified. In children and young adults, emotional factors are thought to be important.[8] Although controlled studies have not proved that mental stress can cause deterioration in diabetic control, these experiments do not come close to simulating the emotional stress experienced by teen-agers in violent and heated confrontations with their parents or the stress experienced by a teen-age girl with diabetes who is sexually abused by her father or other male member of her family. Furthermore, emotional stress is a highly individual matter, and what may be viewed by one person as unimportant is an exquisitely sensitive issue to another. In 25 episodes of DKA developing abruptly in 24 children, emotional factors were thought to be important in about 50%.[4] Many such episodes of DKA begin within 4 to 8 hours after the previous injection of insulin. The increased frequency of DKA in teen-age girls and young women at or before menses also suggests that emotional stress is important. In older patients, DKA may be a result of an underlying but silent or painless myocardial infarction.[4]

Hormonal Basis of Diabetic Ketoacidosis

An absolute or relative deficiency of insulin is the underlying basis for the development of DKA.[9, 10] However, the presence of normal or increased concentrations of the insulin counter-regulatory hormones (ICRHs) is an absolute prerequisite for full expression of gluconeogenesis and ketogenesis.[11] In most settings in which DKA occurs, patients have recently taken their insulin[4] and/or plasma insulin concentrations are in the range 5 to 10 μU/mL, indicating a relative deficiency of insulin.[9, 10] Although insulin levels in this range are normal when the plasma glucose level is normal, they are clearly deficient when there is hyperglycemia. In DKA the concentrations of the ICRHs are increased two- to fivefold above normal basal levels because of insulin deficiency and/or stress- or illness-induced increases in release and/or secretion. Thus, a dose of insulin that may be adequate under ordinary circumstances becomes inadequate when the concentrations of the ICRHs are increased (Fig. 106–1). This concept of the pathogenesis of DKA is supported by studies of patients with type I diabetes mellitus who are under excellent control with continuous intravenous insulin and are challenged with endotoxin while the insulin infusion is continued.[12] Within 2 to 4 hours the concentrations of the ICRHs are increased and plasma levels of glucose and ketones increase. Thus, optimal control of the glucose concentration does not prevent the development of hyperglycemia and ketonemia if stress of the proper magnitude occurs. Administration of the ICRHs alone and in combination to well-controlled diabetics, at rates that produce concentrations similar to those observed during DKA, invariably cause an increase in the glucose concentration.[11, 13] Glucagon is particularly important in the development of DKA.[14] The interaction of the ICRHs and their combined effects on metabolic processes are so potent that it is possible to produce stress hyperglycemia in otherwise normal animals with a "cocktail" of ICRH.[11, 13] When the ICRHs are infused simultaneously, the glycemic response is synergistic rather than simply additive. In fact, most studies of this phenomenon reveal hyper-responsiveness of hormone release, as well as a metabolic hyper-responsiveness in poorly controlled diabetics (Table 106–1). Because most patients who manifest DKA are not optimally controlled, they are more vulnerable to developing DKA. In a sense, patients with poorly controlled diabetes are poised for rapid decompensation and development of DKA. This is probably the explanation of why exercise can precipitate DKA in patients with poor diabetic control.[15]

Biochemistry of Diabetic Ketoacidosis[16–18]

Hyperglycemia and hyperketonemia in DKA are both due to overproduction and underutilization of glucose and ketoacids. The hormonal factors that precipitate these changes were reviewed in the previous section. The relative or absolute deficiency of insulin in peripheral tissues leads to decreased glucose utilization, increased mobilization of adipose tissue free fatty acids (FFAs), and decreased protein synthesis. Increased peripheral release of three-carbon glucose precursors, glycerol, alanine, and other gluconeogenic amino acids provides the substrate for increased glyconeogenesis. Increased FFA flux to the liver provides the substrate for the increase in hepatic ketoacid production.

It was originally thought that the increased supply of FFAs resulting from insulin deficiency was solely responsible for the increase in ketoacid production. Although necessary, increased FFA flux alone is not sufficient to explain the augmentation that occurs in ketoacid production. We now know that changes also occur in critical metabolic pathways in the liver that increase ketogenesis even in the presence of a fixed supply of FFAs. These changes are due to both insulin deficiency and increased release of glucagon. More of the FFAs provided to the liver are channeled into the ketogenic pathway and away from the pathway leading to esterification and triglyceride synthesis. Glucagon is responsible for activating fatty acid oxidation and diverting FFAs from esterification. Glucagon activates the rate-limiting step in mitochondrial fatty acid oxidation by increasing the activity of a mitochondria-bound enzyme, carnitine palmitoyl-transferase I, located on the outer mitochondrial membrane. Many consider that glucagon "turns on" this process and

TABLE 106–1
HORMONAL AND BIOCHEMICAL FEATURES OF DIABETIC KETOACIDOSIS
Insulin concentrations are within normal limits (5 to 15 μU/mL) but inappropriately low.
ICRH concentrations are increased.
ICRH release is provoked by illness or physical and emotional stress.
ICRH release is accentuated in poorly controlled diabetes.
The biologic response to ICRH is exaggerated.
The interaction of ICRH is synergistic.
Insulin and ICRH balance are primary determinants of ketoacidosis.

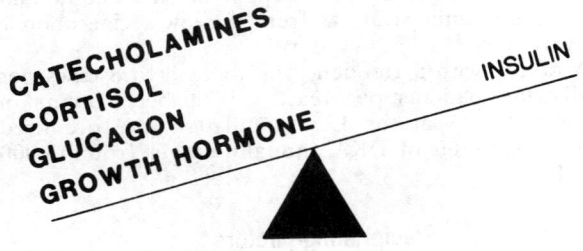

Figure 106–1. Relationship between insulin counter-regulatory hormones and insulin in the pathogenesis of diabetic ketoacidosis. (From Kreisberg RA: Diabetic ketoacidosis: An update. Crit Care Clin 3:817, 1987.)

that it is the primary signal for the increase in hepatic ketogenesis but that it can be expressed only when insulin secretion is impaired.

It is now established that the activity of carnitine palmitoyltransferase I is regulated by malonyl coenzyme A (CoA) levels. Malonyl CoA is the first committed intermediate in the pathway leading to long chain fatty acid synthesis. When the level of fat synthesis is high (insulin-replete, fed state), malonyl CoA levels are also high and inhibit carnitine palmitoyltransferase I, thereby ensuring that newly synthesized fatty acids cannot be oxidized but must enter the esterification pathway. In the starved state with low insulin and high glucagon levels, malonyl CoA concentrations are low, allowing full expression of carnitine palmitoyltransferase I activity and maximal rates of fatty acid entry into mitochondrial oxidative pathways. Glucagon causes such a change in malonyl CoA levels by inhibiting glycolysis (at the step catalyzed by phosphofructokinase) during fasting or uncontrolled diabetes, thereby reducing flux from glucose through pyruvate, citrate, and acetyl CoA to malonyl CoA. Glucagon reduces the concentration of the critical metabolite fructose-2,6-bisphosphate, which is necessary for full expression of phosphofructokinase activity; when the concentration of this intermediate is reduced, phosphofructokinase is deactivated. The ketoacids are synthesized in the liver and are transported to peripheral tissues. However, with a relative or absolute deficiency of insulin the peripheral utilization of ketoacids is inhibited, accentuating the hyperketonemia of DKA. Furthermore, the mitochondrial redox state of the liver is further reduced because of high rates of fatty acid oxidation, and β-hydroxybutyrate levels are increased relative to those of acetoacetate. This is important because during therapy with insulin, peripheral utilization of ketones is restored. Because ketone utilization requires that β-hydroxybutyrate be converted to acetoacetate before oxidation, the acetoacetate levels increase and the nitroprusside color reaction (Acetest reagent) becomes more positive. This suggests worsening of the ketoacidosis at a time when total ketone levels have decreased and the ketoacidosis is improving.

The hyperglycemia of DKA is due in large part to the overproduction of glucose, via gluconeogenesis, by the liver. Insulin deficiency in peripheral tissues increases proteolysis as well as lipolysis, thereby providing increased substrate for the gluconeogenic pathway, which is also activated by glucagon working at the level of the liver. The increased oxidation and conversion of FFAs to ketones provides the hydrogen ions necessary for the increased gluconeogenic activity. However, increased availability of three-carbon substrate, although necessary, is not sufficient to increase gluconeogenesis in the absence of synthesis and full expression of the critical enzymes of the gluconeogenic pathway, particularly pyruvate kinase, the enzyme controlling the rate-limiting step of this process. Hyperglycemia is compounded by reduced peripheral glucose utilization resulting from insufficient insulin. Glucosuria prevents maximal expression of hyperglycemia in DKA. However, when glomerular filtration is compromised because of hypovolemia the plasma glucose rises rapidly to extremely high levels.

Pathogenesis of the Clinical Features of Diabetic Ketoacidosis[19, 20]

Although the metabolism of carbohydrate, fat, and protein is abnormal in patients with DKA symptoms, signs and laboratory abnormalities are due to the alterations that have occurred in carbohydrate and fat homeostasis.

The hyperglycemia leads to a redistribution of water into the extracellular fluid compartment at the expense of the intracellular fluid compartment, and an initial increase in the glomerular filtration rate leads to glucosuria and polyuria. This redistribution of water explains the hyponatremia that exists in most patients with DKA even when their total body water is below normal. It is only when water loss becomes extreme (as in severe DKA or hypernatremia and hyperglycemia) that the serum sodium concentration becomes normal or even elevated. When the hyperglycemia is corrected by therapy, the serum sodium concentration returns toward normal in a manner predictable from the relationship between hyperglycemia and hyponatremia (the serum sodium level should be reduced by approximately 1.6 mmol/L for each increment in glucose of 100 mg/dL).[21] Controlling hyperglycemia in normonatremic patients with DKA predictably leads to hypernatremia; in hypernatremic, hyperglycemic patients the hypernatremia becomes more severe. If the serum sodium is reduced to a level that is lower than can be accounted for by the magnitude of the hyperglycemia, suspect coexistent hypertriglyceridemia[22] or pre-existing syndrome of inappropriate antidiuretic hormone.

The ability of the kidney to filter glucose leads to glucosuria and polyuria. This is an important safety valve that prevents excessive hyperglycemia. Under most circumstances in patients with DKA, the plasma glucose concentration is less than 800 mg/dL (average $\cong$ 500 to 550 mg/dL).[19] In the presence of extensive renal disease or marked hypovolemia, the glomerular filtration rate is further reduced, glucose excretion in the urine is limited, and the plasma glucose increases to extremely high levels (similar to those seen in some hypernatremic, hyperglycemic patients).[20]

Overproduction of ketoacids leads to loss of bicarbonate and other body buffers and the development of an "anion gap" metabolic acidosis.[23] The loss of bicarbonate and ensuing acidemia are compounded by the defect that exists in peripheral utilization of ketones, which limits the potential for regenerating bicarbonate. The net effect is severe metabolic acidosis. Respiratory compensation occurs to limit acidemia, but if the process is extreme the acidemia may be severe. The appropriateness of the respiratory response can be judged from the formula: $Pco_2 = 1.5[HCO_3^-] + 8 \pm 2$.[24] This assessment is important when complex or mixed acid-base disorders are expected. Although the metabolic acidosis is typically of the anion gap type, a continuum of abnormalities has been observed:[25] patients may have primarily a hyperchloremic metabolic acidosis, a mixed anion gap–hyperchloremic acidosis, or an anion gap acidosis. The volume status of the patient determines the pattern of the acidosis. When volume is well maintained, the ketones are filtered and excreted in the urine and chloride is reabsorbed with sodium, leading to the hyperchloremic pattern. When volume contraction is well established, ketones are poorly filtered and maximally reabsorbed by the renal tubule, leading to the classic anion gap pattern. Although it often appears that there is a perfect balance between the bicarbonate lost and ketones retained, no such stoichiometric relationship exists and the apparently perfect reciprocal relationship is an artifact.

In reality, much more buffering capacity has been lost than is apparent from the reduction in the bicarbonate concentration.[25] This is due to the continued excretion of ketoacid anions in the urine, and it explains why hyperchloremia develops during treatment. Fluid resuscitation in patients with DKA increases the loss of substrate ketone that is used to regenerate bicarbonate; as ketones are cleared into the urine, the correction of the deficit in bicarbonate is slowed. Under these circumstances the kidney increases its reabsorption of chloride to balance sodium reabsorption and maintain electrical balance. The net effect is the development of or accentuation of hyperchloremia during the recovery phase of DKA. The kidney adjusts fluid composition over several days, and the chloride level is corrected as bicarbonate synthesis restores the blood bicarbonate level to normal.

A number of important electrolyte abnormalities also occur in patients with well-established DKA.[26] All patients have significant deficiencies of sodium, chloride, potassium, phosphate, and magnesium. With the exception of the low concentrations of sodium and chloride, the concentrations of the other electrolytes are normal or elevated (Table 106–2). During the course of therapy the concentrations decrease dramatically and if appropriate attention is not paid, life-threatening hypokalemia and hypophosphatemia may occur. Potassium, magnesium, and phosphate are the major intracellular cations and anions, and it should not be surprising that their losses are often parallel and balanced. The loss of potassium and phosphate from the intracellular compartment is usually attributed to the metabolic acidosis. However, insulin deficiency may be the most important determinant of intracellular potassium loss.[27, 28] When hyperglycemia occurs after a glucose challenge, the serum potassium level decreases because insulin is released. When hyperglycemia is induced in the presence of insulin deficiency, the serum potassium level increases. This phenomenon is seen commonly in diabetics who also have renal disease and hypoaldosteronism. The shift of potassium from the intracellular fluid compartment to the extracellular fluid compartment can be reproduced by using other nonmetabolizable substances, such as mannitol, that produce hyperosmolality. Thus the hyperkalemia of DKA reflects primarily the effects of insulin deficiency and, if hypovolemia is severe, impaired renal secretion of potassium. The intracellular-extracellular exchange of potassium for hydrogen in metabolic acidosis is relatively unimportant. The deficiencies of calcium and magnesium that exist in DKA are usually of little consequence unless hypocalcemia is induced by inappropriate phosphate replacement during treatment.[29] Symptomatic hypocalcemia may persist because of the state of functional hypoparathyroidism induced by magnesium deficiency.

Diagnosis

The diagnosis of DKA is usually not difficult, but there are some minor pitfalls that may temporarily delay establishing the diagnosis and/or appreciating its severity. These are as follows:

1. The plasma glucose concentration is 350 mg/dL or less in approximately 15% of episodes.[30] Such "euglycemic" DKA should be anticipated in type I diabetic women who are pregnant and in alcoholics. The relatively low plasma glucose concentration in the presence of severe metabolic acidosis is attributed to continued use of glucose by the fetoplacental unit in the absence of insulin in the second and third trimesters of pregnancy and to the inhibitory effects of ethanol on gluconeogenesis in the alcoholic patient.[31, 32] Because insulin deficiency is no less severe in either of these conditions, the ketogenic pathway is maximally active and metabolic acidosis is severe.

2. Occasionally, the plasma and/or urine Acetest reaction is only mildly to moderately positive in patients with well-established DKA.[33] Because the nitroprusside reagent detects primarily acetoacetate and acetone, the intensity of the color reaction is reduced if unusually large amounts of the ketones are in the reduced β-hydroxybutyrate state. This occurs occasionally without explanation, but it should be anticipated in patients in whom alcohol is a complicating problem or in whom low flow and tissue hypoxia exist. The severity of the metabolic acidosis can be documented with arterial blood gas measurements.

3. The severity of the metabolic acidosis may not be fully apparent when other acid-base disturbances coexist in the patient.[24] This is particularly important in the older diabetic who manifests DKA. Pre-existent metabolic alkalosis resulting from thiazide therapy complicated by pneumonia, fever, or other condition and respiratory alkalosis may obscure the diagnosis of DKA or appreciation of its severity. Patients with DKA may have a normal systemic pH or be alkalemic if the magnitude of other acid-base disorders is sufficient to offset the acidosis completely or more than completely. Careful evaluation of the pH, PCO_2, electrolytes, and anion gap should permit proper diagnosis of this problem.

4. Patients with DKA often have severe abdominal pain that resolves with adequate therapy. However, at presentation it is often impossible to know whether the pain reflects an intra-abdominal process that precipitated DKA or is a benign and inconsequential reflection of DKA. This problem is often complicated by the presence of hyperamylasemia.[34] We now know that abdominal pain and hyperamylasemia occur in acute metabolic acidosis of any cause and are not specific for DKA,[35] that the amylase is primarily of salivary origin,[35] and that both pain and hyperamylasemia resolve with correction of the metabolic acidosis. These patients require a thorough initial examination, careful and frequent re-evaluation during therapy, and appropriate diagnostic studies at the outset of therapy or during therapy if there is clinical evidence suggestive of an intra-abdominal process. Do not treat the laboratory, treat the patient.

5. Creatine kinase levels may be elevated or become elevated during therapy.[36] It is not clear why this occurs, but the enzyme is of skeletal muscle origin. However, older diabetics who have sustained a silent or painless myocardial infarction may present with DKA. Be alert to this sequence.

Treatment

The treatment of DKA has been reasonably well standardized[37] and is done well in most institutions because appropriately trained intensive care unit and diabetic care unit specialists (nurses, physicians, and others) manage these patients. Minor differences in protocols and philosophy are probably unimportant as long as there is agreement on certain principles of therapy. There are three elements that must be addressed to treat DKA successfully: (1) use of appropriate doses of insulin, (2) correction of fluid and electrolyte deficits, and (3) careful monitoring of the patient and of the biochemical responses to therapy. Compulsive, meticulous attention to detail is required for successful

TABLE 106–2

SERUM ELECTROLYTE LEVELS AT ENTRY AND AFTER THERAPY IN PATIENTS WITH DIABETIC KETOACIDOSIS

Therapy	% at Entry			% at 12 h		
	Low	Normal	High	Low	Normal	High
Sodium	67	26	7	26	41	33
Chloride	33	45	22	11	41	48
Bicarbonate	100	0	0	46	50	4
Calcium	28	68	4	73	23	4
Potassium	18	43	39	63	33	4
Magnesium	7	25	68	55	24	21
Phosphate	11	18	71	90	10	0

Modified from Martin HE, Smith K, Wilson ML: The fluid and electrolyte therapy of severe diabetic acidosis and ketosis; a study of twenty-nine episodes (twenty-six patients). Am J Med 24:376, 1958.

TABLE 106-3

GUIDELINES FOR THE USE OF INSULIN

1. 10 U of regular insulin IV as a loading dose followed by 5–10 U/h ($0.1\ \mu U/kg$ body weight) thereafter until glucose concentration is 250–300 mg/dL and the pH $\geq$ 7.3 or HCO_3^- $\geq$ 18 mEq/L.
2. 10 U of regular insulin IV as a loading dose followed by 5–10 U/h IM.
3. When control is achieved:
   a. Return to previous regimen, if known and if satisfactory.
   b. Use a modified closed-loop system for the administration of insulin or a perioperative insulin regimen, if an interim strategy is necessary. The rates of insulin, glucose, and potassium administration are ~2–3 U, 10 g, and 2 mEq/h.

TABLE 106-5

GUIDELINES FOR CORRECTION OF ELECTROLYTE ABNORMALITIES

Potassium
1. Measure K^+ and obtain an electrocardiogram before adding K^+ to parenteral fluids.
2. If the K^+ level is 4–5 mEq/L, incorporate 20 mEq K^+ in each liter of isotonic saline and infuse at 1 L/h.
3. Maintain K^+ between 4 and 5 mEq/L.
   a. If 4–5 mEq/L, continue K^+ at rate of 20 mEq/h.
   b. If 5–6 mEq/L, decrease to 10 mEq/h.
   c. If > 6 mEq/L, stop K^+.
   d. If 3–4 mEq/L, increase K^+ to 30 mEq/h.
   e. If $\leq$ 3 mEq/L, increase K^+ to 40–60 mEq/h.

Bicarbonate
1. Not recommended for routine treatment of DKA.
2. Consider if other indications present.

Phosphate
1. Not recommended for routine treatment of DKA.
2. Deficit is approximately 1.0 mmol/kg body weight.
3. Replace 25–50% in first 24 hours if serum phosphate level $\leq$ 1.0 mg/dL.
4. 1.5–2.5 mmol phosphate/h as the potassium salt (some circumstances might justify use of the sodium salt).

Calcium
1. Not recommended for routine treatment of DKA.
2. May be necessary if symptomatic hypocalcemia occurs during phosphate supplementation.

Magnesium
1. Not recommended for routine treatment of DKA.
2. May be necessary if symptomatic hypocalcemia occurs during phosphate supplementation.

---

therapy of DKA. The fact that the outcome is usually good is a reflection of the team approach and the ability to have a physician or nurse on a "one-on-one" basis with the patient. We must guard against complacency and trivialization of this illness, which have been responsible for many of the problems and/or complications that have arisen. A comprehensive plan for the treatment of DKA appears in Tables 106-3 to 106-5. The details are not reviewed here because they should be self-explanatory. However, a number of important matters and subtleties occur during the course of therapy, and these are discussed in the following.

1. Insulin should be administered at a rate of 5 to 10 U/h intramuscularly or by continuous intravenous infusion. A loading dose of 10 U may be given intravenously with either approach but is probably unnecessary with the protocol using continuous infusion of insulin. Rather than calculate the dose based on weight (0.1 U/kg), 10 U may be given arbitrarily. Trying to be more accurate is lending a precision to the selection of the insulin dose that does not exist.

2. Allow approximately 100 mL of the insulin-containing solution to run through its attached tubing to coat all of the plastic surfaces. This is necessary to ensure that the patient receives the amount of insulin he or she should be receiving from the rate of insulin infusion.

3. Infuse the insulin via the line through which parenteral fluids will be administered. Dilute insulin in a small volume (250 U in 250 mL of normal saline) and infuse at a rate of 10 U/h (10 mL/h). In this manner the rate of insulin infusion

---

TABLE 106-4

GUIDELINES FOR FLUID REPLACEMENT

1. Isotonic saline. Infuse at rate of 1–2 L for the first hour and 1 L/h for the second, third, and perhaps fourth hours, based on intake and output measurements and clinical assessment of state of hydration. Where indicated, use hemodynamic monitoring and make decisions based on pressure measurements. Smaller quantities may be indicated in mild to moderate DKA.
2. Hypotonic saline may be alternated with isotonic saline after the first 3 L of fluid at a rate of 500 mL/h. The use of isotonic or hypotonic replacement fluids is determined by clinical and laboratory considerations.
3. When the plasma glucose level reaches 250–300 mg/dL, administer glucose at a rate of 5–10 g/h either as a separate infusion or combined with isotonic saline. If volume requirements remain high give dextrose and water through the same intravenous line; if volume replacement for correction of hypovolemia and dehydration is no longer necessary, use 5–10% dextrose and saline at 100 mL/h.

---

and the rate of fluid and electrolyte replacement are separated and can be varied independently.

4. The glucose concentration decreases at a rate of 75 to 100 mg/dL/h[37] unless there is severe stress and/or infection. Although the rate of decrease varies from patient to patient, it is relatively constant in any one patient, so it is possible to predict when the glucose should reach the target level of 250 to 300 mg/dL. On average, the interval from initiation of treatment to the target is approximately 6 hours. If the glucose concentration does not decrease substantially in the first 2 to 4 hours or if it increases, the rate of insulin infusion should be increased to 50 U/h.[16] Do not lose valuable time trying to titrate the dose. With larger doses of insulin the risks of hypoglycemia and hypokalemia increase[37] but they can be averted if you are vigilant.

5. When the target glucose level is reached, do not reduce the rate of administration of insulin because it takes approximately twice as long for the bicarbonate and pH to reach their target values of about 18 to 20 mmol/L and 7.30, respectively. Premature reduction of the rate of insulin infusion is responsible for no further correction or even worsening of the metabolic acidosis. Hypoglycemia or a further fall in the glucose level is prevented by administering fluids containing glucose at a rate of 5 to 10 g/h (i.e., 100 mL of 5% or 10% dextrose in saline).

6. Despite responsiveness to "low" doses of insulin (5 to 10 U/h), patients with DKA are insulin resistant.[38] Normal subjects receiving insulin at 5 to 10 U/h require about 30 to 40 g of glucose hourly to keep the plasma glucose level constant. In DKA, glucose disappears at a rate of about 15 to 20 g/h and more than half of the glucose that disappears is filtered and excreted in the urine.[39] Approximately 25% of the reduction in glucose concentration can be attributed to dilution of glucose in the extracellular space by infused fluids.[40] As a result, only about 25% or 5 g of glucose per

hour may be metabolized. This suggests that patients with DKA are only 15% as sensitive to insulin as normal subjects. None of this is surprising in view of the high levels of ICRH and perhaps even lymphokines (interleukin-1, tumor necrosis factor) that may independently influence glucose homeostasis.

7. There is now considerable debate about and re-evaluation of the rate at which fluids should be administered.[41] Data from several decades ago indicated that the water deficit in advanced DKA was approximately 100 mL/kg.[42] On the basis of this information and the belief that most patients with DKA had severe hypovolemia, it was routinely recommended that fluids be administered rapidly with replacement of 50 to 60% of the estimated deficit of water in the first 6 to 8 hours and 75% of the deficit by 24 hours.[19] This may no longer be correct because patients generally present themselves to the emergency room or other facilities more quickly now. It was common practice to administer 1 to 2 L of normal saline in the first 2 hours of therapy and 3 to 4 L by the end of the first 4 hours. Fluid administration at these rates led to a decrease in the plasma glucose concentration, for reasons already cited, of approximately 20 to 90 mg/dL/h (average 30 mg/dL/h), in the absence of insulin.[43] Fluid alone, however, did not lead to resolution of the metabolic acidosis. It is clear that the efficacy of fluid administration in reducing the plasma glucose level varies from patient to patient depending on the patient's degree of hypovolemia and glucosuric response to volume expansion. The decrease in plasma glucose concentration in the first 2 hours of therapy may reflect these factors more than the action of insulin. Administration of fluids at 50% of the previously recommended rate in patients with modest volume deficits has been demonstrated to be as effective in reducing the glucose concentration as larger volumes and less likely to be associated with development of a hyperchloremic state during recovery (to be discussed in more detail later).[41] It has also been suggested that excessive rates of fluid administration may predispose the patient to cerebral edema during recovery from DKA.[44]

8. The serum sodium level should increase during therapy as the glucose level is reduced and the gradient for water to be distributed in the extracellular fluid compartment is reversed. The increase in the serum sodium level should be anticipated by calculating how much of the hyponatremia before initiation of therapy is due to coexistent hyperglycemia. The closer the serum sodium level is to normal, the more likely is the development of hypernatremia during recovery, particularly when physiologic saline solution is being administered. More hypernatremic, hyperglycemic patients manifest hypernatremia, often severe, as a result of these changes. A decrease in the serum sodium level during therapy indicates that excessive amounts of free water are being administered or retained. It has been suggested that this may be a factor in the development of cerebral edema; therefore, changes in the serum sodium level during therapy may be important and worth evaluating.[44-46]

9. Potassium stores are markedly reduced in well-advanced DKA; the deficit is approximately 3 to 5 mmol/kg. This may also no longer be true of current patients with DKA. The hyperkalemia is due to deficient insulin action[27, 28] and not to exchange of hydrogen for intracellular potassium. The presence of hypokalemia is a poor prognostic sign because it indicates severe potassium depletion and should suggest pre-existing chloride and potassium loss. Some have suggested initially withholding insulin therapy and aggressively correcting volume and potassium deficits in such individuals.

10. The serum potassium level decreases progressively during the first 4 to 6 hours of therapy and reaches its nadir at this time. The risk of hypokalemia is accentuated with larger doses of insulin.[37] It is traditional to add 20 mmol of potassium chloride to each liter of fluid as soon as it has been established that there is good urine output. The need to use larger supplements of potassium depends on the serum potassium concentration during therapy. When the serum potassium level is less than 3.0 mmol/L, the intravenous fluids should contain 40 to 60 mmol of potassium per liter. The serum potassium level decreases during therapy for several reasons: increased renal potassium excretion with volume expansion, reversal of acidosis, and the direct effects of insulin on cellular entry of potassium. Approximately 20 to 50% of the administered potassium is excreted in the urine.[47] It is still necessary to use potassium supplements in the presence of renal failure; however, reduce the dose by 50% and observe the patient carefully.

11. The concentrations of calcium, magnesium, and phosphate decrease during therapy,[26] usually without clinical signs or symptoms. Prophylactic use of phosphate supplements does not alter morbidity or mortality during recovery from DKA and therefore is not routinely recommended despite several attractive theoretic reasons for doing so.[48, 49] Nonetheless, serious abnormalities in the function of tissues and organs are encountered when the serum phosphate level is 1.0 mg/dL or less. For this reason, monitoring of changes in the serum phosphate level is recommended, as are phosphate supplements when severe hypophosphatemia occurs. The deficit of phosphorus is actually quite mild in DKA (approximately 1 mmol/kg; the total body phosphorus store is about 6000 mmol). Phosphorus should be replaced as potassium phosphate (which contains 5 mmol potassium and 4 mmol phosphorus per milliliter), with the anticipated rate of replacement being 50% of the estimated deficit (about 35 mmol in the first 24 hours of therapy). Aggressive and unwarranted use of phosphate can precipitate symptomatic hypocalcemia.[29] This is due to the "unmasking" of coexistent magnesium deficiency and its effects on parathyroid hormone secretion and action.

12. Metabolic acidosis resolves more slowly than does hyperglycemia. This is not surprising because much of the correction of hyperglycemia is due to glucosuria and dilution. No changes in systemic pH occur before 2 hours.[50] Invariably a hyperchloremic metabolic acidosis replaces the anion gap acidosis of DKA. As a result, the pH approaches 7.30 but is not immediately corrected further. The kidney adjusts body composition over several days and the hyperchloremic metabolic acidosis resolves. The hyperchloremic metabolic acidosis is due to the administration of liberal amounts of chloride and a deficiency of substrate (ketones) from which to regenerate bicarbonate rapidly. The amount of buffering capacity lost during the development of DKA is much greater than indicated by the reciprocal change in the bicarbonate and ketone concentrations reflected by the anion gap. This discrepancy between the amount of substrate needed for bicarbonate regeneration and the actual bicarbonate deficit is aggravated by increased renal ketone excretion during correction of the volume deficit. The kidney reabsorbs sodium with the most plentiful anion, chloride, to maintain electrical neutrality. One should be aware of these evolutionary changes during therapy to recognize when the ketoacidosis has been corrected and then reduce the rate of administration of insulin.

13. Routine use of bicarbonate supplementation has not been demonstrated to confer any therapeutic advantage in the treatment of DKA.[51, 52] The use of bicarbonate should be individualized and reserved for patients with severe acidosis, marked reductions in serum bicarbonate concentrations, and/or maximal respiratory compensation. When bi-

carbonate is used, the quantities administered should be limited and you must be aware of the controversy that exists over the use of bicarbonate in lactic acidosis.[53, 54]

Complications

Cerebral edema is the only complication of the treatment of DKA that is of concern.[44–46, 55] It accounts for approximately 30% of deaths resulting from DKA in young patients with diabetes mellitus.[46] It invariably develops in young patients during their first episode of DKA. No clinical or laboratory features of these patients indicate that they are susceptible to this complication. An increase in cerebral water seems to occur during the course of therapy of all patients with DKA without serious complications. Cerebrospinal fluid pressure, which reflects pressure in the interstitial fluid compartments, increases to levels as high as 600 mm H_2O.[56] There is computed tomographic and echoencephalographic evidence of cerebral swelling during treatment but without adverse effects.[57, 58] This suggests that the difference between the patients who have cerebral edema and those who do not is a quantitative rather than a qualitative one. Several studies have suggested that a falling serum sodium concentration during DKA may be a factor for identification of the patients who are at risk.[44, 45] Several pediatricians have used specially formulated replacement fluids that have lower sodium concentrations for the treatment of DKA, and it may be that this approach has contributed to the problem. Treatment of adults with physiologic saline may circumvent some of these problems. Increased water content of tissues during treatment of DKA is not limited to the brain but also involves other organs; for instance, lung compliance and Po_2 also decrease with therapy.[57]

The causes of development of cerebral edema are poorly and incompletely understood, but most physicians agree that it is probably related to the creation of adverse osmotic gradients that favor excessive movement of water into the intracellular compartment of the brain as the glucose concentration is decreasing.[59] The water content of the brain in established DKA is only slightly decreased relative to normal and to the water content of other cells.[59] This is attributed to the development of osmotically active particles in the brain in hyperosmolar states that minimize the loss of cellular water. The identity of these substances remains unclear, and they are referred to as idiogenic osmoles.[59] Sorbitol and *myo*-inositol, products of the hexose monophosphate shunt, account for only about 35% of the idiogenic osmoles.[60] Cellular *myo*-inositol levels do not decrease promptly as extracellular osmolality is corrected. The decrease in the plasma glucose concentration and extracellular osmolality during therapy occurs more rapidly than the decrease that occurs within the brain cells, leading to cellular re-entry of water. Because the water content of the brain is only slightly reduced before therapy is initiated, the potential exists for development of cerebral edema. A direct effect of insulin on membrane transport of sodium and water and activation of an Na^+,K^+-ATPase have also been implicated in this problem.[61]

Whatever the cause of cerebral edema, the development of headache during treatment of DKA should be a signal that it is developing and should stimulate initiation of preventive therapy that includes the administration of mannitol, dexamethasone, and perhaps loop diuretics. Cerebral edema can lead to death or severe and permanent neurologic damage that leaves the patient in a permanent vegetative state. However, the possibility of recovery with minimal impairment has been suggested.[46] To avoid neurologic impairment, aggressive prophylactic therapy should be instituted at the first appearance of headache.

Mortality

Death is infrequent in young people with DKA but the incidence increases progressively with age.[1–3, 7] In patients 65 years of age or older, the mortality rate from DKA is 15 to 25%. Overall, mortality ranges from 5 to 15% and average mortality rates in two separate contemporary studies were about 8 to 9%. Thus, despite the largely good experience in tertiary care centers, DKA is a serious problem with regard to both recurrent episodes and potential morbidity and mortality. The significance of DKA should not be underestimated. The higher death rate in older patients indicates the seriousness of underlying and precipitating illnesses and does not necessarily indicate that the DKA is different or more difficult to treat. Although most patients with DKA present early with less severe metabolic derangements, for those who present in coma the mortality rate approaches 50%.[1]

HYPOGLYCEMIA

Introduction

Hypoglycemia is diagnosed when a low plasma glucose level is detected during diagnostic evaluation or the patient presents with symptoms and signs compatible with this diagnosis. Hypoglycemia is not a disease but rather a manifestation of a disturbance in glucose homeostasis; it has many causes. Three criteria (Whipple's triad) are required for the diagnosis of hypoglycemia: (1) a low plasma glucose level, (2) symptoms and signs compatible with hypoglycemia, and (3) relief of the symptoms and signs with normalization of the plasma glucose level.[62] Considerable misunderstanding of and controversy about the interpretation of the symptoms of hypoglycemia exist, as well as what constitutes a low plasma glucose level. The most common misattribution is to apply the term hypoglycemia to nonspecific adrenergic symptoms or symptoms of anxiety, which are more appropriately associated with nonhypoglycemia.[63]

Glucose Homeostasis

The regulation of the plasma glucose concentration can be divided into the fasting (postabsorptive) state, which occurs 6 hours or more after feeding, and the fed (postprandial) state. Plasma glucose concentrations are generally maintained within fairly narrow limits, but it is difficult to define precise upper and lower limits of normal in any individual patient.

In the postabsorptive state, at rest, glucose utilization is approximately 2 mg/kg/min, with half of the uptake by non–insulin-dependent tissues such as neural tissue, red blood cells, and the renal medulla and the other half by insulin-dependent tissues such as muscle and fat.[64] Glucose is supplied primarily by glycogenolysis but also by hepatic gluconeogenesis as the fasting state is extended. In the fasting state, approximately 8 to 10 g of glucose per hour is required to prevent hypoglycemia. As fasting is prolonged to 24 to 72 hours, the blood glucose concentration decreases to about 45 to 60 mg/dL and plasma insulin levels decrease (<5 mIU/mL), which reduces the rate of glucose utilization in insulin-dependent tissues. In addition, neural tissue adapts to alternative fuels such as ketones and fatty acids, further reducing glucose utilization to about 1 mg/kg/min or about 5 g/h.[65] Clinical disorders that interfere with glycogenolysis and/or gluconeogenesis, therefore, are central to the pathophysiology of fasting hypoglycemia.

After a mixed meal, the postprandial state is characterized by increasing concentrations of plasma glucose and gut hormones, which stimulate insulin release and suppress glycogenolysis and gluconeogenesis. Glucose utilization increases in the liver and peripheral tissues. As glucose absorption from the gut diminishes, glucose levels begin to fall, leading to a decrease in insulin levels and glucose utilization. Approximately 4 to 6 hours after food ingestion, a transition from the fed to the fasting state begins. A smooth transition from fed to fasting state is mediated by adaptive changes in the hormonal milieu and the secretion of insulin, glucagon, catecholamines, growth hormone, and cortisol. Reactive hypoglycemia occurring 2 to 4 hours after meals can be seen with rare disorders such as galactosemia, hereditary fructose intolerance, and akee fruit poisoning. However, in otherwise healthy adults, reactive hypoglycemia is difficult to demonstrate and most commonly these individuals have nonhypoglycemia. Rarely, insulinomas and the autoimmune insulin syndrome present as reactive hypoglycemia.[66]

Clinical Presentation

Although hypoglycemia can be relatively asymptomatic, a pattern of symptoms tends to occur intermittently. The level of plasma glucose at which symptoms occur varies from individual to individual. The diagnosis of hypoglycemia cannot be based on the level of plasma glucose alone. The value of 50 mg/dL has been used as the lower limit of normal plasma glucose, but this definition is arbitrary because normal healthy women may develop plasma glucose levels of 20 to 30 mg/dL during a 72-hour fast and remain asymptomatic.[67] Marks has defined significant hypoglycemia as a plasma glucose level below 40 mg/dL in persons younger than 60 years and 50 mg/dL in persons older than 60 years.[68] However, for clinical purposes, Whipple's triad must be demonstrated for an unequivocal diagnosis of hypoglycemia.

Symptoms

The symptoms of hypoglycemia are protean and nonspecific. They can be divided into those associated with adrenergic discharge and those associated with lack of glucose supply to the brain (neuroglycopenia) (Table 106–6).

As glucose levels decrease, thresholds are reached that result in release of contrainsulin hormones (epinephrine, norepinephrine, growth hormone, cortisol, and glucagon) and symptoms. There have been conflicting reports about the relationship of the rate of fall of glucose to the hormone release thresholds, but most current data suggest that the rate of fall is not important.[69] The thresholds for activation of glucose counter-regulatory systems are higher than the glycemic threshold for symptoms. Counter-regulatory hormones are released at plasma glucose levels of 60 to 70 mg/dL, whereas symptoms occur generally about 50 to 55 mg/dL.[70] There is evidence, however, that for symptoms the threshold can be altered in diabetics by tight plasma glucose control, giving rise to the concept of "central adaptation" to the perception of hypoglycemia. Cognitive dysfunction might develop without the perception of hypoglycemia in a patient with insulin-dependent diabetes who is tightly controlled clinically and therefore adapted to lower glucose levels.[71]

Common Disorders Causing Hypoglycemia
(Table 106–7)

Endogenous Hyperinsulinism

Hypersecretion of insulin is an important albeit uncommon cause of hypoglycemia. Abnormalities of the islet cells of the pancreas include islet cell adenoma, hyperplasia, carcinoma, and nesidioblastosis. Patients with solitary islet cell adenomas make up about 75% of those with "organic hyperinsulinism." The tumors occur from birth to old age with the majority in young to middle-aged adults (20 to 60 years) and with women affected more commonly than men.[72] The tumors are distributed throughout the pancreas and most are small (0.5 to 2.0 cm). Multiple adenomas occur in 5 to 15% of the patients. Islet cell carcinoma occurs in 5%. Nesidioblastosis (5%) is a condition of proliferation of islet cells in pancreatic ductules and may be diffuse or localized; it seldom, if ever, occurs in adults. Islet cell hyperplasia occurs in about 5 to 6% of patients with organic hyperinsulinism. Combinations of these pathologic entities have been reported. Islet cell adenomas occur as part of the multiple endocrine neoplasia type 1 syndrome in combination with hyperparathyroidism and/or pituitary tumors.

Patients with hyperinsulinism characteristically present with hypoglycemia after an overnight fast, before meals, after a skipped meal, or in a combination of these settings. The presentation can be insidious or rapid and can be progressive in severity and frequency. Neuroglycopenic symptoms are the most common presentation. Most patients learn to prevent or abort their symptoms by eating frequently, and therefore weight gain may occur. The diagnosis of hyperinsulinism is confirmed by finding an inappropriately elevated insulin level in the presence of a low plasma glucose level. Sampling over several days may be required to demonstrate hyperinsulinism. During a prolonged fast, insulin levels normally decline as glucose levels decline. An insulin level higher than 6 μU/ml in the presence of a plasma glucose level less than 40 mg/dL is considered to be diagnostic of hyperinsulinism.[73] Two useful ratios have been suggested. The first, IRI/G, is calculated by dividing the immunoreactive insulin (IRI) level (microunits per milliliter) by the plasma glucose (G) level (milligrams per deciliter); values in normal, healthy, nonobese adults are less than 0.30.[74] The second, the amended IRI/G, has been proposed as a more discriminant ratio. It is calculated as IRI (microunits per milliliter) $\times$ 100 divided by the plasma glucose (milligrams per deciliter) − 30. A normal value is 50 or less.[75] The use of these ratios rather than the criterion of insulin levels higher than 6 μU/mL in the presence of hypoglycemia has not improved diagnostic accuracy. Insulin levels in patients with insulinoma are seldom higher than 100 μU/mL, and higher levels are observed in factitious hyperinsulinemia (surreptitious administration of insulin) and autoimmune hypoglycemia.

Also helpful in the diagnosis of organic hyperinsulinism are measurements of the insulin secretory products C peptide and proinsulin.[76, 77] C peptide is the connecting peptide

---

TABLE 106–6

SYMPTOMS OF HYPOGLYCEMIA

Adrenergic	Neuroglycopenic
Palpitations	Headache
Anxiety	Inability to concentrate
Sweating	Fatigue
Tremulousness	Confusion
Hunger	Blurred vision
Irritability	Incoordination
Nausea	Abnormal behavior
Pallor or flushing	Paresthesias
	Hemiplegias
	Aphonia
	Difficulty awakening
	Convulsions
	Coma

TABLE 106–7

CAUSES OF FASTING HYPOGLYCEMIA

Endogenous hyperinsulinism (islet cell adenoma, hyperplasia, carcinoma, nesidioblastosis)
Endocrine deficiency
    Hypopituitarism (corticotropin or growth hormone)
    Adrenocortical insufficiency
    Hypothyroidism
Liver disease
Alcohol
Non–islet cell neoplasms
Renal disease
Sepsis
Drug-induced
Autoimmune
    Antibodies to insulin receptors
    Antibodies to insulin
Severe inanition or severe exercise
Factitious

of proinsulin, which is released with insulin from the beta cell. It is cleared more slowly than insulin and therefore may reflect increased insulin secretion in borderline situations. Because C peptide is not found in injected formulations of insulin, elevated C peptide levels confirm an endogenous source of the insulin. C peptide levels are suppressed in factitious hypoglycemia. Proinsulin is secreted in excessive amounts (>22% of total IRI) by insulinomas.

A number of provocative and suppression tests have been proposed in the evaluation of insulinoma but are not generally necessary.

Accurate preoperative localization of the adenomas is difficult because of their small size. The methods that have been used include arteriography, computed axial tomography, nuclear magnetic resonance imaging, ultrasonography, transhepatic percutaneous venous sampling, and intraoperative ultrasonography. Treatment is usually surgical for benign lesions, but a number of drugs are useful for symptomatic temporary relief.

Endocrine Deficiencies

Endocrine deficiencies leading to hypoglycemia include hypopituitarism (growth hormone and/or corticotropin deficiency), primary adrenal insufficiency, and possibly severe hypothyroidism. In hypoglycemia resulting from endocrine deficiency, the insulin level is appropriately low (<6 μU/mL). Because hypoglycemia is a stimulus for both growth hormone and corticotropin secretion, measurement of growth hormone and cortisol levels at the time of hypoglycemia is usually adequate to screen pituitary and adrenal function. Treatment is directed at restoring the plasma glucose level to normal and replacing glucocorticoids, when deficient.

Liver Disease

The liver is essential for maintaining glucose during the postprandial state.[78] There is a large reserve, and more than 80% of the liver must be damaged before hypoglycemia ensues. This generally occurs in fulminant hepatic failure, end-stage cirrhosis, and severe congestive heart failure. With liver dysfunction, glycogenolysis and gluconeogenesis fail to provide adequate systemic glucose. Acetaminophen overdosage has been a frequent cause of acute hepatic failure and hypoglycemia. Treatment of the hypoglycemia consists of supplying adequate basal levels of glucose parenterally (at least 10 g/h).

Alcohol

Individuals of all ages are susceptible to the hypoglycemic effects of alcohol. Alcohol metabolism reduces NAD, resulting in diminished access of gluconeogenic precursors to the gluconeogenic pathways. Therefore, alcohol consumption in the absence of adequate food intake results in inhibition of gluconeogenesis and can lead to severe hypoglycemia.[31] Insulin levels are appropriately reduced. Treatment consists of parenteral glucose and abstention from alcohol. The depressed consciousness or coma in patients after an alcohol binge may be mistakenly attributed to the alcohol and the hypoglycemia may be overlooked.

Non–Islet Cell Neoplasm

Various non–islet cell neoplasms have been associated with hypoglycemia.[79] These generally occur in older adults, but a few cases have been reported in children. These patients present with either neuroglycopenic symptoms or symptoms related to the tumor mass. The tumors most commonly are of mesenchymal origin, tend to be quite large, and are located in the abdomen or retroperitoneal spaces. Epithelial neoplasms (such as hepatomas, adrenal carcinomas, hypernephromas, and cervical and breast carcinomas); neuroectodermal neoplasms (such as pheochromocytoma, neurofibromas, and carcinoid); and hematologic malignancies (such as leukemias, lymphomas, and myelomas) have all been reported.

The mechanism of the hypoglycemia in these non–islet cell tumors is not entirely clear. Insulin levels tend to be appropriately low. Speculation has attributed the hypoglycemia to increased uptake of glucose by the tumor, malnutrition, and elaboration of insulin-like growth factors I and II by the tumor. Treatment consists of providing adequate glucose and therapy directed at the tumor (e.g., debulking).

Autoimmune Hypoglycemia

Two forms of autoimmune hypoglycemia have been described, involving autoantibodies directed against insulin and against the insulin receptor.[80] The rare syndrome of acanthosis nigricans with insulin resistance, type B, is due to antibodies against the insulin receptor. Insulin resistance and hyperglycemia are the most common presentation, but patients can manifest severe fasting hypoglycemia or present de novo with hypoglycemia without preceding insulin resistance. These patients frequently have other autoimmune disorders, such as systemic lupus erythematosus and mixed connective tissue disease. It has been suggested that the antibodies mimic the action of insulin. When receptor-mediated degradation of insulin is blocked, insulin levels in the blood are high. C peptide levels are generally low, reflecting suppressed endogenous insulin secretion. Measurement of antireceptor antibody titers is required to confirm this diagnosis.

The second type of immune-mediated hypoglycemia involves the spontaneous development of antibodies to insulin without exposure to exogenous insulin (autoimmune insulin syndrome). This is commonly associated with other autoimmune disorders, particularly Graves' disease, rheumatoid arthritis, and systemic lupus erythematosus. Insulin levels are always elevated in this syndrome. Antiinsulin antibodies are present. This syndrome may suggest surreptitious exogenous insulin injections, and the elevated C peptide levels in autoimmune insulin syndrome differentiate these entities. This disorder is benign and self-limited. The hypoglycemia may occur in a fashion similar to reactive hypoglycemia rather than fasting hypoglycemia.

TABLE 106-8

DIFFERENTIATION OF DISORDERS OF HYPERINSULINEMIA AND HYPOGLYCEMIA

Disorder	Plasma Insulin (μU/mL)	C Peptide (ng/mL)	Anti-Insulin Antibodies	Antireceptor Antibodies
Insulinoma	↑ (<100)	Increased/present	Absent	Absent
Factitious hypoglycemia				
Insulin	↑ (often > 100)	Absent	Present	Absent
Sulfonylurea	↑ (<100)	Increased	Absent	Absent
Autoimmune insulin syndrome	↑ ↑ (often > 100)	Present	Present	Absent
Antireceptor antibodies	↑ (variable)	Absent	Absent	Present

Drug-Induced Hypoglycemia

Extensive reviews of drug-induced hypoglycemia have been published.[81] Sulfonylurea agents alone or in combination with other drugs account for nearly three fourths of drug-induced hypoglycemia. Predisposing risk factors include inadequate nutrition, liver disease, and renal impairment. In addition to the sulfonylureas (particularly those with long half-lives), ethanol, salicylates, and propranolol are commonly involved.

Newer reports of hypoglycemia have implicated quinine, especially when given intravenously in the treatment of malaria; pentamidine, which can cause B cell destruction and insulin release; and ritodrine (beta-adrenergic agonist), used to inhibit premature labor. Other beta$_2$-adrenergic agonists can cause hypoglycemia in both mother and newborn. Finally, disopyramide (Norpace) has been reported to cause hypoglycemia in patients with renal or hepatic impairment.

Vacor, a component in rat poison, which is a B cell toxin, and akee fruit, which contains an inhibitor of gluconeogenesis, cause profound hypoglycemia, especially in undernourished individuals.

Factitious Hypoglycemia

This disorder is due to the surreptitious administration of insulin by the patient.[82] In the past, the presence of anti-insulin antibodies in a patient with hypoglycemia was evidence of this disorder. However, with human insulin preparations, anti-insulin antibodies are produced in low titer, if at all; they may be absent in this disorder but they occur with the autoimmune form of hypoglycemia, so their presence alone is of no diagnostic utility. Differentiation of insulinoma, autoimmune hypoglycemia, factitious hypoglycemia, and antireceptor antibodies is shown in Table 106-8.

Miscellaneous Conditions

A number of other conditions contribute to hypoglycemia. These include renal failure, sepsis, malaria, severe exercise and inanition, discontinuation of hyperalimentation, and spurious hypoglycemia (leukemia, polycythemia).

The mechanism of spontaneous hypoglycemia in renal failure is multifactorial. These patients tend to have chronic malnutrition, reduced clearance of insulin, reduced insulin degradation, and diminished glucose counter-regulation. These defects limit the ability of glycogenolysis and gluconeogenesis to maintain glucose homeostasis. In addition, renal failure predisposes to hypoglycemia in the diabetic treated with insulin or oral sulfonylureas. The hypoglycemia in sepsis is probably the result of glycogen depletion and suppression of gluconeogenesis in addition to possible increased glucose utilization. Hypoglycemia is more likely if sepsis accompanies alcoholism and/or cirrhosis.

Falciparum malaria is frequently complicated by severe hypoglycemia, particularly when treated with intravenous quinine. The mechanism of hypoglycemia involves stimulation of insulin secretion by quinine and possibly large glucose requirements of malaria parasites.

Spurious hypoglycemia caused by in vitro utilization of glucose by white blood cells (leukemia) or red blood cells (polycythemia) occurs if serum is not promptly separated from the cells.

Clinical Approach

Patients with low plasma glucose levels or those suspected of having hypoglycemia must be thoroughly evaluated. A careful description of the symptoms and signs, the timing of the symptoms in relation to food intake, the circumstances under which the symptoms occur, and alleviating factors must be elicited in the history. Current and previous medications, ethanol ingestion, and access to insulin are important. The physical examination should cover the mental status, neurologic findings, evidence of liver disease, and careful palpation of the abdomen for tumors (e.g., hepatoma, adrenal carcinoma, and retroperitoneal fibrosarcoma). A complete blood count should be obtained, and renal and liver function and electrolyes (in addition to the plasma glucose) should be evaluated. If the patient has a low plasma glucose level at the time of the evaluation, insulin, C peptide, growth hormone, and cortisol levels should be measured. If reactive hypoglycemia is suspected, a more conservative approach is recommended (Table 106-9).

If the patient is not hypoglycemic at the time of evaluation, a prolonged fast (48 to 72 hours) in an attempt to test the adequacy of glucose homeostatic mechanisms is the most effective approach to diagnosis. The patient is hospitalized and allowed to consume only noncaloric beverages. Plasma glucose levels are measured every 6 hours and when symptoms develop. If hypoglycemia occurs, plasma insulin, C peptide, growth hormone, and cortisol levels are obtained.

TABLE 106-9

APPROACH TO SUSPECTED REACTIVE HYPOGLYCEMIA

1. Have patient keep a careful diary of type and timing of symptoms.
2. Arrange for plasma glucose determinations during spontaneous symptoms to demonstrate hypoglycemia.
3. Oral glucose tolerance tests are of limited value.
4. If hypoglycemia is demonstrated, perform tests with patient undergoing a prolonged fast (72 h).

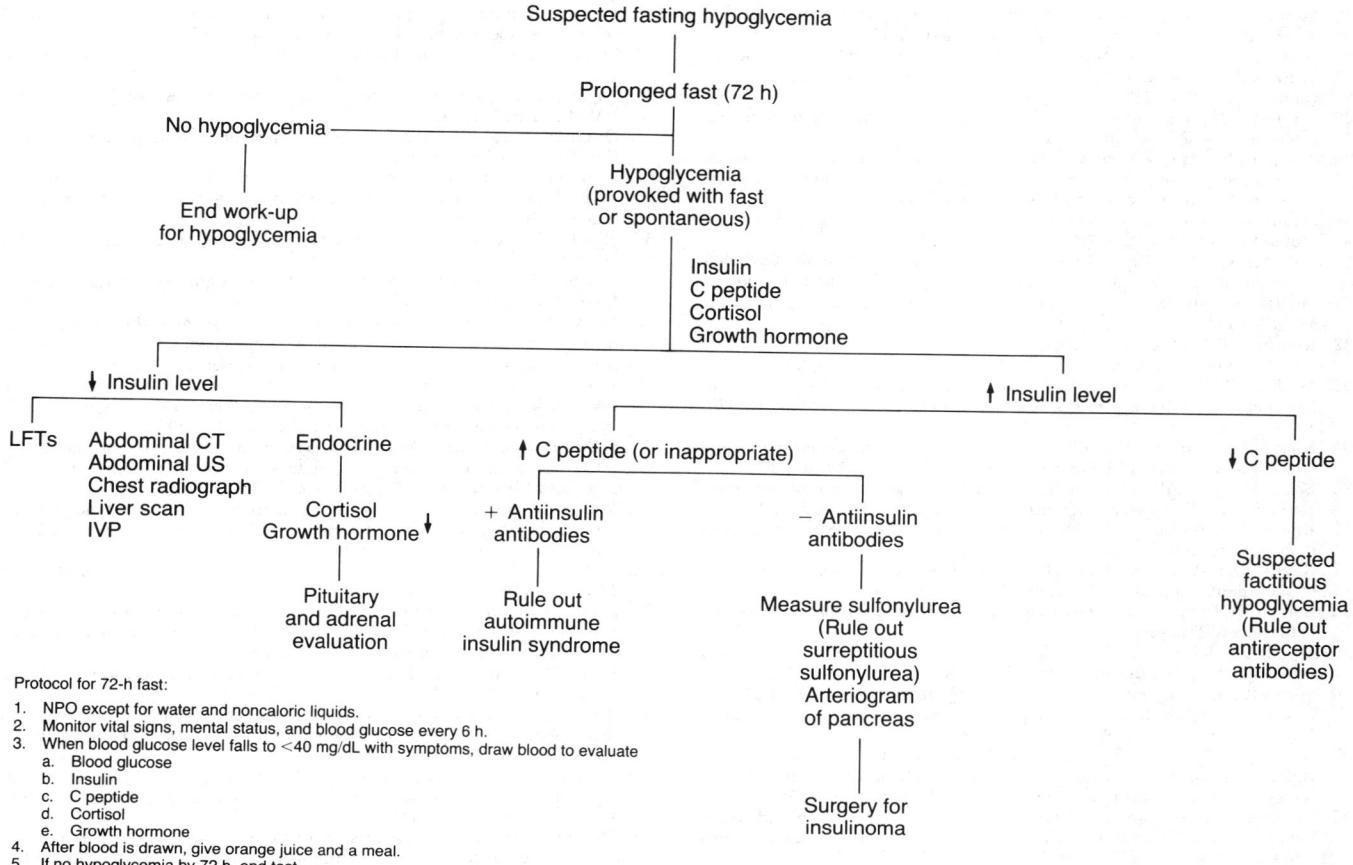

Figure 106–2. Algorithm for evaluation of prolonged fast on suspected fasting hypoglycemia. LFT = liver function test; CT = computed tomography; US = ultrasonography; IVP = intravenous pyelography; NPO = nulla per os.

The patient is then fed and the test ended. Many suggest that exercise be performed at the end of 72 hours if hypoglycemia has not been precipitated. Patients able to tolerate a 72-hour fast without manifesting hypoglycemia have intact glucose homeostatic mechanisms and further diagnostic work-up is not necessary. Most patients (>90%) with fasting hypoglycemia have symptoms within 24 hours. The results of the prolonged fast are evaluated as outlined in Figure 106–2.

References

1. Faich GA, Fishbein HA, Ellis SE: The epidemiology of diabetic acidosis: A population-based study. Am J Epidemiol 117:551, 1983.
2. Holman RC, Herron CA, Sinnock P: Epidemiologic characteristics of mortality from diabetes with acidosis and coma, United States, 1970–78. Am J Public Health 73:1169, 1983.
3. Connell FA, Louden JM: Diabetes mortality in persons under 45 years of age. Am J Public Health 73:1174, 1983.
4. Johnson DD, Palumbo PJ, Chu CP: Diabetic ketoacidosis in a community-based population. Mayo Clin Proc 55:83, 1980.
5. Fulop M: Recurrent diabetic ketoacidosis. Am J Med 78:54, 1985.
6. Flexner CW, Weiner JP, Saudek CD, et al: Repeated hospitalization for diabetic ketoacidosis. Am J Med 76:691, 1984.
7. Centers for Disease Control: Diabetes Control Demonstration Projects, 1978 Phase I Assessment Summary. Atlanta, Centers for Disease Control, June 1979.
8. Macgillivary MH, Bruck E, Voorhess MC: Acute diabetic ketoacidosis in children: Role of stress hormones. Pediatr Res 15:99, 1981.
9. Schade DS, Eaton RP, Alberti KGMM, et al (eds): Diabetic Coma: Ketoacidotic and Hyperosmolar. Albuquerque, University of New Mexico Press, p 59, 1981.
10. Schade DS, Eaton RP, Alberti KGMM, et al (eds): Diabetic Coma:

Ketoacidotic and Hyperosmolar. Albuquerque, University of New Mexico Press, p 72, 1981.
11. Shamoon H, Hendler R, Sherwin R: Synergistic interactions among antiinsulin hormones in the pathogenesis of stress hyperglycemia. J Clin Endocrinol Metab 52:1235, 1981.
12. Schade DS, Eaton RP: Pathogenesis of diabetic ketoacidosis: A reappraisal. Diabetes Care 2:296, 1979.
13. Eigler N, Sacca L, Sherwin R: Synergistic interactions of physiologic increments of glucagon, epinephrine and cortisol in the dog. J Clin Invest 63:114, 1979.
14. Gerich JE, Lorenzi M, Bier DM, et al: Prevention of human diabetic ketoacidosis by somatostatin. N Engl J Med 292:985, 1975.
15. Vranic M, Berger M: Exercise and diabetes mellitus. Diabetes 28:147, 1979.
16. Foster DW, McGarry JD: The metabolic derangements and treatment of diabetic ketoacidosis. N Engl J Med 309:159, 1983.
17. Foster DW: From glycogen to ketones and back. Diabetes 33:1188, 1984.
18. McGarry JD, Foster DW: Ketogenesis. In: Rifkin H, Porte D (eds): Diabetes Mellitus, Theory and Practice. 4th ed. New York, Elsevier, p 292, 1990.
19. Kreisberg RA: Diabetic ketoacidosis: New concepts and trends in pathogenesis and treatment. Ann Intern Med 88:681, 1978.
20. Matz R: Hyperosmolar nonacidotic diabetes (HNAD). In: Rifkin H, Porte D (eds): Diabetes Mellitus, Theory and Practice. 4th ed. New York, Elsevier, p 604, 1990.
21. Katz MA: Hyperglycemia-induced hyponatremia—Calculation of expected serum sodium depression. N Engl J Med 289:843, 1973.
22. Frier BM, Steer CR, Baird JD, et al: Misleading plasma electrolytes in diabetic children with severe hyperlipidemia. Arch Dis Child 55:771, 1980.
23. Emmett M, Narins RG: Clinical use of the anion gap. Medicine 56:38, 1977.
24. Narins RG, Emmett M: Simple and mixed acid-base disorders. A practical approach. Medicine 59:161, 1980.
25. Androgue HJ, Wilson H, Boyd AE, et al: Plasma acid-base patterns in diabetic ketoacidosis. N Engl J Med 307:1603, 1982.

26. Martin HE, Smith K, Wilson ML: The fluid and electrolyte therapy of severe diabetic acidosis and ketosis. Am J Med 20:376, 1958.
27. Androgue HJ, Chap Z, Ishida T, et al: Role of the endocrine pancreas in the kalemic response to acute metabolic acidosis in conscious dogs. J Clin Invest 75:798, 1985.
28. Androgue HJ, Lederer ED, Suki WN: Determinants of plasma potassium levels in diabetic ketoacidosis. Medicine 65:163, 1986.
29. Zipf WB, Bacon GE, Spencer ML, et al: Hypocalcemia, hypomagnesemia and transient hypoparathyroidism during therapy with potassium phosphate in diabetic ketoacidosis. Diabetes Care 2:265, 1979.
30. Munro JF, Campbell IW, McCuish AC, et al: Euglycemic diabetic ketoacidosis. Br Med J 2:578, 1973.
31. Freinkel N, Singer DL, Arky RA, et al: Alcohol hypoglycemia: Carbohydrate metabolism of patients with clinical hypoglycemia and the experimental reproduction of the syndrome with pure ethanol. J Clin Invest 42:112, 1963.
32. Kreisberg RA, Owen WC, Siegal AM: Ethanol-induced hyperlacticacidemia: Inhibition of lactate utilization. J Clin Invest 50:166, 1971.
33. Marliss EB, Ohman JL, Aoki TT, et al: Altered redox state obscuring ketoacidosis in diabetic patients with lactic acidosis. N Engl J Med 283:978, 1970.
34. Knight AH, Williams DN, Ellis G, et al: Significance of hyperamylasemia and abdominal pain in diabetic ketoacidosis. Br Med J 3:128, 1973.
35. Eckfeldt JH, Leatherman JW, Levitt MD: High prevalence of hyperamylasemia in patients with acidemia. Ann Intern Med 104:362, 1986.
36. Knight AH, Williams DN, Spooner RJ, et al: Serum enzyme changes in diabetic ketoacidosis. Diabetes 23:126, 1974.
37. Kitabchi AE, Young R, Sacks H, et al: Diabetic ketoacidosis: Reappraisal of therapeutic approach. Annu Rev Med 30:339, 1979.
38. Barrett EJ, DeFronzo RA, Bevilacqua S, et al: Insulin resistance in diabetic ketoacidosis. Diabetes 31:923, 1982.
39. Owen OE, Light JH, Sapir DG: Renal function and effects of partial rehydration during diabetic ketoacidosis. Diabetes 30:510, 1981.
40. West ML, Marsden PA, Singer GG, et al: Quantitative analysis of glucose loss during acute therapy for hyperglycemic, hyperosmolar syndrome. Diabetes Care 9:465, 1986.
41. Androgue HJ, Barrero J, Eknoyan G: Salutary effects of modest fluid replacement in the treatment of adults with diabetic ketoacidosis. Use in patients without extreme volume deficit. JAMA 262:2108, 1989.
42. Atchley DW, Loeb RF, Richards DW, et al: On diabetic ketoacidosis. A detailed study of electrolyte balances following the withdrawal and reestablishment of insulin therapy. J Clin Invest 12:297, 1933.
43. Meinders AE, Roppeschaar HPF, Sindram EDA, et al: The influence of rehydration in uncontrolled insulin-dependent diabetes mellitus. Neth J Med 21:3, 1978.
44. Duck SC, Wyatt DT: Factors associated with brain herniation in the treatment of diabetic ketoacidosis. J Pediatr 113:10, 1988.
45. Harris GD, Fiordalisi I, Harris WL, et al: Minimizing the risk of brain herniation during treatment of diabetic ketoacidemia: A retrospective and prospective study. J Pediatr 117:22, 1990.
46. Rosenbloom AL: Intracerebral crises during treatment of diabetic ketoacidosis. Diabetes Care 13:22, 1990.
47. Soler NG, Dixon K, Bennett MA, et al: Potassium balance during treatment of diabetic ketoacidosis. Lancet 2:665, 1972.
48. Becker DJ, Brown DR, Steranka BH, et al: Phosphate replacement during treatment of diabetic ketosis. Am J Dis Child 137:241, 1983.
49. Fisher JN, Kitabchi AE: A randomized study of phosphate therapy in the treatment of diabetic ketoacidosis. J Clin Endocrinol Metab 57:177, 1983.
50. King AJ, Cooke NJ, McCuish A, et al: Acid-base changes during treatment of diabetic ketoacidosis. Lancet 1:478, 1974.
51. Hale P, Crase J, Nattrass M: Metabolic effects of bicarbonate in the treatment of diabetic ketoacidosis. Br Med J 289:1035, 1984.
52. Morris L, Murphy M, Kitabchi A: Bicarbonate therapy in severe diabetic ketoacidosis. Ann Intern Med 105:836, 1986.
53. Stacpoole PW: Lactic acidosis: The case against bicarbonate therapy. Ann Intern Med 105:276, 1986.
54. Narins RG, Cohen JJ: Bicarbonate therapy for organic acidosis: The case for its continued use. Ann Intern Med 106:615, 1987.
55. Young E, Bradley RF: Cerebral edema with irreversible coma in severe diabetic ketoacidosis. N Engl J Med 276:665, 1967.
56. Clements RS, Morrison AD, Blumenthal SA, et al: Increased cerebrospinal-fluid pressure during treatment of diabetic ketosis. Lancet 2:671, 1971.
57. Fein LA, Rackow EC, Sprung CL, et al: Relation of colloid osmotic pressure to arterial hypoxemia and cerebral edema during crystalloid volume loading of patients with diabetic ketoacidosis. Ann Intern Med 96:570, 1982.
58. Krane EJ, Rockoff MA, Wallman JK, et al: Subclinical brain swelling in children during treatment of diabetic ketoacidosis. N Engl J Med 312:1147, 1985.
59. Arieff AI, Kleeman CR: Studies on the mechanisms of cerebral edema in diabetic comas. Effect of hyperglycemia and rapid lowering of plasma glucose in normal rabbits. J Clin Invest 52:571, 1973.
60. Lien YH, Shapiro JI, Chan L: Effects of hypernatremia on organic brain osmoles. J Clin Invest 85:1427, 1990.
61. Van Der Meulen JA, Klip A, Grinstein S: Possible mechanism for cerebral edema in diabetic ketoacidosis. Lancet 2:306, 1987.
62. Whipple AO: The surgical therapy of hyperinsulinism. J Int Chir 3:237, 1938.
63. Yager J, Young RT: Non-hypoglycemia is an epidemic condition. N Engl J Med 291:907, 1974.
64. Owen O, Morgan A, Kemp H, et al: Brain metabolism during fasting. J Clin Invest 46:1589, 1967.
65. Randle P, Hales C, Garland P, et al: The glucose fatty acid cycle. Its role in insulin sensitivity and the metabolic disturbances of diabetes mellitus. Lancet 1:785, 1963.
66. Hofeldt FD: Reactive hypoglycemia. Endocrinol Metab Clin North Am 18:185, 1989.
67. Merimee TJ, Tyson JE: Stabilization of plasma glucose during fasting. N Engl J Med 291:1275, 1974.
68. Marks V: The measurement of blood glucose and the definition of hypoglycemia. In: Ancora E, et al: Hypoglycemia: Proceedings of the Rome Symposium. Stuttgart, Georg Thieme Verlag, p 1, 1976.
69. Amiel SA, Simonson DC, Tamborlane WV, et al: Rate of glucose fall does not affect counterregulatory hormone responses to hypoglycemia in normal and diabetic humans. Diabetes 36:518, 1987.
70. Schwartz NS, Clutter WE, Shah SD, et al: Glycemic thresholds for activation of glucose counterregulatory systems are higher than the threshold for symptoms. J Clin Invest 79:777, 1987.
71. Widom B, Simonson DC: Glycemic control and neuropsychologic function during hypoglycemia in patients with insulin-dependent diabetes mellitus. Ann Intern Med 112:904, 1990.
72. Fajans SS, Vinik AI: Insulin-producing islet cell tumors. Endocrinol Metab Clin North Am 18:45, 1989.
73. Service FJ: Clinical presentation and laboratory evaluation of hypoglycemia. In: Service FJ (ed): Hypoglycemic Disorders: Pathogenesis, Diagnosis and Treatment. Boston, GK Hall, p 84, 1983.
74. Fajans SS, Floyd JC Jr: Hypoglycemia: How to manage a complex disease. Mod Med 41:24, 1973.
75. Turner RC, Oakley NW, Nabarro JDN: Control of basal insulin secretion with special reference to the diagnosis of insulinomas. Br Med J 2:132, 1971.
76. Rubenstein AH, Kuzuya H, Horwitz DL: Clinical significance of circulating C-peptide in diabetes mellitus and hypoglycemic disorders. Arch Intern Med 137:625, 1977.
77. Sherman BM, Pek S, Fajans SS, et al: Plasma proinsulin in patients with functioning pancreatic islet cell tumors. J Clin Endocrinol Metab 35:271, 1972.
78. Sherwin RS: Role of the liver in glucose homeostasis. Diabetes Care 3:261, 1980.
79. Daughaday WH: Hypoglycemia in patients with non-islet cell tumors. Endocrinol Metab Clin North Am 18:91, 1989.
80. Taylor SI, Barbetti F, Accili D, et al: Syndromes of autoimmunity and hypoglycemia. Autoantibodies directed against insulin and its receptor. Endocrinol Metab Clin North Am 18:123, 1989.
81. Seltzer HS: Drug-induced hypoglycemia. Endocrinol Metab Clin North Am 18:163, 1989.
82. Greenberger G, Werner JL, Silverman R, et al: Factitious hypoglycemia due to surreptitious administration of insulin. Diagnosis, treatment and long-term follow-up. Ann Intern Med 108:252, 1988.

CHAPTER 107

Acute Renal Failure

H. David Humes

Acute renal failure is a clinical syndrome commonly seen in critically ill patients who require medical intensive care. It is defined as an abrupt decline in renal function. Most nephrologists accept the definition of acute renal failure as a rise in the serum creatinine (SCr) concentration of greater than 0.5 mg/dL/d and a rise in the blood urea nitrogen (BUN) concentration of greater than 10 mg/dL/d over several days. It may occur in a patient with previously normal renal function or may be superimposed on stable but impaired renal function. The clinical manifestations of this disorder arise from the decline in glomerular filtration rate (GFR) and the inability of the kidney to excrete metabolic waste products. Correct diagnosis is important because appropriate management often permits improvement of renal function.

Acute renal failure is best classified in relation to the sequential process of urine formation and excretion. Acute renal failure caused by diminished renal blood flow (RBF) is referred to as prerenal functional acute renal failure; that caused by a sudden, severe renal parenchymal insult is referred to as intrarenal structural acute renal failure; and that caused by obstruction of urine flow is referred to as postrenal obstructive acute renal failure. The initial diagnostic approach, therefore, is to localize the site of dysfunction. If the process is localized to prerenal or postrenal sites, the specific diagnosis and treatment are readily apparent, even though a large number of diseases may alter renal perfusion or urine flow. If the process is localized to an intrarenal site, it is useful to categorize the pathogenetic process further into vascular, glomerular, interstitial, or tubular disease. The most common of these intrarenal processes is acute tubular necrosis (ATN), which develops from ischemic or toxic injury to tubular cells of the kidney.

PRERENAL (FUNCTIONAL) ACUTE RENAL FAILURE

Prerenal acute renal failure, or prerenal azotemia, results from a persistent, significant decline in RBF.[1] Because the GFR is highly dependent on RBF, a decline in RBF results in a decrease in GFR and increases in BUN and SCr. Usually this decline in renal perfusion is part of a generalized condition involving poor tissue perfusion, such as hypotension, volume depletion, congestive heart failure, hepatic cirrhosis, or nephrotic syndrome. However, selective declines in RBF, and hence in GFR, that are disproportionate to changes in blood flow to other tissues may develop as a result of the hepatorenal syndrome, bilateral renal artery stenosis, or the action of certain drugs.

Etiology (Table 107–1)

Hypotension. A decrease in absolute or relative ("effective") arterial blood volume results in a decrease in perfusion of vital tissues and a fall in mean arterial pressure. Central and peripheral baroreceptors are activated to initiate compensatory mechanisms, including increases in cardiac contractility and venous and arteriolar vasoconstriction. Various vasoactive substances are released locally and systemically to promote arteriolar contraction, primarily in the renal, splanchnic, and musculocutaneous circulatory beds. In the kidney, catecholamines and angiotensin II are important hormones released locally for this response. Besides producing a fall in RBF, hypotension is associated with a lowering of the hydrostatic pressure in the glomerular capillary network.[1, 2] Because the glomerular hydrostatic pressure is the major driving force for glomerular filtration, GFR decreases. Thus, a decrease in systemic blood pressure results in both a fall in RBF and a lowering of glomerular capillary hydrostatic pressure, the net effect of which is a decrease in GFR. A similar sequence of events may occur in patients with chronic, uncontrolled hypertension, in which a decrease in GFR (and an increase in BUN and SCr) follows therapy-related acute reductions in systemic blood pressure, even to levels not below normal.[3]

Volume Depletion. Absolute volume depletion secondary to sodium loss may also lead to prerenal azotemia. The

---

TABLE 107–1
ETIOLOGY OF PRERENAL (FUNCTIONAL) ACUTE RENAL FAILURE

Hypotension
Extrarenal sodium loss
  Gastrointestinal loss (vomiting, diarrhea, nasogastric suction, intestinal fistula, bleeding)
  Skin loss (insensible perspiration, burns, inflammatory diseases)
Renal sodium loss
  Extrinsic (osmotic diuresis, diuretic administration, mineralocorticoid deficiency)
  Intrinsic (salt-wasting nephropathy)
Edematous disorders
  Congestive heart failure
  Hepatic cirrhosis
  Nephrotic syndrome
Third-space fluid accumulation
  Gastrointestinal (pancreatitis, peritonitis, bowel obstruction)
  Miscellaneous (crush injury, skeletal fracture)
Hepatorenal syndrome
Bilateral renal artery stenosis
Drugs
  Angiotensin I–converting enzyme inhibitors
  Nonsteroidal anti-inflammatory drugs
  Cyclosporine

---

decrease in extracellular fluid volume results in absolute reductions in intravascular volume, cardiac output, RBF, and GFR. This sequence of events is especially important in patients with underlying intrinsic renal disease. Because of the nonlinear relationship between GFR and SCr, modest reductions in GFR may lead to substantial increases in SCr in patients with already impaired renal function. It is important to rule out superimposed prerenal azotemia in any patient with underlying renal disease, because this reversible condition must be distinguished from progression of the often irreversible intrinsic renal disease. A modest empirical fluid challenge may be required to rule out this possibility but should be considered only for patients who are not volume overloaded.

Edematous Disorders. Prerenal acute renal failure is common in the edematous disorders. In congestive heart failure, prerenal azotemia may result from a reduction in cardiac output secondary to the intrinsic disease phase (with a subsequent decrease in RBF) or, more commonly, from a further reduction in cardiac output related to the use of diuretics to relieve pulmonary congestion in peripheral edema. In the nephrotic syndrome, hypoalbuminemia and the resulting fall in plasma oncotic pressure accelerate the movement of fluid from the intravascular to the interstitial space. In cirrhosis of the liver, elevated portal venous pressure results in sequestration of fluid in the mesenteric vascular system and fluid loss into the peritoneal cavity. Thus, both disorders are associated with decreases in effective circulating blood volume and the potential to develop prerenal azotemia because of a fall in RBF. As is the case in congestive heart failure, this decrease in renal function may be part of the intrinsic renal or hepatic disease but is much more commonly a result of overly aggressive diuretic therapy or paracentesis.

Hepatorenal Syndrome. The hepatorenal syndrome is a form of oliguric acute renal failure occurring in the setting of hepatobiliary disease in which no clinical, laboratory, or anatomic evidence of any recognized cause of renal failure is present.[4] It is most often secondary to alcohol-induced hepatic cirrhosis but occasionally complicates the course of other severe or fulminant liver diseases. The syndrome sometimes develops after decreases in extracellular volume caused by gastrointestinal hemorrhage, aggressive diuresis, large-volume paracentesis, or diarrhea.

Early in the course of the syndrome the urinary sodium concentration is below 10 mEq/L and fractional excretion of sodium is less than 1%. These values may increase with time, which may reflect an element of structural renal damage produced by the persistent reduction in RBF that characterizes this disorder. Because many patients with liver disease have diminished production of urea (secondary to low protein intake and/or impaired hepatic function) and decreased production of creatinine (secondary to reduced muscle mass), BUN and SCr concentrations typically underestimate the reduction in GFR.[5] Progressive renal insufficiency usually occurs, although in a small percentage of patients it may be reversed, especially if liver dysfunction improves. When renal failure develops, however, encephalopathy, gastrointestinal hemorrhage, or sepsis usually develops, and the mortality rate is high.

The pathogenesis of the hepatorenal syndrome appears to be functional rather than structural in nature.[4, 5] When kidneys from patients with hepatorenal syndrome are transplanted into recipients with normal hepatic function, there is a rapid return of renal function.[6] Transplantation of a normal liver into a patient with hepatorenal syndrome reverses the renal dysfunction.[7] The basis of this functional defect is increased renal vascular resistance, which results in a substantial reduction in RBF. The mechanisms responsible for the persistent renal vasoconstriction have not been clearly defined. Angiotensin II and catecholamines do not appear to be involved. An unidentified humoral factor, either formed or not metabolized by the diseased liver, has been postulated to play a major role but has yet to be identified. Severe renal vasoconstriction may well be the end result of the multiple abnormalities, such as hypoalbuminemia, peripheral vasodilatation, arteriovenous shunting, and sequestration of extracellular volume in the peritoneal cavity, that occur in hepatic cirrhosis, decreasing effective arterial blood volume and lowering RBF. The improvement in RBF and renal function after either head-out water immersion or chronic ascites reinfusion via a peritoneovenous shunt suggests that diminished effective arterial blood volume plays an important role in the hepatorenal syndrome.[8]

Bilateral Renal Artery Stenosis. Bilateral renal artery stenosis may not only cause hypertension but also lower RBF sufficiently to decrease GFR, especially in patients with extensive atherosclerotic disease.[9] Acute renal failure occurs when both renal arteries are stenotic or when one kidney is affected in a patient whose other kidney is either absent or already diseased. Treatment of such patients with angiotensin-converting enzyme inhibitors may also cause a dramatic decline in renal function,[10] most likely because of the loss of angiotensin II–induced efferent arteriolar constriction, which maintains glomerular capillary hydrostatic pressure and GFR in the presence of renal ischemia.

Prostaglandin Inhibitors. A decrease in absolute or effective arterial blood volume activates compensatory humoral mechanisms (increased release of vasoconstrictive hormones such as angiotensin II) to maintain blood pressure. These vasoconstrictors participate in a negative feedback loop by promoting the production of vasodilators, primarily prostaglandin E_2, in the kidney to modulate the initial vasoconstrictive response.[11] Because renal prostaglandins have an important role in maintaining RBF and GFR in states of diminished effective arterial blood volume, prostaglandin inhibitors have the potential to lower RBF and GFR significantly in these states and to cause prerenal acute renal failure.[11] Thus, patients receiving aspirin or other nonsteroidal anti-inflammatory drugs may suffer acute declines in renal function, especially if they are salt depleted or edematous (congestive heart failure, nephrotic syndrome, hepatic cirrhosis) or have underlying renal disease.

Cyclosporine. A dose-related decrease in GFR occurs in nearly all cyclosporine-treated patients, including transplant recipients and those with autoimmune diseases, and is frequently seen in the first few weeks or months after initiation of therapy.[12] The most common presentation is a mild-to-moderate, nonprogressive, reversible reduction in GFR with the SCr level rarely rising above 2.5 mg/dL. A less common presentation is a progressive, irreversible renal vasculopathy that is characterized by a rapid deterioration of renal function.[13] The histologic picture is one of intimal proliferation, fibrin deposition, and thrombotic occlusion of the arcuate and interlobular arteries,[12, 14] which can be accompanied by thrombocytopenia and microangiopathic anemia.

Experimental studies have demonstrated a hemodynamic basis for the common type of cyclosporine nephrotoxicity. Cyclosporine has been demonstrated to produce a dose-dependent increase in renal vascular resistance that leads to decreases in RBF and GFR.[15, 16] Stimulation of adrenergic renal nerves may play an important role in these renal hemodynamic effects,[17] but more direct effects on vascular tissue have also been suggested.[18] In addition, there is increasing evidence that alterations in renal prostaglandin metabolism may contribute: cyclosporine increases renal production of the vasoconstrictor prostanoid thromboxane.[19]

Diagnosis

Prerenal (functional) acute renal failure must be distinguished from acute renal failure secondary to intrarenal or postrenal causes by obtaining a careful history, carrying out a careful physical examination, and evaluating certain key laboratory tests. In patients with absolute volume depletion, there may be a history of vomiting, diarrhea, or diuretic use. Physical examination often reveals poor skin turgor, orthostatic hypotension, and tachycardia. On the other hand, patients with effective arterial hypovolemia resulting from congestive heart failure, nephrotic syndrome, or cirrhosis generally have peripheral edema and/or ascites.

The diagnosis of the hepatorenal syndrome is one of exclusion. Various processes may produce simultaneous hepatic and renal disease. These must be excluded because the hepatorenal syndrome is defined as renal failure resulting from, and secondary to, primary hepatic disease. Among the more common causes of simultaneous hepatic and renal dysfunction are biventricular heart failure, collagen-vascular diseases, amyloidosis, Reye's syndrome, and leptospirosis. Other potential causes of acute renal failure such as renal hypoperfusion, urinary tract obstruction, or acute renal interstitial, tubular, or vascular diseases must also be ruled out. Special consideration must always be given to the possibility of typical prerenal azotemia masquerading as hepatorenal syndrome. A patient with cirrhosis and ascites and rising SCr and BUN levels after the use of diuretics may have substantial declines in intravascular volume and diminished renal perfusion. In this circumstance, renal functional parameters stabilize when the diuretics are discontinued and generally return to baseline levels with volume expansion.

The superimposition of ATN may also complicate the diagnosis of acute renal failure in the cirrhotic patient. ATN secondary to aminoglycosides, radiographic contrast agents, ethylene glycol, or rhabdomyolysis occasionally compromises renal function in patients with underlying hepatobiliary disease. However, the hepatorenal syndrome, like other prerenal states, is usually accompanied by a urinary sodium concentration of less than 10 mEq/L and a fractional sodium excretion of less than 1%, whereas values in ATN are much higher. Occasionally, a patient with hepatorenal syndrome presents with a low urinary sodium concentration but over time develops a higher concentration, even without diuretic administration. This may reflect structural ischemic damage associated with persistent renal vasoconstriction, that is, the development of ischemic ATN.

Bilateral renal artery stenosis is most often seen in men older than the age of 50 with atherosclerotic disease. It should be suspected in any patient with renal insufficiency and urinary indices suggestive of prerenal azotemia but no evidence of volume depletion. Hypertension that is difficult to control is usually present. The diagnosis is made with renal arteriography. Because prostaglandin inhibitors cause prerenal azotemia only in the setting of already diminished renal perfusion, the diagnosis is usually based on the history, physical examination, and laboratory data suggesting predisposing conditions.

Functional (prerenal) acute renal failure occurs in a kidney that is not intrinsically diseased, and the urinalysis usually is unremarkable. So-called urinary indices, however, are extremely useful.[20] The renal response to diminished perfusion is avid salt and water reabsorption to defend the circulating blood volume. Increased sodium reabsorption results from hyperaldosteronism, altered renal hemodynamics, and increased sympathetic tone. Increased water reabsorption results from the nonosmotic, hypovolemic stimulus for release of arginine vasopressin. Accordingly, the urine in prerenal acute renal failure is relatively free of sodium and concentrated, so the urinary sodium concentration is less than 10 mEq/L, the fractional excretion of sodium is less than 1%, and the urinary osmolality is greater than 450 mOsm/kg. In addition, the ratio of BUN to SCr usually exceeds 20:1 (normally 10:1 to 15:1). The increase in sodium reabsorption in volume-depleted states, relative or absolute, is accompanied by increased urea reabsorption, a decline in urea clearance that is disproportionate to the fall in GFR, and a rise in BUN. In contrast, creatinine does not undergo tubular reabsorption and the SCr does not rise by an amount out of proportion to the decline in GFR; this results in an increase in the BUN/SCr ratio that often exceeds 20:1. This selective increase in BUN is commonly referred to as prerenal azotemia.

There are several clinical situations, however, in which these urinary indices may be misleading. Individuals with pre-existing renal disease lose the ability to conserve sodium and to concentrate the urine. Furthermore, if volume depletion is the result of renal salt wasting, the urinary sodium concentration may be high. Finally, the BUN/SCr ratio may be normal if urea production is reduced because of a low protein intake or severe liver disease, or the ratio may be greater than 20:1 in obstructive renal disease because of enhanced urea reabsorption arising from low rates of urine flow.

Associated disturbances of plasma electrolytes also may be of assistance in the diagnosis of prerenal states. Volume depletion, absolute or relative, is a strong stimulus of vasopressin release and can override the osmotic control of vasopressin secretion. If water ingestion exceeds water excretion, dilutional hyponatremia develops. In addition, because renal uric acid reabsorption follows sodium reabsorption, increases in sodium reabsorption increase uric acid reabsorption, lower uric acid clearance, and elevate the serum uric acid concentration. Thus, hyponatremia and hyperuricemia may accompany prerenal azotemia.

Treatment

The goal of therapy in prerenal acute renal failure is to improve renal perfusion. The manner in which this goal is achieved depends on the underlying disorder. When volume depletion is the cause of prerenal azotemia, infusion of saline and plasma volume expanders, preferably albumin-containing solution, is indicated. As volume is repleted, the clinical signs of volume depletion disappear and the BUN and SCr concentrations begin to fall within 12 to 24 hours; several days may be necessary to return the BUN and SCr levels to baseline, however.

In the edematous disorders, the development of prerenal azotemia commonly results from excessive diuresis and diminished intravascular volume. This diminution of intravascular volume may occur even though peripheral edema (elevated total body sodium content) persists. In these circumstances, gentle volume repletion improves renal functional parameters. Often all that is needed is to withhold the diuretics and liberalize salt and water intake for a few days. Care must be taken not to expand intravascular volume overzealously, which could cause greater edema formation and congestive heart failure. In critically ill patients with hemodynamic instability, measurement of the pulmonary capillary wedge pressure by means of a Swan-Ganz catheter is indicated.

In the edematous disorders, treatment should also be directed toward the underlying disease process. Cardiac failure can be treated with digitalis and vasodilators, and some forms of nephrotic syndrome are responsive to corticosteroids. When prerenal azotemia is not due to overdiuresis, its presence in patients with congestive heart failure usually reflects severe cardiac dysfunction. Peritoneovenous shunts have been used to treat patients with hepatic cirrhosis and symptomatic ascites. The insertion of such a shunt, most commonly a LeVeen shunt, allows unidirectional drainage of ascitic fluid into the internal jugular vein and expansion of the intravascular space. The result is diminished ascites, improved effective circulating volume, increased renal perfusion, greater urine output, and improved renal function. Although at times dramatically effective, this procedure has potentially serious side effects, including infected shunts, intravascular volume overload, and disseminated intravascular coagulation. Furthermore, portal venous pressure may increase dramatically, thereby increasing the risk of variceal bleeding. The widespread unselective use of shunts to treat symptomatic ascites should be avoided until prospective trials assess the risk/benefit ratio of this procedure.

Therapeutic approaches to the hepatorenal syndrome have been relatively discouraging.[4, 5] Because this disorder occurs in patients with severe liver disease and its associated complications of hepatic encephalopathy and gastrointestinal bleeding, the prognosis is extremely poor. Renal function improves only if hepatic function improves, either spontaneously or after liver transplantation. Treatment is therefore directed toward improvement of liver function. Numerous vasoactive agents, including both vasodilators and vasoconstrictors, have been administered systemically and intrarenally in the hepatorenal syndrome, but results have been disappointing. Hemodialysis has been used as a supportive measure but does not alter the natural history of the disease. Thus, hemodialysis should be considered only for patients who manifest hepatorenal syndrome in association with potentially reversible liver disease. Supportive hemodialysis may allow such patients the opportunity to improve hepatic function and thereby improve renal perfusion and renal function.

The treatment of renal failure secondary to bilateral renal artery stenosis requires either renal artery bypass surgery or percutaneous transluminal angioplasty.[9] If the renal artery occlusions are repaired, hypertension may be ameliorated and renal function stabilized or even improved. Extreme care must be used in the selection of patients for surgery in light of the relatively high morbidity and mortality rates for patients with generalized atherosclerosis undergoing major renal artery bypass surgery.

The treatment of prostaglandin inhibitor–induced prerenal acute renal failure is immediate withdrawal of the offending agent.[11] Because the duration of action of these compounds is only 8 to 12 hours, improvement of renal excretory function is usually apparent within 1 to 2 days. However, the primary abnormality that established the underlying renal vasoconstrictor state may persist after withdrawal of the offending compound, and therapy should also be directed at ameliorating this state; this would include replacement of fluid deficits in sodium-depleted states, discontinuation of diuretics, and treatment of pathologic edematous disorders. Because this drug-induced syndrome is completely reversible, discontinuation of the drug generally returns renal functional indices to baseline. Dialysis should not be required.

The approach to cyclosporine-induced acute renal failure is primarily dose adjustment to minimize the adverse renal effects of this agent.[21] It is now widely accepted that a relationship exists between the serum levels of cyclosporine and its immunosuppressive and toxic effects. Because there is considerable inter- and intrapatient variability in the levels of cyclosporine achieved with any given dose, pharmacokinetic monitoring is useful in determining dosage modifications.

INTRARENAL (STRUCTURAL) ACUTE RENAL FAILURE

Most hospital-acquired intrarenal (structural) acute renal failure is the result of ischemic or nephrotoxic processes (ATN). In many clinical settings, these two processes may be operative simultaneously. For example, ischemic insults often potentiate renal damage produced by nephrotoxins. Atheroembolic disease, renal artery occlusion, rapidly progressive glomerulonephritis, and acute hypersensitivity interstitial nephritis can also present as acute renal failure and must be considered in the differential diagnosis.

Acute Tubular Necrosis

ATN is the most common name given to acute renal failure secondary to either ischemic or toxic processes. Renal failure develops from tubular cell injury that produces necrosis that is limited to certain nephron segments, so only a patchy distribution of necrotic lesions is observed. Even though tubular cell injury is limited to certain nephron segments, substantial renal excretory failure may develop because the nephron functions as a series of segmental units. When more widespread necrosis occurs, an entirely different syndrome (renal cortical necrosis) occurs. This syndrome has causes, pathophysiology, and outcome quite different from those of ATN.

Progressive renal tubular cell injury initiates a series of events that ultimately result in renal excretory failure.[22] These include intratubular obstruction, back leak of glomerular filtrate through damaged tubular epithelium, and a primary reduction in glomerular filtration. Of these three factors, intratubular obstruction and back leak of filtrate appear to be the major mechanisms responsible for the decline in GFR. Intratubular obstruction arises from casts composed of necrotic renal tubular cells that impede the flow of urine. The cells shed into the tubular lumen reduce renal excretory function not only by obstructing urine flow but also by leaving gaps along the tubular epithelium through which glomerular filtrate can re-enter the circulation.

Clinical Course

The decline in renal function observed in ATN may begin abruptly after an ischemic event or develop insidiously as a result of nephrotoxic injury. The problems that may occur during the developing phase of acute renal failure include volume overload; electrolyte disorders, such as hyponatremia, hyperkalemia, hyperphosphatemia, hypocalcemia, and acidemia; and signs and symptoms of uremia, including pericarditis, lethargy, vomiting, and infection. Renal failure predisposes to infectious complications because of poor leukocyte chemotaxis, reduced reticuloendothelial clearance, and diminished lymphocyte responsiveness to antigens. In fact, infection is the most common cause of death in acute renal failure.

The patient usually is oliguric, but urine outputs greater than 500 mL/d may develop in 30 to 40% of patients with ATN. Urine output cannot, and should not, be used as a reflection of GFR. Nonoliguric ATN probably has a better prognosis than oliguric ATN, the consequence, at least in part, of a lesser incidence of hyperkalemia and fluid overload. Moreover, it is likely that nonoliguric renal failure reflects lesser degrees of renal damage, with less frequent progression to symptomatic renal failure requiring dialysis.

Renal excretory failure persists for an average of 7 to 21 days, although durations of several months have been reported. At times, ATN may result in irreversible renal failure, particularly when of multifactorial origin and occurring in the critically ill patient. Reversibility is the result of the regenerative ability of surviving renal epithelial cells. Necrotic areas are replaced with new cells and renal function may return completely, or nearly completely, to baseline. As renal function improves, urine output increases and the BUN and SCr decrease.

The SCr typically follows a triphasic pattern. Initially, in the developing phase of ATN, SCr progressively increases. During the early recovery phase, the improvement in GFR increases creatinine excretion. As the rate of creatinine excretion approaches that of creatinine production, the daily increases in SCr become smaller. Thus, even with an improvement in GFR, SCr still may increase for several days. With further improvements in GFR, creatinine excretion exceeds production so that SCr finally reaches a plateau and then gradually decreases back toward normal.

Diagnosis

Before the diagnosis of ATN can be made, prerenal and postrenal causes of renal insufficiency must be excluded. However, certain key urinary findings may aid in diagnosis.[20] The urine sediment in the early phase of ATN usually contains renal tubular epithelial cells and granular and epithelial cell casts. Because tubular function is impaired, the kidney's ability to conserve sodium and concentrate the urine is diminished.

Urinary indices can be of diagnostic value in differentiating between prerenal azotemia and ATN. In ATN urinary osmolality is usually less than 350 mOsm/kg, urinary sodium concentration is greater than 40 mEq/L, and the urine/plasma creatinine ratio is less than 20. These values discriminate in approximately 80% of patients, leaving approximately 20% with indices in an intermediate, nondiagnostic zone. Further discrimination between these two causes of azotemia can be achieved by using the fractional sodium excretion, which is greater than 1% in patients with ATN and less than 1% in patients with prerenal azotemia. Of note, patients with radiocontrast-induced and rhabdomyolytic acute renal failure may have fractional sodium excretion values less than 1% even in the presence of ATN. Patients receiving large doses of loop diuretics also present a problem. These patients may have fractional sodium excretion greater than 1% and therefore appear to have ATN, even though prerenal azotemia is the underlying problem.

Etiology

Postischemic Acute Renal Failure. Renal ischemia is the most common cause of ATN. Considerable variability in the length and severity of the ischemic insults that produce acute renal failure has been observed. In some patients, a few minutes of ischemia produces ATN. In others, prolonged renal ischemia produces only transient renal dysfunction. The reasons for these differences in susceptibility are unknown. Any prerenal cause of renal excretory function, if prolonged and severe enough, may culminate in structural renal damage. Most cases of ischemic acute renal failure, however, are associated with a period of frank hypotension. Postischemic acute renal failure is seen with higher frequency in patients with sepsis and patients undergoing major surgery.

Nearly half of the clinical cases of ischemic acute renal failure follow surgery. Various processes, including preoperative and intraoperative fluid losses and anesthesia itself, result in intravascular volume depletion and renal hypoperfusion. If an additional hypotensive or other insult is added, susceptible patients may manifest ATN. Abdominal aortic aneurysm repair, open heart surgery, and biliary tract surgery are the surgical procedures associated with the highest incidence of postischemic acute renal failure.[23] In each of these procedures, there is a substantially greater decline in RBF than in other surgical procedures. This may be related to stimulation of nerve inputs to the kidney that control renal arteriolar tone and are activated by manipulation of the biliary tract, abdominal aorta, and heart. The higher frequency of ATN in the septic patient may be related to the hemodynamic effects of endotoxins (systemic hypotension and renal vasoconstriction).

Nephrotoxic Acute Renal Failure. Because the kidney is a major excretory organ, the list of drugs that can induce acute renal failure grows even longer. For now, the causes of nephrotoxic acute renal failure can be categorized into four major groups: antibiotics, heavy metals, radiocontrast agents, and endogenous toxins (Table 107–2).

Aminoglycosides. Aminoglycoside antibiotics are a mainstay of the therapy of gram-negative infections. Because gram-negative organisms account for the majority of hospital-acquired infections, aminoglycoside-induced acute renal failure has become commonplace.[24] Approximately 10% of patients receiving parenteral aminoglycosides develop significant declines in GFR. The aminoglycoside antibiotics that are available clinically include neomycin, streptomycin, kanamycin, gentamicin, tobramycin, amikacin, and netilmicin.

The kidney is the principal route for the elimination of aminoglycosides. These antibiotics accumulate in the renal cortex and produce necrosis exclusively in the proximal tubule. Aminoglycoside nephrotoxicity is classically associ-

TABLE 107–2

ETIOLOGY OF NEPHROTOXIC ACUTE RENAL FAILURE

Antibiotics	Radiocontrast agents
Aminoglycosides	Endogenous toxins
Amphotericin B	Myoglobin
Heavy metals	Hemoglobin
Cisplatin	Myeloma light chains
Mercury	

TABLE 107–3

THERAPEUTIC AND TOXIC SERUM CONCENTRATIONS OF CLINICALLY IMPORTANT AMINOGLYCOSIDES

Aminoglycoside	Recommended Daily Dose (mg/kg body weight)	Therapeutic Concentration (μg/mL)	Toxic Concentration (μg/mL)	
			Peak	Trough
Gentamicin	3–5	4–8	>10	>2
Tobramycin	3–5	4–8	>10	>2
Amikacin	15	8–16	>35	>10

ated with nonoliguric acute renal failure, so excretory failure may develop insidiously in the presence of urine outputs of 1 to 2 L/d or more. Urine output is, therefore, an unreliable marker for aminoglycoside nephrotoxicity. Declines in GFR and elevations in SCr usually are not seen clinically before 5 to 7 days of aminoglycoside treatment. However, the presence of risk factors for aminoglycoside-induced renal injury may condense this time frame.

Risk factors known to predispose to aminoglycoside nephrotoxicity include the dose of drug and duration of therapy, recent aminoglycoside therapy, advanced age, pre-existing renal insufficiency, concomitant nephrotoxin administration, volume depletion, cirrhosis, potassium and magnesium depletion, and metabolic acidosis.[25] The dose and duration of drug administration are probably the two most important factors. A close relationship between serum levels, renal parenchymal concentration, and nephrotoxicity has been described.

The best approach to this serious problem is prevention. The aminoglycosides have a relatively low therapeutic index, so the effective therapeutic dose is quite close to the toxic dose. Because renal function, age, and sodium balance all affect serum aminoglycoside levels, pharmacokinetic monitoring has been utilized to maintain effective, nontoxic antibacterial concentrations and to lower the incidence of nephrotoxicity.[26] Accepted therapeutic and toxic concentrations of the clinically important aminoglycosides are listed in Table 107–3. Peak concentrations are determined 15 to 30 minutes after administration of a dose, and trough concentrations are determined 30 minutes before administration of the next dose.

Numerous formulas have been devised to calculate dose alterations in the presence of renal insufficiency to maintain serum levels below the toxic concentrations. The most useful formula, because of its simplicity, relates dose adjustment to the SCr. In renal insufficiency, the loading dose of aminoglycosides is unchanged. The maintenance dose can be adjusted in either of two ways: the dosing interval may be increased by multiplying the normal dosing interval by the SCr and administering the usual dose, or the usual dose may be decreased by the reciprocal of the SCr and the adjusted dose administered at normal dosing intervals. For example, if a patient's SCr is 2.0, gentamicin dosage can be adjusted from the normal dose of 80 mg every 8 hours to a dose of 80 mg every 16 hours (8 h × 2.0) or to a dose of 40 mg (80 mg × ½) every 8 hours.

Despite the utility of these simple adjustments, pharmacokinetic monitoring should be used to ensure correct dosing in view of the many factors other than level of renal function that influence antibiotic excretion, serum levels, and renal accumulation. Final adjustments in dosage based on serum antibiotic peak and trough concentrations are especially necessary in the elderly, in whom SCr is not as accurate a reflection of renal function as in the younger patient.

Other simple maneuvers to address the risk factors associated with aminoglycoside nephrotoxicity are also worth considering. Patients receiving aminoglycosides should be volume and potassium replete, especially if the clinical setting requires concurrent treatment with potent diuretics. And, if therapy was begun empirically, the culture results should be used to determine whether aminoglycoside therapy needs to be continued. Finally, the potential for nephrotoxicity should always be considered before deciding to utilize an aminoglycoside antibiotic.

If a patient manifests renal insufficiency, the aminoglycoside should be discontinued if a different but equally efficacious antibiotic can be substituted. If the aminoglycoside must be continued despite the acute renal failure, the only reliable guide to dosage is the serum drug level. Even if the antibiotic is discontinued at the time the SCr begins to rise, renal function may continue to worsen inexorably, probably reflecting the continued effects of high tissue levels of the antibiotic. This possibility stresses the need for careful, daily determinations of renal function when using aminoglycosides.

Choice of a particular aminoglycoside should be based, when possible, on the nephrotoxic potential of the different agent.[27] In patients over the age of 55 or with renal insufficiency, tobramycin is the aminoglycoside of choice because it appears to be slightly less nephrotoxic than gentamicin. In other clinical circumstances requiring aminoglycosides, either gentamicin or tobramycin may be used. At present, amikacin and netilmicin should be reserved for treatment of organisms resistant to tobramycin and gentamicin.

Amphotericin B. Amphotericin B is the most effective antibiotic agent for the treatment of deep-seated and disseminated fungal infections. It is a polyene antibiotic and affects microorganisms by interacting with the lipid sterols present in the outer membranes of susceptible cells.[28] Thus, bacteria, which lack sterols as components of their membranes, are not affected by polyenes. Fungal membranes, on the other hand, contain ergosterol and lose their surface integrity after exposure to polyene antibiotics. Mammalian cell membranes contain cholesterol and are also disrupted by polyenes. Not surprisingly, therefore, renal toxicity is a major side effect of this agent.

The cardinal features of amphotericin B renal toxicity are reduced GFR, distal renal tubular acidosis, renal potassium wasting, and vasopressin-resistant nephrogenic diabetes insipidus.[29] The tubular transport abnormalities often precede the reduction in GFR and reflect the fact that renal tubular cell injury is a basis of the developing renal failure. The renal dysfunction produced by amphotericin B is also due to a reduction in RBF, so that both prerenal and intrarenal processes are responsible.

The renal side effects of amphotericin B therapy have important clinical implications because the degree of azotemia, rather than the therapeutic response, dictates both the daily dose and the duration of therapy. During therapy, serum electrolytes, BUN, and SCr should be followed closely. If hypokalemia and acidosis develop, potassium bicarbonate repletion is indicated. Most therapeutic regimens advise either discontinuance or alternate-day therapy when the BUN exceeds 50 mg/dL. When the GFR improves, reinstitution of larger doses may be attempted. It may be necessary, however, to make a judgment as to whether to continue therapy because of the severity of the underlying fungal process or to discontinue therapy and avoid the risk of permanent renal damage. The tubular transport defects and renal insufficiency usually are at least partially reversible, but permanent renal failure has been described with prolonged, large doses of the agent and with multiple courses of amphotericin B therapy.

Heavy Metals. Various heavy metals produce acute renal failure with proximal tubular necrosis. Mercury, platinum, arsenic, bismuth, silver, chromium, and uranium salts are all potent nephrotoxins. Today, ATN secondary to these agents is almost completely confined to occupational exposure or ingestion, either accidental or purposeful. Cisplatin, an inorganic antineoplastic compound containing platinum, is currently the predominant heavy-metal cause of nephrotoxicity in the clinical setting.[30, 31] Several risk factors, including total dose administered, duration of treatment, simultaneous administration of other nephrotoxic agents, and pre-existing renal disease, have been identified in cisplatin nephrotoxicity.

Several therapeutic maneuvers have been demonstrated that minimize the nephrotoxic effects of cisplatin.[29-31] Continuous infusion results in less renal toxicity than intravenous bolus administration of similar doses. Volume expansion (and maintenance of good urine flow) before and during cisplatin administration is also important. Cisplatin is best avoided if the creatinine clearance is below 50 to 60 mL/min, and other nephrotoxic agents, such as the aminoglycosides, should not be used during cisplatin therapy.

Radiocontrast Agents. A significant increase in the incidence of radiocontrast agent–induced ATN has occurred.[21] This is attributable to increased awareness of the problem by physicians and to greater use of radiocontrast agents rather than to an increased nephrotoxic potential of new contrast agents.

Radiocontrast agent–induced acute renal failure is due to combined effects of renal vasoconstriction with resulting ischemia, direct tubular cell toxicity, and intratubular precipitation of the contrast agent with proteins and membrane fragments resulting in intratubular obstruction.[21, 32] The clinical presentation is typical. The patient with radiocontrast agent–induced acute renal failure usually manifests oliguria within the first 24 hours after exposure to the contrast agent, although mild forms of toxicity may be nonoliguric. Oliguria persists for 2 to 4 days. The SCr peaks within 7 days and then returns to baseline in most cases. The process usually is reversible and self-limited, so dialysis rarely is required. However, irreversible renal damage has been described in patients with diabetes mellitus or renal insufficiency.

Although the incidence of nephrotoxicity is relatively low, several risk factors increase the chance of nephrotoxicity developing.[33] Pre-existing renal insufficiency and long-standing insulin-dependent diabetes mellitus are the most important predisposing factors. Renal insufficiency results in a higher plasma level, and a longer plasma half-life, of the contrast agent and a greater exposure time for renal epithelial cells. Diabetes mellitus is a risk factor because the vascular complications so common in this disease result in more prolonged renal ischemia after contrast agent administration. Volume depletion and multiple myeloma are additional important risk factors.

Prevention of radiocontrast agent–induced acute renal failure depends on identification of the patients at high risk. For these individuals, consideration should be given to alternative noninvasive diagnostic studies, including sonography, isotopic scans, retrograde pyelography, and noncontrast computed tomography. If a radiocontrast study cannot be avoided, patients with SCr greater than 1.8 mg/dL should have volume repletion before the contrast load, and urine volume should be maintained for 24 hours after the procedure. The development of newer nonionic radiocontrast agents may lessen the incidence of contrast agent–induced nephrotoxicity, and these agents may be particularly useful for patients at high risk. However, clinical studies are needed to confirm the lower nephrotoxic potential demonstrated in experimental animal studies.

Endogenous Proteins. Several endogenous proteins, including myoglobin and hemoglobin,[34] have been associated with the development of acute renal failure. Myoglobinuric acute renal failure can result from both traumatic and nontraumatic muscle injury. Traumatic muscle injury may be caused by crushing as well as by exertion, ischemia, and seizures. Nontraumatic rhabdomyolytic ATN has been associated with severe (especially alcohol-related) myopathies, drug overdose with pressure-induced myonecrosis, heatstroke, viral infections, potassium depletion, and phosphate depletion.

Hemolysis, with release of free hemoglobin into the circulation, appears to result in ATN only when associated with other systemic abnormalities, especially volume depletion, shock, and acidosis. Hemoglobin-induced ATN has been associated with hemolysis resulting from a variety of chemical compounds, snake and spider venoms, malaria, and transfusion reactions.

The pathophysiology of myoglobin- and hemoglobin-induced ATN is related to the combined effects of accompanying hypotension and shock in these disorders resulting in renal ischemic injury, to the direct nephrotoxic effects of heme pigments, and to intratubular obstruction resulting from the formation of casts composed of these proteins and cellular debris.[35] Myoglobin and hemoglobin are filtered by the glomerulus and reabsorbed by the proximal tubule, where toxic effects are most pronounced. The degree of reabsorption may be enhanced in volume depletion and other states of poor renal perfusion, so that these clinical settings may increase the risk of ATN. Because of its smaller molecular size, myoglobin is more readily filtered than is hemoglobin. Consequently, in the clinical presentation of heme pigment protein–induced ATN, the urine but not the plasma is pigmented in myoglobinuric states, whereas both the urine and the plasma are pigmented in hemoglobinuric states.

Clinically, myoglobinuric acute renal failure is commonly associated with pigmented granular casts, a positive *o*-tolidine reaction in the urine in the absence of red blood cells in the spun urine sediment, and elevation in the plasma level of creatine kinase because of release of this enzyme from damaged muscle cells. A definitive diagnosis can be made by demonstrating myoglobin in the urine. Because skeletal muscle is rich in creatinine and uric acid precursors, potassium, and phosphate, rhabdomyolysis also releases large amounts of these compounds.[36, 37] The release of muscle creatinine precursors can result in a rate of rise of SCr exceeding 2 mg/dL/d. The BUN/SCr ratio is consequently commonly lower than the normal value of 10:1 to 15:1. The serum uric acid concentration is commonly greater than 16 mg/dL, and myoglobinuric ATN must therefore be differentiated from acute acid nephropathy. Severe hyperkalemia occurs frequently and uncontrollable hyperkalemia is an indication for emergency dialysis. Hyperphosphatemia results from the release of phosphate from necrotic muscle and values exceeding 8 mg/dL are common. Hypocalcemia may accompany the hyperphosphatemia because of calcium phosphate deposition in damaged muscle and possibly also decreased synthesis of 1,25–dihydroxycholecalciferol. Although hypocalcemia may be present in the oliguric phase of myoglobinuric acute renal failure, hypercalcemia sometimes develops during the diuretic phase of the disorder. Calcium mobilization from deposits in damaged muscle may contribute to the hypercalcemia, but a complete explanation for this phenomenon is not yet available.

The clinical diagnosis of hemoglobinuric ATN should be considered when a known hemolytic event is followed within minutes to hours by dark urine and a decline in urine output and/or renal insufficiency. Chills and hypotension are common accompanying symptoms and signs.

The most important measure in treating rhabdomyolysis is early and aggressive replacement of intravascular fluid lost into necrotic muscle.[35] Administration of 4 to 12 L of normal saline solution intravenously in the first 24 hours may be necessary to maintain a high urine output. Administration of a single dose of mannitol (25 g) intravenously early in the course of volume replacement is also recommended. Urine output should be maintained at high levels to keep the tubular concentration of myoglobin as low as possible. Similar principles apply to the treatment of hemoglobinuria. It should be remembered that myoglobinuric acute renal failure is often accompanied by severe hyperkalemia, hyperphosphatemia, and hypocalcemia and that early dialysis may be necessary.

General Management Principles in Acute Tubular Necrosis

The therapy of ATN should be directed at ameliorating renal injury during the developing phase of acute renal failure and maintaining fluid and electrolyte homeostasis as close to normal as possible during the later phases of the disorder.[38] Adequate nutrition and treatment of infection, when present, are also important. The use of mannitol or furosemide in the treatment of ATN remains controversial. Although there is no evidence that these diuretic agents can reverse ATN once it has developed, some advocate a trial of furosemide, 80 to 400 mg, or mannitol, 12.5 to 25 g, by intravenous infusion in the early oliguric phase in the hope of inducing a diuresis and decreasing the need for dialysis by limiting hypervolemic and hyperkalemic complications. If no improvement in urine output occurs, the diuretics should be discontinued. Mannitol can cause hyperosmolality, hyponatremia, and intravascular volume expansion. Deafness, which can be irreversible, may follow the use of large doses of furosemide or ethacrynic acid.

Although it does not reverse renal injury, mannitol may be useful in the prevention of nephrotoxic acute renal failure. As an osmotic diuretic, mannitol reduces sodium and water reabsorption in the proximal tubule, thereby lowering the concentration of the nephrotoxin within the tubule lumen and limiting its effect on renal epithelial cells. Thus, mannitol infusion before or during administration of cisplatin, amphotericin B, or radiocontrast agent or during myoglobinuria may be helpful in lessening the degree of renal injury. Mannitol and furosemide have been shown to improve renal function in ischemic acute renal failure, but only if given before the ischemia. Moreover, these diuretics are usually no more beneficial than simple volume repletion.

Prevention of nephrotoxic ATN requires knowledge of the drugs that are nephrotoxic and their correct dosage, selection of nephrotoxic agents only for clearly defined indications, and identification and modulation of factors that increase the risk of nephrotoxicity. Important risk factors include pre-existing renal disease, volume depletion, advanced age, and multiple nephrotoxic drug use. However, even with the most careful use of nephrotoxic agents, acute renal failure may still occur. When it does, the drug or drugs that may be responsible should be discontinued if possible. However, even after the drugs are withdrawn, renal insufficiency may progress for several days because of the persistence of the toxin in the renal parenchyma. Careful monitoring of renal function is therefore mandatory even after the initial recognition of the insult.

Some patients, usually those with oliguric ATN, require dialysis. Either peritoneal dialysis or hemodialysis can be utilized. Indications for dialysis include inability to control hyperkalemia with cation-exchange resins, severe acidemia, intravascular volume overload, and uremic complications such as pericarditis and encephalopathy. Dialysis usually is initiated when the SCr reaches 8 to 10 mg/dL to avoid major uremic problems, which could be life threatening. Furthermore, maintenance of SCr below 8 mg/dL and BUN below 100 mg/dL may improve the general condition of the patient by limiting uremia-related impairment of white blood cell and platelet function. Dialytic therapy is discussed in greater detail in Chapter 109 and nutritional therapy is discussed in Chapter 136.

The prognosis of patients with ATN depends on the causative process. ATN after surgery or trauma has an overall mortality rate of 40 to 75%. The survival rate is much better among patients who do not manifest other complications, such as infection, bleeding, or respiratory failure. Patients with nephrotoxic ATN have an average mortality rate under 10%. Because dialysis can correct most abnormalities associated with renal excretory failure, the dependence of survival on extrarenal complications is not surprising.

Other Intrarenal Processes

Other acute renal parenchymal insults may rapidly diminish excretory function. These include vascular (e.g., atheroembolism), glomerular (e.g., rapidly progressive glomerulonephritis), and interstitial (e.g., acute hypersensitivity interstitial nephritis) processes.

Atheroembolic Disorders

Acute renal failure caused by atheroembolic occlusion of the renal microcirculation occurs spontaneously in the presence of atherosclerotic disease of the aorta and after catheterization and aortic reconstructive surgery.[39, 40] Diagnosis is often difficult but is suggested by livedo reticularis, worsening hypertension, fluctuating azotemia, and emboli in other locations. Management is mainly supportive.[39] The efficacy of anticoagulation is unknown, but it may be beneficial after large-vessel thromboembolic events. Renovascular reconstructive surgery for large-vessel thromboembolism is indicated in patients with bilateral disease and rapidly progressive renal failure.[40] Renal functional recovery may be as high as 70 to 90%, but the operative mortality rate is 10%. Surgery is of no benefit in microvascular disease. A role for streptokinase infusion has not been established.

Rapidly Progressive Glomerulonephritis

Acute renal failure may also develop from inflammation within the glomerulus.[41, 42] Acute glomerulonephritis is generally characterized by hypertension, proteinuria, and hematuria and can be due to primary renal disease or to a systemic disorder such as vasculitis. Absence of significant proteinuria, hematuria, and red blood cell casts virtually excludes this diagnosis. Patients with acute glomerulonephritis usually have low urinary sodium concentration and fractional excretion of sodium, similar to those in prerenal acute renal failure; however, the urine is usually isotonic, whereas it is usually hypertonic in prerenal acute renal failure. These events define a clinical syndrome most commonly referred to as rapidly progressive glomerulonephritis.

Renal biopsy is often required to determine the etiology of rapidly progressive glomerulonephritis and the optimal therapeutic modalities. Some conclusions can be reached, however, without renal biopsy. A low platelet count, evidence of hemolysis, and normal coagulation times are characteristic of the hemolytic-uremic syndrome, thrombotic thrombocytopenic purpura, and postpartum acute renal failure. Poststreptococcal glomerulonephritis may also be diagnosed without renal biopsy by assessing antistreptolysin-O titers and blood or skin cultures.

The renal biopsy in rapidly progressive glomerulonephritis reveals a majority of glomeruli with crescent formation, defined by a collection of proliferating cells within Bowman's space. Crescent formation is initiated by fibrin deposition in Bowman's space resulting from rupture of the glomerular capillary basement membrane because of fulminant inflammation. Fibrin deposition is associated with migration of macrophages into Bowman's space and cellular proliferation, leading to diminished glomerular blood flow and proximal tubular obstruction. Renal excretory function accordingly declines.

The causes of rapidly progressive glomerulonephritis include vasculitis (Wegener's granulomatosis, polyarteritis), systemic lupus erythematosus, Henoch-Schönlein purpura, anti–glomerular basement membrane antibody disease (Goodpasture's syndrome), and primary renal disorders. The approach to the evaluation and treatment of each of these disorders is beyond the scope of this chapter, and the reader is referred to more detailed descriptions elsewhere.[41, 42]

Acute Interstitial Nephritis

Acute hypersensitivity or allergic interstitial nephritis can also present with acute renal failure and always should be considered in the differential diagnosis.[43, 44] This disorder has been associated most frequently with methicillin, but there is a long list of other drugs that may also produce this lesion (Table 107–4). As the name implies, the pathology is characterized by an acute interstitial infiltrate consisting predominantly of lymphocytes and monocytes. Neutrophils and eosinophils may also be present in large numbers, as well as occasional plasma cells and basophils. The infiltrate is predominantly in the renal cortex, is either diffuse or patchy in distribution, and is associated with interstitial edema. Variable degrees of tubular necrosis and renal cell regeneration are present and white blood cell casts can be seen within the tubules.

These pathologic findings strongly suggest an allergic or hypersensitivity reaction. The clinical manifestations, which include a latency period between drug administration and the development of the clinical syndrome, lack of correlation with the drug dose, and the presence of eosinophilia and maculopapular rashes in some patients, provide further evidence for a systemic hypersensitivity reaction. Clinically, the onset of the syndrome is characterized by fever and gross or microscopic hematuria in nearly all patients. Eosinophilia occurs in most patients but may persist for only a day or two and may be missed. Rashes occur in only a minority of patients. The urine usually shows moderate

TABLE 107–4	
DRUGS ASSOCIATED WITH ACUTE INTERSTITIAL NEPHRITIS	
Common	**Rare**
Methicillin	Oxacillin
Penicillin G	Nafcillin
Ampicillin	Carbenicillin
Rifampin	Cephalothin
Phenindione	Cephalexin
Sulfonamides	Cimetidine
Furosemide	Glafenine
Thiazides	Phenylbutazone
Allopurinol	Azathioprine
Phenytoin	Fenoprofen

proteinuria, which only rarely is in the nephrotic range, but always shows pyuria. Eosinophils may be found in the sediment and, when present, are diagnostic of this disorder. A Wright stain of the urine sediment should always be done if this disease is suspected and pyuria (in the absence of bacteriuria) is noted.

Although the differential diagnosis of acute interstitial nephritis includes all other causes of acute renal failure, when fever, hematuria, rash, and eosinophilia or eosinophiluria are present, it is rarely confused with other processes. Renal biopsy is the only means of confirming the diagnosis but is not required if other characteristic clinical signs and symptoms are present. In atypical cases, however, renal biopsy may be more important for diagnosis.

Renal insufficiency occurs in a majority of patients with acute interstitial nephritis, and oliguric acute renal failure develops in 20 to 50%. Most patients recover completely, but the rate of recovery varies considerably. In patients without azotemia, the urine sediment may clear within a few days. In patients who have oliguric acute renal failure, the return to normal renal function may take several weeks.

The mainstay of therapy is identification and discontinuation of the offending drug. Corticosteroids may be of benefit in patients in whom renal failure has persisted for 7 days or more after drug discontinuation.[44, 45] In most studies, steroids, usually prednisone at 60 mg/d, have been associated with a more rapid resolution of the process. Steroids should be discontinued if no measurable response has occurred within 2 to 3 weeks of therapy.

POSTRENAL (OBSTRUCTIVE) ACUTE RENAL FAILURE

Obstruction to urine flow may occur at any site along the urinary tract, including both intrarenal and extrarenal locations (Table 107–5). Because extrarenal urinary tract obstruction is a reversible cause of renal failure, urinary tract obstruction should always be considered as part of the initial differential diagnosis in all patients presenting with renal insufficiency.[46, 47]

Intrarenal Obstruction

Acute renal failure arises from intrarenal obstruction when crystal formation and precipitation occur diffusely along the tubules, as seen in acute uric acid nephropathy and methotrexate-induced acute renal failure. In most cases of intrarenal obstructive acute renal failure the presentation is similar to that in ATN. Because the obstruction is intrarenal rather than extrarenal, the diagnosis is not made by cystoscopy or retrograde pyelography. Awareness of the settings in which intrarenal crystal formation and precipitation may develop is therefore important.

The use of a variety of chemotherapeutic agents in patients

with myeloproliferative or lymphoproliferative disorders results in rapid destruction of neoplastic tissue, elaboration of uric acid from the nucleic acids released from lysed cells, hyperuricemia, uricosuria, intrarenal precipitation of uric acid, and acute renal failure.[48, 49] Clinically, this disorder is characterized by the abrupt onset of oliguria, often leading to anuria, and acute renal failure. The serum uric acid concentration usually exceeds 20 mg/100 mL. In the early phase, uric acid crystals are almost always present in the urine and hematuria may occur. A urinary uric acid/creatinine concentration ratio greater than 1 may aid in the diagnosis.

Treatment is directed toward minimizing uric acid crystallization in the renal collecting ducts. Because the pKa of uric acid is 5.75, increasing urinary pH and increasing urine flow favor excretion of urate salts. Urinary alkalinization is achieved by infusion of sodium bicarbonate and concomitant administration of the carbonic anhydrase inhibitor acetazolamide. Pretreatment of susceptible individuals with allopurinol for at least 24 hours, and preferably for 3 days, decreases the hyperuricemic response and, therefore, the risk of this disorder. Most patients respond to these simple measures. However, patients with persistent renal failure or serum uric acid levels exceeding 25 mg/100 mL may require hemodialysis to lower serum uric acid levels and reverse the renal failure.

Methotrexate nephrotoxicity has become a significant clinical problem with the institution of high-dose (exceeding 50 mg/kg) treatment protocols requiring citrovorin rescue.[50] It is widely accepted that methotrexate (or a metabolite) precipitates in the renal tubules, causing an intrarenal obstructive nephropathy. However, direct epithelial cell injury may also contribute. The problem can be avoided by establishing and maintaining an alkaline diuresis during and after administration of methotrexate.

Extrarenal Obstruction

Extrarenal obstruction to urine flow may occur at the level of the renal pelvis, ureter, urethra, or bladder neck. A wide variety of processes may cause urinary tract obstruction. In young adults, renal stones are the major cause of obstruction. In older adults, benign prostatic hypertrophy, neoplasms, and stones are the most common causes.

If the process is acute, suprapubic or flank pain is common. The location of the pain is determined by the site of obstruction, but if the process is slowly progressive or intrarenal, symptoms may not appear. The urinalysis may be entirely normal, but crystals and hematuria may be present if the renal failure is caused by intratubular crystal deposition or the passage of stones. Of importance, a normal or even high urine output can be seen in obstructive uropathy. Although complete obstruction obviously results in anuria, intermittent and/or partial urinary tract obstruction can cause marked renal insufficiency in the presence of intermittent and variable urine outputs.

In addition to the signs and symptoms directly referable to obstruction, it is important to look for underlying disorders that may be the cause of the obstruction. Clues to the cause may be provided by a history of malignancy; previous abdominal, pelvic, or genitourinary surgery; renal stones; disorders associated with papillary necrosis (diabetes mellitus, analgesic nephropathy, sickle cell disease); or treatment with methysergide, a drug that is used for migraine headache and can cause retroperitoneal fibrosis.

A variety of complications may develop with urinary tract obstruction. With urinary stasis, infection is frequent. Hypertension occasionally develops and is probably volume related. Renal failure occurs only with bilateral obstruction

---

TABLE 107–5

ETIOLOGY OF OBSTRUCTIVE ACUTE RENAL FAILURE

Intrarenal
  Acute uric acid nephropathy
  Methotrexate
  Sulfonamides
Extrarenal
  Renal pelvis: calculus, sloughed papilla, ureteropelvic junction
  Ureter: lymphoma, neoplasia (ureteral, prostate, bladder pelvis), calculus, sloughed papilla, pregnancy, stricture
  Urethra, bladder neck: benign prostatic hypertrophy, neoplasia (prostate, bladder) neurogenic bladder, calculus

or with unilateral obstruction in the case of a solitary kidney. Ischemic papillary necrosis also may develop in patients with acute obstruction.

The search for urinary tract obstruction rests on a high degree of suspicion and begins with catheterization of the urinary bladder. If urethral obstruction or a neurogenic bladder is the cause, urine output increases. If bladder catheterization does not result in a vigorous urine output, the obstruction must be at the level of the ureters or above. In these cases, the diagnosis of obstruction depends on radiologic procedures, including ultrasonography, intravenous pyelography, computed tomographic scanning, and retrograde pyelography. Because of poor renal function, pyelographic visualization of the obstructed collecting system may not occur until 6 to 24 hours after contrast agent administration.

The necessity for and rapidity of treatment of urinary tract obstruction depend on the clinical setting and whether the obstruction is complete or partial. Immediate relief of obstruction is necessary only in patients with generalized sepsis caused by infection proximal to the obstruction. Antibiotic therapy alone in this setting is usually ineffective. Uncontrollable pain, recurrent infections or bleeding, and progressive renal insufficiency are other indications for correction of obstruction, but immediate therapy is not required. A short delay in relieving obstruction does not lead to irreversible deterioration in renal function. For the most part, complete restoration of renal function can occur if obstruction is corrected within 1 week of onset.[51] If obstruction persists for 1 to 4 weeks, some permanent loss of function occurs, although the GFR may return to 30 to 50% of normal. However, after more than 5 weeks of complete obstruction, the damage becomes largely irreversible.

The particular therapeutic intervention for relief of urinary tract obstruction depends on the site and cause of the obstruction. Relief of bilateral complete urinary tract obstruction is often associated with a period of high urine output, referred to as postobstructive diuresis. In most patients, this diuresis is appropriate (and therefore self-limited) and represents the loss of fluid retained during the period of complete obstruction. Rarely, the diuresis is inappropriate and may result in volume depletion if the urinary losses are not replaced. The two can be distinguished by cautiously allowing the patient to go into mild negative fluid balance (by not replacing all ongoing fluid losses). If the diuresis continues, it represents persistent tubular damage. Fluid replacement therapy should then be reinstituted and continued until another trial indicates recovery of tubular function.

References

1. Brenner BM, Humes HD: Mechanics of glomerular ultrafiltration. N Engl J Med 297:184, 1977.
2. Schor N, Ichikawa I, Brenner BM: Glomerular adaptations to chronic dietary salt restriction or excess. Am J Physiol 238:F428, 1980.
3. Woods JW, Blythe WB, Huffines WD: Management of malignant hypertension complicated by renal insufficiency. A follow-up study. N Engl J Med 291:10, 1974.
4. Davidson EW, Dunn MJ: Pathogenesis of the hepatorenal syndrome. Annu Rev Med 38:361, 1987.
5. Gordon JA, Anderson RJ: Hepatorenal syndrome. Semin Nephrol 1:37, 1981.
6. Koppel MH, Coburn JW, Mims MM: Transplantation of cadaveric kidneys from patients with hepatorenal syndrome. N Engl J Med 280:1367, 1969.
7. Iwatsuki S, Popovtzer MM, Corman JL, et al: Recovery from "hepatorenal syndrome" after orthotopic liver transplantation. N Engl J Med 289:1155, 1973.
8. Schroeder ET: Effect of a porta caval and peritoneovenous shunt on renin in the hepatorenal syndrome. Kidney Int 15:54, 1979.
9. Jacobson HR: Ischemic renal disease: An overlooked clinical entity. Kidney Int 34:729, 1988.
10. Hricik DE, Browning PJ, Kapelman R, et al: Captopril-induced functional renal insufficiency in patients with bilateral renal-artery stenoses or renal-artery stenosis in a solitary kidney. N Engl J Med 308:373, 1983.
11. Patrono C, Dunn MJ: The clinical significance of inhibition of renal prostaglandin synthesis. Kidney Int 32:1,1987.
12. Kahan BD (ed): Cyclosporine-associated renal injury. Transplant Proc 17:185, 1985.
13. Sommer BG, Innes JT, Whitehurst RM, et al: Cyclosporine-associated renal arteriopathy resulting in loss of allograft function. Am J Surg 149:756, 1985.
14. Zoja C, Furci L, Ghilardi F, et al: Cyclosporine-induced endothelial cell injury. Lab Invest 55:455, 1986.
15. Jackson NM, Hsu CH, Visscher GE, et al: Alterations in renal structure and function in a rat model of cyclosporine nephrotoxicity. J Pharmacol Exp Ther 242:749, 1987.
16. Murray BM, Paller MS, Ferris TF: Effects of cyclosporine administration on renal hemodynamics in conscious rats. Kidney Int 28:767, 1985.
17. Moss NG, Rowell SL, Falk RJ: Intravenous cyclosporine activates afferent and efferent renal nerves and causes sodium retention in innervated kidneys in rats. Proc Natl Acad Sci USA 82:8222, 1985.
18. Xue H, Bukoski RD, McCarron DA, et al: Induction of contraction in isolated rat aorta by cyclosporine. Transplantation 43:715, 1987.
19. Perico N, Benigni A, Zoja C, et al: Functional significance of exaggerated renal thromboxane A_2 synthesis induced by cyclosporine A. Am J Physiol 251:F581, 1986.
20. Dixon BS, Anderson RJ: Nonoliguric acute renal failure. Am J Kidney Dis 6:71, 1985.
21. Humes HD, Messana JM: Acute renal failure and toxic nephropathy. Contemp Nephrol 5:283, 1989.
22. Humes HD, Weinberg JM: Alterations in renal tubular cell metabolism in acute renal failure. Miner Electrolyte Metab 9:290, 1983.
23. Franklin SS, Merrill JP: Acute renal failure. N Engl J Med 262:711, 1960.
24. Humes HD: Aminoglycoside nephrotoxicity. Kidney Int 33:900, 1988.
25. Moore RD, Smith CR, Lipsky TJ, et al: Risk factors for nephrotoxicity in patients treated with aminoglycosides. Ann Intern Med 100:352, 1984.
26. Dahlgren JG, Anderson ET, Hewlitt WL: Gentamicin blood levels: A guide to nephrotoxicity. Antimicrob Agents Chemother 8:58, 1975.
27. Kahlmeter G, Kahlager J: Aminoglycoside toxicity—A review of clinical studies published between 1975 and 1982. J Antimicrob Chemother 13(suppl A):9, 1984.
28. Andreoli T: On the anatomy of amphotericin B–cholesterol pores in lipid bilayer membranes. Kidney Int 4:337, 1973.
29. Humes HD, Weinberg JM: Toxic nephropathies. In: Brenner BM, Rector FC (eds): The Kidney. 3rd ed. Philadelphia, WB Saunders, p 1491, 1986.
30. Madias NE, Harrington JT: Platinum nephrotoxicity. Am J Med 65:307, 1978.
31. Saffirstein RJ, Winston M, Goldstein D, et al: Cisplatin nephrotoxicity. Am J Kidney Dis 8:356, 1986.
32. Humes HD, Nguyen VD: Acute renal failure and toxic nephropathy. Contemp Nephrol 4:401, 1987.
33. Berns AS: Nephrotoxicity of contrast media. Kidney Int 36:730, 1989.
34. Dubrow A, Flamenbaum W: Acute renal failure associated with myoglobinuria and hemoglobinuria. In: Brenner BM, Rector FC (eds): Acute Renal Failure. 2nd ed. New York, Churchill Livingstone, p 279, 1988.
35. Better OS, Stein JH: Early management of shock and prophylaxis of acute renal failure in traumatic rhabdomyolysis. N Engl J Med 322:825, 1990.
36. Grossman RA, Hamilton RW, Morse BM, et al: Nontraumatic rhabdomyolysis and acute renal failure. N Engl J Med 291:807, 1974.
37. Koffler A, Friedler RM, Massry SG: Acute renal failure due to nontraumatic rhabdomyolysis. Ann Intern Med 85:23, 1976.
38. Kjellstrand CM, Berkseth RO, Klinkman H: Treatment of acute renal failure. In: Schrier RW, Gottschalk CW (eds): Diseases of the Kidney. 4th ed. Boston, Little, Brown, p 1501, 1988.
39. Nicholas GG, Denworth WE Jr: Treatment of renal artery embolism. Arch Surg 119:278, 1984.
40. Henrich WL: Medical considerations in the evaluation of the obstructed renal artery. Am J Med Sci 300:53, 1990.
41. Glassock RJ, Cohen AH, Adler SG, et al: Primary glomerular diseases. In: Brenner BM, Rector FC (eds): The Kidney. 4th ed. Philadelphia, WB Saunders, p 1182, 1986.
42. Glassock RJ, Cohen AM, Adler SC, et al: Secondary glomerular diseases. In: Brenner BM, Rector FC (eds): The Kidney. 4th ed. Philadelphia, WB Saunders, p 1280, 1986.
43. Linton AL, Clark WF, Driedger AA: Acute interstitial nephritis due to drugs. Ann Intern Med 93:735, 1980.
44. Appel GB, Kunis CL: Acute tubulointerstitial nephritis. Contemp Issues Nephrol 10:151, 1983.
45. Neilson BG: Pathogenesis and therapy of interstitial nephritis. Kidney Int 35:1257, 1989.
46. Gillenwater JY: The pathophysiology of urinary obstruction. In: Walsh PC, Gittes RF, Perlmutter AD, et al (eds): Campbell's Urology. 5th ed. Philadelphia, WB Saunders, p 542, 1986.
47. Wilson DR: Urinary tract obstruction. In: Schrier RW, Gottschalk CW (eds): Diseases of the Kidney. 4th ed. Boston, Little, Brown, p 715, 1988.

48. Kjellstrand CM, Campbell DB, von Hartitzsch B, et al: Hyperuricemic acute renal failure. Arch Intern Med 133:349, 1974.
49. Klinenberg JR, Kippen I, Bluesome R: Hyperuricemic nephropathy. Arch Intern Med 138:88, 1978.
50. Jacobs SA, Stoller RG, Chabner BA, et al: 7-Hydroxymethotrexate as a urinary metabolite in human subjects and rhesus monkeys receiving high dose methotrexate. J Clin Invest 57:534, 1976.
51. Gillenwater JY, Westervelt FB Jr, Vaughan E Jr, et al: Renal function after release of chronic unilateral hydronephrosis in man. Kidney Int 7:179, 1975.

CHAPTER 108

Renal Insufficiency

Alan G. Wasserstein

Renal insufficiency adversely affects the prognosis of patients in the intensive care setting. The mortality of patients who require some form of dialysis is 65 to 80%, more than twice that of patients who do not require such support.[1] Despite impressive advances in dialysis technology, this mortality rate is also more than twice that encountered 30 years ago.

Two broad explanations may be offered for these depressing statistics: (1) prognosis is dependent on concomitant or underlying conditions, and (2) renal failure compromises and complicates the management and increases the vulnerability of patients in the intensive care unit. Of these two explanations, the first may be more important. Various modalities to replace renal excretory function are now available; patients do not die of renal failure. However, patients who in the past would have died at an earlier stage of underlying disease, or who would not have been offered surgery, or for whom no surgery was available are now coming to intensive care. In these patients, acute renal failure is often an indicator or marker of the severity of the underlying disease. For example, in patients with prolonged shock and pressor requirements, kidney failure is a predictable complication. In patients with sepsis, kidney failure is a consequence of compromised circulation as well as of the presence of nephrotoxins such as endotoxins and antibiotics. Thus, predisposing factors in the development of renal failure, including circulatory collapse, sepsis, and antibiotic administration, are themselves associated with increased mortality.

In support of this interpretation are the following observations: Isolated renal failure, in the absence of other organ system failure, has a mortality of less than 10%; one additional organ failure increases the mortality to 60%.[2] In one study, for example, the coexistence of severe chronic liver disease with acute renal failure in the intensive care unit was invariably fatal.[3] Factors associated with reduced survival include hypotension, requirement for pressors or inotropes, sepsis, pancreatitis, immunosuppression, and heart failure. Oliguric renal failure has a significantly worse outcome (80% mortality) than nonoliguric renal failure (33% mortality). Although it is easier to manage patients with substantial urine output than those with oliguria, the reason for this difference is likely that oliguric renal failure is typically associated with shock and other severe underlying conditions.

Aside from its significance as a marker of the severity of underlying disease, renal failure can itself contribute to morbidity and mortality in the intensive care setting. Although various modalities of dialytic support are available, they provide an imperfect substitute for the native kidney. Experience with long-term maintenance dialysis makes it clear that dialysis does not restore complete health. There are several possible explanations for this failure: (1) some metabolites or toxins, such as phosphate or so-called middle molecules in the range of 500 to 5000 daltons, are inadequately removed; (2) dialysis may remove some unknown and unmeasured substances to an excessive degree; (3) dialysis support cannot replace endocrine functions of the kidney, including the manufacture of erythropoietin, 1,25-dihydroxycholecalciferol, renin, prostaglandins, and other hormones, some of which may as yet be undescribed; and (4) dialysis may have adverse effects (e.g., exposure to cellulosic hemodialysis membranes may release interleukins and other mediators that favor catabolism or impair white blood cell function).

Important abnormalities persist in even the well-dialyzed patient undergoing long-term dialysis. These include anemia, impaired defenses to bacterial infection and impaired antibody elaboration, catabolic state, bleeding tendency, inability to handle large fluid challenges, bone disease, metastatic calcification, subtle cognitive dysfunction, and neuropathy. Bleeding, infection, and state of nutrition may be of particular relevance in the intensive care setting. In addition, the physiologic demands of that setting may stress the capacity of renal replacement modalities. A highly catabolic state generates waste products of protein metabolism (and uremic toxins) faster than they can be removed. The amount of fluid used in nutritional support, and in antibiotic and pressor therapies, may exceed what can safely be removed at dialysis. Finally, the loss of native ability to regulate body fluids predisposes to electrolyte imbalance.

In summary, in the patient with relatively uncomplicated renal failure, the problems posed by the renal disease are significant but manageable and a good outcome may be expected. This point is supported by the low mortality of uncomplicated renal failure[2] and also by the relatively good outcome of patients undergoing long-term dialysis after coronary arterial bypass grafting.[4] When renal failure supervenes in a patient with multisystem disease, however, it not only is a marker of severity of illness, but also increases significantly the difficulty of management, the risk of complications, and the likelihood of a fatal outcome.

INSULTS TO RENAL FUNCTION

The kidneys receive one fourth of the cardiac output and continuously filter about one fifth of this renal blood flow. These simple facts account, in large part, for their susceptibility to injury. Renal function is critically dependent on adequate perfusion and therefore on adequate systemic circulatory status. The kidneys are also exposed to increased concentrations of exogenous and endogenous toxins in the filtration process.

Impaired renal perfusion can be the consequence of shock (hypovolemic, cardiogenic, or septic shock), extracellular fluid (ECF) volume contraction (salt depletion), congestive heart failure or pericardial tamponade, administration of nonsteroidal anti-inflammatory drugs, liver disease (hepatorenal syndrome), or renovascular disease (including thromboemboli, cholesterol emboli, and dissection). The mechanisms of renal hemodynamic impairment are similar in hypotension, ECF volume contraction, and reduced effective arterial blood volume (congestive heart failure, hepatorenal syndrome): activation of the renin-angiotensin and sympathetic nervous systems causes renal arteriolar vasoconstriction and also reduces the glomerular ultrafiltration coefficient. Low blood flow and (in hypotension) low glomerular hydrostatic pressure reduce the driving force for glomerular filtration while a low ultrafiltration coefficient reduces the glomerular filtration rate (GFR) obtained at any given filtration pressure. Glomerular filtration stops altogether at a mean arterial pressure of about 50 mm Hg.[5]

Renal hemodynamics may be impaired even when blood pressure is in the normal range and the patient is euvolemic. This may occur when, because of large- or small-vessel disease, the patient requires a higher than normal blood pressure to maintain renal perfusion; when the systemic blood pressure is maintained at the expense of vasoconstriction of certain vascular beds, including the renal circulation; or when vascular shunting impairs renal perfusion, as in sepsis.

ECF volume contraction may be due to bleeding, gastrointestinal losses (vomiting, nasogastric suction, fistulas, and diarrhea), or the overzealous use of diuretics. If renal function is intrinsically normal, the renal response is increased tubular sodium reabsorption and the urinary sodium concentration is low (assuming any acute response to diuretics has subsided). Sometimes, volume contraction is a consequence of, or is exacerbated by, renal salt wasting. In these states, which include adrenal insufficiency, certain forms of interstitial renal disease, and the acute response to diuretics, the urinary sodium concentration is inappropriately high.

Similar to true volume contraction are the renal physiologic responses in states of effective arterial hypovolemia, such as congestive heart failure and the hepatorenal syndrome: the renin-angiotensin and sympathetic nervous systems are activated, glomerular perfusion and ultrafiltration are impaired, and the urinary sodium concentration is reduced. In these states, renal perfusion is impaired despite the presence of total body salt and water excess. Correction of effective arterial hypovolemia cannot be accomplished with volume expansion. Rather it requires amelioration of the underlying defect (such as improvement of cardiac performance).

At an early and/or moderate stage of impaired renal perfusion (e.g., caused by ECF volume contraction), renal functional deterioration is quickly reversible if the circulation is restored. However, if hypotension or renal vasoconstriction persists or has been more severe, acute renal failure supervenes and correction of impaired hemodynamics does not immediately restore renal function. A process of renal regeneration, often lasting several weeks, is then necessary. Thus, there is a vulnerable period in renal ischemia, the duration of which depends largely on the severity of the hemodynamic compromise. During this period, the kidneys are most vulnerable to further insults, such as vasoconstriction attributable to pressor agents or nephrotoxins. The transition from the reversible to the irreversible phase is often signaled by a rise in urinary sodium concentration. Low urinary sodium concentration is due to intense sodium reabsorption that characterizes the reversible phase. This is followed by tubular necrosis with resultant failure of sodium reabsorption in the irreversible phase. Prompt restoration of renal perfusion, if possible, before the onset of tubular necrosis should be the goal of therapy.

Nephrotoxins include endotoxin, contrast agents, myoglobin, hemoglobin, and antibiotics (especially aminoglycosides). The acutely ill patient is at risk for exposure to all of these toxins. The adverse effects of nephrotoxins are potentiated, as a general rule, by two factors: ECF volume contraction

and pre-existing renal insufficiency. In radiocontrast nephrotoxicity, other risk factors include diabetes mellitus, albuminuria, hypertension, age over 60 years, dehydration, uric acid level greater than 8 mg/dL, multiple contrast studies, use of more than 2 mg/kg of contrast medium in a single study, and multiple myeloma.[6] In the older patient, renal failure after angiography may be due to cholesterol atheroemboli rather than contrast agent toxicity per se. Aminoglycoside toxicity is favored by hypotension, liver disease, and increased aminoglycoside serum levels (peak level perhaps being more important than trough).[7] Other risk factors include older age, prior exposure, hypokalemia, drug dose and duration of treatment, volume contraction, and concomitant use of cephalothin and other nephrotoxic drugs. Pre-existing renal insufficiency has been assumed to also be a risk factor, but in one study, normal renal function predisposed to toxicity, presumably by increasing renal cortical levels of drug.[7]

PROTECTING RENAL FUNCTION

Insults to the kidneys are virtually inevitable in the acutely ill patient, but their impact can be minimized in a number of ways. First, renal hemodynamics should be optimized and ECF volume contraction avoided. Pressor agents should not be used to support blood pressure in patients with ECF volume contraction; pressors exacerbate renal vasoconstriction, whereas salt and water repletion improve renal blood flow. Second, the incidence of sepsis should be minimized by frequent changing and meticulous care of arterial and venous catheters, endotracheal tubes, and Foley's catheters. Foley's catheters should be avoided if possible. Nephrotoxic antibiotics should also be avoided when possible. Serum levels should always be monitored in patients receiving nephrotoxic antibiotics. Third, the number of contrast studies should be minimized, carefully weighing risk against gain. If these procedures must be performed, the patient should be well hydrated, contrast volume should be minimized, and multiple procedures should be appropriately spaced to allow the serum creatinine concentration to return to baseline before the next study.

Finally, certain pharmacologic agents may be of value in protecting the kidneys if administered before the insult. Mannitol causes a diuresis that may clear cellular debris that would otherwise cause tubular obstruction. Mannitol also restores renal hemodynamics and glomerular filtration pressure and reduces interstitial pressure that might lead to tubular collapse. Furosemide has similar effects on renal blood flow and tubular flow; it also reduces oxygen consumption in the loop of Henle, thereby reducing oxygen demand.

Of the various protective agents, mannitol probably has the most clinical information in its favor, although its superiority over simple saline expansion has not been shown. Mannitol has been reported to protect against acute tubular necrosis after abdominal aortic aneurysm repair, intravenous urography, renal transplantation, and traumatic rhabdomyolysis.[8-11] In patients at high risk (serum creatinine level > 2 mg/dL) who are to be exposed to a potential renal insult, such as contrast agent administration, aortic aneurysm repair, or open heart surgery, a protective regimen is warranted. Normal saline, 500 mL/h for several hours before, during, and after the procedure, and/or 5% mannitol, 500 mL within 60 minutes of the procedure, should be administered. In prevention of acute renal failure after crush injury, a combination of hypotonic saline, sodium bicarbonate, and mannitol has been recommended.[12] Some authors have advised that furosemide be given before contrast agent administration in doses proportional to the severity of renal insufficiency. The use of such regimens may account for the decreasing incidence of oliguric renal failure and the concomitant increasing incidence of nonoliguric renal failure.[6]

AZOTEMIA AND UREMIA

Azotemia refers to a chemical disorder, the accumulation of nitrogenous wastes (urea and creatinine) in the body. *Uremia* is the clinical syndrome that results from the retention of nitrogenous wastes when the chemical disorder is far advanced. *Renal insufficiency* and *renal failure* are vague terms that refer to both the chemical and the clinical disorders, insufficiency usually referring to less severe chemical impairment and failure to more advanced disease. There is a misleading tendency among nephrologists and others to reduce the complexity of renal disease to a single number, the serum creatinine concentration. This is understandable because the simplification of clinical complexities makes them manageable, and the chemical basis of uremia is not understood and so no better available indicator exists. Nevertheless, it should be emphasized that the serum creatinine concentration is an imperfect marker of a complex pathophysiologic state from which it may sometimes be dissociated.

Care of the patient with renal failue is handicapped by inadequate knowledge of what waste products and other substances account for the uremic syndrome. Urea is, at most, a minor toxin, causing perhaps nausea, vomiting, and a bleeding tendency but certainly not central nervous system impairment. Creatinine has no known toxicity. Parathyroid hormone accumulates in renal failure and has diverse toxicities in addition to causing bone disease. Potassium and phosphate, which tend to accumulate in renal failure as well, can also be regarded as uremic toxins. However, in the main, the identity of uremic toxins remains a mystery. I believe that they are products of protein breakdown, and substances such as guanidinosuccinic acid, phenols, and middle molecules have been suggested as putative candidates. The prevailing view is that a variety of nitrogenous wastes, none predominant, account for the syndrome.

Because a specific toxin has not been identified, nephrologists have taken urea to be a surrogate for the true toxins and have tried to optimize its concentration in renal failure. This approach is flawed in that the urea concentration (usually expressed, in the United States, as the blood urea nitrogen [BUN] concentration) is dependent on production as well as excretion, production being a function of protein catabolic rate. Moreover, the production of uremic toxins does not follow the catabolic rate as closely as does the production of urea nitrogen. Therefore, a relatively low BUN level may be found in uremic patients if the patient is malnourished and has a low catabolic rate and consequently a low urea production. Conversely, some patients undergoing long-term dialysis have BUN levels persistently above 100 mg/dL, owing to high protein intake rather than insufficient dialysis, and many of these patients seem to do quite well. Thus, the BUN level is at best a poor marker of uremia. The serum creatinine measurement is also a poor surrogate for the measurement of uremic toxins: patients receiving maintenance dialysis commonly have serum creatinine concentrations of 10 to 15 mg/dL without any overt evidence of uremia. In summary, the BUN and serum creatinine concentrations correlate in general with levels of uremic toxins, but dissociation of the uremic syndrome from circulating concentrations of either of these substances is relatively common.

What the BUN and serum creatinine concentrations really indicate are not so much the circulating amounts of uremic toxins as the level of renal function, with which the accumulation of toxins is inversely correlated. Although the kidney performs multiple functions (some of which may be dissociated in pathologic states), it is traditional and clinically useful to measure renal function in terms of the GFR, which usually correlates well with other functions. However, certain functions may be impaired out of proportion to the decrement in the GFR. For example, some patients are unable to excrete adequate amounts of salt and water, even in response to diuretics, despite relatively well-preserved GFRs. Other patients with only relatively mild renal insufficiency are unable to excrete potassium adequately.

MEASUREMENT OF GLOMERULAR FILTRATION RATE

The BUN level and urea clearance are not useful measures of GFR: the BUN varies with urea production (which depends on the protein catabolic rate) as well as with the GFR, and urea clearance markedly underestimates the GFR because of renal tubular urea reabsorption. Nevertheless, these disadvantages with regard to the measurement of GFR can be of diagnostic utility. For example, a disproportionate rise in the BUN level relative to the serum creatinine concentration may indicate excessive protein breakdown and so be a clue to gastrointestinal bleeding or a catabolic state. Alternatively, it may indicate excessive renal tubular reabsorption of urea, caused by diminished fluid flow rate, and so indicate absolute or effective intravascular volume contraction or urinary tract obstruction. Measurement of the urine urea nitrogen excretion and urea clearance may clarify whether increased production or decreased excretion is responsible for the disproportionate elevation of BUN relative to creatinine.

In clinical practice, GFR is usually estimated from the serum creatinine concentration. Creatinine is produced from the nonenzymatic breakdown of muscle creatine, which occurs at a relatively constant rate that is proportional to muscle mass and age. Hence, for the most part, the use of serum creatinine level to measure GFR is not influenced by variable production such as occurs with urea. An important exception is provided by rhabdomyolysis, in which muscle breakdown releases creatinine at an increased rate and disproportionately elevates the serum creatinine concentration relative to the BUN. Because creatinine production is directly related to muscle mass and inversely related to age, the serum creatinine concentration must be interpreted in light of the patient's age and weight. Equivalent elevations in serum creatinine concentration in an older, smaller person and a younger, more muscular person indicate more renal impairment in the former. These relationships are formalized in the Cockcroft-Gault formulas, in which creatinine clearance (CCr) is estimated from serum creatinine (SCr):

$$CCr = [(140 - age) \times body\ weight\ (kg)/SCr \times 70]$$
in males

$$CCr = [(140 - age) \times body\ weight\ (kg)/SCr \times 70] \times 0.85\ in\ females$$

Whether GFR is estimated from serum creatinine concentration or calculated from the Cockcroft-Gault relations, the result can be interpreted only if renal function is stable. For example, if previously normal renal function suddenly ceases, the serum creatinine concentration rises by 0.5 to 2 mg/dL daily (a higher rate of rise suggests rhabdomyolysis). Calculation of the GFR from the serum creatinine concentration under such circumstances obviously misjudges the true GFR, which is zero.

Creatinine clearance can also be measured directly from timed urine collections. Creatinine clearance in milliliters per minute is given by UCrV/1440 SCr for a 24-hour collection (there are 1440 minutes in 24 hours), where UCrV is urinary creatinine excretion in milligrams and the serum creatinine concentration is expressed in milligrams per milliliter. If the serum creatinine concentration is not stable, the mean of the values at the beginning and end of the collection can be used. In the ambulatory setting, these measurements are flawed by errors in urine collection, but such errors should be avoidable in the intensive care unit, especially if a Foley catheter is in place and the collection period is brief (e.g., 2 hours) and precise.

Whether measured by the Cockcroft-Gault formula or directly, creatinine clearance overestimates the GFR, the degree of overestimation increasing as GFR declines. In advanced renal insufficiency, the creatinine clearance may be as much as twice the GFR. This occurs because creatinine is excreted by tubular secretion as well as by glomerular filtration, and the proportion of creatinine excretion that occurs by secretion increases as renal function worsens.

The best measure of GFR is the inulin clearance, but this test is impractical in the clinical setting. Comparable results can be obtained from excretion of radionuclides such as diethylenetriamine pentaacetic acid and iothalamate, which, like inulin, are filtered by the glomeruli but are neither secreted nor reabsorbed by the renal tubules. These tests require the intravenous injection of the radionuclide and subsequent serum and urine samples during several hours; results correlate well with inulin clearance and are superior to creatinine clearance for measurement of the GFR.[13]

GOALS OF DIALYSIS THERAPY

In the intensive care setting, the presence of uremia is usually judged from its most salient features: altered mental status, fluid overload, pericarditis, acidosis, and hyperkalemia. The decision to initiate dialysis depends on the constellation of these signs and symptoms together with knowledge of the GFR. As a rule, dialysis is often initiated on the basis of the BUN and serum creatinine concentration alone when the BUN exceeds 100 mg/dL and the serum creatinine concentration is 8 to 10 mg/dL. These values generally correspond to a GFR of 5 to 10 mL/min. Earlier dialysis may be required if the patient is oliguric or has fluid overload, hyperkalemia, acidosis, or uremic symptoms. Mental status may, of course, be compromised for reasons other than uremia, but it is customary in patients with impaired mentation to initiate dialysis sooner rather than later because uremic encephalopathy cannot be excluded. On the other hand, dialysis may be deferred despite advanced renal insufficiency if the patient is not oliguric and lacks uremic symptoms. The goal of dialysis is to maintain fluid and electrolyte balance and to avoid cardinal uremic signs and symptoms, including central nervous system depression, pericarditis, and bleeding disorders.

The difficulty of deciding when to initiate dialysis when the nature of uremia is not understood can be illustrated by a frequent problem in the intensive care setting: the patient with BUN elevated out of proportion to serum creatinine concentrations. Most of the time, this constellation is found in the patient receiving enteral or parenteral nutrition, although it may be exacerbated by the presence of volume contraction, poor cardiac output, or gastrointestinal bleeding. The relative contributions of overproduction and underexcretion of urea can be determined from the 24-hour urine urea nitrogen excretion and urea clearance: a urine urea nitrogen level greater than 10 to 15 g/d reflects increased production; a urea clearance less than half of the creatinine clearance reflects impaired excretion. But when and whether to dialyze such patients are problematic. Urea is not a uremic toxin but its levels could possibly rise in

parallel with those of other uremic toxins, some of which derive from protein breakdown. Some investigators have suggested that the GFR be measured by radionuclide technique in this situation, dialysis being performed if the GFR is less than 10 to 15 mL/min.[14] This is a more stringent criterion than is usually utilized and is intended to allow for the possibility that urea accumulation may be a marker of the presence of uremic toxins even when GFR is relatively high.

CENTRAL NERVOUS SYSTEM EFFECTS

Uremia causes central nervous system symptoms ranging from somnolence, fatigue, irritability, depression, inability to concentrate, tremors, and tremulousness to obtundation, seizures, and coma. Signs correlate with these symptoms in roughly the following order of severity: hyperreflexia, asterixis, myoclonus, and seizures. Abnormal mental status in patients undergoing long-term maintenance dialysis should always raise the question of inadequate dialysis, which may occur insidiously: dialysis may be underprescribed, patients may miss cumulative dialysis time, or dialysis access may be stenotic, causing poor removal of uremic toxins. Even patients who are well dialyzed may not have normal cognitive function, as indicated by psychometric testing; hyperparathyroidism and, especially, anemia may contribute to this failure of dialysis to completely normalize mental function, as may unidentified and poorly removed uremic toxins.

The question of dialysis dementia is sometimes raised in patients with renal failure. This syndrome is due to aluminum intoxication, usually because of aluminum-contaminated dialysis water, and is characterized by mutism or dysarthria and characteristic electroencephalographic changes. It is a feature of long-term but not short-term dialysis. However, in long-term dialysis, sepsis may release aluminum into the circulation by an unknown mechanism and precipitate neurologic deterioration.[15]

Dialysis disequilibrium syndrome can also cause mental status changes, as well as headache and cerebral edema; this usually occurs after an initial hemodialysis (but not peritoneal dialysis) treatment. This syndrome, caused by rapid removal of osmotically active particles from the ECF and the subsequent shift of fluid to the intracellular space, occurs during the intitation of dialysis in chronic renal failure but less commonly in acute renal failure. Spontaneous subdural hematoma is another cause of imparied mental status that is well recognized in patients undergoing maintenance dialysis.

The question of the extent to which uremia contributes to mental status changes is often raised in regard to critically ill patients with renal failure, and a trial of dialysis is sometimes initiated despite relatively small elevations of BUN and serum creatinine concentrations. Although uremic mental status changes are difficult to exclude definitively, especially in comatose patients, other causes of mental status impairment, particularly sepsis, impaired cerebral perfusion, hypoxemia, electrolyte abnormalities (hypercalcemia, hyponatremia), and medications (especially narcotics and hypnotics), are more likely offenders in this setting. Patients with renal failure are particularly sensitive to narcotics.

EXTRACELLULAR FLUID VOLUME STATUS AND CARDIOPULMONARY FUNCTION

The patient with renal failure is susceptible to hypovolemia as well as fluid overload. Even in mild-to-moderate renal insufficiency, concentrating ability (i.e., the ability to conserve water during fluid deprivation) is impaired. Particularly in interstitial renal disease, there may also be a tendency to salt wasting, which emerges when salt intake or ECF fluid volume is abruptly reduced. Thus, the kidney in mild-to-moderate renal failure does not conserve salt and water normally in response to hypovolemia, and in consequence, hypovolemia may be exacerbated. In the same fashion, loss of the ability to conserve salt and water during the recovery phase of acute tubular necrosis also predisposes to hypovolemia.

Moderate renal insufficiency should not be regarded as routinely tending to fluid overload; rather it may favor salt and water losses. In general, it is inappropriate to restrict salt and water intake in patients with mild-to-moderate renal failure unless one has a specific goal in mind (e.g., treatment of congestive heart failure, hypertension, or edema) because of the risk of worsening renal function. This is particularly true in the intensive care setting, where patients are exposed to a multitude of potential renal insults, especially when one considers that an adequate state of hydration is protective against many of these insults.

On the other hand, the impaired kidney may not be able to keep pace with the large volumes of fluid typically administered in the intensive care unit. Urine output may be inadequate to maintain fluid balance even when GFR is only mildly to moderately reduced, especially if cardiac performance is impaired. Diuretics are commonly used in such situations but must be administered correctly: the dose of a loop diuretic must be adequate to obtain a significant response, and the adequate dose should be repeated as needed in preference to giving a single massive dose, which does not increase urine output above the maximal response but which may lead to extrarenal toxicity. Ultrafiltration may be necessary to treat fluid overload in patients who are resistant to diuretics; sometimes such ultrafiltration improves cardiac performance (by decreasing left ventricular end-diastolic volume) to the extent that renal salt excretion and water excretion are restored. In patients requiring dialysis, continuous arteriovenous hemofiltration or continuous arteriovenous hemodialysis has emerged as a superior means of dialysis for the patient with high obligatory fluid administration; conventional hemodialysis may have to be performed daily, and aggressive ultrafiltration during the short duration of a standard dialysis session (usually 4 hours) predisposes to hemodynamic instability. Peritoneal dialysis affords the same slow, steady removal of large amounts of fluid as continuous arteriovenous hemodialysis but is impractical in patients with abdominal pathologic changes or after abdominal surgery.

Whether cardiopulmonary function is affected by renal failure itself (rather than by associated fluid retention) is unresolved. Factors in chronic renal failure that may adversely affect cardiac performance include long-standing anemia, iron overload (caused by multiple blood transfusions), elevated levels of parathyroid hormone (shown to be toxic to myocardial cells in tissue culture), myocardial calcification, dialysis fistula (causing high-output failure), long-standing hypertension, and associated coronary artery disease.[16] An unidentified uremic toxin may also play a role, as indicated by observations of dramatic improvement of impaired ejection fraction soon after renal transplantation in patients undergoing maintenance dialysis.[17]

Patients receiving maintenance dialysis have two distinct forms of congestive heart failure that are indistinguishable on clinical grounds: (1) a dilated cardiomyopathy (with reduced ejection fraction) that is best treated with digitalis and vasodilators and (2) a hypertrophic cardiomyopathy (with normal or increased ejection fraction) that is best treated with beta-blockers and calcium channel blockers. Diagnostic discrimination depends on echocardiography.[18] Renal failure has also been said to increase alveolar capillary permeability and thereby cause noncardiogenic pulmonary edema, but there is no evidence to support this conjecture.[19]

BLEEDING

Acute renal failure increases the risk of clinical bleeding in the intensive care setting by three- to fourfold.[20] In renal failure, coagulation factors are normal but platelet function is impaired; bleeding time and platelet adherence are abnormal.[21] The specific cause of the platelet defect is unknown. Abnormal von Willebrand's factor has been suggested but not confirmed. An important element appears to be anemia; both the transfusion of washed red blood cells[22] and the administration of erythropoietin[23] have corrected platelet dysfunction. Higher packed cell volume (>30%) may have a rheological effect to increase platelet proximity to the vascular wall.

Inadequate dialysis exacerbates uremic bleeding, but intensive dialysis does not necessarily correct it, and many apparently well-dialyzed patients with chronic renal failure have abnormal bleeding times. Furthermore, the initiation of dialysis does not improve bleeding time until uremic platelets have been replaced by newly synthesized platelets, which requires a week or more. Hemodialysis or continuous arteriovenous hemodialysis may exacerbate bleeding because of heparin exposure. Consequently, regional heparinization, citrate or prostacyclin anticoagulation, heparin-free dialysis, or peritoneal dialysis may be preferable in the actively bleeding patient.

In addition to blood transfusion, other maneuvers are available to rapidly correct a prolonged bleeding time. Desmopressin, a vasopressin analogue, stimulates the release of factor VIII multimers by endothelial cells.[24] Although these multimers are not deficient in renal failure, the increase improves platelet function and reduces the bleeding time. The effect is maximal within 4 hours of the administration of desmopressin (0.3 µg/kg intravenously) but tachyphylaxis is common. Cryoprecipitate, which contains factor VIII multimers, can be used for the same purpose but carries the risk of transmission of hepatitis or acquired immunodeficiency syndrome. High-dose intravenous conjugated estrogen (0.6 mg/kg intravenously daily for 5 days) reduces the bleeding time by an unknown mechanism.[25]

Renal failure also increases the incidence of gastrointestinal abnormalities associated with bleeding. The incidence of peptic ulcer disease is not increased in patients undergoing maintenance dialysis, but superficial mucosal ulcerations are common. The incidence of arteriovenous malformations in the stomach, the duodenum, and the colon is increased, and arteriovenous malformations may account for a substantial proportion of cases of gastrointestinal bleeding in patients receiving dialysis. Renal failure is associated with a characteristic but asymptomatic gastroenteritis (nodular duodenitis, prominent gastric rugal folds). Diverticulosis is extremely common in polycystic kidney disease. Isolated colonic ulcers of unknown cause may also result in bleeding.[26]

Other manifestations of the bleeding diathesis in renal failure include spontaneous subdural hematoma, spontaneous subcapsular liver hematoma, and retroperitoneal hemorrhage, either spontaneous or after femoral arterial or venous cannulation.

ELECTROLYTE DISORDERS

Renal failure impairs the ability to excrete a water load. Urine-diluting ability is better preserved than is concentrating ability, but the volume of electrolyte-free water that can be excreted is diminished in proportion to the fall in GFR. Hence, administration of hypotonic fluids can lead to hypotonic hyponatremia and its attendant risk of cerebral edema. This problem can be minimized by restricting water intake and limiting hypotonic fluid administration; administered fluids may have to be given as normal saline to achieve this. Dialysis or continuous arteriovenous hemofiltration can be used to help in maintaining water balance, especially if dialysis is performed against a dialysate of high sodium concentration.

In the absence of the nephrotic syndrome, excretion of sodium is often surprisingly well preserved in chronic renal failure until dialysis is needed. Although the filtered load of sodium is reduced, renal tubular reabsorption of sodium falls proportionally, permitting appropriate urinary sodium excretion. However, rapid changes in volume status or the administration of excessive sodium loads may stress the sodium excretory system beyond its capacities. Loop diuretics act from the luminal side of the tubular epithelium, and increased doses are often necessary to achieve the desired effects in patients with renal insufficiency.

Acute renal failure, especially if oliguric, impairs renal potassium excretion. As with sodium excretion, potassium excretion is usually surprisingly well preserved in chronic renal failure (unless hyporeninemic hypoaldosteronism is present) until dialysis becomes necessary. Hyperkalemia can be exacerbated by a high potassium intake and administration of potassium-sparing diuretics; heparin, which inhibits aldosterone biosynthesis; nonselective sympatholytic agents, which inhibit potassium translocation into the intracellular fluid compartment; angiotensin-converting enzyme inhibitors, which reduce aldosterone levels; and nonsteroidal anti-inflammatory agents, because vasodilator prostaglandins promote potassium excretion; as well as tissue breakdown, as in rhabdomyolysis, with release of potassium from intracellular stores, and insulin deficiency, insulin being permissive for the intracellular disposition of potassium. Mineral acidosis, which accompanies renal failure, shifts potassium out of cells and worsens hyperkalemia. In contrast, organic acidosis, as occurs in lactic acidosis and ketoacidosis, has relatively little effect in this regard.

Renal failure reduces the serum calcium concentration, both because of phosphate retention and because of reduced renal synthesis of the active metabolite of vitamin D (1,25-dihydroxycholecalciferol). Although the reduction of the serum calcium concentration is sometimes severe, tetany is unusual, probably because of the concomitant acidosis. Bolus administration of sodium bicarbonate should be avoided; it can unmask tetany in the hypocalcemic patient with renal failure. In acute renal failure, hypocalcemia is generally less severe than in chronic renal failure. An exception is rhabdomyolysis, in which the phosphate released from damaged cells may give rise to dramatic hyperphosphatemia and hypocalcemia as calcium deposits in damaged muscle (dystrophic calcification). The serum phosphate concentration begins to rise in renal failure when GFR falls below 25 to 30 mL/min. Again, the elevation is characteristic of chronic rather than acute renal failure, but rapid rises in the serum phosphate concentration can occur in acute renal failure when phosphate is released from intracellular stores into the ECF (rhabdomyolysis and tumor lysis). Calcium should be administered cautiously in the presence of hyperphosphatemia, and administration of phosphate (including phosphate enemas) should generally be avoided in renal failure. Magnesium is excreted by the kidneys, and mild and asymptomatic hypermagnesemia is a feature of renal failure. Magnesium accumulation is rarely a clinical problem, however, if magnesium-containing compounds, such as certain antacids, are avoided.

Renal failure is generally associated with a moderate anion gap acidosis at serum creatinine concentrations greater than 4 mg/dL. Acidosis is due to diminished ammonia production, which impairs the excretion of fixed acids generated during the metabolism of an acid-ash (protein) diet. The anion gap is due to retention of phosphates and sulfates. The acidosis of renal failure, being due to failure to excrete acids generated in normal metabolism, is gradual in onset and the anion gap rarely exceeds 20 to 25 mEq/L; higher values suggest lactic acidosis, ketoacidosis, or intoxications. Acidosis can be ameliorated by protein restriction, but this is rarely feasible in acutely ill patients. Renal failure limits the amount of alkali that can be given to ameliorate acidemia because of volume overload. If substantial amounts of alkali are required, dialysis is usually necessary.

ANEMIA

The anemia of renal failure correlates with the degree of renal insufficiency (serum creatinine concentration > 2 mg/dL) and is found in approximately 90% of patients undergoing long-term dialysis. However, the correlation is not precise, and among individuals, there is considerable variability in the severity of anemia for a given degree of renal failure. In acute renal failure, the packed red blood cell volume falls by about 1% per day, so that a relatively normal value generally indicates recent onset of renal failure.

The causes of anemia in renal failure are multifactorial: most important is insufficient erythropoietin production;[27] other factors include uremic suppression of the bone marrow, reduced red blood cell survival, and in dialysis patients, chronic gastrointestinal blood loss, loss of blood associated with the dialysis procedure itself, iron deficiency, and aluminum intoxication. Erythropoietin is produced by renocortical interstitial cells in response to oxygen delivery. Circulating levels in patients with renal failure are far below those appropriate for patients with comparable degrees of anemia without renal failure. Treatment with erythropoietin corrects (or markedly ameliorates) anemia in the large majority of patients with renal failure. Such treatment has also revealed that a number of complaints previously attributed to uremia, including somnolence, fatigue, and sexual dysfunction, are, in fact, largely due to anemia.[27, 28]

Patients receiving erythropoietin should continue to receive it in the intensive care unit. However, intercurrent illness, especially infection, sharply impairs the bone marrow response to erythropoietin; this has been attributed to impaired iron utilization. Therefore, a fall in the hemoglobin concentration should be anticipated even if erythropoietin administration is continued or the dosage is increased. Whether a feasible increase in dosing can lessen the need for blood transfusions in this setting is not known. Whether erythropoietin can be used to treat the anemia associated with acute renal failure in the intensive care unit is also unclear. The dose would have to be high to get a response within 1 or 2 weeks, and response to the drug is poor in patients with inflammatory illness, so it seems unlikely.

Patients with chronic renal failure adjust to anemia by various means, including high cardiac output, redistribution of blood flow, and enhanced production of 2,3-diphosphoglycerate (which promotes unloading of oxygen at the tissue level). Hence, the level at which such patients require blood transfusion is usually lower than that in other patients. However, in some patients, maintenance of a relatively high hemoglobin concentration (>10 g/dL) is required for the prevention of angina.

INFECTION

Renal failure predisposes to infection with common bacterial pathogens, including staphylococci and gram-negative rods. Although patients with renal failure are often described as immunosuppressed, infection by opportunistic pathogens is not increased. The susceptibility to bacterial infection is multifactorial. Bacterial portals of entry are increased because of repeated vascular or peritoneal access; skin flora, especially staphylococci, are therefore common pathogens. White blood cell function, including migration and phagocytosis, is impaired. Macrophage Fc receptors, required for clearance of antibody-coated bacteria, are impaired in patients receiving maintenance hemodialysis; this defect is independent of the duration of renal failure and is only partially improved by hemodialysis.[29] Impairment of white blood cell function may be a consequence of dialysis with cellulosic membranes, which may generate various cytokines. Antibody production in dialysis patients is impaired, so that the capacity to develop protective levels after administration of influenza and hepatitis vaccines is diminished.

Infection of the vascular access is usually indicated by local erythema and swelling but may be present even when physical findings are unremarkable. Infection of an arteriovenous fistula may be treated with antibiotics alone with good hope of cure, but infection of a vascular graft (polytetrafluoroethylene) virtually always necessitates removal of the graft. Infection of temporary subclavian and jugular dialysis catheters is a significant problem and necessitates catheter removal. Cuffed Silastic central catheters can, however, sometimes be cured of infection without catheter removal.

Peritonitis in patients receiving peritoneal dialysis is characterized by peritoneal fluid white blood cell counts above 100/mm^3, abdominal pain, and positive cultures; any two of these are sufficient for diagnosis and cultures are negative in 10 to 20% of cases. Mixed flora on Gram's stain or culture of peritoneal fluid indicates a perforated viscus rather than dialysis-related infection.

In addition to dialysis access problems, sources of bacterial infection include pneumonia and urinary tract infection. Patients undergoing dialysis can have purulent infection of the defunctionalized bladder (pyocystis), which may not be obvious on physical examination and which is easily investigated with bladder catheterization. Tuberculosis is more common in the population receiving dialysis than in the general population, and extrapulmonary tuberculosis is disproportionately common. Cutaneous anergy is frequent in dialysis patients and makes the diagnosis more difficult.

Viral infections include hepatitis and human immunodeficiency virus infection. Hepatitis B continues to be a problem in patients undergoing long-term dialysis, but the epidemic of the early 1970s has abated with the introduction of effective screening of transfused blood and the enforcement of universal barrier precautions in dialysis units. Hepatitis C is now the most common form of hepatitis in patients undergoing dialysis and, like hepatitis B, is mainly transmitted through blood transfusions. Chronic hepatitis after hepatitis C exposure is common but usually asymptomatic. Human immunodeficiency virus infection is both a cause of renal failure and a consequence of blood transfusion in dialysis patients (before the introduction of human immunodeficiency virus screening in 1985). Patients with acquired immunodeficiency syndrome who are undergoing dialysis have extremely poor survival (<6 months), but patients with asymptomatic human immunodeficiency virus infection may do well for several years or more.

NUTRITION

Acute renal failure induces a hypercatabolic state, the severity of which varies with underlying disease. Patients with hypotension, sepsis, or rhabdomyolysis break down protein and generate urea at rates three times those of patients with other causes of renal failure. The hypercata-

bolic state is apparently due to uremia per se, but specific mechanisms are unknown. In addition, hemodialysis with cellulosic membranes is itself directly catabolic, probably because of the generation of tumor necrosis factor or other mediators when blood cells interact with the dialysis membrane.

Nitrogen balance cannot be conveniently measured directly. However, nitrogen production is directly proportional to protein intake and provides a convenient estimate of nitrogen balance. Urea nitrogen production (in grams per day) is given by the sum of the urine urea nitrogen excretion, the change in body urea nitrogen, and the dialysate urea nitrogen excretion. Urine urea nitrogen is obtained from a 24-hour urine collection. The change in body urea nitrogen is given by the product of the difference in BUN on successive days and total body water (estimated as 60% of body weight in kilograms). Dialysate urea nitrogen can be ignored if the results are obtained on a nondialysis day. If peritoneal dialysis or continuous arteriovenous hemodialysis is in progress, the dialysate urea nitrogen is given by the product of the final dialysate urea concentration (at the completion of a peritoneal exchange or at the end of the dialysate outflow port of the continuous arteriovenous hemodialysis filter) and the total 24-hour dialysate volume.

Protein catabolic rate can be obtained from the following relationship:

$$6.25[\text{urea nitrogen production (g/d)} + 0.31\text{body weight (kg)}]$$

where nonurea nitrogen production reflects the fixed excretion of nitrogen in forms other than urea, such as creatinine, uric acid, and ammonia. Such nonurea nitrogen excretion is directly proportional to body weight (31 mg/kg of body weight). Using this relationship, it is relatively easy to compare the patient's known protein (or amino acid) intake with the calculated protein catabolic rate. If protein catabolism exceeds intake, the patient is catabolic. Such estimates are helpful in assessing the potential causes of an elevated BUN/serum creatinine concentration ratio; in calculating the amount of dialysis or continuous arteriovenous hemodialysis required to achieve a desired BUN; and in following the effect of treatment on the catabolic state.

Nitrogen balance is maintained at a protein intake of approximately 0.6 g/kg of body weight per day in normal volunteers and in patients with chronic renal failure who are not receiving dialysis therapy. Stable patients receiving maintenance hemodialysis require a protein intake of 1.1 g/kg/d, in part because hemodialysis is a catabolic stimulus; during periods of illness a protein intake of 1.2 to 1.5 g/kg/d is recommended.[30] Stable patients receiving peritoneal dialysis require higher protein intakes (1.2 to 1.3 g/kg/d) than stable patients undergoing hemodialysis because of protein losses across the peritoneal membrane; during acute illness, or with peritonitis (which increases peritoneal protein losses), the protein requirement rises to 1.5 g/kg/d. Thus, in the intensive care setting, where catabolism during renal failure is the rule, the protein requirement generally ranges between 1.2 and 1.5 g/kg/d, the upper end of the range being necessary for extremely catabolic patients.

Patients with acute renal failure who are not acutely ill and not catabolic may benefit from a low nitrogen intake with a high proportion of essential amino acids to minimize the generation of nitrogenous waste products; dialysis may sometimes even be avoided in this way. More catabolic patients require higher nitrogen intakes and a mixture of essential and nonessential amino acids is usually provided. The elevation of BUN is less when essential amino acids alone are given; however, the large quantities of essential amino acids required for catabolic patients lead to marked distortions of the normal amino acid profile and probably do not support protein synthesis.

The energy requirement of patients undergoing maintenance dialysis is approximately 38 kilocalories/kg of body weight per day.[31] However, the average patient undergoing maintenance dialysis consumes even less than the 30 kilocalories/kg/d recommended for normal individuals. This is the main reason for the tendency to wasting and weight loss in the dialysis population. In acutely ill patients with renal failure, the energy requirement is said to rise to 40 to 50 kilocalories/kg/d, the upper end of this range being necessary for patients with severe illness, sepsis, burns, or a urea nitrogen production in excess of intake. However, studies to support these recommendations have not been done. Indeed, provision of a high caloric intake often fails to ameliorate the catabolic state in acutely ill patients with renal failure.

The high energy requirement of catabolic patients with acute renal failure obligates substantial fluid administration. Dextrose (70%) can be employed to minimize fluid volume. Partial parenteral nutrition is generally unable to supply the necessary calories because hyperosmolar solutions (>600 mOsm/kg) cause phlebitis. However, glucose in peritoneal dialysis solutions provides an additional 800 kilocalories daily, which should also be taken into account. Because of high fluid administration, as noted earlier, hemodialysis may have to be performed on a daily basis. Techniques of slow continuous fluid removal, such as continuous arteriovenous hemodialysis or peritoneal dialysis (if possible), are more convenient in this situation.

Lipid infusions are helpful to provide calories and to avoid essential fatty acid deficiency.[30] Excessive glucose administration increases carbon dioxide production (delaying weaning from the ventilator) and also causes fatty liver. Patients with chronic renal failure may have impaired fat utilization; triglyceride levels should be checked after lipid infusion and the frequency of infusion reduced if these levels are excessive.

DRUG DOSING

Renal failure affects drug metabolism in several ways: absorption, volume of distribution, metabolism, protein binding, and excretion may all be affected. The effect of dialysis on drug metabolism must also be assessed. Careful attention to drug dosing is essential in patients with renal failure. Any alteration in renal function should trigger a reassessment of the dosing of all medications. The diverse effects of renal failure on drug dosing are discussed in other chapters within this section.

References

1. Jochimsen F, Schafer JH, Distler A: Impairment of renal function in medical intensive care: Predictability of acute renal failure. Crit Care Med 18:480, 1990.
2. Fisher MM, Raper RF: The optimization of renal function in acute illness. Med J Aust 149:546, 1988.
3. Maher ER, Robinson KN, Scoble JE, et al: Prognosis of critically-ill patients with acute renal failure: APACHE II score and other predictive factors. Q J Med 72:857, 1989.
4. Deutsch E, Bernstein R, Addonizio P, et al: Coronary artery bypass surgery in patients on chronic hemodialysis. A case-control study. Ann Intern Med 110:369, 1989.
5. Myers BD, Moran SM: Hemodynamically mediated acute renal failure. N Engl J Med 314:97, 1986.
6. Berns AS: Nephrotoxicity of contrast media. Kidney Int 36:730, 1989.
7. Moore RD, Smith CS, Lipsky TJ, et al: Risk factors for nephrotoxicity in patients treated with aminoglycosides. Ann Intern Med 100:352, 1984.
8. Barry KG, Cohen A, Knochel JP, et al: Mannitol infusion II. The prevention of acute functional renal failure during resection of an aneurysm of the abdominal aorta. N Engl J Med 264:967, 1961.
9. Anto HR, Chou SY, Porush JG, et al: Infusion intravenous pyelography and renal function. Effect of hypertonic mannitol in patients with chronic renal insufficiency. Arch Intern Med 141:1652, 1981.
10. Weimar W, Geerlings W, Bijnen AB, et al: A controlled study on the effect of mannitol on immediate renal function after cadaver donor kidney transplantation. Transplantation 35:99, 1983.
11. Ron D, Taitelman U, Michaelson M, et al: Prevention of acute renal failure in traumatic rhabdomyolysis. Arch Intern Med 144:277, 1984.
12. Better OS, Stein JH: Early management of shock and prophylaxis of acute renal failure in traumatic rhabdomyolysis. N Engl J Med 322:825, 1990.
13. Wharton WW, Sondeen JL, Gradwohl SE, et al: Assessment of glomerular filtration rate (GFR) in intensive care patients (ICP) with renal dysfunction (RD) using 99mTc diethylenetriaminepentaacetic acid (DTPA). J Am Soc Nephrol 1:297, 1990.
14. Kon V, Ichikawa I: Dialysis for azotemia due to congestive heart failure. Semin Dialysis 3:135, 1990.
15. Davenport A, Williams PS, Roberts NB, et al: Sepsis: A cause of aluminum release from tissue stores associated with acute neurological dysfunction and mortality. Clin Nephrol 30:48, 1988.
16. London GM, Guerin AP, Marchais SJ, et al: Cardiomyopathy in endstage renal failure. Semin Dialysis 2:102, 1989.
17. Burt RK, Gupta-Burt S, Suki WN, et al: Reversal of left ventricular dysfunction after renal transplantation. Ann Intern Med 111:635, 1989.
18. Harnett JD, Grifiths SM, Gault MH, et al: Congestive heart failure in dialysis patients. Arch Intern Med 148:1519, 1988.
19. Morgan AG: Contribution of uremia to pulmonary edema in ESRD. Semin Dialysis 2:192, 1989.
20. Brown RB, Klar J, Teres D, et al: Prospective study of clinical bleeding in intensive care unit patients. Crit Care Med 16:1171, 1988.
21. Remuzzi G: Bleeding in renal failure. Lancet 2:1205, 1988.
22. Livio M, Gotti E, Marchesi D, et al: Uraemic bleeding: Role of anaemia and beneficial effect of red cell transfusions. Lancet 2:1013, 1982.
23. Moia M, Mannucci PM, Vizzotto L, et al: Improvement in the haemostatic defect of uraemia after treatment with recombinant human erythropoietin. Lancet 2:1227, 1987.
24. Mannucci PM, Remuzzi G, Pusineri F, et al: Deamino-8-arginine vasopressin shortens the bleeding time in uremia. N Engl J Med 308:8, 1983.
25. Livio M, Mannucci PM, Vigano G, et al: Conjugated estrogens for the management of bleeding associated with renal failure. N Engl J Med 315:731, 1986.
26. Bills B, Zuckerman G, Sicard G: Discrete colon ulcers as a cause of lower gastrointestinal bleeding and perforation in endstage renal disease. Surgery 89:548, 1981.
27. Eschbach JW, Egrie JC, Downing MR, et al: Correction of the anemia of end-stage renal disease with recombinant human erythropoietin. N Engl J Med 316:73, 1987.
28. Eschbach JW, Kelly MR, Haley NR, et al: Treatment of the anemia of progressive renal failure with recombinant human erythropoietin. N Engl J Med 321:158, 1989.
29. Ruiz P, Gomez F, Schreiber AD: Impaired function of macrophage Fc receptors in end-stage renal disease. N Engl J Med 322:717, 1990.
30. Wolfson M: Parenteral hyperalimentation in dialysis patients. Semin Dialysis 3:254, 1990.
31. Slomowitz LA, Monteon FJ, Grosvenor M, et al: Effect of energy intake on nutritional status in maintenance hemodialysis patients. Kidney Int 35:704, 1989.

CHAPTER 109

Dialysis and Hemoperfusion

Principles of Dialysis Therapy

Richard K. Kasama
Pedro C. Fernandez

Dialysis is the act or process of separating substances in solution by means of a membrane that allows certain constituents of the solution to pass while restricting the passage of others. Several forms of dialysis or closely related treatment modalities are available for the prevention or management of uremia, circulatory overload, and life-threatening electrolyte disturbances and for the removal of exogenous toxic substances. The manner, extent, and rapidity of achieving any of these therapeutic goals vary markedly from one dialysis modality to another, as do the prerequisites, side effects, and complications of the various forms of dialysis. Once the specific circumstances and therapeutic goals are established for a given patient, a dialysis treatment modality should be chosen that best suits that patient's particular condition and needs. Such an approach offers the best chance of success in managing critically ill patients with multiple organ system involvement.

BASIC CONCEPTS

Physicochemical Principles of Solute and Fluid Removal

During dialysis, solutes are removed from plasma across a semipermeable membrane. There are two mechanisms of solute transfer across dialysis membranes: diffusion and convection. Diffusion is the movement of solute from plasma into an artificial electrolyte solution (dialysate), driven by a difference (or gradient) in solute concentration. The rate of solute diffusion (solute flux) is proportional to the solute concentration gradient and to the overall membrane permeability to that solute. Membrane permeability depends on both intrinsic membrane properties and membrane surface area. Convection is the transfer of solute "dragged" along with solvent. Solvent movement occurs when there is ultrafiltration of plasma across a semipermeable membrane in response to transmembrane hydrostatic or osmotic pressure gradients. Convective solute flux depends on the overall membrane permeability to the particular solute and on the rate of ultrafiltration. The ultrafiltration rate is proportional to the hydraulic conductivity of the membrane, usually expressed as its ultrafiltration coefficient, K_{UF}, and to the transmembrane pressure gradient.

Traditionally, the term *dialysis* is employed to describe forms of treatment in which solute removal occurs mostly by diffusion, such as hemodialysis and peritoneal dialysis. By contrast, *hemofiltration* refers to solute removal exclusively by convective transfer (together with replacement of ultrafiltration fluid losses with artificial solutions). Removal of small and highly permeant solutes, such as urea, may be similarly accomplished by both forms of solute transfer. However, hemofiltration is more effective in removing larger and therefore less permeant solutes.

Bioengineering of Artificial Dialyzers

Dialysis Membranes. Dialysis membranes either are derived from the natural D-glucose polymer cellulose or are synthetic polymers. The two kinds of membranes differ in hydraulic conductivity and solute permeability and in their capacity to interact with blood coming in contact with the membrane (biocompatibility).

In general, membranes made of synthetic polymers, such as polyacrylonitrile, polysulfone, poly(methyl methacrylate), and polyamide, have much higher hydraulic conductivity and are more permeable to higher-molecular-weight solutes than are cellulose-derived membranes.[1] Dialyzers incorporating such membranes not only are well suited for hemofiltration but also achieve high clearances of relatively large compounds even when ultrafiltration is kept to a minimum. The ultrafiltration capacity and permeability of cellulose-derived membranes can be increased by reducing membrane thickness and by modifying their basic cellulose structure. The membranes thus achieved (cellulose, cupratetraammonium dihydroxide [cuprophane], cellulose acetate, and other modified or substituted celluloses) also differ from each other in biocompatibility.[1, 2]

Biocompatibility is an extremely complex phenomenon, involving adsorption and/or transformation-activation of both coagulation and complement proteins.[2, 3] Clinically, this may result in clotting of the dialyzer and in release of powerful anaphylatoxins. These reactions are responsible for such untoward intradialytic events as pulmonary hypertension, hypoxemia, and leukopenia and for some of the anaphylactoid reactions that are part of the so-called first-use syndrome. Release of anaphylatoxins is higher with cuprophane than with modified cellulose membranes and is lowest when synthetic membranes are used.[2, 3]

Hemodialysis is also associated with activation of monocytes and lymphocytes, resulting in increased synthesis of such cytokines as interleukin-1, tumor necrosis factor, and possibly interleukin-2.[2] These substances may be responsible for intradialytic pyrogenic reactions, postdialysis lassitude, and accelerated protein catabolism and chronic wasting. The relative contributions of different dialysis membranes and of dialysate bacterial products to cytokine production remain to be elucidated.

The complexity of the biocompatibility problem is exemplified by the fact that adsorption of β_2-microglobulin to a poly(methyl methacrylate) membrane may be desirable because it may prevent the late development of amyloidosis.[4] The same membrane, however, has the undesirable effect of adsorbing erythropoietin, which may exacerbate the anemia of chronic renal failure. How the use of specific membranes and manipulation of biocompatibility-related factors may influence the outcome for critically ill patients awaits further study.

Configuration and Characteristics of Dialyzers. A dialyzer consists of a blood compartment and a dialysate (or ultrafiltrate) compartment, separated from each other by the dialysis membrane. Only two dialyzer designs are in common use.[5, 6] In the hollow-fiber dialyzer (Fig. 109–1), the membrane consists of thousands of capillary tubes, or hollow fibers, each about 200 μm in diameter. A bundle of fibers is encased and sealed at each end into a rigid plastic container. The blood flows inside the fibers and the dialysate circulates outside and around them. In the parallel-plate dialyzer (see Fig. 109–1), sets of two membrane sheets, sandwiched between supporting screens, are stacked on top of each other and enclosed in a rigid casing. Blood flows in thin films between the two membrane sheets and dialysate runs on the outside, along channels sculptured in the supporting screen.

To ensure the largest possible solute transfer, the solute

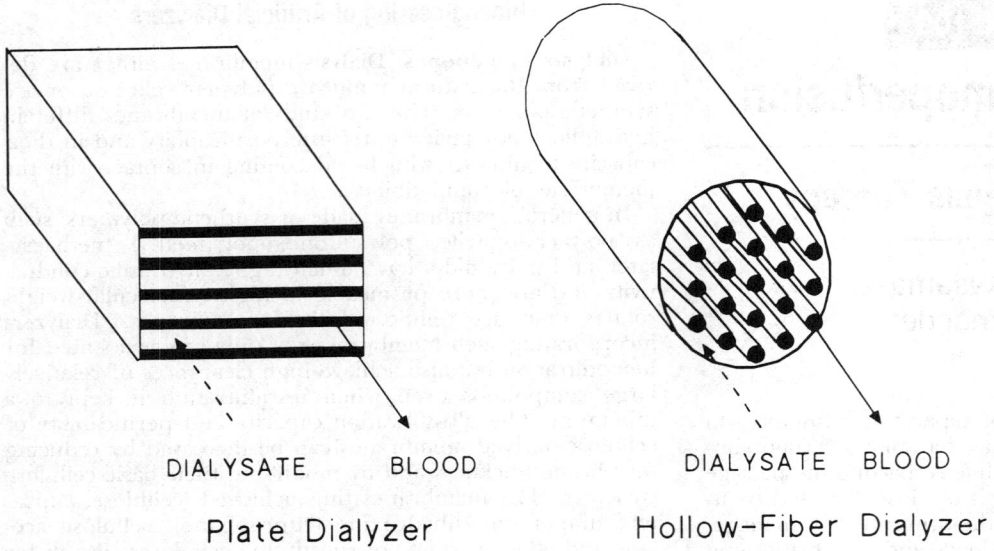

Figure 109–1. Schematic views of parallel-plate and hollow-fiber dialyzers, illustrating the countercurrent flow of blood and dialysate.

DIALYSATE   BLOOD

Plate Dialyzer

DIALYSATE   BLOOD

Hollow-Fiber Dialyzer

concentration gradient between blood and dialysate is kept at a maximum. This is accomplished by having the dialysate flow countercurrent to the flow of blood. Variable rates of ultrafiltration are achieved by altering the hydrostatic pressure across the membrane, usually by creating a negative pressure in the rigid dialysate compartment.

Clinical appraisal of dialyzers involves evaluation of their fluid and solute removal capabilities.[5, 6] Fluid removal capability is given by the ultrafiltration coefficient, K_{UF}, expressed in milliliters per hour per millimeter of mercury of transmembrane pressure. The capacity to remove small solutes is reflected by the urea clearance and the capacity to remove larger solutes ("middle molecules," molecular weight up to 1000 to 1500) by the clearance of vitamin B_{12}. Table 109–1 lists the average in vitro K_{UF} and the clearances of urea and vitamin B_{12} for both hollow-fiber and parallel-plate dialyzers with either cellulose or synthetic membranes. Increasing membrane surface area increases fluid and solute removal capabilities, but it may also impair biocompatibility. The

synthetic membrane dialyzers used in continuous arteriovenous hemofiltration (CAVH) and continuous arteriovenous hemodialysis (CAVHD), described later in this chapter, have smaller surface areas (0.2 to 0.6 m²) than those listed in Table 109–1 and used in conventional hemodialysis.

SOLUTE TRANSFER BY DIALYSIS
Determinants of Solute Transfer by Artificial Dialyzers

During dialysis, solute is transferred across the dialysis membrane, with the amount of solute transferred per unit of time, or solute flux (J), being given by[7, 8]

$$J = K_0 \times A \times C + K_{UF} \times TMP \times C_F \qquad (1)$$

where K_0 = a proportionality factor (= the flux of solute per unit of dialyzer surface area at a solute concentration gradient of unity)

TABLE 109–1

AVERAGE ULTRAFILTRATION COEFFICIENTS AND IN VITRO UREA AND VITAMIN B_{12} CLEARANCES OF CELLULOSE AND SYNTHETIC DIALYZERS*

A (m²)	Type	K_{UF} (mL/mm Hg)	K (mL/min) for Q_B = 200 mL/min		K (mL/min) for Q_B = 300 mL/min	
			UN	B_{12}	UN	B_{12}
0.7–0.8	HF-C	3.1	156	33	187	34
	PP-C	3.0	150	40	180	45
	PP-S	29	142	58	155	59
0.9–1.0	HF-C	4.2	168	44	207	46
	PP-C	8.5	168	61	205	48
	HF-S	21+	170	82	210	106
	PP-S	33+	161	64	194	71
1.1–1.3	HF-C	4.8	176	49	218	49
	HF-S	29+	179	91	236	120
	PP-S	50	171	74	208	84
1.4–1.6	HF-C	5.1	178	50	228	58
	PP-C	6.6	175	55	224	60
	HF-S	25+	180	90	232	138
≥1.7	HF-C	8.5	188	73	249	79
	HF-S	40+	185	108	244	127

*A = membrane surface area; K_{UF} = ultrafiltration coefficient; Q_B = dialyzer blood flow; K = clearance; UN = urea nitrogen; B_{12} = vitamin B_{12}; HF-C = hollow-fiber cellulose dialyzer; PP-C = parallel-plate cellulose dialyzer; HF-S = hollow-fiber synthetic membrane dialyzer; PP-S = parallel-plate synthetic membrane dialyzer.

A = membrane surface area
C = transmembrane solute concentration gradient
K_{UF} = ultrafiltration coefficient
TMP = transmembrane pressure
C_F = concentration of solute in the ultrafiltrate

The first term ($K_0 \times A \times C$) represents the diffusive component and the second term ($K_{UF} \times TMP \times C_F$) the convective component of the solute flux. The product $K_0 \times A \times C$ is a characteristic of a dialyzer and defines the diffusive solute transfer properties of that dialyzer.

The clearance of the dialyzer, K, is given by the solute transfer rate J divided by the concentration of solute in the incoming blood C_{Bi} (i.e., $K = J/C_{Bi}$) and represents the volume of blood completely cleared of a particular solute per unit of time. The following discussion focuses on the factors determining the rate of solute transfer, and consequently the clearance, of the dialyzer.

For mass balance to be maintained across the dialyzer, the amount of solute removed from the blood must equal the amount of solute added to the dialysate. Solute transfer rates are influenced by factors acting on either the blood or the dialysate side of the dialyzer. The flux of solute out of the blood compartment is given by

$$J = Q_{Bi} \times C_{Bi} - Q_{Bo} \times C_{Bo} \qquad (2)$$

where Q_{Bi} and Q_{Bo} are the blood flows in and out of the dialyzer and C_{Bi} and C_{Bo} the concentrations of solute in incoming and outgoing blood, respectively. Because $Q_{Bo} = Q_{Bi} - Q_F$, where Q_F is the ultrafiltration rate, Equation 2 may be rewritten as

$$J = Q_{Bi}(C_{Bi} - C_{Bo}) + Q_F \times C_{Bo} \qquad (3)$$

The first term in Equation 3 represents the flux of solute resulting from diffusion and the second term that resulting from convection. The diffusive and convective clearances are obtained by dividing each of the flux terms by C_{Bi}. These equations allow independent analysis of the factors affecting diffusive and convective solute flux.

Equation 3 explains why diffusive solute flux increases with increasing blood flow, as shown for small, highly diffusible solutes such as urea in Figure 109–2A. At high blood flow, however, urea clearance does not increase in proportion to flow. This is due to the fact that the $K_0 \times A$ value of the dialyzer becomes limiting for solute transfer; increasing A increases $K_0 \times A$ and augments solute transfer and urea clearance. Increasing blood flow does not increase solute flux if the solute diffuses poorly through the membrane, however. Such is the case with vitamin B_{12} and cellulose membranes but not with synthetic membranes. The highly permeable synthetic membranes do display some flow dependence, as shown for a middle molecule such as vitamin B_{12} in Figure 109–2B.

It is also evident from Equation 3 that when C_{Bo} approaches zero, diffusive solute transfer is maximal and the contribution of convection to total solute flux is negligible. As C_{Bo} increases and approaches C_{Bi}, diffusion contributes less and less to solute removal, which then becomes highly dependent on convection. Increasing ultrafiltration also increases convective transfer of small, diffusible solutes, while their transfer by diffusion decreases. Because of these reciprocal changes, total solute removal from the blood remains largely unchanged. However, ultrafiltration, by decreasing the volume of returning blood, may compromise the total rate of transfer of solutes such as buffer anions that normally diffuse from dialysate into blood.

Solute flux into the dialysate compartment is equal to the product $Q_{Do} \times C_{Do}$, where Q_{Do} and C_{Do} are the flow and solute concentration of outgoing dialysate, respectively. Be-

cause Q_{Do} is the sum of the incoming dialysate flow, Q_{Di}, and the ultrafiltration rate, Q_F, the rate of addition of solute to the dialysate is given by

$$J = Q_{Di} \times C_{Do} + Q_F \times C_{Do} \qquad (4)$$

Again, the first and second terms of Equation 4 represent the diffusive and convective solute fluxes, respectively. This equation explains why solute transfer by diffusion is proportional to the dialysate flow. High dialysate flows decrease C_{Do} and cause the concentration gradient for diffusion to be maximal. This is the case during conventional hemodialysis. When Q_{Di} is reduced to a fraction of Q_{Bi}, the rate of solute transfer is limited by Q_{Di}. Under these conditions, C_{Do} tends to equal C_{Bi} and the diffusive clearance of solute approaches the value of Q_{Di}, the dialysate flow. Such low dialysate flow prevails during "continuous" peritoneal dialysis and CAVHD.

Control of Blood Composition by Dialysis

The goals of dialysis are to normalize extracellular fluid content and composition and to maintain low blood levels of metabolic wastes and toxins. In this respect, dialysis prescription is usually guided by the blood urea nitrogen (BUN) concentration, an approach that is based on models of urea kinetics.[8-10] Urea is a small, noncharged solute that equilibrates rapidly across cell membranes. Its volume of distribution (V) is therefore equal to the total body water volume. Because urea is the main metabolic end product of protein catabolism, the generation rate of urea (G, in milligrams per minute) is proportional to the protein catabolic rate (in grams per day).[8, 10] The latter is often markedly increased in critically ill patients.

Dialytic control of the BUN concentration requires that urea be removed at a rate equal to that at which it is being generated. The rate of urea nitrogen removal is equal to the product of the urea clearance and the mean BUN concentration. Disregarding any gastrointestinal contributions, in anuric patients the urea clearance equals the dialytic clearance of urea. However, in nonoliguric patients urea clearance is a composite value, including any residual renal urea clearance in addition to the dialytic clearance of urea.[8-11]

Although the BUN stabilizes whenever urea removal equals urea production (a situation that defines urea balance), the manner in which the BUN is controlled varies according to the form of dialysis used. Dialysis modalities that operate around the clock, such as peritoneal dialysis, CAVH, and CAVHD, result in nearly constant BUN levels when urea balance is achieved. In these cases, an upward trend in the BUN indicates that urea removal is less than urea production. This, or a high BUN level per se, is an indication to search for technical malfunctions or to increase the clearance. The latter may be accomplished either by augmenting dialysate flow or by increasing ultrafiltration-dependent convective solute removal.

By contrast, intermittent hemodialysis results in large and rapid reductions in BUN during the treatment interval, followed by a slow return to the predialysis level during the interdialytic period. In the absence of any residual renal function, the BUN concentration profile during hemodialysis is given by the following exponential equation:[8, 9]

$$C_t = C_0 e^{-(Kt_d/V)} + G/K(1 - e^{-(Kt_d/V)}) \qquad (5)$$

where C_0 = BUN concentration at beginning of dialysis
C_t = BUN concentration at end of dialysis
K = dialyzer urea clearance
t_d = dialysis duration time
and V and G have the meanings given earlier.

A

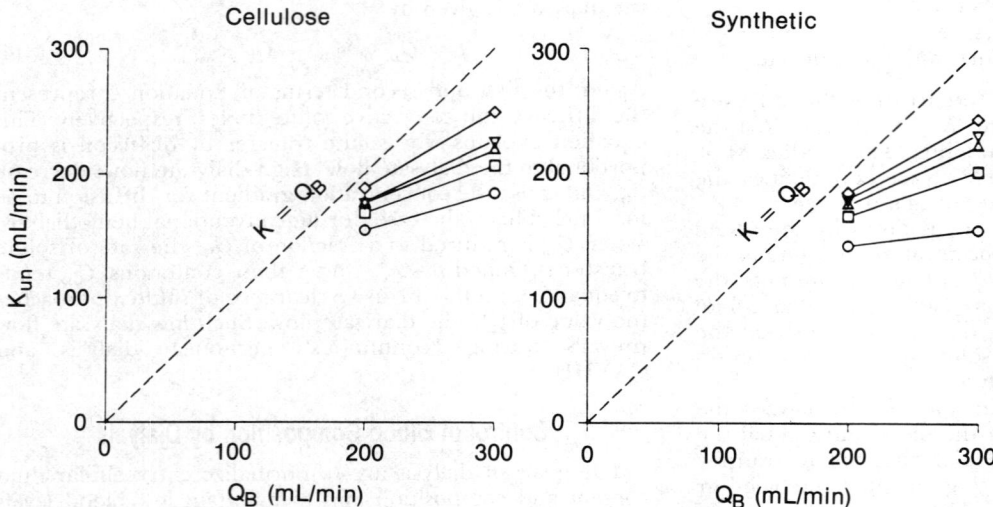

B

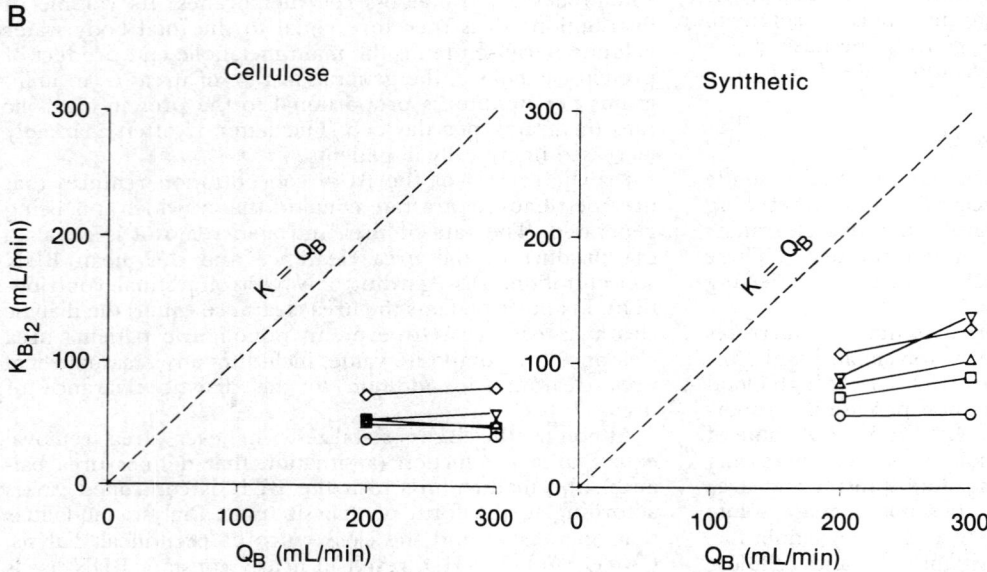

Figure 109–2. Average in vitro clearances of *(A)* urea nitrogen (K_{UN}) and *(B)* vitamin B_{12} (K_{B12}) for cellulose and synthetic membrane dialyzers between blood flow (Q_B) values of 200 and 300 mL/min. Dialyzers were grouped according to their surface areas: (○) 0.7–0.8 m²; (□) 0.9–1.0 m²; (△) 1.1–1.3 m²; (▽) 1.4–1.6 m²; (◇) ≥1.7 m².

During the interdialytic period, the BUN concentration returns from C_t back toward C_0 in accordance with the equation[8, 9]

$$C_0 = C_t + Gt_{id}/V \qquad (6)$$

where t_{id} is the interdialytic time period. The value of *G* can be calculated from Equation 6, assuming that *V* equals 55 to 60% of body weight. Alternatively, more accurate values of *V* and *G* can be obtained by solving Equations 5 and 6 simultaneously.

The characteristic BUN concentration profile described by these equations is depicted graphically in Figure 109–3. Although a "time average" BUN concentration can be calculated by integration and used to determine hemodialysis requirements, such an approach is complex and subject to error if non–steady-state conditions exist. For these reasons, a modified, simpler approach is suggested.

The apparent value of *G* is estimated by means of Equation

6, using BUN determinations done 24 hours apart. A target BUN level (C_{UN}, in milligrams per milliliter) is then chosen empirically to minimize the risk of the patient's developing uremic complications. The continuous urea clearance (K_c, in milliliters per minute) required to maintain the chosen BUN level is given by the ratio G/C_{UN}. The equivalent number of daily hours of hemodialysis required to achieve the same result is approximated by the ratio $1440K_c/K$. If the requirement is less than 150 minutes (2.5 hours) per day, hemodialysis can be given every other day, provided other indications (hyperkalemia, volume overload) are absent.

One of the major sources of error with this approach is the fact that the value of *K*, the hemodialysis urea clearance, is often uncertain and variable—for example, because of hemodynamic instability of the patient or because of temporary access malfunction. For this reason, the adequacy of each hemodialysis treatment should be ascertained by determining whether the predialysis/postdialysis BUN concentra-

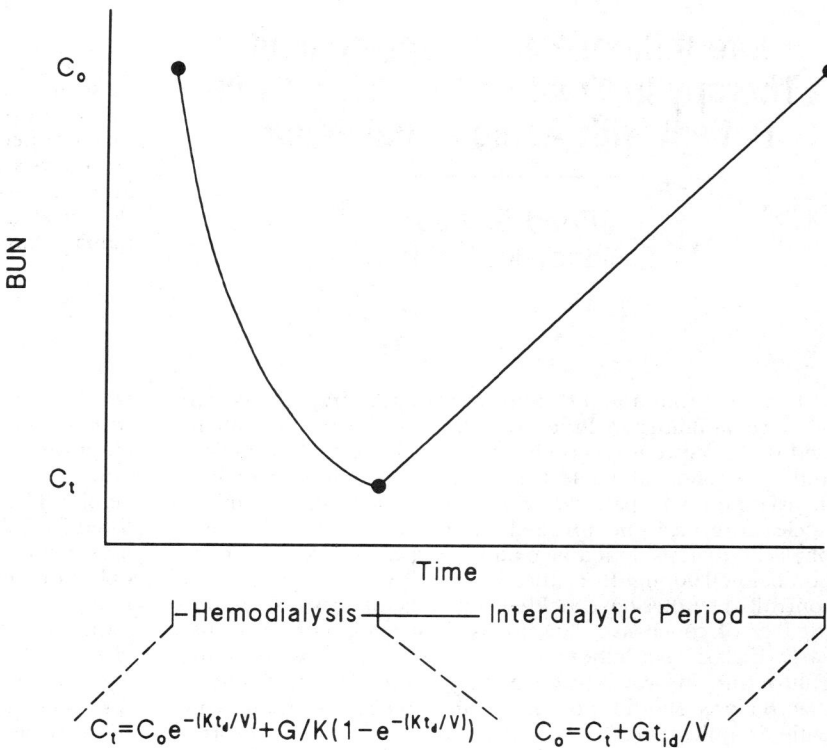

Figure 109–3. BUN concentration profile during intermittent hemodialysis.

$$C_t = C_o e^{-(Kt_d/V)} + G/K(1 - e^{-(Kt_d/V)})$$

$$C_o = C_t + Gt_{id}/V$$

tion ratio closely approaches the expected value of $e^{-(Kt_d/V)}$. If this is not the case, the duration and/or frequency of the hemodialysis must be increased. This hemodialysis treatment assessment plan should be carried out on a regular basis, at least until the patient reaches a stable condition. At that point, dialysis requirements can be reassessed using the models described for end-stage renal disease patients in standard dialysis texts.

Although the classic purpose of dialysis is to remove wastes and toxic substances, it also serves to replenish body buffer stores. Metabolic acidosis and the associated body buffer deficits are corrected by providing a favorable gradient for buffer anions to diffuse from dialysate to blood. Such buffer anions can be either bicarbonate itself or an organic anion, such as acetate, the metabolism of which results in generation of bicarbonate.[12] However, dialysate bicarbonate losses, together with inability to metabolize acetate rapidly, may occasionally result in worsening of the metabolic acidosis during acetate hemodialysis.[12] For this reason, bicarbonate hemodialysis is preferable in the intensive care unit (ICU) setting.[13, 14] This recommendation does not apply to peritoneal dialysis, CAVH, and CAVHD, in which the rate of acetate delivery to the patient is less than the rate of acetate metabolism.

References

1. Mujais SK, Ivanovich P: Membranes for extracorporeal therapy. In: Maher JF (ed): Replacement of Renal Function by Dialysis. 3rd ed. Dordrecht, Kluwer Academic Publishers, p 181, 1989.

2. Henderson LW, Cheung AK, Chenoweth DE: Choosing a membrane. Am J Kidney Dis 3:5, 1983.
3. Cheung AK: Biocompatibility of hemodialysis membranes. J Am Soc Nephrol 1:150, 1990.
4. Chanard J, Lavaud S, Toupance O, et al: Carpal tunnel syndrome and type of dialysis membrane used in patients undergoing long term hemodialysis. Arthritis Rheum 29:1170, 1986.
5. Van Stone JC: Hemodialysis apparatus. In: Daugirdas JT, Ing TS (eds): Handbook of Dialysis. Boston, Little, Brown, p 21, 1988.
6. Hoenich NA, Woffindin C, Ward MK: Dialyzers. In: Maher JF (ed): Replacement of Renal Function by Dialysis. 3rd ed. Dordrecht, Kluwer Academic Publishers, p 144, 1989.
7. Gotch FA, Keen ML: Dialyzers and delivery systems. In: Cogan MG, Garovoy MR (eds): Introduction to Dialysis. New York, Churchill Livingstone, p 1, 1985.
8. Sargent JA, Gotch FA: Principles and biophysics of dialysis. In: Maher JF (ed): Replacement of Renal Function by Dialysis. 3rd ed. Dordrecht, Kluwer Academic Publishers, p 87, 1989.
9. Sargent JA: Control of dialysis by a single-pool urea model. Kidney Int 23:S-26, 1983.
10. Gotch FA, Keen ML: Care of the patient on hemodialysis. In: Cogan MG, Garovoy MR (eds): Introduction to Dialysis. New York, Churchill Livingstone, p 73, 1985.
11. Lowrie EG, Teehan BP: Principles of prescribing dialysis therapy: Implementing recommendations from the National Cooperative Dialysis Study. Kidney Int 23:S-113, 1983.
12. Vreman HJ, Assomull VM, Kaiser BA: Acetate metabolism and acid-base homeostasis during hemodialysis. Influence of dialyzer efficiency and rate of acetate metabolism. Kidney Int 18:S62, 1980.
13. Graefe U, Milutinovitch J, Follette W, et al: Less dialysis-induced morbidity and vascular instability with bicarbonate in dialysate. Ann Intern Med 88:332, 1978.
14. Leunissen KML, Hoorntje SJ, Fiers HA, et al: Acetate versus bicarbonate hemodialysis in critically ill patients. Nephron 42:146, 1986.

Intermittent Renal Replacement Therapy in Treating the Critically Ill Patient with Acute Renal Failure

Fuad Shihab
Sidney M. Kobrin

The most common indications for dialysis in patients with acute renal failure include uremia, fluid overload, metabolic acidosis, persistent bleeding caused by platelet dysfunction, and hyperkalemia (Table 109–2). The value of early dialysis in asymptomatic patients with renal insufficiency remains unclear. Several uncontrolled studies have found that prophylactic dialysis aimed at maintaining the BUN concentration below 100 mg/dL reduced morbidity and mortality, but controlled studies have yielded contradictory results. Despite the lack of conclusive data, many nephrologists believe that early dialysis simplifies the management of acute renal failure and improves survival of patients. We recommend that dialysis should not be commenced in asymptomatic patients unless the BUN and serum creatinine concentrations are greater than 100 and 10 mg/dL, respectively, and are continuing to rise.

Several dialysis modalities are available for use in the intensive care setting, including classic hemodialysis and peritoneal dialysis (intermittent forms of dialysis) and slow, continuous forms of dialysis such as CAVH and CAVHD. The selection of a particular modality depends on a number of factors, such as (1) whether the patient requires fluid removal, solute removal, or both; (2) the experience of the hospital's nephrology team; and (3) the advantages and disadvantages of a particular modality in view of the patient's underlying condition. The various modalities, methods of establishing access, indications, advantages, and disadvantages are compared in Table 109–3. Intermittent forms of dialysis are discussed here; continuous forms of renal replacement therapy are discussed later in the chapter.

TABLE 109–2

INDICATIONS FOR ACUTE DIALYSIS IN THE INTENSIVE CARE UNIT

Presence of uremic syndrome
  Anorexia, nausea, vomiting
  Altered mental status (personality changes, confusion, coma)
  Seizures
  Asterixis, myoclonus
  Pericarditis
Fluid overload
  When resistant to diuretic therapy
Metabolic acidosis
  When additional sodium bicarbonate administration would result in fluid overload
Hyperkalemia
  When unresponsive to other therapy
Persistent bleeding secondary to platelet dysfunction
  When unresponsive to other therapy
Renal insufficiency per se
  BUN and serum creatinine levels greater than 100 and 10 mg/dL, respectively, and rising daily
Drug overdose

HEMODIALYSIS

When this dialysis modality has been selected, the nephrologist, in conjunction with the intensive care team, should establish vascular access, provide the equipment and related material needed for the procedure, prescribe the appropriate dialysis regimen, and monitor the patient during and after dialysis to ensure that the desired treatment has been delivered and that any complications are detected early and managed appropriately.

Vascular Access

Temporary vascular access is used in patients with acute renal failure and in patients with chronic renal failure without a functional permanent vascular access. The device employed is a double-lumen venous catheter placed percutaneously in the femoral, subclavian, or internal jugular vein.[1-3] The advantages and disadvantages[4,5] of each site are listed in Table 109–4. Selection of a particular site is based on the patient's underlying medical condition as well as the operator's experience. The femoral route is the safest and is useful for performing the initial dialysis, particularly in patients with pulmonary edema. Two largely outdated devices, the Scribner shunt and the single-lumen catheter (with a single-line pathway adapter), may be used in the rare instances in which placement of a double-lumen catheter is not feasible. The creation of a native arteriovenous fistula, arteriovenous graft, or right atrial Perma-Cath catheter placement for permanent vascular access is largely limited to patients requiring chronic hemodialysis and is not discussed here.

Equipment and Supplies

The hemodialysis machine consists of a blood pump, dialysis solution delivery system, and safety monitors. The safety-monitoring devices include air bubble detectors in the blood circuit, blood leak detectors in the dialysate circuit, dialysis solution temperature sensors, and conductivity meters and pressure monitors in the blood and dialysate circuits. These monitors may be set either to alert the dialysis staff to problems or to institute automatic countermechanisms, such as shutting off the blood pump when desired pressure limits are exceeded. The features of available dialysis membranes (dialyzers) were discussed earlier in this chapter.

Patients are exposed to 120 L of water during each treatment. All low-molecular-weight substances present in the water have direct access to the patient's blood stream, so it must be ensured that the water is free of contaminants such as copper, chloramine, and bacterial endotoxins.[6] These contaminants are removed by exposing the water to a series of reverse osmosis membranes, ion-exchange resins, activated charcoal, and water-softening procedures.

The choice of acetate or bicarbonate as the dialysate buffer was discussed earlier in this chapter. The remainder of the dialysate is designed to restore or maintain physiologic concentrations of sodium, potassium, calcium, magnesium, and chloride. The composition of standard acetate- and bicarbonate-containing dialysis solutions is shown in Table 109–5. Modern machines have the capacity to perform dialysis with a variety of dialysate compositions, including variable sodium, potassium, and calcium concentrations. The choice of dialysate may therefore be tailored to a patient's specific requirements. For example, a low-potassium or low-calcium dialysate should be used for hyperkalemic or hypercalcemic patients, respectively.

TABLE 109-3

COMPARISON OF THE VARIOUS MODALITIES OF DIALYSIS THERAPY

Characteristic	Isolated Ultrafiltration	Continuous Arteriovenous Hemofiltration	Peritoneal Dialysis	Hemodialysis	Continuous Arterio-venous Hemodialysis
Access	Central vein and femoral vein double-lumen catheter	Femoral arterial catheter plus single-lumen central venous catheter, or Scribner's shunt	Peritoneal dialysis catheter	Central vein and femoral vein double-lumen catheter	Femoral arterial catheter plus single-lumen central venous catheter, or Scribner's shunt
Skilled dialysis nursing requirement	Yes	No	No	Yes	No
Anticoagulation requirements	+*	+*	−	+*	+*
Propensity to induce intradialytic hypotension	+	−	−	+++	−
Solute clearance	Negligible	Negligible	Up to 24 L/d	25 L/d	24–36 L/d
Unique disadvantages	—	Potential complication of femoral artery puncture	May exacerbate pulmonary dysfunction	—	Potential complication of femoral artery puncture

*Rarely, patients may be "autoanticoagulated" and not require anticoagulants. Regional anticoagulation may be utilized when routine anticoagulation is contraindicated.

Anticoagulation

Exposure of blood to dialysis membranes activates the clotting cascade, necessitating the use of anticoagulation to prevent occlusion of the dialyzer. Three anticoagulation regimens are commonly used during hemodialysis in critically ill patients. These are routine heparinization, reduced-dose heparinization, and heparin-free dialysis. The choice of regimen depends on whether the patient has a low, intermediate, or high risk of bleeding. It is important to keep in mind that frequent clotting of the dialyzer because of inadequate anticoagulation is a major source of blood loss that is easily overlooked.

Heparin can be given rather liberally to patients at low bleeding risk. There are two routine techniques of administering heparin. In one, a heparin bolus is followed by a constant heparin infusion. In the second, a heparin bolus is followed by repeated bolus doses as necessary.[7] Two clotting tests, the whole blood partial thromboplastin time and the activated clotting time, are commonly used to monitor the response to heparin. The goal is to maintain the partial thromboplastin time or the activated clotting time 80% above the baseline value during dialysis.

Reduced-dose ("tight") heparinization is recommended for patients who are at slight to moderate risk of bleeding.[8] The target clotting time is set at 40% above the baseline value. A bolus dose followed by a constant infusion of heparin is the best technique for administering a tight heparin prescription, because the rising and falling clotting times that are inevitable with repeated bolus therapy are avoided.

Heparin-free dialysis is the method of choice for patients who are actively bleeding, who are at high risk of bleeding, or in whom the use of heparin is otherwise contraindicated. The success of this technique depends on rinsing the extra-

TABLE 109-4

ADVANTAGES AND DISADVANTAGES OF PERCUTANEOUS VENOUS CATHETERS

Characteristic	Femoral Vein	Subclavian Vein	Internal Jugular Vein
Duration catheter may be left in place	Must be removed within 24–72 h	Can be left in place for several weeks	Can be left in place for several weeks
Patient's position once catheter inserted	Must lie flat while in place	Can be ambulatory	Can be ambulatory; limited neck mobility
Ease of insertion	Inserted easily	Requires a skilled operator	Requires intermediate skills
Position during insertion	Can be inserted in the semirecumbent position	Insertion should not be attempted if patient cannot lie flat	Insertion more difficult, but not impossible, if patient cannot lie flat
Complications	Usually minor: hematomas (groin, retroperitoneal)	Can be major and life threatening: pneumothorax, hemothorax, brachial plexus injury, mediastinal hemorrhage, pericardial tamponade	Usually minor: very low risk of pneumothorax
Risk of thrombosis and stricture of vein	No venographic data	High rate in the subclavian vein and superior vena cava	Low rate in the large veins
Rate of catheter-associated bacteremia	Low rate (provided a new catheter is used for each treatment)	Relatively high rate	No reliable data
Use in bacteremic patients	May be used in bacteremic patients (new catheter for each treatment)	Should not be inserted in bacteremic patients because of risk of catheter seeding	Same as for subclavian catheters

	TABLE 109–5	
COMPOSITION OF STANDARD ACETATE- AND BICARBONATE-CONTAINING DIALYSIS SOLUTIONS		
Component	Acetate Based (mEq/L)	Bicarbonate Based (mEq/L)
Sodium	135–145	135–145
Potassium	0–4.0	0–4.0
Calcium	2.5–3.5	2.5–3.5
Magnesium	0.5–1.0	0.5–1.0
Chloride	100–119	100–124
Acetate	35–38	2–4
Bicarbonate	0	30–38
Dextrose	11	11
P_{CO_2}	0–5	40–100
pH	Variable	7.1–7.3

corporeal circuit with heparinized saline before dialysis, maintaining a blood flow rate of at least 250 mL/min, and performing saline rinses of the dialyzer every 15 to 30 minutes. The periodic rinsing allows inspection of the dialyzer for evidence of clotting and may also reduce the propensity for dialyzer clotting.[9] Rarely, a blood flow rate greater than 250 mL/min may not be achievable or may be contraindicated (e.g., as a precaution against the dialysis disequilibrium syndrome). In these situations, regional citrate anticoagulation may be employed.[10]

Hemodialysis Procedure

The dialyzer should be thoroughly rinsed before initiating hemodialysis. This is important because it reduces the incidence or severity of anaphylactic reactions by removing leachable allergens from the dialyzer (e.g., ethylene oxide, which is used to sterilize dialyzers). Once rinsed, the dialyzer and blood circuit tubing are connected to the vascular access (Fig. 109–4) and the blood flow is set at 50 mL/min and then 100 mL/min until the blood circuit fills with blood. As the blood circuit fills, the priming fluid in the dialyzer is discarded or, for unstable patients, administered to the patient to help maintain blood volume. The blood flow may then be increased to the desired rate, usually 150 to 250 mL/min for acutely ill patients. The dialysate flow can now be initiated. When dialysis is terminated, blood in the extracorporeal circuit is returned to the patient by using isotonic saline. The patient usually receives 100 to 200 mL of this fluid during the rinse-back procedure. The desired ultrafiltration goal should always be adjusted to make allowance for this volume.

Assessment and Monitoring of Patients

The patient should be carefully assessed before ordering the dialysis prescription, the major components of which involve the amount of ultrafiltration required, the composition of the dialysate, the choice of dialyzer, and the amount of urea to be removed.

The desired ultrafiltration volume depends on the degree of circulatory overload and the patient's fluid intake and overall hemodynamic stability. The following guidelines are useful for the initial dialysis. It is rarely necessary to remove more than 5 L of fluid in a single dialysis session; volumes in excess of this are generally best removed in a second session the next day. If pedal edema or anasarca is present, an ultrafiltration goal of 2 to 5 L per treatment is reasonable. When pulmonary edema or jugular venous distention is evident (in the absence of pedal edema or anasarca), an

ultrafiltration goal of no more than 2 L is appropriate. If patients are euvolemic, little or no ultrafiltration is necessary; a dialyzer with an extremely low ultrafiltration coefficient or machines with "ultrafiltration controllers" should be used to forestall excessive fluid removal.

When the patient achieves "dry weight" (the weight at which the patient is free of pulmonary or peripheral edema and is normotensive), the ultrafiltration goal of subsequent treatments can be determined by subtracting the last postdialysis weight from the predialysis weight of the current treatment.

The choice of dialysate should be tailored to the specific needs of the individual patient and is based on the predialysis assessment of potassium, acid-base, and calcium homeostasis. The choice of dialyzer and its effects on urea kinetics can be determined by the methods described earlier in the chapter.

During dialysis, the patient's blood pressure and pulse should be monitored as often as necessary but at least every 30 minutes. Blood gas analysis and/or pulse oximeters should be available for patients with pulmonary dysfunction and those who develop acute dyspnea during the procedure.

Whenever possible, patients should be weighed after dialysis because this weight is important in deciding on the ultrafiltration volume of subsequent treatments. The optimal time for checking blood chemistry after dialysis remains controversial. In general, when bicarbonate is used as the dialysate buffer, blood may be sampled immediately after dialysis to determine the amount of urea nitrogen removed, as well as fluid, electrolyte, and acid-base status. However, when acetate dialysate is used, correction of acidosis may continue for 2 to 4 hours after dialysis while the acetate is metabolized to bicarbonate. Furthermore, because the serum potassium and phosphate concentrations are influenced by acetate metabolism, their true levels may be better reflected in samples drawn 2 to 4 hours after dialysis.

Complications

Several complications may be encountered during or close to a hemodialysis session. The health care team should

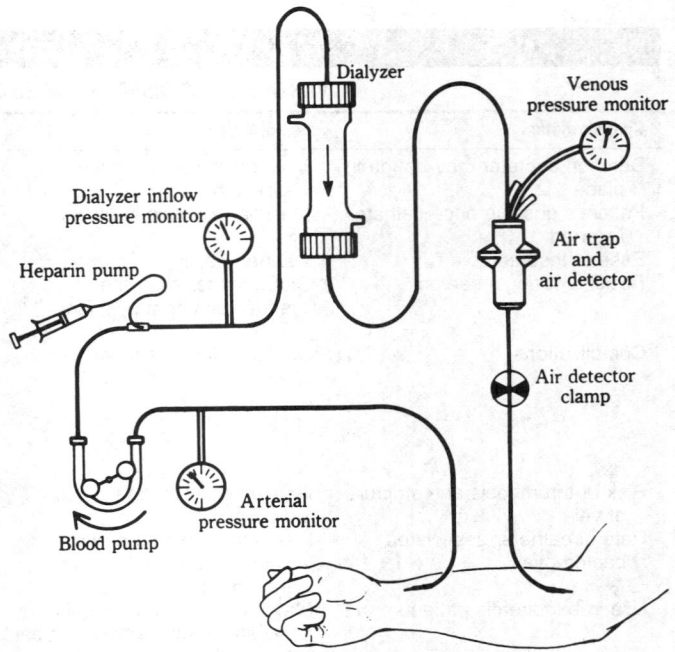

Figure 109–4. The hemodialysis machine blood circuit.

anticipate these problems, institute appropriate prophylactic measures when possible, and administer prompt therapy when they occur. The most common complications are hypotension (20 to 30% of dialyses), cramps (5 to 20%), nausea and vomiting (5 to 15%), chest pain (2 to 5%), back pain (2 to 5%), itching (5%), and fever and chills (<1%).

Intradialytic hypotension is generally due to excessive or unduly rapid decreases in blood volume and/or an inadequate response of the body's defense mechanisms to maintain blood pressure during volume removal. The latter may, in turn, be related to abnormal cardiac function or to lack of appropriate vasoconstriction. The specific causes of intradialytic hypotension and the measures that may prevent or reduce its occurrence are listed in Table 109–6. Unfortunately, acute hypotensive episodes may occur despite extensive precautions. They should be managed by placing the patient in the Trendelenburg position (if pulmonary status permits), reducing the ultrafiltration rate as much as possible, and infusing appropriate amounts of 0.9% saline through the venous line. Alternatives to saline include mannitol and albumin solutions, or packed red blood cells for anemic patients.

The most important factors predisposing to muscle cramps are hypotension, patients' being below their dry weight, and the use of sodium-poor dialysates. If muscle cramps persist despite correction of these underlying conditions, adminis-

---

TABLE 109–6

CAUSES AND PREVENTION OF INTRADIALYTIC HYPOTENSION

Cause	Preventive Measures
Excessive or unduly rapid decreases in blood volume	
Ultrafiltration below the patient's "dry weight"	Reset patient's dry weight upward.
Large interdialytic weight gain	Reduce interdialytic fluid intake or administration, if possible.
Failure to use an ultrafiltration controller	Use machine with an ultrafiltration controller. If not available, use a dialyzer with a low ultrafiltration coefficient.
Short treatment time	Prolong treatment time.
Low dialysate sodium concentration (<140 mEq/L)	Use dialysate with 140–145 mEg/L sodium concentration or sodium modeling machines, if available.
Impaired blood pressure defense mechanisms	
Impaired cardiac function	"Maximize" cardiac function, when possible. Discontinue negatively inotropic drugs, if possible. Treat pericardial effusions, arrhythmias, and other problems.
Impaired vasoconstriction	
Vasodilation caused by eating	Prohibit eating for 1 h before, and during, dialysis.
Vasodilatation caused by anemia	Correct anemia.
Antihypertensive or antianginal drugs	Withhold before and during dialysis.
Acetate dialysate	Use bicarbonate dialysate.
Dialysate endotoxins	Remove endotoxins from dialysate.
Septicemia	Treat appropriately.
Warm dialysate	Use colder dialysate (34–36°C).

---

tration of oral quinine sulfate (260 mg) 2 hours before dialysis may be helpful.[11] Most episodes of nausea and vomiting are probably related to hypotension, and appropriate corrective steps should be instituted as discussed earlier. An antiemetic may be administered in refractory cases. The most common cause of chest pain is probably the first-use syndrome (described later).[12] However, angina may also occur during dialysis and must always be excluded, especially in patients with known coronary artery disease.

The dialysis disequilibrium syndrome occurs commonly during the initial dialysis treatment of markedly uremic individuals when they are dialyzed aggressively. Early manifestations include nausea, vomiting, restlessness, and headache; obtundation, seizures, and even coma may develop in full-blown cases. The cause of this syndrome remains controversial, but fortunately it can be eliminated by preventing rapid decreases in plasma osmolality during the first treatment.[13, 14] This may be achieved with a "gentle" dialysis prescription, infusing hypertonic mannitol or using a high sodium concentration in the dialysate.[15]

A decrease in PO_2 of 5 to 30 mm Hg is a common occurrence during hemodialysis.[16] Dialysis-associated hypoxemia is generally well tolerated by patients with normal cardiopulmonary function but may be clinically significant in patients with pre-existing abnormalities. Various factors, singly or in combination, may account for the hypoxia. This problem has become much less prevalent because bicarbonate dialysate has virtually replaced acetate dialysate in critically ill patients.[17] Nasal oxygen administration is sufficient treatment in most instances.

Rarely, patients may experience an anaphylactic reaction with new dialyzers. This has been linked to residual amounts of ethylene oxide, which is used for sterilization of dialyzers.[18] Another type of first-use syndrome, manifested by chest and back pain, is seen mostly with cellulose dialyzers and has been attributed to complement activation.[19]

Air embolism is a potential catastrophe. Foam is seen in the venous blood line. The air travels to the central nervous system if the patient is seated and to the lungs if the patient is supine. The venous blood line should be clamped immediately, 100% oxygen administered, and the patient placed in the Trendelenburg position.

PERITONEAL DIALYSIS

Peritoneal dialysis is an important modality for the treatment of both acute and chronic renal failure. Survival of patients has been shown to be similar when intermittent peritoneal dialysis and hemodialysis have been compared in the treatment of acute renal failure.[20] Peritoneal dialysis is particularly useful when vascular access cannot be readily established and when anticoagulation is absolutely contraindicated. This relatively slow modality is also advantageous for hemodynamically unstable patients. In contrast to hemodialysis, in which all the ultrafiltration for a 24- to 48-hour period is condensed into 3 to 4 hours of treatment, peritoneal dialysis offers the advantage of slow ultrafiltration during 48 to 72 hours.

Peritoneal Access

All peritoneal catheters have the same basic design: a length of tubing with numerous side holes at the distal end.[21] Traditionally, catheters for acute dialysis are designed to be placed "medically" at the bedside to avoid the delays associated with surgical consultation and implantation. These catheters do not have cuffs to protect against bacterial migration into the peritoneal cavity, and the incidence of peritonitis increases markedly after 3 days of use. These

TABLE 109–7

COMPOSITION OF A TYPICAL PERITONEAL DIALYSIS SOLUTION

Component	Concentration
Sodium	132 mEq/L
Potassium	0
Chloride	96–102 mEq/L
Lactate	35–40 mEq/L
Calcium	3.5 mEq/L
Magnesium	0.5–1.5 mEq/L
Dextrose	1.5% (15 g/L, 347 mOsm/L)
	2.5% (25 g/L, 398 mOsm/L)
	4.25% (42.5 g/L, 486 mOsm/L)

catheters must therefore be removed and replaced at a fresh site if prolonged dialysis is necessary.

Two methods have been described for the nonsurgical placement of cuffed peritoneal dialysis catheters (identical with those used for chronic dialysis) for acute peritoneal dialysis. One method involves a guidewire-directed "blind" placement of the catheter; the other requires the use of a minitrochar and peritoneoscope. With either procedure, the catheter is tunneled into the subcutaneous tissue and a cutaneous exit site is fashioned about 2 inches from the catheter's entry into the peritoneum. Most catheters have two cuffs. The deep cuff is usually embedded in the rectus muscle, the superficial cuff in the subcutaneous tunnel about 0.75 inch from the exit site. The growth of fibrous tissue around the cuffs prevents bacterial migration and protects against peritonitis.[22] These catheters, therefore, have a major advantage over traditional "acute" catheters: they may be used for chronic dialysis if renal function does not recover promptly.

Equipment and Supplies

Peritoneal dialysis is performed by introducing 1 to 3 L of a dextrose-containing salt solution (dialysis solution) into the peritoneal cavity. By diffusion and ultrafiltration, toxic materials move from the blood into the dialysate. Removal from the body of fluid, electrolytes, and waste products occurs when the dialysate is drained. The basic equipment required is dialysis solution (dialysate) and tubing connecting the dialysate container to the peritoneal catheter and the catheter to a drainage bag.

Dialysate solutions are available in 0.5- to 3-L bags. The dialysate has been designed to maintain plasma composition within the physiologic range (Table 109–7). Potassium-free dialysate is often employed because many patients with acute renal failure are hyperkalemic and potassium is cleared slowly by peritoneal dialysis.[23] However, potassium may be added to the dialysate (2 to 4 mEq/L) should hypokalemia develop. The dialysate exerts an osmotic force that results in ultrafiltration of fluid; the greater the concentration, the greater the ultrafiltration rate. Lactate, which is absorbed and converted into bicarbonate, is the most frequently used buffer anion.

Acute peritoneal dialysis can be performed manually by using a long Y transfer set, with one limb of the Y leading to the dialysis solution container for inflow and the other leading to a sterile drainage container. With the manual technique, a new dialysis solution container[24] is attached to one limb of the Y transfer set after each inflow. Alternatively, an automated cycler technique is available. With this method, the desired volume of dialysate for a given period is connected to the cycler machine, which in turn warms the solution, instills set volumes at predetermined times, and

allots time for dwell and drainage of the dialysate. An alarm is activated if inflow or outflow is disrupted. Advantages of the cycler include more efficient use of nursing personnel and fewer breaks in the circuit, which results in a lower incidence of peritonitis.

Principles of Peritoneal Dialysis

Solute clearance during peritoneal dialysis depends on diffusion of solute from blood into the dialysate. In general, the amount of solute removed with each exchange is proportional to the dwell time of that exchange (Fig. 109–5). The degree of ultrafiltration also depends on the dwell time, with peak ultrafiltration occurring at approximately 3 hours (Fig. 109–6). Reabsorption of fluid may occur when the dwell time exceeds 3 hours.

Patients with acute renal failure are frequently uremic, grossly fluid overloaded, acidemic, and hypercatabolic and require a regimen capable of rapid solute removal and ultrafiltration. This is best achieved by frequent exchanges (e.g., hourly exchanges with dwell times of 40 minutes). Even though optimal equilibration between blood and dialysate does not occur with this dwell time, the increased number of exchanges more than compensates for the shortfall.

Assessment and Monitoring of Patients

Before selection of peritoneal dialysis, patients should be evaluated to determine whether any relative or absolute contraindications to this dialysis modality are present. These include multiple abdominal surgeries, compromised respiratory status, placement of abdominal aortic grafts within the past 3 months, and the presence of abdominal wall hernias.

Assessments of the patient's volume status, level of renal function, presence or absence of uremic manifestations, and electrolyte and acid-base status are all necessary to determine the optimal peritoneal dialysis regimen. Appropriate laboratory parameters should be reassessed at least daily during the course of dialysis, and the regimen should be adjusted

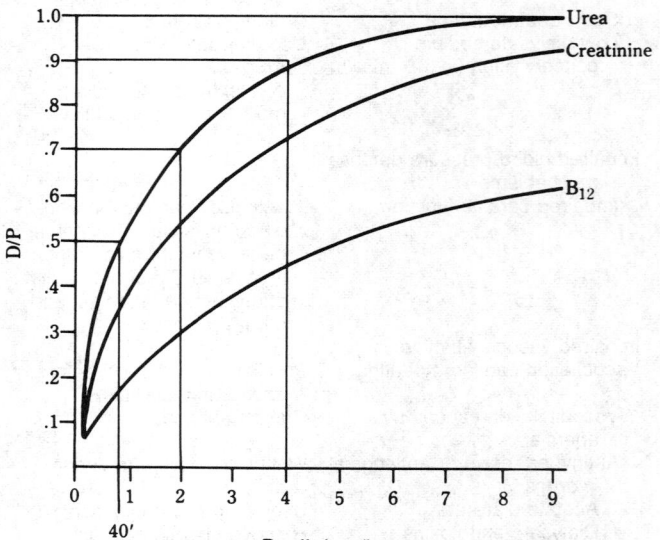

Figure 109–5. Rate of entry of urea, creatinine, and vitamin B_{12} into peritoneal dialysate. Results are expressed as the ratio of the level in dialysate (D) to the level in plasma (P). Typical ratios for urea at time points of 40 minutes, 2 hours, and 4 hours are indicated.

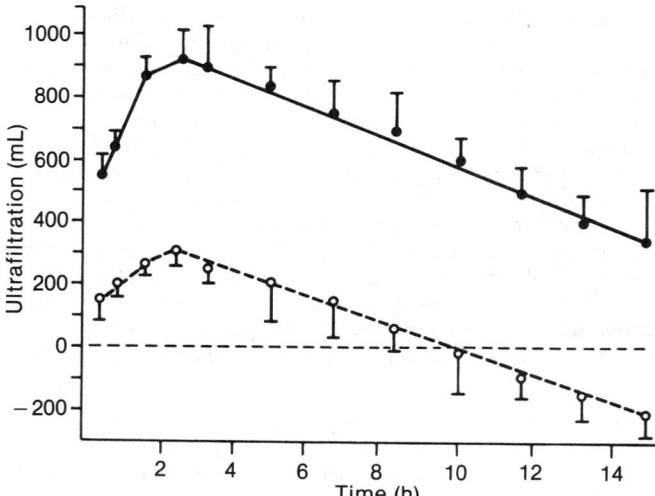

Figure 109–6. Ultrafiltration volume (volume drained minus volume infused) as a function of time after infusion of dialysate containing (○) 1.5% dextrose or (●) 4.25% dextrose.

accordingly. The installation and drainage volumes of each exchange, daily weights, and nature of the effluent (e.g., clear or cloudy, bloody, presence of fibrin) should all be recorded. Particular attention should be paid to the serum glucose and potassium concentrations. Insulin administration may be necessary if hyperglycemia develops, and potassium may have to be added to the dialysate if hypokalemia ensues.

The usual session length for acute peritoneal dialysis is 48 to 72 hours. However, if the acute renal failure is persistent and the patient is hypercatabolic and/or receiving large volumes of fluid, more extended dialysis may be warranted. Because protein loss via the dialysate can be as high as 10 to 20 g/d, nutritional supplementation may be necessary, particularly if the patient is not eating well.[25]

The goals of acute peritoneal dialysis are to eliminate any manifestations of uremia, maintain the BUN less than 100 mg/dL, and correct associated electrolyte and acid-base disorders. By exploiting the principles of ultrafiltration and solute removal illustrated in Figures 109–5 and 109–6 and determining the urea nitrogen generation rate (see earlier in the chapter), the nephrologist can prescribe a regimen for achieving these goals.

Complications (Table 109–8)

Complications Related to Catheter Insertion

Adverse effects can be minimized by ensuring that the bladder is empty before catheter placement and avoiding areas of previous surgery where loops of bowel may be fixed to the anterior peritoneum. Rarely, inadvertent puncture of the urinary bladder, intra-abdominal blood vessels, or bowel may occur.[26] Unexplained polyuria and glycosuria may reflect bladder perforation. Bowel perforation may manifest as abdominal pain, watery diarrhea, and poor dialysate drainage. The effluent may be cloudy or contain feces. Fortunately, the perforation often seals off spontaneously when the catheter is removed. A short course of antibiotics is recommended, and surgery is reserved for occasional patients who do not respond to catheter removal and antibiotic therapy.[27]

Grossly bloody effluent, a fall in the hematocrit, or shock signals that a large intra-abdominal blood vessel has been punctured, necessitating urgent laparotomy. Less severe bleeding resulting in blood-tinged dialysate occurs in up to 30% of cases during the initial three or four exchanges. Such bleeding arises from small vessels in the abdominal wall and may result in clotting of the catheter, a complication that can be prevented by adding heparin at 500 U/L to each exchange until the effluent clears.

Technical Problems

Pericatheter leaks are encountered more commonly with surgically placed chronic peritoneal dialysis catheters than with medically inserted acute catheters. In addition to overt leakage at the skin exit site, leaks may manifest more subtly as subcutaneous swelling and edema, weight gain, and diminished outflow volume. The leakage can generally be controlled by inserting a pursestring suture around the catheter. If this fails, an alternative method of dialysis may be necessary until the site of leakage seals off completely.

Outflow failure is indicated by drainage volume being significantly and persistently less than inflow volume. When this occurs, the first step should be to determine whether plugs or strands of fibrin are present in the dialysate effluent. Heparin should be added prophylactically to the dialysis solution whenever fibrin is evident in the effluent. However, when frank outflow obstruction is present, irrigation of the catheter with heparin is rarely successful. Irrigation with streptokinase or urokinase generally offers a higher success rate under these circumstances. Catheter replacement is necessary if these measures fail to relieve the outflow failure. Constipation has also been associated with outflow failure and laxatives should be employed as appropriate.

Peritonitis

The incidence of infectious peritonitis in patients with acute renal failure treated with peritoneal dialysis is approx-

TABLE 109–8
COMPLICATIONS OF PERITONEAL DIALYSIS
Related to catheter insertion
Bowel, urinary bladder, or blood vessel perforation
Technical
Pericatheter leaks
Leakage of dialysate
Subcutaneous dissection of dialysate
Outflow failure
Outflow obstruction (clots or extrinsic)
Incorrect catheter placement
Loss of siphon effect
Fluid loculation
Infectious
Peritonitis
Wound and catheter infection
Noninfectious peritonitis
Cardiovascular
Hypovolemia or volume overload
Arrhythmias
Respiratory
Pleural effusion
Atelectasis
Pneumonia
Related to abdominal wall
Abdominal hernias
Scrotal or labial swelling
Metabolic
Hyperglycemia
Hypoglycemia
Hypernatremia
Metabolic alkalosis and acidosis
Protein loss

imately 6%.[28] Adherence to strict aseptic technique is mandatory. Prophylactic antibiotics appear to be of no value. The diagnostic criteria for infectious peritonitis include at least two of the following: (1) symptoms and signs of peritoneal inflammation, (2) cloudy peritoneal fluid with an elevated peritoneal fluid leukocyte count ($>100/mm^3$ with $>50\%$ neutrophils), and (3) identification of bacteria in the effluent by Gram's stain or culture.

Empirical antibiotic therapy should be started as soon as the diagnosis is made.[29] A first-generation cephalosporin or vancomycin is generally given parenterally if the Gram stain reveals a gram-positive organism; an aminoglycoside is prescribed for gram-negative organisms. A combination of these antibiotics is prescribed if no organisms are demonstrated by Gram's stain. The final antibiotic regimen is determined by the results of culture and antibiotic sensitivity tests. Treatment should be continued for 10 to 14 days if the catheter is left in place. Failure to respond to the appropriate antibiotics within 2 to 3 days generally necessitates removal of the catheter. When organisms can be identified by Gram's stain and culture, noninfectious peritonitis should be suspected.[30]

"Eosinophilic" peritonitis is diagnosed when the effluent becomes cloudy and the peritoneal fluid eosinophil count is elevated. This problem occurs soon after catheter insertion and is thought to be the result of an irritant effect of either peritoneal air (introduced during catheter insertion) or plasticizers leached into the peritoneum from dialysate containers or tubing. Chemical peritonitis occasionally occurs after the intraperitoneal instillation of vancomycin, an antibiotic commonly used for the treatment of bacterial peritonitis.

Miscellaneous Complications

Hypotension secondary to hypovolemia may occur after excessive ultrafiltration. Orders should always be written to stop dialysis and/or administer intravenous fluid if the blood pressure falls below a predetermined level. Rarely, hypotension may be caused by bradyarrhythmia, which, in turn, results from increased vagal tone caused by abdominal distention.

Respiratory dysfunction is a frequent problem in critically ill patients with acute renal failure and fluid overload. Pulmonary function may be further compromised by peritoneal dialysis. Dialysate may track through channels in the diaphragm and produce large pleural effusions.[31] Abdominal distention after instillation of fluid may also interfere with respiration by causing upward displacement of the diaphragm,[32] thereby interfering with diaphragmatic function. Atelectasis may follow such upward displacement of the diaphragm. As a result of these potential respiratory problems, peritoneal dialysis may be contraindicated in patients with borderline pulmonary function. Furthermore, peritoneal dialysis may have to be discontinued if pulmonary function deteriorates significantly during dwell periods.

Abdominal hernias or scrotal or labial swelling resulting from a patent processus vaginalis may occur as a result of peritoneal dialysis. These complications are encountered more frequently with chronic ambulatory peritoneal dialysis than with acute peritoneal dialysis because intra-abdominal pressure is much less in the latter form of dialysis (which is almost always performed in the recumbent position). Smaller dialysate volumes may be used if hernias or genital edema develops during acute peritoneal dialysis. However, the dialysis must be abandoned if smaller dialysate volumes do not solve the problem.

Hyperglycemia may result from peritoneal absorption of glucose from the dialysate.[33] This problem may be aggravated during episodes of peritonitis because glucose absorption is increased across inflamed membranes. Insulin therapy may be necessary for the duration of the dialysis. Mild degrees of hypernatremia may occur because ultrafiltration with hypertonic solutions results in greater loss of water than sodium from plasma and extracellular fluid.[34] This is easily treated by increasing water intake or administration.

Many patients complain of abdominal pain during dialysate inflow or outflow. Dialysate inflow pain may be secondary to irritation of the peritoneum by the acidity or hypertonicity of the dialysate. This problem is often alleviated by adding alkali or 2 to 5 mL of 2% lidocaine (Xylocaine) to the dialysate. Outflow pain may occur when omentum is drawn into the catheter by a siphoning action during drainage, and it can often be alleviated by a change in position.

References

1. Nelson EW: Venous access techniques. Urol Clin North Am 13:475, 1986.
2. Shaldon S, Chiandussi L, Higgs B: Haemodialysis by percutaneous catheterisation of the femoral artery and vein with regional heparinisation. Lancet 2:857, 1961.
3. Uldall PR, Dyck RF, Woods F, et al: A subclavian cannula for temporary vascular access for hemodialysis or plasmapheresis. Dial Transplant 8:963, 1979.
4. Vanholder R, Hoenich N, Ringoir S: Morbidity and mortality of central venous catheter hemodialysis: A review of 10 years' experience. Nephron 47:274, 1987.
5. Raja RM, Fernandes M, Kramer MS, et al: Comparison of subclavian vein with femoral vein catheterization for hemodialysis. Am J Kidney Dis 2:474, 1983.
6. Bommer J, Ritz E: Water quality—A neglected problem in hemodialysis. Nephron 46:1, 1987.
7. Mingardi G, Perico N, Pusineri F, et al: Heparin for hemodialysis: Practical guidelines for administration and monitoring. Int J Artif Organs 7:269, 1984.
8. Flanigan MJ, Von Brecht J, Freeman RM, et al: Reducing the hemorrhagic complications of hemodialysis: A controlled comparison of low dose heparin and citrate anticoagulation. Am J Kidney Dis 9:147, 1987.
9. Caruana RJ, Raja RM, Bush JV, et al: Heparin free dialysis: Comparative data and results in high risk patients. Kidney Int 31:1351, 1987.
10. Pinnick RV, Wiegmann TB, Diederich DA: Regional citrate anticoagulation for hemodialysis in the patient at high risk for bleeding. N Engl J Med 308:258, 1983.
11. Sherman RA, Goodling KA, Eisenger RP: Acute therapy of hemodialysis-related muscle cramps. Am J Kidney Dis 2:287, 1982.
12. Hakim RM, Breillat J, Lazarus M, et al: Complement activation and hypersensitivity reactions to dialysis membranes. N Engl J Med 311:878, 1984.
13. Arieff AI, Massry SG, Barrientos A, et al: Brain water and electrolyte metabolism in uremia: Effects of slow and rapid hemodialysis. Kidney Int 4:177, 1973.
14. Kleeman CR: Metabolic coma. Kidney Int 36:1142, 1989.
15. Port FK, Johnson WJ, Klass DW: Prevention of dialysis dysequilibrium syndrome by use of high sodium concentration in the dialysate. Kidney Int 3:327, 1973.
16. Vaziri ND, Wilson A, Mukai D, et al: Dialysis hypoxemia. Role of dialyzer membrane and dialysate delivery system. Am J Med 77:828, 1984.
17. Pagel MD, Ahmad S, Vizzo JE, et al: Acetate and bicarbonate fluctuations and acetate intolerance during dialysis. Kidney Int 21:513, 1982.
18. Leitman SF, Bolantsky H, Alter H: Allergic reactions in healthy platelet-pheresis donors caused by sensitization to ethylene oxide gas. N Engl J Med 315:1192, 1986.
19. Craddock PR, Fehr J, Brigham KL, et al: Complement and leukocyte-mediated pulmonary dysfunction in hemodialysis. N Engl J Med 296:769, 1977.
20. Stott RB, Ogg CS, Cameron JS, et al: Why the persistently high mortality in acute renal failure? Lancet 2:75, 1972.
21. Weston RE, Roberts M: Clinical use of stylet catheter for peritoneal dialysis. Arch Intern Med 115:659, 1965.
22. Tenckhoff H, Scheckter H: A bacteriologically safe peritoneal access device. Trans Am Soc Artif Organs 14:181, 1968.
23. Brown ST, Ahearn DJ, Nolph KD: Potassium removal with peritoneal dialysis. Kidney Int 19:564, 1981.
24. Grodstein GP, Blumenkrantz MJ, Kopple JD: Glucose absorption during continuous ambulatory peritoneal dialysis. Kidney Int 19:564, 1981.
25. Dulaney JT, Hatch FE Jr: Peritoneal dialysis and loss of proteins: A review. Kidney Int 26:253, 1984.
26. Similin EP, Wright FH: Perforating injuries of the bowel complicating peritoneal catheter insertion. Lancet 1:64, 1968.
27. Rubin J, Oreopoulos DG, Lios TT, et al: Management of peritonitis and

bowel perforation during chronic peritoneal dialysis. Nephron 16:220, 1976.

28. Vaamonde CA, Perez GO: Peritoneal dialysis today. Kidney Int 10:31, 1977.
29. Keane WF, et al: CAPD related peritonitis management and antibiotic therapy recommendations. Peritoneal Dialysis Bull 7:55, 1987.
30. Karanicolas S, Oreopoulos DG, Izatt S, et al: Epidemic of aseptic peritonitis caused by endotoxin during chronic peritoneal dialysis. N Engl J Med 296:1336, 1977.
31. Edwards SR, Unger AM: Acute hydrothorax—A new complication of peritoneal dialysis. JAMA 199:853, 1967.
32. Berlyne GM, Lee HA, Ralston AJ, et al: Pulmonary complications of peritoneal dialysis. Lancet 2:75, 1966.
33. Grostein GP, Blumenkratz MJ, Kopple JD: Glucose absorption during continuous ambulatory peritoneal dialysis. Kidney Int 19:564, 1981.
34. Nolph KD, Hano JE, Teschan PE: Peritoneal sodium transport during hypertonic peritoneal dialysis: Physiologic mechanism and clinical implications. Ann Intern Med 70:931, 1969.

Continuous Renal Replacement Therapy in Treating the Critically Ill Patient with Acute Renal Failure

Miles H. Sigler
Brendan P. Teehan

Continuous renal replacement therapies have been developed to treat more effectively the uniquely difficult problems presented by the critically ill patient with acute renal failure. In the ICU patient, acute renal failure occurs almost invariably in the setting of sepsis, major surgery, and failure of other organs, such as the heart and lungs. These multiple physiologic disturbances render the patient hemodynamically unstable and may make conventional intermittent hemodialysis technically difficult to accomplish. These patients also have a high obligatory fluid intake, composed of hyperalimentation solutions and intravenous medications, and they are often hypercatabolic and have hour-to-hour changes in their fluid, electrolyte, and acid-base status. The potential advantages of continuous renal replacement therapy in treating these problems are described in this chapter and summarized in Table 109–9.

CONTINUOUS ARTERIOVENOUS HEMOFILTRATION

CAVH, the first continuous therapy to be used for the ICU patient with acute renal failure, utilizes the patient's cardiac output to perfuse blood through a short extracorporeal circuit that consists of blood lines and a hollow-fiber hemofilter (Fig. 109–7). Hydrostatic pressure forces water out the plasma compartment through the large pores of the hemofilter membrane. Typically, these membranes have substantially higher hydraulic permeability than do conventional cellulosic hemodialysis membranes. Hemofiltration membranes are composed of hydrophobic thermoplastics such as polyacrylonitrile, polyamide, and polysulfone. They have improved biocompatibility and do not activate the complement system. As water moves across the membrane it conveys or convects solute, thus cleansing the blood. The filtrate flows through a collecting tube to a closed drainage

container below the level of the patient, creating a siphon effect (see Fig. 109–7). This suction effect or negative pressure adds to the positive arterial pressure exerted across the filter membrane, increasing the transmembrane pressure and enhancing the filtration process.

Factors influencing the efficiency of the filtration process are summarized in Equation 7, which is identical with Starling's law of fluid filtration through capillaries:

$$Q_F = KA(\Delta P - \pi)$$

(7)

where Q_F = device ultrafiltration rate
  K = membrane permeability coefficient after exposure to plasma
  A = membrane surface area
  ΔP = transmembrane hydrostatic pressure
  π = plasma oncotic pressure

Operationally, ΔP and hence Q_F are increased by increasing blood flow, mean arterial blood pressure, and membrane pore size. Factors tending to decrease filtration rate are resistance to blood flow proximal to and in the filter, filter geometry (radius and length of hollow fibers), and high plasma oncotic pressure. The hydraulic and solute permeabilities of the membranes used in continuous therapy are high, and solutes such as urea, creatinine, and glucose are conveyed freely by water through the membrane (solvent drag). The concentration of solute in the filtrate (C_F) in relation to its concentration in plasma water (C_w) is termed the sieving coefficient (S). Thus, $S = C_F/C_w$.

In CAVH, the concentrations of most solutes (creatinine, urea, and glucose) in the filtrate and plasma water are approximately the same, indicating that the sieving coefficient is approximately one. This also means that most low-molecular-weight solutes are isosmotically convected across the membrane with little change in plasma osmolality. This slow isosmotic removal of water and solute that characterizes a convection-based blood-cleansing therapy such as CAVH tends to maintain hemodynamic stability because there is little change in plasma osmolality and thus less osmotic shift of intravascular water to the interstitial and intracellular spaces. In contrast, conventional acute intermittent hemodialysis, a system dependent on diffusion as opposed to convection for solute removal, causes rapid falls in urea and other solute concentrations, resulting in acute lowering of plasma osmolality and osmotic movement of water from the

---

TABLE 109–9

ADVANTAGES OF CONTINUOUS RENAL REPLACEMENT THERAPIES (CAVH AND CAVHD) IN TREATING INTENSIVE CARE PATIENTS

Hemodynamically well tolerated; minimal change in plasma osmolality.

Better control of azotemia and electrolyte and acid-base balance; corrects abnormalities as they are evolving; steady-state chemistries.

Highly effective in removing fluid (pulmonary edema, adult respiratory distress syndrome).

Facilitates administration of parenteral nutrition and obligatory IV medications (i.e., pressors, inotropes) by creating unlimited "space" through continuous ultrafiltration.

Procedure technically simple; no complex machinery needed.

Better membrane biocompatibility, less production of interleukin-1 and tumor necrosis factor, and less dialysis-induced catabolism.

Membranes capable of removing cytokines (interleukin-1, tumor necrosis factor) in septic patients.

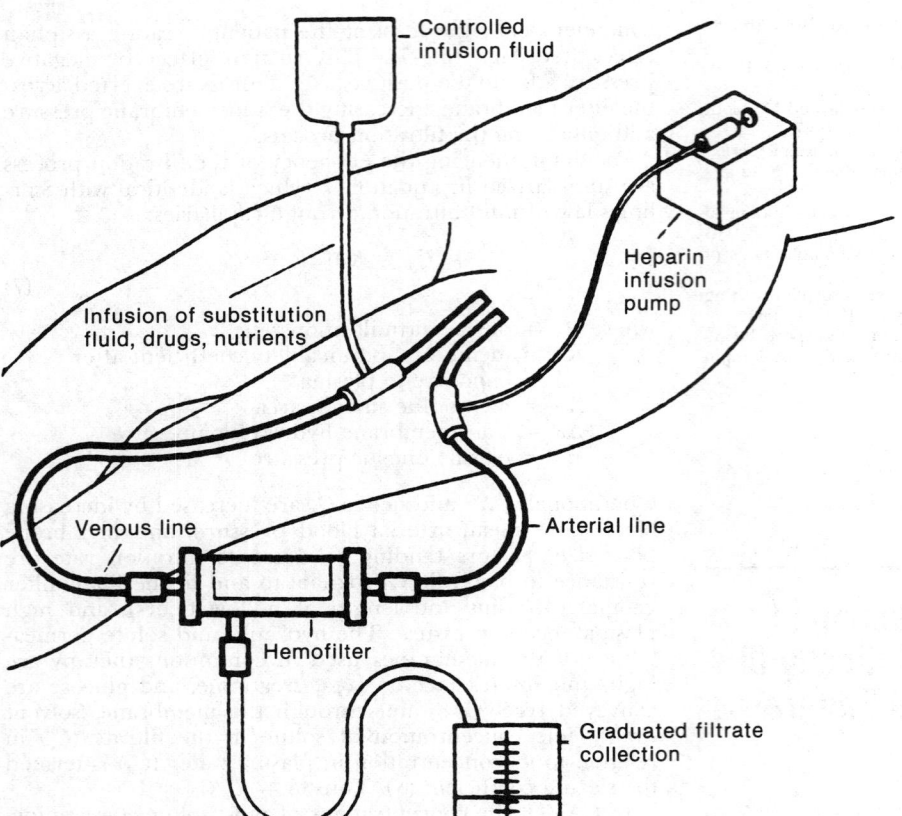

Figure 109–7. Circuitry for CAVH. Access to the circulation is via the femoral artery and femoral vein. Substitution fluid is infused in the venous return distal to the filter (postfilter).

plasma compartment to the more hypertonic intracellular space. In a typical ICU patient, whose circulatory system may already be dependent on pressors and inotropes, such fluid shifts could result in hypotension, arrhythmias, and further multiple-organ ischemia. Although the assumption of greater hemodynamic stability with CAVH (and CAVHD) than with intermittent hemodialysis is based on sound physiologic principles, there have been no published prospective studies that prove or disprove this assumption.

Filtration rates with CAVH using polysulfone hollow-fiber filters average 9 to 10 mL/min or approximately 600 mL/h. With such high fluid losses, a portion of the filtrate must be replaced to avoid hypovolemia. Replacement fluid, a balanced physiologic solution with either acetate or lactate as the buffer base, is given either proximal to the filter (prefilter) or distal to the filter (postfilter). For solutes with sieving coefficients (S) close to unity, the whole blood clearance (CL) of the device is equal to the filtration rate, that is, $CL = (C_F/C_w)Q_F$. Thus, if the filtration rate is 10 mL/min, the urea clearance is also 10 mL/min. Although CAVH is an excellent method for removal of fluid, it can be shown through appropriate kinetic modeling, as well as common clinical experience, that a urea clearance of 10 mL/min is insufficient to control azotemia in patients with hypercatabolic acute renal failure.

CONTINUOUS ARTERIOVENOUS HEMODIALYSIS

To improve solute clearance and better control azotemia, while retaining the advantages of slow continuous therapy, a more efficient diffusion-based therapy known as CAVHD or slow continuous hemodialysis is being used with increasing frequency. This is the current therapy of choice for acute renal failure in the critically ill ICU patient. The extracorporeal circuitry in CAVHD is similar to that in CAVH with one important difference: dialysis fluid is slowly infused through the dialysate compartment of a dialyzer to allow diffusive solute transfer.

A 0.43-m² flat-plate dialyzer (Hospal) with polyacrylonitrile methylsulfonate copolymer membranes is usually employed. The dialysate is sterile, commercially available peritoneal dialysis fluid. The dialysate sodium concentration may be adjusted by addition of hypertonic saline, and potassium can also be added to maintain the serum potassium concentration at any desired level. An I-Med Gemini PCII model dual-channel peristaltic infusion pump propels the dialysate through one channel, while pumping dialysate and ultrafiltrate out through the other channel (Fig. 109–8). Alternatively, the dialysate outflow line can be controlled by gravity drainage.

The dialysate inflow rate of 900 mL/h or 15 mL/min is about 3% of the flow rate used in conventional intermittent hemodialysis. Blood flow from the femoral artery, the most common access site, is usually in excess of 100 mL/min. Thus, blood flow far exceeds dialysate flow, which is the reverse of what occurs in conventional hemodialysis. This results in the presentation of a large quantity of blood solute (i.e., urea) to the highly permeable AN 69S membrane, producing saturation of the small volume of dialysate with blood solute. As a result, the concentration of small blood solutes exiting the dialyzer (i.e., the dialysate urea nitrogen, DUN or C_{Do}) is approximately equal to the concentration of blood solute entering the dialyzer (BUN or C_{Bi}) and the DUN/BUN ratio is 1. If the DUN/BUN ratio is less than 1, the dialyzer is not operating at maximal efficiency and dialyzer clotting must be considered. Hollow-fiber polysulfone and polyamide dialyzers appear to be less efficient than flat-plate dialyzers because DUN/BUN ratios are often less than 1 with the hollow-fiber geometry.[1, 2]

In CAVHD, diffusion and convection occur simultaneously. The diffusive and convective components of clearance

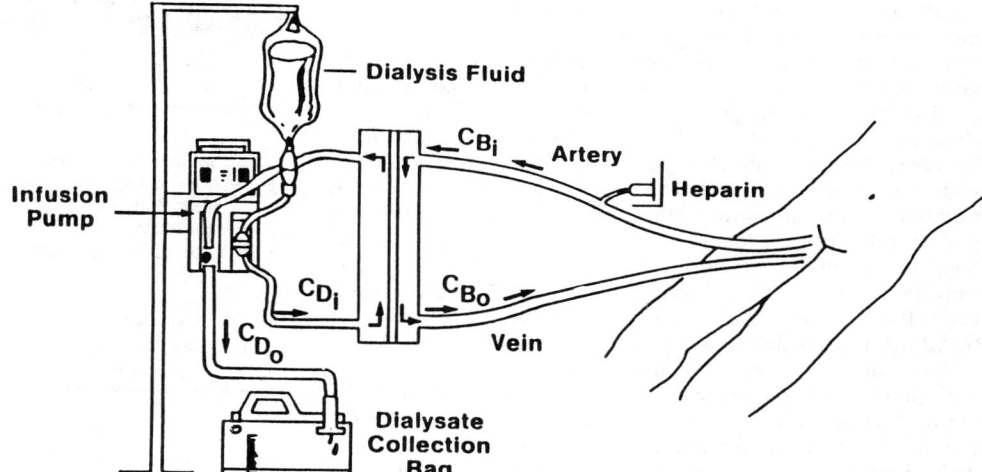

Figure 109–8. Schematic representation of circuitry for CAVHD. Continuous diffusive solute transport is achieved by slowly infusing dialysis fluid countercurrent to blood at 15.0 mL/min or 0.90 L/h.

(K_D) can be calculated in combination or separately as shown in Equations 8a and 8b.[3]

$$K_D = \frac{Q_{Do}C_{Do} - Q_{Di}C_{Di}}{C_{Bi}} \quad (8a)$$

If $Q_{Do} = Q_{Di} + Q_F$ and Q_F is the net ultrafiltration rate, then

$$K_D = \frac{Q_{Di}(C_{Do} - C_{Di})}{C_{Bi}} + \frac{Q_F C_{Do}}{C_{Bi}} \quad (8b)$$

The first term in Equation 8b is the diffusive component of clearance and the second term is the convective component. It has been shown that when CAVHD is performed as outlined earlier, increasing the dialysate flow from 16 to 27 mL/min results in continued saturation of dialysate, that is, $C_{Do} = C_{Bi}$.[4] Inspection of the formula for the diffusive component of clearance in Equation 8b indicates that if saturation of dialysate with blood solute continues as dialysate flow increases from 16 to 27 mL/min and C_{Do} continues to equal C_{Bi} and if C_{Di}, the inflowing dialysate concentration for urea, is 0, then the ratio C_{Do}/C_{Bi} is unity and diffusive clearance continues to equal dialysate inflow, Q_{Di}. At dialysate inflows above 28 to 30 mL/min, diffusive clearance also continues to increase but not in a linear manner. Thus, if BUN in a highly catabolic patient is not well controlled at a dialysate inflow of 16 mL/min, increasing the dialysate flow increases the diffusive clearance as just described. Further

study of the convective component of Equation 8b indicates that if $C_{Do} = C_{Bi}$, or $C_{Do}/C_{Bi} = 1$, then the convective clearance equals the ultrafiltration rate Q_F. The total clearance then, under conditions of dialysate saturation, is the actual dialysate outflow Q_{Do}, which is the sum of the dialysate inflow Q_{Di} and ultrafiltration rate Q_F.

Although CAVHD relies primarily on diffusive clearance, ultrafiltration (convective clearance) is also used but only to the extent necessary to offset obligatory fluid intake associated with hyperalimentation solutions and intravenous drugs (usually 2 to 3 mL/min). Ultrafiltration is kept at the absolute minimum because excessive fluid removal with higher ultrafiltration rates may cause hypovolemia and end-organ (liver, kidney) hypoperfusion even when systemic blood pressure is maintained. Evidence in animal models of acute tubular necrosis suggests that an acutely damaged kidney does not autoregulate its blood flow and episodes of ultrafiltration-induced hypovolemia and renal hypoperfusion could perpetuate tubular damage.[5] However, should clinical circumstances such as pulmonary edema or adult respiratory distress syndrome dictate a need for rapid fluid removal, this is easily achieved with CAVHD by increasing the rate at which fluid is pumped out of the dialyzer. Unlike conventional high-flux hemodialysis, in which changes in convective clearance influence diffusive clearance, in CAVHD changes in ultrafiltration do not affect diffusive clearance.[3] Convective and diffusive clearances can be manipulated separately to achieve either volume or azotemia control, depending on the patient's needs.

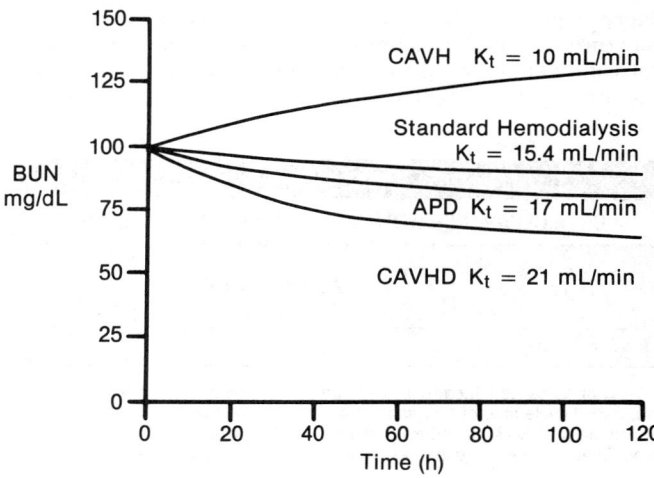

Figure 109–9. Azotemia control for different replacement therapies in acute renal failure. Time course of time-averaged BUN in a hypothetic 70-kg patient with a protein catabolic rate of 2 g/kg/d. Urea generation rate (G) is 13.79 mg/min. K_t = total clearance (mL/min). Standard hemodialysis total clearance (computed from urea clearance of 216 mL/min for 240 minutes three times a week) when distributed during 1 week = 15.4 mL/min. APD = acute peritoneal dialysis. Lines are constructed from a computer solution of the function $C = C_0 e^{-K_t/V} + G/K (1 - e^{-K_t/V})$ at 60-min intervals during dialysis. Net changes in V are assumed to be zero. Duration of acute peritoneal dialysis cycle is 1 hour.

Although clearance in CAVHD, expressed in milliliters per minute, is small compared with that achieved with conventional hemodialysis, the fact that CAVHD is continuous makes the cumulative 24-hour clearance comparable to that of high-efficiency intermittent hemodialysis. The clearances obtained with different blood-cleansing modalities are compared in Table 109–10. The total clearance achieved with hemodialysis three times weekly is distributed over the number of minutes in a week to yield a value, in milliliters per minute, that is less than that obtained with CAVHD (i.e., 15 versus 21 mL/min). If acute intermittent dialysis were performed for 3.5 hours, 5 days a week, the prorated urea clearance over the number of minutes in a week would be 22 mL/min, which is comparable to that of CAVHD.

Based on the urea kinetic modeling equations of Sargent and Gotch[6] and assuming a urea generation rate of 13.79 mg/min (equivalent to a protein catabolic rate of 2 g/kg/d), the levels of azotemic control achievable with different dialysis modalities are depicted in Figure 109–9. The clearances, K_t, from Table 109–10 are used in solving for the values of BUN at 60-minute intervals. The time course of the BUN in a 70-kg patient with oliguric acute renal failure shows that the BUN is approximately 15 to 65 mg/dL lower with CAVHD than with other available renal replacement therapies. Note that azotemia is poorly controlled with CAVH. Published reports of acute renal failure treated with CAVHD in critically ill patients support these calculations.[3, 7–11]

TECHNICAL AND OPERATIONAL CONCERNS

A major technical concern in CAVH and CAVHD is obtaining safe arterial vascular access. CAVH and CAVHD are operated without a blood pump. The preferred access site is the common femoral artery, which is accessed about 2 cm below the inguinal crease by a percutaneous Seldinger cannulation technique using a No. 7 or 8 French catheter with a single hole at the tip. With a mean arterial pressure of 70 to 90 mm Hg, the common femoral artery propels blood at 100 to 120 mL/min through the Hospal parallel-plate dialyzer (see Fig. 109–8). Doppler-audible foot pulses should be present. Vascular bruits over the femoral artery are a relative contraindication. The femoral vein is cannulated in the same way as the artery at the same level. Scribner's shunts in the arm can also be used.

Access complication rates are outlined in Table 109–11; complications consist of arterial and venous hemorrhage, obstruction, thrombosis, and sepsis. The most treacherous complications are line disconnections or accidental removal of the catheter from the femoral artery or vein. Either may result in fatal exsanguination. Long-term use of the femoral artery requires that the patient be immobilized in bed and may threaten the lower limb circulation. Avoidance of arterial cannulation by using a double-lumen catheter in the femoral, internal jugular, or subclavian vein in continuous

renal replacement therapy is rapidly gaining favor. This procedure, termed continuous venovenous hemodialysis, requires a blood pump with associated air and pressure monitors, which increases the technical complexity but avoids arterial access problems.[12]

Clotting in the dialyzer extracorporeal line is also a major problem. Factors causing clotting associated with the extracorporeal circuit include: low blood flow secondary to low mean arterial pressure (<65 mm Hg), low blood flow caused by high resistance within the dialyzer, high filtration fraction with increased plasma protein concentration and hematocrit caused by excessive ultrafiltration, and the intrinsic thrombogenicity of the dialysis membrane. Factors related to the patient that influence clotting include high platelet count, sepsis with disseminated intravascular coagulation, severe liver disease and associated coagulopathy, and inherent variability in heparin sensitivity.

A standard heparin anticoagulation protocol is outlined in Table 109–12. Adding dilute anticoagulant solution, that is, 10,000 U of heparin per liter of saline, prefiltering at a rate of 50 to 75 mL/h, decreases the incidence of clotting. When the DUN/BUN ratio is less than 0.6, it can be assumed that clotting has occurred and the dialyzer must be changed.

Because of the large cumulative clearances obtained with CAVHD, changes in medication doses must always be considered. Table 109–13 shows the changes in antibiotic dosages that are necessary when using CAVHD.[13] CAVHD also has the potential to remove essential nutrients such as amino acids in infused hyperalimentation solutions. When standard hyperalimentation is given at infusion rates of 60 to 100 mL/min, approximately 6 g of the infused protein is lost in dialysate every 24 hours.[14]

Despite these disadvantages, CAVHD is a major therapeutic advance in the management of acute renal failure in the unstable ICU patient. Technical problems, including prolonged arterial cannulation, anticoagulation, variable control

---

TABLE 109–11

BLOOD ACCESS IN CONTINUOUS RENAL REPLACEMENT THERAPY: COMPLICATION RATES

Site	Complication Rate (%)
Femoral artery	
Hemorrhage and obstruction	1–2
Femoral vein	
Short-term complication (bleeding and tear)	0–0.3
Long-term complication (sepsis and thrombosis)	12
Combined artery and vein	
Long- and short-term in CAVHD	15

TABLE 109–10

UREA CLEARANCE WITH VARIOUS DIALYSIS MODALITIES

	CAVHD	CAVH	Acute Peritoneal Dialysis*	Standard Intermittent Hemodialysis†
K_{urea} (mL/min)	21	10	17	15.4

*K_{urea} of acute peritoneal dialysis is computed assuming a dwell time of 30 min, a total cycle time of 1 h, and a dialysate flow rate of 33.3 mL/min.
†Standard dialysis procedure is defined as K_{urea} of 216 mL/min for 240 min three times a week expressed as milliliters per minute for the entire 7-d week.

TABLE 109–12

HEPARIN ANTICOAGULATION PROTOCOL FOR CAVHD

2000 IU heparin in arterial line; start with 500 IU/h constant infusion
PTT arterial and venous* every 4 h
If arterial PTT > 45 s, decrease heparin by 100 IU/h
If venous* PTT < 65 s, increase heparin by 100 IU/h only if arterial PTT < 45 s
Maintain arterial PTT 40–45 s
If arterial PTT < 40 s, increase heparin by 100 IU/h

*"Venous" refers to the line exiting the dialyzer and returning to the patient via the femoral vein. PTT refers to partial thromboplastin time.

TABLE 109-13

APPROXIMATE DOSAGE ADJUSTMENTS OF ANTIBIOTICS IN PATIENTS WITH ACUTE RENAL FAILURE WHILE RECEIVING CAVHD*

Cefuroxime, 500–700 mg q 12 h
Ceftazidime, 1 g q 24 h
Tobramycin, loading dose followed by 60–80 mg/24 h
Gentamicin, loading dose then 80–100 mg/24 h
Ciprofloxacin, 200 mg q 8 h
Vancomycin, 1g q 48 h

*Blood levels should also be determined, if possible.
Modified Davies SP, Brown EA, Knox WJ, et al: Pharmacokinetic studies in patients with acute renal failure treated by continuous arteriovenous hemodialysis. In: Abstracts of the 1990 Interscience Conference on Antimicrobial Agents, p 213, 1990.

of ultrafiltration, and nutrient or drug removal, can all be avoided or controlled with careful monitoring. Continuous venovenous hemodialysis, the natural successor to CAVHD, promises to solve at least some of these problems.

References

1. Jenkins RD, Kacki M, Kahn RJ, et al: Solute clearance of various dialyzers in continuous arteriovenous hemodialysis (CAVHD) (abstract). Blood Purif 7:265, 1989.
2. Yohay DA, Schwab SJ, Quarles LD: Parallel plates are more effective than hollow fiber dialyzers in continuous arteriovenous hemodialysis (CAVHD). J Am Soc Nephrol 1:382, 1990.
3. Sigler MH, Teehan BP, Van Valkenbugh D: Solute transport in continuous hemodialysis: A new treatment for acute renal failure. Kidney Int 32:562, 1987.
4. Sigler MH, Teehan BP: Continuous arteriovenous hemodialysis. In: Nissenson AR, Fine RN, Gentile DE (eds): Clinical Dialysis. 2nd ed. Norwalk, CT, Appleton & Lange, p 726, 1990.
5. Kelleher SP, Robinette JB, Miller F, et al: Effect of hemorrhagic reduction in blood pressure on recovery from acute renal failure. Kidney Int 31:725, 1987.
6. Sargent JA, Gotch FA: Principles of biophysics in dialysis. In: Drukker W, Parsons FM, Maher J (eds): Replacement of Renal Function by Dialysis. 2nd ed. Boston, Martinus Nijhoff, p 59, 1983.
7. Barzilay E, Weksler N, Kessler D, et al: The use of continuous arteriovenous hemodialysis in the management of patients with oliguria associated with multiple organ failure (letter). Intensive Care Med 14:444, 1988.
8. Gibney RT, Stollery DE, Lefebvre RE, et al: Continuous arteriovenous hemodialysis: An alternative therapy for acute renal failure associated with critical illness. Can Med Assoc J 139:861, 1988.
9. Stevens PE, Riley B, Davies SP, et al: Continuous arteriovenous haemodialysis in critically ill patients. Lancet 2:150, 1988.
10. Voerman HJ, Van Schijndel RJ, Thijs LG: Continuous arterial-venous hemodiafiltration in critically ill patients. Crit Care Med 18:911, 1990.
11. Schneider NS, Geronemus R: Continuous arteriovenous hemodialysis. Kidney Int Suppl 24:S159, 1988.
12. Uldall R, Francolur R, Blake P, et al: Improved system for continuous venovenous hemodialysis (CVVHD) in intensive care units (ICU) (abstract). Kidney Int 37:321, 1990.
13. Davies SP, Brown EA, Knox WJ, et al: Pharmacokinetic studies in patients with acute renal failure treated by continuous arteriovenous hemodialysis. In: Abstracts of the 1990 Interscience Conference on Antimicrobial Agents, p 213, 1990.
14. Sigler MH, Snyder S, Teehan BP: Amino acid removal during continuous arteriovenous hemodialysis (CAVHD) in acute renal failure patients receiving total parenteral hyperalimentation (abstract). Blood Purif 6:357, 1988.

Hemoperfusion and the Treatment of Poisoning

Fuad Shihab
Sidney M. Kobrin

Hemoperfusion provides another means of solute removal from the blood by direct adsorption of selected solutes onto a column of activated charcoal or resin.[1] Hemoperfusion has been employed in patients with renal failure and been reported to be effective in removing putative uremic toxins and in improving uremic symptoms.[2] However, the lack of fluid removal has limited its role in the treatment of renal failure per se.[3] To date, its principal role has been in the treatment of certain drug intoxications.[4]

VASCULAR ACCESS

Hemoperfusion requires a reliable vascular access similar to that employed in acute hemodialysis. Femoral catheters are generally preferred in critically ill patients because they can be inserted rapidly and safely without serious complications, and, for the most part, only one or two treatments are performed.

EQUIPMENT AND SUPPLIES

The circuit used for hemoperfusion is similar to that for hemodialysis and includes a blood pump, blood lines, an air detector, and a venous air trap. The hemoperfusion cartridge generally contains a form of activated charcoal (60 to 300 g) or activated carbon coated with polymer membranes. In general, more heparin is needed for a hemoperfusion treatment (approximately 6000 U per session) than for hemodialysis because the charcoal adsorbs heparin. A single 3-hour treatment substantially lowers the blood levels of most poisons for which hemoperfusion is effective. More prolonged use is inefficient because the charcoal becomes saturated. If more prolonged treatment is needed, the cartridge must be replaced.

INDICATIONS

Not all drug intoxications require hemoperfusion. Initial treatment includes cardiorespiratory support, early gastric lavage when indicated and safe, and the administration of activated charcoal and specific drug antagonists. In patients with adequate renal function, forced diuresis (with alkalization or acidification of the urine, depending on the specific poison under consideration) can accelerate removal of certain toxins from the body. The great majority of patients do well with these conservative, nondialytic measures. Serum drug levels may help to determine the severity of toxicity, but the toxic concentration of some drugs remains unknown. However, even in the latter situation, drug levels may be helpful in monitoring the efficacy of therapy.

Hemoperfusion has been successful in removing drugs that are lipid soluble, have relatively high molecular weights, or bind to proteins with high affinity.[5, 6] With this in mind, hemoperfusion has been used successfully to treat intoxications with tricyclic antidepressants,[7] short-acting barbiturates,[8] theophylline,[9] digoxin,[10] glutethemide,[7] and ethchlorvynol.[11] Hemodialysis has been used primarily for removal

TABLE 109–14

DRUGS REMOVED BY HEMOPERFUSION OR HEMODIALYSIS

Better Removed by Hemoperfusion	Better Removed by Hemodialysis
Barbiturates	Alcohols
Tricyclic antidepressants	Ethanol
Nonbarbiturate tranquilizers	Methanol
Ethchlorvynol	Ethylene glycol
Glutethimide	Isopropanol
Methaqualone	Analgesics
Meprobamate	Aspirin
Analgesics	Methylsalicylate
Acetaminophen	Antimicrobial agents
Propoxyphene	Aminoglycosides
Anticancer agents	Penicillins
Methotrexate	Isoniazid
Cardiovascular agents	Electrolytes and metals
Digoxin	Lithium
Procainamide	Bromide
Quinidine	Fluoride
N-Acetylprocainamide	Arsenic
Miscellaneous	Lead
Amanita phalloides	Mercury
(also hemodialysis)	Miscellaneous
Paraquat	*Amanita phalloides*
Theophylline	(also
Phenylbutazone	hemoperfusion)

of drugs of lower molecular weight, drugs that are water soluble, and drugs that are extensively protein bound (e.g., lithium, aspirin, methanol, and ethylene glycol). Peritoneal dialysis is less useful in the treatment of drug intoxications; hemodialysis and hemoperfusion are usually 5 to 20 times more effective in clearing drugs from the circulation.[12] Table 109–14 provides a list of common drug intoxications and indicates whether hemodialysis or hemoperfusion is the therapy of choice.

The most important criteria for intervention with hemoperfusion are severe intoxication with impaired vital functions and progressive deterioration despite aggressive conservative measures. Many consider the presence of potentially lethal drug levels to be another indication. Because many drugs are metabolized or eliminated by the liver or kidney, any acute or chronic damage to these organs may delay recovery from drug overdose and may necessitate early use of dialysis to hasten drug clearance. Furthermore, if a comatose patient also has severe lung or cardiac disease, rapid removal of the drug might decrease the frequency and severity of complications associated with prolonged endotracheal intubation.

TABLE 109–15

COMPLICATIONS OF HEMOPERFUSION

Thrombocytopenia
Leukopenia
Membrane biocompatibility (pyrogen reactions)
Hemorrhage
Microembolization of charcoal particles
Hypoglycemia, hypocalcemia, hypophosphatemia
Removal of hormones, trace elements, and therapeutic drugs
Hypothermia
Hypotension
Anemia
Postperfusion "rebound"

COMPLICATIONS

The potential complications of hemoperfusion are listed in Table 109–15. Profound thrombocytopenia may be encountered,[13] but this problem has been alleviated by using polymer coating techniques[14] and extensive washing procedures and priming the membrane with dilute human albumin solution. The latter is thought to reduce platelet losses to less than 30%.[15] Transient leukopenia also occurs and is thought to be due to complement activation. Problems with membrane biocompatibility may cause typical pyrogen reactions. Adsorption (loss) or activation of coagulation factors may also be seen and are more severe in patients with hepatic failure, in whom platelet aggregation is thought to produce vasoactive amines responsible for hypotension.[16] Hemorrhage is not uncommon in patients treated with hemoperfusion and likely results from the use of heparin and the associated thrombocytopenia.

Microembolization of charcoal particles was common with the early, poorly washed hemoperfusion devices but has been virtually eliminated by the use of polymer coating techniques. Hemoperfusion also removes various plasma constituents such as glucose, calcium, phosphate, and some therapeutic drugs. Trace elements and hormones may also be adsorbed by activated charcoal devices. Reduction of body temperature may result from reinfusion of unheated extracorporeal blood at room temperature. Hypotension may also occur during hemoperfusion, possibly as a result of the large priming blood volume required or removal of catecholamines from the circulation. Anemia may result from large losses of blood in the hemoperfusion device.

Postperfusion "rebound," in which patients deteriorate after termination of the procedure, is due to replenishment of the lowered plasma drug level from body fat depots. This occurs mostly with drugs that have a high volume of distribution, for which the amount of drug present in the blood represents only a small fraction of the total body load.

References

1. Rosenbaum JL, Kramer MS, Raja R: Resin hemoperfusion for acute drug intoxication. Arch Intern Med 136:263, 1976.
2. Chang TMS, Gonda A, Dirks JH, et al: Clinical evaluation of chronic intermittent and short term hemoperfusion in patients with chronic renal failure using semipermeable microcapsules (artificial cells) formed from membrane coated activated charcoal. Trans Am Soc Artif Intern Organs 17:246, 1971.
3. Gelfand MC, Winchester JF: Hemoperfusion results in uremia. Clin Nephrol 1:107, 1979.
4. Gelfand MC, Winchester JF, Knepshield JH, et al: Treatment of severe drug overdosage with charcoal hemoperfusion. Trans Am Soc Artif Intern Organs 23:599, 1977.
5. Winchester JF, Gelfand MC, Knepshield JH, et al: Dialysis and hemoperfusion of poisons and drugs—Update. Trans Am Soc Artif Intern Organs 23:762, 1977.
6. Koffler A, Bernstein M, LaSette A, et al: Fixed-bed charcoal hemoperfusion. Arch Intern Med 138:1691, 1978.
7. Diaz-Buxo JA, Farmer CD, Chandler JT: Hemoperfusion in the treatment of amitriptyline intoxication. Trans Am Soc Artif Intern Organs 24:699, 1978.
8. Trafford JA, Jones RH, Evans R, et al: Haemoperfusion with R-004 Amberlite resin for treating acute poisoning. Br Med J 2:1453, 1977.
9. Russo ME: Management of theophylline intoxication with charcoal column hemoperfusion. N Engl J Med 300:24, 1979.
10. Smiley JW, March NM, Del Guercio ET: Hemoperfusion in the management of digoxin toxicity. JAMA 240:2736, 1978.
11. Lynn RI, Honig CL, Jatlow PI, et al: Resin hemoperfusion for treatment of ethchlorvynol overdose. Ann Intern Med 91:549, 1979.
12. Vale JA, Rees AJ, Widdop B, et al: Use of charcoal haemoperfusion in the management of severely poisoned patients. Br Med J 1:5, 1975.
13. Yatzidis H: A convenient hemoperfusion micro-apparatus over charcoal for the treatment of endogenous and exogenous intoxications. Its use as an artificial kidney. Proc Eur Dial Transplant Assoc 1:83, 1964.
14. Stefoni S, Feliciangeli G, Coli L, et al: Evaluation of a new coated charcoal for hemoperfusion in uremia. Int J Artif Organs 2:320, 1979.

15. Winchester JF: Hemoperfusion in uremia. In: Giordano C (ed): Sorbents and Their Clinical Applications. New York, Academic Press, p 387, 1980.
16. Weston MJ, Langley PG, Rubin MH, et al: Platelet function in fulminant hepatic failure and effect of charcoal haemoperfusion. Gut 18:897, 1977.

CHAPTER 110

Complications of Renal Transplantation

Dale H. Sillix

In the past decade, the number of kidney transplants has increased annually by 10%.[1] This has been accompanied by an improvement in 1-year graft survival. Approximately 10,000 renal transplants are performed each year in the United States. This represents about 10% of patients undergoing dialysis. Transplantation from living related donors accounts for less than 20% of the total. Because the number of cadaveric donors has not increased in proportion to the need, more than 15,000 people now await transplantation in the United States. In financial terms, providing maintenance hemodialysis costs three times more than maintaining a patient with a functioning graft, even considering the high initial cost of transplantation.[2] In terms of quality of life, transplantation again appears to be superior to dialysis.[3–5] As the numbers of older or diabetic patients starting dialysis grow, more of these patients undergo transplantation.[6, 7] Although both patient and graft survival rates in diabetics are lower than those in other patients, transplantation can provide benefits.[8, 9]

As the number of patients with functioning renal allografts grows and selection criteria broaden, more long-term complications are being reported.[10, 11] Although the majority of problems are associated either with end-stage renal disease itself or with the use of immunosuppressive agents, certain technical problems unique to renal transplantation should be kept in mind. During transplantation, reconstruction of the drainage system can lead to several problems. Internal ureteroneocystostomy remains the most common reconstructive procedure, although complication rates may be as high as 10%.[12] Urinary extravasation from the cystostomy and obstruction at the implant site are the most common problems. Obstruction of the ureter may be intrinsic (torsion or necrosis of the ureter) or extrinsic (lymphocele, fibrosis) in origin. Fungus balls, blood clots, renal stones, and papillary necrosis must also be considered.[13] Lymphoceles are common, but the majority are small and resolve without therapy.[14] Before the diagnosis of a lymphocele can be established, a diagnostic aspiration of the fluid should be done to exclude a urinoma. Two thirds of lymphoceles can be managed without surgery, although repeated percutaneous drainage or sclerotherapy may be needed.[14, 15] Vascular complications of renal transplantation are less common but include renal arterial thrombosis, anastomotic aneurysms, renal venous thrombosis, arteriovenous fistulas (after arteriography), and renal arterial stenosis.[16]

IMMUNOSUPPRESSIVE THERAPY

Transplant immunosuppressive protocols vary widely and are too numerous to recount in any detail. Common variations include cyclosporine with high- or low-dose prednisone, triple therapy (cyclosporine, azathioprine, and prednisone), conventional therapy (azathioprine, prednisone) with or without induction with antilymphocyte globulin, or quadruple therapy (induction with antilymphocyte globulin, then maintenance with cyclosporine, azathioprine, and prednisone). Rejection episodes are treated with steroids, antilymphocyte globulin, or monoclonal antibody therapy directed at the pan–T cell receptor T3 (muromonab-CD3, or OKT3). Newer agents such as FK506 or monoclonal antibodies to the interleukin-2 receptor are in development and may soon join the current therapeutic options. For the short-term acute care of transplant patients, focusing on side effects, toxicities and drug interactions of the commonly used immunosuppressive agents is more useful than discussions of long-term immunosuppression strategies.

Glucocorticoids. Glucocorticoids have marked immunosuppressive, anti-inflammatory, and lymphocytolytic effects at pharmacologic doses. The large number of side effects listed in Table 110–1 reflects the wide range of cells that possess glucocorticoid receptors.[17, 18] These receptors transcriptionally regulate a limited number of target genes, and the time to onset of steroid effects as well as the time to dissipation of effects varies with the particular biologic process involved.[19] The major glucocorticoids used in transplantation are prednisone, prednisolone, and methylprednisolone. Substitution of equivalent doses of hydrocortisone or dexamethasone may not provide equivalent immunosuppression because of differences in pharmacokinetic disposition.[18]

Azathioprine. Azathioprine, an analogue of 6-mercaptopurine, has been used in clinical transplantation since 1963. It functions as an antimetabolite and inhibits purine nucleotide synthesis.[20] The major side effect is myelotoxicity, especially leukopenia and thrombocytopenia. Macrocytic anemia can also be seen. Intrahepatic cholestasis and acute pancreatitis have been reported. Interstitial pulmonary fibrosis and bladder carcinoma are rare complications.[21, 22]

Cyclosporine. This fungus-derived agent is remarkably lymphocyte specific, blocking an early stage of lymphocyte activation. Like steroids, it inhibits the entry of activated T cells into the S phase of the cell cycle. It also inhibits interleukin-2 release from activated helper T cells while

TABLE 110–1
GLUCOCORTICOID SIDE EFFECTS
Dermal: acne, wound dehiscence, easy bruising, dermal atrophy, striae
Metabolic: carbohydrate intolerance, diabetes mellitus, truncal fat redistribution, lipid abnormalities, fluid retention, hypertension, hirsutism, atherosclerosis
Musculoskeletal: osteoporosis, proximal myopathy, avascular necrosis of bone
Gastrointestinal: peptic ulcer disease, pancreatitis, oropharyngeal or esophageal candidiasis, colonic ulcerations
Neurologic: sleep disorders, psychiatric symptoms, seizures, epidural lipomatosis, pseudotumor cerebri
Immunologic: increased susceptibility to infections; sequestration of lymphocytes, monocytes, and eosinophils; reduced interleukin-1 production by macrophages; impaired chemotaxis; reduced capillary leak; suppression of inflammatory mediators
Other: growth retardation in children, posterior cataracts, glaucoma

Data from Jusko WJ: Corticosteroid pharmacodynamics: Models for a broad array of receptor-mediated pharmacologic effects. J Clin Pharmacol 30:303, 1990; and Baxter JD: Minimizing the side effects of glucocorticoid therapy. Adv Intern Med 35:173, 1990.

sparing suppressor T lymphocytes. It is neither cytotoxic nor myelotoxic.[23] Table 110–2 lists the wide range of complications seen with cyclosporine.[24–27]

The use of cyclosporine is complicated by tremendous interindividual variation in pharmacokinetics. The hepatic cytochrome P-450 system is responsible for the drug's metabolism. Alterations in bile flow, liver function, or gastric motility can alter a previously stable and therapeutic cyclosporine level.[28, 29] Alterations in medications can likewise affect cyclosporine levels. Table 110–3 lists the more common drug interactions.[30] Further complicating the management of cyclosporine therapy are the variety of assay methods available and the wide range of variables affecting the assay results.[28] Assays can be done on whole blood or serum. Because of extensive binding of cyclosporine to cell membranes, therapeutic whole blood levels are higher and are altered by changes in hematocrit. Hematocrit, sampling time, incubation temperature, and lipoprotein levels all affect cyclosporine concentrations.[31, 32]

One of the more common and serious cyclosporine-associated problems is nephrotoxicity, which may be reversible or irreversible. Functional changes related to afferent arterial vasoconstriction are reversible with a decrease in cyclosporine dose[33–35] and may involve alterations in prostaglandin synthesis in the kidney.[36] Calcium channel blockers have proved beneficial in lessening cyclosporine-induced vasoconstriction.[37] The irreversible vasculopathy of cyclosporine involves afferent arteriole occlusion with ischemia of the associated glomerulus and tubule. Attempts to minimize or avoid chronic irreversible nephrotoxicity include protocols that drastically lower or eliminate cyclosporine at some point after transplantation (commonly 6 to 12 months). With such protocols, there may be increased rates of rejection after conversion.[38] In contrast, long-term use of cyclosporine is not associated with more rapid graft loss.[39–41]

OKT3. This purified murine monoclonal antibody (muromonab-CD3) is directed against the CD3 (T3) antigen found on all mature human T lymphocytes. Within minutes of administration, there is a rapid clearance of T3 cells from the circulation. Daily administration continues this effect and is associated with reversal of most acute rejection episodes, including steroid-resistant rejections.[42] First-dose effects are extremely common and are probably related to release of mediators when the T3 receptor is engaged. The majority of the symptoms are influenza-like. The incidence and severity of these symptoms lessen with the second dose and usually disappear by the third.[43] The most dangerous adverse reaction is severe pulmonary edema. Aseptic men-

TABLE 110–2
CYCLOSPORINE SIDE EFFECTS IN RENAL TRANSPLANT RECIPIENTS

Renal: renal insufficiency, hyperuricemia, hyperkalemia, hypomagnesemia, type IV renal tubular acidosis, interstitial fibrosis, glomerular capillary thrombosis
Vascular: hypertension, arteriolar hyalinosis, vasoconstriction, renal arterial thrombosis, hemolytic-uremic syndrome
Gastrointestinal: hepatotoxicity, cholestasis, cholelithiasis, pancreatitis
Neurologic: tremors, paresthesias, seizures, encephalopathy
Oncogenic: lymphomas, Kaposi's sarcoma
Infectious: bacterial, viral, fungal infections
Metabolic: diabetes, hypercholesterolemia, mammary hyperplasia
Musculoskeletal: gout
Other: hypertrichosis, gingival hyperplasia, acne, mild anemia, thrombocytopenia, leukopenia

Data from refs 24–27.

TABLE 110–3
CYCLOSPORINE INTERACTIONS

Drugs That Increase Cyclosporine Levels
Antibiotics: erythromycin, norfloxacin, imipenem, doxycycline, aminoglycosides
Antifungals: ketoconazole, fluconazole
Antihypertensives: diltiazem, verapamil, nicardipine, acetazolamide
Steroids: methylprednisolone, methyltestosterone, oral contraceptives, danazol
Other: cimetidine, metoclopramide, colchicine
Drugs That Decrease Cyclosporine Levels
Antibiotics: rifampin, nafcillin, trimethoprim-sulfamethoxazole, isoniazid
Anticonvulsants: phenytoin, phenobarbital, carbamazepine
Drugs That Potentiate Cyclosporine Nephrotoxicity
Nonsteroidal anti-inflammatory drugs
Antifungals: amphotericin B
Antibiotics: aminoglycosides, trimethoprim-sulfamethoxazole
Antivirals: ganciclovir, acyclovir
Other: ranitidine, cimetidine

From Yee GC: Pharmacokinetic interactions between cyclosporine and other drugs. Transplant Proc 22:1203, © 1990. Reprinted by permission of Appleton & Lange, Inc.

ingitis has been reported but is mild. More serious long-term consequences of OKT3 use involve increases in the rates and severity of infections, particularly with cytomegalovirus or other herpesviruses.[42]

Antilymphocyte Globulin. The active globulin fraction of antiserum against lymphocytes or thymocytes has been used both as prophylaxis (induction) and as antirejection therapy. Major drawbacks have been a lack of standardization of potency and purity of different preparations. Batch-to-batch variations necessitate daily monitoring of T cells to ensure that the circulating cells have been reduced to less than 10%. Problems of prior sensitization, toxic reactions, and anaphylactic reactions also make these preparations difficult to use. As with OKT3, increased risks of infection pose the greatest late complication.[44]

REJECTION

Immunosuppression protocols are designed to prevent rejection of the transplanted organ. Without administration of immunosuppressive drugs, even human leukocyte antigen–identical kidneys are rejected unless they come from an identical twin. With administration of immunosuppressants, even histoincompatible kidneys can enjoy long-term graft survival. With increasing time after transplantation, the risk of rejection lessens and the dosage of immunosuppressive medications can be decreased. Both host factors (tolerance) and graft factors (adaptation) contribute to long-term graft survival.[45]

Many antigens such as ABO blood type antigens act as histocompatibility antigens, but the major histocompatibility complex on chromosome 6 provides the major barrier to transplantation. These human leukocyte antigens are extremely polymorphic and ensure that there is some degree of major histocompatibility complex incompatibility in recipients of cadaveric donor kidneys. The recipient reaction to this challenge is to mount an immune response involving both the cellular (T cell) and humoral (B cell) arms.

Hyperacute Rejection. Hyperacute rejection occurs if the recipient has preformed cytotoxic circulating antibodies at the time of transplantation. A dramatic destruction of the graft is initiated within minutes, and within hours, the kidney is totally destroyed. No therapy is possible. Only prevention in the form of careful pretransplant cross-matching avoids this type of rejection.

Acute Rejection. Acute rejection occurs typically within the first few months after transplantation. Acute rejection episodes after the first year are unusual and are mostly found in patients noncompliant with their regimen of immunosuppressive medications or after abrupt switches in immunosuppression protocols. Both cellular and humoral patterns occur and often overlap. The antibodies involved are generated after transplantation in response to the allograft but, unlike those responsible for hyperacute rejection, can be controlled and respond to antirejection therapy. Vascular tissue is the usual target of the antibody-mediated attack, with the end result being vessel fibrosis and ischemia. Cell-mediated rejection is characterized by a mononuclear cell infiltrate into the graft with local destruction of tissue leading to interstitial fibrosis. This type of rejection also responds to treatment.[46] The key to successful antirejection therapy is rapid diagnosis and treatment. The longer a rejection episode goes untreated, the less are the chances of complete reversal.[44, 45] Acute rejection must be distinguished from other causes of acute renal failure (Table 110–4). Oliguria after transplantation may be due to hypovolemia, acute tubular necrosis, or problems with the vascular or ureteral anastomosis.[47, 48] Deterioration of renal function after urine flow has been established may be due to acute rejection, even in the absence of typical signs such as graft swelling or tenderness, fever, and hypertension. The diagnosis of acute rejection rests on urinalysis and assessment of renal blood flow and the perinephric bed. Ultrasonography and technetium scans are the most common tools used to assess graft status.[49, 50] Percutaneous renal biopsy may sometimes be necessary to pinpoint the diagnosis.

Chronic Rejection. Chronic rejection occurs 6 months or longer after transplantation and is characterized by a steady deterioration of graft function that is unresponsive to antirejection therapy. Interstitial and glomerular sclerosis are characteristically seen on biopsy. Reversible causes of renal insufficiency must be ruled out before the azotemia is ascribed to chronic rejection. Nonsteroidal anti-inflammatory drugs, angiotensin-converting enzyme inhibitors, and radiographic contrast agents are common offenders. Urinary tract infections and/or obstruction and renal arterial stenosis also need to be considered.[44]

HYPERTENSION

Hypertension is a common complication after renal transplantation and is associated with decreased graft survival and increased rejection episodes.[10, 11, 51–54] Survival of patients is also decreased when hypertension occurs.[52] The incidence of hypertension varies from 20 to 70%, rates generally being higher in the first year. However, even after 10 years, the incidence of hypertension is more than 40%.[10] Table 110–5 lists the multiple causes of post-transplant hypertension.

Etiology

Acute rejection can be associated with the de novo development of hypertension or with worsening of pre-existing hypertension. The renin-angiotensin system is activated by

TABLE 110–4
DIFFERENTIAL DIAGNOSIS OF ACUTE REJECTION

Hypovolemia	Lymphoceles
Acute tubular necrosis	Cyclosporine toxicity
Vascular complications	Urinary tract infection
Urologic complications	Recurrent glomerulopathy

TABLE 110–5
CAUSES OF HYPERTENSION IN RENAL TRANSPLANT PATIENTS

Rejection—acute, chronic	Recurrent renal disease
Drugs—steroids, cyclosporine	Hypertensive donor
Native kidneys	Obstructive uropathy
Renal arterial stenosis	Hyperparathyroidism

ischemic injury of the kidney, and the rapid fall in glomerular filtration rate leads to sodium retention.[53–55] Abrupt rises in blood pressure in the first few months after transplantation can be an important clue to a rejection episode. Prompt antirejection therapy is the most appropriate management. Chronic rejection is commonly associated with hypertension, the blood pressure mirroring increases in the serum creatinine concentration and the irreversible loss of graft function. This type of hypertension is not responsive to antirejection therapy and requires management with standard antihypertensive agents.

Steroids can influence the incidence of hypertension in the early post-transplant period, but steroid therapy is not associated with the long-term occurrence of hypertension.[53–57] The use of cyclosporine has increased the incidence of post-transplant hypertension.[56, 58–62] Cyclosporine-induced hypertension may be mediated by both renal and extrarenal mechanisms. Cyclosporine-induced renal vasoconstriction is associated with decreased renal blood flow despite increased mean arterial pressures, indicating increased renovascular resistance.[60, 63] The hypertension can be seen in the absence of renal insufficiency.[61, 63] Nonrenal mechanisms may include general vasoconstrictor effects, hypomagnesemia, changes in intracellular calcium levels, changes in atrial natriuretic peptide, alterations in the sympathetic nervous system activity, and effects on vasopressin.[59, 63–65] The role of the renin-angiotensin system in cyclosporine-induced hypertension remains unclear. Although studies in several animal models have suggested a therapeutic role for angiotensin-converting enzyme inhibitors in cyclosporine-induced hypertension, clinical studies have found such patients to be resistant to these agents.[66–71]

The presence of the nonfunctioning native kidneys has a profound influence on the development and severity of post-transplant hypertension. Before the introduction of cyclosporine, the incidence of hypertension was closely correlated with the presence of native kidneys. Pretransplant bilateral nephrectomy decreases the prevalence of hypertension after transplantation, and bilateral nephrectomy after transplantation is associated with improvement of hypertension.[51, 53, 72] This three-kidney hypertension model is presumptively mediated by increased renin secretion by the nonfunctioning kidneys and is responsive to angiotensin-converting enzyme inhibition.[51, 53]

The incidence of transplant-associated renal arterial stenosis varies between 1 and 20% but usually falls in the 6 to 10% range.[51, 53, 55] Although angiography may reveal narrowing of the renal artery in a quarter of the cases, this is rarely functionally significant unless at least 60 to 70% of the vessel is occluded.[54] Renal arterial stenosis is usually suspected when the patient has refractory hypertension, mild-to-moderate renal insufficiency, and a localized bruit over the graft within the first year of the transplantation. Unfortunately, these classic findings are not always present, and similar findings can be found in cyclosporine toxicity, obstruction, arteriovenous fistulas, and rejection.[51, 53–55] The captopril challenge test has some support as a noninvasive way of diagnosing significant stenosis of the transplanted renal artery. However, because angiotensin-converting enzyme inhibitors can cause renal insufficiency, especially in patients receiving cyclosporine, this test is no longer recommended.[73, 74] Percutaneous transluminal angioplasty has been useful, but not universally successful, in improving renal arterial stenosis.[75] The indication for surgical correction is influenced by the technical difficulty of the repair, the severity of the hypertension, the degree of renal impairment, and the age or condition of the graft and the patient.

Recurrent (or de novo) glomerulonephritis is associated with decreased graft function, hypertension, and proteinuria.[76, 77] Hypertension in the donor influences the development of hypertension in the recipient.[78] Obstruction of the transplanted kidney is a rare cause of post-transplant hypertension and may be difficult to diagnose.[79] Post-transplant hyperparathyroidism may also influence hypertension.[80]

Treatment

Antihypertensive therapy in the renal transplant patient has no clear-cut directives, but a general scheme is provided in Figure 110–1. Hypertension that occurs early and is associated with large doses of steroid is often volume mediated and responds to salt restriction and administration of diuretics. Acute rejection-associated hypertension can respond to steroids or other antirejection therapies. Cyclosporine-associated hypertension generally responds to adjusting the dose (if blood cyclosporine levels are elevated) or to switching to alternative immunosuppressive protocols.[38] Salt depletion and administration of diuretics are effective in cyclosporine- or rejection-associated hypertension.[68] Cal-

cium channel blockers are also effective in cyclosporine-induced hypertension but in some cases increase cyclosporine levels, requiring further dose adjustments.[81–83] Beta-adrenergic blockers may aggregate hyperlipidemia or fail to improve left ventricular hypertrophy. Intravenous labetalol may induce hyperkalemia.[84] Vasodilators may worsen sodium retention and necessitate treatment with diuretics. Minoxidil may worsen cyclosporine-induced hypertrichosis.[85] Angiotensin-converting enzyme inhibitors may be helpful, especially if the hypertension is related to the presence of native kidneys or is renin related but can cause acute renal failure. Hyperkalemia may be seen with angiotensin-converting enzyme inhibitors, and dose adjustments must be made for renal insufficiency.[73, 74] Alpha-blockers might have special benefit in cyclosporine-induced hypertension.[62] Central alpha-agonists (clonidine) are usually well tolerated. Nitroprusside should be used with a clear understanding that because the serum creatinine concentration may not always be an accurate guide to transplant function,[86] cyanide toxicity may occur unexpectedly.

CARDIOVASCULAR DISEASE

Studies of morbidity in renal transplant recipients show that cardiovascular complications are a leading cause of death after the first 10 years.[11, 16, 87, 88] In those who survive with a functioning transplant for at least 5 years, about 50% of subsequent deaths can be attributed to atherosclerotic heart disease and related vascular complications.[4, 10, 11, 89–91] This is not surprising given the high rate of cardiovascular disease among the general dialysis population.[92–95] Despite

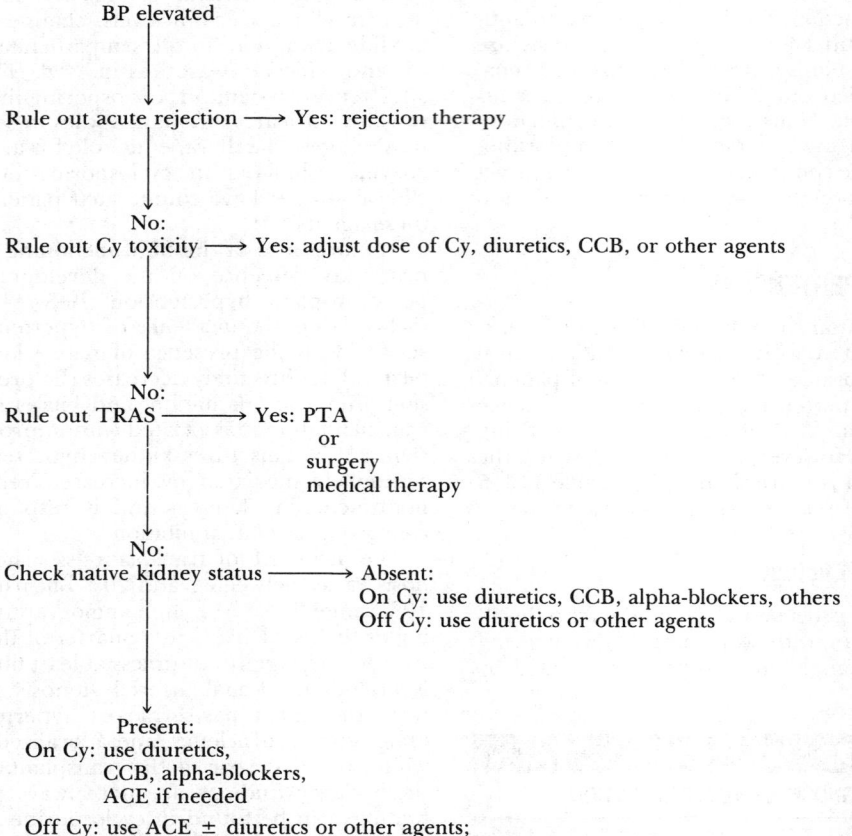

Figure 110–1. Management of elevated blood pressure (BP) in renal transplant patients. CCB = calcium channel blockers; TRAS = transplant renal arterial stenosis; PTA = percutaneous transluminal angioplasty; Cy = cyclosporine; ACE = angiotensin-converting enzyme inhibitors.

this, most patients cleared for transplantation tolerate anesthesia well.[96, 97] Careful pretransplant evaluations are mandatory in patients with cardiovascular risk factors and especially in diabetics, who have a high incidence of silent coronary artery disease.[8]

Many factors are responsible for the high rate of cardiovascular disease in patients undergoing dialysis and renal transplantation (Table 110–6). Although some of these (e.g., left ventricular hypertrophy) can improve after renal transplantation, other factors may worsen and atherosclerosis may accelerate.[4, 11, 98, 99] Glucose tolerance often worsens with steroid and cyclosporine use. Hypertension may be more difficult to control after transplantation. Dialysis-associated hypertriglyceridemia may improve but hypercholesterolemia worsens.[11, 100] Hyperparathyroidism with associated vascular calcification is a significant pretransplant problem that may not resolve completely after transplantation.[11, 89, 93, 94] Aggressive medical and surgical management of these problems is indicated.[89, 101]

DIABETES MELLITUS

Although originally thought to be related to steroid use, the glucose intolerance seen after renal transplantation may also be due to other factors.[102, 103] The incidence of posttransplant diabetes mellitus varies and depends on the definition of abnormal carbohydrate metabolism that is employed and perhaps also on whether cyclosporine is included as part of the immunosuppression protocol.[104–107] Cyclosporine has toxic effects on pancreatic beta-cells and also inhibits glycogen synthesis.[108, 109] Insulin synthesis and secretion are impaired, insulin clearance is increased, and insulin sensitivity is unchanged. Although fasting glucose and insulin levels are not altered by cyclosporine, net glucose disposal is decreased and glucose-stimulated insulin levels are decreased. These findings are especially important to keep in mind when patients receive high intravenous glucose loads, such as during total parenteral nutrition.

HYPERPARATHYROIDISM

Secondary hyperparathyroidism in end-stage renal disease is associated with elevated parathyroid hormone (PTH) levels, hyperphosphatemia, hypocalcemia, and decreased l, 25-dihydroxycholecalciferol production by the kidney. Metastatic calcification, renal osteodystrophy, and pruritus are common. With the introduction of a functioning renal transplant, phosphorus is excreted, vitamin D is metabolized appropriately, and the serum calcium concentration rises. Up to one third of patients become hypercalcemic at some point after successful renal transplantation. This can be seen within days of transplantation and is common within the first month.[110]

Hypercalcemia is due to persistent hyperparathyroidism, although phosphate depletion, mobilization of vascular calcium deposits, and steroid administration may also contribute.[91] The hypercalcemia may persist for months or even years and is not necessarily associated with decreased graft survival.[111] Symptomatic hypercalcemia, nephrolithiasis, nephrocalcinosis, and worsening renal osteodystrophy may necessitate parathyroidectomy.[112]

Elevated PTH levels after transplantation may be due to persistent renal insufficiency or to primary parathyroid abnormalities. In the latter case, elevated PTH levels reflect increased parathyroid tissue mass rather than an autonomous adenoma, and the glands generally slowly involute, although it may take many years.[91, 110, 112, 113] Specialized PTH assays such as NH_2-terminal or intact PTH measurements may be indicated in patients with renal insufficiency to distinguish physiologically important elevations in PTH levels from levels that are high simply because of the retention of inactive metabolic fragments.[114]

Hypophosphatemia may be severe and develop rapidly after transplantation, especially if normal renal function is quickly restored. The persistence of high PTH levels and the presence of renal tubules sensitive to PTH lead to excessive urinary phosphate loss. Continued use of phosphate-binding antacids may aggravate the hypophosphatemia. Renal tubular phosphate leaks unrelated to the high circulating level of PTH have also been described.[115] Phosphorus supplementation should be used to avoid phosphate depletion.[91]

HYPERLIPIDEMIA

Chronic uremia is associated with many alterations in lipid metabolism, which are seen in at least 50% of patients undergoing dialysis and which generally have significant atherogenic potential.[116] Hypertriglyceridemia is the major abnormality seen and occurs in up to 70% of cases. Low-density lipoprotein and very low density lipoprotein levels are increased, and high-density lipoprotein (HDL) levels are decreased. Cholesterol levels are elevated in about 20% of dialysis patients overall, but the incidence of hypercholesterolemia is greater in patients receiving continuous ambulatory peritoneal dialysis than in those receiving hemodialysis. After transplantation, cholesterol levels rise immediately.[100, 116, 117] Variable patterns of hyperlipidemia are seen in renal transplant recipients. Some continue to have hypertriglyceridemia; others have hypercholesterolemia or a mixed picture.[118] HDL levels tend to increase but usually not in proportion to the increase in cholesterol, and an unfavorable high-density–to–low-density lipoprotein ratio develops. The HDL_3 subfraction is responsible for the majority of the rise in HDL, whereas HDL_2 levels remain low. These changes are associated with an increased risk of coronary artery disease.[11, 116, 119]

Cyclosporine therapy may cause additional problems in lipoprotein metabolism, despite its steroid-sparing effect. Hypertriglyceridemia is more common in transplant patients treated with cyclosporine but appears to be correlated with obesity and renal insufficiency rather than with cyclosporine levels or steroid dose.[120–122] Interactions between cyclosporine and lipoproteins are easy to understand given the lipophilic nature of the drug. In whole blood at room temperature, only 5% of the cyclosporine exists in free form; the rest is bound to cells and lipoproteins, principally cholesterol-containing lipoproteins. Hypocholesterolemia is associated with increased cyclosporine toxicity in animal models and in clinical studies, especially in liver transplant recipients. Changes in blood lipids can alter the toxicity and immunosuppressive effects of cyclosporine.[27, 31, 120]

Therapy of hyperlipidemia in the renal transplant recipient can be difficult. Standard dietary therapy can be ineffective, although some success has been reported.[123, 124] Switching to alternate-day steroids is usually not helpful. Lovastatin can cause severe myositis and even rhabdomyol-

TABLE 110–6

RISK FACTORS FOR CARDIAC DISEASE IN DIALYSIS AND RENAL TRANSPLANT PATIENTS

Diabetes mellitus	Hyperparathyroidism
Hypertension	Anemia
Hypertriglyceridemia	Obesity
Hypercholesterolemia	Smoking

ysis in patients taking cyclosporine, whereas gemfibrozil may be ineffective.[100, 116, 117] The rapid changes in lipid levels that can occur in the critically ill patient or patients receiving lipid infusions can alter free cyclosporine levels and/or the cellular uptake of cyclosporine, thus changing its therapeutic and toxic effects.[27, 122, 125]

ERYTHROCYTOSIS

Although the anemia of chronic renal failure is multifactorial in origin, decreased renal erythropoietin production is most important and the anemia can usually be treated successfully with human recombinant erythropoietin.[126] After renal transplantation, serum erythropoietin levels rise within 3 days of surgery and peak by 2 weeks if there is no delay in graft function. Normal feedback mechanisms resume as the hematocrit is normalized.[127] Hemoglobin levels increase within 2 to 6 weeks after successful transplantation and the anemia of chronic renal failure is normalized within a few months.[128, 129] During acute or chronic rejection episodes, erythropoietin levels fall and anemia may return.

Erythrocytosis occurs fairly often after renal transplantation. It can be managed by phlebotomy (for hematocrits > 60%) and usually resolves spontaneously within a few years. Diuretic use, renal artery stenosis, hydronephrosis, and rejection are other potential and correctable causes of erythrocytosis. Erythropoietin levels are not always elevated, and a loss of the normal negative feedback control may be present in a few patients.[130, 131]

ANEMIA

Anemia after renal transplantation must be thoroughly investigated, particularly if renal function is normal. Iron stores may be depleted and serum ferritin levels may be low, although most patients undergoing long-term dialysis have high serum ferritin levels that normalize after transplantation as body iron stores are utilized and the anemia is corrected.[132] Azathioprine may cause anemia as part of a generalized pancytopenia, although pure red blood cell aplasia is also possible.[133] Microangiopathic hemolytic anemia can occur with severe rejection episodes, and the hemolytic-uremic syndrome has been reported with cyclosporine use. The anemia of chronic rejection, like the anemia associated with other causes of chronic renal failure, is responsive to erythropoietin.[134]

RENAL TUBULAR DEFECTS

A variety of abnormalities in tubular function occur in the transplanted kidney. Renal tubular acidosis of either type I (classic distal renal tubular acidosis) or type IV (hyperkalemic renal tubular acidosis) variety can occur transiently in the newly transplanted kidney, especially in grafts with delayed function, ischemia, or acute rejection. A more persistent or later appearing distal renal tubular acidosis usually indicates chronic rejection. Hyperkalemia can be associated with delayed graft function, type IV renal tubular acidosis, or cyclosporine therapy.[91, 135] Glycosuria is common immediately after renal transplantation. Salt-wasting syndromes are rare. Defects in concentrating and diluting capacity may complicate rejection episodes.[91]

SEXUAL DYSFUNCTION

The majority of both men and women report a marked improvement in sexual desire and performance after transplantation.[136] Persistent impotence after transplantation may be due to compromised blood flow because of atherosclerosis and vascular calcification. Diabetes mellitus, antihypertensive medications, and renal insufficiency are also factors that leave up to 40% of men with some degree of impotence.

After successful transplantation in males, previously elevated follicle-stimulating hormone and prolactin levels normalize, but luteinizing hormone levels remain high, indicating that uremic primary hypergonadotropism is not completely reversed. Testosterone levels normalize, but dihydroepiandrosterone levels fall.[137] Chronic uremia causes gonadal damage, and sperm counts may remain low after transplantation, but many successful pregnancies have been reported.[138] In rats, cyclosporine has been reported to decrease testosterone levels, increase gonadotrophin levels, decrease the sperm count and sperm motility, and cause degenerative changes in the testis.[139]

Most women undergoing maintenance dialysis experience amenorrhea or irregular menses. Two thirds of women younger than age 50 years have a return to normal menstrual cycles after transplantation.[136] Pregnancy is best delayed for at least the first year after transplantation. Of pregnancies that go beyond the first trimester, 90% of post-transplantation pregnancies are successful; however, they must be aggressively followed as high-risk pregnancies. One third of these women have preeclampsia, and 15% have some degree of renal insufficiency after delivery. Vaginal deliveries are the rule, as dystocia is uncommon.[140, 141] Pregnancy does not alter long-term graft survival.

LIVER DISEASE

Liver failure and chronic hepatitis are major causes of morbidity and mortality in long-term follow-up studies.[142-144] Hepatitis is present in up to 40% of transplant patients.[10, 11, 142] Hepatitis B infections are the greatest problem because of the high prevalence of chronic antigen carriers in the dialysis population. The rate of hepatitis B virus antigenemia in dialysis patients ranges between 5 and 30%, depending on the geographic area and the use of hepatitis B vaccines.[142-144] Spontaneous seroconversion from positive hepatitis B surface antigen to negative surface antigen status occurs in more than 90% of infected dialysis patients. Of those who are hepatitis B surface antigen–positive at the time of transplant or who are infected later, few convert to an anti–hepatitis B state.[142, 143]

Several large studies of chronic liver disease in renal transplant patients have demonstrated that 40 to 80% of those with chronic liver problems are hepatitis B surface antigen–positive.[142-144] Hepatitis B virus–positive patients are five times more likely to have progressive liver damage than those who have chronic liver disease from other causes.[142, 143] The mortality rates in hepatitis B virus–positive patients were two to five times greater in two of three studies.[142-144]

Hepatitis B is not the only cause of liver disease (Table 110–7). Hepatitis C virus, cytomegalovirus, other herpesvi-

---

TABLE 110–7

CAUSES OF LIVER DYSFUNCTION IN RENAL TRANSPLANT PATIENTS

Acute hepatitis: cytomegalovirus, Epstein-Barr virus, hepatitis B virus, herpesviruses, adenoviruses
Cyclosporine: gallstones, cholestasis
Azathioprine: cholestatic jaundice, peliosis hepatis
Chronic hepatitis: hepatitis B virus infection; non-A, non-B hepatitis
Cirrhosis: chronic hepatitis, alcohol abuse
Other: hemosiderosis, hepatoma, reno-occlusive disease

ruses, and adenoviruses are to blame. Noninfectious causes include hemosiderosis, hemochromatosis, peliosis hepatis, and administration of immunosuppressive drugs.[145–148] Cyclosporine is primarily metabolized in the liver and excreted through the biliary system. Bile and bile salts are required for oral cyclosporine absorption, and cholestasis decreases cyclosporine bioavailability. Drugs metabolized by the P-450 enzyme system are competitive inhibitors of cyclosporine metabolism. Cyclosporine has hepatotoxicity, which usually presents with a cholestatic profile. The intravenous vehicle (polyoxyethylated caster oil) of cyclosporine can also be hepatotoxic.[27] Cyclosporine, however, may decrease the risk of liver disease. Patients receiving azathioprine seem to have a greater incidence of chronic liver disease.[149] Although episodes of hepatotoxicity occur in half of the patients receiving cyclosporine, these are usually self-limited and respond to dose adjustments.[150, 151] High levels of cyclosporine reduce bile flow and inhibit bile acid uptake and excretion by the liver, increasing the risk of cholelithiasis.[152] Gallstones occur in 5% of patients who had cyclosporine hepatotoxicity.[150]

PANCREATITIS

Acute pancreatitis is well described in renal transplant patients.[153, 154] Cytomegalovirus is one of the major causes, but steroids, azathioprine, diuretics, and cyclosporine are others.[150] Asymptomatic hyperamylasemia had been reported in 5 to 10% of renal transplant patients receiving cyclosporine.[150, 153] Patients with post-transplant hypercalcemia may be at increased risk: as many as 20% have hyperamylasemia and 11% have symptomatic pancreatitis.[155]

GASTROINTESTINAL DISORDERS

Gastrointestinal bleeding is common both before and after renal transplantation. Erosive gastritis and peptic ulcer disease are the most likely upper gastrointestinal tract causes and are related to steroid administration, uremia, and hypercalcemia. Precautions that should be taken to minimize these risks include antacids and histamine H_2 receptor antagonists. Dosage adjustments of the H_2 blockers must be made according to the level of renal function.[156, 157] Concerns that cimetidine might facilitate lymphocyte proliferation and augment rejection appear unfounded.[158] Although conservative medical management is successful in uncomplicated cases, an aggressive diagnostic and therapeutic approach, including biopsies for cytomegalovirus and early surgical intervention, may be required in more complicated cases.

Bowel obstruction must always be completely evaluated in the renal transplant recipient. Although small-bowel obstruction often can be nonsurgically treated, bleeding or obstruction of the large bowel necessitates rapid evaluation and serious consideration of surgical intervention.[158, 159] The high morbidity and mortality of colonic complications in these stressed, immunosuppressed individuals are widely recognized. The usual signs and symptoms of perforation may be masked. Cytomegalovirus-induced perforation, pseudomembranous colitis, perforated diverticulitis, ischemic colitis, and serious fecal impaction are all distinct possibilities.[159, 160]

CANCER

An increased rate of malignancy has been reported with all forms of immunosuppression used in transplantation. The more extensive the immunosuppression, the higher the cancer rate is. Malignancy becomes an increasing source of morbidity and mortality in those surviving longer with functioning allografts. For example, 1-year survivors of cardiac transplantation have a 3% incidence of cancer, but this increases to 25% at 5 years.[161] The mean age for the development of cancer is also younger than that of the general population. Although the common malignancies of the general population such as carcinoma of the lung, colon, prostate, breast, and cervix occur with similar incidence in the transplant population, other malignancies are disproportionately more frequent.

In the general population, basal cell carcinoma outnumbers squamous cell carcinoma by a fivefold margin; however, squamous cell skin cancer is almost twice as common as basal cell carcinoma in transplant recipients.[162, 163] Squamous cell carcinomas are more aggressive in transplant recipients, occur at a younger age, are more often multiple, and have a higher mortality rate.[161, 162] Kaposi's sarcoma is extremely rare in the population without acquired immunodeficiency syndrome, but accounts for 6% of malignancies in transplant recipients. Visceral involvement, particularly of the lungs and the gastrointestinal tract, occurs in more than 40%.[161, 162] Renal cell carcinoma is more frequent in patients undergoing long-term dialysis and is associated with acquired renal cystic disease. Successful transplantation seems to slow or even reverse the progression of these cysts.[164] In one group of patients studied more than 7 years after successful transplantation, renal cell carcinoma arising in the native kidneys accounted for less than 5% of all reported malignancies, which was considerably less than projected.[165, 166] Transitional cell carcinoma of the renal pelvis and ureter is common in patients with analgesic abuse nephropathy and can pose a real risk after transplantation in this group.[167]

Lymphoma is four times more likely to occur in transplant recipients than in the general population and is more likely to be of the non-Hodgkin's type. Non-Hodgkin's lymphomas make up more than 90% of post-transplantation lymphomas, instead of the expected 65%.[162, 163, 168] Immunologic markers demonstrate a B cell origin in more than 85% of the non-Hodgkin's lymphomas so far studied, and Epstein-Barr virus infection is a common association. Stimulation of B cell proliferation by Epstein-Barr virus concomitant with suppression of T cell regulatory networks by immunosuppressive therapy provides an attractive explanation for the increased incidence of non-Hodgkin's lymphomas after transplantation.[169, 170]

The role of cyclosporine in the increased risk of non-Hodgkin's lymphomas is also under study. The overall incidence of lymphoma has been reported to be higher in patients receiving cyclosporine than in those receiving conventional (noncyclosporine) immunosuppression.[163, 171, 172] The specific T cell suppressive effects of cyclosporine as well as changes in lymphokine production have been offered as explanations.[161] However, not all groups have noted a difference in the frequency of lymphomas (or other malignancies) in cyclosporine-treated patients compared with that in patients receiving azathioprine.[21, 162, 173–175]

Non-Hodgkin's lymphomas are more likely to have extranodal involvement in transplant recipients. Of particular interest is the unusually high likelihood of multicentric brain involvement.[163] This propensity must be kept in mind in any transplant patient with neurologic symptoms. Lymphoma therapy in transplantation patients commonly includes reduction or elimination of immunosuppressive therapy. In Epstein-Barr virus–associated lymphoproliferative disorders, early use of acyclovir or ganciclovir may be of some benefit.[169, 176] A particularly fulminant post-transplantation lymphoproliferative disorder has been reported after the sequential use of antilymphocyte globulin and OKT3; most of these cases were associated with primary Epstein-Barr virus infections and failed to respond to therapy.[177]

MUSCULOSKELETAL DISORDERS

Musculoskeletal complaints are common in renal transplant recipients. Avascular bone necrosis can occur in the presence or absence of hyperparathyroidism, but the overall incidence is decreasing, possibly because of the smaller doses of steroids used in cyclosporine-containing immunosuppressive protocols.[16] Avascular necrosis occurs in approximately 10% of patients after transplantation and is especially likely to affect the hips. A correlation with total steroid dose is often found.[10, 11] Cyclosporine's steroid-sparing effects are expected to improve the magnitude and incidence of avascular necrosis but severe osteopenia has been reported in animals exposed to cyclosporine.[178, 179] Long-term complications of renal osteodystrophy leading to bone fractures or spinal disk prolapses are also seen in transplant recipients.[10] Patients with maintenance dialysis-associated amyloidosis can show improvement in joint symptoms early after renal transplantation (when steroid doses are high) as well as after 6 months (when steroid doses are lower).[180] New amyloid bone cysts do not form after transplantation and pre-existing cysts do not enlarge; however, preformed cysts do not regress and can cause pathologic fractures.[181]

Although 30 to 50% of patients receiving azathioprine have elevated uric acid levels, clinical gout is rare.[182, 183] In contrast, 50 to 90% of patients receiving cyclosporine have hyperuricemia, and 5 to 12% have gout.[183, 184] Elevated uric acid levels are especially likely in patients taking diuretics. The hyperuricemia results from decreased uric acid excretion rather than from increased production. However, increasing creatinine clearance may not lower uric acid levels.[185] As asymptomatic hyperuricemia does not influence graft survival, therapy should be directed toward management of gout.[183] Gout is especially troublesome to treat in renal transplant recipients because of the risks of using nonsteroidal anti-inflammatory drugs. Treatment generally consists of minimizing diuretic use and administering maintenance doses of colchicine and, if necessary, allopurinol. Allopurinol dosage must be adjusted for the level of renal function. Allopurinol can increase azathioprine toxicity by inhibiting the xanthine oxidase–mediated metabolism of 6-mercaptopurine, the major metabolite of azathioprine.[20] Colchicine can cause a neuromyopathy.[186]

Reports of cyclosporine-induced myopathy are rare but persistent. Even with therapeutic cyclosporine levels, muscle biopsy specimens may show evidence of toxic myopathy.[187] The concomitant use of cyclosporine and lovastatin increases the risk of rhabdomyolysis.[188, 189]

NEUROLOGIC DISORDERS

Neurologic complications of renal transplantation can be divided into those present before transplantation and those associated with transplantation per se. Renal insufficiency is associated with a host of neurologic complications, only some of which are reversed by maintenance dialysis. Patients with chronic renal failure frequently demonstrate disorders of autonomic function such as reduced baroreceptor sensitivity, changes in sweat gland secretion, and abnormal Valsalva's test responses.[190] Autonomic abnormalities generally correct with adequate dialysis, whereas peripheral neuropathies do not. Nerve conduction velocities progressively worsen during maintenance dialysis, but this defect is reversed by transplantation.[190–192] Reversal of dialysis dementia has also been reported after transplantation.[191]

Some neurologic disorders that appear after transplantation may be a carryover of dialysis-related problems. Atherosclerosis remains a risk for cerebrovascular disease in the transplant recipient, and ischemic and thromboembolic cerebrovascular diseases are not uncommon. Other disorders are more clearly related to the operative procedure itself or associated therapy. Femoral nerve damage resulting in sensory or motor problems (e.g., footdrop) is a recognized complication, as is the much rarer risk of distal spinal cord infarction.[191–193] Transplantation-associated infections can lead to seizures, postherpetic neuralgia, or cytomegalovirus retinitis. The propensity for post-transplantation lymphoproliferative disorders to involve the brain has already been mentioned. Abnormalities of water, calcium, phosphorus, magnesium, potassium, and glucose homeostasis can appear rapidly after renal transplantation and can all affect nervous system function.[192, 194] Post-transplant hypertensive encephalopathy can be avoided (or at least ameliorated) by early diagnosis and aggressive treatment.[191]

Immunosuppressive drugs have numerous neurologic effects. Mental status changes, myopathies, and seizures complicate corticosteroid use. Mood swings, sleep disorders, and depression or mania are common. Psychiatric side effects are dose related and are uncommon with prednisone doses less than 40 mg daily.[195] Steroid myopathy is also dose related and usually occurs as a symmetric weakness of the proximal muscles of the shoulder and pelvic girdles.[18, 195] Seizures have been associated with the use of large doses of methylprednisolone, especially in patients also receiving cyclosporine.[194, 196] Less common steroid-associated problems include epidural lipomatosis, pseudotumor cerebri, and persistent hiccups.[195, 197]

Neurologic complications associated with cyclosporine use range from mild tremors to leukoencephalopathy. Paresthesias, flushing, headaches, and peripheral neuropathies have been reported but are usually mild. Most of the seizures reported in patients receiving cyclosporine have occurred in the setting of concurrent high-dose methylprednisolone administration, hypertension, hypomagnesemia, hypocholesterolemia, or aluminum toxicity.[194, 195, 198, 199] Blood cyclosporine levels may be elevated or within the accepted therapeutic range. Neurotoxicity has been variably attributed to changes in tissue binding, cyclosporine metabolites, or alterations in free drug levels.[199–201] Although the seizures are usually grand mal, they may also be localized and present as cortical blindness or hallucinations.[195, 198] Diagnostic studies are generally only nonspecifically abnormal. The cerebrospinal fluid may be normal or show mild protein elevations and mild pleocytosis. The electroencephalogram is usually abnormal but without epileptiform activity. Computed tomography may show a variety of hypodense changes, and magnetic resonance imaging may reveal white matter changes consistent with edema.[195, 198–200, 202]

The neurotoxicity of cyclosporine (or its metabolites) may be related to its highly lipophilic nature and its effect on the blood-brain barrier. Rats treated with progressively increasing doses of cyclosporine have seizures only with the highest doses, but electroencephalographic changes and tremors occur even with low doses.[203] A decrease in the seizure threshold has been found in cyclosporine-treated rats.[203] In humans, cholesterol levels of less than 120 mg/dL have been associated with increased neurotoxicity in liver transplant recipients even in the presence of subtherapeutic cyclosporine levels.[204] Alterations in free cyclosporine levels because of altered lipoprotein binding is a possible explanation.[199]

The treatment of cyclosporine-associated neurotoxicity is to lower the dose of the drug. Phenytoin speeds the hepatic metabolism of cyclosporine, reduces its serum half-life, and decreases cyclosporine levels. When phenytoin is used to treat transplant patients with seizures, cyclosporine levels may rapidly fall and graft rejection may occur. Carbamazepine and phenobarbital also increase cyclosporine metabolism, whereas benzodiazepines and valproic acid have no interactions with cyclosporine.[194, 198]

Antirejection therapy with the OKT3 monoclonal antibody has been associated with aseptic meningitis. This occurs within the first few days of therapy and is self-limited. There is no need to discontinue OKT3 therapy or to treat aseptic meningitis; however, other causes of meningitis must always be eliminated.[42, 43, 198] Seizures have also been reported with prophylactic use of OKT3.[43]

References

1. Evans RW: Organ donation: Facts and figures. Dial Transplant 19:234, 1990.
2. Eggers PW: Effects of transplantation of the Medicare end-stage renal disease program. N Engl J Med 318:223, 1988.
3. Evans RW, Manninen DL, Garrison LP: The quality of life in patients with end-stage renal disease. N Engl J Med 312:553, 1985.
4. Thomson NM, Scott DF, Cesnik B, et al: Morbidity, mortality, and quality of life in long-term survivors of an integrated dialysis renal transplant program. Transplant Proc 21:2184, 1989.
5. Gutmann RA: High-cost life prolongation: The National Kidney Dialysis and Kidney Transplantation Study. Ann Intern Med 108:898, 1988.
6. Kjellstrand CM, Hylander B, Collins AC: Mortality on dialysis—On the influence of early start, patient characteristics, and transplantation and acceptance rates. Am J Kidney Dis 15:483, 1990.
7. Takemot S, Terasaki PI: Donor and recipient age. In: Terasaki PI (ed): Clinical Transplants 1988. Los Angeles, UCLA Tissue Typing Laboratory, p 345, 1989.
8. Heino A: Operative and postoperative non-surgical complications in diabetic patient undergoing renal transplantation. Scand J Urol Nephrol 22:53, 1988.
9. Manninen DL, Evand RW: A longitudinal assessment of the health status of diabetic and nondiabetic renal transplant recipients. In: Terasaki PI (ed): Clinical Transplants 1988. Los Angeles, UCLA Tissue Typing Laboratory, p 345, 1989.
10. Rao KV, Andersen RC: Long-term results and complications in renal transplant recipients. Observations in the second decade. Transplantation 45:45, 1988.
11. Braun WE: Long-term complications of renal transplantation. Kidney Int 37:1363, 1990.
12. Landreneau MD, McDonald JC: Genitourinary complications in renal transplantation. Transplant Rev 1:159, 1987.
13. Reinberg Y, Bumgarner GL, Aliabadi H: Urologic aspects of renal transplantation. J Urol 143:1087, 1990.
14. Pollack R, Veremis SA, Maddux MS, et al: The natural history of and therapy for perirenal fluid collections following renal transplantation. J Urol 140:716, 1988.
15. Cohan RH, Saeed M, Sussman SK, et al: Percutaneous drainage of pelvic lymphatic fluid collections in the renal transplant patient. Invest Radiol 22:864, 1987.
16. Yoshimura N, Oka T: Medical and surgical complications of renal transplantation: Diagnosis and management. Med Clin North Am 74:1025, 1990.
17. Jusko WJ: Corticosteroid pharmacodynamics: Models for a broad array of receptor-mediated pharmacologic effects. J Clin Pharmacol 30:303, 1990.
18. Baxter JD: Minimizing the side effects of glucocorticoid therapy. Adv Intern Med 35:173, 1990.
19. Mucnk A, Mendel DB, Smith LI, et al: Glucocorticoid receptors and actions. Am Rev Respir Dis 141:S2, 1990.
20. Chan GLC, Erdmann GR, Gruber SA, et al: Azathioprine metabolism: Pharmacokinetics of 6-mercaptopurine, 6-thiouric acid and 6-thioguanine nucleotides in renal transplant patients. J Clin Pharmacol 30:358, 1990.
21. Boitard C, Bach JF: Long-term complications of conventional immunosuppressive treatment. Adv Nephrol 18:335, 1989.
22. Chan GL, Canafax DM, Johnson CA: The therapeutic use of azathioprine in renal transplantation. Pharmacotherapy 7:165, 1987.
23. Kerman RH: Effects of cyclosporine immunosuppression in humans. Transplant Proc 20:143, 1988.
24. Cockburn I, Gotz E, Gulich A, et al: An interim analysis of the on-going long-term safety study of cyclosporine in renal transplantation. Transplant Proc 20:519, 1988.
25. Kahan BV, Flechner SM, Lorber MI, et al: Complications of cyclosporine-prednisone immunosuppression in 402 renal allograft recipients exclusively followed at a single center for from one to five years. Transplantation 42:197, 1987.
26. Samara EN, Voss BL, Pederson JA: Renal artery thrombosis associated with elevated cyclosporine levels: A case report and review of the literature. Transplant Proc 20:119, 1988.
27. de Groen PC: Cyclosporine and the liver: How one affects the other. Transplant Proc 22:1197, 1990.
28. Kahan BD, Grevel J: Optimization of cyclosporine therapy in renal transplantation by a pharmacokinetic strategy. Transplant Proc 46:631, 1988.
29. Venkataramanan R, Habucky K, Burckart GJ, et al: Clinical pharmacokinetics in organ transplant patients. Clin Pharmacokinet 16:134, 1989.
30. Yee GC: Pharmacokinetic interactions between cyclosporine and other drugs. Transplant Proc 22:1203, 1990.
31. Awni WM, Heim-Duthoy K, Kasiske BL: Impact of lipoproteins on cyclosporine pharmacokinetics and biological activity in transplant patients. Transplant Proc 22:1193, 1990.
32. Humbert H, Vernillet L, Cabiac MD, et al: Influence of different parameters for the monitoring of cyclosporine. Transplant Proc 22:1210, 1991.
33. Mason J: Renal side-effects of cyclosporine. Transplant Proc 22:1280, 1990.
34. Puschett JB, Greenberg A, Holly J, et al: The spectrum of ciclosporin nephrotoxicity. Am J Nephrol 10:296, 1990.
35. Mihatsch MJ, Thiel G, Ryffel B: Cyclosporine nephrotoxicity. Adv Nephrol 17:303, 1988.
36. Brunner LJ, Vadiei K, Lyer LV, et al: Prevention of cyclosporine-induced nephrotoxicity with pentoxifylline. Ren Fail 11:97, 1989.
37. Dy GR, Raja RM, Mendez MM: The clinical and biochemical effect of calcium channel blockers in organ transplant recipients on cyclosporine. Transplant Proc 23:1212, 1991.
38. Gonwa TA, Nghiem DD, Schulak JA, et al: Results of conversion from cyclosporine to azathioprine in cadaveric renal transplantation. Transplantation 43:225, 1987.
39. Lewis RM, Janney RP, Golden DL, et al: Stability of renal allograft function associated with long-term cyclosporine immunosuppressive therapy—Five year follow-up. Transplantation 47:266, 1989.
40. Delmonico FL, Conti D, Auchincloss H, et al: Long-term, low-dose cyclosporine treatments of renal allograft recipients. Transplantation 49:899, 1990.
41. Ben-Maimon CS, Burke JF, Besarab A, et al: Evidence against chronic progressive cyclosporine toxicity. Transplant Proc 23:1260, 1991.
42. Todd PA, Brogden RN: Muromonab CD3: A review of its pharmacology and therapeutic potential. Drugs 37:871, 1989.
43. Thistlethwaite JR, Stuart JK, Mayes JT, et al: Complications and monitoring of OKT3 therapy. Am J Kidney Dis 11:112, 1988.
44. Rao KV: Mechanism, pathophysiology, diagnosis, and management of renal transplant rejection. Med Clin North Am 74:1039, 1990.
45. Koene RAP: The role of adaptation in allograft acceptance. Kidney Int 35:1073, 1989.
46. Krensky AM, Clayberger C: The molecular basis of renal transplant rejection. Semin Nephrol 9:116, 1989.
47. Olsen S, Burdick JF, Keown PA, et al: Primary acute renal failure ("acute tubular necrosis") in the transplanted kidney: Morphology and pathogenesis. Medicine 68:173, 1989.
48. Finn WF: Prevention of ischemic injury in renal transplantation. Kidney Int 37:171, 1990.
49. Tolkoff-Rubin NE, Rubin RH, Bonventre JV: Noninvasive renal diagnostic studies. Clin Lab Med 8:507, 1988.
50. Letourneau JG, Day DL, Feinberg SB: Ultrasound and computed tomographic evaluation of renal transplantation. Radiol Clin North Am 25:267, 1987.
51. Smith MC, Dunn MJ: Hypertension in renal parenchymal disease. In: Laragh JH, Brenner BM (eds): Hypertension: Pathophysiology, Diagnosis, and Management. New York, Raven Press, p 1583, 1990.
52. Kasiske BL: Possible causes and consequences of hypertension in stable renal transplant patients. Transplantation 44:639, 1987.
53. Curtis JJ: Hypertension in the renal transplant patient. Transplant Rev 2:17, 1988.
54. Olmer M, Noordally R, Berland Y, et al: Hypertension in renal transplantation. Kidney Int 25:S129, 1988.
55. Luke RG: Hypertension in renal transplant recipients. Kidney Int 31:1024, 1987.
56. Chapman JR, Marcen R, Arias M, et al: Hypertension after renal transplantation. A comparison of cyclosporine and conventional immunosuppression. Transplantation 43:860, 1987.
57. Popovtzer MMK, Pinnggera W, Katz FH: Variations in arterial blood pressure after kidney transplantation: Relation to renal function, plasma renin activity, and the dose of prednisone. Circulation 47:1297, 1973.
58. Scherrer U, Vissing SF, Morgan BJ, et al: Cyclosporine-induced sympathetic activation and hypertension after heart transplantation. N Engl J Med 323:693, 1990.
59. Mark AL: Cyclosporine, sympathetic activity, and hypertension. N Engl J Med 323:748, 1990.
60. Tresham JJ, Whitworth JA, Scoggins BA, et al: Cyclosporine-induced hypertension in sheep. The role of thromboxanes. Transplantation 49:144, 1990.
61. Whitworth JA, Mills EH, Coghlan JP, et al: The haemodynamic effects of cyclosporin A in sheep. Clin Exp Pharmacol Physiol 14:573, 1987.
62. Murray BM, Paller MS: Beneficial effects of renal denervation and prozosin on GFR and renal blood flow after cyclosporine in rats. Clin Nephrol 25:S37, 1986.
63. Curtis J: Cyclosporine-induced hypertension. In: Laragh JH, Brenner BM (eds): Hypertension: Pathophysiology, Diagnosis, and Management. New York, Raven Press, p 1829, 1990.
64. Hoover EL, Harrison BS, Williams WW, et al: Decrease in cyclosporin-

mediated prostacyclin production in renal vs carotid arteries: A mechanism for cyclosporin-induced hypertension. J Surg Res 48:481, 1990.

65. Meyer-Lehnert H, Schrier RW: Potential mechanism of cyclosporine A–induced vascular smooth muscle contraction. Hypertension 13:352, 1989.

66. Stanek SJ, Kovarik J, Rasoul-Rockenschaub S, et al: Renin-angiotensin-aldosterone system and vasopressin in cyclosporine treated renal allograft recipients. Clin Nephrol 28:186, 1987.

67. Barros EJG, Boim MA, Ajzen H, et al: Glomerular hemodynamics and hormonal participation on cyclosporine nephrotoxicity. Kidney Int 32:19, 1987.

68. Curtis JJ, Luke RG, Jones P, et al: Hypertension in cyclosporine-treated renal transplant recipients is sodium dependent. Am J Med 85:134, 1988.

69. Bantle JP, Boudreau RJ, Ferris TF: Suppression of plasma renin activity by cyclosporine. Am J Med 83:59, 1987.

70. Clozel JP, Fischli W: Cyclosporine-induced hypertension in marmosets: A new model of hypertension sensitive to angiotensin-converting enzyme inhibition. J Cardiovasc Pharmacol 14:77, 1989.

71. Nahman NS, Cosia FG, Mahan JD, et al: Cyclosporine nephrotoxicity in spontaneously hypertensive rats. Transplantation 45:768, 1988.

72. Yasumura T, Oka T: Beneficial effect of bilateral native nephrectomy on long-term survival of living related kidney allografts. Transplant Proc 21:1967, 1989.

73. Donker AJM: Nephrotoxicity of angiotensin converting enzyme inhibitor. Kidney Int 31:S132, 1987.

74. Ahmad T, Coulthard MG, Eastham EJ: Reversible renal failure due to the use of captopril in a renal allograft recipient treated with cyclosporin. Nephrol Dial Transplant 4:311, 1989.

75. Clements R, Evans C, Salaman JR: Percutaneous transluminal angioplasty of renal transplant artery stenosis. Clin Radiol 38:235, 1987.

76. Mathew TH: Recurrence of disease following renal transplantation. Am J Kidney Dis 12:85, 1988.

77. Troung L, Gelfand J, D'Agati V, et al: De novo membranous glomerulonephropathy in renal allografts: A report of ten cases and review of literature. Am J Kidney Dis 14:131, 1989.

78. Smith RB, Fairchild R, Bradley JW, et al: Cadaver kidney donors with hypertensive histories. Transplant Proc 20:741, 1988.

79. Rettig R, Folbert C, Stauss H, et al: Role of the kidney in primary hypertension: A renal transplantation study in rats. Am J Physiol 258:F606, 1990.

80. Bittar AE, Ratcliffe PJ, Richardson AJ, et al: Hyperparathyroidism, hypertension and loop diuretic medication in renal transplant recipients. Nephrol Dial Transplant 4:740, 1980.

81. Copur MS, Tasdemir I, Turgan C, et al: Effects of nitrendipine on blood pressure and blood ciclosporine A level in patients with posttransplant hypertension. Nephron 52:227, 1989.

82. Chan L, Schrier RW: Effects of calcium channel blockers on renal function. Annu Rev Med 41:289, 1990.

83. Howard RL, Shapiro JI, Babcock S, et al: The effect of calcium channel blockers on the cyclosporine dose requirement in renal transplant recipients. Ren Fail 12:89, 1990.

84. Arthur S, Greenberg A: Hyperkalemia associated with intravenous labetalol therapy for acute hypertension in renal transplant recipients. Clin Nephrol 33:269, 1990.

85. Sever MS, Sonmer YE, Kocak N: Limited use of minoxidil in renal transplant recipients because of the additive side-effects of cyclosporine on hypertrichosis (letter). Transplantation 50:536, 1990.

86. Kasiske BL: Creatinine excretion after renal transplantation. Transplantation 48:424, 1989.

87. Helderman JH: The role of cardiovascular disease in renal transplantation. In: Garovoy MR, Guttman RD (eds): Renal Transplantation, New York, Churchill Livingstone, p 209, 1986.

88. Walker JV, Grove MA: Survival in a community hospital dialysis center. Am J Nephrol 8:40, 1988.

89. Mahony JF, Sheil AGR: Long-term complications of cadaveric renal transplantation. Transplant Rev 1:47, 1987.

90. Toussant C, Kinnaert P, Vereerstraeten P: Late mortality and morbidity five to eighteen years after kidney transplantation. Transplantation 45:554, 1988.

91. Bia MJ, Flye MW: Long-term follow-up of the renal transplant patient. In: Flye MW (ed): Principles of Organ Transplantation. Philadelphia, WB Saunders, p 307, 1989.

92. Collins AJ, Hanson G, Umen A, et al: Changing risk factor demographics in end-stage renal disease patients entering hemodialysis and the impact on long-term mortality. Am J Kidney Dis 15:422, 1990.

93. Parfrey PS, Harnett JD, Griffiths S, et al: Low-output left ventricular failure in end-stage renal disease. Am J Nephol 7:184, 1987.

94. Harnett JD, Parfrey DS, Griffiths SM, et al: Left ventricular hypertrophy in end-stage renal disease. Nephron 48:107, 1988.

95. Painter P, Messer-Rehak D, Hanson P, et al: Exercise capacity in hemodialysis, CAPD, and renal transplant patients. Nephron 42:47, 1986.

96. Linke CL: Anesthesia considerations for renal transplantation. Contemp Anesth Pract 10:183, 1987.

97. Pouttu J: Haemodynamic responses during general anaesthesia for renal transplantation in patients with and without hypertensive disease. Acta Anaesthesiol Scand 33:245, 1989.

98. Teruel JL, Rodriguez Padial L, Quereda C, et al: Regression of left ventricular hypertrophy after renal transplantation. A prospective study. Transplantation 43:307, 1987.

99. Devlin WH, Parfrey PS, Harnett JD, et al: The relationship between hypertension and left ventricular hypertrophy in renal transplant recipients. Transplant Proc 20:1221, 1988.

100. Kasiske BL: Risk factors for accelerated atherosclerosis in renal transplant recipients. Am J Med 84:985, 1988.

101. Albert FW, Seyfert UT, Grossman R, et al: Role of coronary angiography and heart surgery in care of kidney transplant recipients. Transplant Proc 19:3689, 1987.

102. Kokot F, Grzeszczak W, Zukowska-Szczechowska E, et al: Endocrine alterations in kidney transplant patients. Blood Purif 8:76, 1990.

103. Horl WH, Riegel W, Wanner C, et al: Endocrine and metabolic abnormalities following kidney transplantation. Klin Wochenschr 67:907, 1989.

104. Boudreaux JP, McHugh L, Canafax DM, et al: The impact of cyclosporine and combination immunosuppression on the incidence of posttransplant diabetes in renal allograft recipients. Transplant Proc 44:376, 1987.

105. Yoshimura N, Nakai I, Ohmori Y, et al: Effect of cyclosporine on the endocrine and exocrine pancreas in kidney transplant recipients. Am J Kidney Dis 12:11, 1988.

106. Roth D, Milgrom M, Esquenazi V, et al: Posttransplant hyperglycemia. Increased incidence in cyclosporine-treated renal allograft recipients. Transplantation 47:278, 1989.

107. Friedman EH, Shyh T, Beyer MM, et al: Posttransplant diabetes in kidney transplant recipients. Am J Nephrol 5:196, 1985.

108. Dresher LS, Anderson DK, Kahng KU, et al: Effects of cyclosporine on glucose metabolism. Surgery 106:163, 1989.

109. Riegel W, Brehmer D, Thaiss F, et al: Effect of cyclosporin A on carbohydrate metabolism in the rat. Transplant Int 2:8, 1989.

110. David DS, Sakai S, Brennan BL, et al: Hypercalcemia after renal transplantation. Long-term follow-up data. N Engl J Med 289:398, 1973.

111. Garvin PH, Casterneda M, Linderer R: Management of hypercalcemia and hyperparathyroidism after renal transplantation. Arch Surg 120:578, 1985.

112. Sitges-Serra A, Caralps-Riera A: Hyperparathyroidism associated with renal disease. Pathogenesis, natural history, and surgical treatment. Surg Clin North Am 67:359, 1987.

113. McCarron DA, Bennett WM, Muther MD, et al: Posttransplant hyperparathyroidism: Demonstration of retained control of parathyroid function by ionized calcium. Am J Clin Nutr 33:1536, 1980.

114. Blind E, Schmidt-Gayk H, Scharla S, et al: Two-site assay of intact parathyroid hormone in the investigation of primary hyperparathyroidism and other disorders of calcium metabolism compared with a midregion assay. J Clin Endocrinol Metab 67:353, 1988.

115. Ulmann A, Chkoff N, Lacour B: Disorders of calcium and phosphorus metabolism after successful kidney transplant. Adv Nephrol 12:331, 1983.

116. Manske CL: Lipid abnormalities and renal disease. Kidney 20:25, 1988.

117. Management of hyperlipidemia of kidney disease. Kidney Int 37:847, 1990.

118. Kasiske BL, Umin AJ: Persistant hyperlipidemia in renal transplant recipients. Medicine 66:309, 1987.

119. Ettinger WH, Bender WL, Goldberg AP, et al: Lipoprotein-lipid abnormalities in healthy renal transplant recipients: Persistence of low HDL_2 cholesterol. Nephron 47:17, 1987.

120. Vathsala A, Weinberg RB, Schoenberg L, et al: Lipid abnormalities in cyclosporine-prednisone-treated renal transplant recipients. Transplantation 48:37, 1989.

121. Ballantyne CM, Podet EJ, Patche WP, et al: Effects of cyclosporine therapy on plasma lipoprotein levels. JAMA 262:53, 1989.

122. Brenner LJ, Vadiei K, Luke DR: Cyclosporine disposition in the hyperlipidemic rat model. Res Commun Chem Pathol Pharmacol 59:339, 1988.

123. Nelson J, Beauregard H, Gelinas M, et al: Rapid improvement of hyperlipidemia in kidney transplant patients with a multifactorial hypolipidemic diet. Transplant Proc 20: 1264, 1988.

124. Moore RA, Callahan MF, Cody M, et al: The effect of the American Heart Association step one diet for hyperlipidemia following renal transplantation. Transplantation 49:60, 1990.

125. Lindholm A, Dahlquist R, Groth GG, et al: A prospective study of cyclosporine concentration in relation to its therapeutic effect and toxicity after renal transplantation. Br J Clin Pharmacol 30:443, 1990.

126. Eschbach JW: The anemia of chronic renal failure: Pathophysiology and the effects of recombinant erythropoietin. Kidney Int 35:134, 1989.

127. Besarab A, Caro J, Jarrell BE, et al: Dynamics of erythropoiesis following renal transplantation. Kidney Int 32:526, 1987.

128. Brown JH, Lappin TR, Elder GE, et al: The initiation of erythropoiesis following renal transplantation. Nephrol Dial Transplant 4:1076, 1989.

129. Cotorruelo JG, DeFrancisco AL, Canga E, et al: The role of secondary hyperparathyroidism in the recovery of anemia after kidney transplantation. Transplant Proc 22:1412, 1990.

130. Wickre CG, Norman DJ, Bennison A: Post renal transplant erythrocytosis: A review of 53 patients. Kidney Int 23:731, 1983.

131. Pollack R, Maddux MS: Erythrocythemia following renal transplantation: Influence of diuretic therapy. Clin Nephrol 29:119, 1988.
132. Teruel JL, Lamas S, Vila T, et al: Serum ferritin levels after renal transplantation: A prospective study. Nephron 51:462, 1989.
133. Hogge D, Wilson D, Shumak K, et al: Reversible azathioprine-induced aplasia in a renal transplant recipient. Can Med Assoc J 126:512, 1982.
134. Yoshimura N, Oka T, Ohmori Y, et al: Effects of recombinant human erythropoietin on the anemia of renal transplant recipients with chronic rejection. Transplantation 48:527, 1989.
135. Adu D, Turney J, Michael J, et al: Hyperkalemia in cyclosporine-treated renal allograft recipients. Lancet 2:370, 1983.
136. Schover LR, Novick AC, Steinmuller DR, et al: Sexuality, fertility, and renal transplantation: A survey of survivors. J Sex Marital Ther 16:3, 1990.
137. Koutsikos D, Sarandakou A, Agroyannis B, et al: Hormonal profiles in successful renal transplant male recipients. Transplant Proc 22:1399, 1990.
138. Bennett AH: Urological complications of renal transplantation. In: Cerilli GE (ed): Organ Transplantation and Replacement. Philadelphia, JB Lippincott, p 433, 1988.
139. Seethalakshmi L, Menon M, Malhotra RK, et al: Effect of cyclosporine A on male reproduction in rats. J Urol 138:991, 1987.
140. Hou S: Pregnancy in organ transplant recipients. Med Clin North Am 73:667, 1989.
141. Davison JM: Dialysis, transplantation, and pregnancy. Am J Kidney Dis 17:127, 1991.
142. Debure A, Degos F, Pol S, et al: Liver diseases and hepatic complications in renal transplant patients. Adv Nephrol 17:375, 1988.
143. Parfrey PS, Farge D, Forbes CRD, et al: Chronic hepatitis in end-stage renal disease: Comparison of HBsAg-negative and HBsAg-positive patients. Kidney Int 28:959, 1985.
144. Weir MR, Kirkman RL, Strom TB, et al: Liver disease in recipients of long-functioning renal allografts. Kidney Int 28:839, 1985.
145. Boyce NW, Holdsworth SR, Hooke D, et al: Nonhepatitis B–associated liver disease in a renal transplant population. Am J Kidney Dis 11:307, 1988.
146. Venkateswara Rao K, Anderson WR: Hemosiderosis and hemochromatosis in renal transplant recipients. Am J Nephrol 5:419, 1985.
147. Takahara S, Ihara H, Ichikawa Y, et al: Prospective study and long-term follow-up of liver damage in renal transplant recipients. Transplant Proc 19: 2221, 1987.
148. Hankey GJ, Saker BM: Peliosis hepatis in a renal transplant recipient and in a haemodialysis patient. Med J Aust 146:102, 1987.
149. Moreno F, Morales JM, Colina F, et al: Influence of long-term cyclosporine therapy on chronic liver disease after renal transplantation. Transplant Proc 22:2314, 1990.
150. Lorber MI, Van Buren CT, Flechner SM, et al: Hepatobiliary and pancreatic complications of cyclosporine therapy in 466 renal transplant recipients. Transplantation 43:35, 1987.
151. White AG, Kumar MSA, Strannegard O, et al: Renal transplantation in hepatitis B surface antigen–positive patients. Transplant Proc 19:2150, 1987.
152. Stone B, Warty V, Dindzans Y, et al: The mechanism of cyclosporine-induced cholestasis in the rat. Transplant Proc 20:841, 1988.
153. Fernandez-Cruz L, Targarona EM, Cugat E, et al: Acute pancreatitis after renal transplantation. Br J Surg 76:1132, 1989.
154. Prevost X, Myara I, Cosson C, et al: Asymptomatic hyperamylasemia after cyclosporine therapy in patients with renal transplants. Transplant Proc 20:555, 1988.
155. Frick TW, Fryd DS, Sutherland DE, et al: Hypercalcemia associated with pancreatitis and hyperamylasemia in renal transplant patients. Data from Minnesota randomized trial of cyclosporine versus antilymphoblast azathioprine. Am J Surg 154:487, 1987.
156. Ala-kaila K: Upper gastrointestinal findings in chronic renal failure. Scand J Gastroenterol 22:372, 1987.
157. Santiago-Delpin EA, Morales-Otero LA, Gonzales ZA: Gastrointestinal complications and appendicitis after kidney transplantation. Transplant Proc 21:3745, 1989.
158. Gifford RR, Schmidtke JR, Ferguson RM: Cimetidine modulation of lymphocytes from renal allograft recipients. Transplant Proc 13:663, 1981.
159. Stylianos S, Forde KA, Benvenisty AI, et al: Lower gastrointestinal hemorrhage in renal transplant recipients. Arch Surg 123:739, 1988.
160. Ala-Kaila K, Posternack A: Gastrointestinal complications in chronic renal failure. Dig Dis 7:230, 1989.
161. Penn I: Risk of cancer in the transplant patient. In: Flye MW (ed): Principles of Organ Transplantation. Philadelphia, WB Saunders, p 634, 1989.
162. Sheil AGR, Disney APS, Mathew TH, et al: Cancer development in cadaveric donor renal allograft recipients treated with azathioprine (Aza) or cyclosporine (CyA) or Aza/CyA. Transplant Proc 23:1111, 1991.
163. Penn I: The changing pattern of posttransplant malignancies. Transplant Proc 23:1101, 1991.
164. Ishikawa I, Yuri T, Kitada H, et al: Regression of acquired cystic disease of the kidney after successful renal transplantation. Am J Nephrol 3:310, 1983.
165. Almirall J, Ricart MJ, Campistol JM, et al: Renal cell carcinoma and acquired cystic kidney disease after renal transplantation. Transpl Int 3:49, 1990.
166. Noronha IL, Ritz I, Walherr R, et al: Renal cell carcinoma in dialysis patients with acquired renal cysts. Nephrol Dial Transplant 4:763, 1989.
167. Hauser AC, Derfler K, Stockenhuber F, et al: Post-transplantation malignant disease in patients with analgesic nephropathy (letter). Lancet 335:58, 1990.
168. Smith JL, Wilkinson AH, Hunsicker LG, et al: Increased frequency of posttransplant lymphomas in patients treated with cyclosporin, azathioprine, and prednisone. Transplant Proc 21:3199, 1989.
169. Nalesnik MA, Makowka L, Starzl TE: The diagnosis and treatment of posttransplant lymphoproliferative disorders. Curr Probl Surg 25:365, 1988.
170. List AF, Greco FA, Vogler LB: Lymphoproliferative disease in immunocompromised hosts: The role of Epstein-Barr virus. J Clin Oncol 5:1673, 1987.
171. Penn I: Cancers after cyclosporine therapy. Transplant Proc 20:276, 1988.
172. Honda H, Barloon TJ, Franken EA Jr, et al: Clinical and radiologic features of malignant neoplasms in organ transplant recipients: Cyclosporine-treated vs untreated patients. AJR 154:271, 1990.
173. Vogt P, Frei U, Repp H, et al: Malignant tumors in renal transplant recipients receiving cyclosporin: Survey of 598 first-kidney transplantations. Nephrol Dial Transplant 5:282, 1990.
174. Cockburn IT, Krupp P: The risk of neoplasms in patients treated with cyclosporin A. J Autoimmunity 2:723, 1989.
175. Gruber SA, Skjei KL, Sothern RB, et al: Cancer development in renal allograft recipients treated with conventional and cyclosporine immunosuppression. Transplant Proc 23:1104, 1991.
176. Pirsch JD, Stratta RJ, Sollinger HW, et al: Treatment of severe Epstein-Barr virus–induced lymphoproliferative syndrome with ganciclovir: Two cases after solid organ transplantation. Am J Med 86:241, 1989.
177. Cockfield SM, Preiksaitis J, Harvey E, et al: Is sequential use of ALG and OKT3 in renal transplants associated with an increased incidence of fulminant post transplant lymphoproliferative disorder? Transplant Proc 23:1106, 1991.
178. Movsawitz C, Epstein S, Fallon M, et al: Cyclosporin-A in vivo produces severe osteopenia in the rat: Effect of dose and duration of administration. Endocrinology 123:2571, 1988.
179. Movsowitz C, Epstein S, Fallon M, et al: The bisphosphonate 2-PEBP inhibits cyclosporin A induced high-turnover osteopenia in the rat. J Lab Clin Med 115:62, 1990.
180. Campistol JM, Munoz-Gomez J, Sole M, et al: Results of renal transplantation for dialysis arthropathy. Transplant Proc 22:1416, 1990.
181. Jodoul M, Malghem J, Pirson Y, et al: Effect of renal transplantation on the radiological signs of dialysis amyloid osteoarthropathy. Clin Nephrol 32:194, 1989.
182. West C, Carpenter BJ, Hakala TR: The incidence of gout in renal transplant recipients. Am J Kidney Dis 10:369, 1987.
183. Gores PF, Fryd DS, Sutherland DE, et al: Hyperuricemia after renal transplantation. Am J Surg 156:397, 1988.
184. Lin HY, Rocher LL, McQuillan MA, et al: Cyclosporine-induced hyperuricemia and gout. N Engl J Med 321:287, 1989.
185. Morales JM, Hernandez Poblete G, Andres A, et al: Uric acid handling, pregnancy and ciclosporin in renal transplant women. Nephron 56:97, 1988.
186. Rieger EH, Halasz NA, Wahlstrom HE: Colchicine neuromyopathy after renal transplantation. Transplantation 49:1196, 1990.
187. Noppen M, Velkeniers B, Dierckx R, et al: Cyclosporine and myopathy. Ann Intern Med 107:945, 1987.
188. Norman DJ, Illignwork DR, Munson J, et al: Myolysis and acute renal failure in a heart-transplant recipient receiving lovastatin. N Engl J Med 318:46, 1988.
189. East C, Alivizatos PA, Grundy SM, et al: Rhabdomyolysis in patients receiving lovastatin after cardiac transplantation (letter). N Engl J Med 318:47, 1988.
190. Heidbreder E, Schafferhans K, Heidland H: Disturbances of peripheral and autonomic nervous system in chronic renal failure: Effects of hemodialysis and transplantation. Clin Nephrol 23:222, 1985.
191. Moralis-Otero LA, Gonzalez ZA, Santiago-Delpin EA: Neurological complications after kidney transplantation. Transplant Proc 20:443, 1988.
192. Bruno A, Adams HP: Neurologic problems in renal transplant recipients. Neurol Clin 6:305, 1988.
193. Much PR:Femoral neuropathy following renal transplantation. Aust NZ J Surg 60:117, 1991.
194. Gilmore RL: Seizures and epileptic drug use in transplant patients. Neurol Clin 6:279, 1988.
195. Walker RW, Brochstein JA: Neurological complications of immunosuppressive agents. Neurol Clin 6:261, 1988.
196. el-Dahr S, Chevalier RL, Gomez RA, et al: Seizures and blindness following intravenous pulse methylprednisolone in a renal transplant patient. Int J Pediatr Nephrol 8:87, 1987.
197. Tobler WD, Weil S: Epidural lipomatosis and renal transplantation. Surg Neurol 29:141, 1988.
198. Rubin AM: Transient cortical blindness and occipital seizures with cyclosporine toxicity. Transplantation 47:572, 1989.

199. de Groen PC, Aksamit AJ, Rakela J, et al: Central nervous system toxicity after liver transplantation. The role of cyclosporine and cholesterol. N Engl J Med 317:861, 1987.
200. Lane RJ, Roche SW, Leung AA, et al: Cyclosporine neurotoxicity in cardiac transplant recipients. J Neurol Neurosurg Psychiatry 51:1434, 1988.
201. Trull AK, Tan KK, Roberts NB, et al: Cyclosporin metabolites and neurotoxicity (letter). Lancet 2:448, 1989.
202. Berden JHM, Hoitsma AJ, Merx JL, et al: Severe central nervous system toxicity associated with cyclosporin. Lancet 1:219, 1985.
203. Racusen LC, Famiglio LM, Fivush BA, et al: Neurologic abnormalities and mortality in rats treated with cyclosporin A. Transplant Proc 20:934, 1988.
204. Racusen LC, McCrindle BW, Christenson U, et al: Cyclosporine lowers seizure threshold in an experimental model of electroshock-induced seizures in Munich-Wistar rats. Life Sci 46:1021, 1990.

CHAPTER 111

Drug Dosing Adjustments in Renal Failure

David R. Rutledge
Michael A. Geheb
Michael P. Peppers

Excretion of drugs and their active or inactive metabolites in the urine involves three basic processes (glomerular filtration, tubular reabsorption, and tubular secretion). Critically ill patients in an intensive care unit require frequent monitoring of renal function for a variety of reasons. First, they are treated with agents that are either eliminated through the kidney or that alter renal blood flow. Renal function may be affected by changes in blood pressure, which are common in the hemodynamically unstable intensive care unit population. Finally, many patients with renal impairment respond differently to drug regimens when compared with those who have normal renal function because of the biochemical and physiologic changes associated with renal failure. Therefore, attention needs to be given to the appropriate dosing of renally eliminated drugs. Table 111–1 provides general guidelines on which to base initial drug therapy in patients with varying degrees of renal function. The recommendations are derived from a large literature data base, which is often conflicting and seldom based on prospective validation under controlled conditions. Therefore, it is provided as a useful starting point.

Dialysis has become an important therapeutic approach in the treatment of renal failure. Although its main purpose is to remove waste products and water from the body, it also has the effect of removing drugs, although the extent varies (see Table 111–1). Dialysis therapy can be divided into two broad categories: systems filtering the blood stream (hemodialysis) and those performed in the peritoneal cavity (peritoneal dialysis).

MECHANICS OF RENAL DRUG EXCRETION
Serum Creatinine

Creatinine is formed in muscles from creatine and creatine phosphate. Creatine is formed primarily in the liver and is transported to the muscles, where it is phosphorylated to form creatine phosphate, which acts as a storage depot for muscle energy. The enzyme creatine kinase catalyzes the reaction between creatine and creatine phosphate. Creatinine is the metabolic by-product of this reaction. It is excreted through the kidneys at a rate that approximates the glomerular filtration rate, although 20 to 30% is excreted by tubular secretion. Creatinine clearance decreases with age and weight loss and is probably lower in females than in males. There appears to be a circadian rhythm such that clearance is greatest in the afternoon.

TABLE 111–1

DOSING ADJUSTMENTS FOR VARYING DEGREES OF RENAL IMPAIRMENT*

Drug	Half-life (h†) Normal	Half-life (h†) ESRD	Dose Adjustment for Renal Failure Based on C_{cr} (mL/min)‡ >50	10–50	<10	Dialysis§	Comments
Analgesics							
Acetaminophen	2	2	Unch	75	50	Yes (H)	Nephrotoxic as well as hepatotoxic in overdose.
Aspirin	2–30	2–30	Unch	75	Avoid	Yes (H,P)	Salicylate toxicity. Nephrotoxic in large doses. Adds to uremic platelet dysfunction.
Meperidine	2.4–7	2.4–7	Unch	Unch	50–75	No (H)	Active metabolite accumulates, which may produce excessive sedation or seizures.
Methadone	18–97	13–55	Unch	Unch	50–75	No (H,P)	Excessive sedation, respiratory depression.
Morphine	2–2.5	?	Unch	Unch	50–75	No (H,P)	Excessive sedation, respiratory depression. Renal metabolism decreases in ESRD.
Pentazocin	2–3	?	Unch	Unch	50–75	Yes (H)	Respiratory depression.
Analgesics, Antagonists							
Diflunisal	5–20	115	Unch	Unch	50	No (H)	
Fenoprofen	2–3	?	Unch	Unch	Unch	No (H)	May cause sodium retention, reduced GFR.

TABLE 111–1

DOSING ADJUSTMENTS FOR VARYING DEGREES OF RENAL IMPAIRMENT* Continued

Drug	Half-life (h†)		Dose Adjustment for Renal Failure Based on C_cr (mL/min)‡			Dialysis§	Comments
	Normal	**ESRD**	**>50**	**10–50**	**<10**		
Ibuprofen	2.5	2.5	Unch	Unch	Unch	No (H)	May cause sodium retention, reduced GFR.
Indomethacin	4–12	4–12	Unch	Unch	Unch	No (H)	May cause sodium retention, reduced GFR.
Naloxone	1–1.5	?	Unch	Unch	Unch	?	
Naproxen	14–17	15	Unch	Unch	Unch	No (H)	May cause sodium retention, reduced GFR.
Sulindac	7	?	Unch	Unch	Unch	?	Active metabolite (sulfide) $t_{1/2} = 16$ h.
Antianxiety Agents, Hypnotics **Barbiturates**			Unch	Unch	Unch		May increase osteomalacia in patients with ESRD. $t_{1/2}$ decreases with long-term therapy.
Hexobarbital	3.5–5	?				No (H)	
Pentobarbital	18–48	18–48				No (H)	
Phenobarbital	60–150	117–160				Yes (H,P)	Up to 50% excreted unchanged in alkaline urine.
Secobarbital	20–35	?				No (H,P)	
Benzodiazepines							May cause excessive sedation or encephalopathy in dialysis patients.
Chlordiazepoxide	5–30	5–30	Unch	Unch	50	No (H)	Active metabolite accumulates.
Clonazepam	20–60	20–60	Unch	Unch	Unch	?	
Diazepam	24–48	24–48	Unch	Unch	Unch	No (H)	Active metabolite accumulates.
Flurazepam	47–100	47–100	Unch	Unch	Unch	No (H)	
Lorazepam	8–25	32–70	Unch	Unch	50	No (H)	
Oxazepam	6–25	25–90	Unch	Unch	75	No (H)	
Triazolam	2–5	?	Unch	Unch	Unch	?	
Antiarrhythmics (see also beta-adrenergic antagonists)							
Amiodarone	3–100 (d)	3–100 (d)	Unch	Unch	Unch	No (H)	Thyroid dysfunction, peripheral neuropathy. Pulmonary fibrosis.
Bretylium	6–14	16–32	Unch	25–50	Avoid	No (H)	
Disopyramide	5–8	10–18	Unch	50	25	Yes (H)	Urinary retention.
Encainide	1–3	1–3	Unch	Unch	Unch	?	Metabolites accumulate.
Flecainide	12–20	19–38	Unch	Unch	75	Yes (H)	
Lidocaine	1–4	1–3	Unch	Unch	Unch		Active metabolites accumulate.
Lorcainide	7–13	?	Unch	Unch	Unch	?	Active metabolite accumulates.
Mexiletine	8–13	16	Unch	Unch	75	Yes (H)/ No (P)	
Procainamide	3–5	5–6	Unch	50–75	10–25	Yes (H)	Lupus syndrome. Active metabolite accumulates.
Quinidine	3–16	3–16	Unch	Unch	Unch	Yes (H,P)	Active metabolite accumulates.
Antibacterials **Aminoglycosides**							
Amikacin	2–3	30	Pharmacokinetic monitoring			Yes (H,P)	Ototoxic, nephrotoxic.
Gentamicin	2–3	30–50	Pharmacokinetic monitoring			Yes (H,P)	
Kanamycin	2–5	72–96	Pharmacokinetic monitoring			Yes (H,P)	
Netilmicin	2–3	40	Pharmacokinetic monitoring			Yes (H,P)	
Streptomycin	2–3	100	Pharmacokinetic monitoring			Yes (H)	
Tobramycin	2–3	56	Pharmacokinetic monitoring			Yes (H,P)	
Cephalosporins							
Cefaclor	0.6–1	3	Unch	50	33	Yes (H,P)	
Cefamandole	1	11	Unch	Unch	50	Yes (H)	
Cefazolin	1.8–2	2–3	Unch	Unch	50	Yes (H)	
Cefmenoxine	1–2	6–26	Unch	Unch	50	Yes (H)	
Cefonicid	3–5	17–56	Unch	20–50	10–20	Yes (H)	
Cefoperazone	1–3	1–3	Unch	Unch	Unch	Yes (H)	
Cefotaxime	1	2.6	Unch	Unch	50	Yes (H)	
Cefotiam	1	3–13	Unch	Unch	50	Yes (H)	
Cefoxitin	1	13–20	Unch	Unch	50	Yes (H)	
Cefroxadine	1	40	Unch	50	25	Yes (H,P)	
Ceftazidime	1–2	13	Unch	50	25	Yes (H)	

Table continued on following page

TABLE 111–1

DOSING ADJUSTMENTS FOR VARYING DEGREES OF RENAL IMPAIRMENT* Continued

Drug	Half-life (h†) Normal	Half-life (h†) ESRD	Dose Adjustment for Renal Failure Based on C_{cr} (mL/min)‡ >50	10–50	<10	Dialysis§	Comments
Ceftazidime	1–2	13	Unch	50	25	Yes (H)	
Ceftizoxime	1–2	30	Unch	50	25	Yes (H)	
Ceftriaxone	7–9	12–24	Unch	Unch	Unch	Yes (H)	
Cefuroxime	1–2	17	Unch	50	10	Yes (H)	
Cephalexin	1	20–40	Unch	Unch	50	Yes (H,P)	
Cephalothin	1	3–18	Unch	Unch	50	Yes (H)	
Cephradine	1	6–15	Unch	50	25	Yes (H,P)	
Moxalactam	2–3	18–23	Unch	75	50	Yes (H)/ No (P)	
Penicillins							
Amoxicillin	1–2	5–20	Unch	50	25	Yes (H)/ No (P)	
Ampicillin	1–2	7–20	Unch	50	25	Yes (H)/ No (P)	
Azlocillin	1–2	5–6	Unch	Unch	50	Yes (H)/ No (P)	
Carbenicillin	1–2	10–20	Unch	50	25	Yes (H)	
Cloxacillin	0.5	1	Unch	Unch	Unch	No (H)	
Dicloxacillin	1	1–2	Unch	Unch	Unch	No (H)	
Methicillin	1	4	Unch	Unch	50	No (H,P)	
Mezlocillin	1	2–6	Unch	Unch	50	No (H)	
Nafcillin	1	1.2	Unch	Unch	Unch	No (H)	
Penicillin G	0.5	60–85	Unch	75	50	Yes (H)	
Piperacillin	1	3–5	Unch	75	50	Yes (H)	
Ticarcillin	1	16	Unch	50	25	Yes (H)	
Tetracyclines							Potentiates acidosis, raises BUN and phosphorus levels and increases catabolism.
Doxycycline	15–24	18–25	Unch	Unch	50	No (H,P)	
Minocycline	12–16	12–18	Unch	Unch	Unch	No (H,P)	
Tetracycline	6–10	57–108	Unch	75	50	No (H,P)	
Others							
Aztreonam	1–3	6–8	Unch	50	25	Yes (H,P)	
Chloramphenicol	2–4	3–7	Unch	Unch	Unch	No (H,P)	
Cilastatin	1	17.1	Unch	50	25	Yes (H)	
Ciprofloxacin	1–4	1–7	Unch	50	25	Yes (H)	
Clavulanic acid	1	3–4	Unch	Unch	50–75	Yes (H)	
Clindamycin	2–4	3–5	Unch	Unch	Unch	No (H,P)	
Enoxacin	6–9	30	Unch	Unch	25	?	
Erythromycin	1.4	5–6	Unch	Unch	50–75	No (H,P)	
Imipenem	1	3.7	Unch	50	25	Yes (H)	
Metronidazole	6–14	8–15	Unch	75	50	Yes (H)	
Norfloxacin	3–8	6–9	Unch	Unch	75	No (H,P)	
Sulfamethoxazole	9–11	20–50	Unch	75	50	Yes (H)	
Trimethoprim	9–13	20–49	Unch	75	50	Yes (H)	
Vancomycin	6–10	200–250	Pharmacokinetic monitoring			No (H,P)	Ototoxic at serum concentrations > 50 μg/mL. Increased nephrotoxicity when used with aminoglycosides.
Anticoagulants							
Heparin	1–2	0.5–3	Unch	Unch	Unch	No (H,P)	May potentiate uremic bleeding.
Warfarin	42	30	Unch	Unch	Unch	No (P)	Steroisomers. Metabolites accumulate in renal failure and may potentiate uremic bleeding.
Anticonvulsants							
Carbamazepine	12–17	?	Unch	Unch	75	No (H)	May cause inappropriate ADH secretion.
Phenytoin	10–34	8	Unch	Unch	Unch	No (H)	Zero-order kinetics. Decreased protein binding and increased volume of distribution in ESRD. May cause folate deficiency.

TABLE 111–1

DOSING ADJUSTMENTS FOR VARYING DEGREES OF RENAL IMPAIRMENT* Continued

Drug	Half-life (h†)		Dose Adjustment for Renal Failure Based on C_{cr} (mL/min)‡			Dialysis§	Comments
	Normal	*ESRD*	*>50*	*10–50*	*<10*		
Primidone	6–12	12	Unch	Unch	50	Yes (H)	Excessive sedation, folic acid deficiency, nystagmus.
Valproic acid	6–18	10	Unch	Unch	Unch	No (H,P)	
Antidepressants							Agents in this group are anticholinergic and may cause urinary retention. Excessive sedation.
Amitriptyline	21	?	Unch	Unch	Unch	No (H,P)	Metabolized to nortriptyline.
Desipramine	12–54	?	Unch	Unch	Unch	No (H,P)	
Doxepin	8–25	10–18	Unch	Unch	Unch	No (H,P)	
Imipramine	6–20	?	Unch	Unch	Unch	No (H,P)	Metabolized to desipramine.
Lithium carbonate	14–28	> 28	Unch	50–75	25–50	Yes(H,P)	Nephrogenic diabetes insipidus, renal tubular acidosis.
Nortriptyline	15–90	15–66	Unch	Unch	Unch	No (H,P)	
Protriptyline	54–98	?	Unch	Unch	Unch	No (H,P)	
Antifungals							
Amphotericin B	24	24	Unch	Unch	75	No (H,P)	
Fluconazole	20–50	>50	Unch	50	25	Yes (H)	
Flucytosine	3–6	75–200	Unch	Unch	75	Yes (H,P)	Hepatic dysfunction, marrow suppression common in azotemic patients.
Ketoconazole	2–8	2	Unch	Unch	Unch	No (H)	Interferes with cyclosporine metabolism and enhances its nephrotoxicity.
Miconazole	20–24	20–24	Unch	Unch	Unch	No (H,P)	Hyponatremia.
Antihistamines (H₁ Receptor Antagonists)							
Chlorpheniramine	13–31	>31	Unch	Unch	Unch	Yes (H)/ No(P)	Excessive sedation. Anticholinergic effects.
Diphenhydramine	4–7	?	Unch	75	50	?	
Antihypertensives							Blood pressure monitoring is best general guide for dosing.
Captopril	2	21–32	Unch	75	50	Yes (H)	Proteinuria, nephrotic syndrome, hyperkalemia.
Clonidine	6–23	39–42	Unch	Unch	50–75	No (H)	
Diltiazem	2–8	4	Unch	Unch	Unch	No (H,P)	
Endralazine	2	7	Unch	Unch	Unch	?	
Guanabenz	12–14	?	Unch	Unch	Unch	?	
Guanadrel	2–7	19	Unch	50	25	?	
Guanethidine	120–240	?	Unch	Unch	75	?	
Hydralazine	2–3	7–16	Unch	Unch	75	No (H,P)	Slow acetylators. Lupus syndrome.
Methyldopa	1–2	7–16	Unch	75	50	Yes (H,P)	
Minoxidil	3–4	3–4	Unch	Unch	Unch	Yes (H)	
Nifedipine	4–5	5–7	Unch	Unch	Unch	No (H,P)	
Nimodipine	3	22	Unch	Unch	Unch	No (H,P)	
Nitroprusside sodium	<10 min	<10 min	Unch	Unch	Unch	Yes (H)	Toxic metabolite thiocyanate and cyanide.
Prazosin	2–5	?	Unch	Unch	Unch	No (H,P)	
Verapamil	3–7	3–4	Unch	Unch	Unch	No (H,P)	
Antineoplastics and Immunosuppressives							
Azathioprine	1	1	Unch	Unch	75	Yes (H)	Converted to 6-mercaptopurine. Allopurinol increases activity.
Bleomycin	1–9	2–30	Unch	75	50	No (H)	Pulmonary toxicity enhanced.
Busulfan	2–3	?	Unch	Unch	Unch	?	
Cisplatin	2–72	1–240	Unch	75	50	Yes (H)	Nephrotoxic, toxicity decreased by hydration, renal Mg wasting.
Cyclophosphamide	5–7	4–12	Unch	75	50	Yes (H)	Hemorrhagic cystitis, inappropriate ADH secretion.
Cyclosporine	10–24	12–36	Unch	Unch	Unch	No (H,P)	Nephrotoxic, hypertension, hyperkalemia.
Doxorubicin	16–30	16–24	Unch	Unch	75	?	

Table continued on following page

TABLE 111–1

DOSING ADJUSTMENTS FOR VARYING DEGREES OF RENAL IMPAIRMENT* Continued

Drug	Half-life (h†) Normal	Half-life (h†) ESRD	Dose Adjustment for Renal Failure Based on C_{cr} (mL/min)‡ >50	10–50	<10	Dialysis§	Comments
Methotrexate	4–60	>60	Unch	50	Avoid	Yes (H)	Folate deficiency.
Vincristine	1–3	1–3	Unch	Unch	Unch	?	Terminal elimination $t_{1/2}$ 85 h.
Antiparkinsonian Drugs							
Bromocriptine	3	?	Unch	Unch	Unch	?	Orthostatic hypotension.
Levodopa	1–2	?	Unch	Unch	Unch	?	Active metabolites have long $t_{1/2}$.
Antipsychotics							Anticholinergic activity, urinary retention.
Chlorpromazine	16–30	16–30	Unch	Unch	Unch	No (H,P)	
Haloperidol	10–36	?	Unch	Unch	Unch	No (H,P)	
Lithium carbonate	14–28	>28	Unch	50–75	25	Yes (H,P)	Nephrogenic diabetes insipidus, renal tubular acidosis.
Antitrichomonal Drugs							
Chloroquine	6–50 d	?	Unch	Unch	50	No (H)	
Pentamidine	? d	?	Unch	75	50	?	
Pyrimethamine	2–7 d	?	Unch	Unch	Unch	?	
Quinine	4–16	?	Unch	75	30–50	Yes (H)	Marked tissue accumulation.
Antituberculosis Drugs							
Aminosalicyclic acid	1.5	23	Unch	75	Avoid	Yes (H)	Adds to acidosis.
Ethambutol	4	7–15	Unch	75	50	Yes (H,P)	
Isoniazid	1–4	17	Unch	Unch	75	Yes (H,P)	Slow acetylators.
Rifampin	1–5	15–30	Unch	Unch	Unch	No (H)	
Antiulcer Drugs							
Cimetidine	2	5	Unch	75	50	No (H,P)	
Famotidine	3–9	13–18	Unch	50	25	No (H)	
Nizatidine	1.5	7	Unch	50	25	No (H)	
Ranitidine	1–4	20	Unch	75	50	Yes (H)	
Antiviral Drugs							
Acyclovir	2–4	20	Unch	50	25	Yes (H)	
Amantadine	12–15	500	Unch	50	25	No (H,P)	
Beta-Adrenergic Antagonists							
Acebutolol	7–9	7	Unch	50	25	No (H)	Active metabolites (diacetolol) with long $t_{1/2}$.
Atenolol	6–9	15–35	Unch	50	25	Yes (H) No (P)	Accumulates in ESRD.
Bisoprolol	10–12	24	?	?	?		Three inactive metabolites; 10 mg should be maximal dose in ESRD.
Labetalol	3–8	3–8	Unch	Unch	Unch	No (H)	
Metoprolol	3–5	3–5	Unch	Unch	Unch	Yes (H)	
Nadolol	14–24	45	Unch	50	25	Yes (H)	Accumulates in ESRD.
Pindolol	3–4	3–4	Unch	Unch	Unch	?	
Propranolol	2–6	1–6	Unch	Unch	Unch	No (H)	Bioavailability may increase.
Bronchodilators							
Theophylline	3–12	5–9	Unch	Unch	Unch	Yes (H,P)	
Cardiac Glycosides							
Digoxin	30–40	87–100	Unch	25–75	10–25	No (H,P)	
Diuretics							May produce extracellular fluid volume depletion.
Acetazolamide	2–6	?	Unch	50	25	?	Acidosis, urolithiasis.
Amiloride	6–10	8–140	Unch	50	Avoid	?	Hyperkalemia.
Bumetanide	1–1.5	1.5	Unch	Unch	Unch	?	
Ethacrynic acid	1–4	?	Unch	Unch	Avoid	No (H)	
Furosemide	1–2	1–14	Unch	Unch	Unch	No (H)	
Hydrochlorothiazide	6–15	>15	Unch	Unch	Avoid	?	
Indapamide	14–18	14–18	Unch	Unch	Unch	No (H)	
Metolazone	20	?	Unch	Unch	Unch	No (H)	
Gout Drugs							
Allopurinol	1–2	>2	Unch	50	25	Yes (H)	
Colchicine	1	1	Unch	Unch	50	No (H)	
Probenecid	4–12	?	Unch	Unch	Avoid	?	

TABLE 111–1

DOSING ADJUSTMENTS FOR VARYING DEGREES OF RENAL IMPAIRMENT* Continued

Drug	Half-life (h†)		Dose Adjustment for Renal Failure Based on C_{cr} (mL/min)‡			Dialysis§	Comments
	Normal	ESRD	>50	10–50	<10		
Hypoglycemic Drugs							
Acetohexamide	6–8	31	Unch	Avoid	Avoid	No (P)	Hypoglycemia.
Chlorpropamide	24–42	50–200	Unch	Avoid	Avoid	No (P)	Hypoglycemia.
Glipizide	3–7	?	Unch	Unch	Unch	?	
Glyburide	10–16	?	Unch	Unch	Unch	?	
Insulin	2–3	>3	Unch	75	50	?	
Tolazamide	6–8	?	Unch	Unch	Unch	?	
Tolbutamide	4–7	4–7	Unch	Unch	Unch	No (H)	
Muscle Relaxants							
Atracurium	20 min	20 min	Unch	Unch	Unch	?	
Gallamine	2–3	9	Unch	Avoid	Avoid	Yes (H,P)	Prolonged apnea.
Pancuronium	1–2	4	Unch	Unch	Avoid	?	
Succinylcholine	3	?	Unch	Unch	Unch	?	
d-Tubocurarine	1–4	5	Unch	Unch	Unch	?	
Vecuronium	1	1.5	Unch	Unch	Unch	?	
Thyroid and Antithyroid Agents							
Methimazole	2–4	9	Unch	75	50	?	
Propylthiouracil	1–2	8.5	Unch	75	50	?	

*ESRD = end-stage renal disease; C_{cr} = creatinine clearance; Unch = unchanged; H = hemodialysis; P = peritoneal dialysis; $t_{1/2}$ = half-life; GFR = glomerular filtration rate; BUN = blood urea nitrogen; ADH = antidiuretic hormone; ? = unknown or not reported; Mg = magnesium.
†Unless otherwise specified.
‡Percentage of normal daily dose.
Adapted from Mammen GJ (ed): Clinical Pharmacokinetics. Drug Data Handbook 1990. Guide to Drug Dosage in Renal Failure. Auckland, New Zealand, ADIS Press, p 31, 1990.

TABLE 111–2

FACTORS THAT ALTER GLOMERULAR FILTRATION RATE ESTIMATES BASED ON SERUM CREATININE CONCENTRATIONS

Factors That Increase Creatinine Production and/or Excretion
Trauma
Major surgery
Sepsis
Increased body weight

Factors That Decrease Creatinine Production and/or Excretion
Aging
Hepatic diseases
Excessive muscle wasting
Poor protein nutrition
Muscular atrophy or dystrophy
Hyperthyroidism
Paralysis
Glucocorticoids
Decreased body weight

Drug-Induced Decreases in Serum Creatinine Elimination That May Falsely Decrease Filtration Rate Estimates
Cimetidine
Trimethoprim

Drugs That Increase Glomerular Filtration Rate
Dopamine
Isoproterenol
Digoxin
Hydralazine
Nifedipine

Drugs That Decrease Glomerular Filtration Rate
Inhibitors of prostaglandin synthesis (aspirin, indomethacin, ibuprofen)
Thiazide diuretics
Clonidine
Epinephrine
Norepinephrine

Glomerular filtration is limited by the permeability of the capillary endothelium and the ultrafiltration membrane. Only small molecules (<600 Å in diameter) are filtered by the glomeruli into the tubular fluid. Proteins and large macromolecules cannot pass through the filter. Consequently, only unbound (free) drugs can be filtered. Because serum creatinine concentration is used clinically as an index of renal function, factors that can affect serum creatinine concentration and glomerular filtration rate are listed in Table 111–2. Creatinine clearance estimates for the intensive care unit patient are usually poor indicators of actual renal function.

Effects of Renal Failure on Drug Pharmacokinetics

Renal failure has been shown to alter the plasma protein binding of many drugs; generally, the binding of drugs to albumin is decreased. The protein binding of a drug to plasma and tissue proteins affects the intensity of its pharmacologic action, as well as its distribution and elimination from the body. Even for drugs that are primarily eliminated via other routes, renal failure can lead to toxicity through accumulation of toxic metabolites (see Table 111–1). Recommendations based on a fixed dose are subject to error, especially for intensive care unit patients who have variable renal hemodynamics. Therefore, patients must be followed for both efficacy and toxicity.

Bibliography

Bennett WM, Aronoff GR, Morrison G, et al: Drug prescribing in renal failure: Dosing guidelines for adults. Am J Kidney Dis 3:155, 1983.
Cockcroft DW, Gault MH: Prediction of creatinine clearance from serum creatinine. Nephron 16:31, 1976.
Jelliffe RW: Creatinine clearance: A bedside estimate. Ann Intern Med 79:604, 1973.
Levey AS, Perrone RD, Madias NE: Serum creatinine and renal function. Annu Rev Med 39:465, 1988.

Robert S, Zarowitz BJ: Is there a reliable index of glomerular filtration rate in critically ill patients? DICP 25:169, 1991.

Siersbaek-Nielsen K, Hansen JM, Kampmann J, et al: Rapid evaluation of creatinine clearance. Lancet 1:1133, 1971.

Wetzels JFM, Huysmans FTHM, Koene RAP: Creatinine as a marker of glomerular filtration rate. Neth J Med 33:144, 1988.

TABLE 112–1

FACTORS AFFECTING PLASMA CORTISOL-BINDING GLOBULIN

Increase	Decrease
Oral contraceptives	Obesity
Pregnancy	Nephrotic syndrome
Estrogens	Hypothyroidism
Diabetes mellitus	Genetic deficiency
Hyperthyroidism	Multiple myeloma
Genetic excess	
Mitotane	

CHAPTER 112

Disorders of the Adrenal Cortex

Sushma Reddy
Rick J. Schiebinger

A thorough understanding of adrenal function is essential for the management of the critically ill patient. In patients with hypotension, hyperpyrexia, and shock, the diagnosis of acute adrenal insufficiency can be easily overlooked. Unexplained hyperkalemia may be due to unsuspected hypoaldosteronism. Patients with Cushing's syndrome or primary aldosteronism may be admitted to the intensive care unit with a variety of acute illnesses. Management of such patients must include management of the underlying adrenal disorder as well.

The adrenal cortex is composed of three zones, an outer zona glomerulosa, a middle zona fasciculata, and an inner zona reticularis. The zona glomerulosa produces aldosterone. The zona fasciculata produces both cortisol and androgens, cortisol being the major product. The zona reticularis primarily produces androgens and also some cortisol.

PHYSIOLOGY

Glucocorticoid Secretion and Metabolism

Cortisol is the principal glucocorticoid synthesized and secreted by the adrenal cortex. Normally, 15 to 30 mg of cortisol is secreted each day in a diurnal pulsatile fashion, with a peak before awakening and a nadir on retiring. Cortisol circulates in the plasma bound predominantly to cortisol-binding globulin and to a lesser extent to albumin. Less than 10% of plasma cortisol exists in the free form. The plasma free cortisol is the biologically active moiety and is regulated by corticotropin (ACTH). Because plasma cortisol assays measure both bound and free cortisol, changes in cortisol-binding globulin affect plasma cortisol measurements. Factors affecting cortisol-binding globulin concentration, and consequently plasma cortisol levels, are listed in Table 112–1. Plasma cortisol has a half-life of 60 to 100 minutes. Cortisol is inactivated by the liver and excreted by the kidney as a 17-hydroxycorticosteroid.[1] About one half to one third of 17-hydroxycorticosteroids represent cortisol and its metabolites. Only about 1% of circulating cortisol is excreted unchanged in the urine.

Regulation of Cortisol Secretion

The zona fasciculata and the zona reticularis are both regulated by ACTH. ACTH is a 39-amino-acid polypeptide, which is produced by the basophilic cells of the anterior pituitary gland. ACTH has a biologic half-life of less than 10 minutes. It acts rapidly on the adrenal cortex to stimulate the production of cortisol and adrenal androgens via an adenosine 3'5'-cyclic monophosphate–dependent mechanism. ACTH also stimulates aldosterone production, but the effect is not sustained. Increased ACTH production causes hyperplasia of the zona fasciculata and zona reticularis, whereas a deficiency of ACTH leads to atrophy of these zones of the gland.

The major factors controlling ACTH release are corticotropin-releasing hormone (CRH), stress, plasma free cortisol, vasopressin, and the sleep-wake cycle[2] (Fig. 112–1). CRH is a 41-amino-acid hypothalamic peptide that stimulates the synthesis and secretion of ACTH in response to stress and various other stimuli. CRH is secreted in a pulsatile fashion and is responsible for the pulsatile secretion of ACTH and cortisol. Vasopressin also stimulates ACTH release.

Plasma free cortisol exerts inhibitory effects at both the hypothalamic and pituitary levels. However, this negative feedback can be overriden by excessive stimulation of the hypothalamic pituitary axis, as occurs in the early morning and during stress. Stress also abolishes the periodicity of cortisol secretion.[3] A shift in the normal pattern of adrenal steroidogenesis toward the glucocorticoid pathway occurs during severe illness.[4] Critically ill patients lose the diurnal variation of cortisol secretion and may produce as much as 250 to 300 mg of cortisol daily.

Mineralocorticoid Secretion and Metabolism

Aldosterone is the principal mineralocorticoid synthesized and secreted by the adrenal cortex. It is produced solely by the zona glomerulosa. With an average salt intake, 50 to 250 μg of aldosterone is secreted each day. Other steroids—in order of decreasing potency, 11-deoxycorticosterone, 18-oxocortisol, corticosterone, and cortisol—possess mineralocorticoid activity, but aldosterone accounts for more than 50% of plasma mineralocorticoid activity. About 35% of circulating aldosterone exists in a free form; the remainder is bound to albumin, cortisol-binding globulin, and other plasma proteins. The plasma half-life of aldosterone is less than 15 minutes. Aldosterone is inactivated by the liver and excreted by the kidney as a glucuronide.[1] Urinary assays for aldosterone generally measure aldosterone glucuronide. Less than 0.5% of circulating aldosterone is excreted in the unconjugated form.

Regulation of Aldosterone Secretion

The principal factors regulating aldosterone secretion by the zona glomerulosa are the renin-angiotensin system, potassium, and to a lesser extent, ACTH[5] (Fig. 112–2). Renin, a proteolytic enzyme produced by specialized cells of the afferent arterioles (juxtaglomerular cells) of the kidney, acts on angiotensinogen, an alpha-2 globulin produced by the

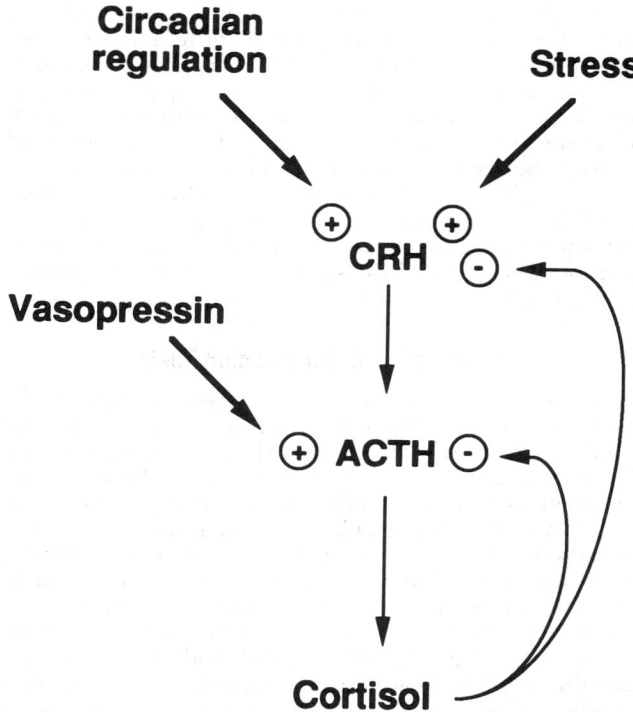

Figure 112-1. Regulation of cortisol secretion.

delivery. Cortisol has a positive inotropic effect, increasing myocardial contractility and cardiac output. It also exerts a permissive effect on the actions of catecholamines, thereby maintaining vascular tone and increasing cardiac output.

Glucocorticoids have potent anti-inflammatory properties and may have a role in immune regulation.[8] Cortisol reduces capillary vascular permeability and blunts phagocytosis and chemotaxis. Glucocorticoids also cause depletion of circulating eosinophils and T lymphocytes, thus depressing cell-mediated immunity.

Cortisol has an important permissive effect on water balance and tonicity homeostasis: in its absence, renal electrolyte-free water clearance is impaired and severe hyponatremia may occur. Cortisol has only weak mineralocorticoid properties, but in large amounts it increases renal tubular sodium reabsorption and potassium and hydrogen ion secretion.

Physiologic Actions of Mineralocorticoids

The mineralocorticoids, principally aldosterone, have major roles in the maintenance of extracellular fluid volume and in potassium and hydrogen ion balance.[9] Aldosterone acts on the renocortical collecting tubule to enhance sodium reabsorption and potassium and hydrogen ion secretion and has effects in the medullary collecting duct as well. In persons with normal renal and cardiac function, chronically elevated circulating mineralocorticoid levels are associated with the so-called mineralocorticoid escape phenomenon in which urinary sodium excretion increases after a few days to equal sodium intake, allowing the kidney to escape from the sodium-retaining effect of these hormones; however, escape from their kaliuretic effect does not occur.

liver, to form angiotensin I. Angiotensin I is converted to the decapeptide angiotensin II by angiotensin-converting enzyme. Angiotensin II is both a potent vasoconstrictor and a potent aldosterone secretagogue. Potassium acts directly on the zona glomerulosa to stimulate aldosterone synthesis and release. ACTH also stimulates aldosterone production, but the effect is not sustained. Dopamine and atrial natriuretic peptide inhibit aldosterone secretion.[6]

The major factors controlling renin secretion are renal afferent arteriolar baroreceptors, the macula densa chemoreceptors, the sympathetic nervous system, and plasma angiotensin II.[7] Volume depletion or decreases in renal perfusion pressure stimulate the afferent arteriolar baroreceptors, causing renin release, from the juxtaglomerular cells via a prostaglandin-dependent mechanism. The macula densa is made up of a group of specialized distal convoluted tubular epithelial cells lying in close apposition to the juxtaglomerular cells of the afferent arteriole. These cells act as a chemoreceptor sensing sodium chloride delivery. Increased delivery, as seen in volume expansion, inhibits renin secretion; decreased delivery, as seen in volume depletion, has the opposite effect. Activation of the sympathetic nervous system increases renin release by stimulating beta-adrenergic receptors in the membrane of the juxtaglomerular cell. In a negative-feedback fashion, angiotensin II acts directly on the juxtaglomerular cell to suppress renin secretion.

Physiologic Actions of Glucocorticoids

Glucocorticoids are essential for survival and the body's response to stress. Glucocorticoids have far-reaching metabolic effects: cortisol increases the release of gluconeogenic substrates from peripheral tissues and stimulates hepatic gluconeogenesis, while at the same time decreasing the uptake of glucose by peripheral tissues. Thus, glucocorticoids mobilize energy stores and maintain cerebral glucose

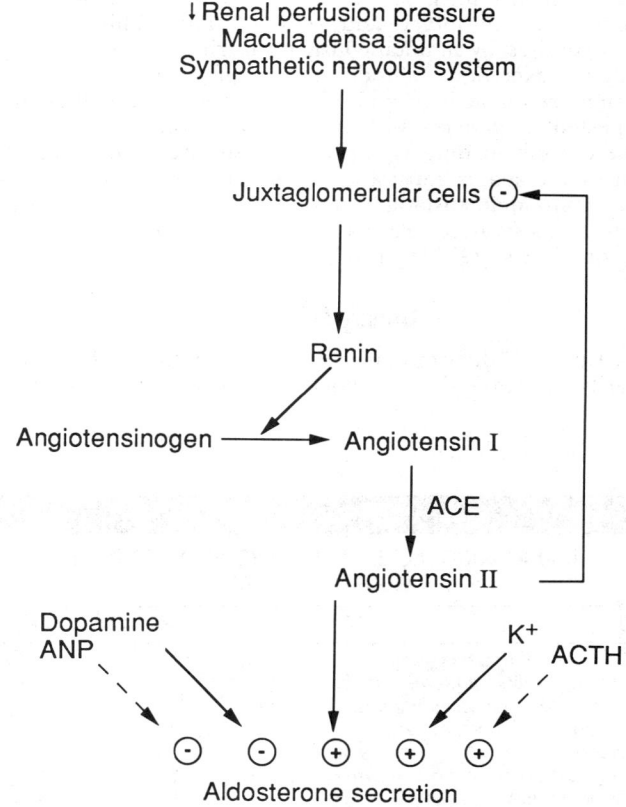

Figure 112-2. Regulation of aldosterone secretion. ANP = atrial natriuretic peptide; ACE = angiotensin-converting enzyme.

LABORATORY EVALUATION OF ADRENAL FUNCTION

Plasma Measurement

Plasma cortisol is measured as total plasma cortisol level and is affected by changes in cortisol-binding globulin levels. In critically ill patients, the plasma cortisol level can vary from 6 to 90 μg/dL.[10] Steroids other than cortisol, such as prednisone and, to a much lesser degree, dexamethasone, may be included in the radioimmunoassay. In critically ill patients suspected of having adrenal insufficiency, a random plasma cortisol level of less than 20 μg/dL is suggestive of adrenal insufficiency; an ACTH stimulation test is necessary to confirm the diagnosis, however. Random plasma cortisol levels are usually not helpful in the diagnosis of Cushing's syndrome.

Plasma ACTH assays may be unreliable, depending on the particular assay used. Two-site immunoradiometric assays, using monoclonal antibodies to the NH_2- and COOH-terminal portions of the molecule, provide a rapid and reliable method for measuring plasma ACTH [11] level. Values greater than 2500 pg/mL are pathognomonic of ectopic ACTH production. Plasma ACTH levels in Cushing's disease are in the high-normal range. In primary adrenal insufficiency, plasma ACTH level is elevated. In patients receiving steroids, plasma ACTH levels are suppressed or undetectable.

Renin is measured by its ability to generate angiotensin I from angiotensinogen. The generated angiotensin I is measured by radioimmunoassay, and plasma renin activity is expressed as nanograms of angiotensin I generated per milliliter of plasma per hour. Blood for plasma renin activity must be collected on ice and the plasma separated within 30 minutes. Plasma aldosterone is also measured by radioimmunoassay. Plasma renin activity and plasma aldosterone measurements must always be interpreted in relation to dietary sodium intake and volume status. This may be accomplished by simultaneously measuring 24-hour urinary sodium excretion. Under physiologic conditions, high plasma renin activity and plasma aldosterone values are expected in patients with intravascular volume depletion, whereas salt loading is expected to suppress these values. Potassium balance must also be considered when evaluating the renin-angiotensin-aldosterone system. Various medications can also affect plasma renin activity and plasma aldosterone levels[12] (Table 112–2).

Urinary Measures

Urinary 17-hydroxycorticosteroid excretion, which primarily measures the metabolites of cortisol and 11-deoxy-cortisol, should be expressed per grams of creatinine to correct for variations attributable to differences in body mass. In a nonstressed individual, urinary 17-hydroxycorticosteroid excretion should be less than 8 mg/g of creatinine daily. Urinary cortisol excretion is also routinely available and is the preferred measurement for the assessment of adrenal hypersecretion: urinary cortisol excretion of greater than 100 μg/24 hours in a nonstressed individual is suggestive of Cushing's syndrome. Urinary aldosterone excretion is measured as aldosterone glucuronide; high aldosterone excretion despite salt loading is characteristic of primary aldosteronism.

Stimulation and Suppression Tests

The cosyntropin (Cortrosyn) test assesses the ability of the adrenal cortex to secrete cortisol in response to ACTH. One ampule (250 μg) of synthetic ACTH (1–24) (cosyntropin) is administered as an intravenous bolus and a plasma cortisol level is measured at 60 minutes. A plasma cortisol level greater than 20 μg/dL is indicative of normal adrenal function, whereas patients with primary or secondary adrenal insufficiency have a blunted response. Thus, the cosyntropin test can establish the diagnosis of adrenal insufficiency but it does not differentiate primary from secondary causes. Measurement of plasma ACTH levels with a reliable assay is helpful in differentiating primary (elevated ACTH) from secondary (low or undetectable ACTH) adrenal insufficiency. Patients may be receiving steroids when the cosyntropin test is performed, although high-dose glucocorticoid treatment for longer than a week may result in a blunted response. The type of glucocorticoid employed is also important: dexamethasone is best because it does not interfere with the cortisol assay.

The results of the cosyntropin test are valid if the patient has chronic adrenal insufficiency. The test may not be valid if the patient is suspected of having acute secondary adrenal insufficiency (e.g., an intracerebral event). Even though such patients may have extensive damage to the hypothalamic-pituitary axis, they may respond normally to cosyntropin because their adrenals have not yet atrophied. In these circumstances, an insulin tolerance test may have to be performed to determine the integrity of adrenal function. This test assesses the ability of the hypothalamic-pituitary-adrenal axis to secrete cortisol in response to the stress of hypoglycemia.[13] The test is dangerous and must be performed with extreme caution. Regular insulin (0.1 U/kg) is administered as an intravenous bolus, and blood is drawn at 0 and 30 minutes for glucose determination. Stimulation is considered adequate if the plasma glucose level is less than 40 mg/dL (<50% of baseline in diabetic patients) or the patient has signs or symptoms of hypoglycemia. A plasma cortisol level greater than 20 μg/dL at 60 minutes is indicative of a normal hypothalamic-pituitary-adrenal axis. The test should not be performed for patients receiving glucocorticoids because steroids blunt the increase in ACTH seen in response to hypoglycemia. Patients should avoid steroids for a minimum of 24 hours before testing.

The high-dose dexamethasone suppression test, metyrapone test, and CRH test are used in the differential diagnosis of Cushing's syndrome. These tests are based on the principle that the pituitary adenomas associated with Cushing's disease do not secrete ACTH autonomously and respond to CRH, whereas ectopic ACTH-secreting tumors are autonomous and unresponsive. ACTH secretion rises in patients with Cushing's disease when plasma cortisol is lowered or when CRH is administered, and ACTH secretion can be suppressed by supraphysiologic doses of dexamethasone.

TABLE 112–2

DRUG-INDUCED ALTERATIONS IN RENIN-ANGIOTENSIN-ALDOSTERONE AXIS

Drug	Renin	Aldosterone
Beta-adrenergic blockers	↓	↓
Prostaglandin synthetase inhibitors (nonsteroidal anti-inflammatory drugs)	↓	↓
Calcium channel blockers	↑	↓
Diuretics	↑	↑
Angiotensin-converting enzyme inhibitors	↑	↓
Cyclosporine	↑	↓ or normal

ADRENOCORTICAL INSUFFICIENCY
Etiology

Adrenocortical insufficiency may be primary or secondary (Table 112–3). Primary adrenal insufficiency (Addison's disease) results from destruction of at least 90% of adrenocortical tissue. Secondary adrenal insufficiency is due to ACTH deficiency. Autoimmune adrenalitis accounts for 70 to 80% of Addison's disease, whereas tuberculosis is the second most common cause. Autoimmune adrenalitis may occur as part of one of the polyglandular autoimmune syndromes.[14]

In patients with acquired immunodeficiency syndrome, destruction of the adrenal glands may result from involvement with cytomegalovirus infection, *Mycobacterium avium-intracellulare* infection, or Kaposi's sarcoma.[15] Adrenal hemorrhage is associated with sepsis (Waterhouse-Friderichsen syndrome) or can be due to anticoagulant therapy.[16, 17] Tumor metastasis to the adrenal is frequent, but adrenal insufficiency is rare because destruction of 90% or more of the gland is required. Any metastatic tumor may be involved, including lymphoma.[18]

Long-term administration of corticosteroids causes suppression of the hypothalamic-pituitary-adrenal axis, resulting in decreased ACTH secretion and adrenal atrophy. Recovery of the axis is related to the dose, duration, and frequency of corticosteroid therapy and may take up to 12 to 18 months.[19, 20]

Pathophysiology

In primary adrenal insufficiency, destruction of the entire adrenal cortex results in combined glucocorticoid and mineralocorticoid deficiency. In contrast, patients with secondary adrenal insufficiency have isolated glucocorticoid deficiency. Corticosteroids maintain the responsiveness of the vasculature to catecholamines, and cortisol deficiency results in hypotension.

Cortisol deficiency also impairs renal electrolyte-free water excretion and may lead to hyponatremia; this is associated with inappropriately elevated vasopressin levels[21] and is promptly corrected by glucocorticoid replacement. Fasting hypoglycemia may occur because of a defect in gluconeo-

TABLE 112–3
ETIOLOGY OF ADRENOCORTICAL INSUFFICIENCY

Primary
Autoimmune adrenalitis: 70%
Tuberculosis: 20%
Other causes: 10%
   Fungal infections—histoplasmosis, blastomycosis, coccidioidomycosis
   Adrenal hemorrhage
      Anticoagulant therapy—heparin or warfarin
      Sepsis (Waterhouse-Friderichsen syndrome)—*Neisseria meningitidis* or *Pseudomonas*
   Infiltrative diseases—sarcoidosis, amyloidosis
   Malignancy—lymphoma; metastatic carcinoma of lung, breast, or colon
   Drugs—mitotane, suramin, ketoconazole
   After adrenal surgery
   Acquired immunodeficiency syndrome—cytomegalovirus infection, Kaposi's sarcoma
   Mycobacterium avium-intracellulare infection

Secondary
Hypopituitarism

TABLE 112–4
SYMPTOMS AND SIGNS OF CHRONIC PRIMARY ADRENAL INSUFFICIENCY

Symptom or Sign	%
Weakness and fatigability	100
Weight loss	100
Anorexia	100
Hyperpigmentation	92
Hyponatremia	88
Hyperkalemia	64
Hypercalcemia	6
Hypotension	88
Gastrointestinal symptoms	56
Postural dizziness	12
Adrenal calcification	9
Muscle and joint pains	6
Vitiligo	4

Adapted from Nerup J: Addison's disease—Clinical studies: A report of 108 cases. Acta Endocrinol 76:127, 1974.

genesis. Hypercalcemia is secondary to decreased renal excretion of calcium, hemoconcentration, and enhanced bone resorption.

Aldosterone deficiency causes renal sodium wasting and decreased urinary potassium and hydrogen ion excretion, leading to volume depletion, hyperkalemia, and metabolic acidosis. The volume depletion exacerbates the hypotensive effect of glucocorticoid deficiency in patients with primary adrenal insufficiency who may exhibit frank shock. Hypotension is less common in secondary adrenal insufficiency and is not a feature of isolated hypoaldosteronism.

Clinical Manifestations

Patients with chronic adrenal insufficiency typically have weakness, easy fatigability, weight loss, anorexia, nausea, vomiting, diarrhea, hypotension, and dizziness[22] (Table 112–4). Electrolyte abnormalities and hypoglycemia may also occur. Hypoglycemia is relatively uncommon but may be easily precipitated by fasting, fever, or infections. Hyperpigmentation on the extensor skin surfaces, creases of the hands, the dentogingival margin, and the lips and buccal mucosa is characteristic of primary adrenal insufficiency, resulting from the melanocyte-stimulating effects of B-lipotropin and ACTH itself. Vitiligo may also occur. In patients with secondary adrenal insufficiency, the classic features of panhypopituitarism may be present.

Acute adrenal insufficiency occurs with nausea, vomiting, hyperpyrexia, and shock. Patients with so-called adrenal crisis may have features of underlying chronic adrenocortical insufficiency. Often, one or more precipitating factors can be identified (Table 112–5). Suspicion of adrenal crisis must be entertained in any patient with septic shock who is not responding to conventional therapy with intravenous fluids and antibiotics. The sudden onset of confusion, nausea, vomiting, hypotension, and tachycardia in a patient receiving anticoagulants may be a manifestation of adrenal crisis. A meticulous drug history is essential. Inhibitors of steroidogenesis such as ketoconazole should be sought. Hepatic oxygenase inducers such as phenytoin, barbiturates, and rifampin may precipitate acute adrenal insufficiency by enhancing corticosteroid metabolism in patients with latent insufficiency.[23, 24] In patients receiving chronic glucocorticoid therapy for nonadrenal disorders (e.g., bronchial asthma), abrupt withdrawal of steroids may precipitate adrenal crisis.

TABLE 112–5

FACTORS PRECIPITATING ACUTE ADRENAL INSUFFICIENCY

Stress (trauma, surgery, acute medical illnesses) in patients with
  chronic (latent) adrenal insufficiency
Abrupt withdrawal of steroid therapy
Adrenal hemorrhage secondary to
  Anticoagulant therapy
  Meningococcemia, pseudomonas sepsis
Drugs
  Steroid synthesis inhibitors—ketoconazole, aminoglutethimide,
    suramin, mitotane
  Hepatic oxygenase inducers—phenytoin, barbiturates, rifampin

---

In a patient with acquired immunodeficiency syndrome, the presence of hypoglycemia, hyponatremia, hyperkalemia, and hypotension unresponsive to volume expansion warrants investigation for adrenal insufficiency.[25, 26]

Diagnosis

The diagnosis of acute adrenal insufficiency is suggested by the clinical picture and laboratory studies revealing hyponatremia, hyperkalemia, hypoglycemia, and eosinophilia. Ideally, plasma ACTH and cortisol levels should be obtained and glucocorticoid replacement therapy initiated without delay. A plasma cortisol level less than 20 μg/dL suggests adrenal insufficiency in a seriously ill patient.

Plasma cortisol levels between 15 and 19 μg/dL should be further evaluated with a cosyntropin stimulation test after the patient's condition has stabilized. The pretreatment plasma ACTH measurement is helpful in differentiating primary from secondary adrenal insufficiency if this is required. An ACTH level obtained after treatment is problematic because glucocorticoid treatment lowers ACTH levels. An elevated plasma ACTH level is diagnostic of primary adrenal insufficiency, whereas a low plasma ACTH level indicates disease of the hypothalamic-pituitary axis.

If the patient has primary adrenal insufficiency, a computed tomographic scan of the adrenal glands may be a useful aid to diagnosis.[27] Enlarged glands suggest adrenal hemorrhage, whereas atrophic glands are consistent with autoimmune adrenalitis. As discussed earlier, the cosyntropin stimulation test is valid only if the patient has chronic adrenal insufficiency. The insulin tolerance test should be performed if the history suggests a recent onset of adrenal insufficiency. Because concurrent steroid therapy invalidates the insulin tolerance test, glucocorticoids must be discontinued for 24 hours before this test.

Treatment

Clinical suspicion of acute adrenal insufficiency mandates immediate therapy. The glucocorticoid of choice is hydrocortisone, particularly if the patient had hyperkalemia suggesting primary adrenal insufficiency. (Hydrocortisone has mineralocorticoid activity, which is maximal at doses greater than 100 mg/d.) A bolus of 10 mg of hydrocortisone is administered intravenously, followed by 10 mg/h as a continuous infusion. No more than 300 mg of hydrocortisone daily is required because this is the maximal amount of cortisol synthesized by the adrenal in 24 hours.[28] Intramuscular cortisone acetate should not be used because its bioavailability is unpredictable.[29] Other glucocorticoids may be used if the patient does not appear to have primary adrenal insufficiency. The doses of methylprednisolone sodium succinate (Solu-Medrol) and dexamethasone need not exceed 60 mg/24 hours or 8 mg/24 hours, respectively.

Hypotensive patients require rapid volume expansion with normal saline, in addition to hydrocortisone administrations. If hypoglycemia is present, glucose should be included, as appropriate, in the intravenous fluids. Patients with acute adrenal insufficiency usually respond, often dramatically, to glucocorticoid replacement and fluid resuscitation within 6 hours. If a response is not seen within this time, the diagnosis of adrenal crisis becomes less likely and other possibilities should be considered. After the crisis resolves, the dosage of hydrocortisone is gradually tapered as the underlying acute illness responds to specific therapy. The usual maintenance dose of hydrocortisone is 20 to 30 mg/d. When patients with primary adrenal insufficiency are able to take oral medication, mineralocorticoid replacement may be provided in the form of 0.05 to 0.3 mg/d of fludrocortisone. Mineralocorticoid replacement is unnecessary in secondary adrenal insufficiency.

In patients who have received long-term glucocorticoid therapy, recovery of the suppressed hypothalamic-pituitary-adrenal axis can be assessed with the cosyntropin test.[30] A peak plasma cortisol level of greater than 20 μg/dL indicates the return of normal adrenal function. Patients with persistently subnormal plasma cortisol responses (plasma cortisol level < 20 μg/dL) require long-term glucocorticoid replacement.

Patients with adrenal insufficiency undergoing surgery should receive stress doses of hydrocortisone during and for a few days after surgery. On the morning of surgery, a 10 mg/h intravenous infusion of hydrocortisone should be started and continued throughout the day of surgery. If the surgery is uncomplicated, the dose may be cut in half each postoperative day until a maintenance dose is achieved.

HYPOALDOSTERONISM

Primary adrenal insufficiency usually results in both hypoaldosteronism and hypocortisolism. Rarely, isolated hypoaldosteronism may occur as an early manifestation of primary adrenal insufficiency, to be followed by cortisol deficiency at a later date. Much more commonly, however, isolated or selective hypoaldosteronism is not a harbinger of generalized adrenal insufficiency, and glucocorticoid synthesis and secretion are normal. Acquired isolated hypoaldosteronism accounts for up to 50% of cases of unexplained hyperkalemia in adult patients. The syndrome is discussed in detail in other chapters in this section; only selected aspects are discussed here.

Etiology

Hypoaldosteronism can result from defects in renin synthesis or release (hyporeninemic hypoaldosteronism), primary defects in the conversion of angiotensin I to angiotensin II or in aldosterone synthesis (hyperreninemic hypoaldosteronism), or unresponsiveness to aldosterone (pseudohypoaldosteronism)[31] (Table 112–6).

The possibility of medications' causing hypoaldosteronism must always be entertained in the intensive care setting.[32] Beta-adrenergic blockers, nonsteroidal anti-inflammatory agents, and calcium channel blockers inhibit renin secretion; these causes of hyporeninemic hypoaldosteronism must be distinguished from the much more common idiopathic variety. Angiotensin-converting enzyme inhibitors block angiotensin II production, and idiopathic (endogenous) causes of decreased angiotensin II production have also been described.[33] Heparin inhibits the enzyme 18-hydroxylase, which is involved in aldosterone biosynthesis.[34] However, this suppression of enzyme activity may be due to the preservative (chlorbutanol) contained in heparin prepara-

TABLE 112–6

ETIOLOGY OF ACQUIRED HYPOALDOSTERONISM

Hyporeninemic Hypoaldosteronism
Idiopathic
Inhibition of renin secretion
   Beta-adrenergic blockers
   Nonsteroidal anti-inflammatory drugs
   Calcium channel blockers
After removal of an aldosteronoma (transient)

Hyperreninemic Hypoaldosteronism
Defects in angiotensin II generation
   Angiotensin-converting enzyme inhibitors
   Idiopathic
Defects in aldosterone synthesis or secretion
   Heparin
   Chlorbutanol (preservative in heparin and certain antimicrobials
     and anesthetics)
   Cyclosporine
   Idiopathic—after prolonged hypotension or hypoxia

Pseudohypoaldosteronism
Renal transplantation
Obstructive neuropathy
Spironolactone, progestins
Triamterene, amiloride

tions rather than to heparin itself.[35] Cyclosporine blocks angiotensin II–mediated aldosterone secretion but not ACTH- or potassium-stimulated secretion.[36, 37]

An idiopathic syndrome of hyperreninemic hypoaldosteronism has been identified in critically ill patients, usually after a prolonged hypotensive episode.[38] The severity of the hypoaldosteronism is related to the duration and severity of the hypotensive episode. Although the exact mechanism is unclear, it is presumed that hypoxia or prolonged ACTH persecretion results in decreased aldosterone biosynthesis.[39, 40] Basal plasma aldosterone levels are reduced and the aldosterone response to angiotensin II and ACTH is impaired.

Transient hyporeninemic hypoaldosteronism may occur after the resection of an aldosteronoma.[41] It is thought to be due to the chronic suppression of plasma renin activity and involution of the zona glomerulosa. Recovery of the zona glomerulosa generally occurs within 6 to 12 weeks. Mineralocorticoid replacement therapy may be required temporarily.

Pseudohypoaldosteronism is characterized by target unresponsiveness to aldosterone and usually occurs in children. However, acquired pseudohypoaldosteronism can be seen after renal transplantation and in obstructive uropathy.[42] Spironolactone and progestins antagonize aldosterone action at the level of the renal tubular mineralocorticoid receptor. Triamterene and amiloride also block the tubular action of aldosterone.

Clinical Manifestations

Aldosterone deficiency results in renal sodium wasting and an inability to secrete potassium and hydrogen ions. Patients typically have volume depletion, hyperkalemia, and metabolic acidosis.

Diagnosis

Unexplained hyperkalemia in the critically ill patient always warrants investigation for mineralocorticoid deficiency. Pharmacologic agents should be excluded. The diagnosis can be confirmed with appropriate measurements of the integrity of the renin-angiotensin-aldosterone axis and the mineralocorticoid responsiveness of the kidney (see other chapters in this section).

Treatment

Administration of any pharmacologic agents that might be contributing to the hypoaldosteronism should be discontinued. In normovolemic or hypovolemic patients, mineralocorticoid replacement with fludrocortisone (0.05 to 3 mg/d orally) is indicated. Volume status, plasma electrolyte concentrations, blood urea nitrogen concentration, serum creatinine concentration, and plasma renin activity can be used to assess the adequacy of replacement. In patients with hypertension or congestive heart failure, fludrocortisone may exacerbate the underlying problem and should be used with caution. In such patients, furosemide or sodium polystyrene sulfonate (Kayexalate) may suffice to control the serum potassium concentration. In patients receiving phenytoin, the dose of fludrocortisone may need to be increased because phenytoin increases the metabolism of corticosteroids via induction of hepatic microsomal enzymes.[23] Patients receiving fludrocortisone who undergo surgery or special procedures should have mineralocorticoid replacement continued and special attention paid to volume status and potassium balance.

CUSHING'S SYNDROME

Etiology

Cushing's syndrome is the clinical manifestation of glucocorticoid excess. Table 112–7 lists the various causes of Cushing's syndrome.[43] The most common cause is exogenous administration of corticosteroids. Cushing's disease accounts for up to 60% of patients with endogenous Cushing's syndrome and is due to an ACTH-secreting pituitary tumor. Ectopic ACTH-secreting tumors and adrenal tumors make up the remainder.

Clinical Manifestations

Patients with Cushing's syndrome typically have weakness, centripetal obesity, moon facies, buffalo hump, increased supraclavicular fat pad, hirsutism, and gynecomastia.[44] Hypertension may also be present. Glucose intolerance results from accelerated gluconeogenesis and decreased uptake of glucose by peripheral tissues (secondary to insulin antagonism). Osteoporosis is common, and patients may have vertebral or rib fractures.[45] Collagen synthesis is inhibited, resulting in purplish abdominal striae, thinning of the skin,

TABLE 112–7

ETIOLOGY OF CUSHING'S SYNDROME

Exogenous—iatrogenic or factitious
   Prolonged use of glucocorticoids
   Prolonged use of ACTH
Cushing's disease
   ACTH-secreting pituitary tumor
Paraneoplastic
   Ectopic ACTH secretion—small cell carcinoma of lung,
     bronchial carcinoid, thymic carcinoid, pancreatic islet cell
     tumor, pheochromocytoma, medullary carcinoma of thyroid
   Ectopic CRH secretion
Adrenal
   Adrenal adenoma
   Adrenal carcinoma
   Micronodular adrenal hyperplasia

easy bruisability, and poor wound healing. Patients with ectopic ACTH secretion typically have hyperpigmentation and hypokalemic alkalosis and lack the more characteristic features of Cushing's syndrome.[46]

Patients with Cushing's syndrome are more susceptible to opportunistic infections such as *Pneumocystis carinii* pneumonia, invasive aspergillosis, nocardiosis, and cryptococcosis.[47] Up to 45% of patients may have superficial cutaneous and mucosal fungal infections. Glucocorticoids can mask the symptoms and signs of infection, and a high index of suspicion must be maintained. The risk of infection is related to the magnitude of the glucocorticoid excess.[48]

Diagnosis

Cushing's syndrome has such protean and typical manifestations that the diagnosis is often suspected. In patients with iatrogenic Cushing's syndrome, the diagnosis is self-evident from the history. The overnight (single-dose) dexamethasone suppression test and urinary free cortisol excretion are of limited value in the intensive care setting.[49, 50] The diagnosis of Cushing's syndrome in the critically ill patient is usually made by performing a low-dose dexamethasone suppression test (dexamethasone, 0.5 mg orally every 6 hours for 2 days). However, false-positive results may occur in the presence of endogenous depression or from the use of anticonvulsants such as phenytoin and phenobarbital.[51] Plasma ACTH levels may be useful in the diagnosis of ectopic ACTH secretion. However, more definitive evaluation (high-dose dexamethasone suppression test or metyrapone test) is generally required to confirm the specific cause of Cushing's syndrome. When the evaluation is equivocal, it should be repeated after the patient recovers from the acute illness.

Treatment

Transsphenoidal adenomectomy is the procedure of choice in patients with Cushing's disease.[52] In patients with an adrenal adenoma or a resectable adrenal carcinoma, surgical removal of the tumor is performed.[53] Ectopic ACTH secretion necessitates therapy directed at the underlying neoplasm.

Patients with Cushing's syndrome may be admitted to the intensive care unit for a variety of acute illnesses. Optimal management may sometimes necessitate medical (as opposed to the standard surgical) treatment of the Cushing's syndrome. Ketoconazole, an inhibitor of adrenal P-450 enzymes; metyrapone, an 11-hydroxylase inhibitor; and aminoglutethimide, an inhibitor of cholesterol side chain cleavage, have been used successfully to lower plasma cortisol levels.[54] Ketoconazole may cause hepatitis, and liver enzyme levels should be monitored closely. Aminoglutethimide interferes with thyroxine production and may produce hypothyroidism; replacement doses of thyroid hormone are recommended when using aminoglutethimide. Inhibitors of adrenal steroidogenesis are less effective in the medical management of Cushing's disease (as compared with other causes of Cushing's syndrome) because the pituitary tumor releases more ACTH when plasma cortisol levels are lowered.[54] This escape from adrenal inhibition may be less prominent with ketoconazole than with metyrapone or aminoglutethimide. Mifepristone (RU 486), an investigational agent, blocks the action of cortisol at the level of the glucocorticoid receptor and is effective in the treatment of all varieties of Cushing's syndrome.[55, 56] Mitotane, an adrenolytic agent, is used primarily in the treatment of Cushing's disease (after unsuccessful surgery) and inoperable adrenal carcinoma.[46] Because adrenal steroidogenesis inhibitors can cause hypoadrenalism, urinary free cortisol measurements should be used to monitor therapy. Because of the danger of adrenal crisis, whenever possible, it is best to delay therapy for Cushing's syndrome until the acute illness has resolved.

The risk of opportunistic infections in patients with Cushing's syndrome mandates more accurate identification of the organism, and prompt and specific antifungal or antibiotic therapy is mandatory. Lowering of the plasma cortisol level into a physiologic range may facilitate the treatment of such opportunistic infections.[48] Glucose intolerance and frank diabetes mellitus may occur in patients with Cushing's syndrome, and large doses of insulin may be required for adequate control. Hypertension must always be controlled, and volume overload, which may reflect excessive mineralocorticoid activity, often responds to spironolactone.

HYPERALDOSTERONISM
Etiology

Primary aldosteronism is found in up to 2% of hypertensive patients. Aldosterone-producing adenomas account for approximately 60% of patients with primary aldosteronism, whereas bilateral adrenal hyperplasia is seen in the majority of the remainder (Table 112–8). Glucocorticoid remediable (suppressible) hyperaldosteronism and aldosterone-producing carcinomas are rare.

Clinical Manifestations

Aldosterone excess results in enhanced renal tubular sodium reabsorption and potassium and hydrogen ion excretion. Patients typically have modest hypertension, hypokalemia, and metabolic alkalosis. However, severe hypertension, with diastolic blood pressure above 110 mm Hg, can occur. Polyuria, polydipsia, impaired glucose tolerance, muscle weakness, and paralysis may result from the hypokalemia.[57]

Diagnosis

The presence of inappropriate kaliuresis in the face of spontaneous hypokalemia of 3.5 mEq/L or less in a hypertensive patient suggests hyperaldosteronism. The definitive diagnosis of primary aldosteronism requires demonstration of nonsuppressible aldosterone secretion and suppressed renin levels, which cannot be stimulated.[58] In practical terms, the lack of suppression of aldosterone secretion with volume expansion and the failure of renin secretion to increase in response to upright posture, salt restriction, or diuretic administration fulfills these criteria. Plasma 18-hydroxycorticosterone levels and the aldosterone response to changes in posture may be useful in distinguishing aldosterone-producing adenomas from bilateral adrenal hyperplasia.[59] Computed tomography and iodocholesterol scans of the adrenals are also helpful.

Treatment

Surgery is the treatment of choice for an aldosterone-producing adenoma. Patients with bilateral adrenal hyper-

---

TABLE 112–8

ETIOLOGY OF PRIMARY ALDOSTERONISM

Aldosterone-producing adenoma
Bilateral adrenal hyperplasia
Glucocorticoid remediable hyperaldosteronism
Aldosterone-producing carcinoma

plasia are treated medically with spironolactone or amiloride.[60] Amiloride is the drug of choice for men because spironolactone can cause impotence and gynecomastia. Triamterene may also be used. Angiotensin-converting enzyme inhibitors[61] and calcium channel blockers[62] have been used in some patients.

Patients with primary aldosteronism may be admitted to the intensive care unit with a variety of acute illnesses. Hypertension is usually controlled with angiotensin-converting enzyme inhibitors or calcium channel blockers. Potassium supplements or potassium-sparing diuretics or both are used to maintain normokalemia.

References

1. Samuels LT, Nelson DH: Biosynthesis of corticosteroids. In: Greep RP, Astwood EB (eds): Handbook of Physiology, Section 7, Endocrinology, Volume VI, Adrenal Gland. Washington, DC, American Physiological Society, p 55, 1975.
2. Antoni FA: Hypothalamic control of adrenocorticotropin secretion: Advances since the discovery of 41-residue corticotropin releasing factor. Endocr Rev 7:351, 1986.
3. Streeten DHP, Anderson GH Jr, Dalakos TG, et al: Normal and abnormal function of the hypothalamic-pituitary-adrenocortical system in man. Endocr Rev 5:371, 1984.
4. Parker LN, Levin ER, Lifrak ET: Evidence for adrenocortical adaptation to severe illness. J Clin Endocrinol Metab 60:947, 1985.
5. Quinn SJ, Williams GH: Regulation of aldosterone secretion. Annu Rev Physiol 50:409, 1988.
6. Carey RM, Thorner MO, Ortt EM: Effects of metoclopramide and bromocriptine on the renin-angiotensin-aldosterone system in man. J Clin Invest 63:727, 1979.
7. Davis JO, Freeman RH: Mechanism regulating renin release. Physiol Rev 56:1, 1976.
8. Munck A, Guyre P, Holbrook NJ: Physiological functions of glucocorticoids in stress and their relation to pharmacological actions. Endocr Rev 5:25, 1984.
9. Morris DJ: The metabolism and mechanism of action of aldosterone. Endocr Rev 2:234, 1981.
10. Drucker D, Shandling M: Variable adrenocortical function in acute medical illness. Crit Care Med 13:477, 1985.
11. White A, Smith H, Hoadley M, et al: Clinical evaluation of a two-site immunoradiometric assay for adrenocorticotrophin in unextracted human plasma using monoclonal antibody. Clin Endocrinol 26:41, 1987.
12. Keeton TK, Campbell WB: The pharmacologic alteration of renin release. Pharmacol Rev 32:91, 1980.
13. Melby JC: Assessment of adrenocortical function. N Engl J Med 285:735, 1971.
14. Loriaux DL: The polyendocrine deficiency syndromes. N Engl J Med 312: 1568, 1985.
15. Glasgow BJ, Steinsapir KD, Anders K, et al: Adrenal pathology in the acquired immune deficiency syndrome. Am J Clin Pathol 84:594, 1985.
16. Siu SCB, Kitzman DW, Sheedy PF, et al: Adrenal insufficiency from bilateral hemorrhage. Mayo Clin Proc 65:664, 1990.
17. Dahlberg PJ, Goellner MH, Pehling GB: Adrenal insufficiency secondary to adrenal hemorrhage. Two case reports and a review of cases confirmed by computed tomography. Arch Intern Med 150:905, 1990.
18. Huminer D, Garty M, Lapidot M, et al: Lymphoma presenting with adrenal insufficiency. Am J Med 84:169, 1988.
19. Axelrod L: Glucocorticoid therapy. Medicine 55:39, 1976.
20. Koch-Weser J, Byyny RL: Drug therapy—withdrawal from glucocorticoid therapy. N Engl J Med 295:30, 1976.
21. Boykin J, deTorrente A, Erickson A, et al: Role of plasma vasopressin in impaired water excretion of glucocorticoid deficiency. J Clin Invest 62:738, 1978.
22. Nerup J: Addison's disease—Clinical studies. A report of 108 cases. Acta Endocrinol 76:127, 1974.
23. Keilholz V, Guthrie GP: Case report: Adverse effect of phenytoin on mineralocorticoid replacement with fludrocortisone in adrenal insufficiency. Am J Med Sci 291:280, 1986.
24. Elias AN, Gwinup G: Effects of some clinically encountered drugs on steroid synthesis and degradation. Metabolism 29:582, 1980.
25. Membreno L, Irony I, Dere W, et al: Adrenocortical function in acquired immunodeficiency syndrome. J Clin Endocrinol Metab 65:482, 1987.
26. Aron DC: Endocrine complications of the acquired immunodeficiency syndrome. Arch Intern Med 149:330, 1989.
27. Doppman JL, Gill JR Jr, Nienhuis AW, et al: CT findings in Addison's disease. J Comput Assist Tomogr 6:757, 1982.
28. Udelsman R, Ramp J, Galluci WT, et al: Adaptation during surgical stress: A reevaluation of the role of glucocorticoids. J Clin Invest 77:1377, 1986.
29. Fariss BL, Hane S, Shinsako J, et al: Comparison of absorption of cortisone acetate and hydrocortisone hemisuccinate. J Clin Endocrinol Metab 47:1137, 1978.
30. Kehlet H, Binder C: Value of an ACTH test in assessing hypothalamic-pituitary-adrenal function in glucocorticoid treated patients. Br Med J 2:147, 1973.
31. Veldhuis JD, Melby JC: Isolated aldosterone deficiency in man: Acquired and inborn errors in the biosynthesis or action of aldosterone. Endocr Rev 2:495, 1981.
32. Ponce SP, Jennings AE, Madias NE, et al: Drug induced hyperkalemia. Medicine 64:357, 1985.
33. Findling JW, Adams AH, Raff M: Selective hypoaldosteronism due to an endogenous impairment in angiotensin II production. N Engl J Med 316:1633, 1987.
34. O'Kelly R, Magee F, McKenna TJ: Routine heparin therapy inhibits adrenal aldosterone production. J Clin Endocrinol Metab 56:108, 1983.
35. Sequeira SJ, McKenna TJ: Chlorbutol, a new inhibitor of aldosterone biosynthesis identified during examination of heparin effect on aldosterone production. J Clin Endocrinol Metab 63:780, 1986.
36. Bantle JP, Nath KA, Sutherland DER, et al: Effects of cyclosporine on the renin-angiotensin-aldosterone system and potassium excretion in renal transplant recipients. Arch Intern Med 145:505, 1985.
37. Stern N, Lustig S, Petrosek D, et al: Cyclosporin A–induced hyperreninemic hypoaldosteronism. A model of adrenal resistance to angiotensin II. Hypertension 9(suppl III):31, 1987.
38. Zipser RD, Davenport MW, Martin KL, et al: Hyperreninemic hypoaldosteronism in the critically ill: A new entity. J Clin Endocrinol Metab 53:867, 1981.
39. Stern N, Beck FWJ, Sowers JR, et al: Plasma corticosteroids in hyperreninemic hypoaldosteronism, evidence for diffuse impairment of the zona glomerulosa. J Clin Endocrinol Metab 57:217, 1983.
40. Davenport MW, Zipser RD: Association of hypotension with hyperreninemic hypoaldosteronism in the critically ill patient. Arch Intern Med 145:735, 1983.
41. Loughlin T, Chrousos GP: Hypoaldosteronism. In: Becker LK (ed): Principles and Practice of Endocrinology and Metabolism. Philadelphia, JB Lippincott, p 643, 1990.
42. Uribarri J, Oh MS, Butt KMH, et al: Pseudohypoaldosteronism following kidney transplantation. Nephron 31:368, 1982.
43. Howlett TA, Rees LH, Besser GM: Cushing's syndrome. Clin Endocrinol Metab 14:911, 1985.
44. Aron DC, Findling JW, Tyrrell JB: Cushing's disease. Clin Endocrinol Metab 16:705, 1987.
45. Hough S, Teitelbaum SL, Bergfeld MA, et al: Isolated skeletal involvement in Cushing's syndrome: Response to therapy. J Clin Endocrinol Metab 52:1033, 1981.
46. Schteingart DE: Cushing's syndrome. Clin Endocrinol Metab 18:311, 1989.
47. Kramer M, Corrado ML, Bacci V, et al: Pulmonary cryptococcosis and Cushing's syndrome. Arch Intern Med 143:2179, 1983.
48. Graham BS, Tucker WS: Opportunistic infections in endogenous Cushing's syndrome. Ann Intern Med 101:334, 1984.
49. Carpenter PC: Diagnostic evaluation of Cushing's syndrome. Clin Endocrinol Metab 17:445, 1988.
50. Connolly CK, Gore MBR, Stanley H, et al: Single dose dexamethasone suppression in normal subjects and hospital patients. Br Med J 2:665, 1968.
51. Crapo L: Cushing's syndrome: A review of diagnostic tests. Metabolism 28:955, 1979.
52. Mampalam TJ, Tyrrell JB, Wilson CB: Transsphenoidal microsurgery for Cushing's disease. Ann Intern Med 109:487, 1988.
53. Bertagna C, Orth N: Clinical and laboratory findings and results of therapy in 58 patients with adrenocortical tumors admitted to a single medical center (1951 to 1978). Am J Med 71:855, 1981.
54. Oates JA, Wood AJJ, Sonino N: The use of ketoconazole as an inhibitor of steroid production. N Engl J Med 317:812, 1987.
55. Nieman LK, Chrousos GP, Kellner C, et al: Successful treatment of Cushing's syndrome with the glucocorticoid antagonist RU 486. J Clin Endocrinol Metab 61:536, 1985.
56. van der Lely A-J, Foeken K, van der Mast RC, et al: Rapid reversal of acute psychosis in the Cushing syndrome with the cortisol receptor antagonist mifepristone (RU 486). Ann Intern Med 114:143, 1991.
57. Bravo EL, Tarazi RC, Dustan HP, et al: The changing clinical spectrum of primary aldosteronism. Am J Med 74:641, 1983.
58. Melby JC: Diagnosis and treatment of primary aldosteronism and isolated hypoaldosteronism. Clin Endocrinol Metab 14:977, 1985.
59. Weinberger MH: Primary aldosteronism: Diagnosis and differentiation of subtypes. Ann Intern Med 100:300, 1984.
60. Loriaux DL, Menard R, Taylor A, et al: Spironolactone and endocrine dysfunction. Ann Intern Med 85:630, 1976.
61. Griffing GT, Melby JC: The therapeutic effect of a new angiotensin-converting enzyme inhibitor, enalapril maleate, in idiopathic hyperaldosteronism. J Clin Hypertens 3:265, 1985.
62. Nadler JL, Asuch W, Horton R: Therapeutic effect of calcium channel blockade in primary aldosteronism. J Clin Endocrinol Metab 60:896, 1985.

CHAPTER 113

Catecholamines and Pressor Agents*

Stephen L. Farrow
Warren E. Lockette
James R. Sowers

PHYSIOLOGY OF THE CATECHOLAMINES

Synthesis

Catecholamines are derived from a hydroxylated aromatic ring with an attached ethylamine (Fig. 113–1). Substitutions can occur on either of the carbon atoms or on the terminal amino group of ethylamine to give compounds with varying

---

*All material in this chapter is in the public domain, with the exception of any borrowed figures or tables.

degrees of sympathomimetic activity.[1] The most important physiologic catecholamines include dopamine, norepinephrine, and epinephrine (Table 113–1). Dopamine and norepinephrine are synthesized from the essential amino acid tyrosine in postganglionic sympathetic neurons of the peripheral nervous system, some fibers of the central nervous system, and the adrenal medulla.

The initial steps in catecholamine synthesis occur in the cytoplasm. Tyrosine is first converted by tyrosine hydroxylase to 3,4-dihydroxyphenylalanine (dopa) in a reaction that is the rate-limiting step in catecholamine synthesis.[1, 2] Next, dopa is converted by dopa decarboxylase.[1, 3] Dopamine is then taken up by intracellular vesicles, where it is converted by dopamine β-hydroxylase to norepinephrine. In the adrenal medulla, norepinephrine is methylated by phenylethanolamine *N*-methyltransferase to epinephrine.[1, 1a] Most plasma norepinephrine comes from sympathetic nerve terminals, and most plasma epinephrine is contributed by the adrenal glands.

Catabolism

After reuptake by prejunctional sympathetic neurons, norepinephrine and epinephrine are degraded by catechol *O*-methyltransferase to normetanephrine and metanephrine, respectively. Catecholamines can also be sequentially metabolized by catechol *O*-methyltransferase and monoamine ox-

(only end products and significant intermediates are shown)

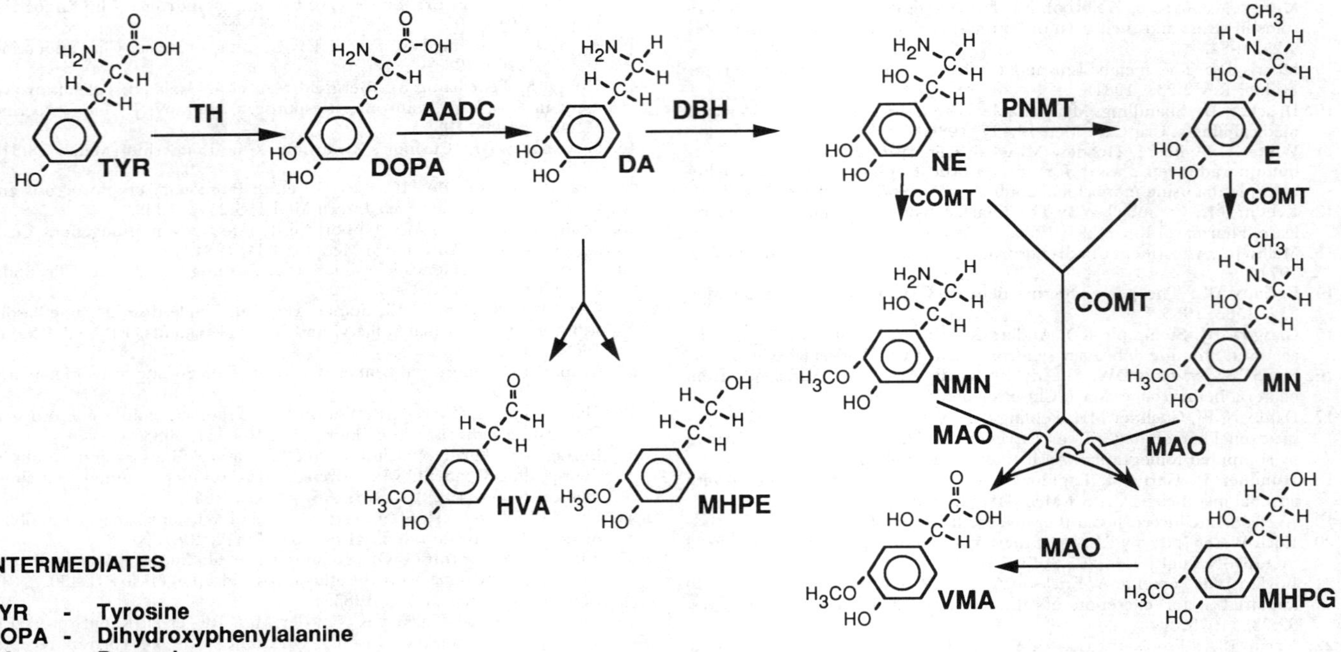

INTERMEDIATES

TYR	-	Tyrosine
DOPA	-	Dihydroxyphenylalanine
DA	-	Dopamine
NE	-	Norepinephrine
E	-	Epinephrine
NMN	-	Normetanephrine
MN	-	Metanephrine
HVA	-	Homovanillylmandelic Acid
VMA	-	Vanillylmandelic Acid
MHPE	-	3-Methoxy-4-hydroxyphenylethanol
MHPG	-	3-Methoxy-4-hydroxyphenylglycol

ENZYMES

TH	-	Tyrosine Hydroxylase
AADC	-	Amino Acid Decarboxylase
DBH	-	Dopamine β-Hydroxylase
PNMT	-	Phenylethanolamine *N*-methyltransferase
COMT	-	Catechol *O*-methyltransferase
MAO	-	Monoamine Oxidase

Figure 113–1. Synthesis of norepinephrine from tyrosine and formation of common metabolites of catecholamine metabolism in humans. Only end products and significant intermediates are shown. Norepinephrine can be subsequently converted to epinephrine by methylation of the amino group. Dopamine may also be metabolized to 3,4-dihydroxyphenylacetic acid. (Adapted from Kagedal B, Goldstein DS: Catecholamines and their metabolites. J Chromatogr 429:177, 1988.)

TABLE 113–1

PHYSIOLOGIC SOURCES OF AND RECEPTORS STIMULATED BY CATIONS OF NOREPINEPHRINE, EPINEPHRINE, AND DOPAMINE

Catecholamine	Sources	Receptors	Actions*	Elimination
Dopamine	Neurons, renal tubule, liver, brain	Alpha₁ (at high concentrations), alpha₂, beta (at high concentrations), D-1, D-2, DA-1, DA-2	Inotrope, vasoconstriction, renal vasodilation	Secreted by renal tubule cells, uptakes 1 and 2
Norepinephrine	Neurons	Alpha₁, alpha₂, beta	Vasoconstriction, − catecholamine release	Adrenal, uptakes 1 and 2, monoamine oxidase secreted by renal tubule cells
Epinephrine	Adrenal	Alpha, beta	Chronotropicity, inotropicity	Uptakes 1 and 2, secreted by renal tubule cells

*The − indicates inhibition of a given action.

idase to form either 3-methoxy-4-hydroxymandelic acid (also known as vanillylmandelic acid) or 3-methoxy-4-hydroxyphenylglycol. Continued release of catecholamines from the prejunctional terminal is inhibited by feedback of already-released catecholamines onto the presynaptic alpha₂-adrenergic receptor (Fig. 113–2). Catechol O-methyltransferase and monoamine oxidase are found in most tissues, and particularly in the liver and the kidneys.[1] Metabolites of catecholamines may also be sulfated in conjugation reactions occurring in the liver. Determinations of metanephrine, normetanephrine, and vanillylmandelic acid are indicators of peripheral catecholamine metabolism. The metabolism of catecholamines to 3-methoxy-4-hydroxyphenylglycol occurs to a greater extent in the central nervous system. Determinations of plasma and central nervous system concentrations of this metabolite remain a research tool.[4]

Measurement

Accurate assessment of catecholamine metabolism is frequently needed in the diagnosis of hyperadrenergic states. Table 113–2 lists normal values for catecholamine concentrations in plasma and urine.[5–7] Drugs can influence plasma catecholamine levels and the excretion of urinary catecholamine metabolites.[5, 7–9] In addition, substances interfere with the assays used to measure catecholamines and catecholamine metabolites. A variety of other factors may also affect catecholamine metabolism. For example, smoking or changes in posture increase the release of catecholamines. Accordingly, plasma and urine for catecholamines and cat-

echolamine metabolite determinations should always be collected under standardized conditions.[5, 7–9]

Whole blood specimens for catecholamine assay are collected in sodium heparin tubes and are stable at room temperature for up to 1 hour.[9] Twenty-four–hour urine samples for catecholamine assay are collected with 15 mL of 6 M hydrochloric acid per liter of sample to prevent degradation of the catecholamines.[8] Both plasma and 24-hour urine samples for catecholamine assay should be stored at 4°C but should be assayed within 24 hours of collection. Liquid chromatography is a low cost, simple procedure that is relatively immune to interference from medications and other substances, which makes it the analytic method of choice.[7, 9–11]

Many drugs can directly affect the release or intraneuronal catabolism of catecholamines and the subsequent concentration of plasma catecholamines. For example, cocaine decreases the uptake and the subsequent metabolism of catecholamines. Reserpine depletes neuronal catecholamine stores. Antidepressants such as tranylcypromine inhibit monoamine oxidase. Tyramine, amphetamines, and yohimbine increase the release of norepinephrine from nerve terminals. Obviously, the use of any of these drugs by patients being evaluated for a hyperadrenergic state can invalidate the results of diagnostic determinations. Table 113–3 lists substances and conditions that may affect accurate determination of catecholamine levels.

Metanephrines and vanillylmandelic acid in the urine are most frequently measured spectrophotometrically. Because many drugs absorb light at similar wavelengths to catechol-

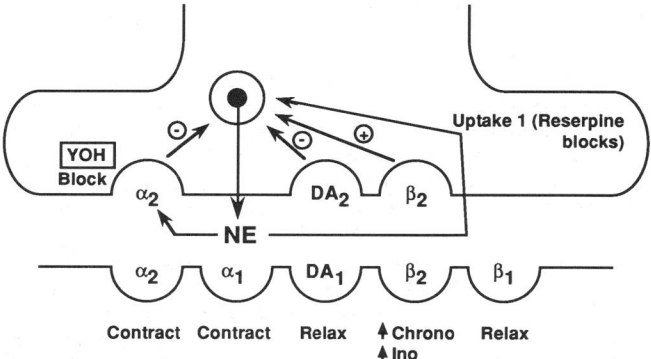

Figure 113–2. Nerve junction. Activation of alpha₂-adrenergic receptors decreases the further release of norepinephrine (NE). YOH = yohimbine; Chrono = chronotropic; Ino = inotropic. (Adapted from M Murphy, W Elliott: Dopamine and dopamine receptor agonists in cardiovascular therapy, Crit Care Med, 18, 1[part 2], S14–S18, © Williams & Wilkins, 1990.)

TABLE 113–2

NORMAL LABORATORY VALUES FOR CATECHOLAMINES AND THEIR METABOLITES

Catecholamine	Normal Range
Plasma	
Dopamine	<100 pg/mL
Norepinephrine	65–400 pg/mL
Epinephrine	15–55 pg/mL
Urine	
Dopamine	25–525 µg/24 h
Norepinephrine	10–64 µg/24 h
Epinephrine	0–36 µg/24 h
Homovanillic Acid	2–13 mg/24 h
Vanillylmandelic acid	2–7 mg/24 h
3-Methoxy-4-hydroxyphenylglycol	1.3–4.3 mg/24 h
Metanephrines	<1.6 ng/24 h

Adapted with permission. Feldman JM: Diagnosis and management of pheochromocytoma. Hospital Practice Volume 24, issue 1, page 178, 1989. Illustration by Hospital Practice.

TABLE 113–3

FACTORS AFFECTING DETERMINATION OF CATECHOLAMINE LEVELS

Increases in Plasma Catecholamines
In Vivo Effect
Ajmaline; aminophylline; chlorpromazine; cocoa; cyclopropane; diazoxide; epinephrine; ethanol; ether; isoproterenol; monoamine oxidase inhibitors; methyldopa; nitroglycerin; perphenazine; phenothiazines; phentolamine; promethazine; stress; bananas; caffeine; calcium channel blockers; vasodilators; hydralazine; yohimbine; luteal phase of menses; increasing age; subclinical hepatic, renal, pulmonary, and cardiac failure; metabolic imbalance; major affective disorders; pheochromocytoma; mitral valve prolapse; pulmonary hypertension; essential hypertension; acute myocardial infarction; neuroblastoma; melanoma
Methodologic Effect
Ampicillin, ascorbic acid, levodopa, methenamine, methyldopa, niacin, oxytetracycline, protamine, quinidine, quinine, riboflavin, sulfamethazine, tea, tetracycline, uremia, vitamin B, vitamin K

Increases in Urine Catecholamines
In Vivo Effect
Ethanol, isoproterenol, muscular exercise, nicotine, nitroglycerin, prochlorperazine, rauwolfia, reserpine, syrosingopine, theophylline
Methodologic Effect
Aspirin, bananas, carbon tetrachloride, chloral hydrate, chlorpromazine, demeclocycline, dihydroxyphenylacetic acid, dopamine, erythromycin, formaldehyde, hydralazine, hydroquinone, isoproterenol, methyldopa, niacin, oxytetracycline, quinidine, riboflavin, tetracycline, vitamin B, labetalol, acetaminophen

Decreases in Plasma Catecholamines
In Vivo Effect
Reserpine, diabetic autonomic neuropathy, idiopathic orthostatic hypotension
Methodologic Effect
Cyclopropane, ether

Decreases in Urine Catecholamines
In Vivo Effect
Clonidine, decaborane, diurnal variation, guanethidine, methyldopa, ouabain, radiographic agents, reserpine, sleep, bretylium tosylate
Methodologic Effect
Chlorpromazine

Modified from Young DS, Pestaner LS, Gibberman V: Effects of drugs on clinical laboratory tests. Clin Chem 21:275D, 1975. Copyright to the American Association of Clinical Chemistry, Inc.

amines, the specificities of these spectrophotometric assays are low. Phenothiazines erroneously increase urinary metanephrine levels, whereas methylglucamine erroneously lowers urinary metanephrine levels. Acetaminophen, clofibrate, methenamine mandelate (Mandelamine), and *p*-aminosalicylic acid interfere with the determination of urinary vanillylmandelic acid.[12]

Norepinephrine and epinephrine are usually measured in the urine by a fluorometric method. Quinidine, quinine, and certain antibiotics and vitamins interfere with these fluorometric determinations. Radioisotopic and enzymatic techniques provide the most reliable estimates of plasma catecholamine levels. However, measurement of plasma and urinary norepinephrine, epinephrine, and dopamine by high-pressure liquid chromatography is accurate. In fact, high-pressure liquid chromatography with electrochemical detection provides the preferred compromise among sensitivity, specificity, speed, cost, and sample requirements among the methods listed in Table 113–4. Thus, the reliability of plasma and urinary catecholamines and catechola-

mine metabolite determinations depends on the assay used. Clinicians must understand the reliability of the particular assays used by their laboratory.[12, 13]

Cellular Action

The physiologic response to catecholamines is determined by the complement of receptors for various catecholamine agonists present in a particular tissue (Table 113–5). Alpha$_1$-adrenergic receptors have their most important role in the control of blood pressure and are found mainly on blood vessels. Norepinephrine is the most potent alpha$_1$-adrenergic receptor agonist (Table 113–6). The activation of alpha$_1$-adrenergic receptors is linked to the hydrolysis of phosphatidylinositol biphosphate to inositol triphosphate and diacylglycerol (Fig. 113–3). Inositol triphosphate induces the release of calcium from intracellular storage sites in the sarcoplasmic reticulum of cardiocytes and skeletal muscle and the endoplasmic reticulum of vascular smooth muscle.[14] Mutations in the gene coding for the calcium release channel that mediates the release of calcium from these intracellular storage sites have been related to the malignant hyperthermia syndrome.[15] Diacylglycerol activates protein kinase C, a ubiquitous enzyme that controls threonine and serine phosphorylation reactions. Inositol triphosphate and diacylglycerol thus serve as intracellular messengers mediating a wide variety of cellular responses.

Alpha$_2$-adrenergic receptors are found on presynaptic neurons and serve as a component of the feedback mechanism that inhibits the further release of norepinephrine from the nerve terminal (see Fig. 113–2). Alpha$_2$-adrenergic agonists such as clonidine decrease blood pressure by inhibiting norepinephrine release from synaptic nerve terminals in the central nervous system. This mechanism is the centerpiece of the clonidine suppression test that is used in the diagnosis of pheochromocytoma. Normal individuals have a decrease in plasma catecholamine levels after administration of clonidine, whereas individuals with autonomously functioning tumors of the adrenal medulla do not respond to clonidine. Alpha$_2$-adrenergic receptors are also found in other tissues and modulate peripheral blood flow and pancreatic insulin release.[16]

Beta-adrenergic agonists are best known for their inotropic and chronotropic effects on the heart. Epinephrine and isoproterenol predominantly activate beta-adrenergic receptors and increase heart rate and myocardial contraction by activating beta$_1$-adrenergic receptors. Activation of beta$_2$-adrenergic receptors induces relaxation of bronchiolar and vascular smooth muscle.

Beta-adrenergic receptors also mediate a number of metabolic effects including catecholamine-related lipolysis and calorigenesis. In addition, activation of beta-adrenergic receptors increases Na$^+$,K$^+$-ATPase activity. Accordingly, it is not unusual for patients treated with adrenergic agonists to have hypokalemia attributable, at least in part, to catecholamine-stimulated cellular potassium uptake. Similarly, postexercise cardiac dysrhythmias may result from catecholamine-induced changes in potassium homeostasis.

The beta-adrenergic receptor is coupled to a guanosine triphosphate–binding protein (G protein). In the presence of the appropriate agonist, G protein binds guanosine triphosphate and dissociates into a guanosine triphosphate-α complex and also a β-γ subunit. In the case of beta-adrenergic receptors, the guanosine triphosphate-α subunit directly activates adenylate cyclase and increases adenosine 3′,5′-cyclic monophosphate (cyclic AMP) production. The resultant increase in cyclic AMP levels is the most likely intracellular mechanism mediating the action of beta-adrenergic agonists.[17]

TABLE 113–4

METHODS OF CATECHOLAMINE ANALYSIS

Method	Characteristics
Liquid chromatography with electrochemical detection	Sensitive, specific, rapid, economical; contamination of detecting electrodes over time (replaceable) less sensitive and specific than mass spectroscopic detection
Colorimetry	Low sensitivity and specificity
Classic fluorometry	Low sensitivity and specificity
Gas chromatography with electrochemical detection	Sample loss caused by volatilization
Gas chromatography with mass spectroscopic detection	Sensitive, specific, rapid; sample loss caused by volatilization, technically complicated, expensive, limited availability
Radioenzymatic assay	Sensitive and specific; expensive, technically complicated
Radioimmunoassay	Primarily a research tool
Immunofluorescence	Primarily for identification of catecholamines in tissues

Beta-adrenergic receptors demonstrate the greatest degree of desensitization of any of the adrenergic receptor family: prolonged stimulation with beta-adrenergic agonists decreases their cellular response. Prolonged exposure activates a specific cyclic AMP–dependent protein kinase, which phosphorylates an adrenergic receptor kinase, which in turn phosphorylates the beta-receptor; the phosphorylated receptor has decreased responsiveness to its activating ligand.[18, 19]

Dopamine receptors are found in the central nervous system where they are classified as either D-1 or D-2 dopamine receptors, and also in the periphery where they are analogously designated as DA-1 and DA-2.[20–24] In general,

stimulation of the D-2 dopamine receptor influences behavior, and in the pituitary gland prevents prolactin release. The role of the D-1 dopamine receptor is not clearly understood.

DA-1 dopamine receptors are found on vascular smooth muscle and mediate relaxation by stimulation of adenylate cyclase. Stimulation of DA-1 dopamine receptors found on renal tubular cells enhances sodium excretion. DA-2 dopamine receptors are found on presynaptic sympathetic neurons of sympathetic ganglia, where they reduce sympathetic outflow and facilitate vascular relaxation. Relaxation is enhanced in tissues that possess DA-1 dopamine receptors in

TABLE 113–5

LOCATIONS AND MINUS EFFECTS OF ADRENERGIC RECEPTORS*

Receptor	Location	Effect	Special Characteristics
Alpha$_1$	Heart (postjunctional)	Inotropicity	Not adenylate cyclase coupled; active at lower heart rates
	Vasculature	Vasoconstriction	
	Renal (vasculature, proximal tubule, thick ascending limb)	Vasoconstriction, − diuresis, − natriuresis	More numerous than alpha$_2$ on vasculature
Alpha$_2$	Heart (prejunctional synaptic terminal)	− Neurotransmission	
	Vasculature (endothelial cells and possibly other sites)	Vasoconstriction, endothelium-derived growth factor release, vasodilation	More numerous on veins than on arteries
	Renal (glomerulus, proximal and collecting tubules)	Diuresis, natriuresis, − renin release	
Beta$_1$	Heart (myocardium)	Inotropicity	Adenylate cyclase coupled
	Renal (juxtaglomerular apparatus, glomerulus, distal collecting tubule)	Renin release, − diuresis, − natriuresis	Predominant over beta$_2$
	Adipocytes	Lipolysis	
Beta$_2$	Heart (myocardium)	Neurotransmission	Adenylate cyclase coupled
	Vasculature	Vasodilation	
	Renal (glomerulus, thick ascending limb, tubule cells)	Na$^+$,K$^+$-ATPase	
	Bronchi	Relaxation	
D-1	Brain	Modulates emesis, psychosis	
D-2	Brain (including pituitary)	Influences behavior, acetylcholine release, − prolactin release, − dopamine neuronal activity	
DA-1	Heart (blood vessels)	Vasodilation	
	Renal (proximal and distal tubules, juxtaglomerular cells)	Diuresis, natriuresis, renin release	
	Mesentery (blood vessels)	Vasodilation	
	? Sympathetic ganglia	Diuresis, natriuresis, − neurotransmission, − afterload	
DA-2	Adrenal (glomerulosa)	Natriuresis, − aldosterone release	
	Sympathetic ganglia	− Neurotransmission	Greatest effects in setting of excessive sympathetic release

*Paradoxical effects for a given receptor are possible, so the net receptor effect for the given system should be considered. The − denotes inhibition of a given action.

TABLE 113–6

ADRENERGIC RECEPTOR ACTIVITY OF COMMONLY USED CATECHOLAMINES*

Catecholamine	Alpha$_1$	Alpha$_2$	Beta$_1$	Beta$_2$	DA-a1	DA-a2
NE	+ + + +	+ + + +	+ + + +	0	0	0
E	+ + + +	+ +	+ + + +	+ +	0	0
DA	+ +	+ +	+ + +	+ +	+ + + +	+ + + +
DB	+	+	+ + + +	+ +	0	0
FD	0	−	0	0	+ + + +	0

*Number of pluses or minuses reflects relative potency of activation of specified receptor at standard agonist infusion rates. NE = norepinephrine; E = epinephrine; DA = dopamine; DB = dobutamine, FD = fenoldopam.

Adapted from H Lollgen, H Drexler, Use of inotropes in the critical care setting, Crit Care Med, 18, 1, S56–S60, © by Williams & Wilkins, 1990.

addition to DA-2 dopamine receptors. As do the alpha- and beta-adrenergic receptors, the dopaminergic receptors mediate their actions through the hydrolysis of phosphatidylinositol biphosphate and G protein–modulated adenylate cyclase activity. Again, the response of a particular organ to dopamine depends on the specific type of dopaminergic receptors present.[25, 26]

PATHOPHYSIOLOGY OF CATECHOLAMINES AND PHARMACOLOGIC INTERVENTION

Details regarding appropriate dosing of medications in Table 113–7 may be found in the text or by consulting the American Hospital Formulary Service Drug Information manual.

Thyroid Hormone–Catecholamine Interactions

The complex interactions between thyroid hormones and catecholamines are incompletely understood. The hypermetabolic clinical features of hyperthyroidism (increased heart rate, cardiac contractility, pulse pressure, and basal metabolic rate) and the hypometabolic features of hypothyroidism suggest increased or reduced adrenergic activity, respectively. Indeed, thyroid hormones may alter the complement of alpha- and beta-adrenergic receptor subtypes in the heart and may also affect the postreceptor cellular response to catecholamines. However, serum and urinary catecholamine levels are generally decreased in the hyperthyroid state and increased in hypothyroidism. Thus, instead of mere augmentation of the effects of catecholamines by thyroid hormone, it has been suggested that similarities in structure between catecholamines and thyroid hormones result in nonselective adrenergic receptor stimulation. Mimicry between these two classes of hormones is also evident because dopamine, like thyroid hormone, inhibits thyroid-stimulating hormone release from the pituitary gland.

Hyperthyroidism and Thyroid Storm

Hyperthyroidism produces hypertension through sympathetic mechanisms, and the inotropic, chronotropic, and vascular effects of catecholamines are potentiated in hyperthyroidism. Consequently, beta-adrenergic antagonists are the first-line treatment for thyroid storm:[27] beta-antagonists decrease cardiac output, heart rate, and pulse pressure in hyperthyroid patients.

In thyroid storm, both the hypermetabolic state in general and the risk of dysrhythmias and congestive heart failure are specific concerns and must be treated. The beta-adrenergic antagonist propranolol is perhaps the most useful of the short-acting agents.[28, 29] However, its mode of action is not completely understood. In addition to reducing the general hypermetabolic state, propranolol also decreases the peripheral conversion of thyroxine (T$_4$) to triiodothyronine (T$_3$), although the clinical significance of this effect is questioned. Propranolol is effective at interrupting superventricular tachycardia and ameliorating congestive heart failure in thyroid storm. In patients with asthma or chronic obstructive pulmonary disease, administration of cardioselective beta-antagonists such as atenolol should be considered.

A variety of other agents has also been advocated for use in thyroid storm. Dexamethasone, 2 mg every 6 hours for four doses, decreases the release of thyroid hormone and reduced peripheral conversion of T$_4$ to T$_3$ and has been found useful. Calcium channel blockers such as verapamil and diltiazem may antagonize some adrenergic effects and decrease ventricular ectopy. In pregnancy, beta-blockade

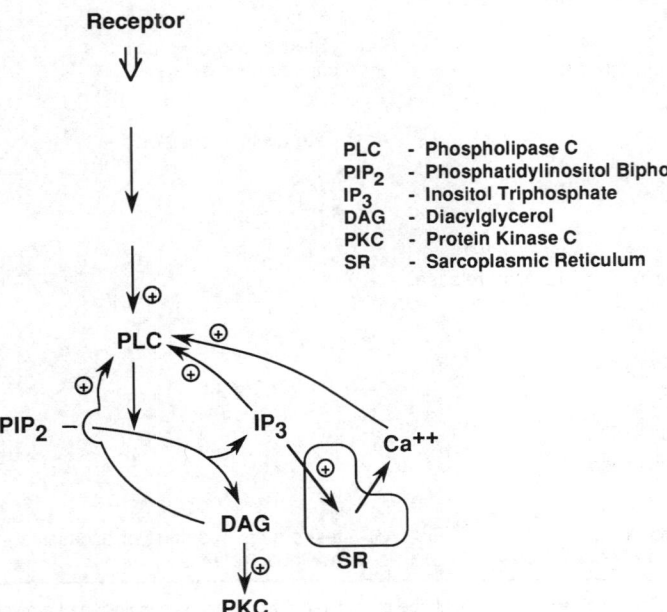

PLC - Phospholipase C
PIP$_2$ - Phosphatidylinositol Biphosphate
IP$_3$ - Inositol Triphosphate
DAG - Diacylglycerol
PKC - Protein Kinase C
SR - Sarcoplasmic Reticulum

Figure 113–3. Putative alpha$_1$-adrenergic postreceptor pathway. Whereas the beta-adrenergic receptors are coupled to either the stimulation or inhibition of adenylate cyclase through GTP-binding proteins, there is evidence that the alpha$_1$-adrenergic receptor is coupled to the hydrolysis of phosphatidylinositol bisphosphate (PIP$_2$), and the subsequent mobilization of intracellular calcium and diacylglycerol. These two intracellular messengers effect their actions by modulating the activity of protein kinases. (Adapted from Cargnelli G, Piovan D, Bova S, et al: Present and future trends in research and clinical applications of inodilators. J Cardiovasc Pharmacol 14[suppl 8]:S124–S132, 1989; and Nahorski SR: Receptors, inositol polyphosphates and intracellular Ca^{2+}. Br J Clin Pharmacol 30:23S, 1990. © by Blackwell Scientific Publications, Ltd.)

TABLE 113-7

AGENTS EMPLOYED IN CRITICAL CARE

Disorder	Agents
Burns	Propranolol
Cardiovascular disorders	
Cardiac arrest	Norepinephrine, epinephrine, dopamine, dobutamine, lidocaine, sodium bicarbonate
Congestive heart failure	Dobutamine, nitroglycerin, nitroprusside, fenoldopam, diuretics, hydralazine, captopril, prazosin, amrinone, digoxin, dopamine, levodopa (with pyridoxine)
Hypertension	
Intracranial hypertension	Urapidil, labetalol
Malignant hypertension	Nitroprusside, phenoxybenzamine, fenoldopam, labetalol, prazosin, propranolol, clonidine, furosemide, urapidil, captopril, phentolamine, nifedipine
Neuroleptic malignant syndrome (acute dopamine depletion syndrome)	Levodopa
Pheochromocytoma	Propranolol, metoprolol, phenoxybenzamine, then propranolol or metoprolol if necessary
Right ventricular insufficiency	Dobutamine, amrinone
Shock and hypotension	
Anaphylactic shock	Epinephrine, histamine H_1 antagonists, dopamine, dobutamine, steroids, volume expansion
Cardiogenic shock	Dopamine, dobutamine, norepinephrine, balloon counterpulsation
Idiopathic orthostatic hypotension	Yohimbine, metoclopramide, domperidone
Septic shock	Dopamine, dobutamine
Pulmonary disease	
Acute respiratory failure	Dobutamine, hydralazine (*warning:* may increase pulmonary edema), amrinone
Chronic obstructive pulmonary disease, pulmonary arterial hypertension	Dobutamine, amrinone
Mechanical ventilation	Dobutamine, dopamine
Pulmonary embolism	Fenoldopam, dobutamine, dopamine, norepinephrine, tissue plasminogen activator
Status asthmaticus	Epinephrine, terbutaline, atropine, ipratropium bromide, albuterol, isoetharine, metaproterenol, steroids
Renal disease	
Acute renal failure	Dopamine, fenoldopam
Thyroid disease	
Hypothyroid disorders	Hydrocortisone, thyroxine, hydralazine, passive warming, pressor support; *avoid* catecholamines unless absolutely necessary
Thyrotoxicosis	Propranolol, dexamethasone, atenolol, Lugol's solution, propylthiouracil, lithium
Caveats	Fenoldopam is a new agent and is not widely used clinically; when using fenoldopam, patients should be euvolemic
	When using dopamine, patients should be euvolemic

should be approached with caution. Calcium channel blockers may be safer agents for treatment of thyroid storm in pregnancy.

Lugol's iodine solution, in conjunction with beta-adrenergic blockade, may also be useful in the short-term treatment of impending thyroid storm.[29] Iodine not only blocks hormone release but also increases thyroid hormone stores by increasing hormone synthesis, so a thiourea should be administered simultaneously with the iodine. The iodine should be continued for several weeks to permit the full effect of the thiourea to develop, after which the iodine can be gradually withdrawn. Ipodate sodium is an iodinated radiocontrast agent that inhibits thyroid hormone secretion and peripheral conversion of T_4 to T_3. Dosages of 0.5 to 1 g/d have been found to be as effective as a thiourea for up to about 30 weeks of treatment. More prolonged use of this agent is not recommended.

Lithium blocks thyroid hormone release at doses of 900 to 1200 mg/d and serum concentrations of 0.6 to 0.8 mEq/L.[29] Unlike iodide, lithium does not promote hormone synthesis, and it may therefore be administered before starting a regimen of thiourea. The effects of lithium are additive to those of iodide. Because of the risk of cardiovascular, renal, and neurologic toxicity, close monitoring of the serum lithium concentration is required, particularly in patients with underlying renal or cardiac failure. The use of lithium, in view of these risks and the availability of several other effective agents, is rarely indicated.

In patients who are not candidates for thyroidectomy because of pregnancy, advanced age, infirmity, or coagulopathy or other contraindications, thioureas and ^{131}I may be considered for definitive treatment of hyperthyroidism. However, it must be remembered that medical ablation of the thyroid takes many weeks, an average of 6 months to achieve remission in most cases, even though some symptoms may be controlled within hours to days.[30]

Hypothyroidism and Myxedema Coma

Patients often come to the critical care unit with depressed sensorium and metabolism. The possibility of hypothyroidism is often raised, especially when there is conflicting evidence as to the cause of the altered mental status. Frequently, measurements of T_4 are low, and the practitioner must decide whether the patient warrants thyroid hormone supplementation or simply has the so-called euthyroid sick syndrome. Nonthyroidal illnesses, including liver failure, renal failure, sepsis, starvation, and a variety of other forms of stress, as well as certain medications, can all depress serum levels of thyroid hormone but do not require hormone supplementation.[31]

Myxedema coma can develop insidiously over several years as a result of undiagnosed and untreated hypothyroidism.[32] A marginal thyroid reserve coupled with severe stress (e.g., cold exposure, infection, surgery, gastrointestinal bleeding, and narcotics) can precipitate coma. A thyroidectomy scar should suggest the diagnosis in any patient with stupor or coma, especially with hypothermia. Facial and pretibial edema, glossomegaly, hypoventilation, bradycardia, low voltage on electrocardiogram, and hyponatremia are other helpful findings. A high index of suspicion clinically and supporting laboratory values (low serum T_4 levels and T_3 resin uptake, with low or high serum thyroid-stimulating hormone levels) allow the diagnosis to be made, but treatment should not await these results.

Because treatment of severe hypothyroidism may precipitate adrenal insufficiency, a serum cortisol level should be obtained and glucocorticoids administered before thyroid hormone. Hydrocortisone (100 mg intravenously every 8 hours), respiratory support, intravenous hydration, passive warming, and monitoring of serum chemistry values and respiratory function are important preludes to the administration of thyroid hormone. T_4 (300 to 500 μg intravenously, then 75 to 100 μg intravenously daily) should then be instituted. T_4 has the advantages over T_3 of being able to be administered intravenously, of having a longer half-life (it can be administered once a day), and of being able to maintain a steady level of T_3 in the serum far better than is the case with frequent administration of T_3. Free T_4 (and thyroid-stimulating hormone) levels should be closely monitored, with conversion to a maintenance dose after the free T_4 level is normal. Except as part of routine cardiopulmonary resuscitation (if this is necessary), administration of catecholamines should be avoided in patients with myxedema coma. Indeed, the overly aggressive use of thyroid supplements may itself precipitate serious dysrhythmias and congestive heart failure.

Hypothroidism may be accompanied by hypertension, which often reverses with correction of the hypothyroid state.[27] In the elderly, hypothyroidism is accompanied by severe diastolic hypertension in approximately one third of these patients. Hypertension may result from unopposed alpha-adrenergic activity associated with increased norepinephrine production. Moreover, tissue myxedema reduces vascular compliance and increases peripheral resistance. Systolic pressure is usually reduced in hypothyroidism so that mean arterial pressure may remain normal.[27]

Catecholamines and Circulatory Hemodynamics
Cardiac Arrest and Cardiogenic Shock

Norepinephrine (Levophed, an alpha-adrenergic agonist) is a commonly used pressor agent. Norepinephrine increases systemic vascular resistance, thereby raising blood pressure, but also flow in the renal and mesenteric circulations. Norepinephrine also possesses inotropic and chronotropic effects by virtue of its weak beta-agonist properties.[33] The combined effects of alpha- and beta-adrenergic stimulation increase myocardial oxygen demand, and this may precipitate or aggravate ventricular ischemia.

The primary indications for norepinephrine are cardiogenic shock refractory to dopamine or dobutamine and cardiogenic shock resulting from pulmonary embolism. Norepinephrine is administered by infusion at 2 to 4 μg/min, and the dosage is titrated to a satisfactory blood pressure. Systemic blood pressure increases, while heart rate is usually unchanged and cardiac output may actually decline. Norepinephrine may induce dysrhythmias, renal and mesenteric ischemia, and if it extravasates, local subcutaneous necrosis.[33]

Epinephrine is an endogenous catecholamine with potent alpha- and beta$_1$-adrenergic agonist effects and more moderate beta$_2$-adrenergic activity.[33] At lower doses (0.04 to 0.1 μg/kg/min), epinephrine has primarily beta-agonist activity and increases heart rate, stroke volume, and cardiac output and decreases peripheral vascular resistance. At higher doses, owing to concomitant stimulation of alpha-adrenergic receptors, peripheral resistance increases. Epinephrine can also increase venous return. Epinephrine is commonly employed in cardiac resuscitation and is generally administered as a 1-mL, 1:1000 ampule, either intravenously or by the endotracheal route.

Evidence suggests that, in the setting of cardiac arrest, norepinephrine may be more beneficial than epinephrine. Alpha-adrenergic agonists improve coronary blood flow by increasing diastolic pressure, whereas beta$_2$-adrenergic agonists possess vasodilatory effects, which may compromise resuscitation attempts by decreasing coronary perfusion pressure.[34] A direct comparison of the two agents in an animal model showed a tendency for norepinephrine to increase coronary blood flow, oxygen delivery, and the myocardial oxygen extraction ratio compared with results achieved with epinephrine.[35] However, the clinical efficacy of norepinephrine versus epinephrine in resuscitation after cardiac arrest remains unclear. After restoration of perfusion after cardiac arrest, dopamine is usually substituted for norepinephrine or epinephrine because of its ability to increase both myocardial contractility and systemic blood pressure. Dopamine activates vasodilatory, DA-1 dopamine receptors, which are found on blood vessels of the coronary, mesenteric, renal, and cerebral circulations. Dopamine also activates presynaptic DA-2 dopamine receptors, which inhibit the release of norepinephrine from sympathetic nerve terminals. Accordingly, at low doses (<2 μg/kg/min), dopamine actually increases blood flow in some vascular beds. At higher doses (2 to 5 μg/kg/min), dopamine activates beta-adrenergic receptors and increases heart rate, stroke volume, and cardiac output, with little effect on peripheral vascular resistance. At even higher doses, by activating alpha-adrenergic receptors, dopamine increases vascular resistance and blood pressure and may decrease tissue perfusion. Myocardial oxygenation may deteriorate if the increase in demand resulting from high-dose dopamine infusion is not matched by an increase in oxygen supply.[33]

Dobutamine is a synthetic catecholamine with significant beta$_1$-adrenergic agonist activity. Dobutamine increases stroke volume and heart rate at lower doses than does dopamine. Because dobutamine has less chronotropic activity than does dopamine (or isoproterenol), it is preferred in the treatment of congestive heart failure after myocardial infarction. However, at higher doses, sinus tachycardia and other dysrhythmias may develop. Because dobutamine is only a weak alpha-adrenergic agonist, it is not recommended as monotherapy of shock. Tissue necrosis after extravasation of the drug is uncommon.[33] The combined use of dopamine and dobutamine has proved effective in the treatment of shock.[36, 37] A relatively new selective DA-1 dopamine receptor agonist, fenoldopam, increases cardiac index, possibly through reduction of systemic vascular resistance.[37–39]

The phosphodiesterase inhibitor is a new class of drugs that increase cyclic AMP levels. Intracellular calcium levels accordingly increase, and this augments myocardial contractility. Although phosphodiesterase inhibitors are not yet recommended as first-line treatment of cardiogenic shock, they do have a role in short-term treatment if more conventional agents have proved ineffective.[33, 40] Unfortunately, at high doses, phosphodiesterase inhibitors may cause hypotension and reduce coronary perfusion pressure, thereby compromising myocardial function. Moreover, titration may be difficult because of the extended plasma half-life of these agents.[33]

Amrinone was the first phosphodiesterase inhibitor used in refractory heart failure. It is a bipyridine derivative with marked vasodilatory and more modest inotropic abilities.[33] It also increases cardiac output and reduces pulmonary capillary wedge pressure and systemic vascular resistance and blood pressure. Although amrinone may be useful for the short-term treatment of heart failure refractory to conventional treatment with digoxin, diuretics, vasodilators, dopamine, or dobutamine, its sometimes pronounced hypotensive effects and long plasma half-life have limited its use to extreme cases. Milrinone, a second-generation congener of amrinone, has many of these same limitations.

Hypovolemic and Septic Shock

Catecholamines are commonly used in the treatment of shock. Shock may occur in two forms: either a low-output state caused by myocardial insufficiency or hypovolemia or a high-output state associated with sepsis and decreased peripheral vascular resistance.[41] Hypovolemic shock may result from hemorrhage, sodium depletion, or massive pulmonary embolism. In many respects, hypovolemic shock resembles cardiogenic shock, with the notable exception that the treatment of the relative hypovolemic state in primary pump failure must avoid anything that would exacerbate the already marginal status of the pump. Hemodynamic support of the patient with cardiogenic shock was discussed earlier.

In either hypovolemic or septic shock, volume expansion (with appropriate intensive hemodynamic monitoring) is always the first priority.[42] Inotropic support is indicated in patients who remain hypotensive despite volume restoration. Dopamine is preferred in septic shock because of its systemic peripheral vasoconstrictive and splanchnic vasodilatory effects.[33, 42] Dopamine may, however, worsen myocardial oxygen balance and cause ischemia and dysrhythmias. Norepinephrine in combination with low-dose dopamine may be also beneficial.[43] Levophed (norepinephrine) or metaraminol (a synthetic alpha-agonist) alone is generally considered in cases of severe, refractory hypotension to maintain perfusion of the brain, the pulmonary system, and the myocardium,[42, 44] but the kidneys and other splanchnic organs may be placed at significant risk of ischemia.

Pheochromocytoma

Pheochromocytomas arise primarily in the adrenal medulla (90%) but may occur in extra-adrenal sites. Peak incidence is in the fourth and fifth decades of life, with 50 to 60% of the tumors occurring in women and 10% of the tumors being bilateral or multiple in origin.[45] Ten percent of pheochromocytomas are malignant. Although only 0.1% of diastolic hypertension results from pheochromocytomas, 50% of pheochromocytomas are not diagnosed in life and untreated hypertension may lead to significant morbidity and mortality.[46]

Pheochromocytomas also occur in patients with multiple endocrine neoplasia syndromes. In addition to pheochromocytoma, multiple endocrine neoplasia type 2A includes medullary carcinoma of the thyroid, parathyroid adenoma or hyperplasia, and (rarely) bilateral adrenocortical hyperplasia; multiple endocrine neoplasia type 2B includes medullary thyroid carcinoma, mucosal neuromas, thickened corneal nerves, alimentary ganglioneuromatosis, and (occasionally) marfanoid habitus. Presenting symptoms include headache, diaphoresis, palpitations, nausea, vomiting, anxiety, constipation, chest and abdominal pain, facial pallor, paresthesias, arm pain, Raynaud's phenomenon, episodic blindness or blurred vision, weight loss, and fatigue. Postural changes, anxiety, pressure in the vicinity of the tumor, smoking, micturition, hyperventilation, or ingestion of al-

cohol or a variety of drugs may precipitate attacks of refractory hypertension or hypotension, as can general anesthesia, endotracheal intubation, operative procedures, angioplasty, and parturition. The long-term exposure to high levels of circulating catecholamines does not always produce characteristic hemodynamic responses in patients with pheochromocytomas; indeed, some patients may be asymptomatic, possibly because of desensitization of the cardiovascular system to catecholamines.[47]

Hypertension may be intermittent or persistent. Orthostatic hypotension in an untreated hypertensive patient should suggest the diagnosis, and a fine tremor, hyperthermia, and glucose intolerance may be also be found. Retinal angiomas, thyroid tumors, mucosal neuromas, neurofibromas, or café au lait spots also occur. Abdominal palpation may precipitate severe hypertension. A palpable abdominal mass is present in 10 to 20% of patients with pheochromocytoma. Transient electrocardiographic changes suggestive of myocardial ischemia and resistant tachydysrhythmias may be present.

A 24-hour urinary metanephrine measurement is the most reliable screening test.[45] A spot urinary metanephrine sample obtained during an acute episode correlates well with the results from 24-hour urine collection. Urinary vanillylmandelic acid determinations have a higher incidence of false-positive and false-negative results.[12, 45] Urinary homovanillylmandelic acid excretion is more likely to be increased in malignant pheochromocytomas (or neuroblastomas) than in nonmalignant pheochromocytomas. Measurement of plasma catecholamines is useful in diagnosing an episodically secreting tumor, but spurious results may be caused by anxiety, smoking, volume depletion, anoxia, exercise, obesity, renal failure, acidosis, increased intracranial pressure, and the use of drugs such as methyldopa and L-dopa.[45]

The clonidine suppression test is used to differentiate pheochromocytoma from essential hypertension.[45, 46] Patients with essential hypertension (and elevated catecholamine levels) suppress plasma norepinephrine levels into the normal range within 3 hours after the oral administration of 0.3 mg of the alpha$_2$-adrenergic agonist clonidine; in contrast, patients with pheochromocytoma show no such suppression. Another suppression test utilizes the preganglionic blocker pentolinium; after administration of 2.5 mg intravenously patients with pheochromocytoma maintain high plasma catecholamine levels.

Computed tomography with contrast agent is the procedure of choice for the localization of pheochromocytomas, and magnetic resonance imaging, which uses nonionizing radiation, is useful in pregnancy.[45, 46, 48–50] Radioisotope scanning with ^{131}I-labeled iodobenzylguanidine can also be utilized. Arteriography and venography have been largely supplanted by these techniques. However, vascular contrast imaging has been used to identify tumors in patients with negative or equivocal noninvasive imaging results, recurrent disease, or persistent symptoms after operation.[49]

Patients with pheochromocytomas should have complete bed rest at 45° head elevation. Phentolamine, an alpha-adrenergic blocker, is administered at 2 to 5 mg intravenously every 5 minutes until blood pressure is stabilized.[45, 48] Sodium nitroprusside may also be useful. Propranolol, 1 to 2 mg intravenously every 5 to 10 minutes, can be used to control dysrhythmias. Intravenous esmolol, a short-acting beta-blocker, is a useful alternative to propranolol. Beta-blockade should be initiated only after adequate alpha-adrenergic blockade is achieved because severe hypertension may result from unopposed alpha-adrenergic receptor stimulation. For long-term therapy, the oral alpha-adrenergic blocker phenoxybenzamine, 10 mg orally twice per day, is gradually titrated to a maintenance dose of 40 to 200 mg/d as needed for blood pressure control. Oral propranolol is used for dysrhythmias, and prazosin can be substituted for the nitroprusside, if necessary.[45, 48]

Preoperative preparation of the patient with pheochromocytoma includes alpha-adrenergic blockade, control of dysrhythmias, and volume repletion. Management may be particularly difficult and prolonged therapy may be necessary in patients with catecholamine cardiomyopathy or recent myocardial infarction and in patients in the third trimester of pregnancy. Alpha-adrenergic blockade is continued until surgery.

Intraoperative hemodynamic and electrocardiographic monitoring is always necessary, and proper volume status must be maintained assiduously. Sodium nitroprusside or phentolamine is used for any acute hypertensive episodes during surgery, and lidocaine can help manage ventricular extrasystole and tachycardia. Beta-blockers are used to treat dysrhythmias. Hypoxia is to be avoided at all costs because it sensitizes the myocardium to catecholamine-induced dysrhythmias. In addition, regional anesthesia may sensitize peripheral alpha-adrenergic receptors to circulating catecholamines.[46] Phenylephrine and norepinephrine are pure adrenergic agonists and cause less myocardial irritability than metaraminol (Aramine); consequently, they should be employed for the treatment of any intraoperative hypotensive episodes.

α-Methyl-*p*-tyrosine (metyrosine), a false substrate for tyrosine hydroxylase,[46] is effective in pheochromocytoma, but its extrapyramidal effects limit its use to metastatic disease or otherwise inoperable cases.[48] Fenoldopam, a selective DA-1 dopamine receptor agonist, has been effective and safe as parenteral monotherapy in patients with severe essential hypertension.[24, 36–39, 51–59] Fenoldopam mesylate is a benzazepine derivative with potent renal and systemic vasodilator properties. Fenoldopam lacks significant alpha- or beta-adrenergic agonist activity and so does not directly increase heart rate or blood pressure.[51] Fenoldopam does increase urinary free water clearance and fractional excretion of sodium even in patients with renal insufficiency.[53, 58] Direct activation of the DA-1 dopamine receptor by fenoldopam results in vasodilation as well.[37, 39, 51, 55] Although not proved effective in patients with pheochromocytoma, fenoldopam has been shown to be as effective as nitroprusside in patients with severe hypertension without nitroprusside's adverse renal effects or potential toxicity.[57, 58]

Orthostatic Hypotension

Idiopathic orthostatic hypotension (the Shy-Drager syndrome) is an uncommon, frustrating disorder with debilitating effects that is frequently resistant to therapy. The inability to maintain systemic blood pressure when the patient in the upright posture has multiple causes, all culminating in a common end: intolerable lightheadedness, syncope, and other manifestations of cerebral ischemia. Minimal changes in heart rate, absence of sympathetic symptoms, narrowing of pulse pressure, and static plasma norepinephrine levels despite severe orthostatic hypotension are all classic concomitants of this syndrome. These characteristics distinguish idiopathic orthostatic hypotension (and similar conditions such as the orthostatic hypotension that follows sympathectomy or tricyclic antidepressant administration) from secondary disorders of orthostasis, such as pheochromocytoma, adrenocortical insufficiency, hypovolemia, and anemia.

Continuing efforts toward characterizing the nature of idiopathic orthostatic hypotension have revealed that most occurrences of insufficient sympathetic response after orthostasis are associated with excessive venous pooling in the lower extremities, which often occurs in the presence of, and is aggravated by, hypovolemia.[59, 60] Plasma norepinephrine levels are often above normal, indicating abnormalities in the responsiveness of the vascular system.

Compression stockings and volume expansion together with synthetic mineralocorticoids have been used to treat idiopathic orthostatic hypotension, but with inconsistent results. Yohimbine, an oral alpha$_2$-adrenergic antagonist, which increases the release of norepinephrine from presynaptic neurons, has yielded gratifying results in some patients.[61] Metoclopramide, a dopamine receptor antagonist, has also been utilized, as has domperidone, although experience and improvement have been greater with the latter.[36, 38, 62–64]

References

1. Innes IR, Nickerson M: Norepinephrine, epinephrine, and the sympathomimetic amines. In: Goodman L, Gilman A (eds): The Pharmacological Basis of Therapeutics. 5th ed. New York, Macmillan, p 477, 1975.
1a. Francis G, Cohen J: Catecholamines in cardiovascular disease. In: Current Concepts. Kalamazoo, MI, Upjohn, 1988.
2. Nagatsu T: The human tyrosine hydroxylase gene. Cell Mol Neurobiol 9:313, 1989.
3. Tanaka T, Horio Y, Taketoshi M, et al: Molecular cloning and sequencing of a cDNA of rat dopa decarboxylase: Partial amino acid homologies with other enzyme synthesizing catecholamines. Proc Natl Acad Sci USA 86:8142, 1989.
4. Charney DS, Heninger GR, Sternberg DE: Assessment of alpha-2 adrenergic autoreceptor function in humans: Effects of oral yohimbine. Life Sci 30:2033, 1982.
5. Feldman JM: Diagnosis and management of pheochromocytoma. Hosp Pract 24:175, 1989.
6. Ratge D, Kohse KP, Steegmuller U, et al: Distribution of free and conjugated catecholamines between plasma, platelets and erythrocytes: Different effects of intravenous and oral catecholamine administrations. J Pharmacol Exp Ther 257:232, 1991.
7. Kagedal B, Goldstein DS: Catecholamines and their metabolites. J Chromatogr 429:177, 1988.
8. Fote A, Kimura S, DeQuattro V, et al: Liquid-chromatographic measurement of catecholamines and metabolites in plasma and urine. Clin Chem 33:2209, 1987.
9. Krstulov AM: Quantitative analysis of catecholamines and related compounds. In: Chalmers RA, Masson M (eds): Analytical Chemistry. New York, John Wiley & Sons, 1986.
10. Pagilari R, Cottet-Emard JM, Peyrin L: Determination of free and conjugated normetanephrine and metanephrine in human plasma by high-performance liquid chromatography with electrochemical detection. J Chromatogr 563:23, 1991.
11. Opacka-Juffry J, Tacconelli F, Coen CW: Sensitive method for determination of picogram amounts of epinephrine and other catecholamines in microdissected samples of rat brain using liquid chromatography with electrochemical detection. J Chromatogr 433:41, 1988.
12. Brown R, Hollifield J: Endocrine hypertension. In: Kohler P (ed): Clinical Endocrinology. New York, John Wiley & Sons, 1986.
13. Moyer TP, Jiang NS, Tyce GM, et al: Analysis for urinary catecholamines by liquid chromatography with amperometric detection: Methodology and clinical interpretation of results. Clin Chem 25:256, 1979.
14. Lockette WL, McCurdy R, Aronow H, et al: Effect of 8-Br-cyclic guanosine monophosphate on intracellular calcium and pH in vascular smooth muscle. Hypertension 13:865, 1989.
15. MacLennan DH, Duff C, Zorzato F, et al: Ryanodine receptor gene is a candidate for predisposition to malignant hypothermia. Nature 343:559, 1990.
16. Farrow S, Mers A, Banta G, et al: Effect of the alpha-2 adrenergic antagonist yohimbine on orthostatic tolerance. Hypertension 15:877, 1990.
17. Johnson GL, Dhanasekaran N: The G-protein family and their interaction with receptors. Endocr Rev 10:317, 1989.
18. Hausdorff WP, Caron MG, Lefkowitz R: Turning off the signal: Desensitization of beta-adrenergic receptor function. FASEB J 4:2881, 1990.
19. Lohse MJ, Benovic JL, Codina J, et al: Beta-arrestin: A protein that regulates beta-adrenergic receptor function. Science 249:1547, 1990.
20. Enjalbert A: Multiple transduction mechanisms of dopamine, somatostatin and angiotensin II receptors in anterior pituitary cells. Horm Res 31:6, 1989.
21. Beaulieu, M: Clinical importance of D-1 and D-2 receptors. Can J Neurol Sci 14:402, 1987.
22. Kohli JD: Peripheral dopamine receptors. Am J Hypertens 3:25S, 1990.
23. Lokhandwala MF, Hedge SS: Cardiovascular pharmacology of adrenergic and dopaminergic receptors: Therapeutic significance in congestive heart failure. Am J Med 90(5B)2S, 1991.

24. The peripheral dopaminergic system: Basic and clinical advances. Am J Hypertens 3:1S, 1990.

25. Vallar L, Muca C, Magni M, et al: Differential coupling of dopaminergic D_2 receptors expressed in different cell types. J Biol Chem 265:10320, 1990.

26. Grandy DK, Marchionni MA, Makam H, et al: Cloning of the cDNA and gene for a human D2 dopamine receptor. Proc Natl Acad Sci USA 86:9762, 1989.

27. Sowers JR, Tuck ML: Hypertension associated with diabetes mellitus, hypercalcaemic disorders, acromegaly and thyroid disease. Clin Endocrinol Metab 10:631, 1981.

28. Levey GS, Klein I: Catecholamine–thyroid hormone interactions and the cardiovascular manifestations of hyperthyroidism. Am J Med 88:642, 1990.

29. Orgiazzi J: Management of Graves' hyperthyroidism. Endocrinol Metab Clin North Am 16:365, 1987.

30. Harada T, Shimaoka K, Mimura T, et al: Current treatment of Graves' disease. Surg Clin North Am 67:299, 1987.

31. Fallon JJ, Yelovich RM, Green PJ: Euthyroid sick syndrome: Association with urosepsis in an elderly man. Postgrad Med 75:117, 1964.

32. Bagdade JD: Endocrine emergencies. Med Clin North Am 70:1111, 1986.

33. Lollgen H, Drexler H: Use of inotropes in the critical care setting. Crit Care Med 18:S56, 1990.

34. Robinson LA, Brown CG, Jenkins J, et al: The effect of norepinephrine versus epinephrine on myocardial hemodynamics during CPR. Ann Emerg Med 18:336, 1989.

35. Linder KH, Ahnefeld FW: Comparison of epinephrine and norepinephrine in the treatment of asphyxial or fibrillatory cardiac arrest in a porcine model. Crit Care Med 17:437, 1989.

36. Murphy MB, Elliott WJ: Dopamine and dopamine receptor agonists in cardiovascular therapy. Crit Care Med 18:S14, 1990.

37. Rajfer SI, Davis FR: Role of dopamine receptors and the utility of dopamine agonists in heart failure. Circulation 82(suppl I):97, 1990.

38. Horn PT, Murphy MB: Therapeutic applications of drugs acting on peripheral dopamine receptors. J Clin Pharmacol 30:674, 1990.

39. Goldberg LI: Pharmacological bases for the use of dopamine and related drugs in the treatment of congestive heart failure. J Cardiovasc Pharmacol 14:S21, 1989.

40. Vincent J-L, Madhoun P, Primo G, et al: Potentiation of the effects of enoximone by a dobutamine infusion. Intensive Care Med 15:530, 1989.

41. Schremmer B, Dhainaut J-F: Heart failure in septic shock: Effects of inotropic support. Crit Care Med 28:S49, 1990.

42. Karakusis PH: Considerations in the therapy of septic shock. Med Clin North Am 70:933, 1986.

43. Desjars P, Pinaud M, Bugnon D, et al: Norepinephrine therapy has no deleterious renal effects in human septic shock. Crit Care Med 17:426, 1989.

44. Goodman L, Gilman A: Norepinephrine, epinephrine, and the sympathomimetic amines. In Goodman L, Gilman A (eds): The Pharmacological Basis of Therapeutics. 6th ed. New York, Macmillan, p 142, 1980.

45. Shapiro B, Fig L: Management of pheochromocytoma. Endocrinol Metab Clin North Am 18:443, 1989.

46. Bravo E, Tarazi R, Fouad F, et al: Clonidine-suppression test: A useful aid in the diagnosis of pheochromocytoma. N Engl J Med 305:623, 1981.

47. Bravo E, Fouad-Tarazi F, Rossi G, et al: A reevaluation of the hemodynamics of pheochromocytoma. Hypertension 15(suppl):128, 1990.

48. Malone MJ, Libertino JA, Tsapatsaris NP, et al: Preoperative and surgical management of pheochromocytoma. Urol Clin North Am 16:567, 1989.

49. Dedrick C: Adrenal arteriography and venography. Urol Clin North Am 16:515, 1989.

50. Greene J, Guay A: New perspectives in pheochromocytoma. Urol Clin North Am 16:487, 1989.

51. Nichols AJ, Ruffolo RR, Brooks DP: The pharmacology of fenoldopam. Am J Hypertens 3:116S, 1990.

52. Carey RM, Siragy HM, Ragsdale NV, et al: Dopamine-1 and Dopamine-2 mechanisms in the control of renal function. Am J Hypertens 3:59S, 1990.

53. Aronson S, Goldberg LI, Roth S, et al: Laboratory investigation: Preservation of renal blood flow during hypotension induced with fenoldopam in dogs. Can J Anaesth 37:380, 1990.

54. Hughes JM, Beck TR, Rose CE, et al: The effect of selective dopamine-1 receptor stimulation on renal and adrenal function in man. J Clin Endocrinol Metab 66:518, 1988.

55. Goldberg LI, Murphy MB: Potential use of DA1 and DA2 receptor agonists in the treatment of hypertension. Clin Exp Hypertens [A] 9:1023, 1987.

56. Hieble JP, Eden RJ, de Mey C: The role of DA-1 and DA-2 receptors in the control of blood pressure. Br J Clin Pharmacol 30:61S, 1990.

57. White WB, Radford MJ, Gonzalez FM, et al: Selective dopamine-1 agonist therapy in severe hypertension: Effects of intravenous fenoldopam. J Am Coll Cardiol 11:1118, 1988.

58. Elliott WJ, Weber RR, Nelson KS, et al: Renal and hemodynamic effects of intravenous fenoldopam versus nitroprusside in severe hypertension. Circulation 81:970, 1990.

59. Holcslaw TL, Beck TR: Clinical experience with intravenous fenoldopam. Am J Hypertens 3:120S, 1990.

60. Streeten DH, Anderson GH, Richardson R, et al: Abnormal orthostatic changes in blood pressure and heart rate in subjects with intact sympathetic nervous function: Evidence for excessive venous pooling. J Lab Clin Med 111:326, 1988.

61. Middeke M, Ittner J, Mezger M, et al: Beta-adrenergic blood pressure regulation in Shy-Drager syndrome and pheochromocytoma. Klin Wochenschr 67:1004, 1989.

62. Lacomblez L, Bensimon G, Isnard F, et al: Effect of yohimbine on blood pressure in patients with depression and orthostatic hypotension induced by clomipramine. Clin Pharmacol Ther 45:241, 1989.

63. Kuchel O, Nguyen TB, Gutkowska J, et al: Treatment of severe orthostatic hypotension by metoclopramide. Ann Intern Med 93:841, 1980.

64. Brown M, Allison D, Jenner D, et al: Increased sensitivity and accuracy of phaeochromocytoma diagnosis achieved by use of plasma-adrenaline estimations and a pentolinium suppression test. Lancet 1:174, 1981.

CHAPTER 114

Hypertensive Urgencies and Emergencies

Linea L. Rydstedt
Warren E. Lockette
James R. Sowers

CLASSIFICATION AND OVERVIEW

Hypertensive crisis can be divided into two categories: hypertensive emergencies (Table 114–1) and hypertensive urgencies. There is no definitive systolic or diastolic blood pressure level that by itself can strictly distinguish a hypertensive emergency from an urgency. Distinction depends instead on the clinical presentation of acute organ damage.

Hypertensive urgency is observed in patients with diastolic pressures greater than 120 mm Hg but without evidence of acute end-organ damage. These patients require a gradual reduction in blood pressure during 24 to 48 hours. This reduction can be accomplished with either parenteral or oral antihypertensive medication.

Hypertensive emergencies can be observed in patients with a diastolic blood pressure greater than 120 to 130 mm Hg with evidence of acute end-organ damage. This end-organ damage commonly involves rapid, progressive deterioration of the central nervous system or myocardial,

TABLE 114–1

HYPERTENSIVE EMERGENCIES

Hypertension (diastolic pressure >120 mm Hg) associated with any of the following:
Encephalopathy
Intracranial hemorrhage or subarachnoid bleed or cerebrovascular accident
Dissecting aortic aneurysm
Acute myocardial infarction
Pulmonary edema
Eclampsia
Adrenergic crisis

hematologic, or renal dysfunction. Delay in appropriate therapy may result in rapid decrement of organ function and permanent damage. Severe pathologic elevations in blood pressure can lead to hypertensive encephalopathy, subarachnoid or intracranial hemorrhage, dissecting aneurysm, acute myocardial infarction, acute pulmonary edema, and eclampsia. Patients with these symptoms require immediate reduction in blood pressure, usually within the hour. This reduction is accomplished by admission to an intensive care unit, administration of parenteral antihypertensive medication, and continuous monitoring of blood pressure.

The clinical features of malignant hypertension, a hypertensive emergency, are significant retinopathy, encephalopathy, encephalopathy, microangiopathic hemolytic anemia, left ventricular failure, renal insufficiency, proteinuria, and hematuria. In the 1940s, less than 1% of hypertensive patients had malignant hypertension. Since then, this percentage has decreased even further. This decrease may be due to two factors. Blood pressure in chronic severe hypertension is more easily controlled with current medications, and also, uncontrolled hypertension is less common. Noncompliance with therapeutic regimens has decreased owing to advances in minimizing the side effects of the available antihypertensive agents, thereby improving overall blood pressure control. At one time, the 5-year mortality rate in patients with malignant hypertension was 99%. More recently, the 5-year mortality rate is 25%.[1] The most common cause of death in those with malignant hypertension is end-stage renal failure.[2]

EPIDEMIOLOGY

Several studies have analyzed the characteristics of patients with malignant hypertension. In a study in New York City, 93% of patients had been previously diagnosed as having hypertension, and 83% of the patients were aware of that prior diagnosis.[3] Another study evaluated the predisposing factors for malignant hypertension by comparing histories of patients with malignant hypertension with those with well-controlled hypertension. Blood pressure of the patients with malignant hypertension was significantly higher at the time of this study, and the number of patients who had discontinued hypertensive drug treatment was greater in the malignant hypertensive group than in the benign hypertensive group.

The presence and extent of organ damage often depend on the degree of blood pressure elevation and the rate of rise of blood pressure. Patients with chronic hypertension are better able to tolerate acute blood pressure elevations than those individuals who were previously normotensive. This is illustrated by patients who develop hypertensive encephalopathy with diastolic pressures of 100 mm Hg or less, such as patients with acute glomerulonephritis or eclampsia.[4]

The brain and kidney are relatively unique because these vascular beds maintain a constant blood flow over the physiologic range of blood pressure. However, the autoregulation curve is shifted with long-standing high blood pressure, and higher arterial pressures are then needed to maintain a constant cerebral or renal blood flow. In the intensive care unit setting, this principle must be remembered. Reduction of blood pressure to normal values may result in a significant reduction in kidney or brain blood flow (Fig. 114–1). The effective treatment of hypertension is a major factor in the declining incidence of stroke in North America. However, for some patients, antihypertensive therapy may actually cause cerebral infarction. These patients often are elderly, and patients with suspected sclerotic stenosis of the cerebral arteries are at increased risk for cerebral ischemic compli-

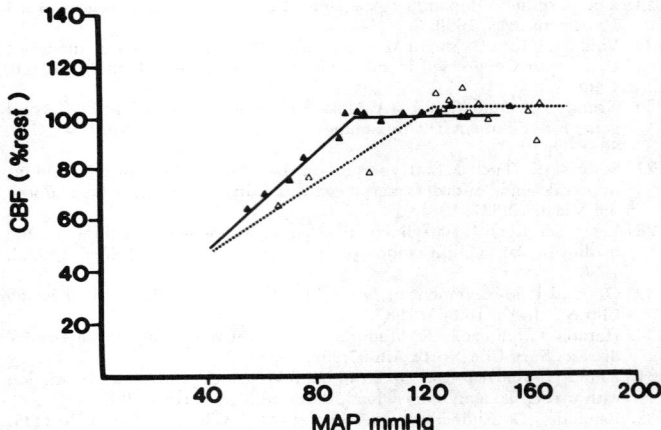

Figure 114–1. Cerebral blood flow (CBF) autoregulation in a normotensive volunteer with resting mean arterial pressure (MAP) of 95 mm Hg *(solid line and filled triangles)* and in a patient with chronic arterial hypertension and resting MAP of 150 mm Hg *(broken line and open triangles).* (From Paulson O, Waldeman G, Schmidt J: Cerebral circulation under normal and pathologic conditions. Am J Cardiol 63:3C, 1989.)

cation if blood pressure is lowered too severely or too rapidly. Blood pressure reduction of 20 to 30% in systolic pressure should be achieved in those who have an initial measurement exceeding 200 mm Hg and to a target of 160/100 in those with lower pressure.

Hypertension in patients with subarachnoid hemorrhage can be protective. Thus, only the most alarming blood pressure in the acute phase should be lowered, and even then, the blood pressure is lowered with caution.

Left ventricular hypertrophy and development of heart failure are a frequent problem in severe hypertension.[5] During a myocardial infarction, one specifically needs to decrease myocardial oxygen demands. This is accomplished by decreasing heart rate, preload, afterload, and wall tension with nitroglycerin, nitroprusside, beta-blockers, angiotensin-converting enzyme (ACE) inhibitors, or calcium channel blockers. One should avoid drugs such as hydralazine, diazoxide, and minoxidil, which can cause more severe reflex tachycardia.

ASSOCIATED CONDITIONS (Table 114–2)

Aortic Dissection

The clinical frequency of systemic hypertension is greater than 90% in patients with aortic dissection.[6] Cystic medial necrosis is a predisposing factor.[7] The drugs of choice for treatment of increased blood pressure in patients with aortic aneurysms are trimethaphan or nitroprusside in combination with a beta-blocker to keep heart rate less than 60 beats/min to decrease shear stress. The reflex tachycardia induced by hydralazine, minoxidil, and diazoxide precludes their use in patients with dissecting aneurysms.

Renal Disease

Patients with Berger's disease, also known as idiopathic immunoglobulin A nephropathy, can have malignant hypertension before the diagnosis of renal disease is made.[8] In addition, they have an increased incidence of accelerated hypertension. On initial evaluation, 36% of the patients with Berger's disease had hypertension. Of these, 15% had malignant or accelerated hypertension.[9]

TABLE 114-2

PRECIPITATING CONDITIONS IN HYPERTENSIVE CRISES

Sudden rise of blood pressure in patient with chronic essential hypertension (most common)[50-52]

Renovascular hypertension[51, 53-55]

Eclampsia[56-58]

Glomerulonephritis, acute[51]

Pheochromocytoma[56, 59-61]

Antihypertensive withdrawal syndromes[56, 62]

Head injuries and central nervous system traumas[56, 63, 64]

Renin-secreting tumors[56, 65]

Ingestion of catecholamine precursors in patients taking monoamine oxidase inhibitors[56, 66-68]

Parenchymal renal disease[53, 69]

Drug induced: Oral contraceptives,[70] tricyclic antidepressants,[71] atropine,[72] fentanyl-diazepam-oxygen,[73] propranolol and nonselective beta-blockers in hypoglycemic patients,[74] monoamine oxidase inhibitors,[56, 66, 67] sympathomimetics (diet pills and amphetamine-like drugs),[56] ergot alkaloids,[56] corticosteroids,[56] nonsteroidal, anti-inflammatory drugs[56]

Burns[56, 75, 76]

Vasculitis[77, 78]

Progressive systemic sclerosis[79] and systemic lupus erythematosus

From Houston MC: Pathophysiology, clinical aspects, and treatment of hypertensive crises. Prog Cardiovasc Dis 32:99, 1989.

Patients with malignant hypertension and renal insufficiency showed that, after control of blood pressure, the renal function nearly stabilized in 10%, progressively deteriorated in 30%, and transiently deteriorated but then improved in 60%. These patients with malignant hypertension and renal insufficiency with good prognosis show improvement with therapy.[10]

Trauma

Treatment of hypertension in patients with head trauma was reviewed by Simard.[11] The incidence of systolic hypertension (>160 mm Hg) is 25% in patients with severe head injuries. These patients have elevated blood pressure, tachycardia, and increases in cardiac output, which are consistent with a hyperadrenergic state. Adequate cerebral blood flow and thus sufficient cerebral perfusion pressure are essential to prevent ischemia. Vasodilating drugs may be dangerous in treatment of hypertension after head injury. These drugs cause cerebral vasodilation and compromise myogenic autoregulation, which can increase cerebral blood volume and capillary pressure. Drugs with these effects include hydralazine, nitroprusside, and nitroglycerin. Because of these concerns, beta-adrenergic blocking agents are often recommended for treatment of hypertension after head injury.

Adrenergic Disorders

Autonomic hyperreflexia occurs in transverse transection of the spinal cord injury. Common in quadriplegic patients, autonomic dysreflexia is characterized by paroxysmal hypertension, headache, vasoconstriction below the cord lesion, flushing of skin above the level of transection, and bradycardia. Trimethaphan (Arfonad) is used to prevent hypertensive crisis intraoperatively in these patients.[12]

Pheochromocytoma is an example of a hyperadrenergic state with excessive catecholamine release. A factor that can induce a crisis is injection of contrast medium during angiography in patients who have pheochromocytoma. In patients undergoing computed tomographic scan with contrast material, plasma catecholamine levels are elevated enough to cause a pressor effect; patients should have an alpha-adrenergic blockade before computed tomographic scan.[13] In addition, there is a hypertensive response associated with tumor manipulation in pheochromocytoma.[14] This becomes important during physical examination of the patient and during surgical removal of the tumor.

Pheochromocytoma is treated preoperatively with phenoxybenzamine[15] (Dibenzyline) and propranolol (Inderal) and intraoperatively with phentolamine (Regitine). Beta-blockers by themselves should be avoided because they can precipitate a hypertensive crisis.

Patients taking monoamine oxidase inhibitors who ingest foods high in tyramine content can develop malignant hypertension. Foods that are high in tyramine include all aged cheeses, concentrated yeast extracts (marmite), sauerkraut, and broad bean pods.[16] The traditional drugs for treatment of these patients are phentolamine, nitroprusside, and labetalol.[17] Administration of α-methyldopa should be avoided because it can potentiate the effects of monoamine oxidase inhibitors.

Drug-Induced Hypertension

Administration of erythropoietin is an effective treatment of anemia associated with chronic renal failure. Approximately 35% of the patients receiving erythropoietin have an increased blood pressure,[18] and 2% of the hypertensive patients have hypertensive encephalopathy and convulsions.[19] The increase in blood pressure is thought to be due to increases in blood viscosity.[20] To avoid this complication, anemia should be corrected slowly during 12 to 16 weeks. The targeted hematocrit level should not exceed 32 to 35% with close monitoring of blood pressure and vital signs during administration of erythropoietin.

Women receiving oral contraceptives are at increased risk for severe hypertension. Contraceptive-induced elevations in blood pressure are relatively easily controlled when the medication is discontinued.

Hypertensive crisis can be precipitated by phencyclidine hydrochloride or cocaine.[21] Labetalol can be used in treatment of cocaine crisis.[22] The observed increased incidence in severe cocaine-induced hypertension and in the development of subarachnoid or intracerebral hemorrhages is perhaps due to the sudden transient increase in blood pressure related to cocaine usage.[23]

The most important toxic effect of over-the-counter stimulants, such as phenylpropanolamine hydrochloride, ephedrine, and pseudoephedrine, is hypertension. In some patients, this can occur after ingestion of only one third of the therapeutic dose of phenylpropanolamine.[24] These patients can have hypertensive encephalopathy or intracerebral hemorrhage. In addition, ephedrine and pseudoephedrine can cause hypertension as well as tachycardia owing to beta-adrenergic stimulation. Treatment of the hypertension is with vasodilators and that for tachycardia is with beta-blockers.

Preeclampsia

Young primigravidas can have severe hypertension, renal failure, proteinuria, edema, convulsions, and other neurologic signs. In treating hypertensive emergencies of pregnancy, one wants to reduce maternal blood pressure without decreasing placental perfusion and compromising the fetus. Recommended treatment is often bed rest and administration of magnesium and hydralazine. Diuretics are not recommended because these patients are often volume depleted and vasoconstricted.

Hypertensive Episodes During Surgery

A specific concern about the presence of hypertension is that the increased blood pressure may cause increased bleeding from vessels at the surgical site. To reduce these risks, one can either attempt to suppress a rise in blood pressure when it occurs or one can prevent the blood pressure rise from occurring at the onset. Hypertension is also a major factor in the etiology of perioperative myocardial ischemia. Nitroglycerin or isosorbide dinitrate has been used in treatment of postoperative hypertension in patients after coronary artery surgery; both are effective agents.[25]

Intravenous labetalol is often used in the management of hypertensive emergencies in postoperative hypertension. Other intravenous agents that are useful are enalapril, nitroprusside, and nitroglycerin.[26]

Rheumatologic Disease

Rheumatologic processes, such as progressive systemic sclerosis (scleroderma) and polyarteritis can present with accelerated hypertension. These patients may have an acute development of accelerated hypertension, hyperreninemia, and acute renal failure even without cutaneous fibrotic manifestations.[27] The malignant hypertension responds to ACE inhibitors; however, control of the blood pressure does not always guarantee that renal failure will not develop.[28]

TREATMENT PRINCIPLES

Hypertensive urgency (diastolic pressure greater than 120 mm Hg without end-organ dysfunction) is more common than hypertensive emergency. Both syndromes necessitate control of blood pressure. Studies have demonstrated a number of alternative approaches to treatment of hypertensive emergency or urgency. A variety of potent antihypertensive drugs can be used to lower blood pressure promptly, but the choice must be individualized. The goal is to lower blood pressure and to stabilize or improve the target organ function without causing hypoperfusion.

When examining a patient, one needs to assess if there is an underlying cause of the malignant hypertension and treat it accordingly. For example, increased volume is a predominant factor contributing to hypertension in cases of acute glomerulonephritis, whereas vasoconstriction is important in renovascular hypertension. Therefore, one must examine each patient and determine the ongoing pathophysiologic mechanisms to decide what treatment would be appropriate.

Treatment involves a balancing act between lowering the blood pressure to prevent endothelial cell damage and fibrinoid necrosis and to avoid too rapid a reduction of blood pressure, which can result in cerebral infarction or myocardial ischemia. One needs to be careful about precipitous decreases in arterial pressure because this may decrease cerebral blood flow below the lower limits of autoregulation and induce cerebral ischemia.[29]

The choice between oral and parenteral drugs depends on the urgency of the situation, the patient's general condition, and the need for close titration of the medications. For example, an asymptomatic patient with a diastolic pressure between 130 and 140 mm Hg may not need parenteral drug therapy. The advantage of parenteral medication is that it allows easy and rapid titration of blood pressure. On the other hand, oral medication does not necessitate admission of the patient to an intensive care unit.[30, 31]

Pharmacologic Agents

The pharmacologic agents used in treatment of malignant hypertension were reviewed by Calhoun and Oparil[32] and Houston.[33] They are listed on Tables 114–3 and 114–4.

Intravenous administration of nitroprusside sodium (Nipride, Nitropress) leads to rapid lowering (1 to 2 minutes) of blood pressure and short duration (1 to 5 minutes) of action and reduces both peripheral arterial vascular resistance and venous tone. Because of its effect on left ventricular function (decreased preload and afterload), it is often the drug of choice in patients with severe hypertension and left ventricular failure. Side effects include nausea, vomiting, headache, disorientation, and thiocyanate toxicity. An in-

---

TABLE 114–3

TYPES OF HYPERTENSIVE EMERGENCY AND TREATMENT RECOMMENDATIONS

Type of Hypertensive Emergency	Recommended Treatment	Drugs To Avoid
Hypertensive encephalopathy	Sodium nitroprusside, labetalol, diazoxide	Beta-adrenergic antagonists, methyldopa, clonidine
Cerebral infarction	No treatment, sodium nitroprusside, labetalol	Beta-adrenergic antagonists, methyldopa, clonidine
Intracerebral hemorrhage, subarachnoid hemorrhage	No treatment, sodium nitroprusside, labetalol	Beta-adrenergic antagonists, methyldopa, clonidine
Myocardial ischemia, myocardial infarction	Nitroglycerin, labetalol, calcium antagonist, sodium nitroprusside	Hydralazine, diazoxide, minoxidil
Acute pulmonary edema	Sodium nitroprusside and loop diuretic, nitroglycerin and loop diuretic	Hydralazine, diazoxide, beta-adrenergic antagonists, labetalol
Aortic dissection	Sodium nitroprusside and beta-adrenergic antagonists, trimethaphan and beta-adrenergic antagonists, labetalol	Hydralazine, diazoxide, minoxidil
Eclampsia	Hydralazine, diazoxide, labetalol, calcium antagonist, sodium nitroprusside*	Trimethaphan, diuretics, beta-adrenergic antagonists
Acute renal insufficiency	Sodium nitroprusside, labetalol, calcium antagonists	Beta-adrenergic antagonists, trimethaphan
Grade 3 or 4 Keith-Wagener funduscopic changes†	Sodium nitroprusside, labetalol, calcium antagonists	Beta-adrenergic antagonists, clonidine, methyldopa
Microangiopathic hemolytic anemia	Sodium nitroprusside, labetalol, calcium antagonists	Beta-adrenergic antagonists

*Because of the potential risk to the fetus, reserve for patients with eclampsia that is refractory to treatment with other agents.
†Grade 3 changes include exudates and hemorrhage, and grade 4 changes, papilledema.
From Calhoun D, Oparil S: Treatment of hypertensive crises. Reprinted with permission from The New England Journal of Medicine 323, 1177–1183, 1990.

TABLE 114-4

PARENTERAL MEDICATIONS USED IN TREATMENT OF HYPERTENSIVE EMERGENCIES

Drug	Administration	Onset	Duration of Action	Dosage	Adverse Effects and Comments
Sodium nitroprusside (initial dose)	IV infusion	Immediate	2–3 min	0.5–10 µg/kg/min (0.25 µg/kg/min for renal insufficiency)	Hypotension, nausea, vomiting. Risk of thiocyanate and cyanide toxicity is increased in renal and hepatic insufficiency, respectively; levels should be monitored. Must be shielded from light.
Diazoxide	IV bolus / IV infusion	1–5 min	6–12 h	50–100 mg every 5–10 min, up to 600 mg / 10–30 mg/min	Hypotension, tachycardia, nausea, vomiting, fluid retention, hyperglycemia. May exacerbate myocardial ischemia, heart failure, or aortic dissection. May require concomitant use of beta-antagonist.
Labetalol	IV bolus / IV infusion	5–10 min	3–6 h	20–80 mg every 5–10 min, up to 300 mg / 0.5–2 mg/min	Hypotension, heart block, heart failure, bronchospasm, nausea, vomiting, scalp tingling, paradoxical pressor response: May not be effective in patients receiving alpha- or beta-antagonists.
Nitroglycerin	IV infusion	1–2 min	3–5 min	5–100 µg/min	Headache, nausea, vomiting. Tolerance may develop with prolonged use.
Phentolamine	IV bolus	1–2 min	3–10 min	5–10 mg every 5–15 min	Hypotension, tachycardia, headache, angina, paradoxical pressor response.
Trimethaphan	IV infusion	1–5 min	10 min	0.5–5 mg/min	Hypotension, urinary retention, ileus, respiratory arrest, mydriasis, cycloplegia, dry mouth. More effective if patient's head is elevated.
Hydralazine (for treatment of eclampsia)	IV bolus	10–20 min	3–6 h	5–10 mg every 20 min (if no effect after 20 mg, try another agent)	Hypotension, fetal distress, tachycardia, headache, nausea, vomiting, local thrombophlebitis; infusion site should be changed after 12 h.
Nicardipine*	IV infusion	1–5 min	3–6 h	5 mg/h increase by 1–2.5 mg/h every 15 min, up to 8 mg/h	Hypotension, headache, tachycardia, nausea, vomiting.

*Not yet approved by the U.S. Food and Drug Administration for this use.
From Calhoun D, Oparil S: Treatment of hypertensive crises. Reprinted with permission from The New England Journal of Medicine 323, 1177–1183, 1990.

crease in thiocyanate level may induce metabolic acidosis. This is often seen in patients with renal insufficiency because thiocyanate is cleared by the kidney. If one needs to infuse nitroprusside for longer than 72 hours or if the patient has renal failure, one must determine blood thiocyanate levels daily and not let the level exceed 12 mg/dL.[34] The cyanide is transformed to thiocyanate by the hepatic enzyme thiosulfate sulfurtransferase[33] (Fig. 114–2), and this reaction requires thiosulfate. The cyanide level can be reduced by simultaneously infusing sodium thiosulfate or hydroxocobalamin,[35] particularly in patients requiring high doses of nitroprusside or in patients with renal failure.

An excessive fall in arterial pressure can be corrected by a head-down tilt of the patient and discontinuation of the infusion. However, nitroprusside results in a decrease in mean cerebral blood flow and an increase in arteriovenous oxygen differences at mean arterial pressures of 80 to 90 mm Hg.[36] Because of these concerns, other antihypertensive agents are gaining favor in patients with severe hypertension with increased cranial pressure.

Nitroglycerin (Nitro-Bid, Nitrostat, Tridil) has a direct vasodilating effect on venous, as well as arterial, circulation. Its primary mode of action is on the venous tone, but at higher infusion rates, nitroglycerin significantly reduces peripheral vascular resistance. It is useful in patients with myocardial damage because it dilates epicardial coronary arteries and collateral vessels, and it improves regional distribution of myocardial blood flow. Common side effects are headache, flushing, dizziness, and tachycardia. Similar to the case with nitroprusside, cerebral autoregulation is impaired during nitroglycerin infusion.[37] Reflex tachycardia can occur.

ACE inhibitors (captopril, enalapril, lisinopril) are often helpful because renin activity is frequently elevated in patients with malignant hypertension. They may cause a precipitous fall in blood pressure, particularly in hypertensive patients with high renin levels (those with renal arterial stenosis or volume depletion). Patients with malignant hypertension attributable to bilateral renal arterial stenosis or unilateral stenosis in a solitary kidney may have acute renal failure in response to treatment with an ACE inhibitor.[38] In response to ACE inhibitors, patients with malignant hypertension show a decrease in total peripheral resistance. This makes this drug attractive in patients with high peripheral resistance, such as those with progressive systemic sclerosis and hypertensive crisis with acute renal failure.[39] The decrease in blood pressure directly correlates with a patient's renin and arterial pressure pretreatment levels. It is generally recommended to start with a small dose to avoid excessive initial fall in blood pressure.

Calcium channel blockers reduce blood pressure predominantly by reducing systemic vascular resistance by direct vasodilator action on arterioles. This vasodilation appears greater with more severe hypertension.[40] The calcium chan-

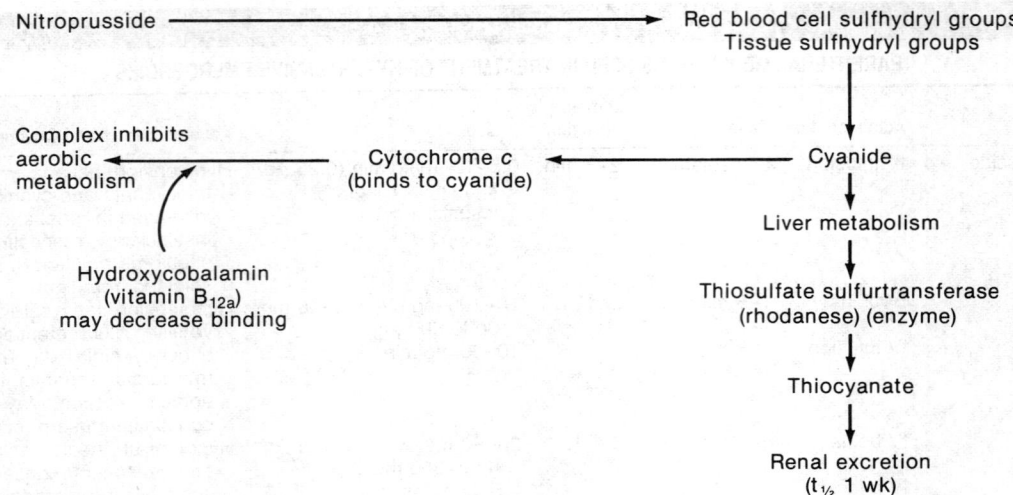

Figure 114–2. Nitroprusside is metabolized to cyanide, which may accumulate in liver disease, and to thiocyanate, which accumulates in renal insufficiency. (From Houston MC: Pathophysiology, clinical aspects, and treatment of hypertensive crises. Prog Cardiovasc Dis 32:99, 1989.)

nel blockers are efficacious in patients with hypertension associated with angina, myocardial infarction, and neurologic defects with decreased cerebral perfusion. One advantage of calcium channel blockers is that cerebral blood flow increases, apparently owing to a spasmolytic effect on the cerebral vessels.[41] Some specific calcium channel blockers currently indicated for treating severe hypertension are discussed.

Nifedipine (Procardia, Adalat), when compared with verapamil and diltiazem, causes the most vasodilation. It also has the greatest potential of the three drugs for causing reflex sinus tachycardia.[42] One concern is that hypotension has been seen with nifedipine after short-term treatment of hypertension.[43]

Nicardipine hydrochloride (Cardene) is similar to nifedipine but has a smaller inotropic effect and causes less reflex tachycardia. Patients may have thrombophlebitis at the site of the infusion when the infusion site is used for more than 14 hours.[44]

Nimodipine (Nimotop) is approved for use in patients with vasospasm after subarachnoid hemorrhage from rupture of an intracranial aneurysm. In a primate model, nimodipine may improve or preserve neurologic outcome after a stroke.[45, 46] Further studies are needed in humans.

Felodipine has renal and hemodynamic effects comparable with those of nitroprusside in hypertensive patients when administered intravenously.[47] Felodipine has been compared with minoxidil in the treatment of severe hypertension.[37] This drug controlled blood pressure as well as minoxidil and therefore holds promise in treatment of severe hypertension.

Verapamil and diltiazem have the most negative chronotropic and inotropic effects compared with those of dihydropyridine calcium antagonists. Verapamil and diltiazem should be used with caution in patients with congestive heart failure or heart block. Common side effects of verapamil are constipation and headache. Neither drug is recommended for the initial management of malignant hypertension because they are difficult to titrate.

Minoxidil (Loniten) administered orally is a potent arterial vasodilator. Because of concern about reflexively increased heart rates and cardiac output and volume overload, it is not used as monotherapy. Side effects include pericardial effusion (3%), which resolves on discontinuing administra-

tion of the drug; hirsutism (80%); and electrocardiographic abnormalities (nonischemic flattening of T waves).

Clonidine (Catapres), by activating presynaptic alpha$_2$-adrenergic receptors and decreasing catecholamine output, is one of the most well tolerated agents used in the oral treatment of hypertensive urgencies.

One advantage of oral clonidine is low overall cost owing to a lessened need for close observation in selected patients with hypertensive urgency. This demonstrates that oral antihypertensives are an alternative treatment to parenteral nitroprusside in patients with hypertensive urgencies and in some patients with hypertensive emergencies.[48]

α-Methyldopa (Aldomet) has a variable absorption and a slow onset of action. Altered mental acuity and impaired judgment cause this drug to be contraindicated for use in patients with hypertensive encephalopathy. Because of these concerns, other drugs are recommended for the initial management of hypertensive crisis.

Alpha-Adrenergic Blocking Agents

Phentolamine mesylate (Regitine) blocks both postsynaptic vascular alpha$_1$-adrenergic receptors. It is often used to control blood pressure at the time of surgery in patients with pheochromocytoma. It is specifically indicated for treatment of hypertensive crisis in association with pheochromocytoma, ingestion of monoamine oxidase inhibitors, and tyramine ingestion or clonidine withdrawal syndrome.

Phenoxybenzamine (Dibenzyline) blocks both alpha$_1$- and alpha$_2$-receptors. The blockade of presynaptic alpha$_2$-receptors inhibits the normal feedback inhibition of norepinephrine release, so extended use leads to marked tachycardia and a loss of antihypertensive effect. Because of these side effects, phenoxybenzamine is not used in chronic hypertension treatment except for pheochromocytoma.

Prazosin (Minipress) decreases total peripheral resistance by dilating both arterioles and veins. Prazosin can be used in the preoperative control of blood pressure for pheochromocytoma.[49] It may cause fluid retention and edema, so a diuretic is often given concomitantly. Occasionally, first-dose syncope occurs. Because this is unpredictable, this drug is used in the long-term rather than the short-term management of pheochromocytoma.

Beta-Blockers

Labetalol (Normodyne, Trandate) is an alpha- and beta-adrenergic receptor blocking agent that is approved for treatment of hypertensive emergencies and urgencies. This medication selectively blocks alpha$_1$-receptors and is non-selective for beta-receptors. Because it is available in both parenteral and oral forms, one advantage is the ease of converting from intravenous to oral administration.

Beta-blockers are contraindicated in pheochromocytoma if an alpha-blocking agent is not administered first. They may precipitate heart failure, increase intracardiac conduction time, or precipitate asthma attack. They have been useful in treatment of malignant hypertension, postoperative hypertension, and hypertension associated with myocardial infarction.

SUMMARY

Severe hypertension can be divided into hypertensive crises or urgencies. The clinical factor that suggests a hypertensive emergency is the presence of acute organ damage. Thus, the presence of rapid deterioration of organ function determines the aggressiveness of therapy.

The current drug of choice in hypertensive emergency is nitroprusside because of its effectiveness and titratability with or without beta-blockade. Hypertensive urgencies can be treated with a number of oral agents.

After the patient has been stabilized, it is mandatory to consider the underlying, treatable causes of the hypertension.

Because the discontinuation of medication is known to be a major precipitating event in malignant hypertension, the patient must be placed on a regimen that will be followed after discharge from the hospital.

References

1. Yu SH, Whitworth JA, Kincaid-Smith PS: Malignant hypertension: Aetiology and outcome in 83 patients. Clin Exp Hypertens [A]8:1211, 1986.
2. Guerin C, Gonthier R, Berthoux FC: Long-term prognosis in malignant or accelerated hypertension. Nephrol Dial Transplant 3:33, 1988.
3. Bennett NM, Shea S: Hypertensive emergency: Case criteria, sociodemographic profile, and previous care of 100 cases. Am J Public Health 78:636, 1988.
4. Finnertz FA Jr: Hypertensive encephalopathy. Am J Med 52:672, 1972.
5. Shepherd RF, Zachariah P, Shub C, et al: Hypertension and left ventricular diastolic function. Mayo Clin Proc 64:1521, 1989.
6. Roberts WC: Frequency of systemic hypertension in various cardiovascular diseases. Am J Cardiol 60:1E, 1987.
7. Roberts WC: Aortic dissection, anatomy, consequences and cause. Am Heart J 101:195, 1981.
8. Perez-Fontan M, Miguel JL, Picaro C: Idiopathic IGA nephropathy presenting as malignant hypertension. Am Med J Nephrol 6:482, 1986.
9. Sublias R, Botey A, Darnell A, et al: Malignant or accelerated hypertension IgA nephropathy. Clin Nephrol 27:1, 1987.
10. Heintz R: The clinical picture of renal hypertension. Clin Nephrol 4:189, 1975.
11. Simard JM, Bellesleur M: Systemic arterial hypertension in head trauma. Am J Cardiol 63:320, 1989.
12. Thorn-Alquist AM: Prevention of hypertensive crises in patients with high spinal lesions during cystoscopy and lithotripsy. Acta Anaesthesiol Scand [Suppl] 79, 1975.
13. Raisanen J, Shapiro B, Glazer GM, et al: Plasma catecholamines in pheochromocytoma: Effect of urographic contrast media. Am J Roentgenol 143:43, 1984.
14. Marty J, Desmonts JM, Chalaux G, et al: Hypertensive responses during operation for pheochromocytoma: A study of plasma catecholamine and haemodynamic changes. Eur J Anaesthesiol 2:257, 1985.
15. Schmucki O: Medical support in surgery for pheochromocytoma [in German]. Helv Chir Acta 46:287, 1979.
16. Shulman KI, Walker SE, MacKenzie S: Dietary restriction, tyramine, and the use of monoamine oxidase inhibitors. J Clin Psychopharmacol 9:397, 1989.
17. Abrams JH, Schulman P, White WB: Successful treatment of a mono-
amine oxidase inhibitor—tyramine hypertensive emergency with intravenous labetalol. N Engl J Med 313:52, 1985.
18. Eschbach JW, Abdulhadi MH, Browne JK, et al: Recombinant human erythropoietin in anemic patients with end-stage renal diseases. Results of a phase III multicenter clinical trial. Ann Intern Med 111:992, 1989.
19. Edmunds ME, Walls J, Tucker B: Seizures in haemodialysis patients treated with recombinant human erythropoietin. Nephrol Dial Transplant 4:1065, 1989.
20. Zehnder C, Blumberg A: Cerebrovascular incidents in four hemodialysis patients treated with erythropoietin [in German]. Schweiz Med Wochenschr 118:1423, 1988.
21. Sioris LJ, Krenzelok EP: Phencyclidine intoxication: A literature review. Am J Hosp Pharm 35:1362, 1978.
22. Gay GR, Loper KA: The use of labetalol in the management of cocaine crisis. Ann Emerg Med 17:292, 1988.
23. Mangiardi JR, Daras M, Geller ME, et al: Cocaine-related intracranial hemorrhage. Report of nine cases and review. Acta Neurol Scand 77:177, 1988.
24. Pentel P: Toxicity of over-the-counter stimulants. JAMA 252:1898, 1984.
25. Durkin MA, Thys D, Morris RB, et al: Control of perioperative hypertension after coronary surgery. A randomized double-blind study comparing isosorbide dinitrate and nitroglycerin. Eur Heart J 9(suppl A):181, 1988.
26. Gonzalez DG, Ram CV: Therapeutic survey: Hypertensive emergencies. Can J Cardiol 3:154, 1987.
27. Sanders PW, Herrera GA, Ball GV: Acute renal failure without fibrotic skin changes in progressive systemic sclerosis. Nephron 48:121, 1988.
28. Whitman HH 3d, Case DB, Laragh JH, et al: Variable response to oral angiotensin-converting-enzyme blockade in hypertensive scleroderma patients. Arthritis Rheum 25:241, 1982.
29. Bauer JH, Reams GP: The role of calcium entry blockers in hypertensive emergencies. Circulation 75:V174, 1987.
30. Bertel O, Marx BE: Hypertensive emergencies. Nephron 47(suppl 1):51, 1987.
31. Gonzalez DG, Ram CV: Therapeutic survey: Hypertensive emergencies. Can J Cardiol 3:154, 1987.
32. Calhoun DA, Oparil S: Treatment of hypertensive crises. N Engl J Med 323:1177, 1990.
33. Houston MC: Pathophysiology, clinical aspect and treatment of hypertensive crisis. Prog Cardiovasc Dis 99:148, 1989.
34. Vesey CJ, Cole PV, Simpson PJ: Cyanide and thiocyanate concentrations following sodium nitroprusside infusions in man. Br J Anaesth 48:651, 1976.
35. Schulz V: Clinical pharmacokinetics of nitroprusside, cyanide, thiosulphate and thiocyanate. J Clin Pharmacokinet 9:239, 1984.
36. Henriksen L, Paulson OB: The effect of sodium nitroprusside on cerebral blood flow and cerebral venous blood gases. Observations in awake man during successive blood pressure reduction. Eur J Clin Invest 12:389, 1982.
37. Wathen CG, Macleod D, Tucker L, et al: Felodipine as a replacement for minoxidil in the treatment of severe hypertension. Eur Heart J 7:893, 1986.
38. Dominiczak A, Isles C, Gillen G, et al: Angiotensin converting enzyme inhibition and renal insufficiency in patients with bilateral renovascular disease. J Hum Hypertens 2:53, 1988.
39. Tharm RH, Alexander JC: Captopril in the treatment of scleroderma renal crisis. Arch Intern Med 144:733, 1984.
40. MacGregor GA: Nifedipine and systemic hypertension. Am J Cardiol 64:46F, 1989.
41. Conen D, Ruttimann S, Noll G, et al: Short- and long-term cerebrovascular effects of nitrendipine in hypertensive patients. J Cardiovas Pharmacol 12(suppl 4):S64, 1988.
42. Dustan HP: Calcium channel blockers. Potential medical benefits and side effects. Hypertension 13:I137, 1989.
43. Wachter RM: Symptomatic hypotension induced by nifedipine in the acute treatment of severe hypertension. Arch Intern Med 147:556, 1987.
44. Wallin JD, Cook ME, Blanski L, et al: Intravenous nicardipine for the treatment of severe hypertension. Am J Med 85:331, 1988.
45. Hadley MN, Zabramski JM, Spetzler RF, et al: The efficacy of intravenous nimodipine in the treatment of focal cerebral ischemia in a primate model. Neurosurgery 25:63, 1989.
46. Gelmers HJ, Gorter K, de Weerdt CJ, et al: A controlled trial of nimodipine in acute ischemic stroke. N Engl J Med 318:203, 1988.
47. Elliott WJ, Weber RR, Nelson KS, et al: Renal and hemodynamic effects of intravenous fenoldopam versus nitroprusside in severe hypertension. Circulation 81:970, 1990.
48. Houston MC: Treatment of hypertensive emergencies and urgencies with oral clonidine loading and titration. Arch Intern Med 146:586, 1986.
49. Nicholson JP Jr, Vaughn ED, Pickering TG, et al: Pheochromocytoma and prazosin. Ann Intern Med 99:477, 1983.
50. Grossman SH, Gannells JC: Recognition and treatment of hypertensive emergencies. Cardiovasc Clin 11:97, 1981.
51. Kincaid-Smith P: Malignant hypertension. Cardiovasc Rev Rep: 42, 1980.
52. Albert MA, Bauer JH: Hypertensive emergencies: Recognition and pathogenesis. Cardiovasc Rev Rep 6:407, 1985.
53. Gudbrandsson T: Malignant hypertension. A clinical follow-up study with

specific reference to renal and cardiovascular function and immunogenetic factors. Acta Med Scand [Suppl] 650:1, 1981.

54. Davis BA, Crook JE, Vestal RE, et al: Prevalence of renovascular hypertension in patients with grade III or IV hypertensive retinopathy. N Engl J Med 301:1273, 1979.
55. Russell GI, Bing RF, Thurston H, et al: Renal artery stenosis in malignant hypertension (letter). Lancet 2:529, 1980.
56. Ram CVS: Hypertensive crises: Parts I and II. Causes. Part III. Drug treatment. J Cardiovasc Med June, July, August: 645, 781, 917, 1983.
57. Lindheimer MD, Katz AI: Hypertension and pregnancy. In: Genest J, Kuchel O, Hamet P (eds): Hypertension (2nd ed). New York, McGraw-Hill, p 889, 1983.
58. Mendlowitz M: Toxemia of pregnancy and eclampsia. Obstet Gynecol Surv 35:327, 1980.
59. Ram CVS, Engleman K: Pheochromocytoma—recognition and management. Curr Probl Cardiol 4:7, 1979.
60. Knapp HR, Fitzgerald GA: Hypertensive crises in prazosin-treated pheochromocytoma. South Med J 77:535, 1984.
61. Swenson SJ, Brown ML, Sheps SG, et al: Use of ^{131}I-MIBG scintigraphy in the evaluation of suspected pheochromocytoma. Mayo Clin Proc 60:299, 1985.
62. Houston MC: Abrupt cessation of treatment in hypertension: Consideration of clinical features, mechanisms, prevention and management of the discontinuation syndrome. Am Heart J 102:415, 1981.
63. Worlsman J, Burns G, Van Beck AL, et al: Hyperadrenergic state after trauma to the neuroaxis. Arch Intern Med 144:1459, 1984.
64. Naftchi NE, Demeny M, Lowman EW, et al: Hypertensive crises in quadriplegic patients. Changes in output, blood volume, serum dopamine–beta-hydroxylase activity. Circulation 57:336, 1978.
65. Kozlowski J, Schaeffer A, DelGreco F, et al: Accelerated hypertension in a 54-year-old woman. J Urol 125:859, 1981.
66. Blackwell B, Marley E, Price J, et al: Hypertensive interactions between monoamine oxidase inhibitors and foodstuffs. Br J Psychiatry 113:349, 1967.
67. Walker JI, Davidson J, Zung WW: Patient compliance with MAO inhibitor therapy. J Clin Psychiatry 45:78, 1984.
68. Smookler S, Bermudez AJ: Hypertensive crises resulting from a MAO inhibitor and an over the counter appetite suppressant. Ann Emerg Med 11:482, 1982.
69. Byrom FB: The evolution of acute hypertensive arterial disease. Prog Cardiovasc Dis 17:31, 1974.
70. Petti DB, Klatsky AI: Malignant hypertension in women aged 15 to 44 years and its relationship to cigarette smoking and oral contraceptives. Am J Cardiol 52:297, 1983.
71. Dunn FG: Malignant hypertension associated with use of amitriptyline hydrochloride. South Med J 75:1124, 1982.
72. Sesoko S, Miyazaki IV, Kato Y, et al: Atropine and a hypertensive crisis. Ann Intern Med 101:720, 1984.
73. Mark JB, Greenberg LM: Intraoperative awareness and hypertensive crisis during high-dose fentanyl-diazepam-oxygen anesthesia. Anesth Analg 62:698, 1983.
74. Mann SJ, Krakoff LR: Hypertensive crisis caused by hypoglycemia and propranolol. Arch Intern Med 144:2427, 1984.
75. Gifford RW Jr: Management and treatment of essential hypertension, including malignant hypertension and emergencies. In: Genest J, Kuchel O, Hamet P (eds): Hypertension (2nd ed). New York, McGraw-Hill, p 1127, 1983.
76. Brizio-Molteni L, Molteni A, Cloutier LC, et al: Incidence of post burn hypertensive crisis in patients admitted to two burn centers and a community hospital in the United States. Scand J Plast Reconstr Surg 13:21, 1979.
77. Wall RA, Sikland PC, Elem B: Malignant hypertension secondary to idiopathic arteritis of the aorta. Br Med J 2:977, 1976.
78. O'Connell MT, Kubrusly DB, Fournier AM: Systemic necrotizing vasculitis seen initially as hypertensive crisis. Arch Intern Med 145:265, 1985.
79. Traub YM, Shapiro AP, Rodnan GP, et al: Hypertension and renal failure (scleroderma renal crisis) in progressive systemic sclerosis. Review of a 25-year experience with 68 cases. Medicine 62:335, 1983.

SECTION NINE

Hematology/Oncology

Section Editors

Lyle L. Sensenbrenner and Judith C. Andersen

CHAPTER 115

Hematology/Oncology: Introduction

Judith C. Andersen
Lyle L. Sensenbrenner

In this section we consider the hematopoietic system, its structure (blood, bone marrow, vessels), self-renewal (hematopoiesis), and functions (carrier of nutritive substances, immune and phagocytic activities, and control of clotting); primary disorders of the hematopoietic system and their manifestations; the hematopoietic system secondarily expressing disorders in other systems; qualitative disorders of the hematopoietic system (failure of one or more of the elements to perform properly); quantitative disorders of the hematopoietic system (an inappropriate quantity of a particular element); the relationship of hematology to medical oncology, historically and therapeutically; the principles of neoplastic proliferation; and the types of disorders neoplasms can produce.

Although we often consider hematology and oncology together as combined disciplines, it is primarily because of historical considerations. Medical oncology as a separate discipline began as a subsection of the hematology division in most medical institutions. The original concerns of medical oncology were almost exclusively the treatment of hematologic neoplasms with cancer chemotherapeutic agents. Hematologic neoplasms were the first and for a long time almost the only malignant disorders in which significant responses to cancer chemotherapy were seen. In addition, it was, and to a great extent still is, true that most of the major limiting toxicities of our useful cancer chemotherapeutic modalities are toxicities expressed by the lymphohematopoietic system. Therefore, it was natural that cancer chemotherapy would be closely allied with hematology. However, as the two disciplines continue to evolve with new techniques and approaches to many of the nonmalignant hematologic disorders and methods of cancer chemotherapy that frequently do not have hematologic toxicity as a major side effect and that have nonhematologic tumors as major targets, the two disciplines are becoming more distinct. Although we consider both hematology and oncology in a single section of this textbook, we treat the disciplines separately within that section.

HEMATOLOGY

The Hematopoietic System: Structure, Self-Renewal, and Function

Hematology, as a discipline, encompasses the study of the circulating blood and its origins, functions, and disorders.[1-7] The blood, a suspension of cells and cellular elements in an aqueous solution of salts and proteins called plasma, makes up 5 to 7% of the body mass. Through a series of conduits called arteries, capillaries, and veins, the blood reaches nearly every tissue and ultimately almost every cell in the body to provide for its nutrition, oxygenation, removal of wastes, and, to a great extent, defense against invading organisms. Thus, disorders of almost any organ in the body are often expressed as alterations in the composition of the blood, and nearly any disorder of the blood is expressed as a disordered function of some other organ of the body.

The major component of the blood is water, and a major function of the blood is to distribute water to and remove excess water from all cells and tissues of the body. Dissolved within the aqueous plasma are various proteins and salts (including sodium, potassium, calcium, iron, and magnesium).

The major proteins are of three types. The first and most abundant are the carrier proteins, which bind various types of molecules and thus prevent nonspecific migration of such substances into the tissues. Plasma proteins bound to a specific molecule of a substance often function to transport and present a needed substance to a cell receptor in a form easily recognized by that cell. This allows uptake by surface receptors of the specific molecules bound to carrier protein, such as iron bound to transferrin, vitamin B_{12} bound to transcobalamin II, and lipids bound to lipoproteins. The transport proteins also frequently bind otherwise toxic substances and prevent them from damaging cells and tissues. Examples are ceruloplasmin, which binds toxic free oxygen radicals; alpha-2 macroglobulin, which binds and neutralizes proteolytic enzymes; and haptoglobin, which binds and carries free hemoglobin.

The second major group of plasma proteins includes the immunoglobulins (primarily immunoglobulins G, A, and M) and the proteins of the complement system, which together function as a major defense against invading organisms.

TABLE 115–1

HEMATOPOIETIC GROWTH FACTORS

Name	Sources	Action
Erythropoietin	Kidney (some liver)	Stimulates proliferation of erythroid precursors and progenitors and release of red blood cells from bone marrow
Granulocyte colony-stimulating factor (G-CSF)	Monocytes, fibroblasts, endothelial cells	Proliferation and activation of granulocytes; increased granulocyte migration
Granulocyte-monocyte colony-stimulating factor (GM-CSF)	Endothelial cells, monocytes, fibroblasts, activated T cells	Activates granulocytes and increases phagocytosis and killing; increased proliferation of granulocytes and monocytes; decreased migration of granulocytes into tissue
Monocyte colony-stimulating factor	Monocytes, stromal cells, lymphocytes	Activates monocytes and stimulates their proliferation
Interleukin-3	Activated T cells	Stimulates early hematopoietic progenitor granulocytes and monocytes and has some effect on early erythroid progenitors
Interleukin-1	Macrophages, endothelial cells, fibroblasts, T cells	Stimulates release of GM-CSF, G-CSF, interleukin-3, monocyte CSF, eosinophil CSF; activates osteoclasts, neutrophils, natural killer cells

The smallest group of plasma proteins includes those that make up the coagulation system. These proteins maintain the integrity of the vasculature by contributing to the formation of gelatinous plugs wherever a break occurs in the conduits through which the blood courses.

Suspended within the plasma are cellular elements that are in many ways the counterparts of the plasma proteins. The first and largest cellular component is the carrier cell fraction, that is, the red blood cells, which are non-nucleated cytoplasmic biconcave disks. They make up about 40% of the blood volume and are primarily responsible for carrying oxygen from the lungs to all cells of the body and carbon dioxide back to the lungs. Their proper size and shape (which results in a large surface area), as well as hemoglobin structure and concentration, are essential for the adequate performance of that function. Too many red blood cells can lead to excessive viscosity of the blood, with subsequent thrombosis and ischemia, and too few can lead to decreased oxygen-carrying capacity and tissue ischemia, resulting in failure of the heart, kidneys, and brain.

The second largest cellular component of the blood is the white blood cell fraction. The white blood cells are divided into two major groups—the phagocytic cells (granulocytes and monocytes), which are capable of engulfing particulate material, and the lymphocytes. The major function of these cells is to defend the body against invading organisms. The granulocytes can be divided into three groups on the basis of the morphologic appearance of their stained cytoplasmic granules—neutrophils, eosinophils, and basophils. The monocytes are the only phagocytes of the peripheral blood capable of dividing. The lymphocytes are nonphagocytic and can be divided into several types according to their cell surface markers. They function to produce antibodies (B cells) or to mediate cellular immunity (T cells). Both the phagocytes and lymphocytes are capable of locomotion and use the peripheral blood channels as conduits to carry them to the various tissues, where they leave the blood stream and perform most of their functions outside the blood vessels. In most medical emergencies involving white blood cells, there are too few white blood cells, allowing microorganisms to invade the body and cause overwhelming sepsis or life-threatening viral infection. Rarely, too many granulocytes (immature forms) produce acute problems of hyperviscosity and occlusion of the blood vessels.

Platelets make up the third and smallest of the cellular compartments and, like the smallest protein fraction of the plasma, have primarily a hemostatic function. Platelets are small disks (7 to 9 fL, 1 to 2 μm in diameter) composed of cytoplasm shed from mature megakaryocytes and released into the blood stream. These anucleate fragments function primarily to plug tiny leaks in the vasculature and initiate clot formation and fibrosis in tears of the larger blood vessels. Most clinical problems are due to too few platelets leading to bleeding problems. Rarely, there are dysfunctional problems of platelets, which most often lead to bleeding. Occasionally, there are clinically significant excessive numbers of platelets. High platelet counts almost never lead to problems unless the platelets are dysfunctional (as in essential thrombocytosis), and even then only rarely does one see thrombosis or bleeding unless the platelet count is greater than 1×10^{12}/L.

The cells and cellular elements of the peripheral blood have a relatively short survival. Red blood cells last approximately 120 days, granulocytes and monocytes spend less than a day in the peripheral blood stream, and platelets last for about 9 days. Thus, relatively massive replacement of these cellular elements by the body takes place continuously. Because of the large turnover of these cells, the bone marrow, which is the source of all hematopoietic cells, is among the most rapidly proliferating organs in the body. Bone marrow in the infant is located in nearly all bones of the body, but as one ages the marrow retreats from the distal bones and remains only in the axial skeleton (spine, ribs, pelvis, sternum, proximal femurs, and humeri). The marrow, a semigelatinous tissue composed of nearly 50% fat cells, is highly vascular. It contains many large venous sinuses around which the marrow elements are dispersed among and between bony trabeculae. The bone marrow itself is a continuously self-renewing system. Within it is a small population of pluripotent stem cells that are capable of producing tremendous numbers of progeny by continuous cell division. With each cell division there is a degree of differentiation and commitment to a variety of cell types including red blood cells, granulocytes, monocytes, platelets, lymphocytes, macrophages, and osteoclasts. This process of proliferation with differentiation is carefully controlled by cellular and humoral growth factors (Table 115–1).[8–13] The mature cells are then released from the bone marrow into the peripheral blood stream, where the cells or cellular elements spend from a few hours (white blood cells) to 4 months (red blood cells). Within the bone marrow, the various growth-regulating factors act on the many blood cell progenitors and precursors, controlling their rate of proliferation and the type of lineage differentiation. Some of these regulatory substances are produced away from the bone marrow and act in an endocrine function on the bone marrow cells (e.g., erythropoietin is produced in the kidney in response to hypoxia and acts in the bone marrow). Other factors appear to be produced and to act locally (granulocyte-monocyte colony-stimulating factor is produced by monocytes of the bone marrow in the response to endotoxin).

In addition to the stem cells of the bone marrow, which make up fewer than 1 in 10,000 of the nucleated cells, there are various progenitor cells (fewer than 1 per 1000 nucleated bone marrow cells). These progenitor cells are not recognizable by light microscopy but are recognizable by in vitro culture techniques. Each of the progenitors, when cultured in vitro with the proper type and concentration of hematopoietic growth factor, produces a colony of mature cells of the lineage or lineages to which the progenitor is committed and in which the available growth factors are capable of stimulating proliferation with differentiation.

The vascular system functions as the conduit through which the blood is delivered and returned from all tissues of the body. Its integrity is maintained by its unique anatomic structure and the cellular (platelets) and soluble (coagulation proteins) factors circulating in the blood, which repair any tears or leaks that develop in the system.

All hematopoiesis in the normal human from infancy on occurs in the bone marrow spaces. However, in times of severe need (severe anemias, especially hemolytic problems such as thalassemia and phthisic disorders such as myelofibrosis), hematopoiesis may again take place in the organs in which it normally occurs during embryonic life, that is, the liver and/or spleen.

Normally, the vascular system remains intact and no leakage of blood elements occurs from its walls. However, in the course of life, trauma or tissue destructive processes (e.g., ulcers, neoplasms, or infectious lesions) may disrupt the vascular conduits, resulting in leakage (bleeding) from the system. The hematopoietic system is well equipped to handle all such vascular insults to any but the largest vessels. The vessels themselves are provided with elastic and smooth muscle cells that allow contraction of the severed ends, providing for some degree of control of bleeding. In addition, the damaged endothelium at the ruptured surface sets off a cascade of events utilizing both the plasma coagulation proteins and the platelets that result in the formation of a gelatinous plug (clot or platelet plug) in the ruptured vessel, which prevents further blood loss.

Because of absence or marked reduction of any of the procoagulants, severe or prolonged bleeding can occur after what appears to be minimal trauma. This occurs when there is a deficiency of factor VIII in classic hemophilia (hemophilia A) and factor IX in hemophilia B. It also occurs in individuals with deficiencies of the vitamin K–dependent factors (prothrombin and factors VII, IX, and X), such as those taking vitamin K antagonists such as warfarin (Coumadin), those taking oral antibiotics that eliminate the normal gut flora, those who have severe liver disease that prevents the synthesis of the coagulation proteins, debilitated patients on a fat-free diet, or patients with severe malabsorption syndromes. The presence of anticoagulants (heparin, lupus anticoagulant, or inhibitors of factor VIII, V, IX, or XIII) can result in a similar picture. On the other hand, the body normally has small amounts of circulating anticoagulants that help prevent intravascular coagulation. These

include antithrombin III and the vitamin K–dependent proteins S and C. Their absence can lead to a marked increase in the incidence of intravascular thrombosis, especially venous thrombosis. The blood must be kept liquid and flowing at all times to maintain an adequate supply of oxygen to all tissues, and clot formation must be allowed to occur only at the site of vessel ruptures.

In addition to the complex, highly regulated process of clot formation, the body maintains an equally complex system for the removal of clots after they have served their purpose in stopping bleeding and the damaged vessel has been repaired. This is the process of fibrinolysis, in which the fibrin clot is digested enzymatically. Clotting factors such as activated Hageman's factor (clotting factor XIIa) act on the circulating plasmin precursor plasminogen to convert it to plasmin, which acts to digest the fibrin clot. Thus, the complex process of clot formation and dissolution is highly regulated by a large series of proteins, excess or deficiency of any one of which can lead to major abnormalities in the clotting process.

Disorders of the Hematopoietic System and Their Manifestation

Because the three major functions of the hematopoietic systems are to distribute oxygen and nutritional elements to all cells of the body, to protect the organism from invading microbes, and to regulate hemostasis, primary and secondary abnormalities of the hematopoietic system are usually manifested by organ and tissue ischemia (anemia), overwhelming infections (neutropenia), and intravascular thrombosis (activation of the clotting cascade) or bleeding (thrombocytopenia or deficiency of one or more of the procoagulants). These are frequently life threatening and require intensive care to maintain life and return the patient to a state of relative good health.

Most disorders manifested by abnormalities of the hematopoietic system are secondary to abnormalities of some other organ system. Thus, severe anemia in the adult is more often due to blood loss secondary to gastrointestinal cancer or an ulcer than to primary failure of the bone marrow as seen in aplastic anemia, leukemia, or myelodysplasia. Because blood perfuses all organs of the body, abnormalities of any organ can be reflected as abnormalities of the blood. Kidney failure can lead to decreased erythropoietin production, which results in severe anemia. Congestion of the spleen can lead to severe reductions in white blood cell (neutropenia) and platelet (thrombocytopenia) counts because of sequestration of those cellular elements in the engorged organ. Parietal cell failure in the stomach secondary to an autoimmune disorder leads to failure of intrinsic factor production and inability to absorb vitamin B_{12}, resulting in severe anemia, leukopenia, and thrombocytopenia. Most of the disorders of the hematopoietic system that are secondary to disease in another organ result in a deficiency of one or more of the normal elements in the peripheral blood. However, occasionally there is secondary overproduction of hematopoietic factors, such as the erythrocytosis associated with increased erythropoietin production by neoplasms of the kidney or cerebellum or the hypoxia of severe chronic lung disease. Neutrophilia frequently accompanies severe infections, and thrombocytosis can be seen with a variety of tumors and after acute bleeding. Except for the erythrocytosis secondary to erythropoietin-producing tumors, these cytoses seldom result in clinically significant problems.

Because blood perfuses all living tissues of the body, disorders of any organ may be reflected as abnormalities of any of the elements of the blood. The most common causes of hematopoietic abnormalities are those secondary to dysfunction of other organs. For example, anemia is one of the most common early signs of a gastrointestinal neoplasm because of blood loss from the tumor's surface. Polycythemia (erythrocytosis) is frequently seen as manifestation of pulmonary disorders. Jaundice (hyperbilirubinemia) may be the first indication of hepatic disorders, and uremia and subsequent platelet dysfunctions may be the first indications of renal disorders.

Primary disorders of the hematopoietic system, which can lead to the need for intensive care, may be divided into qualitative and quantitative disorders and congenital (inherited) and acquired ones. Qualitative disorders of an inherited type include sickle cell disease and thalassemia, in which defective red blood cells are produced; Glanzmann's thrombocytopenia, in which qualitatively defective platelets are produced; and chronic granulomatous disease, in which neutrophils and monocytes can ingest but cannot destroy catalase-positive microorganisms. Qualitative disorders of the hematopoietic system of an acquired type include iron deficiency anemias, in which the lack of iron leads to a deficiency of hemoglobin in the red blood cells and decreased oxygen-carrying capacity. In uremia, platelet aggregation is decreased, resulting in markedly prolonged bleeding times that can result in serious and occasionally life-threatening bleeding problems.

Quantitative disorders of the hematopoietic elements may be hereditary (usually congenital) or acquired. Quantitative hereditary disorders include the severe thalassemias, in which little or no hemoglobin is produced and red blood cells are rapidly lysed by the excess globin chains that are produced, resulting in severe anemia and low red blood cell numbers. Congenital neutropenia (Kostmann's syndrome) was usually fatal early in infancy because of overwhelming bacterial infections but now appears to respond to treatment with exogenous granulocyte-stimulating growth factors. Amegakaryocytic thrombocytopenia, Wiskott-Aldrich syndrome, and the May-Hegglin anomaly result in severe thrombocytopenia in the newborn. In some congenital (inherited) disorders, the cytopenia is manifest long after birth; for example, individuals with Fanconi's anemia appear to inherit a condition predisposing to the development of mono-, di-, or pancytopenia at some time after birth. Acquired deficiencies of cells of any of the hematopoietic lineages can result from a variety of disorders. Failure of production, as in cobalamine or folic acid deficiency, can result in low numbers of red blood cells, platelets, and phagocytic white blood cells. Toxic agents (cancer chemotherapeutic agents, benzene, and many drugs) may inhibit the production of any or all lineages or destroy already formed elements, leading to thrombocytopenia, leukopenia, or erythrocytopenia. Phenylhydrazine lyses red blood cells. Drug-antibody complexes destroy platelets and in some cases neutrophils as well. Benzene and chloramphenicol are two of many agents capable of destroying bone marrow. In some individuals, this leads to severe pancytopenia (aplastic anemia), one of the most life threatening of all hematopoietic disorders.

Of the primary disorders of the hematopoietic system that frequently lead to situations requiring intensive care, neoplastic disorders are perhaps the most common. Because of their nature and the therapies developed for them, acute leukemias of myeloid or lymphoid type and Hodgkin's and non-Hodgkin's lymphomas frequently require and respond well to intensive medical treatment.[14-19] This group of disorders first demonstrated significant responses to the developing armamentarium of anticancer drugs. Even today, they are among the disorders most successfully treated with these agents. Because of the agents' toxicity, especially to the

hematopoietic system, they were originally used primarily by hematologists, and it was in the subspecialty of hematology that much of the early development of medical oncology occurred. Today, medical oncology has developed into a specialty of its own, and most of the tumors that are treated arise from nonlymphohematopoietic tissues. Also, many of the agents and combinations of agents in use today have dose-limiting toxicities associated with damage to nonhematologic organs. However, a strong relationship still exists between the two disciplines. A major factor relating hematology and oncology has to do with our understanding of neoplastic cell growth. Understanding of tumors as well as normal tissues of the hematopoietic system has helped us appreciate many of the basic principles of neoplastic transformation and growth. To a great extent, neoplastic cells share many of the characteristics of normal hematopoietic stem cells. However, unlike normal hematopoietic cells, they are capable of unlimited proliferation without commitment or further differentiation. Both hematopoietic stem cells and cancer cells are capable of metastasis and subsequent clonogenic growth. In the neoplastic cells, unlike all but the most primitive hematopoietic stem cells, proliferation is no longer linked to differentiation, and neoplastic cells are capable of an unlimited number of cell divisions without further maturation toward the terminally differentiated nondividing state.

BASIC PRINCIPLES OF NEOPLASTIC PROLIFERATION[20-25]

As a result of the dissociation of proliferation and differentiation in neoplastic cells, there is poorly controlled or uncontrolled proliferation of clonally derived cells capable of infiltrating surrounding tissues and metastasizing to distant locations. Clonal proliferation ensues when the neoplastic transforming event occurs in one particular cell and endows it with a growth advantage, so that all the neoplastic cells are progeny of (form a clone of) the transformed cell. Studies of the inactivated X chromosome in tumors of women heterozygous for X-linked enzyme defects and studies of visible chromosomal abnormalities demonstrate that all neoplastic cells have the same acquired chromosomally endowed characteristics. This implies clonal origin of the tumor cells. Because the ability to metastasize is also characteristic of neoplastic cells, clonogenic cells can leave the primary site of the neoplasm; migrate via the blood stream, lymphatics, or a cavity (peritoneal or pleural) to another site; take up residence; proliferate; and establish a secondary clone of neoplastic cells.

This unrestricted growth of the neoplastic cells can lead to life-threatening situations that frequently require intensive medical support and care. The disorders fall into three categories. First, the uncontrolled infiltrative growth of the neoplasm can replace and destroy an essential organ (e.g., lung, liver, brain, and bone), impairing its function to the point of serious consequences for the patient. Second, the physical presence of the tumor can disrupt a needed passage; examples are obstruction of the gastrointestinal tract, obstruction of a bronchus, disruption of a major vessel resulting in obstruction or rupture, and compression of a neurologic tract or ureter. Third, tumors may produce substances that cause secondary problems, such as immunoglobulins, leading to hyperviscosity of the blood in multiple myeloma, hyperaldosteronism in small-cell carcinomas of the lung, hypercalcemia in breast cancer, and intravascular thrombosis, seen especially with acute progranulocytic leukemia and pancreatic carcinomas.

Thus, various acute, severe, life-threatening disorders are often observed in patients with neoplastic disorders. In the following chapters we address specific disorders of the hematopoietic system and those secondary to neoplastic disorders requiring intensive medical care, as well as those attributable to abnormalities of the hemostatic system.

References

General Hematology

1. Wintrobe MM, Lee GR, Boggs DR, et al: Clinical Hematology. 8th ed. Philadelphia, Lea & Febiger, 1981.
2. Hoffman R, Benz EJ Jr, Shattil SJ, et al (eds): Hematology: Basic Principles and Practice. New York, Churchill Livingstone, 1991.
3. Williams WJ, Beutler E, Erslev AJ, et al: Hematology. 4th ed. New York, McGraw-Hill, 1990.
4. Nathan DG, Oski FA: Hematology of Infancy and Childhood. 3rd ed. Philadelphia, WB Saunders, 1987.
5. Dacie JV, Lewis SM: Practical Haematology. 6th ed. Edinburgh, Churchill Livingstone, 1984.
6. Babior BM, Stossel TP: Hematology—A Pathophysiological Approach. New York, Churchill Livingstone, 1984.
7. Jandl JH: Blood. Boston, Little, Brown, 1987.

Growth Factors and Regulation of Hematopoiesis

8. Metcalf D: The molecular biology and functions of the granulocyte-macrophage colony stimulating factors. Blood 67:257, 1986.
9. Clark SC, Kamen R: The human hematopoietic colony-stimulating factors. Science 236:1229, 1987.
10. Sieff CA: Hematopoietic growth factors. J Clin Invest 79:1549, 1987.
11. Morstyn G, Burgess AW: Hematopoietic growth factors: A review. Cancer Res 48:5625, 1988.
12. Golde DW (ed): Hematopoietic growth factors. Hematol Oncol Clin North Am 3:369, 1989.
13. Robinson BE, Quesenberry PJ: Hematopoietic growth factors: Overview and clinical applications. Am J Med Sci 300:163, 237, 311, 1990.

Hematopoietic Malignancies

14. Rees JKH, Gray RG, Swirsky D, et al: Principal results of the Medical Research Council's 8th acute myeloid leukaemia trial. Lancet 2:1236, 1986.
15. Yates J, Gledwell O, Wiernik P, et al: Cytosine arabinoside with daunorubicin or adriamycin for therapy of acute myelocytic leukemia: A CALGB study. Blood 60:454, 1982.
16. Bloomfield CD (ed): Adult Leukemias 1. The Hague, Martinus Nijhoff, 1982.
17. Hoelzer D, Thiel E, Loffler H, et al: Intensified therapy of acute lymphoblastic and acute undifferentiated leukemia in adults. Blood 64:38, 1984.
18. Bonadonna G, Santoro A, Viviani S, et al: Treatment strategies for Hodgkin's disease. Semin Hematol 25:51, 1988.
19. DeVita VT, Hubbard SM, Lorgo DL: The chemotherapy of lymphomas: Looking back, moving forward—The Richard and Hinda Rosenthal Foundation Award Lecture. Cancer Res 47:5810, 1987.

General Neoplastic Disorders

20. Ackerman LV, del Regato JH: Cancer: Diagnosis, Treatment, and Prognosis. 6th ed. St Louis, CV Mosby, 1985.
21. DeVita VT Jr, Hellman S, Rosenberg SA (eds): Cancer: Principles and Practice of Oncology. 2nd ed. Philadelphia, JB Lippincott, 1985.
22. Knudson AG Jr: Hereditary cancer, oncogenes, and anti-oncogenes. Cancer Res 45:1437, 1985.
23. Chabner B: Pharmacologic Principles of Cancer Treatment. Philadelphia, WB Saunders, 1982.
24. Vaeth JW (ed): Combined Effects of Chemotherapy and Radiotherapy on Normal Tissue Tolerance. New York, Karger, 1979.
25. Calabresi P, Schein PS, Rosenberg SA (eds): Medical Oncology. New York, Macmillan, 1987.

CHAPTER 116

Bone Marrow Failure and Transplantation

Lyle L. Sensenbrenner

Bone Marrow Failure

Bone marrow failure states are due primarily to a quantitative defect in the production of hematopoietic mature end-stage cells. They have been reviewed by a number of authors.[1-6] Although qualitative defects of the mature cells can lead to similar types of syndromes, we mention them only briefly in this section. Disease processes causing an inordinate demand for or consumption of cellular elements leading to cytopenia are also not considered here.

The production of hematopoietic end-stage mature cells is a dynamic process in which millions of end-stage cells are produced every second.[7] The average adult produces about 2×10^{11} new red blood cells every day, about an equal number of platelets, and about one third as many granulocytes to maintain an adequate number of mature hematopoietic elements in the body to ensure good health. In times of stress, this number can be increased manyfold in response to various humoral stimuli.[8] In this section we consider conditions in which the production of mature hematopoietic end-stage cells is inadequate to meet the normal needs of the individual and a significant decrease or absence of one or more of the formed elements in the blood occurs.

PATHOPHYSIOLOGY

Normal hematopoiesis is an orderly process in which cell proliferation linked with maturation proceeds at a rate capable of maintaining an adequate concentration of end-stage mature cellular elements of each of the various types (red blood cells, granulocytes, monocytes, platelets, and lymphocytes) to maintain a state of good health. This process is controlled by a number of humoral and cellular regulators acting in the delicately structured microenvironment of the bone marrow. The entire hematopoietic system is dependent on the vitality of a small pool of the most primitive stem cells, which give rise to committed early progenitor cells of both the hematopoietic and the lymphoid systems (Fig. 116–1). True self-renewal, possibly even limitless self-renewal, appears to be a property of only the most primitive lymphohematopoietic stem cell. All progeny of that stem cell appear to be significantly limited in their self-renewal capabilities and committed to a degree of maturation with each subsequent division. Only if the stem cell pool remains intact and viable can one have lifelong replacement of the needed number of mature lymphohematopoietic cells.

The progeny of the primitive stem cell are committed to differentiate by a multistep process into the mature cells of each of the various lineages. It has been estimated that between 30 and 40 cell divisions occur between the most primitive stem cell and the final mature cellular element. Each division is associated with a degree of maturation and commitment to a particular lineage. Thus, from a single primitive hematopoietic stem cell, between 10^9 and 10^{12}

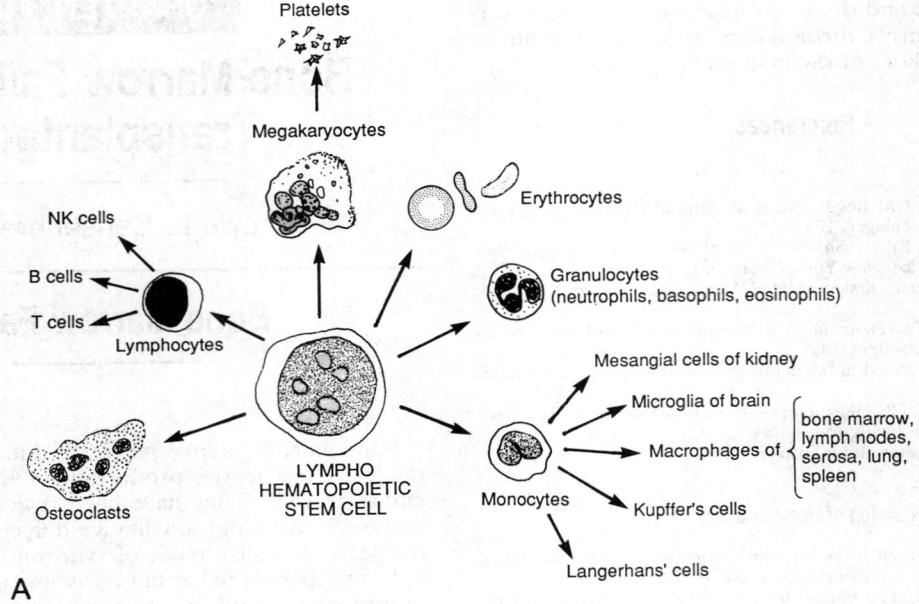

A

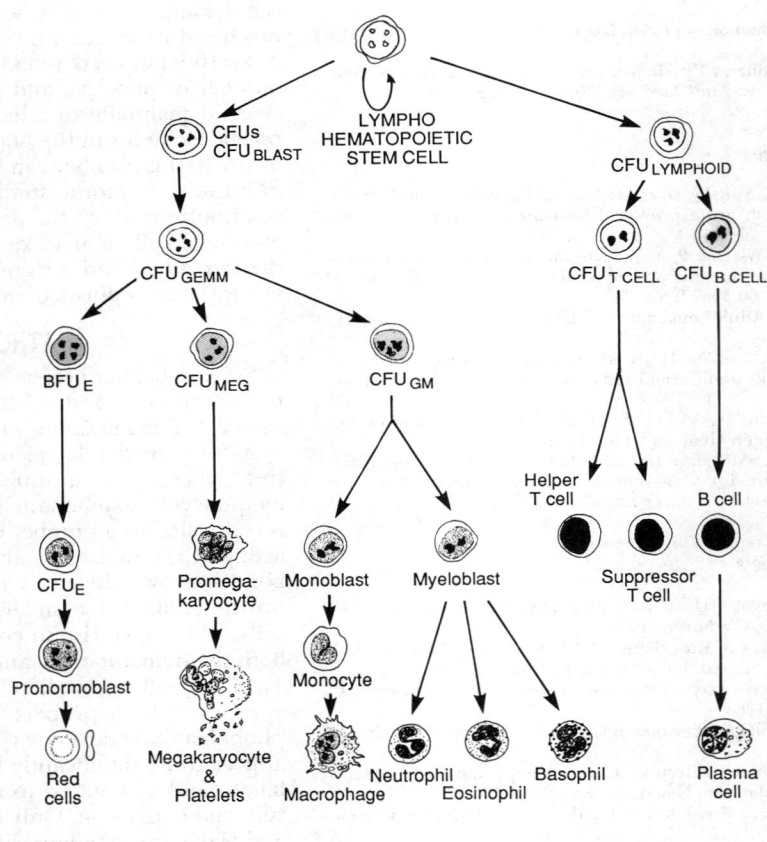

B

Figure 116–1. Hematopoiesis. *A.* End-stage cells derived from the lymphohematopoietic stem cell. *B.* Geneology of the lymphohematopoietic cell system. NK = natural killer; CFU = colony-forming unit; BFU = burst-forming unit; S = spleen; GEMM = granulocyte, erythrocyte, megakaryocyte, monocyte; E = erythrocyte; MEG = megakaryocyte; GM = granulocyte-monocyte.

mature blood cells can be produced. Failure of the primitive hematopoietic stem cell or any of the subsequent progenitor pools can quickly lead to significant numeric deficiencies in one or more of the mature cell populations.

Bone marrow failure can result from a primary or intrinsic defect of the progenitor cells or from a defect in the regulatory microenvironment in which they proliferate and mature. The defects can be either congenital or acquired, and they may be manifested as a deficiency in the mature cellular elements of one or several lineages. Occasionally, it is possible to identify a deficiency (vitamin B_{12} or folate), toxin (benzene exposure or cancer chemotherapeutic agent), or host factor (autoimmune antibody to red blood cell precursors or platelets) that is responsible for the cytopenia, but often no such factor can be delineated. The level of differentiation at which the defect is expressed to a great extent determines which cell lines are deficient. If the defect is manifested at the level of the most primitive stem cell, all lineages are involved and pancytopenia ensues with deficiencies of red blood cells, granulocytes, monocytes, platelets, and eventually lymphocytes. If the defect is at the level of the colony-forming units—granulocyte, erythrocyte, megakaryocyte, monocyte (see Fig. 116–1A), all hematopoietic but no lymphoid lineages are deficient, whereas if the defect is first expressed at the colony-forming units–granulocyte, monocyte level, a deficiency of only granulocytes and monocytes results. The cells at the level of differentiation and maturation at which the defect is initially manifested and all subsequent stages of cells are deficient. Therefore, a defect manifested at the blast-forming units–erythrocyte level results in a deficiency of detectable erythrocyte blast-forming units and colony-forming units and all red blood cell precursors, as well as mature red blood cells.

COMPLICATIONS OF BONE MARROW FAILURE
Red Blood Cell Aplasia or Hypoplasia

The onset of anemia after even sudden complete cessation of red blood cell production tends to be gradual. The hemoglobin level falls about 1 g/wk. With the hemoglobin level falling at this rate, the patient tends to compensate for the decreased oxygen-carrying capacity of the blood until the anemia is extremely severe, resulting in very slow onset of symptoms at a relatively low level of hemoglobin. The intensity of the symptoms and signs seen in any anemia, regardless of the cause, is determined by four major factors: the rate of onset, the extent to which the hemoglobin concentration has been lowered, the degree of blood volume reduction, and the adequacy of cardiorespiratory compensation. Because the onset of the anemia is often gradual, the compensation is great. The patient does not demonstrate any symptoms until the hemoglobin level has reached 5 g or less per deciliter of blood, at which point nearly all patients begin to demonstrate signs and symptoms of tissue hypoxia. The major organs demonstrating this hypoxia are the heart (angina, congestive heart failure), central nervous system (headache, vertigo, tinnitus, faintness, drowsiness, lack of concentration, weakness), kidney (proteinuria, retention of water and sodium), and skin (pallor).

As anemia develops, compensatory mechanisms are set in place. The initial compensatory mechanisms are primarily cardiovascular. Blood is diverted from the skin and kidneys and cardiac output is increased. Initially, the cardiac output is increased primarily by an increase in the stroke volume. As the hemoglobin level drops below 5 g/dL, tachycardia usually accompanies the increased stroke volume to allow greater minute volume. The oxygen dissociation curve is shifted to the right by an increased 2,3-diphosphoglyceric

acid level. This allows the blood to give up its oxygen to the tissues much more easily. As the anemia increases in severity, the arteriovenous differential in oxygen concentration begins to fall as the velocity of the blood flow increases. Decreasing peripheral vascular resistance and increasing respiratory effort to compensate for the decreased pulmonary circulation time, and oxygen-carrying capacity of the blood can eventually lead to a hyperdynamic state whose needs the heart is incapable of meeting. This can lead to congestive failure (high-output failure state), which can readily progress to severe angina caused by left ventricular hypoxia, even though there is frequently a marked increase in coronary blood flow. Pulmonary edema is common and can be precipitated by injudicious administration of blood transfusions in these patients.

The primary approach to therapy of the anemia of these patients is transfusion of plasma-depleted red blood cells. When transfusing, great care must be taken to prevent circulatory overload and acute pulmonary edema. Continuous monitoring of central venous pressure is often necessary when transfusing a severely anemic patient (hemoglobin level less than 5 g/dL). Exchange transfusion is frequently necessary to prevent complications. Whenever the venous pressure begins to rise, the transfusion is stopped and blood is removed from the patient until the venous pressure is reduced, at which time the transfusion can be restarted. The rate of infusion of plasma-depleted red blood cells in these patients should never exceed 1 mL/kg/h and often should be much slower with exchange techniques used to prevent acute, even fatal pulmonary edema. Rapid transfusion of blood is needed only in cases of acute and severe blood loss. When the marrow failure and resulting severe anemia are secondary to a known replaceable defect (e.g., vitamin B_{12} deficiency, iron deficiency, and hemolysis), correction of the underlying defect or replacement of the missing vitamins without transfusing the patient is frequently all that is needed and is much safer for the patient.

White Blood Cell Failure

Here we consider only failure of the phagocytic cell system (granulocytes and monocyte-macrophages). The major clinical manifestations that we recognize at present are acute infections, usually bacterial, related to the severe neutropenia developed by these patients.[9] If the neutrophils produced are normal, these patients usually have no increased infection problems until their neutrophil counts fall below $500/mm^3$ ($5 \times 10^8/L$) of blood. The condition may be the only hematologic abnormality (agranulocytosis) or be part of a full-blown picture of bone marrow failure and pancytopenia. The major problems encountered by patients with severe neutropenia are those of overwhelming bacterial or fungal infections. These infections tend to be bacterial when they occur early in the course of the neutropenia and both bacterial and fungal when the neutropenia has been present for prolonged periods. The onset of drug-induced agranulocytosis is usually fairly abrupt, with a prodromal period that may be accompanied by chills, fever, and a sense of malaise. These are probably the symptoms of initial damage to the granulocytic system. This is followed by a short period (about a week) in which there is relative freedom from symptoms as the granulocyte count falls. Abrupt onset of severe overwhelming symptoms of a rapidly progressive bacterial infection usually follows. These infections most frequently arise in an area that normally harbors bacteria, such as the throat and mouth or the perianal area. Occasionally, the source of infection involves the skin, nose, sinus, or genital area. Sepsis, with shock, often follows rapidly, and septicemia is frequently confirmed.

In patients in whom idiopathic pancytopenia secondary to acquired aplastic anemia results in severe neutropenia, the prodromal symptoms frequently are not seen. In such cases, thrombocytopenia and anemia frequently accompany the severe neutropenia. In isolated agranulocytosis, the peripheral blood examination reveals a low white blood cell count with near absence of neutrophils. The total granulocyte count is usually well under 10^9/L of blood in drug-induced agranulocytosis. In patients with pancytopenia secondary to bone marrow failure, the total neutrophil count is usually less than 300/mm³ (3×10^8/L) at the time overwhelming infection and sepsis are observed. For the therapy of neutropenic infections to be successful, immediate intensive intervention is needed to prevent a rapidly fatal outcome. Patients should immediately be given intravenous broad-spectrum antimicrobial coverage, including at least two antibiotics, usually an aminoglycoside and a cephalosporin, to cover the major gram-negative organisms.[10-12] Cultures of material from all orifices and body fluids should be initiated immediately. If an organism is identified, proper adjustments of the antibiotics should be made. If careful physical examination reveals a potential source of gram-positive organisms (*Staphylococcus aureus* or *Staphylococcus epidermidis*), adequate coverage with vancomycin should be added as well. In cases of isolated agranulocytosis, all potentially causative agents should be withdrawn and scrupulously avoided. Antibiotics should be continued until the patient recovers adequate granulocytes (in cases of agranulocytosis responding to cessation of the offending agent).[13] If there is no recovery of granulocytes, the following guidelines may be used:

1. Start all patients with prolonged granulocytopenia on an oral gut decontamination regimen (e.g., norfloxacin and fluconazole).
2. Continue intravenous antibiotics for 14 days if an infecting organism is found; if the patient is then afebrile, slowly withdraw intravenous antibiotics and watch the patient closely.
3. If no organism has been found and the patient has been afebrile for more than 72 hours, continue oral gut-decontaminating antibiotics and slowly withdraw intravenous antibiotics.
4. If there is no response to antibiotics, no specific organism is found, and fever continues after 72 hours, change the antibacterial coverage. If again after 72 hours there is no response to therapy, consider other types of causative organisms, such as fungi and viruses, and institute coverage for these.

Antibodies to endotoxin are now available for clinical use. Their application in cases of severe gram-negative infections in which endotoxemic shock is imminent or pending appears to be of great value in overcoming and reversing fatal endotoxemic shock. Their use must be initiated early in the course of the infection in the neutropenic patient. Systemic antibiotics must still be used at the same dosage and for the same duration of time.[14-17] In addition, these patients require intensive supportive care—red blood cell transfusions to keep the hemoglobin concentration above 9 g/dL and, if the patient is thrombocytopenic, platelet transfusions to keep the platelet count above 20,000/mm³ (2×10^{10}/L). In the presence of sepsis, platelet survival may be markedly shortened, and increased numbers of transfusions must be given.

Granulocyte transfusions may be considered but should be used only in life-threatening situations in which there is evidence that the period of severe neutropenia (neutrophil count less than 300/mm³ [3×10^8/L]) is probably limited and an organism is causing the infection that antibiotics cannot treat (proved to be unresponsive to appropriate therapy).[18-20] If granulocytes are used, they should be used daily because their half-life is short. There should be about 5×10^{10} neutrophils per transfusion (between 5×10^8 and 10^9/kg body weight) to obtain significant results. Reactions to granulocytes can be severe and even life threatening. Fever and chills are common, and severe respiratory distress may be caused by sequestration of agglutinated granulocytes in the pulmonary circulation. Leukoagglutinins present in the recipient are thought to be a major cause of these reactions. Some decrease in reactions may result if the donor and recipient are human leukocyte antigen (HLA) matched. Like other blood products, granulocytes can transmit bacteria, viruses, or parasitics. Granulocyte transfusions may contain large numbers of contaminating lymphocytes, and immunosuppressed patients receiving them may develop a severe, usually fatal type of graft-versus-host disease (GVHD). Therefore, any cells to be transfused to immunosuppressed patients must be preirradiated with at least 1500 and preferably 3000 rad to prevent engraftment of lymphocytes.

Large amounts of intravenous electrolyte or colloid solutions may be needed to maintain an adequate blood pressure if septic shock ensues. Steroids are frequently of limited value in patients with severe septic shock or evidence of underlying adrenal insufficiency. Reports that compounds that block tumor necrosis factor may be useful in sepsis are encouraging and need confirmation.[21] Granulocyte colony-stimulating factor (G-CSF) and granulocyte-macrophage colony-stimulating factor (GM-CSF) are now available and may be of value for some patients with life-threatening neutropenia.[22-24] They have been shown to shorten the period of neutropenia after bone marrow transplantation and chemotherapy. Their value in treating the pancytopenia of patients with aplastic anemia has been limited. Most patients with the most severe granulocytopenia (granulocyte count less than 200/mm³ [2×10^8/L]) have not shown a significant response. However, G-CSF and GM-CSF have not caused serious toxicity, and their prompt use in these situations is justified.

Failure to Produce Adequate Numbers of Platelets

Platelets are essential elements in normal hemostasis. They adhere to the surface of damaged endothelium and initiate the formation of either an effective platelet plug or a thrombus via the release of platelet products. Normally, the level of circulating platelets ranges between 150,000 and 450,000/mm³ (1.5×10^{11} and 4.5×10^{11}/L). Platelets are cytoplasmic fragments of megakaryocytes, bone marrow cells derived from the hematopoietic stem cell. Megakaryocytes constitute approximately 0.05% of all bone marrow cells.[25] When the number of megakaryocytes in the bone marrow decreases, so does the number of circulating platelets. This decrease in circulating platelets leads to bleeding manifestations whose severity is inversely proportional to the concentration of circulating platelets (Table 116–1).

In cases of bone marrow failure, platelet deficiency (thrombocytopenia) and subsequent hemorrhagic manifestations are frequently the presenting complaints, and hemorrhage is often the cause of death.[26] Thrombocytopenia is defined as a platelet count less than 150,000/mm³ (1.5×10^{11}/L). The defect in thrombocytopenia is either increased destruction or, as with erythrocyte or neutrophil deficiencies, decreased production of the mature cell product. Decreased platelet production may be due to a decreased pool of progenitors, ineffective thrombocytopoiesis despite a normal number of progenitors, or, rarely, abnormal controls of thrombocytopoiesis or may be part of the picture of total bone marrow failure and pancytopenia. In thrombocytopenia caused by hypoproliferation of megakaryocytes, bone

TABLE 116–1
PLATELET LEVELS AND BLEEDING

Level	Signs and Symptoms
>50,000/mm³ (>50 × 10⁹/L)	No signs or symptoms; slight prolongation of bleeding time if less than 100,000/mm³ (1 × 10¹¹/L)
20,000–50,000/mm³ (20–50 × 10⁹/L)	Mild prolongation of bleeding time; increased incidence of bruises, occasional petechiae or epistaxis
10,000–20,000/mm³ (10–20 × 10⁹/L)	Petechiae, sometimes ecchymosis; moderate prolongation of bleeding time; bleeding from pre-existing lesions
5000–10,000/mm³ (5–10 × 10⁹/L)	Severe prolongation of bleeding time; severe ecchymosis and petechiae; frequent uncontrolled bleeding from pre-existing lesions
0–5000/mm³ (0–5 × 10⁹/L)	Severe, life-threatening spontaneous hemorrhage

marrow examination shows a decreased number of megakaryocytes, although the size of those present may be increased. The survival of the platelets produced is normal, but the total platelet mass, production rate, and splenic pool are decreased. The causes of thrombocytopenia are listed in Table 116–2. The manifestation of thrombocytopenia is primary bleeding. The severity and type of bleeding are usually directly related to the platelet count. If the platelets are functioning normally, there are usually no detectable bleeding abnormalities when the platelet count is 50,000/mm³ (5×10^{10}/L) or greater. There may be a slight prolongation of the bleeding time when the platelet count is between 50,000 and 100,000/mm³ (5×10^{10} and 10×10^{10}/L). Most surgery is safe if the platelet count is greater than 50,000/mm³ (5×10^{10}/L).

Megakaryocyte Failure and Subsequent Thrombocytopenia

When the platelet count falls below 50,000/mm³ (5×10^{10}/L), patients experience an increase in bruising and frequently state that they have multiple bruises that cannot be accounted for by trauma. When the platelet count drops to 20,000/mm³ (2×10^{10}/L), the onset of spontaneous petechiae can often be seen. At this level one frequently observes onset of bleeding from pre-existing lesions such as peptic ulcers, mucous membrane abrasions, and skin erosions. As the platelet count decreases further, the severity of the petechiae increases, ecchymoses appear, and more frequent spontaneous bleeding is observed. Epistaxis, bleeding from the gums, and hematuria are frequently seen. Severe, often lethal bleeding can be observed at platelet levels as high as 20,000/mm³ (2×10^{10}/L) but is usually seen at 5000/mm³ (5×10^9/L) or less. At any platelet count, bleeding from pre-existing lesions is more likely than spontaneous bleeding from previously nonbleeding sites. However, at extremely low platelet counts (less than 5000/mm³ [5×10^9/L]) spontaneous, life-threatening bleeding often occurs. Epistaxis, severe diffuse gastrointestinal (GI) hemorrhage, hematuria, and sudden severe fatal intracranial hemorrhage may be observed.

BLOOD PRODUCT SUPPORT
Red Blood Cell Transfusions

Except in cases of acute severe blood loss, patients who are severely anemic should be given packed red blood cells.

If a patient is bleeding severely, transfusion of whole fresh blood is in order. In patients with severe anemia secondary to bone marrow failure syndromes but no severe cardiac or renal disease, one usually tries to maintain a hemoglobin level of at least 8 g/dL. In patients with bleeding associated with extremely low platelet levels, it is suggested that the hemoglobin level be kept above 10 g/dL. If the patient is immunosuppressed and has bone marrow failure, it is essential that all blood products, including red blood cells, be irradiated with at least 1500 rad to prevent the occurrence of GVHD as a result of the transfusion of viable lymphocytes. Frequent transfusions of red blood cells eventually lead to increased body stores of iron and secondary hemochromatosis. To help prevent the development of iron overload syndromes or treating those that develop, the early use of a chelating agent such as deferoxamine to enhance iron excretion is recommended. Caution must be used in transfusing patients who have extremely low hemoglobin levels or evidence of congestive heart failure. In such cases it is frequently necessary to transfuse the patient very slowly (less than 1 mL of red blood cells per kilogram of body weight per hour) while removing an equal volume of whole blood from the patient. Patients who receive many transfusions over a prolonged period, as many bone marrow failure patients do, frequently develop severe reactions to red blood cell transfusion. These reactions are usually due to serum or white blood cell products contaminating the transfusion and can be ameliorated by use of a white blood cell filter and/or washing the red blood cells before transfusion.

White Blood Cell Transfusions

At present, white blood cell transfusions are rarely recommended for patients with bone marrow failure. They are considered only for patients who have a granulocyte count persistently less than 300/mm³ (3×10^8/L) and evidence of an infection that is both life threatening and nonresponsive to antibiotics. Because the complications of white blood cell transfusions are serious and frequent (severe febrile reactions, obstruction of small vessels in the lungs, sensitization and severe allergic reactions, and even anaphylaxis), one must be certain that antibiotics cannot do what one expects from the white blood cells. In some patients with bone marrow failure, the granulocyte count may be elevated in response to a course of either G-CSF or GM-CSF.[27–29] Unfortunately, the patients with the lowest granulocyte counts are usually the ones who respond least.[30] These growth factors have relatively moderate toxicity, and it is worthwhile to use them in such situations. If one does decide to use white blood cell transfusions, they should be given once a day for at least 7 and preferably 14 days. In patients able to tolerate them they can be lifesaving.

Platelet Transfusions

In general, one tries to maintain a platelet level of at least 20,000/mm³ (2×10^{10}/L) in patients with bone marrow failure. The count should be higher if the patient is to undergo a procedure or bleeds spontaneously at a platelet count of 20,000/mm³ (2×10^{10}/L) or greater. For surgical procedures, except superficial ones, the platelet count should be at least 50,000/mm³ (5×10^{10}/L). However, because bone marrow failure states are frequently prolonged, often lasting several months or years, patients treated with platelet transfusions often become sensitized to platelets and fail to respond with an increment in platelet count to all except perfectly matched (HLA class I antigen identical) products. To prevent such sensitization, these patients should be transfused with as few products as possible. Therefore,

TABLE 116–2

CAUSES AND THERAPY OF THROMBOCYTOPENIA

Cause	Therapy

Failure of production
  Bone marrow failure
  Myelophthisis/leukemia, lymphoma, fibrosis, infiltration storage disorders, cancers, osteopetrosis
	Transfuse platelets as necessary to treat underlying disease.

Deficiency disorders (vitamin B₁₂ folic acid)	Replace missing vitamins; rarely need platelet transfusion.
Increased destruction Idiopathic thrombocytopenic purpura	Treat with steroids, intravenous immunoglobulin, and/or splenectomy. Platelet transfusion is of little value.
Immune mediated	Steroids remove offending agent. Transfusion is of little value.
Post-transfusional purpura	Platelets are ineffective and may exacerbate syndrome. Pheresis is of value. Intravenous immunoglobulin is of value. Steroids may be of value.
Disseminated intravascular coagulation	Rarely severe. If patient is bleeding, platelets may be given.
Thrombotic thrombocytopenic purpura	Platelet transfusion is contraindicated. Pheresis, steroids, and anticoagulants are of value.
Platelet sequestration resulting from hypersplenism	Treat underlying cause of splenomegaly if possible. Perform splenectomy if disorder is not responsive to medical therapy.

patients who demonstrate no bleeding at a platelets level as low as 5000/mm³ (5×10^9/L) may not be transfused but rather are carefully watched.

Although it has never been proved, it is theoretically possible that the use of single-donor platelets delays the onset or degree of platelet sensitization. Thus, if possible, one should try to use single donors. The use of leukocyte-poor blood products (both red blood cells and platelets) helps to delay the onset of severe allosensitization because contaminating lymphocytes are the major source of sensitizing antigens.[31, 32] Therefore, one should use as few blood products as possible, as leukocyte-poor blood products as possible, and a white blood cell trap in the administration set. This is especially true for patients who may have bone marrow transplantation in the future because prevention of immunization to potential donors is essential to a successful outcome.[33, 34]

Patients showing no response to platelet transfusions from random donors often respond to platelets from a donor who matches at the HLA-A and HLA-B loci (class I antigens). Platelets express only class I HLA antigens, so only these must be matched to prevent the platelets from being destroyed by antibodies to transplantation antigens. It is thought that other platelet antigens play only a small role in the diminished increments seen in sensitized patients. The HLA matching often need not be perfect. All that is needed is that the platelet donor not have any class I antigens that are not already on the recipient's cells.

Patients with bone marrow failure syndromes who require frequent transfusion support often develop severe reactions to almost any blood product and require large doses of premedications to control these reactions. These patients may have anaphylactoid reactions if they are not properly premedicated.

TREATMENT OF THE UNDERLYING DISORDERS AND THEIR COMPLICATIONS
Bone Marrow Transplantation

This is the definitive therapy for severe bone marrow failure in patients who are younger than 60 years of age and have no other serious organ failures. If no HLA-matched donor is available in the patient's family, unrelated donors can now be found for a fairly high percentage of patients. However, at present, unrelated donor transplantations are usually restricted to patients younger than 40 years of age. Overall, about 80 to 90% of patients who have bone marrow transplantation now have a good outcome.[35, 36]

Immunosuppressive Regimens

For patients for whom bone marrow transplantation is not an option, immunosuppressive regimens have been helpful in 30 to 50%.[37–40] Although most of these patients do not regain normal blood counts, many show enough improvement that they no longer require blood product support. The most commonly used immunosuppressive agent is antithymocyte globulin (ATG). This serum is obtained from horses and often causes severe allergic reactions. Intravenous administration of the agent is associated with fever, chills, rashes (hives), tachycardia, and a delayed serum sickness syndrome. Some patients have even greater reactions, with wheezing, esophageal spasm, edema of the tongue, and sometimes anaphylaxis, and require intensive care monitoring and support. The reaction to ATG should be treated by slowing the infusion rate and giving intravenous hydrocortisone, diphenhydramine hydrochloride (Benadryl), and, if the reaction is extremely severe, epinephrine. When the reaction subsides, the rate of infusion should be advanced slowly to the maximal tolerated rate. Some patients who respond to the antiserum later (months to years) relapse to their state of severe bone marrow failure. In such cases a second course of immunosuppressive therapy can be cautiously instituted. A second course of ATG may result in much more severe reactions than the first course.

Supportive Measures

Prophylactic antibiotics are not routinely recommended except to decontaminate the gut in patients whose granulocyte count is persistently less than 500/mm³ (5×10^8/L). In these patients, routine use of prophylactic oral norfloxacin or trimethoprim-sulfamethoxazole and fluconazole may significantly decrease the incidence of systemic infections. Androgens have been shown in a few patients to increase the production of red blood cells and rarely the blood levels of platelets and granulocytes as well. However, large controlled studies did not demonstrate a significant effect in the treated group compared with the controls. Patients with frequent recurrent herpes simplex infections benefit from the use of prophylactic acyclovir. Patients who also have impaired immune function, decreased levels of immunoglobulins in the serum, and recurrent infections (especially viral or fungal) may benefit greatly from intravenous immunoglobulin support. However, these patients are a small fraction of those with bone marrow failure syndromes.

In general, results obtained with the granulocyte-stimulating growth factors have been disappointing thus far. The patients with the lowest granulocyte counts, who most need an effect, are generally those who are least responsive. There has been virtually no effect of the granulocyte growth factors on red blood cell or platelet levels. However, in patients with severe infection and granulocyte counts less than 500/mm³ (5×10^8/L), they should be tried as an adjunct to eradicate bacterial and fungal infections. G-CSF and GM-CSF are both available and either can be tried. Preliminary results show that interleukin-3 is no better than G-CSF or GM-CSF, and it appears to require a much longer period to raise the counts.[29]

Protective isolation, a laminar airflow room, or a germ-free bubble often markedly reduces the incidence and severity of infection in these patients and should be used if available.

References

1. Alter BP: The bone marrow failure syndromes. In Nathan DG, Oski F (eds): Hematology of Infancy and Childhood. 2nd ed. Philadelphia, WB Saunders, p 159, 1981.
2. Camilta BM, Storb R, Thomas ED: Aplastic anemia: Pathogenesis, diagnosis, treatment and prognosis. N Engl J Med 306:645, 1982.
3. Thomas ED, Storb R: Acquired aplastic anemia: Progress and perplexity. Blood 64:325, 1984.
4. Fohlmeister I, Fischer R, Modder B, et al: Aplastic anemia and the hypocellular myelodysplasias: Histomorphological diagnosis and prognostic features. J Clin Pathol 39:1218, 1985.
5. Lynch RE, Williams DM, Reading JC, et al: The prognosis in aplastic anemia. Blood 45:517, 1975.
6. Bacigalupo A, Van Lint MT, Congier M, et al: Treatment of SAA in Europe 1970–1985: A report of the SAA working party. Bone Marrow Transplant 1(suppl 1):19, 1986.
7. Lajtha LG: The common ancestral cell. In Wintrobe MM (ed): Blood Pure and Eloquent. New York, McGraw-Hill, p 81, 1980.
8. Enslev AJ: Feedback circuits in the control of stem cell differentiation. Am J Pathol 65:269, 1972.
9. Body GP, Buckley M, Sathe YS, et al: Quantitative relationships between circulating leukocytes and infection in patients with acute leukemia. Ann Intern Med 64:328, 1966.
10. Pizzo PA, Hathorn JW, Hiemenz J, et al: A randomized trial comparing ceftazidime alone with combination antibiotic therapy in cancer patients with fever and neutropenia. N Engl J Med 315:552, 1986.
11. Klastersky J: Empiric antimicrobial therapy for febrile granulocytopenic cancer patients: Lessons from four EORTC trials. Recent Results Cancer Res 108:53, 1988.
12. Schimpff SC: Overview of empiric antibiotic therapy for the febrile neutropenic patient. Rev Infect Dis 7(suppl 4):S734, 1985.
13. Pizzo PA, Robichand KJ, Gill FA, et al: Duration of empiric antibiotic therapy in granulocytopenic patients with cancer. Am J Med 67:194, 1979.
14. Ziegler EJ, Fisher CJ Jr, Sprung CL, et al: Treatment of gram-negative bacteremia and septic shock with HA-1A human monoclonal antibody against endotoxin. N Engl J Med 324:429, 1991.
15. Fox JL: Antibodies against sepsis. Biotechnology 8:1240, 1990.
16. Ziegler EJ, McCutchan JA, Fierer J, et al: Treatment of gram negative bacteremia and shock with human antiserum to a mutant *Escherichia coli*. N Engl J Med 307:1225, 1982.
17. Fisher CJ, Zimmerman J, Khazeli MB, et al: Initial evaluation of human monoclonal anti–lipid A antibody (HA-1A) in patients with sepsis syndrome. Crit Care Med 18:1311, 1990.
18. Higby DJ, Yates JW, Henderson ES, et al: Filtration leukapheresis for granulocyte transfusion therapy. N Engl J Med 292:761, 1975.
19. Higby DJ, Burnett D: Granulocyte transfusion: Current status (review). Blood 55:2, 1980.
20. Quie PG: The white cells: Use of granulocyte transfusion. Rev Infect Dis 9:189, 1987.
21. Zabel P, Wolter DT, Schönharting MM, et al: Oxpentifylline in endotoxaemia. Lancet 2:1474, 1989. (Comment in: Lancet 335:543, 1990.)
22. Crawford J, Ozer H, Stoller R, et al: Reduction by granulocyte colony-stimulating factor of fever and neutropenia induced by chemotherapy in patients with small-cell lung cancer. N Engl J Med 325:164, 1991.
23. Metcalf D: The colony-stimulating factors: Discovery, development and clinical applications. Cancer 65:2185, 1990.
24. Groopman JE, Molina J-M, Scadden DT: Hematopoietic growth factors: Biology and clinical applications. N Engl J Med 321:1449, 1989.
25. Levine RF: Isolation and characterization of normal human megakaryocytes. Br J Haematol 45:487, 1980.
26. Stoll DB, Blum S, Pasquale B, et al: Thrombocytopenia with decreased megakaryocytes. Evaluation and prognosis. Ann Intern Med 94:170, 1981.
27. Vadham RS, Buescher S, Le Maistre A, et al: Stimulation of hematopoiesis in patients with bone marrow failure and in patients with malignancy by recombinant human granulocyte-macrophage colony stimulating factor. Blood 72:134, 1988.
28. Champlin RE, Miemer SD, Ireland P, et al: Treatment of refractory aplastic anemia with recombinant human granulocyte-macrophage colony stimulating factor. Blood 73:694, 1989.
29. Ganser A, Lindemann A, Seipelt G, et al: Effects of recombinant human interleukin-3 in aplastic anemia. Blood 76:1287, 1990.
30. Nissen C, Tichelli A, Gratwohl A, et al: Failure of recombinant human granulocyte-macrophage colony stimulating factor therapy in aplastic anemia patients with very severe neutropenia. Blood 72:2045, 1988.
31. Claas FHJ, Smeenk RJT, Schmidt R, et al: Alloimmunization against the MHC antigens after platelet transfusions is due to contaminating leukocytes in the platelet suspension. Exp Hematol 9:84, 1981.
32. Fisher M, Chapman JR, Ting A, et al: Alloimmunization to HLA antigens following transfusion with leukocyte-poor and purified platelet suspensions. Vox Sang 49:331, 1985.
33. Storb R, Prentice RL, Thomas ED: Marrow transplantation for aplastic anemia: Factors associated with rejection. N Engl J Med 296:61, 1977.
34. Storb R, Thomas ED, Buckner CD, et al: Marrow transplantation in 30 "untransfused" patients with severe aplastic anemia. Ann Intern Med 92:30, 1980.
35. Gluckman E: Current status of bone marrow transplantation for severe aplastic anemia: A preliminary report from the International Bone Marrow Transplant Registry. Transplant Proc 19:2597, 1987.
36. Strob R, Thomas ED, Buckner CD, et al: Allogeneic marrow grafting for treatment of aplastic anemia. Blood 43:157, 1974.
37. Frickhofen N, Kaltwasser JP, Schrezenmeier H, et al: Treatment of aplastic anemia with antilymphocyte globulin and methylprednisolone with or without cyclosporine. N Engl J Med 324:1297, 1991.
38. Camitta B, O'Reilly RJ, Sensenbrenner LL, et al: Antithoracic duct lymphocyte globulin therapy of severe aplastic anemia. Blood 62:883, 1983.
39. Hinterberger-Fischer M, Höcker P, Lechner K, et al: Oral cyclosporin-A is effective treatment for untreated and also for previously immunosuppressed patients with severe bone marrow failure. Eur J Haematol 43:136, 1989.
40. Bacigalupo A, Giordano P, Van Lint MT, et al: Bolus methylprednisolone in severe aplastic anemia. N Engl J Med 300:501, 1979.

Medical Intensive Care of the Bone Marrow Transplantation Patient

The bone marrow transplantation patient may require the care of an intensivist for two distinct categories of disorders: those arising primarily as a direct result of the transplantation (toxicity of the preparative regimen, acute GVHD) and those not related etiologically to the transplantation, but frequently occurring after it (opportunistic infections, interstitial pneumonia). Both types of complications may be seen simultaneously in the same patient. In this section we discuss both types of complications and the special consideration they must be given when they occur in a patient who has recently undergone bone marrow transplantation.

TABLE 116–3

TYPES OF BONE MARROW TRANSPLANTATION

Type of Transplantation	Hematopoietic Stem Cells	Complications
Autologous	Patient	Infections with bacteria or fungi during neutropenia; toxicity of preparative regimen; failure or slow engraftment; significant immunosuppression for 2–6 mo
Syngeneic	Identical twin	Infections with bacteria or fungi during neutropenia; toxicity of preparative regimen; significant immunosuppression for 2–4 mo
Allogeneic	Other person, not an identical twin	Infections with bacteria and fungi during neutropenia; toxicity of preparative regimen; failure to engraft; 3–36 mo of severe immunosuppression; acute and chronic GVHD; may last years

BONE MARROW TRANSPLANTATIONS

Many of the problems of transplantation patients are to a great extent determined by the type of bone marrow transplantation the patient has undergone. There are three major groups of bone marrow transplantations: autologous, syngeneic, and allogeneic (Table 116–3). These have been reviewed by a number of authors.[1–4]

Autologous Bone Marrow Transplantation

In autologous bone marrow transplantation,[5–21] used almost exclusively for the treatment of neoplastic disorders, patients have a portion of their own bone marrow (or in some cases peripheral blood) stem cells removed before the intensive pretransplantation conditioning with chemotherapy and/or radiotherapy. The marrow is frequently manipulated after collection to remove any contaminating tumor cells. After manipulation, the marrow is frozen and stored in liquid nitrogen. When the bone marrow–ablating chemo- or radiotherapy regimen has been completed, the marrow is rapidly thawed and reinfused into the patient. Autologous bone marrow transplantation is in many ways an extension of and similar to intensive chemotherapy with or without radiation therapy. In intensive chemotherapy without autologous bone marrow rescue, there is slow recovery of the patient's bone marrow, which has been severely damaged during the therapy, whereas in autologous transplantation, marrow or peripheral blood stem cells are removed before the intensive therapy (thus protected from lethal harm) and replaced afterward. Because the rate and degree of recovery of bone marrow function depend on the number and quality of residual stem and progenitor cells at the time of collection, the amount of prior cytotoxic therapy and the amount and type of prefreezing manipulation significantly influence the kinetics of the patient's bone marrow (hematopoietic) recovery after transplantation. The fewer surviving stem cells infused, the slower the recovery. Recovery may take 6 to 8 weeks in heavily pretreated patients whose marrow has been purged to remove tumor.

Syngeneic Bone Marrow Transplantation

Syngeneic bone marrow transplantation[22–25] is fairly uncommon because the bone marrow used to rescue the patient after the conditioning regimen is obtained from an identical twin (monozygotic). The situation is similar to that in autologous bone marrow transplantation except that the rescue marrow is nearly always obtained from an individual who has never been exposed to bone marrow cytotoxic therapy. In addition, the marrow need not be manipulated before transplantation to purge it of contaminating tumor cells. The donor's bone marrow is usually collected from the monozygotic twin on the day of transplantation. Because

monozygotic twins are truly identical in all genetic respects, a syngeneic bone marrow transplantation is similar to an autologous bone marrow transplantation but without the need to freeze the marrow beforehand, with no risk of tumor contamination, and with a high number of stem cells of good quality.

Allogeneic Bone Marrow Transplantation

Allogeneic bone marrow transplantation[26–33] is similar to syngeneic transplantation except that the donor bone marrow comes from an individual not genetically identical with the recipient of the bone marrow. Because HLAs are determined by genes located on the short arm (p arm) of chromosome 6 and are codominant, siblings of the same set of parents may inherit the same chromosome 6 and thus express the same set of major histocompatibility antigens. Statistically, the chance of siblings being HLA identical is one in four. Thus, about 25% of sibling pairs match for the major HLA antigens.

Most allogeneic bone marrow transplantations are carried out between HLA-identical sibling pairs, but it is sometimes possible to find family member donors who are phenotypically HLA identical with the recipient even though their chromosomes are not genetically identical. There are now international registries of volunteer donors whose HLA type has been determined and who are willing to donate their bone marrow for anyone in need of bone marrow transplantation. As a result, many bone marrow transplantations are now being performed in which the donor is not related to the recipient and there are varying degrees of phenotypic identity between the donor marrow and the recipient. In general, the degree of genotypic and phenotypic disparity between donor and recipient determines the frequency and severity of many of the bone marrow transplantation–related complications, especially recipient rejection of the donor's bone marrow and graft-versus-host reactions (Table 116–4). Thus, special complications rarely seen in autologous or syngeneic bone marrow transplantation patients are seen to varying degrees in allogeneic bone marrow transplantation patients.

Procedure

The bone marrow transplantation procedure involves exposure of a patient to intensive cytotoxic therapy that totally ablates the patient's remaining lymphohematopoietic system. This is followed by the infusion of lymphohematopoietic stem and progenitor cells that repopulate the patient's pools of cells, which are normally derived from the lymphohematopoietic stem cell. One can divide the bone marrow transplantation procedure and the related complications into several phases. During the first, or cytoreductive, phase the

TABLE 116-4

DEGREE OF IDENTITY SEEN IN BONE MARROW TRANSPLANTATIONS

Type of Transplantation	Degree of Identity	Likelihood of Rejection of GVHD
Autologous	Identical	Very unlikely
Syngeneic	Identical	Very unlikely
Allogeneic	Genetically identical siblings	25–35% chance of GVHD
	One chromosome genetically identical but other only phenotypically identical	30–50% chance of GVHD
	Phenotypically but not genotypically identical	60–80% chance of GVHD
	One antigen mismatch	60–90% chance of GVHD
	Two or more antigens mismatch	>80% chance of GVHD

patient is intensively treated with chemotherapy and/or radiotherapy to destroy any defective tissues in the body (neoplastic cells, abnormal bone marrow, abnormal immune system), as well as any remaining normal lymphohematopoietic cells, to provide a disease-free patient with adequate hematopoietic "space" and sufficient immunosuppression to allow acceptance of the donor marrow. The cytoreductive therapy is usually brief (4 to 8 days) and results in complete destruction, without the ability for recovery, of the entire lymphohematopoietic system. The most commonly utilized agent is cyclophosphamide, which is nearly always combined with one or more other agents including total or partial body irradiation, busulfan, etoposide, carmustine (bischloroethylnitrosourea, BCNU), and cytosine arabinoside. All agents are used at doses that can induce life-threatening toxicities.

The cytoreductive phase is followed by infusion of the lymphohematopoietic stem and progenitor cells, usually obtained from the donor's bone marrow. However, an adequate number of stem cells may be obtained from the peripheral or umbilical cord blood of some individuals and may be used in lieu of or in addition to cells obtained from bone marrow. Bone marrow cells from the posterior iliac crests of the donor are obtained under general or spinal anesthesia. Occasionally, the anterior iliac crests and sternum are used as well. The marrow is obtained by aspiration using large, specially adapted needles inserted into the marrow-bearing cavities. The heparinized marrow cells are then manipulated, if necessary, to remove tumor cells, incompatible red blood cells, or plasma before freezing and/or intravenous infusion. Because marrow progenitors and stem cells constantly enter and leave the bone marrow cavities via the blood stream and bone marrow endothelial cells have adhesion molecules that recognize stem cell receptors, allowing them to attach to each other, the stem cells can penetrate the marrow spaces from the blood stream. Thus, intravenous administration of the cell preparation allows the stem cells to seek out and take up residence in the bone marrow cavities.

Pathophysiology of Recovery After Bone Marrow Transplantation

The period after transplantation and the unique transplantation-related complications are best viewed with respect to the two major body systems deliberately destroyed during the transplantation procedure and the secondary disorders observed before their complete recovery. The two systems eradicated are the hematopoietic system and the lymphoid or immune system. Although several of the pretransplantation problems may persist or recur after transplantation (toxicity of preparative regimens used, persistence of the disorder for which the transplantation was done), the major complications in the post-transplantation period are due directly or indirectly to an inadequate or dysfunctional hematopoietic system or lymphoid system. At the time of the bone marrow transplantation, the patient has essentially no lymphohematopoietic system. During this phase, patients are vulnerable to bacterial, fungal, protozoan, and viral infections until both the hematopoietic (phagocytic) cell system and the immune system recover. During the period of neutropenia, which usually lasts from the day of transplantation until 10 to 40 days after transplantation, patients must be protected from pathogenic bacteria and fungi. This is usually accomplished by the use of laminar flow, high-efficiency particulate air–filtered systems; sterile or low-bacteria foods; hand washing and wearing of gloves and masks by all coming near the patient; limited physical contact between the patient and other people; and strict isolation techniques. Oral nonabsorbable antibiotics are frequently used to decrease the number of bacteria in the GI tract, which is the most common source of infecting organisms.[34] Antibiotics used for this purpose include polymyxin, neomycin, norfloxacin, and fluconazole. Because the immune system must be destroyed before infusion of the donor marrow and may take more than 2 years to recover after allogeneic bone marrow transplantation,[35] special precautions for immunocompromised hosts should be utilized during that time period. These include the use of cytomegalovirus (CMV)-negative blood products for all CMV antibody–negative transplantation patients. Acyclovir prophylaxis is frequently used during the first 6 weeks after transplantation for all herpes simplex–positive patients and for patients who have or whose donor has a positive antibody titer to CMV to help prevent resurgence of active infection. In addition, many centers now routinely administer intravenous immunoglobulins to patients after bone marrow transplantation, usually on a weekly basis for the first 2 to 6 months after transplantation. Because the transplanted bone marrow lacks significant "memory" of previous immunizations and the patient's immune capability has been destroyed, it is frequently necessary to reimmunize the patient against poliomyelitis, tetanus, and diphtheria when the new immune system has adequately recovered (usually 1 to 2 years after transplantation). Most patients have poor splenic function for up to 2 years after transplantation and are susceptible to the same kinds of overwhelming infections by encapsulated organisms as patients undergoing splenectomy. These organisms include pneumococci, meningococci, and *Haemophilus influenzae*. Prophylaxis with intravenous immunoglobulins during the early months after transplantation and the use of polyvalent vaccines after the immune system has recovered help to prevent this complication.

The almost total immunosuppression of the host is necessary to ensure engraftment of donor allogeneic bone marrow. Failure to achieve such immunosuppression can result in rejection of the transplanted bone marrow, which fails to engraft at all, or subsequent graft failure with prolonged and possibly permanent lack of bone marrow function (both hematopoietic and immune systems).

After complete destruction of the recipient's lymphohematopoietic system, the newly engrafted bone marrow frequently recovers in a dyspoietic manner. In the hematopoietic system one may observe slow, inadequate recovery of erythropoiesis with marked megaloblastosis and significant dyspoiesis in the bone marrow. The megaloblastosis and dyspoiesis frequently persist for several months after the transplantation, and the resulting red blood cells have a markedly shortened survival in the peripheral blood. Although eosinophilia is a frequent finding in both the bone marrow and peripheral blood for up to a year after bone marrow transplantation, significant qualitative abnormalities of the phagocytic cells are not often observed. Megakaryopoiesis with adequate platelet production may be delayed for weeks or months after transplantation. Platelets are frequently the last of the hematopoietic elements requiring transfusional support. Recovery to normal levels of platelets may take more than a year, although blood platelet counts adequate to allow cessation of transfusions (i.e., >20,000/ mm^3 [2×10^{10}/L]) are usually achieved 3 to 10 weeks after the transplantation.

The most disordered and prolonged recovery is usually noted in the immune system. The recovery of T and B cell functions to normal is markedly delayed. Although this delay is most marked after allogeneic bone marrow transplantation, in which a severe immunodeficiency state can persist for months to years, it is also seen in autologous and syngeneic bone marrow transplantations. In addition, the recovering immune system is frequently in a seriously dysregulated state with abnormal immune responses. One of the most significant of these disordered immune reactions is the graft-versus-host reaction, which, if severe enough to cause clinically significant disease, is known as GVHD.[36-40] Although this disorder is thought to be primarily a reaction of the engrafted immune system against antigens found in the host, there is evidence that dysregulation of the immune system with a disproportionate increase in the ratio of helper to killer cells and a relative deficiency of specific suppressor (veto) cells contributes significantly to the disorder. Graft-versus-host reactions are seen in individuals who are phenotypically and genotypically HLA identical, and they can be induced in patients undergoing autologous and syngeneic bone marrow transplantations[41, 42] as well as by purposely interfering with the recovery of the specific suppressor cells. Thus, a graft-versus-host reaction, a T cell–mediated attack of the engrafting bone marrow against the host, is to a variable degree a reflection of the disordered immune system after bone marrow transplantation.

COMPLICATIONS AFTER BONE MARROW TRANSPLANTATION

Toxicities of the Preparative Regimens

For a successful bone marrow transplantation, it is essential that all recipient lymphohematopoietic tissue be destroyed before infusion of the donor marrow. Supralethal therapy is required to ensure the complete ablation of recipient lymphohematopoietic cells. This produces total and irreversible destruction of the hematopoietic and immune systems. To achieve this destruction of the lymphohematopoietic system, agents such as irradiation, cyclophosphamide, busulfan, carmustine, and etoposide are used at dose levels above those used in the treatment of other disorders. Thus, toxic effects on nonhematopoietic organs are frequently seen that were not encountered or were less severe at lower doses

TABLE 116–5

MOST COMMON AGENTS USED FOR BONE MARROW TRANSPLANTATION AND THEIR LIFE-THREATENING NONLYMPHOHEMATOPOIETIC TOXICITIES

Agent	Toxicity
Irradiation	Burns of the skin; GI tract (severe mucositis with diarrhea), pulmonary fibrosis, veno-occlusive disease of the liver
Cyclophosphamide	Myocardial necrosis and hemorrhage with intractable congestive failure; pulmonary fibrosis; severe chemical burns of renal pelvis, ureters, and bladder; mucositis
Busulfan	Generalized seizures; sloughing of skin, especially in intertriginous areas; severe generalized mucositis; veno-occlusive disease of the liver; pulmonary fibrosis
Etoposide	Severe mucositis; veno-occlusive disease of the liver; severe recall toxicities of the skin and mucous membranes in areas of previous radiation
Carmustine (BCNU)	Veno-occlusive disease of the liver; because carmustine is dissolved in large amounts of alcohol, effects of alcohol overdosage as well

of the agents (Table 116–5). Lethal myocardiopathies[43, 44] and hemorrhagic cystitis[44, 45] can be seen with the doses of cyclophosphamide used. The doses of busulfan used can cause severe intractable generalized seizure disorders and life-threatening mucositis of the GI tract in addition to destruction of the hematopoietic system. The large doses of alkylating agents used either alone or with total body irradiation can result in severe, often fatal veno-occlusive disease of the liver[46, 47] and marked pulmonary fibrosis.[48, 49] Thus, unusual and more severe degrees of nonhematopoietic toxicity accompany the preparative regimens for bone marrow transplantation.

Failure to Engraft or Graft Rejection

One of the most life-threatening complications of bone marrow transplantation is failure of the infused donor bone marrow to engraft and repopulate the lymphohematopoietic system of the recipient. This situation can result from inadequate immunosuppression of the recipient, inadequate numbers of viable hematopoietic stem cells in the marrow inoculum, or, in rare cases, the presence in the recipient of a nonimmune factor lethal to the injected stem cells. It is most frequently seen when the donor marrow has been manipulated to remove either T cells in the allogeneic situation or tumor cells in the autologous situation. Failure of the injected stem cells results in prolonged pancytopenia in the host. Unless a second transplantation can be given, death is likely to result from infections or bleeding a few weeks or months. Occasionally, if the rejection is secondary to inadequate preparation of the recipient, sufficient host marrow function is recovered to allow more prolonged survival when a second transplantation is not possible. Occasionally, especially in patients who have transplantations because of bone marrow failure, there is initial engraftment of the donor bone marrow but, because of persistence of the recipient's immune functions, rejection occurs a few weeks to 6 months after the transplantation. This potentially lethal complication often occurs when the postgrafting immunosuppressive agent being administered to the recipient is decreased or stopped.

Graft-Versus-Host Disease

In GVHD the donor lymphoid cells carry out a T cell–mediated attack against the recipient (host) tissues.[50, 51] This is enhanced by antigenic differences between donor and host cells. The greater the differences, especially in the major HLA antigens, the more severe and prolonged the graft-versus-host reaction. In addition, immunosuppressive agents or infections result in lack of adequate numbers of specific suppressor (or veto) lymphocytes and contribute to the disorder.

The tissues most vulnerable to attack in graft-versus-host reactions are those expressing class II (HLA-DR) histocompatibility antigens. These include cells of epithelial origin in the skin, gut, liver, exocrine glands (lacrimal, salivary), and to some extent the lungs. Although there is tissue destruction by an overactive lymphoid system and lymphoid infiltrates are found in the affected organs, at the time of graft-versus-host reactions the patient is in a state of severe deficiency with regard to many normal immune functions and is susceptible to the many insults experienced by all severely immunosuppressed patients. These include viral (especially herpes simplex, varicella-zoster, and CMV), fungal, protozoan, and some bacterial infections. A further complication is that the primary form of therapy for the disorder is the use of immunosuppressive agents. These agents make the patient more susceptible to many of the infectious complications characteristic of the immunocompromised host.

The organs that are major targets of the graft-versus-host reaction are also major targets of the toxicities of many of the agents used to prepare patients for bone marrow transplantation. Skin, gut, and liver, the most common targets in GVHD, are damaged by the high doses of radiation and alkylating agents used before transplantation. It has been shown that graft-versus-host reactions can be enhanced or even triggered by inducing tissue trauma. Also, trauma to several tissues (the gut, for example) enhances the expression of class II HLA antigens on the cell surface. This helps explain the enhancement of the graft-versus-host reaction seen in many organs associated with drug toxicity or viral enteritis and especially in the gut.

Graft-versus-host reactions have been classified according to three degrees of intensity and clinical presentations: hyperacute, acute, and chronic. Hyperacute reactions occur early after transplantation, progress rapidly, and usually involve the skin and gut[52] (Table 116–6). They are frequently seen 2 to 14 days after infusion of the donor marrow and are more common when there is a major HLA antigenic mismatch between donor and host or when donor-host pairs are well matched but no prophylactic post-transplantation immunosuppression is given. Clinically, hyperacute GVHD is characterized by high fever and rapidly progressive reddening and tenderness of the skin, which is often diffuse from the start. This is accompanied in most cases by the onset of crampy, colicky abdominal pain with copious amounts of watery diarrhea. Bowel sounds are frequently absent or nearly so. Early skin biopsies are often nondiagnostic and should be repeated later. If untreated, the disorder can progress in a few days to overwhelming skin loss similar to that in extensive second-degree burns and massive GI fluid and electrolyte loss (up to 25 L/d in some cases) requiring the most intensive replacement therapy to maintain life. The situation in the gut mimics that seen in severe cholera, and patients must be supported in a similar way.

TABLE 116–6	
MANIFESTATIONS OF CHRONIC GRAFT-VERSUS-HOST DISEASE	
Site	**Manifestations**
Immune system	Severe immunodeficiency, both T cell and B cell; autoantibodies to multiple cells
Skin	Licheniform changes, sclerodermatous changes, alopecia, and scleroderma possibly leading to eventual breakdown of skin
Exocrine glands	Sjögren's syndrome, lacrimal and salivary gland failure; secondary dry ulcerated mouth, loss of teeth
GI mucosa	Inflammation, mucositis, secondary strictures
Liver	Chronic loss of bile ducts leading to liver failure
Lungs	Repeated infection, fibrosis, bronchiolitis obliterans leading to respiratory failure
Muscles	Motor end-plate antibodies (myasthenia gravis)

The therapy for the underlying disorder is intensive immunosuppression[53] with agents such as methylprednisolone at 4 to 20 mg/kg/d, intravenous cyclosporine at 5 to 7.5 mg/kg/d, ATG, and monoclonal anti–T cell antibodies.

The less intense acute GVHD is similar to the hyperacute form except that its onset tends to be later (most often 3 to 6 weeks but occasionally as late as 4 months after transplantation) and its progression less rapid. Classically, the palms of the hands and soles of the feet are first involved with tenderness (occasionally pruritus) and redness that progress proximally over the next few days. Diarrhea with crampy, colicky pain occurs frequently and can become as severe as in the hyperacute form of the disorder. Liver abnormalities often develop early in the disease. The major target of graft-versus-host reactions in the liver appears to be the bile duct epithelium. Thus, intrahepatic cholestasis ensues, and one often sees hyperbilirubinemia (direct) out of proportion to that in most other liver abnormalities.

Although the progression of acute GVHD tends to be somewhat slower than that of the hyperacute form, it can become as severe, with total desquamation of the skin and GI mucosa and liver failure. Biopsy of the skin, gut, or liver usually confirms the diagnosis. Later in the disease, the gut in particular has a totally denuded epithelium and a histologic diagnosis cannot be confirmed. The therapy of acute GVHD is similar to that of the hyperacute form.[53] It can last from a few days to several weeks or months.

The chronic form of GVHD usually develops later (more than 3 months after transplantation) and lasts much longer (months to several years in some cases).[54] It tends to be much more gradual in onset, and, although most patients who develop chronic graft-versus-host reactions have had preceding acute GVHD, it can in some cases arise de novo. Chronic GVHD appears to be a continuum of the acute form of the disorder. The chronic disorder has been associated with a variety of autoimmune-like phenomena from typical Sjögren's syndrome with lacrimal and parotid gland hypofunction to myasthenia gravis or severe scleroderma-like changes of the skin and GI tract (Table 116–7). Typically, it begins slowly as licheniform changes of the skin gradually extend to involve more of the body surface. As the sclerodermatous

TABLE 116–7

MANIFESTATIONS OF CHRONIC GRAFT-VERSUS-HOST DISEASE

Organ or System	Manifestations
Skin	Hyper- and hypopigmentation; lichenoid papules; subcutaneous fibrosis (scleroderma-like changes), local (morphea) or systemic, leading to contractures; alopecia
Liver	Loss of small bile ducts with hyper–alkaline phosphatasemia, obstructive jaundice
Mouth	White, lichen planus–like plaques; ulceration; atrophy of mucosa; patchy erythema; dryness; gum atrophy leading to loss of teeth
Salivary glands	Hyposecretion of saliva, dry mouth, enhanced gum atrophy and dental damage, secretory immunoglobulin A deficiency
Eye	Dry eyes with secondary corneal damage; keratoconjunctivitis sicca secondary to lacrimal gland hypofunction; acute uveitis, lagophthalmos, and ectropion cataracts secondary to steroid therapy
Sinuses	Dry mucosa, gram-positive bacterial infection
Lung	Acute infection secondary to decreased ciliary action; occasional large-airway involvement with bronchorrhea, obliterative bronchiolitis; interstitial pneumonitis, usually viral, *Pneumocystis carinii* or bacterial pathogens associated with it; some lymphoid interstitial pneumonitis, not pathogen related; pulmonary fibrosis
Esophagus	Desquamation of epithelium, web formation, aperistalsis
Intestine	Patchy fibrosis of lamina propria and submucosa and serosa from stomach to colon
Musculoskeletal system	Inflammatory myositis, especially proximal muscles; myasthenia gravis; tendinitis; fasciitis; arthritis
Gynecologic system	Sica syndrome of vagina with strictures
Hematopoietic system	Hypocellularity, plasmacytosis, megaloblastosis, eosinophilia, fibrosis with leukoerythroblastic changes; thrombocytopenia
Immune system	Decreased cellular and humoral immunity; lymphoid hypocellularity and atrophy; antinuclear, anti–smooth muscle, antimitochondrial, antiepidermal antibodies
Kidney	Nephrotic syndrome, membranous glomerulonephritis

changes progress, the patient may develop all the complications of scleroderma, including inability to move air adequately, inability to move the fingers (sclerodactyly), and eventual skin breakdown. The salivary glands are frequently involved with dry, ulcerated mucous membranes of the mouth leading to inability to eat and secondary malnutrition, protein, calorie, and vitamin deficiency syndrome. Involvement of the lacrimal glands can lead to corneal damage, which, left unchecked, can lead to blindness. Repeated pulmonary infections secondary to the combination of pulmonary involvement with GVHD, the accompanying immunodeficiency syndrome, and the restriction of respiratory excursion can lead to secondary pulmonary fibrosis with eventual respiratory failure.

Chronic GVHD, like the acute forms of the disorder, is usually treated with immunosuppressive agents (steroids, azathioprine [Imuran], thalidomide, and cyclosporine).[55] Antibiotics are often given to prevent secondary infections and immunoglobulins are administered intravenously to overcome part of the immunodeficiency.

Recurrence of Disease

Unfortunately, one of the more common and often lethal complications of bone marrow transplantation is recurrence of the underlying disorder for which the transplantation was done. The frequency of this complication varies with the disease treated, being highest for some of the neoplastic disorders and lowest for bone marrow failure states.

COMPLICATIONS FREQUENTLY REQUIRING INTENSIVE CARE AND SUPPORT

Toxicity of Preparative Regimens

Major complications of bone marrow transplantation requiring intensive care are secondary to the drug and/or irradiation therapy used to prepare the patient for transplantation. These include the problems of patients with a totally destroyed bone marrow (immune and hematopoietic system ablation), as well as several non–bone marrow toxicities associated with the preparative regimen at the doses used in bone marrow transplantation recipients. The latter are addressed here.

Cardiac Toxicity

This is most frequently seen in patients being prepared for bone marrow transplantation with large doses of cyclophosphamide (greater than 50 mg/kg per dose). It occurs more often in patients who have underlying cardiac disease or who have been treated with large amounts of anthracycline-type drugs in the past. Cardiac toxicity is more common in patients with acute myelogenous leukemia or one of the high-grade non-Hodgkin's lymphomas because anthracyclines have frequently been used in high doses to treat the underlying disorder. Careful evaluation of ventricular function before transplantation is essential to screen out those who show evidence of pre-existing cardiac disease. Patients who develop cardiac problems after transplantation usually do so during the first 2 weeks after the intensive preparative regimen. The cardiac toxicity often presents as rapidly progressive heart failure, low cardiac output, and a flabby hypodynamic ventricle. The failure is frequently intractable and progressive, resulting in death in a few weeks or months. These patients are prone to develop severe arrhythmias and require intensive support with diuretics, antiarrhythmic agents, and inotropic drugs. However, despite the best supportive care, few recover adequate cardiac function.

Occasionally, patients may present with severe cardiac arrhythmias without evidence of failure. Nearly all such patients, except those with the mildest disorders, eventually progress to intractable heart failure. The major therapy is intensive support where possible, but there is seldom significant improvement and the condition often progresses to death.

Pathologically, one frequently finds a combination of the old changes of anthracycline toxicity and more recent small to large necrotic, hemorrhagic lesions in the myocardium with secondary fibrosis.

Pulmonary Complications

The lungs are particularly vulnerable to certain preparative regimens, especially those in which total body or total lymphoid irradiation is used. Progressive fibrosis with decreasing pulmonary functions may be seen for several months after transplantation. This is especially true in patients whose pretransplantation therapy included mediastinal or pulmonary irradiation and/or the use of bleomycin or busulfan.

A common complication of nearly all preparative regimens for bone marrow transplantation is a severe capillary leak syndrome. This frequently has its onset shortly after bone marrow transplantation and usually reaches its maximal "leak" between 10 and 14 days after the bone marrow infusion. It is characterized by persistent fluid retention (usually without detectable ascites), excessive weight gain, and pulmonary edema with generalized anasarca. The best therapy is prevention with careful attention to fluid intake and output during the first 2 weeks after transplantation. Judicious use of diuretics and restriction of excessive fluid intake can often prevent significant accumulation of fluids and the resulting pulmonary edema. When it does occur, it is treated with vigorous diuresis along with intravenous bolus infusions of albumin, restriction of all fluids to a minimum, endotracheal intubation with positive end-expiratory pressure, and ultrafiltration of the blood to remove excess water. The problem usually clears rapidly 14 to 16 days after the transplantation.

Hepatic Toxicity

Although the preparative regimens can be directly toxic to the hepatocytes, a more frequent toxicity is veno-occlusive disease of the liver, which is seen in a significant number of patients after bone marrow transplantation.[56, 57] It is most commonly seen after total body irradiation but has been observed with all preparative regimens and more often in patients who were heavily treated with chemotherapy or radiotherapy in the past. There also appears to be an increased frequency of this disorder in patients previously treated or prepared for transplantation with one of the nitrosourea compounds.

In veno-occlusive disease of the liver, the endothelial lining of the small venules of the central lobules of the liver appears to be damaged, resulting in occlusion of the vessels. This results in rapid increases in the portal pressure, massive engorgement of the liver and spleen, tender hepatomegaly, marked abdominal venous distention, ascites, secondary liver failure, and frequently encephalopathy. The severity and duration of the disorder vary from mild and barely detectable to overwhelming with severe liver failure and death. In general, the earlier the onset of the veno-occlusive syndrome (e.g., less than 3 weeks after bone marrow transplantation), the more severe and life threatening it is. Episodes of veno-occlusive disease that occur after 3 weeks tend to be less severe, and patients tend to recover with little residual hepatic disorder. A major predisposing factor for veno-occlusive disease appears to be pre-existing hepatic dysfunction. Especially predicative of future trouble are elevated levels of the hepatic transaminases.

Therapy of veno-occlusive disease is conservative, with gentle diureses with an agent such as spironolactone (Aldactone), administration of albumin if necessary, and removal of all hepatotoxic drugs when possible. Heparin therapy has not been clearly shown to be of value. Tapping the ascitic fluid is not indicated unless the ascites progresses to the point of interfering with respiration or there is a question of secondary peritonitis. The use of low doses of dopamine to increase perfusion may be of value.

Mucositis of the Gastrointestinal Tract

Several of the agents used to prepare patients for bone marrow transplantation cause severe mucositis of the entire GI tract. These include irradiation, etoposide, and busulfan. Mucositis tends to be particularly severe in patients who have had mucositis-producing toxicities in the past. Busulfan and etoposide especially appear to evoke a "recall" phenomenon in patients in whom previous therapy (localized irradiation or chemotherapy) caused mucositis in the past. The lesions in the upper GI tract are usually associated with profound difficulty in handling saliva, painful ulcerations, and almost total inability to eat or swallow. Similar lesions continue down much of the GI tract in many patients, at times leading to severe persistent nausea, vomiting, and profound diarrhea. This can rapidly lead to excessive protein loss in the stool and secondary malnutrition unless intravenous supplementations are promptly initiated. Frequently, total parenteral nutrition is indicated for weeks or months. Secondary infections are also frequently seen. Common secondary invaders of the upper GI tract include the herpes simplex viruses or *Candida* organisms. Any area of the GI tract can be involved with CMV, and secondary bacterial infections occur as well. Adenovirus and rotavirus can involve the small intestine and colon, with secondary bacterial infections ensuing. Putting the GI tract at rest while giving adequate parenteral nutrition sometimes allows recovery of the mucosa. However, to be adequately treated secondary infections must be diagnosed (culture for viruses, bacteria, and fungi; direct fluorescent antibody or enzyme-linked immunosorbent assay for herpes simplex and occasionally biopsy). Local anesthetic agents such as viscous lidocaine, local and sometimes systemic antifungals, and systemic acyclovir may be indicated and helpful. Prolonged secondary infections of the esophagus, small intestine, or colon can lead to secondary strictures, which may require future dilatation. Aspiration of infected mucus and regurgitated gastric contents is often a problem in these patients and leads to pneumonia. Mucositis of the lower GI tract is frequently best treated with oral nonabsorbable antibiotics to decrease the bacterial flora and GI rest. Because intensive gut-damaging chemotherapy- or radiotherapy-induced lactase deficiency is common during the first several months after bone marrow transplantation, avoidance of all dairy products is important for many of these patients. A more severe complication of the mucositis and its secondary viral, bacterial, or fungal infection is denudation of the mucosal epithelium resulting in secondary hemorrhage. Hemorrhage can be massive, severe, and difficult to control, especially if there is any underlying platelet or coagulation factor abnormality. On occasion this can lead to fatal exsanguination from the GI tract. Careful attention to platelet and clotting factor levels, bowel rest, and studies to determine whether the bleeding is localized or generalized are often necessary and lifesaving.

Genitourinary Complications

The most frequent form of severe toxicity is the hemorrhagic cystitis associated with cyclophosphamide therapy. This complication can directly result in or contribute markedly to the demise of some patients. The hemorrhagic cystitis is seen almost exclusively in patients treated with high doses of cyclophosphamide. Cyclophosphamide is converted in the body to a variety of substances. One metabolite is acrolein, a toxic compound excreted in the urine and capable of damaging the mucosa of the upper or lower urinary tract, resulting in hemorrhage into the renal pelvis, ureters, or bladder. The hemorrhage can be severe with intraluminal clotting causing obstruction and renal failure. Several cases of bladder rupture secondary to extensive bladder wall damage have been reported. Parenteral N-acetylcysteine provides free sulfhydryl groups in the urine, which readily bind with the acrolein and lessen the likelihood of this toxicity. The use of large volumes of intravenous fluids or continuous bladder irrigation also helps to reduce the concentration of acrolein in the urine and prevents some of the uroepithelial damage. If hemorrhagic cystitis occurs, it is best treated by continuous gentle bladder irrigation with an isotonic solution at a flow rate that results in an effluent with a light pink color. Occasionally, the bleeding sites are relatively few and can be cauterized to help control the hemorrhage. Rupture of the bladder requires immediate surgical intervention if possible. Obstruction of the urinary tract requires cystoscopic removal of the clots when possible. If necessary to maintain urine flow, nephrostomy tubes may have to be placed in the renal pelves to ensure adequate urinary drainage.

Central Nervous System Toxicities

Busulfan has proved to be one of the more useful agents in preparing patients with myeloid disorders for bone marrow transplantation. However, at the doses used, grand mal seizures are frequently seen; these can result in status epilepticus unless patients are heavily pretreated with analeptic agents and adequate levels of the seizure-preventing drugs are maintained during and for 24 hours after busulfan administration. If seizures occur, they can usually be controlled with intravenous phenytoin. Cytosine arabinoside is occasionally used as part of the preparative regimen. At a dose of 2 g/m² or more every 12 hours, severe cerebellar toxicity can be seen. Careful monitoring of the patient during therapy for such cerebellar signs with immediate cessation of therapy if they are seen is necessary to prevent permanent toxicity. Patients with a history of prior central nervous system (CNS) toxicity caused by cytosine arabinoside should not receive the drug again because life-threatening, irreversible cerebellar toxicity may ensue.

Another serious CNS complication is intracranial hemorrhage, which occurs most frequently during the period of severe thrombocytopenia shortly after bone marrow transplantation. Intracranial hemorrhage is not a direct effect of the preparative regimen; it occurs because of the bone marrow suppression induced by the agents used. Patients who fail to respond to platelet transfusions are especially likely to develop serious bleeding, and intracranial hemorrhage is one of the worst consequences. During the preparative therapy, severe nausea and vomiting induced by the chemotherapy or radiotherapy may contribute to this bleeding or to an unsteady gait, which might result in head trauma.

CNS problems are uncommon during the period of pancytopenia. Those seen most often are infections including herpetic (herpes simplex) encephalitis, brain abscess, or fungal infections (especially aspergillus) of the brain, which require adequate antiviral (acyclovir), antibacterial, or antifungal therapy. Toxoplasmosis of the CNS has also been seen 2 to 4 months after bone marrow transplantation. Primary lymphomas and multifocal leukoencephalopathy are two lethal complications of the CNS occasionally seen after bone marrow transplantation. The lymphomas of the CNS tend to be high grade, rapidly progressive, and poorly responsive to therapy. They are often multifocal. Occasionally, they regress on cessation of immunosuppressive therapy, but most frequently they are progressive and relatively resistant to the usual antilymphoma therapies. Multifocal leukoencephalopathy, a progressive multifocal degenerative process of the white matter, is thought, at least in some cases, to be related to viral infections of the CNS in the immunocompromised hosts. If it is diagnosed, every attempt should be made to stop immunosuppressive therapy, but this is usually to no avail and the disease almost invariably progresses rapidly, resulting in death.

Complications of the Period of Pancytopenia

One of the expected, and in fact desired, toxicities of the preparative regimen is total aplasia of the host bone marrow with resulting anemia, leukopenia, and severe thrombocytopenia. The anemia and thrombocytopenia may present transfusion problems. Because of the severe leukopenia, especially of the phagocytic cells (granulocytes and monocyte-macrophages), the host becomes almost completely defenseless against invading microorganisms. As a result, severe and potentially overwhelming bacterial, fungal, and viral infections are a major threat to the bone marrow transplantation patient during this period.[58, 59] Aplasia of the marrow is usually complete at about the time of the bone marrow transplantation. High risk of bacterial and fungal invasion exists when the granulocyte count in the peripheral blood drops to less than 500/mm³ (5 × 10⁸/L) and persists until the granulocyte count again surpasses 500/mm³ (5 × 10⁸/L), which usually occurs 2 to 4 weeks after transplantation. During the period of granulocytopenia, patients are most susceptible to bacterial infections. The organisms most commonly responsible for sepsis during this period are those that make up the normal flora of the skin, respiratory tract, or GI tract. Infections during periods of neutropenia are frequently sudden in onset and severe requiring intensive support and broad-spectrum antibiotic coverage to control the process. Fever, the usual sign of sepsis in these patients, must always be taken seriously. Any neutropenic patient with fever (temperature above 100.5°F [38°C]) must immediately have an adequate physical examination and cultures of stool, urine, sputum, blood, and any intravascular foreign bodies (central venous catheters) for bacteria and fungi. Antibiotics must then be promptly instituted and cover most bacterial organisms, especially the gram-negative bacteria, which are the major cause of rapidly fatal sepsis. Septicemia is the most commonly verified infection in cases of fever during aplasia in these patients.

The cause of a large percentage of the fevers can never be documented by positive cultures from the blood stream or any other source. Despite the lack of a documented infectious agent, intensive antibiotic therapy must be continued until the patient has achieved an afebrile state, completed at least 2 weeks of antibiotic therapy, or recovered adequate granulocytes. If the granulocyte counts have not returned to a level greater than 500/mm^3 (5 × 10^8/L), discontinuation of antibiotics is not advised unless a causative organism was detected, identified, and shown to be susceptible to the therapy administered and the patient has achieved an afebrile state. If no causative organism has been identified but the patient promptly became afebrile, antibiotics may be cautiously discontinued after a 10-day to 2-week course in persistently neutropenic patients. Continued decontamination of the gut with oral antibiotics is recommended for neutropenic patients whose therapeutic antibiotics are being stopped. Bacterial infections in these patients may be rapidly progressive and severe, requiring large amounts of intravenous fluids, including plasma expanders, blood products, and frequently vasopressors, to maintain an adequate blood pressure and proper tissue perfusion.

If a causative organism is identified, specific antibiotics for that organism should be initiated and the systemic broad-spectrum antibiotics stopped unless they are the most appropriate ones for the organism identified. Oral gut-decontaminating antibiotics should be continued as long as the patient is neutropenic.

A common source of infection in these patients is an implanted vascular access device (catheters in large central veins). These should be inspected frequently. At the slightest hint of inflammation or infection they should be cultured to rule them out as a potential source of bacteremia. In general, if a catheter is identified as a potential source of infection, it should be removed and not replaced until it is fairly certain that the sepsis has been terminated. If a catheter is infected with a gram-positive organism, one may try to sterilize the catheter in place by intensive antibiotic therapy for 2 weeks. However, this is unlikely to succeed in the absence of functioning granulocytes. A second episode of infection of a catheter or sepsis with the same organism should always lead to immediate removal of the intravascular device.

Fungal infections, especially with candidal organisms and aspergillosis, present major problems in neutropenic, immunocompromised bone marrow transplantation patients. Fungal infections are usually seen only after prolonged aplasia of the bone marrow in the setting of severe immunosuppression and/or prolonged antibiotic therapy. Fungus is rarely the major cause of problems during the first 2 weeks of bone marrow aplasia except in patients who have received prolonged antibiotic therapy or steroids before the aplasia. The usual signs of fungal infection are persistent fever despite broad-spectrum antibiotic coverage in the absence of any other obvious causative organism. Fevers of 72 hours or more in neutropenic hosts who are receiving broad-spectrum antibiotics are likely to have a fungal cause. Cultures of mouth, sputum, stool, urine, blood, and vascular devices should be carefully assayed for evidence of fungus. The presence of Candida in two or more sites, especially blood or urine in addition to other sites, should be considered evidence of candidal infection and adequately treated. The presence of Aspergillus in any part of the body should be looked on as potential infection and antifungal therapy instituted. In neutropenic patients with fevers persisting beyond 72 hours of antibiotic therapy and no evidence of

fungus, a change in broad-spectrum antibiotics may be tried first. If after 48 hours on the new regimen there is still no response, antifungal therapy should be instituted despite lack of direct evidence that fungus is the cause of the febrile episode.

Prophylaxis against fungi by routine use of fluconazole in neutropenic patients has significantly decreased the incidence of fungal infections after bone marrow transplantation. However, persistence of fever despite broad-spectrum antibiotics in patients with no other cause of temperature elevation should be considered a sign of a possible fungal infection.

Serious complications of candidal infections can result from the seeding of multiple organs during septicemia. Hepatic candidiasis is one of the more common life-threatening fungal infections. It often requires 6 months or more of intensive antifungal therapy to sterilize the host. Seeding of the lungs with Candida, although rare, may cause a severe progressive pneumonia but one that frequently responds to intensive amphotericin therapy. Metastatic candidal lesions of the brain are exceedingly rare, but splenic candidiasis is often seen after prolonged candidal septicemia or hepatic candidiasis. Aspergillus can involve almost any organ of the body. Profoundly neutropenic patients with prolonged aplasia sometimes have Aspergillus infections of the lungs, brain, nasal sinuses, or GI tract that are rapidly progressive despite therapy with amphotericin. Unless the patient can recover significant phagocytic cell function (granulocytes and monocytes) and all immunosuppressive drugs are stopped, most invasive Aspergillus infections progress rapidly and are fatal.

Other fungi rarely cause infections in the immunosuppressed, granulocytopenic patient after bone marrow transplantation. Cryptococcal infections of the respiratory tract and brain are sometimes encountered. Mucormycosis infections are rare but when they do occur are most frequently associated with nasal sinus involvement that progresses to involve the bones of the skull and eventually the brain. Mucormycosis infections that occur after bone marrow transplantation are seldom responsive to treatment unless all immunosuppressive agents are stopped and there is adequate recovery of phagocytic white blood cell function. The use of granulocyte-stimulating factors such as G-CSF or GM-CSF in addition to antifungal agents may be lifesaving in these situations.

Other unusual fungi that occasionally cause life-threatening infections after bone marrow transplantation include *Torulopsis glabrata*, an organism that may often contaminate the GI tract during the early post-transplantation period. It may be responsible for invasive infections of the wall of the GI tract. It is somewhat responsive to amphotericin therapy but much less so than are most strains of *Candida*.

Complication of the Period of Immunosuppression After Recovery of Neutrophil Function

During immunosuppression, patients are susceptible to overwhelming infection by a variety of viruses. The three most common are herpes simplex virus, CMV, and varicella-zoster virus, but adenovirus, respiratory syncytial virus, rotavirus, and the BK viruses present problems as well. Herpes simplex and varicella-zoster infections appear to be almost exclusively due to reactivation of pre-existing infections, whereas CMV infections may be due to reactivation of previous infections (about 60% of cases) or de novo infections thought in most cases to be transmitted by contaminated blood products. Although prophylactic measures have markedly decreased the incidence of herpes simplex and CMV infections after bone marrow transplantation, severe infectious complications still occur. Most herpes simplex problems are manifest during the first 30 days after the transplantation, often while the patient is still neutropenic. Severe oral and esophageal involvement is often seen in patients whose positive herpes simplex antibody titer confirms a previous infection with the virus. Also, the virus may be a secondary invader in the mucosal lesions of patients with severe mucositis caused by the agents used to prepare them for transplantation. Again, the infection is seen almost exclusively in patients already harboring the virus. The infection usually remains superficial but occasionally spreads, probably via aspiration, into the lungs. The most serious herpes simplex infectious complication is involvement of the CNS. Typically, this involves the temporal lobes, producing a characteristic picture on an electroencephalogram. Prompt intensive therapy with acyclovir is essential to reverse the CNS lesions and prevent death. Occasionally, herpes simplex becomes a generalized systemic infection involving the liver (acute viral hepatitis), and lungs (pneumonia) as well. Again, prompt therapy with intravenous acyclovir is essential to arrest the disease.

Nearly all patients likely to develop herpes simplex infections have a pretransplantation antibody titer to the organism. The presence of such an antibody titer along with lesions suspected of harboring herpes simplex should result in prompt therapy with acyclovir, which in most cases eradicates the lesions. In other cases in which one suspects the possibility of herpetic infections, the Tzanck's examination for the characteristic viral inclusion bodies or antiviral fluorescent antibody studies often give a positive diagnosis in a matter of hours. If the fluorescent antibody test fails to give an answer, culture studies of scrapings of the lesion or enzyme-linked immunosorbent assays may be done; especially in early stages of the lesions, these tend to be positive in a high percentage of cases.

The use of moderate doses of acyclovir given prophylactically to patients with a significant antibody titer to herpes simplex has reduced the incidence of clinically significant herpetic lesions to almost zero during the first 6 weeks after bone marrow transplantation.

A far more serious viral infection is seen with CMV. Although it can affect almost any organ, the gut, liver, and lungs are most commonly involved. The organ most frequently involved in fatal infections is the lung. Significant infection of any organ (blood, urinary tract, gut, or liver) may be followed in days to weeks by CMV pneumonia. The patients at greatest risk of CMV infection are those undergoing allogeneic bone marrow transplantation. CMV infection is a rarer and milder complication in autologous or syngeneic bone marrow transplantations. It usually occurs 30 to 90 days after the transplantation but can be seen as much as a year later. The infection may be due to reactivation of a previously acquired virus or may occur de novo. Prophylactic measures have reduced the incidence of severe disease. When only CMV-negative blood products are used and the patients and their bone marrow donors demonstrate no antibody titer to CMV, de novo infections are markedly reduced. CMV antibody–positive blood products appear to be the major route of infection in these patients. When CMV-negative blood products are not available but blood products must be given, the use of leukocyte removal systems to reduce the contamination of the product with white blood cells decreases the chance of transmitting CMV to negative patients. When the transplant recipient or the donor has a pre-existing antibody titer to CMV, the use of high-dose acyclovir (500 mg/m^2 intravenously every 8 hours) prophylactically for the first 6 weeks after transplantation reduces the incidence of clinically significant exacerbations of CMV infection. Some bone marrow transplantation centers use prophylactic ganciclovir for patients who have a positive CMV antibody titer and positive CMV cultures from bronchoalveolar washings 5 to 6 weeks after bone marrow transplantation. They report great success in reducing the incidence of CMV pneumonias in this group of patients.

In addition to prophylactic acyclovir and ganciclovir, weekly or biweekly infusions of intravenous immunoglobulin after transplantation may contribute to the decrease in clinical cases of CMV pneumonia.

Although the liver and GI tract (stomach, small intestine, or colon) may be severely involved with CMV, the most severe and often fatal infections are CMV pneumonias. Confirmation of the diagnosis requires demonstration of the cytopathic changes characteristic of the virus in addition to its isolation. This can sometimes be achieved with bronchoalveolar lavage, but the most reliable method is open lung biopsy. CMV pneumonia usually presents with rapidly progressive bilateral interstitial infiltrates, marked shortness of breath, falling Po$_2$, and early need for respiratory support with intubation and respirator assistance. Prompt intensive therapy with ganciclovir and intravenous immunoglobulin infusions reverses many of these cases. However, the fatality rate for patients with CMV pneumonia less than 4 months after allogeneic bone marrow transplantation is still 50%.

Varicella-zoster is carried by nearly all but the youngest patients undergoing bone marrow transplantation. After primary infection, the virus remains viable but latent in the neural ganglia. In times of immunosuppression, the virus may proliferate and produce an active local (dermatologic zoster) or occasionally generalized systemic infection. After autologous or allogeneic bone marrow transplantation, reactivation of a varicella-zoster infection is common.

Reactivation most often occurs 2 to 9 months after transplantation. The infection is usually cutaneous and localized to one or two dermatomes. When it presents as a rapidly progressive systemic infection, viremia and hepatic, pulmonary, and GI manifestations may be present. In the absence of skin lesions, diagnosis may be difficult. If skin lesions are present, Tzanck's testing of vesicular fluid is usually positive for cells demonstrating a herpes-type infection. In the absence of skin lesions, clinical suspicion leads to prompt intensive use of acyclovir, which must be instituted early to reverse systemic viremia and generalized infection and thus prevent the patient's rapid demise from hepatic failure and/or fatal interstitial pneumonitis.

Other viruses have also caused severe, sometimes fatal, infections in the patient after bone marrow transplantation. Adenovirus causes severe enteritis, lethal viral pneumonitis, and occasionally delayed hemorrhagic cystitis. There is no specific therapy for adenovirus, except for continued intensive support of the involved organ systems and attempted cessation of all immunosuppressive agents. Although never clearly shown to be of value, intravenous immunoglobulins are often used in these patients.

Another major complication of bone marrow transplantation is hemorrhagic cystitis (see earlier). It is nearly always associated with cyclophosphamide therapy in the allogeneic bone marrow transplantation patient but is sometimes delayed in its appearance, developing 2 or 3 months after transplantation. When it occurs late, one can frequently isolate BK-type parvovirus or adenovirus from the urine. Their role in the etiology of the severe, sometimes fatal cystitis is not clear, but decreasing immunosuppression and the use of intravenous immunoglobulins sometimes markedly ameliorate the process.

Rotavirus and respiratory syncytial virus have occasionally been implicated as causative agents in enteritis and pneumonia after bone marrow transplantation.

One of the most serious complications of bone marrow transplantation, and one almost unique to bone marrow transplantation, is the graft-versus-host reaction. (See the earlier discussion of pathophysiology.) It often occurs shortly after the period of pancytopenia. GVHD is manifest primarily in three major organ systems—skin, liver, and GI tract. The hyperacute form of GVHD usually occurs 7 to 21 days and the acute form 30 to 60 days after bone marrow transplantation. However, under special circumstances it can occur much later.

The skin is usually the first site affected. Histopathologically, the reaction is classified as lichenoid. In the hyperacute form of the disease, the initial skin reaction is generalized from the onset with diffuse redness and tenderness throughout much of the body. Nonhyperacute GVHD tends to manifest itself first on the palms of the hands and soles of the feet. The skin over the area becomes red, sometimes pruritic, and is often tender and develops a brawny consistency. Over the next few days, the redness tends to advance proximally, gradually involving the arms, legs, and finally the trunk with a diffuse morbilliform maculopapular erythematous rash, almost indistinguishable from a drug eruption. Early biopsy of the lesion confirms the diagnosis. If the reaction is untreated or fails to respond to therapy, it progresses to vesicle formation (positive Nikolsky's sign). Bullae and ulcerations may form, and if the reaction is unchecked a picture similar to that of toxic epidermal necrolysis may ensue, which can be fatal. The condition resembles diffuse secondary burns over almost the entire body, and supportive therapies similar to those for an acute burn must be instituted, utilizing sterile sheets and frequent sterile whirlpool baths. The skin breakdown may result in loss of large amounts of serum and red blood cells, which must be replaced. The loss of the dermal protective layer frequently results in secondary infections, which must be vigorously treated. Without the protective skin covering, body temperature control mechanisms fail and there is a marked increase in loss of heat from the body. Severe cutaneous GVHD requires intensive support to maintain the patient through the period.

Simultaneous with or shortly after, the skin manifestations, severe GI involvement with GVHD is often seen. At this point early in the post-transplantation period, it is often difficult to distinguish acute GVHD involvement of the gut from the toxic effects of the preparative regimens and/or infections in the neutropenic immunocompromised host. Often two or all three disorders occur simultaneously. One seldom sees acute GVHD of the GI tract without concomitant GVHD of the skin. Thus, the presence or absence of cutaneous manifestations often helps one decide whether the GI signs and symptoms are secondary to GVHD. Histologic confirmation of the diagnosis may be possible by early biopsy of the GI mucosa. However, GVHD damage is usually combined with that of the preparative regimen and/or secondary infections, and shortly after the onset of GVHD total denudation of the gut epithelium occurs with loss of histologic markers of the disorder. The clinical manifestations are usually early onset of profuse watery diarrhea, which may contain leukocytes but no pathogens. This is often accompanied by severe colicky pain and abdominal distention. Bowel sounds are typically hypoactive, and the abdomen frequently has diffuse but not severe tenderness. The volume of diarrhea may be enormous, and there are documented cases of 25 to 30 L of watery stool in less than 24 hours. Barium transit time is markedly shortened and may be only 15 to 30 minutes from mouth to anus. These patients require prompt massive fluid and electrolyte replacement with complete rest of the gut (nothing by mouth). Constant careful monitoring of fluid loss and electrolyte status with prompt, massive replacement is essential to their survival. Radiographic studies show an ileus-type picture with dilated loops of bowel. With the loss of the mucosa, secondary infections and loss of blood from the denuded areas are common. The blood loss can result in fatal hemorrhage. The bleeding sites are often diffuse and in multiple areas of the GI tract. However, occasionally they are localized and amenable to surgical resection. It is imperative to check platelet levels frequently and transfuse if necessary to maintain a level above 50,000/mm^3 (5×10^{10}/L) in the presence of significant GI bleeding. Clotting factors (prothrombin time, partial thromboplastin time, and thrombin time) should be checked frequently and fresh frozen plasma replacement used when necessary. Unless the process can be reversed rapidly and the patient maintained on intensive support systems, death quickly ensues. Because of the extensive damage, secondary scarring and fibrosis can lead to partial or complete obstruction of the GI tract.

The third major organ system damaged in acute GVHD is the liver. Histopathologically, GVHD of the liver produces cholestatic hepatitis secondary to bile duct aplasia as a result of destruction with eventual loss of the duct epithelium. Hepatocytes may become necrotic as well, and one frequently sees lymphocytic infiltrates in the periportal areas on biopsy. Clinically, this is usually manifested by the onset of hepatic functional abnormalities. The major findings are of an obstructive type, with bilirubin and alkaline phosphatase levels rising out of proportion to tests of hepatocyte damage. Conjugated bilirubin levels may reach 30 to 50 mg/dL with little evidence of hepatic failure. One must distinguish hepatic GVHD from veno-occlusive disease, in which the onset is usually before day 35, the liver is tender and enlarged, there is virtually no rise in the alkaline phosphatase level, and ascites and signs of liver failure are more common. Viral hepatitis may also occur in the setting of GVHD and may be confused with it, but viral hepatitis usually results in more hepatocellular damage with markedly elevated transaminase levels. Also, cyclosporine, which is frequently used in these patients, and various other drugs can cause jaundice by several mechanisms. Liver biopsies are most helpful in distinguishing between these disorders if bleeding and clotting parameters allow this to be done.

The specific therapy for acute and hyperacute GVHD is intensive immunosuppression.[53] This is usually done with steroids (methylprednisolone up to 20 mg/kg/d), increasing doses of cyclosporine (up to 7.5 mg/kg/d), ATG, and monoclonal antithymocyte antibodies. Therapy must be rapid, aggressive, and often prolonged, with slow tapering of the therapeutic agents after control of the underlying disease process.

The onset of chronic GVHD is usually later (3 to 6 months after bone marrow transplantation).[54] Chronic GVHD is most frequently seen in patients who are older and/or those who have had previous acute GVHD. It involves many systems.

The major complications requiring intensive medical care[55] and support are infectious and are related to the severe immunodeficiency of these patients and the multiple organs damaged by the autoimmune phenomena in this disorder. Bacterial, viral, fungal, and protozoan (*Pneumocystis*) infections are common, and the target organs are usually the damaged mucosa of the mouth, throat, sinuses, eyes, lungs, and GI tract. With intravenous immunoglobulin therapy, the primary infectious disorders seen are those related to T cell dysfunction. The autoimmune destruction of particular organs makes them targets for secondary infections. These infections are often rapidly progressive and life threatening and require intensive therapy.

Many of the unusual manifestations of chronic GVHD are related to autoimmune dysfunctions and are discussed in the following:

1. *Exocrine gland involvement (Sjögren's syndrome)*: Secondary ulceration of the mouth and throat may lead to severe emaciation, secondary severe infections, and sepsis. Total parenteral nutrition or gastrostomy tube feedings may be necessary to maintain adequate caloric intake. Because of lacrimal gland involvement, administration of artificial tears every half-hour and plugging of the lacrimal ducts may be essential to preserve the cornea and prevent permanent blindness.

2. *Severe sclerodermatous changes of the skin and GI tract*: Progressive systemic sclerotic changes of the skin and GI tract similar to those noted in patients with scleroderma are often seen. Involvement of the chest wall may become so severe that respiratory excursions are impaired, and respiratory failure can ensue. Involvement of the esophagus leading to strictures and secondary obstruction requiring frequent dilatation is often seen.

3. *Pulmonary manifestations of chronic GVHD*: These are often related to the immunosuppression of these patients and direct involvement of the lungs with the GVHD process. A lymphocytic infiltrate in the lungs, secondarily diminished ciliary function, and malfunction of pulmonary alveolar macrophages, when combined with the immunosuppressed state, may lead to repeated bouts of lower respiratory tract infection, damage to terminal bronchi, and secondary pulmonary fibrosis. This condition leads to increased episodes of infection producing progressive pulmonary failure and death. Early therapy of the underlying GVHD and the underlying infections is necessary to break the cycle and prevent respiratory failure. Prophylactic use of antibiotics and intravenous immunoglobulins helps to prevent respiratory infection, and immunosuppressive agents suppress the underlying chronic GVHD.

4. *Hepatic dysfunction*: Chronic GVHD often involves the liver, leading to progressive bile duct destruction. Eventually, liver failure ensues. Other than supportive care and therapy of the underlying GVHD with immunosuppressive agents, little can be done.

5. *Neurologic disorders*: The major neurologic disorders associated with chronic GVHD are multifocal leukoencephalopathy and myasthenia gravis. The multifocal leukoencephalopathy is thought to be related to a viral encephalitis associated with the immunosuppressed state. It is manifested by progressive defects in multiple areas of the brain that can affect motor or sensory tracts. The lesions are multiple and progressive and do not respond to therapy. Stopping immunosuppression is essential but is seldom effective. Myasthenia gravis, an autoimmune disorder mediated by antibodies to the motor end plates, has been reported as a manifestation of chronic GVHD in several patients. Severe myasthenic crisis must be treated in a manner similar to myasthenic crisis in the nontransplantation patient.

6. *Endocrine disorders*: Although multiple endocrine organ dysfunctions have been described as autoimmune disorders, they are not reported direct complications of chronic GVHD. Diabetes induced by steroid therapy or secondary to chronic pancreatitis and thyroid failure are frequently seen and are thought to be more related to previous chemo- or radiotherapy. Adrenal insufficiency after prolonged steroid therapy is frequently seen, but direct autoimmune-mediated endocrine failure syndromes as a result of chronic GVHD have not been reported.

7. *Hemolytic anemia and immune thrombocytopenia*: Acute hemolytic processes and autoimmune thrombocytopenia have been reported after bone marrow transplantation and are probably manifestations of chronic GVHD. The hemolysis may be brisk, severe, and even fatal. Intensive therapy with steroids often reverses it. Immune thrombocytopenia responds to steroids in the same way. A hemolytic process is indicated by the presence of increased reticulocytes in the peripheral blood and red blood cell precursors in the bone marrow, a low haptoglobulin level, increased lactate dehydrogenase activity, and indirect bilirubin in the serum. If this is antibody mediated, warm or cold agglutinins and a positive Coombs' test should be present. In rare cases, the hemolytic process is extreme and does not respond to immunosuppressive agents. Plasmapheresis and cytotoxic chemotherapy may be tried but usually to no avail. Immune thrombocytopenia can be detected by the presence of high numbers of normal-appearing megakaryocytes in the bone marrow but few circulating platelets in the peripheral blood. Those that are present tend to be large and young in appearance. The antibody is usually an immunoglobulin G, which can be found coating any remaining platelets. Platelet transfusions are of little or no value. Immunosuppression with steroids or more potent agents usually controls the problem.

Pulmonary Complications of Bone Marrow Transplantation

Interstitial Pneumonitis

A severe and frequently fatal complication of bone marrow transplantation is the onset of interstitial pneumonitis. This can take an acute, rapidly progressive form with complete failure of the pulmonary system in several hours to a few days, or it may be more chronic with a slow progression over weeks or months.

The acute form of the disorder frequently occurs between 1 and 4 months after bone marrow transplantation and in patients with clinically significant graft-versus-host reactions. Although in most cases a clear-cut causative agent cannot be identified, CMV is found in a significant number of these patients and is the presumed cause in most. Other viruses associated with T cell defects have been implicated, including adenoviruses, herpes simplex virus, and varicella-zoster virus. When markedly immunosuppressed, patients are also susceptible to parasitic infections, the most common being *Pneumocystis carinii*. *Toxoplasma gondii* and *Strongyloides stercoralis* are rare causes of interstitial pneumonias. Fungi must also be considered, especially in patients receiving high doses of steroids or having graft-versus-host reactions. After bone marrow transplantation, patients may have difficulty with opsonization and phagocytosis of encapsulated organisms for up to 2 years. Like patients who have undergone splenectomy, bone marrow transplantation patients sometimes have rapidly progressive, overwhelming pneumonias secondary to infection by *Streptococcus pneumoniae*, *H. influenzae*, or *Staphylococcus aureus*. These patients have difficulty handling gram-negative organisms as well.

When interstitial pneumonia is suspected, a diagnosis should be sought rapidly, including open lung biopsy with smears, silver stains, and cultures for viruses, fungi, and bacteria. Broad-spectrum coverage for *Legionella*, gram-negative bacteria, *P. carinii*, herpes-type viruses (acyclovir), and CMV (ganciclovir plus intravenous immunoglobulins) should be instituted immediately pending the results of diagnostic studies.

The more chronic form of the disorder is seen primarily in patients with chronic graft-versus-host disorders and probably has a variety of causes including toxicity of the preparative regimens (especially in patients who have undergone total body irradiation or had previous radiation therapy of the chest). Previous therapy with busulfan or procarbazine also appears to predispose patients to post-transplantation chronic pulmonary fibrosis. Most of these patients have had, in addition to chronic GVHD, repeated bouts of bacterial bronchitis or pneumonia. This chronic pulmonary fibrosis often leads to progressive respiratory failure. It is seldom reversible, and terminal patients, unless supported by respirators, die of anoxia.

Bronchiolitis Obliterans

Bronchiolitis obliterans is an unusual but severe and often fatal complication of bone marrow transplantation. It is characterized by severe inflammation of the terminal bronchi with formation of secondary fibrinoid nodules in the lumen of the bronchioles leading to airway obstruction, progressive hypoxia, and eventual death. The diagnosis is confirmed by biopsy, and the condition is rarely reversed with high-dose steroid therapy. The use of a respirator is necessary to maintain life. The etiology is unclear but a role of viruses is suspected.

Complications of Therapies Other Than the Bone Marrow Preparative Regimen

Several life-threatening complications of bone marrow transplantation are the result of the therapies instituted after transplantation. Many of these complications are due to the immunosuppressive agents used to treat or prevent GVHD. They include the following:

1. *Cyclosporine*: Cyclosporine causes severe, but reversible, renal tubular damage. Continued use of the drug despite a rising creatinine level may cause complete renal shutdown. Dialysis is essential to maintain the patient until the kidneys can recover. Hepatic toxicity with evidence of acute hepatic damage is also attributed to the use of cyclosporine and is, to a great degree, reversible on cessation of the drug. Extremely high levels or rapid intravenous infusion of cyclosporine can cause severe CNS stimulation with generalized grand mal seizures.

2. *Methotrexate*: Methotrexate is used for postgrafting immunosuppression. Its major life-threatening toxicity is suppression of bone marrow resulting in thrombocytopenia, and granulocytopenia is its major manifestation. Frequently associated with bone marrow toxicity is GI mucositis, which can be severe at times, leading to secondary infection, GI bleeding, and profuse diarrhea. Hepatic damage (fibrosis) and pulmonary fibrosis are extremely rare complications of the use of the drug. A few anaphylactic reactions to the drug have also been reported.

3. *Thalidomide*: The only major toxicity reported for this drug has been the production of congenital abnormalities of the limbs of fetuses of mothers who take the drug during pregnancy, an unlikely concern for bone marrow transplantation patients. Its only other known side effect has been drowsiness.

4. *Azathioprine*: Its major toxicity has been bone marrow suppression, which is reversible on cessation of the drug.

5. *High-dose steroid therapy*: This therapy for severe GVHD causes all of the known complications of steroids and makes these patients susceptible to unusual infections in the damaged organs of the body. Secondary adrenal hypoplasia and necrosis of the femoral head are relatively frequent complications of bone marrow transplantation.

6. *Antithymocyte globulin*: Being a foreign protein, ATG is prone to produce anaphylactic reactions, serum sickness, severe fevers, hives, and angioneurotic edema–type syndromes. In addition, it is a relatively crude preparation and may contain sufficient anti–red blood cell antibodies to cause hemolytic anemias (Coombs' positive) and thrombocytopenia secondary to antiplatelet antibodies. Most of the complications of ATG respond to steroid therapy.

7. *Antiviral agents*: These agents are commonly used in patients undergoing bone marrow transplantation and are also commonly associated with life-threatening complications requiring intensive care.
   a. *Acyclovir*: This effective antiherpes agent has occasionally been associated with renal shutdown, usually in patients who do not receive adequate hydration while receiving acyclovir. At least 1 L of extra fluid should be given for every gram of acyclovir administered.
   b. *Ganciclovir*: This is a potent suppressor of the bone marrow that can result in secondary neutropenia and infection or thrombocytopenia and bleeding.
   c. *Intravenous immunoglobulins*: These proteins are usually well tolerated by patients, but some preparations have been associated with severe, anaphylactoid reactions requiring careful intensive care and support with vasopressors, steroids, and antihistamines to save the patient.

8. *Blood products*: Bone marrow transplantation patients are prone to unusual transfusion-related complications that can be life threatening. Because the genes for the HLA antigens and the red blood cell antigens are not on the same chromosomes, there is frequently a major or minor red blood cell mismatch between the donor and recipient. In the case of a major red blood cell mismatch, reactions can usually be avoided by removing the red blood cells that contaminate the grafting cells. In such cases, the recipient's anti–red blood cell titer prevents the regrowth of erythroid precursors for weeks to months until all circulating antibody has been consumed. During that time, the recipient has pure red blood cell aplasia, with a bone marrow devoid of red blood cell precursors, and requires red blood cell transfusion support.

   In cases in which there is a minor mismatch between donor and recipient (such as an O bone marrow to an A recipient), one need only remove most of the plasma from the bone marrow inoculum to avoid a reaction of the donor antibodies against the recipient's red blood cells. However, the new bone marrow contains antibody-producing cells of donor origin and produces antibodies against the red blood cells of the recipient. At 10 to 14 days after the transplantation, there may be acute, severe hemolytic destruction of the recipient's red blood cells by the donor-derived antibodies. This hemolysis may be life threatening, with the bilirubin level climbing to 30 to 50 mg/dL and hemoglobin level dropping by more than 10 g/dL in only a few hours. Prompt extensive exchange transfusion with red blood cells compatible with the donor serum antibodies is necessary in such cases to prevent death.

   Some patients (e.g., when the donor is B and the recipient is A) are prone to both major and minor mismatch problems.

Third-party GVHD is possible when viable lymphocytes are infused into an immunocompromised host.[60] Because patients are severely immunocompromised after bone marrow transplantation, they must not be given blood products that contain any viable lymphocytes. The usual way to prevent such lymphocytes being infused is to irradiate all blood products. If viable T lymphocytes take up residence in a severely immunocompromised host, they can rapidly replicate and begin attacking the host. In such cases, one sees all the manifestations of an acute graft-versus-host reaction (see earlier) and rapid total destruction of any hematopoietic bone marrow function the patient may have. Because the bone marrow is "foreign" to the lymphocytes causing third-party GVHD, bone marrow is a major target. Total destruction of all granulocytes, platelets, and bone marrow occurs, and despite intensive steroid therapy or the use of other immunosuppressive agents, third-party GVHD is usually a fatal reaction in bone marrow transplantation recipients.

References

1. Champlin RE (ed): Bone Marrow Transplantation. Boston, Kluwer Academic Publishers, 1990.
2. Blume KG, Petz LD (eds): Clinical Bone Marrow Transplantation. New York, Churchill-Livingstone, 1983.
3. Strob R, Buchner CD: Human bone marrow transplantation. Eur J Clin Invest 20:119, 1990.
4. Thomas ED, Storb R, Clift RA, et al: Bone marrow transplantation. N Engl J Med 292:832, 1973.
5. Cheson BD, Locren L, Leyland-Jones B, et al: Autologous bone marrow transplantation: Current grafting and future directions. Ann Intern Med 110:51, 1989.
6. Stewart PS, Buschner CD, Bensenger W, et al: Autologous marrow transplantation in patients with acute non-lymphocytic leukemia in first remission. Exp Hematol 13:267, 1985.
7. Yeager AM, Kaizer M, Santos GW, et al: Autologous bone marrow transplantation in patients with acute nonlymphocytic leukemia using ex vivo marrow treatment with 4-hydroperoxycyclophosphamide. N Engl J Med 315:141, 1986.
8. Yeager AM, Rowley SD, Kaizer H, et al: Autologous bone marrow transplantation in acute non-lymphocytic leukemia: Studies of ex vivo chemopurging with 4-hydroperoxycyclophosphamide. In: Gale RP, Champlin R (eds): Bone Marrow Transplantation: Current Controversies. UCLA Symposia on Molecular and Cellular Biology, New Series, Volume 91. New York, Alan R Liss, p 157, 1989.
9. Ball ED, Mills LE, Coughlin CT: Autologous bone marrow transplantation in acute myelogenous leukemia: In vitro treatment with myeloid cell–specific monoclonal antibodies. Blood 68:1311, 1986.
10. Kersey TH, Weisdorf D, Nesbit ME, et al: Comparison of autologous and allogeneic bone marrow transplantation for treatment of high-risk refractory acute lymphoblastic leukemia. N Engl J Med 317:461, 1987.
11. Ritz J, Sallan SE, Bast RC Jr, et al: Autologous bone-marrow transplantation in CALLA-positive acute lymphoblastic leukemia after in-vitro treatment with J5 monoclonal antibody and complement. Lancet 2:60, 1982.
12. Gorin NC, David R, Strachowiak J, et al: High dose chemotherapy and autologous bone marrow transplantation in acute leukemias, malignant lymphomas and solid tumors. Eur J Cancer 17:557, 1981.
13. Goldstone AM, Griffen JG: The role of autologous bone marrow transplantation in the treatment of malignant disease. Blood Rev 1:193, 1987.
14. Burnett AL: Autologous bone marrow transplantation in acute leukemia. Leuk Res 12:531, 1988.
15. Gorin NC, Aergerter P, Auvert B, et al: Autologous bone marrow transplantation (ABMT) for acute leukemia in remission: Fifth European survey. Evidence in favor of marrow purging. Influence of pretransplant intervals. Bone Marrow Transplant 3(suppl 1):39, 1988.
16. Beron M, Zander AR: Critical issues in autologous bone marrow transplantation. Eur J Haematol 39:97, 1987.
17. Phillips GL, Reece PE: Clinical studies of autologous bone marrow transplantation in Hodgkin's disease. Clin Haematol 15:155, 1986.
18. Applebaum FR, Sullivan KM, Thomas ED, et al: Marrow transplantation as treatment for patients with recurrent malignant lymphoma. Int J Cell Cloning 3:216, 217, 1985.
19. Phillips GL, Herzig RH, Lazarus HM: Treatment of resistant malignant lymphoma with cyclophosphamide, total body irradiation, and transplantation of cryopreserved autologous marrow. N Engl J Med 310:1557, 1984.
20. Gulati SC, Shank B, Black P, et al: Autologous bone marrow transplantation for patients with poor prognosis lymphoma. J Clin Oncol 6:1303, 1988.
21. Barlogie B, Alexanian R, Dicke KA: High-dose chemoradiotherapy with autologous bone marrow transplantation for resistant multiple myeloma. Blood 70:869, 1987.
22. Applebaum FM, Fifer A, Cheever MA, et al: Treatment of aplastic anemia by bone marrow transplantation in identical twins. Blood 55:1033, 1980.
23. Fifer A, Cheever MA, Thomas ED, et al: Bone marrow transplantation for refractory acute leukemia in 34 patients with identical twins. Blood 57:421, 1981.
24. Fefer A, Cheever MA, Thomas ED, et al: Disappearance of Ph[1]-positive cells in four patients with chronic granulocytic leukemia after chemotherapy, irradiation and marrow transplantation from an identical twin. N Engl J Med 300:333, 1979.
25. Santos G, Bias W, Burns W, et al: Syngeneic bone marrow transplantation: The Baltimore experience. Exp Hematol 9(suppl 9):141, 1981.
26. Deeg HJ, Klingemann H-G, Phillips GL: A Guide to Bone Marrow Transplantation. New York, Springer-Verlag, 1967.
27. van Bekkum DW, de Vries JJ: Radiation Chimeras. London, Logos, 1967.
28. Sale GF, Shulman HM (eds): The Pathology of Bone Marrow Transplantation. New York, Masson Publishing USA, 1984.
29. Storb R, Thomas ED: Allogeneic bone marrow transplantation. Immunol Rev 71:77, 1983.
30. Thomas ED: Marrow transplantation for malignant diseases (Karnofsky Memorial Lecture). J Clin Oncol 1:517, 1983.
31. Lenarsky C, Kohn DB, Weinberg KI, et al: Bone marrow transplantation for genetic disease. Hematol Oncol Clin North Am 4:589, 1990.
32. Forman SJ, Blume KG: Allogeneic bone marrow transplantation for acute leukemia. Hematol Oncol Clin North Am 4:517, 1990.
33. Snyder DS, McGlave PV: Treatment of chronic myelogenous leukemia with bone marrow transplantation. Hematol Oncol Clin North Am 4:517, 1990.
34. Vossen JM, Heidt PH, van den Berg M, et al: Prevention of infection and graft-vs-host disease by suppression of the intestinal microflora in children treated with allogeneic bone marrow transplantation. Eur J Clin Microbiol Infect Dis 9:14, 1990.
35. Lum LG: Recapitulation of immune ontogeny: A vital component for the success of bone marrow transplantation. In: Champlin R (ed): Bone Marrow Transplantation. Boston, Kluwer Academic Publishers, p 27, 1990.
36. Barnes DWH, Loutit JF: Spleen protection: The cellular hypothesis. In: Bacq ZM (ed): Radiobiology Symposium. London, Butterworth, p 134, 1955.
37. Billingham RE: The biology of graft-versus-host reactions. Harvey Lect 62:21, 1966–67.
38. Vogelsang GB: Acute graft-versus-host disease. In: Champlin R (ed): Bone Marrow Transplantation. Boston, Kluwer Academic Publishers, p 55, 1990.
39. Sullivan KM: Chronic graft-versus-host disease. In: Champlin R (ed): Bone Marrow Transplantation. Boston, Kluwer Academic Publishers, p 79, 1990.
40. Burakoff SJ, Deeg HJ, Ferrara J, et al (eds): Graft-vs.-Host Disease: Immunology, Pathophysiology, and Treatment. New York, Marcell Decker, 1990.
41. Hess AD: Syngeneic and autologous graft-vs-host disease. In: Burakoff SS, Deeg HJ, Ferrara J, et al (eds): Graft-vs.-Host Disease: Immunology, Pathophysiology, and Treatment. New York, Marcel Dekker, p 95, 1990.
42. Rapperport JM: Syngeneic and autologous graft-vs-host disease. In: Burakoff SS, Deeg HJ, Ferrara J, et al (eds): Graft-vs.-Host Disease: Immunology, Pathophysiology, and Treatment. New York, Marcel Dekker, p 455, 1990.
43. Appelbaum FR, Strauchen JA, Graw RG Jr, et al: Acute lethal carditis caused by high-dose combination chemotherapy. A unique clinical and pathological entity. Lancet 1:58, 1976.
44. Santos GW: Immune suppression for clinical marrow transplantation. Semin Hematol 11:341, 1974.
45. Cox PJ, Abel G: Cyclophosphamide cystitis. Studies aimed at its minimization. Biochem Pharmacol 28:3499, 1979.
46. Beschorner WF, Pino J, Boitnott JK, et al: Pathology of the liver with bone marrow transplantation. Effects of busulfan, carmustine, acute graft-versus-host disease, and cytomegalovirus infection. Am J Pathol 99:369, 1980.
47. Brodsky R, Topolsky D, Crilley P, et al: Frequency of venoocclusive disease of the liver with a modified busulfan/cyclophosphamide preparative regimen. Am J Clin Oncol 13:221, 1990.
48. Krowka MJ, Rosenow EC 3d, Hoaglund HC: Pulmonary complications of bone marrow transplantation. Chest 87:237, 1985.
49. Chan CK, Hyland RH: Pulmonary complications following bone marrow transplantation. Clin Chest Med 11:323, 1990.
50. Deeg J, Cottler-Fox M: Clinical spectrum and pathophysiology of acute graft-vs-host disease. In: Burakoff SJ, Deeg HS, Ferrara J, et al (eds): Graft-vs.-Host Disease: Immunology, Pathophysiology, and Treatment. New York, Marcel Dekker, p 311, 1990.
51. Snover DC: The pathology of graft-vs-host disease. In: Burakoff SJ, Deeg HS, Ferrara J, et al (eds): Graft-vs.-Host Disease: Immunology, Pathophysiology, and Treatment. New York, Marcel Dekker, p 337, 1990.
52. Sullivan KM, Deeg HJ, Sanders J, et al: Hyperacute graft-vs-host disease in patients not given immunosuppression after allogeneic marrow transplantation. Blood 67:1172, 1986.
53. Deeg HJ, Henslee-Downey PJ: Management of acute graft-versus-host disease. Bone Marrow Transplant 6:1, 1990.
54. Atkinson K: Clinical spectrum of human chronic graft-vs-host disease. In: Burakoff SJ, Deeg HS, Ferrara J, et al (eds): Graft-vs.-Host Disease: Immunology, Pathophysiology, and Treatment. New York, Marcel Dekker, p 569, 1990.
55. Atkinson K: Treatment of extensive human chronic graft-vs-host disease. In: Burakoff SJ, Deeg HS, Ferrara J, et al (eds): Graft-vs.-Host Disease: Immunology, Pathophysiology, and Treatment. New York, Marcel Dekker, p 681, 1990.
56. Dulley FL, Kanfer EJ, Applebaum FR, et al: Venoocclusive disease of the liver after chemoradiotherapy and autologous bone marrow transplantation. Transplantation 43:870, 1987.
57. Jones RJ, Lee KSK, Beschorner WE, et al: Venoocclusive disease of the liver following bone marrow transplantation. Transplantation 44:778, 1987.
58. Winston DW, Ho WG, Champlin RE, et al: Infectious complications of bone marrow transplantation. Exp Hematol 12:205, 1984.

59. Wingard JR: Management of infectious complications of bone marrow transplantation. Oncology 4:69, 1990.
60. Spitzer TR: Transfusion-induced graft-vs-host disease. In: Burakoff SJ, Deeg HS, Ferrara J, et al (eds): Graft-vs.-Host Disease: Immunology, Pathophysiology, and Treatment. New York, Marcel Dekker, p 539, 1990.

CHAPTER 117

Bone Marrow Disorders Associated with Excessive Production

Philip J. Burke

NORMAL HEMATOPOIESIS

The bone marrow as an organ maintains the dynamic equilibrium of the formed elements of the peripheral blood within certain effective limits. To buffer rapid change in response to sudden need, masses of cells are available on call in the marrow or marginated in vessels in reserve, with less than 2% circulating in the blood. This bulk effect of constant and immediate supply masks the normally fluctuating levels of red blood cells, granulocytes, and platelets, which oscillate in a menstrual rhythm. This sine wave is identified when magnified by intervention with cytotoxic chemotherapy producing relative bone marrow aplasia. During recovery, the proliferative and subsequent maturative compartments can be distinguished, the progeny determined, and the life cycles mapped.[1] Studies demonstrate positive and negative feedback mechanisms, both cellular and humoral, that control this accentuated growth. When present normally at physiologic levels, these factors maintain cyclic homeostasis.[2]

Hematopoietic cells are produced by activation of a pluripotential stem cell with self-renewal capability whose descendants are committed to mature as a specific cell lineage. The resulting balanced mix of renewing and terminally differentiating elements is kept constant by cytokines elaborated from the cellular microenvironment of the stroma.[2-9] Humoral regulators, acting locally and at a distance, comprise specific lineage glycoproteins (colony-stimulating factors) that affect bone marrow progeny at various levels of proliferation but spare recruitment of the self-renewing primoidial stem cell.[2, 10-13] Through genetic engineering these cell line–specific biomodulators of granulopoiesis have been purified and the genes for their production identified and cloned. These growth factors, interleukin-1, interleukin-3, granulocyte and granulocyte-macrophage colony-stimulating factors, and factors specific for basophils and eosinophils, are being used in clinical trials.[11]

Similarly, lymphokines (e.g., interleukin-1 and interleukin-2), glycoproteins in increasing numbers defined by genetic engineering techniques, stimulate and guide renewal and differentiation of lymphocyte subsets of the immune system. When administered to the intact animal, these specific proteins modulate the effects of a myriad of resident host humoral factors to produce a cascade of effectors involved in function and surveillance.

ABNORMAL HEMATOPOIESIS

Granulocytosis

First-order response to an acute stimulus produces significant fluctuations of the absolute number of blood cells in a brief time. The ripple effect associated with this rapid redistribution of mature cells and products from the marginated to the circulatory pools ensures adequate host defense.

Most benign sources of growth and release of bone marrow products stimulate committed progeny at the distal levels of renewal, and these physiologic causes usually are readily detected and rectified if necessary. For example, strenuous exercise, pregnancy and labor, convulsions, and panic are associated with neutrophilic leukocytosis, and acute blood loss results in a fall and then a rebound of reticulocytes and platelets. Similarly, crises such as allergic reactions or viral infections cause lymphocytic increases, and bacterial infections cause leukemoid reactions.

In this acute response, the primary cell type needed is exaggerated in the differential count, sometimes with lineage crossover, for the duration required to fill the compartment or until cessation of stimulus. The cellular response is restricted to the small portion of the proliferative production pool necessary to replace the mature and immature differentiated cells of the reserve compartment. In cases of more chronic need (e.g., low oxygen saturation in lung disease, congenital hemolytic anemia, or suppurative osteomyelitis), the pluripotential stem cell can continually commit precursors to the specific lineage at risk, either erythroid or myelocytic, until the cause is controlled or compensated without exhaustion of proliferative potential.[14]

When uncovered by drug-induced bone marrow failure, the hematopoietic cycle is quite specific, with 14 days required for white blood cell (WBC) recovery to normal and a subsequent 14 days for rebound WBC and feedback inhibition before the normal muted cycle is re-established.[2] Knowing that this recovery time is predictable is important in accidental impairment of bone marrow function, as with chemotherapy overdose, because methods are readily available for supporting the patient through this short period of remedial aplasia.

Leukemoid Reaction

When a patient presents with a WBC count out of the range of normal reactive levels, identification of cause is critical in view of the high mortality of acute leukocytosis. However, the non-neoplastic causes of a WBC count in the range of 50,000/mm³ are myriad, and the cause is most quickly identified by examination of the peripheral blood. Leukemia and benign disease can virtually always be separated by inspection of stained smears. There are signs of a leukoerythroblastic reaction caused by secondary invasion and disruption of the bone marrow, or a shift to the left, in response to local or systemic infection, acute diabetes, gout, uremia, or other metabolic consequences of organ disease. There is no hiatus between mature and responding immature cells. In most cases, the granulocyte population is involved, with differentiated, nonproliferative, but immature WBCs and nucleated red blood cells. In benign diseases, no blasts are seen. If eosinophils are present, allergic disorders and hypersensitivity states associated with parasitic infestation or drug administration must be excluded. Basophilia can be seen with late-stage chronic granulocytic leukemia and the myeloproliferative disorders but is more likely with allergic reactions and viral infections.

Monocytosis frequently occurs with chronic bacterial, viral, or fungal infections; with debilitating collagen-vascular disorders; and with hematopoietic malignancies. Infection and metabolic diseases are common; leukemia is rare. However, leukemia must be considered and, if it is present, a treatment plan activated.

Hyperleukocytosis

Meaningful survival is possible for most patients with acute leukemia.[15–17] Failure to obtain disease remission late in therapy involves either failure of support or tumor resistance, and early mortality is related to the pathophysiology of the tumor. Included among those with relative biologic resistance are patients with hyperleukocytic leukemia (WBC >100,000/mm³), in whom early death with central nervous system hemorrhage and leakages can often be attributed to delay in treatment.[18–20] Because the early morbid effects of a high WBC count can frequently be ameliorated with expeditious treatment, physicians must be aware of the catastrophic nature and remediability of the syndrome of leukostasis.

In particular, patients with acute myelocytic leukemia (AML) with high blast counts are at grave risk from endarterial and capillary bed sludging and vessel rupture. Although a number of approaches may be used to reduce the cell count acutely, the method used in highly proliferative leukemia must also halt cellular expansion in fragile vessels.

Clinically, high leukemic blast cell counts in AML and chronic myelocytic leukemia (CML) are associated with fever and evidence of functional impairment of the lungs and brain, manifested by dyspnea, shortness of breath, tachy-

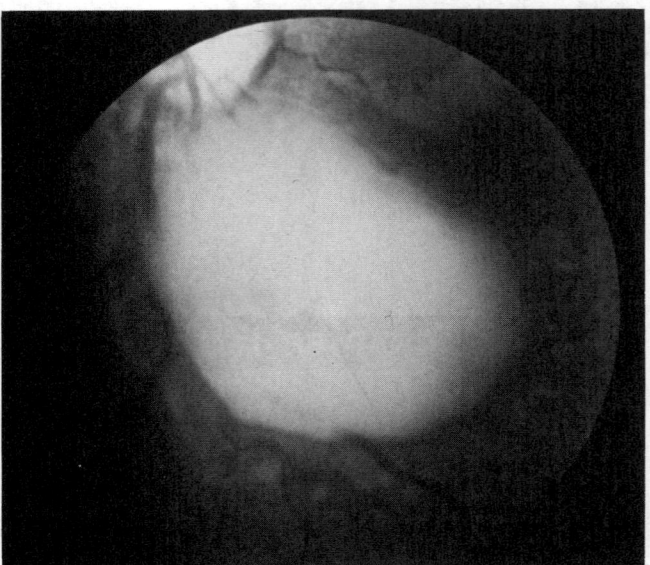

Figure 117–1. Subretinal accumulation of a proliferating leukemic mass at presentation in a patient with more than 100,000 myeloblasts per cubic millimeter.

pnea, confusion, and stupor. Particularly morbid is tissue invasion and extravascular growth of leukemia evidenced by priapism,[21] retinal hemorrhage and Roth's spots[22] (Fig. 117–1), masses at venipuncture and bone marrow biopsy sites, and the most predictive sign of ongoing vascular rupture, target purpura with a single deep central nodule in patients who often have an adequate platelet count (Fig. 117–2).

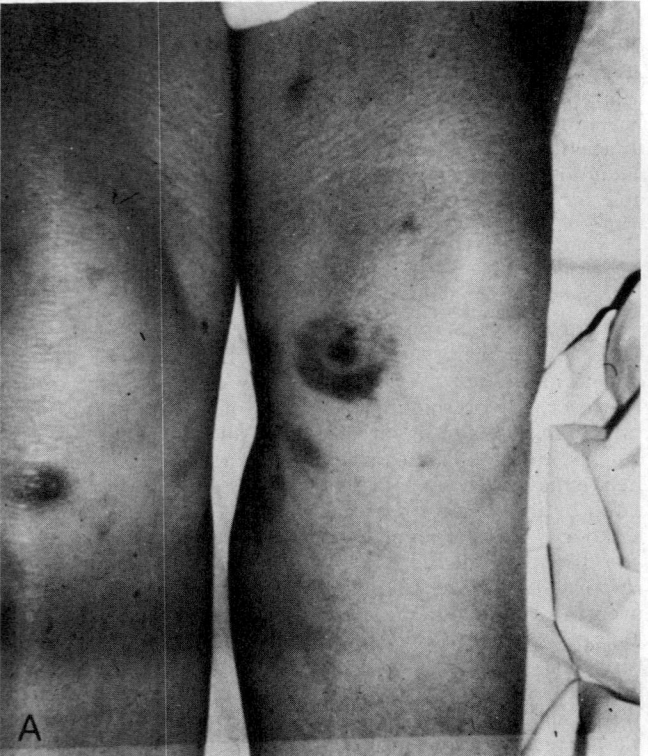

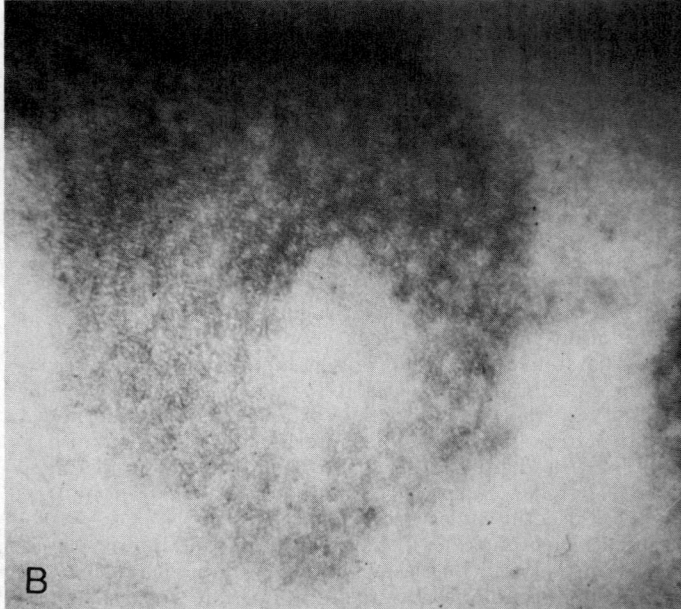

Figure 117–2. *A.* Classic target appearance of purpura formed by infarction of an arteriole by a dividing cluster of leukemic myeloblasts. Typically, a deep, firm nodule can be felt in the pale center of the lesion *(B).*

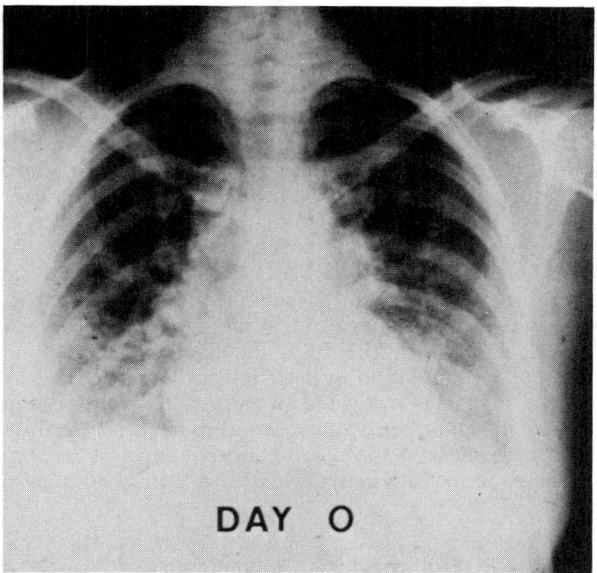

Figure 117-3. Admission chest radiograph of a patient with CML in blastic crisis, WBC count less than 50,000/mm³. The infiltrates and respiratory insufficiency cleared within 3 days of treatment.

Laboratory data confirm the suspicion of imminent catastrophe. Although findings on examination of the lungs may be few, the chest film reveals diffuse fluffy infiltrates (Fig. 117-3), the Po₂ is low, and the WBC count is high.[23-31]

There is evidence that the rigidity of the myeloblast causes stasis, particularly in the low-pressure microcirculation of the lungs and brain, which accounts for the signs of hypoxia in these organs.[30-35] The potential for increased viscosity in the capillaries because of lack of cell deformability is usually offset by a concurrent anemia commensurate with the leukocrit, because the combined hematocrit and leukocrit at presentation is usually not greater than 50%[26] (Fig. 117-4). Because a critical mass is not exceeded unless iatrogenically increased by red blood cell transfusions,[36] unbalanced diuresis, or rapid leukemia cell proliferation, the incidence of clinical leukostasis in patients with WBC counts less than 100,000/mm³ is low.[30]

Clearly, not all patients with an elevated WBC count are at risk for leukostasis. Those with acute lymphocytic leukemia (ALL) and chronic lymphocytic leukemia (CLL), by virtue of the smaller size and deformability and the low mitotic index of these cells, are less likely to be affected,[37, 38] as are those with CML in the chronic stage with a high proportion of mature, nonproliferative cells.[39, 40] In contrast, children with CML, who are prone to have elevated counts and a high leukocrit,[41] and adults with increased numbers of blasts and progranulocytes[24, 37, 42] require effective emergency therapy. Most predictably in jeopardy are patients with blasts with a high proliferative rate and short cell cycle time, evidenced by the presence of mitotic figures in the peripheral blood smear, a rapidly rising WBC count, and evidence of tissue extravasation.[26, 39, 41-44] These patients form thrombi rather than aggregates in the microcirculation, with hemorrhage and necrosis of lung and brain tissue.[18, 37, 45-48] Concomitant decreased oxygen transport and increased consumption by the blasts, as well as release of injurious cellular toxins, may be locally damaging.[45] Such patients commonly have monoblasts as the primary leukemic cells.

Management of Hyperleukocytosis

A successful scheme entails awareness, rapid intervention, aggressive treatment, and critical care management in an emergency situation for all patients with hyperleukocytosis (Table 117-1).

Although the risk rises with the count, it is assumed that all patients with a WBC count greater than 50,000/mm³ are in danger of sudden death, and a plan for immediate treatment of all adults with a high WBC count must be instituted. By the time the patient has been weighed, the drug dose calculated, and the antileukemic drugs readied for infusion, review of the admission blood smear has excluded from this approach patients with CML and a low proliferative/nonproliferative ratio and patients with ALL. Bone marrow aspiration is occasionally needed to substantiate the diagnosis, but treatment should not be delayed if it is not immediately available.

There is less security in the diagnosis of ALL, because M1 and M7 AML and CML in lymphoid blast crisis can appear similar. If there is doubt, all these patients should be treated with active drugs capable of inducing remissions in all acute leukemias.

The immediate goal of therapy is not only abrupt reduction of the WBC count but also arrest of proliferation of aggregates of cells embedded in the small capillaries of the brain, where continued expansion causes endothelial damage and release of intrinsic factor, disseminated intravascular coagulation, vessel rupture, extravasation of tumor, hemorrhage, and irreversible damage. With rapid institution of continuous infusion of high-dose cytosine arabinoside, a cell cycle–dependent DNA synthesis–inhibiting drug, coupled with daunorubicin, an agent highly effective in both AML and ALL, central nervous system damage has been prevented in a high percentage of patients with AML. In

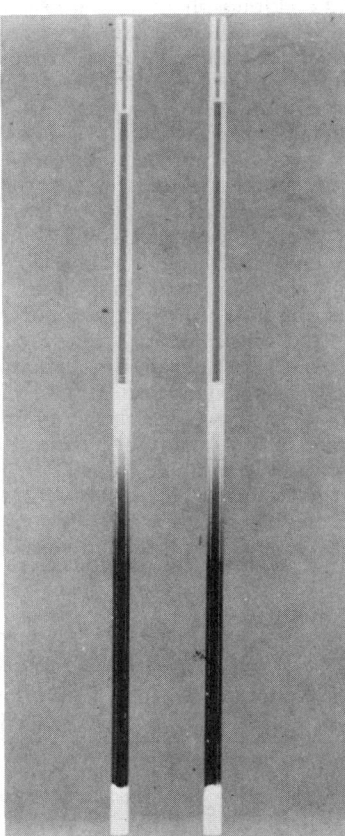

Figure 117-4. Spun leukocrit-hematocrit of a patient with more than 50,000 myeloblasts per cubic millimeter. The combined red blood cell WBC mass must not exceed 45%. Above that level, cellular viscosity increases logarithmically with red blood cell transfusions.

TABLE 117-1

MANAGEMENT OF HYPERLEUKOCYTOSIS*

Institute allopurinol, 600 mg PO immediately, 300 mg PO q. d. × 3

Institute Amphojel, 30 mL PO immediately and q 4 h

Hydrate with 0.45 N NaCl without bicarbonate, 150 mL/h × 5 d

Maintain urine output equal to hydration
Furosemide IV as needed and effective
Dopamine ≤ 3 μg/kg/min infusion

Begin cell cycle–specific antileukemic therapy within 2 h of admission

Transfuse red blood cells only when WBC count < 50,000/mm³ or when clinically imperative

Maintain platelet count > 50,000/mm³

Monitor K⁺, phosphate, creatinine, serum urea nitrogen, blood gases q 12 h until patient's condition is stable

Monitor prothrombin time, partial thromboplastin time, fibrinogen, fibrin degradation products q 12 h until patient's condition is stable

If fibrinogen consumption and fibrin degradation products develop, add heparin

Dialyze early for tumor lysis–related acute renal failure

*The scheme used at the Johns Hopkins Oncology Center to prevent morbidity and mortality associated with leukostasis, tumor lysis, and disseminated intravascular coagulation.

addition, and relative to pulmonary function, viscosity is reduced by the prevention of tumor growth in the bone marrow and lymph nodes, cell loss quickly exceeds cell gain, and the WBC count falls. Other drugs such as hydroxyurea (6 g/m²)[44-54] and cyclophosphamide (3 g/m²) are also of value in reducing the WBC count. In the doses generally used, hydroxyurea is not considered capable of inducing remission, and cyclophosphamide, although useful in tumor reduction in the lymphoid malignancies, is not cell cycle dependent and may lead to hematuria later in the course during aplasia. In our experience, however, its predictable effects on counts and bone marrow recovery make cyclophosphamide the drug of choice in the emergency setting. The mean time to 50% of initial WBC counts is 24 hours and to 10% or less is 48 hours[19] (Table 117-2). With this tumor reduction and decreased sludging in the pulmonary capillary bed, respiratory function is quickly restored and pulmonary infiltrates resolve over a few days.

Additional measures used in the management of this syndrome include cranial irradiation[55] and leukapheresis.[56-60] Effective chemotherapy acts as rapidly as irradiation of a critical organ and permits continued careful medical monitoring. Removing large numbers of cells by pheresis effectively reduces the circulatory blast cell count.[57, 58] However, this mechanical procedure does not affect the proliferation of cells already lodged in tissue and may complicate the management of medically unstable patients if the pheresis

facility is at a distance. Simultaneous leukapheresis and chemotherapy may be of no more value than chemotherapy alone in myeloid tumor reduction. However, particularly in children, in whom ALL is the more likely diagnosis, exchange leukapheresis before treatment is commonly indicated.[61-64] Effectively reducing the tumor load before tumor lysis with chemotherapy reduces the possibility of hyperuricemia and hyperphosphatemia induced by drug therapy. In childhood ALL, the risk of vascular rupture is decreased because the proliferative index is low, and increased viscosity is less likely at high counts because of the relatively small size of the lymphoblast. In adults the risk of error in diagnosis is much higher, and immediate chemotherapy is indicated. Even with the high incidence of disseminated intravascular coagulation in patients with hyperleukocytosis, few die if a plan is instituted promptly. A rapid response, transport by ambulance or helicopter at referral, and increased awareness of the mortal consequences of treatment delay in patients with leukocytosis are critical to survival[19] (Table 117-3).

Erythrocytosis (Polycythemia)

Polycythemia, defined by an increase in the red blood cell mass and a hematocrit higher than 55%, is classified by its pathophysiology. Benign, or secondary, polycythemia results from response to low tissue oxygenation or to increased erythropoietin levels. Stress or relative erythrocytosis occurs with a high hematocrit without an increased red blood cell volume. There are rare familial syndromes as well.

Although a hematocrit greater than 45% indicates improved oxygen-carrying capacity, blood viscosity also increases. With hypervolemia and a hematocrit less than 55%, there is reduced delivery of the excess oxygen to tissues,[65] particularly to low-flow organs and brain.[66] Whereas some patients with secondary polycythemia have an increase in the red blood cell number in response to a physiologic need, those with primary or inappropriate secondary polycythemia are at risk without benefit.

Because of the severe side effects of an elevated red blood cell mass, it is imperative to make a secure diagnosis and develop a management plan early in the course. The most critical diagnosis is that of polycythemia vera (PV). The Polycythemia Vera Study Group[67] has defined criteria and management schemes for PV and nonphysiologic erythrocytosis.

Diagnosis. The red blood cell mass and plasma volume must be determined by ⁵¹Cr measurements. If they are normal, the patient has relative polycythemia. If the red blood cell mass is high, secondary polycythemia must be distinguished from PV. The causes of secondary polycythemia are listed in Table 117-4. In most cases this diagnosis can be made on the basis of history, physical examination, specific radiologic or function tests, and bone marrow examination (Table 117-5). The serum erythropoietin level and arterial oxygen saturation can be measured directly.

TABLE 117-2

EFFECT OF CYTOTOXIC THERAPY ON WHITE BLOOD CELL COUNT IN PATIENTS WITH ACUTE MYELOGENOUS LEUKEMIA PRESENTING WITH HYPERLEUKOCYTOSIS

Total WBC Count (/mm³)	Number of Patients	% of Initial WBCs (Range)			
		24 h*	48 h	72 h	96 h
>100,000	13	53 (37–75)	14 (0.1–36)	4 (0–11)	(0–3)
50,000–100,000	13	48 (31–91)	23 (0.1–61)	10 (0–31)	4 (0–10)

*Hours after treatment.

TABLE 117–3

PRINCIPLES OF MANAGEMENT IN LEUKOCYTOSIS

Prompt referral to treatment center
Immediate measures to lower WBC count (mechanical versus chemical)
Resist temptation to give red blood cell transfusions until WBC count falls
Vigorous supportive care

TABLE 117–5

DIAGNOSIS OF TRUE POLYCYTHEMIA*

A. High red blood cell mass
    Male $\geq$ 36 mL/kg
    Female $\geq$ 32 mL/kg
  PO_2 > 92%
  Splenomegaly
B. Thrombocytosis (>400,000/mm³)
  Leukocytosis (>12,000/mm³)
  Leukocyte alkaline phosphatase level high
  Vitamin B_{12} serum level > 900 pg/mL
  Vitamin B_{12}–binding capacity > 2200 pg/mL

*Diagnosis is based on all three findings in A or the first two in A plus two in B.

Management of Secondary and Relative Polycythemia.

Therapy directed at the secondary causes is the first step. Weight decrease, cessation of smoking, removal of erythropoietin-secreting tumors, and correction of renal disease lead to reduction of the red blood cell mass.

In those with a physiologic need to increase the hematocrit, phlebotomy may not be indicated if the hematocrit is less than 60%.[68] However, a decrease in the hematocrit to 55% is beneficial for patients with chronic lung disease.[69–75] Myelosuppression with hydroxyurea is contraindicated in patients with secondary erythrocytosis. Phlebotomy is indicated before surgery, but this must be balanced with the requirement for increased oxygen-carrying capacity. If needed, isovolemic phlebotomy may avoid acute hemodynamic effects of acute reduced blood volume.[76]

Thrombocytosis

Platelet counts greater than 400,000/mm³ are excessive and have a number of causes. Many benign diseases or specific physiologic events involve stimulation of hematopoiesis with overlap in effect. This overproduction of varying degree of all formed elements of the marrow may be due to acute loss resulting from bleeding or delayed clotting, acute or chronic inflammatory processes of immunity or infection, or acute release of cells held in reserve in response to general stimulants or exercise.

Increased platelet counts are also observed in patients with malignancies not involving the bone marrow, solid tumors and lymphomas, pulmonary involvement in Hodgkin's disease, or delayed removal of senescent platelets after splenectomy. When they are associated with malignancies, the etiology of thrombocytosis is usually overproduction of morphologically normal platelets in response to stimulatory substances released by the tumor itself, with platelet levels decreasing to normal with control of the primary disease.

Although not common with secondary causes of increased platelet numbers, bleeding may occur with intravascular clotting or direct interference with clotting mechanisms, especially at counts greater than 1 million/mm³. Complications are rare and no therapy is indicated unless the patient is symptomatic.

Lymphocytosis

Benign lymphocytosis is seen most commonly in response to acute viral infections and granulomatous diseases. In most cases it involves T or B cells functioning as a host defense mechanism and reorientation of foreign antigen with immunoglobulin production or infiltration and attack. The prominent causes are the acute viral diseases seen in children, infectious mononucleosis, hepatitis, infectious lymphocytosis, chronic infections by myelobacteria and fungus, some endocrine disorders, and collagen-vascular diseases. These are usually self-limited or responsive to correction of the cause.

MALIGNANT HEMATOPOIESIS

The Myeloid Neoplasms

Pathogenesis

The pathogenesis of the myeloid neoplasms can be best understood in light of deviations from the pluripotential stem cell. One class directly evolving by clonal expansion consists of stem cell neoplasms that have various growth advantages and rates of progression while retaining a semblance of response to normal control mechanisms. This group has a morphologic heterogeneity associated with the dominant abnormal cell in the peripheral blood. These diseases are referred to as the myeloproliferative disorders. Erythroid predominance is seen in PV, granulocytic manifestations in chronic granulocytic leukemia and chronic myelomonocytic leukemia, thrombocytosis in essential thrombocythemia, and fibrous bone marrow structure overgrowth in myelofibrosis disease. Each may involve irregular growth of all bone marrow elements because the derivative cell is capable of all directions of myeloid commitment, including lymphoid (Table 117–6).

A similar category, myelodysplastic syndrome (MDS), encompasses entities with neoplastic clonal expansion but with less likelihood of overproduction of circulating terminally differentiated cells. In an attempt to improve our understanding of these disorders, a classification scheme has been devised on the basis of potential for malignant transformation (Table 117–7).

Conditions in each of these classes may terminate with leukemia not dissimilar to de novo AML. De novo leukemia

TABLE 117–4

CLASSIFICATION OF ERYTHROCYTOSES

Primary
  Polycythemia vera
  Pure erythrocytosis
Secondary
  Low tissue oxygen level
    Altitude
    Chronic lung disease
    Right-to-left shunt
    Hemoglobinopathy
    Alveolar hypoventilation
  Normal tissue oxygen level
    Erythropoietin producing tumors
    Renal diseases
    Adrenal hyperplasia
    Androgens
  Stress

TABLE 117–6

DIAGNOSTIC CLASSIFICATION OF MYELOPROLIFERATIVE DISORDERS

FAB Class	Classic Designation	Cytogenetics	Morphology
PV	Polycythemia vera	+8	Hypercellular panmyelopathy
CML	Chronic myelocytic leukemia	t(9;22)	All marrow elements increased
MF	Myelofibrosis		Leukoerythroblastosis, myelofibrosis, extramedullary hematopoiesis
ET	Essential thrombocythemia		Platelet count > 1 million/mm³, moderate increase all elements

is more likely derived from a more committed cell of origin, with residual unaffected normal but functionally suppressed stem cells. This potential for normal reconstitution permits consideration of ablative therapy.

Because of the available therapy, a wider appreciation of the similarities that override the apparent diversity is needed. With the availability of extrinsic hematopoietic support, induced bone marrow failure no longer restricts therapy and is, in fact, necessary if adequate tumor killing is to be achieved. With the drugs now available and concepts of therapy established in the laboratory animal, aggressive therapy of many of these bone marrow neoplasms can be rationally applied and meaningful survival achieved.

New technologies—DNA hybridization, purified specific probes, rapid techniques, monoclonal antibodies marking lineage specificity and maturation antigens, and measures of gene expression—make classification and tracing of tumor origin and progression more accurate and permit prognostication. When these are combined with genetic techniques for characterizing complex chromosomal changes basic to most tumors, new approaches to tumor control can be considered. Single-site genetic mutations, translocations or deletions of chromosomes, loss of suppression or overexpression of gene product, and transcription of an abnormal product that may induce a malignant phenotype are molecular biologic targets. These approaches now include eradication with enhanced chemotherapy, but greater hope for future cancer therapy lies in understanding and controlling pathogenesis with biomodulation to force suppression or stable mutation of the malignant clone.

Classification of the Myeloid Malignancies

Arbitrary classification of these diseases by morphology has led to some confusion. With better definition of these neoplastic diseases by new technologies, the trilineage clonal neoplasms can be unified functionally as a single disease entity displaying a wide spectrum of clinical and laboratory manifestations and a similar outcome.

The hematopoietic neoplasms are classified in the French-American-British (FAB) system by the morphology of the bone marrow elements and their histocompatible characteristics; the subclasses are ordered according to rate of malignant transformation and growth. All subtypes can be considered neoplastic on the basis of evidence of clonal expansion. The classification of the myeloid neoplasms by morphology, maturation, antigen, and cytogenetics is outlined in Tables 117–6 to 117–8.

Polycythemia Vera

PV, characterized by a plethoric appearance, splenomegaly, and an increased red blood cell mass, occurs principally in middle age and is more common in men than in women. Symptoms refer to many different organ systems; many of the clinical manifestations are related to the increased blood volume (increased red blood cell mass), increased blood viscosity, tendency to hemorrhagic and thromboembolic events, and underlying arteriosclerosis.

Constitutional complaints, such as irritability, fatigability, headache, visual disturbances, tinnitus, abdominal fullness, and aching of the lower extremities, are common. Pruritus is experienced by half of the patients and is often severe after bathing. Other symptoms include dyspnea, angina, intermittent claudication, and dependent edema. Less commonly, gout is the initial clinical problem.

The physical findings include ruddy cyanosis, ecchymoses, red mucous membranes, and engorged retinal veins. Hypertension is found in about half of the cases. Peptic ulcer is encountered in 20% of patients and gouty arthropathy in 5%.

TABLE 117–7

DIAGNOSTIC CLASSIFICATION OF THE MYELODYSPLASTIC SYNDROMES

FAB Class	Classic Designation	Cytogenetics	Morphology
RA	Refractory anemia	Normal	Anemia without blasts, cellular bone marrow, moderate dyserythropoiesis
RARS	Refractory anemia with ringed sideroblasts	Normal	Anemia with <5% blasts, >15% nucleated cells are ringed sideroblasts
CMML	Chronic myelomonocytic leukemia	Normal	RAEB plus monocytosis, immature granulopoiesis, monocytosis > 1 million cells per cubic millimeter
RAEB	Refractory anemia with excess blasts	(−5/5q−), (−7/7q−), (20q−), (8+), (Y−)	Cytopenia of two or more elements, dyshematopoiesis 5–20% blasts
RAEB-t	Refractory anemia with excess blasts in transformation		RAEB plus <20%; <30% blasts in bone marrow, <5% blasts in peripheral blood, Auer's rods

TABLE 117–8

DIAGNOSTIC CLASSIFICATION OF ACUTE MYELOCYTIC LEUKEMIA

FAB Class	Classic Designation	Cytogenetics	Morphology
M0	Myelocytic, undifferentiated		100% undifferentiated blasts
M1	Myelocytic, stem cell undifferentiated	Normal, inv(3), +8, 5q/−5, 7q/−7	90% undifferentiated blasts, <10% with granules, Auer's rods
M2	Myelocytic with maturation	Normal, t(8;21), +8, t(3;5), t(9;22)	Maturation to progranulocytes and beyond, >30% primary granules and Auer's rods
M3	Progranulocytic	t(15;17)	Hypergranular, primary granules, Auer's rods, bizarre blasts, disseminated intravascular coagulation
	Progranulocytic variant	t(15;17), +8	Progranulocytes with minimal granulation, bilobed nucleus
M4	Myelomonocytic	t(9;11), +8	20% monoblasts, >20% myeloblasts, monocytosis
M4 BASO		t(6;9)	As in M4, with basophils
M4 EOS	Myelomonocytic	inv(16)	As in M4, with increased eosinophils
M5a	Monocytic	t(9;11), +8	>80% myeloblasts
M5b	Monocytic		Monoblasts with >20% maturation
M6	Erythrocytic	Multiple	Bizarre erythroblasts, dyserythropoiesis, >30% myeloblasts, progranulocytes
M7	Megakaryocytic (acute myelosclerosis)	t(1;3)	Bizarre megakaryocytes with immature lobulation, increased platelets, myelofibrosis with heterogeneous peripheral blasts (confused with L1, L2, M1)

Splenomegaly is a cardinal feature of PV, being present in 75% of cases at presentation. Abdominal discomfort results from massive splenic enlargement and is periodically intensified by the occurrence of splenic infarcts. Modest hepatomegaly is observed in 30 to 50% of patients.

Hematocrit values range between 55 and 80%. The WBC and platelet counts are elevated, the former usually ranging from 10,000 to 50,000/mm³, and the latter from 300,000 to 600,000/mm³. The red blood cells and WBCs appear normal. There is a shift to the left in the granulocytic forms. Nucleated red blood cells and immature myelocytes are encountered occasionally. The granulocyte alkaline phosphatase concentration is high.

The bone marrow is usually hypercellular, consistent with panmyelopathy. Areas of myelofibrosis and osteosclerosis may be seen.

The blood volume is increased, at times being nearly twice normal. Blood viscosity is increased in proportion to the hematocrit. Ferrokinetic studies reveal increased plasma iron turnover and erythrocyte production. The red blood cell life span is normal, as is arterial oxygen saturation. The blood uric acid concentration is high in a significant proportion of patients. Erythropoietin concentrations in serum and urine are usually lower than normal or undetectable. Serum vitamin B$_{12}$ concentrations are usually increased.

Diagnosis. The occurrence of plethora, ruddy cyanosis, splenomegaly, and hepatomegaly, coupled with polycythemia in the absence of detectable cardiac or pulmonary disease, leads promptly to the correct diagnosis in the majority of cases. Increased red blood cell mass, normal arterial oxygen saturation, and splenomegaly establish a firm diagnosis. Thrombocytosis, leukocytosis, elevated granulocyte alkaline phosphatase activity, and increased serum vitamin B$_{12}$ concentration are important secondary criteria (see Table 117–5).

Management of Polycythemia Vera. Phlebotomy is indicated to reduce the hematocrit to 45% over a tolerable period depending on emergency and age, and the hematocrit is then maintained at that level. The PV Study Group guidelines are detailed in Table 117–9.

Phlebotomy alone may not be reasonable because there is a higher risk of thromboembolic coagulation unless myelosuppressive agents are also used. The risk increases with age and history of previous thromboemboli.[77] The treatment of choice based on long-term studies is hydroxyurea, a ribonucleoside inhibitor, given orally at a dose of 1 to 2 g/d.[78, 79] The use of ³²P and chlorambucil is contraindicated because of the incidence of secondary leukemia.[77] Neither aspirin nor dipyridamole is indicated to prevent thromboembolic complications.[80, 81]

Even with control of red blood cell mass, the signs and symptoms of this clonal multiple-organ disease can be significant and should be treated specifically (Table 117–10).

Surgery at presentation is risky because of potential hemorrhage and thrombosis.[82] If possible, the disease should be controlled for 2 months before intervention.[83] If emergency surgery is necessary, the hematocrit should be reduced to 45% by isovolemic phlebotomy.

Patients with PV may be expected to survive for 10 to 20 years. The major medical problems encountered stem from the occurrence of vascular thromboses (and emboli) and hemorrhage. A peptic ulcer, which is common in these individuals, may be the site of gastrointestinal bleeding. Epistaxis, ecchymosis, and bleeding after dental extraction are more common. Intercurrent infections, particularly pulmonary, are a significant but lesser problem.

TABLE 117–9

TREATMENT OF POLYCYTHEMIA VERA

Phlebotomy to hematocrit < 46%
Maintain hematocrit
   Patients older than 50 y: phlebotomy and/or hydroxyurea
   Patients younger than 50 y: phlebotomy alone; hydroxyurea
      when trilineage expression
Risk of thrombosis: hydroxyurea
Symptomatic relief

TABLE 117–10

MANAGEMENT OF COMPLICATIONS OF POLYCYTHEMIA VERA

Symptom	Treatment
Hyperuricemia	Allopurinol
Bleeding	Blood transfusions
Abnormal platelets	Platelet transfusion
Peptic ulcer	Antacids, H$_2$ antagonists
Pruritus	Cyproheptadine
Myelofibrosis or metaplasia	Blood products
Symptomatic splenomegaly	Splenectomy
Acute leukemia	Chemotherapy

The immediate cause of death in this group of patients is principally the associated cardiovascular disease. Cerebral hemorrhage or thrombosis, myocardial infarction, and heart failure are the most frequent terminal events. In 15 to 25% of the patients, the disease pattern changes to one characteristic of granulocytic leukemia or myeloid metaplasia with myelofibrosis. At times, an acute granulocytic leukemia develops toward the end of the disease.

Neoplastic Thrombocytosis

Elevated platelet levels associated with neoplastic disorders of the bone marrow cause problems requiring intervention in some cases. In such instances, platelet counts are seldom the only evidence of the panmyelopathies, and which of the overlapping myeloproliferative disorders is involved can be determined by appropriate studies. Nonetheless, the most significant overt manifestation may require direct action.

Thrombocytosis with abnormal platelet morphology, commonly seen in all cases of the myeloproliferative disorders, is most obvious in patients with CML and essential thrombocythemia. In CML, counts above 1 million/mm³, among other variables, foreshadow a short survival. This predictor reflects the overall momentum of the disease, not necessarily only the damaging effects of the elevated platelet levels. The aim is control of the disease. In essential thrombocythemia, for example, the problems associated with thrombocytosis as a primary manifestation can be significant and the elevated counts should be reduced.

Primary Thrombocythemia (Essential Thrombocythemia)

Primary thrombocythemia is a rare disease characterized by a platelet count of 1 million/mm³, hyperplasia of megakaryocytes, absence of the Philadelphia chromosome, no increase in red blood cell mass, and primary origin. Like the other myeloproliferative disorders, it is a clonal disease, originating in a pluripotential stem cell and occasionally interlinked with CML, PV, and myelofibrosis.[84] Similarly, it is a disease of patients older than 50 years of age and has an insidious onset. Most patients present with bleeding from the gastrointestinal tract, skin, or mucous membranes associated with a high platelet count in the peripheral blood. The bleeding may be due to vascular thrombosis, infection, platelet function abnormalities, and consumption of coagulation factors. Both venous emboli and thromboses occur with gangrene and central venous and arterial thrombosis. Splenomegaly is present at diagnosis in at least 60% of patients. Laboratory features include a markedly elevated platelet count with platelet aggregates, giant platelets, cytoplasmic fragments, and abnormally shaped platelets. The bone marrow aspirate reveals megakaryocytic hyperplasia with a markedly hypercellular marrow. The megakaryocytes are large and abnormal. Because of chronic blood loss, most patients have iron deficiency anemia. Infrequently, an abnormality or deletion of the long arm of chromosome 21 is found. As in the other myeloproliferative disorders, causes of secondary thrombocytosis, including PV and CML, must be ruled out.

Management of Thrombocytosis. Patients with acute thrombocytosis of benign cause should not be treated; those with myeloproliferative diseases should be treated on the basis of clinical findings. Experience dictates that platelet counts above 1 million/mm³ associated with signs and symptoms of impending thrombosis or bleeding offset the risks of therapy. The treatment of choice for reducing morbidity in all patients with myeloproliferative diseases is hydroxyurea. A new agent, anagrelide, has an antiaggregating effect on platelets.[85] In initial studies, a rapid decrease in platelet count in patients with myeloproliferative diseases was seen at effective dose therapy without interruption and sporadic dose adjustment.

Hydroxyurea should be given at 1 to 2 g/m² orally daily. There is evidence of improvement in survival in patients with CML treated over time with this drug, and there have been no observations of induction of secondary malignancies.

Other Therapies. Clinical trials are under way to evaluate the use of interferon in myeloproliferative diseases, and initial results in essential thrombocythemia, PV, and CML appear promising.[86, 87] The doses commonly used are 3 to 5 MU/m² given subcutaneously two or three times a week for months. The patient can be taught to self-administer this biomodulator. Side effects of fatigue and an influenza-like syndrome cause discontinuation in 50% of cases treated over the long term.[80] Because one of the suspected effects of this multifactorial agent is antagonism of platelet-derived growth factor, the onset of myelofibrosis may also be reduced or delayed.

The Myelodysplastic Syndrome

These apparently diverse bone marrow diseases are considered as a group because of their trilineage origin and their ultimate outcome in death from bone marrow failure and/or leukemia. In light of increased cell production, all are associated with hypercellular bone marrow and, if leukemia develops, potentially high peripheral blood cell counts. The terms *myelodysplastic syndrome, smoldering leukemia, preleukemia,* and *refractory anemia with excess blasts* encompass a broad range of patients from those presenting with a low percentage of leukemia cells and a protracted course to those with bone marrow replacement dysplasia and a high percentage of blasts at diagnosis. Over time, however, patients demonstrate continuing progression of a similar neoplastic state. Patients who develop acute leukemia can be managed in a manner similar to that for patients with do novo AML. This designated group is categorized in the FAB system (see Table 117–7).

Clinical Manifestations

MDS is characteristically a disease of the elderly (>70 years), with prominent persistent cytopenia of a single line or all three lineages of the bone marrow elements in spite of hypercellularity of that organ and with conversion to leukemia or death from marrow failure likely within 2 years of diagnosis. MDS is neoplastic and lethal even without manifestation of overt leukemia.

The signs and symptoms of MDS are related to the dominant cell line of the pluripotential clone most detectable at presentation. In half of the cases, the cytopenia is discovered incidentally, with findings dependent on the extent of bone marrow failure and organ invasion commonly associated with infection, bleeding, weakness, and fatigue.

Virtually all patients have refractory anemia and many have pancytopenia, but isolated myeloid cytopenias are rare. The stained smear reveals abnormal red blood cells with macrocytosis and hypochromia and circulating nucleated cells. Neutropenia or thrombocytopenia (or both) is seen in 50% of cases. The hypercellular marrow aspirate reveals abnormal growth and maturation of all elements, with erythroid hyperplasia, megaloblastosis, and marked dyserythropoiesis, sometimes with ringed sideroblasts present. With progression over time and depending on the extent of disease when the patient was first found to have MDS, the picture may change from mild anemia to pancytopenia.

Of these diseases, chronic myelomonocytic leukemia is unique in its association with chronic monocytosis, which abruptly accelerates in its end stage, producing manifestations similar to the blast crisis of CML.

Chronic Myelomonocytic Leukemia

The defining feature is the presence of an absolute monocytosis with more than 1000 cells per cubic millimeter. Often this is associated with an increase in mature granulocytes with or without evidence of dysgranulopoiesis (e.g., hypogranular and/or Pelger's forms). It is a defined disease of the elderly, sometimes confused with CML because of a similar frequent high peripheral WBC count, a differential containing a progressive level of immature cells of the granulocytic series, hepatosplenomegaly, monocytosis, and a markedly hypercellular marrow. It terminates with an aggressive phase, consistent with a multistep evolution and clonal progression characterized by monocytosis with soft tissue invasion, bone pain, hypermetabolism, and leukostasis. However, in contrast to CML, chromosomal abnormalities are infrequent. Palliation can be achieved for variable periods in this fragile elderly population with blood product support and palliative drugs, the most effective being hydroxyurea.

Management of Myelodysplastic Syndrome

Results of therapy other than conservative management of symptoms are dismal, and improved survival awaits new techniques. As in the myeloproliferative diseases, hydroxyurea is the drug of choice for patients with rising counts unless fulminant leukemia evolves. New potential treatments include biomodulation with humoral factors to terminally differentiate leukemic cells and maturation of leukemia with cytotoxic agents. The advent of cloned human colony-stimulating factors suggests a role for growth stimulation of the pluripotential leukemic stem cell to drug sensitivity and of normal splenic colony-forming units to more rapid repopulation with normal marrow elements. These colony-stimulating factors may also force maturation in the neoplastic cell.

In these usually elderly patients, when intensive intervention is unwarranted, allowing the WBC count to rise to leukostatic lethal levels can be considered a humane alternative to palliation and sometimes less than meaningful survival.

Acute Myelocytic Leukemias

These diseases are classified in the FAB system (see Table 117–8). Their overall management is outside the scope of this text. However, immediate recognition of their emergent nature and subsequent skilled management of malignant leukocytosis are critical to the immediate survival of 20% of those presenting with acute leukemia.

Malignant Lymphocytosis

Malignant lymphocytosis may be encountered in virtually all the primary diseases of the lymphoid system. The lymphoid malignancies are a broad spectrum of bone marrow–invading diseases involving the cells of the immune system. At one end is the fulminant, proliferative disease of children and adults, ALL; at the other extreme is the terminally differentiated disease of the elderly, multiple myeloma. Between are myriad diseases that have defied classification by the pathologist and light microscopy. New techniques, as in the myeloid malignancies, define the relationship of these diseases to each other and to normal cells. Use of new investigative techniques has shown that neoplastic cells of B lymphocyte tumors express surface light chain immunoglobulins, which identify these tumors as clonal expansions, with surface phenotype demonstrating clonal excess (Table 117–11).

Chronic Lymphocytic Leukemia

Clinical Manifestations. CLL is the most frequent form of leukemia in elderly people and is usually diagnosed after routine blood examinations in otherwise healthy individuals or on the basis of widespread lymphadenopathy, fatigue, or weight loss. Usually the physical examination reveals no abnormalities, although in some cases generalized lymphadenopathy and splenomegaly are prominent findings. Persistent blood lymphocytosis of more than 15,000 cells per cubic millimeter without apparent cause, with lymphocytic infiltration of the bone marrow, suggests the diagnosis of CLL. It is a neoplasm characterized by proliferation and accumulation of monoclonal small mature-appearing lymphocytes usually of B cell origin.

TABLE 117–11

DIAGNOSTIC CLASSIFICATION OF THE LYMPHOID NEOPLASMS

FAB (Classic)	Immunophenotype	Cytogenetics	Morphology
Chronic lymphocytic leukemia (CLL)			
CLL (B-CLL)	1a⁺, B1⁺, B2⁺, B4⁺, Leu-1⁺, SmIg⁺	+12, 14q+, inv(14)	Small lymphocytes
CLL (T-CLL)	1a⁺, Leu-1⁺, T	Normal	Small lymphocytes
CLL (prolymphocytic)	1a⁺, B4⁺, SmIg⁺	t(6;12), del(3)	Prolymphocytes
CLL (hairy cell) (TRAP+)	1a⁺, B1⁺, Leu-M5, Leu-14, SmIg	Normal	Hairy cells
CLL (plasma cell)	PCA1⁺, B⁺, SmIg, CALLA⁺, Leu-1⁻	Various	Plasma cells
CLL (lymphosarcoma)	1a⁺, B4⁺, B1⁺, SmIg, CALLA⁺, Leu-1⁻	Various	Cleaved lymphocytes
Acute lymphocytic leukemia (ALL)			
L1,L2 (common)	CALLA⁺, tDtk⁺, 1a⁺, B4⁺	t(4;22), t(9;22)	Small lymphocytes
L1,L2 (pre–B cell)	CALLA⁺, tDt⁺, 1a⁺, CLG⁺, B4⁺	t(1;19), t(9;22)	Heterogeneous lymphocytes
L1 (T cell)	tDt, E receptor, Leu-9, Leu-1	t(11;14)	
L3 (B cell)	CALLA⁺, tDt⁻, B4⁺, SmIg⁺, HLA-DR	t(8;14)	Homogeneous large lymphoblasts with vacuoles and cleaved nuclei

Course and Management. CLL may remain indolent for months or years and require no particular therapeutic attention. When it is progressive, the major management problems stem from progressive increase in the size of lymph nodes and lymphoid tumor masses, a progressive anemia that may have a significant hemolytic component, a bleeding diathesis associated with thrombocytopenia, or infectious diseases related to hypogammaglobulinemia and other results of an acquired immunologic deficiency state. The most suitable therapeutic program combines pertinent elements of supportive and specific treatment.

Supportive Care. Systemic complications of CLL are related primarily to manifestations of the disease and not to its management, although tumor lysis and hyperuricemia can occur. The types of treatment used generally do not produce massive killing of tumors immediately, nor is this necessary. True total complete remission or eradication of the disease has been rare in CLL, and attempts to treat aggressively have resulted in depression of normal marrow elements without elimination of the tumor. The systemic complications of CLL include hypogammaglobulinemia and recurrent infections, which can be treated with gamma globulin and appropriate antibiotics. The immune-mediated anemia, thrombocytopenia, and neutropenia respond to prednisone and immunosuppressive agents, occasionally splenectomy, intravenous gamma globulin, and cyclosporine. Hyperviscosity syndrome has been seen with the immunoglobulin M elaboration and treated as is multiple myeloma with plasmapheresis and chemotherapy. Hyperuricemia is rare and hypercalcemia, except in the T cell variant, is uncommon. If it occurs, it is treated primarily with hydration, diuretics, prednisone and calcitonin, and systemic chemotherapy.

Treatment. Alkylating agents (chlorambucil, cyclophosphamide) given for 4 to 8 weeks or more induce good partial remissions in 60 to 70% of the patients. Prednisone has an antitumor effect in about 50%, and combination chemotherapy with drugs such as cyclophosphamide, vincristine, and prednisone may be superior. Adrenal corticosteroids are used frequently to suppress immune hemolysis, bleeding tendencies resulting from thrombocytopenia, or hypercalcemia. Ionizing radiation may induce a marked resolution of lymphoid tumor masses. Interferon-α and pentostatin may play a role in some of the B cell malignancies, but their efficacy is yet to be determined. A new agent, fludarabine, appears to have high activity with a wide therapeutic index.

The course of CLL usually extends for a period of 5 years or longer. One third of patients are alive 10 years after diagnosis. A preterminal acute phase is less common in this disorder than in chronic granulocytic leukemia. Death frequently results from an infectious disease, bleeding, the sequelae of severe anemia, an unrelated disease, or progression of CLL.

B Cell Leukemia. CLL can transform to other varieties of lymphoma including diffuse large-cell lymphoma (Richter's syndrome), a fulminant, debilitating, febrile, and, until recently, rapidly progressive disease. Large-cell lymphoma develops in at least 10% of patients and may be due to a new malignant clone with new genotype and phenotype. Also seen are prolymphoid transformation, lymphoblastic transformation, and even development of multiple myeloma.

Hairy-Cell Leukemia. Hairy-cell leukemia, or leukemic reticuloendotheliosis, a chronic proliferative disease of older men with massive splenomegaly, cytopenia, and fibrotic bone marrows, was previously treated with splenectomy but now responds well to interferon and pentostatin.

Diseases involving lymphadenopathy and splenomegaly mimic many infectious, neoplastic, and immunologic diseases that are relatively benign in their manifestations and out-

come. It is of critical importance to rule out other causes of these findings. With new hybridization techniques, a benign disease is less likely to be confused with a clonal neoplasm.

Acute Lymphocytic Leukemia

Primarily a disease of children, ALL constitutes 15% of adult acute leukemias and is divided into three groups in the FAB classification. Most patients have the common ALL antigen (CALLA) and B cell gene rearrangement. ALL with a T cell phenotype is more common from 15 to 25 years of age, and acute undifferentiated or pre–B cell leukemia, with cells that lack T or B characteristics and are CALLA-negative, is seen more commonly in adults. B lymphocyte antigens are seen in approximately 5% of patients, T lymphocyte antigens in 20%, and neither in 75%. Virtually all patients with ALL have terminal deoxynucleotide transferase.

Clinical Manifestations. As in AML, clinical signs and symptoms are those of bone marrow failure, but there is higher frequency of lymphadenopathy, splenomegaly, mediastinal mass, and associated immunosuppression. This immunosuppression places the patient at risk for infections unique to the immunocompromised host. Nosocomial and parasitic infections, as with *Pneumocystis carinii* and atypical fungal organisms, in addition to those seen in the myeloid malignancies with granulocytopenia but intact immune responsiveness, must be suspected with each new fever. Therapy is prolonged in ALL, and consistent surveillance for pathogenic organisms is necessary even during remission after WBC recovery.

The preferred treatment varies with the phenotype. In all cases, combinations of drugs active against malignant lymphoblasts are required, together with prophylactic treatment of the central nervous system for actual or potential leukemic cell infiltrates. The usual approach consists of a three-phase treatment of induction, central nervous system prophylaxis, and maintenance. Induction therapy includes prednisone, vincristine, L-asparaginase, and daunorubicin.

Management of Lymphocytosis

In most cases, time can be taken to diagnose the cause and classify the disease associated with an elevated WBC count. Acute causes of an increased WBC count that may be mistaken as lymphoid include the FAB classifications M1 and M7 of acute myeloid leukemia. The need for immediate intervention is less urgent with lymphoid cells because they are relatively small and deformable compared with myeloid cells, which lessens the probability of hyperviscosity, and their rupture with chemotherapy releases high levels of phosphates and uric acid unless precautions are taken. An approach to hydration, leukapheresis, and possible dialysis is reviewed in this chapter under Hyperleukocytosis.

References

1. Burke PJ, Diggs CH, Owens AH Jr, et al: Factors in human serum affecting the proliferation of normal and leukemic cells. Cancer Res 33:800, 1973.
2. Burke PJ, Karp JE: Relationship of the hematopoietic cycle to the combined activities of a stimulator and a short-lived inhibitor. Blood 69:513, 1987.
3. Lord BI, Wright EG: Sources of haemopoietic stem cell proliferation: Stimulators and inhibitors. Blood Cells 6:581, 1980.
4. Right EG, Lord BI, Dexter TM, et al: Mechanisms of haemopoietic stem cell proliferation control. Blood Cells 5:247, 1979.
5. Tubina M, Frindel R: Regulation of pluripotent stem cell proliferation and differentiation: The role of long-range humoral factors. J Cell Physiol 1:13, 1982.
6. Gaultieri RJ, Shadduck RK, Baker DG, et al: Hematopoietic regulatory

factors produced in long-term murine bone marrow cultures and the effect of in vitro irradiation. Blood 64:516, 1984.

7. Blackburn MJ, Patt HM: Influence of a marrow stromal factor on survival of hemopoietic stem cells in vitro. Exp Hematol 8:77, 1980.

8. Toksoz D, Dexter TM, Lord BI, et al: The regulation of hemopoiesis in long-term bone marrow cultures. II. Stimulation and inhibition of stem cell proliferation. Blood 55:931, 1980.

9. Schwartz RS, Greenberg PL: Stromal colony-stimulating activity production and myeloid colony-forming cells in human hemopoietic and nonhemopoietic bone marrow. Blood 57:771, 1981.

10. Karp JE, Shadduck RK, Burke PJ, et al: The relationship between humoral stimulating activity and colony stimulating factor. Exp Hematol 11:639, 1983.

11. Metcalf D: The molecular biology and functions of the granulocyte-macrophage colony-stimulating factors. Blood 67:257, 1986.

12. Frindel E, Guigon M: Inhibition of CFU entry into cycle by a bone marrow extract. Exp Hematol 5:74, 1977.

13. Quesenberry P, Levitt L: Hematopoietic stem cells. N Engl J Med 301:755, 1979.

14. Hellman S, Reincke U, Botnick L, et al: Functional organization of the hematopoietic stem cell compartment: Implications for cancer and its therapy. J Clin Oncol 1:277, 1983.

15. Vaughan WP, Karp JE, Burke PJ: Long chemotherapy-free remissions after single cycle timed-sequential chemotherapy of acute myelocytic leukemia. Cancer 45:859, 1980.

16. Vaughan WP, Karp JE, Burke PJ: Two-cycle timed-sequential chemotherapy for adult acute nonlymphocytic leukemia. Blood 64:975, 1984.

17. Geller RB, Burke PJ, Karp JE, et al: A two step timed sequential treatment for acute myelocytic leukemia. Blood 74:1499, 1989.

18. Hug V, Keating M, McCredie K, et al: Clinical course and response to treatment of patients with acute myelogenous leukemia presenting with a high leukocyte count. Cancer 52:773, 1983.

19. Vaughan WP, Kimball AW, Karp JE, et al: Factors affecting survival of patients with acute myelocytic leukemia presenting with high white blood counts. Cancer Treat Rep 65:1007, 1981.

20. Ventura GJ, Hester JP, Smith TL, et al: Acute myeloblastic leukemia with hyperleukocytosis: Risk factors for early mortality in induction. Am J Hematol 27:34, 1988.

21. Suri R, Goldman JM, Catovsky D, et al: Priapism complicating chronic granulocytic leukemia. Am J Hematol 9:295, 1980.

22. Stainsby D, Elleray E, Anderson J, et al: Papilloedema in chronic granulocytic leukaemia. Br J Haematol 55:243, 1983.

23. Bodey GP, Powell RD Jr, Hersh EM, et al: Pulmonary complications of acute leukemia. Cancer 19:781, 1966.

24. Frost T, Isbister JP, Ravich RBM, et al: Respiratory failure due to leukostasis in leukemia. Med J Aust 68:94, 1981.

25. Lester TJ, Johnson JW, Cuttner J: Pulmonary leukostasis as the single worst prognostic factor in patients with acute myelocytic leukemia and hyperleukocytosis. Am J Med 79:43, 1985.

26. Lichtman MA, Rowe JM: Hyperleukocytic leukemias: Rheological, clinical, and therapeutic considerations. Blood 60:279, 1982.

27. Resnick ME, Berkowitz RD, Rodman T: Diffuse interstitial leukemic infiltration of the lungs producing the alveolar-capillary block syndrome. Am J Med 31:149, 1961.

28. Thompson DS, Goldstone AH, Parry HF, et al: Leukostasis in chronic myeloid leukaemia (letter). Br Med J 2:202, 1978.

29. Tryka AF, Godleski JJ, Fanta CH: Leukemic cell lysis pneumopathy. Cancer 50:2763, 1982.

30. Vernant JP, Brun B, Mannoni P, et al: Respiratory distress of hyperleukocytic granulocytic leukemias. Cancer 44:264, 1979.

31. Snyder AB, Barone JG, DiGiacomo JC, et al: Postoperative pulmonary leukostasis. Crit Care Med 18:116, 1990.

32. Lichtman MA: Cellular deformability during maturation of the myeloblast. N Engl J Med 283:943, 1970.

33. Lichtman MA: The relationship of excessive white cell count to vascular insufficiency in patients with leukemia. In: Meiselman JH, Lichtman MA, LaCelle PL (eds): White Cell Mechanics: Basic Science and Clinical Aspects. New York: Alan R Liss, p 295, 1984.

34. Lichtman MA: Rheology of leukocytes, leukocyte suspensions and blood in leukemia: Possible relationship to clinical manifestations. J Clin Invest 52:350, 1973.

35. Groch WN, Sayre GP, Heck FJ: Cerebral hemorrhage in leukemia. Arch Neurol 2:439, 1960.

36. Harris AL: Leukostasis associated with blood transfusion in acute myeloid leukaemia. Br Med J 1:1169, 1978.

37. McKee LC Jr, Collins RD: Intravascular leukocyte thrombi and aggregates as a cause of morbidity and mortality in leukemia. Medicine 53:463, 1974.

38. Wald BR, Heisel MA, Ortega JA: Frequency of early death in children with acute leukemia presenting with hyperleukocytosis. Cancer 50:150, 1982.

39. Lichtman MA, Weed RI: Alteration of the cell periphery during granulocyte maturation: Relationship to cell function. Blood 39:301, 1970.

40. Lichtman MA, Kearney EA: The filterability of normal and leukemic leukocytes. Blood Cells 2:491, 1976.

41. Rowe JM, Lichtman MA: Hyperleukocytosis and leukostasis: Common features of childhood chronic myelocytic leukemia. Blood 63:1230, 1984.

42. Hild DH, Myers TJ: Hyperviscosity in chronic granulocytic leukemia. Cancer 46:1418, 1980.

43. Steinberg MH, Charm SE: Effect of high concentration of leukocytes on whole blood viscosity. Blood 38:299, 1971.

44. Keating MH, Smith TL, Gehan ET, et al: Factors related to length of complete remission in adult acute leukemia. Cancer 45:2017, 1980.

45. Nadel EM, Nelson JS: The pathological characteristics of leukostasis and leukemia nodules occurring in the central nervous system of guinea pigs with LzC/NB leukemia. J Neuropathol Exp Neurol 35:75, 1976.

46. Freireich EJ, Thomas LB, Frei E III, et al: A distinctive type of intracerebral hemorrhage associated with "blastic crisis" in patients with leukemia. Cancer 13:146, 1960.

47. Bloom R, Taveira Da Silva A, Bracey A: Reversible respiratory failure due to intravascular leukostasis in chronic myelogenous leukemia. Am J Med 67:679, 1979.

48. Cuttner J, Conjalka MS, Reilly M, et al: Association of monocytic leukemia in patients who present with extreme leukocytosis. Am J Med 69:555, 1980.

49. Meyer RJ, Ferreira PPC, Cuttner J, et al: Central nervous system involvement at presentation in acute granulocytic leukemia. Am J Med 68:691, 1980.

50. Moore EW, Thomas LB, Shaw RK, et al: The central nervous system in acute leukemia. Arch Intern Med 105:451, 1960.

51. Lisiewicz J: Mechanisms of hemorrhage in leukemias. Semin Thromb Hemost 4:241, 1978.

52. Grund FM, Armitage JO, Burns P: Hydroxyurea in the prevention of the effects of leukostasis in acute leukemia. Arch Intern Med 137:1246, 1977.

53. Schwartz JH, Canellos GP: Hydroxyurea in the management of the hematologic complications of chronic granulocytic leukemia. Blood 41:11, 1975.

54. Fishbein WN, Carbone PP, Freireich EJ, et al: Clinical trials of hydroxyurea in patients with cancer and leukemia. Clin Pharmacol Ther 5:574, 1965.

55. Wiernik PH, Serpick AA: Factors affecting remission and survival in adult acute nonlymphocytic leukemia. Medicine 49:505, 1970.

56. Cuttner J, Holland JF, Norton L, et al: Therapeutic leukapheresis for hyperleukocytosis in acute myelocytic leukemia. Med Pediatr Oncol 11:76, 1983.

57. Eisenstaedt RS, Berkman EM: Rapid cytoreduction in acute leukemia. Management of cerebral leukostasis by cell pheresis. Transfusion 18:113, 1978.

58. Lane TA: Continuous flow leukapheresis for rapid cytoreduction in leukemia. Transfusion 20:455, 1980.

59. Lowenthal RM, Buskard NA, Goldman JM, et al: Intensive leukapheresis as an initial therapy for chronic granulocytic leukemia. Blood 46:835, 1975.

60. Ballas K, Kiesel JK: Leukapheresis for hyperviscosity. Transfusion 19:787, 1979.

61. Kamen BA, Summers CP, Pearson HA: Exchange transfusion as a treatment for hyperleukocytosis, anemia, and metabolic abnormalities in a patient with leukemia. J Pediatr 96:1045, 1980.

62. Bunin NJ, Pui CH: Differing complications of hyperleukocytosis in children with acute lymphoblastic or acute nonlymphoblastic leukemia. J Clin Oncol 3:1590, 1985.

63. Maurer HS, Steinherz PG, Gaynon PS, et al: The effect of initial management of hyperleukocytosis on early complications and outcome of children with acute lymphoblastic leukemia. J Clin Oncol 6:1425, 1988.

64. Saleh RA, Graham-Pole H, Cumming WA: Severe hyperphosphatemia associated with tumor lysis in a patient with T-cell leukemia. Pediatr Emerg Care 5:231, 1989.

65. Murray JF, Gold P, Johnson BL Jr, et al: The circulatory effects of hematocrit variations in normovolemic and hypervolemic dogs. J Clin Invest 42:1150, 1968.

66. Thomas DJ, du Boulay GH, Marshall J, et al: Cerebral blood-flow in polycythaemia. Lancet 2:161, 1977.

67. Berlin NI: Polycythemia vera: An update. Semin Hematol 23:131, 1986.

68. Rosove MH, Perloff JK, Hocking WG, et al: Chronic hypoxaemia and decompensated erythrocytosis in cyanotic congenital heart disease. Lancet 2:313, 1986.

69. Harrison BD, Davis J, Madgwick RG, et al: The effects of therapeutic decrease in packed cell volume on the responses to exercise of patients with polycythemia secondary to lung disease. Clin Sci Mol Med 45:833, 1973.

70. Weisse AB, Moschas CB, Frank MJ, et al: Hemodynamic effects of staged hematocrit reduction in patients with stable cor pulmonale and severely elevated hematocrit levels. Am J Med 58:92, 1975.

71. Segel N, Biship JM: The circulation of patients with chronic bronchitis and emphysema at rest and during exercise with special reference to the influence of changes in blood viscosity and blood volume on the pulmonary circulation. J Clin Invest 45:1555, 1966.

72. Gertz I, Hodensterna G, Webster PO: Improvement in pulmonary function with diuretic therapy in the hypervolemic and polycythemia patients with chronic obstructive pulmonary disease. Chest 75:146, 1979.

73. Cheety KG, Brown SE, Light RW: Improved exercise tolerance of the polycythemia lung patient following phlebotomy. Am J Med 74:415, 1983.
74. Wedzicha JA, Rudd RM, Apps MC, et al: Erythrapheresis in patients with polycythaemia secondary to hypoxic lung disease. Br Med J 286:511, 1983.
75. Wallis PJW, Apps MCP, Newland AC, et al: Calf blood flow and oxygen carriage after reversal of polycythemia secondary to hypoxic lung disease. Thorax 41:306, 1986.
76. Wallis PJW, Skehan JD, Newland AC, et al: Effects of erythrapheresis on pulmonary haemodynamics and oxygen transport in patients with secondary polycythemia and cor pulmonale. Clin Sci 70:91, 1986.
77. Berk PD, Goldberg JD, Donovan PB, et al: Therapeutic recommendations in polycythemia vera based on Polycythemia Vera Study Group protocols. Semin Hematol 23:132, 1986.
78. Kaplan ME, Mack K, Goldberg JD, et al: Long-term management of polycythemia vera with hydroxyurea: A progress report. Semin Hematol 23:167, 1986.
79. Sharon R, Tatarsky I, Ben-Arich Y: Treatment of polycythemia vera with hydroxyurea. Cancer 57:718, 1986.
80. Tartaglia AP, Goldberg JD, Berk PD, et al: Adverse effects of antiaggregating platelet therapy in the treatment of polycythemia vera. Semin Hematol 23:176, 1986.
81. Mulligan DW, MacNamee R, Roberts BE, et al: The influence of iron-deficient indices on whole blood viscosity in polycythaemia. Br J Haematol 50:467, 1982.
82. Rigby PG, Leavell BS: Polycythemia vera. A review of fifty cases with emphasis on the risk of surgery. Arch Intern Med 5:622, 1960.
83. Wasserman LR, Gilbert HS: Surgery in polycythemia. N Engl J Med 5:622, 1963.
84. Murphy S, Iland H, Rosenthal D, et al: Essential thrombocythemia: An interim report from the Polycythemia Study Group. Semin Hematol 23:177, 1986.
85. Silverstein MN, Petitt RM, Solberg LA, et al: Anagrelide: A new drug for treatment of thrombocytosis. N Engl J Med 20:1292, 1988.
86. Talpaz M, Jurzrock R, Kantarjian H, et al: Recombinant interferon-alpha therapy of Philadelphia chromosome–negative myeloproliferative disorders with thrombocytosis. Am J Med 86:554, 1986.
87. Gisslinger H, Ludwig H, Linkesch W, et al: Long-term interferon therapy for thrombocytosis in myeloproliferative diseases. Lancet 1:634, 1989.

CHAPTER 118

Acute Hemolytic Disorders

Charles J. Parker

In hemolysis, the average life span of the red blood cell is reduced because of premature destruction of erythrocytes in the peripheral circulation. However, anemia is not invariably associated with hemolysis, because in some instances the bone marrow can increase erythropoiesis and compensate for the increased destruction. The diagnosis of hemolytic anemia is made by obtaining evidence that peripheral destruction of erythrocytes is either the primary or an important contributing mechanism of the anemia. Hemolytic anemia can be inherited or acquired, but regardless of the cause, if the hemolytic process is present at birth, it is categorized as congenital.

In most types of hemolytic anemia, the erythrocytes are destroyed by the reticuloendothelial system of the spleen and liver, and this mechanism of destruction is called extravascular hemolysis. Two basic pathophysiologic processes cause cells to be removed prematurely by the reticuloendothelial system. First, in immune hemolytic anemias, immunoglobulins or immunoglobulins and complement become

bound to the red blood cells.[1, 2] As a consequence, the erythrocytes undergo phagocytosis because reticuloendothelial cells have specific receptors that recognize both the Fc portion of immunoglobulin G (IgG) and activation and degradation products of the third component of complement (C3). Second, the biophysical properties of the erythrocyte membrane may be altered as a result of certain pathophysiologic processes (e.g., polymerization of sickle hemoglobin) that cause cell deformability to be markedly reduced. As a consequence, the damaged cells are sequestered because they are too rigid to traverse the narrow (3 μm) fenestrations that lead into the splenic sinuses (the diameter of the red blood cell is 7 μm). In addition, significant metabolic stress is placed on the cells by the splenic environment, which is relatively hypoxic, acidic, and hypoglycemic (this process is called splenic conditioning).

In some types of hemolytic anemia, the erythrocytes are directly hemolyzed within the vascular space and free hemoglobin is released into the plasma. Two basic pathophysiologic processes cause cells to undergo intravascular hemolysis. First, red blood cells may be damaged mechanically. This mechanism accounts for the hemolysis that is sometimes associated with prosthetic heart valves or with prolonged marching or running. In disseminated intravascular coagulation (DIC) or microangiopathic hemolytic anemia (MAHA), red blood cells are also damaged mechanically by being forced to flow through small vessels that have been partially occluded by microthrombi. Second, red blood cells may be directly hemolyzed as a result of complement activation. Complement-mediated intravascular hemolysis is uncommon, being the primary mechanism of red blood cell destruction only in major transfusion reactions caused by ABO incompatibility, paroxysmal nocturnal hemoglobinuria (PNH), paroxysmal cold hemoglobinuria (PCH), and in some instances immune hemolytic anemia induced by drugs (e.g., quinidine and quinine).

DIAGNOSIS

When a patient is found to be anemic, hemolytic processes are usually included as part of the differential diagnosis. By determining the reticulocyte count and quantitating the serum bilirubin, haptoglobin, and lactate dehydrogenase levels, hemolysis can be established with relative certainty (Table 118–1).

Reticulocyte Count

The normal reticulocyte count is between 0.5 and 1.5%. An elevated reticulocyte count results from an increase in erythropoiesis and reflects an attempt by the bone marrow

TABLE 118–1
LABORATORY VALUES THAT SUGGEST HEMOLYSIS
Reticulocyte count ≥ 5% (uncorrected*) Indirect bilirubin between 1 and 5 mg/dL† Haptoglobin < 50 mg/dL‡ Lactate dehydrogenase > 100 U/L§

*Uncorrected reticulocyte count is not adjusted for the degree of anemia or premature release of reticulocytes.

†Patients with Gilbert's disease have increased indirect bilirubin in the absence of hemolysis. Unless there is underlying liver disease, the direct bilirubin result is rarely elevated in association with hemolysis.

‡Haptoglobin is an acute-phase reactant. When hemolysis occurs in association with inflammatory processes or with steroid administration, haptoglobin levels may be within the normal range.

§Values are much higher in cases of intravascular hemolysis.

to compensate for increased peripheral destruction of red blood cells. Conventionally, the reticulocyte count is reported as a percentage (number of reticulocytes per 100 red blood cells). Thus, the total number of reticulocytes depends not only on the percentage of reticulocytes but also on the total number of erythrocytes per volume of plasma. For example, a normal individual has approximately 50,000 reticulocytes per cubic millimeter of blood (5 million red blood cells per cubic millimeter × 1.0% reticulocytes). An anemic patient with 2.5 million red blood cells per cubic millimeter and a reticulocyte count of 2% also has a total of 50,000 reticulocytes per cubic millimeter. Thus, when assessing the possibility of a hemolytic process, the reticulocyte count can be corrected for the degree of the anemia by using the following formula:

Corrected reticulocyte count =

$$\frac{\text{patient's hematocrit}}{45(\text{normal hematocrit})} \times \text{patient's reticulocyte count}$$

Hillman and Finch[3] suggested that the reticulocyte count should be further modified to correct for the premature release of reticulocytes that is associated with anemia. They recommended that if the hematocrit is between 25 and 35%, the corrected reticulocyte count should be divided by 1.5; if the hematocrit is between 15 and 25%, the corrected reticulocyte count should be divided by 2.0; and if the hematocrit is less than 15%, the corrected reticulocyte count should be divided by 2.5. If the reticulocyte count is 3% or greater after these corrections are made, hemolysis is likely.

Petz and Garratty[4] suggested that these manipulations may impart a false sense of scientific precision and that patients with "corrected" reticulocyte counts less than 3% may, in some instances, have clinically significant hemolysis. They recommended that hemolysis be suspected in anyone with an uncorrected reticulocyte count of 5% or greater.

Reticulocytosis in the absence of hemolysis may occur as a result of blood loss or after therapy for iron deficiency or for megaloblastic anemia. Distinguishing such conditions from hemolysis, however, rarely presents a problem.

In some instances, hemolysis may be associated with a relative reticulocytopenia. For example, after the abrupt onset of hemolysis, several days are required to mount a reticulocyte response. Hemolysis with reticulocytopenia may also occur in patients who have marrow suppression for unrelated reasons. Nonetheless, provided that significant blood loss is excluded, hemolysis can be inferred in these situations by obtaining serial hematocrit values and reticulocyte counts. If hemolysis is ongoing, the hemoglobin and hematocrit fall rapidly in the absence of a compensatory reticulocytosis.

Aplastic crises characterized by absence of a reticulocyte response are an uncommon but potentially life-threatening complication associated with both inherited and acquired hemolytic anemia.[5] It has become apparent that in many instances these crises are precipitated by infection with the human parvovirus B19.[6] This DNA-containing virus invades hematopoietic stem cells and inhibits their growth. Parvoviral infection usually presents as a febrile illness or as a viral exanthem (fifth disease). Young children are most often affected, but the disease can also affect older children and adults.

Bilirubin

Unless the patient has Gilbert's disease, an elevation of unconjugated (indirect) bilirubin to between 1 and 5 mg/dL strongly suggests hemolysis. On the other hand, the conjugated (direct) bilirubin is rarely elevated in association with hemolysis unless there is underlying liver disease.

Haptoglobin

Serum haptoglobin is a hemoglobin-binding protein, and haptoglobin-hemoglobin complexes are rapidly catabolized. When hemoglobin is released as a result of hemolysis, haptoglobin levels fall because the rate of catabolism of the haptoglobin-hemoglobin complexes exceeds the rate of synthesis of haptoglobin (the normal range for haptoglobin is between 50 and 150 mg/dL). Accordingly, the haptoglobin concentration is a sensitive indicator of hemolysis. It should be kept in mind, however, that haptoglobin is an acute-phase reactant (i.e., synthesis increases in association with certain disease processes or with steroid administration). Thus, in situations in which hemolysis coexists with an inflammatory process, production of haptoglobin may keep pace with increased catabolism of haptoglobin-hemoglobin complexes and, consequently, haptoglobin levels may remain within the normal range.

Lactate Dehydrogenase

When erythrocytes are hemolyzed intravascularly or extravascularly, intracellular lactate dehydrogenase is released into the plasma. Accordingly, plasma lactate dehydrogenase is a useful indicator of hemolysis, with the concentration being markedly elevated in association with intravascular hemolytic processes.

ESTABLISHING THE BASIS OF THE HEMOLYSIS

If the laboratory tests described earlier suggest hemolysis, further investigation is required to determine the nature of the disease process. Keeping the diagnostic possibilities (Table 118–2) in mind helps focus the evaluation.

History and Physical Examination

In many instances, hemolysis may not be suspected at the time of admission. Consequently, it is often necessary to repeat portions of the history and physical examination with emphasis on areas that may be informative about the etiology of the hemolytic process.

Attempts should be made to establish the date of onset of the anemia (by history or by obtaining records of previous blood counts) to distinguish a congenital from an acquired process. A detailed family history may reveal relatives with a history of anemia, jaundice, or splenomegaly and suggest that the patient's anemia is hereditary. The onset of an acute hemolytic crisis may be associated with fever, lethargy, and pain in the back, legs, or abdomen. A history of dark urine is consistent with hemoglobinuria occurring as a sequela of significant intravascular hemolysis. A detailed history of drug use, toxin exposure, and alcohol consumption should be obtained because several types of anemia can be induced by these substances. If a drug-induced mechanism is suspected, establishing concordance between the start of drug ingestion and the onset of the anemia may be informative.

Immune-mediated hemolytic anemia can occur in association with lymphoma, chronic lymphocytic leukemia, and systemic lupus erythematosus. Accordingly, signs and symptoms of these diseases should be sought.

Pallor, jaundice, and splenomegaly are the classic physical findings associated with hemolytic anemia, but the absence of one or all of these signs does not exclude the presence of a clinically significant process. Furthermore, except for thalassemia major, massive splenomegaly is not usually observed in association with hemolytic anemia. When immune hemolytic anemia is secondary to lymphoma or chronic lymphocytic leukemia, a markedly enlarged spleen is most likely due to the primary disease rather than to the hemolytic process.

TABLE 118-2

CLASSIFICATION OF HEMOLYTIC ANEMIAS

Acquired hemolytic anemia
  Immune mediated
    Autoimmune
      Warm antibody
      Cold agglutinin disease
      Paroxysmal cold hemoglobinuria
    Alloimmune
      Acute transfusion reaction
      Delayed transfusion reaction
    Drug induced
  Red blood cell integrity mechanically disrupted
    Microangiopathic hemolytic anemia (see Table 118-3)
    Prosthetic heart valves
  Miscellaneous
    Paroxysmal nocturnal hemoglobinuria
    Infections
      Malaria
      Clostridium perfringens septicemia
    Spur cell anemia associated with severe liver disease

Hereditary hemolytic anemia
  Hemoglobinopathies (e.g., sickle cell anemia)
  Thalassemias
  Hereditary spherocytosis
  Enzyme deficiency
    Glucose-6-phosphate dehydrogenase (G6PD) deficiency
    Pyruvate kinase deficiency

Peripheral Blood Film

A careful review of the morphology of the erythrocytes often suggests a specific diagnosis or at least significantly limits the diagnostic possibilities. The presence of microspherocytes strongly suggests either hereditary spherocytosis or immune hemolytic anemia. Rarely, when spherocytes are seen, the underlying process is burn injury, *Clostridium perfringens (welchii)* septicemia, or hypophosphatemia. Target cells are seen after splenectomy and in association with thalassemia, with some hemoglobinopathies (particularly hemoglobin C), and with liver disease. Acanthocytes (red blood cells with rigid, elongated spicules) are the hallmark of spur cell anemia, a hemolytic process that can complicate the late stages of Laennec's cirrhosis. Fragmented erythrocytes (schistocytes and helmet cells) are consistent with mechanical or microangiopathic processes (Table 118-3). Red blood cells with discrete areas of invagination (bite cells) are observed in hemolytic disorders associated with precipitation of hemoglobins (unstable hemoglobins and deficiency of glucose-6-phosphate dehydrogenase [G6PD]). The hemoglobin precipitate forms Heinz's bodies that are visible in blood films stained with supravital dyes (but not in routine Wright-stained films). Removal of the Heinz bodies by the spleen produces the bite cells.

Distinguishing Between Intravascular and Extravascular Hemolysis

Intravascular hemolysis is associated with the presence of free hemoglobin in the plasma and with hemoglobinuria. Normally, the concentration of serum free hemoglobin is between 2 and 5 mg/dL. Mildly elevated concentrations (10 to 40 mg/dL) may not cause the color of the plasma to change; however, at higher concentrations the plasma becomes pink or red.

Free hemoglobin can cause the urine to be pink, red, or brown. It is critical to distinguish between hemoglobinuria

(free hemoglobin in the urine) and hematuria (red blood cells in the urine). This can usually be done by examining a sample before and after centrifugation. Before centrifugation, microscopic examination reveals red blood cells in cases of hematuria, but erythrocytes are absent in hemoglobinuria. After centrifugation of the urine, the abnormal color is unchanged in hemoglobinuria, but centrifugation eliminates the red blood cells and hence the abnormal color in hematuria.

It is possible to compile a rather long list of processes that can produce hemoglobinemia and hemoglobinuria, but from a practical point of view, significant intravascular hemolysis occurs rarely. This is because the processes that most commonly result in significant intravascular hemolysis (transfusion of ABO-incompatible blood, PNH, PCH, some types of drug-induced immune hemolytic anemia, and *C. perfringens* septicemia) occur rarely. Therefore, unless one of these processes is suspected, quantitation of plasma free hemoglobin as part of the initial evaluation of hemolytic anemia is unlikely to be informative.

Hemosiderin is the storage particle for the iron that is derived from hemoglobin catabolism. As a consequence of hemoglobin accumulation in the renal tubular cells, hemosiderinuria is observed in patients with intravascular hemolysis. Hemosiderinuria is seen primarily in patients with chronic intravascular hemolysis (e.g., PNH). Transient hemosiderinuria may occur in association with acute intravascular hemolysis, but it may not appear until several days after the onset of hemoglobinuria. Hemosiderin particles can be detected by staining the desquamated tubular cells that appear in the urine sediment for iron.

Direct Antiglobulin Test (Coombs' Test)

If hemolysis is present and a review of the peripheral blood film shows microspherocytes, an immune-mediated process should be suspected. The presence of immunoglobulins or complement or both on the patient's erythrocytes can be determined by using the direct Coombs' test. In this assay, the patient's cells are incubated with antiserum against both human IgG and complement component C3. If IgG or complement is bound to the red blood cells, the antiserum cross-links the cells and causes agglutination. The test is scored (from trace to 4+) based on the extent of the

TABLE 118-3

DISEASE PROCESSES ASSOCIATED WITH MICROANGIOPATIC HEMOLYTIC ANEMIA*

Thrombotic thrombocytopenic purpura
Hemolytic-uremic syndrome†
Disseminated intravascular coagulation‡
Drugs§
Disseminated carcinomatosis‖
Pregnancy and the puerperium¶
Transplantation (renal and bone marrow)
Infection
Malignant hypertension
Immune complex or connective tissue diseases

*Fragmented red blood cells (schistocytes and helmet cells) are observed in the peripheral film of patients with MAHA.
†May be primary or drug induced.
‡MAHA is often absent in DIC and when present is usually mild.
§A hemolytic-uremic syndrome can be induced by treatment with cytotoxic chemotherapy, primarily mitomycin C.
‖Most commonly associated with mucin-producing adenocarcinomas (e.g., gastric cancer).
¶Preeclampsia, pregnancy-associated TTP, postpartum hemolytic-uremic syndrome.

agglutination. If the test is positive, monospecific antiserum can be used to determine whether IgG or complement or both are present on the cell.

The indirect assay is designed to determine whether antibody is present in the patient's serum. The test cells (a pool of red blood cells from two or three different donors) used in the indirect assay are selected because of their phenotypic characteristics (i.e., they are type O [to avoid problems with ABO incompatibility] and they express the most common blood group antigens). The patient's serum is incubated with the test cells and, after washing, the cells are incubated with the Coombs' antiserum as described for the direct assay. With rare exception, the indirect test should not be requested unless the direct test is first found to be positive. Even then, before ordering the indirect test, thoughtful consideration should be given to how the results will contribute to the diagnosis or management of the case. The indirect assay is most useful in evaluating drug-induced immune hemolytic anemia or a suspected delayed transfusion reaction.

MICROANGIOPATHIC HEMOLYTIC ANEMIA

The characteristic morphologic feature seen in the peripheral blood film of patients with MAHA is fragmented erythrocytes (schistocytes). The pathophysiologic process (thrombotic microangiopathy) that produces MAHA begins with formation of thrombi in arterioles and capillaries. In passing through the partially occluded small vessels, erythrocytes are caught on fibrin strands, and the resulting shear stress disrupts the structural integrity of the membrane and causes the cell to fragment. Because the underlying pathophysiology involves formation of platelet thrombi, thrombocytopenia resulting from consumption of platelets is a prominent clinical feature of the disease processes associated with MAHA. The clinical spectrum of each disease entity is determined by the extent to which various vital organs are involved. For example, in thrombotic thrombocytopenic purpura (TTP), central nervous system involvement is almost always observed, whereas in hemolytic-uremic syndrome, (HUS), renal involvement is a constant feature. In some instances, thrombotic microangiopathy arises in association with another pathologic process (see Table 118–3).

Thrombotic Thrombocytopenic Purpura

TTP is a rare disease, but prompt recognition and appropriate therapy can be lifesaving. Although the molecular basis of TTP remains to be elucidated, there is evidence that the disease is mediated by a plasma substance that induces platelet aggregation or, alternatively, by the absence of a plasma constituent that inhibits aggregation.[7]

The peak age of incidence is in the fourth decade, but the disease has been reported in essentially all age groups beginning with neonates and including patients 90 years old.[8] The most common presenting symptoms involve disturbances of the central nervous system. Manifestations range from headache and behavioral changes to sensorimotor dysfunction to stupor and coma. Because of the dynamics of formation and dissolution of thrombi, the severity of the symptoms may fluctuate widely. Constitutional symptoms including fever, malaise, weakness, and fatigue are often part of the presenting history.

Patients frequently present with hemorrhagic complications of thrombocytopenia. Petechiae, ecchymoses, and mucosal bleeding are observed most commonly. Most patients with TTP have renal involvement, but gross hematuria is seen in only approximately 15%. Microscopic hematuria and proteinuria are the primary renal manifestations of TTP.

Mildly elevated blood urea nitrogen and creatinine concentrations are also observed frequently, but oliguria and acute renal failure are uncommon.

Most patients with TTP present with the triad of hemolytic anemia, thrombocytopenia, and neurologic symptoms or somewhat less commonly with the pentad of hemolytic anemia, thrombocytopenia, neurologic symptoms, renal involvement, and fever. Neurologic symptoms are essential for the diagnosis, but it is important to remember that the primary pathophysiologic process (microvascular thrombi) can involve virtually any organ system. Consequently, various clinical manifestations have been reported in association with TTP. For example, abdominal pain caused by pancreatic involvement (pancreatitis) or bowel ischemia (microvascular involvement of the bowel wall) is a presenting complaint in 10 to 20% of cases.[8]

Typically, the anemia of TTP is moderate (hemoglobin level > 10 g/dL), but the thrombocytopenia is usually severe (in the range of 20,000 platelets per cubic millimeter). With rare exception, tests for immunoglobulins and complement on red blood cells and platelets are negative because the hemolytic anemia and thrombocytopenia of TTP are not immune mediated. In marked distinction to DIC, abnormalities of the coagulation and fibrinolytic systems are not observed in TTP. Although biopsy of bone marrow, gingiva, or petechial lesion may reveal microthrombi, the diagnosis of TTP is a clinical one and pathologic confirmation is usually not necessary (and in some instances may not be safe).

When the diagnosis of TTP is established, treatment should be initiated promptly. Before 1964, the survival rate for TTP was approximately 5%. With prompt recognition and appropriate therapy, the survival rate has improved dramatically and is now above 80%. The current therapeutic recommendations suggested by the U.S. TTP Study Group[9] are shown in Table 118–4. If plasmapheresis and plasma exchange are not immediately available, infusion of fresh frozen plasma (30 mL/kg/d) can be used. Arrangements for plasmapheresis and plasma exchange, however, should be made as quickly as possible. The molecular basis of the therapeutic efficacy of plasmapheresis and plasma exchange remains to be elucidated. It has been postulated that the plasmapheresis removes a platelet-aggregating substance and that infusion of normal plasma restores the activity of a substance that inhibits platelet aggregation. In general, treatment of TTP is empirical, although the effectiveness of immunosuppressive agents suggests that immune mechanisms may participate in the underlying pathophysiology.

In some patients with TTP, infusion of platelet concentrates has been reported to accelerate the disease and result in clinical deterioration.[10] Accordingly, platelet transfusion should be reserved for use in emergency situations, such as for intracranial bleeding that has been demonstrated by computed tomography or magnetic resonance imaging.

In at least 50% of patients, the TTP episode can be reversed by using the combination of methylprednisolone, plasmapheresis, and plasma exchange. When the episode has remitted, the patient's platelet count should be monitored regularly (weekly until stable for at least 1 month). Relapses usually occur within a few weeks after discontinuation of therapy, but in some cases months or years elapse between recurrences. Patients with chronic relapsing TTP may respond to plasma infusion without concurrent plasmapheresis. Moake and colleagues[11] have presented evidence suggesting a causal relationship between the presence of unusually large multimers of von Willebrand's factor and chronic relapsing TTP. Cryoprecipitate is enriched for large multimers of von Willebrand's factor. Accordingly, it has been suggested that the supernatant (which is relatively

TABLE 118–4

RECOMMENDATIONS* FOR TREATMENT OF THROMBOTIC THROMBOCYTOPENIC PURPURA

Methylprednisolone, 0.75 mg/kg IV every 12 h, and continue until the patient has recovered.
Combined plasmapheresis and plasma exchange (3–4 L/d of fresh frozen platelet-poor plasma).†
Supportive care.
  Transfusion of ↑ed blood cells depending on hematocrit and rate of hemolysis.
  Transfusion of platelets if intracranial bleeding is demonstrated by computed tomography or magnetic resonance imaging.‡
Options for patients who fail to respond to primary therapy.§
  Vincristine (1.4 mg/m² body surface area but not exceeding 2 mg total dosage given IV on d 1, followed by 1 mg on d 4, 7, and 10).
  Substitution of cryosupernatant‖ for fresh frozen plasma in the plasma exchange program.
  Splenectomy.
  Immunosuppressive drugs (e.g., cyclophosphamide or azathioprine).
Agents that are of questionable efficacy, ineffective, or contraindicated.
  Effectiveness of antiplatelet agents (aspirin and dipyridamole) is controversial; aspirin may exacerbate hemorrhagic complications.
  Effectiveness of IV prostacyclin, dextran, and fibrinolytic agents is controversial.
  Substitution of albumin or gamma globulin for plasma as exchange fluid is usually ineffective.
  Heparin in therapeutic dosages is contraindicated.

*Recommendations are those of the U.S. TTP study group.[9]
†The plasmapheresis and plasma exchange should be continued for a minimum of 5 d in patients who respond completely. Complete response is defined as a return to a normal neurologic status, platelet count of greater than 150,000/mm³, rising hemoglobin, and normal serum lactate dehydrogenase. If the patient relapses, the same treatment protocol should be repeated. In patients who achieve a partial response without clinical deterioration, the treatment should be continued for an extended period in an effort to achieve a complete remission.
‡Transfusion of platelets has been reported to exacerbate symptoms in some patients.[10]
§If there is no response within the first 5 d or if there is deterioration within the first 3 d, the patient is considered a treatment failure.
‖Cryosupernatant is plasma from which the cryoprecipitate has been removed.

depleted of large von Willebrand's multimers) from cryoprecipitated plasma may be beneficial as an exchange fluid for treatment of TTP. Furthermore, the presence of unusually large multimers of von Willebrand's factor may serve as an indicator of the propensity of patients to relapse.

Hemolytic-Uremic Syndrome

There are clinical similarities between TTP and HUS, but the natural history of the two diseases and the approach to therapy differ markedly.[12] By giving thoughtful consideration to the history, symptoms, and signs of patients presenting with MAHA, thrombocytopenia, and renal failure, HUS can usually be distinguished from TTP (Table 118–5).

HUS is predominantly a disease of infants and children, although it can also affect adults. A history of a brief prodromal illness (most commonly gastroenteritis) is usually elicited. Patients are often acutely ill with pallor, vomiting, and prostration. Petechiae, ecchymoses, and mucosal bleeding caused by thrombocytopenia are often observed, as are gross hematuria and evidence of renal failure (e.g., edema and hypertension). Neurologic symptoms are observed less often than in TTP, but some patients with HUS present with focal or generalized seizures or alterations in consciousness.

In general, the degree of the anemia parallels the severity of the renal failure. This is not the case, however, with thrombocytopenia. Although thrombocytopenia is a constant feature of HUS, it does not appear to bear any temporal relationship to the course of the renal disease. The urinalysis shows proteinuria, hematuria, and casts, and anuric or oliguric renal failure is relatively common. Compelling evidence for DIC is usually absent, although the concentration of fibrin degradation products may be elevated.

Episodes of HUS may occur in clusters or in small epidemics (usually in association with outbreaks of bacterial gastroenteritis, in which verotoxin-producing *Escherichia coli* O157:H7 is the organism most commonly implicated).[12, 13] The molecular basis of HUS has not been elucidated, although verotoxin has been reported to injure endothelial cells directly. Conceivably, the pathophysiologic process ensues as a result of the loss of antithrombotic properties by damaged endothelium. The noxious effects may not be limited to the kidney, however, because a syndrome resembling TTP has been reported in association with hemorrhagic colitis caused by verotoxin-producing *E. coli*.[14]

HUS is also associated with outbreaks of shigellosis, although most of the reported cases occurred in India and Bangladesh.[12] A relatively uncommon but important variant of HUS is seen in association with infections with *Streptococcus pneumoniae*.[12] An enzyme (neuraminidase) derived from the bacteria cleaves the terminal sialic acid residue from a portion of the carbohydrate moiety of erythrocytes, platelets, leukocytes, and endothelial cells, thereby exposing the Thomsen-Freidenreich antigen. Naturally occurring immunoglobulin M (IgM) antibodies against the Thomsen-Freidenreich antigen are relatively common. If the patient has them a syndrome of polyagglutination with hemolysis,

TABLE 118–5

FEATURES THAT DISTINGUISH HEMOLYTIC-UREMIC SYNDROME FROM THROMBOTIC THROMBOCYTOPENIC PURPURA

Feature	HUS	TTP
Prodrome	Gastroenteritis,* upper respiratory tract infections	Nonspecific constitutional symptoms*
Age	Infants and children	Fourth decade of life
Renal involvement	Dominant feature	Present but not usually dominant
Neurologic symptoms	May be present but not usually dominant†	Dominant feature
Fever	Absent or transient	Relatively common and persistent
Associated with infection	Yes (verotoxin-producing *E. coli*, *Shigella*, *S. pneumoniae*)	Unusual*
Epidemic occurrence	Yes (in association with infections)	Rarely*
Familial occurrence	Yes (autosomal dominant and recessive forms reported)	No

*HUS is associated with hemorrhagic colitis caused by verotoxin-producing *E. coli* O157:H7.[13] Case reports of TTP in association with hemorrhagic colitis caused by verotoxin-producing *E. coli* O157:H7 have been published.[14] Both HUS and TTP have been reported in association with acquired immunodeficiency syndrome.[15, 16]
†In some cases of HUS, neurologic symptoms are a dominant feature. These patients tend to have a worse prognosis than those without significant neurologic involvement.

thrombocytopenia, and intravascular thromboses may develop. Furthermore, the symptoms can be induced or exacerbated by infusion of plasma containing antibodies against the Thomsen-Freidenreich antigen. Accordingly, in a patient who develops HUS in association with *S. pneumoniae* infection, evidence for expression of the Thomsen-Freidenreich antigen should be sought by determining whether the patient's cells are agglutinated by antibodies against the antigen.

Both HUS[15] and TTP[16] have been reported in association with acquired immunodeficiency syndrome.

Both autosomal dominant and autosomal recessive inheritance patterns have been reported for HUS.[12] The autosomal recessive form is associated with high mortality and in some cases may be difficult to distinguish from TTP.

There is no compelling evidence that therapy other than supportive care influences the outcome of HUS.[17] In particular, corticosteroids, anticoagulation with heparin, and antiplatelet agents appear to offer no benefit. Plasmapheresis with plasma exchange should not be used in the treatment of typical HUS of childhood. Aggressive management of the anemia, hypertension, renal failure, and seizures, however, has reduced the HUS mortality rate to less than 5%.

Chemotherapy-Induced Hemolytic-Uremic Syndrome

A syndrome characterized by MAHA, thrombocytopenia, and renal failure has been reported in patients receiving chemotherapy for cancer.[18] Mitomycin C is the drug most commonly involved, and development of the syndrome appears to be dose dependent (>30 mg/m²). The median time from the beginning of therapy with mitomycin C to the onset of HUS is approximately 1 year, and at the time of diagnosis of HUS patients often have no evidence of residual tumor. Chemotherapy-induced HUS indistinguishable from that associated with mitomycin C therapy has also been observed after bleomycin and cisplatin therapy.

The hemolytic anemia is often severe (median hemoglobin level is 7 g/dL), but the thrombocytopenia is usually mild. Evidence supporting a diagnosis of DIC is usually absent. Noncardiogenic pulmonary edema is relatively common and is associated with a poor prognosis. Urinalysis typically shows microscopic hematuria and proteinuria.

The mortality rate of chemotherapy-associated HUS is approximately 70%, with 50% of patients dying within the first 2 months and 75% dying within the first 4 months.[18] Nonetheless, aggressive management is warranted because in some instances complete recovery has been observed and, as noted earlier, patients may have been rendered free of the malignancy. Symptomatic and supportive therapy aimed at controlling hypertension, pulmonary edema, and renal failure should be initiated. Hemodialysis is often required. Careful consideration should be given to transfusion of patients who have chemotherapy-induced HUS for two reasons. First, red blood cell transfusions do not result in a sustained improvement in hematocrit, and second (but more important), the transfusion often exacerbates the symptoms of the syndrome. Although treatment with corticosteroids is ineffective, patients may benefit from the regimen of plasmapheresis and plasma exchange used to treat TTP. A group of patients with chemotherapy-induced HUS were treated with immunoperfusion therapy.[19] The patients' plasma was perfused through a column containing immobilized protein A from *Staphylococcus aureus* to remove immune complexes (the rationale for this therapy is based on studies that implicate immune complexes in the pathophysiology of chemotherapy-induced HUS). Subsequently, the plasma was reinfused into the patients. Long-term benefit was reported for 7 of 11 patients treated in this manner.

These results are encouraging and it is hoped that results from more extensive studies will support them.

Carcinoma-Associated Microangiopathic Hemolytic Anemia

Patients with carcinoma can develop MAHA unrelated to chemotherapy.[20] Unlike the situation in chemotherapy-induced HUS, renal involvement is uncommon in patients with carcinoma-associated MAHA. In the majority of cases, the MAHA is associated with widely metastatic mucin-producing adenocarcinomas (gastric cancer accounts for approximately 50% of the cases). In approximately one third of cases, the metastatic carcinoma is diagnosed after appreciation of the MAHA. Tumor emboli are often observed at autopsy and most frequently involve the microvasculature of the lungs.

The anemia is usually severe, and moderate-to-severe thrombocytopenia is also observed. Renal involvement is uncommon, as are hypertension and pulmonary edema. Neurologic symptoms resulting from intracranial bleeding may be prominent, and evidence of DIC is often present.

The prognosis for patients with carcinoma-associated MAHA is grave. Reducing the tumor burden should be the primary therapeutic goal as it is the only form of treatment that offers the possibility of long-term benefit. Supportive and symptomatic treatment should be undertaken while waiting for the neoplastic process to respond. In contrast to the situation in chemotherapy-induced HUS, red blood cell transfusion of patients with carcinoma-induced MAHA has not been associated with exacerbation of symptoms. Because of the severity of the hemolytic process, patients with carcinoma-associated MAHA often require daily red blood cell transfusion.

Microangiopathic Hemolytic Anemia Associated with Pregnancy and the Postpartum Period

In addition to having hypertension and proteinuria, patients with preeclampsia frequently have MAHA and thrombocytopenia.[21] A syndrome consistent with TTP has been reported in association with pregnancy, although the distinction between pregnancy-associated TTP and preeclampsia may not always be obvious. A causal rather than a temporal relationship between pregnancy and TTP is suggested, however, by the fact that some patients recover rapidly after delivery. Before the advent of plasma therapy, the maternal and fetal mortality rates with pregnancy-associated TTP were extremely high. Plasma therapy can ameliorate symptoms and makes it possible to continue the pregnancy. Postpartum HUS typically follows a symptom-free interval after a normal delivery. In addition to supportive treatment, plasma therapy has been recommended for postpartum HUS.

Other Processes Associated with Microangiopathic Hemolytic Anemia

A syndrome of MAHA and thrombocytopenia associated with histologic evidence of microvascular thrombi has been reported in association with a variety of other processes (see Table 118–3).[22] The association is unusual, however, and distinctions between true thrombotic microangiopathy and more common pathophysiologic features associated with the primary process (e.g., hyperacute rejection of renal allografts, DIC in association with microbial sepsis, or vasculitis in association with systemic lupus erythematosus) may not always be obvious. In general, the consequences of the thrombotic microangiopathy should be managed by using supportive measures while the underlying illness is being treated. The prognosis depends primarily on the nature of the underlying disease and its response to therapy.

Hemolytic Anemia Associated with Cardiovascular Abnormalities

Shear stress caused by turbulent blood flow can disrupt the structural integrity of the membrane and cause erythrocytes to fragment.[23] This process appears to account for the mild hemolysis associated with aortic stenosis, severe aortic regurgitation, ruptured sinus of Valsalva, traumatic arteriovenous fistulas, and aortofemoral bypass procedures.

Clinically significant hemolysis occurs primarily in patients with aortic valve prostheses, and the incidence is greatest when there is ball variance or a paravalvular leak. The severity of the hemolysis is also affected by the valvular material (metal and cloth-covered valves cause more problems than Silastic valves). Because the transvalvular pressure gradient is lower, hemolysis is associated less often with mitral valve than with aortic valve prostheses.

Review of the peripheral blood film shows numerous schistocytes. Occasionally, microspherocytes are observed. Treatment consists of iron replacement in deficient patients and limitations on physical activity to reduce cardiac output. If hemolysis is severe enough to produce a degree of anemia that requires transfusion, replacement of the prosthesis should be strongly considered.

IMMUNE HEMOLYTIC ANEMIA

The three general categories of immune-mediated hemolytic anemia (see Table 118–2) are autoimmune, alloimmune, and drug induced. Autoimmune hemolytic anemia (AIHA) can be further subdivided into three groups, each having idiopathic and secondary forms (Table 118–6).

Warm Antibody Autoimmune Hemolytic Anemia

The criteria for diagnosis of warm antibody AIHA are shown in Table 118–7. In addition to general symptoms and signs of hemolysis (see earlier), patients with warm

---

TABLE 118–6

CLASSIFICATION OF AUTOIMMUNE HEMOLYTIC ANEMIAS

Warm antibody (accounts for approximately 80% of cases)
  Idiopathic
  Secondary—found in association with chronic lymphocytic leukemia, lymphoma (Hodgkin's and non-Hodgkin's), connective tissue diseases (primarily systemic lupus erythematosus), ulcerative colitis, ovarian cysts, immunodeficiency syndromes (including acquired immunodeficiency syndrome)

Cold agglutinin syndrome (accounts for approximately 18% of cases)
  Idiopathic
  Secondary (found in association with *Mycoplasma pneumoniae* infection, infectious mononucleosis, lymphoreticular malignancy, viral infections)

Paroxysmal cold hemoglobinuria (accounts for approximately 2% of cases)
  Idiopathic (associated with a chronic autoimmune disease in adults)
  Secondary (found in association with viral illnesses, typically in children; also associated with syphilis)

TABLE 118–7

DIAGNOSTIC CRITERIA FOR WARM ANTIBODY AUTOIMMUNE HEMOLYTIC ANMEMIA AND COLD AGGLUTININ SYNDROME

Criteria for diagnosis of warm antibody AIHA
  Patient has not been transfused during previous 4 mo*
  Clinical evidence of an acquired hemolytic anemia
  A positive direct Coombs' test for IgG, complement C3, or both
  Absence of a cold agglutinin of high thermal amplitude†
  Patient has a warm antibody with broad reactivity in the serum or eluted from the red blood cell‡

Criteria for diagnosis of cold agglutinin syndrome
  Clinical evidence of acquired hemolytic anemia
  A positive Coombs' test for complement C3
  A negative Coombs' test for IgG§
  The presence of a cold agglutinin with reactivity up to at least 30°C‖

*Patient may still have AIHA, but a delayed transfusion reaction should be excluded.
†Reactivity up to 30°C.
‡If the antibody is not present in the plasma (indirect Coombs' test is negative), it can be eluted from the red blood cell membrane and its reactivity subsequently characterized.
§Cold agglutinins are almost invariably IgM antibodies that activate complement.
‖The antibody causes agglutination up to 30°C.

---

antibody AIHA present with two important laboratory features: (1) the peripheral blood film shows microspherocytes, and (2) the direct antiglobulin (Coombs') test is positive. In approximately 67% of patients, the Coombs' test is positive for both IgG and complement, in 20% the test is positive for IgG but not complement, and in the remaining 13% the test is positive for complement but not IgG.[4] The indirect Coombs' test is positive in approximately 57% of cases.[4] It is uncommon, but not rare, to have cases of Coombs'-negative warm antibody AIHA.[24] In these cases, patients have laboratory evidence of hemolysis and the peripheral blood film shows microspherocytes, but the standard Coombs' test is negative. The presence of IgG or complement or both, however, can often be demonstrated with more sensitive assays (e.g., radioimmunobinding assays using monoclonal antibodies or enzyme-linked antiglobulin tests).

Routinely, the warm antibody is classified as a panagglutinin because it causes agglutination of all of the erythrocytes that are part of the standard test panel used by the blood bank. More detailed characterization often shows that the antibody is directed against antigenic determinants within the Rh system (although many other specificities have been reported).[4]

An approach to treatment of warm antibody AIHA is shown in Table 118–8. In patients who have a secondary form of warm antibody AIHA, effective treatment of the underlying disease usually results in a parallel amelioration of the hemolytic process. Approximately 80% of patients respond to steroids, and the response is usually rapid (within a few days). Unfortunately, permanent remissions are observed in fewer than 20% of cases. The decision to recommend splenectomy should be based on clinical criteria (see Table 118–8), because splenic sequestration studies using radiolabeled erythrocytes have not proved to be predictive of response to splenectomy. In patients who relapse after splenectomy, low doses of steroids may be effective in controlling the hemolytic process. Immunosuppressive therapy (see Table 118–8) is often beneficial in patients who have not responded to splenectomy. Plasmapheresis with plasma exchange is not standard therapy but offers the

---

TABLE 118–8

TREATMENT OF WARM ANTIBODY HEMOLYTIC ANEMIA

Prednisone (1.0–1.5 mg/kg/d)*
Splenectomy†
Immunosuppressive therapy‡
Other§

*Patients who fail to respond after 3 wk are considered to be treatment failures. If patients respond, steroids should be tapered gradually (during 3–4 mo).

†Indications: (1) failure to respond to steroids; (2) steroid dose required to maintain remission unacceptably high (>10 mg/d or 15 mg q.o.d.)

‡Indications: (1) failure to respond to splenectomy (or a combination of splenectomy and low-dose prednisone); (2) patients who cannot tolerate splenectomy. Cyclophosphamide (1.5–2.0 mg/kg/d) or azathioprine (2.0–2.5 mg/kg/d) is recommended. Treatment should continue for at least 3 mo.

§Plasmapheresis with plasma exchange may be beneficial in emergency situations.

---

possibility of rapidly ameliorating the hemolysis in emergency situations.[25] In contrast to immune thrombocytopenia, AIHA appears not to respond to intravenous immunoglobulin therapy and in some instances such treatment may exacerbate the disease.[25] Anecdotal reports suggest that some patients with AIHA may respond to immunoadsorbent therapy using immobilized protein A from *S. aureus*.[25]

It is not necessary that the hematocrit be normal for the patient to be classified as a treatment success. The goal of therapy is to restore the hematocrit to a level that provides adequate oxygenating capacity (usually higher than 30% unless there are attendant problems). Furthermore, although the titer of the direct antiglobulin test may decrease in response to therapy, it is unusual for the test to become negative. Thus, a goal of therapy should not be normalization of the Coombs' test.

Transfusion of patients with warm antibody AHIA should be undertaken with caution.[26, 27] It is important to remember that response to steroid therapy is usually rapid. Thus, in most instances, transfusion can be avoided by reducing oxygen demand by placing the patient at rest. Nonetheless, in cases of fulminant hemolysis or when a patient at rest becomes symptomatic while awaiting a response to therapy (e.g., a patient with AIHA and reticulocytopenia), transfusion can be lifesaving.[5] Careful consideration should be given to the volume of blood to be infused because overtransfusion can have two dangerous effects: patients may become volume overloaded, causing further cardiopulmonary embarrassment, and the rate of hemolysis of donor red blood cells is exponentially related to the amount of blood infused.[26] Consequently, problems associated with acute hemolysis are more likely to occur in patients who have received relatively large amounts of blood. Accordingly, the amount of blood transfused should be the minimum required to control the patient's symptoms (e.g., 100 mL of packed cells twice a day may be effective in preventing high-output heart failure).

Inasmuch as the autoantibody is almost always a panagglutinin, it is virtually impossible to find donor cells that are not recognized by the patient's antibody. Therefore, the goal of the blood bank staff is not to find donor cells that are unreactive in the cross-matching studies but rather to ensure that the patient's ABO and Rh phenotypes are properly determined and that the patient does not have an alloantibody in addition to an autoantibody. A detailed history of previous pregnancies and transfusions is important because patients with warm antibody AIHA who have never been pregnant or transfused would be unlikely to have become alloimmunized. A number of assays are available that allow identification of a concurrent alloantibody, but these types

of studies are usually not performed routinely. Accordingly, it is important that the blood bank have a level of sophistication and experience that ensures competence in the performance and interpretation of these critical studies.

Some immunohematologists advocate studies to determine the relative specificity of the autoantibody so that donor cells that lack the antigen can be transfused.[4] For example, the antibody may react more strongly with cells that have the e antigen than with those that have the E antigen (E and e are part of the Rh antigen system). In this case, the antibody is said to have relative specificity for the e antigen. Data from limited studies suggesting that a clinical benefit results from transfusing cells that lack the antigen of relative specificity, however, are not compelling. Nonetheless, it seems prudent to determine the relative specificity of the antibody and avoid transfusing cells that express the antigen, especially if in vitro studies indicate a strong degree of specificity (e.g., if the antibody induces hemolysis of antigen-positive but not antigen-negative cells).

Patients with AIHA who are being transfused should be monitored closely during and after the infusion. Laboratory studies should be carried out to document the extent of hemolysis (e.g., lactate dehydrogenase, haptoglobin, plasma free hemoglobin, and hemoglobinuria) and the development of renal compromise.

Cold Agglutinin Syndrome

Cold agglutinins are relatively common in the plasma, but cold agglutinins that produce clinically significant hemolysis are relatively uncommon. A cold agglutinin titer of less than 1:64 is normal. Patients with cold agglutinin syndrome may complain of Raynaud's phenomenon or of acrocyanosis of the ears, nose tip, fingers, and toes that occurs at low temperatures and vanishes quickly on warming. These symptoms arise because, as the blood flows through skin capillaries, the intravascular temperature drops to levels at which the cold agglutinin is functional. As a consequence of the agglutination, blood flow through the small vessels is restricted. Hemoglobinuria after exposure to cold may be part of the history, but in general this symptom is unusual. Hepatosplenomegaly is not usually prominent, and lymphadenopathy is uncommon. Agglutination of the red blood cells at room temperature is an obvious consequence of the disease.

The criteria for diagnosis of cold agglutinin syndrome are shown in Table 118–7. It should be emphasized that mere observance of cold agglutination is not diagnostic of cold agglutinin disease. The antibodies of cold agglutinin disease are almost invariably IgM and, in the majority of cases, they are directed against determinants of the I antigen system. Although in most instances the cold agglutinin titer in cold agglutinin syndrome is above 1:1000, the titer at 4°C does not correlate well with the hemolytic potential of the antibody. A more useful characterization is determination of the thermal amplitude of the antibody (defined as the highest temperature at which the antibody causes agglutination). Most cold agglutinins that produce clinically significant hemolysis have a thermal amplitude of at least 30°C; if the thermal amplitude is less, the antibody lacks the capacity to activate complement significantly.

Treatment of cold agglutinin syndrome is mainly supportive because patients tend to have a low-grade, compensated anemia and, in general, the available therapeutic modalities (i.e., corticosteroids, splenectomy, and alkylating agents) are ineffective. A small minority of patients appear to benefit from chlorambucil or cyclophosphamide, and these agents should be tried if the disease is complicated by severe anemia. In situations in which the cold agglutinin syndrome arises in association with underlying neoplasia, the hemolytic process often ameliorates in response to treatment of the underlying disease. Patients should avoid cold conditions, and in some instances it may be necessary for the patient to move to a warm climate. Inasmuch as the antibody is an IgM, plasmapheresis offers the opportunity to lower the antibody concentrations in emergency situations.

The I antigen is present on all adult red blood cells. Thus, it is not possible to transfuse unreactive donor cells. Difficulties in establishing ABO and Rh phenotypes and in identifying alloantibodies are usually not encountered, however, because tests can be performed at a temperature above that at which the cold agglutinin is active. The clinical benefit of using in-line blood warmers during transfusion of patients with cold agglutinin disease (or with PCH; see later) has not been clearly established.[4] In general, properly cross-matched blood can be transfused safely if it is warmed to room temperature and infused slowly. In cases of particularly severe cold agglutinin syndrome or PCH, however, it seems prudent to use an in-line warmer.

Secondary Cold Agglutinin Syndrome

Although the finding of cold agglutinins in association with infectious processes is relatively common (particularly for *Mycoplasma pneumonia* infections and infectious mononucleosis), clinically significant hemolysis in this setting is unusual. The association of cold agglutinin disease with lymphoproliferative neoplasias is also uncommon. Some of the features of secondary cold agglutinin disease are shown in Table 118–9.

Paroxysmal Cold Hemoglobinuria

PCH is an uncommon disease that can be dramatic in presentation. Patients with PCH (usually children) experience acute attacks of shaking chills, fever, malaise, and aching pains involving the abdomen, back, and legs. Hemoglobin is usually present in the first urine passed after the attack. A history of exposure to cold is usually elicited, although the extent of the exposure may be modest. In rare instances, cold exposure is not part of the presenting history.

TABLE 118–9

SECONDARY CHRONIC COLD AGGLUTININ DISEASE

Mycoplasma pneumoniae infections.
  Approximately 50% of patients have elevated cold agglutinin titers, but overt hemolysis is rare.
  When it does occur, the hemolytic process begins in the second or third week of the infection and the onset is rapid. Fatalities have been reported.
  Characteristically, the cold-reacting antibody is an IgM that recognizes I antigens. The antibody may cross-react with mycoplasmal antigens.
  The hemolysis is self-limited and steroids are ineffective.
Infectious mononucleosis.
  Clinically significant hemolysis occurs infrequently.
  Hemolysis occurs 1–2 wk after onset of the infection.
  The antibody may be IgM anti-i, IgM anti-I, or IgG anti-i.*
  Hemolysis is usually self-limited, but steroids may be of benefit.
Association with reticuloendothelial neoplasia is unusual.

*The I antigen is found predominantly on adult red blood cells, and the i antigen is found primarily on fetal red blood cells. In primary cold agglutinin disease, the antibody is almost invariably IgM anti-I. The cold agglutinins associated with infectious mononucleosis are unusual in that they may have specificity for the i antigen and they may be IgG.

TABLE 118–10

DRUGS REPORTED TO INDUCE AUTOIMMUNE HEMOLYTIC ANEMIA

α-Methyldopa	L-Dopa	Mefenamic acid*
Procainamide	Phenacetin†‡	Chlorpromazine‡
Streptomycin		

*Other nonsteroidal anti-inflammatory drugs (ibuprofen, naproxen, tolmetin, feprazone, and fenoprofen) have caused immune hemolysis but the mechanism is not clear.
†Also may cause hemolysis by immune complex or drug adsorption mechanisms.
‡Only one case associated with autoantibodies has been reported.
Adapted from Petz LD: Drug-induced immune hemolytic anemia. In: Nance SJ (ed): Immune Destruction of Red Blood Cells. Arlington, VA, American Association of Blood Banks, p 53, 1989.

Often there is a history of an influenza-like prodromal illness. The anemia is usually moderate to severe at the time of presentation and may be progressive even though the patient is kept warm.

The diagnosis of PCH is made by finding the Donath-Landsteiner antibody in the patient's plasma. This IgG antibody is directed against the P blood group antigen and is identified by using a bithermic assay. First, the patient's serum is incubated with erythrocytes at 4°C. Under these conditions, the cold-reacting antibody binds to the red blood cells. Subsequently, the reaction mixture is warmed to 37°C, and the cells hemolyze as a result of complement activation initiated by the Donath-Landsteiner antibody.

Most patients with PCH require only supportive care because the process is usually transient. The patient should be kept warm at all times. Guidelines for transfusion are the same as those for patients with cold agglutinin syndrome. In severe cases, an empirical trial of corticosteroids is warranted. Although the association is now rare, patients with PCH should be evaluated for evidence of syphilis. PCH has also been reported as part of a chronic autoimmune process in adults.

Drug-Induced Immune Hemolytic Anemia

In previous reviews of drug-induced hemolytic anemia, methyldopa (Aldomet) was reported to be the responsible agent in the majority of cases.[28] Because the use of methyldopa as an antihypertensive has declined markedly over the past several years, the incidence of drug-induced hemolytic anemia has probably fallen. Nonetheless, drug-induced hemolytic anemia continues to account for a significant proportion of all cases of acquired immune hemolytic anemia[29, 30] (Table 118–10). Accordingly, when evaluating patients with evidence of immune hemolysis, eliciting a detailed drug history is essential. In addition, a temporal relationship between drug administration and the development of hemolysis should be sought. Unfortunately, such relationships are often rendered inconclusive because patients are taking multiple drugs. Although some drugs induce immune hemolytic anemia more frequently than others, in any one patient any drug must be considered potentially culpable.

Quinine and Quinidine

There are several mechanisms by which drugs can induce immune hemolysis (Table 118–11). In susceptible individuals, ingestion of small amounts of quinine and quinidine can cause severe thrombocytopenia or hemolytic anemia or both. The molecular basis of the immune thrombocytopenia has been extensively investigated, and it seems likely that similar

---

TABLE 118-11

CHARACTERISTICS OF DRUG-INDUCED HEMOLYTIC ANEMIAS

Quinidine-quinine
  Proposed mechanism: The drug acts as a hapten after binding to a cell membrane protein. Consequently, antibodies against
    constituents of the drug–membrane protein complex arise.
  Clinical characteristics
    Small doses of drug induce the process.
    Intravascular hemolyis is common; hemolysis may be severe and life threatening.
  Laboratory findings
    Direct Coombs' test positive for complement but not IgG.
    Antibody may be IgG or IgM.
    Positivity of the indirect Coombs' test depends on having the drug present in the reaction mixture, demonstrating the drug-dependent
      nature of the antibody.
Pencillin*
  Proposed mechanism: Drug binds tightly to the red blood cell. Antidrug antibody binds to the drug on the red blood cell surface.
  Clinical characteristics
    Large doses of drug are required (10 million U or more per day).
    Hemolysis is usually subacute, developing during 1–2 wk.
    Patients may have a positive Coombs' test without clinical evidence of hemolysis.
  Laboratory findings
    Direct Coombs' test is positive for IgG but is rarely positive for complement.
    Patient's serum reacts in the indirect Coombs' test with red blood cells coated with drug.
Methyldopa
  Proposed mechanism: Speculative, but may alter the immune system resulting in a pathophysiologic process similar to that observed in
    idiopathic autoimmune hemolytic anemia.
  Clinical characteristics
    Dose and time dependent (patient will have taken drug for at least 3 mo).
    Hemolysis is usually mild and resolves gradually during several weeks after cessation of the drug.
    Patients may have a positive Coombs' test without clinical evidence of hemolysis.
  Laboratory findings
    Direct Coombs' test is positive for IgG but is rarely positive for complement. When hemolysis is present, the indirect Coombs' test is
      invariably positive.
    Positivity of Coombs' test is not dependent on having the drug in the reaction mixture.
    Coombs' test may be positive for months after cessation of drug.
Cephalosporin*
  Proposed mechanism: Interaction of drug with the cell alters properties of the membrane, causing plasma proteins to be nonspecifically
    adsorbed.
  Clinical characteristics: There is no evidence of hemolysis.
  Laboratory findings: Specific antisera demonstrate the presence of both immunologic (e.g., IgG and complement) and nonimmunologic
    (e.g., albumin and fibrinogen) proteins.

*Cephalosporins can induce hemolytic anemia in the same way as penicillin. In some cases, the antibody is cephalosporin specific. In other cases, antipenicillin antibodies cross-react with the cephalosporin.

---

mechanisms account for the drug-dependent sensitization of erythrocytes. Available evidence supports the hypothesis that drug interactions with the red blood cell induce antibody formation.[30] According to this hypothesis, in combination with a membrane protein, the drug acts as a hapten (Table 118–12). Consequently, the following three types of antibodies may be formed: (1) antibodies against the membrane protein–drug complex, (2) antibodies against the drug, and (3) antibodies against the membrane protein. The fact that quinidine- and quinine-dependent antibodies bind to the cell via the Fab portion of the immunoglobulin molecule provides evidence in support of the hapten hypothesis. Also in support of this hypothesis is the finding that "autoantibodies" with specificity for a membrane constituent may appear simultaneously along with drug-dependent antibodies. A plausible explanation for this observation is that the drug binds to a specific membrane protein and that the "autoantibodies" are direct against the drug-binding protein. Previously, the cells were considered to be "innocent bystanders" in that the drug-antibody complex was thought to bind to the cell membrane either nonspecifically in the case of erythrocytes or via the Fc receptor in the case of platelets (erythrocytes do not have an Fc receptor). The observations described, however, provide compelling evidence that antibody binding is specific and suggest that the concept of the cell as innocent bystander is incorrect.

Binding of antibody to the drug–membrane protein complex initiates complement activation, and as a consequence the cells undergo immune destruction. Thus, patients with hemolytic anemia induced by quinidine or quinine (or other drugs that act by the same mechanism) often present with hemoglobinemia and hemoglobinuria resulting from intravascular hemolysis. Renal failure is relatively common. The antibody may be IgM or IgG. Cell-bound immunoglobulins are usually not detected, but the Coombs test is positive because of the binding of complement components. For the indirect Coombs' test to be positive, the drug must be present. If the drug has been stopped before testing, adding the drug to the patient's serum in vitro causes the indirect test to be positive.

In patients presenting with acute intravascular hemolysis, aggressive supportive care is essential. The offending drug must be stopped and adequate renal blood flow must be maintained. Transfusion may be necessary. Guidelines for compatibility testing and transfusion are similar to those for idiopathic AIHA (see earlier). In cases of severe hemolysis, an empirical trial of steroids is warranted. Inasmuch as antibody binding to cells is drug dependent, the sensitization process should resolve once the drug has been metabolized. Accordingly, the duration of the hemolysis depends primarily on the half-life of the drug (or its active metabolite).

TABLE 118–12

DRUGS THAT HAVE BEEN REPORTED TO INDUCE IMMUNE HEMOLYTIC ANEMIA BY THE HAPTEN MECHANISM

Acetaminophen	Aminopyrine	p-Aminosalicylic acid
Antazoline	Butizide	Carbimazole
Cefotaxime*	Ceftriaxone*	Chlorpromazine
Chlorpropamide	Cinanidanol	Dipyrone*
Fluorouracil	Hydralazine	Hydrochlorothiazide†
9-Hydroxy-2-methylellipticinium	Insulin*	Isoniazid*
Melphalan	Nomifensine‡	Methotrexate
Nalidixic acid	Quinidine*	Phenacetin§
Probenecid	Stibophen	Quinine
Rifampicin	Teniposide (VM-26)‡	Streptomycin*‡
Sulfonamides	Zomepirac sodium (Zomax)	Tolmetin
Triamterene*		

*May also bind to red blood cells, and hemolysis may be caused in part by the drug adsorption mechanism.
†Intravascular hemolysis and renal failure were reported only with an overdose of the drug.
‡Also causes development of red blood cell autoantibodies.
§May also cause hemolysis by the drug adsorption mechanism and has been associated with the development of AIHA.
Adapted from Petz LD: Drug-induced immune hemolytic anemia. In: Nance SJ (ed): Immune Destruction of Red Blood Cells. Arlington, VA, American Association of Blood Banks, p 53, 1989.

Penicillin

When used in high doses (at least 10 million U/d for a week or more), penicillin can induce immune hemolytic anemia. In this case, the drug is first adsorbed onto the cell membrane.[30] Subsequently, antipenicillin antibodies bind to the membrane-bound penicillin, thereby sensitizing the cells. The same mechanism appears to be operative for cephalosporin-induced hemolytic anemia (Table 118–13). The direct Coombs' test is usually positive because of the presence of cell-bound IgG. It is uncommon, however, for complement components to be detected. The penicillin-dependent nature of the antibody can be demonstrated by incubating donor cells with the drug. Addition of the patient's serum to the penicillin-coated cells produces a positive indirect Coombs' test.

Penicillin-induced hemolytic anemia is usually gradual in onset, developing during 7 to 10 days; in rare instances, the process may be life threatening. Other manifestations of penicillin allergy are not necessarily present. In cases of overt hemolysis, cessation of the drug is necessary. It is not imperative, however, to stop the drug if the direct Coombs' test becomes positive but there is no evidence of clinically significant hemolysis. Under these circumstances the drug can be continued while the patient is closely monitored for evidence of hemolysis.

In addition to mechanisms described for penicillin, cephalosporins can cause the development of a positive direct Coombs' test that is nonimmunologic in nature. In this case, the drug alters the biochemical properties of the cell causing plasma proteins to be nonspecifically adsorbed onto the membrane.[30] Specific antiserum can be used to demonstrate the presence of nonimmunologic proteins such as albumin and fibrinogen in addition to immunoglobulins and complement proteins. This type of cephalosporin-induced abnormality is not associated with hemolysis but may cause problems during compatibility testing. Furthermore, it should be distinguished from cases in which cephalosporin administration produces immune hemolytic anemia as a result of the development of anticephalosporin antibodies or antipenicillin antibodies that cross-react with cephalosporin.

Methyldopa

The mechanism by which methyldopa induces immune hemolytic anemia has not been definitively established.[30, 31] The fact that the direct Coombs' test may be positive for up to 2 years after stopping the drug, however, suggests that the pathophysiologic process may involve an alteration in lymphocyte function.

Apparently, L-dopa induces immune hemolytic anemia by the same mechanism as methyldopa (the two compounds are structurally related). In the case of methyldopa, antibody development is dose and time dependent, usually occurring 3 to 6 months after starting the drug. Although as many as 36% of patients taking methyldopa develop a positive direct Coombs' test, only about 1% develop clinically significant hemolysis. The direct Coombs' test is strongly positive for IgG, but it is uncommon for complement proteins to be detected. In patients with overt hemolysis, the indirect Coombs' test is invariably positive. Inasmuch as antibody binding is not drug dependent, methyldopa-induced hemolytic anemia cannot be diagnosed using the indirect Coombs' test in the way described earlier for quinidine, quinine, or penicillin. The diagnosis is presumptive because, based on laboratory studies, methyldopa-induced hemolytic anemia cannot be distinguished from AIHA. Indeed, it has been suggested that methyldopa induces the development of AIHA.

After cessation of the drug, signs and symptoms of hemolysis regress within a few weeks. During the same period, the indirect Coombs' test reverts to negative, but the direct test usually remains positive for several months. Although it is not absolutely necessary, the availability of other effective agents makes it prudent to switch antihypertensives even in patients who have a positive Coombs' test but no evidence of clinical hemolysis.

TABLE 118–13

DRUGS THAT BIND TIGHTLY TO RED BLOOD CELLS AND INDUCE HEMOLYSIS BY THE DRUG ADSORPTION MECHANISM

Penicillins	Cephalothin	Cephaloridine
Cephalexin	Cefazolin	Cefamandole
Tolbutamide	Erythromycin	Cisplatin
Tetracycline		

Adapted from Petz LD: Drug-induced immune hemolytic anemia. In: Nance SJ (ed): Immune Destruction of Red Blood Cells. Arlington, VA, American Association of Blood Banks, p 53, 1989.

Numerous other drugs have been reported to induce immune hemolytic anemia. For patients with newly diagnosed acquired immune hemolytic anemia, all drugs that are not absolutely essential should be discontinued. If temporal events implicate a drug (particularly one previously reported to induce immune hemolysis), that drug should be stopped and alternative therapy using a structurally unrelated compound should be initiated. A causative role for a particular drug may be established by using in vitro tests similar to those described earlier for quinidine or quinine and penicillin. The basis of these types of assays is the indirect Coombs' test modified to determine whether antibody binding to the red blood cell is drug dependent. The technical aspects of the test (particularly the concentration of drug to use) can be obtained from published reports if studies have been done on a particular drug. If a drug that has not been shown to induce immune hemolysis is suspected, experiments are required to establish the optimal conditions for testing. Unfortunately, drug-related antibodies cannot be conclusively demonstrated in many cases in which the clinical suspicion is strong. Adding to the problem is the fact that antibodies may be directed against metabolites rather than the whole drug.[32] In these cases, ex vivo antigens (present in the serum or urine of the patient) may be required to demonstrate the drug-dependent nature of the antibody.

Immune Hemolytic Anemia Caused by Alloantibodies

The development of alloantibodies requires exposure to foreign antigens. Individuals who have the O blood group phenotype develop anti-A and anti-B antibodies because these blood group antigens are polysaccharides that are present on a number of substances found in the environment. Allosensitization can also occur as a result of pregnancy or transfusion. In the case of pregnancy, the mother may become sensitized because of exposure to "foreign" antigens (primarily Rh) present on the small amounts of fetal red blood cells that cross the placenta at parturition. Because of the vast number of different membrane constituents, transfusion recipients are exposed to many foreign antigens. The relatively low incidence of alloimmunization after transfusion is due to the fact that most red blood cell constituents are not strongly immunogenic.[33] An exception is the Rh antigen, but in this case allosensitization is eliminated by the cross-matching process that ensures that only Rh-compatible blood is transfused.

Major Transfusion Reactions

Acute, major transfusion reactions are almost always due to infusion of ABO-incompatible blood, and transfusion of ABO-incompatible blood is almost always the result of clerical rather than technical errors (in most cases, the blood is given to the wrong patient). Major transfusion reactions are rare events, having an incidence of 1 per 10,000 to 20,000 transfusions.[34]

The potentially devastating consequences of transfusion of ABO-incompatible blood are the result of massive, complement-mediated intravascular hemolysis. The pathophysiologic processes that accompany the reaction are due primarily to formation of immune complexes and to complement activation rather than to release of hemoglobin. As a consequence of complement activation, C3a and C5a are generated, and these vasoactive peptides appear to be responsible for the vascular instability that is a critical part of the pathophysiology of major transfusion reactions. Con-

ceivably, complement activation may also be responsible in part for the association of DIC with major transfusion reactions because complement activation can initiate activation of the coagulation system. Anti-A and anti-B antibodies have the capacity to mediate intravascular hemolysis for the following reasons: (1) they are present in high titer, (2) they efficiently activate complement because they are usually IgM, and (3) the antigen recognized by the antibodies is present in high density on the red blood cell surface.

In some cases, symptoms may be relatively subtle, but major transfusion reactions are usually associated with sudden, dramatic clinical deterioration of the recipient. Patients complain of chest pain (frequently substernal), back pain (frequently paravertebral), leg pain, dyspnea, anxiety, flushing, chills, and diaphoresis. Hypotension and renal failure are frequently observed, and evidence of intravascular hemolysis (hemoglobinuria and serum free hemoglobin) is apparent. In patients who have evidence of intravascular hemolysis in the absence of symptoms of a transfusion reaction, care should also be taken to investigate the possibility of nonimmunologic causes of hemolysis. For example, if solutions containing 5% dextrose are added to the blood bag or infused concomitantly in the same tubing as the transfused red blood cells, hemolysis may ensue.

Diagnosis of acute hemolytic transfusion reactions in patients undergoing surgery may be difficult because under anesthesia the usual symptoms are not manifested. Because of lack of untoward signs and symptoms, infusion of the incompatible blood is likely to continue, increasing the severity of the episode. Unexplained hypotension or generalized bleeding may be the first evidence of a major transfusion reaction in the anesthetized patient. It is important, however, to document that incompatible blood has been transfused because a number of other pathologic processes can result in hypotension and bleeding during surgery.

When a hemolytic reaction is suspected, the transfusion should be stopped immediately because the severity of the injury is in part related to the volume of blood infused. Plasma and urine should be examined for evidence of hemoglobin, and the blood from the transfusion set along with that of the recipient should undergo compatibility testing. Evidence for immune-mediated cell destruction should be sought by testing the patient's blood for immunoglobulin (both IgG and IgM because anti-A and anti-B antibodies are usually IgM). A "mixed field" reaction is observed in the microscopic Coombs' assay because only the transfused cells are coated with immunoglobulins and complement. The term mixed field is used to describe the observation that the agglutination is heterogeneous; that is, only some of the cells (those from the donor) are agglutinated. The standard direct Coombs' test is negative if all of the donor cells have been destroyed, although this is not usually the case.

Treatment of major acute hemolytic transfusion reactions is primarily supportive.[34] Once the diagnosis is established, or if there is a high degree of suspicion, the patient should receive furosemide (80 to 120 mg intravenously) and urine output should be maintained at more than 100 mL/h. Nonblood volume expanders (e.g., colloid and crystalloid) can be used to help maintain renal perfusion (the use of mannitol in this setting is controversial), but patients must be closely monitored for signs of volume overload. Based on the observation that hemoglobin is more soluble in alkaline solutions, it has been suggested that alkalinization of the urine may ameliorate the renal damage associated with a major transfusion reaction. Evidence supporting this hypothesis, however, is not compelling. Vasopressors may be required to maintain blood pressure, but agents that have the attendant feature of restricting renal blood flow are contraindicated. In patients who develop renal failure, short-term dialysis may be required while waiting for the damaged kidneys to recover.

The DIC that arises as part of a major transfusion reaction is usually self-limited. Accordingly, overzealous treatment should be avoided and therapeutic intervention should be reserved for patients who exhibit evidence of uncompensated disease. Platelet transfusion and fresh frozen plasma as a source of coagulation factors may be beneficial, but the use of heparin (either low doses or therapeutic amounts) is controversial. Moderate-to-severe hypofibrinogenemia can be treated by using cryoprecipitate.

Delayed Transfusion Reactions

Delayed transfusion reactions (those occurring 3 to 21 days after infusion of the blood) are usually the result of an anamnestic immune response.[33] In these cases, the initial allosensitization most likely occurred as a result of pregnancy or prior transfusion, but at the time the compatibility testing is done the presence of the alloantibody is not observed because the titer is too low. Thus, unlike major transfusion reactions, which are almost always the result of human error, delayed transfusion reactions are usually unavoidable.

The transfused cells bearing the alloantigen stimulate an anamnestic immune response that generates a marked increase in the titer of the alloantibody. As a consequence, the donor cells become sensitized and subsequently undergo immune destruction. Depending on the characteristics of the antibody and antigen, either intravascular or extravascular hemolysis may be the predominant process. Symptoms are usually mild (often low-grade fever only, but chills, pallor, and jaundice may be observed). In rare instances, renal failure and DIC have been observed in association with delayed transfusion reactions.

The diagnosis is made by demonstrating an alloantibody in the patient's serum. The indirect Coombs' test is usually strongly positive because the antibody must be present in relatively high concentrations for clinically significant hemolysis to be apparent. The need to distinguish a delayed transfusion reaction from AIHA, however, may create a dilemma (Table 118–14). The problem is complicated by the observation that transfusion can stimulate development of AIHA.

Standard laboratory tests (see Table 118–1) document hemolysis but do not differentiate between AIHA and delayed transfusion reaction. The direct Coombs' test is positive for both AIHA and delayed transfusion reaction, but microscopic examination reveals a mixed field reaction (see earlier) in the case of delayed transfusion reaction. The indirect Coombs' test is almost invariably positive in delayed transfusion reactions. Although the test is also positive in approximately 50% of the cases of AIHA, it may be informative to compare the relative strength of the direct and indirect tests.

In AIHA, the direct test is usually stronger for two reasons. First, because the antibody is a panagglutinin, all red blood cells bear the antigen recognized by the autoantibody (as opposed to only the donor cells in the case of delayed transfusion reactions). Second, the high affinity of the antibody and the presence of large amounts of antigen result in most of the autoantibody being adsorbed from the plasma onto the red blood cells (thus weakening the indirect assay).

In contrast, the indirect test is usually stronger in cases of delayed transfusion reaction. Inasmuch as the antigen is present only on donor cells, the patient's own cells do not react in the direct assay. Thus, the strength of the direct test is dependent on the proportion of donor cells that are present in the test sample. Furthermore, as the donor cells are destroyed, the direct assay becomes weaker, and the mixed field pattern of the reaction becomes more apparent. Also favoring a stronger indirect test in cases of delayed transfusion reaction is the fact that alloantibody binds only to donor cells. Consequently, if the amount of blood transfused was small or most of the donor cells have been destroyed, there is relatively less antigen to which the antibody can bind and therefore less antibody is adsorbed from the plasma.

Determination of antibody specificity may also help differentiate AIHA from delayed transfusion reactions. As discussed earlier, autoantibodies are usually panagglutinins, and although they may show some specificity for antigens of the Rh system, this specificity is relative. In cases of relative specificity, the antibody reacts more strongly with cells expressing a particular antigen, but reactivity with cells lacking the antigen is also observed. In contrast, alloantibodies are truly specific in that they fail to react with cells that lack the antigen. The antigen systems most frequently involved in delayed transfusion reaction are Rh (34%), Kidd (30%), Duffy (14%), Kell (13%), and MNSs (4%).

If the reticulocyte count is relatively high (≥10%), separation of donor from recipient cells can be accomplished by taking advantage of the fact that reticulocytes are less dense than more mature cells. Accordingly, reticulocytes can be isolated by density centrifugation and used for testing in the direct and indirect Coombs' assays. Because the reticulocytes are of recipient origin, they do not react with alloantibodies. On the other hand, if the patient has an autoantibody, the direct Coombs' tests using reticulocytes are positive.

Delayed transfusion reactions usually require only minimal symptomatic and supportive treatment. If the anemia is severe, however, transfusion may be necessary. Kidney function should be monitored. In the unusual circumstance in which there is evidence of renal impairment, treatment should be initiated using the management guidelines provided earlier for acute major transfusion reactions.

	TABLE 118–14	
METHODS FOR DIFFERENTIATING BETWEEN DELAYED TRANSFUSION REACTIONS AND AUTOIMMUNE HEMOLYTIC ANEMIA		
Parameter	**Delayed Transfusion Reaction**	**AIHA**
Direct Coombs' test	Positive, with mixed field reaction	Positive, with homogeneous agglutination
Indirect Coombs' test	Positive in virtually all cases	Positive in ~ 50% of cases
Relative strength of Coombs' tests	Indirect > direct	Direct > indirect
Specificity of antibody	True specificity for cells expressing alloantigen	Panagglutinin, may have *relative* specificity for Rh antigens
Reactivity of reticulocytes	Coombs'-negative	Coombs'-positive

MISCELLANEOUS CAUSES OF ACQUIRED HEMOLYTIC ANEMIA

Paroxysmal Nocturnal Hemoglobinuria

PNH is an uncommon disease in which the hemolytic anemia is due to the exquisite sensitivity of the red blood cells to the lytic effects of complement.[33, 35] The blood cells are deficient in a group of membrane proteins that share the common biochemical feature of being anchored to the cell through a glycosylphosphatidylinositol moiety, and two of these proteins, decay-accelerating factor and membrane inhibitor of reactive lysis, are critically important regulators of complement activity. In PNH, complement is not activated by the classic pathway because antibody is almost never present. Rather, the lack of the membrane inhibitory proteins allows the alternative pathway of complement to undergo spontaneous activation on the cell surface. As a consequence, the erythrocytes are hemolyzed.

Although some patients may give a history consistent with recurrent episodes of hemoglobinuria, it is a presenting symptom in only 25% of cases. In most instances, patients with PNH present with anemia of uncertain etiology. Hemolytic crises are, however, associated with intercurrent illnesses and particularly with trauma. Thus, PNH should be suspected in a critically ill patient who has evidence of intravascular hemolysis with a negative Coombs' test. The Coombs test is negative for immunoglobulin because antibody is not present, and the test is negative for complement because the cells on which complement is activated are hemolyzed and lost from the circulation. For unexplained reasons, thrombotic events often complicate PNH. Other associated symptoms include esophageal spasm, abdominal pain, and impotence. Evidence of renal dysfunction may be apparent. The diagnosis can be made by showing that the red blood cells are abnormally susceptible to complement-mediated hemolysis. Both Ham's test (also called acidified serum lysis) and the sucrose lysis test detect the presence of the abnormal cells.

Corticosteroids (prednisone at 1 mg/kg/d) should be given in an attempt to ameliorate the severity of a hemolytic crisis. Transfusion may be necessary. In general, patients with PNH tolerate transfusion without untoward consequences, although in rare instances hemolytic crises have been reported in association with transfusion. The problem can usually be circumvented by giving washed cells. Thromboses should be treated aggressively. Patients should be fully anticoagulated with heparin, followed by chronic therapy with warfarin. Thrombolytic therapy has been used without complication. Patients with PNH are often iron deficient because of urinary loss in association with hemoglobinuria. Iron should be replaced. As a consequence of iron repletion, however, erythropoiesis increases and so does the number of complement-sensitive cells in the peripheral circulation. Accordingly, after initiation of iron therapy, patients should be carefully monitored for evidence of a hemolytic crisis (and worsening of other symptoms).

Hemolytic Anemia Resulting from Infections

On a worldwide basis, malaria is the most common cause of hemolytic anemia. Merozoites from infected tissues invade erythrocytes and parasitize constituents that are critical for normal metabolic function. As a consequence, the osmotic fragility and cation permeability are altered. In some cases, neoantigens are expressed by infected red blood cells. This observation provides a plausible explanation for the development of a positive Coombs' test in some cases of falcipa-

rum malaria. The red blood cells are destroyed primarily by the spleen, and splenomegaly is observed in virtually all cases of malaria. Characterized by pyrexia and hemoglobinuria, blackwater fever is a term used to describe an acute hemolytic crisis sometimes seen in association with treatment of falciparum malaria. The complication is no longer common, and it remains unclear whether the phenomenon is produced by the infection or by the antimalarial (usually quinine). The diagnosis of malaria is made by demonstrating the parasites in the peripheral blood film. If it is treated promptly, the prognosis is excellent. It is important to remember, however, that certain antimalarials (primaquine, quinacrine, and various sulfones and sulfonamides) should not be given to patients with G6PD deficiency because these drugs evoke severe hemolysis by inducing oxidant stress (see later).

Babesia, a protozoan that parasitizes red blood cells, can induce hemolytic anemia.[36] The infection is transmitted to humans by the wood tick or through transfusion of infected cells. Most cases have come from the northeastern United States, particularly Nantucket and Martha's Vineyard, MA. The disease appears to be particularly fulminant in patients who have been previously splenectomized. Such patients may present with DIC and renal insufficiency. The diagnosis of babesiosis is made by demonstrating the organism in the peripheral blood film. A combination of quinidine and clindamycin has been used successfully to treat transfusion-related babesiosis.[37]

Acute hemolytic anemia is associated with infections with *Bartonella bacilliformis*, a bacterial species endemic to South America.[36] The disease is transmitted by the bite of the sandfly. Apparently the organism grows on the surface of the red blood cell, and the diagnosis can be made by observing red-violet rods in Giemsa-stained peripheral blood films. Bartonellosis can be effectively treated by using penicillin, streptomycin, chloramphenicol, or tetracyline.

Severe intravascular hemolysis with striking hemoglobinemia and hemoglobinuria can complicate sepsis caused by *C. perfringens*.[36] The alpha toxin of *C. perfringens* is a phospholipase that can induce hemolysis through enzymatic degradation of the glycerophosphoryl bond of membrane lecithin. Microspherocytes are observed in the peripheral blood film. Renal failure and hepatic failure often supervene. Treatment of the infection and aggressive supportive management of these severely ill patients are mandatory. Unfortunately, even with intensive treatment, half of the patients die.

A mild, transient hemolytic anemia may be seen in association with bacteremia caused by pneumococci, staphylococci, and *E. coli*.[36]

Toxin-Induced Hemolytic Anemia

Intravascular hemolysis has been reported in association with spider bites, with the brown recluse (*Loxosceles reclusa*, endemic to the central and southern portions of the United States) being most frequently implicated.[38] The hemolysis can last from several days up to 1 week. Bee stings are a rare cause of hemolysis. Cobra venom contains phospholipases that can induce hemolysis in vitro, but clinically significant hemolytic anemia is an uncommon complication of snake bites.

Patients who have extensive burn injuries may develop hemoglobinemia and occasionally hemoglobinuria.[38] Review of the peripheral blood film shows microspherocytes. The pathophysiologic basis of the spherocytic hemolytic anemia associated with severe burns has been elucidated by observing the effects of heat on red blood cells in vitro. At temperatures above 49°C, the erythrocyte cytoskeletal protein, spectrin, becomes unstable. As a consequence, the integrity of the cell is disturbed, and microspherocytes are created when portions of the membrane are lost as a result of vesiculation.

The hemolytic anemia associated with toxic amounts of copper salts appears to be the result of oxidative stress.[38] The hemolysis of Wilson's disease has been attributed to elevated plasma copper levels, and patients undergoing hemodialysis have experienced acute hemolysis when the dialysis fluid became contaminated by copper pipes.[38] Inhalation of arsine gas (formed in the course of many industrial processes) has been reported to cause massive hemolysis.[38] Hemolysis makes only a minor contribution to the anemia associated with lead intoxication.[38]

Spur Cell Anemia

The anemia associated with liver disease is usually multifactorial (nutritional deficiencies, toxic effects of alcohol on erythropoiesis, splenomegaly, and bleeding from gastritis, esophageal varices, and duodenal ulcers).[39] An unusual, but dramatic, hemolytic process called spur cell anemia may be observed in association with advanced Laennec's cirrhosis.[39] The diagnosis should be suspected in cirrhotic patients who experience a sudden fall in hematocrit. The diagnosis is made by observing erythrocytes with elongated spicules (acanthocytes, spur cells) in the peripheral blood film. These cells contain a 50 to 70% excess of cholesterol, but the phospholipid content is normal. Spur cells can be induced in vitro by incubating normal erythrocytes with the patient's plasma. The disturbance in lipid content results from passive incorporation into the red blood cell of an abnormal low-density lipoprotein containing an increased cholesterol/phospholipid ratio. The excess cholesterol markedly reduces red blood cell deformability, and consequently the spur cells become sequestered in the spleen.

Transfusion is of little benefit to patients with spur cell anemia because the donor cells rapidly acquire the abnormality.[39] Splenectomy has been reported to be beneficial in reducing the severity of the hemolysis, but the severity of the liver disease and its attendant complications usually make the morbidity and mortality associated with the procedure unacceptably high. Cholesterol-lowering agents appear to be of no benefit. Patients with spur cell anemia have a 1-year mortality rate greater than 90%.

HEREDITARY HEMOLYTIC ANEMIAS

Inherited Hemolytic Anemia Associated with Membrane Abnormalities

Patients with hereditary spherocytosis (HS) have an inherited genetic defect that is manifested as a quantitative or, less commonly, both a quantitative and a qualitative abnormality of spectrin.[40–42] Because it is a critically important part of the cytoskeleton, even subtle abnormalities of spectrin produce changes in the structural integrity and biophysical properties of the red blood cell that are clinically apparent. The nature and extent of the spectrin defect determine the severity of the hemolytic process. Approximately 75% of cases are inherited in an autosomal dominant fashion, and the remaining 25% have a nondominant (probably recessive) pattern. Patients with dominant HS have mild deficiencies of spectrin (75 to 90% of normal), whereas the deficiency is more severe (30 to 50% of normal) in the recessive form. A subset of patients with dominant HS also have a qualitative

defect, and as a consequence a portion of the spectrin lacks the capacity to combine properly with band 4.1, another important component of the cytoskeleton.

Although definitive proof is lacking, available evidence is most consistent with the hypothesis that the spherocytes are formed because HS red blood cells gradually lose the portions of the membrane that overlie the spectrin-deficient regions. Membrane loss is accentuated by the conditioning that occurs when the cells become sequestered in the spleen. As discussed earlier, the splenic microenvironment is relatively hypoxic, acidic, and hypoglycemic, and these conditions are particularly toxic to HS red blood cells. Splenic conditioning is the basis of the incubated osmotic fragility test that is useful in diagnosing HS. When HS cells are incubated in solutions of graded hypotonicity in the absence of glucose, they hemolyze more extensively than normal erythrocytes. HS red blood cells are more osmotically fragile than normal even when the test is done in the presence of glucose, but the specificity of the test is higher when the cells are placed under greater metabolic stress (by omitting the glucose).

The clinical severity of HS varies widely (even among affected family members). In rare instances, patients have life-threatening hemolysis and are transfusion dependent. In many patients, however, the hemolytic process is fully compensated, and anemia is absent except when other pathologic processes supervene. Hemolytic crises frequently occur in association with infection, probably because the attendant inflammatory process induces reticuloendothelial hyperplasia. Aplastic crises occur when patients acutely become reticulocytopenic. As discussed earlier, this potentially life-threatening event is usually due to infection with human parvovirus. Supportive measures are required until the infection resolves. Because of the chronic hemolysis, patients with HS have a propensity to develop bilirubinate gallstones. Ultrasonography is the most reliable method for detecting cholelithiasis in patients with HS because only 50% of bilirubin stones are radiopaque.

The following findings are consistent with the diagnosis of HS: (1) evidence of hemolysis, (2) splenomegaly, (3) microspherocytes in the peripheral blood film, (4) a negative Coombs' test, and (5) a positive family history. The incubated osmotic fragility test is almost invariably abnormal and should be performed if confirmatory evidence of HS is needed. Close relatives should be evaluated for HS and affected individuals treated appropriately.

Splenectomy is recommended for all HS patients with anemia or significant hemolysis (to prevent gallstones). For young children the operation is usually delayed until age 5 or 6 years. Preoperatively, patients should receive pneumococcal vaccine, but the use of prophylactic antibiotics after splenectomy remains controversial. Folic acid (1 mg/d) should be given to all unsplenectomized patients.

Hereditary elliptocytosis is inherited in an autosomal dominant fashion.[43] The disease is noteworthy because it is relatively common (1 in 2500) but rarely causes clinically significant hemolysis. The molecular defect usually involves spectrin, but in some cases the cytoskeletal protein, band 4.1, may be partially absent. The diagnosis is made by observing more than 40% elliptocytes on the peripheral film (normal < 15%).

A rare variant of hereditary elliptocytosis, called hereditary pyropoikilocytosis, is associated with moderate-to-severe hemolysis.[43] The diagnosis should be suspected if the blood film shows bizarre poikilocytosis (marked red blood cell fragmentation). Splenectomy ameliorates the hemolytic process.

Inherited Hemolytic Anemia Associated with Enzyme Deficiencies

Because red blood cells are present at sites of inflammation, they are exposed to powerful oxidants such as superoxide anion, hydrogen peroxide, and hydroxyl radicals that are produced by activated phagocytic cells in response to infection. In addition, certain drugs (Table 118–15) induce an oxidative stress that is potentially harmful. Reduced glutathione is primarily responsible for protecting red blood cells against oxidant injury. During the detoxification reaction, reduced glutathione is converted to oxidized glutathione. Restoration of reduced glutathione levels is accomplished enzymatically by glutathione reductase, and in the process NADPH is oxidized to NADP. Red blood cell NADPH is generated by the hexose monophosphate shunt, and G6PD is a critically important component of the process by which NADP is converted to NADPH. Thus, maintenance of red blood cell reduced glutathione levels is tightly coupled to the activity of the hexose monophosphate shunt.

The most common enzyme abnormality associated with hemolytic anemia is G6PD deficiency, a disease that affects millions of people worldwide.[44-46] The normal enzyme (G6PD type B) is found in 99% of American whites and 70% of American blacks. Approximately 20% of American blacks have the A+ form. A+ is functionally normal but differs from the wild type in electrophoretic mobility because of a single amino acid substitution (asparagine for aspartic acid). The A— type is found in 10% of American blacks and in many African black populations. The A— enzyme has the same electrophoretic mobility as A+, but the catalytic activity is abnormal. The Mediterranean variant (G6PD Med) has a normal electrophoretic mobility, but its catalytic activity is markedly reduced. G6PD Med is the second most common abnormal variant and is found in peoples of the Mediterra-

nean region (particularly Sephardic Jews), in India, and in southeast Asia. A third relatively common abnormal variant (G6PD Canton) occurs in China and produces a clinical syndrome similar to that of the A— variant. The prevalence of the gene in many geographic areas has been attributed to a selective advantage it is thought to provide against malarial infection.

Because the G6PD gene is located on the X chromosome, the inheritance pattern is sex linked. Females who are heterozygous for an abnormal variant are usually asymptomatic except in cases of extreme lyonization.

The half-life of normal G6PD is 60 days. Because the life span of a red blood cell is 120 days, the concentration of G6PD declines significantly by the time the cell reaches senescence. However, even the amount of enzyme present in senescent cells (approximately 50% of that found in reticulocytes) is enough to prevent oxidant injury under all but the most extreme conditions. In contrast, the half-life of the A— variant is only 13 days. Consequently, the red blood cells of patients with A— exhibit a marked heterogeneity of G6PD activity. Young cells have normal or nearly normal activity, but older cells are grossly deficient. This heterogeneity of expression accounts for the clinical observation that when A— patients are exposed to an oxidant challenge, only some of the cells (those that are grossly deficient) are hemolyzed. Hemolysis is more severe in patients with G6PD Med because the enzyme is more unstable than that in A—. As a consequence, more of the red blood cells are markedly deficient and therefore susceptible to oxidant-induced injury.

Normally, even patients with G6PD Med manifest no evidence of clinically significant hemolysis. Implicit in this observation is the suggestion that red blood cells are ordinarily subject to little oxidant stress. Hemolytic episodes are triggered most commonly by viral or bacterial infections. Drugs or toxins that serve as oxidation-reduction catalysts impose an oxidant stress that induces hemolysis in patients with G6PD deficiency (see Table 118–15). Hemolysis can also be precipitated by diabetic ketoacidosis and by accidental ingestion of naphthalene (found in moth balls). Some patients with G6PD Med (but not A—) experience severe hemolysis after exposure to fava beans. Although aspirin is frequently implicated, it appears that high doses are required to generate enough oxidant stress to induce hemolysis in patients with G6PD Med (patients with A— are not affected).

Susceptible patients may experience a hemolytic crisis within hours of exposure to an oxidant stress. In severe cases, signs of intravascular hemolysis and vascular instability may be evident. Inasmuch as only the older, grossly deficient cells are susceptible, however, the hemolytic crisis is self-limited (e.g., 25 to 30% of cells are vulnerable in patients with A—). Oxidation of hemoglobin produces intracellular precipitates called Heinz's bodies. These red blood cell inclusions are not seen on routine Wright's staining of the peripheral blood film, but they may be visualized by using supravital stains such as methyl violet. Heinz's bodies are usually not seen after the first day or so of the crisis, however, because they are rapidly removed by the spleen. In the process of removal of the Heinz body, a portion of the membrane is lost, resulting in the formation of bite cells. A small number of spherocytes may also be observed.

Several assays are available for the diagnosis of G6PD deficiency. In general, the sensitivity of these tests is such that 20 to 40% of the cells must be deficient for the tests to be positive. Inasmuch as only young cells with relatively normal G6PD are left after a hemolytic crisis, false-negative results may be obtained if the assay is done during or shortly after the episode. Accordingly, it may be necessary to repeat the studies when the patient has recovered.

TABLE 118–15

DRUGS IMPLICATED IN HEMOLYTIC EPISODES ASSOCIATED WITH GLUCOSE-6-PHOSPHATE DEHYDROGENASE DEFICIENCY

Antimalarials
   Primaquine
   Quinacrine (Atabrine)
Sulfonamides
   Sulfanilamide
   Salicylazosulfapyridine (Azulfidine)
   Sulfisoxazole (Gantrisin)*
Other antibacterials
   Nitrofurantoin (Furadantin)
   Nitrofurazone (Furacin)
   Chloramphenicol
   p-Aminosalicylic acid
   Nalidixic acid
Analgesics
   Acetanilide
   Acetylsalicylic acid*
   Acetophenetidin (phenacetin)*
Sulfones
   Diaminodiphenylsulfone (Dapsone)
Miscellaneous
   Dimercaprol (British Anti-Lewisite)
   Naphthalene (moth balls)
   Methylene blue*
   Vitamin K (water-soluble analogues)*
   Ascorbic acid*

*Possible risk in patients with Med variant but not in those with A— or Canton variant.

Adapted from Lux SE: Hereditary defects in the membrane or metabolism of the red cell. In: Wyngaarden JB, Smith LH Jr, Bennett JC (eds): Cecil Textbook of Medicine. 19th ed. Philadelphia, WB Saunders, p 857, 1988.

Specific therapy is usually not necessary because hemolysis is self-limited. Rarely, patients with the Med variant require transfusion. Emphasis should be placed on prevention of hemolytic episodes by screening any black patients to be given an oxidant drug for G6PD deficiency.

Congenital Heinz's body hemolytic anemia caused by unstable hemoglobin variants may clinically resemble G6PD deficiency.[43] Hemolysis is exacerbated by infections and by drugs that induce an oxidant stress on red blood cells (see Table 118–15), and Heinz's bodies can be visualized when the red blood cells are treated with a supravital stain. More than 100 unstable hemoglobin variants have been reported. In many cases, the abnormality is due to a single amino acid substitution that greatly affects the stability and solubility of hemoglobin. The disorders of unstable hemoglobin are inherited in an autosomal dominant fashion, with only heterozygotes having been reported.

The diagnosis is established if the following are demonstrated: (1) a precipitate when the red blood cell hemolysate is incubated at 50°C or in the presence of 17% isopropanol, (2) an abnormal component on hemoglobin electrophoresis, (3) Heinz's bodies, and (4) an abnormal oxygen dissociation curve.

The hemolysis associated with congenital Heinz's body hemolytic anemia is rarely severe enough to require blood transfusion. As with all patients who experience chronic hemolysis, supplemental folate should be given to cover the needs associated with increased erythropoiesis. In severe cases, patients may benefit from splenectomy, but the procedure is not curative.

Deficiencies of enzymes of the Embden-Meyerhof (glycolytic) pathway are thought to cause hemolysis by limiting ATP production.[45, 46] Pyruvate kinase deficiency is responsible for 90 to 95% of the hemolytic anemias associated with abnormalities of glycolytic enzymes. Compared with G6PD deficiency, which affects millions of people, pyruvate kinase deficiency is a rare disease affecting hundreds or perhaps thousands of patients worldwide. The disease is inherited in an autosomal recessive pattern. Heterozygotes are asymptomatic despite the fact that their red blood cells contain less than normal amounts of pyruvate kinase. Among homozygotes, the severity of the hemolysis varies dramatically, with some patients having a mild, compensated process and others requiring frequent transfusion. Hemolysis is not exacerbated by drugs. Splenomegaly is common, but red blood cell morphology is unremarkable. The deficiency can be demonstrated by using specific assays that measure enzymatic activity. Most patients do not require therapy, but in those who do, splenectomy is usually beneficial.

Thalassemias and Hemoglobinopathies

The thalassemias and hemoglobinopathies (particularly sickle cell anemia) are important causes of hemolysis, but a detailed discussion of the pathophysiology and treatment of the protean manifestations of these diseases is beyond the purview of this chapter.

References

1. Rosse WF: Autoimmune hemolytic anemia. Hosp Pract 20:105, 1985.
2. Frank MM, Schreiber AD, Atkinson JP, et al: Pathophysiology of immune hemolytic anemia. Ann Intern Med 87:210, 1987.
3. Hillman RS, Finch CA: Erythropoiesis: Normal and abnormal. Semin Hematol 4:327, 1967.
4. Petz LD, Garratty G: Acquired Immune Hemolytic Anemia. New York, Churchill Livingstone, 1980.
5. Conley CL, Lippman SM, Ness PM, et al: Autoimmune hemolytic anemia with reticulocytopenia and erythroid marrow. N Engl J Med 306:281, 1982.
6. Young N: Hematologic and hematopoietic consequences of B19 parvovirus infection. Semin Hematol 25:159, 1988.
7. Lian EC-Y: Pathogenesis of thrombotic thrombocytopenic purpura. Semin Hematol 24:82, 1987.
8. Kwaan HC: Clinicopathologic features of thrombotic thrombocytopenic purpura. Semin Hematol 24:71, 1987.
9. Roberts HR, Moake JL, Murphy S: Pathogenesis and management of some acquired bleeding disorders. In: McArthur JR (ed): Hematology—1988. Education Program of the American Society of Hematology, American Society of Hematology, p 54, 1988.
10. Gordon LI, Kwaan HC, Rossi EC: Deleterious effects of platelet transfusions and recovery thrombocytosis in patients with thrombotic microangiopathy. Semin Hematol 24:197, 1987.
11. Moake JL, Byres JJ, Troll KH, et al: Effects of fresh-frozen plasma and its cryosupernatant fraction on von Willebrand factor multimeric form in chronic relapsing thrombotic thrombocytopenic purpura. Blood 65:1232, 1985.
12. Kaplan BS, Proesmans W: The hemolytic uremic syndrome of childhood and its variants. Semin Hematol 24:148, 1987.
13. Griffin PM, Ostroff SM, Tauxe RV, et al: Illnesses associated with Escherichia coli O157:H7. Ann Intern Med 109:705, 1988.
14. Kovacs MJ, Roddy J, Grégoire S, et al: Thrombotic thrombocytopenic purpura following hemorrhagic colitis due to Escherichia coli O157:H7. Am J Med 88:177, 1990.
15. Farina C, Gavazzeni G, Caprioli, A, et al: Hemolytic uremic syndrome associated with verocytotoxin-producing Escherichia coli infection in acquired immunodeficiency syndrome (letter). Blood 75:2465, 1990.
16. Leaf AN, Laubenstein LJ, Raphael B, et al: Thrombotic thrombocytopenic purpura associated with human immunodeficiency virus type 1 (HIV-1) infection. Ann Intern Med 109:194, 1988.
17. Siegler RL: Management of hemolytic-uremic syndrome. J Pediatr 112:1014, 1988.
18. Murgo AJ: Thrombotic microangiopathy in the cancer patient including those induced by chemotherapeutic agents. Semin Hematol 24:161, 1987.
19. Korec S, Schein PS, Smith FP, et al: Treatment of cancer-associated hemolytic syndrome with staphylococcal protein A immunoperfusion. J Clin Oncol 4:210, 1986.
20. Antman KH, Skarin AT, Mayer RJ, et al: Microangiopathic hemolytic anemia and cancer: A review. Medicine 58:377, 1979.
21. Weiner CP: Thrombotic microangiopathy in pregnancy and the postpartum period. Semin Hematol 24:119, 1987.
22. Kwaan HC: Miscellaneous secondary thrombotic microangiopathy. Semin Hematol 24:141, 1987.
23. Rosse WF: Traumatic cardiac hemolytic anemia. In: Williams WJ, Beutler E, Drslev DJ, et al: (eds): Hematology. 3rd ed. New York, McGraw-Hill, p 618, 1983.
24. Issitt PD, Gutgsell NS: Clinically significant antibodies not detected by routine methods. In: Nance SJ (ed): Immune Destruction of Red Blood Cells. Arlington, VA, American Association of Blood Banks, p 77, 1989.
25. Sokol RJ, Hewitt H: Autoimmune hemolysis: A critical review. CRC Crit Rev Oncol Hematol 4:125, 1985.
26. Rosenfield RE, Jagathambal R: Transfusion therapy for autoimmune hemolytic anemia. Semin Hematol 13:311, 1976.
27. Kruskall MS: Clinical management of transfusions to patients with red cell antibodies. In: Nance SJ (ed): Immune Destruction of Red Blood Cells. Arlington, VA, American Association of Blood Banks, p 263, 1989.
28. Worlledge SM: Immune drug-induced haemolytic anaemias. Semin Hematol 6:181, 1969.
29. Petz LD: Drug-induced immune hemolysis. N Engl J Med 313:510, 1985.
30. Petz LD: Drug-induced immune hemolytic anemia. In: Nance SJ (ed): Immune Destruction of Red Blood Cells. Arlington, VA, American Association of Blood Banks, 53, 1989.
31. Dameshek W: Alpha-methyldopa red-cell antibody: Cross-reaction or forbidden clones? N Engl J Med 276:1382, 1967.
32. Salama A, Müeller-Eckhard C: The role of metabolite-specific antibodies in nomifensine-dependent immune hemolytic anemia. N Engl J Med 313:469, 1985.
33. Rosse WF: Clinical Immunohematology: Basic Concepts and Clinical Applications. Boston, Blackwell Scientific Publications, 1990.
34. Popovsky MA: Immune-mediated transfusion reactions. In: Nance SJ (ed): Immune Destruction of Red Blood Cells. Arlington, VA, American Association of Blood Banks, p 201, 1989.
35. Parker CJ: Paroxysmal nocturnal hemoglobinuria. Clin Aspects Autoimmun 5:8, 1990.
36. Beutler E: Hemolytic anemia due to infections with microorganisms. In: Williams WJ, Beutler E, Drslev DJ, et al: (eds): Hematology. 3rd ed. New York, McGraw-Hill, p 628, 1983.
37. Wittner M, Rowin KS, Tanowitz HB, et al: Successful chemotherapy of transfusion babesiosis. Ann Intern Med 96:601, 1982.
38. Beutler E: Hemolytic anemia due to chemical and physical agents. In: Williams WJ, Beutler E, Drslev DJ, et al (eds): Hematology. 3rd ed. New York, McGraw-Hill, p 625, 1983.
39. Cooper RA: Hemolytic syndromes and red cell membrane abnormalities in liver disease. Semin Hematol 17:103, 1980.
40. Becker PS, Lux SE: Hereditary spherocytosis and related disorders. Clin Haematol 14:15, 1985.

41. Agre P, Asimos A, Casella JF, et al: Inheritance pattern and clinical response to splenectomy as a reflection of erythrocyte spectrin deficiency in hereditary spherocytosis. N Engl J Med 315:1579, 1986.
42. Lux SE: Disorders of the red cell membrane. In: Nathan DG, Oski FA (eds): Hematology of Infancy and Childhood. 3rd ed. Philadelphia, WB Saunders, p 443, 1987.
43. Lux SE: Hereditary defects in the membrane or metabolism of the red cell. In: Wyngaarden JB, Smith LH Jr, Bennett JC (eds): Cecil Textbook of Medicine. 19th ed. Philadelphia, WB Saunders, p 857, 1992.
44. Luzzatto L, Testa U: Human erythrocyte glucose-6-phosphate dehydrogenase: Structure and function in normal and mutant subjects. Curr Top Hematol 1:1, 1978.
45. Valentine WN, Tanaka KR, Paglia DE: Hemolytic anemias and erythrocyte enzymopathies. Ann Intern Med 103:245, 1985.
46. Beutler E: Red cell enzyme defects as nondiseases and diseases. Blood 54:1, 1979.

Blood Banking and Transfusion Principles in Critical Care

Thomas S. Kickler

Providing compatible blood starts with ensuring that the correct ABO group is given to a patient. The concept of universal donor (group O) or universal recipient (group AB) is relevant only in extreme emergencies or where technical support is unavailable (mass casualties or battlefield situations). For elective transfusions, it is preferable to provide group-specific blood so that scarcer group O blood is not used indiscriminately. In emergency situations in which the blood type is unknown and there is no time to test the patient's blood type or perform compatibility testing, giving group O packed red blood cells is a safe and well-accepted policy.

ABO SYSTEM

The ABO system was the first blood group recognized and is of unparalleled importance in matching blood for transfusion. A reciprocal relationship exists whereby the presence of an antigen on the red blood cell prohibits the presence of an antibody against that antigen in the serum. This reciprocal relationship is the basis of routine serologic practice in the blood bank. Two antisera, anti-A and anti-B, are used to test the patient's red blood cells, a practice known as front-typing or forward grouping. The patient's serum is also tested with cells of known ABO group, known as back-typing or reverse grouping. These results are compared and should not be discrepant before a blood type is assigned to an individual.

The large number of ABO antigens present on the red blood cell membrane are ready targets for anti-A or anti-B. Their reaction with incompatible red blood cells usually causes significant red blood cell destruction. ABO-incompatible blood transfusions remain the most common cause of fatal transfusion reactions.

Patients who are of the uncommon AB type were considered universal recipients in the past because they lack anti-A and anti-B; likewise, group O red blood cells (universal donor) are considered safe to administer to all patients. Blood supplies are generally adequate to avoid using universal donor blood except in cases of major trauma in which transfusion is required before blood grouping can be completed. Group O blood is administered as red blood cells in these emergencies to avoid the potential problem of anti-A and anti-B in the donor plasma. If one wishes to switch such a patient to group-specific blood, it is necessary to confirm that the patients' plasma contains no detectable passively administered anti-A or anti-B, which would cause hemolysis of the transfused red blood cells. ABO-incompatible plasma products should be avoided if large volumes are to be administered to recipients with a small blood volume.[1]

THE RH SYSTEM

Although the Rh blood group system contains at least 40 different specificities, the original specificity identified, Rh_oD, remains the most important. In the Rh system, unlike the ABO system, antibodies to the D antigen form only after stimulation by incompatible pregnancies or transfusions. The D antigen is clinically second to ABO because of its immunogenicity.[2] It has been found that aliquots of less than 1 mL of D-positive red blood cells can immunize Rh-negative recipients and that 50% of the 75% of Rh-negative patients receiving Rh-positive blood produce anti-D antibody. Because the Rh_oD antigen is highly immunogenic and the 85% of donors who have the antigen can readily immunize the 15% of patients who lack the antigen, Rh-negative red blood cell products should be administered to Rh-negative recipients. If the patient's Rh type is unknown, it is preferable to give Rh-negative blood, especially if the patient is a female with the potential of having children. If Rh-positive blood must be given to an Rh-negative individual, passive administration of Rh immune globulin may prevent the recipient from forming anti-D.[3]

The Rh antigen is not expressed as a plasma antigen and is not located on platelet or leukocyte membranes. However, red blood cells contaminate platelet and leukocyte transfusions. Therefore, Rh-positive platelets or granulocytes should be avoided for Rh-negative recipients. Frozen plasma products do not contain enough red blood cells to cause Rh immunization.

PRINCIPLES OF TRANSFUSION THERAPY

The safe and effective use of blood products requires that one know the available blood products and their respective therapeutic advantages. With all transfusions there is some risk of alloimmunization and incompatibility as well as a risk of virus transmission. As with any potent therapy, the potential benefit of the transfusion should outweigh any potential risk. Physicians ordering transfusions can minimize transfusion-associated complications by following two basic transfusion principles. First, patients should receive only specific blood components to correct the deficiency without supplying unnecessary cells or plasma-derived products that may lead to complications. Second, it is unnecessary to correct a deficiency to normal levels. Physiologic levels need only be restored, allowing the patient's own homeostatic mechanisms to make any additional correction after acute treatment. Adherence to these principles minimizes the number of transfusions received and reduces the risk.

A decade ago, there was little debate about when red blood cell transfusions should be administered. If a patient's hemoglobin level fell below 10.0 g/dL, red blood cells were almost routinely given. With the realization that human immunodeficiency virus and other viruses could be transmitted by transfusion, there has been much closer review of the indications for transfusion.[4]

Writing guidelines for any form of therapy is relatively simple if there are well-controlled trials on which to base critical assessment of a therapeutic maneuver. Unfortunately, in developing guidelines for red blood cell transfusion therapy, there is a lack of well-designed transfusion trials to indicate when transfusions should be given.

The main function of red blood cells is to deliver oxygen to the tissues. It follows that the purpose of red blood cell transfusion is to improve the oxygen-carrying capacity of blood, not to treat hypovolemia. Numerous mechanisms exist for maintaining oxygen delivery. These mechanisms involve control of pulmonary ventilation and perfusion, diffusion of oxygen into the blood, characteristics of the red blood cells and hemoglobin (including the effect of plasma pH), cardiac function, perfusion of the tissue, oxygen consumption by the tissue, and perhaps the pattern of oxygen utilization within the tissue. There is no experimental model or single parameter with which to measure these homeostatic mechanisms. Sole reliance on the hemoglobin concentration, which is easy to measure, oversimplifies a complex phenomenon.

In deciding when to transfuse, the physician must decide whether the anemia is chronic or acute. Generally, in the former situation the clinician must rely on clinical judgment in deciding whether oxygen delivery needs improvement. If the anemia cannot be corrected by iron or folate replacement and the patient is showing signs or symptoms of decompensation (such as fatigue, dyspnea, tachycardia, or tachypnea), red blood cell transfusions are justified. In these chronic situations, unaccompanied by volume loss, hemoglobin values of 7 g/dL or less may be tolerated.

When managing anemias of more acute onset, such as that seen in intensive care units, invasive hemodynamic monitoring may provide a more comprehensive physiologic measure of oxygen delivery. These physiologic measurements include the mixed venous oxygen content, the extraction ratio, and the oxygen consumption along with the cardiac output. Agreement on what constitutes impaired oxygen delivery and which measurements best reflect this derangement is needed.[5]

RED BLOOD CELL PRODUCTS

Various red blood cell products are available for transfusion. Each product has particular characteristics that determine its effectiveness in a given clinical situation.[1]

Whole Blood

Massive hemorrhage is best treated with whole blood because red blood cells and plasma are replaced simultaneously. Prompt correction of intravascular volume depletion is important to prevent the sequelae of prolonged hypotension (acidosis, disseminated intravascular coagulation, and renal failure). Other red blood cell products may be used instead of whole blood in combination with volume expanders (i.e., crystalloid, plasma, or plasma derivatives such as albumin or plasma protein fraction).

After 24 hours of storage, whole blood contains few viable platelets. Replacement of blood loss with platelet-free blood could result in dilutional thrombocytopenia. In the massively transfused patient, this dilutional thrombocytopenia has not been found to be clinically significant until 15 or 20 U of blood has been given. If thrombocytopenia does develop,

platelet concentrates can be given to raise the platelet count above 50,000/mm³.

The other hemostatic change that occurs on storage is a gradual decrease in levels of coagulation factors V and VIII. By 3 weeks of storage, factor V levels range from 20 to 60%. Factor VIII levels are between 20 and 50%. The clinical significance of these deficiencies is minimal because only about 15% is needed for hemostasis. In general, factor VIII levels of 30 to 40% are satisfactory for maintaining clotting. The other coagulation factors are stable in stored blood. Hence, in the uncompromised recipient, whole blood maintains clotting factors at adequate levels for hemostasis.

Despite these considerations, one should still monitor the coagulation profiles of massively transfused patients. When bleeding develops, therapy is best assessed by monitoring the platelet count, prothrombin time, partial thromboplastin time, and fibrinogen level. If urgent situations require empirical transfusion therapy, platelet concentrates (6 to 8 U) should be given after transfusion of 15 U of whole blood. Although routine administration of fresh frozen plasma has also been advocated, no evidence strongly supports this recommendation.[6, 7]

Red Blood Cell Concentrates

Red blood cells are the component of choice when restoration of oxygen-carrying capacity alone is required. If the patient has chronic anemia or congestive heart failure or is elderly, transfusing with red blood cells minimizes volume expansion and maximally improves oxygen delivery. Packed red blood cells are obtained from a unit of whole blood by removing the plasma and are preserved for 35 to 42 days. The resulting unit of red blood cells has a volume of approximately 300 mL and a hematocrit of 65 to 80%. Some concentrates are collected in an extended preservative solution that allows storage for up to 42 days. These red blood cells have virtually all of the plasma removed and have a volume of 350 mL because of the additive solution used.[1]

Frozen Red Blood Cells

Red blood cells can be frozen effectively with a cryoprotective agent such as glycerol and stored for several years. The indications for this product are limited. Freezing red blood cells can provide an inventory of phenotyped cells for transfusion to patients with complex antibody problems or patients requiring rare blood types. Freezing also provides a mechanism for storing autologous units that may be used for future surgery or for patients who are unlikely to have compatible blood available. The freezing and subsequent deglycerolization procedure remove immunoglobulin A (IgA) protein and leukocyte antigens; frozen cells are, therefore, useful in reducing immunologic reactions.[8]

Leukocyte-Poor Blood

Patients receiving multiple transfusions or multiparous women may develop antibodies to leukocytes. When they are transfused with incompatible leukocytes contained in red blood cell units, febrile reactions may occur. To prevent these reactions, leukocyte-poor red blood cells prepared by differential centrifugation, filtration, or cell washing are recommended. By removing at least 70% of leukocytes, most reactions are prevented.[9]

Washed Red Blood Cells

Washing red blood cells with isotonic saline solution removes almost all plasma and non–red blood cell constituents.

This product is indicated for patients with severe allergic reactions to plasma constituents. In particular, patients with absent IgA and antibodies to IgA who are at risk for anaphylactic transfusion reactions should receive washed cells.

CLINICAL CONSIDERATIONS WHEN TRANSFUSING STORED BLOOD

Preservation of blood in the liquid state is achieved by storage at 1 to 6°C and by addition of anticoagulant preservatives that allow red blood cells to maintain ATP. Until recently, the only available preservative solutions were acid-citrate-dextrose and citrate-phosphate-dextrose (CPD). Citrate-phosphate-dextrose-adenine (CPDA) is now the standard anticoagulant preservative and extends available storage time to 35 days. These storage conditions lead to several biochemical and functional changes in the red blood cells that may affect the recipient. Hence, it is important to know the altered characteristics of stored blood so that the potential adverse effects of transfusion can be monitored.

Hemoglobin Function

The pH of blood collected in CPDA is initially 7.55 and falls to 6.71 by day 35 as a result of accumulation of hydrogen ions generated in the metabolism of glucose to lactate. As pH decreases, the 2,3-diphosphoglycerate (2,3-DPG) level falls because of the decreased enzymatic activity of hexokinase, phosphofructokinase, and DPG mutase. The 2,3-DPG plays an important role in oxygen delivery to the tissues because it stabilizes the deoxyhemoglobin conformation of hemoglobin and facilitates oxygen delivery to tissue.

When blood is stored in CPDA, 2,3-DPG levels are adequate for 12 to 14 days and then gradually decline to less than 5% of the initial value. This stored blood, depleted of 2,3-DPG, has increased oxygen affinity and is less efficient in delivery of oxygen. However, the clinical importance of transfused erythrocytes with low 2,3-DPG levels is not clear.

In the recipient, transfused red blood cells regenerate 2,3-DPG levels to at least 50% of normal within several hours. By 24 hours, the oxygen-hemoglobin affinity is nearly normal. In patients who are able to increase this cardiac output, adequate oxygen delivery is maintained despite these biochemical changes that affect hemoglobin function. Studies of resuscitation of seriously injured male soldiers showed adequate oxygen delivery to tissue after three blood volume exchanges of 2,3-DPG–depleted red blood cells. On the other hand, it has been suggested that patients with compromised homeostatic mechanisms may be adversely affected by transfusion of red blood cells with increased oxygen affinity. Further work is needed to clarify these theoretic concerns. At present, it appears that transfusion with stored blood is adequate to meet oxygen delivery requirements for the vast majority of transfused patients.[10, 11]

Acid Load

The metabolic component or acid load has been of concern. When blood was stored in acid-citrate-dextrose, the hydrogen ion load was sufficiently great that administration of sodium bicarbonate was advocated if several units were rapidly transfused. This practice is no longer necessary because of the lower acid load of CPD blood. If a patient is massively transfused and there is concern about the patient's ability to buffer the acid load of stored blood, close monitoring of the acid-base status is recommended rather than blind administration of sodium bicarbonate.

Potassium

The plasma potassium concentration in packed cells stored in CPDA for 35 days is approximately 78 mEq/L, in contrast to 5 mEq/L in freshly collected blood. This accumulation of potassium results from intracellular leakage because of inhibition of ion transport during storage. A second contribution to the potassium load is made by the early destruction of nonviable red blood cells. The potassium value at 35 days may appear dangerously high. However, it should be recalled that the total plasma volume in red blood cell concentrates is less than 70 mL. Therefore, the total load of potassium per unit of red blood cells is only 5.5 mEq. Whole blood at expiration date has a slightly higher load, 8.2 mEq, than packed cells. Because of these factors, patients who cannot tolerate an excess potassium load should be transfused with blood less than 5 days old.[10–12]

Citrate Toxicity

Citrate, being an active binder of calcium, may decrease the blood recipient's ionized calcium concentration. This depletion may cause problems after rapid infusions of blood in patients with hepatic dysfunction or neonatal immaturity. Citrate toxicity has, therefore, been of great concern to physicians carrying out massive transfusions or exchange transfusions. However, there has been no demonstration of citrate toxicity in massively transfused patients. The occurrence of citrate toxicity in neonates is well documented, particularly in exchange transfusions. This problem can be minimized by carrying out exchanges at low rates.

Beside citrate's effect on calcium, its administration affects acid-base balance. Citrate is metabolized to bicarbonate, and 1 U of whole blood generates 22.8 mEq of this base. This contribution has a positive effect in counterbalancing the effect of administering blood of a low pH. Also, the resulting mild metabolic alkalosis mitigates the tendency toward transfusion-induced hyperkalemia.[13, 14]

PLATELET TRANSFUSION THERAPY

In critically ill patients with multiple organ system failure, sepsis, and hypotension, thrombocytopenia is commonly encountered. For platelet counts above 50,000/mm³, surgical hemostasis can usually be maintained. Therefore, not all patients with thrombocytopenia require platelet transfusions. As the platelet count falls to 20,000/mm³, the risk of spontaneous hemorrhage increases, and at this level prophylactic platelet transfusions should be considered. If invasive procedures are planned, platelets should be transfused to increase the platelet count to more than 50,000/mm³ or, in situations such as major surgery, to approximately 100,000/mm³. Even with normal platelet counts, platelet function may be impaired because of uremia or medications.

Platelet transfusions may be obtained by pooling platelets from several whole blood donors or collected from a single donor by apheresis, which enables the collection of several units of platelets. Each unit equivalent of platelets (5.5 × 10¹⁰) may be expected to increase the platelet count by 10,000/mm³. Because patients may become immunized to platelet alloantigens through multiple blood product transfusions or pregnancy, careful monitoring of platelet counts 1 hour after transfusion is necessary. If a patient becomes alloimmunized to routine platelet transfusions, human leukocyte antigen–matched platelet transfusions should be given.[15]

PLASMA PRODUCTS

Various plasma products are available for replacing clotting factors. These include fresh frozen plasma, cryoprecipitate, serum immunoglobulin, albumin, and plasma protein fraction. In addition, various purified plasma concentrates are available for the treatment of congenital coagulation deficiency states. The latter specialized plasma products are covered elsewhere in this text.

Fresh Frozen Plasma

A unit of fresh frozen plasma has a volume of 200 to 250 mL and contains all of the labile and stable plasma constituents if maintained frozen. One unit contains approximately 400 mg of fibrinogen and 1 U of clotting activity per milliliter. Appropriate uses of fresh frozen plasma include massive transfusion with hemorrhage, liver disease with bleeding and multiple coagulation defects uncorrected by vitamin K, emergency reversal of warfarin treatment, disseminated intravascular coagulation and bleeding, and thrombotic thrombocytopenic purpura. Fresh frozen plasma is not recommended as a volume expander, as a nutritional source, for correction of coagulation abnormalities in an otherwise stable patient, or for prophylactic administration in multiply transfused patients without documented coagulation abnormalities.

Cryoprecipitate

Cyroprecipitate is prepared from a cold insoluble precipitate of plasma. It contains therapeutic levels of clotting factor VIII (contains both the procoagulant activity and von Willebrand's factor) and fibrinogen. Insufficient amounts of the other clotting factors are present to be of therapeutic value. Cyroprecipitate can be used to treat hemophilia A and von Willebrand's disease. The amount of fibrinogen present in a bag of cyroprecipitate is approximately 200 mg. For hypofibrinogenemic states, cyroprecipitate can be used for replacement therapy. The amount given depends on the severity of the hypofibrinogenemia with the goal of increasing the fibrinogen concentration to 100 to 150 mg/dL. Fibronectin, an opsonic protein important in promoting phagocytosis, is also present in cyroprecipitate. Some patients with multiple organ system failure have low fibronectin levels, leading to increased risk of sepsis. Some investigators have suggested that cyroprecipitate may be beneficial for these patients. Uremic platelet dysfunction may be temporarily corrected by cyroprecipitate infusions. However, this usefulness in uremic bleeding should be considered variable.[1]

Blood Derivatives

Human serum albumin is the most commonly used plasma volume expander. It is produced by fractionating plasma and collecting Cohn's fraction V. The most widely available product is a 25% solution. In the manufacturing process, heating inactivates any viruses, so there is no risk of hepatitis. The primary indication for its administration is a need for volume expansion. There is much debate about whether crystalloid solutions alone are equally effective in correcting hypovolemia. Other possible indications for albumin administration are cardiac bypass pump priming, fluid replacement for burn patients, adult respiratory distress syndrome, and acute nephrosis.[16, 17]

If in the fractionation of plasma both Cohn's fraction V (albumin) and Cohn's fraction IV are not further separated, the product is known as plasma protein fraction. This product can be used for the same indications as albumin. Plasma protein fraction has been implicated in causing severe hypotension when rapidly infused. This hypotensive effect is mediated by prekallikrein activator, which acts on kininogen to produce bradykinin.[18]

ADVERSE EFFECTS OF TRANSFUSION
Transfusion Reactions
Acute Hemolytic Transfusion Reactions

The signs and symptoms of an acute hemolytic transfusion reaction are triggered by the interaction of an antibody, generally of the immunoglobulin M class, with transfused red blood cells, leading to the activation of complement and intravascular hemolysis. This type of hemolytic reaction most frequently occurs when ABO-incompatible blood is mistakenly transfused. The most serious sequelae of hemolytic transfusion reactions are acute renal failure, hypotension, and disseminated intravascular coagulation. The disseminated intravascular coagulation is most likely initiated by intravascular hemolysis of the incompatible red blood cells and by antigen-antibody complex activation of the coagulation process. Despite intensive study of the pathogenesis of the acute renal failure, some uncertainty remains. In general, there is agreement that it is postischemic in origin and etiologically unrelated to hemoglobin toxicity. The decreased renal blood flow, particularly to the cortical area, may be related to release of vasoconstrictor substances that lead to decreased microcirculation and increased stasis. It is not clear whether disseminated intravascular coagulation plays a major role in inducing the renal failure associated with acute hemolytic reactions.

The initial signs and symptoms of a hemolytic transfusion reaction are variable. The most frequent ones are fever and chills. Vague symptoms of backache or flushing may be the only initial manifestation. In unconscious patients, the only signs may be hypotension and bleeding at surgical or venipuncture sites. If sufficient incompatible red blood cells are transfused, hypotension and oliguria progressing to anuria may ensue.

When a hemolytic reaction is suspected, the transfusion should be stopped and samples of the blood and the patient's post-transfusion blood sent to the blood bank for investigation. In general, two simple tests are sufficient to confirm or exclude acute hemolysis: (1) visual inspection of the patient's serum for hemoglobin and (2) a direct Coombs' test, the results of which should be available in approximately 30 minutes. Initial treatment should not be delayed pending these results.

Aggressive treatment of hypotension and maintenance of adequate renal blood flow are the goals of the therapy for hemolytic transfusion reactions. To promote urine output, 0.9% saline should be administered along with intravenous furosemide, which improves cortical blood flow. Previously, mannitol, an osmotic diuretic, was frequently used, but there is some debate concerning its usefulness. If anuria develops, the patient should be managed for acute renal failure (i.e., fluid restriction, observation of electrolytes, and dialysis may be required).

The management of the hemorrhagic complications of a hemolytic reaction should be individualized. It has been recommended that heparin be used for the treatment of disseminated intravascular coagulation. However, most patients with severe reactions improve without any heparin therapy. If severe coagulation deficiencies develop with clinical bleeding, appropriate blood component therapy should be given.[19, 20]

Delayed Transfusion Reactions

This type of hemolytic reaction is usually mild and occurs 7 to 10 days after the transfusion. The hemolysis results from an anamnestic response to transfused red blood cell antigens in a previously immunized recipient. The alloantibody, usually an immunoglobulin G, formed after the primary response may decrease to undetectable levels. As the rechallenged recipient develops an anamnestic immune response, the newly produced alloantibody binds to the transfused red blood cells that provoked the immune response. These red blood cells are then destroyed in the reticuloendothelial system. The most frequent presenting symptoms of a delayed immune hemolytic transfusion reaction are fever, unexplained fall in the patient's hemoglobin level, and jaundice. Renal failure is unusual. The direct Coombs' test is positive until the transfused blood is destroyed. Serum alloantibody usually becomes detectable. Blood that lacks the antigens against which the alloantibodies have formed is required for future transfusions.[19, 20]

Nonhemolytic Febrile Transfusion Reactions

Recipients who have been multiply transfused or have had multiple pregnancies may develop febrile transfusion reactions. These reactions occur because patients become sensitized to leukocyte antigens. The development of fever and/or chills during transfusion is an indication to stop the transfusion because an acute hemolytic transfusion may first present as fever. A second possible but rare cause of fever during transfusion is bacterial contamination of the blood product. Therefore, it is best that these conditions be ruled out before proceeding with the transfusion. After the initial febrile reactions, not all patients experience similar reactions. However, if a patient has had two or more reactions, leukocyte-poor red blood cells should be administered.[9]

Noncardiogenic Pulmonary Edema

The occurrence of pulmonary edema in the absence of left ventricular failure is a well-recognized complication of blood transfusion. When blood products containing antileukocyte antibodies are transfused to a recipient whose leukocytes contain the epitopes against which the passively administered antibodies are directed, acute systemic symptoms of fever, chills, and hypotension may be seen. Clinical findings include pulmonary edema without cardiac enlargement, cough, dyspnea, and tachycardia. Hemodynamic monitoring studies show normal left end-diastolic pressures and significant pulmonary vascular hypertension occurring before deterioration in oxygenation. Work in experimental animals has demonstrated large increases in pulmonary vascular resistance occurring acutely after complement-induced granulocyte aggregation and pulmonary sequestration of granulocytes. Aggressive pulmonary support is frequently required to maintain oxygenation. Corticosteroids are frequently used for patients who have developed respiratory failure. It is not known whether corticosteroids are beneficial.[21]

Urticaria

The etiology of urticarial reactions is not clear. If hives are not accompanied by any other symptom or sign, the transfusion may be resumed without any laboratory testing. It is suggested that if hives develop the transfusion should be slowed or stopped and antihistamines administered. When the patient has improved, the transfusion may resume. Pretreatment with antihistamines is usually adequate to prevent future occurrences.

Anaphylactic Transfusion Reactions

Anaphylactic reactions to blood products are rare. They most commonly occur in IgA-deficient patients who have antibodies to IgA. About 1 in 700 people is IgA deficient. When absence of IgA is demonstrated in an individual who has experienced an anaphylactic transfusion reaction, measurement of anti-IgA can further confirm the hypersensitivity. To prevent further reactions in these sensitized patients, only blood products free of IgA should be transfused. Washed or frozen-deglycerolized red blood cells may be used for red blood cell replacement. If plasma is required, it must be obtained from IgA-deficient donors. Small amounts of IgA are present in albumin preparations and significantly larger amounts are present in plasma protein fractions. These blood derivatives should, therefore, be avoided in IgA-deficient, sensitized patients.

Microaggregates

In stored blood, aggregates of leukocytes and platelets up to 200 μm form. Patients who have received a massive transfusion of blood commonly develop hypoxia proportional in severity to the volume of blood transfused. A possible cause is pulmonary deposition of debris from stored transfused blood. In a series of severely traumatized patients given stored blood administered through microaggregate filters to eliminate the aggregates, it was shown that pulmonary insufficiency could be reduced. Animal studies have led to questions concerning the relationship of pulmonary insufficiency and microaggregates found in stored blood. Opinions vary about the necessity for administering blood through special filters when giving a large volume of blood.[22-25]

Infectious Agents Transmitted by Transfusion
Viral Hepatitis

Viral hepatitis is one of the most serious post-transfusion complications. Despite the elimination of commercial blood donors and screening of donor blood for hepatitis B surface antigen, post-transfusion hepatitis still develops in as many as 10% of transfusion recipients. Type B hepatitis accounts for only 10% of cases; the remaining cases are attributed to non-A, non-B hepatitis. Although transmitted in a similar fashion to hepatitis B, non-A, non-B hepatitis is subclinical and anicteric in most cases. Post-transfusion non-A, non-B hepatitis may become a chronic infection. Since the introduction of an antibody test for non-A, non-B hepatitis in 1990, units of blood have been screened for this agent.[26-29]

Cytomegalovirus

After transfusion of blood, recipients may develop a mild febrile illness, splenomegaly, and reactive lymphocytes in the blood. This mononucleosis-like syndrome was originally described in cardiac surgery patients who had received large amounts of fresh blood; hence, it was called postperfusion syndrome. Subsequently, cytomegalovirus (CMV) was implicated as the etiologic agent. Although CMV infection was initially described after fresh blood transfusions, it also occurs after the transfusion of stored blood. Patients who are immunosuppressed, such as patients undergoing solid organ or bone marrow transplantation, are at greatest risk of CMV infection. To prevent CMV transmission to patients at high risk for post-transfusion CMV infection, blood components from donors who are negative for CMV antibodies should be transfused.[30]

Acquired Immunodeficiency Syndrome

The transmission of acquired immunodeficiency syndrome (AIDS) by blood transfusion accounts for 2% of reported AIDS cases associated with blood transfusion. AIDS has also occurred in many hemophiliacs who have been treated with factor VIII concentrates. These events occurred before a test for antibody to human immunodeficiency virus type 1 became available in 1985. At present, the risk of transmission of AIDS by transfusion has been reduced to 1 in 50,000 to 1 in 150,000 U. Heat-treated factor concentrates as well as solvent- or detergent-treated and monoclonal factor VIII concentrates have eliminated the risk of AIDS for hemophiliacs. Because the incubation period for AIDS may be quite long, a thorough transfusion history should be obtained from any patient who develops AIDS.[31, 32]

Human T Cell Lymphotropic Virus Type I

Human T cell lymphotropic virus type I is a retrovirus associated with cases of adult T cell leukemia-lymphoma and tropical spastic paraparesis. Because asymptomatic blood donors can transmit this virus, resulting in seroconversion in recipients, screening for the virus in blood donors was initiated in 1989. Several cases of neuropathy have been reported in recipients of transfused blood before the availability of testing.[33]

Other Delayed Complications of Blood Transfusion
Transfusion Hemosiderosis

Each unit of blood contains about 250 mg of iron. In patients chronically transfused for congenital anemias or aplastic anemia, the iron load can become deleteriously high. Accumulation of iron in the heart, liver, and endocrine organs eventually leads to organ dysfunction. Iron chelation may reduce deposited iron.

Graft-Versus-Host Disease

Immunocompetent donor lymphocytes may survive storage of red blood cell products and are in greatest numbers in white blood cell or platelet products. These lymphoid cells may engraft in immunosuppressed recipients, leading to graft-versus-host disease. The hazard is eliminated by irradiation of blood products to be used for recipients who are considered susceptible to graft-versus-host reactions. If transfusions from related blood donors are given to normal recipients with human leukocyte antigen types similar to those of the donor, transfused lymphocytes may engraft, leading to graft-versus-host disease. For this reason, when transfusions from close relatives are used, irradiation of the transfusion product is recommended.[34]

REDUCING THE RISK OF TRANSFUSION
Red Blood Cell Transfusion

With the growing awareness of the risks of transfusion, especially risks of virally transmitted diseases, approaches to reducing the number of transfusion exposures have become popular. Autologous blood transfusions can effectively eliminate the risks of transfusion. The most widely used form of autologous transfusion involves presurgical blood donation. Autologous blood donation is generally well tolerated and usually leads to the collection of as many as 4 to 6 U of blood. Blood shed intraoperatively from sterile sites can also be used. A third approach to autologous transfusion is hemodilution. Just before surgery, units of blood can be collected and the reduced blood volume replaced with crystalloid. When bleeding occurs, the autologous blood may be transfused.[1]

With the availability of recombinant erythropoietin, pa-

tients who have hypoproliferative anemias caused by deficiency of endogenous erythropoietin may have their anemia treated by the administration of recombinant erythropoietin. This approach has been especially effective in patients with the anemia of end-stage renal failure. It appears that patients with other forms of anemia associated with malignancy or anemia of chronic disease may also benefit from erythropoietin administration. Preliminary studies suggest that the amount of autologous blood donated before surgery may be increased by recombinant erythropoietin treatment. In addition, patients treated with recombinant erythropoietin enter surgery with higher hemoglobin values. Even patients who have anemia associated with inflammatory states have increased erythropoiesis with recombinant erythropoietin administration.[35, 36]

Hemoglobin-based substitutes free of red cell stroma have been investigated for more than 50 years. The human hemoglobin gene has been incorporated into animals, which allows the production of large quantities of stroma-free hemoglobin. It remains to be determined whether this approach will be more successful than previous attemps at finding a blood substitute.[37] No blood substitutes are currently available.

Platelet Disorders

Patients may develop dysfunctional platelets because of treatment with a drug such as aspirin, uremia, or exposure to cardiopulmonary assist devices such as bypass machines or intra-aortic balloon pumps. Various approaches have been tried to correct the platelet dysfunction in these conditions. Pharmacologic approaches have been investigated.

Patients with uremia may develop diffuse mucocutaneous bleeding. Serious hemopericardium may develop in patients with uremic pericarditis. Although hemodialysis can partly correct the bleeding disorder, 1-deamino-(8-D-arginine)-vasopressin (DDAVP or desmopressin) and conjugated estrogens may correct the abnormality. DDAVP at 0.3 μg/kg given intravenously corrects the platelet abnormality within 2 hours of administration. The bleeding time remains corrected for up to 4 to 12 hours. Estrogens given at a dose of 0.6 mg/kg/d can also correct the bleeding time prolongation seen in uremia. The mechanism of action is not known.

There have been reports concerning the use of DDAVP after cardiopulmonary bypass surgery and even after extensive surgery such as placement of Harrington's spinal fusion rods.[38]

References

1. Widmann FK (ed): Technical Manual of the American Association of Blood Banks. 8th ed. Washington, DC, American Association of Blood Banks, p 105, 1981.
2. Landsteiner K, Wiener AS: An agglutinable factor in human blood recognized by immune sera for rhesus blood. Proc Soc Exp Biol (NY) 43:223, 1940.
3. Bowman JM: Suppression of Rh isoimmunization, a review. Obstet Gynecol 52:384, 1978.
4. Perioperative Red Cell Transfusion. National Institutes of Health Consensus Development Conference Statement, Volume 7, Number 4, p 1, June 27–29, 1988.
5. Gould SA, Rice CL, Moss GS. The physiologic basis of the use of blood products. Surg Annu 16:13, 1984.
6. Counts RB, Haisch C, Simon TL, et al: Hemostasis in massively transfused trauma patients. Ann Surg 190:91, 1979.
7. Murray DJ, Olson J, Strauss R, et al: Coagulation changes during packed red cell replacement of major blood loss. Anesthesiology 69:839, 1988.
8. Meryman HT: The cryopreservation of blood cells for clinical use. Prog Hematol 11:193, 1979.
9. Perkins HA, Payne R, Ferguson J, et al: Non-hemolytic febrile transfusion reactions. Quantitative effects of blood components with emphasis on isoantigenic incompatibility of leukocytes. Vox Sang 11:578, 1966.
10. Zuck TF, Bensinger TA, Peck CC, et al: The in vivo survival of red blood

cells stored in modified CPD with adenine: Report of a multi-institutional cooperative effort. Transfusion 17:374, 1977.

11. Valeri CR, Hirsch NM: Restoration in vivo of erythrocyte adenosine triphosphate, 2,3-diphosphoglycerate, potassium ion, and sodium ion concentrations following the transfusion of acid-citrate-dextrose–stored human red blood cells. J Lab Clin Med 73:722, 1969.

12. Moore GL, Peck CC, Sohmer PR, et al: Some properties of blood stored in anticoagulant CPDA-1 solutions. A brief summary. Transfusion 21:135, 1981.

13. Collins JA: Problems associated with the massive transfusion of stored blood. Surgery 75:274, 1974.

14. Howland WS, Bellville JW, Zucker MB, et al: Massive blood transfusion. V. Failure to demonstrate citrate intoxication. Surg Gynecol Obstet 105:529, 1957.

15. Slichter SJ: Controversies in platelet transfusion therapy. Annu Rev Med 31:509, 1980.

16. Tullis JL: Albumin 1. Background and use. JAMA 237:335, 1977.

17. Tullis JL: Albumin 2. Guidelines for clinical use. JAMA 237:460, 1977.

18. Alving B, Hojima Y, Pisano JJ, et al: Hypotension associated with prekallikrein activator in plasma protein fraction. N Engl J Med 299:66, 1978.

19. Pineda AA, Brzica SM, Taswell H: Hemolytic transfusion reaction. Mayo Clin Proc 53:378, 1978.

20. Goldfinger D: Acute hemolytic transfusion reactions—A fresh look at pathogenesis and considerations regarding therapy. Transfusion 17:85, 1977.

21. Latson T, Kickler TS, Baumgartner W: Pulmonary hypertension and non-cardiogenic pulmonary edema associated with anti-granulocyte antibody. Anesthesiology 64:106, 1986.

22. Swank RL: Alterations of blood on storage: Measurement of adhesiveness of aging platelets and leukocytes and their removal by filtration. N Engl J Med 265:728, 1961.

23. Reul GJ, Beall AC, Greenfield SD: Protection of the pulmonary vasculature by fine screen blood filtration. Chest 66:4, 1974.

24. Tobey RE, Kopriva CJ, Homer LD, et al: Pulmonary gas exchange following hemorrhagic shock and massive transfusion in the baboon. Ann Surg 179:316, 1974.

25. Solis RT, Walker BD: International forum: Does a relationship exist between massive blood transfusion and the adult respiratory distress syndrome? Vox Sang 32:319, 1977.

26. Aach RD, Lander JJ, Sherman LA, et al: Transfusion-transmitted viruses: Interim analysis of hepatitis among transfused and nontransfused patients. In: Vyas GN, Cohen SN, Schmid R (eds): Viral Hepatitis. Philadelphia, Franklin Institute Press, p 383, 1978.

27. Aach RD, Kahn RA: Post-transfusion hepatitis: Current perspectives. Ann Intern Med 92:539, 1980.

28. Choo QL, Kuo G, Weiner AJ, et al: Isolation of a cDNA clone derived from a blood-borne non-A, non-B hepatitis genome. Science 244:359, 1989.

29. Alter HJ, Purcell RH, Shih JW, et al: Detection of antibody to hepatitis C virus in prospectively followed transfusion recipients with acute and chronic non-A, non-B hepatitis. N Engl J Med 321:1494, 1989.

30. Yeager AS, Grumet FC, Hafleigh EB, et al: Prevention of transfusion-acquired cytomegalovirus infections in newborn infants. J Pediatr 98:281, 1982.

31. Possible transfusion-associated acquired immune deficiency syndrome (AIDS)—California. MMWR 31:652, 1982.

32. Eyster ME, Goedert JJ, Sarngadharau MG, et al: Development and early natural history of HTLV-III antibodies in persons with hemophilia. JAMA 253:2219, 1985.

33. Cohen ND, Munoz A, Ness PM, et al: Transmission of human T-cell leukemia virus type I (HTLV-I) by transfusion among patients undergoing cardiac surgery. N Engl J Med 320:1172, 1989.

34. Vogelsang G: Transfusion associated graft versus host disease in nonimmunocompromised hosts. Transfusion 30:101, 1990.

35. Eschback JW, Egrie JC, Downing MR, et al: Correction of the anemia of end stage renal disease with recombinant human erythropoietin. Results of a combined phase I and II clinical trial. N Engl J Med 316:73, 1987.

36. Spivak JL: The mechanism of action of erythropoietin. Int J Cell Cloning 4:139, 1986.

37. Zuck TF: The quest for a blood substitute: In 1990, an unfulfilled promise. In: Nance SJ (ed): Transfusion Medicine in the 1990's. Arlington, VA, American Association of Blood Banks, p 181, 1990.

38. Bolan CD, Alving BM: Pharmacologic agents in the management of bleeding disorders. Transfusion 30:541, 1990.

CHAPTER 120

Acute Effects of Neoplastic Disease

Elizabeth Poplin
Antoinette Wozniak

Neoplastic disease, by virtue of the protean possibilities conferred by its transformed phenotype, can create novel and complex clinical problems in its host. Although a discussion of the properties characteristic of transformed cells is beyond the scope of this chapter, consideration of the clinical complications of neoplasia is of great relevance to the practice of intensive care medicine. Indeed, many admissions to the intensive care unit are occasioned by acute metabolic or anatomic problems caused by malignancy. Although often approached as merely temporary "patching" of an ultimately hopeless clinical condition, prompt recognition and treatment of these problems may allow a cancer patient to return to a previously good performance status, with preservation of a good quality of life for a prolonged period. Occasionally, resolution of an acute complication may provide a temporal window through which definitive curative treatment may be accomplished.

Acute problems attributable to malignancy may be categorized by the organ system in which clinical manifestations are most prominent and are discussed in this chapter in that order, that is, problems affecting the cardiovascular, pulmonary, neurologic, and urologic systems. Metabolic abnormalities attributable to neoplastic disease are dealt with in the final section of this chapter.

CARDIOVASCULAR EFFECTS

Superior Vena Cava Syndrome

Superior vena cava (SVC) syndrome is a clinical entity that results from the obstruction of blood flow through the SVC. It was first described in 1757 by William Hunter[1] in a patient with a syphilitic aortic aneurysm. This syndrome can result from external compression, invasion, thrombosis, or stenosis of the SVC. The causes of the syndrome have changed over the years from syphilitic aneurysms and tuberculous mediastinitis before 1954[2] to malignancy as the foremost etiology.

Pathophysiology

The SVC is a thin-walled, low-pressure vessel that accounts for the primary venous drainage from the upper torso including the head, neck, upper extremities, and thorax. It is surrounded by a number of structures including the aorta, pulmonary artery, sternum, trachea, right mainstem bronchus, thymus and lymph nodes (perihilar, paratracheal, anterior mediastinal nodes). The position of the SVC in the mediastinum makes it an ideal candidate for compression when any of the surrounding structures become enlarged. When the SVC becomes obstructed, collateral venous circulation usually develops. The azygous system is probably the most important collateral pathway. The internal mammary, lateral thoracic, paraspinous, and subcutaneous veins are alternative collateral pathways.[3]

TABLE 120–1

CAUSES OF SUPERIOR VENA CAVA SYNDROME

Malignant (78–97%)
　Bronchogenic carcinoma
　　Small-cell carcinoma (most common)
　　Non–small-cell carcinoma
　Lymphoma
　　Diffuse large-cell lymphoma (most common)
　　Lymphoblastic lymphoma
　　Hodgkin's lymphoma (rarely)
　Germ cell cancer
　Thymoma
　Neuroblastoma
　Kaposi's sarcoma
　Metastases (breast cancer most common)
Benign
　Mediastinitis
　　Histoplasmosis, tuberculosis, other infectious causes
　　Radiation therapy
　Aortic aneurysm (atherosclerotic, syphilitic)
　Benign tumors of the mediastinum
　　Thymoma
　　Teratoma
　　Dermoid cyst
　　Bronchogenic cyst
　　Substernal thyroid goiter
　Thrombosis
　　Indwelling catheter or pacemaker wire
　　Idiopathic
　Other
　　Sarcoidosis
　　Behçet's disease
　　Trauma

Data from refs 3, 5, 9.

Etiology

Some of the benign and malignant causes of SVC syndrome are listed in Table 120–1. Malignancy is the most common cause of SVC syndrome, accounting for 78 to 97% of the cases.[4, 5] Bronchogenic carcinoma accounts for approximately 85% of the malignancies.[6] Small-cell carcinoma is the most frequent histologic type (40%). Squamous cell carcinoma accounts for 18% of the cases. Lymphomas usually make up the remainder of malignant causes of SVC syndrome, with the most common histologies being diffuse large-cell and lymphoblastic lymphoma.[7] Hodgkin's lymphoma is a rare cause of SVC syndrome. Other malignancies, such as germ cell tumors, thymomas, mesotheliomas, and metastatic disease, have been reported.[8] Breast cancer is the most common metastatic malignancy known to cause SVC obstruction.

Although benign causes of SVC obstruction are uncommon, it is important to recognize them when they do occur. Mahajan and colleagues reviewed the experience at the Cleveland Clinic.[9] In this series, mediastinitis caused by various granulomatous processes (i.e., histoplasmosis) was the most common cause of the benign syndrome. Two important features distinguish benign etiologies: the insidious onset and slow progression of the illness and the relatively young age of the patients. With the use of indwelling catheters for hyperalimentation and chemotherapy, SVC syndrome has been observed secondary to thrombosis of the vessel.[10]

Clinical Features

The most common presenting symptoms are dyspnea, facial swelling, cough, arm and trunk swelling, chest pain, dysphagia, headache, dizziness, visual changes, hoarseness, and syncope.[4, 5] Symptoms, particularly dyspnea, are likely to be exaggerated if the patient is in the supine position or leaning forward. The most common physical findings are facial edema and plethora, distention of neck veins, cyanosis, edema of the arm and chest wall, and dilatation of the veins on the chest and abdominal wall. The development of the collateral circulation depends on how rapidly the SVC obstruction has developed. Findings of stridor and/or increased intracranial pressure are ominous and indicate emergent treatment.

Diagnosis

SVC syndrome at one time was always considered to be an emergency. Diagnostic procedures were avoided for fear they would lead to life-threatening complications such as hemorrhage and respiratory failure, resulting in treatment delay.[11] Radiation therapy was usually used to treat SVC syndrome without the benefit of histologic diagnosis. In actuality, patients rarely die of symptoms related to SVC obstruction. SVC syndrome most of the time is not a medical emergency and there is sufficient time to make a diagnosis before treatment.[6, 8]

The clinical presentation of the patient is unmistakable. A chest x-ray film is positive in most cases and may show a widened mediastinum, a lung mass (most often on the right side), or a pleural effusion. Computed tomography (CT) with contrast enhancement is usually helpful and provides information about the mediastinum, the lung parenchyma, and the SVC and its collateral circulation.[5] Venography is of questionable value but is required if surgery is being considered.[3] Its use in determining the area of obstruction and in differentiating tumor from thrombus is still under investigation.[12]

It is important to establish a histologic diagnosis because there are benign causes of SVC syndrome and treatment of malignancies varies. Because the most common malignancy associated with SVC obstruction is lung cancer, diagnosis can often be made with sputum cytology. When this is not helpful, more invasive procedures such as thoracocentesis in the presence of a pleural effusion, supraclavicular or axillary node biopsy, bronchoscopy, mediastinoscopy, and even thoracotomy can be performed with few complications.[6, 8, 13]

Treatment

Treatment (Table 120–2) depends on the etiology of the SVC obstruction. Some general measures can be utilized, including elevation of the head of the bed and oxygen administration. Diuretics may be helpful in relieving the edema temporarily; however, care should be taken not to deplete the patient intravascularly and reduce cardiac output. The use of steroids is of questionable benefit, but they may help reduce associated inflammation and edema.

Experience with surgery is limited, and it is not generally the mode of treatment. Bypass grafts between the innominate or jugular vein on the left and the right atrial appendage have been reported to be successful.[3] Surgery has been used when symptoms are rapidly progressive in benign or malignant etiologies and when other therapeutic measures have failed.

Chemotherapy is the treatment of choice when the SVC obstruction results from small-cell lung carcinoma or malignant lymphoma. In patients with small-cell carcinoma, symptomatic relief provided by chemotherapy is equivalent to that which can be obtained with radiation therapy alone[14] and is more appropriate because of the systemic nature of the disease. Chemotherapy alone or in combination with

TABLE 120–2

TREATMENT OF SUPERIOR VENA CAVA SYNDROME

Chemotherapy
  Small-cell carcinoma of the lung
  Malignant lymphoma
  Chemosensitive malignancies
Radiation therapy
  Emergently when diagnosis not obtained
  Chemoresistant malignancies
    Non–small-cell carcinoma of the lung
  In combination with chemotherapy
Surgery
  Rapid progression of symptoms
  Occasionally in benign conditions
Anticoagulants
  Thrombosis associated with benign or malignant conditions
    (use not well established)
  Thrombolytic therapy: catheter- or wire-associated thrombosis
Percutaneous angioplasty
  SVC stenosis
General measures
  Elevate head
  Oxygen
  Diuretics
  Steroids

radiotherapy is effective in the treatment of lymphomas.[7] It is preferable that the upper extremities not be used for administration of the chemotherapy because of the decreased blood flow and the higher probability of phlebitis and extravasation of the drugs.

Radiation therapy is the modality used in nonchemosensitive malignancies such as non–small-cell carcinoma. It is the treatment of choice when SCV syndrome is seen as an emergency and histologic diagnosis has not been established (tracheal obstruction, respiratory failure). Treatment often consists of 400 cGy given daily for 3 days and then 150 cGy/d to a total dose of 3000 to 5000 cGy, depending on the malignancy being treated.[15] Subjective improvement usually occurs in 3 to 4 days and objective improvement in 7 days.

The use of anticoagulants is controversial. It has been suggested that they may be helpful because thrombosis often accompanies the obstruction, but this has not been proved.[16] In catheter-induced SVC syndrome, thrombolytic therapy (streptokinase and urokinase) has been used successfully to relieve symptoms.[17, 18] Percutaneous transluminal balloon angioplasty has been used when stenosis of the SVC is present.[19, 20]

Cardiac Tamponade

In patients with malignancies, metastases to the heart and pericardium are not an uncommon finding (0.1 to 21%) at autopsy.[21] Patients who have pericardial disease and/or pericardial effusions are usually asymptomatic, and the diagnosis is not suspected. Thurber and colleagues reviewed 189 patients with pericardial metastases.[22] The diagnosis of cardiac involvement was suspected in 16 patients ante mortem but was thought to have contributed to the death of 53 patients. It is important to recognize the symptoms of cardiac tamponade because it requires urgent attention and with treatment can result in prolonged survival for the cancer patient.

Pathophysiology

The pericardial sac normally contains a small amount of fluid (<50 mL) that serves as a lubricant. The excess fluid in malignant pericardial effusion usually results from the obstruction of venous and lymphatic drainage of the heart. As the amount of fluid increases, the intrapericardial pressures also increase. There is equalization of intracardiac and intrapericardial pressures resulting in a decreased cardiac output and cardiac tamponade. The development of tamponade also depends on how rapidly the fluid accumulates, the cardiac function of the patient, and the pliability of the pericardium. When the pericardium is thickened secondary to tumor infiltration or fibrosis (i.e., after radiation therapy), cardiac tamponade can result from constriction in the absence of a significant fluid collection.

Etiology

Lung and breast carcinomas, leukemias, lymphomas, and melanoma account for 80% of the malignancies that metastasize to the pericardium,[23] although virtually any malignancy can be responsible. Primary tumors of the pericardium, such as mesothelioma, sarcoma, and teratoma, are much less common. Benign causes of pericardial effusions should always be considered in patients with malignancies. These include infections; hypothyroidism; congestive heart failure; and drug-related, autoimmune, and postirradiation etiologies.[24] Radiation-induced chronic pericardial disease has been reported to occur as long as 124 months after radiotherapy for Hodgkin's disease.[25]

Clinical Features

The most common symptoms related to cardiac tamponade are dyspnea, anxiety, cough, chest pain, orthopnea, and weakness (Table 120–3).[23] The patient is usually more comfortable in a sitting position. Symptoms may be vague, and the patient may even be relatively asymptomatic.

Physical findings frequently include tachycardia, jugular venous distention, pleural effusion, hypotension, and hepatomegaly. More classic signs such as pulsus paradoxus (drop of >10 mm Hg in systolic pressure during inspiration), Kussmaul's sign, distant heart sounds, and Ewart's sign may not be present.[23]

Diagnosis

The chest x-ray film may be normal or may show an enlarged cardiac silhouette ("water bottle heart"), particularly when the pericardial effusion is large. Pleural effusions are a common finding, and there may also be an abnormal space between the pericardium and epicardial fat pad on a lateral chest film.[26] The most common electrocardiographic

TABLE 120–3

SIGNS AND SYMPTOMS OF CARDIAC TAMPONADE

Symptoms	
Dyspnea	Hiccups
Anxiety	Nausea
Cough	Abdominal pain
Chest pain	Hoarseness
Orthopnea	Dysphagia
Weakness	Impaired consciousness

Physical Findings	
Tachycardia	Kussmaul's sign
Jugular venous distention	Distant heart sounds
Pleural effusion	Ewart's sign
Hypotension	Pericardial friction rub
Hepatomegaly	Tachypnea
Pulsus paradoxus	

TREATMENT OF CARDIAC TAMPONADE AND PERICARDIAL EFFUSION

Method	Indication	Advantage	Disadvantage or Complication
Pericardiocentesis–pericardial catheter drainage	Relief of cardiac tamponade	Local anesthesia	Arrhythmias, chamber puncture, coronary artery laceration, recurrence of fluid
Instillation of tetracycline and other agents	Prevention of recurrence of pericardial fluid	Local anesthesia, 10% recurrence	Chest pain, fever, minor arrhythmias
Subxyphoid pericardiotomy	Relief of cardiac tamponade, prevention of recurrence of pericardial fluid	Low recurrence, cytologic and tissue diagnosis, local anesthesia	May be difficult in patients with poor performance status
Pericardiectomy	Constrictive pericarditis	Tissue diagnosis, almost no recurrence	Large procedure with significant morbidity and mortality

findings are ST-T wave abnormalities, low voltage, and sinus tachycardia. Both atrial and ventricular arrhythmias can occur. Electrical alternans (alternating high and low voltage) of the P waves, QRS complexes, or both (total alternans) are more pathognomonic of cardiac tamponade but less frequent in occurrence.

Two-dimensional echocardiography is probably the most important diagnostic technique available for evaluating pericardial effusion with regard to size and position of the fluid.[27] Cardiac function can be evaluated and even the presence of pericardial metastases can be detected.[28] The hemodynamic significance of the pericardial effusion is much more difficult to recognize. Assessing the extent and timing of the right atrial and ventricular collapse may be helpful.[29]

CT may be of particular value in assessing malignant pericardial disease. The CT criteria that suggest malignant pericardial disease include pericardial effusion with high CT density, localized or diffuse pericardial thickening, masses arising from or contiguous with the pericardium, and obliteration of normal tissue planes between a paracardiac mass and the heart or pericardium.[30]

Right-sided heart catheterization is used primarily in evaluating constrictive pericarditis. The presence of cardiac tamponade is demonstrated when right atrial, right ventricular end-diastolic, pulmonary atrial diastolic, and pulmonary wedge pressures increase and equalize.

Treatment

Cardiac tamponade as a result of a benign or malignant pericardial effusion is a medical emergency. Percutaneous pericardiocentesis guided by two-dimensional echocardiography provides almost instantaneous relief and can be life-saving. Complications of the technique include arrhythmias, cardiac chamber puncture, and coronary artery laceration, but they have been minimized with the use of echo guidance and the controlled environment of the catheterization suite.[31] More complications can occur if the effusion is small or if it has a posterior location. Fluid obtained via pericardiocentesis should always be sent for cytology and culture. Negative cytologic results do not necessarily mean that the effusion is not malignant.

The pericardial effusion can be drained during several days by placement of a catheter. Catheter drainage is usually not adequate for long-term therapy of malignant effusions because of the high recurrence rate. Shepard and coworkers instilled tetracycline (after lidocaine hydrochloride) into the pericardial sac after catheter drainage and the effusions were controlled in 74% of the patients.[32] Side effects were

mild and included arrhythmias, fever, and chest pain. Other agents such as nitrogen mustard, cisplatin, thiotepa, and methotrexate have been used for this purpose.

Creation of a pericardial window through a subxiphoid approach or a limited anterior thoracotomy has been used in the treatment of cardiac tamponade and malignant pericardial effusions.[33, 34] The subxiphoid pericardiotomy is usually preferred because it is less invasive and can be done under local anesthesia. There is some controversy as to whether catheter drainage with tetracycline instillation or subxiphoid pericardiotomy should be the treatment of choice for the management of malignant effusions. Decisions should be made by taking the patient's overall clinical situation into consideration. Pericardiectomy with total removal of the pericardium results in the lowest recurrence rate. This is a major procedure with high morbidity and mortality. It is most useful in the treatment of constrictive pericarditis.

Radiotherapy should not be used for the management of cardiac tamponade; however, it is of value in the treatment of malignant pericardial effusions or pericardial metastases.[35] It is more likely to be used in the treatment of lymphoma, leukemia, and other radiosensitive tumors. Systemic chemotherapy should be used when appropriate in the treatment of the malignancy when the cardiac tamponade is relieved. Table 120–4 summarizes the treatment modalities.

PULMONARY EFFECTS
Massive Hemoptysis

Hemoptysis is a frequent occurrence in patients with malignancies. It is often insignificant and not cause for emergent treatment. The definition of massive hemoptysis is expectoration of 600 mL or more of blood within 24 hours. Asphyxiation is the most common cause of death. An episode of massive hemoptysis is a medical emergency that requires urgent treatment. Mortality rates can vary from 50 to 100 % with conservative management alone.[36]

Infection is one of the more common causes of hemoptysis and can result from tuberculosis, lung abscess, bronchiectasis, fungal pneumonia, and fungus balls.[37] Bronchogenic carcinoma is the most common malignancy that can result in massive bleeding. Squamous cell lung cancers are associated with a greater incidence of massive hemoptysis than other tumor types because of their propensity to cavitate, cause tissue necrosis, and involve the main bronchi.[38] When patients with hematologic malignancies experience life-threatening bleeding, a fungal pneumonia is often the culprit. The fungi can invade blood vessels, resulting in vascular thrombosis and hemorrhagic pulmonary infarction.[39]

Patients who fit the criteria for massive hemoptysis should be monitored in an intensive care unit. Basic support measures include keeping the patient in a semiupright position, oxygen, correction of abnormal clotting parameters, transfusion, and tracheal intubation as needed. It is important to try to determine the source of bleeding. This can usually be accomplished by bronchoscopy. Many bronchoscopists prefer the rigid bronchoscope because it allows better suctioning if the procedure is done during a bleeding episode.

Surgery remains the most definitive treatment for massive hemoptysis. It essentially removes the source of bleeding and decreases the likelihood of recurrence. In a series of 67 patients, Crocco and associates demonstrated that mortality could be reduced from more than 50% with conservative management to 18.8% with surgical intervention.[36] Operative mortality in this series was 23%. Although it appears that surgery offers the best treatment alternative, many patients with malignancies have inadequate lung function and/or extensive disease so that surgery becomes technically impossible. Iced saline lavage has been used to cause bronchial artery constriction and hypothermic vasospasm of areas of inflammatory neovascularization.[37] This procedure cannot be used in patients with bronchovascular fistulas and relieves the bleeding temporarily. A technique using a No. 8 or 9 venous Fogarty's catheter balloon can block the bleeding bronchus and the hemorrhage.[40, 41] Selective bronchial arteriography and embolization of the bronchial artery have been used to control massive hemoptysis. Uflacker and coworkers achieved adequate hemostasis in 27 of 33 patients (81.8%) with follow-up ranging from 1 to 24 months.[42] Risks include spinal cord injury because of the proximity of the anterior spinal artery and downstream embolization. The neodymium:yttrium-aluminum-garnet (Nd:YAG) laser has been used to coagulate sites of bronchial bleeding.[43, 44] Complications of this procedure include hemorrhage, pneumothorax, endobronchial combustion, smoke inhalation, and bronchoesophageal fistula.

Airway Obstruction

Airway obstruction can occur in patients with malignancies, particularly bronchogenic carcinomas. The patient may present with symptoms of dyspnea, cough, and hemoptysis. The situation may be emergent with nearly complete obstruction and respiratory collapse. External beam radiotherapy can be used but does not provide rapid relief of the obstruction in an emergent situation. The Nd:YAG laser can provide immediate relief of obstructive symptoms. It is most successful when there is partial obstruction. Complete obstruction usually indicates more extensive disease and is technically more difficult to treat.[44] The laser must be maintained along the linear axis of the trachea and bronchus to avoid perforation. For the same reason, right upper lobe and peripheral obstructions are more difficult to treat. Complications are noted in the section on massive hemoptysis. Treatment with the laser usually provides only temporary relief and must be repeated or supplemented with radiotherapy or brachytherapy when the obstruction recurs.

NEUROLOGIC COMPLICATIONS

Neurologic problems are frequent complications of cancer. Both primary brain disease and metastases from systemic cancers can cause neurologic syndromes. Some of these neurologic complications are slow in onset, diagnosed during routine management, and are treatable in either an outpatient setting or during short routine hospitalizations. However, many problems present as emergencies and are life threatening. Involvement of brain by tumor, metabolic en-

TABLE 120–5
CAUSES OF ALTERED MENTAL STATUS IN PATIENTS WITH CANCER

Mass lesion, intracranial
   Tumor, primary or metastatic
   Hemorrhage, intraparenchymal
   Hematoma, subdural abscess
Seizure disorder
Leptomeningeal
   Carcinomatosis
   Infection
Paraneoplastic syndrome
   Encephalitis
   Dementia
   Cerebellar degeneration
Vascular stroke
   Embolic
   Thrombotic
Infection
   Abscess: bacterial or fungal
   Meningitis: viral, bacterial, fungal
   Encephalitis: herpetic
Metabolic encephalopathy
   Hypercalcemia
   Hypoglycemia
   Hyponatremia
   Hypomagnesemia
   Uremia
   Hepatic encephalopathy
Treatment-related toxicity
   Narcotic analgesia
   Antiemesis medication
   Chemotherapy
   Radiation

cephalopathy, cerebrovascular events, infection, paraneoplastic syndromes, and treatment-induced (chemotherapy, narcotics) neurologic deterioration (Table 120–5) may all have a catastrophic presentation.

Increased Intracranial Pressure

Of the multiple etiologies of altered mental status and obundation, only a few are unique to cancer patients. Tumors can involve the neurologic system, presenting as a mass lesion in the brain or as meningeal disease. Both primary malignancies and metastatic cancer, usually from lung or breast (Table 120–6), involve brain substance.[45]

The onset of symptoms resulting from a tumor mass is

TABLE 120–6
COMMON INTRACRANIAL MALIGNANCIES

Primary
   Glioma
   Glioblastoma multiforme
   Astrocytoma
   Anaplastic astrocytoma
   Meningioma
   Lymphoma
Metastatic
   Lung
   Breast
   Kidney
   Melanoma
   Colorectum
   Prostate
   Pancreas

usually insidious with a low-grade morning headache, occasionally vomiting, and evidence of slowing of intellectual facility and responsiveness. Rarely, a seizure or rapid deterioration in neurologic function resulting from hemorrhage into a tumor or rapid development of paratumoral cerebral edema is the first sign.

Increased intracranial pressure results from the combined effects of tumor mass and cerebral edema adjacent to the tumor. Vasogenic edema occurs in the area of the tumor, resulting from transudation of proteins and capillary leakiness. With the build-up of sufficient focal pressure, herniation of brain substance can occur laterally and caudally. Herniation can occur as brain substance translocates across the falx, downward through the tentorium, and through the foramen magnum. Papilledema may or may not be seen. With rising intracranial pressure, systolic and diastolic arterial blood pressures often rise with concurrent bradycardia (Cushing's effect). Signs of herniation include pupillary and eye movement abnormalities, paresis, and alterations in respiratory pattern (Cheyne-Stokes breathing, central neurogenic hyperventilation, Biot's breathing).

When rapid deterioration in neurologic status is evident, immediate intervention must be undertaken to stabilize and reverse the patient's problems. When herniation is suspected or anticipated, the following measures should be rapidly instigated. Tracheal intubation and respiratory control with hyperventilation to decrease the $PaCO_2$ to 25 to 30 mg Hg immediately cause cerebral vasoconstriction and lower the intracranial pressure. Raising the position of the patient's head relative to the chest also facilitates cerebral venous return and is considered helpful. Mannitol, 0.5 to 2.0 g/kg, is given intravenously for 15 minutes and can be followed by a mannitol drip. Mannitol and similar agents, urea and glycerol, are isosmotic. Water is drawn from the brain's extracellular space across the blood-brain barrier to decrease extracellular fluid volume and presumably cerebral edema.

Steroids decrease cerebral edema. Steroid therapy, usually intravenous dexamethasone, should be initiated immediately although the benefits, apparent in the majority of patients, are not manifested for hours or days. Dexamethasone, 16 to 100 mg/d, is given intravenously. Higher doses are considered more efficacious, especially in emergent circumstances. Gastric hyperacidity should be suppressed prophylactically with antacids and histamine H_2 blockers.

If the acute manifestations of increased intracranial pressure are reversed and the patient is stabilized, more definitive management of the patient's tumor can be initiated. For the majority of patients, the brain neoplasm is a metastatic focus of a non-neurologic primary tumor. Therefore, radiation therapy to the brain should be initiated immediately. Steroids should be continued.

Under certain circumstances, however, surgical intervention is more appropriate than initial radiation therapy. Primary brain neoplasms and tumors of unknown histologic type should be resected. When the known primary tumor is considered radioresistant (e.g., melanoma, renal cell cancer), consideration should be given to resecting metastatic brain lesions because the expected response to radiation of these metastatic tumors would be modest and of short duration. A solitary metastasis of a non-neurologic primary tumor should be resected with subsequent radiation therapy to the brain because the outcome for such patients is particularly promising. Other circumstances that require surgical intervention include decompression of hemorrhage, hydrocephalus, or abscess; the outcome in latter circumstances depends on the patient's underlying problem.

Seizures

Seizures pose an emergent problem in a cancer patient and should be treated in the standard fashion. Metabolic, vascular, and infectious etiologies must be investigated and if present, corrected. A CT scan or magnetic resonance image must be obtained. If a mass lesion is discovered, steroids, as part of the definitive treatment, should be initiated to decrease edema. Surgery or radiation should follow to control the tumor. When a tumor is observed with or is complicated by seizures, permanent control of the seizures is needed. Acute control of the seizures consists of diazepam at 5 mg intravenously every 5 to 10 minutes until control is obtained. Phenytoin can be given as an intravenous loading dose at 15 mg/kg at a rate of not more than 50 mg/min. Subsequent oral or intravenous administration should be dictated by serum levels of free phenytoin.

Leptomeningeal Disease[46, 47]

Leptomeningeal carcinomatosis is seen in 5 to 8% of patients with solid tumors, most commonly in patients with lung or breast cancer. It is also seen less frequently in patients with melanoma or gastric or other cancers. Leukemia and lymphoma can also involve the leptomeninges.

In patients with leptomeningeal disease, tumor studs the brain surface, cranial nerves, and spinal roots. Patients develop multifocal neurologic abnormalities not explainable by a focal neurologic injury. Altered sensorium, headaches, nausea, diplopia, weakness, and paresthesias may be noted. On examination, patients have abnormalities at multiple levels with cerebral dysfunction, cranial nerve paresis, sensory loss, motor weakness, and/or reflex asymmetry.

In the absence of evidence of a mass lesion and midline shift in a patient with cancer and altered mental status, a lumbar puncture for cerebrospinal assessment is mandatory. Characteristically, if leptomeningeal carcinomatosis is present, cerebrospinal fluid pressure is 160 mm H_2O or more and the fluid shows increased cellularity. The protein level is elevated and the glucose level decreased. Malignant cells are seen on cytologic analysis. Unfortunately, rarely is the analysis so classic. More often, only one or two of these positive findings are present. When the suspicion of leptomeningeal cancer is high but the initial cerebrospinal fluid assay is nondiagnostic, a spinal tap for cytology evaluation should be repeated one or two additional times because the yield increases with multiple sampling.

Therapy of leptomeningeal carcinomatosis depends on the etiology of the cancer. In adult patients with leptomeningeal leukemia, brain and neuraxis radiation is helpful, especially when patients have symptomatic nerve or root disease. Systemic or intrathecal therapy with methotrexate or cytosine arabinoside may induce remission of the leptomeningeal disease. Resolution of meningeal leukemia is frequent and responses are often prolonged. Patients with meningeal solid tumor carcinomatosis are treated with intrathecal methotrexate, cytosine arabinoside, or thiotepa. Unfortunately, clearing of malignant cells from the cerebrospinal fluid in the latter circumstance occurs only in a minority of patients and the overall median survival is under 3 months. In rare instances, however, a patient with a highly sensitive tumor such as breast cancer may have a prolonged remission after radiotherapy and intrathecal therapy.

Cord Compression[48, 49]

Spinal cord compression occurs in patients with cancer. Because this problem can often be treated directly, rapidly, and successfully and is not necessarily associated with rapidly progressive terminal cancer, aggressive attempts should be made to identify patients who develop cord compression at the earliest and most reversible stage. Tumor may involve

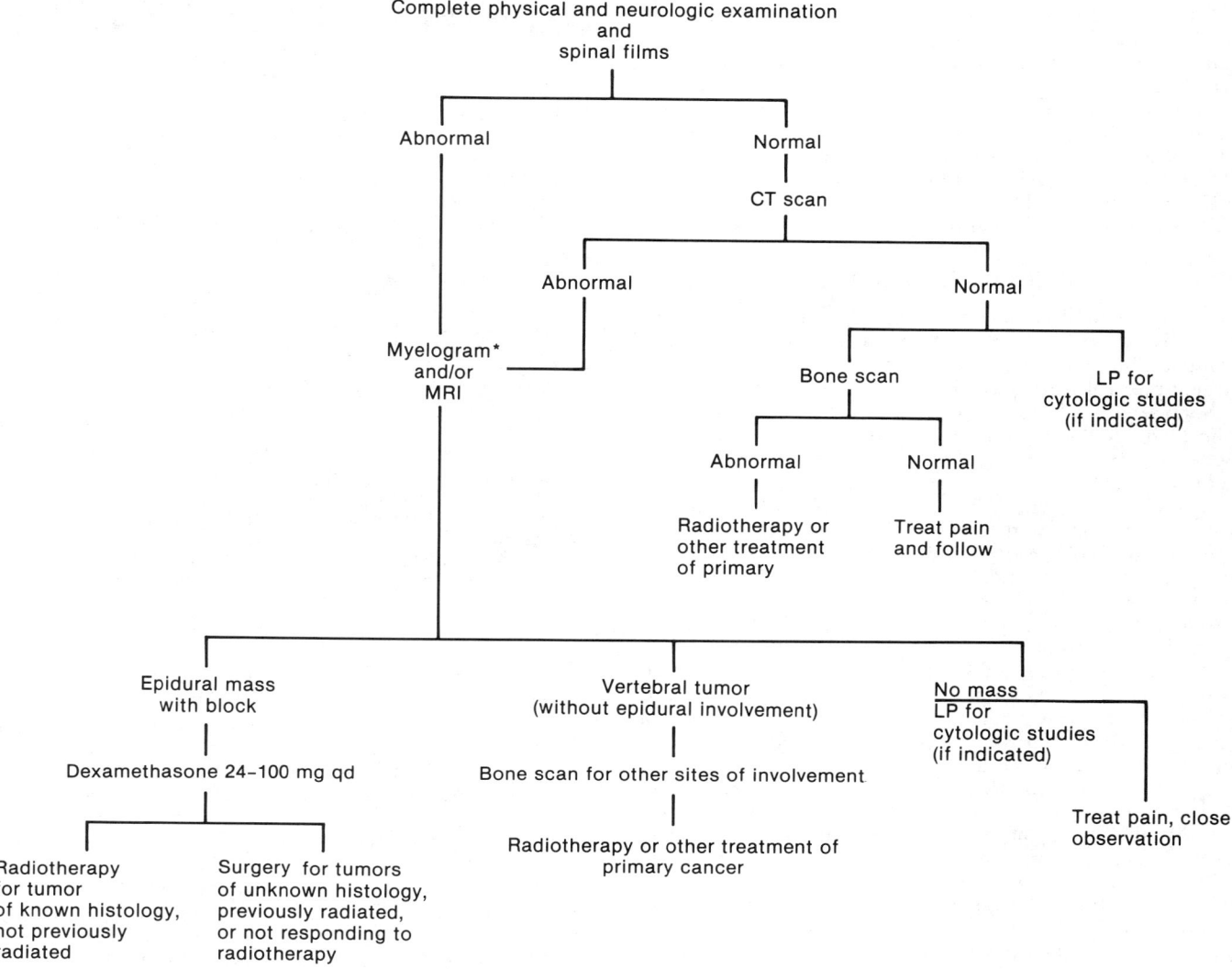

Figure 120–1. Evaluation of spinal cord compression back pain.

the cord itself or more commonly impinges on the cord extradurally from an expanding paraspinal mass.

Patients tend to present with back pain and weakness. Breast, lung, and prostate cancers are responsible for most spinal cord compression. Myeloma and lymphoma account for compression caused by hematologic malignancy. Compression is seen most often in the thoracic vertebrae, with cervical and lumbosacral involvement less frequent.

Multiple algorithms have been developed to identify patients with emergent impending cord compressions. Patients with rapidly progressing symptoms and signs must be considered emergencies in need of rapid evaluation and treatment. Patients with back pain and sensory, motor, or autonomic deficits require immediate evaluation. Patients with back pain and radiculopathy or with back pain and vertebra collapse or erosion of pedicle on plain spine films also need rapid evaluation (Fig. 120–1).

After careful neurologic examination to assess neurologic deficits, if cord compression is suspected, patients should undergo diagnostic radiologic evaluation for epidural block. Myelography is the "gold standard," providing definition of the suspected block as well as any additional areas of com-

promise. CT and magnetic resonance imaging may be useful, and the latter may ultimately supplant myelography as the diagnostic test of choice. However, any radiologic assessment requires documentation not only of the suspected block but also of the length of the compression, which is needed for radiotherapy port planning. At present, the latter is best achieved with a myelogram.

When cord compression has been documented, corticosteroids should be initiated immediately. Doses of dexamethasone of up to 100 mg intravenously have been used to decrease spinal cord swelling acutely. The initial bolus dose of dexamethasone is followed by dexamethasone in divided doses of up to 100 mg/d. Murine data and retrospective analyses of outcome of patients support the use of high-dose dexamethasone. However, a study comparing this dose to lower doses has not been carried out.

Definitive therapy of the compression depends on the etiology. In patients with a known primary tumor and other evidence of metastatic disease, radiation therapy should be initiated immediately. Neurosurgical consultation should be obtained. If symptoms progress despite radiotherapy and steroids, decompression laminectomy is required.

When the tissue diagnosis is unclear, the diagnosis cannot be made rapidly by needle biopsy, the tumor is known to be radioresistant, or the tumor has caused an unstable vertebral body, surgical decompression is required.

The prognosis of spinal cord compression is directly related to the level of disability with which the patient presents. Ambulatory patients tend to remain ambulatory. Patients with compression and paresis of several days' duration are highly unlikely to respond to treatment. Hence, early effective intervention is essential.

UROLOGIC EMERGENCIES

Multiple complications exist, including hemorrhagic cystitis, obstructive uropathy, and uric acid nephropathy. Any complication may be acute in presentation and require urgent medical management.

Severe hemorrhagic cystitis is seen after high-dose cyclophosphamide therapy, more often in patients who have had bone marrow transplantation. Such a problem is best prevented by aggressive hydration concurrent with therapy and with bladder catheter placement and bladder irrigation. Intravenous mesna (mercaptoethanesulfonate) is used in some centers to prevent cystitis. Prostaglandins are being studied for the same purpose. Should hemorrhagic cystitis occur, formalin instillation into the bladder may control the problem.[50]

Obstructive uropathy, with outflow impaired at the ureteral, bladder, or urethral level, is noted in conjunction with lymphomas and carcinomas of cervix, ovary, prostate, and colorectum or with primary ureteral, bladder, or urethral tumors. Rarely, other tumors cause obstruction. Obstruction may also be seen as a result of surgery or radiation therapy.

The problem is simply evaluated in a patient presenting with uremia and an elevated serum creatinine level. A Foley catheter should be placed in the bladder if possible. Inability to introduce a catheter suggests lower urinary obstruction. Ultrasonographic evaluation of the upper urinary tract identifies upper tract obstruction. When complete obstruction has occurred, acute management consists of urinary diversion above the obstruction, (i.e., suprapubic bladder catheterization or percutaneous nephrostomy).

Diuresis after relief of the obstruction should be anticipated, and lost fluid and electrolytes should be replaced vigorously. When the obstruction has been relieved, the cause of the obstruction should be identified and treated.

Uric acid nephropathy may result from disease or, more usually, treatment. Patients with leukemia and lymphoma may be expected to develop uric acid nephropathy immediately after the initiation of treatment. Hence, such patients should receive prior therapy with allopurinol and be aggressively hydrated during initial therapy. Supplementation with intravenous bicarbonate may be required.

METABOLIC EMERGENCIES
Hypercalcemia

Hypercalcemia is one of the common and serious metabolic disorders associated with malignancy, occurring in 10% of patients. Cancer is the most frequent cause of hypercalcemia in hospitalized patients, and primary hyperparathyroidism is the most likely cause in ambulatory patients.[51]

Etiology

Only a few malignancies account for most of the hypercalcemia that is seen in cancer patients. In a review by Mundy and Martin,[52] the types of cancer associated with hypercalcemia are divided into three categories:

TABLE 120–7
CAUSES OF HYPERCALCEMIA

Malignant
  Lung cancer
  Breast cancer
  Multiple myeloma
  Lymphoma (Burkitt's, adult T cell lymphoma)
  Head and neck cancer
  Renal cell carcinoma
  Other (gastrointestinal, prostate)
Benign
  Primary hyperparathyroidism
  Immobilization
  Drugs (thiazide diuretics, hormone therapy of breast cancer, lithium, theophylline)
  Sarcoidosis
  Tuberculosis
  Hypervitaminosis A and D
  Adrenal insufficiency
  Hyperthyroidism
  Severe liver or renal disease
  Milk-alkali syndrome
  Acquired immunodeficiency syndrome
  Rhabdomyolysis
  Idiopathic hypercalcemia of infancy

Data from refs 51, 52.

1. Solid tumors without metastases (i.e., humoral hypercalcemia). Lung cancer usually falls into this group, with squamous cell being the most common histologic type. It is almost always associated with advanced disease.[53] Hypercalcemia rarely occurs in small-cell carcinoma even though other paraneoplastic syndromes are common in this malignancy.[54] Carcinomas of the head and neck, kidney, and ovary are often included in this group.

2. Solid tumors with metastases. This category includes patients whose primary cancer has metastasized to the bone and accounts for 70% of cancer-associated hypercalcemia. Breast cancer makes the largest contribution to this group. Hypercalcemia occurs late in the disease, often accompanied by osteolytic metastases. Carcinomas of the lung may also fall into this group. As suggested by Mundy and Martin, there is overlap between the categories and the fact that a patient has bone metastases does not mean that this is the direct cause of the hypercalcemia.

3. Hematologic malignancies. Patients with multiple myeloma often have osteolytic bone destruction and 20 to 40% of the patients develop hypercalcemia.[51] Hypercalcemia can also occur in patients with lymphomas (Burkitt's or adult T cell lymphoma).

One must not lose sight of the fact that benign conditions may be responsible for the hypercalcemia in cancer patients. Primary hyperparathyroidism can coexist with a malignancy, but there is no increase in the incidence of this condition over that found in the general population.[55] Table 120–7 lists many additional benign causes of hypercalcemia.

Pathophysiology

Calcium is controlled by the interaction of parathyroid hormone (PTH), 1,25-dihydroxyvitamin D, and calcitonin on the bone, kidney, and gastrointestinal tract. Dietary calcium is absorbed through the intestine primarily under the influence of 1,25-dihydroxyvitamin D. PTH stimulates bone resorption, renal calcium reabsorption, and production of vitamin D by the kidney. Calcium reabsorption occurs in the distal renal tubules under the influence of PTH, and in

TABLE 120–8

TREATMENT OF HYPERCALCEMIA

Agent	Dose	Indication	Toxicity or Disadvantage
Normal saline	250–400 mL/h	Dehydration	Fluid overload; congestive heart failure
Furosemide	20–40 mg IV	Promotes calcium excretion	Hypovolemia
Plicamycin	25 µg/kg IV	Decreases bone resorption	Nausea, vomiting, bone marrow suppression, renal and hepatic dysfunction
Etidronate disodium	7.5 mg/kg/d IV up to 7 d	Decreases bone resorption	Contraindicated in renal failure; limited utility as oral agent
Calcitonin	2–8 IU/kg IM or SC every 6 h	Decreases bone resorption	Rare allergic reaction; effect not complete and wears off rapidly
Steroids: prednisone	40–100 mg/d	Hematologic malignancies, breast cancer	Steroid-associated toxicities (i.e., gastritis, hyperglycemia)
Oral phosphate	1–3 g/d divided doses	Maintenance therapy	Diarrhea, must monitor renal function

the proximal tubule it is related to sodium and fluid reabsorption.[56] Calcitonin counteracts the effect of PTH on bone and has limited importance in normal calcium regulation in adults.

Several pathogenic mechanisms have been postulated as causes of hypercalcemia of malignancy. In patients with no obvious bone metastases, humoral factors are thought to be the etiology of hypercalcemia. These include a PTH-related hormone, transforming growth factor α, and cytokines such as interleukin-1 and tumor necrosis factor. PTH-related hormone bears some resemblance to the NH_2-terminal portion of PTH and probably mimics some of its actions. Bone resorption is much higher than might be expected, and there are differences in renal and gut reabsorption of calcium. It has been suggested that other humoral factors modify the effect of PTH-related hormone.[57]

In a large number of patients hypercalcemia is related to bone destruction by the metastatic cancer. Prostaglandins, transforming growth factor α, and procathepsin D could all be involved in the osteolytic process.[56] Osteoclast-activating factor has been implicated as the cause of hypercalcemia in hematologic malignancies. Osteoclast-activating factor represents cytokines such as lymphotoxin, tumor necrosis factor, and interleukin-1, which are powerful stimulators of osteoclast bone resorption.[57]

Clinical Features

Clinical symptoms vary depending on the level of serum calcium and how rapidly it was achieved. Patients with a high serum calcium level (>14 mg/dL) are symptomatic. Often the manifestations of hypercalcemia are nonspecific (i.e., nausea, fatigue, weakness, and anorexia) and can easily be related to the existing malignancy. If the signs of hypercalcemia are not recognized, severe dehydration and neurologic, cardiac, and renal dysfunction can result. Poor performance status, advanced age, and renal and hepatic dysfunction can add to the effects of the hypercalcemia.[58]

Patients are usually markedly dehydrated. There is a reversible defect in the kidney that results in loss of urine-concentrating ability and polyuria.[59] Glomerular filtration is also decreased and can result in renal insufficiency. Abdominal pain, nausea and vomiting, anorexia, and obstipation are frequent gastrointestinal symptoms that contribute to the dehydration. Neurologic manifestations include lethargy, weakness, confusion, and coma. Electrocardiographic changes can occur with prolongation of the PR and QRS intervals. High calcium levels (>16 mg/dL) can result in a widening of the T wave and an increased QT interval. Bone pain is common because of metastases and increased bone resorption. Nephrocalcinosis and calcium deposition are more common in hyperparathyroidism than in hypercalcemia of malignancy.

The serum calcium level should be elevated but is not specifically correlated with the etiology of the hypercalcemia. Because 55% of calcium is bound to albumin and serum proteins, a correction must be made for the serum albumin level. An ionized calcium level may be helpful in certain situations. Hyperkalemia and hypercalciuria are usually associated. Other laboratory tests are of marginal assistance in making the diagnosis.[60] There is no ideal PTH assay that can be used when PTH-related hormone is thought to be the cause of the hypercalcemia;[61] however, there are some new labeled-antibody assays that may prove to be useful.[62]

Treatment

Patients who exhibit the signs of hypercalcemia or have serum calcium levels higher than 13 mg/dL require emergent treatment. Goals include hydration, inhibition of bone resorption, promotion of calcium excretion, and treatment of the underlying malignancy.

Vigorous hydration with isotonic saline (250 to 400 mL/h) should be used to restore intravascular volume and glomerular filtration and promote calcium excretion.[63] Dialysis should be considered for patients who have renal and/or cardiac failure and cannot tolerate excessive fluid. Furosemide may help promote calcium excretion by interfering with calcium reabsorption in the ascending limb of Henle's loop. Diuretics should be used judiciously only after hydration, and thiazide diuretics should be avoided. Usually, hydration alone is not sufficient to treat severe hypercalcemia and an agent that reduces bone resorption is required.

Plicamycin (mithramycin) is an antineoplastic agent that is toxic to osteoclasts, resulting in reduction of bone resorption. The dose is 25 µg/kg as an intravenous bolus or short infusion. The effect occurs within 24 to 48 hours and can last up to 2 weeks. Toxicities include tissue necrosis if injected subcutaneously, renal and hepatic insufficiency, bone marrow suppression, and nausea and vomiting. The dose should be reduced or the drug avoided in patients with hepatic or renal insufficiency.

The bisphosphonates, relatively new compounds that are structural analogues of pyrophosphate, bind to hydroxyapatite and are potent inhibitors of bone crystal dissolution and osteoclast resorption.[63] The only available bisphosphonate is etidronate disodium, which is administered intravenously at 7.5 mg/kg/d for up to 7 days.[64] The drug is contraindicated in patients with renal failure. Etidronate disodium has limited value as an oral agent.[65]

Calcitonin, which inhibits bone resorption and promotes calcium excretion, can be used safely in patients with renal insufficiency.[52] The maximal recommended dose is 8 IU/kg intramuscularly or subcutaneously every 6 hours.[58] A test dose of 1 IU should be given initially because of the rare chance of a hypersensitivity reaction. It acts in 2 to 4 hours; however, the hypocalcemic effect is usually not complete and wears off rapidly.

Steroids at doses of 40 to 100 mg/d are of benefit in hypercalcemia related to hematologic malignancies and occasionally for breast cancer. Although prostaglandins are implicated as causative agents of hypercalcemia, prostaglandin inhibitors such as indomethacin are disappointing. Inorganic phosphates have dangerous side effects when administered by the intravenous route to a patient with hypercalcemia. Oral phosphates at a dose of 1 to 3 g/d may be helpful as maintenance therapy. Side effects include dose-limiting diarrhea and occasional azotemia. Several new agents are being evaluated, including other bisphosphonates and gallium nitrate.[66] The various treatments for hypercalcemia are summarized in Table 120–8. Every effort should be made to treat the malignancy that is the source of the hypercalcemia.

Hyponatremia

The syndrome of inappropriate antidiuretic hormone (SIADH) is most commonly associated with small-cell carcinoma of the lung. Other cancers of the prostate, adrenal cortex, esophagus, pancreas, colon, and head and neck; carcinoid tumors; thymoma; lymphoma; and mesothelioma have also been reported to cause SIADH.[67] Drugs such as cyclophosphamide, vincristine, and narcotics have also been implicated. There are other conditions associated with hyponatremia such as cardiac, liver, and renal disease; adrenal insufficiency; hypothyroidism; and gastrointestinal and renal losses.

Examination of serum and urinary electrolytes and osmolality and renal function as well as other parameters helps determine whether SIADH is the etiology of the hyponatremia.

Symptoms associated with hyponatremia are usually nonspecific, such as nausea, generalized weakness, anorexia, and lethargy.[68] When the serum sodium level falls below 115 mEq/L, altered mental status, psychosis, seizures, focal neurologic signs, and coma can result.[51]

A serum sodium level less than 115 mEq/L associated with symptoms requires emergent treatment with 3% hypertonic saline or normal saline and diuretic therapy. Less severe SIADH-related hyponatremia can be treated with fluid restriction or demeclocycline. Demeclocycline at 600 mg/d partially inhibits the action of Vasopressin (antidiuretic hormone) by producing a reversible diabetes insipidus.[69] Primary therapy of the cancer as in the case of small-cell lung cancer, if successful, should treat the hyponatremia.[70]

Hypoglycemia

Hypoglycemia is usually caused by insulin-producing islet cell tumors (i.e., insulinomas). Non–islet cell malignancies, including large mediastinal or retroperitoneal mesenchymal tumors (mesotheliomas, sarcomas), hepatomas, adrenal carcinomas, gastrointestinal cancers, leukemias, and lymphomas, can also cause hypoglycemia.[51] Insulin-like growth factor II, loss of mechanisms normally compensatory for hypoglycemia, and increased utilization of glucose by the tumor are thought to be responsible for the hypoglycemia.[71, 72]

Symptoms are related to the serum glucose level and include weakness, fatigue, confusion, seizure, and coma. Acute therapy includes intravenous infusion of glucose (initially 50% dextrose followed by an infusion of 10% dextrose). Treatment should ultimately be directed at managing the tumor and may include surgery, chemotherapy, and/or radiation therapy. Frequent small meals, steroids, and glucagon may be of some benefit.[51] Diazoxide may be helpful in patients with insulinoma but not in those with non–islet cell cancers.

References

1. Hunter W: The history of an aneurysm of the aorta, with some remarks on aneurysms in general. Med Obser Inq 1:323, 1757.
2. Schechter MM: The superior vena cava syndrome. Am J Med Sci 227:46, 1954.
3. Nieto AF, Doty DB: Superior vena cava obstruction: Clinical syndrome, etiology, and treatment. Curr Probl Cancer 10:443, 1986.
4. Yahalom J: Oncologic emergencies: Superior vena cava syndrome. In: DeVita VT Jr, Hellman S, Rosenberg SA (eds): Cancer: Principles and Practice of Oncology. 3rd ed. Philadelphia, JB Lippincott, p 1971, 1989.
5. Helms SR, Carlson MD: Cardiovascular emergencies. Semin Oncol 16:463, 1989.
6. Ahmann FR: A reassessment of the clinical implications of the superior vena cava syndrome. J Clin Oncol 2:961, 1984.
7. Perez-Soler R, McLaughlin WS, Velasquez FB, et al: Clinical features and results of management of superior vena cava syndrome secondary to lymphoma. J Clin Oncol 2:260, 1984.
8. Schraufnagel DE, Hill R, Leech JA, et al: Superior vena cava obstruction. Is it a medical emergency? Am J Med 70:1169, 1981.
9. Mahajan V, Strimlan V, Van Ordstrand HS, et al: Benign superior vena cava syndrome. Chest 68:32, 1975.
10. Bertrand M, Presant CA, Klein L, et al: Iatrogenic superior vena cava syndrome. A new entity. Cancer 54:376, 1984.
11. Lokich JJ, Goodman R: Superior vena cava syndrome: Clinical management. JAMA 231:58, 1975.
12. Stanford W, Jolles H, Ell S, et al: Superior vena cava obstruction: A venographic classification. AJR 148:259, 1987.
13. Lewis RJ, Sisler GE, Mackenzie JW: Mediastinoscopy in advanced superior vena cava obstruction. Ann Thorac Surg 32:458, 1981.
14. Sculier JP, Evans WK, Feld R, et al: Superior vena caval obstruction syndrome in small cell lung cancer. Cancer 57:847, 1986.
15. Davenport D, Ferree C, Blake D, et al: Radiation therapy in the treatment of superior vena caval obstruction. Cancer 42:2600, 1978.
16. Adelstein DJ, Hines JD, Carter SG, et al: Thromboembolic events in patients with malignant superior vena cava syndrome and the role of anticoagulation. Cancer 62:2258, 1988.
17. Dajee H, Deutsch LS, Benson LN, et al: Thrombolytic therapy for superior vena caval thrombosis following superior vena cava–pulmonary artery anastomosis. Ann Thorac Surg 38:637, 1984.
18. Katz PO, Hackshaw BT, Barish CF, et al: Venous thrombosis as a cause of superior vena cava syndrome. Arch Intern Med 143:1050, 1983.
19. Capek P, Cope C: Percutaneous treatment of superior vena cava syndrome. AJR 152:183, 1989.
20. Walpole HT, Lovett KE, Chuang VP, et al: Superior vena cava syndrome treated by percutaneous transluminal balloon angioplasty. Am Heart J 115:1303, 1988.
21. Pass HI: Treatment of metastatic cancer: Treatment of malignant pleural and pericardial effusions. In: DeVita VT Jr, Hellman S, Rosenberg SA (eds): Cancer: Principles and Practice of Oncology. 3rd ed. Philadelphia, JB Lippincott, p 2317, 1989.
22. Thurber DL, Edwards JE, Achor RWP: Secondary malignant tumors of the pericardium. Circulation 26:228, 1962.
23. Press OW, Livingston R: Management of malignant pericardial effusion and tamponade. JAMA 257:1088, 1987.
24. Buzaid AC, Garewal HS, Greenberg BR: Managing malignant pericardial effusion. West J Med 150:174, 1989.
25. Applefeld MM, Cole JF, Pollock SH, et al: The late appearance of chronic pericardial disease in patients treated by radiotherapy for Hodgkin's disease. Ann Intern Med 94:338, 1981.
26. Carsky EW, Mauceri RA, Azimi F: The epicardial fat pad: Analysis of frontal and lateral chest radiographs in patients with pericardial effusion. Radiology 137:303, 1980.
27. Friedman MJ, Sahn DJ, Haber K: Two-dimensional echocardiography and B-mode ultrasonography for the diagnosis of loculated pericardial effusion. Circulation 60:1644, 1979.
28. Chandraratna PAN, Aronow WS: Detection of pericardial metastases by cross-sectional echocardiography. Circulation 63:197, 1981.

29. Gaffney FA, Keller AM, Peshock RM, et al: Pathophysiologic mechanisms of cardiac tamponade and pulsus alternans shown by echocardiography. Am J Cardiol 53:1662, 1984.

30. Johnson FE, Wolverson MK, Sundaram M, et al: Unsuspected malignant pericardial effusion causing cardiac tamponade: Rapid diagnosis by computed tomography. Chest 82:501, 1982.

31. Wong B, Murphy J, Chang CJ, et al: The risk of percardiocentesis. Am J Cardiol 44:1110, 1979.

32. Shepherd FA, Morgan C, Evans WK, et al: Medical management of malignant pericardial effusion by tetracycline sclerosis. Am J Cardiol 60:1161, 1987.

33. Hankins JR, Satterfield JR, Aisner J, et al: Pericardial window for malignant pericardial effusion. Ann Thorac Surg 30:465, 1980.

34. Alcan KE, Zabetakis PM, Marino ND, et al: Management of acute cardiac tamponade by subxiphoid pericardiotomy. JAMA 247:1143, 1982.

35. Cham WC, Freiman AH, Carstens PHB, et al: Radiation therapy of cardiac and pericardial metastases. Radiology 114:701, 1975.

36. Crocco JA, Rooney JJ, Fankushen DS, et al: Massive hemoptysis. Arch Intern Med 121:495, 1968.

37. Conlan AA, Hurwitz SS, Krige L, et al: Massive hemoptysis. J Thorac Cardiovasc Surg 85:120, 1983.

38. Miller RR, McGregor DH: Hemorrhage from carcinoma of the lung. Cancer 46:200, 1980.

39. Panos RJ, Barr LF, Walsh TJ, et al: Factors associated with fatal hemoptysis in cancer patients. Chest 94:1008, 1988.

40. Garzon AA, Cerruti MM, Golding ME: Exsanguinating hemoptysis. J Thorac Cardiovasc Surg 84:829, 1982.

41. Gourin A, Garzon AA: Control of hemorrhage in emergency pulmonary resection for massive hemoptysis. Chest 68:120, 1975.

42. Uflacker R, Kaemmerer A, Neves C, et al: Management of massive hemoptysis by bronchial artery embolization. Radiology 146:627, 1983.

43. Brutinel WM, Cortese DA, McDougall JC, et al: A two-year experience with the neodymium-YAG laser in endobronchial obstruction. Chest 91:159, 1987.

44. Gelb AF, Epstein JD: Neodymium-yttrium-aluminum-garnet laser in lung cancer. Ann Thorac Surg 43:164, 1987.

45. Posner JB, Chernik NL: Intracranial metastases from systemic cancer. Adv Neurol 19:579, 1978.

46. Bleyer WA, Byrne TN: Leptomeningeal cancer in leukemia and solid tumors. Curr Probl Cancer 12:181, 1988.

47. Wassestrom WR, Glass JP, Posner JB: Diagnosis and treatment of leptomeningeal metastases from solid tumors. Experience with 90 patients. Cancer 49:759, 1982.

48. Posner J: Back pain and epidural spinal cord compression. Med Clin North Am 71:185, 1987.

49. Greenberg HS, Kim JH, Posner JB: Epidural spinal cord compression from metastatic tumor: Results from a new treatment protocol. Ann Neurol 8:361, 1980.

50. Spiro LH, Hecht H, Horowitz A, et al: Formalin treatment for massive bladder hemorrhage. Urology 2:699, 1983.

51. Silverman P, Distelhorst CW: Metabolic emergencies in clinical oncology. Semin Oncol 16:504, 1989.

52. Mundy GR, Martin TJ: The hypercalcemia of malignancy: Pathogenesis and management. Metabolism 31:1247, 1982.

53. Coggeshall J, Merrill W, Hande K, et al: Implications of hypercalcemia with respect to diagnosis and treatment of lung cancer. Am J Med 80:325, 1986.

54. Hayward ML, Howell DA, O'Donnell JF, et al: Hypercalcemia complicating small-cell carcinoma. Cancer 48:1643, 1981.

55. Farr HW, Fahey TJ Jr, Nash AG, et al: Primary hyperparathyroidism and cancer. Am J Surg 126:539, 1973.

56. Mundy GR: Pathophysiology of cancer-associated hypercalcemia. Semin Oncol 17:10, 1990.

57. Mundy GR: Hypercalcemia of malignancy revisited. J Clin Invest 82:1, 1988.

58. Warrell RP, Bockman RS: Oncologic emergencies: Metabolic emergencies. In: DeVita VT Jr, Hellman S, Rosenberg SA (eds): Cancer: Principles and Practice of Oncology. 3rd ed. Philadelphia, JB Lippincott, p 1986, 1989.

59. Bajorunas DR: Clinical manifestations of cancer-related hypercalcemia. Semin Oncol 17:16, 1990.

60. Boyd JC, Ladenson JH: Value of laboratory tests in the differential diagnosis of hypercalcemia. Am J Med 77:863, 1984.

61. Lufkin EG, Kao PC, Heath H: Parathyroid hormone radioimmunoassays in the differential diagnosis of hypercalcemia due to primary hyperparathyroidism or malignancy. Ann Intern Med 106:559, 1987.

62. Endres DB, Villanueva R, Sharp CF Jr, et al: Measurement of parathyroid hormone. Endocrinol Metab Clin North Am 18:611, 1989.

63. Ritch PS: Treatment of cancer-related hypercalcemia. Semin Oncol 17:26, 1990.

64. Jacobs TP, Gordon AC, Silverberg SJ, et al: Neoplastic hypercalcemia: Physiologic response to intravenous etidronate disodium. Am J Med 82:42, 1987.

65. Schiller JH, Rasmussen P, Benson AB, et al: Maintenance etidronate in the prevention of malignancy-associated hypercalcemia. Arch Intern Med 147:963, 1987.

66. Warrell RP, Skelos A, Alcock NW, et al: Gallium nitrate for acute treatment of cancer-related hypercalcemia: Clinicopharmacological and dose response analysis. Cancer Res 46:4208, 1986.

67. Glover DJ, Glick JH: Metabolic oncologic emergencies. CA 37:302, 1987.

68. Trump DL: Serious hyponatremia in patients with cancer: Management with demeclocycline. Cancer 47:2908, 1981.

69. Cherrill DA, Stote RM, Birge JR, et al: Demeclocycline treatment in the syndrome of inappropriate antidiuretic hormone secretion. Ann Intern Med 83:654, 1975.

70. Hainsworth JD, Workman R, Greco A: Management of the syndrome of inappropriate antidiuretic hormone secretion in small cell lung cancer. Cancer 51:161, 1983.

71. Axelrod L, Ron D: Insulin-like growth factor II and the riddle of tumor-induced hypoglycemia (editorial). N Engl J Med 319:1477, 1988.

72. Unger RH: The riddle of tumor hypoglycemia (editorial). Am J Med 40:325, 1966.

CHAPTER 121

Complications of Therapy of Neoplastic Disease: An Overview

Michael M. Millenson
Steven E. Come

The care of patients with neoplastic disorders presents a great challenge, given the difficulties posed both by the disease process and by the complex, often toxic therapies employed. The clinician must often distinguish between morbidity caused by the malignancy and that resulting from its treatment. New therapies (e.g., biologicals) and new uses of established agents (e.g., dose-intensive chemotherapy with autologous bone marrow transplantation) are appearing in practice at an ever-increasing rate. Thus, physicians caring for cancer patients must understand the acute and long-term effects of both standard and novel treatments. Although many of these toxicities are managed primarily by the specialist in hematology/oncology, the focus of this chapter is on complications likely to be encountered by the physician in the intensive care unit (ICU) or critical care setting.

THERAPY-INDUCED CYTOPENIAS

The most common and predictable complication of cancer therapy is myelosuppression. Chemotherapeutic agents are usually directed against, but not selective for, the proliferative capacity of tumor cells. Normal bone marrow progenitors, engaged in a continuous process of cell renewal, are extremely sensitive to the same medications. Indeed, treatment-induced myelosuppression is the anticipated dose-limiting toxicity of many regimens.

The bone marrow consists of a slowly proliferating pluripotential stem cell compartment and a rapidly proliferating progenitor cell compartment. The former compartment has a high fraction of cells in G_0 (resting) phase, although they may be recruited into active cell cycling under appropriate circumstances. This compartment plays a critical role in

TABLE 121–1

LOCALIZATION OF CELL CYCLE ACTIVITY AND DEGREE OF CHEMOTHERAPY-RELATED MYELOSUPPRESSION

Therapy	Degree of Myelosuppression*
I. Cell cycle active	
A. Phase specific	
1. S phase	
a. 5-Fluorouracil	+
b. Methotrexate	+ +
c. 6-Mercaptopurine, 6-thioguanine	+ +
d. Cytosine arabinoside	+ + (+)
2. G₂ phase	
a. Bleomycin	+
b. Etoposide (VP-16)	+ +
3. M phase	
a. Vincristine	+
b. Vinblastine	+ +
B. Phase nonspecific	
1. Intercalating agents	
a. Anthracyclines	+ +
b. Actinomycin D	+ +
2. Some alkylating agents	
a. Cyclophosphamide	+ + (+)
b. Ifosfamide	+ + (+)
II. Non–cell cycle active	
1. Most alkylating agents	
a. Cisplatin	+ +
b. Carboplatin	+ + (+)
c. Nitrogen mustard	+ + +
d. Mitomycin C	+ + +
e. Melphalan (L-phenylalanine mustard)	+ + +
f. Busulfan	+ + +
g. Chlorambucil	+ + +
2. Nitrosoureas	
a. Carmustine (BCNU)	+ + +
b. Lomustine (chloroethylcyclohexylnitrosourea, CCNU)	+ + +
c. Semustine (methyl CCNU)	+ + +
3. Miscellaneous	
a. L-Asparaginase	+
b. Steroids (prednisone, dexamethasone)	0
c. Hormones (tamoxifen, megestrol)	0
d. Procarbazine	+

*Key: 0 = none; + = mild; + + = moderate; + + + = severe.

replenishing the ranks of committed progenitor cells. The rapidly proliferating compartment has a high fraction of dividing progenitor cells as well as committed, nondividing cells that are maturing.

When considering treatment-induced myelosuppression, it is useful to group cancer therapies according to their effects on these marrow compartments (Table 121–1). The agents that affect nonpoliferating cells (non–cell cycle–active drugs) are capable of affecting the relatively quiescent pluripotential stem cell compartment, causing severe myelosuppression that is often cumulative because of stem cell depletion. As a rule, the agents that principally affect proliferating cells (cell cycle–active drugs) produce only mild-to-moderate myelosuppression that is short-lived and not cumulative. Radiation is thought to inhibit target cells by directly affecting DNA and by creating free radicals, which damage important cellular macromolecules.[1] Radiation resembles cell cycle–active chemotherapy in its toxicity to rapidly dividing progenitor cells. However, myelosuppression associated with radiation results not only from direct injury to proliferating elements in the marrow but also from damage to the hematopoietic marrow stroma, which provides the appropriate microenvironment for hematopoietic growth and differentiation.[2] Therefore, radiation therapy to fields overlying sizable areas of active marrow such as the pelvic bones or spine may result in profound and prolonged myelosuppression that reflects stem cell and stromal injury.

The degree to which a patient develops treatment-related cytopenias depends on a number of factors,[3, 4] including (1) the intrinsic myelosuppressive activity of the chemotherapy involved; (2) concomitant or prior exposure to radiation therapy; (3) the age and nutritional status of the patient (elderly patients and those in negative nitrogen balance may tolerate therapy less well); and (4) the extent of bone marrow reserve, which depends on the intensity of prior therapy and the integrity of the pluripotential marrow stem cell compartment. Cytopenias may also be related to the neoplastic process itself, as in myelophthisis secondary to marrow replacement by tumor cells, sequestration in a massively enlarged spleen, or cell destruction associated with autoantibodies.

Neutropenia

The postmitotic marrow phase of myeloid differentiation from myelocyte to mature neutrophil takes about 6.5 days,[5] providing a 7-day reserve of neutrophils after exposure of the dividing committed progenitor cells to cell cycle–active chemotherapy. Thereafter, a fairly rapid decline in the peripheral blood neutophil count occurs because the half-life of neutrophils in the peripheral blood is approximately 6 hours. Neutrophils are generally the first of the peripheral blood elements to decrease and to recover after myelosuppressive therapy.

The morbidity and mortality associated with therapy-induced neutropenia are directly related to the depth and duration of the neutropenic nadir.[6] Because of the crucial role of neutrophils and monocytes as mediators of microbial surveillance and defense, a deficiency in these cells places the patient at increased risk for bacterial and fungal infections. Relative neutropenia is generally defined as an absolute neutrophil count of less than 1000/mm³, and absolute neutropenia is typically regarded as an absolute neutrophil count of less than 500/mm³. However, these definitions are somewhat arbitrary, and the risk of infectious complications is a continuum related to the degree of neutropenia, rather than an all-or-nothing phenomenon.[6] Most patients with an absolute neutropenia of more than 7 days' duration experience febrile episodes; of these patients, approximately 40 to 60% have an identifiable microbial pathogen found by appropriate evaluation.[7–9] Many of these patients develop hypotension and other features of the septic syndrome and require ICU monitoring and care.

In general, bacterial and fungal infections in neutropenic patients arise from within the host at areas of normal bacterial or fungal colonization, such as oral mucosa and periodontal tissues, gastrointestinal (GI) tract, perianal area, and skin. Cancer patients tend to have multiple potential portals of entry for such organisms; in particular, cutaneous organisms may enter via permanent vascular access devices (Porta-A-Cath, Hickman's, and Broviac's catheters) and GI organisms via oropharyngeal or intestinal mucous membrane injury resulting from chemotherapy. In several series in the literature, gram-negative bacilli and gram-positive cocci have been identified as preponderant microbial causes of febrile episodes in neutropenic cancer patients,[10, 11] and *Staphylococcus epidermidis* is a prominent pathogen associated with the increased use of vascular access devices.[12]

An algorithm for the management of the febrile, neutropenic patient has been developed and is discussed in detail elsewhere in this section. Briefly, the treating physician should obtain a thorough history and physical examination, including a detailed inspection of the skin, vascular access devices, oropharyngeal mucosa, and perianal region. The patient should be "pancultured," with blood cultures drawn via both peripheral venipunctures and indwelling catheters.[13] Although chest roentgenograms are usually obtained in this setting, radiographic abnormalities are unusual in the absence of clinical symptoms or signs.[14] Febrile, neutropenic patients should be maintained in isolation, with institution of scrupulous hand washing and "neutropenic precautions" in an effort to minimize colonization with nosocomial pathogens, which may be a particular concern in the ICU setting.

Evaluation of patients with neutropenia and fever should be expeditious, and intravenous broad-spectrum antibiotics that empirically cover gram-negative bacilli and gram-positive cocci should be started quickly. The ideal choice for such empirical broad-spectrum coverage continues to evolve as newer antimicrobial agents become available. The traditional combination of a semisynthetic penicillin and an aminoglycoside (e.g., mezlocillin and gentamicin) has been compared with monotherapy with newer agents (ceftazidime, imipenem-cilastatin), and the results have been fairly comparable.[15–17] If a source of infection is identified on physical examination or a specific organism on panculturing, tailored antibiotic coverage should be added to the usual empirical regimen, because such patients remain at risk of infection with multiple pathogens and/or sites.[18] Persistence of fever and neutropenia for several days despite these measures raises the possibility of invasive fungal infections, which are discussed in this section.

The increasing use of growth factors that stimulate marrow recovery after chemotherapy may alter the prevalence and management of fevers in the oncology population. Several studies have shown that recombinant human granulocyte-macrophage colony-stimulating factor and granulocyte colony-stimulating factor may significantly reduce the number of days of absolute neutropenia, number of days of empirical antibiotic therapy, and incidence of mucositis in patients treated with standard doses of chemotherapy for solid tumors.[19, 20] Numerous studies are under way to define the optimal uses of these and newer agents in managing this serious and frequent complication of antineoplastic therapy.

Thrombocytopenia

Thrombocytopenia, arbitrarily defined as a platelet count of less than 150,000/mm³, is also commonly encountered in patients being treated for neoplastic disorders. Platelets normally have a life span in the peripheral circulation of approximately 10 days, after a compartment transit time in the bone marrow of about 5 to 7 days.[21] Thus, thrombocytopenia tends to develop somewhat later than neutropenia after chemotherapy. Likewise, recovery of platelet counts to pretreatment levels tends to lag slightly behind recovery from neutropenia. Again, the distinction between cell cycle–active and non–cell cycle–active chemotherapy applies, with the latter tending to cause more profound and prolonged thrombocytopenia.

The depth and duration of the platelet count nadir, as is the case with the neutrophil count, depend on a number of independent factors, including (1) the type, dose, and schedule (i.e., dose intensity) of chemotherapy administered; (2) the extent of prior treatment with chemotherapy and/or radiation therapy; (3) the presence of underlying fever and infection; (4) concomitant use of drugs that may suppress platelet counts, such as semisynthetic penicillins, amphotericin B, or heparin; (5) coexistent consumptive coagulopathy;

and (6) the presence of splenomegaly with hypersplenism and sequestration.[22] It is necessary to exclude the presence of any of these confounding factors before ascribing thrombocytopenia to chemotherapy alone. This is particularly important in view of the high prevalance of both disseminated intravascular coagulation and heparin use in the ICU setting. Of note, thrombocytopenia occurs in 5 to 8% of patients exposed to heparin and may occur even when so-called minidoses are used.[23]

The normal number of circulating platelets in peripheral blood (250,000 ± 100,000/mm³) is approximately 10 times the number needed to provide adequate hemostasis in most situations.[21] Thanks to this hemostatic reserve, the bleeding time remains normal until the platelet count drops to about 100,000/mm³, below which there is a linear increase in bleeding time as the platelet count continues to drop. As the count falls below 50,000/mm³, patients may manifest ecchymoses at sites of trivial incidental soft tissue trauma and may develop spontaneous dependent petechial lesions as counts approach 20,000 to 30,000/mm³. The risk of serious spontaneous hemorrhage begins to increase as the platelet count falls below 20,000/mm³. In most series, spontaneous intracranial hemorrhage is rarely the first manifestation of bleeding unless the platelet count is less than 10,000/mm³.[24–27]

Proper management of the thrombocytopenic cancer patient in the ICU depends on a sound understanding of the foregoing principles. Every effort should be made to search for the confounding causes of thrombocytopenia. Coexisting coagulopathies must be identified and corrected. "Bleeding precautions" should be instituted, with prolonged pressure over venipuncture sites, avoidance of repeated arterial punctures if possible, minimization of heparin use including catheter flushes, and avoidance of potential platelet toxins such as nonsteroidal anti-inflammatory agents and β-lactam antibiotics. Actively bleeding patients should initially be managed as nonthrombocytopenic patients would be, with expeditious identification and correction of the source of bleeding, if possible.

Platelet transfusions are the primary approach when reversal of thrombocytopenia is necessary. In general, actively bleeding patients should be transfused as needed to maintain a platelet count above 50,000/mm³ while local measures are undertaken, if possible, to control bleeding. In nonbleeding patients whose counts are less than 50,000/mm³ for whom surgical or other invasive procedures are planned (e.g., central lines, arterial lines, lumbar punctures, and thoracenteses), platelets should be transfused just before the procedure to achieve a post-transfusion platelet count greater than 50,000/mm³.[28, 29] Nonbleeding patients with counts greater than 20,000/mm³ for whom no invasive procedures are planned can probably be observed without prophylactic platelet transfusions. However, for patients with counts less than 10,000 to 20,000/mm³, the standard practice has been to transfuse platelet concentrates routinely to achieve post-transfusion counts above this level to avoid the small but finite risk of spontaneous intracranial hemorrhage. Most chemotherapy programs produce dose-limiting neutropenia and, therefore, such severe thrombocytopenia is infrequent, sparing patients the well-known risks associated with platelet transfusions (see Chapter 119 for further details).

Anemia

In contrast to the abrupt development of neutropenia and thrombocytopenia after cytotoxic chemotherapy, the onset of anemia tends to be relatively delayed and gradual. This is attributable to the relatively long average life expectancy of approximately 120 days for the mature red blood cell in the peripheral circulation. Thus, for most cyclic programs of cytotoxic chemotherapy, it takes two or three cycles of therapy, during which erythroid progenitors are repeatedly suppressed, to allow the normal senile decay of preformed red blood cells to outpace red cell renewal and produce anemia. Acute anemia, conversely, rarely occurs on the basis of myelosuppression by chemotherapy alone.[30]

As with neutropenia and thrombocytopenia, it is important to exclude the many possible coexistent etiologies of anemia in the critically ill cancer patient. Acute blood loss resulting from hemorrhage secondary to thrombocytopenia or coagulopathy must always be ruled out. Microangiopathic hemolytic anemia associated with disseminated intravascular coagulation may be encountered in these patients. Autoimmune hemolysis should be considered in patients with underlying lymphoproliferative disorders. Myelophthisic anemia secondary to marrow infiltration by tumor and fibrous tissue may be suspected in the presence of characteristic findings on the peripheral blood smear (a "leukoerythroblastic" pattern with prominent "teardrop" red blood cells). Finally, chronically ill patients with advanced cancer may be malnourished and hence at risk for vitamin (in particular, folate) deficiencies.

When deciding on the appropriate management of the anemic cancer patient, it is important to bear in mind that the hemoglobin and hematocrit levels are merely laboratory values that may be tolerated quite differently by different patients. In general, young patients without underlying cardiopulmonary or cerebrovascular disease may chronically tolerate hemoglobin levels as low as 6 or 7 g/dL with few symptoms, whereas elderly or acutely ill patients may be symptomatic or develop complications in the 8 to 9 g/dL range.[28] For acutely ill patients in the ICU, who may require higher cardiac outputs to meet the demands of an intercurrent febrile illness or cardiopulmonary compromise, packed red blood cell transfusions should be used judiciously to maintain a hemoglobin level of 9 to 10 g/dL. (For a more detailed discussion of red blood cell transfusion therapy in the anemic cancer patient, see Chapter 119.)

The role of recombinant human erythropoietin in the management of anemic cancer patients is expanding.[31] Several studies have demonstrated efficacy in correcting hemoglobin levels, reducing transfusion requirements, and improving the overall sense of well-being in patients with a variety of underlying neoplastic disorders.[32–34]

RENAL AND METABOLIC ABNORMALITIES

Patients with malignancies who are treated with chemotherapy may develop a number of metabolic and renal abnormalities that require monitoring and treatment in the ICU. These disorders result from the neoplastic process itself, the direct effects of the antineoplastic drugs on renal function, or the consequences of treatment-induced lysis of tumor cells.

Acute Urate Nephropathy and Acute Tumor Lysis Syndrome

A distinctive syndrome of acute renal insufficiency associated with multiple metabolic abnormalities has been well described in the setting of cytoreductive treatment of high-grade lymphoid malignancies,[35, 36] such as Burkitt's lymphoma, and some rapidly progressive solid tumors.[37, 38] This syndrome is characterized by variable degrees of hyperuricemia, hyperphosphatemia, hyperkalemia, and hypocalcemia along with progressive azotemia, and it occurs during the first 3 to 5 days after initiation of chemotherapy. Abrupt release of large quantities of intracellular contents (uric acid, phosphorus, and potassium) into the blood stream results

from rapid tumor cell lysis. These materials overwhelm normal renal clearance mechanisms and result in renal damage, leading to further decrement in clearance and the establishment of a vicious circle culminating in acute renal failure. When this syndrome was first recognized, patients succumbed to complications of uncontrolled hyperkalemia and hypocalcemia, including lethal arrhythmias, tetany, seizures, and other complications of acute renal failure.

Many patients with highly proliferative malignancies have baseline hyperuricemia and established urate nephropathy before receiving any chemotherapy. Presumably, this reflects a high volume of spontaneous tumor cell turnover, producing excessive uricosuria with precipitation of uric acid crystals in the distal tubules and collecting ducts. Without appropriate prophylaxis, these patients are at particularly high risk for development of the full-blown acute tumor lysis syndrome when chemotherapy is commenced.

The relative contribution of excessive uricosuria versus phosphaturia to the ensuing development of renal failure is debated.[36] Some patients who develop acute renal failure in this setting have profound hyperphosphatemia with little or no uricosuria, suggesting that excessive phosphaturia with intrarenal precipitation of calcium phosphate crystals may be the primary mechanism of renal injury in these cases. Both mechanisms probably contribute in a synergistic fashion to the development of renal insufficiency in the majority of patients with this syndrome.

Essential to proper management of the acute tumor lysis syndrome is timely recognition of patients at risk for its development. In addition to the characteristic types of neoplasms involved, other specific pretreatment predictors have been identified. These include (1) large tumor burden (frequently associated with a marked increase in lactate dehydrogenase level; (2) obstructive uropathy (particularly common in high-grade lymphoma patients with bulky abdominal disease); (3) baseline oliguria or renal insufficiency (as a result of either intravascular volume depletion or baseline urate nephropathy associated with rapid tumor cell turnover); and (4) excessive hyperuricemia before initiation of chemotherapy.[35] If the pace of tumor progression allows, it is prudent in such high-risk patients to withhold administration of cytoreductive chemotherapy for the first 24 to 48 hours of hospitalization to correct hyperuricemia and/or oliguric renal insufficiency.

The single most important intervention for the prevention and management of the acute tumor lysis syndrome is provision of adequate intravenous hydration to induce a brisk flow of dilute urine through the distal tubules and collecting ducts and thereby decrease the concentration of solutes (especially uric acid and phosphorus) and prevent precipitation and subsequent injury to the nephron.[39] In general, hydration with 3 L/m²/d is given; a urine flow of at least 100 mL/h is desirable. Failure to diurese in response to aggressive hydration may indicate obstructive uropathy and requires further investigation. The solubility of uric acid in the urine is enhanced by urinary alkalization (pH > 7) because the pKa of uric acid is 5.7; an alkaline solution, therefore, promotes the maintenance of urate in the ionized, more highly soluble dissociated form.[40] This degree of alkalization is generally achievable by adding 50 to 100 mEq of $NaHCO_3$ to each liter of intravenous fluid. The load of filtered uric acid should be diminished simultaneously by administration of allopurinol, a xanthine oxidase inhibitor that prevents conversion of the purine precursors (hypoxanthine and xanthine) to uric acid. Allopurinol should generally be started at a loading dose of 600 to 900 mg/d in divided doses and should be reduced to a maintenance dose of 100 to 300 mg/d when hyperuricemia is corrected, because xanthine itself may precipitate and cause a "xanthine nephropathy" analogous to urate nephropathy. Also, because xanthine is poorly soluble in alkaline solution, bicarbonate infusions should be discontinued when uric acid levels are consistently normal.

While these measures are ongoing, patients should have frequent monitoring of electrolytes, blood urea nitrogen, creatinine, calcium, phosphorus, and uric acid, preferably every 8 to 12 hours during the prechemotherapy period and for the first 3 to 5 days after its initiation. Development of severe hypocalcemia or hyperkalemia should prompt immediate evaluation for electrocardiographic (ECG) changes and institution of corrective measures. Early institution of hemodialysis should be considered for patients with progressive or refractory renal insufficiency or oliguria or electrolyte abnormalities that are not corrected with more conservative measures. Likewise, patients with cardiac or pulmonary compromise who cannot tolerate vigorous hydration may benefit from early hemodialysis. With prompt institution of the appropriate preventive measures, however, the great majority of patients at risk for developing this syndrome can be managed successfully without dialysis.[36]

Divalent Cation Wasting

Severe hypomagnesemia with mild-to-moderate hypocalcemia may complicate therapy with platinum-containing compounds (cisplatin and carboplatinum).[41–43] A series from the National Cancer Institute combining retrospective and prospective analyses of patients treated with cisplatin identified hypomagnesemia in 23 of 44 evaluatable patients (52%), most of whom were completely asymptomatic.[40, 41] Two patients had symptomatic tetany, however, and four of seven studied prospectively had inappropriate wasting of magnesium in the urine (with abnormally high fractional excretion of magnesium). In several additional series, a dose-response relationship has been demonstrated, indicating that virtually all patients treated with repeated cycles of cisplatin eventually develop hypomagnesemia.[44, 45] A persistent and selective defect in renal tubular reabsorption of magnesium may last for months to a few years after discontinuation of chemotherapy.[46] The specific site and mechanism of this defect produced by platinum remain unclear, but injury to the distal tubules, where magnesium is normally reabsorbed, is likely. Divalent cation wasting may be transiently exacerbated by the forced diuresis that frequently precedes and accompanies cisplatin administration (see later). In addition, many patients receiving this agent have severe nausea, vomiting, and/or diarrhea, contributing to depletion of total body magnesium stores.

Because the majority of patients treated with platinum compounds develop divalent cation wasting, routine measurement of serum levels of magnesium and calcium in this group is essential. Life-threatening complications may occur in previously asymptomatic patients. The value of routine magnesium supplementation is controversial, however, because normal serum levels are generally unattainable in the presence of persistent urinary magnesium wasting.[45] Many oncologists undertake a trial of routine supplementation with oral magnesium salts for asymptomatic hypomagnesemic patients, but these salts frequently cause diarrhea and may worsen magnesium depletion. Most patients who develop symptoms, particularly children, have moderate hypocalcemia (presumably resulting from defective parathyroid hormone secretion or action associated with magnesium depletion); consequently, administration of calcium salts is frequently ineffective in correcting hypocalcemia until the deficit in magnesium is also corrected. Clearly, serious complications such as seizures or tetany are an indication for intravenous $MgSO_4$ administration, which usually results in

prompt resolution of symptoms and transient correction of hypomagnesemia.

Nephrotoxicity of Antineoplastic Agents

Cisplatin. In addition to its effect on renal handling of divalent cations, cisplatin is a potent nephrotoxin. Many studies suggest a cumulative dose-toxicity relationship, particularly with repeated cycles at doses above 50 mg/m^2 given at short intervals.[47–50] The mechanism of renal injury by cisplatin is not fully understood, but the effect is considered to be analogous to the direct nephrotoxicity seen with other heavy metals, particularly mercury.[51] Like other metals, cisplatin is excreted primarily by the kidneys and may be concentrated in the renal medulla and distal tubules. Renal biopsy and autopsy light microscopic data have revealed morphologic changes in patients who develop renal insufficiency after cisplatin therapy, with prominent distal tubular necrosis and dilatation of tubules but relative sparing of glomeruli.[52] Numerous studies have been undertaken in both animals and humans to devise ways to minimize the concentration of cisplatin in the renal medulla and distal tubules and to promote rapid elimination of the drug without compromising its antitumor effects.

Induction of a brisk saline diuresis before, during, and after cisplatin administration results in marked attenuation of the nephrotoxic effects of this drug.[47, 53] The recommended practice is to provide "prehydration" during several hours before administration of cisplatin to ensure a urine output of at least 100 mL/h, thus decreasing the potential transit time of platinum through the tubules and collecting ducts and minimizing local platinum concentrations. This often requires administration of intravenous fluids (saline or half-normal saline) at rates of 250 mL/h or more, usually continued for several hours after the last dose of cisplatin and frequently necessitating judicious use of diuretics to avoid fluid overload. With appropriate hydration, nephrotoxicity occurs in only 5 to 10% of treated patients and may be relatively mild and transient.[47, 48]

There is experimental evidence to suggest that induction of chloruresis in particular provides specific protection against platinum-induced nephrotoxicity by altering the "aquation equilibrium," thereby decreasing the concentration of the toxic aquated species of platinum. This has provided the rationale for the use of hypertonic saline and furosemide in patients receiving high doses of cisplatin.[53] The use of mannitol for induction of an osmotic diuresis (12.5 g intravenous bolus just before platinum administration) has also been advocated, and many studies have documented its efficacy in conjunction with vigorous hydration and diuresis.[47–53] The relative renal protection afforded by brisk saline diuresis alone versus diuresis in conjunction with furosemide and/or mannitol has not been well studied in randomized trials, however.

The schedule of cisplatin administration may also influence the subsequent development of nephrotoxicity, with divided doses during 3 to 5 days being preferable to a single bolus of equivalent total dose. There is evidence that higher peak plasma levels of platinum are a stronger predictor of subsequent azotemia than the area under the curve (plasma platinum level versus time).[54] Consequently, the use of small, divided doses or longer-term infusions may further attenuate the nephrotoxic potential of platinum compounds. Finally, uncorrectable pretreatment azotemia and concurrent use of aminoglycosides during platinum administration increase the risk of nephrotoxicity and should be avoided if possible.

Methotrexate. In conventional doses, methotrexate is rarely associated with alterations in renal function. With more recent use of intermediate-dose (200 mg/m²) and high-dose (1.0 to 7.5 g/m²) regimens, however, renal injury has become a significant dose-limiting toxicity, despite the use of rescue techniques such as leucovorin administration. Methotrexate is excreted primarily by the kidneys, and unusually high concentrations may result in precipitation of the drug or its metabolites (7-hydroxy methotrexate) in the renal tubules and collecting ducts.[50] In addition, the drug may have direct toxic biochemical effects on renal tubular cells. By any mechanism, an abrupt decline in creatinine clearance results in decreased elimination of methotrexate in the urine, with establishment of a vicious circle leading to higher serum methotrexate levels and further renal injury.

The occurrence of nephrotoxicity with methotrexate administration is unpredictable. It depends in part on the integrity of renal function before treatment, the dose of methotrexate administered, and the timely institution of preventive measures. Patients with a baseline creatinine clearance of less than 60 mL/min and those with "third space" fluid collections (e.g., effusions, ascites, and edema) should not receive intermediate or high doses of methotrexate. Patients receiving high doses of methotrexate (>500 mg/m²) should be vigorously hydrated to promote a urine flow of at least 100 mL/h beginning several hours before and continuing for 2 to 3 days after initiation of therapy. In addition, because methotrexate is a weak acid, the urine should be alkalized to maintain a pH greater than 7 by adding 50 to 100 mEq NaHCO₃ to each liter of intravenous fluid (0.5 normal saline solution or 5% dextrose in water). With institution of alkaline diuresis, the incidence of nephrotoxicity resulting from high-dose methotrexate may be reduced from approximately 60% of patients to 15% or less.[55, 56]

During therapy with high-dose methotrexate, serum creatinine and methotrexate levels should be monitored at 24-hour intervals. Normally, leucovorin (10 to 20 mg/m² every 6 hours) is started 24 hours after infusion of methotrexate and continued until methotrexate levels are less than 5×10^{-8} mol/L. If renal insufficiency develops during the first 24 to 48 hours after methotrexate administration or if the methotrexate level is inappropriately high, it is crucial to provide increased doses and duration of leucovorin rescue to protect normal tissues (bone marrow, GI mucosa) from the toxic effects of these higher, sustained methotrexate levels.

Patients receiving intermediate-dose methotrexate seldom require continued intravenous hydration and have a lower incidence of renal complications. Serum creatinine should be measured 24 hours after administering the methotrexate dose, and intravenous hydration and alkalization should be instituted only in patients who sustain a 50% or greater increase from baseline. These patients should have methotrexate levels checked and may require increased doses of leucovorin.

Mitomycin C. A clinical picture indistinguishable from the hemolytic-uremic syndrome has been described during mitomycin C therapy for a variety of adenocarcinomas, particularly of the GI tract (gastric, colonic, and pancreatic). This syndrome is characterized by the clinical triad of microangiopathic hemolytic anemia, progressive renal insufficiency, and thrombocytopenia. It has generally developed in patients with minimal tumor burden who have received mitomycin C for 6 to 12 months. Estimates of the incidence of this syndrome in all patients receiving mitomycin C range from 4 to 15%.[57]

A national registry for this complication was established in 1984 and has identified 85 patients with suspected mitomycin-associated hemolytic-uremic syndrome and better defined the syndrome.[58, 59] This study identified a probable dose-toxicity relationship, because most patients who developed the syndrome received more than 60 mg/m² cumulatively. One third of the patients had no evidence of cancer at the time the syndrome became manifest, supporting a direct pathogenetic role of chemotherapy administration. The overall mortality rate exceeded 50%, with most patients dying of complications of renal failure within 8 weeks of diagnosis. Renal biopsy and autopsy data have confirmed the presence of fibrin thrombi along with intimal hyperplasia and fibrinoid necrosis of arterioles.[57]

As in other patients with thrombotic microangiopathy, the specific cause of mitomycin-associated hemolytic-uremic syndrome remains undefined. Several authors have speculated on the role of circulating immune complexes in the pathogenesis of this syndrome, finding them present in virtually all cases in which they are measured. Nonetheless, studies of immune reactivity fail to reveal detectable binding of the antibodies in these complexes to mitomycin C in vitro. Investigational therapy directed at selective removal of circulating immune complexes in these patients, however, has had anecdotal success.[57]

Conventional therapies for this syndrome have had limited success, as evidenced by the high overall mortality rate. As with other forms of thrombotic microangiopathy, the cornerstones of therapy are plasma exchange, immunosuppressive agents (primarily corticosteroids), and antiplatelet agents, with dialytic support of patients who develop profound renal failure. With greater awareness of this syndrome and more careful monitoring of patients exposed to mitomycin, it is hoped that further exposure may be avoided and corrective therapy instituted early in the course, with prevention of the full-blown syndrome. All patients receiving mitomycin should have regular monitoring of blood smears and renal function in addition to complete blood counts. The high incidence of this syndrome after therapy with mitomycin also calls into question the wisdom of using this agent in adjuvant settings where its efficacy appears to be only marginal.

Radiation. Almost all patients who receive radiation exposure totaling more than 2300 to 2500 cGy to the kidney have detectable histopathologic changes and may develop alterations in renal function. Fortunately, because of improved methods of shielding and limitation of scatter, bilateral renal exposures to these doses are uncommon. A syndrome of radiation nephritis has been described, however, and consists of progressive renal insufficiency, hypertension, and proteinuria occurring from 6 months to many years after radiation of fields that include the kidneys. The clinical spectrum of radiation nephritis is broad, with some patients having only mild asymptomatic proteinuria, whereas others have malignant hypertension and chronic renal failure with a mortality rate approaching 50%.[50]

The correlation between clinical dose and renal toxicity is loose, although a threshold of about 2000 cGy appears to exist. It is likely that radiation causes direct damage to renal vascular structures, resulting in pathologic findings consisting of hyalinization and occlusion of efferent and afferent arterioles and glomerular capillary loops.[40] Injury to the juxtaglomerular apparatus and abnormalities of renin release may mediate some of the morbid cardiovascular features of this syndrome. It is important to maintain a high index of suspicion for subclinical abnormalities in renal function in certain patients who may have had significant radiation exposures to the kidneys (e.g., patients with germ cell tumors and Hodgkin's disease) and to limit exposure of these patients to other nephrotoxins.

PULMONARY TOXICITY

One of the most frequent and serious complications of antineoplastic therapy encountered by the ICU physician is

Adapted from Cooper JAD, White DA, Matthay RA: Drug-induced pulmonary diseases. Part I: Cytotoxic drugs. Am Rev Respir Dis 133:321, 1986.

TABLE 121-2

ANTINEOPLASTIC AGENTS COMMONLY ASSOCIATED WITH PULMONARY INJURY

Antibiotics	Nitrosoureas
Bleomycin	Carmustine (BCNU)
Mitomycin C	Lomustine (CCNU)
Alkylating agents	Semustine (methyl CCNU)
Busulfan	Miscellaneous
Chlorambucil	Procarbazine
Cyclophosphamide	Vinblastine
Melphalan	Vindesine
Antimetabolites	Interleukin-2
Methotrexate	
Cytosine arabinoside	

pulmonary toxicity. The cancer patient developing respiratory compromise often presents a difficult differential diagnosis, which may, in addition to treatment-related toxicity, include (1) pulmonary progression of the underlying neoplasm, (2) pulmonary infection, (3) pulmonary edema (either cardiogenic or noncardiogenic), (4) pulmonary hemorrhage, (5) pulmonary emboli, and (6) leukoagglutinin reactions. It is important to maintain a high index of suspicion for treatment-induced lung disease because withdrawal of the offending agent(s) may be lifesaving. This section reviews the clinical features of treatment-related pulmonary toxicity, the mechanisms of lung injury involved, and the individual agents of greatest importance.

Chemotherapy-Related Pulmonary Toxicity

There is a growing list of chemotherapeutic agents that have been recognized as causing pulmonary toxicity on the basis of multiple well-documented case reports; the most significant of these are listed in Table 121-2.[60] It is important to realize that associations between cytotoxic drug exposures and subsequent lung disease are sometimes difficult to substantiate because multiple drugs may be used simultaneously and there are no specific markers or pathognomonic histologic findings. Despite subtle differences among these agents with respect to mechanisms of lung injury and dose-toxicity responses, four basic patterns of clinical pulmonary dysfunction are encountered: (1) chronic pneumonitis with pulmonary fibrosis, (2) hypersensitivity pneumonitis, (3) noncardiogenic pulmonary edema, and (4) acute chest pain syndromes (Table 121-3).

The most common form of chemotherapy-induced lung

TABLE 121-3

CLINICAL SYNDROMES ASSOCIATED WITH CHEMOTHERAPY-RELATED PULMONARY DISEASE

Syndrome	Drugs Implicated
Chronic pneumonitis with fibrosis	All categories, but especially bleomycin, mitomycin C, alkylating agents, and nitrosoureas
Hypersensitivity pneumonitis	Bleomycin, methotrexate, and procarbazine
Noncardiogenic pulmonary edema	Cytosine arabinoside, interleukin-2, methotrexate, cyclophosphamide
Acute chest pain syndrome	Bleomycin, methotrexate

disease is the syndrome of chronic pneumonitis with pulmonary fibrosis. Most of the agents listed in Table 121-2 have been associated with this type of lung injury, suggesting that it may represent a final common pathway by which diverse types of damage become clinically manifest. The prototype for this pattern of pulmonary toxicity is bleomycin, which has been the agent most extensively studied both in vitro and in animal models. Several lines of evidence suggest that bleomycin and other cytotoxic drugs may cause direct generation of reactive oxygen metabolites[60] that overwhelm the normal pulmonary antioxidant defense systems. These oxygen free radicals damage the alveolar capillary endothelium, with subsequent interstitial fibrinous edema, recruitment of mononuclear cells and fibroblasts, loss of type I pneumocytes, and hyperplasia of atypical type II pneumocytes resulting in irreversible alveolar septal thickening.[61]

Clinically, patients with chemotherapy-induced chronic pneumonitis present with the insidious onset of progressive dyspnea, nonproductive cough, fatigue, and malaise, which typically evolve during a period of several weeks. Physical findings may include tachypnea with fine, crackling bibasilar rales and, rarely, a pleural friction rub. Laboratory evaluation usually reveals hypoxemia and hypocapnia, and chest radiographs show a diffuse reticular or reticulonodular pattern progressing to bibasilar alveolar and interstitial infiltrates. Lung volume may be diminished, and pulmonary function studies classically demonstrate a restrictive ventilatory defect, with a diminished carbon monoxide diffusion capacity.

Although chronic pneumonitis is often diagnosed presumptively, the establishment of a firm diagnosis may require a lung biopsy because of the need to exclude neoplastic and infectious etiologies that could result in similar signs and symptoms. However, open biopsy should be undertaken only after careful consideration because any perioperative increase in fraction of inspired oxygen or barotrauma resulting from artificial ventilation may exacerbate the underlying interstitial pneumonitis. When there is a history of bleomycin therapy, past or present, the fraction of inspired oxygen should be maintained at 21% unless increases are absolutely necessary.

The cornerstone of therapy for chronic pneumonitis consists of prompt withdrawal of the offending agent, followed by a judicious trial of steroids in doses equivalent to a prednisone dose of 1 mg/kg/d. The likelihood of steroid responsiveness varies according to the particular cytotoxic drug involved and appears to depend on the degree of fibrosis at presentation. Most authors believe there is little role for steroids when the pulmonary parenchymal process has evolved to fibrosis. Nonetheless, a trial is often undertaken in view of the numerous anecdotal reports of dramatic responses to such therapy in the literature. In addition, many of these patients require ICU monitoring and support because of the usually profound abnormalities in gas exchange seen with this complication.

The other clinical syndromes of chemotherapy-related pulmonary toxicity are less common. Hypersensitivity pneumonitis is a syndrome that typically develops within several hours to days of cytotoxic drug administration and is characterized by the subacute onset of dyspnea, nonproductive cough, fever, and occasionally rash.[62] Laboratory evaluation may be notable for a marked eosinophilia (up to 20% of total white blood cells), and lung biopsy occasionally reveals patchy eosinophilic infiltration of pulmonary parenchyma. This subtype of lung injury tends to respond to administration of steroids and, overall, has a much better prognosis than chronic pneumonitis with fibrosis. Hypersensitivity pneumonitis has been most frequently reported in association with bleomycin, methotrexate, and procarbazine.

TABLE 121-4

RISK FACTORS FOR CYTOTOXIC DRUG-INDUCED PNEUMONITIS

Risk Factor	Drugs
Cumulative dose	Carmustine (BCNU), ? bleomycin
Patient age	Bleomycin
Concurrent or prior radiotherapy	Bleomycin, busulfan, mitomycin C
Combined use with other drugs	Bleomycin, cyclophosphamide, BCNU, methotrexate, mitomycin C
Oxygen therapy	Bleomycin, cyclophosphamide, mitomycin C
Pre-existing pulmonary disease	BCNU
Renal insufficiency	Bleomycin

Adapted from Stover DE: Pulmonary toxicity. In: DeVita VT, Hellman S, Rosenberg SA (eds): Cancer: Principles and Practice of Oncology. 3rd ed. Philadelphia, JB Lippincott, p 2165, 1989.

Noncardiogenic pulmonary edema has been described after administration of several chemotherapeutic agents, including cytosine arabinoside,[63] methotrexate, cyclophosphamide, and biologic agents such as interleukin-2[64] and colony-stimulating factors. The "capillary leak syndrome" associated with interleukin-2 therapy has been particularly well studied and occurred in up to 10% of patients receiving this therapy in a National Cancer Institute series.[64] The signs and symptoms associated with this syndrome are indistinguishable from those seen with noncardiogenic pulmonary edema of other causes and are managed similarly after withdrawal of the offending agent (see Chapter 73 for details of the management of noncardiogenic pulmonary edema).

Acute chest pain has been described in association with administration of some chemotherapeutic agents, including bleomycin[65] and methotrexate.[66] The pain is often described as pleuritic in nature, but many patients experience retrosternal pressure instead. Physical examination is typically unrevealing, although rare patients have a pleural or pericardial friction rub. Chest radiographs and ECGs generally do not show acute changes. These episodes resolve spontaneously during a few hours without long-term sequelae. Some authors recommend slowing the rate of drug infusion and managing the pain with analgesics. Drug administration should be stopped in the event of ECG abnormalities or intractable pain.

Several risk factors for the development of chemotherapy-induced pulmonary toxicity have been identified, and these are summarized in Table 121–4. Unfortunately, these risk factors are not completely predictive for the development of severe, even fatal, pneumonitis in individual patients. For instance, although the incidence of fatal pulmonary toxicity associated with bleomycin appears to increase greatly beyond a cumulative dose of 400 to 500 mg, many patients with no identifiable risk factors develop this toxicity at total doses below 200 mg.[67]

Pulmonary Toxicity of Antineoplastic Drugs

Bleomycin. Bleomycin is the best-described and best-studied cause of chemotherapy-induced pneumonitis, occurring in 2 to 40% of exposed patients. The consensus of multiple studies is that symptomatic, nonlethal pulmonary fibrosis occurs in 2 to 3% of patients, and fatal pulmonary toxicity is seen in an additional 1 to 2% of patients.[61] A higher incidence of lung injury (most of which is subclinical)

is detected if all patients undergo routine serial pulmonary function testing. Most studies show a dose-related decline in carbon monoxide diffusion capacity over time, and some suggest that bleomycin should be discontinued if the diffusion capacity falls to 40% or less of the pretreatment value, because of the subsequent high risk of developing fatal pulmonary toxicity.[68] Other studies indicate that serial monitoring of the carbon monoxide diffusion capacity is a poor predictor of bleomycin lung, and it had a sensitivity of only 17% in one study.[69] Many authors also recommend routine serial chest roentgenography to monitor for early signs of pulmonary toxicity, such as the development of Kerley's B lines at the costophrenic angles. The drug should certainly be discontinued at the earliest sign or symptom of pulmonary disease, and caution should be excercised earlier if any of the risk factors enumerated in Table 121–4 are present.

Bleomycin pneumonitis may follow either a fulminant, fatal course with progressive respiratory failure or one of gradual resolution during a period of several months to a few years.[70] The overall mortality rate is probably about 50%, with substantial variation between series.[61, 67–70] The role of steroids is uncertain in the chronic pneumonitis variant of bleomycin lung, although a few studies clearly demonstrate a benefit to some patients.[67] The more unusual hypersensitivity pneumonitis associated with bleomycin responds more reliably to steroid administration and has a favorable prognosis.

Mitomycin C. A syndrome of chronic interstitial pneumonitis with fibrosis has been described in association with mitomycin exposure in at least 30 well-documented cases.[60] This complication has a reported frequency ranging from 3 to 12%[60] and appears to share many of the clinical features of bleomycin lung. The risk factors for development of this complication after mitomycin exposure are not as well established as with bleomycin; however, there is no evidence of a dose-toxicity relationship, and some patients develop pulmonary toxicity with cumulative doses as low as 20 to 30 mg.[71] The mortality rate is about 50%. As in the case of bleomycin, there are no randomized, controlled trials examining the role of corticosteroids, although dramatic responses have been described anecdotally.[72] A therapeutic trial of steroids is probably indicated in all patients with this complication of mitomycin therapy.

BCNU. Carmustine (bischloroethylnitrosourea, BCNU) is used chiefly in the treatment of intracranial tumors of childhood. Many such patients survive for prolonged periods after receiving large cumulative doses, and there are convincing data supporting a linear dose-toxicity relationship beginning at a cumulative dose of about $1000 \ mg/m^2$.[73] Early reports suggested a frequency of pulmonary toxicity of 20 to 30% in exposed patients, but a study of long-term survivors evaluated 14 years after treatment indicates a much higher incidence in that subgroup.[74] In addition, pre-existing pulmonary disease seems to be a strong predictor of subsequent BCNU-induced lung injury and is considered a relative contraindication to such therapy. The benefit of steroids in the treatment of this complication is unclear, and many of these patients concurrently receive steroids for management of intracranial tumors.

Methotrexate. More than 50 cases of pulmonary toxicity related to methotrexate therapy in patients treated for both malignant and nonmalignant disorders have been described.[60] Although progressive pulmonary fibrosis has been seen with methotrexate therapy, the most typical presentation is that of subacute hypersensitivity pneumonitis. Noncardiogenic pulmonary edema has also been described after intrathecal administration of methotrexate, suggesting a possible neurogenic mechanism.[60] The overall frequency of pulmonary complications related to methotrexate treatment is difficult to determine from the literature but is probably 5 to 10%.[62] No clear risk factors for lung injury from methotrexate have been identified. In general, the prognosis for recovery from methotrexate-induced lung injury is quite good; the mortality rate is about 1%. Steroids appear to be particularly beneficial in patients manifesting hypersensitivity pneumonitis, although numerous patients have been found to recover spontaneously, in some instances even despite continuation of methotrexate therapy.

Radiation-Related Pulmonary Toxicity

Radiation therapy to the thorax may result in significant lung injury with considerable morbidity and, rarely, mortality. Lung tissue appears to be particularly vulnerable to radiation damage because of high ambient Po_2 levels and local generation of toxic oxygen free radicals. Radiation lung injury appears to be almost universal with doses in excess of 6000 cGy but seldom occurs with doses below 2000 cGy; this dose-dependent damage is attenuated by delivering radiation in multiple small fractions, which may allow repair of sublethal damage between treatments.

The evolution of radiation pneumonitis has classically been divided into three phases.[75] The initial or early phase occurs during the first 2 months after initiation of radiation therapy and is characterized by damage to alveolar capillary endothelial cells, with leakage of fibrin-rich exudates and formation of hyaline membranes. The second or intermediate phase occurs from 2 to 9 months after radiation and is typified by proliferation of type II pneumocytes and infiltration by mononuclear cells and fibroblasts, with resulting thickening of alveolar walls. These first two phases are thought to be potentially reversible. During the third or late phase, which occurs beyond 9 months after radiation, irreversible dense collagen fibrosis and scarring develop.

Clinically, these phases are manifest as syndromes of acute radiation pneumonitis (corresponding to the early and intermediate histologic phases) and chronic radiation fibrosis (corresponding to the late histologic phase).[75] These syndromes occur in 5 to 15% of patients who receive pulmonary radiation, but the occurrence of asymptomatic radiologic changes is much more frequent.

Acute radiation pneumonitis develops within 2 to 3 months after initiation of radiation therapy and is characterized by the insidious onset of dyspnea, an irritating, hacking cough, and occasionally fever with other constitutional symptoms. The cough may be so severe as to induce chest pain and small amounts of blood-tinged sputum. Physical examination is often unrevealing, although rare patients may have localizing pulmonary signs such as rales or a pleural friction rub. Chest radiographs may demonstrate a reticular interstitial pattern with progression to alveolar infiltrates and dense consolidation. The radiographic changes are almost always limited to the outlines of the radiation field, allowing the physician to make a presumptive diagnosis if the clinical context is appropriate.[76]

Most patients with acute radiation pneumonitis improve clinically over the course of a few months, while developing characteristic x-ray findings of chronic radiation fibrosis overlying the area of previous pneumonitis. Many of these patients are asymptomatic unless they have substantial volume loss and coexistent lung disease. These roentgenographic changes typically occur from 6 to 24 months after completion of radiation, with stabilization thereafter. Rarely, patients have presented with symptoms of chronic radiation fibrosis without a prior history of acute radiation pneumonitis.

The use of corticosteroids, either prophylactically or therapeutically, in the management of radiation pneumonitis has not been adequately studied in a randomized, controlled fashion. There have been anecdotal reports of dramatic improvement after initiation of steroids at the earliest signs of acute radiation pneumonitis,[77] and this has become the standard practice. The patient is usually given prednisone 1 mg/kg/d until symptoms resolve, at which time a cautious and gradual tapering is undertaken. Most authors agree, however, that there is no role for steroids when the injury has evolved to the chronic radiation fibrosis phase. In fact, great caution must be exercised whenever patients who have developed prior radiation pneumonitis must receive steroids for any reason, because sudden withdrawal of steroids may result in a dramatic flare of pulmonary symptoms related to previous radiation injury. It is generally recommended that steroid use be avoided if possible in these patients, and physicians caring for these patients must remain alert to the potential development of this complication.

CARDIAC TOXICITY

Cardiac toxicities resulting from therapy of neoplastic disorders are commonly encountered in the intensive care setting and are often difficult to distinguish from non–treatment-related cardiac disorders. The cardiac complications of therapy may occur acutely after drug administration, as in the case of acute arrhythmias and ECG abnormalities associated with anthracycline administration. Conversely, cancer patients may manifest cardiac injury many months to years after their treatment, when the index of suspicion for such disorders may be low. This situation is exemplified by radiation-induced pericarditis and ischemia, as well as by anthracycline cardiomyopathy.

The various syndromes of cardiac toxicity associated with antineoplastic therapy and the agents most commonly implicated as causing them are summarized in Table 121–5.[78] This section focuses on the clinical features of these syndromes, mechanisms of cardiac injury, strategies for evaluation and prevention, and individual agents of greatest significance.

Anthracycline Cardiotoxicity

The most clinically important chemotherapeutic cardiotoxins are the anthracyclines doxorubicin and daunorubicin. These agents have been implicated in the entire spectrum of cardiac disorders from acute arrhythmias and sudden death to chronic congestive cardiomyopathy. The mechanism responsible for this cardiac toxicity is not completely understood but probably involves generation of free radicals in cardiac muscle cells when anthracyclines are reduced by cytochrome P-450. The free radicals may then cause lipid peroxidation with damage to mitochondrial and sarcolemmal membranes, manifest morphologically as swelling of the sarcoplasmic reticulum with vacuolization, myofibrillar dropout, and ultimately frank necrosis.[79] These histologic changes are easily detected on tissue obtained by endomyocardial biopsy and are seen in virtually all patients receiving more than 240 mg/m^2 cumulatively, even when all other tests of cardiac function are within normal limits.[79] The heart may be particularly susceptible to injury by free radicals because it is relatively lacking in mechanisms (e.g., catalase and glutathione peroxidase) that are normally protective.[78]

Acute and Subacute Toxicity. Administration of anthracyclines has been associated with the development of acute toxicities ranging from benign ECG abnormalities to various arrhythmias and rare reports of sudden death.[80] The overall incidence of ECG changes is difficult to quantify because of variations in the extent of monitoring but has been reported

TABLE 121–5

SUMMARY OF TREATMENT-RELATED CARDIAC TOXICITY

Therapy	Arrhythmias	Pericarditis	Ischemia	Cardiomyopathy
Amsacrine	+		+/−	+
Cyclophosphamide		+		+
Cytosine arabinoside		+/−		
Daunorubicin	+	+	+	+
Doxorubicin	+	+	+	+
5-Fluorouracil			+	
Interleukin-2			+	
Radiation	+	+	+	+
Vinca alkaloids			+	

Adapted from Torti FM, Lum BL: Cardiac toxicity. In: DeVita VT, Hellman S, Rosenberg SA (eds): Cancer: Principles and Practice of Oncology. 3rd ed. Philadelphia, JB Lippincott, p 2154, 1989.

to range from 0 to 41%.[81] The most common findings are self-limited ST segment and T wave abnormalities, which occur within hours of drug administration and seem to be more common in patients with baseline ECG abnormalities. These abnormalities are not related to the dose of anthracycline, do not necessarily predict later development of cardiomyopathy, and are generally not an indication to discontinue anthracycline use.[78]

An acute pericarditis-myocarditis syndrome has been reported in association with anthracycline administration but appears to be quite rare.[82] Several patients have been described with subacute onset of myocardial dysfunction secondary to an inflammatory myopathy, and some patients died of intractable heart failure. This syndrome has occurred in the setting of relatively low cumulative doses of anthracycline (60 to 180 mg/m²).

Chronic Toxicity. The most prominent cardiac toxicity associated with anthracycline therapy is chronic cardiomyopathy, which occurs with an overall frequency of 0.4 to 9%.[78] The onset of clinical findings is highly variable; they usually occur in the context of ongoing anthracycline therapy but occasionally begin many years after exposure.[83] In the past, the development of congestive heart failure secondary to anthracycline therapy was an ominous finding and the mortality rate exceeded 60%.[84] More recent series suggest a much better prognosis, with return of normal cardiac function in the majority of patients resulting from earlier detection, discontinuation of anthracycline use (if ongoing), and appropriate supportive care. Such care entails the judicious use of inotropic agents, diuretics, and afterload-reducing agents, as would be the case for congestive cardiomyopathy resulting from other causes.

Although histologic abnormalities are seen on endomyocardial biopsy after relatively small cumulative exposures (200 to 240 mg/m²), it is unusual for patients to develop clinically detectable anthracycline cardiomyopathy below a cumulative dose of 450 mg/m² in the absence of other risk factors. Above this threshold, the cumulative probability of developing chronic heart failure increases rapidly, perhaps reaching 30% at 700 mg/m².[84] Thus, routine use of anthracycline should be limited to a cumulative dose not exceeding 450 mg/m². However, with the realization that the majority of patients do not develop heart failure even at cumulative doses as high as 700 mg/m² and may benefit from continuation of anthracycline therapy, monitoring strategies have evolved for selecting patients who may safely continue to receive the drug (see later).

In addition to cumulative dose, numerous studies have identified other risk factors for the development of anthracycline cardiotoxicity. Prior or concurrent cardiac irradiation lowers the threshold for development of cardiomyopathy.[78]

Administration of anthracyclines in the setting of prior mediastinal irradiation is common in patients with Hodgkin's and non-Hodgkin's lymphomas, lung cancers, breast cancers, germ cell tumors, and some upper GI malignancies. Cumulative dose limits should be reduced in these individuals, and a higher level of concern and vigilance is necessary. Among other risk factors, the schedule of anthracycline administration is important, because high peak levels resulting from bolus administration may be responsible for much of the cardiac toxicity. Indeed, data suggest that weekly treatment with low doses[85] or prolonged infusions during 72 to 96 hours[86] may result in less cardiac toxicity than equivalent cumulative doses given in standard bolus fashion.

Various strategies for the prevention of anthracycline cardiomyopathy have been devised. Serial resting radionuclide angiography, with specific guidelines for discontinuing further anthracycline administration in the event of significant absolute or relative decline in left ventricular ejection fraction, may reduce the incidence of anthracycline cardiotoxicity as much as fourfold.[87] Attempts to improve on this reduction by incorporating exercise radionuclide angiography and endomyocardial biopsy have met with mixed success and are the subject of continuing study.[88] More invasive evaluation (e.g., endomyocardial biopsy and cardiac catheterization) should be reserved for selected high-risk patients at centers where these are performed with particular expertise. With earlier detection of cardiac toxicity using these measures and with institution of standard supportive therapy including digoxin, diuretics, angiotensin-converting enzyme inhibitors, and vasodilators, the outcome for these patients has significantly improved.

5-Fluorouracil–Induced Ischemia

The temporal association between 5-fluorouracil (5-FU) administration and acute cardiac ischemia, both in patients with pre-existing heart disease and in those with no prior cardiac history, is well recognized. The clinical spectrum of 5-FU–induced ischemic heart disease ranges from silent ischemia to symptomatic angina pectoris to acute myocardial infarction and sudden death. Numerous case reports suggest that 5-FU induces coronary vasospasm and that appropriate prophylaxis with calcium channel blockers may prevent episodes on subsequent re-exposure.[89, 90] Typically, patients who develop this complication experience anginal symptoms within minutes to several hours after drug administration and respond to treatment with nitrates and calcium channel blockers. Most studies fail to demonstrate a dose-toxicity relationship; however, patients with pre-existing heart disease may be more sensitive to the drug.

A prospective study using continuous ambulatory ECG

monitoring found that 5-FU–induced ischemia may be much more common than previously recognized.[91] Among 25 patients monitored, 68% had ischemic changes during or after 5-FU therapy, one patient had symptomatic angina, and two patients had sudden death. Thus, 5-FU should be administered with caution to patients with a history of ischemic heart disease, and a high index of suspicion for silent ischemia in these patients is warranted.

Cyclophosphamide-Induced Myocardial Necrosis

A distinctive syndrome of acute pericarditis-myocarditis associated with administration of high-dose cyclophosphamide in preparation for bone marrow transplantation is well described. Most of these patients received doses of cyclophosphamide between 120 and 270 mg/kg,[92, 93] although a few patients developed fatal myocardial necrosis with doses as low as 90 to 120 mg/kg.[94] Typically, affected patients develop impaired systolic function, pericardial effusion, and decreased voltage on ECG beginning 5 to 16 days after initiation of cyclophosphamide therapy. Some patients develop only pericarditis without evidence of myocardial dysfunction; this subgroup appears to have a relatively good prognosis.

Among the patients who develop cardiac toxicity, the overall mortality rate ranges from 10 to 20% and most deaths result from myocardial failure. Autopsy findings are characterized by the presence of hemorrhagic myopericarditis in the majority of cases. Most series suggest that patients with a history of anthracycline and/or radiation exposure are at increased risk of developing this complication; patients undergoing autologous bone marrow transplantation for Hodgkin's disease and non-Hodgkin's lymphomas may, therefore, be at particularly high risk. There is no specific treatment for this complication other than supportive care, with invasive monitoring and use of inotropic agents as needed.

Radiation-Induced Cardiac Toxicity

As indicated in Table 121–5, radiation therapy to fields overlying the heart may result in a variety of cardiac complications that may be difficult to distinguish from preexisting heart disease (e.g., ischemia), or progression of the underlying neoplastic disorder (e.g., pericardial effusion). Much of the experience with cardiac toxicity of radiation therapy predates the use of modern shielding techniques, simulated planning, and higher-energy radiation. These technical changes may alter the spectrum and reduce the frequency of cardiac toxicity resulting from radiotherapy.[95]

Radiation-Induced Pericarditis. Pericarditis and pericardial effusions occur commonly in cancer patients as a result of the neoplastic process. No specific clinical features allow a reliable distinction between radiation-induced pericarditis and that resulting from other causes. Radiation-induced injury to the pericardium ranges from acute pericarditis with cardiac tamponade to chronic pericarditis with an incidentally discovered pericardial effusion or to chronic constrictive pericarditis. The cumulative incidence of radiation-induced pericarditis is approximately 5%, although the actual incidence may be lower with use of modern techniques.[78]

Acute pericarditis secondary to radiation therapy generally develops within the first 6 to 24 months after treatment and may be associated with a significant pericardial effusion and the risk of tamponade.[96] Evaluation including echocardiography and right-sided heart catheterization may suggest urgent need for pericardiocentesis. Generally, patients with this entity can be managed successfully with catheter drain-

age and careful serial follow-up. Occasional patients with recurrent or refractory pericardial effusion despite percutaneous drainage require partial pericardiectomy. It is important to distinguish this entity from a malignant pericardial effusion because the latter has a much poorer prognosis and may necessitate antineoplastic therapy. The yield of pericardial fluid cytology in establishing a malignant etiology in this setting is approximately 85%.[96] When cytology is equivocal, an open procedure with biopsy and creation of a pericardial window for drainage is the alternative.

Chronic pericarditis resulting from radiation therapy is generally benign and discovered incidentally on routine follow-up chest roentgenography. Most patients are asymptomatic and present 2 to 15 years after therapy. Many of these patients may be managed expectantly with serial physical examinations and echocardiography and do not require invasive treatment. Rare patients with a history of acute or chronic radiation pericarditis develop a chronic constrictive pericarditis for which pericardiectomy must be performed.

Radiation-Induced Myocardial Ischemia and Fibrosis. The association between radiation therapy to fields overlying the heart and the subsequent development of ischemic heart disease has been well documented in both animal studies and autopsy series in humans.[95, 97, 98] It is postulated that radiation may cause both microvascular and macrovascular injury directly, resulting pathologically in intimal fibrosis of the epicardial arteries in addition to generalized myocardial fibrosis. Excess mortality related to coronary artery disease in relatively young patients, such as those treated with mediastinal radiation for Hodgkin's disease, has been reported.[97, 98] The consensus of these studies is that the overall incidence of radiation-related coronary artery disease in young patients receiving more than 3500 cGy of mediastinal radiation is 5 to 20%, with a latency period of about 8 to 10 years. Currently, radiation exposure to the heart is greatly reduced by using equally weighted posteroanterior ports (as opposed to anterior ports alone) and incorporating subcarinal blocks after a cumulative dose of approximately 3000 cGy. Studies using these newer techniques have thus far failed to reveal a clear association between mediastinal irradiation and ischemic heart disease, but the follow-up has been relatively short.[95] Nevertheless, the ICU physician treating a critically ill patient with a history of mediastinal irradiation should maintain a high index of suspicion for subclinical left ventricular dysfunction and ischemic heart disease and should manage the patient accordingly.

GASTROINTESTINAL AND HEPATIC TOXICITY
Gastrointestinal Toxicity

The GI toxicities of antineoplastic therapy are often the most distressing to the cancer patient. These range from mild anorexia to nausea and vomiting to widespread mucositis manifesting as ulcerative stomatitis, esophagitis, or enteritis, which in rare circumstances may be lethal. As is true for the evaluation of other toxicities, it is necessary to exclude many other potential causes in the cancer patient undergoing treatment. For instance, anorexia, nausea, and vomiting may be early manifestations of progression of the underlying neoplasm, with occult metastases involving the liver or brain, or may be a side effect of narcotic analgesics. Emesis and mucositis are the two major forms of GI toxicity most likely to be encountered by ICU physicians.

Treatment-Related Emesis. This troublesome side effect of antineoplastic therapy is becoming more manageable through improved understanding of its pathogenesis and more aggressive prophylactic treatment. The reflex resulting in emesis involves the coordinated activities of two centers

TABLE 121–6

POTENTIAL GASTROINTESTINAL TOXICITY OF COMMONLY USED CHEMOTHERAPEUTIC AGENTS

Drug	Emesis*	Mucositis*
Actinomycin D	+ + +	+ + +
Bleomycin	+	+ +
Carmustine (BCNU)	+ +	+
Cisplatin	+ + +	+
Cyclophosphamide	+ +	+
Cytosine arabinoside (high dose)	+ +	+ +
Dacarbazine	+ + +	+
Daunorubicin	+ +	+ +
Doxorubicin	+ +	+ +
Etoposide (VP-16)	+(+)	+ +(+)
Fluorouracil	+	+ + +†
Lomustine (CCNU)	+ +	+
Methotrexate	+	+ + +
Mitomycin C	+ +	+ +
Nitrogen mustard	+ + +	+
Radiation	+	+ + +
Streptozocin	+ + +	+
Vinblastine	+	+(+)

*Key: + = mild; + + = moderate; + + + = severe.
†Increased when concurrent leucovorin used.

in the medulla, the vomiting center and the chemoreceptor trigger zone, which integrate afferent signals from the cerebral cortex, the GI tract, and the vestibular apparatus.[99] Because these centers are rich in receptors for dopamine and serotonin, attempts to design rational antiemetic therapy have focused on antagonists of these substances.

The degree to which an individual patient experiences emesis resulting from a given chemotherapeutic regimen depends on a number of factors, the most important of which are the intrinsic emetic properties of the drugs involved, the dosage and schedule of drug administration, and the degree of emesis control during prior courses of chemotherapy. Because the cerebral cortex supplies major afferent input to the vomiting center, anticipatory emesis in response to stimuli associated with prior bouts of emesis (e.g., the sight of the syringe containing the chemotherapy agent to be administered) may be a serious problem. The severity of this problem may be minimized by appropriate use of prophylactic antiemetic medications.

The chemotherapeutic agents with the greatest emetogenic potential are listed in Table 121–6.[100] Those classified as severe produce vomiting in virtually 100% of patients unless prophylactic antiemetic therapy is given. Intractable nausea and vomiting caused by these or other agents may require hospitalization for intravenous replacement of fluid and electrolytes. The agents in the moderate category cause nausea and vomiting in at least 50% of patients, depending on the dose and schedule of administration. Smaller doses given by slow infusions or in divided fashion tend to have a lower emetic potential. Nausea and vomiting typically begin within a few hours of chemotherapy administration and may last up to several days in the absence of effective antiemetic therapy, particularly after cisplatin therapy. The pathogenesis of this delayed emesis associated with cisplatin therapy has not been well established and has proved difficult to treat effectively.

The cornerstone of management of chemotherapy-related emesis is prophylactic use of combinations of antiemetic agents that work by different and, therefore, complementary mechanisms. In patients receiving the most highly emetogenic agents, it is particularly important to minimize nausea and vomiting during the first few courses in an effort to prevent subsequent anticipatory nausea.

With cisplatin-induced emesis as the prototype, the most effective antiemetic regimens have employed combinations of (1) high-dose metoclopramide (1 to 3 mg/kg intravenously 30 minutes before treatment and every 2 hours thereafter, or infusion of 0.5 mg/kg/h), (2) dexamethasone (10 to 20 mg intravenously before treatment), and (3) lorazepam (1.5 mg intravenously every 6 hours) or diphenhydramine (50 mg intravenously every 6 hours). The last two agents are important in minimizing the incidence of extrapyramidal side effects associated with the antidopaminergic properties of metoclopramide. These combination regimens offer complete protection from nausea and vomiting in 60 to 70% of initial courses.[101]

Unfortunately, these regimens have proved to be less effective in preventing emesis with subsequent courses of chemotherapy and in controlling the delayed emesis characteristic of cisplatin therapy.[102] Therefore, attempts have been made to develop new therapies that suppress the emesis reflex by alternative mechanisms. One such approach involves the use of serotonin receptor antagonists exemplified by ondansetron.[103] Phase III trials comparing ondansetron with standard combination antiemetic regimens have demonstrated equivalent or superior efficacy with diminished toxicity, particularly extrapyramidal effects.[104] Tetrahydrocannabinol, the active ingredient of marijuana, is also available but has seldom been found superior to the more commonly employed antiemetic agents and may result in a variety of unpleasant side effects such as dysphoria.

The development of extrapyramidal side effects during antiemetic therapy is problematic, particularly in younger patients. These are most commonly acute dystonic reactions (torticollis, trismus, or oculogyric crises) or akathisia (restlessness). Because these symptoms are most common in patients receiving metoclopramide, phenothiazine derivatives (e.g., prochlorperazine, thiethylperazine, and perphenazine) are often used as an alternative. However, these agents may be less effective antiemetics and still cause dystonia with considerable frequency. Fortunately, periodic administration of antihistamines and/or benzodiazepines may make these unpleasant side effects more tolerable.

Mucositis. Another common and distressing toxicity of antineoplastic therapy is injury to the epithelium of the GI mucosa. The renewal time of cells in the GI epithelium ranges from 2 to 6 days, depending on the location in the GI tract.[99] Cell cycle–specific chemotherapy may result in clinically evident injury to these rapidly proliferating tissues within a few days of drug administration. This injury may be manifest as stomatitis, glossitis, cheilosis, esophagitis, and enteritis resulting in odynophagia, diarrhea, and considerable disruption of normal alimentation. If particularly severe, such injury may result in denudation and ulceration of tissues at multiple locations throughout the GI tract, allowing endogenous flora to enter the blood stream. Patients experiencing septicemia secondary to mucositis are often concurrently neutropenic, and this combination of problems has a significant mortality rate.

The agents with the greatest propensity for causing mucositis are also enumerated in Table 121–6. For some of these agents, there are mitigating factors that determine the severity of mucositis associated with their use. Methotrexate is a common cause of mucositis if administration results in prolonged exposure of mucosal tissues to this antimetabolite. Because methotrexate is excreted primarily by the kidneys, patients with renal insufficiency may have delayed clearance of the drug with prolonged elevation of plasma levels, resulting in severe mucositis even after relatively low doses. Similarly, patients with significant peritoneal or pleural fluid accumulations or edema may experience profound mucositis as a result of distribution of methotrexate into third-space fluid reservoirs, with prolonged elevation of plasma levels. Patients with these risk factors should, in general, not receive methotrexate. When methotrexate is given in intermediate (e.g., 200 mg/m²) or high doses, it is imperative to "rescue" the normal tissues (such as the GI mucosa) with leucovorin given every 6 hours beginning 24 hours from the time of methotrexate administration. Plasma methotrexate levels should be monitored in these situations, and leucovorin rescue should generally be continued until the levels are 5×10^{-8} mol/L or less. Failure to provide such rescue has resulted in occasional toxic deaths resulting from severe mucositis.

5-FU is also a frequent cause of mucositis, particularly when used in combination with leucovorin. The GI toxicity of 5-FU appears to be both dose and schedule dependent, with more profound mucositis resulting not only from high doses but also from prolonged exposure. Also, because 5-FU is a radiation sensitizer, it is often administered in conjunction with radiation therapy for certain tumors (e.g., esophageal, rectal, and head and neck), with the combination being especially injurious to the exposed GI mucosa. Many studies have reported mortality resulting from severe mucositis related to 5-FU therapy, and care must be taken to withhold or reduce doses if patients are experiencing significant GI toxicity.

In general, the management of mucositis is supportive. Patients should be maintained with intravenous fluids, with careful attention to correcting fluid and electrolyte deficits and replacing ongoing losses from diarrhea. Patients should receive nothing by mouth or be maintained on a liquid diet as tolerated in the event of severe stomatitis, glossitis, or esophagitis with odynophagia. Palliative mouth care with warm saline rinses, viscous lidocaine (Xylocaine), or dyclonine HCl may help to alleviate mouth pain if systemic analgesics are not effective. Chlorhexidine gluconate rinses may help to reduce oral colonization with bacteria and fungi and may thereby minimize the severity of stomatitis if initiated early in the course.[105] The development of fevers in the neutropenic patient with mucositis should be managed as described at the beginning of this chapter, with initiation of broad-spectrum antibiotics covering for the gram-positive cocci and gram-negative bacilli that normally inhabit the compromised sites along the GI tract. Fortunately, most patients recover completely after appropriate supportive care, with renewal of the GI epithelium occurring more or less in conjunction with recovery of the peripheral blood cell counts.

Hepatic Toxicity

As is often the case with toxicities involving the other organ systems, the adverse effects of antineoplastic therapies on the liver frequently occur in the setting of multiple, confounding toxic events in otherwise ill cancer patients. Several of these confounding variables are listed in Table 121–7 and are likely to be encountered in the ICU setting. It is important when assessing the hepatotoxic potential of a given antineoplastic agent in an individual patient to exclude as many of these factors as possible. This is particularly true if the patient is considered to be responding to the antineoplastic therapy and would benefit from its continued use.

The antineoplastic agents that are most associated with liver injury are listed in Table 121–8. Occasional reports of hepatic toxicity have been described with almost all chemotherapeutic agents, and because combinations of these drugs may be synergistic in causing liver damage, the clinician must remain vigilant for the possibility of chemotherapy-induced hepatotoxicity.

TABLE 121–7

CONFOUNDING FACTORS IN THE ASSESSMENT OF HEPATOTOXICITY OF ANTINEOPLASTIC THERAPIES

Progression of underlying neoplasm with liver metastases
Primary infection of the liver
   Viral hepatitis (hepatitis B, hepatitis C, cytomegalovirus related to transfusion)
   Bacterial or fungal infections (from prolonged immunosuppression)
Systemic infections (sepsis) and septic shock
Hepatic congestion secondary to right-sided heart failure
Concomitant use of multiple nonchemotherapeutic hepatotoxic drugs (e.g., acetaminophen, allopurinol, diphenylhydantoins, and sulfonamides)
Acute or chronic graft-vs.-host disease (after allogeneic transplantation)
Hepatic complications of total parenteral nutrition

The spectrum of liver injury caused by antineoplastic drug exposure is quite broad, ranging from mild and transient elevation of liver enzyme levels to acute parenchymal necrosis to chronic fibrosis and cirrhosis. The best-studied agent in the last regard is methotrexate, particularly as it is used for non-neoplastic indications such as severe psoriasis and rheumatoid arthritis. Several studies suggest that chronic exposure to small daily or weekly doses (resulting in a large area under the curve of concentration versus time) is particularly likely to cause liver injury culminating in cirrhosis. The incidence of progression to cirrhosis after chronic methotrexate exposure has not been accurately determined but was as high as 24% in one series[106] and appears to be directly related to cumulative dose. Unfortunately, careful monitoring of liver function does not always reflect ongoing hepatic injury, and liver biopsy is routinely recommended at a cumulative methotrexate dose of 1.5 g. The drug should be discontinued if cirrhosis or moderate fibrosis is found, and this usually results in subsequent stabilization or regres-

---

TABLE 121–8

ANTINEOPLASTIC AGENTS CAUSING HEPATIC TOXICITY

Agent	Biochemical or Histologic Abnormality
Antimetabolites	
Methotrexate	Fibrosis, cirrhosis
6-Mercaptopurine	Cholestasis, parenchymal necrosis
Azathioprine	Cholestasis, parenchymal necrosis
Cytosine arabinoside	Transient elevation of liver enzymes
Nitrosoureas	
BCNU	Transient elevation of liver enzymes
CCNU	Transient elevation of liver enzymes
Streptozocin	Transient elevation of liver enzymes
Enzymes	
L-Asparaginase	Fatty transformation
Antibiotics	
Mithramycin	Transaminitis, acute necrosis
Biologicals	
Interleukin-2	Transient cholestatic hepatitis
Interferon-α	Transient transaminitis

sion of the process. Another liver biopsy is usually undertaken in 6 months if mild fibrosis is evident on the initial biopsy. When used as antineoplastic therapy, however, methotrexate rarely results in permanent liver injury, although transient liver function test abnormalities are common.

The antimetabolites 6-mercaptopurine and its metabolic derivative, azathioprine, are well-described hepatotoxins, with 6-mercaptopurine being the more common and serious of the two. Hepatic toxicity associated with 6-mercaptopurine typically occurs in the setting of chronic maintenance therapy for acute lymphoblastic leukemia in adults, and the incidence may be as high as 40 to 50%.[107] Both drugs may cause transient elevation of bilirubin, alkaline phosphatase, and transaminase levels, with liver biopsy demonstrating variable degrees of both intrahepatic cholestasis and parenchymal cell necrosis. These drugs are relatively contraindicated in patients with pre-existing liver disease and should be discontinued in the presence of persisting liver function test abnormalities. Concomitant use of other drugs known to cause hepatic toxicity should be minimized in patients requiring these antineoplastic agents.

Cytosine arabinoside and BCNU may cause moderate elevation of the liver enzymes, which tend to return to baseline with time; failure to return to baseline should raise suspicion of another process, such as transfusion-associated hepatitis, veno-occlusive disease (VOD), or graft-versus-host disease. To date, there have been rare reports of permanent liver injury documented by liver biopsy associated with either of these two drugs in nontransplantation doses.

Veno-Occlusive Disease. A distinct clinicopathologic entity has been described in patients manifesting liver injury after exposure to various combinations of antineoplastic agents in the bone marrow transplantation setting. VOD is characterized by a clinical syndrome of right upper quadrant tenderness, hepatomegaly, jaundice, and ascites, usually occurring within 40 days of marrow reinfusion (peak incidence at approximately 16 days).[108] These patients frequently develop progressive hepatic failure requiring supportive care in the ICU. Pathologic findings include subintimal thickening and occlusion of small to medium-sized hepatic venules with subsequent engorgement of sinusoids, centrilobular congestion, and hemorrhage, culminating in hepatocellular degeneration and necrosis.[109] These findings are distinct from those in hepatic graft-versus-host disease, which may also occur after allogeneic bone marrow transplantation, albeit usually somewhat later than is typical of VOD.

The incidence of VOD varies depending on the intensity of the preparative regimen, the disease for which transplantation is undertaken, and the integrity of hepatic function before transplantation. Most series involving significant numbers of patients receiving transplants because of a diagnosis of leukemia suggest an incidence of VOD of approximately 20%,[110] and a series in which patients with solid tumors or lymphomas were selected found an incidence of only 4%.[108] Liver metastases or abnormal liver function tests at baseline are predictive of a higher incidence of VOD.[108] The mortality rate varies depending on the method of case selection but is on the order of 40 to 70%.[108–110]

The diagnosis of VOD is often made clinically in the appropriate setting. It is important to exclude the other causes of hepatic injury enumerated in Table 121–7. The management of VOD is primarily supportive, because no specific treatment has reversed the process of liver injury. Treatment consists of careful fluid management (intravascular volume expanders when needed and spironolactone to control extravascular fluid accumulation), along with measures to minimize encephalopathy (e.g., protein restriction, lactulose, and avoidance of sedatives).

TABLE 121–9	
SPECTRUM OF CHEMOTHERAPY-RELATED NEUROTOXICITY	
Syndrome	**Responsible Agents**
Acute encephalopathies	Intrathecal methotrexate ± cranial radiation, intrathecal ara-C ± cranial radiation, ifosfamide-mesna
Chronic encephalopathies	Intrathecal methotrexate ± cranial radiation, intrathecal ara-C ± cranial radiation, high-dose IV methotrexate
Leukoencephalopathy	
Cerebral atrophy	
Somnolence syndrome	
Pontine myelinolysis	
Acute cerebellar syndrome	ara-C, fluorouracil
Cranial neuropathies	Cisplatin, vinca alkaloids
Ototoxicity	Cisplatin
Autonomic neuropathy	Vinca alkaloids
Peripheral neuropathy	Cisplatin, vinca alkaloids
Pure sensory	
Sensorimotor	

Adapted from Kaplan RS, Wiernik PH: Neurotoxicity of antineoplastic drugs. Semin Oncol 9:103, 1982.

NEUROTOXICITY

Neurologic symptoms occur frequently in the setting of neoplastic disease and its treatment and present a great challenge to physicians because of the multiplicity of pathogenetic processes that may be etiologic. The spectrum of neurologic disorders arising in cancer patients includes central nervous system (CNS) metastases, carcinomatous meningitis, spinal cord or nerve root compression, paraneoplastic neuropathic disorders, metabolic or nutritional disturbances, CNS infections, radiation myelopathy, and drug toxicity. The protean toxic effects of antineoplastic agents range from mild peripheral neuropathy to severe acute encephalopathy culminating in seizures, coma, and rarely even death (Table 121–9).[111] The neurotoxicities most likely to require ICU care are acute and chronic encephalopathies and acute cerebellar syndromes. The chemotherapeutic drugs of greatest concern in these particular neurotoxicities are methotrexate, ifosfamide, and cytosine arabinoside (ara-C).

Methotrexate Neurotoxicity

Several distinct neurologic syndromes have been described in association with methotrexate administered either systemically or intrathecally. Acute aseptic meningitis or arachnoiditis associated with intrathecal administration occurs in up to half of patients shortly after injection and resolves within a few days. These episodes are typically self-limited and of little consequence. However, a syndrome of paraplegia or acute encephalomyelopathy resulting from intrathecal methotrexate has been described in more than 20 patients to date[111] and in some cases involved prophylactic administration of the drug for leukemia or lymphoma. In most of these cases, the neurologic deficits have resolved spontaneously; however, rare patients have been left with permanent disability or have suffered progressive, lethal encephalomyelopathy.[112] The mechanism by which intrathecal methotrexate causes this toxicity remains unclear, but it may involve either primary demyelination or direct axonal injury by methotrexate with secondary demyelination.

Methotrexate has also been implicated in a syndrome of chronic encephalopathy that ranges from mild, subclinical intellectual impairment to debilitating dementia characterized pathologically as disseminated necrotizing leukencephalopathy. This encephalopathy may appear several months after intrathecal administration of methotrexate, high-dose systemic methotrexate, or, more commonly, either of these types of exposure after a course of cranial irradiation. It has been suggested that radiation to the brain may result in endothelial or ependymal cell injury and compromise the integrity of the blood-brain or blood–cerebrospinal fluid barrier. Methotrexate administered after this may gain easier access to the CNS and result in greater neurotoxicity.[113]

Several authors have identified factors that predict the development of this syndrome. Treatment with methotrexate at a young age may expose the developing brain to injury at a particularly critical time. Long-term follow-up of children with leukemia and lymphoma receiving CNS prophylaxis suggests that 5 to 50% may develop clinical leukoencephalopathy, depending on the doses of methotrexate used and the degree of prior cranial irradiation.[114] Formal neuropsychiatric testing, however, may detect an even higher prevalance of intellectual impairment. Another potential risk factor for methotrexate-induced leukoencephalopathy is the presence of cerebrospinal fluid outflow obstruction, which may result in prolonged exposure of neural tissue to toxic levels of the drug. This may account for the higher incidence of leukoencephalopathy in patients being treated for leukemic or lymphomatous meningitis than in patients receiving prophylactic methotrexate.[113]

The diagnosis of this disorder is presumptive and may be supported by compatible findings on electroencephalography, computed tomography, and magnetic resonance imaging. It is important to exclude other more common causes of confusion and somnolence in these patients, including metastases to brain or meninges, CNS hemorrhage, hypercalcemia, and sedative or narcotic overdosage. There is no specific therapy for disseminated necrotizing leukoencephalopathy other than discontinuation of further methotrexate administration and supportive care as needed. Some patients die of complications of progressive neurologic deterioration, but many experience partial improvement with time. Rarely, complete recovery has been described.[111]

Ifosfamide Encephalopathy

An acute, transient encephalopathy coincident with the administration of ifosfamide has been reported in both children and adults.[115] This will probably be seen with greater frequency because the use of ifosfamide is increasing. The syndrome is characterized clinically by the abrupt onset of mental status changes ranging from irritability, confusion, personality changes, and psychosis to drowsiness, somnolence, stupor, and frank coma. Other neurologic manifestations may be seen as well, including cerebellar dysfunction, cranial nerve palsies, and seizures. The rapidity and severity of these changes are alarming, but they have readily reversed after discontinuation of the drug in the majority of instances.

Clinically apparent ifosfamide neurotoxicity occurs in 15 to 20% of courses of therapy.[115–118] The incidence of electroencephalographic abnormalities is even higher. The development of neurotoxicity with a single course predicts similar problems with subsequent courses, although several patients have been reported to tolerate further ifosfamide exposure without additional neurotoxicity.[116] The cause of this toxicity remains uncertain, but it may result from the accumulation of neurotoxic metabolites of ifosfamide, in particular, chloracetaldehyde. Several risk factors have been identified for the development of ifosfamide-induced encephalopathy, including impaired renal function, impaired hepatic function, bulky pelvic tumor burden, high previous cumulative dose of cisplatin, and rapid infusion of the drug. Selection of

patients and slow drug administration may help to minimize the risk of encephalopathy.[118]

As with other forms of chemotherapy-related neurotoxicity, the diagnosis of ifosfamide encephalopathy is made by exclusion, with acute toxic-metabolic disorders and CNS hemorrhage being the major alternative diagnoses in these acutely deteriorating patients. Because the prognosis for full recovery is generally quite good, it is important to support these patients as needed through the acute episode. There is no specific therapy for this disorder other than discontinuation of the ifosfamide and use of anticonvulsant medications if seizures occur.

Cytosine Arabinoside Neurotoxicity

ara-C has been used as a chemotherapeutic agent in the treatment of hematologic malignancies for many years, but it is only with the use of this agent in extremely high doses (2 to 3 g/m^2 × 10 to 12 doses) that significant neurotoxicity has been encountered. A distinctive syndrome of acute cerebellar dysfunction beginning 3 to 8 days after initiation of high-dose ara-C has been described,[119–123] characterized by varying degrees of dysarthria, dysdiadochokinesia, and truncal ataxia. Less commonly recognized but also occurring with considerable frequency is a syndrome of acute encephalopathy manifest as lethargy, disorientation, somnolence, and, if particularly severe, seizures and coma. These two syndromes frequently coexist and may run a similar course.[119, 123] The overall frequency of CNS neurotoxicity after high-dose ara-C therapy is 5 to 20%, depending on the population of patients, and is irreversible or fatal in 10 to 20% of those in whom it develops.[121]

Several risk factors may help to predict the likelihood of developing serious neurotoxicity with this agent. These include age greater than 50 years, cumulative dose greater than 48 g/m^2, individual dose greater than 3 g/m^2, pre-existing renal insufficiency, pre-existing hepatic dysfunction, and antecedent neurologic disease. Among these, age of the patient appears to be the risk factor of greatest single importance. The mechanism of CNS injury remains uncertain but may involve direct injury to neurons resulting from high levels of ara-CTP (cytosine arabinoside triphosphate, the activated metabolite of ara-C) in the cerebrospinal fluid.[119] Pharmacokinetic data suggest that high levels are likely to occur if large individual doses of ara-C are administered in the setting of renal insufficiency because the drug and its metabolites are excreted in the urine. Dose reduction, when appropriate, and careful selection of patients are critical when ara-C is used in high doses.

The same diagnostic and therapeutic considerations discussed for the other chemotherapy-related neurotoxicities apply to patients who develop these syndromes in the setting of treatment with ara-C. Other acute toxic-metabolic disorders, as well as CNS hemorrhage or tumor, must be excluded and further ara-C withheld. Because 80% of patients who develop neurotoxicity resulting from ara-C recover fully, aggressive supportive care is justified, particularly if the patient is likely to achieve remission of the underlying neoplastic disorder. Patients who achieve full recovery and require further antineoplastic therapy have received subsequent courses of ara-C without experiencing recurrent neurotoxicity,[119] but the dose should be reduced to 2 g/m^2 or less and reversible risk factors (such as renal insufficiency) should be corrected.

References

1. Hellman S: Principles of radiation therapy. In: DeVita VT, Hellman S, Rosenberg SA (eds): Cancer: Principles and Practice of Oncology. 3rd ed. Philadelphia, JB Lippincott, p 254, 1989.

2. Fried W, Alder S: Late effects of chemotherapy on hematopoietic progenitor cells. Exp Hematol 13(suppl 16):49, 1985.

3. Hoagland HC: Hematologic complications of cancer chemotherapy. Semin Oncol 9:95, 1982.

4. Creaven PJ, Mihich E: The clinical toxicity of anticancer drugs and its prediction. Semin Oncol 4:147, 1977.

5. Bainton DF: Morphology of neutrophils and neutrophil precursors. In: Williams WJ, Bentler E, Erslev AJ, et al (eds): Hematology. 4th ed. New York, McGraw-Hill, p 761, 1990.

6. Bodey GP, Buckley M, Sathe YS, et al: Quantitative relationship between circulating leukocytes and infection in patients with acute leukemia. Ann Intern Med 64:328, 1966.

7. Pizzo PA, Robichaud KJ, Gill FA, et al: Duration of empiric antibiotic therapy in granulocytopenic patients with cancer. Am J Med 67:194, 1979.

8. Pizzo PA, Robichaud KJ, Gill FA, et al: Empiric antibiotic and antifungal therapy for cancer patients with prolonged fever and granulocytopenia. Am J Med 72:101, 1982.

9. Pizzo PA, Commers J, Cotton D, et al: Approaching the controversies in antibacterial management of cancer patients. Am J Med 76:436, 1984.

10. Brown AE: Neutropenia, fever and infection. Am J Med 76:421, 1984.

11. Schimpff SC, Young VM, Green WH, et al: Origin of infection in acute nonlymphocytic leukemia: Significance of hospital acquisition of potential pathogens. Ann Intern Med 77:707, 1972.

12. Wade JC, Schimpff SC, Newman KA, et al: *Staphylococcus epidermidis*: An increasing cause of infection in patients with granulocytopenia. Ann Intern Med 97:503, 1982.

13. Kramer BS, Pizzo PA, Robichaud KJ, et al: Role of serial microbiologic surveillance and clinical evaluation in the management of cancer patients with fever and granulocytopenia. Am J Med 72:561, 1982.

14. Jochelson MS, Altschuler J, Stomper PC: The yield of chest radiography in febrile and neutropenic patients. Ann Intern Med 105:708, 1986.

15. Pizzo PA, Hathorn JW, Hiemenz J, et al: A randomized trial comparing ceftazidime alone with combination antibiotic therapy in cancer patients with fever and neutropenia. N Engl J Med 315:552, 1986.

16. Bodey GP, Alvarez ME, Jones PG, et al: Imipenem-cilastatin as initial therapy for febrile cancer patients. Antimicrob Agents Chemother 30:211, 1986.

17. Wade JC, Johnson DE, Bustamante CI: Monotherapy for empiric treatment of fever in granulocytopenic cancer patients. Am J Med 80:85, 1986.

18. Pizzo PA, Ladisch S, Robichaud KJ: Treatment of gram positive septicemia in cancer patients. Cancer 45:206, 1980.

19. Gabrilove JL, Jakubowsky A, Scher H, et al: Effect of granulocyte colony-stimulating factor in neutropenia and associated morbidity due to chemotherapy for transitional-cell carcinoma of the urothelium. N Engl J Med 318:1414, 1988.

20. Antman KS, Griffin JD, Elias A, et al: Effect of recombinant human granulocyte-macrophage colony-stimulating factor on chemotherapy-induced myelosuppression. N Engl J Med 319:593, 1988.

21. Jandl JH: Disorders of platelets. In: Jandl JH (ed): Blood: Textbook of Hematology. Boston, Little, Brown, p 1041, 1987.

22. Schiffer CA, Wade JC: Supportive care: Issues in the use of blood products and treatment of infection. Semin Oncol 14:454, 1987.

23. Heeger PS, Backstrom JT: Heparin flushes and thrombocytopenia (letter). Ann Intern Med 105:143, 1986.

24. Consensus development conference on platelet transfusion therapy. JAMA 257:1777, 1987.

25. Hasker LA, Slichter SJ: The bleeding time as a screening test for evaluation of platelet function. N Engl J Med 287:155, 1972.

26. Gaydos LS, Freireich EJ, Mantel N: The quantitative relation between platelet count and hemorrhage in patients with acute leukemia. N Engl J Med 266:905, 1962.

27. Menitove JE, Aster RH: Transfusion of platelets and plasma products. Clin Haematol 12:239, 1983.

28. Deisseroth A, Wallerstein R Jr: Use of blood and blood products. In: DeVita VT, Hellman S, Rosenberg SA (eds): Cancer: Principles and Practice of Oncology. 3rd ed. Philadelphia, JB Lippincott, p 2051, 1989.

29. O'Connell B, Lee EJ, Schiffer CA: The value of 10-minute posttransfusion platelet counts. Transfusion 28:66, 1988.

30. Gerson SL, Lazarus HM: Hematopoietic emergencies. Semin Oncol 16:532, 1989.

31. Bunn HF: Recombinant erythropoietin in cancer patients. J Clin Oncol 8:949, 1990.

32. Oster W, Herrmann F, Gamm H, et al: Erythropoietin for the treatment of anemia of malignancy associated with neoplastic bone marrow infiltration. J Clin Oncol 8:956, 1990.

33. Miller CB, Jones RJ, Piantadosi S, et al: Decreased erythropoietin response in patients with the anemia of cancer. N Engl J Med 322:1689, 1990.

34. Ludwig H, Fritz E, Kotzmann H, et al: Erythropoietin treatment of anemia associated with multiple myeloma. N Engl J Med 322:1693, 1990.

35. Cohen LF, Balow JE, Magrath IT, et al: Acute tumor lysis syndrome: A review of 37 patients with Burkitt's lymphoma. Am J Med 68:486, 1980.

36. Tsokos GC, Balow JE, Spiegel RJ, et al: Renal and metabolic complica-

tions of undifferentiated and lymphoblastic lymphomas. Medicine 60:218, 1981.

37. Vogelzang NJ, Nelimark RA, Nath KA: Tumor lysis syndrome after induction chemotherapy of small-cell bronchogenic carcinoma. JAMA 249:513, 1983.

38. Cech P, Block JB, Cone LA, et al: Tumor lysis syndrome after tamoxifen flare (letter). N Engl J Med 315:263, 1986.

39. Silverman P, Distelhorst CW: Metabolic emergencies in clinical oncology. Semin Oncol 16:504, 1989.

40. Schilsky RL: Renal and metabolic toxicities of cancer chemotherapy. Semin Oncol 9:75, 1982.

41. Schilsky RL, Anderson T: Hypomagnesemia and renal magnesium wasting in patients receiving cisplatin. Ann Intern Med 90:929, 1979.

42. Lyman NW, Hemalatha C, Viscuso RL, et al: Cisplatin-induced hypocalcemia and hypomagnesemia. Arch Intern Med 140:1513, 1980.

43. Gonzalez C, Villasanta U: Life-threatening hypocalcemia and hypomagnesemia associated with cisplatin chemotherapy. Obstet Gynecol 59:732, 1982.

44. Buckley JE, Clark VL, Mayer TJ, et al: Hypomagnesemia after cisplatin combination chemotherapy. Arch Intern Med 144:2347, 1984.

45. Vogelzang NJ, Torkelson JL, Kennedy BJ: Hypomagnesemia, renal dysfunction, and Raynaud's phenomenon in patients treated with cisplatin, vinblastine, and bleomycin. Cancer 56:2765, 1985.

46. Schilsky RL, Barlock A, Ozols RF: Persistent hypomagnesemia following cisplatin chemotherapy for testicular cancer. Cancer Treat Rep 66:1767, 1982.

47. Chiuten D, Vogl S, Kaplan B, et al: Is there cumulative or delayed toxicity from cis-platinum? Cancer 52:211, 1983.

48. Hayes DM, Cvitkovic E, Golbey RB, et al: High-dose cis-platinum diammine dichloride: Amelioration of renal toxicity by mannitol diuresis. Cancer 39:1372, 1977.

49. Dentino M, Luft FC, Yum MN, et al: Long term effects of cis-diammine-dichloride platinum on renal function and structure in man. Cancer 41:1274, 1978.

50. Goldberg ID, Garnick MB, Bloomer WD: Urinary tract toxic effects of cancer therapy. J Urol 132:1, 1984.

51. Madias NE, Harrington JT: Platinum nephrotoxicity. Am J Med 65:307, 1978.

52. Gonzalez-Vitale JC, Hayes DM, Cvitkovic E, et al: The renal pathology in clinical trials of cis-platinum II diammine dichloride. Cancer 39:1362, 1977.

53. Ozols RF, Corden BJ, Jacob J, et al: High-dose cisplatin in hypertonic saline. Ann Intern Med 100:19, 1984.

54. Reece PA, Stafford I, Russell J, et al: Creatinine clearance as a predictor of ultrafilterable platinum disposition in cancer patients treated with cisplatin: Relationship between peak ultrafilterable platinum plasma levels and nephrotoxicity. J Clin Oncol 5:304, 1987.

55. Pittman SW, Frei E III: Weekly methotrexate–calcium leucovorin rescue: Effect of alkalinization on nephrotoxicity, pharmacokinetics in the CNS, and use in CNS non-Hodgkin's lymphoma. Cancer Treat Rep 61:695, 1977.

56. Frei E III, Blum RH, Pittman SW, et al: High dose methotrexate with leucovorin rescue: Rationale and spectrum of antitumor activity. Am J Med 68:370, 1980.

57. Hanna WT, Kraus S, Regester RF, et al: Renal disease after mitomycin C therapy. Cancer 48:2583, 1981.

58. Lesesne JB, Rothschild N, Erickson B, et al: Cancer-associated hemolytic-uremic syndrome: Analysis of 85 cases from a national registry. J Clin Oncol 7:781, 1989.

59. Cantrell JE, Phillips TM, Schein PS: Carcinoma-associated hemolytic-uremic syndrome: A complication of mitomycin C chemotherapy. J Clin Oncol 3:723, 1985.

60. Cooper JAD Jr, White DA, Matthay RA: Drug-induced pulmonary disease. Part I: Cytotoxic drugs. Am Rev Respir Dis 133:321, 1986.

61. Ginsberg SJ, Comis RL: The pulmonary toxicity of antineoplastic agents. Semin Oncol 9:34, 1982.

62. Sostman HD, Matthay RA, Putnam CE: Methotrexate-induced pneumonitis. Medicine 55:371, 1976.

63. Haupt HM, Hutchins GM, Moore GW: Ara-C: Non-cardiogenic pulmonary edema complicating cytosine arabinoside therapy of leukemia. Am J Med 70:256, 1981.

64. Lee RE, Lotze MT, Skibbler JM, et al: Cardiorespiratory effects of immunotherapy with interleukin-2. J Clin Oncol 7:7, 1989.

65. White DA, Schwartzberg LS, Kris MG, et al: Acute chest pain syndrome during bleomycin infusions. Cancer 59:1582, 1987.

66. Haworth E, Burroughs AK: Pleurisy and methotrexate treatment. Br Med J 2:867, 1977.

67. White DA, Stover DE: Severe bleomycin-induced pneumonitis: Clinical features and response to corticosteroids. Chest 86:723, 1984.

68. Comis RL: Detecting bleomycin pulmonary toxicity: A continued conundrum. J Clin Oncol 8:765, 1990.

69. McKeage MJ, Evans BD, Atkinson C, et al: Carbon monoxide diffusing capacity is a poor predictor of clinically significant bleomycin lung. J Clin Oncol 8:779, 1990.

70. van Barneveld PWC, Sleijfer DTH, van der Mark THW, et al: Natural course of bleomycin-induced pneumonitis. Am Rev Respir Dis 135:48, 1987.

71. Buzdar AU, Legha SS, Luna MA, et al: Pulmonary toxicity of mitomycin. Cancer 45:236, 1980.
72. Orwell ES, Kiessling PJ, Patterson JR: Interstitial pneumonia from mitomycin. Ann Intern Med 89:352, 1978.
73. Aronin PA, Mahaley MS, Rudnick SA, et al: Prediction of BCNU pulmonary toxicity in patients with malignant gliomas: An assessment of risk factors. N Engl J Med 303:183, 1980.
74. O'Driscoll OR, Hasleton PS, Taylor PM, et al: Active lung fibrosis up to 17 years after chemotherapy with carmustine (BCNU) in childhood. N Engl J Med 323:378, 1990.
75. Gross NJ: Pulmonary effects of radiation therapy. Ann Intern Med 86:81, 1977.
76. Stover DE: Pulmonary toxicity. In: DeVita VT, Hellman S, Rosenberg SA (eds): Cancer: Principles and Practice of Oncology. 3rd ed. Philadelphia, JB Lippincott, p 2162, 1989.
77. Castellino RA, Glatstein E, Turbow MM, et al: Latent radiation injury of lungs or heart activated by steroid withdrawal. Ann Intern Med 80:593, 1974.
78. Torti FM, Lum BL: Cardiac toxicity. In: DeVita VT, Hellman S, Rosenberg SA (eds): Cancer: Principles and Practice of Oncology. 3rd ed. Philadelphia, JB Lippincott, p 2153, 1989.
79. Bristow MR, Mason JW, Billingham ME, et al: Doxorubicin cardiomyopathy: Evaluation by phonocardiography, endomyocardial biopsy, and cardiac catheterization. Ann Intern Med 88:168, 1978.
80. Wortman JE, Lucas SL, Schuster E, et al: Sudden death during doxorubicin administration. Cancer 44:1588, 1979.
81. Von Hoff DD, Rozencweig M, Piccart M: The cardiotoxicity of anticancer agents. Semin Oncol 9:23, 1982.
82. Bristow MR, Billingham ME, Mason JW, et al: Clinical spectrum of anthracycline antibiotic cardiotoxicity. Cancer Treat Rep 62:873, 1978.
83. Freter CE, Lee TC, Billingham ME, et al: Doxorubicin cardiac toxicity manifesting seven years after treatment: Case report and review. Am J Med 99:483, 1986.
84. Von Hoff DD, Layard MW, Basa P, et al: Risk factor for doxorubicin-induced congestive heart failure. Ann Intern Med 91:701, 1979.
85. Torti FM, Bristow MR, Howes AE, et al: Reduced cardiotoxicity of doxorubicin delivered on a weekly schedule: Assessment by endomyocardial biopsy. Ann Intern Med 99:745, 1983.
86. Legha SS, Benjamin RS, Mackay B, et al: Reduction of doxorubicin cardiotoxicity by prolonged continuous infusion. Ann Intern Med 96:133, 1982.
87. Schwartz RG, McKenzie WB, Alexander J, et al: Congestive heart failure and left ventricular dysfunction complicating doxorubicin therapy: Seven year experience using serial radionuclide angiography. Am J Med 82:1109, 1987.
88. McKillop JH, Bristow MR, Goris ML, et al: Sensitivity and specificity of radionuclide ejection fraction in doxorubicin cardiotoxicity. Am Heart J 106:1048, 1983.
89. Burger AJ, Mannino S: 5-Fluorouracil–induced coronary vasospasm. Am Heart J 114:433, 1987.
90. Kleiman NS, Lehane DE, Geyer CE Jr, et al: Prinzmetal's angina during 5-fluorouracil chemotherapy. Am J Med 82:566, 1987.
91. Rezkalla S, Kloner RA, Ensley J, et al: Continuous ambulatory ECG monitoring during fluorouracil therapy: A prospective study. J Clin Oncol 7:509, 1989.
92. Gottdiener JS, Appelbaum FR, Ferrans VJ, et al: Cardiotoxicity associated with high-dose cyclophosphamide therapy. Arch Intern Med 141:758, 1981.
93. Cazin B, Gorin NC, Laporte JP, et al: Cardiac complications after bone marrow transplantation: A report on a series of 63 consecutive transplantations. Cancer 57:2061, 1986.
94. Trigg ME, Finlay JL, Bozdech M, et al: Fatal cardiac toxicity in bone marrow transplant patients receiving cytosine arabinoside, cyclophosphamide, and total body irradiation. Cancer 59:38, 1987.
95. Corn BW, Trock BJ, Goodman RL: Irradiation-related ischemic heart disease. J Clin Oncol 8:741, 1990.
96. Posner MR, Cohen GI, Skarin AT: Pericardial disease in patients with cancer: The differentiation of malignant from idiopathic and radiation-induced pericarditis. Am J Med 71:407, 1981.
97. Brosius FC III, Waller BF, Roberts WC: Radiation heart disease: Analysis of 16 young (aged 15 to 33 years) necropsy patients who received over 3500 rads to the heart. Am J Med 70:519, 1981.
98. Boivin JF, Hutchinson GB: Coronary heart disease mortality after irradiation for Hodgkin's disease. Cancer 49:2470, 1982.
99. Mitchell EP, Schein PS: Gastrointestinal toxicity of chemotherapeutic agents. Semin Oncol 9:52, 1982.
100. Gralla RJ: Nausea and vomiting. In: DeVita VT, Hellman S, Rosenberg SA (eds): Cancer: Principles and Practice of Oncology. 3rd ed. Philadelphia, JB Lippincott, p 2137, 1989.
101. Roila F, Tonato M, Basurto C, et al: Protection from nausea and vomiting in cisplatin-treated patients: High-dose metoclopramide combined with methylprednisolone versus metoclopramide combined with dexamethasone and diphenhydramine: A study of the Italian Oncology Group for Clinical Research. J Clin Oncol 7:1693, 1989.
102. Kris MG, Gralla RJ, Tyson LB, et al: Controlling delayed vomiting: Double-blind, randomized trial comparing placebo, dexamethasone alone, and metoclopramide plus dexamethasone in patients receiving cisplatin. J Clin Oncol 7:108, 1989.
103. Einhorn LH, Nagy C, Werner K, et al: Ondansetron: A new antiemetic for patients receiving cisplatin chemotherapy. J Clin Oncol 8:731, 1990.
104. DeMulder PMH, Seynaeve C, Vermorken JB, et al: Ondansetron compared with high-dose metochlopramide in prophylaxis of acute and delayed cisplatin-induced nausea and vomiting: A multicenter, randomized, double-blind crossover study. Ann Intern Med 113:834, 1990.
105. Sonis ST: Oral complications of cancer chemotherapy. In: DeVita VT, Hellman S, Rosenberg SA (eds): Cancer: Principles and Practice of Oncology. 3rd ed. Philadelphia, JB Lippincott, p 2151, 1989.
106. Perry MC: Hepatotoxicity of chemotherapeutic agents. Semin Oncol 9:65, 1982.
107. Menard DB, Gisselbrecht C, Marty M, et al: Antineoplastic agents and the liver. Gastroenterology 78:142, 1980.
108. Ayash LJ, Hunt M, Antman K, et al: Hepatic venoocclusive disease in autologous bone marrow transplantation of solid tumors and lymphomas. J Clin Oncol 8:1699, 1990.
109. Woods WG, Dehner LP, Nesbit ME, et al: Fatal veno-occlusive disease of the liver following high-dose chemotherapy, irradiation, and bone marrow transplantation. Am J Med 68:285, 1980.
110. Shulman HM, McDonald GB, Matthews D, et al: An analysis of hepatic veno-occlusive disease and centrilobular hepatic degeneration following bone marrow transplantation. Gastroenterology 79:1178, 1980.
111. Kaplan RS, Wiernik PH: Neurotoxicity of antineoplastic drugs. Semin Oncol 9:103, 1982.
112. Ten Hoeve RFA, Twijnstra A: A lethal neurotoxic reaction after intraventricular methotrexate administration. Cancer 61:2111, 1988.
113. Gilber MR, Harding BL, Grossman SA: Methotrexate neurotoxicity: In vitro studies using cerebellar explants from rats. Cancer Res 49:2502, 1989.
114. Aur RJA, Simone JV, Verzosa MS, et al: Childhood lymphocytic leukemia—Study VIII. Cancer 42:2123, 1978.
115. Pratt CB, Green AA, Horowitz ME, et al: Central nervous system toxicity following treatment of pediatric patients with ifosfamide/mesna. J Clin Oncol 4:1253, 1986.
116. Pratt CB, Goren MP, Meyer WH, et al: Ifosfamide neurotoxicity is related to previous cisplatin treatment for pediatric solid tumors. J Clin Oncol 8:1399, 1990.
117. Meanwell CA, Blake AE, Blackledge G, et al: Encephalopathy associated with ifosfamide/mesna therapy (letter). Lancet 1:406, 1985.
118. Meanwell CA, Kelly KA, Blackledge G: Avoiding ifosfamide/mesna encephalopathy (letter). Lancet 2:406, 1986.
119. Damon LE, Mass R, Linker CA: The association between high-dose cytarabine neurotoxicity and renal insufficiency. J Clin Oncol 7:1563, 1989.
120. Herzig RH, Herzig GP, Wolff SN, et al: Central nervous system effects of high-dose cytosine arabinoside. Semin Oncol 14:21, 1987.
121. Herzig RH, Hines JD, Herzig GP, et al: Cerebellar toxicity with high-dose cytosine arabinoside. J Clin Oncol 5:927, 1987.
122. Lazarus HM, Herzig RH, Herzig GP, et al: Central nervous system toxicity of high-dose systemic cytosine arabinoside. Cancer 48:2577, 1981.
123. Baker WJ, Royer GL, Weiss RB: Cytarabine and neurologic toxicity. J Clin Oncol 9:679, 1991.

CHAPTER 122

Clinical Apheresis

Irene Zielinski
Judith C. Andersen

Clinical apheresis, a subspecialty of blood banking and hematology, has arisen from the need for and availability of mechanical devices for efficient extracorporeal separation of an individual's whole blood into cellular and liquid components with rapid return of one or more components to the individual. Apheresis is a general procedural term derived by familiar usage from the parent noun plasmapheresis, meaning to effect separation (pheresis) of plasma from whole blood. It now refers specifically to clinical procedures, as opposed to procedures used in the laboratory to separate components of biologic fluids by mechanical or electrical means (e.g., protein electrophoresis). Apheresis, as it is now practiced, relies on semiautomated instruments, which accomplish removal, extracorporeal separation, and return of appropriate blood components to the donor or patient.[1]

Apheresis can be divided, at present, into two broad categories, cytapheresis and plasmapheresis, each comprising several subcategories.[2] Both categories of apheresis may be employed for either direct therapeutic benefit to a patient or preparation of a blood component product for transfusion therapy. Emphasis throughout this chapter is placed on direct therapeutic applications of apheresis to the care of critically ill patients, but it should be remembered that the techniques involved are frequently applicable to routine or emergency preparation of blood products as well. Photopheresis is a specialized form of apheresis that involves extracorporeal exposure of plasma or plasma-suspended cells to ultraviolet A light.[3] Ex vivo activation of orally or parenterally administered photosensitive nucleic acid–binding compounds such as 8-methoxypsoralen or merocyanin derivatives may then be employed to inhibit nucleic acid synthesis in replication-competent cells or organisms.[4, 5] This technique has been approved for use in cutaneous T cell lymphomas[6, 7] and is being studied for efficacy in disorders such as scleroderma, graft-versus-host disease in transplant recipients, and acquired immunodeficiency syndrome. Although there are no current critical care indications for photopheresis, its principle may be of future value in targeting systemically toxic therapies to specific cell populations ex vivo.

Cytapheresis is a procedure in which blood cells are separated and removed from whole blood, and plasma is returned to the patient with or without the replacement of cellular elements. White blood cell removal and platelet removal (leukapheresis and thrombocytapheresis) are typically undertaken for relief of symptoms of hyperviscosity or leukostasis related to excessively high numbers of cells in neoplastic disorders of hematopoiesis. Because simple phlebotomy is usually efficacious for relief of hyperviscosity symptoms resulting from erythrocytosis, erythrocytapheresis is usually reserved for partial or total exchange transfusion, in which volume-for-volume exchange of a patient's red blood cell mass is undertaken, as in preparation of a patient with sickle cell disease for surgery.

Therapeutic plasmapheresis, frequently called plasma exchange, refers to the extracorporeal separation of a patient's whole blood into cellular and plasma components in which the plasma is removed and cellular elements are returned to the patient with a suitable replacement fluid. It is most frequently employed in clinical situations in which a plasma component such as an immunoglobulin is known to be injurious to the patient's tissues—for instance, by impairing blood flow (as in the immunoglobulin M [IgM]–mediated hyperviscosity syndrome of Waldenström's macroglobulinemia[8]) or directly interfering with or injuring a physiologic structure (such as the neuromuscular acetylcholine receptor in myasthenia gravis or myelin basic protein in autoimmune polyneuropathy[9])—or when the target of a plasma component is ill defined but empirical use of plasma exchange has led to clinical benefit (as in thrombotic thrombocytopenic purpura [TTP][10–23]). In these situations, plasma exchange is often used as an adjunct to medical therapies, employed to remove injurious molecules while pharmacologic measures are directed at their source. Plasmapheresis has been refined by the interposition of affinity binding materials in the extracorporeal circuit, allowing removal of specific plasma components such as immunoglobulin G (IgG)[24] or low-density lipoproteins.[25, 26] Many more such applications are being explored to allow greater specificity of therapy and decrease the potential morbidity of repetitive whole plasma removal.

HISTORY

Mechanical extracorporeal separation of blood into components for the direct benefit of patients as well as for preparation of therapeutic blood components has been practiced since the early years of the 20th century. Introduction of citrate anticoagulation and nutrient blood storage solutions, corresponding temporally roughly to the occurrence of World Wars I and II, led to increased separation efficiency. The forerunner of one type of apheresis device, the centrifugal separator, was a dairy cream separator patented in Sweden in 1878 by Delaval. Techniques for large-scale centrifugal separation of whole blood were developed to satisfy the demand for plasma in World War II by E. J. Cohn, best known for his scheme of combined physicochemical and mechanical fractionation of blood and plasma introduced in the postwar years and still in use for preparation of commercial plasma fractions. Manual centrifugation of blood was widely used in blood banks in the 1950s and served as the basis for manual plasmapheresis and partial exchange transfusion, in which individual units of blood were drawn sequentially from donors or patients and processed by centrifugation and the plasma or red blood cell component was returned to the patient by gravity methods using an appropriate diluent.[27]

George Judson, an engineer for International Business Machines (IBM), observed manual leukapheresis of a white blood cell donor with chronic granulocytic leukemia in 1962 during treatment of a family member at the National Cancer Institute. Recognizing the need for a method to harvest non-neoplastic granulocytes from individuals with normal white blood cell counts, he conceived the idea for automated extracorporeal blood cell separation. The instrument developed by Judson at IBM and introduced less than 1 year later incorporated the principles of continuous flow centrifugation and was the prototype for subsequent apheresis technology development.[28]

In the past 30 years, quantum increases in the efficacy of apheresis devices have been achieved, drawing on technologies developed in the fields of agriculture, physical chemistry, electronics, and immunobiology. Sophisticated automated extracorporeal separation instruments suitable for treatment of children and adults are now widely available in developed countries. Although there have been many refinements in instrumentation, centrifugal separation of whole blood as Judson first engineered it remains one of the two major methods for clinical apheresis.[29]

PRINCIPLES OF APHERESIS

All apheresis instruments use disposable "software," plastic separation chambers connected by tubing to venous needles or cannulas, to remove whole blood from and to return recombined blood elements to the apheresis patient. Although many instruments require cannulation of two peripheral veins or the use of a double-lumen catheter with an "arterialized" return lumen, several modern instruments allow the use of a "single-needle" technique, permitting both withdrawal and return of blood elements to a single large vein, usually an antecubital or femoral vein.

Most currently available apheresis instruments achieve physical separation of withdrawn whole blood into its liquid and cellular components by application of one of two principles: centrifugation or ultrafiltration.

Centrifugation utilizes centrifugal force to separate blood components by buoyant density, taking advantage of the principle, useful in both clinical and laboratory settings, that plasma, platelets, white blood cells, and erythrocytes differ from one another in buoyant density and separate into layers under the influence of an applied centrifugal force, with plasma "floating" above layers of leukocytes, platelets, and erythrocytes, respectively. Apheresis instruments may employ continuous flow or interrupted flow centrifugation techniques. Continuous flow refers to a separation procedure in which whole blood is drawn continuously from the patient and centrifuged in a continuously rotating ring from which individual components are allowed to flow according to their buoyant density and the setting of outflow parameters.[30, 31] Separation in current instruments is achieved according to algorithms preset in the instrument electronics, with the appropriate elements returned continuously to the patient as separation is achieved. Cobe Spectra, Fenwal CS 3000, and Haemonetics V50 instruments are examples of state-of-the-art instruments employing continuous flow methodology, the Spectra representing an updated version of the original IBM design.[29] An example of a current continuous flow centrifugation instrument is shown in Figure 122–1.

Interrupted flow refers to a procedure in which a preset volume of blood is withdrawn from the patient and separated into its components; the appropriate components, combined with replacement fluid, are reinfused to the patient; and the process is repeated until the desired volume of blood has been processed. Earlier Haemonetics instruments and the Green Cross Knightmage instrument employed interrupted flow centrifugation techniques.[29] Although, on theoretic grounds, continuous flow centrifugation offers increased separation efficiency and economy of time, both techniques have strong proponents in the apheresis community and are widely used in both therapeutic and preparative settings. Centrifugation techniques are useful for both cytapheresis and plasmapheresis.

Ultrafiltration apheresis devices separate whole blood into formed elements and plasma by application of pressure across a membrane filter of uniform pore size that is incorporated in a disposable unit.[29, 32–34] Such a membrane allows passage of fluid and macromolecules but prevents passage of cellular elements. The physical principle is similar to that used in dialysis machines, but membrane pore size allows passage of larger molecules.[32] Ultrafiltration efficiency is greatest for blood with a high ratio of plasma to packed cell volume, such that fluid access to the membrane is maximal, and least efficient and most time consuming for blood with normal to increased hematocrit values.[34] Currently, ultrafiltration is of little use for collection of formed elements or removal of specific populations of formed elements because it does not allow fractionation of cellular elements by size or buoyant density. Its use is restricted to situations in which plasma removal or collection is indicated. It does allow the collection of cell-free plasma, even from patients with anomalously light or fragmented cells, which is of some importance for critically ill patients or those for whom transfusion is proscribed by medical condition or religious persuasion.[32] An example of an ultrafiltration apheresis instrument, the Cobe TPE (total plasma exchanger), is shown in Figure 122–2.

CYTAPHERESIS

The use of apheresis for removal of white blood cells or platelets is most appropriate when rapid reduction of cell volume is required but cannot be achieved safely by phar-

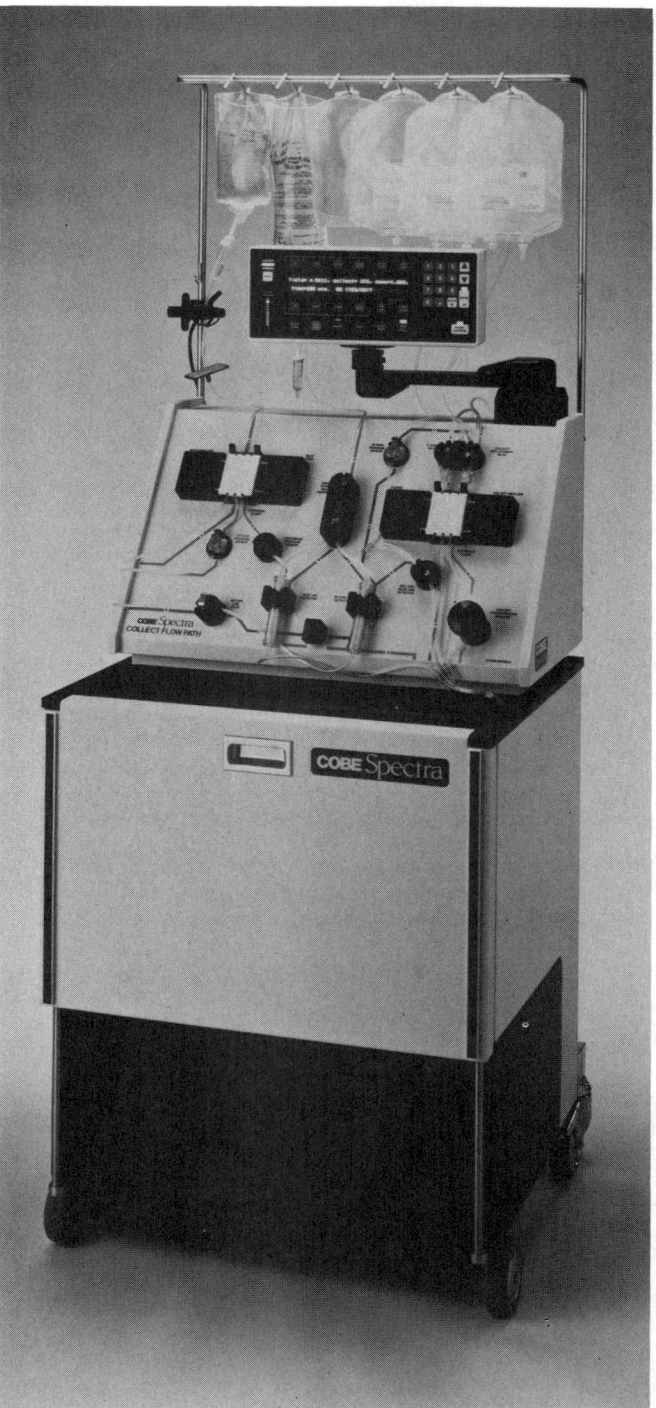

Figure 122–1. Cobe Spectra continuous flow centrifugation instrument.

macologic means. With rare exception, this occurs in patients who have neoplastic disorders of the bone marrow or lymphoid tissues, often in circumstances in which symptoms of hyperviscosity elevate a previously undiagnosed disorder to the threshold of clinical recognition or in which the metabolic and circulatory consequences of rapid pharmacologic cytoreduction might prove life threatening. Cell type, rate of accumulation, and turnover time, as well as the patient's performance status, general clinical condition, renal function, and special considerations (e.g., pregnancy), determine

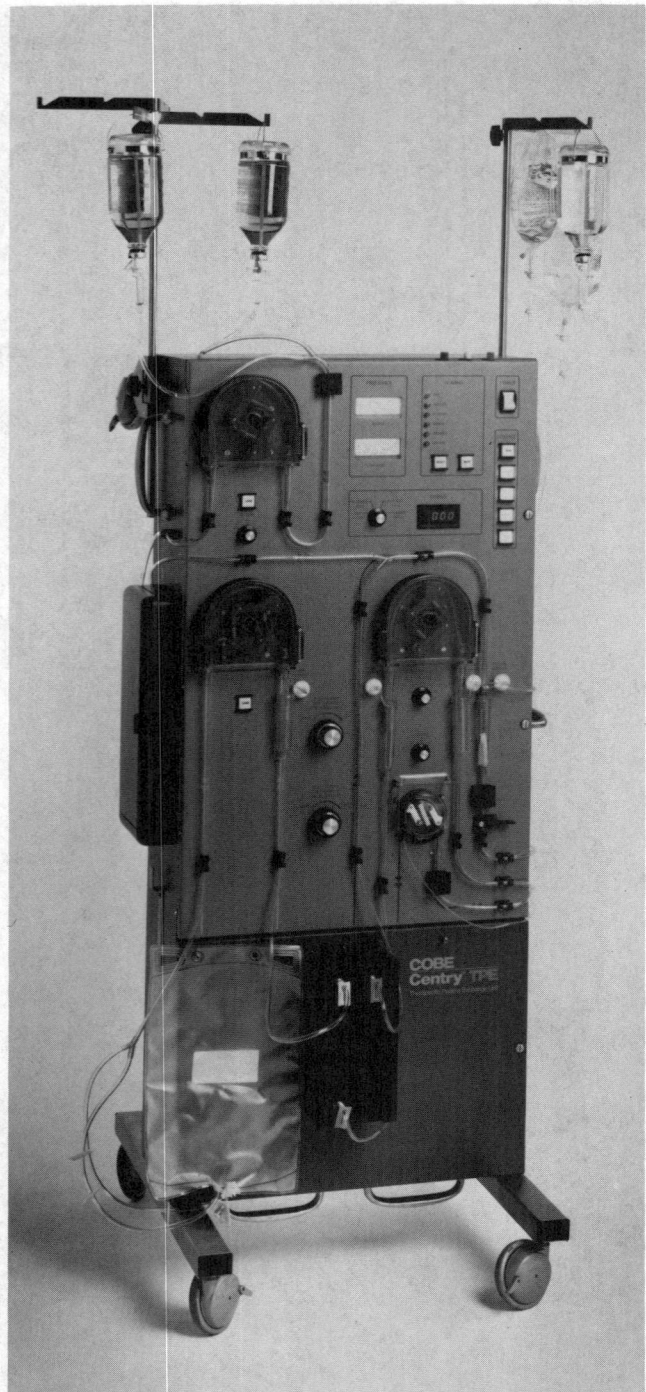

Figure 122–2. Cobe Centry total plasma exchanger.

of cell reaccumulation in the vascular compartment then depend on cell size and type,[36] kinetics of cell turnover and tissue distribution, presence or absence of underlying vascular disease, and the timeliness of cytapheresis.[2] Cytapheresis does not reverse a completed occlusive vascular accident but may alter tissue fate in areas adjacent to an infarct, limiting infarct size and allowing improved recovery. Specific applications and examples are described in the following.

Because circulating platelets have a plasma survival of 8 to 10 days and are anucleate, thus inaccessible to rapid control by DNA-targeted antineoplastic agents such as hydroxyurea, thrombocytapheresis ("plateletpheresis") is the only method currently capable of relieving symptoms of extreme thrombocytosis.[37–40] Organ dysfunction (e.g., myocardial ischemia), bleeding, and impending cerebrovascular accident caused by thrombocytosis in disease states such as essential thrombocythemia, chronic granulocytic leukemia, or polycythemia rubra vera or in inflammatory disorders with extreme thrombocytosis can be palliated effectively with thrombocytapheresis. Peripheral platelet counts requiring intervention usually exceed $1.0 \times 10^6/mm^3$ ($1.0 \times 10^{12}/L$) but must be considered in an individual patient's clinical context. Elderly patients or those with underlying atherosclerotic vascular disease are at particular risk and may exhibit symptoms with platelet counts that would not prove troublesome to younger individuals. A single cell collection, lasting 2 to 4 hours depending on the patient's size, reduces cell number by 50%[37] and usually provides symptomatic relief, but one to five additional procedures per week[38, 41] may be required to ensure freedom from recurrence until pharmacologic control of the underlying disease process can be achieved (often 2 to 3 weeks).[2]

Therapeutic leukapheresis is useful in alleviating symptoms of vascular leukostasis in both acute and chronic leukemias and, in occasional circumstances, in promoting reduction of lymph node and organ size and relief of B symptoms in chronic lymphoid disorders poorly responsive to other therapies. In acute myeloid leukemias, leukapheresis is also of value in ameliorating the unique form of tumor lysis syndrome that occurs when large numbers of nucleated procoagulant-rich cells are destroyed pharmacologically in the vascular system.

In patients with acute myeloid leukemias, chronic granulocytic leukemia in blast phase, and acute lymphoblastic leukemia, high peripheral white blood cell numbers (> $100,000/mm^3$ [$1.0 \times 10^{11}/L$]) are associated with respiratory distress and cerebrovascular symptoms attributed to occlusion of microvasculature by large, poorly deformable immature white blood cells.[42–44] Myeloid and monocytic precursors are capable of synthesizing cell surface tissue factor when stimulated by inflammatory mediators such as interleukin-1 and tumor necrosis factor and may initiate a cascade of reactions leading to vascular endothelial procoagulant synthesis with intravascular coagulation. Symptoms arising from such a sequence may appear abruptly in a leukemic patient and, because of coexistent thrombocytopenia, result in lethal vascular occlusion with periocclusion hemorrhage.[42–44] Intravascular destruction of these cells by cytotoxic chemotherapeutic agents may transiently worsen this situation by increasing the amount of procoagulant available to the extrinsic clotting system and loading the extracellular fluid compartment with the metabolic products of cell destruction, leading to extreme hyperkalemia, hyperphosphatemia, and hyperuricemia.

Rapid reduction of circulating blast numbers by leukapheresis ameliorates symptoms of leukostasis,[45] reduces the numbers of potential sources of tissue factor and nuclear debris, and allows time for adjunctive measures such as hydration, urine alkalization, and use of xanthine oxidase

the suitability of apheresis for a given clinical situation, as well as the value of and appropriate interval for repetitive treatment. Cytapheresis should be regarded solely as palliation, a means of achieving temporary control of symptomatic cell excess, while definitive therapy is being undertaken.

Although earlier studies suggested 20 to 36% cell removal efficiency from a single cytapheresis procedure,[35] a skilled apheresis clinician using current instrumentation to process one patient's blood volume can achieve 40 to 60% removal of a selected circulating cell population.[31] The degree of resulting symptomatic relief, duration of relief, and kinetics inhibitors to provide protection against metabolite excess. Leukapheresis should be contemplated for all patients with acute or chronic granulocytic leukemia with blast-progranulocyte numbers in excess of 100,000/mm³ (1.0 × 10¹¹/L) and patients with acute lymphoblastic leukemias with similar blast numbers and symptoms suggestive of leukostasis (dyspnea, tachypnea, headache, mental status changes, or renal dysfunction).[2, 42–44] The patient's age, vascular status, and duration of symptoms should, as always, be considered in decision making, but the relative ease of the procedure and its low morbidity weight the decision in favor of leukapheresis in marginal cases. In patients distant from an apheresis facility, hydration, urine alkalization, and allopurinol administration should be initiated before transfer, which should be accomplished with a skilled nurse or physician in attendance.

Leukapheresis for chronic granulocytic leukemia in chronic phase is less frequently required but may be necessary when diagnosis of the disorder is suggested by leukostasis-associated symptoms (leukocyte numbers usually greater than 250,000/mm³ [2.5 × 10¹¹/L]),[43] when a patient has uncomfortable organ enlargement and wasting with relatively low peripheral white blood cell counts or severe anemia,[46] or when the diagnosis is made during pregnancy, with its relative contraindications to chemotherapy and potential fetal compromise resulting from maternal leukostasis.[47] With currently available apheresis techniques, leukapheresis once or twice weekly controls leukocyte counts and, when performed during a period of weeks to months, may promote decrease in organ size, improvement of performance status, and possible long-term (2 to 6 months) remission of leukocytosis. The costs of repetitive leukapheresis in equipment, staff, and the patient's time seem especially justified during pregnancy, when fetal wastage resulting from uncontrolled leukocytosis or fetal abnormality resulting from chemotherapy represents an unacceptable loss of inestimable magnitude. They are rarely reasonable in routine chronic-phase chronic granulocytic leukemia, in which chemotherapeutic control is usually easily achieved.

Leukapheresis is less frequently employed in chronic B cell lymphoproliferative disorders because peripheral blood involvement is unusual in most non-Hodgkin's lymphomas and the high circulating numbers of long-lived small lymphocytes characteristic of chronic lymphocytic leukemia are usually well tolerated. Occasional patients with organ enlargement or skin involvement caused by low-grade lymphomas poorly responsive to conventional therapy or patients with chronic lymphocytic leukemia with organomegaly or cell numbers greater than 500,000/mm³ (5.0 × 10¹¹/L) respond favorably to repetitive cytoreductive procedures performed two or three times weekly for several weeks.[48, 49] In these patients, little reduction in circulating cell number is seen after the first several procedures because of tissue redistribution; measurable results, however, are often seen in lymph node and organ size or in severity of skin involvement. Chronic T cell disorders are a special subcategory of lymphoid disorders for which leukapheresis is occasionally useful[50] and for which the efficacy of photopheresis is being explored (see earlier).

Erythrocytapheresis, or "total" red blood cell exchange, is a useful technique for prevention and treatment of the complications of sickle cell disease, as well as treatment of other rarer disorders such as parasitic infestations of red blood cells and acquired red blood cell membrane abnormalities.

Symptoms in sickle cell disease are created by a complex cycle of blood flow degradation caused by rheologic abnormalities associated with irreversibly sickled erythrocytes, tissue hypoxia and acidosis, further erythrocyte sickling, com-

plete vascular occlusion, and infarction, all triggered by intracellular polymerization of deoxygenated hemoglobin S molecules during physiologic fluctuations of tissue P_{O_2} and pH. The empirical observation that patients with sickle cell trait, heterozygotes with approximate relative proportions of hemoglobins A and S of 50 and 40%, respectively, are virtually symptom free suggested that decreasing by transfusion the proportion of circulating cells containing hemoglobin S to below 50% might prevent the majority of sickling episodes. In practice, despite the severe anemia characterizing most sickle cell disease, achievement of this goal by transfusion alone is hindered by a short-term unfavorable alteration in P_{50} and an increase in viscosity occasioned by increased red blood cell mass, as well as the long-term problem of transfusional iron overload. Thus simple transfusion for relief of sickle cell complications is rarely effective and is recommended only when anemia is worsened acutely by blood loss or erythrocyte production is impaired by viral infection or intoxication (aplastic crisis).

Partial exchange transfusion,[51, 52] achieved by sequential manual removal of units of whole blood, centrifugation and discarding of removed SS erythrocytes, and return of plasma and normal AA erythrocytes, is a cumbersome and time-consuming process, limited by staff time and the patient's tolerance. Furthermore, it is made inefficient in SS erythrocyte removal by rapid mixing of AA and SS erythrocytes in vivo such that all units after the first represent significant admixtures of transfused and SS cells. Automated erythrocytapheresis of one red cell mass, in which the patient's red blood cell volume is removed and replaced by an equal volume of hemoglobin A–containing cells, allows more effective replacement of the patient's SS cells by AA erythrocytes. Although some admixture of the patient's cells and transfused cells occurs during the procedure, precluding more than 70% efficiency, the speed of the exchange, particularly when performed with a continuous flow centrifugal device, allows uniform reduction of hemoglobin S to below 50%.[53–56]

Additional exchanges may be performed during 48 to 72 hours for a patient who has impending stroke or incompletely resolved priapism and during 2 to 3 weeks for a pregnant patient to maintain hemoglobin S levels below 30%. For a severely anemic patient (hemoglobin level < 70 g/L) with potent hypoxic stimulation of red blood cell production, transfusion of additional red blood cells after erythrocytapheresis decreases erythropoietin secretion, damping bone marrow production of SS reticulocytes and enhancing both the antisickling effect and its duration. In chronic erythrocytapheresis programs, such transfusion is rarely necessary beyond the first two exchange procedures.

When performed without additional red blood cell transfusion, automated erythrocytapheresis promotes neutral iron balance, removing and replacing equal volumes of iron-containing red blood cells. Simple transfusion of red blood cells results in an iron increment of 1 mg/mL of packed cells. Thus transfusion of one unit of packed erythrocytes (250 mL) per month would result in total body iron increments of approximately 170 mg/mo for a menstruating or gravid female and 210 mg/mo for a male or postmenopausal female, increases of 75 to 100% per year over normal total body iron stores.

Erythrocytapheresis has been of value in shortening sickle cell–associated painful crises,[52, 57] alleviating priapism,[58] and preventing threatened stroke, as well as in promoting successful pregnancy,[51] preventing surgical complications, and decreasing the morbidity associated with radiologic studies using radiocontrast agents.[53]

Potentially life-threatening red blood cell disorders caused by red blood cell parasitism with hemolysis can be diminished in severity or eradicated by erythrocytapheresis. Oroya fever (*Bartonella bacilliformis*), babesiosis (*Babesia microti*), and falciparum malaria (*Plasmodium falciparum*) are examples of such illnesses,[59-62] and others may exist. Preoperative erythrocytapheresis in paroxysmal nocturnal hemoglobinuria has been reported to decrease surgical morbidity caused by increased red blood cell complement sensitivity.[63] Erythrocytapheresis of rapidly engrafting recipients of ABO-incompatible bone marrow transplants (O to A, B, or AB donation) may be useful in diminishing hemolytic consequences (see later for plasmapheresis of reverse donations). Automated red blood cell exchange may also be of value for Rh-negative young women who, after acute major trauma or hemorrhage, receive group- but not type-specific whole blood or red blood cells. Rapid recognition of the incompatibility, erythrocytapheresis with antigen-negative cells, and large-volume anti-Rh$_o$ immunoglobulin use may prevent sensitization and allow subsequent successful pregnancy.

Erythrocytapheresis offers significant advantages over conventional transfusion for sickle cell disease as well as relief of morbidity associated with other disease states. Problems associated with its use include the need for large quantities of red blood cells for chronic exchange programs, the potential for infection of exchange recipients with blood-borne pathogens, the risk of alloimmunization to red and white blood cell antigens with the potential for severe transfusion reaction, the expense in time and money of multiple exchange procedures, and problems of vascular access. None of these problems is insuperable.

Addressing the blood supply requirements for a chronic red blood cell exchange program is a significant problem, particularly for adult patients whose red blood cell mass ranges from 500 to 2000 mL (2 to 8 units of packed red blood cells). Individualizing the frequency of erythrocytapheresis based on careful evaluation of hemoglobin S levels rather than maintaining a routine exchange interval may help to reduce blood needs. For the present, blood availability can be improved both by notifying local blood suppliers of a continuing or regularly recurring need and by encouraging the patient's family members and coworkers to join blood donation programs where appropriate.

Exclusion of infected units by current testing for blood-borne pathogens is excellent, and further reduction in infectivity as well as alloimmunization likelihood can be achieved by the use of leukocyte-poor erythrocytes (washed, antigen matched, in the case of already alloimmunized patients). The theoretic concern that exposure to multiple units of packed red blood cells during each exchange procedure would lead to broad alloimmunization has proved unfounded. Severe transfusion reactions during erythrocytapheresis, although theoretically possible,[64] have been extremely rare. The high apparent procedural expense must be compared with the potential costs of hospitalization for painful crisis or other sickle cell complications, as well as societal loss through lost work time, analgesic addiction, and fetal wastage.

Vascular access remains problematic when approached for the first time in adult sickle cell patients. Severely symptomatic patients often have had peripheral veins damaged by years of frequent venipuncture and intravenous therapy and may require periodic insertion of vascular cannulas, creation of arteriovenous fistulas, or Gore-Tex shunts for erythrocytapheresis. Instructing pediatric patients and their families that peripheral veins are precious and must be protected even from well-meaning care givers (similar to the instruction given to hemophilic patients) may prove useful in preserving vascular access in the next generation of sickle cell patients. Problems of catheter-associated infection and thrombosis may be significant in sickle cell patients with indwelling cannulas; meticulous in-hospital care, thorough instruction of the patient, home care nursing, and frequent follow-up are necessary to prevent morbidity with these devices.

PLASMAPHERESIS

The rationale for therapeutic plasma exchange is best established in disease states in which pathophysiologic evidence exists for the targeted toxicity of large molecules such as immunoglobulins. (Disease states in which symptoms are caused by "physiologic" or pharmacologic molecules of less than 10,000 daltons are better treated by dialysis or hemoperfusion procedures.) Effective reduction of the concentration of these molecules might be expected to allow healing of damaged organs and alleviate symptoms. As mentioned earlier, there are few controlled studies that establish incontrovertibly the value of plasma exchange in human disease. Those studies,[22] however, as well as the accumulation of reports of efficacy from clinicians treating serious illnesses for which either no other effective therapies exist or conventional therapies are poorly tolerated, have allowed the definition of specific indications for plasma exchange therapy[65-67] and permitted hypothesis development for future areas of clinical study.

The efficacy of a single procedure in diminishing the plasma concentration of a pathogenic material, assuming no diffusion from an extravascular compartment during the procedure, has been described by Nusbacher[2] on the basis of literature considerations[68-70] in the following formula:

$$C_t = C_0 e^{-b/vt}$$

where C_t = concentration of pathogen in patient's plasma at time t
C_0 = concentration in patient's plasma before exchange
b = volume of plasma exchange
v = patient's plasma volume
t = duration of exchange

Although most substances removed by plasma exchange are distributed extravascularly and diffuse into the plasma space during the procedure along the concentration gradient established by the exchange, the formula indicates that the efficacy of a procedure in removing a pathogen decreases with exchanges exceeding one plasma volume. Because logistics of plasma exchange require the patient to be reclining, the patient's tolerance for time-consuming large-volume exchanges is limited. Thus, most plasma exchange recommendations are for single exchanges of one plasma volume, with the frequency of repetition dictated by the type and severity of illness.

Many of the disorders for which plasma exchange therapy is thought to be effective are of immune etiology, either alloimmune (i.e., appropriate but potentially problematic response to a nonself antigen) or autoimmune (inappropriate synthesis of antiself immunoglobulin). Examples of the former include "post-transfusion purpura," a syndrome of severe thrombocytopenia caused by sensitization to a transfused platelet antigen not shared by the transfusion recipient;[71-73] hemolysis caused by residual isoagglutinins in bone marrow transplant recipients receiving human leukocyte antigen–compatible but ABO-incompatible bone marrow;[74-76] human leukocyte alloimmunization of potential organ transplant recipients such that hyperacute rejection of the donated organ is likely;[77] or uncontrollable hemorrhage caused by factor VIII or IX "inhibitors," antibodies to factor VIII or IX arising in transfused hemophilic patients with specific types of inherited molecular defects in these coagulation factors.[78, 79] Simple plasmapheresis is particularly useful in post-transfusion purpura, because it is typically self-limited and responds definitively to a short series of plasma exchanges. Treatment of either alloimmune transplant recipients[80–82] or patients with anti–factor VIII or IX inhibitors[83–86] appears to be most effective when plasma exchange is combined with IgG and/or IgM immunoadsorption and immunomodulation techniques.[87, 88]

Plasma exchange has been widely used to achieve short-term relief from the clinical manifestations of autoimmune disorders such as myasthenia gravis;[9, 89] acute (Guillain-Barré syndrome)[9, 90] and chronic[91] inflammatory demyelinating polyneuropathy;[9, 92, 93] neuropathies caused by myelin-toxic IgG or IgM paraproteins;[92, 93] autoimmune hemolytic anemias and their cold agglutinin variants;[94, 95] idiopathic thrombocytopenic purpura;[96, 97] Evans' syndrome (concomitant autoimmune hemolytic anemia and idiopathic thrombocytopenic purpura);[98] fulminant systemic or cerebral vasculitides as in systemic lupus erythematosus;[99] and the manifold disorders resulting from human immunodeficiency virus–mediated immune dysregulation.[100] The therapeutic goal in each is similar: removal of pathogenic immunoglobulin so that symptomatic disease activity subsides quickly. Short-term success is commonplace. Long-term success in disease control typically depends on use of immunomodulators such as corticosteroids and intravenous gamma globulin preparations.[101] Plasma exchange may be used as an adjunctive therapy when only partial success is achieved by other measures or a patient cannot tolerate effective doses of available agents. It may also serve as a primary reinduction measure when an acute severe relapse punctuates an otherwise symptom-free interval in a patient with one of these chronic illnesses.

A non-"immune" disorder caused by immunoglobulins and amenable to improvement with plasma exchange is that of hyperviscosity caused by paraproteinemia accompanying plasma cell dyscrasia.[102] Hyperviscosity occurs most frequently in multiple myeloma, typically when IgG paraproteins are present in high concentration in plasma[102, 103] or when self-associating paraproteins, typically immunoglobulin A (IgA), are produced.[104] It has been suggested that excessive plasma levels of kappa light chain may induce symptoms of hyperviscosity.[105, 106] Waldenström's macroglobulinemia, a neoplastic disorder of relatively well-differentiated B cells, although less common than multiple myeloma, is frequently implicated in hyperviscosity syndromes; the IgM macroglobulin secreted by its plasmacytoid lymphocytes, a molecule approximately five times larger than IgG, contributes to whole blood and plasma viscosity.[107] Hyperviscosity symptoms are effectively relieved by plasmapheresis[108–111]—IgM with one or two procedures because it is distributed chiefly within the vascular space[8, 108, 109] and IgG or IgA with three to six, depending on the initial plasma concentrations.[110, 111] Long-term relief is achieved with cytotoxic chemotherapy directed toward the underlying neoplastic disorder.

TTP is a lethal disorder of disputed etiology, characterized by microvascular thrombosis and secondary hemolytic anemia and thrombocytopenia. The low frequency and high mortality of the untreated disease have discouraged the performance of randomized controlled therapeutic trials.[112] Whole blood and plasma exchange became established empirically as effective therapy[10–12] but dispute about the comparative efficacy of plasma exchange[14] and plasma infusion[13] continued until 1991, when results of the Canadian Plasmapheresis Study Group established the superiority of plasma exchange for TTP.[22] A simultaneously reported, uncontrolled but extensive companion study has lent support to its efficacy.[23] Hemolytic-uremic syndrome (HUS), regarded by many as a TTP-like syndrome with manifestations restricted to the renal vasculature, has not been studied in this fashion, but literature reports of effective treatment by plasmapheresis have guided clinicians toward its use.[113] Uncontrolled studies have suggested that plasma immunoadsorption therapy, an immunoaffinity variant of conventional plasma exchange, may have some efficacy in ameliorating HUS;[114, 115] controlled studies to evaluate efficacy are in the planning stages.

A valuable review of apheresis practice in Canada from 1982 to 1987 by the Canadian Apheresis Study Group established that neurologic disease had superseded hematologic disease as the most frequent indication for plasmapheresis in 1987 and accounted for 60% of all procedures.[116] The procedure numbers include multiple sclerosis, for which plasmapheresis is undergoing controlled study in Canada but no consensus for plasmapheresis has developed in the United States. However, exclusion of multiple sclerosis does not alter the primacy of neurologic diseases, chiefly myasthenia gravis and acute and chronic inflammatory polyneuropathy (Guillain-Barré syndrome), as an indication for therapeutic plasma exchange. Clinical trials comparing the efficacy of intravenous immunoglobulin administration with that of plasma exchange in myasthenia gravis and Guillain-Barré syndrome are in progress. Although flawed by methodologic inconsistencies and poor overall response rates compared with previous studies,[117, 118] one study suggests that immunoglobulin may be as effective as or more effective than plasma exchange for Guillain-Barré syndrome.[119] Current studies are helping to establish the relative values of these therapies for debilitating neurologic illness. The potential value of plasmapheresis in other conditions is therefore becoming more clear. Two studies of plasmapheresis for severe lupus nephritis and for corticosteroid-resistant polymyositis and dermatomyositis indicated that the procedure was not more effective than the standard or sham therapy.[120, 121] Accordingly, the effectiveness of plasmapheresis in altering the course of disease is limited to a restricted number of disorders, and the procedure is no longer widely used or recommended for a variety of desperate disorders.[122]

Tables 122–1 and 122–2 outline representative treatment regimens for various disorders in which plasma exchange may be effective.

VASCULAR ACCESS

The requirements for vascular access for therapeutic apheresis are similar to those for successful hemodialysis: cannulas used for blood outflow from the patient must be sufficiently rigid to withstand substantial negative "draw" pressure from the apheresis instrument and of sufficiently great diameter to permit rapid blood flow, and those used for blood return, although not necessarily as sturdy, must still permit rapid enough flow to prevent development of high back pressures in the instrument. For short-term or intermittent use in patients with large accessible peripheral veins, standard steel needles or plastic cannulas of adequate diameter may be inserted into antecubital or large forearm veins (No. 14 to 18 French for the draw, No. 19 to 21 French for the return line, based on the patient's size).[123, 124] Repetitive procedures, chronic or maintenance apheresis regimens, or single procedures in patients with inaccessible or sclerotic peripheral veins may necessitate the use of double-lumen intravenous catheters. Scalp vein infusion sets, soft polyethylene central venous catheters, and the Silastic catheters and infusion port devices used for long-term chemotherapy or blood product administration are not useful for apheresis because they collapse with machine-gener-

TABLE 122–1

TREATMENT REGIMENS FOR IMMUNOGLOBULIN-MEDIATED DISORDERS

Disorder	Putative Target	Replacement Fluid	Exchange Schedule (at 1 Plasma Volume)
Myasthenia gravis	Anti–acetylcholine receptor antibody	5% albumin	Induction: six q.o.d. exchanges
Guillain-Barré syndrome	Myelin-toxic antibody (?)	5% albumin	q.o.d. exchange until rate of improvement stable
Chronic relapsing polyneuropathy	Myelin-toxic immunoglobulin	5% albumin	Induction: six q.o.d. exchanges, then weekly to monthly
Myelin-toxic gammopathy	Myelin-toxic paraprotein	5% albumin	IgM: three q.o.d. exchanges, then monthly IgG: six q.o.d. exchanges, then monthly
Hyperviscosity syndromes	IgG, IgA, IgM paraproteins	5% albumin	IgM: two or three exchanges IgG, IgA: six q.o.d. exchanges
Myeloma kidney	IgG, IgA, free light chains	5% albumin	Six to nine q.o.d. exchanges
Idiopathic thrombocytopenic purpura	Platelet-associated immunoglobulin	5% albumin Immunoglobulin-depleted plasma	Six to nine q.o.d. exchanges or staphylococcal protein A adsorption

ated suction and have narrow lumens permitting only moderate flow rates.

Two catheter types have been found suitable for patients with inadequate peripheral veins or those requiring frequent apheresis over a prolonged time. The Quinton-Mahurkar catheter,[125] a rigid double-lumen plastic catheter suitable for insertion into either the subclavian or femoral vein, can be used for up to 2 weeks after aseptic bedside insertion. The Quinton Perma-Cath and the Davol/Bard Perma-Cath, slightly more flexible double-lumen catheters that are inserted into the subclavian vein in the operating suite with mild sedation and local anesthesia, are useful for several months, available for both pediatric and adult patients, and particularly suitable for chronic outpatient apheresis. Both types of catheters must be dressed aseptically and flushed with heparinized saline (2500 U of 1:1000 heparin/mL saline, the volume used dependent on catheter gauge and length) in meticulous fashion two or three times weekly, using precautions appropriate for all central venous catheters and following any additional instructions provided in the product inserts. Because of the size and rigidity of these catheters, caps must be replaced firmly on catheter ports and clamps must remain closed while the catheter is not in use to prevent air embolism, thrombosis in the catheter lumen, or serious hemorrhage resulting from catheter leak. Patients should be instructed in proper catheter care, even if care is to be given by a home care agency, to ensure that proper technique and heparin solutions of the correct concentration are used.

Clotted catheters can be declotted using thrombolytic agents. A poorly functioning catheter, unilateral arm swelling, or tenderness suggests subclavian and/or axillary venous thrombosis. Noninvasive and radiocontrast imaging techniques may be necessary to define the extent of thrombus, and moderate-dose thrombolytic therapy or systemic heparin administration may be required for relief of symptomatic venous obstruction.

The value of surveillance blood cultures for chronic venous catheters has not been established, but apheresis personnel should be vigilant for early signs of catheter bacterial colonization or infection: erythema or tenderness at the insertion site; fever, chills, or sweats within hours of catheter flushing; unexplained malaise, arthralgias, or myalgias; and normocytic or microcytic anemia out of proportion to blood loss from apheresis and blood sampling. Chronic catheters may be sterilized with appropriate systemic antibiotic therapy. Continued symptoms or positive blood cultures despite adequate blood levels of appropriate antibiotic, however, necessitate catheter removal and a 7- to 14-day course of systemic antibiotics when negative cultures have been achieved. Continued bacteremia implies a septic focus, possibly endocarditis; appropriate diagnostic procedures should be undertaken to evaluate this possibility.

Long-term access in some patients is best achieved by surgical creation of arteriovenous fistulas[126, 127] or insertion of prosthetic vascular segments.[128, 129] Because healing and "maturation" of these constructs require 6 to 8 weeks, the need for chronic apheresis should be anticipated to allow their creation while a semipermanent catheter is still useful

TABLE 122–2

TREATMENT REGIMENS FOR THROMBOTIC THROMBOCYTOPENIC PURPURA AND HEMOLYTIC-UREMIC SYNDROME

Disorder	Putative Target	Replacement Fluid	Exchange Schedule
TTP	Endothelium-toxic immunoglobulin (?) Ultra–high-molecular-weight von Willebrand's factor (?) Platelet-aggregating factor (?)	Fresh frozen plasma	Daily until lactate dehydrogenase and platelets normal, then q.o.d. Corticosteroids, dipyridamole adjunctive prescription
HUS	Endothelium-toxic immune complexes	Fresh frozen plasma or plasma-albumin mixture	Daily or q.o.d. until platelets normal, creatinine decreasing; hemodialysis often necessary

and reduce the number of invasive procedures a patient must undergo. Complications of arteriovenous fistulas and vascular grafts include vascular scarring, thrombosis, infection, aneurysm and pseudoaneurysm formation, and arterial steal and high-output cardiac failure,[126, 127] and these must be weighed against the potential benefit of long-term apheresis therapy.

ANTICOAGULATION

The anticoagulant used obligatorily during apheresis is acid-citrate-dextrose, formula A, or a variant thereof, a compound in routine blood bank use. This agent, a nutrient calcium-chelating solution, is used in the extracorporeal circuit of the apheresis instrument and is administered as a continuous intravenous solution throughout the apheresis procedure. Its composition per liter of solution is 4.90 g dextrose, 4.40 g sodium citrate, and 1.46 g citric acid, and its major side effect is symptomatic hypocalcemia.[130, 131] Because citrate metabolism is hepatocellular, use in patients with severely impaired hepatic function may necessitate a decreased infusion rate[132] or careful attention to calcium replacement.[133] In practice, despite continuing literature dialogue about its advisability,[132, 133] calcium gluconate is often added to replacement fluids in the amount of 3.76 mEq (8.0 mL) per 0.5 L of fluid.[134] Alternatively, when addition to the replacement fluid is not feasible (e.g., when fresh frozen plasma is used), calcium gluconate can be administered by slow intravenous push. Infusion rate of a 10% calcium gluconate solution should not exceed 0.5 mL/min, to avoid cardiac rhythm abnormalities.

For many patients, simple anticoagulation with acid-citrate-dextrose, formula A, is sufficient for uneventful apheresis and circumvents the possibility of clinical bleeding or sensitization with thrombocytopenia and leukopenia caused by proteoglycan anticoagulants.[135] In others, however, particularly those with hyperviscosity syndromes, sickle cell disease, and myasthenia gravis, additional anticoagulation with heparin sodium may be necessary to maintain fluid instrument circuits. In these cases, careful attention must be paid to heparin pharmacokinetics (half-time, 60 to 120 minutes; pseudo–first-order kinetics) and observation of the patient. Routine heparin monitoring techniques are rarely useful because of the relatively short duration of most apheresis procedures, but in patients in whom lengthy procedures are necessitated by large plasma volumes, activated clotting time monitoring of heparin concentration may be useful in adjusting dosage.

REPLACEMENT FLUIDS

To maintain hemodynamic stability in a patient undergoing therapeutic apheresis, the volume of cell suspension or plasma withdrawn mechanically during a continuous procedure must be replaced with a fluid appropriate to the clinical situation. Replacement fluids should be administered through a carefully calibrated blood warming device, especially when returning processed blood through a subclavian line or treating pediatric patients.[1] Mild electrolyte or mineral imbalance before the procedure may be addressed with in-line supplementation of the deficient element, but this should not be undertaken without careful consideration of flow rate, particularly when return is through a central venous catheter.

In cytoreduction procedures such as leukapheresis or thrombocytapheresis for relief of symptomatic hyperviscosity in neoplastic hematologic disorders, decreased total packed cell volume is a therapeutic goal. Because the material removed by apheresis consists chiefly of cells suspended in relatively small amounts of plasma, simple crystalloid replacement results in mild hemodilution and is thus recommended. Special circumstances, such as the coexistence of disseminated intravascular coagulopathy with extreme leukocytosis, may warrant fresh frozen plasma replacement.

Cell replacement during erythrocytapheresis is achieved with the use of packed red blood cells. Because red blood cell removal and replacement are quite rapid ($\geq$40 mL/min), allowing little time to respond to early manifestations of a transfusion reaction, careful cross-matching is essential, and removal of white blood cell and platelet contamination by washing or filtration leukocyte depletion is recommended.[136]

Plasmapheresis, or plasma exchange, often results in removal of one or more plasma volume equivalents, necessitating replacement by colloid with an oncotic pressure similar to that of plasma. Fresh frozen plasma was the early replacement fluid, but because of the risk of plasma-borne infections such as the viral hepatitides and human immunodeficiency virus, high cost per volume unit, and possible allergic reactions, plasma replacement is now usually reserved for clinical syndromes such as TTP, HUS, and occasionally leukostasis with consumptive coagulopathy, in which its use has specific, often empirical, therapeutic justification. Because fresh frozen plasma contains citrate anticoagulant, symptomatic hypocalcemia may be more prominent with plasma replacement than with crystalloid or albumin, especially with the large-volume exchanges performed in anemic patients with TTP and HUS.[132]

Human serum albumin, a pasteurized semipurified product known to be free of identified transmissible pathogenic organisms, has proved most useful as a plasma replacement solution. Solutions of 5% (w/v) albumin in saline are available from several manufacturers of biologicals and may be used without further modification. In routine clinical practice, particularly for patients with large plasma volumes, potassium chloride replacement by addition of 1 to 2 mEq of KCl per 0.5 L of 5% albumin—not to exceed a total of 20 mEq of KCl per plasma exchange—(amount based on patient's prepheresis serum potassium concentration and adjusted based on estimation of total body potassium status) may be useful in preventing clinically significant potassium depletion after the procedure. Calcium replacement during the procedure may be necessary to prevent symptoms of citrate-mediated hypocalcemia and can be accomplished either by intermittent intravenous injection of calcium gluconate or by oral administration of calcium carbonate wafers.

CALCULATIONS

Simple calculations are used to determine whole blood volume, plasma volume, and red blood cell mass before an apheresis procedure. Simple formulas in general use are stated in the following; additional nomograms are described in the literature.[1, 137, 138] Current apheresis instrument software contains algorithms for specific procedures such that the patient's height, weight, hematocrit (Hct) value, and so forth are entered and the instrument calculates anticoagulant, blood product, and fluid replacement needs. The apheresis clinician must still be proficient in determining these parameters to estimate fluid or blood product replacement needs for a procedure, validate the instrument algorithms, and manually override present instrument parameters in unique situations.

$$\text{Total blood volume (TBV)} = \text{patient's weight (kg)} \times 70 \text{ mL/kg}$$

$$\text{Plasma volume} = \text{TBV} \times (100 - \text{Hct})$$

$$\text{Red cell volume} = \text{TBV} \times \text{Hct}/100$$

Quantities of replacement materials for plasma exchange and erythrocytapheresis can be calculated by using the following volume approximations:

One unit of fresh frozen plasma = 250 mL

One unit of packed red blood cells = 250 mL

Exchange of one plasma volume removes approximately 60% of a molecule distributed exclusively in the intravascular compartment (e.g., IgM). Concentration gradient–directed diffusion of molecules with extracellular fluid compartment distribution results in vascular reaccumulation of these molecules over 24 to 72 hours, and five to nine additional exchanges of one plasma volume each are needed to achieve more than 90% depletion, assuming no significant resynthesis during the period of plasma exchange.[137] Little apparent benefit results from exchange of more than one plasma volume per procedure, because of decreasing yield of pathogenic molecules in removed plasma, increased infused citrate load, and the patient's intolerance for long exchange times.[1, 133, 134, 136, 137]

Cytapheresis (e.g., leukapheresis or thrombocytapheresis) performed by a skilled apheresis clinician processing one blood volume removes 40 to 60% of circulating cells.[31] Erythrocytapheresis with exchange of 1 to 1.5 red blood cell volumes can be expected to decrease a sickle cell patient's pretreatment hemoglobin S concentration by approximately 50%.[54, 56, 58]

COMPLICATIONS

Compared with many other modern medical procedures, therapeutic apheresis is rather uncomplicated. A solitary leukapheresis or thrombocytapheresis, performed using needle access to peripheral veins, may result in such dramatic relief of hyperviscosity symptoms that the discomfort of venipuncture seems trivial. The complications that occur are related to the establishment of vascular access; use of a calcium-binding anticoagulant; altered plasma pharmacokinetics for essential medications; removal of protective serum immunoglobulins and coagulation factors with frequently repeated plasmapheresis; hypersensitivity to a component of the replacement material—albumin, fresh frozen plasma, or erythrocytes; possible activation of inflammatory cells or plasma components on ultrafiltration membranes or extracorporeal affinity-binding materials; and the volume of the extracorporeal circuit in patients with severe anemia or a small blood volume.

Achievement of vascular access may be difficult in pediatric patients, patients with small or fragile peripheral veins, or patients who have undergone repetitive intravenous fluid or drug administration with venous sclerosis. In these patients, insertion of a Quinton catheter or its equivalent into a femoral site may be accompanied by bleeding and hematoma formation, pain, or arterial laceration and, because of catheter size and rigidity, may make it necessary for patients to remain at bed rest while it is in place. Subclavian insertion may be complicated by venous or arterial laceration with hematoma formation, hemothorax, or pneumothorax. Poor insertion technique, inadequate catheter care, or failure to replace a temporary catheter in timely fashion may result in either local infection or bacteremia with sepsis. Catheter occlusion by thrombus may occur and, if unrecognized, result in venous thrombosis with limb pain, swelling, and possible embolization. Proper care in insertion, dressing, flushing, and removal of these catheters, as well as good general care of the patient, renders these complications infrequent.

Complications related to the use of citrate-based anticoagulants may be minimized by cautious use in patients with hepatic insufficiency, decreased flow rates in patients with symptomatic hypocalcemia, and either oral or intravenous calcium supplementation during the apheresis procedure.

Altered plasma levels of critical medications may affect disease outcome, if not properly addressed. All plasma protein–bound agents are removed by plasma exchange, with both short-term depletion of circulating agent and long-term undermedication if apheresis losses are not considered in the dosing regimen.[137] Of particular concern are cardiac medications, anticonvulsants, and cholinergic medications used in the treatment of myasthenia gravis, because all are susceptible to rapid fluctuation during plasma exchange.[65, 139–141] Myasthenic patients and those with seizure disorders often require additional or larger doses before apheresis. Medications given once daily should be administered after plasma exchange to ensure that adequate stable tissue distribution occurs.

Frequent repetition of plasma exchange with albumin replacement may result in serum immunoglobulin and coagulation factor depletion. Clinically significant depletion of coagulation factors is not observed if large-volume exchange procedures are separated by 36 to 48 hours, allowing reequilibration of vascular and intravascular components and repletion by new protein synthesis.[137] Progressive immunoglobulin depletion is, in many disease states, both a therapeutic goal (e.g., the removal of a myelin-toxic IgG) and a potential complication, increasing susceptibility to bacterial or fungal infection in an often already seriously ill patient. Because plasma exchange regimens are designed to enhance pathogenic immunoglobulin removal, administration of a pasteurized intravenous pooled normal immunoglobulin preparation at a dose of 0.4 to 1.0 g/kg after an "induction" series of plasma exchange procedures may be beneficial in preventing infection and enhancing immunomodulation of the underlying disease state.

Hypersensitivity to albumin or plasma components may become evident during a procedure by the appearance of urticaria, fever, dyspnea, hypertension, or hypotension and should be treated aggressively with antihistamines, meperidine, corticosteroids, additional fluids, and vasopressors, if extreme. Such reactions are more common with plasma replacement and occur more frequently in alloimmunized patients, that is, multigravid patients or those who have received blood products previously. Patients with a history of hypersensitivity should receive premedication with corticosteroids and antihistamines, have resuscitation equipment in readiness nearby, and, if severely symptomatic despite premedication, receive plasma prepared from units of blood depleted of leukocytes immediately after being drawn.

Transfusion reactions may occur in patients undergoing erythrocytapheresis and may be severe because the apheresis instrument's rapid flow rate may result in a large-volume infusion of incompatible cells before the reaction is recognized. Meticulous blood banking technique and adherence to nursing routine prevent all but the most unusual reactions. Occurrence of a hemolytic transfusion reaction during erythrocytapheresis is a medical emergency requiring immediate cessation of the procedure, rapid fluid and mannitol infusion to enhance renal blood flow and glomerular filtration rate, obtaining of both plasma and urine specimens for blood bank analysis, and other emergency support measures as judged by the apheresis physician. Use of leukocyte-poor or washed red blood cells minimizes the incidence of human leukocyte antigen alloantibody-mediated transfusion incidents and obviates the need for sedating premedication.[136]

Activation of platelets and white blood cells on apheresis ultrafiltration membranes with febrile reactions and respiratory distress, such as may occur on hemodialysis or cardiopulmonary bypass instrument membranes, has not been reported in patients undergoing plasma exchange. Should it occur, substitution of a centrifugal method of apheresis would be curative. Anaphylactoid reactions have been reported in patients undergoing immunoadsorption plasmapheresis using a staphylococcal protein A–silica gel affinity column (Prosorba, Imre, Seattle, WA). These have been attributed to complement activation by the protein A–silica gel, although the possibility of leaching of protein A from the column into the returned plasma has not been disproved. Reactions are ameliorated by antihistamines, corticosteroids, and meperidine and become less severe with repetitive immunoadsorption procedures, but they are still a cause for concern in fragile, seriously ill patients.

The volume of the extracorporeal circuit in apheresis instruments varies from approximately 170 to 250 mL and may present a problem in a pediatric patient with a small blood volume, a severely anemic adult patient, or one who is hemodynamically unstable. Priming the extracorporeal circuit with albumin or saline-diluted packed compatible red blood cells has allowed successful apheresis in pediatric patients as small as 2 kg[142] and virtually any adult patient with adequate left ventricular function.

COST-BENEFIT CONSIDERATIONS

The cost of apheresis therapy is a composite of instrument expense and depreciation and costs for instrument disposable "software"; anticoagulant and diluent solutions; albumin, plasma, or erythrocyte replacement fluids; clinical laboratory tests; nursing and physician time; and hospital or blood bank overhead. These costs are somewhat variable between and within geographic regions but are considerable. They must be balanced, however, against both the social costs of morbidity and mortality resulting from life-threatening disorders and the costs of prolonged provision of critical care and extended rehabilitation programs. The value of apheresis techniques in preventing morbidity from genetic disorders such as sickle cell disease and enhancing recovery from various serious or disabling acquired illnesses can be expressed in terms of medical care dollars saved or, more important, in terms of the return to health and productive life of patients with these disorders. It is hoped that all invasive therapeutic procedures, particularly those involving infusion of blood or blood products, will eventually be replaced with more specific, less hazardous, and less costly therapies. Until they are, therapeutic apheresis can provide rapid and unique benefits in a variety of critical disease states[143, 144] and should be a familiar technique in the repertoire of the critical care physician.

References

1. Gianino NJ: American Red Cross Blood Services Directive 4.47—Therapeutic apheresis. J Clin Apheresis 2:290, 1985.
2. Nusbacher J: Therapeutic hemapheresis: Indications, efficacy, complications. In: Williams WJ, Beutler E, Erslev AJ, et al (eds): Hematology. 4th ed. New York, McGraw-Hill, p 1686, 1990.
3. Knober RM: Photopheresis: Extracorporeal irradiation of 8-MOP containing blood, a new therapeutic modality. Blut 54:247, 1987.
4. Santella RM, Dharmaraja N, Gasparro FP, et al: Monoclonal antibodies to DNA modified by 8-methoxypsoralen and ultraviolet A light. Nucleic Acids Res 13:2533, 1985.
5. Edelson RL: Light-activated drugs. Sci Am 259(2):68, 1988.
6. Honigsmann H, Brenner W, Rauschmeier W, et al: Photochemotherapy for cutaneous T-cell lymphoma. J Am Acad Dermatol 10:238, 1984.
7. Edelson R, Berger C, Gasparro F, et al: Treatment of cutaneous T-cell lymphoma by extracorporeal photochemotherapy. N Engl J Med 316:297, 1987.
8. Lawson NS, Nosanchuk JS, Oberman HA, et al: Therapeutic plasmapheresis in treatment of patients with Waldenström's macroglobulinemia. Transfusion 8:174, 1968.
9. Lisak R: Plasma exchange in neurologic diseases. Arch Neurol 41:654, 1984.
10. Rubenstein MA, Kagan EM, MacGillivray MH: Unusual remission in a case of thrombotic thrombocytopenic purpura syndrome following fresh blood exchange transfusions. Ann Intern Med 51:1409, 1959.
11. Pisciotta AV, Garthwaite T, Darin J, et al: Treatment of thrombotic thrombocytopenic purpura by exchange transfusion. Am J Hematol 3:73, 1977.
12. Bukowski RM, King JW, Hewlett JS: Plasmapheresis in the treatment of thrombotic thrombocytopenic purpura. Blood 50:413, 1977.
13. Byrnes JJ, Khurana M: Treatment of thrombotic thrombocytopenic purpura with plasma. N Engl J Med 297:1386, 1977.
14. Taft EG: Thrombotic thrombocytopenic purpura and dose of plasma exchange. Blood 54:842, 1979.
15. Lian EC, Harkness DR, Byrnes JJ: Presence of a platelet aggregating factor in the plasma of patients with thrombotic thrombocytopenic purpura (TTP) and its inhibition by normal plasma. Blood 53:333, 1979.
16. Byrnes JJ, Lian EC: Recent therapeutic advances in treatment of thrombotic thrombocytopenic purpura. Semin Thromb Hemost 5:199, 1979.
17. Myers TJ, Wakem CJ, Ball ED, et al: Thrombotic thrombocytopenic purpura: Combined treatment with plasmapheresis and antiplatelet agents. Ann Intern Med 92:149, 1980.
18. Rossi EC, DelGreco F, Kwaan HC, et al: Hemodialysis-exchange transfusion for treatment of thrombotic thrombocytopenic purpura. JAMA 244:1466, 1980.
19. Breckenridge RL, Solberg LA, Pineda AA: Treatment of thrombotic thrombocytopenic purpura with plasma exchange, antiplatelet agents, corticosteroids and plasma infusion: Mayo Clinic experience. J Clin Apheresis 1:6, 1982.
20. Machin SJ: Thrombotic thrombocytopenic purpura. Br J Haematol 56:191, 1984.
21. Blitzer JB, Granfortuna JM, Gottlieb AJ: Thrombotic thrombocytopenic purpura: Treatment with plasmapheresis. Am J Hematol 24:329, 1987.
22. Rock GA, Shumak KH, Buskard NA, et al: Comparison of plasma exchange with plasma infusion in the treatment of thrombotic thrombocytopenic purpura. N Engl J Med 325:393, 1991.
23. Bell WR, Braine HG, Ness PM, et al: Improved survival in thrombotic thrombocytopenic purpura–hemolytic uremic syndrome. N Engl J Med 325:398, 1991.
24. Snyder HW, Balint JP, Jones FR: Modulation of immunity in patients with autoimmune disease and cancer treated by extracorporeal immunoadsorption with Prosorba columns. Semin Hematol 26(suppl 1):10, 1989.
25. Yokoyama S, Hayashi R, Satani M, et al: Low-density lipoprotein (LDL) apheresis using dextran sulfate–cellulose in familial hypercholesterolemia. Ther Plasmapheresis 5:325, 1985.
26. Riesen WF: Experience with low-density lipoprotein apheresis by polyclonal and monoclonal antiOapolipoprotein B antibodies and by dextran sulfate cellulose. Curr Stud Hematol Blood Transfus 57:208, 1990.
27. Milleward B, Hueltg G: The historic development of automated hemapheresis. J Clin Apheresis 1:25, 1982.
28. Jones A: The IBM Blood Cell Separator and Blood Cell Processor: A personal perspective. J Clin Apheresis 4:171, 1988.
29. Sawada K, Malchesky PS, Nose Y: Available removal systems: State of the art. Curr Stud Haematol Blood Transfus 57:51, 1990.
30. Samtleben W, Ronderson D, Blumenstein M: Apheresis: Principles and application techniques. J Clin Apheresis 2:163, 1984.
31. Culotta E: Apheresis. In: Harmenin D (ed): Modern Blood Banking and Transfusion Practices. 2nd ed. Philadelphia, FA Davis, p 276, 1989.
32. Smith J, Malchesky P, Nose Y: Membrane plasma separation: Current clinical uses and future directions. Plasma Ther Transfus Technol 5:283, 1984.
33. Farrell P: Apheresis using membrane systems: Physical principles, problems, and applications. Plasma Ther Transfus Technol 5:291, 1984.
34. Malchesky P, Smith J, Nose Y: Membrane separators: Which one to choose. Plasma Ther Transfus Technol 5:299, 1984.
35. Lichtman MA, Heal J, Rowe JM: Hyperleukocytic leukemia: Rheological and clinical features and management. Ballieres Clin Hematol 1:725, 1987.
36. Lichtman MA: Rheology of leukocytes, leukocyte suspensions and blood in leukemia. J Clin Invest 52:350, 1973.
37. Taft EG, Babcock RB, Scharfman WB, et al: Plateletpheresis in the management of thrombocytosis. Blood 50:927, 1977.
38. Younger J, Umlas J: Rapid reduction of platelet count in essential hemorrhagic thrombocythemia by discontinuous flow plateletpheresis. Am J Med 64:659, 1978.
39. Panlilio AL, Reiss RF: Therapeutic plateletpheresis in thrombocythemia. Transfusion 19:147, 1979.
40. Taft EG: Apheresis in platelet disorders. Plasma Ther Transfus Technol 2:181, 1982.
41. Goldfinger D, Thompson R, Lowe C: Long-term plateletpheresis in the management of primary thrombocytosis. Transfusion 19:336, 1979.
42. Fritz RD, Forkner GE, Freireich EJ: The association of fatal intracranial hemorrhage and "blastic crisis" in patients with acute leukemia. N Engl J Med 261:59, 1959.

43. McKee LC, Collins RD: Intravascular leukocyte thrombi and aggregates as a cause of morbidity and mortality in leukemia. Medicine 53:463, 1974.

44. Ventura GJ, Hester JP, Smith TL, et al: Acute myeloblastic leukemia with hyperleukocytosis: Risk factors for early mortality in induction. Am J Hematol 27:34, 1988.

45. Eisenstadt RS, Berkman EM: Rapid cytoreduction in acute leukemia: Management of cerebral leukostasis by cell pheresis. Transfusion 18:113, 1978.

46. Vallejos GS, McCredie KB, Britten GM, et al: Biological effects of repeated leukapheresis of patients with chronic myelogenous leukemia. Blood 45:925, 1973.

47. Caplan SM, Coco FV, Berkman EM: Management of chronic myeloid leukemia in pregnancy by cell pheresis. Transfusion 18:120, 1978.

48. Curtis JE, Hersh EM, Freireich EJ: Leukapheresis therapy of chronic lymphocytic leukemia. Blood 39:163, 1972.

49. Fay JW, Moore JO, Logue GL, et al: Leukopheresis therapy of leukemic reticuloendotheliosis (hairy cell leukemia). Blood 54:747, 1979.

50. Bongiovanni MB, Katz RS, Tomaszewski JE: Cytapheresis in a patient with Sézary syndrome. Transfusion 21:332, 1981.

51. Ricks P: Further experience with exchange transfusion in sickle cell anemia and pregnancy. Am J Obstet Gynecol 100:1087, 1968.

52. Brody JI, Goldsmith MH, Park SK, et al: Symptomatic crisis of sickle cell anemia treated by limited exchange transfusion. Ann Intern Med 72:327, 1970.

53. Kernoff LM, Botha MB, Jacobs P: Exchange transfusions in sickle cell disease using a continuous-flow blood separator. Transfusion 17:269, 1977.

54. Klein HG, Garner RJ, Miller DM, et al: Automated partial exchange transfusion in sickle cell anemia. Transfusion 20:578, 1980.

55. Miller DM, Winslow RM, Klein HG, et al: Improved exercise performance after exchange transfusion in subjects with sickle cell anemia. Blood 56:1127, 1980.

56. Castro O, Finke CH, Coats D: Improved method for automated red cell exchange in sickle cell anemia. J Clin Apheresis 3:93, 1986.

57. Kleinman S, Thompson-Breton R, Hurvits C, et al: Exchange red blood cell pheresis in a pediatric patient with severe complications of sickle cell anemia. Transfusion 21:443, 1981.

58. Lanzowsky P, Shende A, Karayalcin G: Partial exchange transfusion in sickle cell anemia. Am J Dis Child 132:1206, 1978.

59. Yarrish RL, Janas JS, Nosanchuk JS: Transfusion-acquired falciparum malaria: Treatment with exchange transfusion following delayed diagnosis. Arch Intern Med 142:187, 1982.

60. Kramer SL, Campbell CC, Moncreif RE: Fulminant *Plasmodium falciparum* infection treated with exchange blood transfusion. JAMA 249:244, 1983.

61. Jacoby GA, Hunt JV, Kosinski KS: Treatment of transfusion-transmitted babesiosis by exchange transfusion. N Engl J Med 303:1098, 1980.

62. Cahill KM, Benach JL, Reich LM: Red cell exchange treatment of babesiosis in a splenectomized patient. Transfusion 21:193, 1981.

63. Cundall JR, Moore WH, Jenkins DE: Erythrocyte exchange in paroxysmal nocturnal hemoglobinuria prior to cardiac surgery. Transfusion 18:626, 1978.

64. Miller W: Adverse effects of blood transfusion. In: Rutman R, Miller W (eds): Transfusion Therapy: Principles and Procedures. Rockville, MD, Aspen Systems, p 297, 1981.

65. Shumak KH, Rock GA: Therapeutic plasma exchange. N Engl J Med 310:762, 1984.

66. Rock GA, Pineda AA: Controlled clinical trials: necessity and progress. In: MacPherson J, Kasprisin D (eds): Therapeutic Hemapheresis. Boca Raton, FL, CRC Press, p 179, 1985.

67. Klein H, Balow J, Dau P, et al: Clinical applications of therapeutic apheresis. Report of the Clinical Applications Committee, American Society for Apheresis. J Clin Apheresis 3:1, 1986.

68. Marsaglia G, Thomas ED: Mathematical consideration of cross circulation and exchange transfusion. Transfusion 11:216, 1971.

69. Collins JA: Problems associated with the massive transfusion of stored blood. Surgery 75:274, 1971.

70. McCullough J, Chopek M: Therapeutic plasma exchange. Lab Med 12:745, 1981.

71. Ziegler A, Murphy S, Gardner FH: Post-transfusion purpura: A heterogeneous entity. Blood 45:529, 1975.

72. Kickler TS, Ness PM, Herman HJ, et al: Studies on the pathophysiology of posttransfusion purpura. Blood 68:347, 1986.

73. Cimo PL, Aster RH: Post-transfusion purpura. Successful treatment by exchange transfusion. N Engl J Med 6:290, 1972.

74. Berkman EM, Caplan W, Kim GS: ABO-incompatible bone marrow transplantation: Preparation by plasma exchange and in vivo antibody absorption. Transfusion 18:504, 1978.

75. Bensinger WJ, Baker DA, Buckner CD: Immunoadsorption for removal of A and B blood group antibodies. N Engl J Med 304:160, 1981.

76. Buckner CD, Clift PA, Sanders JE: ABO-incompatible marrow transplants. Transfusion 26:335, 1981.

77. Taube D, Palmer A, Welsh K, et al: Removal of anti-HLA antibodies prior to transplantation: An effective and successful strategy for highly sensitized renal allograft recipients. Transplant Proc 21:694, 1989.

78. Roberts HR: Overview of inhibitors to factor VIII and IX. In: Hoyer LW (ed): Factor VIII Inhibitors. New York, Alan R Liss, p 1, 1984.

79. McMillan CW, Shapiro SS, Whitehurst D, et al: The natural history of factor VIII-C inhibitors in patients with hemophilia A. A national cooperative study. Blood 71:344, 1988.

80. Hakim RM, Milford E, Himmelfard J, et al: Extracorporeal removal of anti-HLA antibodies in transplant candidates. Am J Kidney Dis 16:423, 1990.

81. Taube D: Immunoadsorption in the sensitized transplant recipient. Kidney Int 38:350, 1990.

82. Kupin WL, Venkat KK, Hayashi H, et al: Removal of lymphocytotoxic antibodies by pretransplant immunoadsorption therapy in highly sensitized renal transplant recipients. Transplantation 51:324, 1991.

83. Nilsson IM, Berntorp E, Zettervall O: Induction of split tolerance and clinical cure in high-responding hemophiliacs with factor IX antibodies. Proc Natl Acad Sci USA 83:9169, 1986.

84. Freiburgshaus C, Ohlson S, Nilsson IM: Extracorporeal systems for adsorption of antibodies in hemophilia A and B. Methods Enzymol 137:458, 1988.

85. Nilsson IM, Berntorp E, Zettervall O: Induction of immune tolerance in patients with hemophilia and antibodies to factor VIII by combined treatment with intravenous IgG, cyclophosphamide, and factor VIII. N Engl J Med 318:947, 1988.

86. Uehlinger J, Button GR, McCarthy J, et al: Immunadsorption for coagulation factor inhibitors. Transfusion 31:265, 1991.

87. Freiburgshaus C, Larsson LA, Sundqvist SB, et al: A summary of five years' clinical experience with extensive removal of immunoglobulins. Plasma Ther Transfus Technol 7:545, 1986.

88. Gjorstrup P, Watt RM: Therapeutic protein A immunoadsorption. A review. Transfus Sci 11:281, 1990.

89. Seybold M: Plasmapheresis in myasthenia gravis. Ann NY Acad Sci 505:587, 1987.

90. Khann G, Griffin J, Cornblath D, et al: Plasmapheresis and Guillain-Barré syndrome: Analysis of prognostic factors and the effect of plasmapheresis. Ann Neurol 23:347, 1988.

91. Heininger K, Gibbels E, Besinger UA: Role of therapeutic plasmapheresis in chronic inflammatory demyelinating polyneuropathy. Prog Clin Biol Res 8:275, 1990.

92. Consensus conference: The utility of therapeutic plasmapheresis for neurologic disorders. JAMA 256:1333, 1986.

93. Uldry PA, Steck AJ: Plasma exchange in neurology. Curr Stud Hematol Blood Transfus 57:167, 1990.

94. Branda RF, Moldow CF, McCullough JJ, et al: Plasma exchange in the treatment of immune disease. Transfusion 15:570, 1975.

95. Taft EG, Propp RP, Sullivan SA: Plasma exchange for cold agglutinin hemolytic anemia. Transfusion 18:172, 1977.

96. Branda RF, Tate DY, McCullough JJ, et al: Plasma exchange in the treatment of fulminant idiopathic (autoimmune) thrombocytopenic purpura. Lancet 1:688, 1978.

97. Williams C, Buskard N, Bussel J: Plasma exchange in idiopathic thrombocytopenic purpura. In: Nydegger UE (ed): Therapeutic Hemapheresis. Basel, Karger, p 131, 1990.

98. Patten E, Reuter FP, Castle R, et al: Evans syndrome: Benefit from plasma exchange. Transfusion 18:383, 1978.

99. Jones J: Plasma exchange in systemic lupus erythematosus. In: Nose Y, Malchesky P, Smith J, et al (eds): Plasmapheresis: Therapeutic Applications and New Techniques. New York, Raven Press, p 273, 1983.

100. Kiprov DD, Kwiatkowska BJ, Miller RG: Therapeutic apheresis in human immunodeficiency virus–related syndromes. Curr Stud Hematol Blood Transfus 57:184, 1990.

101. Nydegger UE: Immunoglobulin adjuvant therapy to plasmapheresis in immunopathologic disorders. Plasma Ther Transfus Technol 6:197, 1986.

102. Bloch K, Maki DG: Hyperviscosity syndromes associated with immunoglobulin abnormalities. Semin Hematol 10:113, 1973.

103. McGrath MA, Penny R: Paraproteinemia blood hyperviscosity and clinical manifestations. J Clin Invest 58:1155, 1976.

104. Chandy KG, Stockley RA, Leonard RCF, et al: Relation between hyperviscosity syndrome and intravascular IgA polymer concentration in IgA myeloma. Clin Exp Immunol 46:653, 1981.

105. Carter PJ, Cohen HJ, Crawford J: Hyperviscosity syndrome in association with kappa light chain myeloma. Am J Med 86:591, 1989.

106. Bachrach HJ, Myers JB, Bartholomer WR: A unique case of kappa light-chain disease associated with cryoglobulinemia, pyroglobulinemia, and hyperviscosity syndrome. Am J Med 86:596, 1989.

107. Somer T: Hyperviscosity syndrome in plasma cell dyscrasia. Adv Microcirc 6:1, 1975.

108. Solomon A, Fahey JL: Plasmapheresis therapy in macroglobulinemia. Ann Intern Med 58:789, 1963.

109. Schwab PJ, Fahey JL: Treatment of Waldenström's macroglobulinemia by plasmapheresis. N Engl J Med 263:574, 1960.

110. Powles R, Smith CR, Hamilton-Fairley G: Method of removing abnormal protein rapidly from patients with malignant paraproteinemias. Br Med J 2:664, 1871.

111. Beck JR, Quinn BM, Meier FA, et al: Hyperviscosity syndrome in paraproteinemia. Managed by plasma exchange, monitored by serum tests. Transfusion 22:51, 1982.

112. Amorosi EL, Ultmann JE: Thrombotic thrombocytopenic purpura: Report of 16 cases and review of the literature. Medicine 45:139, 1966.

113. Kalmin ND, Himot ED: Plasmapheresis in a child with the hemolytic-uremic syndrome. Transfusion 23:139, 1983.
114. Mittelman A, Bertram J, Snyder HW Jr, et al: Treatment of patients with HIV thrombocytopenia and hemolytic uremic syndrome with protein A immunoadsorption. Semin Hematol 26(suppl 1):15, 1989.
115. Korec S, Schein P, Smith F, et al: Treatment of cancer-associated hemolytic uremic syndrome with staphylococcal protein A immunoperfusion. J Clin Oncol 4:210, 1986.
116. Rock GA, Tricklebank GW, Kasaboski CA: Plasma exchange in Canada. The Canadian Apheresis Study Group. Can Med Assoc J 142:557, 1990.
117. Guillain-Barré Study Group: Plasmapheresis and acute Guillain-Barré syndrome. Neurology 35:1096, 1984.
118. Osterman PO, Fagius J, Lundemo G, et al: Beneficial effects of plasma exchange in acute inflammatory polyradiculoneuropathy. Lancet 2:1296, 1984.
119. van der Meche FGA, Schmitz PIM, Dutch Guillain-Barré Study Group: A randomized trial comparing intravenous immune globulin and plasma exchange in Guillain-Barré syndrome. N Engl J Med 326:1123, 1992.
120. Miller FW, Leitman SF, Cronin ME, et al: Controlled trial of plasma exchange and leukapheresis in polymyositis and dermatomyositis. N Engl J Med 326:1380, 1992.
121. Lewis EJ, Hunsicker LG, Lan S-P, et al: A controlled trial of plasmapheresis therapy in severe lupus nephritis. N Engl J Med 326:1373, 1992.
122. Campion EW: Desperate diseases and plasmapheresis. N Engl J Med 326:1425, 1992.
123. Reimann P, Mason P: Plasmapheresis: Technique and complications. Intensive Care Med 16:3, 1990.
124. Button G: Vascular access. In: MacPherson J, Kasprisin D (eds): Therapeutic Hemapheresis. Boca Raton, FL, CRC Press, p 29, 1988.
125. Graber D, Dinerstein C: The Quinton-Mahurkar dual lumen subclavian catheter: Preliminary evaluation. Dial Transplant 12:847, 1983.
126. Wilson S, Williams R: Vascular access for hemodialysis. In: Massky S, Glassock R (eds): Textbook of Nephrology. 2nd ed. Baltimore, Williams & Wilkins, p 1362, 1989.
127. Wyman C, Lindbloom L: Hemodialysis: Fistulas. In: Larson E, Lindbloom L, Davis K (eds): Clinical Nephrology Practitioner. St Louis, CV Mosby, p 226, 1982.
128. Schanzer H, Kaplan S, Bosch J, et al: Double lumen rubber indwelling venous catheters. Arch Surg 121:229, 1986.
129. Schwab S, Buller G, McCann R, et al: Prospective evaluation of a Dacron cuffed hemodialysis catheter for prolonged use. Am J Kidney Dis 1:166, 1988.
130. Olson P, Cox C, McCullough J: Laboratory and clinical effects of the infusion of ACD solution during platelet pheresis. Vox Sang 33:79, 1977.
131. Walton D, Penny A, Marshall R, et al: Citrate-induced hypocalcemia during cell separation. Br J Haematol 44:505, 1980.
132. Silberstein L, Naryshil S, Haddad J, et al: Calcium homeostasis during therapeutic plasma exchange. Transfusion 26:151, 1986.
133. Morse E, Hohnadel D, Genco P, et al: Decreased ionized calcium during therapeutic plasma exchange pheresis and platelet pheresis. Johns Hopkins Med J 146:260, 1980.
134. Cobe BCT: Operation. In: Cobe TPE Operator's Handbook. Lakewood, CO, Cobe Laboratories, p 1, 1983.
135. Pinnick R, Wiegmann T, Drederich D: Regional citrate anticoagulation for hemodialysis in the patient at high risk for bleeding. N Engl J Med 316:260, 1983.
136. Goldfinger D, Lowe C: Prevention of adverse reactions to blood transfusion by the administration of saline-washed red blood cells. Transfusion 21:277, 1981.
137. Klein HG: Effect of plasma exchange on plasma constituents: Choice of replacement solutions and kinetics of exchange. In: MacPherson J, Kasprisin D (eds): Therapeutic Hemapheresis. Boca Raton, FL, CRC Press, 1983.
138. Sprenger K, Huber-Kratz W: Nomograms for the prediction of patient plasma volume in plasma exchange therapy from height, weight, and hematocrit. J Clin Apheresis 3:185, 1987.
139. Keller F, Hauff A, Schultze G, et al: Effect of repeated plasma exchange on steady state kinetics of digoxin and digitoxin. In: Nose Y, Malchesky P, Smith J, et al (eds): Plasmapheresis: Therapeutic Applications and New Techniques. New York, Raven Press, p 183, 1983.
140. Buffalo G, Dau P, Erickson R, et al: Technical considerations. In Cobe BCT: Therapeutic Plasma Exchange Disease Compendium. Lakewood, CO, Cobe Laboratories, p 3, 1983.
141. Lai C, Leppik I, Jenkins D, et al: Epilepsy, myasthenia gravis, and the effect of plasmapheresis on antiplatelet drug concentrations. Arch Neurol 47:68, 1990.
142. Kevy S, Fosburg M: Therapeutic apheresis in childhood. J Clin Apheresis 5:87, 1990.
143. Klein HG: Therapeutic apheresis in perspective: Apheresis in transition. In: Nydegger UE (ed): Therapeutic Hemapheresis in the 1990s. Basel, Karger, p 1, 1990.
144. Isbister JP: The risk/benefit equation for therapeutic plasma exchange. In: Nydegger UE (ed): Therapeutic Hemapheresis in the 1990s. Basel, Karger, p 10, 1990.

SECTION TEN

The Gastrointestinal System

Section Editor

Rosemarie L. Fisher

CHAPTER 123

Esophageal Emergencies

Harold M. Schwartz
Morris Traube

Few esophageal disorders are truly emergencies, but knowledge of their presentation and management is essential. Certainly, hemorrhage from esophageal varices, Mallory-Weiss tears, or other disorders is an emergency, but this is discussed in other chapters in this section. The medical intensivist must be familiar with the potentially life-threatening consequences of caustic injury and foreign body ingestion. The physician must also be able to recognize acute obstruction or perforation of the esophagus; delay in diagnosis of the latter is particularly associated with high morbidity and mortality. These true esophageal emergencies are the focus of this chapter.

Symptoms of various esophageal disorders include dysphagia, odynophagia, heartburn, and chest pain. They may be most confusing in the intensive care unit, where cardiac and respiratory diseases are more prevalent. Although it is important to recognize and consider esophageal disorders, most are not true emergencies and can be dealt with in more resolute manner, after more serious conditions are treated or excluded. Only brief mention of some of these disorders is made in this chapter.

CAUSTIC INGESTIONS
Pathophysiology

Although caustic ingestions are underreported, it is estimated that 5000 to 15,000 cases occur in the United States annually.[1, 2] Children account for up to 80% of reported incidents. Among adults, the majority are suicide attempts or accidental ingestions in alcoholics. The location, severity, and extent of injury are related to numerous factors, including the chemical nature (acid vs. alkali, solids vs. liquids) (Table 123-1), concentration, and quantity of the ingestant, as well as the duration of contact.[2]

Commonly ingested alkalis include sodium and potassium hydroxide, sodium and potassium carbonate, ammonium hydroxide, and potassium permanganate. The most damaging ingestions are of concentrated liquid alkali (lye), which cause extensive injury to the esophagus and often to the gastric mucosa.[2] Mucosal damage occurs through liquefaction necrosis, with dissolution of protein and collagen, saponification of fat, and thrombosis of blood vessels.[3] Rapid penetration of successive tissue layers has been demonstrated in animal experiments, in which just a few milliliters of concentrated sodium hydroxide caused transmural burns within seconds of contact.[4] The heat of hydration generated by neutralization, when the ingestant is mixed with gastric

TABLE 123-1
COMMON CORROSIVES

Alkali
Sodium and potassium hydroxide (drain and oven cleaners)
Sodium and potassium carbonate (household cleaners)
Ammonium hydroxide and chloride (toilet bowl, metal, and jewelry cleaners)
Potassium permanganate (topical medications)
Clinitest tablets
Disk (button) batteries

Acids
Hydrochloric and sulfuric acids (drain and toilet bowl cleaners)
Nitric acid
Miscellaneous: oxalic, acetic, carbolic, formic acids; sodium bisulfate

Bleaches
Sodium and calcium hypochlorite (chlorine and household bleaches)
Sodium and hydrogen peroxide
Sodium perborate (commercial bleaches)

Detergents
Sodium phosphates (laundry, dishwasher, and scouring powder cleansers)

Miscellaneous
Iodine
Tablets: potassium, ascorbic acid, chloral hydrate, doxycycline

and intestinal secretions, also contributes to injury. Pyloric spasm and esophageal regurgitation, accompanied by cricopharyngeal spasm, may lead to periods of to-and-fro washing of the ingestant over the esophagus with resultant increased damage.[5] This abnormal motility is often succeeded by esophageal or gastric atony.

It has been claimed that ingestants with an initial pH of greater than 12 are responsible for most serious injury, whereas weak bases such as household bleaches with pH of less than 11 rarely cause similar injury.[2, 6] One study, however, indicated that the extent of injury is more related to the amount of titratable acid or alkali reserve than to the initial pH of the ingested compound.[7] Solid alkalis (crystals, pellets) tend to adhere to the oropharyngeal mucosa and are usually expectorated with the onset of severe local pain.[1] As such, there is usually limited, if any, damage distal to the pharynx. Weaker alkali (e.g., ammonia) is less likely to cause serious long-term damage.

Acid intake is involved in only about 5% of reported caustic ingestions.[8] The most commonly implicated ingestants that cause injury are hydrochloric and sulfuric acids. In contrast to alkali, acids extend their damaging effects via coagulation necrosis, with the formation of a protective superficial eschar, so there is usually less penetration into deeper layers and typically less injury.[9] However, some surveys of concentrated acid ingestion have demonstrated esophageal injury with severity similar to that of alkali ingestion.[8, 10] Indeed, sloughing of mucosa in acid-induced injury can lead to shock and sepsis; as such, acid ingestions should not be treated lightly. Nevertheless, partially because of neutralization in the esophagus and incapacity for penetrating necrosis, most damage occurs not in the esophagus but in the stomach, predominantly along the lesser curvature and antrum. Localization of injury may depend on the patient's position and the amount of pre-existing food in the stomach at the time of ingestion. Esophageal involvement is reported in only 6 to 20% of acid ingestions, usually with concomitant severe gastric injury.[9]

Bleaches (pH ~ 7; sodium hypochlorite and peroxide), soap, and detergents, which are involved in most of the remainder of ingestions, almost never cause serious injury.

The depth of injury to the esophagus is usually graded as in thermal injury to skin.[5] First-degree burns are limited to the mucosa and are manifested by hyperemia, edema, vascular dilation, desquamation, and perhaps tiny superficial punctate ulcers. Second-degree burns extend through the mucosa into the muscularis and are seen grossly as friable lesions with white membranes and deeper ulcers. Third-degree burns are transmural and often extend into the periesophageal and mediastinal tissue. They are almost always circumferential in nature. Prognostic factors are directly related to depth of damage.

Although there is variability in the extent and location of injury, as seen especially with liquid ingestions, damage tends to occur at areas of anatomic narrowing within the esophagus, specifically the cricopharyngeus muscle, aortic arch, left mainstem bronchus, and diaphragmatic pinch.[1]

Acute sequelae of ingestion can include glottic and laryngeal damage leading to airway obstruction; there can often be concurrent damage to skin, eyes, and lungs. Third-degree burns may lead to perforation, periesophagitis and mediastinitis, pericarditis, tracheoesophageal or bronchoesophageal and aortoesophageal fistulas, and in the case of gastric perforation, injury to spleen, pancreas, and other intra-abdominal organs.

First-degree burns heal without scar or stricture formation. In second- and third-degree alkali burns, substantial inflammation and granulation occur within 1 week of ingestion, with early fibroblast activity, thrombosis, and neovas-cularization. Within the second to third weeks, there is collagenogenesis, which leads, during the subsequent few weeks, to fibrous tissue formation, contraction and epithelialization, and in severe cases, shortening of the entire esophagus and dysmotility. Strictures form in approximately 20 to 30% of cases of penetrating injury and are evident as early as 3 weeks after ingestion.[2, 5] Acid ingestions tend to cause gastric stricture, achlorhydria, and dysmotility, and patients may later have gastric outlet obstruction.

Disk, or button, batteries, as used in watches or cameras, can cause corrosive injury to the gastrointestinal tract when ingested.[11] The overwhelming majority of ingestions are by children. Injury usually occurs with batteries greater than 21 mm in diameter because they lodge within the esophagus. Injury probably results from chemical leak of the sodium or potassium hydroxide and mercury oxide, as well as from pressure necrosis and electrical burn from contact with conducting gastrointestinal fluids. Clinitest tablets contain 40 to 50% potassium or sodium hydroxide; after ingestion, severe burns, usually circumferential and often localized to the level of the carina, are seen.[12]

Presentation

The patient may have a variety of signs and symptoms after an acute ingestion, but the severity of injury often does not correlate well with the complaints.[1, 13] Lesions in the buccal mucosa and oropharynx include edema, hyperemia, ulcerations, and friability and may appear as white mucosal plaques or brown-to-black ulcerations. Perioral pain is, of course, the predominant symptom. However, dysphagia, odynophagia, chest pain, and sialorrhea suggest substantial esophageal damage. Fever is common, as is vomiting, and indeed one may see hematemesis. Hoarseness, dyspnea, and stridor all suggest hypopharyngeal and laryngeal or even tracheobronchial involvement. Epigastric pain suggests damage to the stomach or gastroesophageal junction and is often seen in acid ingestion. Rebound tenderness may occur even in the absence of transmural gastric involvement or perforation.[2] One should be alert for symptoms suggesting esophageal perforation, including chest pain, dyspnea, and the presence of subcutaneous emphysema. Perforation may not develop for 48 hours.[14] Table 123–2 summarizes some of the clinical manifestations of caustic ingestion.

TABLE 123–2
COMPLICATIONS OF CAUSTIC INGESTION

Acute
Hemorrhage
Perforation
Mediastinitis or peritonitis
Glottic or laryngeal edema
Aspiration or adult respiratory distress syndrome
Skin and eye injury
Shock

Latent
Strictures
Dysmotility
Infection or abscess
Enteral fistulas: aortoesophageal, tracheoesophageal or bronchoesophageal, gastrocolic

Long-Term
Strictures
Gastric outlet obstruction
Malnutrition (resulting from poor intake)
Aspiration (caused by dysmotility, strictures)
Esophageal carcinoma

Diagnosis

It is important to obtain information from both the patient and the family about the type and amount of ingestant, the time of ingestion, and whether the ingestion was accidental or intentional. Whenever possible, one should obtain the original container. Some authors advocate testing the pH of the substance to help predict the severity of injury.[15]

After vital signs are obtained and the patient is stabilized, the focus should be on possible airway damage, as evidenced by stridor or dyspnea, and on possible perforation. A thorough oral examination should be performed to assess the extent and depth of pharyngeal damage. Radiographs of the neck, the chest, and the abdomen should be obtained to rule out perforation. Indeed, if perforation is suspected, a contrast study should be performed for localization and delineation of extent.

Endoscopy should be performed, as it helps to guide therapy and determine prognosis. If there is suspicion of perforation, evidence of shock, respiratory distress, or airway instability, the procedure should be delayed until it is considered less risky. Some authors also consider high suspicion of third-degree injury as a contraindication.

Controversy exists as to the degree of correlation of esophageal injury with the presence of pharyngeal damage. With acid ingestion, there may be little or no oral abnormalities but much gastric damage. With alkali ingestion, there is almost always pharyngeal damage if esophageal injury has occurred. However, in up to 10% of esophageal injuries, there are less extensive, if any, pharyngeal burns.[16] Contrariwise, in 20 to 60% of pharyngeal burns, there is no esophageal injury.[17] We suggest that there is no need for esophagoscopy in the patient without oropharyngeal lesions, provided (1) there are no symptoms of esophageal injury, such as chest pain or sialorrhea; (2) the ingestant is not a strong acid corrosive; and (3) one is confident that the ingestant has been weak in nature or of small volume.

Endoscopy should otherwise be done within the first 24 hours with a flexible instrument. Although one can usually evaluate safely as distal as the duodenum, the procedure should be terminated when severe circumferential injury is encountered. Introduction of the endoscope should be with direct visualization of the hypopharynx, the larynx, and the proximal esophagus to minimize the risk of perforation. Disk batteries should be removed if entrapped within the esophagus.

Unfortunately, there is no standardized system of interpreting endoscopic findings and of correlating them with pathologic injury. One can attempt to estimate burn depth by the mucosal appearance, but there is great overlap between second- and third-degree burns. First-degree burns usually appear as friable, hyperemic lesions with erythema and perhaps small ulcerations, whereas deep ulcerations and black eschar of gangrene suggest the transmural injury of third-degree burns. Second-degree burns, however, are most difficult to correlate with endoscopic findings. The endoscopist should keep in mind that almost all strictures form within an area of circumferential injury.

Management

There is much confusion in the literature concerning treatment, and many published studies involve only small numbers of patients. Although there is little consensus about treatment, the stated goal is to prevent stricture formation.

Initial management should consist of stabilization of the patient and control of the airway. If there is respiratory compromise, the patient should be endotracheally intubated via the oral approach with direct visualization, but cricothyrotomy may be indicated. Intravenous catheters should be inserted and the patient given crystalloid, and perhaps colloid in the event of severe gastrointestinal hemorrhage. Nothing should be administered by mouth, at least until the evaluation is complete. Emetic agents and charcoal are always contraindicated, as is nasogastric lavage in cases of lye ingestion. Immediate surgery is necessary if there is perforation. There has been debate concerning the administration of diluent or neutralizing liquids. Because severe injury occurs within the first minute after ingestion of strong alkali, and because fluid administration may induce emesis and thus increase injury, this option may be futile and even dangerous. However, in stable patients who have ingested a small amount of mild alkali (bleaches), milk, dilute vinegar, or citrus juice may be carefully administered. In pure acid ingestion, vigorous gastric aspiration followed by cold fluid lavage (with the tube placed under endoscopic visualization) may be of use; antacids are contraindicated because of the heat of neutralization.

After stabilization of the patient and endoscopy, patients with minimal or no damage to mucosa may be discharged with careful medical and psychiatric follow-up, and they may advance their diet as tolerated. On the other side of the spectrum, esophagectomy or gastrectomy or both are indicated for diffuse third-degree burn. Although some authors advocate early exploration in any patient with the mere suspicion of transmural involvement,[3] this approach is controversial and appears institution dependent. Surgery is also necessary in cases complicated by tracheoesophageal or aortoesophageal fistulas.

The management of moderate-to-severe (second-degree) injury remains the most controversial. Administration of steroids with antibiotics had been the mainstay of therapy for years;[18] therapy was usually initiated within 24 hours of ingestion and extended to a complete course of 4 weeks, presumably to prevent extensive fibrosis and stricture formation and to combat secondary mural infection leading to pyogenic granulation. However, more recent studies have not shown benefit from corticosteroids,[15, 19] and their use cannot be universally recommended, except in the presence of laryngeal edema. Antibiotics must be administered only in suspected perforation or aspiration.

Some authors have advocated the use of early, frequent dilation of the esophagus beginning 1 week after ingestion, again presumably to retard stricture formation. This has often been preceded by insertion of a nasogastric tube or string during initial stages of management to ensure luminal patency.[20] Because of lack of good evidence for efficacy, prophylactic bougienage cannot be routinely recommended.

Patients with severe cicatricial injury should be treated with early institution of total parenteral nutrition. They may benefit from insertion of intraluminal Silastic stents,[3] although their role remains unproved.

Diet can be advanced over time, to liquid and then soft, as tolerated. The use of histamine H_2 antagonists or slurried sucralfate has been suggested.[17]

Otorhinolaryngologic consultation should be obtained in the majority of cases, as pharyngolaryngoscopy is often indicated, and treatment of oral lesions, including potential reconstructive surgery, may be necessary.[21] Psychiatric consultation may also be warranted.

In cases of ingestion of a disk battery, plain films help in localization. If lodged within the esophagus, the battery should be removed via endoscopy, which may also allow assessment of local damage. If it is in or distal to the stomach, serial plain films help to assess progress, and after 1 week, strong cathartics may be given. Surgery should be reserved for intestinal perforation or obstruction, or retarded evacuation.

The major long-term complication of caustic injury to the esophagus is the formation of strictures, 80% of which develop within 2 months of ingestion.[17] After strictures have formed, frequent dilation with mercury-weighted bougies or with endoscopically guided devices may be necessary. One must be vigilant in monitoring for dysphagia. Endoscopy, or at least contrast radiography, should routinely be performed 3 weeks after ingestion to assess healing and locate early strictures; dilation is often begun at this point. These studies should be repeated at least at 6 weeks and at 6 months, or when symptoms develop. In cases of multiple or long strictures and bougienage failures, isoperistaltic colonic interposition or insertion of a feeding gastrostomy tube is indicated.

There is an estimated 1000-fold increase in incidence of squamous cell carcinoma in affected areas of the esophagus.[22] As such, the development of dysphagia decades after injury should be anticipated and investigated.

FOREIGN BODY INGESTION
Pathophysiology

Foreign body ingestion is an emergency (1) when there is acute obstruction of the esophagus, which may lead to aspiration, necrosis, or perforation; (2) when the foreign body is sharp or irregular, with potential for bleeding or perforation; or (3) when disk batteries are ingested, as discussed earlier.

Foreign bodies can be classified as either food or nonfood (true) in nature. With the former, impaction in the esophagus leads to the so-called steakhouse syndrome. Typically, the impaction develops in an elderly patient or someone with pre-existing esophageal disease, such as a stricture, ring, or web. Other predisposing factors include an ectatic aorta, decreased oral tactile sensitivity from use of dental prostheses, improper mastication from poor dentition, and esophageal diverticuli. In one study of patients older than 60 years of age, 72% had concomitant esophageal disease; dentures were used by 28% of the patients.[23]

Most nonfood foreign body ingestions are by children. They may also be seen in adults, particularly with psychiatric disease, alcohol abuse, or mental retardation. Ingestions by prisoners are also common. Ingestions are often intentional in these groups. Common accidental ingestants in adults include coins, bones, pits, dentures, and nails or tacks (Table 123–3).

Objects that obstruct the esophagus tend to be either large (as in food impaction) or angulated and sharp (bones, pins). Although 80 to 90% of foreign bodies pass through the gastrointestinal tract without difficulty,[24–26] certain anatomic locations are predisposed as sites of obstruction. These include the cervical esophagus at the lower border of the cricopharyngeus muscle, where there is a transition from striated to smooth muscle; the level of the aortic arch; and the gastroesophageal junction.[24]

Morbidity and mortality are related to the location, the type, and the duration of impaction of the foreign body. Objects that lodge within the esophagus may predispose to a number of complications, including (1) respiratory compromise attributable to aspiration of secretions or the object itself, or from anterior pressure on the trachea at the level of the cricopharyngeal muscle; (2) perforation and fistula formation; and (3) pressure necrosis or local ischemia, as occurs when large food objects are present for longer than 24 hours within the lumen.[25] Rarely, penetration to great vessels may lead to hemorrhage.[27] Although less than 1% of all objects perforate the gastrointestinal tract, one may see perforation rates as high as 15 to 35% with sharp foreign bodies, such as pointed toothpicks, pins, and bones.[25, 28] Finally, even objects that have passed the esophagus may cause injury to the more distal gastrointestinal tract, such as perforation (manifested by abscess formation, peritonitis, or sepsis) and obstruction.

Presentation

Patients with food obstruction usually give a clear history of ingestion. Almost all patients with substantial food bolus or bone impaction have symptoms. These are the sense of choking, distress, the acute onset of dysphagia, odynophagia, and sialorrhea, the latter of which occurs especially in either proximal or complete obstruction. Patients may have symptoms of aspiration or respiratory obstruction, and indeed respiratory signs may be the only manifestation in some cases.[29] Most patients can describe a sensation of obstruction at a certain level in the neck or the chest; in truth, the object may be trapped anywhere distal to this. Many patients have experienced prior similar episodes. Indeed, the patient may have come to expect transient symptoms and rapid improvement, and delay in presentation may result. These patients may be dehydrated and even have orthostatic hypotension.

Only half of patients with true foreign body ingestions have such symptoms.[23] In addition, suicidal and cognitively impaired patients may not relay a history of ingestion. These patients may receive medical attention after substantial delay, and the symptoms and signs will include those of serious complications of the ingestion.

Diagnosis

A complete history should include an evaluation for risk factors in both accidental and intentional ingestions. In the case of food boluses, onset is usually obvious. The patient who has acute dysphagia should be questioned about previous episodes, brief or extended, and any previous esophageal abnormalities. In the case of true foreign bodies, circumstances of previous ingestions should be determined.

The physical examination is generally not helpful, although signs of perforation (see later) should be sought. Distress, fever, and oropharyngeal abrasions or erythema may be present. Pulmonary signs of consolidation, stridor, wheezing, and decreased breath sounds should be sought. The abdomen should be palpated for a mass and for signs of perforation. Sialorrhea suggests either proximal or complete obstruction.

Chest and abdominal radiographs may show evidence of perforation. They should be done to help identify and locate a true foreign body. Cervical soft tissue films may be obtained if proximal impaction or perforation is suspected. Repeated examinations are helpful when symptoms change or disappear.

Endoscopy is the diagnostic method of choice in most

TABLE 123–3
COMMONLY INGESTED FOREIGN BODIES IN ADULTS*

Food boluses
Bones (fish, chicken) or pits
True foreign bodies
  Coins
  Sharp objects: safety pins, razor blades, toothpicks, pins, nails, tacks, needles, glass, wire, paper clips, aluminum can pull-tabs
  Miscellaneous: spoons, dentures, cocaine packets, bottle caps, pen caps, disk batteries

*In order of descending frequency.

patients. Aside from locating and identifying the foreign body, endoscopy allows for its removal, as well as for evaluation of underlying esophageal lesions. Contrast radiography should first be obtained in suspected perforation. It may also be useful if the foreign body is radiolucent (e.g., food, fish bones, glass, aluminum, plastic, and wood) *and* there is either (1) doubt of its continued presence within the esophagus or (2) suspicion of a proximal obstruction, because of known prediagnosed lesion, presence of sialorrhea, or a description of immediate onset of dysphagia. Flexible esophagoscopy may be hazardous in the latter case; otorhinolaryngologic evaluation is warranted when the ingestant is in the proximal esophagus. Contrast studies are best done with water-soluble agents, unless aspiration risk is high, because barium may interfere with subsequent endoscopy.

Management

The patient should be kept in an upright position, frequent suctioning of oral secretions should be performed as needed, and airway stability should be guaranteed and maintained. In the absence of perforation, an individual case approach is used. In general, sharp, irregular, edged, or angulated objects that may cause perforation should be removed immediately via endoscopy. Other objects and food may be removed within 12 to 24 hours after ingestion, unless there is evidence of complete obstruction (e.g., sialorrhea and inability to swallow sip of water) or potential for aspiration. Flexible fiberoptic endoscopy has supplanted rigid esophagoscopy as the method of choice for retrieval, because of its safety and ease of performance.[25] General anesthesia may be necessary for the very young or uncooperative patient, as well as in cases of proximal impaction, the latter of which remains most often treated by rigid esophagoscopy. Foreign bodies at the level of the pharynx or the cricopharyngeus muscle (commonly fish bones) necessitate removal by laryngoscopic approach.

Pharmacologic agents may be given while awaiting endoscopy or in food bolus impaction. Although there have been no controlled studies performed to confirm efficacy, smooth muscle relaxants such as sublingual nifedipine (up to 20 mg), or intravenous diazepam, glucagon, or anticholinergics may be carefully administered. The risk of aspiration, and that of gastric outlet obstruction if atropine is chosen, should be kept in mind. There is no role for this type of therapy with sharp objects, which may cause perforation.

Glucagon is the most useful of these agents and is most appropriate when foreign bodies lie in the distal esophagus. By relaxing smooth muscle, it decreases lower esophageal sphincter tone, although it has no effect on the strictures and rings associated with most cases of meat impaction. A dose of 0.5 mg is injected intravenously, and this may be repeated twice at 10- to 20-minute intervals. Aspiration precautions must be used as glucagon may stimulate nausea.

Enzymatic digestion of boneless meat with papain, administered orally or by catheter, is controversial. There have been reports of esophageal perforations and aspiration-induced hemorrhagic pulmonary edema.[25] Its use is no longer recommended, except where endoscopy is not available, and then only when the bolus impaction is confirmed by a contrast study and of short duration. Likewise, we do not recommend the use of effervescent agents in distending the esophagus (as has been advocated in the radiology literature),[30] because of risk of perforation.

Balloon- or basket-tipped catheters (e.g., Foley's catheter) have been passed under fluoroscopic guidance to help in the removal of blunt foreign bodies. Their use should best be limited to experienced practitioners, particularly if there is no endoscopist and no underlying esophageal disorder.[31]

By and large, however, endoscopic removal of foreign bodies is recommended.

Endoscopic removal of sharp and pointed foreign bodies may be impossible to accomplish, and surgical management is then usually required. If sharp or angulated foreign bodies spontaneously pass the esophagus and stomach into the small bowel, one should monitor carefully for signs of bowel perforation, hemorrhage, or obstruction, in which cases surgery is necessary.[26] Laxatives should not be administered.

After the acute episode of foreign body obstruction has passed, radiographic or endoscopic evaluation of the esophagus may need to be performed to evaluate for the presence of underlying esophageal disease. One should also continue to monitor for evidence of perforation.

PERFORATION

Pathophysiology

Although perforation of the esophagus is an uncommon occurrence, it is associated with high morbidity and mortality. Lack of suspicion of the diagnosis, as from decreased recognition of associated symptoms, too often leads to delay in proper management.

The causes of esophageal perforation can be divided into three broad categories[32] (Table 123-4). These are (1) intraluminal trauma, (2) extraluminal trauma, and (3) spontaneous causes.

The majority of cases of intraluminal trauma are iatrogenic or due to foreign bodies. Although fiberoptic flexible endoscopy is safer than the previously commonplace rigid endoscopy, the increased utilization of therapeutic techniques, such as dilation or sclerotherapy, has maintained the

TABLE 123-4
CAUSES OF ESOPHAGEAL PERFORATION

Intraluminal Trauma
Iatrogenic
  Esophagoscopy
    Sclerotherapy[33, 34]
    Esophageal dilation, especially pneumatic[35]
    Electrocautery
    Biopsy
  Esophageal tubes or stents
    Nasogastric[36]
    Sengstaken-Blakemore
    Prosthetic
    Obturator airway placement
  Endotracheal intubation
  Surgical anastomotic leaks
Foreign bodies
Caustic ingestions
Pneumatic
  Compressed gas
Medications
  Aspirin, doxycycline, potassium chloride, quinidine

Extraluminal Trauma
Penetrating
  Gunshot, stab wounds
Blunt
  Motor vehicle accidents, external barotrauma
Heimlich's maneuver
Paraesophageal surgery
  Vagotomy, hiatal hernia repair
Cervical spinal fracture with anterior dislocation

Spontaneous (Boerhaave's)
Usually with vomiting (i.e., barogenic)
With or without underlying esophageal disease

overall perforation rate for endoscopy at somewhat less than 1%.[37, 38] Some interventional techniques used in palliation of neoplastic disease, such as laser photocoagulation, dilation, and prosthetic stent placement, have an associated perforation rate of about 5 to 10%.[39]

The majority of perforations of the esophagus occur in patients with pre-existing esophageal disease, such as strictures, webs, rings, ulcerations (e.g., Barrett's), cancer, and diverticuli. Other associated conditions include patient agitation, cervical vertebral spurs (especially in endotracheal or esophageal obturator intubation),[40] caustic burns, foreign bodies, mediastinal disease (tumors, cysts, and abscesses), recent surgical anastomoses, and recent use of steroids or digestants.[38] Although primary neoplasms may spontaneously undergo fistulization to other nearby organs, they rarely perforate freely unless manipulated.

Causes of extraluminal traumatic perforations include penetrating and blunt trauma, cervical spinal fracture and dislocation, and pneumatic injury or barotrauma. These perforations tend to be within the cervical esophagus, whereas iatrogenic ruptures are both cervical and thoracic.

Spontaneous ruptures (Boerhaave's syndrome) are often not truly spontaneous but the result of barotrauma during episodes of intense retching, as seen for example in alcohol ingestion. Here too an underlying esophageal disorder often exists. It is in this category that missed diagnoses are more common, because perforations are often not suspected. Spontaneous perforations are almost always within the thorax and commonly near the gastroesophageal junction on the left side, where the esophagus is intrinsically weakest and unsupported.[41]

If left untreated, perforation is a fatal event. The prognosis of esophageal perforation, as has been determined in a number of series, is most related to the patient's age and the time lapse before treatment. Although most studies have concluded that spontaneous perforation is associated with higher morbidity and mortality than iatrogenic cases, this difference can be accounted for by longer delay in recognition and onset of treatment.[32, 37, 42]

Overall mortality of esophageal perforation is estimated at greater than 20%.[43] Mortality is higher in thoracic involvement than in cervical, in cases of delayed diagnosis, and in patients with other medical disease.[44]

The prognosis is also related to the severity of mediastinal contamination and infection. Perforation allows for contamination of mediastinal tissues with oral secretions and gastric contents (acid, bile, food, digestive enzymes), with a resultant necrotizing chemical mediastinitis. Aerobic and anaerobic bacterial mediastinitis is superimposed within 12 hours.[37] Although cervical perforation may at times cause only a localized periesophageal abscess, it too can cause mediastinal contamination, spread either by swallowing or by negative intrathoracic pressure on inspiration. Suppurative damage may extend to the pleural space, especially in large or long-standing perforations.[38]

Presentation

The presenting signs and symptoms are essentially the same for both iatrogenic and spontaneous perforations. Chest pain is the most common symptom, although ruptures may initially be painless and their recognition delayed. The pain is often severe and continuous. Its onset is often acute (30%),[43] but it may be gradual. It may be aggravated by inspiration, swallowing, or alteration in position, and it may radiate to the interscapular area. Other symptoms include dyspnea, dysphagia, hematemesis, and neck or abdominal pain. Signs of perforation include fever, tachycardia, crepitus, leukocytosis, pleural effusion (with pH < 7), and pneu-mothorax. The findings at presentation depend on the site of perforation: cervical perforation occurs more often with neck pain and subcutaneous emphysema; thoracic involvement may be associated with abdominal and back pain, as well as wheeze, pulmonary crackles, hydrothorax, and auscultated mediastinal crunch (Hamman's sign); and abdominal involvement may cause epigastric pain and demonstrate retroperitoneal air.

Any of the above-mentioned presentations occurring during or after instrumentation or trauma should suggest the possibility of esophageal perforation. The onset of acute pain after an episode of forceful vomiting suggests spontaneous perforation.

Substantial perforations may be associated with mediastinitis, empyema, and if delayed in presentation, mediastinal abscesses and pleuropulmonary changes. Sepsis and indeed frank shock are not uncommon.

A rarer form of perforation involves intramural dissection of the esophageal wall, or so-called double-barreled esophagus, also known as esophageal apoplexy or hematoma.[45-47] These perforations may be iatrogenic, secondary to foreign bodies, or spontaneous.[48] They have been described in patients with bleeding diatheses or those receiving anticoagulants. Presentation is similar to that of transmural rupture, although hematemesis is more common and sepsis unusual.

Diagnosis

The key to proper diagnosis of esophageal perforation lies in (1) consideration of its existence in the setting of a potential cause, if any; (2) recognition of symptoms and signs; and (3) the prompt use of confirmatory radiologic techniques. One must recognize the possible presentations, suspect perforation, and proceed to prove or disprove it. An initial history should establish heralding events and procedures.

The differential diagnosis of esophageal perforation is large and includes dissecting aneurysm, myocardial infarction, pneumothorax, pulmonary embolism, pericarditis, lung abscess, and acute pancreatitis.

Findings on plain radiographs may include mediastinal or subcutaneous air, pneumothorax, pleural effusion, and pulmonary infiltrates. In cervical perforations, lateral hyperextended neck films may demonstrate free air, esophageal displacement, and widened retropharyngeal spaces. The overall sensitivity of plain films may be greater than 80%, but contrast radiography must be used to disprove or confirm the presence of perforation and determine its extent and severity. Iodinated water-soluble agents (e.g., meglumine diatrizoate [Gastrografin]) in small quantities should be introduced while precautions against aspiration are taken. False-negative rates with these agents may be 20% in thoracic and up to 50% in cervical perforations.[48] If the result of the study is negative or equivocal, one should give barium sulfate because of its higher sensitivity and ability to better define the extent of disease. Barium should probably not be initially used because of its propensity to cause mediastinitis. In rare cases of perforation with high-risk for aspiration, dilute barium, or even the newer but expensive low-osmolality water-soluble agents such as iohexol, is recommended.[49] Because false-negative results may occur with contrast radiography, repeated examinations or even surgical exploration may be required if perforation remains a clinical suspicion.[50]

Computed tomography may be used in patients too ill to undergo an oral esophagogram and to confirm the presence of a mediastinal abscess. It is increasingly being utilized to define the site and mediastinal involvement of perforations.

The radiographic appearance of intramural perforation,

whether spontaneous or acquired, is that of a mucosal tear of the esophagus with some mucosal dissection, often appearing as a false or double-barreled lumen. If radiography is equivocal or unrevealing, careful endoscopy can be performed; the tears and hematomas are usually visualized.[46]

Management

Again, a high index of suspicion of perforation and early diagnosis and treatment are paramount. Although management of esophageal perforation demands an individual approach with regard to the site, the cause, the severity, and the underlying disease, one may make generalizations. In a selected group of patients, one may use medical therapy (e.g., allowing nothing by mouth, careful monitoring, administration of intravenous fluids and antibiotics, hyperalimentation, and nasogastric suction). These patients include those with relatively asymptomatic small, contained perforations, usually pharyngeal but sometimes cervical, without sepsis or communication to the pleura. There should be only a small degree of extravasation of contrast material. These are often small instrumental tears.

Most perforations should be treated surgically. Options for surgery include drainage procedures, primary closure, esophagectomy, and exclusion or diversion techniques.[37, 50, 51] Within the first 24 hours, most thoracic perforations can be treated with thoracotomy and primary suture repair and drainage. Most authors now advocate buttressing of the repair with a pleural or muscular flap.[32] In these cases, there should be greater than 90% survival. Cervical esophageal tears can often be treated with drainage and antibiotics alone; repair can be reserved for larger perforations. Exclusion procedures are recommended if there are large tears with substantial pleural and mediastinal contamination.[52] Esophagectomy should be used only in selected cases, such as in caustic injury or in neoplastic or other severe primary esophageal disease.[53]

More than 24 hours after perforation, the recommended management remains more controversial, although primary closure remains most popular. Surgery should still be prompt in cases of shock, sepsis, respiratory failure, pneumothorax or pneumoperitoneum, and abscess formation. If diagnosis has been delayed because of a relative lack of symptoms, some clinicians advocate careful medical management while watching for continued leak or abscess formation. However, progression to more severe disease is unpredictable, and overall mortality in these cases tends to remain higher than in surgically managed patients. Percutaneous or transesophageal drainage has been advocated but is not yet widely used.

In patients who have experienced perforations during palliative intubation of neoplastic strictures, an aggressive nonsurgical approach is often favored.[39] Continuous mediastinal irrigation and drainage via chest or neck tubes is then often necessary.

It is important to exclude the existence of intrinsic esophageal disease, such as Barrett's esophagus or neoplasia, in the stable patient postoperatively. This is best accomplished by endoscopy.

The management of incomplete or intramural perforation is usually conservative. Surgery is reserved for those cases with incomplete resolution or complications.[54] Localized perforations, as in aortoesophageal and other fistulas, are usually surgically repaired.

MISCELLANEOUS

A number of disorders, although often not life-threatening emergencies, are encountered in the intensive care setting.

Chest pain of noncardiac origin remains a frequent cause of admission to intensive care units, as myocardial ischemia is first excluded. The esophagus may be responsible for 20 to 60% of all noncardiac pain.[55] Disorders responsible for presentations that simulate angina include esophageal reflux, esophageal dysmotility, and mucosal irritation, as in infectious esophagitis. Pain from motor disorders may be relieved by nitroglycerin and calcium channel antagonists, further challenging the diagnostician. After being convinced that coronary or other cardiac disease is nonexistent, the physician may pursue an elective evaluation for esophageal causes.[56, 57]

Acquired tracheoesophageal fistulas of nonmalignant cause occur rarely in ventilator-dependent patients, especially those with high cuff pressures, elevated airway pressures, and prolonged duration of intubation. Other associations include esophageal infections and long-standing nasogastric tubes. Recognition of these factors and their elimination are important. The patient with decreased alveolar ventilation may benefit from use of a high-frequency jet ventilator.[58] Infectious esophagitis must be sought and treated if present.

Esophageal infection in critically ill patients is indeed common, especially in those who are immunocompromised, diabetic, or receiving antibiotics or steroids. Fungal (usually candida) and viral (herpes virus, cytomegalovirus) infections may be the cause of dysphagia and, more often, odynophagia, and they may also occur with hemorrhage, chest pain, fever, or malnutrition. Endoscopy may be required for pathologic and microbiologic diagnosis, because treatment is organism directed, but empirical treatment may often be initiated.

Patients who have nasogastric tubes for extended periods may develop elongated strictures secondary to local inflammation and reflux. Only flexible narrow-bore tubes should be placed for long-term enteral feeding. Alternatively, percutaneous gastrostomy tube placement may be of benefit in patients requiring extended nutritional support. When gastroesophageal reflux and aspiration are of concern, endoscopic techniques may be used to pass a percutaneous feeding tube more distally in the jejunum.

References

1. Moore WR: Caustic ingestions: Pathophysiology, diagnosis and treatment. Clin Pediatr 25:192, 1986.
2. Howell JM: Alkaline ingestions. Ann Emerg Med 15:820, 1986.
3. Estrera A, Taylor M, Mills LJ, et al: Corrosive burns of the esophagus and stomach: A recommendation for an aggressive surgical approach. Ann Thorac Surg 41:276, 1986.
4. Leape LL, Ashcraft RW, Scarpelli DG, et al: Hazard to health: Liquid lye. N Engl J Med 248:578, 1971.
5. Goldman LP, Weigart JM: Corrosive substance ingestion: A review. Am J Gastroenterol 79:85, 1984.
6. Vancuro EM, Clinton JE, Ruiz E, et al: Toxicity of alkaline solutions. Ann Emerg Med 9:118, 1980.
7. Hoffman RS, Howland MA, Kamerow HN, et al: Comparison of titratable acid/alkaline reserve and pH in potentially caustic household products. Clin Toxicol 27:241, 1989.
8. Zargar SA, Kochhar R, Nagi B, et al: Ingestion of corrosive acids: Spectrum of injury to upper gastrointestinal tract and natural history. Gastroenterology 97:702, 1989.
9. Penner GE: Acid ingestion: Toxicology and treatment. Ann Emerg Med 9:374, 1980.
10. Dilawavi JB, Singh S, Rao PN, et al: Corrosive acid ingestion in man—A clinical and endoscopic study. Gut 25:183, 1984.
11. Litovitz TL: Button battery ingestions: A review of 56 cases. JAMA 249:2495, 1983.
12. Lacouture PG, Gaudreault P, Lovejoy FH Jr: Clinitest tablet ingestion: An in vitro investigation concerned with initial emergency management. Ann Emerg Med 15:143, 1986.
13. Friedman EM, Lovejoy FH Jr: The emergency management of caustic ingestions. Emerg Med Clin North Am 2:77, 1984.
14. Postlethwait RW: Chemical burns of the esophagus. Surg Clin North Am 63:915, 1983.

15. Ferguson MK, Migliore M, Staszak VM, et al: Early evaluation and therapy for caustic esophageal injury. Am J Surg 157:116, 1989.
16. Sarfati E, Gossot D, Assens P, et al: Management of caustic ingestion in adults. Br J Surg 74:146, 1987.
17. Neimark S, Rogers AI: Chemical injury of the esophagus. In: Berk JE, Haubrich WS, Kaiser MH, et al (eds.): Bockus Gastroenterology. 4th ed. Philadelphia, WB Saunders, p 769, 1985.
18. Haller JA Jr, Andrews HG, White JJ, et al: Pathophysiology and management of acute corrosive burns of the esophagus: Results of treatment in 285 children. J Pediatr Surg 6:578, 1971.
19. Anderson KD, Rouse TM, Randolph JG: A controlled trial of corticosteroids in children with corrosive injury of the esophagus. N Engl J Med 323:637, 1990.
20. Wijburg FA, Beukers MM, Heymans HS, et al: Nasogastric intubation as sole treatment of caustic eosphageal lesions. Ann Otol Rhinol Laryngol 94:337, 1985.
21. Rubin MM, Jui V, Cozzi GM: Treatment of caustic ingestion. J Oral Maxillofac Surg 47:286, 1989.
22. Appelqvist P: Lye corrosion carcinoma of the esophagus: A review of 63 cases. Cancer 45:2655, 1980.
23. Vizcarrondo FJ, Brady PG, Nord HJ: Foreign bodies of the upper gastrointestinal tract. Gastrointest Endosc 29:208, 1983.
24. Taylor RB: Esophageal foreign bodies. Emerg Med Clin North Am 5:301, 1987.
25. Webb WA: Management of foreign bodies of the upper gastrointestinal tract. Gastroenterology 94:204, 1988.
26. Selivanov V, Sheldon GF, Cello JP, et al: Management of foreign body ingestion. Ann Surg 199:187, 1984.
27. Scher RL, Tegtmeyer CJ, McLean WC: Vascular injury following foreign body perforation of the esophagus. Ann Otol Rhinol Laryngol 99:698, 1990.
28. Henderson CT, Engel J, Schlesinger P: Foreign body ingestion: Review and suggested guidelines for management. Endoscopy 19:68, 1987.
29. Handler SD, Beaugard ME, Canalis RF, et al: Unsuspected esophageal foreign bodies in adults with upper airway obstruction. Chest 80:234, 1981.
30. Rice BT, Spiegel PK, Dombrowski PJ: Acute esophageal food impaction treated by gas-forming agents. Radiology 146:299, 1983.
31. Ginaldi S: Removal of esophageal foreign bodies using a Foley catheter in adults. Am J Emerg Med 3:64, 1985.
32. Attar S, Hankins JR, Suter CM: Esophageal perforation: A therapeutic challenge. Ann Thorac Surg 50:45, 1990.
33. Perino LE, Gholson CF, Goff JS: Esophageal perforation after fiberoptic variceal sclerotherapy. J Clin Gastroenterol 9:286, 1987.
34. Korula J, Pandya K, Yamada S: Perforation of esophagus after endoscopic variceal sclerotherapy: Incidence and clues to pathogenesis. Dig Dis Sci 34:324, 1989.
35. Kozarek RA, Phelps JE, Partyka EK, et al: Intraluminal pressures generated during esophageal bougienage. Gastroenterology 81:833, 1981.
36. Jackson RH, Payne DK, Bacon BR: Esophageal perforation due to nasogastric intubation. Am J Gastroenterol 85:439, 1990.
37. Sarr MG, Pemberton JH, Payne WS: Management of instrumental perforations of the esophagus. J Thorac Cardiovasc Surg 84:211, 1982.
38. Atkins JP Jr, Keane WM, Rowe LD: Foreign bodies in the esophagus: Esophageal perforation. In: Berk JE, Haubrich WS, Kaiser MH, et al (eds): Bockus Gastroenterology. 4th ed. Philadelphia, WB Saunders, p 777, 1985.
39. Hine KR, Atkinson M: The diagnosis and management of perforations of the esophagus and pharynx sustained during intubation of neoplastic esophageal strictures. Dig Dis Sci 31:571, 1986.
40. Wright RA: Upper-esophageal perforation with a flexible endoscope secondary to cervical osteophytes. Dig Dis Sci 25:66, 1980.
41. Henderson JAM, Peloquin AJM: Boerhaave revisited: Spontaneous esophageal perforation as a diagnostic masquerader. Am J Med 86:559, 1989.
42. Graeber GM, Niezgoda JA, Albus RA, et al: A comparison of patients with endoscopic esophageal perforations and patients with Boerhaave's syndrome. Chest 92:995, 1987.
43. Michel L, Grillo HC, Malt RA: Operative and nonoperative management of esophageal perforations. Ann Surg 194:57, 1981.
44. Flynn AE, Verrier ED, Way LW, et al: Esophageal perforation. Arch Surg 124:1211, 1989.
45. Pellicano A, Watier A, Gentile J: Spontaneous double-barrelled esophagus: Report of two cases and review of the literature. J Clin Gastroenterol 9:149, 1987.
46. Steadman C, Kerlin P, Crimmins F, et al.: Spontaneous intramural rupture of the oesophagus. Gut 31:845, 1990.
47. Berliner L, Redmond P, Pachter HL: Spontaneous intramural perforation of the esophagus: Case report and review of the literature. Am J Gastroenterol 77:355, 1982.
48. Phillips LG, Cunningham J: Esophageal perforation. Radiol Clin North Am 22:607, 1984.
49. Brick SH, Caroline DF, Levy-Toaff AS, et al: Esophageal disruption: Evaluation with iohexol esophagography. Radiography 169:141, 1988.
50. Bladergroen MR, Lowe JE, Postlethwait RW: Diagnosis and recommended management of esophageal perforation and rupture. Ann Thorac Surg 42:235, 1986.
51. Goldstein LA, Thompson WR: Esophageal perforations: A 15 year experience. Am J Surg 143:495, 1982.
52. Brewer LA, Carter R, Mulder GA: Options in the management of perforations of the esophagus. Am J Surg 152:62, 1986.
53. Orringer MB, Stirling MC: Esophagectomy for esophageal disruption. Ann Thorac Surg 49:35, 1990.
54. Barone JE, Robilotti JG, Comer JV: Conservative treatment of spontaneous intramural perforation (or intramural hematoma) of the esophagus. Am J Gastroenterol 74:165, 1980.
55. Nevens F, Janssens J, Piessens J, et al: Prospective study on prevalence of esophageal chest pain in patients referred on an elective basis to a cardiac unit for suspected myocardial ischemia. Dig Dis Sci 36:229, 1991.
56. Richter JE, Bradley LA, Castell DO: Esophageal chest pain: Current controversies in pathogenesis, diagnosis, and therapy. Ann Intern Med 110:66, 1989.
57. Rothstein RD, Ouyang A: Chest pain of esophageal origin. Gastroenterol Clin North Am 18:257, 1989.
58. Payne DK, Anderson WM, Romero MD, et al: Tracheoesophageal fistula formation in intubated patients: Risk factors and treatment with high-frequency jet ventilation. Chest 98:161, 1990.

CHAPTER 124

Upper Gastrointestinal Tract Hemorrhage

Rosemarie L. Fisher

Hemorrhage from the upper gastrointestinal tract is common, accounting for approximately 50 to 150 hospital admissions per 100,000 patients per year. In 1984, bleeding caused by gastric or duodenal ulcer was the discharge diagnosis for 47 patients per 100,000 admissions.[1] Overall, the hemorrhage itself is usually self-limited and stops spontaneously in approximately 80% of cases.[2, 3] The remaining 20%, which either fail to stop or rebleed, have various causes, and the morbidity and mortality in these patients depend on the source of the bleeding episode (e.g., peptic ulcer disease, esophageal or gastric varices, and gastritis) and on other comorbid factors (e.g., age, coagulopathy, and coexistent diseases). Unfortunately, the overall mortality of 10% has not changed during the past 30 years. Data collected by the American Society of Gastrointestinal Endoscopy, in 1979, on 2225 patients with upper gastrointestinal tract hemorrhage, showed that the most common sites of bleeding were gastric erosions (29.6%), duodenal ulcer (22.8%), gastric ulcer (21.9%), varices (15.4%), and esophagitis (12.8%)[4-7] (Table 124–1). In this group, surgery was required in 15.6% of patients (22.6% of duodenal ulcers, 17.3% of gastric

TABLE 124–1

ETIOLOGY OF UPPER GASTROINTESTINAL TRACT HEMORRHAGE

Site	%
Gastric erosions	29.6
Duodenal ulcer	22.8
Gastric ulcer	21.9
Gastroesophageal varices	15.4
Esophagitis	12.8

ulcers). Overall mortality was 10.8 and 30.1%, respectively, in patients with varices. Since that time, however, various endoscopic therapeutic interventions have been introduced that may be able to alter the morbidity and mortality rates.

Although the majority of patients with upper gastrointestinal tract hemorrhage in intensive care units (ICU) are there because of that diagnosis, other patients experience upper gastrointestinal tract hemorrhage in the ICU. Stress-related mucosal damage is found in nearly 100% of patients admitted to an ICU, when it is looked for endoscopically.[8-11] Although the incidence of severe hemorrhage is low (2 to 5%) in these patients, when it does occur, it carries an 80% mortality rate.[12-14]

MANAGEMENT

The management of the patient with upper gastrointestinal tract hemorrhage revolves around resuscitation and general supportive measures, general and specific localization of the site, and then site-directed therapy. Surgical consultation should be considered as part of the resuscitative measures and should be performed simultaneously.

Although this approach is clearly indicated in the patient with active bleeding, the approach to the patient who has ceased bleeding may not be as clearly defined; it is similar, although the rapidity with which the procedures are performed may be based more on the clinical prognostic factors.

Resuscitation

Resuscitation first includes an assessment of blood loss. If signs of shock are present, it is estimated that there has been a 20 to 25% loss of total blood volume. The presence of postural hypotension, postural pulse changes, acidosis, or decreased urine output may indicate severe volume loss. One should not depend on the presence or absence of a decreased hematocrit to predict the amount of blood loss—it is the least sensitive of measures of bleeding and may take up to 72 hours to reach equilibration.[15] The clinician must also be aware of concomitantly administered medications, such as beta-blockers, which might mask the presence of postural changes.

The establishment of vascular access is clearly one of the first steps in the resuscitative process. Large-bore catheters, preferably two, are necessary for the delivery of large volumes of replacement fluid. Although the placement of central venous catheters for pressure monitoring, or a Swan-Ganz catheter, may be necessary in a patient with cardiovascular disease or pulmonary disease, these devices have small-dimension lumina and are not as useful in delivering large volumes, as a 16-gauge peripheral catheter. Fluid replacement should be performed immediately with either normal saline or Ringer's solution. If the blood loss is severe, and compatible blood is not readily available, type O-negative or -positive blood may be administered. If the bleeding is suspected to be from esophageal or gastric varices, volume replacement should proceed cautiously, as overexpansion of the vascular space may result in increased portal pressures, and recurrence or persistence of hemorrhage. Fresh frozen plasma or vitamin K or both may need to be administered, pending the return of laboratory evaluations, or a knowledge of the clinician of previous abnormalities in clotting disorders.

Initial laboratory evaluation should include a measurement of hematocrit, prothrombin time, partial thromboplastin time, and platelet count; blood type and cross-match; blood urea nitrogen level; electrolyte determinations and liver function tests. If one obtains a history of aspirin or nonsteroidal anti-inflammatory drug ingestion, one may want to consider obtaining a bleeding time to decide on the possible benefits of the administration of platelets.

Identification of Bleeding Site
General Localization

Initially, one must assess whether the point of hemorrhage is from an upper or a lower gastrointestinal tract source. The history and physical examination give clues as to the possible origin of the hemorrhage—if the patient has had previous bleeding episodes, the nature and origin of these episodes are useful; the presence of symptoms related to acid-peptic disorders leads to a possible diagnosis of ulcer or esophagitis; the ingestion of ethanol, aspirin, or nonsteroidal anti-inflammatory drugs raises the possibility of gastritis or duodenitis; an antecedent history of nausea or vomiting may indicate a Mallory-Weiss tear; previous aortic graft surgery should suggest an aortoenteral fistula; a history of a bleeding disorder or warfarin (Coumadin) ingestion may suggest a diffuse bleeding disorder; a prior history of inflammatory bowel disease or liver disease suggests other possible sources of hemorrhage. In addition, findings of systemic diseases, such as Osler-Weber-Rendu or pseudoxanthoma elasticum, may suggest other bleeding sites within the gastrointestinal tract.

The presentation of the bleeding episode may not be as helpful to the general localization of a bleeding site as the clinician may desire. Although hematemesis is clearly indicative of an upper gastrointestinal tract hemorrhage, the presence of melena, in a subacute hemorrhage, may not be as reliable, as bleeding colonic lesions may occasionally occur with melena. In addition, the presence of hematochezia may not imply a lower gastrointestinal tract hemorrhage, even in the presence of a clear nasogastric aspirate.

Rapid hemorrhage from a duodenal ulcer might result in rapid gastrointestinal transit to produce hematochezia, with little gastroduodenal reflux to give a positive nasogastric aspirate. In one study, 16% of patients with a clear nasogastric aspirate had active bleeding at the time of endoscopy, with 10% of that group requiring surgery, with a mortality rate of 6% in that group.[4-6] The utilization of a nasogastric tube in these patients has been widely debated among clinicians. Clearly, the placement of a nasogastric tube if the patient has hematemesis is unnecessary. Another study, however, suggested that one may be able to predict the severity of the hemorrhage, and the possible need for transfusion and/or surgery, depending on the rapidity of clearing of the aspirate[16] (Table 124–2).

In the American Society of Gastrointestinal Endoscopy survey, the presence of a coffee grounds aspirate resulted in a 30% incidence of active bleeding at the time of endoscopy, with 13% of the group requiring surgery, and a 10% mortality rate, whereas bright red blood in the aspirate resulted in a 48% incidence of active bleeding at the time of endoscopy, a 23% incidence of surgical intervention, and an 18% mortality rate.[4-6] This same study was able to correlate the appearance of the nasogastric aspirate with the stool color as a predictor of mortality[4-6] (Table 124–3).

The nasogastric tube may thus be useful only to look for obvious bleeding from the upper gastrointestinal tract, if the patient has not vomited blood, or to empty the stomach to prevent the patient from further vomiting and possible aspiration. The disadvantages of nasogastric tube intubation, however, include not only patient discomfort but also aspiration. There is no evidence that the placement of a nasogastric tube initiates hemorrhage from esophageal varices. To clear the stomach before endoscopic evaluation, the standard No. 16 to 18 French nasogastric tubes are inade-

TABLE 124-2

TABLE 124-2

NASOGASTRIC ASPIRATE AS PREDICTOR OF SEVERITY OF UPPER GASTROINTESTINAL TRACT HEMORRHAGE

Nasogastric Aspirate	Number	% of Patients		
		Needing Transfusion	Undergoing Surgery	Dead
Clear	15	40	0	0
Coffee grounds	47	47	11	0
Red-clear, <1 L of fluid	13	54	8	8
Clear, 1–6 L of fluid	16	81	25	25
No clearing	10	100	50	50

Data from McLaughlin WD, Kolts BE, Achem SR: Nasogastric lavage compared with outcome in 101 patients seen in an emergency room for upper gastrointestinal hemorrhage. Gastroenterology 92:1529, 1987.

quate; large-bore tubes are required. The use of iced saline to lavage the stomach has not been proved to be superior to room temperature saline, and in fact, iced fluids may impair coagulation.[17] The use of vasoconstrictive agents in the lavage fluid, such as levarterenol, have not been uniformly successful.

Specific Localization

Studies have shown that the diagnosis predicted by the evaluations discussed earlier are correct in approximately 40% of cases. To allow further definition of the bleeding site, and perhaps direct specific therapy, other modalities must be used.

Barium Contrast Studies. Multiple studies have shown that endoscopy is clearly diagnostically superior to barium contrast studies, even double-contrast studies. Barium studies may show more than one lesion and not be able to identify which lesion is bleeding, and mucosal lesions (such as in stress-related mucosal disease) may be missed in up to 50% of the cases. Further, the introduction of barium into the upper gastrointestinal tract may obscure the identification of lesions if bleeding continues and endoscopy is attempted, or if angiography is required.

Panendoscopy. It is clear that panendoscopy is the most sensitive and specific method to identify the origin of an upper gastrointestinal tract hemorrhage and to evaluate the presence or absence of bleeding and or nonbleeding lesions.[18] However, the introduction of urgent endoscopy into the management scheme did not appear to affect mortality rates, and several controlled studies have confirmed this.[19–22] This absence of benefit may be due to many factors, including lack of stratification of patients according to risk of bleeding site (e.g., varices vs. acid-related causes); inadequate study size; and the failure to use the diagnostic information therapeutically. Since the majority of these studies in the late 1970s and the early 1980s, many endoscopic therapeutic measures have been developed. These measures, along with increasing knowledge of the pathophysiology of bleeding ulcers and the identification of prognostic risk factors for

ongoing bleeding or rebleeding, have led to increased information on the benefits and risks of therapeutic endoscopy. Overall, the American Society of Gastrointestinal Endoscopy survey showed a 0.9% incidence of complications, with a 0.1% mortality attributable to endoscopic complications.[4–6]

The clinician should thus attempt to identify the patients who have a worse prognosis with their hemorrhage and might most benefit from the early identification of and directed therapy to a bleeding site. Patients with cirrhosis, a history of duodenal ulcer disease, or a history of gastric surgery are candidates for early endoscopy, based on the inability of other studies to identify the lesion. Multiple studies have shown that between 30 and 60% of patients with known esophageal varices are bleeding from a second lesion at the time of endoscopy. In addition, specific endoscopic therapy of esophageal variceal hemorrhage has been shown to be clearly effective in stopping the hemorrhage (see Chapter 125). Patients with a history of peptic ulcer disease are likely to have a deformed duodenal bulb on barium study, which makes it difficult to identify a lesion. Patients with a history of gastric surgery (partial gastrectomy) may have a marginal ulcer; this lesion is missed in 60% of the cases by barium studies. Multiple prognostic risk factors have been identified (both clinical and endoscopic) that help to identify the patients who might most benefit from endoscopic intervention (Table 124–4).

The origin of the bleeding site itself is predictive of the incidence of rebleeding and the mortality rate. The 1984 World Organization of Gastroenterology international survey of more than 4000 patients showed that patients with esophageal varices had a rebleeding rate of approximately 60%, with a mortality rate of 30%; patients with gastric cancer had a 50% rebleeding rate and a 14% mortality rate, whereas patients with gastric or duodenal ulcer had a rebleeding rate of approximately 25% and a mortality rate of approximately 5%.[23] Patients older than the age of 60 years have demonstrated a mortality rate of 13.4%, whereas those

TABLE 124-3

CORRELATION OF STOOL AND NASOGASTRIC COLOR WITH PERCENTAGE OF MORTALITY

Nasogastric Aspirate	% Mortality	
	Black Stool	Red Stool
Clear	5	7
Coffee grounds	9	20
Red	12	30

TABLE 124-4

ADVERSE PROGNOSTIC FACTORS OF UPPER GASTROINTESTINAL TRACT HEMORRHAGE

Site of hemorrhage (e.g., varices > cancer > ulcer)
Elderly patient
Severe initial bleed
Onset or recurrence in hospital
Coincidental disease (e.g., cardiac, pulmonary)
Endoscopic stigmata of recent hemorrhage
    Active bleeding
    Visible vessel
Need for emergency surgery

younger than 60 years have a 8.7% mortality rate.[4–6] The severity of the initial hemorrhage, based on the appearance of the nasogastric aspirate, the presence of shock, and the transfusion requirement, has also correlated with the mortality rate. Transfusion of 1 to 3 U of blood was associated with a mortality rate of approximately 8%, whereas a transfusion requirement of greater than 10 U of blood was associated with a 58.7% mortality rate.[4–6] Recurrence of hemorrhage in the hospital has been associated with a four to seven times increase in the mortality rate, and onset of bleeding in the hospitalized patient was associated with a mortality rate of 33%, as opposed to 7% in those with pre-existing upper gastrointestinal tract hemorrhage.[4–6] The presence of other medical diseases also increased the mortality rate significantly—from 2.6% with no concomitant diseases to 66.7% with six concomitant diseases.[4–6, 24]

The classification of endoscopic stigmata of hemorrhage has helped not only to define the risk of rebleeding and predict mortality but also to define when endoscopic therapy should be utilized. In one study of patients with hemorrhage from ulcer disease, the presence of active arterial spurting was not seen commonly during endoscopy (approximately 8% of the time) but was associated with an 85 to 100% rebleeding rate. The presence of a visible vessel that was oozing or had fresh clot attached to it was seen about 10% of the time and had a 42% rebleeding rate; an organized clot with no visible vessel seen was present in about 26% of the cases, with a 24% rebleeding rate, whereas no stigmata of recent hemorrhage were seen in 10% of the cases and no incidence of rebleeding.[25] Several other studies have shown similar results. The utilization of these predictive factors, in addition to the clinical risk factors, helps to define further those patients who may benefit from the therapeutic endoscopic maneuvers.[26–29]

Radionuclide Imaging Studies. Although the use of technetium-labeled sulfur colloid and technetium- or indium-labeled red blood cells may be of benefit in the localization of bleeding from a lower gastrointestinal or small intestinal site (see Chapter 126), there are few data that these are beneficial in the identification of an upper gastrointestinal tract source of hemorrhage.

Angiography. Occasionally, the rapidity of the hemorrhage may preclude the visualization of a bleeding site by endoscopy. It is then that the utilization of angiography may be helpful in defining the site of hemorrhage, either before surgery or for specific therapeutic intervention, with vasoconstrictive substances or thrombotic agents.

Site-Directed Specific Therapy
Gastroesophageal Varices

The treatment of hemorrhage from gastroesophageal varices has been well researched and refined during the past several years, including endoscopic and pharmacologic methods, and is discussed thoroughly in Chapter 125.

Gastritis

Gastritis consists of the occurrence of superficial mucosal lesions in the presence of ingestion of alcohol or administration of nonsteroidal anti-inflammatory agents and, more commonly within the ICU, in patients with multiple organ system failure or multiple stress factors, such as, burns, head trauma, and sepsis. If patients are examined endoscopically, these lesions are present in 60 to 100% of patients, although clinical evidence of hemorrhage is seen in only 20% of these cases. More important, serious hemorrhage is seen to occur in only 2 to 7% of patients but is then associated with an 80% mortality rate.[30]

The cause of these lesions is thought to be due to multiple factors, all relating to a breakdown in the gastric mucosal barrier, with the subsequent reflux of gastric acid across the mucosal barrier. It is believed by some investigators that the primary insult is a breakdown of the mucosal barrier and the secondary insult is the reflux of acid. Decreased mucosal blood flow and subsequent ischemia of the gastric mucosa are considered to be the primary insult in these patients. With lower perfusion rates of the mucosa, there is a decreased delivery of oxygen and other nutrients to maintain the superficial epithelial cells, as well as an inability to maintain rapid epithelial cell renewal, and a lower production of bicarbonate within the mucosal cell, allowing greater injury by the refluxed acid. Other factors in the causation of stress-related mucosal disease (SRMD) have included a decreased production of gastric mucus and a decreased production of endogenous prostaglandins.[31]

Prevention of SRMD in critically ill patients is considered to be the first step in the treatment of this lesion.[32] However, as the severity of the process and the incidence of hemorrhage appear to be directly related to the severity of the primary illness, therapy should be to correct the metabolic and physiologic abnormalities in the patient. Not every patient who is admitted to an ICU is a candidate for therapy to prevent SRMD. In fact, with the improvement in ICU care of these critically ill patients, the incidence of SRMD-related hemorrhage may be declining. The addition of other medications to some of these patients may be more harmful than beneficial.

Multiple studies have shown that the administration of antacids to maintain an intragastric pH above 4 significantly reduces the incidence of mucosal disease and blood loss.[30] However, the amount of antacids required to do this may result in diarrhea, pulmonary aspiration, and metabolic abnormalities, such as hypophosphatemia or hypermagnesemia. The use of histamine (H_2) receptor antagonists has also been shown in multiple studies (primarily performed with cimetidine) to prevent the incidence of mucosal abnormalities and decrease the amount of blood loss. Dosing regimens using both bolus and continuous infusions have been studied and have not been shown to be significantly different. Even in the presence of these data, the only H_2 receptor antagonist that has been approved at this time for use for this purpose by the U.S. Food and Drug Administration is cimetidine. It is of interest that, in the studies presented to support the application, there appeared to be little relationship between the development of the lesions and the intragastric pH, as a large percentage of these patients had pH values greater than 5. The approved dosing regimen is for 50 mg/h, without a bolus dose.[33] Lastly, sucralfate has been shown to be as effective as antacids in preventing macroscopic bleeding in ICU patients.[34]

Concern has been raised about the possibility of an increased incidence of nosocomial pneumonia related to the use of acid-suppressive therapy.[35] Although an increased incidence was seen in patients receiving antacids or H_2 receptor antagonists, this was not seen in patients receiving sucralfate. If one, however, separates the patients into those having received only H_2 receptor antagonists and not antacids, versus those receiving antacids or sucralfate, the patients receiving only H_2 receptor antagonists had a lower incidence of nosocomial pneumonia. A great deal of uncertainty still revolves around this topic, and these results have not been duplicated.

After hemorrhage has started from SRMD, 75 to 80% of episodes stop spontaneously. Although all of these measures have been used to attempt to stop the bleeding, none have shown a great deal of effect. Again, the approach should be to attempt to correct the underlying illness in the patient, including any coagulopathy. Therapeutic endoscopic measures have not been effective, as the lesions are usually multiple and necessitate a great deal of endoscopic manipulation.[32] Angiographic pharmacotherapy has been suggested in cases of persistent hemorrhage from SRMD. Although there have not been large, controlled studies to definitively show a benefit to this technique, early results with intra-arterial vasopressin have suggested a decrease in the amount of blood loss, perhaps allowing more time for stabilization and possible surgical intervention.[32]

The prognosis for the patient with recurrent or continuous bleeding from SRMD is poor, and although surgical intervention, ranging from vagotomy and pyloroplasty with oversewing of the bleeding lesions, to total gastrectomy, has not been shown in prospective studies to be of benefit, it may be the only possible therapy.[32] The mortality with bleeding from SRMD is approximately 10%, whereas the overall mortality in these patients is 33 to 100%, reflecting the severity of illness of these patients.[30, 31]

Peptic Ulcer Disease

The major cause of upper gastrointestinal tract hemorrhage is peptic ulcer disease, primarily duodenal ulcer. The majority of bleeding episodes from duodenal ulcer stop spontaneously, requiring no active intervention and only supportive therapy and prophylactic administration of acid-suppressive therapy, to initiate the healing process of the ulcer. There have been no studies to show that the administration of these therapies has decreased the incidence of rebleeding.

The clinician must attempt to identify those patients at a high risk for persistent bleeding, or rebleeding, to determine further therapy. As stated earlier, several clinical and endoscopic factors assist the clinician in predicting these patients[4–6, 36] so that endoscopic therapy can be utilized. Multiple endoscopic modalities have been developed, including topical, mechanical, injection, and thermal. These therapies have been utilized at the endoscopic lesions that are associated with the highest risk of rebleeding: the active bleeding site (the spurter), the visible vessel with oozing or a bright red clot, the oozing site without a visible vessel, and the nonbleeding visible vessel (in some studies).[26–29]

The most commonly used methods at present are the injection and thermal methods.[37, 39] Laser therapy, both neodymium:yttrium-aluminum-garnet and argon, was initially utilized for control of bleeding from ulcer sites.[39–42] Neodymium:yttrium-aluminum-garnet laser was shown to be safer and decreased the rebleeding rate, the need for urgent surgery, transfusion requirements, and mortality. However, the lasers were expensive, not portable, and not easy to use and did not show an advantage over thermal therapies.

At present, the most widely used thermal therapies are multipolar electrocoagulation and heater probes. Both methods can be utilized through standard endoscopes, are portable, and are relatively inexpensive. When compared with standard therapy, multipolar electrocoagulation has been shown to increase significantly the incidence of hemostasis (90% vs. 13%), decrease the transfusion requirement (2.4 U vs. 5.4 U of packed red blood cells), decrease the need for surgical intervention (14% vs. 57%), decrease the length of hospital stay (4.4 days vs. 7.2 days), and decrease the cost of hospitalization by more than one half. However, even though there was a trend to a decrease in the mortality rate (0% vs. 13%) in one study, this did not reach statistical significance.[43, 45] A higher rate of hemostasis (95%), a lower rebleeding rate (23%), lower transfusion requirement (1.4 U of packed red blood cells), shorter stay in the ICU (2.4 days),

and a lower incidence of surgery (11%) in patients with active bleeding who were treated with the heater probe was noted when compared with control, standard therapy (14% hemostasis, 93% continued or rebleeding, 4.6 U of packed red blood cells, 8.4 ICU days, 57% required surgery), or the use of multipolar electrocoagulation (47% continued or rebleeding, 2.5 U of packed red blood cells, 4.7 ICU days, and 29% required surgery).[45] Only the initial rate of hemostasis was similar between the two thermal methods. However, the mortality rates, although showing a trend in favor of the thermal methods, were not significantly different among the three therapies (21% with control therapy, 7% with multipolar electrocoagulation therapy, 5% with heater probe therapy). Other studies have demonstrated no major differences in results between heater probes and multipolar electrocoagulation.[46, 47]

Although thermal methods are readily available and easy to use, the adaptation of injection methods from variceal sources of hemorrhage to ulcers has shown them to be equally safe and effective when compared with thermal methods.[47, 48] The use of either epinephrine[48] or absolute alcohol,[49] injected into the vessel directly or around the vessel, has been shown to be effective in producing similar rates of hemostasis, length of hospitalization, need for surgery, need for transfusion, and rebleeding rates as mentioned earlier.[47] A study using injection therapy, followed by neodymium:yttrium-aluminum-garnet laser therapy, in a small group of patients, showed marginal improvement in efficacy.[50]

One must be aware, however, that the safety of these modalities depends on the endoscopist's experience and the milieu in which the procedure is performed. There has been reported a 10 to 30% incidence of the precipitation of rebleeding with endoscopic therapy. This complication appears to be related to the size of the visible vessel, the size of the ulcer, a false aneurysm in the ulcer, the operator's experience, other factors such as the number of previous transfusions, concomitant medications, or the position of the ulcer, with ulcers high on the lesser curve or on the posterior duodenal bulb having a higher incidence of rebleeding. The risk of precipitating rebleeding in large vascular malformations has been as high as 50%. Another complication is perforation, which occurred in approximately 1% of cases.

Published recommendations from a National Institutes of Health Consensus Conference on Therapeutic Endoscopy and Bleeding Ulcers[51] stated that endoscopic hemostatic therapy should be used only in patients at high risk for persistent or recurrent bleeding and death. The procedure should be done by experienced endoscopists, because of the complication rate. Multipolar electrocoagulation and heater probe are presently the most promising therapies. The available data on injection therapy were not sufficient to recommend it strongly at this time. In addition, the recommendations concluded that there was a need for further research to be performed in randomized controlled multicenter, trials to standardize terminology, quantitate different rebleeding risks, develop a composite predictive risk profile, develop optimal treatment regimens, and explore new therapeutic and diagnostic modalities.

One letter has outlined two meta-analyses, which showed a beneficial effect of all these therapies not only on rebleeding rates and the need for emergency surgery, but also on decreasing mortality.[51a]

Occasionally, the rate of bleeding may be severe enough to preclude endoscopic visualization and therapy. In these cases, if the patient is not a candidate for surgery or is not believed to be stable enough for surgery, angiography may be utilized first to visualize the bleeding site and then therapeutically either to deliver vasoconstrictive drugs[52, 53] to the site or to achieve thrombosis of the bleeding vessel. Although this procedure controls the bleeding in 35 to 45% of cases, approximately 30 to 40% rebleed owing to multiple collaterals and the inadequacy of the hemostatic technique.[54-56]

Surgical therapy of bleeding peptic ulcers, although not as frequently used, because of endoscopic hemostatic measures, is still indicated in the therapy of recurrent or continued hemorrhage from either a duodenal or a gastric ulcer.[57]

Rarer Causes

Mallory-Weiss Tear. This lesion is known to occur in approximately 10% of upper gastrointestinal tract hemorrhages. The presentation usually occurs after an episode of vomiting, although the patient may vomit bright red blood with the first emesis. The bleeding is usually self-limited and stops spontaneously. If this does not occur, other therapeutic measures have included endoscopic hemostatic methods,[58] Sengstaken-Blakemore balloon tamponade, angiographic pharmacotherapy or embolic therapy, systemic administration of vasopressin, and surgery.

Esophagitis. Massive hemorrhage from esophagitis is rare. Therapy includes antireflux measures, as well as the reduction of intragastric acidity by pharmacologic measures.

Arteriovenous Malformations. Vascular malformations in the upper gastrointestinal tract can occur in the elderly (angiodysplasia), in uremic patients, or in patients with Osler-Weber-Rendu disease. Although general supportive measures, including correction of coagulation abnormalities, are helpful, therapeutic endoscopic hemostatic maneuvers, as well as angiographic hemostatic measures, may be helpful before the consideration of surgery.[52-54]

Aortoenteral Fistula. One must remember the possible diagnosis of aortoenteral fistula in a patient with upper gastrointestinal tract hemorrhage with an aortic graft in place. The severity of the hemorrhage may vary, with several small, heralding episodes occurring before the major episode. Although endoscopy is the first procedure to be performed in an attempt to localize a bleeding site in the distal duodenum,[59] further diagnostic procedures, such as computed tomographic imaging, magnetic resonance imaging, and angiography, may be necessary to make the diagnosis.[60] Therapy of this lesion is surgical repair.

SUMMARY

Upper gastrointestinal tract hemorrhage is a common diagnosis in patients admitted to the ICU, as well as in a proportion of patients with multiple illnesses who are already in the ICU. The etiology of the hemorrhage is varied, and the majority of hemorrhagic episodes stop spontaneously. The mortality from upper gastrointestinal tract hemorrhage has not changed during the past 30 years. The initial therapeutic thrust in all patients is resuscitation, with the restitution of the intravascular volume and correction of any concomitant complicating diagnoses, including coagulopathy. Therapy is then based on further diagnostic evaluation of a specific site of hemorrhage. It is hoped that, with the development of predictive risk factors for the severity of a hemorrhage and the refinement of newer modalities to treat the bleeding sites, it may be possible to alter the mortality rates for upper gastrointestinal tract hemorrhage.

References

1. Booker JA, Johnston M, Booker CI, et al: Prognostic factors for continued or rebleeding and death from gastrointestinal hemorrhage in the elderly. Age Ageing 16:208, 1987.
2. Allan R, Dykes P: A study of factors influencing mortality rates from gastrointestinal hemorrhage. Q J Med 45:533, 1976.
3. Kang JY, Piper DW: Improvement in mortality rates in bleeding peptic ulcer disease. Med J Aust 1:213, 1980.
4. Silverstein FE, Gilbert DA, Tedesco FJ, et al: The national ASGE survey on upper gastrointestinal bleeding. I. Study design and baseline data. Gastrointest Endosc 27:73, 1981.
5. Silverstein FE, Gilbert DA, Tedesco FJ, et al: The national ASGE survey on upper gastrointestinal bleeding. II. Clinical prognostic factors. Gastrointest Endosc 27:80, 1981.
6. Silverstein FE, Gilbert DA, Tedesco FJ, et al: The national ASGE survey on upper gastrointestinal bleeding. III. Endoscopy in upper gastrointestinal bleeding. Gastrointest Endosc 27:94, 1981.
7. Gilbert DA, Silverstein FE, Tedesco FJ, et al: National ASGE survey on upper gastrointestinal bleeding: Complications of endoscopy. Dig Dis Sci 26(suppl 7):27S, 1981.
8. Kitamura T, Ho K: Acute gastric changes in patients with acute stroke. I. With reference to gastroendoscopic findings. Stroke 7:460, 1976.
9. Lucas CE: Prevention and treatment of acute gastric erosions and stress ulcerations. In: Fiddian-Green RG, Turcotte JG (eds): Gastrointestinal Hemorrhage. New York, Grune & Stratton, p 167, 1980.
10. Czaja AF, McAlhand JC, Pruitt BA Jr: Acute gastroduodenal disease after thermal injury. N Engl J Med 291:925, 1974.
11. Peura DA, Johnson LF: Cimetidine for prevention and treatment of gastroduodenal mucosal lesions in patients in an intensive care unit. Ann Intern Med 103:173, 1985.
12. Schuster DP, Rowley H, Feinstein S, et al: Prospective evaluation of the risk of upper gastrointestinal bleeding after admission to a medical intensive care unit. Am J Med 76:623, 1984.
13. Lucas CE: Stress ulceration: The clinical problem. World J Surg 5:139, 1981.
14. Lucas CE, Riddle J, Rosenberg B, et al: Natural history and surgical dilemma of "stress" gastric bleeding. Arch Surg 4:266, 1971.
15. Ebert RV, Stead EA, Gibson JG: Response of normal subjects to acute blood loss. Arch Intern Med 68:578, 1941.
16. McLaughlin WD, Kolts BE, Achem SR: Nasogastric lavage compared with outcome in 101 patients seen in an emergency room for upper gastrointestinal hemorrhage. Gastroenterology 92:1529, 1987.
17. Ponsky JL, Hoffman M, Swaygim DS: Saline irrigation in gastric hemorrhage: The effect of temperature. J Surg Res 28:204, 1980.
18. Morrissey JF: Clinical approach to diagnostic endoscopy in patients with upper gastrointestinal bleeding. Dig Dis Sci 26(suppl 7):6s, 1981.
19. Schrock TR: Does endoscopy affect the surgical approach to the patient with upper gastrointestinal bleeding? Dig Dis Sci 26(suppl 7):27s, 1981.
20. Eastwood GL: Does the patient with upper gastrointestinal bleeding benefit from endoscopy? Reflections and discussions of recent literature. Dig Dis Sci 26(suppl 7):22S, 1981.
21. Graham DY: Limited value of early endoscopy in the management of acute upper gastrointestinal bleeding: Prospective controlled trial. Am J Surg 140:284, 1980.
22. Peterson WL, Barnett CC, Smith HJ, et al: Routine early endoscopy in upper-gastrointestinal-tract bleeding: A randomized controlled trial. N Engl J Med 304:925, 1981.
23. Morgan AG, Clamp SE: O.M.G.E. International Upper Gastro-intestinal Bleeding Survey 1978–1982. Scand J Gastroenterol Suppl 95:41, 1984.
24. Pimpl W, Boeckl O, Waclawiczek HW, et al: Estimation of the mortality rate of patients with severe gastrointestinal hemorrhage with the aid of a new scoring system. Endoscopy 19:101, 1987.
25. Wara P: Endoscopic prediction of major rebleeding—A prospective study of stigmata of hemorrhage in bleeding ulcer. Gastroenterology 88:1209, 1985.
26. Griffiths WH, Neumann DA, Welsh JD: The visible vessel as an indicator of uncontrolled or recurrent gastrointestinal hemorrhage. N Engl J Med 300:1411, 1979.
27. Foster DN, Miloszewski K, Losowsky MS: Stigmata of recent haemorrhage in diagnosis and prognosis of upper gastrointestinal bleeding. Br Med J 1:1173, 1978.
28. Swain CP, Storey DW, Brown SG, et al: Nature of the bleeding vessel in recurrently bleeding gastric ulcers. Gastroenterology 90:595, 1986.
29. Wara P: Endoscopic treatment of bleeding peptic ulcer. J Gastroenterol Hepatol 5(suppl 1):22, 1990.
30. Brown KE, Peura DA: Stress-related mucosal damage. Which ICU patients are at greatest risk? J Crit Illness 5:1215, 1991.
31. Schiessel R, Feil W, Wenzl E: Mechanisms of stress ulceration and implications for treatment. Clin Gastroenterol North Am 19:101, 1990.
32. Cheung LY: Pathogenesis, prophylaxis and treatment of stress gastritis. Am J Surg 156:437, 1988.
33. Lewis JH: Proceedings of the 35th GI Drugs Advisory Committee of the Food and Drug Administration. Am J Gastroenterol. In press.
34. Cannon LA, Heiselman D, Gardner W, et al: Prophylaxis of upper gastrointestinal tract bleeding in mechanically ventilated patients. A randomized study comparing the efficacy of sucralfate, cimetidine, and antacids. Arch Intern Med 147:2101, 1987.
35. Dirks MR, Craven DE, Celli BR, et al: Nosocomial pneumonia in intubated patients given sucralfate as compared with antacids or histamine type 2 blockers. The role of gastric colonization. N Engl J Med 317:1376, 1987.

36. Bornman PC, Theodorou NA, Shuttleworth RD, et al: Importance of hypovolemic shock and endoscopic signs in predicting recurrent hemorrhage from peptic ulceration: A prospective evaluation. Br Med J 29:245, 1985.
37. Kovacs TOG, Jensen DM: Endoscopic control of gastroduodenal hemorrhage. Annu Rev Med 38:267, 1987.
38. Kovacs TOG, Jensen DM: Electrothermal modalities in the treatment of non-variceal upper gastrointestinal bleeding. Eur J Gastroenterol Hepatol 2:87, 1990.
39. Swain CP, Brown SG, Storey DW, et al: Controlled trial of argon laser photocoagulation in bleeding peptic ulcers. Lancet 2:1313, 1981.
40. Swain CP, Kirkham JS, Salmon PR, et al: Controlled trial of Nd-Yag laser photocoagulation in bleeding peptic ulcers. Lancet 1:1113, 1986.
41. Brown SG: Controlled studies of laser therapy for hemorrhage from peptic ulcers. Acta Endosc 15:1, 1985.
42. Krejs GJ, Little KH, Westergaard H, et al: Laser photocoagulation for the treatment of acute peptic-ulcer bleeding: A randomized controlled clinical trial. N Engl J Med 316:1618, 1987.
43. Laine L: Multipolar electrocoagulation in the treatment of active upper gastrointestinal tract hemorrhage: A prospective controlled trial. N Engl J Med 316:1613, 1987.
44. Laine L: Multipolar electrocoagulation in the treatment of peptic ulcer with nonbleeding visible vessels. Ann Intern Med 110:510, 1989.
45. Jensen DM, Machicado GA, Kovacs TOG, et al: Controlled randomized study of heater probe and BICAP for hemostasis of severe ulcer bleeding. Gastroenterology 94:A208, 1988.
46. Jensen DM: Heat probe for hemostasis of bleeding peptic ulcers: Techniques and results of randomized controlled trials. Gastrointest Endosc 36:S42, 1990.
47. Chung SCS, Leung JWC, Sung JY, et al: Injection or heat probe for bleeding ulcer. Gastroenterology 100:33, 1991.
48. Chung SCS, Leung JWC, Steele RJC, et al: Endoscopic adrenaline injection for actively bleeding ulcer: A randomised trial. Br Med J 296:1631, 1988.
49. Sugawa C, Fujita Y, Ikeda T, et al: Endoscopic hemostasis of bleeding of the upper gastrointestinal tract by local injection of 98 per cent dehydrated ethanol. Surg Gynecol Obstet 162:159, 1986.
50. Loizou LA, Brown SG: Endoscopic treatment for bleeding peptic ulcers: Randomised comparison of adrenaline injection and adrenaline injection + Nd:YAG laser photocoagulation. Gut 32:1100, 1991.
51. NIH Consensus Development Conference—Therapeutic endoscopy and bleeding ulcers. JAMA 262:1369, 1989.
51a. Henry D, Cook D: Meta-analysis workshop in upper gastrointestinal hemorrhage. Gastroenterology 100:1481, 1991.
52. Eckstein MR, Kelemouridis V, Athanasoulis CA, et al: Gastric bleeding: Therapy with intraarterial vasopressin and transcatheter embolization. Radiology 152:643, 1984.
53. Stump DL, Hardin TC: The use of vasopressin in the treatment of upper gastrointestinal hemorrhage. Drugs 39:38, 1990.
54. Lieberman DA, Keller FS, Katon RM, et al: Arterial embolization for massive upper gastrointestinal tract bleeding in poor surgical candidates. Gastroenterology 86:876, 1984.
55. Gomes AS, Loin JF, McCoy RD: Angiographic treatment of gastrointestinal hemorrhage: Comparison of vasopressin infusion and embolization. AJR 146:1031, 1986.
56. Dempsey DT, Burke DR, Reilly RS, et al: Angiography in poor-risk patients with massive nonvariceal upper gastrointestinal bleeding. Am J Surg 159:282, 1990.
57. Murray WR: Surgical management of haemorrhage from peptic ulceration. Br J Surg 73:947, 1986.
58. Jensen DM, Kovacs TOG, Freeman M, et al: A multicenter randomised prospective study of gold probe versus heater probe for hemostasis of very severe ulcer or Mallory-Weiss bleeding. Gastroenterology 100:A92, 1991.
59. Martin J, Cano N, Di-Costanzo J, et al: Aortoduodenal fistula: Endoscopic diagnosis. Dig Dis Sci 26:956, 1981.
60. Gregson R, Craig O: Aorto-enteric fistulae: The role of radiology. Clin Radiol 34:65, 1983.

CHAPTER 125

Portal Hypertension and Variceal Hemorrhage

Jacob Korula

PORTAL HYPERTENSION

Portal hypertension is an inevitable complication of progressive chronic liver disease but may rarely develop in the absence of liver disease. The overt presentation of complications of portal hypertension, such as ascites, variceal hemorrhage, and hepatic encephalopathy, heralds the development of advanced liver disease and usually signifies a nonreversible state.

Anatomy of Portal Circulation

A brief review of the anatomy of the portal circulation is pertinent to understanding the derangements that occur and the pathophysiologic approach to management. The portal vein, formed by the confluence of the splenic and superior mesenteric veins at the level of the second lumbar vertebra and posterior to the head of the pancreas, is about 1.2 cm in diameter, contains no valves, and runs for about 6 to 8 cm before it enters the substance of the liver. At the hilum, the portal vein divides into the right branch, which supplies the right lobe, and the left branch, which supplies the left, caudate, and quadrate lobes of the liver. Remnants of the fetal circulation such as the umbilical and paraumbilical veins extend from the umbilicus and are contained in the ligamentum teres, connecting to the left branch of the portal vein. The inferior mesenteric vein drains the entire colon and rectum, excluding the ascending colon, and may occasionally drain into the superior mesenteric vein instead of into the splenic vein. The short gastric and left gastro-epiploic veins drain into the splenic vein at the level of the splenic hilum, whereas the left gastric, or coronary, vein usually drains into the portal vein or, infrequently, into the splenic vein[1] (Fig. 125–1). Thus, the portal venous circulation is composed of venous blood from the stomach, the intestine, and the pancreas and is unique because it originates in one capillary bed and terminates in another, the hepatic sinusoids. The hepatic artery, a branch of the celiac artery, supplies arterial blood at systemic pressure to the liver but unites with the low-pressure portal venous blood at the level of the hepatic sinusoids.[2] The intercommunicating sinusoidal network is lined by a single layer of endothelial cells and is separated from hepatocytes by a potential space, called the space of Disse. Blood from the sinusoidal network drains into terminal hepatic veins, which are tributaries of the right, middle, and left hepatic veins, which in turn collectively drain through the main hepatic vein into the inferior vena cava.[1] Both hepatic arterial and portal venous flow constitute hepatic blood flow, which approximates 1500 mL/min. To overcome sinusoidal vascular resistance, portal venous pressure is slightly higher than that in the systemic veins; in addition, the portal vein has a mean flow velocity of 16 cm/s and accounts for about 60 to 70% of the hepatic blood flow and 50% of the oxygen supply.[3]

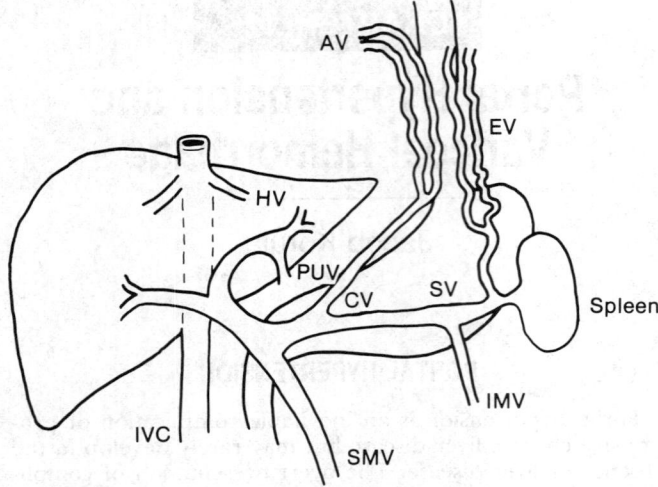

Figure 125—1. Anatomy of the portal circulation depicting esophagogastric collaterals that develop with portal hypertension. PV = portal vein; SV = splenic vein; PUV = paraumbilical vein; HV = hepatic vein; IVC = inferior vena cava; CV = coronary vein; SG = short gastric veins; EV = esophageal varices.

Pathophysiologic Events

As portal pressure rises, potential communications between the portal and systemic circulations open up at the level of the gastroesophageal junction, the anorectum, the bare area of the liver, the retroperitoneum, and the region of the splenic and left renal veins. Consequently, tortuous veins, or varices, develop in these locations, with those occurring at the gastroesophageal junction being most important clinically. In addition, recanalization of the paraumbilical vein may occur in some cases and is identified by an audible continuous venous hum (Cruveilhier-Baumgarten murmur), confirming the existence of intrahepatic portal hypertension.[3]

In most forms of liver disease, an increase in portal pressure occurs at the level of the hepatic sinusoids, referred to as sinusoidal hypertension. A good example of this lesion is the type that occurs in alcoholic liver disease. An increase in sinusoidal fibrosis leads to an increase in sinusoidal resistance.[4] An increment in portal pressure ensues, because pressure is directly related to resistance and flow. As liver disease progresses, an exponential rise in portal pressure leads to the establishment of portal-systemic collaterals, collectively called collateral circulation, which is formed to reduce the elevations in portal pressure. Portal inflow via the splanchnic arteries increases as collateral circulation develops, presumably in an effort to maintain portal flow into the liver. Ultimately, portal hypertension and the collateral circulation become irreversibly established.

An increase in collaterals is evidenced by visible collaterals in the abdominal and thoracic wall. Large collections of veins (caput medusae) are sometimes observed, with centrifugal direction of blood flow radiating from the umbilicus.[3] The recognition of large collaterals in the lumbar region and inferior to the umbilicus with cephalad direction of blood flow should raise the possibility of concomitant chronic obstruction of the inferior vena cava at the level of the hepatic veins, such as membranous occlusion of the vena cava.[5]

Large intra-abdominal and splanchnic collaterals are seen in extrahepatic portal hypertension, owing to obstructive lesions in the portal vein (usually remote, such as cavernous transformation of the portal vein).[6] Thrombosis of the splenic vein resulting from pancreatitis, trauma, or carcinoma (because the splenic vein courses the superior border of the pancreas) leads to hypertension of the left side of the portal circulation, or sinistral portal hypertension.[7] In this condition, gastric varices are prominent and are usually the source of hemorrhage. Esophageal varices (and to a lesser extent, gastric varices) develop in all types of portal hypertension, whether intrahepatic or extrahepatic (Table 125–1).

With progression of liver disease, an increase in the

TABLE 125–1
CAUSES OF PORTAL HYPERTENSION

Acute Liver Disease
Fulminant or submassive hepatic necrosis*
Alcoholic hepatitis
Acute fatty liver of pregnancy

Chronic Liver Disease
Active hepatitis or cirrhosis
   Alcoholic (includes alcoholic fibrosis and cirrhosis and
     chronic sclerosing hyaline necrosis)
   Hepatitis viruses (hepatitis B virus, hepatitis C virus)*
   Autoimmune lupoid conditions*
   Cryptogenic conditions*
Hepatic fibrosis
   Schistosomiasis†
   Noncirrhotic portal fibrosis*
   Vitamin A toxicity
Biliary diseases*
   Primary biliary cirrhosis
   Primary sclerosing cholangitis
   Secondary biliary cirrhosis
Congenital or hereditary diseases
   Copper overload: Wilson's disease
   Iron overload: idiopathic hemochromatosis
   Congenital hepatic fibrosis: microcystic disease†
   α_1-Antitrypsin deficiency
   Cystic fibrosis
   Gaucher's disease
   Biliary atresia
Miscellaneous diseases
   Nodular regenerative hyperplasia†
   Partial nodular transformation†
   Sarcoidosis
   Hepatic metastases

Diseases of Hepatic Venous Outflow
Budd-Chiari syndrome
Veno-occlusive disease
Membranous obstruction of vena cava

Diseases of Extrahepatic Portal Circulation†
Portal venous thrombosis (cavernous malformation of portal
   vein)
Splenic venous thrombosis

Diseases Not Primarily Affecting the Liver
Increased splanchnic flow
   Hematologic factors (increased portal blood flow)
     Myelofibrosis, agnogenic myeloid metaplasia
   Splanchnic arteriovenous fistula
   Hereditary hemorrhagic telangiectasia (Rendu-Osler-
     Weber syndrome)
Cardiac conditions
   Cardiomyopathy, right-sided failure
   Constrictive pericarditis
Arsenic poisoning, vinyl chloride†
Idiopathic portal hypertension†

*Conditions in which good correlation between hepatic venous pressure gradient and portal venous pressure gradient is not observed.

†Conditions with presinusoid portal hypertension (i.e., normal hepatic venous pressure gradient).

sinusoidal hydrostatic pressure leads to edema of the hepatic interstitium (in the space of Disse) and the need for removal of increased amounts of interstitial fluid by hepatic lymphatics. The ability of these lymphatics to remove fluid is soon exceeded as more fluid accumulates with increasing sinusoidal pressure, resulting in leakage of the excessive interstitial fluid from the surface of the liver into the peritoneal cavity and the appearance of ascites. In addition, renal retention of sodium and an increase in plasma volume perpetuate ascites formation.[8] Thus, ascites is a harbinger of significant intrahepatic portal hypertension; ascites is not usual in extrahepatic or idiopathic portal hypertension, except in advanced stages of the disease.[9]

In chronic liver disease, hepatic encephalopathy occurs with the development of portal-systemic collaterals and shunting of portal blood into the systemic circulation. The presence of such shunts in the region of the spleen and the left kidney or the adrenal gland can lead in some patients to spontaneous encephalopathy without common precipitating factors such as sepsis and gastrointestinal hemorrhage.[10]

Investigation

Because portal hypertension develops as a consequence of chronic liver disease in most instances, investigation is related largely to the search for the cause of liver disease (see Table 125-1).

Portal hypertension is suspected or identified when there is clinical evidence of an increase in abdominal collaterals or when patients exhibit consequences such as ascites, portal-systemic encephalopathy, and variceal hemorrhage. Esophageal or gastric varices can be detected with ease by fiberoptic esophagogastroduodenoscopy, in which size of the varices[11] and characteristics such as red wale signs, cherry red spots, and hemocystic spots on varices can be recognized.[12] Barium esophagogram is not sensitive for detection of small esophageal or gastric varices or varices in the antrum or the duodenum. Although hemorrhoids are seen in patients with portal hypertension, their occurrence is not specific, because a large proportion of individuals without liver disease have this problem. Rectal varices, on the other hand, are related to portal hypertension and can be identified by either flexible sigmoidoscopy or colonoscopy; the latter method is also useful to detect varices in the colon.[13]

Deep abdominal sonography with color flow imaging is a noninvasive modality that delineates the main portal vein, right and left branches, and the splenic vein. In addition to determining the presence of thrombus, color flow imaging can provide information regarding hepatofugal or hepatopetal flow.[14] The superior mesenteric vein, the left gastric vein, and collaterals in the gastrohepatic ligament may be seen by abdominal sonography, although less consistently. The ability to carry out serial studies noninvasively is a distinct advantage, however. Esophagogastric collaterals are not well characterized by this method; the availability of endoscopic ultrasonography shows some promise in the delineation of gastric and periesophageal collaterals, but its role in the assessment of submucosal varices of the esophagus is not known.[15] Large collaterals intra-abdominally can be seen with computed tomography or magnetic resonance imaging; collaterals are better characterized by the latter, if they appear as masses in the region of the splenic hilum on computed tomographic scan. Other methods of visualization of the portal and collateral circulation such as transhepatic portography[16] and splenoportography[17] are invasive and associated with complications; the former is not popular in the United States, and the risk of hemorrhage and splenic rupture limits the widespread use of the latter.[18] The venous phase of angiography after superior mesenteric arterial injection or splenic arterial injection is often adequate to visualize the portal and splenic veins and collaterals.[19] Digital subtraction is an improvement and provides better sequential images.

The measurement of portal pressure is usually not essential in the investigation of portal hypertension. There are a number of methods, however, by which portal pressure can be measured. Pressure in the portal vein or in the main tributaries can be measured at the time of surgery by placing a needle in these veins and connecting it to a water-filled manometer.[20] Portal pressure can also be measured at hepatic vein catheterization, in which a catheter introduced through the femoral or antecubital vein is deflected into the hepatic vein at the site of its entry into the inferior vena cava and wedged in a peripheral hepatic vein.[21] Pressure is recorded with a strain gauge transducer. In normal individuals, because of the intercommunicating sinusoidal network, the wedged pressure is low (<4 mm Hg). In diseases such as alcoholic liver disease, in which fibrosis of the sinusoids limits the extent of the intercommunications, wedging the catheter records pressure (wedged hepatic venous pressure) in a static column that reflects pressure in a portal vein branch. Withdrawal of the catheter from a wedged position records free hepatic venous pressure. The difference between the wedged pressure and the free hepatic vein pressure (or intra-abdominal inferior vena caval pressure) provides the hepatic venous pressure gradient, which approximates portal pressure. The free hepatic venous pressure, or inferior vena caval pressure, provides an internal zero reference. Wedged pressures can also be recorded by using a balloon catheter, which functions as a wedged catheter when the balloon is inflated in a hepatic vein branch; free hepatic venous pressure is obtained by deflating the balloon.[22] The normal hepatic venous pressure gradient is less than 4 mm Hg. The hepatic venous pressure gradient is approximately equal to portal pressure in alcoholic liver disease. In other types of liver disease, it may be 10 to 30% lower than portal pressure.

Portal pressure can be measured directly by using a transhepatic approach.[23] A thin needle is inserted into the liver under fluoroscopic guidance and contrast is injected as the needle is withdrawn. Entry of the needle into a portal vein radicle is confirmed if arborization is observed. Portal venous pressure is recorded only if blood is aspirated freely. At a separate puncture, the needle is directed toward the hepatic outflow and, by a similar technique, a hepatic vein branch is entered; no arborization is noted, but instead contrast in the vessel is observed to stream toward the hepatic outflow. The hepatic venous pressure serves as the internal zero reference, and the difference between the portal and hepatic venous pressures is the portal venous pressure gradient. The normal portal venous pressure gradient is less than 5 mm Hg. The reliability of intrahepatic (parenchymal) pressure achieved by transhepatic puncture of the liver and considered to reflect sinusoidal pressure has not been proved.[24] Pressure in the portal system can also be measured at splenoportography, in which a needle is inserted into the spleen; splenic pulp pressure that is recorded reflects pressure in the splenic and in turn the portal vein. The normal portal pressure by this method is less than 17 mm Hg.[17] The most popular method to measure pressures is hepatic venous catheterization. Entry into the hepatic vein is possible in more than 95% of cases and has little morbidity. This method is useful in the diagnosis of Budd-Chiari syndrome, which is confirmed by an inability to enter the hepatic veins.[25] This method is also used to distinguish presinusoidal (in which hepatic venous pressure gradient is usually normal) from sinusoidal portal hypertension. Hepatic venous catheterization is employed by researchers studying the pathophysiology of the portal circulation and in assessing the response of patients with portal hypertension to pharmacologic therapy.

The measurement of hepatic blood flow is used primarily for research purposes and has little clinical utility. Hepatic blood flow comprises both the hepatic arterial and portal venous flows. Measurements of flow do not specifically separate either component but rather assess total flow. Hepatic blood flow can be measured at surgery using electromagnetic flowmeters. Blood flow can be measured via microspheres[26] or by the infusion of an inert dye, indocyanine green, that is cleared only by the liver. In the latter method, blood flow is calculated by using the Fick principle.[27] Portal blood flow can be measured by deep abdominal sonography with pulsed Doppler flowmeter and determination of portal blood velocity at the main portal vein.[28] Portal blood flow is calculated by multiplying the peak portal blood velocity by the cross-sectional area of the portal vein (which is assumed to be elliptic or circular in shape). Because the Doppler technique measures the maximal blood velocity in the central part of the vessel, various experimentally determined correction factors are used to calculate mean portal blood velocity.[29] Improvements in technology may soon permit accurate measurements of portal blood flow.

VARICEAL HEMORRHAGE
Mechanism of Variceal Rupture

The factors leading to hemorrhage from esophageal and gastric varices are not known. Two mechanisms, namely erosion and explosion, have been proposed.[30] The erosion theory was based on the finding of esophagitis in the distal esophagus of patients with variceal hemorrhage, in endoscopic[31] and autopsy studies.[32] Evidence, however, does not suggest a role for gastroesophageal reflux, as lower esophageal sphincter pressures were normal in those who bled from varices; the administration of cimetidine also did not affect the rate of variceal rebleeding.[33] Histologic examination of a cuff of esophageal tissue obtained at esophageal transection performed for variceal hemorrhage did not confirm esophagitis, providing additional evidence against this mechanism.[34]

Most of the evidence tends to support explosion as a cause of rupture. Varices developing in the esophageal submucosa are considered elastic structures and consequently, structural abnormalities or the tension on the variceal wall may be important factors leading to the explosion of the varix. Wall tension of the varix is a function of the transmural pressure, radius, and wall thickness and is derived from the Laplace law:

$$T = TP \times r/w$$

where T is wall tension; TP represents transmural pressure; r indicates radius; and w is wall thickness.

Polio and Groszmann examined this relationship in artificial varices.[35] They proposed that this concept relates size of varices and intravarix pressures to bleeding risk; larger varices bleed at lower transmural pressures, and conversely, hemorrhage from smaller varices may occur at higher transmural pressures. By measuring intravarix pressure and determining varix size at endoscopy, Rigau and colleagues calculated wall tension and found a higher wall tension in those who bled from varices.[36] In another study, higher intravarix pressures were observed in patients who bled compared with those without history of hemorrhage.[37] Bleeding from esophageal varices rarely occurs when portal pressure is less than 12 mm Hg. Hemorrhage is frequently seen in patients with large varices, and in these patients,

portal pressure is usually greater than 12 mm Hg.[38] Patients who bleed tend to have higher portal pressure than those who do not. This relationship is not absolute, because patients have been observed with pressures in excess of 12 mm Hg who have not bled, whereas other patients with lower portal pressures have recurrent hemorrhage. Thus, there may be only a weak correlation between the risk of bleeding and the level of portal pressure.

It is suggested that increases in plasma volume in patients with chronic liver disease[8] may lead to elevations in portal venous pressure, contributing to bleeding risk. Studies in an animal model of portal hypertension showed that repletion of intravascular volume leads to increments in portal pressure over control values.[39] If data from experimental animals can be extrapolated to humans, there appears to be some basis for avoiding overexpansion of intravascular volume in patients who have bled, possibly reducing rebleeding risk. The role of ascites in precipitating variceal hemorrhage is also not certain. It is suggested that ascites formation leads to increased portal blood flow and pressure in the esophageal varices. This observation was not borne out in clinical studies by Iwatsuki and Reynolds, who demonstrated that portal pressure and hepatic blood flow were unchanged when intraabdominal pressure was lowered with therapeutic paracentesis.[40]

To select patients at risk for bleeding, one must determine the natural history of bleeding varices. When patients who had their varices endoscopically graded and had not bled were followed for periods ranging from 6 to 86 months, bleeding was found to occur in 30% of those with large varices and in 10% of patients with small varices.[41] Thus, size of varices and portal and intravarix pressures may be important to bleeding risk. The presence of red wale markings on large varices was reported to identify patients most likely to bleed.[42] However, problems with interobserver agreement make selection of patients solely on the basis of endoscopic signs somewhat unreliable.[43]

Management
Acute Hemorrhage

Hemorrhage from esophageal varices is a potentially fatal complication of portal hypertension with a mortality that exceeds 50% in patients with acute severe or chronic advanced liver disease. The goal of therapy is to control the acute bleeding episode and to prevent the recurrence of hemorrhage.

The first step is to assess the severity of the bleed (see Chapter 124). It should be noted that, specifically with regard to patients with liver failure and variceal hemorrhage, gastric lavage has not been shown to precipitate variceal hemorrhage and may be useful in preventing hepatic encephalopathy. In addition, lavage with tap water is preferred, as the use of saline should be avoided because of the risk of accumulating ascites. Patients with chronic liver disease usually have increased cardiac output and decreased peripheral vascular resistance;[44] consequently, monitoring of central venous pressure, cardiac output, and pulmonary capillary wedge pressure may not accurately reflect the volume status of these patients.

Although intravenous saline is readily used to replete volume, injudicious saline infusions must be avoided to prevent the subsequent development of ascites and edema. The infusion of colloid (5% human plasma protein fraction [Plasmanate]) in isotonic saline provides less sodium for the volume administered. With the restitution of blood volume and hemodynamic stability, the rate and type of fluid infused should be changed to an infusion of 0.45% saline or 5%

TABLE 125-2

POTENTIAL RISKS OF VASOPRESSIN THERAPY

Clinical Effects
Skin pallor
Abdominal cramps*
Decreased intestinal transit time*
Bradycardia
Hyponatremia, antidiuretic effect

Complications
Angina
Myocardial ischemia
Arrhythmia
Mesenteric ischemia or infarction
Ischemia of extremities
Renal insufficiency
Cerebrovascular accident
Activation of fibrinolysis

*Caused by increased peristaltic activity of smooth muscle (effects on V_2 receptor).

dextrose in water; unlimited volumes of these fluids may add to the problem of hyponatremia. The latter problem is compounded if vasopressin is administered for control of hemorrhage. For an actively bleeding patient, one must be vigilant to ensure that the airway is patent; however, it is not essential to carry out endotracheal intubation in all patients with variceal hemorrhage. Patients at high risk of aspiration, such as those with brisk bleeding, tense ascites, and encephalopathy during hemorrhage, must be electively intubated before endoscopy or inflation of tamponading balloon. Blood loss is replaced with transfusion of packed red blood cells or, rarely, whole blood; infusion of fresh frozen plasma either to replace colloid or to replenish clotting factors is not recommended and usually not needed; the latter may be necessary only when massive blood transfusions result in a washout phenomenon. Overexpansion of intravascular volume by overtransfusion should be discouraged to reduce the risk of recurrent hemorrhage; consequently, maintenance of hematocrit between 25 and 30% is adequate and permits optimal oxygen delivery to the tissues.

Diagnostic endoscopy should be carried out only when a patient with a protected airway is hemodynamically stable. In a patient with stigmata of chronic liver disease and ascites, hemorrhage is most likely from esophageal varices, and systemic vasoconstrictor therapy can be initiated even before confirmation of the diagnosis; in an individual with occult liver disease, however, therapy must be delayed until the diagnosis is made.

Pharmacologic Management. After a variceal source of hemorrhage is confirmed, three choices of therapy are available. The first is pharmacologic therapy and has the advantage that initiation of therapy does not require special equipment or expertise. Arginine vasopressin, the naturally occurring nonapeptide secreted by the posterior pituitary, has potent constrictor effects on splanchnic arterioles and to a lesser extent on the venules (effects on the V_1 receptor) and prokinetic actions on the smooth muscle (effects on the V_2 receptor).[45] Vasopressin decreases portal pressure by splanchnic arteriolar vasoconstriction and consequent decreased portal venous flow, hence the basis for its use in variceal hemorrhage. Although vasopressin causes a decrease in variceal pressure, this drug is effective in only 50% of patients with bleeding varices, and randomized controlled trials have not confirmed a beneficial effect.[46] The drug is usually administered at a dose of 0.4 U/min. A number of side effects (Table 125-2) have been reported with its administration. Although intra-arterial vasopressin demonstrated similar efficacy with a lower dose when compared

with intravenous infusion, delays in instituting therapy, the radiologic equipment, and personnel required for intra-arterial infusion make intravenous administration preferable.[47] With cessation of hemorrhage, vasopressin administration can be discontinued, as no data support the need for tapering the infusion. The benefits of longer-acting analogues of vasopressin, such as triglycyllypressin (Glypressin, terlipressin), which have been touted to reduce side effects and improve efficacy, have not been conclusively proved.[48]

Groszmann and associates reported that the addition of nitroglycerin mitigated the deleterious cardiovascular effects of vasopressin.[49] Subsequently, three independent controlled studies confirmed the beneficial effects of nitrites when used concomitantly with vasopressin, regardless of sublingual, intravenous, or transdermal route of administration.[50-52] In a patient who is not in shock, concomitant use of a nitroglycerin patch (10 cm, 5 mg) is simple and probably beneficial. When nitrites are absorbed into the systemic circulation, vasodilatation leads to reflex splanchnic vasoconstriction and reduction in portal pressure.[53] Because of systemic vasodilatation, intravenous administration of this drug should be avoided during acute hemorrhage, because potentiation of hypotension could occur.

Somatostatin is an octopeptide that decreases splanchnic blood flow and reduces portal pressure.[54] This drug has fewer systemic vasoconstrictor effects, which makes it more desirable than vasopressin; controlled studies have not conclusively established efficacy. In a multicenter study in the United States, control of hemorrhage occurred in 80% of controls compared with 67% of patients receiving somatostatin.[55] In another study, somatostatin was found in one center to control hemorrhage in 64% of patients who received the drug compared with 41% patients receiving placebo.[56] The large variability in the cessation of bleeding in the control groups in both studies attests to the problem of interpreting results.

Balloon Tamponade. An alternative to pharmacologic therapy is tamponade, which is aimed at compressing varices with balloons that are inflated in the esophagus or the stomach. Three types of tubes are available (Fig. 125-2) and are of comparable efficacy. The Sengstaken-Blakemore tube is a three-lumen tube that consists of an esophageal balloon, inflated with 40 mm Hg pressure (using a sphygmomanometer), and a gastric balloon that is inflated with 100 to 200 mL of air.[57] A third lumen allows aspiration of gastric contents. The high risk of pulmonary aspiration of oral and esophageal secretions with the use of this tube can be reduced by taping a small catheter to the esophageal tube and connecting it to suction. The Minnesota tube is a modification of the Sengstaken-Blakemore tube and has four lumina with ports in the esophageal tube to facilitate aspiration of pharyngeal secretions.[58] The Linton-Nachlas tube, reported to be more effective in controlling bleeding from gastric varices, consists of only a gastric balloon that is inflated with 500 to 600 mL of air.[59] Multiple openings in the esophageal and gastric lumina allow aspiration of secretions and blood. In some centers, traction (200 g to 1 kg depending on the tube) is used in the belief that compression on the varices is improved; the use of a helmet placed over the face has avoided the need for a pulley and a supporting frame over the bed. Despite modifications of these tubes, in the technique of insertion and in the efforts to reduce complications, efficacy of this modality was not changed during three decades of its use.[60] Complications seen with this tube (Table 125-3) do not favor its use as initial treatment currently.

Endoscopic Sclerotherapy and Variceal Ligation. The most promising of treatments in the management of acute variceal hemorrhage is endoscopic sclerotherapy. The original technique, described in 1939, was carried out with a

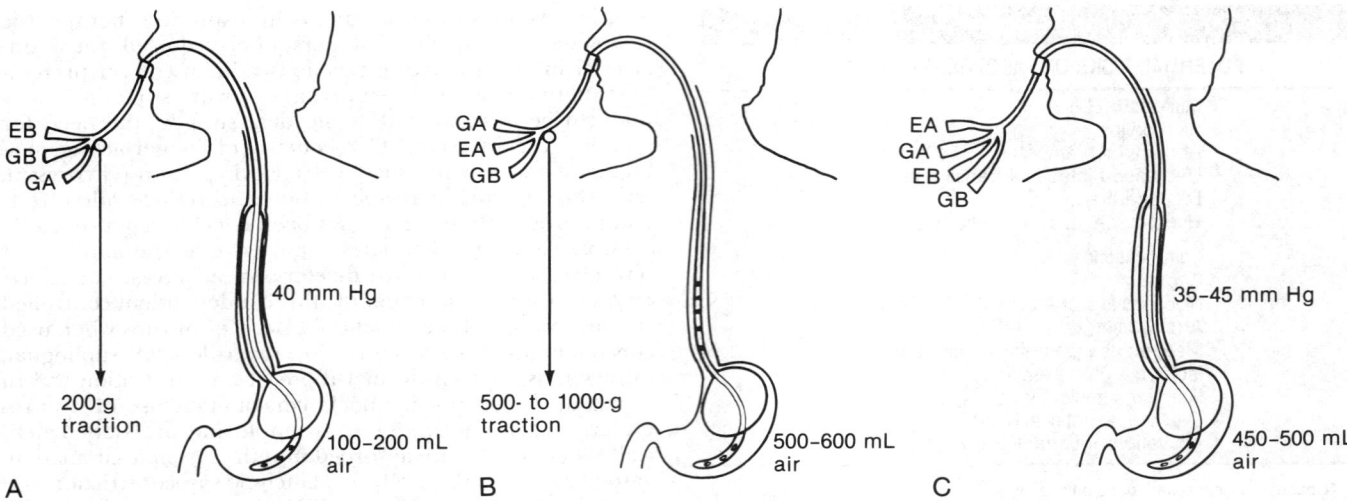

Figure 125–2. Types of balloon tubes for tamponade therapy. *A.* Sengstaken-Blakemore tube. *B.* Linton-Nachlas tube. *C.* Minnesota tube. GB = gastric balloon; EB = esophageal balloon; GA = gastric aspirate; EA = esophageal aspirate.

rigid endoscope.[61] The present availability of fiberoptic endoscopes has allowed the performance of this procedure emergently at the bedside or electively in ambulatory patients. Injection of sclerosants into submucosal veins leads to thrombosis and necrotizing inflammation; eventually, varices become obliterated with the development of fibrosis.[62] The injection of small volumes of sclerosants paravariceally by some endoscopists results in mucosal fibrosis without obliteration of esophageal varices and also leads to comparable reductions in rebleeding risk.[63] Acute thrombotic occlusion appears to be the mechanism by which intravariceal injection causes a varix to cease bleeding.[62] A number of sclerosants are available, and only a few studies comparing their relative efficacy have been reported. The three most commonly used sclerosants in the United States of seemingly comparable efficacy are 5% sodium morrhuate, 5% ethanolamine oleate, and 3% sodium tetradecyl sulfate.[64–66] Ethanol absolute or 50% is an effective sclerosant, although ulcerogenic, and is popular in developing countries because of its low cost.[67]

Short-term sclerotherapy is about 60 to 70% effective in controlling active bleeding[68] (Fig. 125–3). The risk of complications rises if the frequency of treatments is increased[69] and if visibility is decreased in an actively bleeding patient.[70] Considerably more expertise and technical skill are required in carrying out sclerotherapy in an actively bleeding, compared with a nonbleeding, patient. When endoscopic examination is obscured by brisk bleeding, temporizing with balloon tamponade for a few hours, until blood from the

stomach is cleared, allows satisfactory injection of varices subsequently. A number of complications have been reported with sclerotherapy[71] (Table 125–4) and are seen more frequently in patients with severe or advanced liver disease. Controlled trials of short-term sclerotherapy, although clearly showing a decrease in early rebleeding and superiority over vasopressin[72] and balloon tamponade,[73] have not demonstrated improved short-term survival in patients who received this treatment compared with controls.

Ligation of varices by a technique similar to rubber band ligation of hemorrhoids has been reported by Steigmann and colleagues.[74] Release of O rings (stretched onto a capsule that slips into a cylindric attachment at the distal aspect of the endoscope) over a bolus of esophageal mucosa and varices that is suctioned into the distal cylindric chamber causes strangulation of the varix (Fig. 125–4). The O rings are eliminated intestinally with sloughing of the mucosa. Mucosal ulceration is mostly superficial, and preliminary results of a controlled comparison with chronic sclerotherapy showed significantly fewer complications with this technique; survival was similar, however.[75] Because this technique necessitates the suction of the esophageal varix into the distal chamber for an optimal ligation, the ability to carry this out successfully may be limited with brisk bleeding. Results of controlled studies comparing sclerotherapy with variceal ligation in acute variceal hemorrhage are awaited.

Portal-Systemic Shunt Surgery. Despite the widespread use of endoscopic sclerotherapy (or the anticipated success of variceal ligation), there is a role for emergency portal-systemic shunt surgery in patients in whom sclerotherapy fails to control variceal hemorrhage.[76, 77] Patients with good-risk liver disease determined by using Child's classification[78] or modifications[79] (Table 125–5) in whom bleeding cannot be controlled with endoscopic sclerotherapy must be offered surgery. The morbidity and mortality of the surgery, however, are significantly increased in patients with severe-risk liver disease, such as Child's class C patients. The portacaval type of shunt is preferred because it can be carried out expeditiously. In centers in which expertise is available, esophageal transection[79, 80] and esophageal devascularization[81] (disconnection of periesophageal and gastric veins) are considered suitable alternatives to portal-systemic shunt surgery. Anastomotic leak is the most frequent complication with esophageal transection. Obliteration of esophageal and gastric varices can also be achieved by transhepatic catheterization of the portal vein. Thrombophlebitis and sepsis occur

TABLE 125–3
COMPLICATIONS OF BALLOON TAMPONADE

Improper Tube Placement
Esophageal rupture or perforation
Asphyxiation

Prolonged Placement
Gastroesophageal ulceration
Aspiration pneumonia
Esophageal perforation
Periesophageal inflammation and abscess

Devices Used to Retain Tamponade Tube
Pressure necrosis of nasal ala
Pressure necrosis over forehead and chin (from helmet)

in about 25%, although cessation of hemorrhage may be seen in almost 75% of patients offered this therapy.[82] These three latter approaches, however, provide temporary benefit only. Ultimately, the choice of alternatives in patients in whom sclerotherapy fails is determined by the severity of the liver disease and the expertise available at each center.

Transjugular Intrahepatic Portal-Systemic Shunt (TIPS). Successful insertion of expandable metallic stents in the liver bridging the hepatic and portal veins and resulting in an intrahepatic portal-systemic shunt has been reported (Fig. 125–5).[83a] With the percutaneous transjugular approach, a needle is advanced through the hepatic parenchyma into a branch of the portal vein proximal to its bifurcation and guided by transabdominal ultrasonography or by placement of a transhepatic needle or guidewire in a portal vein branch. The needle track is then dilated with a balloon before insertion of a self-expanding stent. Although results from controlled studies are not yet available, this nonsurgical procedure appears to be promising and has been found useful in controlling variceal hemorrhage before hepatic transplantation.[83b]

Prevention of Rebleeding

The risk of rebleeding from esophagogastric varices is not abolished with methods used to control acute hemorrhage, except with emergency portal-systemic shunt surgery (in which decompression of the portal circulation is adequate). A number of therapeutic options are available to reduce the subsequent risk of rebleeding and potential mortality related to the hemorrhage. Of the options available, however, endoscopic sclerotherapy or variceal ligation and portal-systemic shunt surgery appear the most promising. Beta-blocking drugs such as propranolol are not recommended because controlled trials have shown conflicting results, and these agents are not considered beneficial.[83]

Endoscopic Sclerotherapy. A number of controlled trials of long-term sclerotherapy have demonstrated a significant decrease in rebleeding when patients treated with sclerotherapy were compared with those who received standard medical therapy for bleeding with balloon tamponade and/or vasopressin administration.[84, 85] Survival of patients who received sclerotherapy was not improved, except at one cen-

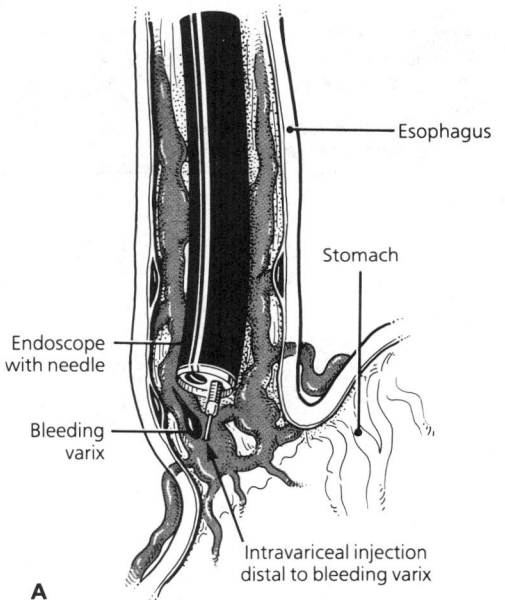

A
Esophagus
Stomach
Endoscope with needle
Bleeding varix
Intravariceal injection distal to bleeding varix

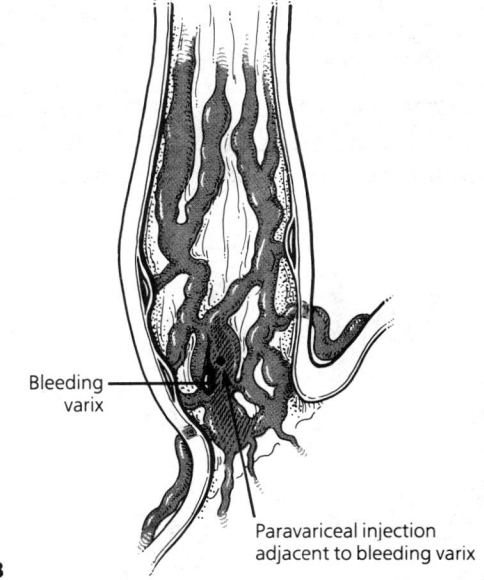

B
Bleeding varix
Paravariceal injection adjacent to bleeding varix

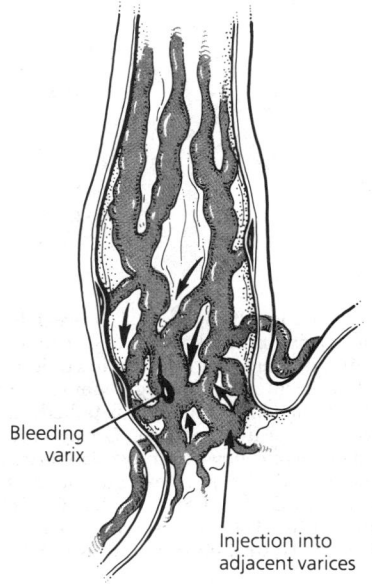

C
Bleeding varix
Injection into adjacent varices

Figure 125–3. Several maneuvers may help slow or stop blood flow from esophageal varices. *A.* If blood is seen spurting or oozing from a varix, inject distal to the bleeding site because variceal flow is usually proximal or cephalad. *B.* If bleeding continues, try to raise a small bleb adjacent to the site of spurting with a paravariceal injection. *C.* If both of these techniques fail to slow or halt bleeding, try injecting into large varices that lie adjacent to the bleeding varix. Communication between variceal columns may occasionally allow the sclerosant to traverse these columns and to stop the bleeding. If bleeding continues despite these measures, balloon tamponade is indicated. (From Korula J, Yamada S: Technique of endoscopic sclerotherapy for esophageal varices. J Crit Illness 2[2]:53, 1987.)

TABLE 125–4
COMPLICATIONS OF ENDOSCOPIC SCLEROTHERAPY

Esophageal
Perforation
Stricture
  Rarely refractory
Ulceration
  Superficial
  Deep (± plaques)
Mucosal bridges
Mucosal defects
Intramural hematoma
Esophagoesophageal fistula
Dysmotility
  Decrease lower esophageal sphincter
    pressure
  Delayed clearance

Cardiorespiratory
Pleural effusion (exudative)
Pneumonia
  Usually aspiration
Adult respiratory distress syndrome
  (? related)
Fistula
  Esophagopleural
  Esophagobronchial
Mediastinitis
Chylothorax
Pericarditis

Systemic, Other
Bacteremia
  Streptococcus
  Staphylococcus
  Enterococci
  Serratia
Fungemia
  Candidiasis
Spinal cord paralysis
  ? Venous infarction (subsequent thrombosis
    of anterior spinal artery)
Spontaneous bacterial peritonitis
Portal venous thrombosis

Gastric
Ulceration
Thrombosis
Uncertain
Laceration
Pseudodiverticula
Cardiac arrhythmias
Aneurysm of aorta
Rupture of aorta
Thrombosis of vasa vasorum
Pulmonary emboli
Coagulopathy
Acute gastric dilatation (? symptoms of
  esophageal perforation, sepsis)

Adapted from Korula JJ: Endoscopic variceal sclerotherapy. J Clin Gastroenterol 10:588–590, 1988.

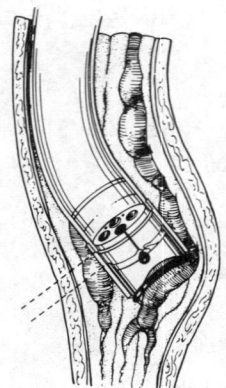
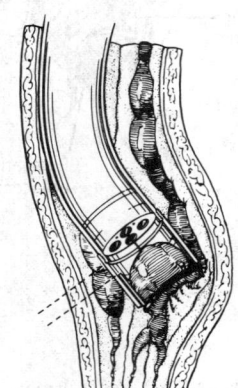
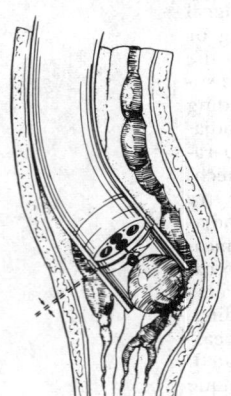
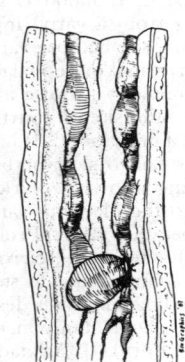

Figure 125–4. The technique of endoscopic variceal ligation. The endoscopist approaches a target varix and makes full 360° contact between the varix and the end of the ligating device *(upper left)*. Endoscopic suction is activated, gently drawing the target varix into the ligating chamber *(upper right)*. The trip wire (which passes through the biopsy channel) is pulled, moving the inner cylinder toward the endoscope, releasing the elastic O ring around the neck of the varix *(lower left)*. The target varix is now securely ligated *(lower right)*. The endoscope is removed, the ligating device is reloaded, and further varices are ligated. (From GV Steigmann, JS Goff, JH Sun, et al, Endoscopic variceal ligation: An alternative to sclerotherapy, Gastrointestinal Endoscopy, 35, 431–434, 1989, © by American Society for Gastrointestinal Endoscopy.)

TABLE 125–5

CRITERIA FOR CHILD'S CLASSIFICATION

	Child's Class		
	A	B	C
Variable	1	2	3*
Serum bilirubin level (mg/dL)	<2	2–3	>3†
Serum albumin level (g/dL)	>3.5	2.8–3.5	<2.8
Ascites	None	Slight	Large
Encephalopathy	None	Grades 1 and 2	Grades 3 and 4
Prothrombin time (s)	1–4	4–6	>6‡
Nutrition§	Excellent	Good	Poor, wasting

*A scoring system first reported by Pugh and colleagues[79] allocates from 1 to 3 points for each of five variables. Thus, Child's class A has a score of 5–8; class B, 9–11; and class C, 12–15.[79]

†In patients with primary biliary cirrhosis, serum bilirubin is allocated 1 point if < 4 mg/dL, 2 points if between 4 and 10 mg/dL, and 3 points if > 10 mg/dL.[79]

‡May be modified using prothrombin activity in which 4 using Quick time is approximately equivalent to 40% activity.

§Assessment of nutrition was included in the original criteria by Child but is not commonly used because of difficulty in distinguishing classes A and B.

ter.[86] Obliteration of varices appears to be the end point of sclerotherapy.[86, 87] A study has challenged this concept by demonstrating that rebleeding risk in patients who received only short-term sclerotherapy for rebleeding episodes was no different when compared with that in those in whom obliteration of varices was achieved.[88] Unless additional evidence supports this view, sclerotherapy must be continued to variceal obliteration. Obliteration can be achieved in more than 70% of cases, provided treatments are repeated regu-

larly, unless esophageal ulceration, stricture, or ulcer-related rebleeding precludes achieving this objective. The reasons for sclerotherapy failure are not known; inability to obliterate varices completely,[62] hemorrhage from gastric varices,[89] ulceration overlying incompletely sclerosed varices,[62] and bleeding from portal hypertensive gastropathy[90] are presumed causes. Technical modifications to improve the rate of variceal obliteration and reduction of sclerotherapy-related ulceration may decrease failure rate. Gastric varices developed in only 15% of patients receiving sclerotherapy, in whom gastric varices were not present at inception of sclerosing treatment, and only 4% were large fundal varices.[89] Patients with fundal varices must be referred for portal-systemic shunt surgery because results of sclerosis of large fundal varices are poor. The precise incidence of bleeding from portal hypertensive gastropathy is not known, and it is not clear if sclerotherapy increases the risk of this complication. Although variceal ligation is expected to decrease the risk of esophageal and pulmonary complications, the overall efficacy when compared with that of sclerotherapy is similar. It is not known if variceal ligation results in a lower rebleeding rate.

Portal-Systemic Shunt Surgery. The construction of a portal-systemic shunt was considered a major advance in surgery for the management of variceal hemorrhage. Initial enthusiasm for this procedure led to the performance of shunts prophylactically; controlled trials demonstrated no benefit by this approach.[91] In patients who bleed from varices, controlled trials of portal-systemic shunts have shown a significant reduction in rebleeding, although a fivefold to sixfold increase in the incidence of encephalopathy was seen in the shunted patients when compared with patients who were managed medically.[85, 92–95] These results prompted modifications of the portacaval or total shunt (end to side, side to side) and led to the introduction of the distal

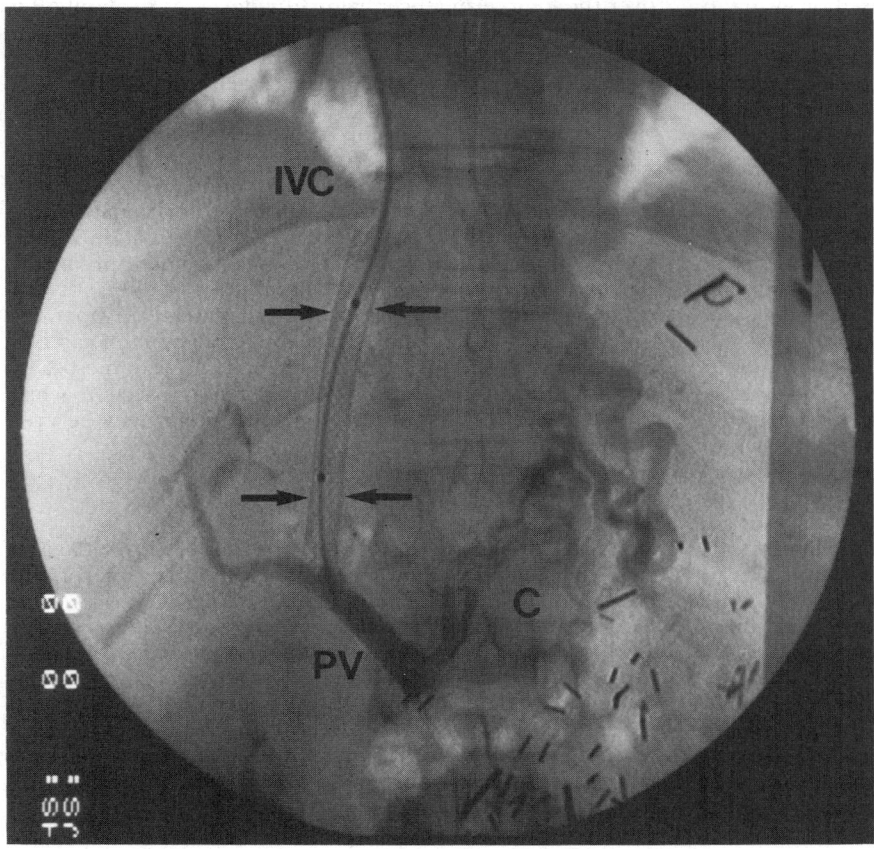

Figure 125–5. Radiograph showing the stent *(arrows)* within the liver. The catheter was inserted through the jugular vein, entering the liver via the inferior vena cava *(IVC)* and allowing cannulation and opacification of the portal vein *(PV)*. Note large collaterals *(C)*, which were later embolized with coils.

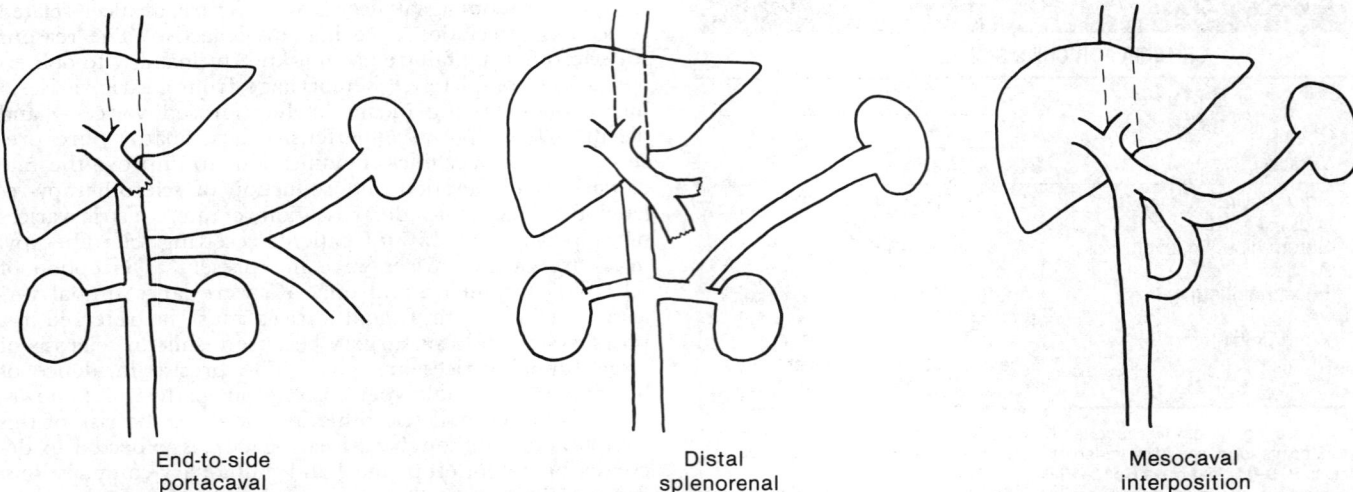

End-to-side
portacaval

Distal
splenorenal

Mesocaval
interposition

Figure 125–6. Common types of surgical portal-systemic shunts placed for management of variceal hemorrhage.

splenorenal or selective shunt.[96] In this latter shunt, the distal splenic vein is anastomosed to the left renal vein, resulting in decompression of the short gastric and left gastroepiploic veins and consequent drainage of blood from the esophageal and gastric collaterals into the systemic circulation. The rationale of this innovative surgery is to preserve superior mesenteric venous flow, which transports hepatotropic factors from the pancreas to the liver, reducing perhaps the long-term risk of hepatic hypoperfusion and failure reported with the total shunts.[97] Because decompression of the portal circulation is only partial with selective shunts, rebleeding rate is higher than that seen with the portacaval shunt, probably owing to thrombosis of the shunt from the small caliber of the veins anastomosed or owing to inadequate decompression of esophagogastric collateral flow. In addition, a patent coronary vein or collaterals in the region of the pancreatic bed may require disconnection from the portal circulation to further reduce the rebleeding risk after this surgery.[98]

In alcoholic liver disease, controlled comparisons between portacaval (total) and distal splenorenal (selective) shunts showed no difference in the incidence of encephalopathy.[99–102] Over the long term, in these patients, selective shunts function as total shunts, perhaps explaining the lack of difference between the two types of shunts. There are insufficient data to determine if distal splenorenal shunt has advantages in nonalcoholic liver disease.

Sarfeh and colleagues have shown that small-caliber (8- to 12-mm) portacaval H grafts preserve prograde portal flow while effectively reducing variceal hemorrhage and decreasing postshunt encephalopathy; a 16% shunt thrombosis rate is a drawback of this type of surgery.[103] Mesocaval shunt consists of anastomosis between the superior mesenteric vein and the inferior vena cava by means of a venous or prosthetic graft.[104] Interposition of a graft (H graft) sometimes facilitates this anastomosis;[105] infrequently, anastomosis of a large coronary vein to the inferior vena cava (coronocaval shunt) achieves the same result. Thrombosis of the graft may complicate surgery with consequent rebleeding. A mesocaval shunt is useful as a temporizing procedure and could be considered in a patient with bleeding varices who may require hepatic transplantation later. Of the different types of shunts available, portacaval, mesocaval, and distal splenorenal shunts are the most frequently performed; both portacaval and mesocaval shunts can be performed emergently (Fig. 125–6). In cases of Budd-Chiari syndrome, side-to-side shunt is performed;[25] if venous pressures are elevated

in the inferior vena cava, the lack of a significant gradient precludes flow through the shunt. An end-to-side portacaval shunt could prove fatal if performed in Budd-Chiari syndrome because of the lack of venous outflow from the liver. Mesoatrial or mesoinnominate shunts are placed if side-to-side shunts are not possible for this condition.[25]

Ascites may develop transiently after portal-systemic shunt surgery and may be chylous in nature when a distal splenorenal shunt is placed. Although shunt thrombosis is uncommon, this complication occurs more frequently with the distal splenorenal shunt, related perhaps to the smaller caliber of the veins anastomosed. Encephalopathy that develops soon after shunt surgery portends a poor prognosis; over the long term, encephalopathy develops in about 20 to 30% of shunted patients. There are few substantive data to support an increased incidence of acid-pepsin disease after shunt surgery and the cause of increased iron overload seen rarely is not clear.

In patients who develop recurrent hemorrhage after TIPS, placement of a second stent within the liver or embolization of large collaterals is an option.

A patient who is a potential candidate for hepatic transplantation should be considered for transplantation if satisfactory options are unavailable for management of variceal hemorrhage. Although prior shunt surgery does not preclude subsequent transplantation, an increase in operative time resulting from dissection at the hepatic hilum can be a disadvantage. Therapeutic options such as TIPS, mesocaval, or distal splenorenal shunt, or esophageal transection, which avoid surgical anastomosis at the liver hilum, may be preferable choices.

Prophylactic Therapy

A brief discussion of therapy directed to prophylaxis of variceal bleeding is appropriate. The desirable concept, that the first episode of bleeding from esophageal varices could be prevented with a view to improving survival, was considered in the 1960s when the technique of shunt surgery was evolving. Controlled studies with prophylactic shunts, however, did not demonstrate improved survival of patients who received these shunts.[91] Enthusiasm for prophylactic therapy was renewed when preliminary results of propranolol and endoscopic sclerotherapy showed some benefit in the treatment of variceal hemorrhage. A number of controlled trials ensued; results of trials using selective and nonselective beta-blockers demonstrated a significant decrease in the incidence of first hemorrhage[106–108] and, in some studies, even showed a lower mortality in those who received these drugs.[106] On the other hand, results of controlled studies with sclerotherapy were not as encouraging; in some European studies, sclerotherapy was found beneficial,[109–112] whereas studies in the United States showed sclerotherapy to be deleterious, not only increasing the frequency of bleeding but also decreasing survival.[113, 114] Thus, on the basis of this evidence, some clinicians favor the administration of prophylactic propranolol in patients with large esophageal varices who have not bled, whereas others prefer to await additional evidence from controlled trials. Certainly, endoscopic sclerotherapy should not be carried out except in the setting of controlled trials.

Summary (Fig. 125–7)

When a patient with large esophagogastric varices is identified, particularly if there are red wale signs, propranolol may be administered at a dose that decreases resting heart rate by 25%. If acute hemorrhage develops, intravenous vasopressin is administered with transdermal nitroglycerin, while the patient is made hemodynamically stable and prepared for endoscopy. Emergency endoscopic sclerotherapy (or ligation if efficacy of this modality is proved) should be offered to control bleeding. If bleeding continues, balloon tamponade (used concomitantly with vasopressin and nitroglycerin if bleeding is severe) may be attempted initially, followed by one or two attempts at sclerotherapy. The ability to inject varices, without the development of extensive ulceration and rebleeding, determines if a patient should continue to receive sclerotherapy. Good-risk patients in whom sclerotherapy fails must be offered TIPS or portal-systemic shunt surgery, the choice of which is determined by the expertise available at each center, or considered for hepatic transplantation, provided that the patient is stable.

After acute hemorrhage is controlled, a program of long-term sclerotherapy is started to obliterate esophageal and gastric varices. Recurrent variceal hemorrhage on this regimen, especially after obliteration of esophageal and gastric varices, should lead to a consideration of alternative therapy such as TIPS, portal-systemic shunt, esophageal transection, and devascularization. In potential candidates for hepatic transplantation, referral for transplantation should be considered at the time of sclerotherapy failure. In poor-risk patients, regardless of the type of alternative therapy offered, treatment is usually unsatisfactory and the outcome poor.

References

1. Douglass BC, Bagenstoss A, Holinshead W: The anatomy of the portal vein and its tributaries. Surg Gynecol Obstet 91:562, 1950.
2. Lautt WW: Hepatic vasculature: A conceptual review. Gastroenterology 73:1163, 1977.
3. Reynolds TB: Portal hypertension. In: Schiff L, Schiff E (eds): Diseases of the Liver. 6th ed. Philadelphia, JB Lippincott, p 875, 1987.
4. Reynolds TB, Redeker AG, Geller HM: Wedged hepatic vein pressure. Am J Med 22:341, 1957.
5. Rector WG, Xu Y, Goldstein L, et al: Membranous obstruction of the inferior vena cava in the United States. Medicine 64:134, 1985.
6. Lindsay J, Webb J, Sherlock S: The aetiology, presentation and natural history of extra-hepatic portal venous obstruction. Q J Med 48:627, 1979.
7. Turrill FL, Mikkelsen WP: "Sinistral" (left sided) extrahepatic portal hypertension. Arch Surg 99:365, 1969.
8. Levy M: Pathogenesis of ascites. In: Epstein M (ed): The Kidney in Liver Disease. 2nd ed. New York, Elsevier, p 209, 1983.
9. Boyer JL, Gupta KPS, Biswas SK, et al: Idiopathic portal hypertension. Comparison with the portal hypertension of cirrhosis and extrahepatic portal vein obstruction. Ann Intern Med 66:41, 1967.
10. Lam KC, Juttner HU, Reynolds TB: Spontaneous portosystemic shunt. Relationship to spontaneous encephalopathy and gastrointestinal hemorrhage. Dig Dis Sci 26:346, 1981.
11. Lebrec D, DeFleury P, Rueff B, et al: Portal hypertension, size of esophageal varices and risk of gastrointestinal bleeding in cirrhosis. Gastroenterology 79:1139, 1980.
12. Beppu K, Inokuchi K, Koyanagi N, et al: Prediction of variceal hemorrhage by esophageal endoscopy. Gastrointest Endosc 27:213, 1981.
13. Weinshel E, Chein W, Falkenstein DB: Hemorrhoids or rectal varices:

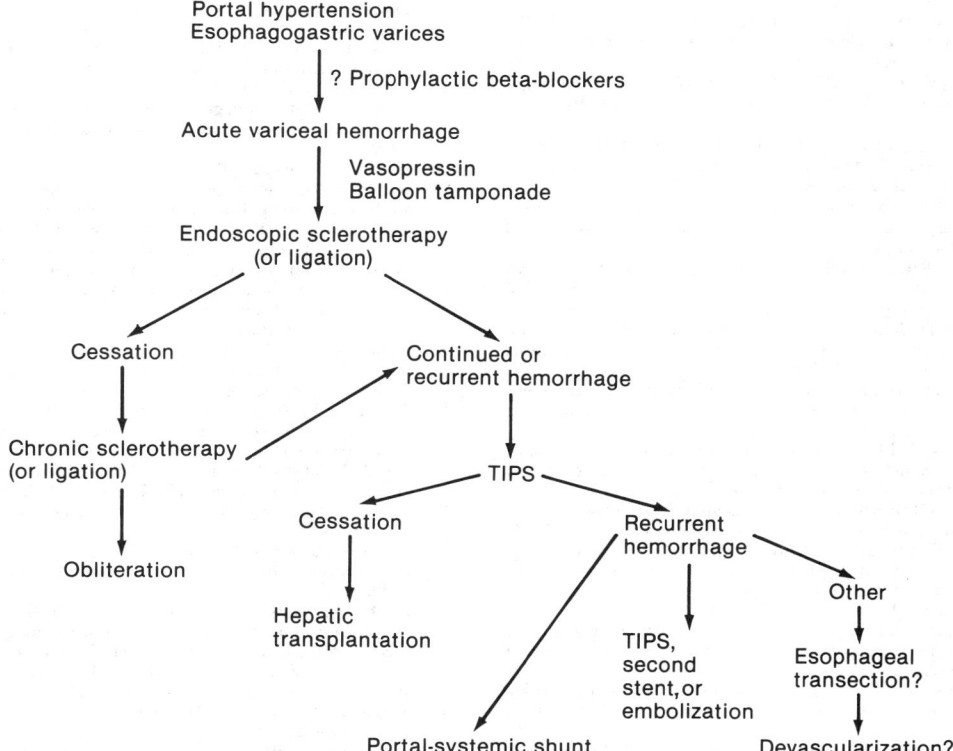

Figure 125–7. Algorithm for the management of variceal hemorrhage.

Defining the cause of massive rectal hemorrhage in patients with portal hypertension. Gastroenterology 90:744, 1986.

14. Ralls PW: Color doppler sonography of the hepatic artery and portal venous system. AJR 155:517, 1990.

15. Caletti G, Brocchi E, Baraldini M, et al: Assessment of portal hypertension by endoscopic ultrasonography. Gastrointest Endosc 36:S21, 1990.

16. Okuda K, Suzuki K, Musha H, et al: Percutaneous transhepatic catheterization of the portal vein for the study of portal hemodynamics and shunts: A preliminary report. Gastroenterology 73:279, 1977.

17. Turner M, Sherlock S, Steiner R: Splenic venography and intrasplenic pressure measurement in the clinical investigation of the portal venous system. Am J Med 23:846, 1957.

18. Panke W, Bradley E, Moreno A, et al: Technique, hazards and usefulness of percutaneous splenic portography. JAMA 169:1032, 1959.

19. Viamonte M, Warren W, Fomon J, et al: Angiographic investigations in portal hypertension. Surg Gynecol Obstet 128:37, 1970.

20. Schenk WG, MacDonald J, McDonald K, et al: Direct measurement of hepatic blood in surgical patients with related observations on hepatic flow dynamics in experimental animals. Ann Surg 156:166, 1968.

21. Myers JD, Taylor WJ: Estimation of hepatic sinusoid pressure by means of venous catheters and estimation of portal pressure by hepatic vein catheterization. Am J Physiol 165:527, 1951.

22. Groszmann R, Glickman M, Blei A, et al: Wedged and free hepatic venous pressure measured with a balloon catheter. Gastroenterology 76:253, 1979.

23. Boyer TD, Triger D, Horisawa M, et al: Direct transhepatic measurement of portal vein pressure using a thin needle: Comparison with wedged hepatic vein pressure. Gastroenterology 72:584, 1977.

24. Orruego H, Blendis LM, Crossley IR, et al: Correlation of intrahepatic pressure with collagen in the Disse space and hepatomegaly in humans and in the rat. Gastroenterology 80:546, 1981.

25. Mitchell MC, Boitnott JK, Kaufman S, et al: Budd-Chiari syndrome: Etiology, diagnosis and management. Medicine 61:199, 1982.

26. Huet PM, Marleau D, Lavoie P, et al: Extraction of 125 I-albumin microaggregates from portal blood. Gastroenterology 70:74, 1976.

27. Bradley SE, Ingelfinger FJ, Bradley GP, et al: The estimation of hepatic blood flow in man. J Clin Invest 24:890, 1945.

28. Ohnishi Y, Saito M, Koen H, et al: Pulsed Doppler flow as a criterion of portal venous velocity: Comparison with cineangiographic measurements. Radiology 154:495, 1985.

29. Sabba C, Weltin GC, Cicchetti DV, et al: Observer variability in the echo-Doppler measurements of portal flow in cirrhotic patients and normal volunteers. Gastroenterology 98:1603, 1990.

30. Liebowitz HR: Pathogenesis of esophageal varix rupture. JAMA 175:138, 1961.

31. Polish E, Sullivan BG: Esophagitis associated with hemorrhage from esophageal varices. Ann Intern Med 54:908, 1961.

32. Chiles NH, Bagenstoss A, Butt HR, et al: Esophageal varices: Comparative incidence of ulceration and spontaneous rupture as a cause of fatal hemorrhage. Gastroenterology 25:565, 1953.

33. MacDougall BRD, Williams R: A controlled trial of cimetidine in the recurrence of variceal hemorrhage. Implications about the pathogenesis of hemorrhage. Hepatology 3:69, 1983.

34. Spence RAJ, Sloan JM, Johnston GW: Oesophagitis in patients undergoing oesophageal transection for varices—A histological study. Br J Surg 70:332, 1983.

35. Polio J, Groszmann RJ: Hemodynamic factors involved in the development and rupture of esophageal varices: A pathophysiologic approach to treatment. Semin Liver Dis 6:318, 1986.

36. Rigau J, Bosch J, Bordas JM, et al: Endoscopic measurement of variceal pressure in cirrhosis: Correlations with portal pressure and variceal hemorrhage. Gastroenterology 96:873, 1989.

37. Sarin SK, Sundaram KR, Ahuja RK: Predictors of variceal bleeding: An analsyis of clinical, endoscopic and hemodynamic variables with special reference to intravariceal pressure. Gut 30:1757, 1989.

38. Viallet A, Marleau D, Huet PM, et al: Relationship between portal hypertension and bleeding from ruptured varices in alcoholic cirrhosis patients. Gastroenterology 69:1297, 1975.

39. Kravetz D, Sikuler E, Groszmann RJ: Splanchnic and systemic hemodynamics in portal hypertensive rats during hemorrhage and blood volume restitution. Gastroenterology 90:1232, 1986.

40. Iwatsuki S, Reynolds T: Effects of increased intra-abdominal pressure on hepatic hemodynamics in patients with chronic liver disease and portal hypertension. Gastroenterology 65:294, 1973.

41. Rector WG, Reynolds TB: Risk factors for haemorrhage from oesophageal varices and acute gastric erosions. Clin Gastroenterol 14:139, 1985.

42. The North Italian Endoscopic Club for the Study and Treatment of Esophageal Varices: Prediction of the first variceal hemorrhage in patients with cirrhosis of the liver and esophageal varices: A prospective multicenter study. N Engl J Med 319:983, 1988.

43. Bendtsen F, Skovgaard LT, Sørensen TIA, et al: Agreement among multiple observers on endoscopic diagnosis of esophageal varices before bleeding. Hepatology 11:341, 1990.

44. Mashford M, Mahon W, Chalmers T: Studies of the cardiovascular system in the hypotension of liver failure. N Engl J Med 267:1071, 1962.

45. Laird J-F: Vasopressin in cardiovascular regulation. In: Lebrec D, Blei AT (eds): Vasopressin Analogs and Portal Hypertension. London, John Libbey Eurotext, p 1, 1987.

46. Fogel MR, Knauer M, Lyudevit L, et al: Continuous intravenous vasopressin in upper gastrointestinal bleeding. Ann Intern Med 96:565, 1982.

47. Chokjier M, Groszmann RJ, Atterbury CE, et al: A controlled comparison of continuous intra-arterial infusions of vasopressin in hemorrhage from esophageal varices. Gastroenterology 77:540, 1979.

48. Walker S, Stiehl A, Raedsch R, et al: Terlipressin in bleeding esophageal varices: A placebo controlled double blind study. Hepatology 6:112, 1986.

49. Groszmann RJ, Kravetz D, Bosch J, et al: Nitroglycerin improves the hemodynamic response to vasopressin in portal hypertension. Hepatology 2:757, 1982.

50. Gimson AES, Westaby D, Hegarty J, et al: A randomized trial of vasopressin and vasopressin plus nitroglycerin in the control of acute variceal hemorrhage. Hepatology 6:410, 1986.

51. Tsai Y-T, Lay C-S, Lai K-H, et al: Controlled trial of vasopressin plus nitroglycerin vs vasopressin alone in the treatment of bleeding esophageal varices. Hepatology 6:406, 1986.

52. Bosch J, Groszmann RJ, Garcia-Pagan JC, et al: Association of transdermal nitroglycerin to vasopressin infusion in the treatment of variceal hemorrhage: A placebo controlled clinical trial. Hepatology 10:962, 1989.

53. Vatner SF, Pagani M, Rutherford JD, et al: Effects of nitroglycerin on cardiac function and regional blood flow distribution in conscious dogs. Am J Physiol 234:H244, 1978.

54. Sonneberg GE, Keller U, Perruchoud A, et al: Effect of somatostatin on splanchnic hemodynamics in patients with cirrhosis of liver and normal subjects. Gastroenterology 80:526, 1981.

55. Valenzuela JE, Shubert T, Fogel MR, et al: A multicenter randomized double blind trial of somatostatin in the management of acute hemorrhage from esophageal varices. Hepatology 10:958, 1989.

56. Burroughs AK, McCormack PA, Hughes MD, et al: Randomized double blind placebo controlled trial of somatostatin for variceal bleeding. Emergency control and prevention of early variceal rebleeding. Gastroenterology 99:1388, 1990.

57. Sengstaken RW, Blakemore AH: Balloon tamponade for the control of hemorrhage from esophageal varices. Ann Surg 131:781, 1950.

58. Boyce HW: Modification of the Sengstaken-Blakemore balloon tube. N Engl J Med 267:195, 1960.

59. Teres J, Cecilia A, Bordas JM, et al: Esophageal tamponade for bleeding varices. Controlled trial between Sengstaken-Blakemore tube and the Linton-Nachlas tube. Gastroenterology 75:566, 1978.

60. Chokjier M, Conn HO: Esophageal tamponade in the treatment of bleeding varices. A decadal progress report. Dig Dis Sci 25:267, 1980.

61. Crafoord C, Frenckner P: New surgical treatment of varicose veins of the esophagus. Acta Otolaryngol (Stockh) 27:422, 1939.

62. Kage M, Korula J, Harada A, et al: The effects of endoscopic variceal sclerotherapy on the esophagus. A clinical, endoscopic and histopathological study. J Clin Gastroenterol 9:639, 1987.

63. Paquet KJ: Endoscopic paravariceal injection sclerotherapy of the esophagus—Indications, technique, complications, results of a period of 14 years. Gastrointest Endosc 29:310, 1983.

64. McClave SA, Kaiser SC, Wright RA, et al: Prospective randomized comparison of esophageal variceal sclerotherapy agents: Sodium tetradecyl sulfate versus sodium morrhuate. Gastrointest Endosc 36:567, 1990.

65. Kochhar R, Goenka MK, Mehta S, et al: A comparative evaluation of sclerosants for esophageal varices. A prospective randomized controlled study. Gastrointest Endosc 36:127, 1990.

66. Kitano S, Iso Y, Koyanagi N, et al: Ethanolamine oleate is superior to polidocanaol (Aethoxysclerol) for endoscopic injection sclerotherapy of esophageal varices. Hepatogastroenterology 34:19, 1987.

67. Sarin SK, Nanda R, Sachdev GK, et al: Relative efficacy and safety of absolute alcohol and 50% alcohol as variceal sclerosants. Gastrointest Endosc 33:362, 1987.

68. Larson AW, Cohen H, Zweiban B, et al: Acute esophageal variceal sclerotherapy. Results of a prospective randomized controlled trial. JAMA 255:497, 1986.

69. Akriviadis E, Korula J, Ko Y, et al: Frequent endoscopic sclerotherapy increases risk of complication. A prospective randomized controlled trial of two treatment schedules. Dig Dis Sci 34:1068, 1989.

70. Korula J, Pandya K, Yamada S: Perforation of the esophagus. Incidence and clues to pathogenesis. Dig Dis Sci 34:324, 1989.

71. Korula J: Endoscopic variceal sclerotherapy. J Clin Gastroenterol 10:589, 1988.

72. Westaby D, Hayes PC, Gimson AES, et al: Controlled clinical trial of injection sclerotherapy for active variceal bleeding. Hepatology 9:274, 1989.

73. Paquet KJ, Feussner H: Endoscopic sclerosis and esophageal balloon tamponade in acute hemorrhage from esophagogastric varices: A prospective controlled randomized trial. Hepatology 5:580, 1985.

74. Steigmann GV, Goff JS, Sun JH, et al: Endoscopic variceal ligation: An alternative to sclerotherapy. Gastrointest Endosc 35:431, 1989.

75. Steigmann GV, Goff JS, Michaeletz P, et al: Endoscopic variceal ligation vs sclerotherapy for bleeding esophageal varices: Early results of a prospective randomized trial. Gastrointest Endosc 36:188, 1990.

76. Orloff MJ, Charters AC, Chandler JG, et al: Portacaval shunt as an emergency procedure in unselected patients with alcoholic cirrhosis. Surg Gynecol Obstet 141:59, 1975.
77. Sarfeh IJ, Rypins EB: The emergency portacaval H graft in alcoholic cirrhotic patients: Influence of shunt diameter on clinical outcome. Am J Surg 152:290, 1986.
78. Conn HO: A peek at the Child-Turcotte classification. Hepatology 1:673, 1981.
79. Pugh RNH, Murray-Lyon IM, Dawson JL, et al: Transection of the esophagus for bleeding esophageal varices. Br J Surg 60:646, 1976.
80. Burroughs AK, Hamilton G, Phillips A, et al: A comparison of sclerotherapy with staple transection of the esophagus for the emergency control of bleeding from esophageal varices. N Engl J Med 321:857, 1989.
81. Sugiura M, Futugawa S: Further evaluation of the Sugiura procedure in the treatment of esophageal varices. Arch Surg 112:1317, 1977.
82. Galambos JT: Portal hypertension. Semin Liver Dis 5:277, 1985.
83. Rector WG: Drug therapy for portal hypertension. Ann Intern Med 105:96, 1986.
83a. Zemel G, Katzen BT, Becker GJ, et al: Percutaneous transjugular portosystemic shunt. JAMA 266:390, 1991.
83b. Ring, EJ, Lake JR, Roberts JP, et al: Using transjugular intrahepatic portosystemic shunts to control variceal bleeding before liver transplantation. Ann Intern Med 116:304, 1992.
84. Infante-Rivard C, Esnaola S, Villeneuve JP: Role of endoscopic variceal sclerotherapy in the long term management of variceal bleeding. A meta-analysis. Gastroenterology 96:1087, 1989.
85. Pagliaro L, Burroughs AK, Sorensen TIA, et al: Therapeutic controversies and randomised controlled trials (RCTs): Prevention of bleeding and rebleeding in cirrhosis. Gastroenterol Int 2:71, 1989.
86. Westaby D, MacDougall BRD, Williams R: Improved survival following injection sclerotherapy for oesophageal varices. Final analysis of a controlled trial. Hepatology 5:827, 1985.
87. Korula J, Balart LA, Radvan G, et al: A prospective randomized controlled trial of chronic endoscopic variceal sclerotherapy. Hepatology 5:584, 1985.
88. Burroughs AK, McCormack PA, Siringo S, et al: Prospective randomized trial of long term sclerotherapy for variceal rebleeding using the same protocol to treat rebleeding in all patients. Final report. Hepatology 10:579, 1989.
89. Korula J, Chin K, Ko Y, et al: The demonstration of two distinct subsets of gastric varices: Observations during a seven year study of endoscopic variceal sclerotherapy. Dig Dis Sci 36:303, 1991.
90. D'Amico G, Montalbano L, Traina M, et al: Natural history of congestive gastropathy in cirrhosis. Gastroenterology 99:1558, 1990.
91. Conn HO, Lindenmuth WW, May CJ, et al: Prophylactic portacaval anastomosis. Medicine 51:27, 1972.
92. Jackson FC, Perin EB, Felix RW, et al: A clinical investigation of the portacaval shunt: Survival analysis of the therapeutic operation. Ann Surg 174:672, 1971.
93. Resnick RH, Iber FL, Ishiara A, et al: A controlled study of the therapeutic portacaval. Lancet 2:655, 1974.
94. Rueff B, Prandis D, Degos F, et al: A controlled study of therapeutic portacaval shunt in alcoholic cirrhosis. Lancet 2:655, 1976.
95. Reynolds TB, Donovan AJ, Mikkelsen WP, et al: Results of a 12 year randomized trial of portacaval shunt in patients with alcoholic liver disease and bleeding varices. Gastroenterology 80:1005, 1981.
96. Warren WD, Zeppa R, Fomon J: Selective trans-splenic decompression of gastroesophageal varices by distal splenorenal shunt. Ann Surg 166:437, 1967.
97. Mutchnick MG: Portal systemic encephalopathy and portal anastomosis. A prospective, controlled investigation. Gastroenterology 66:1005, 1974.
98. Warren WD, Abu-El Magd KM, Richards WO, et al: Splenopancreatic disconnection: Improved selectivity of distal splenorenal shunt. Ann Surg 204:346, 1986.
99. Conn HO, Resnick RH, Grace ND, et al: Distal splenorenal shunt versus portal systemic shunt: Current status of a controlled trial. Hepatology 1:151, 1981.
100. Langer B, Taylor R, Mackenzie DR, et al: Further report of a prospective randomized trial comparing distal splenorenal shunt with end to side shunt. Gastroenterology 88:424, 1985.
101. Millikan WJ Jr, Warren WD, Henderson JM, et al: The Emory prospective randomized trial: Selective versus nonselective shunt to control variceal bleeding. Ten year follow-up. Ann Surg 201:712, 1985.
102. Harley HAJ, Morgan T, Redeker AG, et al: Results of a randomized trial of end-to-side portacaval shunt and distal splenorenal shunt in alcoholic liver disease and variceal bleeding. Gastroenterology 91:802, 1986.
103. Sarfeh IJ, Rypins EB, Mason GB: A systematic appraisal of portacaval H-graft diameters: Clinical and hemodynamic perspectives. Ann Surg 204:356, 1986.
104. Drapanas T: Interposition mesocaval shunt for the treatment of portal hypertension. Ann Surg 176:435, 1972.
105. Thompson BW, Read RC: Interposition "H" grafting for portal hypertension. Arch Surg 108:502, 1974.
106. Pascal JP, Cales P: Multicenter study group: Propranolol in the prevention of first upper gastrointestinal hemorrhage in patients with cirrhosis of the liver and esophageal varices. N Engl J Med 317:856, 1987.
107. Italian multicenter project for propranolol in prevention of bleeding. Propranolol for prophylaxis of bleeding in cirrhotic patients with large varices: A multicenter, randomized, clinical trial. Hepatology 8:1, 1988.
108. Ideo G, Bellati G, Fesca E, et al: Nadolol can prevent the first gastrointestinal bleeding in cirrhotics: A prospective randomized study. Hepatology 8:6, 1988.
109. Paquet KJ: Prophylactic endoscopic sclerosing treatment of esophageal wall in varices. A prospective controlled trial. Endoscopy 14:4, 1982.
110. Witzel L, Wolbergs E, Merki H: Prophylactic endoscopic sclerotherapy of esophageal varices. A prospective controlled study. Lancet 1:773, 1985.
111. Koch H, Henning H, Grimm H, et al: Prophylactic sclerosing of esophageal varices—Results of a prospective controlled study. Endoscopy 18:40, 1986.
112. Piai G, Cipolletta L, Claar M, et al: Prophylactic sclerotherapy of high risk esophageal varices: Results of a multicenter prospective controlled trial. Hepatology 8:1495, 1988.
113. Santangelo W, Dueno MI, Estes BL, et al: Prophylactic sclerotherapy of large esophageal varices. N Engl J Med 318:814, 1988.
114. Gregory P, Hartigan P, Amodes D, et al: Prophylactic sclerotherapy for esophageal varices in alcoholic liver disease: Results of the VA cooperative randomized trial. Gastroenterology 92:1414, 1987.

CHAPTER 126

Lower Gastrointestinal Tract Hemorrhage

Kim L. Isaacs
Eugene M. Bozymski

Bleeding from the lower gastrointestinal tract is associated with significant morbidity and mortality. An estimated 5% of emergency hospital admissions are for lower gastrointestinal tract bleeding requiring 2 U or more of blood.[1] Lower gastrointestinal tract bleeding is defined as bleeding originating from beyond the ligament of Trietz. The volume and rapidity of the blood loss may vary from intermittent, slow bleeding to acute loss of blood. The rate and amount of blood loss affect critical care in terms of diagnosis and management of lower gastrointestinal tract hemorrhage. The addition of colonoscopy, nuclear medicine scans, and visceral arteriography as diagnostic tools has added greatly to the localization of the bleeding site in these patients. Among the causes of lower gastrointestinal tract bleeding, diverticular bleeding is thought to be most common, being responsible for more than 50% of cases of lower gastrointestinal tract hemorrhage. Arteriovenous malformations are found in this group of patients with increasing frequency, whereas other causes of lower gastrointestinal tract bleeding are less common[2] (Table 126–1).

INITIAL MANAGEMENT

Patients with gastrointestinal bleeding often present as medical emergencies. Resuscitation and stabilization are necessary while one is obtaining historical data and performing a physical examination. Laboratory investigation is carried out simultaneously. Surgical consultation should be obtained from the onset. In less urgent situations (patients who are hemodynamically stable or those with chronic blood loss), a more systematic approach may be taken (Fig. 126–1).

TABLE 126–1

CAUSES OF LOWER GASTROINTESTINAL TRACT BLEEDING

Diverticular disease
Angiodysplasia or vascular ectasia
Colitis
  Inflammatory bowel disease
  Infection
  Ischemia
  Vasculitis
  Radiation
Malignancy
Polyps
Rectal ulcers
Aortoenteral fistulas
Anastomotic bleeds
Anorectal disease
  Hemorrhoids
  Anal fissure
Trauma
Coagulopathy

Assessment

History

Certain aspects of the patient's history may provide clues to the cause of the current gastrointestinal blood loss. The character of the blood may indicate the site of blood loss. Bright red blood per rectum is characteristically due to distal gastrointestinal disease (e.g., hemorrhoids and other distal lesions). If the transit time is rapid, more proximal lesions (diverticulosis, angiodysplasia) may also lead to a red rectal effluent. On occasion, patients with an upper gastrointestinal tract source (e.g., varices) may have red blood per rectum if the bleeding is brisk. Such patients generally show the effects of volume depletion. Melena is characteristically seen with upper gastrointestinal tract blood loss, whereas maroon stool is typically seen in colonic bleeding.[3] Occasionally, patients bleeding from a right-sided colonic source may have melena.

The cause of any past gastrointestinal bleeding may be relevant in the assessment of the current situation. For example, ulcerative colitis, diverticular disease, and angiodysplastic lesions may be associated with recurrent bleeding. Medication history is important both in terms of etiology of gastrointestinal tract bleeding (nonsteroidal anti-inflammatory drugs and upper gastrointestinal tract blood loss) and in terms of management (coagulopathy caused by anticoagulant, platelet defect caused by aspirin). Associated symptoms such as pain may lead to early consideration of ischemia as a possible cause. Painless bleeding is more characteristic of a diverticular site, angiodysplastic lesions, or neoplasms. A change in bowel habits or a family history of polyps or cancer may likewise suggest carcinoma, whereas the presence of a vascular graft or an abdominal aortic aneurysm raises the consideration of an aortoenteral fistula.

Physical Examination

Vital signs (pulse and blood pressure) are important in assessing the significance of the hemorrhage and predicting ongoing bleeding. Changes in orthostatic blood pressure and pulse rate occur when there has been acute blood loss leading to decreased intravascular volume. Changing the patient from a supine to a sitting position that is associated with a pulse rate increase greater than 20 beats/min or a systolic blood pressure drop of greater than 10 mm Hg is suggestive of the loss of at least 1 L of blood. Other signs of hypovolemia include poor capillary refill and decreased distal blood flow leading to pallor and cool extremities.

Stigmata of chronic liver disease such as spider angiomas, palmar erythema, splenomegaly, and gynecomastia may suggest a coagulopathy or variceal bleeding (right-sided colonic varices, rectal varices). Other skin lesions such as telangiectasia of the lips, mouth, or extremities raise the possibility of Osler-Weber-Rendu disease, or hereditary hemorrhagic telangectasia. A murmur consistent with aortic valvular disease may suggest an angiodysplastic lesion in the colon. The presence of an abdominal bruit suggests vascular disease and raises the possibility of ischemic colitis. The presence of a palpable aorta alerts one to the possibility of an abdominal aortic aneurysm and an aortoenteral fistula.

Rectal examination and anoscopy provide the initial access to the lower gastrointestinal tract. A rectal mass may be palpable. Hemorrhoids and fissures can be identified.

As part of the physical examination, nasogastric lavage should be considered. An upper gastrointestinal tract hemorrhage with rapid transit can present with red blood per rectum. Even with a normal nasogastric lavage result, approximately 1 of 100 patients is found to have a duodenal ulcer as the source of what appears to be lower gastrointestinal tract bleeding.[4]

Laboratory Evaluation

In the case of rapid blood loss, hemoglobin level and hematocrit may be normal. As extravascular fluid enters the vascular space in an attempt to restore volume, the hematocrit falls. Equilibration of extravascular and intravascular volume (reflected by the hematocrit) may require 24 to 72 hours. The mean corpuscular volume may provide a clue to chronic versus acute blood loss. It is low if the blood loss has been chronic, indicating an iron deficiency anemia.

Coagulation studies, prothrombin time, partial thromboplastin time, platelet count, and bleeding time may help to detect a coagulopathy and guide therapy.

Blood urea nitrogen and creatinine determinations may help to delineate upper versus lower gastrointestinal tract bleeding. Blood urea nitrogen level is increased out of proportion to creatinine level in upper gastrointestinal tract bleeding caused by the absorption of nitrogenous products from digestion of blood in the small intestine. Electrolyte levels may be altered because of rapid fluid shifts. Calcium levels may decrease after blood transfusion owing to binding by citrate, which is a common component of transfused blood.

Volume Replacement

Large-bore intravenous lines for rapid fluid resuscitation should be placed. Blood can be drawn during intravenous catheter placement and sent for complete blood count, type and cross-match, coagulation studies, and determination of electrolytes, blood urea nitrogen, creatinine, calcium, and glucose, as well as other studies thought to be necessary in the individual case. Crystalloid should be isotonic (e.g., normal saline and lactated Ringer's solution) and infused to restore volume. Volume is assessed by blood pressure and pulse measurements.[5] In elderly patients or those with underlying cardiac disease or renal disease, central venous pressure monitoring may be required to help guide fluid resuscitation. Urine output is a good measure of tissue perfusion. In hypovolemic shock, urine output is markedly decreased.

Packed red blood cells are transfused as necessary on the basis of general physical status, hematocrit, ongoing blood loss, and underlying disease. Fresh frozen plasma may be required to correct a coagulopathy. Platelet transfusion may be needed with massive hemorrhage (>10 U) or in a patient

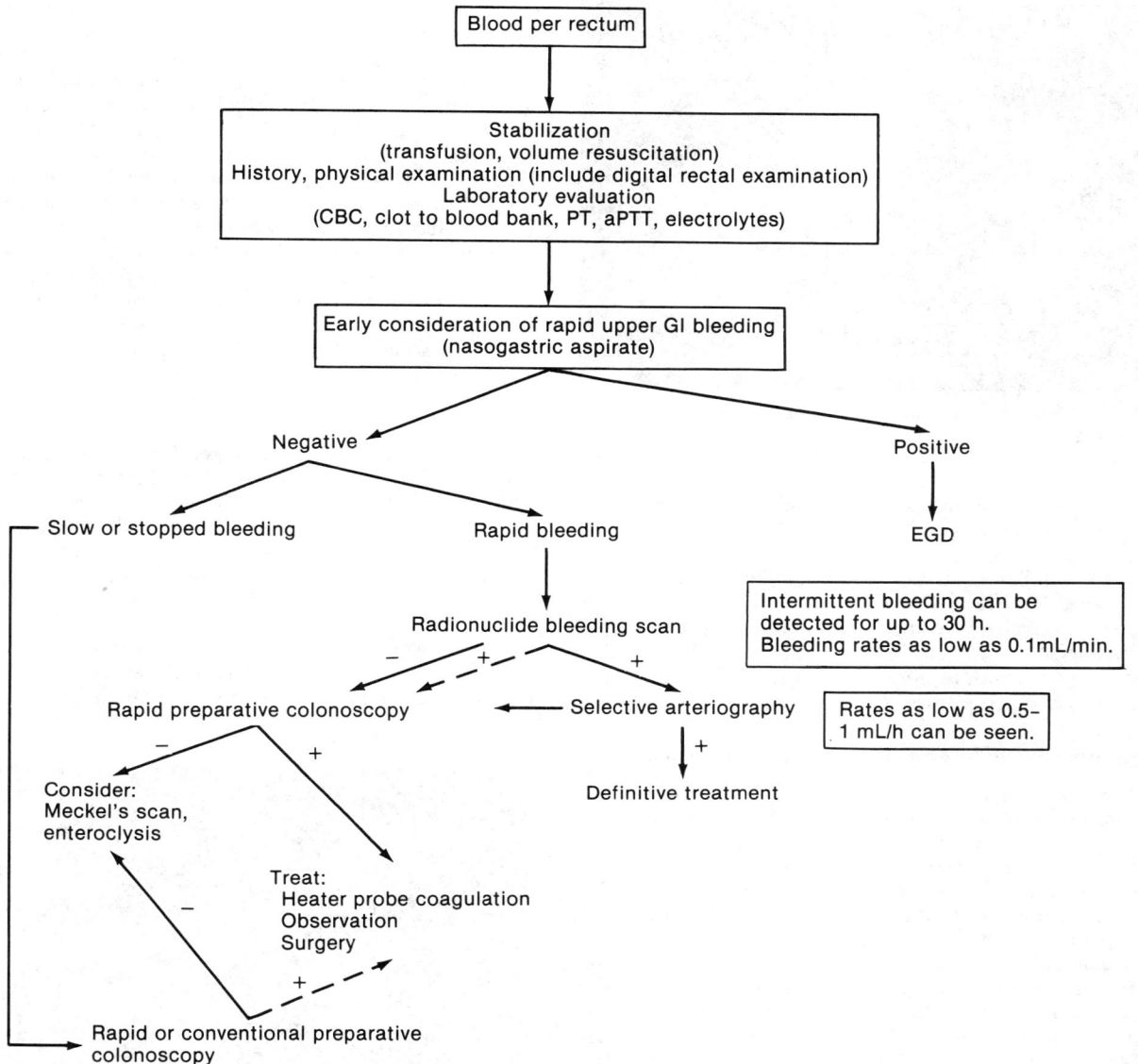

Figure 126–1. Diagnosis and management of lower gastrointestinal tract bleeding. CBC = complete blood count; PT = prothrombin time; aPTT = activated partial thromboplastin time; GI = gastrointestinal; EGD = esophagogastroduodenoscopy; + = positive; − = negative.

with thrombocytopenia or a platelet defect. After the decision to transfuse is made, transfusion to a hematocrit of near 30% allows for adequate tissue oxygenation.

ETIOLOGY

Diverticular Bleeding

In the United States, diverticular disease of the colon has a prevalence of 50% at autopsy.[6] Most patients are asymptomatic. It is estimated that approximately 5% of patients with diverticular disease have severe lower gastrointestinal tract blood loss attributed to diverticula, with 10 to 15% of people with diverticula having less severe lower gastrointestinal tract bleeding. Because diverticula are so common, other causes of rectal bleeding should be strongly considered before the bleeding is attributed to diverticular disease. With current diagnostic techniques, angiodysplastic lesions are being recognized as a source of lower gastrointestinal tract bleeding more frequently. In earlier reports, much of the

bleeding attributed to diverticular disease may have been secondary to angiodysplasia.

Although there is a greater incidence of left-sided diverticula, it is thought that most diverticular bleeding is from the right side of the colon. Intramural arterial branches are close to the necks and domes of diverticula. The blood vessel is exposed between the mucosa and the serosa, and bleeding occurs through a noninflammatory local erosion into the diverticulum.[7]

The bleeding may go undetected for several days while blood fills the right side of the colon. If the hemorrhage is large, the patient has hypovolemic symptoms, possibly abdominal cramps, and passes maroon or red blood per rectum. Bleeding typically stops spontaneously and conservative management (bed rest, clear liquid diet, and transfusion as necessary) usually suffices. The recurrence rate is estimated at 25% after the first hemorrhage and 50% after a second episode of bleeding.[5]

When conservative measures fail to control hemorrhage from a diverticular site, other options include selective intra-

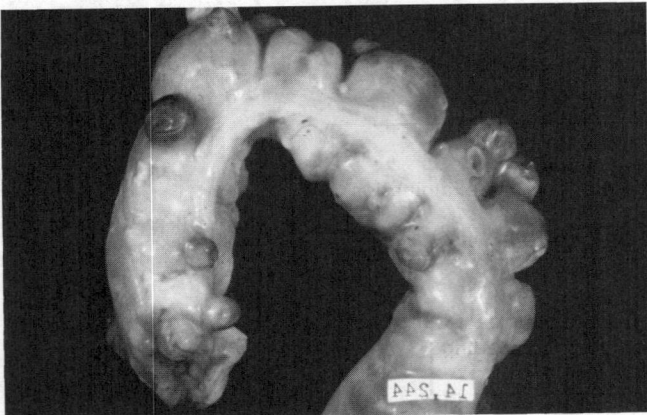

Figure 126-2. Colonic resection specimen from a patient with diverticular bleeding.

arterial infusion of vasopressin. The catheter is placed during angiography and vasopressin at 0.2 U/min is infused for 6 to 12 hours.

A small number of patients require surgery to control hemorrhage. The site of bleeding should be determined as accurately as possible by using a combination of colonoscopy, radionuclide scanning, and arteriography. This helps guide colonic resection, and, as noted earlier, right hemicolectomy is frequently the procedure of choice (Fig. 126-2).

Arteriovenous Malformations or Angiodysplasia

With the use of colonoscopy and angiography in the early evaluation of lower gastrointestinal tract bleeding, angiodysplastic lesions and arteriovenous malformations have been demonstrated with increased frequency[8] (Fig. 126-3). Angiodyplasias are acquired dilatations of normal vascular structures of the colon and may be seen in up to 25% of elderly patients.[9] The terms *angiodysplasia* and *arteriovenous malformation* are often used interchangeably, although some authors reserve the term arteriovenous malformation for the congenital vascular abnormality. Angiographically, the appearance of the presumed, acquired, and congenital lesions is similar. In some series, bleeding from an arteriovenous malformation was up to 10 times more common than diverticular bleeding.[4] When demonstrated at angiography, the location of arteriovenous malformations is usually the right side of the colon or the cecum. The jejunum is the next most frequent site. At colonoscopy, smaller angiodys-

plastic lesions can be demonstrated in the left side of the colon as well and appear as red patches of dilated vessels. These are thought not to contribute as significantly to lower gastrointestinal tract bleeding as do right-sided lesions. Angiographically, angiodysplasia is seen as a densely opacified intramural vein; a vascular tuft (degenerated mucosal venules) and an early filling vein may also be seen (Fig. 126-4). Extravasation of contrast from this lesion may be seen if there is ongoing bleeding. It is estimated that there is up to 85% rebleeding rate in patients who have bled from an arteriovenous malformation. There appears to be an increased risk of arteriovenous malformations in patients with aortic stenosis and those with renal disease.[10] Therapy consists of thermal coagulation during colonoscopy and occasionally resection of the involved segment.

Colitis

Inflammatory Bowel Disease. Ulcerative colitis usually presents with bloody loose stool. Bleeding is due to diffuse mucosal inflammation. Uncommonly, the bleeding may be sufficient to necessitate transfusion, and rarely, it is associated with an abrupt exsanguinating hemorrhagic event. Diagnosis is based on clinical course, sigmoidoscopic findings, and negative stool cultures for gastrointestinal pathogens.

Gross lower gastrointestinal tract bleeding is seen in 1 to 15% of patients with Crohn's disease. Angiography may demonstrate inflammatory neovascularity in the terminal

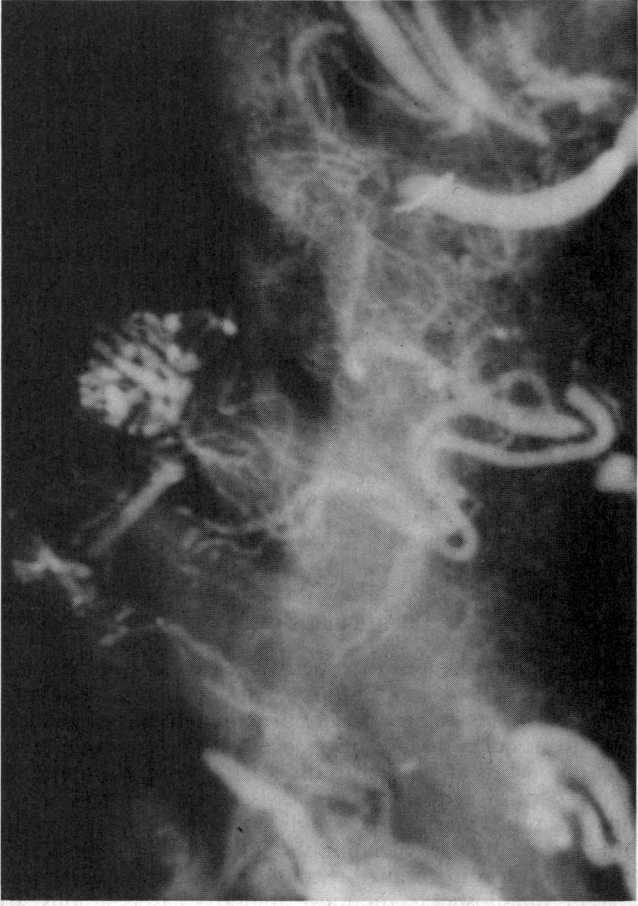

Figure 126-4. Arteriographic appearance of a large colonic arteriovenous malformation.

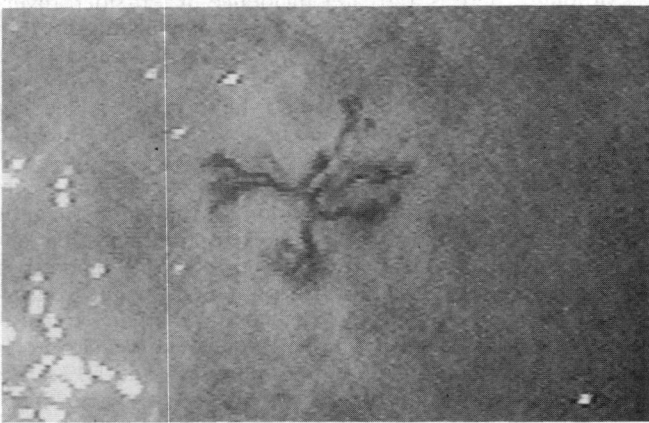

Figure 126-3. Endoscopically viewed arteriovenous malformation.

ileum or the colon. Patients with Crohn's disease who have lower gastrointestinal tract bleeding tend to have recurrent bleeding and may require surgical resection.[11]

Infectious Colitis. Invasion of the colonic mucosa by infectious agents may also lead to bleeding per rectum. There is associated abdominal cramping and diarrhea. Colitis is evident on sigmoidoscopic examination and may be indistinguishable grossly from the changes seen in ulcerative colitis. Positive stool cultures are diagnostic. Blood in the stool is common in *Shigella* and *Campylobacter jejuni* infections. Blood may be seen less commonly with enteropathogenic *Escherichia coli* and *Salmonella* and in pseudomembranous colitis attributable to *Clostridium difficile*.[12]

Ischemic Colitis. The bleeding seen in ischemic colitis is usually associated with abdominal pain. The pain may be out of proportion to findings on abdominal examination. Ischemic colitis is often seen in the setting of a low-flow state (e.g., cardiogenic shock, hypovolemia, sepsis, hemodialysis, and vasoconstrictive drugs, and after cardiac surgery). In these conditions, there is a decreased blood supply to the bowel wall. Other conditions that may lead to mesenteric ischemia are arterial occlusion or vasculitis and venous occlusion. No specific features of mesenteric ischemia allow for an early definitive diagnosis. Radiographic studies may show thumbprinting (evidence of mucosal edema), but this is nonspecific. Angiographic studies are usually not helpful. Colonoscopy may show the result of decreased mucosal blood flow (e.g., edema, purple or red discoloration, necrosis, and aperistalsis). Colonoscopy is generally not helpful in delineating the severity of ischemia, as the mucosal surface is the first layer of bowel affected and is the only layer seen at endoscopy unless ulceration is present. Therapy includes treatment of the underlying process, restoration of blood flow if possible, and resection of nonviable bowel.[13]

Radiation Enteritis. Radiation enteritis is seen in the setting of pelvic irradiation, most commonly for gynecologic or prostatic cancer. The rectum is usually affected, although fixed parts of the colon and the ileum may also be damaged. Bleeding may be severe enough to necessitate transfusion. In acute radiation injury, bleeding is secondary to ulceration. Spotty ulcers may coalesce to form large ulcers. In chronic or delayed radiation injury, there may be a latent period after radiation of a few months to 30 years.[14] Telangiectasia of the mucosal and submucosal vessels occurs. Severe bleeding occurs when there is rupture of these thin-walled vessels. Treatment includes stool softeners and steroid enemas. Sulfasalazine has been used with some success in a small number of patients. Surgical intervention is reserved for patients with refractory bleeding. Diversion of the fecal stream without rectal resection and rectal resection are the two main procedures used.[14] Difficulties arise when operating on previously irradiated bowel.

Vasculitis. Vasculitis may cause colitis and bleeding through a variety of mechanisms. In vasculitis involving large vessels (e.g., polyarteritis nodosa), the patient may have ischemic bowel resulting from large-vessel occlusion. Vasculitis involving the vasa recta and intramural vessels (e.g., systemic lupus erythematosus, polyarteritis, dermatomyositis, Henoch-Schönlein purpura, rheumatoid vasculitis) leads to ulceration and edema of the mucosal surface.[15] Bleeding is usually occult. The abdominal findings are nonspecific. Diagnosis is made by the combination of clinical course, associated symptoms, and laboratory features of the disease process. Management is dependent on the underlying disease and on findings that suggest the need for surgical exploration.

Other Lesions of the Colon

Polyps may cause occult blood loss from the colon but are less likely to cause severe acute blood loss.

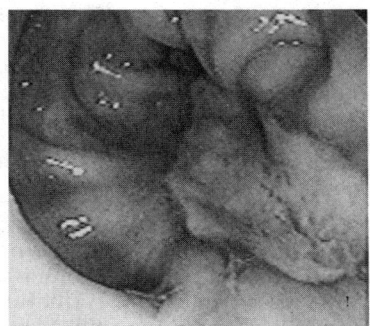

Figure 126–5. Rectal ulcer.

Solitary rectal ulcers occur on the anterior or anterolateral wall of the rectum between 4 cm from the anal verge to 15 cm from the anal verge at the rectosigmoid junction. On histologic evaluation, there is replacement of the normal lamina propria by fibroblasts. These ulcers may bleed massively, necessitating transfusion[16] (Fig. 126–5).

Dieulafoy's ulcer of the colon was first described in the stomach, and the associated bleeding is generally abrupt and brisk. The lesion is a small mucosal erosion into a submucosal artery. Detection may be difficult.[17]

Although an unusual cause of hemorrhage, an aortoenteral fistula should be considered in any patient with an aortic graft and lower gastrointestinal tract bleeding. The majority have bleeding into the third and fourth portions of the duodenum. A long endoscope (pediatric colonoscope) should be used so that the distal duodenum can be examined.[18] Computed tomographic scan of the abdomen with special attention to the aortoduodenal area may be helpful in diagnosis. Angiography is generally not helpful. Surgical exploration may be required if no other source of bleeding is identified.

Malignancy

Carcinoma of the colon is an important cause of bleeding. As many as one half to two thirds of patients with colorectal cancer have bleeding as their presenting complaint.[1] Gross hemorrhage may be seen with rectosigmoid cancer, whereas occult bleeding is seen with cecal or right-sided colonic cancer.

Hemorrhoids

Hemorrhoids are a common cause of gastrointestinal bleeding. Typically, blood loss is small and clinically seen as bright red blood occurring on toilet tissue, dripping into the commode, or coating formed stool. Occasionally, massive bleeding may occur. A careful anorectal examination helps identify this cause.[19]

DIAGNOSTIC MEASURES
Immediate or Urgent Colonoscopy

With ongoing active lower gastrointestinal tract bleeding, emergency colonoscopy can be difficult in the unprepared colon. Anoscopy may reveal an anorectal source such as hemorrhoids or a fissure. Flexible or rigid sigmoidoscopy should be performed early in the evaluation.[20] This examination may allow for the detection of a rectal mass or diffuse colitis and may augment anoscopy in the detection of anorectal disorders. More proximal lesions are not detected. In addition, in an unprepared colon, it is difficult to identify small arteriovenous malformations. Urgent colonoscopy can be performed safely in patients with severe hematochezia after a rapid oral purge.[21] By cleaning the colon, there is an increased frequency of detection of a variety of lesions, including angiodysplasia, and therapeutic endoscopic intervention is possible.

Barium Enema

In the face of acute ongoing lower gastrointestinal tract bleeding, barium studies of the colon are not useful and are detrimental to further evaluation.[22] Mucosal lesions may easily be missed, and arteriography and colonoscopy are not possible with a barium-filled colon. If bleeding has slowed or stopped, an air-contrast barium enema may detect a probable lesion responsible for bleeding; however, colonoscopy is usually necessary to detect synchronous lesions, detect mucosal pathologic changes, obtain biopsy specimens, or intervene therapeutically such as with thermal coagulation of a bleeding site.

Radionuclide Scans

Radionuclide scans are noninvasive and relatively simple to perform in the face of acute gastrointestinal blood loss. Bleeding can be detected at a rate as low as 0.1 mL/min.[23] Scans using technetium Tc 99m sulfur colloid and autologous technetium Tc 99m red blood cells are the two most commonly performed bleeding scans. Technetium-labeled sulfur colloid is useful for immediate evaluation of acute blood loss. Delayed evaluation is not possible owing to the extensive uptake of the technetium Tc 99m sulfur colloid by the reticuloendothelial system. Bleeding scans with autologous technetium Tc 99m red blood cells may allow for delayed identification of a bleeding site up to 30 hours after infusion.[24] The bleeding scan is used to aid in localizing the site of blood loss and guiding selective angiography. Bleeding scans can help to guide therapy; however, it has been demonstrated that surgical therapy relying solely on localization of bleeding site by a radionuclide bleeding scan leads to surgical error in approximately 42% of patients.[23]

Radiolabeled technetium can also be used to identify Meckel's diverticulum, which, even in the elderly, is an occasional source of lower gastrointestinal tract bleeding. Technetium-99m pertechnetate is taken up by ectopic gastric mucosa.[25]

Arteriography

Selective visceral arteriography may help to detect the site of bleeding when the rate of bleeding exceeds 0.5 mL/min[3] (Fig. 126–6). Arteriography also allows the possibility of therapeutic intervention. For angiography to be most useful, the patient must be actively bleeding at the time of the study. If that is the case, angiography has been reported to be diagnostic in 40 to 70% of patients studied.[3] In addition to extravasation of blood from a bleeding vessel, nonbleeding lesions such as angiodysplasia or a vascular neoplasm can also be identified by arteriography. There is a 9% incidence of complications, including thrombosis, embolization, and contrast-induced renal failure.[21]

THERAPEUTIC OPTIONS
Therapeutic Colonoscopy

Electrocoagulation. Several types of probes are available for electrocoagulation of a bleeding vessel. These include the heat probe (pulsed thermal energy), bipolar or multi-

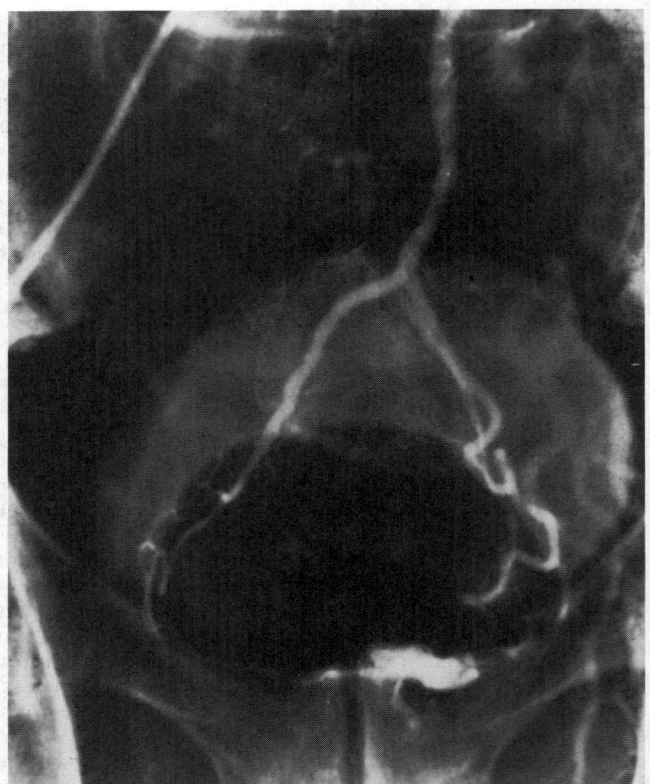

Figure 126–6. Abnormal arteriogram from inferior mesenteric arterial injection in a patient with lower gastrointestinal tract hemorrhage.

polar electrocoagulation, and electrohydrothermal electrocoagulation.[26] Monopolar electrocoagulation is not recommended in colonic bleeding owing to its propensity to cause deep necrosis and perforation. Hot biopsy forceps are monopolar.[27] Most commonly used are the heat probe and bipolar or multipolar electrocoagulation. Care must be taken with any form of electrocoagulation in the colon because of the thin colonic wall and the risk of perforation, which is problematic in the right side of the colon.

In lower gastrointestinal tract bleeding, electrocoagulation is often a successful approach to the control of bleeding from arteriovenous malformations[28] (Fig. 126–7). Rebleeding rates range from 20 to 50% and are thought in part to be related to the number of arteriovenous malformations in the bowel. Ulceration with an obvious bleeding site may also be amenable to electrocoagulation. Diverticular bleeding, colitis, and carcinoma are usually not responsive to electrocoagulation.[3]

Photocoagulation. Endoscopic laser therapy has been used in lower gastrointestinal tract bleeding predominately for the treatment of arteriovenous malformations. Both argon and neodymium:yttrium-aluminum-garnet lasers have been used. No large trials have been performed comparing the efficacy of laser treatment of arteriovenous malformations with other treatment modalities. Many reports support the use of laser therapy for treating bleeding arteriovenous malformations. In one study, 52 patients were treated with an argon laser; 2 to 5 watts was continuously applied until the lesion blanched. In this series, there was a statistically significant decrease in the number of bleeding episodes and number of blood transfusions per year. No laser complications were reported. The argon laser penetration is shallow. The laser light is selectively absorbed by the hemoglobin pigment in the arteriovenous malformation. Alternatively,

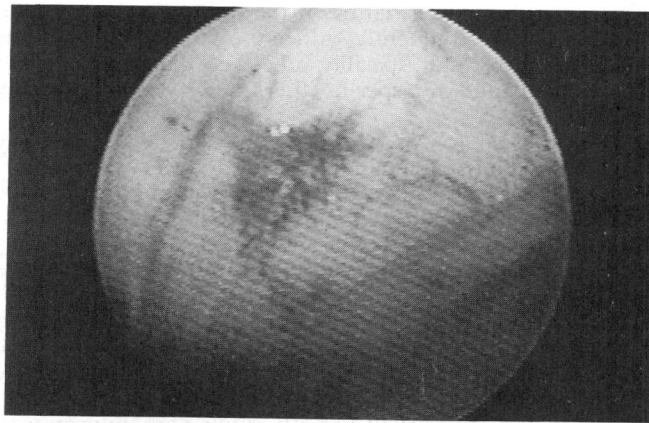

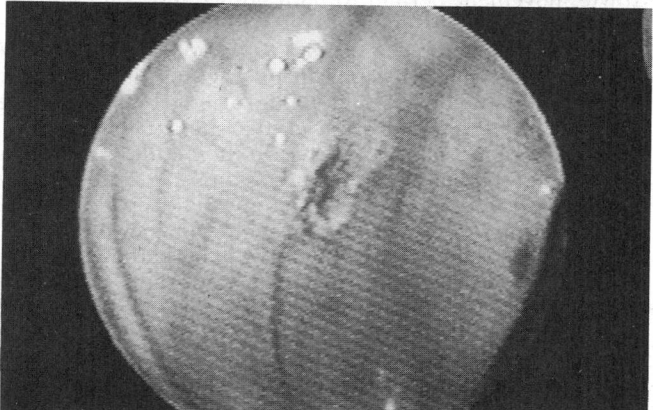

Figure 126–7. Colonic arteriovenous malformation before *(A)* and after *(B)* thermal coagulation.

neodymium:yttrium-aluminum-garnet laser therapy has been used in treating arteriovenous malformations. Transmural injury with the need for surgical intervention has been reported. It is advised that the neodymium:yttrium-aluminum-garnet laser not be used for flat lesions in the right side of the colon because of these complications.[29]

Laser treatment may also be useful in the palliative treatment of a bleeding cancer in a patient who is not a surgical candidate. The higher-power neodymium:yttrium-aluminum-garnet laser is most commonly used for this application.

Interventional Radiology

Angiographic localization of a bleeding site opens the avenue for possible therapeutic intervention. Intra-arterial vasopressin administration and embolization therapy have both been used successfully in upper gastrointestinal tract bleeding.[30] The vascular supply of the colon has less redundancy, and the use of these techniques in the colon carries with it a greater risk of bowel infarction.

After identification of a bleeding vessel by arteriography, the use of intra-arterial vasopressin is possible. Selective vasopressin infusion (i.e., infusion into the bleeding vessel) decreases the risk of bowel ischemia seen with nonselective administration. The recommended dose is 0.2 U/min.[31] If continued bleeding is documented angiographically, the rate is increased to 0.4 U/min. The infusion is continued for 12 to 24 hours. If bleeding stops, the vasopressin dosage is tapered during 12 to 24 hours by decreasing the dose every 6 to 8 hours. Reported efficacy is from 65 to 85%, depending on vessel size. Rebleeding rates are dependent on the underlying disease process. Intra-arterial vasopressin may also

be useful in bleeding associated with diverticular disease. It is less likely to be helpful in bleeding from arteriovenous malformations or angiodysplastic lesions owing to the presence of abnormal blood vessels.[30] Bleeding from carcinoma likewise may not be controlled with vasopressin infusions because of the poor response of tumor vessels to vasoconstrictive agents. In inflammatory bowel disease, the usually diffuse nature of the mucosal disease makes bleeding less likely to be adequately controlled by selective vasopressin infusion.

Embolization has been reported to be successful in a few case reports, but again owing to the limited collateral blood flow in the colon, there is a high risk of bowel ischemia.[32] Use of embolization for lower gastrointestinal tract bleeding is usually not done because of that risk, but it may be considered in selected cases.

Surgical Therapy

If nonoperative measures fail to control bleeding, surgical intervention is required. In one large study of hospital admissions for lower gastrointestinal tract bleeding, it was found that, if patients needed more than 4 U of blood in the first 24 hours, they had a 50% likelihood of requiring surgery.[1] Ideally, the bleeding site should be identified preoperatively so that a segmental resection may be performed. In cases in which preoperative localization of the bleeding site is not possible, resection limited to an area of diverticulosis, presumed to be the site, is not advised because of the high rebleeding rate. Some reports suggest that, if a bleeding site cannot be identified and surgery is required, a subtotal colectomy with an ileorectal anastomosis be performed. Others advocate right hemicolectomy owing to the high incidence of right-sided bleeding from angiodysplasia and from right-sided diverticula.[33]

SUMMARY

Lower gastrointestinal tract hemorrhage is a common reason for hospital admission, with most bleeding attributed to diverticular disease and angiodysplasia. Early management consists of resuscitation and stabilization of the patient followed by diagnostic studies. Useful studies in the evaluation of lower gastrointestinal tract bleeding are emergent colonoscopy, radionuclide scans, and arteriography. Therapy is dependent on the lesion responsible for the hemorrhage.

References

1. Farrands PA, Taylor I: Management of acute lower gastrointestinal hemorrhage in a surgical visit over a 4-year period. J R Soc Med 80:79, 1987.
2. Bope E: Lower gastrointestinal bleeding. Prim Care 15:93, 1988.
3. Schrock T: Colonoscopic diagnosis and treatment of lower gastrointestinal bleeding. Surg Clin North Am 69:1309, 1989.
4. Potter GD, Sellin JH: Lower gastrointestinal bleeding. Gastroenterol Clin North Am 17:341, 1988.
5. Buchman TG, Bulkley GB: Current management of patients with lower gastrointestinal bleeding. Surg Clin North Am 67:651, 1987.
6. Almy TP, Howell D: Diverticular disease of the colon. N Engl J Med 302:324, 1980.
7. Thompson WG, Patel DG: Clinical picture of diverticular disease of the colon. Clin Gastroenterol 15:903, 1986.
8. Spencer J: Lower gastrointestinal bleeding. Br J Surg 76:3, 1989.
9. Meyer C, Troncale F, Galloway S, et al: Arteriovenous malformations of the bowel: An analysis of 22 cases and a review of the literature. Medicine 60:36, 1981.
10. Cappel M, Lebwohl O: Cessation of recurrent bleeding from gastrointestinal angiodysplasia after aortic valve replacement. Ann Intern Med 105:54, 1986.
11. McGarrity T, Manasse J, Koch K, et al: Crohn's disease and massive lower gastrointestinal bleeding: Angiographic appearance and two case reports. Am J Gastroenterol 82:1096, 1987.

12. Plotkin G, Kluge R, Waldman R: Gastroenteritis: Etiology, pathophysiology and clinical manifestations. Medicine 58:95, 1979.
13. Williams L: Mesenteric ischemia. Surg Clin North Am 68:331, 1988.
14. Cunningham I: The management of radiation proctitis. Aust NZ J Surg 50:172, 1980.
15. Grendell J, Ockner R: Vascular diseases of the bowel. In: Sleisenger M, Fordtran J (eds): Gastrointestinal Disease: Pathophysiology, Disease, Management. 4th ed. Philadelphia, WB Saunders, p 1916, 1989.
16. Rutter KR, Riddell RH: The solitary ulcer syndrome of the rectum. Clin Gastroenterol 4:505, 1975.
17. Richards W, Grove-Mahoney D, Williams L: Hemorrhage from a Dieulafoy type ulcer of the colon: A new cause of lower gastrointestinal bleeding. Am Surg 54:121, 1988.
18. O'Donnell T, Scott G, Shepard A, et al: Improvements in the diagnosis and management of aortoenteric fistula. Am J Surg 149:481, 1985.
19. Lieberman D: Common anorectal disorders. Ann Intern Med 101:837, 1984.
20. The role of endoscopy in the patient with lower gastrointestinal bleeding: Guidelines for clinical application. Gastrointest Endosc 34(suppl):23S, 1988.
21. Jensen D, Machicado G: Diagnosis and treatment of severe hematochezia: The role of urgent colonoscopy after purge. Gastroenterology 95:1569, 1988.
22. Peterson W: Gastrointestinal bleeding. In: Sleisenger M, Fordtran J (eds): Gastrointestinal Disease: Pathophysiology, Diagnosis, Management. 4th ed. Philadelphia, WB Saunders, p 412, 1989.
23. Hunter JM, Pezim ME: Limited value of technetium 99m–labeled red cell scintigraphy in localization of lower gastrointestinal bleeding. Am J Surg 159:504, 1990.
24. Nicholson ML, Neoptolemos J, Sharp J, et al: Localization of lower gastrointestinal bleeding using in vivo technetium-99m–labelled red blood cell scintigraphy. Br J Surg 76:358, 1989.
25. Gelfand MJ, Silberstein EB, Cox J: Radionuclide imaging of Meckel's diverticulum in children. Clin Nucl Med 3:4, 1978.
26. Jiranek G, Silverstein F: Introduction to endoscopic therapy for bleeding peptic ulcers. Gastrointest Endosc 36:S25, 1990.
27. Wadas D, Sanowski R: Complications of the hot biopsy forceps technique. Gastrointest Endosc 34:32, 1988.
28. Trudel J, Fazio V, Sivak M: Colonoscopic diagnosis and treatment of arteriovenous malformations in chronic lower gastrointestinal bleeding: Clinical accuracy and efficacy. Dis Colon Rectum 31:107, 1988.
29. Hunter JG: Endoscopic laser applications in the gastrointestinal tract. Surg Clin North Am 69:1147, 1989.
30. Cardella JF, Tadavarthy S, Castaneda F, et al: Vasoactive drugs and embolotherapy in the management of gastrointestinal bleeding. In: Castaneda-Zuniga WR, Tadavarthy SM (eds): Interventional Radiology. Baltimore, Williams & Wilkins, p 164, 1988.
31. Athanasoulis C, Baum S, Rosch J, et al: Mesenteric arterial infusions of vasopressin for hemorrhage from colonic diverticulosis. Am J Surg 129:212, 1975.
32. Goldberger L, Bookstein J: Transcatheter embolization for treatment of diverticular hemorrhage. Radiology 122:613, 1977.
33. Eaton A: Emergency surgery for acute colonic haemorrhage—A retrospective study. Br J Surg 68:109, 1981.

CHAPTER 127

Pathophysiology of Acute Diarrhea in the Intensive Care Unit

Uma Sundaram
Henry J. Binder

Diarrhea is not a frequent problem in an intensive care unit (ICU) setting, but when diarrhea does occur, often because of the serious nature of the patient's other medical problems, it is frequently difficult to establish a specific diagnosis. As a result, specific and effective therapy may not be initiated, and nonspecific therapy may not be totally effective.

It is unusual for diarrhea in adults to be the primary reason for admission to a medical ICU. However, the occurrence of severe ulcerative colitis, with or without the presence of toxic megacolon, necessitates the expert care provided in an ICU. In contrast, in infants and children, the dehydration and metabolic acidosis resulting from volume depletion are not an infrequent reason for admission to a pediatric ICU. Although discussion of the particular problems associated with diarrhea in a pediatric age population is beyond the scope of this chapter, most of the general principles of the physiology and pathophysiology of intestinal fluid and electrolyte movement pertain to both adults and children with diarrhea.

To provide a rational basis for a discussion of the diagnosis and treatment of diarrhea in an ICU setting, it is useful to review briefly the normal physiology of fluid and electrolyte transport and the pathogenesis of diarrhea in general.

First, it is important to emphasize the definitions of *diarrhea*, which is both a symptom and a sign. The term diarrhea may be used to describe the symptom of a decrease in stool consistency and/or an increase in stool frequency or volume. Specific questioning is required to establish the subjective character of each patient's diarrhea. As a sign, diarrhea is best defined as an increase in stool weight (or volume) to more than 200 to 225 g (or mL) per 24 hours. For a typical Western diet, normal stool weight is 100 to 150 g/d. Seventy-five percent or more of the wet weight of stool represents water content. Because there is no evidence of active water transport and because water movement is coupled to solute movement, it is necessary to review the regulation of normal intestinal electrolyte transport to understand the mechanisms responsible for the development of diarrhea.

OVERALL FLUID AND ELECTROLYTE MOVEMENT

As mentioned earlier, fluid movement in the intestine parallels solute movement. Thus, solute movement is the driving force for water movement in the small and large intestine. The characteristics of fluid and electrolyte movement in the small and large intestine have both similarities and distinct differences. The ability to conserve Na^+ differs in the jejunum and the colon. When the jejunum is perfused with an isosmolar solution, Na^+ is absorbed only if the luminal Na^+ concentration is greater than 133 mEq/L. When the luminal Na^+ concentration is less than 133 mEq/L, net Na^+ secretion is observed. In contrast, Na^+ is absorbed in the colon in this experimental setting when the luminal concentration of Na^+ is reduced to as low as 30 mEq/L. As a consequence, the colon, but not the jejunum, is able to absorb Na^+ when luminal concentrations of Na^+ are low and, therefore, is important in Na^+ conservation.

The response of the small and large intestine to aldosterone also differs. Aldosterone markedly enhances Na^+ absorption in the colon but has little effect in the small intestine. As aldosterone is secreted in response to Na^+ depletion, the colon contributes to the adaptive response that occurs in the dehydration that is a consequence of diarrhea.

Another difference in small and large intestinal function is the ability to absorb dietary nutrients, which is a small-intestinal, not colonic, function. Thus, glucose and amino acids are actively absorbed and stimulate water and Na^+ absorption in the jejunum and the ileum but not in the colon.

A fourth difference in function is found in the permea-

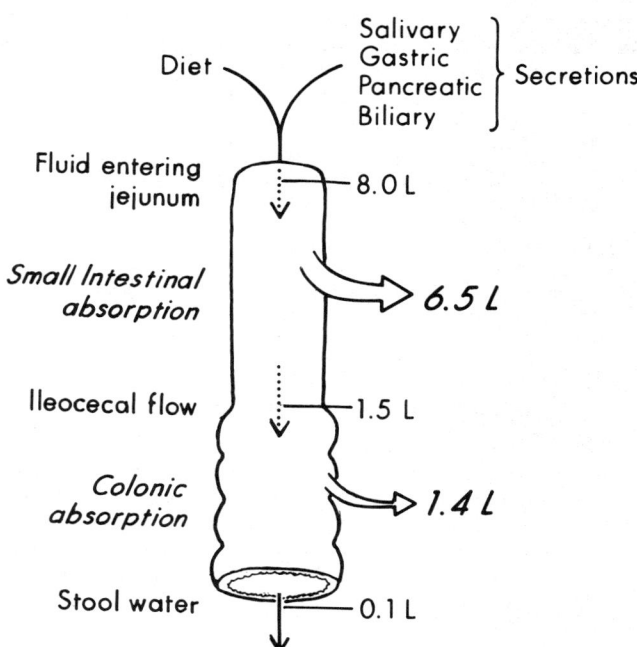

Figure 127–1. Overall fluid balance in the gastrointestinal tract. See text for discussion. (From Binder HJ: Absorption and secretion of water and electrolytes by small and large intestine. In: Sleisenger M, Fordtran JJ [eds]: Gastrointestinal Disease: Pathophysiology, Diagnosis, Management. 4th ed. Philadelphia, WB Saunders, p 1022, 1989.)

bility of the small- and large-intestinal epithelium. The permeability characteristic of the intestinal epithelium is most likely related to the tight junctions between epithelial cells. The permeability is substantially greater in the jejunum than the colon, which probably explains, at least in part, the inability of the jejunum to absorb Na$^+$ against an Na$^+$ gradient. However, when there is a favorable Na$^+$ gradient, the leaky nature of the jejunum is responsible for passive Na$^+$ absorption; this so-called solvent drag phenomenon occurs to a lesser extent in the ileum and not at all in the colon.

When one considers fluid movement in the intestine as a whole, approximately 8 L of fluid enters the jejunum daily. Only 1.5 L of this is due to daily oral intake; the remainder comes from salivary, gastric, pancreatic, and biliary secretions (Fig. 127–1). It must be emphasized that these values at best represent approximations. The small intestine absorbs 6.5 L, whereas only 1.5 to 2 L crosses the ileocecal valve. The colon absorbs at least 1.4 L of the colonic load. Therefore, the efficiency of absorption is about 75% in the small intestine and more than 90% in the colon. Probably more important is that the colon has the capacity to absorb up to 4 to 5 L of fluid a day. This point is critical to understand because a decrease in small-intestinal absorption does not result in diarrhea as long as the maximal absorptive capacity of the colon is not exceeded. However, a relatively small decrease in colonic absorption results in diarrhea even with normal small-intestinal function.

SPECIFIC TRANSPORT MECHANISMS

There are several different cellular mechanisms for electrolyte absorption in the intestine, and the characteristics of ion transport processes present in the jejunum, the ileum, and the colon reflect both the specific transport processes present in that segment and the permeability properties of the mucosa.

Sodium and Chloride Absorption

There are at least five transport mechanisms for Na$^+$ absorption, but these are not present in all segments of the small and large intestine. In the jejunum, Na$^+$ is absorbed via both active and passive transport processes. Glucose and amino acids stimulate Na$^+$ and water absorption at least in part via the glucose (or amino acid)–Na$^+$ cotransport process. This is probably the most important mechanism for fluid and electrolyte absorption in this portion of the small intestine. Although there is controversy regarding the specific details of glucose, Na$^+$, and water absorption, enhancement of water absorption by actively absorbed dietary nutrients (glucose or amino acid) is the physiologic basis for oral rehydration solution therapy. Another mechanism of Na$^+$ absorption in the jejunum is via solvent drag, as mentioned earlier. A third mechanism of Na$^+$ absorption in the jejunum is HCO$_3^-$-stimulated Na$^+$ absorption. This enhancement of Na$^+$ absorption by luminal HCO$_3^-$ is a consequence of a Na$^+$-H$^+$ exchange in the jejunum. Na$^+$-H$^+$ exchange is also important in the ileum and the proximal portion of the colon, but in these segments Na$^+$-H$^+$ exchange often is coupled to Cl$^-$-HCO$_3^-$ exchange, resulting in overall electroneutral NaCl absorption.

In the distal colon, a different Na$^+$ transport mechanism predominates, electrogenic Na$^+$ absorption. This process is inhibited by the diuretic amiloride and is responsible for significant conservation of Na$^+$ (i.e., the ability of the colon to absorb Na$^+$ against steep electrochemical gradients). Aldosterone stimulates electrogenic Na$^+$ absorption and contributes to the overall fluid conservation in dehydration.

The small and large intestines absorb large quantities of Na$^+$ and Cl$^-$. In general, the movements of these two ions are approximately equal and are coupled by two primary mechanisms. Some Na$^+$ absorptive processes (e.g., electrogenic and glucose stimulated) result in the development of a serosal positive electrical potential difference that serves as a driving force for Cl$^-$ absorption (i.e., potential-dependent Cl$^-$ absorption). As a result, Cl$^-$ is absorbed by a passive transport mechanism that is linked to active Na$^+$ absorption. In addition, Cl$^-$ absorption may also be coupled to active Na$^+$ absorption via intracellular pH. In this setting, parallel Na$^+$-H$^+$ and Cl$^-$-HCO$_3^-$ exchanges result in overall electroneutral NaCl absorption and are especially important in the ileum and the proximal colon. Cl$^-$-HCO$_3^-$ exchange may also be present without a parallel Na$^+$-H$^+$ exchange in the distal colon. In congenital chloridorrhea, there is absence of this exchange, resulting in high fecal Cl$^-$ concentrations.

Chloride Secretion

During the past two decades, multiple studies have contributed to the establishment of a model of secretagogue-induced Cl$^-$ secretion to explain anion secretion in most diarrheal disorders. In this model, based in part on experiments in the T$_{84}$ colon carcinoma cell line that has been used as a model for secretory epithelia, Cl$^-$ uptake across the basolateral membrane occurs via an Na$^+$-K$^+$-2Cl$^-$ transport process driven by an Na$^+$ gradient, which is maintained by the Na$^+$ pump (i.e., Na$^+$,K$^+$-ATPase). As the normal apical membrane is relatively impermeable to Cl$^-$, there is little Cl$^-$ movement across the apical membrane. However, several agonists activate Cl$^-$ secretion (i.e., secretagogues) in these cells and mediate this effect via intracellular second messengers. These intracellular mediators activate one or more protein kinases that phosphorylate membrane proteins, resulting in an apical membrane Cl^- channel, with the outcome that Cl^- enters the intestinal lumen. The mechanism by which Cl^- movement is stimulated is unknown but probably represents either insertion of a Cl^- channel into the apical membrane or activation of an inactive apical channel. Of great significance is that the defect in cystic fibrosis appears to represent an abnormality in postreceptor activation of this Cl^- channel. Stimulation of active Cl^- secretion is also associated with activation of a basolateral K^+ channel. Active Cl^- secretion is associated with a luminal negative potential difference, which is the primary driving force for Na^+ secretion, resulting in overall fluid and Na^+ and Cl^- secretion.

Potassium Movement

K^+ movement in the small intestine is generally believed to be passive, as it responds to changes in fluid movement and electrical potential difference. In the colon, net K^+ secretion is always observed in vivo and is largely potential dependent as a result of the existing luminal negative potential difference. In the absence of a potential difference, active K^+ secretion has been identified in the proximal colon, whereas both active K^+ secretory and absorptive processes are located in distal colon. Because dietary K^+ intake can affect the direction of K^+ transport, the distal colon may function to modulate overall K^+ balance. Cyclic nucleotides stimulate active K^+ secretion, which could contribute to enhanced K^+ losses in several diarrheal disorders (e.g., cholera). However, it is rare to observe significant K^+ depletion in most acute diarrheal illness in adults. K^+ depletion is more often found in children and some adults with chronic diarrheal disorders.

Bicarbonate Secretion

The large intestine and the ileum normally secrete HCO_3^- via a Cl^--HCO_3^- exchange. Although in vitro studies with several secretagogues demonstrate active Cl^- secretion, in vivo studies invariably reveal active HCO_3^- (not Cl^-) secretion. Although an excellent model exists to explain Cl^- secretion, similar understanding of active electrogenic HCO_3^- secretion is not available. However, studies using isolated cells from the ileum support the hypothesis that HCO_3^- secretion may occur via stimulation of the luminal Cl^--HCO_3^- exchange in crypt but not villus cells. In any event, enhanced colonic losses of HCO_3^- lead to HCO_3^- depletion with ensuing metabolic acidosis.

REGULATION OF INTESTINAL ION TRANSPORT PROCESSES

Both the enteral nervous system and the central nervous system control intestinal fluid and electrolyte absorption and secretion by a variety of neurohumoral agents. These agents in turn mediate their effect via intracellular second messengers (adenosine 3',5'-cyclic monophosphate [cyclic AMP], guanosine 3',5'-cyclic monophosphate [cyclic GMP], and Ca^{2+}). In general, agents that increase cyclic nucleotides and Ca^{2+} inhibit fluid and electrolyte absorption and may induce net fluid and electrolyte secretion. In contrast, agents that decrease the levels of these intracellular second messengers stimulate absorption. Table 127–1 lists some of the neurohumoral agents and the second messengers that mediate their effects on intestinal electrolyte transport. Phosphoinositide metabolites are another class of second messengers whose actions are not fully understood, except that their stimulation of Cl^- secretion is by increasing intracellular Ca^{2+} and by stimulating protein kinase C.

TABLE 127–1

NEUROHUMORAL SECRETAGOGUES AND THEIR SECOND MESSENGERS

Neurohumoral Agents	Second Messenger
Vasoactive intestinal polypeptide, secretin, adenosine, porcine intestinal peptide	Cyclic AMP
Atrial natriuretic factor	Cyclic GMP
Acetylcholine, serotonin, neurotensin, substance P	Ca^{2+}
Calcitonin, angiotensin, histamine, cholecystokinin	Not known

MECHANISMS OF DIARRHEA

Alterations in fluid and electrolyte movement have been identified in almost all diarrheal disorders that have been studied, and in many, net fluid secretion has been observed. Several different mechanisms can alter fluid and electrolyte movement. In many disorders, however, more than one mechanism may be responsible for the development of diarrhea.

Increased Luminal Osmolality

Diarrhea attributable to increased luminal osmolality is invariably a result of impaired digestion—absorption of dietary carbohydrates, which may be due to either inadequate hydrolysis or incomplete absorption (Table 127–2). Lactose intolerance resulting from primary lactase deficiency is the best example of a diarrheal disorder caused by increased luminal osmolality. After intake of lactose, individuals with diminished jejunal lactase activity often (but not always) have diarrhea, cramps, and flatus. Not understood has been the frequent lack of direct correlation between jejunal lactase activity and the occurrence or severity of symptoms. Factors that influence the development of symptoms include the rate of gastric emptying, small-bowel transit, and colonic compensation.

In any case, colonic bacteria metabolize nonabsorbed lactose presented to the colon to short chain fatty acids. Although these fatty acids were initially thought to stimulate fluid secretion, data indicate that they enhance colonic Na^+ and water absorption. Such colonic absorption represents a compensatory mechanism for conservation of carbohydrate calories and fluid and electrolytes. As a result, changes in colonic bacterial flora may result in variable rates of short chain fatty acid production and thus may account for the unpredictable occurrence of symptoms after lactose ingestion in patients with lactase deficiency. Indeed, it is not unlikely that antibiotic-associated diarrhea may in part be related to antibiotic suppression of colonic flora, thus resulting in reduced short chain fatty acid production and diminished absorption of fluid and electrolytes.

TABLE 127–2

CAUSES OF OSMOTIC DIARRHEA

Cause	Example
Reduced hydrolysis	Lactose intolerance, intestinal resection
Reduced absorption	Glucose-galactose malabsorption
Intake of carbohydrate without intestinal hydrolysis or absorption system	Lactulose therapy, sorbitol

Decreased Absorption

Most of the acquired diarrheal disorders with altered mucosal function are associated with intestinal inflammation and alteration of surface epithelial cells and mucosal permeability, factors that may also contribute to diarrhea. There are few examples of diarrheal disorders in which diminished absorptive function is the primary explanation for changes in fluid and electrolyte movement. Most of the diarrheal disorders usually associated with decreased absorption are also associated with mucosal inflammation. Studies have emphasized the role of immune products released by lamina propria cells in inflammation in the genesis of diarrhea (see later).

Celiac sprue, which has often been considered an excellent example of diarrhea that occurs as a result of decreased absorption, has at least four different mechanisms: (1) net fluid secretion in basal state that is probably due to crypt hyperplasia, (2) secondary lactase deficiency, (3) immune-inflammatory mediators, and (4) induction of colonic fluid secretion by nonabsorbed long chain fatty acids.

The examples of diarrhea largely caused by decreased absorption are the rare congenital absence of a specific transport process: (1) congenital chloridorrhea represents the deletion of Cl^--HCO_3^- exchange in ileal and colonic mucosa, (2) glucose-galactose malabsorption represents an inability to absorb actively transported monosaccharides owing to a congenital absence of the glucose transport protein in the jejunum, (3) congenital secretory diarrhea represents diminished or absent Na^+-H^+ exchange in the jejunal mucosa, and (4) primary bile acid malabsorption represents a congenital deficiency of the ileal bile acid transport protein.

Increased Secretion

Agents that induce net fluid and electrolyte secretion in the intestine can be classified in four general categories: bacterial enterotoxins, neurohumoral agents, immune-inflammatory mediators, and detergents.

Bacterial Enterotoxins

Many bacteria produce exotoxins that elicit intestinal fluid and electrolyte secretion (thus, the term *enterotoxin*). Some of these agents produce their effect via stimulation of one or more intracellular second messengers (Table 127–3), whereas the second messenger for others has not yet been identified. The classic example of an enterotoxin-induced diarrhea is cholera or the diarrhea produced by the heat-labile toxin of *Escherichia coli*. Cholera enterotoxin binds to

a receptor, GM_1 ganglioside, on the brush border membrane, resulting in stimulation of adenylate cyclase with a resulting increase in intracellular cyclic AMP. Cyclic AMP alters fluid and electrolyte transport, leading to net fluid and electrolyte secretion without any evidence of mucosal damage or injury. Not all enterotoxins mediate their effect via cyclic AMP. For example, heat-stable enterotoxin of *E. coli* increases intracellular cyclic GMP, and *Clostridium difficile* enterotoxin probably mediates its effects by increasing intracellular Ca^{2+}.

The diarrhea produced by microorganisms is not always the result of enterotoxin production. Other mechanisms include (1) direct tissue invasion with activation of inflammatory cells in the lamina propria, (2) production of cytotoxins that cause tissue damage and also may activate lamina propria cells, and (3) release of serotonin and other secretagogues from an invading microorganism (e.g., *Entamoeba histolytica*).

Neurohumoral Agents

Neurohumoral agonists influence ion transport in physiologic as well as pathologic situations. These neurohumoral agents (see Table 127–1) may affect transport while acting as endocrine or paracrine transmitters or neurotransmitters. An excellent example is vasoactive intestinal polypeptide (VIP), which is present normally in the gut and the brain. In the watery diarrhea syndrome caused by an islet cell adenoma, serum VIP levels are elevated and result in intestinal secretion and severe diarrhea. Cyclic AMP, the intracellular second messenger for VIP, is responsible for VIP's stimulation of fluid and electrolyte secretion. Serotonin, which is also a neurotransmitter and produces diarrhea in carcinoid syndrome, acts via a different second messenger, Ca^{2+}.

Immune-Inflammatory Mediators

Many studies have established that products of lamina propria cells alter epithelial cell ion transport. When the intestine of sensitized animals is re-exposed to the sensitizing antigen, serotonin, histamine, and other immune mediators are released from mast cells and are most likely responsible for the ensuing stimulation of Cl^- secretion (Fig. 127–2). Other stimuli also activate lamina propria cells (e.g., mast cells and neutrophils) to release multiple agents that affect ion transport. These experimental observations may well explain the changes in fluid and electrolyte transport that occur in several inflammatory diarrheal illnesses, including ulcerative colitis. Mesalamine, the active moiety of sulfasalazine, and glucocorticoids may be effective in diarrheal diseases as a consequence of their inhibition of release of these immune mediators. Development of new therapeutic approaches to alter the release of these lamina propria substances will undoubtedly be important in the future treatment of diarrhea in these conditions.

Detergents

Detergents that induce diarrhea include most commercial laxatives, bile acids, and long chain fatty acids. Although there is some controversy as to their exact mechanism of action to produce net secretion, it is fairly well accepted that detergents both induce anion secretion and increase mucosal permeability. Ca^{2+} mediates the laxative action of senna laxatives and bile acids; however, the specific intracellular second messenger has not been established for other laxatives.

TABLE 127–3

ENTEROTOXINS AND THEIR SECOND MESSENGERS

Agent	Second Messenger
Cholera toxin, heat-labile *E. coli* enterotoxin, *Salmonella* enterotoxin, *Campylobacter jejuni* enterotoxin, *Pseudomonas aeruginosa* enterotoxin, *Shigella* enterotoxin	Cyclic AMP
Heat-stable *E. coli* enterotoxin, *Yersinia enterocolitica* enterotoxin, *Klebsiella pneumoniae* enterotoxin	Cyclic GMP
Clostridium difficile enterotoxin (toxin A)	Ca^{2+}
Clostridium perfringens, *Bacillus cereus* enterotoxin, *Staphylococcus aureus* enterotoxin, *Vibrio parahaemolyticus* enterotoxin	Unknown

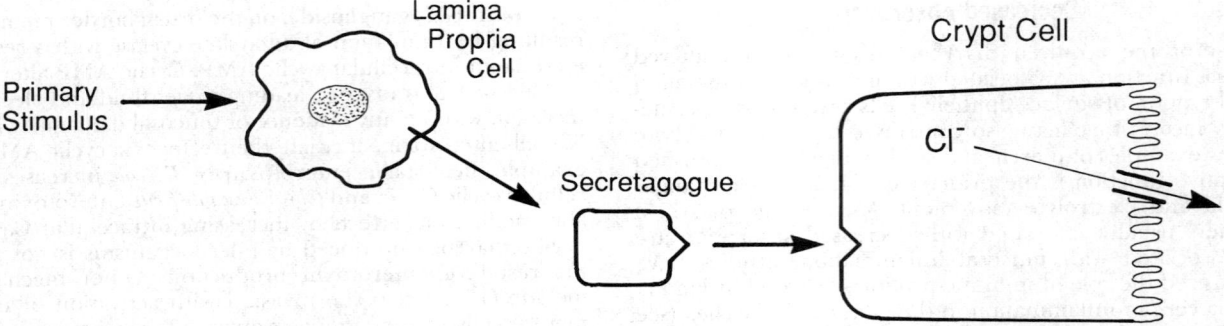

Figure 127–2. Role of products of lamina propria cells in stimulation of active Cl⁻ secretion. Several stimuli, including cytokines and antigens (in sensitized animals), induce mast cells (and other cells in lamina propria) to release agonists (e.g., histamine, eicosanoids) to stimulate active Cl⁻ secretion by crypt cells.

Altered Intestinal Motility

There is a considerable controversy regarding the role of intestinal motility in diarrheal conditions. A role for altered motor activity in diarrheal disorders has frequently been emphasized, but it is highly unlikely that increased transit alone alters fluid absorption. In contrast, there is speculation that many of the agonists derived from the lamina propria cells affect both epithelial cells and smooth muscle cells simultaneously, which may account for the net observed fluid secretion and coordinated propulsive muscle contractions, respectively, in several diarrheal disorders.

DIARRHEA IN THE INTENSIVE CARE UNIT

Almost all established causes of diarrhea may occur in a patient in an ICU. In general, however, four categories of patients most often may be in a medical ICU with diarrhea: (1) patients in whom severe diarrhea is the primary illness that caused significant metabolic abnormalities requiring admission to the ICU (e.g., severe ulcerative colitis); (2) hospitalized patients in whom diarrhea complicates their other medical problems, necessitating transfer to the ICU (e.g., antibiotic-associated diarrhea in patients with meningitis); (3) patients in whom diarrhea is a part of their disease process (e.g., acquired immunodeficiency syndrome); and (4) patients in an ICU with a serious medical or surgical illness who have diarrhea.

It is extremely unlikely that a previously healthy young or middle-aged adult experiences diarrhea of such magnitude to necessitate admission to an ICU. In contrast, elderly individuals with multiple medical problems or the very young can have diarrhea of any cause resulting in severe fluid and electrolyte loss, with associated metabolic abnormalities, and requiring an ICU admission. For example, the severe electrolyte abnormalities and metabolic acidosis that may result in cardiovascular collapse in the elderly with traveler's diarrhea is not uncommon. Similarly, diarrhea necessitating an ICU admission occurs frequently in the pediatric age population, but consideration of this is beyond the scope of this chapter.

The severity of the diarrheal illness per se, regardless of the age of the patient, at times necessitates the expert care provided in an ICU. Some such examples include patients with thromboembolic disease with ischemic bowel; patients with inflammatory bowel disease, with or without toxic megacolon, whose fluid and electrolyte losses may be so great as to necessitate admission to an ICU; and patients with *Shigella* dysentery. Obviously, this list is not all-inclusive.

Another class of patients who are admitted to the ICU with diarrhea is those who are already in the hospital with other medical problems. Although diarrhea itself may not be the sole reason that these hospitalized patients may require transfer to the ICU, it may complicate and cause significant deterioration in a previously ill patient.

The most common cause of acute diarrhea in the hospitalized patient is drug related. Many classes of drugs can cause diarrhea, but the most common are antibiotics, magnesium-containing antacids, other laxatives, and chemotherapeutic agents (e.g., 5-fluorouracil). Some commonly prescribed cardiovascular drugs have been associated with diarrhea and include quinidine and beta-blockers. The most likely way to identify a drug as the cause of diarrhea is to review the patients' records for those drugs that may induce diarrhea. Proof of the role of the drug rests on cessation of the diarrhea when administration of the drug is discontinued.

Diarrhea in ICU patients resulting from antibiotic use is not unexpected in view of the frequent use of antibiotics in such patients. Two different types of diarrhea are usually recognized: (1) pseudomembranous enterocolitis, which is frequently associated with bloody diarrhea, evidence of colitis on sigmoidoscopy (with or without demonstration of pseudomembranes), and the presence of *C. difficile* toxin in stool, and (2) diarrhea without evidence of colitis. The latter syndrome occurs more frequently than pseudomembranous enterocolitis and may not necessarily be related to the production of *C. difficile* cytotoxin and/or enterotoxin. Virtually all antibiotics, except vancomycin, have been associated with diarrhea, but it is uncertain whether there is a single (or multiple) pathogenic mechanism responsible for its development. One such mechanism, as mentioned earlier, is antibiotic suppression of colonic flora resulting in reduced short chain fatty acid production and diminished absorption of fluid and electrolytes after oral carbohydrate intake.

Enteral feeding formulas are commonly associated with diarrhea. This cause should be suspected if there is cessation of the diarrhea after discontinuation of these oral feedings. The mechanism of diarrhea that occurs with enteral feedings is not entirely clear. Because reducing the osmolarity of the enteral solutions (e.g., half-strength solutions) frequently reduces diarrhea, it is likely that the reason for diarrhea in these patients is related, at least in part, to an increase in the osmotic load.

An additional group of patients includes those in whom diarrhea is a part of their disease process. In patients with malignancies, the tumor, the therapy, or the immunocompromised state may cause diarrhea. The patient may have a rare paraneoplastic syndrome (e.g., small-cell cancer of the lung that produces VIP) or tumors (e.g., carcinoid) that are known to cause diarrhea. Carcinoid tumors release serotonin, a bioactive amine normally present in the enteral nervous system, into the circulation. This hormone, a potent secretagogue, inhibits coupled NaCl absorption by the villus cells and stimulates HCO₃⁻ secretion by the crypt cells in the rabbit ileum. Its exact role in patients with carcinoid syndrome remains to be established.

Diarrhea in a patient with a neoplasm may be due to the therapy that he or she is receiving. Chemotherapeutic agents such as 5-fluorouracil not infrequently cause diarrhea. The mechanism by which the chemotherapeutic agent induces diarrhea is probably secondary to the fact that most chemotherapeutic agents impair cell division and the intestinal tract has rapid cell turnover; thus, diarrhea may be most likely a consequence of loss of absorptive cells. It is possible that such therapies also result in an immunocompromised state (see later). Radiation therapy can also cause either acute or chronic diarrhea. Finally, because of the immunocompromised status of these patients, usual infectious causes as well as opportunistic pathogens should be considered. In any immunocompromised patient, such organisms as *Mycobacterium avium-intracellulare*, cytomegalovirus, adenovirus, *Giardia, Cryptosporidium, Aeromonas,* and *Strongyloides* should be considered. Often, treatable causes are not found or when a cause is found (e.g., *M. avium-intracellulare*), treatment may be ineffective.

In patients with acquired immunodeficiency syndrome, diarrhea is the most common gastrointestinal complication. These patients are particularly susceptible to opportunistic enteral infections by the agents mentioned earlier. Unfortunately, only infrequently is there a treatable infectious cause in patients with acquired immunodeficiency syndrome. These patients often have diarrhea that is not associated with an infectious agent, and, as a result, this entity has often been called acquired immunodeficiency syndrome enteropathy.

The status of the bowel rather than the immune status of the host may be compromised in certain situations that result in significant fluid and electrolyte loss from diarrhea. For example, the patient with an ileostomy whose colonic ability to conserve Na^+ is lost may have a considerably higher morbidity from a diarrheal illness and even require an ICU admission. Similarly, any patient with resection of a significant length (>100 cm) of the bowel for any reason may be particularly susceptible to significant fluid and electrolyte losses from diarrheal illnesses. Finally, the patient with inflammatory bowel disease may have diarrhea not only from immune-inflammatory mediators and altered motility, but also from loss of absorptive surface area caused by villus cell denudation.

DIAGNOSIS

The diagnosis and treatment of diarrhea in the first three categories (see earlier) are not altered by hospitalization in an ICU. The usual problems associated with obtaining stool specimens, however, are almost invariably compounded by the nature of a patient's illness that required hospitalization in an ICU. The approach to such patients is well outlined in standard texts of medicine and gastroenterology. Comments regarding diagnosis are limited to the group of patients already in an ICU who experience diarrhea.

Assessment of diarrhea in a patient hospitalized in an ICU is no different from that in non-ICU patients. The etiology of diarrhea outside of an ICU is most often determined on the basis of history alone. Important information leading to identification of the cause is provided by data such as the age of the patient, recent travel history, duration of diarrhea, epidemiologic nature of companions with diarrhea, character and description of diarrhea, past medical history, and past and present drug use. History is also extremely important for ICU patients, except that it may be more difficult to obtain.

Characterization of a patient's diarrhea is invariably diffi-

cult in an ICU, frequently as a result of the patient's inability to ambulate and to cooperate fully with the nursing staff. The nursing staff, in turn, often views changes in bowel function as a major nursing problem that complicates care of patients. Nonetheless, examination of stool is imperative. Presence of blood, occult blood, or leukocytes is evidence of colonic inflammation. Conversely, their absence may suggest a small-intestinal, not colonic, cause of the diarrhea.

It is also critical to determine which medications that the patient is receiving (or has received). Specific attention must be directed to present or past antibiotic use. Although it is well recognized that antibiotics may cause diarrhea, diarrhea may not occur for several days after antibiotic administration has been discontinued. The primary therapeutic approach to antibiotic-associated diarrhea is discontinuation of the antibiotic and examination of stool for *C. difficile* and *C. difficile* toxin. Persistence or severity of diarrhea necessitates further diagnostic studies, including flexible sigmoidoscopy, stool cultures for bacterial pathogens, and examination for ova and parasites. It is important to emphasize that the majority of pathogens (especially in the immunocompromised patient) are not identified by the usual standard hospital bacteriologic procedures.

Medications other than antibiotics are also not infrequent causes of diarrhea. It is essential to determine whether such patients have received magnesium-containing antacids, laxatives, and certain cardiotropic drugs (e.g., calcium channel blockers). Diarrhea in a patient with a neoplasm who had recently received a course of chemotherapy may be a result of either altered epithelial cell function or opportunistic infections.

Another cause of diarrhea that must be considered, especially in the elderly patient with cardiovascular disease, is ischemic injury to the intestine. Most such patients have bloody stools (with or without diarrhea). Patients who have diarrhea after a period of prolonged hypotension may have had ischemic injury to the intestine.

INTERPRETATION OF STOOL ELECTROLYTES

There has been much emphasis on analysis of stool electrolytes. Usually, these studies are not performed for patients with acute diarrhea but rather for individuals who have had unexplained chronic diarrhea after an initial evaluation. Determination of stool osmolality and Na^+ and K^+ concentrations can be helpful (together with determination of the effect of fasting on stool output) in establishing the diagnosis of unexplained chronic diarrhea. Rarely, if ever, should such studies be performed for individuals who have acute diarrhea (i.e., duration of less than 2 to 3 weeks). The stool osmolality should be compared with twice the concentration of the stool Na^+ and K^+ concentrations. (An important caveat is that a stool osmolality greater than 310 mOsm/kg most likely represents degradation of nonabsorbed carbohydrate by fecal bacteria in the collection bottle after defecation and should be considered an artifact.) When the stool osmolality approximates $2([Na^+] + [K^+])$, it is likely that a dietary nutrient is not the cause of diarrhea. In such patients, it is likely that fasting does not result in a significant decrease in stool output and that either a luminal (e.g., bacterial enterotoxin) or a humoral (i.e., circulating) secretagogue is responsible for the diarrhea.

In contrast, when diarrhea is a result of a dietary nutrient, a substantial decrease in stool output is observed, and a significant difference (osmotic gap) is present between the stool osmolality and twice the stool Na^+ plus K^+ concentrations. Although it is readily evident that a difference of more than 50 represents a gastroenterologist's stool osmotic gap, whereas one of 0 to 5 does not, there is a paucity of data available to help evaluate intermediate values. Determination of stool electrolytes is rarely an important study in the initial evaluation of diarrhea in a patient in an ICU under most circumstances.

TREATMENT

Ideally, the most effective therapy is one that results in cure (i.e., elimination of the underlying cause). Treatment of diarrhea in the ICU is no different and depends on accurate diagnosis.

Frequently, primary attention must be directed toward correction of dehydration and any electrolyte imbalance that may be present. However, in view of the frequent multitude of other medical problems, a delicate balance of fluid replacement requires individual tailoring of therapy.

Diarrhea caused by *C. difficile* most often resolves when treated with vancomycin or metronidazole. Alternatively, establishment of the pathogenic process responsible for diarrhea may lead to a reduction or elimination of the specific mechanism responsible for the alteration in intestinal fluid and electrolyte movement. Thus, the patient with lactase deficiency who has diarrhea after administration of lactose in an enteral feeding improves when the lactose is removed from the enteral feeding solution.

When the cause of diarrhea cannot be established or when the pathogenic mechanism cannot be identified, nonspecific therapy should be instituted. Frequently, judicious use of loperamide and other opiate-related compounds may be of temporary benefit.

Bibliography

Binder HJ: Absorption and secretion of water and electrolytes by small and large intestine. In: Sleisenger M, Fordtran JJ (eds): Gastrointestinal Disease: Pathophysiology, Diagnosis, Management. 4th ed. Philadelphia WB Saunders, p 1022, 1989.

Binder HJ, Sandle GI: Electrolyte absorption and secretion in the mammalian colon. In: Johnson LR (ed): Physiology of the Gastrointestinal Tract. 2nd ed. New York, Raven Press, p 1389, 1987.

Castro GA: Immunological regulation of electrolyte transport. In: Lebenthan E, Duffey ME (eds): Textbook of Secretory Diarrhea. New York, Raven Press, p 31, 1990.

Dobbins JW: Approach to the patient with diarrhea. In: Kelley WM (ed): Textbook of Internal Medicine. Philadelphia, JB Lippincott, p 669, 1989.

Donowitz M, Welsh MJ: Regulation of mammalian small intestinal electrolyte secretion. In: Johnson LR (ed): Physiology of the Gastrointestinal Tract. 2nd ed. New York, Raven Press, p 1351, 1987.

Field ME, Rao MC, Chang EB: Intestinal electrolyte transport and diarrheal diseases. N Engl J Med 321:800, 879, 1989.

Fine KD, Krejs GJ, Fordtran JJ: Diarrhea. In: Sleisenger M, Fordtran JJ (eds): Gastrointestinal Disease: Pathophysiology, Diagnosis, Management. 4th ed. Philadelphia, WB Saunders, p 290, 1989.

Purdue MH, Gall DG: Intestinal anaphylaxis in the rat: Jejunal response to in vitro antigen exposure. Am J Physiol 250:G427, 1986.

CHAPTER 128

Inflammatory Bowel Disease

Stephen B. Hanauer

Ulcerative colitis and Crohn's disease encompass the idiopathic inflammatory bowel diseases (IBDs). They are chronic and uncommonly necessitate treatment in the critical care setting, except in a few complicating situations. These disorders are not rare and the critical care physician will likely encounter such patients and must be aware of the course and prognosis of each situation to determine optimal therapeutic approaches.

Ulcerative colitis is an inflammatory disease confined to the colon. In the usual course, the inflammation occurs as a diffuse, continuous, superficial process confined to the mucosa and may extend to a variable extent proximally in individual patients. The symptoms depend on the extent and severity of colonic involvement, which always occurs in the rectum but may include any contiguous proximal segment of colon. Hence, ulcerative proctitis is confined to the rectum, proctosigmoiditis to the sigmoid colon, and left-sided colitis to the splenic flexure; extensive colitis or pancolitis pertains to inflammation extending proximal to the transverse colon. The small intestine is not involved, except occasionally when a similar superficial inflammation is present in the most distal terminal ileum as an extension of pancolitis. The severity of the inflammatory process remains relatively constant along the entire extent and typically determines the severity of symptoms and the likelihood of intestinal complications. Serious acute complications of ulcerative colitis include intestinal hemorrhage, fulminant colitis or toxic megacolon, and perforation. Colonic carcinoma is a long-term sequela that may manifest as bleeding or obstruction.

Crohn's disease is a more protean form of IBD that may involve any segment of the digestive tract in a focal, discontinuous, transmural manner. Acute and chronic mucosal inflammation manifests grossly as aphthoid ulcerations that can extend along the mucosal surface as linear ulcerations or deeper into the submucosa and serosa as fissures or sinus tracts that can produce inflammatory mesenteric masses, abscesses, or fistulas into adjacent organs. Most commonly, the ileum alone (ileitis) or along with the right side of the colon (ileocolitis) is inflamed, but Crohn's disease may also be limited to the small bowel (jejunoileitis) or colon (colitis). The stomach and the duodenum are less commonly involved and, if so, usually in conjunction with another segment. The transmural nature of Crohn's disease accounts for both the short-term and long-term intestinal complications. Acutely, mural thickening and luminal narrowing are due to edema, but fibrosis is a chronic sequela that may also produce obstruction. Deep ulcerations can invade arteries, leading to profuse hemorrhage, or as fissures can evolve into abscesses or occasionally perforations. Toxic megacolon may also occur in Crohn's disease involving a limited colonic segment or the entire colon.

Initial diagnostic measures for patients with acute ulcerative colitis or Crohn's disease must determine whether the situation can be treated with medical management alone or whether surgical intervention is necessary. In any case, immediate supportive therapy must include fluid and electrolyte repletion according to predicted enteral and insensible losses and administration of blood products in the case of hemorrhage and antibiotics if a septic complication is suspected. Patients who have been treated with corticosteroids are susceptible to adrenal insufficiency and require stress doses of parenteral steroids to prevent addisonian crisis. Patients with IBD must be observed for consequences of chronic diseases. Stress ulceration may manifest as upper gastrointestinal tract bleeding (aggravated by long-term steroid therapy); hypercoagulability and thrombocytosis increase the likelihood of phlebitis and pulmonary emboli; and rarely, immunosuppression (owing to therapy or malnutrition) can potentiate abdominal, pulmonary, hepatic, central nervous system, or vascular infections.

COMPLICATIONS

Hemorrhage

Rectal bleeding is a common manifestation of both ulcerative colitis and Crohn's disease, but profuse or acute hemorrhage is infrequent.[1] Ulcerative colitis is associated with blood in the stool attributable to superficial mucosal ulceration or friability. Blood typically coats the stool, is mixed with loose stools, or is passed within mucopus. The most common complication of bleeding in ulcerative colitis is chronic iron deficiency that improves with iron supplementation after the acute inflammation resolves. More profound bleeding may occur in the setting of severe colitis in the presence of other symptoms of acute disease (fever, tachycardia, more than six bowel movements a day, abdominal tenderness).[2] Intensive intravenous therapy with corticosteroids[3, 4] or corticotropin[5] is indicated for the severe disease with maintenance of the hematocrit above 30% until the control of bowel frequency and blood loss is achieved. The need for continued transfusions in the setting of acute ulcerative colitis is an ominous sign that colectomy may be necessary.[6]

Rectal bleeding is also a common symptom in Crohn's disease and may contribute to chronic anemia, although other nutritional anemias such as folate and vitamin B_{12} deficiency should be considered when there is small-bowel disease.[7] Deeper ulceration may produce arterial bleeding in Crohn's disease associated with profuse gastrointestinal hemorrhage. Profound hemorrhage usually occurs as an uncommon manifestation within the course of Crohn's disease, although it occasionally is the initial or single manifestation of disease activity.[8] Nonsteroidal anti-inflammatory drug therapy is a predisposing factor,[9] as is anticoagulation that may occur as a complication of malabsorption of fat-soluble vitamins or prolonged antibiotic therapy.

The source and rapidity of bleeding determine the nature of the blood loss. Ileal bleeding begins as melena or maroon stools, quickly turning red, with clots. Colonic bleeding may begin with bowel movements, but the purgative properties of blood quickly turn the bowel movements to mainly blood and clots. The general location of bleeding can be estimated by tagged red blood cell scanning, although colonoscopy is a better means of identifying the exact site as well as determining the status of mucosal changes along the colon and the distal ileum. When colonoscopic visualization is technically not feasible owing to the rapidity of hemorrhage, arteriography may be required. In patients with previous bowel resections for Crohn's disease, the anastomotic site is a common location for hemorrhage, even in the absence of other symptoms of active disease.

Management includes having the patient take nothing by mouth while intravenous fluids and packed red blood cells are replenished. In the absence of other manifestations of active disease (e.g., fever, prior diarrhea, and abdominal

tenderness), most bleeding stops spontaneously. Intensive doses of corticosteroids are not of proven value, although the greater the suspicion that the bleeding is a manifestation of more extensive disease, the greater is the empirical indication to introduce a short-term course of steroids. Colonoscopic electrocoagulation and injection therapy around anastomotic ulcers has been described, but controlled trials have not been performed. Rarely, intra-arterial vasopressin administration may control bleeding. Surgical resection may be necessary for persistent or uncontrolled hemorrhage,[10] and the focus should be on a prior anastomotic site, although intraoperative endoscopy may assist in defining the extent of resection that is required. Recurrent hemorrhage may be a pattern in some patients, especially if bleeding is the solitary indication for intestinal resection.

Fulminant Colitis and Toxic Megacolon

Extension of the inflammatory process into the submucosa leads to severe or fulminant ulcerative colitis.[10–12] With disease progression, the muscular layers of the bowel become necrotic and the entire thickness of the bowel wall becomes tissue paper thin and is associated with colonic dilatation with a serious risk of perforation. The latter status is deemed toxic megacolon and, although most often seen with ulcerative colitis, can also occur in Crohn's disease[13–15] and other acute colitides (e.g., infections).[16–18] Precipitating factors include severe and extensive disease activity,[19] instrumentation of the colon with either endoscopy or barium enemas in patients with severe disease[12] (possibly related to vigorous laxative preparations), electrolyte imbalance (especially hypokalemia),[19, 20] and the use of anticholinergic or antidiarrheal agents in patients with severe disease.[20] Although toxic megacolon sometimes occurs during the first attack of colitis, in most cases, chronic colitis has been present for years.[20–22]

Toxic megacolon typically occurs with progressive symptoms of diarrhea, bloody stools, and tenesmus. Localizing lower abdominal pain and tenderness herald the transmural and serosal extension of inflammation, and some patients may paradoxically report a noticeable improvement of diarrhea with the passage of only blood or bloody membranes without fecal material. Clinical signs of toxemia, including fever, tachycardia, and leukocytosis, develop as abdominal pain and distention become progressive and bowel sounds diminish or cease. Peritoneal signs of rebound tenderness and abdominal guarding may be subtle or absent in elderly patients or those receiving high-dose corticosteroid therapy.[12, 20] In some cases, the loss of hepatic dullness may be the first clinical indication of perforation, and mental status changes, including confusion, agitation, and apathy, are occasionally noted. Leukocytosis with a left shift generally is present along with anemia, hypokalemia, and hypoalbuminemia.

Diagnostic studies should be limited to plain films of the abdomen, which demonstrate loss of haustration with segmental or total colonic dilatation.[23] The magnitude of dilatation need not be severe, averaging 8 to 9 cm (normal < 5 to 6 cm) to diagnose toxic megacolon. Maximal dilatation may exceed 15 cm and may occur in any part of the colon where thumbprinting or pneumatosis cystoides coli documents the transmural extension. Free peritoneal air, retroperitoneal tracking of air, or pneumomediastinum documents perforation. Small-intestinal ileus may accompany colonic dilatation or perforation.[24]

In situations in which the diagnosis of colitis has not been confirmed, a limited proctoscopic examination shows the extensive ulcerations with friable, bleeding mucosa, and a subsequent abdominal radiograph can provide a partial air-contrast study to define the proximal extent of disease. More extensive sigmoidoscopic or colonoscopic studies should be undertaken only in the most experienced hands with a clear understanding of the potential benefits versus the risk of these procedures.[12] Scans after reinjection of radiolabeled white blood cells have demonstrated the extent of intestinal inflammation and may, on occasion, be useful when the diagnosis or possible involvement of the small intestine is in question.[25]

The management of fulminant colitis and toxic megacolon entails close cooperation between medical and surgical services. Any evidence of worsening, failure to improve, or perforation necessitates immediate colectomy. Early recognition and management have substantially lowered the mortality from as high as 50% in the presence of perforation to less than 15%.[24, 26] Mortality is higher if patients are older than the age of 40 years, when perforation has occurred, and when surgery has been delayed.[27]

After fulminant colitis has been recognized, oral intake should be discontinued, and a nasogastric tube is indicated in the presence of small-bowel ileus or vomiting. Colonic dilatation alone, without other indications of toxicity, may improve with initiating oral intake or rolling the patient from front to back to redistribute colonic air and assist in decompression. Administration of anticholinergic medications and narcotics should be discontinued and narcotic pain medications restricted to patients on their way to the operating room. Vigorous replacement of fluid, electrolytes, and blood is paramount to restore previous losses and to continue replenishing ongoing losses from diarrhea, fever, and third spacing of fluids. Transfusions of packed red blood cells should be instituted to maintain the hematocrit above 30%.

Total body potassium stores are commonly depleted and, despite normal serum potassium levels, necessitate replacement along with replenishment of phosphate, calcium, and magnesium. Severe hypoalbuminemia (<2 g/dL) may benefit from perioperative albumin transfusion to maintain serum oncotic pressure, although it must be recognized that the effects are transient owing to the rapid metabolism and excretion of infused albumin.

Specific medical therapy is limited to parenteral corticosteroids or corticotropin in patients who have not previously been receiving corticosteroids.[3, 12, 28] Although the efficacy of steroid therapy to abort progressive dilatation in patients with toxic megacolon has been controversial, continuation of therapy is essential in the majority of patients who have already been receiving these drugs and augmented doses should be administered owing to the additional toxic stress. Doses equivalent to hydrocortisone, 100 mg every 6 to 8 hours, or methylprednisolone, 15 mg every 6 hours, should be administered as an intermittent or continuous infusion. Intravenous infusion of corticotropin, 100 to 150 U daily, may be preferable in patients not previously exposed to corticosteroids.

Although antibiotic therapy has not been useful as a primary therapy for ulcerative colitis, in the setting of fulminant colitis or toxic megacolon, broad-spectrum antibiotic treatment with adequate gram-negative and anaerobic coverage should be instituted if transmural inflammation or toxic megacolon is suspected.[3, 12, 28] Antibiotic therapy should be continued during several days to a week, until the patient stabilizes or through the initial postoperative period. Continued surveillance for *Clostridium difficile* colitis, a potentially complicating condition in the severely ill patient with colitis, is important whenever prolonged hospitalization or antibiotic exposure has occurred.

Surgical intervention is necessary for any evidence of perforation, uncontrolled hemorrhage, suspicion of septic shock, imminent transverse colonic rupture, or either worsening or failure of the patient to improve during the initial 12 to 24 hours of intensive therapy.[3, 12, 29] Severely malnourished patients and pregnant women with toxic megacolon have potential for increased morbidity and are candidates for emergent colectomy.[30] Patients with toxic megacolon should be monitored with complete blood count and electrolyte evaluations every 12 hours and radiographic surveys of the abdomen every 12 to 24 hours. Continued transfusion requirements, persistent white blood cell counts greater than 20,000/mm³ (and greater than 80% neutrophils), or deteriorating vital signs necessitate immediate surgical intervention. Progressive colonic dilatation or colonic diameter greater than 12 cm is an ominous finding of imminent rupture.

A team approach between internists and surgeons is essential to determine optimal timing (or delay) of surgery. The decision must be individualized for each patient according to the gravity of the condition, age of the patient, duration of colitis, and psychologic status of the patient and the family. Some physicians advocate early surgical intervention to avoid postoperative morbidity[31] and the inevitability of eventual colectomy in patients progressing to toxic megacolon.[32] This conviction is supported by the possibility of eventual ileoanal procedures to avoid the previous necessity of ileostomy. However, patients who respond to aggressive medical management have the potential for prolonged remission or, at least, elective colectomy under more optimal circumstances.

The choice of operation depends on the diagnosis (ulcerative colitis, Crohn's disease, or indeterminant colitis), the medical condition of the patient, and the experience of the surgical team. Options now include subtotal colectomy with ileocolonic anastomosis, mucous fistula, or Hartmann's pouch; proctocolectomy; and colectomy and mucosal proctectomy or ileoproctectomy via stapling.[33, 34] Subtotal colectomy is the procedure of choice for the majority of patients in whom the diagnosis remains in question or if Crohn's disease with rectal sparing is suspected, for patients who are critically ill in whom prolongation of pelvic dissection is not desired, or for patients who may opt for an eventual ileoanal anastomosis under more elective conditions. Rectal sparing offers the option of an ileorectal anastomosis if the surgical procedure is without complication and the resected margins are free from disease. Total proctocolectomy can occasionally be performed by experienced surgeons in stable patients who have elected against potential sphincter-saving procedures.

Postoperative Complications

Postoperative complications should be anticipated in critically ill patients who are undergoing operations and who have IBD.[35, 36] Malnourishment, prolonged corticosteroid therapy, and abdominal sepsis are predisposing factors for anastomotic leakage, residual abscess, pneumonia, or pulmonary emboli. The last is a common complication of colectomy and pelvic dissection that has led some surgeons to recommend prophylactic vena caval clipping or the placement of a caval filter in patients with extensive colitis who are undergoing colectomy.[35] High-dose corticosteroid therapy predisposes to poor wound healing and often masks infections by inhibiting immediate fevers or typical pain. Persistence of an elevated white blood cell count, low-grade fever, prolonged ileus, and development of drainage from wounds are sentinel signs of intra-abdominal septic complications that may be subtle in patients who undergo diversion procedures. Pelvic abscesses are not rare in patients undergoing colectomy owing to anastomotic leakage attributable to pelvic sepsis or torsion from pulling down bowel and mesentery. Occasionally, suture line breakdown of retained rectum or inadequate closure of the pelvic musculature leads to pelvic abscess formation with persistent drainage through the rectal wound or even to the abdominal wound.[36] Computed tomographic scanning or pelvic ultrasonography can identify the presence of an abscess when the postoperative recovery is prolonged or complicated.

ASSOCIATED CONDITIONS
Malnutrition

Nutritional complications are also common in patients with chronic intestinal disease.[37] Many patients have malnourishment and weight loss and a kwashiorkor-like picture of protein-calorie malnutrition owing to reduced intake of nutrients (to avoid symptoms) or prolonged diarrhea that is often associated with protein-losing enteropathy. These features, along with the heightened caloric needs caused by inflammation and the catabolic effects of steroid therapy, significantly increase the calorie and protein requirements of seriously ill patients. Despite the presence of intestinal inflammation, enteral feeding remains a preferred method of replenishing nutrient needs and is as efficacious as parenteral feeding in patients with uncomplicated Crohn's disease (in the absence of obstruction, stricture formation, or sepsis) and ulcerative colitis when patients can tolerate oral intake or tube feeding without nausea, vomiting, or increasing abdominal pain or diarrhea. Elemental feeding via nasoenteral tube can be efficacious and has a demonstrable therapeutic role equivalent to that of steroids in uncomplicated Crohn's disease.[38] However, most patients in the critical care unit also require supplemental or primary parenteral nutrition to maintain or replenish nutrient stores. Calorie demands on the order of 40 to 60 kilocalories/kg are common in these patients, with protein requirements of 1 to 2 g/kg.[37] Potassium requirements should be expected to be increased owing to losses from diarrhea and steroid-induced urinary excretion. Magnesium and phosphate depletion is also predictable, as is zinc deficiency in patients with chronic diarrhea or fistulizing Crohn's disease.

Parenteral nutrition via central catheters has the usual risks of infection in patients with IBD,[37, 39] but the risk of *Candida* sepsis is increased owing to the concurrent use of steroids and antibiotics. Subclavian venous thrombosis is an additional risk owing to the hypercoagulable state of chronic inflammation.

Pregnancy

Pregnant patients with IBD present additional, not rare problems for the critical care team. The potential problems of bleeding, obstruction, abscess formation, and toxic megacolon can occur during any stage of pregnancy.[40] Early during gestation, the major concern is the likelihood of miscarriage owing to the medical complications, whereas by the third trimester, the primary objective is to maintain the fetus in utero as long as possible to ensure adequate fetal growth and development sufficient for neonatal viability. For the most part, fertility is normal for men and women with IBD and the likelihood of pregnancy, in general, is related to the health of the woman.[41] The effect of pregnancy on IBD is usually more important than the effect of IBD on the pregnancy. In other words, women with IBD who become pregnant usually have a good outcome with full-term, healthy neonates. However, many pregnant women have flare-ups of IBD during pregnancy. When the active disease is treated in an appropriate manner, the fetus tends to do well without apparent adverse outcomes in the absence

of premature labor. The latter can be induced by severe illness in the mother, such as abdominal sepsis and toxic megacolon, or the need for abdominal surgery.

Active IBD during pregnancy, with few exceptions, should be treated in the same manner as in the nonpartum state. Nutritional support is important for the woman, as fetal growth usually takes precedence over maintenance of maternal nutritional stores. Hence, the fetus may continue to grow at the expense of the mother's muscle mass and fat stores. Either enteral or parenteral support may be necessary and is safe during gestation. Sulfasalazine and corticosteroids are safe to use during pregnancy[42] to support maternal well-being, and stress doses of steroids should be administered to severely ill women who have been receiving ongoing steroid therapy to prevent an adrenal crisis. Neonates should be observed for adrenal insufficiency if the mother had been treated with significant doses of preterm steroids. In the first trimester, administration of metronidazole[43] should be avoided because of potential teratogenic effects but may be administered, if necessary, in the latter stages of pregnancy.

Complications of IBD during pregnancy should be treated aggressively with monitoring of the mother and the fetus. Intestinal obstruction should be treated with nasogastric suction and steroids in the setting of Crohn's disease. Women who have undergone previous abdominal surgery (resection or ileostomy) may be predisposed to adhesive obstructions during pregnancy as the uterus expands. Most patients respond to conservative management with nasogastric decompression and fluid and electrolyte support. Parenteral nutritional support should be provided in the case of prolonged obstruction, and surgery should be deferred as long as there are no signs of impending perforation (rebound tenderness or peritoneal signs) or sepsis (fever, leukocytosis). Intra-abdominal sepsis (perforation or abscess) necessitates surgical exploration and drainage. In this setting, the most expeditious surgical approach is to treat the acute complication and limit the operation by diverting the proximal segment to an ileostomy or colostomy for future (postpartum) reanastomosis. Perioperative monitoring of the fetus is essential, and premature labor should be treated aggressively by the obstetric team. Likewise, toxic megacolon should be treated with aggressive medical therapy as with nonpregnant women. The indications for colectomy are the same; however, premature labor should be treated concurrently, and if colectomy is indicated, subtotal colectomy and creation of mucous fistula are the procedures of choice to limit anesthesia and reduce postoperative morbidity.

References

1. Farmer RG: Clinical features and natural history of inflammatory bowel disease. Med Clin North Am 64:1103, 1980.
2. Smith JN, Winship DH: Complications and extraintestinal problems in inflammatory bowel disease. Med Clin North Am 64:1161, 1980.
3. Jarnerot G: Intensive treatment. In: Gitnick G (ed): Inflammatory Bowel Disease: Diagnosis and Treatment. New York, Igaku-Shoin Medical Publishers, p 403, 1991.
4. Jarnerot G, Rolny P, Sandberg-Gertzen H: Intensive intravenous treatment of ulcerative colitis. Gastroenterology 89:1005, 1985.
5. Meyers S, Sachar D, Goldberg J, et al: Corticotropin versus hydrocortisone in the intravenous treatment of ulcerative colitis. A prospective, randomized, double-blind clinical trial. Gastroenterology 85:351, 1983.
6. Robert JH, Sachar DB, Aufses AH Jr, et al: Management of severe hemorrhage in ulcerative colitis. Am J Surg 159:550, 1990.
7. Phillips SF: Pathophysiology of symptoms and clinical features of inflammatory bowel disease. In: Kirsner JB, Shorter RG (eds): Inflammatory Bowel Disease. 3rd ed. Philadelphia, Lea & Febiger, p 239, 1988.
8. Janowitz HD, Mauer K: Crohn's disease. In: Gitnick G (ed): Inflammatory Bowel Disease: Diagnosis and Treatment. New York, Igaku-Shoin Medical Publishers, p 101, 1991.
9. Kaufmann HJ, Taubin HL: Nonsteroidal anti-inflammatory drugs activate quiescent inflammatory bowel disease. Ann Intern Med 107:513, 1987.

10. Huizenga KA, Schroeder KW: Gastrointestinal complications of ulcerative colitis and Crohn's disease. In: Kirsner JB, Shorter RG (eds): Inflammatory Bowel Disease. 3rd ed. Philadelphia, Lea & Febiger, p 257, 1988.
11. Riddell RH: Pathology of idiopathic inflammatory bowel disease. In: Kirsner JB, Shorter RG (eds): Inflammatory Bowel Disease. 3rd ed. Philadelphia, Lea & Febiger, p 329, 1988.
12. Krawitt EL, Vecchio JA, Heilman RS: Toxic dilatation. In: Gitnick G, (ed): Inflammatory Bowel Disease: Diagnosis and Treatment. New York, Igaku-Shoin Medical Publishers, p 479, 1991.
13. Greenstein AJ, Kark AE, Dreiling DA: Crohn's disease of the colon. III. Toxic dilatation of the colon in Crohn's colitis. Am J Gastroenterol 63:117, 1975.
14. Grieco MB, Bordan DL, Greiss AC, et al: Toxic megacolon complicating Crohn's colitis. Ann Surg 191:75, 1980.
15. Whorwell PJ, Isaacson P: Toxic dilatation of colon in Crohn's disease. Lancet 2:1334, 1981.
16. Stein D, Bank S, Louw JH: Fulminating amoebic colitis. Surgery 85:349, 1979.
17. Brown CH, Ferrante WA, Davis WD: Toxic dilatation of the colon complicating pseudomembranous enterocolitis. Am J Dig Dis 13:813, 1968.
18. Schofield PF, Mandal BK, Ironside AG: Toxic dilatation of the colon in salmonella colitis and inflammatory bowel disease. Br J Surg 66:5, 1979.
19. Caprilli R, Vernia P, Colaneri O, et al: Risk factors in toxic megacolon. Dig Dis Sci 25:817, 1980.
20. Norland CC, Kirsner JB: Toxic dilatation of colon (toxic megacolon): Etiology, treatment and prognosis in 42 patients. Medicine 48:229, 1969.
21. Jalan KN, Sirues W, Card WI, et al: An experience of ulcerative colitis. I. Toxic dilatation in 55 cases. Gastroenterology 57:68, 1969.
22. Binder SC, Miller HH, Deterling RA: Emergent and urgent operations for ulcerative colitis. Arch Surg 110:284, 1975.
23. Halpert RD: Toxic dilatation of the colon. Radiol Clin North Am 25:145, 1987.
24. Caprilli R, Vernia P, Latella G, et al: Early recognition of toxic megacolon. J Clin Gastroenterol 9:160, 1987.
25. Campieri M, Gionechetti P, Belluzzi A, et al: Management of severe attacks of ulcerative colitis with new technologies. Can J Gastroenterol 4:347, 1990.
26. Katzka I, Katz S, Morris E: Management of toxic megacolon: The significance of early recognition in medical management. J Clin Gastroenterol 1:307, 1979.
27. Greenstein AJ, Sachar DB, Gibas A, et al: Outcome of toxic dilatation in ulcerative and Crohn's colitis. J Clin Gastroenterol 7:137, 1985.
28. Hanauer SB, Kirsner JB: Medical therapies in ulcerative colitis. In: Kirsner JB, Shorter RG (eds): Inflammatory Bowel Disease. 3rd ed. Philadelphia, Lea & Febiger, p 431, 1988.
29. Danovitch ST: Fulminant colitis and toxic megacolon. Gastroenterol Clin North Am 18:73, 1989.
30. Soyer MT, Aldrete JS: Surgical treatment of toxic megacolon and proposal for a program of therapy. Am J Surg 140:421, 1980.
31. Vickers CR, Gallagher ND, Glenn DC, et al: A reappraisal of the management of severe colitis in its fulminant phase. J Gastroenterol Hepatol 2:217, 1987.
32. Grant CS, Dozois RR: Toxic megacolon: Ultimate fate of patients after successful medical management. Am J Surg 147:106, 1984.
33. Smith LE: Surgery therapy in ulcerative colitis. Gastroenterol Clin North Am 18:99, 1989.
34. Glotzer DJ: The surgical management of idiopathic inflammatory bowel disease. In: Kirsner JB, Shorter RG (eds): Inflammatory Bowel Disease. 3rd ed. Philadelphia, Lea & Febiger, p 585, 1988.
35. Block GE, Schraut WH: Complications of the surgical treatment of ulcerative colitis and Crohn's disease. In: Kirsner JB, Shorter RG (eds): Inflammatory Bowel Disease. 3rd ed. Philadelphia, Lea & Febiger, p 685, 1988.
36. Gelernt IM, Gorfine SR: Management of postsurgical problems. In: Gitnick G (ed): Inflammatory Bowel Disease: Diagnosis and Treatment. New York, Igaku-Shoin Medical Publishers, p 451, 1991.
37. Seidman EG: Nutritional management of inflammatory bowel disease. Gastroenterol Clin North Am 18:129, 1989.
38. O'Morain C, Segal AW, Levi AJ: Elemental diet as primary treatment of acute Crohn's disease: A controlled trial. Br Med J 288:1859, 1984.
39. Rhodes J, Compston JE, Clements DG: Diet, nutrition, and oral and parenteral therapy. In: Gitnick G (ed): Inflammatory Bowel Disease: Diagnosis and Treatment. New York, Igaku-Shoin Medical Publishers, p 241, 1991.
40. Darvasi RS: Pregnancy. In: Gitnick G (ed): Inflammatory Bowel Disease: Diagnosis and Treatment. New York, Igaku-Shoin Medical Publishers, p 517, 1991.
41. Hanan IM, Kirsner JB: Inflammatory bowel disease in the pregnant woman. Clin Perinatol 12:669, 1985.
42. Nielsen OH, Andreasson B, Bondesen S, et al: Pregnancy in ulcerative colitis. Scand J Gastroenterol 18:735, 1983.
43. Ursing B: Metronidazole in Crohn's disease. In: Gitnick G (ed): Inflammatory Bowel Disease: Diagnosis and Treatment. New York, Igaku-Shoin Medical Publishers, p 347, 1991.

CHAPTER 129

The Acute Abdomen

Alexander J. Walt
Scott Dulchavsky

The diagnosis of acute abdomen has challenged physicians and surgeons alike ever since laparotomy became a reasonably safe procedure about the turn of this century after general anesthesia and antisepsis had been well established. Although definitions of the acute abdomen vary, the term fundamentally refers to the patient with abdominal pain of a type and degree that makes it essential to exclude the need for surgical intervention. The penalty for delayed or inaccurate diagnosis may be avoidable death, either because of neglect when surgical intervention is called for or because of injudicious surgical exploration when the lesion should be treated by nonsurgical means. In practice, 40% or fewer of patients with an acute abdomen have lesions that mandate an operation.[1] Diagnosis can be extremely difficult, but accuracy may be greatly enhanced by the use of modern technology. Nevertheless, it cannot be too strongly stressed that technology has not in any way supplanted the essential need for detailed clinical history and meticulous physical examination. Furthermore, examination may need to be repeated hourly or more often during an extended period of observation to detect slight changes in clinical course.

Although the core definition of the acute abdomen remains unchanged, a much expanded spectrum of causes continues to evolve. In parallel, clinical presentations have increased in variety, in complexity, and often in urgency. Modern illnesses and techniques such as those associated with cardiopulmonary bypass, chemotherapy, administration of powerful antibiotics, and acquired immunodeficiency syndrome (AIDS) have brought new challenges, and the dividing line between critical medical and surgical options is often unclear. At one time, clinical precision was often little more than an intellectual exercise until lifesaving therapies for these previously hopeless conditions made prompt and accurate diagnosis vital. For example, when the techniques of vascular surgery matured and could cure patients, the need to diagnose the leaking aortic aneurysm or mesenteric occlusion became urgent if the then existing 100% mortality rate was to be reduced. Similarly, the deceptive abdominal pain encountered in patients who are immunosuppressed by chemotherapeutic drugs or who have antibiotic- or immunosuppressant-related intestinal lesions became important as therapy grew in sophistication and efficacy. In more recent years, the abdominal complications associated with AIDS, the transplantation of organs, and the use of illicit drugs have seriously challenged clinical judgment and decisions.

Accurate diagnosis is central to rational therapy. Unnecessary operations, apart from being painful and expensive, may lead in the depleted patient to avoidable death. Technologic advances such as ultrasonography, computed tomography (CT), peritoneal cytology, upper and lower intestinal tract endoscopy, isotopic imaging, arteriography, and laparoscopy exercise an increasingly striking impact on the decision-making process.[2-9] In addition, the use of computer-assisted systems is being explored and sometimes advocated.[10]

This chapter defines the acute abdomen in modern terms with particular reference to newer syndromes and draws

TABLE 129–1

DIAGNOSIS IN HOSPITAL ADMISSIONS FOR ABDOMINAL PAIN*

Diagnosis	Number of Admissions (%)		
	Total	Age ≥ 60 y	Age < 60 y
Nonspecific abdominal pain	415 (34.9)	106 (22.5)	309 (43.0)
Acute appendicitis	200 (16.8)	20 (4.2)	180 (25.0)
Intestinal obstruction	176 (14.8)	132 (28.0)	44 (6.1)
Urologic disorders	70 (5.9)	15 (3.2)	55 (7.6)
Cholelithiasis	61 (5.1)	42 (8.9)	19 (2.6)
Colonic diverticular disease	46 (3.9)	40 (8.5)	6 (0.8)
Abdominal trauma	37 (3.1)	2 (0.4)	35 (4.9)
Abdominal malignancy	36 (3.0)	26 (5.5)	10 (1.4)
Perforated peptic ulcer	30 (2.5)	20 (4.2)	10 (1.4)
Pancreatitis	29 (2.4)	18 (3.8)	11 (1.5)
Exacerbated peptic ulcer	17 (1.4)	9 (1.9)	8 (1.1)
Ruptured aortic aneurysm	15 (1.3)	14 (3.0)	1 (0.1)
Gynecologic disorders	13 (1.1)	1 (0.2)	12 (1.7)
Inflammatory bowel disease	10 (0.8)	5 (1.1)	5 (0.7)
Medial conditions (e.g., pneumonia, pulmonary embolism, myocardial infarction)	10 (0.8)	5 (1.1)	5 (0.7)
Mesenteric vascular occlusion	7 (0.6)	7 (1.5)	0
Gastroenteritis	4 (0.3)	0	4 (0.6)
Miscellaneous	14 (1.2)	9 (1.9)	5 (0.7)
TOTAL	1190 (100)	471 (100)	719 (100)

*Age-separated summary of causes of acute abdominal pain of 1190 hospitalizations in a British district hospital.
From Irving TT: Abdominal pain: A surgical audit of 1190 emergency admissions. Br J Surg 76:1121, 1989. By permission of the publishers, Butterworth-Heinemann Ltd.

attention to the potential of newer technology. The problems of trauma are not explored, as the cause of the abdominal pain associated with trauma is almost always obvious. In hospitals with a large geriatric population, obtunded patients, severely ill patients in critical care units, patients receiving intensive chemotherapy, and transplant recipients, the clinical complexities of the acute abdomen are magnified. Space precludes detailed discussion of the clinical features and treatment of individual lesions and the list of causes considered is by no means exhaustive; only the salient features or deceptive aspects are delineated.

OVERVIEW

The long-recognized common causes of the acute abdomen such as appendicitis, gallbladder disease, obstruction and perforation of the gastrointestinal tract, pelvic inflammations, and gynecologic emergencies still dominate any list of etiologic incidence.[3]

The distribution of the acute abdomen in Western society is reflected in a study by Irvin of consecutive admissions to a British district hospital (equivalent to a U.S. community hospital) during a 4-year period[1] (Table 129–1). A number of observations can be made on this excellent survey. (1) Increasing regionalization of high-intensity illness is occurring, and data collected from district or community hospitals do not embrace the tremendously complicated presentations seen in hospitals that are referral centers for immunocompromised, transplant recipient, or addicted patients or in major cardiologic and oncologic centers. Thus, the pattern of the acute abdomen varies considerably in different types of hospitals, and the problems of the acute abdomen in hospitals specializing in the critically ill patient have been given only sporadic attention. (2) The high incidence of nonspecific abdominal pain (NSAP) as the most common cause of hospital admission in many geographic areas is still often overlooked. Today, in cases of doubt, the rush to surgery has been slowed and can often be avoided by extended clinical observation with the patient under anti-

biotic cover and by information derived from adjunctive technology. (3) The marked discrepancies in the frequency of individual lesions in different age groups encourages a selective clinical approach to children (not reviewed here), geriatric patients, and women in their childbearing years. (4) The causes of intestinal obstruction have changed during the past decades, as hernias are less often neglected and the occurrence of abdominal carcinoma and carcinomatosis has increased as longevity is extended.

DIAGNOSIS
Clinical History Taking

Technologic improvements have not supplanted the essential need for meticulous history. It remains essential to record the duration of pain; its site, specific nature, mode of onset, and pattern of persistence or fluctuation; and the occurrence of similar episodes in the past. Details of nausea, vomiting, distention, and bowel movements are vital. A complete history of drug ingestion, legal and illegal, must be elicited. Family history and the presence of associated diseases are important, and the elucidation of any concomitant symptom that may relate to the cardiopulmonary, vascular, urologic, cerebral, or gynecologic systems is essential. The relevance of these historical details is referred to in discussion of individual disease entities.

Physical Examination

Cope, whose classic Early Diagnosis of the Acute Abdomen was first published in 1921 and is now in its 18th edition,[11] taught that the optimal sequence in evaluating the acute abdomen was first to exclude any hernias (directing particular attention in the obese woman to a Richter hernia in the femoral canal); then to eliminate any extra-abdominal cause (e.g., myocardial infarction, pulmonary embolism, pneumonia, and diabetes); and lastly, to concentrate on thorough palpation and auscultation of the abdomen itself. This examination of the abdomen can be divided into four main areas: (1) the central abdomen, including the liver, the gallbladder, the intestines, and the appendix; (2) the pelvic organs (rectal and vaginal examinations are integral); (3) the retroperitoneal organs, such as the aorta, the pancreas, the kidneys, and the spine; and (4) the skin and the body wall (e.g., herpes zoster, purpura, hematomas, and ecchymoses).

Caveats

We have not aimed to provide an exhaustive list of potential causes of abdominal pain that may mimic the acute abdomen and in which surgery is both contraindicated and potentially lethal. It is, however, always vital to keep in mind the following conditions, especially when the clinical picture does not readily fit pattern recognition: (1) myocardial infarction; (2) pneumonia; (3) aortic dissection; (4) renal calculus or pyelonephritis; (5) hemolytic crisis, as may be seen in sickle cell crisis, Hodgkin's disease (pseudoacute abdomen), narcotic withdrawal, and Henoch's syndrome; and (6) acute intermittent porphyria (especially in endemic areas) and diabetes (especially in children).

Laboratory Investigations

Basic blood studies should include determination of hemoglobin, hematocrit, differential and total leukocyte counts, and serum electrolyte levels and multiphasic tests, including serum amylase and liver function tests. Coagulation studies, peripheral blood smear, and special tests for amebic or viral disease or human immunodeficiency virus antibodies (with the patient's consent) may be necessary.

Urine and stool tests may be performed.

ETIOLOGY

Nonspecific Abdominal Pain and Acute Appendicitis

The classic picture of cramping periumbilical pain accompanied by anorexia, nausea, vomiting, and fever, with initial cramping and subsequent rebound tenderness, guarding, and finally sharp persisting pain in the right lower quadrant remains the hallmark of acute appendicitis. One encounters many variations on this symptom complex. Unfortunately, a general attenuation of all these clinical features characterizes both the appendicitis that is difficult to diagnose and NSAP. NSAP is more common in children than in adults, which accounts for the greater number of nonindicated or unnecessary appendectomies performed in children (up to 40% in some series). A second group at disproportionate risk of ill-advised appendectomy are women between the ages of 18 and 35 years in whom gynecologic disorders are misdiagnosed as appendicitis, with a consequent unnecessary appendectomy rate of up to 30%.[6]

Until recent times, an unnecessary appendectomy rate of about 15 to 20% was regarded as acceptable to audit committees. The general thesis has been that when any doubt exists, appendectomy is preferable to observation because of the morbidity and even mortality of perforated appendicitis. Better understanding of the spectrum of intra-abdominal pathologic changes and their natural history, together with a more demanding surgical audit, have led to serious challenge of this traditional figure. Unquestionably, acute appendicitis can still be a difficult clinical diagnosis. Before the advent of antibiotics, intravenous fluids, electrolyte replacement, and support systems, delayed diagnosis too often led to death. Today, with these adjuncts available, close and more extended observation in cases of doubt is accepted, provided that intervention takes place before perforation. During this time of indecision, many technical aids are now available to increase the accuracy of diagnosis. These include barium enema study, ultrasonography, laparoscopy, diagnostic peritoneal aspiration, computer-aided diagnosis, and imaging with radioactive isotopes.[6-10]

In practice, barium enema examination, ultrasonography, and laparoscopy have been of most value in helping to refine the accuracy of diagnosis. Their sensitivity, specificity, and costs vary, whereas their applicability obviously depends on their ready availability and on the skill of the operator. Barium enema studies, which exclude appendicitis when they unequivocally fill the appendix, have the disadvantage of being technically unsatisfactory in about 15% of patients. For the remaining 85%, however, they provide a sensitivity of about 95% and a specificity of about 85%. Ultrasonography has slightly lower sensitivity and specificity than a barium enema study but has the advantage of delineating the adjacent pelvic organs, which is of great assistance in women, especially in those of childbearing age. Few surgeons are trained in ultrasonography as yet, and reports should be accepted only from skilled ultrasonographers with the recognition that even they may misinterpret shadows, which may lead to inappropriate clinical decisions.

The laparoscope is currently the instrument of revolution in abdominal surgery, and the definition of its future role in the acute abdomen is still unfolding. Laparoscopy may be invaluable to exclude appendicitis when the entire appendix is visualized as being normal. In addition, laparoscopy can identify nonappendiceal lesions such as gynecologic abnormalities, Crohn's disease, perforated ulcers, and cholecystitis. Unfortunately, the appendix cannot be fully visualized in about 40% of laparoscopies, and the procedure has the disadvantage of being invasive while adding expense and diagnostic time. Furthermore, performance of laparoscopy requires experience and has the potential to cause complications, although these are usually minor. Nevertheless, the potential benefit of avoiding unnecessary appendectomy often overrides these negative factors, and more recently, the ability to remove the appendix laparoscopically in selected patients is a bonus. At this time, the extent to which the acute appendix may be safely removed laparoscopically is being assessed.

Aspiration cytology of the peritoneal cavity through a catheter inserted via a 12- or 14-gauge needle with examination of the aspirate and observation of the number and percentage of neutrophils in the specimen has been enthusiastically proposed as being helpful in determining the need for surgery in uncertain cases.[9] A neutrophil percentage of greater than 50% indicates the presence of an inflammatory process but, unfortunately, does not indicate its source nor whether the offending lesion may better be treated nonsurgically, as in the case of acute salpingitis. The main value of aspiration cytology in selected cases is the identification of peritonitis. Aspiration cytology is of most value in focusing observation, promoting frequent re-examination, and recording accurate data, but its ultimate value is inversely proportional to the experience of the attending physician. As yet, aspiration cytology has not gained widespread acceptance among trained clinicians.

Small-Intestinal Obstruction

Obstruction of the small intestine is most often due to adhesions now that hernias and carcinoma of the colon are less often neglected than in the past. Intestinal obstruction is the most common single cause of the acute abdomen in patients older than the age of 60 years but may occur at any age. Small-bowel obstruction usually, but not necessarily, follows a previous laparotomy. The clinical picture has not changed through the years and reflects the level and the acuteness of the obstruction. Colicky pain dominates, although it may be minimal in high small-bowel obstructions, the hallmarks of which are intense vomiting and dehydration. In contrast, obstructions lower in the intestine are marked by increasing distention, abdominal tenderness, and increased bowel sounds.

Intestinal obstruction is not an emergency, except in cases of impending or established strangulation, and may be managed conservatively, especially in patients in the immediate postoperative period and in those with previous episodes of adhesive obstruction or known carcinomatosis. However, in view of the markedly increased mortality rate after strangulation occurs, early recognition of its threat or its presence is vital. Fever, tachycardia, leukocytosis, and localized pain are early signs of strangulated obstruction, with pallor and shock the ultimate hallmarks of nonviable bowel. Unfortunately, many of these clinical signs are deceptively absent in about 10% of patients with proven strangulation.

Erect and supine abdominal radiographs remain the cornerstone of diagnosis in suspected intestinal obstruction. The distribution of intestinal distention and fluid levels, the presence of a closed loop of distended bowel, and visualization of a foreign body (e.g., gallstone) are significant.

Gynecologic Causes

Next to NSAP, gynecologic lesions cause the most widespread clinical confusion. Pain of gynecologic origin accounts for up to 15% of the admissions to surgical units of patients with acute abdominal pain. This pain may originate from the ovaries, the fallopian tubes, the uterus, or pelvic infection. In the past, many young women have undergone unnecessary laparotomies when the fundamental condition did not warrant surgical treatment; others have had unnecessary removal of some or all pelvic reproductive organs. Consequently, inappropriate diagnosis or treatment may ultimately be responsible for preventing future reproduction.

The most frequently encountered difficulty is the distinction between acute appendicitis and acute salpingitis. With the increase in sexually derived disease (mostly caused by *Neisseria, Chlamydia, Trachomatis,* or *Bacteroides fragilis*) and the use of intrauterine devices, acute pelvic infection remains a common cause of acute abdominal pain. In most cases, the bilaterality of the lower abdominal pain, the guarding on palpation, the pyrexia (temperature in excess of 101°F), and pain on movement of the fornix make a diagnosis reasonably straightforward. Specimens for aerobic and anaerobic cultures should be taken from the vagina, the cervix, and the urethra, and Gram's stain smears made for rapid examination. If the distinction from acute appendicitis is difficult or if uncertainty exists as to whether a palpable mass is due to a tubo-ovarian abscess or pyosalpinx, laparoscopy may be invaluable. Acute salpingitis is confirmed by a swollen and inflamed tube in which frank pus is often visualized. Alternatively, some other gynecologic lesion may be revealed, and the laparoscopic information is likely to direct appropriate treatment.

Pain Related to Ovarian Function

Acute abdominal pain may be associated with ovulation in which transient pain (mittelschmerz) occurs but soon recedes. In a few patients, the pain persists when bleeding into the peritoneal cavity occurs after hemorrhage from the follicular wall. In these circumstances, symptoms may suggest a ruptured ectopic pregnancy. Occasionally, pain associated with menstruation attributable to concomitant endometriosis or retrograde menstruation may be so severe as to produce an acute abdomen, but the temporal relationship to the menses together with physical examination should resolve this diagnostic problem. In cases of doubt, ultrasonography may be invaluable.[2]

Ectopic Pregnancy

The possibility of ectopic pregnancy should be considered in any woman of childbearing age who has lower abdominal pain and amenorrhea or who has abnormal vaginal bleeding, even when this is minimal. Subjective symptoms of pregnancy are present in only 50% of these patients. Suspicion is compounded if the patient has had a previous ectopic pregnancy, salpingitis, or tubal surgery or if she uses an intrauterine device.

A ruptured ectopic pregnancy occurs as an obvious emergency with acute diffuse peritoneal pain and signs of blood loss mandating emergency laparotomy. In contrast, a leaking ectopic pregnancy may have subtle symptoms. In the past, palpation of an adnexal mass by vaginal examination (present in only about 40% of ectopic pregnancies was the only objective evidence obtainable. Today, the diagnosis, if considered, is easily confirmed by the use of (1) assay of the beta-subunit of human chorionic gonadotropin, which identifies the presence, although not the site, of any pregnancy; (2) transvaginal or abdominal ultrasonography, which provides an accurate outline of pelvic structures; or (3) laparoscopy, which provides direct visualization of the tubes and may permit definitive treatment by linear salpingostomy.

A special caveat concerns the widespread use of birth control pills and the development of hepatic adenomas, which may rupture and hemorrhage acutely, producing a clinical picture of severe abdominal pain and blood loss into the peritoneal cavity indistinguishable from that of a ruptured ectopic pregnancy. A similar clinical picture is presented by ruptured splenic and hepatic aneurysms. Consequently, the presence of free blood in the peritoneal cavity at laparotomy in the absence of an ectopic pregnancy must always prompt an immediate search for these lesions in the upper abdomen. A second incision is often necessary.

Torsion of Fallopian Tubes

Acute abdominal pain may follow torsion of a tube, with or without torsion of the ovary, and is most often seen in children and adolescents who suddenly double up with pain, vomit, and have tenderness and marked guarding of the lower abdomen, most often unilateral. The intensity of the pain may be disproportionate to the paucity of physical findings. A mass may or may not be palpable but its presence is easily confirmed by ultrasonography. This clinical picture closely resembles that of torsion of an ovarian cyst. Treatment of both these lesions is surgical, as rapid correction of the torsion may permit salvage of the tube and/or the ovary before ischemic necrosis occurs.

Rupture of a cyst, with or without associated endometriosis, may result in sudden generalized lower peritoneal irritation and acute pain. Ultrasonography may not be helpful in these circumstances, as the cyst has decompressed on rupture. Operation is necessary, and future treatment depends on the nature of the original lesion, its benignity, and the degree of importance of trying to preserve future fertility.

Gallbladder Disease

Gallbladder disease is a frequent cause of the acute abdomen, especially in elderly patients.[12] Classically, patients with acute calculous cholecystitis have a history of previous dyspepsia or biliary colic. The acute clinical syndrome varies, but guarding and tenderness in the right upper quadrant associated with nausea and vomiting dominate the picture. A history of previous flatulence and fatty food intolerance, with or without abnormal ultrasonography or cholecystography, may be elicited. Jaundice (serum bilirubin level usually <4 mg/dL), positive Murphy's sign, and fever may or may not be present. Ultrasonography, the diagnostic investigation of choice, demonstrates the presence of stones and possibly thickening of the gallbladder wall in virtually all cases of acute calculous cholecystitis. Nevertheless, acute attacks caused by small stones may occur initially in the absence of objective radiologic evidence. A classic clinical picture of biliary colic should not be lightly set aside just because the radiologic findings are not confirmatory.

Less well recognized is the ominous modern problem of acalculous cholecystitis. Acalculous cholecystitis is the new deceiver of the 1990s. Although in the past most attacks of right upper quadrant pain were due to acute calculous cholecystitis or to biliary colic, the incidence of acalculous cholecystitis has risen markedly during the past decade. This entity is increasingly seen in critically ill patients in critical care units. Many with this lesion are patients with sepsis, burns, recent large vascular operations, or multiple organ system failure; a large percentage are receiving intravenous hyperalimentation.[13] Multiple etiologic mechanisms have been postulated (e.g., dehydration, fasting, ileus, and diminished oxygen delivery), but the central clinical fact is the importance of early diagnosis. The development of acalculous cholecystitis may be overshadowed by the severity of the illness that brought the patient to the critical care unit initially. The pain in the right upper quadrant may be deceptively mild, but the degree of septic illness that develops is often disproportionately greater than the physical findings.

The most confusing cases, however, are patients in the process of recovering from abdominal sepsis who deteriorate again, misleadingly suggesting a flare-up of the original infection. This problem is compounded if the patient is obtunded or undergoing mechanical respiration when it may be difficult to elicit any clear symptoms or signs. In such cases, the possibility of acute acalculous cholecystitis must always be considered. Ultrasonography, which has a sensitivity of 80% and a specificity of 98%, showing a thickened gallbladder wall (>3.5 mm) and pericholecystic fluid is invaluable in helping to confirm the diagnosis and a ^{99m}Tc-labeled acetanilid or similar isotopic scan (with cholecystokinin stimulation if necessary) is diagnostic in virtually all cases of doubt. Cholecystectomy with a minimum of delay may be lifesaving, as gangrene and perforation advance rapidly in many of these patients.

Perforated Peptic Ulcer

With the advent of histamine H_2 receptor blockers, perforated peptic ulcer is a less common cause of the acute abdomen than in the past but continues to carry a high mortality rate (up to 30%), largely because it occurs predominantly in older patients who often have concomitant cardiac, pulmonary, and renal disease. The differential diagnosis of perforated peptic ulcer includes myocardial infarction, acute pancreatitis, biliary or renal colic, and rarely, dissecting aortic aneurysm. Perforation may occur without any previous history of dyspepsia but the patient is often taking nonsteroidal anti-inflammatory drugs. In older patients, delay in calling a physician is not infrequent, so that sepsis may already be established in this group when the patient is first examined.[12]

The clinical picture is usually classic (acute epigastric pain, which may radiate along the abdominal gutter to the right hypogastrium, and abdominal wall rigidity), but some patients have partially sealed perforations, in which case distention and discomfort rather than rigidity and pain may predominate. Perforated gastric ulcers are more likely to be insidious in onset than duodenal perforations. The diagnosis is made by radiographs, which show air under the diaphragm in 70% of perforated duodenal ulcers and in most perforated gastric ulcers. In cases of doubt, meglumine diatrizoate (Gastrografin) may be instilled into the stomach through a nasogastric tube for radiographic confirmation of the perforation.

Most surgeons favor laparotomy and operative closure of the perforation with an omental patch, or resection and anastomosis. There have been reports of diagnosis and successful closure through the laparoscope. For older patients, especially those with cardiac abnormalities or in whom the perforation appears clinically sealed, a rekindled enthusiasm is discernible for a nonoperative approach of systemic support, administration of antibiotics and intravenous parenteral nutrition, and nasogastric decompression through a large nasogastric tube. A decision to treat nonsurgically must be made selectively and the clinical progress meticulously monitored.

Acute Pancreatitis

The diagnosis of acute pancreatitis must always be entertained in any alcoholic patient or in a patient with gallstones who suddenly has acute upper abdominal pain, usually in conjunction with nausea and vomiting. The differential diagnosis from a perforated peptic ulcer may be difficult to make early, but the degree of abdominal rigidity tends to be appreciably less in acute pancreatitis. In addition, pain in the back is a more pronounced feature of acute pancreatitis and the abdominal pain is poorly localized. The possibility of acute pancreatitis as the cause of acute abdominal pain must also be entertained in postoperative patients with upper abdominal pain, especially those who have undergone cardiopulmonary bypass during which there may have been episodes of hypotension or in patients who have undergone organ transplantation with administration of large amounts of immunosuppressant drugs.

The diagnosis of acute pancreatitis is partly one of exclusion by noting the absence of free air on abdominal radiographs or the presence of a sentinel loop of bowel. Ultrasonography and CT may be of considerable assistance in demonstrating pancreatic edema, peripancreatic fluid, and subsequently pancreatic necrosis, if hemorrhage and ischemia occur. In the presence of ileus or obesity, CT is unquestionably more accurate. The presence of elevated serum amylase and, later, serum lipase levels is helpful. Nevertheless, hyperamylasemia itself is not pathognomonic of acute pancreatitis and may be found in patients with ruptured ectopic pregnancy, acute hepatitis and cholecystitis, acute erosive gastritis, trauma, mesenteric infarction, perforated peptic ulcer, strangulated obstruction, and many other conditions.

Perforation of a pseudocyst in the peritoneal cavity occurs in about 2 to 3% of patients. The clinical picture is that of acute generalized abdominal pain followed by hypotension owing to a third-space effect as the peritoneum reacts by a pouring of fluid into the peritoneal cavity. These patients rapidly become distended, and emergency drainage of the peritoneal cavity may be lifesaving.

Colonic Perforation

Apart from trauma, there are many causes of acute colonic perforation such as diverticular disease, carcinoma, rupture of ischemic bowel proximal to an obstruction (mostly in the cecum), or perforation of inflamed and distended bowel as in ulcerative colitis. Colonic perforation, whatever the cause, is a potential catastrophe. The patient has acute abdominal pain, guarding and rigidity, fever, leukocytosis, and rapid distention and soon becomes septic. The clinical picture reflects the degree of peritoneal contamination and consequently may be subacute and localized or acute and generalized. In most circumstances, a predisposing cause is easily elicited by the history, but in the case of colonic diverticula, perforation may be sudden and unanticipated, resembling the initial symptoms of a perforated peptic ulcer. In geriatric patients, the symptoms and signs of a perforated sigmoid perforation may develop slowly.

The diagnosis is usually easily made by demonstration of free air in the peritoneal cavity on radiography, but the specific site may be less obvious. Brief comments on selected clinical entities follow.

Acute diverticulitis most often occurs in the sigmoid colon but is occasionally found in the cecum. Most patients never have an acute abdomen unless an acute peridiverticulitis from a localized perforation results in widespread sepsis or a large perforation produces massive fecal contamination. Patients with symptomatic diverticular disease are usually older than 60 years of age and, although most give a previous history of gastrointestinal difficulties, a few have perforation without any previous warning.

Inflammatory bowel disease, including chronic ulcerative colitis, Crohn's disease (less frequent), pseudomembranous colitis, and the colitis of *Clostridium difficile*, may be accompanied by toxic colitis and megacolon, with or without perforation. The disease is often brief, and the clinical picture is characterized by fever, leukocytosis, abdominal pain, and diarrhea. In most cases, the underlying condition has been previously diagnosed and treated or the patient is known to have recently had broad-spectrum antibiotics.

Iatrogenic perforation of the prepared bowel in the course of colonoscopy by a rent through excessive pressure or by overenthusiastic biopsy of the colonic wall is increasingly encountered. Pain in these circumstances may be insidious, but any pain after colonoscopy should be suggestive of perforation. In highly selected cases, observation under intensive antibiotic coverage without surgery may be successful, but such an approach must be followed with great caution. Laparoscopic repair of iatrogenic colon perforation has been reported and may be efficacious in selected cases.

Colonic Pseudo-obstruction

An uncommon entity, which may be difficult to differentiate from large-bowel obstruction requiring operation, is pseudo-obstruction. Clinical presentation is seldom acute, but by the time the patient is seen, the abdomen may be painful, grossly distended, and tender. Although the syndrome was popularized by Ogilvie[13a] in 1948, who described it in two patients with retroperitoneal malignancy, pseudo-obstruction is most often encountered in elderly patients who are dehydrated and frequently verging on renal or cardiac failure. Increased bowel sounds may be heard, but although the overall picture closely resembles that of classic large-bowel obstruction, a few discrepancies may be noted, such as the presence of gas in the rectum suggesting an incomplete obstruction. A barium enema examination shows a patent colon, and decompression by either colonoscope or indwelling rectal tube is effective in producing temporary relief.

Fulminating Pseudomembranous Colitis

Fulminating pseudomembranous colitis is an increasingly common nosocomial infection, which can be deceptive. Pa-

tients with fulminating pseudomembranous colitis may have acute abdominal pain, distention, ileus, and a leukocytosis, which in some may have leukemoid characteristics. The lesion originates on medical and surgical wards in equal numbers and is frequently encountered in immunosuppressed patients, especially those older than the age of 60 years. Fulminating pseudomembranous colitis is basically a pancolonic disease, although the initial impression at laparotomy may be that of a segmental lesion. CT reveals a greatly thickened colonic wall and free peritoneal fluid. Sigmoidoscopy and colonoscopy are invaluable in making the definitive diagnosis. Tests for *C. difficile* should be done, although fulminating pseudomembranous colitis can occur in the absence of clostridia. Treatment is medical, including oral vancomycin or intravenous metronidazole administration. If the patient's condition deteriorates, surgery becomes unavoidable and subtotal colectomy may be necessary.[14] Every effort should be made, however, to make the diagnosis by means other than laparotomy.

Vascular Causes

Mesenteric Ischemia

Acute mesenteric ischemia threatening infarction of large segments of the small and/or large bowel is increasingly encountered as the population ages and as more extensive surgical procedures such as cardiopulmonary bypass and aortic resection are performed.[15–18] The main causes in approximate descending order of frequency are extensive nonocclusive ischemia associated most often with congestive cardiac failure, digitalis administration, and hypoperfusion attributable to low flow or vasoconstriction; embolism or thrombosis of the superior mesenteric artery; thrombosis of the superior mesenteric vein; and aortic dissection and arteritis, as in systemic lupus erythematosus.

History is of vital importance in this group of patients, and intervention is urgent as the margin of reserve is small. Because the mortality rate approaches 100%, any hope of salvage depends on rapid and appropriate diagnosis.

Mesenteric ischemia should be immediately suspected in the presence of a recent myocardial infarction, atrial fibrillation, hypovolemia or dehydration, recent cardiopulmonary bypass or resection of an aneurysm, or any hypercoagulation state such as polycythemia vera. Whenever such a patient has acute abdominal pain, the possibility of mesenteric ischemia must be entertained, even as one is excluding the more common entities such as cholecystitis, pancreatitis, and diverticulitis.[19] Suspicion should always be heightened when the degree of pain significantly exceeds the demonstrable abdominal physical signs such as distention and rebound, which are often absent in the early stages. Furthermore, with the rapid shift of blood volume that occurs, signs of impending shock soon appear, often accompanied by bloody diarrhea. Radiographs are likely to show an airless intestinal pattern and thumbprinting. In addition, ultrasonography and CT may be helpful, demonstrating thickening of the bowel wall with intramural and portal vein gas as a later sign. Ultimately, aortography is the study most likely to provide a definitive diagnosis and guide to optimal therapy, although false-negative results occur in up to 40%. Superior mesenteric arterial emboli are usually distinguishable from thrombosis, especially on selective arteriographic studies.

The need for surgical intervention is generally clarified by the aortogram, but in cases of doubt, laparotomy is advisable. At operation, determination of bowel viability and the ultimate extent of resection necessary may be helped by the use of fluorescein dye or Doppler techniques. Small-bowel ischemia after aortic surgery is rare and is related to prolonged suprarenal clamp time, embolus, retractor trauma, or visceral steal syndrome.

Intestinal ischemia after cardiopulmonary bypass has a 94% mortality owing partly to delay in diagnosis. Hypoperfusion of the viscera during bypass and a prolonged pump time correlate with intestinal ischemia. Patients with operations necessitating an open cardiac procedure also have an increased risk of ischemia attributable to embolization.

Clinically significant intestinal ischemia occurs in 1 to 2% of patients after abdominal aortic aneurysm surgery. The ischemia is almost exclusively confined to the distal colon supplied by the inferior mesenteric artery. The incidence of postoperative intestinal ischemia is much higher after emergency operations and after repeated aortic procedures. Patients requiring operation for aneurysmal or atherosclerotic disease have an equal frequency of intestinal ischemia. Prior abdominal or colonic surgery appears to increase the risk of intestinal ischemia, as collateral circulation to the distal colon may be interrupted. Bloody diarrhea, leukocytosis, thrombocytopenia, and acidosis are noted in the majority of patients with ischemic colitis after aortic surgery.[4, 15, 17] Sepsis and clinical signs of peritonitis suggest full-thickness injury. The diagnosis is confirmed by sigmoidoscopy; a friable mucosa suggests partial-thickness injury, whereas grayish black firm tissue is present in full-thickness injury. The management of postoperative colonic ischemia is based on clinical presentation and extent of injury. Medical management is successful in patients with partial-thickness injury in the absence of clinical signs of sepsis. Full-thickness injury or peritoneal signs demand colon resection with a Hartmann procedure.

Abdominal Aortic Aneurysms

Abdominal aortic aneurysms are common and, when larger than 5 cm in diameter, become a distinct threat to life by their propensity to rupture. Whereas the mortality rate for elective aortic aneurysmectomy is 2 to 5%, the figure exceeds 40% for ruptured aneurysms in most institutions. Most leaks or ruptures of the abdominal aortic aneurysm occur in older patients, but the method of presentation varies widely. At its most dramatic, the abdominal aortic aneurysm that has ruptured produces agonizing pain in the flank and is associated with classic signs of shock. The possibility of a leaking aneurysm must always be entertained when any older patient has abdominal pain but particularly when there is no evidence of sepsis or a previous gastrointestinal disturbance. Careful palpation of the abdomen usually reveals a tender pulsatile mass, provided the blood pressure is not too low. Flank ecchymoses may be present. Most patients have palpable peripheral pulses.

Some patients may exhibit a more deceptive picture, especially when the aneurysm is leaking slowly and is contained. In these circumstances, pain may be maximal in the back or present in the sciatic, inguinal, or testicular regions depending on the distribution of the compression neuropathy.

The dominating clinical factor of importance is recognition of the possibility of the presence of a leaking aneurysm. Ultrasonography rapidly confirms the diagnosis, but operation should not be delayed for this confirmatory test in the unstable patient.

Time is of the essence and the patient must be stabilized by the administration of appropriate blood, fluid, and electrolytes and then taken to the operating room. Resuscitation is continued on the operating room table with attempts made to restore the blood pressure to about 100 mm Hg systolic. With all preparations made, the abdomen is opened and the aorta is controlled immediately so that as little blood as possible is lost after the tamponading effect of the abdominal wall is removed.

Other Ruptured Abdominal Aneuryms

Rupture of splenic artery, hepatic artery, and mesenteric arteries is uncommon and is seldom diagnosed preoperatively. The splenic artery is the site of rupture in more than 50% of these cases, which are most common in women and are most likely to rupture during pregnancy. A history of previous pain in the left upper quadrant may be present. This catastrophe is usually recognized by the clinical picture of acute intraperitoneal blood loss with guarding and rebound tenderness. The potential confusion with ruptured ectopic pregnancy was discussed earlier.

Aortic Dissection

Aortic dissection causes abdominal pain by direct aortic afferent pain fibers and secondarily by occlusion of the superior and inferior mesenteric arteries, causing intestinal ischemia. Patients with aortic dissection generally have a history of poorly controlled hypertension and abrupt onset of severe, unrelenting mid-scapular and abdominal pain. Differential blood pressures, mid-scapular bruit, and abdominal pain with a paucity of abdominal findings support the diagnosis. The diagnosis is confirmed by CT of the abdomen and arteriography. Management is by medical control of hypertension in the absence of renal or visceral ischemia.

Urologic Causes

Referred pain originating from the genitourinary tract may occasionally simulate the acute abdomen so closely as to trap the unwary physician into performing an unnecessary laparotomy. Passage of a ureteral stone and obstruction associated with this may cause sudden and excruciating pain with concomitant vomiting, distention attributable to ileus, guarding, and a low-grade fever. A clinical clue is usually provided by the concentration of pain in the flank, but occasionally, the pain may be diffuse and involve the entire abdomen with local tenderness on palpation. Radiography should rapidly dispel confusion, as 90% of calculi are opaque. Small impacted stones may not be easily appreciated, but intravenous pyelography provides a firm diagnosis. Consequently, if adequate renal function is present, intravenous pyelography should be ordered for all patients in whom it is necessary to exclude a ureteral calculus or obstruction. In patients allergic to contrast materials, ultrasonography or radionuclide renography may be helpful. The radiographs also delineate the presence of any hydronephrosis as a contributor to the abdominal pain.

Renal or perinephric (and less often, pylonephritic) abscesses may present with acute abdominal pain. These patients are usually febrile, and the clinical picture is more likely to resemble that of cholecystitis, appendicitis, or diverticulitis. Contrast-enhanced CT provides the most rapid and accurate information in such cases.

Intrascrotal lesions, notably testicular torsion in adolescents and acute epididymitis in adults, may cause sudden and severe pain radiating into the lower abdomen. The diagnosis is obvious, however, if the scrotum is examined and may be confirmed by urinalysis and more definitively by ultrasonography.

ASSOCIATED CONDITIONS
Immunocompromised Patients

Immunocompromised patients are common in hospitals that provide services for AIDS patients, patients undergoing cancer chemotherapy, and patients undergoing organ transplantation.

Acute abdominal pain is frequent in these patients and the need for urgent surgery may be difficult to determine.[20, 21] The decision is of obvious importance, as a nontherapeutic laparotomy may lead to significant morbidity or death.[22] Although these patients are subject to standard intra-abdominal lesions such as appendicitis, their ability to mount a systemic response is limited by their disease, which complicates successful diagnosis and subsequent treatment. The patients are, however, also subject to additional lesions directly related to their immune dysfunction.

The successful diagnosis of the acute abdomen in an immunosuppressed patient demands an aggressive diagnostic approach.[23] Because these patients frequently have a paucity of abdominal findings despite widespread peritonitis, minimal abdominal pain in these debilitated patients should be regarded as a potential acute abdomen. Diagnostic tests such as the indium or gallium scan, which rely on an intact immune system, are subject to a high rate of error. Results of paracentesis may be falsely negative in neutropenic patients and falsely positive in lymphoma patients owing to the altered white blood cell count. A polymicrobial bacterial aspiration constitutes definitive evidence of a surgical abdominal disorder.

Immunocompromised patients may also harbor a variety of conditions mimicking an acute abdomen, which are best managed medically. These disorders include cytomegalovirus (CMV) infection, neutropenic enterocolitis, and a graft-versus-host reaction.[24]

Finally, therapies, including chemotherapy or steroids, designed to favorably alter the original disease process may predispose the patient to abdominal complications such as perforation. An appreciation of the diverse nature of abdominal abnormalities in these difficult patients allows the rapid diagnosis and treatment necessary for a favorable outcome.

Cytomegalovirus Infection

CMV infection is the most significant viral infection in the compromised host. The infection may be primary by exposure to a carrier or occur through reactivation during immune suppression, as 60 to 90% of normal adults have been exposed or infected. The symptoms associated with CMV infection include an influenza-like prodrome or a syndrome resembling mononucleosis. One quarter of immunocompromised patients with CMV require hospitalization for fever and leukopenia. After it is established, CMV infection may cause interstitial pneumonia, cholecystitis, hepatitis, pancreatitis, or gastrointestinal ulceration. The diagnosis of CMV superinfection relies on tissue biopsy of the infected site with isolation of the virus or inclusion cells. Anti-CMV titers are not diagnostic of acute infection. Treatment consists of a reduction in immunosuppressive drugs to allow natural defense; acyclovir is minimally active against CMV but may be indicated, as 50% of patients have a dual viremia. A favorable clinical trial of 9-(1,3-dihydroxyl-2-propoxlymethyl) guanine has been reported and may reduce the disability of CMV infection in immunocompromised hosts.

Neutropenic Enterocolitis

Neutropenic enterocolitis (NEC) is the most common cause of the acute abdomen in leukemic patients and is noted in 12 to 46% of these patients in autopsy series.[22] NEC may also complicate the treatment of lymphomas, aplastic anemia, and solid tumors. The pathophysiology of NEC involves localized bacterial overgrowth with mucosal invasion in the colon and terminal ileum; more than 70% of patients have *Klebsiella, Pseudomonas,* or *Enterobacter* septicemia. The mortality rate of NEC remains 50 to 100% if treatment is not instituted promptly.

Patients with NEC frequently have dull hypogastric pain and a moderate fever. Abdominal roentgenograms are nonspecific, with decreased bowel gas, thickened loops of intestine, and occasionally pneumatosis intestinalis. Early diagnosis of NEC in the compromised patient depends on a high clinical suspicion. Patients with NEC by definition have neutropenia; the onset of the syndrome does not appear to correlate with the nadir of white blood cell count.

The majority of patients with NEC do not require operation and are best managed medically. Patients should undergo bowel rest with nasogastric decompression, judicious fluid management, and administration of antibiotics to cover enteric organisms. The role of granulocyte transfusions is unproved. Operation is undertaken for increasing tenderness when perforation is feared or when systemic symptoms progress and consists of resection of the involved segment. The operative treatment of nonperforated bowel during exploration is controversial. Alt and associates[24a] advocated resection of the involved segment with primary anastomosis or ileostomy and mucous fistula, whereas continued medical management has been used successfully by other authors. The small numbers and diverse nature of these patients make valid comparisons difficult, but it is clear that not all patients with NEC require bowel resection.

Graft-Versus-Host Reaction

The graft-versus-host reaction is an infrequent cause of the acute abdomen in leukemic patients after bone marrow transplantation.[25] Three to four weeks after transplantation, the patients are noted to have a gradual onset of diffuse abdominal pain progressing to peritoneal irritation. The abdominal pain is caused by transmural small-bowel edema resulting from increased permeability. Patients with graft-versus-host reaction exhibit a red maculopapular rash on the trunk, the palms, the soles, and the ears, which facilitates the diagnosis. Management of these difficult patients consists of increasing dosages of immunosuppressant drugs after excluding other causes of the acute abdomen.

Fungal Hepatosplenic Abscess

Patients with hepatosplenic abscess are a newly recognized variant of the immunocompromised host with fungemia. Predisposing factors include immunosuppressive chemotherapy, prednisone administration for prolonged periods, neutropenia, administration of antibiotics for longer than 3 weeks, and gastrointestinal colonization with candida. Patients typically have fever, chills, malaise, and bilateral upper quadrant pain.[24] CT may show multiple defects in the liver and the spleen; however, small miliary abscesses are frequently overlooked. Serial examinations by CT at weekly intervals may aid the diagnosis in difficult cases. The diagnosis of these hepatosplenic abscesses is confirmed by percutaneous aspiration of an abscess cavity; routine blood cultures are positive in less than 30% of patients. The treatment of hepatosplenic abscess is by a prolonged regimen of antifungal agents, often exceeding 2 g of amphotericin B. Splenic lesions generally regress in 6 to 8 weeks, but the hepatic lesions may persist for longer than 6 months. Splenectomy is reserved for refractory abscesses and deterioration in the clinical course, despite optimal therapy.

Renal Failure and Renal Transplant Patients

An acute abdomen that tests clinical judgment severely is often seen in patients after organ transplantation.[26] The pseudoacute abdomen may be associated with renal failure and consists of a functional colonic obstruction mimicking Ogilvie's syndrome. Small-bowel motility dysfunction may also be noted with electrolyte abnormalities. Decreased platelet numbers and function may lead to petechial irritation of the small bowel, causing abdominal pain.

Peptic ulcer disease occurs more frequently in the renal transplant patient and can be lethal. Hemorrhage is more frequent than perforation in these patients. A high incidence of CMV inclusions in post-transplant gastric and duodenal ulcers may be etiologically related.

Historically, colonic perforation from diverticulitis or ischemia was the most common colonic abnormality in the renal transplant patient. The mortality of colonic perforation in these compromised patients approached 60%, causing some authorities[26a] to recommend barium enema examination before transplant. Fecal impaction leading to ischemia, primarily in the right side of the colon, may also be seen in these patients owing to dehydration, administration of narcotics, and prolonged bed rest.[27] Alterations in the immunosuppression schedules and improved perioperative care have greatly reduced the colonic morbidity in renal transplant patients.

Small-bowel obstruction may occur in renal transplant patients, especially after pelvic surgery. Fever and leukocytosis associated with small-bowel strangulation are often absent in these patients. Special attention should be directed to the transplant site, as small-bowel herniation with obstruction may occur in this region.

Patients with renal insufficiency may have an elevated serum amylase level in the absence of pancreatic irritation because renal clearance of the enzyme is decreased. Administration of steroids and azathioprine and CMV infection may, however, predispose these patients to a particularly virulent pancreatitis. The diagnosis is often made by raised serum lipase levels and occasionally by CT and ultrasonography, which confirm pancreatic edema. Treatment is supportive with judicious fluid management.

Hepatitis, caused by hepatitis A, B, and non-A, non-B viral strains, is a common cause of right upper quadrant pain in the transplant patient. The concomitant immunosuppression may lead to Epstein-Barr viral hepatitis or hepatosplenic abscess.

Leukemia and Lymphoma Patients

The acute abdomen in leukemia and lymphoma patients is most frequently caused by chemotherapy-induced neutropenia.[22, 24] Small-bowel perforation after induction or prolonged chemotherapy for patients with stage III and IV non-Hodgkin's lymphoma is a recognized complication. A relationship with cytosine arabinoside use has been noted and should suggest the diagnosis.

Splenic rupture is occasionally noted in leukemic patients owing to acute sequestration of white blood cells. Patients with leukemic rupture of the spleen have hypotension, tachycardia, fever, and shoulder tip pain. Diagnosis is confirmed by ultrasonography, CT, or peritoneal lavage; therapy consists of prompt splenectomy.

Acute appendicitis is most commonly caused by lymphocytic obstruction of the appendiceal lumen and is therefore rarely noted in immunosuppressed adult hosts. However, an increased incidence of appendicitis is noted in children with acute leukemia caused by lymphocytic infiltration of the terminal ileum and appendiceal base. The diagnosis of acute appendicitis is particularly difficult in these patients and is often not made before gangrene with perforation occurs.

Acquired Immunodeficiency Syndrome

AIDS may frequently lead to abdominal pain, which is estimated to occur in about 12% of AIDS patients but necessitates surgery in only 5% of these.[28] As the incidence of the disease increases, the number of patients who may need emergency laparotomy is also increasing. The determination of whether the acute abdomen necessitates surgical treatment in these patients can be difficult. Concomitant ethical and social considerations may complicate the clinical decision in assessing whether intervention significantly benefits the patient. Because the great majority have been previously diagnosed as being infected with the human immunodeficiency virus, most patients are receiving drug treatment for AIDS. Many of these patients are infected with a variety of other organisms, including CMV, *Mycobacterium avium-intracellulare*, cryptococcus, *Helicobacter pylori*, hepatitis B virus, and *C. difficile*.

Abdominal pain may be mild initially or severe, may be local or generalized, and may be associated with rebound tenderness and guarding or a rigid abdomen. In addition, about one third of these patients have diarrhea that may be bloody, reflecting mucosal changes caused by the associated opportunistic organisms.

It must always be kept in mind that patients with AIDS may have non-AIDS–related lesions such as appendicitis, cholecystitis, or pancreatitis. The standard radiologic investigation for signs of obstruction, free air, and masses is essential. In selected cases, CT may be helpful in delineating masses.[5] Although Kaposi's sarcoma is common and has been noted on endoscopy in about one third of the patients, complications of the sarcoma are uncommon and seldom precipitate an acute abdomen.

The lesions more specific to AIDS can be broadly divided into three main groups. (1) Acute toxic entercolitis associated with AIDS has a clinical picture similar to that of acute ulcerative colitis in which the large bowel is grossly distended, ischemic, infected by CMV, and likely to perforate. These patients require colonic resection with ileostomy in most cases, as primary anastomosis is not feasible. (2) B cell lymphomas may be in the small or large bowel and produce symptoms of intestinal obstruction or, less often, perforation. (3) A miscellaneous group of patients have disseminated lymphoma, or gross splenic enlargement with or without rupture, or *M. avium-intracellulare* infection affecting the intra-abdominal reticuloendothelial system.

Perioperative mortality of AIDS patients with abdominal pain is high and the benefit of operation is often questionable. Consequently, preoperative diagnosis must be extremely accurate and the scope of operation carefully defined.

Illicit Drug Use

The acute abdomen is seen with increased frequency in illicit drug users.[29] Whereas intravenous drug abuse and septic complications were common in the 1970s and early 1980s, cocaine and crack usage is now more prevalent. Cocaine hydrochloride powder has limited systemic absorption because of an intense vasoconstriction of the nasal and mucosal membranes. In contrast, crack cocaine relies on pulmonary absorption, resulting in higher systemic levels and enhanced effects. Intestinal ischemic sequelae of cocaine use are increasingly reported.[30-33] Whereas small-bowel ischemia and colonic ischemia occasionally occur after exces-

TABLE 129–2
TOXICOLOGIC CAUSES OF ACUTE ABDOMINAL PAIN

Agent	Exposure	Toxicity	Symptoms	Treatment
Therapeutic Agents				
Acetylsalicylic acid	Aspirin-containing tablets	Gastrointestinal ulceration and perforation	Tinnitus Epigastric pain Peritonitis Bleeding	Rehydration Potassium supplementation Alkalization of urine
Acetaminophen	Tablets	Hepatic Central nervous system	Right upper quadrant pain	Gastric lavage Hydration N-Acetylcysteine
Heavy Metals				
Iron	Iron supplements Multivitamins	Gastritis Perforation Pyloric stenosis Obstruction	Nausea Vomiting Bleeding Epigastric pain	Gastric lavage Deferoxamine
Mercury	Industrial exposure	Gastric erosions Membranous colitis Central nervous system	Diffuse abdominal pain Nausea Vomiting Central nervous system abnormalities	Gastric lavage Charcoal Chelation therapy
Arsenic	Occupational exposure Attempted homicide	Gastrointestinal ulceration	Esophageal pain Vomiting Cholera-like symptoms	Gastric lavage Fluid resuscitation Chelation therapy Exchange transfusion
Lead	Occupational exposure Lead paint ingestion	Central nervous system	Colicky abdominal pain Constipation	Gut decontamination Chelation therapy
Environmental Exposure				
Latrodectus mactans venom	Black widow spider bite	Central nervous system	Colicky abdominal pain Pseudoacute abdomen	Tetanus prophylactic Calcium gluconate Muscle relaxants
Amanita phalloides mushroom	Mushroom ingestion	Hepatic	Right upper quadrant pain	Hydration Gastric lavage

sive use of crack cocaine, a great increase in the incidence of ischemic perforation of the stomach and duodenum has been noted.

Cocaine-induced ulcer perforation can sometimes be differentiated from standard peptic ulcer disease by the location of the ulcer, which tends to be in the mid-gastric region. The symptoms of cocaine-induced perforation may have an insidious onset owing to the altered mental state of the patient or the gradual nature of the perforation. In addition, the white blood cell count in drug-induced perforation is frequently not elevated in contrast to the case in classic perforation.

Intestinal pain from obstruction of the gastrointestinal tract may be noted in enteral drug smugglers, or "mules."[29, 34] Swallowing of packets containing 3 to 12 g of cocaine per packet has increased. These smugglers may have perforation of the packet and cocaine overdose, or obstruction of the stomach, the distal ileum, and the splenic flexure resulting from foreign body impaction. Refinements in packing technique have reduced the incidence of toxic manifestations of cocaine overdose, but the obstructive symptoms continue to occur.

Patients suspected of enteral cocaine trafficking may be examined radiologically, as 80% of swallowed cocaine packets are visible on abdominal radiographs. Type I packets consist of finger cots or condoms and are prone to rupture; an aggressive surgical approach to their removal for any symptoms is warranted, as more than 50% of these rupture in transit. A halo around the packet identifies leakage of one of the layers and is consistent with imminent rupture. Type II packets are machine packaged and rarely rupture; surgical treatment of these individuals is reserved for obstructive symptoms.

Toxicologic Causes

Abdominal pain attributable to chemicals or medications should always be considered when the clinical diagnosis remains uncertain[35] (Table 129–2).

Mercury. Although the primary toxicity of mercuric poisoning involves the central nervous system, gastrointestinal symptoms may predominate in some patients. Nausea and vomiting with gastrointestinal erosions and severe abdominal pain may occur in selected patients, mandating surgical evaluation.

Arsenic. The gastrointestinal manifestations of arsenic exposure are similar to those of cholera, with rice water diarrhea, nausea, vomiting, and severe, colicky abdominal pain. Patients exposed to arsenide gas generally have a 24-hour lag phase before gastrointestinal symptoms occur. Surgical intervention is not necessary after arsenic poisoning.

Acid or Alkali Ingestion. The injury associated with acid or alkali ingestion is dependent on the amount, strength, and form of the preparation. Crystalline preparations are associated with less severe injury, as ingestion is limited and the primary injury is oropharyngeal. Highly concentrated forms of acid and alkali are associated with more severe injury that reaches the stomach and the proximal intestine. Acid products cause mucosal coagulation necrosis, which limits the depth of injury but may cause gastric ulceration and perforation. Alkali ingestion leads to liquefaction necrosis. Although gastric injury caused by alkali is not common, the increased depth of oropharyngeal and esophageal injury may cause immediate and irreparable damage. The history and local evidence on inspection or careful esophagoscopy give the diagnosis.

Aspirin. Aspirin-containing products are well-established gastrointestinal irritants; a dose-dependent increase in gastric and duodenal erosions is noted with prolonged usage. Although enteric-coated products have limited this toxicity, occasional cases of gastrointestinal ulceration and perforation are reported.

Iron. The gastrointestinal toxic manifestations of iron ingestion are dose related and consist of corrosive gastrointestinal injury. Patients with iron toxicity exhibit nausea, vomiting, and hemorrhagic gastritis. Gastrointestinal perforation after iron ingestion has been reported; late manifestations of iron injury include gastric scarring and pyloric stenosis. Occasional patients may have gastric or small-bowel obstruction as a result of ingestion of iron tablet bezoars.

Organ-Specific Toxicologic Injury

Intestinal Ischemia. Sympathomimetic drugs, including cocaine, amphetamines, and catecholamines, can cause intestinal ischemia by increasing splanchnic resistance and decreasing intestinal blood flow. Gastrointestinal ischemic necrosis and consequent acute abdominal pain are reported with many of these agents.

Digoxin has been implicated in colonic and small-bowel ischemic injury by decreasing and redistributing splanchnic blood flow, leading to nonocclusive vascular ischemia. Elderly patients requiring digoxin are at higher risk.

Phenobarbital has been reported to cause intestinal ischemia, primarily through a depression in arterial pressure. Phenobarbital-induced intestinal injury is rare at recommended dosages.

Hepatitis or Hepatic Necrosis. Acetaminophen, copper, and iron overdose and ingestion of carbon tetrachloride, phosphorus, or *Amanita phalloides* mushrooms may cause direct hepatotoxicity. Idiopathic hepatic necrosis may follow re-exposure to halothane anesthesia. Patients with severe right upper quadrant pain and exposure to these substances should have liver function tests to exclude hepatic injury.

Pancreatitis. Pancreatic toxicity has been noted after ingestion of acetaminophen, steroids, furosemide (Lasix), methanol, insecticides, sulfonamides, thiazide diuretics, and tetracycline. A particularly virulent pancreatitis may be seen after scorpion envenomation. Surgical intervention is rarely necessary, except to exclude other conditions in occasional patients.

Antibiotic-Associated Colitis. *Clostridium*-associated colitis has been reported after administration of most antibiotics; development of the toxin-associated disorder is dependent on the duration of antimicrobial use and colonization of the colon with *C. difficile*. The diagnosis is entertained after endoscopic documentation of colonic pseudomembrane in a patient with abdominal pain and diarrhea. Conformation of *Clostridium* colitis is made by endotoxin assay. Treatment consists of enteric or parenteral administration of vancomycin or metronidazole (Flagyl).

Toxicologic Causes of Pseudoacute Abdomen

A variety of agents can cause extra-abdominally mediated abdominal pain that mimics the surgical abdomen. Care must be exercised to avoid unnecessary laparotomy in these instances.

Vinca Alkaloid Neuropathy. Neurotoxicity is the major side effect and limitation of vincristine; vinblastine may also exhibit this toxicity. Enteric neuropathy may lead to constipation and ileus in 10% of recipients. Occasionally, patients have severe, colicky abdominal pain mimicking the acute abdomen; treatment is supportive.

Black Widow Spider Bite. The black widow spider, *Latrodectus mactans,* is endogenous to the Southwest United States and, to a lesser extent, the Southeast. After significant envenomation, abdominal muscle spasm and pain may ensue and resemble the acute abdomen. A history of exposure and the absence of peritoneal signs help to exclude surgical causes of the disorder. Treatment consists of tetanus prophylaxis and administration of calcium gluconate and muscle relaxants.

Anticoagulants. Bleeding into the rectus sheath or the abdominal wall may occur in patients receiving anticoagulant therapy.[36] The abdominal pain associated with this may be abrupt in onset and severe. Careful physical examination may allow palpation of the hematoma or elicit Fothergill's sign, which is worsening of abdominal pain on tightening of the abdominal wall. Care must be taken to exclude intra-abdominal bleeding or enteric hematoma formation in these patients. Treatment is supportive, with reversal of anticoagulation if possible; occasionally, surgical evacuation of the hematoma is necessary.

SUMMARY

Diagnosis of the acute abdomen remains an almost incomparable test of clinical acumen. The spectrum of etiologic factors and the complexity of clinical presentation have broadened significantly with the advent of immunologically depressed patients, expanded surgical operations, more potent antibiotics, and changing behavior patterns. The diagnosis and management of abdominal pain in the critically ill patient are particularly challenging. New technology has permitted more accurate diagnosis, resulting in fewer avoidable operations and also fewer delays when operation is needed.

References

1. Irvin TT: Abdominal pain: A surgical audit of 1190 emergency admissions. Br J Surg 76:1121, 1989.
2. Coleman B, Arger PH, Grumback K, et al: Transvaginal and transabdominal sonography: Prospective comparison. Radiology 168:639, 1989.
3. Gottlieb JE, Menashe PI, Cruz E: Gastrointestinal complications in critically ill patients: The intensivists' overview. Am J Gastroenterol 81:227, 1986.
4. Iberti TJ, Salky BA, Onofrey D: Use of bedside laparoscopy to identify intestinal ischemia in postoperative cases of aortic reconstruction. Surgery 105:686, 1989.
5. Kuhlman JE, Fishman EK: Acute abdomen in AIDS: CT diagnosis and triage. Ragiographics 10:621, 1990.
6. Ooms HWA, Koumans RKJ, Ho Kan You PJ, et al: Ultrasonography in the diagnosis of acute appendicitis. Br J Surg 78:315, 1991.
7. Paterson-Brown S, Vipond MN: Modern aids to clinical decision-making in the acute abdomen. Br J Surg 77:13, 1990.
8. Shaff MI, Tarr RW, Partain CL, et al: Computed tomography and magnetic resonance imaging of the acute abdomen. Surg Clin North Am 68:233, 1988.
9. Vipond MN, Paterson-Brown S, Tyrrell MR, et al: Evaluation of fine catheter aspiration cytology of the peritoneum as an adjunct to decision making in the acute abdomen. Br J Surg 77:86, 1990.
10. Paterson-Brown S, Vipond MN, Gatzen C, et al: Clinical decision making and laparoscopy versus computer prediction in the management of the acute abdomen. Br J Surg 76:1011, 1989.
11. Silen W (ed): Cope's Early Diagnosis of the Acute Abdomen. 18th ed. New York, Oxford University Press, 1991.
12. Wroblewski M, Mikulowski P: Peritonitis in geriatric inpatients. Age Ageing 20:90, 1991.
13. Scher KS, Sarap MD, Jaggers RL: Acute acalculous cholecystitis complicating aortic aneurysm repair. Surg Gynecol Obstet 163:475, 1986.
13a. Ogilvie H: Large intestine colic due to sympathetic deprivation. A new clinical syndrome. Br Med J 2:671, 1948.
14. Triadafilopoulos G, Hallstone AE: Acute abdomen as the first presentation of pseudomembranous colitis. Gastroenterology 101:685, 1991.
15. Brewster DC, Franklin DP, Cambria RP, et al: Intestinal ischemia complicating abdominal aortic surgery. Surgery 109:447, 1991.
16. Huddy SPJ, Joyce WP, Pepper JR: Gastrointestinal complications in 4473 patients who underwent cardiopulmonary bypass surgery. Br J Surg 78:293, 1991.

17. Jonung T, Ribbe E, Norgren L, et al: Visceral ischemia following aortic surgery. Vasa 20:125, 1991.
18. Leitman IM, Paull DE, Barie PS, et al: Intra-abdominal complications of cardiopulmonary bypass operations. Surg Gynecol Obstet 165:251, 1987.
19. Desai MH, Herndon DN, Rutan RL, et al: Ischemic intestinal complications in patients with burns. Surg Gynecol Obstet 172:257, 1991.
20. Kemeny MM, Brennan MF: The surgical complications of chemotherapy in the cancer patient. Curr Probl Surg 24:613, 1987.
21. Wilson SE, Robinson G, Williams RA, et al: Acquired immune deficiency syndrome (AIDS). Indications for abdominal surgery, pathology and outcome. Ann Surg 210:428, 1989.
22. Nylander WA Jr: The acute abdomen in the immunocompromised host. Surg Clin North Am 68:457, 1988.
23. Wade DS, Douglass H Jr, Nava HR, et al: Abdominal pain in neutropenic patients. Arch Surg 125:1119, 1990.
24. Bodey GP, McKenna RJ Jr: Surgical considerations in the immunocompromised cancer patient. In: McKenna RJ, Murphy GP (eds): Fundamentals of Surgical Oncology. New York, Macmillan Publishing, p 114, 1986.
24a. Alt B, Glass NR, Sollinger H: Neutropenic enterocolitis in adults: Review of the literature and assessment of surgical intervention. Am J Surg 149:405, 1985.
25. Ferrara JIM, Deeg HJ: Mechanisms of disease: Graft vs. host disease. N Engl J Med 324:667, 1991.
26. Komorowski RA, Cohen EB, Kauffman HM, et al: Gastrointestinal complications in renal transplant recipients. Am J Clin Pathol 86:161, 1986.
26a. Misra MK, Pinkus GS, Birtch AG: Major colonic diseases complicating renal transplantation. Surgery 73:942, 1973.
27. Digenis GE, Abraham G, Savin E, et al: Peritonitis-related deaths in continuous ambulatory peritoneal dialysis (CAPD) patients. Peritoneal Dialysis Int 10:45, 1990.
28. Katz MH, French DM: AIDS and the acute abdomen. Emerg Med Clin North Am 7:575, 1989.
29. Lancashire MJR, Legg PK, Lowe M, et al: Surgical aspects of international drug smuggling. Br Med J 296:1035, 1988.
30. Abramson DL, Gertler JP, Lewis T, et al: Crack-related perforated gastropyloric ulcer. J Clin Gastroenterol 13(1):17, 1991.
31. Hon DC, Salloum LJ, Hardy HW, et al: Crack-induced enteric ischemia. NJ Med 87:1001, 1990.
32. Lee HS, LaMaute HR, Pizzi WF, et al: Acute gastroduodenal perforations associated with use of crack. Ann Surg 211:15, 1990.
33. Yang RD, McCarthy JH: Ischemic colitis in a crack abuser. Dig Dis Sci 36:238, 1991.
34. Trent MS, Kim U: Cocaine packet ingestion. Surgical or medical management? Arch Surg 122:1179, 1987.
35. Mueller PD, Benowitz NL: Toxicologic causes of acute abdominal disorders. Emerg Med Clin North Am 7:667, 1989.
36. Euhus DM, Hiatt JR: Management of the acute abdomen complicating oral anticoagulation therapy. Am Surg 56:582, 1990.

CHAPTER 130

Acute Mesenteric Ischemia

Lawrence J. Brandt

Intestinal ischemia produces a broad spectrum of disorders, ranging from completely reversible functional changes to total hemorrhagic necrosis. The end result of ischemic injury depends on many variables, including the mechanism of ischemia (embolus, spasm, or thrombosis), the vessel involved (artery or vein), the onset and duration of the injury (acute or chronic), and the area and length of bowel affected (small intestine or colon). To enable a practical approach to the management of patients with the various forms of bowel ischemia, they can be divided into four broad categories, each with a general pattern of clinical presentation that can be correlated with the nature of the ischemic involvement. In three of these, there is a single episode of

TABLE 130–1

INCIDENCE OF INTESTINAL ISCHEMIA AT MONTEFIORE MEDICAL CENTER

Type of Ischemia	Incidence (%)
Acute mesenteric ischemia	30
Superior mesenteric arterial embolus	50
Nonocclusive mesenteric ischemia	25
Superior mesenteric arterial thrombosis	10
Mesenteric venous thrombosis	5
Miscellaneous (e.g., vasculitis)	5
Colonic ischemia	60
Focal segmental ischemia	5
Chronic mesenteric ischemia	5

acute ischemia, whereas in the fourth, chronic mesenteric ischemia, there are multiple recurrent attacks. As a rule, the clinical presentation and natural history of each group are different, although some overlap is inevitable.

In the past 10 years, the incidence of acute mesenteric ischemia (AMI) at Montefiore Medical Center has plateaued at about 1 per 100 hospital admissions and approximately one new case of ischemia of the large or small bowel is seen each week (Table 130–1). Although AMI is second to colonic ischemia in frequency, it is the most life threatening of the ischemic disorders involving the intestine. In the intensive care unit, a bout of ischemia is much more likely to involve the small intestine than the colon. Thus, it is crucial to understand the pathophysiology of AMI and to be able to differentiate it from colonic ischemia. Only by prompt diagnosis and aggressive therapy can the unacceptably high mortality of this intra-abdominal catastrophe be reduced.

AMI may be caused by a superior mesenteric arterial (SMA) embolus or thrombus, by nonocclusive mesenteric ischemia's producing a low-flow state with associated vasoconstriction, or by mesenteric venous thrombosis. SMA embolus is the most common cause of AMI and accounts for approximately 50% of such cases.[1] Nonocclusive ischemia, which previously was more common, is now being reported less often, presumably because of better monitoring in intensive care units, prompt correction of hemodynamic abnormalities before hypotension occurs, and the widespread use of systemic unloading (vasodilating) agents in the management of congestive heart failure and myocardial ischemia.

Regardless of the changing distribution of causes of AMI, in most series, this intra-abdominal catastrophe is as lethal today as in 1933, when Hibbard and colleagues reported a mortality rate of 70%.[2, 3] The lack of improvement in survival with these vascular accidents can be attributed to three main factors: (1) an inability to make the diagnosis before intestinal gangrene develops, (2) a progression of bowel infarction after the primary initiating vascular or systemic cause has been corrected, and (3) a lack of appreciation of the deleterious role of vasospasm in cases of occlusive mesenteric ischemia. In 1973, Boley and colleagues proposed an aggressive plan of management employing early angiography and the intra-arterial infusion of the vasodilator papaverine to interrupt splanchnic vasoconstriction[4] (Fig. 130–1). This approach has resulted in the salvage of compromised bowel and a dramatic improvement in survival.[5, 6]

PATHOPHYSIOLOGY

The intestines are protected from ischemia by an abundant collateral circulation. Collateral pathways open immediately on occlusion of a major vessel in response to arterial hypotension distal to the obstruction. Increased blood flow

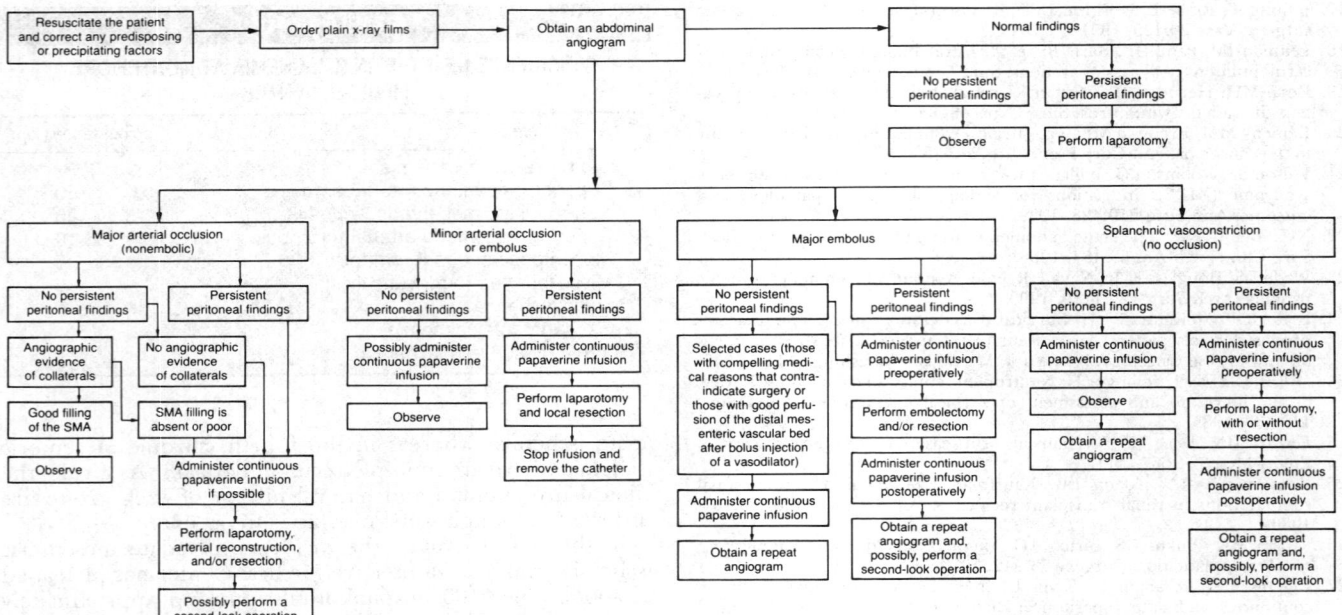

Figure 130–1. Management of the patient with suspected AMI. (From Reinus JF, Brandt LJ, Boley SJ: Ischemic diseases of the bowel. Gastroenterol Clin North Am 19:319, 1990.)

through collateral pathways maintains adequate perfusion for a variable, but brief, period. If blood flow is diminished for a prolonged period, vasoconstriction in the affected bed develops and may persist even after the primary cause of mesenteric ischemia has been corrected. Such vasoconstriction, or nonocclusive mesenteric ischemia, was first described by Ende in 1958[7] and may occur in response to a variety of systemic insults that diminish mesenteric blood flow. These include decreased cardiac output (pump failure or arrhythmias), hypovolemia (dehydration, bleeding), hypotension (shock, sepsis), rapid digitalization, or use of vasopressors. Persistent vasoconstriction can also follow SMA occlusion by embolus or thrombus and can occur after SMA occlusion in the absence of shock. Vasoconstriction increases resistance, producing a rise in arterial pressure in the dependent segment, which in turn impairs collateral blood flow. Splanchnic blood flow and mesenteric ischemia thus reflect the state of the systemic circulation, the degree of functional or anatomic vascular compromise, the number and caliber of vessels affected, the response of the vascular bed to diminished perfusion, the nature and capacity of the collateral circulation, the duration of the ischemic insult, and the metabolic needs of the involved segment of bowel.

The mechanism whereby ischemic necrosis occurs is poorly understood. For many years, such necrosis was simply thought to be caused by diminished blood flow and tissue hypoxia. More recent studies suggest that a reperfusion injury, mediated in part by oxygen free radicals derived from oxidant enzymes, as well as phagocytes, may contribute to the ischemic damage.[8, 9] In this concept, intestinal xanthine oxidase is converted to xanthine dehydrogenase under conditions of hypoxemia. On reperfusion, this enzyme acts on hypoxanthine, produced from the metabolism of ATP during the ischemic event, to produce xanthine and uric acid, during which superoxide and hydrogen peroxide are generated. The latter two are largely responsible for lipid peroxidation and damage to biologic membranes. During reperfusion, leukocyte adherence and extravasation occur in the mesenteric venules along with increased microvascular permeability, further contributing to tissue damage.

DIAGNOSIS

In 1973, an aggressive approach to the management of AMI was presented, with the hope of decreasing the extremely high mortality rate reported with this entity.[4] The essential features in this approach are (1) the earlier and more extensive use of angiography to diagnose mesenteric ischemia before the development of gangrene and also to determine its cause and (2) interruption of the splanchnic vasoconstriction that persists after successful management of its underlying local or systemic cardiovascular cause by the intra-arterial infusion of papaverine. The proper incorporation of these concepts in a comprehensive radiologic and therapeutic plan for the management of patients with suspected AMI has resulted in a significant improvement in both survival of patients and salvage of compromised bowel. Prompt recognition and early treatment are the keys to the successful management of patients with nonocclusive mesenteric ischemia. Experience with AMI indicates not only that diagnosis within the initial 24 hours of the development of symptoms is crucial, but also that the aggressive use of mesenteric angiography and vasodilators improves outcome twofold over that in cases managed by more traditional methods.[5, 6, 10]

Early diagnosis of AMI depends on the identification of individuals at risk and the recognition that the disparity between the severity of the abdominal pain and the absence of significant abdominal findings is characteristic of early AMI. Patients at risk are usually older than age 50 years and have congestive heart failure, cardiac arrhythmias, recent myocardial infarction, hypovolemia, hypotension, or sepsis. Therapy with digitalis or its derivatives may play an adjunctive role in the development of mesenteric ischemia, because these drugs are potent splanchnic vasoconstrictors. Patients with AMI usually report severe abdominal pain, which may be localized or diffuse; the severity of the pain helps to differentiate AMI from colonic ischemia, in which pain is a much less prominent symptom. The combination of severe abdominal pain and a paucity of significant abdominal findings in a patient at risk demands that AMI be excluded if another cause of the pain is not discovered on plain film study of the abdomen. Reluctance to undertake early angiography in these often critically ill patients is the primary cause of continuing high mortality. Improved survival will come only when it is recognized that the dangers of waiting for definite physical signs (the acute abdomen) or roentgenologic signs of ischemia (ileus, thumbprinting, free or intramural air) outweigh the risks of early invasive studies in patients in whom AMI is a real possibility.

Abdominal pain may be absent in 15 to 25% of patients with AMI; lack of pain is especially common in those with nonocclusive mesenteric ischemia. Unexplained abdominal distention or gastrointestinal bleeding may be the only indication of acute intestinal ischemia, and distention may be the first sign of impending intestinal infarction. As infarction develops, increasing tenderness, rebound tenderness, and muscle guarding become more prominent. Significant abdominal findings are strong evidence of the presence of nonviable bowel. Nausea, vomiting, fever, rectal bleeding, hematemesis, intestinal obstruction, back pain, shock, and increasing abdominal distention are other late signs.

Leukocytosis greater than 15,000 cells per cubic millimeter occurs in approximately 75% of patients with AMI, and a metabolic acidosis with increased base deficit is present in about 50%. Elevations in levels of serum and peritoneal fluid amylase, alkaline phosphatase, and inorganic phosphates have been reported, but the consistency and specificity of these findings have not been established. Leukocytosis, especially if out of proportion to the physical findings, an elevated hematocrit, and blood-tinged peritoneal fluid, often with a high amylase content, are signs of advanced intestinal necrosis.

An important clinical problem in evaluating a patient with suspected intestinal ischemia is the differentiation of AMI from colonic ischemia.[11] The pathophysiology, clinical presentation, approach to diagnosis, therapy, and prognosis are distinctly different for these entities. In brief, patients with colonic ischemia usually do not appear ill, have only mild abdominal pain, and predominantly have rectal bleeding and bloody diarrhea. The diagnosis is supported by gentle colonoscopy or barium enema study demonstrating submucosal hemorrhage or segmental colitis. Angiography plays a small role in the examination of patients suspected of having colonic ischemia, because even at this early stage of clinical presentation, colonic blood flow has already returned to normal, the mucosa is no longer ischemic, and the outcome of the involved segment of colon is already determined. In contrast, as described earlier, patients with AMI usually have a precipitating cause of the ischemic episode and are often ill with marked abdominal pain. In this disorder, the small bowel is affected by an ongoing and evolving acute ischemic injury; angiography is crucial in defining its cause (embolus, thrombosis, nonocclusive mesenteric ischemia) and enabling a rational therapeutic approach combining administration of intra-arterial vasodilators and surgery.

MANAGEMENT

The initial treatment of any patient at risk who is suspected of having AMI is to correct predisposing or precipitating causes. Relief of acute congestive heart failure, correction of new or unstable cardiac arrhythmias, and replacement of blood volume precede any diagnostic studies. In general, efforts at increasing intestinal blood flow are futile if low cardiac output, hypotension, or hypovolemia persists. Patients who are hypotensive, hypovolemic, or in shock should not have angiography, because mesenteric vasoconstriction is always evident, even without intestinal ischemia. Such patients should not receive intra-arterial papaverine because this increases the size of the mesenteric vascular bed, aggravates hypovolemia, and lowers blood pressure.

The management of associated congestive heart failure or shock may be especially difficult, because digitalis preparations have a direct vasoconstrictor action on SMA smooth muscle[12] and therefore should be avoided in AMI, if possible. Vasopressors are also contraindicated in the treatment of shock if mesenteric ischemia is suspected. A helpful development is increased use of systemic vasodilators in the therapy of congestive heart failure and myocardial infarction. These drugs (e.g., hydralazine, prazosin, nitroglycerin, and nitroprusside) reduce arterial impedance by diminishing preload and/or afterload and theoretically are ideal agents to treat the low mesenteric flow syndromes associated with congestive failure.

When intestinal ischemia has progressed to the extent that systemic alterations are present, correction of plasma volume deficits, gastrointestinal decompression, and administration of parenteral antibiotics are essential before any roentgenologic studies are undertaken. The value of both systemic and locally administered antibiotics in preserving the viability of compromised bowel is well established. Thus, broad-spectrum systemic antibiotics are given intravenously as soon as the diagnosis of AMI is established. After these initial measures, roentgenologic studies are undertaken, regardless of the abdominal physical findings or the surgeon's decision whether to operate.

Plain film examination of the abdomen is performed not to identify signs of intestinal ischemia but to exclude other diagnosable causes of abdominal pain (e.g., a perforated viscus or intestinal obstruction). If the plain films do not reveal another cause of the pain, angiography is performed. Patients suspected of having AMI, with the combination of severe abdominal pain lasting several hours, an unimpressive abdominal examination, and a normal plain film of the abdomen, are prime candidates for angiography; for these are the patients with possible AMI who probably do not have infarcted bowel and who may therefore survive the ischemic episode. Signs of intestinal ischemia on plain film studies occur late and usually indicate bowel infarction.

A normal plain film does not exclude a diagnosis of AMI. Early emergency splanchnic angiography is the keystone of an aggressive approach (see Fig. 130–1). Even when the decision to operate has been made, an angiogram must be obtained to manage the patient properly at operation. Emboli, thromboses, and mesenteric vasoconstriction can be diagnosed, and the adequacy of the splanchnic circulation can be evaluated. The angiographic catheter provides a route for the administration of intra-arterial vasodilators, such as papaverine, which relieve the mesenteric vasoconstriction of both nonocclusive and occlusive forms of mesenteric ischemia (Figs. 130–2 and 130–3). Intra-arterial papaverine has been used to improve mesenteric perfusion in the nonoperative management of patients with AMI, as well as preoperatively, intraoperatively, and postoperatively. Depending on the angiographic findings and the presence or absence of peritoneal signs, the patient can be managed according to a therapeutic algorithm incorporating surgery, intra-arterial infusions of vasodilators, and serial angiographic studies.

Papaverine is infused through the angiography catheter, which is left in the SMA, at a constant rate of 30 to 60 mg/h. To prevent dislodgment, the catheter is sutured to the skin at its point of entry into the thigh. The drug usually is diluted in saline to a concentration of 1 mg/mL, but this may be varied with the fluid limitations or requirements of the patient. Continuous monitoring of systemic arterial pressure and cardiac rate and rhythm is indicated, because this amount of papaverine theoretically could have systemic

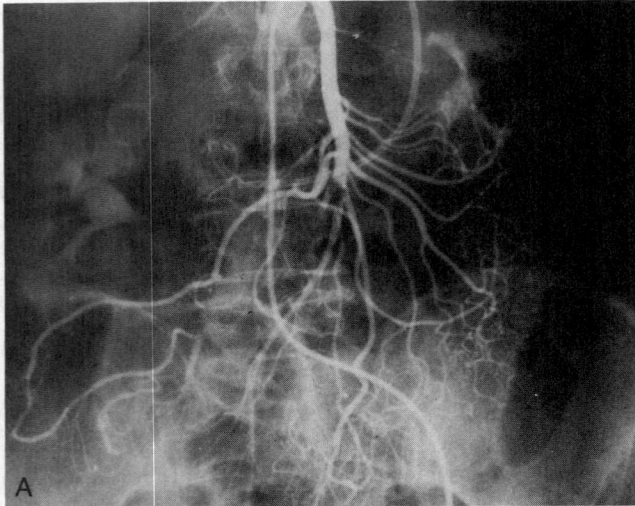

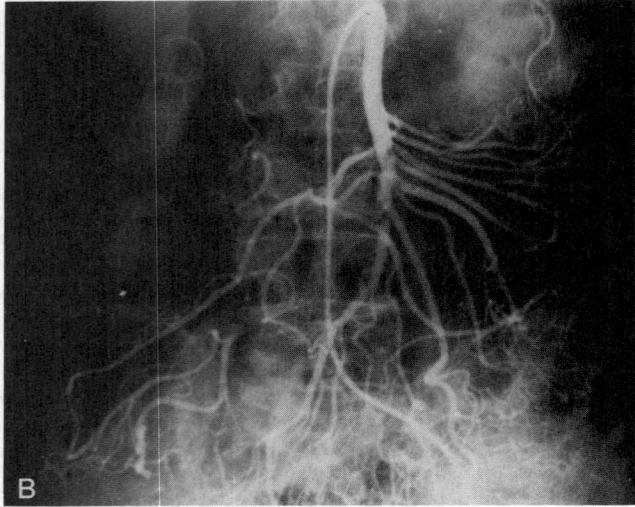

Figure 130–2. Patient with nonocclusive mesenteric ischemia after an episode of hemorrhage and shock. *A.* Initial superior mesenteric angiogram showing diffuse vasospasm. *B.* Angiogram performed after 36 hours of papaverine infusion shows dilation of all vessels. Study was obtained 30 minutes after papaverine was replaced with saline. At this time, the patient's abdominal symptoms and signs were absent. (From Boley SJ, Brandt LJ, Veith FJ: Ischemic disorders of the intestine. Curr Probl Surg 15[4]:1–85, 1978.)

effects. I have not observed such effects in either experimental or clinical studies, probably because the drug is metabolized in the liver before it reaches the general circulation. A sudden decrease in blood pressure should suggest the possibility that the angiographic catheter has been dislodged from the SMA and that the papaverine is being infused into the aorta. In such cases, saline should be substituted for papaverine and a plain film obtained. If the catheter is not in the SMA, it should be correctly repositioned and papaverine reinfused.

Heparin is not added to the infusion, because it is not compatible with papaverine hydrochloride and it is not necessary to prevent thrombus formation within the SMA. No other medications or fluids should be administered through the arterial catheter.

When papaverine infusion is used as the primary treatment of nonocclusive mesenteric ischemia (see Fig. 130–2), it is continued for approximately 24 hours and then another angiogram is obtained 30 minutes after changing the infu-

sion to isotonic saline. On the basis of the clinical course of the patient and the response of the vasoconstriction to therapy, as revealed by the angiogram, the infusion is discontinued or maintained for another 24 hours. The patient's status then is re-evaluated. If at any time peritoneal signs develop, operation is performed promptly. Infusions may be continued for up to 5 days but usually can be stopped after 24 hours. When papaverine is used in conjunction with laparotomy for nonocclusive disease, a second-look operation frequently is necessary. In such cases, the infusion is continued postoperatively and is discontinued only when the patient's abdominal findings have returned to normal and when no signs of vasoconstriction remain on an angiogram that is obtained 30 minutes after the vasodilator infusion has been replaced by saline alone. The SMA catheter is removed as soon as the intra-arterial infusion is stopped.

When papaverine is used in the treatment of SMA embolus (see Fig. 130–3), the infusion is given through a catheter placed selectively in the SMA proximal to the occlusion. The patient is then managed according to the algorithm in Figure 130–1 on the basis of the presence or absence of peritoneal signs, the site of the embolus, the adequacy of collateral blood flow, and the degree of vasospasm in the vascular bed distal to the embolus after administration of an intra-arterial bolus of 25 mg of tolazoline. Although SMA embolus is conventionally treated by surgery, some high-risk patients may be candidates for angiographic therapy alone. To be considered for such therapy, these individuals must not have signs of peritonitis and their vascular bed distal to the embolus must show adequate perfusion after administration of the tolazoline bolus.

Laparotomy is performed to restore intestinal blood flow obstructed by an embolus or by thrombosis or to resect necrotic bowel. Revascularization should precede evaluation of intestinal viability because bowel that initially appears infarcted may show surprising recovery after restoration of blood flow. Early in the course of an intestinal ischemic insult, serosal blood flow is preserved, despite injury to the mucosa and the submucosa, often making inspection of the external surface of the bowel inaccurate. Nonetheless, assessment of the color of the bowel and the presence of pulsations, bleeding, and peristalsis remain the clinical criteria for the judgment of tissue viability. Doppler ultrasonography,[13] laser Doppler velocimetry,[14] and perfusion fluorometry[15] show promise of aiding in this determination. If there is any question as to the viability of unresected intestine, a planned re-exploration, or second-look operation, is performed within 12 to 24 hours. The purpose of the second look, as proposed by Shaw, is "not just to allow a clear definition between dead and live bowel to take place, but to allow time for the institution of supportive measures which may render more of the bowel viable."[16]

The use of anticoagulants in the management of AMI is controversial. To prevent the occurrence of thrombosis late in the postoperative period, however, while avoiding an increased risk of early gastrointestinal or intraoperative bleeding, anticoagulation is begun 48 hours after embolectomy or arterial reconstruction, except for patients with mesenteric venous thrombosis in whom immediate anticoagulation is essential.

OUTCOME

Although survival of 10 to 30% of patients has been reported with conventional methods of evaluation and therapy, the approach outlined here has substantially improved outcome. Of the first 50 patients managed at Montefiore Medical Center in this fashion, 35 (70%) proved to have

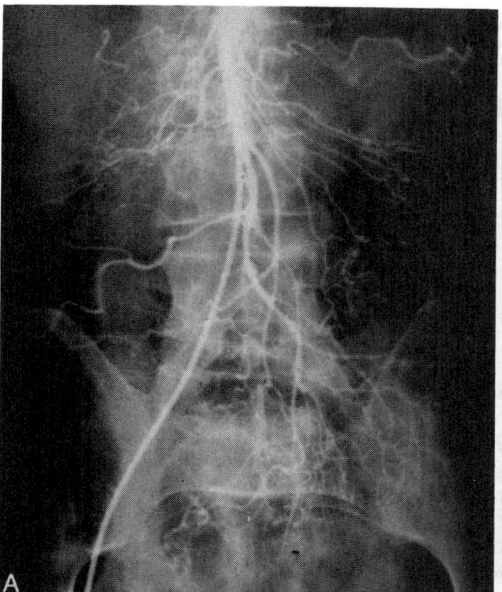
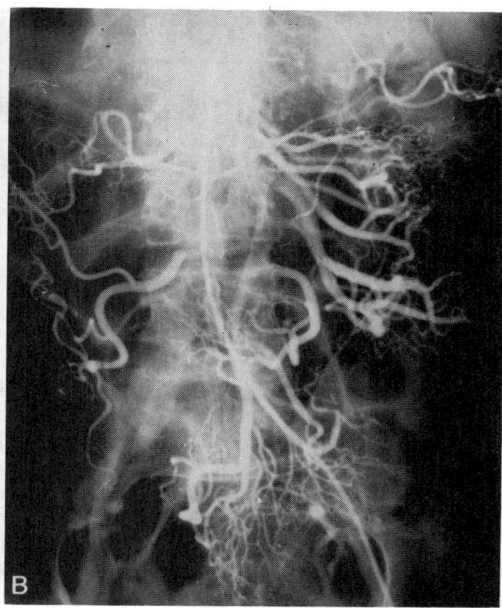

Figure 130–3. SMA angiogram in a 52-year-old woman admitted to the hospital with emboli to the right arm and left leg. *A.* The development of abdominal pain led to mesenteric angiography, which shows emboli in the SMA at the level of the ileocolic artery. *B.* Papaverine was infused into the SMA for 54 hours, resulting in good filling of the SMA and some retraction of the embolus. Subsequent laparotomy revealed normal bowel, and no resection of either embolus or bowel was performed. (From Boley SJ, Brandt LJ, Veith FJ: Ischemic disorders of the intestine. Curr Probl Surg 15[4]:1–85, 1978.)

AMI and 19 (54%) of these survived. Eighty-five percent of the survivors did not lose any bowel or had excision of less than 3 ft of small intestine, thus permitting the preservation of relatively normal bowel function. Similar survival statistics have been reported by the group at the University of Cincinnati[6] utilizing this protocol.

In a review from Montefiore Medical Center of 47 patients with intestinal ischemia resulting from SMA emboli, a survival rate of 55% was obtained in those patients managed according to the aggressive protocol, whereas only 20% of those treated by traditional methods survived.[10] Intra-arterial papaverine as the primary treatment was successful in four patients, two of whom were not operated on and two of whom had normal intestines at the time of delayed laparotomy.

The complications of the angiographic studies and prolonged infusions of vasodilator drugs have not been excessive. Three of the first 50 patients had transient acute tubular necrosis after angiography and treatment of their mesenteric ischemia. One patient had arterial occlusions in both lower extremities during a papaverine infusion for an SMA embolus. These probably represented additional emboli from the primary source of embolization, but the SMA catheter could not be excluded as a factor. There were several instances of local hematomas at the arterial puncture site, but no other major problems were encountered with blood flow to the lower extremities.

CONCLUSION

Although AMI is being recognized more frequently than previously and the mechanisms of ischemic injuries are the subject of intense research efforts, patients with these catastrophic disorders have unacceptably high mortality rates. There are promising new therapies on the horizon, but for now an approach using early angiography, administration of intra-arterial vasodilators, and prompt surgery appears to yield the best survival data.

References

1. Reinus JF, Brandt LJ, Boley SJ: Ischemic diseases of the bowel. Gastroenterol Clin North Am 19:319, 1990.
2. Vellar ID, Doyle JC: Acute mesenteric ischemia. Aust NZ J Surg 47:54, 1977.
3. Hibbard JS, Swenson JC, Levin AG: Roentgenology of experimental mesenteric vascular occlusion. Arch Surg 26:20, 1933.
4. Boley SJ, Sprayregen S, Veith FJ, et al: An aggressive roentgenologic and surgical approach to acute mesenteric ischemia. Surg Annu 5:355, 1973.
5. Boley SJ, Sprayregen S, Seigelman SJ, et al: Initial results from an aggressive roentgenological and surgical approach to acute mesenteric ischemia. Surgery 82:848, 1977.
6. Clark RA, Gallant TE: Acute mesenteric ischemia: Angiographic spectrum. AJR 142:555, 1984.
7. Ende N: Infarction of the bowel in cardiac failure. N Engl J Med 258:879, 1958.
8. Koningsberger JC, Marx JJM, Van Hattum J: Free radicals in gastroenterology. A review. Scand J Gastroenterol 23(suppl 154):30, 1988.
9. Hernandez LA, Grisham MB, Twohig B, et al: Role of neutrophils in ischemia-reperfusion–induced microvascular injury. Am J Physiol 253:H699, 1987.
10. Boley SJ, Feinstein FR, Sammartano R, et al: New concepts in the management of superior mesenteric artery embolus. Surg Gynecol Obstet 153:561, 1981.
11. Boley SJ, Brandt LJ, Veith FJ: Ischemic disorders of the intestines. Curr Probl Surg 15:1, 1978.
12. Harrison LA, Blaschke J, Phillips RS, et al: Effects of ouabain on the splanchnic circulation. J Pharmacol Exp Ther 169:321, 1969.
13. Hartnell GG, Gibson RN: Doppler ultrasound in the diagnosis of intestinal ischemia. Gastrointest Radiol 12:285, 1987.
14. Johansson K, Ahn H, Lindhagen J: Assessment of small bowel ischemia by laser Doppler flowmetry. Scand J Gastroenterol 21:1147, 1986.
15. Carter MS, Fantini GA, Sammartano RJ, et al: Qualitative and quantitative fluorescein fluorescence in determining intestinal viability. Am J Surg 147:117, 1984.
16. Shaw RS: The "second look" after superior mesenteric arterial embolectomy or reconstruction for mesenteric infarction. In: Ellison EH, Friesen SR, Mulholland JH (eds): Current Surgical Management. Philadelphia, WB Saunders, p 389, 1965.

CHAPTER 131

Endoscopic Management of Biliary Emergencies

Jerome H. Siegel
Annamalai Veerappan

Biliary emergencies include acute cholangitis, acute pancreatitis, and acute cholecystitis. Because acute cholecystitis remains a surgical disease, it is not discussed here. Since the introduction of endoscopic retrograde cholangiopancreatography (ERCP) and its rapid development as a therapeutic modality, the management of gallstone pancreatitis and acute suppurative cholangitis has changed dramatically. This chapter focuses on these two conditions and discusses in detail the pros and cons of the various treatment modalities currently being utilized.

GALLSTONE PANCREATITIS

Acute pancreatitis is defined as an acute inflammatory process involving the pancreas, which is manifested by the sudden onset of upper abdominal pain, tenderness, and distention and corroborated by an elevated serum amylase and/or lipase level. Gallstone disease and alcohol abuse are the two most common etiologic factors and inciting causes responsible for the development of pancreatitis.[1, 2] The presence of gallstone disease and the absence of other etiologic factors associated with pancreatitis clinically define and confirm the diagnosis of gallstone pancreatitis.[3]

Incidence

In the United States, the incidence of gallstone pancreatitis varies with the population studied. Its occurrence is estimated to be 50 to 60% in community hospitals and only 10 to 20% in city, county, and Veterans Administration hospitals, where alcoholic pancreatitis is more prevalent. Gallstone pancreatitis is more common than alcoholic pancreatitis in Europe, except for France, where the reverse is true.[4]

Pathogenesis

The pathogenesis of gallstone pancreatitis is not absolutely definitive; however, various hypotheses, including the common channel, pancreatic duct obstruction, duodenopancreatic reflux, and pancreatic hypersecretion theories, have been proposed. Each theory has validity and proponents, but there is a great deal of evidence to support the common channel theory.

Common Channel Theory

The association of biliary and pancreatic inflammatory disease was first made in 1856 by Claude Bernard, who was able to induce pancreatitis in dogs by injecting bile and other substances into the pancreatic duct.[5] This concept was confirmed a few years later when Lancereaux suggested that pancreatitis was the direct result of reflux of bile into the pancreatic duct.[6] In 1901, Opie proposed the common channel theory as the basis of gallstone pancreatitis.[7] This latter theory suggested that the offending gallstone became impacted at the distal end of a common biliary-pancreatic duct or channel. Distal common bile duct obstruction then permitted bile reflux from the biliary tree into the pancreatic ductal system, inducing inflammation.

It is generally believed that pure, uninfected bile does not provoke or induce inflammation of the pancreas when it is allowed to flow without pressure into the pancreatic duct.[8] However, under increased pressure, such as might be created by ampullary obstruction in the presence of an impacted stone in a common channel, pancreatic ductal permeability increases and interstitial edema occurs.[9] In addition, the bile of patients with common bile duct stones is usually infected, and the infected bile activates an enzyme cascade, which is initiated by a powerful proteolytic enzyme, bacterial amidase.[10, 11] In addition, lysolecithin, the major phospholipid in bile, participates as a mediator of bile-induced pancreatitis. Lysolecithin, a cytotoxic agent, is the end product of the conversion of lecithin by pancreatic phospholipase A and lipase. During the conversion cascade, release of lysolecithin produces injurious effects to the pancreas.

The fact that gallstones can be recovered from the stools in some 90% of patients in the first few days after an attack of pancreatitis[12, 13] is supportive evidence that a gallstone passed through the common channel induces the enzyme cascade and clinical pancreatitis. A report by Acosta and colleagues that 72% of patients with gallstone pancreatitis, who were operated on within 48 hours of the onset of symptoms, were found to have a stone impacted in the ampulla of Vater[14] was supportive evidence of the common channel–bile reflux theory. It has been shown, during operative cholangiography, that reflux of contrast material into the pancreatic duct occurs in about 60% of patients with a history of pancreatitis compared with only 15% of controls.[15–17] A long common channel was also found in 72% of patients with pancreatitis compared with only 20% of control subjects.[17] Jones and associates corroborated this theory when they reported more frequent occurrence of a common channel in patients with gallstone pancreatitis (67%) than in those with other forms of biliary tract disease (32%).[18] Jones and associates also demonstrated that patients who experienced gallstone pancreatitis were found to have a longer common channel and that the length of the common channel exceeded the stone diameter. This finding and its correlation with disease were not found in other biliary diseases.[18]

A number of studies have raised doubts and conflicting data concerning the common channel theory. Anatomic studies have shown that the common channel of sufficient length, which would allow reflux of bile at the time of ampullary obstruction caused by a stone, occurs in only a minority of patients.[19] Usually, pancreatic secretory pressure exceeds biliary secretory pressure,[20] which favors egress or flow of pancreatic juice into the biliary tree rather than the reverse.

Finally, bile itself does not activate pancreatic digestive enzymes. This was confirmed by an experimental surgical procedure that deliberately diverted bile flow into an unobstructed pancreatic ductal system. Pancreatitis did not occur in this situation.[21] Although there are opinions and data opposed to the common channel theory, it remains the most viable of the hypotheses with the qualification that obstruction of the channel (short-term or long-term) occurs in the presence of infection.

Duodenopancreatic Reflux Theory

The observation that retrograde injection of activated digestive enzymes, duodenal contents, or even mixtures of bile and trypsin into the pancreatic ductal system could cause experimental pancreatitis prompted some to suggest that reflux of duodenal contents through an incompetent sphincter of Oddi could be the triggering mechanism for an attack of pancreatitis.[22] Advocates of the duodenal reflux theory suggest that passage of a stone through the sphincter renders the sphincter incompetent, and in this manner, pancreatitis occurs. However, duodenal reflux has not been widely accepted as a cause of most attacks of pancreatitis, although it might explain the occasional occurrence of pancreatitis in association with afferent loop obstruction after Bilroth's type II gastrectomy. The most serious objection to this theory is that pancreatitis does not occur in patients who have undergone sphincterotomy, surgical or endoscopic, or in patients with a surgical pancreaticojejunostomy in whom gastrointestinal reflux into the pancreatic duct does occur.

Pancreatic Ductal Obstruction and Ductal Hypertension

The final theory proposed to explain gallstone pancreatitis suggests that pancreatic ductal obstruction triggers pancreatitis. Presumably, continued acinar secretion into the obstructed pancreatic ductal system, under either normal physiologic conditions or a hypersecretory state, induces ductal hypertension, rupture of small ducts, and extravasation of pancreatic juice rich in enzymes into the parenchyma of the gland. To refute this, experimental ligation of the pancreatic duct actually induces pancreatic atrophy rather than acute pancreatitis. Furthermore, extravasated ductal fluid is in an inactive form, and parenchymal injury is unlikely to occur when exposed to this fluid. This latter issue might be resolved by studies that suggest that pancreatic ductal obstruction may lead to activation of digestive enzymes within the acinar cells.[23] More work is needed to confirm these findings.

Risk Factors

Several characteristics of gallstones and anatomic features have been described as risk factors for gallstone pancreatitis. Armstrong and coworkers, in a prospective study of 764 patients, found that, in patients with gallstone pancreatitis on operative cholangiogram, the cystic duct measured 4 mm or more in 52% of these patients, but this greater diameter was present in only 19.5% of controls.[17] The wider cystic duct may allow stones less than 4 mm in diameter to pass spontaneously into the common bile duct. These stones then may produce obstruction at the papilla, which has a diameter of approximately 2 mm. Certain stone characteristics have also been identified as causative of or associated with pancreatitis: small size[17, 24, 25] and facets.[26]

Clinical Features

The signs and symptoms of gallstone pancreatitis are ubiquitous and nonspecific and are described in detail elsewhere in this chapter. Characteristically, pain associated with pancreatitis is usually epigastric or located in the right upper quadrant. Radiation of pain to the back, which is usually thought to be associated with pancreatitis, occurs in approximately half of the patients with pancreatitis. The pain is exacerbated by eating and leaning forward. Peritoneal irritation is found in one third of these patients, and tenderness is appreciated on deep palpation in the remaining two thirds of patients. Clinically, jaundice is evident in about 60 to 70% of patients with gallstone pancreatitis, and biochemical determinants corroborate elevations of levels of transaminases,

alkaline phosphatase, bilirubin, and serum amylase and the white blood cell count.

Diagnosis

Although elevation of serum amylase levels is one of the most reliable diagnostic indicators for confirming pancreatitis, the degree of elevation does not correlate with the severity of an attack.[27] Scoring systems based on multivariate laboratory criteria are used for predicting the severity of the attack with a high degree of certainty and are described in detail in Chapter 132. The Acute Physiology and Chronic Health Evaluation (APACHE) scoring system has been found to be useful in assessing the clinical severity of pancreatitis when used shortly after admission of the patient to the hospital.[28] An elevated serum bilirubin level, usually present shortly after hospital admission, was found by Neoptolemos and associates to be a good predictor of persistent common bile duct stones.[29] Persistence of common bile duct stones is associated with increased morbidity and mortality,[30] and immediate relief of common bile duct obstruction improves the outcome and prognosis.

Clinical signs and symptoms and routine laboratory studies including amylase and lipase determinations and liver function tests are helpful but not specific for confirming the diagnosis of gallstone pancreatitis. No single biochemical test is currently considered a reliable indicator of gallstone pancreatitis.

Sonography and Radioscintigraphy

An abdominal sonogram usually can demonstrate gallstones (cholelithiasis); however, the diagnostic accuracy of sonography is limited and nonspecific for common bile duct stones. In a study by Stone and associates, ultrasonography correctly identified gallbladder stones in 31 of 33 (93%) patients who submitted to early biliary surgery for acute pancreatitis.[31] Dilatation of the common bile duct and the presence of stones in the gallbladder are considered compatible with gallstone pancreatitis. Ultrasonography, however, is not always reliable, and its ability to detect stones is compromised in the presence of paralytic ileus[32] because the overlying bowel containing air obscures the area. The diagnostic value of abdominal computed tomographic scans and their value in the management of subsequent complications such as pancreatic abscess and necrosis are undisputed.[33, 34] Radionuclide scanning (lidofenin, or HIDA) is of little value, and although some investigators suggest a strong association between obstruction of the cystic duct and gallstone pancreatitis, this finding has not been confirmed by others.[31]

Cholangiography

None of the investigations just mentioned can compare with direct cholangiography for the identification of stones in the common bile duct. Oral cholecystography and intravenous cholangiography are inappropriate examinations, especially in acute disease, and are not utilized in acute pancreatitis. ERCP provides the most information concerning both the pancreatic and biliary ductal systems. There is no evidence that ERCP exacerbates pancreatitis; in fact, its utility in gallstone disease is critical. Exacerbation of pancreatitis does not occur if contrast material is injected with low pressure and in low volume. In a study by Neoptolemos and coworkers, which included 131 patients with pancreatitis, 100 of whom had gallstones, a higher incidence of choledocholithiasis was found in the first 3 days of the attack (63 to 78%) compared with a lower incidence when ERCP was performed within a few days or months (3 to 33%).[29]

The following observations also were made: (1) patients with severe attacks had a greater incidence of common bile duct stones; (2) patients with common bile duct stones had significantly larger common bile duct diameters, even after corrections were made for age (concurring with the study of Faris and associates[35]); and (3) the incidence of pancreatic duct filling was lower in patients with predicted severe attacks and common duct stones. Although percutaneous transhepatic cholangiography provides information comparable with that obtained with ERCP, the complications associated with this procedure are greater (including hemorrhage, biliary peritonitis, and sepsis), making it an undesirable procedure. Pancreatography is rarely provided by percutaneous transhepatic cholangiography.

The association of common bile duct stones and pancreatitis was reported by Acosta and colleagues describing the presence of gallstones in strained stools.[36] These investigators found that a high percentage of patients recovering from pancreatitis had gallstones in their stools.

Natural History

There is a spectrum of severity of the attack in patients with gallstone pancreatitis ranging from hyperamylasemia with or without mild edema of the pancreas to diffuse hemorrhagic necrosis of the gland. About 20 to 25% of patients with gallstone pancreatitis are seriously ill, half of them having hemorrhagic necrosis of the gland.[14, 37, 38] Most patients (75 to 80%) pass the stones spontaneously from the bile duct (ampulla) and recover with no complications.[37, 38] An attack of gallstone pancreatitis is potentially lethal, but if the patient recovers, few significant sequelae result. However, mild pancreatic dysfunction may occur in as many as 25% of patients.[39] In spite of modern treatment, the mortality of gallstone pancreatitis remains significant (approximately 10%).[30, 37, 40] If the patient does not undergo cholecystectomy after the initial attack, recurrent pancreatitis is likely to occur within 6 to 12 months in one third to two thirds of patients.[14, 30, 38] Obviously, there is no benefit in performing cholecystectomy or common bile duct exploration in patients without gallstone disease such as alcoholic or idiopathic pancreatitis.[38, 41] It is essential that gallstone disease is confirmed before subjecting the patient to surgery.

The incidence of hemorrhagic necrosis (10%) is about the same whether pancreatitis is due to gallstone disease or alcohol.[4] However, a greater proportion of patients with gallstone pancreatitis (hemorrhagic type) have abscesses because of concomitant infection associated with gallstone disease.[42] The incidence of pseudocyst formation involving the pancreas is greater in patients with alcoholic pancreatitis than in those with gallstone or idiopathic pancreatitis; the reason for this is unclear.

Treatment

Most patients make an uneventful recovery with supportive, conservative therapy. Patients with severe, unremitting attacks and those who fail to improve or respond to conservative measures require intervention, either surgical or endoscopic. Because the complications are fewer and less severe with the endoscopic techniques, they are preferred over surgical intervention.

Surgery

The role of early surgery in the management of gallstone pancreatitis has prompted a number of reports with conflicting and opposing opinions. With the exception of two prospective reports, all other studies were retrospective.

Acosta and associates compared the results and outcome of early surgical intervention (mean, 28 hours) in 46 patients with those in historical controls treated medically.[14] They reported a mortality of 2% in the surgically treated group compared with 16% in the control group. The shortcomings of this study were that (1) it compared historical controls rather than randomized, matched controls and (2) the severity of pancreatitis was not defined.

In a group of 23 patients reported by Ranson in whom severe attacks were predicted (three to five of Ranson's criteria [see Table 132–4]), 9 patients underwent urgent surgery (<7 days) and 14 were treated conservatively. There were four deaths in the surgical group (44%), whereas none of the controls died. As a result of this study, Ranson recommended deferring surgery until the acute pancreatitis had subsided completely (usually after 7 days). An objection raised to this study was directed to the differences in the severity of pancreatitis in the two groups; the surgical group had a higher Ranson's score than the nonsurgical group, thus predicting a poorer outcome.[37]

Stone and colleagues reported the only randomized, controlled, and prospective study of early (<72 hours) versus delayed surgery (3 months). Both groups of patients underwent cholecystectomy, sphincteroplasty, and pancreatic duct septotomy. Morbidity and mortality were not statistically different between the two groups. The early-surgery group had a higher incidence of common bile duct stones and a significantly shorter hospitalization. The authors described a striking "gush" of pancreatic juice when sphincteroplasty was performed during early surgery. They also thought that sphincteroplasty could reverse the pathologic events and subsequent complications of gallstone pancreatitis. Again, this study did not stratify the severity of pancreatitis according to Ranson's criteria.[37]

Kelly and Wagner, in a prospective and randomized study, showed that the timing of surgery appeared to have little effect on the outcome of mild pancreatitis (fewer than three of Ranson's criteria), whereas early surgery resulted in an excessively high mortality rate of 48% in patients with severe pancreatitis (more than three of Ranson's criteria).[43]

Other studies have shown higher mortality rates for urgent surgery in gallstone pancreatitis,[44–46] but these studies, although poorly controlled, deserve recognition and comment.

At present, cholecystectomy is the definitive treatment of gallstone pancreatitis and is best performed after recovery from pancreatitis but during the same hospital admission. Emergency surgery during the acute episode, undertaken in patients who are deteriorating with conservative therapy, carries a high mortality rate of 2 to 48%,[14, 31, 37, 43–46] and these patients are probably best treated endoscopically.

Endoscopic Sphincterotomy

ERCP and sphincterotomy in the setting of acute pancreatitis are associated with technical difficulty and are best attempted and performed by an experienced biliary endoscopist. The difficulties encountered are technical and result from edema and ulceration of the papilla and impaction of the stone in the ampulla, prohibiting introduction of the sphincterotome. Selective cannulation of the common bile duct is desirable, although cannulation and controlled injections of contrast media into the pancreatic duct contribute to lower morbidity rates.[47]

Safrany and Cotton were the first to report the use of endoscopic sphincterotomy in patients with gallstone pancreatitis who were critically ill.[47] All 11 patients in their series demonstrated common bile duct stones, and 6 were found to have stone impaction at the papilla. All patients underwent endoscopic sphincterotomy, but only 9 of 11 had successful

TABLE 131-1

ENDOSCOPIC TREATMENT OF GALLSTONE PANCREATITIS

Number of patients	53
Males	22
Females	31
Age range	22–91 y
Mean age	65.5 y
Previous cholecystectomy	41 patients (71%)
Mean hospital stay	4.5 d
Emergency surgery	0 patients
Deaths	0 patients

From Siegel JH: Endoscopic Retrograde Cholangiopancreatography: Technique, Diagnosis, and Therapy. New York, Raven Press, p 141, 1991.

extraction of the stones. Although one of the two required a second procedure, the other patient passed the stone spontaneously. Ten of the 11 patients promptly defervesced, and these ten patients experienced clinical and biochemical improvement after the procedure.[47]

In another endoscopic series, Rosseland and Solhaug reported two groups of patients who were studied at different intervals.[48] Of the first group, 14 patients underwent ERCP, endoscopic sphincterotomy, and stone extraction 1 to 8 weeks after clinical recovery. Surgery was required in two of these patients to accomplish bile duct clearance. The second group of 15 patients was treated within 48 hours of hospital admission. There were no complications associated with the endoscopic procedure. All patients promptly benefited with immediate relief of symptoms. One patient died 5 days after the procedure because of myocardial infarction.

In a personal series (Table 131–1), 53 patients underwent endoscopic sphincterotomy and stone extraction (Fig. 131–1) within 72 hours of presentation with no mortality.

Van der Spuy reported the successful performance of

endoscopic sphincterotomy in 10 patients with gallstone pancreatitis without mortality or morbidity.[49] Active stone extraction was not attempted in these patients, and the stones were permitted to pass spontaneously.

The largest series of endoscopic sphincterotomy in gallstone pancreatitis was reported by Escourrou and coworkers.[50] ERCP was performed in 118 patients early in the course of acute pancreatitis (<72 hours). Common bile duct stones were present in 78% of patients. Endoscopic sphincterotomy was successful in 95% of these patients, and stone clearance was accomplished in 85%. The procedure-associated mortality was 1.7%. There was no control group in this series; however, the complication rate was lower than predicted for patients managed conservatively.

Neoptolemos and associates conducted a 5-year prospective randomized controlled study, which included 131 patients with gallstone pancreatitis.[51] Two groups were randomized, one receiving conventional treatment, with the other group undergoing urgent ERCP (<72 hours). Endoscopic sphincterotomy and stone extraction were performed only if common bile duct stones were found at the time of ERCP. The following important conclusions were drawn from this trial: (1) ERCP can safely be performed in patients with acute gallstone pancreatitis, provided that it is performed by an experienced endoscopist; (2) there was a significant reduction in complication rates in patients who underwent ERCP and endoscopic sphincterotomy compared with controls (24% vs. 61%); (3) there was a statistically significant reduction in mortality in patients with predicted severe attacks (1.7% vs. 17.9%); (4) there was a significant reduction in the hospital stay of those with severe attacks who underwent ERCP and endoscopic sphincterotomy (9.5 vs. 17 days); and (5) finally, because patients with mild disease do so well (historical controls), it is unlikely that any urgent therapeutic modality is superior to conventional therapy.[51]

Thus, the following recommendations may be made: (1) gallstone pancreatitis should be classified as mild or severe according to prognostic criteria; (2) patients with mild disease should be managed conservatively unless they deteriorate, at which time ERCP should be performed; (3) endoscopic sphincterotomy and stone extraction are recommended if common bile duct stones are identified; (4) patients with severe disease, who are more likely to have common bile duct stones, should undergo ERCP within 24 to 72 hours, and endoscopic sphincterotomy and stone extraction are performed if common bile duct stones are identified (early surgery in acute severe cases is associated with an unacceptably high mortality and morbidity); (5) ERCP and endoscopic sphincterotomy are recommended electively for postcholecystectomy patients after recovery from the acute attack; and (6) the same recommendation can also be made for elderly, poor surgical risk patients with an intact gallbladder[52, 53] (Table 131–2). It should be emphasized that performance of ERCP, endoscopic sphincterotomy, and stone extraction in acute gallstone pancreatitis constitutes only one component of management. Conservative, supportive management provides the best results. Elective cholecystectomy in patients considered good surgical risks is recommended during the same hospitalization. Laparoscopic cholecystectomy has been shown to reduce the hospital stay and costs and is more acceptable to patients. However, one must understand that general anesthesia is required for laparoscopic cholecystectomy, and the attendant risks of anesthesia must be taken into consideration. Last, it is essential that ERCP and endoscopic sphincterotomy should be undertaken only by experienced interventional endoscopists.

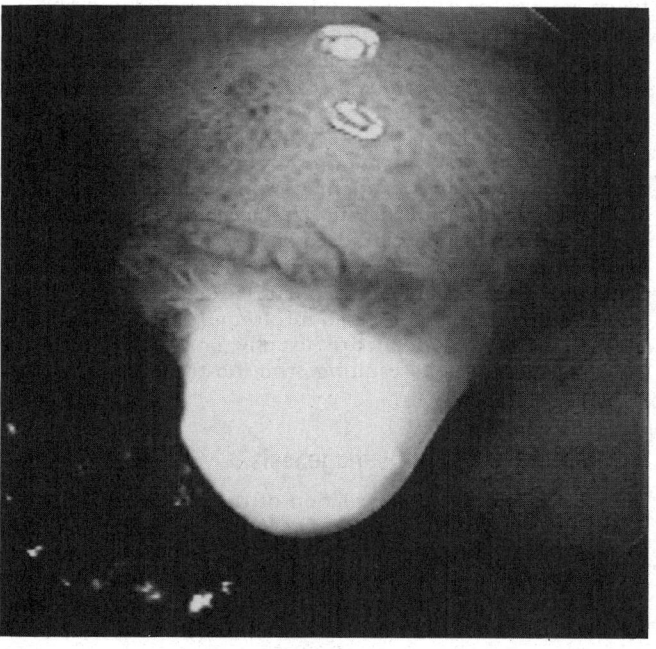

Figure 131–1. Stone impacted in the ampulla, common channel, producing pancreatitis. After sphincterotomy and stone removal, pancreatitis subsided. (From Siegel JH: Endoscopic Retrograde Cholangiopancreatography: Technique, Diagnosis, and Therapy. New York, Raven Press, p 142, 1991.)

TABLE 131-2

PROPHYLACTIC SPHINCTEROTOMY (MEDICAL CHOLECYSTECTOMY) FOR GALLSTONE PANCREATITIS

Number of patients	15
Males	11
Females	4
Mean age	59 y
Age range	43–83 y
Chronic obstructive pulmonary disease	5 patients
Arteriosclerotic heart disease	10 patients
Complications	0 patients
Surgery	0 patients
Deaths	0 patients

From Siegel JH: Endoscopic Retrograde Cholangiopancreatography: Technique, Diagnosis, and Therapy. New York, Raven Press, p 144, 1991.

ACUTE SUPPURATIVE CHOLANGITIS

Acute cholangitis, a potentially life-threatening disease, is manifested clinically by fever (and chills), right upper quadrant pain, and jaundice (Charcot's triad). These classic manifestations were first described by Charcot in 1877.[54] In 1959, Reynolds and Dargan characterized acute suppurative cholangitis as a distinct clinical entity manifested by a pentad consisting of Charcot's three signs plus shock and an abnormal mental status.[55] Biliary obstruction and sepsis are the clinical characteristics of cholangitis.

Cholangitis, however, is not a single disease with a distinct, well-recognized appearance but, instead, is a spectrum of diseases associated with multivariate features and degrees of severity. The severity of the disease varies from a mild form responding to antibiotics alone to a severe suppurative form that necessitates immediate decompression. Failure to provide immediate decompression may result in death, as mortality rates of acute cholangitis range from 13 to 88%. Acute suppurative cholangitis, fortunately, remains uncommon, accounting for only 15% of all cases.[56] Acute suppurative cholangitis is defined as a syndrome resulting from obstruction and resultant infection (with pus) of the bile duct, and the full-blown syndrome is manifested systemically by hypotension and death unless it is treated promptly.

Clinical Features

The symptoms and signs of cholangitis vary in intensity and severity from mild right upper quadrant abdominal pain and low-grade fever to septicemia and concomitant shock. Charcot's triad is associated with the clinical presentation in approximately 70% of patients.[56] Abdominal pain may be absent in acute cholangitis, but when present, it may vary from mild to moderate. Severe pain, especially with colicky characteristics, is more suggestive of acute cholecystitis. Often, mild upper quadrant tenderness is evident on physical examination. If severe, generalized abdominal tenderness or peritoneal signs are present, other diagnoses should be considered, including acute cholangitis. The presence of peritoneal signs is unusual, unless a hepatic abscess is present. This distinction is important because, often, the immediate treatment of acute cholangitis is medical, whereas for other diseases with an acute abdomen, the treatment is surgical.

Often considered distinct clinical entities, suppurative cholangitis and nonsuppurative cholangitis are differentiated by the presence or absence of pus within the bile duct. Obstructive suppurative cholangitis is a more critical entity, which occurs as complete ductal obstruction and is so severe that it usually is associated with shock and mental confusion.[55, 57–62] In a series of 99 patients, Boey and Way found that clinical severity frequently did not correlate with the finding of suppurative cholangitis at surgery.[56] Eight percent of patients with nonsuppurative disease required emergency laparotomy for manifestations of sepsis, whereas as many as 36% of their patients were found to have suppurative disease at surgery. It appears that the degree of clinical toxicity represents the balance between host resistance (determined by age, nutrition, and concurrent medical illnesses), the pathologic pyogenesis, and the virulence of the organisms involved. The lack of correlation between the clinical presentation and the presence of pus in the bile duct was reported by O'Connor and colleagues in a retrospective study of 65 patients with biliary sepsis,[63] making the diagnosis difficult to confirm.

Most patients have abnormal liver function test results, which include elevated bilirubin, alkaline phosphatase, and transaminase levels. During the initial, early evaluation of a patient, liver function studies should be obtained because the diagnosis is frequently corroborated by biochemical abnormalities. It is unusual not to find abnormal liver function test results with cholangitis.

Etiology

Partial or complete obstruction of the bile duct is necessary for the development of cholangitis. At least 80% of patients with cholangitis have associated common bile duct stones.[59, 62–66] However, only 6 to 9% of patients with acute cholangitis are admitted to the hospital with cholelithiasis and concomitant cholecystitis.[66, 67] Most common duct stones migrate from the gallbladder into the bile duct, whereas a small number of stones form primarily in the duct. The question of the form of entry of gallstones into the bile duct and their exit remains unanswered, and why some common duct stones remain silent is not well understood.[68] Choledocholithiasis is not uncommon, as duct stones are found in as many as 15% of patients undergoing cholecystectomy.[69, 70]

Malignant obstruction of the biliary tree may contribute to cholangitis and, surprisingly, constitutes about 10% of cases. The most common neoplasms causing biliary obstruction are carcinomas of the bile duct, the pancreas, and the papilla of Vater. However, even though the degree of obstruction of the biliary tree is complete in malignant disease, the incidence of infection is lower than with stone disease. More often, infection occurs in patients with malignant obstruction after instrumentation such as after ERCP or percutaneous transhepatic cholangiography when concomitant drainage of this closed space is not provided.

Cholangitis occurs in association with benign strictures, congenital abnormalities, papillary stenosis, choledochoduodenostomy, choledochojejunostomy, sclerosing cholangitis, blood clots (which are usually iatrogenic), and the presence of parasites resulting from obstruction and bacterial contamination.

Pathogenesis

Partial or complete obstruction of the biliary tree leads to biliary stasis and favors aerobic and anaerobic bacterial proliferation.[71] Infection of stagnant bile probably occurs via the portal circulation[72–75] in the majority of cases, although direct ascent from the gut and the lymphatics and systemic arterial dissemination are alternative routes.[76] The microorganisms responsible for infection typically constitute the usual gut flora, and these pathogens can be cultured from bile aspirates in the majority of cases. It has been shown that the mechanism of bacteremia occurs as a result of a raised intrabiliary pressure (>250 mm H_2O) and the cholangiovenous reflux of bacteria and endotoxins. The severity of the subsequent clinical syndrome is then dependent on the degree of endotoxemia and bacteremia, the virulence of the organisms, and the effectiveness of host resistance.[75, 77] Persistent elevation of intrabiliary pressure and delay in decompression allows for the development of multiple abscesses, which are disseminated throughout the liver parenchyma. When centrilobular degeneration and pyelophlebitis develop, the patient's condition rapidly deteriorates and survival is in doubt. When all of these events occur concomitantly and abscesses become established, combined aggressive surgical and antimicrobial therapies are usually ineffective in changing the persistent septic course.

Bacteriology

The most common microorganisms isolated during the acute suppurative phase of cholangitis are enteric flora and pathogens. Mixed infections are quite common.[60] *Escherichia coli*, *Klebsiella* species, *Enterobacter* species, and *Streptococcus faecalis* (enterococcus) are the organisms most commonly isolated.[60, 62, 78–80] Anaerobes, including *Clostridium perfringens* and *Bacteroides fragilis*, are not uncommon.[78, 81, 82] In a few reported series, the incidence of sepsis from *B. fragilis* was as high as 40%.[81, 82] Other organisms such as *Pseudomonas* species, *Proteus* species, and *Staphylococcus aureus* have been identified, but these are rare.

Diagnostic Studies

In addition to routine blood counts, biochemical studies, and blood cultures, certain noninvasive imaging studies are helpful in establishing the diagnosis and arriving at a treatment plan for cholangitis. Sonographic studies are useful because the equipment is portable, the test is inexpensive, and there is no exposure to radiation. The sonogram detects the presence of extrahepatic obstruction in 96% of cases in which the biliary tree is dilated.[83] Dilatation may not be present, either because of spontaneous stone clearance before the diagnostic study or because of an accelerated syndrome that develops before dilatation occurs. Ultrasound detection of stones in the common bile duct is not reliable.[84] Computed tomographic scanning is useful in detecting mass lesions, especially of the pancreatic duct, and computed tomographic scans are considered more accurate than ultrasound scans in detecting common bile duct stones, especially calcium bilirubinate stones, when closer cuts (5 mm) are made. Both ultrasonography and computed tomography may detect hepatic abscesses, although these are usually small and not appreciated early.

Radionuclide scanning has been reported to demonstrate bile duct obstruction and dilatation earlier than ultrasonography. Two retrospective studies supported these findings,[85, 86] but prospective studies are needed before making any firm recommendations because radionuclide scans are not as specific as ultrasound scans.

Cholangiography, percutaneous or endoscopic, provides an immediate, direct, and most often, accurate diagnosis to support the impression of acute cholangitis. The choice or preference of either modality, percutaneous or endoscopic, depends on the availability of the facilities and the expertise of the particular specialists. Coagulopathy and massive ascites are contraindications to percutaneous transhepatic cholangiography and favor endoscopy, whereas anatomic variations such as previous gastric surgery favor the percutaneous route. Cholangiographic studies also can detect hepatic microabscesses that are not appreciated by other modalities.[87] Microabscesses appear as multiple small ectatic

areas affecting the smaller intrahepatic ducts. The choice of procedures is also influenced by the local expertise

Treatment
Medical Therapy

Initially, if the patient is hypotensive, he or she must be stabilized hemodynamically. To achieve stabilization, correcting the fluid and electrolyte imbalance is accomplished by administering large volumes of intravenous fluids. Specific antibiotics are started immediately. Close clinical and laboratory monitoring is essential. In mild cases, a single antibiotic, cefoxitin or cefotetan, should be sufficient. In more severe cases, triple antibiotic therapy (a combination of a third-generation cephalosporin, ampicillin, and metronidazole) is essential. Additional coverage for gram-negative organisms is recommended when these specific organisms are isolated, sepsis is documented, and there is little or no response using triple therapy. Aminoglycosides are specific for gram-negative organisms and should be started early if the patient's clinical course does not improve. Eighty-five percent of patients with cholangitis have a mild case and respond to the conservative measures mentioned earlier. Approximately 15% of cases do not respond to aggressive medical therapy, and without intervention, death may ensue.[59, 62, 67] Those patients who are severely ill must undergo immediate decompression of the biliary tree, which can be achieved by surgery, percutaneous transhepatic biliary drainage (PTBD), or endoscopic methods (Fig. 131–2).

Surgical Decompression

Operative therapy for cholangitis was first advocated as early as 1903 when Rogers placed a glass tube within the bile duct of a patient with common bile duct stones and cholangitis, providing decompression and drainage.[88] Independently, in 1945, Grant and Cole published their small series of patients who benefited from surgical decompres-

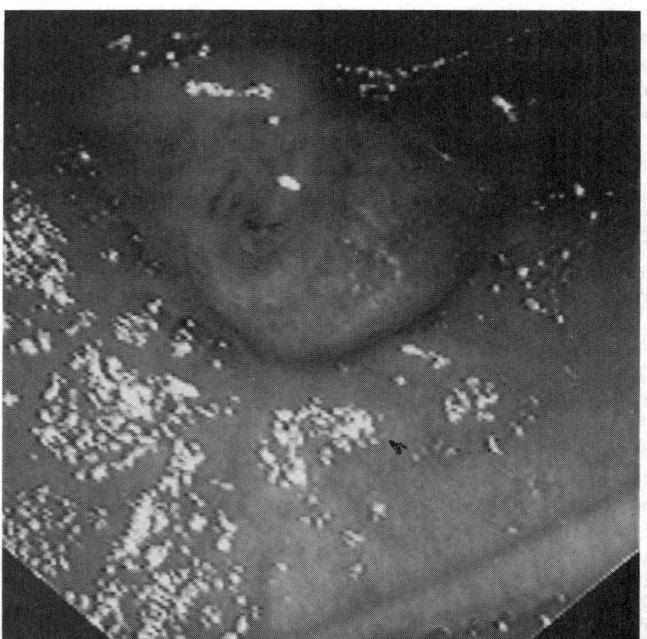

Figure 131–2. Papilla seen endoscopically after stone passage. (From Siegel JH: Endoscopic Retrograde Cholangiopancreatography: Technique, Diagnosis, and Therapy. New York, Raven Press, p 145, 1991.)

sion, reporting 100 and 85% survival rates, respectively.[89, 90] Results of emergency surgery for cholangitis, however, have been disappointing, as surgery in a patient requiring vasopressors carries a high morbidity and mortality. The mortality rate after early surgical decompression varies from 7 to 40%.[59, 60, 62, 64, 65, 67, 91, 92] Higher mortality rates are associated with comorbid conditions, including advanced age; intercurrent, chronic medical illnesses; and delay in surgical decompression.

The surgical approach to cholangitis, which may also include endoscopy and percutaneous transhepatic cholangiography, is dictated by the clinical status of the patient. In patients who are critically ill, the procedure should be limited to choledochotomy and T tube drainage with or without concomitant cholecystostomy. If the patient survives this operative approach, elective common bile duct clearance and cholecystectomy, common bile duct exploration, and T tube drainage or a biliary enteric anastomosis are indicated. In patients who are moribund, cholecystostomy with local anesthesia is an alternative approach, provided the cystic duct is patent.[79] However, the mortality after cholecystostomy alone is extremely high owing to ineffective drainage of the biliary system[59, 62, 64] and associated comorbid conditions. Currently, with the availability of percutaneous and endoscopic techniques, surgical decompression in extremely high-risk conditions may be obviated in favor of the less morbid, nonsurgical procedures.

Percutaneous Transhepatic Biliary Drainage

Since its introduction more than 50 years ago, percutaneous transhepatic cholangiography has become an important and universally available diagnostic modality in the clinical work-up of patients with jaundice.[93] The therapeutic dimensions of percutaneous transhepatic cholangiography were first introduced by Molnar and Stockhum in 1974.[94] Their method of drainage was successful in more than 90% of attempts, especially in the presence of a dilated biliary tree. Proximal bile duct lesions are managed more easily by the percutaneous route than by endoscopic means because of the easier access presented by proximal dilatation. The percutaneous approach, however, has increased morbidity and mortality[95–98] when compared with endoscopy. Frequent complications that are associated with the percutaneous method include bleeding, biliary leak and peritonitis, liver abscess, pneumothorax, catheter dislodgment, biliary-portal fistula, and bacteremia. Catheter-related sepsis is the most frequent (40%) of all these complications, particularly when prolonged drainage is necessary.[95] Percutaneous sessions often require additional procedures to clear the ducts when stones are demonstrated, which include percutaneous catheter extraction[75, 99, 100] and dissolution methods.[101]

In 1985, Gould and colleagues reported their results in treating seven patients with acute cholangitis using PTBD. Two patients (29%) died after manipulation.[99] Kadir and colleagues reported morbidity and mortality rates of 33 and 17%, respectively, in a group of 18 patients undergoing PTBD for the treatment of obstructive jaundice.[100] In a retrospective study, Kinoshita and coworkers reported a decreased mortality rate in patients who underwent PTBD (14%) instead of urgent surgery (20%), but these data were not statistically significant.[75] McPherson and associates conducted a controlled prospective randomized trial incorporating PTBD followed by surgery.[97] In their study, they found a significantly higher postoperative mortality rate (32% vs. 19%) in the PTBD group than in patients who underwent surgical intervention without prior percutaneous drainage of the biliary tract.[97]

The percutaneous approach is not recommended as the

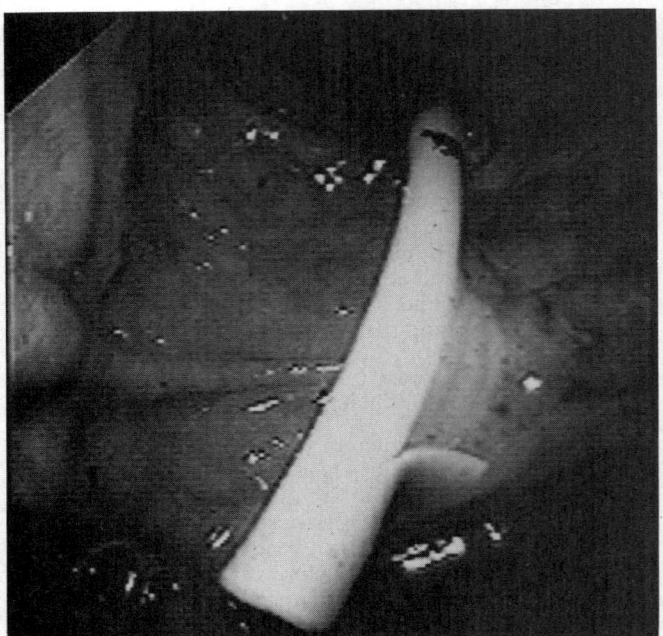

Figure 131–3. Stent placed into the bile duct for treatment of cholangitis. Note the white, purulent material flowing from the stent. (From Siegel JH: Endoscopic Retrograde Cholangiopancreatography: Technique, Diagnosis, and Therapy. New York, Raven Press, p 215, 1991.)

first choice or definitive treatment if endoscopic drainage is available. PTBD is recommended only when the endoscopic approach fails to establish drainage or is not available.

Endoscopic Therapy

Endoscopic sphincterotomy, stone extraction, and placement of either prostheses or nasobiliary drains are well established as safe and effective therapeutic procedures[102, 103] (Fig. 131–3). The overall success rate for sphincterotomy and ductal clearance of stones exceeds 90%.[104, 105] The 30-day mortality experienced in the authors' personal series of more than 5000 sphincterotomies is only 0.09%, with a morbidity of 5.5%[106] (Table 131–3).

Most reports of endoscopic therapy for the management of acute suppurative cholangitis have been retrospective. In 1980, Siegel reported the use of sphincterotomy in managing 83 patients with acute cholangitis.[107] In 1982, Vallon and coworkers reported success in treating 12 of 14 patients

TABLE 131–3

COMPLICATIONS OF ENDOSCOPIC SPHINCTEROTOMY
(N = 5370)

Complication	Number of Patients	Percentage
Bleeding	94	
Cholangitis	53	>5.2
Pancreatitis	103	
Perforation, pain	21	
Emergency surgery	15	0.28
Deaths	5	0.09
Transfusion	35	0.7

Adapted from Siegel JH: Endoscopic Retrograde Cholangiopancreatography: Technique, Diagnosis, and Therapy. New York, Raven Press, p 216, 1991.

ENDOSCOPIC MANAGEMENT OF CHOLANGITIS
(947 Patients)

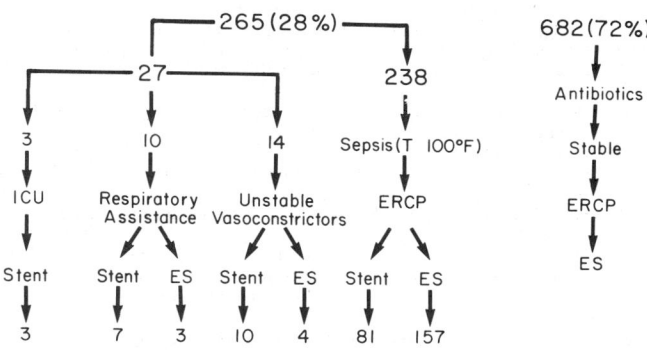

Figure 131–4. Endoscopic management of cholangitis (947 patients). T = temperature; ICU = intensive care unit; ES = endoscopic sphincterotomy. (From Siegel JH: Endoscopic Retrograde Cholangiopancreatography: Technique, Diagnosis, and Therapy. New York, Raven Press, p 212, 1991.)

using endoscopic sphincterotomy, stone extraction, or biliary prostheses placement.[108] Similarly encouraging results were reported by Delmott and colleagues.[109]

Gogel and associates managed 13 high-risk patients utilizing ERCP and endoscopic sphincterotomy and successfully extracted stones in 10 patients who experienced immediate improvement. Three patients of this group required surgery, and one of these patients died.[110]

Siegel and associates tabulated their experience in managing 947 patients with cholangitis[111] (Fig. 131–4). Six hundred eighty-two patients (72%) were stable with either a low-grade fever or no fever and were maintained on antibiotics. Two hundred sixty-five (28%) of the total were unstable, with a temperature greater than 100°F; 27 of these required vasopressors, 10 were undergoing mechanical respiration, and 3 were treated in the intensive care unit. Most patients improved with endoscopic sphincterotomy, stone extraction, or prosthesis placement. A low morbidity rate (6%) was experienced. There were no procedure-related deaths. In this study, the overall mortality (deaths occurring in 30 days after drainage and not procedure related) was 0.42% (4 of 947); the mortality, however, for the acutely ill patients was 7.4% (2 of 27), and the mortality for those who were more stable but ill was 1.5% (4 of 265).

Leese and coworkers, in a retrospective study of 82 patients with acute cholangitis, reported the successful use of endoscopic therapy.[112] All patients in this study were treated with antibiotics. Endoscopic sphincterotomy was selected in 43 patients and surgery in 28, and 11 patients had neither. Four of the latter group were moribund and died before they could be stabilized for decompression therapy (mortality rate, 36.4%), 6 of 28 surgical patients (21.4%) died, and only 2 of 43 patients in the endoscopic sphincterotomy group (4.7%) died. These data were achieved despite the greater risk for the patients in the endoscopic group who were older and had a higher number of medical risk factors. A morbidity rate of 57% occurred in the surgically treated patients compared with 28% in the endoscopic group. Although the study was retrospective and nonrandomized, the results remain impressive.

Similarly encouraging reports have been published by Leung and colleagues, who treated 105 patients with acute suppurative cholangitis.[113] In their series, the success rate of endoscopic therapy was 97% and the overall mortality was 4.7%.

Thus, it has been shown that endoscopic therapy offers a safer and effective therapeutic option for patients with acute suppurative cholangitis who fail to respond to conservative and supportive measures, which include administration of antibiotics and intensive supportive therapy. No data are available for the timing of endoscopic interventional decompression, but on the basis of surgical series, early (<24 hours) intervention is associated with decreased mortality.[62] In treating stone disease, if extraction techniques fail, or if the procedure time is limited and an expeditious regimen is favored, drainage can be provided by either a nasobiliary catheter or internal biliary stents. If endoscopic drainage fails in calculous or noncalculous biliary disease, PTBD is recommended first before surgery especially in patients who are not stable. If both nonsurgical modalities fail, the patient should be referred for surgery, accepting the known higher mortality and morbidity rates. Early surgery may be necessary for patients who fail to improve after successful endoscopic or percutaneous drainage. Further therapy for patients who improve after endoscopic drainage is dependent on the patient's suitability as a surgical candidate. Younger patients and low surgical risk patients should undergo cholecystectomy. On the other hand, patients who are older or at greater risk because of comorbid medical problems should not undergo surgery. Leaving the gallbladder in situ in such patients has been shown not to increase risks, morbidity, or mortality.[114] The decision to pursue further therapy largely depends on the state of health of the patient and should be arrived at after careful and thorough discussions with all parties concerned. A clear understanding of all risks and alternatives must be taken into consideration.

References

1. Paloyan D, Simonowitz D: Diagnostic considerations in acute alcoholic and gallstone pancreatitis. Am J Surg 132:329, 1976.
2. McMahon M, Pickford IR: Biochemical prediction of gallstones early in an attack of acute pancreatitis. Lancet 2:541, 1979.
3. Classen M: Endoscopic papillotomy—New indications, short and long term results. Clin Gastroenterol 15:446, 1986.
4. Frey CF: Gallstone pancreatitis. Surg Clin North Am 61:923, 1981.
5. Bernard C: Lecors de Physiologie Experimental. Paris, JB Bailliere, 1856.
6. Lancereau E: Traité des Maladies du Foie et du Pancreas. Paris, O Poin, 1899.
7. Opie EL: The relationship of cholelithiasis to disease of the pancreas and fat necrosis. Am J Med Surg 12:27, 1901.
8. Poncelet P, Thompson AG: Action of bile phospholipids on the pancreas. Am J Surg 123:196, 1972.
9. Elliott W, Williams RD, Ollinger RM: Alteration in pancreatic resistance to bile in the pathogenesis of acute pancreatitis. Ann Surg 14:669, 1957.
10. Dragstedt LR, Haymond HE, Ellis C: Pathogenesis of pancreatitis (acute pancreatic necrosis). Arch Surg 28:232, 1934.
11. Siegel JH, Tone P, Menikem D: Gallstone pancreatitis: Pathogenesis and clinical forms—The emerging role of endoscopic management. Am J Gastroenterol 81:744, 1986.
12. Acosta JM, Ledesma CL: Gallstone migration as a cause of acute pancreatitis. N Engl J Med 290:484, 1974.
13. Kelly TR, Swaney PE: Gallstone pancreatitis: The second time around. Surgery 92:571, 1982.
14. Acosta JMO, Rossi R, Galli OMR, et al: Early surgery for acute gallstone pancreatitis: Evaluation of a systematic approach. Surgery 83:367, 1978.
15. Cuschieri A, Hughes JH: Pancreatic reflux during operative choledochography. Br J Surg 60:933, 1973.
16. Kelly TR: Gallstone pancreatitis: Pathophysiology. Surgery 80:488, 1976.
17. Armstrong CP, Taylor TV, Jeacock J, et al: The biliary tract in patients with acute gallstone pancreatitis. Br J Surg 72:551, 1978.
18. Jones BA, Salsberg BB, Mehta MH, et al: Common pancreaticobiliary channels and their relationship to gallstone size in gallstone pancreatitis. Ann Surg 205:123, 1987.
19. Mann FC, Giordano AS: The bile factor in pancreatitis. Arch Surg 6:1, 1923.
20. Manguy RB, Hallenbeck GA, Bollman JC, et al: Intraductal pressures and sphincteric resistance in canine pancreatic and biliary ducts after various stimuli. Surg Gynecol Obstet 106:306, 1958.
21. Robinson TM, Dunphy JE: Continuous perfusion of bile protease activators through the pancreas. JAMA 183:530, 1963.
22. McCutcheon AD: Reflux of duodenal contents in the pathogenesis of pancreatitis. Gut 9:296, 1968.

23. Saluja A, Saluja M, Rutledge PL, et al: Effect of pancreatic duct obstruction on the subcellular distribution of lysosomal enzymes in rabbit pancreas. Dig Dis Sci 32:1186, 1987.

24. Houssin D, Castaing D, Lemoine J, et al: Microlithiasis of the gallbladder. Surg Gynecol Obstet 157:20, 1983.

25. McMahon MJ, Shefta JR: Physical characteristics of gallstone and the calibre of the cystic duct in patients with acute pancreatitis. Br J Surg 67:6, 1980.

26. Kelly TR: Gallstone pancreatitis: Local predisposing factors. Ann Surg 200:479, 1984.

27. Williamson RCN: Early assessment of severity in acute pancreatitis. Gut 25:1331, 1984.

28. Knaus WA, Draper EA, Wagner DI, et al: APACHE II: A severity of disease classification system. Crit Care Med 13:818, 1985.

29. Neoptolemos JP, Carr-Locke DL, London NJ, et al: ERCP findings and the role of endoscopic sphincterotomy in acute gallstone pancreatitis. Br J Surg 10:954, 1988.

30. DeBolla AR, Obeid ML: Mortality in acute pancreatitis. Ann R Coll Surg Engl 66:184, 1984.

31. Stone HH, Fabian TC, Dunlop WE: Gallstone pancreatitis. Ann Surg 194:305, 1981.

32. McKay AJ, Duncan JG, Imrie CW, et al: A prospective study of clinical value and accuracy of grey scale ultrasound in detecting gallstones. Br J Surg 65:330, 1978.

33. Maier W: Early objective diagnosis and staging of acute pancreatitis by contrast-enhanced computed tomography. In: Beger HG, Buchler M (eds): Acute Pancreatitis. New York, Springer-Verlag, p 132, 1987.

34. Aldridge MC: Diagnosis of pancreatic necrosis. Br J Surg 75:99, 1988.

35. Faris I, Thompson JPS, Grundy DJ, et al: Operative cholangiography: A reappraisal based on a review of 400 cholangiograms. Br J Surg 62:966, 1975.

36. Acosta JM, Rossi R, Ledesma CL: The usefulness of stool screening for diagnosing cholelithiasis in acute pancreatitis. A description of the technique. Am J Dig Dis 22:168, 1977.

37. Ranson JHC: The timing of biliary surgery in acute pancreatitis. Ann Surg 189:654, 1979.

38. Frey CF: The operative treatment of pancreatitis. Arch Surg 98:406, 1969.

39. Sato T, Saiton Y, Noto N, et al: Clinicopathological studies on the relationship between cholelithiasis and chronic pancreatitis. Ohoku J Exp Med 113:97, 1974.

40. Medical Research Council Multicenter Trial of Glucagon and Aprotinin. Death from acute pancreatitis. Lancet 2:632, 1977.

41. Glen FG, Frey CF: Re-evaluation of the treatment of pancreatitis associated with biliary tract disease. Ann Surg 160:723, 1964.

42. Frey CF, Lindenauer SW, Miller TA: Pancreatic abscess. Surg Gynecol Obstet 149:722, 1979.

43. Kelly TR, Wagner DS: Gallstone pancreatitis: A prospective randomized trial of the timing of surgery. Surgery 4:600, 1988.

44. Kelly TR: Gallstone pancreatitis. The timing of surgery. Surgery 88:345, 1980.

45. Osborne DH, Imrie CW, Carter DC: Biliary surgery in the same admission for gallstone associated acute pancreatitis. Br J Surg 68:758, 1981.

46. Tondelli P, Stutz K, Harder F, et al: Acute gallstone pancreatitis. Best timing for biliary surgery. Br J Surg 69:709, 1982.

47. Safrany L, Cotton PB: A preliminary report. Urgent duodenoscopic sphincterotomy for acute gallstone pancreatitis. Surgery 89:424, 1981.

48. Rosseland AR, Solhaug JH: Early or delayed endoscopic papillotomy (EPT) in gallstone pancreatitis. Ann Surg 199:165, 1984.

49. van der Spuy S: Endoscopic sphincterotomy in the management of gallstone pancreatitis. Endoscopy 13:25, 1981.

50. Escourrou J, Liguory C, Boyer J, et al: Emergency endoscopic sphincterotomy in acute biliary pancreatitis: Results of a multicenter study (abstract). Gastroenterology 92:1385, 1987.

51. Neoptolemos JP, Carr-Locke DL, London NJ, et al: Controlled trial of urgent endoscopic retrograde cholangiopancreatography and endoscopic sphincterotomy versus conservative treatment for acute pancreatitis due to gallstones. Lancet 2:979, 1988.

52. Siegel JH: Endoscopic management of patients with intact gallbladders and gallstone pancreatitis: Controversy or reality? In: Syllabus: Proceedings of the American Society for Gastrointestinal Endoscopy's Fourth National Postgraduate Course. Advances in Therapeutic Endoscopy. Washington, DC, January 30–February 1, 1987.

53. Siegel JH: Endoscopic sphincterotomy: When is it appropriate? In: Barkin JS, Rogers AI (eds): Difficult Decisions in Digestive Diseases. Boca Raton, FL, Year Book Medical Publishers, p 551, 1989.

54. Charcot JM: Leçon sur les Maladies du Foie des Voies Filiares et des Reins. Paris, Faculté de Médecine de Paris, 1877.

55. Reynolds BM, Dargan EL: Acute obstructive cholangitis: A distinct clinical syndrome. Ann Surg 150:299, 1959.

56. Boey JH, Way LW: Acute cholangitis. Ann Surg 191:264, 1980.

57. Dow RW, Lindenauer SM: Acute obstructive suppurative cholangitis. Ann Surg 169:272, 1969.

58. Glenn F, Moody FG: Acute obstructive suppurative cholangitis. Surg Gynecol Obstet 113:265, 1961.

59. Hinchey EJ, Couper CE: Acute obstructive suppurative cholangitis. Am J Surg 117:62, 1969.

60. Haupert AP, Carey LC, Evans WE, et al: Acute suppurative cholangitis. Arch Surg 94:460, 1967.

61. Longmire WP Jr: Suppurative cholangitis. In: Hardy JD (ed): Critical Surgical Illness. Philadelphia, WB Saunders, 1971.

62. Welch JP, Donaldson GA: The urgency of diagnosis and surgical treatment of acute suppurative cholangitis. Am J Surg 131:527, 1976.

63. O'Connor MJ, Schwartz ML, McQuarrie DG, et al: Acute bacterial cholangitis, an analysis of clinical manifestations. Arch Surg 117:437, 1982.

64. Leese T, Neoptolemos JP, Baker AR, et al: The management of acute cholangitis and the impact of endoscopic sphincterotomy. Br J Surg 73:988, 1986.

65. Saharia PC, Cameron JL: Clinical management of acute cholangitis. Surg Gynecol Obstet 142:369, 1976.

66. Saik RP, Greenburg AG, Farris JM, et al: Spectrum of cholangitis. Am J Surg 130:143, 1975.

67. Andrew DJ, Johnson SE: Acute suppurative cholangitis; A medical and surgical emergency. Am J Gastroenterol 54:141, 1970.

68. Vennes JA: Management of calculi in the common duct. Semin Liver Dis 3:162, 1983.

69. Pitkin H, Beal JM: Choledocholithiasis associated with acute cholecystectitis. Arch Surg 114:887, 1979.

70. Stubbs RS, McLoy RF, Blumgart LH: Cholelithiasis and cholecystitis: Surgical treatment. Clin Gastroenterol 12:179, 1983.

71. Lygidakis NJ: Bile infection: Its incidence and significance in biliary lithiasis. Am J Gastroenterol 77:210, 1982.

72. Schotton WE, Desprez JD, Holden WA: A bacteriological study of portal vein blood in man. Arch Surg 71:404, 1955.

73. Dineen P: The importance of the route of injection in experimental biliary tract obstruction. Surg Gynecol Obstet 119:1001, 1964.

74. Ong GB: A study of recurrent pyogenic cholangitis. Arch Surg 84:199, 1962.

75. Kinoshita H, Hitohashi K, Igawa S, et al: Cholangitis. World J Surg 8:963, 1984.

76. Edlung YA, Mollstedt BO, Ouchterlony O: Bacteriological investigation of the biliary system and liver in biliary tract disease correlated to clinical data and microstructure of the gallbladder and liver. Acta Chir Scand 116:461, 1959.

77. Huang T, Bass JAB, Williams RD, et al: The significance of biliary pressure in cholangitis. Arch Surg 98:629, 1969.

78. Finegold SM: Anaerobes in biliary tract infections. Arch Intern Med 139:1338, 1979.

79. Hinshaw DB: Acute obstructive suppurative cholangitis. Surg Clin North Am 53:1089, 1973.

80. Keighley MRB, Drysdale RB, Quoraishi AH, et al: Antibiotic treatment of biliary sepsis. Surg Clin North Am 55:1379, 1975.

81. Bourgault AM, England DM, Rosenblatt FE: Clinical characteristics of anaerobic bacterobilia. Arch Intern Med 139:1346, 1979.

82. Shimada K, Inamatsu T, Yamashiro M: Anaerobic bacteria in biliary disease of elderly patients. J Infect Dis 135:850, 1977.

83. Taylor KJW, Rosenfield AT, Spiro HM: Diagnostic accuracy of gray scale ultrasonography for the jaundiced patient. Arch Intern Med 139:60, 1979.

84. Einstein DM, Lapin SA, Ralls PW, et al: The insensitivity of sonography in the detection of choledocholithiasis. AJR 143:725, 1984.

85. Kaplun L, Weisman HS, Rosenblatt RR, et al: The early diagnosis of common bile duct obstruction using cholescintigraphy. JAMA 254:2431, 1985.

86. Miller DR, Egbert RM, Braunstein P: Comparison of ultrasound and hepaticobiliary imaging in the early detection of acute total common bile duct obstruction. Arch Surg 119:1233, 1984.

87. Neoptolemos JP, Macpherson DS, Holm J, et al: Pyogenic liver abscess: A study of forty-four cases in two centres. Acta Chir Scand 148:415, 1982.

88. Rogers L: Biliary abscess of the liver with operation. Br Med J 2:706, 1903.

89. Grant HD: Acute suppurative cholangitis. Permanente Found Med Bull 3:175, 1945.

90. Cole WN: Suppurative cholangitis. Surg Clin North Am 27:23, 1947.

91. Thompson JE, Tompkins RK, Longmire WP: Factors in management of acute cholangitis. Ann Surg 195:137, 1982.

92. Lygidakis NJ, Brummelkamp WH: The significance of intrabiliary pressure in acute cholangitis. Surg Gynecol Obstet 161:465, 1985.

93. Dodd GD: Percutaneous transhepatic cholangiography. Surg Clin North Am 47:1095, 1967.

94. Molnar W, Stockhum AE: Relief of obstructive jaundice through percutaneous transhepatic catheter: A new therapeutic method. AJR 122:356, 1974.

95. Joseph PK, Bizer LS, Sprayregen SS, et al: Percutaneous transhepatic biliary drainage: Results and complications in 81 patients. JAMA 255:2763, 1986.

96. Smith RC, Pooley M, George CR, et al: Preoperative percutaneous transhepatic internal drainage in obstructive jaundice: A randomized, controlled trial examining renal function. Surgery 97:641, 1985.

97. McPherson GA, Benjamin IS, Hodgson HJ, et al: Pre-operative percutaneous biliary drainage: The results of a controlled trial. Br J Surg 71:371, 1984.

98. Audiosio A, Bozzetti F, Severini A, et al: The occurrence of cholangitis after percutaneous drainage: Evaluation of some risk factors. Surgery 103:507, 1988.

99. Gould RJ, Vogelzang RL, Nieman HL, et al: Percutaneous biliary drainage as an initial therapy in sepsis of the biliary tract. Surg Gynecol Obstet 160:523, 1985.

100. Kadir S, Baassiri A, Barth KH, et al: Percutaneous biliary drainage in the management of biliary sepsis. AJR 138:25, 1982.

101. Allen MJ, Borody TJ, Bugliosi TF, et al: Rapid dissolution of gallstones by methyl ter-butyl ether. N Engl J Med 321:217, 1985.

102. Kawai K, Akasaka Y, Murakami K, et al: Endoscopic sphincterotomy of the ampulla of Vater. Gastrointest Endosc 20:148, 1974.

103. Classen M, Demling L: Endokopische Sphinkterotomie der Papilla Vateri und Steinextraktion aus dem Ductus choledochus. Dtsch Med Wochenschr 99:496, 1974.

104. Siegel J: Endoscopic papillotomy: Sphincterotomy or sphincteroplasty. Am J Gastroenterol 72:511, 1979.

105. Cotton PB: Endoscopic management of bile duct stones—Apples and oranges. Gut 25:587, 1984.

106. Siegel JH: Endoscopic Retrograde Cholangiopancreatography: Technique, Diagnosis, and Therapy. New York, Raven Press, 1991.

107. Siegel JH: Endoscopic papillotomy. A definitive treatment for cholangitis. Gastroenterology 78:1259, 1980.

108. Vallon AG, Shorvon PJ, Cotton PB: Duodenoscopic treatment of acute cholangitis (abstract). Gut 23:A915, 1982.

109. Delmott JS, Pommelet P, Houcke P, et al: Initial duodenoscopic sphincterotomy in patients with acute cholangitis or pancreatitis complicating biliary stones (abstract). Gastroenterology 82:1042, 1982.

110. Gogel HK, Runyon B, Volpicelli NA: Acute suppurative obstructive cholangitis due to stones: Treatment by urgent endoscopic sphincterotomy. Gastrointest Endosc 33:210, 1987.

111. Siegel JH, Ramsey WH, Pullano W: Endoscopic management of 947 patients with cholangitis: Proven safety and efficacy (abstract). Gastrointest Endosc 32:154, 1986.

112. Leese T, Neoptolemos JP, Baker AR, et al: Management of acute cholangitis and the impact of endoscopic sphincterotomy. Br J Surg 73:988, 1986.

113. Leung JWC, Chung SCS, Sung JJY, et al: Urgent endoscopic drainage for acute suppurative cholangitis. Lancet 1:1307, 1989.

114. Siegel JH, Safrany L, Ben-Zvi JS, et al: Duodenoscopic sphincterotomy in patients with gallbladder in situ: Report of a series of 1272 patients. Am J Gastroenterol 83:1255, 1988.

CHAPTER 132

Pancreatitis

Dean Railey
Jamie S. Barkin

The goal of this chapter is to update clinicians on this common condition and further the readers' understanding of acute pancreatic inflammation and its sequela. The authors try to take a balanced approach summarized as never being the first to embrace the new or the last to throw the old aside.

Acute pancreatitis typically occurs with abdominal pain, nausea with vomiting, and elevated pancreatic enzyme levels.[1] The pathogenesis of acute pancreatitis is activation of pancreatic enzymes with resulting parenchymal autodigestion, which by definition results in no permanent functional or morphologic damage to the gland.[2] Chronic pancreatitis, however, by conventional definition has permanent morphologic damage. The relationship between acute pancreatitis and chronic pancreatitis remains unclear. Acute pancreatitis rarely leads to chronic pancreatitis, except that originating from alcohol. In patients with acute alcoholic pancreatitis, pathologic evidence of chronic pancreatitis is present at the initial clinical episode of acute pancreatitis. Clinically, exacerbations of chronic pancreatitis mimic acute episodes of pancreatitis.

The incidence of acute pancreatitis varies in smaller cities depending on the population studied, whereas in larger cities, it was found to be 10 per 100,000 with a mortality of 1 per 100,000.[3] There is no sexual predominance, and the incidence rises from the fourth to seventh decade (median age, 53 years), which most likely reflects the increasing incidence of cholelithiasis with increasing age.[4] In the majority of patients, acute pancreatitis is a self-limiting disease that responds to medical management, whereas in the remaining 5 to 15%, the disease is fulminant and has an associated mortality of up to 20%, and 60% of this small group may have potentially lethal complications.[5] One of the initial goals of the clinician is the early identification of these patients, in the hope of improving their survival.[6]

PATHOGENESIS

Acute pancreatitis is usually an isolated episode resulting from autodigestion. Normally, pancreatic enzymes are secreted in an inactive form (proenzymes) and are activated in the duodenum by enterokinase originating from the intestinal mucosa as well as trypsin. However, in acute pancreatitis, the inactive enzymes are prematurely transformed within the pancreas into active enzymes. Although the exact sequence of events leading to this premature activation has not been elucidated, it is believed that minute amounts of trypsin activate the proenzymes of phospholipase A and elastase.[7] The leading hypothesis of events that result in this proenzyme activation include (1) outflow obstruction of pancreatic secretions;[8] (2) reflux of duodenal contents through the sphincter of Oddi, into the pancreatic duct;[9] and (3) the common channel theory of Opie with bile reflux into the pancreatic duct resulting from gallstone obstruction of the ampulla of Vater.[10] However, whether one or all are applicable is unclear.

ETIOLOGY

The conditions that are associated with acute pancreatitis are listed in Table 132–1.[11–18] Gallstones remain the most common cause (55%) of acute pancreatitis in private hospitals and the second most common cause (30%) in city hospitals.[19] There is a well-established association of pancreatitis with gallstones, especially with stones less than 3 mm in diameter.[20] Episodes of recurrent pancreatitis occur in approximately 50% of patients whose gallstones are left untreated.[21] Alcohol-related pancreatitis is the most common type of acute pancreatitis in public hospitals. The mortality rate in patients with alcohol-related pancreatitis is lower than that in patients with gallstone pancreatitis, probably because these patients are younger and many have underlying chronic pancreatitis.[19, 22]

Multiple medications have been associated with acute pancreatitis (Table 132–2), and it is imperative that a drug-induced or -associated cause is not overlooked.[23] A drug may produce pancreatitis, even though the patient has been ingesting it for some time. Postoperative pancreatitis may develop after a variety of intra-abdominal surgical procedures, and although the mechanism of injury has been believed to be due to direct operative trauma, it may result from vascular compromise with the development of ischemic pancreatitis. Pancreatitis may occur after cardiopulmonary bypass and has been described as severe with an associated high mortality. However, this was due to study bias.[24] A

TABLE 132–1

CONDITIONS ASSOCIATED WITH ACUTE PANCREATITIS*

70% of Cases
Gallstones (number 1 in private hospitals)
Alcohol (number 1 in public hospitals)

20% of Cases
Medications (see Table 132–2)
Postoperative (abdominal, cardiac, transplant surgery)
Trauma (number 1 in young people)
Post-ERCP (1% of ERCPs)
Hyperlipidemia (types I, IV, and V)
Hypercalcemia (hyperparathyroidism, myeloma, TPN)
? Pancreas divisum
Infectious agents
   Viral: mumps, coxsackie B, CMV, Epstein-Barr, hepatitis
   Bacterial: *Mycoplasma, Campylobacter, Legionella*
   Parasitic: *Clonorchis sinensis,* ascaris worms
Pregnancy (90% gallstone associated, third trimester)
Scorpion bite (Trinidad, West Indies)
Ampullary disease: ampulloma
Hereditary
Penetrating duodenal ulcer
Connective tissue disorders with vasculitis
Eating disorders (anorexia nervosa, bulimia)

10% of Cases
Idiopathic

*ERCP = endoscopic retrograde cholangiopancreatography; TPN = total parenteral nutrition; CMV = cytomegalovirus.

prospective evaluation of the occurrence of pancreatitis after cardiopulmonary bypass found that chemical pancreatitis occurred in more than 50% of patients. Clinical pancreatitis was rare and had no effect on mortality (Barkin JS, unpublished data).

Trauma is the most common cause of pancreatitis in young people. Blunt trauma (resulting from automobile steering wheels and bicycle handlebars) as well as penetrating injuries is responsible.[25] It is important to suspect acute pancreatitis in this setting and document main ductular rupture. This can be accomplished only preoperatively by endoscopic retrograde cholangiopancreatography (ERCP). Clinically evident pancreatitis develops in approximately 1% of patients after ERCP.[26] Precipitating factors that have been implicated include the speed, volume, and pressure of injection as well as the underlying pancreatic anatomy, the presence of a patent minor ampulla, and the type of contrast material used.

Patients with Fredrickson's types I, IV, and V hyperlipoproteinemia are at risk for the development of acute pancreatitis.[27] Pancreatitis occurs in 27 to 41% of patients with the type IV pattern.[28] Hypercalcemia of any origin, including total parenteral nutrition (TPN) and familial hypocalciuric

TABLE 132–2

MEDICATIONS ASSOCIATED WITH ACUTE PANCREATITIS

Antimetabolites	Hormonal agents
Azathioprine	Estrogen
L-Asparaginase	Anticonvulsants
Antibiotics	Valproic acid
Sulfonamides	Others
Tetracycline	Phenformin
Metronidazole (Flagyl)	Procainamide
Diuretics	
Hydrochlorothiazide	
Furosemide	

hypercalcemia, may lead to acute pancreatitis.[29, 30] Pancreas divisum is a congenital condition in which there is nonfusion of the dorsal with the ventral pancreatic ducts.[31] It is found in up to 10% of the population.[32] Controversy exists regarding whether it is associated with pancreatitis. There seems to be a subgroup of patients with pancreas divisum who have changes of chronic pancreatitis in their main pancreatic duct, originating from the dorsal pancreatic bed embryologically and connecting to the minor ampulla. Therefore, it is essential to visualize the dorsal duct at ERCP when pancreatic divisum is present.

There is a 2 to 7% incidence of acute pancreatitis in patients who have undergone renal transplantation.[33] This group has many possible predisposing factors, including drugs, such as the immunosuppressant agents (e.g., azathioprine and L-asparaginase); secondary hyperparathyroidism with hypercalcemia; vasculitis; and superimposed viral infections. Acute pancreatitis is also seen often in patients who have undergone cardiac transplantation, in which intraoperative hypotension may be contributory,[34] as well as the factors seen in renal transplantation.

Infectious causes are frequently unrecognized and commonly include viral, bacterial, and parasitic origins. These causes are especially prominent in immunocompromised patients. Pancreatitis occurring during pregnancy originates from gallstones in 90% of patients.[19] These are most likely to occur in the third trimester or post partum and are believed to be secondary to the lithogenic effects of pregnancy.[35, 36] The overall prognosis is good and the treatment is elective, postpartum cholecystectomy. ERCP with endoscopic sphincterotomy and stone removal can be safely performed during pregnancy but should be utilized only in selected patients. Similarly to gallstones, other causes of obstruction of the ampulla of Vater may result in acute pancreatitis. These processes include congenital abnormalities such as duodenal duplication, annular pancreas, and periampullary diverticula;[37, 38] inflammatory and neoplastic diseases such as Crohn's disease and non-Hodgkin's lymphoma;[39] and mechanical obstruction, such as a trichobezoar[40] or afferent loop obstruction after gastrojejunostomy. Primary ampullary disease such as hypertensive sphincter of Oddi[41] and ampullary tumors[42] can also cause pancreatitis.

Hereditary pancreatitis is an autosomal dominant condition with incomplete penetrance that has been documented in at least 19 families.[43, 44] This disease usually occurs in the second decade of life and may progress to chronic pancreatitis. It may be due to a stricture in the postampullary area, which, if confirmed, lends itself to endoscopic therapy.[45] Unfortunately, there is an association between hereditary pancreatitis and an increased incidence of pancreatic adenocarcinoma. It is unclear whether there is an increased incidence of pancreatic adenocarcinoma with chronic pancreatitis.[46] Anorexia nervosa and bulimia have been associated with the occurrence of acute pancreatitis.[47] A proposed mechanism is the variation of pancreatic secretory output resulting from fasting and binge eating.

CLINICAL PRESENTATION

Mid-epigastric and periumbilical abdominal pain with radiation to the back is the hallmark symptom of acute pancreatitis.[48, 49] The pain is often more intense when the patient is in the supine position and may range from mild to severe. It should be noted that pancreatitis occurs without pain in up to 2% of patients and that this presentation carries a poor prognosis.[50] Associated symptoms include nausea, vomiting, and abdominal distention. The temperature may increase up to 101°F. However, beyond this level, superimposed sepsis should be investigated. Hypotension occurs in 30 to 40% of patients. Less commonly encountered findings on physical examination include tetany from hypocalcemia, subcutaneous nodules caused by fat necrosis from circulating lipase,[51] a hemorrhagic bluish discoloration of the flanks (Grey Turner's sign), and discoloration of the periumbilical region (Cullen's sign). Phlegmon, pseudocyst, or abscess may cause palpable abdominal masses in up to 15% of patients.[52]

Mild jaundice (bilirubin level < 2.5 mg/dL) is seen in 40% of cases, and although this is usually due to an inflamed, enlarged pancreas' causing partial bile duct obstruction, it may result from primary hepatocellular disease, especially in an alcoholic population, or primary or secondary ampullary disease. The latter is due to an impacted stone in the distal common bile duct. In this situation, bilirubin levels are frequently increased and signs and symptoms of cholangitis may be present. Pulmonary complications, including hypoxemia, pleural effusions, atelectasis, pneumonia, and adult respiratory distress syndrome, are the most commonly encountered systemic complications. These may result either from pulmonary compromise secondary to abdominal distention from ileus or from a primary insult to the pulmonary parenchyma.[53]

LABORATORY STUDIES

Serum Amylase

Elevation of the serum amylase level, although a sensitive marker, is not specific for acute pancreatitis. It may be elevated in numerous nonpancreatic abdominal diseases as well as several nonabdominal diseases.[54] Increased specificity for amylase can be achieved by using a higher cutoff level, as values greater than five times normal are infrequently due to an extrapancreatic origin.[55] Whereas elevated levels of cardiac enzymes in a patient with an acute myocardial infarction portend a poor prognosis, the amylase level bears no relation to the severity of acute pancreatitis and, in fact, a normal serum amylase level may occur in 10% of cases of fatal pancreatitis.[56] A variety of conditions that simulate acute pancreatitis may cause an elevation in serum amylase levels.[57, 58] Nonpancreatic conditions associated with increased serum amylase activity (Table 132–3) include biliary colic, perforated peptic ulcer, mesenteric infarction, salivary gland dysfunction, renal insufficiency, macroamylasemia, and tumors (especially of the lung and the ovary).

Measurement of serum amylase isoenzymes has been developed in an attempt to improve the specificity for the diagnosis of acute pancreatitis. In normal subjects, 40% of total serum amylase is composed of pancreatic-type isoamylases and 60% is composed of salivary-type isoamylases.[59] In acute pancreatitis, most amylase in serum is pancreatic-type isoamylase.[60, 61] Unfortunately, pancreatic-type isoamylase is also released in other abdominal illnesses, such as perforated peptic ulcer and mesenteric infarction.[58] Thus, although isoamylase determinations appear to be of some clinical value, they probably cannot distinguish between acute pancreatitis and acute abdominal surgical catastrophes.

Serum Lipase

Serum lipase levels are usually increased in acute pancreatitis and remain elevated longer than total serum amylase levels.[62] Lipase levels have been found to be more sensitive and specific than amylase levels for the diagnosis of acute pancreatitis. However, lipase levels may also be elevated in abdominal conditions such as perforated ulcer, intestinal obstruction and infarction, acute cholecystitis, and afferent

TABLE 132–3

NONPANCREATIC CONDITIONS ASSOCIATED WITH INCREASED SERUM AMYLASE ACTIVITY

Intra-abdominal Diseases
Biliary tract disease, including acute cholecystitis and spasm or stenosis of sphincter of Oddi
Perforation of esophagus, stomach, small intestine, or colon
Intestinal ischemia or infarction
Intestinal obstruction
Appendicitis, acute
Diverticulitis, acute
Gynecologic conditions, acute (salpingitis, ruptured ectopic pregnancy)

Abnormalities of Salivary Glands
Mumps
Calculous obstruction of salivary glands
Scorpion sting
Effects of alcohol

Tumors
Lung carcinoma
Papillary cystadenocarcinoma of ovary
Ovarian cysts

Renal Insufficiency

Macroamylasemia

Miscellaneous
Head trauma with intracranial bleeding
Diabetic ketoacidosis
Anorexia nervosa
Prostatic disease
Peroral endoscopy
Drugs (morphine, for example)
Pneumonia

From Fayne SD, Barkin JS: Acute pancreatitis: Update 1986. Mt Sinai J Med 53(S):396–403, 1986.

loop syndrome. A normal serum lipase level helps to exclude such processes as macroamylasemia, some tumors, pelvic inflammatory disease, and salivary gland dysfunction. Macrolipasemia has been described,[63] in which the lipase is bound to a macroglobulin and is not excreted by the kidneys.

Urinary Amylase

The determination of urinary amylase has a limited diagnostic role. The urinary amylase clearance is increased in patients with acute pancreatitis and may remain elevated for 9 to 15 days. It is also increased in patients with renal tubular disease (e.g., diabetic ketoacidosis, burns, neoplasms, renal failure, chronic hemodialysis, and fulminant alcoholic liver disease).

IMAGING STUDIES

The flat plate of the abdomen may reveal the following findings that suggest the presence of acute pancreatitis: (1) a sentinel loop, which is a dilated jejunal loop, adjacent to the pancreas; (2) the colon cutoff sign, which consists of an air-filled transverse colon with no colonic gas distally; (3) paralytic ileus; (4) indistinct outline of the kidneys and psoas muscles; and (5) the presence of ascites.[64] Chest x-ray findings reflect the infradiaphragmatic inflammatory process and may consist of (1) elevation of one or both hemidiaphragms; (2) pleural effusion, usually left sided; (3) pericardial effusion; (4) plate-like atelectasis; and (5) pulmonary edema.

Ultrasonography may be useful in the diagnosis of acute pancreatitis. However, its major limitation is a high incidence of technically unsatisfactory examinations, primarily because of an ileus with overlying excessive bowel gas, ascites, or obesity.[65] When visualized, the pancreatic gland in patients with acute pancreatitis appears edematous and sonolucent when compared with the liver. An abnormally dilated pancreatic duct may indicate chronic pancreatitis.[66] Ultrasonography has a predominant role in diagnosing cholelithiasis and is also useful for imaging pancreatic pseudocysts. The advantage of abdominal computed tomography over ultrasonography is its ability to define the pancreas, even when it is surrounded by a large amount of adipose tissue, as in obese patients or in acutely ill patients with an ileus.[67] In addition, abdominal computed tomographic pancreatic imaging allows accurate depiction of the presence of complications of pancreatitis, such as fluid collections, and, when used with rapid bolus contrast injection, can determine the presence of pancreatic necrosis.[68] It can suggest the presence of superinfection but cannot be utilized alone to diagnose its presence. Suggestive features include changing density of pseudocyst fluid (although this can also be found in intracystic bleeding) and the presence of air in a pseudocyst (the latter can be seen in pseudocysts that have decompressed or ruptured into adjacent bowel).

PROGNOSIS

Multiple criteria have been developed to attempt early identification of patients who pursue a malignant course. These criteria mainly reflect the presence of multisystem disease. The most frequently used prognostic signs are those developed by Ranson (Table 132–4). Originally based on alcoholic pancreatitis alone, they have now been broadened to include all causes of pancreatitis.[69] The overall mortality rate of acute pancreatitis is approximately 1% in patients with fewer than three signs, 15% if three or four signs are present, 40% if five or six signs are positive, and 100% if seven or more criteria are met. The major concern in applying these criteria is that they utilize not only determinations at the time of hospital admission, but also criteria obtained up to 48 hours after admission. During this latter period, therapy may produce alterations. Hypoxemia, for example, may be induced by overhydration with subsequent pulmonary edema. These criteria have been simplified by Bank and colleagues; they found that, in patients with acute pancreatitis or acute relapsing pancreatitis, if one or more organ systems in addition to the pancreas were affected, the

TABLE 132–5

THREE GLASGOW MULTIFACTORIAL PROGNOSTIC SCORING SYSTEMS

Prognostic Factors*	Imrie et al (1978)	Osborne et al (1981)	Blamey et al (1984)
Age (y)	>55	Omitted	>55
Serum transaminase (U/L)	>100	>200	Omitted
White blood cell count (× 10/L)	>15	>15	>15
Blood glucose (mmol/L)	>10	>10	>10
Serum urea (mmol/L)	>16	>16	>16
Arterial oxygen saturation (kPa)	<8	<8	<8
Serum calcium (mmol/L)	<2	<2	<2
Serum albumin (g/L)	<32	<32	<32
Serum lactate dehydrogenase (U/L)	>600	>600	>600

*Zero to two adverse factors indicate mild disease; three or more adverse factors predict severe disease.

Adapted from Leese T, Shaw D: Comparison of three Glasgow multifactor scoring systems in acute pancreatitis. Br J Surg 75:460, 1988 by permission of the publishers Butterworth-Heinemann Ltd.

mortality was 56%.[70] Conversely, with the lack of involvement of any organ system outside the pancreas, the mortality rate was only 2%.

The Glasgow multifactorial scoring system of Imrie and colleagues (Table 132–5) is another prognostic scoring system used in patients with acute pancreatitis. Leese and Shaw assessed these factors in patients with 198 attacks of acute pancreatitis, who were treated in the standard fashion.[71] Multivariate analysis showed that PaO_2, white blood cell count, and lactate dehydrogenase and blood urea nitrogen levels each had independent significance in projecting severity of the attack. Conversely, serum glucose, albumin, and transaminase levels were the least useful. The omission of either age or transaminase level improved the predictive value of the scoring system. The advantage of this scoring system is that all eight factors are available for assessment at the time of hospital admission and thus may be simpler to apply than the Ranson criteria.

Computed tomography of the pancreas is important for predicting the prognosis of patients with acute pancreatitis.[72] The presence of a normal pancreas is indicative of edematous mild pancreatitis. However, an abnormal pancreas may be found in either edematous or necrotizing pancreatitis. Clavien and coworkers confirmed the predictive value of early computed tomography and recognized that the extrapancreatic spread of pancreatic inflammation is the best early predictor of the severity of acute pancreatitis.[73] In addition, both the extent and the localization of the extrapancreatic spread correlated with morbidity and mortality rates.[73]

The volume and the color of peritoneal lavage fluid have been shown to correlate with the severity of acute pancreatitis.[74] Dark-colored free fluid, mid–straw-colored lavage return fluid, and more than 20 mL of free fluid, regardless of color, indicate severe pancreatitis. This method has the advantage of providing immediate results but is not sensitive for predicting the severity of gallstone-induced disease from alcoholic pancreatitis.[75]

MEDICAL TREATMENT
Fluid Resuscitation

The initial approach to the management of patients with acute pancreatitis should be assessment of its severity and

TABLE 132–4

SIGNS FOR CLASSIFICATION OF SEVERITY OF ACUTE PANCREATITIS

At time of admission or diagnosis
  Age > 55 y
  White blood cell count > 16,000/mm³
  Blood glucose level > 200 mg/dL
  Serum lactate dehydrogenase level more than twice normal
  Serum glutamic-oxaloacetic transaminase level more than six times normal

During initial 48 h
  Decrease in hematocrit of > 10%
  Serum calcium level < 8 mg/dL
  Increase in blood urea nitrogen level of > 5 mg/dL
  Arterial Po_2 < 60 mm Hg
  Base deficit > 4 mEq/L
  Estimated fluid sequestration > 6000 mL

Adapted from Ranson JH, Rifkind KM, Turner JW: Prognostic signs and nonoperative peritoneal lavage in acute pancreatitis. Surg Gynecol Obstet 143:209, 1976. By permission of Surgery, Gynecology & Obstetrics.

confirmation of its cause, as both of these influence the therapeutic approach. It was thought that the goal of therapy for acute pancreatitis is to place the pancreas at rest. However, this is probably done by the pathologic process, as pancreatic secretion was markedly depressed in the single patient with acute pancreatitis in whom it was measured. Therefore, the goal should be restated to institute supportive measures that allow the inflammatory process to subside. These include volume and electrolyte replacement and pain relief, using meperidine hydrochloride intramuscularly, in preference to morphine, as the former may induce less spasm of the sphincter of Oddi. Nasogastric suction is useful only for the patient with an ileus or who has nausea and/or vomiting. Otherwise, the patient is given nothing by mouth.[76]

In 75% of patients, acute pancreatitis resolves with these supportive measures.[77] Steinberg and Schlesselman emphasized that drug therapy for patients with acute pancreatitis has a limited role.[78] They reviewed the outcome of 25 studies of experimentally induced pancreatitis in animals and 13 studies of human acute pancreatitis in which the same therapeutic agents were utilized. A positive effect on survival was found in 81% of the animal studies and in only 8% of the human studies. The major reason for this discrepancy is that drugs are administered immediately after the induction of pancreatitis in animals, whereas in human patients, there is a variable period of disease before they receive the drug therapy. Therefore, after the damage has been done, there is little role for applying a pharmacologic agent. However, there may be a role for these agents for the prevention of pancreatitis.

Nutritional Support

In patients with delayed resolution of symptoms that precludes oral alimentation, peripheral parenteral nutrition or central parenteral nutrition should be considered. Although it may seem logical that improving nutrition improves the outcome of acute pancreatitis, this has never been fully established. Sax and colleagues showed that the early use of TPN was not advantageous.[79] Interestingly, the TPN group had a significantly higher rate of catheter-related sepsis than did another group of patients who received TPN but who did not have pancreatitis; it is unclear why this occurred. Sitzmann and coworkers showed that, if positive nitrogen balance can be achieved in patients with acute severe pancreatitis, mortality can be significantly decreased.[80] In addition, the administration of lipid emulsion twice a week with a hypertonic glucose solution resulted in a lower mortality rate than either glucose-based TPN alone or with daily lipid administration. Obviously, further studies need to be performed.

Peritoneal Dialysis

Peritoneal lavage has been used in patients with necrotizing pancreatitis in an attempt to remove vasoactive substances from the peritoneal cavity, before their absorption and systemic effects. Initial uncontrolled trials appeared promising. However, a multicenter randomized controlled clinical trial of therapeutic peritoneal lavage in 91 patients showed no benefits.[81] This may have occurred because of the incorrect location of the dialysate, which was infused into the peritoneal cavity, and not into the peripancreatic area in the retroperitoneum. Lavage has been found to be useful when combined with surgical débridement.

Fluid Resuscitation

Restoration of intravascular volume in patients with acute pancreatitis is an important critical care maneuver, as the basic pathophysiology of acute pancreatitis is a retroperitoneal burn leading to large third-space losses. If intravenous fluid replacement does not compensate for these losses, the resulting systemic hypotension could theoretically lead to stasis within the microcirculation of the pancreas, causing intensification of pancreatic inflammation. In patients who require large volumes of fluid resuscitation, this should be guided by either central venous monitoring or Swan-Ganz catheter insertion.

Respiratory Monitoring

Respiratory complications are common sequelae of acute pancreatitis, occurring in 15 to 55% of cases. They range from subclinical arterial hypoxemia to the full-blown adult respiratory distress syndrome. Some of these may be difficult to recognize by physical examination and chest x-ray film in patients with acute pancreatitis. Therefore, arterial blood gases should be measured every 12 hours during the initial 48 to 72 hours of treatment in severely ill patients.

Management of Complications

The systemic complications of acute pancreatitis have been reviewed by Pitchumoni and colleagues[82] (Table 132–6).

Pseudocysts

Pseudocyst formation occurs in approximately 25% of patients with acute pancreatitis. Fortunately, almost 85% spontaneously resolve with no intervention during the first few weeks after the acute episode.[83] Pseudocysts should be suspected in the patient with persistent pain, nausea, vomiting, or elevated serum amylase level that persists for more

---

TABLE 132–6

COMPLICATIONS OF ACUTE PANCREATITIS

Pancreatic
1. Sterile collections
   a. Fluid: pseudocysts
   b. Solid lesions: pancreatic necrosis (phlegmon)
2. Infected collections
   a. Fluid: infected pseudocysts
   b. Solid: pancreatic abscess

Local—Nonpancreatic
1. Involvement of contiguous organs (intraperitoneal hemorrhage, gastrointestinal bleeding, thrombosis of splenic vein, bowel infarction)
2. Pancreatic ascites
3. Obstructive jaundice

Systemic
1. Pulmonary
   a. Arterial hypoxia to adult respiratory distress syndrome
   b. Atelectasis, pneumonia, pleural effusion, mediastinal abscess
2. Cardiac: shock, pericardial effusion, electrocardiographic changes, arrhythmias
3. Hematologic: disseminated intravascular coagulation
4. Gastrointestinal: gastrointestinal bleeding (portal-splenic vein thrombosis, colonic infarction)
5. Renal: azotemia, oliguria
6. Metabolic: hypocalcemia, hyperglycemia, hypertriglyceridemia, acidosis, elevation of free fatty acids
7. Central nervous system: psychosis, encephalopathy, Purtscher's retinopathy
8. Peripheral: fat necrosis (skin and bones), arthritis

Adapted from CS Pitchumoni, N Agarwal, NK Jain, Systemic complications of acute pancreatitis, Am J Gastroenterol, 83, 6, 597–606, 1988, © by The American College of Gastroenterology.

than 5 days. Potential complications directly related to pseudocysts include (1) spontaneous rupture into the peritoneum or pleural cavity, (2) obstruction of adjacent organs such as common bile duct or stomach, and (3) erosion into the gastrointestinal tract, which results in bleeding.

The natural history of the majority of pseudocysts is spontaneous resolution within 6 weeks. Therefore, definitive therapy should not be instituted until after this period of observation. If the pseudocyst is greater than 6 cm in diameter and unchanged or increasing in size, decompression is probably indicated. If the cyst is asymptomatic and less than 6 cm in diameter, a more prolonged period of observation is reasonable. Pseudocysts were observed for 1 year and 60% resolved.[84] However, 10% of patients had complications, and those pseudocysts greater than 6 cm were more likely to necessitate decompression. The decompression can be performed via percutaneous aspiration at 6 weeks, guided by ultrasonography or computed tomography, or with endoscopic or surgical methods.[85, 86] We favor the use of percutaneous guided aspiration and catheter drainage. Up to 80% of pseudocysts can be successfully treated with this modality.[87] The major complication is superimposed infection, necessitating catheter drainage for an average of 3 weeks. If attempts at percutaneous or endoscopic drainage are unsuccessful, surgical internal drainage via cystogastrostomy or Roux-en-Y drainage is the procedure of choice.

Infection

The presence of superimposed bacterial infection should be sought in the appropriate clinical setting. This evidence includes fever (>101°F), leukocytosis, persistent tachycardia, hypotension, and positive blood cultures. In these patients, it is mandatory to obtain a computed tomography–guided percutaneous aspiration of fluid collections, or of areas with decreased perfusion, as it is clinically impossible to distinguish a sterile from an infected area.[87, 88] Gram's stain and aerobic and anaerobic cultures of the aspirate should be obtained. If bacteria with leukocytes are present in the aspirate, or cultures become positive, which occurs in 10% of patients, an additional catheter drainage with appropriate antibiotic therapy should be utilized. If percutaneous catheter drainage is unsuccessful in the infected pseudocyst, or if the lesion is predominantly infected solid material, surgical therapy is required in the majority of patients.

SURGICAL TREATMENT
Acute Pancreatitis

In the setting of an uncertain diagnosis, deteriorating clinical condition, biliary pancreatitis, pancreatic abscess, or colonic necrosis, surgical intervention may be indicated.[89]

The surgical treatment of gallstone pancreatitis deserves special mention, because overall mortality is 10% or greater[90] (see Chapter 131). The first decision is the timing of operative intervention. It has been shown that urgent operations are associated with increased mortality, compared with surgical intervention performed after 3 to 5 days of hospitalization.[91, 92] Therefore, in the absence of cholangitis or empyema, elective intervention is planned. An alternative decompressive modality is ERCP with sphincterotomy, which has played an increasing role in the management of biliary pancreatitis. In a trial of 121 patients with acute biliary pancreatitis who were randomly assigned to undergo urgent ERCP with sphincterotomy versus conservative treatment, the patients with severe pancreatitis who underwent endoscopic decompression had a lower mortality rate and shorter hospital stay.[93]

Management of patients who are at high surgical risk after endoscopic sphincterotomy with removal of common bile duct stones may not require cholecystectomy. Only 10% of high-risk patients need elective cholecystectomy when followed for 2 to 9 years.[94] However, this may change because of the widespread availability of laparoscopic cholecystectomy, and its attendant decreased mortality. Cholecystectomy is not essential, provided an adequate endoscopic sphincterotomy has been performed.[95]

Necrotizing Pancreatitis

Necrotizing pancreatitis is the most serious form of pancreatitis, with mortality approaching 100% with nonsurgical management.[96] Distal or total pancreatectomy for necrotizing pancreatitis results in a high complication rate and a mortality in excess of 40%.[97] Necrosectomy is an alternative approach in which only necrotic pancreatic or extrapancreatic tissue is removed and viable islands of pancreatic tissue are conserved. Necrosectomy combined with local lavage was shown to have a lower mortality rate of 84% compared with that in historical controls.[98] Necrosectomy and open drainage has been reported to yield similarly good results, especially in patients with infected necrosis.[99]

Severe acute pancreatitis presents the clinician with a formidable disease process, which may progress rapidly to multiple organ system failure. Unfortunately, the management at this time still consists of primarily supportive measures. Interventional measures are focused more on the complications.

References

1. Sarner M, Cotton PB: Classification of pancreatitis. Gut 25:756, 1984.
2. Fayne SD, Barkin JS: Acute pancreatitis: Update 1986. Mt Sinai J Med 53:396, 1986.
3. Langman MJS: The Epidemiology of Chronic Digestive Disease. Chicago, Year Book Medical Publishers, 1979.
4. O'Sullivan JW, Nobrega FT, Marlock CG, et al: Acute and chronic pancreatitis in Rochester, Minnesota 1940–1969. Gastroenterology 62:373, 1972.
5. Dammann HG, Dreyer M, Walter TA, et al: Prognostic indicators in acute pancreatitis: Clinical experience and limitations. In: Beger HG, Buchler M (eds): Acute Pancreatitis. New York, Springer-Verlag p 181, 1987.
6. Wilson C, Imrie CW, Carter DC: Fatal acute pancreatitis. Gut 29:782, 1988.
7. Geokas MC, Rinderkaecht H, Swanson V, et al: The role of elastase in acute hemorrhagic pancreatitis in man. Lab Invest 19:235, 1968.
8. McDermott WV Jr, Bartlett MK, Culver PJ: Acute pancreatitis after prolonged fast and subsequent surfeit. N Engl J Med 254:379, 1956.
9. Creutzfeldt W, Schmidt H: Aetiology and pathogenesis of pancreatitis. Scand J Gastroenterol 5(suppl 6):47, 1979.
10. Opie EL: The etiology of acute hemorrhagic pancreatitis. Bull Johns Hopkins Hosp 12:182, 1901.
11. Feldstein JD, Johnson FR, Kallick CA, et al: Acute hemorrhagic pancreatitis due to mumps. Ann Surg 180:85, 1974.
12. Ursing B: Acute pancreatitis in coxsackie-B infection. Br Med J 3:524, 1973.
13. Lech A, Montesi G, Solbiati M, et al: Serum pancreatic enzyme alterations in acute viral hepatitis. Hepatogastroenterology 30:233, 1983.
14. Geokas MC, Olson H, Swanson V, et al: The association of viral hepatitis and acute pancreatitis. Calif Med 117:1, 1972.
15. Freeman R, McMahon M: Acute pancreatitis and serological evidence of infection with *Mycoplasma pneumoniae*. Gut 19:367, 1978.
16. Pönkä A, Kosonew T: Pancreatitis affection in association with enteritis due to *Camphylobacter fetus* ssp. *jejuni*. Acta Med Scand 209:239, 1981.
17. Winters C Jr, Chobanian SJ, Benjamin SB, et al: Endoscopic documentation of *Ascaris*-induced pancreatitis. Gastrointest Endosc 30:83, 1984.
18. Bartholomew C: Acute scorpion pancreatitis in Trinidad. Br Med J 1:666, 1970.
19. Trapnell JE, Duncan EHL: Patterns of incidence in acute pancreatitis. Br Med J 2:179, 1975.
20. McMahon MJ, Shetta JR: Physical characteristics of gallstones and the

calibre of the cystic duct in patients with acute pancreatitis. Br J Surg 67:6, 1980.

21. Howard MJ: Pancreatitis associated with gallstones. In: Howard MJ, Jordan GL Jr (eds): Surgical Diseases of the Pancreas. Philadelphia, JB Lippincott, p 169, 1960.

22. Medical Research Council Multicenter Trial of Glucagon and Aprotinin. Death from acute pancreatitis. Lancet 2:632, 1977.

23. Mallory A, Kern F Jr: Drug-induced pancreatitis: A critical review. Gastroenterology 78:813, 1980.

24. Hanks JB, Curtis SE, Hanks BB, et al: Gastrointestinal complications after cardiopulmonary bypass. Surgery 92:394, 1982.

25. Northrop WF III, Simmons RL: Pancreatic trauma. A review. Surgery 71:27, 1972.

26. Bilbao MK, Dotter CT, Lee TG, et al: Complications of endoscopic retrograde cholangiopancreatography (ERCP). Gastroenterology 70:314, 1976.

27. Herfort K, Sobra J, Frie P, et al: Familial hyperlipoproteinemia and exocrine pancreas. Scand J Gastroenterol 6:139, 1971.

28. Buch A, Buch J, Carlsen A, et al: Hyperlipidemia and pancreatitis. World J Surg 4:307, 1980.

29. Izsak EM, Shike M, Roulet M, et al: Pancreatitis in association with hypercalcemia in patients receiving total parenteral nutrition. Gastroenterology 79:555, 1980.

30. Davies M, Klimuk PS, Adams PH, et al: Familial hypocalciuric hypercalcemia and acute pancreatitis. Br Med J [Clin Res] 282:1023, 1981.

31. Warshaw AL, Richter JM, Shapiro RH: The cause and treatment of pancreatitis associated with pancreas divisum. Ann Surg 198:443, 1983.

32. Delhaye M, Engelholm L, Cremer M: Pancreas divisum: Congenital anatomic variant or anomaly? Contribution of endoscopic retrograde dorsal pancreatography. Gastroenterology 89:951, 1985.

33. Corrodi P, Knoblauch M, Binswanger V, et al: Pancreatitis after renal transplantation. Gut 16:285, 1975.

34. Adiseshiah M, Wells FC, Cury-Pearce R, et al: Acute pancreatitis after cardiac transplantation. World J Surg 7:519, 1983.

35. Harary A, Barkin JA: Acute pancreatitis. In: Gleicher N (ed): Principles of Medical Therapy in Pregnancy. New York, Plenum Publishing, p 853, 1985.

36. Young KR: Acute pancreatitis in pregnancy. Two case reports. Obstet Gynecol 60:653, 1982.

37. Abrahms J, Cannon JJ: Duodenal duplication presenting as relapsing pancreatitis in an adult. Am J Gastroenterol 79:360, 1984.

38. Chevillotte G, Shael J, Raillat A, et al: Annular pancreas. Report of one case associated with acute pancreatitis and diagnosed by endoscopic retrograde pancreatography. Dig Dis Sci 29:75, 1984.

39. Freed JS, Dreiling DH, Reiner MA: Non-Hodgkin's lymphoma of the pancreas producing acute pancreatitis and pancreatic abscess. Mt Sinai J Med 50:424, 1983.

40. Shawis RN, Doig CM: Gastric trichobezoar associated with transient pancreatitis. Arch Dis Child 59:944, 1984.

41. Guelrud M, Siegel JH: Hypertensive pancreatic duct sphincter as a cause of pancreatitis. Successful treatment with hydrostatic balloon dilation. Dig Dis Sci 39:225, 1984.

42. Moosa MR, Segal I: Tumor-associated acute pancreatitis (letter). J Clin Gastroenterol 6:188, 1984.

43. Sata T, Saitah Y: Familial chronic pancreatitis associated with pancreatic lithiasis. Am J Surg 127:511, 1974.

44. McCannel RB: Genetic aspects of gastrointestinal cancer. Clin Gastroenterol 5:483, 1976.

45. Renner IG, Wisner JR, Rosenthal P, et al: Hereditary pancreatitis: Evidence of primary pancreatic ductal lesion in a family (abstract). Pancreas December, 1990.

46. Ammann RW, Akovbiantz A, Largiader F, et al: Course and outcome of chronic pancreatitis: Longitudinal study of a mixed medical-surgical series of 245 patients. Gastroenterology 86:820, 1984.

47. Marano AR, Sangree MH: Acute pancreatitis associated with bulemia. J Clin Gastroenterol 6:245, 1984.

48. White TT: Pancreatitis. Baltimore, Williams & Wilkins, 1966.

49. Gambill EE: The clinical manifestations of pancreatitis. In: Gambill EE (ed): Pancreatitis. St Louis, CV Mosby, p 83, 1973.

50. Toffler AH, Spiro HM: Shock or coma as the predominant manifestation of painless acute pancreatitis. Ann Intern Med 57:655, 1962.

51. Dhawan SS, Acosta FJ, Poppiti R, et al: Subcutaneous fat necrosis associated with pancreatitis: Histochemical and electron microscopic findings. Am J Gastroenterol 85:1025, 1990.

52. Warshaw AL: Inflammatory masses following acute pancreatitis: Phlegmon, pseudocyst and abscess. Surg Clin North Am 54:621, 1974.

53. Roseman DM, Kowlessar OD, Sleisenger MH: Pulmonary manifestations of pancreatitis. N Engl J Med 265:294, 1960.

54. Tietz NW: Amylase measurements in serum—Old myths die hard (editorial). J Clin Chem Clin Biochem 26:251, 1988.

55. Steinberg WM, Goldstein SS, Davis ND, et al: Diagnostic assays in acute pancreatitis. A study of sensitivity and specificity. Ann Intern Med 102:576, 1985.

56. Peterson LM, Brooks JR: Lethal pancreatitis: A diagnostic dilemma. Am J Surg 137:491, 1979.

57. Levitt MD, Ellis CJ, Meier PB: Extrapancreatic origin of chronic unexplained hyperamylasemia. N Engl J Med 302:670, 1980.

58. Bank PA, Warshaw AL, Wolfe GZ, et al: Identification of amylase isoenzymes in intestinal contents. Dig Dis Sci 29:297, 1984.

59. Warshaw AL, Lee KH: The mechanism of increased renal clearance of amylase in acute pancreatitis. Gastroenterology 71:388, 1976.

60. Weaver DW, Bouwman DL, Walt AJ, et al: A correlation between clinical pancreatitis and isoenzyme patterns of amylase. Surgery 92:576, 1982.

61. Koehler DF, Eckfeldt JH, Levitt MD: Diagnostic value of routine isoamylase assay of hyperamylasemic serum. Gastroenterology 82:887, 1982.

62. Kolars JC, Ellis CJ, Levitt MD: Comparison of serum amylase, pancreatic isoamylase and lipase in patients with hyperamylasemia. Dig Dis Sci 29:289, 1984.

63. Bode CH, Riederer J, Brauner B, et al: Macrolipasemia: A rare course of persistently elevated serum lipase. Am J Gastroenterol 85:412, 1990.

64. Mitchell JR: Significance of roentgen findings in pancreatitis. J Chronic Dis 15:1077, 1962.

65. Cox KL, Ament ME, Sample WF, et al: The ultrasonic and biochemical diagnosis of pancreatitis in children. J Pediatr 96:407, 1980.

66. Bryan PJ: Appearance of normal pancreatic duct: A study using real-time ultrasound. JCU 10:63, 1982.

67. Mendez G Jr: CT of acute pancreatitis: Interim assessment. AJR 135:463, 1980.

68. Block S, Maier W, Bittner R, et al: Identification of pancreas necrosis in severe acute pancreatitis: Imaging procedures versus clinical staging. Gut 27:1035, 1986.

69. Ranson JH, Rifkind KM, Turner JW: Prognostic signs and nonoperative peritoneal lavage in acute pancreatitis. Surg Gynecol Obstet 143:209, 1976.

70. Bank S, Wise L, Gerstein M: Risk factors in acute pancreatitis. Am J Gastroenterol 78:637, 1983.

71. Leese T, Shaw D: Comparison of three Glasgow multifactor scoring systems in acute pancreatitis. Br J Surg 75:460, 1988.

72. Hill MC, Barkin JS, Isikoff MD, et al: Acute pancreatitis. Clinical vs CT finding. AJR 139:262, 1982.

73. Clavien PA, Hauser H, Meyer P, et al: Value of contrast-enhanced computerized tomography in the early diagnosis and prognosis of acute pancreatitis. Am J Surg 155:457, 1988.

74. McMahon MJ, Pickford A, Playforth MJ: Early prediction of severity in acute pancreatitis using peritoneal lavage. Acta Chir Scand 146:171, 1980.

75. Corfield AP, Cooper MJ, Williamson RCN, et al: Prediction of severity in acute pancreatitis. A prospective comparison of three prognostic indices. Lancet 2:403, 1985.

76. Field BE, Hepner GW, Shabat MM, et al: Nasogastric suction in alcoholic pancreatitis. Dig Dis Sci 24:339, 1979.

77. Soergel KH: Medical treatment of acute pancreatitis. Gastroenterology 74:620, 1978.

78. Steinberg WM, Schlesselman SE: Treatment of acute pancreatitis: Comparison of animal and human studies. Gastroenterology 93:1420, 1987.

79. Sax HC, Warner BW, Talamini MA, et al: Early total parenteral nutrition in acute pancreatitis. Lack of beneficial effects. Am J Surg 155:117, 1987.

80. Sitzmann JV, Steinborn PA, Zinner MJ, et al: Total parenteral nutrition and alternate energy substrates in treatment of severe pancreatitis. Surg Gynecol Obstet 168:311, 1989.

81. Mayer AD, McMahon MJ, Corfield AP, et al: Controlled clinical trial of peritoneal lavage for the treatment of severe acute pancreatitis. N Engl J Med 312:399, 1985.

82. Pitchumoni CS, Agarwal NM, Jain NK: Systemic complications of acute pancreatitis. Am J Gastroenterol 83:597, 1988.

83. Czaja AS, Fisher M, Marin GA: Spontaneous resolution of pancreatic masses (pseudocysts?) appearing after acute alcoholic pancreatitis. Arch Intern Med 135:558, 1975.

84. Yeo CJ, Bastidas JA, Lynch-Nyham, et al: The natural history of pancreatic pseudocysts documented by computed tomography. Surg Gynecol Obstet 170:411, 1990.

85. Barkin JS, Smith FR, Pereiras R, et al: Therapeutic percutaneous aspiration of pancreatic pseudocysts. Dig Dis Sci 26:585, 1981.

86. Karlson KB, Martin EC, Fankuchen EI, et al: Percutaneous drainage of pancreatic pseudocysts and abscesses. Radiology 143:619, 1982.

87. van Sonnenberg E, Wittich GR, Casola G, et al: Percutaneous drainage of infected and non-infected pancreatic pseudocysts: Experience in 101 cases. Radiology 170:757, 1989.

88. Hill MC, Dach JL, Barkin JS, et al: The role of percutaneous aspiration in the diagnosis of pancreatic abscess. Am J Radiol 141:1035, 1983.

89. Martin JK Jr, van Heerden JH, Besse MA: Surgical management of acute pancreatitis. Mayo Clin Proc 59:259, 1984.

90. DeBolla AR, Oseid MC: Mortality in acute pancreatitis. Ann R Coll Surg Engl 66:184, 1984.

91. Ranson JHC: Timing of biliary surgery in acute pancreatitis. Ann Surg 189:654, 1979.

92. Osborne DH, Imrie CW, Carter DC: Biliary surgery in the admission for gallstone associated pancreatitis. Br J Surg 68:758, 1981.

93. Neoptolemos JP, Carr-Locke DL, London NJ, et al: Controlled trial of urgent endoscopic retrograde cholangiopancreatography and endoscopic sphincterotomy versus conservative treatment for acute pancreatitis due to gallstones. Lancet 2:979, 1988.

94. Cotton PB: 2–9 year follow-up after sphincterotomy for stones in patients with gallbladders. Gastrointest Endosc 2:157, 1986.

95. Davidson BR, Neoptolemos JP, Carr-Locke DL: Endoscopic sphincterotomy for common bile duct calculi in patients with gallbladder in situ considered unfit for surgery. Gut 29:114, 1988.

96. Roscher R, Beger HG: Bacterial infection of pancreatic necrosis. In: Beger HC, Buchler M (eds): Acute Pancreatitis. New York, Springer-Verlag, p 314, 1987.
97. Alexander JH, Guerreri MT: Role of total pancreatectomy in the treatment of necrotizing pancreatitis. World J Surg 5:369, 1981.
98. Beger HG, Buchler M, Bittner R, et al: Necrosectomy and postoperative local lavage in necrotizing pancreatitis. Br J Surg 75:207, 1988.
99. Bradley EL: Management of infected pancreatic necrosis by open drainage. Ann Surg 206:542, 1987.

CHAPTER 133

Hepatic Emergencies

Gabriel Garcia
Daniel Luba

Although abnormal results of liver function tests (aminotransferase, alkaline phosphatase, and bilirubin levels) may be common in the intensive care unit (ICU) setting, there are several scenarios in which the primary hepatic problem places the patient in the ICU. Acute variceal hemorrhage, as a complication of portal hypertension, is one of these situations and may occur either on presentation or while the patient is in the ICU (see Chapter 125). Hepatic encephalopathy is often encountered by the intensivist and is common in patients with any form of severe liver disease. The complexities of its pathogenesis and its therapy are discussed fully in Chapter 135. The final therapy of end-stage liver disease (liver transplantation) is becoming more common and is encountered by most intensivists in academic tertiary care medical centers. The nuances of the care of patients both before and after transplantation are the subject of Chapter 134. In addition, three clinical presentations are of concern to the intensivist: spontaneous bacterial peritonitis (SBP), severe alcoholic hepatitis, and fulminant hepatic failure (FHF). The recognition, diagnosis, and management of these disorders are the subject of this chapter.

SPONTANEOUS BACTERIAL PERITONITIS

SBP is a common and frequently lethal complication of end-stage liver disease. When cirrhotic patients with ascites undergo paracentesis at the time of routine or emergency hospital admission, between 10 and 27% are found to have SBP.[1] SBP can be defined as an ascitic fluid infection in which (1) the ascitic fluid culture is positive, (2) the ascitic fluid polymorphonuclear (PMN) cell count is greater than 250/mm³, and (3) there is no intra-abdominal source of infection. Culture-negative neutrocytic ascites (CNNA) is defined as the presence of ascitic fluid with a negative culture but a PMN cell count greater than 500/mm³, no intra-abdominal source of infection, and no recent antibiotic therapy.[2] Although the ascitic fluid culture is negative in this disorder, CNNA is nonetheless believed to be caused by bacterial infection and necessitates the same treatment as for SBP. Bacterascites is defined as the presence of ascitic fluid with a PMN count less than 250/mm³ but a positive culture. Bacterascites probably represents transient colonization, and

treatment should be based on the PMN count and bacterial culture results of repeated paracentesis.

Pathogenesis

The pathogenesis of SBP is multifactorial. Cirrhotic patients are more prone to bacteremia because of impaired hepatic reticuloendothelial system function. In addition, they have neutrophil dysfunction, complement deficiency, and impaired ascitic fluid opsonic activity.[3] When bacteria seed the ascitic fluid during a bacteremic episode, they must be engulfed and killed by phagocytic cells. Before this can occur, the bacterial cell surface must be coated with immunoglobulin G and/or the third component of complement. However, the complement levels and opsonic activity in patients with cirrhotic ascites are often low and correlate with ascitic fluid total protein level.

In a series of 24 cases of SBP, the opsonic activity in the ascitic fluid was significantly lower than that found in patients with sterile ascites.[2] Patients with a low ascitic fluid total protein, complement, and opsonic activity have a higher risk of SBP. In a prospective study of 125 patients with ascites who underwent routine admission paracentesis, 15% of those patients with initially sterile ascitic fluid and protein level less than 1 g/dL had SBP, compared with 1.5% of patients with an ascitic fluid protein level greater than 1 g/dL.[4] In general, patients with cirrhotic and nephrotic ascites have low ascitic fluid protein levels and a high risk of SBP, whereas patients with malignant and cardiac ascites have higher ascitic fluid protein levels and develop SBP infrequently.

Clinical Presentation and Laboratory Analysis

Patients with SBP classically exhibit fever and abdominal pain. A significant proportion of patients, however, are asymptomatic. In a series of 224 patients with cirrhosis and ascites who had routine paracentesis on admission to the hospital, 27 patients (12%) had SBP. In this group of 27 patients, 4 patients were totally asymptomatic, and 5 patients had only one feature of SBP, such as fever or abdominal pain without rebound tenderness.[5] Therefore, to make the diagnosis of SBP, clinical suspicion must be high. The diagnosis can be made only by examination of ascitic fluid. Paracentesis should be performed routinely on admission to the hospital and with onset of any symptoms suggestive of SBP such as abdominal pain, fever, confusion, hypotension, and hypothermia.

Paracentesis is a safe procedure. There is only a 0.6% rate of needle perforation of the gut leading to peritonitis[6] and a 1% risk of bleeding.[7] Prophylactic transfusions of either fresh frozen plasma or platelets are not indicated because the risk of post-transfusion hepatitis is greater than the risk of bleeding. Bleeding is likely to occur, regardless of coagulopathy, if a needle enters an artery or a high-pressure venous system.

When analyzing ascitic fluid, the most important test is the white blood cell count with differential and culture. A PMN cell count greater than 250/mm³ has a sensitivity of 81% and a specificity of 95% in diagnosing SBP.[8] Ascitic fluid pH, lactate level, and serum–to–ascitic fluid pH ratio are all less sensitive and less accurate. Culture technique has proved to be of utmost importance in isolating an organism. Ten milliliters of ascitic fluid should be inoculated into each of two blood culture bottles at the patient's bedside. Inoculating ascitic fluid on agar plates and broth in the bacteriology laboratory results in positive cultures only 43% of the time. In contrast, when 10 mL of ascitic fluid is inoculated into blood culture bottles at the patient's bedside, 93% of cases of SBP are culture-positive.[9, 10] In a large proportion of cases diagnosed in the past as CNNA, negative culture results were probably due to inadequate culture technique. Blood cultures are positive in 60% of patients with SBP.[10]

Ascitic fluid total protein level has prognostic importance because patients with ascitic fluid total protein levels less than 1 g/dL are at greater risk for SBP.

Differentiating SBP from secondary peritonitis is difficult. Physical findings are not helpful. Patients with 10 to 20 L of ascitic fluid do not have a rigid abdomen, even with free perforation. In SBP, ascitic fluid total protein level is usually less than 1 g/dL, glucose concentration is similar to simultaneous serum values, lactate dehydrogenase level is less than the upper limits of normal for serum, and cultures grow a single organism. In contrast, patients with intestinal perforation have multiple organisms on culture, and two of the following three criteria: protein level greater than 1 g/dL, glucose level less than 50 mg/dL, and lactate dehydrogenase level greater than the upper limit of normal for serum.[7] In addition, the PMN count decreases significantly and ascitic fluid becomes sterile within 48 hours of antibiotic treatment in SBP, whereas in secondary peritonitis, the PMN count increases and cultures remain positive. Because the mortality rate of exploratory laparotomy is 80% in patients with SBP,[11] patients with ascites and peritonitis should go to the operating room only if there is convincing evidence.[7] This generally necessitates radiographic studies to determine whether there is extravasation of intraluminal contrast material from the gut.

Treatment

All patients with ascites and a PMN cell count greater than 250/mm³ should be treated for SBP. *Escherichia coli*, streptococcal species, and *Klebsiella pneumoniae* account for more than 80% of the organisms isolated. Other enteric gram-negative bacteria complete the list.[9, 12–14] Aminoglycosides should not be used in treating SBP because their volume of distribution is unpredictable in ascitic patients, and they are nephrotoxic. Cefotaxime has been shown to be more efficacious and to have fewer side effects than ampicillin or tobramycin.[7, 15]

Paracentesis should be performed 48 hours after initiation of antibiotic treatment and then every 3 or 4 days to document a decrease in PMN cell count. Treatment should be discontinued when the ascitic fluid PMN cell count drops below 250/mm³.[16] This usually takes about 5 days.

Prognosis

Patients with SBP have a mortality rate of 30 to 40% during the index hospitalization[7, 16] and a recurrence rate of 69% by 1 year.[17] The mortality rate increases to 50% at 1 month, 60% at 6 months, and 75% at 1 year[18] and correlates with the severity of the underlying disease. CNNA seems to be a less severe form of SBP. These patients have a 20% 1-month mortality, which increases to 40% by 1 year.[16, 18] The majority of deaths in patients with SBP and CNNA are caused by liver failure, hepatorenal syndrome, and gastrointestinal bleeding. Patients with non-neutrocytic bacterascites have an 18% in-hospital mortality rate, which is no different from that of patients with sterile ascites.[5] In view of the significant 1-year mortality rate in patients with SBP, one must consider any patient with cirrhosis and SBP for liver transplantation if he or she is otherwise a good candidate for this therapy.

Summary

Infections of ascitic fluid in patients with cirrhosis frequently have a silent clinical presentation but can have grave immediate consequences and are a sign of advanced liver disease. The clinician must have a low threshold for performing a diagnostic paracentesis in any patient admitted to the ICU with ascites. Although therapy with cefotaxime leads to rapid resolution of SBP, plans for appropriate therapy of the underlying liver disease, including liver transplantation in patients who are appropriate candidates, must be started as soon as the diagnosis of SBP is made.

ALCOHOLIC HEPATITIS

Damage to the liver from alcohol ingestion, generally caused by an alcohol intake greater than 80 g daily for more than 15 years,[19] can result in three distinct syndromes of alcoholic liver disease: fatty liver, alcoholic hepatitis, and cirrhosis. Alcoholic hepatitis is a potentially life-threatening form of toxic liver injury resulting from alcohol consumption; the pathophysiology of the injury is unclear. Its true incidence is unknown, because many patients are asymptomatic and formal diagnosis necessitates a liver biopsy. However, approximately 20% of patients admitted to a hospital with alcoholism have alcoholic hepatitis, two thirds of whom already have histologic evidence of cirrhosis.[20] It is estimated that 33% of chronic alcoholics experience alcoholic hepatitis.[21] With approximately 17 million alcoholics in the United States, it is not surprising that death resulting from liver disease is common in urban adults.

Clinical Presentation

The presentation of alcoholic hepatitis varies from a mild, asymptomatic illness to one of fulminant, life-threatening liver failure. Patients who are admitted to an ICU and have alcoholic hepatitis are likely to have anorexia, vomiting, jaundice, and right upper quadrant abdominal pain. Because this presentation is also compatible with cholangitis, it is imperative that patients with alcoholic hepatitis be not misdiagnosed as having biliary tract disease, as operative procedures in this setting have serious morbidity and mortality. Alternatively, patients may present to the ICU because of complications of portal hypertension or cirrhosis (gastrointestinal bleeding, hepatic encephalopathy, hepatorenal syndrome, or SBP). The physical examination is likely to show hepatomegaly (an early sign of alcoholic hepatitis, present in more than 85% of cases), jaundice, asterixis, and ascites. In a Veterans Administration cooperative study, ascites was present in 39% of cases in which there was no histologic evidence of cirrhosis.[22] Portal hypertension and varices may be present without cirrhosis.

Results of laboratory studies can be characteristic of alcoholic hepatitis, but none are diagnostic. The white blood cell count can be markedly elevated. A macrocytic anemia is usually present. Patients are often folate deficient, and there may be gastrointestinal blood loss as well. There is no correlation between the level of the aminotransferases (aspartate aminotransferase [AST] and alanine aminotransferase [ALT]) and the severity of the illness; in fact, a high AST (greater than 300 IU/L) makes the diagnosis of alcoholic hepatitis unlikely. The AST value is often elevated to twice the level of the ALT. As a rule, the bilirubin level is markedly elevated, and hepatic synthetic function is diminished, as manifested by a prolonged prothrombin time and a low serum albumin level. Occasionally, a predominantly cholestatic picture with a markedly elevated serum alkaline phosphatase level is seen; this may make differentiation between alcoholic hepatitis and ascending cholangitis even more difficult.

If the liver is examined histologically, three features allow the diagnosis of alcoholic hepatitis to be made: (1) liver cell necrosis with ballooning degeneration; (2) a lobular inflammatory infiltrate, predominantly polymorphonuclear; and (3) fibrosis, particularly around the terminal hepatic vein.

Other features commonly present include fatty change (in more than 95% of the cases but not specific), Mallory's bodies, intrahepatic cholestasis, and excessive iron deposits. Occasionally, features suggestive of chronic hepatitis (a portal mononuclear infiltrate with a variable amount of piecemeal necrosis) may be present; coinfection with the hepatitis C virus may be responsible for this finding.

Diagnosis

The diagnosis of alcoholic hepatitis is made when a patient has characteristic symptoms and signs. Patients may have anorexia, vomiting, jaundice, right upper quadrant pain, ascites, spider angiomas, encephalopathy, leukocytosis, coagulopathy, hyperbilirubinemia, and hypertransaminasemia. The AST value is usually less than 300 IU/L, and the ratio of AST to ALT is often 2:1. Patients with ascites should have a paracentesis to rule out SBP. If necessary, an ultrasound scan help differentiate obstructive jaundice from hepatocellular jaundice.

Course and Prognosis

Differences in the severity of alcoholic hepatitis account for published survival figures of 0 to 100% in patients hospitalized with this condition. Many patients with alcoholic hepatitis have a mild disease, which responds merely to abstinence and supportive care. Other patients may experience an increase in the severity of illness during the initial 2 weeks after hospitalization; they may continue to deteriorate for as long as 3 weeks before either improvement or death. Measures that can predict mortality include the levels of bilirubin, creatinine, and albumin; prothrombin time; the age of the patient; and the presence of hepatic encephalopathy or ascites. Prognostic indices have been proposed to identify patients who may be at greatest risk of death resulting from alcoholic hepatitis. The highest correlation has been found with Maddrey's discriminant function (DF):

$$DF = 4.6 \times [\text{prothrombin time (s)} - \text{control}] + \text{bilirubin (mg/dL)}$$

When the discriminant function is greater than 32, patients have a mortality of approximately 35%.[23, 24] Other more complicated indices, such as Pugh's modification of the Child-Turcotte classification or the University of Toronto's combined clinical and laboratory index, do not appear to predict survival any better.[24]

Treatment

Good general supportive care is an essential part of the management of patients with alcoholic hepatitis but may not be sufficient to prevent death in those with more serious disease. Several studies have examined the effects of various therapeutic modalities for severe alcoholic hepatitis, including steroids, propylthiouracil (PTU), and nutritional therapy.[23–38] There have been two major difficulties in designing these trials. The first difficulty has been deciding which patients to treat. Many patients have mild disease and improve whether or not therapy is given. Other patients are so severely ill that no therapy is beneficial. Finding the subgroup of patients who are neither too ill to benefit nor too well to require therapy is important. The use of prognostic indices in the admission criteria for studies of drug therapy allows the identification of patients at highest risk for death and may allow smaller differences in outcome between treated and untreated groups to be evident. The second problem has been enrolling a large enough number of patients in the study so that a benefit of small magnitude is not missed through a type 2 error. Most studies of appropriate magnitude need to be multi-institutional.

The rationale for the use of corticosteroids in patients with alcoholic hepatitis is based on the assumption that alcohol damage to the liver induces liver neoantigens, that alcoholic hepatitis can result from an immune response to these liver antigens, and that suppression of this immune attack can be of benefit. Many studies of the use of prednisolone in the treatment of patients with alcoholic hepatitis have had conflicting results, but interpretation of their results is hampered by the difficulties in study design as outlined earlier. In a randomized, double-blind, placebo-controlled, multicenter study on the effects of a 4-week course of prednisolone (32 mg daily) in patients with serious alcoholic hepatitis (discriminant function > 32), the mortality in the treatment group was 6% versus 35% in placebo recipients.[24]

On the basis of this and other studies, the following conclusions can be drawn. Patients with mild-to-moderate disease receive no benefit from steroid therapy. Because there appears to be no long-term effect of steroids on the development of cirrhosis,[33] therapy should not be prolonged. The subgroup of patients who are likely to benefit from steroid treatment consists of patients with serious alcoholic hepatitis, as defined by a discriminant function greater than 32 or particularly by the presence of spontaneous hepatic encephalopathy. One should exclude from steroid therapy patients who have gastrointestinal hemorrhage, diabetes, active infection, clinical evidence of acute pancreatitis, recent head trauma, or pre-existing chronic renal disease with a creatinine concentration greater than 175 μmol/L; these patients are likely either to be too ill to benefit from therapy or to have specific difficulties with the use of corticosteroids.

Protein-calorie malnutrition is a universal finding in patients hospitalized with alcoholic hepatitis, and its severity correlates with the severity of the disease and the mortality rate. Nutritional support can achieve positive nitrogen balance and improve nutritional status in patients with alcoholic hepatitis.[37, 38] Although it has been difficult to prove that a nutritional intervention (through enteral or parenteral means) leads to improved survival in patients with alcoholic hepatitis, some studies have shown that mortality is much lower in patients in whom a positive nitrogen balance is achieved than in those with a negative nitrogen balance.[39] The literature also supports the safety of dietary or parenteral protein administration in patients with hepatic encephalopathy;[37, 38] thus, there is no reason to restrict protein intake in patients with alcoholic hepatitis. There is no clear benefit of the initial use of special formulations of amino acids (such as those enriched in branched chain amino acid), and their use should be reserved for those patients whose encephalopathy worsens with protein feeding.[39]

The use of PTU in alcoholic hepatitis is controversial. It is based on studies finding an ethanol-induced hypermetabolic state and increased liver oxygen consumption, a predominantly centrilobular pattern of injury common to both hypoxia and alcoholic liver injury, and a protective effect of thyroidectomy or PTU in preventing hypoxic injury in animals with alcoholic liver disease. One group of investigators found a small reduction in the cumulative mortality rate and an improvement in a prognostic index score in patients with severe alcoholic liver disease given 300 mg daily of PTU for up to 6 weeks.[34, 35] However, another large and well-designed study showed no difference in mortality rate between the use of PTU and placebo in patients with alcoholic hepatitis.[36] More studies need to be performed before PTU can be recommended for the treatment of alcoholic hepatitis.

The use of anabolic steroids in alcoholic hepatitis is also controversial. The rationale for the use of anabolic steroids is that they may facilitate improvement in the formation of coagulation factors and accelerate the removal of excessive hepatic fat. In addition, a delayed, long-term therapeutic effect is hypothesized to occur by inducing expression of fetal gene products that result in liver regeneration. In a randomized trial comparing prednisolone, oxandrolone, and placebo, there was no statistically significant difference in mortality among the treatment and placebo groups. However, there was a stabilization in the 6-month conditional death rate, defined as the probability of dying in a 6-month period given that a patient has survived for 1 to 5 months after initiation of treatment, in the group with moderately severe alcoholic hepatitis.[25] However, because most deaths occur during the index hospitalization and in patients with severe disease, anabolic steroid therapy cannot be recommended at this time.

Experience with liver transplantation has increased significantly since Starzl pioneered it. There were 1700 liver transplants in the United States in 1988. The overall 5-year survival is 70%.[40] In patients with end-stage alcoholic liver disease, the 1-year survival is about 70 to 80%.[41-44] Patients with alcoholic liver disease may be considered candidates for liver transplantation if they have progressive liver disease that has proved resistant to other therapeutic modalities and have no absolute contraindication to transplantation, such as sepsis or malignancy outside the hepatobiliary system. One must carefully seek evidence of serious cardiomyopathy or irreversible central nervous system disease in all potential candidates. Patients undergoing transplantation must have a strong social support system and be compliant with follow-up care. The question of whether to consider transplantation in patients with acute alcoholic hepatitis is controversial. Although the length of abstinence may not be a prognostic factor in patients with end-stage liver failure who undergo transplantation, there are no comparable data in patients with acute alcoholic hepatitis.[41, 45]

Summary

Alcoholic hepatitis may be an acute, life-threatening toxic liver disorder. In patients with signs and symptoms of alcoholic hepatitis, it is imperative to make an accurate diagnosis to prevent unnecessary exploratory surgery. Patients with severe alcoholic hepatitis should receive supportive therapy, including enteral or parenteral nutrition. Treatment with prednisolone should be reserved for patients with a discriminant function greater than 32 or spontaneous encephalopathy, in the absence of gastrointestinal hemorrhage, diabetes, active infection, acute pancreatitis, recent head trauma, or chronic renal disease. There is currently not enough evidence to support the use of PTU or oxandrolone in acute severe alcoholic hepatitis. Although patients with end-stage liver disease may benefit from liver transplantation, there is a paucity of data regarding liver transplantation in acute alcoholic hepatitis.

FULMINANT HEPATIC FAILURE

FHF is a syndrome in which there is severe hepatic injury resulting in encephalopathy within 8 weeks of onset of illness in a patient without evidence of previous liver disease.[46] There are fewer than 2000 cases of FHF per year in the United States.[47] The prognosis of FHF is related to both the cause of the liver injury and the severity of the encephalopathy on presentation.

TABLE 133–1

CAUSES OF FULMINANT HEPATIC FAILURE

Viral Hepatitis
Hepatitis A, B, C, D, and E virus infection
Cytomegalovirus and herpes simplex virus infections
Viral hemorrhagic fevers (yellow fever virus, Ebola and Marburg viruses, Rift Valley fever virus)

Drug or Toxic Hepatitis
Acetaminophen, isoniazid, halothane, valproic acid, *Amanita phalloides,* carbon tetrachloride

Hemodynamic Injury
Heat stroke, shock, hepatic venous thrombosis or veno-occlusive disease

Miscellaneous Disorders
Microvesicular steatosis (fatty liver of pregnancy, Reye's syndrome)
Wilson's disease
Autoimmune chronic active hepatitis

Etiology

The many causes of FHF are outlined in Table 133–1. Viral hepatitis is the most common cause of FHF; some viral infections cause it more frequently than others. Hepatitis A is usually a benign, self-limited disease, but it is complicated by FHF between 0.01 and 0.1% of the time and, in most series of FHF, accounts for approximately 5% of cases.[48] Hepatitis B is the most common cause of FHF and accounts for between 30 and 65% of cases in some series.[48, 49] In patients who survive FHF caused by hepatitis B, development of the hepatitis B carrier state is unusual. Hepatitis D virus superinfection or coinfection can increase the severity of hepatitis B; its presence should be sought in all patients with FHF who are hepatitis B surface antigen–positive. Non-A, non-B hepatitis (generally attributable to the hepatitis C virus) can cause FHF, is associated with a particularly poor prognosis, and can lead to aplastic anemia and bone marrow failure, particularly in patients who undergo liver transplantation. Hepatitis E is an epidemic form of hepatitis similar to hepatitis A. It is spread through contamination of drinking water by raw sewage and is common in India and Southeast Asia. It is generally benign and does not cause chronic liver disease. However, it is a particularly serious disease in pregnant women, with a 20% mortality rate when women are infected in the third trimester of pregnancy.[50] Other viral infections can cause FHF; these occur generally in immunocompromised hosts (e.g., with infection by cytomegalovirus, herpes simplex virus, or Epstein-Barr virus) or in travelers to tropical areas where hemorrhagic fevers are endemic (e.g., yellow fever virus, Ebola and Marburg viruses, or Rift Valley fever virus).

Drug-induced FHF is generally due to either a hypersensitivity reaction or direct hepatotoxicity. Drugs that cause hypersensitivity do so through a direct or indirect allergic reaction; such hypersensitivity reactions are not dose dependent, are species specific, and can be accompanied by other features of an allergic reaction, such as fever, rash, eosinophilia, granulomas, or atypical lymphocytosis. Isoniazid, halothane, and valproic acid all cause FHF through hypersensitivity reactions. On the other hand, intrinsic hepatotoxins cause a dose-related liver injury in many species. Acetaminophen, a common cause of FHF in England, is frequently ingested in a suicide attempt.

Administration of hepatotoxic drugs should be discontinued when liver abnormalities become manifest, because the risk of FHF is increased when the administration of hepatotoxic drugs is continued.[48] Other drugs that have been implicated in FHF include tricyclic antidepressants, cocaine,[61] and nonsteroidal anti-inflammatory agents.

Consumption of poisonous mushrooms is one of the most dramatic causes of FHF. *Amanita phalloides* is the most common mushroom implicated in FHF, although other *Amanita* species may be implicated. Multiple patients often present at the same time, all having eaten the same batch of mushrooms. There are four characteristic stages:

1. A latent, asymptomatic period, which lasts 6 to 24 hours
2. A gastrointestinal phase, which is marked by severe crampy abdominal pain, nausea, vomiting, and profuse watery diarrhea, and lasts 12 to 24 hours
3. A second latent phase, which lasts 12 to 24 hours, but during which time there is laboratory evidence of subclinical hepatic injury
4. A hepatic phase, which is notable for rising aminotransferase levels, coagulopathy, jaundice, hypoglycemia, acidosis, encephalopathy, and renal failure

Without hepatic transplantation, about 20 to 30% of all patients with severe poisonous mushroom ingestion die within 6 to 16 days.[52]

Pathology

Two different types of hepatic lesions are seen in patients with FHF. The first type consists of massive hepatocellular necrosis, either centrilobular or diffuse. There is marked loss of hepatocytes, with confluent necrosis involving adjacent lobules. Extensive necrosis may cause disruption of the reticular framework of the lobule. The remaining hepatocytes may appear shrunken, swollen, or vacuolated. In addition, there may be a variable inflammatory infiltrate. Viral hepatitis and most cases of drug-induced FHF are characterized by this pathologic lesion.

The second type of lesion is one of microvesicular steatosis. The hepatocytes are filled with small fat-laden vesicles. There is minimal necrosis. Fatty liver of pregnancy, tetracycline toxicity, and Reye's syndrome are characterized by microvesicular steatosis.

Clinical Manifestations and Treatment

The clinical manifestations of FHF are protean and involve nearly all organ systems. In the absence of specific therapy for FHF, treatment consists of intensive supportive care, treatment of the complications of acute liver failure, and possibly liver transplantation. If the cause of FHF is unknown, serologic studies for hepatitis A, B (if positive, D), and C viruses, Epstein-Barr virus, herpes simplex virus, and cytomegalovirus should be done. In addition, a urine screen for toxins and copper and serum ceruloplasmin and copper levels should be obtained. Intense hemolysis in the setting of FHF is suggestive of Wilson's disease or hepatitis associated with glucose-6-phosphate dehydrogenase deficiency; the latter may be seen in the sulfone syndrome associated with dapsone hypersensitivity. Granulocytopenia, with or without lymphocytosis, is suggestive of fulminant non-A, non-B hepatitis.[53]

General Management and Transfer

All patients with FHF should be admitted to an ICU. Because of the potential for cerebral edema to complicate FHF, certain simple measures should be taken. The patient's upper body should be kept 30 to 40° to the horizontal to decrease cerebral edema. Extreme flexion, extension, or rotation of the head should be avoided, because this can decrease venous return and exacerbate cerebral edema. Movement during routine nursing can also increase intracranial pressure (ICP) and should be avoided in patients with deep coma.

Other general measures are important. Blood and body fluid precautions should be instituted. Urine output should be monitored, and central venous pressure should be followed, preferably with a Swan-Ganz catheter. Hypoglycemia should be prevented by infusion of either 5 or 10% dextrose in water. Patients should be transferred to a liver transplant center after they have reached stage 2 encephalopathy or if the prothrombin time is prolonged to greater than 30 seconds.[54] The mode of transportation is important because appreciable gravitational forces may be generated during high-speed road transfer, especially around corners, and during takeoff and landing of aircraft. These forces can increase ICP. Helicopter is the safest option over long distances. Patients in stage 3 or 4 hepatic encephalopathy should be intubated to protect their airway before transfer, and if they are hypoxemic or hypercapnic, they should be ventilated.[54]

Treatment of Encephalopathy

Hepatic encephalopathy is a necessary condition for the diagnosis of FHF. Encephalopathy is divided into four stages:

Stage 1: Patient shows mild confusion, slowed mentation, slurred speech, disordered sleep rhythm, and mild asterixis.
Stage 2: Patient shows drowsiness, inappropriate behavior, incontinence, marked asterixis.
Stage 3: Patient sleeps most of the time but is rousable, speech is incoherent, and confusion is marked. Asterixis is present.
Stage 4: Deep coma. Patient may or may not respond to deep pain. Asterixis is absent.[47]

Although portal-systemic shunting plays an important role in the pathophysiology of encephalopathy in chronic liver disease, it is not important in the encephalopathy of FHF. It is essential to rule out secondary causes of encephalopathy, including hypoglycemia, hypoxemia, hemorrhage, sepsis, sedative or hypnotic drugs, electrolyte imbalance, acid-base disturbance, reduced cerebral perfusion pressure, and cerebral edema. There is little evidence that lactulose prevents the development of stage 3 or 4 encephalopathy, but it may be useful in the early stages. The dose of lactulose should be adjusted to result in two to four loose bowel movements per day. If patients are confused and unable to take lactulose orally, a nasogastric tube can be placed and the lactulose administered per nasogastric tube. It is important to avoid excessive loss of free water caused by excessive diarrhea, as often happens when more than 30 ml three times daily is used, because of the potential for severe hypernatremia.[54]

Administration of neomycin should be avoided because of its propensity to cause ototoxicity and nephrotoxicity. Plasmapheresis has been reported to decrease encephalopathy and improve hemostasis, especially when coupled with plasma exchange. Although it has no effect on mortality, it may be useful in stabilizing patients who have significant bleeding or require invasive procedures (liver biopsy, central venous catheter or ICP monitor placement) before transplantation.[55]

Treatment of Cerebral Edema

Cerebral edema is the major cause of mortality in patients with FHF. It usually occurs in patients who are in stage 4 coma. The earliest sign of increased ICP is an increase in muscle tone in the extremities. Patients can progress to full decerebrate posturing, with hyperpronation and adduction of the arms. Hyperventilation occurs, and the pupils become dilated and react sluggishly to light. As the ICP continues to rise, trismus and opisthotonos occur. Failure to arrest the process at this point often results in respiratory arrest and brain stem herniation. Changes in pupillary light reflexes are particularly reliable in diagnosing elevated ICP, especially when patients are ventilated and paralyzed. Bilateral dilated, unresponsive pupils often imply irreversible brain stem herniation, but can be caused by increased sympathetic tone. Patients with FHF are usually hypotensive, and transient hypertension can be a manifestation of increased ICP. Treating hypertension in this situation is inappropriate, because it may critically reduce cerebral perfusion pressure.[47, 54]

The routine use of ICP monitors in patients with FHF is controversial. They allow early detection of increased ICP and rapid calculation of cerebral perfusion pressure, defined as the mean arterial pressure minus the ICP. Elevated ICP should be treated when it has reached a persistent level of 30 mm Hg. Cerebral perfusion pressure must be maintained at 40 mm Hg or more if brain stem herniation is to be prevented.[54] In addition, ICP monitors allow physicians to see the dramatic effects of seemingly innocuous procedures on ICP. Simple turning of the patient's head may increase ICP because of increased resistance to venous flow in the neck combined with reduced intracranial compliance.[56] The complications of ICP monitors are low and include oozing from the implantation site, displacement of the monitor by clot, infection, and rarely intracranial hemorrhage.[54, 56] On the other hand, ICP monitoring has not been shown to reduce mortality in patients with head injury [57, 58] or in patients with FHF (the latter in a prospective study).[59] In addition, clinical signs become present when the ICP remains at 30 mm Hg for approximately 5 minutes.[59] In conclusion, ICP monitoring should be used when evaluating new treatments for cerebral edema and considered when cerebral edema is difficult to control or when it is likely to be prolonged, as in Reye's syndrome.[54]

Mannitol administration has been shown to be effective[60] and is the mainstay of treatment for increased ICP. It should be infused rapidly, preferably through a central catheter as a 20% solution, at a dose of 0.5 to 1 g/kg of body weight, and repeated as necessary. Urine output, blood pressure, and serum osmolarity should be monitored. Because mannitol can increase ICP as a result of fluid overload and hyperosmolarity, it should be used only in patients with adequate renal function, or when ultrafiltration or hemodialysis is in progress in patients with renal failure. Rapid removal of urea and other solutes during hemodialysis can precipitate hyposmolar edema and even brain stem herniation. Serum osmolarity should be checked immediately before dialysis, and if it is low, it should be corrected by infusion of 20% mannitol as soon as dialysis is commenced. Osmolarity should then be checked every 1 to 2 hours, and kept in the high-normal range.[54]

Several other modalities have been investigated in the treatment of cerebral edema. Steroids have been shown to be ineffective in several randomized, prospective trials.[61–64] An uncontrolled study of charcoal hemoperfusion done in 1982 suggested that early charcoal hemoperfusion reduced the incidence of cerebral edema.[65] However, a later randomized, prospective study did not support these findings.[66]

Although controlled, mechanical hyperventilation may delay the onset of brain stem herniation, it does not decrease the incidence of cerebral edema or affect the mortality rate. In addition, it causes vasoconstriction and may lead to decreased hepatic blood flow.[59] Thiopental and pentobarbital have been shown to be effective in reducing ICP in small groups of patients who were refractory to conventional therapy.[67, 68] The reduction in ICP is believed to be due to its anesthetic effect and cerebral vasoconstriction. Toxicity included systemic hypotension and decreased cerebral perfusion pressure, which responded to discontinuing infusion.

Hemostasis

The coagulopathy that occurs in FHF is multifactorial. The platelet count is low as a result of hypersplenism, bone marrow suppression, increased consumption of platelets, and loss of platelets in extracorporeal hemoperfusion. There is diminished production of coagulation factors in the liver, including fibrinogen; prothrombin; factors V, VII, IX, and X; antithrombin III; protein C; and protein S. Low-grade disseminated intravascular coagulation is present, and the circulating fibrin degradation products serve as circulating inhibitors. Bleeding usually occurs from the gastrointestinal tract and is often severe. Histamine H_2 receptor antagonists have been shown to decrease the incidence of gastrointestinal bleeding.[69]

When managing a patient with FHF, the platelet count, prothrombin time, partial thromboplastin time, fibrinogen, and fibrin degradation products should be followed frequently. Vitamin K should be administered parenterally for the first 3 days and intermittently thereafter, in an attempt to correct any potential deficiency. Clotting factor concentrates should not be given because they can exacerbate disseminated intravascular coagulation. Administration of fresh frozen plasma prophylactically is not recommended but may be used with platelet infusions or plasma exchange to cover surgical procedures.[55, 70]

Management of Other Complications

Patients with FHF often have multiple organ system failure. Cardiac arrhythmias are common. Sinus tachycardia occurs most commonly. Heart block, ventricular ectopy, and bradycardia usually occur in the setting of hypoxemia, acidosis, electrolyte disturbances, or elevated ICP. Patients are often hypotensive. The systemic vascular resistance is usually inappropriately low, which may be due to diminished hepatic clearance of endogenous vasodilators, and the cardiac output is increased. Hypotension with a hyperdynamic circulation results. It may be difficult to distinguish this from sepsis, and a high level of suspicion should be maintained. Unless volume depletion is evident and systolic blood pressure is consistently less than 90 mm Hg, volume expansion and pressors should be withheld. A decrease in heart rate suggests central vasomotor depression and is often caused by cerebral edema.[71]

Pulmonary complications are frequently present. Patients may have hypoxemia as a result of intrapulmonary arteriovenous shunting, pulmonary edema, adult respiratory distress syndrome, aspiration pneumonia, and atelectasis. Patients with stage 4 encephalopathy should be intubated prophylactically to protect their airway and prevent aspiration of blood or stomach contents. Ventilatory correction of hypocapnia is contraindicated, as it may exacerbate cerebral edema.

As the patients' defense mechanisms become impaired, infections can set in. There are decreased ventilatory and cough reflexes, poor clearance of secretions, and endotracheal tubes, all of which set the stage for pneumonia. Urinary catheters predispose to urinary tract infections and intravenous and dialysis catheters put patients at risk for systemic infections. It is important to obtain cultures frequently, because many of the signs of infection may be obscured.

Renal failure is a poor prognostic sign. It may be caused by prerenal factors, acute tubular necrosis, or hepatorenal syndrome. Hypokalemia is common and may be due to increased losses, inadequate replacement, and secondary hyperaldosteronism. Hyponatremia is often dilutional. Total body sodium level is elevated from secondary hyperaldosteronism, but free water secretion is impaired. Hypoglycemia may result from impaired gluconeogenesis, and all patients should be maintained on a 5 or 10% dextrose infusion. If hypoglycemia is severe, 20 or 50% dextrose solutions can be used.

Specific Therapy

Although therapy directed at the underlying disease is generally not helpful in patients with FHF, in rare circumstances it may be critical. Patients with FHF caused by acetaminophen administration should be treated with N-acetylcysteine, even if the ingestion occurred up to 36 hours before the initiation of therapy, as this therapy may replete the liver with glutathione and protect the liver against the epoxide metabolite injury.[72] Patients with a fulminant presentation of Wilson's disease should be stabilized using postdilutional hemofiltration to lower the serum copper levels initially, followed by prompt liver transplantation.

Prognostic Factors

The prognosis of patients with FHF depends on the cause of the disease and on the severity of the presenting clinical manifestations. Patients with FHF secondary to acetaminophen administration and hepatitis A and hepatitis B have a survival rate between 40 and 60%, whereas those with FHF attributable to non-A, non-B hepatitis, halothane administration, and other drug reactions have a survival rate between 12 and 20%.[66] In patients with acetaminophen toxicity, poor prognostic factors include a serum pH less than 7.3, a prothrombin time longer than 100 seconds, and a serum creatinine concentration greater than 300 μmol/L. When FHF occurs in the setting of viral hepatitis or drug reactions, poor prognostic factors include younger age than 11 years or older than 40 years, jaundice of more than 7 days' duration before the onset of encephalopathy, bilirubin level greater than 300 μmol/L, and prothrombin time longer than 50 seconds.[73] In patients with hepatitis B, survival is increased in the absence of hepatitis B surface antigen, with increased factor V levels, with increased serum α-fetoprotein levels, and with young age.[74]

Liver Transplantation

Before the development of liver transplantation, the mortality in FHF was high. Patients with stage 4 encephalopathy had a survival rate between 10 and 30%.[75, 76] Survival rates in patients undergoing transplantation in stage 3 or 4 encephalopathy are approximately 60%.[49, 53, 56, 77, 78] Patients with FHF should be transfered to a liver transplantation center as soon as possible, because deterioration can be rapid, and it is essential for patients to be put on the donor list as early as possible. The indications for transplantation are still evolving and have been discussed elsewhere (see Chapter 134).

Because outcome worsens as hepatic failure increases, transplant teams are caught in the dilemma of performing transplantation before patients become too ill versus waiting to see if they recover on their own. Some groups recommend transplantation for patients with rapidly progressing encephalopathy, severe hemolysis, cerebral edema, or a rapidly shrinking liver.[53] Others recommend transplantation for patients on the basis of the severity of illness and the cause of FHF. Patients with acetaminophen hepatotoxicity generally undergo transplantation if they are acidotic, if the prothrombin time is prolonged, or if the creatinine concentration is elevated, in the face of stage 3 or 4 encephalopathy. In non–acetaminophen-induced FHF, transplantation is recommended if the prothrombin time is longer than 100 seconds, or if patients have poor prognostic factors as given earlier.[73]

Contraindications to transplantation include extrahepatic malignancy, active extrahepatic sepsis, thrombosis of the entire mesenteric venous system, and irreversible brain damage caused by intracranial hemorrhage or cerebral edema.[56] In patients with FHF from hepatitis B, the hepatitis B surface antigen generally clears after liver transplantation, contrary to the usual recurrent hepatitis B when patients with hepatic failure and chronic hepatitis B undergo transplantation.

Summary

FHF should always be managed in the ICU. Patients with FHF represent a major challenge to the intensivist, as any organ system can and frequently does fail. General measures of support should be started in all patients. Attention to the potential development of hypoglycemia, acid-base disorders, hypoxemia attributable to noncardiogenic pulmonary edema, and aspiration of blood or stomach contents in patients in deep coma is necessary. Specific consideration should be given to the administration of histamine H_2 receptor blockers to prevent gastrointestinal bleeding and to the use of mannitol infusions to treat increased ICP. Therapy with N-acetylcysteine should be given to patients with acetaminophen toxicity. Failure to respond to supportive measures and to specific therapy when available should prompt transfer of the patient to a liver transplantation center.

Measures to protect the ICU staff against viral hepatitis should be instituted when appropriate, and all ICU staff should be encouraged to undergo hepatitis B vaccination and to report any potential critical exposure to a patient with FHF, such as a needle stick. The possibility that secondary cases of viral hepatitis can be prevented in household or sexual contacts of the patient should also be explored.

References

1. Runyon BA, Antillon MR, Montano AA: Effect of diuresis versus therapeutic paracentesis on ascitic fluid opsonic activity and serum complement. Gastroenterology 97:158, 1989.
2. Runyon BA: Patients with deficient ascitic fluid opsonic activity are predisposed to spontaneous bacterial peritonitis. Hepatology 8:632, 1988. (Published erratum in: Hepatology 8:1184, 1988.)
3. Runyon BA, Morrissey RL, Hoefs JC, et al: Opsonic activity of human ascitic fluid: A potentially important protective mechanism against spontaneous bacterial peritonitis. Hepatology 5:634, 1985.
4. Runyon BA: Low-protein-concentration ascitic fluid is predisposed to spontaneous bacterial peritonitis. Gastroenterology 91:1343, 1986.
5. Pinzello G, Simonetti RG, Craxi A, et al: Spontaneous bacterial peritonitis: A prospective investigation in predominantly nonalcoholic cirrhotic patients. Hepatology 3:545, 1983.
6. Runyon BA, Hoefs JC: Spontaneous vs secondary bacterial peritonitis. Differentiation by response of ascitic fluid neutrophil count to antimicrobial therapy. Arch Intern Med 146:1563, 1986.
7. Runyon BA: Spontaneous bacterial peritonitis: An explosion of information. Hepatology 8:171, 1988.
8. Reynolds TB: Rapid presumptive diagnosis of spontaneous bacterial peritonitis. Gastroenterology 90:1294, 1986.
9. Runyon BA, Canawati HN, Akriviadis EA: Optimization of ascitic fluid culture technique. Gastroenterology 95:1351, 1988.
10. Runyon BA, Umland ET, Merlin T: Inoculation of blood culture bottles

with ascitic fluid. Improved detection of spontaneous bacterial peritonitis. Arch Intern Med 147:73, 1987.

11. Garrison R, Cryer H, Howard D: Clarification of risk factors for abdominal operations in patients with hepatic cirrhosis. Ann Surg 199:648, 1984.

12. Pinzello G, Virdone R, Lojacono F, et al: Is the acidity of ascitic fluid a reliable index in making the presumptive diagnosis of spontaneous bacterial peritonitis? Hepatology 6:244, 1986.

13. Runyon BA, Hoefs JC: Ascitic fluid analysis in the differentiation of spontaneous bacterial peritonitis from gastrointestinal tract perforation into ascitic fluid. Hepatology 4:447, 1984.

14. Yang CY, Liaw YF, Chu CM, et al: White count, pH and lactate in ascites in the diagnosis of spontaneous bacterial peritonitis. Hepatology 5:85, 1985.

15. Felisart J, Rimola A, Arroyo V, et al: Cefotaxime is more effective than is ampicillin-tobramycin in cirrhotics with severe infections. Hepatology 5:457, 1985.

16. Fong TL, Akriviadis EA, Runyon BA, et al: Polymorphonuclear cell count response and duration of antibiotic therapy in spontaneous bacterial peritonitis. Hepatology 9:423, 1989.

17. Tito L, Rimola A, Gines P, et al: Recurrence of spontaneous bacterial peritonitis in cirrhosis: Frequency and predictive factors. Hepatology 8:27, 1988.

18. Pelletier G, Salmon D, Ink O, et al: Culture-negative neutrocytic ascites: A less severe variant of spontaneous bacterial peritonitis. J Hepatol 10:327, 1990.

19. Lelbach WK: Epidemiology of alcoholic liver disease. Prog Liver Dis 5:494, 1976.

20. Goldberg SJ, Mendenhall CL, Connell AM, et al: "Nonalcoholic" chronic hepatitis in the alcoholic. Gastroenterology 74:598, 1977.

21. Mendenhall CL: Alcoholic hepatitis. Clin Gastroenterol 10:417, 1981.

22. Mendenhall C: Alcoholic hepatitis. In: Schiff ER, Schiff L (eds): Diseases of the Liver. 6th ed. Philadelphia, JB Lippincott, p 669, 1987.

23. Maddrey WC, Boitnott JK, Bedine MS, et al: Corticosteroid therapy of alcoholic hepatitis. Gastroenterology 75:193, 1978.

24. Carithers RJ, Herlong HF, Diehl AM, et al: Methylprednisolone therapy in patients with severe alcoholic hepatitis. A randomized multicenter trial. Ann Intern Med 110:685, 1989.

25. Mendenhall CL, Anderson S, Garcia PP, et al: Short-term and long-term survival in patients with alcoholic hepatitis treated with oxandrolone and prednisolone. N Engl J Med 311:1464, 1984.

26. Porter HP, Simon FR, Pope C 2nd, et al: Corticosteroid therapy in severe alcoholic hepatitis. A double-blind drug trial. N Engl J Med 284: 1350, 1971.

27. Campra JL, Hamlin EJ, Kirshbaum RJ, et al: Prednisone therapy of acute alcoholic hepatitis. Report of a controlled trial. Ann Intern Med 79:625, 1973.

28. Blitzer BL, Mutchnick MG, Joshi PH, et al: Adrenocorticosteroid therapy in alcoholic hepatitis. A prospective, double-blind randomized study. Am J Dig Dis 22:477, 1977.

29. Depew W, Boyer T, Omata M, et al: Double-blind controlled trial of prednisolone therapy in patients with severe acute alcoholic hepatitis and spontaneous encephalopathy. Gastroenterology 78:524, 1980.

30. Lesesne HR, Bozymski EM, Fallon HJ: Treatment of alcoholic hepatitis with encephalopathy. Comparison of prednisolone with caloric supplements. Gastroenterology 74:169, 1978.

31. Schlichting P, Juhl E, Poulsen H, et al: Alcoholic hepatitis superimposed on cirrhosis. Clinical significance and effect of long-term prednisone treatment. Scand J Gastroenterol 11:305, 1976.

32. Shumaker JB, Resnick RH, Galambos JT, et al: A controlled trial of 6-methylprednisolone in acute alcoholic hepatitis. With a note on published results in encephalopathic patients. Am J Gastroenterol 69:443, 1978.

33. Helman RA, Temko MH, Nye SW, et al: Alcoholic hepatitis. Natural history and evaluation of prednisolone therapy. Ann Intern Med 74:311, 1971.

34. Orrego H, Kalant H, Israel Y, et al: Effect of short-term therapy with propylthiouracil in patients with alcoholic liver disease. Gastroenterology 76:105, 1979.

35. Orrego H, Blake JE, Blendis LM, et al: Long-term treatment of alcoholic liver disease with propylthiouracil. N Engl J Med 317:1421, 1987.

36. Hallé P, Paré P, Kaptein E, et al: Double-blind, controlled trial of propylthiouracil in patients with severe acute alcoholic hepatitis. Gastroenterology 82:925, 1982.

37. Mendenhall C, Bongiovanni G, Goldberg S, et al: VA Cooperative Study on Alcoholic Hepatitis. III: Changes in protein-calorie malnutrition associated with 30 days of hospitalization with and without enteral nutritional therapy. JPEN 9:590, 1985.

38. Johnson RD, Williams R. Nutritional support in alcoholic liver disease. Acta Med Scand Suppl 703:209, 1985.

39. McCullough A, Mullen K, Smanik E: Nutritional therapy in liver disease. Gastroenterol Clin North Am 18:619, 1989.

40. Starzl TE, Demetris AJ, Van Thiel D: Liver transplantation (2). N Engl J Med 321:1014, 1989.

41. Kumar S, Stauber RE, Gavaler JS, et al: Orthotopic liver transplantation for alcoholic liver disease. Hepatology 11:159, 1990.

42. Doffoel M, Wolf P, Ellero B, et al: Results of orthotopic liver transplantation (OLT) in alcoholic cirrhosis. Hepatology 9:527, 1989.

43. Brems J, Joshi S, Kane R, et al: Orthotopic liver transplantation: Primary therapy for alcoholic cirrhosis. Hepatology 10:658, 1989.

44. Lucey M, Merion R, Henley K, et al: Selection of patients with alcoholic liver disease for orthotopic liver transplantation. Hepatology 10:572, 1989.

45. Schenker S, Perkins HS, Sorrell MF: Should patients with end-stage alcoholic liver disease have a new liver? Hepatology 11:314, 1990.

46. Trey C, Davidson C: The management of fulminant hepatic failure. Progr Liver Dis 3:282, 1970.

47. Katelaris PH, Jones DB: Fulminant hepatic failure. Med Clin North Am 73:955, 1989.

48. Bernuau J, Rueff B, Benhamou JP: Fulminant and subfulminant liver failure: Definitions and causes. Semin Liver Dis 6:97, 1986.

49. Emond JC, Aran PP, Whitington PF, et al: Liver transplantation in the management of fulminant hepatic failure. Gastroenterology 96:1583, 1989.

50. Ramalingaswami V, Purcell RH: Waterborne non-A, non-B hepatitis. Lancet 1:571, 1988.

51. Kanel GC, Cassidy W, Shuster L, et al: Cocaine-induced liver cell injury: Comparison of morphological features in man and in experimental models. Hepatology 11:646, 1990.

52. Pinson CW, Daya MR, Benner KG, et al: Liver transplantation for severe *Amanita phalloides* mushroom poisoning. Am J Surg 159:493, 1990.

53. Stieber AC, Ambrosino G, Van TD, et al: Orthotopic liver transplantation for fulminant and subacute hepatic failure. Gastroenterol Clin North Am 17:157, 1988.

54. Ede RJ Williams RW: Hepatic encephalopathy and cerebral edema. Semin Liver Dis 6:107, 1986.

55. Winikoff S, Glassman MS, Spivak W: Plasmapheresis in a patient with hepatic failure awaiting liver transplantation. J Pediatr 107:547, 1985.

56. Schafer DF, Shaw BJ: Fulminant hepatic failure and orthotopic liver transplantation. Semin Liver Dis 9:189, 1989.

57. Bowers SA, Marshall LF: Outcome in 200 consecutive cases of severe head injury treated in San Diego County: A prospective analysis. Neurosurgery 6:237, 1980.

58. Stuart GG, Merry GS, Smith JA, et al: Severe head injury managed without intracranial pressure monitoring. J Neurosurg 59:601, 1983.

59. Ede RJ, Gimson AE, Bihari D, et al: Controlled hyperventilation in the prevention of cerebral oedema in fulminant hepatic failure. J Hepatol 2:43, 1986.

60. Canalese J, Gimson AE, Davis C, et al: Controlled trial of dexamethasone and mannitol for the cerebral oedema of fulminant hepatic failure. Gut 23:625, 1982.

61. Randomised trial of steroid therapy in acute liver failure. Report from the European Association for the Study of the Liver (EASL). Gut 20:620, 1979.

62. Rakela J: A double-blinded, randomized trial of hydrocortisone in acute hepatic failure. Gastroenterology 76:1297, 1979.

63. Redeker A, Schweitzer I, Yamahiro H: Randomization of corticosteroid therapy in fulminant hepatitis. N Engl J Med 294:728, 1976.

64. Ware AJ, Jones RE, Shorey JW, et al: A controlled trial of steroid therapy in massive hepatic necrosis. Am J Gastroenterol 62:130, 1974.

65. Gimson AE, Braude S, Mellon PJ, et al: Earlier charcoal haemoperfusion in fulminant hepatic failure. Lancet 2:681, 1982.

66. O'Grady JG, Gimson AE, O'Brien CJ, et al: Controlled trials of charcoal hemoperfusion and prognostic factors in fulminant hepatic failure. Gastroenterology 94:1186, 1988.

67. Rockoff MA, Marshall LF, Shapiro HM: High-dose barbiturate therapy in humans: A clinical review of 60 patients. Ann Neurol 6:194, 1979.

68. Forbes A, Alexander GJ, O'Grady JG, et al: Thiopental infusion in the treatment of intracranial hypertension complicating fulminant hepatic failure. Hepatology 10:306, 1989.

69. Macdougall BR, Bailey RJ, Williams R: H2-receptor antagonists and antacids in the prevention of acute gastrointestinal haemorrhage in fulminant hepatic failure. Two controlled trials. Lancet 1:617, 1977.

70. Munoz SJ, Ballas SK, Moritz MJ, et al: Perioperative management of fulminant and subfulminant hepatic failure with therapeutic plasmapheresis. Transpl Proc 21: 3535, 1989.

71. Bihari DJ, Gimson AE, Williams R: Cardiovascular, pulmonary and renal complications of fulminant hepatic failure. Semin Liver Dis 6:119, 1986.

72. Harrison PM, Keays R, Bray GP, et al: Improved outcome of paracetamol-induced fulminant hepatic failure by late administration of acetylcysteine. Lancet 335:1572, 1990.

73. O'Grady JG, Alexander GJ, Hayllar KM, et al: Early indicators of prognosis in fulminant hepatic failure. Gastroenterology 97:439, 1989.

74. Bernuau J, Goudeau A, Poynard T, et al: Multivariate analysis of prognostic factors in fulminant hepatitis B. Hepatology 6:648, 1986.

75. Tygstrup N, Ranek L: Assessment of prognosis in fulminant hepatic failure. Semin Liver Dis 6:129, 1986.

76. Pappas SC: Fulminant hepatic failure and the need for artificial liver support. Mayo Clin Proc 63:198, 1988.

77. Bismuth H, Samuel D, Gugenheim J, et al: Emergency liver transplantation for fulminant hepatitis. Ann Intern Med 107:337, 1987.

78. Iwatsuki S, Stieber AC, Marsh JW, et al: Liver transplantation for fulminant hepatic failure. Transplant Proc 21:2431, 1989.

CHAPTER 134

Liver Transplantation

Rowen K. Zetterman

In the past, the prolongation of life of patients with end-stage liver disease was limited by the capacity to manage or prevent the complications as they occurred. The success of liver transplantation has dramatically changed the management of these patients, bringing with it a new series of questions and management problems. In this brief discussion, some of these problems are addressed, including pretransplant issues of selection and evaluation of patients, problems of pretransplant care, and some clinical care issues that occur in the immediate post-transplant period.

LIVER TRANSPLANT CANDIDATE

For many physicians, the most difficult decision is the proper timing of referral for liver transplant evaluation. In most transplant centers, the answer would be to send them early. It is obviously better to see a patient too early and wait for the proper time than to see a patient in extremis with advanced complications and little chance of survival. For patients with cirrhosis, the first significant complication of portal hypertension, including variceal or portal hypertensive gastropathy bleeding, ascites, and encephalopathy, should be a reason to refer the patient. Although there have not been (nor are there likely to be) any comparison trials of liver transplantation and portal-systemic shunts for management of variceal hemorrhage, the growing consensus is that liver transplantation is the appropriate therapy for some patients who bleed. Furthermore, there may be an increased risk of portal venous thrombosis after liver transplantation in those who have had a prior shunt.[1] For patients with primary biliary cirrhosis, referral should also be considered because of advancing bone disease or alteration of life style because of severe lethargy. If the transplant center decides that a patient has been referred too early, an evaluation will have been completed that prepares the patient for the eventuality of transplantation when additional complications supervene.

The age limits for transplantation have been extended for both the donor[2] and the recipient.[3] For the transplant candidate, age alone is no longer a sole criterion. One patient 76 years of age and many patients in their 60s have undergone liver transplantation. There does not appear to be any significant difference in outcome for those adults older than age 60 years when compared with that in those younger.[4] Prior intra-abdominal surgery also does not interfere with transplantation. The scarring of the right upper quadrant of the abdomen after abdominal surgery with formation of portal-systemic collaterals may increase blood loss during transplantation but does not significantly affect overall mortality. How to handle the positive human immunodeficiency virus status of the potential liver transplant recipient is unresolved. At present, human immunodeficiency virus positivity alone may not be a contraindication,[3] although patients with evidence of pretransplant immunodeficiency have a greater likelihood of infection with the additional immunosuppression after liver transplantation.[5]

Indications

The majority of patients who come to transplantation have one of the chronic necroinflammatory or cholestatic diseases of the liver[6] (Table 134–1). The most common indications in adults are the causes of postnecrotic cirrhosis (e.g., chronic viral hepatitis and autoimmune chronic hepatitis), primary biliary cirrhosis, or sclerosing cholangitis. The majority of pediatric patients undergo transplantation for biliary atresia. Unfortunately, there is little role for liver transplantation in the management of patients with primary tumors of the liver. Only those with incidental (unsuspected until the liver is removed at transplantation) or coincidental (found during the immediate preoperative evaluation but not the reason for consideration of transplantation) tumors have done well with little likelihood of recurrence.[7]

Acute hepatic diseases may also necessitate liver transplantation for survival of patients. Most of these patients have fulminant hepatic failure (FHF) that is due to viral hepatitis and come to medical attention within 2 to 3 weeks of onset of symptoms. Drug injury of the liver and Wilson's disease may also occur as acute hepatic failure. The timing of liver transplantation in patients with a fulminant course can be difficult. In general, those with progressive encephalopathy and severe coagulopathy who reach deep stage 2 or stage 3

TABLE 134–1

SOME INDICATIONS FOR LIVER TRANSPLANTATION

A. Diseases associated with fulminant hepatic failure
  1. Viral hepatitis A, B, or B plus D, or non-A, non-B; unknown agents
  2. Wilson's disease
  3. Drug-induced or toxin-induced liver disease
    a. Acetaminophen
    b. Valproic acid
    c. Isoniazid
    d. *Amanita phalloides*
    e. Disulfiram
  4. Acute fatty liver of pregnancy
B. End-stage liver diseases
  1. Hepatocellular disorders
    a. Chronic viral hepatitis B, B plus D, non-A, non-B
    b. Autoimmune chronic hepatitis
    c. Wilson's disease
    d. Alcoholic cirrhosis
    e. Chronic drug-induced disorders
    f. α_1-Antitrypsin deficiency
    g. Congenital hepatic fibrosis
  2. Cholestatic disorders
    a. Primary biliary cirrhosis
    b. Sclerosing cholangitis
    c. Arteriohepatic dysplasia (Alagille's syndrome)
    d. Secondary biliary cirrhosis
  3. Vascular disorders
    a. Budd-Chiari syndrome
    b. Veno-occlusive disease
  4. Miscellaneous diseases
    a. Polycystic liver disease
C. Metabolic disorders
  1. Tyrosinemia
  2. Glycogen storage disease
  3. Primary hyperoxaluria
  4. Homozygous familial hypercholesterolemia
  5. Erythropoietic protoporphyria
D. Primary hepatic malignancy
  1. Hepatocellular carcinoma, incidental and coincidental
  2. Selected ductular and parenchymal cholangiocarcinomas
  3. Selected hemangioendotheliomas
  4. Selected angiosarcomas
  5. Selected metastatic diseases (e.g., carcinoid tumors)

TABLE 134–2

STAGES OF HEPATIC COMA

Stage	Consciousness	Asterixis	Reflexes	Electroencephalogram
0	Normal	None	Normal	Normal
1	Agitation, personality changes	None	Increased	Normal to slow waves
2	Lethargic, arousable	Present	Increased	Slow waves
3	Poorly arousable	Variable	Decreased	Slow waves, triphasic waves
4	Unarousable	Absent	Flaccid	Slow waves, triphasic waves

encephalopathy (Child-Pugh scale)[8] (Table 134–2) should be considered for transplantation.[9, 10]

Contraindications

There are few absolute contraindications to liver transplantation. Patients with acquired immunodeficiency syndrome, extrahepatic metastatic primary hepatic carcinomas, most metastatic diseases to the liver, ongoing sepsis, or advanced, uncorrectable cardiovascular diseases are generally considered not to be candidates for liver transplantation.[6] Patients who are human immunodeficiency virus–positive but who lack signs of immunosuppression may be candidates.[3] Selected patients with metastatic diseases to the liver may also be candidates, such as those with carcinoid tumors.[11]

One of the persisting questions is the status of the patient with alcoholism. Although there is an increasing consensus that the patient with end-stage alcoholic liver disease who has stopped drinking is a good candidate,[12, 13] the patient with active alcoholism and life-threatening complications such as hepatic failure from acute alcoholic hepatitis continues to be excluded from transplantation in many centers. This question may be resolved only by a careful study of patients with acute alcoholic hepatitis who undergo liver transplantation with outcome assessments that include both medical survival and recidivism.

Evaluation

The transplant evaluation of the patient can generally be completed in 2 days on an outpatient basis. A thorough evaluation process is necessary to determine the candidacy of the patient. It is designed to confirm the indications for transplantation, determine if contraindications exist, assess psychosocial factors that may interfere with postoperative care, determine the degree of operative risk, establish the timing of liver transplantation, and diagnose diseases that may necessitate pretransplant correction or treatment.

The coexistence of malnutrition increases postoperative mortality,[14] and any deficiencies should be treated before transplantation. Ultrasonography of the liver and Doppler ultrasonography of the hepatic artery and portal vein address questions of vessel patency.[15] If there is additional concern about vessel patency, arteriography should be completed.[16] Ultrasonography can also assist in exclusion of coincidental hepatocellular carcinomas, bile duct abnormalities, ascites, and other intra-abdominal complications of end-stage liver disease.

The cardiopulmonary evaluation should include pulmonary function studies, arterial blood gas determinations, an electrocardiogram, and if there is any additional question of significant heart disease, echocardiography and/or heart catheterization. Peripheral vascular Doppler studies can also assist in exclusion of significant peripheral vascular disease.

Hypoxemia may occur in conjunction with advanced liver disease and can be a difficult problem to control. It has been suggested that octreotide (somatostatin analogue) infusion improves oxygenation by reduction of right-to-left shunts.[17] This effect has not been observed by all (Shaw BW Jr, personal communication). When the arterial P_{O_2} on room air is less than 50 mm Hg and worsens with standing, it may be a relative contraindication to liver transplantation.[18] Hypoxemia may be a consequence of hypoventilation, arteriovenous shunting of blood, impairment of alveolar capillary diffusion of oxygen, and/or ventilation-perfusion inequality.[19] A routine chest x-ray film, pulmonary function studies, and arterial blood gas determinations with and without 100% oxygen inhalation assist in evaluation of these problems.

Psychosocial evaluation is indicated in the majority of patients undergoing liver transplant evaluation. The psychiatrist can determine the presence of premorbid psychiatric diseases, evaluate and initiate treatment recommendations for chemical dependency, and assist in the selection process of transplant candidates.[20] The social worker determines the ability of the family to provide continuing care for the patient after transplantation.

Specialized studies may be needed for selected patients, including esophagogastroduodenoscopy and endoscopic retrograde cholangiography. Patients with end-stage liver disease have an increased prevalence of acute mucosal disease of the stomach and the duodenum[21] and may have continuing needs for sclerotherapy to control the risk of variceal hemorrhage. The evaluation of biliary tract disorders, including complicating bile duct carcinomas, may necessitate endoscopic retrograde cholangiography. Spontaneous bacterial peritonitis frequently occurs in the presence of low-protein ascites and should be excluded by paracentesis.

The stratification of risk for liver transplantation can be determined by a combination of pretransplant and intraoperative factors, including level of encephalopathy, presence of ascites, nutritional status, bilirubin level, prothrombin time, patient's age, and intraoperative blood loss.[22] Preoperative multiple organ system failure, including renal failure, sepsis, and simultaneous central nervous system disorders, is also a poor prognostic indicator.[23] Indications of a poor outcome in patients with coexisting renal failure include a serum creatinine level greater than 3 mg/dL, the continuing need for dialysis after transplantation, and the requirement for multiple liver transplants.[23] However, renal failure alone does not appear to increase the risk of transplantation.[24] Acute tubular necrosis and hepatorenal syndrome are the most frequent causes of acute renal failure, occurring in association with the complications of end-stage liver disease.

PRE–LIVER TRANSPLANTATION CARE
Complications of Cirrhosis

After the decision has been made to perform a liver transplant in the patient with end-stage liver disease, existing and new complications of cirrhosis must be controlled until a suitable donor organ can be identified. Hepatic encephalopathy may develop as a result of infection, gastrointestinal bleeding, dietary excesses, constipation, dehydration, and metabolic abnormalities such as azotemia, hypokalemia, and hypomagnesemia. In these patients, cultures of sputum, blood, urine, and ascitic fluid; examination of gastrointestinal aspirates and stool samples for the presence of blood; determination of serum electrolytes; and renal function studies should be performed. While the initiating event is being corrected lactulose can be administered to control encephalopathy. It may increase colonic gas at eventual transplantation, although it usually does not interfere with the operation. Although many clinicians avoid neomycin administration because of its potential for ototoxicity and nephrotoxicity, it may assist in reducing the risk of spontaneous peritonitis in patients with end-stage liver disease while controlling encephalopathy.[25]

Ascites can usually be managed by sodium restriction, diuretic therapy, and/or large-volume paracentesis. Sodium restriction to 500 mg/d (approximately 22 mEq/d) is usually recommended. If ascites is difficult to control, diuretic therapy with spironolactone plus a loop diuretic (or hydrochlorothiazide), if necessary, is added. Renal function must be regularly assessed. If large-volume paracentesis is required, administration of an equivalent amount of intravenous albumin to that removed may reduce problems with albumin depletion, hypotension, and azotemia.[26] Although a prior study suggested that albumin replacement is not required in the usual patient with cirrhosis and ascites treated by paracentesis,[27] patients with end-stage disease awaiting transplantation were not studied. Peritoneovenous shunts are rarely utilized to control ascites while a patient is awaiting transplantation. Water restriction is generally not required unless severe hyponatremia is present. In pretransplant patients, there should be an attempt to keep the serum sodium level near normal, as rapid correction of hyponatremia at the time of transplantation may precipitate central pontine myelinolysis.[28]

Spontaneous bacterial peritonitis may be present in up to 25% of patients who are hospitalized with ascites.[29] It is more frequent in those with the low-protein ascites typical of end-stage liver disease and should be considered in anyone who develops encephalopathy or azotemia, increasing ascites, fever, abdominal pain, persistent nausea, diarrhea, or ileus, and a diagnostic paracentesis should be completed. The organisms are typically *Escherichia coli*, enterobacter, pneumococcus, or other streptococci. Up to 50% of patients have associated bacteremia. Spontaneous bacterial peritonitis must be treated before transplantation. If there are more than 500 polymorphonuclear leukocytes per milliliter of ascitic fluid, treatment should be initiated while awaiting culture results.[30]

Pleural effusions are present in up to 5% of patients with ascites owing to passage of abdominal ascites through transdiaphragmatic channels. Although such effusions may contribute to hypoventilation, they are generally of little clinical importance and are usually controlled by ascites management.

All patients with evidence of upper gastrointestinal tract bleeding should have endoscopy for determination of cause and for treatment. Hemorrhage from varices and acute mucosal disease continues to be a potentially life-threatening event for patients with end-stage liver disease. Some groups advocate prophylactic sclerotherapy for all patients awaiting liver transplantation.[31] I utilize sclerotherapy for those with recent variceal bleeding. If surgical portal-systemic shunting is required because of uncontrolled life-threatening hemorrhage, distal splenorenal shunts are preferred.[32]

Hyponatremia is frequent in the patient with cirrhosis as a consequence of impaired free water clearance, increased vasopressin activity, and alterations of renal prostaglandin levels.[33] Ascites is usually present, and sodium depletion is not a consideration. Because the decline in serum sodium level is gradual in the cirrhotic patient, symptoms of hyponatremia are typically absent. Initial treatment should consist of water restriction. If symptoms of hyponatremia occur, correction of serum sodium levels should be gradual, as central pontine myelinolysis may develop.[34] Central pontine myelinosis is associated with the rapid correction of hyponatremia, and signs of tetraparesis, pseudobulbar palsy with dysarthria and dysphagia, seizure disorders, behavior disturbances, or coma may develop 1 to 3 days later. Computed tomography of the brain may not show signs of central pontine myelinolysis for up to 4 weeks after it is clinically detectable. Central pontine myelinosis can develop in severe end-stage liver disease of any kind but is especially likely in the alcoholic and those who are malnourished. There is also a risk of central pontine myelinolysis during liver transplantation because of the large volumes of administered fluid, which can result in rapid correction of low serum sodium levels.[28]

It has been suggested that hyponatremia should not be corrected at a rate faster than 0.5 mEq/L/h if possible.[34] If more rapid correction is needed, the rate should not exceed 1 to 2 mEq/L/h, and the level of increase should be limited to that necessary to control symptoms, usually 5 to 6 mEq/L.[35] Demeclocycline should not be used in cirrhosis because of the risk of renal failure.[36] Hypokalemia is common in patients with cirrhosis owing to total body potassium depletion.[37] In general, it is best to keep the serum potassium levels at the lower limit of normal while awaiting liver transplantation. During transplantation, the sudden increase of serum potassium level after reperfusion of the donor liver with efflux of high-potassium preservation fluid into the systemic circulation can result in substantial rises of serum potassium level.[38]

Fulminant Hepatic Failure

The traditional definition of FHF is the development of encephalopathy and impaired coagulation within 8 weeks of onset of symptoms of acute hepatic injury.[10] Typically, the signs of FHF develop within 14 days of initial symptoms. These patients need intensive management with prevention of potential complications, the details of which have been described elsewhere in this section. However, despite careful medical therapy, up to 70% of patients with FHF have an adverse outcome.[39] Because of the potential for rapid clinical deterioration and death, it is suggested that all patients with signs of FHF be referred and managed in a liver transplant center. Survival of patients with FHF after liver transplantation is approximately 50 to 74%.[40]

The proper timing of liver transplantation in the patient with FHF is a difficult decision. Although it must be completed before irreversible central nervous system injury develops, the desire is also to wait as long as possible to permit any chance of spontaneous recovery. Recovery is more likely in acetaminophen hepatotoxicity than in acute viral hepatitis. If signs of clinical improvement such as a spontaneous decline in intracranial pressure or prothrombin time occur, it may be worthwhile to wait and see if improvement is sustained. In those with progressive encephalopathy that has reached stage 3, however, liver transplantation should be considered.

POST–LIVER TRANSPLANTATION CARE

Initial evidence of graft function after revascularization is observed in the operating room with the resumption of bile flow. After return of the patient to the intensive care unit, the early awakening of the patient and normalization of the prothrombin time are also good signs of graft function. Assessment of graft function should begin immediately after liver transplantation and include assessment of mental status; laboratory variables, including prothrombin time and levels of hepatocellular enzymes; and adequacy of urine and bile flow.

Primary graft failure develops in up to 10% of patients after liver transplantation.[41] Although its mechanism is unknown, it seems to be more common in donor livers exhibiting fatty metamorphosis of hepatocytes. With the development of improved preservation solutions and more time before donor organs must be implanted, a liver biopsy may be done on the donor liver, with rapid processing of the specimen and exclusion of any livers with significant fatty change. This seems to have decreased the risk of primary graft dysfunction.[42]

In the first hours after transplantation, potent hyperaldosteronism persists, resulting in sodium retention and little requirement for sodium-containing intravenous solutions. Serum sodium and potassium levels should be determined and fluid administration modified as needed. Calcium levels may be diminished because of the citrate received with blood transfusion and magnesium and phosphate levels decreased owing to preoperative malnutrition. Alkalosis is also frequent after liver transplantation and is, in part, related to blood transfusion.[43]

Patients should be maintained by assisted ventilation until fully awake. Coexisting pulmonary conditions such as pneumonia, hypoxemia, and graft dysfunction may produce hypoventilation and necessitate continuing ventilator support.[44] Bronchoalveolar lavage should be considered for any persisting pulmonary infiltrate, especially in those who received preoperative corticosteroids or had a prolonged pretransplant hospitalization. For patients with symptomatic right-sided pleural effusions after liver transplantation, placement of a pigtail intrathoracic catheter may permit adequate control of the effusion without significant discomfort.

Prophylaxis for stress-related mucosal disease should include routine administration of either intermittent or continuous infusion of histamine H_2 blockers or of sucralfate at 1 g orally every 4 hours. If upper gastrointestinal tract bleeding develops, likely causes include stress-related mucosal disease, recurrent peptic ulcer, and variceal bleeding or bleeding at sites of Roux-en-Y anastomoses for biliary enterostomy. If varices rebleed, it may mean that portal venous thrombosis has occurred at the anastomosis.

Complications

Systemic arterial hypertension is frequent after liver transplantation.[45] It is more common in children than in adults but up to 60% of adult patients can expect to leave the hospital while receiving antihypertensive medication. The etiology of hypertension is unknown, appears to be multifactorial, and is in part, due to the effect of cyclosporine and the initial sodium retention postoperatively. Nitroprusside administration is preferred as the initial management because of the familiarity of intensive care nurses with the medication, its rapid onset of action, and its short half-life. The initial dose is 0.5 µg/kg/min, with the dose titrated to keep the mean arterial pressure at 80 to 90 mm Hg (usually about 1 to 3 µg/kg/min). Thiocyanate toxicity can occur. As soon as wedge pressure, renal function, and heart rate permit, the patient should be switched to a combination of beta-blockers, prazocin, and loop diuretics[46] (Table 134–3).

TABLE 134–3
ARTERIAL HYPERTENSION MANAGEMENT
Immediate Postoperative Period
Step 1: Nitroprusside IV at 0.5 µg/kg/min and adjust as needed for control of blood pressure up to a maximum of 10 µg/kg/min. Change to prazosin at 1–3 mg t.i.d. when feasible.
Step 2: Give furosemide at 10–20 mg IV if pulmonary capillary wedge pressure is adequate. Switch to oral when feasible.
Step 3: Propranolol at 10–20 mg orally q.i.d. when feasible, if no evidence of bronchoconstriction.
Step 4: Hydralazine at 5–20 mg IV q 4 h if needed for acute elevations of blood pressure. Can switch to 25 mg orally q.i.d. for long-term control.
Management of Chronic Hypertension
Step 1: Dietary sodium restriction.
Step 2: Loop diuretic such as furosemide.
Step 3: Addition of a beta-blocker.
Step 4: Addition of a vasodilator. Addition of calcium channel blocker.
Step 5: Use of an angiotensin-converting enzyme inhibitor.
Step 6: Use of other agents such as minoxidil or clonidine.

Adapted from Shaw BW, Stratta RJ, Donovan JP, et al: Postoperative care after liver transplantation. Reprinted with permission from Seminars in Liver Disease, volume 9, pages 202–230, 1989, Thieme Medical Publishers, Inc.

Intravenous hydralazine may also be used for its effects of vasodilation with reduction of afterload.

Infection is the most frequent complication after liver transplantation, occurring in up to 70 to 80% of patients.[47, 48] In the intensive care setting, bacterial and fungal infections predominate. Up to 50% of all infections develop in the first month. Bacterial infections include pneumonia, catheter sepsis, wound infections, urinary tract infections, and intra-abdominal abscesses. Early, gram-negative organisms and staphylococcal species account for most pneumonias. Later infections are frequently due to *Streptococcus pneumoniae*, and immunization is recommended for all transplant recipients. Wound infection is generally polymicrobial. Hepatic arterial infections may occur, causing pseudoaneurysm formation with rupture and life-threatening hemorrhage.[49]

Symptomatic cytomegalovirus (CMV) infection occurs in approximately 35% of patients.[50] It is most likely in those who initially have CMV antibody–negative status and receive a CMV-positive donor organ, those who receive antilymphocyte therapy, and those who receive multiple liver transplants. It usually develops in the first 2 months after liver transplantation, with a mean onset time of 38 days.[51] CMV hepatitis is the most frequent invasive event. CMV pneumonitis and enteritis also occur. Ganciclovir is effective treatment for systemic CMV infection.[52] Herpes simplex infection is generally mucocutaneous, although visceral infections can occur.

Fungal infections are usually due to *Candida* or *Aspergillus* and develop in the first 2 months. Invasive *Candida* infection occurs in 31% of patients, typically involving the abdominal cavity or urinary tract.[53] *Aspergillus* infections usually occur as lung infection but can also involve the brain, the peritoneum, the gastrointestinal tract, and the kidney.[54] *Nocardia* infections of the lung may also occur.[55]

Pneumocystis carinii pneumonia is uncommon, usually occurring in the first 6 months after transplantation.[48] Monthly aerosol treatments with pentamidine, 300 mg, are effective prophylaxis and avoid the potential nephrotoxicity of trimethoprim-sulfamethoxazole combinations.[56]

Hepatic arterial occlusion develops in 8 to 10% of patients after liver transplantation, is more likely to occur in children than adults, and accounts for up to 40% of retransplantations in children.[57] Potential causes include protein C deficiency, kinking or stricture of the hepatic artery, an unrecognized intimal tear that developed during organ harvest, infection, or the small size of vessels in young recipients. After hepatic arterial occlusion occurs, severe hepatocellular necrosis, rapid enzyme level rise, and potential loss of the graft may ensue. Infection of the damaged graft can develop, and any patient with recurring bacteremia after transplantation should be examined for hepatic arterial occlusion. Biliary leaks also develop with hepatic arterial thrombosis owing to loss of perfusion of the donor common bile duct.[58] Because of the severity of potential consequences of unrecognized hepatic arterial occlusion, frequent hepatic arterial evaluation by Doppler ultrasonography should be routinely completed postoperatively.[59]

Surgical complications develop in up to 55% of patients after liver transplantation and include intra-abdominal infections, postoperative bleeding, biliary leaks, and strictures.[60, 61] Biliary leaks may occur spontaneously or as a consequence of hepatic arterial loss.[62] Biliary leaks may be controlled by placement of nasobiliary tubes for bile drainage, intraductal biliary stents, or reoperation.[60, 61, 63] Biliary leaks may also develop at the time of removal of T tubes because of limited formation of a T tube tract. Control of the leak by intraductal stenting or nasobiliary drainage should be attempted, although some patients require reoperation.

SUMMARY

Liver transplantation has been a significant advance in therapy for end-stage liver disease and has changed the management of the complications of cirrhosis. Patients with complications of cirrhosis should be referred early to a transplant center. Those with FHF should also be managed at a center capable of liver transplantation because of the potential for sudden deterioration. Progressive encephalopathy that reaches stage 3 and progressive hypoprothrombinemia are indications for liver transplantation in patients with FHF. Cerebral edema is a common cause of death in FHF and usually necessitates placement of an intracerebral pressure monitor with administration of mannitol or pentobarbital for control. After liver transplantation, up to 60% of patients require long-term antihypertensive medications. Infection is the most frequent complication and generally develops in the first 2 months after transplantation. Surgical complications can also occur, including hepatic arterial occlusion, biliary leaks, intra-abdominal infections, and bile duct strictures.

References

1. Lerut J, Tzakis AG, Bron K, et al: Complications of venous reconstruction in human orthotopic liver transplantation. Ann Surg 205:404, 1987.
2. Wall WJ, Mimeault R, Grant DR, et al: The use of older donor livers for hepatic transplantation. Transplantation 49:377, 1990.
3. Starzl TE, Demetris AJ, Van Thiel D: Liver transplantation. N Engl J Med 321:1014, 1989.
4. Castaldo P, Langnas AN, Stratta RJ, et al: Liver transplantation in patients over 60 years of age. Unpublished results.
5. Rubin RH, Jenkins RL, Shaw BW, et al: The acquired immunodeficiency syndrome and transplantation. Transplantation 44:1, 1987.
6. Donovan JP, Zetterman RW, Burnett DA, et al: Preoperative evaluation, preparation and timing of orthotopic liver transplantation in the adult. Semin Liver Dis 9:168, 1989.
7. Starzl TE, Demetris AJ, Van Thiel D: Rejection and histocompatibility. N Engl J Med 321:1019, 1989.
8. Pugh RN, Murry-Lyon JM, Dawson JL, et al: Transection of the oesophagus for bleeding oesophageal varices. Br J Surg 60:646, 1973.
9. O'Grady JG, Alezander GJ, Hagllar KM, et al: Early indicators of prognosis in fulminant hepatic failure. Gastroenterology 97:439, 1989.
10. Schafer DF, Shaw BW: Fulminant hepatic failure and orthotopic liver transplantation. Semin Liver Dis 9:189, 1989.
11. O'Grady JG, Polson RJ, Rolles K, et al: Liver transplantation for malignant disease. Ann Surg 207:373, 1988.
12. Kumar S, Stauber RE, Gavaler JS, et al: Orthotopic liver transplantation for alcoholic liver disease. Hepatology 11:159, 1990.
13. Peabody FW: Should patients with end-stage alcoholic liver disease have a new liver? (editorial). Hepatology 11:314, 1990.
14. Johnson PJ, O'Grady J, Calvey H, et al: Nutritional management and assessment. In: Calne CY (ed): Liver Transplantation. 2nd ed. Orlando, FL, Grune & Stratton, p 103, 1987.
15. Morton MJ, James M, Wiesner RH, et al: Applications of duplex ultrasonography in the liver transplant patient. Mayo Clin Proc 65:360, 1990.
16. Cardella JF, Amplatz K: Preoperative angiographic evaluation of prospective liver recipients. Radiol Clin North Am 25:299, 1987.
17. Salem O, Dindzans V, Freeman J, et al: Liver transplantation following postoperative closure of intrapulmonary shunts. Hepatology 10:569, 1989.
18. Van Thiel DH, Schade RR, Gavaler JB, et al: Medical aspects of liver transplantation. Hepatology 4(suppl): 79, 1984.
19. Agusti AGN, Roca J, Bosch J, et al: The lung in patients with cirrhosis. J Hepatol 10: 251, 1990.
20. Greiner CB, Roccaforte W: Psychiatric issues in liver transplantation. Semin Liver Dis 9:184, 1989.
21. Rabinovitz M, Schade RR, Dindzans V, et al: Prevalence of duodenal ulcer in cirrhotic males referred for liver transplantation: Does the etiology of cirrhosis make a difference? Dig Dis Sci 35:321, 1990.
22. Shaw BW Jr, Wood RP, Gordon RD, et al: Influence of selected patient variables and operative blood loss on six-month survival following liver transplantation. Semin Liver Dis 5:385, 1985.
23. Esquivel CO, Koneru B, Todo S, et al: Is multiple organ failure a contraindication for liver transplantation in children? Transplant Proc 19:47, 1987.
24. Gonwa TA, Klintonalm GB, Husberg BS, et al: Liver transplantation in patients with preexisting acute and chronic renal failure. Transplant Proc 20:561, 1988.
25. Rimola A, Borg F, Teres J, et al: Oral, nonabsorbable antibiotics prevent infection in cirrhotics with gastrointestinal hemorrhage. Hepatology 5:463, 1985.
26. Gines P, Tito L, Arroyo V, et al: Randomized comparative study of therapeutic paracentesis with and without intravenous albumin in cirrhosis. Gastroenterology 94:1493, 1988.
27. Antillon MR, Runyon BA, Steindel H, et al: Is albumin infusion needed after large volume paracentesis in patients with refractory ascites? Gastroenterology 98:A565, 1990.
28. Wsolek ZK, McComb RD, Pfeiffer RF, et al: Pontine and extrapontine myelinolysis following liver transplantation. Transplantation 48:1006, 1989.
29. Runyon BA: Low protein concentration ascites is predisposed to spontaneous bacterial peritonitis. Gastroenterology 91:1343, 1986.
30. Jones SR: The absolute granulocyte count in ascites fluid. West J Med 126:344, 1977.
31. Van Thiel DH, Schade RR, Dindzans VJ, et al: Prophylactic versus emergency sclerotherapy of large esophageal varices prior to liver transplantation. Gastroenterology 96:A670, 1989.
32. Lerut J, Tzakis AG, Bron K, et al: Complications of venous reconstruction in human orthotopic liver transplantation. Ann Surg 205:404, 1987.
33. Vaamonde CA: Renal water handling in liver disease. In: Epstein M (ed): The Kidney in Liver Disease. 3rd ed. Baltimore, Williams & Wilkins, p 31, 1988.
34. Cluitmans FHM, Meinders AE: Management of severe hyponatremia: Rapid or slow correction? Am J Med 88:161, 1990.
35. Sterns RH: The treatment of hyponatremia: First do no harm (editorial). Am J Med 88:557, 1990.
36. DeTroyer A, Pillou W, Broeckaert I, et al: Demeclocycline treatment of water retention in cirrhosis. Ann Intern Med 85: 336, 1976.
37. Mas A, Bosch J, Piera C, et al: Intracellular and exchangeable potassium in cirrhosis. Dig Dis Sci 26:723, 1981.
38. Chapin JW, Newland MC, Hurlbert BJ: Anesthesia for liver transplantation. Semin Liver Dis 9:195, 1989.
39. Ward ME, Trewby PN, Williams R, et al: Acute liver failure. Anaesthesia 32:228, 1977.
40. O'Grady JG, Alexander GJ, Thick M, et al: Outcome of orthotopic liver transplantation in the aetiological and clinical variants of acute liver failure. Q J Med 69:817, 1988.
41. Grenvik A, Gordon R: Postoperative care and problems in liver transplantation. Transplant Proc 19: 26, 1987.
42. Markin RS, Wood RP, Stratta RJ, et al: Histopathologic analysis of primary allograft failure: Evaluation of pretransplant biopsies and explanted allografts. Transplant Proc 22:418, 1990.
43. Fortunato FL, Kang Y, Aggarwal JA, et al: Acid-base status during and after orthotopic liver transplantation. Transplant Proc 19:59, 1987.
44. Jensen WA, Rose RM, Hammer SM, et al: Pulmonary complications of orthotopic liver transplantation. Transplantation 42:484, 1986.
45. Rine R, Bechstein WO, Bunzendahl, et al: Chronic renal dysfunction and hypertension after hepatic transplantation in adults treated with cyclosporine A. Transplant Proc 20:639, 1988.

46. Shaw BW, Stratta RJ, Donovan JP, et al: Postoperative care after liver transplantation. Semin Liver Dis 9:202, 1989.
47. Markin RS, Stratta RJ, Woods GL: Infection after liver transplantation. Am J Surg Pathol 17(suppl 1):64, 1990.
48. Colonna JO, Winston DJ, Brill JE, et al: Infectious complications in liver transplantation. Arch Surg 123:360, 1988.
49. Lerut JP, Gordon RD, Iwatsuki S, et al: Human orthotopic-liver transplantation: Surgical aspects in 393 consecutive grafts. Transplant Proc 20:603, 1988.
50. Barkholt LM, Ericzon B-G, Ehrnst A, et al: Cytomegalovirus infections in liver transplant patients: Incidence and outcome. Transplant Proc 22:235, 1990.
51. Stratta RJ, Shaefer MS, Markin RS, et al: Clinical patterns of cytomegalovirus disease after liver transplantation. Arch Surg 124:1443, 1989.
52. Salmela K, Höckerstedt, Lautenschlager I, et al: Ganciclovir in the treatment of cytomegalovirus disease in liver transplant patients. Transplant Proc 22:238, 1990.
53. Tollermar J, Ericzon B-G, Holberg K, et al: The incidence and diagnosis of fungal infection in liver transplant recipients. Transplant Proc 22:242, 1990.
54. Boon AP, Adams DH, Buckels J, et al: Cerebral aspergillosis in liver transplantation. J Clin Pathol 43: 114, 1990.
55. Raby N, Forbes G, Williams R: *Nocardia* infection in patients with liver transplants or chronic liver disease: Radiologic findings. Radiology 174:713, 1990.
56. Leoung GS, Feigal DW, Montgomery AB, et al: Aerosolized pentamidine for prophylaxis against *Pneumocystis carinii* pneumonia. N Engl J Med 323:769, 1990.
57. Yanaga K, Lebeau G, Marsh JW, et al: Hepatic artery reconstruction for hepatic artery thrombosis after orthotopic liver transplantation. Arch Surg 125:628, 1990.
58. Kaplan SB, Zajko AB, Koneru B: Hepatic bilomas due to hepatic artery thrombosis in liver transplant recipients: Percutaneous drainage and clinical outcome. Radiology 174:1031, 1990.
59. Flint EW, Sumkin JH, Zajko AB, et al: Duplex sonography of hepatic artery thrombosis after liver transplantation. Am J Radiol 151:481, 1988.
60. Lebeau G, Yanaga K, March JW, et al: Analysis of surgical complications after 397 hepatic transplantations. Surgery 170:317, 1990.
61. Lerut J, Gordon RD, Iwatsuki S, et al: Biliary tract complications in human orthotopic liver transplantation. Transplantation 43:47, 1987.
62. Evans RA, Raby ND, O'Grady JG, et al: Biliary complications following orthotopic liver transplantation. Clin Radiol 41:190, 1990.
63. Ostroff JW, Robert JP, Gordon RL, et al: The management of T tube leaks in orthotopic liver transplant recipients with endoscopically placed nasobiliary catheters. Transplantation 49:922, 1990.

CHAPTER 135

Pathophysiology and Therapy of Hepatic Encephalopathy

Andres T. Blei

Intensive care is required for patients with liver disease who are comatose. In fulminant hepatic failure, the neurologic status is a key element for the prognosis and management of these critically ill subjects.[1] In patients with cirrhosis, the degree of encephalopathy is among the five criteria that compose the modified Child's classification,[2] a widely used prognostic index. The mechanisms that account for changes of mental state in acute and chronic liver disease may be similar in some respects but differ in others. Clinical management also has distinct features. The organization of this chapter responds, therefore, to the main dividing line that

TABLE 135–1

ETIOLOGY OF FULMINANT HEPATIC FAILURE

Fulminant failure (course < 2 wk)
 Viral hepatitis: A, B, D, E
 Mushroom poisoning
 Acute fatty liver of pregnancy
 Intoxication with acetaminophen
 Hepatic ischemia

Subfulminant failure (course 2 wk–3 mo)
 Drug-induced hepatitis
 Acute manifestation of chronic hepatitis
  Autoimmune chronic hepatitis
  Wilson's disease
 Hepatic venous obstruction
  Budd-Chiari syndrome
  Veno-occlusive disease

From Bernuau J, Rueff B, Benhamou JP: Fulminant and subfulminant liver failure: Definitions and causes. Reprinted with permission from Seminars in Liver Disease, volume 6, pages 97–106, 1986, Thieme Medical Publishers, Inc.

the intensivist initially faces: is this coma in acute or in chronic liver disease?

ENCEPHALOPATHY IN ACUTE LIVER FAILURE

Acute liver failure may be severe, as evidenced by jaundice and a marked drop in the liver's synthetic capacity (e.g., levels of coagulation factor V).[3] Changes in mental state may develop within 2 weeks of the onset of illness (fulminant hepatic failure) or after 2 weeks to 3 months (subfulminant liver insufficiency).[3] The etiology of acute liver failure can be grouped according to this classification (Table 135–1), and this may help in the differential diagnosis.

Regardless of the etiology, all forms of acute liver failure may be accompanied by changes in mental state. Neurologic symptoms have been classified according to clinical criteria (Table 135–2), although the Glasgow criteria for classification of coma have been increasingly used.[4] The unique aspect of encephalopathy in this syndrome is the development of brain edema and intracranial hypertension in its terminal phase. The demonstration of brain herniation at the time of autopsy indicates that intracranial hypertension is a direct cause of death.[5] Series confirm that cerebral edema is still a leading factor in the mortality of this disorder.[6]

Pathophysiology

Massive hepatic necrosis results in loss of liver function. This led to the hypothesis that encephalopathy occurs as a result of the deprivation from the brain of a trophic factor synthesized in the liver.[7] Cross-circulation studies in experimental animals have cast doubt on this mechanism,[8] and current views highlight the role of different neurotoxins that reach the brain via the systemic circulation.[9] In acute

TABLE 135–2

CLINICAL SYMPTOMS IN HEPATIC ENCEPHALOPATHY

Stage	Symptoms
1	Confusion, altered behavior and mood
2	Drowsiness, inappropriate behavior, slurred speech
3	Stupor and/or marked confusion; obeys simple orders but inarticulate speech
4	Coma, unarousable; in fulminant hepatic failure at this stage, possibly additional symptoms related to intracranial hypertension

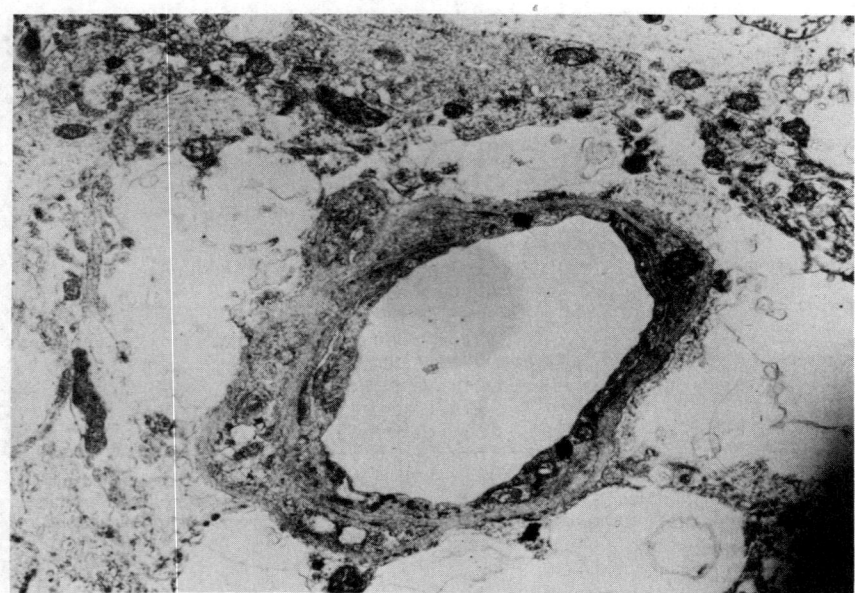

Figure 135–1. Swollen astrocyte foot processes surround a capillary endothelial cell in rats with ischemic fulminant hepatic failure. Electron micrograph, × 24,000, after perfusion fixation of the brain. (Courtesy of Mauro DalCanto, Northwestern University.)

liver failure, without functional exchange across sinusoids, portal blood flow traverses the liver as one large and complete intrahepatic shunt. In addition, compounds released from the necrotic liver may influence the mental state; in human observations, uncontrollable intracranial hypertension could be temporarily managed by removing the liver while keeping patients on an extracorporeal venous-venous bypass (Shaw BW Jr, personal communication).

Brain Edema

The mechanisms that account for the increase in brain water in acute liver failure are poorly understood. Brain edema has traditionally been viewed as the result of either a cytotoxic injury (in which cellular swelling is produced by impaired osmoregulation) or a vasogenic mechanism (in which the blood-brain barrier is disrupted).[10] Clinical evidence in human disease argues against a gross breakdown of the barrier, as evidenced by the lack of an increase in cerebrospinal fluid protein level and the absence of focal abnormalities on brain imaging.[11] Current views of the molecular mechanisms that account for water movement across the endothelial cell suggest similar pathways for both vasogenic and cytotoxic edema.[12] Still, evidence in experimental animals suggests that a cytotoxic injury may be the initial lesion.[13]

In rabbits with galactosamine-induced injury, swelling of the cortical gray matter, rich in cells, progresses with evolution of the encephalopathy, while white matter is unaffected.[14] In all neuropathologic studies in experimental acute liver failure, swelling of cortical astrocytes appears as the dominant feature (Fig. 135–1) and raises the possibility that this cell may be the initial site of injury. Several possibilities could account for preferential swelling of this cellular element. Ammonia combines with glutamate to form glutamine, a reaction catalyzed by glutamine synthetase, an enzyme mainly localized within astrocytes.[15] Accumulation of osmogenic amino acids, such as glutamine[16] and alanine,[17] could account for water accumulation within glial cells.

One laboratory has suggested that inhibition of Na^+,K^+-ATPase in the brain may also be present.[18] This membrane pump facilitates sodium extrusion from cells, and an increase in Na^+ cellular content results from its inhibition. The source of this effect may be present in the serum of these patients[19] and could be related to the measurable digoxin-like immunoreactivity present in these subjects.[20] It is unclear how to reconcile the possible inhibition of this membrane pump with the observed effects on glial cells.

After edema progresses, changes in the permeability of the blood-brain barrier may be detectable. Injections of horseradish peroxidase (molecular weight 44,000)[21] or microperoxidase (molecular weight 5000)[22] indicate the presence of vesicles containing this material within endothelial cells of experimental models. Rather than a breakdown of the integrity of the capillary endothelial cell, this transcellular pathway may be the route for water movement in many instances of brain edema.[12] As an intimate anatomic relation exists between the end-foot processes of astrocytes and the capillary endothelial cell, the noted abnormalities in glial cells may be related to the subsequent changes in permeability of the barrier. In cell cultures, full expression of endothelial cell properties can be achieved only when the latter are cocultured with glial cells.[23]

Intracranial Hypertension

Intracranial pressure may rise as a result of the expansion of the brain blood volume, cerebrospinal fluid space, or brain tissue. Brain blood volume has not been measured, but cerebral blood flow is decreased in encephalopathic patients.[24] Expansion of the cerebrospinal fluid space is not a feature of patients with intracranial hypertension, as seen by computed tomography.[11] Intracranial hypertension evolves as brain compliance is progressively reduced by the development of brain edema (Fig. 135–2).

An elevation of arterial pressure, coupled with bradycardia, is observed during the rise in intracranial pressure (the Cushing reflex). In both animals and humans with acute liver failure, a more pronounced elevation of arterial pressure appears to offer a protective effect.[25, 26] This rise maintains cerebral perfusion pressure, the difference between mean arterial pressure and intracranial pressure, and thus diminishes the risk of a secondary ischemic injury.

Pressure waves have been described in the terminal phase of intracranial hypertension in both animal[25] and human[27] acute liver failure. They signal a critical period in the course of an elevated intracranial pressure, with an imminent risk of brain herniation. Cerebral perfusion pressure is critically

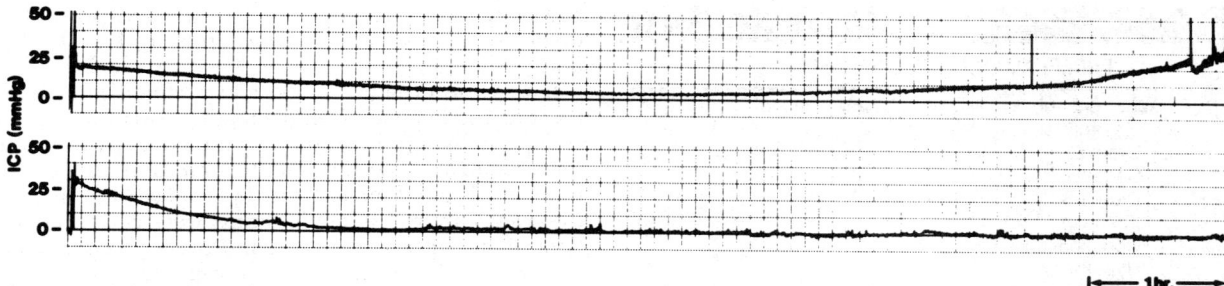

Figure 135–2. Intracranial pressure progressively rises in rats with ischemic fulminant hepatic failure. At time 0, an intracranial pressure monitor is placed, accounting for an initial elevation of intracranial pressure. *(Top)* Intracranial pressure rises in the last 2 hours of the course, punctuated by marked elevations (pressure spikes). *(Bottom)* Unchanged values are seen in a normal animal. (From Webster S, Gottstein J, Levy R, et al: Intracranial pressure-waves and intracranial hypertension in rats with ischemic fulminant hepatic failure. Hepatology 14:715, 1991.)

reduced during these episodes and may add an important component of ischemic injury to the original lesion.

Brain herniation and intracranial hypertension have been described in patients with cirrhosis.[28] This phenomenon was observed in cirrhosis of different causes; patients were in deep coma, and measurements of intracranial pressure in vivo showed elevated values. In patients who underwent autopsy, herniation of the temporal lobe could be detected. These results suggest that, in hepatic encephalopathy, abnormalities in the regulation of brain water may be more prevalent than previously thought.

Clinical Aspects

General aspects of the clinical presentation of acute liver failure are discussed in this section. Neurologically, patients may exhibit subtle changes in mental state or may be in deep coma. Early manifestations may include a period of excitation and delirium, which is rare in patients with cirrhosis and encephalopathy. In many instances, the progression toward overt encephalopathy is rapid, in a course that can be counted in hours. Asterixis, a common physical sign in cirrhotic patients at early stages of encephalopathy, is seldom elicited. Speech becomes unintelligible and stupor quickly ensues. After the patient is in coma, respiratory arrest can be sudden, and these patients should be carefully monitored. Symptoms and signs of intracranial hypertension, when present, are not seen at an early stage; pressure elevations of up to 60 mm Hg may go undetected by clinical observation.[29] Myoclonic seizures, decerebrate posturing, loss of vestibular reflexes, and poorly reacting pupils can be observed at a late stage. Papilledema is seldom noted; the rapid evolution of the neurologic picture does not allow time for this manifestation to develop.

Management of Brain Edema and Intracranial Hypertension

Only recently have intracranial pressure monitors been used to follow the course of brain edema and intracranial hypertension. Cerebral edema is not detected by computed tomography, although this test is useful in excluding other pathologic processes.[11] The monitors used have included epidural, subdural, and intraventricular catheters.[30] The coagulopathy of these patients can be corrected temporarily during placement of these monitors by administration of fresh frozen plasma or plasmapheresis.[31] Still, there is concern about the risks of intracranial hemorrhage with subdural and intraventricular catheters, especially in children.[32] An increasing experience with epidural transducers has shown them to enhance the predictability of neurologic

outcome.[33] Management of these patients is greatly simplified with such monitors; this is especially the case in patients with renal failure, in whom repeated injections of mannitol may induce a hyperosmolar state.

Mannitol is used for the treatment of brain edema in this condition. The usual dose is 1 g/kg administered intravenously during 30 minutes. When administered without intracranial pressure monitoring, it should not be given at fixed intervals. Rather, a careful neurologic follow-up is required to minimize side effects, including hyperosmolarity (which aggravates the neurologic picture) and a rebound effect.[34] In patients with renal failure, dialysis may be required to allow excretion of mannitol and subsequent administration of the drug.

Mechanical hyperventilation provides only marginal benefit in the management of brain edema and intracranial hypertension;[35] these patients already exhibit respiratory alkalosis and spontaneously experience a reduced cerebral blood flow.[24] Thiopental may be of benefit in extreme cases,[36] although a decision to use barbiturates to reduce the brain metabolic needs removes neurologic assessment as a clinical tool to follow these patients; intracranial pressure monitoring is extremely helpful in the case of barbiturate therapy. Finally, hypothermia, widely used to treat vasogenic brain edema, has been shown to improve brain edema in an experimental model of acute liver failure.[23] Prophylactic tracheal intubation is recommended at stage 2 encephalopathy, as respiratory arrest may occur suddenly.

Some of the measures used in the treatment of encephalopathy in cirrhosis (see later) are also applicable to fulminant hepatic failure. Sedation must be avoided if at all possible. Catharsis can be induced by nonabsorbable disaccharides, but care should be taken to avoid excessive diarrhea. Correction of hypoxia, hypotension, and hypokalemia should be undertaken.

The timing of liver transplantation in fulminant hepatic failure is dependent on the liver's synthetic ability (as assessed by several laboratory measures, such as the levels of factor V[37]) and the evolution of the neurologic picture.[37] This is discussed in more detail in Chapter 134. Intracranial hypertension may be a major management problem during the operative procedure itself,[38] and the patients should have monitors placed preoperatively. Several cases of postoperative neurologic deficits after a technically successful liver transplant have been reported.[39]

ENCEPHALOPATHY IN CHRONIC LIVER DISEASE

Changes in mental state in cirrhosis (Table 135–3) can occur as a precipitant-induced event. This is by far the most common presentation of hepatic encephalopathy; a common

TABLE 135-3
ENCEPHALOPATHY IN CIRRHOSIS
Acute encephalopathy (precipitant induced)
Gastrointestinal bleeding
Uremia
Sedatives
Diuretics
Infection
Constipation
Hypokalemia
Chronic encephalopathy
Recurrent
Chronic hepatocerebral degeneration
Latent portal-systemic encephalopathy

misconception is to attribute the appearance of changes in mental state to a terminal stage of chronic liver disease. This can occur and is suspected in patients with deep jaundice and a severe coagulopathy. However, in most instances, cirrhotic subjects with a previously stable course have symptoms and signs of encephalopathy within a variable period owing to an intercurrent event. In a large series, gastrointestinal bleeding, uremia, and use of sedatives were the most common precipitants.[40] Other causes include infection (encephalopathy can be a presenting symptom of spontaneous bacterial peritonitis[41]), hypokalemia (many times induced by diuretics), constipation, and excessive protein consumption.

The term *portal-systemic encephalopathy* has been coined to reflect a variable state of consciousness that occurs when portal venous blood bypasses the liver;[9] intestinal contents are not metabolized by the hepatic parenchyma and the brain is exposed to the deleterious effects of these neurotoxins. Cirrhotic patients with extensive portal-systemic shunts (e.g., large splenorenal collateral[42]) may have spontaneous episodes of overt encephalopathy. Such spontaneous episodes may also be seen after portacaval shunts, with which, in addition, a chronic derangement of mental state may ensue. The crippling nature of these symptoms has been the major stimulus for the development of alternative therapies to prevent recurrent hemorrhage from portal hypertension.

Rarely, patients with long-standing portacaval shunts exhibit a distinct neurologic picture, termed *acquired hepatocerebral degeneration*. The main neuropathologic finding is the cavitation and degeneration of the lenticular nucleus.[43] Changes in gait, ataxia, and mood, seen in this condition, can be crippling.

Pathophysiology

Splanchnic Territory

Hepatic encephalopathy results from the exposure of the brain to the deleterious effects of neurotoxins arising from the gut. Two factors combine in chronic liver disease to increase such an exposure: portal-systemic shunting and a decrease in liver function.

Portal-systemic shunts develop as a result of portal hypertension. In alcoholic cirrhosis, a critical portal venous pressure, which is estimated to be 12 mm Hg[44] (measured as hepatic venous pressure gradient: hepatic vein wedge pressure minus hepatic vein free pressure), results in the opening of embryonic venous channels or redirects blood via existing vessels. The likelihood of developing spontaneous episodes of encephalopathy is higher when most portal venous blood is redirected via a large shunt (e.g., splenorenal) rather than through a network of collaterals. This clinical observation suggests that the rate of toxin delivery from the splanchnic

bed to the systemic circulation is affected not only by the toxin load (its portal vein concentration) but also by blood flow.[45]

Is the sole presence of portal-systemic shunts enough to account for hepatic encephalopathy? It is rare for patients with portal-systemic shunting and no hepatic dysfunction (schistosomiasis, portal vein thromboses) to be in coma; however, brain function can be abnormal.[46] In an earlier experience, portal-systemic shunts were constructed for patients with pancreatic cancer, and overt encephalopathy was detected in the presence of a normal liver.[47] Such patients tend to be of older age; portal-systemic shunts in younger patients are better tolerated. Age is an additional factor influencing the expression of encephalopathy.

Loss of hepatocellular function occurs in cirrhosis as a consequence of a decrease in cellular mass rather than a reduction in cellular function. The intact hepatocyte theory suggests that, in cirrhosis, individual cells function appropriately; architectural distortion with loss of hepatic parenchyma and the development of intrahepatic portal-systemic shunts account for the progressive deterioration of liver function.[48] The capacity to synthesize urea in periportal hepatocytes decreases, and the reduction of the maximal rate of synthesis of this compound may predict the development of encephalopathy after portacaval anastomosis.[49] Loss of pericentral hepatocytes may impair the formation of glutamine, as the amidation of glutamate with ammonia is catalyzed by glutamine synthetase in the last rim of perivenous hepatocytes.[50]

Nature of the Neurotoxin

Several substances have been incriminated in the pathogenesis of encephalopathy. Clinical observations provide clues to the nature of these compounds. The neurotoxin must be of intestinal origin, as constipation can precipitate encephalopathy and purging the bowel improves the mental state. It is related to protein metabolism, as diets low in protein improve encephalopathy, whereas the reverse may occur with a high protein ingestion. Intestinal bacteria play a pathogenic role, as poorly absorbable antibiotics improve the clinical picture. Finally, the neurotoxin should be highly extracted by the liver on first pass, as precipitation of encephalopathy by portal-systemic shunts indicates that the bioavailability of such substances is low under normal conditions.

Ammonia. Ammonia has been the most extensively incriminated neurotoxin.[51] As a nitrogenous product, it is generated from glutamine within the intestinal mucosa by the action of glutaminase and from the urease-splitting activity of intestinal bacteria. Its first-pass extraction is high, close to 90%.[50] Other hyperammonemic conditions, such as congenital deficiencies of the urea cycle enzymes, Reye's syndrome, and a post–chemotherapy-induced change in mental state,[52] are all associated with encephalopathy, with similarities and differences with the classic symptoms of hepatic encephalopathy.

Arguments have been raised against the ammonia hypothesis. These include the lack of correlation between blood levels of ammonia and the degree of encephalopathy (Fig. 135–3), the frequent presence of seizures seen with urea cycle enzyme deficiencies (seldom, if ever, seen in hepatic encephalopathy), and the difficulty in ascribing to hepatic encephalopathy the multiple neurochemical mechanisms altered by hyperammonemia. However, each of these arguments has a counterpoint. The lack of relation between blood and brain levels can be explained by simultaneous changes in the permeability of the blood-brain barrier to ammonia.[53] Ammonia intoxication seldom causes seizures in

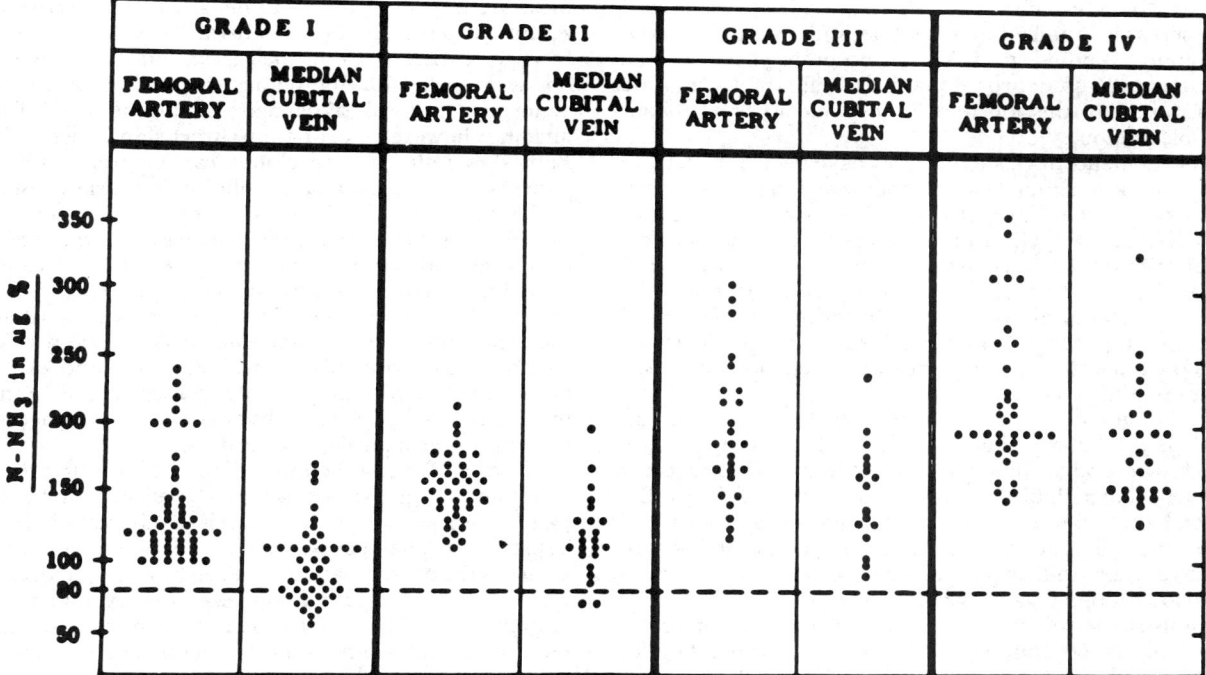

Figure 135–3. Arterial ammonia levels are slightly higher than venous values at different stages of encephalopathy. The lack of relation between ammonia values and stages of coma has been a major criticism of the ammonia hypothesis. (Reproduced, with permission, from Stahl J: Studies of blood ammonia in liver disease. Its diagnostic, prognostic, and therapeutic significance. Ann Intern Med. 1963; 53:1–24.)

the experimental animal.[54] For those investigators who lend support to the ammonia hypothesis, it is the complex nature of its effects that lends credence to a pathogen ic role in hepatic encephalopathy[55] (Table 135–4). These include inhibition of chloride extrusion from neurons, effects on the exchange of amino acids at the level of the blood-brain barrier, and more important, the generation of metabolites, such as glutamine, that may mediate some of its deleterious effects.[16, 17] When balanced against all factors, reproduction by chronic hyperammonemia of Alzheimer's type II astrocytosis (the only pathologic feature seen in patients dying in hepatic coma) suggests that ammonia is still a key feature in the pathogenesis of hepatic encephalopathy.[51]

Two other hypotheses include ammonia or its metabolic effects but add new elements. The synergistic neurotoxin hypothesis suggests that other products of intestinal bacterial metabolism potentiate the neurotoxic effects of ammonia.[56] These include octanoic acid (a medium chain fatty acid), mercaptans (products of methionine metabolism), and phenol. In experimental animals, ammonia induces coma in a dose-dependent fashion; the synergistic neurotoxins, individually and in combination, shift the dose-response curve to the left. The exact role of these neurotoxins in human encephalopathy has not been well defined; however, some antibiotics improve hepatic encephalopathy without changing blood levels of ammonia.[57] It is possible that their beneficial effect is mediated via suppression of synergistic toxins.

The second hypothesis suggests that the neuroinhibition seen in hepatic encephalopathy occurs as the result of the accumulation of false neurotransmitters. Glutamine, whose levels increase as a result of ammonia metabolism in the brain, is transported out of the brain via the neutral amino acid carrier at the level of the blood-brain barrier.[58] In exchange, aromatic amino acids (whose plasma levels are increased as a result of decreased hepatic catabolism) enter the brain, also favored by the decrease in competing plasma branched chain amino acids (whose lower levels may be explained by increased insulin resistance[59]) with concomitant uptake into muscle. In the brain, aromatic amino acids are converted to false neurotransmitters, which exert a deleterious effect on mental state. This line of thought has led to the extensive testing of dietary formulations rich in branched chain amino acids, with the hope that the excess in brain aromatic amino acids could be corrected.[60, 61] A conclusive beneficial effect has not been demonstrated.

γ-Aminobutyric Acid. In 1982, it was proposed that γ-aminobutyric acid (GABA), the main inhibitory neurotransmitter in the brain, may account for the development of encephalopathy.[62] On the basis of studies in an animal model of fulminant hepatic failure, it was suggested that GABA gained access to the brain as a result of increased blood levels (from portal-systemic shunting) and an abnormally

---

TABLE 135–4

POSTULATED MECHANISMS OF AMMONIA NEUROTOXICITY

1. *Changes in blood-brain barrier carriers*
   Increased uptake of aromatic amino acids
   Increased permeability: surface product to ammonia
2. *Electrophysiologic effects*
   Inhibition of chloride extrusion from neurons
3. *Interference with neurotransmitter function*
   Decrease in brain glutamate and aspartate (excitatory neurotransmitters)
4. *Morphologic changes in astrocytes*
   Alzheimer's type II astrocytes
5. *Interference with biochemical pathways*
   Increased glycolysis
   Reduced α-ketoglutarate dehydrogenase (Krebs' cycle)
   Interference with malate-aspartate shuttle
6. *Effects on brain water*
   Accumulation of glutamine exerts osmotic effect

From Copper AJ, Plum F: Biochemistry and physiology of brain ammonia. Physiol Rev 67:440, 1987.

permeable blood-brain barrier. In the brain, it was bound to an increased number of receptors and resulted in neuroinhibition. Binding to $GABA_A$ receptors increases the permeability of the neuronal plasma membrane to chloride ion with entry of this ion into the cell and its concomitant hyperpolarization.

All the elements of this hypothesis have been subjected to intensive experimental testing, and many have not been confirmed by other investigators. The increased levels of plasma GABA may reflect other compounds,[63] the permeability of the barrier to GABA may not be increased,[64] and the initial observation of an increase in receptors may be related to technical factors.[65] However, an increased GABAergic tone may still be involved in the pathogenesis of encephalopathy if the presence of endogenous benzodiazepines is confirmed.

The endogenous benzodiazepine hypothesis is a variant of the GABA theory. Postsynaptic $GABA_A$ receptors are coupled to benzodiazepine receptors so that benzodiazepines exert their neuroinhibitory effect via activation of the GABA channel.[66] Preliminary observations suggest that the mental state of cirrhotic patients improves with administration of flumazenil, a benzodiazepine receptor antagonist.[67] If there is a benzodiazepine ligand, what is its source?

Administration of this family of drugs is common in subjects receiving endoscopy or other instrumentations. However, endogenous ligands can be detected in animal models reared in the laboratory.[68] In addition, studies in human brains of patients dying with acute liver failure revealed the presence of compounds that were identified as 1,4-benzodiazepines.[69] The possibility that they may be of plant origin has been raised.[70] Whether they are present at sufficiently high concentration to induce encephalopathy is still unclear. Cirrhotics may be more prone to the sedative effects of benzodiazepines[71] but also appear more susceptible to the effects of other sedative medication.

As with many of the hypotheses proposed for hepatic encephalopathy, removal of the offending neurotoxin via a clinical experience solidifies a thesis or leaves it on the wayside. In the case of benzodiazepine antagonists, randomized clinical trials are awaited with interest. In one preliminary report, patients at early stages of encephalopathy did not particularly benefit from 1 mg of flumazenil,[72] a dose used for benzodiazepine intoxication. Additional studies are awaited with great interest.

MANAGEMENT
Differential Diagnosis

Encephalopathy in a patient with cirrhosis may result from other causes (Table 135–5). A meningeal infection is suspected when fever and leukocytosis are present, because

---

TABLE 135–5

DIFFERENTIAL DIAGNOSIS OF ENCEPHALOPATHY IN A CIRRHOTIC PATIENT

Search for precipitant (most important)
Smoldering meningeal infection (tuberculosis, cryptococcosis)
In alcoholics
  Subdural hematoma
  Wernicke's encephalopathy
  Withdrawal
Vitamin E deficiency (in chronic cholestatic disorders)
  Posterior column dysfunction, cerebellar ataxia
Hepatolenticular degeneration (Wilson's disease)
  Choreoathetosis, extrapyramidal symptoms

---

these are unusual features in hepatic coma; performance of a lumbar puncture in an individual with a coagulopathy from liver disease should be carried out by an experienced operator and with temporary correction of the clotting abnormality. Focal signs may signal the need for brain imaging; however, fleeting long-tract signs (such as bilateral Babinski's reflexes) and clonus can be transiently seen in patients in hepatic coma. Alcohol withdrawal presents with excitation and tremulousness, signs seldom seen in liver insufficiency. Oculomotor disturbances in a confused patient may reflect thiamine deficiency (Wernicke's encephalopathy). The discovery of a precipitating event responsible for the development of hepatic coma serves as a reassurance that encephalopathy is not due to other causes. When a cirrhotic has compatible neurologic signs and evidence of gastrointestinal bleeding, an infected ascitic fluid, or a history of recent sedative use, additional tests are unnecessary to rule out other neurologic disorders.

Asterixis (the so-called liver flap), which is the inability to maintain an agonist position and is elicited by holding the palms with wrists dorsiflexed, is a characteristic sign of hepatic encephalopathy. It can be obtained from other muscle groups, such as an outstretched tongue or a maneuver in which the patient squeezes the examiner's fingers. However, asterixis is not unique to liver disease. It can be seen in patients with uremia, carbon dioxide narcosis, hypomagnesemia, and phenytoin intoxication.

Treatment of Acute Encephalopathy

Treatment of an episode of acute encephalopathy is based on the combination of removal of the precipitating stimulus, when identifiable, and several measures to reduce the neurotoxin load. These include restriction of dietary protein, increased catharsis, and administration of nonabsorbable disaccharides or poorly absorbable antibiotics.

Removal of the Precipitating Stimulus

A vigorous diagnostic search is pursued to detect a precipitating event. Antagonists are administered for suspected overdoses of opioids and, if available, flumazenil for excessive benzodiazepine effects. Potassium is replaced and diuretics discontinued if renal function has deteriorated; this may also necessitate volume expansion. Parenteral antibiotics are administered if findings at paracentesis suggest an infected ascitic fluid. Gastrointestinal bleeding resulting in encephalopathy is an emergency in which control of hemorrhage should be approached first.

Removal of Neurotoxin Load

Diet. Dietary protein intake is suspended until recovery has ensued. Dextrose is the main source of calories during the period of acute encephalopathy. Controversy has risen about the potential benefits of branched chain amino acid therapy in this acute condition. Two studies have shown equivocal benefits in accelerating recovery;[73, 74] because of uncertainty, the cost of the product, and the availability of other therapies, intravenous branched chain amino acids are not indicated in this situation. As a source of protein, other products are available for intravenous supplementation, which in most cases are unnecessary in the acute setting.

Nonabsorbable Disaccharides. A key element in the treatment of hepatic encephalopathy is the administration of nonabsorbable disaccharides, such as lactulose or lactitol; in the presence of lactose malabsorption, a common finding in certain parts of the world,[75] lactose can be used. Randomized double-blind studies have shown that lactulose is an effective treatment of acute encephalopathy.[76] Lactitol, currently available in Europe but not in North America, is more palatable, results in a more prompt awakening from coma than does lactulose, and may cause less abdominal discomfort.[77, 78]

Lactulose acts via multiple mechanisms. The drug is a synthetic disaccharide (galactose-fructose) that arrives undigested at the cecum; anaerobic species in the cecum break down this sugar to lactic acid and other organic acids. The accumulation of these products results in catharsis; however, other cathartics do not decrease the urea production rate as lactulose does.[79] The latter reflects profound effects on the movement of ammonia from blood to the intestinal lumen and back to portal blood.

The reduction in colonic pH can reach values of 4.5 to 5.0 in the cecum.[80] This colonic acidification favors movement of ammonia from the blood stream to the intestinal lumen. This ammonia nitrogen is incorporated into fecal bacteria, as the major portion of the increased fecal nitrogen seen with lactulose is found in the bacterial fraction of stool.[81] In addition, an acidic pH reduces the amount of ammonia produced by intestinal bacteria. These two mechanisms combine to reduce the amount of ammonia entering the portal blood. The bacterial production of medium chain fatty acids that may act synergistically with ammonia is also reduced.[81]

A dose of 15 to 30 mL is administered orally every 1 to 2 hours until catharsis is obtained. In controlled trials, the range of required doses was from 45 to 200 mL/d. After catharsis is obtained, the dose is adjusted to result in two or three soft bowel movements per day. The clinical response is not immediate; 24 to 48 hours may elapse before resolution of encephalopathy occurs. Side effects include flatulence and abdominal cramping. Some patients find the sweet taste of lactulose unpalatable, but this is of greater concern for long-term therapy. Rarely, profuse diarrhea occurs, with loss of the normally hypotonic colonic fluid; hypernatremia develops, and plasma hyperosmolarity results in additional changes in mental state.[82] If hyperosmolarity is erroneously attributed to hepatic encephalopathy, and more lactulose is administered, the hyperosmolarity can be potentially fatal.

Death resulting from hepatic coma in cirrhosis is rare, although a report suggested that intracranial hypertension may be present in prolonged, deep coma.[83] However, cirrhotic patients in coma may need to be resuscitated promptly if the precipitating event is still uncontrolled. Few options are available for this situation. A lactulose enema (200 to 300 mL in a total volume of 1 L) is given by retention. As the drug is metabolized by intestinal bacteria, the patient is placed in Trendelenburg's position to maximize contact with right-sided colonic contents. Lactose enemas can be administered for a fraction of the cost.[84]

Retention of lactulose enemas for a short period (30 to 60 minutes) allows continuation of purgative therapy. Care should be exercised with magnesium enemas, as they may cause severe hypermagnesemia in patients who also exhibit renal failure.[85]

Oral Antibiotic Treatment. The combination neomycin-sorbitol is as effective as lactulose in the management of acute encephalopathy.[76] Antibiotics reduce the population of urease-containing bacteria, and less ammonia is produced in the intestinal lumen. Effects on the small-bowel mucosa, where ammonia is formed from glutamine, may also reduce the generation of ammonia from this source and explain the inconsistent effect of neomycin on bacterial flora.[86] A similar clinical response can be observed with other antibiotics, such as metronidazole[57] and vancomycin.[87] In the case of metronidazole, care should be exercised with the dose, as elimination of the drug is impaired in liver disease; 250 mg twice daily is a safe initial dose.

In acute encephalopathy, doses of neomycin of 2 to 4 g are administered daily. A small fraction of this aminoglycoside is absorbed, and care should be exercised in patients with underlying renal failure. Long-term use is associated with other side effects: ototoxicity, diarrhea, and malabsorption (owing to effects on the intestinal mucosa as well as changes in the intestinal microflora). Addition of neomycin to lactulose does not impair the survival of disaccharide-metabolizing bacteria, which explains the additive effect of this combination in chronic hepatic encephalopathy.[88] The effect of combined therapy in acute encephalopathy has not been systematically studied.

Other Treatments

The use of flumazenil in the treatment of acute encephalopathy is uncertain. Uncontrolled studies indicate a marked arousal effect,[67] but whether controlled double-blind studies will confirm this efficacy is still unclear.[72] It is certainly indicated when a history of benzodiazepine administration is present; the elimination of the drug is markedly prolonged in liver disease[89] and doses of 1 mg[72] to 15 mg[67] have been administered.

Occlusion of a portal-systemic shunt may provide relief from intractable encephalopathy;[90] in this case, care should be exercised in preventing gastrointestinal bleeding from portal hypertension. Liver transplantation has been shown to correct advanced encephalopathy, including that in subjects with hepatocerebral degeneration.[91]

References

1. Ede RS, Williams RJ: Hepatic encephalopathy and cerebral edema. Semin Liver Dis 6:352, 1986.
2. Pugh RN, Murray-Lyon IM, Dawson JL, et al: Transection of the oesophagus for bleeding oesophageal varices. Br J Surg 60:646, 1973.
3. Bernuau J, Rueff B, Benhamou JP: Fulminant and subfulminant liver failure: Definitions and causes. Semin Liver Dis 6:97, 1986.
4. Schafer DF, Shaw BW Jr: Fulminant hepatic failure and orthotopic liver transplantation. Semin Liver Dis 9:189, 1989.
5. Gazzard BG, Portmann B, Murray-Lyon IM, et al: Causes of death in fulminant hepatic failure and relationship to quantitive histological assessment of parenchymal damage. Q J Med 44:615, 1975.
6. O'Grady JG, Alexander GJ, Hayllar KM, et al: Early indicators of prognosis in fulminant hepatic failure. Gastroenterology 97:439, 1989.
7. Geiger A, Magnes J, Taylor RM, et al: Effect of blood constituents on uptake of glucose and metabolic rate of the brain in perfusion experiments. Am J Physiol 177:138, 1954.
8. Roche-Sicot J, Sicot C, Peignou M, et al: Acute hepatic encephalopathy in the rat: The effect of cross circulation. Clin Sci Mol Med 47:609, 1974.
9. Conn HO, Lieberthal MM (eds): The Hepatic Coma Syndromes and Lactulose. Baltimore, Williams & Wilkins, 1979.
10. Klatzo I: Neuropathological aspects of brain edema. J Neuropathol Exp Neurol 26:1, 1967.
11. Munoz SJ, Robinson M, Northrup B, et al: Elevated intracranial pressure and computed tomography of the brain in fulminant hepatocellular failure. Hepatology 13:209, 1991.
12. Joo F: A unifying concept on the pathogenesis of brain oedemas. Neuropathol Appl Neurobiol 13:161, 1987.
13. Blei AT, Traber PG: Brain edema in experimental fulminant hepatic failure. In: Butterworth RF, Pomier-Layrargues G (eds): Hepatic Encephalopathy: Pathophysiology and Treatment. Clifton, NJ, Humana, p 231, 1989.
14. Traber PG, Ganger DR, Blei AT: Brain edema in rabbits with galactosamine-induced fulminant hepatitis. Gastroenterology 91:1347, 1986.
15. Martinez-Hernandez A, Bell KP, Norenberg MD: Glutamine synthetase: Glial localization in brain. Science 195:1356, 1977.
16. Takahashi H, Koehler RC, Brusilow SW, et al: Effect of glutamine accumulation on cerebral edema formation during hyperammonemia. FASEB J 4:A955, 1990.
17. Swain M, Butterworth RF, Blei AT: Ammonia and related amino acids in the pathogenesis of brain edema in acute ischemic liver failure in rats. Hepatology 15:449, 1992.
18. Ede RJ, Gove CD, Hughes RD, et al: Reduced brain NA^+,K^+-ATPase activity in rats with galactosamine-induced hepatic failure: Relationship to encephalopathy and cerebral oedema. Clin Sci 72:365, 1987.
19. Seda HMW, Hughes RD, Gove CD, et al: Inhibition of rat brain Na^+-K^+

ATPase activity by serum from patients with fulminant hepatic failure. Hepatology 4:74, 1984.

20. Yang SS, Hughes RD, Williams R: Digoxin-like immunoreactive substances in severe acute liver disease due to viral hepatitis and paracetamol overdose. Hepatology 8:93, 1990.

21. Traber P, DalCanto M, Ganger D, et al: Effect of body temperature on brain edema and encephalopathy in the rat after hepatic devascularization. Gastroenterology 96:885, 1989.

22. Livingstone AS, Potvin M, Goresky CA, et al: Changes in the blood-brain barrier in hepatic coma after hepatectomy in the rat. Gastroenterology 73:697, 1977.

23. Dehouck MP, Meresse S, Delorme P, et al: An easier, reproducible and mass-production method to study the blood-brain barrier in vitro. J Neurochem 54:1798, 1990.

24. Almdal T, Schroeder T, Ranek L: Cerebral blood flow and liver function in patients with encephalopathy due to acute and chronic liver diseases. Scand J Gastroenterol 24:299, 1989.

25. Webster S, Gottstein J, Levy R, et al: Intracranial pressure-waves and intracranial hypertension in rats with ischemic acute hepatic failure. Hepatology 15:715, 1991.

26. Keays R, Alexander G, Williams R: Intracranial pressure rises and its association with clinical signs and prognosis in fulminant hepatic failure (abstract). J Hepatol 9:548, 1989.

27. Hanid MA, Davies M, Mellon PJ, et al: Clinical monitoring of intracranial pressure in fulminant hepatic failure. Gut 21:866, 1980.

28. Donovan JP, Quigley EMM, Sorrell MF, et al: Cerebral edema as a complication of chronic liver disease (abstract). Hepatology 12:860, 1990.

29. Langfitt TW: Increased intracranial pressure. Clin Neurosurg 16:436, 1969.

30. Blei AT: Cerebral edema and intracranial hypertension in acute liver failure: Distinct aspects of the same problem (editorial). Hepatology 13:376, 1991.

31. Munoz SJ, Ballas SK, Moritz MJ, et al: Perioperative management of fulminant and subfulminant hepatic failure with therapeutic plasmapheresis. Transplant Proc 21:3535, 1989.

32. Lidofsky SD, Lake JR, Read AE, et al: Liver transplantation for fulminant hepatic failure: The role of intracranial pressure monitoring (abstract). Gastroenterology 98:A604, 1980.

33. Inagaki M, Shaw B, Schafer D, et al: Advantages of intracranial pressure monitoring in patients with fulminant liver failure. Gastroenterology 102:A826, 1992.

34. Node Y, Nakazawa S: Clinical study of mannitol and glycerol on raised intracranial pressure and on their rebound phenomenon. Adv Neurol 52:359, 1990.

35. Ede RJ, Gimson AE, Bihari D, et al: Controlled hyperventilation in the prevention of cerebral oedema in fulminant hepatic failure. J Hepatol 2:43, 1986.

36. Forbes A, Alexander GJM, O'Grady JG, et al: Thiopental infusion in the treatment of intracranial hypertension complicating fulminant hepatic failure. Hepatology 10:306, 1989.

37. Bismuth H, Samuel D, Gugenheim J, et al: Emergency liver transplantation for fulminant hepatitis. Ann Intern Med 107:337, 1987.

38. Brajtbord B, Parks R, Ramsay M, et al: Management of acute elevation of intracranial pressure during hepatic transplantation. Anesthesiology 70:139, 1989.

39. O'Brien CJ, Wise RJ, O'Grady JG, et al: Neurological sequelae in patients recovered from fulminant hepatic failure. Gut 28:93, 1987.

40. Conn HO: A rational program for the management of hepatic coma. Gastroenterology 57:715, 1969.

41. Munoz SJ, Maddrey WC: Major complications of acute and chronic liver disease. Gastroenterol Clin North Am 17:265, 1988.

42. Takashi M, Igarashi M, Hino S, et al: Portal hemodynamics in chronic portal-systemic encephalopathy. Angiographic study in seven cases. J Hepatol 1:467, 1985.

43. Victor M, Adams RD, Cole M: The acquired (non-wilsonian) type of chronic hepatocerebral degeneration. Medicine 44:345, 1965.

44. Garcia-Tsao G, Groszman RJ, Fisher RL, et al: Portal pressure—Presence of gastroesophageal varices and variceal bleeding. Hepatology 5:419, 1985.

45. Coy DL, Srivastava A, Gottstein J, et al: The postoperative course after portacaval anastomosis in rats is determined by the portacaval pressure gradient. Am J Physiol 261:G1072, 1991.

46. Hawey A, Massoud A, Badr el Din N, et al: Bacterial flora in hepatic encephalopathy in bilharzial and non-bilharzial patients. J Egypt Soc Parasitol 19(suppl 2):797, 1989.

47. McDermott WV Jr, Adams RD: Episodic stupor associated with an ECK fistula in the human with particular reference to the metabolism of ammonia. J Clin Invest 33:1, 1954.

48. Wood AJ, Villeneuve JP, Branch RA, et al: Intact hepatocyte theory of impaired drug metabolism in experimental cirrhosis in the rat. Gastroenterology 76:1358, 1979.

49. Rudman D, DiFulco TJ, Galambos JT, et al: Maximal rates of excretion and synthesis of urea in normal and cirrhotic subjects. J Clin Invest 52:2241, 1973.

50. Haussinger D: Nitrogen metabolism in liver: Structural and functional organization and physiological relevance. Biochem J 135:199, 1991.

51. Butterworth RF, Giguere JF, Michaud J, et al: Ammonia: Key factor in the pathogenesis of hepatic encephalopathy. Neurochem Pathol 6:1, 1987.

52. Watson AJ, Chambers T, Karp JE, et al: Transient idiopathic hyperammonaemia in adults. Lancet 2:1271, 1985.

53. Lockwood AH, Yap EW, Wong WH: Cerebral ammonia metabolism in patients with severe liver disease and minimal hepatic encephalopathy. J Cereb Blood Flow Metabol 11:337, 1991.

54. Raabe W: Seizures in hyperammonemic encephalopathy (abstract). J Hepatol 10:S20, 1990.

55. Cooper AJ, Plum F: Biochemistry and physiology of brain ammonia. Physiol Rev 67:440, 1987.

56. Zieve L: Pathogenesis of hepatic encephalopathy. Metab Brain Dis 2:147, 1987.

57. Morgan MH, Read AE, Speller DC: Treatment of hepatic encephalopathy with metronidazole. Gut 23:1, 1982.

58. Fischer JE, Baldessarini RJ: False neurotransmitters and hepatic failure. Lancet 2:75, 1971.

59. Blei AT, Robbins DC, Drobny E, et al: Insulin resistance and insulin receptors in hepatic cirrhosis. Gastroenterology 83:1191, 1982.

60. Eriksson LS, Conn HO: Branched-chain amino acids in the management of hepatic encephalopathy: An analysis of variants. Hepatology 10:228, 1989.

61. Naylor CD, O'Rourke K, Detsky AS, et al: Parenteral nutrition with branched-chain amino acids in hepatic encephalopathy. A meta-analysis. Gastroenterology 97:1033, 1989.

62. Schafer DR, Jones EA: Hepatic encephalopathy and gamma-aminobutyric acid neurotransmitter system. Lancet 1:18, 1982.

63. Ferenci P, Ebner J, Zimmerman C, et al: Overestimation of serum concentrations of gamma-aminobutyric acid in patients with hepatic encephalopathy by the gamma-aminobutyric acid–radioreceptor assay. Hepatology 8:69, 1988.

64. Knudsen GM, Poulsen HE, Paulson OB: Blood-brain barrier permeability in galactosamine-induced hepatic encephalopathy: No evidence for increased GABA transport. J Hepatol 6:187, 1988.

65. Rossie M, Deckert J, Jones EA: Autoradiographic analysis of GABA-benzodiazepine receptors in an animal model of acute hepatic encephalopathy. Hepatology 10:143, 1989.

66. Sieghart W: Heterogeneity of $GABA_A$-benzodiazepine receptors. Biochem Soc Trans 19:129, 1991.

67. Grimm G, Ferenci P, Katzenschlanger R, et al: Improvement of hepatic encephalopathy treated with flumazenil. Lancet 2:1392, 1988.

68. Olasmaa M, Rothstein JD, Guidotti A, et al: Endogenous benzodiazepine receptor ligands in human and animal hepatic encephalopathy. J Neurochem 55:2015, 1990.

69. Basile AS, Hughes RD, Harrison PM, et al: Elevated brain concentrations of 1,4-benzodiazepines in fulminant hepatic failure. N Engl J Med 325:473, 1991.

70. Mullen KD: Benzodiazepine compounds and hepatic encephalopathy. N Engl J Med 325:509, 1991.

71. Bakti G, Fisch HU, Karlaganis G, et al: Mechanism of the excessive sedative response of cirrhotics to benzodiazepines: Model experiments with triazolam. Hepatology 7:629, 1987.

72. Vander Rijt CC, Schalm SW, Meulstee J, et al: Flumazenil therapy for hepatic encephalopathy: A double-blind cross-over study. Hepatology 10:590, 1989.

73. Wahren J, Denis J, Desurmont P, et al: Is intravenous administration of branched chain amino acids effective in the treatment of hepatic encephalopathy? A multicenter study. Hepatology 3:475, 1983.

74. Michel H, Bories P, Aubin JP, et al: Treatment of acute hepatic encephalopathy in cirrhotics with a branched-chain amino acids enriched versus a conventional amino acids mixture. A controlled study of 70 patients. Liver 5:282, 1985.

75. Uribe M: Treatment of chronic portal-systemic encephalopathy with lactose in lactase-deficient patients. Dig Dis Sci 25:924, 1980.

76. Atterbury CE, Maddrey WC, Conn HO, et al: Neomycin-sorbitol and lactulose in the treatment of acute portal-systemic encephalopathy. Am J Dig Dis 23:398, 1978.

77. Patil DH, Westaby D, Mahida YR, et al: Comparative modes of action of lactitol and lactulose in the treatment of hepatic encephalopathy. Gut 28:255, 1987.

78. Uribe M, Campollo O, Vargas F, et al: Acidifying enemas (lactitol and lactose) vs. nonacidifying enemas (tap water) to treat acute portal systemic encephalopathy: A double blind randomized clinical trial. Hepatology 7:639, 1987.

79. Weber FL Jr, Fresard KM: Comparative effects of lactulose and magnesium sulfate on urea metabolism and nitrogen balance in cirrhotic subjects. Gastroenterology 80:994, 1981.

80. Weber FL Jr: Treatment of hepatic encephalopathy with lactulose and antibiotics. In: Butterworth RF, Pomier-Layrargues G (eds): Hepatic Encephalopathy: Pathophysiology and Treatment. Clifton, NJ, Humana, p 483, 1989.

81. Mortensen PB, Holtug K, Bonnen H, et al: The degradation of amino acids, proteins, and blood to short-chain fatty acids in colon is prevented by lactulose. Gastroenterology 98:353, 1990.

82. Conn HO: Adverse reactions and side-effects of lactulose and related agents. In: Conn HO, Bircher J (eds): Hepatic Encephalopathy: Management with Lactulose and Related Carbohydrates. East Lansing, MI, Medi-Ed Press, p 199, 1988.

83. Donovan JP, Quigley MM, Sorrell MF, et al: Cerebral edema as a complication of chronic liver disease (abstract). Hepatology 12:860, 1990.

84. Uribe M, Moreno BJ, Lewis H: Lactose enemas plus placebo tablets vs. neomycin tablets plus starch enemas in acute portal systemic encephalopathy. Gastroenterology 81:101, 1981.

85. Collinson PO, Burroughs AK: Severe hypermagnesaemia due to magnesium sulfate enemas in patients with hepatic coma. Br Med J 293:1013, 1986.

86. Dawson AM, McLaren J, Sherlock S: Neomycin in the treatment of hepatic coma. Lancet 2:1263, 1957.

87. Tarao K, Ikeda T, Hayashi K, et al: Successful use of vancomycin hydrochloride in the treatment of lactulose resistant chronic hepatic encephalopathy. Gut 31:702, 1990.

88. Weber FL Jr, Fresard KM, Lally BR: Effects of lactulose and neomycin on urea metabolism in cirrhotic subjects. Gastroenterology 82:213, 1982.

89. Pomier-Layrargues G, Giguère JF, Lavoie J, et al: Pharmacokinetics of benzodiazepine antagonist Ro 15-1788 in cirrhotic patients with moderate or severe liver dysfunction. Hepatology 10:969, 1989.

90. Potts JR III, Henderson JM, Millikan WJ Jr, et al: Restoration of portal venous perfusion and reversal of encephalopathy by balloon occlusion of portal-systemic shunt. Gastroenterology 87:208, 1984.

91. Powell EE, Pender MP, Chalk JB, et al: Improvement in chronic hepatocerebral degeneration following liver transplantation. Gastroenterology 98:1079, 1990.

SECTION ELEVEN

Nutrition

Section Editor

John L. Rombeau

Indications for and Administration of Enteral and Parenteral Nutrition in Critically Ill Patients

John L. Rombeau

Advances in the monitoring and support of vital organ systems have led to improved survival of critically ill patients. Patients now survive life-threatening conditions such as overwhelming sepsis and acute episodes of respiratory, cardiac, renal, and hepatic failure. Because of the inordinate number of personnel, extensive resources, and increased length of hospital stay required in the care of the critically ill, aggressive life support of these patients has become one of the most challenging and controversial issues in modern medicine.

Nutritional support is now an integral part of the complete care of hospitalized patients. It is defined as the provision of specialized diets via either an enteral or parenteral route (enteral nutrition [EN] and parenteral nutrition [PN]). The role of nutritional support in critically ill patients, however, is often unclear. Some of these patients are either too ill or their life expectancy is too short to permit the initiation of nutritional support. Other critically ill patients are subject to so many forms of invasive monitoring and therapy that nutritional intervention has low priority. The widespread use of PN has demonstrated that the nutritional status of these patients can be supported temporarily until the critical illness subsides.[1] Of greater concern is whether the provision of nutritional support prevents the adverse clinical outcome due to malnutrition. This chapter reviews the following with particular emphasis on the critically ill patient: nutritional assessment, determination of nutrient requirements, and indications for and administration of EN and PN.

NUTRITIONAL ASSESSMENT

Nutritional assessment, as commonly performed for hospitalized patients, is imprecise. Various indices are measured

to obtain a general impression of whether a patient suffers from protein-energy malnutrition; however, the cutoff points for establishing degrees of malnutrition in critically ill patients have yet to be standardized. There is still a major need to identify more specific means of assessment. In large population studies, the parameters commonly used appear to be useful in defining malnutrition; however, the appropriateness of applying these measurements to individual patients remains to be proved. Nutritional assessment usually includes history, physical examination, laboratory tests, and special tests.

Nutritional History

Perhaps the most important component of the nutritionally oriented history is related to assessing gastrointestinal (GI) function. The physician should question the patient carefully about possible symptoms of GI disease, such as nausea, vomiting, or diarrhea. Factors that limit food intake—anorexia, dysphagia, disorders in chewing or swallowing, and food allergies—should be uncovered, as should factors that increase metabolic needs, such as recent illnesses, surgery, trauma, or sepsis. The patient should be asked about the ingestion of medications that interfere with appetite or the absorption and use of nutrients. Examples of these medications are laxatives, antineoplastics, antibiotics, and antacids. Chronic illnesses, such as alcoholism, diabetes, severe congestive heart failure, and GI disorders, affect nutritional status. Psychosocial problems—advanced age, psychosis, drug addiction, poverty—also affect the patient's general nutritional status.

For the critically ill patient, the primary diagnosis or reason for hospitalization in the intensive care unit is often the major determinant of the need for nutritional support because of predisposing to protein-energy malnutrition. Protein-energy malnutrition in the hospitalized patient is defined as either nonvolitional loss of 10% of usual body weight or a serum albumin level less than 3.5 g/dL when the patient is in a euvolemic state. It is particularly significant in critically ill patients because it has a major adverse effect on clinical outcome[2] and it is difficult to correct in the presence of severe stress or sepsis.

Protein-energy malnutrition is subclassified as marasmus, kwashiorkor, or a combination of the two. Marasmus is the wasting of energy reserves in adipose tissue and somatic muscle that occurs with prolonged starvation. Marasmus is associated with an acceptable protein/calorie intake ratio but inadequate total intake of these nutrients. Most critically ill patients ultimately suffer from marasmic protein-energy malnutrition. Kwashiorkor occurs when a diet provides adequate calories but insufficient total protein. Clinically, patients with kwashiorkor have increased extracellular fluid with pitting edema, occasional ascites, and anasarca. Levels of liver-dependent transport proteins such as albumin, transferrin, and thyroxine-binding prealbumin are decreased, but skeletal muscle mass is normal or only slightly depleted. In addition to protein-energy malnutrition, critically ill patients may suffer from selective vitamin or mineral deficiencies; however, these are usually treated without major difficulty.

It is neither cost-effective nor possible to do a complete nutritional assessment of all critically ill patients, using all the tests that are currently available. Reasonable methods of initial nutritional assessment consist of taking a history and performing a physical examination with emphasis on the changes described earlier, including the patient's weight and height.[3] However, it may be difficult to obtain accurate measurements of weight and height, particularly for critically ill patients.

Physical Examination

When marasmic patients are examined, they appear to have wasting of both muscle and fat. Patients with kwashiorkor have decreased skin turgor, ascites, liver enlargement, and occasionally parotid gland hypertrophy.

Critically ill patients with chronic malnutrition may be deficient in trace elements or vitamins. These deficits may be worsened during the course of the critical illness. Patients with vitamin, trace element, or mineral deficiencies may have a number of related physical signs (Table 136–1).

The integument is an important component of the nutritionally oriented physical examination. Examination of the hair may reveal alopecia, hypopigmentation, dryness, brittleness, and easy loss, which can be symptoms of protein-energy malnutrition or a deficiency of zinc, vitamin E,

vitamin A, or biotin. The skin may be extremely dry. Follicular keratosis or acneiform lesions, associated with vitamin A deficiency, may be seen. Vitamin C or vitamin K deficiency may cause petechiae and ecchymoses. Iron, folate, or vitamin B_{12} deficiency may cause pallor. Scrotal dermatitis, erythema, and hyperpigmentation are associated with niacin deficiency. Scaly skin lesions over the trunk of the body, accompanied by alopecia, may indicate a deficiency of an essential fatty acid, zinc, or biotin.

Patients with vitamin A deficiency commonly have xerosis and white exudates outside the limbus of the eye (Bitot's spots). Vitamin C deficiency may also cause xerosis of the eyes. Optic neuritis and ophthalmoplegia may result from thiamine deficiency. Riboflavin deficiency can cause increased vascularity of the bulbar conjunctivae and angular blepharitis. Riboflavin and pyridoxine deficiencies are associated with nasolabial exfoliation, inflammation, and seborrhea.

The mouth may reveal angular stomatitis and cheilosis. These symptoms are characteristically associated with riboflavin deficiency, although they may occur with a deficiency of any of the B complex vitamins. Interdental gingival hypertrophy or gingivitis is associated with vitamin C, vitamin A, niacin, and riboflavin deficiencies. An atrophic tongue or glossitis is associated with iron, folate, niacin, or pyridoxine deficiency or a combination of these. It should be noted that physical signs of malnutrition and vitamin deficiencies usually appear only in advanced cases.

Body Weight

Measurements of body weight are usually compared with ideal body weights in tables such as those derived by the Metropolitan Life Insurance Company. Ideal body weights are based on frame size. In the Metropolitan Life tables, ideal weights for individuals with small, medium, and large frames are arbitrarily assigned by quartiles—that is, the

TABLE 136–1		
SOME PHYSICAL SIGNS OF NUTRITIONAL DEFICIENCY		
Site	Signs	Deficiencies
Hair	Alopecia	Protein-calorie malnutrition
	Brittleness	
	Color change	Biotin
	Dryness	Zinc
	Easy pluckability	Vitamins E and A, zinc (?)
Skin	Acneiform lesions	Vitamin A
	Follicular keratosis	
	Xerosis (dry skin)	
	Ecchymosis	Vitamin C or K
	Intradermal petechia	
	Erythema	Niacin
	Hyperpigmentation	
	Scrotal dermatitis	
Eyes	Angular palpebritis	Vitamin B_2
	Bitot's spots	Vitamin A
	Conjunctival xerosis	Vitamin A
Mouth	Angular stomatitis	Vitamin B_{12}
	Atrophic papillae	Niacin
	Bleeding gums	Vitamin C
	Cheilosis	Vitamin B_2
	Glossitis	Niacin, folate, vitamin B_{12}
	Magenta tongue	Vitamin B_2
Extremities	Genu valgum or varum	Vitamin D
	Loss of deep tendon reflexes of the lower extremities	Vitamins B_1 and B_{12}

Adapted in part from Rombeau JL, Richter GC, Forlaw L: Practical aspects of nutritional assessment. Pract Gastroenterol 8:43, 1984.

lower fourth of the range of average weight for a particular age and height is assigned to a small frame. Unfortunately, there is no uniformly accepted method for accurately measuring frame size.

Other ways in which body weight may be used to assess a patient's degree of malnutrition include evaluation of current weight as a percentage of ideal body weight, current weight as a percentage of usual weight, and recent weight change. The following formulas were devised by Blackburn and colleagues:[4]

$$\text{Percentage of ideal body weight} = \text{(current weight/ideal body weight)} \times 100$$

with 80–90% = mild malnutrition
70–79% = moderate malnutrition
0–69% = severe malnutrition

$$\text{Percentage of usual weight} = \text{(current weight/usual weight)} \times 100$$

with 85–95% = mild malnutrition
75–84% = moderate malnutrition
0–74% = severe malnutrition

$$\text{Percentage of recent weight change} = [\text{(usual weight} - \text{current weight)} / \text{usual weight}] \times 100$$

with significant weight loss = ≥1–2 % over 1 wk
≥5% over 1 mo
≥7.5% over 3 mo
≥10% over 6 mo or more

Among these measurements, the percentage of recent weight change correlates best with ultimate morbidity and mortality in individual patients. This is because many patients have a usual weight above the ideal weight for their height. Patients with certain illnesses lose 20 to 25% of their usual body weight. Morbidity and mortality of these patients are significantly greater than those of patients with the same diagnosis without such severe weight loss.[2]

LABORATORY MEASUREMENTS

Serum Albumin

Measurements of this serum protein have classically been used in population studies as an indicator of visceral protein depletion. An outstanding review of this subject has been published.[5] Albumin is a poor indicator of early protein malnutrition because serum levels fall and recover slowly with changes in nutritional status. This slow response is a result of the body's large albumin pool and albumin's long serum half-life of 20 days. As with other plasma proteins, a decrease in the serum albumin level generally indicates a decrease in liver protein synthesis caused by a limited supply of substrate. Albumin synthesis usually decreases during fasting and protein deprivation, and there is a decrease in catabolism in several days. These are frequent findings in critically ill patients who have exacerbation of a chronic illness. However, factors other than nutrient supply can affect the serum albumin level (and levels of other plasma proteins). Increased extracellular fluid frequently causes an artifactual decrease in the serum albumin level. The stresses of critical illness, surgery, trauma, and sepsis can lead to decreased albumin levels as a consequence of increased peripheral breakdown and extravasation.[6] Liver and kidney disease can also lower the serum albumin level through decreased synthesis and increased excretion, even when there is adequate provision of nutrients.

Serum albumin levels lower than 3 g/dL have been cor-related with increased morbidity and mortality of hospitalized patients.[2] In general, it is thought that serum albumin concentrations indicate various degrees of visceral protein depletion: mild depletion is associated with 2.8 to 3.5 g/dL, moderate depletion with 2.1 to 2.7 g/dL, and severe depletion with less than 2.1 g/dL.

Serum Transferrin

This beta globulin, synthesized by the liver, transports iron in the plasma. The normal serum concentration ranges from 250 to 300 mg/dL. The serum half-life of transferrin is 8 to 10 days. Thus, the serum transferrin level reflects acute changes in visceral protein status more accurately than the serum albumin level.

Serum transferrin levels can be measured directly by radial immunodiffusion. In addition, a close estimate of the serum transferrin level is obtained from the more clinically available measurement of total iron-binding capacity (TIBC), using the following formula:

$$\text{Serum transferrin level} = 0.8(\text{TIBC}) - 43$$

A serum transferrin concentration determined from the TIBC can be altered by iron deficiency; thus, the degree of transferrin depletion is frequently underestimated in moderately iron-depleted patients. Studies have shown that the derived transferrin level is routinely lower than the directly measured level, so the levels obtained by the two methods cannot be compared.[7] However, derived transferrin levels followed serially in a single patient can serve as indicators of the patient's response to nutritional therapy. Transferrin values between 150 and 200 mg/dL, as measured by radial immunodiffusion, are considered to represent mild visceral protein depletion, values between 100 and 150 mg/dL represent moderate depletion, and levels below 100 mg/dL reflect severe depletion.

Creatinine-Height Index

Urinary creatinine excretion in 24 hours may be used to evaluate skeletal muscle mass. The quantity of creatinine excreted from the body is directly proportional to skeletal muscle mass. In the presence of rapid loss of skeletal muscle with critical illness, measured creatinine excretion is an index of skeletal muscle proteolysis. Creatinine is derived from the breakdown of creatine, an energy depot molecule synthesized by the liver. Creatinine excreted in a 24-hour urine collection directly reflects the level of total body creatine and thus indicates total body muscle mass. Creatinine excretion in the human is a reasonable predictor of lean body mass, even when compared with more sophisticated measurements of skeletal muscle (see later under Body Composition Studies).

To determine the degree of somatic protein depletion in hospitalized patients, Bistrian and colleagues[8] used the creatinine-height index, the ratio of a patient's 24-hour creatinine excretion to the expected 24-hour creatinine excretion of a normal adult. The expected 24-hour creatinine excretion for individuals of various heights was calculated from the mean creatinine excretion of healthy young males and females; the ideal weight for a person of medium frame at each height was taken from Metropolitan Life standards. Creatinine-height index values between 60 and 80% are thought to indicate moderate somatic protein depletion and values lower than 60%, severe depletion. However, these levels of protein malnutrition have not been validated in studies of the correlation between depressed creatinine-height index levels and the incidence of morbidity and mortality.

There are several problems with determination of the creatinine-height index. Accurate 24-hour urine collections are difficult to obtain even from patients in intensive care units. In addition, prediction of creatinine excretion from data based on ideal body weight and medium frame involves all of the difficulties related to determining frame size. Problems also arise because the available standards have been applied to young and old patients alike. Because creatinine excretion decreases with increasing age, these standards are likely to overestimate protein depletion in elderly patients.

Thyroxine-Binding Prealbumin

This carrier protein for retinol-binding protein also plays a major role in the transport of thyroxine. Its serum half-life is estimated to be as short as 2 days. In addition, the body pool of thyroxine-binding prealbumin is small. For these reasons, sudden demands for protein synthesis that occur with infection and stress rapidly depress serum prealbumin levels. The normal mean serum concentration is 22.4 $\pm$ 7 mg/dL. Lower levels are consistent with different degrees of visceral protein depletion: 10 to 15 mg/dL indicates mild depletion; 5 to 10 mg/dL, moderate depletion; and less than 5 mg/dL, severe depletion. As with the other acute-phase proteins, wide variations occur in normal thyroxine-binding prealbumin levels. Therefore, this parameter may not be extremely sensitive to mild protein depletion. Serum prealbumin is best measured by radial immunodiffusion.

Retinol-Binding Protein

This is the specific protein for vitamin A alcohol transport. It is linked with prealbumin in a constant molar ratio. It is filtered by the glomerulus and metabolized by the kidney; therefore, it may be elevated in kidney disease despite visceral protein compartment depletion. Normal serum concentrations are 5.1 $\pm$ 2.5 mg/dL. Because of its 10-hour half-life, retinol-binding protein reflects acute changes in protein malnutrition.

Urinary 3-Methylhistidine Excretion

This amino acid is present almost exclusively in myofibrillar protein. On breakdown of myofibrillar protein, 3-methylhistidine is released but not recycled and is excreted almost entirely in the urine. A measurement of 3-methylhistidine excretion in a 24-hour urine sample therefore approximates total muscle turnover during the time of collection. Problems with this technique include the difficulty of sample collection and the lack of sensitivity to breakdown of sarcoplasmic protein, which constitutes about 35% of muscle protein. Many other factors, including age, sex, dietary intake, starvation, trauma, and infection, may also influence 3-methylhistidine excretion.

24-Hour Urinary Nitrogen Excretion

The urinary excretion of nitrogen as urea nitrogen is often measured to assess the adequacy of protein repletion during nutritional therapy. Urea nitrogen excretion represents approximately 85 to 90% of total nitrogen excretion if there are no abnormal sources of nitrogen loss (e.g., protein-losing gastroenteropathy, nephropathy, burns, or desquamative skin disease). In critically ill patients with protein depletion who are receiving nutritional support, the goal is usually achievement of nitrogen equilibrium (see the section on protein requirements). In routine clinical practice, fecal

and integumentary losses of nitrogen are not measured; however, many intensive care units are acquiring the capacity to measure total nitrogen content in urine, feces, and fistula effluent by the Kjeldahl technique. Nitrogen balance may be calculated as follows:

$$N \text{ balance (g)} = \frac{\text{24-h protein intake (g)}}{6.25} - \text{24-h urinary urea nitrogen (g)} + 4\text{g}$$

where 4 g is an estimate of fecal and integumentary losses. This measurement is still the "gold standard" of assessing nitrogen losses in the intensive care setting.

FURTHER NUTRITIONAL TESTING

Patients whose history, physical examination, or weight change and standard laboratory tests are consistent with malnutrition and for whom more nutritional-metabolic information is desired may benefit from a more complete nutritional assessment. Various tests may be used in this assessment. There is not a close correlation between different parameters used for nutritional assessment, and no one parameter necessarily predicts a patient's nutritional status. However, lack of correlation between parameters may simply suggest different degrees of sensitivity. The results of multiple nutritional tests given at the initial assessment may be useful in serial monitoring of a patient's response to nutritional therapy. Of the many parameters listed in this chapter, the only ones that consistently correlate with morbidity and mortality are recent loss of more than 10 to 15% of usual body weight and a serum albumin level less than 3 g/dL.

Plasma Vitamin Levels

Vitamin deficiencies in plasma are common in chronically malnourished patients; however, acute vitamin deficiencies in critically ill patients are uncommon. This may be because serum vitamin levels can be decreased by stress or infection without reflecting a true total body depletion of vitamins. Despite these concerns, critically ill patients should be given routine supplementation with a multiple-vitamin preparation. In contrast to exogenous proteins and calories, vitamins (and minerals) are needed in small quantities that are often easily provided by giving vitamins and minerals orally or parenterally. Nonetheless, it is becoming increasingly popular to monitor levels of vitamins (and some minerals) in hospitalized patients receiving nutritional support.[9]

Measurements of Immunocompetence

Malnutrition is frequently associated with depression of the patient's immunologic responsiveness. Decreases in the total lymphocyte count, impairment of lymphocyte responses to phytohemagglutinin, depressed neutrophil chemotaxis, deficiencies in immunoglobulin G and C3, and depression of reactivity to various allergens in skin tests have all been observed as malnutrition progresses.[10] These changes are often reversible with nutritional repletion. However, the tests of immune function are nonspecific and have minimal clinical utility, and most clinical laboratories are not equipped to do extensive evaluations of the immune system. Therefore, standard nutritional assessment in most institutions does not include measurements of immunocompetence.

Hand Grip Dynamometry and Muscle Function Testing

Hand grip strength and other forms of skeletal muscle testing have been used as functional measurements of nutritional status. Hand muscle strength or more general muscle function is usually tested by a trained physical therapist. Results are relatively reproducible if performed by experienced personnel and with the patient's cooperation. The different instruments used for hand grip dynamometry, however, are not strictly comparable. Muscle function testing is potentially an appealing way to monitor responses to nutritional therapy because it is a functional measure and can be performed serially. More extensive evaluation of standards is needed according to age and gender and the relationship of abnormalities to prognosis.

Plasma and Muscle Amino Acid Patterns

Plasma and muscle amino acid patterns have been proposed as aids in the diagnosis of malnutrition and evaluation of the response to nutritional treatment. These tests are difficult to obtain and are usually not clinically feasible. It has been demonstrated that these patterns are influenced by recent protein intake and by renal and hepatic failure.[11] Levels of essential amino acids are more depressed than those of nonessential amino acids in childhood protein malnutrition. Plasma amino acids have not yet been found helpful in predicting nutritional status or prognosis.

Muscle amino acid patterns may correlate more strongly with a patient's actual nutritional status than do plasma amino acid profiles.[12] At present, however, assessment of muscle amino acid patterns is still a research technique. Thus far, the expense and complexity of the technique and its lack of validation make it less attractive as a routine nutritional assessment tool.

PROGNOSTIC INDICES

Several attempts have been made to correlate multiple measurements of nutritional status with morbidity and mortality. An early composite measurement in surgical patients was the prognostic nutritional index based on measurements of albumin, transferrin, and skin test reactivity.[13] This index has not been uniformly accepted because not all the variables are independent (e.g., albumin and transferrin), the variables are not solely affected by nutritional status (e.g., delayed hypersensitivity), and subsequent studies have shown the index not to be predictive of outcome in critically ill postoperative patients[14] and patients with acute abdominal trauma. Finally, it has not been demonstrated that the improvement in the prognostic nutritional index with nutritional support correlates with decreased morbidity and mortality.

A subjective global assessment of nutritional status has been developed and validated in hospitalized patients (Table 136–2).[15] This assessment is based on nutritionally relevant features of the medical history and physical examination and classifies a patient's nutritional status into one of three categories: (1) well nourished, (2) moderately malnourished, and (3) severely malnourished. It is emphasized that the subjective global assessment is indeed subjective, and there are no absolute values for its measurement. Consideration of the complete clinical picture and the physician's experience and judgment determine the value of this assessment. The subjective global assessment combined with measurement of serum albumin levels is superior or equal to single-objective parameters in predicting the development of nutrition-related complications in hospitalized patients.[16]

BODY COMPOSITION STUDIES

Because of the expense of the equipment and the complexity of the techniques, these studies are usually performed as research procedures. The following are examples of body composition studies undergoing investigation:

Isotope dilution with ^{42}K to determine total exchangeable potassium and therefore body cell mass

Whole body ^{40}K counting to determine total exchangeable potassium by assessing naturally occurring ^{40}K, which exists in a fixed ratio to ^{39}K in body tissue

In vivo neutron activation analysis to measure total body nitrogen and thereby establish the amount of total body protein

Computed tomography to measure fat, skeletal muscle, bone, and visceral organ mass

Nuclear magnetic resonance to measure fat, fat-free body mass, and skeletal muscle

Nuclear magnetic resonance spectroscopy to measure high-energy phosphates in skeletal muscle

Ultrasonography to measure fat, skeletal muscle, and visceral organs

Magnetic resonance imaging to measure fat and fat-free body mass

Biostereometrics to measure fat and fat-free body mass

DETERMINATION OF NUTRIENT REQUIREMENTS

Determination of nutrient requirements is an important component of nutritional assessment in the critically ill patient. There has been considerable research on the best ways to determine calorie and protein requirements. Before

---

TABLE 136–2

CLASSIFICATION OF NUTRITIONAL STATUS: SUBJECTIVE GLOBAL ASSESSMENT

Criteria	Well Nourished	Moderately Malnourished	Severely Malnourished
Medical history			
Body weight change in the last 6 mo	Loss < 5%	Loss 5–10%	Loss > 10%
Dietary intake	Balanced diet that meets requirements	70–90% of required	<70% of required
GI symptoms (vomiting, diarrhea)	No	Intermittent	Daily for >2 wk
Functional capacity	Full capacity	Reduced	Bedridden
Physical examination			
Subcutaneous fat	Normal	↓	↓↓
Muscle mass (quadriceps, deltoids)	Normal	↓	↓↓
Edema (ankle, sacral)	No	+	+
Ascites	No	+	+
Serum albumin	>4.0 g/dL	3.0–4.0 g/dL	<3.0 g/dL

Data from Baker JP, Detsky AS, Wesson DE, et al: Nutrition assessment: A comparison of clinical judgment and objective measurements. N Engl J Med 306:969, 1982.

making these determinations, it is important to decide whether the overall goal of nutritional support is maintenance or repletion. Because the hormonal milieu (increased levels of catabolic cytokines, catecholamines, cortisol, and glucagon) during the catabolic phase of illness impairs nitrogen retention, the initial goal of nutritional support for a critically ill patient should be to provide enough calories and protein to maintain, not replete, lean body mass.[17] Nutritional repletion can be expected to occur only when the acute, catabolic phase of the illness has subsided and the patient is in the anabolic phase of recovery. Nutritional support per se does not convert a patient from catabolism to anabolism. Furthermore, the provision of inordinate amounts of protein and calories to a critically ill patient may actually enhance the stress response.

Giving calories in excess of requirements is of questionable value in the critically ill patient because it increases lipogenesis and the deposition of fat in the liver.[17] Delivery of excessive calories may produce a respiratory quotient greater than 1.0, which implies fat synthesis and suggests that the extra calories are not required. Therefore, there is enough evidence to support the conclusion that hyperalimentation is not clinically efficacious.

Determination of Energy Requirements

Energy requirements are based on age, sex, body build, activity level, and disease state. There is no single formula or test to determine energy needs for all patients. Energy requirements are usually estimated by standard equations. Occasionally, energy requirements are measured by indirect calorimetry.

In most clinical settings, energy requirements are based on energy expenditure estimated or predicted from formulas derived from multiple measurements. The formula most widely used to predict resting metabolic expenditure (RME) is the Harris-Benedict equation:

$$\text{RME (male)} = 66 + 13W + 5H - 6.8A$$
$$\text{RME (female)} = 655 + 9.6W + 1.7H - 4.7A$$

where RME = resting metabolic expenditure (kcal/d)
  W = weight (kg)
  H = height (cm)
  A = age (years)

After determination of the RME, energy requirements are adjusted according to the patient's activity and illness, as indicated in Table 136–3. Patients are given some increment above the estimated RME depending on their degree of stress and on whether there is a need for weight maintenance or repletion. The percentages by which calorie requirements are increased for patients with various critical illnesses have been determined by measurements by indirect calorimetry[18] (see Table 136–3). These percentages have not been as well established for groups of patients other than those listed.

In the absence of significant weight loss or sepsis, many diseases do not significantly alter basal metabolism, and calculations of RME based on the Harris-Benedict equation are as good as the energy expenditures measured by indirect calorimetry.

Indirect calorimetry can be performed with a metabolic measuring cart or with equipment attached to a ventilator provided by a respiratory therapy department.[19] In this technique, the energy expended with oxygen consumption and carbon dioxide production is calculated from measurements of respiratory gas exchange. Indirect calorimetry is frequently helpful for critically ill patients with sepsis and multiple organ system failure and when there is an insufficient response to "appropriate" nutritional support.

TABLE 136–3

CORRECTION FACTORS FOR PREDICTING ENERGY REQUIREMENTS FOR HOSPITALIZED PATIENTS

Clinical Condition	Correction Factor (× RME*)
Physical activity	
Confined to bed	1.2
Out of bed	1.3
Starvation	0.7
Fever	1.0 + 0.13 per °C
Elective surgery	1.0–1.2
Peritonitis	1.2–1.5
Soft tissue trauma	1.1–1.3
Major sepsis	1.4–1.8

*RME = resting metabolic expenditure.
Adapted from Bernard MA, Jacobs DO, Rombeau JL: Nutritional and Metabolic Support of Hospitalized Patients. Philadelphia, WB Saunders, p 13, 1986.

Determination of Protein Requirements

Protein needs are increased in critically ill patients because of decreased intake and increased demands for tissue synthesis and repair. Protein and amino acid requirements are difficult to estimate during the catabolic phase of illness. Table 136–4 provides estimates of protein needs for several examples of critical illness. The stress of trauma and sepsis increases nitrogen requirements, and a tumor, especially with associated antineoplastic therapy, may cause similar metabolic stress.

Protein requirement is influenced to a great extent by energy intake. To some extent, the more calories given, the better the nitrogen retention. However, nitrogen retention also depends on the nonprotein calorie/nitrogen ratio, which is influenced by different clinical conditions. In general, for the nonstressed patient the optimal nonprotein calorie/nitrogen ratio is approximately 150:1. For critically ill patients, the nonprotein calorie/nitrogen ratio decreases (~100:1) because these patients have a greater need for amino acids to support the synthesis of acute-phase proteins (which have a shorter half-life than structural proteins) for tissue healing and energy.

The exact quantity of protein needed with the various levels of caloric intake has not been clearly defined. Useful general guidelines are noted in Table 136–4. These guidelines allow an initial estimate of appropriate quantities of calories and protein. The quantities should be altered during the course of nutritional therapy depending on the results of nitrogen balance studies and other studies performed to demonstrate nutritional progress.

TABLE 136–4

PROTEIN REQUIREMENTS AND NONPROTEIN CALORIE/NITROGEN RATIO IN HOSPITALIZED PATIENTS

Clinical Condition	N (g/kg/d)*	NPC/N†
Nonstress		
N maintenance	0.6–0.8	150:1
N repletion	1.0–1.2	150:1
Stress		
Active inflammation	1.2–1.5‡	150:1
Major surgery	1.2–1.5	120:1
Sepsis	2.0–2.5	80:1

*N (g/kg/d) = grams of nitrogen per kilogram of body weight per day.
†NPC/N = nonprotein calorie/nitrogen ratio.
‡Add fecal losses.

Determination of Requirements for Electrolytes and Micronutrients

Requirements for sodium, potassium, bicarbonate, chloride, magnesium, calcium, and phosphate should be based on the patient's baseline levels, estimates of daily requirements, and ongoing losses. These requirements have been reviewed extensively.[20]

Vitamins should be administered daily in amounts recommended by the Nutritional Advisory Group of the American Medical Association.[21] Standard amounts of commercial trace element mixes are usually adequate for short-term parenteral feeding. Copper and manganese should be omitted from total parenteral nutrition (TPN) because they are predominantly excreted in the bile in patients with liver disease.

ENTERAL NUTRITION

Rationale

EN is the provision of liquid formula diets either orally or by tube into the GI tract. EN preserves intestinal structure and function and facilitates nutrient utilization. Safety, convenience, and economy of delivery further justify the administration of such therapy in the absence of contraindications.

The trophic effects on gut structure and function are a major reason for providing EN.[17] The presence of luminal nutrients preserves the integrity of the intestinal mucosa, including absorptive cells (enterocytes), mucus-secreting cells, gut-associated lymphoid tissue, and brush border enzymes.[22, 23] Both brush border enzymes and enterocyte replication are essential for digestion and absorption, and mucus and gut-associated lymphoid tissue are key components of the intestinal barrier. Bacteria, endotoxins, and antigenic substances are contained in the intestinal lumen by this barrier. Enteral feedings may also buffer the gastric acidity, thereby avoiding the need for H_2 blockers and maintaining normal motility.[24]

The liver, by first-pass processing of nutrients, regulates both the plasma concentration of metabolic substrates and the chemical form in which nutrients are presented to target organs. For instance, lipids administered via the enteral route are processed by the intestine into chylomicrons and then by the liver into lipoproteins. Lipid emulsions administered directly into the blood stream by PN are associated with abnormal fractions in the plasma lipid profile. Disorders of lipid, carbohydrate, and amino acid metabolism have been implicated in the occurrence of fatty liver during administration of PN.[25] Whatever the cause of TPN–induced fatty liver, it is not associated with EN.

Improved safety further supports the use of EN. EN avoids complications caused by insertion of central venous catheters and eliminates the risk of catheter sepsis. Although not without its own risks, EN may be safer than the parenteral technique.

Finally, EN is less expensive and easier to administer than TPN.[26] It does not require the extensive sterile techniques used during parenteral feedings, and there is less need for a trained maintenance team. Furthermore, the minimal daily requirements of various vitamins and nutrients are well established for enteral feeding, whereas parenteral requirements are not as well known.

Indications

General indications for EN in critically ill patients include malnutrition, insufficient volitional intake of food, and a GI

TABLE 136–5

INDICATIONS FOR ENTERAL NUTRITION IN CRITICALLY ILL PATIENTS

Hypermetabolism	Organ system failure
Trauma	Respiratory (producing
Burn	ventilator dependence)
Sepsis	Cardiac (resulting in
Postoperative major	cardiac cachexia)
surgeries	Intestinal (caused by
	short-bowel syndrome)
Gastrointestinal disease	Hepatic (resulting in
Esophageal obstruction	hepatic encephalopathy)
Pancreatitis	Renal (producing uremia)
Inflammatory bowel	Central nervous system
disease	(resulting in coma)
Fistulas	Multiple organ system
	failure

From Rolandelli RH, Koruda MJ, Guenter P, et al: Enteral nutrition: Advantages, limitations, and formula selection. J Crit Illness 3(10):93, 1988.

tract that can be used safely and effectively. Malnutrition is defined as either recent nonvolitional loss of at least 10% of usual body weight or a serum albumin level less than 3.3 g/dL. Insufficient volitional intake of food is arbitrarily defined as less than 50% of intake to meet nutritional requirements. Safe usage of the GI tract is defined as absence of abdominal distention, obstruction, diarrhea, and hemorrhage.

The American Society for Parenteral and Enteral Nutrition has listed a number of conditions grouped in categories of responsiveness to EN. Unfortunately, in critically ill patients the indications for EN are not as clear as in stable hospitalized patients. The indications have therefore been modified as shown in Table 136–5.

As described previously, critical illnesses are associated with numerous GI disorders in which EN may be beneficial in one patient and deleterious in another, even when both patients have the same GI disorder. For instance, stress gastritis, acalculous cholecystitis, ileus, and mild diarrhea are not absolute contraindications for EN. Furthermore, one could postulate that EN instituted early in the course of critical illnesses might help prevent these complications. However, the decision to initiate EN in these patients should be based on a thorough clinical and biochemical examination and clinical projection of anticipated outcome as described previously.

Certain types of patients are conditional candidates for EN. For example, a patient with mild bleeding stress ulceration and hemodynamic stability may benefit from EN.[24] Patients with postoperative ileus can be fed with EN as long as mechanical obstruction has been eliminated and there is access to the small bowel for feedings with simultaneous gastric decompression.

Patients with neurologic disorders that prevent satisfactory oral intake and those with oropharyngeal or esophageal disorders who cannot eat are excellent candidates for EN. Ventilation-dependent patients and patients with obtundation caused by sepsis, sedation, or metabolic disorders are the primary candidates for enteral feedings in the intensive care unit. Enteral feedings can also be used during the transition from TPN to combined PN and EN to oral intake.

Contraindications to use of the enteral route include vomiting, intestinal obstruction, severe ileus, and upper GI bleeding. New distal enteric anastomoses also contraindicate use of this route.

It has been hypothesized that the GI tract participates in the body's response to stress and may become the source of sepsis and multiple organ system failure syndrome.[27] Although provision of nutrients may attenuate the deleterious effects of stress on the GI tract, critical illnesses are commonly associated with GI disorders that make it difficult, if not impossible, to administer EN. To determine the need for and feasibility of providing EN to critically ill patients, it is essential to understand the body's response to stress, as well as the pathophysiology of the GI tract during critical illness.

Enteral Nutrition and the Gastrointestinal Barrier

EN is contraindicated if the patient has failure of more than two organ systems, with ongoing sepsis unresponsive to therapy and cardiopulmonary instability. In these patients, it is unlikely that a hyperpermeable small bowel populated by bacteria would benefit from EN. Moreover, intraluminal nutrients may increase bacterial overgrowth and worsen the situation. However, it is also unlikely that bowel rest would reduce bacterial translocation and endotoxin transmigration.

Nutritional intervention and management of the patient with intestinal barrier failure are controversial and the subject of research in many medical centers. To enhance barrier function, research groups are working on providing intestinal fuels such as glutamine,[28] short chain fatty acids,[29] and ketones.[30] Hormones such as epidermal growth factor with trophic effects on the intestine are also being investigated.[31]

The sequential responses of the GI tract and potential therapeutic interventions during critical illnesses are shown in Figure 136–1. At the onset of most critical illnesses, oral intake is significantly decreased, so the intestine "rests." The lack of intraluminal nutrients leads to mucosal atrophy and diminished digestive secretions. Continued stress and progressive deficits of intestinal fuels lead to further atrophy of the gut mucosa. This initial phase of gut atrophy is reversed or ameliorated by administration of early enteral feedings, as shown by a series of experiments with animal models of stress.[32] Intestinal fuels such as short chain fatty acids added to enteral diets significantly reduce the atrophy caused by lack of luminal nutrients and may further increase intestinal trophism.[33]

As the critical illness progresses, the blood flow to the intestine is compromised, the lumen of the small intestine becomes colonized by bacteria, and the colonic microflora is disrupted. These derangements lead to increased permeability of the gut mucosa with translocation of bacteria and transmigration of endotoxins. This stage is known as barrier failure. The vertical dashed line in Figure 136–1 represents an arbitrary point after which intraluminal manipulations may be not only ineffective but also deleterious.

Many intensive care specialists are now aware of the possibility of the gut's being the origin of sepsis and multiple organ system failure.[34] The suspicion arises when a patient develops enteric bacteremia and sepsis without discernible evidence of the source of sepsis. These patients may be traversing any phase of the multiple organ system failure with varying compromise of other organ systems. On the basis of clinical data,[35] one can predict that a patient with isolated pulmonary failure is at an early stage of this syndrome, whereas a patient with renal failure and two or more organ failures is at an end stage of the spectrum.

The presence of gut barrier breakdown and bacterial translocation is difficult to diagnose. The problem is compounded by the lack of confirmatory tests to aid in diagnoses of bacterial translocation and endotoxin transmigration. For the purpose of deciding to provide EN to maintain barrier function, it may suffice to know whether or not there is underlying bacterial overgrowth of the small bowel. Breath hydrogen analysis is a simple, noninvasive test designed to assess bacterial overgrowth of the small bowel in a variety of chronic GI diseases. At a few research centers, this test is being employed to diagnose bacterial overgrowth in critically ill patients. The results of this test are confounded by motility disorders, and the test is somewhat cumbersome in intubated patients. However, preliminary results with the breath hydrogen test are promising, and it may become a useful measurement for the critically ill patient. Other methods are being tested for assessing intestinal permeability, such as urinary excretion of lactulose and fecal clearance of α_1-antitrypsin.

If the patient is stable, only one organ system is affected, and bacterial overgrowth cannot be demonstrated, a trial of EN is warranted. These patients tolerate hyperosmolar and high-fat diets poorly; therefore, an isotonic carbohydrate-based diet is administered by continuous infusion into the stomach at a rate of 40 mL/h. The patient should be closely monitored not only for signs of diet intolerance but also for

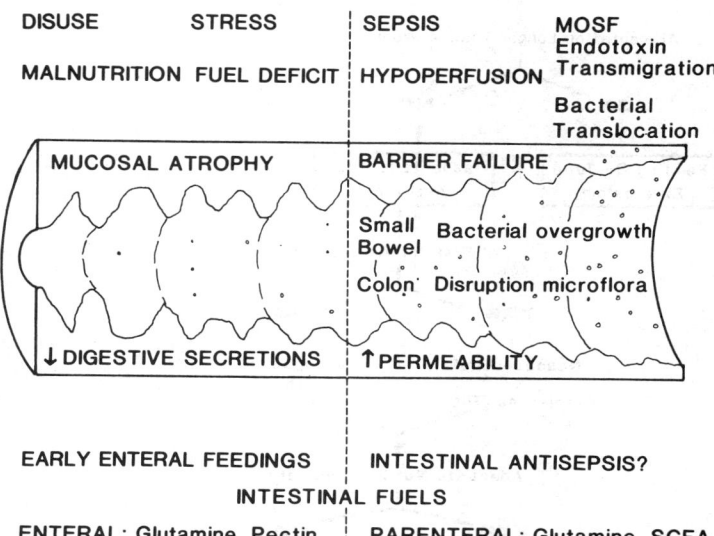

Figure 136–1. Responses of the gastrointestinal tract and potential therapeutic interventions during critical illness. MOSF = multiple organ system failure; SCFA = short-chain fatty acids. (From Rolandelli RH, Rombeau JL: Enteral nutrition in critically ill patients. Perspect Crit Care 2:1, 1989.)

worsening of the organ failure syndrome. If the patient develops ileus, diarrhea worsens, or the organ failure syndrome continues to involve more systems, EN should be withheld. Intolerance to EN is associated with increased mortality in critically ill patients.[36, 37] Therefore, EN may be considered a "stress test" in critically ill patients. The development of symptoms of "gut failure" usually indicates a poor prognosis.

Regardless of the tolerance to EN, in the critically ill patient one should not plan to meet all nutritional requirements immediately via the GI tract. Supplemental parenteral feeding is usually necessary to meet the patient's needs while concurrent delivery of EN provides progressive stimulation of the GI tract.

A prerequisite for initiating EN in critically ill patients is adequate cardiopulmonary stability. As mentioned previously, provision of EN in shock states may actually be harmful. For practical purposes, cardiac stability is defined as a cardiac index of more than 2 L/m², with a mean arterial blood pressure of more than 70 mm Hg and without the need for alpha sympathetic stimulation. Adequate pulmonary function is defined as arterial oxygen saturation of more than 95% with inspired concentrations of oxygen of

less than 60% and with less than 5 cm of positive end-expiratory pressure. These are some arbitrary criteria that indicate acceptable oxygen delivery to the intestine, which seems to correlate with tolerance to EN.

ASSESSMENT AND SELECTION OF PATIENTS

Selection of patients for EN is based on the algorithm shown in Figure 136–2. Before initiating nutritional therapy, baseline nutritional assessment is performed; a medical and dietary history, physical examination, and laboratory evaluation (complete blood count, analysis of serum electrolyte and albumin levels, and liver function tests) are obtained as discussed previously. With most critically ill patients, the primary reasons for admission to the intensive care unit influence conventional nutritional assessment indices, such as serum albumin level, TIBC, and body weight. Therefore, recent dietary history, physical examination, and the nature and course of the illness are given major consideration when assessing the nutritional status of a critically ill patient.

As mentioned previously, to establish the need for supplementary EN the nutritional assessment should demonstrate that the patient's volitional intake of food is insufficient to

DECISION MAKING FOR ENTERAL FEEDING

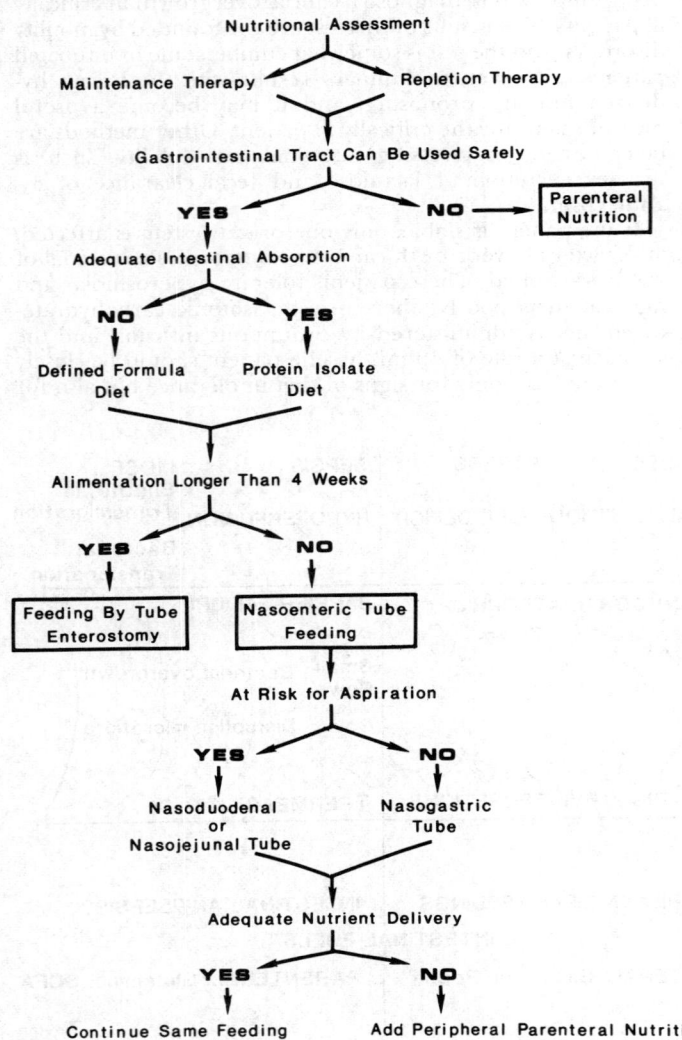

Figure 136–2. Selection of patients for enteral nutrition. (From Guenter P, Jones S, Jacobs DO, et al: Administration and delivery of enteral nutrition. In: Rombeau JL, Caldwell MD [eds]: Clinical Nutrition: Enteral and Tube Feeding. 2nd ed. Philadelphia, WB Saunders, p 192, 1990.)

meet at least 50% of his or her needs. Patients whose oral intake provides 50% or more of their needs can be managed with oral balanced nutritional supplements.

Feeding into the GI tract is generally safe in the absence of distention, diarrhea, vomiting, or GI bleeding. However, clinical judgment determines whether the GI tract is functioning adequately and can be used safely. Most reports show that a maximum of 3000 kcal/d can be delivered enterally; however, it may take as long as 5 days to reach this goal. In critically ill patients, it is common for significantly fewer calories to be delivered than are prescribed, and the actual time to reach the caloric goal is often nearly twice as long as anticipated. (Repeated interruptions resulting from other diagnostic and therapeutic priorities frequently impair nutrient delivery.) Thus, patients with excessive nutrient requirements or for whom an extended period is needed to reach adequate EN intake usually require supplemental intravenous feedings.

Enteral Dietary Formulations

When the decision to provide EN is made, the proper dietary formulation must be selected. Because of the frequent changes in existing commercial formulations and the increasing availability of new products, only the major classifications of dietary formulations with examples of each are presented here. An extensive discussion of this topic has been reported.[38]

In general, diet selection is based on the following factors:

1. The ability of the GI tract to digest and absorb major nutrients
2. The patient's total nutrient requirements
3. Fluid-electrolyte restrictions

A typical decision tree for the selection of an initial dietary formula is depicted in Figure 136–3.

The nutrient needs of the critically ill patient are determined during the initial nutritional assessment as discussed previously. Consideration is given to conditions such as severe hypercatabolism, renal or hepatic failure, pulmonary insufficiency, and the severity of malnutrition in the critically ill. These disorders may alter nutrient needs and thereby necessitate the administration of a more specific dietary formulation.

Several classifications of enteral dietary formulations have been proposed.[38, 39] Unfortunately, none of these is completely satisfactory. The problem with existing classifications is that the dietary categories are often intermingled in terms of both composition and clinical use. The following classification of formulas, which is based on nutrient composition, is used: (1) polymeric, (2) elemental, (3) immune-enhanced, and (4) modular.

Polymeric Formulas

In polymeric formulas, the three basic nutrients—proteins, carbohydrates, and fats—are in complex forms (i.e., polymers). Carbohydrates are present in the form of oligosaccharides, maltodextrins, or polysaccharides; fats consist of medium or long chain triglycerides. The protein source is a natural protein, which may be intact or partially hydrolyzed. In general, these diets are isotonic, lactose free, "ready to use," and available in liquid form. Many polymeric diets can be used either for tube feedings or for oral supplementation. These diets are selected on the basis of calorie, protein, and fluid requirements. Polymeric diets can be further divided according to their caloric density, which may be 0.6, 1.0, 1.5, or 2.0 kcal/mL (Table 136–6). The group with 1 kcal/mL includes the largest number of commercially available diets. The nonprotein caloric content in these diets is derived from either carbohydrates or lipids. Polymeric diets formulated with carbohydrates as the main caloric source have higher osmolality than isocaloric diets containing lipids. Hypertonic diets, which are carbohydrate based, are well tolerated when infused intragastrically and reasonably well tolerated when administered directly into the small

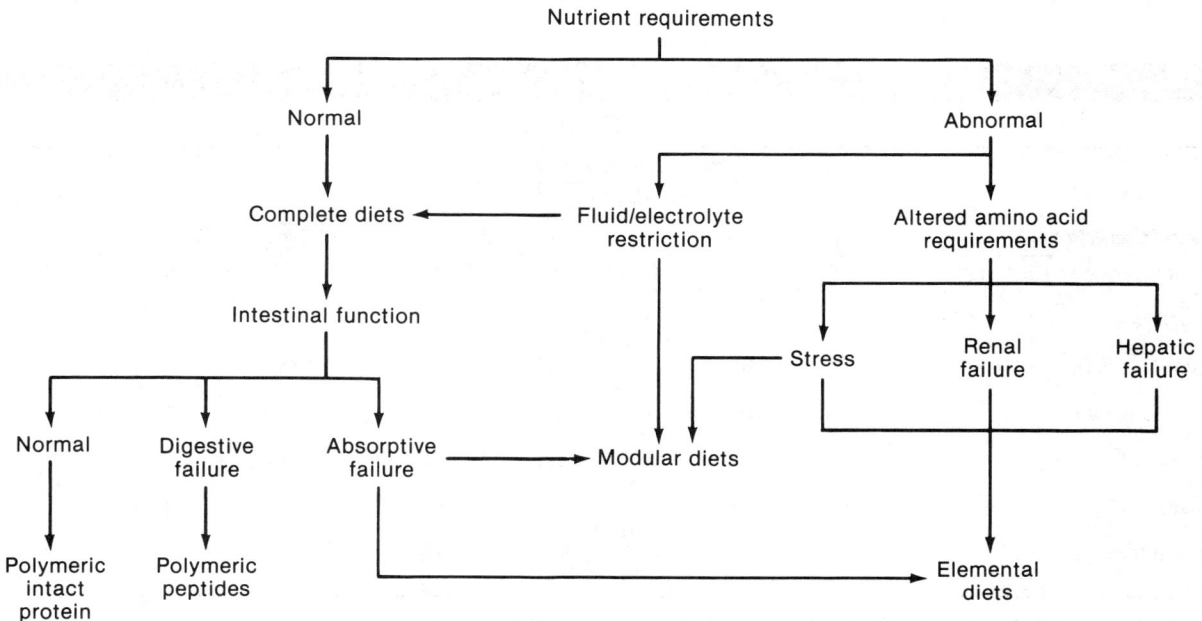

Figure 136–3. Selection of initial dietary formula. (From Rolandelli RH, Rombeau JL: Enteral feeding: Liquid formula diets. In: Bayless T [ed]: Current Therapy in Gastroenterology and Liver Disease–2. Toronto, BC Decker, p 206, 1986.)

TABLE 136–6

POLYMERIC DEFINED FORMULA DIETS*

Kilocalories	Protein (g/L)	Carbohydrate (g/L)	Fat (g/L)	Product
0.66	40	121	1.7	Citrotein
	26–45	217–249	1.3–13.5	Criticare, Precision LR and HN, Vital HN, Travasorb HN and STD
1	25–49	115–176	25–40	Isocal, Ensure, Enrich,† Precision Isotonic, Osmolite, Travasorb MCT, Renu, Vipep
	60	130	23	Sustacal
1.5	55–61	190–200	53–57	Ensure Plus, Sustacal HC
	62	105	92	Pulmocare
	83	143	68	Traumacal
2.0	70–75	225–250	80–91	Magnacal, Isocal HCN

*Caloric density and nutrient contents are based on the information provided in the product literature.
†Enrich includes 21 g of soy polysaccharide per liter of diet as a fiber source.
From Rolandelli RH, Rombeau JL: Enteral feeding: Liquid formula diets. In: Bayless T (ed): Current Therapy in Gastroenterology and Liver Disease–2. Toronto, BC Decker, p 206, 1986.

---

bowel. Carbohydrate-based diets are advantageous for patients with steatorrhea and hyperlipidemia. Polymeric diets, which are fat based, may be more appropriate for patients who have diarrhea associated with tube feedings, especially when the feedings are infused directly into the small bowel. High-fat diets are useful for patients receiving mechanical ventilatory assistance because they reduce carbon dioxide production and thereby facilitate ventilator weaning. Most polymeric diets are formulated to provide approximately 6.25 g of protein (1 g of nitrogen) for every 150 kcal. Concomitant provision of sufficient calories at this ratio promotes the utilization of nitrogen for synthesis of structural compounds (i.e., visceral and muscle protein). If the caloric content of the diet does not meet the patient's requirements, the protein content is utilized as an energy source and the nitrogen intake results in increased ureagenesis. Diets with high calorie/nitrogen ratios are recommended for patients with renal and hepatic insufficiency. Diets with higher caloric density, 1.5 and 2.0 kcal/mL, are used for patients with increased energy requirements (e.g., hypercatabolism) or fluid restrictions (e.g., respiratory distress syndrome) and renal failure.

Elemental Formulas

Elemental formulas, also called chemically defined or synthetic diets, include basic nutrients in monomeric forms. All elemental diets contain crystalline amino acids as the protein source, but the composition of these amino acids is variable. The source of carbohydrates varies from dextrose to oligosaccharides, and fats are usually in the form of medium chain triglycerides. Elemental diets are hypertonic, are usually in powder form, and are not palatable. Because of this lack of palatability, they are rarely used for oral supplements. Elemental diets were initially formulated with a ratio of essential to nonessential amino acids of 35:65. This ratio was chosen because the high biologic value of the diet resembled that of proteins such as egg albumin and human milk.

In addition to this standard formulation of amino acids, new "specialized" elemental diets have been developed with different compositions of amino acids (Table 136–7). Specialized formulas have been designed for patients with diseases in which nutrient requirements are specifically altered. In three of these states—hepatic failure, renal failure, and

---

TABLE 136–7

ELEMENTAL DIETS*

Product Formula Name	Total	Essential TOTAL	Essential BC	Essential A	Nonessential	CHO (g/L)	Fat (g/L)	Caloric Density kcal/g N	Caloric Density kcal/mL
Standard Vivonex T.E.N. (stress)	38	20.1	12.6 (33%)	3.8	18.2	206	3	164	1.0
Stresstein	37	23.2	16.4 (44%)	3.4	14.0	140	23	90	1.2
Traum-Aid HBC	28	18.4	13.9 (50%)	2.7	9.6	166	12	87	1.0
Amin-Aid (renal)	19	18.3	6.4 (33%)	6.0	0.6	366	19	380	1.9
Travasorb Renal	23	14.5	5.9 (25%)	3.9	8.4	274	18	362	1.3
Hepatic-Aid	43	24.4	13.8 (32%)	1.3	18.5	289	36	215	1.7
Travasorb Hepatic	29	20.7	12.5 (43%)	0.8	7.8	210	15	218	1.1

*Nutrient contents and caloric density are based on the information provided in the product literature.
†BC = branched chain. The numbers in parentheses refer to the percentages of essential amino acids provided as BC. A = aromatic amino acids, including methionine. The amount given for nonessential amino acids includes histidine, which may be regarded as an essential amino acid for renal patients.
From Rolandelli RH, Rombeau JL: Enteral feeding: Liquid formula diets. In: Bayless T (ed): Current Therapy in Gastroenterology and Liver Disease–2. Toronto, BC Decker, p 206, 1986.

stress—amino acid needs appear to be altered. In a few patients with chronic pulmonary insufficiency, a particular caloric substrate profile may be indicated. A new formula has been developed that contains nutrients chosen to enhance the immune response during critical illness.

Formulas for Hepatic Failure. Specialized formulas for patients with hepatic encephalopathy contain high quantities of branched chain amino acids (BCAAs) and low quantities of aromatic amino acids and methionine. An abnormal plasma ratio of these amino acids in patients with liver failure is thought to be partially responsible for the encephalopathy.[40] Critical analysis of the prospective, randomized studies of patients with hepatic encephalopathy suggests that intravenous hepatic formulations improve encephalopathy and nutritional status; however, they do not improve survival.[41]

It is recommended that these formulas be restricted to patients with hepatic encephalopathy who have an acceptable hepatic reserve and who do not respond to administration of standard polymeric formulations. Formulas enriched in BCAAs are more expensive than polymeric diets and are not recommended for patients who have nonencephalopathic manifestations of liver disease or end-stage liver failure.

Formulas for Renal Failure. The aim of EN in acute renal failure is to minimize the abnormal accumulations of nitrogenous compounds, electrolytes, and fluid without adversely affecting, and perhaps even improving, nutritional status and outcome. The specialized formulas for renal failure contain crystalline essential amino acids as the sole nitrogen source. These formulas attempt to decrease urea production by recycling urea nitrogen into the synthesis of nonessential amino acids. Such formulas are lactose free, contain little or no electrolyte, are hyperosmolar, and are not palatable; therefore, they are usually given by tube.

The theory behind the design of these products is novel; however, clinical trials of these formulas given intravenously have not shown that they are superior to products containing essential and nonessential amino acids. Survival and improvement in renal function are not enhanced by use of these formulas; however, dialysis requirements may be reduced.[42] Because of this and because of the relatively high cost of these formulas, their administration during *acute* renal failure is recommended when attempting to avoid dialysis. When dialysis is ongoing the use of standard polymeric or modular formulas is recommended.

Stress Formulas. The hormonal response to stress (caused by trauma or sepsis) promotes early increased proteolysis in skeletal muscle. This process leads to irreversible combustion of BCAAs, which skeletal muscle oxidizes for energy. The stress of critical illness also makes available other amino acids (alanine and glutamine) for gluconeogenesis, enzyme synthesis, wound healing, and immune function.[43]

The enteral diets formulated for stressed patients are high in BCAAs (44 to 50% of total amino acids, compared with 25 to 33% in standard polymeric or elemental formulas). Nonprotein calories are provided as carbohydrate (maltodextrins) and fat (medium chain triglycerides and soy oil) at a calorie/nitrogen ratio of 80:1 to 100:1 (compared with about 150:1 for standard formulas). These diets have a caloric density of 1.0 to 1.2 kcal/mL, are hyperosmolal (675 to 910 mOsm/kg), and are expensive.

In theory, BCAAs, especially leucine, may stimulate protein synthesis and reduce proteolysis in the stress state. Although several studies have shown that high-BCAA diets promote nitrogen retention in stressed patients, none has documented improved clinical outcome.[44] Thus, these products are restricted to patients who are highly stressed, as shown by markedly negative nitrogen balance, an increased

blood urea nitrogen (BUN) level, or intolerance to standard diets.

Formulas for Respiratory Failure. Nutritional support is an important consideration for the critically ill patient with respiratory insufficiency. Maintenance of nutritional status is associated with enhanced ability to wean patients from ventilator support.[45] High-carbohydrate diets, either enteral or parenteral, increase carbon dioxide production, oxygen consumption, and ventilatory requirements.[46] In patients with compromised pulmonary function, these sequelae can precipitate respiratory failure and complicate weaning.

Complete oxidation of fat produces less carbon dioxide on a per calorie basis than does complete oxidation of either glucose or protein. Replacing carbohydrate calories with fat calories reduces carbon dioxide production, oxygen consumption, and minute ventilation. These effects imply that patients may be rapidly weaned from ventilatory support, but more data are needed to confirm these observations. Also, enteral diets with high-fat content are not well tolerated and tend to produce diarrhea in critically ill patients.

Because of the lack of conclusive evidence to support the use of high-fat diets and the frequent intolerance of critically ill patients to these formulas, patients with respiratory failure are initially fed a 30% fat polymeric diet and arterial blood gas levels are monitored. If arterial carbon dioxide levels increase, the dietary fat content is increased to 50% of total calories and arterial blood gases are monitored accordingly. If the high-fat diet reduces carbon dioxide retention but produces diarrhea, the fat content in the enteral formula is decreased and fat emulsions are provided intravenously.

Immune-Enhanced Formulas

The normal immune system has local and systemic components, both of which are affected by the nutritional status of the host. Impaired host immunity is seen in the critically ill, in patients with extensive neoplasia or protein-calorie malnutrition, and in those who are receiving immunosuppressive drugs. An enteral diet supplemented with arginine, RNA, and the omega-3 fatty acids has been formulated and marketed as enhancing the immune status of the host. This diet was studied in a prospective controlled trial in surgical patients with upper GI tract cancer.[47] Patients were assigned randomly to receive the supplemented diet or a similar diet without arginine, RNA, and the omega-3 fatty acids (control group). Infections and wound complications were significantly less frequent in patients receiving the enhanced diet. Unfortunately, the nitrogen intake of the control group was significantly less than that of the patients receiving the supplemented diet, and the study was not "double blinded." A further concern was that many of the patients were not malnourished at the time of entering the study. Thus, this diet can be recommended only for research purposes at this time. This concept is an interesting one, and further studies will be made of the abilities of various nutrients to provide pharmacologic immune enhancement.

Modular Formulas

Even though there are many formulated enteral diets, for some patients the use of standard, fixed-ratio formulas may not be optimal. For these patients, the use of modular formulas may obviate the need for PN. Modular diets are formulated as separately packaged nutrient sources for each substrate. The modules consist of single or multiple nutrients that can be combined to produce a nutritionally complete feeding or used individually to enhance an existing fixed-ratio formula, such as a polymeric or elemental diet. The modular system allows the physician to alter the ratio of a constituent nutrient without affecting the concentrations of other constituents. One can select not only the amount of each nutrient, substrate, mineral, vitamin, and so forth but also the type of nutrients most appropriate for the patient (e.g., whole protein vs. partially hydrolyzed vs. crystalline amino acids). If adequate facilities for compounding these formulas are available, administration of modular diets provides "prescription nutrition" to meet the specific requirements of the critically ill patient.

Formula Selection

It is often difficult to select the appropriate enteral formula, although choices may be limited because of an incomplete selection at any one institution. A decision algorithm is summarized in Figure 136–3. Polymeric diets are the first choice for patients who have normal intestinal function and no dietary restrictions and in whom standard-sized feeding tubes have been placed. Elemental diets are usually given for specific disease-related indications, such as impaired enzymatic digestion, reduced absorptive surface, renal or hepatic failure, and hypercatabolic states. Modular diets are reserved for the rare patient who cannot be fed with the two previously mentioned formulas.

Approximately 90% of our critically ill patients receive standard polymeric diets. These diets are inexpensive and well tolerated by most patients. Furthermore, there is little evidence that the more expensive specialized formulations are superior to polymeric diets in effect on clinical outcome. However, critically ill patients occasionally need specialized diets.

ACCESS AND DELIVERY
Access

Enteral formulas are administered by mouth, nasoenteric tube, and tube enterostomy. Nasoenteric tubes are most commonly used to administer EN to critically ill patients (Fig. 136–4). Nasoenteric tubes are preferred for short-term EN (less than 4 weeks) because the soft tubes (composed of nonreactive materials, such as silicone rubber or polyurethane) are reasonably well tolerated for 3 to 4 weeks. These tubes are in some instances weighted on the tip to help the tube pass through the pylorus; however, the importance of the weight has been questioned.[48]

Nasoenteric tubes are placed in the stomach or advanced into the jejunum. In most patients, the stomach is the preferred site for nutrient delivery. However, critically ill patients have a high incidence of gastroparesis and aspiration, and every attempt should be made to feed into the jejunum.

Critically ill patients are often unable to tolerate the right lateral decubitus position, which facilitates advancement of the tube out of the stomach. Therefore, transpyloric advancement is usually accomplished with the aid of fluoroscopy or endoscopy (Fig. 136–5). Administration of metoclopramide (10 mg intravenously) aids in the transpyloric passage of the tube in a few patients.

Patients who need long-term EN (more than 4 weeks) are fed by tube enterostomy. Tube enterostomy sites include the pharynx, esophagus, stomach, and jejunum. Most postoperative critically ill patients in need of feeding by tube enterostomy have the tubes placed either endoscopically or operatively.

Jejunostomy is used as a feeding route for patients undergoing gastroesophageal surgery or surgery for abdominal trauma and for those at increased risk of gastric aspiration. A combined gastrostomy-jejunal feeding tube has

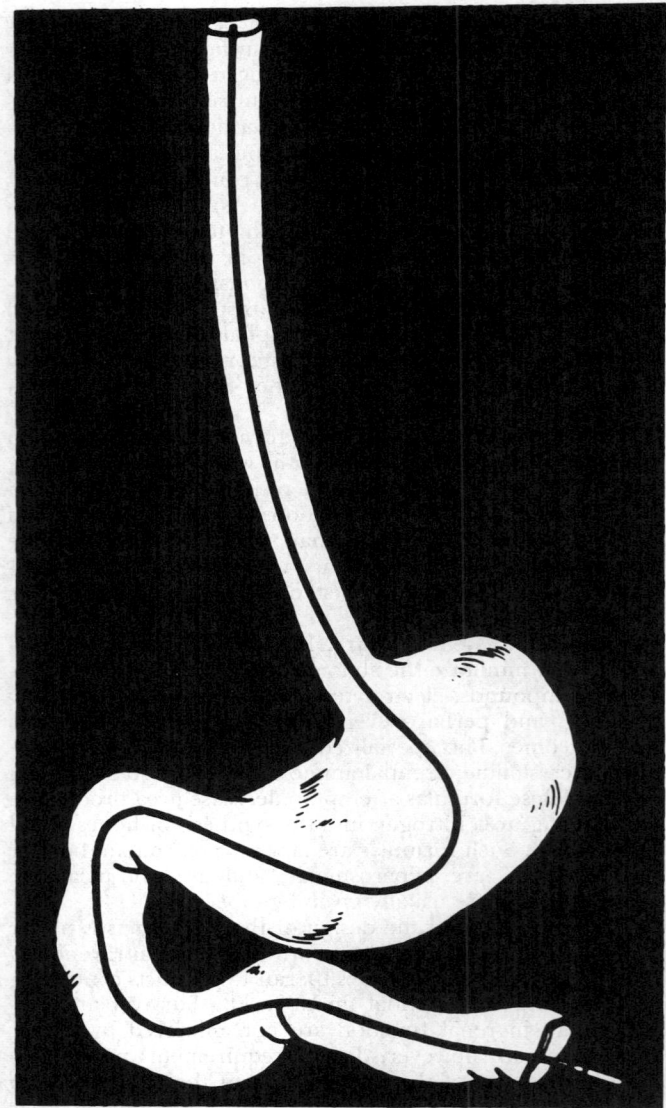

Figure 136–4. Optimal site for placement of nasoenteric tubes in critically ill patients. (From Guenter P, Jones S, Jacobs DO, et al: Administration and delivery of enteral nutrition. In: Rombeau JL, Caldwell MD [eds]: Clinical Nutrition: Enteral and Tube Feeding. 2nd ed. Philadelphia, WB Saunders, p 192, 1990.)

been developed that permits concurrent gastric decompression and jejunal feeding.[49] Even in the presence of mild paralytic ileus, low volumes of EN can be given by delivering diet into the duodenum or jejunum while the stomach is vented to remove swallowed air. Concomitant decompression of the stomach is an important part of feeding critically ill patients with intestinal ileus. This can be performed by a combined nasogastric-jejunal feeding tube (Fig. 136–6).

Delivery Methods

For critically ill patients, continuous feeding is preferred because it is better tolerated, it is associated with smaller residual volumes of formula, and it reduces the possibility of aspiration of formula when compared with intermittent feeding. In addition, continuously fed patients generally require less supervision (particularly if an infusion pump is used) than those fed intermittently.[50]

Improved weight gain and positive nitrogen balance occur

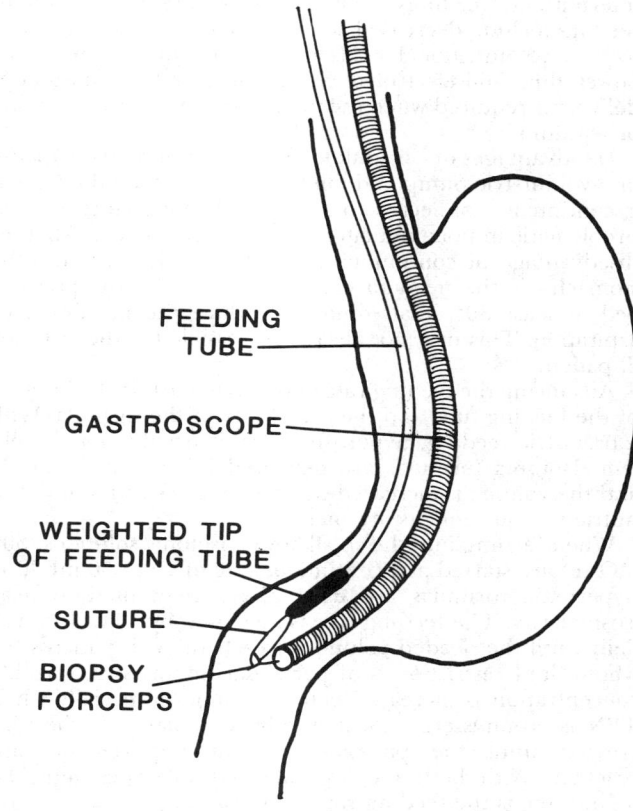

GASTROSCOPE AIDED PASSAGE OF FEEDING TUBE

Figure 136–5. Transpyloric endoscopic placement of nasoenteric tubes. (From Rolandelli RH, DePaula JA, Guenter P, et al: Critical illness and sepsis. In: Rombeau JL, Caldwell MD [eds]: Clinical Nutrition: Enteral and Tube Feeding. 2nd ed. Philadelphia, WB Saunders, p 288, 1990.)

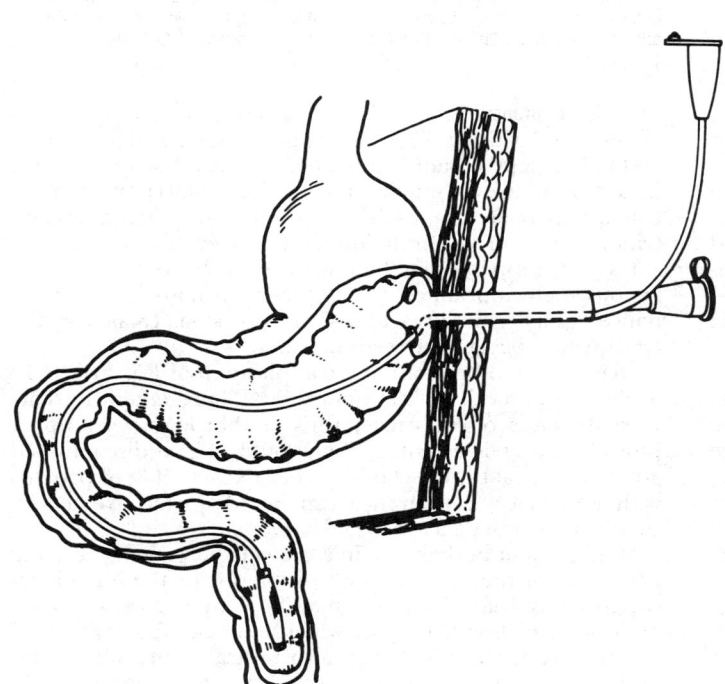

Figure 136–6. Combined nasogastric-jejunal feeding tube for concurrent gastric decompression and jejunal feeding. (From Rombeau JL: Enteral feeding into the jejunum with combined gastric decompression. Nutr Clin Pract 1:205, 1986.)

in critically ill children receiving continuous, rather than intermittent, feedings.[51] Other advantages of continuous feeding include decreased stool frequency and shorter time to achieve nutritional goals.[52] To avoid distention of the bowel, fluid and electrolyte shifts, and diarrhea, continuous delivery is required when the tube is placed in the duodenum or jejunum.

Disadvantages of continuous feedings include the expense of a volumetric pump and limited mobility when the patient is continually connected to a pump. These factors are less problematic in nonambulatory critically ill patients. Another disadvantage of continuous feedings—particularly into the stomach—is the need to elevate the head of the patient's bed at least 30° at all times to reduce the likelihood of aspiration. This may not always be possible for the critically ill patient.

Advancing the feeding rate depends in part on the location of the feeding tube and the osmolarity of the formula. With intragastric feeding, hyperosmolarity is usually not a problem. Isotonic formulas are delivered initially at 30 mL/h, and the volume is increased during 48 to 96 hours until full nutrient requirements are met.

When feeding into the small bowel, isotonic solutions (300 mOsm) are started at a continuous rate of 25 to 50 mL/h. If hypertonic formulas are used, they are diluted to near isosmolarity. The feeding rate is increased by 10 to 15 mL/h daily until the needed volume is reached. With patients for whom fluid restriction is of particular importance, formula concentration is increased before volume—especially when TPN is administered concurrently. Osmolarity is then increased until the patient's nutrient requirements are reached. With both feeding sites, GI tolerance must be monitored as the feeding rate is increased.

Monitoring

Patients who receive EN require the same careful monitoring as those who receive PN. A monitoring protocol helps to ensure that the specified nutritional goals are met (Table 136–8). A protocol is especially needed in institutions in which physicians with various levels of experience are responsible for writing orders.

Critically ill patients commonly have overlying or secondary dysfunction of the GI tract, which may result in intolerance to enteral diets. Daily evaluation is essential to ascertain the presence of diarrhea, constipation, nausea, abdominal distention, high gastric residuals, and vomiting.

In patients with an endotracheal tube who are at risk for aspiration, addition of food coloring to the diet may help to identify episodes of aspiration. With all critically ill patients, careful attention to the patient's metabolic status and fluid and electrolyte balance is especially important. With standardized monitoring, potential complications can be averted—in many cases, by simple maneuvers such as changing the infusion rate, caloric density, or formulation.

Periodic assessment is required to evaluate the adequacy of the nutritional support. Nitrogen balance, weight change, and serum protein status are routinely monitored, and the nutrient prescription is amended when indicated. We have found that hospitalized patients receiving EN actually received only 70 to 85% of their ordered calories;[53] as a result, we frequently supplement EN with parenteral feeding until a satisfactory EN intake is obtained.

Complications

Adverse effects of EN in the critically ill are classified as gastrointestinal, metabolic, aspiration, and mechanical.

Gastrointestinal Complications. In enterally fed patients,

TABLE 136–8
ENTERAL FEEDING STANDARD ORDERS

Feeding tube type and location of tip_____

Check items to be completed:

_____ 1. Obtain chest x-ray film after placement to confirm position.

_____ 2. Before feeding, confirm placement of tube by aspiration of gastric contents.

_____ 3. Elevate head of bed 30° when feeding into the stomach.

_____ 4. Name of the formula _____
    a. Intermittent: Give _____mL during 30 min every _____h at _____strength.
    b. Continuous: Give _____mL/h for _____h at _____ strength.

_____ 5. Check for residual _____h with gastric feedings. Return residual to stomach. Hold feedings for 1 h if residual is greater than _____mL and recheck in 1 h. Notify physician if this occurs on two consecutive measurements of residual.

_____ 6. Weigh patient Monday and Thursday and record on chart.

_____ 7. Record intake and output daily. Chart volume of formula separately from water or other oral intake for each shift. Record number, volume, and consistency of bowel movements.

_____ 8. Change administration tubing and feeding bag daily.

_____ 9. Irrigate feeding tube with 20 mL of water at the completion of each intermittent feeding, when tube is disconnected, after delivery of medications, and when the feeding is stopped for any reason.

_____ 10. Obtain complete blood count, complete serum chemistry profile, and total iron-binding capacity (transferrin) weekly.

_____ 11. Obtain basic chemistry profile every Monday and Thursday.

_____ 12. Begin 24-h urine collection for urea nitrogen and creatinine at 7:00 AM on _____.

_____ 13. Notify physician of nausea, vomiting, severe diarrhea, or shortness of breath.

From Guenter P, Jones S, Jacobs DO, et al: Administration and delivery of enteral nutrition. In: Rombeau JL, Caldwell MD (eds): Clinical Nutrition: Enteral and Tube Feeding. 2nd ed. Philadelphia, WB Saunders, p 192, 1990.

---

most complications are GI.[54] Delayed gastric emptying is common in critically ill patients and is exacerbated by intra-abdominal sepsis, pancreatitis, peptic ulcer disease, trauma, laparotomy, head injury, myocardial infarction, hepatic coma, hypercalcemia, diabetes mellitus, myxedema, malnutrition, mechanical ventilation, and a variety of medications.

Gastric emptying may be improved with the use of intravenous metoclopramide (10 mg every 6 hours), which enhances gastric motility. This drug occasionally aids in the transpyloric passage of feeding tubes.

Diarrhea, another common complication of EN, affects 40 to 60% of all critically ill patients.[55, 56] Management of diarrhea depends on its cause; thus, a thorough work-up of possible causes is essential. EN should not be discontinued automatically at the onset of diarrhea. Nearly 50% of patients with EN-associated diarrhea can be adequately treated by correcting dietary factors.[57]

Management of diarrhea in a critically ill patient receiving EN is one of the most difficult problems for the nutritional support physician. Diarrhea may be simply a consequence of prolonged bowel rest, in which case careful delivery of EN is warranted, but it may also indicate gut failure with underlying ischemia and bacterial overgrowth, wherein EN is contraindicated.

GI bleeding may occur in the stressed critically ill patient. One study concluded that EN may protect the mechanically ventilated patient against stress-induced hemorrhage.[24]

Metabolic Complications. In critically ill patients, metabolic complications of EN are common and are usually managed with ease when patients are properly monitored. Complications include abnormalities in fluid balance, glucose metabolism, electrolyte levels, and protein tolerance.

Aspiration. This is a potentially fatal complication of EN. Witnessed episodes confirm its occurrence. The prevalence of witnessed episodes in patients who receive EN varies from 1 to 44%.[57]

The influence of feeding methods and sites on aspiration has not been studied in a controlled manner. Standard clinical teaching is that the likelihood of aspiration can be decreased in patients fed beyond the pylorus. Our experience has been in accord with this teaching. Preventive measures to decrease the risk of aspiration include elevating the head of the bed to 30°, periodically measuring gastric residuals, and inflating endotracheal tube cuffs.

Methods for detecting "silent" aspiration of enteral formulas in intubated patients include checking tracheal aspirates for presence of glucose with glucose oxidant reagent strips. Food coloring can also be added to the formula and the tracheal aspirate monitored.

Mechanical Complications. Most mechanical complications of EN are related to the EN tube or its anatomic position. Nasoenteric tubes can cause nasopharyngeal erosions and discomfort, sinusitis, otitis media, gagging, esophagitis, esophageal reflux, tracheoesophageal fistulas, and rupture of esophageal varices. Clogging of the tubes is fairly common and can be prevented by routine irrigation of the tube with 30 mL of water at the completion of the feeding.

Gastrostomy or jejunostomy tubes can cause obstruction of the pylorus or small bowel. Several reports have noted the passage of nasoenteric tubes to areas outside the GI tract, such as the submucosa of the pharynx and the pleural space, with subsequent pneumothorax.[58]

Despite these reports, small-bore feeding tubes can be passed safely in most patients. In patients who are at increased risk for aspiration or who are obtunded, feeding tubes can be placed distally and more safely with the aid of fluoroscopy or endoscopy.

PARENTERAL NUTRITION*

PN is the administration of nutrients into a peripheral or central vein. Peripheral PN is the administration of water, electrolytes, protein, and caloric substrates through a peripheral vein to meet partial nutrient requirements. Central venous nutrition is the administration of greater quantities of the same nutrients because of the hyperosmolarity of the solution into a large-bore central vein.

Central Parenteral Nutrition

Central PN is indicated in most critically ill patients receiving intravenous nutrition. These patients usually require considerable amounts of energy and cannot tolerate excessive fluid volumes, and solutions of high caloric density and tonicity can be infused without adverse effects only into central veins. The solutions usually contain hypertonic glucose (25%), amino acids (5%), and other essential nutrients.

As a result of the hypertonicity of the solutions (greater than 2000 mOsm/kg), administration of the mixture into peripheral veins causes severe thrombophlebitis. When the solution is delivered into a central vein at a continuous rate, the nutrients are rapidly diluted to near isotonicity to be cleared from the blood stream. The standard central peripheral nutrition solutions contain at least 1 kcal/mL; therefore a solution given at 2.0 to 2.5 L/d provides 2000 to 2500 kcal and additional nutrients essential for critically ill patients. This energy load is sufficient for the complete energy needs of most nontrauma patients admitted to intensive care units.

Indications

As a rule, PN is indicated for a malnourished critically ill patient when the GI tract cannot or should not be used. Careful consideration should be given to the nutritional status, clinical condition, and GI function of the patient to assess whether PN or another type of nutritional support should be used. The indications for TPN are either absolute or relative (Table 136–9).

Access for Central Parenteral Nutrition

As mentioned previously, the hypertonicity of the nutrient admixtures mandates central venous access. This is best achieved by percutaneous cannulation of the subclavian vein with placement of the catheter tip into the superior vena cava. Alternative access routes into the superior vena cava include the internal or external jugular veins. These veins are not as desirable as the subclavian vein because of difficulty in maintaining adequate sterility of dressings in the neck over the catheter access site. Most intensive care physicians should be able to cannulate the superior vena cava safely by using at least two different approaches (both subclavian and internal jugular venipuncture) because situations may require the need for more than one route of venous access.

Catheterization of central veins should be done or at least supervised by physicians who are experienced with the procedure. To become experienced, it is suggested that more than 50 successful cannulations be performed.

TABLE 136–9

INDICATIONS FOR PARENTERAL NUTRITION

Central Venous Infusions
   To provide adequate IV nutritional support for 10 d or more
   To satisfy nutrient requirements in patients with increased energy needs and normal or decreased fluid requirements
   To support the patient with single-organ failure or multiple organ system failure by infusing modified nutrient solutions in a limited fluid volume

Peripheral Venous Infusions
   To provide initial feeding (<5 d) before catheter insertion in a patient who will require central venous feedings
   To infuse less concentrated solutions via a multiuse central catheter (i.e., a line for blood drawing, medication, and nutrients) into an individual in whom other venous access cannot be easily or safely obtained
   To supplement enteral feedings that are inadequate because of GI dysfunction
   To satisfy energy requirements that are nearly basal (1500–1800 kcal/d) in a nondepleted patient who can tolerate 2.5–3.0 L IV solution each day

---

Percutaneous puncture of the central vein should not be attempted if platelet counts are below 50,000/mm³ or if the bleeding time is prolonged. In such a case, the patient should be transfused with platelets or fresh frozen plasma (or specific plasma components) before catheter insertion. Alternatively, a jugular vein cutdown may be performed. Insertion of a central venous line requires strict aseptic technique. For the right-handed physician, cannulation of the right subclavian vein is generally easier and avoids potential injury to the thoracic duct. If intrathoracic or extrathoracic pathologic changes and anatomic abnormalities exist, however, they should be avoided in the catheterization attempt and the contralateral side should be selected for venipuncture. If a chest tube is in place and the upper thoracic anatomy is relatively normal, the catheterization should take place on the side where intrathoracic decompression is present.

Triple-lumen catheters are commonly inserted using the Seldinger guidewire technique in critically ill patients. This is a safe way to provide central venous access and includes additional ports for fluid administration if needed. This technique has been reviewed.[59] The patient is placed in the supine Trendelenburg's position, with the head tilted 10 to 20° and turned to the side opposite the insertion site. A rolled towel is placed between the scapulae to push the clavicles forward and shoulders backward. The person inserting the catheter should use appropriate sterile technique including cap, mask, gown, and gloves. The anterior chest is prepared with an antiseptic solution and the anatomic landmarks are identified. The suprasternal notch and anterior border of the sternocleidomastoid muscle should be visible in the prepared field. The proposed site of needle insertion is identified and 1% lidocaine local anesthetic is injected with a 22-gauge by 1.5-inch needle. A 14-gauge needle is attached to a 3-mL non–Luer-Lok syringe, and the needle is inserted slightly lateral to the junction of the proximal and middle third of the clavicle and 1 cm caudal to the clavicle so that it passes under the clavicle (Fig. 136-7). The needle is inserted with the calibrations of the syringe aligned with the bevel of the needle to identify the direction of the bevel. The direction of the needle insertion is slightly cephalad to the suprasternal notch. The syringe is kept in a

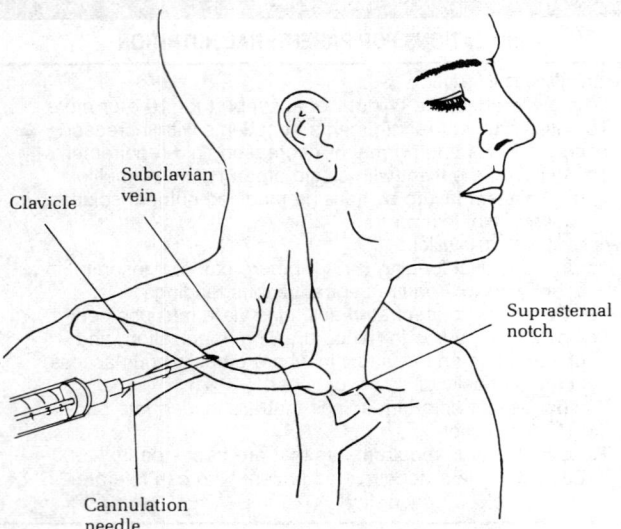

Figure 136–7. Subclavian venipuncture. (From Caldwell MD, Pomp A: Percutaneous central venous cannulation. In: Rombeau JL, Caldwell MD, Forlaw L, et al [eds]: Atlas of Nutritional Support Techniques. Boston, Little, Brown, p 208, 1989.)

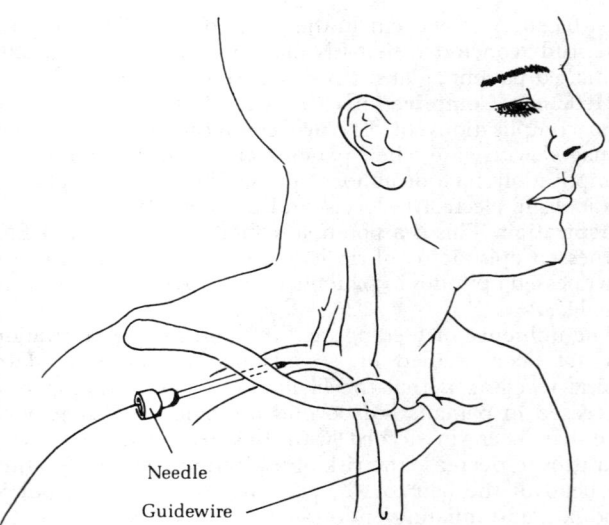

Figure 136–8. Insertion of central catheter into subclavian vein. (From Caldwell MD, Pomp A: Insertion of triple-lumen catheter using Seldinger wire technique. In: Rombeau JL, Caldwell MD, Forlaw L, et al [eds]: Atlas of Nutritional Support Techniques. Boston, Little, Brown, p 213, 1989.)

plane parallel to the anterior chest wall. The needle is advanced while aspirating gently on the syringe. When venous blood returns freely, intravenous location is confirmed. If pulsatile flow occurs, the subclavian artery has been entered and the needle should be withdrawn and reinserted. The syringe is removed and the needle hub occluded with a finger to prevent air embolus while preparing to insert the guidewire. The guidewire is inserted through the needle into the subclavian vein. The guidewire is advanced into the superior vena cava, a distance of approximately 15 cm in the adult (Fig. 136–8). If resistance is encountered, the guidewire should not be advanced, and if resistance continues to be encountered, the guidewire and needle should be removed together. When the guidewire has been inserted into the subclavian vein with adequate ease, the needle is removed and the dilator is inserted over the guidewire into the subclavian vein to dilate the tract from the skin to the vein. The dilator is withdrawn, and the catheter is inserted over the guidewire so that the tip lies in the junction of the superior vena cava and right atrium (Fig. 136–9). The catheter is then attached to the intravenous tubing, and the intravenous fluid container is lowered beneath the patient's heart to ensure good return of blood. Intravenous infusion is begun. The catheter is then sutured to the skin, and routine catheter dressing is applied. The patient is returned to a head-up position and assessed for respiratory difficulties.

After catheter insertion, the position of the catheter tip in the superior vena cava is verified by chest x-ray study. If the catheter tip is in the right atrium or ventricle, the catheter should be pulled back an appropriate distance so that the tip is positioned in the superior vena cava. If the catheter tip is in the contralateral subclavian vein or directed upward into veins of the neck, attempts can be made to reposition the catheter into the superior vena cava by using blind manipulation. This step can also be performed by using fluoroscopy and image intensification to visualize the intravascular portion of the catheter.

After the catheter has been positioned correctly, it is used exclusively for administering central parenteral nutrition. Drawing blood, monitoring central venous pressure, and

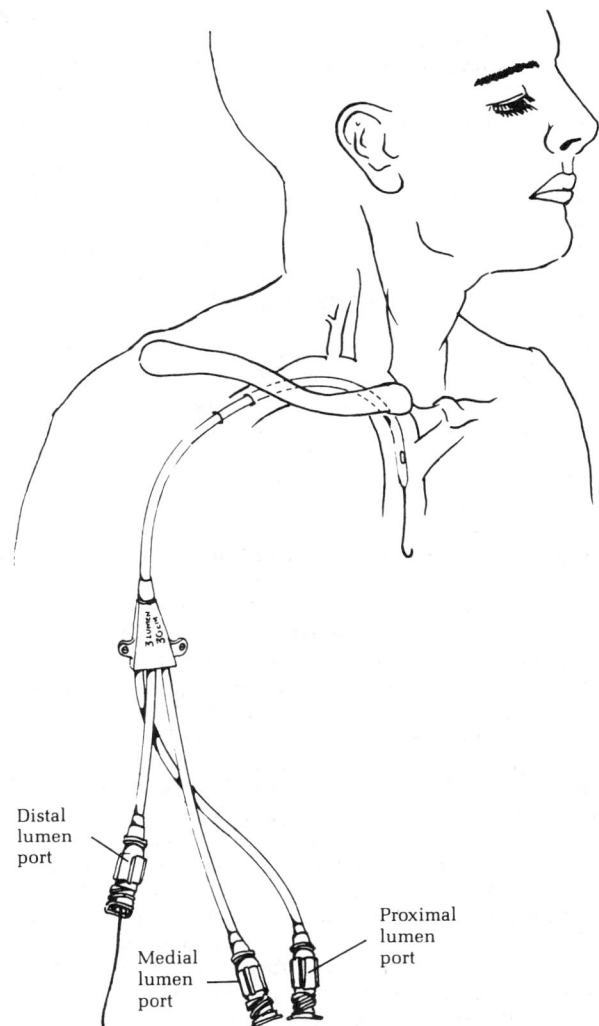

Figure 136–9. Position of central venous catheter. (From Caldwell MD, Pomp A: Insertion of triple-lumen catheter using Seldinger wire technique. In: Rombeau JL, Caldwell MD, Forlaw L, et al [eds]: Atlas of Nutritional Support Techniques. Boston, Little, Brown, p 214, 1989.)

administering medication through this dedicated line are prohibited. Manufacturers suggest that at least one port be devoted to infusion of the nutrient solutions and additional ports be used for drawing blood, monitoring pressure, and infusing medications. Reports suggest that the rate of catheter sepsis associated with the use of these lines is the same as[60] or greater than[61] rates of infection associated with single-lumen catheters. Removal of the multiple-lumen catheters is indicated when multiple central access ports are no longer required or when one of the lumina becomes clotted or malfunctions. Multiple-lumen catheters can be used in the intensive care unit for central venous nutrient infusions if strict protocols are maintained to ensure that one lumen is dedicated to nutrient infusion, other lumina are handled safely, and catheters are removed when they are no longer required.

Occasionally, a patient may require infusion of hypertonic nutrient solutions but percutaneous puncture of central veins is impossible or contraindicated. In these individuals, catheterization of an antecubital vein and insertion of a 24-inch catheter with the tip position in the superior vena cava can be performed. These lines should be removed after 5 days because they are associated with a high risk of infection. Catheterization of the femoral vein may provide a route for central venous access in some situations. Because of the high density of skin pathogens in the groin area, these catheters should be replaced every 2 or 3 days. If the catheter tip is positioned in the iliac vein or inferior vena cava, the concentration of solution infused through the catheter should not exceed 15%. Strict care of the entrance site of the catheter should be maintained because of the high complication rate associated with lines placed in the groin.[62]

Central Parenteral Nutrition Solutions

Central parenteral nutrition solutions are formulated in the hospital pharmacy. These solutions usually include combinations of 500 mL of 50% dextrose and 500 mL of a 10% amino acid mixture (Table 136–10) to which electrolytes, vitamins, and trace elements are added.

Usually, 2 L of this solution is infused daily. Administration of fat emulsion (500 mL, 20%) 1 day each week meets essential fatty acid requirements. Alternatively, the three major nutrients may be mixed together in a 3-L bag (triple or three-in-one mix) and the entire contents of the single bag infused during the 24-hour period (see Table 136–10). An additional innovation is the use of an automatic mixing device (Auto-mix, Travenol Laboratories, Clintech Nutrition, Deerfield, IL) that compounds various portions of glucose, amino acids, and fat emulsions in 3-L bags. This device allows the hospital pharmacy to manufacture various nutrient combinations with minimal effort. This approach provides the opportunity to tailor various nutrient admixtures to the metabolic needs of the critically ill patient.

Electrolytes are added to the base formula as required (Table 136–11). Sodium and potassium salts are added as chloride or acetate, depending on the specific requirements of the patient. The solution should usually consist of approximately equal quantities of chloride and acetate. If chloride losses are excessive, as in the patient with large fluid losses resulting from nasogastric tube decompression, most salts should be administered as chloride. Sodium bicarbonate is incompatible with the nutrient solutions, and acetate is administered when additional base is required (when metab-

TABLE 136–10		
COMPOSITION OF CENTRAL VENOUS SOLUTIONS		
Component	**Standard Solution**	**Triple-Mix Solution**
Volume		
Amino acids 10% (mL)	500	1000
Dextrose 50% (mL)	500	1000
Fat emulsion 20% (mL)	—	250
Total (mL)	1000	2250
Contents		
Amino acids (g)	50	100
Dextrose (g)	250 (25%)	500
Total nitrogen (g)	8.4	16.8
Total kcal	1050	2600
Nitrogen/kcal ratio	1:125	1:154
kcal/mL	1.0	1.15
mOsm/L	≈1970	≈1900

From Rombeau JL, Rolandelli RH, Wilmore DW: Nutritional support. In: Wilmore DW, Brennan MF, Harken AH (eds): American College of Surgeons Care of the Surgical Patient, Volume 1, Critical Care, Section II, Chapter 10. A Publication of the Committee on Pre and Postoperative Care. New York, Scientific American, p 16, 1989. © 1989 Scientific American, Inc. All rights reserved.

olized, acetate generates bicarbonate); sodium phosphate is used when potassium is contraindicated. Phosphate is also present in fat emulsions.

Commercially available preparations of vitamins, minerals, and trace elements are also added to the nutrient mix for daily administration unless they are contraindicated. Both fat- and water-soluble vitamins should be added daily. Vitamin K_1 (phytonadione), 10 mg, is given once a week but is contraindicated in patients receiving warfarin.

Trace elements are usually given daily. Usual requirements are satisfied by adding commercially available mixtures either to 1 L of standard solution or to the triple-mix bag each day. Trace elements are indicated for all patients receiving central PN, except those with chronic renal failure or severe liver disease. At especially high risk for zinc deficiency are alcoholics and patients with pancreatic insufficiency, malabsorption, massive small-bowel resection, renal failure with dialysis, or nephrotic syndrome; at high risk for copper deficiency are patients with short-bowel syndrome, malabsorptive conditions, or nephrotic syndrome. Copper and manganese are excreted primarily via the biliary tract. Therefore, in patients with biliary tract obstruction, excess retention of copper and manganese should be avoided by either decreasing intake of these ions or monitoring blood levels or both. Although the main excretory route for zinc and chromium is also via the feces, renal excretion minimizes dangers from modest excesses of these elements. In patients with renal insufficiency, however, daily zinc and chromium administration may be contraindicated. Critically ill patients usually do not require iron. This element is not readily compatible with amino acid solutions and may cause anaphylactic reactions in some individuals. Iron may be required to treat iron deficiency anemia, particularly during convalescence from critical illness. Rarely does the anemia that is associated with chronic disease and inflammation respond to iron therapy during the active stages of disease.

Solutions for Patients with Organ Dysfunction

Several solutions are now commercially available for patients with various forms of organ dysfunction. Many critically ill patients have dysfunction of more than one major organ system, and changes in metabolic status require frequent alterations in nutrient admixtures. Currently available solutions have been formulated for patients with acute renal failure, hepatic dysfunction, cardiac failure, pulmonary insufficiency, and severe metabolic stress.

Acute Renal Failure. Patients with renal failure are unable to excrete the end products, primarily urea, of nitrogen metabolism. Urea is generated from dietary amino acids and endogenous body protein breakdown. Urea production can be regulated by modifying nutrient intake: restriction of dietary amino acids decreases urea production from ingested protein, and provision of calories primarily in the form of carbohydrate limits breakdown of body protein. In general, the immediate goal of treating the acutely ill patient with renal failure is to provide an optimal combination of nutrients that prevents symptoms of uremia and the metabolic complications associated with acute renal failure. A secondary goal is to achieve energy balance and facilitate protein synthesis.

In planning nutritional therapy for patients with acute renal failure, three factors are important: BUN concentration, fluid requirements, and dialysis. Inasmuch as the BUN reflects the balance between production and excretion of urea, it serves as an index of the quantity and quality of amino acids that should be provided (Table 136–12). In general, the BUN should not be greater than 100 mg/dL. As the BUN rises, the quantity of amino acids in the nutrient solution is reduced and the quality of amino acids is modified. As the BUN falls, nitrogen administration is increased and the more balanced amino acid solution is administered. The BUN can be controlled not only by adjusting dietary protein but also by providing exogenous energy to decrease protein breakdown and satisfy energy requirements. Glucose should be the primary energy source because it has a much greater protein-sparing effect than fat, especially in the catabolic patient.[63] Furthermore, glucose is available in high concentrations (50 to 70%) and can be delivered when fluid requirements are limited. Although fat emulsion (20%) is a good source of calories, it is not as effective as carbohydrate in reducing protein breakdown in the catabolic patient and hence in reducing urea production. Fat emulsion also contains phosphate (15 mmol/L), which may be contraindicated in the patient with renal failure and hyperphosphatemia. Fat is a good source of concentrated energy in patients with fluid restrictions, however, and can be given in amounts up to 30 or 40% of the total caloric requirement if at least 60 to 70% of energy requirement has been provided as carbohydrate.

In the anuric phase of acute renal failure, fluid requirements are generally reduced unless the patient is undergoing dialysis. Nutritional support is provided if 1.0 to 1.5 L of the daily fluid requirement is allocated for this purpose. During the polyuric phase of acute renal failure, the nutrient mix is infused at a constant rate and additional quantities of free water are administered by a second infusion route to balance the fluid losses, which vary from day to day. If the patient is undergoing hemodialysis and fluid and nitrogen restrictions are not as stringent, fluid at approximately 2 L/d and protein at 1 g/kg/d are allowed if the BUN is maintained between 60 and 80 mg/dL. Stable dialysis patients often tolerate 2 L of standard central venous solution that is modified only by the addition of electrolytes. On the basis of the BUN concentration, energy requirements, and fluid restrictions, the appropriate nutrient mix can be selected (Table 136–13). These formulas are virtually free of electrolytes, and sodium, potassium, and chloride can be added to the nutrient mixes in the amounts required. Serum electrolyte levels should be monitored at least daily because potassium, phosphate, and magnesium levels often decline rapidly if a high glucose load is infused. Acetate salts of sodium and potassium can be added to correct metabolic acidosis. Standard vitamin mixtures are administered daily. Additional folate and water-soluble vitamins may be added if the patient requires hemodialysis because these substrates are lost into the dialysate bath. Trace elements should initially be omitted from solutions for an anuric patient. After about 2 weeks,

TABLE 136–12

COMPOSITION OF AMINO ACID SOLUTIONS FOR PATIENTS WITH RENAL FAILURE

Component	BUN 40–60 mg/dL		BUN 60–80 mg/dL		BUN 80–100 mg/dL	
	Moderate Calories	High Calories	Moderate Calories	High Calories	Moderate Calories	High Calories
Volume						
Amino acids (mL)	500 (mixture high in essential amino acids*)	500 (mixture high in essential amino acids*)	250 (mixture high in essential amino acids*)	250 (mixture high in essential amino acids*)	400 (essential amino acids only)	400 (essential amino acids only)
Dextrose (mL)	500 (50%)	500 (70%)	500 (50%)	500 (70%)	500 (50%)	500 (70%)
Total (mL)	1000	1000	750	750	900	900
Contents						
Amino acids (g)	32.5 (3.2%)	32.5 (3.2%)	16.3 (2.1%)	16.3 (2.1%)	20.8 (2.3%)	20.8 (2.3%)
Dextrose (g)	250 (25%)	350 (35%)	250 (33%)	350 (47%)	250 (28%)	350 (39%)
Total nitrogen (g)	5	5	2.5	2.5	3.3	3.3
Nonprotein N kcal/g	170	238	340	476	258	360
Total kcal	875	1315	913	1253	932	1273
kcal/mL	0.9	1.3	1.2	1.7	1.0	1.4

*70% essential amino acids and 30% nonessential amino acids.
From Rombeau JL, Rolandelli RH, Wilmore DW: Nutritional support. In: Wilmore DW, Brennan MF, Harken AH (eds): American College of Surgeons Care of the Surgical Patient, Volume 1, Critical Care, Section II, Chapter 10. A Publication of the Committee on Pre and Postoperative Care. New York, Scientific American, p 18, 1989. © 1989 Scientific American, Inc. All rights reserved.

these substances are provided every other day to hemodialysis patients on the days when they are not undergoing dialysis.

Hepatic Dysfunction

Hepatic dysfunction in critically ill patients varies from mild abnormalities in liver function tests, such as in the patient with sepsis, to the overt signs of acute liver failure observed in the end-stage cirrhotic patient with jaundice, ascites, GI bleeding, and severe wasting. Critically ill patients frequently present with liver dysfunction associated with sepsis. In these individuals nutrient requirements depend on the primary disease and on the cause of liver failure. If bilirubin concentrations rise as a result of primary hepatic injury (but not hepatitis), limitation of protein intake is not usually necessary unless encephalopathy develops. In contrast, patients with acute fulminant viral hepatitis require protein restriction.

TABLE 136–13

MODIFICATION OF NUTRITIONAL SOLUTIONS* FOR PATIENTS WITH FLUID INTOLERANCE

Component	Solution 1	Solution 2	Solution 3
Volume			
Amino acids†	250	250	500
Dextrose (mL)	500 (50%)	500 (70%)	500 (70%)
Total (mL)	750	750	1000
Contents			
Amino acids (g)	21	21	42.5
Total nitrogen (g)	3.4	3.4	6.6
Total kcal	935	1275	1358
kcal/mL	1.3	1.7	1.4

*250 mL of 20% fat emulsion may be added to these formulas if additional calories are required and the fat emulsion and extra fluid volume are tolerated.
†Specialized amino acid solutions can be used for patients with hepatic or renal failure.
From Rombeau JL, Rolandelli RH, Wilmore DW: Nutritional support. In: Wilmore DW, Brennan MF, Harken AH (eds): American College of Surgeons Care of the Surgical Patient, Volume 1, Critical Care, Section II, Chapter 10. A Publication of the Committee on Pre and Postoperative Care. New York, Scientific American, p 19, 1989. © 1989 Scientific American, Inc. All rights reserved.

Most stable patients with chronic liver disease can tolerate dietary protein administered at a rate of 1.0 to 1.5 g/kg body weight/d. Anorexia, nausea, and vomiting may preclude enteral feedings in patients who have acute alcoholic hepatitis. In these individuals, PN has been associated with increased survival.[64]

Protein intake must be altered in patients with advanced hepatic failure and impending encephalopathy. In general, amino acids given intravenously are better tolerated than the equivalent amount of protein administered enterally. These patients have elevated blood levels of aromatic amino acids and low levels of BCAAs. Possible therapeutic approaches are to reduce the quantity of dietary amino acid to 20 to 40 g/d and to administer a solution that corrects the altered concentration of amino acids in the blood stream. Such a solution contains high concentrations of BCAAs and no aromatic amino acids. Infusion of this solution may allow administration of more nitrogen than can be administered with standard formulas. If this solution is used, central nervous system function may not be disturbed with large protein loads. The effects of large protein loads, however, are controversial.[65] Because of the relative high cost of solutions containing high levels of BCAAs, some physicians use a more balanced and moderately priced formula that has only slightly elevated concentrations of BCAAs (Aminosyn 8.5%, Abbott Laboratories, Abbott Park, IL).

Fluid restriction may be necessary in some patients. In such cases of fluid intolerance, several solution mixtures can be administered; the sodium content in the nutrient mix should be reduced. The standard quantity of vitamins is given daily, and additional folic acid is recommended. Administration of all trace elements is often contraindicated; the main excretory route for copper is via the biliary system, and excesses may occur in patients with jaundice. Zinc deficiency is commonly observed in cirrhotic patients; supplementation of this mineral may be required, depending on the concentration in serum.

Cardiac Failure

For patients with cardiac failure, the goals of PN are to provide nutrient requirements in a limited fluid volume and to restrict sodium intake. The appropriate nutrient solution is similar to that provided to patients with renal or hepatic failure, especially if prerenal acidemia is present.

Pulmonary Insufficiency

Most parenteral formulas prescribed for critically ill patients contain moderate to large quantities of carbohydrate. This carbohydrate is oxidized to carbon dioxide, which is excreted by the lungs. If the patient does not have adequate respiratory reserve, as in the presence of chronic obstructive pulmonary disease, or if carbon dioxide excretion is fixed by mechanical ventilation, carbon dioxide will be retained if large carbohydrate loads are administered. In a nonventilated patient with some degree of respiratory compromise, increased carbon dioxide production may precipitate respiratory failure. In the patient being mechanically ventilated, the rate of gas exchange can usually be adjusted while feedings are varied to maintain a normal PCO_2. Increased carbon dioxide production, however, may delay or prevent weaning from the respirator.[45] In the individual with respiratory insufficiency, only maintenance calories are administered to avoid overfeeding. The caloric source can be equally divided between glucose and fat calories, and amino acid loads are reduced to approximately 1 g/kg body weight (Table 136–14). It should be emphasized that less than 10% of individuals needing mechanical ventilation require this modified formula. When a patient is weaned from a mechanical ventilator, the infusion rate is stabilized to provide maintenance calories or even reduced to provide only 60 to 70% of the maintenance calories. Alternatively, the nutrient solution can be temporarily discontinued overnight and weaning attempted the next morning. Fluid restriction may also be necessary in these patients.

High–Branched Chain Amino Acid Solutions for Stressed Patients. The BCAAs are essential amino acids that may be used primarily by skeletal muscle. They serve as an oxidizable fuel for this tissue. Leucine in particular stimulates protein synthesis and inhibits protein degradation in muscle in a dose-dependent manner.[66] It has therefore been proposed that amino acid solutions for stressed patients be fortified with the BCAAs. Solutions containing 40 to 50% BCAAs are now commercially available. Some clinical studies have found improved nitrogen retention with use of BCAA-enriched solutions, but little major effect on outcome has

been demonstrated. After reviewing the experimental and clinical data, one panel of experts concluded[67] that "greater benefits must be demonstrated in man before any widespread application of the use of BCAA formulations, alone or as supplements, can be endorsed."

Peripheral Parenteral Nutrition

Solutions that are slightly hypertonic (approximately 600 to 900 mOsm/kg) can be prepared for peripheral venous infusions from commercially available amino acid mixtures (5%), dextrose solutions (10%), and fat emulsions (20%). These nutrient mixtures have a low caloric density (approximately 0.3 to 0.6 kcal/mL) and thus provide only 1200 to 2300 calories in 2000 to 3500 mL of solution. Large volumes of fluid are required.

The solutions are compounded in the pharmacy in two ways (Table 136–15). In one method, all nutrients are placed in the same bag (triple mix) along with electrolytes, vitamins, and trace elements and the admixed contents are administered during 24 hours. Alternatively, the glucose, amino acids, electrolytes, vitamins, and minerals are mixed together in separate 1-L bags, and this solution is infused during the 24-hour period. Fat emulsion is simultaneously administered during a period of 8 to 12 hours by means of a "piggyback" technique (infusion of the fat through a Y connector along with the dextrose–amino acid mixture).

These dilute nutrient mixtures can be infused through plastic cannulas placed in large-bore peripheral veins. The catheter insertion site and surrounding tissue should be inspected routinely for signs of phlebitis or infiltration, and the infusion site should be rotated every 48 to 72 hours to prevent thrombophlebitis. Only fat emulsion should be administered simultaneously through the same intravenous site as a peripheral venous solution. The nutrient solution should be stopped temporarily if the catheter is used for administration of antibiotics, chemotherapy, blood, or blood products. The infusion line should then be flushed with saline and infusion of the nutrient solution resumed. If the fat

---

TABLE 136–15

COMPOSITION OF PERIPHERAL VENOUS SOLUTIONS

Component	1 L of Peripheral Venous Solution*	2 L of Peripheral Venous Solution* Plus 500 mL 20% Fat Emulsion†
Volume		
Amino acids 5% (mL)	500	1000
Dextrose 10% (mL)	500	1000
Fat emulsions 20% (mL)	—	500
Contents		
Amino acids (g)	25 (2.5%)	50
Dextrose (g)	50 (5%)	100
Fat (g)	—	100
Total nitrogen (g)	4.2	8.2
Total kcal	275	1550
Nitrogen/kcal ratio	1:65	1:189
kcal/mL	0.3	0.62
mOsm/kg	655	~600

*Electrolytes, vitamins, and minerals are added as indicated.
†Administered either separately or from a 3-L bag as a mixture.
From Rombeau JL, Rolandelli RH, Wilmore DW: Nutritional support. In: Wilmore DW, Brennan MF, Harken AH (eds): American College of Surgeons Care of the Surgical Patient, Volume 1, Critical Care, Section II, Chapter 10. A Publication of the Committee on Pre and Postoperative Care. New York, Scientific American, p 20, 1989. © 1989 Scientific American, Inc. All rights reserved.

TABLE 136–14

COMPOSITION OF CENTRAL VENOUS SOLUTIONS FOR PATIENTS WITH PULMONARY INSUFFICIENCY

Component	Volume Tolerated by Patient	
	1 L	2 L
Volume		
Amino acids 8.5% (mL)	500	1000
Glucose 50% (mL)	250	500
Fat emulsion 20% (mL)	250	500
Total (mL)	1000	2000
Contents		
Amino acids (g)	42	85
Total nitrogen (g)	6.8	13.6
Total kcal	1042	2084
Nitrogen/kcal ratio	1:153	1:153
kcal/mL	1	1

From Rombeau JL, Rolandelli RH, Wilmore DW: Nutritional support. In: Wilmore DW, Brennan MF, Harken AH (eds): American College of Surgeons Care of the Surgical Patient, Volume 1, Critical Care, Section II, Chapter 10. A Publication of the Committee on Pre and Postoperative Care. New York, Scientific American, p 19, 1989. © 1989 Scientific American, Inc. All rights reserved.

emulsion is infused in the piggyback manner, it should be administered during 8 to 12 hours ending in the early morning to allow clearance of the emulsion from the blood. Blood sampling should be avoided during short-term periods of fat infusion because the associated hypertriglyceridemia interferes with many of the serum measurements. In patients receiving peripheral venous solutions by triple mix, hypertriglyceridemia is rare because the rate of infusion has been reduced and the infusion is extended during a 24-hour period. Intensive care unit patients receiving peripheral venous feeding should be monitored as suggested for individuals receiving central venous feedings. Mechanical and septic complications are uncommon. Fluid imbalances and alterations in serum electrolyte concentrations are similar to those seen with standard intravenous infusions, and corrections are made by altering the volume of the infusion or adding or omitting electrolytes. Hyperglycemia and glycosuria are rarely observed unless the patient is diabetic. In patients receiving peripheral venous feedings, the BUN may be mildly elevated (20 to 35 mg/dL). This elevation may be related to mild renal insufficiency, inadequate hydration, or inadequate nonprotein calories. An increase in calories or additional non–protein-containing fluid usually corrects this abnormality. Because of the moderate nitrogen load, peripheral venous solutions are contraindicated in patients with severe renal failure or hepatic insufficiency.

Metabolic Monitoring

Many metabolic complications may occur during parenteral feeding. They are minimized by frequent metabolic monitoring and adjustment of nutrients in the infusion. Table 136–16 lists a suggested regimen for metabolic monitoring. The most common metabolic problems occurring in critically ill patients receiving PN are hyperglycemia and glucosuria. Initially, increased blood levels of glucose should be treated by administration of subcutaneous insulin (5.0 U every 4 to 6 hours for glucose 200 to 250 mg/dL, 7.5 U for glucose 250 to 300 mg/dL, 10.0 U for glucose 300 to 350 mg/dL). When the nutritional solution is ordered for the next 24-hour period, half the quantity of insulin administered subcutaneously is added to the bag. At least 10 U of regular insulin per liter of solution should be used as the initial dose, and in some cases as much as 40 U/L may be required. If larger doses of insulin are needed (more than 100 U/d), a separate insulin infusion drip should be used. Blood glucose levels can be monitored at the bedside by using a small meter with finger-stick techniques, and the insulin infusion can be adjusted hourly, if necessary, to control blood glucose concentration. In most critically ill patients with severe glucose intolerance, the rate of glucose administration should not exceed 5 mg/kg/min (approximately 500 g/d).[68]

Additional calories should be administered as fat emulsion. The commercially available fat emulsions are all generally well tolerated by critically ill patients. Triglyceride levels should be monitored, and the rate of administration of the emulsion should be decreased or the emulsion temporarily discontinued if levels exceed 500 mg/dL. Fat emulsion should be used with caution in patients with known hypertriglyceridemia or in those with gram-negative septicemia associated with hyperlipidemia.

Infusion of excess calories as either glucose or lipid may alter pulmonary function and in some patients prevent weaning from a mechanical ventilator. Excessive carbohydrate loads (greater than 500 g/d) increase carbon dioxide production. If the quantity of carbon dioxide produced exceeds the ability of the lungs to excrete this oxidative end product, hypercapnia results. Carbon dioxide production

can be greatly reduced by decreasing the carbohydrate load; if the patient receives less than 5 mg/kg/min of carbohydrate and cannot be weaned from the ventilator, one approach is to administer only 5% glucose solution overnight and then attempt weaning the next morning. If the patient can be removed from the ventilator, parenteral feedings may be gradually reinstituted. Fat emulsions may also interfere with diffusion of gas across the alveolar membranes. This interference is generally related to the concentration of the

TABLE 136–16

METABOLIC MONITORING FOR PARENTERAL NUTRITION

Variable	Suggested Monitoring Frequency	
	First Week	Later
Energy balance		
Weight	Daily	Daily
Metabolic variables		
Blood measurements		
Plasma electrolytes (Na⁺, K⁺, Cl⁻)	Daily	3× weekly
BUN	3× weekly	2× weekly
Plasma osmolarity	Daily	3× weekly
Plasma total calcium and inorganic phosphorus	3× weekly	2× weekly
Blood glucose	Daily	3× weekly
Plasma transaminases	3× weekly	2× weekly
Plasma total protein and fractions	2× weekly	Weekly
Blood acid-base status	As indicated	As indicated
Hemoglobin	Weekly	Weekly
Ammonia	As indicated	As indicated
Magnesium	2× weekly	Weekly
Triglycerides	Weekly	Weekly
Urine measurements		
Glucose	4–6× daily	2× daily
Specific gravity or osmolarity	Daily	Daily
General measurements		
Volume of infusate	Daily	Daily
Oral intake (if any)	Daily	Daily
Urine output	Daily	Daily
Prevention and detection of infection		
Clinical observations (activity, temperature, symptoms)	Daily	Daily
White blood cell and differential counts	As indicated	As indicated
Cultures	As indicated	As indicated

From Wilmore DW: Metabolic Management of the Critically Ill. New York, Plenum Publishing, p 231, 1977.

emulsion in the blood stream; hence, monitoring triglyceride levels and preventing hypertriglyceridemia minimize this complication.

Catheter Care and Catheter Sepsis

One of the most common problems associated with central PN is catheter sepsis. Primary catheter sepsis is defined as the signs and symptoms of infection (usually a febrile episode) with the indwelling catheter being the only anatomic focus of sepsis. After removal of the catheter, the symptoms and fever usually resolve. Cultures of the catheter tip with semiquantitative techniques yield at least 10^3 organisms.[69] The organisms are the same as those recovered from cultures of blood drawn from a peripheral vein during the initial evaluation of the infection.

Secondary catheter infection, in contrast to primary catheter sepsis, is associated with a second infectious focus that causes bacteremia and thus seeds or contaminates the catheter. The microorganisms cultured from the catheter tip are similar to those cultured from the primary source. The infection resolves after specific treatment of the primary infection.

Primary catheter sepsis is prevented or at least greatly reduced by following strict protocols. These protocols provide guidelines for the use and manipulation of the central venous feeding catheter and include a systematic method of care and surveillance of the catheter entrance site. Usually, catheter care is performed by a nurse with expertise in maintenance of long-term intravenous access (the nurse may be assigned to the nutrition support service or may be experienced in intravenous access or infection control). Every 48 to 72 hours, the dressing that covers the entrance site of the catheter is removed, the site inspected, the area around the entrance site cleaned, a topical antibiotic or antiseptic ointment applied, and the site redressed with a new sterile dressing. This procedure is documented in the clinical record; if drainage or crusting appears at the catheter entrance site, appropriate culture samples are taken. In addition, the dressing is changed if it becomes wet or soiled or no longer remains intact. The entire dressing should be covered with a transparent barrier drape to minimize contamination in patients who have either draining wounds close to the catheter entrance site or tracheostomies.

If signs and symptoms of infection develop in a recipient of central PN, a history should be taken and a thorough physical examination should be performed to evaluate the potential source of sepsis. Appropriate tests (complete blood count and urinalysis) and diagnostic studies (including chest roentgenogram) should also be performed. If blood cultures are needed, the blood should be drawn from a peripheral vein. If trained nurses have maintained the catheter and no evidence of infection at the exit site has been noted, the catheter dressing should not be removed and the catheter should not be manipulated. Blood for cultures should almost never be taken through the catheter. The one possible exception to this rule is the case in which the initial presentation of infection is characterized by marked hyperpyrexia or hypotension or both. If no other focus of sepsis is identified, the physician should remove all indwelling lines, including the feeding catheter. In addition, either drainage around the catheter or a previous positive culture from the catheter exit site may indicate immediate removal. If another primary source of the infection is diagnosed, specific therapy should be instituted and the PN continued. If no source of infection is identified, the catheter should be removed and the catheter tip cultured. Occasionally, another source of infection is identified and signs and symptoms of infection persist despite what appears to be appropriate therapy. If blood cultures are positive, it is recommended that the catheter be removed to avoid complications associated with the contaminated indwelling catheter (e.g., septic emboli and endocarditis). If peripheral blood cultures are negative, the catheter can be changed over a guidewire and the catheter tip cultured to confirm that catheter infection does not exist. Central venous feeding can be continued during this interval. If the catheter tip culture is positive ($>10^5$ organisms), the catheter should be removed.

Changing the central venous catheter over the guidewire can aid in the diagnosis of primary catheter infection.[70] Because most critically ill patients have multiple potential sources of infection, this technique allows culture of the catheter tip but minimizes the risk associated with insertion of a new central catheter. Strict aseptic technique is used. The area surrounding the catheter entrance site is sterilized, the intravenous tubing is disconnected from the catheter, the guidewire is passed into the catheter, and the catheter is removed over the guidewire. A new catheter is inserted over the wire and sutured in place. The tip of the old catheter is cut, placed in a transfer vessel, and taken to the microbiology laboratory for semiquantitative culture. With strict aseptic care of catheters, the incidence of sepsis should be less than 5%. Septicemia is most commonly caused by growth and invasion of organisms along the catheter tract. Occasionally, bacteria are infused through the catheter because of a breach in sterility during the care of the infusion apparatus. The most common bacterial organisms causing catheter sepsis are the skin contaminants *Staphylococcus epidermidis*, *Staphylococcus aureus*, *Klebsiella pneumoniae*, and *Candida albicans*. In rare cases, the intravenous solutions may be contaminated. Moreover, most patients who require central PN are immunocompromised; their resistance is lowered further by disease, severe malnutrition, or treatment, or by some combination of these factors. Coexisting conditions such as urinary tract infection, abscess, pneumonia, or mucositis secondary to the chemotherapy predispose the patients to bacteremia, which may contaminate the central venous catheter.

Immunosuppressed critically ill patients receiving multiple broad-spectrum antibiotics are also at risk for *Candida* septicemia. Blood cultures positive for *C. albicans* in a critically ill patient are an indication for catheter removal and treatment with amphotericin. An ophthalmologist should examine the retinas of patients with proven candidemia to exclude metastatic *Candida* ophthalmitis.

SUMMARY

Nutritional support is a mandatory component of the complete care of critically ill patients. Nutritional assessment, including determination of nutrient requirements, should be performed before prescribing EN or PN. The goal of nutritional support in this setting is maintenance of nutrient balances and not repletion of existing deficits. Because of the well-documented enterotrophic effects of intraintestinal nutrients, routine use of small amounts of enteral nutrients is recommended. Most malnourished critically ill patients require both EN and PN to meet nutrient requirements and minimize complications of malnutrition.

References

1. Cerra FB: Hypermetabolism, organ failure, and metabolic support. Surgery 101:1, 1987.
2. Apelgren KN, Rombeau JL, Twomey PL et al. Comparison of nutritional indices and outcome in critically ill patients. Crit Care Med 10:305, 1982.
3. Rombeau JL, Richter GC, Forlaw L: Practical aspects of nutritional assessment. Pract Gastroenterol 8:34, 1984.
4. Blackburn GL, Bistrian BR, Maini BS, et al: Nutritional and metabolic assessment of the hospitalized patient. JPEN 1:11, 1977.

5. Dowelko JP, Nompleggi DJ: Role of albumin in human physiology and pathophysiology. JPEN 15:207, 1991.
6. Deysine M, Lieblich N, Aufses AH: Albumin changes during clinical septic shock. Surg Gynecol Obstet 137:475, 1973.
7. Morgan EH: Transferrin and transferrin iron. In: Jacobs A, Worwood M (eds): Iron in Biochemistry and Medicine. London, Academic Press, p 29, 1974.
8. Bistrian BR, Blackburn GL, Sherman M, et al: Therapeutic index of nutritional depletion in hospitalized patients. Surg Gynecol Obstet 141:512, 1975.
9. Dempsey DT, Mullen JL, Rombeau JL, et al: Treatment effects of parenteral vitamins in total parenteral nutrition. JPEN 11:229, 1987.
10. Buzby GP, Mullen JL: Nutritional assessment. In: Rombeau JL, Caldwell MD (eds): Clinical Nutrition, Volume I, Enteral and Tube Feeding. Philadelphia, WB Saunders, p 127, 1984.
11. Alvestrand A, Bergstrom J: Renal diseases. In: Kinney JM (ed): Nutrition and Metabolism in Patient Care. Philadelphia, WB Saunders, p 531, 1988.
12. Lopes J, Russell DM, Whitewell J, et al: Skeletal muscle function in malnutrition. Am J Clin Nutr 36:602, 1982.
13. Mullen JL, Buzby GP, Waldman MT: Prediction of operative morbidity and mortality by preoperative nutritional assessment. Surg Forum 30:82, 1979.
14. Ryan JA, Taft DA: Preoperative nutritional assessment does not predict morbidity and mortality in abdominal operations. Surg Forum 31:96, 1980.
15. Jeejeebhoy KN: Assessment of nutritional status. In: Rombeau JL, Caldwell MD (eds): Clinical Nutrition, Volume I, Enteral and Tube Feeding. 2nd ed. Philadelphia, WB Saunders, p 118, 1990.
16. Baker JP, Detsky AS, Wesson DE, et al: Nutritional assessment: A comparison of clinical judgement and objective measurements. N Engl J Med 306:969, 1982.
17. Rombeau JL, Rolandelli RH, Wilmore DW: Nutritional support. In: Wilmore DW (ed): American College of Surgeons Care of the Surgical Patient, Volume I, Critical Care. A Publication of the Committee on Preoperative and Postoperative Care. New York, Scientific American, p 1, 1990.
18. Kinney JM: The application of indirect calorimetry to clinical studies. In: Kinney JM (ed): Assessment of Energy Metabolism in Health and Disease. Columbus, OH, Ross Laboratories, p 151, 1980.
19. Kinney JM: Energy metabolism: heat, fuel and life. In: Kinney JM (ed): Nutrition and Metabolism in Patient Care. Philadelphia, WB Saunders, p 3, 1988.
20. Albina JE, Melnik G: Fluids, electrolytes and body composition. In: Rombeau JL, Caldwell MD (eds): Clinical Nutrition, Volume II, Parenteral Nutrition. Philadelphia, WB Saunders, p 135, 1988.
21. Vitamin preparations as dietary supplements and as therapeutic agents. JAMA 257:1929, 1987.
22. Leohane GM, Deren JJ, Steiger E, et al: Role of oral intake in maintenance of gut mass and disaccharidase activity. Gastroenterology 67:975, 1974.
23. Raul F, Noriegar R, Doffeol M, et al: Modification of brush border enzyme activities during starvation in the jejunum and ileum of adult rats. Enzyme 28:328, 1982.
24. Pingleton SK, Hodzima SK: Enteral alimentation and gastrointestinal bleeding in mechanically ventilated patients. Crit Care Med 11:13, 1983.
25. Lowery SF, Brennan MF: Abnormal liver function during parenteral nutrition. Relation to infusion excess. J Surg Res 26:300, 1979.
26. Twomey PL, Patching SC: Cost-effectiveness of nutritional support. JPEN 9:3, 1985.
27. Marshall JC, Christou NV, Horn R, et al: The microbiology of multiple organ failure. Arch Surg 123:309, 1988.
28. Hwang TL, O'Dwyer ST, Smith RJ, et al: Preservation of small bowel mucosa using a glutamine enriched parenteral nutrition. Surg Forum 37:56, 1986.
29. Koruda MJ, Rolandelli RH, Settle RG, et al: The effect of parenteral nutrition supplemented with short-chain fatty acids on adaptation to massive small bowel resection. Gastroenterology 95:710, 1988.
30. Kripke SA, Fox AD, Berman JM, et al: Inhibition of TPN-associated intestinal mucosal atrophy with monoacetoacetin. J Surg Res 44:436, 1988.
31. Jacobs DO, Evans DA, Mealy K, et al: Combined effects of glutamine and epidermal growth factor on the rat intestine. Surgery 104:358, 1988.
32. Rolandelli RH, Koruda MJ, Settle RG, et al: Comparison of parenteral nutrition and enteral feeding with pectin in experimental colitis in the rat. Am J Clin Nutr 47:715, 1988.
33. Rolandelli RH, Koruda MJ, Settle RG, et al: Effect of intraluminal short chain fatty acids on healing of colonic anastomosis in the rat. Surgery 100:198, 1986.
34. Rolandelli RH, Rombeau JL: Enteral nutrition in critically ill patients. Perspect Crit Care 2:1, 1989.
35. Fry DE: Multiple system organ failure. Surg Clin North Am 68:107, 1988.
36. Chang RWS, Jacobs S, Lee B: Gastrointestinal dysfunction among intensive care unit patients. Crit Care Med 15:909, 1987.
37. Border JR, Hassett J, Laduca J, et al: The gut origin of septic states in blunt multiple trauma (ISS = 40) in the ICU. Ann Surg 206:427, 1987.
38. MacBurney M, See-Young L, Russell C: Enteral nutrition formula. In:

39. Heimburger DC, Weinsier RL: Guidelines for evaluating and categorizing enteral formulas according to therapeutic equivalence. JPEN 9:61, 1985.
40. Horst D, Grace ND, Conn HO, et al: Comparison of dietary protein with an oral branched-chain enriched amino acid supplement in chronic portal systemic encephalopathy: A randomized controlled trial. Hepatology 4:279, 1984.
41. Cerra FB, Cheung NK, Fischer JE, et al: Disease-specific amino acid infusion (FO80) in hepatic encephalopathy: A prospective, randomized double-blind controlled trial. JPEN 9:288, 1985.
42. Feinstein E, Blumenkrantz M, Healy H, et al: Clinical and metabolic responses to parenteral nutrition in acute renal failure. A controlled double blind study. Medicine 60:124, 1981.
43. Wilmore DW, Smith RH, O'Dwyer ST, et al: The gut: A central organ of surgical stress. Surgery 104:917, 1988.
44. Cerra FB, Mazuki J, Teasley K, et al: Nitrogen retention in critically ill patients is proportional to the branched-chain amino acid load. Crit Care Med 11:775, 1983.
45. Askanazi J, Weissman C, Rosenbaum SH, et al: Nutrition and the respiratory system. Crit Care Med 10:163, 1982.
46. Al-Saady N, Blackmore C, Bennett ED: High fat, low carbohydrate enteral feeding reduces $PACO_2$ and the period of ventilation in ventilated patients. Chest 94(suppl):49S, 1989.
47. Daly JM, Lieberman M, Goldfine J, et al: Enteral nutrition with supplemental arginine, RNA and omega-3 fatty acids: A prospective clinical trial. JPEN 15:19S, 1991.
48. Levenson R, Turner WW, Dyson A, et al: Do weighted nasogastric tubes facilitate duodenal intubations? JPEN 12:135, 1988.
49. Rombeau JL, Twomey PL, McLean GK, et al: Experience with a new gastrostomy-jejunal feeding tube. Surgery 93:574, 1983.
50. Orr G, Wade J, Bothe A, et al: Feeding alternatives in the critically ill patient. Crit Care Med 8:29, 1980.
51. Parker P, Stroop S, Greene H: A controlled comparison of continuous versus intermittent feeding in the treatment of infants with intestinal disease. J Pediatr 99:360, 1981.
52. Hiebert JM, Brown A, Anderson RG, et al: Comparison of continuous vs intermittent tube feeding in adult burn patients. JPEN 5:73, 1981.
53. Evans D, DiSipio M, Barot L, et al: Comparison of gastric and jejunal tube feedings. JPEN 4:79, 1980.
54. Heimberger DC, Weinsier RL: Guidelines for evaluating and categorizing enteral feeding formulas according to therapeutic equivalence. JPEN 9:61, 1985.
55. Heymsfield SB, Bethel RA, Ansley JE, et al: Enteral hyperalimentation: An alternative to central venous hyperalimentation. Ann Intern Med 90:63, 1979.
56. Keohane PP, Attrill H, Love M, et al: Relation between osmolality of diet and gastrointestinal side effects in enteral nutrition. Br Med J 288:678, 1984.
57. Cataldi-Belcher EL, Seltzer MH, Slocum BA, et al: Complications occurring during enteral nutrition support: A prospective study. JPEN 7:546, 1983.
58. Aronchik JM, Epstein DM, Gefter WB, et al: Pneumothorax as a complication of placement of a nasoenteric tube. JAMA 252:3207, 1984.
59. Caldwell MD, Pomp A: Seldinger wire technique. In: Rombeau JL, Caldwell MD, Forlaw L, et al: (eds): Atlas of Nutritional Support Techniques. Boston, Little, Brown, p 213, 1989.
60. Pemberson LB, Lyman B, Lander V, et al: Sepsis from triple- versus single-lumen catheters during total parenteral nutrition in surgical or critically ill patients. Arch Surg 121:591, 1986.
61. Miller JJ, Venus B, Mathru M: Comparison of the sterility of long-term central venous catheterization using single lumen, triple lumen, and pulmonary artery catheters. Crit Care Med 12:634, 1984.
62. Moncrief JA: Femoral catheters. Ann Surg 147:166, 1958.
63. Long JM, Wilmore DW, Mason AD Jr, et al: Effect of carbohydrate and fat intake on nitrogen excretion during total intravenous feeding. Ann Surg 185:417, 1977.
64. Galambos JT, Hersh JT, Fulenwider JT, et al: Hyperalimentation in alcoholic hepatitis. Am J Gastroenterol 72:535, 1979.
65. Wahren J, Demis J, Desurmont P, et al: Intravenous administration of branched-chain amino acids effective in the treatment of hepatic encephalopathy? A multicenter trial. Hepatology 3:475, 1983.
66. Buse MG, Reid SS. Leucine: A possible regulator of protein turnover in muscle. J Clin Invest 56:1250, 1975.
67. Brennan MF. Report of a research workshop: Branched-chain amino acids in stress and injury. JPEN 10:446, 1986.
68. Black PR, Brooks DC, Bessey PQ, et al: Mechanisms of insulin resistance following injury. Ann Surg 196:420, 1982.
69. Maki DG, Weise CE, Saarafin HW: A semiquantitative culture method for identifying intravenous catheter related infections. N Engl J Med 296:1305, 1977.
70. Pettigrew RA, Lang SDR, Haydock DA, et al: Catheter-related sepsis in patients on intravenous nutrition: A prospective study of quantitative catheter cultures and guidewire changes for suspected sepsis. Br J Surg 74:52, 1985.

SECTION TWELVE

Special Topics

Section Editors

Richard W. Carlson and Michael A. Geheb

CHAPTER 137

Preoperative Care

John M. Oropello
Thomas J. Iberti

PREOPERATIVE CONSIDERATIONS FOR THE INTENSIVIST

As the field of intensive care expands, intensivists are increasingly taking part in the evaluation of high-risk patients before major nonemergent (as well as emergent) operative procedures. Intensivists are well suited for this role because they administer postoperative care in the intensive care unit (ICU) and are aware of postoperative complications and how they can be reduced with appropriate preoperative management. Even if patients do not require intensive care preoperatively, it is desirable to become involved in their management before surgery. In this way the intensivist and the patient become acquainted, and the patient becomes informed about the anticipated ICU stay. Although it has not been proved, this may result in reduced anxiety and improved cooperation of the patient postoperatively.

Although most of the preoperative evaluation of the high-risk patient is performed outside the ICU by the internist, anesthesiologist, and surgeon, the intensivist should be equipped to assess risks and to decide which patients require preoperative ICU admission, invasive hemodynamic monitoring, postponement of surgery, and further preoperative testing, as well as to provide preoperative therapeutic recommendations.

The following sections deal with general preoperative considerations, specific preoperative considerations in major organ system disease, high-risk preoperative management, and other situations commonly encountered by the consulting intensivist. The emphasis of this chapter is on the assessment of operative risks and ways of reducing these risks preoperatively.

GENERAL PREOPERATIVE CONSIDERATIONS

Recommendations for routine preoperative screening have included a chest roentgenogram, electrocardiogram, electrolyte profile (e.g., sequential multiple analysis), creatinine, blood urea nitrogen, urinalysis, complete blood count, platelet count, and prothrombin time (PT). However, routine preoperative screening tests ordered without clinical indication are inefficient and costly.[1, 2] They rarely (0.22% of the time)[2] provide information that influences management. No test is routinely indicated for every patient or all operations, and no known tests can preoperatively screen for unsuspected disease while maintaining cost-effectiveness. Despite this, many anesthesiologists may require the foregoing preoperative testing for all patients as a routine.

The best preoperative screening strategy is a thorough history and physical examination followed by preoperative testing directed toward determining the severity of any known or suspected conditions that may adversely affect surgical morbidity and mortality. The history and physical examination together are diagnostic in 75 to 90% of patients.[3]

The decision making involved in ordering consultations or more specialized tests (e.g., thyroid function, stress testing, echocardiography, cardiac catheterization, and pulmonary function testing) depends on a systematic operative risk assessment. These matters are discussed in more detail in the sections on general and specific preoperative considerations. Preoperative assessment and treatment of the stable high-risk or critically ill patient are then considered.

SPECIFIC PREOPERATIVE CONSIDERATIONS

Preoperative Neurologic Considerations

Cerebrovascular Disease

The best predictors of cerebral ischemic events in patients with asymptomatic carotid bruit are ischemic heart disease and male sex. Neurologically asymptomatic patients with carotid bruit who have other surgical procedures are at significant risk for perioperative mortality principally because of coexisting coronary artery disease (CAD).[4] The correlation between carotid bruit and demonstrable carotid artery disease is approximately 60%.[5] A minority of such patients have high-grade carotid stenosis. In these patients, the annual stroke rate is as high as 3 to 5%.[4] Patients with completed strokes or transient ischemic attacks who undergo noncardiovascular surgery have a high incidence of CAD. Heart disease is the most common cause of death in such patients. Appropriate preoperative cardiac screening is indicated (see under Preoperative Cardiac Considerations).

Regardless of the type of stroke, elective surgery should

be postponed for at least 2 weeks after an acute event.[5] This recommendation is based on data showing that patients undergoing carotid endarterectomy had 34% mortality when surgery was performed within 24 hours of a stroke, 15% after 1 to 13 days after a stroke, and 0% after 2 weeks.[6] The major causes of death were myocardial infarction (MI) and stroke.

Patients with embolic disease who are taking anticoagulants need adjustment of therapy before surgery (see under Preoperative Cardiac Considerations).

Carotid Doppler studies may be done to assess the degree of carotid disease in patients with frequent transient ischemic attacks or recurrent strokes. The indications for carotid endarterectomy have been questioned. Clinical trials are ongoing to evaluate clinical efficacy.[7] At this time, significant ipsilateral carotid artery stenosis in the setting of a carotid-distribution transient ischemic attack (in a patient without multi-infarct dementia) remains the principal indication for this procedure.[4]

Parkinson's Disease

Patients with Parkinson's disease can have restrictive lung impairment secondary to rigidity and bradykinesia of the respiratory muscles. They may also have kyphosis. Preoperative arterial blood gas and pulmonary function tests can be done to assess the degree of impairment. Incentive spirometry should be taught preoperatively. These patients may need hydration because of abnormal sweating secondary to autonomic dysfunction.

Antiparkinsonian medications can cause hypotension (bromocryptine, levodopa), hypertension (levodopa), and arrhythmias (levodopa) in the perioperative period. Such medication should be continued until the evening before surgery and restarted when oral intake resumes postoperatively.[5]

Myasthenia Gravis

Patients with myasthenia gravis are at increased risk of postoperative respiratory failure. Factors predictive of the need for postoperative mechanical ventilation are duration of myasthenia for 6 years or more, chronic respiratory disease, the need for more than 750 mg of pyridostigmine per day, and vital capacity less than 2.9 L.[8] Patients should be at their optimal strength before elective surgery. Pyridostigmine, an anticholinesterase drug, is the treatment most frequently used for myasthenia gravis. One thirtieth of the oral dose can be used intravenously until oral intake is resumed. Other treatments include thymectomy, steroids, azathioprine, and plasmapheresis. Aminoglycoside antibiotics can reduce acetylcholine release and should be avoided. Beta-blockers, morphine, quinidine, and procainamide can worsen transmission across the neuromuscular junction and should be used with caution.[5]

Seizure Disorders

There are four major categories of seizures: generalized (tonic-clonic), simple partial (focal), complex partial (temporal lobe, psychomotor), and absence (petit mal). Patients with seizure disorder can be classified as well or poorly controlled. Stage I (excitation) and stage II (delirium) of anesthesia are risk periods for seizure activity. Seizure disorders, except for absences, can be controlled with phenytoin or phenobarbital, which are the only available parenteral anticonvulsants. Before elective surgery, patients should be checked for evidence of drug toxicity (liver function tests, complete blood count, and creatinine level). Therapeutic serum levels of anticonvulsants should be achieved and maintained preoperatively.

Absence-type seizures do not pose a serious risk and oral medications may be resumed postoperatively. Perioperative seizure prophylaxis with phenytoin is recommended for patients with head trauma, brain tumors, and brain abscesses.[5]

Preoperative Pulmonary Considerations

The goal of preoperative pulmonary evaluation is to identify patients who are at increased risk for postoperative respiratory complications and to attempt to minimize the risk. Pulmonary complications can result in respiratory failure with significant morbidity and mortality and prolongation of hospital stay with increased costs. They are the most frequent causes of postoperative complications.

The most common is atelectasis, which is responsible for about 90% of all pulmonary complications. Other problems include retained secretions, bronchitis, pneumonia, bronchospasm, hypoxemia, hypercapnia, pulmonary hypertension, and right-sided heart failure. Any of these alone or in combination may lead to respiratory failure. Depending on the preoperative respiratory status, how complications are defined, and the type of surgery performed, the incidence ranges from 2.9 to 70%.[9] Although such complications cannot be completely eliminated even in patients with normal preoperative lung function, they may be reduced.

Information from the history and physical examination regarding the type of surgery being performed should guide the ordering of preoperative pulmonary function tests. A careful history with specific questions regarding cough, sputum production, wheezing, dyspnea on exertion, effort tolerance, cigarette smoking, and a past medical history of asthma, emphysema, or bronchitis is required. The physical examination is performed with particular attention to weight, evidence of tobacco stains, auscultation for rales and rhonchi on deep rapid breathing as well as during normal respirations, and evidence of pulmonary hypertension, cor pulmonale, or right-sided heart failure.

Basic Pathophysiology

Postoperative pulmonary pathophysiologic changes occur in patients with and without pre-existing lung disease.[10] The incidence of complications depends on the extent of these changes and the degree of underlying lung disease. These changes are caused by pain, sedation, the surgical incision site, the length of anesthesia, the supine position, and endotracheal intubation. Normally these changes resolve within 2 weeks postoperatively. Static lung volumes including the total lung capacity, vital capacity, residual volume, functional residual capacity, and the expiratory reserve volume may be reduced 20 to 60%.[10] Greater reductions occur with upper abdominal and thoracic surgery than with lower abdominal surgery. Virtually no reductions occur in nonthoracic, nonabdominal surgery.

Ventilatory patterns show an approximately 20% reduction in tidal volume, with a 26% increase in respiratory rate and no change in respiratory minute volume.[9] Deep breathing and coughing are also reduced. These changes may decrease end-tidal lung volumes into the range of closing lung volume, resulting in an increased number of collapsed airways. This promotes airway closure and decreases lung compliance, leading to microatelectasis (not seen on chest x-ray film), macroatelectasis (e.g., subsegmental and lobar), and decreased PaO_2 secondary to ventilation-perfusion inequalities.

Diaphragmatic dysfunction can occur, especially after thoracic or upper abdominal surgery. Increases in $Paco_2$ postoperatively are usually due to depression of central drive resulting from narcotics or muscle paralysis. Increases in $Paco_2$ resulting from pulmonary parenchymal disease itself occur only in patients with advanced lung disease. They often have preoperative carbon dioxide retention. In addition to fever, sepsis, and other catabolic states, increased carbon dioxide production can be caused by carbohydrate overfeeding with total parenteral nutrition (TPN) formulations. This may add significantly to the work of breathing in patients with borderline pulmonary function and interfere with weaning efforts. Reducing the caloric intake and increasing the percentage of calories given via lipids can decrease the carbon dioxide load.

Reduced pulmonary defense mechanisms can result in retained secretions and may worsen the degree of atelectasis and promote infection. Clearance of bacteria and other particles is reduced by a decreased cough reflex, depression of mucociliary transport, changes in mucous secretions, development of atelectasis, and arterial hypoxemia. In the presence of pre-existing lung disease, such as asthma, chronic bronchitis, emphysema, and bronchiectasis, these risks are increased.

Preoperative Predictors of Postoperative Pulmonary Complications

Postoperative pulmonary complications can be predicted by the assessment of age, weight, smoking history, operative factors, and preoperative pulmonary function.

Age. Increasing age is associated with a higher incidence of postoperative pulmonary complications such as atelectasis and hypoxemia. The normal effects of aging include decreases in lung volume, elastic recoil, flow rates, and upper airway reflexes.

Weight. Obesity predisposes to postoperative hypoxemia and atelectasis. The functional residual capacity and expiratory reserve volume are decreased, resulting in end-tidal breaths occurring below the closing volume. Obesity is not a contraindication to surgery in most cases; however, weight reduction before elective surgery is advisable.

Smoking. Postoperative complications are twice as great in smokers as in nonsmokers.[11] There is an association between cigarette smoking, increased closing volume, decreased mucociliary activity, and postoperative atelectasis. Smoking is associated with a fourfold increase in postoperative atelectasis if more than one pack per day is smoked.[11]

Operative Factors. The type of surgery greatly influences the risk of postoperative complications (Table 137–1). The duration of anesthesia and the degree of skill with which it is administered may be more important than the anesthetic method (i.e., spinal or general) in producing postoperative pulmonary complications. Surgeries lasting more than 3.5

hours are associated with higher rates of atelectasis and other complications.[9]

Preoperative Pulmonary Function

Preoperative evaluation of pulmonary function has been primarily concerned with patients who have obstructive lung disease rather than restrictive disorders in which flow rates and cough are maintained. Patients with chronic obstructive pulmonary disease, especially if they have pulmonary hypertension and cor pulmonale, are at higher risk for postoperative pulmonary complications.

A number of studies have identified pulmonary function parameters that predict increased postoperative risk (Table 137–2). These values provide only guidelines for the estimation of risk. Advances in surgical and anesthetic techniques coupled with improvements in postoperative intensive care continue to reduce the incidence of postoperative pulmonary complications. Therefore, statistical data from many older studies may overestimate the current risks. If such preoperative tests are normal, the postoperative pulmonary complication rate may be 3% or less, but abnormal tests may be associated with a 70 to 80% chance of pulmonary complications.

Preoperative Pulmonary Function Tests (Table 137–3)

Arterial Blood Gases. An arterial blood gas analysis is recommended for all patients who have evidence of pulmonary disease as well as patients undergoing pulmonary resection or coronary artery bypass surgery. An elevated

---

TABLE 137–2

PULMONARY FUNCTION PARAMETERS THAT PREDICT INCREASED POSTOPERATIVE RISK

Parameter	Value
Arterial blood gas	
$Paco_2$	>45 mm Hg
Spirometric data*	
FEV_1	<2.0 L or <50% FVC
FVC	<50%
MVV	<50% predicted
RV/TLC ratio	>50%

*FEV_1 = forced expiratory volume in 1 s; FVC = forced vital capacity; MVV = maximal voluntary ventilation; RV = residual volume; TLC = total lung capacity.

TABLE 137–1

RISK OF POSTOPERATIVE PULMONARY COMPLICATION FOR VARIOUS TYPES OF SURGERY

Surgery	Postoperative Risk of Pulmonary Complications
Thoracic surgery with lung resection	Highest
Thoracic surgery without lung resection	•
Upper abdominal surgery	•
Lower abdominal surgery	•
Nonabdominal, nonthoracic procedures	Lowest (<1%)

TABLE 137–3

PULMONARY FUNCTION PARAMETERS COMMONLY USED FOR PREDICTING INCREASED RISK OF POSTOPERATIVE MORBIDITY AND MORTALITY AFTER LUNG RESECTION

Parameter	Value
Arterial blood gas	
$Paco_2$	>45 mm Hg
Spirometric data	
Predicted postoperative FEV_1	<0.8 L
Exercise physiology	
Hemodynamic	
Pulmonary vascular resistance	>190 dyne · s/cm^5 during exercise
Oxygen consumption $\dot{V}o_2$max	<1.0 L/min

resting $Paco_2$ greater than 45 mm Hg in the absence of acute exacerbation of chronic obstructive pulmonary disease, neuromuscular disease, severe metabolic alkalosis, or drug-induced central hypoventilation predicts increased mortality in these patients. There are many patients with an elevated $Paco_2$ who can successfully undergo coronary artery bypass surgery and other major procedures, and an elevated $Paco_2$ is a contraindication to surgery only in patients who do not have reversible hypercapnia and are scheduled for lung resection.

The Pao_2 is not a reliable indicator of postoperative complications. Some patients may have an improved Pao_2 postoperatively if an area of right-to-left shunting (perfusion without ventilation) is removed. This may occur in patients with lung carcinomas.

Spirometry. The incidence of postoperative complications is correlated with the degree of spirometric abnormality.[10] The forced vital capacity (FVC), forced expiratory volume in 1 second (FEV_1), FEV_1/FVC ratio, and maximal voluntary ventilation are parameters that are commonly assessed. There is wide variation in the normal values for these tests, about $\pm 20\%$ predicted. For the forced expiratory flow of 25 to 75%, the variation is $\pm 40\%$ predicted, which limits the value of this parameter in estimating postoperative risk. Spirometry should be performed before and after testing with a bronchodilator, and the best result obtained should be used.

Split Perfusion Lung Scanning. In patients undergoing pulmonary resection, the postoperative FEV_1 can be accurately and reliably determined by using ventilation-perfusion or perfusion lung scanning to determine the amount of functioning lung to be removed.[12, 13] This predicted FEV_1 is probably less than that actually observed postoperatively, providing a margin of safety.

The FEV_1 can be used in postpneumonectomy as well as postlobectomy cases. Formulas for predicting the postoperative FEV_1 are as follows for postpneumonectomy and postlobectomy, respectively:

Postpneumonectomy FEV_1 =
    preoperative FEV_1 × percent function of remaining lung
    from ventilation-perfusion scan

Postlobectomy FEV_1 =
    preoperative FEV_1 × number of functional segments
    in lobe to be resected/total number of functional
    segments in both lungs

The predicted postoperative FEV_1 is an acceptable indicator of success after lung resection if it is greater than 0.8 L. However, if it is less than 0.8 L successful pulmonary resection may still be possible. Women may tolerate a lower absolute postoperative FEV_1. It has been suggested that FEV_1 as a percentage of normal (e.g., >30%) would be more appropriate in determining postoperative risk in such patients.[14]

Exercise Testing. Several studies suggest that measurements of cardiopulmonary function during exercise are better predictors of postoperative morbidity and mortality that spirometry or split function studies in patients undergoing pulmonary resection. A pulmonary vascular resistance greater than 190 dyne · s/cm[5] during exercise may be a better predictor of death after pulmonary resection than the arterial blood gas and spirometric data.[15]

The preoperative maximal oxygen consumption ($\dot{V}o_2max$) during exercise (bicycle ergometry) has also been related to postoperative complications and mortality. One study showed that if the $\dot{V}o_2max$ was less than 15 mL/kg/min the incidence of postoperative complications was 100% but if it was greater than 20 mL/kg/min the incidence was 10%.[16]

This noninvasive test was found to be superior to use of split perfusion lung scanning to calculate the postoperative FEV_1.[16] Another study showed that if the $\dot{V}o_2max$ was less than 1 L/min the mortality was 75%, but there were no deaths if the $\dot{V}o_2max$ was greater than 1 L/min.[17] Further investigations with greater numbers of patients are needed to determine the role of invasive and noninvasive exercise testing in assessing the postoperative risks of pulmonary resection.

Indications for Preoperative Pulmonary Function Testing

1. General surgery. Any patient with evidence of lung disease in the history or physical examination (e.g., heavy smoking, dyspnea, and wheezing) should have preoperative blood gas analysis and spirometry.

2. Lung resection. Current data support routine use of pulmonary function testing for all patients undergoing pulmonary resection. Patients undergoing resection should have preoperative arterial blood gas analysis and spirometry. In addition, if the preoperative FEV_1 is less than 2.0 L, split perfusion lung scanning is necessary for prediction of the postoperative FEV_1. Predicted postoperative FEV_1 values less than 0.8 L do not unequivocally rule against a pulmonary resection. If the predicted postoperative FEV_1 is less than 0.8 L (or <30% of normal) and the patient has a surgically curable lesion, consideration should be given to performing an exercise test or right-sided heart catheterization.

3. Thoracic surgery without lung resection. Patients undergoing coronary artery bypass surgery who are smokers or have a history of dyspnea or obstructive lung disease should have preoperative arterial blood gas testing and spirometry.

4. Upper or lower abdominal surgery. Although the incidence of postoperative pulmonary complications is greater after upper abdominal surgery, preoperative spirometry or blood gas analysis is not necessary unless there is evidence for a pulmonary problem.

5. Morbidly obese patients.
6. Patients older than 70 years.

The role of preoperative pulmonary function testing in nonabdominal, nonthoracic surgery (e.g., orthopedic or head and neck surgery) has not been adequately studied.[18]

Preoperative Intervention

The following measures are helpful in minimizing postoperative complications.

1. Weight reduction if obese.
2. Smoking cessation. For at least 3 weeks if possible. The longer a patient abstains from smoking before surgery, the lower the risk of pulmonary complications.[11]
3. Respiratory therapy. The incentive spirometer is a device that encourages a patient to perform voluntarily a hyperinflation maneuver that is sustained at peak inspiration for 5 to 10 seconds. Incentive spirometry was shown to decrease postoperative pulmonary complications after abdominal and thoracic surgery in patients with normal or abnormal lung function.[18] It is simple and inexpensive and should be provided to all of these patients. It may shorten the length of hospital stay.

Chest physical therapy, intermittent positive pressure breathing, and continuous positive pressure breathing are no more beneficial than incentive spirometry.[19] Patients should be trained in proper use preoperatively, not postoperatively when the patient is sedated and in pain.

4. Pharmacotherapy. Bronchodilators and antibiotics should be given as indicated to maximize preoperative pulmonary function in patients with obstructive lung disease, bronchitis, or bronchiectasis. Antibiotics useful in the treatment of patients with bronchitis, sinusitis, or bronchiectasis include ampicillin, amoxicillin–clavulanic acid (Augmentin), trimethoprim-sulfamethoxazole (Bactrim), and erythromycin.

Elective surgery should never be performed for a patient who is wheezing. First-line bronchodilator therapy should consist of an inhaled beta$_2$-selective agent such as metaproterenol or albuterol. For acute episodes, subcutaneous epinephrine or terbutaline may be beneficial. Inhaled corticosteroids or cromolyn is indicated for certain patients, but these take several weeks to achieve a therapeutic effect. Systemic corticosteroids are used if indicated for more severe, refractory cases.

There is a trend away from the use of aminophylline. Aminophylline is not more beneficial in relieving bronchospasm than the inhaled beta$_2$-agonists and is associated with variable pharmacokinetics and a greater incidence of toxic effects such as nausea, vomiting, cardiac arrhythmias, and seizures. Intravenous use occasionally results in hypotension. For selected patients who are already taking aminophylline or who are not controlled with other agents, sustained-release oral preparations may be used to achieve fairly constant serum levels or the intravenous route may be used. Rectal administration may lead to erratic absorption and should be avoided.

5. Patients with recent exacerbations of chronic obstructive pulmonary disease or pneumonia should have postponement of elective surgery for approximately 6 weeks.

6. Careful selection of the patient with borderline lung function to undergo pulmonary resection. In selected cases in which cure of disease is possible and postoperative FEV$_1$ predicted by spirometry and ventilation-perfusion scan is less than 0.8 L, exercise testing for pulmonary vascular resistance or $\dot{V}o_2$max may be indicated.

Preoperative Cardiac Considerations

In 1977 Goldman and colleagues[20] prospectively studied 1001 patients undergoing major noncardiac surgery and identified nine independent risk factors for the development of life-threatening cardiac complications (Table 137–4). Patients were grouped into high- and low-risk categories by assigning points to each risk factor. A cardiac risk index score was generated and later modified[21] (Table 137–5). It should be noted that in the Goldman study, only cardiac outcome was assessed. Forty patients died postoperatively of noncardiac causes, but only their cardiac complications were included in the analysis.

After the Goldman study, it was found that symptomatic peripheral vascular disease in the patient with chronic angina predicts an increased risk of perioperative cardiac complication.[22] In addition, the rate of cardiac complications for patients undergoing abdominal aortic surgery is perhaps 40% greater than that predicted in the Goldman study.[23] Several prospective studies have provided some degree of validation for this predictive index.[24] Others have attempted to tailor the index to their own hospital and improve risk stratification based on the type of surgical procedure.[25] There is evidence that the identification and aggressive perioperative care of high-risk patients (Goldman class IV) have reduced perioperative cardiac complications 40% or more.[26] Factors found not to be independent risk factors for perioperative cardiac complications were smoking, hypertension, diabetes, cardiomegaly, mitral valve disease without heart failure, compensated heart failure (no jugular venous

TABLE 137–4
CARDIAC RISK INDEX

Risk Factor	Points
Signs of CHF (S$_3$ gallop, jugular venous distention)	11
MI within previous 6 mo	10
Rhythm other than sinus or premature atrial contractions	7
>5 premature ventricular contractions/min*	7
Age > 70 y	5
Emergency operation	4
Significant aortic stenosis	3
Intraperitoneal, intrathoracic, or aortic† operation	3
Poor general medical condition‡	3

*Premature ventricular contractions in the otherwise healthy patient with a normal heart are probably not associated with increased cardiac risk.

†Since the Goldman study, it has been found that elective abdominal aortic surgery carries a higher risk than predicted by the original index. Also, symptomatic peripheral vascular disease in the patient with stable angina is associated with increased cardiac risk.

‡For example, respiratory failure (Pao$_2$ < 60 mm Hg or Paco$_2$ > 50 mm Hg); renal failure (blood urea nitrogen > 50 or creatinine > 3 mm/dL); chronic liver disease; bedridden for a noncardiac cause.

From Goldman L, Caldera DL, Nussbaum SR, et al: Multifactorial index of cardiac risk in noncardiac surgical procedures. Reprinted with permission from The New England Journal of Medicine, 297, 845–850, 1977.

distention or S$_3$ gallop), ST-T changes on the electrocardiogram, chronic stable angina, MI more than 6 months before surgery, and bundle branch block.

Anesthesia

Spinal anesthesia has no demonstrable advantage over general anesthesia for patients with ischemic heart disease.[27] For patients with aortic stenosis, general anesthesia is, in fact, preferred. In lower abdominal and extremity surgery, spinal anesthesia results in sympathetic blockade that may produce hemodynamically detrimental hypotension and tachycardia in these patients.

Arrhythmias

Preoperative cardiac rhythms other than sinus or premature atrial contractions are associated with increased perioperative risks of ischemia or hemodynamic instability caused by underlying heart disease rather than sustained arrhythmia. Also, premature ventricular contractions in the otherwise healthy patient with a normal heart are probably not associated with increased cardiac risk. For this reason, antiarrhythmic medications do not alter perioperative risk and should be avoided because of their arrhythmogenic potential.[27] However, for patients with a history of sustained ventricular tachycardia or cardiac arrest, perioperative antiarrhythmic therapy is recommended.[27]

TABLE 137–5
RISK ESTIMATES BY GOLDMAN CLASS

Goldman Class	Point Total	Life-Threatening Complications (%)	Death (%)
I	0–5	0.6	0.2
II	6–12	3	1
III	13–25	11	3
IV	>26	12	39

Adapted from Weitz HH, Goldman L: Noncardiac surgery in the patient with heart disease. Med Clin North Am 71:413, 1987.

Heart Blocks and Pacemakers

Patients with conduction system disease have a higher incidence of underlying heart disease and a higher perioperative risk of cardiac complications. Development of complete heart block, however, is rare. Temporary pacemakers are not recommended and probably should be inserted in the operating room only as needed. Transvenous or external pacemakers may be utilized. In patients requiring hemodynamic monitoring and pacing, a Paceport-type pulmonary arterial catheter can be inserted preoperatively.

Electrocautery devices can cause unpredictable malfunction of permanent pacemakers, resulting in irregular impulse generation. Unipolar-type pacemakers are more susceptible to external electromagnetic interference than bipolar types.

Hypertension

In patients with mild-to-moderate hypertension, the preoperative systolic and diastolic blood pressures have not been correlated with the development of postoperative congestive heart failure (CHF), myocardial ischemia, or infarction.[28] Consequently, surgery need not be delayed for mild or moderate hypertension. However, preoperative control of hypertension is recommended because it helps prevent perioperative hypertension and hypotension.

Preoperative antihypertensive medications should be continued until the day of surgery. Evidence of secondary hypertensive end-organ damage, particularly left ventricular hypertrophy, should be sought preoperatively. Left ventricular hypertrophy results in a thick, noncompliant ventricle that may require higher filling pressures for optimal function.

Congestive Heart Failure

CHF is an independent risk factor for the development of perioperative cardiac complications and is the major predictor of postoperative pulmonary edema. Elective surgery should be postponed until the CHF is controlled. Preload and afterload reduction, inotropic support, and diuretics are the major modalities of current treatment.

Patients with signs of left ventricular dysfunction who are not in overt CHF are optimally managed with invasive hemodynamic monitoring. Patients with overt CHF requiring emergent surgery are best managed by invasive monitoring of hemodynamic parameters (via arterial and pulmonary arterial catheters) to be treated preoperatively, intraoperatively, and postoperatively.

Postoperative pulmonary edema most often occurs on the day of surgery when large volumes of fluid are given or on the second or third postoperative day when third-space fluid is reabsorbed into the intravascular space.[27] For this reason, perioperative hemodynamic monitoring should continue until the third postoperative day. Younger patients with mild left ventricular dysfunction who are not having thoracic, abdominal, or aortic surgery may not require invasive monitoring.

Hypertrophic Cardiomyopathy

Patients with hypertrophic cardiomyopathy have a low risk of perioperative complications, but associated CAD increases the risk. Hypovolemia- and hypotension-inducing drugs should be avoided. Spinal anesthesia is therefore relatively contraindicated.[27]

Valvular Disease

Systolic Murmur. The presence of a non–aortic stenosis systolic murmur (i.e., mitral regurgitation), in the absence of left ventricular failure, does not predispose to postoperative cardiac complications.

Aortic Stenosis. If the murmur of aortic stenosis is apparent preoperatively in an asymptomatic patient, two-dimensional echocardiography and Doppler flow echocardiography are necessary to identify significant stenosis. If significant stenosis is present, further study with cardiac catheterization is needed to determine the valve area, ventricular function, and status of the coronary circulation. Patients who are symptomatic (angina, syncope, dyspnea) and have an aortic stenosis murmur require cardiac catheterization[27] and possibly surgery.

Patients who do not have a significant gradient across the valve and have normal left ventricular function are not at a greater risk of perioperative cardiac complications.[27] Most asymptomatic patients with mild aortic stenosis tolerate surgical intervention well. Those with significant stenosis require valve replacement before surgery. Percutaneous valvuloplasty may be beneficial in elderly patients who are not candidates for open heart surgery. As mentioned earlier general anesthesia is better tolerated than spinal anesthesia.

Mitral Stenosis. Elective surgery should be delayed if critical mitral stenosis is present. Invasive hemodynamic monitoring is suggested if emergent surgery is necessary. These patients are particularly prone to the adverse hemodynamic effects of supraventricular tachycardia. Cardiac evaluation and valvuloplasty or replacement may be indicated before the proposed surgery.[27]

Mitral Regurgitation. This lesion does not increase the risk of perioperative cardiac complications unless left ventricular failure is also present.[27]

Prosthetic Valves. A major concern is adequate anticoagulation in patients with mechanical prosthetic valves. The newer low-profile mechanical valves are less prone to thromboembolic complications than the older caged-ball valves. The risk of thromboembolic complication is about 2% for aortic mechanical prostheses and 5% for mitral prostheses.[27]

For aortic valves, oral anticoagulation is stopped 3 days preoperatively and resumed on the second postoperative day. In patients with mitral valve prostheses, oral anticoagulants may be stopped and reversed with vitamin K 36 hours before operation unless there is a large left atrium or a history of previous thromboembolic disease. In these cases, heparin should be continued until 4 to 6 hours before operation. Heparin is begun 12 to 24 hours postoperatively and continued until the PT is sufficiently elevated with warfarin.[27]

Angina Pectoris

Elective surgery should not be performed for patients with unstable angina.[27] They are at significant risk of developing an MI and require intensive medical therapy, stabilization, and further preoperative evaluation. Patients with chronic stable angina are not at increased risk for perioperative myocardial infarction unless they also have symptomatic peripheral vascular disease (PVD). Such patients need a thorough preoperative evaluation (see next section). Clinically silent ischemia can occur in patients with CAD; it is not known whether this alters perioperative risk.

Peripheral Vascular Disease

Patients with stable angina and symptomatic PVD have a high rate of perioperative cardiac complications (10 to

30%).[24-26, 29, 30] This is due to the high frequency of CAD in patients with vascular disease. Further preoperative evaluation of these high-risk patients is necessary to identify patients with significant CAD. Perioperative intervention can significantly reduce the complication rate. (See under Preoperative Evaluation for Coronary Artery Disease.)

Patients undergoing abdominal aortic aneurysm repair also can benefit from invasive preoperative hemodynamic optimization in the ICU. After insertion of a pulmonary arterial catheter, the effects of fluid challenges on cardiac output, systemic vascular resistance, stroke volume, and pulmonary capillary wedge pressure are assessed. (See under Preoperative Preparation of the Stable High-Risk or Critically Ill Patient in the Intensive Care Unit.) Use of intravenous nitroglycerin to lower the systemic vascular resistance and permit further fluid loading may be helpful.

These preoperative interventions can reduce cardiac and renal stress during aortic cross-clamping and unclamping and have contributed to the reduction of perioperative cardiac and renal complications.[31-33]

Myocardial Infarction

The overall risk of developing a perioperative MI in patients 30 years of age or older undergoing general anesthesia and without a prior history of MI is less than 1% (about 0.1 to 0.7%).[27] If there is a history of previous MI the risk increases to about 6 to 7%. Of particular importance is the elapsed time between MI and surgery.

A Mayo Clinic study in 1972 found that patients who have had an MI within the 3 months before surgery have a 37% rate of postoperative MI.[34] Those who have had infarcts 3 to 6 months before surgery have a 16% incidence of postoperative MI. After 6 months, the risk of postoperative MI levels off to about 5% and does not decrease further. This 6-month risk "cutoff" was also supported by the data of Goldman and colleagues discussed earlier.

There have been reports of markedly reduced reinfarction rates in patients with recent MIs undergoing major surgery.[35, 36] In patients who have surgery within 6 months of MI, reinfarction rates are reduced to about 5%. Surgery after 6 months is associated with a reinfarction rate of about 3%.[35-37] Patients with PVD and those having aortic surgery have higher rates of cardiac complications than other groups.

It still seems prudent to postpone elective surgery until more than 6 months have elapsed after an MI, especially in patients with PVD and/or those undergoing aortic surgery. If it is urgent to operate sooner, these data suggest that the current risk of reinfarction is less. Anesthetic techniques and aggressive perioperative identification and treatment of cardiac risk factors aided by invasive hemodynamic monitoring have probably contributed to the decline in perioperative cardiac complications.

Preoperative Evaluation for Coronary Artery Disease

The cardiac risk associated with noncardiac surgery is most often determined by the degree of CAD.[38] The CAD may be clinically silent, stable, or unstable. Perioperative intervention (such as medical therapy, invasive hemodynamic monitoring, and coronary artery bypass grafting [CABG]) in patients with significant CAD can considerably reduce cardiac complications.[38]

Consideration is given to the type of surgery, probability of CAD before surgery, utility of available preoperative tests, and therapeutic options. The types of surgery most likely to cause significant cardiac stress are major abdominal and thoracic operations, aortic surgery, and orthopedic procedures. They involve prolonged surgery, anesthesia, postoperative pain, mechanical ventilation, and greater hemodynamic alterations secondary to blood loss and fluid shifts. Head and neck, prostate, and ophthalmologic surgeries cause less cardiac stress and fewer perioperative cardiac complications. Vascular surgery is associated with a greater cardiac risk because of the high incidence of CAD.

Young men and especially women without angina are at the lowest risk. Patients with unstable angina, recent MI, or uncompensated heart failure are at the highest risk of perioperative cardiac complications. Older men with typical angina, previous MI, or compensated heart failure have a medium to high risk. Patients with stable angina and PVD are also at intermediate risk. These patients may appear to be stable, but the severity of underlying CAD is not clinically apparent.

Patients at moderate-to-high risk of CAD who undergo major surgery should have preoperative testing. Those at low cardiac risk probably do not need testing.

Additional studies are needed to determine the usefulness of preoperative testing in patients with multiple risk factors for CAD (e.g., diabetes, smoking, and PVD) who do not have clinical evidence of CAD and patients at high cardiac risk undergoing less hazardous surgery.[38]

Testing for Coronary Artery Disease. Coronary angiography is not routinely indicated because of the risk and cost incurred if all patients are studied. Noninvasive tests are sensitive enough to select most of the patients who would benefit from more invasive study. Even noninvasive studies such as stress testing are cost-ineffective if performed for all patients.[38] In addition, specificity is reduced when patients with low cardiac risk are studied. Testing should be reserved for patients in the intermediate- to high-risk groups as outlined earlier.

The standard method for detecting myocardial ischemia is exercise testing, but it is often poorly tolerated by patients who are older, chronically ill, or have PVD. Arm exercise is also difficult for most patients. They often exercise submaximally, thereby reducing the sensitivity.

The dipyridamole–thallium-201 stress test uses dipyridamole to increase coronary blood flow several times, producing a "steal" of blood away from the areas supplied by stenotic vessels. It is safe and involves no exercise. Two minutes after dipyridamole injection, thallium-201 is injected and the heart is scanned for perfusion ("cold") defects. Reperfusion studies are performed several hours later. Cold areas that later reperfuse suggest the presence of coronary artery stenosis. Studies have shown that the dipyridamole–thallium-201 stress test is useful in stratifying patients into higher-risk groups. Abnormal tests in patients undergoing vascular surgery are associated with risks of a postoperative ischemic event of 30%[30] to 50%.[22]

In one study, ambulatory Holter's monitoring before peripheral vascular surgery[29] demonstrated myocardial ischemia in 18% of patients, 38% of whom developed a postoperative cardiac complication (unstable angina, MI, or pulmonary edema). It is less costly and more widely available than dipyridamole–thallium-201 stress testing and may be an attractive alternative for selected patients. Holter's monitoring is limited to patients with normal baseline ST-T segments. Further studies are necessary.

Patients in high-risk groups after noninvasive testing should have coronary angiography if they are candidates for CABG.

Preoperative Coronary Artery Revascularization. Several studies have evaluated the impact of preoperative CABG on perioperative MI or cardiovascular mortality. The incidence of perioperative MI is significantly reduced in patients with critical CAD who have had prior CABG.[39-41] The risk of the noncardiac surgery versus the risk of coronary angiography and CABG must be determined at each specific institution. Percutaneous transluminal angioplasty may protect against perioperative cardiac complications. Further studies are needed to compare its effectiveness to that of CABG.

Preoperative Pharmacotherapy

The goal is to provide optimal myocardial oxygenation by maintaining adequate oxygen delivery and limiting oxygen demand. Maintenance of normal heart rate and rhythm, correction of anemia and hypoxemia, control of blood pressure and pain, and relief of ventricular dysfunction are important. Patients receiving beta-blockers and nitrates should continue to receive them throughout the preoperative, intraoperative, and postoperative periods. Beta-blockers may be continued intravenously, or a long-acting oral preparation may be given on the morning of surgery.

Beta-blockers should be restarted 24 to 48 hours postoperatively to avoid beta-blocker withdrawal syndrome or prolonged tachycardia. Intravenous short-acting beta-blockers (e.g., esmolol) may be used in unstable situations when beta-blockade may have to be discontinued suddenly. Nitrates may be continued intravenously. Patients receiving calcium channel blockers can have nitrates and/or beta-blockers substituted perioperatively.

Indications for Invasive Perioperative Hemodynamic Monitoring

Hemodynamic data can be useful for optimizing cardiovascular and volume status of some patients in the ICU before operation, intraoperatively, and postoperatively. Such perioperative hemodynamic monitoring via the pulmonary arterial catheter has probably contributed to the lower incidence of perioperative cardiac complications reported in more recent studies (Table 137–6).

Preoperative Considerations in the Patient with Gastrointestinal or Hepatic Disease

Gastrointestinal Disease

Gastritis, peptic ulcer disease, and reflux esophagitis are often exacerbated by the stresses of surgery. Elective surgery should be postponed for patients with an active ulcer disease until it is fully healed.[42] The healing rates for peptic ulcer are similar for antacids, H_2 blockers, and sucralfate. There has been concern that H_2 blockers may increase the risk of nosocomial pneumonia resulting from aspiration of bacteria that overgrow in the alkaline stomach.

Intravenous H_2 blockers can be used in the perioperative period. The risks and benefits of such therapy must be addressed on an individual basis. Ulcer complications that require surgical intervention include uncontrolled bleeding, perforation, gastric outlet obstruction, or an ulcer unresponsive to medical therapy. Reflux esophagitis should be aggressively treated preoperatively with diet, antacids, H_2 blockers, or sucralfate.

When there is major gastrointestinal tract bleeding the main concerns are providing adequate volume resuscitation, determining the site of hemorrhage, and deciding the need for endoscopic and surgical interventions. Invasive hemodynamic monitoring with the pulmonary arterial catheter can be useful in guiding optimal preoperative resuscitation, especially of elderly patients or those with heart disease.

In upper gastrointestinal tract bleeding involving hemodynamic changes, early endoscopy is valuable in identifying the cause of bleeding, determining the need for early surgical intervention (e.g., arterial bleeding from a peptic ulcer, visible vessel, aortoenteric fistula), and controlling hemorrhage.

When there is lower gastrointestinal tract bleeding after an upper gastrointestinal tract source has been ruled out, proctosigmoidoscopy may be done to exclude hemorrhoids, fissures, rectal ulcers, and tumors. If the results are negative, the most common causes of bleeding in adults are angiodysplasia, diverticular disease, polyps, carcinoma, and inflammatory bowel disease.[42] The incidence of angiodysplastic lesions increases with age.

If proctosigmoidoscopy is negative and the rate of bleeding is greater than 1 mL/min, angiography is the procedure of choice for diagnostic and therapeutic reasons.[42] Angiodysplasia can be identified even if there is no active bleeding. If the rate of bleeding is insufficient for angiographic visualization, a bleeding scan using radionuclide-tagged red blood cells may identify the bleeding site. If hemorrhage has slowed or stopped, colonoscopy may be performed to identify the lesion and to control bleeding via polypectomy, electrocoagulation, heater-probe thermal coagulation, or laser photocoagulation.

Surgery is indicated for nonvariceal bleeding from any site that results in hemorrhagic shock, loss of 30% of the estimated blood volume within 24 hours, requirements of 3 or more units of transfused blood per day to maintain hemodynamic stability, and rebleeding despite therapeutic endoscopy or angiography.[42]

Patients with unexplained hemorrhage and an aortic prosthesis need urgent surgical evaluation.

Preoperative management of cholecystitis consists of nasogastric suction, fluid and electrolyte balance, and antibiotics. Surgery is indicated in those with frequent biliary colic and for acute cholecystitis. In acute cholecystitis there may be no benefit in delaying surgery. Emergency surgery is needed if complications such as gallbladder empyema, pericholecystic abscess or perforation, emphysematous cholecystitis, or suppurative cholangitis are present.[42] Patients with acute pancreatitis that requires emergent surgery are critically ill and should be optimally resuscitated preoperatively with invasive hemodynamic monitoring.

Patients with inflammatory bowel disease are often steroid dependent. They require perioperative steroid replacement. Patients taking maintenence sulfasalazine or metronidazole usually tolerate short-term discontinuation of these medications.[42]

Acute mesenteric ischemia is associated with a high mortality rate, which may be reduced by aggressive diagnostic measures, perioperative resuscitation, and early surgery. When the diagnosis is considered, angiography should be performed to determine whether occlusive arterial or venous disease is present. This provides information about the suitable type of surgical procedure: bowel resection, embolectomy, or endarterectomy.[43]

TABLE 137–6

INDICATIONS FOR INVASIVE PERIOPERATIVE HEMODYNAMIC MONITORING

Unstable angina
Recent myocardial infarction
Moderate-to-severe valvular heart disease
Goldman's cardiac risk class III or IV
Intra-abdominal, intrathoracic, or abdominal aortic surgical procedures in patients older than 70 y
Emergent surgery in critically ill patients requiring resuscitation before operation (e.g., intra-abdominal catastrophes)

Modified from Deron SJ, Kotler MN: Noncardiac surgery in the cardiac patient. Am Heart J 116:831, 1988.

If nonocclusive disease is present, angiography is both diagnostic and therapeutic; infusion of the superior mesenteric artery with vasodilators such as papaverine can improve mesenteric blood flow and protect the bowel.

Before going to the operating room, aggressive ICU resuscitation consisting of invasive hemodynamic monitoring with optimization of volume status, cardiac output, and mesenteric flow and correction of arrhythmias and electrolyte abnormalities can improve the outcome.

Patients with inflammatory bowel disease, gastrointestinal malignancies, and malabsorption syndromes are often malnourished. They may benefit from preoperative nutritional intervention.

Hepatic Disease

Patients with preoperative clinical or laboratory evidence of liver disease must be thoroughly evaluated before undergoing elective surgery. The extent of investigation depends on the severity of the derangement and may include a liver biochemical profile, viral studies, coagulation profile, abdominal ultrasonography, diagnostic or therapeutic paracentesis, assessment of renal function, and liver biopsy.[44]

Important preoperative goals include preventing dehydration, hypokalemia, and alkalosis; reducing ascites; treating infection; correcting coagulopathy; controlling gastrointestinal bleeding; improving nutritional status; and reducing ammonia absorption from the bowel.

Hypoglycemia requiring dextrose infusions may occur with severe liver failure.

The coagulopathy of liver disease is multifactorial and involves reduced synthesis of all clotting factors (except factor VIII) and increased fibrinolytic activity (disseminated intravascular coagulation). Depending on the severity of the underlying liver disease, patients may have varying degrees of prolongation of PT, activated partial prothromboplastin time (aPTT), and thrombin time. Hypofibrinogenemia may also be present.

Patients who have a prolonged PT secondary to poor nutrition or obstructive jaundice (bile salt deficiency) may respond to vitamin K, but patients with coagulopathy caused by more severe degrees of hepatic dysfunction require fresh frozen plasma. The PT should be corrected to within 3 seconds of control.[44] The effects of fresh frozen plasma are transient, and it may be difficult to correct the PT, especially if severe hypofibrinogenemia is present. In certain cases the addition of cryoprecipitate may be helpful.

Thrombocytopenia may occur in patients with hypersplenism, folate deficiency, significant disseminated intravascular coagulation, or alcohol-induced bone marrow suppression. Platelet dysfunction and prolonged bleeding time may be present despite normal platelet counts. 1-Deamino-(8-D-arginine)-vasopressin (DDAVP) can shorten the bleeding time in cirrhotic patients. For major surgery, platelet counts should be at least 50,000/mm^3. Platelet transfusion is indicated if the platelet count is below 50,000/mm^3.[44]

Renal insufficiency often develops in patients with severe hepatic dysfunction. Hepatorenal syndrome is the most severe expression of this phenomenon. It is a severe form of prerenal azotemia possibly induced by renal vasoconstriction secondary to increased angiotensin levels coupled with a decrease in levels of compensatory renal vasodilatory prostaglandins (e.g., prostaglandin E$_2$). Nonsteroidal antiinflammatory agents and aminoglycosides can reduce the prostaglandin E$_2$ level and should be avoided in patients with severe liver dysfunction. Preliminary data show that infusion of vasodilatory prostaglandins may help reverse hepatorenal syndrome in certain instances.[44] Perioperative hemodynamic monitoring is helpful in assessing and adjusting the volume status of patients with significant liver and renal dysfunction.

When diagnostic paracentesis or treatment of ascites with diuretics or paracentesis is performed, the removal of volume should be gradual in patients without peripheral edema to avoid precipitating renal failure or encephalopathy. Patients with peripheral edema may well tolerate rapid removal of large volumes of fluid.[44] Potassium-sparing diuretics (e.g., spironolactone) may be used for patients with hypokalemia and acceptable renal function. A more potent diuretic such as furosemide can be added. For patients with bleeding gastroesophageal varices, prophylactic sclerotherapy before elective surgery may reduce the subsequent risk of bleeding.[44]

It is often difficult to predict the response of the patient with liver disease to the stresses of surgery and anesthesia.[44] Most surgical procedures are associated with clinically insignificant elevations of liver biochemical parameters (serum glutamic-oxaloacetic transaminase, serum glutamic-pyruvic transaminase, alkaline phosphatase, or bilirubin) even in patients without liver disease. During surgery, intraoperative traction, fluid shifts, blood loss, changes in cardiac output, anesthetic agents, hypoxemia, hypercapnia, vasoactive drugs, and positive pressure mechanical ventilation can reduce hepatic blood flow and oxygenation.[44] In patients with liver disease, these factors may precipitate clinically significant hepatic dysfunction or frank hepatic failure. Such patients have a higher than normal risk of postoperative hepatic complications (worsening ascites, encephalopathy, renal failure, pulmonary insufficiency, sepsis, gastrointestinal bleeding) and death after surgery. The risk is related to the severity of the underlying liver disease and the type of surgery.

Hepatitis caused by modern anesthetic agents is extremely rare and has not been reported with isoflurane.[44]

Patients with acute viral hepatitis (e.g., hepatitis A, B, non-A, non-B) or hepatitis attributable to cytomegalovirus or Epstein-Barr virus infection have an increased risk of perioperative complications and mortality. It is recommended that elective surgery be postponed until the liver biochemical results have returned to normal for at least 1 month.[44]

Patients without abnormal preoperative liver biochemical results may have an early viral hepatitis that can become clinically apparent postoperatively and be erroneously attributed to the surgery or anesthesia. A full work-up and follow-up are indicated before elective surgery. Asymptomatic chronic carriers of hepatitis B virus are not at greater risk if preoperative liver biochemistry tests are normal.

Chronic hepatitis is chronic inflammation of the liver for at least 3 to 6 months and may be diagnosed and characterized by clinical and laboratory findings and liver biopsy. In chronic persistent hepatitis, there is no need to postpone elective surgery. These patients are usually asymptomatic or minimally symptomatic with mildly elevated liver biochemical values. They have well-preserved liver function and do not progress to cirrhosis. Chronic active hepatitis is associated with a greater degree of liver dysfunction.

Data are limited, but surgery is usually well tolerated in mild or asymptomatic cases. Patients with symptomatic chronic active hepatitis may have increased surgical mortality; therefore, elective surgery should be delayed.

Alcoholism may predispose the liver to the hypoxic insults and stresses of surgery and anesthesia. Elective surgery should be postponed until after abstinence from alcohol and after alcohol-induced nutritional deficiencies are corrected. Alcoholism can result in several degrees of liver disease. Fatty liver is associated with slight liver enzyme elevations and hepatomegaly. It is not a precursor of cirrhosis and resolves with abstinence from alcohol. Acute alcoholic hepatitis is a serious condition associated with significant liver dysfunction. The mortality rate for this condition alone is significant. Surgery should be postponed until clinical resolution and the return of bilirubin levels to normal. The patient may have to discontinue alcohol intake for several months.[44] A preoperative liver biopsy may be performed if there is suspicion of continued alcoholic hepatitis.

Obstructive jaundice is associated with a surgical mortality of 5 to 60%.[44] Anemia (hematocrit < 30%), hyperbilirubinemia (serum bilirubin level > 11 mg/dL), malignancy (as a cause of obstruction), hypoalbuminemia, and renal failure all increase the postoperative morbidity and mortality. Preoperative transhepatic or endoscopic biliary decompression is a good alternative to surgery for palliation of incurable disease, but it probably does not lower the mortality resulting from subsequent surgery.

Cirrhosis is an irreversible lesion of the liver characterized by fibrosis, necrosis, and nodular regeneration resulting in disorganization of the hepatic lobular architecture. It is most commonly caused by alcoholism and hepatitis B infection. Although the risk of surgery in cirrhotic patients has been studied more than that in patients with other hepatic conditions, precise estimates of risk are not available.[44] This is because the available data are derived from small, retrospective studies of limited design. From this culmination of information, several deductions are possible.[44]

Surgical risk is increased in patients with cirrhosis, and emergent or abdominal procedures enhance the risk. Child's classification (Table 137–7) of liver disease was originally devised to predict mortality after portosystemic shunt surgery. It has also been shown to predict mortality in patients with hepatic disease undergoing nonportosystemic shunt surgery. The surgical mortality figures given in Table 137–7 are derived from a retrospective study of 100 cirrhotic patients undergoing abdominal surgery.[45] Child's class also correlates with postoperative morbidity, which increases from class A to class C. Patients in Child's class A generally tolerate surgery well. Elective surgery should be delayed in patients in classes B and C. They need thorough preoperative preparation. The aim is to treat any reversible aggravating precipitants of liver failure. This is important because Child's class at the time of surgery rather than at the time of admission predicts overall morbidity and mortality.[44]

Surgery of the biliary tree may result in massive hemorrhage in part because of the hypervascularity of the gallbladder bed. In certain cases a subtotal cholecystectomy or a cholecystotomy may be preferable. Hepatic resection is generally contraindicated in the presence of significant liver dysfunction.

Significant advances in immunosuppressive therapy and surgical technique have made liver transplantation a viable option for many patients with significant irreversible liver failure. The quality of life after liver transplantation is similar to that of the normal population, and the 5-year survival is generally greater than 75%.

TABLE 137–7
CHILD'S CLASSIFICATION

Factor	Class A	Class B	Class C
Albumin (g/dL)	>3.5	3.0–3.5	<3.0
Bilirubin (mg/dL)	<2.0	2.0–3.0	>3.0
Ascites	None	Mild	Severe
Encephalopathy	None	Mild	Severe
Nutritional status	Normal	Good	Poor
Surgical mortality (%)[45]	10	30	>70

Preoperative Renal Considerations

Patients with renal failure often undergo elective and emergent surgery. Elective surgery should be postponed for patients with acutely worsening renal function or acute renal failure. Prompt diagnosis and treatment have priority.

Renal failure results in an impaired response to operative stresses and an increased incidence of perioperative complications. The risk of developing such complications is closely related to the glomerular filtration rate. A serum creatinine level greater than 3.0 mg/dL is a cardiac risk factor in patients undergoing noncardiac surgery.[46] There is a high incidence of arteriosclerosis in patients with renal failure. Diabetics with chronic renal failure have an even higher risk of coronary atherosclerosis. They also have autonomic dysfunction that makes them further susceptible to the fluid shifts and the stresses of surgery.

When the glomerular filtration rate is reduced to 25% of normal, fluid and electrolyte homeostasis is significantly impaired.[46] Salt and water retention may lead to hypertension and peripheral edema. Treatment may consist of fluid and salt restriction and diuretics. Fluid overload may require dialysis. Hypertension usually responds to correction of hypervolemia.

Patients with chronic pyelonephritis and polycystic kidney disease have a propensity for salt wasting and a tendency toward fluid and salt depletion. Renovascular hypertension usually leads to a hypovolemic state because of increased renin secretion. Such patients often require careful preoperative hydration.

Pancreatitis, bowel obstruction, inflammatory bowel disease, and other disorders can result in large losses of fluid and electrolytes through vomiting, fistula output, diarrhea, or sequestration in the abdomen. Adequate preoperative resuscitation is essential. Invasive hemodynamic monitoring is helpful in providing the information necessary for precise fluid management.

Prevention of the sequelae of intraoperative hypotension (MI, stroke, further deterioration of renal function, and mesenteric ischemia) is critical in any severely ill patient and magnified in the presence of renal failure. In patients with hypotension and adequate intravascular volume, low-dose (2 to 5 μg/kg/min) dopamine may be helpful in maintaining renal perfusion.[46]

Impaired excretion of hydrogen ion and potassium occurs as the glomerular filtration rate falls. The degree of acidosis and hyperkalemia is variable, depending on many renal and extrarenal factors. Attainment of a pH of 7.25 or more preoperatively is recommended.[46] This may be accomplished by bicarbonate administration or in more severe cases by dialysis.

Hyperkalemia can be controlled with dietary restriction, diuretics, and bicarbonate administration in some patients. The greater the degree of illness and underlying renal dysfunction, the more likely that dialysis will be necessary to control hyperkalemia.

Dialysis-dependent patients should be dialyzed 24 hours before operation.[46] The serum potassium level should again be checked before surgery because equilibration takes several hours after dialysis. The preoperative potassium level should be less than 6 mEq/L.

Patients with vomiting, diarrhea, and other gastrointestinal losses of fluid may be hypokalemic. The serum potassium level should be interpreted with respect to the pH; total body potassium stores are less at any given potassium level if acidosis is present.

Hypocalcemia is common in patients with chronic renal failure. It is treated with calcium carbonate and phosphate binders. Patients with renal failure are partially protected from tetany by acidosis. Acute intravenous administration of calcium is rarely necessary because tetany is unusual.

Preservation of residual renal function is a major goal in patients undergoing surgery.[46] This is best attained by avoidance of renal toxic substances and the careful preoperative optimization of fluid and electrolyte balance, cardiac output, and renal perfusion before operation.

Some patients with chronic renal failure have loss of concentrating ability, and good urine output is not an indicator of hydration. The use of invasive hemodynamic monitoring is indicated in selected patients. Nephrotoxic drugs should be minimized. Modification of drug dosage is often necessary, using blood levels when appropriate. The use of radiopaque iodinated dye for angiographic and other radiographic purposes should be minimized. Patients with diabetic nephropathy are particularly sensitive. If a contrast agent is used, it is important to maintain fluid balance both before and after administration to prevent dehydration resulting from the brisk dye-induced osmotic diuresis.

Anemia is common in patients with chronic renal failure, and it is not necessary to transfuse unless significant blood loss is expected. In this case transfusion to a hematocrit of 25% is advised. Ideally, this can be done during the preoperative hemodialysis so that fluid balance can be adjusted.

Platelet function is abnormal because of uremia-induced abnormalities in circulating von Willebrand's factor. This is particularly marked when the serum creatinine level exceeds 6 mg/dL.[46] Both adhesion and aggregation are reduced. The best indicator is an increased bleeding time. The treatment for uremic platelet dysfunction is frequent dialysis, which improves the bleeding time in some patients. If dialysis is required on the day of surgery, 2 hours should elapse for the heparin effect to diminish before operating. In patients who still have prolonged bleeding times, cryoprecipitate containing von Willebrand's factor can correct the platelet dysfunction. DDAVP causes release of endogenous von Willebrand's factor from the vascular endothelium and can be helpful for short-term improvement. The dose is 0.3 μg/kg. Conjugated estrogens have a more prolonged effect but have a delayed onset of action. Blood transfusions to a hematocrit of 30% may help to control uremic bleeding, probably by increasing blood viscosity.

Protein-calorie malnutrition is present in approximately 20% of patients with chronic renal failure. It is due to malabsorption and anorexia secondary to accumulation of nitrogenous metabolic by-products. It is important to recognize and treat malnutrition before surgery to improve wound healing and immunocompetence. Protein requirements can be met with a 40-g diet in stable patients, but critically ill patients require protein geared toward meeting the increased catabolic demands associated with inflammation and infection.

Preoperative Endocrinologic Considerations
Diabetes Mellitus

Patients with diabetes mellitus often have atherosclerotic disease, autonomic dysfunction, and renal disease. The stress of surgery and anesthesia causes increased catecholamine, glucagon, cortisol, and growth hormone release. They antagonize the release and action of insulin as well as promoting gluconeogenesis and glycogenolysis. Such mechanisms cause hyperglycemia in normal patients and worsen hyperglycemia in diabetics. Patients undergoing elective procedures should have stable blood glucose control with levels less than 250 mg/dL.[47] Hyperglycemia may predispose to infection and poor wound healing.

Electrolyte abnormalities are common. Significant hyper-natremia, hyponatremia, hyperkalemia, and hypokalemia must be corrected preoperatively. Diabetics are also prone to hypophosphatemia, which can lead to postoperative respiratory muscle weakness.

Elective surgery should not be performed in the presence of diabetic ketoacidosis or a hyperosmolar state.[47]

For all patients, careful perioperative monitoring of blood glucose is needed, and the physician should be aware of the development of ketoacidosis. Recommendations for preoperative glucose control can be divided into four categories.[47, 48]

1. Diet-controlled diabetes mellitus. There are no special recommendations. Intravenous solutions lacking glucose may be used.

2. Oral hypoglycemic–controlled diabetes mellitus. Oral hypoglycemics should be discontinued on the day before surgery to prevent hypoglycemia when the patient is not eating. Drugs with a long half-life such as chlorpropamide (36 hours) should be discontinued 3 days before surgery. If blood glucose levels rise above 250 mg/dL, regular insulin coverage on a sliding scale can be instituted. Most patients undergoing prolonged surgery require insulin during the operation. Regular insulin, 0.1 U/kg/L 5% dextrose, is usually sufficient.[48]

3. Insulin-controlled diabetes mellitus. It is helpful to operate early in the day to avoid wide swings in blood glucose in patients who have received insulin and intravenous glucose and are not eating. Most patients are receiving a regimen of neutral protamine Hagedorn or Lente insulin with added doses of regular insulin. There are several methods for providing glucose control in this setting. If the patient is well controlled (i.e., blood glucose level less than 250 mg/dL), one half of the normal daily insulin dose as neutral protamine Hagedorn can be given on the morning of surgery. If the blood glucose level is consistently greater than 250 mg/dL, two thirds of the normal daily insulin dose may be given. In both cases, an infusion of 5% dextrose at 10 g/h (200 mL/h) is given to replace the carbohydrate intake. Another regimen consists of a continuous infusion of regular insulin in place of the adjusted morning neutral protamine Hagedorn.

4. Emergent operation in uncontrolled diabetes mellitus. These patients often need correction of electrolyte and acid-base abnormalities, dehydration, and hyperglycemia. A bolus dose of 5 to 10 U of regular insulin followed by a continuous infusion is recommended. When the blood glucose level is less than 250 mg/dL, a dextrose infusion is started.

Thyroid Disorders

Patients with a history of hyperthyroidism or hypothyroidism are not at increased operative risk as long as they are euthyroid at the time of surgery. Large goiters may make endotracheal intubation difficult.

Hypothyroidism. Hypothyroidism was once thought to contraindicate surgery, but this perspective has been altered. Intraoperative hypotension, postoperative ileus, and neuropsychiatric complications may be more common, but there is no difference in postoperative pulmonary complications, recovery from anesthesia, electrolyte disturbances, arrhythmias, or death for these patients compared with matched controls.[47]

Thyroid replacement therapy may unmask silent CAD. Patients requiring coronary artery bypass should have it performed before thyroid replacement is begun. In other patients, elective surgery should be postponed and thyroid replacement done gradually over several months. This is especially true in the elderly, who are often given levothyroxine sodium (Synthroid) started at 25 μg/d and increased by 25 μg every 2 weeks as needed.

Emergent surgery can be performed without thyroid replacement in patients with mild-to-moderate hypothyroidism. Replacement therapy can be started postoperatively. Severely hypothyroid, myxedematous patients should be treated with a slow intravenous dose of 200 to 400 μg of Synthroid followed by 50 to 100 μg/d.[47] With this regimen, thyroxine levels may be restored to about normal in 24 hours. Such patients need close hemodynamic monitoring for arrhythmias, MI, and hypotension. If any complications develop, the dose of Synthroid must be reduced. Myxedematous patients may also have a reduced adrenal reserve that cannot respond to the increased stress of surgery and return to the euthyroid state. Hydrocortisone, 100 mg intravenously every 8 hours, is the standard replacement therapy.[47]

Sick Euthyroid State. Critically ill patients often have low thyroid hormone levels, but this may be a physiologic response to reduce oxygen consumption and catabolism during stress. This is called a sick euthyroid state. A commonly seen pattern is a fall in triiodothyronine with a normal or slightly reduced thyroxine level. Treatment of this condition with thyroid hormone may be harmful.

The differentiation from primary hypothyroidism can usually be made by the level of thyroid-stimulating hormone, which is high in hypothyroid states but usually normal or slightly elevated in the sick euthyroid state.[49] Also, in sick euthyroid states the reverse triiodothyronine level is elevated but in hypothyroidism it is low. Patients suspected of having secondary hypothyroidism may need further evaluation of anterior pituitary function with a thyrotropin-releasing hormone stimulation test or adrenocorticotropic stimulation.

Hyperthyroidism. The chance of precipitating a thyroid storm by operating on a patient with hyperthyroidism is 10 to 32%.[47] Elective surgery should be postponed until antithyroid medications render the patient euthyroid. If emergent surgery is necessary, there are various recommended regimens. The objectives are to block the peripheral effects of thyroid hormone (beta-blockade), decrease its production (propylthiouracil, methimazole), and limit its release (steroids, iodide) and peripheral conversion to triiodothyronine (steroids, beta-blockers, propylthiouracil). A recommended regimen[47] consists of the following:

1. Propranolol 10 to 40 mg orally or 2 to 10 mg by slow intravenous infusion every 6 hours to decrease the heart rate to less than 90 beats/min. Longer-acting beta-blockers such as atenolol or nadolol may be used to reduce the dosing schedule.

2. A 1-g oral loading dose of propylthiouracil followed by 100 to 300 mg every 8 hours. Methimazole can be used in place of propylthiouracil but does not block peripheral conversion of thyroxine to triiodothyronine.

3. Potassium iodide (saturated solution) 1 hour after propylthiouracil. Give five drops orally, three times a day. Sodium iodide, 1 g every 8 to 12 hours, can be given intravenously if the potassium iodide cannot be taken.

4. Hydrocortisone, 100 mg intravenously every 8 hours.

Adrenal Insufficiency

The stress of anesthesia and surgery evokes a dramatic rise in corticosteroid requirements and cortisol production. If the postoperative course is uncomplicated, cortisol levels usually fall to normal values within 72 hours. The most frequent perioperative adrenal problem is iatrogenic, secondary adrenal insufficiency. It occurs most commonly in patients receiving long-term steroid therapy when periop-erative requirements for corticosteroids are not met. Primary adrenal insufficiency (Addison's disease) is much less common. Patients should be presumed to have significant suppression of the pituitary-adrenal axis if they have received more than 2 weeks of adrenal-suppressing doses of steroid in the previous 6 months or they are currently taking steroids.

Perioperative coverage for surgical stress is achieved by using intravenous hydrocortisone at 100 mg the evening before surgery, 100 mg 1 hour before surgery, 100 mg during surgery, and 100 mg every 6 hours after surgery for 24 hours or until postoperative complications resolve. For uncomplicated cases, steroid tapering is not necessary. In patients who are maintained with steroids chronically, the dose may be decreased by 50% each day until the regular dosage is reached. Hydrocortisone given at doses greater than 25 mg/d usually provides adequate mineralocorticoid activity.[50]

Pheochromocytoma

Patients with pheochromocytoma often have low circulating volumes because of high output of catecholamines.[51] Long-standing hypercatecholamine secretion may result in a cardiomyopathy.

Patients with active tumors can benefit from perioperative pulmonary arterial catheterization. It can be used to guide hemodynamic optimization, which includes volume expansion, alpha- and beta-blockade, and assessment of cardiac output. Intraoperatively, it can be useful for monitoring and treatment of significant hemodynamic fluctuations that may occur when the tumor mass is removed.

Care must be taken not to trigger a hypertensive crisis (catecholamine surge) preoperatively. This can be done by providing adequate analgesia and sedation before performing any procedures on the patient (e.g., catheter insertion).

Preoperative Hematologic Considerations
Red Blood Cell Disorders

Anemia. The major reason for blood transfusion (packed red blood cells) is to provide adequate oxygen delivery. Neither the hematocrit nor the hemoglobin level is the sole determinant of the need for blood transfusion.[52] Other more critical factors (although not all are readily determined) include the volume of distribution, oxygen delivery, oxygen consumption, cardiopulmonary status, age, ongoing metabolic demands, type of operative procedure, and chronicity of the anemia.

Hemodynamically stable patients with adequate oxygen delivery and stable hematocrits of 20 to 30% generally tolerate major surgery well.[52] They do not routinely require preoperative transfusion. It should be noted that patients with chronic anemia show evidence of compromised oxygen delivery when the hematocrit falls below 18%. Hemodynamically unstable anemic patients with significant blood loss (more than 20 to 30% of their blood volume) obviously need transfusion. In the ICU setting, hemodynamic monitoring with determination of volume status, cardiac output, oxygen delivery, and oxygen consumption should guide blood transfusion.

For elective surgery when there is a significant potential for perioperative blood transfusion, preoperative collection of autologous blood should be seriously considered. Autologous blood transfusion is retransfusion of blood that has been previously collected from the same patient. Increased recognition of the hazards of homologous blood transfusion, principally the acquired immunodeficiency syndrome and non-A, non-B hepatitis, has led to efforts to increase the availability and utilization of autologous blood.[53, 54]

Elective surgery should be postponed until the etiology of anemia is determined. This may uncover certain disorders (e.g., malignancy, liver disease, vitamin deficiencies) that can affect the perioperative course.

Hemolytic anemias present special perioperative problems.[55] Sickle cell anemia may be associated with an increased risk of vaso-occlusive episodes (sickle crisis) during general anesthesia or regional anesthesia done under tourniquet (bloodless field). In addition, these patients often have significant cardiopulmonary and renal dysfunction. These patients have chronic severe anemia (hemoglobin level of 5 to 10 g/dL) with adequate circulating volume. They usually tolerate anemia of this magnitude well. Preoperative transfusions are not routinely indicated. In major surgery when significant hemodynamic instability resulting in hypoxia and acidosis is anticipated, preoperative exchange transfusion may help reduce the incidence of sickle crisis. The level of hemoglobin S should be reduced to less than 20 to 30%.[55] Other measures include adequate hydration and oxygenation. Sickle cell trait does not result in an increase in surgical morbidity.

Immune hemolytic anemias should be treated and stabilized before elective surgery. In the "warm"-type, immunoglobulin G–mediated variety, blood transfusions should be given slowly with caution because it may be difficult to determine compatibility. When surgery is emergent, prednisone at 1 mg/kg should be started immediately.[55] In "cold"-type, immunoglobulin M–mediated hemolytic anemia, washed red blood cells (to reduce complement-aggravated hemolysis) should be given through a blood warmer.

Erythrocytosis. As the hematocrit rises above 50%, blood viscosity increases significantly and oxygen transport decreases regardless of the underlying cause. The hematocrit may rise because of a reduction in plasma volume (relative erythrocytosis) or an increase in red blood cell mass (absolute erythrocytosis).

Relative erythrocytosis is usually a chronic condition seen in older hypertensive male smokers. Absolute erythrocytosis is termed polycythemia. Patients with uncontrolled polycythemia vera have a high incidence of thromboembolic events.

Diagnosis of the underlying cause of polycythemia is important because the approach to preoperative reduction in hematocrit depends on whether the polycythemia is physiologically inappropriate (e.g., polycythemia vera; cysts or tumors of the kidney, liver, or uterus; or cerebellar hemangioblastoma) or physiologically appropriate (e.g., secondary to chronic hypoxemic states like chronic obstructive pulmonary disease).

In otherwise healthy patients, blood may be removed in 300- to 500-mL increments every other day. In the elderly and patients with cardiac disease, it is best to remove blood slowly in 200-mL increments.[55] When surgery is emergent, rapid phlebotomy along with colloid or plasma volume resuscitation can be used for rapid reduction in the hematocrit.

In cases of physiologically inappropriate polycythemia, the hematocrit should be reduced to 45 to 50% preoperatively.[55] In polycythemia vera, the hematocrit should be reduced to less than 45% preoperatively. When thrombocytosis is present, reduction of the platelet count may be advantageous.

If polycythemia is physiologically appropriate, a preoperative hematocrit of 50 to 60% is accepted.[55] Although further reductions in hematocrit may reduce viscosity, a decrease in oxygen delivery caused by a reduction in oxygen-carrying capacity may not be well tolerated.

Platelet Disorders

Platelet abnormalities are associated with an increased risk of intraoperative and postoperative bleeding complications. In general, if platelet function is normal, the risk of bleeding is proportional to the platelet count.[55] The risk of bleeding is increased if fever, infection, anemia, or coexistent coagulopathies are present.

Thrombocytopenia. Normal platelet counts are greater than 150,000/mm³, and thrombocytopenia is defined as a platelet count below 150,000/mm³. Platelet counts of at least 80,000 to 100,000/mm³ are desirable in patients undergoing major surgical procedures. Adequate hemostasis for most procedures is usually provided if the platelet count is above 50,000/mm³. For central nervous system and cardiac surgery, platelet counts greater than 100,000/mm³ are preferable.[55] Minor surgery not involving the airway or blood vessels can usually be performed with a platelet count of 30,000/mm³.

When platelet counts are less than 50,000/mm³, major surgery may precipitate excessive bleeding, but this is not a consistent finding; it depends on the degree of platelet function that is present. When platelet counts drop below 10,000/mm³, major spontaneous gastrointestinal or central nervous system bleeding may occur.[55]

Any patient with a platelet count less than 100,000/mm³ needs a thorough preoperative evaluation before elective surgery is performed. If a treatable cause is found, it should be corrected before surgery. In cases of immune thrombocytopenia, steroids may induce a remission. If this fails, splenectomy should be performed along with the planned procedure. Intravenous gamma globulin infusions have been used in conjunction with platelet transfusions to raise the platelet level transiently in patients with severe, refractory immune thrombocytopenia.

One unit of platelet transfusion generally raises the platelet count from 5000 to 10,000/mm³. However, in immune thrombocytopenia the platelets are rapidly destroyed, and a platelet count 1 hour after transfusion is useful for evaluating the response to transfusion.

Thrombocytosis. Primary thrombocytosis is seen in myeloproliferative disorders such as essential thrombocytosis, myeloid metaplasia, and polycythemia vera. Platelet counts are often greater than 1 million/mm³, and platelet function is abnormal. The disorders are associated with increased risks of thrombohemorrhagic events; essential thrombocytosis and myeloid metaplasia are more commonly associated with hemorrhagic events and polycythemia vera with thrombotic complications.[55] Some patients have both types of complication.

The risks of such complications increase with increasing age and prior history of thrombohemorrhage. The complications include venous thromboembolism (deep venous thrombosis, pulmonary embolism, mesenteric thrombosis) and arterial thromboembolism (stroke, MI, peripheral arterial occlusion).

Secondary thrombocytosis is seen in a variety of inflammatory and neoplastic states. Platelet counts are usually less than 1 million/mm³ and platelet function is normal. Patients with secondary thrombocytosis or primary thrombocytosis associated with chronic myelogenous leukemia are not predisposed to thrombohemorrhagic events.[55]

Preoperative platelet reduction below 1 million/mm³ may be beneficial for certain patients with primary thrombocytosis. This includes elderly patients with vascular disease and prior thrombotic history. In addition, patients undergoing splenectomy may have postoperative platelet counts of 2 million/mm³ that are associated with increased risk of thrombosis.

Such high platelet counts also occur in patients with secondary thrombocytosis; however, the patients are not at increased thrombotic risk and do not require therapy.[55]

When necessary, platelet reduction may be achieved emergently via plasmapheresis. Chemotherapeutic agents (e.g., hydroxyurea and phosphorus-32) can also be used, but they act more slowly. Aspirin is not recommended for patients with primary thrombocytosis because abnormal platelet function may lead to hemorrhagic complications.[55]

Platelet Dysfunction. Patients with primary bone marrow disorders (e.g., essential thrombocytosis and myeloid metaplasia), dysproteinemia (e.g., multiple myeloma), liver failure, von Willebrand's disease, uremia, or aspirin use have varying degrees of platelet dysfunction and a higher incidence of postoperative bleeding complications regardless of the platelet count. Platelet aggregation studies, ristocetin cofactor measurement, and renal function studies are helpful for diagnostic purposes.

A prolonged bleeding time identifies a qualitative platelet abnormality. A bleeding time longer than 20 minutes is clinically significant.[55] Although the bleeding time normally ranges from 3.5 to 7.5 minutes, moderately increased bleeding times do not reliably predict an abnormal hemostatic response to surgery. Younger platelets may function better than older ones. If there is an intrinsic platelet defect, the most valuable indicator of bleeding risk is a prior history of the degree of bleeding, if any, after surgery.

Treatment of significant platelet dysfunction depends on the etiology of the disorder, prior bleeding history, and the type of surgery. Measures taken may include discontinuing aspirin, dialysis for renal failure, and plasmapheresis in dysproteinemias. Intravenous infusion of 0.3 $\mu g/kg$ of DDAVP is helpful in reversing platelet dysfunction associated with aspirin, uremia, or liver failure and is useful before emergent surgery.

Platelet transfusions can also transiently improve hemostasis and should be available during and after surgery if bleeding occurs. Platelet transfusions are used prophylactically in patients with platelet dysfunction who have a significant bleeding history or are to have ophthalmologic and neurologic procedures in which even a small amount of bleeding can be detrimental.

Hemostatic Disorders

Platelet disorders have just been discussed.

Factor Deficiencies. Factor deficiencies can cause prolongation of the PT and/or the aPTT, but not all are associated with a clinically significant bleeding risk. Elevation of the aPTT resulting in increased bleeding is caused by deficiencies of factor VIII, IX, or XI; von Willebrand's disease; or the presence of specific factor inhibitors. Other causes of increased aPTT, such as deficiencies in contact factors (factor XII, high-molecular-weight kininogen, prekallikrein) or presence of lupus anticoagulant, are not associated with increased bleeding.[55] The presence of lupus anticoagulant may be associated with thrombosis.

Isolated elevation of the PT can be caused by a deficiency of factor VII; this is rare and does not result in bleeding diathesis. Prolongation of the PT associated with a clinically significant bleeding risk may be caused by vitamin K deficiency or liver disease.

Patients with clinically significant factor deficiencies need factor replenishment, usually with fresh frozen plasma, but rarely need specific factor infusion before surgery. Isolated factor deficiencies are quite rare (1 in 1 million).

Prolongation of both the PT and aPTT is most commonly secondary to liver disease, vitamin K deficiency, or disseminated intravascular coagulation. The coagulopathy of liver disease is discussed under Preoperative Considerations in the Patient with Gastrointestinal or Hepatic Disease.

Hemophilia A is an X-linked recessive disorder caused by a deficiency in factor VIII coagulant activity. The aPTT is elevated and the PT is normal. The degree of bleeding depends on factor VIII levels and can be mild (factor VIII: >6% normal), moderate (factor VIII: 1 to 6% normal), or severe (factor VIII: <1% normal). All patients should be tested for antibodies to factor VIII. Even minor surgery in patients with factor VIII antibodies is potentially hazardous and should be performed in centers that have considerable experience.

The type of therapy depends on the severity of hemophilia and the type of surgery. Severe hemophiliacs undergoing major procedures should be given 40 U/kg of factor VIII concentrate immediately before surgery.[55] The concentrate has a half-life of 8 to 12 hours and raises factor VIII levels to normal. Factor levels are kept at more than 30% of normal by infusing 20 U/kg of factor VIII every 8 to 12 hours. This is continued for about 1 week postoperatively but may be given for as many as 6 weeks after orthopedic procedures.

For minor procedures in severe hemophiliacs, the same protocol is followed but continued for only 1 to 2 days postoperatively. Factor VIII may be given as factor VIII concentrate or cryoprecipitate, which contains about 100 U of factor VIII activity per bag. Cryoprecipitate exposes the patient to fewer donors than pooled factor VIII concentrate, reducing the risk of hepatitis. DDAVP (0.4 $\mu g/kg$) given 30 minutes before a minor procedure can release enough factor VIII from the vascular endothelium to prevent bleeding complications in mild hemophiliacs.

Hemophilia B is caused by an X-linked deficiency of factor IX and is clinically similar to hemophilia A. The aPTT is elevated with a normal PT. In severe factor IX deficiency, prothrombin complex concentrates rich in factor IX are used. The dose of factor IX is 50 U/kg immediately before surgery and 25 U/kg every 24 hours postoperatively.[55] Factor IX infusions are continued according to the recommendations given for factor VIII infusion. Prothrombin complex concentrates have variable levels of activated coagulation factors and the risk of thrombosis is increased, especially in patients with liver disease in whom the clearance of activated factors is reduced.

Von Willebrand's disease is a group of related quantitative or qualitative disorders of factor VIII–associated antigen (von Willebrand's factor). Abnormalities in von Willebrand's factor result in platelet dysfunction and an elevated aPTT. For major surgery, the treatment consists of cryoprecipitate. DDAVP infusion alone may suffice for minor surgery. It causes the release of factor VIII–von Willebrand's factor from the vascular endothelium.

White Blood Cell Abnormalities

The effect of white blood cell disorders on the perioperative course depends on underlying diseases, which must be identified and appropriately treated before elective surgery. Leukocytosis may be seen with neoplasms, myeloid malignancies, infections, bleeding, steroids, and chronic inflammatory disorders.

Neutropenia is usually seen after radiotherapy or chemotherapy. In patients undergoing such treatments, elective surgery should be planned so that the perioperative period does not coincide with the nadir of the blood count (peak bone marrow suppression). Neutropenia is associated with an increased incidence of infection.

Elective surgery should be postponed until neutropenia resolves; if emergent operation is necessary, surveillance for infection is important. Prophylactic antibiotics are used as appropriate to the surgical procedure. Granulocyte transfusions are not indicated.

Idiopathic neutropenia is uncommon, occurs more often in black persons, and does not predispose to infection.

PREOPERATIVE PREPARATION OF THE STABLE HIGH-RISK OR CRITICALLY ILL PATIENT IN THE INTENSIVE CARE UNIT

Preoperative admission of a high-risk surgical candidate to the ICU is a relatively new practice that is becoming more widespread. As more major surgical procedures are carried out in high-risk patients, this type of admission will probably continue to increase.

Currently, many centers do not routinely provide such care because of personnel, bed capacity, and financial constraints. At present, good prospective studies of the clinical usefulness of preoperative admission and its influence on morbidity, mortality, and length of hospital stay are needed. The additional expense makes it necessary to identify patients who will benefit from such care.[56]

The intensivist should participate in the final determination of operative risk. Only patients for whom active intervention or alteration in therapy (e.g., fluid loading) is planned should be considered for preoperative admission to the ICU. This includes patients with unstable angina, recent MI, decompensated or recent CHF, severe hypertension, moderate to severe valvular disease, sepsis, and aortic vascular diseases. Patients with severe hypertension or angina may benefit from preoperative admission to allow safe replacement of oral therapy by intravenous medications. Patients with pheochromocytoma, subarachnoid hemorrhage, and morbid obesity may also warrant preoperative ICU admission.

Patients who are hemodynamically stable and need no preoperative therapy but require intraoperative hemodynamic monitoring can be managed by the anesthesiologist in the operating room. Other patients are high surgical risks but do not have underlying diseases that benefit from preoperative intensive care. Examples include those with severe chronic pulmonary disease, chronic renal insufficiency, malnutrition, remote MI, or chronic ventricular dysrhythmias. In such patients, the risks of invasive hemodynamic and pharmacologic therapy outweigh the benefits.

Age alone is not a criterion for preoperative intensive care.

Before any invasive procedure or therapeutic intervention, clearly defined goals or end points should be established with consideration of the risk/benefit ratio. No absolute policy regarding any generalized profile of patients should be established. Each request for ICU admission should be evaluated on an individual basis.

If preoperative intervention is used, the patient should receive the full advantage of such an admission. In addition to advanced monitoring and therapeutic interventions, this includes familiarization with the surroundings and staff of the unit, a discussion of what to expect postoperatively, and answers to any questions. Pertinent family members should also be acquainted with these issues. Such actions may reduce the anxiety of the patient and family and improve postoperative cooperation.

Elective surgical patients should be admitted no sooner than the day before scheduled surgery. This approach is cost-effective, reduces the use of a limited number of ICU beds, and decreases the number of hours of invasive monitoring, which may reduce the risk of catheter infections. It is almost useless to admit a high-risk yet stable patient for preoperative ICU intervention if the time available for hemodynamic optimization is limited to a few hours. At least 12 hours is required to evaluate the effects of therapeutic interventions satisfactorily, because if abnormalities are found and changes in therapy are made, several hemodynamic profiles over time are necessary. Also, the initial hemodynamic profile may not reflect the patient's true baseline because of anxiety.

For emergency surgical procedures, the operative delays incurred with preoperative ICU intervention must be weighed against the urgency of the surgery. The minimal amount of time required to admit a patient to the ICU, evaluate routine blood studies, and insert arterial and pulmonary arterial catheters is about 1 to 2 hours. Trauma patients rarely, if ever, benefit from preoperative ICU management. However, critically ill patients benefit from a 2- to 4-hour resuscitation-stabilization period in the ICU before going to the operating room.[56] In these patients it seems that the benefits outweigh the risks of delaying surgery.

Hemodynamic "Optimization"

ICU intervention geared toward optimizing the cardiovascular status preoperatively is referred to as hemodynamic optimization. This involves monitoring vital signs and collecting pulmonary arterial catheter data (including oxygen delivery and consumption) before and after therapy with fluid challenges, inotropes, and vasodilators. It is done to determine whether therapy has had a favorable, detrimental, or insignificant hemodynamic effect.

The information obtained with the pulmonary arterial catheter can be useful only if strict attention is focused on accurate calibration, positioning, technique, and rational appraisal of the data.[57] Collection of the data can be facilitated by keeping a timed flow sheet or computer trend of hemodynamic variables and therapy.

If a therapy has no effect or a detrimental effect, it should be discontinued. Frequently, medications are used preoperatively without determination of effect. Every medication, especially the inotropes, may have markedly different effects in different patients. If therapy results in an improved hemodynamic profile, efforts should be made to maintain this effect throughout the perioperative period.

Although the pathophysiology of cardiac disease, sepsis, and other disorders varies greatly, the preoperative determinations and optimization strategies have similar predetermined goals. However, there is a need to individualize the preoperative preparation of each patient. A "cookbook" approach is not recommended.

It is crucial at this point to define the term "optimization." The quotation marks are placed to emphasize that it has been defined as maximal cardiac output, oxygen delivery, and wedge pressure, but these may not be the best parameters for all patients. Despite attempts by numerous authors to establish an optimal range of filling pressures and cardiac output, this should not be the goal of preoperative intervention.[56]

Contrary to the maximization philosophy, it is better to have patients meet their oxygen requirement using the least amount of cardiac work. This is especially true for patients with heart disease. An attempt should be made to establish each patient's oxygen demand using all the hemodynamic data. This approach may be controversial, but it is consistent with the approach used for all types of chronic heart disease including ischemic heart disease. In such an approach, beta-blocker medications that decrease myocardial oxygen consumption and stroke work have been shown to improve postinfarction survival.

It should also be pointed out that in the patient with heart disease, regardless of the etiology, the pulmonary capillary wedge pressure has little relationship to the left ventricular end-diastolic volume. This is due to marked changes in ventricular compliance or valvular disease.

Cardiac output should be deemed insufficient only when used in conjunction with other easily obtained data. If the mixed venous oxygenation, lactate level, and oxygen delivery and consumption are normal, cardiac output should be interpreted as adequate. Maximizing a cardiac output that is currently satisfying oxygen demands increases myocardial oxygen consumption and stroke work. This is exactly opposite to the goal of hemodynamic optimization.

Along the same lines, in cardiac and most other patients, an attempt should not be made to optimize urine output.[56] Before pulmonary arterial catheterization and other determinations of systemic perfusion, the urine output served as a guide, although poor, to perfusion. Although an adequate urine output probably indicates sufficient perfusion, a low urine output does not necessarily indicate that perfusion is poor at that point in time. Oliguria, particularly in elderly patients with coexisting heart disease, may not be secondary to low renal blood flow but may be due to pre-existing renal disease, sepsis, acute tubular necrosis, drugs, or other etiologies.

Before fluid challenges to treat oliguria, preoperative hemodynamic data, basic kidney function tests, urinary electrolytes, and urinary osmolality should be determined to ascertain whether oliguria is secondary to low flow, volume depletion, or an etiology unrelated to perfusion. The pulmonary arterial catheter determines systemic flow, which may be normal and therefore fail to detect regional renal blood flow abnormalities. Despite this, oliguria per se should no longer be used as a determinant of systemic perfusion in the perioperative patient.

When fluid loading is used in preoperative optimization, it is important to tailor this intervention to each patient's individual myocardial compliance characteristics. This is done by closely monitoring the response of the pulmonary capillary wedge pressure during the administration of fluid; a disproportionately large rise (e.g., >5 mm Hg) should alert the physician to the presence of a noncompliant ventricle. If this happens, the fluid challenge should be stopped and hemodynamics observed.

Measurements of heart rate, respiration, cardiac output, arterial and mixed venous blood gases, and pulmonary capillary wedge pressure are taken at regular intervals to determine the effect of the volume administered. It is never acceptable to administer volume until signs of heart failure appear and then taper off.

Previous studies have concentrated on volume loading until the maximal cardiac index is achieved for a given volume load or until a specified pulmonary capillary wedge pressure is reached (i.e., 12 to 18 mm Hg).[32, 33] As stated earlier, it is potentially deleterious to maximize the cardiac output for cardiac output's sake. It is better to look at both cardiac output and systemic oxygen dynamics (supply and demand) to determine the adequacy of circulatory performance. Further interventions are based on these data.

Hemodynamic Optimization of Critically Ill Patients

In general, the hemodynamic principles discussed for the preoperative management of the cardiac patient also apply to other situations. Although it is ineffective to attempt preoperative ICU hemodynamic optimization in a stable but high-risk cardiac patient in only a few hours, patients in septic shock requiring emergency surgery can benefit from even only a few hours of intensive care resuscitation. These patients are suspected of having a perforated viscus, abdominal abscess, peritonitis, or bowel ischemia.

Despite the apparent urgency to operate, it is better to postpone surgery for a few hours while the hemodynamics, perfusion, and acid-base status are corrected. It seems simplistic to think that delaying surgery for 1 to 2 hours necessarily worsens the outcome for a patient who already has an endotoxin-induced systemic inflammatory process. The goal in such patients is to ensure a safe operative course and to limit the end-organ damage by correcting hypoxemia, acidosis, and hypoperfusion, which can lead to multiple organ system failure.

Emergent admission to the ICU, intubation, and hyperventilation to help correct the usual metabolic acidosis are the first steps. These are followed by insertion of arterial and pulmonary arterial catheters and assessment of hemodynamics and oxygen transport.

Volume expansion is important in the initial resuscitation of patients with septic shock, but it is not necessary to administer 8 to 10 L of fluid as is commonly advocated because (1) many patients have already been volume loaded in the emergency room, (2) septic patients, especially if elderly, have noncompliant ventricles and may develop pulmonary congestion, (3) massive edema may worsen oxygen delivery at the tissue level, and (4) few studies have demonstrated a beneficial effect of massive volume loading.

This volume-limiting approach may be viewed as radically different from most recommended approaches, but the mortality resulting from septic shock is still about 50% and has not changed in the past 20 years. As stated earlier, hemodynamic and oxygen transport trends (e.g., lactate, metabolic acidosis, oxygen delivery-consumption, mixed venous oxygen) are the best measures for determining the adequacy of systemic perfusion; they dictate the combination of volume, blood, and inotropic support that is necessary. If the septic patient remains markedly hypotensive, acidotic, and hyperlactemic despite resuscitation, surgical intervention is invariably in vain.

SPECIAL CONSIDERATIONS

Preoperative Considerations in the Cancer Patient

Preoperative preparation of the oncology patient should take into account the effects of previous chemotherapeutic agents and radiotherapy, as well as the effects of malignancy itself on organ function. The toxic effects of chemotherapy can be delayed in onset, acute, or chronic. A thorough history includes the names, dates, and dosages of all drugs and radiotherapy[58] and the recognition that any organ system can be affected.

The cancer patient with central nervous system symptoms should have a work-up for brain metastasis, which may alter plans for surgical intervention. Postoperative weaning from the ventilator may be difficult in patients with neuromuscular syndromes.

Acute cerebellar syndromes and ataxia may occur after 5-fluorouracil, procarbazine, hexamethylmelamine, and nitrosoureas. Methotrexate given intrathecally can produce signs and symptoms of acute bacterial meningitis. Acute paralysis caused by spinal cord demyelination has also been reported with intrathecal use. Chronic encephalopathy can result if methotrexate is combined with radiotherapy or intrathecal cytosine arabinoside.

Ototoxicity and peripheral neuropathies have been described with cisplatin. Vincristine can cause severe peripheral and autonomic neuropathy. Muscle weakness and paralytic ileus may result. Other drugs that can cause peripheral neuropathy include procarbazine, 5-azacytidine, VP-16, and cytosine arabinoside. Hyponatremia resulting from syndrome of inappropriate antidiuretic hormone may occur with cyclophosphamide or the vinca alkaloids.

Neuromuscular weakness may also result from the Eaton-Lambert syndrome (oat cell carcinoma), dermatomyositis (adenocarcinoma of the gastrointestinal tract), or myasthenia gravis (thymoma). Increased sensitivity to aminoglycoside antibiotics and muscle relaxants is seen in the Eaton-Lambert syndrome and in myasthenia.

The two agents that most commonly cause pulmonary toxicity are bleomycin and the nitrosoureas, which may cause interstitial fibrosis.[58] Bleomycin toxicity is associated with cumulative doses of greater than 450 U, but can occur at lower doses. Pre-existing lung disease, age greater than 70, high doses of inspired oxygen, and prior radiotherapy lower the dose needed to produce toxicity. Patients with a history of bleomycin exposure should receive the lowest possible oxygen concentration. Nitrosourea causes interstitial fibrosis in 20 to 30% of patients treated with cumulative doses greater than 1000 mg/m^2. Methotrexate may result in a delayed form of toxicity characterized by fever, dyspnea, hypoxemia, interstitial infiltrates on the chest roentgenogram, and restrictive lung disease.[58]

Other drugs that cause pulmonary toxicity include busulfan, cyclophosphamide, procarbazine, and cytosine arabinoside. Patients with a history of significant exposure to the agents just discussed should have preoperative pulmonary function assessment.

Doxorubicin (Adriamycin) and daunorubicin are the two most important chemotherapeutic agents that can cause acute or chronic cardiotoxicity. The acute toxicities are usually transient but sometimes produce life-threatening arrhythmias. Nonspecific ST-T segment changes and a decreased QRS voltage may also be seen. Congestive heart failure (cardiomyopathy) may result from chronic administration of cumulative doses greater than 550 mg/m^2 and mediastinal radiation, and cyclophosphamide may potentiate this chronic complication.[58] Patients at risk for cardiomyopathy should have a preoperative cardiac evaluation (e.g., echocardiogram). Perioperative invasive hemodynamic monitoring is indicated if significant cardiac dysfunction is present. Hematologic disturbances are common (see under Preoperative Hematologic Considerations).

Preoperative evaluation of hormonal function is indicated in patients who have had endocrine glands exposed within radiotherapy fields. Hypothyroidism or adrenal insufficiency can result from such radiation exposure.

Attention should be paid to possible electrolyte, hepatic, and renal disturbances that may result from chemotherapeutic agents or paraneoplastic syndromes. Nephrotoxicity, hypocalcemia, and hypomagnesemia can complicate cisplatin treatment. Methotrexate may cause renal dysfunction. Cyclophosphamide and oat cell carcinoma can produce hyponatremia associated with the syndrome of inappropriate antidiuretic hormone secretion. Hypercalcemia may result from breast carcinoma or squamous cell lung cancer. Many chemotherapeutic agents are metabolized in the liver, but clinically significant hepatotoxicity is unusual. Mild elevations in liver function tests may occur. Methotrexate may lead to hepatic fibrosis after chronic use, but hepatic failure is unusual.

Preoperative Considerations in the Geriatric Patient

The elderly population in the United States is continuing to increase. The literature concerning surgery in the elderly patient is growing. The life expectancy and tolerance of surgery in the elderly are often underestimated. With careful planning and care, the elderly can undergo surgery safely

TABLE 137–8

AMERICAN SOCIETY OF ANESTHESIOLOGY PHYSICAL STATUS CLASSIFICATION

Class*	Description
1	Healthy normal
2	Mild systemic disease or normal, age > 80 y
3	Severe systemic disease that is nonincapacitating
4	Incapacitating systemic disease that is a constant threat to life
5	Moribund, not expected to survive for 24 h with or without surgery

*In emergency surgery cases, an "E" is assigned to the class number.

and with risks similar to those seen in younger patients.[59] The American Society of Anesthesiology physical status classification system (Table 137–8) is useful for identifying high-risk patients. Patients older than 80 years in class 2 have less than 1% mortality; however, those in class 4 have 25% mortality.[60]

The aging cardiovascular system has been well studied. The relaxation phase of heart muscle is prolonged, although contractility is not affected. There are decreases in maximal heart rate and cardiac output with exercise. This is due in part to a decrease in responsiveness to catecholamines and an increase in afterload because of noncompliant arteries. Blood pressure tends to increase with age but is normal in many elderly patients, especially those who are physically active.[59]

The lungs lose their elasticity with age and become more compliant, with increases in closing volume. These changes result in increased residual volume and ventilation-perfusion mismatching. There is a linear decrease in PaO_2 with age. The vital capacity decreases by about 25 mL/y starting at about age 30.[59] There are also decrements in maximal voluntary ventilation, FEV_1, and maximal midexpiratory flow rate.

The kidneys lose about 20 to 30% of their weight from age 30 to 80.[59] The number of glomeruli decreases and interstitial fibrosis increases. Creatinine clearance also decreases without an increase in serum creatinine level because the lean body mass is also decreased. An estimate of creatinine clearance (CC) is roughly possible, based on age, weight, and serum creatinine (SCr):

$$CC \ (mL/min) = (140 - age) \times \frac{weight \ (kg)}{SCr \times 72}$$

Decreases in creatinine clearance are important and should be taken into account when administering drugs such as digoxin and antibiotics. The tubular function of the kidneys is also reduced with age, resulting in decreases in concentrating and diluting ability.

There is also a decreased thirst awareness. Abnormalities in arginine vasopressin secretion in some elderly patients may lead to decreased free water clearance and hyponatremia. These factors make the elderly more prone to dehydration or fluid overload and hypernatremia or hyponatremia.

Skin and bone changes result in fragile bones and skin prone to decubitus ulcers. Lean body mass, plasma volume, and total body water decrease. Extracellular water decreases 40% and body fat increases 35%.[59] These changes alter drug action depending on the drug's relative water and lipid solubility. For water-soluble drugs, a decrease in the volume of distribution results in a higher concentration of drug. For lipid-soluble drugs, there is a relatively higher volume of distribution, often resulting in a prolonged action. Drug metabolism by the liver is altered in complex, variable ways. Some important drugs that have decreased metabolic clearance in the elderly are warfarin, benzodiazepines, and phenytoin.

The most common medical problems in the elderly are dementia, chronic obstructive pulmonary disease, diabetes, CAD, heart failure, and hypertension.[58]

If viable elderly patients are studied, the mortality resulting from surgery may approximate that of younger patients. Surgery in the elderly has been proved to be safe in cardiopulmonary bypass, resection of abdominal aneurysms, lung resection, abdominal surgery, orthopedic procedures, and major gynecologic surgery. In the younger population, the mortality for emergency surgery is much greater than that for elective surgery. This is especially so in the elderly. It has been suggested that in as many as 33% of cases, surgery is delayed in the elderly until it becomes emergent. This may result in increased mortality in some cases.[60]

The frequency of surgery in patients older than 80 years is increasing.[60] Mortality is from 30 to 40% for emergency surgery and about 10% for elective surgery, with several reports of less than 5% mortality. Surgery may result in long-term improvement in survival in the elderly. A large study in 1979 of surgical mortality in the elderly[61] found 33% of mortality resulting from pulmonary emboli, 20% from pneumonia, 11% from cardiovascular collapse (without evidence of MI), and 9% from the primary illness. Aspiration, strokes, and gastrointestinal bleeding accounted for 6% each and MI only 2%. The highest death rates were in patients having abdominal procedures because of perforation, obstruction, or bowel infarction. In this study, cardiac disease was common; cardiac disease alone or in combination with diabetes, gangrene, dementia, or pulmonary disease accounted for 44 of the 54 deaths. Heart failure, MI, pulmonary complications, and pulmonary embolism are the most common postoperative problems.

Preoperative care of the elderly differs little from that of younger patients except that the physician must be aware of the physiologic decrements of aging. Although the elderly can often withstand the initial stress of surgery, if a complication ensues they have less physiologic reserve and are much less likely to survive.

Preoperative Considerations in the Pregnant Patient

The rate of nonobstetric surgery during pregnancy has remained low at about 2 per 1000 pregnancies.[62] The surgical problems that occur most commonly during pregnancy are acute appendicitis (1 of 1500 pregnancies) and intestinal obstruction (1 to 3 per 10,000 pregnancies). Other surgical problems include cholecystitis, spontaneous visceral rupture, and perforated duodenal ulcer, but these are rare.[63]

In addition to the usual measures commensurate with the severity and type of underlying condition, the preoperative management of the pregnant patient must take into account the presence of an additional patient—the fetus. Maternal physiology and alteration of anatomic landmarks often cause delay in diagnosis and misdiagnosis of surgical problems in pregnant patients.[64]

During pregnancy there are major increases in alveolar ventilation, cardiac output, oxygen consumption, and glomerular filtration rate. Increased blood volume, decreased systemic vascular resistance, and impaired venous return also occur.[62] The stresses of pregnancy and childbirth may unmask certain underlying pathologic conditions. When possible, it is preferable to identify conditions that may lead to intrapartum surgical complications before pregnancy (e.g., symptomatic gallstones and congenital heart disease).

As soon as an acute surgical problem has been identified, operative intervention is urgent. Delayed intervention, not pregnancy itself, contributes to increased fetal and maternal mortality. Preservation of maternal oxygen delivery to the placenta is of paramount importance. The severity of the underlying disease, intraoperative hypoxia, and hemodynamic instability are more important than the surgery itself in predicting fetal and maternal morbidity and mortality. In addition to continuous blood pressure and urine output measurements, pulmonary arterial catheterization is helpful for guiding preoperative resuscitation and monitoring the status of oxygen delivery in patients with hemodynamic instability. Perioperative nasogastric suctioning is helpful in preventing aspiration secondary to delayed gastric emptying. After the 26th week of gestation, fetal heart monitoring should be employed.[63] Radiographic and radionuclide studies should be minimized, especially during the first trimester, when the fetus is most susceptible. Ultrasonography is safe and useful for both fetal and maternal evaluations. Drugs that may be teratogenic should be avoided whenever possible.

Less acute surgical problems that arise during pregnancy should be addressed during the second trimester because uterine size, fetal stability, and placental stability are optimal compared with those in the third trimester. Premature labor may occur during the third trimester. The risk of spontaneous abortion is greatest during the first trimester.

An effort should be made to avoid surgery during pregnancy if medical management of the condition will suffice. Such conditions may include cholecystitis, peptic ulcer disease, pancreatitis, and inflammatory bowel disease.

Preoperative Considerations in the Transplant Recipient

Advances in immunosuppression (e.g., cyclosporine, FK 506) and perioperative care have made organ transplantation an important modality in the treatment of many end-stage diseases. Specific issues regarding the transplantation of particular organs are beyond the scope of this chapter. Some general guidelines are given here.

Pretransplantation evaluation should consist of a full work-up of the primary disease necessitating transplantation, optimization of physiologic status, treatment of infections, work-up for occult malignancies, minimization of risk of post-transplantation complications, and the need for preoperative ICU care and monitoring.[65] The patient's mental ability to handle the stress of transplantation must be evaluated. Psychosocial, family, and financial support systems are important.

A thorough pretransplantation evaluation of major organ systems is required for selecting the best transplantation candidates and effectively treating correctable problems, such as significant CAD, preoperatively. Active infection or malignancy (uncontrolled primary tumor or metastatic disease) must be treated and eradicated before transplantation so that immunosuppressive therapy can be given. A thorough evaluation for sites of infection is essential. In addition to the usual respiratory tract, urinary tract, and blood assessment, diagnosis and treatment of dental and skin infection are important. Isoniazid is given postoperatively to those with evidence of tuberculosis infection (a positive purified protein derivative test). Titers of viruses (e.g., human immunodeficiency virus, cytomegalovirus, herpes simplex virus, and Epstein-Barr virus) are determined preoperatively and compared postoperatively in diagnosing postoperative viral infections.

Relative contraindications to transplantation include acquired immunodeficiency syndrome, hepatitis, advanced disease in another organ system, and a history of substance abuse.

Preoperative care of patients before liver and heart transplantation often takes place in the ICU, whereas renal and pancreatic transplantation candidates are often managed preoperatively on the ward. Patients undergoing liver or heart transplantation routinely receive invasive perioperative hemodynamic monitoring and optimization via arterial and pulmonary arterial catheters.

Preoperative Nutritional Support

It is beyond the scope of this section to discuss nutritional support in detail. What follows are some general guidelines and considerations for preoperative nutritional support.

Improvement of the nutritional status before undertaking major surgical procedures can be beneficial. Preoperative malnutrition is associated with higher surgical morbidity (infection, poor wound healing) and mortality.[66, 67] This is related to the severity of underlying conditions contributing to malnutrition as well as to malnutrition itself.

Postoperative complications that increase catabolism and prevent enteral intake worsen the nutritional status. Elective, major surgical procedures should therefore be postponed if a poor nutritional state can be improved preoperatively. This depends on the underlying disorder, the integrity of the gastrointestinal tract, and the urgency for operation (i.e., the length of time available for preoperative nutritional support).

Although extensive anthropometric and immunologic tests have been used to classify degrees of malnutrition, as a group they lack adequate sensitivity and specificity.[68] Patients can be better separated into risk groups on the basis of a thorough history and physical examination and a serum transferrin or albumin determination.[69] In this scheme, patients are grouped into three categories: normal status, mild-to-moderate malnutrition, or severe malnutrition.

1. Severe malnutrition is defined as greater than 12% loss of the usual body weight along with a serum albumin level less than 3.5 g/dL and serum transferrin level less than 220 mg/dL.
2. Mild-to-moderate malnutrition is defined as a recent weight loss of 6 to 12% of usual body weight when the serum albumin level is greater than 3.5 g/dL and the serum transferrin level is greater than 220 mg/dL.
3. Patients with a normal status have a serum albumin level greater than 3.5 g/dL and a serum transferrin level greater than 220 mg/dL and have lost less than 6% of their usual body weight.

The well-nourished patient does not require any preoperative dietary intervention other than an ad libitum diet. There is no demonstrable benefit in giving preoperative intravenous nutrition (TPN) to these patients.[70, 71]

In the malnourished patient, the benefit of preoperative TPN versus enteral feeding is controversial.[72] In one study, 34 malnourished patients with a prognostic nutritional index above 30% who were about to undergo major gastrointestinal surgery were randomized to 10 days of preoperative TPN or a standard diet. In the TPN group, there were significant improvements in weight gain, triceps skin fold, and prognostic nutritional index, but there were no significant differences in the number of major complications (TPN, 6; control, 3) or mortality (TPN, 1; control, 3). The overall hospital stay was 38 days in the control group and 44 days in the TPN group.[73] In another prospective study, 459 moderately malnourished patients undergoing major operations were randomized to receive TPN for 10 days before surgery or ad libitum diets.[74] There was no significant difference in

terms of mortality (TPN, 13%; control, 11%) or complications (TPN, 26%; control, 25%), but the incidence of sepsis was higher in the TPN group (TPN, 14%; control, 6%). Perioperative TPN may not provide any advantages over enteral feeding, is more costly, and may lead to more septic complications.

The studies cited compared TPN with enteral feeding, not with complete starvation. It is probable that in cases of little or no oral intake, TPN is better than no caloric intake at all. The length of time that TPN can be given before surgery may be important for deriving significant nutritional benefits. Further studies are needed to determine the timing, clinical situations, and benefits derived from preoperative TPN.

Prophylactic Antibiotics for Surgery

Antimicrobial prophylaxis can decrease the incidence of infection after certain operations. It is particularly effective in preventing wound infection.[75] Prophylaxis, although routinely used, is not routinely indicated because of cost and potential toxic and allergic side effects.

The type of surgery and the presence of structural heart disease are the major factors determining the selection of antimicrobial prophylaxis:

1. Clean surgery occurs when there are no major breaks in surgical technique and the gastrointestinal, respiratory, and genitourinary tracts are not penetrated. The risk of infection in this group is less than 5%.[76] Prophylaxis is generally not indicated for clean surgery unless prosthetic implants are involved. Routine prophylaxis is also not indicated in cardiac catheterization, endoscopy of the gastrointestinal tract, repair of simple lacerations, outpatient treatment of burns, or placement of "lines" (e.g., central venous catheter and arterial line).[75]
2. Clean-contaminated surgery occurs when the gastrointestinal, respiratory, or genitourinary tract is entered but the surgical fields remain relatively uncontaminated. The rate of infectious complications in this group is about 10%.[76] Antibiotics aimed at the surgical site and flora are started at the time of surgery and continued for not more than 24 hours.
3. Contaminated procedures occur during major gastrointestinal spillage, surgery through traumatic wounds, and major breaks in surgical technique. The incidence of infection in this group is about 20%.[76] Antibiotics are started at the time of surgery and continued for not more than 48 hours.
4. "Dirty" procedures are those done in the presence of an established infection (e.g., abscess and gangrene). The risk of wound infection is high in this group: 30 to 40%.[76] Antibiotics in this group constitute treatment rather than prophylaxis and are continued until the disease is cured.
5. Endocarditis prophylaxis is indicated in patients with previous endocarditis, prosthetic heart valves, rheumatic heart disease, congenital heart disease (excluding uncomplicated ostium secundum defect), idiopathic hypertrophic subaortic stenosis, and mitral valve prolapse with regurgitation.[75] There are no controlled trials of antibiotic regimens for endocarditis prophylaxis. Recommendations are based on indirect information.[76] In a small number of cases, antimicrobial prophylaxis may not prevent endocarditis.
6. Immunosuppressed patients undergoing transplantation are often given perioperative antibiotic prophylaxis to cover organisms likely to cause postoperative infection.[65]
7. Antimicrobial prophylaxis is not routinely indicated for cardiac catheterization, gastrointestinal endoscopy, thoracocentesis, or line insertion (e.g., arterial and central venous).

TABLE 137-9

ANTIBIOTIC PROPHYLAXIS IN SURGERY

Clean Surgery

Type of Operation	Likely Pathogens	Drugs of Choice	Adult Dosage*
Cardiac: open heart surgery, prosthetic valve surgery	*Staphylococcus epidermidis, S. aureus, Corynebacterium,* enteric gram-negative bacilli	Cefazolin or vancomycin† (some experts prefer cefuroxime [Zinacef] to cefazolin)	1 g IV 1 g IV
Thoracic noncardiac	Pulmonary resection: conflicting results in controlled trials; some show a reduction in wound infection, but not in pneumonia or empyema Closed tube thoracostomy for chest trauma or spontaneous pneumothorax: no decrease in infection rate with prophylactic antibiotics		
Vascular Abdominal aortic surgery or prosthesis	*S. aureus, S. epidermidis,* enteric gram-negative bacilli	Cefazolin or vancomycin	1 g IV
Lower extremity amputation for ischemia	*S. aureus, S. epidermidis,* enteric gram-negative bacilli, *Clostridium*	Cefazolin	1 g IV
Orthopedic: total joint replacement, internal fixation of fractures	*S. aureus, S. epidermidis*	Cefazolin or vancomycin	1 g IV
Neurosurgery	Cerebrospinal fluid shunt: no decrease in infection rate with prophylactic antibiotics Spinal surgery: postoperative rate of infection so low that prophylactic antibiotics are unjustified Craniotomies: an antistaphylococcal antibiotic may decrease the incidence of wound infection; further studies are needed		
Ocular surgery	*S. aureus, S. epidermidis,* streptococci, enteric gram-negative bacilli, *Pseudomonas*	Gentamicin or tobramycin or neomycin + gramicidin + polymyxin B	Multiple drops topically over 2 to 24 h

Clean-Contaminated Surgery

Colorectal	Enteric gram-negative bacilli, anaerobes	Oral: neomycin plus erythromycin base	1 g of each at 1 PM, 2 PM, and 11 PM on day before surgery
Appendectomy	Enteric gram-negative bacilli, anaerobes	Cefoxitin	1 g IV
Hysterectomy: vaginal or abdominal	Enteric gram-negative bacilli, anaerobes, group B streptococci, enterococci	Cefazolin	1 g IV
Cesarean section: only for high-risk patients: active labor, ruptured membranes	Enteric gram-negative bacilli, anaerobes, group B streptococci, enterococci	Cefazolin	1 g IV after cord clamping
Abortion: first-trimester abortion with history of pelvic inflammatory disease	Enteric gram-negative bacilli, anaerobes, group B streptococci, enterococci	Aqueous penicillin G or doxycycline	1 million U IV 300 mg PO
After second-trimester abortion		Cefazolin	1 g IV
Urology	Antimicrobial prophylaxis is not recommended in patients with sterile urine. If urine cultures are positive, antibiotics should be given until the urine cultures are negative, or a single preoperative dose of an appropriate antibiotic may be given at the time of surgery.		

Dirty Surgery

Ruptured viscus	Enteric gram-negative bacilli, anaerobes, enterococci	Cefoxitin with or without gentamicin or clindamycin + gentamicin	Cefoxitin: 1 g q 6 h IV Gentamicin: 1.5 mg/kg q 8h IV Clindamycin: 600 mg IV q 6 h
Traumatic wound	*S. aureus,* group A streptococci, clostridia	Cefazolin	1 g q 8h IV
Bite wounds	Above + oral anaerobes: human, *Eikenella corrodens;* dog or cat, *Pasteurella multocida*	Amoxicillin–clavulanic acid (Augmentin) or ampicillin-sulbactam (Unasyn)	500 mg PO q 8 H 2 g q 6 h IV

*Cefazolin may be given IM.

†Use vancomycin if rate of methacillin-resistant wound infection is high, or allergy to penicillin or cephalosporin.

Adapted from Antimicrobial prophylaxis. In: Abramowicz M (ed): Handbook of Antimicrobial Therapy. New Rochelle, NY, The Medical Letter, p 76, 1990.

TABLE 137-10

RECOMMENDED ANTIBIOTIC PROPHYLAXIS FOR ENDOCARDITIS

Type of Procedure	Pathogens	Drugs of Choice	Adult Dosage
Dental and upper respiratory tract procedures	Streptococcus viridans	Oral	
		Amoxicillin	3 g before procedure, 1.5 g 6 h later
		Erythromycin (if penicillin allergic)	1 g 2 h before procedure and 500 mg 6 h later
		Parenteral	
		Ampicillin and	2 g IV or IM 30 min before procedure
		Gentamicin	1.5 mg/kg IV or IM 30 min before procedure
		Vancomycin alone (if penicillin allergic)	1 g infused slowly over 1 h, 1 h before procedure
Gastrointestinal and genitourinary procedures	Enterococci	Oral	
		Amoxicillin	3 g before procedure, 1.5 g 6 h later
		Parenteral	
		Ampicillin and	2 g IV or IM 30 min before procedure
		Gentamicin	1.5 mg/kg IV or IM 30 min before procedure
		Vancomycin and	1 g infused slowly over 1 h, 1 h before procedure
		Gentamicin (if penicillin allergic)	1.5 mg/kg IV or IM 30 min before procedure

Adapted from Antimicrobial prophylaxis. In: Abramowicz M (ed): Handbook of Antimicrobial Therapy. New Rochelle, NY, The Medical Letter, p 76, 1990.

One dose of a parenteral antibiotic given within 30 minutes before surgery usually provides adequate tissue concentrations for several hours.[75] During prolonged surgery or massive blood loss, a second dose is advisable. Postoperative antibiotics are not necessary unless an infection is thought to be present.

The clinical data regarding optimal antibiotic prophylactic regimens for every situation are not clear. Such studies are difficult to perform and interpret. Currently recommended antimicrobial prophylactic regimens are summarized in Tables 137–9 and 137–10.

Preoperative Prophylaxis for Venous Thromboembolism

The highest incidence of venous thromboembolism is seen in the postoperative period (Table 137–11).[77] Patients undergoing orthopedic surgery on the lower extremities or those with hip fracture have the greatest risk of thromboembolism: a 40% chance of developing deep venous throm-

TABLE 137-11

RISK GROUPS FOR VENOUS THROMBOEMBOLISM

Treatment Group	Incidence of Deep Venous Thrombosis (%)	Site	Incidence of Fatal Pulmonary Embolism (%)
Orthopedic surgery (hip fracture, total hip replacement, total knee replacement)	40–70	Thigh or calf	1–5
Neurosurgery	15–20*	Calf	1
General and gynecologic surgery	15–20	Calf	1
Urologic surgery	15–20	Calf	5
Medical patients	15	Calf	1

*Some studies report up to a 43% incidence of deep venous thrombosis in neurosurgery patients.[82]

Modified from Hyers TM, Hull RD, Weg JG: Antithrombotic therapy for venous thromboembolic disease. Chest 95:37S, 1989.

bosis, 20% in the calf and 20% in the thigh.[77] Thrombi in the proximal veins are more likely to embolize to the lungs, resulting in pulmonary embolism. The major risk factors for the development of venous thromboembolism are prevalent in this population and include venous stasis (bed rest, immobility, CHF) and trauma (surgery, childbirth). The other risk factors are old age, estrogen intake, and carcinoma (especially adenocarcinoma of breast, lung, and viscera).

The goal is primary prevention of thromboembolism. Current prophylactic regimens can reduce the incidence of thromboembolic disease by 50 to 60%.[77]

Preoperative Measures

Patients undergoing elective hip surgery should be pretreated prophylactically with adjusted-dose heparin to prolong the aPTT in the upper half of the normal range or moderate-dose warfarin to prolong the PT to 1.3 to 1.5 times control (using rabbit brain thromboplastin).[77-79] Patients undergoing surgery for hip fracture should be pretreated with moderate-dose warfarin to prolong the PT to 1.3 to 1.5 times control.[77] Future prophylactic therapies may include low-dose warfarin at 1 mg/d for 3 weeks preoperatively[80] or low-molecular-weight heparin,[81] but further studies are needed.

Postoperative Measures

The preventive treatment of choice for moderate-risk patients is low-dose subcutaneous heparin at a dose of 5000 U every 8 to 12 hours or intermittent pneumatic compression. They are effective in preventing deep venous thrombosis after general surgery, acute MI, respiratory failure, elective thoracic or abdominal surgery, stroke, and acute spinal syndromes resulting in para- or quadriplegia.[77]

Intermittent pneumatic compression is recommended for patients undergoing major knee surgery, urologic surgery, and neurosurgery.[77] Heparin is not as effective in these patients and may be dangerous in neurosurgical patients, in whom even a minimal amount of bleeding can be harmful.

References

1. Blery C, Charpak Y, Szatan M, et al: Evaluation of a protocol for selective ordering of preoperative tests. Lancet 1:139, 1986.

2. Kaplan EB, Boeckman MF, Roizen MF, et al: Elimination of unnecessary preoperative laboratory tests. Anesthesiology 57:A445, 1982.
3. Hampton JR, Harrison MJG, Mitchell JRA, et al: Relative contributions of history-taking, physical examination, and laboratory investigation to diagnosis and management of medical outpatients. Br Med J 2:486, 1975.
4. Cebul RD, Whisnant JP: Indications for carotid endarterectomy. Ann Intern Med 111:675, 1989.
5. Merli GJ, Bell RD: Preoperative management of the patient with neurologic disease. Med Clin North Am 71:511, 1987.
6. DeWeese JA, Rob CG, Satran R, et al: Surgical treatment for occlusive disease of the carotid artery. Ann Surg 168:85, 1968.
7. Cebul RD, Whisnant JP: Carotid endarterectomy. Ann Intern Med 111:660, 1989.
8. Leventhal SR, Orkin FK, Hirsch RA: Prediction of the need for postoperative mechanical ventilation in myasthenia gravis. Anesthesiology 53:26, 1980.
9. Latimer RG, Dickman M, Clinton Day WC, et al: Ventilatory patterns and pulmonary complications after upper abdominal surgery determined by preoperative and postoperative computerized spirometry and blood gas analysis. Am J Surg 122:622, 1971.
10. Tisi GM: Preoperative evaluation of pulmonary function: Validity, indications, and benefits. Am Rev Respir Dis 119:293, 1979.
11. Collins CD, Drake CS, Knowelden J: Chest complications after upper abdominal surgery: Their anticipation and prevention. Br Med J 1:401, 1968.
12. Wernly JA, DeMeester TR, Kirchner PT, et al: Clinical value of quantitative ventilation-perfusion lung scans in the surgical management of bronchogenic carcinoma. J Thorac Cardiovasc Surg 80:535, 1980.
13. Olsen GN, Block AJ, Tobias JA: Prediction of postpneumonectomy pulmonary function using quantitative macroaggregate lung scanning. Chest 66:13, 1974.
14. Gass GD, Olsen GN: Preoperative pulmonary function testing to predict postoperative morbidity and mortality. Chest 89:127, 1986.
15. Fee JH, Holmes EC, Gerwirtz HS, et al: Role of pulmonary vascular resistance measurements in preoperative evaluation of candidates for pulmonary resection. J Thorac Cardiovasc Surg 75:519, 1978.
16. Smith TP, Kinasewitz GT, Tucker WY, et al: Exercise capacity as a predictor of post-thoracotomy morbidity. Am Rev Respir Dis 129:730, 1984.
17. Eugene J, Brown SE, Light RW, et al: Maximum oxygen consumption: A physiology guide to pulmonary resection. Surg Forum 33:260, 1982.
18. Zibrak JD, O'Donnell CR, Marton K: Indications for pulmonary function testing. Ann Intern Med 112:763, 1990.
19. Celli BR, Rodriguez KS, Snider GS: A controlled trial of intermittent positive pressure breathing, incentive spirometry, and deep breathing exercises in preventing pulmonary complications after abdominal surgery. Am Rev Respir Dis 130:12, 1984.
20. Goldman L, Caldera DL, Nussbaum SR, et al: Multifactorial index of cardiac risk in noncardiac surgical procedures. N Engl J Med 297:845, 1977.
21. Weitz HH, Goldman L: Noncardiac surgery in the patient with heart disease. Med Clin North Am 71:413, 1987.
22. Boucher CA, Brewster DC, Darling RC, et al: Determination of cardiac risk by dipyridamole-thallium imaging before peripheral vascular surgery. N Engl J Med 312:389, 1985.
23. Jeffrey CC, Kunsman J, Cullen D, et al: A prospective evaluation of cardiac risk. Anesthesiology 58:462, 1983.
24. Gerson MC, Hurst JM, Hertzberg VS, et al: Cardiac prognosis in noncardiac geriatric surgery. Ann Intern Med 103:832, 1985.
25. Detsky AS, Abrams HB, McLaughlin JR, et al: Predicting cardiac complications in patients undergoing noncardiac surgery. J Gen Intern Med 1:211, 1986.
26. Zeldin RA: Assessing cardiac risk in patients who undergo noncardiac surgical procedures. Can J Surg 27:402, 1984.
27. Deron SJ, Kotler MN: Noncardiac surgery in the cardiac patient. Am Heart J 116:831, 1988.
28. Goldman L, Caldera DL: Risks of general anesthesia and elective operation in the hypertensive patient. Anesthesiology 50:285, 1979.
29. Raby KE, Goldman L, Creager MA, et al: Correlation between preoperative ischemia and major cardiac events after peripheral vascular surgery. N Engl J Med 321:1296, 1989.
30. Eagle KA, Coley CM, Newell JB, et al: Combining clinical and thallium data optimizes preoperative assessment of cardiac risk before major vascular surgery. Ann Intern Med 110:859, 1989.
31. Bernstein EF, Dilley RB, Randolph HF III: The improving long-term outlook for patients over 70 years of age with abdominal aortic aneurysms. Ann Surg 207:318, 1988.
32. Grindlinger GA, Armando MV, Manny J, et al: Volume loading and vasodilators in abdominal aortic aneurysmectomy. Am J Surg 139:480, 1980.
33. Bush HL, LoGerfo FW, Weisel RD, et al: Assessment of myocardial performances and optimal volume loading during elective abdominal aortic aneurysm resection. Arch Surg 112:1301, 1977.
34. Tarhan S, Moffitt EA, Taylor WF, et al: Myocardial infarction after general anesthesia. JAMA 220:1451, 1972.
35. Rao TL, Jacobs KH, El-Etr AA: Reinfarction following anesthesia in patients with myocardial infarction. Anesthesiology 59:499, 1983.
36. Shah KB, Kleinman BS, Sami H, et al: Reevaluation of perioperative myocardial infarction in patients with prior myocardial infarction undergoing noncardiac operations. Anesth Analg 71:231, 1990.
37. Shah K, Kleinman B, Rao T, et al: Reduction in mortality from cardiac causes in Goldman class IV patients. J Cardiothoracic Anesth 2:789, 1988.
38. Eagle KA, Boucher CA: Cardiac risk of noncardiac surgery (editorial). N Engl J Med 321:1330, 1989.
39. Mahar LJ, Steen PA, Tinker JH, et al: Perioperative myocardial infarction in patients with coronary artery disease with and without aorta-coronary bypass grafts. J Thorac Cardiovasc Surg 76:533, 1978.
40. Scheppel SL, Wilkinson C, Waters J, et al: Effects of myocardial infarction on perioperative cardiac complications. Anesth Analg 62:493, 1983.
41. Foster ED, Davis KB, Carpenter JA, et al: Risk of noncardiac operation in patients with defined coronary artery disease: The coronary artery surgery study (CASS) registry experience. Ann Thorac Surg 41:42, 1986.
42. Gordon SJ, Chatzinoff M, Peikin SR: Medical care of the surgical patient with gastrointestinal disease. Med Clin North Am 71:433, 1987.
43. Benjamin E, Iberti TJ: Visceral ischemia and sepsis. In: Kaplan JA (ed): Vascular Anesthesia. New York, Churchill Livingstone, p 417, 1991.
44. Friedman LS, Maddrey WC: Surgery in the patient with liver disease. Med Clin North Am 71:453, 1987.
45. Garrison RN, Cryer HM, Howard DA, et al: Clarification of risk factors for abdominal operations in patients with hepatic cirrhosis. Ann Surg 199:648, 1984.
46. Burke JF, Francos GC: Surgery in the patient with acute or chronic renal failure. Med Clin North Am 71:489, 1987.
47. Goldmann DR: Surgery in patients with endocrine dysfunction. Med Clin North Am 71:499, 1987.
48. Caldwell MD: Diabetes mellitus. In: Wilmore DW, Brennan MF, Harken AH, et al (eds): Care of the Surgical Patient, Volume 2, Elective Care, Section VII, Chapter 1. New York, Scientific American, p 1, 1988.
49. Siddiq KY, Gebhart SSP: Disorders of the thyroid gland. In: Lubin MF, Walker HK, Smith RB (eds): Medical Management of the Surgical Patient. 2nd ed. Stoneham, MA, Butterworth, p 292, 1988.
50. Siddiq KY, Watts NB: Disorders of the adrenal gland. In: Lubin MF, Walker HK, Smith RB (eds): Medical Management of the Surgical Patient. 2nd ed. Stoneham, MA, Butterworth, p 301, 1988.
51. Siddiq KY, Watts NB: Pheochromocytoma. In: Lubin MF, Walker HK, Smith RB (eds): Medical Management of the Surgical Patient. 2nd ed. Stoneham, MA, Butterworth, p 305, 1988.
52. Greenberg GA. Indications for transfusion. In: Wilmore DW, Brennan MF, Harken AH, et al (eds): Care of the Surgical Patient, Volume 1, Critical Care. New York, Scientific American, p 1, 1988.
53. Toy PT, Strauss RG, Stehling LC, et al: Predeposited autologous blood for elective surgery. A national multicenter study. N Engl J Med 316:517, 1987.
54. Sandler SG, Naiman JL, Fletcher JL: Alternative approaches to transfusion: Autologous blood and directed blood donations. Prog Hematol 15:183, 1987.
55. Fellin F, Murphy S: Hematologic problems in the preoperative period. Med Clin North Am 71:477, 1987.
56. Amin DN, Iberti TJ: Use of the surgical intensive care unit in the preoperative preparation of the high-risk patient. J Cardiothorac Anesth 4(suppl 1):13, 1990.
57. Iberti TJ, Fischer EP, Leibowitz AB, et al: A multicenter study of physician's knowledge of the pulmonary artery catheter. JAMA 264:2928, 1990.
58. McClay EF, Bellet RE: Preoperative evaluation of the oncology patient. Med Clin North Am 71:529, 1987.
59. Lubin MF: Preoperative considerations in the elderly patient. In: Lubin MF, Walker HK, Smith RB (eds): Medical Management of the Surgical Patient. 2nd ed. Stoneham, MA, Butterworth, p 381, 1988.
60. Keating HJ III: Preoperative considerations in the geriatric patient. Med Clin North Am 71:568, 1987.
61. Palmberg S, Hirsjarvi E: Mortality in geriatric surgery. Gerontology 25:103, 1979.
62. Barron WM: The pregnant surgical patient: Medical evaluation and management. Ann Intern Med 101:683, 1984.
63. Brooks DC: Pregnancy. In: Wilmore DW, Brennan MF, Harken AH, et al (eds): Care of the Surgical Patient, Volume 2, Elective Care, Section VII, Chapter 11. New York: Scientific American, p 1, 1988.
64. Kammerer WS: Nonobstetric surgery in pregnancy. Med Clin North Am 71:551, 1987.
65. Gruber SA, Cerra FB: General principles of perioperative transplant care. Crit Care Clin 6:893, 1990.
66. Mullen JL, Gertner MH, Buzby GP, et al: Implications of malnutrition in the surgical patient. Arch Surg 114:121, 1979.
67. Muller JM, Brenner U, Dienst C, et al: Preoperative parenteral feeding in patients with gastrointestinal carcinoma. Lancet 1:68, 1982.
68. Weiss SM: Nutritional aspects of preoperative management. Med Clin North Am 71:369, 1987.
69. Daly J: Malnutrition. In: Wilmore DW, Brennan MF, Harken AH, et al (eds): Care of the Surgical Patient, Volume 2, Elective Care, Section VII, Chapter 12. New York, Scientific American, p 1, 1988.
70. Detsky AS, Baker JP, O'Rourke K, et al: Perioperative parenteral nutrition: A meta-analysis. Ann Intern Med 107:195, 1987.

71. American College of Physicians: Position paper: Perioperative parenteral nutrition. Ann Intern Med 107:252, 1987.
72. Zaloga GP, MacGregor DA: What to consider when choosing enteral or parenteral nutrition. J Crit Illness 5(11):1180, 1990.
73. Smith RC, Hartemick R: Improvement of nutritional measures during preoperative parenteral nutrition in patients selected by the prognostic nutritional index: A randomized controlled study. JPEN 12:587, 1988.
74. The Veterans Affairs Total Parenteral Nutrition Cooperative Study Group: Perioperative total parenteral nutrition in surgical patients. New Engl J Med 325:525, 1991.
75. Antimicrobial prophylaxis. In: Abramowicz M (ed): Handbook of Antimicrobial Therapy. New Rochelle, NY, The Medical Letter, p 76, 1990.
76. Bergquist EJ, Murphey SA: Prophylactic antibiotics for surgery. Med Clin North Am 71:357, 1987.
77. Hyers TM, Hull RD, Weg JG: Antithrombotic therapy for venous thromboembolic disease. Chest 95:37S, 1989.
78. Francis CW, Marder VJ, McCollister EC, et al: Two step warfarin therapy. JAMA 249:374, 1983.
79. Leyvraz PF, Richard J, Bachmann F, et al: Adjusted versus fixed dose subcutaneous heparin in the prevention of deep vein thrombosis after total hip replacement. N Engl J Med 309:954, 1983.
80. Poller L, McKernan A, Thompson JM, et al: Fixed mini-dose warfarin: A new approach to the prophylaxis of venous thrombosis after major surgery. Br Med J 295:1309, 1987.
81. Turpie AGC, Levine MN, Hirsh J, et al: A randomized controlled trial of a low molecular weight heparin (enoxaparin) to prevent deep vein thrombosis in patients undergoing elective hip surgery. N Engl J Med 315:925, 1986.
82. Skillman JJ, Collins R, Coe N, et al: Prevention of DVT in neurosurgical patients: A controlled, randomized, trial of external pneumatic compression. Surgery 83:354, 1978.

CHAPTER 138

Care of the Trauma Patient

Edmund J. Rutherford
Loren D. Nelson

More than 140,000 Americans die of injury each year, making injury the fourth leading cause of death overall and the leading cause of death in individuals up to the age of 44 years.[1] The cost is estimated at $75 to $100 billion a year, and trauma surpasses all major disease groups in terms of loss of productive life with more than 4 million years of future work life lost to death and disability each year. Because of this impact, injury has been dubbed "the neglected epidemic."[2]

Deaths resulting from trauma can be categorized into a trimodal distribution.[3] The majority of deaths occur within the first few minutes after injury and are usually due to lacerations of the brain, the brain stem, the high spinal cord, the heart, and the aorta or other large vessels (Figure 138–1). The second peak occurs within the first few hours and is usually due to subdural and epidural hematomas, hemopneumothorax, ruptured spleen, lacerations of the liver, pelvic fractures, or multiple injuries associated with significant blood loss. Because quick and systematic management of these injuries can be lifesaving for the majority of these patients, this population of patients makes up the thrust of the Advanced Trauma Life Support Course as put forth by the American College of Surgeons.[4] This period has been referred to as the "golden hour." The third peak occurs days to weeks after injury and represents patients in the intensive care unit (ICU) who succumb to closed head injury,

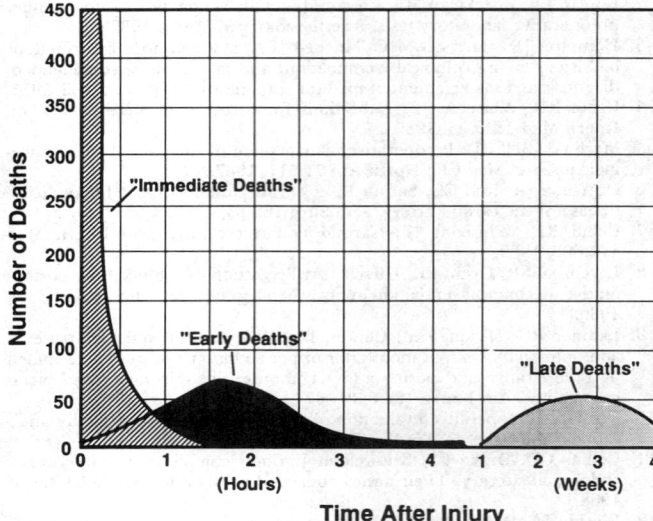

Figure 138–1. Trimodal distribution of trauma deaths. (From Trunkey DD: Trauma. Copyright © 1983 by Scientific American, Inc. All rights reserved.)

sepsis, and late organ failure. Review of this trimodal curve demonstrates some variation in the distribution of deaths for certain subpopulations such as the elderly, patients with head injuries, and persons with burns.[5]

Although not a priority, tetanus prophylaxis should be addressed in the emergency department. Recommendations by the American College of Surgeons are based on the condition of the wound and previous immunization.[4] Wounds are categorized according to low risk and high risk of tetanus (Table 138–1). In addition to immunization (Table 138–2), all high-risk wounds should be débrided of all devitalized tissue and foreign bodies.

An objective assessment of the severity of trauma can be based on one of many scoring systems. The two most common scoring systems in trauma are the Trauma Score and the Injury Severity Score.[6, 7] The Trauma Score has subsequently been revised and now only includes the Glasgow Coma Scale (Table 138–3), systolic blood pressure, and respiratory rate[8, 9] (Table 138–4). The Revised Trauma Score directly correlates with survival (Fig. 138–2) and can be used as a triage tool.[10]

TABLE 138–1
WOUND CHARACTERISTICS AND TETANUS RISK

Parameter	Low Risk	High Risk
Mechanism	Sharp (e.g., knife, glass)	Burn, missile, crush, frostbite
Time	≤6 h	>6 h
Wound type	Linear	Abrasion, stellate, puncture, avulsion
Depth	≤1 cm	>1 cm
Contaminants	None	Dirt, soil, feces, saliva
Devitalized, denervated, or ischemic tissue	Absent	Present
Infection	Absent	Present

Adapted from Committee on Trauma of the American College of Surgeons: Tetanus immunization. In: Advanced Trauma Life Support Course. Chicago, American College of Surgeons, p 272, 1989.

TABLE 138-2
RECOMMENDATIONS FOR TETANUS IMMUNIZATION

Previous Immunization	Low Risk of Tetanus*	High Risk of Tetanus*
Unknown or ≤3	Td†	Td and TIG
>3	Td if >10 y since last dose	Td if >5 y since last dose

*Td = tetanus and diphtheria toxoids; TIG = tetanus immune globulin.
†For children younger than 7 y of age, diphtheria, tetanus, and pertussis vaccine is preferred unless pertussis vaccine is contraindicated.
Adapted from Committee on Trauma of the American College of Surgeons: Tetanus immunization. In: Advanced Trauma Life Support Course. Chicago, American College of Surgeons, p 273, 1989.

The Injury Severity Score is based on the three worst injuries.[7] These injuries are graded on a scale of 1 to 5 using the Abbreviated Injury Scale[11] (Table 138-5). Each individual score is squared, and the sum is the Injury Severity Score. The Revised Trauma Score and Injury Severity Score can then be combined to give the TRISS probability of survival.[12] Other trauma scoring systems have been proposed and include the Anatomic Index,[13] the Triage Index,[14] and the Penetrating Abdominal Trauma Index.[15] Another commonly used scoring system is the Acute Physiology and Chronic Health Evaluation II (APACHE II).[16] The use of APACHE II in surgical patients, however, has been questioned.[17, 18]

The role of the ICU in the care of the critically injured patient includes continuation of the resuscitation and evaluation initiated in the emergency department and the operating room. This chapter focuses on the care of the trauma patient in the ICU after the initial resuscitation. It is essential that ongoing resuscitation be continuously evaluated and appropriate adjustments made.

TABLE 138-3
GLASGOW COMA SCALE

Category	Response	Points
1. Eyes open	Spontaneously	4
	To verbal command	3
	To pain	2
	No response	1
2. Best verbal response	Oriented and converses	5
	Disoriented and converses	4
	Inappropriate words	3
	Incomprehensible sounds	2
	No response	1
3. Best motor response	Obeys verbal commands	6
	Purposefully localizes pain	5
	Flexion—withdrawal to pain	4
	Flexion—abnormal to pain (decorticate rigidity)	3
	Extension to pain (decerebrate rigidity)	2
	No response to pain	1
Total score (minimum = 3, maximum = 15)		

TABLE 138-4
REVISED TRAUMA SCORE

Measure	No. of Points	Trauma Score
Glasgow Coma Scale	13–15	4
	9–12	3
	6–8	2
	4–5	1
	3	0
Systolic blood pressure (mm Hg)	>90	4
	70–89	3
	50–69	2
	1–49	1
	0	0
Respiratory rate (breaths/min)	10–24	4
	25–35	3
	>35	2
	1–9	1
	0	0
TOTAL		0–12

GENERAL APPROACH

There is a general misconception among physicians that trauma patients are generally young and healthy and therefore have tremendous physiologic reserves. In fact, greater numbers of older patients who have sustained major injuries are now surviving to the ICU phase of their care. These patients as well as younger patients with pre-existing medical conditions[19] have an increased mortality. Furthermore, the young and healthy trauma patient who is involved in a high-speed motor vehicle crash with severe multisystem injuries is no longer healthy.

Trauma is a multisystem disease that results in a loss of normal homeostatic mechanisms and places the patient in a situation of increased and abnormal physiologic demands. At the same time, access to normal metabolic substrates is removed. Pain, blood loss, fluid shifts, and sepsis all compound the physiologic abnormalities of injury.

The earliest abnormality is an increased pulmonary vascular resistance, which correlates with survival.[20] Right ventricular dysfunction also occurs early and may not affect left ventricular function.[21] Because of this discrepancy, a pul-

Text continued on page 1582

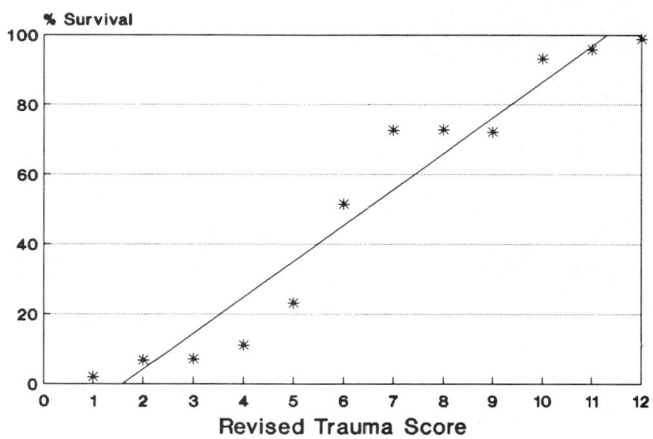

Figure 138-2. Revised trauma score and survival. Data on 7657 admissions from the Vanderbilt University Trauma Registry.

TABLE 138–5		
ABBREVIATED INJURY SCALE		
	1 **Minor**	**2** **Moderate**
External	Abrasion/contusion 　Superficial or unspecified/≤25 cm² on 　　face or 50 cm² on body Superficial or unspecified laceration 　Not into subcutaneous tissue regardless 　　of length 　Into subcutaneous tissue but ≤5 cm on 　　face or ≤10 cm on body 1° burn up to 100% 2° or 3° burn <6% total body	Major abrasion/contusion 　>25 cm² on face 　>50 cm² on body Deep laceration (into subcutaneous tissue) 　and >10 cm on body or >5 cm on face 2° or 3° burn to 6–15% total body
Head (includes face [F])	Awake on admission or initial observation 　No prior unconsciousness but may have 　　headache/dizziness resulting from 　　head trauma Ear canal injury Eyes (F) 　Conjunctival abrasion/contusion/ 　　laceration 　Corneal abrasion/contusion 　Lid abrasion/contusion/laceration 　Vitreous/retina/canaliculis (tear duct) 　　laceration 　Choroid rupture 　Uvea injury Gingiva (F) (gum) contusion/laceration Lip (F) contusion/laceration (no matter how 　extensive) Mandible (F) 　Fracture unspecified 　Ramus fracture Nose (F) fracture Teeth (F) avulsion/dislocation (loosened)/ 　fracture Superficial tongue (F) laceration	Awake on admission or initial observation 　Prior unconsciousness but length of time 　　unspecified 　Amnesia (no recollection of crash) 　Unconsciousness <15 min Lethargic, stuporous, obtunded on 　admission or initial observation (can 　be aroused by verbal stimuli) 　No prior unconsciousness 　Unconsciousness <15 min When level of consciousness on admission 　or initial observation is unknown 　Unconsciousness <15 min Medical diagnosis listed as concussion with 　no other description Fracture of vault (frontal, occipital, parietal 　sphenoid, temporal or unspecified) 　closed, undisplaced, diastatic, linear, 　simple, unspecified Ear 　Inner/middle-ear injury 　Ossicular bone dislocation 　Tympanic membrane rupture 　Avulsion of pinna (outer ear) Eye (F) 　Cornea laceration 　Sclera laceration/rupture Alveolar ridge (bone) (F) fracture with or 　without tooth injury Avulsion gingiva/lid/lip (F) Mandibular fracture (F) 　Ramus if open/displaced/comminuted 　Body with or without ramus involvement 　Subcondylar Maxilla fracture (F) closed/unspecified/Le 　Fort I/zygomatic fracture Tongue (F) deep and/or extensive 　laceration Nose (F) fracture open/displaced/ 　comminuted

TABLE 138–5

ABBREVIATED INJURY SCALE *Continued*

3 Severe, Not Life Threatening	4 Severe, Life Threatening	5 Critical, Survival Uncertain
2° or 3° burn to 16–35% total body	2° or 3° burn to 26–35% total body	2° or 3° burn to 36–90% total body

Awake on admission or initial observation
  Prior unconsciousness but length unspecified/amnesia
  Unconsciousness 15 min with neurologic deficit
  Unconsciousness 15–59 min
Lethargic, stuporous, obtunded on admission or initial observation (can be aroused by verbal stimuli)
  No prior unconsciousness/ unconsciousness <15 min with neurologic deficit
  Unconsciousness 15–59 min
  Prior unconsciousness/loss of consciousness unspecified
Unconsciousness on admission or initial observation (unresponsive to verbal commands)
  Length of unconsciousness unspecified
  Unconsciousness <1 h
When level of consciousness on admission or initial observation is unknown
  Unconsciousness 15–59 min
  Unconsciousness <15 min with neurologic deficit
Fracture of base (basilar ethmoid, orbital roof, sphenoid, temporal) without CSF leak
Comminuted compound, depressed, or displaced fracture of vault
Cerebellum or cerebrum
  Contusion
  Injury involving any of the following but no further anatomic description (subarachnoid hemorrhage, edema, brain swelling, subpial hemorrhage, hygroma, ischemia, infarction)
Zygomatic fracture (F) open/displaced/ comminuted
Eye (F)
  Avulsion
  Optic nerve avulsion/laceration
  Tear
Mandibular fracture (F)
  Ramus involvement/mandible fracture
  Subcondylar/body with or without ramus
  Involvement for any one displaced/ comminuted
Orbit fracture open/displaced, comminuted (F)
Le Fort II (F)
	Awake on admission or initial observation
	  Unconscious 15–59 min with neurologic deficit
	  Lethargic, stuporous, obtunded on admission or initial observation (can be aroused by verbal stimuli)
	  Unconsciousness 15–59 min/prior unconsciousness for unspecified length of time/unspecified loss of consciousness involving neurologic deficit
	Unconscious on admission or initial observation (unresponsive to verbal commands)
	  1–24 h (includes 1 calendar day when hours cannot be estimated)
	  Appropriate movements but only on painful stimuli (no matter the length of unconsciousness)
	  Length of unconsciousness unspecified/ unconscious <1 h involving neurologic deficit
	When level of consciousness on admission or initial observation is unknown, but unconscious for
	  1–24 h (includes 1 calendar day when hours cannot be estimated)
	  15–59 min involving neurologic deficit
	Fracture of base (basilar ethmoid, orbital roof, sphenoid, temporal) with CSF leak or pneumocephalus
	Fracture of vault (frontal occipital, parietal, sphenoid, temporal, unspecified) open/ dura torn/CSF leak/pneumocephalus or brain exposed
	Cerebellum or cerebrum
	  Laceration
	  Hematoma, epidural/subdural ≤100 mL or unspecified
	  Hematoma, intracerebral, intracerebellar (including petechial and subcortical hematoma)
	Le Fort III (F)
		Unconscious on admission or initial observation (unresponsive to verbal stimuli)
		  Inappropriate movements (decerebrate, decorticate, flaccid, no response to pain—no matter the length of unconsciousness) 1–24 h (includes 1 calendar day when hours cannot be estimated)/appropriate movements but only on painful stimuli (no matter the length of unconsciousness) with neurologic deficit
		When level of consciousness on admission or initial observation is unknown, but unconscious for
		  1–24 h (includes 1 calendar day when hours cannot be estimated) with neurologic deficit >24 h
		Brain stem
		  Compression/contusion/injury involving hemorrhage
		Cerebellum or cerebrum
		  Hematoma, epidural/subdural, >100 mL
		  Diffuse brain injury (white matter shearing injury)

Table continued on following page

	1 Minor	2 Moderate
TABLE 138–5		
ABBREVIATED INJURY SCALE *Continued*		
Neck	Pharynx contusion/laceration/puncture/ rupture Throat (inner soft tissue) abrasion/ contusion/laceration (not involving major artery) Tracheal contusion	Pharynx contusion with hematoma/ laceration with hemorrhage Contusion of esophagus/larynx/thyroid gland
Thorax	Rib contusion/fracture	Rib fracture open/displaced/>2 adjacent ribs up to flail chest Sternum fracture
Abdomen/pelvic contents (includes all described in parentheses)	Superficial or unspecified laceration/ perforation of abdominal wall (no organ involvement) Abrasion/contusion/superficial or unspecified laceration or perforation of scrotum/vagina/vulva/perineum Penis contusion Scrotum rupture	Abdominal wall avulsion Deep and/or extensive laceration or perforation of abdominal wall (no organ involvement)/scrotum Stomach contusion Ureter contusion/superficial or unspecified laceration
Spine	Acute strain with no fracture or dislocation of cervical/thoracic/lumbar spine	Dislocation (subluxation) and/or fracture spinous or transverse process (or unspecified) of cervical/thoracic/lumbar spine Minor compression fracture T1-12/L1-5 (≤20% loss in height of anterior vertebral body/unspecified)

TABLE 138–5

ABBREVIATED INJURY SCALE *Continued*

3 Severe, Not Life Threatening	4 Severe, Life Threatening	5 Critical, Survival Uncertain
Trachea crush Thyroid gland laceration	Laceration of trachea/carotid artery/ subclavian artery Larynx crush/fracture/laceration	Esophagus/larynx/trachea avulsion/rupture

Lung/pericardium contusion with or without
  unilateral hemothorax
Lung laceration superficial or unspecified
Unilateral hemothorax/pneumothorax with
  rib cage or thoracic cavity injury
Sternum fracture open/displaced/
  comminuted
	Chest wall (soft tissue) perforation/puncture
	Lung contusion with hemomediastinum/
	  pneumomediastinum/bilateral
	  hemothorax or pneumothorax
	Myocardium contusion
	Pericardium contusion with
	  hemomediastinum/pneumomediastinum
	  or tamponade/perforation/puncture/
	  rupture/laceration/bilateral hemothorax or
	  pneumothorax
	Bilateral hemothorax/pneumothorax
	Hemomediastinum/pneumomediastinum
	Flail chest ("sucking chest" wound)
	Lung laceration superficial or unspecified
	  with hemothorax/pneumothorax
	Inhalation burn
		Laceration of aorta/bronchus/coronary
		  artery/lung (deep and/or extensive)/
		  myocardium (including multiple
		  chambers)/pulmonary artery or vein/
		  superior or inferior vena cava/
		  pericardium if involving
		  hemomediastinum/pneumomediastinum
		  or tamponade
		Puncture/rupture of aorta/intracardiac valve
		  or septum/myocardium (involving
		  multiple chambers)/superior or inferior
		  vena cava/pericardium if involving
		  hemomediastinum/pneumomediastinum
		  or tamponade
		Perforation of aorta/bronchus/myocardium/
		  pericardium if involving
		  hemomediastinum/pneumomediastinum/
		  tamponade
		Rupture of bronchus
		Inhalation burn requiring mechanical
		  respiratory support
		Myocardium contusion if severe or
		  involving hemomediastinum or
		  pneumomediastinum

Abdominal wall musculature rupture
Contusion of biliary tract (gallbladder,
  hepatic, cystic, and common bile ducts)/
  colon/duodenum/jejunum/ileum/kidney
  (with or without hematuria)/liver/bladder/
  mesentery (omentum)/pancreas/
  peritoneum/rectum/spleen/urethra/uterus
Superficial or unspecified laceration/
  perforation of bladder/penis/ureter/
  diaphragm
Deep and/or extensive laceration/
  perforation of perineum/ureter/vagina/
  vulva
Avulsion of scrotum/ureter
Retroperitoneal injury involving hemorrhage
  or hematoma
	Superficial or unspecified laceration/
	  perforation of biliary tract/colon/
	  duodenum/jejunum/ileum/kidney/liver/
	  pancreas/peritoneum/rectum (superficial
	  over entire rectal wall, extraperitoneal)
	Deep and/or extensive laceration/
	  perforation of bladder/mesentery/penis/
	  stomach/urethra/uterus
	Avulsion of bladder/mesentery/penis/
	  spleen/stomach/testes/urethra/uterus
	  (unpregnant or first trimester)/ovary
	Rupture of spleen/stomach/urethra/uterus
	  (unpregnant or first trimester)/bladder
	  (intraperitoneal)
	Rupture/tear ovarian/fallopian tube
	Spleen laceration
		Avulsion/deep and/or extensive laceration/
		  perforation/rupture of biliary tract/colon/
		  duodenum/jejunum/ileum/kidney/liver/
		  pancreas (with or without duodenum
		  involvement)
		Deep and/or extensive laceration/rupture of
		  peritoneum/rectum
		Intra-abdominal or intrapelvic major vessel
		  laceration
		Uterus (in second or third trimester)
		  avulsion/rupture

Cervical cord contusion with transient
  neurologic signs (muscle weakness,
  paralysis, loss of sensation)
Disk herniation (rupture) with nerve root
  damage of cervical/thoracic/lumbar spine
Dislocation (subluxation) and/or fracture of
  lamina/body/facet/pedicle/odontoid of
  cervical/thoracic/lumbar spine
Nerve root/trunk brachial plexus/lumbar
  plexus/sacral plexus avulsion/laceration/
  rupture, injury with unknown lesion
Compression fracture of more than one
  vertebra and/or >20% loss of height of
  anterior body T1-12/L1-5
	Cervical cord lesion incomplete with
	  preservation of significant sensation and/
	  or motor function
		Cervical cord crush/laceration or total
		  transection with or without fracture and/
		  or dislocation C-4 or below
		Complete cervical cord lesion (quadriplegia
		  or paraplegia)
		Crush/laceration/total transection
		  (paraplegia) of cord/cauda equina

Table continued on following page

TABLE 138–5

ABBREVIATED INJURY SCALE *Continued*

	1 Minor	2 Moderate
Extremities and bony pelvis	Contusion/sprain of acromioclavicular joint/ elbow/shoulder (glenohumeral joint)/ sternoclavicular joint/wrist (carpus)/ankle Contusion fibula/knee Sprain finger/foot/hip/toe Fracture/dislocation finger/toe	Dislocation/laceration into joint of acromioclavicular joint/elbow (dislocation of radial head)/hand (laceration involving flexor or extensor tendons)/ sternoclavicular joint/wrist/heel (dislocation subtalar; laceration involving Achilles' tendon)/patella (laceration or rupture patellar tendon) Fracture of clavicle/acromion/hand (carpal or metacarpal)/humerus/radius (including Colles')/scapula/ulna/fibula (head, neck, shaft, or lateral malleolus)/foot (metatarsal talar, tarsal or unspecified)/ heel (calcaneous) patella/pelvis (closed or unspecified with or without dislocation of any of the combination of the ilium, ischium, coccyx, sacrum, pubic ramus)/ tibia (shaft, malleolus, plateau, condyles) Laceration into joint of shoulder/ankle/knee Muscle avulsion or laceration of major muscle tendon of upper and lower (except patella and Achilles) extremities Nerve laceration of upper (median, radial, ulnar) or lower (femoral, tibial, sciatic or peroneal) extremity Dislocation of foot (subtalar, transtarsal, or transmetatarsal) Laceration or rupture of distal biceps tendon Biceps muscle rupture Amputation/crush of finger/toe Acromioclavicular separation Contusion of fibula with peroneal nerve injury ("footdrop") Rupture of collateral or cruciate ligaments of the knee

From L Greenspan, BA McLellan, H Greig, Abbreviated Injury Scale and Injury Severity Score: A scoring chart, J Trauma, 25, 60–64, © by Williams & Wilkins, 1985.

TABLE 138–5

ABBREVIATED INJURY SCALE *Continued*

3 Severe, Not Life Threatening	4 Severe, Life Threatening	5 Critical, Survival Uncertain
Crush of acromioclavicular joint/arm/ forearm/elbow/hand/shoulder/ sternoclavicular joint/wrist/ankle/foot/heel/ knee/below knee Amputation upper extremity above or below elbow/hand/foot/heel/lower extremity below knee (traumatic; partial or complete) Dislocation of shoulder/wrist (radiocarpal, intercarpal, pericarpal)/ankle/knee/elbow (if involving olecranon)/hip (with or without fracture of acetabulum, femoral head, neck or intertrochanteric) Fracture of humerus/radius (including Colles')/ulna (with any one or combination of open, displaced, comminuted, or involving radial nerve)/ femur (condyle, head, neck, shaft with or without sciatic nerve involvement) Fracture of tibia/fibula/or pelvis (closed or unspecified with or without dislocation, of any one or combination of the following: ilium, ischium, coccyx, sacrum, pubic ramus) with any one or combination of open, displaced, or comminuted Sacroiliac fracture and/or dislocation Symphysis pubis separation (fracture) Knee rupture of collateral or cruciate ligaments Ankle rupture of collateral ligaments and/or Achilles' tendon Laceration of axillary/brachial/femoral/ popliteal artery Nerve laceration of upper (median, radial, ulnar) or lower (femoral, tibial, sciatic or peroneal) extremity involving ≥ 2 nerves in same extremities Muscle avulsion or laceration of multiple major muscle tendons in upper and lower (except patella or Achilles') extremities Complete patellar tendon laceration or rupture	Pelvis crush Above knee crush/amputation (traumatic partial or complete)	

monary arterial catheter may be necessary for evaluation of the hemodynamic status.

Historically, it was believed that trauma patients had an initial period (48 hours) of low oxygen consumption (the ebb phase) followed by a time of increased oxygen consumption (the flow phase).[22] However, oxygen consumption is not reduced after major trauma.[23] An elevated oxygen consumption is expected with this hyperdynamic state and release of the stress hormones: corticotropin, glucagon, and the catecholamines. Therapy should be directed at this increased demand and prevention or correction of any oxygen debt, anaerobic metabolism, and lactic acidosis.

Nearly all injured patients at some time in their ICU course are physiologically unstable and are prone to sudden occurrences of previously unsuspected problems. Goal-directed physiologic monitoring is necessary to provide an early warning to the potential problems of missed vascular or neurologic injuries, bleeding, peritonitis, sepsis, pancreatitis, pneumothorax, atelectasis, pulmonary embolism, and other life-threatening complications.

Monitoring of the injured patient should include a goal-directed survey of all organ systems and a more in-depth review of systems most likely to be adversely affected by direct trauma or secondary injury related to hypoxia, hypoperfusion, or sepsis.

TRAUMA

Closed Head Injuries

Head injuries are a major contributor to the morbidity and mortality of trauma patients. Patients with a Glasgow Coma Scale score of 8 or less have a mortality of 18 to 30%, whereas those with a Glasgow Coma Scale score greater than 8 have a mortality of 1 to 6%.[24, 25] This increased mortality is independent of extracranial injuries.[25]

Intracranial pressure (ICP) monitoring measures the pressure within the skull exerted by the brain, cerebral blood, and cerebrospinal fluid (CSF). According to the Monro-Kellie doctrine, the quantity of blood (not blood flow) is approximately constant at all times. Therefore any increase in ICP is due to either an increase in CSF or an increase in brain volume. An increase in ICP may reduce cerebral perfusion pressure (CPP) to the point that cerebral blood flow is reduced and cerebral oxygen delivery is inadequate.

CPP can be calculated from the difference between mean arterial pressure (MAP) and ICP (CPP = MAP − ICP). An inadequate CPP may be treated by raising MAP or decreasing ICP. ICP can be monitored by an epidural monitor, a subarachnoid bolt, an intraparenchymal monitor, or an intraventricular catheter (Fig. 138–3). The relative merits and disadvantages of various ICP monitors are listed in Table 138–6. Fiberoptic technology has been applied to ICP monitoring. Comparison of fiberoptic systems with fluid-filled systems is depicted in Table 138–7. Any patient with a Glasgow Coma Scale score of 8 or less should be considered

TABLE 138–6

INTRACRANIAL PRESSURE MONITORS

Monitor	Advantages	Disadvantages
Epidural monitor	Ease of insertion No dural penetration Low risk of infection	Unable to drain CSF Questionable accuracy
Subarachnoid bolt	Useful if ventricles are small No penetration of brain Decreased risk of infection	Unable to drain CSF Requires intact skull
Intraventricular catheter	Reliable measurement Access to CSF	Difficulty locating ventricle Risk of infection Risk of intracerebral bleeding or edema
Intraparenchymal monitor	Ease of insertion Low risk of infection Useful if ventricles are small May be most accurate ICP	Unable to drain CSF Risk of bleeding

Adapted from Hollingsworth-Fridlund P, Vos H, Daily EK: Use of fiber-optic pressure transducer for intracranial pressure measurements: A preliminary report. Heart Lung 17:111, 1988.

TABLE 138–7

SYSTEMS FOR MEASURING INTRACRANIAL PRESSURE

Parameter	Fluid Filled	Fiberoptic
Placement	Subarachnoid or intraventricular	Subarachnoid, intraventricular epidural, or intraparenchymal
CSF	Unable to monitor while draining ventricular catheter	Able to drain from ventricular catheter while continuously monitoring
Infection	Static fluid column with stopcocks	Lack of fluid column may reduce risk
Artifact	Dampening, air bubbles, kinking, movement of patient	Minimal or none
Calibration	Required	Factory set

Adapted from Hollingsworth-Fridlund P, Vos H, Daily EK: Use of fiber-optic pressure transducer for intracranial pressure measurements: A preliminary report. Heart Lung 17:111, 1988.

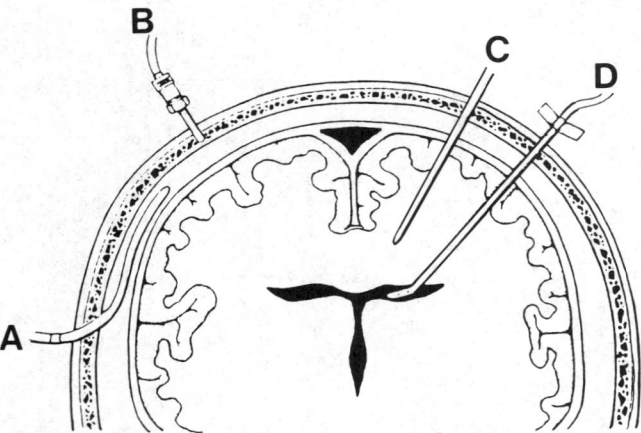

Figure 138–3. Intracranial pressure monitors: *A.* Subdural cup catheter. *B.* Subarachnoid screw. *C.* Intraparenchymal monitor. *D.* Ventriculostomy catheter. (Adapted from Aucoin PJ, Kotilainen HR, Gantz NM, et al: Intracranial pressure monitors: Epidemiologic study of risk factors and infections. Am J Med 80:369, 1986.)

for ICP monitoring. The normal ICP is 10 to 15 mm Hg, and concern should arise when the ICP is greater than 20 mm Hg. This must be evaluated in the context of the CPP, which should be maintained at greater than 50 mm Hg and possibly as high as 70 to 80 mm Hg.[26]

As with all monitors, placing a foreign body into a sterile environment is associated with a risk of infection. The infectious risk of ICP monitors is about 10 to 11% and varies with several factors, including the type and duration of monitoring.[27-30] The infectious risk increases after 3 to 5 days and therefore prophylactic antibiotics have been proposed if the anticipated duration is more than 3 days.[30] Although the most common organism has been gram-positive bacteria, with staphylococcus as a predominant organism, certain series have found slightly more infectious complications attributable to gram-negative organisms.[28, 29] With this variation in infecting organism and the lack of a benefit of prophylactic antibiotics,[27-29] the use of prophylactic antibiotics should be individualized.

The principal method of decreasing ICP is through hyperventilation. Decreasing the $PaCO_2$ to between 25 and 30 mm Hg causes alkalosis, cerebral vasoconstriction, and decreased intracranial blood volume. This degree of hyperventilation can bring about a 12% decrease in vessel diameter[31] and reduce ICP as much as 30%.

Mannitol is an osmotic agent that has several potential benefits for patients with head injuries. As an osmotic agent, its first potential benefit may be a short-term increase in intravascular volume and thereby an increase CPP because of increased MAP. Mannitol also improves cerebral blood flow by decreasing blood viscosity.[31] Although mannitol is generally believed to have a dehydrating effect on the brain, there is no evidence that it decreases brain water content.[26] Mannitol enhances renal excretion of water and increases serum sodium concentration, which further raises serum osmolality. Rapid infusions of up to 1 g/kg of body weight are recommended. Mannitol is often used to raise the serum osmolality to 310 mOsm/kg and the serum sodium level to 155 mEq/L. The effect of mannitol can be estimated by calculating the osmolar gap (measured osmolality minus calculated osmolality).

Calculated osmolality =
[2 × sodium (mEq/L)] + [glucose (mg/dL)/18] +
[urea (mg/dL)/2.8]

Finally, mannitol is a free radical scavenger and may play a role in limiting reperfusion injury.[32]

The effect of steroids in the management of brain malignancies is well established. The effects, however, with experimental models and human brain injury have been contradictory. Three prospective double-blind studies have shown no effect of either low-dose or high-dose dexamethasone on morbidity or mortality.[33-35] In one study, there was a worse outcome in patients with an increased ICP who received steroids.[33]

Hyperglycemia with or without diabetes has been related to poor neurologic outcome in patients after cardiac arrest and ischemic stroke.[36, 37] The mechanism is unknown but appears to be related to brain tissue lactic acidosis. Therefore, the blood glucose level should be monitored and hyperglycemia avoided.

After an ischemic injury, cerebral blood flow follows a no reflow phenomenon (Fig. 138–4). This is characterized by a hyperemic response followed by a gradual decrease until there is again virtually no flow.[38] Because this may be due to cerebral vasospasm, the efficacy of calcium channel blockers to block this response has been studied. Nimodipine has been shown to produce a statistically significant improvement

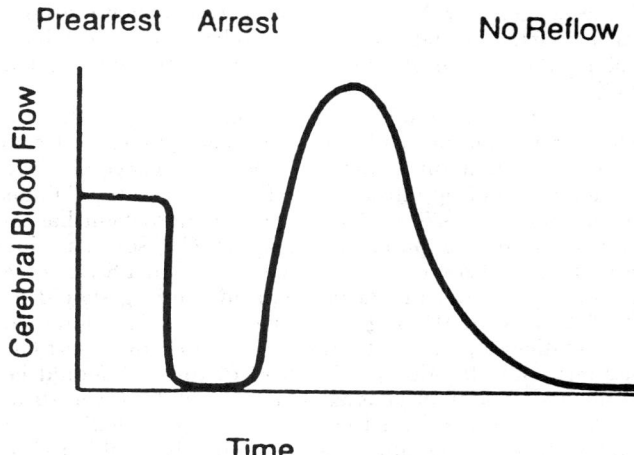

Figure 138–4. The temporary interruption of cerebral blood flow produces a transient hyperemic response followed by a gradual decline in cerebral blood flow called the no reflow phenomenon. (From Rogers MC, Kirsch JR: Current concepts in brain resuscitation. JAMA 261:3143, 1989. Copyright 1989, American Medical Association.)

in cerebral blood flow. The improvement, however, is only 30 to 35% above control values and may be clinically insignificant. In addition, cerebral metabolism does not appear to be improved. An improved outcome after nimodipine administration to reduce spasm has been demonstrated after subarachnoid hemorrhage.[39, 40]

Barbiturates have been suggested to decrease cerebral metabolism; however, they also lower cerebral blood flow. Because barbiturates do not lower metabolism selectively, any benefit from decreasing metabolism is countered by a decrease in blood flow. At present, barbiturates are generally restricted to the effect of lowering ICP.[38]

Naloxone (Narcan) and thyrotropin-releasing hormone are endorphin antagonists. Both have been shown to improve cardiovascular measures, perfusion pressures, arterial blood gas levels, and cerebral electrical activity.[41] Clinical studies, however, are contradictory. Studies of septic shock suggest that the β-endorphin release is a consequence rather than a cause of shock and that the beneficial effect of naloxone may be due to nociceptive stimulation.[42]

Patients with head injuries are at increased risk for infectious complications. This may be due to their altered level of consciousness as well as their need for long-term ventilator support. Pulmonary infection is the most common source of sepsis and necessitates early recognition and treatment.[43] These patients are also at a low but increased risk for post-traumatic seizures, which can be improved with phenytoin administration during the first week.[44] Although these patients are still at an increased risk for post-traumatic seizures after the first week, there is no improvement with phenytoin at 1 or 2 years and there is a negative cognitive effect with impaired neurobehavior performance in the severely injured.[45]

Another medication dilemma is the choice of sedation and pain control in the obtunded, and often combative, patient. Although the importance of the ability to perform the neurologic examination cannot be overemphasized, withholding analgesics from these patients, who often have other significant injuries, can worsen their agitation. Adequate pain control and sedation can be accomplished with narcotics, which can be reversed with narcotic antagonists. The use of benzodiazepines should be individualized because reversal of these agents with antagonists may precipitate seizure activity. Active metabolites of benzodiazepines may have prolonged effects in patients with organ dysfunction related to injury.

To summarize, the initial management of the patient with suspected significant head injury with altered consciousness is tracheal intubation, hyperventilation to a $PaCO_2$ of 25 to 30 mm Hg, and administration of minimal isotonic fluids (normal saline at 0.75 to 1 mL/kg/h). If the patient has an abnormal brain computed tomographic (CT) scan showing focal or generalized injury and a Glasgow Coma Scale score of 8 or less without intoxicants, ICP monitoring should be introduced. If the ICP is greater than 20 mm Hg, continued hyperventilation, fluid restriction with isotonic or hypertonic solutions, and elevation of the head of the bed should be maintained. Mannitol (1 g/kg) is given rapidly (over 10 to 15 minutes) and repeated every 4 to 6 hours (0.25 to 0.5 g/kg) while serum sodium concentrations (the goal is 150 to 155 mEq/L) and serum osmolality (the goal is 310 to 320 mOsm/kg) are monitored every 6 hours. Administration of cerebral vasodilators (nitroprusside, nitroglycerin, and others) is avoided. If treatment is needed for a significant period or must be maximized in a potentially unstable patient, pulmonary arterial catheterization is used to optimize systemic oxygen transport. If ICP is still not controlled, consideration may be given to inducing barbiturate coma to make the patient areflexic with an isoelectric electrocardiogram. This may necessitate administration of inotropes to maintain systemic oxygen transport.

Spinal Cord Injuries

All trauma patients should be considered to have a spinal cord injury until proved otherwise. This is particularly problematic for those patients who are unresponsive and unable to be assessed clinically. The lateral cervical spine film, even when demonstrating all seven vertebrae, has a sensitivity of only 0.83 to 0.85 for detecting significant injury.[46, 47] An anteroposterior and open mouth odontoid view must be used to rule out more than 99% of bony cervical injuries.

The care of patients with a cord injury begins with rapid identification and initiation of methylprednisolone administration within 8 hours of injury.[48] A bolus of 30 mg/kg followed by 5.4 mg/kg/h for 23 hours resulted in a statistically significant improvement in motor function, sensation to pinprick and touch at 6 months. The same study demonstrated no effect with naloxone.

Patients with a neurologic deficit have unique hemodynamic problems. Because of the unopposed parasympathetic outflow, these patients are vasodilated with a low systemic vascular resistance, low blood pressure, and at times, bradycardia. In high cervical cord injuries, cardiac sympathetics are lost and bradycardia and low cardiac output may occur. Cardiac output may be elevated in low cord injuries. The low systemic vascular resistance places these patients at risk for uncontrolled heat loss, and attention to temperature is critical, particularly in patients with other injuries.

If perfusion is inadequate, sympathomimetics with both alpha- and beta-effects such as dopamine are usually effective. Pure alpha-antagonists have a role in low cord injuries when the heart rate and contractility are not problematic.

Because of the loss of intercostal function, there is a decrease in tidal volume and negative inspiratory force. This, coupled with difficulty mobilizing secretions, makes the patient prone to atelectasis and pulmonary infection. Prophylactic intubation can be avoided with early and aggressive pulmonary toilet. Oscillating beds such as the RotoRest kinetic treatment table not only improve pulmo-

nary toilet, but also improve pulmonary shunt fraction.[49–51] When intubation is necessary, minimal support should be used to maximize spontaneous ventilatory activity and preserve ventilatory muscle strength.

Neck Injuries

Neck injuries can be dramatic or subtle but are equally lethal. This is particularly true of blunt laryngeal injuries, which account for the second most common cause of death in head and neck trauma.[52] After the airway has been established, there must be constant attention to keep it secured, as loss of the airway can have devastating consequences.

Evaluation of all penetrating injuries of the neck should include an examination of the great vessels, either by surgical exploration or arteriography. With both these modalities, follow-up should include serial neurologic examinations as well as evidence of bleeding and hematoma formation, which can compromise the airway. Another feature to note on physical examination is evidence of infection. This may represent an unrecognized esophageal injury, which is unusual in blunt trauma, or an esophageal fistula, which is common with extensive esophageal injuries.[53]

Chest Trauma

Twenty-five percent of trauma deaths are caused by chest injuries.[4] Because of the potential substantial impact of intervention, the chest x-ray film is of critical importance in the trauma patient. In addition to identification of a hemopneumothorax, important findings must be sought and ruled out on the trauma chest x-ray film (Table 138–8; see Figs. 138–5 to 138–9). Certain fractures (see Table 138–8), mediastinal changes (see Table 138–8), and a mechanism of injury associated with rapid deceleration are associated with injuries to the aorta and the great vessels. If these findings

---

TABLE 138–8

TRAUMA CHEST X-RAY FINDINGS

1. Fractures
   a. Ribs (Fig. 138–5)
      i. First or second
      ii. Segmental, flail segment
   b. Sternum
   c. Scapula
   d. Clavicle
2. Thorax
   a. Pneumothorax
   b. Hemothorax
   c. Integrity of diaphragm (Fig. 138–6)
   d. Pulmonary contusion (Fig. 138–7)
3. Mediastinum
   a. Widening (Fig. 138–8)
   b. Obscure aortic knob
   c. Shift of nasogastric tube to right
   d. Shift of trachea to right
   e. Depression of the left mainstem bronchus
   f. Apical cap
   g. Displacement of paraspinous stripe
   h. Obliteration of aortopulmonary clear space
   i. Pneumomediastinum
   j. Pneumopericardium (Fig. 138–7)
4. Tube placement (Fig. 138–9)
   a. Endotracheal tube
   b. Central venous pressure catheter
   c. Pulmonary arterial catheter
   d. Chest tube

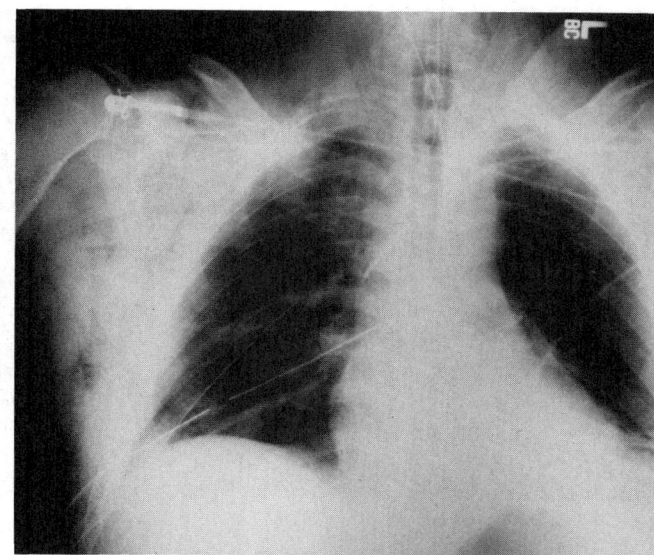

Figure 138–5. Multiple rib fractures. Note the subcutaneous emphysema outlining the pectoralis major.

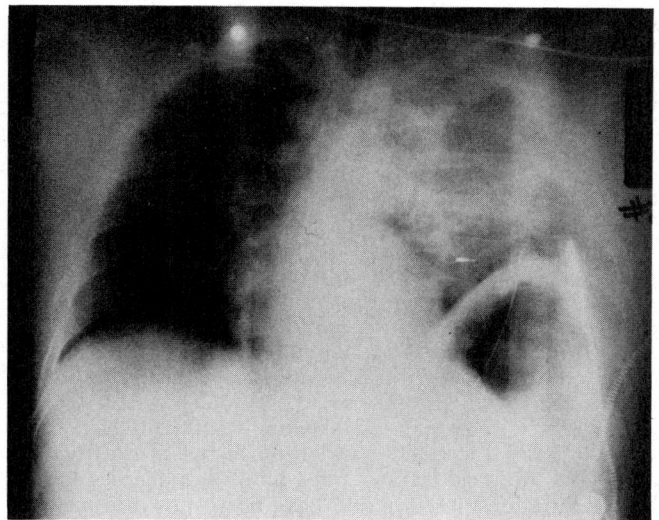

Figure 138–6. Rupture of the left hemidiaphragm. Note the position of the nasogastric tube and gastric bubble in the left hemithorax.

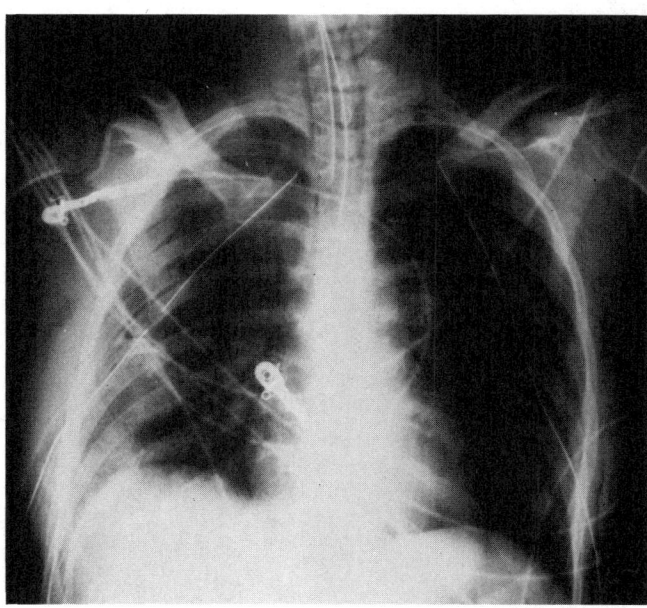

Figure 138–7. Pulmonary contusion, multiple rib fractures, and subcutaneous emphysema. Note the pneumopericardium along the left-sided heart border.

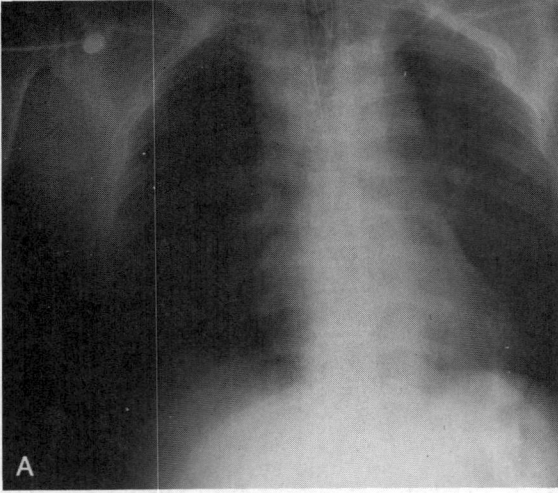
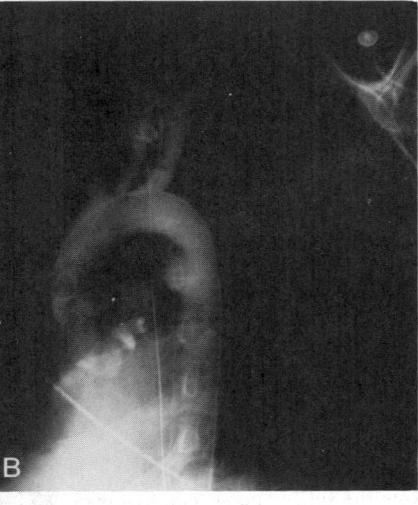

Figure 138–8. *A.* Widening of the mediastinum. Note the malposition of the nasogastric tube. *B.* Traumatic disruption of the aorta just distal to the ligamentum arteriosum.

are manifested in the first 24 hours after injury, an arch aortogram should be considered.

Rib fractures are the most common thoracic injury, and the presence of multiple rib fractures increases the likelihood of other injuries and complications and the need for possible operative intervention and intensive care management.[54] The absence of injury to the bony thorax, however, does not rule out significant underlying injury.[55] The most common clinical consequence of rib fractures or penetrating chest trauma that necessitates intervention is a pneumothorax and/or hemothorax. The majority of pneumothoraces and hemothoraces only necessitate placement of a large-bore (e.g., No. 38 French) chest tube connected to an underwater seal and collection system (e.g., Pleurovac). A large-bore chest tube is preferred because of the propensity for smaller tubes to become obstructed by clot. Operative intervention may rarely be required for large air leaks, which may signal major tracheobronchial injuries, or persistent air leaks. A hemothorax that initially drains more than 1500 mL of blood or continues to drain more than 200 mL/h may require a thoracotomy.[4] The most common ICU problems in patients with chest trauma include pain control, management of pulmonary contusion, and flail chest.

Pain control has a major impact on patients with chest

injuries and allows improved pulmonary toilet. Because many ICU trauma patients are unable to take enteral analgesics in doses necessary to achieve pain control, parenteral routes must be used. For patients who are awake and oriented, a patient-controlled analgesia device may provide adequate pain control with minimal invasiveness and personnel resources. Intercostal nerve blocks have been used for many years but entail multiple injections and carry a small risk of pneumothorax.[56] Other newer techniques include intrapleural and epidural analgesia. Intrapleural analgesics can be administered via a previously placed chest tube or by way of a catheter placed specifically for this purpose.[57] This technique has been shown to be effective in patients with thoracic trauma.[58, 59] There is, however, no difference in postoperative narcotic requirement, recovery room time, length of hospital stay, or time to ambulation compared with those of patients receiving intramuscular narcotics.[60]

Epidural narcotics in the treatment of pain have been used clinically since 1979[61] and are effective in rib fractures and other thoracic trauma.[62–66] Epidural analgesics have a longer duration of action and have been shown to improve forced expiratory volume in 1 second, PaO_2, and alveolar-arterial oxygen tension difference compared with intrave-

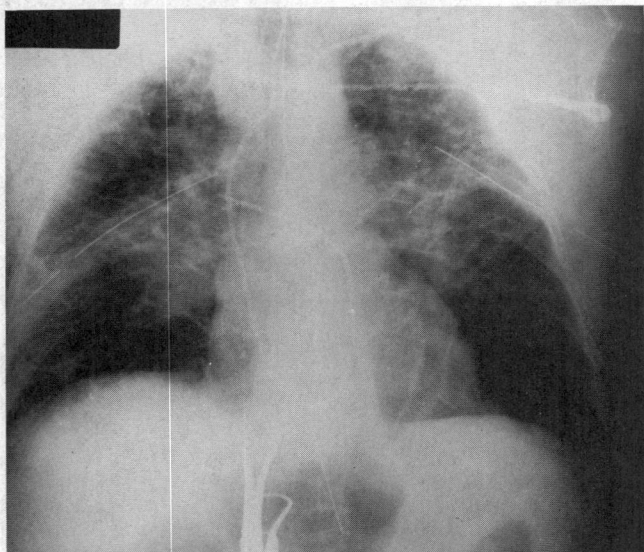

Figure 138–9. Malposition of the endotracheal tube, pulmonary arterial catheter, left chest tube, and nasogastric tube. Note the temporary abdominal closure utilizing towel clips.

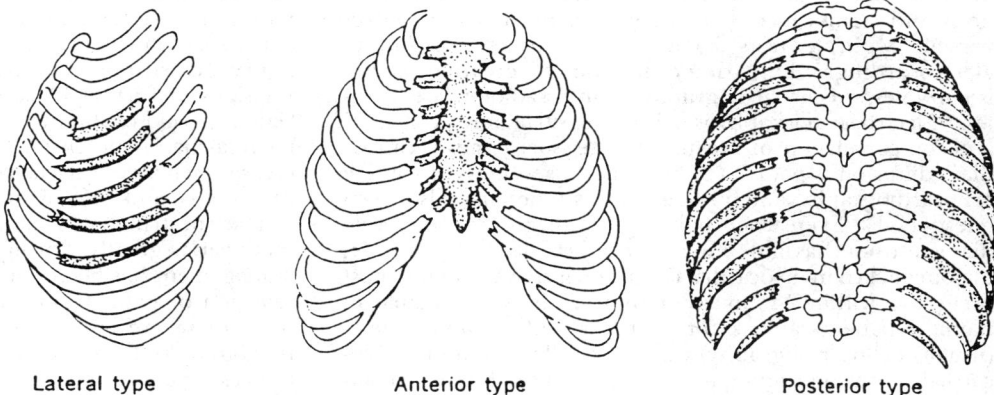

Figure 138–10. Types of flail chest. (From Naclerio EA: Chest Injuries; Physiologic Principles and Emergency Management. Orlando, FL, Grune & Stratton, p 217, 1971.)

Lateral type   Anterior type   Posterior type

nous or intramuscular analgesics.[67, 68] Narcotics can be given via this route by either bolus or continuous administration. Side effects include pruritus, urinary retention, hypotension, and respiratory depression. Continuous administration of epidural narcotics has fewer side effects than bolus administration.[69] The narcotic agent also has an effect on the response and is related to its lipid solubility. Lipophilic drugs such as fentanyl appear to have a better efficacy/safety ratio and a lower incidence of side effects.[70]

Pulmonary contusion (see Fig. 138–7) is a major factor in the morbidity and mortality of patients with chest trauma.[71, 72] Although the number of fractures does not correlate with the severity of the pulmonary injury,[73] rib, scapular, and sternal fractures are important markers of the magnitude of injury and should increase the suspicion of underlying injury. Likewise, the extent of pulmonary contusion on the initial chest x-ray film does not correlate with the need for intubation or mortality.[74] Patients with pulmonary contusion should be intubated and ventilatory support instituted on the basis of their clinical status. Arterial blood gas analysis and pulse oximetry may be helpful. Nonventilating oxygenation support and continuous positive airway pressure by mask may be useful in selected patients. Risk factors that have been shown to increase the likelihood of the need for tracheal intubation are (1) an initial respiratory rate of more than 25 breaths/min, (2) pulse greater than 100/min, (3) systolic blood pressure less than 100 mm Hg, and (4) the presence of other injuries.[73] Ventilatory support includes increasing levels of positive end-expiratory pressure until oxygen saturation is satisfactory. Fluid resuscitation should be tempered but not at the expense of restoring adequate perfusion.

Like pulmonary contusion, flail chest has been associated with an increased mortality.[71] Defined as paradoxical ventilatory movement, a *flail chest* generally involves at least two segmental fractures in each of three adjacent ribs (Fig. 138–10). The treatment of flail chest has evolved during the past 35 years from towel clip traction (Fig. 138–11) to nonselective internal pneumatic stabilization to selective ventilator therapy.[75, 76] The emphasis in the management of patients with flail chest is on the underlying pulmonary injury, pulmonary toilet, and pain control. The instability of the chest wall does not preclude adequate spontaneous ventilation when adequate pain control is achieved. The paradoxical movement may even increase with adequate pain control. For those patients requiring ventilatory support, intermittent mandatory ventilation and positive end-expiratory pressure have been shown to improve the functional residual capacity and oxygenation, and decrease the mean length of mechan-

ical ventilatory support.[77, 78] Operative stabilization of the chest wall is rarely necessary. Long-term disability after flail chest injury is significant, with the majority of patients having persistent pain and dyspnea.[79, 80]

The spectrum of cardiac injuries ranges from concussion (injury without demonstrable pathologic changes) and contusion to rupture of the papillary muscles or any of the cardiac chambers or septae.[81] Myocardial injury is believed

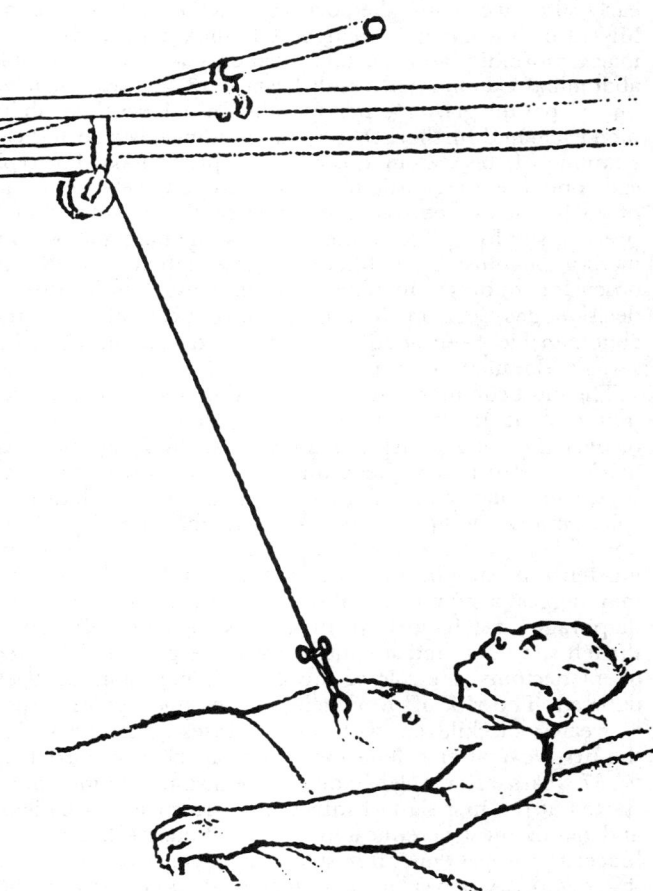

Figure 138–11. Towel clip traction (historical interest only). (From Nealon TF Jr: Fundamental Skills in Surgery. 3rd ed. Philadelphia, WB Saunders, p 284, 1979.)

to be common, often with minimal morbidity.[82] The diagnosis and significance of myocardial contusion are controversial. Multiple tests have been advocated, including electrocardiography,[83] determination of creatine kinase isoenzymes,[84] echocardiography,[85] and radionuclide studies.[86] Electrocardiography is neither sensitive nor specific,[86, 87] and the correlation of creatine kinase isoenzymes with cardiac contusion is poor.[88, 89] The clinical usefulness of routine echocardiography and radionuclide studies has also been questioned.[90] Even when positive, the diagnosis of myocardial contusion has little impact on morbidity.[91] Because the major concern in myocardial contusion is dysrhythmias, most occurring within 12 hours of injury,[92] it is reasonable to monitor patients at risk for 24 hours with additional tests (usually echocardiography) when clinically indicated.[93] Myocardial contusion leading to left ventricular failure is uncommon but is associated with a high mortality. Pulmonary arterial catheterization may be necessary for the titration of inotropes and vasodilators when ventricular dysfunction is suspected.

Creatine kinase isoenzymes may be of value in detecting peritraumatic myocardial infarction in high-risk patients. Total creatine kinase determination is of little value in detecting myocardial necrosis because most injured patients have high total creatine kinase as a result of their skeletal muscle injuries.

Abdominal Trauma

Abdominal trauma is the most frequent cause of treatable, early, life-threatening hemorrhage in the injured patient. Missed or inadequately treated abdominal injuries result in major morbidity and mortality. Patients with an unreliable abdominal examination result because of intoxicants, head injury, paraplegia, or other reasons must have their abdomen evaluated further. Diagnostic peritoneal lavage and CT scanning of the abdomen can be complementary, but typically only one diagnostic test is utilized. The relative merits of each test are beyond the scope of this chapter, but a prerequisite for CT scanning is hemodynamic stability. Pain medication must be withheld in these patients to prevent obscuring findings on physical examination until either a decision has been made for operative exploration or the abdomen has been adequately evaluated and the need for serial abdominal examinations excluded.

The most common injury necessitating operative intervention in blunt trauma is injury to the spleen. Since the report of overwhelming postsplenectomy sepsis by King and Shumacker,[94] efforts have been directed toward splenic salvage by splenorrhaphy or partial splenectomy rather than total splenectomy. Drains may be left in the left upper quadrant but, if kept in place for an extended period, increase the incidence of subphrenic abscess. Signs and symptoms that may suggest a subphrenic abscess include an elevated hemidiaphragm, a left-sided pleural effusion, pain referred to the left shoulder, and singultus. For those patients subjected to splenectomy, the role of prophylactic penicillin has been debated. The risk of overwhelming postsplenectomy sepsis is greatest in children, with 50% of cases occurring within the first year after splenectomy, but has been reported up to 37 years after splenectomy.[95] Penicillin administration started at the first sign of infection is effective, but patients and family must be educated.[96] Medical alert (Medic Alert) bracelets for patients after splenectomy may be helpful in this regard. A polyvalent pneumococcal vaccine is available and should be administered to patients requiring a splenectomy.[97] Although more effective if given before splenectomy, this is possible only for elective procedures. No information is available regarding the best time of administration after a splenectomy. We prefer to give pneumococcal vaccine (Pneumovax) before the patient is discharged from the hospital.

Patients who have undergone splenorrhaphy or splenic injury treated nonoperatively need to be closely monitored for signs of further bleeding or delayed bleeding after the "latent period of Baudet." Bleeding is usually manifested by tachycardia, hypotension, oliguria, and eventually a decreased hematocrit. Delayed bleeding occurs in less than 1% of patients, and 75% of cases occur within 2 weeks.

The spectrum of liver injuries and subsequent management varies greatly. For limited blunt injuries, nonoperative management has been demonstrated to be safe with proper selection of patients and close follow-up.[98, 99] The management of severe injuries is more complex and ranges from tractotomy with ligation of vessels and bile ducts to resection to packing of the abdomen with laparotomy packs (Fig. 138–12), temporary closure of the abdomen (see Fig. 138–9), and planned re-exploration when hypothermia and coagulopathy have been corrected.[100–102] Hypothermia and coagulopathy represent the most common complications.

Hypothermia is a major contributor to coagulopathy and mortality.[103–106] Correction of hypothermia can be difficult. Useful techniques include warming the external environment (turning the room temperature up), using heat shields and warming blankets, closing body cavities and covering exposed body areas to decrease further heat loss, adding a humidifier to the ventilator circuit, and warming all intravenous fluids. Rarely, irrigation of body cavities with warm fluid via chest tubes or peritoneal lavage or cardiopulmonary bypass is necessary.[107–108]

The most common late complication of liver injury is sepsis. Postoperative fever is common and is usually due to the bodily reaction to small amounts of necrotic liver and residual hematoma. The rate of intra-abdominal abscess varies, and the relationship to drains is controversial.[109, 110] Risk factors for intra-abdominal abscess include gunshot wounds, shock, blood transfusion of more than 6 U, major liver injuries, and injury of three or more abdominal organs.[111] Other complications of major hepatic trauma include

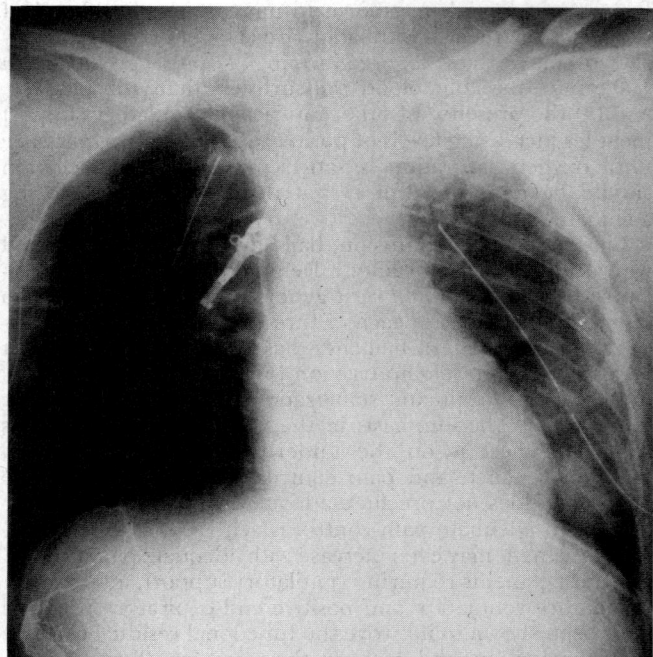

Figure 138–12. Laparotomy packs in the right upper quadrant.

hyperpyrexia, prolonged biliary leak, late hemorrhage, and hypoglycemia.[112]

Renal contusion is one of the most common urinary tract injuries after blunt trauma. The majority of renal contusions resolve without intervention or sequelae. The most common manifestation is hematuria, but significant injuries can occur in the absence of hematuria.[113] Patients with blood at the urethral meatus, scrotal hematoma, or high-riding prostate should have a retrograde urethrogram before insertion of a Foley catheter to evaluate the possibility of urethral disruption (Fig. 138–13). Patients with hematuria, particularly with pelvic fractures, may need a cystogram to rule out a bladder disruption. The immediate treatment of urethral and bladder injuries is to provide adequate drainage, but operative repair may be required.

The upper urinary tract is evaluated by either intravenous pyelography or CT scan with intravenous contrast material. The CT scan assesses parenchymal injuries as well as providing information about other retroperitoneal structures.[114] A nonperfused kidney should be revascularized as soon as possible because the long-term function is related to the warm ischemic time.[115]

The magnitude of renal injury correlates with the incidence of complications, the presence of renal failure, and death.[116, 117] The most common causes of renal failure are hypoperfusion and nephrotoxic drugs. Another cause to be kept in mind in trauma patients is rhabdomyolysis from crush injuries and ischemia. The most common cause of death in a patient with acute renal failure is sepsis and multiple organ system failure. Renal failure may also be associated with decreased filtration caused by increased intra-abdominal pressure.[118] The increased pressure may be due to edema, ongoing bleeding, ascites, or placement of laparotomy packs and may necessitate opening of the abdomen (Fig. 138–14). Adequate volume resuscitation and maintenance of renal oxygen delivery remain the key to preventing post-traumatic renal failure.

Small-bowel and colon injuries are less frequent than solid viscus injuries but are becoming more common with increased use of seat belts. The most common site of the injury is the proximal jejunum, the distal ileum, or the sigmoid colon.[119] The evaluation of these injuries can be difficult, as CT scanning is neither sensitive nor specific.[120] Results of diagnostic peritoneal lavage may also be normal.

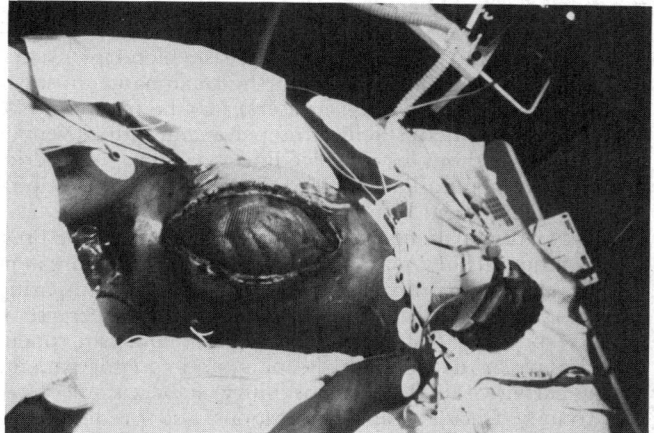

Figure 138–14. An open abdomen. Note the distended, edematous loops of bowel, which prevented closure without greatly increasing intra-abdominal pressure.

Delayed diagnosis increases morbidity. Timely intervention necessitates a high index of suspicion, particularly in patients with a seat belt contusion. Findings of increased abdominal pain, abdominal tenderness, and fever, especially in the first 24 hours after injury, should raise suspicion and prompt the use of enteral and possibly colonic contrast material to confirm the diagnosis.

Pancreatic injuries can be difficult to diagnose and contribute significantly to morbidity and mortality. Because the pancreas is a retroperitoneal organ, peritoneal lavage may not show any evidence of pancreatic injury. Amylase and lipase determinations are also of limited usefulness.[121] Successful treatment entails a high index of suspicion, identification of ductal injuries, and appropriate resection and drainage.[122] Closed suction drains have been shown to have a lower incidence of intra-abdominal abscesses than sump drains.[123] Other complications include fistulas, pseudocysts, and pancreatic insufficiency. Fistulas in the absence of obstruction usually close spontaneously with adequate drainage. Somatostatin may increase the rate of closure by decreasing pancreatic secretion.[124] Pancreatitis and pseudocysts are managed in a similar fashion to nontraumatic pancreatitis and pseudocysts. Exocrine and endocrine insufficiency is unusual, except after near-total pancreatectomies.

Duodenal injuries can also be difficult to diagnose. A nondiagnostic peritoneal lavage and delayed diagnosis can result in increased morbidity and mortality.[125] A CT scan with enteral contrast media may demonstrate extravasation as well as extraluminal gas. The operative management incorporates the same principles as in pancreatic injuries: débridement of devitalized tissue, closure, and adequate drainage and diversion of enteral flow when indicated. Rarely (<5%), a combined pancreaticoduodenectomy is required.[126] Postoperative complications are similar to those with pancreatic injuries, most commonly fistulas and intra-abdominal abscesses. Central parenteral nutrition is an important adjunct in the treatment of pancreatic and duodenal injuries.

Orthopedic and Extremity Injuries

Pelvic fractures are common and may be a source of potential morbidity as well as mortality (see Fig. 138–13). For this reason, an anteroposterior view of the pelvis is included in the routine radiographs of the trauma patient. Bleeding from pelvic fractures can be massive. Because of the difficulty in controlling the source of bleeding, opening

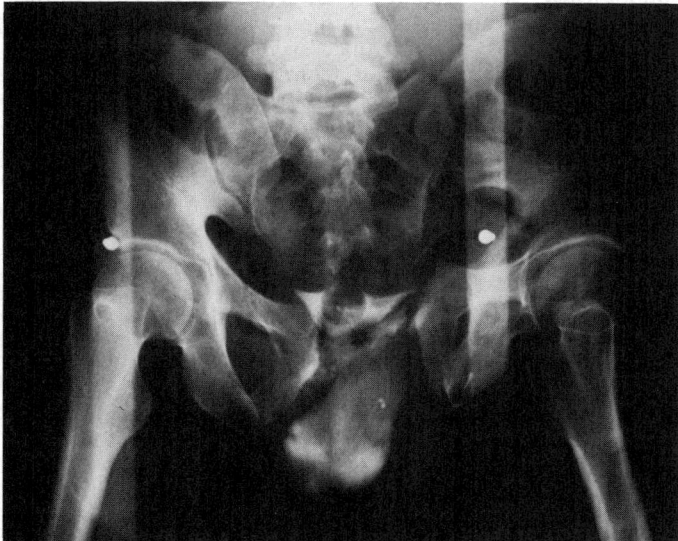

Figure 138–13. Open book pelvic fracture with urethral disruption.

the retroperitoneal hematoma from a pelvic fracture during a celiotomy is to be avoided. Placement of an external fixator stabilizes the bone fragments and decreases blood loss. When external fixation is not indicated, the pneumatic antishock garment (military antishock trousers) may be inflated to 30 to 40 mm Hg to help stabilize the pelvis and induce venous tamponade. Although most bleeding is venous, an arteriogram with embolization of bleeding points may be helpful in cases of persistent bleeding (usually >6 U).[127, 128]

Many trauma patients have associated extremity fractures, which although they may not be immediately life threatening, have a major impact on outcome. Studies comparing early versus delayed stabilization demonstrate a decrease in adult respiratory distress syndrome, fat embolism, pneumonia, days in the ICU and hospital, and cost for patients having early (within 24 hours of injury) stabilization.[129-133]

Extremity fractures and dislocations also predispose to vascular injuries. Perfusion of the extremity and signs of compartment syndromes must be monitored. An arteriogram is the "gold standard," but Doppler examination may be a good screening modality. Revascularization must be accomplished rapidly, and caution should be used in attributing a defect to spasm in trauma.[134] Follow-up with Doppler-derived ankle/brachial indices allows early recognition of graft failure and the opportunity for graft and limb salvage.[135] Neurologic deficits are the most common long-term sequelae.[136] Other complications include pseudoaneurysms and arteriovenous fistulas. If a compartment syndrome is suspected, the compartmental pressures should be measured, and if elevated, fasciotomies performed. Normal compartmental pressures range from 0 to 8 mm Hg.[137] Decompression should be considered for pressures greater than 30 mm Hg.[138] Prolonged compartmental syndromes may result in permanent muscle or nerve injury, rhabdomyolysis, or loss of the extremity.

Other Critical Care Issues

Trauma patients are at an increased risk for many of the same problems that plague other ICU patients. Immobilization predisposes these patients to deep venous thrombosis and pressure ulcers. Prophylactic measures for deep venous thrombosis using anticoagulants many be contraindicated by other injuries, such as intracranial bleeding. Pneumatic compression stockings may not be effective when their use is started after the onset of immobilization. Pressure ulcers can occur early, even in young patients, particularly when they are kept on back boards because a spinal injury has not been excluded. Patients should be taken off the back board and spinal precautions instituted utilizing in-line stabilization and log-rolling until a spinal injury can be excluded.

Trauma patients are also at risk for infectious complications. This is due in part to the multitude of invasive devices and in part to the nonelective and sometimes less than sterile circumstances in which they were placed. All central catheters placed in the emergency department should be considered contaminated and replaced or removed within the first 24 hours. Other causes of infectious processes to be considered include pneumonia, urinary tract infection, sinusitis (particularly with nasal endotracheal tubes), intra-abdominal abscesses, and acalculous cholecystitis.

Trauma itself is a risk factor for acalculous cholecystitis. Other risk factors include shock, increased bile pigment load, drugs, surgery, parenteral nutrition, sepsis, multiple transfusions, prolonged fasting, ventilatory support, vascular disease, and narcotic-induced biliary stasis.[139-142] There are no pathognomonic laboratory studies. Fever is usually the first sign. Right upper quadrant tenderness may be difficult to elicit. A high index of suspicion and a bedside ultrasound

scan can be diagnostic. Findings diagnostic by ultrasound scan include a gallbladder wall thickness of 3.5 mm or greater, pericholecystic fluid, subserosal edema, intramural gas, and a sloughed mucosal membrane.[143-145] A percutaneous cholecystostomy may be therapeutic and can be done at the bedside.[146] Cholecystectomy is required for extensive gallbladder necrosis. The syndrome may be preventable by the stimulation of gallbladder emptying.[138]

Multiple organ system failure may be the ultimate expression of infectious complications. The development of multiple organ system failure has a high mortality and should initiate a search for occult infection.[147, 148] Because the gastrointestinal tract appears to be the reservoir for the pathogens of multiple organ system failure, strategies to prevent breakdown of mucosal barriers and translocation include a regimen of antacids, oral nystatin administration, and enteral nutrition.[149, 150]

Nutritional support is an integral component of the ICU care of the trauma patient and should be instituted as soon as the patient is hemodynamically stable. Although the enteral route is preferred, the gastrointestinal tract may not be accessible or functional. Central parenteral nutrition should be infused via a dedicated port in a multilumen catheter or preferably through a dedicated single-lumen catheter. The subclavian approach is preferred because of patient comfort and the capability of maintaining an occlusive dressing. For patients having an exploratory celiotomy with a prolonged convalescence expected, placement of an enteral feeding access such as a jejunostomy or gastrostomy is helpful. Using the gastrointestinal tract buffers against stress gastritis and reduces septic complications.[151, 152] Because nutritional requirements vary greatly in injured patients, metabolic monitoring may be of value to estimate actual energy expenditure.[153]

SUMMARY

Because of the magnitude of trauma and the population affected, ICU care of the injured patient has a great and positive potential impact both in economic terms and on morbidity. To avoid missed injuries and to enhance a positive outcome, care should be systematic and goal directed. The most common injuries and potential complications should be kept in mind. Because trauma management is a multidisciplinary field, communication among all parties (personnel of the trauma team, ICU service, subspecialties, nursing, and ancillary services and the family) is crucial. Care of the injured patient can be challenging, rewarding, and satisfying. It must be kept in mind that, even in those instances of brain death, societal benefits from these young and previously healthy patients can be significant, as they provide an important source of donor organs. Families receive comfort knowing that some good can come from a tragic event. All families should be given this opportunity to donate organs.[154]

References

1. Committee on Trauma Research of the National Research Council: Injury in America: A Continuing Public Health Problem. Washington, DC, National Academy Press, 1985.
2. Baker SP: Injuries: The neglected epidemic: Stone lecture, 1985 American Trauma Society Meeting. J Trauma 27:343, 1987.
3. Trunkey DD: Trauma. Sci Am 249(2):28, 1983.
4. Committee on Trauma of the American College of Surgeons: Advanced Trauma Life Support Course. Chicago, American College of Surgeons, 1989.
5. Floccare DJ, MacKenzie EJ, Ramzy AI: The trimodal curve revisited. Personal communication.
6. Champion HR, Sacco WJ, Carnazzo AJ, et al: Trauma score. Crit Care Med 9:672, 1981.
7. Baker SP, O'Neill B, Haddon W Jr, et al: The Injury Severity Score: A

method for describing patients with multiple injuries and evaluating emergency care. J Trauma 14:187, 1974.

8. Teasdale G, Jennett B: Assessment of coma and impaired consciousness. Lancet 2:81, 1974.

9. Champion HR, Sacco WJ, Copes WS, et al: A revision of the Trauma Score. J Trauma 29:623, 1989.

10. Morris JA Jr, Auerbach PS, Marshall EA, et al: The Trauma Score as a triage tool in the prehospital setting. JAMA 256:1319, 1986.

11. Committee on Medical Aspects of Automotive Safety: Rating the severity of tissue damage: I. The Abbreviated Scale. JAMA 215:277, 1971.

12. Boyd CR, Tolson MA, Copes WS: Evaluating trauma care: The TRISS method. J Trauma 27:370, 1987.

13. Champion HR, Sacco WJ, Lepper RL, et al: An Anatomic Index of injury severity. J Trauma 20:197, 1980.

14. Champion HR, Sacco WJ, Hannan DS, et al: Assessment of injury severity: The Triage Index. Crit Care Med 8:201, 1980.

15. Moore EE, Dunn EL, Moore JB, et al: Penetrating Abdominal Trauma Index. J Trauma 21:439, 1981.

16. Knaus WA, Draper EA, Wagner DP, et al: APACHE II: A severity of disease classification system. Crit Care Med 13:818, 1985.

17. Cerra FB, Negro F, Abrams J: APACHE II score does not predict multiple organ failure or mortality in postoperative surgical patients. Arch Surg 125:519, 1990.

18. Civetta JM, Hudson-Civetta JA, Nelson LD: Evaluation of APACHE II for cost containment and quality assurance. Ann Surg 212:226, 1990.

19. Morris JA Jr, MacKenzie EJ, Edelstein SL: The effect of pre-existing conditions on mortality in trauma patients. JAMA 263:1942, 1990.

20. Sturm JA, Lewis FR Jr, Trentz O, et al: Cardiopulmonary parameters and prognosis after severe multiple trauma. J Trauma 19:305, 1979.

21. Eddy AC, Rice CL, Anard DM: Right ventricular dysfunction in multiple trauma victims. Am J Surg 155:712, 1988.

22. Cuthbertson DP: Observations on the disturbance of metabolism produced by injury to the limbs. Q J Med 1:233, 1932.

23. Edwards JD, Redmond AD, Nightingale P, et al: Oxygen consumption following trauma: A reappraisal in severely injured patients requiring mechanical ventilation. Br J Surg 75:690, 1988.

24. Baxt WG, Moody P: The differential survival of trauma patients. J Trauma 27:602, 1987.

25. Gennarelli PA, Champion HR, Sacco WJ, et al: Mortality of patients with head injury and extracranial injury treated in trauma centers. J Trauma 29:1193, 1989.

26. Rosner MJ, Daughton S: Cerebral perfusion pressure management in head injury. J Trauma 30:933, 1990.

27. Aucoin PJ, Kotilainen HR, Gantz NM, et al: Intracranial pressure monitors: Epidemiologic study of risk factors and infections. Am J Med 80:369, 1986.

28. Mayhall CG, Archer NH, Lamb VA, et al: Ventriculostomy-related infections: A prospective epidemiologic study. N Engl J Med 310:553, 1984.

29. Clark WC, Muhlbauer MS, Lowrey R, et al: Complications of intracranial pressure monitoring in trauma patients. Neurosurgery 25:20, 1989.

30. Wyler AR, Kelly WA: Use of antibiotics with external ventriculostomies. J Neurosurg 37:185, 1972.

31. Muizelaar JP, Wei EP, Kontos HA, et al: Mannitol causes compensatory cerebral vasoconstriction and vasodilation in response to blood viscosity changes. J Neurosurg 59:822, 1983.

32. Little JR: Treatment of acute cerebral ischemia with intermittent, low dose mannitol. Neurosurgery 5:687, 1979.

33. Dearden NM, Gibson JS, McDowell DG, et al: Effect of high-dose dexamethasone on outcome from severe head injury. J Neurosurg 64:81, 1986.

34. Braakman R, Schouten HJA, Blaauw-Van Dishoeck M, et al: Megadose steroids in severe head injury: Results of a prospective double-blind clinical trial. J Neurosurg 58:326, 1983.

35. Cooper PR, Moody S, Clark WK, et al: Dexamethasone and severe head injury: A prospective double-blind study. J Neurosurg 51:307, 1979.

36. Longstreth WT, Inui TS: High blood glucose level on hospital admission and poor neurological recovery after cardiac arrest. Ann Neurol 15:59, 1984.

37. Pulsinelli WA, Levy DE, Sigsbee B, et al: Increased damage after ischemic stroke in patients with hyperglycemia with or without established diabetes mellitus. Am J Med 74:540, 1983.

38. Rogers MC, Kirsch JR: Current concepts in brain resuscitation. JAMA 261:3143, 1989.

39. Pickerd JD, Murray GD, Illingworth R, et al: Effect of oral nimodipine on cerebral infarction and outcome after subarachnoid haemorrhage: British aneurysm nimodipine trial. Br Med J 298:636, 1989.

40. Allen GS, Ahn HS, Reziosi TJ, et al: Cerebral arterial spasm—a controlled trial of nimodipine in patients with subarachnoid hemorrhage. N Engl J Med 308:619, 1983.

41. Faden AI: Opiate antagonist and thyrotropin-releasing hormone: II. Potential role in the treatment of central nervous system injury. JAMA 252:1452, 1984.

42. Bonnet F, Bilaine J, Lhoste F, et al: Naloxone therapy of human septic shock. Crit Care Med 13:972, 1985.

43. Helling TS, Ebans LL, Fowler DL, et al: Infectious complications in patients with severe head injury. J Trauma 28:1575, 1988.

44. Temkin NR, Dikmen SS, Wilensky AJ, et al: A randomized, double-blind study of phenytoin for the prevention of post-traumatic seizures. N Engl J Med 323:497, 1990. (Comment in: N Engl J Med 323:540, 1990.)

45. Dikmen SS, Temkin NR, Miller B, et al: Neurobehavioral effects of phenytoin prophylaxis of posttraumatic seizures. JAMA 265:1271, 1991. (Comment in: JAMA 265:1307, 1991.)

46. MacDonald RL, Schwartz ML, Mirich D, et al: Diagnosis of cervical spine injury in motor vehicle crash victims: How many x-rays are enough? J Trauma 30:392, 1990.

47. Ross SE, Schwab CW, David ET, et al: Clearing the cervical spine: Initial radiologic evaluation. J Trauma 27:1055, 1987.

48. Bracken MB, Shepard MJ, Collins WF, et al: A randomized, controlled trial of methylprednisolone or naloxone in the treatment of acute spinal cord injury. N Engl J Med 322:1405, 1990.

49. Gentilello L, Thompson DA, Tonnesen AS, et al: Effect of a rotating bed on the incidence of pulmonary complications in critically ill patients. Crit Care Med 16:783, 1988.

50. Nelson LD, Anderson HB: Physiologic effects of steep positioning in the surgical intensive care unit. Arch Surg 124:352, 1989.

51. Fink MP, Helsmoortel CM, Stein KL, et al: The efficacy of an oscillating bed in the prevention of lower respiratory tract infection in critically ill victims of blunt trauma: A prospective study. Chest 97:132, 1990.

52. Myers EM, Iko BO: The management of acute laryngeal trauma. J Trauma 27:448, 1987.

53. Felciano DV, Bitonda CG, Mattox KL, et al: Combined tracheoesophageal injuries. Am J Surg 150:710, 1985.

54. Lee RB, Morris JA Jr, Parker RS: Presence of three or more rib fractures as an indicator of need for interhospital transfer. J Trauma 29:795, 1989.

55. Shorr RM, Crittenden M, Indeck M, et al: Blunt thoracic trauma: Analysis of 515 patients. Ann Surg 206:200, 1987.

56. Moore DC: Intercostal nerve block for postoperative somatic pain following surgery of thorax and upper abdomen. Br J Anaesth 47:284, 1975.

57. Kvalheim L, Reiestead F: Intrapleural catheter in the management of postoperative pain. Anesthesiology 61:A231, 1984.

58. Rocco A, Reiestead F, Gudman J, et al: Intrapleural administration of local anesthetics for pain relief in patients with multiple rib fractures; Preliminary report. Reg Anaesth 12:10, 1987.

59. Carli PA, Mazoit X, Zetlaoui J, et al: Intrapleural administration of lidocaine for treatment of post traumatic thoracic pain. Anesthesiology 67:A241, 1987.

60. Frank ED, McKay W, Rocco A, et al: Comparison of intrapleural bupivacaine versus intermuscular narcotic for treatment of subcostal incisional pain. Anesth Analg 67:S62, 1988.

61. Behar M, Magora F, Olshwang D, et al: Epidural morphine and treatment of pain. Lancet 1:527, 1979.

62. Wright RMB, Goroszeniuk T: Epidural fentanyl for pain of multiple fractures. Lancet 2:1033, 1980.

63. Johnston JR, McCaughey W: Epidural morphine: A method of management of multiple fractured ribs. Anaesthesia 35:155, 1980.

64. Mackersie RC, Shackford SR, Hoyt DB, et al: Continuous epidural fentanyl analgesia: Ventilatory function improvement with routine use in treatment of blunt chest injury. J Trauma 27:1207, 1987.

65. Wisner DH: A stepwise logistic regression analysis of factors affecting morbidity and mortality after thoracic trauma: Effect of epidural analgesia. J Trauma 30:799, 1990.

66. Mackersie RC, Karagianes TG, Hoyt DB, et al: Prospective evaluation of epidural and intravenous opiates for pain control and restoration of ventilatory function following multiple rib fractures. J Trauma 30:925, 1990.

67. Bromage PR, Camporesi E, Chestnut D: Epidural narcotics for postoperative analgesia. Anesth Analg 59:473, 1980.

68. Rybro L, Schurizek BA, Petersen TK, et al: Postoperative analgesia and lung function: A comparison of intramuscular with epidural morphine. Acta Anaesth Scand 26:514, 1982.

69. Staren ED, Cullen ML: Epidural catheter analgesia for the management of postoperative pain. Surg Gynecol Obstet 162:389, 1986.

70. Cousins MJ, Mather LE: Intrathecal and epidural administration of opioids. Anesthesiology 61:276, 1984.

71. Clark GC, Schecter WP, Trunkey DD: Variables affecting outcome in blunt chest trauma: Flail chest vs. pulmonary contusion. J Trauma 28:298, 1988.

72. Gaillard M, Herve C, Mandin L, et al: Mortality prognostic factors in chest injury. J Trauma 30:93, 1990.

73. Barone JE, Pizzi WS, Nealon TF Jr, et al: Indications for intubation in blunt chest trauma. J Trauma 26:334, 1986.

74. Johnson JA, Cogbill TH, Winga ER: Determinants of outcome after pulmonary contusion. J Trauma 26:695, 1986.

75. Cohen EA: Treatment of flail chest by towel clip traction. Am J Surg 90:517, 1955.

76. Trinkle JK, Richardson JD, Franz JL, et al: Management of flail chest without mechanical ventilation. Ann Thorac Surg 19:355, 1975.

77. Sladen A, Aldredge CF, Albarran R: PEEP vs. ZEEP in the treatment of flail chest injuries. Crit Care Med 4:187, 1973.

78. Cullen P, Modell JH, Kirby RR, et al: Treatment of flail chest: Use of intermittent mandatory ventilation and positive end-expiratory pressure. Arch Surg 110:1099, 1975.

79. Landercasper J, Cogbill TH, Lindesmith LA: Long-term disability after flail chest injury. J Trauma 24:410, 1984.

80. Beal FL, Oreskovich MR: Long-term disability associated with flail chest injury. Am J Surg 150:324, 1985.

81. Bright EF, Beck CS: Nonpenetrating wounds of the heart: A clinical and experimental study. Am Heart J 10:293, 1935.

82. Parmley LF, Manion WC, Mattingly TW: Nonpenetrating traumatic injury of the heart. Circulation 18:371, 1958.

83. Jones JW, Hewitt RL, Drapanas T: Cardiac contusion: A capricious syndrome. Ann Surg 181:567, 1975.

84. Fabian TC, Mangiante EC, Patterson CR, et al: Myocardial contusion in blunt trauma: Clinical characteristics, means of diagnosis, and implications for patient management. J Trauma 28:50, 1988.

85. Tenzer ML: The spectrum of myocardial contusion: A review. J Trauma 25:620, 1985.

86. Harley OP, Mena I, Narahara KA, et al: Traumatic myocardial dysfunction. J Thorac Cardiovasc Surg 87:386, 1984.

87. Blair E, Topuzlu C, Davis JH: Delayed or missed diagnosis in blunt chest trauma. J Trauma 11:129, 1971.

88. Keller KD, Shatney CH: Creatine phosphokinase-MB assays in patients with suspected myocardial contusion: Diagnostic test or test of diagnosis? J Trauma 28:58, 1988.

89. Fabian TC, Sicicala RS, Croce MA, et al: A prospective evaluation of myocardial contusion: Relationship between CPK and cardiac dysfunction. J Trauma 30:920, 1990.

90. Hossack KF, Moreno CA, Vanway CW, et al: Frequency of cardiac contusion in nonpenetrating chest injury. Am J Cardiol 61:391, 1988.

91. Ross P Jr, Degutis L, Baker CC: Cardiac contusion: The effect on operative management of the patient with trauma injuries. Arch Surg 124:506, 1989.

92. Baxter BT, Moore EE, Moore FA, et al: A plea for sensible management of myocardial contusion. Am J Surg 158:557, 1989.

93. Beresky R, Klingler R, Peake J: Myocardial contusion: When does it have clinical significance? J Trauma 28:64, 1988.

94. King H, Shumacker HB Jr: Splenic studies; Susceptibility to infection after splenectomy performed in infancy. Ann Surg 136:239, 1952.

95. Pearce WH, Moore EE, Moore FA: Injury to the spleen. In: Mattox KL, Moore EE, Feliciano DV (eds): Trauma. East Norwalk, CT, Appleton & Lange, p 443, 1988.

96. Powell RW, Blaylock WE, Hoff CJ, et al: The efficacy of post-splenectomy sepsis prophylactic measures: The role of penicillin. J Trauma 28:1285, 1988.

97. Scher KS, Wroczynski FAS, Jones CW: Protection from post-splenectomy sepsis: Effect of prophylactic penicillin and pneumococcal vaccine on clearance of type 3 pneumococcus. Surgery 93:792, 1983.

98. Meyer AA, Crass RA, Lin RC Jr, et al: Selective nonoperative management of blunt liver injury using computed tomography. Arch Surg 120:550, 1985.

99. Farnell MB, Spencer MP, Thompson E, et al: Nonoperative management of blunt hepatic trauma in adults. Surgery 104:748, 1988.

100. Carmona RH, Peck DZ, Lin RC Jr: The role of packing and planned reoperation in severe hepatic trauma. J Trauma 24:779, 1984.

101. Moore FA, Moore EE, Seagraves A: Nonresectional management of major hepatic trauma; An evolving concept. Am J Surg 150:725, 1985.

102. Feliciano DV, Mattox KL, Burch JM, et al: Packing for control of hepatic hemorrhage. J Trauma 26:738, 1986.

103. Valeri CR, Cassidy G, Khuri S, et al: Hypothermia-induced reversible platelet dysfunction. Ann Surg 205:175, 1987.

104. Slotman GJ, Jed EH, Burchard KW: Adverse effects of hypothermia in postoperative patients. Am J Surg 149:495, 1985.

105. Ferrara A, MacArthur JD, Wright HK, et al: Hypothermia and acidosis worsen coagulopathy in the patient requiring massive transfusion. Am J Surg 160:515, 1990.

106. Jurkovich GJ, Greiser WB, Luterman A, et al: Hypothermia in trauma victims: An ominous predictor of survival. J Trauma 27:1019, 1987.

107. Jurkovich GJ: Hypothermia in the trauma patient. Adv Trauma 4:111, 1989.

108. Gentillo LM, Cortes V, Moujaes S, et al: Continuous arteriovenous rewarming: Experimental results and thermodynamic model simulation of treatment for hypothermia. J Trauma 30:1436, 1990.

109. Cox EF, Flancbaum L, Dauterive AH, et al: Blunt trauma to the liver; Analysis of management and mortality in 323 consecutive patients. Ann Surg 207:126, 1988.

110. Gillmore D, McSwain NE Jr, Browder IW: Hepatic trauma: To drain or not to drain? J Trauma 27:898, 1987.

111. Noyes LD, Doyle DJ, McSwain NE Jr: Septic complications associated with use of peritoneal drains in liver trauma. J Trauma 28:337, 1988.

112. Cogbill TH, Moore EE, Jurkovich GJ, et al: Severe hepatic trauma: A multi-center experience with 1,335 liver injuries. J Trauma 28:1433, 1988.

113. Clark DE, Georgitis JW, Ray FS: Renal artery injuries caused by blunt trauma. Surgery 90:87, 1981.

114. Vieira J, Smith CS, Cass AS, et al: Diagnosis of renal injury with computed tomography. Minn Med 69:207, 1986.

115. Spirnak JP, Resnick MI: Revascularization of traumatic thrombosis of the renal artery. Surg Gynecol Obstet 164:22, 1987.

116. Carroll PR, Klostermen PW, McAninch JW: Surgical management of renal trauma: Analysis of risk factors, technique, and outcome. J Trauma 28:1071, 1988.

117. Narrod JA, Moore EE, Posner M, et al: Nephrectomy following trauma—Impact on patient outcome. J Trauma 25:842, 1985.

118. Richards WO, Scovill W, Shin B, et al: Acute renal failure associated with increased intra-abdominal pressure. Ann Surg 197:183, 1983.

119. Wisner DH, Chun Y, Blaisdell W: Blunt intestinal injury: Keys to diagnosis and management. Arch Surg 125:1319, 1990.

120. Sherck JP, Oakes DD: Small bowel injuries missed by computed tomography. J Trauma 28:1096, 1988.

121. Buechter KJ, Arnold M, Steele B, et al: The use of serum amylase and lipase in evaluating and managing blunt abdominal trauma. Am Surg 56:204, 1990.

122. Smego DR, Richardson JD, Flint LM: Determinants of outcome in pancreatic trauma. J Trauma 25:771, 1985.

123. Fabian TC, Kudsk KA, Croce MA, et al: Superiority of closed suction drainage for pancreatic trauma: A randomized, prospective study. Ann Surg 211:724, 1990.

124. Pederzoli P, Bassi C, Falconi M, et al: Conservative treatment of external pancreatic fistulas with parenteral nutrition alone or in combination with continuous intravenous infusion of somatostatin, glucagon or calcitonin. Surg Gynecol Obstet 163:428, 1986.

125. Levinson MA, Petersen SR, Sheldon GF, et al: Duodenal trauma: Experience of a trauma center. J Trauma 24:475, 1984.

126. Cogbill TH, Moore EE, Kashuk JL: Changing trends in the management of pancreatic trauma. Arch Surg 117:722, 1982.

127. Ayella RJ, DuPriest RW Jr, Khaneja SC, et al: Transcatheter embolization of autologous clot in the management of bleeding associated with fractures of the pelvis. Surg Gynecol Obstet 147:849, 1978.

128. Panetta T, Sclafani SJA, Goldstein AS, et al: Percutaneous transcatheter embolization for massive bleeding from pelvic fractures. J Trauma 25:1021, 1985.

129. Johnson KD, Cadambi A, Seibert GB: Incidence of adult respiratory distress syndrome in patients with multiple musculoskeletal injuries; Effect of early operative stabilization of fractures. J Trauma 25:375, 1985.

130. Lozman J, Deno DC, Feustel PJ, et al: Pulmonary and cardiovascular consequences of immediate fixation or conservative management of long-bone fractures. Arch Surg 121:992, 1986.

131. Ten Duis HJ, Nijsten MWN, Klassen HJ, et al: Fat embolism in patients with an isolated fracture of the femoral shaft. J Trauma 28:383, 1988.

132. Bone LB, Johnson KD, Weigelt J, et al: Early versus delayed stabilization of femoral fractures: A randomized study. J Bone Joint Surg [Am] 71:336, 1989.

133. Behrman SW, Fabian TC, Kudsk KA, et al: Improved outcome with femur fractures: Early versus delayed fixation. J Trauma 30:792, 1990.

134. Brink BE: Vascular trauma. Surg Clin North Am 57:189, 1977.

135. Bishara RA, Pasch AR, Lim LT, et al: Improved results in the treatment of civilian vascular injuries associated with fractures and dislocations. J Vasc Surg 3:707, 1986.

136. Feliciano DV, Herskowitz K, O'Gorman RB, et al: Management of vascular injuries in the lower extremities. J Trauma 28:319, 1988.

137. Mubarak SJ, Hargens AR, Owen CA, et al: The wick catheter technique for measurement of intramuscular pressure: A new research and clinical tool. J Bone Joint Surg [Am] 58:1016, 1976.

138. Mubarak SJ, Owen CA, Hargens AR, et al: Acute compartment syndromes: Diagnosis and treatment with the aid of the wick catheter. J Bone Joint Surg [Am] 60:1091, 1978.

139. DuPriest RW Jr, Khaneja SC, Cowley RA: Acute cholecystitis complicating trauma. Ann Surg 189:84, 1979.

140. Petersen SR, Sheldon GF: Acute acalculous cholecystitis: A complication of hyperalimentation. Am J Surg 138:814, 1979.

141. Gately JF, Thomas EJ: Acute cholecystitis occurring as a complication of other diseases. Arch Surg 118:1137, 1983.

142. Flancbaum L, Majerus TC, Cox EF: Acute posttraumatic acalculous cholecystitis. Am J Surg 150:252, 1985.

143. Deitch EA, Engel JM: Acute acalculous cholecystitis: Ultrasonic diagnosis. Am J Surg 142:290, 1981.

144. Johnson LB: The importance of early diagnosis of acute acalculus cholecystitis. Surg Gynecol Obstet 164:197, 1987.

145. Cornwell EE III, Rodriguez A, Mirvis SE, et al: Acute acaluous cholecystitis in critically injured patients. Preoperative diagnostic imaging. Ann Surg 210:52, 1989.

146. Eggermont AM, Lameris JS, Jeekel J: Ultrasound-guided percutaneous transhepatic cholecystostomy for acute acalculous cholecystitis. Arch Surg 120:1354, 1985.

147. Fry DE, Pearlstein L, Fulton RL, et al: Multiple system organ failure: The role of uncontrolled infection. Arch Surg 115:136, 1980.

148. Polk HC Jr, Shields CL: Remote organ failure: A valid sign of occult intra-abdominal infection. Surgery 81:310, 1977.
149. Marshall JC, Christou NV, Horn R, et al: The microbiology of multiple organ failure: The proximal gastrointestinal tract as an occult reservoir of pathogens. Arch Surg 123:309, 1988.
150. Baker CC, Degutis LC: Trauma and multiple organ failure: The clinical challenge. In: Kreis DJ Jr, Gomez GA (eds): Trauma Management. Boston, Little, Brown, p 473, 1989.
151. Kudsk KA, Stone JM, Carpenter G, et al: Enteral and parenteral feeding influences mortality after hemoglobin–E. coli peritonitis in normal rats. J Trauma 23:605, 1983.
152. Moore FA, Moore EE, Jones TN, et al: TEN versus TPN following major abdominal trauma—Reduced septic morbidity. J Trauma 29:916, 1989.
153. Cortes V, Nelson LD: Errors in estimating energy expenditure in critically ill surgical patients. Arch Surg 124:287, 1989.
154. Morris JA Jr, Slaton J, Gibbs D: Vascular organ procurement in the trauma population. J Trauma 29:782, 1989.

CHAPTER 139

Obstetrics and Gynecology in the Intensive Care Unit

Michael A. Belfort
Gary A. Dildy
David B. Cotton

Modern technology and practices have greatly reduced the incidence of emergencies requiring intensive care in the field of obstetrics and gynecology. However, death and serious morbidity, although less common in current times, are still prevalent, and it is to these emergent situations that this chapter is directed.

There has been a steady decline in maternal mortality in the United States since 1915, when national vital statistics were first reported.[1] Of the 321 maternal deaths in 1978, 19% were due to toxemia, 19% to sepsis, 12% to ectopic pregnancy, and 11% to obstetric hemorrhage.[2] Kaunitz and associates reviewed the causes of maternal mortality in the United States (1974 to 1978) and noted that of 2475 maternal deaths, 2067 (84%) were pregnancy related, not including previable pregnancies.[3]

The most frequent causes of death were embolism, hypertensive disease, obstetric hemorrhage, and infection, and the most common cause in the previable group was ectopic pregnancy. This study showed an overall decrease in maternal death resulting from all of the foregoing causes except embolism, which may be less preventable and relatively over-reported. In a review of 501 consecutive maternal deaths in Texas between 1969 and 1973, Gibbs and Locke demonstrated that most deaths occurred in the postpartum period (297 postpartum deaths vs. 155 antepartum deaths).[4] There were 309 maternal deaths secondary to direct obstetric causes: hemorrhage (36%), pregnancy-induced hypertension (PIH) (23%), infection (21%), amniotic fluid embolism (7%), and anesthesia (5%). Several studies have shown a markedly increased risk of death with advancing maternal age.[5]

The final common denominator of many of the conditions described in this chapter is the appearance of various forms of shock, defined here as a condition in which circulation fails to meet the nutritional needs of the cell and fails to remove metabolic wastes. When the circulating blood volume is less than the capacity of the vascular bed, hypotension with diminished tissue perfusion results, leading to cellular hypoxia and ultimately cell death. Depending on the duration and severity of the insult, irreversible organ damage or death may ensue. We deal initially with shock in general, giving a brief outline of the most commonly encountered situations and the supportive measures that can be broadly applied. Then, specific conditions and their management are dealt with in a little more detail.

GENERAL SUPPORTIVE MEASURES IN OBSTETRIC AND GYNECOLOGIC PATIENTS IN SHOCK

Etiology of Shock in Obstetric and Gynecologic Patients

Shock in the obstetric patient may be subdivided by cause, including hypovolemia, sepsis, neurogenic causes, or cardiogenic causes (Table 139–1). Although the causes are quite different, there is often a common pathophysiologic pathway ultimately leading to hypoperfusion at the tissue level. This decreased perfusion, secondary to hypovolemia or cardiac pump failure, results in hypoxia and acidosis and finally clinical shock.

Hypovolemic shock is usually the result of hemorrhage secondary to disruption of a closed cardiovascular circuit or less commonly to a coagulopathy or intravascular depletion associated with increased capillary permeability. Causes of the former include uterine atony, abnormal placentation or development (placenta previa, abruptio placentae, placenta accreta, ectopic pregnancy, spontaneous abortion, and hydatidiform mole), and trauma (accidental or obstetric). Obstetric trauma refers to lacerations of the cervix, vagina, and perineum; episiotomy; forceps delivery; cesarean section; dilatation and curettage; and abortion and loosely includes rupture of the uterus or liver. Gynecologic surgical procedures may result in severe blood loss, particularly in oncology cases, in which major vessels are frequently encountered during the node dissection. These patients may also spend many hours on the operating table and lose a large amount of interstitial fluid into the third space.

Coagulopathies causing hemorrhage may be acquired or hereditary and, although uncommon, may follow abortion induced with hypertonic saline,[6] sepsis,[7] retained dead fetus syndrome,[8] abruptio placentae,[9] amniotic fluid embolism,[10] preeclampsia or eclampsia,[11–14] intravascular hemolysis,[15] or trauma[16] (Table 139–2). Coagulopathy may also be precipitated by hemorrhage managed with massive volume replacement with crystalloid and packed red blood cells.

Sepsis may precipitate shock via several pathophysiologic pathways usually mediated by intravascular volume depletion and myocardial depression. Septic shock in obstetrics can occur in association with many conditions (Table 139–3), some of which are unique to obstetrics. Septic abortion,[17] pyelonephritis,[18] appendicitis,[19, 20] chorioamnionitis,[21] toxic shock syndrome,[22] and septic pelvic thrombophlebitis[23, 24] are

TABLE 139–1
COMMON CAUSES OF SHOCK IN OBSTETRICS AND GYNECOLOGY
Hypovolemia
Sepsis
Neurogenic causes
Cardiogenic causes
Anaphylaxis

TABLE 139–2

COMMON CAUSES OF COAGULOPATHY IN OBSTETRICS AND GYNECOLOGY

Abruptio placentae
Pregnancy-induced hypertension and HELLP* syndrome
Sepsis
Amniotic fluid embolism
Retained dead fetus syndrome
Massive blood transfusion
Induced abortion using intra-amniotic hypertonic saline

*HELLP = hemolysis, elevated liver enzymes, and low platelet count.

---

all well described in the obstetric literature. Septic shock secondary to chorionic villus sampling has also been reported.[25, 26]

Cardiogenic shock occurs secondary to ventricular dysfunction or cardiac compression. Unique to the obstetric patient are such conditions as amniotic fluid embolism and peripartum cardiomyopathy. Certain structural cardiac defects can be lethal during pregnancy, especially in the peripartum period.

General Supportive Measures

The diagnosis of shock in the obstetric patient should initiate several important actions. Placement of two large-bore intravenous catheters for rapid intravascular volume expansion with infusion of 1 L of balanced salt solution during the first 15 minutes is essential while further diagnostic and therapeutic measures are taken. An indwelling bladder catheter is placed for determination of urine output. An arterial catheter allows continuous measurement of systemic blood pressure, as well as easy access for laboratory investigations. In cases requiring massive transfusion or infusion of fluids, invasive hemodynamic monitoring should be instituted to follow cardiac and respiratory parameters. Oxygen should be administered via nasal prongs or face mask at 6 to 8 L/min, and the fraction of inspired oxygen should be adjusted according to arterial blood gas results to maintain the PaO_2 within acceptable limits. If the ability to maintain an adequate tidal volume or if oxygen and carbon dioxide gas exchange is impaired or if the airway is obstructed, endotracheal intubation and positive pressure ventilation may be required.

Initial laboratory investigation should include blood type and cross-match, complete blood count, platelet count, prothrombin time, partial thromboplastin time, fibrinogen, electrolytes, blood urea nitrogen and creatinine, and arterial blood gases. A urine specimen obtained via catheter should be sent for analysis and microscopic evaluation. If sepsis is suspected, when the patient is stabilized, cultures of blood, urine, sputum, amniotic fluid, endometrial cavity, and stool should be made, as indicated.

Controversy still exists regarding the use of crystalloids or colloids for initial treatment. One study showed that two to four times as much 0.9% saline was required to reach the same hemodynamic end points as 6% hetastarch and 5% albumin. Colloid osmotic pressure (COP) rose when albumin and hetastarch were administered but fell with saline. Resuscitation with normal saline also resulted in a higher incidence of pulmonary edema. Standard dextran with a molecular weight averaging 75,000 may initiate intravascular coagulation but has been used without complication in the volume expansion of patients with PIH.[27] Low-molecular-weight dextran, with a molecular weight averaging 40,000, is less likely to initiate disseminated intravascular coagulation (DIC) but also has less tendency to "pull" fluid into the intravascular space.[28]

In 1984 the American College of Obstetricians and Gynecologists recommended avoidance of dextran because of its anticoagulant effects and risks of anaphylaxis.[29] If initial crystalloid therapy does not result in the desired clinical improvement, administration of colloids for further volume expansion is advisable. In cases of hemorrhagic hypovolemic shock and DIC, blood component therapy is indicated; bear in mind that, grossly, the degree of hemorrhage is often underestimated by as much as 50%.[30] "Relative bradycardia," a sign of acute intraperitoneal bleeding, may accompany hypotension, giving the false impression of a normal pulse rate as opposed to the tachycardia expected with blood loss.[31] The term massive blood replacement is used when at least one total volume is replaced during a 24-hour period.[30] In patients who need urgent or massive transfusion and for whom blood typing and screening have already been done, the risk of abbreviating the major cross-match after the "immediate spin" phase is low.[32] Liberal use of fresh frozen plasma is now under scrutiny and requires specific indications, as noted in Table 139–4.[33, 34]

In addition to containing the components of the coagulation, fibrinolytic, and complement systems, fresh frozen plasma contains proteins that maintain oncotic pressure and modulate immunity. Because of risks, including disease transmission, anaphylactoid reactions, alloimmunization, and volume overload, alternative therapy with crystalloids and other colloids is encouraged. This aspect of fluid replacement is discussed at greater depth in Chapter 12.

Because pathologic hemorrhage in the patient receiving massive transfusion is usually due to thrombocytopenia (rather than depletion of coagulation factors), only when factor deficiencies are presumed to be the cause of the bleeding should patients receive empirical administration of fresh frozen plasma.[33] In most cases of massive transfusion with uncontrolled hemorrhage, concentrated platelet infu-

---

TABLE 139–3

INFECTIONS ASSOCIATED WITH SEPTIC SHOCK IN THE OBSTETRIC AND GYNECOLOGY PATIENT

Chorioamnionitis
Postpartum endometritis
Urinary tract infections including pyelonephritis
Appendicitis
Necrotizing fasciitis (postoperative)
Septic abortion
Septic pelvic thrombophlebitis
Toxic shock syndrome

TABLE 139–4

INDICATIONS FOR THE USE OF FRESH FROZEN PLASMA IN THE CRITICALLY ILL OBSTETRIC PATIENT

Replacement of isolated factor deficiencies
Reversal of warfarin effect
Antithrombin III deficiency
Immunodeficiencies
Thrombotic thrombocytopenia purpura
Massive blood transfusion when factor deficiencies are the sole or principal derangements

Adapted from Consensus Conference: Fresh-frozen plasma. Indications and risks. JAMA 253:551, 1985.

TABLE 139–5

INDICATIONS FOR PLATELET TRANSFUSION IN AN OBSTETRIC PATIENT

Platelet count below 20,000/mm³ without evidence of active bleeding
Platelet count below 50,000/mm³ with evidence of bleeding
Platelet count below 50,000/mm³ before surgery
Massive transfusion of over 20 U of blood in a 12-h period

sions are appropriate (Table 139–5). No evidence exists that the prophylactic transfusion of a unit of fresh frozen plasma every 5 or 6 U of packed red blood cells decreases transfusion requirements in massively transfused patients, unless coagulation factor defects have been found.[35] The most useful values for predicting abnormal bleeding and guiding therapy in massively transfused trauma patients are the platelet count and fibrinogen level.[36] Adults have a limited mobilizable platelet pool and a limited ability to increase production acutely, and platelets in refrigerated blood quickly become nonviable,[37] making acute correction of thrombocytopenia difficult without platelet component transfusion.

Blood product transfusion can be minimized by selective correction of thrombocytopenia and specific coagulation factor defects.[30] In trauma patients, platelets are usually required after more than 20 U of blood is given in a 12-hour period;[36] however, in obstetric patients with thrombocytopenia secondary to preeclampsia, platelet transfusion may be indicated much earlier in the treatment. Cryoprecipitate should be administered instead of fresh frozen plasma when the calculated coagulation factor defect based on blood fibrinogen levels may result in volume overload.

Inotropic Agents

If adequate intravascular volume replacement is not successful in supporting blood pressure (a systolic blood pressure of at least 80 mmHg), advancing shock should be suspected and inotropic therapy may be required. Dopamine, one of the first-line inotropic agents, increases myocardial contractility and heart rate via beta-adrenergic receptors releasing norepinephrine from myocardial storage sites. Its action is dose dependent, resulting in beta-adrenergic receptor–mediated vasodilation of renal, mesenteric, coronary, and intracerebral vessels. In higher doses dopamine causes vasoconstriction of all vascular beds via alpha-adrenergic receptors.[38] Dopamine should be started at 2 to 5 μg/kg/min and titrated to the desired clinical effect.[38] Doses between 2 and 5 μg/kg/min result in vasodilation of renal and mesenteric vasculature via beta$_2$-adrenergic and dopaminergic receptors, and doses between 5 and 10 μg/kg/min result in increased myocardial contractility and cardiac output via beta$_1$-adrenergic receptors.[39] Doses higher than 20 μg/kg/min result in generalized vasoconstriction via alpha-adrenergic receptors. If an adequate hemodynamic response has not been achieved, dobutamine should be added to the dopamine regimen at 2 to 10 μg/kg/min.[40] Dobutamine increases cardiac output with minimal tachycardia by acting as a myocardial beta-receptor stimulant. If the addition of dobutamine still does not provide adequate support, isoproterenol, a beta-adrenergic agonist, may be added. Increased heart rate and increased contractility are achieved at the risk of ventricular ectopy, excessive tachycardia, and peripheral vasodilation. Other inotropic agents, such as digoxin and amrinone (Inocor), may also be used to improve myocardial contractility.[41] Digoxin is usually administered under contin-

uous electrocardiographic monitoring with an initial bolus of 0.5 mg by intravenous push, followed by 0.25-mg doses every 4 hours for a total loading dose of 1.0 mg. The maintenance dosage in pregnant patients is usually 0.25 to 0.37 mg/d, depending on the plasma levels.[40] Amrinone, an inotropic agent with vasodilatory activity, is indicated for the short-term management of cardiac failure.[41] A bolus of 0.75 mg/kg over 2 to 3 minutes followed by an infusion of 5 to 10 μg/kg/min should be given. Vasodilation may be undesirable in septic shock, and vasodilators should be used only when absolutely indicated and in appropriately monitored circumstances.

Vasopressor Agents

If blood pressure does not respond to inotropic therapy, a peripheral vasoconstrictor should be started to maintain systemic vascular resistance. Before potent inotropic agents (Table 139–6) or vasopressor agents are used, it is advisable to have available the appropriate invasive monitoring device, preferably a pulmonary arterial catheter. Phenylephrine, an alpha-adrenergic agonist, may be initiated at 1 to 3 μ/kg/min. Norepinephrine, a mixed alpha- and beta-agonist with powerful vasoconstrictive properties, may be added to provide generalized vasoconstriction and increased systemic vascular resistance. This agent should be utilized only when blood pressure is dangerously low in spite of other inotropic therapy, because perfusion of vital organs (kidneys and lungs) may be reduced by the vasoconstriction. Caution must be exercised in use of these agents in gravid patients. Dopamine has the capacity to reduce uteroplacental perfusion. When it was administered to the normotensive pregnant ewe at more than 10 μg/kg/min, there was a significant reduction in uterine blood flow.[42] Furthermore, pregnant ewes subjected to spinal hypotension showed further reduction in uteroplacental blood flow and a higher uterine vascular resistance than normotensive controls when dopamine was administered in sufficient doses to maintain normal blood pressure.[43] Greiss and Van Wilkes also noted a marked increase in uterine vascular resistance, out of proportion to the increase in blood pressure, resulting in decreased uterine blood flow in pregnant ewes.[44] They concluded that these vasopressors are indicated only in cases in which they are essential for maternal survival. When these agents are required, fetal distress should be anticipated and, if possible, arrangements for emergency delivery should be made while the maternal condition is stabilized.

Invasive Monitoring

Since its introduction in 1970 by Swan, Ganz, and coworkers,[45] the pulmonary arterial catheter, used for determina-

TABLE 139–6

DOSAGE REGIMENS OF THE COMMONLY USED INOTROPES

Agent	Loading Dose	Maintenance Dose
Dopamine	—	2–5 μg/kg/min (renal) 5–10 μg/kg/min (cardiac)
Dobutamine	—	2–10 μg/kg/min
Digoxin	0.5 mg IV push followed by 0.25 mg IV push q 4 h × 2	0.25–0.375 mg/d PO
Amrinone	0.75 mg/kg slow IV push	5–10 μg/kg/min IV
Phenylephrine	—	1–5 μg/kg/min IV

TABLE 139–7

INDICATIONS FOR INVASIVE MONITORING IN OBSTETRIC AND GYNECOLOGY PATIENTS

Pulmonary edema or adult respiratory distress syndrome associated with severe PIH
Oliguria or anuria associated with severe PIH
Severe hypertension unresponsive to vasodilator therapy in patients with severe PIH
Critical maternal cardiac disease (New York Heart Association classes III and IV) during labor, delivery, and early puerperium
Severe PIH with suspicion of tissue-level ischemia
Endotoxic shock

tion of cardiac output and right-sided heart and pulmonary capillary wedge pressures, has become increasingly important to clinicians managing critically ill patients. Invasive monitoring of this nature is indicated in many clinical situations (Table 139–7),[46] some of which are unique to obstetrics.[29, 47, 48] In many instances, pathophysiologic conditions secondary to or associated with the pregnant state may be diagnosed and treated more appropriately with the Swan-Ganz catheter. Kirshon and Cotton found that hydrostatic pulmonary edema may develop at a lower pulmonary capillary wedge pressure during pregnancy than in the nonpregnant state, probably because of a lower COP during pregnancy.[47] In a study of 18 patients with severe PIH, Cotton and coworkers found central venous pressure to be a poor predictor of pulmonary capillary wedge pressure.[49] Packman and Rackow found an inconstant correlation between central venous pressure and wedge pressure during fluid loading in patients with hypovolemia and septic shock.[50] In addition, these authors stated that left-sided heart filling pressure during fluid resuscitation should not exceed 12 mm Hg.[50] Belfort and colleagues, however, showed that the pulmonary capillary wedge pressure may be safely elevated to as much as 16 mm Hg by using low volumes (400 to 600 mL) of high-molecular-weight colloids in the management of severe PIH.[27, 51] Clark and associates suggested that the Swan-Ganz catheter is particularly helpful in managing patients with severe preeclampsia and patients who have structural cardiac defects during the peripartum period.[48] This subject is discussed more completely in the section on invasive monitoring in severe PIH.

An alternative approach to invasive monitoring is pulsed Doppler ultrasonography,[52] which yields results that correlate closely with thermodilution-derived estimates of stroke volume and cardiac output. Noninvasive methods of cardiac output determination may be beneficial when invasive monitoring is not feasible, such as in severe maternal thrombocytopenia, or when the facility of hemodynamic monitoring is not available. In addition, cardiac output measurements by the thermodilution technique are misleading in some patients (those with tricuspid insufficiency or pulmonic insufficiency),[52] and in these cases noninvasive monitoring may aid in management. Bioimpedance plethysmography[53] has been used to monitor cardiac output continuously; although it is not accepted as a clinical tool at this time, this method, in association with other noninvasive methods of monitoring, may provide more controlled management of the severely hypertensive gravida.

Surgical Therapy

In conjunction with medical therapy and support, surgical therapy is an integral part of managing the critically ill obstetric patient. It is important that surgical intervention in the shocked obstetric patient be well timed. The specific surgical procedures indicated are discussed with each condition in the following.

Perimortem Cesarean Section

One of the more dramatic, although infrequently performed, emergency surgical procedures in obstetric practice is perimortem cesarean section, and this operation may be indicated on occasion in the intensive care unit setting. Katz and colleagues stressed that, today, most maternal deaths occur acutely and the chances of fetal survival when perimortem cesarean section is initiated are improved if maternal death is sudden.[54] If the procedure is begun within 4 minutes of maternal cardiac arrest, both fetal and maternal outcomes are improved.[54] When cardiopulmonary resuscitation of a pregnant woman is undertaken, cesarean section is indicated to improve maternal survival because effective cardiopulmonary resuscitation is often impossible in the third trimester without reduction of the abdominal distention.[54] Fetal outcome is related to fetal gestational age and the amount of time that elapses between maternal death and delivery. The longest documented time interval from maternal death to delivery with fetal survival is 25 minutes.[55] In cases of moribund patients suffering from chronic disease, preparation for perimortem cesarean section should be planned well in advance. In the rare cases in which the operation is performed electively before death of the mother, the operator should address the appropriate medicolegal questions. Katz and colleagues have concluded that there is minimal legal risk for the physician in performing a perimortem section.[54] The possible benefits include survival of the infant and improved maternal cardiopulmonary resuscitation. Removal of the placenta at the time of delivery is encouraged because postoperative placental expulsion has been known to occur.

SPECIFIC ETIOLOGIES AND THEIR DIAGNOSES, PATHOPHYSIOLOGIES, AND TREATMENTS

Hemorrhagic shock is often easy to control and reverse, but hemorrhage is still one of the leading causes of death in the obstetric population.[3] Pritchard has shown that the average blood volume expansion induced by pregnancy is about 1500 mL.[56] The average amount of blood lost during a vaginal delivery is 500 mL and during elective repeated cesarean section is 1000 mL.[56] No physiologic compromise should be encountered if the volume of blood lost at delivery does not exceed the amount added during pregnancy.

Treatment of hemorrhagic shock involves correcting the initiating process and instituting general supportive measures, as previously discussed. If medical therapy is unsuccessful, surgical procedures such as uterine artery ligation,[57, 58] internal iliac artery ligation,[59] and emergency hysterectomy[60] may be required.

Uterine Atony

Uterine atony occurs in 1 of 20 deliveries and is the most common cause of postpartum hemorrhage.[29] These patients may rapidly decompensate and frequently require intensive care unit management for attendant problems complicating the resuscitation and stabilization efforts (Table 139–8).

Factors associated with atony include precipitous or prolonged labor, use of oxytocin or magnesium sulfate, chorioamnionitis, overdistention of the uterus, fetal macrosomia, and operative delivery.[60] The diagnosis is usually made after delivery of the placenta when excessive bleeding is noted per vaginam in the absence of vaginal or cervical laceration. The uterine fundus is invariably poorly con-

TABLE 139-8

MANAGEMENT PLAN FOR UTERINE ATONY AND POSTPARTUM HEMORRHAGE

Large-bore IV line with balanced salt solution at 250 mL/h and 20–30 U of oxytocin (Syntocinon, Pitocin) added to each liter of fluid

Exclude other causes of hemorrhage (see text)

If uterus still remains atonic, administer 0.2 mg methylergonovine maleate (Methergine) IM (or if peripheral perfusion is impaired, IV)

If uterus still remains atonic, administer a solution of 15-methyl $PGF_{2\alpha}$ (Prostin 15/M, Hemabate: 20 mg in 20 mL of 0.9% NaCl) into the myometrium (transabdominally or transvaginally) in several separate areas

If bleeding continues, consider surgical options (see text)

tracted. The uterine cavity should be explored to rule out retained placenta, retained blood clot, and disruption of the uterine wall. Initial management includes bimanual fundal massage and administration of oxytocin (Pitocin, Syntocinon), 20 to 30 U/L, at a high intravenous rate or via direct intramyometrial injection. Methylergonovine maleate (Methergine), 0.2 mg, may be given intramuscularly except in those patients with antepartum hypertension, in whom it may precipitate a hypertensive crisis with severe vasospasm.

Prostaglandin derivatives have been effective in treating postpartum uterine atony when other modalities have failed. Takagi and associates showed that intramyometrial administration of prostaglandin $F_{2\alpha}$ ($PGF_{2\alpha}$) was superior to both intravenous or intramuscular injection.[61] They noted that intramyometrial $PGF_{2\alpha}$ was associated with increased oxytocin levels, possibly via the Ferguson reflex, with enhanced release of oxytocin from the pituitary. Hayashi and others evaluated the 15-methyl analogue of $PGF_{2\alpha}$, (15S)-15-methyl $PGF_{2\alpha}$ tromethamine salt (Prostin 15/M), in the management of uterine atony unresponsive to conventional therapy.[62] Control was successful in 44 of 51 patients (86%). Four of the seven patients who did not respond to therapy had chorioamnionitis. The intramyometrial route may be preferable to peripheral intramuscular injection, especially in patients who are in shock and have compromised circulation. Side effects were infrequent and mild in degree.[62] Caution is indicated when considering the use of this agent for patients with pulmonary compromise. Hankins and coworkers reported marked transient arterial desaturation secondary to intrapulmonary shunting in five women treated with 15-methyl $PGF_{2\alpha}$ for severe postpartum hemorrhage resulting from uterine atony.[63]

If hemorrhage persists despite medical therapy, surgical intervention is mandated.[58–60] Clark and colleagues considered that hypogastric artery ligation should be reserved for stable patients of low parity who strongly desire further childbearing, as they found a high complication rate and a low success rate with hypogastric artery ligation in obtaining control of uterine hemorrhage.[60] Percutaneous transcatheter hypogastric artery embolization[64] may be considered in certain situations. Hysterectomy, as a last resort, is clearly indicated for profound intractable hemorrhage if the patient is unstable, multiparous, or not desirous of future childbearing.[57] Over the years, uterine atony and placenta accreta have replaced uteroplacental apoplexy (Couvelaire's uterus) and simple dehiscence of a uterine scar as major indications for hysterectomy at the time of cesarean section.[57]

Placenta Previa

Placenta previa may be classified as marginal, partial, or total, depending on the relationship of the placenta to the internal os of the cervix. The overall incidence near term is 1 in 200 pregnancies.[65] The major hazards associated with placenta previa are profound maternal hemorrhage and shock, with significant perinatal morbidity and mortality. Risk factors associated with the development of placenta previa include high parity, advanced maternal age, previous history of abortions, and previous history of cesarean section. Clark and coworkers noted that the incidence of placenta previa was 0.26% with an unscarred uterus and increased linearly to 10% in patients with four or more cesarean sections.[66]

Diagnosis is best made by ultrasonography, which may also be useful in predicting, during the early second trimester, which patients will be at risk for total placenta previa at term. If the diagnosis cannot be made with certainty based on ultrasonography, a double-setup examination should be performed, with preparations for blood transfusion and cesarean section. The "conservative aggressive management" of placenta previa, utilizing expectant management, has resulted in a reduction of perinatal mortality to approximately 12.6%.[67] This approach includes antenatal transfusions, tocolytic agents for preterm labor, and elective termination of pregnancy based on amniotic fluid maturity studies.

Placenta previa is also associated with placenta accreta, increta, and percreta, especially when the patient had a previous cesarean section.[66] Profuse bleeding secondary to placenta previa requires immediate cesarean section and in some cases, especially if complicated by placenta accreta, progression to hysterectomy after less radical surgical maneuvers, such as uterine artery ligation and hypogastric artery ligation, have failed. Rare cases of invasion into extrauterine structures such as the bladder, requiring bladder resection and massive transfusion, have been reported.[68] Improved maternal and fetal outcomes are thought to result from improved antenatal surveillance, increased use of cesarean section, and better neonatal care.

Abruptio Placentae

The incidence of abruptio placentae is estimated to be 1 in every 120 deliveries.[69] The exact etiology is unknown, but associated conditions include hypertensive disorders, parity, and history of previous abruption. Although the incidence is relatively low, abruption accounts for 15 to 25% of all perinatal deaths and has a perinatal mortality rate of 25 to 50%.[69–71]

Patients usually present with abdominal pain, which may be associated with vaginal bleeding. The fetal condition depends on the duration and degree of the placental separation. Amniotomy may reveal bloody amniotic fluid. Antenatal ultrasonographic evidence of a retroplacental blood clot or subchorionic hematoma is rarely seen. At the time of delivery, adherent hematoma and compression of placental tissue are usually noted.

Abdella and associates studied 265 cases of abruption and noted that 26.8% were complicated by a hypertensive disorder.[72] There was a correlation between the incidence of abruption and the severity of hypertension, with 2.3, 10.0, and 23.6% incidences of abruption among preeclamptics, chronic hypertensives, and eclamptics, respectively.[72] Pritchard and Brekken noted that between 1956 and 1965 the incidence of abruption resulting in fetal death was 1 per 433 deliveries (0.2%).[9] They estimated that at least 2 L of blood must be lost to result in fetal death. In 38% of the patients, the fibrinogen level was below 150 mg/100 mL and in 28%, below 100 mg/100 mL.[9]

An increasingly seen risk factor for abruption is cocaine abuse during pregnancy.[73] Cocaine causes placental vasoconstriction, decreased blood flow to the fetus, and increased uterine contractility.[74] A comparison of cocaine and methadone users showed a significant difference in the complication rate during labor and delivery, with a 17.3% abruption rate among cocaine users and a 1.3% rate in the methadone users.[74] With more common usage of cocaine, an increased incidence should be expected during pregnancy in the future. Little and colleagues reported a 9.8% prevalence of cocaine abuse during pregnancy in an indigent population.[75] The exact impact on the incidence of abruption is still unknown.

Abruption also follows abdominal trauma and sudden decompression of the uterus and may occasionally result from rupture of the membranes in cases of polyhydramnios.

The management of abruption still has controversial aspects. Initial treatment includes establishment of large-bore intravenous access, supplementary oxygen, cross-matching of red blood cells, hematologic and coagulation laboratory studies, fetal heart rate monitoring, maternal urine output via an indwelling catheter, and amniotomy with use of oxytocin in some cases.[76] Simultaneous correction of anemia and coagulation defects should be instituted.

The decision to allow vaginal delivery or to proceed with cesarean section when the fetus is still alive has been facilitated with the advent of electronic fetal monitoring. In most situations, consideration of maternal hemodynamic and coagulation status and fetal well-being guides clinical decision making. Cesarean section is reserved for usual obstetric indications, as well as for severe hemorrhage or worsening coagulopathy developing at a time remote from expected delivery. When severe abruption has resulted in fetal demise associated with coagulopathy, vaginal delivery should be attempted with appropriate blood component replacement and oxytocic augmentation as required. There are cases in which the uterus appears resistant to augmentation and labor does not progress despite maternal resuscitation and correction of the coagulopathy. In these cases infusion of aprotinin has been reported to be of use.[77] Application of a bone screw to the fetal cranium (after decompression of the fetal head) followed by traction on the fetal skull has also been reported to effect vaginal delivery in cases with protracted or arrested labor curves and avoids potentially life-threatening surgery in cases complicated by DIC.[78]

Anemia and infection are commonly encountered during the postpartum period in patients who have experienced severe abruptio placentae,[76] and anticipation and early intervention are important.

Ectopic Pregnancy

Ectopic pregnancy continues to have a major influence on maternal morbidity and mortality in the United States. The incidence is said to be 1 per 100 pregnancies.[79] The usual symptoms associated with ectopic pregnancy include a classic triad of abdominal pain, a period of amenorrhea, and irregular vaginal bleeding. This triad is often associated with symptoms of pregnancy and occasionally with syncope and shoulder pain secondary to intraperitoneal bleeding. Commonly elicited signs include adnexal tenderness, a slightly enlarged uterus, and, in patients who have sustained significant blood loss, tachycardia and hypotension. In this condition, definitive palpation of an adnexal mass is uncommon.

The diagnosis is made by further evaluation utilizing urine or serum human chorionic gonadotropin beta-subunit testing, culdocentesis, and ultrasonography. When positive, culdocentesis is accurate in predicting the presence of ectopic pregnancy. Quantitative beta-subunit levels usually double during a 48-hour period in the first 6 weeks of pregnancy. If a rise of less than 66% occurs in a 2-day period, a high probability of ectopic pregnancy is considered.[80] Ultrasonography has improved our ability to diagnose ectopic pregnancies at an early stage; an intrauterine sac should be observed at a beta-subunit level of 6500 mIU with transabdominal ultrasonography and at 3600 mIU with transvaginal ultrasonography.[81] Absence of a gestational sac at these levels is strongly suggestive of ectopic pregnancy.

Depending on available information, dilatation and curettage, laparoscopy, or exploratory laparotomy may be indicated to make the diagnosis. If an ectopic pregnancy is confirmed, there are various surgical options, ranging from conservative (laparoscopic salpingostomy, "milking out" the ectopic sac, linear salpingostomy, partial salpingectomy) to radical (salpingo-oophorectomy, uterine wall excision). In the rare cornual and cervical ectopics, hysterectomy is often indicated. The main goals of treatment are to remove the trophoblastic tissue, control bleeding, and minimize damage to the reproductive tract, especially in patients of low parity. Ovarian, interstitial, and abdominal pregnancies are associated with greater blood loss and higher morbidity and mortality than tubal pregnancies, which make up the vast majority (97.7%) of ectopic pregnancies.[82]

Methotrexate is being evaluated as a potential chemotherapeutic treatment for ectopic pregnancies.[83, 83a] Even with improved early diagnosis and a decreased ratio of death rate to case rate, the overall number of maternal deaths resulting from hemorrhage would not be expected to fall as long as the overall incidence of ectopic pregnancy continues to increase. There should be a high index of suspicion when women in the reproductive age group present with lower abdominal pain, abnormal vaginal bleeding, and the other associated signs and symptoms.

Trauma

Obstetric trauma includes laceration of the cervix and lower genital tract during the second stage of labor, spontaneous uterine rupture, and spontaneous rupture of the liver, which may occur in patients with PIH. Obstetric trauma may also occur during surgical procedures such as episiotomy, forceps operations, cesarean section, dilatation and curettage, and induced abortion. Nonobstetric trauma may be further subdivided into blunt trauma, as occurs during a fall or a motor vehicle accident, and penetrating trauma resulting from gunshots and stabs.

The pathophysiologic significance of trauma is usually related to hypovolemia. However, tissue damage and necrosis may also play an important role.

Spontaneous Obstetric Trauma

Lacerations of the Lower Genital Tract. Spontaneous lacerations of the lower genital tract may occur with ensuing blood loss. The amount of blood lost is related to the degree and depth of the laceration and the time elapsed before the repair is completed. Severe bleeding may result from obstetric lacerations, and vaginal hematomas may account for significant blood loss into the tissue and retroperitoneum with little revealed hemorrhage. Vulval and vaginal hematomas should always be excluded in patients complaining of vaginal pain in the postpartum period, especially when the clinical condition does not correlate with the measured blood loss.

Uterine Rupture. Spontaneous rupture of the gravid uterus is still associated with significant maternal and fetal mortality. The incidence is approximately 1 in 2000 deliveries, with a 9.7% maternal mortality rate and a fetal wastage of 56%.[84] Uterine rupture may be spontaneous, secondary to trauma, or caused by rupture of a previous uterine scar.

Prolonged or obstructed labor is thought to be the predominant causative factor for spontaneous rupture.[85] Conditions associated with uterine rupture include use of oxytocin, cephalopelvic disproportion, grand multiparity, trauma, external and internal podalic version, and abruption.[84] Dehiscence of a previous cesarean section scar, with extension, is probably the most frequent etiology in modern obstetrics.[84, 85]

The most common clinical presentation is that of vaginal bleeding, shock, and lower abdominal pain.[84] In some instances, the area to which the fetal heart tones were initially localized is noted to have shifted. Sometimes acute bradycardia or sudden profound fetal distress is noted. In cases of catastrophic rupture and fetal demise, inability to detect fetal heart tones may be concomitant with acute abdominal pain, hypotension, vaginal bleeding, appearance of frank blood in the urinary catheter (indicative of anterior rupture into the bladder), and retraction of the fetal presenting part (indicative of fetal expulsion into the abdomen).[84]

Treatment of uterine rupture should be individualized. Abdominal hysterectomy is no longer advocated in all cases. If the fetus is still undelivered or if uterine bleeding is thought to be secondary to a uterine or cervical defect, immediate laparotomy is indicated. If a defect is found at the time of examination after a vaginal birth after cesarean section but no bleeding is noted and the patient is hemodynamically stable, close observation is warranted, with resort to laparotomy only if the patient shows signs of decompensation.

Spontaneous Hepatic Rupture. Spontaneous rupture of the liver during pregnancy was first described in 1844 by Abercrombie.[86] Since then, reported cases have usually been associated with PIH and have occurred in multiparous patients.[87, 88] In the typical scenario, the patient, often considered preeclamptic, develops epigastric or right upper quadrant pain associated with nausea and vomiting. Right upper abdominal tenderness may be elicited on examination.[89] If the subcapsular hepatic hemorrhage has extended beyond Glisson's capsule and intraperitoneal bleeding occurs, signs and symptoms of shock follow. Laboratory values may show evidence of a falling hematocrit, elevated liver enzyme and serum bilirubin levels, and a developing coagulopathy. The diagnosis is often made on clinical grounds; however, paracentesis, liver scan, ultrasonography, and computed tomography may be helpful for confirmation.[88] Also of note is the occasional finding of a right pleural effusion in patients with spontaneous liver rupture.[90] Liver biopsy usually reveals fibrin thrombi extending up the hepatic arterioles to the periportal sinusoids and periportal hemorrhagic necrosis.[90]

Expedient exploratory laparotomy is mandated for a patient in shock with evidence of intraperitoneal bleeding, because delay has been associated with increased mortality. Packing the liver and upper abdomen with abdominal lap packs and adequate drainage of the abdomen are recommended in the initial management.[89] The patient may be returned to the operating room at a later time to remove the packs when her condition has stabilized. Death usually results from massive hemorrhage. In cases in which bleeding is controlled by hepatic artery ligation or lobectomy, postoperative mortality is still high, secondary to hepatic failure and multiple organ system failure. In such cases, after arterial occlusion or partial liver resection, hepatic reserve is presumed to be insufficient to sustain life.[91]

Surgical Obstetric Trauma

Forceps Operations. Forceps delivery may result in a variety of complications including uterine rupture, cervical laceration, vaginal lacerations, pelvic hematomas, and episiotomy extensions. The significance of any associated bleeding is relative to the pre-existing hematocrit and cardiovascular status, the extent of the injury, the rate of blood loss, and the time taken to complete surgical repair. Fortunately, lacerations of this type are rarely of major clinical significance if correctly repaired and can usually be avoided by good judgment and clinical skill. It is always wise to observe patients who have had particularly difficult forceps deliveries for an appropriate amount of time to exclude the development of a vaginal hematoma, which may form insidiously and result in significant occult blood loss. Any patient complaining of undue vaginal or vulvar pain after delivery should be examined vaginally to exclude this potentially devastating complication.

Legal Abortion. Maternal death resulting from legal abortion remains a problem in modern obstetrics. Statistics from the Centers for Disease Control in Atlanta reveal that 24 deaths resulted from hemorrhage and 132 deaths from other causes after 7,298,000 legal abortions performed between 1972 and 1979.[21] The most common cause of death was infection (23%), followed by anesthetic complications (17%) and hemorrhage (15%). Hemorrhage may result from retained products of conception, consumptive coagulopathy related to the use of chemical abortifacients,[15] or uterine perforation during abortion induced in midtrimester. Clinical features common to these cases of lethal hemorrhage included uterine trauma, inadequate postoperative monitoring, delayed surgical intervention, and delayed blood transfusions.

Management of overt bleeding includes early recognition, surgical intervention, and volume replacement, utilizing blood components as necessary.[21] If unusual postabortal bleeding does not resolve, diagnostic laparoscopy and/or exploratory laparotomy should be performed without delay.[21]

In cases of suspected uterine perforation, close attention must be paid to the site of presumed perforation. Some authors recommend conservative monitoring of a patient who is suspected of having a perforation in the fundal region with no obvious bleeding and hospitalization with laparoscopy for a patient with a suspected lateral perforation.[92] At our institution, any patient with suspicion of a lateral perforation is admitted for observation with serial hematocrit determinations and examinations. Laparoscopy or laparotomy is performed when persistent bleeding is suspected or cannot be ruled out, when damage to intraperitoneal organs is suspected, or when pain is thought to be excessive or worsening.

Other Surgery-Related Causes of Bleeding. Dilatation and curettage for missed abortion or incomplete abortion is not usually associated with significant blood loss unless uterine perforation has occurred, and when this happens it is usually a lateral perforation. Cesarean section, in general, is associated with loss of approximately 1000 mL of blood unless associated with extensions or postpartum atony. Extensions are managed by identifying anatomic landmarks and reapproximating the separated tissue edges. Often, the bladder must be dissected inferiorly to identify the apical margin of a lower uterine segment extension. Hysterectomy is rarely required for control of extensions associated with cesarean section.

Nonobstetric Trauma

The subject of trauma during pregnancy has been comprehensively discussed in the literature.[93–95] The incidence of accidental injury during pregnancy is estimated to be 6 to 7%.[96] In most cases, injury is minor and not associated with a significant increase in perinatal mortality. An increased incidence of minor trauma has been observed as pregnancy progresses. Major trauma, however, may place the mother and infant at severe risk.

The initial management of a pregnant woman who has sustained severe trauma is essentially the same as that of a nonpregnant person. Crosby has described in detail the initial evaluation of the gravid trauma patient.[97] Maternal stabilization often leads to fetal stabilization. Delivery of the fetus before stabilization of the mother may worsen the mother's condition and result in delivery of a premature fetus. Electronic fetal monitoring during maternal evaluation provides information about fetal and maternal well-being because deteriorating maternal cardiovascular status may be reflected by the appearance of fetal distress.[97]

Animal studies have shown that maternal hypoxia results in a reduction of uterine and placental blood flow via the liberation of catecholamines.[98] Fetal well-being usually reflects maternal cardiovascular stability. Blunt trauma caused by falls and motor vehicle accidents is often managed differently from the penetrating injuries of stab wounds and projectiles such as bullets.

Blunt Trauma. There are reports of fetal and neonatal death secondary to in utero traumatic splenic rupture, placental laceration, and contusion with hemorrhage of the liver, adrenal gland, and kidney. Rose and associates found evidence of fetomaternal hemorrhage in 28% of pregnant trauma patients.[99] They recommended a protocol consisting of electronic fetal monitoring, Kleihauer-Betke analysis (with another analysis, if positive, to rule out chronic fetomaternal hemorrhage), and determination of the Rh status of the mother, with appropriate Rh immune globulin therapy for the Rh-negative mother.

Simple falls that do not result in loss of consciousness or bruises are unlikely to produce significant injury to the mother or the fetus.[97] We recommend early fetal assessment (nonstress test or biophysical profile) to provide reassurance to a concerned mother and her physician. Maternal Rh status should be checked and a Kleihauer-Betke test performed. Clotting studies are indicated if placental abruption is suspected.

Diagnostic peritoneal lavage for blunt trauma in pregnant women has been found to be both safe and accurate in diagnosing intra-abdominal injuries.[100] Physical examination of the abdomen is thought to be less reliable in the pregnant patient. Splenic rupture has been postulated to occur more commonly in the pregnant state, and Buchsbaum noted a 15.4% mortality rate associated with splenic rupture.[101] A typical clinical pattern of biphasic rupture or delayed hemorrhage, with a prolonged latent period before massive hemorrhage, has been described and mandates close prolonged surveillance in any patient suspected of having splenic rupture.[101] Pelvic fractures are commonly associated with motor vehicle accidents, and serious complications may result from urologic and vascular damage. Retroperitoneal hemorrhage may be massive, the result of minor pelvic fractures with minimal bone displacement. Nonexpanding retroperitoneal hematomas found at laparotomy should probably be managed expectantly to prevent further hemorrhage.[97]

Penetrating Trauma. The gravid uterus is the most frequently injured organ in cases of penetrating abdominal trauma.[95] As the uterus expands, the bowel is compartmentalized into the upper abdomen. Because of the physical forces involved, gunshot wounds result in a substantially higher mortality rate than stab wounds. Nance and colleagues reported a 12.5% mortality rate in the civilian population after gunshot wounds, compared with a 1.4% mortality rate related to stab wounds.[102] Gunshot wounds are also the most common penetrating injury during preg-

nancy.[93] An 89% incidence of fetal injury and a 66% perinatal mortality rate were noted in a series reported by Buchsbaum.[94] Prematurity contributed significantly to the perinatal mortality. In all cases of gunshot wounds to the abdomen, exploratory laparotomy should be performed to determine the extent of visceral injury.[94] However, exploratory laparotomy is not a reason for routinely performing a cesarean section.[97] Maternal indications for delivery include severe compromise of the maternal cardiovascular status and obstruction of the operating field by the gravid uterus limiting the required surgical exposure of damaged vital structures. Fetal indications for delivery include fetal hemorrhage and distress and intra-amniotic infection.[93] Suspected fetal injury and fetal distress must be balanced against the likelihood of fetal immaturity. Even if labor has begun, some authors think that vaginal delivery after exploratory laparotomy is preferable to hysterotomy.[97]

Stab wounds of the abdomen present a somewhat more complicated problem for clinical management. It is often difficult to determine whether the peritoneal cavity has been violated. Fistulograms using Hypaque and peritoneal lavage have been promoted in the management of stab wounds.[93, 100] Stab wounds require surgical repair in about 50% of reported cases.[93] As with gunshot wounds, if the wound is confined to the lower abdomen, the uterus usually sustains the most damage and the other viscera may be spared. Because of the high incidence of upper abdominal wounds, the decision to perform an exploratory laparotomy should be individualized.[93]

A rare but lethal complication of blunt or penetrating trauma to the chest or upper abdomen is delayed traumatic rupture of the diaphragm.[103] Mortality is related to the number of herniated organs, strangulation of such herniated organs, and the time lapse from rupture to surgical intervention. Most of these hernias occur on the left side, probably because the presence of the liver prevents herniation on the right. The patient commonly presents with pain, fever, and dyspnea. The diagnosis is made radiologically. Treatment is surgical via a thoracotomy incision. Some authors recommend routine baseline chest x-ray study of all prenatal patients with a history of penetrating wounds and suggest that cesarean section be performed if labor begins within 4 weeks of reparative surgery.[103]

Acquired Coagulopathy

Acquired coagulation defects in pregnancy are common. Clinical states associated with coagulopathy include sepsis, retained dead fetus syndrome, abruptio placentae, amniotic fluid embolism, preeclampsia or eclampsia, intravascular hemolysis, trauma, and induced abortion by hypertonic saline. Other cases have involved afibrinogenemia secondary to a degenerating leiomyoma,[104] placenta previa accreta with afibrinogenemia,[105] hydatidiform mole,[106] and ovarian vascular accidents secondary to anticoagulation therapy.[107]

Sepsis and Disseminated Intravascular Coagulation

DIC may be triggered in patients with septic shock; however, the exact mechanism remains to be elucidated.[15] Platelets are thought to be important in the development of DIC secondary to sepsis.[108] Endotoxins administered to baboons led to a hypercoagulable state, followed by depletion of platelets and clotting factors and ultimately resulting in DIC. The first organism associated with DIC was meningococcus, but many other organisms have been isolated in obstetric patients with sepsis. Obstetric infections are usually of the mixed polymicrobial variety.[7] Gram-negative enteric bacteria such as *Escherichia coli, Klebsiella, Enterobacter, Pseudomonas,* and *Serratia* have been the most commonly isolated organisms.[108] Gram-negative anaerobes (*Bacteroides*), gram-positive organisms, viruses (varicella), and fungal infections may all lead to septic shock and DIC.[15, 108] Therefore, the triggering stimulus of DIC may not always be an endotoxin but may involve the presence of exotoxins, antigen-antibody complexes, or other mediators.[15] Treatment of DIC in sepsis includes general supportive measures, antibiotics, correction of any underlying coagulopathy, and, if possible, removal of the source of infection.

Retained Dead Fetus Syndrome

With the advent of ultrasonography, improved methods of labor induction, and aggressive management, the retained dead fetus syndrome is rarely encountered in obstetric practice today. The association of fetal death and coagulopathy, not Rh sensitization and coagulopathy, was made in 1953 after a bleeding disorder was identified in an Rh-positive patient with a long-standing fetal demise.[109] Data published in 1959 showed that the process is slowly progressive and unlikely to develop sooner than 5 weeks after fetal death; 26% of patients would then go on to develop a coagulopathy if delivery did not occur.[110]

The cause of the coagulopathy is postulated to be release of tissue thromboplastin from the fetus or placenta, activating the extrinsic pathway and resulting in DIC and secondary activation of the fibrinolytic system.[8] Patients may present in a compensated or decompensated hemostatic state, as manifested by clinical evidence of bleeding and laboratory studies. Romero and associates stressed the need for coagulation screening of all patients with intrauterine fetal demise before attempting to deliver the fetus to detect a potentially lethal coagulopathy.[8] Laboratory studies should include a complete blood count, platelet count, fibrinogen, fibrin split products, prothrombin time, and partial thromboplastin time.

Thrombin time is prolonged when (1) the fibrinogen level is less than 100 mg/dL; (2) qualitative disorders of fibrinogen are present; (3) fibrin split products are elevated, resulting in inhibition of fibrin polymerization; and (4) the thrombin inhibitor heparin has been exogenously administered.[8]

If the patient is found to have DIC and is in labor, fibrinogen is replaced by administration of cryoprecipitate, as the volume of fresh frozen plasma may be excessive and result in volume overload. If the patient is not in labor, heparin may be administered by continuous intravenous infusion until fibrinogen levels rise to 200 to 300 mg/dL and platelet counts are greater than 60,000/mm³. Heparin is then discontinued and induction of labor is instituted 6 hours after discontinuation of heparin.[8]

In modern obstetrics, prompt termination of the pregnancy in cases of fetal demise by cervical ripening and dilatation with prostaglandin agents should avoid the dead fetus syndrome.

Abruptio Placentae and Disseminated Intravascular Coagulation

Abruptio placentae and its relationship to hemorrhagic shock have been discussed. Pritchard and Brekken noted a 38% incidence of hypofibrinogenemia complicating abruption severe enough to result in fetal death.[9] DIC probably results from the release of an unidentified thrombogenic substance into the circulation. Hypofibrinogenemia and the presence of fibrin split products correlate closely with postpartum hemorrhage.[111] Treatment consists of prompt blood transfusion, replacement of clotting factors, and delivery of the products of conception.

Amniotic Fluid Embolism and Disseminated Intravascular Coagulation

The clinical diagnosis of amniotic fluid embolism is rare, estimated to be 1 in 20,000 to 1 in 80,000 deliveries.[112, 113] Of great significance is an overall mortality rate of approximately 80%.[112, 113] Risk factors include advanced maternal age, multiparity, vigorous uterine contractions, meconium in the amniotic fluid, large fetal size, and fetal demise.[112] Fetal death before the acute episode occurs in 40% of cases, and abruptio placentae may accompany 50% of cases.[112, 113] Passage of amniotic fluid into the maternal vasculature results in cardiopulmonary compromise mimicking pulmonary hypertension and cor pulmonale. Later, DIC results from the coagulant activity of amniotic fluid.[31] Microemboli may pass through the pulmonary capillary bed and into the systemic vessels. The patient classically develops chills, restlessness, dyspnea, cyanosis, nausea, vomiting, altered mental status, and then hypotension and tachycardia. Cardiorespiratory arrest follows. Hemodynamic findings in humans with documented amniotic fluid embolism show a mild-to-moderate rise in mean pulmonary arterial pressure, a variable rise in central venous pressure, and a high pulmonary capillary wedge pressure with evidence of left ventricular failure.[114] Clark and coworkers[114] have proposed a biphasic hemodynamic alteration in which the initial episode of hypoxia is secondary to transient pulmonary arterial vasospasm. This event is followed by left ventricular and pulmonary capillary injury, possibly secondary to the initial episode of hypoxia, or a direct effect of the amniotic fluid on the myocardium.[10] The mortality rate during the first hour is 25 to 50%.[115] In 40% of survivors of the initial event, coagulopathy and subsequent hemorrhagic shock may ensue.[115] Uterine atony may accompany the coagulopathy, which is thought to result from release of thromboplastin or some other powerful anticoagulant into the maternal circulation.[115] Diagnosis is traditionally made at autopsy, with fetal squames, mucin, and amorphous debris found in arteries under 1 mm in diameter, arterioles, and capillaries of the pulmonary vasculature.[37] Evidence suggests that the presence of trophoblastic or squamous cells in maternal pulmonary circulation may not be pathognomonic of clinically significant amniotic fluid embolism.[116] Gregory and Clayton proposed the use of lung scans in the diagnosis of amniotic fluid embolism.[117] It appears that the diagnosis is usually made on clinical grounds in survivors and on both clinical and histologic grounds in nonsurvivors. Treatment includes cardiovascular resuscitation, respiratory support, and correction of the abnormal coagulation state. Intravenous heparin has been used in the treatment of amniotic fluid embolism but has not gained widespread acceptance. Inotropic support is warranted in the presence of left ventricular failure and pulmonary edema,[114] and Clark and colleagues suggested that inotropic support may be the critical therapeutic modality in patients diagnosed with amniotic fluid embolism.[114]

Intravascular Hemolysis

DIC can be triggered by intravascular hemolysis, perhaps via release of red blood cell adenosine diphosphate or red blood cell membrane phospholipoprotein.[15] Intravascular hemolysis of any etiology, including frank hemolytic transfusion reactions and minor hemolysis secondary to multiple transfusions of banked whole blood, may initiate activation of the coagulation cascade and result in DIC.

Trauma and Disseminated Intravascular Coagulation

DIC may result from trauma in several ways. Massive crushing injuries cause release of substances, probably from

---

TABLE 139–9

CURRENTLY HELD HYPOTHESES ON THE ETIOLOGY OF PREGNANCY-INDUCED HYPERTENSION

Prostacyclin or thromboxane imbalance[121]
Immunologic mechanism[122]
Increased vascular sensitivity to angiotensin II[123]
Hyperdynamic disease model[124]

---

damaged tissue, into the circulation, activating the coagulation cascade.[16] Massive hemorrhage resulting from injury may deplete coagulation factors. Trauma to the uterus may result in abruption or amniotic fluid embolism, which are both known to cause DIC. Treatment includes replacement of blood and coagulation products, general supportive care, and measures to correct the inciting factors.

Inherited Coagulopathies

Hereditary disorders of coagulation occur in approximately 1 to 2 per 10,000 persons and, therefore, are rarely encountered in obstetric practice.[115] A deficiency of any factor in the intrinsic, extrinsic, or common pathways of blood coagulation may result in a clotting disorder.[115] Screening tests include platelet count, prothrombin time, partial thromboplastin time, bleeding time, thrombin clotting time, and clot stability test. Depending on the results of these studies, specific clotting factor assays may be indicated.[115] Von Willebrand's disease is the most common coagulation defect encountered by obstetricians. It is typically an inher-

---

TABLE 139–10

DIAGNOSTIC CRITERIA FOR PREGNANCY-INDUCED HYPERTENSION ACCORDING TO RECOMMENDATIONS OF THE AMERICAN COLLEGE OF OBSTETRICIANS AND GYNECOLOGISTS

Pregnancy-Induced Hypertension*
1. Blood pressure
   Systoloic blood pressure of at least 140 mm Hg
   Diastolic blood pressure of at least 90 mm Hg
   or
   Increase in blood pressure from the systolic baseline pressure of 30 mm Hg or from the diastolic baseline pressure of 15 mm Hg on two separate occasions at least 2 h apart
2. Proteinuria
   More than 300 mg in a 24-h period
   or
   Urine protein concentration of at least 1 g/L in two random urine specimens collected at least 6 h apart
3. Edema
   Generalized
   Weight gain of more than 5 lb in 1 wk

Severe Pregnancy-Induced Hypertension
1. Blood pressure > 160/110 on two occasions 6 h apart
2. More than 5 g of protein in a 24-h specimen or 3+ to 4+ proteinuria noted on semiquantitative assay
3. Oliguria, defined as <500 mL urine in 24 h
4. Cerebral and visual disturbances
5. Pulmonary edema or cyanosis
6. Epigastric or right upper quadrant pain
7. Impaired liver function of unclear etiology
8. Thrombocytopenia

*These changes must be shown to have occurred after 20 wk of gestation or, if noted before 20 wk, must be associated with extensive hydatidiform changes in the chorionic villi.
From American College of Obstetricians and Gynecologists: Management of Preeclampsia. ACOG Technical Bulletin # 91. Washington, DC, 1986.

---

ited autosomal dominant disorder manifested by mucocutaneous, post-traumatic, and postoperative bleeding.[118] Close monitoring for a rise in factor VIII–related activities (factor VIII coagulant activity, factor VIII–related antigen, and factor VIII ristocetin cofactor) during the antepartum period detects developing coagulopathy.[118] Cryoprecipitate, containing all forms of the factor VIII macromolecular complex, is preferred over commercial factor VIII concentrates, which do not provide the high-molecular-weight forms of the macromolecular complex.[118] Management of cryoprecipitate transfusion in pregnancy is outlined by Caldwell and coworkers[115] and Lipton and coworkers.[118]

There is an increased risk of thromboembolism associated with antithrombin III deficiency,[119] factor XII deficiency,[120] and the dysfibrinogenemias.[115] Inheritance of coagulation factor defects may be autosomal dominant, autosomal recessive, or X-linked recessive. Diagnosis is based on screening tests and specific factor assays. Treatment, specific for each entity, may require cryoprecipitate, fresh frozen plasma, factor concentrates, 1-deamino-(8-D-arginine)-vasopressin, ε-aminocaproic acid, or heparin.

Pregnancy-Induced Hypertension

PIH is a complex and diverse syndrome involving almost every maternal organ system. It is still one of the major causes of maternal and fetal morbidity and mortality, and although great strides have been made in the diagnosis and management of this condition, the basic underlying etiology remains unclear. Approximately 5% of all pregnancies in the United States are affected by PIH in one form or the other, and it is the second most common cause of maternal death in late pregnancy in the United States.[3]

Various causes have been proposed in an attempt to explain the etiology of this disease, and the most current of these are shown in Table 139–9.[121–124] A more detailed discussion of these hypotheses is beyond the scope of this chapter.

Diagnosis

The criteria for the diagnosis of this disease have been strictly outlined by the American College of Obstetricians and Gynecologists[125] and are presented in Table 139–10.[125]

Differential Diagnosis

PIH may masquerade as many other conditions and the initial diagnosis may on occasion be a challenge. Conditions that should be excluded when diagnosing PIH are listed in Table 139–11.

TABLE 139–11

SOME CONDITIONS TO BE CONSIDERED IN THE DIFFERENTIAL DIAGNOSIS OF PREGNANCY-INDUCED HYPERTENSION

Chronic essential hypertension
Chronic renal disease
Severe urinary tract infection
Gestational trophoblastic disease (especially in patients at less than 20 wk of gestation)
Pheochromocytoma
Idiopathic thrombocytopenic purpura
Thrombotic thrombocytopenic purpura
Hemolytic-uremic syndrome
Acute fatty liver of pregnancy
Viral hepatitis
Gallbladder disease

TABLE 139–12

COMPLICATIONS OF SEVERE PREGNANCY-INDUCED HYPERTENSION

Cardiovascular: hypertension, dysrhythmias, congestive heart failure, cardiomyopathy, pulmonary edema
Respiratory: abnormal oxygen delivery and consumption
Renal: oliguria, renal failure, nephrotic syndrome
Hematologic: hemolysis, thrombocytopenia, disseminated intravascular coagulation
Neurologic: eclampsia, cerebral edema, cerebral hemorrhage, visual disturbances
Hepatic: elevated enzyme levels, liver rupture
Uteroplacental: abruption, intrauterine growth retardation, fetal distress, fetal death
Soft tissue: laryngeal edema, massive vulval edema

Complications

Severe PIH may have a devastatingly rapid and malignant course, and all pregnant patients with progressively worsening hypertension and proteinuria should be treated as potential candidates for developing the sequelae of end-stage PIH. In this way the complications of the disease (Table 139–12) may be minimized.

Hemodynamic and Respiratory Profile of Pregnancy-Induced Hypertension

The use of the pulmonary arterial catheter,[45] introduced nearly 20 years ago, has greatly helped in defining the hemodynamic and respiratory profile of patients with severe PIH. Many of the early studies employing central hemodynamic monitoring in pregnancy, and specifically in PIH, were complicated by confounding factors, making them unreliable. In many instances, the data were collected from patients in labor or in the postpartum period, and in most cases the patients had been given fluid and/or medications before the data collection. More recent studies[27, 51, 126, 127] of carefully selected patients have allowed the definition of the typical central hemodynamics in severe preeclampsia. These hemodynamic findings are listed in Table 139–13.

Although the hemodynamic findings in severe PIH are well defined, the respiratory function remains unclear. Invasive monitoring has been used to clarify the respiratory parameters in untreated severely hypertensive gravidas.[127] Expected baseline levels of oxygen delivery and utilization have not been established in severe PIH. Data for six severely hypertensive patients suggest, however, that untreated PIH is associated with critical tissue-level hypoxia and may help to explain why severe end-stage PIH is frequently associated with multiple organ dysfunction (see Table 139–13).

TABLE 139–13

HEMODYNAMIC FINDINGS IN SEVERE PREGNANCY-INDUCED HYPERTENSION

Elevated mean arterial pressure
Normal or elevated heart rate
Normal or low central venous pressure
Normal or low cardiac output
Low pulmonary capillary wedge pressure
Elevated mean pulmonary arterial pressure
Hyperdynamic ventricular function
Increased pulmonary shunt fraction
Reduced oxygen consumption index
Reduced oxygen availability index

TABLE 139–14

RECOMMENDED WORK-UP OF PATIENTS WITH PREGNANCY-INDUCED HYPERTENSION

Complete blood count with blood smear and platelet count
Clot observation for evidence of prolonged coagulation or lysis
Serum electrolytes and renal function tests
Liver function tests
Baseline coagulation studies (prothrombin time, partial thromboplastin time, fibrinogen)
Urine sample for protein estimation and microscopy; if delivery is not imminent, a 24-h urine collection should be initiated
Left lateral recumbent positioning and fetal assessment with nonstress test, oxytocin challenge test, or biophysical profile

Prolonged exposure of cells to ischemia eventually leads to organ failure and the typical lesions of end-stage PIH. This may explain the rapid maternal and fetal hemodynamic and metabolic decompensation frequently witnessed when the stresses of blood pressure control, labor, and delivery are superimposed on an underlying state of chronic tissue-level hypoxia.

Management of Pregnancy-Induced Hypertension

Management of the patient with PIH requires the simultaneous initiation of several steps. A peripheral large-bore intravenous line is inserted and samples for blood tests as detailed in Table 139–14 should be drawn.

The management of patients with severe PIH is controversial at present, with some authors recommending immediate delivery regardless of gestational age[12] and others advising conservative management, with delay in delivery to achieve fetal lung maturity.[128] Most would agree that delivery is mandated by worsening of the maternal or fetal condition. A practical approach is to deliver in cases of PIH with worsening maternal clinical or biochemical parameters, fetal distress, or documented fetal lung maturity. In those cases in which the maternal-fetal unit is in stable condition without evidence of severe PIH, steroid therapy should be considered if amniocentesis reveals an immature fetal lung profile. Delay or inappropriate therapy exposes the patient to the complications of PIH, as listed in Table 139–12. The issue of whether to use invasive monitoring with a pulmonary arterial catheter is controversial, but most would agree on the indications listed in Table 139–15.

For the purposes of this chapter, the discussion of the management of severe PIH is restricted to the following subjects: fluid therapy, antiseizure prophylaxis, antihypertensive therapy, and common complications of PIH—pulmonary edema, oliguria, hematologic disturbances (particularly the syndrome of hemolysis, elevated liver enzymes, and low platelet count [HELLP syndrome]), and eclampsia and cerebral edema.

TABLE 139–15

INDICATIONS FOR INVASIVE MONITORING IN PATIENTS WITH PREGNANCY-INDUCED HYPERTENSION

Pulmonary edema or adult respiratory distress syndrome
Oliguria or anuria unresponsive to initial volume expansion
Severe hypertension unresponsive to vasodilator therapy
Critical maternal cardiac disease (New York Heart Association classes III and IV) during labor, delivery, and early puerperium
Severe PIH with suspicion of tissue-level ischemia
Endotoxic shock

Fluid Therapy. This is a controversial subject with drastically divergent approaches ranging from severe fluid restriction[129] to volume expansion.[27, 51, 127] As with most controversies in medicine, the truth probably lies in the middle, and the most appropriate course of action is still to individualize the management plan for the particular situation.

Fluid therapy in severe PIH is usually initiated with balanced salt crystalloid solution at a rate of 75 to 125 mL/h, depending on the perceived degree of hemoconcentration. In most cases, this is all that is required to maintain adequate volume status. In patients with previously untreated severe PIH, additional bolus volumes of fluid (1000 to 1500 mL of crystalloid) may be required before the use of epidural anesthesia or vasodilator therapy to prevent maternal hypotension and/or fetal distress.[27, 51, 127, 130]

Intravenous fluids cause a decrease in COP in patients in labor.[131] The COP may also decrease in the postpartum period as a result of the mobilization of third-space fluids, and this may be important in the development of pulmonary edema in patients with severe PIH.[132] Volume expansion in patients with PIH has been extensively studied, and opinions differ as to the amount of fluid to be given as well the most appropriate volume expander. Kirshon and colleagues placed pulmonary arterial catheters in 15 primigravid patients with severe PIH during labor and monitored COP, pulmonary capillary wedge pressure, and mean arterial pressure throughout labor, delivery, and the postpartum period.[133] Low COP and pulmonary capillary wedge pressure were corrected by administration of albumin. They found that the only benefit of volume expansion was the avoidance of sudden profound drops in systemic blood pressure during antihypertensive therapy. The overall incidence of fetal distress during labor was not affected. Because of a significant requirement for pharmacologic diuresis to prevent pulmonary edema in the study group, these investigators recommend that the COP should not be corrected with colloidal solution unless it is markedly decreased (less than 12 mm Hg).[133]

A more aggressive approach has been proposed by Belfort and associates in severe previously untreated PIH.[27, 51] These workers showed that small volumes of colloidal solution could be safely used to effect volume expansion before vasodilation in patients with severe PIH. Volume expansion with small volumes of high-molecular-weight solutions avoided excessive volume infusion, resulting in a positive inotropic effect and a beneficial effect on respiratory function. None of their patients developed pulmonary edema. The data are presented in Table 139–16.[127] This study shows the importance of managing the patient on the basis of end-organ respiratory function rather than simply using cardiac output and pulmonary capillary wedge pressure.

Failure to use volume expansion for the critically ill patient with untreated PIH before instituting blood pressure reduction with a potent vasodilator may worsen the underlying tissue hypoxia and potentiate progressive organ dysfunction. This was shown in a study by Cotton and colleagues in which vasodilatation without volume expansion resulted in a statistically significant reduction in oxygen delivery (617 ± 78 to 491 ± 106 mL/min/m²) and a fall of 12 mL/min/m² in oxygen consumption from 123 ± 30 to 111 ± 30 mL/min/m².[134] Judicious use of fluid and vasodilators (and possibly even inotropic agents such as dobutamine) may be indicated to achieve this end, with the indicator of optimal resuscitation being normal respiratory function parameters and not simply an apparently adequate cardiac output.

Although volume expansion before blood pressure reduction has been shown to have a beneficial effect, such management should be undertaken only in an appropriate setting with an appropriate monitoring capability and with expert perinatal consultation.

TABLE 139–16

RESPIRATORY DATA FOR SIX PATIENTS WITH SEVERE PREGNANCY-INDUCED HYPERTENSION AT BASELINE AND AFTER VOLUME EXPANSION WITH DEXTRAN 70 (400 ± 116 mL)

Measure*	Baseline	Postdextran	P
Respiratory rate	16 ± 4†	19 ± 6†	NS
Pao₂ (mm Hg)	115 ± 7	110 ± 6	NS
Paco₂ (mm Hg)	30 ± 1	30 ± 2	NS
Pv̄o₂ (mm Hg)	43 ± 2	44 ± 2	NS
% So₂	99 ± 1	98 ± 1	NS
Pao₂ − Pao₂ (mm Hg)	9 ± 5	11 ± 5	NS
Ḋo₂ (mL/min/m²)	484 ± 119	643 ± 102‡	<.05
V̇o₂ (mL/min/m²)	102 ± 22	133 ± 21‡	<.05
Qs/Qt (%)	6.9 ± 1.4	8.9 ± 2.3	NS

*Pao₂ = arterial oxygen tension; Paco₂ = arterial carbon dioxide tension; Pv̄o₂ = mixed venous oxygen tension; % So₂ = percent oxygen saturation; Pao₂ − Pao₂ = alveolar-arterial oxygen tension difference; Ḋo₂ = oxygen availability (delivery) index; V̇o₂ = oxygen consumption index; Qs/Qt % = percent arteriovenous shunt; NS = not statistically significant.
†Mean ± SD (N = 6).
‡Significantly different from baseline.
Data from Belfort M, Anthony J, Kirshon B: Respiratory function in severe pregnancy induced hypertension: The effects of volume expansion and subsequent vasodilatation with verapamil. Br J Obstet Gynaecol 98:904, 1991.

Antiseizure Prophylaxis: Magnesium Sulfate. Magnesium sulfate has long been the standard treatment of preeclampsia and eclampsia in the United States.[135] The mechanism of action of magnesium sulfate remains controversial.[136] Many investigators think that magnesium sulfate acts primarily via neuromuscular blockade.[137] Others consider it to act centrally.[138] Abnormal electroencephalographic findings were reported to be common in humans with preeclampsia or eclampsia and are not altered by levels of magnesium considered by most to be in the therapeutic range.[139] Magnesium sulfate has been shown to cross the blood-brain barrier in patients with PIH, but the significance of this is unknown.[140]

Magnesium sulfate acts as a cerebral vasodilator in PIH and has been shown to cause a significant increase in the pulsatility index of the middle cerebral artery, as measured by transcranial Doppler ultrasonography. This is unlikely to be the result of generalized vasodilation because there was no concomitant increase in the pulsatility index of the common carotid artery or internal carotid artery over the same time period.[140a] This finding lends credence to the theory that eclampsia is caused by cerebral ischemia and that magnesium sulfate reduces ischemia by decreasing small-vessel resistance and thus improving peripheral brain perfusion.

The efficacy and safety of magnesium sulfate have been proved empirically by using a protocol that includes a combined intravenous-intramuscular loading dose of magnesium sulfate, followed by intramuscular injections pending patellar reflex checks.[141] Because magnesium sulfate is cleared by the kidneys, magnesium levels should be determined and patellar reflex checks made before administering repeat intramuscular maintenance doses, to avoid toxic side effects.[142]

Magnesium levels maintained at 4 to 7 mEq/L are thought to be therapeutic in the prevention of eclamptic seizures.[141] Patellar reflexes are usually lost at 8 to 10 mEq/L, respiratory depression occurs at levels above 11 mEq/L, and respiratory arrest may occur at 13 mEq/L.[143] Urine output, patellar reflexes, respiratory rate, and serum magnesium levels should be closely monitored in patients with renal impairment and volume contraction. The ability to perform emergency endotracheal intubation should be available when magnesium sulfate is administered in this dosage range.

Sibai and associates compared the original Pritchard regimen to a regimen employing a 4-g intravenous loading dose, followed by continuous intravenous maintenance infusion at 1 or 2 g/h.[144] These investigators determined that the intravenous loading dose with a maintenance dose of 1 g/h does not produce adequate serum levels of magnesium (4 to 7 mEq/L). They recommended a 2 g/h maintenance dose.[144] A regimen of a 6-g loading dose infused during 20 minutes, followed by continuous intravenous infusion of 2 g/h has been used with success at our institution. The maintenance infusion is adjusted according to clinical parameters and serum magnesium levels. Pruett and coworkers found no significant effects on the neonatal Apgar scores with this regimen.[145] Although magnesium sulfate is used to prevent and treat eclamptic seizures, the drug is not considered an antihypertensive agent.[143] Studies have, however, demonstrated a transient decrease in blood pressure related to bolus infusion, but not continuous infusion, in severe preeclampsia.[146]

Antihypertensive Therapy. Markedly elevated systemic arterial blood pressure is one of the definitive signs of severe PIH. Careful control of blood pressure must be achieved to prevent the complications of this disease. Medical intervention is usually recommended when systolic blood pressure exceeds 160 to 170 mm Hg or diastolic blood pressure exceeds 110 mm Hg.[147]

Hydralazine Hydrochloride (Apresoline). Hydralazine hydrochloride is the principal antihypertensive agent used in patients with PIH in the United States. Hydralazine reduces vascular resistance by direct relaxation of arterial smooth muscle. This affects the precapillary resistance vessels more than postcapillary capacitance vessels.[148] Reports of hydralazine causing severe hypotension, uteroplacental insufficiency, fetal distress, and fetal death have been published.[149] Hydralazine has been administered as a continuous intravenous infusion, as well as by bolus dose injection. A useful regimen is an initial intravenous dose of 5 mg, followed by additional 5- to 10-mg doses intravenously at 20-minute intervals (to a total dose of 40 mg) to effect blood pressure control. Patients with hypertension that does not respond to this approach warrant central hemodynamic monitoring and the use of more potent antihypertensive agents.[150]

Nifedipine. Nifedipine is a calcium channel blocker and lowers blood pressure primarily by relaxing arterial smooth muscle. An initial oral dose of 10 mg is administered, and this may be repeated after 30 minutes, if necessary, in the acute management of severe hypertension. Then 10 to 20 mg may be administered orally every 3 to 6 hours as needed.[151] Care should be taken when administering this drug to patients receiving concomitant magnesium sulfate because of the possibility of a hypotensive response and of cardiac arrhythmias.[152] Initial studies in animals using calcium antagonists raised concerns that fetal acidosis and death could occur with these drugs. Follow-up studies in humans have not confirmed this, and fetal blood gas analysis of patients being treated with nifedipine for preterm labor did not demonstrate any adverse effect.

Verapamil. Verapamil has also been used in the management of severe PIH.[27, 153] This agent has the advantage of being administered intravenously and having a shorter half-life than nifedipine. Belfort and associates showed that with careful volume expansion and administration of verapamil, severe hypertension could be controlled in a smooth manner without maternal or fetal side effects.[27, 127] Initial concern that the drug would depress myocardial function was not supported by data derived from invasive monitoring during the blood pressure reduction. In addition, careful examination of the neonate in the immediate postpartum period and again 24 hours post partum, did not show any detrimental effects of the drug.[27]

Labetalol. Labetalol is a combined alpha- and beta-adrenergic receptor antagonist that may be used to induce a controlled rapid decrease in blood pressure in patients with severe hypertension.[154] There are many reports of the efficacy and safety of labetalol in the treatment of hypertension during pregnancy. Mabie and coworkers compared bolus intravenous labetalol with intravenous hydralazine in the treatment of severe PIH.[155] They noted a quicker onset of action with labetalol and absence of a reflex tachycardia. In addition, a positive effect on early fetal lung maturation in patients with severe hypertension remote from term has been reported.[156] Labetalol is given as an initial dose of 10 mg intravenously followed by progressively increasing doses (20, 40, 80 mg) every 10 minutes to a total dose of 300 mg. A constant intravenous infusion may be started at 1 to 2 mg/min and continued until the therapeutic goals are achieved. This infusion should then be decreased to 0.5 mg/min as a maintenance dose or completely stopped.[151] Lunell and colleagues studied the effects of labetalol on the uteroplacental vasculature in hypertensive pregnant women and showed an increase in uteroplacental perfusion with a decrease in uterine vascular resistance.[157]

Angiotensin-Converting Enzyme Inhibitors. Angiotensin-converting enzyme inhibitors are not in general use in pregnant hypertensive patients. Experience is limited and the risk of inducing neonatal renal failure has not been determined.[158] Data for pregnant rabbits suggest that fetal abortion, secondary to reduced uterine blood flow resulting from the decreased prostaglandin E_2 synthesis, may occur. The angiotensin-converting enzyme inhibitors are not useful in the acute treatment of hypertension in pregnancy because of a 1- to 4-hour delay in the achievement of peak serum levels after ingestion.[159] It is recommended that this class of drugs not be used in the management of pregnant patients with hypertension.

Management of Some Common Complications of Severe Pregnancy-Induced Hypertension

Pulmonary Edema. The etiology of pulmonary edema in preeclampsia appears to multifactorial, as demonstrated by Benedetti and Carlson, who showed that an abnormal COP–pulmonary capillary wedge pressure gradient, pulmonary capillary permeability, and left ventricular failure all play a role.[160]

Pregnancy is known to lower COP, and the COP has been shown to be lower in preeclampsia than in normal pregnancy. Factors that may additionally reduce the COP include supine positioning in the postpartum period, bleeding at the time of parturition, and overzealous infusion of crystalloid solutions.[160]

Sibai and colleagues reported a 2.9% incidence of pulmonary edema in severe preeclampsia-eclampsia.[161] Of the 37 cases, 70% developed pulmonary edema in the postpartum period. In patients who developed pulmonary edema before delivery, chronic hypertension was identified as an underlying factor. Patients at high risk for pulmonary edema include older multigravid patients with a history of underlying chronic hypertension.[161] These patients need careful management of their volume status to ensure that excess fluid is not administered.

The diagnosis of pulmonary edema is made on clinical grounds, and any sudden onset of dyspnea, chest discomfort, tachycardia, tachypnea, and rales should mandate chest x-ray examination and arterial blood analysis. Cotton and coworkers showed that the central venous pressure does not correlate well with pulmonary capillary wedge pressure in severe PIH, and when it is critical to know the true pulmonary status a pulmonary arterial catheter is important.[49]

Other conditions that may present in a similar manner, such as pulmonary thromboembolism and amniotic fluid embolus, should be excluded before making the diagnosis of pulmonary edema.

Initial management of pulmonary edema includes administration of oxygen, restriction of fluids, and diuresis. A pulse oximeter should be placed, if available, and continuous monitoring of peripheral oxygen saturation should be initiated. Many authorities recommend the placement of a pulmonary arterial catheter in patients with severe preeclampsia and pulmonary edema, especially when the intravenous fluid intake has been carefully managed. It is critical to distinguish between fluid overload and left ventricular failure.[150, 162] In addition, for patients who do not immediately respond to oxygen therapy and diuresis, invasive pulmonary arterial monitoring should be instituted. Intravenous furosemide, in a dosage of 10 to 40 mg during 1 to 2 minutes, is the first line of conventional therapy. When immediate diuresis is not apparent within 1 hour, a further 80-mg dose may be slowly given. Most cases of severe pulmonary edema require diuresis of at least 2 to 3 L before discernible improvement in oxygenation. For patients who are thought to have pulmonary edema secondary to left ventricular failure, resulting from increased afterload, Straus and coworkers have advocated the use of peripheral arterial vasodilators such as sodium nitroprusside.[163] Continuous arterial blood pressure monitoring is essential when using such potent agents. When hypoxemia and impaired respiratory functions persist after initial treatments, mechanical ventilation may be required for cardiopulmonary support, pending correction of the underlying problem.

Cardiac glycosides are rarely indicated, except when left ventricular failure can be demonstrated. In patients with severe PIH who develop pulmonary edema, fluid balance must be carefully maintained and fluid intake and output should be monitored on an hourly basis. Serum electrolytes should be closely monitored and frequent blood gas analyses should be performed in the absence of peripheral arterial pulse oximetry.

Oliguria. Renal plasma flow and glomerular filtration are diminished in preeclampsia.[164] Renal biopsy of patients with PIH often demonstrates a distinctive glomerular capillary endothelial cell change termed glomerular endotheliosis.[165] Such glomerular membrane damage often results in renal dysfunction. Acute renal failure secondary to PIH is, however, uncommon with current methods of management[166] and is usually the result of acute tubular necrosis. The precipitating factors include abruptio placentae, coagulopathy, severe hemorrhage, and hypotension.[167] Renal failure in association with PIH may be the result of an underlying renal condition, especially in the older multiparous patient.[168]

Renal cortical necrosis may be associated with eclampsia, and these patients usually present with anuria or oliguria. In cases in which acute renal failure does occur, hemodialysis or peritoneal dialysis is required until adequate renal function is restored.[166]

Renal depression in preeclampia is more commonly manifested as oliguria than as renal failure. Oliguria is defined as urine output of less than 30 mL/h in two consecutive hours. It is usually associated with increases in the serum uric acid, creatinine, and blood urea nitrogen levels and a fall in creatinine clearance.[169]

When oliguria develops, close monitoring of fluid intake and output is of paramount importance. The cause of the renal failure should initially be considered to be prerenal, because preeclampsia is known to be a plasma volume–constricted state.[51, 127, 170] A fluid challenge of 500 to 1000 mL of normal saline or lactated Ringer's solution should be administered during 20 minutes. If the urine output does

TABLE 139–17

CLASSIFICATION AND MANAGEMENT OF OLIGURIA IN PREGNANCY-INDUCED HYPERTENSION

Group	Hemodynamic Profile	Management
1	Low pulmonary capillary wedge pressure Hyperdynamic left ventricular function Moderate increase in systemic vascular resistance	Volume replacement
2	Normal or increased pulmonary capillary wedge pressure Normal left ventricular function Normal systemic vascular resistance	Preload reduction Afterload reduction
3	Markedly increased pulmonary capillary wedge pressure Decreased left ventricular function Markedly increased systemic vascular resistance	Volume restriction Afterload reduction

From Clark SL, Greenspoon JS, Aldahl D, et al: Severe preeclampsia with persistent oliguria: Management of hemodynamic subsets. Am J Obstet Gynecol 154:490, 1986.

not respond to this, pulmonary arterial catheterization is usually indicated.[50] Repetitive fluid challenges should be avoided in the absence of invasive monitoring because pulmonary edema can evolve quickly. With continuous monitoring of the peripheral arterial oxygen saturation, it may be possible to allow further volume expansion before having to resort to invasive monitoring. Preeclamptic or eclamptic patients with persistent oliguria may be divided into three categories based on invasive monitoring data, as shown in Table 139–17:[171]

1. A group with a low pulmonary capillary wedge pressure, hyperdynamic left ventricular function, and moderately increased systemic vascular resistance. These patients respond to volume replacement, and the oliguria is thought to be the result of intravascular volume depletion in conjunction with systemic arterial vasospasm.

2. A second group with normal or increased pulmonary capillary wedge pressure, normal cardiac output, and normal systemic vascular resistance. These patients respond to pharmacologic preload and/or afterload reduction. The oliguria in this group is thought to be secondary to renal arteriovasospasm.

3. A third group with markedly elevated pulmonary capillary wedge pressure and systemic vascular resistance associated with depressed ventricular function. These patients respond to volume restriction and afterload reduction. Renal arterial spasm and decreased cardiac output are the cause of the oliguria in this group. These patients should ideally be managed with the use of invasive hemodynamic monitoring because they are very likely to have incipient pulmonary edema with fluid accumulation in the pulmonary interstitial space.[171]

Low-dose dopamine (1 to 5 μg/kg) has been shown to produce a significant rise in urine output in severe preeclampsia. Such management is especially appropriate for patients with oliguria and depressed ventricular function.[172]

TABLE 139–18

SYMPTOMS, SIGNS, AND LABORATORY VALUES HELPFUL IN THE DIAGNOSIS OF HELLP SYNDROME

Clinical indices
  Hypertension
  Proteinuria
  Facial or extremity edema
  Hyperreflexia
  Epigastric or right upper quadrant pain
  Nausea and vomiting
  Lethargy and confusion
  Jaundice
  Hematuria and occasionally oliguria
Laboratory findings
  Hemolysis
    Hemoglobinuria
    Reduced haptoglobin level
    Reticulocytosis
    Anemia
    Increased indirect bilirubin
    Abnormal peripheral smear with schistocytes or burr cells
  Elevated liver enzyme levels
    Increase in serum glutamic-oxaloacetic transaminase or
      serum glutamic-pyruvic transaminase levels
    Increase in lactate dehydrogenase levels
    Increase in bilirubin levels
  Low platelet count
    Platelet count often < 100,000/mm³
  Electolyte abnormalities
    Hyponatremia
    Hypoglycemia
    Elevated creatinine
    Elevated uric acid

Hematologic Complications. In 1954 Pritchard and colleagues reported an association of intravascular hemolysis, hepatic dysfunction, coagulation defects, and thrombocytopenia with eclampsia.[11] In 1982 Weinstein described the same syndrome complex, which he termed the HELLP syndrome.[12] It is thought that HELLP syndrome complicates between 3 and 12% of all preeclamptic gestations.

Thrombocytopenia is thought to be secondary to the increased consumption of platelets, possibly resulting from adherence to the exposed collagen of damaged vascular endothelium. Hemolytic anemia is also thought to be secondary to red blood cell destruction in small blood vessels. Burr cells, schistocytes, and polychromasia are seen on peripheral blood smears. Serum haptoglobin may help identify cases of hemolytic anemia in patients with HELLP syndrome.

The usual presentation of patients with HELLP syndrome is that of a pregnant primigravida, remote from term, with hypertension and proteinuria (Table 139–18). Epigastric pain or right upper quadrant pain should always alert the clinician to the possibility of the HELLP syndrome. Some patients complain of symptoms suggestive of a viremia, and a few have severe nausea and vomiting. The variable presentation of this condition has led to delay in its recognition and confusion with other diagnoses such as hepatitis, cholelithiasis, alloimmune thrombocytopenia, thrombotic thrombocytopenia, hemolytic-uremic syndrome, and peptic ulcer disease.

Sibai and colleagues reviewed 112 patients with HELLP syndrome treated during an 8-year period and showed that the incidence was significantly higher in white multiparous patients with severe PIH in whom diagnosis and delivery was delayed.[173] There were two maternal deaths, two patients had ruptured liver hematomas, nine developed acute renal failure, 20% had abruptio placentae, and 34% developed evidence of intravascular coagulopathy. The perinatal mortality rate was 367 per 1000. Of the 38 patients followed in subsequent pregnancies, only 1 developed the HELLP syndrome again.

Delivery of the products of conception is the only known definitive treatment for patients with HELLP syndrome. The appearance of the clinical and biochemical markers of the disease should prompt early termination of the pregnancy. Platelet counts lower than 30,000/mm³ mandate platelet transfusion before delivery (either vaginal or by cesarean section) even in the absence of evidence of active bleeding. There is ample evidence that blood loss at the time of delivery is significantly higher in patients who are not transfused. In patients with platelet counts higher than 30,000/mm³, a conservative and expectant transfusion policy is advisable. Martin and coworkers showed that all forms of hemotherapy in patients with HELLP syndrome are associated with a significantly increased risk of postpartum infection, regardless of delivery route or receipt of prophylactic antibiotics.[174] Steroids have not been shown to be of any use in elevating the maternal platelet count.[60] Plasma exchange transfusion has been of use in the management of persistent postpartum thrombocytopenia and is advised when platelet counts remain depressed for longer than 72 hours.[61]

Hematologic Markers of Pregnancy-Induced Hypertension

Further hematologic changes in preeclampsia include elevated beta-thromboglobulin levels,[175] an increased ratio of factor VIII antigen to activity,[176] and decreased antithrombin III levels.[177] Levels of fibronectin have been found to be increased in the serum of pregnant women who develop preeclampsia.[178] Rodgers and colleagues reported the identification of a serum factor that is cytotoxic to human endothelial cells in vitro and decreases in concentration 24 to 48 hours post partum.[179] The exact role of this factor (endothelin) in the pathophysiology of PIH is, however, still uncertain.[179]

Use of Blood Products in Pregnancy-Induced Hypertension

Hemolysis in preeclampsia usually does not require red blood cell transfusion. Severe thrombocytopenia, however, may result in severe hemorrhage, especially when associated with delivery and/or abruptio placentae. The development of hemorrhage and thrombocytopenia necessitates termination of the pregnancy. Therapy with specific blood products based on specific laboratory parameters is indicated at this time. The exact hemoglobin level at which packed red blood cells should be infused has not been determined; it depends on the patient's current condition, the hemoglobin level at the time, and the estimated rate of blood loss. Two points should be remembered: (1) the degree of blood loss at the time of delivery is frequently underestimated by as much as 50%, and (2) the blood loss at the time of delivery in patients with preeclampsia is significantly higher than that in a normal pregnancy.[180]

Data on blood replacement products are useful to remember when planning requirements (Table 139–19). The fibrinogen level should be maintained above 100 mg/dL, and fresh frozen plasma or cryoprecipitate should be transfused to correct a prolonged prothrombin time or partial thromboplastin time.

Neurologic Complications

Cerebral hemorrage and cerebral edema are the two major causes of maternal mortality in preeclampsia.[181] Cerebral

TABLE 139-19
USEFUL DATA ON BLOOD PRODUCTS
Each unit of packed red blood cells increases the hematocrit between 3 and 4%.   Platelet concentrates (30–50 mL) contain at least 5–6 × 10¹⁰ platelets.   A unit of fresh frozen plasma (220–250 mL) provides 500 mg of fibrinogen.   One unit of cryoprecipitate (10–25 mL) contains approximately 200 mg of fibrinogen.

hemorrhage, cerebral edema, amaurosis, and eclamptic seizures are separate but related neurologic conditions that may all occur in preeclampsia. Intracranial hemorrhage is thought to result from a combination of severe hypertension and hemostatic compromise. Cerebral edema is thought to be secondary to anoxia associated with eclamptic seizures but may be due to the loss of cerebral autoregulation in severe hypertension.[182] Signs of diffuse cerebral edema may be seen in eclampsia by using computed tomography of the brain.[183] Magnetic resonance imaging has also been useful in providing an index of the water content in select areas of the brain.

Temporary blindness (amaurosis) may be seen in 1 to 3% of patients with preeclampsia or eclampsia. Pregnancy-related blindness has been associated with eclampsia, cavernous sinus thrombosis, and hypertensive encephalopathy.[184] Hill and coworkers noted that recovery of vision correlated with the return to a normal pulmonary capillary wedge pressure in patients with severe preeclampsia and amaurosis.[185]

The cause of seizures in preeclampsia remains undetermined. Hypertensive encephalopathy, hemorrhage, ischemia, and edema of the cerebral hemispheres have all been proposed as etiologic factors.[186] Thrombotic and hemorrhagic lesions have been identified at autopsy in patients with severe preeclampsia.

The standard therapy for management of eclampsia in the United States is magnesium sulfate to control the seizures, hydralazine to control any concomitant hypertension, and delivery of the fetus.[180] The administration of these drugs was discussed earlier in this chapter. If control of the seizures has not been accomplished after the initial intravenous dose, a second 2-g dose of magnesium sulfate may be cautiously given. No more than 8 g of magnesium sulfate should be given as an intravenous loading dose. Seizures unresponsive to the standard magnesium sulfate regimen may be treated with a slow 100-mg intravenous injection of thiopental sodium. Alternatively, sodium amobarbital may be administered intravenously in a dosage of 250 mg.[135, 141] Patients with eclampsia who experience repetitive seizures despite therapeutic levels of magnesium sulfate should have computed tomographic evaluation of the head. Dunn and colleagues found that five of seven such patients had abnormalities such as cerebral edema, cerebral venous thrombosis, and low-density white matter.[187]

Amaurosis usually resolves spontaneously after delivery of the fetus.[184] Focal neurologic deficits such as this require ophthalmologic evaluation and computed tomography of the brain. The management of cerebral edema should follow general principles and include correction of hypoxemia and hypercarbia, avoidance of volatile anesthetic agents, control of body temperature, and control of blood pressure.[188] Hyperventilation reduces intercranial hypertension and the Paco₂ should be maintained between 25 and 30 mm Hg.[188] Hyperbaric oxygen therapy is aimed at maintaining a Pao₂ of 1000 mm Hg using an ambient pressure of 2 to 2.5 atm

to effect cerebral vasoconstriction. This therapy is still considered experimental.[188] Administration of hypertonic solutions such as mannitol is thought to increase cerebral serum osmolality and withdraw water from the brain into the vascular compartment. A 20% solution of mannitol is given as a dose of 0.5 to 1 g/kg during 10 minutes or as a continuous infusion of 5 g/h. The serum osmolality should be checked and maintained in the range 305 to 315 mOsm/kg.[188] Steroid therapy is not thought to be beneficial in cases of global cerebral edema.[188]

Anaphylactic Shock

Anaphylactic reactions may be fatal in as many as 10% of cases.[18a] Obstetric patients are also at risk because they may, at some point during pregnancy, receive some form of pharmacologic therapy. Antibiotics, nonsteroidal anti-inflammatory agents, narcotics, local anesthetics, iodinated radiocontrast agents, hormones, blood products, colloid solutions, and antivenins may result in anaphylactic reactions. There are few reports in the current obstetric literature regarding this subject. Entman and Moise reported a case of anaphylactic shock resulting from administration of a horse serum–based antivenin after a snake bite.[189] Clinical manifestations may be mild to severe.

Life-threatening events include airway obstruction and cardiovascular collapse. The first priorities in the management are ventilation, oxygenation, and external cardiac massage, which, in general, are followed by subcutaneous administration of epinephrine in 0.2-mg increments up to a total dose of 1.0 mg.[190] In obstetric patients, ephedrine, 25 to 50 mg by intravenous push, has been recommended because other vasoactive agents have detrimental uteroplacental effects.[189] However, failure to achieve an adequate clinical response with ephedrine should not contraindicate the use of other more potent agents, such as epinephrine, dopamine, norepinephrine, and isoproterenol. Other drugs, such as aminophylline, antihistamines, and corticosteroids, have been recommended to enhance clinical response.

Aggressive fluid replacement is required. In severe cases of anaphylactic shock, colloid volume expanders are preferred because crystalloids have been ineffective in volume replacement.[190]

Septic Shock

Septic shock is a rare condition in obstetrics, but it is still one of the most frequent contributory causes of maternal mortality in the United States.[4] Many infections in obstetric patients may result in septic shock, but endometritis, chorioamnionitis, and pyelonephritis are the most common.[110] Before the legalization of abortion, criminal abortion resulting in septic shock was common. Risk factors for septic shock include prolonged rupture of membranes, retained products of conception, and instrumentation of the genitourinary tract.[40] Serious infections that may develop in obstetric patients include pneumonia, appendicitis, septic abortion, toxic shock syndrome, septic pelvic thrombophlebitis, and endocarditis.

Bacteremia was found in 9.7% of obstetric patients for whom blood cultures were obtained.[191] Interestingly, the mortality resulting from septic shock in the general population (40 to 90%) is significantly higher than the 3% reported in obstetric and gynecologic patients.[192] This may be explained by the relative good health and youth of obstetric patients, prompt vigorous treatment, and infrequent underlying disease processes.[191] Paradoxically, animal studies demonstrate increased susceptibility to complications in pregnant versus nonpregnant subjects after intravenous injection of endotoxin. Endotoxin administered to pregnant baboons caused increased uterine activity and severe fetal distress with intrauterine death.[193]

Obstetric infections are usually caused by organisms normally found in the genital tract and are thus often polymicrobial.[18] Common organisms include *E. coli, Klebsiella, Enterobacter, Pseudomonas,* and *Serratia*.[108] Most cases of bacterial infection complicated by shock are caused by gram-negative enteric organisms. Gram-negative infections are usually systemic, whereas gram-positive infections tend to be suppurative.[194]

Septic shock usually results from a combination of events. The release of bacterial endotoxins and intracellular mediators causes increased capillary permeability with fluid shifts, leading to intravascular hypovolemia. The endotoxin itself may depress myocardial function. Endotoxin has been shown to cause metabolic and membrane transport abnormalities at a cellular level in the lungs, resulting in pulmonary edema.[195] Renal, gastrointestinal, metabolic, and coagulation involvements are well documented.[108] Septic shock has classically been described in three phases: an early warm-hypotensive phase, a late cold-hypotensive phase, and a terminal irreversible phase.[108] Flushed warm skin, fever, chills, diaphoresis, and tachycardia are representative of the reversible early warm-hypotensive phase, during which the pulse pressure and urine output remain stable. The late cold-hypotensive phase is characterized by cool and clammy skin, a drop in body temperature, and an obtunded mental state. Although hypotension, tachycardia, and oliguria invariably follow, this phase is still reversible with treatment. If medical intervention is not initiated, however, cellular hypoxia and anaerobic metabolism continue and the irreversible phase of septic shock develops. Metabolic acidosis, anuria, respiratory distress, cardiac failure, and coma are ominous signs.

Lee and coworkers found that 80% of cases of septic shock in pregnancy occurred during the postpartum period.[40] Significant hemodynamic observations included decreased peripheral vascular resistance and left ventricular function. The source of infection in obstetric patients is usually identified as the genital or urinary tract.[23] Routine laboratory evaluation of patients with suspected septic shock includes complete blood count with differential, platelet count, coagulation studies, urinalysis, and electrolyte, blood urea nitrogen, creatinine, lactate, and arterial blood gas levels. Laboratory evidence of infection may include leukocytosis on peripheral blood smear; pyuria and bacteriuria on urinalysis; blood gas aberrations, typically metabolic acidosis with compensatory respiratory alkalosis; and, in some patients, evidence of coagulopathy with abnormalities in platelet count, fibrinogen, prothrombin time, and partial thromboplastin time and the presence of fibrin split products. Cultures of urine, blood, and, if possible, amniotic fluid or endometrium should be obtained for all patients. Other specific sources, such as stool, wound, and sputum, are cultured as indicated. Lumbar puncture should be considered in patients with altered mental status.[194] A chest x-ray study should be done to rule out infiltrates, evidence of pulmonary edema, and adult respiratory distress syndrome. Abdominal x-ray films should be obtained to rule out free air under the diaphragm or a foreign body.

Treatment of septic shock requires general supportive measures, including restoration of intravascular volume and often inotropic support (see the section on general supportive measures). Adequate oxygenation is essential. Antibiotic therapy for sepsis should be tailored to the suspected source guided by information obtained with a Gram stain. In cases of septic shock, however, we usually institute intravenous broad-spectrum antibiotics with ampicillin, 2 g every 6 hours;

clindamycin, 900 mg every 8 hours; and gentamicin, 1.5 mg/kg every 8 hours. Gentamicin dosage is guided by serum peak and trough levels. Failure to respond promptly to simple volume resuscitation warrants transfer to an intensive care setting. If response to treatment is not satisfactory, close examination for abscesses or necrotic tissue should be initiated and appropriate surgical intervention instituted. Timely drainage of abscesses and removal of necrotic tissue should be done early rather than late and may require extirpative surgery with hysterectomy. In postpartum patients with refractory fevers, septic pelvic vein thrombophlebitis must be excluded. Computed tomographic scanning may be helpful in making the diagnosis.[108] In a patient who does not respond to medical therapy with antibiotics and heparin, exploratory laparotomy with ligation of the inferior vena cava and ovarian veins may be mandated.[24] Isolation of *Clostridium perfringens* in blood cultures does not warrant surgical intervention unless myonecrosis is present.[191]

Septic Abortion

Before the availability of legalized abortions, septic shock and death after criminal abortion were not uncommon. Septic abortion rarely complicates spontaneous incomplete abortion. Today, sepsis is still the most common complication of legal abortion resulting in maternal death in the United States.[21]

Treatment includes general supportive measures, antibiotics, and removal of the infected necrotic tissue. Broad coverage with an aminoglycoside, clindamycin, and penicillin or ampicillin is recommended because the infection is usually of a mixed aerobic-anaerobic type. Dilatation and curettage is performed to remove the infectious nidus in the uterus. Antibiotic therapy and evacuation of uterine contents successfully control infection in approximately 95% of all cases. If the infection has progressed beyond the endometrium and is not responsive to conservative therapy, exploratory laparotomy, hysterectomy, and possibly removal of the adnexae are required.

Chorionic villus sampling, a relatively new procedure used in the prenatal diagnosis of genetic abnormalities, carries a risk of fetal loss as well as maternal infection.[26] Others have reported septic shock unresponsive to uterine evacuation, antibiotics, and vasopressor therapy and complicated by renal failure after chorionic villus sampling.[25] Clinical improvement followed exploratory laparotomy, total abdominal hysterectomy, and bilateral salpingo-oophorectomy.

Septic pelvic vein thrombophlebitis, which may complicate pelvic sepsis and does not respond to antibiotics and intravenous heparin therapy, requires surgical therapy with exploratory laparotomy and ligation of the inferior vena cava and the ovarian vessels.

Chorioamnionitis

Uterine infections in pregnancy may be grouped into three categories: septic abortion before 20 weeks of gestation, chorioamnionitis after the 20th week, and puerperal sepsis (postpartum endometritis) after delivery. Chorioamnionitis follows approximately 1% of deliveries.[196] Although maternal and fetal complications are significant, the overall clinical outcome is usually good.[17] The diagnosis is usually made on clinical grounds based on evidence of leakage of fluid from the vagina, fever, maternal and/or fetal tachycardia, leukocytosis, uterine tenderness, and foul-smelling amniotic fluid.[17] Gram's staining of amniotic fluid obtained by transabdominal amniocentesis or intrauterine pressure catheters may be helpful. Bacteremia was observed in 12% of patients with chorioamnionitis in one series.[17] Septic shock is rarely seen.[17] Today, maternal death is rare; however, earlier reviews demonstrated significant mortality associated with chorioamnionitis.[4] Maternal morbidity was more significant in patients who delivered by cesarean section than those who delivered vaginally.[17] Perinatal mortality is increased sixfold in near-term fetuses of mothers with chorioamnionitis, but this increased perinatal mortality may be related more to prematurity than to sepsis.

Treatment consists of hydration, administration of parenteral antibiotics, and prompt delivery of the fetus. Time limits from diagnosis to delivery should not be set because vaginal delivery is still preferable to cesarean section in the presence of chorioamnionitis. Obviously, if the maternal condition deteriorates, fetal distress ensues, or any of the usual obstetric indications for cesarean section apply, the operation should not be delayed.

Endometritis

Endometritis is rare after vaginal delivery and is more often encountered after cesarean section. The incidence varies widely and is related to the population of patients studied. After blood, urine, and endometrial cultures are obtained, broad-spectrum antibiotic coverage of aerobic and anaerobic organisms is instituted. Most patients respond to antibiotic therapy; hysterectomy may be necessary for nonresponders because of the potential for the formation of intramyometrial abscesses. Septic pelvic thrombophlebitis must also be considered in patients who do not respond to medical therapy. Gas gangrene of the uterus, caused by *C. perfringens,* requires supportive medical therapy, surgical removal of infected tissue, and broad antibiotic coverage.[197] Abdominal radiography may reveal physometra (gas in the uterus), aiding in the diagnosis of gas gangrene.

Pyelonephritis

Acute pyelonephritis complicates 1 to 2% of all pregnancies and usually occurs in the latter half of pregnancy.[198] The incidence of asymptomatic bacteriuria in pregnancy is 5 to 6%. Untreated asymptomatic bacteriuria progresses to pyelonephritis in 30% of patients.[198] Presenting symptoms include back pain, fever, chills, lower urinary tract symptoms, nausea, and vomiting. The usual clinical findings are fever and costovertebral angle tenderness. Diagnosis is confirmed by bacteriuria and pyuria on urinalysis. The organism is identified by urine culture in 90% of cases. *E. coli* is isolated in the majority of these patients. Duff found that 7.2% of patients with pyelonephritis developed bacteremia and that septic shock supervened in 1.3 to 3% of patients hospitalized for acute pyelonephritis.[198] Cunningham and colleagues reported four cases of respiratory insufficiency with multiple organ system derangement associated with pyelonephritis in pregnancy.[199] Treatment of pyelonephritis necessitates early administration of an antibiotic to which the organism is susceptible. If urosepsis is suspected, broad-spectrum antibiotics are recommended.

The choice of antibiotic should be based on the known bacterial drug resistance profile at each individual hospital.[198] Because of a high incidence of *E. coli* resistance to ampicillin at our institution, we begin therapy with cefazolin, 1 g intravenously every 8 hours. If severe infection or urosepsis is suspected, we administer an aminoglycoside plus ampicillin. Hydration with crystalloid solutions is another crucial aspect of therapy. After the patient is afebrile for 24 hours, intravenous antibiotics are discontinued and we start an oral antibiotic to which the organism is sensitive.

Gilstrap and coworkers demonstrated significant transient renal dysfunction in 21% of women with pyelonephritis;[200]

TABLE 139–20
DIFFERENTIAL DIAGNOSIS OF APPENDICITIS IN PREGNANCY

Cholecystitis	Abruptio placentae
Torsion of an adnexa	Preterm labor
Degenerating leiomyoma	Pneumonia
Ruptured corpus luteum cyst	Urinary tract infection
Ruptured dermoid cyst	Nephrolithiasis
Infarction of an ovary	Acute salpingitis

for this reason, therapy with nephrotoxic drugs and intravenous fluids should be closely monitored. If the patient remains febrile after 72 hours of treatment, antibiotic resistance, urinary tract obstruction, or misdiagnosis should be suspected. Intravenous pyelography should be performed to exclude renal or ureteral stones or extrinsic obstruction.[198]

Appendicitis

Appendicitis is the most common nonobstetric indication for exploratory laparotomy in the obstetric patient. The incidence is 1 per 1500 deliveries. Appendicitis may occur at any age, but 90% of patients are less than 30 years old and 75% of patients are between 20 and 30 years old. As gestational age advances, the diagnosis becomes more difficult because of anatomic and physiologic changes associated with the pregnancy (Table 139–20).[19] Delays in diagnosis and treatment increase the fetal and maternal mortality and morbidity.[201] Because the risk of a negative laparotomy is not significant to either mother or fetus, especially when compared with that of a neglected diagnosis of appendicitis, exploratory laparotomy is mandated in all cases of suspected appendicitis.[201] Babler stated that "the mortality of appendicitis complicating pregnancy is the mortality of delay," and this as true today as it was in 1908.[202] Delay in diagnosis is related to gestational age and has been found to be 0, 18, and 75% in the first, second, and third trimesters, respectively.[201] The classic signs and symptoms of appendicitis are less frequently obvious in the pregnant patient[201] because the enlarging uterus displaces of the appendix into the mid-abdomen. This often results in atypical symptoms, sometimes confused with some of the more benign complaints of pregnancy such as round ligament tendonitis and muscle cramps. Cunningham and McCubbin's retrospective review of 34 cases demonstrated that abdominal pain and nausea were reliably present, whereas diarrhea and urinary symptoms were not.[201] Anorexia was common early in pregnancy but occurred less frequently as pregnancy progressed. Reliable signs included direct abdominal tenderness and low-grade fever. Rebound tenderness and rectal tenderness were common early in pregnancy but became less frequent with the more advanced state. In addition, localization of abdominal tenderness may change as gestation progresses.[20]

Useful laboratory values include leukocytosis with counts in the range of 10,000 to 15,000/mm³, with 25% of patients having a white blood cell count less than 10,000/mm³ and 25% having a white blood cell count greater than 15,000/mm³. Urinalysis may reveal pyuria without bacteriuria but is usually normal in 91% of cases.[201] Differential diagnoses include cholecystitis, torsion of an adnexa, degenerating myoma, ruptured corpus luteum cyst, ruptured dermoid, infarction of an ovary, preterm labor, abruptio placentae, and pneumonia.[19] Pyelonephritis is the most commonly confused diagnosis.

Treatment is surgical. When a normal-appearing appendix is encountered, most authorities recommend removal because some appendices are still found to be histologically abnormal, suggesting early appendicitis. Future diagnostic dilemmas may thus be avoided.[201]

Routine use of postoperative antibiotic therapy is controversial. The visual appearance of the appendix may guide in the decision-making process. Maternal mortality was found to be 2% overall and 7.3% in the last trimester. This high mortality rate is related to gestational age and delay in diagnosis.[201] Perinatal mortality is 8.7 to 17.3% and is related to prematurity in approximately one third of cases.[201] The perforated appendix follows a less benign course in the pregnant patient because the omentum, confined to the upper abdomen by the uterus, cannot adequately wall off the affected area. The appendix itself may lie outside the pelvic cavity and cause generalized peritoneal contamination. Uterine contractions may also inhibit the localization process, and elevated maternal adenocorticosteroid levels may decrease inflammatory response and mask signs of infection.

In conclusion, appendicitis, although not rare in pregnancy, is a difficult diagnosis to confirm. Confirmation relies on surgical exploration, which, if delayed, may result in severe maternal and fetal compromise.

Toxic Shock Syndrome

Toxic shock syndrome has been reported to occur in association with vaginal delivery, spontaneous abortion, cesarean section, and mastitis.[203] The exact incidence of nonmenstrual toxic shock syndrome is unknown.[203] Mortality may be as high as 5%. Toxic shock syndrome is characterized by a temperature greater than 102°F, a diffuse macular erythrodermal rash with desquamation, hypotension, and evidence of multiple organ system dysfunction. It is caused by systemic absorption of exotoxin produced by certain strains of *Staphylococcus aureus*.[22] Vasodilation with loss of intravascular fluid and plasma into the extravascular compartment results in oliguria, hypotension, edema, low central venous pressure, hypoproteinuria, and hypoalbuminemia.[22]

Initial clinical management requires aggressive fluid replacement to correct systemic hypotension. Invasive monitoring in an intensive care unit is necessary in most instances. Cultures should be obtained of the blood and urine, as well as the genital tract and other suspected areas (e.g., surgical wound, cutaneous lesion, or throat). β-Lactamase–resistant antistaphylococcal antibiotics (oxacillin, dicloxacillin, nafcillin), first-generation parenteral cephalosporins, and aminoglycosides may be used for treatment, although they usually do not have a significant effect on the course of the acute disease. Administration of dopamine was required to maintain a low-normal blood pressure in 7 of 22 patients with toxic shock syndrome reported by Chesney and associates.[22] If the diagnosis is in question, an aminoglycoside should be added to cover gram-negative organisms. Irrigation of the vagina, and other possible sources of bacteria and exotoxins, may be helpful but is not of proven benefit.

Suppurative Pelvic Thrombophlebitis

Septic or suppurative pelvic thrombophlebitis describes a condition in which septic thrombosis occurs in the pelvic veins.[79] Genital tract trauma is thought to be the stimulus inciting thrombosis and infection.[204] In addition to bacteremia and sepsis, thromboembolism may occur, with pulmonary infarction occurring in 45% of patients.[205]

Presenting symptoms include temperature as high as 106°F, chills, and tachycardia. Pelvic examination is essentially normal except for palpation of tender thrombosed veins in 30% of cases.[24] Chest x-ray study may reveal pulmonary infiltrates suggestive of infarction.[205] A 35% incidence of positive blood cultures is reported.[24] Diagnosis may

be difficult and is often one of exclusion. Computed tomography of the pelvis has been proposed for detection of venous thrombosis.[108] Medical therapy with broad-spectrum antibiotics (e.g., gentamicin, clindamycin, and ampicillin) for suspected endometritis is often instituted before the diagnosis of suppurative pelvic thrombophlebitis is made. Intravenous heparin is then begun and clinical improvement within 48 hours is anticipated. In the absence of pulmonary emboli, heparin should be continued for 10 days.[23] Surgical therapy, once the mainstay of treatment, is still indicated if medical management is unsuccessful, if pulmonary infarction develops during medical therapy, or if the patient presents before therapy with pulmonary infarction. Surgery usually involves ligation of the inferior vena cava and both ovarian veins.[24] Collins recommended discontinuation of all medical therapy after completion of surgery.[24] Mortality ranged from 52% in the early part of this century to 10% in a series of 202 cases between 1941 and 1969.[24] Death often results from septic complications rather than thromboembolism.

Burns

Each year in the United States approximately 2,200,000 people suffer burns that require medical treatment.[206] Maternal mortality, fetal mortality, and the incidence of premature labor are all directly proportional to the extent of maternal injury. Maternal mortality was found to be 3% and fetal mortality from 17 to 27% if the burn involved less than 40% of the total body surface.[206] Because experience with pregnant burn patients is limited, few specific treatment guidelines beyond electrolyte and fluid replacement, adequate ventilatory support, and antibiotic therapy have been proposed. Tocolytic therapy is complex because beta-mimetic therapy may result in further electrolyte imbalance and cardiopulmonary complications and magnesium sulfate may produce unwanted vasodilatory effects. Indomethacin has been proposed for acute temporary management of premature labor, which may then be managed expectantly, or by conventional means, after the patient's condition has stabilized.[207] As in other instances of maternal injury, maternal stability, fetal well-being, and fetal maturity must all be considered in making decisions regarding delivery. The route and timing of delivery should be based on obstetric indications.[207]

Necrotizing Fasciitis

Necrotizing fasciitis, a suppurative bacterial infection of the superficial and deep fasciae, is a rare but deadly complication in obstetrics. Only two of four patients reported by Golde and Ledger survived.[208] Treatment requires prompt diagnosis, wide surgical débridement of necrotic tissue, drainage, and parenteral antibiotics with emphasis on anaerobic coverage.[208]

Ventricular Dysfunction
Peripartum Cardiomyopathy

Cardiomyopathy refers to a disease that directly affects one or both cardiac ventricles in a diffuse fashion and may lead to congestive heart failure.[209] Peripartum cardiomyopathy is defined as cardiomyopathy developing during the final month of pregnancy or within the first 6 postpartum months in a patient who is known to have been cardiovascularly normal before pregnancy.[210] The incidence in the United States is estimated to be 1:1500 to 1:4000 deliveries.[211] The peak incidence occurs in the second postpartum month, and older, black, multiparous patients (often with a family history of the disease) are most frequently affected.[212] Multiple pregnancy and PIH have also been associated with this condition.[212, 213] Nutritional, autoimmune, and hormonal theories of the etiology of this condition have been advanced, but none has, so far, been substantiated. Myocarditis has been associated with peripartum cardiomyopathy,[214] and viral particles (enterovirus RNA) have been found in biopsy specimens.[215] Although it is possible that pregnancy somehow renders these patients more vulnerable to a cardiotropic viral infection, the precise connection between pregnancy and viral myocarditis is unknown.

An unfortunate but important point about peripartum cardiomyopathy is its tendency to recur in subsequent pregnancies, and this is apparently related to the resolution of the cardiac size in the postpartum period. Patients whose heart size returned to within normal limits by 12 months had an 11 to 14% maternal mortality rate in a subsequent pregnancy, whereas persistent cardiomegaly was associated with 40 to 80% maternal mortality.[210]

The clinical picture of this condition is characterized by fatigue, dyspnea, and edema, both peripheral and pulmonary. Congestive cardiac failure develops with an elevated jugular venous pressure, rales, an S_3 gallop, and the classic electrocardiographic and chest x-ray findings of congestive failure. Up to 50% of these patients have evidence of peripheral or pulmonary embolic phenomena. Overall mortality ranges from 25 to 50%.[211, 212]

In patients developing this complication before delivery, spontaneous vaginal delivery is indicated except when obstetric indications mandate cesarean section. Epidural anesthesia is safe and may help the management of the condition. Management of peripartum cardiomyopathy includes prolonged bed rest in Fowler's position and the use of digitalis, diuretics, and vasodilators. Improvement usually occurs during the ensuing weeks but may be as rapid as a week. Approximately 50% of these patients achieve normal heart size and left ventricular function within 6 months of their illness[210] and continue to be in good health up to a decade later. Many of these women have subsequent pregnancies without difficulty. However, patients who do not have a reduction in heart size do not tolerate subsequent pregnancy well.[210] When spontaneous improvement has not occurred within 30 days of the illness, other modes of therapy should be tried. These include treatment with immunosuppressants such as azathioprine or prednisone, particularly if there is biopsy-proven myocarditis,[216] and, in intractable heart failure, heart transplantation. There are patients who have had successful pregnancies after transplantation, but current opinion is that patients should be advised against this course of action.

Beta-Adrenergic Agents

Ventricular dysfunction, manifested by arrhythmias, angina pectoris, pulmonary edema, or cardiovascular collapse, has been reported with the use of terbutaline, salbutamol, hexoprenaline, and ritodrine in the tocolytic therapy of premature labor.[216–218] Immediate cessation of the tocolytic agent, close monitoring, and treatment of any associated maternal arrhythmia or cardiopulmonary abnormality are essential to prevent further complications.

Thrombotic Pulmonary Embolism

Obstruction of the pulmonary vessels may result in pulmonary hypertension, right-sided heart failure, cardiogenic shock, and frequently death. Massive embolization, defined as greater than 40 to 50% obstruction of the pulmonary

vascular bed, may result in depression of cardiac output in normal patients.[219] Kaunitz and colleagues[3] found embolism to be the leading cause of maternal death in the United States, with thrombotic, amniotic fluid, and air emboli constituting 55, 39, and 5% of cases, respectively.

Treatment of thrombotic pulmonary embolism consists of cardiopulmonary support and heparin anticoagulation to prevent progressive formation of thrombus. The efficacy and safety of thrombolytic agents, such as streptokinase, urokinase, and tissue plasminogen activator, remain unproved, especially in obstetrics.[220] Urokinase has been utilized in pregnancy with success,[221] and it is known that neither urokinase nor streptokinase crosses the placenta. Recent surgery or delivery is a contraindication to thrombolytic therapy.[222] Surgical embolectomy is indicated in rare cases.[220, 222]

Cardiogenic Shock

A review of maternal mortality in California between 1960 and 1968 showed that heart disease was the most common nonobstetric cause of maternal death, being responsible for 77 of 348 (22%) nonobstetric deaths.[223] Rheumatic heart disease was the most frequent cardiac condition, with congenital heart disease, peripartum cardiomyopathy, and coronary heart disease also contributing significantly to mortality. The relative frequency of disease entities changes with advancing technology, and for this reason the ratio of rheumatic heart disease to congenital heart disease is decreasing with time. Patients with congenital heart disease now survive into their reproductive years as a result of surgery. Nevertheless, rheumatic heart disease is still sufficiently prevalent and complications such as pulmonary congestion, pulmonary edema, right-sided heart failure, dysrhythmias, and embolism still occur in pregnancy.[224]

Severe Anemia

When chronic blood loss results in a drop in hemoglobin to 4.4 g/dL or hematocrit to 14%, profound circulatory changes develop and cardiac failure may follow.[225] Patients with chronic severe anemia require slow transfusion with packed red blood cells in combination with potent, rapidly acting diuretics to prevent volume overload. In emergency situations, such as labor or surgery, severe anemia may be corrected rapidly via partial exchange transfusion to avoid volume overload.[225]

PREVENTIVE MEASURES

In many cases, the development of shock is unforeseeable and unavoidable. However, clinical suspicion and preparation may decrease the morbidity and mortality in obstetric or gynecologic emergencies. All obstetric patients should be considered potential victims of hemorrhage. Certain patients present with conditions that place them in a high-risk category. These include placenta previa, multiple previous cesarean sections, intrauterine fetal demise near term, and PIH. In these situations adequate preparation should include ensuring good venous access, the availability of volume expanders and blood products, anesthesia, and uterotonic agents. These steps may allow prompt and effective treatment in the event of acute blood loss and may prevent further blood loss and subsequent complications. In general, preparedness and identification of patients at risk for shock may minimize or prevent maternal and fetal life-threatening events.

References

1. National Center for Health Statistics: Vital Statistics of the United States, 1982, Volume II, Mortality, Part A. Washington, DC, US Government Printing Office, p 64, 1986. US Department of Health and Human Services publication (PHS) 86–1122.
2. National Center for Health Statistics: Vital Statistics of the United States, 1978, Volume II, Part A. Washington, DC, US Government Printing Office, p 1, 1982. US Department of Health and Human Services publication (PHS) 83–1101.
3. Kaunitz AM, Hughes JM, Grimes DA, et al: Causes of maternal mortality in the United States. Obstet Gynecol 65:605, 1985.
4. Gibbs CE, Locke WE: Maternal deaths in Texas, 1969 to 1973. Am J Obstet Gynecol 126:687, 1976.
5. Hansen JP: Older maternal age and pregnancy outcome: A review of the literature. Obstet Gynecol Surv 41:726, 1986.
6. Laros RK, Collins J, Penner JA, et al: Coagulation changes in saline-induced abortion. Am J Obstet Gynecol 116:277, 1973.
7. Gonik B: Septic shock in obstetrics. Clin Perinatol 13:741, 1986.
8. Romero R, Copel JA, Hobbins JC: Intrauterine fetal demise and hemostatic failure: The fetal death syndrome. Clin Obstet Gynecol 28:24, 1985.
9. Pritchard JA, Brekken AL: Clinical and laboratory studies on severe abruptio placentae. Am J Obstet Gynecol 97:681, 1967.
10. Clark SL: Amniotic fluid embolism. In: Clark SL, Phelan JR, Cotton DB (eds): Critical Care Obstetrics. Oradell, NJ, Medical Economics Books, p 315, 1987.
11. Pritchard JA, Weisman R Jr, Ratnoff OD, et al: Intravascular hemolysis, thrombocytopenia and other hematologic abnormalities associated with severe toxemia of pregnancy. N Engl J Med 250:89, 1954.
12. Weinstein L: Syndrome of hemolysis, elevated liver enzymes and low platelet count: A severe consequence of hypertension in pregnancy. Am J Obstet Gynecol 142:159, 1982.
13. Pritchard JA, Cunningham FG, Mason RA: Coagulation changes in eclampsia: Their frequency and pathogenesis. Am J Obstet Gynecol 124:855, 1976.
14. Weinstein L: Preeclampsia/eclampsia with hemolysis, elevated liver enzymes, and thrombocytopenia. Obstet Gynecol 66:657, 1985.
15. Bick RL: Disseminated intravascular coagulation and related syndromes: Etiology, pathophysiology, diagnosis, and management. Am J Hematol 5:265, 1978.
16. Blaisdell FW: Traumatic shock: The search for a toxic factor. ACS (Am Chem Soc) Bull 68:2, 1983.
17. Yoder PR, Gibbs RS, Blanco JD, et al: A prospective, controlled study of maternal and perinatal outcome after intra-amniotic infection at term. Am J Obstet Gynecol 145:695, 1983.
18. Cunningham FG, Morris GB, Mickal A: Acute pyelonephritis of pregnancy: A clinical review. Obstet Gynecol 42:112, 1973.
19. DeVore GR: Acute abdominal pain in the pregnant patient due to pancreatitis, acute appendicitis, cholecystitis, or peptic ulcer disease. Clin Perinatol 7:349, 1980.
20. Baer JL, Reis RA, Arens RA: Appendicitis in pregnancy, with changes in position and axis of the normal appendix in pregnancy. JAMA 98:1359, 1932.
21. Grimes DA, Kafrissen ME, O'Reilly KR, et al: Fatal hemorrhage from legal abortion in the United States. Surg Gynecol Obstet 157:461, 1983.
22. Chesney PJ, Davis JP, Purdy WK, et al: Clinical manifestations of toxic shock syndrome. JAMA 246:741, 1981.
23. Gibbs RS: Treatment of refractory postpartum fever. Clin Obstet Gynecol 19:83, 1976.
24. Collins CG: Suppurative pelvic thrombophlebitis: A study of 202 cases in which the disease was treated by ligation of the vena cava and ovarian vein. Am J Obstet Gynecol 108:681, 1970.
25. Barela AI, Kleinman GE, Golditch IM, et al: Septic shock with renal failure after chorionic villus sampling. Am J Obstet Gynecol 154:1100, 1986.
26. Cowart V: NIH considers large-scale study to evaluate chorionic villi sampling. JAMA 252:11, 1984.
27. Belfort MA, Anthony J, Buccimazza A, et al: Verapamil in the treatment of severe gestational proteinuric hypertension. Obstet Gynecol 75:970, 1990.
28. Hardaway RM: Coagulation disorders and hemorrhagic shock in the parturient. Int Anesthesiol Clin 6:743, 1968.
29. American College of Obstetricians and Gynecologists: Hemorrhagic Shock. Washington, DC, American College of Obstetricians and Gynecologists, p 1, 1984. ACOG Technical Bulletin 82.
30. Hayashi RH: Hemorrhagic shock in obstetrics. Clin Perinatol 13:755, 1986.
31. Jansen RPS: Relative bradycardia: A sign of acute intraperitoneal bleeding. Aust NZ J Obstet Gynaecol 18:206, 1978.
32. Oberman HA, Barnes BA, Friedman BA: The risk of abbreviating the major crossmatch in urgent or massive transfusion. Transfusion 18:137, 1978.
33. Consensus Conference: Fresh-frozen plasma. Indications and risks. JAMA 253:551, 1985.
34. Oberman HA: Uses and abuses of fresh frozen plasma. In: Garratty A

(ed): Current Concepts in Transfusion Therapy. Arlington, VA, American Association of Blood Banks, p 109, 1985.
35. Mannucci PM, Federici AB, Sirchia G: Hemostasis testing during massive blood replacement: A study of 172 cases. Vox Sang 42:113, 1982.
36. Counts RB, Haisch C, Simon TL, et al: Hemostasis in massively transfused trauma patients. Ann Surg 190:91, 1979.
37. Murphy S, Gardner FH: Platelet preservation: Effect of storage temperature on maintenance of platelet viability—Deleterious effect of refrigerated storage. N Engl J Med 280:1094, 1969.
38. Goldberg LI: Dopamine—Clinical uses of an endogenous catecholamine. N Engl J Med 291:707, 1974.
39. Abboud FM: Shock. In: Wyngaarden JB, Smith LH (eds): Cecil Textbook of Medicine. 17th ed. Philadelphia, WB Saunders, p 211, 1985.
40. Lee W, Clark SL, Cotton DB, et al: Septic shock during pregnancy. Am J Obstet Gynecol 159:410, 1988.
41. Goenen M, Pedemonte O, Baele P, et al: Amrinone in the management of low cardiac output after open heart surgery. Am J Cardiol 56:33B, 1985.
42. Callender K, Levinson G, Shnider SM, et al: Dopamine administration in the normotensive pregnant ewe. Obstet Gynecol 51:586, 1978.
43. Rolbin SH, Levinson G, Shnider SM, et al: Dopamine treatment of spinal hypotension decreases uterine blood flow in the pregnant ewe. Anesthesiology 51:36, 1979.
44. Greiss FC, Van Wilkes D: Effect of sympathomimetic drugs and angiotensin on the uterine vascular bed. Obstet Gynecol 23:925, 1964.
45. Swan HJC, Ganz W, Forrester J, et al: Catheterization of the heart in man with use of a flow-directed balloon-tipped catheter. N Engl J Med 283:447, 1970.
46. Swan HJC, Ganz W: Use of balloon flotation catheters in critically ill patients. Surg Clin North Am 55:501, 1975.
47. Kirshon B, Cotton DB: Invasive hemodynamic monitoring in the obstetric patient. Clin Obstet Gynecol 30:579, 1987.
48. Clark SL, Horenstein JM, Phelan JP, et al: Experience with the pulmonary artery catheter in obstetrics and gynecology. Am J Obstet Gynecol 152:374, 1985.
49. Cotton DB, Gonik B, Dorman K, et al: Cardiovascular alterations in severe pregnancy-induced hypertension: Relationship of central venous pressure to pulmonary capillary wedge pressure. Am J Obstet Gynecol 151:762, 1985.
50. Packman MI, Rackow EC: Optimum left heart filling pressure during fluid resuscitation of patients with hypovolemic and septic shock. Crit Care Med 11:165, 1983.
51. Belfort MA, Uys PC, Dommisse J, et al: Haemodynamic changes in gestational proteinuric hypertension: The effects of rapid volume expansion and vasodilator therapy. Br J Obstet Gynaecol 96:634, 1989.
52. Lee W, Rokey R, Cotton DB: Noninvasive maternal stroke volume and cardiac output determinations by pulsed Doppler echocardiography. Am J Obstet Gynecol 158:505, 1988.
53. Masaki DI, Greenspoon JS, Ouzounian JG: Measurement of cardiac output in pregnancy by thoracic electrical bioimpedance and thermodilution. A preliminary report. Am J Obstet Gynecol 161:680, 1989.
54. Katz VL, Dotters DJ, Droegemueller W: Perimortem cesarean delivery. Obstet Gynecol 68:571, 1986.
55. Ritter JW: Postmortem cesarean section. JAMA 175:715, 1961.
56. Pritchard JA: Changes in the blood volume during pregnancy and delivery. Anesthesiology 26:393, 1965.
57. Clark SL, Phelan JP: Surgical control of ob hemorrhage. Contemp Ob/Gyn 24:70, 1984.
58. Waters EG: Surgical management of postpartum hemorrhage with particular reference to ligation of uterine arteries. Am J Obstet Gynecol 64:1143, 1952.
59. Clark SL, Phelan JP, Yeh S-Y, et al: Hypogastric artery ligation for obstetric hemorrhage. Obstet Gynecol 66:353, 1985.
60. Clark SL, Yeh S-Y, Phelan JP, et al: Emergency hysterectomy for the control of obstetric hemorrhage. Obstet Gynecol 64:376, 1984.
61. Takagi S, Yoshida T, Togo Y, et al: The effects of intramyometrial injection of prostaglandin $F_{2\alpha}$ on severe postpartum hemorrhage. Prostaglandins 12:565, 1976.
62. Hayashi RH, Castillo MS, Noah ML: Management of severe postpartum hemorrhage with a prostaglandin $F_{2\alpha}$ analogue. Obstet Gynecol 63:806, 1984.
63. Hankins GDV, Berryman GK, Scott RT Jr, et al: Maternal arterial desaturation with 15-methyl prostaglandin $F_{2\alpha}$ for uterine atony. Obstet Gynecol 72:367, 1988.
64. Smith DC, Wyatt JF: Embolization of the hypogastric arteries in the control of massive vaginal hemorrhage. Obstet Gynecol 49:317, 1977.
65. Hibbard LT: Placenta previa. Am J Obstet Gynecol 104:172, 1969.
66. Clark SL, Koonings PP, Phelan JP: Placenta previa/accreta and prior cesarean section. Obstet Gynecol 66:89, 1985.
67. Cotton DB, Read JA, Paul RH, et al: The conservative aggressive management of placenta previa. Am J Obstet Gynecol 137:687, 1980.
68. Aho AJ, Pulkkinen MO, Vaha-Eskeli K: Acute urinary bladder tamponade with hypovolemic shock due to placenta percreta with bladder invasion. Case report. Scand J Urol Nephrol 19:157, 1985.
69. Knab DR: Abruptio placentae: An assessment of the time and method of delivery. Obstet Gynecol 52:625, 1978.
70. Pritchard JA: Genesis of severe placental abruption. Am J Obstet Gynecol 108:22, 1970.

71. Golditch IM, Boyce NE: Management of abruptio placentae. JAMA 212:288, 1970.

72. Abdella TN, Sibai BM, Hays JM Jr, et al: Relationship of hypertensive disease to abruptio placentae. Obstet Gynecol 63:365, 1984.

73. Acker D, Sachs BP, Tracey KJ, et al: Abruptio placentae associated with cocaine use. Am J Obstet Gynecol 146:220, 1983.

74. Chasnoff IJ, Burns KA, Burns WJ: Cocaine use in pregnancy: Perinatal morbidity and mortality. Neurotoxicol Teratol 9:291, 1987.

75. Little BB, Snell LM, Palmore MK, et al: Cocaine use in pregnant women in a large public hospital. Am J Perinatol 5:206, 1988.

76. Hurd WW, Miodovnik M, Hertzberg V, et al: Selective management of abruptio placentae: A prospective study. Obstet Gynecol 61:467, 1983.

77. Sher G: Pathogenesis and management of uterine inertia complicating abruptio placentae with consumptive coagulopathy. Am J Obstet Gynecol 129:164, 1977.

78. Belfort MA, Moore PJ: The use of a cephalic perforator for delivery of the dead fetus in cases of severe abruptio placentae. S Afr Med J 77:80, 1990.

79. American College of Obstetricians and Gynecologists: Ectopic Pregnancy. Washington, DC, American College of Obstetricians and Gynecologists, 1989. ACOG Technical Bulletin 126.

80. Kadar N, Caldwell BV, Romero R: A method of screening for ectopic pregnancy and its indications. Obstet Gynecol 58:162, 1981.

81. Shapiro BS, Cullen M, Tayler KJ, et al: Transvaginal ultrasonography for the diagnosis of ectopic pregnancy. Fertil Steril 50:425, 1988.

82. Dorfman SF, Grimes DA, Cartes W Jr, et al: Ectopic pregnancy mortality, United States, 1979 to 1980: Clinical aspects. Obstet Gynecol 64:386, 1984.

83. Ory SJ, Villanueva AL, Sand PK, et al: Conservative treatment of ectopic pregnancy with methotrexate. Am J Obstet Gynecol 154:1299, 1986.

83a. Stovall TG, Ling FW, Gray LA, et al: Methotrexate treatment of unruptured ectopic pregnancy: A report of 100 cases. Obstet Gynecol 77:749, 1991.

84. Golan A, Sandbank O, Rubin A: Rupture of the pregnant uterus. Obstet Gynecol 56:549, 1980.

85. Krishna Menon MK: Rupture of the uterus: A review of 164 cases. J Obstet Gynaecol Br Commonw 69:18, 1962.

86. Abercrombie J: Case of hemorrhage of the liver. London Med Gaz 34:792, 1844.

87. Owen A, Kandalaft E: Spontaneous subcapsular hematoma and rupture of the liver during pregnancy. Br J Obstet Gynaecol 80:852, 1973.

88. Jewett JF: Eclampsia and rupture of the liver. N Engl J Med 297:1009, 1977.

89. Smith LJ Jr, Moise KJ Jr, Dildy GA III, et al: Spontaneous rupture of liver during pregnancy: Current therapy. Obstet Gynecol 77:171, 1991.

90. Mokotoff R, Weiss LS, Brandon LH, et al: Liver rupture complicating toxemia of pregnancy. Arch Intern Med 119:375, 1967.

91. Aziz S, Merrell RC, Collins JA: Spontaneous hepatic hemorrhage during pregnancy. Am J Surg 146:680, 1983.

92. Freiman SM, Wulff GJL Jr: Management of uterine perforation following elective abortion. Obstet Gynecol 50:647, 1977.

93. Buchsbaum HJ: Penetrating injury of the abdomen. In: Buchsbaum HJ (ed): Trauma in Pregnancy. Philadelphia, WB Saunders, p 82, 1979.

94. Buchsbaum HJ: Diagnosis and management of abdominal gunshot wounds during pregnancy. J Trauma 15:425, 1975.

95. Crosby WM: Trauma during pregnancy: Maternal and fetal injury. Obstet Gynecol Surv 29:683, 1974.

96. Buchsbaum HJ: Traumatic injury in pregnancy. In: Barber HRK, Garber EA (eds): Surgical Disease in Pregnancy. Philadelphia, WB Saunders, p 184, 1974.

97. Crosby WM: Traumatic injuries during pregnancy. Clin Obstet Gynecol 26:902, 1983.

98. Karlsson K: The influence of hypoxia on uterine and maternal placental blood flow, and the effect of alpha-adrenergic blockade. J Perinat Med 2:176, 1974.

99. Rose PG, Strohm PL, Zuspan FP: Fetomaternal hemorrhage following trauma. Am J Obstet Gynecol 153:844, 1985.

100. Rothenberger DA, Quattlebaum FW, Zabel J, et al: Diagnostic peritoneal lavage for blunt trauma in pregnant women. Am J Obstet Gynecol 129:479, 1977.

101. Buchsbaum HJ: Splenic rupture in pregnancy. Obstet Gynecol Surv 22:381, 1967.

102. Nance FC, Wennar MH, Johnson LW, et al: Surgical judgment in the management of penetrating wounds of the abdomen: Experience with 2,212 patients. Ann Surg 179:639, 1974.

103. Dudley AG, Teaford H, Gatewood TS Jr: Delayed traumatic rupture of the diaphragm in pregnancy. Obstet Gynecol 53:25s, 1979.

104. Glueck HI, Burket RL, Sutherland JM, et al: Afibrinogenemia in pregnancy apparently due to a degenerating leiomyoma. Obstet Gynecol 18:285, 1961.

105. Koren Z, Zuckerman H, Brzezinski A: Placenta previa accreta with afibrinogenemia: Report of three cases. Obstet Gynecol 18:138, 1961.

106. Henderson SR, Lund CJ: Severe preeclampsia, disseminated intravascular coagulopathy and hydatidiform mole complicating a 20-week pregnancy with a fetus. Obstet Gynecol 37:722, 1971.

107. Goldman JA, Dekel A, Peleg D: Ovarian vascular accidents: A complication of anticoagulant therapy. Eur J Obstet Gynecol Reprod Biol 8:163, 1978.

108. Knuppel RA, Rao PS, Cavanagh D: Septic shock in obstetrics. Clin Obstet Gynecol 27:3, 1984.

109. Reid DE, Weiner AE, Roby CC, et al: Maternal afibrinogenemia associated with long-standing intrauterine fetal death. Am J Obstet Gynecol 66:500, 1953.

110. Pritchard JA: Fetal death in utero. Obstet Gynecol 14:573, 1959.

111. Basu HK: Fibrinolysis and abruptio placentae. Br J Obstet Gynaecol 76:481, 1969.

112. Morgan M: Amniotic fluid embolism. Anaesthesia 34:29, 1979.

113. Courtney LD: Amniotic fluid embolism. Obstet Gynecol Surv 29:169, 1974.

114. Clark SL, Montz FJ, Phelan JP: Hemodynamic alterations associated with amniotic fluid embolism: A reappraisal. Am J Obstet Gynecol 151:617, 1985.

115. Caldwell DC, Williamson RA, Goldsmith JC: Hereditary coagulopathies in pregnancy. Clin Obstet Gynecol 28:53, 1985.

116. Lee W, Ginsburg KA, Cotton DB, et al: Squamous and trophoblastic cells in the maternal pulmonary circulation identified by invasive hemodynamic monitoring during the peripartum period. Am J Obstet Gynecol 155:999, 1986.

117. Gregory MG, Clayton EM Jr: Amniotic fluid embolism. Obstet Gynecol 42:236, 1973.

118. Lipton RA, Ayromlooi J, Coller BS: Severe von Willebrand's disease during labor and delivery. JAMA 248:1355, 1982.

119. Nelson DM, Stempel LE, Brandt JT: Hereditary antithrombin III deficiency and pregnancy: Report of two cases and review of the literature. Obstet Gynecol 65:848, 1985.

120. McPherson RA: Thromboembolism in Hageman trait. Am J Clin Pathol 68:420, 1977.

121. Friedman SA: Preeclampsia: A review of the role of prostaglandins. Obstet Gynecol 71:122, 1988.

122. Redman CWG: Immunologic factors in the pathogenesis of preeclampsia. Contrib Nephrol 25:120, 1981.

123. Gant NF, Daley GL, Chand S, et al: A study of angiotensin II pressor response throughout primigravid pregnancy. J Clin Invest 52:2682, 1973.

124. Easterling TR, Benedetti TJ: Preeclampsia: A hyper-dynamic disease model. Am J Obstet Gynecol 160:1447, 1989.

125. American College of Obstetricians and Gynecologists: Management of Preeclampsia. Washington, DC, American College of Obstetricians and Gynecologists, p 1, 1986. ACOG Technical Bulletin 91.

126. Groenendijk R, Trimbos JBMJ, Wallenburg HCS: Hemo-dynamic measurements in preeclampsia: Preliminary observations. Am J Obstet Gynecol 150:232, 1984.

127. Belfort M, Anthony J, Kirshon, B: Respiratory function in severe pregnancy induced hypertension: The effects of volume expansion and subsequent vasodilatation with verapamil. Br J Obstet Gynaecol 98:904, 1991.

128. Thiagarajah S, Bourgeois FJ, Harbert GM, et al: Thrombocytopenia in preeclampsia: Associated abnormalities and management principles. Am J Obstet Gynecol 150:1, 1984.

129. Hankins GDV, Wendel GD, Cunningham FG, et al: Longitudinal evaluation of hemodynamic changes in eclampsia. Am J Obstet Gynecol 150:506, 1984.

130. Wasserstrum N, Cotton DB: Hemodynamic monitoring in severe pregnancy-induced hypertension. Clin Perinatol 13:781, 1986.

131. Gonik B, Cotton DB: Peripartum colloid osmotic pressure changes: Influence of intravenous hydration. Am J Obstet Gynecol 150:99, 1984.

132. Cotton DB, Gonik B, Spillman T, et al: Intrapartum to postpartum changes in colloid osmotic pressure. Am J Obstet Gynecol 149:174, 1984.

133. Kirshon B, Moise KJ Jr, Cotton DB, et al: Role of volume expansion in severe pre-eclampsia. Surg Gynecol Obstet 167:367, 1988.

134. Cotton DB, Longmire S, Jones MM, et al: Cardiovascular alterations in severe pregnancy-induced hypertension: Effects of intravenous nitroglycerin coupled with blood volume expansion. Am J Obstet Gynecol 154:1053, 1986.

135. Pritchard JA, Pritchard SA: Standardized treatment of 154 consecutive cases of eclampsia. Am J Obstet Gynecol 123:543, 1975.

136. Shelley WC, Gutsche BB: Magnesium and seizure control. Am J Obstet Gynecol 136:146, 1980.

137. Hilmy MI, Somjen GG: Distribution and tissue uptake of magnesium related to its pharmacological effects. Am J Physiol 214:406, 1968.

138. Borges LF, Gucer G: Effect of magnesium on epileptic foci. Epilepsia 19:81, 1978.

139. Sibai BM, Spinnato JA, Watson DL, et al: Pregnancy outcome in 303 cases with severe preeclampsia. Obstet Gynecol 64:319, 1984.

140. Moore PJ, Belfort MA, Bryant SS: Cerebrospinal fluid magnesium levels in gestational proteinuric hypertension patients on magnesium sulphate therapy (abstract). In: Proceedings of the South African Pharmacological Society, October 10–12, 1989, p 12.

140a. Belfort MA, Moise KJ: The effect of magnesium sulfate on maternal brain blood flow in pregnancy induced hypertension: A randomized placebo controlled study. Am J Obstet Gynecol (in press).

141. Pritchard JA, MacDonald PC, Gant NF: Hypertensive disorders in pregnancy. In: Williams Obstetrics. 17th ed. Norwalk, CT, Appleton-Century-Crofts, p 525, 1985.

142. Chesley LC: Parenteral magnesium sulfate and the distribution, plasma levels, and excretion of magnesium. Am J Obstet Gynecol 133:1, 1979.
143. Pritchard JA: The use of the magnesium ion in the management of eclamptogenic toxemias. Surg Gynecol Obstet 100:131, 1955.
144. Sibai BM, Graham JM, McCubbin JH: A comparison of intravenous and intramuscular magnesium sulfate regimens in preeclampsia. Am J Obstet Gynecol 150:728, 1984.
145. Pruett KM, Kirshon B, Cotton DB, et al: The effects of magnesium sulfate therapy on Apgar scores. Am J Obstet Gynecol 159:1047, 1988.
146. Cotton DB, Gonik B, Dorman KR: Cardiovascular alterations in severe pregnancy-induced hypertension: Acute effects of intravenous magnesium sulfate. Am J Obstet Gynecol 148:162, 1984.
147. Lubbe WF: Hypertension in pregnancy: Whom and how to treat. Br J Clin Pharmacol 24:15S, 1987.
148. Kock-Weser J: Hydralazine. N Engl J Med 295:320, 1976.
149. Spinnato JA, Sibai BM, Anderson GD: Fetal distress after hydralazine therapy for severe pregnancy-induced hypertension. South Med J 79:559, 1986.
150. Clark SL, Cotton DB: Clinical indications for pulmonary artery catheterization in the patient with severe preeclampsia. Am J Obstet Gynecol 158:453, 1988.
151. Naden RP, Redman CWG: Antihypertensive drugs in pregnancy. Clin Perinatol 12:521, 1985.
152. Waisman GD, Mayorga LM, Camera MI, et al: Magnesium plus nifedipine: Potentiation of hypotensive effect in preeclampsia? Am J Obstet Gynecol 159:308, 1988.
153. Belfort MA, Moore P: Verapamil in the treatment of severe post partum hypertension. S Afr Med J 74:265, 1988.
154. Lund-Johansen P: Short- and long-term (six-year) hemodynamic effects of labetalol in essential hypertension. Am J Med 75:24, 1983.
155. Mabie WC, Gonzales AR, Sibai BM, et al: A comparative trial of labetalol and hydralazine in the acute management of severe hypertension complicating pregnancy. Obstet Gynecol 70:328, 1987.
156. Michael CA: The evaluation of labetalol in the treatment of hypertension complicating pregnancy. Br J Clin Pharmacol 13:127S, 1982.
157. Lunell NO, Lewander R, Mamoun I, et al: Uteroplacental blood flow in pregnancy induced hypertension. Scand J Clin Lab Invest Suppl 169:28, 1984.
158. Schubiger G, Flury G, Nussberger J: Enalapril for pregnancy-induced hypertension: Acute renal failure in a neonate. Ann Intern Med 108:215, 1988.
159. Oates JA, Wood AJJ: Converting-enzyme inhibitors in the treatment of hypertension. N Engl J Med 319:1517, 1988.
160. Benedetti TJ, Carlson RW: Studies of colloid osmotic pressure in pregnancy-induced hypertension. Am J Obstet Gynecol 135:308, 1979.
161. Sibai BM, Mabie BC, Harvey CJ, et al: Pulmonary edema in severe preeclampsia-eclampsia: Analysis of thirty-seven consecutive cases. Am J Obstet Gynecol 156:1174, 1987.
162. Benedetti TJ, Kates R, Williams V: Hemodynamic observations in severe preeclampsia complicated by pulmonary edema. Am J Obstet Gynecol 152:330, 1985.
163. Strauss RG, Keefer, JR, Burke T, et al: Hemodynamic monitoring of cardiogenic pulmonary edema complicating toxemia of pregnancy. Obstet Gynecol 55:170, 1980.
164. Chesley, LC, Duffus GM: Preeclampsia, posture, and renal function. Obstet Gynecol 38:1, 1971.
165. Spargo B, McCartney CP, Winemiller R: Glomerular capillary endotheliosis in toxemia of pregnancy. Arch Pathol 68:593, 1959.
166. Krane NK: Acute renal failure in pregnancy. Arch Intern Med 148:2347, 1988.
167. Grunfeld J-P, Pertuiset N: Acute renal failure in pregnancy. Am J Kidney Dis 9:359, 1987.
168. Fisher KA, Luger A, Spargo BH, et al: Hypertension in pregnancy: Clinical-pathological correlations and remote prognosis. Medicine 60:267, 1981.
169. Redman CWG, Beilin LJ, Bonnar J: Renal function in preeclampsia. J Clin Pathol 10:91, 1976.
170. Gallery EDM, Hunyor SN, Gyroy AZ: Plasma volume contraction: A significant factor in both pregnancy associated hypertension (preeclampsia) and chronic hypertension in pregnancy. Q J Med 48:593, 1979.
171. Clark SL, Greenspoon JS, Aldahl D, et al: Severe preeclampsia with persistent oliguria: Management of hemodynamic subsets. Am J Obstet Gynecol 154:490, 1986.
172. Kirshon B, Lee W, Mauer MB, et al: Effects of low-dose dopamine therapy in the oliguric patient with preeclampsia. Am J Obstet Gynecol 159:604, 1988.
173. Sibai BM, Taslimi MM, El-Nazer A, et al: Maternal-perinatal outcome associated with the syndrome of hemolysis, elevated liver enzymes, and low platelets in severe preeclampsia-eclampsia. Am J Obstet Gynecol 155:501, 1986.
174. Martin JN Jr, Blake PG, Lowry SL, et al: Pregnancy complicated by preeclampsia-eclampsia with the syndrome of hemolysis, elevated liver enzymes, and low platelet count: How rapid is postpartum recovery? Obstet Gynecol 76:737, 1990.
175. Socol ML, Weiner CP, Louis G, et al: Platelet activation in preeclampsia. Am J Obstet Gynecol 151:494, 1985.
176. Redman CWG, Beilin LJ, Stirrat GM, et al: Factor VIII consumption in pre-eclampsia. Lancet 2:1249, 1977.
177. Weiner CP, Kwaan HC, Xu C, et al: Antithrombin III activity in women with hypertension during pregnancy. Obstet Gynecol 65:301, 1985.
178. Lazarchick J, Stubbs TM, Romein L, et al: Predictive value of fibronectin levels in normotensive gravid women destined to become preeclamptic. Am J Obstet Gynecol 154:1050, 1986.
179. Rodgers GM, Taylor RN, Roberts JM: Preeclampsia is associated with a serum factor cytotoxic to human endothelial cells. Am J Obstet Gynecol 159:908, 1988.
180. Pritchard JA, Stone SR: Clinical and laboratory observations on eclampsia. Am J Obstet Gynecol 99:754, 1967.
181. Hibbard, LT: Maternal mortality due to acute toxemia. Obstet Gynecol 42:263, 1973.
182. Benedetti TJ, Quilligan EJ: Cerebral edema in severe pregnancy-induced hypertension. Am J Obstet Gynecol 137:860, 1980.
183. Kirby JC, Jaindl JJ: Cerebral CT findings in toxemia of pregnancy. Radiology 154:114, 1984.
184. Beck RW, Gamel JW, Willcourt RJ, et al: Acute ischemic optic neuropathy in severe preeclampsia. Am J Ophthalmol 90:342, 1980.
185. Hill JA, Devoe LD, Elgammal TA: Central hemodynamic findings associated with cortical blindness in severe preeclampsia. A case report. J Reprod Med 30:435, 1985.
186. Sheehan HL: Pathological lesions in the hypertensive toxaemias of pregnancy. In: Hammond J, Browne FJ, Walstenholme GEW (eds): Toxaemias of Pregnancy, Human and Veterinary. Philadelphia, Blakiston, p 16, 1950.
187. Dunn R, Lee W, Cotton DB: Evaluation by computerized axial tomography of eclamptic women with seizures refractory to magnesium sulfate therapy. Am J Obstet Gynecol 155:267, 1986.
188. Miller JD: The management of cerebral oedema. Br J Hosp Med 21:152, 1979.
189. Entman SS, Moise KJ: Anaphylaxis in pregnancy. South Med J 77:402, 1984.
190. Smith BE: Anesthetic emergencies. Clin Obstet Gynecol 28:391, 1985.
191. Blanco JD, Gibbs RS, Castaneda YS: Bacteremia in obstetrics: Clinical course. Obstet Gynecol 58:621, 1981.
192. Ledger WJ, Norman M, Gee C, et al: Bacteremia on an obstetric gynecologic service. Am J Obstet Gynecol 121:205, 1975.
193. Morishima HO, Niemann WH, James LS: Effects of endotoxin on the pregnant baboon and fetus. Am J Obstet Gynecol 131:899, 1978.
194. Rackow EC: Clinical definition of sepsis and septic shock. In: Sibbald WJ, Sprung CL (eds): Perspectives on Sepsis and Septic Shock. Fullerton, CA, Society of Critical Care Medicine, p 1, 1986.
195. Sayeed MM: Pulmonary cellular dysfunction in endotoxin shock: Metabolic and transport derangements. Circ Shock 9:335, 1982.
196. Gibbs RS, Blanco JD, St Clair PJ, et al: Quantitative bacteriology of amniotic fluid from women with clinical intraamniotic infection at term. J Infect Dis 145:1, 1982.
197. Mariona FG, Ismail MA: *Clostridium perfringens* septicemia following cesarean section. Obstet Gynecol 56:518, 1980.
198. Duff P: Pyelonephritis in pregnancy. Clin Obstet Gynecol 27:17, 1984.
199. Cunningham FG, Leveno KJ, Hankins GDV, et al: Respiratory insufficiency associated with pyelonephritis during pregnancy. Obstet Gynecol 63:121, 1984.
200. Gilstrap LC, Cunningham FG, Whalley PJ: Acute pyelonephritis in pregnancy: An anterospective study. Obstet Gynecol 57:409, 1981.
201. Cunningham FG, McCubbin JH: Appendicitis complicating pregnancy. Obstet Gynecol 45:415, 1975.
202. Babler EA: Perforative appendicitis complicating pregnancy. JAMA 51:1310, 1908.
203. Petitti D, D'Agostino RB, Oldman MJ: Nonmenstrual toxic shock syndrome. Methodologic problems in estimating incidence and delineating risk factors. J Reprod Med 32:10, 1987.
204. Collins CG, MacCallum EA, Nelson EW, et al: Suppurative pelvic thrombophlebitis. I. Incidence, pathology and etiology. Surgery 30:298, 1951.
205. Collins CG, Nelson EW, Collins JH, et al: Suppurative pelvic thrombophlebitis. II. Symptomatology and diagnosis. Surgery 30:311, 1951.
206. Smith BK, Rayburn WF, Feller I: Burns and pregnancy. Clin Perinatol 10:383, 1983.
207. Gonik B: Intensive care monitoring of the critically ill pregnant patient. In: Creasy RK, Resnik R (eds): Maternal-Fetal Medicine: Principles and Practice. 2nd ed. Philadelphia, WB Saunders, p 845, 1989.
208. Golde S, Ledger WJ: Necrotizing fasciitis in postpartum patients. Obstet Gynecol 50:670, 1977.
209. Johnson RA, Palacios I: Dilated cardiomyopathies of the adult. N Engl J Med 307:1051, 1982.
210. Demakis JG, Rahimtoola SH, Sutton GC, et al: Natural course of peripartum cardiomyopathy. Circulation 44:1053, 1971.
211. Homans DC: Peripartum cardiomyopathy. N Engl J Med 312:1432, 1985.
212. Veille JC: Peripartum cardiomyopathies: A review. Am J Obstet Gynecol 148:805, 1984.
213. Pierce JA, Price BO, Joyce JW: Familial occurrence of postpartal heart failure. Arch Intern Med 111:651, 1963.
214. Melvin KR, Richardson PJ, Olsen EGJ, et al: Peripartum cardiomyopathy due to myocarditis. N Engl J Med 307:731, 1982.
215. Meany BT, Richardson PJ, Archard LC, et al: Clinical presentation and

follow-up of patients with enterovirus RNA myocarditis (abstract). Circulation 80 (suppl):11, 1989.

216. Carpenter RJ, Decuir P: Cardiovascular collapse associated with oral terbutaline tocolytic therapy. Am J Obstet Gynecol 148:821, 1984.

217. Michalak D, Klein V, Marquette GP: Myocardial ischemia: A complication of ritodrine tocolysis. Am J Obstet Gynecol 146:861, 1983.

218. Tye KH, Desser KB, Benchimol A: Angina pectoris associated with use of terbutaline for premature labor. JAMA 244:692, 1980.

219. McIntyre KM, Sasahara AA: Hemodynamic and ventricular responses to pulmonary embolism. Prog Cardiovasc Dis 17:175, 1974.

220. Billhardt RA, Rosenbush SW: Cardiogenic and hypovolemic shock. Med Clin North Am 70:853, 1986.

221. Delclos GL, Davila F: Thrombolytic therapy for pulmonary embolism in pregnancy. Am J Obstet Gynecol 155:375, 1986.

222. Bonnar J: Venous thromboembolism and pregnancy. Clin Obstet Gynaecol 8:455, 1981.

223. Hibbard LT: Maternal mortality due to cardiac disease. Clin Obstet Gynecol 18:27, 1975.

224. Szekely P, Turner R, Snaith L: Pregnancy and the changing pattern of rheumatic heart disease. Br Heart J 35:1293, 1973.

225. Harrison KA: Anaemia, malaria and sickle cell disease. Clin Obstet Gynaecol 9:445, 1982.

CHAPTER 140

Burn Injury

Joseph A. Moylan

A burn patient injured by a thermal, electrical, or chemical agent presents the intensivist with a clinical challenge involving multisystem pathophysiologic potential secondary to surface damage plus major metabolic, cardiovascular, and organ dysfunction. Annually, 2 million people incur burn injuries, of whom 20 to 30% require hospitalization.[1] The intensive care unit with its professional staff is involved in the lengthy management of patients with major burn injuries in many areas of the United States. It is not unusual for an individual with full-thickness burn injuries covering 30% of the body surface to require intensive care for up to 60 days. Understanding the pathophysiology of burn injury with its initial evaluations, resuscitation, and systems monitoring of complications is essential for the intensive care physician. A team approach to in-depth care, including the surgeon, intensivist, nurses, physical therapist, occupational therapist, laboratory personnel, and religious leader, has long been a supported concept.[2] The specific role of the intensive care physician should be defined on the basis of the level of expertise and specialty of the surgical physician treating the patient. Various treatment models have been developed and applied successfully through the understanding and close working relationships of these medical groups.

PATHOPHYSIOLOGY

Burn injuries can be divided into three types based on the mechanism of injury: thermal, chemical, and electrical. Each type of injury produces some surface damage. Adverse effects involving other organ systems may be injury specific and are discussed separately.

Thermal Injury

After a thermal accident, the extent and depth of the burn injury depend on the temperature of the heat source and the duration of exposure. It is estimated that exposure for as little as 1 to 2 seconds to a 170°F heat source at the skin surface can produce a full-thickness injury. Factors modifying the depth of the injury include the distance of the heat source from the surface of the skin and insulating effects of clothing and air.

Pathophysiologic changes caused by a thermal accident can be divided into early, intermediate, and late. Early effects of a major burn develop primarily in the cardiovascular and pulmonary systems. There is increased capillary permeability, resulting in loss of fluids and proteins from the intervascular space to the extravascular compartment. This transudation of fluid is caused by cellular disruption and release of vasoactive substances. Edema may occur in both burned and unburned areas. There is a fall in the cardiac output that continues until resuscitation has begun. As effective resuscitation begins, cardiac output returns to normal and even supernormal levels. However, the plasma volume falls behind cardiac output and may not return to normal until 36 to 48 hours after the injury even though adequate blood pressure and cardiac output are maintained through arterial-venous shunting (Fig. 140–1).

Thermal injury also causes destruction of red blood cells. Approximately 8 to 10% of the red blood cell mass may be destroyed, depending on the size of the burn injury. The cell count continues to fall during 24 to 48 hours after the injury because of sequestration of injured cells. There may also be coagulation changes, including depressed platelet and fibrinogen levels, as well as disseminated intravascular coagulation associated with sepsis in the later period.

Burn patients have a higher incidence of infection because of both the skin destruction and altered levels of immunoglobulins.[3] Humoral factors are depressed in the early and intermediate postburn period but return to normal levels.[4] Cellular components of the infectious response, including lymphocyte and neutrophil functions, are also impaired after thermal injury and may remain so for weeks.[5] Alterations in the pulmonary and metabolic systems are discussed in the section on organ systems monitoring.

Chemical Burns

Chemical burns occur at work and at home, where there is a potential for exposure to a wide variety of chemical agents including lye and acid in industry and similar compounds used in home cleaning and agricultural preparations.[6] In addition, sanitizers and disinfectants contain phenols, which are capable of producing significant surface damage. The pathophysiology of tissue damage caused by a chemical agent depends on the strength and concentration of the agent, the quantity of the agent on the skin surface, the duration of exposure, the penetration of the agent into the tissue, and the mechanism of the agent's action.[7] Various mechanisms for chemical burns have been described, including oxidation, corrosion, protein denaturation, desiccation, and surface blistering. Specific agents may have caused not only surface damage but also disruption of the underlying tissues; for example, fluoride and hydrochloric acid can penetrate the soft tissue and cause liquefaction of fat and decalcification of bone. Inhalation of a chemical gas such as ammonia may produce inhalation injury. Hepatotoxic damage has been due to inhalation of similar agents. Treatment is directed at early and vigorous irrigation to dilute and neutralize the toxic substances.

Electrical Burns

Electrical burns occur frequently and may cause either immediate death through cardiopulmonary arrest or cere-

PERCENT

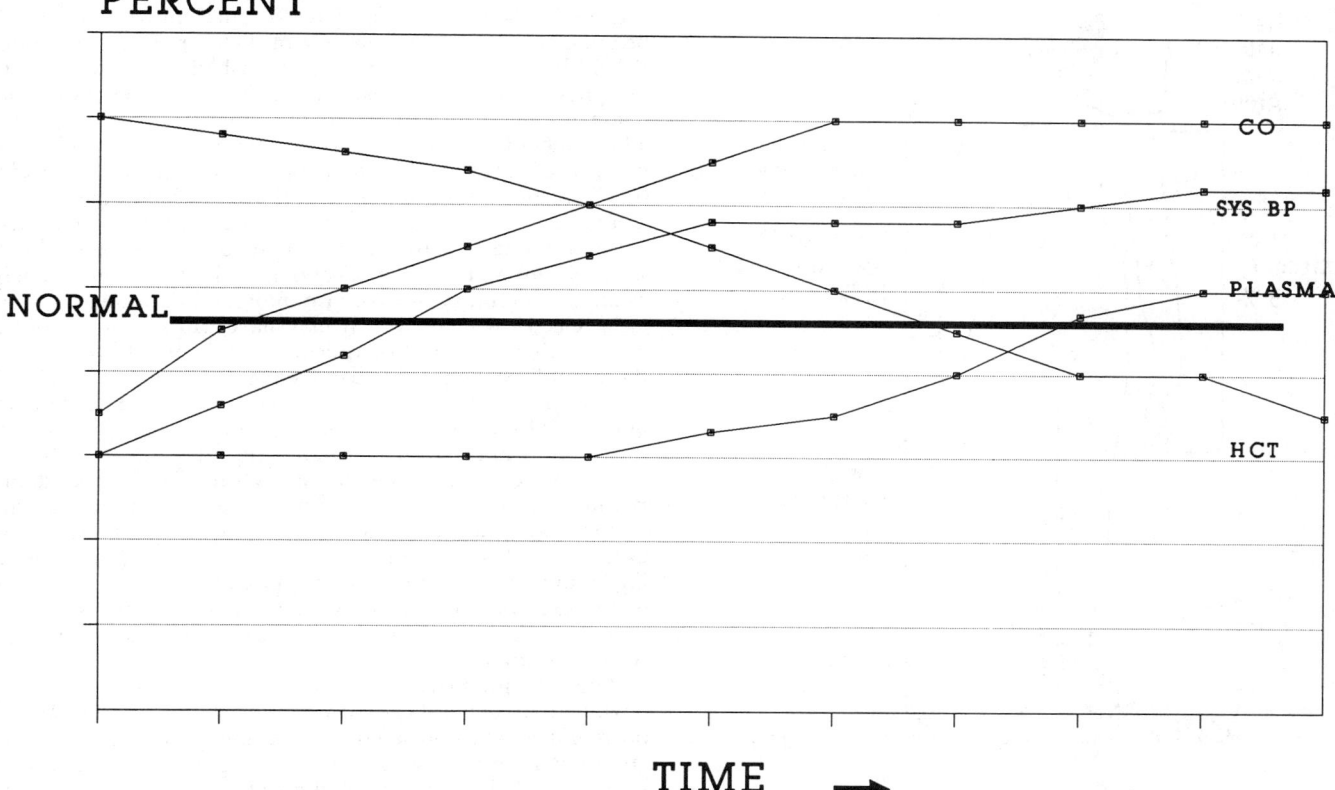

Figure 140–1. Hemodynamic aberrations in thermal injury. CO = cardiac output; SYS BP = systemic blood pressure; PLASMA = plasma volume; HCT = hematocrit.

bral damage or insults involving the circulatory, neurovascular, and skeletal systems. The magnitude of the injury depends on the type of circuit and the voltage at the time of electrical contact.[8] Amperage of 15 mA or more is associated with significant damage. The pathophysiology of an electrical injury is such that the pathway of the current determines the type of injury. Passage of the current through vital organs, such as the heart and brain, may result in immediate death. The damage also depends on the duration of contact and the resistance of the tissue through which the current passes. Resistance is greatest in bone, fat, and tendon; less in skin and muscle; and least in nerve and blood vessels. The current usually travels along the neurovascular bundles but may be transmitted through other more resistant tissues, causing significant damage.

Electrical accidents produce three types of injuries. The actual electrical injury caused by the path of the current to the skin produces characteristic entrance and exit wounds with local disruption. Because the current travels preferentially along blood vessels, there may be extensive intimal damage resulting in progressive thrombosis and spasm of blood vessels with subsequent skin and muscle ischemia. The second type of injury is an arc burn produced by the current temporarily coursing external to the body surface across a joint. This type of injury is commonly seen in high-tension accidents and may involve severe and deep skin damage because electrical arc temperatures frequently exceed 2500°C. The third type of injury is a typical thermal injury caused by ignition of clothing by an electrical spark. Understanding of the three different types of mechanisms of electrical injuries helps resuscitation to proceed in a more organized way.

INITIAL EVALUATION OF THE BURN PATIENT IN THE INTENSIVE CARE UNIT

Although evaluation and treatment have usually been started in the emergency department, it is incumbent on the intensive care physician to undertake a complete assessment of the severely burned patient during the initial phase of burn therapy. The burn patient undergoes rapid physiologic changes and is most unstable. In addition, it is not unusual for subtle injuries and important aspects of the past medical history of the patient to be overlooked at the initial presentation of the patient in the emergency department. Frequently these patients are in shock, in severe pain, minimally responsive, and extremely agitated. With resuscitation, they become physiologically more stable, have relief of their pain and anxiety, and are able to provide a more accurate history. In addition to making a head-to-toe assessment and recording the past and current medical history, the intensivist should document the extent and depth of the injury.

The assessment of the severity of a burn injury is based on the extent of the body surface involved and the depth of the burn injury. Evaluation of the size and depth of the burn is applicable to thermal and chemical injuries; electrical injuries are assessed using a different approach. The size of the burn injury is the most important aspect in determining the outcome as well as the initial resuscitation. The assessment tool most commonly used for estimating the size of the injury is the "rule of nines," as shown in Figure 140–2. By using this approach, portions of the body surface are divided up into multiples of 9%, such that a burn of the upper extremities alone would be an 18% burn. A burn of the torso circumferentially would be a 36% burn. A burn of

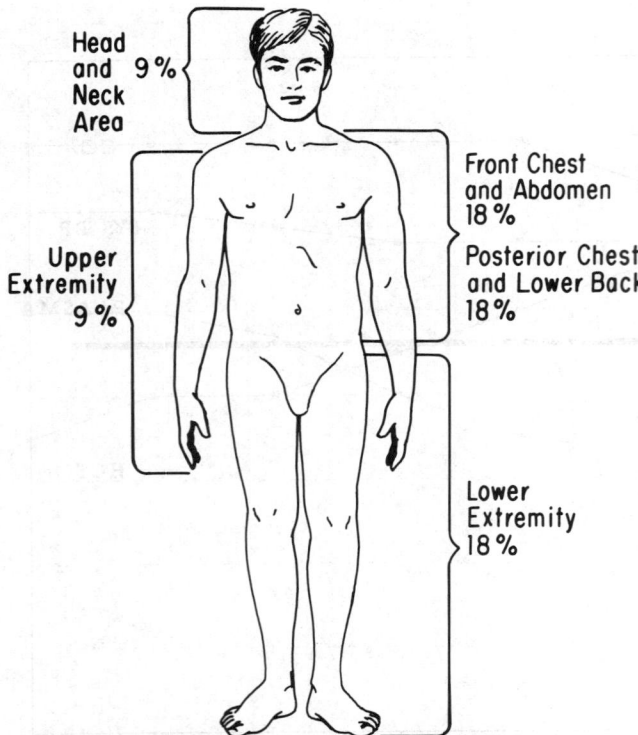

Figure 140–2. Rule of nines for estimating size of an injury.

the upper and lower extremities would be a 54% total body surface burn. For assessment of small and irregular burns, the palmar surface of the hand is approximately 1% of the body surface and can be used to calculate the size of these irregular injuries.

The depth of the burn is categorized as first, second, or third degree or, in more current terminology, partial thickness or full thickness. First- and second-degree burns are partial-thickness injuries; they damage a portion of the dermis but there is residual dermis capable of producing an epithelial covering over the damaged area. Third-degree burns are full-thickness injuries extending totally through the dermis into the subcutaneous space, resulting in a wound that requires skin graft for healing. Characteristics of partial-thickness and full-thickness injuries are shown in Table 140–1.

When the intensivist has calculated and recorded the size, depth, and areas of the burn injury, the patient should be accurately weighed because most of burn resuscitative formulas are based on not only the size of the burn but also the weight of the patient. Special attention is then turned to

TABLE 140–1		
CHARACTERISTICS OF BURN INJURIES		
	Depth of Burn	
Characteristic	**Second Degree**	**Third Degree**
Mechanisms	Liquids, explosion, flames heating skin surface to less than 170°F	Liquids, flame, electricity, chemicals heating skin surface to more than 170°F
Appearance	Swollen, pink to red	Pale, ischemic
Wound surface	Blisters, weeping	Dry
Sensation	Able to perceive pin prick	Unable to perceive pin prick

associated injuries. If fiberoptic bronchoscopy has not been carried out in patients who have thermal injuries, it should be done at this time. Assessment of the extremity circulation should be carefully recorded as described in the section on peripheral circulation. Baseline laboratory studies should be made if not already done in the emergency department. These include hematocrit, white blood cell count, electrolytes, creatinine, blood urea nitrogen, partial thromboplastin time, prothrombin time ratio, and arterial blood gas assays. These tests are usually normal initially after burn injury except in patients with pre-existing medical diseases or those with serious systemic complications of the burn injury, such as inhalation injury or carbon monoxide poisoning.

An electrical burn, which may have caused more severe damage than chemical or thermal burns, may have little in the way of external evidence, frequently only entrance and exit wounds. (Please refer to Chapter 143.) The contact point usually shows some charring and is the smaller of the two surface injuries. In addition, there may be skin burns caused by ignition of the clothes by the electrical accident. Because the incidence of cardiac damage is substantial, an electrocardiogram is a mandatory component of the initial evaluation of all patients with electrical injury, no matter how minimal the accident may appear. Careful examination of the extremity bones is also part of the initial evaluation of an electrical injury because fractures are a sequela of this type of accident.

When the intensivist has completed the assessment of the burn patient, general care orders should be recorded. Major burn injuries are associated with significant pain, and careful attention should be given to the analgesic regimen. Intravenous narcotic should be employed initially because intramuscular drugs are poorly absorbed during the shock phase of the resuscitation. The intensivist should obtain adequate intravenous access, selecting nonburned sites after a major burn. A Foley catheter should be placed in the bladder to monitor urine output. Patients with electrical injuries should have continuous electrocardiographic monitoring because the risk of dysrhythmia is significant.[9]

BURN SHOCK AND FLUID RESUSCITATION

Burn shock and effective resuscitation of the patient present the intensivist with some of the components of the traditional understanding of shock and its treatment. However, the pathophysiologic abnormalities may last beyond the expected time periods. Initially, the patient with major burns has a classic hypovolemic presentation with increased capillary permeability resulting in inadequate plasma volumes and loss of fluids and protein from the intravascular to the extravascular space.[10] The patient demonstrates the complications of the decreased cardiac output, including low blood pressure, inadequate urine output, confusion, hypoxia, poor capillary refill, and peripheral vasoconstriction. The translocation of fluid from the vascular compartment to its extravascular location is secondary to either cell disruption or liberation of vasoactive materials.[11] This edema phenomenon develops in both burned and unburned areas. The loss of vascular volume increases proportionally with the size of the injury; that is, the larger the burn injury, the more profound the loss of plasma volume. The interval of capillary leaking may last up to 36 hours, although reversal of this phenomenon usually begins in major burn injuries as early as 8 to 12 hours after insult.

With resuscitation, the cardiac output usually exceeds normal levels to a hyperdynamic state such as that seen in sepsis. Blood pressure remains normal; however, measurements of the intervascular volume during this period of hyperdynamic outputs remain low. In spite of adequate

TABLE 140-2

ELECTROLYTE SOLUTIONS

Resuscitative Technique	Sodium Concentration (mEq/L)	Solution	Rate of Administration (mL/kg/% burn)	Advantages	Complications
Hypotonic	130–140	Ringer's lactate	4	Safe, effective	Fluid overload, excessive edema
Isotonic	150–160	Ringer's lactate plus one fourth ampule of NaHCO₃ per liter	3	Safe, effective	May underestimate burns less than 25% of total body surface
Hypertonic	225–250	Addition of sodium to base solution to provide 225–250 mEq/L	2–2.5	Limits amount of fluid	Hypernatremia, under-resuscitation, renal failure

tissue perfusion, plasma volumes usually do not return to normal for 48 to 72 hours after injury. The primary mechanism of adequate output appears to be arterial-venous shunting.

The focus of burn shock resuscitation is rapid return of cardiac output, reversal of burn shock, and preservation of organ function, especially renal, gastric, pulmonary, cerebral, and cardiac function. Historically, various formulas have been utilized, including Moore's formula, Brooke's formula, and Evans' formula. Current approaches include electrolyte solutions that are hypotonic, isotonic, or hypertonic in composition (Table 140–2). Use of colloid in the first 24 hours is limited, deviating from the classic approaches of the past. Because of persistent capillary leaking during the initial postburn phase, colloid solutions have limited effectiveness and do not remain in the intravascular space.

Patients with burn injuries involving more than 15% of the total body surface are at risk for the complications of burn shock, including ileus, vomiting, and inadequate tissue perfusion. Oral intake may be ineffective in reversing burn shock because of vomiting; therefore, intravenous access and intravenous resuscitation should be implemented early in the care of these patients.

Modern resuscitation approaches are based on the use of solutions with various concentrations of sodium to improve cardiac output according to the formula cardiac output = $K(\text{Na} + \text{H}_2\text{O})$ (where K = constant).[12] By varying the sodium concentrations and quantities of water in solutions, effective resuscitation can be accomplished; the complications and safety factors of the various formulas are proportional to the ratio of sodium and water. One milliequivalent of sodium has a resuscitative effect equivalent to that of 13 mL of water. The volume of fluid utilized for resuscitation in each approach is determined by the size of the burn injury and the initial weight of the patient. Hypotonic resuscitation involves larger volumes because a more dilute sodium solution is employed, and hypertonic techniques involve smaller volumes with more sodium provided per milliliter.

Hypotonic Resuscitation

The Parkland formula utilizing 4 mL of Ringer's lactate per kilogram per percent burn is the most commonly employed electrolyte resuscitation formula for burn patients.[13] An example of its use is as follows. A patient weighing 60 kg and having a 70% burn would receive 16.8 L in the first 24 hours. Classically, half or 8.4 L is provided in the first 8 hours after burn insult. The remaining 8.4 L is given in the second 16 hours after injury.[14] This is based on experience indicating that capillary leaking in the first phase is more significant. With hypotonic resuscitative approaches, large volumes of resuscitation fluids are employed; therefore, the incidence of tissue swelling including nonburned areas, lung,

and cerebral and intestinal tissue is much higher. There may be a higher incidence of pulmonary edema, prolonged ileus, and cerebral edema after this resuscitative technique. It is not unusual for patients receiving the Parkland formula to gain 20 to 25% of their baseline weight by 48 hours after the burn. However, extensive experience with the formula and a wide margin of safety in terms of preventing renal failure have made its use widespread.[15] It should be remembered that all formulas suggested for burn shock resuscitation provide only estimates of the volumes of solutions that will be required and that there is wide variation in individual responses. Careful monitoring of the initial cardiovascular and pulmonary responses in terms of readjusting the amount of fluid is mandatory.

Isotonic Resuscitation

Electrolyte solutions containing 150 to 160 mEq of sodium per liter have been used in burn shock resuscitation. The addition of one half an ampule of sodium bicarbonate to a liter of Ringer's lactate yields a solution containing 152 mEq of sodium per liter. This approach, which utilizes 3 mEq/kg/% body burn, results in effective burn shock resuscitation.[16] A patient who weighs 60 kg and has a 70% total body surface burn would receive 12.6 L in the initial 24-hour period, with half of that being administered in the first 8 hours. Although the primary factor in isotonic resuscitation is the sodium concentration, the bicarbonate may be beneficial during the initial resuscitation when the patient has a base deficit resulting from metabolic acidosis. Unlike patients given hypotonic resuscitation, who gain between 20 and 25% of their preinjury weight, burn patients receiving isotonic resuscitation usually gain only 10% of their preinjury weight because of the early natriuresis effected by this solution. The mechanism of this is unclear; however, extensive clinical experience demonstrates that the incidence of edema in the lung, gut, and brain is less with this resuscitative approach than with hypotonic solutions. In addition, the incidence of renal failure is low and there is a wide margin of safety as seen with the Parkland formula.

Hypertonic Resuscitation

Electrolyte solutions containing 225 to 250 mEq of sodium per liter have been employed in an effort to limit the total volume of resuscitation fluid and the subsequent complications of tissue edema.[17] In this approach, a hypertonic solution is administered at 2 to 2.5 mL/kg/% body burn, although no definite resuscitative formula has been established.[18] Thus a 60-kg individual with a 70% burn would receive approximately 8.4 to 10.5 L of this solution during the first 24 hours after the burn. As with all resuscitative formulas, careful attention to hemodynamics, urine output, and the individual patient's response is essential during this period. Experience with this approach has shown that effectively resuscitated patients gain between 7 and 9% of their preburn weight by recruiting fluids from the intracellular and extravascular spaces. Because there is a smaller margin of safety in using endogenous fluid for intravascular expansion, careful attention to organ dysfunction is essential. As with isotonic resuscitation, significant natriuresis occurs with this resuscitative technique.

Colloid Solutions

At present, colloids are not routinely employed in the first 24 hours with any of these resuscitative techniques. Current therapy favors the use of colloids after 24 hours, when capillary permeability returns toward normal.[19, 20] With the Parkland formula, plasma or plasmanate is commonly used during the second 24 hours to replace 20 to 60% of the calculated plasma volume based on the size of the burn. In the isotonic and hypertonic techniques, colloids are usually employed during the second 24 hours only if the serum albumin level falls below 2.5 g/100 mL or commonly below 2 g/100 mL.

During the second 24 hours, it is common to decrease the amount of electrolyte-containing fluid regardless of the type of resuscitative technique. As urine output increases to above 75 mL/h, the volume of solution is significantly decreased to allow the patient to diurese and return gradually to his or her preburn weight. After 48 hours, it is common to use salt-free solutions because the patient's total body sodium content is increased.

SYSTEMS MONITORING

Monitoring of the severely burned patient in the intensive care unit is based on anticipation, intervention, diagnosis, and treatment of complications that are specific to the burn injury. This chapter emphasizes this aspect of the management of burn injuries, describing problems specific to major burn injuries rather than complications common to intensive care of severely stressed or injured patients.

The Wound

After the initial burn injury, the wound evolves over the course of the hospitalization. Monitoring of the burn wound begins with assessment of the burn injury in terms of magnitude and depth. As discussed in the section on the initial evaluation in the intensive care setting, careful evaluation of the burn wound is continuous. Daily evaluation of the burn wound is necessary because unexpected changes related to hemodynamics and infectious and mechanical alterations are possible even after the wound is totally healed.[21] It is mandatory that the intensivist look at every aspect of the surface because minimal changes may precede catastrophic systemic complications.

The topical antibacterial agent is usually removed once each day, and this is a convenient time for the intensive care physician to assess the wound. The wound should be inspected for (1) conversion from partial thickness to full thickness, (2) the presence of new hemorrhage after initial stabilization, and (3) increased surface inflammatory reaction as indicated by pus and the odor of the discharge from the wound.

During the early phase of hemodynamic instability, which is the first 24 to 36 hours, lack of perfusion may cause the wound to convert from a partial-thickness injury to a full-thickness injury.[22] This is indicated by changes in cutaneous perfusion resulting in increased pallor, whiteness of the wound, absence of sensation in an area where pain was

initially present after the burn injury, and cold and clammy extremities. Changes such as these in the initial resuscitative phase usually indicate inadequate cardiac output and perfusion of these tissues. Reassessment of the resuscitative program is necessary and, when these changes are coupled with other signs of inadequate perfusion such as low urine output, indicates the need for additional resuscitative fluids.

Development of hemorrhage in burn wound areas that were initially stable is indicative of bacterial invasion from the eschar (previously damaged tissue) into the viable interface beneath it. This characteristic change is one of the early indicators of burn wound sepsis and demands immediate therapy. Both surface cultures and burn wound biopsies should be used to evaluate the penetration of bacteria or fungi into the viable tissue. The treatment of burn wound sepsis is discussed in a later section.

It is normal for the burn eschar to separate from the underlying viable tissue.[23] The rate of separation varies with the type of topical antibacterial agent used. The antibacterial agent is used to control colonization to prevent organism overgrowth and invasion into the underlying viable tissue. Normally, separation begins approximately 10 days after injury and continues for up to 3 weeks. Careful assessment of the wound eschar during this time is necessary to débride any pockets of suppuration to assist in the débridement. Because the eschar in full-thickness injuries is without nerve interaction, this débridement process is accomplished with forceps and scissors at the time of daily wound cleaning. Débriding these suppurative areas allows penetration of the antibacterial agent and prevents overgrowth.[24] Many physicians caring for severely burned patients obtain quantitative wound cultures on a weekly basis to evaluate the types and concentrations of bacterial organisms present. The characteristic color and odor of the suppuration also provide the experienced physician with information about the colonizing organism. Bacteria such as *Pseudomonas* have a characteristic color and odor.

After eschar separation, the exposed underlying granulation tissue requires increased care to prevent desiccation. Biologic dressings in the form of homografts and heterografts are commonly used with major third-degree burn injuries. These dressings require inspection either daily or every other day during the early period after eschar separation. Because suppuration is common under biologic dressings, they are changed frequently based on the presence of colonization underneath. Knowledge of wound care techniques is necessary for the medical intensivist who is participating in the management of a major burn injury with the surgical staff.

Cardiovascular Monitoring

The focus of cardiovascular monitoring is similar to that for any patient in shock, although specific sequelae of burn shock make interpretation more difficult, particularly in the first 24 to 48 hours after injury. Frequently, patients with major burns are managed without invasive monitoring because of the risk of systemic sepsis via invasive instruments. Standard cardiovascular assessments, such as blood pressure, pulse, respiratory rate, and urine output, are made for a large percentage of patients with major burn injuries. Decrease in blood pressure, decrease in urine output, and increase in pulse rate in the first 24 hours are indicators of inadequate fluid resuscitation and the need for increased fluid replacement, as discussed earlier. Excessive urine output without glucosuria indicates overresuscitation and increased risk of tissue edema; a decrease in the resuscitative fluid volume is then required.

Because the usual sites for placement of invasive monitors

may be involved in the burn wound itself, placement of arterial and venous lines may be difficult. As a rule, an unburned site should be selected for placement of these lines. If common sites are involved in the burn injury, more frequent changes of the intravenous line and removal as early as possible are indicated. Although it appears that arterial lines involve only a slightly increased risk of infection in the burn patient compared with the nonburned patient, early removal of arterial catheters is advised after the need for continuous arterial monitoring or blood samples has decreased. In patients with circumferential full-thickness burns of the limb, it is ill advised to use that extremity for an arterial monitoring site. Any proximal or peripheral decrease in flow caused by the presence of an intra-arterial catheter may compromise the survival of that limb.

Although Swan-Ganz catheters have revolutionized monitoring of hemodynamically unstable patients, their use in patients with major burns requires some caution in terms of both interpretation and risk of infection. Capillary leaking and cell permeability occur in both the involved and uninvolved burn areas. They reach their peak in the initial period after the burn injury and slowly improve during a 36- to 48-hour period.[25] During this initial phase, devices such as the Swan-Ganz catheter, which measures intravascular volume in terms of central venous and wedge pressures, may indicate lower than expected levels in the presence of adequate cardiac output and tissue perfusion. It is not unusual for an adequately resuscitated burn patient to have a central venous pressure of zero or less, pulmonary wedge pressures in the low single digits, and cardiac outputs of 8 to 10 L/min, as well as satisfactory urine outputs. The tendency to resuscitate based on the measurement rather than the clinical situation must be resisted because fluid overload in these patients is extremely hazardous. On the other hand, the presence of low central venous and wedge pressures in the presence of low cardiac output is indicative of the need for more fluid resuscitation. As with other kinds of shock monitoring, high filling pressures and a low cardiac output indicate poor cardiac function and the need for pharmacologic support.

As the capillary leak phenomenon improves, the Swan-Ganz catheter becomes an effective monitoring tool as it is for other seriously hemodynamically compromised patients. However, bacteremias are common in burn patients because of the large surface injury and presence of a variety of bacteria, so long-term use of central monitoring is hazardous. The incidence of tricuspid and pulmonary valve vegetation is manyfold higher in burn patients than in other critically ill individuals. Therefore, the Swan-Ganz catheter should be removed as soon as feasible.

Peripheral Circulation

The thermally injured patient with a full-thickness circumferential extremity burn is at risk of peripheral circulatory compromise because of increasing edema under the burn. Full-thickness damage to the skin changes its elasticity, producing a nonyielding tourniquet when the burn wound is circumferential. Careful monitoring of the peripheral circulation for adequate arterial inflow and venous outflow is mandatory during the initial phase of the resuscitation up to 72 hours after injury. As intercellular and interstitial pressures increase under a full-thickness circumferential burn, venous return may initially be compromised and the compartment pressure may exceed the venous pressure. Ultimately, arterial inflow ceases as complete venous congestion and obstruction occur.[26]

It may be inaccurate to monitor peripheral circulation using the usual clinical signs, such as the presence of capillary refill, distal sensation, and joint motion. These are late signs of circulatory inadequacy that occur just before irreversible change. Commonly, the Doppler flowmeter is used to measure extremity circulation by placing the instrument over the palmar arch for the upper extremity and the posterior tibial or dorsal pedal artery for the lower extremity. Presence of arterial flow detected with this tool indicates adequate distal circulation.

Elevation of the burned limb to augment venous return is helpful in preventing edema. Loss of flow shown by the Doppler flowmeter is an indication to decompress the full-thickness circumferential burn using escharotomies. This involves an incision on the medial and lateral aspect of the extremity through the full-thickness or third-degree burn into the subcutaneous space. It is effective in returning circulation to an adequate level.

Electrical injuries present a special problem in monitoring peripheral circulation because electrical current travels preferentially along the intimal surface of blood vessels as well as nerves. This is associated with delayed thrombosis, which may occur 24 hours after the initial injury. The electrical current itself produces disruption of the intimal lining and swelling, which result in progressive ascending thrombosis. When initially seen, patients with major electrical injuries may have palpable peripheral pulses that disappear acutely. Therefore, continuous monitoring of involved extremities is essential. In addition, there may be a progressive increase in compartment pressures resulting in decreased arterial flow because of pressure differentials as the compartment pressure exceeds the arterial inflow pressure. This also occurs progressively during the first 24 hours and is associated with edema development within the compartment. Changes in pulses may occur before ischemic damage to muscles and nerves. Monitoring of compartment pressures by direct measurement should be considered with major electrical burns of the extremities. With progressively rising compartment pressures, fasciotomy is indicated.

Pulmonary Monitoring

Monitoring of the pulmonary system focuses on the mechanical aspects of ventilation, gas exchange, and infectious complications. Initially, the burn victim is at risk of effects of inhalation injury and carbon monoxide poisoning. Inhalation injury produces damage to the airway itself, which results in swelling, potential obstruction, ulceration, and, infrequently, immediate alveolar membrane compromise. With airway surface damage caused by inhalation injury, there is loss of ciliary action and the normal protective barrier of the pulmonary lining. This may lead to increased infectious complications including bronchial pneumonia and tracheal bronchitis, usually developing late in the first postburn week.[27] For additional information on inhalation injury, please refer to Chapter 79. Carbon monoxide poisoning, the other immediate complication, produces binding of hemoglobin, displacement of oxygen, and risk of significant tissue anoxia.[28]

Bronchoscopy is the primary procedure for the initial pulmonary evaluation to determine the presence or absence of an inhalation injury.[29] Edema, particularly involving the true and false vocal cords, may cause airway occlusion, and at some institutions an endotracheal tube is placed prophylactically for 24 to 48 hours. If upper airway edema is minimal, it is safe to monitor the patient closely for laryngeal occlusion utilizing respiratory rate, stridor, and the ability to move adequate tidal volumes as indicators of a patent airway. An increase in respiratory rate or stridor or decrease in tidal volume necessitates the placement of an endotracheal tube. The initial blood gas analysis is used to evaluate the presence of carbon monoxide poisoning as well as hypoxia caused by severe inhalation injury involving the capillary alveolar membrane.

Carboxyhemoglobin, particularly at levels over 20%, necessitates intubation, rapid ventilation, a tidal volume of 15 mL/kg, the use of 5 to 8 cm H_2O of positive end-expiratory pressure, and a fraction of inspired oxygen of 100%.[30] Rapid displacement of the carbon monoxide from hemoglobin by oxygen is mandatory to minimize the complications of carbon monoxide poisoning. The magnitude of the damage is proportional to the level and duration of occurrence of carbon monoxide poisoning. The value of hyperbaric oxygenation when carbon monoxide levels have returned to less than 4% is questionable, although supporters of this technique think that it minimizes the incidence of carbon monoxide rebound as well as the central nervous system demyelination process. Controlled clinical studies are not available to support these theses.

Serial chest x-ray studies are an important component of the pulmonary monitoring. With inhalation injury the initial chest x-ray film may be normal, but when there is significant damage to the tracheal bronchial tree pneumonia may develop within 4 to 5 days after the injury because of colonization of the airway and inability to clear insipid secretions. In addition, the chest x-ray film is used to obtain information about cardiac performance, because there is a risk of pulmonary edema, particularly in elderly patients.

Bacteremia is common in burn patients during their hospitalization, particularly at the time of separation of eschar, and hematogenous pneumonia resulting from seeding of the lung is a common sequela in this type of injury.[31] Close monitoring of the daily chest x-ray film, particularly during febrile episodes, is essential.

Many suggest that serial culturing of the endobronchial secretions, particularly when the diagnosis of inhalation injury has been made, provides accurate data on bacterial colonization of the airway and antibiotic sensitivities that are helpful when pneumonia develops. Use of broad-spectrum antibiotics in the treatment of pneumonia is associated with rapid development of resistant organisms in burn patients. Prophylactic antibiotics have not been helpful in preventing pulmonary infectious complications after inhalation injury.

Central Nervous System Monitoring

Monitoring of the central nervous system is a general aspect of the evaluation of the initial fluid resuscitation. Improvement in mental status in terms of alertness, responsiveness, and appropriateness of behavior is indicative of adequate return of circulatory stability. Sudden decrease in central nervous system function during the first 24 hours is usually due to inadequate fluid resuscitation and necessitates an increase in the volume of resuscitation fluid. However, caution must be used in evaluating children younger than 3 years of age who have head and neck burns because cerebral edema occurs frequently in this group of patients. This occurs 24 to 36 hours after burn injury and resuscitation. Changes in mental status in young burned children necessitate careful assessment of fluid balance because they may be due to cerebral edema and diureses, and hyperventilation may be required to minimize cerebral perfusion. The presence of adequate cardiac output, high filling pressures, and a good urine output indicates cerebral edema in this group of patients.

Central nervous system damage resulting from electrical injury may be due to entry or exit of current through the brain. Damage to the respiratory center may be temporary or permanent; therefore, vigorous respiratory support of the apneic patient is necessary after electrical burn. When

the patient is stabilized, a brain computed tomographic scan may demonstrate irreversible central nervous system damage, particularly when there is hemorrhage in the fourth ventricle after an electrical accident.

Gastrointestinal Monitoring

Early gastrointestinal monitoring focuses on the complications of ileus after a burn injury. Edema in the gastrointestinal tract is a common sequela of burn resuscitation, particularly when hypotonic resuscitation formulas are used. Ileus may persist for 2 to 3 days after injury. Decompression of the gastrointestinal tract using a nasogastric tube should be done to prevent vomiting and aspiration until the presence of bowel sounds and adequate passage of intestinal secretions are observed.

Stress ulceration is a frequent complication in this type of injury. Serial monitoring of the nasogastric aspirate, frequent hematocrit determinations, and stool guaiac testing for evidence of blood loss should be routine components of systems monitoring in burn patients. Stress ulceration prophylaxis, including early feeding and use of an H_2 blocker or sucralfate (Carafate), minimizes the incidence of this complication.

BURN COMPLICATIONS
Inhalation Injury

Inhalation injury, which is a chemical burn of the airway caused by inhaling incomplete products of combustion, is a primary determinant of survival. This complication occurs in approximately 30% of patients with thermal burns and should be distinguished from carbon monoxide poisoning.[32] Inhalation injury is an anatomic injury of the airways and pulmonary parenchyma, whereas carbon monoxide poisoning is an oxygen-binding abnormality caused by displacement of oxygen from hemoglobin by carbon monoxide. These two phenomena may occur simultaneously, but they are unrelated in terms of pathophysiology and therapy. Inhalation injuries can be divided into three anatomic areas: upper airway (damage involving the pharynx and larynx to the level of the vocal cord), major airway (damage involving the tracheobronchial tree), and parenchyma (damage involving the capillary alveolar pulmonary membrane) (Fig. 140–3).[33] Inhalation of the incomplete products of combustion produces chemical damage resulting in mucosal disruption, progressive swelling, plugging of the airway, tracheobronchitis, and pneumonia. The injury progresses during an 18- to 24-hour period.

Even though the patient may be free of any signs and symptoms initially, all patients involved in major thermal accidents should be evaluated for inhalation injury. Clinical signs include head and neck burns, singeing of the nasal vibrissae, coughing with sooty sputum, hoarseness, wheezing, and bronchorrhea. Absence of these clinical signs does not rule out inhalation injury. Currently, two techniques are commonly used to diagnose inhalation injury: fiberoptic bronchoscopy and ^{133}Xe lung scans.

Fiberoptic bronchoscopy affords an opportunity for direct examination of the airway and can be accomplished at the bedside. The patient should be adequately oxygenated before the examination and the nasal mucosa anesthetized with a topical anesthetic. Because upper airway edema is frequently present, early intubation should be anticipated and it is often helpful to place a No. 7 or 8 nasotracheal tube over the bronchoscopy before beginning the examination. Evidence of inhalation injury includes swelling, mucosal disruption, ulceration, and deposition of carbonaceous par-

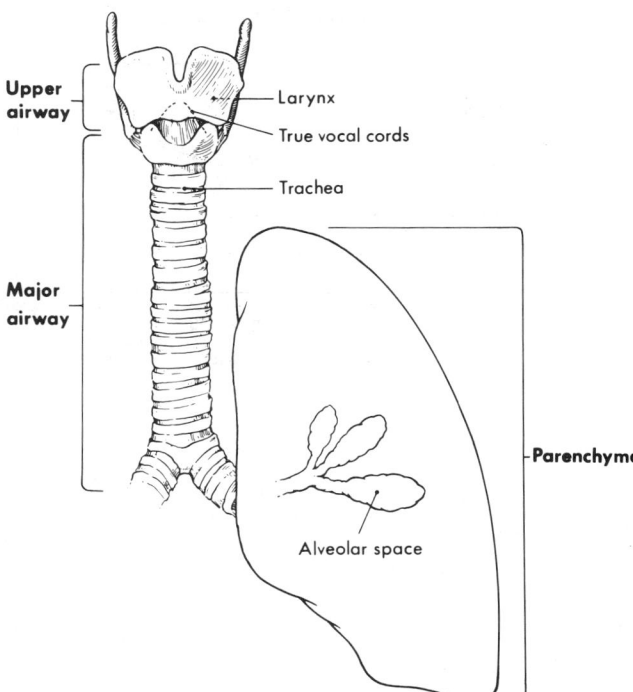

Upper airway — Larynx, True vocal cords
Major airway — Trachea
Parenchyma
Alveolar space

Figure 140–3. Three anatomic areas of inhalation injury.

ticles in the airway. These findings are diagnostic of inhalation injury. The technique is extremely accurate and has few false-positive or false-negative results.

A ^{133}Xe lung scan is also another objective means of diagnosing inhalation injury.[34] This test involves intravenous injection of the insoluble gas ^{133}Xe, which is cleared by ventilation through the lung. After inhalation injury, the isotope is trapped and is not cleared from damaged segments. This test is also highly accurate; however, false-positives and -negatives can occur because of hyperventilation and pre-existing bronchitis. Pulmonary function testing is useful in following the course of the disease itself; however, it has limited applications in early postburn diagnosis.

The treatment of inhalation injury is directed at the severity of the disease process. Patients with inhalation injury should be carefully observed for progressive hypoxia and upper airway occlusion. Both may require insertion of a nasotracheal tube and positive ventilation. For patients with mild inhalation injury, the use of warm, humidified, oxygen-rich air helps to mobilize the inspissated secretions and prevent cast formation. Incentive spirometry is also valuable in clearing these airway plugs. Repeated bronchoscopy may be necessary when the usual techniques of tracheal toilet are unsuccessful in preventing occlusion and atelectasis. Severe inhalation injury produces an adult respiratory distress–like syndrome, and mechanical ventilation with positive end-expiratory pressure is frequently employed when respiratory failure develops.[35] Prophylactic antibiotics have not been helpful and may cause superinfections. Also, systemic steroid treatment for patients with surface burns and inhalation injuries has caused an increased incidence of infections, bacteremia, pneumonia, and septic mortality.[36]

Because patients with inhalation injuries are at a higher risk for pulmonary edema, careful regulation of fluid resuscitation for burn shock is essential. These patients require special attention to minimize positive fluid balance while maintaining adequate renal function. Patients requiring intubation and mechanical ventilation benefit from central venous volume monitoring with a Swan-Ganz catheter.

Pneumonia frequently occurs after this burn complication.[37] Serial chest x-ray studies, as pointed out before, are essential for this group of patients. Frequent culturing of the airway to determine which types of bacteria are colonizing this damaged surface allows appropriate antibiotic choice if an infiltrate develops. The organisms most frequently seen are *Staphylococcus, Pseudomonas,* and gram-negative bacteria.

Burn Wound Sepsis

The goal of burn wound care is a rapid separation of the burn tissue (eschar) and creation of a granulation bed so that skin grafts can be placed where full-thickness injury has occurred or epithelialization of secondary partial-thickness injury can take place as rapidly as possible. Conventional burn wound care includes daily washing and removal of the topical agent. The eschar begins to separate in the second to third week after the burn, necessitating sharp débridement to remove the nonviable tissue.

Topical antibacterial agents, such as mafenide (Sulfamylon) and silver sulfadiazine (Silvadene), are applied to control bacterial growth. The burn wound is rich in protein and moisture because of the fluid and serum transudation and provides an excellent microbiologic culture medium. Topical agents do not sterilize the wound; they are utilized to maintain minimal colonization levels to prevent invasion of viable nonburned tissue by the bacteria.[38] Multiple host factors influence the ability to prevent bacterial invasion, including local circulation, cardiac and renal disease, and systemic immune response. Many microbiologic factors influence the burn wound interphase, including the density of the bacteria, the variety of species, and specific factors such as the ability of bacteria to produce both endo- and exotoxins as well as enzymes such as proteases and elastase. Certain species of bacteria such as *Pseudomonas* are more virulent and are associated with conversion of partial-thickness to full-thickness injuries by invasion of the viable underlying tissue.

Burn wound sepsis is a term used to describe bacterial invasion of otherwise healthy or partially injured tissue. It occurs when wound microbial factors, such as increased colonization, are combined with a depressed immune response.[39] The wound should be inspected for changes in appearance, one of the earliest signs of burn wound sepsis. Conversion of the area of partial-thickness to full-thickness necrosis and the presence of black or dark hemorrhagic discolorations are the most common findings indicative of burn wound sepsis. Others include unusually rapid eschar separation, bleeding into subeschar fat, and marked erythema and edema at the edge of the wound. When these clinical findings occur, burn wound sepsis can be confirmed by analysis of a lens-shaped biopsy including both the eschar and the underlying unburned tissue.[40] One half of the specimen is sent for quantitative cultures and the other half is examined under the microscope, where microbial organisms can be seen to invade the unburned viable tissue. Serial swab quantitative cultures of burn surface may be misleading, although they give some information about the type and relative density of bacteria on the surface wound. Clinical attention to the appearance of the wound and full-thickness biopsy appears to constitute the optimal approach to the early diagnosis of this major complication.

When major burn sepsis develops, vigorous therapy is indicated. Frequently, this involves changing the topical agent being used. Parenteral antibacterial therapy should be instituted immediately, utilizing specific antibiotics effective against the microflora on the burn wound surface. Infusion of antibiotic solution directly into the infected tissue, called subeschar infusion, has been suggested. Agents such as

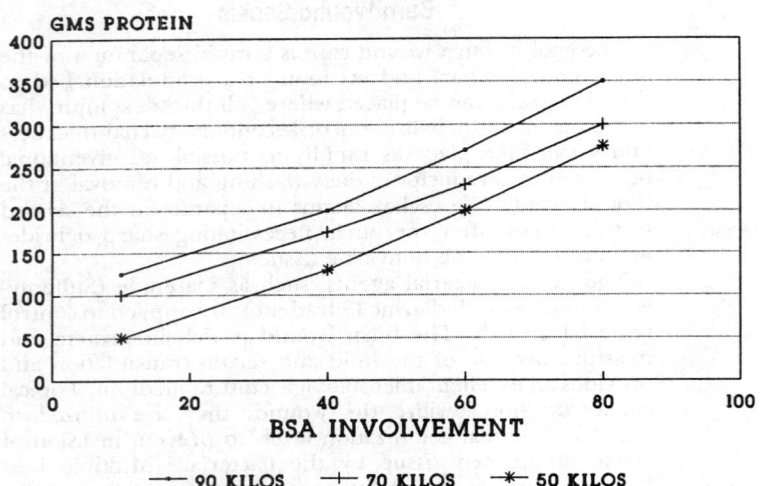

Figure 140–4. Protein and calorie requirements of a patient in the hypermetabolic state. BSA = body surface area.

carbenicillin have been effective when used every 12 hours. Total excision of the area of burn wound sepsis has also been beneficial, particularly when the involved area is relatively localized. Amputation has been necessary to control the process if it extends into the fascia and muscle of an extremity. Adequate preoperative levels of antibacterial agents are essential, and the agents should be continued into the postsurgical period when excision or amputation is employed.

The most commonly used topical agent is Silvadene burn cream.[41] It is a 1% cream of silver sulfadiazine that is bacteriostatic. The agent rapidly penetrates the eschar and covers a broad spectrum of bacteria.[42] Thrombocytopenia may be seen with Silvadene use, although many investigators have not found a cause-and-effect relationship.

Another agent commonly utilized is Sulfamylon cream, which is also a bacteriostatic agent that is water soluble and diffuses readily through the eschar.[43] Its major limitations include wound pain and carbonic anhydrase inhibition; the latter results in bicarbonate excretion with secondary hyperventilation and carbon dioxide retention, a particular problem for patients with inhalation injury. Allergies to both agents have been reported in 3 to 5% of the patients, probably because of the sulfa component of the drugs.

Hypermetabolism

After a major burn injury, there is a significant increase in metabolism, causing an increase in oxygen consumption over the cardiac output, an elevated core temperature, and significant catabolism.[44] Catechol production and excretion, accompanied by low thyroid hormone levels, appear to account for this supermetabolic state early in the course of the injury.[45] Gradually, catechol levels decrease and thyroid hormone levels return toward normal. However, an elevated metabolic state may persist until the burn wound is completely healed. This catabolic state results in major muscle breakdown through the gluconeogenic pathway to produce

energy, and there is significant muscle wasting unless careful attention is paid to nutritional support. Attempts at pharmacologic manipulation of the hypermetabolic state have resulted in a decrease in metabolic rate but also significant complications.[46] Early estimation of protein replacement and caloric needs is essential to prevent major complications related to malnutrition.[47] A convenient formula is presented in Figure 140–4. Because these patients have continuous pain, a sense of chronic illness, and depression, feeding is often difficult by the oral route. Supplements are helpful, but many patients with major burns require feeding through a tube to prevent weight loss. Losses of more than 10% of the preburn weight are associated with many infectious complications and with death.[48] Early feeding also minimizes stress ulceration and bleeding.[49] Every effort should be made to prevent this catastrophe. Intravenous parenteral feeding may be helpful, but the high incidence of catheter-related sepsis limits its use. Addition of antacids in the early phase before feeding can be instituted is also beneficial. No distinct advantage of H_2 antagonists versus an early feeding and antacid program has been found in treating burn patients.

Renal Dysfunction

Acute tubular necrosis associated with hypoperfusion and burn shock is rare with modern resuscitation, although renal failure was previously a common cause of mortality in burn-injured patients. The modern incidence of this problem after thermal injury is less than 1%. However, electrical burns with concurrent muscular damage and myoglobinuria may cause renal failure. Attention to adequate urine flow and pH is critical after electrical injury. When myoglobinuria occurs, urine output should be in excess of 2 mL/kg/h and the urine should be alkalized with sodium bicarbonate to minimize the risk of myoglobin precipitation. The diuresis should be continued for 48 to 72 hours after injury until the myoglobinuria stops.

Neuromuscular Damage

Neuromuscular damage is uncommon with thermal and chemical burns but is usual after an electrical injury. Electrical injuries have both entrance and exit wounds, and the passage of current along the neurovascular pathway may produce extensive underlying damage. Muscular disruption causes myoglobinuria, and damage to the intima of blood vessels produces progressive thrombosis and muscular ischemia. Significant edema in muscle tissue results in high compartment pressures necessitating fasciotomy. Careful monitoring of compartment pressures by both invasive and noninvasive measurements is essential after this injury.

In addition, contact near the brain causes significant cerebral damage, especially to the respiratory center. Damage to the spinal cord occurs frequently and may not be evident initially. Careful neurologic examination for both motor and sensory function may elucidate subtle findings. Spastic paresis with little sensory deficit may be a delayed phenomenon.

Fractures, primarily of the humerus and femur, are caused by tetanic contracture of muscles at the time of the electrical injury. Careful assessment of the extremity with plain x-ray films of the bones may be indicated because of the pathway of the current.

Damage to the muscles by progressive necrosis may require either excision of the muscle groups or amputation of the extremity because of the danger of ischemic gangrene and its systemic complications. Persistence of acidosis and myoglobinuria in the early period after electrical burn should alert the intensivist to underlying muscular damage even though the skin surface may appear viable.

Ocular Injury

Ocular damage occurs in all types of burn injuries. In thermal injuries, ocular damage may be caused initially by the accident itself. Exposure of the conjunctiva to the heat source may produce a surface burn of the eye, although this type of injury is rare because the natural impulse is to close the eyelids at the time of heat exposure. People with carbon monoxide poisoning, however, may have ocular exposure during the comatose period. Examination of the conjunctiva at the time of initial assessment may show the usual signs of surface injury including erythema, swelling, and surface disruption. However, subtle injuries may occur, necessitating examination with fluorescein under the slit lamp. This examination should be carried out as early as possible during the resuscitation period after stabilization.[50]

Late damage to the ocular surface may occur when the cornea is constantly exposed by scar contraction of the lids caused by deep burns in this area. The exposed cornea may dry out and undergo desiccation with development of infection and ulceration. Careful attention with placement of eye drops and other liquefying solutions and early use of tarsorrhaphies minimizes exposure damage.

Cataract development has been noted after electrical injuries. Progressive clouding of the lens occurs as late as 3 to 4 months after the electrical injury. The patient should have a follow-up evaluation, particularly after electrical injuries involving head and neck contact points have occurred.

Chemical burns are frequently associated with ocular damage.[51] Immediate treatment includes copious irrigation with water at the time of the accident and during transport.[52] Physical examination may show tearing, conjunctivitis, blepharospasm, and uncontrolled rubbing of the eyes. Initial ophthalmologic examination using a slit lamp may show corneal swelling, ulceration, and potential clotting of the anterior chamber. Late sequelae of a chemical burn include ulceration and scarring of the cornea. Topical antibiotics should be used early when there is evidence of ocular damage. Failure to control bacterial infection results in perforation of the cornea or sclera. Cycloplegics are frequently helpful if iritis occurs, and the intraocular pressure should be monitored for potential glaucoma after chemical burns of the eye. Early involvement of an ophthalmologist after completion of the initial emergent treatment is mandatory.

References

1. US Department of Health and Human Services: Detailed Diagnoses and Surgical Procedures for Patients from Short-Stay Hospital: United States, 1979. Washington, DC, US Government Printing Office, 1985. Department of Health and Human Services publication (PHS) 1:82.
2. Pruitt BA Jr, Moylan JA: Current management of thermal burns. Adv Surg 6:237, 1972.
3. O'Mahony J, Palder S, Wood J, et al: Depression of cellular immunity after multiple trauma in the absence of sepsis. J Trauma 24:830, 1984.
4. Constantin M: Association of sepsis with an immunosuppressive polypeptide in the serum of burn patients. Ann Surg 188:209, 1978.
5. Wolfe JHN, Wu AVO, O'Connor NE, et al: Anergy, immunosuppressive serum and impaired lymphocyte blastogenesis in burn patients. Arch Surg 117:1266, 1982.
6. Burgess WA: Potential exposures in industry—Their recognition and control. In: Clayton GD, Clayton FE (eds): Patty's Industrial Hygiene and Toxicology, Volume 1. 3rd ed. New York, John Wiley & Sons, p 1149, 1978.
7. Klaassen CD: Absorption, distribution and excretion of toxicants. In: Doull J, Klaassen CD, Amdur MO (eds): Toxicology: The Basic Science of Poisons. 2nd ed. New York, Macmillan, p 35, 1980.
8. Hunt JL, Sato RM, Baxter CR: Acute electric burns. Current diagnostic and therapeutic approaches to management. Arch Surg 115:434, 1980.
9. Schenk WG III, Alexander LG Jr, Moylan JA: Burn care updated: Initial management and prevention of complications. Crit Care Update 5:5, 1978.
10. Demling RH: Burn edema: Pathophysiology and treatment. Surg Rounds 6(7):32, 1983.
11. Harms BA, Bodai B, Demling RH: Microvascular fluid and protein flux in pulmonary and systemic circulations after thermal injury. Microvasc Res 23:77, 1982.
12. Moylan JA, Mason AD, Rogers P, et al: Postburn shock, a critical evaluation of resuscitation. J Trauma 13:354, 1973.
13. Scheuler JJ, Munster AM: The Parkland formula in patients with burns and inhalation injury. J Trauma 22:869, 1982.
14. Baxter CR: Crystalloid resuscitation of burn shock. In: Stone H, Polk HA (eds): Contemporary Burn Management. Boston, Little, Brown, p 7, 1971.
15. Caldwell FT, Bowser BH: Critical evaluation of hypertonic and hypotonic solutions to resuscitate severely burned children. Ann Surg 189:546, 1979.
16. Moylan JA: Resuscitation and early management of the acutely burned child. In: Serafin D, Georgiade N (eds): Pediatric Plastic Surgery. Philadelphia, WB Saunders, p 112, 1984.
17. Moylan JA, Rickler JA, Mason AD: Resuscitation with hypertonic lactate saline in thermal injury. Am J Surg 125:580, 1973.
18. Monato WW, Chunktrasakul C, Ayvazian VH: Hypertonic sodium solutions in the treatment of burn shock. Ann Surg 126:778, 1973.
19. Demling RH: Fluid resuscitation after major burns. JAMA 250:1438, 1983.
20. Goodwin C, Dorethy J, Pruitt B: Randomized trial of efficacy of crystalloid and colloid resuscitation on hemodynamic response and lung water following thermal injury. Ann Surg 197:520, 1983.
21. Pruitt BA Jr: The burn wound. In: Cameron JL (ed): Current Surgical Therapy. Philadelphia, BC Decker, p 513, 1984.
22. Teplitz C: The pathology of burns and the fundamentals of burn wound sepsis. In: Artz CP, Moncrief JA, Pruitt BA (eds): Burns: A Team Approach. Philadelphia, WB Saunders, p 45, 1979.
23. Wolfe R, Roi L, Flora J, et al: Mortality differences and speed of wound closures among specialized burn care facilities. JAMA 250:763, 1983.
24. Georgiade GS, Moylan J: Burns. In: Mayer TA (ed): Emergency Management of Pediatric Trauma. Philadelphia, WB Saunders, p 413, 1985.
25. Tranbaugh RF, Lewis FR, Christensen J, et al: Lung water changes after thermal injury: The effects of crystalloid resuscitation and sepsis. Ann Surg 192:479, 1980.
26. Moylan JA Jr, Inge WW Jr, Pruitt BA Jr: Circulatory changes following circumferential extremity burns evaluated by the ultrasonic flowmeter: An analysis of 60 thermally injured limbs. J Trauma 11:763, 1971.
27. Moylan JA, Alexander LG: Diagnosis and treatment of inhalation injury. World J Surg 2:185, 1978.
28. Zikria BA, Weston GC, Chodoff M, et al: Smoke and carbon monoxide poisoning in fire victims. J Trauma 12:641, 1972.

29. Moylan JA, Birnbaum M, Adib K: Fiberoptic bronchoscopy following thermal injury. Surg Gynecol Obstet 140:541, 1975.
30. Larkin JM, Brahos GJ, Moylan JA: Treatment of carbon monoxide poisoning: Prognostic factors. J Trauma 16:111, 1976.
31. Nishimura N, Hiranuma N: Respiratory changes after major burn injury. Crit Care Med 10:25, 1982.
32. Moylan JA, Chan CK: Inhalation injury—An increasing problem. Ann Surg 188:34, 1978.
33. Moylan JA: Smoke inhalation and burn injury. Surg Clin North Am 60:1533, 1980.
34. Moylan JA, Wilmore DW, Mounton DE, et al: Early diagnosis of inhalation injury using xenon 133 lung scan. Ann Surg 176:477, 1972.
35. Venus B, Matsuda T, Copiozo J: Prophylactic intubation and continuous positive airway pressure in the management of inhalation injury in burn victims. Crit Care Med 9:519, 1981.
36. Moylan JA: Smoke inhalation: Diagnostic techniques and steroids. J Trauma 19:917, 1979.
37. Pruitt BA Jr, Erickson DR, Morris A: Progressive pulmonary insufficiency and other pulmonary complications of thermal injury. J Trauma 15:369, 1975.
38. Ollstein R, Symonds FC, Crikelair GF, et al: Alternate case study of topical sulfamylon and silver sulfadiazine in burns. Plast Reconstr Surg 48:311, 1971.
39. Teplitz C: The pathology of burns and the fundamentals of burn wound sepsis. In: Artz CP, Moncrief JA, Pruitt BA (eds): Burns: A Team Approach. Philadelphia, WB Saunders, p 45, 1979.
40. Pruitt B, Foley F: The use of biopsies in burn patient care. Surgery 73:887, 1973.
41. Curreri PW, Luterman A, Braun DW Jr, et al: Burn injury. Analysis of survival and hospitalization time for 937 patients. Ann Surg 192:472, 1980.
42. Baxter CR: Topical use of 1.0% silver sulfadiazine. In: Polk HC, Stone HH (eds): Contemporary Burn Management. Boston, Little, Brown, p 217, 1971.
43. Moncrief JA: Topical antibacterial therapy of the burn wound. Clin Plast Surg 1:563, 1974.
44. Wilmore DW, Long JM, Mason AD Jr, et al: Catecholamines: Mediator of the hypermetabolic response to thermal injury. Ann Surg 180:653, 1974.
45. Wilmore D, Aulick L, Mason A: Influence of the burn wound on local and systemic responses to injury. Ann Surg 156:444, 1977.
46. Wilmore DW, Moylan JA, Bristow BF, et al: Anabolic effects of human growth hormone and high caloric feedings following thermal injury. Surg Gynecol Obstet 138:875, 1974.
47. Schenk WG III, Moylan JA: Nutritional aspects of burn care. In: Practical Approaches to Burn Management. Deerfield, IL, Flint Laboratories, p 42, 1977.
48. Matsuda T, Kagan RJ, Jonasson O: The importance of burn wound size in determining the optimal calorie:nitrogen ratio. Surgery 94:562, 1983.
49. Dominioni L, Trocki O, Mochizuki H, et al: Prevention of severe postburn hypermetabolism and catabolism by immediate intragastric feeding. J Burn Care Rehab 5:106, 1984.
50. Moylan JA: Considerations in care of the eye. In: Feller I, Grabb WC (eds): Reconstruction and Rehabilitation of the Burned Patient. Ann Arbor, MI, National Institute for Burn Medicine, p 114, 1980.
51. Curreri PW: Chemical burns. In: Artz CP, Moncrief JA, Pruitt BA (eds): Burns: A Team Approach. Philadelphia, WB Saunders, p 363, 1979.
52. Leonard LG, Scheuler JJ: Chemical burns—Effect of prompt first aid. J Trauma 22:420, 1982.

CHAPTER 141

Heat Injuries

Ernest L. Yoder
Michael A. Geheb

Hyperthermia is said to be present at any core body temperature above the normal range.[1] Heat injury syndromes frequently result in body temperatures in excess of 40°C, temperatures frequently associated with protein denaturation and tissue damage. Multiple organ system failure is a regular concomitant of several of these disease states; hence, there is a significant mortality and morbidity. Patients with the heat injury syndromes usually require admission to the intensive care unit. After a discussion of the physiology of temperature homeostasis and the pathogenesis of fever, the important heat injury syndromes are discussed in detail.

PHYSIOLOGY OF THERMAL REGULATION

Humans are homeothermic organisms and thermal homeostasis is maintained through a highly integrated neuroendocrine system. Equilibrium between heat gained and heat lost must be maintained to prevent the organism from becoming either hyperthermic or hypothermic.[1, 2] Lysis of high-energy phosphate bonds during all energy-requiring body functions results in net heat production. Heat loss to the environment is dependent on the existence of a temperature gradient between the body and its milieu. When ambient temperatures are excessive, body temperature may rise. Mechanisms of heat transfer to the environment are radiation, conduction, convection, and evaporation.[1, 2] Radiation, which is responsible for approximately 50 to 70% of the body's heat loss, involves transfer of heat between two bodies not in direct contact. Conduction is exchange of heat between objects in direct contact. Muscle, fat, and skin insulate against this type of heat loss and are effective in air. However, these tissues are relatively ineffective in water, so there is greater heat exchange during immersion. Convection involves exchange of heat with the warmer (or cooler) moving particles of air flowing over the skin. The temperature difference between the two determines the magnitude of heat loss to or gain from the environment. Because evaporation is an energy-requiring process, heat is lost when water is lost from the skin to the surrounding air. Approximately 0.6 kcal is lost per gram of water evaporated.[1] Evaporation is the only mechanism that can result in net heat loss against a temperature gradient; thus, the body can lose heat to a warmer environment.[1]

Information from peripheral (skin and viscera) and central receptors is integrated by the hypothalamus, which effects changes in autonomic tone and endocrinologic function to maintain stable body temperature. In hyperthermic states the hypothalamus causes increased sweat production, cutaneous vasodilation, and decreased muscle tone to increase heat loss through evaporation, conduction, and radiation.[2] Central mediators to which the hypothalamus responds include dopamine and norepinephrine.

Voluntary responses are also important in prevention of hyperthermia and include moving to a cooler environment, removing of clothing, decreasing level of activity, and increasing exposed skin area. Endocrinologic changes are integrated with the neurologic adjustments but are slower to develop and are sustained for longer periods. Hence, the endocrinologic system is more important to long-term acclimatization than to the immediate response to temperature change.[1, 3, 4]

FACTORS PREDISPOSING TO HYPERTHERMIA

Elderly individuals are more susceptible to both hyperthermia and hypothermia. Aging results in impaired ability to detect small changes in body temperature, impaired ability to produce adequate volumes of sweat, and an increased threshold for sweating.

Drugs may also affect the body's temperature regulation mechanisms. The body's ability to dissipate heat is impaired by volume depletion associated with diuretics, impaired cutaneous vasodilation with beta-blockers, impaired hypo-

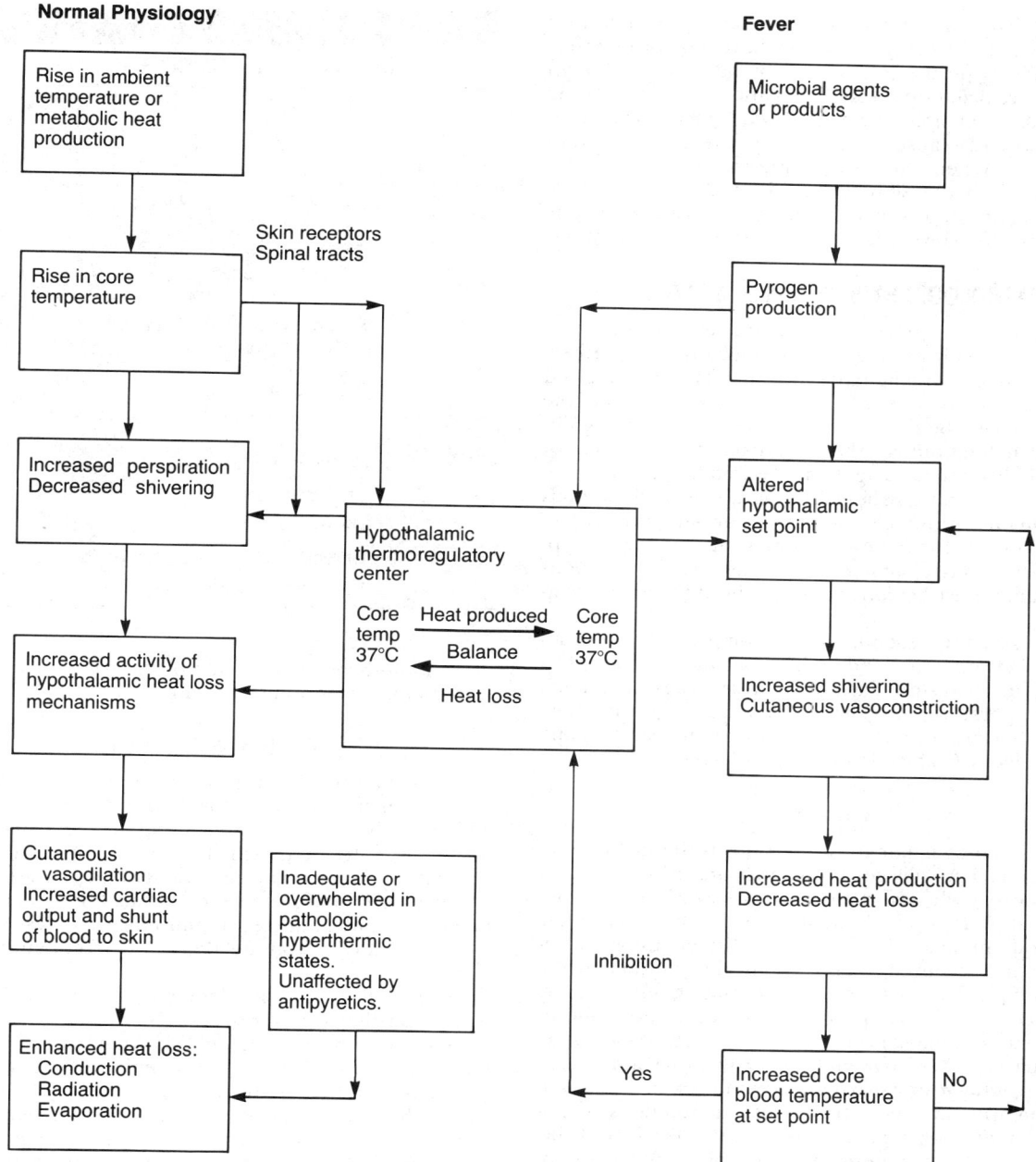

Figure 141–1. Physiologic responses in fever and pathologic hyperthermic states.

thalamic function with major tranquilizers, and impaired sweating with anticholinergic drugs.[3, 5]

Acclimatization results in improved ability of the body to eliminate heat. Adaptive responses include increases in cardiac output (including stroke volume), volume of sweat, and intravascular volume (mediated through increased aldosterone secretion) and decreases in peak heart rate, threshold to sweating, and concentration of sodium in sweat (mediated through increased aldosterone levels). These changes result in increased heat tolerance and ability to dissipate heat.[1, 3, 4, 6] These adaptive changes may be inadequate in the elderly or if heating is sudden. Heat waves in normally cool regions have been associated with significantly greater mortality than even higher temperatures in areas that are normally hot.[7, 8] Acute physiologic responses to heat are illustrated in Figure 141–1. It is clear that sudden heating produces severe cardiovascular stress.

FEVER

Fever is the highly integrated biologic response of the human body to nearly all classes of infective organisms and is considered by most experts to be protective.[9–11] Leukocytic pyrogen, a polypeptide of phagocytic origin, is the primary mediator of fever. Mononuclear phagocytes are the most important source of this inducible protein. After microbial stimulation, leukocytes elaborate the pyrogenic peptide, which causes resetting of the hypothalamic thermoregulatory center. Resetting is thought to be mediated by metabolites of arachidonic acid.[9] Heat production is increased through shivering, and heat loss is mitigated by peripheral vasoconstriction. Figure 141–1 details the physiologic differences between fever and pathologic hyperthermic states. Vascular and muscular responses to the two states are clearly different, as is the mechanism of temperature increase. Whereas antipyretic drugs are effective in reducing temperature during normal febrile responses, they have little or no effect in pathologic hyperthermic states. In addition, although fever may have deleterious effects in patients with borderline cardiovascular function, the pathologic hyperthermic syndromes frequently cause significant dysfunction of various body systems. When the core temperature reaches 42°C, normal cells are irreversibly damaged, resulting in cerebral, cardiac, hepatic, and renal dysfunction. Skeletal muscle necrosis (rhabdomyolysis) is another frequent complication.

PATHOLOGIC HYPERTHERMIC STATES

Heat injury syndromes to be discussed include heat cramps, heat exhaustion, heatstroke, malignant hyperthermia, and neuroleptic malignant syndrome. Heat cramps and heat exhaustion are milder forms of heatstroke, but the other two seem to be distinct syndromes. There are significant commonalities among these syndromes in the areas of mechanism, differential diagnosis, precipitating events, predisposing factors, pathogenesis, complications, and methods of management. Although the clinical presentation is frequently diagnostic for these syndromes, thyroid storm, sepsis, central nervous system infection, and central nervous system tumors must be considered in the differential diagnosis.

In each case, the heat injury syndrome results from an imbalance between the body's heat-producing and heat-dissipating mechanisms. Factors such as drugs, humidity, ambient temperature, muscular exertion, and age have been identified as causing such imbalances or at least making them more likely (Tables 141–1 and 141–2).

Heat Cramps

Painful spasm of major muscle groups is the hallmark of this syndrome. Typically seen in young, unacclimatized athletes or laborers who exert themselves excessively in a hot climate, heat cramps are thought to be related to excessive losses of sodium, chloride, and water. Patients usually complain of nausea, vomiting, and fatigue in addition to the muscle cramps. The onset of symptoms frequently occurs several hours after cessation of exercise. Laboratory abnormalities include hemoconcentration and rarely rhabdomyolysis. Clinically, these patients show signs of volume contraction. Therapy consists of volume expansion and rehydration with oral or intravenous salt solutions. Previously recommended prophylaxis with salt tablets is probably ineffective.[3, 4, 6] Heat cramps are probably a precursor of heat exhaustion and heatstroke, and the best approach is

TABLE 141–1
FACTORS PREDISPOSING TO HEAT INJURY
Patient-related factors
Lack of acclimatization
Dehydration
Exercise when poorly trained
Fever, infection
Obesity
Fatigue, exhaustion
Excessive clothing
Advanced age
Living on higher floors of buildings
Environmental factors
High ambient temperature
High humidity
Lack of wind

TABLE 141–2
MEDICAL CONDITIONS PREDISPOSING TO HEAT INJURY
Alcoholism
Neurologic disorders
Stroke
Dementia
Autonomic dysfunction
Hypothalamic lesions
Cardiovascular diseases
Cardiomyopathy
Class III–IV angina
Skin or sweat gland diseases
Cystic fibrosis
Scleroderma
Ectodermal dysplasia
Extensive burn scars
Miliaria
Diabetes mellitus
Thyrotoxicosis
Hypokalemia
Chronic obstructive pulmonary disease
Psychiatric illness

prevention through education of the patient concerning the early signs related to heat cramps.

Heat Exhaustion

Heat exhaustion is the most common heat injury syndrome seen in athletes and is probably due to severe dehydration and electrolyte loss.[3, 6] In the young, heat exhaustion usually occurs after strenuous activity in a hot, humid environment. Typically, young, novice, unacclimatized runners attempt to increase their performance or distance in a warm environment.[12, 13] Under these circumstances, excessive sweating results in severe volume depletion (frequently in excess of 8 L).

In the elderly, the problem is usually related to an inadequate cardiovascular response to heat with disruption of the normal circulatory changes shown in Figure 141–1. Aged individuals have impaired autonomic responses, which may be further altered by drugs (Table 141–3).[6] Epidemics of heat exhaustion, especially in elderly patients, have been reported during heat waves.[4] Patients frequently complain of cramps, headache, fatigue, nausea, and vomiting. They appear listless and have pallor of the skin and profuse sweating. Other clinical findings include orthostatic hypotension, core temperatures of 37.5 to 39°C, altered mental

TABLE 141–3
DRUGS PREDISPOSING TO HEAT INJURY
Amphetamines
Anticholinergics
Antidepressants
Antihistamines
Antiparkinsonian medications
Barbiturates
Beta-blockers
Butyrophenones
Diuretics
Ethanol
Hallucinogens
Phenothiazines

status, incoordination, and diffuse weakness. They produce scant amounts of concentrated urine, and laboratory values may demonstrate hemoconcentration and hypernatremia.

Therapy includes slow correction of the volume deficit with room temperature saline solution and gradual cooling through exposure of large areas of skin. Significant complications are unusual, but cardiac failure, rhabdomyolysis, and renal failure have been reported.[3, 4, 6]

Heatstroke

Heatstroke is a syndrome attributable to acute thermoregulatory decompensation occurring in a warm environment and is associated with central nervous system depression, hypohidrosis (decreased sweating), core temperatures in excess of or equal to 41°C, and severe physiologic and biochemical abnormalities.[1]

Pathogenesis

Heatstroke is classified as exertional or nonexertional. Exertional heatstroke occurs in people working or exercising in a warm environment who have an overwhelmed but unimpaired central thermoregulatory center. The problem is overproduction of heat coupled with poor dissipation. The normal response to rising temperature is cutaneous vasodilation so that warm central blood is brought to the surface, maximizing heat loss by radiation, conduction, and convection. Increased blood flow to the skin also ensures that metabolic needs are met for enhanced sweat production and evaporation. Even when these mechanisms function normally, heat production may exceed dissipation. Environmental factors that impede heat loss include high ambient temperature, lack of wind, excessive clothing, and high humidity.[1, 3, 6, 14]

Nonexertional heatstroke occurs most frequently in elderly, debilitated, schizophrenic, intoxicated, paraplegic, or quadriplegic patients.[15, 16] These patients have impaired central and/or peripheral thermoregulatory mechanisms. In addition, they have impaired awareness of or inability to leave a hot environment. They also have poor acclimatization with an inadequate ability to increase cardiac output in response to heat. Typically, these patients have a decreased threshold for sweating and a decreased volume of sweat. The hallmark of these groups of patients is autonomic instability. Many of these patients are given medications with anticholinergic effects, which further compromises their thermoregulatory response. As a result, when they are faced with a thermal challenge (e.g., a heat wave), core temperature rises excessively and heatstroke may result (see Tables 141–1 and 141–2).

Clinical Features and Diagnosis

Heatstroke should be considered when the clinical setting is suggestive. Exertional heatstroke is manifested by core temperatures equal to or greater than 41°C, altered mentation, hyperhidrosis (sweating), and elevated serum creatine kinase. Patients with nonexertional heatstroke typically have core temperatures equal to or greater than 41°C, coma or somnolence, anhidrosis (dry skin), and elevated serum creatine kinase. In both exertional and nonexertional heatstroke, care must be taken to rule out primary hypothalamic disease, thyroid storm, severe infection (including meningitis), and encephalitis, all of which must be considered in the differential diagnosis.[1]

Pathophysiology

The mechanism of injury is direct cellular damage, which occurs when the core temperature exceeds 41°C. Enzymes are denatured, mitochondrial function is disturbed, cell membranes are destabilized, and oxygen-dependent metabolic pathways are disrupted.

Skeletal muscle necrosis (rhabdomyolyis) occurs commonly, especially in the exertional form of heatstroke. Cardiac muscle is affected similarly. As temperature increases and cutaneous vasodilation occurs, systemic vascular resistance falls with a reflex increase in cardiac output. Hypotension eventually develops and is exacerbated by dehydration and volume depletion. Tachyarrhythmias, including ventricular tachycardia, are common. Myocyte necrolysis occurs and is associated with subepicardial, subendocardial, and intramuscular hemorrhage. Cardiac failure can result and recovery may be delayed.[17, 18] Because of cell membrane damage (with disruption of Na^+,K^+-ATPase activity), cytotoxic cerebral edema can occur.

Focal parenchymal hemorrhages and petechiae may also develop because of capillary fragility and platelet dysfunction. Rhabdomyolysis may precipitate acute renal failure. This is seen more commonly in the exertional form (35%) and is further potentiated by dehydration, volume depletion, hypotension, and cardiac failure. Urinalysis usually reveals low osmolality, 2 to 3+ proteinuria, and an active sediment containing red blood cells, white blood cells, and granular casts.[1, 3, 4, 6] When rhabdomyolysis occurs, the urine dipstick is markedly positive for hemoglobin out of proportion to the number of red blood cells seen on the microscopic examination, indicating the presence of myoglobin in the urine.

Uncomplicated hyperthermia is typically associated with depletion of total body potassium and hypokalemia. Early in the condition, serum levels of phosphate and calcium are usually normal.

When rhabdomyolysis supervenes, especially when it leads to renal failure, cellular release of potassium frequently results in hyperkalemia. Although hypophosphatemia (caused by intracellular trapping)[18a] can be seen initially in heatstroke, once renal failure occurs, severe hyperphosphatemia can occur (secondary to tissue phosphate release). Hypocalcemia (typically without severe clinical findings) is frequently associated with heat injury when rhabdomyolysis occurs. In this setting, hypocalcemia is secondary to sequestration of calcium in the injured muscle and to the massive phosphate release associated with myonecrosis.[1, 3, 4, 6]

Thus, the classic electrolyte patterns associated with acute renal failure (hyperkalemia, hypocalcemia, hyperphosphatemia, and rising creatinine level) are exaggerated in rhabdomyolysis. Hyperkalemia may be quite severe and hypocalcemia and hyperphosphatemia can be prolonged. Dialysis is usually necessary.

Stress leukocytosis is common, as are anemia and thrombocytopenia. Consumptive coagulopathy may develop 24 to 72 hours into the course, but bleeding occurs early because of thrombocytopathy and impaired hepatic coagulation factor synthesis.

Heat is also directly toxic to megakaryocytes and vascular endothelium, the latter resulting in coagulopathy, microangiopathy, and capillary leak.[1, 3, 4, 6]

Both cardiac and noncardiac pulmonary edemas are common in heatstroke. In addition to cardiac failure, the pulmonary vascular bed is affected directly, leading to the adult respiratory distress syndrome.[1, 18, 19] Respiratory alkalosis occurs early in the course because of increased oxygen demand.

Heat damage and ischemia cause gastrointestinal ulceration, and frank bleeding is common. Hepatic necrosis and cholestasis (which peaks 48 to 72 hours after the insult) are associated with a 5 to 10% mortality rate and contribute to the metabolic and coagulation disorders. Lactic acidosis may be quite severe, and hypoglycemia (caused by continued metabolic demand and glycogen depletion) is common in exertional heatstroke.[20]

Work-up and Laboratory Findings

Baseline studies aimed at identifying complications are indicated in Table 141–4. Arterial blood gas values should be corrected for core temperature because patients are usually more acidotic and less hypoxic than uncorrected values indicate: for each degree above 37°C, PaO_2 should be increased by 4.4% and pH should be decreased by 0.015 unit. In addition, a drug screen and blood cultures should be obtained to rule out drug overdose (see Table 141–3) and infection. If meningitis is suspected, lumbar puncture should be performed immediately.

To monitor for hepatic necrosis, consumption coagulopathy, developing renal failure, and rhabdomyolysis, appropriate laboratory values should be followed serially (see Table 141–4).

Serum potassium, calcium, phosphorus, and glucose levels should be checked frequently until the patient is euthermic and stable. This is particularly true if rhabdomyolysis is present. Frequent blood pH determinations are necessary to titrate bicarbonate therapy.[4, 21] Table 141–5 contains a suggested monitoring protocol.

Management

The primary goal of therapy is rapid cooling. Three initial steps to be undertaken include removal from the hot environment, inhibition of thermogenesis, and active cooling. Table 141–6 shows methods of cooling. In the emergency room, the patient should have continuous core temperature and electrocardiographic monitoring. Active cooling should be continued until the core temperature reaches 39°C. If the patient is shivering, thus inhibiting cooling, chlorpromazine, 25 to 50 mg every 6 hours intramuscularly, may be administered. The clinical condition of the patient dictates the aggressiveness of cooling techniques. Immersion techniques make continuous monitoring difficult but work more rapidly than evaporation methods. Hemodialysis and cardiopulmonary bypass require special equipment, expertise, and trained personnel. After initial steps in the emergency room, patients should be admitted to an intensive care unit at the first opportunity.[1, 6, 21]

A practical approach is to combine several methods of cooling while constantly monitoring core temperature. Maximal exposure of skin surface, wetting with water, and fanning help to reduce core temperature quickly. Axillary and perineal ice packs are safe, as is iced saline lavage. All five of these modalities can be initiated simultaneously, and none of them impedes monitoring of the patient.

Initial therapy should include central venous access with infusion of room temperature saline or colloidal solutions. Bicarbonate should be supplied as an approximately isotonic solution (e.g., two ampules, 100 mEq in 5% dextrose with 0.3 N saline) with frequent pH monitoring. Blood pH should be maintained at 7.30 or above. Phosphates should be replaced if the level is less than 1 mg/dL. If tetany (or other sign of neuromuscular instability) occurs, calcium should be infused and ionized calcium should be monitored.[1, 4, 6, 21]

For hypotension, small doses of isoproterenol may be infused (2 to 20 μg/min). Because they impede heat loss, alpha-agonists should be avoided. Isoproterenol at excessive doses may produce resistant ventricular arrhythmias (including ventricular fibrillation). Supraventricular tachycardia is common with severe hyperthermia, is resistant to therapy, and usually resolves spontaneously as the core temperature returns toward normal. Digoxin should be avoided because hyperkalemia is common in these patients and the risk of heart block is high. If hypotension persists,

---

TABLE 141–5

MONITORING PROTOCOL

1. Protect the airway
2. Insert at least two large-bore intravenous tubes
3. Monitor core temperature
   a. Pulmonary arterial catheter
   b. Rectal probe
   c. Esophageal probe
4. Actively cool the skin
   a. Exposure
   b. Wetting with water (avoid alcohol rubs)
   c. Fanning
   d. Ice baths
   e. Axillary or perineal ice packs
   f. Upper gastrointestinal iced saline lavage
   g. Peritoneal lavage
5. Monitor for seizures
6. Monitor electrocardiogram for dysrhythmias
7. Obtain serial diagnostic studies (see Table 141–4)

TABLE 141–4

DIAGNOSTIC STUDIES FOR ASSESSMENT OF THE HYPERTHERMIC PATIENT

Electrocardiography
Chest x-ray study
Complete blood count
Platelet count
White blood cell count with differential
Serum studies
    Lactate dehydrogenase
    Transaminases
    Alkaline phosphatase
    Bilirubin
    Creatine kinase
    Blood urea nitrogen
    Creatinine
    Phosphate
    Calcium
    Glucose
    Electrolytes
Partial thromboplastin time
Uric acid time
Prothrombin time
Fibrin split products
Fibrinogen
Arterial blood gas assays
Urinalysis

TABLE 141–6

METHODS OF COOLING

1. Place in cool environment, remove clothing
2. Wet skin with cool water, continuously fan air across exposed skin with constant massage
3. Immersion in cold water (22°C)
4. Peritoneal lavage with cool saline (22°C)
5. Gastric or colonic lavage with cool saline (15–20°C)
6. Hemodialysis
7. Cardiopulmonary bypass
8. Axillary or perineal ice packs
9. Infusion of room temperature saline

arterial and pulmonary arterial catheters should be inserted to determine ventricular function, filling pressures, and hemodynamic parameters. Calcium infusion may help support blood pressure if ionized calcium levels are low (<0.8 mmol/L).[1, 4, 6, 15, 17, 18, 21]

Corticosteroids and antibiotics are not a part of routine therapy and should be used only when clearly indicated. Dantrolene has been used to facilitate temperature reduction in heatstroke victims. Although cooling occurred more rapidly in the dantrolene group, the expense of this drug makes routine use prohibitive.[22] All medications should be given with great care because impaired hepatic and renal functions alter drug metabolism. Blood products should be supplied only if active bleeding occurs.

Course and Prognosis

In most cases, mild-to-moderate neurologic, hepatic, and renal dysfunctions resolve after return to normothermia.[1] Muscle weakness may persist for several months when rhabdomyolysis has been severe. The more severe the injury, the greater the likelihood of permanent sequelae.

Mortality rates as high as 70% have been reported.[1, 6] Factors that determine mortality are peak temperature, delay in therapy, and advanced age. Ventricular fibrillation, consumption coagulopathy, prolonged coma, and severe lactic acidosis indicate a poor immediate prognosis. One occurrence of heatstroke may indicate a tendency toward heatstroke in individual patients. Patients so identified should be cautioned to avoid the behavioral and environmental risk factors that may lead to a recurrent event.[23]

Malignant Hyperthermia

Malignant hyperthermia is a hypermetabolic, myopathic syndrome, chemically or stress induced, and is manifested by an abrupt rise in core temperature, vigorous muscle contractions, metabolic and respiratory acidosis, and ventricular arrhythmias. The syndrome occurs in approximately 1 of 15,000 anesthetic events and is thought to be a result of a genetic predisposition.[24] Autosomal dominance with multiple gene loci and alleles and variable penetrance has been postulated.[24–27a] Human leukocyte antigen typing has not been of value in identifying patients at risk,[28] and serum creatine kinase is not an adequate screening test.[29] A high index of suspicion when taking a family history is the best approach to identifying these patients. The most reliable way to diagnose susceptibility in patients at risk is to immerse muscle fibers obtained from muscle biopsy into caffeine-containing solutions. Fibers from malignant hyperthermia–susceptible patients contract, whereas those from normal individuals do not.[30]

Pathogenesis

In susceptible individuals, the sarcoplasmic reticulum appears defective in its ability to take up and sequester calcium. The consequence is an increased cellular concentration of calcium, resulting in sustained contraction. Other theories include enhanced calcium release and a defect in calcium-mediated electromechanical coupling. In the presence of an inciting agent or event, sustained or repetitive muscular contractions occur. ATP hydrolysis increases and remains constant, with heat and lactate production similar to that occurring in sustained exercise. Thermogenesis overwhelms the body's ability to dissipate heat. In response to the muscular activity, catecholamines are released, resulting in increased substrate turnover and further heat production.

TABLE 141–7
DRUGS AND AGENTS THAT TRIGGER MALIGNANT HYPERTHERMIA
Anesthetic agents
Halogenated hydrocarbons: enflurane, halothane, methoxyflurane
Neuromuscular blocking agents
Depolarizing: succinylcholine, decamethonium, gallamine
Nondepolarizing; *d*-tubocurarine, curare
Local anesthetics: carbocaine, lidocaine
Arylcycloalkylamines: ketamine, phencyclidine
Older, flammable anesthetics: diethyl ether, ethylene, ethyl chloride, cyclopropane
Thiopentone
Spinal anesthesia
Caffeine
Sympathomimetic agents
Parasympatholytic agents
Cardiac glycosides
Calcium salts
Other: stress, excitement, infection, lymphoma, muscle injury

Glycogenolysis in liver and skeletal muscle also produces heat.[25, 26]

No evidence for allergic or primary thermoregulatory problems exists.[26] Table 141–7 lists drugs and other precipitating factors for malignant hyperthermia.[30a, 30b]

Clinical Features and Diagnosis

Diagnosis is based primarily on the typical clinical presentation with a closely associated trigger, anesthetic agents being the most common. The full-blown syndrome of rapid temperature rise and vigorous muscle contraction is easily diagnosed but difficult to reverse. Associated signs include muscular rigidity, tachycardia, mottled and cyanotic skin, and hypertension. Soon thereafter, hypotension develops, with falling pH, rising potassium level, peaked T waves on the electrocardiogram, and ventricular arrhythmias. Early signs that occur during anesthesia induction and are suggestive of the diagnosis are an early rise in end-tidal CO_2 and masseteric spasm. End-tidal CO_2 is most reliably measured in intubated patients with fixed minute ventilation and should be measured in all patients at risk.[31, 32] The differential diagnosis includes thyroid storm, pheochromocytoma, and infection.

Work-up and Laboratory Findings

The work-up and laboratory findings are similar to those for heatstroke (see Table 141–4) and should be followed in much the same way in anticipation of the complications of malignant hyperthermia.

Management

Succinylcholine produces masseteric spasm in approximately 1% of patients. Thirty-six percent of patients with malignant hyperthermia develop spasm, and 61% of children who developed masseteric spasm during anesthesia had muscle biopsy findings compatible with malignant hyperthermia.[24, 30, 33, 34] If masseteric spasm or rising end-tidal CO_2 is noted in early anesthesia, most believe that the procedure should be aborted and the operation postponed.[24, 30, 33, 34] Cessation of anesthesia when masseteric spasm occurs is therefore advisable. If the procedure must continue, a temperature probe (esophageal, axillary, or rectal) should be inserted and end-tidal CO_2 monitored continuously. Anesthetic agents selected for continuation should be a combination of nitrous oxide, barbiturates, diazepam, pancuronium, and/or opiates.[24-26]

If thermogenesis begins, treatment should be immediately begun with dantrolene, which disrupts electromechanical coupling and lowers cytoplasmic calcium. The dosage is 100 mg/kg intravenously every 5 to 10 minutes to a maximal dose of 10 mg/kg. After this, dantrolene at 100 mg/kg should be administered intravenously every 6 hours for 24 to 48 hours to prevent relapse.[35] Generally, temperature rapidly declines. The anesthesia apparatus should be changed as soon as possible to remove all drug traces, and routine cooling methods should be instituted (see Table 141–6).

Management also includes anticipation of complications (as described under Heatstroke) should temperatures exceed 42°C. Ventricular fibrillation is common, and prophylaxis with procainamide is recommended. The loading dose is 30 to 50 mg/min to a total dose of 15 to 20 mg/kg, followed by a maintenance infusion of 2 to 6 mg/min. Procainamide stimulates calcium uptake from the cytoplasm to sarcoplasmic reticulum and may actually help decrease thermogenesis. As in the case of heatstroke, digoxin should be avoided because of hyperkalemia, and an isoproterenol infusion may be required to support blood pressure temporarily. Alpha-agonists should be avoided because they impair heat dissipation.[15, 25, 26]

Because seizures are quite common, prophylaxis with phenobarbital has been suggested.[24] Phenytoin (Dilantin) should probably be avoided because of impaired hepatic function. The patient should be carefully observed for gastrointestinal bleeding, which may be massive.[15, 25, 26]

Prognosis and Prevention

With aggressive treatment, the mortality rate for malignant hyperthermia has been reduced to 30%.[24] A careful history of anesthesia including past operations and family history is a must. Muscle biopsy and in vitro testing for at-risk individuals is recommended. If general anesthesia is necessary without preoperative evaluation of a patient at potential risk, the following anesthetics have been recommended as safe: nitrous oxide, barbiturates, diazepam, pancuronium, and opiates.

Neuroleptic Malignant Syndrome

Neuroleptic malignant syndrome (hyperpyretic-rigidity syndrome) is a complex of extrapyramidal muscular rigidity, high core temperature, altered level of consciousness, and elevated creatine kinase levels occurring as an acute or subacute reaction to therapy with neuroleptic medications. This combination of findings must occur in the absence of infections, hyperactivity, heatstroke, thyrotoxicosis, and anesthesia.[36] Neuroleptic malignant syndrome was first described in the United States in 1959 and is thought to occur in 0.2 to 1% of patients receiving such medications.[36-48] Its detailed pathogenesis and therapy are described in Chapter 61. The diagnosis of neuroleptic malignant syndrome must always be considered in any differential diagnosis of heat injury.

References

1. Curley FJ, Irwin RS: Disorders of temperature control. Part I. J Intensive Care Med 1:5, 1986.
2. Cabanac M: Temperature regulation. Annu Rev Physiol 37:415, 1975.
3. Stine RJ: Heat illness. JACEP 8:154, 1979.
4. Anderson RJ, Reed G, Knochel J: Heatstroke. Adv Intern Med 29:115, 1983.
5. Rosenberg J, Pentel P, Pond S, et al: Hyperthermia associated with drug intoxication. Crit Care Med 14:964, 1986.
6. Geis P, Marr JJ: Management of heat injury syndromes. In: Shoemaker WC, Thompson WL (eds): Critical Care: State of the Art, Volume 3. Fullerton, CA, Society of Critical Care Medicine, p K1, 1982.
7. Stevens WK: Heat is more lethal when it is unusual, researchers find. New York Times, p B8, July 31, 1990.
8. Jones TS, Liang AP, Kilbourne EM, et al: Morbidity and mortality associated with the July 1980 heat wave in St. Louis and Kansas City, MO. JAMA 247:3327, 1982.
9. Dinarello CA, Wolff SM: Molecular basis of fever in humans. Am J Med 72:799, 1982.
10. Styrt B, Sugarman B: Antipyresis and fever. Arch Intern Med 150:1589, 1990.
11. Burnheimmm HA, Block LH, Atkins E: Fever: Pathogenesis, pathophysiology and purpose. Ann Intern Med 91:261, 1979.
12. Hanson PG, Zimmerman SW: Exertional heatstroke in novice runners. JAMA 242:154, 1979.
13. Rose RC, Hughes RD, Yarbrough DR, et al: Heat injuries among recreational runners. South Med J 73:1038, 1980.
14. Tucker LE, Stanford J, Graves B, et al: Classical heatstroke: Clinical and laboratory assessment. South Med J 78:20, 1985.
15. Sprung CL: Hemodynamic alterations of heat stroke in the elderly. Chest 75:362, 1979.
16. Kilbourne EM, Choi K, Jones TS, et al: Risk factors for heatstroke. JAMA 247:3332, 1982.
17. Costrini AM, Pitt HA, Gustafson AB, et al: Cardiovascular and metabolic manifestations of heat stroke and severe heat exhaustion. Am J Med 66:296, 1979.
18. Zagher D, Moses A, Weiss AT: Evidence of prolonged myocardial dysfunction in heat stroke. Chest 95:1089, 1989.
18a. Knochel JP, Caskey JH: The mechanism of hypophosphatemia in acute heatstroke. JAMA 238:425, 1977.
19. El-Kassimi FA, Mashhadani SA, Abdullah AK, et al: Adult respiratory distress syndrome and disseminated intravascular coagulation complicating heat stroke. Chest 90:571, 1986.
20. Rubel LE: Hepatic injury associated with heatstroke. Ann Clin Lab Sci 14:130, 1984.
21. Hart GR, Anderson RJ, Crumpler CP, et al: Epidemic classical heat stroke: Clinical characteristics and course of 28 patients. Medicine 61:189, 1982.
22. Channa AB, Seraj MA, Saddique AA, et al: Is dantrolene effective in heatstroke patients? Crit Care Med 18:290, 1990.
23. Shapiro Y, Magazanik A, Udassin R, et al: Heat intolerance in former heatstroke patients. Ann Intern Med 90:913, 1979.
24. Curley FJ, Irwin RS: Disorders of temperature control. Part II. J Intensive Care Med 1:91, 1986.
25. Gronert GA: Malignant hyperthermia. Anesthesiology 53:395, 1980.
26. Aldrete JA: Advances in the diagnosis and treatment of malignant hyperthermia. Acta Anaesthesiol Scand 25:477, 1981.
27. Adams BE, Manoguerra AS, Lilja GP, et al: Heat stroke associated with medications having anticholinergic effects. Minnesota Med 60:103, 1977.
27a. McPherson E, Taylor CA: The genetics of malignant hyperthermia: Evidence for heterogeneity. Am J Med Genet 11:273, 1982.
28. Lutsky I, Witkowski J, Henschel ED: HLA typing in a family prone to malignant hyperthermia. Anesthesiology 56:224, 1982.
29. Paasuke RT, Brownell AKW: Serum creatine kinase as a screening test for susceptibility to malignant hyperthermia. JAMA 255:769, 1986.
30. Rodgers IR: Malignant hyperthermia: A review of the literature. Mt Sinai J Med 50:95, 1983.
30a. Gallant EM, Ahern CP: Malignant hyperthermia: Response of skeletal muscles to general anesthetics. Mayo Clin Proc 58:758, 1983.
30b. Denborough MA: The pathopharmacology of malignant hyperpyrexia. Br J Anaesth 48:357, 1976.
31. Baudendistel I, Goudsouzian N, Cote C, et al: End-tidal CO2 monitoring: Its use in the diagnosis and management of malignant hyperthermia. Anaesthesia 39:1000, 1984.
32. Triner L, Sherman J: Potential value of expiratory carbon dioxide measurement in patients considered to be susceptible to malignant hyperthermia. Anesthesiology 55:482, 1981.
33. Byrd JP: Malignant hyperthermia. South Med J 76:890, 1983.
34. Nelson TE, Flewellen EH: The malignant hyperthermia syndrome. N Engl J Med 309:416, 1983.
35. Kolb ME, Horne ML, Martz R: Dantrolene in human malignant hyperthermia. Anesthesiology 56:254, 1982.
36. Gibb WRG, Lees AJ: The neuroleptic malignant syndrome: A review. Q J Med 56:421, 1985.
37. Guze BH, Baxter LR: Neuroleptic malignant syndrome. N Engl J Med 313:163, 1985.
38. Levenson JL: Neuroleptic malignant syndrome. Am J Psychiatry 142:1137, 1985.
39. Smego RA, Durack DT: The neuroleptic malignant syndrome. Arch Intern Med 142:1183, 1982.
40. Caroff SN: The neuroleptic malignant syndrome. J Clin Psychol 41:79, 1980.
41. Tollefson GD, Garvey MJ: The neuroleptic syndrome and central dopamine metabolites. J Clin Psychopharmacol 4:150, 1984.

42. Morris HH, McCormick WF, Reinarz JA: Neuroleptic malignant syndrome. Arch Neurol 37:462, 1980.
43. Eles GR, Songer JE, DiPette DJ: Neuroleptic malignant syndrome complicated by disseminated intravascular coagulation. Arch Intern Med 144:1296, 1984.
44. Eiser AR, Neff MS, Slifkin RF: Acute myoglobinuria renal failure: A consequence of the neuroleptic malignant syndrome: Review of response to therapy. Arch Intern Med 142:601, 1982.
45. Rosenberg MR, Green M: Neuroleptic malignant syndrome: Review of response to therapy. Arch Intern Med 149:1927, 1989.
46. Granato JE, Stern BJ, Ringel A, et al: Neuroleptic malignant syndrome: Successful treatment with dantrolene and bromocriptine. Ann Neurol 14:89, 1983.
47. Mueller PS, Vester JW, Fermaglich J: Neuroleptic malignant syndrome: Successful treatment with bromocriptine. JAMA 249:386, 1983.
48. May DC, Morris SW, Stewart RM, et al: Neuroleptic malignant syndrome: Response to dantrolene sodium. Ann Intern Med 98:183, 1983.

CHAPTER 142

Cold Exposure Injuries

T. M. Jiva
Ernest L. Yoder
Richard W. Carlson

Humans are homeothermic. Core temperature is therefore maintained at a constant temperature of approximately 37°C plus or minus 1°, despite variations in ambient temperature. Thermoregulatory, physiologic, and behavioral responses come into play when individuals are exposed to changes in ambient temperature. These thermoregulatory defense mechanisms may be deranged by disease states and a variety of drugs. In addition, exposure of healthy subjects to cold environments for excessive lengths of time also results in cold injury.

Cold injuries may be classified as local (e.g., frostbite) or systemic (hypothermia). It is not infrequent for the patient with hypothermia also to sustain local injuries, particularly of the hands, the feet, or the face. Hypothermia is defined as a core body temperature less than 35°C (95°F) and results from prolonged exposure to cold environment, drugs, and underlying pathologic conditions.[1]

Reports of skiers, mountain climbers, and persons engaged in Arctic expeditions, as well as military literature, document many tragic cases of hypothermia. Military personnel are particularly likely to be exposed to extremes of environmental temperature.[2] Accordingly, hypothermia and frostbite have often dictated the outcome of military campaigns in history. From Hannibal's crossing of the Alps and Napoleon's campaign in Russia, winter and cold have been wartime enemies, and many a soldier has succumbed to hypothermia. Dominique Jean Larrey, Napoleon Bonaparte's surgeon, witnessed the effects of hypothermia on his troops, with frostbite that progressed to gangrene, amputation, and loss of life.[3] Immersion foot (or trench foot), leading to gangrene, was a common and devastating experience for infantry soldiers in World War I and World War II.[4]

In civilian life, persons interested in outdoor sports such as skiing, mountaineering, hiking, and hunting are also at risk for cold injuries. Others prone to cold injury include the poor and homeless without adequate clothing and shelter, the elderly, and those intoxicated by alcohol or other drugs. In winter months, hypothermia is commonly encountered in the emergency room. Intentional induction of hypothermia is used routinely in cardiothoracic surgery.

The mortality rate in treated accidental hypothermia ranges from 30% to more than 80%, but may be as low as 6% in young individuals.[5, 6] Although severe underlying disease and old age are poor prognostic factors, the depth and duration of hypothermia are among the most important factors affecting outcome.[1] In 135 cases of urban accidental hypothermia, the overall mortality rate was 12%, but increased to 50% in cases with severe underlying disease. It was also observed that mortality increased 1.8% for each 1° decrement in temperature.[7] The mortality from hypothermia in the United States has been estimated at 17 deaths per million population per year.[8]

This chapter reviews the physiology of thermoregulation, as well as the cause, pathogenesis, pathophysiology, clinical features, diagnosis, and management of hypothermia. Local cold injuries and their management are also examined.

PHYSIOLOGY OF TEMPERATURE HOMEOSTASIS

Body temperature is normally regulated between 35.8 and 37.2°C (96.5 and 99°F). This tight control of body temperature is achieved by the hypothalamic thermostat, which has an extremely high feedback gain for a biologic system.[9]

Physics of Heat Loss

Heat is continually produced in the body as a by-product of metabolism. The body dissipates this heat to the environment by three mechanisms: radiation, conduction, and evaporation.[10] The amount of heat dissipation by any of these mechanisms is proportional to the temperature difference between the body and the environment.[11]

Radiation. All objects that are not at absolute zero temperatures release heat by radiation to their surroundings. This loss is in the form of electromagnetic (infrared) rays. A significant amount of heat is lost by this mechanism. At 4°C, heat loss from an unprotected head may account for one half of the body's total heat production.[11] Heat loss by radiation can account for up to 70% of the heat produced at an ambient temperature of 20°C.[11]

Conduction. Heat loss by conduction occurs by transfer of kinetic energy from molecules with a higher kinetic energy to molecules with lower kinetic energy by direct collision. Therefore, if the skin is warmer than surrounding objects in immediate contact, heat is transferred by conduction to these objects. Under normal conditions, loss of heat by conduction to air represents a sizable proportion of body's heat loss (12%), whereas only 3% of the total heat loss is by conduction to objects.[11] There is a rapid loss of body heat with sharp decline in body temperature during immersion in cold water, because the thermal conductivity of water is 32 times that of air.[11] Heat loss by conduction can be augmented by convection. This implies replacement of air warmed by the skin with cooler air by air currents. Wind chill causes heat to be lost from the body faster than would be the case in still air. The faster the wind, the greater the wind chill is. With a wind velocity of 12 mph, the rate of convective heat loss is five times that in still air.[12]

Evaporation. Evaporation takes place when water molecules with high kinetic energy vaporize into the surrounding air. This high energy is needed to overcome the intermolecular forces of the other water in the skin. Loss of these high–kinetic energy molecules reduces the average kinetic energy of the remaining molecules in the skin. This results

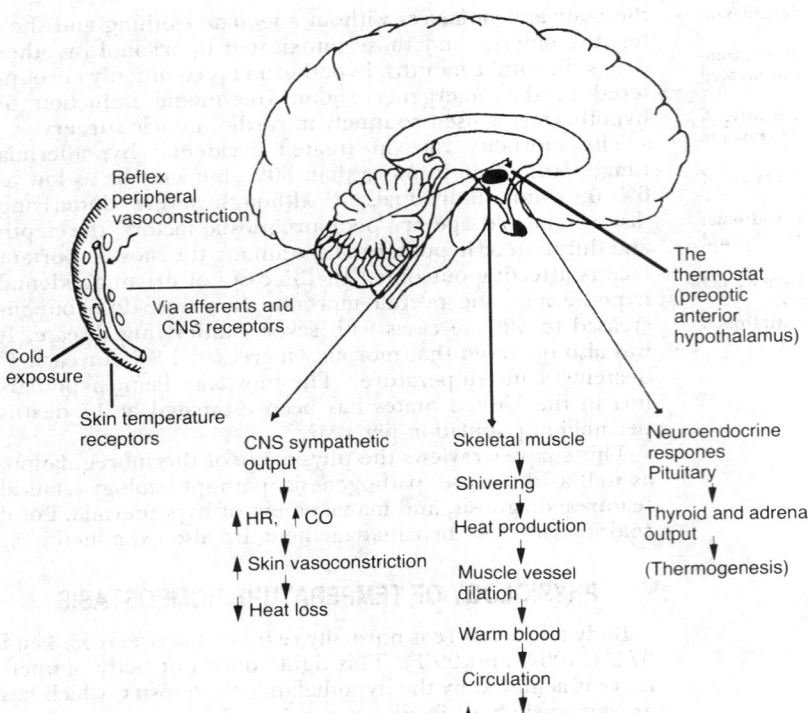

Figure 142–1. Normal physiologic response to cold exposure. CNS = central nervous system; HR = heart rate; CO = cardiac output.

in the loss of 0.6 kcal of heat for each gram of water that evaporates from the skin, the oral cavity, or the respiratory tract.[13]

Mechanism of Temperature Regulation

The temperature of the body is regulated by complex nervous feedback mechanisms. These involve an afferent system, a central processing unit, and an efferent system. The afferent system can be divided into central and peripheral sensors. The principal central sensor is the preoptic anterior hypothalamus.[14] This thermostat is set to a precise reference temperature, usually close to 37°C (98°F)[11] (Fig. 142–1). Changes in the temperature of the blood bathing this area generate corresponding impulses, which are relayed to the central processing unit. The principal peripheral sensors include cold and warm receptors of the skin. Impulses from here are also eventually relayed to the central processing unit. The posterior hypothalamus is the central processing unit of this feedback loop. After information processing occurs here, efferent impulses are relayed to the efferent terminals and various heat conservation and production mechanisms are activated. The efferent system is executed by control of (1) sweating, (2) piloerection, (3) shivering, (4) cutaneous vasomotor tone, (5) hormonal thermogenesis by adrenergic and thyroid hormones, and (6) behavioral responses.

HYPOTHERMIA

Causes and Pathogenesis

"Let there be sought for my lord the king a young virgin: and let her stand before the king, and let her cherish him, and let her lie in by bosom, that my lord the king may get heat" (I Kings 1:1–2). This biblical verse refers to hypothermia of old age and the use of passive rewarming techniques. The causes of hypothermia are either primary (accidental) or secondary. The accidental form is defined as a sponta-

neous decrease of core temperature to less than 35°C, usually in a cold environment, often but not necessarily associated with an acute medical problem, and without a primary disturbance of the temperature-regulating center.[15]

Secondary hypothermia is characterized by dysfunction of hypothalamic thermoregulation. An underlying illness or alcohol consumption may be the predisposing factor. Alcohol ingestion leads to altered consciousness, lack of natural protective behavior, a proclivity to trauma, and cutaneous vasodilation, which enhances heat loss. There is also loss of shivering with alcohol intoxication.[16]

Three clinical forms of hypothermia have been identified: cold exposure, exhaustion hypothermia, and subclinical chronic hypothermia[17] (Table 142–1).

The elderly and very young are prone to hypothermia because of decreased muscle mass, lessened ability to increase basal metabolic rate (thermogenesis), decreased peripheral vasoconstrictive responses, and inability or lack of inclination

---

TABLE 142–1

CLINICAL FORMS OF ACCIDENTAL HYPOTHERMIA

1. *Cold exposure* is hypothermia in a usually healthy individual who is accidentally exposed to a cold environment without adequate protection. Cold water immersion hypothermia is that which develops rapidly as a result of the high heat conductivity of water.
2. *Exhaustion hypothermia* develops because energy stores are depleted and heat production is diminished (e.g., in mountain climbers).
3. *Subclinical chronic hypothermia* occurs in patients with underlying disorders such as infection, malnutrition, endocrine or metabolic disorders, strokes, and one or more precipitating factors, such as mental impairment, administration of sedatives and hypnotics, and an adverse climatic factor.*

*See Tables 142–2 and 142–4 for conditions and risk factors.
Adapted from Lloyd EL: Hypothermia and Cold Stress. London, Croom Helm, 1986.

TABLE 142–2

RISK FACTORS FOR HYPOTHERMIA

Exposure to cold environment, inadequate clothing
Extremes of age (e.g., elderly and infants)
Mental impairment, altered level of consciousness
Immobility
Debility and exhaustion
Wet clothing
Wind chill factor
Acute intoxication or drug overdose
Acute or chronic alcoholism
Chronic metabolic diseases
Trauma and accidents
Malnutrition

to leave or defend against a cold environment.[18] It should be emphasized that the environment need not be bitterly cold for severe hypothermia to develop. Household temperatures of 60 to 65°F during the winter months are well within the range that can result in severe hypothermia. Therefore, an elderly person with altered mental status is prone to have hypothermia in such circumstances.

There are several other risk factors for hypothermia (Table 142–2). A variety of drugs such as alcohol and sedatives affect normal protective mechanisms, leading to impairment of behavior that would lead to voluntary departure from a hostile environment. Other agents suppress hypothalamic mechanisms and sensory afferents and inhibit shivering[19–22] (Table 142–3).

Pathophysiology

Hypothermia affects virtually every body system (Fig. 142–2). There is generalized slowing of enzymatic activity, peripheral vasoconstriction, and uncoupling of oxygen-dependent metabolism, resulting in metabolic acidosis. Furthermore, perfusion of peripheral tissues is compromised owing to decreased blood volume, a fall in cardiac output, and increased blood viscosity.[23]

Cardiovascular Function

Alterations in cardiovascular physiology include an early catecholamine-mediated increase in heart rate, cardiac out-

TABLE 142–3

DRUGS RELATED TO OR CAUSING HYPOTHERMIA

Alcohol
Phenothiazines
Narcotics (e.g., morphine)
Anesthetic agents (e.g., halothane and ether)
Sedatives
Tricyclic antidepressants
Barbiturates
Hypnotics
Lithium
Hypoglycemic agents
Antithyroid medications
Paralytic agents
Prazosin
Reserpine
Glutethimide
Meprobamate
Methaqualone
Heroin
Cannabis
Ethylene glycol
Organophosphates

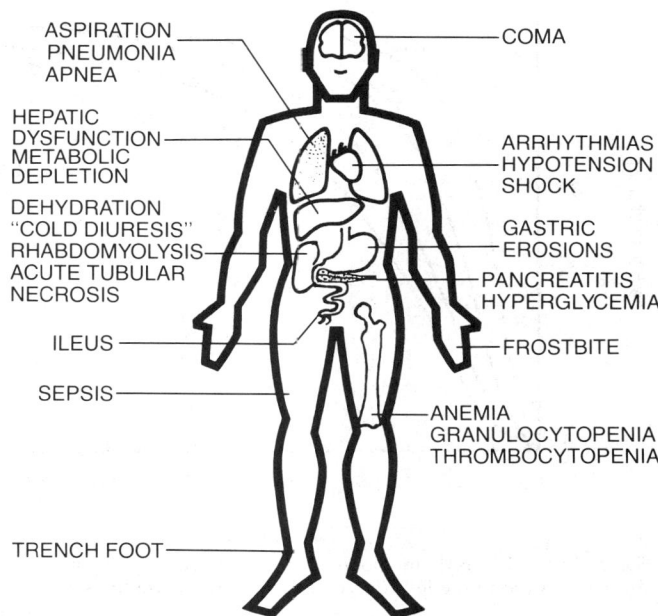

Figure 142–2. Complications of hypothermia and local cold injuries.

put, and mean arterial pressure. Arterial pressure remains elevated, resulting in a reflex decline in heart rate and cardiac output, with subsequent hypotension. The negative inotropic and chronotropic effects of hypothermia and decreased effective blood volume have further deleterious effects on cardiac output.

The electrocardiogram (ECG) may demonstrate sinus bradycardia and slowing of conduction with prolonged PR interval, QRS axis, and QT interval; atrioventricular block; and T wave inversion. P waves may be absent.[24–26] After core temperature reaches 32°C, the classic Osborn, or J wave appears. This acute elevation of ST segment is pathognomonic of hypothermia when associated with decreased body core temperature[27, 28] (Fig. 142–3). However, the J wave is not specific for hypothermia. J waves have also been reported

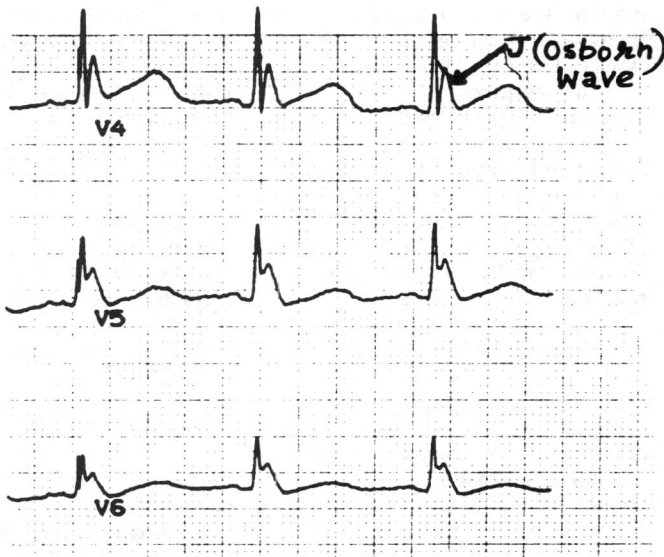

Figure 142–3. Electrocardiographic tracing illustrating the J (Osborn) wave of hypothermia.

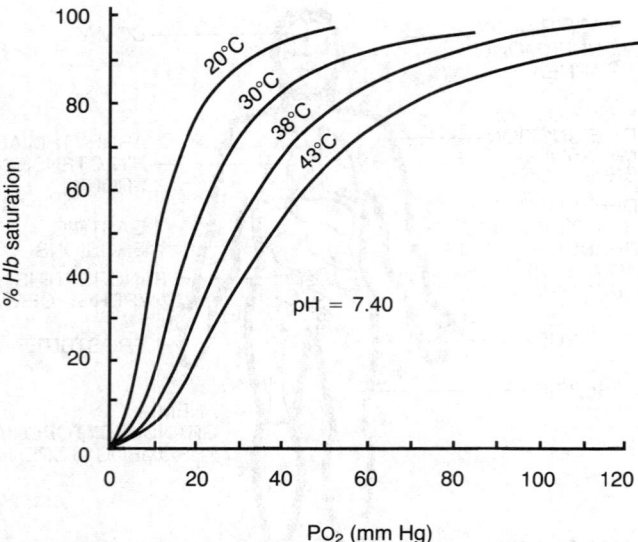

Figure 142–4. The oxyhemoglobin dissociation curve. Hypothermia shifts the curve to the left, decreasing oxygen release to tissues.

in normothermic young patients with massive cerebral injury.[29] Further cooling of core temperature to less than 30°C (86°F) may result in supraventricular tachyarrhythmias, including atrial fibrillation and, eventually, ventricular fibrillation and asystole.

The cold heart is highly irritable and any physical stimulation may lead to ventricular fibrillation. A myocardial temperature gradient of greater than 2°C is associated with increased risk of ventricular fibrillation.[30]

Pulmonary Function

Central stimulation frequently results in tachypnea, but as hypothermia becomes pronounced, there is depression of the respiratory center with a decrease in respiratory rate, tidal volume, and alveolar ventilation. The $Paco_2$ and the physiologic dead space initially increase. These changes, together with shivering, induce an increase in oxygen consumption. Because of a decrease in alveolar ventilation, Pao_2 may decline to subnormal levels. Hypoxemia may also result from aspiration pneumonia, pulmonary edema, or other causes. The ventilatory response to carbon dioxide retention may be blunted.[31] At temperatures below 24°C, there is failure of respiratory drive and apnea may ensue.[32]

Hypothermia causes generalized slowing of enzymatic activity and decreases metabolic rate and oxygen consumption.

Van't Hoff's law indicates that oxygen consumption changes by a factor of 2 for each 10°C change from normal temperature. As body temperature decreases, there is also a marked leftward shift of the oxyhemoglobin dissociation curve, resulting in decreased oxygen release to the tissues (Fig. 142–4) (see Chapter 21). This shift of the oxyhemoglobin dissociation curve may be partially offset by metabolic acidosis resulting from poor tissue perfusion. Other factors are the solubility of oxygen and tissue binding, which are also affected by temperature.[33]

Altered mental status, depressed cough and gag reflexes, bronchorrhea, and impaired mucociliary activity caused by hypothermia predispose the patient to aspiration pneumonia and bronchitis.[15] Edema of bronchiolar and alveolar membranes develops and may be followed by adult respiratory distress syndrome.

Renal Function and Electrolyte Abnormalities

As hypothermia develops, peripheral vasoconstriction is observed initially. This leads to increases in central intravascular volume, renal perfusion, and urine output.[34] However as hypothermia deepens and is prolonged, a cold diuresis continues, despite hypotension, decreased renal blood flow, and glomerular filtration rate. At 30°C, the glomerular filtration rate is approximately 50% of normal.[21, 35, 36] Hypothermia directly depresses renal tubular enzymatic activity, which results in a renal concentration defect and reduced absorption of sodium and water in the proximal and distal tubules and diuresis.[37, 38]

The other mechanisms involved in cold diuresis are direct suppression of vasopressin release and the insensitivity of the nephron to vasopressin.[39] The net result is a maximally dilute urine with low specific gravity and osmolality. Therefore, in the presence of hypothermia, specific gravity and osmolality are insensitive indicators of intravascular volume. If protracted, cold diuresis leads to further volume depletion and a hyperosmolar state. The result is oliguria, azotemia, and an increased risk of acute tubular necrosis.

Electrolyte abnormalities associated with hypothermia include hyperkalemia and hyponatremia attributable to inhibition of cell membrane Na^+,K^+-ATPase. Metabolic acidosis may further increase the serum potassium level. The serum phosphorus level may also rise, which may be associated with hypocalcemia. Impaired excretion of hydrogen ions occurs and is related to the tubular defect discussed earlier. Most authorities do not recommend treatment of the acidemia if pH is greater than 7.2. Patients with hypothermia are particularly susceptible to rhabdomyolysis; the cause is often multifactorial. Immobilization, decreased peripheral perfusion, and local compression may all play roles in the development of rhabdomyolysis. In the setting of a decrease in glomerular filtration rate, myoglobinuria may lead to acute tubular necrosis.[40]

Hepatic and Gastrointestinal Function

Gastrointestinal motility is inhibited by temperatures less than 34°C, resulting in ileus and abdominal distention. Acute dilatation of the stomach, which may be massive, may also occur.

Multiple punctate erosions known as Wischnevsky's ulcers form in the upper gastrointestinal tract.[41] Duodenal ulcerations and perforation have also been described. Although significant gastrointestinal bleeding is rare, autopsy studies frequently reveal gastric submucosal hemorrhages.[42] Pancreatitis of varying severity, from subclinical pancreatitis with high amylase values to hemorrhagic pancreatitis, has commonly been observed.[43]

Hepatic dysfunction also leads to impaired ability to metabolize and conjugate a variety of toxins and drugs. The synthetic ability of the liver is compromised, with a reduction of bile flow. Accordingly, drugs that are primarily detoxified and excreted in bile may rapidly reach toxic plasma levels.[21, 44] The hepatic metabolism of lactate is compromised in severely hypothermic patients and may aggravate metabolic acidosis and hyperlactatemia. Hypothermia leads to depletion of glycogen stores and hypoglycemia.[33]

Endocrine and Metabolic Function

Glucose metabolism is altered in hypothermia.[33] Initially, the cold stress induces increases in levels of growth hormone, glucagon, cortisol, and catecholamines. These changes result in glycogenolysis and hyperglycemia. Hypothermia directly inhibits insulin release from the pancreas. Moreover, the peripheral utilization of glucose is severely reduced at core temperatures below 30°C, despite the presence of circulating insulin.[45, 46] This insulin resistance probably results from the inhibition of the cell membrane glucose carrier system.

Therefore, hyperglycemia persists and is usually associated with mild ketosis. With rewarming and depletion of glycogen stores, life-threatening hypoglycemia may occur.[15]

In the absence of pre-existing hormonal deficiency, plasma thyroxine and cortisol levels are usually normal or increased.[11, 47–49] At low temperatures, the free fractions of cortisol and thyroxine are progressively protein bound. Therefore, less thyroxine is available to stimulate heat production.[50] Although serum thyrotropin (thyroid-stimulating hormone) levels increase as body temperature falls, there is a blunted response to thyrotropin.[35]

In hypothermia, catecholamines are potent mediators of thermogenesis after the shivering phase is over. They increase the rate of lipolysis, leading to high plasma free fatty acid levels.[50, 51]

Hematologic Status

Cold diuresis and loss of plasma to extravascular space lead to volume depletion and hemoconcentration. Changes in hematocrit may therefore provide the clinician with estimates of plasma volume, although splenic contraction may also contribute to the increase in hematocrit. However, in humans, the effects of splenic constriction are usually not pronounced.[52] After rewarming and volume repletion, mild anemia often supervenes. This may result from maturation arrest, which may have been observed in hypothermic patients.[53] As core temperature falls, blood viscosity increases. This finding is usually observed at temperatures less than 27°C.[52, 54] The elevation of hematocrit magnifies the effect of low temperature on blood viscosity. Increased blood viscosity causes stasis of red blood cells in the microcirculation, leading to tissue hypoxia. Microthrombi with embolization may result. Prolongations of bleeding time and thrombocytopenia are caused by intravascular clumping and splenic and hepatic sequestration. These changes are reversible on rewarming.[55, 56] Severe leukopenia with granulocytopenia may occur at temperatures lower than 28°C.[55] The peripheral blood smear and other laboratory studies may demonstrate evidence of microangiopathy and disseminated intravascular coagulation.[57–60] Hemolysis may be caused by cold agglutinins.

Immune System

Infectious complications are frequent with cold injuries, result from abnormalities of host defense mechanisms, and account in part for the increased mortality of hypothermic patients. Atelectasis, aspiration pneumonia, bronchitis, and bacterial invasion of ischemic regions of the skin and intestine are common. In vitro studies have demonstrated impaired bactericidal activity of alveolar macrophages during exposure to cold.[1] Cold induces granulocytopenia, impaired neutrophil chemotaxis, phagocytosis, and bactericidal function.[61, 62] These alterations of immune function may result in ineffective bacterial clearance and persistent lowgrade bacteremia. Delayed clearance of staphylococcal bacteremia has been demonstrated in hypothermic animals.[63, 64]

Neurologic Function

During mild hypothermia, a variety of physiologic and behavioral changes are utilized in an attempt to conserve and regenerate heat. The awake and alert individual seeks shelter from the cold. Shivering occurs during this excitation stage, which is characterized by increased muscle tone, rhythmic contraction of skeletal muscles, and intense heat production.[65] However, as core temperature decreases to less than 33°C (91°F), central nervous system depression occurs with attendant alteration of mental status. This may include apathy, confusion, dysarthria, incoordination, poor judgment, and bizarre behavior. Amnesia occurs at a temperature of approximately 34°C. Consciousness may be maintained to a core temperature as low as 29°C. At a core temperature of 25°C, the patient becomes areflexic and atonic, with dilated and nonreactive pupils and infrequent shallow respirations, which progress to apnea. The electroencephalogram is usually isoelectric at or below core temperatures of 18°C. The severely hypothermic patient appears lifeless; he or she is comatose, cold, and without palpable pulse. However, hypothermic patients with core temperatures as low as 17°C and with prolonged periods of cardiac arrest have been successfully revived with subsequent recovery of intellectual and physical functions.[66–68]

Cold appears to have a protective effect on the brain. As core temperature declines, cerebral metabolic rate decreases, although metabolic pathways are unchanged.[69] In concert with the decrease in metabolic activity, the electroencephalogram exhibits diminished electrical cortical activity during progressive hypothermia.[21] Several factors account for a decrease in cerebral blood flow during hypothermia. These include the fall in cardiac output and systemic arterial pressure, an increase in blood viscosity, and an increase in cerebrovascular resistance. With each 1°C drop of core temperature, cerebral blood flow decreases by 6 to 7%. This can lead to cerebral hypoxia and subsequently altered mental status.[21, 70]

With the decline in brain blood flow, there is a concomitant reduction in cerebral oxygen consumption and cerebrospinal fluid pressure. For each 10°C drop in temperature, the cerebral oxygen consumption decreases by approximately 55%.[69] Thus, the decrease in blood flow and nutrient availability to the brain is compensated by a reduction in brain metabolic rate and oxygen consumption. There is experimental evidence that the intracellular pH of brain remains unchanged in severe hypothermia, even after prolonged periods of anoxia. This compensatory mechanism may account for the resistance of the brain to cold injury.[71, 72]

Clinical Features and Diagnosis

The diagnosis of hypothermia is straightforward for patients with a history of cold exposure or immersion. However, for others, the diagnoses may be less obvious. Subclinical, chronic hypothermia seen in elderly and alcoholic patients is usually precipitated by factors other than cold. This may mask the underlying disease process and make the diagnosis of hypothermia more difficult. Hypothermia should be considered in the differential diagnoses of any hypotensive, comatose patient.[73, 74]

Hypothermia should be also suspected in any patient with pale or cyanotic cold skin, altered mentation, and bradycardia, with or without characteristic ECG changes. Proof of a body core temperature of less than 35°C establishes the diagnosis. In the emergency room it is important to utilize thermometers that record low temperatures. Electronic thermometers with digital readouts or electronic thermistors may be placed and maintained in the lower esophagus, the rectum, or the urinary bladder. These reflect core temperature. Other sites that are less acceptable or prone to complications include the tympanic membrane and nasopharynx. Temperature can also be measured by the thermistor on a pulmonary arterial catheter. However, because of the risk of cardiac arrhythmias, it is hazardous to insert

TABLE 142-4

STATES ASSOCIATED WITH OR CAUSING HYPOTHERMIA

Endocrine and metabolic abnormalities
  Hypoglycemia, hypopituitarism, hypoadrenalism, myxedema, hyperosmolar coma, diabetic ketoacidosis, uremia, hepatic failure
Central nervous system diseases
  Cerebrovascular accident, head trauma, spinal cord transection (e.g., in quadriplegia), syncope, acute confusional states, subdural hematoma, tumors, Alzheimer's disease
Cardiovascular conditions
  Acute myocardial infarction, cardiogenic shock, congestive heart failure, prolonged cardiopulmonary resuscitation
Severe infections
  Pneumonia, sepsis, peritonitis, meningitis
Gastrointestinal and nutritional conditions
  Acute pancreatitis, malnutrition, cirrhosis of liver, gastrointestinal bleeding
Hypothalamic dysfunction and diseases
  Severe thiamine deficiency, Wernicke's encephalopathy, anorexia nervosa, pinealoma, luetic gliosis, sarcoidosis, carbon monoxide poisoning, tumors
Dermal conditions
  Severe burns, erythroderma, psoriasis, ichthyosis
Iatrogenic or therapeutic factors
  Cancer chemotherapy, prolonged surgery or anesthesia, cardiopulmonary bypass
Debilitating illness
  Cachexia caused by metastatic malignancy, Hodgkin's disease, systemic lupus erythematosus, tuberculosis

central venous and pulmonary arterial catheters or pacemakers in the severely hypothermic patient.

History and Physical Examination

A detailed medical history and physical examination are essential to unearth precipitating causes, underlying diseases, end-organ failure, or signs of impending morbidity (Table 142-4).

Important historical items include age, previous neuropsychiatric illness, prior health problems, drug overdose, and ethanol ingestion, as well as the circumstances under which the patient is found and the probable duration of exposure. The physical examination should include a search for signs and symptoms of head trauma, underlying diseases, and frostbite. The cardiovascular, pulmonary, and neurologic systems merit thorough examination. Neurologic and cardiovascular signs depend on the depth of hypothermia. Altered mental status is an important clue to the diagnosis of hypothermia. Profound hypothermia may mimic death.

Classification by Severity

Hypothermia has been classified on the basis of core temperature; these categories have prognostic implications (Table 142-5). The classification of hypothermia into mild, moderate, and severe is useful and has implications for management and prognosis.

During mild hypothermia, the individual is conscious, although there may be slight confusion, incoordination, and a withdrawn behavior. Memory may be impaired. There is uncontrollable shivering, tachypnea, tachycardia, urinary urgency, and polyuria. Shivering may not occur during heavy physical exertion.

Moderate hypothermia is characterized by increasing confusion, fatigue, weakness, apathy, dysarthria, and muscular

incoordination. The patient is usually drowsy or stuporous. Vision and hearing are impaired, and hallucinations may supervene. Amnesia, poor judgment, and inappropriate, combative, and at times bizzare behavior, including paradoxical undressing, occur. Severe bradycardia, hypotension, and shallow and infrequent respirations may result. The fingers and toes are cold and numb with loss of function. The skin is pale, cyanosed, cold, and edematous.

In severe hypothermia with a core temperature less than 27°C, 83% of patients are comatose, with a glassy stare and fixed dilated pupils.[75] There is complete loss of shivering. The facies may resemble that in myxedema.[42, 76] Pulse is absent, blood pressure may be inaudible, and there may be apnea. The patient appears to be in rigor mortis, with areflexia, although plantar responses are upgoing.[77–79] There is a markedly increased risk of cardiac dysrhythmias. At core temperatures less than 25°C, the ECG may be flat. Deep hypothermic coma is indistinguishable from death.[75] However, patients have been reported to survive after prolonged cardiac arrest.[26, 58, 66] Hence, patients should not be pronounced dead until the core temperature has been restored to near 37°C.

Management

The basic goals of management are to maintain cell viability, prevent further heat loss, increase core temperature toward normal, restore the normal internal milieu, and recognize and treat any underlying disease, as well as prevent or treat anticipated complications (Table 142-6).

Management of hypothermic patients therefore involves five areas of priority: (1) initial field care and transport, (2) initial management in the emergency room, (3) laboratory studies, (4) recognition and treatment of any underlying cause of hypothermia, (5) prevention and treatment of anticipated complications, and (6) rewarming.

Initial Field Care and Transportation

If hypothermia is a likely diagnosis, the patient should be moved to any available shelter, wet clothing removed, and insulation from the environment supplied by dry clothing, blankets, sleeping bags, and so on. If the patient is alert and awake with an intact gag reflex, glucose drinks may be helpful, but alcohol should be avoided.

Cardiopulmonary resuscitation (CPR) should be initiated if the person is without vital signs. CPR should be continued until ECG and arterial pressure monitoring are initiated. When facilities are available, intravenous normal saline administration should be started, oxygen supplied, and naloxone and dextrose given. If appropriate, endotracheal intubation should be performed.

Even minor manipulations can induce ventricular fibrillation in a hypothermic patient. Therefore, rough handling of the patient must be avoided and transport should be accomplished as gently as possible with the patient in the supine position.[80–82] Seizure activity has been reported for upright patients, presumably from orthostatic hypotension.[83]

TABLE 142-5

CLASSIFICATION OF HYPOTHERMIA BY SEVERITY

Class	Core Temperature
Normothermia	36–37.5°C (98–99.5°F)
Mild hypothermia	34–36.5°C (93–98°F)
Moderate hypothermia	28–33.5°C (82–92°F)
Severe hypothermia	<27°C (<80°F)

TABLE 142–6

MANAGEMENT OF HYPOTHERMIA

Basic Principles

1. The goal is to rewarm the heart (0.5–1°C/h).
2. Avoid rewarming the extremities before the heart (because of risk of afterdrop).
3. Avoid unnecessary movement of the patient.
4. Avoid irritating the cold heart (<32°C) with central venous pressure and pulmonary arterial catheters and/or pacemakers.
5. Use rectal or other core temperature measurements with low reading instruments.
6. Hypovolemia is common; causes are multifactorial.
7. Drug and toxin metabolism is markedly reduced.

Mild Hypothermia (34–36.5°C)

1. Use gentle passive rewarming techniques.
2. Give warm (40°C) oxygen through a mask or an endotracheal tube.
3. Give warm (40°C), dextrose-containing intravenous fluids.
4. Warm the environment (thermostat, overhead lights).
5. Do not overtreat hyperglycemia.

Moderate (<33.5°C) and Severe (<27°C) Hypothermia

1. Intensive care unit admission indicated; mortality is up to 80%.
2. Gentle rewarming is performed; active rewarming may be considered.
3. Focus active warming processes on the trunk; warm the heart before the periphery.
4. Consider special beds and protect against pressure necrosis.
5. If the patient is not warming at 0.5–1.0°C/h, consider peritoneal dialysis or other techniques.
6. Anticipate multiorgan dysfunction and secondary infection.

Cardiac Arrest in Hypothermic Patients

1. The cold heart (<30°C) may be refractory to interventions.
2. Continue cardiopulmonary resuscitation in all cases of ventricular fibrillation and asystole as patient is warmed.
3. For ventricular fibrillation, follow advanced cardiac life support algorithm. If rhythm is refractory to one course of medication and four attempts at defibrillation, continue cardiopulmonary resuscitation and warm the patient. If the rhythm does not revert spontaneously at a temperature of 30–32°C, use medications and defibrillation per advanced cardiac life support standards.
4. For asystole, one course of medications can be used. If unsuccessful, continue cardiopulmonary resuscitation until the patient is warm and repeat. Avoid pacemakers if temperature <30°C, if possible.
5. Abnormal rhythms associated with perfusion (e.g., sinus bradycardia, atrial fibrillation, and nodal rhythms) should not be treated; a trial of atropine may be considered for severe bradycardia.

Initial Management in Emergency Room

After the patient reaches an emergency facility, advanced treatment modalities should be instituted. Early death from hypothermia is due to shock and dysrhythmias. Therefore, a primary objective is to stabilize the cardiopulmonary status. Initial management should include infusion of large amounts of warmed fluids (38 to 40°C), inhalation of warmed oxygen (38 to 40°C), continuous ECG monitoring, and continuous core temperature monitoring with CPR until a state of normothermia or normal blood pressure and pulse have been obtained.

In mild-to-moderate hypothermia, shock is due to hypovolemia caused by cold diuresis. Slightly hypotonic crystalloid fluid such as lactated Ringer's solution is preferred, because most patients exhibit hemoconcentration and hyperosmolarity. Some authors have suggested that fluids containing lactate should be avoided because of impaired hepatic function. However, this has not been proved to be a practical problem in management. Fluid resuscitation via a central catheter permits monitoring of right-sided heart filling pressure as a guide to fluid management. However, if possible, intracardiac catheters should be avoided before establishing normothermia. Furthermore, because of peripheral vasoconstriction, insertion of a peripheral intravenous catheter may be difficult and delivery of peripherally injected medications may be impaired. Femoral venous access may be therefore considered as an alternative to jugular or subclavian sites in this setting.

Intravenous fluids should be warmed to at least room temperature before infusion. Thermal injury to organs may occur if overheated fluids or inhaled gases are utilized. Because of hypotension and the need for frequent pH determinations, insertion of an arterial catheter should be considered. Urine output should be monitored and kept at or above 0.5 to 1 mL/kg/h.

If fluid resuscitation does not restore hemodynamic stability, pressor agents may be added. Although vasoactive agents may increase the risk of ventricular dysrhythmias, they are commonly employed in hypothermia.[84, 85]

The use of pharmacologic agents in the management of arrhythmias associated with hypothermia is complicated and controversial. If possible, digitalis should be avoided for supraventricular arrhythmias, because the efficacy is unclear and there is a risk of toxicity as the patient is rewarmed. Atrial arrhythmias and heart block generally resolve spontaneously on rewarming.[28, 86, 87] The efficacy of calcium channel blockers is not known in the treatment of supraventricular arrhythmias associated with hypothermia.[1] In the face of ventricular and supraventricular tachyarrhythmias, lidocaine and propranolol are helpful and are commonly employed, whereas some reports suggest that procainamide is not as useful.[85] Bretylium may be the drug of choice in this situation. Bretylium has been demonstrated to decrease the incidence of ventricular fibrillation and increase the likelihood of successful cardioversion in experimental hypothermic dogs.[81, 88–90] Electrical defibrillation is unlikely to succeed until core temperature is greater than 30°C.[30, 91] Pacemakers should not be inserted prophylactically because of the risk of fibrillation; attempts at pacing human hearts during asystole have usually been unsuccessful.[92]

Intubation and mechanical ventilation should be carried out with care in obtunded or comatose patients to ensure adequate ventilation and gas exchange and to minimize the risk of aspiration. Orotracheal intubation may be difficult because of rigidity of muscles of the jaw, and nasotracheal intubation may be required.[84] Admission chest x-ray films should be obtained to rule out adult respiratory distress syndrome or aspiration pneumonia.[42, 93] As manipulation of the patient and airway may induce dysrhythmias, the clinician may elect to utilize local anesthetic spray or gels before intubation or premedication with intravenous lidocaine. If possible, preparation should also include facilities for ECG monitoring and CPR.

When the core temperature is greater than 33°C, passive rewarming is usually adequate and is associated with few complications. More severe hypothermia usually necessitates one or more active means of increasing core temperature (described later). Problems associated with rewarming techniques include afterdrop, worsening metabolic acidosis, severe hyperkalemia, hypotension, and cardiovascular collapse. Afterdrop is a fall in temperature as rewarming is begun and movement or muscular activity increases. As peripheral dilation of blood vessels occurs and cardiac output increases, cold peripheral blood moves centrally, causing core temperature to fall.

TABLE 142–7
EFFECT OF HYPOTHERMIA ON BLOOD GAS CORRECTIONS AND DIRECTIONAL CHANGES

Variable	Change per 1° from 37°C
pH	0.015
Pco_2 (mm Hg)	4.4%
Po_2 (mm Hg)	7.2%

Patients with significant cold injury, and particularly those with moderate or severe hypothermia, should be admitted to an intensive care unit.

Laboratory Studies

A battery of baseline studies should be obtained, including ECG, chest x-ray films, complete blood count with differential leukocyte count, platelet count, prothrombin and partial thromboplastin times, and determination of serum electrolytes, blood urea nitrogen, creatine, arterial blood gases, lactate, glucose, amylase, creatine kinase, lactate dehydrogenase, alkaline phosphatase, transaminase (aminotransferase), fibrinogen, and fibrin split products. Levels of serum cortisol, triiodothyronine, thyroxine, and thyrotropin may be measured to rule out myxedema and adrenal insufficiency. The blood ethanol level should be quantitated to identify alcohol ingestion and to assess for osmolar disturbances. It may be appropriate to perform serum and urine toxicology analyses. Blood cultures should be obtained for all serious cold injuries. The physician should consider serial monitoring of variables such as hematocrit, white blood cell and platelet counts, glucose and amylase levels, serum electrolyte levels, renal function, and arterial blood gas concentrations. If the patient's temperature is provided, most laboratories correct measured values to the patient's temperature. For each 1°C decline in body temperature, $Paco_2$ declines by 7.2%, and pH increases by 0.015 units[94, 95] (Table 142–7).

Computed tomography of the head should be performed for any patient who fails to improve neurologically with normalization of temperature or if seizure or focal neurologic deficits are observed. Closed head trauma or cerebral edema must be strongly considered in such instances. Although cervical muscle rigidity may mimic meningitis, lumbar puncture should be considered if there is clinical suspicion of infection.

Recognition and Treatment of Underlying Cause

The successful management of hypothermia depends on establishment of the diagnosis and a thorough consideration of underlying disorders. A comprehensive diagnostic evaluation is therefore warranted.

Hypoglycemia should be treated with 25 to 50 g of glucose given intravenously in a 50% dextrose solution. Naloxone should be administered to a comatose patient. Thiamine should be administered with glucose to prevent Wernicke's syndrome. If myxedema is suspected in a hypothermic comatose patient, thyroxine, 100 mg intravenously followed by 50 mg every 24 hours, is administered. The patient is then maintained with 0.05 to 0.1 mg of thyroxine intravenously daily until clinically stable.[96]

Moderate hyperglycemia should not be treated in the hypothermic patient. If possible, administration of insulin should be delayed until the patient's temperature is 30°C; below this level, there is marked insulin resistance.[7] If large doses of insulin are given to the hypothermic patient, severe hypoglycemia may result as temperature is raised.

Debilitating disease such as congestive heart failure and hepatic or renal failure should be treated in the conventional manner. Infection or underlying sepsis should be treated aggressively with appropriate antibiotic coverage. However, the routine use of prophylactic antibiotics in hypothermic patients should be avoided if possible.

Prevention and Treatment of Complications

Morbidity and mortality of hypothermia can be significantly reduced by prevention and early treatment of complications.

Infectious complications occur commonly and account for substantial morbidity and mortality in these patients. Appropriate positioning of the patient and suctioning and protection of the airway by intubation may prevent aspiration. Vigorous pulmonary toilet and periodic hyperinflation have been shown to decrease the incidence of pneumonia.[97] The efficacy of prophylactic antibiotics for pulmonary complications has not been demonstrated.

Invasive vascular procedures should be undertaken with great caution because of the risk of bleeding attributable to hypothermia-induced thrombocytopenia, prolonged bleeding time, and disseminated intravascular coagulation.

Electrolyte levels must be carefully monitored at frequent intervals as hyperkalemia and hypophosphatemia are commonly encountered during treatment.[98] Hypermagnesemia has been shown to lower temperatures in hypothermic patients with renal failure and should be avoided.[99]

Elderly patients who have had one episode of hypothermia may relapse. Therefore, they should be monitored closely for recurrent episodes. They are also at greater risk for future episodes of hypothermia.[100]

Rewarming

The choice of rewarming techniques should include consideration of available equipment and resources, experience, expertise, clinical course, and the gravity of the situation. Three categories of rewarming techniques have been defined: passive external rewarming, active external rewarming, and active central rewarming (Table 142–8). These techniques vary in invasiveness and in the speed with which they warm the patient.

Passive Rewarming. Passive measures to rewarm may be initiated at the scene and continued during transfer to an acute care setting. Wet garments should be removed from the patient. The patient should be placed in dry, layered garments, such as a sleeping bag. A normothermic volunteer may huddle with the patient. These techniques are the least invasive and the slowest, with an average rate of temperature rise of 0.38°C/h.[101] Passive techniques are associated with minimal complications. Passive measures are appropriate for patients with core temperatures above 30°C and stable hemodynamic status, as the patient is rewarmed by his or her endogenous heat production.

Active External Rewarming. Active rewarming involves raising the core temperature by heating the skin with heating blankets, hot water bottles, warm water immersion, and so on. This technique is controversial and is associated with higher morbidity and mortality than with other modalities.[102] The peripheral vasodilation results in the afterdrop effect (see earlier). Furthermore, the hyperkalemic and acidotic blood from underperfused peripheral areas returns centrally and may precipitate ventricular arrhythmias and cardiac arrest.[67] Heating blankets and other warm objects in contact with the patient may produce serious burns. The water

TABLE 142–8

REWARMING METHODS IN HYPOTHERMIA

Passive Rewarming
1. Removal from environmental exposure
2. Removal of wet clothing
3. Insulating material (e.g., blankets, sleeping bag)

Active External Rewarming
1. Heating blankets
2. Electric heating pads
3. Hot water bottles
4. Warming lights
5. Warm water bath or immersion
6. Normothermic rescuer

Active Core or Central Rewarming
1. Inhalation rewarming with heated humidified oxygen
2. Lavage via intragastric or esophageal balloons
3. Colonic irrigation
4. Warm peritoneal lavage
5. Urinary bladder lavage
6. Warm intravenous fluids
7. Hemodialysis
8. Cardiopulmonary bypass pump
9. Extracorporeal blood rewarming
10. Thoracotomy with warm mediastinal lavage
11. Arteriovenous shunt warmers
12. Experimental therapy with microwave or ultrasonic diathermy

Adapted, with permission, from Reuler JB, Hypothermia: Pathophysiology, clinical settings, and management. Ann Intern Med 1978; 89:519–527.

immersion technique is difficult, inconvenient, and inappropriate for patients who require cardiac monitoring. In view of these risks, external rewarming techniques should be avoided if possible.

Active Core Rewarming. Inhalation rewarming with heated, humidified gases (40 to 45°C [104 to 174°F]) via face mask or endotracheal tube is a safe and effective technique. The increase in temperature is usually less than 1°C/h. Poor temperature control of the inspired air may lead to mucosal burns.

Peritoneal lavage with warm saline or dialysate raises temperature at rates of up to 4 to 6°C/h. It may be the best method of rewarming for patients with temperatures below 33°C but with stable hemodynamic status. This method may be advantageous in the management of intoxicated, hypothermic patients, as the lavage removes toxins as well as raises core temperature.

Cardiopulmonary bypass pump oxygenators offer the advantage of extremely rapid rewarming rates between 3 and 10°C/h, as well as hemodynamic support for patients with cardiovascular collapse.[103, 104] However, cardiopulmonary bypass necessitates specialized equipment and personnel and is associated with significant risks. Cardiopulmonary bypass should be considered only in the management of severe hypothermic injuries. Systemic anticoagulation is required for cardiopulmonary bypass, which may limit its use in patients who are bleeding or have coagulation defects.

LOCAL COLD INJURIES

Accidental hypothermia may be accompanied by frostbite that involves the ears, the nose, the scrotum, the penis, or the extremities. At the time of hospital admission, the diagnosis of frostbite and the assessment of the extent of tissue damage may be difficult. An understanding of the pathophysiologic mechanisms is essential for appropriate management of local cold injuries.

Frostbite

Frostbite is defined as a freezing type of local injury that involves skin and subcutaneous tissue. Frostbite results from direct cellular injury and ice crystal formation. There is also a delayed indirect damage to the microcirculation.

Clinical Features. A tingling sensation or pain is experienced initially in the exposed body parts, followed by numbness and loss of sensation. The frozen tissue appears gray, white, or waxy. On rewarming, the skin may become edematous with blisters or hemorrhagic vesicles (Fig. 142–5). On the basis of the extent of tissue damage and the duration of injury, frostbite is classified into four degrees of severity (Table 142–9).

Pathophysiology. The mechanism of tissue injury is ice crystal formation and microvascular damage. In frostbite, direct cellular injury results from freezing of extracellular water with formation of ice crystals. Interstitial solutes become concentrated, raising the osmotic pressure. This results in intracellular dehydration and hypertonicity, as water moves from the intracellular compartment to the extracellular space. The cell membrane is damaged and cell rupture occurs. Toxic intracellular concentrations of electrolytes may also result in cell necrosis.[105] During thawing of frostbitten tissues, a reversal of this phenomenon may occur. Frostbite also incurs a delayed indirect injury to the microcirculation.[106] This can occur weeks or months after the freezing. The microvascular changes include red blood cell sludging and microthrombi formation, resulting in local tissue hypoxia and necrosis. Radionuclide scans and serial angiograms of frostbitten extremities have demonstrated de-

TABLE 142–9

CLASSIFICATION OF FROSTBITE SEVERITY AND SEQUELAE

Severity	Initial Findings	Rewarming
First degree	Hyperemia and edema.	Mottled and cyanotic; intense burning sensation. Superficial tissue may desquamate after 5–10 d.
Second degree (clear)	Hyperemia, edema, and large blisters or vesicles.	Skin is red, hot, and dry; swelling of tissues occurs within 2–3 h. Blebs form after 6–12 h with clear fluid.
Third degree (hemorrhagic)	Vesicles filled with fluid. Necrosis of underlying tissues.	Within 6 d of rewarming, region is edematous. Early anesthesia followed by severe aching or throbbing sensation in the involved area within 2 wk.
Fourth degree (gangrene)	Complete necrosis, dry mummification, and autoamputation.	

Late sequelae include cold sensitivity, skin color changes, pain with activity or at rest, ulcerations, muscle atrophy, osteoarthritis, hyperhidrosis, and vasomotor instability.

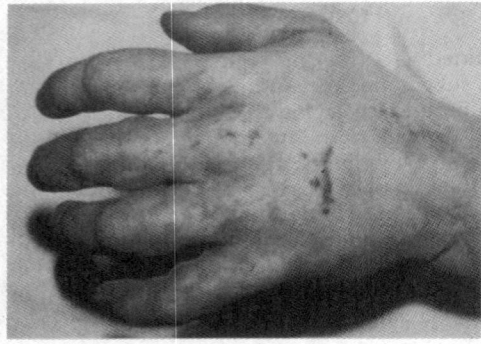
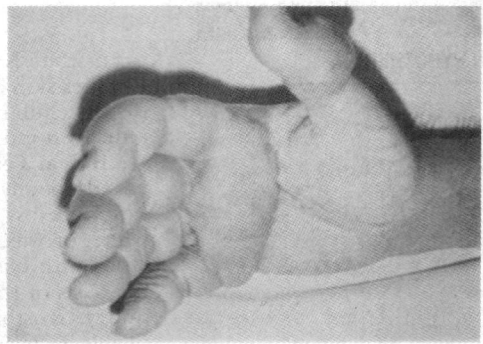
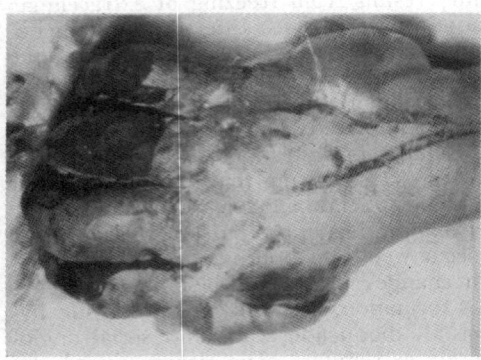
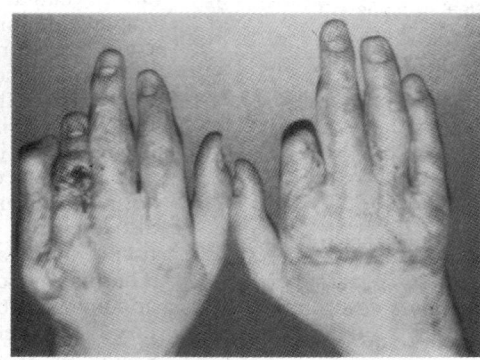

Figure 142–5. The degrees of frostbite injury. (From Barish RA: Frostbite damage may not be immediately apparent. Intern Med News 24[3]:9, 1991.)

creased local blood flow. Microthrombi are observed within 1 to 2 hours after thawing frostbitten tissue. Increased blood viscosity is probably responsible for the vascular stasis, sludging, and formation of microthrombi. Release of prostaglandins and thromboxane leads to tissue ischemia.[107] Experimental studies have shown that antiprostaglandin agents and thromboxane inhibitors are beneficial in prolonging tissue survival.

There is also dysfunction of sympathetic vasomotor reflexes with dilated arterioles and venules. Tissue edema may result from increased hydrostatic pressure, vascular permeability, and damage of the endothelium.

Degenerative changes in myelin may occur in peripheral nerves and may result in sensory and/or motor neuropathies. Vascular thrombosis leading to gangrene may also occur.

Partially rewarmed frostbitten tissue should not be allowed to refreeze. A freeze-thaw-freeze cycle produces massive tissue damage that is cumulatively far greater than the initial injury.

Predisposing Factors. Some individuals are more prone to experience frostbite. Patients with peripheral vascular disease and the malnourished are at increased risk (Table 142–10). A variety of climatic factors such as wind velocity, humidity, ambient temperature, and duration of exposure are important determinants of the extent and depth of local cold injury. In civilian life, 90% of frostbite injuries occur at a temperature below —6.7°C (20°F) and after 7 to 10 hours of exposure.[4] Microvascular damage from previous cold injury makes tissue more prone to subsequent frostbite with increased morbidity. Local cold injury is aggravated in patients with peripheral vascular disease, and particularly those with microvascular disease, diabetes mellitus, Raynaud's disease, and the presence of drugs such as nicotine. Agents such as alcohol and narcotics that impair mental status and heat-productive mechanisms also increase the risk of cold injuries.

Immersion (Trench) Foot

Immersion foot is a nonfreezing cold injury that usually occurs in lower extremities that have been exposed for prolonged periods to a cold, wet environment with temperatures that usually range from just above freezing to approximately 10°C (50°F). The duration of exposure usually exceeds 10 to 12 hours.[4] Trench foot is well known in soldiers and shipwreck survivors whose feet are wet and cold but without freezing of tissues.[108] Additional factors may be the constriction of a limb by tight-fitting clothes and boots, as well as immobile, dependent positions of the involved extremity. In civilian life, trench foot is often seen in fishers and hunters.

The individual initially experiences tingling sensations, itching, numbness, and leg cramps, which progress to a total lack of sensation in the feet. The skin has a waxy gray pallor with a blotchy, mottled cyanosis. Subsequently, limb edema occurs, and large epidermal vesicles or bullae appear. These are attributed to vasodilation and increased permeability of blood vessels, leading to exudation of proteinaceous fluid

TABLE 142–10
PREDISPOSING FACTORS FOR FROSTBITE
Adverse climatic factors related to ambient temperature, wind chill factor, humidity, duration of exposure, and high altitude
Inappropriate clothing, tight clothing or boots
Poor nutrition
Use of alcohol, tobacco
Pre-existing arterial disease (e.g., arteriosclerosis, Raynaud's disease, thromboangiitis obliterans)
Previous history of frostbite
Hypovolemic shock and decreased peripheral circulation
Concurrent injuries

TABLE 142–11

STAGES IN PROGRESSION OF IMMERSION INJURY

Prehyperemic Phase
Persists for hours to days. The limb is cold, slightly swollen, discolored, and numb. Pulses are barely palpable because of vasospasm. Tissue ischemia and edema are primary factors in this phase.

Hyperemic Phase
Hyperemia follows rewarming of the involved extremity. This phase may last 2–6 wk. It is characterized by a hot, red, and swollen foot with bounding, pulsatile circulation. There may be severe pain. Bullae may form, which may persist for 4–10 d. Repeated exposure can result in gangrene and extensive tissue loss.

Posthyperemic Phase
This phase persists for weeks to months. The limb may be warm with increased sensitivity to cold. There may be maceration of tissue with superficial, moist, liquefied gangrene.

Recovery Phase
In uncomplicated cases, this phase is characterized by decreasing edema and return of pulses. Late sequelae include cold sensitivity, depigmentation, hyperhidrosis, and pain on weight bearing. These symptoms may persist for years.

and edema. Extreme tissue maceration and gangrene can lead to loss of limb with permanent disability. There are three stages in the progression of this cold injury (Table 142–11).

Other Local Cold Injuries

A variety of other cold injuries have been described, including frostnip, chilblains, and snow blindness.

Frostnip. Frostnip describes early and mild frostbite. Ice crystals form on the skin surface, but freezing of tissue does not take place. It involves apical structures (nose, ears, hands, feet, chin, cheeks) and is most often seen in skiers exposed to fast-moving, extremely cold air. It is characterized by numb whitening or blanching of the skin with a frosted appearance.

Subsequently there may be pain in the involved area. On rewarming, the skin may turn red with tingling sensations.

Chilblains. Chilblains is commonly seen in climates that are damp and cool for long periods. A localized nodule, probably representing a vasculitis and edema of the papillary dermis, forms on the skin and superficial fatty tissue. It is primarily seen on the face and dorsum of hands and feet and develops after repeated exposure. There is usually moderate-to-severe pruritus with red, dry, and roughened skin. These lesions are self-limiting and heal within a few days. The elderly and those with vascular disorders are predisposed and may have ulcerated areas. Patients with Raynaud's phenomenon are particularly likely to develop these lesions.

Ophthalmic Injuries. Freezing of the corneas is frequently reported in skiers, snowmobilers, and others without protective goggles who are exposed to high wind chill situations. Corneal flare and pain may occur during rewarming. Complications include keratitis and corneal opacification.

Ultraviolet solar radiation reflected from snow or ice may cause snow blindness. A painful red eye may develop after exposure to ultraviolet radiation. Corneal pitting and retinal damage have been described.[11]

Management

Proper management, including protection of the frostbitten extremity from trauma, rapid rewarming, and long-term follow-up care of an affected extremity can significantly reduce morbidity and mortality.

Superficial frostbite (frostnip) can be managed by simply warming the extremity by steady pressure of a warm hand (without rubbing) or by placing the affected fingers in the axilla.

In cases of frostbite, removal of the patient from the cold environment and treatment of hypothermia must be initiated. The extremity should be handled gently to avoid trauma, such as pressure injury or friction. Rewarming by rubbing with snow or exercising is contraindicated. Weight bearing on the affected part may result in further damage to the tissues.

The frostbitten limb should not be thawed if there is any possibility of refreezing, as this may result in increased tissue injury. Rapid rewarming is best accomplished by immersion of the frozen extremity in a water bath heated to a temperature of 38 to 42°C. Hot liquids, blankets, or other hot objects should not be used, as they may induce greater damage. Rewarming is continued until the frostbitten tissue has a flushed appearance; this usually takes 30 to 60 minutes. Administration of narcotic analgesics may be necessary to relieve pain during this procedure. After thawing, the skin is carefully dried with fine-pore cell sponges and the affected part is elevated to minimize edema and is left uncovered at room temperature. A protective cradle may be used to avoid trauma. Gentle whirlpool débridement at 37°C is instituted twice daily, with active range of motion of all joints.

After initiation of the rewarming process, prevention of infectious complications is of paramount importance. Therefore, strict aseptic technique should be employed. Tetanus prophylaxis is indicated[109] for all local cold injuries in which there is breakdown of skin or other barriers. Minor localized infections may be treated with soaks of soapy water or betaine. Antibiotics may be required for deep tissue infections. Surgical consultation is indicated for management of significant local cold injuries.

Ibuprofen and *Aloe vera*, a topical antithromboxane agent, used in combination, have been shown to prevent the progressive ischemia in frostbite and reduce morbidity.[110] Anticoagulation with heparin, warfarin, or dextran is controversial but may be helpful to prevent secondary thromboses.[4]

In cold injuries, there is intense vasoconstriction because of increased sympathetic tone. Intra-arterial reserpine and tolazoline administration has been used for sympathetic blockade. Early regional sympathectomy is ineffective in the acute phase but has been reported to be protective against late sequelae of frostbite and the deleterious effects of subsequent cold injuries.[111]

Fasciotomy may be required if a compartmental syndrome develops in the frostbitten extremity. Measurement of tissue pressure is indicated in a suspected compartmental syndrome. Amputation should be delayed, as tissue necrosis (even with black eschar formation) may be quite superficial and the underlying skin may subsequently heal. Scintigraphy may be of benefit in frostbite injuries to assess the degree of severity and tissue viability.[112, 113] Severe infection with sepsis that is refractory to débridement and antibiotic administration is an indication for amputation. In immersion foot injury, the extremity should be protected from trauma after gentle washing and drying. Gradual rewarming by exposure to cool air (not ice or heat) is initiated during the hyperemic phase. Water immersion of the affected part is contraindicated.

Bed rest and slight elevation of the extremity to decrease tissue edema is required. After all ulcers have healed, physical therapy may be initiated. Precautions should be taken for bed sores, and pressure sites such as the heels should be protected. Antibiotics are necessary if infection develops.

References

1. Curley FJ, Irwin RS: Disorders of temperature control: Hypothermia. Part III. J Intensive Care Med 1:270, 1986.
2. Barber FA: Cold injury in the military. Med Bull US Army, Europe 37:22, 1980.
3. Paton BC: Accidental hypothermia. Pharmacol Ther 22:331, 1983.
4. Christenson C, Stewart C: Frostbite. Am Fam Pract 30(6):111, 1984.
5. Hudson LD, Conn RD: Accidental hypothermia: Associated diagnoses and prognosis in a common problem. JAMA 227:37, 1974.
6. McNicol MW, Smith R: Accidental hypothermia. Br Med J 1:19, 1964.
7. Miller JW, Danzl DF, Thomas DM: Urban accidental hypothermia: 135 cases. Ann Emerg Med 9:456, 1980.
8. Kurtz KJ: Hypothermia in the elderly: The cold facts. Geriatrics 17:85, 1982.
9. Guyton AC: Body temperature, temperature regulation and fever. In: Guyton AC (ed): Textbook of Medical Physiology. Philadelphia, WB Saunders, p 849, 1986.
10. Benzinger TR: Heat regulations: Homeostasis of central temperature in man. Physiol Rev 40:672, 1969.
11. Edlich RF, Chang DE, Birk KA, et al: Cold injuries. Compr Ther 15(9):13, 1989.
12. Fritz RL, Perrin DH: Cold exposure injuries: Prevention and treatment. Clin Sports Med 8(1):111, 1989.
13. Moore RE: Physiology of the response to low temperature. In: Mountain Medicine and Physiology. Clarke C, Ward M, Williams E (eds): London, Alpine Club, p 9, 1975.
14. Hammel HT: Regulation of internal body temperature. Annu Rev Physiol 30:641, 1968.
15. Reuler JB: Hypothermia: Pathophysiology, clinical settings, and management. Ann Intern Med 89:519, 1978.
16. Weyman AE, Greenbaum DM, Grace WJ: Accidental hypothermia in an alcoholic population. Am J Med 56:13, 1974.
17. Lloyd EL: Treatment of accidental hypothermia. Br Med J 1:413, 1979.
18. Collin KJ, Exton-Smith AN, Dore C: Urban hypothermia. Preferred temperature and thermal perception in old age. Br Med J 282:175, 1981.
19. Whittle JL, Bates JH: Thermoregulatory failure secondary to acute illness, complications and treatment. Arch Intern Med 139:418, 1979.
20. Prescott LF, Peard MC, Wallace IR: Accidental hypothermia: A common condition. Br Med J 2:1367, 1962.
21. Vandam LD, Burnap TK: Hypothermia. N Engl J Med 261:546, 1959.
22. Duff RS, Farrant PC, Leveaux VM, et al: Spontaneous periodic hypothermia. Q J Med 30:329, 1961.
23. McNicol NW, Smith R: Accidental hypothermia. Br Med J 1:19, 1964.
24. Cooper KE: The circulation in hypothermia. Br Med Bull 17:48, 1961.
25. Trevino A, Rasi B, Beller BM: The characteristic electrocardiogram of accidental hypothermia. Arch Intern Med 127:470, 1971.
26. Southwick FS, Dalglish PH: Recovery after prolonged asystolic cardiac arrest in profound hypothermia. JAMA 243:1250, 1980.
27. Thompson R, Rich J, Chmelik F, et al: Evolutionary changes in the electrocardiogram of severe progressive hypothermia. J Electrocardiol 10:67, 1977.
28. Rankin AC, Rae AP: Cardiac arrhythmias during rewarming of patients with accidental hypothermia. Br Med J 289:874, 1984.
29. Abbott JA, Cheitlin MD: The nonspecific camel-hump sign. JAMA 235:413, 1976.
30. Mouritzen CV, Andersen MN: Myocardial temperature gradients and ventricular fibrillation during hypothermia. J Thorac Cardiovasc Surg 49:937, 1965.
31. Blair ET, Esmond WG, Attar S, et al: The effect of hypothermia on lung function. Ann Surg 160:814, 1964.
32. Martyn JW: Diagnosing and treating hypothermia. Can Med Assoc J 124:1089, 1981.
33. Holdcroft A: Control of body temperature. In: Holdcroft A (ed): Body Temperature Control: In Relation to Anesthesia, Surgery and Intensive Care. New York, Macmillan, p 1, 1980.
34. Hervey GR: Hypothermia. Proc R Soc Med 66:1055, 1973.
35. Hardy JD, Bard P: Body Temperature Regulation in Medical Physiology. St Louis, CV Mosby, p 1305, 1974.
36. Morales P, Carbery W, Morello A, et al: Alterations in renal function during hypothermia in man. Ann Surg 145:488, 1957.
37. Moyer JH, Morris C, DeBakey ME: Hypothermia: I. Effect on renal hemodynamics and on excretion of water and electrolytes in dog and man. Ann Surg 145:26, 1957.
38. Segar WE, Riley PA, Barila TG: Urinary composition during hypothermia. Am J Physiol 185:528, 1956.
39. Rosenfeld JB: Acid-base and electrolyte disturbances in hypothermia. Am J Cardiol 12:678, 1963.
40. McKean WI, Dixon SR, Gwynne JF, et al: Renal failure after accidental hypothermia. Br Med J 2:463, 1970.
41. Hirvonen J, Elefving R: Histamine and serotonin in the gastric erosions of rats dead from exposure to cold: A histochemical and quantitative study. Z Rechtsmed 74:273, 1974.
42. Mant AK: Autopsy diagnosis of accidental hypothermia. J Forensic Med 16:126, 1969.
43. Maclean D, Murison J, Griffiths PD: Acute pancreatis and diabetic ketoacidosis in accidental hypothermia and hypothermic myxoedema. Br Med J 4:757, 1973.
44. Blair E: Clinical Hypothermia. New York, McGraw-Hill, 1964.
45. Curry DL, Curry KP: Hypothermia and insulin secretion. Endocrinology 87:750, 1970.
46. Baum D, Dillard DH, Porte D: Inhibition of insulin release in infants undergoing deep hypothermic cardiovascular surgery. N Engl J Med 279:1309, 1968.
47. Stoner HB, Frayn KN, Little RA, et al: Metabolic aspects of hypothermia in the elderly. Clin Sci 59:19, 1980.
48. Maclean D, Browning MC: Plasma 11 hydroxycorticosteroid concentrations and prognosis in accidental hypothermia. Resuscitation 42:249, 1974.
49. Woolff PD, Hollander CS, Mitusma T, et al: Accidental hypothermia: Endocrine function during recovery. J Clin Endocrinol Metab 34:460, 1972.
50. Wilson O, Hedner P, Laurell S, et al: Thyroid and adrenal response to acute cold exposure in man. J Appl Physiol 28:543, 1970.
51. Masoro EJ: The effect of cold on the metabolic use of lipid. Physiol Rev 46:67, 1966.
52. Kanter GS: Hypothermic hemoconcentration. Am J Physiol 214:856, 1968.
53. O'Brien H, Amess JAL, Mollin LD: Recurrent thrombocytopenia, erythroid hypoplasia and sideroblastic anaemia associated with hypothermia. Br J Haematol 51:451, 1982.
54. Rand PW, Lancombe E, Hunt HE, et al: Viscosity of normal human blood under normothermic and hypothermic conditions. J Appl Physiol 19:117, 1964.
55. Blair E: A physiologic classification of clinical hypothermia. Surgery 58:607, 1965.
56. Thomas RT, Hessel EA, Harker LA, et al: Platelet function during and after deep surface hypothermia. J Surg Res 31:314, 1981.
57. Koeppen AH, Daniels JC, Baroron KD: Subnormal body temperatures in Wernicke's encephalopathy. Arch Neurol 21:493, 1969.
58. Schissler P, Parker MA, Scott SJ: Profound hypothermia: Value of prolonged cardiopulmonary resuscitation. South Med J 74:474, 1981.
59. Chadd MA, Gray OP: Hypothermia and coagulation defects in the newborn. Arch Dis Child 47:819, 1972.
60. Cohen IJ: Cold injury in early infancy: Relationship between mortality and disseminated intravascular coagulation. Isr J Med Sci 13:405, 1977.
61. Bohn D, Barker C, Kent G, et al: Accidental and induced hypothermia: Effects on neutrophil migration in vivo. Crit Care Med 129:A112, 1984.
62. Biggar WD, Bohn DJ, Kent G, et al: Neutrophil migration in vitro and in vivo during hypothermia. Infect Immun 46:857, 1984.
63. Fedor EJ, Fisher ER, Lee SH, et al: Effect of hypothermia upon induced bacteremia. Proc Soc Exp Biol Med 93:510, 1956.
64. deGuzman VC, Webb WR, Grogan JB: The effect of hypothermia on clearance of staphylococcal bacteremia. Clin Res 10:58, 1962.
65. Hemingway A: Shivering. Physiol Rev 43:397, 1963.
66. Jessen K, Hagelsten JO: Search and rescue service in Denmark with special reference to accidental hypothermia. Aerospace Med 43:787, 1972.
67. Pickering BG, Bristow GK, Craig DB: Core rewarming by peritoneal irrigation in accidental hypothermia with cardiac arrest. Anesth Analg 56:574, 1977.
68. Anderson S, Herbring BG, Widman B: Accidental profound hypothermia. Br J Anaesth 42:653, 1970.
69. Michenfelder JD, Theye RA: Hypothermia: Effect on canine brain and whole-body metabolism. Anesthesiology 29:1107, 1965.
70. Ehrmantraut WR, Ticktin HE, Fazekras JF: Cerebral hemodynamics and metabolism in accidental hypothermia. Arch Intern Med 99:57, 1957.
71. Norwood WI, Norwood CR: Influence of hypothermia on intracellular pH during anoxia. Am J Physiol 243:C62, 1982.
72. Norwood WI, Norwood CR, Castaneda AR: Cerebral anoxia: Effect of deep hypothermia and pH. Surgery 86:203, 1979.
73. Tolman KG, Cohen A: Accidental hypothermia. Can Med Assoc J 103:1357, 1970.
74. Sheehan HL, Summers VK: Treatment of hypopituitary coma. Br Med J 1:1214, 1952.
75. Fischbeck KH, Simon RP: Neurologic manifestations of accidental hypothermia. Ann Neurol 10:384, 1981.
76. Rosin AJ, Exton-Smith AN: Clinical features of accidental hypothermia, with some observations on thyroid function. Br Med J 1:16, 1964.
77. Hansen B, Larrson C, Wiren J, et al: Hypothermia and infection in Wernicke's encephalopathy. Acta Med Scand 215:185, 1984.
78. Stoner HB: Mechanism of body temperature changes after burns and other injuries. Ann NY Acad Sci 150:722, 1968.
79. FitzGibbon T, Hayward JD, Walker D: EEG and visual evoked potential of conscious man during moderate hypothermia. Encephalogr Clin Neurophysiol 58:48, 1984.
80. Althaus U, Aeberhard T, Schupbach P, et al: Management of profound accidental hypothermia with cardiorespiratory arrest. Ann Surg 195:492, 1982.
81. Carden D, Doan L, Sweeney PJ, et al: Hypothermia. Ann Emerg Med 11:497, 1982.

82. Towne WD, Geiss WP, Yanes HO, et al: Intractable ventricular fibrillation associated with profound accidental hypothermia—Successful treatment with partial cardiopulmonary bypass. N Engl J Med 287:1135, 1972.
83. Milner JE: Hypothermia. Ann Intern Med 89:565, 1978.
84. DaVee TS, Reineberg EJ: Extreme hypothermia and ventricular fibrillation. Ann Emerg Med 9:100, 1980.
85. Nicodemus HF, Chaney RD, Herold R: Hemodynamic effects of inotropes during hypothermia and rapid rewarming. Crit Care Med 9:325, 1981.
86. Angelakos ET, Torres J, Driscoll R: Ouabain on the hypothermic dog heart. Am Heart J 56:458, 1958.
87. Maclean D, Griffiths PD, Emslie-Smith D: Serum-enzymes in relation to electrocardiographic changes in accidental hypothermia. Lancet 2:1266, 1968.
88. Danzl DF, Sowers MB, Vicario SJ, et al: Chemical ventricular defibrillation in severe accidental hypothermia. Ann Emerg Med 11:698, 1982.
89. Dronen S, Nowak RM, Tomlanovich MC: Bretylium tosylate and hypothermic ventricular fibrillation. Ann Emerg Med 9:335, 1980.
90. Buckley JJ, Bosch OK, Bacaner MB: Prevention of ventricular fibrillation during hypothermia with bretylium tosylate. Anesth Analg 50:587, 1971.
91. Alexander L: The treatment of shock from prolonged exposure to cold, especially in water. London, Combined Intelligence Objectives Subcommittee, APO 413, C105 Item 24, Her Majesty's Stationery Office, 1945.
92. Severinghaus JW: Respiration and hypothermia. Ann NY Acad Sci 80:384, 1959.
93. Fitzgerald FT, Jessop C: Accidental hypothermia: A report of 23 cases and review of the literature. Adv Intern Med 27:128, 1982.
94. Bradley AF, Stupfel M, Severinghaus JW: Effect of temperature on Pco₂ and Po₂ of blood in vitro. J Appl Physiol 9:201, 1956.
95. Kelman GR, Nunn JF: Nomograms for correction of blood Po₂, Pco₂, pH and base excess for time and temperature. J Appl Physiol 21:1484, 1966.
96. Emerson CH: Myxedema coma. In: Rippe JM, Irwin RS, Alpert JS, et al (eds): Intensive Care Medicine. Boston, Little, Brown, p 802, 1985.
97. Hedley-Whyte J, Pontoppidan H, Laver MB, et al: Arterial oxygenation during hypothermia. Anesthesiology 26:595, 1965.
98. Levy LA: Severe hypophosphatemia as a complication of the treatment of hypothermia. Arch Intern Med 140:128, 1980.
99. Freeman RM: The role of magnesium in the pathogenesis of azotemic hypothermia. Proc Soc Exp Biol Med 137:1069, 1971.
100. Arnold JW, Eichenberger CH: The hydraulic sarong: Emergency treatment device for accidental hypothermia. JACEP 4:438, 1975.
101. MacLean D, Griffiths PD, Browning MCK, et al: Metabolic aspects of spontaneous rewarming in accidental hypothermia and hypothermic myxedema. Q J Med 43:371, 1974.
102. Gregory RT, Doolittle WH: Accidental hypothermia. II. Clinical implications of experimental studies. Alaska Med 15:48, 1973.
103. Truscott DG, Frior WB, Clein LJ: Accidental profound hypothermia: Successful resuscitation by core rewarming and assisted circulation. Arch Surg 106:216, 1973.
104. Rodriguez JL, Weissman C, Damask MC, et al: Morphine and postoperative rewarming in critically ill patients. Circulation 68:1238, 1983.
105. Mazur P: Cryobiology: The freezing of biological systems. The responses of living cells to ice formation are of theoretical interest and practical concern. Science 168:939, 1970.
106. Gage AW, Gage AA: Frostbite. Compr Ther 7(9):25, 1981.
107. Purdue GF, Hunt JL: Cold injury: A collective review. J Burn Care Rehabil 7:331, 1986.
108. Ungley CC, Blackwood W: Peripheral vasoneuropathy, after chilling. "Immersion foot and immersion hand." Lancet 2:447, 1942.
109. Committee on Trauma: Prophylaxis against tetanus in wound management. Bull Am Coll Surg 69(10):22, 1984.
110. Heggers JP, Robson MC, Manvalenk K, et al: Experimental and clinical observations on frostbite. Ann Emerg Med 16:1056, 1987.
111. Bouwmann DL, Morrison S, Lucas CE, et al: Early sympathetic blockade for frost bite—Is it of value? J Trauma 20:744, 1980.
112. Salimi Z: Frostbite: Assessment of tissue viability by scintigraphy. Postgrad Med 77:133, 1985.
113. Bangs C, Hamelt M: Out in the cold—Management of hypothermia, immersion and frostbite. Top Emerg Med 2:19, 1980.

CHAPTER 143

Electrical and Lightning Injuries

Bassam N. Helou
Richard W. Carlson

ELECTRICAL INJURIES

Since the commercial use of electricity in 1849, there has been a progressive increase in the incidence of electrical injuries. In 1987, 760 deaths in the United States were attributed to electrical accidents.[1] Electrical injuries account for approximately 3% of admissions to burn units.[2] Exposure to electric current results in a wide variety of injuries that prompt evaluation in emergency rooms. As critical care physicians become involved in the management of many of these patients, they should have a working knowledge of the pathophysiology, clinical manifestations, and treatment of electrical injuries. Lightning injuries constitute a special form of electrical injuries (see later).

Physics and Pathophysiology

Direct contact with an energized conductor is the most common mechanism of electrical injury. However, other mechanisms play important roles and frequently complicate the clinical presentation. Arcing of the electric current from a high-voltage line to a grounded victim may result in severe thermal burns, as the temperature of the arc may exceed 3000°C.[3] Flame burns may occur if clothing is ignited by the intense heat generated by the current. Skeletal trauma caused by violent muscular contraction or falls after electrocution is also common.[4] Therefore, electrically injured patients should be regarded as potentially having multisystem trauma.

The majority of electrical injuries in the United States occur after exposure to alternating current, as this is widely used for domestic and industrial purposes. Alternating current has a tetanizing effect on muscles, which may result in locking of the victim's hand to the source of the current. This prolongs the time of exposure, which in turn increases the severity of injury.[5] In contrast, direct current often leads to a single muscular contraction, which forces the victim away from the current.[5, 6] Household alternating current, at a frequency of 60 cps and 110 to 120 V, is more likely to cause serious cardiac arrhythmias and respiratory arrest than is direct current or alternating currents of higher frequencies.[5, 7]

When the body becomes a conduit for electric current, the injury produced results from conversion of electrical energy to heat. The amount of heat generated by an electric current is described by Joule's law and is related to the triple product of the square of the current intensity, resistance, and time:

$$J = I^2 \times R \times T$$

where J = amount of heat in joules
I = current intensity (amperage) in amperes
R = resistance in ohms
T = duration in time unit

The extent of the resultant damage therefore depends on many factors, including amperage, voltage, tissue resistance, tissue susceptibility to electrical injury, duration of contact, and current pathway.

Amperage, or current intensity, is one of the most critical factors affecting deep tissue injury and mortality.[8] Amperage may be calculated by Ohm's law as the voltage/resistance ratio. Tissue resistance at the time of injury is not easily measured. Accordingly, amperage cannot be calculated in most instances.[8] Electrical injuries are therefore classified by voltage, which is usually the only known factor at the time of exposure. In most series, currents of less than 1000 V are considered low tension whereas those greater than 1000 V are classified as high tension.[9-11] Because the heat generated is proportional to the square of voltage, severe burns tend to be limited to high-tension injuries.

For a current to cause tissue injury, it must overcome the resistance of the skin, which acts as a barrier. Normal skin resistance is approximately 5000 Ω, but this is affected by many factors, chiefly skin thickness and wetness. The resistance of callused skin may reach 1 million Ω, whereas that of moist skin can be as little as 1000 Ω.[12] After the current penetrates the skin, the amount of heat generated, as described by Joule's law, is directly proportional to the resistance offered by underlying tissues. Bones offer the highest resistance of body tissues. Accordingly, osseous tissues may become hot, causing extensive damage by conduction to the surrounding muscles and other adjacent structures. Deep tissue injury may therefore exceed superficial damage, which frequently leads to an initial underestimation of the extent of injury.[3, 5] Some tissues, such as nerves and blood vessels, are inherently susceptible to damage by electric current, despite their relatively low resistance. Peripheral neuropathy and coagulation of vessels are common after exposure to electricity.[13-15]

Other factors that play important roles in determining the severity of injury are the density of the current and the pathway of current through the patient. Current density, in turn, is inversely related to the cross-sectional diameter of the conductor.[5] This explains why tissue damage is most prominent at the sites of entry and exit and more severe in extremities than in the trunk. Current pathways involving the thorax or the head are more likely to cause cardiac dysrhythmias or central nervous system dysfunction.[7, 10, 16]

Clinical Manifestations

The clinical manifestations of electrical injuries are both complex and varied. Multiple organ systems are frequently involved (Table 143–1).

Cutaneous and Musculoskeletal Effects

Burns, which may range from 1 to 90% of body surface area,[2, 10] are the most striking features of electrical injuries. Burns are typically observed at entrance and exit sites of the electric current. The usual entrance site is either in an upper extremity or the skull,[10, 15, 17] with the exit sites in the lower extremities.

High-tension injuries may result in massive muscle destruction that resembles crush trauma.[18] These injuries may necessitate extensive débridement and amputation. The characteristic pathologic change is coagulation myonecrosis.[19] In addition, compartmental syndromes may result from severe tissue swelling in areas bound by fascia, with consequent disruption of blood and nerve supply.[20]

Secondary orthopedic complications include fractures and dislocations, which are usually due to falls that follow electrocution. Occasionally, compression fractures of the spine have been observed and have been attributed to intense muscular contractions.[10, 16] Direct injury to bone may occur;

TABLE 143–1
MAJOR CLINICAL MANIFESTATIONS OF ELECTRICAL INJURY
Musculoskeletal
Myonecrosis, compartmental syndromes, bony fractures, compression fractures
Vascular
Arterial and venous thrombosis, arterial rupture, aneurysms
Cardiac
Ventricular fibrillation, asystole, sinus tachycardia, atrial fibrillation, myocardial infarction, ECG abnormalities, creatine kinase isoenzyme (MB) level elevation
Neurologic
Loss of consciousness, confusion, seizures, paralysis, transverse myelitis, peripheral neuropathy
Renal or metabolic
Acute tubular necrosis, lactic acidosis
Gastrointestinal
Nausea or vomiting, stress ulcers, ileus, intestinal perforation
Ophthalmic
Cataracts

periosteal necrosis and subsequent sequestral formation may result from the intense heat produced when the current passes through the highly resistant bony structures.[4] It is necessary to remove dead periosteum to minimize further damage to bone.

Vascular Effects

Small muscular arteries are extremely susceptible to thrombosis when exposed to high temperatures. Thrombosis may lead to ischemic gangrene, necessitating amputation.[10, 13] Damage to the medial layer of arteries may result in the formation of aneurysms with immediate or delayed life-threatening hemorrhages.[10, 17] Prolonged immobilization predisposes to deep venous thrombosis.[10]

Cardiac Abnormalities

The heart is remarkably sensitive to the effects of electric current, particularly when the current pathway involves the thorax. Cardiac arrhythmias are the most frequent cause of immediate death in electrical injuries.[5, 21] Currents of greater than 0.1 A may induce ventricular fibrillation, whereas cardiac standstill may occur if the amperage is greater than 2 A.[21] The onset of arrhythmias is usually immediate, although on occasion it may be delayed up to 12 hours after injury.[22] Supraventricular tachycardia, atrial fibrillation, and frequent premature ventricular contractions have also been recorded.[10]

The electrocardiogram (ECG) obtained at the time of hospital admission is abnormal in up to 36% of patients.[8] A wide spectrum of ECG disturbances may be found. The most frequent findings are nonspecific ST and T wave changes and sinus tachycardia, which may persist for several weeks.[4]

Myocardial infarction, although uncommon, may follow high-voltage injuries.[10, 15, 23, 24] Two aspects differentiate this type of infarction from the ischemic type:

1. Serious arrhythmia is an infrequent complication.[23]
2. Damage to the coronary arteries has not been reported, and only occasional endocardial and pericardial petechial hemorrhages have been found on pathologic examination.[8, 25] The diagnosis of infarction is often difficult, as classic ECG changes may not develop until 4 days after hospital admission,[24] and creatine kinase isoenzyme CK_2 (MB) activity is often falsely positive in electrical injuries.[21, 26] The latter is

due to the release of CK$_2$ (MB) enzyme from damaged skeletal muscles.[24] In this setting, the technetium Tc 99m pyrophosphate myocardial scan may be particularly helpful for establishing the diagnosis.[23]

Neuropsychiatric Disorders

Neurologic dysfunction is the most common nonlethal complication in electrical injury.[4, 10] Many of these patients experience a variety of cerebral abnormalities immediately after electrocution, including loss of consciousness, obtundation, amnesia, and transient blindness.[4, 8] Seizures may occur and are thought to be related either to the direct effect of the current on the brain or to cerebral anoxia caused by ventricular fibrillation.[8]

Injury to the spinal cord may be immediate or delayed. In the immediate type, symptoms of spastic paralysis and sensory deficits usually resolve within 24 hours.[27] However, delayed cord injuries, which may take days to years to develop, are usually irreversible and only rare recoveries have been reported.[28] The clinical presentation may resemble that of incomplete cord transection, ascending paralysis, amyotrophic lateral sclerosis, or transverse myelitis.[19, 29] These injuries are unpredictable, as the pathway of the current correlates poorly with the level of the lesion.[4] The diagnosis of spinal cord lesions is often difficult and frequently delayed until the patient is ambulatory.[4]

Peripheral nerve damage occurs most frequently in association with extensive burns.[29] The median and ulnar nerves are the most commonly injured.[8, 10] Three mechanisms may produce neuropathy: (1) direct injury from the heat generated by the current,[15] (2) mechanical injury resulting from trauma during débridement or from compression attributable to a compartment syndrome, and (3) delayed injury (months to years) caused by perineural scarring and neural ischemia.[8, 29] The prognosis for peripheral nerve injury is guarded; functional recovery is often absent or incomplete.[8]

Finally, a variety of psychiatric disturbances have been described after electrocution. These include depression, insomnia, anxiety, and fear of electricity, which may necessitate a change of occupation.[10]

Renal and Metabolic Effects

Acute renal failure may occur in electrical injury and carries a poor prognosis.[2, 30] Renal failure is caused either by myoglobinuria attributable to muscle necrosis or, less commonly, by hemoglobinuria resulting from hemolysis. Fortunately, the incidence of renal failure appears to be declining, which may be related to a greater recognition of pigmenturia and more aggressive fluid therapy.[8, 9]

Metabolic disturbances consist of hyperkalemia and lactic acidosis.[3, 31] The former results from potassium leakage from damaged cells; the latter is due to lactic acid production by seizures or to devascularized ischemic tissues. The magnitude of the acidosis correlates poorly with the extent of injury. This may be explained, in part, by the occlusion of vessels that prevents ischemic tissue products from reaching the circulation.[3]

Infections

Sepsis is the leading cause of death in electrical injury after initial resuscitation.[4, 10] Deep necrotic tissue is the usual source of infection.[4, 8] Accordingly, the detection of occult deep tissue damage coupled with adequate débridement and amputation are crucial aspects of therapy. The most commonly involved pathogens are *Pseudomonas* and gram-positive cocci.[4, 15] Clostridial myositis is common in cases of inadequate débridement and may necessitate amputation.[2, 3] Other reported infectious complications include pneumonia, septicemia, osteomyelitis,[9, 10] and meningitis.[8, 9]

Gastrointestinal Effects

Abdominal symptoms are observed in as many as 25% of cases and usually include nausea and vomiting. Stress ulceration, or Curling's ulcer, is the most frequent serious gastrointestinal complication and may affect 13% of patients.[4] Bleeding occurs in a high percentage of these ulcers[4, 10] and may necessitate surgical intervention.

Perforation of the small or large bowel may occur after electrocution with either low- or high-voltage current.[2, 32] The mechanisms that lead to perforation have not been clarified. Adynamic ileus,[10] hemorrhagic necrosis of the gallbladder,[2] and pancreatitis[4] have also been reported.

Ophthalmic Consequences

Cataracts are a well-known late complication of electrical injury and may affect up to 6% of victims of severe electrical injuries.[8, 33] Most cataracts are bilateral and are more common afer high-tension injuries, especially when the current traverses the head.[17]

Management

Prehospital Management

The immediate course of action is removal of the victim from the current source, preferably by shutting off the power. Extreme caution must be exercised when using nonconductive tools to extricate a victim. Far too often, rescuers have become additional victims.

Conventional cardiopulmonary resuscitation should be initiated at the scene for patients who have experienced cardiopulmonary arrest. In cases of electrocution involving line maintainers on utility poles, mouth-to-mouth breathing should be started before the victim is lowered to the ground.[34] If the possibility of a fall exists, a cervical collar is applied and other orthopedic injuries are splinted. As soon as possible, the patient should be transported to a hospital for definitive therapy.

Hospital Management

Electrical injuries cause considerable multisystemic responses, which require aggressive resuscitative therapy. For comatose or post-cardiac resuscitation patients, patency of the airway must be ensured. The next goal is to establish hemodynamic stability. For high-tension injuries, large volumes of intravenous fluids may be needed, as massive fluid losses can occur owing to exudation into damaged areas. Conventional formulas used to estimate fluid requirements in burn injuries are of little value in guiding fluid replacement because extensive deep tissue damage may underlie minimal surface burns. Physiologic goals are therefore preferred to preselected volumes. Establishing a urine output of at least 1 mL/kg/h has been recommended.[3] Invasive hemodynamic monitoring is suggested for severe injuries to titrate physiologic responses and to avoid fluid overload.

Arterial pH should be determined and closely followed by serial blood gas determinations. It has been recommended that sodium bicarbonate be administered to achieve a near-normal pH for patients with severe acidemia and for cases in which myoglobinuria complicates acidosis.[3, 4] Hyperkalemia is treated in the usual fashion using dextrose and insulin, sodium bicarbonate, and cation-exchange resins.

Urine should be tested for myoglobin; a positive result is managed by increasing urine output above 1 mL/kg/h by fluid loading. Persistent myoglobinuria despite aggressive fluid therapy warrants urine alkalinization with sodium bicarbonate, osmotic diuresis with mannitol,[9, 20] and a careful search for devitalized tissues.[3, 9]

Electrical burns should be managed in consultation with an experienced surgeon. Indications for immediate decompression by fasciotomy include extensive limb burns, severe limb swelling, diminished distal pulses and neurologic function, and increased compartmental pressure measured by the wick catheter.[3, 11] Injuries that do not meet these criteria should be observed closely. Multiple techniques have been recommended to guide further surgical interventions. Technetium Tc 99m stannous pyrophosphate scintigraphy is useful for identifying occult necrotic muscles and for assessing the extent of débridement or amputation.[9, 11, 35] Repeated ^{99m}Tc scanning may be performed, as the isotope has a short half-life (6 hours). Serial muscle biopsies have been advocated by some authors to evaluate tissue viability. However, the inaccuracy of biopsy results during the first day after injury and the need for multiple biopsies make this technique impractical.[11, 36] Arteriography has been of limited value because of its inability to visualize small muscular arteries.[14, 35]

Controversy surrounds the need for routine ECG monitoring for high-tension injuries. Purdue and Hunt recommended specific criteria for monitoring, as they found no serious delayed arrhythmias in patients with a normal ECG.[23] However, other writers documented dangerous arrhythmias as well as delayed myocardial infarction.[22, 24] Until this issue is settled, it is prudent to monitor the ECG of patients with high-tension injury for at least 48 hours. However, urgent surgical procedures should not be delayed until a myocardial injury has been excluded. In this regard, surgery appears to be well tolerated, even in the setting of abnormal ECG findings and elevated CK_2 (MB) levels.[10, 21, 24] Currently, the recommended indications for ECG monitoring for patients with low-tension injuries include a history of loss of consciousness, documented serious arrhythmias, and an abnormal ECG on hospital admission.

A detailed neurologic examination should be performed on hospital admission and repeated frequently during the hospital course. Most patients who are obtunded or comatose show a steady improvement in mental status. The lack of such improvement should prompt a careful search for complicating factors such as intracranial hemorrhage attributable to blunt trauma or cerebral anoxia caused by cardiac arrest. Seizures must be treated aggressively to avoid further neurologic damage. Dysfunction of peripheral nerves should be identified, and aggravating factors such as compartmental syndrome or vascular insufficiency should be addressed. The relief of increased compartmental pressure is of the utmost importance. Major peripheral nerves that are exposed during débridement should be preserved if the nerve sheath is intact.[4] Nerve grafting may be required when neurologic improvement is unsatisfactory.[3]

Every effort should be made to prevent infection. Adequate débridement of necrotic tissues is a guiding principle, as devitalized tissue serves as a medium for bacterial overgrowth. Prophylactic treatment with anticlostridial antibiotics, such as high-dose penicillin G or chloramphenicol, and tetanus toxoid is recommended for cases that involve significant tissue injury.[9, 18, 37] Topical antimicrobial agents are used for local wound care. Silver sulfadiazine and mafenide (Sulfamylon) are the most commonly used agents. However, when the latter is applied to a large surface area, a non–anion gap metabolic acidosis may develop because of inhibition of carbonic anhydrase.[38]

TABLE 143–2

HIGH-VOLTAGE VERSUS LIGHTNING INJURIES

Parameter	High-Voltage	Lightning
Voltage	Variable, usually several thousand volts	10^5–10^8 V
Current	Alternating or direct current	Direct current
Duration	Variable, usually seconds	0.01–0.001 s
Flashover	Not observed	Frequent
Deep tissue injury	Frequent	Uncommon

Other aspects of management of electrical burns utilize techniques that are similar to those used for other burn injuries (see Chapter 140). Prophylaxis for deep venous thrombosis should be considered for nonambulatory patients. The high incidence of stress ulcerations in electrical victims warrants empirical treatment with antacids or histamine H_2 blockers.

In the past, the hospital mortality of patients with severe electrical injury was approximately 15%.[2] However, aggressive management has led to a marked decrease in mortality to 2%.[8, 9, 20] Intensive therapy for patients with electrical injury is warranted, as most survivors return to a productive life after recovery.[20]

LIGHTNING INJURIES

Lightning, which was considered to be of divine origin, has been feared since early history. In Greek mythology, lightning was thought to have come from the hand of Zeus, so that the places it struck were considered sacred. In fact, lightning is the electrical discharge occurring between the negatively charged lower layers of the clouds and the earth, which is positively charged.[39] Each year, lightning kills more people than any other natural phenomenon.[40] The National Center for Health Statistics reported 99 deaths attributable to lightning in 1987.[1]

Although the same physical laws apply to both lightning and high-voltage injuries, several distinct differences exist between these two forms of electrical injury (Table 143–2).

Lightning is a direct current of several hundred million volts or more, with an amperage of 5000 to 200,000 A.[41] Despite this awesome power, deep tissue damage and subsequent myoglobinuria are less frequently encountered than in conventional high-voltage injuries.[6] Two major factors may be cited to explain this paradox: (1) lightning is associated with an extremely brief exposure time, and (2) the bulk of the current flows around the outside of the patient's body.[6, 39] This unique phenomenon is known as flashover.

Lightning may induce injuries by various mechanisms. One dramatic example is a direct strike by a lightning bolt. Injury may also occur owing to current's splashing from its primary target, such as a tree or another person, to the individual.[42] In addition, serious injuries may result if the lightning bolt strikes the ground near the individual.[39] Telephone-mediated lightning injuries have been reported in areas where telephone wires lack lightning protection.[43] Finally, explosions caused by the intense heat produced by lightning may result in blunt trauma.[6] Often, more than one person is involved in a lightning strike.

Clinical Manifestations

The most dramatic effects of lightning involve the heart and the central nervous system. The extremely high amperage results in forceful contraction of the myocardium in systole, producing cardiac arrest.[44] In most instances, this is followed by spontaneous return of sinus rhythm. Unfortunately, lightning also causes respiratory arrest, possibly through its effect on the nervous system, which outlasts the asystole.[39, 42] Apnea and subsequent myocardial hypoxia may lead to secondary cardiac arrhythmias and possible death if cardiopulmonary resuscitation is not initiated promptly. Ventricular fibrillation has also been reported after lightning injury.[45] However, it is not clear if ventricular fibrillation is the result of the direct effect of lightning or is caused by hypoxia.[41] In rare instances, myocardial infarction has been reported[44, 46] and may lead to hemodynamic compromise owing to left ventricular dysfunction.[44]

The neurologic effects of a lightning strike are multiple. Loss of consciousness, prolonged amnesia, or confusion occurs in more than 70% of cases.[39] Transient paralysis that usually involves the lower extremities is not uncommon.[39] Of special interest is autonomic dysfunction attributable to sympathetic discharge that follows the strike. This dysfunction may be manifested by transient hypertension and peripheral vasoconstriction. The latter effect causes the extremities to appear mottled and pulseless.[45, 47] Fortunately, these findings are usually reversible within a few hours.[47]

Cutaneous burns are present in the majority of lightning

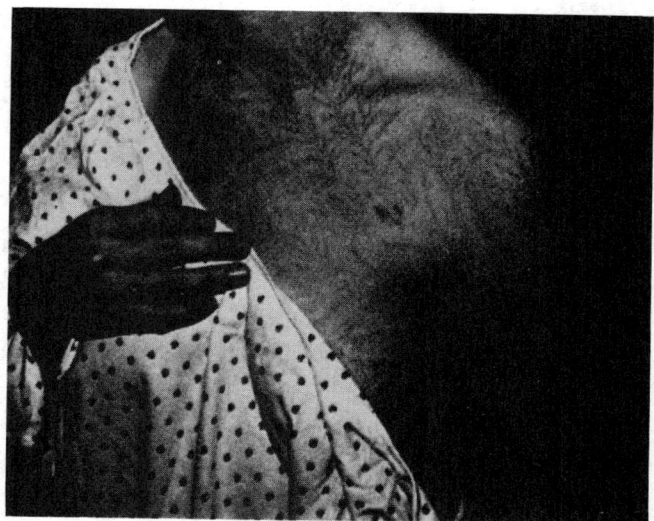

Figure 143–2. Feathering pathognomonic of lightning injury. (From Bartholome CW, Jacoby WD, Ramchand SC: Cutaneous manifestations of lightning injury. Arch Dermatol 111:1466–1468, 1975. Copyright 1975, American Medical Association.)

injury patients. The pathognomonic lesion consists of linear, fern-like, superficial skin markings that usually disappear in several days[48] (Figs. 143–1 and 143–2). This lesion has been variously labeled as feathering or lightning prints. Blistering may occur but late scarring is rare.[47] The site of the burn has a prognostic significance. Patients with burns of the head or the leg have a mortality rate three to five times higher than that of patients with lightning injury without such burns.[39]

A variety of other injuries have been associated with lightning strikes. Rupture of the tympanic membrane may occur owing to the thunder that accompanies lightning.[39, 49] Cataracts may develop days to years after injury.[41, 50] Myoglobinuria, although uncommon, has also been reported.[41, 45] Lightning strikes involving pregnant women may result in fetal or neonatal death in approximately 50% of cases.[39]

Treatment

In the case of cardiac arrest, cardiopulmonary resuscitation should be initiated promptly and continued aggressively. Complete recoveries have been documented repeatedly after a prolonged arrest.[41, 47, 51] Patients who do not experience immediate cardiac arrest have an excellent prognosis.[39] Therefore, when multiple persons are simultaneously struck by lightning, initial attention should be directed to those who appear clinically dead.[34, 42]

Survivors of lightning strike should be admitted to the intensive care unit for cardiac monitoring and supportive care. Serial ECGs and cardiac enzyme determinations should be followed. Arrhythmias are treated by conventional techniques. Further management consists of general supportive measures, including fluid resuscitation, tetanus prophylaxis, and management of burns and other associated injuries. As deep tissue injury is infrequent after lightning strikes, aggressive fluid therapy should be reserved for cases in which urine tests are positive for myoglobin.[50] Mottled extremities are treated conservatively, as improvement generally occurs spontaneously;[47] fasciotomy is rarely necessary.[41]

Approximately two thirds of lightning victims survive their injuries. However, many survivors sustain a variety of permanent sequelae such as cataracts, hearing loss, and paresis.[39]

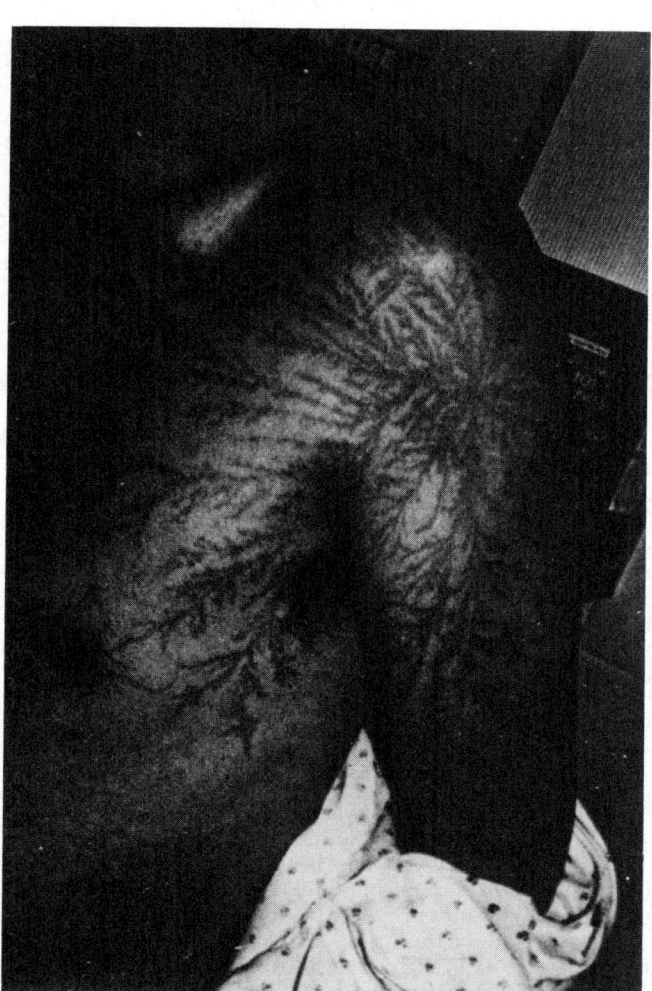

Figure 143–1. Fern-like lesions of lightning injury. (From Bartholome CW, Jacoby WD, Ramchand SC: Cutaneous manifestations of lightning injury. Arch Dermatol 111:1466–1468, 1975. Copyright 1975, American Medical Association.)

References

1. US Department of Health and Human Services: Vital Statistics of the United States. II, Part A. Washington, DC, US Government Printing Office, p 34, 1987.
2. DiVincenti FC, Moncrief JA, Pruitt BA Jr: Electrical injuries: A review of 65 cases. J Trauma 9:497, 1969.
3. Kay NRM, Boswick JA: The management of electrical injuries of the extremities. Surg Clin North Am 53:1459, 1973.
4. Baxter CR: Present concept in the management of major electrical burns. Surg Clin North Am 53:1459, 1973.
5. Sances A Jr, Larson SJ, Myklebust J, et al: Electrical injuries. Surg Gynecol Obstet 149:97, 1979.
6. Cooper MA: Electrical and lightning injuries. Emerg Med Clin North Am 2:489, 1984.
7. Sturim HS: The treatment of electrical burns. J Trauma 11:959, 1971.
8. Solem L, Fischer RP, Strate RG: The natural history of electrical injury. J Trauma 17:487, 1977.
9. Hunt JL, Sato RM, Baxter CR: Acute electric burns. Arch Surg 115:434, 1980.
10. Butler ED, Gant TD: Electrical injuries, with special reference to the upper extremities. A review of 182 cases. Am J Surg 134:95, 1977.
11. Holliman CJ, Saffle JR, Kravitz M, et al: Early surgical decompression in the management of electrical injuries. Am J Surg 144:733, 1982.
12. Pearl FL: Electric shock: Presentation of cases and review of literature. Arch Surg 27:227, 1933.
13. Hunt JL, Mason AD, Masterson TS, et al: The pathophysiology of acute electric injuries. J Trauma 16:335, 1976.
14. Hunt JL, McManus WF, Haney WP, et al: Vascular lesions in acute electric injuries. J Trauma 14:461, 1974.
15. Wilkinson C, Wood M: High voltage electric injury. Am J Surg 136:693, 1978.
16. Skoog T: Electrical injuries. J Trauma 10:816, 1970.
17. Robinson DW, Masters FW, Forrest WJ: Electrical burns: A review and analysis of 33 cases. J Surg 57:385, 1965.
18. Rouse RG, Dimick AR: The treatment of electrical injury compared to burn injury: A review of pathophysiology and comparison of patient management protocols. J Trauma 18:43, 1978.
19. Hartford CE, Ziffren SE: Electrical injury. J Trauma 11:331, 1979.
20. Hammond JS, Ward CG: High-voltage electrical injuries: Management and outcome of 60 cases. South Med J 81:1351, 1988.
21. Hammond J, Ward CG: Myocardial damage and electrical injuries: Significance of early elevation of CPK-MB isoenzymes. South Med J 79:414, 1986.
22. Jensen PJ, Thomson PE, Bagger JP, et al: Electrical injury causing ventricular arrhythmias. Br Heart J 57:279, 1987.
23. Purdue GF, Hunt JL: Electrocardiographic monitoring after electrical injury: Necessity or luxury. J Trauma 26:166, 1986.
24. McBride JW, Labrosse KR, McCoy HG, et al: Is serum creatine kinase–MB in electrically injured patients predictive of myocardial injury? JAMA 255:764, 1986.
25. Ku CS, Lin SL, Hsu TL, et al: Myocardial damage associated with electrical injury. Am Heart J 118:621, 1989.
26. Housinger TA, Green L, Shahangian S, et al: A prospective study of myocardial damage in electrical injuries. J Trauma 25:122, 1985.
27. Levine NS, Atkins A, McKeel DW, et al: Spinal cord injury following electrical accidents: Case report. J Trauma 15:459, 1975.
28. Christensen JA, Sherman RT, Balis GA, et al: Delayed neurologic injury secondary to high-voltage current, with recovery. J Trauma 20:166, 1980.
29. Farrell DF, Starr A: Delayed neurologic sequelae of electrical injuries. Neurology 18:601, 1968.
30. Haberal M: Electrical burns: A five-year experience—1985 Evans lecture. J Trauma 26:103, 1986.
31. Kobernick M: Electrical injuries: Pathophysiology and emergency management. Ann Emerg Med 11:633, 1982.
32. Williams DB, Karl RC: Intestinal injury associated with low-voltage electrocution. J Trauma 21:246, 1981.
33. Saffle RS, Crandall A, Warden GD: Cataract: A long-term complication of electrical injury. J Trauma 25:17, 1985.
34. Ornato JP: Special resuscitation situations: Near drowning, traumatic injury, electric shock, and hypothermia. Circulation 74(suppl IV):23, 1986.
35. Hunt J, Lewis S, Parkey R, et al: The use of technetium-99m stannous pyrophosphate scintigraphy to identify muscle damage in acute electric burns. J Trauma 19:409, 1979.
36. Quinby WC, Burke JF, Trelstad RL, et al: The use of microscopy as a guide to primary excision of high-tension electrical burns. J Trauma 18:423, 1978.
37. Dixon GF: The evaluation and management of electrical injuries. Crit Care Med 11:384, 1983.
38. Moncrief JA, Lindberg RB, Switzer WE, et al: The use of a topical sulfonamide in the control of burn wound sepsis. J Trauma 6:407, 1966.
39. Cooper MA: Lightning injuries: Prognostic signs for death. Ann Emerg Med 9:134, 1980.
40. Weigel EP: Lightning, the underrated killer. NOAA 6:2, 1976.
41. Apfelberg DB, Masters FW, Robinson DW: Pathophysiology and treatment of lightning injuries. J Trauma 14:453, 1974.
42. Taussig HB: "Death" from lightning—and the possibility of living again. Ann Intern Med 68:1345, 1968.
43. Andrews CJ, Darveniza M: Telephone-mediated lightning injury: An Australian survey. J Trauma 29:665, 1989.
44. Kleiner JP, Wilkin JH: Cardiac effects of lightning stroke. JAMA 240:2757, 1978.
45. Yost JW, Holmes FF: Myoglobinuria following lightning stroke. JAMA 228:1147, 1974.
46. Amy BW, McManus WF, Goodwin CW, et al: Lightning injury with survival in five patients. JAMA 253:243, 1985.
47. Strasser EJ, Davis RM, Menchey MJ: Lightning injuries. J Trauma 17:315, 1977.
48. Bartholome CW, Jacoby D, Ramchand SC: Cutaneous manifestations of lightning injury. Arch Dermatol 111:1466, 1975.
49. Peters WJ: Lightning injury. Can Med Assoc J 128:148, 1983.
50. Ghezzi KT: Lightning injuries: A unique treatment challenge. Postgrad Med 85:197, 1989.
51. Ravitch MM, Lane R, Safar P, et al: Lightning stroke. N Engl J Med 264:36, 1961.

CHAPTER 144

Anaphylaxis

Marilyn T. Haupt
Richard W. Carlson

Anaphylaxis refers to an acute, life-threatening, frequently explosive clinical response to environmental stimuli. In susceptible individuals, these stimuli elicit a complex sequence of cellular and biochemical events that produce life-threatening clinical sequelae. The cumulative effects of these events may lead to upper airway edema, bronchospasm, vascular permeability increases, acute respiratory failure, and circulatory shock. Untreated or improperly treated reactions are likely to be fatal, but prompt recognition and early treatment may be lifesaving. It is therefore essential that physicians be able to identify the acute presentation of anaphylaxis and to distinguish anaphylaxis from similar acute conditions. The immediate management of these events should proceed rapidly and automatically. After the initial management of patients with anaphylaxis, the critical care specialist must be prepared to manage the advanced manifestations using a rational therapeutic approach.

The list of agents producing anaphylaxis is extensive. Some of the more commonly implicated agents are cited in Table 144–1.

HISTORICAL BACKGROUND

The first record of anaphylaxis was believed to have been carved in wood in the form of hieroglyphics in 2641 BC (Fig. 144–1). Although there has been controversy about the interpretation of this writing, one theory is that King Menes of Egypt died suddenly after receiving a wasp sting.[1-3] A more basic understanding of anaphylaxis was imparted by the work of two French investigators, Portier and Richet.[4] While on a Mediterranean cruise, these physiologists demonstrated in the dog that, although a first injection of sea anemone venom was innocuous, a subsequent injection was fatal. They used the term *anaphylactique,* or reverse protection, to describe this reaction, and contrasted these reactions

TABLE 144–1

AGENTS COMMONLY IMPLICATED IN ANAPHYLACTIC AND ANAPHYLACTOID REACTIONS

Class	Agent
Antibiotics	Penicillin and penicillin analogues, cephalosporin, tetracyclines, erythromycin
Nonsteroidal anti-inflammatory agents	Salicylates, aminopyrine
Narcotic analgesics	Morphine, codeine, meprobamate
Local anesthetics	Procaine, lidocaine, cocaine
General anesthetics	Thiopental
Anesthetic adjuncts	Succinylcholine, tubocurarine
Blood products and antisera	Red blood cell, white blood cell, and platelet transfusions; gamma globulin; rabies, tetanus, and diphtheria antitoxin; snake and spider antivenom
Diagnostic agents	Iodinated radiographic contrast agents
Foods	Eggs, milk, nuts, legumes (peanuts, soybeans, kidney beans), fish, shellfish
Venoms	Bees, wasps, hornets, fire ants, scorpions
Enzymes and other biologicals	Acetylcysteine, pancreatic enzyme supplements, chymopapain
Extracts of potential allergens used in desensitization	Pollen, food, venoms
Chemotherapeutic agents	Cisplatin, cyclophosphamide, daunorubicin, methotrexate
Other drugs	Protamine, chlorpropamide, parenteral iron, iodides, thiazide diuretics

with the attenuated or tachyphylactic response that commonly protects subjects from reintroduced antigens.

Subsequent laboratory experiments and clinical studies further defined the histopathologic and gross anatomic changes associated with anaphylactic reactions as well as the complex sequence of immunologic, cellular, and biochemical events. More recent landmarks in the understanding of this acute allergic emergency include the identification and recognition of the role of the immunoglobulin (Ig) E,[5] the characterization of slow reacting substance of anaphylaxis into a group of mediators that are now known to be leukotrienes,[6, 7] and the characterization of granule- and membrane-derived mediators from mast cells and basophils.[8]

DEFINITIONS

The *classic anaphylactic response* refers to an IgE-mediated allergic response, which is also referred to as a type I reaction

according to the classification of Gell and Coombs. Type I reactions have also been referred to as reagin-dependent reactions, immediate hypersensitivity reactions, and cytotropic responses. The anaphylactic reaction has similarities to other type I reactions such as allergic rhinitis, hives and urticaria, and allergic asthma. In these reactions, an immunologic sequence of events involving antigen and IgE-specific effector cells (tissue-based mast cells and circulating basophils) results in the release of inflammatory mediators. However, unlike other type I reactions, anaphylaxis is generalized rather than restricted to local sites such as the nasal mucosa, the airways, and the skin. Agents that typically produce classic anaphylactic reactions include the penicillins, Hymenoptera stings (bees, wasps, hornets, and fire ants), and egg albumin.

Anaphylactoid reactions have clinical manifestations identical with those of classic anaphylactic reactions. However, a nonimmune release of mast cell– and basophil-derived mediators has been implicated in these disorders. Typical agents producing anaphylactoid reactions include radiographic contrast dyes, opiates, salicylates, and other nonsteroidal anti-inflammatory agents. Exercise has also been associated with an anaphylactoid clinical response.[9]

Idiopathic anaphylactoid reactions may also be clinically identical with anaphylactic reactions. However, a specific inciting agent as well as immune mediation has not been demonstrated. These events are rare and seldom fatal. Nighttime and postprandial occurrences are typical. Idiopathic anaphylactoid reactions typically occur in young adults who frequently have multiple allergies. Complete remissions are common.[10–12]

Factitious anaphylaxis refers to the factitious simulation of anaphylaxis. This illness is believed to represent a type of Munchausen's syndrome. In some instances, a response to an antigen such as bee venom is claimed by the patient. In other instances, the syndrome is confused with idiopathic anaphylaxis because an inciting agent is not identified.[13, 14]

INCIDENCE AND SIGNIFICANCE

The true incidence of anaphylactic and anaphylactoid reactions is difficult to determine because of their spontaneous, unpredictable nature and because of the failure to distinguish these reactions from other acute events such as vasovagal episodes and acute cardiac, pulmonary, and metabolic crises (Table 144–2). The most frequently reported anaphylactic episodes involve antibiotics, which are usually of the penicillin and cephalosporin β-lactam varieties.[15–19] Approximately 0.01% of patients have anaphylactic reactions to penicillin, and 9% of these reactions are fatal. It thus has been estimated that several hundred fatal reactions to penicillin take place annually in the United States.[15–17]

Anaphylaxis caused by the cephalosporins has also been described.[18, 19] In patients with a history of allergic reactions to penicillin, a 3 to 7% allergic reaction rate to cephalosporin is expected.[19] Precise information on the incidence of anaphylaxis in response to newer β-lactam antibiotics (e.g.,

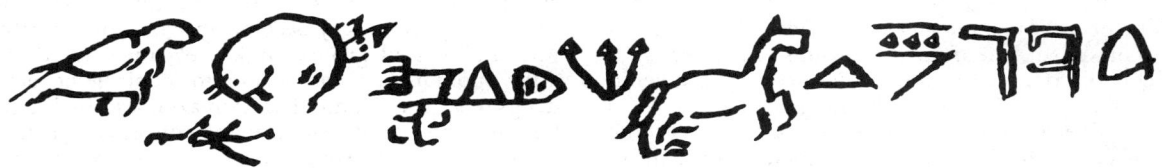

Figure 144–1. The death of the King of Egypt, Menes, is depicted in hieroglyphs carved in wood. Translation: "Fate Pierced [him] by a wasp, the King of the Two Crowns of Manshu. This board tablet set up of hanging wood is dedicated [to his memory]." (From Haupt MT, Carlson RW: Anaphylactic and anaphylactoid reactions. In: Shoemaker WC, Ayres S, Grenvik A, et al [eds]: The Society of Critical Care Medicine: Textbook of Critical Care. 2nd ed. Philadelphia, WB Saunders, p 993, 1989.)

TABLE 144-2
CONDITIONS THAT SIMULATE ANAPHYLACTIC AND ANAPHYLACTOID REACTIONS
Vasovagal episodes
Acute pulmonary events
Asthmatic attacks
Pulmonary edema
Pulmonary embolus
Spontaneous pneumothorax
Foreign body aspiration
Acute cardiac events
Supraventricular and ventricular tachycardias
Acute myocardial infarction
Acute drug overdose
Insulin shock
Carcinoid syndrome attacks

aztreonam and imipenem) awaits additional clinical experience with these drugs. However, extensive in vivo cross-reactivity with penicillins characterizes the bicyclic carbapenem drugs, which are represented by imipenem.[19] Therefore, a significant incidence of anaphylaxis from this class of antibiotics can be anticipated in patients who have had allergic reactions to penicillin. In contrast, the monocyclic β-lactam antibiotics represented by aztreonam show no cross-reactivity with penicillin.[19] The incidence of anaphylaxis in penicillin-allergic patients receiving these antibiotics is thus expected to be minimal.

Approximately 200 to 800 deaths per year from acute reactions to iodinated radiographic contrast agents have been estimated.[20] Most of these reactions are characterized by typical symptoms of anaphylaxis.[21] Although these reactions characterize less than 2% of individuals taking these agents, the high mortality rate is attributed to the large number of contrast agents used each year.[22]

Insect stings account for more deaths resulting from anaphylaxis in the United States than all other types of venoms. Annually, approximately 60 to 80 deaths are reported from insect stings. However, many deaths are probably unreported or fail to be identified as caused by insect stings. Most fatal stings are caused by insects from the order Hymenoptera, which includes bees, wasps, hornets, and fire ants.[23] Fire ants are insects imported from South America to the United States that have proliferated in the rural and urban portions of the Southern Gulf states. These insects have been responsible for a significant number of immediate hypersensitivity reactions. Fire ants are aggressive and sting up to 58% of residents yearly in a some areas. It has been estimated that anaphylaxis occurs in up to 1% of fire ant stings.[24]

Snake bites probably account for approximately a dozen deaths per year in the United States. Snake venom poisoning produces clinical signs and symptoms that are similar to those of anaphylaxis, especially from pit vipers (rattlesnakes, moccasins, and copperheads). Often, however, patients experience additional problems related to the variety of enzymes, proteins, and peptides contained in the venoms. These problems may include local tissue necrosis, coagulopathies, hemolysis, and neurologic transmission defects.[25, 26] Anaphylactic reactions may also be induced by antivenin used in the treatment of venom poisoning.

Although adverse reactions to food are frequent, the incidence of type I allergic reactions to foods is difficult to ascertain because many reported reactions are probably nonallergic in nature. However, allergic reactions to food have been estimated to characterize 1 to 2% of adverse food reactions in children.[27] Lower estimates for adult food hy-persensitivity have been suggested.[28] A small number of these allergic reactions may have features of systemic anaphylaxis.

Anaphylactic reactions, as well as other type I allergic reactions, are characteristically observed in susceptible, genetically predisposed individuals. The evolution of these complex IgE-mediated reactions has been a subject of considerable speculation. A popular theory is that a system of localized IgE-mediated reactions to parasitic antigens conveyed a survival advantage to individuals exposed to parasites. Several studies and observations support this view. In one study, children infected with a wide variety of helminthic parasites exhibited elevated serum IgE concentrations.[29] In another study, humans infected with *Ascaris* worms were demonstrated to have decreased worm burdens if they were capable of synthesizing large quantities of IgE.[30] In a laboratory study, rats infected with *Trichinella* larvae harbored more larvae if treated with anti-IgE than did untreated controls.[31] In addition, the sites of IgE synthesis demonstrated in laboratory subjects correspond to the sites of entry of many parasites. These sites include the lymphoid tissue of the respiratory tract, gastrointestinal tract, and skin, typical sites of parasitic entry and infestation. Eosinophils, which migrate to the site of antigen introduction in anaphylaxis, elaborate mediators that have specific toxicity to parasitic components.

These observations suggest that, when localized, IgE-mediated reactions may be important in combating parasitic antigens as well as other antigens. Anaphylaxis, a systemic reaction, may thus represent a failure to restrict the IgE-mediated reactions to local areas. This failure may be genetically determined or acquired. The resultant generalized release of mediators, triggered by the IgE interaction with antigens, mast cells, and basophils, leads to increases in vascular permeability, vasodilation, and impaired gas exchange. These effects are clearly decompensatory and threaten survival.

SEQUENCE OF EVENTS LEADING TO ANAPHYLAXIS

Immunologic Events

The sequence of immunologic events leading to the classic form of anaphylaxis is initiated when an antigen, to which an individual has been previously sensitized, is reintroduced. At least several weeks is required between the initial and subsequent exposure to antigen for a clinically significant reaction to develop. The site of reintroduction may be the skin or the respiratory or gastrointestinal tracts. Introduction of antigen by intramuscular and intravenous routes may characterize the administration of drugs or venoms.

The antigens that produce classic anaphylaxis are usually small bivalent proteins with molecular weights of 10,000 to 70,000. Haptens, small chemicals that combine with a host protein, may also function as antigens.[32] The reactive anhydrides or quinones found in industrial chemicals as well as the β-lactam group of the penicillins and cephalosporins appear to function as haptens by directly conjugating to protein. Penicillin may become antigenic by directly reacting with amino acid groups or by reacting with these groups after spontaneous conversion to penicillenic acid. Other drugs (e.g., acetaminophen, isoniazid, and hydralazine) may become haptens after enzymatic conversion in the liver or in other organs.[33] Anaphylactic reactions to polysaccharides (e.g., dextrans and hydroxyethyl starches) have also been described but are infrequent.

After reintroduction into the host, the antigen encounters IgE, which was previously synthesized by plasma cells after

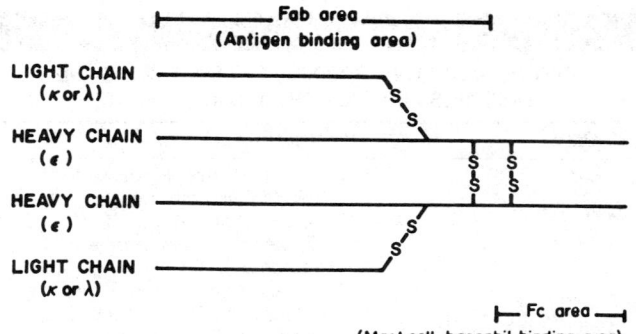

Figure 144-2. An IgE molecule, composed of four polypeptide chains linked by disulfide bonds, is illustrated. The heavy chains, or epsilon (ε) chains, are unique to IgE. The light chains may be kappa (κ) or lambda (λ) chains and are also characteristic of other immunoglobulins. Antigen binding takes place at the Fab area. The Fc area binds to mast cells or basophils. (From Haupt MT, Carlson RW: Anaphylactic and anaphylactoid reactions. In: Shoemaker WC, Ayres S, Grenvik A, et al [eds]: The Society of Critical Care Medicine: Textbook of Critical Care. 2nd ed. Philadelphia, WB Saunders, p 993, 1989.)

the initial encounter. IgE, like other immunoglobulins, is composed of two heavy chains and two light chains linked by disulfide bonds (Fig. 144–2). The Fab portion of the IgE molecule recognizes and binds the antigen. The Fc portion of the molecule binds reversibly to high-affinity receptors on the surface of mast cells and basophils (Fig. 144–3).

The combination of IgE with antigen sets the stage for a sequence of events leading to the release of biochemical mediators that produce the clinical syndrome of anaphylaxis. The bivalent antigen, by cross-bridging two IgE molecules, facilitates the approximation of Fc surface receptor areas on mast cells and basophils. This cross-bridging reaction triggers the release of mediators from intracellular granules and from membrane-based phospholipids (see Fig. 144–3).

An immunologic basis for anaphylaxis without mediation by IgE has also been described. Immunoglobulins of the IgG class may combine with antigens to produce an antigen-antibody complex, which activates complement. Activated complement results in the generation of C3a and C5a. These components are called anaphylatoxins because they stimulate the release of mediators from mast cells and produce clinical symptoms typical of anaphylaxis. These IgG-mediated reactions are classified as type III reactions according to the classification of Gell and Coombs and have previously been termed Arthus' reactions. IgA-deficient individuals may exhibit these reactions after blood transfusions. When blood is transfused, anti-IgA (of the IgG class) to the IgA in the blood product is formed. The anti-IgA–IgA combination produced after a subsequent transfusion leads to the activation of complement, generation of C3a and C5a, and anaphylactic symptoms. Because approximately 1 in 700 individuals is IgA deficient and 40% have class-specific anti-IgA, a sizable number are susceptible to anaphylactic reactions to blood transfusion.[32, 34] Anaphylaxis to protamine is also thought to be an IgG-mediated response.[35–37]

Anaphylaxis as well as other type I allergic reactions may be followed by late-phase reactions. These reactions may occur from 6 to 12 hours after the immediate reaction and are characterized by the infiltration of a variety of cells into areas of antigen introduction. The cells include polymorphonuclear cells as well as mast cells and basophils. A second wave of mediator release ensues and may lead to a recurrence or exacerbation of anaphylactic symptoms.[38–40]

Nonimmunologic Events in Anaphylactoid Reactions

It is currently believed that nonimmunologic stimuli initiate anaphylactoid reactions. The mechanisms leading to the nonimmunologic release of mediators, however, remain poorly defined. There is emerging evidence that several pathways from stimulus to mediator release may characterize the anaphylactoid response.

In some reactions, the surface receptors of mast cells and basophils appear to be directly activated by the offending agent. A direct stimulation of these cells is believed to initiate the anaphylactoid response to iodinated radiographic contrast agents, opiates, curare, tubocurarine, and highly charged polyanionic antibiotics. Physical stimuli (heat, cold, exercise) and hyperosmolar stimuli (radiographic contrast agents, mannitol, 50% dextrose) may also produce anaphylaxis by directly stimulating mast cells and basophils.

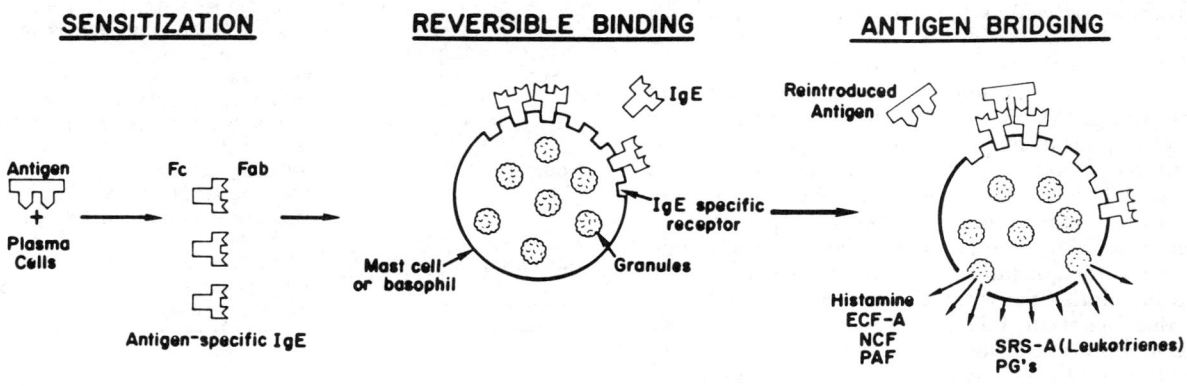

Figure 144-3. The sequence of events leading to mediator release. The initial exposure of antigen to plasma cells is termed sensitization and leads to the synthesis of antigen specific IgE. The Fc portion of the IgE molecule binds reversibly to receptors on mast cells and basophils. When antigen is reintroduced, it cross-links two cell-bound IgE molecules (also termed antigen bridging). This bridging initiates a sequence of biochemical events in the cell leading to the release of mediators from granules and from the cell wall. ECF-A = eosinophil chemotactic factor of anaphylaxis; NCF = neutrophil chemotactic factor; PAF = platelet-activating factor; SRS-A = slow reacting substance of anaphylaxis; PG's = prostaglandins. (From Haupt MT, Carlson RW: Anaphylactic and anaphylactoid reactions. In: Shoemaker WC, Ayres S, Grenvik A, et al [eds]: The Society of Critical Care Medicine: Textbook of Critical Care. 2nd ed. Philadelphia, WB Saunders, p 993, 1989.)

Aspirin and other nonsteroidal anti-inflammatory drugs are thought to produce anaphylactoid reactions through the inhibition of cyclooxygenase. It has been postulated that this inhibition facilitates the production of lipoxygenase-derived mediators. These mediators, known as leukotrienes (LTs), produce bronchospasm and vascular permeability defects that are typical of anaphylaxis. However, this theory does not account for the observation that most individuals treated with aspirin and other nonsteroidal anti-inflammatory drugs fail to exhibit anaphylactic symptoms in spite of drug–induced cyclooxygenase blockade. Other theories to account for aspirin sensitivity have been proposed and include the direct stimulation of mast cells, platelets, or eosinophils and the direct activation of the complement cascade.[41] Up to 50% of patients with sensitivity to aspirin exhibit sensitivity to the yellow dye tartrazine, which is frequently used as food coloring (FD&C Yellow No. 5).[42] Although the chemical structure of tartrazine is similar to that of several nonsteroidal anti-inflammatory drugs, the mechanism for anaphylaxis to this chemical also remains unclear.[42]

Cellular Characteristics, Actions, and Interactions

Mast cells and basophils are important components of the anaphylactic response because of their role in the release of biochemical mediators that produce both local and systemic abnormalities. There are characteristic differences between these cells. Mast cell precursors can be found in embryonic tissue and the thymus. Basophil precursors are found in the bone marrow. Mast cells are more abundant than basophils and reside in the connective tissue of submucosal and subcutaneous tissues. Basophils are usually found circulating in the blood but have also been identified in the nasal and bronchial mucosa in patients with hypersensitivity disease of the respiratory tract.[43]

In spite of these differences in origin and location, major functional differences between mast cells and basophils have not been identified. The cells have many structural and biochemical similarities. In addition to having specific receptors for the Fc portion of IgE, both cells have granules that bind basic dyes. These granules contain histamine, a major mediator in anaphylaxis, as well as histidine decarboxylase, an enzyme responsible for the synthesis of histamine. Histamine and many other mediators released from these cells initiate the anaphylactic response. The mediators are derived from the granules as well as the membranes of these cells (Table 144–3).

Eosinophils are bone marrow–derived leukocytes with acidophilic granules. They migrate to the site of allergen introduction in anaphylaxis as well as in other type I allergic reactions. Eosinophils dwell primarily in tissues but may also be found in the blood. A variety of chemotactic factors attract eosinophils, including mast cell– and basophil-derived chemotactic factors, antigen-antibody complexes, complement, and histamine. The granules of eosinophils contain a variety of mediators, including the cationic proteins, which are toxic to helminthic parasites. Eosinophils also elaborate substances that inactivate LTs and histamine.[43–45] The role played by eosinophils in acute allergic emergencies remains unclear. Although the inactivation of LTs and histamine may dampen the inflammatory response associated with anaphylaxis, the antiparasitic properties of eosinophilic granular proteins may exacerbate local tissue injury.

Platelets and polymorphonuclear neutrophils respond to the release of mast cell– and basophil-derived chemotactic factors, as well as to the tissue injury produced during the anaphylactic response. These cells also release an abundant variety of inflammatory mediators. The significance and extent of the participation of these cells in anaphylaxis

remains poorly defined. However, polymorphonuclear neutrophils may be responsible, in part, for recurrent or late-phase anaphylactic episodes.

Primary Mediators of Anaphylaxis

Mediators derived from mast cell and basophils are often termed primary mediators to distinguish them from secondary mediators. Secondary mediators are released from

TABLE 144–3

PRIMARY MEDIATORS PRODUCED BY MAST CELLS AND BASOPHILS AND THEIR PHYSIOLOGIC EFFECTS

Mediator	Physiologic Effect
Histamine	Histamine H_1 receptor stimulation
	Bronchial smooth muscle contraction
	Increased vascular permeability
	Cardiac arrhythmias
	Increased mucus secretion
	Vasoactive effects (vasodilation, vasoconstriction)
	Histamine H_2 receptor stimulation
	Increased vascular permeability
	Increased mucus and gastric acid secretion
	Activation of inhibitory lymphocytes
	Histamine H_3 receptor stimulation
	Inhibition of histamine synthesis and release
Platelet-activating factor	Increased vascular permeability
	Bronchospasm
	Aggregation and activation of platelets
	Attracts neutrophils and eosinophils
Eosinophil chemotactic factors	Attract eosinophils
Neutrophil chemotactic factors	Attract neutrophils
Arachidonic acid metabolites	
Prostaglandin D_2	Bronchoconstriction
	Potentiates leukocyte migration
Prostaglandin E_2	Bronchodilation
Prostaglandin $F_{2\alpha}$	Bronchoconstriction
LTC_4, LTD_4, LTE_4	Bronchoconstriction
	Increased vascular permeability
LTB_4	Attracts neutrophils and eosinophils
Enzymes	
Hydrolytic enzymes	Degradation of parasitic and host tissue
Proteases	Degradation of parasitic and host tissue
	Interact with complement components, the coagulation cascade, and the kinin system
Oxidative enzymes	
Superoxide dismutase	Inactivates O_2^- and associated cytotoxic effects
Peroxidase	Inactivates cytotoxic effects of H_2O_2
	May inactivate LTC_4
Heparin	Anticoagulant activity
	Anticomplement activity
	May assist in the repair of injured tissues
Adenosine	Bronchospasm
	Regulates mast cell degranulation
Serotonin	Vasoactive effects

other leukocytes and from cascading biochemical pathways after primary mediator release. Primary mediators may be further classified into preformed mediators, which are stored in the intracellular granules, and newly synthesized mediators, which are derived from the metabolism of arachidonic acid, a cell membrane–derived phospholipid. The physiologic characteristics of the major primary mediators are listed in Table 144–3.

Histamine is a primary granule-derived mediator that has been studied extensively. Histamine stimulates both histamine H_1 and H_2 receptors located on the surfaces of vascular and bronchial smooth muscle cells. Stimulation of histamine H_1 receptors causes precapillary arteriolar dilation, contraction of postcapillary venules, and the formation of intercellular gaps between capillary endothelial cells. These changes, by increasing capillary hydrostatic pressure and permeability, encourage the movement of plasma from the intravascular space to the interstitium. Histamine H_1 receptor stimulation is also associated with bronchial smooth muscle contraction. Histamine H_2 receptor stimulation is associated with vasodilation, enhanced mucus secretion, increase in heart rate and myocardial contractility, inhibition of eosinophils, increased gastric acid secretion, and inhibition of T cells. The vasoactive and cardiac effects of histamine H_2 receptor stimulation are believed to play an important role in the clinical manifestations of anaphylaxis. Arachidonic acid metabolism via the lipoxygenase pathway leads to the LTs, a family of potent mediators formerly known as slow reacting substance of anaphylaxis. LTC_4, LTD_4, and LTE_4, in addition to the intermediate lipoxygenase products hydroxyeicosatetraenoic acid and hydroperoxyeicosatetraenoic acid, are potent vascular permeability agents and mediators of bronchoconstriction. LTs may be more important than histamine in producing the clinical manifestations of anaphylaxis. They have been estimated to be 1000 times more potent than histamine in producing bronchospasm. Another LT, LTB_4, has eosinophil and neutrophil chemotactic properties.

Arachidonic acid metabolism via the cyclooxygenase pathway leads to the production of prostaglandins D_2 and $F_{2\alpha}$, which have bronchoconstrictive effects. Prostaglandin E_2 is also produced and is associated with bronchodilation. The relative contributions of these opposing effects of prostaglandins in anaphylaxis are unknown.

Additional primary mediators modulate the cellular response in anaphylaxis and have hydrolytic, proteolytic, and cytotoxic activity. A description of these activities is provided in Table 144–3.

Regulation of Primary Mediator Release

The release of primary mediators from mast cells and basophils is an energy-requiring process, which may be modified by intracellular levels of adenosine $3',5'$-cyclic monophosphate (cAMP), guanosine $3',5'$-cyclic monophosphate (cGMP), calcium and other bivalent cations, and agents that affect microtubular function. Pharmacologic agents that favorably alter the levels of these modulators are used in the treatment of anaphylaxis (Table 144–4).

Agents that increase intracellular levels of cAMP, for example, inhibit the release of mediators and are associated with clinical improvement. These include beta$_2$-agonists such as epinephrine and metaproterenol, which increase cAMP by stimulating adenylate cyclase. Methylxanthines such as aminophylline and theophylline increase intracellular cAMP levels by inhibiting phosphodiesterase, although experimental data suggested that this effect is minimal at therapeutic concentrations.[46]

cGMP antagonizes the action of cAMP. Therefore, phar-

TABLE 144–4
PHARMACOLOGIC MODULATION OF MEDIATOR RELEASE
Inhibit release
Beta-adrenergic drugs (↑ cAMP)
Phosphodiesterase inhibitors (↑ cAMP)
Anticholinergic drugs (↓ cGMP)
Enhance release
Beta-blockers (↓ cAMP)
Alpha-adrenergic drugs (↓ cAMP)
Cholinergic drugs (↑ cGMP)

macologic agents that decrease intracellular cGMP levels inhibit mediator release. Anticholinergic agents decrease cGMP levels and may have a role in the treatment of anaphylaxis.

Mediator release from mast cells and basophils is associated with an influx of calcium and may be inhibited by calcium channel–blocking agents. Other bivalent cations such as magnesium and manganese may also enhance mediator release.[40]

Secondary Mediators

The release of primary mediators from mast cells and basophils sets the stage for involvement by secondary mediators. Secondary mediators of anaphylaxis include products of enzyme-dependent, cascading biochemical pathways. In addition, the products of neutrophils, platelets, and eosinophils activated by mast cell– and basophil-derived chemotactic factors function as secondary mediators.

The activated complement system generates highly reactive mediators with a variety of pathophysiologic effects. Activation of both the classic and alternative pathways has been observed in anaphylaxis. The anaphylatoxins C3a and C5a are potent mediators, which contract smooth muscle; increase vascular permeability; attract neutrophils, macrophages, and monocytes; and injure cellular membranes. C3a and C5a also stimulate additional mediator release from mast cells and basophils.[47, 48] Complement components C6 through C9 also cause further membrane damage. C3 binds to receptors on eosinophils and may modulate the effector functions of these cells.[49]

The coagulation cascade and fibrinolytic systems are activated during anaphylaxis when factor XII (Hageman's factor) is exposed to the subendothelial collagen of injured vessels. Activation of these cascades produces intravascular coagulation and additional tissue injury. Activated factor XII also stimulates the kinin system to produce bradykinin, a potent mediator of vascular permeability.

Pathophysiologic Effects of Mediators

Although the mediators released and synthesized during an anaphylactic crisis have a variety of actions, the acute clinical presentation of this disorder suggests that the major effects are due to sudden increases in vascular permeability, systemic arteriolar vasodilation, and bronchial smooth muscle contraction. Autopsies in fatal cases of anaphylaxis reveal edema of the lungs, the larynx, the epiglottis, the skin, and the viscera. In one study, 36 of 40 fatalities exhibited gross pulmonary congestion, with fluid-filled alveoli apparent on light microscopy.[50] Another autopsy study revealed that almost half of anaphylactic fatalities exhibited acute pulmonary emphysema with hyperdistended alveoli and thinning of alveolar septae.[51] Because of the association of acute pulmonary emphysema with upper airway edema, especially involving the larynx, these anaphylactic deaths appear to result from complete upper airway obstruction.[51] Alveolar rupture caused by forced exhalation against the obstruction and inability to ventilate may thus be preterminal events.

Although cardiac dysfunction, especially dysrhythmias, reduced contractility, and myocardial ischemia and necrosis have characterized anaphylaxis in laboratory animals,[52] evidence of cardiac abnormalities in the autopsies of fatal cases of human anaphylaxis appear to be minimal.[50, 51] Nevertheless, dysrhythmias, myocardial infarction, and coronary artery vasospasm have been documented in isolated instances.[52] Although reduced cardiac contractility may characterize the effects of histamine and LTs on the myocardium in laboratory studies, the majority of patients with anaphylaxis show no evidence of impaired cardiac function as assessed by routine clinical tests.[52–54]

CLINICAL AND HEMODYNAMIC FEATURES

The clinical presentation of anaphylaxis is highly variable. However, most patients have severe rapidly progressive symptoms after exposure to antigen. The symptoms may be modified by the portal of entry for the antigen as well as by the rate of absorption and degree of hypersensitivity to the antigen. Accordingly, gastrointestinal symptoms may precede more severe systemic symptoms after ingestion of an antigen. These symptoms may include nausea, vomiting, abdominal cramps, and diarrhea. Inhalation of an antigen may produce nasal coryza, a sensation of tightness or a lump in the throat, hoarseness, stridor, wheezing, and dyspnea. Introduction of antigen through the skin may produce local pruritus, urticaria, and swelling before the development of systemic symptoms.

The most life-threatening reactions are usually explosive, often within minutes of exposure to the antigen. Patients with these reactions may describe a feeling of impending doom before more defined symptoms develop. Generalized cutaneous abnormalities may be observed and include erythema, urticaria, and flushing. Swelling of the periorbital and perioral areas is characteristic. Upper and lower airway abnormalities are frequently observed and pose a major threat to life. Swelling of the posterior pharynx, the uvula, the tonsils, and the vocal cords may develop rapidly. Auscultation may reveal generalized wheezing and prolongation of expiration. Auscultatory and radiographic signs of pulmonary edema may be present and are often severe. Signs of circulatory shock, including progressive hypotension, oliguria, and lactic acidosis, emerge as plasma continues to escape the circulation. In some instances, such as the intravenous injection of venom, circulatory shock may develop without preceding cutaneous and respiratory abnormalities. The clinical features of anaphylaxis may respond quickly to treatment or, in the most severe cases, may last for several hours to several days. An initial favorable response to treatment may be followed by a late-phase reaction, a recurrence of symptoms approximately 6 to 12 hours after the initial reaction.[38, 40]

Hemodynamic descriptions of human anaphylaxis are limited to the detailed studies of a few cases. The loss of circulating plasma volume is a characteristic feature and may be associated with hemoconcentration, hypotension, tachycardia, decreased cardiac filling pressures, and decreased cardiac output.[55, 56] Vasodilation may contribute to the reduction in venous return and cardiac output and is associated with decreased systemic vascular resistance. Lactic acidosis emerges and has been attributed to the activation of anaerobic metabolic pathways.[57] Changes in myocardial contractility are minimal in human anaphylaxis when assessed in studies employing routine hemodynamic monitoring. Most patients with anaphylaxis respond favorably to fluid therapy and do not require inotropic support.[55–59] In a few instances, reduced contractility was observed in association with myocardial ischemia and infarction.[60–65] Some of these adverse cardiac effects have been associated with epinephrine administration but have also been noted before the administration of this drug.[60–65]

Laboratory studies provide more detailed descriptions of the hemodynamic features of anaphylaxis, although there is considerable variation, which is dependent on the type of animal model utilized. Nevertheless, hemodynamic characteristics in primate models of anaphylaxis are the most similar to those in humans and may reflect the clinical changes observed in anaphylaxis in humans. After antigenic challenge in primates, a transient increase in cardiac output is observed and is followed by decreases in arterial pressure, right and left ventricular filling pressures, and peripheral vascular resistance.[65] The transient increase in cardiac output has been attributed to left ventricular unloading from vasodilation and/or an increase in cardiac contractility. Elevated plasma levels of epinephrine, norepinephrine, and histamine have been observed in laboratory animals as well as humans[67–69] and may contribute to this increase in contractility. When hypotension and shock become established, cardiac output decreases because of a decrease in venous return from decreased plasma volume. In the canine model of anaphylaxis, splanchnic vasodilation and pooling of blood contributes to the decrease in venous return.[70, 71]

Pulmonary edema fluid sampled from the airway of patients with anaphylaxis is characterized by albumin concentrations and oncotic pressures that are virtually identical with plasma values. An association of pulmonary edema with low pulmonary arterial wedge pressures is also characteristic.[55] These findings suggest that the pulmonary edema in anaphylaxis is noncardiogenic and secondary to increased microvascular permeability. Transient pulmonary hypertension and increased pulmonary vascular resistance have been observed in primates immediately after antigen challenge.[67] It is not known, however, whether this effect characterizes human anaphylaxis.

In summary, the major hemodynamic characteristics of human anaphylaxis are determined by a decrease in vascular tone as well as an increase in vascular permeability. These effects lead to the venous pooling of blood and loss of circulating plasma volume. The lung responds to the permeability effects of mediators with the development of noncardiogenic pulmonary edema. Changes in cardiac contractility are usually not observed in human anaphylaxis using routine hemodynamic measurements, although elevated plasma catecholamine and histamine levels suggest that contractility may be increased. Infrequently, however, reduced contractility may characterize patients who exhibit signs of myocardial ischemia or infarction, especially in association with epinephrine therapy.

MANAGEMENT

Initial Management

A brief initial assessment of the patient with suspected anaphylaxis is important because immediate therapeutic interventions are often required. Because a variety of conditions simulate anaphylaxis (see Table 144–2), appropriate evaluations should be quickly performed. One of the conditions most frequently confused with anaphylaxis is the vasovagal episode. A bradycardic rhythm, pale skin, and diaphoresis in an acutely ill patient are suggestive of a vasovagal attack and contrast with the tachycardic, flushed appearance typical of anaphylaxis.

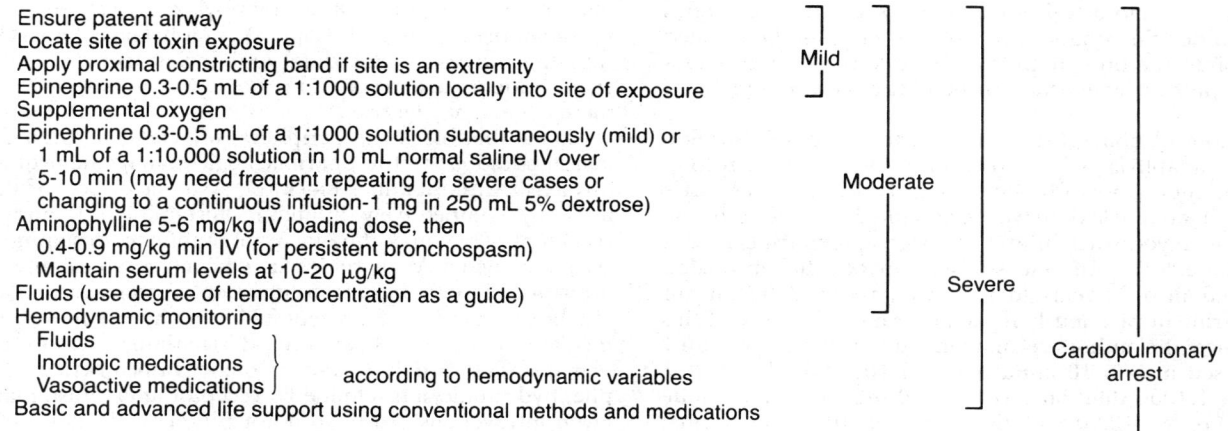

Ensure patent airway
Locate site of toxin exposure
Apply proximal constricting band if site is an extremity
Epinephrine 0.3-0.5 mL of a 1:1000 solution locally into site of exposure — Mild
Supplemental oxygen
Epinephrine 0.3-0.5 mL of a 1:1000 solution subcutaneously (mild) or
   1 mL of a 1:10,000 solution in 10 mL normal saline IV over
   5-10 min (may need frequent repeating for severe cases or — Moderate
   changing to a continuous infusion-1 mg in 250 mL 5% dextrose)
Aminophylline 5-6 mg/kg IV loading dose, then
   0.4-0.9 mg/kg min IV (for persistent bronchospasm)
   Maintain serum levels at 10-20 μg/kg — Severe
Fluids (use degree of hemoconcentration as a guide)
Hemodynamic monitoring
   Fluids
   Inotropic medications } according to hemodynamic variables — Cardiopulmonary arrest
   Vasoactive medications
Basic and advanced life support using conventional methods and medications

Figure 144-4. Initial treatment of anaphylactic and anaphylactoid reactions. See text for a detailed description of initial and follow-up management.

When a diagnosis of anaphylaxis is secure or reasonably certain, the treatment should proceed rapidly (Fig. 144–4). This includes (1) the provision of a patent airway, (2) the removal of toxin at the site of introduction and/or an attempt to delay the systemic absorption of toxin, (3) the establishment of intravenous access for fluid therapy, and (4) the initiation of pharmacologic support with epinephrine. A team approach is important in severe cases of anaphylaxis because these initial interventions must proceed rapidly and, if possible, simultaneously.

Admission to the hospital is necessary for all serious cases of anaphylaxis. The hospital should be equipped with personnel skilled in advanced airway management and in advanced treatment guided by hemodynamic monitoring. Hospitalization should not be precluded for patients with severe symptoms who exhibit a favorable response to therapy. These patients are susceptible to late-phase reactions, and severe symptoms may occur up 12 hours after the initial attack. While in the hospital, the patient should be monitored for signs of circulatory shock and respiratory failure. Accordingly, blood pressure, urine output, and heart and respiratory rates should be evaluated at frequent intervals.

The electrocardiogram should be monitored continuously during the initial period because anaphylaxis has been associated with serious dysrhythmias and cardiac ischemia. These cardiac problems may also be secondary to drugs used to treat anaphylaxis, including epinephrine, other catecholamines such as dopamine, dobutamine, and levarterenol, beta-agonistic bronchodilators, and phosphodiesterase inhibitors such as aminophylline and theophylline.

When signs of circulatory shock and impaired pulmonary gas exchange develop, advanced monitoring with intra-arterial and pulmonary arterial catheters is required. As with other types of circulatory shock, fluid therapy, inotropic and vasopressor therapy, and ventilatory support are adjusted according to hemodynamic measurements to maintain organ perfusion, pulmonary gas exchange, and systemic oxygen delivery.

Close attention to the airway is important. Frequent assessment for hoarseness, stridor, and upper airway obstruction is required for patients who do not have their airway protected with an endotracheal tube. If consciousness is altered, the head and neck should be positioned so that the airway is not obstructed by the tongue. If stridor caused by laryngeal or upper respiratory tract edema develops, endotracheal intubation should be attempted. Because intubation may be difficult in the presence of laryngeal edema, skilled personnel capable of performing an emergency cricothyrotomy should be available.

If spontaneous ventilation is uncertain or impaired, mechanical ventilation should be implemented. Supplemental oxygen should be provided as needed. Positive end-expiratory pressure is frequently necessary when hypoxemia, pulmonary edema, and reduced lung compliance develop.

The site of antigen introduction should be identified whenever possible. If the patient is unconscious or unaware of the site of antigen introduction, a thorough search of skin surfaces should proceed. Retained stingers from Hymenoptera may be found and necessitate complete and immediate removal. If the site of envenomization is an extremity, a constricting band should be applied to delay the absorption of the venom. This band should be sufficiently tight to delay venous absorption of venom but should not interrupt arterial flow to the distal extremity. A dilute solution of epinephrine (1:10,000 solution) may be injected locally to retard systemic absorption of venom through alpha-adrenergic–mediated vasoconstriction. Sequestered snake venom may be removed with the use of suction kits or by surgical techniques. However, these removal practices are controversial and may actually enhance the absorption of venom and exacerbate local tissue injury. Thorough washing of the skin should follow exposure to antigen that has contacted the skin surface.

The mainstay of pharmacologic therapy for anaphylaxis is epinephrine. This drug is of proven efficacy in reversing bronchoconstriction and hypotension associated with anaphylaxis. The beta-adrenergic effects of epinephrine inhibit mediator release by increasing intracellular levels of cAMP. In addition, beta-adrenergic stimulation decreases bronchospasm, increases myocardial contractility, and increases heart rate. The alpha-adrenergic properties of epinephrine are associated with constriction of systemic arterioles. This property of epinephrine leads to an elevation of diastolic pressure and may thus increase reduced coronary flow.

Medical personnel should be aware that two dilutions of epinephrine are commonly available: a 1:1000 and a 1:10,000 dilution. Epinephrine in the 1:10,000 dilution is available in the form of prefilled syringes for rapid intravenous injection and is frequently employed for cardiopulmonary resuscitation. Most authors recommend that, for mild cases, 0.3 to 0.5 mL of the 1:1000 solution (0.3 to 0.5 mg) be given subcutaneously. This dose may be repeated at 5- to 10-minute intervals if symptoms do not improve. For severe cases of anaphylaxis, a dilute solution of epinephrine should be given intravenously (see next paragraph for dose and concentration). When conventional intravenous access routes are difficult to obtain, alternative routes should be explored. Epinephrine may be administered intravenously through the femoral vein or through a vein in the venous plexus under the tongue. Epinephrine may also be instilled directly into the bronchopulmonary tree through an endotracheal tube or by injection through the cricothyroid membrane.

The dose of epinephrine for intravenous administration in severe anaphylaxis is controversial. Most authors recommend an initial dose of 0.3 to 0.5 mg. However, several case reports of anaphylaxis have documented cardiac ischemia and acute myocardial infarction after epinephrine in this dose range.[61, 64, 68] In one study, a myocardial infarction developed in a 34-year-old man who received 0.5 mg of epinephrine intravenously for anaphylaxis.[64] Because of this experience, the authors recommended a starting dose of 0.1 mg infused in 5 to 10 minutes at a 1:100,000 dilution (0.1 mL of a 1:1000 dilution mixed in 10 mL of normal saline or 1 mL of a 1:10,000 dilution mixed in 10 mL of normal saline).[64] This cautious starting dose may need to be repeated at frequent intervals if symptoms do not improve. Alternatively, a continuous infusion of epinephrine may be started after the initial dose of epinephrine. The infusion (1 mg in 250 mL of 5% dextrose in water) is similar to infusions recommended in advanced cardiac life support protocols. The infusion may be started at 1 μg/min and increased to 4 μg/min if symptoms persist.[64, 72] The cardiac rhythm should be monitored in all patients who receive epinephrine.

Fluid therapy is also an important component of the initial treatment of anaphylaxis. Fluids effectively reverse the intravascular volume deficits produced by increased vascular permeability. They also counteract the effects of mediator-induced vasodilation by increasing venous return. One approach to fluid therapy is to replace estimated plasma losses with a plasma substitute. Colloid fluids such as 5% human serum albumin or 6% hydroxyethyl starch are rational choices because they mimic the oncotic properties and electrolyte concentrations of plasma. Clinicians should be aware that considerably more crystalloid than colloid is required to achieve comparable intravascular volume repletion in anaphylaxis. In one laboratory study of severe anaphylaxis produced by the intravenous injection of rattlesnake venom, six times more crystalloid was required to produce volume expansion similar to that in colloid-resuscitated animals.[73] Reversal of hemoconcentration is a reasonable resuscitative goal for stable patients. However, in unstable patients with wide fluctuations in vital signs and worsening pulmonary function, fluid therapy should be administered according to hemodynamic measurements. Monitoring with a pulmonary arterial catheter may be necessary so that the effect of fluid therapy on systemic and pulmonary hemodynamic variables can be determined.

If hypotension and other signs of circulatory shock persist after the initial administration of epinephrine and fluids, inotropic support is required. In general, the continuous infusion of a catecholamine is employed. Some authorities recommended a continuous infusion of epinephrine (2 to 4 mg in 1 L of saline at 2 to 4 mg/min). Others suggested norepinephrine for use in this condition (4 to 8 mg in 1 L of saline at 4 to 8 μg/min). Dopamine has also been used in anaphylaxis in doses up to 15 μg/kg/min. However, dopamine has been ineffective in at least one reported case of anaphylaxis.[74]

Additional Therapeutic Options

When symptoms of anaphylaxis persist after initial treatment with epinephrine and fluids, other pharmacologic agents may be tried. The rationale for the use of these agents is based on a basic knowledge of their pharmacologic actions in the laboratory setting and in clinical conditions that usually do not include anaphylaxis. Because of the sporadic presentation of clinical anaphylaxis, experience with these drugs is anecdotal and inconclusive. However, when patients are responding poorly to initial treatment, these agents may be tried.

Agents that block the peripheral effects of histamine are logical additions to the pharmacologic management of anaphylaxis. Antihistamines block the systemic effects of histamine by competitively inhibiting histamine (H_1 and H_2) receptors. They may thus favorably influence histamine H_1 receptor–mediated increases in vascular permeability and bronchial smooth muscle contraction. Antihistamines may also block histamine H_2 receptors in the myocardium, which mediate increases in heart rate, dysrhythmias, atrioventricular conduction delays, and coronary vasoconstriction. Diphenhydramine, a histamine H_1 receptor antagonist, may be given intravenously at 4- to 6-hour intervals in doses of 25 to 50 mg. Three hundred milligrams of the histamine H_2 receptor blocker cimetidine (in 50 mL of normal saline) may be infused intravenously during 5 minutes and repeated at 6- to 8-hour intervals.

Aminophylline and theophylline are methylxanthines that are frequently employed in anaphylaxis. Although these agents inhibit phosphodiesterase and may thus decrease mediator release by increasing intracellular cAMP concentrations, there is evidence that this effect is minimal at therapeutic concentrations.[46] Nevertheless, these agents are effective in alleviating bronchospasm, probably because of direct effects on smooth muscle.[46] A loading dose of 5 to 6 mg/kg is infused during 20 minutes and followed by a continuous infusion of 0.2 to 0.9 mg/kg/h. Mild bronchospasm may be treated with anhydrous theophylline, 200 to 400 mg by mouth twice daily.

Corticosteroids should be administered in severe cases of anaphylaxis because they increase tissue responsiveness to beta-agonists and inhibit the synthesis of histamine. These agents also prevent or attenuate late-phase reactions by inhibiting the characteristic secondary wave of mediator release. Hydrocortisone, 100 to 200 mg, should be given intravenously in severe cases, repeated at 4- to 6-hour intervals for 24 hours, and rapidly tapered.

Inhalation drugs have a limited role in the treatment of anaphylaxis. They may be useful, however, in patients with persistent bronchospasm. An inhaled beta-agonist that may be used is metaproterenol, 0.2 to 0.3 mL of a 5% solution in 2.5 mL of saline administered by nebulization and repeated every 2 to 4 hours. Ipratropium bromide is a bronchodilator with anticholinergic properties; 36 μg may be inhaled and repeated at 2-hour intervals as needed. If 12 inhalations during 24 hours is not exceeded, the anticholinergic side effects of these agents should be minimal. Laryngeal edema, if mild, may respond to nebulized racemic epinephrine. It is believed that localized vasoconstriction from the alpha-adrenergic properties of these drugs minimizes edema formation in the laryngeal area. Racemic epinephrine, 0.5 mL of a 2.25% solution diluted in 3.5 mL of distilled water, may be administered by nebulization. Severe laryngeal edema associated with respiratory distress or stridor should always be treated with intubation of the trachea.

Several other agents have been used in cases of human anaphylaxis or in laboratory models of anaphylaxis with apparent success. Glucagon, a pancreatic hormone that increases intracellular cAMP levels through the activation of adenylate cyclase, was effective in a case report of a patient with anaphylaxis who was receiving beta-blocker therapy.[75] Because of the role of calcium in enhancing mediator release, it has been speculated that calcium channel blockers might be useful in anaphylaxis. Although calcium channel blockers have been demonstrated to prevent histamine-induced symptoms, their use has not been investigated in clinical studies of anaphylaxis. These agents have proved to be disappointing in alleviating bronchospasm in clinical trials of asthma, however.[76] In addition, calcium channel–blocking agents have negative inotropic effects, which may be undesirable in severe anaphylaxis associated with circulatory shock. The opiate antagonist naloxone reverses the inhibitory effects of endogenous opiates on the sympathetic nervous system. This agent has been shown to be effective in laboratory models of anaphylaxis.[77] Glucagon, calcium channel–blocking agents, and opiate antagonists have a limited role in the treatment of anaphylaxis. Additional understanding of the physiologic and clinical effects of these drugs in anaphylaxis is required before their routine use is recommended.

Management After Anaphylactic Episode: Prophylaxis and Immunotherapy

Because of the life-threatening nature of anaphylaxis, arrangements must be made for patients who have experienced anaphylaxis to receive follow-up by a physician experienced in the management of acute allergic events. Skin testing may be required to identify the inciting agent. Instructions in self-treatment of subsequent events is often necessary. Kits are available with self-injectable epinephrine and oral antihistamines for patients to take immediately after exposure to antigen.

Agents that produce anaphylaxis should be avoided whenever possible. However, if a patient must receive an agent that has previously produced anaphylaxis or severe allergic symptoms and no alternative exists, premedication should be implemented. Although the effectiveness of premedication has not been conclusively demonstrated, most authorities recommend premedication with histamine H_1 and H_2 receptor blockers and corticosteroids in this situation. Several studies suggested that premedication may decrease the anaphylactoid reaction to radiographic contrast media.[78-81] For high-risk patients, some authorities believe that epinephrine or isoproterenol should be included as premedication.[82] Because fatal anaphylaxis has been described in spite of premedication, it remains preferable, if clinically possible, to avoid all medications associated with anaphylaxis.

Methods to desensitize individuals immediately before the administration of a drug have been described in detail,[32] especially for penicillin,[83] aspirin,[84] and insulin.[85] However, these techniques, which involve exposure to antigen in increments every 20 to 30 minutes, may be unsuccessful and occasionally fatal.[86-88]

Long-term desensitization may be useful in patients who have experienced anaphylaxis to antigens that may be difficult to avoid, especially foods and venoms. This type of immunotherapy involves an initial injection of a minute dose of antigen followed by a gradual increases in dose at weekly or biweekly intervals according to the tolerance of the patient.[24, 89-91] The exact mechanisms for the effectiveness of desensitization is unclear but appears to involve the formation of non-IgE blocking antibodies, a decline in IgE antibody, and a reduction in the reactivity of mast cells and basophils to antigen.

Education of the patient as well as short-term and long-term desensitization should be the responsibility of physicians experienced in the management of immediate hypersensitivity disorders. It is the responsibility of the critical care physician to ensure the referral of patients who have experienced anaphylaxis to the care of suitable specialists.

Acknowledgment. The authors would like to thank Norma Padilla and Renita Braxton for their help in the preparation of this manuscript.

References

1. Waddell LA: Egyptian Civilization: Its Sumerian Origin and Real Chronology and Sumerian Origin of Egyptian Hieroglyphs. London, Luzac and Company, 1930.
2. Chafee F: Insect-sting allergy. J Allergy 43:309, 1969.
3. Cohen SG: The pharaoh and the wasp. Allergy Proc 10:149, 1989.
4. Portier P, Richet C: De l'action anaphylactique de certains venins. C R Soc Biol Paris 54:170, 1902.
5. Ishizaka T: IgE and mechanisms of IgE-mediated hypersensitivity. Ann Allergy 48:313, 1982.
6. Murphy RC, Hammarstrom S, Samuelsson B: Leukotriene C: A slow-reacting substance from murine mastocytoma cells. Proc Natl Acad Sci USA 76:4275, 1979.
7. Lewis RA, Austen KF, Soberman RJ: Leukotrienes and other products of the 5-lipoxygenase: Biochemistry and relation to pathobiology in human diseases. N Engl J Med 323:645, 1990.
8. Serafin WE, Austen KF: Mediators of immediate hypersensitivity reactions. N Engl J Med 317:30, 1987.
9. Sheffer AL, Austin KF: Exercise-induced anaphylaxis. J Allergy Clin Immunol 66:106, 1980.
10. Boxer M, Greenberger PA, Patterson R: Clinical summary and course of idiopathic anaphylaxis in 73 patients. Arch Intern Med 147:269, 1987.
11. Wiggins CA, Dykewicz MS, Patterson R: Idiopathic anaphylaxis: A review. Ann Allergy 62:1, 1989.
12. Wong S, Dykewicz MS, Patterson R: Idiopathic anaphylaxis: A clinical summary of 175 patients. Arch Intern Med 150:1323, 1990.
13. Hendrix S, Sale S, Zeiss CR, et al: Factitious hymenoptera allergic emergency: A report of a new variant of Munchausen's syndrome. J Allergy Clin Immunol 67:8, 1981.
14. McGrath KG, Greenberger PA, Zeiss CR: Factitious allergic disease: Multiple factitious illness and familial Munchausen's stridor. Immunol Allergy Pract 6:41, 1984.
15. Idsoe O, Guthe T, Willcox RR, et al: Nature and extent of penicillin side-reactions with particular reference to fatalities from anaphylactic shock. Bull WHO 38:159, 1968.
16. Parker CW: Penicillin allergy. Am J Med 34:747, 1963.
17. Parker CW: Allergic drug responses—Mechanisms and unsolved problems. Crit Rev Toxicol 1:261, 1972.
18. Kabins SA, Eisenstein B, Cohen S: Anaphylactoid reaction to an initial dose of sodium cephalothin. JAMA 193:165, 1965.
19. Saxon A, Beall GN, Rohr AS, et al: Immediate hypersensitivity reactions to beta-lactam antibiotics. Ann Intern Med 107:204, 1987.
20. Kellerman R: Reactions to radiographic contrast media. Am Fam Physician 23:149, 1981.
21. Cohan RH, Dunnick NR, Bashore TM: Treatment of reactions to radiographic contrast material. AJR 151:263, 1988.
22. Lasser EC, Lang J, Slovak M, et al: Steroids: Theoretical and experimental basis for utilization in prevention of contrast media reactions. Radiology 125:1, 1977.
23. Barnard JH: Studies of 400 hymenoptera sting deaths in the United States. J Allergy Clin Immunol 52:259, 1973.
24. DeShazo RD, Butcher BT, Banks WA: Reactions to the stings of the imported fire ant. N Engl J Med 323:462, 1990.
25. Russell FE, Carlson RW, Wainschel J, et al: Snake venom poisoning in the United States. Experiences with 550 cases. JAMA 233:341, 1975.
26. Kunkel DB: Bites of venomous reptiles. Emerg Med Clin North Am 2:563, 1984.
27. Bock SA: Prospective appraisal of complaints of adverse reactions to foods in children during the first three years of life. Pediatrics 79:683, 1987.
28. Metcalfe DD: Diseases of food hypersensitivity. N Engl J Med 321:255, 1989.
29. Johansson SGO, Melvin T, Vahlquist B: Immunoglobulin levels in Ethiopian preschool children with special reference to high concentrations of immunoglobulin E (IgND). Lancet 1:1118, 1968.
30. Phils JA, Harrold AJ, Whiteman GV: Pulmonary infiltrates, asthma, and eosinophilia due to Ascaris suum infestation in man. N Engl J Med 286:965, 1972.
31. Dessein AJ, Parker WL, James SL, et al: IgE antibody and resistance to infection. I. Selective suppression of the IgE antibody response in rats diminishes the resistance and eosinophil response to Trichinella spiralis infection. J Exp Med 153:423, 1981.
32. Austen KF: The anaphylactic syndrome. In: Samter M, Talmadge DW, Frank MM, et al (eds): Immunological Diseases. Boston, Little, Brown, p 1119, 1988.
33. VanArsdel PP: Diagnosing drug allergy. JAMA 247:2576, 1982.
34. Vyas GN, Holmdahl L, Perkins HA: et al: Serologic specificity of human anti-IgA and its significance in transfusion. Blood 34:573, 1969.
35. Lakin JD, Blocker TJ, Strong DM, et al: Anaphylaxis to protamine sulfate mediated by a complement dependent IgG antibody. J Allergy Clin Immunol 61:102, 1978.

36. Best N, Sinosich MJ, Teisner B, et al: Complement activation during cardiopulmonary bypass by heparin-protamine interaction. Br J Anaesth 56:339, 1984.

37. Sharath MD, Metzger WJ, Richerson HB, et al: Protamine-induced fatal anaphylaxis. J Thorac Cardiovasc Surg 90:86, 1985.

38. Gleich GJ: The late phase of the immunoglobulin E mediated reaction: A link between anaphylaxis and common allergic disease? J Allergy Clin Immunol 70:160, 1982.

39. Naclerio RM, Proud D, Togias AC, et al: Inflammatory mediators in late antigen-induced rhinitis. N Engl J Med 313:65, 1985.

40. Kaliher M: Hypotheses on the contribution of late-phase allergic responses to the understanding and treatment of allergic diseases. J Allergy Clin Immunol 73:311, 1984.

41. Samter M, Stevenson DD: Reactions to aspirin and aspirin-like drugs. In: Samter M, Talmage DW, Frank MM, et al (eds): Immunological Diseases. Boston, Little, Brown, p 1135, 1988.

42. Juhlin L, Michaelsson G, Zetterstron D: Urticaria and asthma induced by food-and-drug additives in patients with aspirin hypersensitivity. J Allergy Clin Immunol 50:92, 1972.

43. Sullivan TJ, Kulczycki A: Immediate hypersensitivity responses. In: Parker CW (ed): Clinical Immunology. Philadelphia, WB Saunders, p 115, 1980.

44. Butterworth AE, David JR: Eosinophil function. N Engl J Med 304:154, 1981.

45. Weller PF: The immunobiology of eosinophils. N Engl J Med 324:1110, 1991.

46. Persson CG: Overview of effects of theophylline. J Allergy Clin Immunol 78:780, 1986.

47. Duorak AM, Lett-Brouns M, Thueson D, et al: Complement induced degranulation of human basophils. J Immunol 126:523, 1981.

48. Hugli TE, Muller-Eberhard HJ: Anaphylatoxins: C3a and C5a. Adv Immunol 26:1, 1978.

49. David JR, Butterworth AE: Immunity to Schistosoma mansoni: Antibody-dependent eosinophil-mediated damage to schistosomula. Fed Proc 36:2176, 1977.

50. Delage C, Irey NS: Anaphylactic deaths: A clinicopathologic study of 43 cases. J Forensic Sci 17:525, 1972.

51. James LP, Austen KF: Fatal systemic anaphylaxis in man. N Engl J Med 270:597, 1964.

52. Fisher MM: Anaphylaxis. Acute Care 14–15:47, 1988–1989.

53. Graver LM, Robertson DA, Levi R, et al: IgE-mediated hypersensitivity in human heart tissue: Histamine release and functional changes. J Allergy Clin Immunol 77:709, 1986.

54. Burke JA, Levi R, Guo Z-G, et al: Leukotrienes C4, D4, and E4: Effect on human and guinea-pig cardiac preparations in vitro. J Pharmacol Exp Ther 221:235, 1982.

55. Carlson RW, Schaeffer RC, Puri VK, et al: Hypovolemia and permeability pulmonary edema associated with anaphylaxis. Crit Care Med 9:883, 1981.

56. Silverman HJ, Van Hook C, Haponik EF: Hemodynamic changes in human anaphylaxis. Am J Med 77:341, 1984.

57. Hanashiro PK, Weil MH: Anaphylactic shock in man. Report of two cases with detailed hemodynamic and metabolic studies. Arch Intern Med 119:129, 1967.

58. Fisher M: Blood volume replacement in acute anaphylactic cardiovascular collapse related to anaesthesia. Br J Anaesth 49:1023, 1977.

59. Fisher MM, Dix I: Blood volume replacement in acute anaphylactoid reactions. Anesth Intensive Care 7:373, 1979.

60. Booth BH, Patterson R: Electrocardiographic changes in human anaphylaxis. JAMA 211:627, 1970.

61. Levine HD: Acute myocardial infarction following a wasp sting. Am Heart J 91:365, 1976.

62. Sullivan TJ: Cardiac disorders in penicillin induced anaphylaxis. JAMA 248:2161, 1982.

63. Austin SM, Banajit B, Kim CS: Reversible acute cardiac injury during cefoxitin induced anaphylaxis in a patient with normal coronary arteries. Am J Med 77:729, 1984.

64. Barach EM, Nowak RM, Lee TG, et al: Epinephrine for treatment of anaphylactic shock. JAMA 251:2118, 1984.

65. Raper RF, Fisher MM: Profound reversible myocardial depression after anaphylaxis. Lancet 1:368, 1988.

66. Smedegard G, Revenas B, Lundberg C: Anaphylactic shock in monkeys passively sensitized with human reaginic serum. I. Hemodynamics and cardiac performance. Acta Physiol Scand 111:239, 1981.

67. Moss J, Fahmey NR, Sunder N, et al: Hormonal and hemodynamic profile of an anaphylactic reaction in man. Circulation 63:210, 1981.

68. Hamberger B, Fredholm BB, Farnebo LO: Anaphylaxis and plasma catecholamine. Life Sci 26:1465, 1980.

69. Olinger GN, Becker RM, Bonchek LI: Non-cardiogenic pulmonary edema and peripheral vascular collapse following cardiopulmonary bypass: Rare protamine reaction? Ann Thorac Surg 29:20, 1980.

70. Enjeti S, Bleeker ER, Smith PL, et al: Hemodynamic mechanisms in anaphylaxis. Circ Shock 11:297, 1983.

71. Kapin MA, Ferguson JL: Hemodynamic and regional circulatory alterations in dog during anaphylactic challenge. Am J Physiol 249:H430, 1985.

72. Standards and guidelines for cardiopulmonary resuscitation (CPR) and emergency cardiac care (ECC). JAMA 255:2905, 1986.

73. Haupt MT, Teerapong P, Green D, et al: Increased pulmonary edema with crystalloid compared to colloid resuscitation in shock associated with increased vascular permeability. Circ Shock 12:213, 1984.

74. Sullivan TJ, Stark HJ: Drug reactions. In: Bayless TM, Brain MC, Cherniak RM (eds): Current Therapy in Internal Medicine. St Louis, CV Mosby, p 24, 1984.

75. Zaloga GP, Delacey W, Holmboe E, et al: Glucagon reversal of hypotension in a case of anaphylactoid shock. Ann Intern Med 105:65, 1986.

76. Kaliner MA, McFadden ER: Bronchial asthma. In: Samter M, Talmage DW, Frank MM, et al (eds): Immunological Diseases. Boston, Little, Brown, p 1067, 1988.

77. Gullo A, Romano E: Naloxone and anaphylactic shock. Lancet 1:819, 1983.

78. Lalli AE: Urography shock reaction and repeated urography. Am J Roentgenol 125:264, 1975.

79. Lasser EC, Berry CC, Talner LB, et al: Pretreatment with corticosteroids to alleviate reactions to intravenous contrast material. N Engl J Med 317:845, 1987.

80. Miller WL, Doppman JL, Kaplan AP: Renal arteriography following systemic reaction to contrast material. J Allergy Clin Immunol 56:291, 1975.

81. Zweiman B, Mishkine MM, Hildreth EA: An approach to the performance of contrast studies in contrast material–reactive person. Ann Intern Med 83:159, 1975.

82. Watkins J: Adverse anaesthetic reactions. Anaesthesia 40:797, 1985.

83. Weiss ME, Adkinson NF: Immediate hypersensitivity reactions to penicillin and related antibiotics. Clin Allergy 18:515, 1988.

84. Pleskow WN, Stevenson DD, Mathison DA, et al: Aspirin desensitization in aspirin sensitive asthmatic patients: Clinical manifestations and characterization of the refractory period. J Allergy Clin Immunol 69:11, 1982.

85. Mattson JR, Patterson R, Roberts M: Insulin therapy with systemic insulin allergy. Arch Intern Med 135:818, 1975.

86. Blankenhorn MA: Anaphylactic shock and failure of desensitization after administration of pneumococcus type I serum. JAMA 85:325, 1925.

87. Grieco MH, Dubin MR, Robinson JL, et al: Penicillin hypersensitivity in patients with bacterial endocarditis. Ann Intern Med 60:204, 1964.

88. Tuft L: Fatalities following the reinjection of foreign serum: With report of an unusual case. Am J Med Sci 175:325, 1928.

89. Norman PS, Lichtenstein LM: Allergic rhinitis. In: Samter M, Talmage DW, Frank MM, et al (eds): Immunological Diseases. Boston, Little, Brown, p 1047, 1988.

90. Graft DF: Venom immunotherapy for stinging insect allergy. Clin Rev Allergy 5:149, 1987.

91. Lockey RF: Immunotherapy for allergy to insect stings. N Engl J Med 323:1627, 1990.

CHAPTER 145

Injuries by Venomous and Poisonous Animals

Richard W. Carlson

Poisonous and venomous animals are numerous and varied. Throughout the world, thousands of species among several phyla are toxic, and hundreds of thousands of people are injured each year. The severity of these poisonings ranges from minor irritation to fulminant multiple organ system failure and death.

These organisms have been worshiped, feared, and viewed with awe throughout history. Many misconceptions about these animals and their toxins have therefore been perpetuated. Some of these misconceptions persist in current medical literature and lead to controversies in management. In addition, both lay and medical personnel are likely to have only fragmentary knowledge of the organisms responsible for these injuries. Accurate, up-to-date information on the chemistry, pharmacology, clinical manifestations, and principles of management of these intoxications is not familiar to most practitioners. Misconceptions and gaps in knowledge of these animals and their toxins may be complicated by the wide variability in the severity of intoxications, even by the same species. Treatments that were apparently effective for one patient may be of little value in the management of subsequent cases. Some treatments are dangerous and are associated with considerable risk that may result in death. Accordingly, for injuries by these animals, mistaken diagnoses and incorrect estimates of severity are often compounded by errors in therapy.

For these reasons, it is important for the intensive care clinician to have a fundamental understanding of these animals, their toxins, and the injuries they produce. Many patients who come in contact with these forms are referred to an intensive care unit (ICU) for monitoring and definitive care. Fortunately, the vast majority of these injuries do not result in death. However, *all* envenomations and poisonings by animals should be regarded as potentially lethal. The intensivist should be familiar with the nature of the toxins, which organ systems are likely to be affected, the priorities of management, and how to assess the progression of signs and symptoms to determine the severity of injury. In addition, the intensivist should be able to summon expert help to identify the offending organism, secure appropriate consultation for the management of specific aspects of the intoxication, and obtain unique medications such as antivenin.

This chapter includes a description and classification of some venoms and animal poisons and general principles for the management of these injuries. Selected toxic marine and terrestrial organisms are reviewed. Emphasis is placed on serious intoxications and those that may be encountered in North America. However, several of the dangerous species found elsewhere in the world are described, as travel to virtually all areas of the world is now possible within hours. Furthermore, the number of rare animals maintained as pets or in private collections is substantial. The intensive care practitioner must be prepared to manage a life-threatening injury by an exotic species or a poisoning with an unusual presentation.[1-7]

For more detailed information on specific organisms and their toxins, the reader is referred to standard texts and monographs on dangerous marine and terrestrial animals.[8-11] Poison control centers can provide immediate assistance in the identification and management of these intoxications and may direct the physician to recognized consultants with expertise, as well as providing current information on diagnosis and treatment. Local zoos, aquaria, universities and colleges, and other authoritative sources may also give valuable assistance. A nearby zoo may be the only local source of antivenin for management of a bite or sting by an exotic species.

There are a number of regional sources for expert advice. The American Association of Zoological Parks and Aquaria (Ogleby Park, Wheeling, WV 26003) prepares a worldwide antivenin index, which is updated periodically, and can provide further information. Additional sources of information include the Arizona Poison and Drug Information Center at the University of Arizona, Tucson, AZ (telephone: (602) 626–6016), which maintains a 24-hour service to provide information on venomous and poisonous animals, and the pediatric service of the Los Angeles County/University of Southern California Medical Center.

PRINCIPLES OF MANAGEMENT

The general principles of management of intoxications by poisonous and venomous animals are depicted in Figure

1. CONFIRM AND QUANTITATE ENVENOMATION
2. IDENTIFY OFFENDING SPECIES
3. INITIATE FIRST AID
4. TRANSPORT TO HOSPITAL
5. GENERAL &/OR SPECIFIC THERAPY:
   A. REMOVE VENOM FROM WOUND
   B. RETARD ABSORPTION OF VENOM
   C. NEUTRALIZE VENOM (ANTIVENIN)
   D. COMBAT EFFECTS OF VENOM
   E. TREAT LATE OR SECONDARY EFFECTS

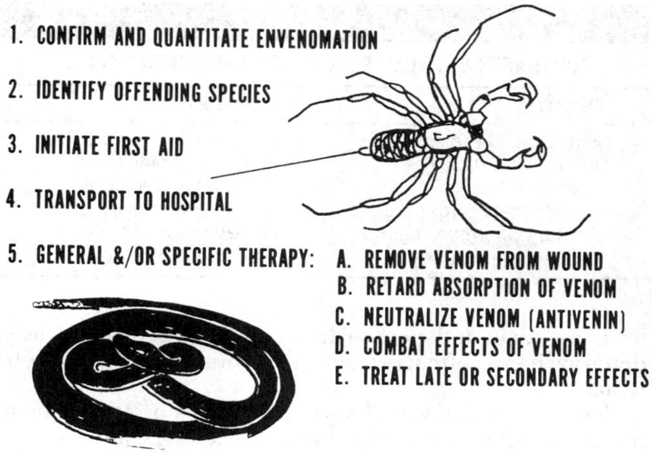

Figure 145–1. Management of suspected venom injuries.

145–1. These include identification of the offending organism, first-aid measures and ongoing assessment of the severity of the injury, transport to an ICU for monitoring, and measures to treat local and life-threatening systemic toxicity.

A guiding theme in treating venom injuries is to do no harm. In most instances, the patient survives the intoxication. However, some treatments may cause death or serious injury. The intensivist's role should be to evaluate and quantitate the severity of intoxication as monitoring and life-support measures are employed as needed. If no signs or symptoms of significant local or systemic toxicity develop, management should be conservative. A risk-benefit evaluation should be considered for any specific therapy that is contemplated.

VENOMS VERSUS POISONS

The word *poison* is often used to describe any toxic substance. However, not all poisons are venoms. Poisons typically cause injury when ingested via the enteral route, although some poisons are toxic when injected or administered in other ways. A *venom* is an animal poison that may or may not be toxic when ingested but causes local and/or systemic toxicity when administered parenterally. A venomous animal produces a venom by a specialized group of secretory cells or gland and possesses a venom apparatus to deliver the toxin into the victim via a stinger, fang, spine, barb, jaw, or other device. Poisonous animals are forms that are toxic when ingested.[12-17] Some animals are both venomous and poisonous.

A poison usually consists of a single or few toxic components, whereas venoms are invariably mixtures of multiple substances. For example, a rattlesnake venom may contain more than 20 individual fractions, including proteins, peptides, amines, metals, lipids, and other substances.[9, 18] Many of the toxins in a venom have effects on several organ systems, so that a specific neurotropic fraction of a snake venom may also exert adverse effects on the myocardium, the vascular endothelium, the coagulation cascade, and other organs or cells. Poisons, on the other hand, are likely to consist of one or only a few toxic components and have more restricted pharmacologic properties (Table 145–1).

Venoms from closely related forms generally share certain chemical and pharmacologic features. However, toxins from unrelated organisms may occasionally have similar or identical properties and/or chemical structure.[19-21] Finally, toxins used by an animal to capture and/or ingest its prey tend to share similar features, whereas toxins used defensively often have other properties. Venoms used offensively are likely to

TABLE 145–1

CONTRASTS BETWEEN POISONINGS AND ENVENOMATION

Poisoning	Envenomation
Single or few toxins	Multiple toxic components
Intoxication usually enteral	Parenteral administration
Few primary target organs	Multiple organs affected
Primary pharmacologic effects of toxins	Prominent secondary and tertiary responses (auto-pharmacologic)

be more toxic and potentially fatal. Toxins that are used defensively are often painful or irritating but may also be lethal.

Venoms may activate a variety of mediators and inflammatory systems within the victim. Mediators and systems that have been linked to venoms and venom fractions include bradykinin and bradykinin-potentiating peptides, slow reacting substance of anaphylaxis (leukotrienes), angiotensin-converting enzyme inhibitors, thrombin-like enzymes, factors that activate specific coagulation factors, fractions that affect plasminogen, complement and lytic systems, and others. Some of these compounds were first isolated or described in association with venoms. These secondary and tertiary autopharmacologic effects of venoms may be extremely complex and increase the danger of the envenomation. Reactions of this type are infrequently encountered with poisonings.

PHYLUM CHORDATA, CLASS REPTILIA, ORDER SQUAMATA, SUBORDER SERPENTES: SNAKES

Snakes have been the subject of fear and superstition for thousands of years. Cobras were worshipped in ancient India; the Mayans and Aztecs duplicated images of rattlesnakes on temple walls; and the early Greeks and Romans prominently featured vipers in mythology. Snakes were considered to be the embodiment of evil in early Judeo-Christian literature, and serpents have been the subject of prose and poetry throughout history.[9, 17, 18]

There are approximately 3000 species of snakes, of which 10% are venomous.[9, 22, 23] The venomous snakes are found in five families: Hydrophiidae (sea snakes), Viperidae (vipers), Elapidae (elapids), Crotalidae (pit vipers), and Colubridae (rear-fanged snakes) (Table 145–2).

It has been estimated that there may be as many as 300,000 snakebites each year throughout the world, which lead to 30,000 to 40,000 fatalities, although Russell suggests that this number may be too high.[9] In many countries, reports of the incidence and morbidity and mortality of these injuries are inaccurate. In the United States, it is estimated that 45,000 snakebites occur each year, of which approximately one fifth are by venomous forms.[24] In Australia, venomous snakes outnumber nonvenomous forms, and Australia is the home of several of the most venomous snakes in the world. A few thousand bites occur in the Australian subcontinent each year, although mortality is low because of the widespread availability of antivenin and other therapy and a more consistent approach to the management of these injuries.

Several factors complicate the initial evaluation and estimation of severity of snakebites (Table 145–3). First, for 20% or more of pit viper bites and a greater percentage of bites by elapids and sea snakes, there is no injection of venom.[25–27] The management of these dry bites should be conservative observation. It is likely that several folk remedies and medical and surgical approaches to management may have had their origins in application of these treatments to patients who were not envenomated or only minimally

TABLE 145–2

CLASSIFICATION OF SELECTED VENOMOUS SNAKES

Family	Genus and Species	Common Names
Hydrophiidae		Sea snakes
Viperidae		Vipers
	Echis carinatus	Saw-scaled vipers
	Echis coloratus	Carpet vipers
	Vipera russelli	Russell's viper
	Bitis gabonica	Gaboon viper
	Bitis arietans	Puff adder
Elapidae		Elapids
	Ophiophagus hannah	King cobra
	Naja	Cobras
	Bungarus	Kraits
	Dendroaspis	Mambas
	Notechis scutatus scutatus	Tiger snake
	Acanthophis antarcticus	Death adder
	Oxyuranus scutellatus	Taipan
	Demansia	Brown snakes
	Denisonia	Copperheads (Australia)
	Micruroides euryxanthus	Western coral snake
	Micrurus fulvius fulvius	Eastern coral snake
	Micrurus fulvius tenere	Texas coral snake
Crotalidae		Pit vipers
	Crotalus	Rattlesnakes
	Sistrurus	Pigmy rattlesnakes and massasaugas
	Agkistrodon	Cottonmouths, copperheads, and Asiatic pit vipers
	Bothrops	Lance-headed vipers
	Trimeresurus	Asiatic lance-headed vipers
	Lachesis	Bushmaster
Colubridae		Rear-fanged snakes
	Dispholidus typus	Boomslang

TABLE 145–3
ESTIMATING SEVERITY OF SNAKEBITES

1. At least 20% of bites do not involve envenomation.
2. The medical status and the age of the patient must be considered to gauge the severity of the poisoning.
3. The size and condition of the snake affect the dose and quality of venom injected during a bite.
4. The location of the wound and the proportion of venom injected intravenously influence the balance of local versus systemic injury.
5. The physical activity of the patient and the effects of first-aid measures may modify the progression of signs and symptoms.
6. Systemic toxicity may be life threatening, despite minimal local injury.

envenomated. The condition and age of the patient affect the seriousness of the injury. The condition of the snake and the location of the wound as well as the predominant route of injection (subcutaneous, intramuscular, intravenous) play important roles in the development of local and systemic toxicity. The activity of the patient and the effects of first-aid measures may alter the progression of signs and symptoms. Increased local or general physical activity tends to increase absorption and systemic effects of the toxins. The assessment of severity may be complicated because some poisonings lead to marked local changes, whereas in other injuries systemic toxicity may be the first manifestation of a severe envenomation. Death caused by snake venom poisoning may result from a single critical organ failure, from the simultaneous effects of the venom on several organ systems, or from a complication of therapy (Table 145–4).

Many misconceptions about snake venoms have been perpetuated in medical as well as lay literature. For example, it is commonly believed that bites by cobras and other elapids are almost exclusively associated with neurologic changes and that local tissue injury or other deleterious effects are not typical features of these injuries. Similarly, it is widely held that bites by vipers and pit vipers lead to severe local injury and that these local changes can reliably be used to gauge the severity of the poisoning. Although these concepts have some validity when discussing these venoms in general terms, such conclusions may lead to dangerous errors in diagnosis and management. Bites by elapids may be associated with tissue injury, coagulation changes, and other effects, as well as neuromuscular findings. Similarly, evaluation of a viper or pit viper injury that is based on only local signs and symptoms may lead to serious errors in the

assessment of severity. A venom fraction frequently exerts multiple simultaneous pharmacologic properties.

It was commonly believed that the predominant cause of toxicity of snake venoms was associated with the enzymatic components of these venoms. However, it is now known that several of the lower-molecular-weight proteins and peptides, many of which have no enzymatic activity, are among the most toxic fractions.

Chemistry of Snake Venoms

Snake venoms are mixtures of multiple toxic and nontoxic substances that are produced by glandular structures that are homologous to salivary glands.[28–30] Enzymes, and other proteins, peptides, carbohydrates, lipids, amines, ions, and other substances are found in these venoms (Table 145–5). The quantity of venom that a snake delivers during a strike varies greatly, and the snake can adjust the amount of venom during a bite when hunting a prey. However, it is impossible to predict the amount of venom that is given for bites involving humans. The size and condition of the snake and other factors also affect the quantity and quality of the venom administered. The dose may vary from a few to several hundred milligrams.

The quantity of venom yielded from a snake is usually expressed in dry weight. Toxicity is typically quantitated by lethality. A common method is to give the milligrams of venom per kilogram of body weight that cause death of 50% of test animals subjected to intravenous, intramuscular, or intraperitoneal doses of venom. This expression is the median lethal dose (LD_{50}), and the value varies among the venomous snakes from a few micrograms to more than 10 mg/kg. The most lethal venoms are found among the elapids and sea snakes. However, some viper and pit viper venoms are also toxic. In this regard, the venoms of the Mojave rattlesnake (*Crotalus scutulatus scutulatus*) and the tropical rattlesnake (*Crotalus durissus*) are the most lethal snake venoms in the Western Hemisphere.[11]

Although enzymatic components, and particularly phospholipase A_2, and various proteases contribute to the toxicity of snake venoms, many of the lethal and other deleterious properties are related to smaller proteins and peptides.[19, 31–33] A number of these substances interact with specific receptor sites on various cells of the patient. For example, several postsynaptic neurotoxins have been isolated

TABLE 145–4
POTENTIALLY FATAL CONDITIONS ASSOCIATED WITH SNAKE VENOM POISONING AND/OR TREATMENT

Circulatory shock
Hemorrhage, hypovolemia
Respiratory and ventilatory failure
Coagulopathy, disseminated intravascular coagulation, thrombocytopenia
Hemolysis, thrombolysis, thromboembolism
Coma, seizures, intracranial hemorrhage
Cranial nerve dysfunction
Rhabdomyolysis, renal failure, hyperkalemia
Sepsis, secondary infection
Gastrointestinal bleeding
Anaphylaxis to venom components or to antivenin

TABLE 145–5
SOME COMPONENTS OF SNAKE VENOMS

Proteins
Enzymes
  Thrombin-like enzymes
  Phospholipases A_2, B, and C
  Collagenase
  L-Amino-acid oxidase
  Phosphodiesterase
  Acetylcholinesterase
  Proteolytic enzymes
  Prothrombin activators
  Factor V, IX, and X activators
  Ribonuclease I
  5′-Nucleosidase
Peptides
Electrolytes
Carbohydrates
Lipids
Amino acids
Metals

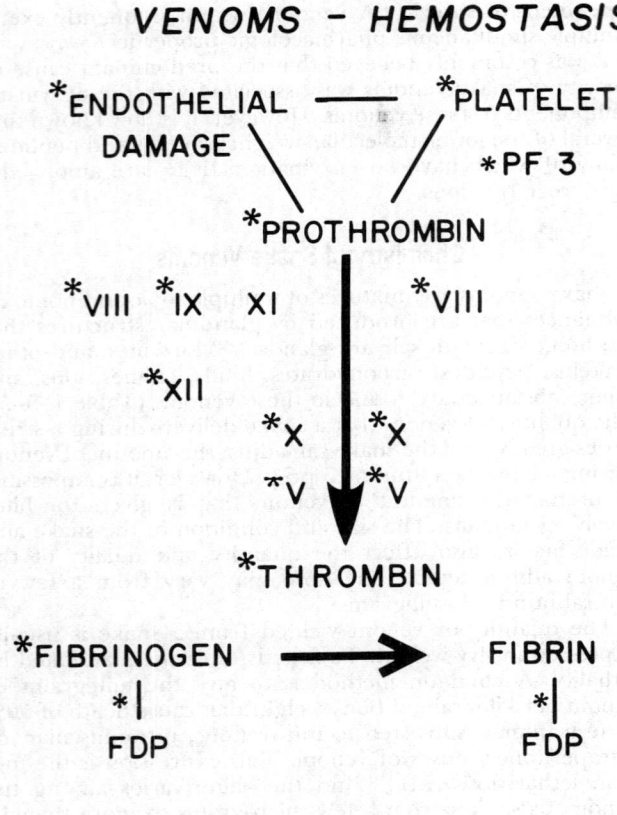

*= POTENTIAL SITE
OF ACTION

Figure 145–2. Potential sites of action of snake venoms and venom fractions on coagulation, hemostasis, and fibrinolysis. PF = platelet factor; FDP = fibrin degradation products.

from elapid and other forms. These toxins bind to nicotinic acetylcholine receptors, producing a nondepolarizing block. Presynaptic neurotoxins, on the other hand, have also been isolated from various snakes. These toxins inhibit release of acetylcholine. Several toxins of this variety have phospholipase A_2 activity.[19, 34, 35]

Many venoms contain fractions that alter hemostasis. One of the most common findings after envenomation is hypofibrinogenemia, caused by consumption of fibrinogen in the clotting process; fibrinogenolysis by direct or indirect activation of factors V, IX, and X and prothrombin; or other procoagulant or anticoagulant actions[9, 36–44] (Fig. 145–2). The effects of snake venoms on coagulation, hemostasis, and fibrinolysis are extremely complex.

Family Hydrophiidae: Sea Snakes

These animals are found in the Pacific and Indian oceans, including the waters of Hawaii, and as far north as Baja, California. Sea snakes are particularly dangerous and are closely related in many ways to the elapids. There are approximately 50 species of sea snakes within two subfamilies, Laticaudinae and Hydrophiinae.[45] The animals may reach lengths of more than 6 ft and are characterized by a flat tail, which is used for swimming.

Sea snakes are relatively docile animals and do not usually attack humans. Many bites occur as a result of attempts to capture or handle animals or when snakes are caught in fishing nets. The fangs are short, and fortunately many bites do not result in envenoming. However, the venom is extremely toxic.

The venom of sea snakes contains potent fractions with both presynaptic and postsynaptic activity, in addition to other components. The presynaptic toxins inhibit release of the neurotransmitter acetylcholine and are generally more lethal than the postsynaptic neurotoxins.[34, 46] Hemotoxic and myotoxic compounds are also present and account for the frequent development of hemolysis and rhabdomyolysis after sea snake poisoning.

Tissue edema around the wound and local pain are not usually prominent features after sea snake envenomation. Symptoms typically occur after a few hours, although in some cases life-threatening neuromuscular signs may develop within minutes. These include pain on motion, ascending paralysis, cranial nerve dysfunction, and respiratory distress. When present, these are indicative of severe sea snake poisoning, which may be fatal if not treated promptly with intensive management.[47–51] Death soon after envenomation is due to respiratory failure; death several days after envenoming is usually caused by renal failure and associated complications.

Management is similar to that for elapid bites and includes immobilization and transport to a hospital as quickly as possible. Sutherland proposed the use of a pressure-immobilization dressing for elapid and sea snake poisonings to delay systemic absorption of venom.[52, 53] However, he cautioned that this intervention might lead to further local damage and that release of the pressure dressing may result in sudden deterioration of the patient's condition. He recommended leaving the dressing in place until the patient reaches a hospital. Incision and suction over the fang marks is not recommended for sea snake bites. An enzyme-linked immunosorbent assay (ELISA) venom detection kit may be helpful to confirm envenomation.

Detection of venom in the patient and the development of systemic findings, and especially neurotropic signs and symptoms, are the most frequent indications for the administration of antivenin. Sea snake antivenin, tiger snake antivenin, or polyvalent elapid antivenin may be used, depending on the location, the species, and availability of antivenin. Skin testing is not highly predictive of acute allergic reactions and is therefore not recommended by some authors. However, physicians should be prepared to manage anaphylaxis, and serum sickness develops in a substantial number of individuals treated with these sera. Antihistamines or epinephrine or both given before or concomitantly with antivenin may prevent or ameliorate serious, acute systemic reactions, but do not alter the incidence of serum sickness. Corticosteroids are useful to treat late serum reactions.

An initial battery of laboratory studies for a suspected envenomation should include a venom detection assay if available, urinalysis with assay for hemoglobin (myoglobin), a complete blood count, serum electrolyte determination, and measurements of blood urea nitrogen and creatinine, together with baseline studies of muscle enzymes and a coagulation profile (Table 145–6). Assessment of respiratory and ventilatory adequacy is indicated for sea snake bites. Other tests should be selected in response to specific organ system dysfunction.

During the first 24 hours, it is important to closely monitor neurologic function as well as adequacy of ventilation. Monitoring may include serial arterial blood gas measurements and assessments of vital capacity, peak flow rates, and other measures of respiratory motor function. The electrocardiogram should be monitored. The ability of the patient to handle secretions and to develop an effective cough should

TABLE 145–6

HOSPITAL EVALUATION AND MANAGEMENT OF SUSPECTED VENOMOUS SNAKEBITE*

1. History and physical examination, with particular attention to
   a. Age and cardiopulmonary, neurologic, or hemostatic disturbances
   b. Medications: anticoagulants, cardiac medications
   c. Allergies—horse serum
   d. Time and nature of injury
   e. Accurate identification of snake; obtain snake if possible
   f. Initial signs and symptoms: swelling, pain, paresthesias, fasciculations, ecchymoses, weakness or paralysis, disturbances of vision, respiratory distress, nausea or vomiting
   g. First-aid measures and other therapy before hospital admission
   h. Symptoms on admission
   i. Description of wound, with attention to
      (1) Edema (grade), ecchymoses or bullae or petechiae
      (2) Pulses, skin color and temperature, capillary refill
      (3) Local sensory and motor examination, including range of motion
      (4) Fang marks or lacerations
      (5) Regional edema, adenopathy, ecchymoses, hemorrhage
   j. Cardiorespiratory: vital signs, postural changes
   k. Neurologic, including cranial nerve and mental status
2. Initial laboratory evaluation
   a. Complete blood count, including platelet, red and white blood cell counts, hemoglobin, and hematocrit
   b. Urinalysis, including blood and microscopic examination
   c. Electrolytes, blood urea nitrogen, and creatinine levels
   d. Electrocardiogram
   e. Baseline coagulation profile: prothrombin and partial thromboplastin times, fibrinogen titer; fibrin or fibrinogen degradation assays and titers of specific coagulation factors as needed
   f. Creatine kinase (MM and MB fractions) assays
   g. Type and cross-match for blood, haptoglobin levels
   h. Venom detection assay, if available
3. Selected additional procedures and monitoring
   a. Skin test for antivenin; antivenin IV with appropriate monitoring for anaphylaxis
   b. Vital signs, urine output
   c. Respiratory: vital capacity, peak flow rates, negative inspiratory force
   d. Evaluation of progression of local and regional edema, ecchymoses, and bullae
   e. Periodic evaluation of local and systemic perfusion, as well as neurologic function, including cranial nerves; consider noninvasive studies of region of wound (ultrasound)
   f. Serial assays of coagulation and hemostatic function and bleeding and creatine kinase, renal function assessment, pigmenturia
   g. Chest radiograph and examination of area of injury (embedded fangs; osteomyelitis)
   h. Photographs of injury
   i. Wick tissue pressure measurements for suspected compartmental syndrome
   j. Tetanus prophylaxis or therapy
   k. Computed tomography of head for altered mental status, seizures, cranial nerve dysfunction
   l. Arterial blood gas determination
   m. Central venous and/or arterial catheters (correct hemostatic defects first, if possible)
   n. Surgical consultation; débridement as needed

*Note: No one protocol is appropriate for all snake venom poisoning; the clinician is advised to consult additional references or experts, especially for bites by exotic species or unusual or severe injuries.

be evaluated at frequent intervals. Indications for intubation and mechanical ventilation are similar to those for patients with myasthenia gravis or Guillain-Barré syndrome.

Fluid therapy during the first 24 hours should be guided by hemodynamic stability, as determined by arterial pressure, urine output, and other measures of cardiovascular function. Coagulopathies, bleeding hemolysis, and loss of plasma volume may lead to marked changes in hematocrit. Fluid loading should utilize physiologic end points such as oxygen transport, improvements in cardiac output, and serial changes in cardiac filling pressures. Colloid fluids may be needed for hemodynamic support. Crystalloid fluids are indicated to maintain urine output and to manage rhabdomyolysis.

Edrophonium hydrochloride (Tensilon), 10 mg intravenously after 0.6 mg of atropine, may be considered to treat neurotropic alterations that threaten respiratory function.[54] If improvement is observed with edrophonium, neostigmine may be given, 0.25 to 0.5 mg intramuscularly every 30 minutes.

Cardiac arrhythmias may be a manifestation of neuromuscular toxicity. Electrocardiographic monitoring is therefore indicated for at least 24 hours after confirmed sea snake envenomation.

Other aspects of management of sea snake bites are similar to those for serious elapid envenomations.

Family Viperidae: Vipers

The family Viperidae includes a large number of snakes that inhabit the Old World, including all of the European and Asiatic mainlands and Africa. These forms are closely related to the pit vipers, and some authorities include the pit vipers (Crotalidae) as a subfamily of Viperidae.

The vipers and pit vipers have large, mobile front fangs (Fig. 145–3). These are folded against the upper jaw at rest and moved perpendicularly to the erect position for use against prey. There is full control of this process by the snake, which may also adjust the amount of venom injected during a bite.

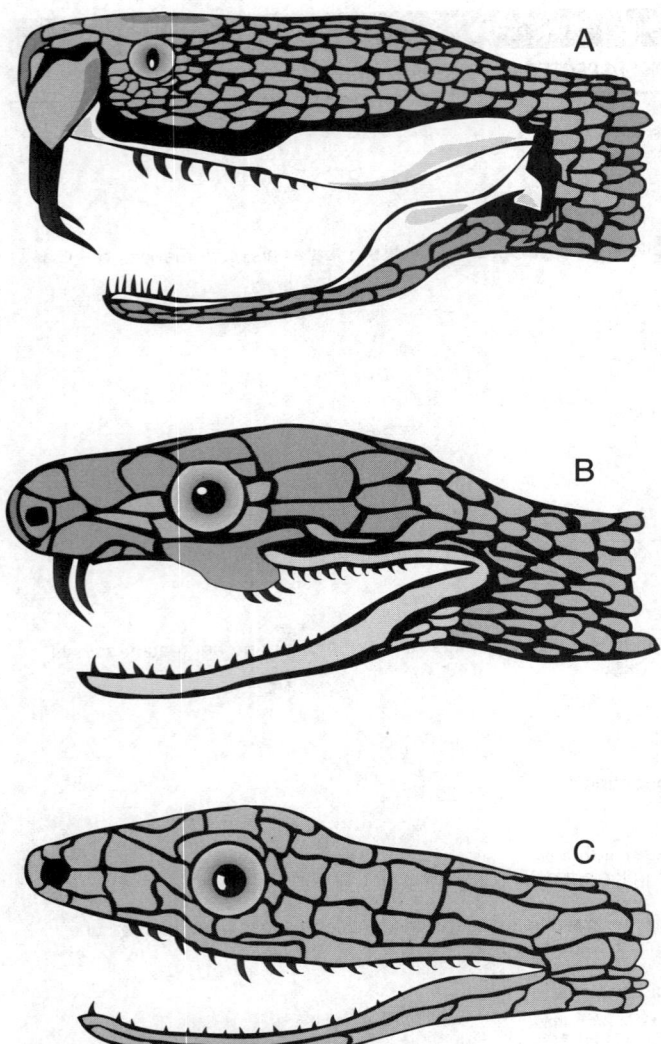

Figure 145–3. Anatomy of mouth and fangs of pit vipers *(A)*, elapids or sea snakes *(B)*, and rear-fanged snakes *(C)*.

Some vipers are large, such as the Gaboon viper, *Bitis gabonica,* a heavy-bodied snake that may exceed 6 ft in length. Other vipers are small but equally dangerous. The saw-scaled vipers (*Echis carinatus*) and carpet vipers (*Echis coloratus*) are typically less than 2 ft in length but cause many serious and often fatal envenomations. All vipers are dangerous to humans. The volume of venom that a viper delivers is related to the species and the size of the snake.

Viper venoms contain a number of enzymes and other components that alter hemostasis. Edema, tissue destruction, hemorrhage, and coagulation defects are commonly observed after viper bites. In some instances, the coagulopathy produced by procoagulant and other venom fractions leads to disseminated intravascular coagulation with defibrinogenation.[55, 56] Other common causes of viperid defibrination syndromes are Russell's viper, *Vipera russelli,* and the crotalid Malayan pit viper, *Agkistrodon rhodostoma.*[57]

Genus Echis: Saw-Scaled or Carpet Vipers

The saw-scaled or carpet vipers account for a substantial proportion of snakebite mortality in the Afro-Asian region. In Nigeria and other areas, thousands of people are bitten by these snakes, with considerable loss of life.[58–61] Management of *Echis* bites is controversial, and the use of heparin was previously recommended. Bites of these snakes cause extensive local effects, as well as serious and often life-threatening bleeding complications.[62–65]

Antivenin is indicated for all serious envenomations, particularly when blood is incoagulable[65–67] and patients have progressive local signs. However, antivenin therapy is associated with the risk of anaphylaxis; at least 20% of patients treated with antivenin experience serum sickness.

Echis bites are common. It is likely that *Echis* species bite and kill more people in the world than any other snake.[58, 60] In some parts of Africa, the annual incidence is six bites per thousand population, with a mortality of 12%.[59, 61] In the savanna region of Nigeria, as many as 10,000 snakebite deaths occur annually, and *Echis* species are the predominant offending organisms. Another 23,000 deaths from snakebites are estimated in West Africa.[61] Persons with *Echis* bites occupy as many as 10% of all hospital beds in Nigeria. Furthermore, health statistics in these areas may underestimate the magnitude of the problem.

Echis venom contains a mixture of proteins and peptides, some of which possess enzymatic activity. One of these fractions activates prothrombin to thrombin by a mechanism that is distinct from the factor Xa complex process. The venom prothrombin activator first cleaves the Arg-Ile-peptide bond of prothrombin to form meizothrombin.[68, 69] The result is ultimately the formation of thrombin. The venom activator does not require calcium, phospholipid, or factor Xa.[40] Infusion of *Echis* venom in animals leads to activation of prothrombin and disseminated intravascular coagulation with afibrinogenemia, thrombocytopenia, and marked declines in the activities of factors II, VIII:C, and XII.[70] The defibrination syndrome persists for 5 to 6 days.[55, 56] In addition to local and systemic bleeding, experimental subjects have an increase in pulmonary microvascular permeability to fluid and protein and pulmonary hypertension,[71, 72] along with other findings similar to those of the adult respiratory distress syndrome.

Heparin was previously proposed as a treatment for the defibrination caused by *Echis* species.[62–64] The rationale was based on the notion that heparin inhibits thrombin produced by the venom-induced activation of prothrombin and that fibrinogen is therefore preserved. However, the meizothrombin produced by *Echis* venom may react differently to heparin. In a prospective study in patients bitten by *E. carinatus,* Warrell and colleagues showed no difference in the speed of resolution of the coagulopathy among those patients treated with heparin or with antivenin.[65] There was no effect of heparin on the local effects of the poisoning. The authors concluded that there appears to be no place for heparin in the treatment of *Echis* poisoning if antivenin is available. Because intracranial hemorrhage is one of the most common mechanisms of death after *Echis* envenomation, there is considerable risk in the use of an anticoagulant such as heparin, and it is no longer recommended as standard therapy.

In the future, other techniques may be considered to counter the coagulation changes induced by these toxins. Schaeffer and associates tested the effects of a synthetic inhibitor of thrombin on the coagulopathy and microembolic damage produced by an infusion of *Echis* venom in dogs.[70] The agent D-phenylalanyl-L-propyl-L-arginine-L-chloromethyl ketone (PPACK) has a high affinity for thrombin but a lower affinity for kallikrein or plasmin. Antagonism of the thrombin released by venom was observed, without any major deleterious clotting abnormalities, in the animals treated with PPACK. PPACK also inhibited the marked hemolysis usually observed after venom, although PPACK did not prevent the thrombocytopenia induced by venom. In a separate study, the pulmonary fibrin microembolism and edema associated with *Echis* venom were inhibited by the use of the thrombin inhibitor PPACK.[71] However, it is not clear if the use of synthetic thrombin inhibitors such as PPACK will have a role in the clinical management of patients poisoned by these snakes.

Other fractions isolated from *Echis* venom include a variety of proteolytic enzymes, including L-amino-acid oxidase, phospholipase, and hyaluronidase.[72, 73]

Except for animals in zoos or collections elsewhere in the world, the majority of *Echis* bites in the Afro-Asian region occur in rural areas. The bite is usually on the foot, and pain and swelling are almost universally found shortly after the envenoming. Within the next few hours, 50% of patients experience spontaneous bleeding from remote sites such as the gums or injection sites.[60] A small percentage of patients have altered consciousness, which may progress to coma and death. Hypotension and signs of hypovolemia are seen in approximately 5% of cases. Tissue necrosis may be massive. Hemolysis and thrombocytopenia are also observed, but incoagulable blood, together with a reliable history and evidence of local findings, predicts severe *Echis* envenomation. The use of a micro-ELISA for detecting venom in urine, serum, aspirated fluid, or other body fluids is highly accurate for diagnosis.[74, 75] Despite a 3% risk of anaphylaxis and a significant chance of serum sickness, antivenin treatment is indicated for *Echis* bites associated with hemostatic failure. The untreated mortality of these bites exceeds 10%,[60] whereas the death rate falls to 3% with antivenin therapy. Antivenin may be given several days after envenomation if systemic envenoming is present. Death is usually from central nervous system bleeding or hemorrhagic shock.[58, 60, 65, 66]

Management of a suspected *Echis* bite should include admission to an ICU setting. Progressive local signs and coagulation alterations are indications for the use of antivenin. A battery of laboratory studies are indicated at the time of hospital admission, with special attention to assessment of hemostasis.

Antivenin is helpful for the bleeding complications of these bites but is often less effective to combat the progression of tissue injury. Marked destruction of superficial and deep structures with rhabdomyolysis may occur. The tissue damage and necrosis are likely to require débridement. However, if possible, surgical procedures should be performed after the hemostatic defects have subsided. Transfusion with fresh frozen plasma, cryoprecipitate, platelets, and red blood cells may be required. The clinician should be particularly alert for central nervous system disturbances, as these may herald the development of intracranial hemorrhage.

Vipera russelli: *Russell's Viper*

This snake is found from northern Eurasia into and throughout Asia, including India, Sri Lanka, Bangladesh, Southeast China, Burma, Thailand, Indonesia, and Taiwan, as well as North Africa and the East Indies. The animal may reach a length of 4 ft and possesses up to 250 mg of venom with an intravenous LD_{50} of 0.08 mg/kg.[11] Russell's viper and other venomous snakes are the fifth leading cause of death in Burma, and in Sri Lanka the snake causes five deaths per 100,000 people per year.[75, 76] The venom contains a protein that activates factor X, as well as a number of other proteins, peptides, and enzymes.

Incoagulable blood is a consistent feature of patients with systemic Russell's viper envenoming. A micro-ELISA is available to detect venom in the serum or other body fluids of victims. In one study of 123 Burmese patients, 25% showed

no evidence of envenoming, another 25% had only local findings, but nearly one half of patients exhibited serious toxicity with marked coagulation changes that included thrombocytopenia, spontaneous bleeding, and shock.[77] Several antivenins are available, and antivenin is usually effective to treat the coagulation defects. Antivenin may also have some effects on tissue damage and other findings. However, the effectiveness of different antivenin preparations varies considerably.[76–79]

In one study, administration of antivenin within 4 hours did not prevent the development of renal failure. This may be related to the fact that oliguria and renal failure in these injuries is multifactorial. Oliguria resulting from perfusion failure, pigmenturia, and renal microthrombotic changes may also lead to renal dysfunction.[80] Fluid loading is usually effective to combat hypotension. Eight percent of patients may die as a result of renal failure, central nervous system hemorrhage, or shock.[77] An increase in vascular permeability may also be observed. Some patients have hemoconcentration, hypoalbuminemia, and pleural and peritoneal effusions similar to those observed in animal models of crotalid venom shock.[81]

Bitis gabonica: *Gaboon Viper and* Bitis arietans: *Puff Adder*

Several vipers in tropical and southern Africa are dangerous to humans. These include the puff adder, the Gaboon viper, and other closely related snakes. These animals are large, heavy snakes that possess fangs that may exceed 2 inches in length. The venom is toxic, and untreated cases are usually fatal.[11] These snakes account for a substantial proportion of fatal snakebites in Africa. A large puff adder possesses enough venom to kill several humans.

The venoms of these animals contain hemorrhagic components,[82] as well as factors that affect both intrinsic and extrinsic coagulation pathways and enhance the activation of plasminogen. A thrombin-like but not a fibrinolytic enzyme has been isolated from *B. gabonica* venom.[38, 83–85] Accordingly, severe and potentially fatal regional as well as systemic bleeding, together with tissue destruction, is common after bites by these snakes. Hemorrhage is consistently observed after injection of these toxins into experimental subjects.[37, 39, 85–87] In addition to the coagulation changes, a direct cardiotoxic fraction may also contribute to shock.[88] In a study of the circulatory, respiratory, metabolic, lethal, and tissue permeability effects of *Bitis* venom in rats, venom led to perfusion failure with hypotension, hemodilution, hypoproteinemia, and marked hyperventilation.[89] Total blood volume as well as red blood cell and plasma volumes were critically reduced, together with an increase in the transvascular escape of albumin. The study concluded that the venom leads to an increase in vascular permeability to albumin, as well as bleeding.

Treatment of these injuries includes prompt administration of antivenin, infusion of fluid and blood products that may include fresh frozen plasma and platelets, and management of tissue damage, which may be massive.[3]

Family Elapidae: *Elapids*

These snakes are found in many regions of the globe, from the New World to Australia and New Guinea, Africa, southern Asia and the Malay archipelago, the Philippines, and the Fiji Islands.[90] All members of this large family are venomous and include the cobras, mambas, coral snakes, death adders, kraits, taipans, and the tiger snake. Elapids are among the most lethal snakes in the world. The venom apparatus of the elapids includes a venom gland, duct, and fangs. In contrast to the fangs of the vipers and the pit vipers, those of the elapids are shorter and are fixed in position (see Fig. 145–3). The largest venomous snake in the world is an elapid. The king cobra (*Ophiophagus hannah*) is found in Southeast Asia and the Philippines and may reach a length of 18 ft.[7] The venom of many elapids has a variety of fractions that affect neuromuscular function, and elapid envenomations often include prominent neurotropic findings. However, these venoms also may lead to hemotoxic, cardiotoxic, and other disturbances and to substantial tissue damage.[91]

Although many toxins isolated from elapid venoms have action on other organ systems, certain purified basic proteins and polypeptides that are devoid of enzymatic activity have been shown to act selectively on the neuromuscular junction.[19, 34] The neurotoxins can be classified as presynaptic or postsynaptic in action (Table 145–7). Cobra toxin and α-bungarotoxin derived from krait venom produce an antidepolarizing block by acting on the postsynaptic end plate. Other toxins, such as β-bungarotoxin, are presynaptic. These affect the release of acetylcholine. Carbohydrates, free amino acids, nucleic acids, and lipids are also present.[33] Many of the venoms are yellow owing to the presence of L-amino-acid oxidase, which contains riboflavin. This component is a nonhydrolytic enzyme that converts free amino acids into alpha-keto acids.[9, 19] One of the most common enzymes in many snake venoms is phospholipase A_2 or lecithinase. Disruption of the electron transport chain and mitochondrial integrity are two of the deleterious properties of this material.

The neurotoxin isolated from the Australian tiger snake *Notechis scutatus scutatus* is a presynaptic compound that inhibits release of acetylcholine.[19, 34] The substance accounts for 6% of the weight of the crude venom and is also myonecrotic.

Mamba (genus *Dendroaspis*) venoms are neurotoxic, myonecrotic, and anticoagulant.[92, 93] Poisoning by mambas typically produces diaphoresis, hypotension, coma, vomiting, and respiratory arrest. Four species of mambas are found in tropical Africa. These animals are slender, are fast moving, and may be aggressive. Because of their toxic venom, speed, and aggressiveness, the mambas are extremely dangerous. A large mamba possesses sufficient venom to kill several people, and untreated mamba bites are often fatal. There are many reports of serial bites by one snake. Death is usually due to respiratory depression or cardiac arrhythmias. Pain and swelling at the site of the wound are less prominent with mamba bites, and tissue necrosis is usually minimal. However, respiratory paralysis may occur within minutes of the bite. Many elapids grasp the victim during biting and chew, rather than quickly releasing after the bite.

This action may introduce more venom into the wound. There are several species of kraits (genus *Bungarus*) in Southeast Asia. These animals may reach 7 ft in length and are nocturnal. They are usually less aggressive than mambas, although envenomation may be fatal. Respiratory paralysis may occur within minutes or develop after several hours; and fatalities are often associated with complications of prolonged mechanical ventilation.[94] Pain and local findings are moderate to severe.

α-Bungarotoxin, isolated from krait venom, has a molecular weight of 7000 and is a competitive postsynaptic neurotoxin that causes a nondepolarizing neuromuscular block.[7, 19, 34, 93, 95] Although it competes for the postsynaptic receptor, the blockade is irreversible and leads to a flaccid paralysis. The postsynaptic toxins may account for earlier symptoms than the presynaptic fractions, but the postsynaptic fractions appear to be more responsive to the effects of antivenin. The ptosis and ophthalmoplegia seen early after envenomation may therefore be due predominantly to the postsynaptic toxins. The presynaptic neurotoxins inhibit release of acetylcholine and are thought to be more lethal[34] than the postsynaptic compounds. β-Bungarotoxin and other similar toxins isolated from the tiger snake and taipan are typical presynaptic neurotoxins. They have molecular weights of 13,000 to 22,000 and resemble phospholipase A_2 in structure.

Closely related to the mambas and kraits are the cobras. These animals are dangerous. There are at least six species of the cobra genus *Naja*. Cobras are widely distributed in Africa and Asia.

Edrophonium, 10 mg intravenously after 0.6 mg of atropine, is useful in the management of neurotoxic envenoming by cobras and related species.[54, 94] Edrophonium is a short-acting anticholinesterase, which has been shown to help reverse signs and symptoms such as cranial nerve dysfunction. The careful use of this agent may improve swallowing, coughing, and speaking after envenomation. If the response is successful, a longer-acting preparation such as neostigmine may be considered. In studies comparing edrophonium with antivenin, edrophonium was more successful in reversing these symptoms.[96]

Anticholinesterases have been reported to be helpful for other elapid bites and for sea snake envenomations, but responses are variable. For example, in bites by kraits, the results are often less dramatic than for cobra envenomings.[34, 97–99] Therefore, antivenin should not be withheld if available. Guidelines for the use of antivenin for serious elapid poisonings include a documented envenomation by history, signs and symptoms, and/or ELISA test results, and the development of systemic evidence of poisoning, such as cranial nerve dysfunction, respiratory distress, alterations in speech, and/or dysphagia.

Attempts to remove elapid venom from the wound have not been successful, although a number of devices have been utilized to aspirate venom from the wound.[100]

North American Elapids

There are three species of elapids in the United States. All are brightly colored coral snakes, which may be confused with several nonvenomous snakes. The most dangerous is the Eastern coral snake, *Micrurus fulvius fulvius*, which may reach a length of 3 ft. This animal is found in the southern states to Mississippi. The Texas coral snake, *M. fulvius tenere*, is primarily confined to that state. The smaller Western or Sonoran coral snake, *Micruroides euryxanthus euryxanthus*, is common in Arizona and surrounding regions of New Mexico and Mexico.

Few deaths are reported from coral snakes, although

TABLE 145–7

EXAMPLES OF SNAKE VENOM NEUROTOXINS

Site and Action	Examples	Effects
Postsynaptic Compete for postsynaptic receptor	α-Bungarotoxin Tiger snake neurotoxin Sea snake toxin	Early paralysis Early symptoms may be more responsive to antivenin
Presynaptic Inhibit release of acetylcholine	β-Bungarotoxin Sea snake neurotoxin Taipan neurotoxin	Potentially more lethal

Modified from Minton SA: Neurotoxic snake envenoming. Reprinted with permission from Seminars in Neurology, volume 10, pages 52–61, 1990, Thieme Medical Publishers, Inc.

envenomation occurs in up to 75% of bites, and serious neurotoxic symptoms are common after contact with the Eastern coral snake.[101] Symptoms may be delayed for up to 12 hours. Most bites occur on the hand or the foot and usually occur in the spring or fall. Local findings are seen in 40% of patients but may be mild. A variety of neurotropic changes are likely to develop, including cranial nerve dysfunction and respiratory failure that may require endotracheal intubation and mechanical ventilation. These complications develop in approximately 5% of cases of bites by the Eastern species. Antivenin is available for the Eastern coral snake and is helpful in management, although its effectiveness to reverse or prevent severe neurotropic dysfunction has not been clarified. A significant number of patients treated with antivenin experience urticaria and/or serum sickness, and anaphylactic reactions are always a risk when antivenin is given. In one study of 39 patients, up to 15 vials of antivenin were given, although the average dose was approximately 6 vials.[101] Findings of neuromuscular toxicity may be manifested by fasciculations, paresthesias, and increases in creatine kinase levels.

Bites by the Sonoran and Texas coral snakes are generally less dangerous than those by the Eastern coral snake.[102] No antivenin is available for these injuries, and Eastern coral snake antivenin is not effective for these bites.[9]

Australian Elapids

Sutherland estimated that 3000 snakebites occur each year in Australia, of which 300 necessitate antivenin therapy.[53] Despite the extreme danger of these snakes, only a few deaths occur. There are many dangerous snakes in Australia, and the venomous forms outnumber nontoxic snakes in this subcontinent. In addition to the dangerous tiger snake (*N. scutatus scutatus*) and taipan (*Oxyuranus scutellatus*), several species of brown snakes (genus *Demansia*) and copperheads (genus *Denisonia*) and the death adder (*Acanthophis antarcticus*), a viper-like elapid, are found. Venom detection kits using ELISA technology are available to confirm envenomation and to help identify the species.[53, 103–105] Local therapy is of little aid in the early management of these injuries, although Sutherland has popularized the use of a compression dressing if a delay is anticipated in the transport of the patient to a hospital. Incision and suction and other local measures are not effective. Scrubbing or washing the area of the wound is also not recommended. These measures may also remove material that could be used for venom detection studies by ELISA kits. First-aid measures should therefore concentrate on efforts to immobilize the patient and to rapidly transport the victim to a hospital.

Local reactions to Australian elapid bites are often mild. However, severe tissue damage that may be associated with myonecrosis, rhabdomyolysis, and renal failure may supervene. Systemic effects, particularly neurologic toxicity, are among the most dangerous effects of envenomation. Frequently reported findings include nausea, vomiting, hypotension, weakness, cranial nerve dysfunction, abdominal pain, hematuria, coagulation changes, and systemic bleeding as well as bleeding from the wound. In addition, intracranial hemorrhage may be the first manifestation of a severe envenomation and the associated coagulopathy.

A swab should be obtained from the site of the bite, as well as a sample of blood for venom detection studies. Arterial blood gas studies, assessment of respiratory muscle function, and an electrocardiogram, together with a coagulation profile; determination of electrolytes, blood urea nitrogen, and serum creatinine; and assays of muscle enzymes (creatine kinase), should be obtained on admission. These studies should be repeated at intervals, particularly during the first 24 hours.

Highly effective antivenin to the various species of Australian elapids is produced by the Commonwealth Serum Laboratories, Melbourne. However, most authorities recommend that these sera should not be given in the field, but only in an intensive care setting that is equipped to manage potentially fatal allergic reactions. A subcutaneous test dose of antivenin may be given, but the results do not accurately predict an acute allergic reaction. Premedication with antihistamines and occasionally catecholamines may be considered. Antivenin is given intravenously.

Death resulting from these snakebites is usually caused by respiratory depression, but bleeding, renal failure, and other multisystem disturbances complicate these bites. Plasma volume repletion using colloid fluids may be needed, as well as red blood cell infusions and fresh frozen plasma and platelet transfusions to correct hemostatic defects.[53, 106]

Family Crotalidae: Pit Vipers

Although there are a number of injuries by exotic snakes maintained in zoos or as pets, the overwhelming majority of snakebites in North America are due to pit vipers. These include the various rattlesnakes (genus *Crotalus*), pygmy rattlesnakes and massasaugas (genus *Sistrurus*), and the cottonmouths and copperheads (genus *Agkistrodon*). Approximately 8000 people are treated for snake venom poisoning in the United States each year.[107, 108] Russell estimated that an additional 1000 snake bites are not reported.[107] However, fewer than 10 deaths result annually from snake venom poisoning in the United States. There are several pit vipers in Asia, including the Malayan pit viper, *A. rhodostoma*, and the sharp-nosed pit viper, *Agkistrodon acutus*.

Pit vipers are similar to vipers in many respects but also possess a loreal pit behind each nostril. These structures are thermosensitive organs and are thought to be used in conjunction with the other senses to localize prey and enemies. Pit vipers and most vipers have vertically elliptic pupils, whereas elapids and most nonvenomous snakes have round pupils. Crotalids possess a well-developed venom apparatus that includes long, erectile fangs and the ability to deliver a considerable dose of venom during a strike. In approximately 20% of bites, there is no evidence of envenoming, although for patients who are subsequently referred to a tertiary care center, the percentage of patients without envenomation is less.[108] For bites in the United States, most injuries involve males, usually involve a hand or a foot, and are most common in spring and summer. More than one half of bites involve attempts by the patient to capture or handle the snake.

Bites by vipers and pit vipers produce tissue damage as well as disturbances that may affect hemostatic, cardiopulmonary, metabolic, and neuromuscular function. Local symptoms are typically prominent. A simplified grading system for snake bites is depicted in Table 145–8. Pain is a variable symptom after crotalid envenoming. Some patients report numbness. Pain may also be related to the development of edema and local hemorrhage. Regional pain may involve the axilla or inguinal sites.

The venom of *C. scutulatus scutulatus* is among the most toxic of that of any snake in North America.[9, 11, 109] Therefore, this snake is particularly dangerous and accounts for significant morbidity and mortality among snakebites in the Southwest.[110–113] Injuries by the Mojave rattlesnake have been described in which local symptoms were minimal, despite serious systemic neurologic toxicity.[110, 111, 113] However, more recent reports of bites by this species suggest that marked local tissue changes and symptoms are more common than previously observed and that severe neurologic dysfunction occurs relatively infrequently.[114, 115] Coagulation changes may also be observed with this species. The tropical rattlesnake,

TABLE 145–8

SIMPLIFIED GRADING SYSTEM FOR CROTALID AND VIPERID SNAKEBITES

No Envenomation
Bites by venomous (or unknown) species; no local or systemic findings after several hours of observation

Minimal Envenomation
Bite
Local findings (edema, ecchymoses, and so on) without progression
No systemic signs or symptoms

Moderate Envenomation
Bite
Progressive local and regional findings and/or systemic toxicity that is not life threatening
Moderate disturbances of laboratory assays

Severe Envenomation
Bite
Large or dangerous species or high-risk victim
Marked local and regional findings and/or serious cardiopulmonary or metabolic derangements
Marked laboratory abnormalities

C. durissus, also possesses an extremely potent venom, and bites by this snake are particularly dangerous.

For other pit viper bites, local edema and hemorrhage are characteristic and may progress rapidly (Fig. 145–4). In some instances, edema may be associated with the development of blebs, which may be hemorrhagic. These usually develop within the first 24 hours. If venom is injected into a vascular structure, local findings may be minimal or absent, despite significant systemic toxicity. Paresthesias and pain may supervene and may be accompanied by fasciculations. Analogous findings of muscular irritability may be manifested as cardiac arrhythmias. Some patients complain of a rubbery or metallic taste in the mouth. This has been particularly observed after bites by the Southern Pacific rattlesnake, *Crotalus viridis helleri.*[9, 116]

Although pit viper envenomation is a medical emergency, it is important to remember that only a few deaths result from these injuries. Accordingly, the intensive care practitioner must recognize the most dangerous signs and symptoms of a severe envenoming but should avoid unnecessary treatment. Restraint should also be exercised in the use of new or provocative therapies. In particular, the management of the wound and surrounding tissue injury has undergone considerable re-evaluation during the past several years. A variety of treatments have been shown to be ineffective or dangerous, and recommendations for the first aid of these injuries have been modified and updated.

Initial enthusiastic reports of incision and suction, excision of the wound, use of constricting bands and tourniquets, local application of ice, administration of various solutions, and inhalation of oxygen have yielded to the conclusion that, in most situations, early local therapy is of little value and may be hazardous. The most efficacious initial treatment is immobilization. Cryotherapy (application of cold) and use of tourniquets are no longer recommended for these injuries, and most authorities do not recommend early aggressive surgical procedures.

The most recent therapy that has emerged is the application of high-voltage direct current to the wound by a stun gun.[117–119] Initial reports of the effectiveness of this treatment were based on the theory that the high-voltage current neutralized or denatured venom toxins. Analogous ill-founded theories were cited as rationale for the use of a number of other maneuvers that have been subsequently abandoned, such as cryotherapy, excision of the wound, or extensive débridement. In an experimental study to test the effectiveness of high-voltage current, no beneficial results could be demonstrated.[120]

Coagulation studies may demonstrate a variety of hemostatic defects, in addition to local and systemic bleeding.[39, 43] Thrombocytopenia may develop within hours. In one study of experimental rattlesnake venom poisoning, the severity of thrombocytopenia was related to the dose of venom.[121] Fibrinogen levels may also decline, in part owing to the fibrinogenolysis associated with the thrombin-like serine esterase venom fractions, as well as other components that affect intrinsic and extrinsic clotting pathways.[9, 23, 122–128]

In severe cases, perfusion failure occurs. There are marked changes in vascular resistance, although the cause of shock is multifactorial[129–131] (Fig. 145–5). The venom of *Bothrops jararaca* and *Agkistrodon halys blomhoffi* contains peptides that inhibit angiotensin-converting enzyme and may lead to a marked decrease in vascular pressure and resistance.[132–134] Shock may be related in part to toxicity of venom fractions on the myocardium.

Hypovolemia is consistently observed in experimental models of rattlesnake venom poisoning.[81] Venom leads to a marked increase in vascular permeability to red blood cells and plasma. The critical defect in experimental models is a deficit of plasma volume, and shock is neither prevented nor altered by large doses of corticosteroids or antivenin.[135] Prompt fluid loading, particularly with colloid fluids, restores vascular volume in experimental venom shock.[136] If crystalloid fluids are given, at least six times the volume deficit must be given to restore plasma volume.[137]

For patients with hemodynamic instability after pit viper envenomation, the intensive care specialist is well advised to evaluate vascular volume and hemostasis. Fluid loading may be required to achieve acceptable end points for oxygen transport, arterial pressure, and systemic perfusion. I utilize colloid fluids; fresh frozen plasma, red blood cells, and platelets may be needed. If fluid resuscitation does not lead to restoration of hemodynamic competence, vasoactive agents may be needed.[137] If arterial or central venous access is needed for monitoring or therapy, disturbances of hemostasis should be addressed before vascular catheterization.

Polyvalent antivenin for American pit vipers (Antivenin [Crotalidae] polyvalent, Wyeth-Ayerst Laboratories, Philadelphia) is prepared against the venoms of the Eastern diamondback (*Crotalus adamanteus*), Western diamondback (*Crotalus atrox*), South American or tropical rattlesnake or Cascabel (*Crotalus durissus terrificus*), and the fer-de-lance (*Bothrops atrox*). This product is the only antivenin currently available for treatment of pit viper bites in the United States. Unfortunately, this serum has limited effectiveness against many of the lethal and other deleterious crotalid venom fractions. Use is associated with a significant risk of acute and subacute allergic reactions. Immediate hypersensitivity reactions to antivenin may be seen in as many as 25% of patients, and the incidence of delayed serum reactions appears to correlate with the dose of antivenin given.[108, 138, 139] The polyvalent antivenin contains equine antibodies that predominantly bind to large (>30,000 daltons) venom fractions but has minimal antibody titers to the smaller basic proteins and peptides in pit viper venoms.[140] These smaller molecules are associated with many of the most deleterious properties of the venoms. In the future, antivenin may be available that is prepared in vitro in sheep, chickens, or other species, using techniques that may enable the production of sera with high titers of antibodies against specific, deleterious venom fractions but with a reduced risk of allergic reactions.[141, 142]

Some clinicians have cautioned against the routine use of

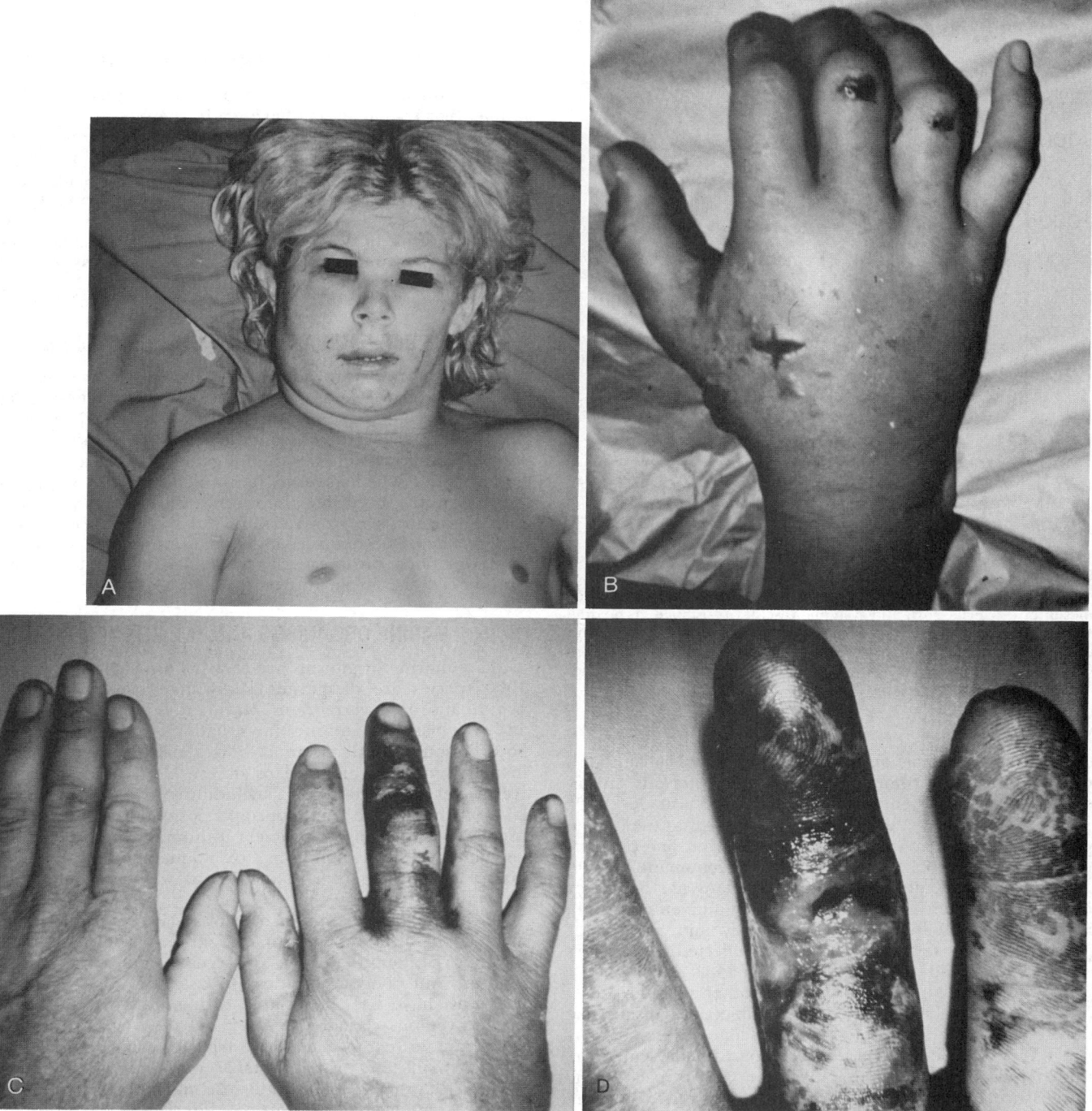

Figure 145–4. Edema, hemorrhage, and tissue injury resulting from crotolid envenomation of the face (*A*), hand (*B*), and finger (*C* and *D*).

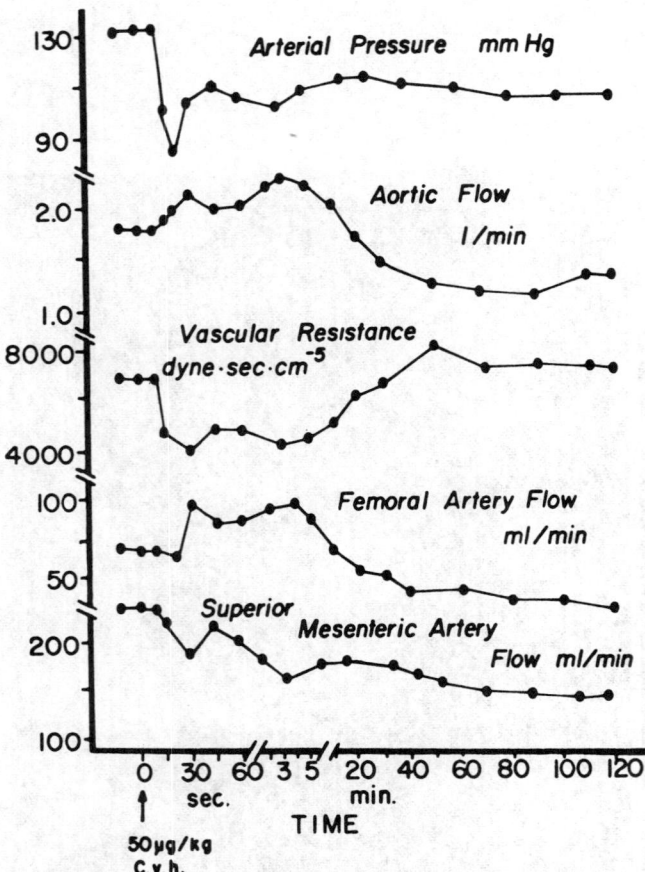

Figure 145-5. Effects of a rapid, intravenous, sublethal injection of rattlesnake venom on arterial pressure; aortic, femoral, and superior mesenteric arterial flow; and systemic vascular resistance in the dog. Initial increases in flow are followed by a subsequent decline and are accompanied by a biphasic response of vascular resistance. (From Carlson RW, Bowles AL, Haupt MT: Anaphylactic, anaphylactoid, and related forms of shock. Crit Care Clin 2:347, 1986.)

the currently available antivenin in pit .viper bites, although most authorities recommend antivenin for serious envenomings after a risk-benefit evaluation has been made.[9, 108, 114, 138, 143–151] Accordingly, any suggestions regarding the appropriate dose of antivenin are controversial, but one protocol recommends up to 5 vials for minimal envenomation, up to 10 vials for moderate injuries, and as many as 15 vials or more for severe envenomations.[23, 108, 144] If antivenin is given, it should be administered intravenously and as soon as practicable. The serum should not be injected into fingers or toes and should not be used in the field.

The indications for fasciotomy and other surgical procedures in crotalid bites have been the subject of considerable debate.[23, 27, 144, 152–163] Although marked edema and hemorrhage may occasionally lead to a compartmental syndrome, this complication develops in only a few patients, particularly if measurements of tissue pressure are used to confirm compartmental hypertension.[152, 162–165] It is difficult to assess the adequacy of vascular supply in a tense, edematous extremity. These findings may lead the clinician to suspect a compartmental syndrome on the basis of clinical signs and symptoms. However, despite considerable edema, blood flow is usually adequate. In one study in which several patients exhibited local edema and bleeding, blood flow to the region determined by noninvasive techniques was normal to increased.[166] The wick technique to measure tissue pressure is

recommended in situations in which a compartmental syndrome is suspected. Surgical consultation is indicated for crotalid bites and other snakebites for management of tissue injury. In my experience, a conservative approach is warranted in most injuries. Secondary infection develops in many wounds after snakebites, but prophylactic antibiotics are not indicated in most cases. Appropriate therapy for tetanus should be given.

Family Colubridae: Rear-Fanged Snakes

Many nonvenomous snakes belong to the large Colubridae family. Because all snakes have teeth, the bite of any snake can lead to local and occasionally systemic signs and symptoms, as well as secondary infection and direct injury by the bite. The most dangerous colubrid is the boomslang (*Dispholidus typus*), a tree-dwelling snake found in tropical and southern Africa.[9, 167–169] The venom is extremely toxic and bites may result in death. Marked coagulation changes typically occur, as well as other systemic effects. Antivenin is available for treatment of these injuries.

SUBORDER SAURIA, FAMILY HELODERMATIDAE

Heloderma horridum (beaded lizard) and *Heloderma suspectum* (Gila monster) are two lizards in the Southwest United States and Mexico that are venomous. These animals have grooved mandibular teeth and submandibular venom glands. These stout, slow-moving animals do not generally pose a threat to humans, but when aroused bite and grasp the victim as venom is introduced into the wound. Fortunately, bites are rare. Signs and symptoms resemble those of a crotalid bite and include pain, edema, coagulation changes, and in serious envenomations, cardiovascular instability.[9, 170–173] There is no commercially available antivenin.

MARINE ORGANISMS AND THEIR TOXINS

Many marine organisms are toxic to humans. More than 1000 species are dangerous and range from unicellular protozoans to the vertebrates. Marine toxins include poisons and venoms;[12, 15, 17] and in some situations, an animal may be both poisonous and venomous. Toxic organisms are found in all of the seas and oceans of the world and in many freshwater bodies of water, including rivers, streams, and lakes. Although the venomous and poisonous forms do not usually present a major problem to humans, in some areas, and under certain conditions, toxic aquatic organisms may pose a risk to the local population as well as a danger to individuals.

Marine toxins are complex mixtures that vary considerably in their chemical and pharmacologic properties. Some are proteins, although amines, quaternary ammonium compounds, mucopolysaccharides, lipids, and other unique chemicals have been associated with these forms. Several marine venoms contain enzymes, but these substances are less common than in many terrestrial venoms. A number of marine toxins are highly unstable, and after they are removed from the animal, rapidly lose many of their chemical and/or pharmacologic properties. Many of these poisons are heat labile.

PHYLUM PROTOZOA, ORDER DINOFLAGELLATA
Paralytic Shellfish Poisoning

Paralytic shellfish poisoning is related to ingesting shellfish that contain toxic unicellular organisms. These dinoflagellates bloom during changes in water and weather conditions.

When these blooms occur, high concentrations of these organisms in the water cause red tide or brown water conditions. The large numbers of these protists may lead to death of fish and other marine life, but the danger to humans is when the organisms are ingested by mollusks, echinoderms, or arthropods. The toxins are concentrated in the tissues of these animals, which subsequently eaten by humans.

The most common form of this poisoning is termed paralytic shellfish poisoning. It has been reported worldwide and is most common in spring and fall months.[8, 174-176] The capture or sale of shellfish during these seasons may be prohibited in some areas to prevent human poisoning. Bivalved mollusks such as mussels and clams are most commonly involved, although other animals may become contaminated. Boiling, freezing, steaming, frying, or other techniques of preservation and cooking do not destroy the toxin, and many poisonings occur after consumption of meat or broth of contaminated shellfish that have been steamed.

The genus most commonly associated with these outbreaks is *Gonyaulax*.[15] Species of this genus have been responsible for poisonings in North and South America and Japan and other Pacific regions, as well as several areas in the Atlantic. *Pyrodinium* and *Gymnodinium* are other genera that have been implicated in human poisonings.[177, 178]

The toxin associated with these poisonings is termed *saxitoxin*. A number of similar saxitoxin molecules have been identified. The structure is a tetrahydropurine derivative, and one saxitoxin has the following chemical composition: $C_{10}H_{17}N_7O_4 \cdot 2HCl$, with a molecular weight of 372. The material is highly toxic and the purified toxin has an LD_{50} of approximately 3 μg/kg.[178-181] The pharmacology of this material is similar to that of another marine toxin. Tetrodotoxin and faxitoxin interfere with the early, transiently open channel that admits sodium ions in excitable membranes.[182, 183] Potassium conductance is not altered. Therefore, these toxins block action potentials in nerves and muscles. Death is usually related to respiratory failure, although direct cardiotoxicity may be seen, as well as hypotension caused by changes in vascular resistance.

Clinical features are primarily related to neurologic signs and symptoms. Symptoms usually develop within minutes to hours after ingestion of contaminated shellfish. Paresthesias and dysesthesias occur often initially around the mouth and progress to involve the limbs. Muscle paralysis may supervene, and cranial nerve dysfunction may be a prominent feature in some poisoning.[184, 185] Respiratory insufficiency is a common problem, which provokes admission to hospital. Approximately 50% of patients seek hospitalization, and a significant number may require ventilatory support. Hypotension may also be observed. Mortality has decreased with aggressive ICU supportive care, but previously ranged from 5 to 18%.[185] Death usually occurs within the first few hours. If the patient is maintained with supportive measures, the illness subsides within 3 to 5 days.

There is no antidote or immunity, although the diagnosis may be confirmed in some instances by detecting the toxin in gastric fluid or in the suspected food.

Ciguatera Poisoning

Ciguatera poisoning is also caused by eating seafood that has been contaminated by a dinoflagellate. In this case, the toxin is concentrated in a variety of coral reef fishes and eels. The benthic dinoflagellate *Gambierdiscus toxicus* is incorporated into the food chain from fish that feed on algae and debris around tropical reefs. These herbivores such as the surgeonfish and parrotfish are subsequently eaten by reef carnivores and omnivores. These include moray eels, jacks and amberjacks, snappers, some tunas, groupers, and barracuda. The meat of these fish contains the toxin, which, when ingested by humans, leads to the typical symptoms of the poisoning. This form of fish poisoning is termed *ichthyosarcotoxism*, as it involves the viscera, flesh, muscle, and skin of fish. The brain, intestines, liver, and gonads of the fish contain substantially higher concentrations of the toxin than does muscle.

Ciguatera poisoning occurs in tropical and subtropical areas throughout the world. It is particularly common in the waters of the Caribbean and around Florida, the South Pacific, and Hawaii. Ciguatera poisoning is probably the most common form of marine intoxication in the United States.[177, 186, 187]

There is more than one ciguatera toxin, and the chemical structures of these molecules have not been completely characterized. Ciguatoxins are lipid soluble, colorless, odorless, and heat stable with a molecular weight of approximately 1100. The material is toxic. Like saxitoxin, ciguatoxins primarily affect neuromuscular transmission. Sodium permeability of excitable membranes is increased, causing depolarization.[188, 189] The depolarization induced by ciguatoxin is blocked by tetrodotoxin. Symptoms typically include paresthesias, peripheral muscle weakness, respiratory distress, myalgias, pruritus, diaphoresis, headache, and ataxia, as well as gastrointestinal symptoms such as cramps, abdominal pain, diarrhea, nausea, and vomiting. Two frequently reported symptoms are heat-cold dysesthesia and altered taste. Cardiovascular findings may be observed, such as hypotension, tachycardia, and marked sinus bradycardia. Some complaints, particularly neurologic symptoms, may persist for protracted intervals.[178, 190-194]

Treatment is supportive. For management of the more severe neurologic and cardiovascular findings, admission to an ICU is warranted. A variety of agents have been suggested to be helpful: calcium salts, mannitol, atropine, magnesium, tricyclic antidepressants, and calcium channel–blocking agents.[195-199] Some patients report an increase in symptoms with consumption of alcohol. The toxin may be detected in contaminated fish by an enzyme-linked assay.[200]

Scombroid Fish Poisoning
Scombrotoxism

Scombrotoxism is a form of ichthyosarcotoxism caused by bacteria in spoiled fish that produce a toxin. The syndrome results from the ingestion of improperly preserved fish. Dark meat fish are most commonly implicated, such as bonito, skipjack, mackerels, dolphin, albacore, and tuna. Scombroid poisoning may be the most common form of fish poisoning in the world. Symptoms develop within an hour after ingestion of the fish and include flushing, nausea, diaphoresis, vomiting, diarrhea, palpitations, rash, and occasionally edema of the face and tongue. Hypotension and respiratory distress with bronchospasm may occur.

It has now been established that this poisoning appears to be due to the production of histamine in spoiled fish by bacteria because of inadequate cooling.[201-204] Histamine content of affected tissues is high. Symptoms are improved by treatment with histamine H_1 and H_2 receptor antagonist drugs.[205] Signs and symptoms may be severe and may warrant admission to an ICU, but the syndrome generally resolves within hours.

Clupeotoxism

Clupeotoxism is another form of ichthyosarcotoxic poisoning that is seen after eating herring, anchovies, bonefishes,

TABLE 145-9
CLASSIFICATION OF VENOMOUS COELENTERATES

Phylum Cnidaria (Coelenterata)
 	
Class Hydrozoa: hydroids; stinging, fire or false coral
  Order Siphonophora: free-floating siphonophores
    Family Physaliidae
      Physalia physalis—Portuguese man-of-war,
        bluebottle Caravelle, vissie de mer, galere
Class Anthosoa: sea anemones, sea fans, corals
Class Scyphozoa (Scyphomedusae): jellyfish
  Family Chirodropidae: sea wasps, box jellyfish
    Chironex fleckeri—sea wasp
    Chiropsalmus quadrigatus, C. quadrumanus—
      sea wasp

and tarpons. The origin of the toxin appears to be derived from the ingestion of dinoflagellates by these fishes. The poisoning is fatal in many cases. Signs and symptoms resemble those of severe paralytic shellfish poisoning, and the syndrome develops rapidly.[8] In some reports, death occurred before the victim had finished eating the fish.[206] There is no specific treatment, but the poisoning may require immediate application of life-support measures.

PHYLUM PORIFERA: SPONGES

Although there are more than 5000 species of sponges, only limited numbers of tropical and subtropical forms are toxic to humans. Intoxication occurs through skin abrasions by spicules of the sponge. A variety of toxic substances have been isolated from sponges, including histamine, acetylcholine, nitrogenous bases, and steroids. Contact with some sponges may cause severe skin and local reactions, as well as anaphylactoid reactions.[207–210] Aside from management of the life-threatening allergic reactions, therapy is primarily directed to local signs and symptoms. Treatments that have been reported to be effective include soaks or application of acetic acid (5%) or isopropyl alcohol to affected parts. Topical corticosteroid preparations are helpful. Another syndrome associated with contact with sponges is sponge-diver's disease, caused by a coelenterate envenomation from contact with anenomes attached to or near the sponge.[8, 211]

PHYLUM CNIDARIA (COELENTERATA): JELLYFISH, ANEMONES, AND PORTUGUESE MAN-OF-WAR

The coelenterates include vast numbers of animals that are found throughout the seas of the world. At least 70 species are toxic to humans and are found in three classes: Hydrozoa (including the hydroids and the free-floating siphonophores or *Physalia*, commonly termed the Portuguese man-of-war); the Anthozoa (anemones, sea fans, and corals); and the Scyphozoa, or Scyphomedusae (true jellyfish)[15] (Table 145–9).

The venom apparatus of coelenterates is the nematocyst, although not all nematocysts are able to puncture human skin. The nematocyst is a highly sophisticated device, which fires a hollow tube containing venom into a person on contact (Fig. 145–6). Activation may be induced by a variety of chemical and mechanical stimuli, a point that has clinical and therapeutic significance. There is a high concentration of nematocysts in coelenterates, particularly on the surface of tentacles and other structures. Hence, the dose of venom is related to the surface area of the animal in contact with the person. Literally hundreds of thousands of nematocysts may be discharged into a person.

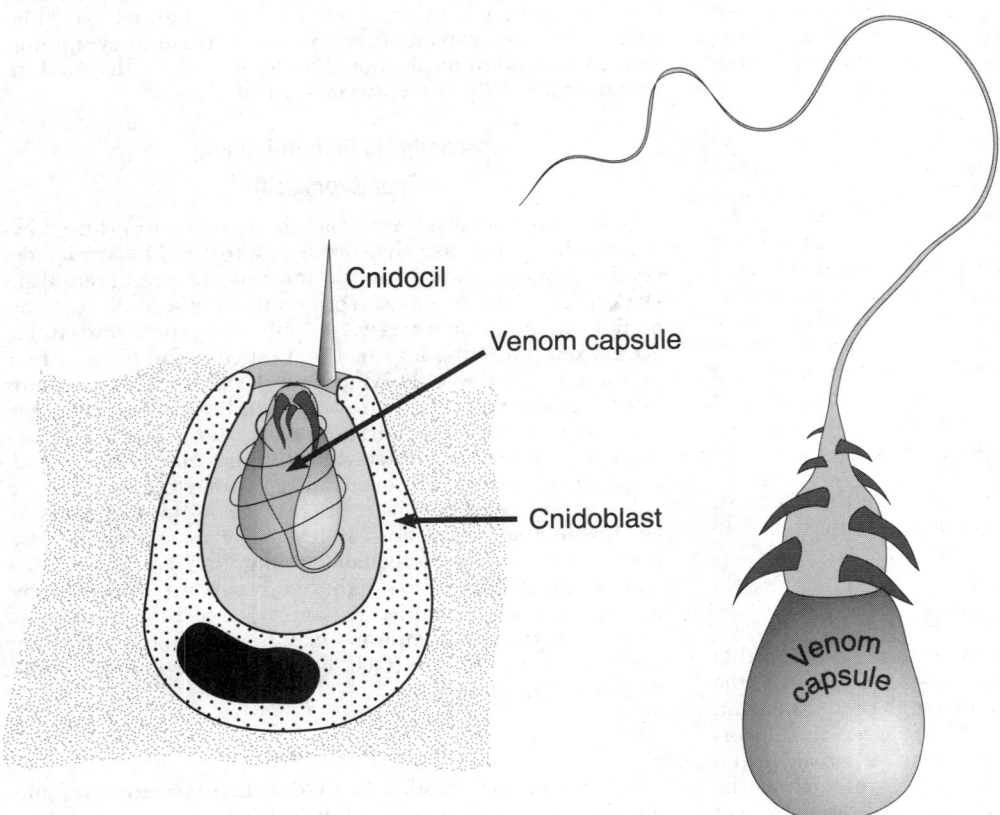

Figure 145–6. Nematocyst, showing the cnidocil, cnidoblast, and venom capsule.

Interrelationships and similarities between anaphylaxis and venom injuries have been the subject of many studies, particularly of coelenterate envenomations. In the early portion of this century, anaphylactic and tachyphylactic responses to the venom of a sea anenome were noted.[212, 213] In describing human envenomations with various cnidarians, it may be difficult to separate allergic reactions from the primary effects of the toxins, as the responses may be similar. There are reports of anaphylactic reactions to coelenterates.[214]

The venom of coelenterates contains a variety of low- and high-molecular-weight substances. Proteins, amines, hydroxyproline, amino acids, minerals, and other substances have been isolated. The lethal components are proteins,[12, 176, 215–217] some of which have enzymatic activities. Proteins with cardiotoxic properties are thought to be among the most lethal components of the dangerous cnidarians such as the box jellyfish or sea wasp, *Chironex fleckeri* and *Chiropsalmus quadrigatus*.[214, 218]

Envenomations range from minor skin irritation to a rapidly fatal syndrome. Immediate pain is characteristic of these injuries. Dermal reactions include pruritus, paresthesias, pain, bullae, secondary infection, local hemorrhage, desquamation, and other changes.[219–223] A variety of other systemic findings may develop.

Attempts to remove the patient from tentacles or other parts should be accomplished quickly. Care should be exercised to avoid additional discharge of nematocysts into the patient or rescuers. The tentacles may be scraped from the wound or removed with forceps. The area should be rinsed with salt water, alcohol, shaving cream, a slurry of baking soda, acetic acid, or alcohol. Freshwater should not be used, as it causes firing of nematocysts. Sea sand may be used to help remove the animal and prevent further discharge of stinging units[224–226] (Table 145–10).

TABLE 145–10

EMERGENCY TREATMENT OF COELENTERATE STINGS

1. Remove victim from water or exposure
2. Disengage from tentacles
   - Gently scrape with sea sand or salt water
   - Avoid contact with rescuers
   - Remove tentacles with forceps or other instruments
3. Irrigate and cleanse affected area
   - Baking soda powder or slurry
   - Shaving cream
   - Vinegar, meat tenderizer
   - *Note:* Do not use ammonia, liquid bleach, fresh water, mineral spirits; these may result in firing of nematocysts
4. Treat local lesions
   - Corticosteroid cream or spray (severe reactions may necessitate systemic steroids)
   - Antibiotics as needed
   - Pain: opiates often required
5. Antitetanus therapy
6. Treat systemic reactions
   - Cardiopulmonary arrest
   - Shock, respiratory arrest, bronchospasm
   - Arrhythmias: consider verapamil, 5–10 mg IV, with repeated doses as needed
   - Gastrointestinal: pain, nausea or vomiting
   - Hematologic: hemolysis, coagulopathy
   - Ophthalmic: irrigate; consider ophthalmology evaluation
   - Neuromuscular: altered sensorium, pain on motion, spasm arthralgia, seizures, coma
   - Constitutional: fever, chills, leukocytosis
   - Anaphylaxis or cardiac arrest
   - Consider antivenin for severe reactions to *C. fleckeri*

For contact with coral, it is important to remove tiny fragments from the wound with hydrogen peroxide and vigorous cleansing. These injuries are particularly likely to become infected and heal slowly.

Steroid cream or sprays are helpful to manage the skin lesions after initial treatment. Tetanus prophylaxis is indicated. An ice pack may also help relieve local symptoms.[226]

The pain associated with coelenterate stings may be excruciating and may be aggravated by movement. Pain may be accompanied by systemic symptoms such as nausea, vomiting, muscle cramps, hypotension, urticaria, bronchospasm, and respiratory distress. Hypotension and other signs such as hemolysis may herald a severe response to the venom. Verapamil given intravenously has been used with good results to combat life-threatening cardiotoxicity and may potentiate the effects of antivenin.[227–230]

It is possible that skin divers, swimmers, and surfers who experience repeated contact with coelenterates may develop immunoglobulin E antibodies followed by anaphylaxis. It is likely therefore that some reports of drowning may actually be caused by such reactions.[215, 230, 231]

Hospital admission is indicated for patients with marked signs and symptoms. Observation and ICU management of life-threatening cardiopulmonary changes may be necessary.

The box jellyfish or sea wasp (*C. fleckeri*) is a scyphozoan that is found off the northeast coast of Australia. This organism has an extremely toxic venom, and cardiopulmonary collapse and death may occur after contact within minutes. Aside from first-aid measures and cardiopulmonary resuscitation, an antivenin is available for intravenous use in life-threatening reactions.[215, 220, 230, 232, 233]

PHYLUM ECHINODERMATA: ECHINODERMS

Many echinoderms are venomous or poisonous. The venomous species are found in three classes: Asteroidea (starfishes), Echinoidea (sea urchins), and Holothuroidea (sea cucumbers).[15]

Most starfishes are not dangerous to humans, although contact with slime or spines may lead to local, and occasionally systemic, toxicity. The only venomous starfish is the *Acanthaster planci*. This animal may reach 60 cm in diameter and is found along the Great Barrier Reef of Australia. Contact with spines of this animal may lead to painful wounds, together with nausea, vomiting, and paralysis.[8, 12, 15] There is no specific therapy.

The sea urchins possess two types of spines: primary spines and the smaller, secondary spines. The primary spines produce puncture wounds and often troublesome foreign body reactions. The secondary spines include the venomous, globiferous pedicellariae.[233–235]

Several toxins have been isolated from echinoderms, including steroid glycosides, serotonin, and acetylcholine-like compounds.[12, 15, 17, 178, 236] Hemolytic and hypotensive activities as well as release of histamine and neurologic alterations have been described for these toxins.[237] The steroid molecules and attached sugars are anionic saponins that cause irreversible changes of cholinergic neuromuscular junctions.[237] Immediate pain, edema, and other local findings may be accompanied by syncopy, respiratory paralysis, and paralysis. Secondary infection of these wounds is common, and the lesions may cause considerable irritation. Therapy is supportive. Local heat may be helpful to combat pain. Pedicellariae and embedded spines should be removed, if possible. There is no antivenin. The venomous sea urchins are widely distributed throughout many seas of the world.

The class Holothuroidea includes the sea cucumbers. These are free-living, bottom-dwelling echinoderms that produce a toxin excreted as a defensive maneuver. Toxicity

TABLE 145–11
VENOMOUS AND POISONOUS MOLLUSKS

Phylum Mollusca

Class Gastropoda: univalve snails and slugs
  Family Conidae: cone shells
Class Pelecypoda: bivalves (scallops, clams, oysters) (paralytic
  shellfish poisoning)
Class Cephalopoda: squid, octopus, nautilus, cuttlefish
  Octopus maculosus—blue-banded octopus, ringed octopus

may follow contact or ingestion. The poison is known as holothurin.[176, 236–238] Holothurians may also contain intact nematocysts from ingested coelenterates. Local and/or systemic findings may occur. One toxin isolated from sea cucumbers is holothurin A. The empirical chemical composition is $C_{50-52}H_{81-85}O_{25-26}$, with a molecular weight of approximately 1100. It is a mixture of several closely related sulfate ester glycosides that have hemolytic and neurotropic effects. Therapy is similar to that for contact with other echinoderms and should include removal of slime with sea sand, vinegar, or alcohol and immersion in hot water.

PHYLUM MOLLUSCA: MOLLUSKS

Although there are thousands of species of mollusks, fewer than 100 may be toxic to humans.[8, 17] These are found in three classes of this phylum: Gastropoda (snails, slugs, and cone shells), Cephalopoda (squids and octopuses), and Pelecypoda (bivalves, including scallops, oysters, and clams)[12] (Table 145–11).

Cone shells possess a sophisticated venom apparatus that can induce a puncture wound and injection of venom if the animal is disturbed, and the most dangerous species are found in the Indo-Pacific and are often highly sought for their shells. A variety of toxic substances have been isolated from cone shells, including proteins, amines, lipoproteins, and carbohydrates. Cardiovascular and neurologic effects may be life threatening, and the LD_{50} of the venoms ranges from 0.2 to 2.4 mg/kg.[179] Therapy is supportive but may include intubation, mechanical ventilation, and cardiovascular support with fluids and/or vasoactive agents. In addition to respiratory failure, severe envenomings may be characterized by paralysis, dysphagia, areflexia, weakness, coagulopathies, coma, hypotension, and death.[207, 209, 224, 239] There is limited information on the ICU management of these poisons. Some components of the venom may be heat sensitive; local application of warm soaks may therefore be helpful.

The bites of certain cephalopods are dangerous.[240, 241] In severe cases of bites by Australian octopuses *Octopus maculosus* and *O. lunulatus,* respiratory distress and cardiovascular collapse may occur and deaths have been reported. The venom contains a number of small peptides, which affect vascular resistance, and one component may have actions similar to those of tetrodotoxin.[224] There is no specific therapy, and management of the wound may be difficult. Excision of the wound has been recommended in severe intoxications. Antivenin is not available.

PHYLUM CHORDATA, CLASSES OSTEICHTHYES AND CHONDRICHTHYES
Tetrodotoxic Fishes

One of the most interesting stories in the history of poisons was the discovery that two toxins from unrelated organisms were remarkably similar. Saxitoxin, a poison derived from a protozoa, and tetrodotoxin, an ichthyosarcotoxin, have virtually identical pharmacologic properties, despite differences in origin and chemical structure.[12, 15, 17] Tetrodotoxin is a perhydroquinazoline ichthyosarcotoxin found in puffer fish, ocean sunfishes, and certain other fish. This molecule has an empirical chemical structure of $C_{11}H_{17}N_3O_8$ and exists as a zwitterion.[175–178] Saxitoxin and tetrodotoxin both affect sodium conductance of excitable membranes. Both compounds are extremely toxic, and only a few molecules are needed to disrupt transmission. The flesh, and especially the viscera of fugu or puffer fish, is poisonous, producing tetrodotoxin poisoning. The onset may be dramatic, with paresthesias about the mouth and lips within minutes, followed by salivation, marked weakness, nausea, vomiting, and progressive paralysis of systemic and respiratory muscles. Coma and seizures have been reported, and up to 50% of severe poisonings may be fatal.[8] There is no antidote; treatment is supportive. Intubation and mechanical ventilation, as well as hemodynamic support with fluids and/or vasoactive agents, are frequently required to manage these patients. However, with intensive care, complete recovery is possible.

Venomous Fishes: Stingrays, Scorpion Fishes, Catfishes, Weevers, and Others

There are more than 200 species of fish that possess a venom apparatus.[8, 12, 15, 17] These animals are widely distributed among fresh and marine forms and include bony fishes such as catfish, scorpion fish, stargazers, toadfishes, surgeonfishes, and weevers. Many elasmobranch fishes, chiefly stingrays, are also venomous. The venom apparatus, with the exception of the weevers, is used defensively. Therefore, people are likely to become injured by contact with the animals while swimming, wading, fishing, or performing other activities. Injuries are either lacerations or puncture wounds[242–246] (Fig. 145–7). In some cases, the wounds are life threatening.[247–249]

Fish venoms are characterized by instability. Toxicity is rapidly lost when the venom or venom apparatus is exposed to heat.[12, 17, 250, 251] The venoms are mixtures of many compounds, although the most deleterious materials are proteins of 50 to 800 kd that are extremely heat labile.[251] Proteins isolated from the venom of *Scorpaena guttata* produce marked respiratory and hemodynamic changes, including bronchoconstriction, hypotension, and alterations in heart rate[252, 253] (Fig. 145–8). The venom has a muscarinic action and a secondary beta-adrenergic stimulating action. In experimental subjects, atropine partially counteracts the effects of acetylcholine, which is released in response to venom components.[253]

Pain is a consistent and prominent feature of fish envenomings. The pain is excruciating and may involve an entire extremity. Other symptoms include local edema, vomiting, nausea, diaphoresis, hypotension, and bradyarrhythmias.[208, 254] The most lethal venomous fishes are the stonefish, members of the genus *Synanceja,* found in the Indo-Pacific, Australia, Indian Ocean, China Sea, and Red Sea. The venom apparatus of the stonefish, although more highly developed, is similar to that of the other scorpion fishes, and consists of dorsal and pelvic spines in which an integumentary sheath covers the venom tissue located in grooves or either side of the spine. As the spine punctures the person, the integumentary sheath is ruptured and the glandular tissue in the grooves is introduced into the wound. Stonefish venom is extremely toxic. An antivenin to stonefish venom is prepared by the Commonwealth Serum Laboratories, Melbourne. Injuries by other scorpion fish are common throughout the world, as many scorpion fish are caught

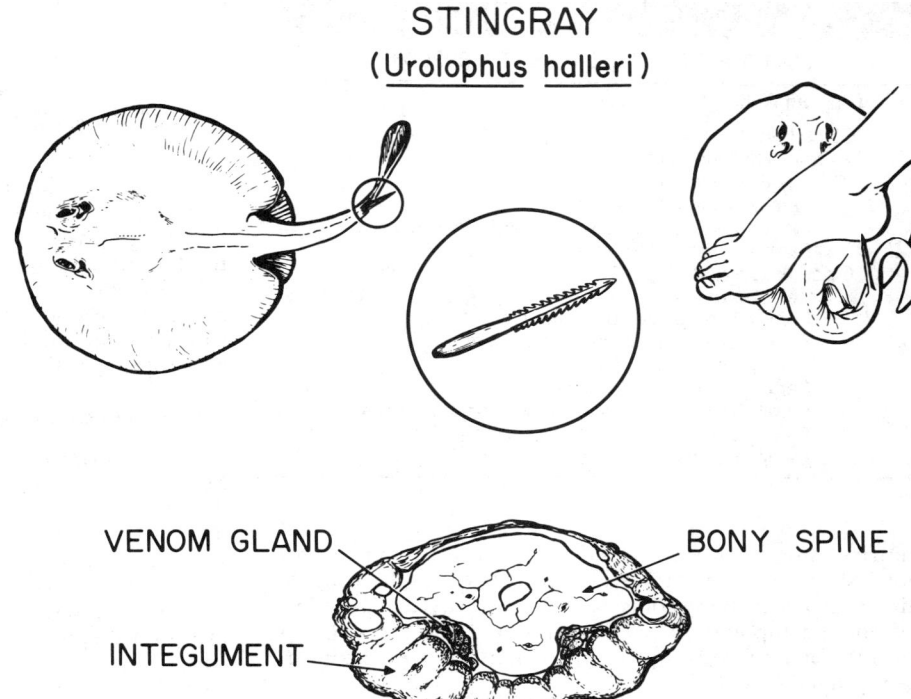

Figure 145–7. Stingray venom apparatus and mechanisms of envenomation.

as food fish or maintained in aquaria. In particular, lion-fish or zebra fish (genus *Pterois*) are highly prized for saltwater aquaria and result in many stings each year.[255, 256] Although large proteins are contained in the venom, fluid aspirated from the blisters after a lion-fish sting includes prostaglandin F_2 and small amounts of prostaglandin E_2.[257]

There are three priorities in the management of these injuries: (1) treatment of the wound, (2) relief of pain, and (3) therapy for the systemic effects of the envenomation. For stingray injuries, the wound may be extensive and lacerated. It is important to clean the wound thoroughly and to remove any remaining portions of the venom apparatus. Débridement may be required. Secondary infection and sloughing are common.[247, 258] For puncture wounds of

scorpion fish and other forms, the clinician must ensure that the sting has been removed. Immersion of the affected part in warm soaks is helpful to treat the pain of these injuries. Application of cold may intensify the pain. Local anesthetic agents and/or systemic analgesic agents are often required. Lidocaine has been reported to be effective for immediate relief of pain of these injuries. Stonefish antivenin is effective for these injuries and may have some effectiveness against other scorpion fish venoms such as lion-fish or zebra fish. Patients with severe envenomations should be observed in an ICU for cardiopulmonary instability (Table 145–12).

PHYLUM ARTHROPODA: ARTHROPODS

There are approximately 1 million species of arthropods, and these animals cause more envenomations than any other group of animals. Several thousand venomous arthropods are dangerous to humans (Table 145–13). The spiders, scorpions, and the Hymenoptera account for most human

SCORPIONFISH
(*Scorpaena guttata*)

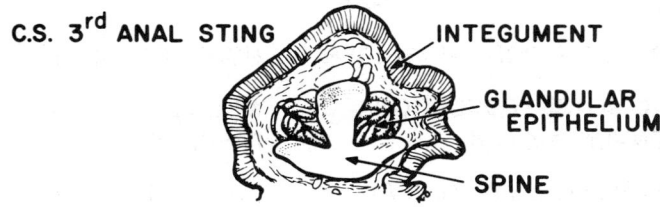

C.S. 3rd ANAL STING

INTEGUMENT

GLANDULAR EPITHELIUM

SPINE

Figure 145–8. California scorpion fish and a cross-section (C.S.) of an anal spine.

TABLE 145–12
PRINCIPLES OF TREATMENT OF FISH STINGS
1. Treat the wound
Warm soaks
Remove *all* components of venom apparatus and venom
Laceration: débride, ensure adequate drainage;
wounds often heal slowly
2. Provide relief of pain
Opiates may be required
Local lidocaine (Xylocaine) may be helpful
3. Treat secondary infection
4. Give appropriate tetanus therapy
5. Manage cardiopulmonary crises
Atropine
Vasoactive agents or volume loading
Antivenin for stonefish or lion-fish poisonings
Intubation, mechanical ventilation for respiratory failure

<table>
<tr><td>

TABLE 145–13

SOME IMPORTANT VENOMOUS ARTHROPODS

Phylum Arthropoda

Class Insecta
  Order Hymenoptera
    Family Apidae: bees
    Family Bonidae: bumblebees
    Family Vespidae: wasps, hornets, yellow jackets
    Family Formiciadae: ants
Class Arachnida
  Order Araneae: Spiders
    Family Theraphositae: tarantulas
    Family Clubonoidae: running spiders
    Family Salticidai: jumping spiders
    Family Araneidae: orb weavers
    Family Theridiidae: comb-footed spiders (widows)
    Family Loxoscelidae: brown (violin) spiders
    Family Buthidae: scorpions

</td></tr>
</table>

injuries. Most of these envenomings are irritating but are not life threatening. However, death may result from the direct effects of the venoms as well as anaphylactic reactions to venom components.[259–267] The reader is referred to Chapter 144 for a more complete discussion of anaphylaxis and its management.

Arthropod poisonings pose several problems in diagnosis and management. Many of these venoms contain substances that cause signs and symptoms that resemble anaphylaxis. True anaphylactic reactions are also encountered, as repeated contact with an animal may induce the production of immunoglobulin E antibodies by the patient. Certain arthropod injuries are characterized by distinctive features, such as necrotic lesions. However, other species may induce a similar response. Finally, identification of the offending animal is not possible in many cases because the animal is destroyed, not observed, or confused with another species. Therefore, the intensive care practitioner must often provide empirical therapy for a presumed bite or sting by an arthropod. This uncertainty may create practical problems when one is contemplating specific therapy such as antivenin or other potentially dangerous treatments.

Arthropod venoms are complex mixtures and consist of multiple components that have a wide variety of chemical and pharmacologic properties. Neurologic toxicity is common among arthropod injuries. Proteins, enzymes, peptides, amines, sugars, free bases, and alkaloids are among the many components that have been isolated from these venoms.

Class Arachnida, Order Araneae: Spiders

There are several families of spiders of clinical importance.[13, 268–270] Virtually all spiders are venomous, but only a few have chelicerae that can inflict a bite in humans. There are approximately 60 species of spiders in the United States that cause envenomations.

Family Theraphosidae: Tarantulas and Family Lycosidae: True Tarantulas, or Wolf Spiders

The spiders commonly known as tarantulas in the United States are mygalomorphs, members of the family Theraphosidae. These large animals are not particularly dangerous, although they bite when provoked. Envenomation leads to local pain, urticaria, edema, and other local signs and symptoms. Therapy is symptomatic. Secondary infection may occur. The wolf spiders, or true tarantulas, are also

large, hairy spiders that may cause a painful bite. Necrotic lesions or systemic effects are uncommon.

Family Clubionoidae: Running Spiders, Family Salticidae: Jumping Spiders, and Family Araneidae: Golden Orb Weavers

Running and jumping spiders are found in many gardens and yards and fields. They account for many painful bites. A variety of reactions may occur, but the bites are usually not life threatening. Necrotic lessions may develop.

The golden orb weavers are large, often colorful spiders that spin large webs to hunt insects. The bites are associated with pain and local findings. Systemic toxicity is uncommon, although necrotic lesions have been reported.

Family Theridiidae: Comb-Footed or Cobweb Spiders

The genus *Latrodectus* is a member of the Theridiidae family and includes the most dangerous spiders in the world. These animals have large, globular bodies and long legs. They are usually black or brown and typically have distinctive red markings on the abdomen. *Latrodectus* species are found worldwide and are known by many names, including black or brown widows, red back, and shoe button spiders. There are several species of *Latrodectus* in the United States. The species name *mactans* means murderer. These animals are typically encountered on or close to the ground, in woodpiles, under stones or logs, and in sheds, garages, and privies. There are eight eyes, and the lateral eyes are widely separated. The term comb footed refers to the hind pair of legs, which are used for ensnaring its prey with silk. The animal is usually not aggressive but may vigorously attack those who disturb its web.

The venom contains several peptide and protein fractions from 5000 to more than 100,000 daltons.[271–274] Among other properties of these fractions are neuromuscular conduction disturbances with an initial release of acetylcholine and/or catecholamines. Postsynaptic depolarization and morphologic changes occur at the end plate.[275–277]

Clinical features are distinctive. The bite produces some initial pain, although local features are usually minimal. There may be paresthesias locally. Local and regional muscle irritation develops with fasciculations and spasms. Deep tendon reflexes are increased, and there may be marked pain and spasm of muscle groups (Fig. 145–9). When this involves the abdominal muscles, the findings may resemble those of an acute abdomen. A variety of other findings may

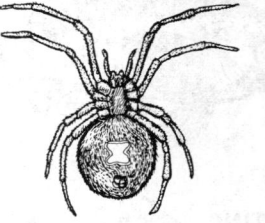

LATRODECTUS ENVENOMATION

Clinical   Features

DESCRIPTION OF SPIDER	HYPERTENSION
LOCATION-CONDITIONS OF ENVENOMATION	MUSCLE SPASMS-FASCICULATIONS
PARESTHESIAS (LOCAL)	LACK OF EDEMA, ERYTHEMA

Figure 145–9. Important clinical features of *Latrodectus* envenomation.

be observed, including headache, dysesthesias with burning of plantar surfaces, diaphoresis, urinary retention, ptosis, salivation, respiratory distress, nausea, and vomiting. Sharp increases in arterial pressure may lead to a hypertensive crisis. Increases or decreases of heart rate may be observed. The increase in blood pressure, muscle tone, and reflexes may progress to generalized seizures and coma. Intracranial hemorrhage may be found in fatal envenomings. Laboratory findings and the electrocardiogram are usually nonspecific, although increases in the white blood cell count, increased muscle enzyme levels, hemolysis, pigmenturia, and the development of progressive azotemia may result.[259, 268, 269, 276–282]

The elderly, the young, and those with underlying cardiopulmonary or neurologic disorders are particularly prone to complications of these envenomations. The venom is sufficiently toxic that the bite may be lethal for a small child. Accordingly, for cases of suspected *Latrodectus* envenomation, it is prudent to observe the patient in an emergency room setting for several hours. If systemic symptoms do not develop within this interval, the patient may be discharged. If signs of serious toxicity develop, the patient should be admitted to an ICU.

Local therapy consists of application of an ice cube or a cooling pack over the bite. A variety of agents have been used to treat the muscle spasms and pain: intravenous calcium gluconate, diazepam, magnesium sulfate, methocarbamol, and a variety of sedatives. Beta-blocking agents or other antihypertensive agents have been used. There is no consensus on the optimal drug therapy to control the hypertensive crisis. Caution should be exercised if the patient exhibits respiratory distress. Seizures should be managed with conventional therapy (administration of diazepam and phenytoin [Dilantin] and protection of the airway). It is important to monitor arterial pressure and neurologic findings closely. Dantrolene (Dantrium), a direct muscle relaxant, has also been used to treat muscle spasms,[242] although this is not one of the indicated uses of this agent, and the drug is associated with more toxicity than other agents. There is no apparent benefit from the use of corticosteroids.

An antivenin (Antivenin [*Latrodectus mactans*], Merck Sharp & Dohme) prepared with horse serum is available and is highly effective. It may be given intravenously or intramuscularly. Administration of one vial (2.5 mL) is usually sufficient. Serum sickness and anaphylaxis are considerations that should temper use of the serum. Most authorities recommend antivenin for severe poisoning or in a high-risk patient.

Family Loxoscelidae: Fiddleback, Brown, Violin, and Recluse Spiders

Spiders of the Loxoscelidae family are commonly found in North and South America and are frequently incriminated in lesions with dermal necrosis (necrotic arachnidism, also termed loxoscelism). There are several species of the genus *Loxosceles* in the United States and all are dangerous to humans (Fig. 145–10). They are widely distributed, particularly in the South Central regions of the country. The animals are nocturnal and reclusive but bite when provoked.

The animals may be identified by a tan, yellowish, or gray body of 10 to 15 mm, with a violin-shaped marking on the dorsal surface of the cephalothorax, six eyes (most spiders have eight), and long, spindly legs that may be 25 mm in length.[13, 267, 268]

The venom has not been fully characterized but includes a number of proteins, some with enzymatic activity, such as phospholipase D (sphingomyelinase), which may be important in the development of dermonecrotic lesions; hyaluron-

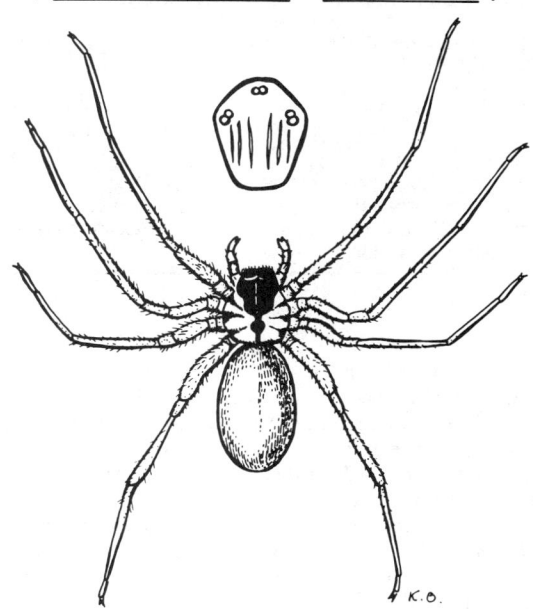

BROWN RECLUSE SPIDER
(Loxosceles reclusa)

Figure 145–10. The brown recluse spider, showing location of the three pairs of eyes on the head.

idase; 5'-ribonuclease; collagenase; and others. Several lytic factors, peptides, and other components are present.[283–285]

The bite may be only mildly painful. Within a few hours, however, increasing pain and local findings become prominent. A central blister or bleb may develop, which may have a central blue-black region, surrounded by peripheral erythema. The lesion may progress with alarming speed, with an expanding area of central necrosis. This process usually begins within 12 hours, although great variations in the sequence of the local necrosis and dermal changes have been reported. Additional bullae or blebs may develop regionally. The central necrosis frequently leads to scar formation. Systemic findings may be minimal, but chills, fever, nausea, vomiting, arthralgias, coagulation changes, rash, thrombocytopenia, hemolysis, hemoglobinuria, renal failure, and seizures have been documented.[286–294] Coma and seizures have also been reported, although these findings may be secondary to other systemic changes, rather than primary effects of the envenoming.

Because other animal bites and stings may lead to necrotic lesions, it is important to describe an injury as cutaneous necrosis, necrotic insect bite, or presumptive, clinically typical, or documented recluse spider bite with loxoscelism.[286, 287] Precise descriptions of the lesion and the spider, together with the clinical course, should be entered in the medical record. If the offending animal cannot be identified, this should be recorded.

Management is often unsatisfactory and several techniques have been recommended to treat these lesions (Table 145–14). There is no widely available test to confirm *Loxosceles* envenomation, nor is there currently a commercially prepared antivenin for this venom. *Latrodectus* antivenin is not effective against *Loxosceles*. Management should be directed to the local changes, which may be dramatic, as well as to systemic toxicity. The wound should be cleansed and tetanus prophylaxis administered. If the characteristic lesion is iden-

---

TABLE 145–14

MANAGEMENT OF LOXOSCELISM AND DERMONECROTIC ARTHROPOD REACTIONS

1. Observe progression of local findings
   Frequent examinations, especially during initial 24 h
   Consider early curettage of lesion
   Cleanse
2. Tetanus prophylaxis
3. Treat secondary infection
4. Steroids of dubious value
5. Laboratory studies: complete blood count; tests for hemolysis, electrolytes, renal function, and muscle enzymes
6. Dapsone, 50–200 mg/d in divided doses PO, for developing dermonecrotic lesion

---

tified quickly, some authorities recommend curettage of the necrotic material within the wound.[296] Earlier reports of excision of the wound suggested that this helped prevent progression of the necrotic lesion. However, excision is no longer recommended by most authorities, and may complicate the disfigurement created by these bites.[269, 287, 295–298] Antibiotics may be needed but should not be given prophylactically. Steroids are of no proven benefit, but some authors continue to recommend local and/or systemic corticosteroid preparations.[286, 299]

Alpha-adrenergic blocking agents or other vasodilators are of no proven benefit, even though the necrotic lesion is in part due to intensive local vasospasm with ischemic necrosis.[300] Heparin is not indicated. Dapsone (4,4-diaminodiphenylsulfone) has been recommended and has been subjected to clinical and experimental trials.[144, 269, 287, 288, 294, 300, 301] This agent is an inhibitor of white blood cell function and may limit necrosis. However, this drug is associated with significant side effects such as hemolysis and methemoglobinemia. Dosage is 50 to 200 mg/d orally in divided doses. It is recommended by several authors for severe, developing dermonecrotic lesions. Wilson and King have popularized the mnemonic RICE for rest, ice, and elevation to emphasize the other maneuvers that can be utilized in the care of these patients.[270] Monitoring renal and hemostatic variables should be undertaken in serious envenomings. Surgical consultation is indicated for patients with marked necrotic lesions, particularly for injuries that involve the face.

Class Arachnida, Family Buthidae: Scorpions

There are approximately 650 species of scorpions within this family, but only two species in North America are associated with fatal poisoning in humans. These animals are found in Arizona and Mexico. However, in tropical and subtropical regions of the world, including the Middle East and South America, several dangerous species are found, and severe envenomings are reported.[302–304] Life-threatening syndromes are particularly likely to occur in children or patients with cardiovascular disease. Tachycardia, seizures, hypertension, pulmonary edema, coma, vomiting, hyperreflexia, diaphoresis, cardiac injury and arrhythmias, and a variety of other findings have been documented.[305–307]

The venoms contain several potent protein neurotoxins, which may also affect the cardiovascular system.[308–311]

In the United States and Mexico, the genus *Centruroides* accounts for dangerous stings[312–314] (Fig. 145–11). The venom contains several basic proteins that are relatively resistant to proteolytic enzymes. Grading of these injuries is difficult, but one scheme is grade I for pain and local findings

only; grade II for pain and paresthesias remote from the sting, in addition to local findings; grade III for cranial nerve or somatic neuromuscular dysfunction, in addition to the local changes; and grade IV for both cranial nerve and somatic changes.[312] The site of envenomation is characteristically hypersensitive and tapping over the region may elicit severe pain. Antivenin made using goat serum is available for serious envenomations. Patients should be observed closely and admitted to an intensive care environment if the syndrome progresses to grade II or higher.

Antivenin is available for some species, but vasodilators such as nitroprusside, prazosin, hydralazine, and calcium channel–blocking agents are often used to combat the left ventricular failure and hypertension. It is thought that the cardiovascular manifestations of scorpion envenomation are related to increased levels of angiotensin, renin, and catecholamines. In experimental studies with scorpion toxin, researchers observed increases in left ventricular contractility and systemic hypertension, together with increases in left ventricular diastolic pressure.[307] The authors concluded that there was a rapid decrease in left ventricular compliance with improved diastolic filling, that is accompanied by a marked increase in systemic impedance. Cardiac arrhythmias are not uncommon, and myocarditis or a picture that resembles myocardial infarction may supervene. Antivenin may prevent cardiovascular alterations when given before venom in experimental studies. However, the effects of antivenin given after envenomation are less dramatic.

SCORPION
(<u>Centruroides</u> <u>sculpturatus</u>)

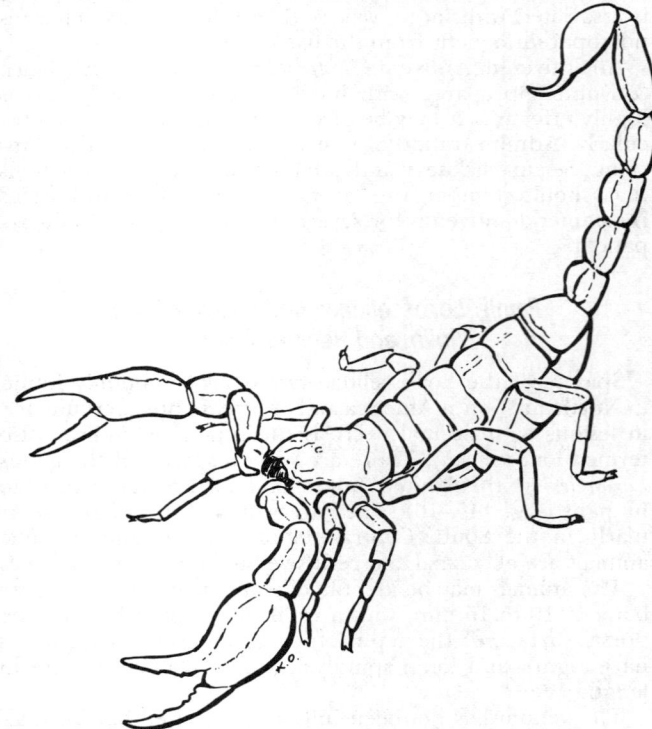

Figure 145–11. The *Centruroides* scorpion, which is a dangerous and common hazard in the Southwest United States and portions of Mexico.

HONEYBEE (worker)
(<u>Aspis</u> <u>mellifera</u>)

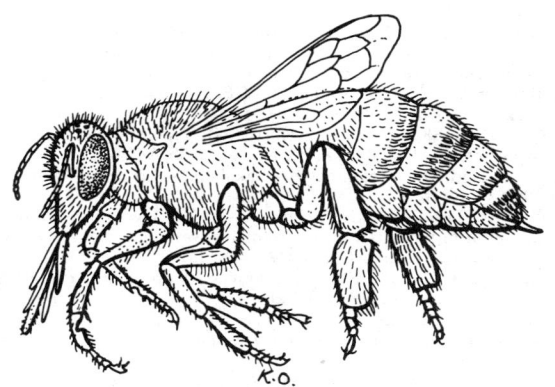

Figure 145–12. Honeybee.

Class Insecta, Order Hymenoptera: Bees, Wasps, Hornets, and Ants

The Hymenoptera include more than 16,000 species in the United States, but four families of this order account for the majority of insect stings: Apidae (honeybees) (Fig. 145–12), Bomidae (bumblebees), Vespoidae (wasps, yellow jackets, and hornets), and Formicadae (fire and harvester ants) (Fig. 145–13).

The venoms of the bees, wasps, and related forms have been studied extensively and contain a variety of proteins and low-molecular-weight substances that are toxic[17, 20, 21, 260, 318–322] (Table 145–15). However, these venoms are not toxic to humans unless many stings occur simultaneously. In most instances, therefore, the greatest danger from these envenomations is anaphylaxis. Desensitization with extracts of bee venom is indicated for patients who demonstrate marked sensitivity to these venoms.[268, 322–325]

Many species of ants possess venoms that are painful or irritating. Formic acid may account for pain and local find-

FIRE ANT
(<u>Solenopsis</u> <u>saevissima</u>)

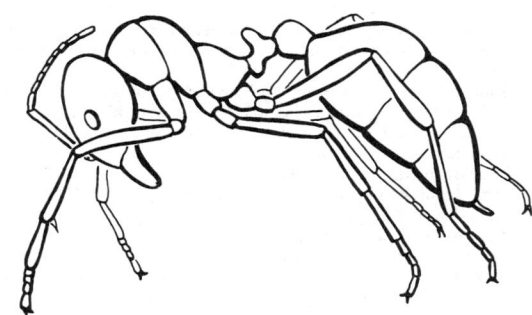

Figure 145–13. One species of fire ant (*Solenopsis saevissima*).

TABLE 145–15
SOME IMPORTANT COMPONENTS OF HYMENOPTERA VENOMS

Bee	Wasp, Yellow Jacket, Hornet	Fire Ant
Histamine	Histamine	Disubstituted
Apamin	Kinins	piperidines
Melittin*	Serotonin	Phospholipase A,
Mast cell–degranulating substance	Phospholipase A, B*	B*
	Other peptides, including those that degranulate mast cells	Other allergenic proteins
Hyaluronidase*		
Acid phosphatase*		
Norepinephrine		
Dopamine		
Allergen C*		
Other peptides		

*Documented allergies to these substances.
Adapted from Wright DN, Lockey RF: Local reactions to stinging insects (Hymenoptera). Allergy Proc 11:23, 1990.

ings, and the venom of several ants contains a high percentage of this compound.

The imported red fire ant, *Solenopsis invicta*, and the imported black fire ant, *Solenopsis richteri*, have become a public health problem as well as a threat to individuals and animals in many areas of the Gulf South.[326, 327] Fatal envenomations have been described.[328–332] These ants are aggressive, and many ants are typically involved in these injuries. Up to 95% of the venom is an alkaloid, although proteins and peptides are also present. The predominant alkaloids are piperidines with hemolytic, antibacterial, and cytotoxic properties.[333, 334] Repeated exposure to the protein components of fire ant venom may induce immunoglobulin E–mediated allergic reactions.

A variety of skin and systemic responses may occur. Pustular and occasionally necrotic lesions often develop. When multiple stings occur, or if an anaphylactic reaction develops, the injury may be fatal. A survey of physicians found 32 deaths attributable to allergic reactions to fire ants.[329]

Immunotherapy to fire ant extract may be useful prophylaxis for patients who have experienced serious allergic reactions.[335] Venom is preferred to whole body extracts for desensitization.[336] The initial treatment of the sting is empirical. No antivenin is available. A number of therapies have been suggested, including local agents, meat tenderizer containing papain, and other folk remedies. However, these maneuvers are probably of limited value. Corticosteroids and other agents may be helpful, particularly for late reactions. In cases of multiple stings, close observation is indicated, with monitoring of cardiopulmonary and neurologic function.

Acknowledgment. This chapter is dedicated with appreciation to my instructor, Findlay E. Russell, who introduced me to the field of toxinology, and in friendship to my colleague, Richard C. Schaeffer, Jr.

References

1. Wetzel WW, Christy NP: A king cobra bite in New York city. Toxicon 27:393, 1989.
2. Trestrail JH: The underground zoo. Vet Hum Toxicol 24(suppl):144, 1982.
3. Brown R, Brasch L, Leichter D, et al: Gaboon viper envenomation: An unexpected big-city emergency. Pediatr Emerg Care 5:248, 1989.
4. Schelstraete E, Vercruysse P, Lust P: Exotic snakebite, an unusual emergency. Acta Anaesth Belg 36:407, 1985.

5. Crane DB, Irwin JS: Rattlesnake bite of the glans penis. Urology 26:50, 1985.

6. Pfeiffer RB, Price VG: Case report: Recovery from Western diamond-back rattler bite to mouth. Postgrad Med 59:283, 1976.

7. Gerkin R, Sergent KC, Curry SC, et al: Life-threatening airway obstruction from rattlesnake bite to the tongue. Ann Emerg Med 16:813, 1987.

8. Halstead BW: Poisonous and Venomous Marine Animals of the World (Revised). Princeton, NJ, Darwin Press, 1978.

9. Russell FE: Snake Venom Poisoning. Philadelphia, JB Lippincott, 1980.

10. Klauber LM: Rattlesnakes: Their Habits, Life Histories, and Influence on Mankind, Volumes 1 and 2. Berkeley, University of California Press, 1972.

11. Minton SA, Dowling HG, Russell FE (eds): Poisonous Snakes of the World. 2nd ed. Washington, DC, US Government Printing Office, 1968.

12. Russell FE: Marine toxins and venomous and marine plants and animals. Adv Mar Biol 21:60, 1984.

13. Gertsch WJ: American Spiders. Princeton, NJ, D Van Nostrand, 1949.

14. Sutherland SK: Australian Animal Toxins. The Creatures, Their Toxins and Care of the Poisoned Patient. Melbourne, Oxford University Press, 1983.

15. Halstead BW: Poisonous and Venomous Marine Animals, Volumes 1–3. Washington, DC, US Government Printing Office, 1965–1970.

16. Minton SA: Venom Diseases. Springfield, IL, Charles C Thomas, 1974.

17. Russell FE: Comparative pharmacology of some animal toxins. Fed Proc 26:1206, 1967.

18. Minton SA, Minton MR: Venomous Animals. New York, Charles Scribner's Sons, 1969.

19. Tu AT: Venoms: Chemistry and Molecular Biology. London, John Wiley & Sons, 1977.

20. Russell FE, Saunders PR (eds): Animal Toxins. Oxford, Pergamon Press, 1967.

21. Bucherl W, Buckley EE, Deulofeu V (eds): Venomous Animals and Their Venoms, Volume 2. New York, Academic Press, 1968.

22. Swaroop S, Grab B: The snakebite mortality problem in the world. Bull WHO 10:35, 1954.

23. Russell FE: Snake Venom Poisoning. Great Neck, NY, Scholium International, 1983.

24. Parrish HM: Mortality from snakebite. Public Health Rep 72:1027, 1966.

25. Russell FE, Carlson RW, Wainschel J, et al: Snake venom poisoning in the United States: Experiences with 550 cases. JAMA 233:341, 1975.

26. Myint-Lwin, Warrell DA, Phillips RE, et al: Bites by Russell's viper (*Vipera russelli siamensis*) in Burma: Haemostatic, vascular and renal disturbances and response to treatment. Lancet 2:1159, 1985.

27. Kunkel DB, Curry SC, Vance MV, et al: Reptile envenomations. J Toxicol Clin Toxicol 21:503, 1984.

28. Kochva E, Gans C: Histology and histochemistry of venom glands of some crotaline snakes. Copeia 3:506, 1966.

29. Schaeffer RC Jr, Bernick S, Rosenquist TH, et al: The histochemistry of the venom glands of the rattlesnake *Crotalus viridis helleri*. I. Lipid and nonspecific esterase. Toxicon 10:183, 1972.

30. Schaeffer RC Jr, Bernick S, Rosenquist TH, et al: The histochemistry of the venom glands of the rattlesnake *Crotalus viridis helleri*. II. Monoamine oxidase, acid and alkaline phosphatase. Toxicon 10:295, 1972.

31. Iwanaga S, Suzuki T: Enzymes in snake venoms. In: Lee CY (ed): Handbook of Experimental Pharmacology, Volume 52, Snake Venoms. Berlin, Springer-Verlag, 1979.

32. Schaeffer RC Jr, Pattabhiraman T, Carlson RW, et al: Cardiovascular failure produced by a peptide from the venom of the Southern Pacific rattlesnake, *Crotalus viridis helleri*. Toxicon 17:447, 1979.

33. Russell FE: Pharmacology of animal venoms. Clin Pharmacol Ther 8:849, 1967.

34. Minton SA: Neurotoxic snake envenoming. Semin Neurol 10:52, 1990.

35. Harris JB: Phospholipases in snake venoms and their effects on nerve and muscle. Pharmacol Ther 31:79, 1985.

36. Markland FS, Damus PS: Purification and properties of a thrombin-like enzyme from the venom of *Crotalus adamanateus* (Eastern diamondback rattlesnake). J Biol Chem 21:6460, 1971.

37. Brink S, Steytler JG: Effects of puff-adder venom on coagulation, fibrinolysis and platelet aggregation in the baboon. S Afr Med J 48:1205, 1974.

38. MacKay N, Ferguson JC, McNichol GP: Effects of the venom of the rhinoceros horned viper (*Bitis nasicornis*) on blood coagulation, platelet aggregation and fibrinolysis. J Clin Pathol 23:789, 1970.

39. Bajwa SS, Russell FE, Markland FS: Thrombolytic agents in snake venoms. Proc West Pharmacol Soc 25:353, 1982.

40. Schieck A, Kornalick F, Habermann E: The prothrombin-activating principles from *Echis carinatus* venom. Naunyn Schmiedebergs Arch Pharmakol 272:402, 1972.

41. Huang S-Y, Perez, JC: Comparative study on hemorrhagic and proteolytic activities of snake venoms. Toxicon 18:421, 1980.

42. Nahas L, Denson KWE, MacFarlane RG: A study of the coagulant action of eight snake venoms. Thromb Diath Haemorrh 12:355, 1964.

43. Denson KWE, Russell FE, Alveagro D, et al: Characterization of the coagulant activity of some snake venoms. Toxicon 10:557, 1972.

44. Kornalik F, Blombach B: Prothrombin activation induced by ecarin—A prothrombin converting enzyme from *Echis carinatus* venom. Thromb Res 6:53, 1975.

45. Tu AT: Biotoxicology of sea snake venoms. Ann Emerg Med 16:1023, 1987.

46. Tu AT: Sea snakes and their venoms. In: Tu AT (ed): Handbook of Natural Toxins, Volume 3, Marine Toxins and Venoms. New York, Marcel Dekker, 1987.

47. Reid HA: Myoglobinuria and sea snake poisoning. Br J Med 1:1284, 1961.

48. Reid HA: Diagnosis, prognosis and treatment of sea-snake bite. Lancet 2:399, 1961.

49. Audley I: A case of sea-snake envenomation. Med J Aust 143:532, 1985.

50. Reid HA: Antivenom in sea-snake poisoning. Lancet 1:622, 1975.

51. Reid HA: Epidemiology and clinical aspects of sea snake bites. In: Dunson WA (ed): The Biology of Sea Snakes. Baltimore, University Park Press, 1975.

52. Sutherland SK, Coulter AR, Harris RD: The rationalisation of first aid measures for elapid snakebite. Lancet 1:183, 1979.

53. Sutherland SK: Treatment of snakebite. Austr Fam Physician 19:21, 1990.

54. Watt G, Theakston RDG, Hayes CG, et al: Positive response to edrophonium in patients with neurotoxic envenoming by cobras (*Naja naja philippinensis*). N Engl J Med 315:1444, 1986.

55. Kornalik F, Pudlak FP: A prolonged defibrination caused by *Echis carinatus* venom. Life Sci 10:309, 1971.

56. Fairnaru M, Eisenberg S, Manny N: The natural course of defibrination syndrome caused by *Echis colorata* venom in man. Thromb Diath Haemorrh 31:420, 1974.

57. Reid HA, Chan KE, Thean PC: Prolonged coagulation defect (defibrination syndrome) in Malayan viper bite. Lancet 1:621, 1963.

58. Warrell DA, Arnett C: The importance of bites by the saw-scaled or carpet viper (*Echis carinatus*): Epidemiological studies in Nigeria and a review of the world literature. Acta Trop 33:307, 1976.

59. Pugh RNH: Bites by the carpet viper in the Niger valley. Lancet 2:625, 1979.

60. Warrell DA, Davidson NMcD, Greenwood BM, et al: Poisoning by bites of the saw-scaled or carpet viper (*Echis carinatus*) in Nigeria. J Med 46:133, 1977.

61. Pugh RNH, Theaksston RDG: Incidence and mortality of snakebite in savanna Nigeria. Lancet 2:1181, 1980.

62. Weiss HJ, Phillips LL, Hopewell WS, et al: Heparin therapy in a patient bitten by a saw-scaled viper (*Echis carinatus*), a snake whose venom activates prothrombin. Am J Med 54:653, 1973.

63. DeVries A, Rechnic Y, Moroz C, et al: Prevention of *Echis colorata* venom–induced afibrinogenemia by heparin. Toxicon 1:241, 1963.

64. Schulchynska-Castel H, Dvilansky A, Keynan A: *Echis colorata* bites: Clinical evaluation of 42 patients. Isr J Med Sci 22:880, 1986.

65. Warrell DA, Pope HM, Prentice CRM: Disseminated intravascular coagulation caused by the carpet viper (*Echis carinatus*): Trial of heparin. Br J Haematol 33:335, 1976.

66. Gilon D, Shalev O, Benbassat J: Treatment of envenomation by *Echis coloratus* (mid-east saw scaled viper): A decision tree. Toxicon 27:1105, 1989.

67. Warrell DA, Davidson NMcD, Omerod LD, et al: Bites by the saw-scaled or carpet viper (*Echis carinatus*): Trial of two specific antivenoms. Br Med J 4:437, 1974.

68. Morita T, Iwanaga S, Suzuki T: The mechanism of activation of bovine prothrombin by an activator isolated from *Echis carinatus* venom and characterization of the new active intermediates. J Biochem 79:1089, 1976.

69. Rhee M-J, Morris S, Kosow DP: Role of meizothrombin and meizothrombin-(des F1) in conversion of prothrombin to thrombin by *Echis carinatus* coagulant. Biochemistry 21:3437, 1982.

70. Schaeffer RC Jr, Briston C, Chilton SM, et al: Disseminated intravascular coagulation following *Echis carinatus* venom in dogs: Effects of a synthetic thrombin inhibitor. J Lab Clin Med 107:488, 1986.

71. Schaeffer RC Jr, Chilton SM, Hadden TJ, et al: Pulmonary fibrin microembolism following infusion of *Echis carinatus* venom in dogs: Effects of a synthetic thrombin inhibitor. J Appl Physiol 57:1824, 1984.

72. Schaeffer RC Jr, Barnhart MI, Carlson RW: Pulmonary fibrin deposition and increased microvascular permeability to protein following fibrin microembolism in dogs: A structure-function relationship. Microvasc Res 33:327, 1987.

73. Bouquet P: Pharmacology and toxicology of snake venoms of Europe and the Mediterranean regions. In: Bucherl W, Buckley EE, Deulofeu V (eds): Venomous Animals and Their Venoms, Volume 1. New York, Academic Press, p 340, 1968.

74. Theakston RDG, Jones MJL, Reid HA: Micro-ELISA for detecting and assaying snake venom and venom antibody. Lancet 2:639, 1977.

75. Aung-Khin: The problem of snakebites in Burma. Snake 12:125, 1980.

76. Phillips RE, Theakston RDG, Warrell DA, et al: Paralysis, rhabdomyolysis and haemolysis caused by bites of Russell's viper (*Vipera russelli pulchella*) in Sri Lanka: Failure of Indian (Haffkine) antivenom. Q J Med 68:691, 1988.

77. Myint-Lwin, Warrell DA, Phillips RE, et al: Bites by Russell's viper (*Vipera russelli siamensis*) in Burma: Haemostatic, vascular, and renal disturbances and response to treatment. Lancet 2:1259, 1985.

78. Than T, Khin EH, Hutton RA, et al: Evolution of coagulation abnormalities following Russell's viper bite in Burma. Br J Haematol 65:193, 1987.

79. Aung-Khin: Histological and ultrastructural changes of the kidney in renal failure after viper envenomation. Toxicon 16:71, 1977.

80. George A, Tharakan VT, Solez K: Viper bite poisoning in India: A review with special reference to renal complications. Ren Fail 10:91, 1987.

81. Carlson RW, Schaeffer RC Jr, Whigham H, et al: Rattlesnake venom shock in the rat: Development of a method. Am J Physiol 229:1668, 1975.

82. Mebs D, Panholzer F: Isolation of a hemorrhagic principles from *Bitis arietans* (puff adder) snake venom. Toxicon 20:509, 1982.

83. Phillips LL, Weiss HJ, Pessar L, et al: Effects of puff adder venom on the coagulation mechanism: I. In vivo. Toxicon 11:423, 1973.

84. Phillips LL, Weiss HJ, Christy NP: Effects of puffer adder venom on the coagulation mechanism: II. In vitro. Thromb Diath Haemorrh 30:499, 1973.

85. Tu AT, Homma M, Hong B: Hemorrhagic, myonecrotic, thrombotic and proteolytic activities of viper venoms. Toxicon 6:175, 1969.

86. Osman OH, Gumaa KA: Pharmacologic studies on snake (*Bitis arietans*) venom. Toxicon 12:569, 1974.

87. Chapman DS: The symptomatology, pathology and treatment of bites of venomous snakes of Central and Southern Africa. In: Bucherl W, Buckley E, Deulofeu V (eds): Venomous Animals and Their Venoms, Volume 1. New York, Academic Press, p 463, 1968.

88. Adams ZS, Gattullo D, Losano G, et al: The effect of *Bitis gabonica* (Gaboon viper snake venom) on blood pressure, stroke volume and coronary circulation in the dogs. Toxicon 19:263, 1981.

89. Schaeffer RC Jr, Chilton SM, Carlson RW: Puff adder venom shock: A model of increased vascular permeability. J Pharmacol Exp Ther 233:312, 1985.

90. Pope CH: The Reptile World. New York, Alfred A. Knopf, 1955.

91. Reid HA: Cobra bites. Br J Med 2:540, 1964.

92. Hilligan R: Black mamba bites. A report of 2 cases. S Afr Med J 72:220, 1987.

93. Narita K, Mebs D, Iwanaga S, et al: Primary structure of α-bungarotoxin from *Bungarus multicinctus* venom. J Formosan Med Assoc 71:336, 1972.

94. Looareesuwan S, Viravan C, Warrell DA: Factors contributing to fatal snake bite in the rural tropics: Analysis of 46 cases in Thailand. Trans R Soc Trop Med Hyg 82:930, 1988.

95. Endo T, Tamiya N: Current view on the structure-function relationship of postsynaptic neurotoxins from snake venoms. Pharmacol Ther 34:403, 1987.

96. Watt G, Meade BD, Theakston RDG, et al: Comparison of Tensilon and antivenom for the treatment of cobra-bite paralysis. Trans R Soc Trop Med Hyg 83:570, 1989.

97. Warrell DA, Looareesuwan S, White NJ, et al: Severe neurotoxic envenoming by the Malayan krait, *Bungarus candidus* (Linnaeus): Response to antivenom and anticholinesterase. Br Med J 286:678, 1983.

98. Mitrakul C, Dhamkrong-at A, Futrakul P, et al: Clinical features of neurotoxic snake bite and response to antivenom in 47 children. Am J Trop Med Hyg 33:1258, 1984.

99. Theakston RDG, Phillips RE, Warrell DA, et al: Envenoming by the common krait (*Bungarus caeruleus*) and Sri Lankan cobra (*Naja naja naja*): Efficacy and complications of therapy with Haffkine antivenom. Trans R Soc Trop Med Hyg 84:301, 1990.

100. Reitz CJ, Goosen DJ, Odendaal MW, et al: Evaluation of the venom ex apparatus in the treatment of Egyptian cobra envenomation. S Afr Med J 66:135, 1984.

101. Kitchens CS, Van Mierop LHS: Envenomation by the Eastern coral snake (*Micrurus fulvius fulvius*). JAMA 258:1615, 1987.

102. Russell FE: Bites by the Sonoran coral snake *Micruroides euryxanthus*. Toxicon 5:39, 1967.

103. Jamieson R, Pearn J: An epidemiological and clinical study of snake-bites in childhood. Med J Aust 150:698, 1989.

104. Parrish HM: Mortality from snake bites, United States, 1950–54. Public Health Rep 72:1027, 1957.

105. Parrish HM: Incidence of treated snakebites in the United States. Public Health Rep 81:269, 1966.

106. Fisher MMD, Dieks I: Volume replacement in acute anaphylactoid reactions. Anesth Intensive Care 7:375, 1979.

107. Russell FE: Snake venom poisoning in the United States. Annu Rev Med 31:247, 1980.

108. Wingert WA, Chan L: Rattlesnake bites in Southern California and rationale for recommended treatment. West J Med 148:37, 1988.

109. Pattabhiraman TR, Russell FE: Isolation and purification of the toxic fractions of Mojave rattlesnake venom. Toxicon 13:291, 1975.

110. Russell FE, Puffer H: Pharmacology of snake venoms. In: Minton SA (ed): Snake Venoms and Envenomation. New York, Marcel Dekker, p 87, 1971.

111. Russell FE, Puffer H: Pharmacology of snake venoms. Clin Toxicol 3:433, 1970.

112. Minton SA, Parrish HM, Talley JH, et al: Snakebite? Get the facts, then hurry. Patient Care June 1:48, 1976.

113. Russell FE: Pharmacology of animal venoms. Clin Pharmacol Ther 8:849, 1967.

114. Hardy DL: Fatal rattlesnake envenomation in Arizona: 1969–84. Clin Toxicol 24:1, 1986.

115. Hardy DL: Envenomation by the Mojave rattlesnake (*Crotalus scutulatus scutulatus*) in Southern Arizona, USA. Toxicon 21:111, 1983.

116. Russell FE: Medical problems of snakebite. In: Russell FE (ed): Snake Venom Poisoning. New York, Harper & Row, p 229, 1980.

117. Osborn CD: Treatment of venomous bite by high voltage direct current. J Okla State Med Assoc 83:9, 1990.

118. Guderian RH, Mackenzie CD, Williams JF: High voltage shock treatment for snakebite (letter). Lancet 2:229, 1986.

119. Russell FE: Another warning about electric shock for snake bite. Postgrad Med 82:32, 1987.

120. Howe NR, Meisenheimer JL: Electric shock does not save snake bitten rats. Ann Emerg Med 17:245, 1988.

121. La Grange RG, Russell FE: Blood platelet studies in man and rabbits following *Crotalus* envenomation. Proc West Pharmacol Soc 13:99, 1970.

122. Weiss HJ, Allan S, Davidson E, et al: Afibrinogenemia in man following the bite of a rattlesnake (*Crotalus adamanteus*). Am J Med 47:625, 1969.

123. Amaral CFS, Da Silva OA, Lopez M, et al: Afibrinogenemia following snake bite (*Crotalus durissus terrificus*). Am J Trop Med Hyg 29:1453, 1980.

124. Hasiba U, Rosenbach LM, Rockwell D, et al: DIC-like syndrome after envenomation by the snake, *Crotalus horridus horridus*. N Engl J Med 292:505, 1975.

125. Kamiguti AS, Cardoso JLC: Haemostatic changes caused by the venoms of South American snakes. Toxicon 27:955, 1989.

126. Tu AT: Blood coagulation. In: Tu AT (ed): Venoms, Chemistry and Molecular Biology. New York, John Wiley & Sons, p 329, 1977.

127. Ruiz C, Schaeffer RC Jr, Carlson RW, et al: Hemostatic changes following rattlesnake (*Crotalus viridis helleri*) venom in the dog. J Pharmacol Exp Ther 213:414, 1980.

128. Simon TL, Grace TG: Envenomation coagulopathy in wounds from pit vipers. N Engl J Med 305:443, 1981.

129. Schaeffer RC Jr, Pattabhiraman T, Carlson RW, et al: Cardiovascular failure produced by a peptide from the Southern Pacific rattlesnake *Crotalus viridus helleri*. Toxicon 17:447, 1979.

130. Schaeffer RC Jr, Carlson RW, Whigham H, et al: Acute hemodynamic effects of rattlesnake, *Crotalus viridis helleri*, venom. In: Rosenaberg P (ed): Toxins: Animal, Plant and Microbial. Oxford, Pergamon Press, p 383, 1978.

131. Schaeffer RC Jr, Briston C, Chilton SM, et al: Hypotensive and hemostatic properties of rattlesnake venom (*Crotalus viridis helleri*) venom and venom fractions in dogs. J Pharmacol Exp Ther 230:393, 1984.

132. Ondetti MA, Williams NJ, Sabo EF, et al: Angiotensin-converting enzyme inhibitors from the venom of *Bothrops jararaca*: Isolation, elucidation of structure, and synthesis. Biochemistry 22:4033, 1971.

133. Ferreira SH, Bartlet, DC, Greene LJ: Isolation of bradykinin-potentiating peptides from *Bothrops jararaca* venom. Biochemistry 9:2583, 1970.

134. Kato H, Suzuki T: Bradykinin-potentiating peptides from the venom of *Agkistrodon halys blomhoffi*. Experientia 25:694, 1969.

135. Schaeffer RC Jr, Carlson RW, Weil MH: Effects of antivenin and corticosteroid analogues on rattlesnake venom shock in the rat. J Pharmacol Exp Ther 211:409, 1979.

136. Schaeffer RC Jr, Carlson RW, Puri V, et al: The effects of colloidal and crystalloidal fluids on rattlesnake venom shock in the rat. J Pharmacol Exp Ther 206:687, 1978.

137. Haupt MT, Teerapong P, Green D, et al: Increased pulmonary edema with crystalloid compared to colloid resuscitation of shock associated with increased vascular permeability. Circ Shock 12:213, 1984.

138. Burch JM, Agarwal R, Mattox KL, et al: The treatment of crotalid envenomation without antivenin. J Trauma 28:35, 1988.

139. Otten EJ, McKimm D: Venomous snakebite in a patient allergic to horse serum. Ann Emerg Med 12:624 1983.

140. Schaeffer RC Jr, Randall H, Resk J, et al: Enzyme-linked immunosorbent assay (ELISA) of size-selected crotalid venom antigens by Wyeth's polyvalent antivenin. Toxicon 26:67 1988.

141. Russell FE, Sullivan JB, Egen NB, et al: Preparation of a new antivenin by affinity chromatography. Am J Trop Med Hyg 34:141, 1985.

142. Russell FE, Timmerman WF, Meadows PE: Clinical use of antivenin prepared from goat serum. Toxicon 8:63, 1970.

143. Wagner CW, Golladay ES: Crotalid envenomation in children: Selective conservative management. J Pediatr Surg 24:128, 1989.

144. Pennell TC, Babu SS, Meredith JW: The management of snake and spider bites in the Southeastern United States. Am Surg 53:198, 1987.

145. White BD, Rodger GC Jr, Matyunas NJ, et al: Copperhead snakebites reported to the Kentucky regional poison center 1986: Epidemiology and treatment suggestions. J Ky Med Assoc 86:61, 1986.

146. Hankin FM, Smith MD, Penner JA, et al: Eastern massasuaga rattlesnake bites. J Pediatr Orthop 7:201, 1987.

147. Jurkovich GJ, Lutterman A, McCullar K, et al: Complications of Crotalidae antivenin therapy. J Trauma 28:1032, 1988.

148. Kunkel DB: Bites of venomous reptiles. Emerg Med Clin North Am 2:563, 1984.

149. Russell FE, Ruzic N, Gonzales H: Effectiveness of antivenin (Crotalidae) polyvalent following injection of *Crotalus* venom. Toxicon 11:461, 1973.

150. Butner AN: Rattlesnake bites in Northern California. West J Med 139:179, 1983.

151. Sabback MS, Cunningham ER, Fitts CT: A study of the treatment of pit viper envenomization in 45 patients. J Trauma 17:569, 1977.
152. Garfin SR, Mubarak SJ, Davidson TM: Rattlesnake bites—Current concepts. Clin Orthop 140:50, 1979.
153. Grace TG, Omer GE: Management of upper extremity pit viper wounds. J Hand Surg 5:168, 1980.
154. Glass TG: Early debridement in pit viper bites. JAMA 235:2513, 1976.
155. Arnold RE: Controversies and hazards in the treatment of pit viper bites. South Med J 72:902, 1979.
156. Snyder CC, Knowles RP: Snakebites, guidelines for practical management. Postgrad Med 83:52, 1988.
157. Clement JF, Pietrusko RG: Pit viper snakebite in the United States. J Fam Pract 6:269, 1978.
158. Stewart ME, Greenland S, Hoffman JR: First aid treatment of poisonous snakebite: Are currently recommended procedures justified? Ann Emerg Med 10:331, 1981.
159. Durand LS, Hiebert JM, Rodeheaver GT, et al: Snake venom poisoning. Comp Ther 7:51, 1981.
160. Huang TT: Surgical management of poisonous snakebite. J Miss State Med Assoc 28:65, 1987.
161. Watt CH: Treatment of poisonous snakebite with emphasis on digit dermotomy. South Med J 78:694, 1985.
162. Roberts RS, Csencsitz TA, Heard CW: Upper extremity compartment syndromes following pit viper envenomation. Clin Orthop 193:184, 1985.
163. Mubarak SJ, Hargens AR, Owen CA, et al: The wick catheter technique for measurement of intramuscular pressure: A new research and clinical tool. J Bone Joint Surg [Am] 58:1016, 1976.
164. Garfin SR, Castiliona RR, Mubarak SJ, et al: Role of surgical decompression in treatment of rattlesnake bites. Surg Forum 30:502, 1979.
165. Clayton JM, Hayes AC, Barnes RW: Tissue pressure and perfusion in the compartment syndrome. J Surg Res 22:333, 1977.
166. Curry SC, Kraner JC, Kunkel DB, et al: Noninvasive vascular studies in management of rattlesnake envenomation to extremities. Ann Emerg Med 14:1081, 1985.
167. Blaylock RS: Time of onset of clinical envenomation following snakebite. S Afr Med J 64:357, 1983.
168. Reitz CJ: Boomslang bite—time of onset of clinical envenomation. S Afr Med J 76:39, 1989.
169. Aitchison JM: Boomslang bite: Diagnosis and managment. S Afr Med J 78:39, 1990.
170. Du Toit DM: Boomslang (Dispholidus typus) bite: Case report and review of diagnosis and managment. S Afr Med J 57:507, 1980.
171. Russell FE, Bogert CM: Gila monster: Its biology, venom and bite—A review. Toxicon 19:341, 1981.
172. Stahnke HL, Heffron WA, Lewis DL: Bite of the Gila monster. Rocky Mt Med J 67:25, 1970.
173. Streiffer RH: Bite of the venomous lizard, the Gila monster. Postgrad Med 79:297, 1986.
174. Placentine J, Curry SC, Ryan PJ: Life-threatening anaphylaxis following Gila monster bite. Ann Emerg Med 15:959, 1989.
175. Provasoli L: Recent progress—an overview. In: Taylor DL, Seliger HH (eds): Toxic Dinoflagellate Blooms. New York, Elsevier/North Holland, p 1, 1979.
176. Sakamoto Y, Lockey RF, Krzanowski, JJ: Shellfish and fish poisoning related to the toxic dinoflagellates. South Med J 80:866, 1987.
177. Halstead BW: Dangerous Marine Animals. Centerville, MD, Cornell Maritime Press, 1980.
178. Sweeney BM: The organisms. In: Taylor DL, Seliger HH (eds): Toxic Dinoflagellate Blooms. New York, Elsevier/North Holland, p 23, 1979.
179. Sanders EW Jr: Intoxications from the seas: Ciguatera, scombroid and paralytic shellfish poisoning. Infect Dis Clin North Am 1:665, 1987.
180. Russell FE, Carlson RW: Animal toxins: Marine organisms. In: Altman PL, Dittmer DS (eds): Biology Data Book, Volume II. 2nd ed. Bethesda, MD, Federation of American Societies for Experimental Biology, p 726, 1973.
181. Ritchie JM: Binding of tetrodotoxin and saxitoxin to sodium channels. Philos Trans R Soc Lond 270:319, 1975.
182. Kao CY: Pharmacology of tetrodotoxin and saxitoxin. Fed Proc 31:1117, 1972.
183. Narahashi T: Mechanism of action of tetrodotoxin and saxitoxin on excitable membranes. Fed Proc 31:1124, 1972.
184. Hughes JM: Epidemiology of shellfish poisoning in the United States, 1971–1977. In: Taylor DL Seliger HH (eds): Toxic Dinoflagellate Blooms. New York, Elsevier/North Holland, p 23, 1979.
185. Long RR, Sargent JC, Hammer K: Paralytic shellfish poisoning: A case report and serial electrophysiologic observations. Neurology 40:1310, 1990.
186. Meyer KF: Food poisoning. N Engl J Med 249:843, 1953.
187. Withers NW: Ciguatera fish poisoning. Annu Rev Med 33:97, 1982.
188. Morris PD, Campbell DS, Freeman JI: Ciguatera fish poisoning: An outbreak associated with fish caught from North Carolina coastal waters. South Med J 83:379, 1990.
189. Rayner MD: Mode of action of ciguatoxin. Fed Proc 31:1139, 1972.
190. Ogura Y, Nara J, Yoshida T: Comparative pharmacological actions of ciguatoxin and tetrodotoxin, a preliminary account. Toxicon 6:131, 1968.
191. Russell FE: Ciguatera poisoning: A report of 35 cases. Toxicon 13:383, 1975.
192. Morris JG Jr, Lewin P, Hargrett NT, et al: Clinical features of ciguatera fish poisoning. Arch Intern Med 142:1090, 1982.
193. Hashmi MA, Sorokin JJ, Levine SM: Ciguatera fish poisoning. N J Med 86:469, 1989.
194. Lawrence DL, Enriquez MB, Lumish RM, et al: Ciguatera fish poisoning in Miami. JAMA 244:254, 1980.
195. Ho AM, Fraser IM, Todd EC: Ciguatera poisoning: A report of three cases. Ann Emerg Med 15:1225, 1986.
196. Palafox NA, Jain LG, Pinano AZ, et al: Successful treatment of ciguatera fish poisoning with intravenous mannitol. JAMA 259:2740, 1988.
197. Calvert GM, Hryhorczuk DO, Leikin JB: Treatment of ciguatera fish poisoning with amitriptyline and nifedipine. Clin Toxicol 25:423, 1987.
198. Pearn JH, Lewis, RJ, Ruff T, et al: Ciguatera and mannitol: Experience with a new treatment regimen. Med J Aust 151:77, 1989.
199. Williamson J: Ciguatera and mannitol: A successful treatment. Med J Aust 153:306, 1990.
200. Sims JK: A theoretical discourse on the pharmacology of toxic marine ingestions. Ann Emerg Med 16:1006, 1987.
201. Hokama Y, Abad MA, Kimura LH: A rapid enzyme-immunoassay for the detection of ciguatoxin in contaminated fish tissues. Toxicon 21:817, 1983.
202. Morrow JD, Margolies GR, Rowland J, et al: Evidence that histamine is the causative toxin of scombroid-fish poisoning. N Engl J Med 324:716, 1991.
203. Clifford RN, Walker R, Wright J, et al: Studies with volunteers on the role of histamine in suspected scombrotoxicosis. J Sci Food Agric 47:365, 1985.
204. Lange WR: Scombroid poisoning. Am Fam Physician 37:163, 1990.
205. Dickinson G: Scombroid fish poisoning syndrome. Ann Emerg Med 11:487, 1982.
206. Blakesley ML: Scombroid poisoning: Prompt resolution of symptoms with cimetidine. Ann Emerg Med 12:104, 1983.
207. Ferguson W: On the poisonous fishes of the Caribbee Islands. Trans R Soc Edinburgh 9:65, 1823.
208. Kizer KW: Marine envenomations. J Toxicol Clin Toxicol 21:527, 1984.
209. Sims JK, Irei MY: Human Hawaiian marine sponge poisoning. Hawaii Med J 38:263, 1979.
210. Auerbach PS: Hazardous marine animals. Emerg Clin North Am 2:531, 1984.
211. Southcott RV, Coulter JR: The effects of the Southern Australian marine stinging sponges, Neofibularia mordens, and Lissodendoryx sp. Med J Aust 2:895, 1971.
212. Zervos SG: La maladie des pêcheurs d'éponges nus. Paris Med 93:89, 1934.
213. Portier P, Richet C: De l'action anaphylactique de certains venins. C R Soc Biol Paris 54:170, 1902.
214. Richet C: Anaphylaxie par la mytilo-congestive. C R Soc Biol Paris 62:358, 1907.
215. Togias AG, Burnett JW, Kagey-Sobotka A, et al: Anaphylaxis after contact with a jellyfish. J Allergy Clin Immunol 75:672, 1985.
216. Burnett JW, Calton GJ: Venomous pelagic coelenterates: Chemistry, toxiciology, immunology and treatment of their stings. Toxicon 25:581, 1987.
217. Cobbs CS, Gaur PK, Russo AJ, et al: Immunosorbent chromatography of sea nettle (Chrysaora quinquecirrha) venom and characterization of toxins. Toxicon 21:385, 1983.
218. Burnett JW, Calton GJ: The chemistry and toxicology of some venomous pelagic coelenterates. Toxicon 15:177, 1977.
219. Freeman SE, Turner RJ: Cardiovascular effects of toxins isolated from the cnidarian Chironex fleckeri southcott. Br J Pharmacol 41:154, 1971.
220. Martin JC, Audley I: Cardiac failure following Irukandji envenomation. Med J Aust 153:164, 1990.
221. Burnett JW, Calton GJ: Jellyfish envenomation syndromes updated. Ann Emerg Med 16:100, 1987.
222. Stein MR, Marraccini JV, Rothschild NE, et al: Fatal Portuguese man-o'-war (Physalia physalis) envenomation. Ann Emerg Med 18:312, 1989.
223. Lumley J, Williamson JA, Fenner PJ, et al: Fatal envenomation by Chironex fleckeri, the North Australian box-jellyfish. The continuing search for lethal mechanisms. Med J Aust 128:527, 1988.
224. Auerbach PS, Hays JT: Erythema nodosum following a jellyfish sting. J Emerg Med 5:487, 1987.
225. Auerbach PS, Hays JT: Current concepts: Marine envenomations. N Engl J Med 325:486, 1991.
226. Burnett JW, Rubinstein H, Calton GJ: First aid for jellyfish envenomation. South Med J 76:870, 1983.
227. Exton DR, Fenner PJ, Williamson JA: Cold packs: Effective topical analgesia in the treatment of painful stings by Physalia and other jellyfish. Med J Aust 151:625, 1989.
228. Burnett JW, Gean CJ, Calton GJ, et al: The effect of verapamil on the cardiotoxic activity of Portuguese man-o'-war (Physalia physalis) and sea nettle (Chrysaora quinquecirrha) venoms. Toxicon 23:681, 1985.
229. Burnett JW, Calton GJ: Response of the box-jellyfish (Chironex fleckeri) cardiotoxin to intravenous administration of verapamil. Med J Aust 2:192, 1983.
230. Endean R, Sizemore DJ: The effectiveness of antivenom in countering

the actions of box-jellyfish (*Chironex fleckeri*) nematocyst toxins in mice. Toxicon 26:425, 1988.

231. Burnett JW, Othman IB, Endean R, et al: Verapamil potentiation of *Chironex* (box-jellyfish) antivenom. Toxicon 28:242, 1990.

232. Hartman K, Calton GJ, Burnett JW: Use of the radioallergosorbent test for the study of coelenterate toxin-specific immunoglobulin E. Int Arch Allergy Appl Immunol 61:389, 1980.

233. Williamson JA, LeRay LE, Wohlfahrt M, et al: Acute management of serious envenomation by box-jellyfish (*Chironex fleckeri*). Med J Aust 141:851, 1984.

234. Baden HP, Burnett JW: Injuries from sea urchins. South Med J 70:459, 1977.

235. Cracchiolo A III, Goldberg L: Local and systemic reactions to puncture injuries by the sea urchin spine and the data palm thorn. Arthritis Rheum 20:1206, 1977.

236. Fries SL, Standaert FG, Whitcomb ER, et al: Some pharmacological properties of holothurian. J Pharmacol Exp Ther 126:323, 1959.

237. Strauss MB, MacDonald RI: Hand injuries from sea urchin spines. Clin Orthop 114:216, 1976.

238. Friess SL: Mode of action of marine saponins on neuromuscular tissues. Fed Proc 31:1146, 1972.

239. Fries SL, Standaert FG, Whitcomb ER, et al: Some pharmacologic properties of holothurian A. Ann NY Acad Sci 90:893, 1960.

240. Hinegardner RT: The venom apparatus of the cone shell. Hawaii Med J 17:533, 1958.

241. Sutherland SK, Lane WR: Toxins and mode of envenomation of the common ringed or blue-banded octopus. Med J Aust 1:893, 1969.

242. Edmonds CG: Non-fatal case of blue-ringed octopus bite. Med J Aust 2:601, 1969.

243. Bitseff EL, Garoni WJ, Hardison CD, et al: The management of stingray injuries of the extremities. South Med J 63:417, 1970.

244. Russell FE: Stingray injuries. Public Health Rep 74:855, 1959.

245. Cross TB: An unusual stingray injury. Med J Aust 2:947 1976.

246. Grainger CR: Occupational injuries due to stingrays. Trans R Soc Trop Med Hyg 74:408, 1980.

247. Grainger CR: Stingray injuries. Trans R Soc Trop Med Hyg 79:443, 1985.

248. Fenner PJ, Williamson JA, Skinner RA: Fatal and non-fatal stingray envenomation. Med J Aust 151:621, 1989.

249. Rathjen WJ, Halstead BW: Report on two fatalities due to stingray. Toxicon 6:301, 1969.

250. Russell FE, Panos TC, Kang XW, et al: Studies on the mechanism of death from stingray venom: A report of two fatal cases. Am J Med Sci 235:566, 1958.

251. Saunders PR: Pharmacological and chemical studies of the venom of the stonefish (genus *Synanceja*) and other scorpionfishes. Ann NY Acad Sci 90:798, 1960.

252. Schaeffer RC Jr, Carlson RW, Russell FE: Some chemical properties of the venom of the scorpionfish *Scorpaena guttata*. Toxicon 9:69, 1971.

253. Carlson RW, Schaeffer RC Jr, La Grange RG, et al: Some pharmacological properties of the venom of the scorpionfish *Scorpaena guttata*. I. Toxicon 9:379, 1971.

254. Carlson RW, Schaeffer RC Jr, Whigham H, et al: Some pharmacological properties of the venom of the scorpionfish *Scorpaena guttata*. II. Toxicon 10:167, 1973.

255. Kizer KW, McKinney HE, Auerbach PS: Scorpaenidae envenomation. JAMA 253:807, 1985.

256. Trestrail JH, Al-Mahasneh QM: Lionfish string [sic] experience of an inland poison center: A retrospective study of 23 cases. Vet Hum Toxicol 31:173, 1989.

257. Kasdan ML, Kasdan AS, Hamilton DL: Lionfish envenomation. Plast Reconstr Surg 80:613, 1987.

258. Auerbach PS, McKinney HE, Rees RS, et al: Analysis of vesicle fluid following the sting of the lionfish *Pterois volitans*. Toxicon 25:1350, 1987.

259. Barss P: Wound necrosis caused by the venom of stingrays. Med J Aust 141:354, 1984.

260. Binder LS: Acute arthropod envenomation: Incidence, clinical features and management. Med Toxicol Adverse Drug Exp 4:163, 1989.

261. Stawiski MA: Insect bites and stings. Emerg Med Clin North Am 3:785, 1985.

262. Golden DBK, Marsh DG, Kaghey-Sobotka A, et al: Epidemiology of insect venom sensitivity. JAMA 262:240, 1989.

263. Lanter R, Reisman RE: Clinical and immunologic features and subsequent course of patients with severe insect-sting anaphylaxis. J Allergy Clin Immunol 84:900, 1989.

264. Valentine MD, Lichenstein LM: Anaphylaxis and stinging insect hypersensitivity. JAMA 258:2881, 1987.

265. Paull BR: Imported fire ant allergy: Perspectives on diagnosis and treatment. Postgrad Med 76:155, 1984.

266. Settipane GA, Boyd GK: Anaphylaxis from insect stings: Myths, controversy and reality. Postgrad Med 86:273, 1989.

267. Oertel T, Loehr MM: Bee-sting anaphylaxis: The use of medical antishock trousers. Ann Emerg Med 13:459, 1984.

268. Gupta S, O'Donnell J, Kupa A, et al: Management of bee-sting anaphylaxis. Med J Aust 149:602, 1988.

269. Wong RC, Hughes SE, Voorhees JJ: Spider bites. Arch Dermatol 123:98, 1987.

270. Wilson DC, King LE Jr: Spiders and spider bites. Dermatol Clin 8:277, 1990.

271. Russell FE, Gertsch WJ: Letter to editor. Toxicon 21:337, 1983.

272. McCrone JE, Netzloff ML: An immunological and electrophoretical comparison of the venoms of the North American *Latrodectus* spiders. Toxicon 3:107, 1965.

273. Granata F, Paggi P, Frontali N: Effects of chromatographic fractions of black widow spider venom on in vitro biological systems. Toxicon 10:551, 1972.

274. Okamoto M, Longnecker HE, Riber WF, et al: Destruction of mammalian motor nerve terminal by black widow spider venom. Science 172:733, 1971.

275. Gorio A, Mauro A: Reversibility and mode of action of black widow spider venom on the vertebrate neuromuscular junction. J Gen Physiol 73:245, 1979.

276. Griffiths DJG, Smyth T Jr: Action of black widow spider venom at insect neuromuscular junctions. Toxicon 11:369, 1973.

277. Longnecker HE Jr, Hurlbut WP, Mauro A, et al: Effect of black widow spider venom on the frog neuromuscular junction. Nature 225:701, 1970.

278. Pinto JEF, Rothlin, RP, Dagrosa EE, et al: Peripheral adrenergic effect of *Latrodectus mactans* venom. Toxicon 11:395, 1973.

279. Rauber A: Black widow spider bites. J Toxicol Clin Toxicol 21:473, 1984.

280. Sutherland SK, Trinca JC: Survey of 2144 cases of red-back spider bites. Australia and New Zealand 1963–1976. Med J Aust 2:620, 1978.

281. Maretic Z: Latrodectism: Variations in clinical manifestations provoked by *Latrodectus* species of spiders. Toxicon 21:457, 1983.

282. Kunkel DB: Arthropod envenomations. Emerg Med Clin North Am 2:579, 1984.

283. Ryan PJ: Preliminary report: Experience with the use of dantrolene sodium in the treatment of bites by the black widow spider *Latrodectus hesperuss*. J Toxicol Clin Toxicol 21:487, 1984.

284. Geren CR, Chan TK, Howell DE, et al: Isolation and characterization of toxins from brown recluse spider venom (*Loxosceles reclusa*). Arch Biochem Biophys 174:90, 1976.

285. Geren CR, Chan TK, Howell DE, et al: Partial characterization of the low molecular weight fractions of the extract of the venom apparatus of the brown recluse spider and of its hemolymph. Toxicon 13:233, 1975.

286. Forrester LJ, Barrett JG, Campbell BJ: Red blood cell lysis induced by the venom of the brown recluse spider: The role of sphingomyelinase D. Arch Biochem Biophys 187:355, 1978.

287. Wasserman GS, Anderson PC: Loxoscelism and necrotic arachnidism. J Toxicol Clin Toxicol 21:451, 1984.

288. Russell FE, Waldron WG, Madon MB: Bites by the brown spiders *Loxosceles unicolor* and *Loxosceles arizonica* in California and Arizona. Toxicon 7:109, 1969.

289. Young VL, Pin PL: The brown recluse spider bite. Ann Plast Surg 20:447, 1988.

290. Majeski JA, Durst GG: Necrotic arachnidism. South Med J 69:887, 1976.

291. Hobbs GD, Harrell RE: Brown recluse spider bites: A common cause of necrotic arachnidism. Am J Emerg Med 7:309, 1989.

292. Nance W: Hemolytic anemia of a necrotic arachnidism. Am J Med 31:801, 1961.

293. Rees R, Campbell D, Rieger E, et al: The diagnosis and treatment of brown recluse spider bites. Ann Emerg Med 16:945, 1987.

294. DeLozier JB, Reaves L, King LE, et al: Brown recluse spider bites of the upper extremity. South Med J 81:181, 1988.

295. Gutowicz M, Fritz RA, Sonoga AL: Brown recluse spider bite. J Am Podiatry Med Assoc 79:142, 1979.

296. Hollabaugh RS, Fernandes ET: Management of the brown recluse spider bite. J Pediatr Surg 24:126, 1989.

297. Auer AI, Hershey FB: Proceedings: Surgery for necrotic bites of the brown spider. Arch Surg 108:612, 1974.

298. Fardon DW, Wingo CW, Robinson DW, et al: The treatment of brown spider bite. Plast Reconstr Surg 40:482, 1967.

299. Rees RS, Altenbern DP, Lynch JB, et al: Brown recluse spider bites. Ann Surg 202:659, 1985.

300. Rees R, Shack B, Withers E, et al: Management of the brown recluse spider bite. Plast Reconstr Surg 68:768, 1981.

301. King LE Jr, Rees RS: Dapsone treatment of a brown recluse bite. JAMA 254:2895, 1985.

302. Efrati P: Epidemiology, symptomatology and treatment of Buthidae stings. In: Bettini S (ed): Handbook of Experimental Pharmacology, Volume 40, Arthropod Venoms. Berlin, Springer-Verlag, p 312, 1978.

303. Guyffon M, Vachon M, Broglio N: Epidemiological and clinical characteristics of scorpion envenomation in Tunisia. Toxicon 20:337, 1982.

304. Rimsza ME, Zimmerman DR, Bergeson PS: Scorpion envenomation. Pediatrics 66:298, 1980.

305. Gueron M, Yarom R: Cardiovascular manifestations of severe scorpion sting. Chest 57:156, 1970.

306. Campos JA, Silva OA, Lopez M, et al: Signs, symptoms and treatment of severe scorpion sting in children. Toxicon 17(suppl 1):19, 1979.

307. Gueron M, Adolph R, Grupp TL, et al: Hemodynamic and myocardial consequences of scorpion venom. Am J Cardiol 45:979, 1980.

308. Amitia Y, Mines Y, Aker M, et al: Scorpion sting in children. A review of 51 cases. Clin Pediatr 24:136, 1985.
309. Freire-Maia L, Diniz CR: Pharmacological action of a purified scorpion toxin in the rat. Toxicon 8:132, 1970.
310. Wang GK, Strichartz GR: Purification and physiological characterization of neurotoxins from venoms of the scorpions *Centruroides sculpturatus* and *Leiurus quinquestriatus*. Mol Pharmacol 23:519, 1983.
311. Moss J, Thoa NB, Kopin IJ: On the mechanism of scorpion toxin-induced release of norepinephrine from peripheral adrenergic neurons. J Pharmacol Exp Ther 190:39, 1974.
312. Curry SC, Vance MV, Ryan PJ, et al: Envenomation by the scorpion *Centruroides sculpturatus*. J Toxicol Clin Toxicol 21:417, 1984.
313. McIntosh ME, Watt DD: Purification of toxins from the North American scorpion *Centruroides sculpturatus*. In: Russell F, Saunders P (eds): Animal Toxins. New York, Pergamon Press, p 529, 1967.
314. Meves H, Rubly N, Watt DD: Effect of toxins isolated from the venom of the scorpion *Centruroides sculpturatus* on the Na currents of the node of Ranvier. Pflugers Arch 393:56, 1982.
315. Rahay G, Weiss AT: Scorpion sting induced pulmonary edema. Chest 97:1478, 1990.
316. Bawaskar HS, Bawaskar PH: Prazosin for vasodilator treatment of acute pulmonary oedema due to scorpion sting. Ann Trop Med Parasitol 81:719, 1987.
317. Gueron M, Sofer S: Vasodilators and calcium blocking agents as treatment of cardiovascular manifestations of human scorpion envenomation. Toxicon 28:127, 1990.
318. Freire-Maia L, Campos JA: What is the treatment for the cardiovascular manifestations of scorpion envenomation? Toxicon 25:121, 1987.
319. Habermann E: Bee and wasp venoms: The biochemistry and pharmacology of their peptides and enzymes are reviewed. Science 177:314, 1972.
320. Piek T: Neurotoxins from venoms of the Hymenoptera—Twenty-five years of research in Amsterdam. Comp Biochem Physiol [C] 96:223, 1990.
321. Bochner BS, Lightenstein LM: Anaphylaxis. N Engl J Med 324:1785, 1991.
322. Wright DN, Lockey RF: Local reactions to stinging insects (Hymenoptera). Allergy Proc 11:23, 1990.
323. Lantner R, Reisman RE: Clinical and immunological features and subsequent course of patients with severe insect-sting anaphylaxis. J Allergy Clin Immunol 84:900, 1989.
324. Golden DBK, Marsh DG, Kagey-Sobotka A, et al: Epidemiology of insect venom sensitivity. JAMA 262:240, 1989.
325. Valentine MD, Schuberth KC, Kagey-Sobotka A, et al: The value of immunotherapy with venom in children with allergy to insect stings. N Engl J Med 323:160l, 1990.
326. Stafford CT, Hutto LS, Rhoades RB, et al: Imported fire ant as a health hazard. South Med J 82:515, 1989.
327. Owens VJ, Malloy C, Schuman S, et al: Underrecognition of morbidity from stings of the red imported fire ant in the Southeastern United States. Public Health Nurs 7:88, 1990.
328. Triplett RF: The imported fire ant: Health hazard or nuisance? South Med J 69:258, 1976.
329. Rhoades RB, Stafford CT, James FK Jr: Survey of fatal anaphylactic reactions to imported fire ants stings: Report of the Fire Ant Subcommittee of the American Academy of Allergy and Immunology. J Allergy Clin Immunol 84:159, 1989.
330. Bloom FK, Del Mastro PL: Imported fire ant death: A documented case report. J Fla Med Assoc 71:87, 1984.
331. Hensel AE, Schutze WH, Lockey RF: Death from imported fire ant, *Solenopsis invicta* Buren, confirmed by insect identification and autopsy. Ann Allergy 50:359, 1983.
332. deShazo RD, Butcher BT, Banks WA: Reactions to the stings of the imported fire ant. N Engl J Med 323:462, 1990.
333. MacConnell JG, Blum MS, Fales HM: Alkaloid from fire ant venom: Identification and synthesis. Science 168:840, 1970.
334. MacConnell JG, Blum MS, Buren WF, et al: Fire ant venoms: Chemotaxonomic correlations with alkaloidal compositions. Toxicon 14:69, 1976.
335. Stafford CT, Rhoades RB, Bunker-Soler AL, et al: Survey of whole body extract immunotherapy for imported fire ant–and other Hymenoptera-sting allergy: Report of the Fire Ant Subcommittee of the American Academy of Allergy and Immunology. J Allergy Clin Immunol 83:1107, 1989.
336. Stroom GB Jr, Boswell RN, Jacobs RL: In vivo and in vitro comparison of fire ant venom and fire ant whole body extract. J Allergy Clin Immunol 72:46, 1983.

CHAPTER 146

Pharmacologic Agents and Poisoning

Pharmacokinetics in Critically Ill Patients

David R. Rutledge
Michael A. Geheb
Simon Cronin
Michael P. Peppers

Critically ill patients are at great risk for sustaining physiologic insults that may result in organ failure or death. Counteractive measures should be taken to prevent and eliminate as many insults as possible, thus ensuring optimal care of patients. Therapeutic drug monitoring has found its way into the critical care arena for this reason.

Pharmacokinetic monitoring is a branch of therapeutic drug monitoring that encompasses the science of analyzing serum drug concentrations for predicting absorption, distribution, metabolism, and excretion of drugs by the body. Patients who undergo proper pharmacokinetic monitoring via pharmacokinetic services have serum drug samples drawn more appropriately, have therapeutic serum drug concentrations attained more quickly and maintained in the therapeutic range more often, and experience fewer adverse drug effects than patients who are not adequately monitored.[1–4] Several studies have documented adverse clinical events, including cardiac arrest and intractable seizures, in patients receiving drugs for which pharmacokinetic monitoring was not adequately performed.[5–15] In addition to preventing or correcting toxic drug concentrations, one can correct subtherapeutic concentrations by using a formal pharmacokinetic service.

MULTIDISCIPLINARY APPROACH TO THERAPEUTIC DRUG MONITORING

Effective drug monitoring entails the employment of various health care disciplines. Benefits gained via a multidisciplinary effort include systematic pharmacokinetic approaches; better communication among physicians, pharmacists, nurses, and laboratory personnel; and the capture of data that are important for determining pharmacokinetic estimates that are clinically relevant for a specific population. A well-coordinated service ensures that quality drug monitoring occurs. An efficient pharmacokinetic service should evaluate drugs by considering the various factors listed in Tables 146–1 and 146–2.

PHARMACOKINETIC PRINCIPLES

Clinical pharmacokinetics is the application of pharmacokinetic concepts for the rational design of an individualized dosage regimen.[4, 16–21] A therapeutic design may need to be changed frequently owing to multiple-organ diseases that cause rapid changes in the critically ill patient's pharmaco-

TABLE 146–1

FACTORS TO BE CONSIDERED FOR EFFICIENT THERAPEUTIC DRUG MONITORING

Patient-related factors: age, weight, height, sex
Prior drug exposure
Dose of drug administered
Time of drug administration
Route of drug administration
Precision and accuracy of analytic methods
Sample handling
Sample storage conditions
Time of sample collection
Transportation of sample to laboratory
Validity of pharmacokinetic models used for each drug
Assumptions made for each model used
Concomitant therapies (drug, fluid, nutrition)
Concurrent disease processes
Pharmacologic response
Therapeutic end points

kinetic variables. Regardless of the specific circumstance, an understanding of the basic principles of pharmacokinetics is a must. Table 146–3 outlines some basic pharmacokinetic terminology.

Absorption

Drugs can reach the systemic circulation through intravenous administration or via absorption through various anatomic sites such as the gastrointestinal tract, the mucous membranes, the skin, and the lungs. *Bioavailability* denotes the fraction of drug that reaches the systemic circulation after absorption (see Table 146–3).

After intravenous administration, the bioavailability of any drug should be 1, representing 100% drug absorption and delivery into the systemic circulation. Drugs that undergo hepatic metabolism on their first pass through the body, known as the *first-pass effect*, generally have an oral bioavailability of less than 1. A drug that undergoes a significant first-pass effect acts more efficiently when given by a route that allows it to bypass the liver on its first pass through the body. Sublingual administration of nitroglycerin for acute anginal pain is an example of this concept. Nitroglycerin undergoes significant first-pass metabolism in the liver, thus exhibiting a low systemic bioavailability when absorbed through the gastrointestinal tract. Nitroglycerin exhibits a greater bioavailability and greater pharmacodynamic action when metabolism by the liver is circumvented by sublingual administration.

Distribution

Drugs are distributed into various tissues following absorption. The *apparent volume of distribution* is a fictitious space required to account for the total amount of drug in

TABLE 146–2

FACTORS AFFECTING DRUG CONCENTRATION INTERPRETATION

Failure to draw sample at specified time
Sample not drawn at appropriate time in relation to dose
Drug administration time not documented
Sampling time not documented
Improper sample handling
Delays in assay turnaround time
Assay results not recorded in patient's chart

TABLE 146–3

BASIC PHARMACOKINETIC TERMINOLOGY

Term	Meaning
Bioavailability	Percentage of drug that reaches the systemic circulation after administration.
Absolute bioavailability	Fraction of a drug reaching the systemic circulation from dosage form compared with the fraction of the same drug given IV.
Relative bioavailability	Term used when two or more dosage forms are being compared with a standard dosage form for the same drug; the bioavailability of a drug from a given dosage form compared with the bioavailability of the same drug when used in an accepted standard dosage form. Area under the concentration-time curves for each dose form is used for determining relative bioavailability.
Apparent volume of distribution	Size of compartment necessary to account for the total amount of drug in the body if it were present throughout the body at the same concentration found in plasma; not a true value.
Half-life	For first-order reactions, it is the time required for the concentration of drug to decline by 50%.
Steady state	Point in time at which drug intake equals drug excretion; only mild fluctuations should occur in the serum concentration when analyzed at the same time each day.
First-pass effect	Extensive metabolism by the liver on first pass.
Clearance	The volume of blood (serum, bile, etc.) that can be completely cleared of a drug per unit of time. This removal can occur through distribution to tissues, metabolism, or excretion.

the body if the drug is present throughout the body at the same concentration observed in the plasma. Apparent volume of distribution is used to calculate the loading dose of a drug required to achieve a desired plasma concentration. To attain an immediate therapeutic concentration of theophylline, the clinician must administer a loading dose (LD) equal to the product derived from the desired plasma concentration (Cp) times the volume of distribution (V).

$$LD = Cp \text{ (desired)} \times V$$

For example, for a patient weighing 70 kg, if the volume of distribution of theophylline is 0.45 L/kg of body weight and the desired initial serum concentration is 10 mg/L, then

$$LD = (10 \text{ mg/L}) (0.45 \text{ L/kg}) (70 \text{ kg})$$
$$LD = 315 \text{ mg}$$

Thus, an initial 315-mg intravenous loading dose of theophylline is required to obtain an immediate therapeutic serum concentration in a lean 70-kg patient.

The extent to which a drug distributes depends on the lipophilic versus hydrophilic properties and plasma- versus tissue protein–binding properties possessed by the drug. A drug with good lipophilic properties and low plasma protein binding exhibits a large apparent volume of distribution because it is easily distributed into various tissues other than serum. Generally, it follows that a drug with low lipophilic and high plasma protein–binding properties exhibits a small volume of distribution because most of the drug remains in the serum. Thus, the critical care patient who has changing hydration status with varying concentrations of serum proteins may exhibit periodic shifts in serum drug concentrations owing to frequently changing volumes into which the drug may distribute. As a result, the serum drug concentration fluctuates from time to time. This basic concept must always be considered when making dosage adjustments in the critically ill patient.

For a more detailed discussion on the apparent volume of distribution, including that of various compartments within the body, the reader is referred to specialized reference texts.[9, 10]

Clearance

Clearance can be defined as the intrinsic ability of the body to clear drugs from body fluids. This pharmacokinetic concept defines a theoretic volume of fluid (serum) that is completely cleared of a drug per unit of time; clearance does not define a true amount of drug removed from the body. Drugs may be cleared from the blood via distribution into tissues, metabolism, and/or excretion. Clearance is an important concept used to determine the amount of drug required to maintain a steady-state serum concentration (see later).

Each organ that has the capability of metabolizing a drug or eliminating it from the serum has an inherent clearance value. The two major organs responsible for clearing drugs from the serum are the kidneys and the liver.

Renal clearance is the volume of serum cleared of drug by the kidneys per unit of time. Drugs that are polar, water soluble, or have a low molecular weight (<500) are eliminated primarily by the kidneys via glomerular filtration and active tubular secretion. Dosages of drugs that undergo extensive elimination via the kidneys must be adjusted in renal failure to prevent toxic effects resulting from drug accumulation. Equations designed to estimate creatinine clearance can be used for proper drug dosing in patients with kidney dysfunction.[10, 11] Dosing guidelines can be found in Chapter 111.

Hepatic clearance is the volume of serum cleared of drug by the liver per unit of time. The liver metabolizes drugs via phase I and phase II reactions. Phase I reactions involve chemical oxidation, hydrolysis, and reduction to produce polar molecules that are then easily excreted by the kidneys. Phase II reactions involve conjugation to form inactive glucuronides, sulfates, and acetates, which are either secreted into the bile for removal by the gastrointestinal tract or excreted by the kidneys.[12]

Liver blood flow is approximately 1.5 L/min. Conditions that alter liver blood flow such as changes in cardiac output, sepsis, altered nutritional (protein) status, and concomitant administration of drugs can affect intrinsic hepatic drug clearance. Hepatic drug clearance can be increased via enzyme induction by coadministration of drugs (phenobarbital, carbamazepine, rifampin), by tobacco smoking, or by improved physiologic variables such as liver blood flow and oxygenation. Drug clearance can be decreased via hepatic enzyme inhibition by drugs such as cimetidine or by physiologic factors that adversely affect tissue blood flow and oxygenation.

Various drugs may undergo a metabolic process known as *enterohepatic circulation*, which occurs when a parent drug is conjugated by the liver in a phase II reaction, secreted into the bile as the conjugate or parent form, and then reabsorbed by the gastrointestinal tract as the parent compound. Enteric bacteria are responsible for cleaving the conjugate from the parent compound, thus allowing reabsorption to occur. This metabolic phenomenon is extremely important in the critical care unit when evaluating certain drug overdoses. For example, in glutethimide overdose, the patient may intermittently go into and out of coma as the drug is absorbed, excreted, and then reabsorbed via enterohepatic circulation.

Patients who exhibit liver dysfunction should have their drug dosage regimens modified. Table 146–4 can be used as a guide for dosage adjustment in patients with liver dysfunction. Specialized references should also be reviewed.[15]

Half-Life

Half-life is defined as the time required for a drug to decrease in concentration by 50% (provided that no drug absorption is occurring during the decline). For a drug exhibiting linear pharmacokinetics (see later), it takes the same amount of time to decrease from a serum concentration of 50 mg/L to 25 mg/L as it does to decline from a serum concentration of 25 mg/L to 12.5 mg/L. For drugs exhibiting zero-order pharmacokinetics (e.g., phenytoin), half-life is a function of plasma concentration; the half-life of elimination changes as the concentration of drug changes. The half-life value can be used to estimate the time required for a drug to reach a steady-state serum concentration; at steady-state concentration, drug intake equals drug excretion, thus producing only mild fluctuations in serum concentration if analyzed at the same time each day (i.e., drug intake is in equilibrium with drug excretion). Generally, four to five half-lives are required for a drug to reach greater than 90% of its steady-state concentration, if a loading dose is not given. Loading doses achieve the desired steady-state drug concentration more rapidly.

Pharmacokinetic Order

Drugs are assumed to follow either first-order, zero-order (Michaelis-Menton), or mixed-order pharmacokinetic profiles. First-order pharmacokinetics means that the serum drug concentration and elimination are in linear proportion to the amount of drug within the body; for example, a patient who exhibits a steady-state serum concentration of 10 mg/L while receiving 300 mg of continuous intravenous drug per day would be expected to exhibit a steady-state serum concentration of 20 mg/L if the intravenous infusion was increased to 600 mg daily. The metabolizing organs have the capability of increasing or decreasing the metabolic rate of drugs, depending on the amount available.

Zero-order pharmacokinetics is in effect when drug elimination occurs at a constant rate, regardless of the drug amount available. Drugs exhibiting this order of pharmacokinetics display disproportionate changes in serum concentration with respect to changes in dosage. This is due to saturable enzyme systems responsible for drug metabolism. As the enzymes become saturated, only a fixed amount of drug can be eliminated from the body, regardless of how much drug is present. Other terms used to describe this type of pharmacokinetic profile include capacity-limited,

TABLE 146–4
DOSING ADJUSTMENTS FOR VARIOUS DEGREES OF HEPATIC DYSFUNCTION*

Drug	Disease	Half-Life (h)	Fraction Unbound (%)	Comment and Dosage Adjustment
Beta-Adrenergic Receptor Antagonists				Reduced dose probably necessary. Stereoisomers exist for many compounds.
Atenolol	C	6.0 ± 1.4 (5.0 ± 1.4)	?	
Esmolol	C	4.4 ± 0.89	?	Unchanged in chronic stable hepatic disease.
Labetalol	C	2.8 ± 1.15 (3.1 ± 1.3)	?	
Metoprolol	C	7.2 ± 3.8 (4.2 ± 2.7)	?	
Propranolol	C	11.8 ± 8.5 (3.9 ± 0.85)	10.2 ± 4.2 (6.6 ± 1.2)	
Anesthetics				Owing to increased cerebral sensitivity, these agents should be used cautiously in liver disease.
Fentanyl	C	5.07 ± 3.5 (4.38 ± 3.0)	?	Unchanged.
Thiopentone	C	11.9 ± 11.9 (8.8 ± 4.9)	25.2 ± 11.0 (41.5 ± 10.2)	Unchanged.
Analgesics				
Acetaminophen	C	2.9 ± 0.3 (2.0 ± 0.4)	?	Appears to be well tolerated in cirrhosis. Serum levels may need to be monitored with long-term use.
Aspirin	ALD	7.3 ± 2.3 (7.9 ± 2.0)	18.6 ± 10.5 (8.5 ± 2.6)	Avoid in severe liver disease. Values are for salicylates.
Meperidine	AVH	7.0 ± 2.7 (3.4 ± 0.8)	44.0 ± 12.0 (42.0 ± 9.0)	Reduction in dose is more important after oral dosing than IV dosing.
	C	7.0 ± 0.9 (3.2 ± 0.8)	35.0 ± 6.0 (36.0 ± 14.0)	R. Increased narcotic effect in cirrhosis.
Methadone	CLD, severe	35.5 ± 17.0 (18.9 ± 6.7)	?	Avoid in severe liver disease.
Morphine	C	2.2 ± 1.3 (2.5 ± 1.5)	84.0 ± 24.0 (80.0 ± 6.1)	Unchanged in mild liver disease. Substantial extrahepatic metabolism may occur. Excessive sedation may occur in cirrhosis.
Pentazocine	C	6.6 ± 1.9 (3.8 ± 0.5)	?	R.
NONSTEROIDAL ANTI-INFLAMMATORY DRUGS				
Ibuprofen	ALD, severe	2.6 ± 0.6 (2.2 ± 0.4)	?	Avoid in severe liver disease.
Antianginal Agents (See Also Beta-Adrenergic Receptor Antagonists)				
Isosorbide mononitrate	C	4.6 (4.77)	?	Unchanged.
Antianxiety Drugs and Hypnotics				
BARBITURATES				
Hexobarbital	AVH	8.2 ± 3.1 (4.3 ± 1.1)	?	Avoid in severe liver disease.
	C	17.0 ± 7.5 (5.7 ± 1.8)	?	R.
	IC	5.9 ± 2.5	?	
	OJ	5.7 ± 1.9 (5.4 ± 1.4)	?	
BENZODIAZEPINES				These drugs may exacerbate or precipitate hepatic encephalopathy in patients with cirrhosis or severe acute liver disease. They are best avoided or used with care and in reduced doses. Oxazepam and lorazepam appear safe in cirrhosis.
Alprazolam	C	19.7 ± 14.3 (11.4 ± 4.9)	23.2 ± 4.2 (29.0 ± 2.5)	R.
Chlordiazepoxide	C	62.7 ± 27.3 (23.8 ± 11.6)	5.4 ± 3.0 (3.5 ± 1.8)	Avoid.
	ALD	40.1 ± 16.9 (16.5 ± 8.0)	?	Avoid.
Diazepam	C	105 ± 15.2 (46.6 ± 14.2)	4.7 ± 0.2 (2.2 ± 0.1)	Reduce dose by 50%.
Lorazepam	AVH	28.3 ± 8.9	9.0 ± 1.9	Unchanged.
	C	41.2 ± 24.5 (21.7 ± 7.6)	11.0 ± 2.5 (6.8 ± 1.8)	Unchanged.
Temazepam	C	12.8 ± 5.7 (15.9 ± 5.8)	5.5 ± 1.7 (3.8 ± 0.4)	May be safe at usual doses.
Antiarrhythmic Drugs				
Encainide	C	3.6 ± 1.2 (2.7 ± 0.8)	24 (30)	No increase in effect in cirrhosis because of reduced formation of active metabolites.
Lidocaine	AVH	2.67 (1.5)	?	R.
	C	5.7 ± 3.9 (1.8 ± 0.1)	?	R.
Quinidine	CAH	41.5 (6.3 ± 1.7)	?	Reduce dose by 70% in severe liver disease.
	C	9.0 ± 2.8 (6.0 ± 1.4)	†5.0–55.0 (11.0–65.0)	R.
Tocainide	C	27.4 ± 15.4 (13.5 ± 2.3)	?	Unchanged.

Table continued on following page

TABLE 146–4

DOSING ADJUSTMENTS FOR VARIOUS DEGREES OF HEPATIC DYSFUNCTION* Continued

Drug	Disease	Half-Life (h)	Fraction Unbound (%)	Comment and Dosage Adjustment
Antibacterial Drugs				
CEPHALOSPORINS				
Cefoperazone	C	4.5 ± 2.7 (1.5 ± 0.2)	?	R.
Cefotaxime	C	2.3 (1.1–4.1)	?	R.
Ceftazidime	IC	1.7 ± 0.08	?	Unchanged.
Ceftriaxone	C with ascites	9.7 ± 1.8 (8.4 ± 1.8)	75.0 ± 4.0 (46.0 ± 7.0)	Unchanged.
Cefuroxime	C	1.0 ± 0.3 (1.8 ± 0.4)	?	Unchanged.
PENICILLINS				
Ampicillin	C	1.9 ± 0.6 (1.3 ± 0.2)	?	Unchanged.
Mezlocillin	C	2.6 ± 0.5 (1.0 ± 0.1)	?	Reduce dose by 50%.
Nafcillin	C	1.2 ± 0.3	?	R.
	OJ	1.7 ± 0.4 (1.0 ± 0.2)	?	R.
OTHERS				
Aztreonam	C	3.2 ± 0.6	?	Unchanged.
	PBC	2.2 ± 0.1 (1.9 ± 0.2)	?	Unchanged.
Chloramphenicol	C	10.5 ± 2.8 (4.6 ± 0.9)	?	Avoid. Increased toxicity may occur in cirrhosis.
	AH	11.6 ± 1.6	?	Avoid.
Clindamycin	AH	2.6	?	Unchanged.
	CAH	2.1	?	Unchanged.
	C	2.5 (1.8)	?	Unchanged.
Erythromycin	C	3.2 ± 0.4 (2.0 ± 0.7)	?	Unchanged.
	C	2.2 ± 0.9 (1.4 ± 0.4)	58.3 ± 17.7 (30.5 ± 2.8)	
Metronidazole	C	10.8 ± 5.9 (7.4 ± 0.7)	?	Reduce dose in severe liver disease.
Norfloxacin	C	5.47 ± 0.8 (4.3 ± 1.3)	?	Unchanged.
Vancomycin	LD	37.0 ± 74.3 (2.6 ± 1.3)	?	Reduce dose by 60%.
Anticoagulants				
Heparin	C	1.96 ± 0.06 (1.2 ± 0.5)	?	Monitor effect. Anticipate lower dose to be used.
Warfarin	AVH	23.0 ± 5.0 (25.0 ± 3.0)	?	The response may be enhanced in OJ owing to reduced vitamin K absorption. In hepatitis and cirrhosis, there is a decreased production of vitamin K–dependent clotting factors. Bleeding times should be monitored closely.
Anticonvulsants				
Phenobarbital	C	130.0 ± 36.7 (86.0 ± 7.3)	?	R. Increased side effects may occur in severe liver disease.
Phenytoin	AVH	13.2 ± 6.5 (13.5 ± 5.7)	?	Safe in usual doses in mild liver disease.
Primidone	AVH	17.4 ± 2.4 (18.0 ± 3.1)	?	Unchanged.
Valproic acid	C	18.9 ± 5.1 (12.2 ± 3.7)	29.0 (11.0)	R.
Antidepressants				
Amitriptyline	C	Unchanged.	?	Cerebral depressant effect in cirrhosis; therefore, use with caution.
Antihistamines (Histamine, Receptor Antagonists)				
Diphenhydramine	C	15.2 ± 4.4 (9.3 ± 2.0)	33.3 (21.9)	Unchanged.
Antihypertensives				
Nifedipine	C	7.0 ± 4.2 (1.8 ± 0.4)	8.5 ± 2.5 (4.4 ± 0.8)	Reduce oral dose by 50%.
Verapamil	C	14.2 (3.7)	?	Reduce oral dose by 25%.
Antineoplastic Drugs				
Cyclophosphamide	LF	12.5 ± 1.0 (7.6 ± 1.4)	87.5 (87.5)	R.
Antituberculosis Drugs				
Aminosalicylic acid	C, AVH	0.45 ± 0.09 (0.44 ± 0.09)	?	Unchanged.
Isoniazid	C	6.74 ± 1.2 (3.24 ± 1.0)	?	Reduce dose in severe liver disease.
Rifampin	C	5.4 ± 1.98 (2.8 ± 0.76)	?	R. Increased risk of hepatotoxicity if usual doses used.
Antiulcer Drugs				
Cimetidine	CLD	2.9 ± 1.1 (2.3 ± 0.7)	?	Usual dose safe in mild liver disease, but use with caution and in a reduced dosage in severe liver disease. Increased risk of CNS side effects.
	C	1.97 ± 0.4 (2.3 ± 0.4)	?	Same as above.
Ranitidine	C	2.77 ± 0.65 (2.06 ± 0.26)	?	Unchanged.

TABLE 146–4

DOSING ADJUSTMENTS FOR VARIOUS DEGREES OF HEPATIC DYSFUNCTION* Continued

Drug	Disease	Half-Life (h)	Fraction Unbound (%)	Comment and Dosage Adjustment
Bronchodilators				
Theophylline	C	25.6 (6.7)	63.2 (47.4)	Higher incidence of toxicity (seizures) in cirrhosis. Monitor drug levels and decrease dose.
Cardiac Glycosides				
Digoxin	C	Unchanged.	?	Unchanged.
	AVH	Unchanged.	?	Unchanged.
Corticosteroids				
Prednisolone	CAH	3.4 ± 0.56 (3.58 ± 0.35)	?	Unchanged.
Prednisone	CAH	3.0 ± 1.0 (3.3 ± 1.0)	?	Unchanged.
Diuretics				
Bumetanide	C	2.3 ± 1.0 (1.1 ± 0.7)	?	Unchanged.
Furosemide	C	0.87 ± 0.1 (0.85 ± 0.1)	?	Diminished natriuretic effect with increased sensitivity to hypokalemia and volume depletion in cirrhosis. Increased risk of HE. Monitor effects, especially at higher doses.
Spironolactone	C	10.0 (6.0)	?	Unchanged.
Hypoglycemics				
Tolbutamide	C	9.26 (4.4 ± 0.7)	?	Use with caution in cirrhosis. Increased risk of hypoglycemia.
Muscle Relaxants				
Pancuronium	C	3.47 ± 1.55 (1.9 ± 0.55)	?	Patients with liver disease may show resistance to nondepolarizing muscle relaxants. Large doses may be required and problems may arise in antagonizing their effects postoperatively.
Miscellaneous Drugs				
Cyclosporine	LD	8.7 (3.5)	?	R. Monitor levels.

*Values in parentheses indicate data obtained from healthy subjects for comparison. C = cirrhosis; LD = undefined liver disease; ALD = alcoholic liver disease; AVH = acute viral hepatitis; CLD = chronic liver disease; IC = intrahepatic cholestasis; OJ = obstructive jaundice; CAH = chronic active hepatitis; PBC = primary biliary cirrhosis; AH = acute hepatitis; ? = unknown or not reported for the specific liver disease state; R = reduced.
Adapted from Bass NM, Williams RL. Guide to drug dosage in hepatic disease. In: Mammen GJ (ed): Clinical Pharmacokinetics. Drug Data Handbook 1990. Mairang, Bay Auckland 10, New Zealand, ADIS Press, p 85, 1990.

dose-dependent, and saturation pharmacokinetics. It is difficult to accurately predict the time at which a desired concentration will be achieved for a drug exhibiting zero-order pharmacokinetics. The most useful measures to use in calculating the rate or velocity (V) at which an enzyme system can metabolize a drug are the maximal drug-metabolizing capacity (V_{max}) and a constant with a value equal to the plasma concentration at which the rate of metabolism is one half the maximal (K_m). For further information, specialized references are recommended.[9, 10, 12] Phenytoin and ethanol are examples of drugs that exhibit Michaelis-Menton pharmacokinetics (see later).

Drugs that exhibit mixed-order pharmacokinetics follow a linear pattern of elimination at low concentrations but have the potential of overwhelming the enzymatic systems to produce a Michaelis-Menton pharmacokinetic profile at higher doses, generally in the toxic range. Theophylline and salicylate are examples of drugs that exhibit mixed-order pharmacokinetics.

Plasma Protein Binding

Drugs may bind to various plasma proteins such as albumin, α_1-acid glycoprotein, lipoprotein, gamma globulin, transcortin, fibrinogen, and thyroid-binding globulin. The extent of plasma protein binding depends on the specific drug and circumstance. Acidic drugs are primarily bound to albumin (Table 146–5), whereas basic drugs bind to α_1-acid glycoprotein and lipoprotein (Table 146–6). The other proteins have a smaller capacity for drug binding and are highly specific with respect to which drugs they bind to.

Plasma protein binding strongly influences drug distribution, clearance, and serum drug analysis. Hypoproteinemia results in a lower percentage of bound drug and a greater percentage of free drug (active portion) in the serum. In hypoproteinemia, there is a greater amount of free drug that leaves the intravascular space and distributes into the tissues, thus producing a greater than expected volume of distribution for the drug. For some drugs, clearance also increases in the hypoproteinemic patient because a larger amount of drug is free for metabolism and excretion; drugs bound to proteins are not metabolized or excreted until the drug is released from the protein.

TABLE 146–5

DRUGS PRIMARILY BOUND TO ALBUMIN

Warfarin	Sulfa drugs
Valproic acid	Phenytoin
Furosemide	Benzodiazepines
Ethacrynic acid	Clofibrate
Probenecid	

TABLE 146–6

DRUGS BINDING TO α_1-ACID GLYCOPROTEIN AND LIPOPROTEINS

α_1-Acid Glycoprotein	Lipoproteins
Quinidine	Cyclosporine
Nortriptyline	Chlorpromazine
Lidocaine	Quinidine
Erythromycin	Probucol
Chlorpromazine	
Propranolol	
Methadone	
Bupivacaine	
Disopyramide	
Metoprolol	
Meperidine	
Imipramine	
Dipyridamole	

TABLE 146–7

FACTORS THAT SHIFT THERAPEUTIC RANGES

Stage of disease (acute seizure treatment vs. prophylactic treatment)

Pre-existing disease (moderate renal disease and aminoglycoside therapy)

Concurrent therapy (loop diuretic and digoxin therapy with or without potassium supplementation)

Acute increases in α_1-acid glycoprotein concentration from trauma, surgery, or an acute myocardial infarction leading to a decrease in drug free fraction (lidocaine, verapamil, propranolol).

Prior drug exposure (increased probability of antimicrobial resistance)

Cardiovascular stability (hemodynamic changes and their effect on renal and liver blood flow, dopamine or norepinephrine infusions and their effects on organ blood flow and drug distribution and/or elimination)

Nutritional status (decrease in serum albumin level and increase in free drug fraction).

Serum drug levels may actually decline in the hypoproteinemic patient owing to the increases in volume of distribution and clearance. Although the total serum drug level (protein bound plus free) may decline, it is not indicative that a therapeutic failure will occur if the level drops below the customary therapeutic window. This is because the free drug fraction (active portion) increases with hypoproteinemia; in the hypoproteinemic patient, it is possible for drug toxicity to occur even when the serum drug concentration appears to be subtherapeutic by laboratory analysis (most laboratories analyze total drug in serum [protein bound plus free]). If possible, free drug levels should be monitored in such situations.

Therapeutic Window (Therapeutic Range)

Therapeutic window is defined as the range of serum concentrations within which a drug elicits a desired clinical response with minimal toxicity.[16] Therapeutic drug ranges are derived from average population outcomes and should be used as guidelines only. A therapeutic range should never be considered in absolute terms. Clinical assessment is a must; some drugs such as phenytoin may be toxic to a patient, even though serum analysis reflects subtherapeutic concentrations, whereas other drugs such as digoxin may

TABLE 146–8

PHARMACOKINETICALLY MONITORED DRUGS IN THE CRITICALLY ILL PATIENT

Drug	Half-Life (h)	Desired Concentration	Sample Collection Times
Antibiotics			
Amikacin	2–3	Peak: 20–35 μg/mL	0.5–1.0 h after the end of the 0.5- to 1.0-h infusion
		Trough: 2–8 μg/mL	0.5 h before the infusion
Gentamicin or tobramycin	2–3	Peak: 4–10 μg/mL	0.5–1.0 h after end of the 0.5- to 1.0-h infusion
		Trough: <2 μg/mL	0.5 h before the infusion
Vancomycin	6–10	Peak: 25–40 μg/mL	1 h after the end of 1-h infusion
		Trough: <10 μg/mL	15 min before next dose
Antiepileptics			
Carbamazepine	12–17	Steady state: 4–12 μg/mL	15 min before next dose
Phenobarbital	75–126	Steady state: 10–30 μg/mL	15 min before next dose
Phenytoin	10–34	Steady state: total—10–20 μg/mL; free—1–2 μg/mL	15 min before next dose
Valproic acid	6–18	Steady state: 50–100 μg/mL	15 min before next dose
Bronchodilator			
Theophylline	8–9	Steady state: 10–20 μg/mL	24–36 h after beginning of constant infusion; if oral dosing regimen, 15 min before next dose
Cardiovascular Agents			
Digoxin	36–48	Steady state: 1–2 ng/mL	15 min before next dose or 8–12 h after dose
Lidocaine	1.5–2	Steady state: 1–5 μg/mL	4–8 h after beginning of constant infusion
Quinidine	6–7	Steady state: 1–4 μg/mL	15 min before next dose after steady state is achieved
Procainamide or N-acetylprocainamide	3–4 / 6–7	Steady state: 4–8 μg/mL Steady state: 10–20 μg/mL	15 min before next dose after steady state is achieved
Immunosuppressant			
Cyclosporine	18–36	Trough: 100–300 ng/mL	15 min before next dose

appear toxic by serum analysis when levels are actually subtherapeutic or absent.

The therapeutic range has not been well defined for most drugs when used in critically ill patients. In this population, the therapeutic window may vary from hour to hour owing to fluid and protein shifts, differing ventilator settings, and various interacting drugs that may be added to the regimen. Table 146–7 lists other factors that may alter the therapeutic range for drugs. Therapeutic decisions should not be based solely on serum concentrations but should incorporate pharmacodynamic outcomes as well.

SPECIFIC DRUGS

Table 146–8 gives general information related to the pharmacokinetics of commonly monitored drugs. Table 146–4 gives guidelines for dosage adjustment in hepatic failure. Table 146–9 lists common intravenous infusion rates. Guidelines for dosage adjustment in patients with varying degrees of renal function can be found in Chapter 111.

Antibiotics

Aminoglycosides

Gentamicin, tobramycin, amikacin, and neomycin are the most frequently used aminoglycosides. With the exception of neomycin, these antibiotics are used to treat serious gram-negative and some gram-positive infections.

Aminoglycosides follow first-order pharmacokinetics, and each has essentially the same pharmacokinetic profile with regard to absorption, distribution, and elimination. These drugs are not well absorbed by the gastrointestinal tract and thus necessitate parenteral administration for systemic activity; neomycin exhibits a great deal of systemic toxicity and is therefore primarily used as an oral antibiotic for gastrointestinal sterilization before gut surgery. Aminoglycosides distribute rapidly into extracellular, synovial, peritoneal, ascitic, and pleural fluids, and they distribute slowly into bile, feces, and prostatic and amnionic fluids. Aminoglycosides distribute poorly into the central nervous system (CNS) and vitreous humor. Their volume of distribution ranges from 0.1 to 0.5 L/kg, depending on the hydration status of the patient;[10] the critically ill patient generally has an increased volume of distribution compared with that of less seriously ill patients.[22-27] These antibiotics are eliminated unchanged by glomerular filtration in the kidney. The elimination half-life can range from 2 to 60 hours, depending on renal function. Clearance is increased in burn and cystic fibrosis patients; as a result, these patients may require a higher dose at more frequent intervals than other types of patients.

Clinical cure of gram-negative bacteremia is best achieved when peak serum concentrations, 1 hour after infusion, are greater than 5 µg/mL for gentamicin or tobramycin and greater than 20 µg/mL for amikacin.[19] Aminoglycoside concentration in pulmonary fluid is approximately 40% of serum concentration; for adequate treatment of pulmonary infections, peak serum concentrations should exceed 8 µg/mL for gentamicin or tobramycin and 25 µg/mL for amikacin.[9]

The aminoglycosides appear to exhibit a postantibiotic effect. As the aminoglycoside concentration falls below what is considered therapeutic, it continues to elicit bactericidal effects. This is probably due to sustained drug concentrations within the bacteria, even though serum concentrations appear subtherapeutic.

Systemic toxicity from the aminoglycosides correlates with

TABLE 146–9

DOSING RATES FOR COMMONLY USED INTRAVENOUS DRUGS

Analgesics	
Morphine	2–10 mg during 2 min.
Antianxiety Agents	
Lorazepam	1–4 mg during 2 min.
Midazolam	1–2.5 mg during 2 min.
Cardiovascular Agents	
Adenosine	6 mg as a rapid bolus q 1–2 s, followed by two 12-mg doses at 2-min intervals if needed.
Amrinone	0.75 mg/kg during 2–3 min, then 5–10 µg/kg/min.
Bretylium	5–10 mg/kg during 2 min. May repeat q 15–30 min up to a total dose of 30 mg. For refractory dysrhythmias, 5–10 mg/kg during 10 min q 2 h.
Dopamine	1–4 µg/kg/min, 5–10 µg/kg/min, 10–20 µg/kg/min for renal, inotropic, and vascular effects, respectively.
Dobutamine	1–20 µg/kg/min.
Hydralazine	10–20 mg q 4–6 h.
Isoproterenol	1–5 µg/min initially, then titrate to effect.
Lidocaine	1–2 mg/kg loading dose, then 1–4 mg/min.
Nitroprusside	0.5–10 µg/kg/min.
Norepinephrine	2–4 µg/min.
Procainamide	100 mg q 5 min up to 1000 mg, then 1–4 mg/min.
Phenytoin	100 mg q 5 min up to 1000 mg, then 300–400 mg/d.
Propranolol	1 mg q 3–5 min up to 10 mg, then 10–20 mg/d.
Verapamil	5–10 mg. May repeat every 30 min to a total of 30 mg.
Gastrointestinal Agents	
Cimetidine	37.5 mg/h (900 mg/d) or 300 mg q 6–8 h.
Ranitidine	6.25 mg/h (150 mg/d) or 50 mg q 6–8 h.
Vasopressin	0.25–0.5 U/min.
Narcotic Antagonists	
Naloxone	0.4–2 mg repeated q 2–3 min.
Neuromuscular Blocking Agents	
Atracurium	Intubating dose of 0.4–0.5 mg/kg, with repeated doses of 0.08–0.1 mg/kg q 25–45 min.
Pancuronium	Intubating dose of 0.07–0.1 mg/kg, with repeated doses if desired.
Vecuronium	0.08–0.1 mg/kg initially, with repeated doses of 0.01–0.015 mg/kg q 25–40 min.

serum concentrations. An increased incidence of reversible renal dysfunction occurs when trough serum concentrations exceed 2 µg/mL for gentamicin or tobramycin or 10 µg/mL for amikacin. Factors that may contribute to aminoglycoside-induced renal toxicity include increasing age, total daily dose, cumulative dose, concurrent use of nephrotoxic drugs (amphotericin B, cisplatin, and contrast media), duration of therapy, prior aminoglycoside exposure, pre-existing renal dysfunction, hypovolemia, and gram-negative sepsis.[9]

Ototoxicity has occurred when trough serum gentamicin concentrations exceeded 4 µg/mL for 10 days.[10] Factors that may contribute to aminoglycoside-induced ototoxicity are similar to those that contribute to renal toxicity. Concurrent administration of ototoxic drugs (furosemide) and dialysis may contribute to ototoxicity.

Serum peak concentration samples should be drawn 1 hour after infusion to ensure that the drug is in its postdistributive phase. If the sample is drawn before the postdistributive phase, the peak represents a clinically false value. The trough serum concentration sample should be drawn immediately before a subsequent dose. Depending on the values obtained, the dosage regimen may or may not require altering.

Pharmacokinetic computer programs use logarithmic equations to predict the dose and dosing interval required to maximize therapeutic outcome and minimize toxicity. These are fairly accurate and should be utilized. Hand-held computers can be used for quick pharmacokinetic analysis. Initial estimates of loading dose and maintenance regimens have been suggested and are based on estimates of creatinine clearance.[28–30] Critically ill patients possess significantly different dosing variables.

Cephalosporins

Parenteral cephalosporins are generally not well absorbed compared with oral cephalosporins. Exceptions include cefuroxime and cephradine, which can be taken via both routes. The major route of elimination and half-life for commonly used cephalosporins can be found in Table 146–10. With the exception of cefotaxime and cephalothin, cephalosporins are not extensively metabolized. Cephalosporins have a large volume of distribution, and their degree of protein binding ranges from 17 to 90%.

First- and second-generation cephalosporins (see Table 146–10) do not penetrate well into the CNS. Consequently, these generations have limited use for treating CNS infections. Third-generation cephalosporins penetrate well into the CNS and are considered the antibiotics of choice for CNS infections with pathogens sensitive to them.

Glycoproteins

Vancomycin, teicoplanin, and daptomycin are glycoprotein antibiotics that routinely undergo pharmacokinetic monitoring. These drugs exhibit low systemic bioavailability when administered orally and elicit severe pain at the injection site when administered intramuscularly.[31] Therefore, the glycoprotein antibiotics are generally administered intravenously when systemic activity is desired.

TABLE 146–10

CEPHALOSPORINS AND ELIMINATION CHARACTERISTICS

Cephalosporin	Half-Life (h)	Primary Route of Elimination	Central Nervous System Penetration
First generation			
Cefazolin	1.4–2.2	Renal	Poor
Cephalexin	0.8	Renal	Poor
Cephalothin	0.5	Renal/metabolism	Poor
Cephradine	0.8	Renal	Poor
Cefadroxil	1.5	Renal	Poor
Second generation			
Cefaclor	0.7	Renal/biliary	Poor
Cefamandole	0.9–1.5	Renal	Poor
Cefotetan	2.8–4.6	Renal/biliary	Poor
Cefoxitin	0.7	Renal	Poor
Cefuroxime	1.0–2.0	Renal	Poor
Third generation			
Ceftriaxone	5.4–10.9	Renal/biliary	Good
Cefotaxime	0.8–1.4	Renal/metabolism	Moderate*
Cefoperazone	1.6–2.6	Biliary	Moderate*
Ceftazidime	1.4–2.0	Renal	Good
Ceftizoxime	1.4–1.9	Renal	Moderate*

*CNS penetration improves with inflamed meninges.

Vancomycin distributes into various compartments and has a volume of distribution that ranges between 0.5 and 1 L/kg, approximating that of total body water.[10] Plasma protein binding is approximately 55%. Vancomycin is excreted unchanged via glomerular filtration. Its elimination half-life ranges between 6 and 10 hours with normal renal function but may increase to as long as 7 days in the renally impaired patient.

Vancomycin elicits bactericidal effects when peak serum concentrations are between 30 and 50 μg/mL. Because vancomycin distributes into various compartments, it is important that peak serum concentration samples be drawn in the postdistributive phase, 1 to 3 hours after its 1-hour infusion. This should minimize inaccurate interpretation of the serum concentration while the drug is in its distributive phase. Vancomycin has been associated with renal toxicity when trough serum concentrations exceed 10 μg/mL, especially when used in combination with other nephrotoxic drugs.[13, 31] Ototoxicity has occurred with sustained elevated serum concentrations. Most clinicians administer vancomycin so that peak concentrations fall between 30 and 40 μg/mL and trough concentrations fall below 10 μg/mL.

Teicoplanin is a newer glycopeptide antibiotic that has a large volume of distribution, is 90% bound to plasma proteins, and has an elimination half-life of 40 to 162 hours.[32] This drug is generally administered once daily, and dosage adjustments are necessary in patients with renal dysfunction. Therapeutic serum concentrations are not yet established. Teicoplanin can be administered intramuscularly or intravenously.

Daptomycin represents a new class of compounds known as peptolides.[33] This antibiotic can be given intravenously, is 80% bound to serum proteins, and has a half-life of approximately 6 to 9 hours.[32] Dosage adjustment is required in renal failure.

Penicillins

Gastrointestinal absorption of the various penicillins and penicillin salts depends on their relative susceptibility to acid hydrolysis in the stomach. Penicillin V, ampicillin, cloxacillin, dicloxacillin, and oxacillin are acid stable and are well absorbed. Other penicillins such as penicillin G, timentin, and piperacillin are not well absorbed in the gastrointestinal tract and must be given parenterally. In general, penicillin antibiotics have a large volume of distribution and minimal protein binding. However, cloxacillin, dicloxacillin, and oxacillin are greater than 90% bound to plasma proteins. Distribution into the CNS depends on the specific penicillin and the degree of meningeal inflammation. With inflamed meninges, penicillin G, ampicillin, carbenicillin, and ticarcillin distribute into the CNS at a concentration approximately 25 to 30% that of serum concentration.

Penicillins are primarily eliminated via glomerular filtration and renal tubular secretion; however, cloxacillin, dicloxacillin, and nafcillin undergo some hepatic metabolism. Most penicillins have an average elimination half-life of less than 1 hour; probenecid can be used to block the tubular secretion of penicillins, resulting in a longer penicillin half-life. Dosage may require downward adjustment in patients with renal impairment to prevent drug accumulation and adverse CNS effects such as seizures.

Quinolones

Nalidixic acid was the first quinolone antibiotic. Since its inception, microorganisms have grown extremely resistant. However, norfloxacin, enoxacin, and ciprofloxacin are newly developed fluoroquinolones that have extended antibacterial activity. Fluoroquinolone antibiotics are well absorbed by the gastrointestinal tract and, as a result, are frequently used orally to treat serious systemic infections such as osteomyelitis. These drugs distribute well into most body fluids. Fluoroquinolones are eliminated via hepatic and renal mechanisms and have an average elimination half-life of 4 hours. Significant drug-drug interactions may occur between fluoroquinolones and other drugs that are metabolized by the liver such as theophylline, propranolol, and metoprolol; extreme caution and close monitoring should be used with these combinations.

Antiepileptics
Phenytoin

Phenytoin is a frequently monitored anticonvulsant that is available in parenteral, capsule, chewable tablet, and suspension dosage forms. The capsules and parenteral solution consist of phenytoin sodium, which is 92% phenytoin, whereas the chewable tablet and suspension contain 100% phenytoin acid.[34] The amount of phenytoin in each of these dosage forms must be recalled and incorporated into dosing calculations when switching a patient from one form to another.

The bioavailable fraction for most oral and parenteral phenytoin preparations approaches 1.[35] However, this fraction may significantly decrease when there is an increase in gastrointestinal transit time, as is seen with catharsis or when the patient is receiving enteral nutrition.

Phenytoin is metabolized by the liver and follows Michaelis-Menton pharmacokinetics. Less than 5% of the drug is excreted unchanged in the urine. After an intravenous dose, phenytoin distributes rapidly into tissues, achieving equilibrium within 60 minutes. At equilibrium, phenytoin appears to possess a volume of distribution equal to that of total body water (0.5 to 1.0 L/kg).

Phenytoin is 90% bound to plasma proteins (primarily albumin) and tissues. Therefore, the active portion of phenytoin is approximately 10% of the total drug present. This should be kept in mind when patients have conditions that alter the binding of phenytoin to plasma proteins (see later).

The therapeutic concentration for phenytoin is generally quoted to range between 10 and 20 μg/mL.[34] However, some patients may have therapeutic serum concentrations ranging from 5 to 10 μg/mL. (For a discussion of phenytoin concentration as it correlates with toxicity, see later.) In the critically ill patient, the generally accepted therapeutic range may be inaccurate owing to factors that alter the binding of phenytoin to plasma proteins. Disease states that are associated with a decreased serum albumin concentration (burns, hepatic cirrhosis, pregnancy, cystic fibrosis, and nephrotic syndrome) or that decrease the affinity of albumin for phenytoin (renal failure, severe jaundice, and drug interactions) can potentially lead to an increase in the free phenytoin fraction. In these situations, both therapeutic and toxic effects may occur at lower than expected total phenytoin serum concentrations. Monitoring the free phenytoin concentration is recommended in clinical situations that are expected to alter the serum protein–binding properties of phenytoin. It is accepted that the therapeutic window for free phenytoin ranges between 1 and 2 μg/mL (10% of the therapeutic window for total phenytoin concentration in the normal individual). However, little information exists that adequately correlates free drug concentrations with effect.

Factors that may alter the clearance of phenytoin include changes in plasma protein binding and hepatic enzyme induction or inhibition. A decrease in plasma protein binding results in a larger fraction of free phenytoin available for

TABLE 146–11

DRUGS THAT ALTER HEPATIC METABOLISM OF PHENYTOIN

Drug	Effect on Metabolism	Effect on Serum Level	Mechanism
Barbiturates	Increase	Decrease	Enzyme induction
Chloramphenicol	Decrease	Increase	Inhibition
Disulfiram	Decrease	Increase	Inhibition
Ethanol	Increase	Decrease	Enzyme induction
Folic acid	Increase	Decrease	Enzyme induction
Isoniazid	Decrease	Increase	Inhibition
Phenylbutazone	Decrease	Increase	Competition
Rifampin	Increase	Decrease	Enzyme induction
Trimethoprim	Increase	Decrease	Enzyme induction

Adapted by permission from Drug Interactions & Updates, edited by Philip D. Hansten and John R. Horn, published by Applied Therapeutics, Inc., Vancouver, WA, © 1991.

enzymatic degradation, whereas increases in plasma protein binding result in the opposite effect. Drugs that cause autoinduction of hepatic enzymes increase phenytoin clearance, whereas drugs that inhibit hepatic enzymes cause phenytoin clearance to decline[14] (Table 146–11).

The rate of clearance for phenytoin depends on the serum concentration. As serum concentration increases, enzymes responsible for phenytoin metabolism become saturated, thus causing the rate of clearance from the body to decrease. Saturated enzymes can metabolize only a set amount of phenytoin. Any amount presented for metabolism that is in excess of metabolic capacity is not metabolized. This metabolic phenomenon renders the pharmacokinetic concept of half-life unusable for predictions of phenytoin clearance.

Estimates of phenytoin clearance are best performed by calculating the velocity (V) or rate at which an enzyme system can metabolize a drug. The velocity can be calculated by using the pharmacokinetic measures of V_{max} (maximal rate of phenytoin metabolism by the enzyme system) and K_m (the plasma phenytoin concentration at which the rate of metabolism is one half the maximum).[34] This is best illustrated by the following equation:

$$V = \frac{(V_{max})\,(\text{phenytoin concentration at steady state})}{K_m + \text{phenytoin concentration at steady state}}$$

This equation can be rearranged to the following:

$$\text{Phenytoin concentration at steady state} = \frac{(K_m)\,(V)}{V_{max} - V}$$

Clinical use of this equation for predicting daily dose of phenytoin required to achieve a desired serum concentration can be performed as follows:

1. Substitute the daily dose of phenytoin for V, taking into account the amount of phenytoin available from the dosage form used (see earlier).

$$\text{Phenytoin dose/d} = \frac{(V_{max})\,(\text{phenytoin concentration at steady state})}{K_m + \text{phenytoin concentration at steady state}}$$

2. Use the population estimates for V_{max} and K_m.[10, 34]

$$V_{max} = 7\ \text{mg/kg/d}$$
$$K_m = 4\ \text{mg/L}$$

3. Decide on the desired serum phenytoin concentration and insert the value into the equation. For example, to achieve a desired serum phenytoin concentration of 10 to 20 μg/mL in the average 70-kg adult:

$$\text{Phenytoin dose/d} = \frac{(V_{max})\ (\text{phenytoin concentration at steady state})}{K_m + \text{phenytoin concentration at steady state}}$$

$$= \frac{(7\ \text{mg/kg/d} \times 70\ \text{kg})\ (10\ \mu\text{g/mL})}{(4\ \text{mg/L} + 10\ \mu\text{g/mL})}$$

$$= 350\ \text{mg/d}$$

Repeat this process for a serum concentration of 20 μg/mL:

$$\text{Phenytoin dose/d} = 408\ \text{mg/d}$$

Use a dosage regimen that consists of a daily phenytoin dose between 350 and 408 mg (e.g., 400 mg of phenytoin sodium once daily or 200 mg of phenytoin sodium twice daily for a total of 368 mg of phenytoin per day, 400 mg times 0.92 [percentage of pure phenytoin in phenytoin sodium]).

The above-described methods for predicting serum concentration data in the critically ill should be used as a guideline only. Phenytoin dosing in the critically ill patient should be approached with caution, as these patients generally have concurrent pathophysiologic factors that alter the accuracy of prediction as compared with that for the normal individual. Hepatic cirrhosis decreases V_{max}, whereas hepatic enzyme induction increases V_{max}. Drugs that inhibit hepatic enzyme function can increase K_m, whereas hypoproteinemia decreases K_m. Because of these multiple factors affecting drug metabolism, few patients achieve a true steady-state serum phenytoin concentration during their stay in the critical care unit. Phenytoin dosing requirements should be re-evaluated after the patient is discharged from the critical care unit to prevent potential toxicity (see phenytoin in the section on drug poisoning later in this chapter).

Phenobarbital

Phenobarbital is available in tablet, oral solution, and parenteral dosage forms. The oral bioavailability of phenobarbital approaches 100%.[36] Phenobarbital possesses a volume of distribution of approximately 0.7 L/kg. This drug distributes rapidly into well-perfused organs, except the brain, where it penetrates slowly. Phenobarbital is 60% bound to serum proteins (mainly albumin) and has an elimination half-life ranging from 75 to 126 hours in adults. Phenobarbital is eliminated primarily by hepatic metabolism. Approximately 20% is excreted unchanged in the urine. Renal clearance of phenobarbital can be increased by increasing urine flow or by alkalizing the urine.

The therapeutic serum concentration for phenobarbital ranges from 10 to 40 μg/mL. Increased CNS depression and ataxia are associated with a serum concentration that approaches the upper end of the therapeutic window. Levels exceeding 100 μg/mL are potentially lethal.[10]

Phenobarbital stimulates autoinduction of cytochrome P-450 mixed-function oxidase enzyme and therefore enhances the clearance of drugs metabolized by this enzyme.

Valproic Acid

Valproic acid is rapidly and completely absorbed after oral administration.[36] It is 90% bound to plasma proteins (primarily albumin). Protein binding of valproic acid is a saturable process, therefore resulting in fluctuations in the fraction that is bound to plasma proteins; this occurs within the therapeutic range. The apparent volume of distribution of valproic acid ranges from 0.1 to 0.5 L/kg. Approximately 95% of valproic acid is eliminated by hepatic metabolism; 5% is excreted unchanged in the urine. The elimination half-life of valproic acid ranges from 4 to 8 hours.

The therapeutic serum concentration for valproic acid ranges between 50 and 100 μg/mL. Levels exceeding 100 μg/mL are not necessarily associated with increased toxicity, but dose-dependent side effects such as nausea, vomiting, diarrhea, and cramps limit the use of large doses.

Bronchodilators

Theophylline

Theophylline is a methylxanthine generally used for treating bronchoconstrictive airways disease. This drug is available in various oral preparations and as an intravenous solution; aminophylline is a theophylline ethylenediamine product that contains approximately 80% theophylline. Gastrointestinal absorption of theophylline is rapid and complete. The rate of gastrointestinal absorption can be accelerated when theophylline is taken with a meal that is high in fat content; consequently, this can result in a dose dumping and acute transient toxicity when some sustained-release products are taken with fat.[37] Theophylline distributes into fat-free body mass and body water at a volume of distribution of 0.45 L/kg. It is 40% bound to plasma proteins (albumin) and exhibits pH- and temperature-dependent binding; a decrease in serum pH or an increase in body temperature or both increase the free fraction of theophylline. Alteration in plasma protein binding has been reported in mechanically ventilated patients.

Theophylline has a therapeutic window that ranges from 10 to 20 μg/mL. Within the therapeutic range, theophylline exhibits first-order (linear) pharmacokinetics. However, when concentrations exceed the therapeutic maximum, theophylline may elicit zero-order (Michaelis-Menton) pharmacokinetics; in the child, zero-order pharmacokinetics may occur within the therapeutic range. Severe toxicity is associated with theophylline concentrations that exceed the therapeutic range. Nausea, vomiting, diarrhea, headache, cardiac dysrhythmias, and seizures are among the most severe symptoms of toxicity (for a complete discussion of serum concentrations as they correlate with toxicity, see later).

Theophylline is metabolized (cleared) in the liver via cytochrome P-450 enzyme.[38-40] Drugs that can significantly decrease theophylline clearance include allopurinol, cimetidine, erythromycin, oral contraceptives, propranolol, troleandomycin, ciprofloxacin, and enoxacin. Drugs that increase theophylline clearance include rifampin, phenytoin, phenobarbital, isoproterenol, carbamazepine, and tobacco. If a patient is started on a theophylline regimen while regularly indulging in tobacco use, the clearance is rapid. After approximately 6 months of no tobacco use, theophylline clearance declines. This is an important consideration in a patient who decides to quit smoking while being treated with theophylline. Theophylline dosage may require downward adjustment to prevent chronic toxicity.

Making adjustments for attaining theophylline concentrations in the therapeutic range requires a proportional dose change. For every 1 mg/kg change in dose, there is generally a 2 μg/mL change in serum concentration. To convert from intravenous to oral administration, a zero-order sustained-release tablet is the best product to use. The total daily oral dose is the same as the total daily intravenous dose; the total daily oral dose should be divided into two or three doses given every 8 to 12 hours. The intravenous theophylline should be discontinued after conversion.

Sympathomimetics

Epinephrine is a nonselective sympathomimetic agent that can be used to improve airflow by decreasing airway edema through vasoconstriction of arterioles and by inducing bronchodilation.[38, 39] Epinephrine has a short duration of action of 20 minutes. Both the gastrointestinal mucosa and the liver rapidly metabolize epinephrine via conjugation and oxidation reactions; therefore, epinephrine is not effective when given orally. Concentrated solutions that are nebulized and inhaled have both local actions in the lung and systemic actions attributable to good absorption via the pulmonary route; epinephrine is systemically effective when given via endotracheal tube in cardiac arrest. Systemic and pulmonary pharmacologic effects decrease rapidly through metabolism by intracellular and circulating monoamine oxidase (MAO) and catechol O-methyl transferase (COMT) enzymes. Only small amounts of epinephrine appear in the urine. Dosing adjustments are based on pharmacologic effect.

Ephedrine is the oldest of the nonspecific beta-sympathomimetic bronchodilators and is found in many over-the-counter preparations. Unlike epinephrine, it is effective when taken orally. Ephedrine has a slower onset of action than epinephrine, but its pharmacologic effects persist for several hours.

Isoproterenol is another nonspecific beta-adrenergic agonist that can be given parenterally or as an aerosol when bronchodilation is required. Isoproterenol has also been used intravenously for treatment of various cardiovascular conditions such as third-degree heart block and asystole; these uses are controversial at this time owing to the adverse effect profile of the drug. It is metabolized primarily in the liver by COMT. Isoproterenol is a relatively poor substrate for MAO and is not taken up by sympathetic neurons to the same extent as epinephrine and norepinephrine.

Isoetharine is a short-acting beta$_2$-selective catecholamine. Although it is resistant to metabolism by MAO, it is a catecholamine and therefore is a good substrate for COMT metabolism. It is used only by inhalation for the treatment of acute episodes of bronchoconstriction.

Metaproterenol is an analogue of isoproterenol with beta$_2$-specificity that exerts a moderately long duration of action. The therapeutic action may last up to 4 hours. Metaproterenol can be administered either orally or by inhalation. It is resistant to methylation by COMT. A substantial fraction (40%) is absorbed in active form after oral administration. After metabolism in the liver, metaproterenol is eliminated in the urine.

Terbutaline and albuterol have a slightly greater selectivity for beta$_2$-adrenergic receptors. Therapeutic effect lasts from 4 to 8 hours. Terbutaline is effective when taken orally, by inhalation, or intravenously. Albuterol can be administered either by inhalation or orally for the symptomatic relief of bronchoconstriction.

Cardiovascular Drugs

The critically ill patient often requires treatment with drugs possessing positive inotropic effects to help maintain adequate tissue perfusion. Natural and synthetic catecholamines are generally used in the critical care unit for this purpose. The pharmacologic action of these drugs depends on the degree of receptor stimulation produced at the specific adrenergic receptor site (Table 146–12). The underlying cardiovascular disorder may necessitate the use of more than one inotropic agent with different receptor sensitivities to achieve therapeutic efficacy; combination therapy may also help to minimize potential adverse effects that occur when a single agent is increased to its maximal dose.

Receptors are susceptible to up-regulation (externalization) or down-regulation (internalization). Prolonged therapy with agents that stimulate adrenergic receptors may result in physiologic down-regulation of the number or density of the receptors. This theoretically results in decreased effectiveness of the agent that stimulates the receptors. Conversely, prolonged use of adrenergic receptor blockers may result in up-regulation, leading to an increased number or density of adrenergic receptors. This theoretically results in an increased pharmacologic effect for agents that stimulate the receptors; rebound hypertension after abrupt clonidine or beta-blocker withdrawal is thought to result from this type of phenomenon. These phenomena in critically ill patients have received relatively little attention yet could potentially have major effects on therapeutic considerations.

Pressor Agents

Epinephrine is an important endogenous catecholamine that stimulates both alpha- and beta-adrenergic receptors.[40] Pharmacologic effects of epinephrine are dose dependent.

TABLE 146–12

RELATIVE ADRENERGIC RECEPTOR SELECTIVITY AND PHARMACOLOGIC EFFECTS OF INTRAVENOUS CATECHOLAMINES

Drug	Relative Receptor Selectivity*			
	Beta$_1$-Inotropic	Chronotropic	Beta$_2$-Vasodilation	Alpha-Vasoconstriction
Dopamine†	+ + +	+ +	+ +	0 (up to + + + with higher rates)
Dobutamine‡	+ + +	+	+	+
Epinephrine	+ + +	+ + +	+ + +	+ + +
Isoproterenol	+ + +	+ + +	+ + +	0
Norepinephrine	+ +	+	0	+ + +

Drug	Dose§	Relative Hemodyamic Effects*				
		HR	MAP	PCWP	CO	SVR
Dopamine	10.0–20.0 μg/kg/min	+ + +	+ + +	+ +	+ + +	+ + +
Dobutamine	10.0–20.0 μg/kg/min	+	+	−	+ + +	0
Epinephrine	0.02–0.2 μg/kg/min	+ +	0	+	+ +	−
Isoproterenol	0.02–0.2 μg/kg/min	+ +	−/+	−	+	−
Norepinephrine	2.0–16.0 μg/min	+	+ + +	+	−/+	+ + +

*HR = heart rate; MAP = mean arterial pressure; PCWP = pulmonary capillary wedge pressure; CO = cardiac output; SVR = systemic vascular resistance; +, + +, + + + = degree of increase; − = decrease; 0 = no change; −/+ = variable.

†Dopamine has dose-dependent effects; at low doses (0.5–3.0 μg/kg/min), the dopaminergic effects predominate and there is vasodilation of the renal and mesenteric vessels. At intermediate doses (3.0–10.0 μg/kg/min), the beta$_1$-adrenergic effects predominate. At higher doses (>10.0 μg/kg/min), the alpha-adrenergic effects predominate. The results in this chart are given for the 10 μg/kg/min rate.

‡Dobutamine is a racemic mixture. This table lists the net effect of this mixture at a rate of 10 μg/kg/min.

§The usual adult dosing ranges are compared.

Low doses predominantly stimulate the beta-adrenergic receptors, whereas high doses elicit greater alpha-receptor stimulation. Beta-receptor stimulation results in widening of the pulse pressure, decreased systemic and pulmonary vascular resistance, and increases in cardiac contractility, output, conduction, and rate. Alpha-receptor stimulation results in increased systemic vascular resistance and increased blood pressure. Hemodynamic effects may also depend on the fluid status of the patient. Other direct and indirect pharmacologic effects of epinephrine include glycogenolysis, lactate production, increases in β-hydroxybutyrate and free fatty acids, hypokalemia, and hypophosphatemia. Epinephrine is cleared from the serum via neuronal reuptake mechanisms and via metabolism by COMT and MAO. Figure 146–1 shows the degradative pathways of catecholamines such as epinephrine. Epinephrine has a half-life of elimination of approximately 2 to 3 minutes.

Norepinephrine is a precursor of epinephrine that stimulates alpha$_1$-, alpha$_2$-, and beta$_1$-adrenergic receptors.[40] Low doses produce mainly beta$_1$-adrenergic effects, whereas high doses produce alpha-adrenergic effects. Norepinephrine has a half-life of elimination of approximately 2 to 3 minutes.

Dopamine is the immediate precursor of norepinephrine.[40] Hemodynamic effects attributed to dopamine are dose dependent and are the direct result of adrenergic receptor stimulation or the indirect result of norepinephrine release from neurons. Dopamine receptors are stimulated at low doses (<4 μg/kg/min), resulting in renal, mesenteric, coronary, and cerebral arterial vasodilation. Intermediate doses (5 to 10 μg/kg/min) result in greater beta-receptor stimulation, and high doses (greater than 10 μg/kg/min) result in alpha-receptor stimulation. Therefore, cardiovascular effects depend on the dose of dopamine and the specific receptors that are stimulated. Cardiovascular effects may include changes in heart rate, mean arterial pressure, cardiac output, pulmonary capillary wedge pressure, central venous pressure, and systemic vascular resistance. Low-dose dopamine has been used in combination with norepinephrine to reverse or combat the renal vasoconstriction seen with norepinephrine. Dopamine is metabolized in the liver by COMT and MAO. Its half-life of elimination is approximately 2 to 3 minutes.

Dobutamine is an enantiomer consisting of a 50:50 racemic mixture of the (−) and (+) stereoisomers.[40] Each stereoisomer elicits a different pharmacologic effect on the adrenergic receptors. The (−) isomer stimulates the alpha$_1$-receptor, whereas the (+) isomer competitively blocks it. In addition, the (+) isomer stimulates the beta-adrenergic receptors. Therefore, the ultimate hemodynamic effect that occurs during dobutamine administration is consistent with beta$_1$-receptor stimulation. Dobutamine generally increases cardiac output and lowers pulmonary capillary wedge pressure. Dobutamine is metabolized by COMT, MAO, and conjugation in the liver and other tissues. The half-life of elimination of dobutamine is approximately 2 to 3 minutes.

Isoproterenol is a synthetic catecholamine similar in structure to epinephrine. It is a potent nonspecific beta-adrenergic receptor agonist. Its pharmacologic actions are similar to those seen when dobutamine is used in combination with nitroglycerin. Isoproterenol is eliminated in a similar fashion to other catecholamines.

Digoxin

Digoxin, a cardiac glycoside, is available as a conventional tablet, injectable solution, and soft gelatin capsule.[41] The bioavailability of oral digoxin ranges from 70 to 80% with tablets to greater than 90% with the gelatin capsule; the digoxin content of the gelatin capsule is 20% less than that in the conventional tablet, thus compensating for the difference in bioavailability between dosage forms. Digoxin is 20 to 30% bound to albumin. Digoxin distributes widely into tissues and possesses a volume of distribution of approximately 7.3 L/kg. After distribution, digoxin concentration is greatest in the heart, the kidneys, the intestines, the stomach, the liver, and the skeletal muscle and least in the plasma, the brain, and fat. Digoxin is usually distributed 6 hours after a dose. Serum digoxin concentration does not accurately reflect pharmacologic effect until distribution is complete; therefore, the serum concentration sample should be drawn at least 6 hours after dose.

The serum digoxin concentration correlates with its inotropic effects, but less so with its atrioventricular nodal blocking effects. The therapeutic range for treating congestive heart failure is between 0.8 and 2.0 ng/mL. Therapeutic concentrations that approach 3 ng/mL may be required when digoxin is used to control the ventricular response to atrial fibrillation; however, the incidence of toxicity may increase.

When analyzing the serum digoxin concentration, the clinician must be aware that a digoxin-like immunoreactive substance is released into the serum of pregnant patients, neonates, and patients with renal and/or liver failure. Certain assays falsely report this substance as digoxin. Inappropriate adjustments in dosing may be ordered if the clinician is unfamiliar with the specific assay used. Consult the specific laboratory to see if its assay reports this substance as a positive digoxin concentration.

Hypokalemia enhances digoxin binding in myocardial and skeletal muscle tissues and may cause an apparent digoxin toxicity, even when the serum digoxin concentration appears to be within the therapeutic range. Digoxin toxicity may occur in the malnourished patient owing to lack of sufficient muscle mass for digoxin binding, thus causing greater binding in other tissues such as the heart. Hypomagnesemia, hypercalcemia, and hypothyroidism may also potentiate digoxin toxicity. Downward adjustments in dosing may be required with these various conditions. (For further discussion of digoxin toxicity and treatment, see later.)

The elimination half-life of digoxin is approximately 36 hours in the average adult. Approximately 75% of digoxin is excreted unchanged in the urine, whereas 25% is metabolized in the intestinal wall and the liver. Enteric bacteria are responsible for digoxin metabolism in the intestinal wall. The inactive metabolites produced from enteral metabolism account for about 12% of digoxin clearance in the average patient. However, a subgroup of individuals metabolize 30 to 40% of digoxin by this mechanism; this difference is probably due to variations in the make-up of intestinal flora. Erythromycin and tetracycline antibiotics can alter intestinal flora, thus reducing the amount of digoxin metabolized via this mechanism; this can result in increased digoxin bioavailability and higher serum concentrations. The liver metabolizes digoxin to a small extent and plays little role in clearance.

Both the volume of distribution and the clearance of digoxin are decreased in patients with chronic renal dysfunction. Elimination half-life may approach 5 days in these patients, thus necessitating downward dosage adjustment.

Concomitant administration of quinidine or verapamil can decrease digoxin clearance by more than 50%. Serum digoxin concentrations may increase more than twofold after several days of combined therapy. If these drugs are used in combination with digoxin, doses should be initiated at 50% of normal. The serum digoxin concentration should be reassessed 5 days after quinidine or verapamil has been added to the regimen.

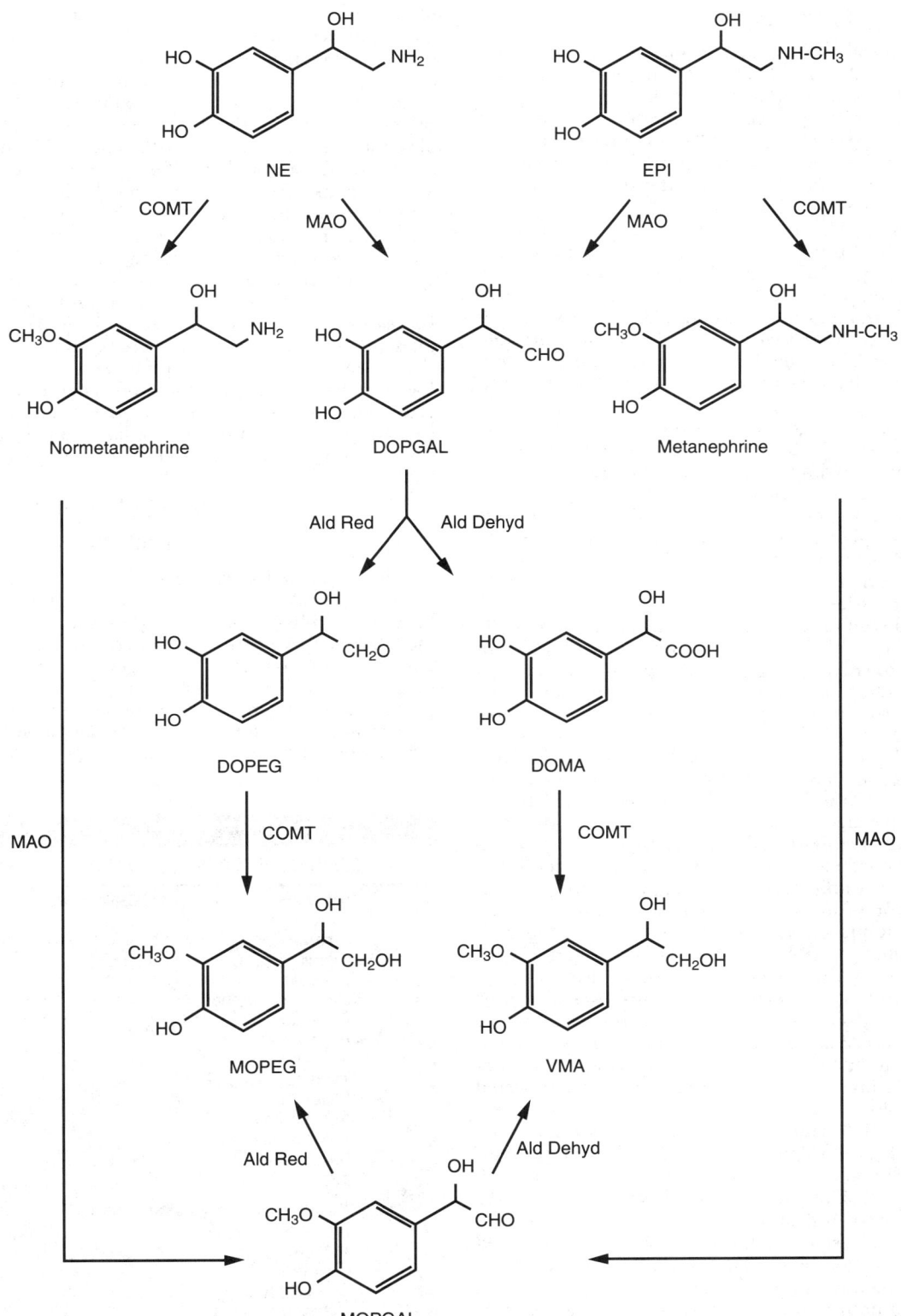

Figure 146–1. Degradative pathways of catecholamine. Both epinephrine (EPI) and norepinephrine (NE) can have a methyl group attached to the -OH in the 3 position with the enzyme COMT producing metanephrine and normetanephrine, respectively. When oxidized by MAO, these become converted to 3-methoxy-4-hydroxyphenylglycoaldehyde (MOPGAL). Aldehyde reductase (Ald Red) then produces 3-methoxy-4-hydroxyphenylethyleneglycol (MOPEG) or aldehyde dehydrogenase (Ald Dehyd) produces vanillylmandelic acid (VMA). The same enzymes may act in a different sequence to produce the same products. Both epinephrine and norepinephrine can be oxidized by MAO to form 3,4-dihydroxyphenylglycolaldehyde (DOPGAL). Aldehyde reductase and aldehyde dehydrogenase then act to form 3,4-dihydroxyphenylethyleneglycol (DOPEG) and 3,4-dihydroxymandelic acid (DOMA), respectively. Addition of the methyl group to the 3 -OH position by COMT then produces MOPEG (from DOPEG) and VMA (from DOMA).

Antiarrhythmics

Lidocaine is a common antiarrhythmic used in the critical care unit. The oral bioavailability of lidocaine is poor. Lidocaine distributes into lung, heart, kidney, muscle, and adipose tissues.[42] Fifty per cent of lidocaine is bound to serum α_1-acid glycoprotein, and 20% is bound to albumin. Conditions that alter serum α_1-acid glycoprotein concentration (e.g., trauma, surgery) may alter the free fraction and pharmacologic potency of lidocaine.

Lidocaine has an elimination half-life of 1.5 to 2 hours and is metabolized primarily by the liver to monoethylglycinexylidine and glycinexylidide. The monoethylglycinexylidine metabolite appears to have activity similar to that of lidocaine and is thought to be responsible for acute seizures that have occurred after several days of lidocaine infusion. Congestive heart failure or liver disease can decrease lidocaine clearance, thus necessitating downward dosage adjustments.

The therapeutic range for lidocaine is 1 to 5 μg/ml. Lidocaine must be given by the intravenous route to achieve predictable antiarrhythmic effects. A bolus dose of 1 to 2 mg/kg is required to obtain an immediate response. An infusion of 1 to 4 mg/min should be started at the same time the bolus dose is given. Breakthrough arrhythmias, necessitating a second bolus dose, may occur 10 to 15 minutes into the infusion period; lidocaine rapidly distributes out of serum and into tissues early in therapy.

Procainamide can be administered orally, intramuscularly, and intravenously.[10, 43] The oral bioavailability of procainamide is approximately 85%.[43] Gastrointestinal absorption may be slow and incomplete in patients with congestive heart failure. Oral procainamide preparations contain 87% procainamide base.

Procainamide has a volume of distribution of 2 L/kg. Low cardiac output may decrease the volume of distribution of procainamide by 25%. Procainamide is metabolized by the liver to the active metabolite N-acetylprocainamide (NAPA); NAPA may enhance both efficacy and toxicity of procainamide. Acetylator phenotype differs among patients but remains constant within each individual. Consequently, empirical prediction of metabolizing capability cannot be made with accuracy. Rapid acetylators convert approximately 30% of procainamide to NAPA. Slow acetylators convert 15% of procainamide to NAPA. NAPA has a renal clearance rate that is 1.6 times that of creatinine clearance. Renal or liver dysfunction may result in accumulation of procainamide or NAPA, thus necessitating therapeutic monitoring and dosage adjustment in the critical care unit patient. Procainamide is also cleared via renal excretion and nonacetylated hepatic metabolism.

The therapeutic serum concentration for procainamide ranges from 4 to 8 μg/mL. Some patients with resistant ventricular arrhythmias may require levels approaching 20 μg/mL. Toxicity is likely to occur at levels greater than 12 μg/mL. The therapeutic and toxic serum concentrations of NAPA are not well established. It is generally recommended that NAPA levels not exceed 30 μg/mL. The oral or intramuscular loading dose for procainamide is 50 mg/kg divided into an every-3-hour regimen, not to exceed a loading dose of 1000 mg. The loading dose can be given via intravenous infusion at a rate not exceeding 50 mg/min. Sustained-release products or an intravenous drip may then be used to supply the patient with approximately 50 mg/kg/d in divided doses.

Immunosuppressive Agents: Cyclosporine

Cyclosporine is an immunosuppressive agent available as an oral and a parenteral solution. This drug is only 20 to 50% absorbed after oral or intramuscular administration.[44] Cyclosporine is lipophilic and requires bile for gastrointestinal absorption to occur. Factors that alter bile flow can alter the absorption of cyclosporine in the gut. It is highly tissue bound. In plasma, approximately 98% is bound to plasma protein, mostly lipoproteins. It is extensively metabolized in the liver via the cytochrome P-450 enzyme system. Liver dysfunction and interfering drugs that are concomitantly metabolized by cytochrome P-450 enzyme may decrease the clearance of cyclosporine. The pronounced differences in pharmacokinetic variables, such as bioavailability and clearance, result in marked variations in blood cyclosporine concentrations. Cyclosporine is distributed 50% into erythrocytes, 10% into leukocytes, and 40% into plasma. Increases in leukocyte number (infections) can lead to an increase in cyclosporine-leukocyte binding.

Cyclosporine-induced renal failure occurs during the first few months of therapy. In addition, nephrotoxic antibiotics are frequently used to prevent infections in cyclosporine-treated patients. Dosing of cyclosporine is generally decreased by 50% when amphotericin B is given concomitantly.

FUTURE RESEARCH

Polymorphism

Pharmacogenetics deals with genetic variations in drug disposition and effect. Genetic polymorphic drug metabolism (Table 146–13) is drawing attention.[45–47] Genetic polymorphism exists when an inherited trait is maintained in the general population because the gene controlling that trait is present at greater than 1%.[48] The three types of polymorphism undergoing most study are the debrisoquin/sparteine, N-acetylation, and mephenytoin oxidative polymorphisms.[47]

Debrisoquin/sparteine oxidative polymorphism, com-

TABLE 146–13

GENETIC POLYMORPHISMS OF DRUG METABOLISM

Debrisoquin/Spartein Type of Oxidative Polymorphism
Alprenolol
Amitriptyline
Clomipramine
Codeine
Dextromethorphan
Encainide
Flecainide
Imipramine
Methoxyamphetamine
Metoprolol
Nortriptyline
Propafenone
Propranolol
Timolol

N-Acetylation Type of Polymorphism
Aminobenzoic acid
Amrinone
Caffeine
Clonazepam
Dapsone
Hydralazine
Isoniazid
Procainamide
Sulfadiazine
Sulfamethazine
Sulfapyridine
Sulfasalazine

Mephenytoin Type of Oxidative Polymorphism
Mephobarbital
Propranolol

monly referred to as debrisoquin polymorphism, accounts for the metabolism of more than 20 agents.[47] The prevalence of poor or slow metabolizers is approximately 2 to 10%. *N*-Acetylation polymorphism accounts for poor or slow drug acetylation in 50% of black and white Americans, 50% of European whites, 5% of Canadian Eskimos, and 80 to 90% of Egyptian and Moroccan subjects. Mephenytoin-type polymorphism accounts for 5% of poor metabolizers in the general population; the prevalence is 20% in Japanese subjects.

Pharmacokinetics in Critically Ill Patients

Much of the information about drug disposition and effect for many of the agents used in the critical care unit has not come from this population. A fruitful area of research is the use of this population to determine the limits on the rates at which the body can eliminate drugs. Because many patients are monitored aggressively, studies evaluating physiologic variables as potential markers of pharmacokinetic or pharmacodynamic effects would be valuable.

CONCLUSION

Critically ill patients are at risk for physiologic insults that can lead to organ damage or death. Clinical pharmacokinetics has evolved as a method to monitor drug therapy to potentially prevent these insults. In the critical care environment, pharmacokinetic monitoring should be applied with great dedication and vigor. There is much research left to be performed in the arena of clinical pharmacokinetics as it relates to the critically ill patient.

References

1. Ried LD, McKenna DA, Horn JR: Effect of therapeutic drug monitoring services on the number of serum drug assays ordered for patients: A meta-analysis. Ther Drug Monit 11:253, 1989.
2. Ried LK, McKenna DA, Horn JR: Meta-analysis of research on the effect of clinical pharmacokinetics services on therapeutic drug monitoring. Am J Hosp Pharm 46:945, 1989.
3. Ried LK, McKenna DA, Horn JR: Therapeutic drug monitoring reduces toxic drug reactions: A meta-analysis. Ther Drug Monit 12:72, 1990.
4. Crisp CB, Lane JR, Murray W: Audit of serum drug concentration analysis for patients in the surgical intensive care unit. Crit Care Med 18:734, 1990.
5. Bedell SE, Deitz DC, Leeman D, et al: Incidence and characteristics of preventable iatrogenic cardiac arrests. JAMA 265:2815, 1991.
6. Brennan TA, Leape LL, Laird NM, et al: Incidence of adverse events and negligence in hospitalized patients: Results of the Harvard Medical Practice Study I. N Engl J Med 324:370, 1991.
7. Leape LL, Brennan TA, Laird N, et al: The nature of adverse events in hospitalized patients: Results of the Harvard Medical Practice Study II. N Engl J Med 324:377, 1991.
8. Schiff GD, Hegde HK, LaCloche L, et al: Inpatient theophylline toxicity: Preventable factors. Ann Intern Med 114:748, 1991.
9. Evans WE, Schentag JJ, Jusko WJ (eds): Applied Pharmacokinetics: Principles of Therapeutic Drug Monitoring. 2nd ed. Spokane, WA, Applied Therapeutics, 1986.
10. Winter ME (ed): Basic Clinical Pharmacokinetics. 2nd ed. Spokane, WA, Applied Therapeutics, 1988.
11. Cockcroft DW, Gault MH: Prediction of creatinine clearance from serum creatinine. Nephron 16:31, 1976.
12. DiPiro JT, Talbert RL, Hayes PE, et al (eds): Pharmacotherapy: A Pathophysiologic Approach. New York, Elsevier Science Publishing, 1989.
13. Rybak MJ, Albrecht LM, Boike SC, et al: Nephrotoxicity of vancomycin alone and with an aminoglycoside. J Antimicrob Chemother 25:679, 1990.
14. Hansten PD (ed): Drug Interactions. 5th ed. Philadelphia, Lea & Febiger, 1985.
15. McEvoy GK, Litvak K, Welsh OH, et al (eds): AHFS Drug Information. Rev. ed. Bethesda, American Society of Hospital Pharmacists, 1991.
16. Evans WE: General principles of applied pharmacokinetics. In: Evans WE, Schentag JJ, Jusko WJ (eds): Applied Pharmacokinetics: Principles of Therapeutic Drug Monitoring. 2nd ed. Spokane, WA, Applied Therapeutics, p 1, 1986.
17. Dasta JF, Armstrong DK: Pharmacoeconomic impact of critically ill surgical patients. Drug Intell Clin Pharm 22:994, 1988.
18. Bootman JL, Wertheimer AI, Saske D, et al: Individualizing gentamicin dosage regimens in burn patients with gram-negative septicemia: A cost-benefit analysis. J Pharm Sci 68:267, 1979.
19. Moore RD, Smith CR, Lietman PS: Association of aminoglycoside plasma levels with therapeutic outcome in gram-negative pneumonia. Am J Med 77:657, 1984.
20. Jusko WJ: Guidelines for collection and analysis of pharmacokinetic data. In: Evans WE, Schentag JJ, Jusko WJ (eds): Applied Pharmacokinetics. Principles of Therapeutic Drug Monitoring. 2nd ed. Spokane, WA, Applied Therapeutics, p 9, 1986.
21. Peck CC, Rodman JH: Analysis of clinical pharmacokinetic data for individualizing drug dosage regimens. In: Evans WE, Schentag JJ, Jusko WJ (eds): Applied Pharmacokinetics: Principles of Therapeutic Drug Monitoring. 2nd ed. Spokane, WA, Applied Therapeutics, p 55, 1986.
22. Gibaldi M, Perrier D (eds): Pharmacokinetics. 2nd ed. New York, Marcel Dekker, 1982.
23. Chelluri L, Jastremski MS: Inadequacy of standard aminoglycoside loading doses in acutely ill patients. Crit Care Med 15:1143, 1987.
24. Dasta JF, Armstrong DK: Variability in aminoglycoside pharmacokinetics in critically ill surgical patients. Crit Care Med 16:327, 1988.
25. Hassan E, Ober JD: Predicted and measured aminoglycoside pharmacokinetic parameters in critically ill patients. Antimicrob Agents Chemother 31:1855, 1987.
26. Townsend PL, Fink MP, Stein KL, et al: Aminoglycoside pharmacokinetics: Dosage requirements and nephrotoxicity in trauma patients. Crit Care Med 17:154, 1989.
27. Rodvold KA, Pryka RD, Kuehl PG, et al: Bayesian forecasting of serum gentamicin concentrations in intensive care patients. Clin Pharmacokinet 18:409, 1990.
28. Sawchuk RJ, Saske DE: Pharmacokinetics of dosing regimens which utilize multiple intravenous infusions: Gentamicin in burn patients. J Pharmacokinet Biopharm 4:183, 1976.
29. Sawchuk RJ, Zaske DE, Cipolle RJ, et al: Kinetic models for gentamicin dosing with the use of individual patient parameters. Clin Pharmacol Ther 21:360, 1977.
30. Zaske DE: Aminoglycosides. In: Evans WE, Schentag JJ, Jusko WJ (eds): Applied Pharmacokinetics: Principles of Therapeutic Drug Monitoring. 2nd ed. Spokane, WA, Applied Therapeutics, p 331, 1986.
31. Matzke GR: Vancomycin. In: Evans WE, Schentag JJ, Jusko WJ (eds): Applied Pharmacokinetics: Principles of Therapeutic Drug Monitoring. 2nd ed. Spokane, WA, Applied Therapeutics, p 399, 1986.
32. Rotschafer JC, Garrison MW, Rodvold KA: Therapeutic update on glycopeptide and lipopeptide antibiotics. Pharmacotherapy 8:211, 1988.
33. Eliopoulos GM, Thauvin C, Gerson B, et al: In vitro activity and mechanism of action of A21978C₁, a novel cyclic lipopeptide antibiotic. Antimicrob Agents Chemother 27:357, 1985.
34. Winter ME, Tozer TN: Phenytoin. In: Evans WE, Schentag JJ, Jusko WJ (eds): Applied Pharmacokinetics: Principles of Therapeutic Drug Monitoring. 2nd ed. Spokane, WA, Applied Therapeutics, p 331, 1986.
35. Jusko WJ, Koup JR, Alvan G: Nonlinear assessment of phenytoin bioavailability. J Pharmacokinet Biopharm 4:327, 1976.
36. Levy RH, Wilensky AJ, Friel PN: Other antiepileptic drugs. In: Evans WE, Schentag JJ, Jusko WJ (eds): Applied Pharmacokinetics: Principles of Therapeutic Drug Monitoring. 2nd ed. Spokane, WA, Applied Therapeutics, p 540, 1986.
37. Hendeles L, Massanari M, Weinberger M: Theophylline. In: Evans WE, Schentag JJ, Jusko WJ (eds): Applied Pharmacokinetics: Principles of Therapeutic Drug Monitoring. 2nd ed. Spokane, WA, Applied Therapeutics, p 1105, 1986.
38. Iafrate RP, Hendeles L: Asthma. In: Herfindal ET, Gourley DR, Hart LL (eds): Clinical Pharmacy and Therapeutics. 4th ed. Baltimore, Williams & Wilkins, p 354, 1988.
39. Kelly HW, Davis RL: Asthma. In: DiPiro JT, Talbert RL, Hayes PE, et al: Pharmacotherapy, A Pathophysiologic Approach. New York, Elsevier Science Publishing, p 347, 1989.
40. Zaritsky AL, Chernow B: Catecholamines and other inotropes. In: Chernow B (ed): The Pharmacologic Approach to the Critically Ill Patient. 2nd ed. Baltimore, Williams & Wilkins, p 584, 1988.
41. Reuning RH, Geraets DR: Digoxin. In: Evans WE, Schentag JJ, Jusko WJ (eds): Applied Pharmacokinetics: Principles of Therapeutic Drug Monitoring. 2nd ed. Spokane, WA, Applied Therapeutics, p 570, 1986.
42. Pieper JA, Rodman JH: Lidocaine. In: Evans WE, Schentag JJ, Jusko WJ (eds): Applied Pharmacokinetics: Principles of Therapeutic Drug Monitoring. 2nd ed. Spokane, WA, Applied Therapeutics, p 639, 1986.
43. Coyle JD, Lima JJ: Procainamide. In: Evans WE, Schentag JJ, Jusko WJ (eds): Applied Pharmacokinetics: Principles of Therapeutic Drug Monitoring. 2nd ed. Spokane, WA, Applied Therapeutics, p 682, 1986.
44. Yee GC, Kennedy MS: Cyclosporine. In: Evans WE, Schentag JJ, Jusko WJ (eds): Applied Pharmacokinetics: Principles of Therapeutic Drug Monitoring. 2nd ed. Spokane, WA, Applied Therapeutics, p 826, 1986.
45. Eichelbaum M: Defective oxidation of drugs: Pharmacokinetic and therapeutic implications. Clin Pharmacokinet 7:1, 1982.
46. Meyer UA, Gut J, Kronbach T, et al: The molecular mechanisms of two common polymorphisms of drug oxidation: Evidence for functional changes in cytochrome p450 isozymes catalysing bufuralol and mephenytoin oxidation. Xenobiotica 5:449, 1986.
47. Relling MV: Polymorphic drug metabolism. Clin Pharm 8:852, 1989.
48. Weinshilboum RM: Human pharmacogenetics, an introduction. Fed Proc 43:2295, 1984.

Pharmacologic Poisoning

Michael P. Peppers

The diagnosis and management of the poisoned patient entail an understanding of physical assessment, laboratory analysis, pharmacology, pharmacodynamics, pharmacokinetics, and toxicokinetics. Well-designed clinical trials cannot be ethically performed in humans to assess the toxicity of substances when taken in massive amounts. Therefore, the clinician must rely on the analysis of individual case studies, retrospective data, and epidemiologic data for developing treatment strategies. Information gathered from these sources is important for predicting trends in human exposure to toxic agents and for determining the potential for many substances to cause toxicity in humans.

This discussion concerns general principles needed to correctly diagnose toxicity and treat the poisoned patient. Emphasis is placed on describing clinical toxic syndromes, laboratory use, and treatment issues for the more commonly encountered drugs responsible for admission of patients to the critical care unit.

EPIDEMIOLOGY

A nationwide survey of 72 poison control centers conducted by the American Association of Poison Control Centers revealed that in 1990 there were 1,713,462 reported human exposures to toxic substances, which represents a mean of 9 exposures per 1000 population.[1, 2] An extrapolated estimate is that more than 2.2 million toxic exposures occurred in the United States in 1990. The National Center for Health Statistics, Mortality Statistics Branch, estimated that approximately 13,000 deaths occur each year as a result of toxic exposures. In the American Association of Poison Control Centers' survey, there were 612 fatalities reported, with the majority (87%) occurring in people older than 17 years of age. Approximately 57% of the fatal exposures resulted from a suicidal intent. The routes of exposure most often associated with mortality were ingestion (77%), inhalation (13%), and injection (6%). The substances that led to death were antidepressants (26%), analgesics (22%), stimulants (8%), sedative-hypnotics (12%), cardiovascular drugs (13%), volatile alcohols (13%), gases or fumes (6%), antiasthmatics (6%), chemicals (6%), cleaning agents (4%), and pesticides (2%). These statistical data tend to change from year to year, with an increase in numbers reported. This is probably due to the increased public awareness of poison control centers and the increased participation in the National Data Collection System by poison control centers.[1, 3–7] European data are similar to U.S. data.[8]

Self-poisoning appears to be most frequent in people 15 to 30 years of age who are prescribed psychiatric medications, who have no job, or who have a drug abuse problem.[9, 10] Factors that may increase the likelihood of fatal outcome are old age, psychosocial stress, concurrent illness, drug abuse, psychosis, depression, and lack of family support.

INITIAL APPROACH TO MANAGEMENT
Stabilization

Many overdose poisonings involve agents that rapidly cause respiratory depression and cardiac dysrhythmias; thus,

it is not surprising that the majority of deaths attributable to poisoning are a result of cardiorespiratory arrest.[1] Ensuring that the poisoned patient has adequate cardiorespiratory function is by far the most important task the clinician should perform. The patient should undergo cardiac monitoring, have vital signs checked frequently (every 10 minutes), have an intravenous access established as soon as possible, and have serum blood samples drawn for laboratory assessment.

An important note regarding cardiopulmonary resuscitation in the poisoned patient is that the drugs most often associated with overdose fatality are the antidepressants. Antidepressants are effective alpha-receptor blockers, which can lead to significant hypotension when taken in large quantities.[11–14] In resuscitation efforts, the clinician must remember that epinephrine, the first-line sympathomimetic agent used in advanced cardiac life support, nonselectively stimulates both types of alpha-receptors and both types of beta-receptors. Administering epinephrine in the presence of an alpha-receptor blocker can potentially result in a noncompetitive beta$_2$-receptor stimulation in the vascular smooth muscle, thus resulting in an active vasodilatory response; this is opposite from the desired action of increasing mean arterial pressure that one wishes to obtain from epinephrine when used in treating cardiac arrest.[15] An agent such as dopamine or norepinephrine, which does not stimulate beta$_2$-receptors yet does stimulate alpha$_1$-receptors, is preferred for use in the resuscitation of a patient with cardiac arrest resulting from an overdose of an alpha-receptor–blocking drug. Table 146–14 lists some drugs that block alpha-receptors.

Many poisonings can result in seizure activity, which should be treated with standard seizure management. If seizures continue to be uncontrolled and are the result of a drug with anticholinergic properties (antidepressants and antipsychotics, for example), physostigmine can be tried (see later). However, controversy exists regarding the use of physostigmine because of its adverse effect profile, which includes life-threatening cholinergic crisis, seizures, cardiac dysrhythmias, and pulmonary edema.[14]

During the stabilization period, a history detailing the events of poisoning should be solicited from all persons (patient, relatives, friends, and emergency personnel) present at the scene of the poisoning. Although important for subjective assessment, histories obtained from those involved with the poisoned patient can be unreliable.[16, 17] Therefore, the history should be used as an adjunct to, rather than in place of, clinical and laboratory assessment. Information to be obtained from the history includes the substance involved, the amount of substance exposed to, the route of exposure, the time course of exposure, the reason for exposure, any symptoms such as vomiting and seizures that occurred before arrival at the emergency department, any treatment already initiated, concurrent medical problems, and all medications taken on a regular basis. If available, all substance containers should be inspected for contents and all intact dosage forms should be identified by using appropriate resources (POISINDEX, Identidex, Drugdex, Physicians' Desk Reference, poison control center, and pharmacy personnel, for example).

Diagnosis

When diagnosing poisoning, the clinical laboratory should be utilized in a cost-efficient manner. Laboratory indices and toxicology screens should be ordered in accordance with their ability to contribute to overall management of and outcome for patients. Routine laboratory assessment of serum electrolytes, renal function tests, liver function tests,

TABLE 146–14

COMMON AGENTS RESPONSIBLE FOR SYMPATHETIC OR SYMPATHOLYTIC TOXIC SYNDROMES

Alpha-Receptor Stimulation	Beta-Receptor Stimulation
Stimulants	Stimulants
Amphetamines	Amphetamines
Catecholamines	Catecholamines
Cocaine	Cocaine
Decongestants	Decongestants
Alpha-Receptor Blockade	**Beta-Receptor Blockade**
Antidepressants	Beta-blockers
Amoxapine	Acebutolol
Desipramine	Atenolol
Imipramine	Betaxolol
Nortriptyline	Esmolol
Trazodone	Labetolol
Antihypertensives	Metoprolol
Phenoxybenzamine	Nadolol
Phentolamine	Propranolol
Prazosin	Timolol
Terazosin	
Antipsychotics	
Chlorpromazine	
Haloperidol	
Prochlorperazine	
Thiothixene	
Thioridazine	
Trifluoperazine	

and determination of serum glucose, ketones, anion gap, serum osmolarity, and blood gases are of significant benefit in contributing to overall management and may alter the ultimate outcome in the majority of poisoned patients. All patients with suspected poisoning should have samples for routine laboratory indices taken and analyzed.

Toxicology Screens

Toxicology screens are either qualitative or quantitative and can be of great help when used properly. Before obtaining a toxicology screen, the clinician should first decide which type of screen, if any, is most beneficial for guiding therapy to improve the outcome of the poisoned patient.

Qualitative toxicology screens utilize a body fluid sample, such as urine or gastric contents, for analysis to determine the presence of unknown potential toxins. Results generated by this type of screen are used primarily to confirm a diagnosis of poisoning or to rule out possible causes of psychosis, seizures, or coma. There is no good correlation between the toxins found to be present by qualitative analysis and the clinical effects elicited by the toxins.

When there is a strong suspicion of either intentional or accidental poisoning, the qualitative toxicology screen is of minimal use in guiding therapy to improve patient outcome because the majority of toxicities are treated by supportive care alone. In fact, test results may not be available until after therapy has been initiated. When a positive history of toxicity is obtained, the greatest diagnostic tool available to the clinician is the appearance of toxic syndromes on physical examination.

CLINICAL TOXIC SYNDROMES
Autonomic Nervous System Effects

The autonomic nervous system is composed of both parasympathetic (cholinergic) and sympathetic (adrenergic) nerve fibers, which in concert maintain body homeostasis (respiration, thermoregulation, metabolism, and circulation). Various autonomic nervous system receptor effects are outlined in Table 146–15. Most organs in the body are innervated by both parasympathetic and sympathetic nerves. Parasympathetic stimulation and sympathetic stimulation antagonize one another, and the predominant effect elicited by the organ depends on the degree of stimulation produced by each branch of the autonomic nervous system. Many of the toxins involved in severe poisonings affect the autonomic nervous system by either stimulating or inhibiting one or both of its branches.

Cholinergic Poisoning

Cholinergic poisoning resembles an overabundance of acetylcholine stimulating both nicotinic and muscarinic receptors.[8] Peripheral symptoms of muscarinic stimulation include defecation, urination, miosis, bradycardia, bronchorrhea, emesis, lacrimation, and sweating. This constellation of symptoms can be remembered by the mnemonic *dumbbels*.

Hypotension and decreased myocardial contractility and conduction may also occur as a result of muscarinic stimulation. Low doses of cholinergic poison stimulate nicotinic receptors to produce skeletal muscle fasciculations; however, high doses of cholinergic poison block nicotinic receptors and produce muscular weakness and paralysis. Table 146–16 outlines various agents responsible for producing a cholinergic crisis under toxic conditions.

Anticholinergic toxicity manifests clinical symptoms opposite from those of the cholinergic poisons. Parasympatholytic agents block the actions of acetylcholine. Clinical signs of anticholinergic poisoning include increased blood pressure, tachycardia, warm dry skin, mydriasis, erythema, delirium, hallucinations, urinary urgency and retention, and

TABLE 146–15

PHYSIOLOGIC RESPONSE TO AUTONOMIC NERVOUS STIMULATION OF VARIOUS RECEPTORS

Autonomic Nervous System Receptor Type	Organ Effects
Alpha	Mydriasis; arteriolar and venous constriction; gastrointestinal and urinary sphincter contraction; uterine contraction; pilomotor contraction in skin; sweat gland secretion; decreased secretion from the acini and islet cells of the pancreas; salivation
Beta	Increased heart rate, myocardial contractility, conduction velocity, automaticity, and rate of intraventricular pacemakers; arteriolar dilation; bronchial relaxation; decreased gastrointestinal motility and tone; uterine relaxation; glycogenolysis and gluconeogenesis; increased pancreatic cell secretion; lipolysis; salivation
Cholinergic	Miosis; decreased heart rate, contractility, and conduction velocity; arteriolar dilation, bronchial muscle contraction and gland secretion; gastrointestinal peristalsis and secretion; gastrointestinal sphincter relaxation; urinary bladder contraction with sphincter relaxation; generalized secretion by sweat glands; glycogen synthesis; salivation

TABLE 146–16

COMMON AGENTS RESPONSIBLE FOR CHOLINERGIC AND ANTICHOLINERGIC TOXIC SYNDROMES

Cholinergic Crisis	Anticholinergic Syndrome
Acetylcholine	Antidepressants
Black widow spider	Amitriptyline
Insecticides	Amoxipine
Organophosphates	Desipramine
Carbamates	Imipramine
Nicotine	Nortriptyline
Mushrooms (some species)	Trazodone
Nicotine	Antihistamines
Pilocarpine	Chlorpheniramine
Tobacco	Diphenhydramine
	Antipsychotics
	Butyrophenones
	Phenothiazines
	Belladonna alkaloids
	Atropine
	Homatropine
	Hyoscine
	Scopolamine
	Jimson weed
	Mushrooms (some species)

minimal or absent bowel sounds. Anticholinergic toxicity can be remembered by the phrase *hot as Hades, blind as a bat, red as a beet, dry as a bone, mad as a Hatter.* Table 146–16 outlines various agents responsible for producing an anticholinergic syndrome under toxic conditions.

Sympathetic Nervous System Effects

Toxic agents that affect the sympathetic nervous system can do so by either agonizing or antagonizing the various adrenergic receptors.[8] They may also act by increasing or decreasing sympathetic outflow from the CNS. The clinical picture may vary, depending on the receptors or systems affected most by the toxin. Symptoms such as mydriasis (dilated pupils), hypertension, decreased gastrointestinal motility, and bladder incontinence may suggest poisoning with an alpha-receptor stimulant. Beta-receptor stimulants may result in miosis, tachycardia, hypertension, hypotension, accelerated atrioventricular conduction, bladder incontinence, hyperglycemia, and decreased gastrointestinal motility. Signs suggestive of alpha-receptor blockade include miosis, postural hypotension, reflex tachycardia, angina, and gastric hyperactivity. Beta-receptor blockade results in hypotension, cardiac dysrhythmias such as heart block and bradycardia, bronchospasm, pulmonary edema, hypoglycemia with hypertension, and hyperkalemia. Table 146–14 lists some common drugs that stimulate or block the various adrenergic receptors.

Temperature Regulation Alterations

Many drugs can produce problems in thermoregulation.[8] Hyperthermia may result with the ingestion of stimulants, antipsychotics, barbiturates, anticonvulsants, salicylates, antiarrhythmics, antibiotics, nonsteroidal anti-inflammatory drugs, allopurinol, and clofibrate. Table 146–17 lists some drugs commonly associated with hyperthermia. Other causes of hyperthermia such as infection, which might be seen in aspiration, should also be ruled out. The reader is referred to Chapter 141 for a complete discussion of the etiology of hyperthermia.

Core temperatures greater than 41°C (106°F) constitute a medical emergency. Survival from probable cocaine-induced hyperthermia with a temperature of 46°C (114°F) has been reported.[18] Aggressive treatment with cardiorespiratory support, ice water baths, thermorectal probing, and warm water gastric lavage may be needed to correct the hyperthermic event. If uncorrected, extreme hyperthermia may result in rhabdomyolysis, organ failure (kidneys, heart, lungs, liver), electrolyte disturbances, and convulsions.[8]

Hypothermia, a core temperature less than 35°C (95°F), most commonly results from ingestion of ethanol.[8] Other agents responsible for hypothermia include narcotics, sedative-hypnotics, phenothiazines, tricyclic antidepressants, general anesthetics, carbon monoxide, and insulin (hypoglycemia). Hypothermia attributable to other causes, such as occult infections, should be ruled out. The reader is referred to Chapter 142 for a complete discussion of the etiology of hypothermia.

Central Nervous System Effects

Coma is a nonspecific sign of toxicity and occurs with most drugs if consumed in large enough quantities.[8] Caution should be taken to rule out all possible reasons for coma, including structural damage and drugs. Rapid onset of coma generally occurs after poisoning with cyanide, hydrogen sulfide, carbon monoxide, narcotics, barbiturates, and nicotinic acid. Alternating levels of consciousness suggest a drug with enterohepatic circulation such as phencyclidine or glutethimide; as the drug is excreted into the gastrointestinal tract by the liver, the patient may become more alert, but as the gastrointestinal tract reabsorbs the drug, the patient may again go into coma. Table 146–18 lists other common agents responsible for inducing coma.

Seizures are also a nonspecific sign of drug toxicity.[8] Drug-induced seizures are almost always of the grand mal type. Focal or absence seizures generally suggest a cause other than drug ingestion or drug withdrawal. Drugs most com-

TABLE 146–17

COMMON AGENTS RESPONSIBLE FOR DISORDERS OF TEMPERATURE REGULATION

Hyperthermia	Hypothermia
Allopurinol	Antipsychotics
Anesthetics	Phenothiazines
Halothane	Antidepressants
Phencyclidine	Desipramine
Antiarrhythmics	Imipramine
Procainamide	Nortriptyline
Quinidine	Carbon monoxide
Antibiotics	Ethanol
Isoniazid	General anesthetics
Penicillins	Insulin
Sulfonamides	Sedative-hypnotics
Anticonvulsants	Barbiturates
Phenytoin	Chloral hydrate
Antipsychotics	Glutethimide
Butyrophenones	
Phenothiazines	
Thioxanthenes	
Barbiturates	
Clofibrate	
Nonsteroidal anti-inflammatory drugs	
Salicylates	
Aspirin	
Methylsalicylate	
Stimulants	
Amphetamines	
Cocaine	

TABLE 146–18

COMMON AGENTS RESPONSIBLE FOR CENTRAL NERVOUS SYSTEM TOXIC SYNDROMES

Seizures	Coma
Anesthetics	Alcohols
Bupivacaine	Anticholinergics
Enflurane	Anticonvulsants
Halothane	Antidepressants
Ketamine	Antihistamines
Lidocaine	Antipsychotics
Phencyclidine	Barbiturates
Procaine	Benzodiazepines
Antibiotics	Bromides
Carbapenems	Carbon monoxide
Isoniazid	Cyanide
Penicillins	Hydrogen sulfide
Anticonvulsants	Nicotinic acid
Phenytoin	Opiates
Antihypertensives	Insulin
Beta-blockers	Sulfonylureas
Clonidine	
Hypoglycemics	
Insulin	
Sulfonylureas	
Insecticides	
Carbamates	
Organophosphates	
Lithium	
Methylxanthines	
Caffeine	
Pentoxifylline	
Theophylline	
Narcotics	
Meperidine	
Propoxyphene	
Stimulants	
Amphetamines	
Cocaine	
Strychnine	

monly associated with seizures include anticholinergics (antidepressants, antihistamines, antipsychotics), hypoglycemics (insulin, sulfonylureas), lidocaine and other local anesthetics, and methylxanthines (theophylline, caffeine, pentoxifylline). Seizures with an alert sensorium suggest strychnine poisoning. Other drugs that may cause seizures are listed in Table 146–18.

SPECIFIC TOXINS

A complete discussion of all possible toxins that a patient may be exposed to is beyond the scope of this chapter. The following discussion considers 10 of the most common drug toxins encountered in critical care practice. The clinician should consult specialized references for a complete discussion of the many potential toxins.[8]

Theophylline

Theophylline is an effective drug with a small therapeutic window (10 to 20 µg/mL) used for the treatment of hyperactive airways disease. In toxic doses, however, theophylline can lead to significant morbidity and mortality.[9, 10, 19–27] Theophylline poisoning may produce any or all of the following symptoms: nausea, vomiting, diarrhea, abdominal pain, tremors, headache, cardiac dysrhythmias, hypotension, sei-

zures, coma, and death. Unfortunately, the least severe of these may not always be the presenting symptoms in patients with toxicity; seizures may be the first and only symptom manifested by some. Theophylline-induced seizures can result in long-term neurologic damage or death.[22]

The severity of symptoms may differ in acute and chronic toxicity.[10, 19, 20] Patients with acute toxicity most often have a greater number of the aforementioned symptoms. In addition, they may have hypokalemia and low serum bicarbonate levels. Cardiac dysrhythmias noted during acute toxicity include sinus tachycardia, supraventricular tachycardia, and rarely, premature ventricular contractions.[10, 19, 28] In chronic intoxication, all symptoms may occur, but it is also possible that seizures may be the only presenting sign of toxicity.[10]

Analysis of the serum theophylline concentration may offer great benefit in patient management. Life-threatening events have been reported after acute ingestion of theophylline with serum levels in the range of 30 to 100 µg/mL.[19, 21, 23–25] Evidence suggests, however, that patients with acute theophylline toxicity and a serum theophylline concentration less than 100 µg/mL are at lower risk for experiencing severe or life-threatening symptoms such as seizures. If predisposing factors such as idiopathic seizure disorder or alcohol withdrawal are present, however, the seizure threshold may be lower.[10, 20]

With chronic intoxication, patients without predisposing problems have a 50% chance of eliciting seizure activity when serum levels exceed 40 µg/mL.[10, 20] In patients with predisposing conditions, seizure activity may ensue with serum levels less than 40 µg/mL.

When assessing serum theophylline levels in cases of acute toxicity, the clinician must obtain serial levels so as not to miss the peak. In massive overdose, theophylline time-release tablets may form a gastrointestinal bezoar, which continuously releases drug for absorption into the body and may not peak for up to 18 hours after ingestion.[19–22] This is much longer than the 4- to 6-hour time to peak expected after therapeutic ingestion. Failure to recognize this toxicokinetic phenomenon can lead to gross misinterpretation of the serum theophylline level, with serious toxicity possibly going undetected and untreated.

Frequent monitoring of vital signs and neurologic status is recommended. Gastric decontamination should be performed regardless of the time of ingestion. This ensures that any prolonged absorption resulting from bezoar formation of sustained-release products is prevented. Using repeated doses (1 g/kg) of activated charcoal increases theophylline clearance by as much as 50%.[29–31] A cathartic such as sorbitol (0.5 mL/kg) or magnesium citrate (4 mL/kg) may accompany the first dose of charcoal.

Historically, prophylactic charcoal hemoperfusion was recommended when the serum theophylline concentration exceeded 30 µg/mL to minimize the potential for seizure activity and subsequent morbidity and mortality.[22] Other investigators have stated that prophylactic charcoal hemoperfusion should be considered on a patient-specific basis when concentrations exceed 60 to 80 µg/mL.[21, 23, 29] Because of data assessing differences between acute and chronic toxicity, as well as differences between patients with and without predisposing factors for seizure activity, charcoal hemoperfusion may not be indicated for theophylline toxicity until concentrations approach or exceed 100 µg/mL in the acute setting or 40 µg/mL in the chronic setting.[10] Additional research is needed to determine the place of prophylactic charcoal hemoperfusion. Charcoal hemoperfusion should be considered in any case of serious, life-threatening, toxic manifestation regardless of the serum theophylline concentration.[10, 19–24]

Phenytoin

Phenytoin is an effective anticonvulsant medication possessing a narrow therapeutic window, ranging between 10 and 20 µg/mL. Phenytoin undergoes capacity-limited metabolism in the liver. As phenytoin enters the liver for metabolism, sites for metabolism may become saturated with the drug. On saturation of these metabolic sites, only a fixed amount of phenytoin can be eliminated by the liver. Consequently, a disproportionate rise in serum concentration with regard to dose occurs. This unique pharmacokinetic profile, commonly refered to as Michaelis-Menton pharmacokinetics, is responsible for the potential toxicity that can result even from normal therapeutic doses of phenytoin.[32]

Toxic manifestations of phenytoin correlate to some degree with serum phenytoin concentrations.[33] Mild nystagmus begins to appear at a concentration of 15 to 25 µg/mL. This is intensified with a lateral gaze induced at a 45° deviation from the midline when the serum phenytoin concentration approaches or exceeds 30 µg/mL. Ataxia, slurred speech, and some disorientation also begin to appear. At concentrations exceeding 40 µg/mL, marked ataxia, unsteadiness on sitting, severe nystagmus, and mental confusion may be prevalent. With chronic intoxication, paradoxical seizure activity has been reported at levels of 35 µg/mL or greater.[34]

Phenytoin is highly bound to serum proteins (primarily albumin); therefore, care should be taken when using serum phenytoin levels as an index of toxicity in the hypoproteinemic patient. The free phenytoin level (active portion) may be in the toxic range (>2 µg/mL), while the total phenytoin level (albumin bound plus free) appears to be normal or subtherapeutic. Failure to recognize this can lead to misinterpretation of phenytoin concentration and potentially an iatrogenic overdose. To avoid this pitfall, the clinician should monitor free phenytoin levels (if available) when making therapeutic decisions on the basis of serum blood levels.[9, 32]

Phenytoin absorption is extensively delayed in acute overdoses.[35-37] Peak concentrations may not occur until 4 days after ingestion, even when gastric lavage is performed. It is therefore recommended that repeated doses of activated charcoal follow gastic lavage regardless of time of ingestion. Serial phenytoin levels should be obtained to make sure that the concentration is declining. If phenytoin levels are greater than 30 µg/mL, a minimum of 23 hours' hospital observation may be warranted to watch for possible paradoxical seizures.

The elimination half-life of phenytoin in a therapeutic setting averages 22 hours. In the toxic setting, however, phenytoin may exhibit a serum half-life as long as 200 hours.[32, 38, 39] It is thus hard to predict, from a pharmacokinetic viewpoint, how fast the serum levels will fall.

Gastric lavage, repeated doses of activated charcoal (1 g/kg), and frequent neurologic monitoring are the mainstays of treating phenytoin toxicity. Dialysis and hemoperfusion are not expected to offer much to therapy, as phenytoin is highly protein bound and possesses a large volume of distribution.[32]

Digitalis Glycosides (Digoxin)

Toxicity can occur with any of the digitalis preparations, including digoxin, digitoxin, ouabain, and digitalis leaf. Each of these cardiac glycosides produces a similar clinical picture when toxicity occurs. Because digoxin is more widely used than others in its class, it is discussed as the class prototype.

Individual sensitivity to digoxin depends on underlying problems such as cardiac condition, coronary artery disease, pulmonary disease, thyroid disease, altered serum electrolyte concentrations (potassium, magnesium, calcium), and age of the patient.[40] Any of these problems may increase the toxic potential of digitalis.

A serum digoxin concentration may be of some help in determining toxicity, but caution should be used when trying to correlate toxicity with serum concentration. Although the majority of patients who exhibit toxic signs do so when the serum concentration exceeds 2 ng/mL, a small percentage show signs of toxicity at levels below this.[41] On the other hand, some populations of patients may have falsely elevated serum digoxin levels. Pregnant patients, neonates, and patients with renal failure all produce and release into the blood stream an endogenous digoxin-like immunoreactive substance that may interfere with some digoxin assays.[42] This interference can lead to a falsely elevated digoxin level. Levels as high as 1 ng/mL have been reported in patients not receiving digoxin, but experiencing renal failure. Each laboratory should know its own sensitivities to digoxin and digoxin-like immunoreactive substances. Communication with the laboratory regarding this point is important.

Regardless of the serum level, the overall clinical picture is most important for determining digoxin toxicity. Non–life-threatening symptoms of digoxin toxicity include (1) gastrointestinal complaints such as nausea, vomiting, and diarrhea; (2) CNS symptoms such as fatigue, malaise, neuralgia, headache, confusion, delusions, and hallucinations; and (3) visual disturbances, including blurred vision, green-yellow color perception, and visualization of halos around objects.[43] Serious and potentially life-threatening signs of digoxin toxicity include those that are associated with the electrical activity of the myocardium and abnormalities in the serum potassium concentration. Digoxin toxicity may produce dysrhythmias of all known types. Acute digoxin toxicity generally occurs with dysrhythmias resulting from conduction disturbances in the sinoatrial or atrioventricular nodes such as bradycardia or varying degrees of heart block.[40] Hyperkalemia is often present with acute digoxin toxicity. This is primarily due to Na^+,K^+-ATPase inhibition by digoxin, which results in an intracellular leakage of potassium into the serum.[41] If the ingestion is recent, however, the serum potassium level may be normal owing to the lack of significant digoxin tissue distribution, given the time course of ingestion. Digoxin may display a decreased serum half-life from a mean of 31 hours to as low as 6 hours in the patient with acute toxicity.[44]

Chronic digoxin intoxication most typically produces disturbances of ventricular electrical impulse formation such as premature ventricular contractions, ventricular tachycardia, and ventricular fibrillation.[43] Occasionally, disturbances in sinus impulse conduction such as premature atrial contractions or asystole may occur. A rule of thumb is that toxicity may be present when there is any change in a previously stable cardiac rhythm, even if a previously stable abnormal rhythm changes to a normal rhythm. With chronic toxicity, the serum potassium concentration is often either normal or decreased, most likely related to concomitant diuretic therapy.[40, 41, 43]

General management of digoxin toxicity includes gastric decontamination for the acute ingestion, continuous cardiac monitoring, evaluation of old electrocardiographic tracings for comparison, administration of atropine for conduction disturbances, administration of phenytoin or lidocaine for dysrhythmias of impulse formation, placement of a pacemaker for arrhythmias that are resistant to atropine or antiarrhythmics, and digoxin-specific antigen-binding (Fab) fragments for cases resistant to all other therapies.

When significant rhythm disturbances such as bradycardia or heart block are present, methods used to decontaminate the gastrointestinal system may lead to an increase in vagal tone and a worsening of the dysrhythmia; asystole has been reported.[45] One reviewer suggested that pretreatment with atropine may be warranted before gastrointestinal decontamination.[40]

Ventricular ectopy should be treated first by correcting any electrolyte disturbances.[40] Lidocaine can be used safely in atrioventricular block as long as care is taken not to abolish escape rhythms. Phenytoin reverses digitalis-induced atrioventricular block and can terminate supraventricular arrhythmias resulting from digitalis intoxication. Atropine blocks the vagal effects that digoxin places on the sinoatrial and atrioventricular nodes and should be considered as first-choice therapy for a hemodynamically compromised patient with high-degree heart block or bradycardia. Isoproterenol may worsen ectopy and is therefore not recommended. Cardiac pacing with a temporary transvenous ventricular pacemaker is recommended if the patient is unresponsive to atropine and has decreased organ perfusion.

When all else has failed or if the patient exhibits acute accidental or suicidal overdose, digoxin-specific antibody (Fab) fragments may be used to reverse the toxic effects of digoxin.[46, 47] These antibody fragments bind free serum digoxin and produce a concentration gradient that results in egress of digoxin from tissues. The Fab fragment continues to bind digoxin as it is released into the serum.

Caution must be taken when considering Fab therapy in patients with renal failure or in patients with underlying congestive heart failure or atrial fibrillation. The Fab-digoxin complex is excreted via the kidneys; therefore, the possibility exists for dissociation of digoxin from the Fab fragment with recurring toxicity over time if renal function is significantly depressed. Patients who require digoxin for therapeutic reasons have the therapeutic value abolished when digoxin-specific Fab fragment is used; alternative measures should be available to treat underlying disorders such as atrial fibrillation with rapid ventricular response and congestive heart failure if they occur after Fab therapy.

Fab fragments are produced by injecting sheep with digoxin so that antibodies against the digoxin are produced. The sheep serum with the antibodies is then put through a process of immunoadsorption to separate specific fragments of the digoxin antibodies, thus rendering the Fab fragment less immunogenic than the whole sheep-derived antibody.

Each vial of digoxin-specific Fab (Digibind) contains 40 mg of Fab, which binds 0.6 mg of digoxin or digitoxin. Dosage calculation for digoxin-specific Fab is based on total body load of digitalis. The following formulas give an estimate of the number of vials required to treat the toxicity:

Digoxin:

$$\text{Body load (mg)} = \text{(serum digoxin concentration)} \\ (5.6) \text{ (weight in kg)}/1000$$

$$\text{Dose (vials)} = \text{body load}/0.6 \text{ (mg/vial)}$$

Digitoxin:

$$\text{Body load (mg)} = \text{(serum digitoxin concentration)} \\ (0.56) \text{ (weight in kg)}/1000$$

$$\text{Dose (vials)} = \text{body load}/0.6 \text{ (mg/vial)}$$

If the decision is made to administer Fab fragments, the clinician should be aware that subsequent digoxin blood levels represent both free drug and antibody-bound drug and thus are extremely elevated and have little clinical utility.[46, 47] It is suggested that serum levels not be monitored after administration of digoxin-specific Fab fragments, for this is an expensive waste of resources.

Acetaminophen

Acetaminophen, an analgesic or antipyretic used in many over-the-counter and prescription drug products, may cause significant morbidity and mortality when overdosed.[48–50] Regardless of history obtained, it is of paramount importance to consider the possibility of acetaminophen toxicity in all patients who attempt suicide by overdose.

In therapeutic doses, acetaminophen is converted in the liver to glucuronide and sulfate conjugates, which are then excreted in the urine. In large doses, acetaminophen is additionally metabolized via the cytochrome P-450 mixed-function oxidase system to a toxic, intermediate metabolite (N-acetylimidoquinone). This metabolite is further metabolized by glutathione reductase to a nontoxic compound. Sulfhydryl groups are required for glutathione reductase to perform its metabolic function. When toxic amounts of acetaminophen are presented to the liver for metabolism, the glutathione system becomes overwhelmed, is depleted of sulfhydryl groups, and subsequently loses metabolic activity. Unless these sulfhydryl groups are repleted with antidotal therapy, the liver is unable to detoxify the intermediate metabolite, which may eventually produce hepatic necrosis, renal failure, and cardiac damage. N-Acetylcysteine is the antidote of choice for replenishing the glutathione system with sulfhydryl groups. This then allows further metabolism of the intermediate acetaminophen metabolite to a nontoxic compound. There are also data suggesting that cimetidine can be protective against acetaminophen toxicity by inhibiting the cytochrome P-450 enzyme system and thus preventing the formation of the toxic intermediate metabolite.[51–54] This therapy, however, must be in place before the formation of the toxic intermediate metabolite; therefore, clinical utility after overdose is questionable.

Acetaminophen toxicity occurs in three stages. Stage 1 occurs within 12 to 24 hours after ingestion and consists of either mild gastrointestinal distress or no symptoms at all. Stage 2 occurs 24 to 48 hours after ingestion with resolution of all previous symptoms. Liver enzymes begin to elevate in stage 2. This stage may linger for up to 4 days before the third stage appears. In stage 3 the patient either improves, with normalization of liver enzyme levels, or progresses to acute hepatic necrosis, liver failure, and potential demise.[48–50]

Analyzing the serum acetaminophen concentration may be the only reliable tool for diagnosing toxicity early in the presentation.[48, 49] From an assessment standpoint, it would be sensible to obtain routine serum acetaminophen concentrations on all suspected overdoses because there is no obvious or reliable clinical presentation with acute toxicity.

If possible, serum acetaminophen concentrations should be obtained no sooner than 4 hours after ingestion to use the Rumack-Matthew nomogram to help guide therapy (Fig. 146–2). Obtaining an accurate time course of ingestion is critical because the nomogram is based on serum concentration versus hours after ingestion; it is best to err on the side of caution by overestimating the time since ingestion. High potential for toxicity exists when the serum concentration is 200 μg/mL at 4 hours, 50 μg/mL at 12 hours, and 7 μg/mL at 24 hours after ingestion. N-Acetylcysteine should be administered as soon as possible within the first 24 hours of ingestion. However, antidotal therapy is optimal when given within 12 hours (stage 1) of acetaminophen ingestion.[48, 49] The dose of N-acetylcysteine is 140 mg/kg as an initial oral loading dose, followed by 70 mg/kg every 4 hours for a total of 17 doses.[48, 49] This drug has a putrid taste and odor and may necessitate placing the dose in a glass of orange juice or cola to mask its full flavor. In situations in which acetaminophen concentrations are not readily available, antidotal

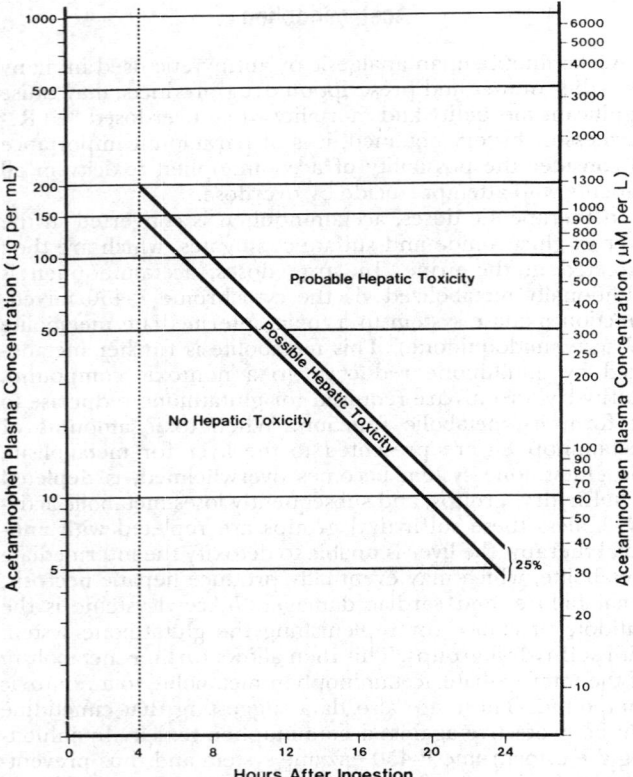

Figure 146–2. Rumack-Matthew nomogram for acetaminophen poisoning. Semilogarithmic plot of plasma acetaminophen levels versus time. The cautions for the use of this chart are (1) the time coordinates refer to time of ingestion, (2) serum levels analyzed before 4 hours may not represent peak levels, (3) the graph should be used only in relation to a single acute ingestion, and (4) the lower solid line 25% below the standard nomogram is included to allow for possible errors in acetaminophen plasma assays and estimated time from ingestion of an overdose. (Rumack-Matthew Nomogram for Acetaminophen Poisoning, copyright Micromedex, Inc., 1974–1993, adapted from Pediatrics 1975; 55:871–876.)

therapy is recommended. Similarly, in situations in which there is an extensive delay in obtaining results of the acetaminophen analysis, it is wise to initiate *N*-acetylcysteine treatment, then reassess when concentrations are available.

Frequently encountered is the desire to stop antidotal therapy prematurely as the acetaminophen concentration falls to zero. This is discouraged because it is not the acetaminophen that is toxic, but its metabolite. To avoid this potential problem, it is recommended that no further acetaminophen levels be analyzed after the decision has been made to treat the patient; the full course of antidote should be administered.

Salicylates

Salicylates are encountered in a variety of forms such as aspirin, methylsalicylate (oil of wintergreen), and bismuth subsalicylate. Although serum concentrations do not correlate well with clinical symptoms, they are useful in determining the course of therapy. Unlike the case with acetaminophen, there are some clinical measures that facilitate evaluation of salicylate toxicity. Useful clues for making the diagnosis include the patient's history, an anion gap metabolic acidosis, and respiratory alkalosis, as well as clinical signs such as gastric upset and tinnitus. Other symptoms

include increased depth of respirations, a feeling of fullness in the ears, headache, seizures, and coma.[55]

Obtaining a serum salicylate concentration provides information to assess overall toxicity. The Done nomogram (Fig. 146–3) uses a serum concentration at least 6 hours after ingestion so as not to miss the peak after an acute ingestion. However, the Done nomogram is of limited use in assessing chronic toxicity.[55, 56] A serum concentration can be obtained at any time in a case of chronic salicylism. Levels greater than 30 μg/mL are potentially toxic in the chronic setting.

Serial serum concentrations at 6-hour intervals, after acute ingestion, characterize an absorption-elimination profile and can indicate a concretion that continues to release aspirin in the stomach. This finding should be suspected when the patient's clinical status does not appear to improve despite appropriate intervention.

Routine management of salicylate toxicity includes supportive care, gastrointestinal decontamination, multiple-dose activated charcoal, and forced alkaline diuresis (alkalinizing the urine with sodium bicarbonate produces ion trapping and increases elimination). In cases of severe toxicity (seizures, coma), emergent dialysis is useful. The decision to dialyze is based solely on clinical grounds, but blood level monitoring is useful to monitor drug elimination.[55, 56]

Antidepressants

Tricyclic antidepressant poisoning results in a disproportionate number of both critical care unit admissions and

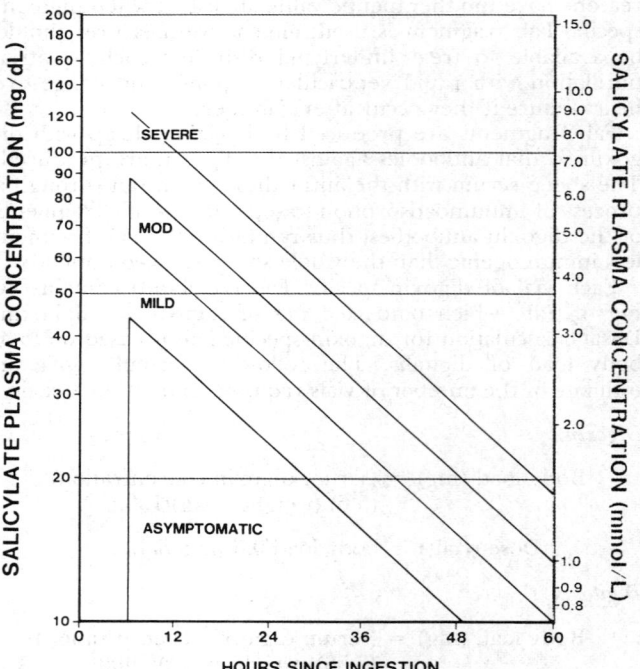

Figure 146–3. Done nomogram for salicylate poisoning. The Done nomogram should be used with the following cautions: (1) the patient has taken a single acute ingestion and is not experiencing chronic toxicity, (2) the blood level to be plotted on the nomogram was analyzed 6 hours after ingestion, (3) levels in the toxic range found before 6 hours should be treated, and (4) levels in the nontoxic range analyzed before 6 hours should be repeated to see if the level is increasing. (Adapted from Done AK: Salicylate intoxication. Significance of measurements of salicylate in blood in cases of acute ingestion. Reproduced by permission of Pediatrics, vol 26, page 800, copyright 1960.)

fatalities when compared with those associated with other drugs used in suicide attempts.[1, 2, 11] Antidepressants initially undergo rapid gastrointestinal absorption and can result in toxic serum concentrations during a short time. Eventually, however, the anticholinergic action of these drugs slows both gastrointestinal peristalsis and the rate of drug absorption. Antidepressants are highly bound to plasma proteins and have a large volume of distribution that ranges from 10 to 50 L/kg. Hypoalbuminemia and acidosis both lead to decreased plasma protein binding and thus may free up a larger proportion of active drug.[11, 57] Antidepressant serum concentrations do not correlate well with toxic symptoms in overdose.[58, 59] Therefore, analysis of antidepressant serum concentration is of minimal clinical value in known antidepressant overdose.

Antidepressant toxicity occurs rapidly after ingestion and produces clinical effects on the CNS, parasympathetic nervous system, and cardiovascular system.[11] Signs of anticholinergic poisoning occur early and include mydriasis, blurred vision, dry mucous membranes, tachycardia, hyperpyrexia, urinary retention, decreased gastrointestinal motility, agitation, and mental confusion. Rapidly after the initial phase, the patient may experience extreme somnolence, respiratory depression, seizures, and coma.

Antidepressants elicit anticholinergic effects on the pacemakers of the heart and quinidine-like activity on the His-Purkinje conduction system.[11–13, 59, 60] Sinus tachycardia with rates greater than 100 beats/min is indicative of anticholinergic activity. The quinidine-like effects may produce a widened QRS, PR, and QT interval as well as a right bundle branch block pattern on the electrocardiogram resulting from inhibition of sodium flux across the cell membrane. Ventricular dysrhythmias are rare but are an ominous sign if they occur. Torsades de pointes has been reported.[61] The best predictor of both seizures and cardiac dysrhythmias is a QRS complex that is greater than 0.1 second on the limb leads of the electrocardiogram.[59] Hypotension may occur owing to drug-induced alpha-receptor blockade, vasodilation, or cardiac depression. Eventually, cardiovascular collapse occurs if intervention is unsuccessful.

Treatment necessitates careful evaluation of neurologic and cardiorespiratory status with proper supportive care, including provision of intravenous access and secured airways and cardiac monitoring. Decontamination should be carefully approached by performing gastric lavage using a large-bore orogastric tube. Activated charcoal, 1 g/kg (50 to 100 g) should be given via lavage tube to bind any drug remaining in the gastrointestinal tract. A suitable cathartic such as sorbitol (0.5 mL/kg) or magnesium citrate (4 mL/kg) should accompany the first dose of charcoal, as peristalsis may be impaired because of anticholinergic activity of the poison. Repeated oral doses of charcoal every 2 to 4 hours may be of benefit in removing the antidepressant from the circulation. Charcoal administration should be continued only if the patient is passing stool, as impaction can develop. Ipecac syrup is not generally recommended for treatment of tricyclic antidepressant overdose because the patient may become obtunded before the emetic effects occur. Aspiration of vomitus could then lead to secondary problems.

Seizures and cardiac dysrhythmias are the most dangerous of all toxic sequelae. Seizures have been effectively treated using either intravenous diazepam or intravenous phenobarbital.[14] Phenytoin is ineffective and may actually be dangerous in antidepressant overdose. When maximal diazepam or phenobarbital regimens fail, physostigmine may be of benefit. However, one is cautioned against the routine use of physostigmine because of its potent cholinergic activity and toxic potential. Physostigmine can produce a cholinergic crisis with seizures. Physostigmine is administered as 2 mg

intravenously over 2 minutes and repeated every 20 to 30 minutes or 2 mg intramuscularly and repeated every 2 to 3 hours. If a cholinergic crisis results from physostigmine use, glycopyrrolate, 0.4 to 1.0 mg intravenously, can be used to reverse the crisis. Glycopyrrolate is preferred over atropine because atropine does not reach the CNS as easily.

Cardiac dysrhythmias may be suppressed by increasing the serum pH in the range of 7.45 to 7.55.[11] This can be performed by hyperventilating the patient or by using intravenous infusions of sodium bicarbonate.[62–64] Increasing the serum pH increases plasma protein binding and thus decreases the total amount of free active drug. In addition, when sodium bicarbonate is used, the sodium load may possibly antagonize the quinidine-like effects seen at the His-Purkinje system. These measures reverse the widening of the QRS, PR, and QT intervals.

For life-threatening ventricular dysrhythmias, lidocaine can be used.[11] Some success has been reported with beta-blockers, but increased cardiovascular collapse has also been reported; caution is therefore advised.

Hypotension is best treated with fluid therapy and selective alpha-receptor stimulators such as phenylephrine and norepinephrine (see earlier).

Cocaine

Cocaine is a naturally occurring alkaloid, which is extracted from the South American plants *Erythroxylon coca* and *Erythroxylon novogranatense*. This potent CNS stimulant possesses great abuse potential and—with the exception of local anesthetic effects in eye, ear, nose, and throat surgery—has little medical use. Illicit cocaine comes in various forms, is cut with many different adulterants, and has various names (Table 146–19).

Cocaine is rapidly and well absorbed via oral, intranasal, and intravenous routes.[65–69] Maximal euphoric effects occur at 45 to 90 minutes, 15 to 20 minutes, and 6 to 11 minutes after oral administration, nasal insufflation, and free base smoking, respectively.[68, 70] Intravenous administration produces a similar euphoric onset as free base smoking.

Cocaine is hydrolized by plasma and liver cholinesterases to the metabolites ecgonine methyl ester and benzoylecgonine.[71–73] These metabolites make up the majority of cocaine derivatives excreted in the urine. Only a small fraction of cocaine undergoes *N*-methylation to form norcocaine. The elimination half-life of cocaine is approximately 48, 75, and 54 minutes for oral, intranasal, and intravenous administration, respectively.[65] Cocaine elimination half-life may vary between individuals depending on liver and plasma cholinesterase level. Cocaine remains detectable in urine for only 12 hours after exposure. The benzoylecgonine metabolite, however, remains detectable in urine for up to 144 hours, depending on the type of assay used, and is therefore the substance most often screened for.[67, 74, 75]

Cocaine produces sympathomimetic effects by blocking the reuptake of norepinephrine at the presynaptic nerve terminal.[77] Norepinephrine accumulates within the synaptic cleft, thus giving rise to great sympathomimetic stimulation at the postsynaptic effector site. With long-term use, CNS dopamine stores can become depleted, thus giving rise to a biochemical mechanism for both drug craving and seizure activity.[77–79] These may also be the result of pharmacologic stimulation of the limbic system.

Clinical effects after acute cocaine poisoning include (1) CNS stimulation leading to euphoria, hyperactivity, restlessness, and garrulity; (2) peripheral sympathomimetic stimulation leading to increased blood pressure and pulse rate, tachycardia, vasoconstriction, and hypertension; (3) myocardial depression with depressed conduction and contractility,

TABLE 146–19

COMMON FORMS, NAMES, AND ADULTERANTS FOR COCAINE

Forms of Illicit Use	Time to Maximal Euphoria (min)
Oral	45–90
Insufflation	15–20
Free base	6–11
Coca paste	6–11
Intravenous	6–11

Common Names

Bernice	Lady
Blow	Liquid lady (alcohol and cocaine)
C	
Cadillac	Nose candy
Champagne	Pimp's drug
Coke	Rock
Crack (free base)	She
Dama blanca	Snow
Flake	Speedball (heroin and cocaine)
Gold dust	
Green gold	Star-spangled powder
Happy trails	Toot
Her	White girl
Jam	White lady

Common Adulterants

Sugars (mannitol, lactose, glucose, inositol, maltose, sucrose)

Local anesthetics (procaine, lidocaine, tetracaine, benzocaine)

Stimulants (theophylline, strychnine, ergotamine, methylphenidate, caffeine, amphetamine)

Hallucinogens (phencyclidine, marijuana, hashish, lysergic acid diethylamide)

Opioids (codeine, heroin)

Depressants (alcohol, methapyrilene)

Anticholinergics (atropine)

Inert substances (magnesium silicate [talc], flour, cornstarch)

Miscellaneous (quinine, magnesium sulfate, thiamine, tyramine, sodium bicarbonate, salicylamide)

cardiac standstill, and ventricular dysrhythmias; (4) increased ventilation followed by respiratory depression; (5) mydriasis and cycloplegia; (6) hyperthermia from psychomotor hyperactivity, vasoconstriction, direct pyrogenic action, and/or increased calorigenic activity in the liver; (7) gastrointestinal symptoms, including nausea, vomiting, and diarrhea; and (8) anaphylactic reactions attributable to adulterants. These clinical effects develop rapidly after exposure, except in those who smuggle drugs via body packing (ingestion of cocaine-filled balloons). In the body packer, acute clinical effects appear after rupture of the container while in transit through the gastrointestinal tract. Several cases of anginal pain and myocardial infarction have been reported after cocaine use and may be the result of increased coronary artery tone or thrombogenesis.[80–84] Status epilepticus, hyperthermia, respiratory arrest, and ventricular dysrhythmias represent the most dangerous of clinical sequelae. Most cocaine-related deaths are the result of tonic-clonic seizures followed by respiratory arrest.[85]

Most patients who die of cocaine overdose do so before reaching the hospital. Treatment of cocaine overdose should begin with supportive measures. Naloxone should not be ignored (see later) in the lethargic or comatose patient, as opioids are commonly used in conjunction with cocaine. Seizures should be controlled using diazepam as the first-line agent; phenobarbital and phenytoin are not well tested in cocaine overdose. Hyperthermia with core temperatures exceeding 40.5°C (105°F) should be treated with immersion in an ice bath or cooling blankets, and vital signs should be monitored frequently. Less severe elevations of temperature should be treated by minimizing the patient's activity, placing the patient in a cool room, removing the patient's clothes, and giving tepid sponging. Hypertension may necessitate the use of sodium nitroprusside.[86] Beta-adrenergic blockers can be used for treating ventricular bigeminy and multifocal premature ventricular contractions.[87] Lidocaine should probably not be used, as it is commonly an adulterant, and it has similar action to cocaine; lidocaine may potentially worsen the condition. Hypotension may necessitate dopamine or norepinephrine infusions, as fluids often do not correct this late complication.

Body packers should be monitored by radiograph to determine the need for surgical removal.[88, 89] Bags located in the upper gastrointestinal tract indicate a need for surgical removal. Newer body packing methods have resulted in stronger bags, which do not easily deteriorate on transit through the gastrointestinal tract. If this is the case, surgery may not be warranted. All ingestions should be treated with oral activated charcoal and a cathartic to bind the drug and aid its transit through the gastrointestinal tract.

Lithium

Lithium salts have a narrow therapeutic range (0.6 to 1.5 mEq/L) and are used primarily for treating unipolar and/or bipolar affective disorders. Lithium is rapidly absorbed in the gastrointestinal tract, but absorption may be delayed for up to 72 hours in massive overdose. Distribution into tissues is slow and may take up to 10 days to equilibrate among serum, CNS, bone, and muscle; serum concentrations may not accurately reflect CNS concentrations owing to slow equilibration, thus explaining continued CNS effects even in the absence of significant serum levels. Lithium is eliminated entirely via glomerular filtration. Hyponatremia decreases elimination, whereas alkalizing the urine enhances it.[90]

Generally expected adverse effects that may appear on initiation of lithium therapy include fine motor tremor of the hands, dry mouth, increased thirst, mild polyuria, and transient mild nausea. These effects can be seen within the therapeutic range of lithium. As lithium concentration exceeds the therapeutic range, there appears to be some correlation between toxic effects and serum concentrations in most patients. Mild-to-moderate toxicity occurs when the serum lithium concentration is between 1.5 and 2.5 mEq/L and includes nausea, vomiting, diarrhea, polyuria; these lead to greater lithium toxicity resulting from sodium and water depletion—blurred vision, muscular weakness, drowsiness, dizziness, vertigo, confusion, slurred speech, scotomas, blackouts, fasciculations, and increased deep tendon reflexes. Severe toxicity occurs when serum concentration is between 2.5 and 4 mEq/L and includes myoclonus or movements of the entire limb, choreoathetoid movements, urinary and fecal incontinence, increased restlessness, stupor, coma, epileptiform seizure, and cardiac dysrhythmias including ST-T wave changes, sinoatrial block, sinus and junctional bradycardia, first-degree atrioventricular block, intraventricular conduction delay, and QT prolongation.[91–94] Potentially life-threatening toxic effects occur at serum concentrations greater than 4 mEq/L and include hypotension followed by peripheral vascular collapse. Death resulting from lithium-induced renal failure has also been reported.[95]

After acute ingestion, the onset of all aforementioned symptoms may be delayed. Similarly, blood concentration determinations may take up to a week to reflect peak levels.

Development of a therapeutic plan for treating lithium toxicity is complicated by a paucity of information regarding outcome as assessed by serum levels or clinical presentation. Unfortunately, lithium toxicity can have serious sequelae, so treatment should be aggressive. Management of acute ingestion should begin with good supportive therapy and gastric lavage, regardless of time after ingestion; activated charcoal is not effective for adsorbing lithium but may be indicated if an ingestion of multiple drugs has occurred. Establishing a sodium diuresis increases the elimination of lithium, as sodium excretion and lithium excretion are linked in the nephron. Hemodialysis effectively removes lithium from the serum and is indicated in those with lithium levels greater than 4 mEq/L, in those receiving long-term lithium therapy, and in those with serum levels between 2 and 4 mEq/L with signs of serious toxicity.[90]

Opioids

Narcotic analgesics and illicit opiate derivatives are responsible for a large number of overdose fatalities.[96, 97] A list of common opiate derivatives and their common trade or street name can be found in Table 146–20. In general, overdose with the opiate derivatives produces constricted pupils (pinpoint pupils), bradycardia, hypotension, hypothermia, pulmonary edema, respiratory depression, and coma.[98] Morphine, meperidine, and propoxyphene may also produce seizures. Propoxyphene as well as its metabolite has resulted in rapid deaths attributable to cardiac dysrhythmias.

In general, treatment of opiate overdose consists of good supportive care and administration of the opiate antagonist naloxone (Narcan).[98] In suspected opiate overdose or in any patient coming to the emergency department in a comatose or semicomatose state with miosis and respiratory depression, naloxone should be administered. Naloxone antagonizes all known opiate receptor sites (mu, kappa, sigma), and its rapid administration may be lifesaving after overdose of all the drugs listed in Table 146–20 or derivatives thereof. Higher than normal doses may be required in codeine, propoxyphene, pentazocine, methadone, and meperidine overdose. Naloxone reverses the respiratory depression, hypotension, and comatose state in opiate overdose.

Naloxone should be administered as an initial intravenous bolus of 0.4 to 2 mg in the adult (0.01 to 0.03 mg/kg in the child). This dose can be repeated every 3 to 5 minutes up to a total of 10 mg. If no response is seen after 10 mg, it is likely that opiates are not the main complicating source. If response is noted, a continuous naloxone infusion may be prepared by placing 8 mg into 1000 mL of 5% dextrose in water and infusing at a rate of 0.4 to 0.8 mg/h (50 to 100 mL/h) titrated to effect. For overdose with some agents, naloxone infusion may be required for up to 48 hours. Naloxone has an approximate duration of effect equal to 45 to 70 minutes. When discontinuing naloxone administration, frequent assessments should be made for relapsing coma and respiratory depression.

Nitroprusside

Nitroprusside is used primarily for the treatment of hypertensive emergencies and to provide controlled hypotension during anesthesia so that minimal hemorrhage occurs.[99] Nitroprusside has also been used for improving left ventricular function in refractory heart failure. The hypotensive effects of nitroprusside occur primarily via direct vasodilatory action on vascular smooth muscle, whereas improvement in left ventricular function occurs as a result of decreased afterload.

Nitroprusside contains five cyanide (CN^-) molecules within its chemical structure ($Na_2Fe(CN)_5NO$).[99] On metabolism, these molecules are released; one CN^- molecule attaches to the ferric ion of hemoglobin to produce cyanhemoglobin, and the other four molecules are taken up by tissues and red blood cells. Rhodanase enzyme, located in tissues and red blood cells, then utilizes sulfhydryl groups to convert CN^- to the less toxic form thiocyanate, which is easily excreted by the kidneys. Significant accumulation of either metabolite can result in tissue toxicity.

Cyanogenic substances rapidly penetrate tissues, bind to ferric ions of mitochondrial cytochrome oxidase, and cause inhibition of oxidative phosphorylation, which ultimately leads to respiratory paralysis and death of the cell.[100–102] Clinical toxicity from nitroprusside therapy occurs most often as a result of rapid infusions (>10 µg/kg/min) and in those with liver and renal dysfunction. In addition, it is possible that some patients may have a genetic lack of rhodanase enzyme or sulfhydryl groups, thus predisposing them to cyanide poisoning. To avoid potential toxicity, many investigators recommend that serum thiocyanate levels be maintained below 10 mg/dL.[99] However, this type of monitoring does not rule out the possibility of pure cyanide poisoning in those who lack the ability to convert cyanide to thiocyanate; one fatality has been reported to result from nitroprusside-induced cyanide poisoning, even though serum thiocyanate levels were undetectable.[104] Patients who are resistant to the hypotensive effects of nitroprusside should have administration of this drug discontinued, as resistance or tachyphylaxis may be a sign of cyanide or thiocyanate toxicity.

Cyanide toxicity affects the respiratory system in two phases.[100–102] Initially, there is increased ventilatory drive via hypoxic stimulation of the respiratory center in the medulla oblongata. This is followed by depressed respirations, owing to hypoxic nerve damage in the central respiratory center, which leads to apnea. In addition, pulmonary edema may

TABLE 146–20

COMMON NARCOTIC ANALGESICS AND ILLICIT OPIATE DRUGS

Generic Name	Common Trade or Street Name
Alphaprodine	Nisentil
Anileridine	Leritine
Butorphanol	Stadol
Buprenorphine	Buprenex
Codeine	Schoolboy, cough syrup, number 4s
Diphenoxylate	Lomotil
Fentanyl	Innovar, Sublimaze, China white
Heroin	Smack, TNT, white junk, noise, dujie, horse, stuff, junk, snow, Harry, H, crap, Mexican brown, Persian, Rufus, Dana, and others
Hydrocodone	Percodan, Pecocet, Vicodin, and others
Hydromorphone	Dilaudid
Loperamide	Imodium
L-α-Acetyl-methadol	LAAM
Morphine	M, dreamer, Ms Emma, cube juice, hard stuff, hocus, morph, morpho, unkie, and others
Meperidine	Demerol, Pethidine
Methadone	Dolly, Dolophine
Nalbuphine	Nubaine
Oxymorphone	Numorphan
Paregoric	Blue velvet
Pentazocine	Talwin, Talacen, loads, Ts and blues
Propoxyphene	Darvocet, Darvon

occur, thus causing a ventilation-perfusion mismatch. Cyanosis is an ominous sign of end-stage toxicity.

Cyanide toxicity also affects the cardiovascular system in a biphasic manner.[100–102] Flushing, hypertension with reflex bradycardia, sinus dysrhythmias, and atrioventricular nodal and/or idioventricular dysrhythmias constitute the early phase of toxicity, whereas hypotension, tachycardia, and electrical abnormalities ultimately lead to cardiovascular collapse.

Helpful laboratory variables for assessing toxicity include venous and arterial oxygen concentrations and serum lactate and serum thiocyanate levels.[99–102] Venous oxygen tension approaching that of arterial oxygen tension suggests that tissues may not be extracting oxygen for use. A rise in serum lactate levels is indicative of metabolic acidosis, which has appeared in all reported cases of cyanide toxicity from nitroprusside. Serum thiocyanate levels greater than 10 mg/dL may indicate potential toxicity; however, cyanide toxicity may ensue at even lower levels (see earlier).

Management of nitroprusside-induced cyanide toxicity begins with discontinuing the nitroprusside infusion. General treatment should include proper airway support using 100% oxygen via endotracheal tube if necessary, cardiac monitoring, and frequent checks of vital signs. Blood pressure should be supported with fluid and vasopressor therapy as required.

A Cyanide Antidote Package marketed by Eli Lilly and Co. has proved beneficial in treating cyanide poisoning; this kit should be available and used when there is a high suspicion of cyanide poisoning.[104] This kit contains 12 amyl nitrite aspirol inhalants, two 300 mg/10 mL sodium nitrite 3% ampules, and two 12.5 g/50 mL sodium thiosulfate 25% ampules. The antidote should be administered as follows:

1. Crush amyl nitrite ampules into gauze and hold gauze under the patient's nose for 30 seconds every minute until an intravenous line is established (use a new ampule every 3 minutes).
2. Administer the entire contents (300 mg/10 mL) of one sodium nitrite ampule intravenously over at least 5 minutes (the pediatric dose is 0.22 to 0.39 mL/kg, not exceeding 10 mL).
3. Administer the entire contents (12.5 g/50 mL) of one sodium thiosulfate ampule intravenously immediately after the sodium nitrite (pediatric dose is 1.1 to 1.95 mL/kg, not exceeding 50 mL).[105]

Nitrites (amyl nitrite and sodium nitrite) induce an approximate 20% methemoglobinemia (if at least 20% methemoglobinemia does not occur, one half of the original nitrite dose can be administered 30 minutes later). Cyanide then releases itself from the cytochrome oxidase enzyme and attaches to methemoglobin, for which it has greater affinity, thus producing cyanomethemoglobin. The sodium thiosulfate then supplies sulfhydryl groups to which the CN^- attaches after releasing from the methemoglobin. The end product after administration of the antidote is a thiocyanate molecule that is less toxic than cyanide and is excreted in the urine.

Methemoglobin levels should be monitored and maintained at concentrations less than 40%. Too rapid infusions of nitrites can also lead to excessive hypotension for which support may be required.[106]

Use of hyperbaric oxygen therapy is controversial in cyanide-poisoned patients but may be considered if the patient does not respond to other treatment modalities. This therapy, however, has not been proved to have additional benefit to normal oxygen therapy.[107]

Hydroxocobalamin (vitamin B_{12a}) is used in Europe for cyanide poisonings but is not yet approved for this in the United States. This vitamin interacts with CN^- to form cyanocobalamin (vitamin B_{12}). The major problem with use of this agent is that the dosage form available in the United States is much too small for clinical utility. The hydroxocobalamin dose for treating cyanide toxicity is 4 g combined with 8 g of sodium thiosulfate; in the available dosage form (10 mg/10 mL), it would require 4000 mL, or 400 vials, to treat a cyanide poisoning.

Another agent available in Europe to treat cyanide poisoning is dicobalt editate (Kelocyanor).[102, 103] This drug is a chelating agent that binds free cyanide to form cobalticyanide, a nontoxic compound. A major advantage this drug has over the nitrites is that no methemoglobinemia is produced. Disadvantages include cardiac dysrhythmias; severe hypertension, which can occur in the absence of cyanide; and anaphylactic reactions.

CONCLUSION

Well-controlled clinical trials cannot ethically be performed on human subjects to uncover the toxic effects that may result from drugs taken in massive amounts. Epidemiologic data, case reports, and retrospective data can, however, give insight into the potential for drugs to cause toxicity.

Clinical diagnosis and treatment of poisonings must be performed by utilizing clinical assessment skills in conjunction with knowledge of pharmacology, pharmacodynamics, and pharmacokinetics. With this approach, the majority of patients arriving at the hospital alive with a diagnosis of poisoning should leave the hospital alive.

References

1. Litovitz TL, Bailey KM, Schmitz BF, et al: 1990 annual report of the American Association of Poison Control Centers National Data Collection System. Am J Emerg Med 9:461, 1991.
2. Litovitz TL, Schmitz BF, Holm KC: 1988 annual report of the American Association of Poison Control Centers National Data Collection System. Am J Emerg Med 7:495, 1989.
3. Veltri K, Litovitz TL: 1983 annual report of the American Association of Poison Control Centers National Data Collection System. Am J Emerg Med 2:420, 1984.
4. Litovitz TL, Veltri JC: 1984 annual report of the American Association of Poison Control Centers National Data Collection System. Am J Emerg Med 3:423, 1985.
5. Litovitz TL, Normann SA, Veltri JC: 1985 annual report of the American Association of Poison Control Centers National Data Collection System. Am J Emerg Med 4:427, 1986.
6. Litovitz TL, Martin TG, Schmitz B: 1986 annual report of the American Association of Poison Control Centers National Data Collection System. Am J Emerg Med 5:405, 1987.
7. Litovitz TL, Schmitz BF, Matyunas N, et al: 1987 annual report of the American Association of Poison Control Centers National Data Collection System. Am J Emerg Med 6:479, 1988.
8. Ellenhorn MJ, Barceloux DG: General approach to the poisoned patient. In: Ellenhorn MJ, Barceloux DG (eds): Medical Toxicology: Diagnosis and Treatment of the Poisoned Patient. New York, Elsevier Science Publishing, p 4, 1988.
9. Opheim KE, Raisys VA: Therapeutic drug monitoring in pediatric acute drug intoxications. Ther Drug Monit 7:148, 1985.
10. Olson KR, Benowitz ML, Woo OF, et al: Theophylline overdose: Acute single ingestion versus chronic repeated overmedication. Am J Emerg Med 3:386, 1985.
11. Frommer DA, Kulig KW, Marx JA, et al: Tricyclic antidepressant overdose: A review. JAMA 257:521, 1987.
12. Nictora MB, Rivera M, Pool JL, et al: Tricyclic antidepressant overdose: Clinical and pharmacologic observations. Clin Toxicol 18:599, 1981.
13. Biggs JT, Spiker DG, Petit JM, et al: Tricyclic antidepressant overdose: Incidence of symptoms. JAMA 238:135, 1975.
14. Callaham M: Tricyclic antidepressant overdose. J Am Coll Emerg Physicians 8:413, 1979.
15. Gonzalez ER, Ornato JP, Garnett AR, et al: Dose-dependent vasopressor response to epinephrine during CPR in human beings. Ann Emerg Med 18:920, 1989.

16. Olson KR, Pentel PR, Kelley MT: Physical assessment and differential diagnosis of the poisoned patient. Med Toxicol 2:52, 1987.
17. Goldberg MJ, Spector R, Park GD, et al: An approach to the management of the poisoned patient. Arch Intern Med 146:1381, 1986.
18. Roberts JR, Quattrocchi E, Howland MA: Severe hyperthermia secondary to intravenous drug abuse. Am J Emerg Med 2:373, 1984.
19. Buckley BM, Braithwaite RA, Vale JA: Theophylline poisoning. Lancet 2:618, 1983.
20. Gaudreault P, Wason S, Lovejoy FGH: Acute pediatric theophylline overdose: A summary of 28 cases. J Pediatr 102:474, 1983.
21. Paloucek FP, Rodvold KA: Evaluation of theophylline overdoses and toxicities. Ann Emerg Med 17:135, 1988.
22. Park GD, Spector R, Roberts RJ, et al: Use of hemoperfusion for treatment of theophylline intoxication. Am J Med 74:961, 1983.
23. Bertino JS, Walker JW: Reassessment of theophylline toxicity: Serum concentrations, clinical course, and treatment. Arch Intern Med 127:757, 1987.
24. Yarnell PR, Chu N-S: Focal seizure and aminophylline. Neurology 25:819, 1975.
25. Aiken ML, Martin TR: Life-threatening theophylline toxicity is not predictable by serum levels. Chest 91:10, 1987.
26. Coupe M: Self-poisoning with sustained release aminophylline: A mechanism for observed secondary rise in serum theophylline. Hum Toxicol 5:341, 1986.
27. Connell JMC, McGeachie JF, Knepil J, et al: Self-poisoning with sustained release aminophylline: Secondary rise in serum theophylline concentration after charcoal haemoperfusion. Br Med J 284:943, 1982.
28. Sessler CN, Cohen MD: Cardiac arrhythmias during theophylline toxicity: A prospective continuous electrocardiographic study. Chest 98:672, 1990.
29. Goldberg MJ, Park GD, Berlinger WG: Treatment of theophylline intoxication. J Allergy Clin Immunol 78:811, 1986.
30. Berlinger WG, Spector R, Goldberg MJ, et al: Enhancement of theophylline clearance by oral activated charcoal. Clin Pharmacol Ther 33:351, 1983.
31. Park G, Redomski L, Goldberg M, et al: Effect of size and frequency of multiple oral charcoal doses on theophylline clearance. Clin Pharmacol Ther 34:663, 1983.
32. Winter ME, Tozer TN: Phenytoin. In: Evans WE, Schentag JJ, Jusko WS (eds): Applied Pharmacokinetics: Principles of Therapeutic Drug Monitoring. 2nd ed. Spokane, WA, Applied Therapeutics, p 493, 1986.
33. Kutt H, Winters W, Kokenge R, et al: Diphenylhydantoin metabolism, blood level, and toxicity. Arch Neurol 11:642, 1964.
34. Troupin AS, Moretti Ojemann L: Paradoxical intoxication—A complication of anticonvulsant administration. Epilepsia 16:752, 1975.
35. Chaikin P, Adir J: Unusual absorption profile of phenytoin in a massive overdose case. J Clin Pharmacol 27:70, 1987.
36. Halcomb R, Lynn R, Harvey B, et al: Intoxication with 5,5-diphenylhydantoin (Dilantin). J Pediatr 80:627, 1972.
37. Pruitt AW, Zwiren GT, Patterson JH, et al: A complex pattern of disposition of phenytoin in severe intoxication. Clin Pharmacol Ther 18:112, 1975.
38. Wilder BJ, Buchanan JRA, Cerrano EE: Correlation of acute diphenylhydantoin intoxication with plasma levels and metabolite excretion. Neurology 23:1329, 1973.
39. Albertson TE, Fisher CJ, Shragg TA, et al: A prolonged severe intoxication after ingestion of phenytoin and phenobarbital. West J Med 135:418, 1981.
40. Sharff JA, Bayer MJ: Acute and chronic digitalis toxicity: Presentation and treatment. Ann Emerg Med 11:327, 1982.
41. Ekins BR, Watanabe AS: Acute digoxin poisonings: Review of therapy. Am J Hosp Pharm 35:268, 1978.
42. Pleasants RA, Gadsden RH, McCormack JP, et al: Interference of digoxin-like immunoreactive substances with three immunoassays in patients with various degrees of renal function. Clin Pharm 5:810, 1986.
43. Smith TW, Antman EM, Friedman PL, et al: Digitalis glycosides: Mechanisms and manifestations of toxicity. Prog Cardiovasc Dis 27:21, 1984.
44. Smith TW, Willerson JT: Suicidal and accidental digoxin ingestion: Report of five cases with serum digoxin level correlations. Circulation 44:29, 1971.
45. Hobson JD, Zettner A: Digoxin serum half life following suicidal digoxin poisoning. JAMA 223:147, 1978.
46. Wenger TL, Butler VP, Haber E, et al: Treatment of 63 severely digitalis-toxic patients with digoxin-specific antibody fragments. J Am Coll Cardiol 5(suppl):118A, 1985.
47. Cole PL, Smith TW: Use of digoxin-specific Fab fragments in the treatment of digitalis intoxication. Drug Intell Clin Pharm 20:267, 1986.
48. Rumack BH, Peterson RC, Koch GG, et al: Acetaminophen overdose. Arch Intern Med 141:380, 1981.
49. Rumak BH: Acetaminophen overdose in children and adolescents. Pediatr Clin North Am 33:691, 1986.
50. Blake KV, Bailey D, Zientek GM, et al: Death of a child associated with multiple overdoses of acetaminophen. Clin Pharm 7:391, 1988.
51. Ruffalo RL, Thompson JF: Cimetidine and acetylcysteine as antidote for acetaminophen overdose. South Med J 75:954, 1982.
52. Chen MM, Lee CS: Cimetidine-acetaminophen interaction in humans. J Clin Pharmacol 25:227, 1985.
53. Mitchell MC, Schenker S, Avant GR, et al: Cimetidine protects against acetaminophen hepatotoxicity in rats. Gastroenterology 81:1052, 1981.
54. Abernethy DR, Greenblatt DJ, Divoll M, et al: Differential effect of cimetidine on drug oxidation (antipyrine and diazepam) vs. conjugation (acetaminophen and lorazepam): Prevention of acetaminophen toxicity by cimetidine. J Pharmacol Exp Ther 224:508, 1983.
55. Done AK, Temple AR: Treatment of salicylate poisoning. Mod Treat 8:528, 1971.
56. Temple AR: Acute and chronic effects of aspirin toxicity and their treatment. Arch Intern Med 141:364, 1981.
57. Van Brunt N: The clinical utility of tricyclic antidepressant blood levels: A review of the literature. Ther Drug Monit 5:1, 1983.
58. Perry PJ, Pfohl BM, Hostad SG: The relationship between antidepressant response and tricyclic antidepressant plasma concentrations: A retrospective analysis of the literature using logistic regression analysis. Clin Pharmacokinet 13:381, 1987.
59. Boehnert MT, Lovejoy FH: Value of the QRS duration versus the serum drug level in predicting seizures and ventricular arrhythmias after an acute overdose of tricyclic antidepressants. N Engl J Med 313:474, 1985.
60. Bessen H, Niemann JT, Rothstein RJ, et al: Electrocardiographic criteria for tricyclic antidepressant cardiotoxicity, abstracted. Ann Emerg Med 16:650, 1986.
61. Hermann HC, Kaplan LM, Bierer BE: QT prolongation and torsade de pointes ventricular tachycardia produced by the antidepressant agent maprotiline. Am J Cardiol 51:904, 1983.
62. Brown TCK, Barker GA, Dunlop ME, et al: The use of sodium bicarbonate in the treatment of tricyclic antidepressant–induced arrhythmias. Anaesth Intensive Care 1:203, 1973.
63. Molloy DW, Penner SB, Rabson J, et al: Use of sodium bicarbonate to treat tricyclic antidepressant–induced arrhythmias in a patient with alkalosis. Can Med Assoc J 130:1457, 1984.
64. Hoffman JR, McElroy CR: Bicarbonate therapy for dysrhythmia and hypotension in tricyclic antidepressant overdose. West J Med 134:60, 1981.
65. Wilkinson P, Van Dyke C, Jatlow P, et al: Intranasal and oral cocaine kinetics. Clin Pharmacol Ther 27:386, 1980.
66. Van Dyke C, Barash PG, Jatlow P, et al: Cocaine: Plasma concentrations after intranasal application in man. Science 191:859, 1976.
67. Hamilton HE, Wallace JE, Shimak EL, et al: Cocaine and benzoylecgonine excretion in humans. J Forensic Sci 22:697, 1977.
68. Van Dyke C, Jatlow P, Ungerer CJ, et al: Oral cocaine: Plasma concentrations and central effects. Science 200:211, 1978.
69. Perez-Reyes M, Diguiseppi S, Ondrusek G, et al: Free base cocaine smoking. Clin Pharmacol Ther 32:459, 1982.
70. Javaid JI, Fischman MW, Schuster CR, et al: Cocaine plasma concentrations. Relation of physiological subjective effects in humans. Science 202:227, 1978.
71. Misra AL, Nayak PK, Block R, et al: Estimation and disposition of (^{3}H)-I-benzoylecgonine and pharmacological activity of some metabolites. J Pharm Pharmacol 27:784, 1975.
72. Stewart DJ, Inaba T, Tang BK, et al: Hydrolysis of cocaine in human plasma by cholinesterases. Life Sci 20:1557, 1977.
73. Inaba T, Stewart DJ, Kalow W: Metabolism of cocaine in man. Clin Pharmacol Ther 23:547, 1978.
74. Wallace JE, Hamilton HE, Christenson JG, et al: An evaluation of selected methods for determining cocaine and benzoylecgonine in urine. J Anal Toxicol 1:20, 1977.
75. Budd RD, Mathis DF, Yang FC: TLC analysis of urine for benzoylecgonine and norpropoxyphene. Clin Toxicol 16:1, 1980.
76. Ellenhorn MJ, Barceloux DG: Cocaine. In: Ellenhorn MJ, Barceloux DG (eds): Medical Toxicology: Diagnosis and Treatment of the Poisoned Patient. New York, Elsevier Science Publishing, p 644, 1988.
77. Wise RA: Action of drugs of abuse on brain reward systems. Pharmacol Biochem Behav 13(suppl):213, 1980.
78. Gold MS, Dackis CA: New insights and treatments: Opiate withdrawal and cocaine addiction. Clin Ther 7:6, 1984.
79. Post RM, Kopandra RT: Cocaine, kindling and reverse tolerance. Lancet 1:409, 1975.
80. Coleman DL, Ross TF, Naughton JL: Myocardial ischemia and infarction related to recreational use of cocaine. West J Med 136:444, 1982.
81. Schachne JS, Roberts BH, Thompson PD: Coronary artery spasm and myocardial infarction associated with cocaine use. N Engl J Med 310:1665, 1984.
82. Howard RE, Hueter DC, Davis GJ: Acute myocardial infarction following cocaine abuse in a young woman with normal coronary arteries. JAMA 254:95, 1985.
83. Cregler LL, Mark H: Relation of acute myocardial infarction to cocaine abuse. Am J Cardiol 56:794, 1985.
84. Gould L, Gopalaswamy C, Patel C, et al: Cocaine-induced myocardial infarction. NY State J Med 85:660, 1985.
85. Finkle DS, McCloskey KL: The forensic toxicology of cocaine (1971–1976). J Forensic Sci 23:173, 1978.
86. Ramoska E, Sacchetti AD: Propranolol-induced hypertension in treatment of cocaine intoxication. Ann Emerg Med 14:1112, 1985.

87. Rappolt RT, Gay GR, Soman M, et al: Treatment plan for acute and chronic adrenergic poisoning crisis utilizing sympatholytic effects of the beta$_1$-beta$_2$ receptor site blocker propranolol (Inderal) in concert with diazepam and urine acidification. Clin Toxicol 14:55, 1979.

88. McCarron MM, Wood JD: The cocaine 'body packer' syndrome. JAMA 250:1417, 1983.

89. Carvana DS, Weinbach B, George D, et al: Cocaine packet ingestion. Diagnosis, management and natural history. Ann Intern Med 100:73, 1984.

90. Ellenhorn MJ, Barceloux DG: Lithium. In: Ellenhorn MJ, Barceloux DG (eds): Medical Toxicology: Diagnosis and Treatment of the Poisoned Patient. New York, Elsevier Science Publishing, p 1042, 1988.

91. Hall NC, Perl M, Pfefferbaum B: Lithium therapy and toxicity. Am Fam Pract 19:133, 1979.

92. Wilson JR, Kraus ES, Bailas MM, et al: Reversible sinus node abnormalities due to lithium carbonate therapy. N Engl J Med 294:1223, 1976.

93. Fenves AZ, Emmett M, White MG: Lithium intoxication associated with acute renal failure. South Med J 77:1472, 1984.

94. Mateer JR, Clark NR: Lithium toxicity with rarely reported ECG manifestations. JAMA 251:1680, 1984.

95. Rutherford RS, Klein-Schwartz W, Oderda GM, et al: Lithium intoxication with acute renal failure and death. Drug Intell Clin Pharm 22:691, 1988.

96. Ellenhorn MJ, Barceloux DG: Opiate, opioids, and designer drugs. In: Ellenhorn MJ, Barceloux DG (eds): Medical Toxicology: Diagnosis and Treatment of the Poisoned Patient. New York: Elsevier Science Publishing, p 689, 1988.

97. Hine CH, Wright JA, Allison DJ, et al: Analysis of fatalities from acute narcotism in a major urban area. J Forensic Sci 27:372, 1982.

98. Ellenhorn MJ, Barceloux DG: Opioid antagonists. In: Ellenhorn MJ, Barceloux DG (eds): Medical Toxicology: Diagnosis and Treatment of the Poisoned Patient. New York, Elsevier Science Publishing, p 752, 1988.

99. Greiss L, Tremblay NAG, Davies DW: The toxicity of sodium nitroprusside. Can Anaesth Soc J 23:480, 1976.

100. Holland M, Kozlowoski L: Clinical features and management of cyanide poisoning. Clin Pharm 5:737, 1986.

101. Hall A, Rumack B: Clinical toxicology of cyanide. Ann Emerg Med 15:1067, 1986.

102. Ellenhorn MJ, Barceloux DG: Cyanide. In: Ellenhorn MJ, Barceloux DG (eds): Medical Toxicology: Diagnosis and Treatment of the Poisoned Patient. New York, Elsevier Science Publishing, p 78, 1988.

103. Davies DW, Kadar D, Steward DJ, et al: A sudden death associated with the use of sodium nitroprusside for induction of hypotension during anaesthesia. Can Anesth Soc J 22:547, 1975.

104. Chen K, Rose C, Clowes G: Methylene blue, nitrites and sodium thiosulfate against cyanide poisoning. Proc Soc Exp Biol Med 31:250, 1933.

105. PoisIndex. Denver, CO, Micromedex, June 1990–August 1990 update.

106. Vogel S, Sultan T, Ten Eyck R: Cyanide poisoning. Clin Toxicol 18:367, 1981.

107. Kizer K: Hyperbaric oxygen and cyanide poisoning. Am J Emerg Med 2:113, 1984.

Methanol, Ethylene Glycol, and Related Intoxications

James A. Kruse

Although not among the most commonly encountered poisonings, methanol and ethylene glycol intoxications are not rare. Uncovering these diagnoses is sometimes straightforward but at other times elusive. Timely recognition allows institution of specific therapeutic measures and, in many cases, may mitigate the potential for morbidity and mortality.

METHANOL POISONING

Methanol, also known as methyl alcohol or wood alcohol, is a volatile liquid with a mild odor that resembles that of ethanol. It has a broad range of commercial and industrial uses as a solvent and a synthetic precursor, and methanol-containing products are widely available (Table 146–21).

The lethal dose is frequently cited as approximately 100 mL but is highly variable, reportedly ranging from less than 10 mL to more than 500 mL.[1-9] In one early review, the mortality rate associated with methanol ingestion was more than 50%, and nearly 30% of the surviving patients experienced blindness during the acute phase of poisoning.[10] Methanol-induced blindness has been widely reported and has occurred after ingestion of as little as 4 mL.[11] The majority of patients who survive regain most or all of their visual acuity, although permanent sight impairment may occur.[12] A syndrome akin to parkinsonism has also been described among survivors.[13-15]

Methanol intoxication may result from either intentional or accidental ingestion. Intentional consumption often occurs in alcoholics who have access to a methanol-containing product and ingest it as a substitute for ethanol. Large epidemics, sometimes involving hundreds of individuals and dozens of fatalities, have been reported after widespread distribution of illicit alcoholic beverages made from methanol.[2, 4, 16-20]

Methanol is metabolized to formaldehyde and formic acid (Fig. 146–4). Although the alcohol itself is relatively innocuous,[11, 21] its metabolites are highly toxic and interfere with mitochondrial respiration.[6, 22-25] The ocular toxicity can be directly attributable to formic acid.[22, 26] It has been demonstrated that animals injected with formic acid have optic nerve damage.[27] The slow metabolic conversion of methanol to formic acid results in a time lag between ingestion and development of toxicity, typically ranging from 12 to 24 hours.[1, 2, 6, 7, 21, 22, 28-30] The poisoned patient may appear inebriated but otherwise normal during this interval. Although the odor of methanol may be detectable on the patient's breath, it is sufficiently mild that it may go unnoticed or be confused with the odor of ethanol. It is also masked if the patient has ingested ethanol in addition to methanol. A variety of ocular symptoms have been reported, including blurred vision, scintillations, and partial or complete loss of sight. Unreactive pupils, scotomas, and papilledema may be noted on physical examination.[2, 18, 19, 31] Vomiting, epigastric pain, and gastritis frequently occur and pancreatitis has also been described.[2, 4, 18, 32] Meningeal signs, convulsions, and coma may occur.[2, 6] Infarction of the basal

TABLE 146–21
COMMON COMMERCIAL PRODUCTS THAT MAY CONTAIN METHANOL

Denatured alcohol	Furniture refinishers
Windshield washer fluids	Dry gas
Windshield deicers	Some gasolines (gasohol)
Sterno (canned heat)	Dyes
Antifreeze	Duplicating fluids
Paints	Carburetor cleaners
Wood stains	Adhesives
Paint removers	Glass cleaners
Shellacs	Dewaxing preparations
Varnishes	Pipe sweetener
Lacquer thinners	Embalming fluids
Paint thinners	Various other solvents and cleaners

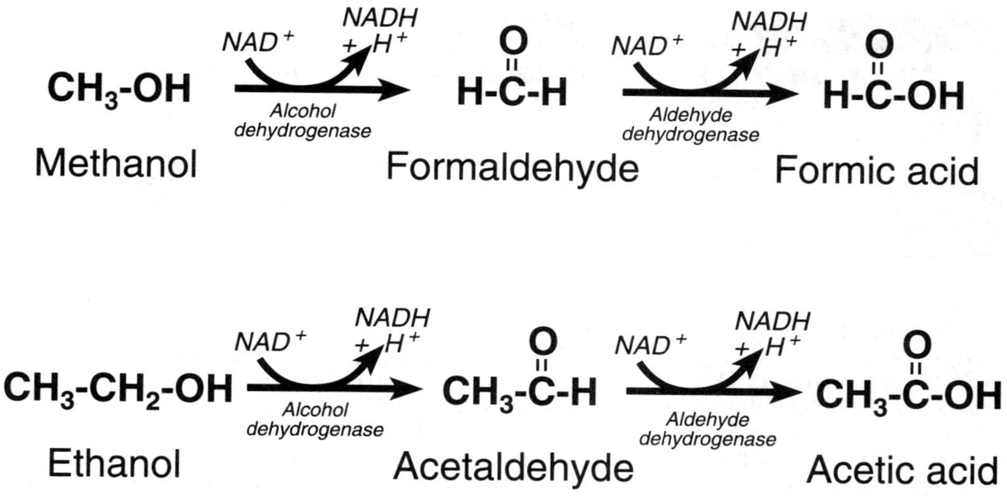

Figure 146–4. Metabolism of methanol *(top)* and ethanol *(bottom).* Note that because the two alcohols are metabolized by the same enzymes they can act as competitive substrates.

ganglia can also occur and may be visualized by computed tomography of the brain.[6, 13, 14, 33–36]

The production of formic acid results in metabolic acidosis.[22, 23, 28, 30, 37] The serum anion gap is increased owing to the accumulation of formate anions. In cases of severe poisoning, the acidosis can be profound and the anion gap correspondingly high. Because methanol and its metabolites are of low molecular weight and may be present in high concentration, serum osmolality may be strikingly increased. Normally serum osmolality is slightly higher than osmolality estimated from blood urea nitrogen (BUN) and serum glucose (in milligrams per deciliter) and serum sodium (Na$^+$) (measured in millimoles per liter) by the following formula:[38, 39]

$$\text{Calculated osmolality} = 2 \times [\text{Na}^+] + \frac{[\text{BUN}]}{2.8} + \frac{[\text{glucose}]}{18}$$

In methanol poisoning the measured osmolality is often strikingly higher than calculated osmolality. This discrepancy, known as the *osmole gap*, can be represented as the following:[38, 40–42]

Osmole gap = measured osmolality − calculated osmolality

The normal osmole gap is less than about 10 to 15 mOsm/kg. Although any toxic solute theoretically raises the osmole gap, only low-molecular-weight substances present in relatively high concentration have a measurable effect on this value. Ethanol intoxication is the most common cause of an increased osmole gap.[43] The serum ethanol concentration should therefore be assessed before ascribing an elevated osmole gap to methanol poisoning. When ethanol is present, its effect on the osmole gap can be taken into account by dividing its serum concentration (expressed in milligrams per deciliter) by 4.6 and subtracting this quotient from the osmole gap. If the osmole gap remains abnormally high, the presence of an additional toxic solute is suggested. Methanol, isopropanol, and ethylene glycol are the only common toxic solutes fulfilling the above criteria. A few other low-molecular-weight hydrocarbons may also be associated with an abnormal osmole gap, including acetone, trichloroethane, and diethyl ether, but these poisonings are comparatively rare.[42, 44] The osmole gap may also be increased in patients with severe hypoperfusion. The cause of this increase has not been fully elucidated, but it has been observed in both animal experiments and clinical cases of circulatory shock.[39, 45–48] Small increases in the osmole gap have also

been described infrequently in some patients with hyperosmolar nonketotic coma, diabetic and alcoholic ketoacidosis, and renal failure.[39, 49–51]

In using the osmole gap to detect methanol poisoning, the measured serum osmolality must be determined by the freezing point depression method.[40, 52, 53] Some clinical laboratories employ instruments that use the dew point or vapor pressure techniques. With these methods, volatile solutes result in a falsely lowered value for osmolality, obscuring the utility of the osmole gap.[41, 54–56]

The diagnosis of methanol intoxication is straightforward when an accurate history is available. In some cases, often attributable to the patient's altered sensorium and inability to give a reliable history, the diagnosis is not obvious. Except perhaps for certain of the ocular manifestations, most of the physical findings seen in methanol poisoning are rather nonspecific. Although serum assays for methanol are diagnostic, this test may not be promptly available in all institutions. Unless it can be ensured that this test result is immediately obtainable, it is necessary to make a presumptive diagnosis and initiate treatment pending quantitative blood levels. Because both the anion gap and the osmole gap are readily available and easily calculated at the bedside, they serve as important diagnostic tools in cases of suspected methanol poisoning. Examining these markers in all cases of otherwise unexplained metabolic acidosis allows early recognition of occult methanol intoxication and enables the clinician to begin specific therapy promptly.

ETHYLENE GLYCOL POISONING

Ethylene glycol is a clear, colorless, viscous liquid that is essentially odorless and has a sweet taste. It is used industrially as a solvent and antifreeze and as a synthetic precursor (e.g., in the production of synthetic fibers and plastics). It is also used in a variety of products that may be found in the home (Table 146–22), but in this setting it is most widely available as automotive antifreeze. The lethal human dose is generally estimated at 1 to 2 mg/kg, but fatal intoxication has reportedly occurred at much lower doses.[5, 7, 11, 20, 44, 57–69] Although the renal failure caused by this substance is usually reversible, permanent renal failure has occurred.[59, 62, 70, 71] Some survivors have also sustained permanent CNS damage.[71, 72]

In common with methanol, ethylene glycol itself appears rather nontoxic and its metabolites are responsible for the toxicity.[59, 68, 69, 73–75] Ethylene glycol is metabolized to several

TABLE 146–22

COMMON COMMERCIAL PRODUCTS THAT MAY CONTAIN ETHYLENE GLYCOL

"Permanent" antifreeze	Inks
Paints	Cosmetics
Lacquers	Hydraulic brake fluids
Polishes	Solar collector fluids
Detergents	Car wash fluids

aldehydes including glycoaldehyde and glyoxal and several carboxylic acids, including glycolic, glyoxylic, and oxalic acid[59, 76] (Fig. 146–5). These intermediates inhibit cellular respiration, protein synthesis, and nucleic acid replication.[77–83] Oxalic acid may crystallize as calcium oxalate within many tissues and organs, including the brain, the heart, the liver, and the kidney[20, 44, 59, 71, 84–87] and can result in sufficient sequestration of calcium to cause hypocalcemia. Although formerly attributed to oxalic acid, most of the acidosis is now known to be due to accumulation of glycolic acid.[59, 71, 74, 76, 88–90] The corresponding anion, glycolate, is responsible for the increased anion gap that is characteristically seen.

The initial phase may start within 30 minutes of ingestion and manifests as confusion and lethargy and may progress to coma and/or seizures.[44, 67, 87, 91–93] Ocular manifestations have infrequently been described in ethylene glycol poisoning and are not characteristic. After approximately 12 hours, the patient typically has signs of pulmonary edema, which may lead to respiratory failure requiring mechanical ventilation.[44, 59, 94] The pulmonary edema may be cardiogenic or noncardiogenic. Circulatory shock is not infrequent and severely poisoned patients may succumb at this stage. The final stage is heralded by the development of acute renal failure, usually occurring between 1 and 3 days of the ingestion.[59] Originally attributed to precipitation of oxalate crystals within the renal tubules, this form of acute tubular necrosis is more likely caused by the direct toxic effects of other intermediates (e.g., glycolic and glyoxylic acids).[64, 73, 76, 89, 95–97]

When the history is inadequate, laboratory findings are critical to identifying this intoxication. Ethylene glycol assays are not routinely available in many hospital laboratories. Therefore, a presumptive diagnosis and initiation of treatment are frequently based on demonstrating a high-anion-gap metabolic acidosis in conjunction with an increased osmole gap, findings that are essentially identical with those seen in methanol ingestions.[3, 44, 98] The excretion of large amounts of calcium oxalate leads to microscopic crystalluria, a finding not observed in methanol poisoning. Although not universally present in ethylene glycol poisoning, the appearance of characteristic octahedral crystals on urinalysis can be a helpful diagnostic clue in cases of occult poisoning. Calcium oxalate can also appear in a variety of other crystal configurations, so any type crystalluria should be construed as possible corroborating evidence, unless the crystals can be positively identified.[44, 60, 99] Hippuric acid crystals have also been described, but it is likely that other forms of calcium oxalate were mistakenly identified as hippurate in many of these cases.[60, 66, 89, 99–104] It is worth emphasizing that oxalate crystalluria is not always present, even in confirmed cases of ethylene glycol poisoning, and their absence does not rule out this diagnosis.[44, 61, 64, 67, 87, 98, 105]

Because pure ethylene glycol is nearly odorless, another clue is provided by patients who appear inebriated but have no odor of ethanol on their breath. However, the converse finding does not rule out ethylene glycol ingestion because ethanol is not infrequently consumed along with the ethylene glycol. A final clue may be observed by exposing the patient's urine to ultraviolet light. Fluorescein dyes are added to many (but not all) automotive antifreeze solutions to facilitate locating cooling system leaks, and this yellow-green substance brightly fluoresces under ultraviolet light.[11, 106]

TREATMENT OF METHANOL AND ETHYLENE GLYCOL POISONING

Treatment of methanol and ethylene glycol poisoning consists of general supportive care common to that of all poisoned patients, and specific measures to delay the metabolism of the compounds, increase the metabolism of their toxic by-products, correct the metabolic acidosis, and hasten elimination of both the parent compounds and their metabolites. Initial general measures include ensuring that ventilation and circulation are adequate, establishing intravenous access, administering glucose and thiamine if the sensorium is abnormal and the etiology still unclear, and performing gastric lavage.[3, 18] Syrup of ipecac is hazardous because the patient's level of consciousness may be depressed or become depressed after emesis is induced, risking aspiration pneumonitis. Activated charcoal is frequently recommended, although its efficacy is controversial.[11, 69, 107–111] If significant metabolic acidosis is present, sodium bicarbonate should be given to partially correct the acidemia.[1, 2, 4, 12, 112] This may have a favorable effect on symptoms[2, 113–116] including the ocular manifestations in the case of methanol poisoning. In

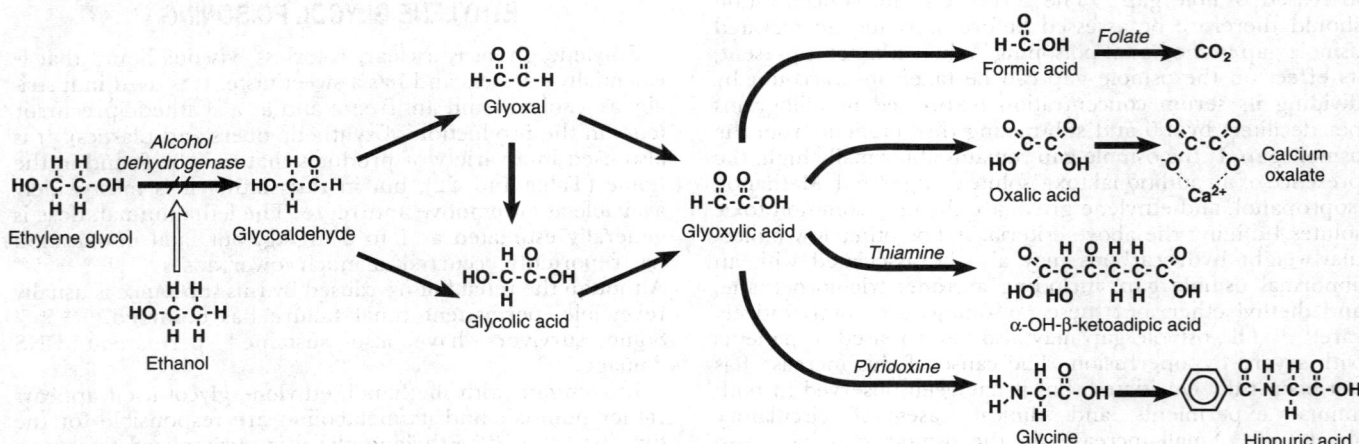

Figure 146–5. Metabolism of ethylene glycol. "Broken" arrow depicts competitive inhibition of alcohol dehydrogenase by ethanol.

ethylene glycol poisoning, it has been shown to favorably affect survival in laboratory animals.[117]

Because the metabolites of methanol and ethylene glycol rather than the parent compounds are toxic, delaying their breakdown should facilitate excretion instead of metabolic conversion and thereby mitigate toxicity. To accomplish this, ethanol is administered to competitively inhibit the enzyme alcohol dehydrogenase, which catalyzes the initial catabolic reaction of ethanol, methanol, and ethylene glycol.[118–120] Laboratory investigations have demonstrated the effectiveness of ethanol at reducing the mortality of rats poisoned with ethylene glycol.[117] Ethanol therapy should be instituted in all methanol-poisoned patients with either ocular manifestations or metabolic acidosis. If a serum methanol concentration is immediately available, treatment with ethanol should be started in all patients with levels greater than 20 mg/dL, even if asymptomatic and free of acidosis. The same applies to ethylene glycol. The serum methanol concentration ([MeOH]), in units of milligrams per deciliter, may be estimated from the serum glucose, ethanol (EtOH), and BUN levels (also in milligrams per deciliter) and the serum sodium (in millimoles per liter) and measured serum osmolality (Osm$_s$), by the formula

$$[MeOH] = 3.2 \times$$

$$\left(Osm_s - 2 \times [Na^+] - \frac{[BUN]}{2.8} - \frac{[glucose]}{18} - \frac{[EtOH]}{4.6} - 10 \right)$$

In ethylene glycol intoxication, the factor 6.2 is substituted for the factor 3.2 in this equation.

A loading dose of ethanol, consisting of 600 mg/kg, is administered and followed by a maintenance regimen. The maintenance dose varies with the patient's underlying degree of tolerance to ethanol. For patients who are not long-term ethanol consumers, a typical maintenance dose is approximately 100 mg/kg/h.[119, 121, 122] Higher maintenance doses, typically ranging from 150 to 200 mg/kg/h, are frequently required in chronic alcoholics who metabolize ethanol at higher than normal rates.[119, 121, 122]

Ethanol can be administered enterally (by mouth or nasogastric tube) or parenterally by intravenous infusion. Commercially available whiskey can be used for enteral administration. For example, 80 proof whiskey contains 40% ethanol by volume, or 31.7 g/dL. The drawback to enteral administration is that many individuals do not tolerate these doses of ethanol, and vomiting may occur. This can be minimized but not necessarily prevented by diluting the ethanol as much as is practical. Intravenous administration may be preferable, particularly because many patients have a depressed sensorium (if not before ethanol administration then after) and thus are at increased risk for aspiration if emesis occurs.

Sterile ethanol for parenteral administration is available in 5 and 10% (volume/volume) solutions containing 3.9 and 7.9 g/dL, respectively. The 10% solution is generally recommended because of the relatively large volumes that are required. These solutions are hyperosmolar and should therefore be routinely administered by central venous catheter.[18] The goal is rapidly to achieve and maintain a serum ethanol level of 100 to 150 mg/dL to ensure a maximal yet safe degree of enzyme inhibition.[1, 3, 59, 69, 119, 121–123] Because some patients have also ingested ethanol, it is important to determine the serum ethanol concentration before initiating this treatment and, if necessary, adjust the loading dose accordingly. Serum ethanol levels should be repeated hourly to confirm the adequacy of the dosing and provide feedback for titrating the maintenance infusion to achieve a stable target serum level. This task is frequently difficult, especially in patients who are chronic drinkers.

The experimental compound 4-methylpyrazole has been shown to competitively inhibit alcohol dehydrogenase in vitro and in vivo.[124–130] This agent has been used to treat methanol and ethylene glycol intoxication in animal models and given investigationally in patients, and it will likely prove useful as a therapeutic alternative to ethanol.[58, 76, 88, 90, 95, 131]

Alkaline diuresis is probably not helpful in methanol poisoning, although it may be of minor utility in some cases of ethylene glycol poisoning until dialysis can be instituted.[58, 92] Hemodialysis facilitates removal of methanol, ethylene glycol, and their metabolites and is probably indicated in all patients with serum levels greater than 50 mg/dL.[5, 11, 22, 28, 67, 69, 75, 85, 89, 107, 115, 119, 120, 132–136] It should be used in all methanol-poisoned patients with ocular symptoms, and in all methanol- and ethylene glycol–poisoned patients with significant metabolic acidosis. Note that the serum levels of these solvents may underestimate the degree of intoxication if the patient presents many hours following ingestion. In this situation much of the solvent may have already been converted to its acid metabolites. Consideration for dialysis should therefore be entertained when there is an elevated anion gap along with significant metabolic acidosis, even though the serum methanol or ethylene glycol concentration is below 50 mg/dL. In patients with renal insufficiency, whether pre-existing or attributable to the acute effects of ethylene glycol, dialysis is of critical importance because normal urinary elimination of the toxins is impaired, thus increasing the propensity for toxicity. Peritoneal dialysis also eliminates the toxins and facilitates correction of the fluid and acid-base imbalances but is substantially slower than hemodialysis.[11, 71, 92, 120, 132, 137] Nevertheless, it should be used if hemodialysis is unavailable. Hemoperfusion, on the other hand, should not be employed because it is less effective at removing these toxins, and furthermore it does not assist with correction of the metabolic acidosis.[11, 92, 109] The ethanol maintenance infusion rate should be increased during dialysis because ethanol is removed in addition to the methanol or ethylene glycol. Typically, the infusion rate needs to be doubled or even tripled to maintain the target serum concentration.[69, 119–122, 132, 133] Ethanol titration is thus particularly difficult during and immediately after dialysis.

In animal models, folic acid has been shown to be an important cofactor necessary for the metabolism of formic acid to carbon dioxide.[29, 138, 139] Its utility in clinical methanol poisoning is unproved, but because it may be efficacious, either folic or folinic acid should be administered at doses of 50 to 100 mg every 4 hours.[3, 11, 28, 69] The toxic effects of formic acid may be mitigated if folate actually does increase the rate of conversion of formic acid to carbon dioxide in humans. There is some evidence that minor amounts of formic acid may be generated in ethylene glycol intoxication from the breakdown of glyoxylic acid (see Fig. 146–5). Thus, folic acid may be given in this poisoning as well. Minor fractions of glyoxylic acid are also converted to glycine and α-hydroxy-β-ketoadipic acid.[44, 59, 92, 97, 99, 101] Because these pathways require pyridoxine and thiamine as cofactors, administration of these vitamins might be of some, albeit probably limited, therapeutic value in ethylene glycol poisoning. Although some authors have advocated calcium administration as a means of sequestering oxalic acid, it is not clear whether this is beneficial or harmful. Therapeutic calcium administration should probably be limited to cases of symptomatic hypocalcemia.[3, 11, 44, 140]

POISONING WITH SELECTED OTHER AGENTS

The number of organic solvents and other liquid hydrocarbons is extremely large. A few selected agents that have caused clinical poisonings and that share certain properties

---

TABLE 146–23

IMPORTANT CLINICAL FINDINGS IN TOXIC ALCOHOL AND RELATED POISONINGS*

Agent	Breath Odor†	Metabolic Acidosis	Increased Anion Gap	Increased Osmole Gap	Serum Acetone	Urine Crystals
Methanol	±	+	+	+	−	−
Ethylene glycol	−	+	+	+	−	±
Isopropanol	+	−	−	+	+	−
Acetone	+	−	−	+	+	−
Paraldehyde	+	+	+	−	±	−
Propylene glycol	−	+	+	+	−	−
Toluene	+	+	±	−	−	±

*+ = characteristically present; − = characteristically absent; ± = sometimes present.
†Concomitant ethanol intoxication may be present and cause breath odor in glycol intoxication, or mask the characteristic odor of the toxic ingestant in other poisonings.

in common with methanol and ethylene glycol are briefly described here. Table 146–23 compares certain key clinical features that may be helpful in differentiating these forms of intoxication.

Isopropanol

Isopropanol (isopropyl alcohol, 2-propanol) is a clear, colorless, three-carbon alcohol with a distinctive odor and a bittersweet, burning taste. It is most widely known for its use as rubbing alcohol but is also a common constituent of many readily available commercial products that can be found in the home (Table 146–24). It has been ingested accidentally and intentionally, the latter frequently representing use as an alcohol substitute and in suicide attempts. Although toxic blood concentrations have resulted from extensive topical application, this may have been related more to inhalation than to cutaneous absorption.[11, 141–143] Toxicity has also been reported after rectal administration as an enema.[144, 145] Although as little as 10 to 20 mL of pure isopropanol has been associated with symptoms,[69, 146, 147] survival has been reported after consumption of as much as 1 L of rubbing alcohol.[148] Ingestion of 16 oz has been associated with both death and survival.[142, 149, 150] In general, it is less toxic than either methanol or ethylene glycol.[151] Its chief clinical manifestations are neurologic and hemodynamic. Among its CNS effects are confusion, dizziness, slurred speech, headache, miosis, ataxia, lethargy, stupor, and coma. Gastrointestinal symptoms include nausea, vomiting, abdominal pain, hemorrhagic gastritis, and diarrhea. Other manifestations include flushing, hypotension, bradycardia, pulmonary edema, respiratory failure, renal dysfunction,

myopathy, rhabdomyolysis, hypothermia, and hemolysis.[142, 150, 152, 153] A greater degree of inebriation and more severe gastric symptoms are seen with isopropanol ingestion compared with that of a similar quantity of ethanol.

Isopropanol is metabolized in the liver to acetone, which represents the only important metabolic by-product of the alcohol (Fig. 146–6). The alcohol and acetone are slowly eliminated by the kidney and the lungs. Because the parent compound and its metabolite are not acids, metabolic acidosis is not characteristic of this intoxication. Neither is the anion gap elevated because both are uncharged molecules. However, a high-anion-gap acidosis may be seen in cases in which significant hemodynamic derangement occurs, leading to hypoperfusion and lactic acidosis from tissue hypoxia. As the alcohol is metabolized to acetone, the serum ketone assay becomes strongly positive. In a study of healthy volunteers consuming subtoxic amounts of isopropanol, both serum isopropanol and acetone were detectable within 30 minutes after ingestion.[154] However, other reports indicate that serum acetone levels may not be measurable until several hours after ingestion.[155] Spurious elevation of serum creatinine levels may occur because acetone interferes with the colorimetric assay for creatinine employed by certain autoanalyzers.[156] Because isopropanol has a low molecular weight and relatively low toxicity, serum osmolality and the osmole gap may be increased. Thus, in the appropriate setting, an elevated osmole gap (not attributable to ethanol) accompanied by ketosis, normal acid-base status, and a normal anion gap strongly suggests isopropanol poisoning. The odor of acetone and/or isopropanol may be detectable on the patient's breath.

Isopropanol can be quantitatively assayed by gas-liquid chromatography. This method is preferable to enzymatic assays utilizing alcohol dehydrogenase because the latter do not differentiate between ethanol and isopropanol.[157] Blood concentrations greater than 400 mg/dL are generally associated with severe intoxication manifested by coma and hypotension,[153] but coma has occurred at concentrations of

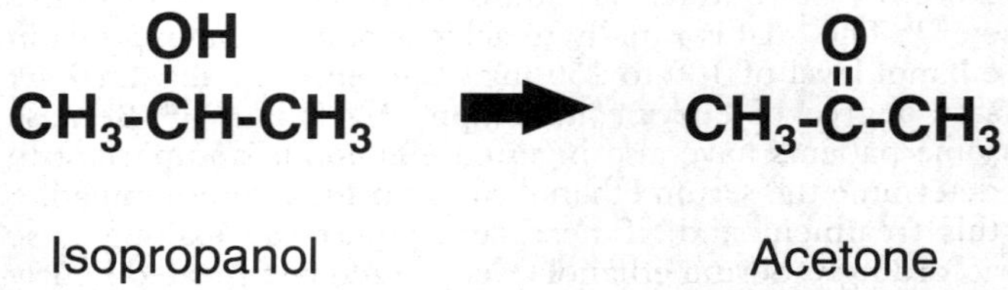

TABLE 146–24

COMMON COMMERCIAL PRODUCTS THAT MAY CONTAIN ISOPROPANOL

Rubbing alcohol	Mouthwash
Alcohol sponges	Adhesives
Antiseptics, disinfectants	Aerosol products
Pharmaceuticals	Dog and cat repellents
Hair tonics	Rust preventives
Permanent wave preparations	Acne remedies
Skin lotions, liniments	Cosmetics
Perfumes, aftershave	Rug and upholstery cleaners
Window cleaners	Jewelry cleaners
Liquid detergents	Frost removers
Dyes	Antifreeze
Lacquers	Gasket cements
Paint removers	Radiator stopleak
Windshield deicers	Stain, spot, and rust removers

$$\underset{\text{Isopropanol}}{CH_3\text{-}\overset{\displaystyle OH}{\underset{|}{C}H\text{-}CH_3}} \quad \longrightarrow \quad \underset{\text{Acetone}}{CH_3\text{-}\overset{\displaystyle O}{\overset{\|}{C}}\text{-}CH_3}$$

Figure 146–6. Metabolism of isopropanol to acetone. Note that the parent compound and its metabolite are neither acids nor anions and isopropanol therefore does not per se cause metabolic acidosis or an increased anion gap.

approximately 120 mg/dL.[142, 158, 159] Treatment is mainly supportive. Syrup of ipecac should not be given because the patient is at risk for sensorial depression. Gastric lavage has reportedly been effective even when there has been a significant delay between ingestion and presentation.[160] This might be explained by enterohepatic recirculation of the alcohol via salivary and gastric secretion, and it suggests that continuous nasogastric aspiration might be of therapeutic benefit.[161] Activated charcoal is given, although its efficacy is doubtful.[69, 107] Endotracheal intubation, mechanical ventilation, hemodynamic monitoring, and vasoactive pharmacotherapy may be required. Hemodialysis and peritoneal dialysis have been recommended in severe poisonings, particularly those associated with hypotension.[11, 75, 142, 153, 158, 162] Peritoneal dialysis is less effective.[142] High serum levels (e.g., 400 mg/dL or more) and coma have also been cited as indications for dialysis, but more specific criteria remain controversial.[69, 107]

Acetone

Acetone (dimethyl ketone, 2-propanone) is a volatile and highly flammable liquid with a characteristic odor. It is used in a variety of commercial and industrial solvents and in chemical synthesis. It is most well known as the main component of many nail polish remover products. Acetone is much less toxic than methanol and ethylene glycol. Ingestions of as much as several hundred milliliters have been reported without serious consequences, as have doses of 80 mg/kg administered to volunteers.[163] Principal effects include nausea, vomiting, inebriation, drowsiness, slurred speech, stupor, and coma. Significant exposure by inhalation may cause respiratory irritation and cough. In general, serious manifestations are rare.

In cases of occult poisoning, the diagnosis is suspected by finding any of the above-mentioned manifestations along with a strongly positive serum ketone test result and lack of a pathophysiologic process that would explain the ketosis (e.g., diabetic or alcoholic ketoacidosis). Both diabetic ketosis and alcoholic ketosis are associated with metabolic acidosis and an elevated anion gap. Although acetone intoxication has been reported to be associated with acidosis, this may have been due to associated respiratory depression.[164] Most cases are not associated with acidosis. Quantitative serum acetone levels are helpful. Acetone concentrations are typically less than 70 mg/dL in diabetic ketoacidosis, whereas in acetone ingestions, much higher levels can be achieved.[165] In the setting of poisoning, the half-life of acetone may be as long as 30 hours. Treatment consists of respiratory support, consideration of gastric lavage, and other supportive measures.

Paraldehyde

Paraldehyde is neither an alcohol nor a glycol but rather a cyclic polyether (Fig. 146–7). However, it is considered here because intoxication with this substance shares some similarities with methanol and ethylene glycol poisoning. First introduced into medicine in the 1880s, it is a colorless liquid with a strong and characteristic odor.[166, 167] It has been used primarily as a sedative-hypnotic, as an anticonvulsant, and in the treatment of alcohol withdrawal. In the past, it was abused by some as an alcohol substitute. As with other sedative-hypnotic agents, a drug dependency syndrome may develop with long-term use and symptoms similar to those of ethanol withdrawal occur after discontinuation. Acute overdose causes respiratory depression and hemodynamic derangements. Metabolic acidosis in this setting is probably due mainly or entirely to lactic acidosis from hypoxia.

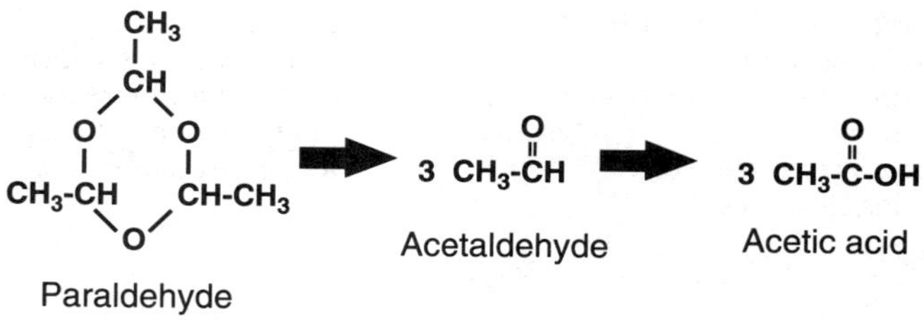

Figure 146–7. Metabolism of paraldehyde, a cyclic trimer of acetaldehyde.

Habituated subjects have tolerance to the drug, allowing larger doses to be consumed without development of these cardiopulmonary effects. In this setting a form of high-anion-gap metabolic acidosis can occur, the cause of which has never been completely elucidated.

The compound is oxidized to acetaldehyde and acetic acid in vivo (see Fig. 146–7), but this does not appear to account fully for either the increased unmeasured anion concentration or the acidosis. The drug decomposes with prolonged storage, especially if exposed to light or if not tightly sealed. Decomposed paraldehyde has been reported to contain as much as 40% acetic acid and has caused severe corrosive effects when given by mouth or per rectum.[151] Although it has been suggested that the acidosis is predominantly due to use of the decomposed drug, this is probably not the case because the acidosis has not correlated with blood acetate concentrations.[151, 167, 168] It has been hypothesized that overdose concentrations of paraldehyde may somehow interfere with intermediary metabolism and result in increased production of certain undetermined endogenous organic acids.[168-170]

Hepatic and renal dysfunction, pulmonary edema, and gastritis have been reported in cases of paraldehyde poisoning.[171] Acetaldehyde reportedly reacts with nitroprusside, a reagent commonly used in clinical chemistry laboratories to test for ketones. Thus, paraldehyde ingestion can potentially produce a false-positive test result for serum ketones.[172] A substantial minority of ingested paraldehyde is eliminated by the lungs and, because of the strong characteristic odor, provides an important diagnostic clue to this intoxication. The osmole gap is probably not appreciably affected in this overdose because paraldehyde has a relatively high molecular weight.[42] Management is similar to that of other sedative-hypnotic overdoses. Ipecac-induced emesis is contraindicated because CNS depression is expected. Hemodialysis and peritoneal dialysis have been employed in severe cases.[169] Although responsible for many deaths during the 1950s,[171] paraldehyde intoxication is chiefly of historical interest because the drug is seldom used today.

Propylene Glycol

Propylene glycol (1,2-propanediol) is a colorless and nearly odorless three-carbon glycol used as an antifreeze, plasticizer, solvent, and synthetic precursor.[151] It is also widely used in pharmaceuticals as a vehicle and diluent, including certain parenteral preparations of nitroglycerin, phenytoin, diazepam, digoxin, antibiotics, and many other commonly used drugs.[11, 173-178] Although it is generally safe if limited to low dosage levels, cases of intoxication have been reported with the use of some of these medicinals. Significant systemic accumulation has also occurred with cutaneous administration in the form of topical antibiotics used in burn patients.[179] CNS manifestations predominate, particularly seizures.[180] Tachypnea, tachycardia, and diaphoresis have also been reported.[151] As with ethylene glycol and other lower-molecular-weight toxins, high serum propylene glycol concentrations result in increased serum osmolality and an increase in the osmole gap.[178, 179] Because propylene glycol is metabolized to lactate (see Fig. 105–8), a high-anion-gap metabolic acidosis can result.[174, 181, 182]

Toluene

Toluene (toluol, methylbenzene) is a clear, colorless, flammable, aromatic hydrocarbon with a molecular weight of 92, used extensively as a solvent and in industrial processes, but best known for its use in model airplane glues. Occupational exposures may occur, but most clinical presentations have involved intentional abuse by adolescents. Toluene-containing model airplane cements have been one of the most commonly abused organic solvents. One survey noted that more than 10% of high school seniors had reported abusing organic solvents and aerosols by inhalation or sniffing.[183] Two methods are commonly used: "huffers" apply the solvent onto a rag, and "baggers" place a quantity inside a plastic or paper bag. The bag or rag is applied over the mouth and/or nose, and the subject repeatedly inhales the vapors.

Visual hallucinations, excitement, euphoria, dizziness, and ataxia can occur acutely. More severe manifestations include seizures, coma, and death. Long-term abuse has led to serious renal, cardiac, and gastrointestinal disorders and a variety of CNS and peripheral nervous system derangements.[184] Serious electrolyte disturbances, including hypokalemia and hypophosphatemia, may be seen.[185, 186]

Toluene is oxidized in the liver to benzoic acid, which is then metabolized to hippuric acid[184, 187, 188] (Fig. 146–8). Cresol and benzoylglucuronide are also produced.[151, 184, 189] The metabolic acidosis resulting from benzoic and hippuric acid production may lead to an increased anion gap owing to hippurate accumulation, but it is more frequently associated with a normal anion gap.[188] Rapid renal elimination of the hippurate anion probably explains the normal anion gap observed in most reported cases. Subjects who maintain adequate renal perfusion probably are able to excrete most of the hippurate, whereas those with substantial dehydration accumulate the anion. There is evidence that this solvent can cause direct renal tubular damage, leading to renal tubular acidosis.[185, 186] Hippurate crystalluria can occur and might be helpful diagnostically in cases of occult toluene intoxication. Changes in erythrocyte volume and mean corpuscular hemoglobin concentration have also been reported.[190]

Other compounds reportedly abused by inhalation include a variety of aliphatic and aromatic hydrocarbons, petroleum distillates, and related organic compounds such as benzene, xylene, naphthalene, gasoline, kerosene, ethyl acetate, acetone, methyl ethyl ketone, trichloroethane, carbon tetrachloride, chloroform, and many others. Not infrequently, the abused substance consists of a mixture of toluene and other

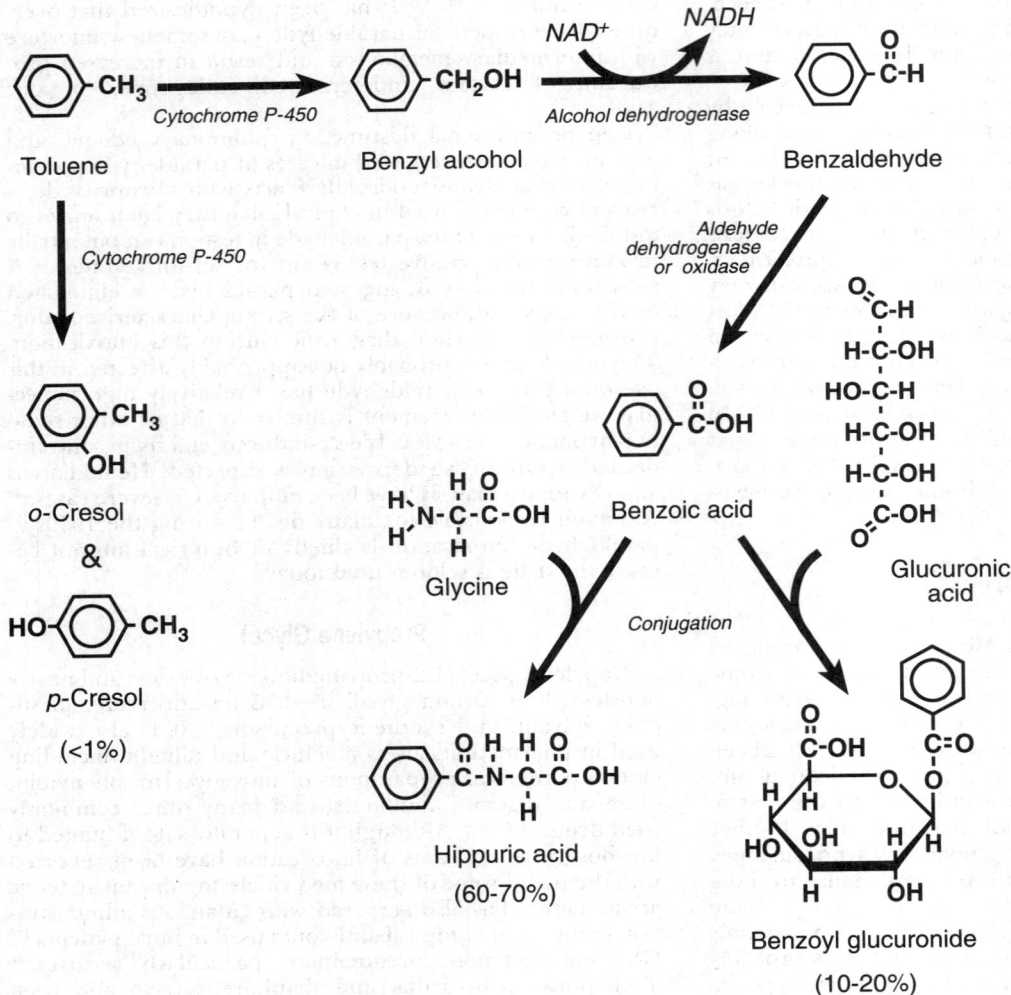

Figure 146–8. Metabolism of toluene.[151, 184, 187–189] Numbers in parentheses indicate the quantitative relationship among the metabolites. The ortho and para cresol metabolites also appear as sulfate and glucuronide conjugates.

hydrocarbon constituents.[184] In addition to the CNS manifestations, acute poisoning with these hydrocarbons may lead to pulmonary edema, arrhythmias, or circulatory shock. Treatment consists primarily of removal of the agent and institution of respiratory and other supportive measures as required. In the case of hydrocarbon ingestions, induced emesis is inadvisable owing to the danger of aspiration. Gastric lavage may be indicated for ingestions of agents that have inherent toxicity and those that are used as solvents for another toxic agent, as in certain pesticides.[5] Toluene may fall within this category if the volume consumed is more than a few milliliters.[191]

References

1. Roe O: Methanol poisoning. Acta Med Scand 126(suppl 182):1, 1946.
2. Bennett IL Jr, Cary FH, Mitchell GL, et al: Acute methyl alcohol poisoning: A review based on experiences in an outbreak of 323 cases. Medicine 32:431, 1953.
3. Jacobsen D, McMartin KE: Methanol and ethylene glycol poisonings: Mechanism of toxicity, clinical course, diagnosis and treatment. Med Toxicol 1:309, 1986.
4. Naraqi S, Dethlefs RF, Slobodniuk RA, et al: An outbreak of acute methyl alcohol intoxication. Aust NZ J Med 9:65, 1979.
5. Dreisbach RH, Robertson WO: Handbook of Poisoning: Prevention, Diagnosis and Treatment. 12th ed. East Norwalk, CT, Appleton & Lange, pp 168, 189, 1987.
6. Suit PF, Estes ML: Methanol intoxication: Clinical features and differential diagnosis. Cleve Clin J Med 57:464, 1990.
7. Tong TG: The alcohols. Crit Care Q 4:75, 1982.
8. Ziegler SL: The ocular menace of wood alcohol poisoning. JAMA 77:1160, 1921.
9. Roe O: Species differences in methanol poisonings. Crit Rev Toxicol 10:275, 1982.
10. McNally WD: Medical Jurisprudence and Toxicology. Philadelphia, WB Saunders, 1939.
11. Bryson PD: Comprehensive Review in Toxicology. 2nd ed. Rockville, MD, Aspen Publishers, p 284, 1989.
12. Chew WB, Berger EH, Brines OA, et al: Alkali treatment of methyl alcohol poisoning. JAMA 130:61, 1946.
13. McLean DR, Jacobs H, Mielke BW: Methanol poisoning: A clinical and pathological study. Ann Neurol 8:161, 1980.
14. Ley CO, Gali FG: Parkinsonian syndrome after methanol intoxication. Eur Neurol 22:405, 1983.
15. Guggenheim MA, Couch JR, Weinberg W: Motor dysfunction as a permanent complication of methanol ingestion. Arch Neurol 24:550, 1971.
16. Kane RL, Talbert W, Harlan J, et al: A methanol poisoning outbreak in Kentucky. Arch Environ Health 17:119, 1968.
17. Pinkus F: Die Massenerkrankungen im Städtischen Asyl für Obdachlose in Berlin, 24. bis 31. December 1911. Med Klin 1:41, 1912.
18. Swartz RD, Millman RP, Billi JE, et al: Epidemic methanol poisoning: Clinical and biochemical analysis of a recent episode. Medicine 60:373, 1981.
19. Benton CD Jr, Calhoun FP Jr: The ocular effects of methyl alcohol poisoning: Report of a catastrophe involving 320 persons. Am J Ophthalmol 36:1677, 1953.
20. Goldsher M, Better OS: Antifreeze poisoning during the October 1973 war in the Middle-East: Case reports. Milit Med 144:314, 1979.
21. Riley LJ, Ilson BE, Narins RG: Acute metabolic acid-base disorders. Crit Care Clin 5:699, 1987.
22. McMartin KE, Ambre JJ, Tephly TR: Methanol poisoning in human subjects. Role for formic acid accumulation in the metabolic acidosis. Am J Med 68:414, 1980.
23. Shahangian S, Ash KO: Formic and lactic acidosis in a fatal case of methanol intoxication. Clin Chem 32:395, 1986.
24. Nicholls P: Formate as an inhibitor of cytochrome c oxidase. Biochem Biophys Res Commun 67:610, 1975.
25. Nicholls P: The effect of formate on cytochrome aa and on electron transport in the intact respiratory chain. Biochim Biophys Acta 430:13, 1976.
26. McMartin KE, Martin-Amat G, Noker PE, et al: Lack of a role for formaldehyde in methanol poisoning in the monkey. Biochem Pharmacol 28:645, 1979.
27. Martin-Amat G, McMartin KE, Hayreh SS, et al: Methanol poisoning. Ocular toxicity produced by formate. Toxicol Appl Pharmacol 45:201, 1978.
28. Osterloh JD, Pond SM, Grady S, et al: Serum formate concentrations in methanol intoxication as a criteria for hemodialysis. Ann Intern Med 104:200, 1986.
29. National Institute of Health: Use of folate analogue in treatment of methyl alcohol toxic reactions is studied. JAMA 242:1961, 1979.
30. Clay KL, Murphy RC, Watkins WD: Experimental methanol toxicity in the primate: Analysis of metabolic acidosis. Toxicol Appl Pharmacol 34:49, 1975.
31. Hayreh MS, Hayreh SS, Baumbach GL, et al: Methyl alcohol poisoning III. Ocular toxicity. Arch Ophthalmol 95:1851, 1977.
32. Kaplan K: Methyl alcohol poisoning. Am J Med Sci 244:170, 1962.
33. Orthner H: Methylalkoholvergiftung mit besonders schweren Hirnoeranderungen: Ein Beitrag zur Permeabilitatspathologie des Gehirns. Virchows Arch Pathol Anat 323:442, 1953.
34. Erlanson P, Fritz H, Hagstam K-E, et al: Severe methanol intoxication. Acta Med Scand 177:393, 1965.
35. Aquilonius SM, Askmark H, Enoksson P, et al: Computed tomography in severe methanol intoxication. Br Med J 2:929, 1978.
36. Aquilonius SM, Bergstrom K, Enoksson P, et al: Cerebral computed tomography in methanol intoxication. J Comput Assist Tomogr 4:425, 1980.
37. Sejersted OM, Jacobsen D, Ovrebo S, et al: Formate concentrations in plasma from patients poisoned with methanol. Acta Med Scand 212:105, 1983.
38. Gennari FJ: Serum osmolality. Uses and limitations. N Engl J Med 310:102, 1984.
39. Dorwart WV, Chalmers L: Comparison of methods for calculating serum osmolality from chemical concentrations, and the prognostic value of such calculations. Clin Chem 21:190, 1975.
40. Smithline N, Gardner KD: Gaps—anionic and osmolal. JAMA 236:1594, 1976.
41. Weisberg HF: Osmolality—calculated, "delta," and more formulas. Clin Chem 21:1182, 1975.
42. Glasser L, Sternglanz PD, Combie J, et al: Serum osmolality and its applicability to drug overdose. Am J Clin Pathol 60:695, 1973.
43. Robinson AG, Loeb JN: Ethanol ingestion—commonest cause of elevated plasma osmolality? N Engl J Med 284:1253, 1971.
44. Haupt MC, Zull DN, Adams SL: Massive ethylene glycol poisoning without evidence of crystalluria: A case for early intervention. J Emerg Med 6:295, 1988.
45. Rubin AL, Braveman WS, Dexter RL, et al: The relationship between plasma osmolality and concentration in disease states. Clin Res Proc 4:129, 1956.
46. Boyd DR, Mansberger AR Jr: Serum water and osmolal changes in hemorrhagic shock: An experimental and clinical study. Am Surgeon 34:744, 1968.
47. Boyd DR, Folk FA, Condon RE, et al: Predictive value of serum osmolality in shock following major trauma. Surg Forum 21:32, 1970.
48. Hirasawa H, Odaka M, Sugai T, et al: Prognostic value of serum osmolality gap in patients with multiple organ failure treated with hemoperfusion. Artif Organs 12:382, 1988.
49. Sulway MJ, Malins JM: Acetone in diabetic ketoacidosis. Lancet 2:736, 1970.
50. Sklar AH, Linas SL: The osmolal gap in renal failure. Ann Intern Med 98:481, 1983.
51. Mattar JA, Weil MH, Shubin H: A study of the hyperosmolal state in critically ill patients. Crit Care Med 1:293, 1973.
52. Juel R: Serum osmolality. A CAP survey analysis. Am J Clin Pathol 68:165, 1977.
53. Epstein FB: Osmolality. Emerg Med Clin North Am 4:253, 1986.
54. Rocco RM: Volatiles and osmometry. Clin Chem 22:399, 1976.
55. Preuss HG, Podlasek SJ, Henry JB: Evaluation of renal function and water, electrolyte, and acid-base balance. In: Henry JB (ed): Clinical Diagnosis and Management by Laboratory Methods. 18th ed. Philadelphia, WB Saunders, p 126, 1991.
56. Barlow WK: Volatiles and osmometry. Clin Chem 22:1230, 1976.
57. Gaultier M, Cosno F, Bismuth C, et al: Ethylene glycol poisoning. Acta Pharm Toxicol 41(suppl):339, 1977.
58. Porter GA: The treatment of ethylene glycol poisoning simplified. N Engl J Med 319:109, 1988.
59. Parry MG, Wallach R: Ethylene glycol poisoning. Am J Med 57:143, 1974.
60. Cadnapaphornchai P, Taher S, Bhathena D, et al: Ethylene glycol poisoning: Diagnosis based on high osmolal and anion gaps and crystalluria. Ann Emerg Med 10:94, 1981.
61. Moriarty RW, McDonald RH: The spectrum of ethylene glycol poisoning. Clin Toxicol 7:583, 1974.
62. Frommer JP, Ayus JC: Acute ethylene glycol intoxication. Am J Nephrol 2:1, 1982.
63. Brown CG, Trumbull D, Klein-Schwartz JD: Ethylene glycol poisoning. Ann Emerg Med 12:501, 1983.
64. Levinsky NG, Ropper AH, Robert NJ, et al: Case records of the Massachusetts General Hospital. Case 38–1979. N Engl J Med 301:650, 1979.
65. Eckfeldt JH, Kershaw MJ: Hyperamylasemia following methyl alcohol intoxication. Source and significance. Arch Intern Med 146:193, 1986.
66. Field DL: Acute ethylene glycol poisoning. Crit Care Med 13:872, 1985.
67. Stokes J: Prevention of organ damage in massive ethylene glycol ingestion. JAMA 243:2065, 1980.
68. Olson E, McEnrue J, Greenbaum DM: Alcohols and miscellaneous agents. Heart Lung 12:127, 1983.

69. Kulig K, Duffy JP, Linden CH, et al: Toxic effects of methanol, ethylene glycol, and isopropyl alcohol. Topics Emerg Med 6:14, 1984.
70. Gutman RA, Hamon CB, Striker GE: Recovery after prolonged oliguria. Arch Intern Med 126:914, 1970.
71. Jacobsen D, Ovrebo S, Ostborg J, et al: Glycolate causes the acidosis in ethylene glycol poisoning and is effectively removed by hemodialysis. Acta Med Scand 216:409, 1984.
72. Jacobsen D, Ostby N, Bredesen JE: Studies on ethylene glycol poisoning. Acta Med Scand 212:11, 1982.
73. Bove KE: Ethylene glycol toxicity. Am J Clin Pathol 45:46, 1966.
74. Hewlett TP, McMartin KE: Ethylene glycol poisoning. The value of glycolic acid determinations for diagnosis and treatment. Clin Toxicol 24:389, 1986.
75. Smith SS: Solvent toxicity: Isopropanol, methanol, and ethylene glycol. Ear Nose Throat J 62:126, 1983.
76. Clay KL, Murphy RC: On the metabolic acidosis of ethylene glycol intoxication. Toxicol Appl Pharmacol 39:39, 1977.
77. De Breyer IJJ, Ortiz A, Soehring K: The effects of aldehydes on serotonin metabolism in rat liver slices. Pharmacology 3:85, 1970.
78. Klamerth OL: Influence of glyoxal on cell function. Biochim Biophys Acta 155:271, 1968.
79. Bowes JH, Cater CW: The interaction of aldehydes with collagen. Biochim Biophys Acta 168:341, 1968.
80. McChesney EW, Golberg L, Parekh CK, et al: Reappraisal of the toxicology of ethylene glycol. II. Metabolism studies in laboratory animals. Food Cosmet Toxicol 9:21, 1971.
81. Bachmann E, Golberg L: Reappraisal of the toxicology of ethylene glycol. III. Mitochondrial effects. Food Cosmet Toxicol 9:39, 1971.
82. Lamothe C, Thuret F, Laborit H: Action de l'acide glyoxylique, de l'acide glycolique et du glycoaldéhyde, in vivo et in vitro, sur quelques étapes du métabolisme énergétique de coupes de cortex cérébral, de foie, et de myocarde de rat. Agressologie 12:233, 1971.
83. Laborit H, Baron C, London A, et al: Activité nerveuse centrale et pharmacologie générale comparée du glyoxylate, du glycolate et du glycoaldéhyde. Agressologie 12:187, 1971.
84. Smith DE: Morphologic lesions due to acute and subacute poisoning with antifreeze. Arch Pathol 51:423, 1951.
85. Michelis MF, Mitchell B, Davis BB: "Bicarbonate resistant" metabolic acidosis in association with ethylene glycol intoxication. Clin Toxicol 9:53, 1976.
86. Friedman EA, Greenberg JB, Merril JP, et al: Consequences of ethylene glycol poisoning. Report of four cases and review of the literature. Am J Med 32:891, 1962.
87. Berger J: Neurological complications of ethylene glycol intoxication. Arch Neurol 38:724, 1981.
88. Baud FJ, Bismuth C, Garnier R, et al: 4-Methylpyrazole may be an alternative to ethanol therapy for ethylene glycol intoxication in man. J Toxicol Clin Toxicol 24:463, 1986–1987.
89. Gabow PA, Clay K, Sullivan JB, et al: Organic acids in ethylene glycol intoxication. Ann Intern Med 105:16, 1986.
90. Chou JY, Richardson KE: The effect of pyrazole on ethylene glycol toxicity and metabolism in the rat. Toxicol Appl Pharmacol 43:33, 1978.
91. Kassirer JP, Kopelman RI: A comatose alcoholic. Hosp Pract 20:26, 1985.
92. Verrilli MR, Deyling CL, Pippenger CE: Fatal ethylene glycol intoxication. Cleve Clin Med J 54:289, 1987.
93. Miskovitz PF: Metabolic acidosis in a somnolent alcoholic. Drug Ther 10:33, 1980.
94. Catchings TT, Beamer WC, Lundy L, et al: Adult respiratory distress syndrome secondary to ethylene glycol ingestion. Ann Emerg Med 14:594, 1985.
95. Van Stee EW, Harris AM, Horton ML, et al: The treatment of ethylene glycol toxicosis with pyrazole. J Pharmacol Exp Ther 192:251, 1975.
96. Sanyer JL, Oehme FW, McGavin MD: Systematic treatment of ethylene glycol toxicosis in dogs. Am J Vet Res 34:527, 1973.
97. Beasley VR, Buck WB: Acute ethylene glycol toxicosis: A review. Vet Hum Toxicol 22:255, 1980.
98. Heckerling PS: Ethylene glycol poisoning with a normal anion gap due to occult bromide intoxication. Ann Emerg Med 16:1384, 1987.
99. Godolphin W, Meagher EP, Sanders HD, et al: Unusual calcium oxalate crystals in ethylene glycol poisoning. Clin Toxicol 16:479, 1980.
100. Hagemann PO, Chiffelle TR: Ethylene glycol poisoning. J Lab Clin Med 33:573, 1948.
101. Riley JH: Urine and tissue oxalate and hippurate levels in ethylene glycol intoxication in the dog. Vet Hum Toxicol 24:331, 1982.
102. Kramer JW, Bistline D, Sheridan P, et al: Identification of hippuric acid crystals in the urine of ethylene glycol–intoxicated dogs and cats. J Am Vet Med Assoc 184:584, 1984.
103. Terlinsky AS, Grochowski J, Geoly KL, et al: Identification of atypical calcium oxalate crystalluria following ethylene glycol ingestion. Am J Clin Pathol 76:223, 1981.
104. Jacobsen D: Organic acids in ethylene glycol intoxication. Ann Intern Med 105:799, 1986.
105. Palmer BF, Eigenbrodt EH, Henrich WL: Cranial nerve deficit: A clue to the diagnosis of ethylene glycol poisoning. Am J Med 87:91, 1989.
106. Winter ML, Ellis MD, Snodgrass WR: Urine fluorescence using a Wood's lamp to detect the antifreeze additive sodium fluorescein: A qualitative adjunctive test in suspected ethylene glycol ingestions. Ann Emerg Med 19:663, 1990.
107. Ellenhorn MJ, Barceloux DG: Medical Toxicology: Diagnosis and Treatment of Human Poisoning. New York, Elsevier Science Publishing, p 800, 1988.
108. Decker WJ, Corby DG, Hilburn RE, et al: Adsorption of solvents by activated charcoal, polymers, and mineral sorbents. Vet Hum Toxicol 23(suppl 1):44, 1981.
109. Whalen JE, Richards CJ, Ambre J: Inadequate removal of methanol and formate using the sorbent based regeneration hemodialysis delivery system. Clin Nephrol 11:318, 1979.
110. Szabuniewicz M, Bailey EM, Wiersig DO: A new regimen for the treatment of ethylene glycol poisoning. IRCS Med Sci 3:102, 1975.
111. Cooney DO: The treatment of ethylene glycol poisoning with activated charcoal. IRCS Med Sci 5:265, 1977.
112. Branch A, Tonning DJ: Acute methyl alcohol poisoning: Observations in some thirty cases. Can J Public Health 36:147, 1945.
113. Nadeau G, Cote R, Delaney FJ: Two cases of ethylene glycol poisoning. Can Med Assoc J 70:69, 1954.
114. Flanagan P, Libcke JH: Renal biopsy observations following recovery from ethylene glycol nephrosis. Am J Clin Pathol 41:171, 1964.
115. Pendras J: Ethylene glycol poisoning as an indication for hemodialysis. Clin Res 11:249, 1963.
116. Wacker WEC, Haynes H, Druyan R, et al: Treatment of ethylene glycol poisoning with ethyl alcohol. JAMA 194:1231, 1965.
117. Borden TA, Bidwell CD: Treatment of acute ethylene glycol poisoning in rats. Invest Urol 6:205, 1968.
118. Agner K, Hook O, von Porat B: The treatment of methanol poisoning with ethanol. Q J Stud Alcohol 9:515, 1949.
119. McCoy HG, Cipolle RJ, Ehlers SM, et al: Severe methanol poisoning. Application of a pharmacokinetic model for ethanol therapy and hemodialysis. Am J Med 67:804, 1979.
120. Keyvan-Larijarni H, Tannenberg AM: Methanol intoxication. Comparison of peritoneal dialysis and hemodialysis treatment. Arch Intern Med 134:293, 1974.
121. Peterson CD: Oral ethanol doses in patients with methanol poisoning. Am J Hosp Pharm 38:1024, 1981.
122. Peterson CD, Collins AJ, Himes JM, et al: Pharmacokinetics during therapy with ethanol and hemodialysis. N Engl J Med 304:21, 1981.
123. Vestal RE, McGuire EA, Tobin JD, et al: Aging and ethanol metabolism. Clin Pharmacol Ther 21:343, 1977.
124. McMartin KE, Hedstrom K-G, Tolf B-R, et al: Studies on the metabolic interactions between 4-methylpyrazole and methanol using the monkey as an animal model. Arch Biochem Biophys 199:606, 1980.
125. Jacobsen D, Sebastian S, Blomstrand R, et al: 4-Methylpyrazole: A controlled study of safety in healthy human subjects after single, ascending doses. Alcoholism 12:516, 1988.
126. Blomstrand R, Ostling-Wintzell H, Lof A, et al: Pyrazoles as inhibitors of alcohol oxidation and as important tools in alcohol research: An approach to therapy against methanol poisoning. Proc Natl Acad Sci USA 76:3499, 1979.
127. Bloomstrand R, Ellin A, Lof A, et al: Biological effects and metabolic interactions after chronic and acute administration of 4-methylpyrazole and ethanol to rats. Arch Biochem Biophys 199:591, 1980.
128. McMartin ME, Jacobsen D, Sebastian S, et al: Safety and metabolism of 4-methylpyrazole in human subjects. Vet Hum Toxicol 29:471, 1987.
129. Wilson WL, Bottiglieri NG: Phase I studies with pyrazole. Cancer Chemother Res 21:137, 1962.
130. Weintraub M, Standish R: 4-Methylpyrazole: An antidote for ethylene glycol and methanol intoxication. Hosp Forum 23:960, 1988.
131. Baud FJ, Galliot M, Astier A, et al: Treatment of ethylene glycol poisoning with intravenous 4-methylpyrazole. N Engl J Med 319:97, 1988.
132. Gonda A, Gault H, Churchill D, et al: Hemodialysis for methanol intoxication. Am J Med 64:749, 1978.
133. Tobin M, Lianos E: Hemodialysis for methanol intoxication. J Dial 3:97, 1979.
134. Humphreys TJ: Methanol poisoning: Management of acidosis with combined haemodialysis and peritoneal dialysis. Med J Aust 1:833, 1974.
135. Schreiner GE, Maher JF, Marc-Aurele J, et al: Ethylene glycol—Two indications for hemodialysis. Trans Am Soc Artif Intern Organs 5:81, 1959.
136. Underwood F, Bennett WM: Ethylene glycol intoxication. Prevention of renal failure by aggressive management. JAMA 226:1453, 1973.
137. Vale J, Prior J, O'Hare J, et al: Treatment of ethylene glycol poisoning with peritoneal dialysis. Br Med J 284:557, 1982.
138. McMartin KE, Martin-Amat G, Makar AB, et al: Methanol poisoning. V. Role of formate metabolism in the monkey. J Pharmacol Exp Ther 201:564, 1977.
139. Noker PE, Eells JT, Tephly TR: Methanol toxicity: Treatment with folic acid and 5-formyl tetrahydrofolic acid. Alcoholism 4:378, 1980.

140. Levy R: Renal failure secondary to ethylene glycol intoxication. JAMA 173:1210, 1976.
141. Litovitz T: The alcohols: Ethanol, methanol, isopropanol, ethylene glycol. Pediatr Clin North Am 33:311, 1986.
142. Mecikalski M, Depner T: Peritoneal dialysis for isopropanol poisoning. West J Med 137:322, 1982.
143. Lewin GA, Oppenheimer PR, Winger WA: Coma from alcohol sponging. J Am Coll Emerg Physicians 6:165, 1977.
144. Corbett J, Meier G: Suicide attempted by rectal administration of drug. JAMA 206:2320, 1968.
145. Barnett JM, Plotnick M, Fine KC: Intoxication after an isopropyl alcohol enema. N Engl J Med 113:638, 1990.
146. Grant DH: The pharmacology of isopropyl alcohol. J Lab Clin Med 8:382, 1923.
147. Fuller HC, Hunter OB: Isopropyl alcohol—An investigation of its physiologic properties. J Lab Clin Med 12:326, 1927.
148. King LH, Bradley KP, Shires DL: Hemodialysis for isopropyl alcohol poisoning. JAMA 211:1855, 1970.
149. Adelson L: Fatal intoxication with isopropyl alcohol (rubbing alcohol). Am J Clin Pathol 38:144, 1962.
150. Chapin MA: Isopropyl alcohol poisoning with acute renal insufficiency. J Maine Med Assoc 40:288, 1949.
151. Gosselin RE, Smith RP, Hodge HC, et al: Clinical Toxicology of Commercial Products. 5th ed. Baltimore, Williams & Wilkins, p II–153, II–179, II–368, III–217, III–397, 1984.
152. Juncos L, Taguchi T: Isopropyl alcohol intoxication—Report of a case associated with myopathy, renal failure and hemolytic anemia. JAMA 204:186, 1968.
153. Lacouture PG, Wason S, Abrams A, et al: Acute isopropyl alcohol intoxication. Diagnosis and management. Am J Med 75:680, 1983.
154. Lacouture PG, Heldreth DD, Shannon M, et al: The generation of acetonemia/acetonuria following ingestion of a subtoxic dose of isopropyl alcohol. Am J Emerg Med 7:38, 1989.
155. Gaudet MP, Fraser GL: Isopropanol ingestion: Case report with pharmacokinetic analysis. Am J Emerg Med 7:297, 1989.
156. Hawley PC, Falko JM: "Pseudo" renal failure after isopropyl alcohol intoxication. South Med J 75:630, 1982.
157. Vasiliades J, Pollock J, Robinson CA: Pitfalls of the alcohol dehydrogenase procedure for the emergency assay of alcohol—A case study of isopropanol overdose. Clin Chem 24:383, 1978.
158. Freireich AW, Cinque TJ, Xanthaky G, et al: Hemodialysis for isopropanol poisoning. N Engl J Med 277:699, 1967.
159. Visudhiphan P, Kaufman H: Increased cerebrospinal fluid protein following isopropyl alcohol intoxication. NY State J Med 71:887, 1971.
160. Light FB, Marx GF: The value of gastric aspiration in a comatose child. Anesthesiology 31:478, 1969.
161. Lehman AJ, Schwerma H, Rickards E: Isopropyl alcohol: Rate of disappearance from the blood stream of dogs after intravenous and oral administration. J Pharmacol Exp Ther 82:196, 1944.
162. Depner TA, Mecikalski MB: Peritoneal dialysis for isopropanol poisoning. West J Med 137:322, 1981.
163. Haggard HW, Greenberg LA, McCullough-Turner J: The physiological principles governing the action of acetone together with determination of toxicity. J Indust Hyg Toxicol 26:133, 1944.
164. Winchester JF: Methanol, isopropyl alcohol, higher alcohols, ethylene glycol, cellosolves, acetone, and oxalate. In: Haddad LM, Winchester JF (eds): Clinical Management of Poisoning and Drug Overdose. 2nd ed. Philadelphia, WB Saunders, p 701, 1990.
165. Ramu A, Rosenbaum J, Blaschke TF: Disposition of acetone following acute acetone intoxication. West J Med 129:429, 1978.
166. Sharpless SK: Hypnotics and sedatives. II. Miscellaneous agents. In: Goodman LS, Gilman A (eds): The Pharmacological Basis of Therapeutics. 3rd ed. New York, Macmillan, p 134, 1965.
167. Seyffart G: Paraldehyde. In: Haddad LM, Winchester JF (eds): Clinical Management of Poisoning and Drug Overdose. Philadelphia, WB Saunders, p 410, 1983.
168. Harrington JT, Cohen JJ: Metabolic acidosis. In: Cohen JJ, Kassirer JP (eds): Acid-Base. Boston, Little, Brown, p 168, 1982.
169. Beier LS, Pitts WH, Gonick HC: Metabolic acidosis occurring during paraldehyde intoxication. Ann Intern Med 58:155, 1963.
170. Kittel J: Paraldehyde toxicity. Hosp Pharm 8:263, 1973.
171. Hayward JN, Boshell BR: Paraldehyde intoxication with metabolic acidosis. Am J Med 23:965, 1957.
172. Hadden JW, Metzner RJ: Pseudoketosis and hyperacetaldehydemia in paraldehyde acidosis. Am J Med 47:642, 1969.
173. Klaassen CD: Nonmetallic environmental toxicants: Air pollutants, solvents and vapors, and pesticides. In: Gilman AG, Rall TW, Nies AS, et al (eds): Goodman and Gilman's The Pharmacological Basis of Therapeutics. 8th ed. New York, Pergamon Press, p 1625, 1990.
174. Kelner MJ, Bailey DN: Propylene glycol as a cause of lactic acidosis. J Anal Toxicol 9:40, 1985.
175. Martin G, Finberg L: Propylene glycol: A potentially toxic vehicle in liquid dosage form. J Pediatrics 77:877, 1970.
176. Bossaert LL, Demey HE: Propylene glycol intoxication. Arch Intern Med 147:611, 1987.
177. Demey H, Daelemans R, De Broe ME, et al: Propyleneglycol intoxication due to intravenous nitroglycerin. Lancet 1:1360, 1984.
178. Huggon I, James I, Macrae D: Hyperosmolality related to propylene glycol in an infant treated with enoximone infusion. Br Med J 301:19, 1990.
179. Kulick MI, Lewis NS, Bansal V, et al: Hyperosmolality in the burn patient: Analysis of an osmolal discrepancy. J Trauma 20:223, 1980.
180. Arulanantham K, Genel M: Central nervous system toxicity associated with ingestion of propylene glycol. J Pediatrics 93:515, 1978.
181. Huff E: The metabolism of 1,2-propanediol. Biochim Biophys Acta 48:505, 1961.
182. Cate JC, Hedrick R: Propylene glycol intoxication and lactic acidosis. N Engl J Med 303:1237, 1980.
183. Smart RG: Solvent use in North America: Aspects of epidemiology, prevention and treatment. J Psychoactive Drugs 18:87, 1986.
184. McCormick MJ, Mogabgab E, Adams SL: Methanol poisoning as a result of inhalational solvent abuse. Ann Emerg Med 19:639, 1990.
185. Streicher HZ, Gabow PA, Moss AH, et al: Syndromes of toluene sniffing in adults. Ann Intern Med 94:758, 1981.
186. Voigts A, Kaufman CE Jr: Acidosis and other metabolic abnormalities associated with paint sniffing. South Med J 76:443, 1983.
187. Fishman CM, Oster JR: Toxic effects of toluene. JAMA 241:1713, 1979.
188. Carlisle EJF, Donnelly SM, Vasuvattakul S, et al: Glue-sniffing and distal renal tubular acidosis: Sticking to the facts. J Am Soc Nephrol 1:1019, 1991.
189. Life Systems, Inc: Toxicological Profile for Toluene. Atlanta, GA, Agency for Toxic Substances and Disease Registry, p 58, 1989.
190. Greenburg L, Mayers MR, Heimann R, et al: The effects of exposure to toluene in industry. JAMA 118:573, 1942.
191. Rocky Mountain Poison Center, Barone JA, Marcus SM, et al: In: POISINDEX, Volume 70. Denver, CO, Micromedex, 1991.

SECTION THIRTEEN

Ethics

Section Editor

Charles L. Sprung

CHAPTER 147

Ethical Decision Making in Critical Care

H. Tristram Engelhardt, Jr.

Critical care medicine provokes moral concerns because it is costly (it consumes nearly 1% of the U.S. gross national product) and because it involves decisions made in the face of death. The moral questions are many and pressing, but the answers are more numerous and often in conflict: there is no universal agreement about the proper allocation of resources or the morally correct point at which a patient should decline further treatment. In a secular pluralist context, in which one cannot appeal to divine authority or rely on a particular established tradition or precedent, the challenge is to find an authoritative or canonic basis for moral judgments. The field of secular bioethics has arisen in great measure as a systematic attempt to guide medical decision making in the face of such moral controversy and ambiguity. Although critical care has its special moral puzzles, problems, and controversies, these are a function of underlying moral puzzles in ethics itself. This chapter first explores foundational ethical issues and their implications for critical care. It then concludes with an application to problems of everyday practice.

SECULAR BIOETHICS AS A MODE OF DISPUTE RESOLUTION

The term *ethics* is ambiguous. First, ethics, reflecting its Greek etymology, identifies the customs of a group, as does the Latin *mos,* mores. Medicine is always practiced within a set of customary expectations, obligations, and rights. These constitute the informal moral world of everyday life and provide the background for medical decision making. Second, ethics has the sense of etiquette, identifying the formal and informal canons of civil probity of a community, class, or profession. Unlike mores, canons of professional etiquette are more explicitly formulated. In medicine, with the American Medical Association's eschewal (May 1847) of the old rubric "code of medical etiquette" in favor of the "code of medical ethics," the latter became fashionable. Third, ethics is often used also to include compliance with legal constraints, including administrative law. However, what is legal is not necessarily ethical; legal issues fall beyond the scope of this chapter. Yet it is important to distinguish legal and ethical issues. Just because an act is morally justifiable does not mean that it is legally allowable, making consultation with a lawyer imperative when concerns of legality arise. Fourth, ethics can identify particular religious or moral rules. Much of the literature of medical ethics in fact developed out of religious communities. Finally, for more than two and a half millennia there has been recognition of a need for a moral language to span particular customary expectations and religious beliefs and provide a basis for common critical assessment of codes of mores, etiquette, and law. This final sense identifies a secular understanding of ethics in general and of medical ethics or bioethics in particular, and it is the focus of this chapter.

Because all human decision making is directed by values, no critical care choice is value free. For example, a decision that an intervention is indicated usually reflects an assessment of whether treatment will on balance be useful or harmful. But judgments of usefulness are judgments about a likely balance of benefits over harms. Judgments about benefits and harms are value judgments. Indeed, all human judgments are value infected because they occur within a context of human expectations, which are themselves framed by human values. Thus, claims that critical care is indicated or unwarranted, futile or useful, are not value-free descriptions of the world but the results of particular value judgments.

In all of this, secular bioethics functions not to disclose a particular body of moral doctrine but to (1) clarify the values of the participants in a moral dispute, (2) indicate the possible bases for solutions to such disputes, and (3) determine the lines of moral authority.

PRINCIPLES OF SECULAR BIOETHICS
Respect for Autonomy and Beneficence

The principles of bioethics can be understood either (1) as general summaries of secular morality or (2) as foundational sources for moral justification. Either way, respect for autonomy and beneficence are cardinal principles. The principle of respect for autonomy is best understood as the principle of authority through consent. It is the central moral principle because ethics has failed to discover a concrete, morally authoritative vision of the good life or of proper action. The difficulty for contemporary ethics can be put succinctly: there are numerous possible accounts of the good life or proper action. These accounts differ even if one agrees on the general goals of life but disagrees regarding their ranking. Thus, there will be substantial disagreements regarding the kind of society one ought to establish (and, therefore, regarding the resources that should be made available for critical care), depending on the ranking of such social desiderata as liberty, equality, security, and prosperity. Nor is there a way to select definitively among competing visions of the good, alternative accounts of proper action, and various possible moral senses, because to do so one must already possess a morally authoritative, higher-level account or vision of the good in order to choose correctly.

Appeals to consequences do not resolve the difficulty because one must know how to rank consequences (for example, how to rank liberty, equality, security, and prosperity consequences). Nor is a mere appeal to satisfying preferences sufficient, because one needs to know how to rank emotionally emphatic preferences versus rationally well-considered preferences, present preferences versus future preferences, and so forth. However, even if one cannot discover an authoritative view of proper action, based on the authority of God or on the authority of a rationally canonical vision of proper conduct, one can still justify a morality and create policy for directing critical care based on the authority of mutual consent. Respect for autonomy is central, not because one values liberty but because individual agreement is the only source of common authority when one cannot appeal to God or to a concrete, morally authoritative view of proper action. Consent, agreement, and therapeutic contract constitute the cardinal sources of moral authority for critical care because they function even when there is no consensus with regard to an independent authoritative moral vision. Even when one cannot discover the unambiguously right choice, one can commonly choose or agree about what will be done.

The second principle, the principle of beneficence, identifies morality's focus on achieving the good of others, including their liberty, goods, or interests. Critical care is developed to benefit patients. Stated in such general terms, the principle of beneficence is unproblematic but not useful clinically, because one cannot uncontroversially specify the good of others. The good of a patient (e.g., whether admission to an intensive care unit offers sufficient benefits to justify the morbidity and economic costs involved) can be specified in terms of the patient's interpretation of that good, in terms of the family's interpretation of the patient's good, in terms of a proxy decision maker's interpretation of the patient's good, in terms of the attending physician's interpretation of that good, in terms of the interpretation provided by the director of the critical care unit, and so on. The interpretation of the patient's good also varies depending on the vision of proper action by which the patient's good is defined. For example, a patient who truly believes in an afterlife may not think it worth expending all available resources in clinging to this one. This reintroduces the principle of respect for autonomy. To manage the treatment of patients in a critical care unit, the physicians, nurses, and others engaged in providing care, as well as the hospital, need to fashion agreements with patients and/or their proxies regarding the patients' good. This often requires establishing formal policies and guidelines for admission to, and continued treatment in, a critical care unit.

In all of this, bioethical controversies occur on two levels of moral discussion, that of particular concrete moral communities and that of general secular moral discourse. The first is defined by a concrete moral vision accepted in whole or in part by the members of a particular moral community.

Thus, views of proper medical treatment may differ depending on whether one is a Christian Scientist, a Jehovah's Witness, an orthodox Catholic, or an atheist. For members of a particular moral community, a concrete moral framework can determine what limits are appropriate in providing critical care. Moreover, a concrete moral community may provide moral authorities (e.g., rabbis, priests, and ministers) for specific moral guidance. But such communities of vision do not meet the needs of the larger society that spans a number of such communities. When patients, the families of patients, physicians, nurses, and hospital administrators encounter the problem of providing good critical care in a secular pluralist context, they must create a fabric of agreements establishing the goals and limits of critical care.

Nonmaleficence and Justice

Some might add other principles in addition to respect for autonomy and beneficence. However, these can be reduced to either or both of autonomy and beneficence. For example, the principle of nonmaleficence expresses the notion either that it is wrong to harm people (i.e., to be radically nonbeneficent to them) or that it is wrong to do things to others that they believe would injure them (e.g., to provide medical treatment that a physician knows is indicated but a patient refuses). A similar reduction can be provided for the principle of justice. The principle of justice can be understood either as giving to persons that which would meet their basic needs (i.e., being basically beneficent to them) or as returning to persons that which they possess as a fundamental right (i.e., not keeping what belongs to others without their permission). Given the diverse views of justice, one is forced to establish distributive schemes (i.e., an investment in a basic level of critical care available for all when particular indications are met) by general agreement out of commonly owned resources. One is not able to discover *the* just system. Instead, one needs to create a generally acceptable system within the limits of claims to privacy and private ownership.

PROVIDING CRITICAL CARE: GAINING AUTHORITY TO TREAT

There are no unambiguous or uncontroversial definitions of good conduct. The first strategy in secular bioethics is to determine who is in authority and with respect to what issues. In so doing, one must attend to the following sources of moral authority in approaching the delivery of critical care.

The Autonomy of Patients

As far as possible, patients should be asked to participate in determining the character of their own care. Patients should also be free to rely fully on their physicians' recommendations and to convey authority to their physicians. In limiting treatment, patients withdraw authority to be treated, mirroring the basic principle in the law of battery that a competent innocent person may not be touched without consent. In demanding treatment (e.g., to be admitted to critical care when this offers very little, if any, therapeutic benefit), patients require others to act on their behalf. The right to be left alone (e.g., to be removed from critical care so that one can die in the presence of one's family) can be justified negatively by bringing the would-be intervener's authority in question. But, to justify a right to a particular treatment or to a level of treatment, one must justify a particular concrete view of proper action that warrants constraining others to provide a service.

Autonomy of Physicians

Physicians, just as much as patients and their surrogates, have the right to determine how they will be used. In particular, physicians have a moral right to refuse to be involved in procedures or endeavors that violate their own moral and professional integrity (e.g., providing critical care for a persistently vegetative patient because they hold such to be a misuse of resources). However, because there are numerous visions of proper moral conduct and of proper medical deportment, physicians must place patients, families of patients, their colleagues, other health professionals, and institutions on notice with respect to the circumstances under which they feel themselves morally bound not to participate in the usual range of medical treatment or professional conduct (e.g., they should warn patients in advance if they feel committed to saving life at any cost). In establishing the therapeutic contract honestly, all parties should disclose the moral, medical, and other restrictions they intend to place on its usual scope.

Autonomy of Nurses and Other Health Professionals

What is true for physicians is true for other health professionals as well: they have a right to their moral and professional integrity. However, they must disclose the ways in which their integrity is likely to circumscribe usual expectations (e.g., nurses should inform the health care institution in which they work, should they have difficulties in carrying out orders to limit care). The difficulty for nurses and many other health care professionals lies in the fact that they have generally not practiced as independent professionals but rather as professionals hired by hospitals and other institutions, working in part under the direction of physicians. This description is increasingly true of physicians as well. Physicians and other health care professionals may be employed by institutions that have established bioethical policies for critical care. At the least, the decisions of health professionals must be made against a background of institutional policy and group concerns.

Institutional Autonomy

Health care institutions are complex creatures of human invention. They have special obligations to those who provide professional care under their aegis, to patients and their families who come for care, to those who pay for the care, and to those who have established the institution. Health care institutions should articulate policy that makes clear to providers, patients, families, and payers the moral limits and conditions of care. For example, in institutions affiliated with religions that have significant and substantial moral commitments in the area of bioethics, there may be constraints on the character of care that may be provided without violating the fundamental beliefs and moral commitments of the institution. In many areas these constraints are obvious (e.g., Roman Catholic hospitals adamantly forbid direct euthanasia). In other areas these constraints are less apparent and there is an obligation on the part of the institution to make them clear (e.g., there is a long history in Roman Catholic moral theology of allowing patients to refuse any life-sustaining support that involves an undue inconvenience, including the refusal of natural hydration and nutrition; however, some Roman Catholic institutions may nevertheless hold themselves to be obliged to provide artificial hydration and nutrition to patients despite the wishes of families and the prior statements of patients).

In institutions without a guiding religious or moral commitment, moral policy must be created. Even in institutions with a guiding religious or moral commitment, there are probably many areas in which its implications for health care, and critical care in particular, are unclear and in need of clarification. Bioethics committees have played an important role in such fashioning and clarification, both through education and through policy formation. Establishing institutional policy with regard to triage in critical care units, the writing of do-not-resuscitate orders, and the identification of appropriate surrogate decision makers is an important step not only toward moral clarity but also toward creating a policy with moral authority. However, one must take care not to create policy that adversely restricts the choices of patients already admitted to a hospital. It must be possible for patients to have known in advance about hospital policies, and for this reason hospital policies regarding the use of critical care units must be publicly available (e.g., that a hospital will not honor proxy refusals for critical care on behalf of patients with advanced Alzheimer's disease or that a hospital will not provide critical care if the likely benefits are marginal).

PROVIDING CRITICAL CARE: ACHIEVING THE GOOD WHILE RESPECTING THE PATIENT
Free and Informed Consent

From a moral point of view, the practice of free and informed consent serves both to gain authority for diagnostic and therapeutic interventions and to protect the various goods that are associated with individual liberty. Concern with free and informed consent thus involves issues of respect for autonomy and beneficence. To convey permission, an individual must understand and appreciate that about which permission is given and convey the permission without coercion. But an individual need not be fully informed to give permission with moral validity. Patients may agree to therapeutic interventions, relying fully on their faith in their physician. The law has tended to impose particular disclosures of information not so much to honor the principle of autonomy as a source of authority but rather to achieve particular values associated with liberty. This is especially the case in jurisdictions that require disclosure of the information that reasonable and prudent individuals would need to decide whether to refuse a treatment, to accept a treatment, or to choose an alternative. In terms of the moral concern to honor the patient's right to consent (i.e., autonomy), it would be enough if physicians informed patients that they will be told only what physicians generally take to constitute an appropriate disclosure and that additional information will be available only on request.

In contrast, from the perspective of the principle of beneficence, of achieving the good of patients, one wants to disclose sufficient information so that (1) patients have their liberty interests, desires, and/or preferences satisfied and (2) they can choose in a way that maximizes their own long-term interests, desires, and/or preferences. Finally, for consent to be valid, a person must be free to give (or withhold) consent (e.g., young children and individuals awaiting execution, even if competent, may not be able to refuse lifesaving treatment validly) and the consent must be uncoerced. In summary, the general elements required for valid consent are (1) competence, (2) disclosure of adequate information, (3) communication of this information so that it is understood, (4) absence of coercion (i.e., voluntariness), and (5) appropriate status (e.g., being of an age adequate to give consent).

There are four general exceptions to the practice of free and informed consent, all of which are important for critical care. The first is the failure to give valid consent, because of lack of either competence or appropriate status. In either case, an appropriate surrogate or proxy decision maker must be found. The second is that of an emergency. When life, limb, or serious health interests are at stake and there is not time to gain consent from a patient or a patient's surrogate, physicians are under the general moral obligation to provide the kind of care a reasonable and prudent person would be likely to wish under the circumstances. The moral criterion becomes not actual consent but presumed consent on the basis of an ideal construct. The third exception is that of therapeutic privilege. When a patient is so ill that either (1) the stress of the disclosure of information would render the patient incompetent or (2) the stress would itself do serious damage to the patient, one may then morally turn to a surrogate to direct care. The fourth exception hinges on the circumstance that not all may value freedom and autonomy. Instead, a patient may wish to forgo the stress of a full disclosure of risks and therapeutic choices and rely on the physician's judgment. From a moral point of view, if the physician is willing to accept this responsibility, the patient passes responsibility to the physician. In this case, the physician becomes a special surrogate decision maker for the patient. If one forced a patient to face unwanted information (i.e., if one forced a patient to act freely), one would act paternalistically on behalf of a value assigned to liberty.

Advance Directives and Surrogate Decision Makers: Respecting Autonomy and Protecting Best Interests

In critical care, when patients are often of compromised competence, it is important to have at least informal, if not formal, therapeutic agreements and authorizations of proxy decision makers. Advance directives allow patients to consent in advance in an informed fashion (or refuse treatment in an informed fashion). Advance directives can take the form of oral statements, written statements (i.e., living wills), formal written statements under the color of law (e.g., natural death acts), and the appointment of proxies. The physician should be acquainted with local legal requirements that may encumber the moral rights of patients to make advance directives (e.g., by requiring clear and convincing evidence of a patient's wishes). In identifying an appropriate proxy, the patient should consider whether the next of kin (e.g., spouse) will be able to make difficult, emotionally laden decisions or whether some other proxy should be sought (e.g., a son or daughter). Thought should also be given to identifying back-up proxies in the event that the proxy of first choice is not available or is unwilling to serve. Concerns of beneficence support giving special attention to patients with fractured social lives (e.g., who are estranged from their spouses) so that appropriate proxies are identified and appointed and customary but inappropriate proxies avoided.

The creation of understandings in advance is a prophylactic measure against familial conflict, as well as against failure to respect the wishes and interests of patients adequately. It serves also as a prophylaxis against overtreating seriously ill patients because there is no available appropriate proxy or record of the patient's wishes. Whenever appropriate, physicians should encourage patients to create advance directives that specify their wishes, indicate the range of actions physicians should take, and appoint proxy decision makers to clarify the many points that cannot be anticipated in advance. So that such documents can be accessible when needed, a number of original copies should be made so that patients will have at least one readily available (e.g., not only in a safe deposit box) to be taken to the hospital on admission.

In approaching surrogates or proxy decision makers, one should note that not all have the same kind of moral authority. Indeed, the status of the surrogate or proxy can be of four general varieties. First, the patient may explicitly convey moral authority to a surrogate, morally authorizing the surrogate to act in accord with previously expressed wishes or to act as the surrogate determines is best in light of the surrogate's own vision of proper conduct. In this case, the surrogate is made a moral extension of the patient with respect to defining the patient's best interests and approving treatment decisions.

Second, members of the family or the patient's acquaintanceship may know what the patient would have wanted. Such a reporter or historian of the patient's judgments can, by substituted judgment, choose in ways that honor the patient's wishes and the patient's view of the patient's good. In accepting such surrogates, physicians should carefully evaluate choices that seem to serve the interests of the surrogate rather than the patient. The surrogate in these circumstances should be reporting the patient's view of the patient's best interests; the surrogate should be conveying what is tantamount to an oral advance directive.

Third, society may recognize particular individuals as surrogates who, according to broadly accepted criteria, may make judgments to limit care on the basis of what will harm or benefit the patient. In this case, the surrogate acts to resolve ambiguities regarding the patient's best interests, where the notion of best interests accords at least minimally with the preponderant societal view in the matter. In ignorance of the patient's own view of the patient's best interests, a view is adopted that is most likely to accord with the patient's viewpoint (i.e., the surrogate substitutes the judgment of a hypothetical patient to define the patient's best interests). The surrogate acts to apply a general model of best interests to a particular case. When law or custom establishes presumptive surrogate decision makers, individuals are put on notice that they should by explicit advance directives state their own view of their best interests and select surrogates of their own choice, if they are not willing to accept those who are otherwise provided. With respect to surrogates, it is important to note that surrogates need not be family members, nor need family members always be recognized as the proper surrogates for patients.

Finally, a surrogate may have special moral rights with respect to a patient, as where custom and some legal traditions recognize parents as having special rights related to their children, such that parents are at liberty to choose among courses of treatment as long as the choices agree with some generally accepted body of medical opinion. In this model, the surrogate's choices should not be interfered with unless a choice clearly falls beyond the pale of any generally accepted vision of the good or of proper action within the society.

Special Concerns About Competence

Patients in critical care are usually severely ill and as a result are often compromised in whole or in part in their capacity to make competent decisions. Competence can be totally absent (i.e., general incompetence) or can exist in different areas of an individual's life and to different degrees and at different times. Competence is not an all-or-none phenomenon.

From a moral point of view, one's concern about determining the competence of a patient should rise in proportion to the costs of false-positive and false-negative determinations. Thus, if a patient is facing imminent death, appears competent, and requests nonstandard but harmless treatment, the request may be accepted with little moral concern. If the patient were in fact incompetent, if the judgment of competence were a false-positive, little harm is likely to have been done to the patient, in that the patient would have died in any event. However, if a patient who would benefit significantly from aggressive critical care refuses needed treatment, one must take care not to harm interests (e.g., in lifesaving treatment) that the patient would have affirmed had the patient been competent.

This attention to the costs of false-positive and false-negative determinations of competence should not make the patient's autonomy hostage to the physician's view of the therapeutic best interests of the patient. Patients should remain those who have the prima facie right to make decisions regarding their own treatment. However, in a world of scarce time, energy, and resources, one cannot maximally assess competence on all occasions. Physicians and other health professionals who are dedicated to achieving the good of patients, but who are also restrained by the moral authority of patients over themselves, quite reasonably come to a moral double standard with regard to competence decisions: (1) if the patient appears competent and accepts the treatment needed to achieve the physician's best professional understanding of the patient's therapeutic needs, the patient's decision should usually be accepted as competent; (2) if the patient appears competent and refuses treatment that in the physician's best professional understanding is necessary to meet the patient's substantial therapeutic needs (e.g., the patient is not terminally ill and not likely to die in any event), the patient's decision should not be accepted as competent until thoroughly assessed.

Withholding Versus Withdrawing Treatment

From considerations of both autonomy and beneficence, it should be as easy to withdraw treatment as to withhold or decline it. Insofar as the authority to treat emanates from the consent of the patient or the patient's surrogate, all else being equal, this authority is as easily withdrawn as withheld or provided. Insofar as the authority to treat emanates from the pursuit of the patient's good, treatment should be as easy to withdraw as withhold, if the grounds for withdrawing treatment are that the treatment would not any longer sustain, or would indeed harm, the patient's interests. That is, considerations of the patient's good can properly work to stop treatment and to block its initiation. If withdrawing treatment were more difficult than withholding it, patients, patients' surrogates, and physicians would be tempted to hold back from providing trials of aggressive treatment in the fear that, once treatment is initiated (e.g., artificial ventilatory support), it could not be withdrawn. The goal of encouraging the aggressive exploration of all therapeutic options argues against making the withdrawal of treatment more difficult than the withholding of treatment.

Ordinary Versus Extraordinary Care: No Obligation to Save Life Is Absolute

Obligations of beneficence are prima facie obligations. They oblige unless they are defeated by other considerations. The notion of ordinary versus extraordinary care developed out of Roman Catholic moral theologic reflections at the end of the 16th and the beginning of the 17th century. In these discussions, "ordinary" and "extraordinary" identified not simply usual versus unusual treatment but rather appropriate or proportionate treatment on the one hand (i.e., ordinate treatment) versus inappropriate or disproportionate treatment on the other (i.e., inordinate treatment). The distinction recognizes that undue inconvenience, undue burden, or undue cost (including social and psychologic, not merely monetary, costs) could defeat the obligation of a patient to accept treatment or of a physician, family, or group to provide treatment.

Beyond recognizing the nonabsolute character of the obligation to save lives, the distinction is part of a larger moral concern not to absolutize or idolatrize mere human physical existence. If one seeks to save human life at any cost, one makes human physical life tantamount to the highest good. Yet, even within many nonreligious moral frameworks, many goods are acknowledged to be worth more than mere extension of physical existence. This moral distinction between ordinary (i.e., appropriate or obligatory) treatment and extraordinary (i.e., inappropriate or nonobligatory) treatment can support discussions between physicians and patients, as well as with family members, regarding the proper emphasis that should be placed on postponing death versus accepting death and planning for an exit from this life with dignity. These discussions are often burdened by an informal expectation that dying in a critical care unit is an element of our culture's required rites of death. For a patient or a patient's family to accept less than full aggressive efforts to postpone death, the physician may need to reassure all that accepting supportive care can be morally appropriate, in fact, morally praiseworthy, insofar as this supports comfort and dignity of death. Finally, after the death of the patient, it is often helpful for the physician to remind the family members that they have done everything appropriate. Even in high-technology medicine, physicians must often play the ancient sacerdotal role of the physician-priest by giving appropriate absolution from guilt.

Clarifying the Virtues of Supportive Care

It is important that the patient and/or the family of the patient acknowledge that high-technology medicine cannot forever postpone death and cannot always restore function. Toward this goal, unrealistic expectations should be brought within realistic parameters as early in the hospitalization as possible, so that patients and/or their families can accept the fact that aggressive efforts at curative or death-postponing care are inappropriate if the hope of success is slim and the likelihood of suffering by the patient considerable. Misunderstandings can at times be avoided by eschewing such phrases as "treatment should be stopped" or "further treatment is not warranted" because these expressions suggest that the patient will be abandoned and will no longer receive medical or nursing attention. Understandably, patients do not want to be abandoned. Moreover, families may want to go to the graveside saying that they have done all possible for their beloved. When attempts at cure or restoration of function are no longer appropriate, it is important for the physician not to refer to "stopping treatment" but to indicate that full energies should now be devoted to providing the best of comfort care. In short, the focus should be on helping patients and their families to understand that the meaning of appropriate care changes with the condition of the patient and may warrant discharge from the critical care unit.

Ethics Consultants and Ethics Committees

A bioethicist should be consulted when there is moral unclarity regarding the provision of critical care. The expertise of the bioethicist is primarily that of a geographer and clarifier of values, rights, duties, and virtues. Bioethicists should not be viewed as individuals who supplant the authority of the physician or who interfere with the physician-patient relationship. At times, bioethicists can help mediate conflicts between physicians and patients or between physicians and other health care professionals. This role of mediation is often performed through the consultative role of bioethics committees. In all of this, the themes of beneficence and respect for autonomy are central; the accent should be on determining lines of authority and/or a proper definition of the patient's therapeutic good.

Bioethics committees can play the special role of creating institutional health care policy. As official hospital committees, they can directly or indirectly fashion triage policies, policies for the writing of do-not-resuscitate orders, and policies for acquainting patients with the availability of advance directives. Bioethics committees can create forms that encourage clear and specific decisions about the kind of treatment to be provided or withheld. Rather than, for instance, simply recording a do-not-resuscitate order on the chart, one may require an explicit decision, recorded on a specially colored order sheet, indicating whether to use or to forgo external compression, intubation, and mechanical ventilation, electrocardioversion, the use of antiarrhythmic drugs, and so forth. By using such a sheet, which optimally includes a menu or checklist of possible interventions, one encourages detailed and careful discussions with the patient and/or family (or other surrogate decision makers), leading to a decision recorded in a way that allows quick retrieval when a split-second decision must be made by hospital staff about whether and to what extent to attempt resuscitation.

ESTABLISHING APPROPRIATE LEVELS OF CARE

If the demand for critical care is likely to exceed the available resources, criteria must be established for admission to and discharge from critical care units. In all areas of medicine, indications for treatment incorporate subtle judgments about whether the benefits of the treatment contemplated are worth the costs likely to be entailed. There have always been informal considerations, not only of costs of morbidity and mortality but also of financial costs. Generally, health care systems have focused not on providing the best of care for all who might benefit but instead on defining and guaranteeing a basic adequate level of care. In addition, in most countries, those with resources can buy additional luxury care on the model that even the cheapest automobiles must meet certain safety requirements but that people with resources can purchase more expensive crashproof luxury vehicles. In industrialized countries, some access to critical care has become part of the basic health care package. The moral and public policy challenge in critical care is to define a concept of basic access to critical care that takes into account likelihood of success, life expectancy, quality of life, and costs. The fundamental moral challenge is to determine the extent to which private resources can be considered public resources to support critical care and the extent to which unfortunate circumstances of illness and poverty may be considered unfair circumstances so as to generate claims against the community and create duties to meet health needs.

The general problem in ethics of discovering a correct moral vision or account of proper action is replayed once again. There is no unanimity or likely theoretic basis for unanimity regarding the various accounts of how resources should be distributed, allocated, or rationed, or regarding the extent to which needs generate rights. Nor is there a generally accepted view of the line between private and public resources. In the presence of such theoretic unclarity, one must abandon totalizing moral claims, accept the existence of both private and public resources, and eschew the language of justice in favor of the language of a social insurance policy against losses at the natural and social lotteries. Because a noncontroversial account of the proper ownership and distribution of resources is not available, moral claims must be moderated and health care policy must be created through democratic discussions regarding the proper scope of a society's view of social insurance. Under such circumstances, citizens must decide whether they want communal resources invested in critical care for themselves, should they become patients with Alzheimer's disease, be in a persistent vegetative state, or have other conditions of compromised quality of life. They must recognize, as in other areas of public policy, that one cannot prudently invest resources to save lives at any cost and likelihood of success (e.g., if one expends $500,000 per patient for a class of patients likely to survive only 1% of the time, one has committed the community to saving lives at the cost of $50 million per life saved). Moreover, if resources are not all public, individuals and communities with special moral and other commitments to saving life should not be disbarred from creating their own institutions for treatment in ways that others find disproportionate.

Because there is no canonical guide to the weight that should be given to costs, quality of life considerations, length of life expectancy, and chance of success, institutional guidelines for admission and continued intensive treatment must be created. Physicians involved in critical care as members of a learned profession thus have a special role to play in helping frame such criteria and in having the community accept these guidelines as establishing the limits of obligations at civil and criminal law. In so doing, physicians can better discharge their duties to provide announced standards of care. For example, physicians and institutions have an obligation not to overadmit to critical care units if this compromises the standard of care. In the absence of community guidelines (e.g., set by third-party payers), institutions must create and announce their own procedures for discharging patients who are either too ill to benefit significantly from critical care or well enough that such care does not provide a significant contribution to their well-being.

RULES OF THUMB FOR ETHICAL DECISION MAKING IN CRITICAL CARE

The strategies of ethical decision making in critical care can be summarized under four rubrics.

The first is prophylaxis. Physicians should reduce the possibility of significant moral puzzles and controversies by determining in advance of a loss of competence the wishes of the patient and by encouraging the patient to identify an appropriate proxy decision maker. This is especially urgent if the patient suffers from a terminal disease or a disease likely to lead to incompetence. This is first and foremost the obligation of the primary care physician, not the intensivist. Still, the responsibility often falls on the shoulders of physicians in critical care.

1. The physician should determine the patient's view about treatment, especially about the use of high-cost, high-technology medicine, before the patient is critically ill.

2. If the patient's view of proper treatment collides with usual understandings, the physician should be sure that the patient realizes the implications of the choice, that the patient is in fact competent, and that the patient has the status to make such determinations validly.

3. When the physician is convinced that the patient has competently and validly expressed an advance directive, this should be formally recorded, if possible.

4. Finally, the physician should endeavor to amplify the advance directive with the appointment of a proxy, along with back-up proxies.

Second, the physician should rely on the patient's wishes as far as possible in limiting care and choosing levels of treatment. If the physician approaches the patient for the first time in the critical care unit:

1. The physician should determine whether the patient is competent and whether an advance directive exists.

2. If the patient is competent and no advance directive exists, the physician should proceed as when helping a patient devise an advance directive before hospitalization.

3. If the patient is incompetent and there is no formal directive, the physician should ascertain whether someone in the family or acquaintanceship is an adequate historian of the patient's previous wishes and may function as an informal surrogate decision maker.

4. If no advance directive of a formal or informal nature exists, one should then turn to the proxies provided by law, custom, or hospital policy.

Third, physicians should help their patients, the patients' families, and society accept the finitude of the human condition. In the face of death, one should attempt to avoid the distortions in care arising from unrealistic expectations, guilt expressed in overtreatment, or an absolutization of the value of saving lives.

1. Physicians should help patients and their families to recognize that trying to save life at any cost often costs the patient financial and other goods, including a good death.

2. In writing orders that limit care, the physician should clearly specify the meaning of "limiting care" or "do-not-resuscitate orders."

3. Physicians should work with their hospitals to fashion institutional health care policies that establish forms and procedures requiring clear expressions by physicians of decisions with regard to levels of care.

4. Physicians should never, while withdrawing or withholding curative treatment, suggest to the patient or the patient's family that all treatment is being stopped. Instead, physicians should ascertain that other appropriate treatment continues to be provided, even when the only appropriate treatment is comfort care, and assure the patient and family of this.

Finally, physicians and other health care professionals involved in critical care should help their institutions and society to fashion policy that recognizes the finitude of human life and that postponing death and saving lives at any price can be extremely costly, both financially and culturally.

1. Policies must be established that maintain the announced standards of care, even if this involves discharging patients who are so ill that they are not likely to benefit from critical care, as well as those well enough to derive only a marginal benefit.

2. If the establishment of policies for the allocation or rationing of health care is understood under the metaphor of framing a social insurance policy, one can approach limiting care, when the care would be costly, have only a small likelihood of success, or secure only a limited quality of life, in terms of whether one wishes to purchase such care for oneself in the event that one is impecunious and in need of treatment.

3. The insurance metaphor can help to democratize the framing of health care policy.

4. Insofar as resources and energies are not all publicly owned, there is always the moral possibility of a second tier of health care, including institutions that provide forms of critical care that many find disproportionate or inordinate (e.g., the admission of individuals with advanced Alzheimer's disease for critical care).

Critical care confronts physicians, patients, nurses, and individuals generally with one of the exemplar challenges of a high-technology civilization: choosing limits against images of god-like powers. In particular, critical care forces individuals and societies to recognize that, although high-technology medicine promises the allure of postponing death and miraculously restoring health, it does so only under some circumstances and usually only at significant costs. Because humans cannot do all that they would want, health care policies must set limits to what is done. Such limit setting requires the consent of those who participate and the public definition of goals for common endeavors. In the end, this means that patients must decide how they want to die, whom they want to make choices for them when they become incompetent, and how they wish to have communal resources invested in critical care. If one invests all disposable resources in the endeavor of postponing and avoiding death, one will have no resources available to enjoy a much protracted life.

Bibliography

Aaron HJ, Schwartz WB: The Painful Prescription. Washington, DC, Brookings Institution, 1984.

Berenson RA: Intensive Care Units (ICUs): Clinical Outcomes, Costs, and Decision Making. Washington, DC, Office of Technology Assessment, 1984. Health Technology Case Study 28.

Brody BA: Life and Death Decision Making. New York, Oxford, 1988.

Callahan D: Setting Limits. New York, Simon & Schuster, 1987.

Callahan D: What Kind of Life. New York, Simon & Schuster, 1990.

Chang RWS, Jacobs S, Lee B: Use of APACHE II severity of disease classification to identify intensive-care-unit patients who would not benefit from total parenteral nutrition. Lancet 1:1483, 1986.

Eagle KA, Mulley AG, Skates SJ, et al: Length of stay in the intensive care unit. JAMA 264:992, 1990.

Engelhardt HT Jr: Bioethics and Secular Humanism. Philadelphia, Trinity Press International, 1991.

Engelhardt HT Jr, Rie MA: Intensive care units, scarce resources, and conflicting principles of justice. JAMA 255:1159, 1986.

Faden RR, Beauchamp TL: A History and Theory of Informed Consent. New York, Oxford University Press, 1986.

King NMP: Making Sense of Advance Directives. Dordrecht, Kluwer, 1991.

Luce JM: Ethical principles in critical care. JAMA 263:696, 1990.

Morreim EH: Balancing Act. Dordrecht, Kluwer, 1991.

Moskop JC, Kopelman L (eds): Ethics and Critical Care Medicine. Dordrecht, Reidel, 1985.

Pellegrino ED, Thomasma DC: For the Patient's Good. New York, Oxford University Press, 1988.

President's Commission for the Study of Ethical Problems in Medicine and Biomedical and Behavioral Research: Securing Access to Health Care. Washington, DC, US Government Printing Office, 1983.

Shelp EE: Born to Die? New York, Free Press, 1986.

Sprung CL: Surrogate decision-making in critical care medicine. In: Lumb PD, Shoemaker WC (eds): Critical Care: State of the Art. Fullerton, CA, Society of Critical Care Medicine, p 367, 1990.

Task Force on Ethics of the Society of Critical Care Medicine: Consensus report on the ethics of foregoing life-sustaining treatments in the critically ill. Crit Care Med 18:1435, 1990.

Veatch RM: A Theory of Medical Ethics. New York, Basic Books, 1981.

Weir RF: Abating Treatment with Critically Ill Patients. New York, Oxford University Press, 1989.

Weir RF: Selective Nontreatment of Handicapped Newborns. New York, Oxford University Press, 1984.

Welch HG: Health care tickets for the uninsured. N Engl J Med 321:1261, 1989.

Zimmerman JE, Knaus WA, Sharpe ST, et al: The use and implications of do not resuscitate orders in intensive care units. JAMA 255:351, 1986.

CHAPTER 148

Ethical and Legal Aspects of Forgoing Life-Sustaining Treatments

Thomas A. Raffin

GOALS OF CRITICAL CARE MEDICINE

Four decades ago, postoperative recovery rooms and specialized care units devoted to patients with burns, trauma, war-related injuries, and poliomyelitis gave rise to intensive care units (ICUs).[1] In the early 1960s, only 10 to 20% of acute care hospitals in the United States had ICUs. However, by 1990, 90 to 100% of the more than 6000 acute care hospitals had designated ICUs. Some of these ICUs are specialty units such as medical, surgical, cardiac, neurosurgical, cardiovascular surgical, trauma, or burn units. Other ICUs are more general and bring together the full spectrum of critically ill patients.

In the United States, there are approximately 65,000 ICU beds, and the range of overall average charges for intensive care is from $2,000 to $8,000 per day. Thus, it has been estimated that intensive care costs in the United States are more than $50 billion per year. Because total health care expenditures were more than $600 billion in 1990 (and might climb to $1.5 trillion by the year 2000), intensive care expenditures now account for approximately 10% of health care costs in the United States.[2] The gross national product of the United States is close to $6 trillion. Thus, total health care expenditures are approximately 13%, and the cost of intensive care is almost 1% of the gross national product.[1]

During the past two decades there has been a remarkable expansion in lifesaving technologies and treatment modalities in intensive care medicine. These increased abilities have resulted in significant dilemmas in ethical decision making. In the middle to late 1970s, stimulated by the national publicity received by the 1976 Karen Ann Quinlan case in New Jersey, there began a national dialogue about how to make ethical decisions concerning critically ill patients who are hopelessly ill.

Physicians, nurses, respiratory therapists, and all other members of the ICU health care team have two major goals when caring for patients in ICUs. The first goal is to save the salvageable. A medical judgment must be made about whether a patient is salvageable; then, if the patient appears to be savable, the health care providers do all in their power to save the patient as long as this is in concert with what the patient desires. Essentially, the health care team is following two age-old tenets of medicine: (1) to restore health and (2) to relieve suffering. These key goals of medicine have been handed down through the centuries from Hippocrates, Galen, Maimonides, clinicians, philosophers, and ethicists who have attempted to define the goals of medicine. Fundamentally, the goal of an intensive care practitioner is to stop a patient from dying by using life-support measures such as mechanical ventilation, massive fluid resuscitation with inotropic support, dialysis, or total parenteral or nasogastric tube feeding. When the patient is stable and the illnesses or injuries are being treated, the intensive care team waits for the patient to heal and regain strength. In effect, it is the wisdom of the body that decides which organ system heals and which patient survives. Intensive care team members can do only so much. Even with great knowledge, judgment, and technology, it is still up to the wisdom of the body to determine whether the patient gets better.

The second major goal of intensive care medicine is to help the dying have a peaceful and dignified death. There is no question that this is a vitally important goal because many patients who are admitted to ICUs die there. In fact, many patients are inappropriately admitted to ICUs because the mortality rates of such patients before admission are close to 100%. To gain insight into this, one must review mortality rates of specific subpopulations of patients admitted to ICUs. This is covered shortly. Because many patients admitted to ICUs have, in essence, no chance to leave the unit alive, it is important for intensive care team members to understand that death is both an enemy and a colleague. In other words, it is appropriate and, in fact, a thoughtful and sensitive act to assist a hopelessly ill patient to die with peace and dignity. It is not the goal of intensive care to prolong the process of dying. Life support should be withdrawn if the patient has, in essence, no chance to regain a reasonable quality of life and the decision is one with which the patient agrees. It takes skill and sensitivity to work with patients, their families, their surrogates, and other health care team members in managing death with sensitivity and compassion. Close attention to the needs of family members results in an appropriate grieving process and, it is hoped, a healthier return to a functional life.

The overall death rate for all patients admitted to ICUs in the United States is approximately 15 to 20%.[3] However, this death rate is misleadingly low because it includes large numbers of patients admitted to ICUs who have low mortality rates. For example, patients who have had coronary artery bypass graft surgery are admitted to ICUs for several-day stays. In 1989 more than 300,000 Americans had coronary artery bypass graft procedures; the mortality rate was approximately 4 to 6% and the overall cost $4 billion to $6 billion. Another low-mortality-rate group admitted to ICUs is patients who have attempted suicide and need either close cardiologic monitoring or respiratory support. Of the hundreds of thousands of Americans who take overdoses each year, only 5 to 10% need to be admitted to ICUs, and the overall mortality rate of this group is as low as 5 to 6%.[3] Such low mortality rates are also seen in other surgical patients who require intensive care after carotid endarterectomies, aneurysm repairs, or other vascular surgeries. When low-mortality-rate subpopulations such as those just described are excluded from the calculation, the overall mortality rate of patients in ICUs is closer to 30 to 40%.

ICU mortality rate statistics have been published since the mid-1970s.[3] For example, in 1984 Cullen and coworkers updated a 1976 study and identified a current overall ICU mortality rate of 69% compared with the 1976 mortality rate of 73%.[4] Interestingly, in 1984 the survivors' quality of life appeared to be significantly better. A study by LeGall and coworkers from France showed that 66% of patients were discharged from the ICU alive. However, the survival rate fell to 50% at 6 months and to 49% at 1 year.[5]

During this time, there was a strong emphasis on developing a classification system to standardize data concerning critically ill patients. One of the best-known and most utilized classification systems was the APACHE (Acute Physiology Assessment and Chronic Health Evaluation) system developed by Knaus and colleagues.[6] The APACHE II classification system, derived from the original APACHE study, uses a point score based on admission values of 12 routine physiologic measurements, age, and previous health status to compute a measure of the severity of disease.[7] Investigators demonstrated that an increasing score was closely correlated with the subsequent risk of hospital death for 5815 patients from 13 hospitals.[7] In 1985, the APACHE II study identified the prognosis of critically ill patients with single or multiple organ system failure.[8] Objective definitions for five organ system failures were developed (cardiovascular, respiratory, renal, hematologic, and neurologic), and these systems were monitored during ICU admissions. The number and duration of organ system failures were linked to outcome at hospital discharge for each of 2719 ICU patients (48%) who developed them. The ICU prognosis data from the APACHE II study provided information that is of significant assistance when obtaining informed consents from patients, surrogates, and families. These data revealed that, for all ICU medical and most surgical admissions, a single organ system failure lasting more than 1 day was associated with a mortality rate approaching 40%. For two organ system failures lasting more than 1 day the death rate increased to 60%. The mortality rate for 99 patients with three or more organ system failures persisting after 3 days was 98%. Advanced chronologic age was associated with both an increased probability of developing organ system failure and an increased probability of death when organ system failure occurred. The APACHE II classification system has provided important data, and important new research projects are ongoing as part of APACHE III.

Many subpopulations of critically ill patients in ICUs have mortality rates as high as 80 to 100%. Patients with adult respiratory distress syndrome (ARDS) have death rates ranging from 65 to 100%.[3, 9] The prognosis is markedly worse when the ARDS is secondary to bacterial sepsis. Schuster and Marion performed a classic study of ICU outcome in patients with hematologic malignancies.[10] For 77 patients who were admitted to a medical ICU over a 21-month period, the overall hospital mortality rate was 80%. Sixteen patients (21%) were discharged from the ICU but died in the hospital. Only 4 of 52 patients who required mechanical ventilation left the hospital alive. Any patient receiving mechanical ventilation for more than 5 days died.

Several studies have shown that critically ill patients who develop renal failure have a greater mortality rate than those who do not.[3, 8, 11] Liver failure has also been associated with a high mortality rate in ICU patients.[3, 12] In a 1977 study by Imbus and Zawacki, the decision-making autonomy of burn patients was maximized when it was clear from their presentation that survival was unprecedented.[13] The authors believed that when burns are extremely severe, survival is unprecedented, and thus an aggressive approach to decision making should be invoked to preserve the patient's autonomy. While still legally competent and with sufficient data, the patient was asked whether he or she wished to choose between a full therapeutic regimen and ordinary care. Their wishes were then carried out. These patients had no reasonable chance to survive.

A general statement can be made about a critically ill patient who is admitted to an ICU: The longer the patient is in the ICU, the greater the likelihood of severe morbidity or death. This seems like a paradoxical statement because there is no safer place for a critically ill patient than an ICU. However, there is also no more dangerous a place. The leading cause of death of critically ill patients is infection, and it is easy to become infected in the ICU because of the multiple invasive procedures used and the highly resistant microorganisms found there. For example, in a 1985 study Montgomery and colleagues determined that 47 patients with ARDS who were in ICUs had a 68% mortality rate.[9] Only 16% of the ARDS patients died because of unmanageable respiratory failure; 73% died because of nosocomial sepsis and multiple organ system failure. The leading infections in critically ill patients in ICUs are sepsis, pneumonia,

and other nosocomial infections such as catheter-induced urinary tract infections.[14] It is estimated that patients with ARDS have a 60% incidence of nosocomial pneumonia.[15] Severe organ infections with or without sepsis can lead to multiple organ system failure and a poor prognosis. Other key factors that can lead to high mortality rates in critically ill patients include cardiac arrhythmias, gastrointestinal bleeding, acute airway problems, abdominal catastrophes, pneumothorax, and pulmonary embolism.[16]

For patients and families, the ICU is a foreign, frightening, and bewildering environment. Non–health care professionals visiting loved ones or friends clearly feel out of place. Odd and unusual noises assault their ears: high-pitched regular beeps, buzzers, alarms, and the deep rhythmic swooshing sounds of machines that aid breathing. Intravenous bottles with tubes dangle from the ceiling like vines. Patients and family members feel that the situation is out of their control. In view of all the difficulties of intensive care for patients and their families, what are the survivors' preferences regarding intensive care? In 1988 a study was made of patients' and families' preferences for medical intensive care.[17] Patients who were 55 years of age or older and had been in an ICU were interviewed. Family members were interviewed if the patient had died. Of interest, 70% of the patients and families said they would be 100% willing to undergo intensive care again to achieve even a 1-month survival. Only 8% were completely unwilling to undergo intensive care to achieve any prolonged survival. The preferences of the patient or family were not well correlated with functional status or quality of life for 82% of the respondents. Willingness to undergo intensive care was not influenced by age, severity of critical illness, length of stay, or charges for care. In 1986, the preferences of homosexual men with acquired immunodeficiency syndrome for life-sustaining treatment were reported; many were willing to forgo life-sustaining treatment if the prognosis was extremely poor.[18] More studies are needed to evaluate the preferences of patients or family members for intensive care, especially among the many cultural and ethnic groups in our pluralistic society.

Many people who have never been admitted to an ICU are frightened and hesitant about being given life support in an effort to save their lives. It is important to educate the lay public about the benefit of intensive care, that is, saving certain subpopulations of patients and returning them to a good quality of life. It is also important for both the lay public and health care professionals to have insight into what patients and their families want. The results of the 1988 study mentioned earlier would not have been predicted by many health care providers. Thus, "substituted judgments" made for incompetent patients concerning whether to provide or continue intensive care must be made with objectivity and thoughtfulness to ensure that they reflect only the values of the patient.

LEGAL PRECEDENTS IN ETHICAL DECISION MAKING

Many state legislatures and courts have handed down decisions that have built the legal framework in our nation's approach to biomedical ethical issues. It is important to remember that a legislative action or court decision in one state does not make precedent or law for any other state. Furthermore, just as individual concepts and insights into morality and ethics differ, so too do the arbitrary judgments of different state and federal legislatures and courts. There is no question that the family histories, life experiences, politics, and personal feelings and prejudices of individual legislators and jurists play a role in forming their decisions.

Thus, there is an arbitrary component in legislative and judicial action, but, taken as a whole, the ultimate evolution of decisions reflects our society's morality.

When studying legal precedents in ethical decision making, it is important to keep in mind the four major biomedical ethical principles that have been discussed in another chapter: beneficence, nonmaleficence, autonomy, and justice.[1] The U.S. Supreme Court has rendered its first decision on life-sustaining treatment in the Cruzan case. This is discussed shortly. In 1891 the U.S. Supreme Court recognized the legality of a citizen's right of autonomy when it stated:[19]

No right is held more sacred or is more carefully guarded by the common law than the right of every individual to the possession and control of his own person, free from all restraints or interference by others, unless by clear and unquestionable authority of law.

Thus, autonomy is not only an ethical principle but also a vital legal principle in the United States.

The ground-breaking Karen Ann Quinlan case, adjudicated in 1976, dealt with a 22-year-old woman who became comatose after the probable ingestion of alcohol and drugs.[20] She was maintained with mechanical ventilation and, although not brain dead, appeared to have a terrible prognosis. Her father had himself appointed her legal guardian and asked her physicians to remove her from the ventilator and allow her to die because he believed that she would not want to live under such circumstances. The physicians refused, and the Quinlan case went to court.

The New Jersey Supreme Court examined "the reasonable possibility of return to cognitive and sapient life as distinguished from . . . biological vegetative existence."[20] The court suggested that a benefit exists when life-sustaining treatment contemplates "at very least, a remission of symptoms enabling a return toward a normal functioning, integrated existence." In addition, the court felt that these ethical decisions should be made by the physician and family.

The New Jersey Supreme Court ruled that Ms. Quinlan had a constitutional "right to privacy" to be removed from the ventilator if the family, the physicians, and the hospital ethics committee agreed. The court implied that, in some situations, the family's wishes could overrule the physician's concerns. Thus, "substituted judgment" could be made for an incompetent patient. Because Ms. Quinlan was not brain dead but was in a persistent vegetative state, she continued to live when the ventilator was removed. One decade after the removal of her ventilator, she finally died.

The Massachusetts Supreme Court ruled on the *Saikewicz v Superintendent of Belcher State School* case in 1977. The court stated that, without information from the patient and the patient's family, only the court—and not the physician and family—has a right to make substituted judgments.[21] Thus, the Massachusetts Supreme Court implied that courts must be involved in decision making to withhold or withdraw life support. The impact of this ruling was powerful in the state of Massachusetts, where health care professionals became worried about how to make decisions in cases involving withholding and withdrawing life support without the assistance of the courts. In 1978 the Massachusetts Court of Appeals ruled in the Dinnerstein case that family members and physicians could make a thoughtful judgment concerning withholding life support in a case involving an incompetent patient without having to bring the case to the courts.[22]

In California in 1981, Clarence Herbert, a 55-year-old patient, had a myocardial infarction after surgery that left him with severe brain damage. Two days after the sudden event, his family agreed with his physicians that life support should be withdrawn. The family based their agreement on the fact that the patient had earlier made comments that he did not wish to be kept alive artificially. After the removal of mechanical ventilation, Mr. Herbert did not die. Two days later, his family agreed that routine life support should be stopped, including intravenous fluid and nutrition. One week later, Mr. Herbert died. The two physicians who cared for Mr. Herbert were charged with murder by the Los Angeles District Attorney in 1983 in the well-known case *Barber v Superior Court*.[23] After much debate and many conflicting opinions, the California Superior Court dismissed the charges. In its ruling, the court relied on the vital concept of proportionality as the key criterion to be used in deciding whether to withdraw life support. The court stated, "Proportionate treatment is that which, in the view of the patient, has at least a reasonable chance of providing benefits to the patient which outweigh the burdens attendant to the treatment."[23] The Barber court decision relied heavily on the Quinlan decision in attempting to define terms such as benefits and burdens. In addition, the Barber court ruled that nutrition and hydration were medical procedures and should be evaluated by health care professionals:[23]

Medical procedures to provide nutrition and hydration are more similar to other medical procedures than to typical human ways of providing nutrition and hydration. Their benefits and burdens ought to be evaluated in the same manner as any other medical procedure.

The Barber court decision went on to discuss who can appropriately decide for incompetent patients. The court emphasized that when patients are incompetent, physicians must identify a surrogate to make a substituted judgment on the patient's behalf. The California court, with the proviso that there was no legislation to the contrary, considered it legal to bypass formal conservatorship proceedings. The court reasoned that the spouse and children are the most appropriate surrogates because they are in the best position to know the patient's feelings and desires regarding treatment, would be affected by the treatment decision, and have a concern for the patient's comfort and welfare.

Another California case, *Bartling v Superior Court*, affirmed the right of competent adult patients with imminently fatal diseases to refuse treatment over the objection of physicians and hospitals.[24] Mr. Bartling was legally competent. He and his family wished to have him removed from a ventilator because his prognosis was extremely poor. The physicians and hospital refused, but eventually the California Appeals Court ruled in favor of Mr. Bartling and his family after Mr. Bartling's death. The appeals court stated:[24]

If the right of the patient to self-termination as to his own medical treatment is to have any meaning at all, it must be paramount to the interest of the patient's hospital and doctors. The right of a competent ill patient to refuse medical treatment is a constitutionally guaranteed right which must not be abridged.

Bouvia v Superior Court, a 1986 California decision, established the right of a patient to refuse both nourishment and hydration.[25] This was a well-publicized case in which an intelligent young quadriplegic woman with cerebral palsy demanded that the hospital treating her halt all food and water so that she could die because she was in constant pain, was totally dependent on others, and found her quality of life unacceptable. In April 1986, the California State Court of Appeals overturned a lower court's decision and held that state policy does not require that "all and every life must be preserved against the will of the sufferer." Bouvia was allowed to leave the hospital. At the time of this writing, she remains alive.

Brophy v New England Sinai Hospital, Inc., a 1986 Massachusetts case, supported the withholding of nutrition and hydration from a patient in a persistent vegetative state.[26] The Massachusetts court made this ruling because the evidence demonstrated that the patient would never regain cognitive behavior, the ability to communicate, or the capability of interacting purposefully with his environment. The Massachusetts Supreme Judicial Court observed in the Brophy case:[26]

> In certain, thankfully rare circumstances, the burden of maintaining the corporeal existence degrades the very humanity it was meant to serve. The law recognizes the individual's right to preserve his humanity even if to preserve his humanity to allow processes of a disease or affliction to bring about a death with dignity.

In 1987, the New Jersey Supreme Court ruled on new cases concerning withholding and withdrawing life support and took the position that a person's right to determine his or her own fate took precedence over even the state's interests.[27, 28] These rulings were the first that specifically provided immunity from liability for relatives or friends who made decisions on behalf of a patient "in good faith."

In the Drabick case in California in 1988 it was ruled that mentally incapacitated patients are entitled to have appropriate decisions made in their behalf by surrogate decision makers.[29] The family wanted nutrition and hydration withdrawn from Mr. Drabick, who was in a persistent vegetative state. The court supported the Drabick family, and life support was withdrawn. The report of the President's commission in 1983 urged adoption of the "proportionate treatment test" in situations in which an individual did not make his or her wishes known in a legally acceptable writing or by some other reliable means such as a living will.[30] The 1983 *Barber v Superior Court* decision relied on a proportionate treatment analysis. The Drabick court also focused on the question of whether the benefits of the treatment outweigh the detriments. Specifically, the Drabick court stated:[29]

> Proportionate treatment is that which, in the view of the patient, has at least a reasonable chance of providing benefits to the patient, which benefits outweigh the burdens attendant to the treatment. Thus, even if a proposed course of treatment might be extremely painful or intrusive, it would still be proportionate treatment if the prognosis was for complete cure or significant improvement in the patient's condition. On the other hand, a treatment course which is only minimally painful or intrusive may nonetheless be considered disproportionate to the potential benefits if the prognosis is virtually hopeless for any significant condition.

At the same time that the Drabick court made a progressive decision concerning the withholding of nutrition and hydration for patients in persistent vegetative states in California, the state courts in New York and Missouri made it more difficult to withhold or withdraw life-sustaining treatment from incompetent patients.[31, 32] In the New York case concerning Mary O'Connor, the court ruled that treatment must be given unless there is clear evidence the patient would have chosen to refuse it.[31] This rigid and strict decision set a standard of proof that few patients are likely to be able to meet. In the Missouri case of Nancy Cruzan, the court declared that the state had an "unqualified" interest in prolonging life.[32] Thus, the Missouri court severely limited the right of families to make decisions on behalf of incompetent patients. Furthermore, the court stated that families cannot make the decision to have treatment stopped without "the most rigid of formalities." The type of data the court discussed that would assist in making the decision to withdraw care from incompetent patients included a living will or clear and convincing evidence of a patient's refusal to be treated. However, in the same ruling, the Missouri court undermined the power of living wills (advance directives):

"It is definitionally impossible for a person to make an informed decision—either to consent or refuse—under hypothetical circumstances."[32] Of note, Missouri's living-will law does not permit refusal of artificial feedings. In addition, the court determined that continued tube feedings were "not heroically invasive" because the "invasion took place when the gastrostomy tube was inserted."[32]

In June 1990 the Supreme Court of the United States made its landmark ruling on the Nancy Cruzan case, which had been appealed from the state of Missouri.[32-35] This was the first case dealing with withholding and withdrawing life support ever heard by the Supreme Court of the United States. The Supreme Court voted to uphold the state of Missouri and its position that a state can prohibit families from withdrawing life support from a legally incompetent loved one if there is not definite and convincing data clearly supporting the fact that the patient wanted life support to be withheld or withdrawn. The U.S. Supreme Court voted five to four in upholding the Missouri ruling. At first glance, the decision might appear to have sweeping implications. However, it is a narrow ruling that simply upholds the rights of a specific state to decide what type of evidence it will require when considering the withholding and withdrawing of life support from incompetent patients. It must be emphasized that many states already support the right of families and physicians to withhold or withdraw life support. In addition, a number of states have supported the withdrawing of nutrition and hydration from patients in persistent vegetative states.[29]

Chief Justice William Rehnquist of the U.S. Supreme Court wrote, "There is no automatic assurance that the view of close family members will be necessarily the same as the patient's would have been had she been confronted with her situation while competent." Chief Justice Rehnquist's opinion implied that if Ms. Cruzan had filled out a living will, the U.S. Supreme Court might have honored such a statement signed by her. Thus, the Cruzan decision both supported states' rights to decide how to handle withholding and withdrawing life support and upheld the importance of advance directives that could determine whether life support could be withheld or withdrawn from an incompetent patient. Chief Justice Rehnquist wrote, "For purposes of this case, we assume that the United States Constitution would grant a competent person a constitutionally protected right to refuse life saving hydration and nutrition."

There is no question that there will be many future state decisions concerning these issues and perhaps even more U.S. Supreme Court decisions. Withholding and withdrawing life support is one of the most important biomedical ethical issues in intensive care medicine. Other key ethical issues in intensive care include the extent of health care rationing and the just distribution of ICU resources.

LIVING WILL LEGISLATION AND ETHICAL DECISION MAKING

In the early 1980s, state legislatures began to pass liberal legislation that allowed citizens the right to dictate what type of health care they would receive if they became legally incompetent.[36] Fundamentally, three types of living wills or advance directive documents have been passed by individual states: living wills, natural death act directives, and durable powers of attorney for health care.[37] Generic living wills (not necessarily passed by specific state legislatures) are available from the Society for the Right to Die or Concern for Dying.[19] It is important to remember that if a living will has not been approved by a specific state legislature, it is not legally binding. In other words, if you have a durable power of attorney for health care from California and become critically ill and lose your legal competence in Missouri, the California living will document does not have legal validity in Missouri. However, living will documents are still of significant value to families, loved ones, surrogates, and health care providers in determining what the patient would have wanted. It is better to have filled out a living will document even if it is not legally valid in a particular state than not to have filled one out. At present, more than 44 states have passed living will legislation.

The most effective type of advance directive is a durable power of attorney for health care. The first durable power of attorney for health care was passed in Pennsylvania in 1982. The California legislature passed the California Durable Power of Attorney for Health Care in 1984. This document enables the individual to indicate treatment preferences in various situations and designate an "attorney in fact" who is empowered to make decisions should the patient become legally incompetent.[37]

In the same way that a will guarantees the person's wishes concerning his or her estate after death, a living will document (which all adult Americans should fill out) guarantees the person's wishes concerning the quality or quantity of health care to be delivered if he or she becomes legally incompetent. Extensive court precedents and legislative actions support the view that life-sustaining treatments can be withheld if it can be determined that the incompetent patient would not have wanted them.[1, 23, 29, 30, 38]

It is not necessary for a person filling out a living will to list all the specific management approaches he or she would prefer in a variety of possible illness scenarios. Because different individuals would develop different lists and each individual's medical problems are unique, it is preferable to complete a living will with a generic statement such as, "If I have, in essence, no chance to regain a reasonable quality of life, please withhold and withdraw life support (including nutrition and hydration) from me so I can die with peace and dignity." If a standard list of scenarios and management approaches was developed in the future for use throughout the country, this approach might be reasonable.

KEY PRACTICAL PRINCIPLES IN ETHICAL DECISION MAKING

Four practical principles should be followed when considering withholding or withdrawing life support or other biomedical ethical issues in care of patients (Table 148–1).[1, 38] Probably the most important key practical principle in ethical decision making in the ICU is the identification of the true source of authority for decision making. Physicians guide patients through decisions; they are not in charge of decision making. The actual authority over the patient never resides with the physician. Patients have the ethical and legal autonomy to decide what type of health care they wish to receive. If the patient is incompetent, appropriately identified family or other surrogates (e.g., "attorney in fact" identified in a durable power of attorney for health care) have the right to

decide what happens to them. Many of the ethical problems and controversies in intensive care are a result of overt or covert violations of this principle. Physicians are consultants engaged to evaluate their patient's problems; present reasonable options for diagnosis and management in clear, understandable language; and assist in thoughtful decision making. Except in emergencies, doctors should not proceed with management plans until those with the true authority (i.e., patients) have clearly decided.

The second key practical principle in ethical decision making in intensive care medicine is that health care providers should be excellent communicators with patients and families. Communication skills vary considerably among intensive care providers, from physicians to nurses. Especially in critical care situations, stress, fear, intimidation, and unfamiliarity with the setting can overwhelm even sophisticated patients and families. Intensive care professionals are responsible not merely for attempting to communicate but also for ensuring that effective communication takes place. In essence, solutions to difficult problems involving withholding and withdrawing life support evolve through effective communication with patients, families, and surrogate decision makers. There is no skill more important in the ICU setting.

Some physicians communicate better than others. When physicians are told about communication problems by patients, families, surrogates, or members of the health care team, they should quickly obtain the assistance of an effective communication facilitator—a social worker, religious leader, ethicist, or psychotherapist, for example. Communication in the intensive care setting is difficult for a physician for a number of reasons. First, each case is stressful and emotionally wrenching and takes a major physical and psychologic toll on physicians. Second, the accumulation of many such cases exacts a high price from physicians in terms of emotional fatigue, personal fear of death, guilt, insecurity, and anxiety. In fact, it is probable that many intensive care providers "burn out" because of the high stress levels of their jobs. Third, effective communication in catastrophic situations requires time, a scarce commodity among physicians. With the demands, stress, and time commitments in such a work environment, it is understandable that physicians often have difficulty in nurturing their personal lives. Again, outside facilitators can be extremely valuable to the health care team because they have superior communication skills and the time to use them. Unfortunately, physicians and other intensive care providers sometimes feel a loss of control when they ask facilitators to help them in handling difficult cases, which often concern withholding or withdrawing life support. It should be a rule rather than an exception to bring in a facilitator at an early stage whenever ethical decision making appears difficult.

A number of actions can be taken to optimize effective communication: (1) create an environment that fosters communication. Rushed or chaotic settings, such as hospital corridors, hinder optimal decision making. (2) Remember that stress often impairs the reasonableness of patients, families, and health care providers. Keep communication simple until it is clear that more medical detail will be helpful rather than intimidating or overwhelming. (3) Encourage patients, families, and surrogates to ask questions and express their feelings. This helps to counteract the intimidation many people experience in dealing with health care providers and ICUs.

Remember to present information in the language and at the level of detail that best enables patients or surrogates to decide. It is not helpful to keep people at a distance with an esoteric medical vocabulary, unnecessary details, or an inappropriate or standoffish emotional tone. Ask patients and

---

TABLE 148–1

FOUR KEY PRACTICAL PRINCIPLES FOR ETHICAL DECISION MAKING IN INTENSIVE CARE MEDICINE

1. Identify the source of authority for decision making.
2. Achieve effective communication with patients and families.
3. Carry out early determination and ongoing review of patients' desires.
4. Clearly recognize patients' rights.

families to summarize what has been said to check the accuracy of communication, correct misunderstandings, and assess the level of comprehension and reasoning. All intensive care providers should make an effort to gain insight into and optimize their communication skills. Colleagues who act as observers can be most helpful in this situation.

An example of poor communication in an intensive care setting would be telling a family that their critically ill loved one is "stable" without any further explanation. A more truthful report to the family might be: "Your husband is as sick as any person can be, and the odds are overwhelming he will not survive. His status has not changed in the last 24 hours, and if he does not improve over the next several days, we might have to begin to discuss decreasing our level of intensive care support."

Another example of poor communication is telling a family that a critically ill patient has improved after 4 days, whereas, in fact, the patient's overall status still carries a dismal prognosis and only one relatively unimportant physiologic criterion has mildly improved. Although this type of misleading good news may make the health care provider feel better, it inappropriately alters the expectations of the patient's family. Care must be taken at all times to state the true prognosis for any patient before discussing daily, often unimportant, fluctuations in status.

The third key practical principle in ethical decision making is the necessity for early determination and ongoing review of quality of life values. Physicians must learn, whenever possible, the views of each patient or surrogate on the balance between quality and mere prolongation of life—this is the concept of proportionality that was discussed in the previous section on legal precedents. Health care professionals should avoid making assumptions in this area, especially with patients who have different religious, cultural, or ethnic backgrounds. The balance between the probable extension of life and the reduction of quality of life resulting from any treatment must be clearly described and discussed with each patient.

When physicians were more paternalistic several decades ago, as compared with being partners in health care in today's practice of intensive care, they also painted an unduly optimistic picture. This was a mistake then and certainly would be one now, because physicians who unintentionally do this appear untrustworthy at a time when the ability to trust one's physician is critical. The same applies to families who want to withhold information from their loved ones who are patients. In almost all cases, it is the physician's duty to be honest and straightforward with the patient concerning diagnosis, treatment options, and prognosis. Specific treatment options for probable complications should be explored as early as possible to avoid unnecessary guilt when surrogates are forced to decide for incompetent patients. After permission from patients, family members should be included in anticipatory decision making so that they have no doubt about the patient's wishes. For example, having a patient agree with a do-not-resuscitate (DNR) order without informing the family might result in a situation in which the patient becomes legally incompetent and the family refuses to allow a DNR order even though the patient's wishes were stated in front of several health care providers. This can result in a complex, highly emotional, adversarial relationship between the patient's surrogates and the health care team. As an illness progresses, patients commonly reassess the relative cost and benefits of treatments as they gain insight into available therapies. Thus, it is important to understand the patient's feelings about proportionality if there is any significant change in status. Such reassessment also requires active and careful exploration of the thoughts and feelings of families as they might participate in or influence the patient in decision making.

Any medical intervention should be oriented toward the patient's goals as well as toward solving a clinical dilemma. In many cases, there is a point beyond which medical interventions act less to prolong life than to extend a miserable dying process.[1, 30, 38-40] Professionals cannot expect patients or families to take the lead in asking these questions.

The fourth key practical principle in ethical decision making is the recognition that patients have significant rights. Most physicians do not realize that the American Hospital Association developed a code of patients' rights and this code has been enacted into law in many states.[41] When intensive care practitioners observe the spirit of these rights, ethical decision making is not a major difficulty. Some of the most important of these patients' rights are: (1) to receive considerate and respectful care; (2) to receive information about the illness, the course of treatment, and the prospects for recovery in terms the patient can understand; (3) to receive as much information about any proposed treatment or procedure as the patient may need in order to give informed consent or to refuse this course of treatment (except in emergencies, this information should include a description of the procedure or treatment, the medically important risks involved in the treatment, alternative courses of treatment or nontreatment and the risks involved in each, and the name of the person who will carry out the treatment or procedure); (4) to participate actively in decisions regarding the medical care (to the extent permitted by law, this includes the right to refuse treatment); and (5) to have patients' rights applied to the person who may have legal responsibility to make decisions about medical care on behalf of the patient.[38]

WITHHOLDING BASIC LIFE SUPPORT

Forgoing basic life support such as food, water, and supplementary oxygen is difficult in clinical practice. Usually, these basics of care are provided as a reflex, without carefully considering whether a truly caring act is being performed.

When patients are critically ill, health care providers must replace such impulses with a careful decision-making process that takes into account a number of important points. (1) Every medical intervention should serve what patients define to be in their best interest. This can be determined only through optimal communication among patients, families, surrogates, and health care providers. (2) It is wise to include close family members in the decision-making process whenever possible. This minimizes the possibility of emotional and adversarial conflicts at times of significant stress. (3) Health care providers should anticipate the likely medical course or courses and obtain clearly in advance the specific choices the patient wishes to make for each major situation. (4) When a medical intervention is begun during a grave illness, withdrawing it to avoid an agonizing dying process requires a direct action that may result in a death. However necessary and humane such an action may be, those forced to make such decisions and those who carry them out are inevitably left with disturbing feelings.

The types of medications used in caring for critically ill patients must be evaluated carefully. For example, patients who are terminally ill, suffering, and awaiting death might be better served by not having infections treated with antibiotics or cerebral edema treated with steroids. It is horrible to observe comatose, hopelessly ill patients being pulled back needlessly from a painless death to live out several more days or weeks in pain, misery, and indignity. When this situation occurs, it may be due to frustrated health care providers attempting to gain a sense of control by treating conditions as opposed to treating patients. If family members or legal surrogates for the patient want every possible measure taken to keep the patient alive, professionals should comply with this request. If the desire to persist in treatment seems inappropriate to the intensive care providers, a direct, logical challenge often fails, whereas a sensitive and compassionate exploration of underlying feelings often results in more thoughtful ethical decision making.[38]

It is important for health care providers to clarify the purpose of placing intravenous catheters in patients with bleak prognoses. Unless a patient-oriented goal has been defined, it is not acceptable to begin intravenous therapy for hydration and nutrition. As with all forms of active therapy, when an intravenous line is in place, it becomes more difficult to stop treating infections and electrolyte imbalances that might provide a humane death. The same reasoning applies to ordering laboratory tests or assessing vital signs. When a treatment problem is identified, it becomes harder not to act, especially when one considers plaintiff's attorneys and legal liability. Obviously, cautions similar to those related to placing intravenous lines apply to the placement of feeding tubes, especially in patients in persistent vegetative states.

WITHHOLDING ADVANCED LIFE SUPPORT

The application of cardiopulmonary resuscitation (CPR) raises many ethical issues. A patient in cardiac or pulmonary arrest presents professionals with an emergency requiring a set of automatic responses if function is to be restored before severe organ damage or death occurs. Unless they are aware of the patient's previously expressed wishes about resuscitation, physicians must act first and evaluate later. No one is interested in training paramedics to delay CPR while studiously analyzing the ethics of the situation.

A 1983 study of all the resuscitations in 1 year at a major medical center revealed that only 14% of those who received CPR survived to leave the hospital.[42] Only 19% of all patients discussed the procedure with their physicians, and in only 32% of the cases was the family consulted about resuscitation, even though more than 95% of the physicians claimed to believe such consultations appropriate. In a 1986 study, 22% of patients and 86% of families were involved in decisions not to resuscitate.[43] The families identified the attending physician as a source of help in making their decisions. Other useful factors included the presence of coma or brain death, indicating a hopeless prognosis; support and reassurance from physicians and nurses that the decision was appropriate; assurances from the staff that care and comfort would be maintained; and previous conversations with the patient about CPR.

The success rate of CPR in 503 consecutive patients aged 70 and older in five Boston hospitals was published in 1989.[44] Twenty-two percent of the patients survived initially but only 3.8% survived to hospital discharge. Only 2 of 244 patients with out-of-hospital cardiopulmonary arrest left the hospital alive. Only 17 of 259 patients with in-hospital arrest survived to discharge. Most of these survivors had ventricular arrhythmias and were resuscitated within minutes. The poorest outcomes were for patients with unwitnessed arrests, terminal arrhythmias such as electromechanical dissociation and asystole, and patients with CPR lasting more than 15 minutes.

These studies show the poor survival and ethical dilemmas inherent in CPR. In view of the invasive and, at times, almost brutal nature of the procedure, it is difficult to reconcile the small chance of a successful outcome in certain subpopulations with the loss of a more dignified death. This is especially so in the setting of chronic, severely debilitating, or terminal conditions. In attempting to minimize this type of dilemma, the intensive care provider should focus on several important points: (1) because cardiopulmonary arrest is likely to occur

during the hospitalization of an elderly, chronically ill, or terminally ill person, there is little ethical justification for not discussing it in advance. This imperative applies to similar patients who remain at home or in nursing homes. (2) The code status of patients should be identified early and conveyed to patients, families, and all health care providers. (3) Prominent signs at the front of medical charts or records should be mandatory. (4) Attending physicians and other health care providers must take the lead in bringing up this matter. If they neglect to do so, everyone pays a high price. Physicians or other health care providers who feel uneasy with such decision making or who are not fully prepared to support it have an obligation to seek education or counseling to prepare them to perform this duty effectively. All intensive care medicine training programs should devote a component of their educational program to this area. When the critical care team has any doubt or lack of unanimity, it is often of significant help to enlist the aid of a facilitator to discuss the thoughts and feelings of each member of the team.

Some physicians have difficulty in asking patients whether they want a DNR order written in the chart. The reasons for this were discussed earlier and include stress, time limitations, and the emotional difficulty of having such a discussion with a patient—especially a long-term patient who might even be a friend. Another reason why some physicians do not regularly discuss potential DNR orders with their patients is that many severely ill patients, when asked whether they want a DNR order, decide not to have one written in the chart. The main reason for this is human tenacity in holding on to life. Facing death is something we attempt to avoid at all costs, even when death is near. However, physicians should not be dissuaded from asking patients about DNR orders. In fact, to make this type of discussion with patients, relatives, or surrogates more productive, physicians should always ask two questions:

1. "Would you like us to write a DNR order in your medical chart? This means, if you have a cardiopulmonary arrest, you will not be resuscitated, and therefore, you will probably not survive."

2. [To be asked if the patient wants CPR] "Let's presume you are successfully resuscitated and admitted to the ICU on life support. If the critical care team determines after 72 hours of doing all in their power to save your life that you have, in essence, no chance to regain a reasonable quality of life, would you agree to let us withdraw life support and let you die with peace and dignity?"

Most patients who do not agree to a DNR order do agree to this second proposal. If the patient agrees to the second proposal, it should be documented in the medical chart in front of witnesses, and the family and legal surrogates should be notified immediately to make sure they are aware of the patient's plan. Thus, talking with patients about whether they want CPR is vitally important and, in almost all cases, assists health care providers in determining how to care for their patients.

In the late 1980s, biomedical ethicists began to address the obligations of the physician to provide care when, in fact, it would be medically futile. In 1988 Tomlinson and Brody stated, "The right of self-determination, as well as the patient's preferences, is irrelevant to the determination that resuscitation would be of no medical benefit. When this is the rationale for a DNR decision, the physician has no duty to ascertain the patient's preferences."[45] Although the health care provider should always make an effort to ascertain the patient's preferences in order to optimize sensitive and thoughtful communication, the underlying point is that, if a diagnostic or therapeutic management option is medically futile, the intensive care team is not clearly obligated to pursue the option. Some hospitals in the United States have policies stating that CPR does not have to be administered if it is deemed to be medically futile by the physician(s) of record.

The key problem is, what is the definition of medical futility? Many believe three criteria must be met to establish medical futility: (1) the disease process must be terminal, (2) the disease process must be irreversible, and (3) death must be imminent. However, the definition of imminent is not clear. Most health care providers, patients, jurists, and ethicists would agree that imminent could easily be defined as 24 to 48 hours. However, does imminent death mean within 7 days, 2 weeks, or 2 months? In addition, there have not been enough significant court cases to help us define medical futility. Health care providers should be careful not to claim care is medically futile as an excuse not to communicate effectively with the patient, family, or legal surrogates. Thoughtful decision making comes only through effective communication.

Lantos and colleagues, in 1989, wrote an article concerning the illusion of futility in clinical practice.[46] They stated that a physician is under no obligation to offer, or even discuss, futile therapies. They showed how this concept is supported by moral reasoning in ancient and modern medical ethics, by public policy, and by case law. However, they emphasized that there are no strict criteria for defining futility. They stated that it is important for health care providers to follow both clinical judgment and an explicit consideration of the patient's goals for therapy. They underscored the point that claims of medical futility should not be used to avoid difficult discussions with patients, their families, or surrogates.

Schneiderman and colleagues, in 1990, attempted to find a practical way of using the concept of medical futility in clinical practice.[47] They proposed, "When physicians conclude (either through personal experience, experiences shared with colleagues, or consideration of published empiric data) that, in the last 100 cases a medical treatment has been useless, they should regard that treatment as futile. If a treatment merely preserves permanent unconsciousness or cannot end dependence on intensive medical care, the treatment should be considered futile."[47] This provocative proposal will, in all likelihood, be one of many discussed in the next decade. Eventually, the definition of medical futility must be arrived at by state judicial or legislative decisions. The issue of medical futility will be one of the most important biomedical ethical issues in the next several years.

WITHDRAWING ADVANCED LIFE SUPPORT

One of the most difficult decisions made by intensive care providers, family members, or surrogates is whether or not to withdraw advanced life support.[1, 38, 48–50] Ideally, if effective communication has taken place before a patient is given advanced life support, the guidelines for withdrawal have already been defined by health care providers, patients, families, or surrogates. Unfortunately, such clear definition is more the exception than the rule. The following are suggestions for intensive care providers when considering withdrawal of advanced life support.

Carefully judge the likelihood of the medical benefit of intensive care using published data from studies such as APACHE II.[3]

Assess whether a patient is legally competent. A sound evaluation of mental status is key to decision making, and psychiatric consultation should be sought when the state of competence cannot be clearly identified.

Always seek unanimity among members of the intensive care team. When team members feel excluded from the decision-making process, problems arise. Because intensive care nurses provide most of this care, they often have information about patients and families that is available only to those who spend long hours at the bedside.

Vigorously solicit the patient's judgment regarding withdrawal of life support. Although most individuals receiving life support are legally incompetent, many are legally competent and have the right to make health care decisions. For example, in the California court case discussed earlier, even though Mr. Bartling was receiving ventilation, he had the right to demand that life support be stopped.[24] However, competent patients receiving life support who request that their support be stopped must be evaluated carefully. It is difficult to discriminate between a patient who is severely depressed (which interferes with reasonable decision making) and one who is making a thoughtful and reasonable request. In this type of situation, it is important to call in a facilitator. Patients receiving life support have a legal right to control their health care, and professionals who do not comply may be committing battery.

Do not rush decision making with families. These are delicate processes that have their own timing and often are not worked out for many days. Facilitators can be invaluable. Calling in facilitators early rather than late is a wise choice. The health care team should work with the family toward making a unanimous decision regarding life support for incompetent patients.

The establishment of time-limited goals based on clinical judgment and information from published studies is valuable. After being advised that life support should be discontinued, families are often overwhelmed with confusion and guilt and may resist the advice. They can be helped in decision making if concrete, temporal milestones can be identified that herald improvement or failure. For example, the physician might say to the adult children of a patient who has respiratory failure and renal failure and has been receiving ventilation for 2 weeks, "If we see no signs that your father has improved over the next 72 hours, then we believe you should consider withdrawing life support. We believe that your father is suffering and has essentially no chance to regain a reasonable quality of life. To withdraw life support would allow him a more peaceful and dignified death."[38]

Time-limited goals for decision making can involve times ranging from several days to many days. If one attempts to make decisions on a day-by-day basis, it is difficult to step back and gain a broad perspective and insight into the true prognosis. The interlude provided by time-limited goals is a period for families to give up unrealistic expectations and begin to accept the sad situation. Sometimes, before patients and families can come to a thoughtful decision, they need to express anger and mistrust generated by suboptimal communication with health care providers. Regularly, physicians must tolerate expressions of hostility without becoming defensive. The anger of patients and family members usually subsides when they understand that intensive care team members are sensitive and supportive. Even if patients or families do not express anger, it is wise to explore these feelings. Statements such as, "This may have turned out to be a lot more than you bargained for. It wouldn't surprise me if you are angry about it," can open the way to the expression and resolution of such feelings.

An effective way to tell a family that you believe life support should be withdrawn from their relative is to say, "It is my best judgment, and that of the other doctors and nurses, that your relative has essentially no chance to regain a reasonable quality of life. I am saying this based on what I understand to be your relative's desires for quality of life. We believe that life support should be withdrawn, which means your relative will probably die." There are two important components in this statement. First, the statement is realistically qualified in a way that implies a decision must be shared. Second, it makes clear that death is the probable result of the recommended course. Without this knowledge, there is no true informed consent, and emotional and legal liability is possible.

It is not uncommon for grief-stricken or guilty family members to attempt to relieve their distress at the patient's expense by pressing for disproportionate treatment (i.e., prolonging the process of dying). A good example of this would be a son returning home to visit his critically ill mother who is receiving ventilation and has, in essence, no chance to regain a reasonable quality of life. Because the son has not written to or talked with his mother for years, he is overwhelmed by guilt. It is common in such a situation for the son to be strongly against withdrawing life support. Such insistence usually dissolves when the underlying feelings are acknowledged and understood.

As a general principle, health care professionals should avoid becoming involved in cases that are inconsistent with their ethical principles. Resentment inevitably arises under such circumstances and may compromise reasonable clinical judgment. If the intensive care professional wishes, the care of the patient can be transferred in an appropriate fashion to another professional. This should be an unusual event. If involvement with the patient cannot be avoided by the intensive care professional, frequent ventilation of feelings with understanding colleagues makes optimal care more likely.

If patients are legally incompetent and there has been no documented written or oral communication about withdrawal of treatment, the problem is greater. This was true in the U.S. Supreme Court decision about Nancy Cruzan and the New York ruling on the O'Connor case.[31, 32] However, in these two cases the key issue was withdrawing basic life support—that is, hydration and nutrition—compared with withdrawing advanced life support. Intensive care providers must be knowledgeable about the laws of the state they practice in when attempting to care for incompetent patients with no written or oral communication about withdrawal of treatment. Overall, the most satisfactory resolution of such cases occurs when professionals and families carefully explore the quality-of-life values previously held by the patient. When family members have agreed that the patient would not have wanted to go on, consent to withdraw treatment usually follows. If no one knows the patient well enough to provide information about his or her quality-of-life values, professionals can establish an interdisciplinary group composed of physicians, nurses, families or friends, and two or three patient advocates (at least two of whom represent an organized religion, preferably that of the patient). This group identifies what it believes to be the most thoughtful "substituted judgment." Decisions should be made by family, friends, health care providers, and facilitators. Only rarely is legal assistance necessary.

WITHDRAWING BASIC LIFE SUPPORT

The withdrawal of basic life support, such as hydration or nutrition by intravenous catheters or feeding tubes, is legally controversial. This has been covered in the section on legal precedents and is of much current interest because of the U.S. Supreme Court ruling on the Cruzan case. Because the legality of withdrawing basic life support from patients who have not left clear instructions such as in an advance directive is now a state's rights issue, all intensive care providers should be familiar with their own state's laws. For example, to withdraw basic life support from a patient who did not leave "clear instructions" in Missouri would be against the law.

The key to resolving ethical problems in this area lies in clarifying the patient's interests. With truly informed consent and sensitive psychosocial management of decision making, most painful ambiguities can be resolved. Communication, as always, is the key. The patient's wishes regarding withdrawal of treatment should be in writing. If possible, conflicts between the patient's wishes and those of the family should be mediated toward a consensus, although the patient's wishes must be controlling. Families need assurance that comfort and caring will be maintained and intensive care providers will not abandon their loved ones.

References

1. Raffin TA, Shurkin J, Sinkler WS: Intensive Care: Facing the Critical Choices. New York, W.H. Freeman, 1988.
2. Ginzberg E: US health policy: Expectations and realities. JAMA 260:3647, 1988.
3. Raffin TA: ICU survival of patients with systemic illness. Am Rev Respir Dis 140:S28, 1989.
4. Cullen DJ, Keene R, Waternaux C, et al: Results, charges and benefits of intensive care for critically ill patients: Update 1983. Crit Care Med 12:102, 1984.
5. LeGall J, Brun-Buisson C, Trunet P, et al: Influence of age, previous health status and severity of acute illness on outcome from intensive care. Crit Care Med 10:575, 1982.
6. Knaus WA, Zimmerman JE, Wagner DP, et al: APACHE. Acute physiology and chronic health evaluation: A physiologically based classification system. Crit Care Med 9:591, 1980.
7. Knaus WA, Draper EA, Wagner DP, et al: APACHE II: A severity of disease classification system for acutely ill patients. Crit Care Med 6:685, 1985.
8. Knaus WA, Draper EA, Wagner DP, et al: Prognosis in acute organ-system failure. Ann Surg 202:685, 1985.
9. Montgomery AB, Stager MA, Carrico CJ, et al: Causes of mortality in patients with ARDS. Am Rev Respir Dis 132:485, 1985.
10. Schuster DP, Marion JM: Precedents for meaningful recovery during treatment in a medical intensive care unit: Outcome in patients with hematologic malignancy. Am J Med 75:402, 1983.
11. Fowler AA, Hammon RF, Zerbe GO, et al: Adult respiratory distress syndrome. Prognosis after onset. Am Rev Respir Dis 132:472, 1985.
12. Goldfarb G, Noel O, Poynard T, et al: Efficiency of respiratory assistance in cirrhotic patients with liver failure. Intensive Care Med 9:271, 1983.
13. Imbus SH, Zawacki BE: Autonomy for burn patients when survival is unprecedented. N Engl J Med 297:308, 1977.
14. Pinilla JC, Ross DF, Martin T, et al: Study of the incidence of intravascular catheter infection in associated septicemia in critically ill patients. Crit Care Med 11:21, 1983.
15. Tobin MJ, Grenvik A: Nosocomial lung infection and its diagnosis. Crit Care Med 12:191, 1984.
16. Girard K, Raffin TA: The chronically critically ill: To save or let die? Respir Care 30:339, 1985.
17. Danis M, Patrick DL, Sutherland LI, et al: Patients' and families' preferences for medical intensive care. JAMA 260:797, 1988.
18. Steinbrook R, Lo B, Moulton J, et al: Preferences of homosexual men with AIDS for life sustaining treatment. N Engl J Med 314:457, 1986.
19. Society for the Right to Die: The Physician and the Helplessly Ill Patient. New York, Society for the Right to Die, 1985.
20. In re Karen Quinlan, 70 NJ 10, 355 A2d 647 (1976).
21. *Saikewicz v Superintendent of Belcher State School*, 373 Mass 728, 370 NE2d 417 (1977).
22. In re Dinnerstein, 380 NE2d 134 (1978).
23. *Barber v Superior Court of Los Angeles*, 195 Cal Rptr 484, 147 Cal App 3d 1006 (1983).
24. *Bartling v Superior Court*, 209 Cal Rptr 220, 163 Cal App ed 196 (1984).
25. *Bouvia v Superior Court*, 225 Cal Rptr 297, 179 Cal App 3d 1127 (1986).
26. *Brophy v New England Sinai Hospital Inc.*, 390 Mass 417, 497 NE2d 626 (1986).
27. In re Farrell, 108 NJ 335, 529 A2d 404 (NJ 1987).
28. In re Jobes, 108 NJ 394, 529 A2d 434 (1987).
29. In re Drabick, 200 Cal App 3d 185, 245 Cal Rptr 840 (Cal Ct App 1988), *reviewed denied* (Cal, July 28, 1988), *cert denied*, 109 S Ct 399 (1988).
30. President's Commission for the Study of Ethical Problems in Medicine and Biomedical and Behavioral Research: Deciding to Forego Life-Sustaining Treatment. Washington, DC, US Government Printing Office, 1983.
31. In re O'Connor, 72 NY2d 517, 531 NE2d 607, 534 NYS2d 886 (1988).
32. *Cruzan v Harmon*, 760 SW2d 408 (1988).
33. Lo B, Rouse F, Dornbrand L: Family decision making on trial: Who decides for incompetent patients? N Engl J Med 322:1228, 1990.

34. Angell M: Prisoners of technology: The case of Nancy Cruzan. N Engl J Med 322:1226, 1990.
35. Snyder L: Life, death, and the American College of Physicians: The Cruzan case. Ann Intern Med 112:802, 1990.
36. Raffin TA: Value of the living will. Chest 90:444, 1986.
37. Gilfix M, Raffin TA: Withholding or withdrawing extraordinary life support: Optimizing rights and limiting liability. West J Med 141:387, 1984.
38. Ruark JE, Raffin TA, and the Stanford University Medical Center Committee on Ethics: Initiating and withdrawing life support: Principles and practices in adult medicine. N Engl J Med 318:25, 1988.
39. Luce JM, Raffin TA: Withholding and withdrawal of life support from critically ill patients. Chest 94:621, 1988.
40. Luce JM: Ethical principles in critical care. JAMA 263:696, 1990.
41. Title 22, §70707, Cal Admin Code (1991).
42. Bedell SE, Delbanco TL, Cook EF, et al: Survival after cardiopulmonary resuscitation in the hospital. N Engl J Med 309:569, 1983.
43. Bedell SE, Pelle D, Maher PL, et al: Do-not-resuscitate orders for critically ill patients in the hospital: How are they used and what is their impact? JAMA 256:233, 1986.
44. Murphy DJ, Murray AM, Robinson BE, et al: Outcomes of cardiopulmonary resuscitation in the elderly. Ann Intern Med 111:199, 1989.
45. Tomlinson T, Brody H: Ethics and communication in do-not-resuscitate orders. N Engl J Med 318:43, 1988.
46. Lantos JD, Singer PA, Walker RM, et al: The illusion of futility in clinical practice. Am J Med 87:81, 1989.
47. Schneiderman LJ, Jecker NS, Johnsen AR: Medical futility: Its meaning and ethical implications. Ann Intern Med 112:949, 1990.
48. NIH Workshop Summary: Withholding and withdrawing mechanical ventilation. Am Rev Respir Dis 134:1327, 1986.
49. Hastings Center: Guidelines on the termination of life-sustaining treatment in the care of the dying: A report. Hastings Cent Rep 1987.
50. Dracup K, Raffin TA: Withholding and withdrawing mechanical ventilation: Quality of life considerations. Am Rev Respir Dis 140:S44, 1989.

CHAPTER 149

The Future of Ethical Issues in Critical Care Medicine

Charles L. Sprung

During the last few decades, major alterations have occurred in the practice of medicine. These changes have been secondary to major advances in science, together with changes in the law and society. Only 30 years ago, physicians believed they had "to do everything" for their patients. This stemmed from the ethical belief in the infinite worth of a human being. Death was to be prevented at all costs. These were times of seemingly limited medical capabilities and unlimited resources.

Advances in medical technology and practices have led to a vast array of new and previously inconceivable possibilities that have been developed at a price. This price has included not only great financial costs but also the cost of human suffering. U.S. society today realizes that human finitude is a reality, that physicians cannot cure all patients, that many patients are "saved" but remain with severe disabilities, and that we possess only finite resources. Physicians have been forced to make difficult medical and ethical decisions in allocating society's scarce health care resources. They have had to decide who shall live when not all can live. This chapter traces the changes that have occurred in the practice of medicine in the last few decades and the relation of these

changes to the ethical decisions that will be made by physicians practicing critical care medicine in the future. The chapter focuses primarily on the two most common ethical issues in critical care medicine today: forgoing life-sustaining treatments and "triaging" the scarce resource of critical care beds.

HISTORICAL PERSPECTIVE

Only three decades ago, when a person ceased to breathe for several minutes, insufficient amounts of oxygen were delivered to the heart and brain and these organs stopped functioning almost immediately. The lungs, heart, and brain are interdependent, and loss of function of any one of these vital organs caused irreversible failure of the other two, leading to death within minutes.[1] In 1956, Zoll and colleagues[2] described the use of externally applied countershock to terminate ventricular fibrillation. By 1960, mouth-to-mouth ventilation and closed chest massage had also been described.[3, 4] The widespread application of these techniques, currently termed cardiopulmonary resuscitation, and the use of mechanical respirators, which were introduced in the 1950s during a catastrophic poliomyelitis epidemic,[5] have altered the previous natural sequence of events. Physicians now routinely interrupt the dying process by performing cardiopulmonary resuscitation and providing patients with respiratory assistance. Unfortunately, many patients have cardiac and respiratory function restored but remain with irreversible damage to the brain.

In the early 1960s, there was little debate about the definition of death. The traditional definition of death that was accepted by physicians and the lay public was the cessation of function of both the lungs and the heart. In 1968, the Ad Hoc Committee of the Harvard Medical School published their now famous report "to define irreversible coma as a new criterion for death."[6] The Harvard criteria for brain death determination include unreceptivity and unresponsitivity, no movements or breathing, and no reflexes. Patients who meet the Harvard criteria for brain death typically meet the traditional heart and lung criteria for death shortly thereafter—usually within 24 to 48 hours. The fact that somatic death follows brain death has led to the acceptance by the medical profession, the courts, and the public of brain death as an alternative means of diagnosing death. Several states have enacted statutory definitions of death that allow the application of brain death criteria as an alternative means of determining an individual's death.[1] The fact that brain death is now accepted has not fully solved the problem. Most unconscious patients do not meet the criteria for brain death and may still have irreversible central nervous system injury. Decisions for these patients were typically made by physicians and families and only rarely by the courts before 1975. The Quinlan case changed this and is a landmark case in the evolution of medical practice as we know it.

LEGAL PERSPECTIVE ON FORGOING LIFE-SUSTAINING TREATMENT

Karen Ann Quinlan was a 22-year-old woman who became comatose after the alleged ingestion of alcohol and tranquilizers. Her father requested that she be disconnected from her respirator. The physicians and hospital refused because they believed that she would die if she were removed from the respirator. Karen Ann Quinlan did not meet the Harvard brain death criteria and was not terminally ill. For most medical professionals at that time, withdrawing medical treatment was more difficult than withholding treatment before it had commenced.[7] It was the consensus not only of the treating physicians but also of several experts who testified in the case that removal of a patient who was not brain dead from a respirator would not conform to medical practices, standards, and traditions.[8] The New Jersey Supreme Court gave Ms. Quinlan's father the authority to remove the ventilator.[8] The court ruled that "the state's interest [in the preservation of life] contra weakens and the individual's right to privacy grows as the degree of bodily invasion increases and the prognosis dims." The court justified its decision by using the principle of "substituted judgment." Ms. Quinlan's right to refuse treatment could be exercised by her father to decide whether she would have refused therapy under these circumstances. She had previously stated that she would not want to live if she had to be confined to a ventilator.

The court had decided a matter that had previously been decided only by the medical profession, on whose authority the lower court refused to tread:[8]

> Doctors . . . to treat a patient, must deal with medical tradition and past case histories. They must be guided by what they do know. The extent of their training, their experience, consultation with other physicians, must guide their decision-making processes in providing care to their patient. The nature, extent and duration of care by societal standards is the responsibility of a physician. The morality and conscience of our society places this responsibility in the hands of the physician. What justification is there to remove it from the control of the medical profession and place it in the hands of the courts?

Several states have enacted statutes that establish procedures for forgoing life-sustaining procedures or treatments when individuals have a terminal condition. The first statute, enacted in California in 1976, was labeled a "natural death" act, and this term has been used to describe other similar state statutes.[7] Many of the statutes have a clause that gives immunity from civil or criminal liability to physicians who execute a document under the statute and in good faith withhold or withdraw life-sustaining procedures or treatments. The statutes are usually binding only when signed by a "qualified patient" or the person's legal representative. The patient must have a terminal illness, which is usually defined as an incurable condition in which death is imminent regardless of the life-prolonging procedures used. Despite the fact that many of these statutes were inspired by the Quinlan case, they usually do not apply to a patient, such as Karen Ann Quinlan, who is in a persistent vegetative state and whose death is not imminent. Many physicians have, however, considered such patients to fall within the meaning of the statutes.

MEDICAL AND LEGAL PERSPECTIVE ON FORGOING NUTRITION AND HYDRATION

Several more recent opinions have addressed not only the discontinuation of ventilators but also the issue of discontinuing artificial feeding and intravenous fluids. In a survey in 1983, physicians were presented with a hypothetic patient. The patient had incurable cancer, remained comatose after a cardiac arrest, and had no hope of recovery. Physicians were asked to note the type of intravenous fluid therapy they would give this terminally ill patient.[9] Seventy-nine of 103 physicians (73%) stated that they would administer sufficient intravenous fluids to maintain adequate hydration of the patient. Of these physicians who would initially maintain adequate hydration, 84% stated they would restart the intravenous fluid therapy if it infiltrated and 71% stated they would continue the use of the intravenous fluid therapy after the patient had remained in a coma for 3 days. Forty percent of the physicians stated they would even use invasive means to secure an intravenous route. Twenty-seven percent

of the surveyed physicians, however, would not give adequate intravenous fluids to hydrate the patient. Despite the differences of opinion among the physicians in this study, the large majority of the physicians still believed that intravenous fluids should be provided to a comatose, dying patient without any hope of survival. In addition, intravenous fluids appeared to be different from other medical treatments and their use seemed to be standard therapy entrenched in medical practice.

Several court decisions have dealt with the problem of withdrawing intravenous fluids and nutrition. In 1981, Clarence Herbert suffered a postoperative myocardial infarction that left him with severe brain damage. Because the likelihood of his recovery was poor, the family requested that all machines sustaining life be withdrawn.[10] The patient's respirator and other life-prolonging equipment were then removed. After several days and further discussions with the family, the physicians ordered the removal of the catheters that provided hydration and nourishment. Mr. Herbert died of dehydration and pneumonia approximately 1 week later, and his physicians were prosecuted for murder by the Los Angeles District Attorney. The California trial court acquitted the physicians and ruled that the cessation of life-sustaining measures "is not an affirmative act but rather a withdrawal or omission of further treatment."[10] The court stated that "medical procedures to provide nutrition and hydration are more similar to other medical procedures than to typical human ways of providing nutrition and hydration. Their benefits and burdens ought to be evaluated in the same manner as any other medical procedure." This case demonstrates that only a decade ago, the removal of life-prolonging treatments such as intravenous fluids and nutrition was considered such a gross deviation from legal and ethical standards that physicians were tried for murder for such actions. Today, almost 90% of critical care professionals state that they are withholding and withdrawing life-sustaining treatment from their patients whom they deem to have irreversible and terminal diseases.[11]

In contrast to physicians' previously held idea that continuation of intravenous fluid therapy and nutrition in patients in a persistent vegetative state is required and the opinions of district attorneys that physicians who withdraw such therapy should be prosecuted, a new medical and legal consensus on the withdrawing of artificial feeding and fluids has emerged. Several court decisions have changed the old philosophies. In *Brophy v New England Sinai Hospital Inc.*, a patient remained in a persistent vegetative state after unsuccessful surgery.[12] After 2 years, his wife requested that the feedings he was receiving through a gastrostomy be stopped. The hospital refused. The Massachusetts Supreme Judicial Court, in a four-to-three decision, ruled that Mr. Brophy's feeding tube could be removed and the patient could be allowed to die.[12]

The court rejected the argument that artificial feeding should be continued because it was ordinary and not extraordinary care. The court stated that "to be maintained by such artificial means over an extended period is not only intrusive but extraordinary." The court also rejected a difference between withholding and withdrawing treatments, including artificial feeding. It concluded that if withdrawing therapy was more difficult than withholding treatment, the distinction could discourage attempts at lifesaving medical treatments and could lead to premature decisions to allow patients to die. The President's Commission for the Study of Ethical Problems in Medicine and Biomedical and Behavioral Research had previously come to a similar conclusion.[7] Mr. Brophy had stated, "If I am ever like that, just shoot me, pull the plug."[12] The court reasoned that the state had no duty to preserve life when a patient believed that the means of prolonging life was inappropriate. This decision was made despite the fact that Mr. Brophy was not terminally ill. The court did not believe the discontinuation of feeding was suicide or direct killing but rather that it allowed the underlying disease to take its natural course. Finally, the court decided that the ethical integrity of the medical profession would not be violated if health care professionals were not forced to discontinue feedings when such behavior was contrary to their "view of their ethical duty toward their patients."[12]

Another case involving the withdrawal of nutrition was the Bouvia decision.[13] In April 1986, a California court of appeals ordered physicians to remove a nasogastric tube from Elizabeth Bouvia, a 28-year-old quadriplegic woman with severe cerebral palsy and severe arthritic pain. The court held that her refusal of treatment was not suicide and rejected the hospital's contention that removing the feeding tube would make it a party to suicide. The court did not require that a patient be comatose or terminally ill to refuse treatment. A patient could refuse treatment even if the therapy could save his or her life and its refusal would lead to an earlier death. One of the opinions in the Bouvia decision recognized a right to die with assistance.

In its first decision involving the right to refuse life-sustaining treatments or the right to die, the U.S. Supreme Court did not allow the discontinuation of tube feedings from Nancy Cruzan, a young woman in a persistent vegetative state.[14] The court held that the U.S. Constitution does not forbid the state of Missouri from requiring clear and convincing evidence of an incompetent's wishes concerning the withdrawal of life-sustaining treatments. Important, however, was the court's affirmation of the right of a competent patient to refuse life-sustaining treatments based on the due process clause of the Fourteenth Amendment. In addition, the court did not distinguish between forgoing artificial nutrition and hydration and other types of medical treatments.

Many of the court decisions noted previously cited the opinion of the Council on Ethical and Judicial Affairs of the American Medical Association that "it is not unethical to discontinue all means of life prolonging medical treatment" for patients in irreversible comas.[15] The council specifically included nutrition and hydration among other life-prolonging medical treatments.

CHANGING ATTITUDES AND PRACTICES OF PHYSICIANS

As can be seen, there has been a movement to include patients in a persistent vegetative state in the natural death statutes and to allow the withdrawal of life-support treatments from these patients. Prominent legal and medical scholars have gone one step further and have suggested that a reformulation of the definition of death criteria is warranted.[16] They assert that we should move away from the whole brain death criteria to the recognition that patients who are in a persistent vegetative state are actually dead. This redefinition is proposed despite the fact that the patients in a persistent vegetative state are in fact alive and breathing. In view of the facts that keeping these patients alive requires large expenditures and that limited health care dollars are available, this proposed change may receive added support.

Not only has there been action to discriminate against patients in a persistent vegetative state, but also evidence of discrimination against the elderly is becoming apparent. It has been proposed that age alone should be used as a standard for terminating treatment.[17] After a person has lived most of his or her natural life span, medical care should not be oriented to resisting death and should be limited to the relief of suffering.[17]

The previously discussed cases have been thought to represent passive euthanasia. In these circumstances, the patient does not receive medical treatment because it is withheld or the patient receives a medical treatment that is later withdrawn. Active euthanasia, or mercy killing, occurs when individuals take an active role in killing a patient.[18] In its 1977 policy statement on the physician and the dying patient, the American Medical Association condemned mercy killing as "contrary to the most fundamental measures of human value and worth."

Although active euthanasia remains a criminal offense in The Netherlands, the Dutch Medical Association suggested guidelines for the medical practice of euthanasia in 1984.[19] These guidelines require three "necessary conditions" for a physician to participate in euthanasia: (1) the request for euthanasia must be made consistently and freely by the patient, (2) the patient's state of illness and prognosis must be unbearable and beyond recovery, and (3) the physician must consult a colleague to "confirm the correctness of diagnosis and prognosis, to support and verify the correct medical performance of euthanasia, and to check if all (legal) requirements are met."[19] No official statistics on the incidence of euthanasia in The Netherlands are available, but a frequency of 2000 to 10,000 cases per year has been estimated.[19]

Although active euthanasia may be considered by many Americans as something that could not occur in the United States and that is impossible at the present time, the seeds of active euthanasia have already been planted in this country. Prominent physicians with an interest in ethics have stated that they believe it is not immoral for a physician to assist in the rational suicide of a terminally ill patient.[20] A 20-year-old woman with terminal ovarian cancer was killed by a physician who wanted to put her out of her misery.[21] A proposal to place a new law for active euthanasia for terminally ill patients on the November 1988 ballot in California was unsuccessful.[22] This initiative failed because of organizational problems and not because of voter sentiment. In fact, public opinion polls show that approximately 60% of the American public favor legalizing active euthanasia under certain circumstances.[23] Therefore, during the past 15 years we have evolved from situations in which it was a deviation from the medical and ethical standard to withdraw a respirator, nutrition, or intravenous fluids from a non–brain-dead patient to the present environment, in which it is accepted practice and becoming the norm to withdraw such medical treatments from certain groups of patients. We are inching closer to active euthanasia in this country, much as has already occurred in The Netherlands.

In the past two decades, we have seen a shift in the attitudes and practices of physicians.[24] There has been a movement away from the autonomy of physicians as more and more physicians become salaried employees and fewer are independent practitioners.[25] As availability of scarce resources continues to decrease, physicians have become more concerned with societal needs as opposed to the needs of individual patients. The great economic burdens posed by patients in persistent vegetative states, the elderly, and individuals with acquired immunodeficiency syndrome have worsened. Physicians are performing active euthanasia in The Netherlands, and U.S. society has become more complacent about procedures that were considered unconscionable about a decade ago.

Many individuals may believe that many of the changes that have been discussed are appropriate and ethically sound. Decisions to terminate life-sustaining treatments are made by patients and their families in an effort to exert the patient's autonomy and self-determinism, not because of the unilateral decisions of physicians. Changes in behavior are an appropriate response to the altered public perception of life-sustaining treatment as prolonging suffering and to increased recognition of the autonomy of patients. Some argue that suggestions of a "slippery slope" and movement toward active euthanasia for certain classes of patients are absurd. But even if one disagrees with these opinions, the facts clearly reveal a change in physicians' attitudes and practices during the last 15 years.

It can be inferred from the foregoing discussion that patients in chronic vegetative states and the elderly and perhaps now patients with acquired immunodeficiency syndrome are being discriminated against.[26, 27] These classes of patients represent groups of people who may be viewed by some as having lives not worth living. If a treatment is deemed futile not because it will fail technically but rather because the life saved is deemed not worthy of being saved, a moral judgment and not a medical judgment has been made. Judgments concerning the social worth of a patient's life have traditionally been considered unacceptable criteria for triage and forgoing care, yet these factors appear to be considered in some decisions.

RATIONING INTENSIVE CARE

In addition to the problem of forgoing life-sustaining treatments, the issue of triage of intensive care unit (ICU) beds is and will continue to be a most difficult problem for critical care professionals. The problem includes the allocation and triage of scarce resources, the definition of nonbeneficial or futile therapy, and the identification of who should decide and how they should decide. Triage and rationing should be distinguished from allocation. Allocation concerns the distribution of different resources and typically involves decisions made by the government, municipality, or a hospital; rationing is usually done by physicians, who determine which individual patient receives treatment or a bed when there are insufficient resources to treat all patients. Allocation decisions usually precede rationing or triage decisions. If the government decided it wanted to spend more than 12% of the gross national product on health care, many life-and-death triage decisions made by physicians on a daily basis would disappear. As the federal deficit remains significant, this is most unlikely. Therefore, the need to make triage decisions for ICU beds will more than likely continue and even increase.

There are data suggesting that physicians can ration ICU beds by adjusting admission and discharge thresholds without adversely affecting patients' outcomes.[28, 29] These changes in admission and discharge criteria included restricting ICU admissions to more severely ill patients, reducing the proportion of patients admitted primarily for monitoring, and discharging more severely ill patients earlier.[28, 29] When physicians do make triage decisions and especially when they alter their criteria for admitting and discharging patients, it is hoped that their decisions remain objective and are not based on value judgments. Unfortunately, despite certain good predictive scoring systems[30] and risk stratification, medical uncertainty persists. A physician's ability to predict accurately a patient's survival and benefit from critical care remains inadequate. This ability will probably improve in the future, but accuracy of 100% is still unlikely.

Physicians have no ethical, medical, or legal obligation to provide futile treatment.[31] Unfortunately, there is a lack of consensus in defining futility. Physicians appear to disagree about several elements of medical futility, including the likelihood of treatment success and the goals of therapy.[32] Futility as an expression of probability means different things to different individuals. Some strictly define it in terms of a moribund patient who will die within hours or days no matter what treatment is given,[31] whereas others are less strict and use the term futile for situations in which success rates are as high as 13%.[33] Disagreements about the chances of success may also be related to incorrect medical knowledge and different clinical assessments secondary to medical uncertainty.[31] Physicians can also disagree with patients, families, and colleagues about the goals of treatment. Physicians may consider treatment futile if it merely allows a patient to survive for a few weeks in an ICU,[34] whereas a patient may view such an outcome as an opportunity to see loved ones or to get his or her affairs in order. Therefore, in a pluralistic American society based on individualism, it may be extremely difficult to define treatment success, goals of therapy, or absolute triage criteria for admission to and discharge from the ICU.

Who should decide which patients are to be admitted to critical care? If a patient with acquired immunodeficiency syndrome, multiple organ system failure, or metastatic carcinoma desires a chance to live and demands admission to an ICU, but the ICU physicians believe that admission would be futile or not beneficial, should the patient be admitted? Should there be any difference if the patient's physicians agree with the patient and family? Even if curative therapy is not an option, should the ICU be used to alleviate suffering and provide care that cannot be given on a hospital ward? Some advocate treatment even when the chance of success is low if the patient requests treatment and the alternative is death.[31] But does this treatment include a scarce resource such as a bed in an ICU? Does nonadmission to an ICU mean death? Should this patient be admitted if it will take away from the care of patients already present in the ICU? When demand for these beds threatens the capability of the ICU to provide care, treatment decisions should be based on the relative needs of all patients.[35] Therefore, the easy way, which is usually just admitting another patient, is not in the best interests of the patients already being treated in the ICU. The President's commission[36] described an adequate level of medical care below which no one should fall, not a ceiling above which no one may rise. What is adequate, however, may vary depending on the availability of scarce resources such as critical care beds, the effectiveness of different types of care, or the priorities set by society.[36]

If the patient and family do not decide, should the physician alone decide? In most circumstances, physicians do make these decisions based on objective criteria. For practical decision making, guidelines must be flexible, which may allow unfair, subjective decisions. Ideally, medical inclusion and exclusion criteria should be established and any patient meeting inclusion criteria should be admitted on a first come, first served basis. Physicians and our society would be much better off if allocation and triage decisions were explicitly made on the basis of objective guidelines developed by a consensus panel of experts after public debate. Until public discussion occurs and guidelines are developed, controversy will continue. With the increasing power of hospital committees and administrators, it would not be surprising if ICU triage decisions were made by them and not by physicians in the future. In the future, physicians will be called on more and more to make difficult ethical decisions for institutions and society rather than just for their individual patients.

CONCLUSIONS

Physicians are having and will continue to have difficulty in treating their patients on the basis of their ethical standards. They have been forced to worry too much about legal liability. At times, the courts, hospital administrators, risk managers, hospital attorneys, and insurance companies dictate the practice of medicine more than physicians. Unfortunately, these problems will become worse in the future. Physicians must become more active in advocating and publicizing medical standards. Our society must recognize that physicians can act prospectively to define what is best for patients and society, whereas the legal system merely reacts to a specific case. In addition, what is legal may not be ethical. What lies ahead for physicians practicing critical care medicine is uncertain but is sure to be challenging. Only by being true to our ethical standards and continuing to advocate for our individual patients will we survive as true physicians.

"The purely scientific issues pale by comparison to highly sensitive issues of law, ethics, economics, morality and social cohesion that are beginning to surface."[37]

References

1. President's Commission for the Study of Ethical Problems in Medicine and Biomedical and Behavioral Research: A Report on the Medical, Legal and Ethical Issues in the Determination of Death: Defining Death. Washington, DC, US Government Printing Office, 1981.
2. Zoll P, Linenthal A, Gibson W, et al: Termination of ventricular fibrillation in many by externally applied electric countershock. N Engl J Med 254:727, 1956.
3. Safar P: Mouth-to-mouth airway. Anesthesiology 18:904, 1957.
4. Kouwenhoven W, Jude J, Knicherbocker G: Closed-chest cardiac massage. JAMA 173:1064, 1960.
5. Engstrom CG: Treatment of severe respiratory paralysis by the Engstrom Universal Respirator. Br Med J 2:666, 1954.
6. Ad Hoc Committee of the Harvard Medical School to Examine the Definition of Brain Death: A definition of irreversible coma. JAMA 205:337, 1968.
7. President's Commission for the Study of Ethical Problems in Medicine and Biomedical and Behavioral Research: A Report on the Ethical, Medical, and Legal Issues in Treatment Decisions: Deciding to Forego Life-Sustaining Treatment. Washington, DC, US Government Printing Office, 1983.
8. In re Quinlan, 70 NJ 10, 355 A2d 647 (1976).
9. Micetich KC, Steinnecker PH, Thomasma DC: Are intravenous fluids morally required for a dying patient? Arch Intern Med 143:975, 1983.
10. Barber v Superior Court, 195 Cal Rptr 484, 147 Cal App 3d 1006 (1983).
11. The Society of Critical Care Medicine Ethics Task Force: Attitudes of critical care medicine professionals concerning foregoing life-sustaining treatments. Crit Care Med 20:320, 1992.
12. Brophy v New England Sinai Hospital Inc., 497 NE2d 626 (Mass 1986).
13. Bouvia v Superior Court, 225 Cal Rptr 297, Cal App 2d Dist (1986).
14. Cruzan v Director, Missouri Department of Health, 110 S Ct 2841 (1990).
15. Current Opinions of the Council on Ethical and Judicial Affairs of the American Medical Association—1986: Withholding or Withdrawing Life-Prolonging Medical Treatment. Chicago, American Medical Association, 1986.
16. Schaffner KF, Snyder JV, Abramson NS, et al: Philosophical, ethical, and legal aspects of resuscitation medicine, III: Discussion. Crit Care Med 16:1069, 1988.
17. Callahan D: Terminating treatment: Age as a standard. Hastings Cent Rep 17:21, 1987.
18. Rachels J: Active and passive euthanasia. N Engl J Med 292:78, 1975.
19. De Wachter MAM: Active euthanasia in The Netherlands. JAMA 262:3316, 1989.
20. Wanzer SH, Federman DO, Adelstein SJ, et al: The physician's responsibility toward hopelessly ill patients. N Engl J Med 320:844, 1989.
21. It's over, Debbie. JAMA 259:272, 1989.
22. The Humane and Dignified Death Act, Cal Civ Code 10.5.
23. Roper Organization of New York City: The 1988 Roper Poll on Attitudes Toward Active Voluntary Euthanasia. Los Angeles, National Hemlock Society, 1988.
24. Sprung CL: Changing attitudes and practices in foregoing life-sustaining treatments. JAMA 263:2211, 1990.
25. Starr P: The Social Transformation of American Medicine. New York, Basic Books, p 420, 1982.
26. Brandt A: AIDS: From social history to social policy. Law Med Health Care 14:231, 1986.
27. Skeel JD, Self DJ: AIDS and the allocation of limited resources: Admissions to intensive care units. J Crit Care 3:195, 1988.
28. Singer DE, Carr PL, Mulley AG, et al: Rationing intensive care—Physician responses to a resource shortage. N Engl J Med 309:1155, 1983.
29. Strauss MJ, LoGerfo JP, Yeltatzie JA, et al: Rationing of intensive care unit services. JAMA 255:1143, 1986.
30. Knaus WA, Draper EA, Wagner DP, et al: APACHE II: A severity of disease classification. Crit Care Med 13:818, 1985.
31. Lo B, Raffin TA, Cohen NH, et al: Ethical dilemmas about intensive care for patients with AIDS. Rev Infect Dis 9:1163, 1987.
32. Lantos JD, Singer PA, Walker RM, et al: The illusion of futility in clinical practice. Am J Med 87:81, 1989.
33. Wachter RM, Cooke M, Hopewell PC: Attitudes of medical residents regarding intensive care for patients with the acquired immunodeficiency syndrome. Arch Intern Med 148:149, 1988.
34. Danis M, Patrick DL, Southerland LI, et al: Patients' and families' preferences for medical intensive care. JAMA 260:797, 1988.
35. Engelhardt HM, Rie MA: Intensive care units, scarce resources, and conflicting principles of justice. JAMA 255:1159, 1986.
36. President's Commission for the Study of Ethical Problems in Medicine and Biomedical and Behavioral Research: A Report on the Ethical, Medical, and Legal Issues in Treatment Decisions. Securing Access to Health Care. Washington, DC, US Government Printing Office, 1983.
37. Koop CE: Medical news and perspectives. JAMA 258:2023, 1987.

INDEX

Note: Page numbers in *italics* refer to illustrations;
page numbers followed by t refer to tables.

A

A wave, atrial, *1017*, 1017–1018, *1079*,
  1079–1080, *1080*
  giant, 1080, *1080*
Abbreviated Injury Scale, 1575, 1575t–
  1581t
Abdomen. See also *Pain, abdominal.*
  acute, 1474–1484
  binding of, 122–123
  CPR role of, 122–123
  emergent disorders in, 1133–1142, 1145
  paracentesis of, 168t, 168–169
  trauma injury to, 892–893, 1145, 1578t,
    1579t, 1588–1589, *1589*
  vascular disorders in, 1133–1142, 1145
  wall of, bleeding in, 1484
Aberrant air, thoracic trauma and, 889
ABO system, 1387
Abortion, septic, 1609
Abscess. See also *Fasciitis, necrotizing.*
  brain, drug abuse patient and, 567, 567t
    sinusitis and, 475t, 476, *476*
  cutaneous, 450
  drug abuse patient and, 567, 570–571
  fungus infection and, 1481
  gas, 450
  hepatosplenic, 1481
  intra-abdominal, 516, 516t, 518, 518t,
    561–562
  lung, 570–571
  muscle, 452
  neck, *477*, 477–479
  parapharyngeal, 478–479
  peritoneal, 516, 516t, 518, 518t
  peritonsillar, *477*, 478
  spinal epidural, 567
  subperiosteal, 473
Abulia, Wernicke-Korsakoff syndrome and,
  710
Acanthocytes, hemolytic anemia and, 1372,
  1384
Accidents, disasters caused by, 32, 32t, 33t
  transportation and, 32, 32t, 33t
ACE inhibitors, cough and, 900
  heart failure and, 1044–1045
  hypertensive emergency and, 1331
  pregnancy and, 1605
Acetaldehyde, ethanol metabolized to, *1715*
  paraldehyde metabolized to, *1719*
Acetaminophen, abdominal pain due to,
  1483t
  lactic acidosis caused by, 1238–1239
  poisoning due to, 1707–1708, *1708*

Acetate, dialysis solution of, 1280–1282,
  1282t
Acetazolamide, diuresis due to, 1164–1165,
  1165t
Acetone, *1718*
  isopropanol metabolized to, 1718, *1718*
  poisoning due to, 1718t, 1719
Acetylcholine, motor neuron and, 673–674
Acetylcholinesterase, nerve agent inhibition
  of, 48, 51–52
  organophosphate inhibition of, 48, 51–52
Acetylcysteine, asthma treated with, 810
  oxygen toxicity treated with, 955, 955t
  sputum viscosity and, 810, 962
Acetylsalicylic acid. See *Aspirin (acetylsalicylic
  acid).*
Acid-base balance, 1219–1229. See also
  Acidosis; Alkalosis.
  heart affected by, 1038–1048
  hydrogen ion and, 1220–1222, *1221*,
    1222
  kidney role in, 1219–1221, *1221*
  nomogram for, *1222*
  regulatory mechanisms for, 1219–1221,
    1221, *1222*
Acidosis, 1038–1048
  alcoholic, 1223–1224
  anion gap and, 1223–1224
  bicarbonate therapy and, 1042–1044,
    1042–1044
  causes of, *1221*, 1223t, 1223–1226, 1224t,
    1225t
  COPD and, 798
  deficient ammonia excretion and, 1225t,
    1225–1226
  diagnosis of, *1222*, 1229t
  hyperchloremic, 1223t, 1224
  hypoxia with, 1041–1044, *1041–1044*
  impaired acid excretion in, 1225t, 1225–
    1226
  kidney transplant and, 1298
  lactic, 1231–1242. See also *Lactic acidosis.*
  metabolic, 1038–1042, *1222*, 1222–1226,
    1223t
  myocardium affected by, *1039*, 1039t,
    1039–1041, *1040*, 1040t
  nomogram for, *1222*
  potassium level and, 1180, 1180t, 1181
  renal tubular, 1220–1222, *1221*, 1224t,
    1224–1225
  respiratory, 1039–1040, *1040*, *1222*
  shock and, 980, *980*, 985
  treatment of, 1041–1044, *1041–1044*,
    1226, 1229t

Acids, corrosive ingestion and, 1432t,
  1432–1435, 1434t
  dietary source of, 1220
  esophageal injury caused by, 1432t,
    1432–1435, 1434t
  impaired excretion of, 1221, *1221*, 1225–
    1226
Acinus, 719, *720*, *721*
Acquired immunodeficiency syndrome
  (AIDS). See also *HIV infection.*
  abdominal pain with, 1482
  bronchoalveolar lavage in, 199, 589–598
  diarrhea and, 511–512
  epidemiology of, 591t, 591–592, *592*,
    592t
  global aspects of, 591t, 591–592, *592*
  ocular infections and, 472
  pathophysiology of, 589–591, *590*
  prevention of, 564, 596–598, 598t
  prognosis and, 596, 597t
  pulmonary disorders with, 595, 595t
  staging of, 597t
  transfusion and, 1391–1392
  transmission issues and, 591t, 591–592,
    592t, 596–598
  trauma patient with, 564
  treatment of, 593–594
  tuberculosis with, 430, 571
ACTH. See *Adrenocorticotropic hormone
  (ACTH).*
Action potential, heart cells and, *1050*,
  1050–1051
  motor neuron and, 673
  refractory period and, 1051
Activated charcoal. See *Charcoal.*
Acute Physiology and Chronic Health
  Evaluation (APACHE), 82–86
  format for, 84t
  II version, 83, 83t, 84t
  III version, 83–84
  mortality rates and, 83, 83t
  original, 82
  simplified, 82–83, 83t
  trauma patient and, 1575
Acyclovir, 405
  varicella treated with, 395
Addison's disease, diagnosis of, 1313t, 1314
  etiology of, 1313, 1313t
  hyperkalemia and, 1184
  precipitating factors in, 1314t
  symptoms and signs of, 1313t, 1313–
    1314
  treatment of, 1313t, 1314
Adenosine, arrhythmia treated with, 1057t
  drug interactions of, 1057t

Adenosine monophosphate (AMP), immune response role of, 1655, 1655t
Adenosine triphosphate (ATP), brain metabolism and, 632–633
cell metabolism and, 354, *355*
energy and, 354, *355*
glucose metabolism and, 1231–1233, *1232, 1233*
sepsis and, 354–357, *355, 357*
transport of, 358, *358*
Adenylate kinase, ATP production and, *355*
Adhesin, staphylococcal slime and, 604–605
Adhocracy, ICU management and, 63–64
Adipose tissue, TNF effects in, 317t
Administration, expert systems role in, 102–103
ICU and, 59–66, 60t
Admission and discharge, 1743–1744
ethical issues and, 1731–1732, 1743–1744
ICU and, 62–65, 1731–1732, 1743–1744
standards for, 74t
Adrenal glands, 1310–1317. See also *Epinephrine.*
catecholamine secretion by, 1318
hyperfunction of, 1315–1317, 1316t
hypofunction of, 1313t–1315t, 1313–1315, 1563
laboratory evaluation of, 1312
preoperative care and, 1563
secretory function of, 1310–1311, *1311*
Adrenergic agents, CPR and, 124
inhalation delivery of, 961, 961t
Adrenocorticotropic hormone (ACTH), 1310–1317
glucocorticoids and, 1310–1311, *1311*
laboratory test for, 1312
mineralocorticoids and, 1310–1311, *1311*
regulatory role of, 1310–1311, *1311*
releasing hormone for, 1310, *1311*
Adult respiratory distress syndrome (ARDS). See *Respiratory distress syndrome (adult).*
Aerobes, burn injury and, 524
granulocytopenia and, 533t
peritonitis and, 514–515
Aerosols, adrenergic agents in, 961t, 961–962
jet nebulizer and, 960, *960*
particle size in, 959–960, 960t
production of, *960*, 960–961, *961*
therapy using, 959t, 959–963
ultrasonic nebulizer and, 960–961, *961*
Afterload, 1081–1082, *1082*
heart failure and, 1018–1019, *1019, 1023*
Age, CPR and, 126–127
endocarditis and, 492
preoperative care and, 1568t, 1568–1569
tuberculosis and, *424*
Agglutinins, hemolytic anemia and, 1376t, 1377–1378, 1378t
AIDS. See *Acquired immunodeficiency syndrome (AIDS).*
Air. See also *Embolism, air.*
aberrant, 889
extrarespiratory, 889
Airplane transport, 43t, 43–45, *44*, 45t, 54, 54t
crashes and, 32, 32t, 33t
Airway. See also *Respiratory tract.*
acinar, 719, *720, 721*
anatomy of, 195–196, *196*, 719, *720, 721*
convective acceleration in, *725*
cross-sectional area of, 719, *720, 721*

Airway *(Continued)*
management of, 109–116. See also *Endotracheal intubation*; *Ventilation.*
algorithm for, *36*
chemical exposure and, 49–50
disasters and, 35, *36*
dust protection in, 35
equipment for, 111t, 111–113, *112*
historical aspects of, 3
indications for, 110
Mallampati classification and, 109–110, 110t
prehospital care and, 14–15, 17, 18
obstruction of, asthma causing, 805–808, 807t
chronic, 793–803, 805–813
cor pulmonale and, 841
fixed, 727, *728*
flow-volume loop in, 727, *728*
foreign bodies and, 1435t, 1435–1436
intubation complications and, 115–116, 968–976, *969, 970, 972, 975*
laryngospasm causing, 116
neoplasia causing, 1397
pulmonary hypotension and, 841
sleep apnea and, 778–781, *779*
trauma injury and, 890
variable, 727, *728*
resistance in, 724, *724–726*
alveolar, *730*, 730–731
bronchiolar, 724, *725*
expiration and, 726–731
flow patterns and, *724*
lung volume and, 724, *726*
ventilation and, 735–737, *736, 737*
tracheobronchial tree and, 195–196, *196*
Akathisia, 699
Akee fruit, hypoglycemia caused by, 1254
Albumin, drug binding by, 1691t, 1691–1692
fluid resuscitation using, 132–133, *137*, 146
hepatic failure grading and, 79t, 1452t, 1561t
malnutrition and, 1530
metabolism of, 132–133
osmotic pressure due to, 130
pharmacokinetics of, 132–133
side effects of, 133, 146
volume expansion with, 1390
Albuterol, asthma treated with, 809t, 809–810
Alcohol. See *Ethanol*; *Isopropanol*; *Methanol.*
Alcohol dehydrogenase, ethanol and, 1715, *1715, 1717*
ethylene glycol and, *1716*, 1717
methanol and, 1715, *1715*, 1717
propylene glycol and, 1239, *1239*
Alcoholism, 706–712
acidosis of, 1223–1224, 1236, 1239
amnesia of, 707
blood alcohol levels and, 706t, 706–707
clinical features of, 706t, 706–708
collateral vessels in, 1445
drug interactions and, 707
hepatitis and, 1507–1509
ketoacidosis of, 710–712
lactic acidosis due to, 1236, 1239
magnesium depletion in, 1207–1208
myopathy of, 685
nutritional deficiencies in, 710–712
phosphate deficit in, 1214–1215
portal hypertension and, 1445, 1446t
thiamine deficiency in, 1236
treatment of, 707t, 707–710

Alcoholism *(Continued)*
Wernicke-Korsakoff syndrome and, 710–711
withdrawal syndromes of, 708t, 708–710
Aldehydes, smoke inhalation and, 884
Aldosterone, 1310–1317
deficiency of, 1314–1315, 1315t
drug-induced changes in, 1312t
excess of, 1316t, 1316–1317
metabolism of, 1310, *1311*
physiologic actions of, 1311, *1311*
potassium level and, 1181, 1184–1185
regulatory factors for, 1310–1311, *1311*
Alertness, 631. See also *Consciousness disorders.*
Alkalemia. See *pH.*
Alkalis, corrosive ingestion and, 1432t, 1432–1435, 1434t
esophageal injury caused by, 1432t, 1432–1435, 1434t
Alkalosis, 1226–1229
base excess and, 246, 1226–1227
causes of, 1227t, 1227–1228
diagnostic approach in, 1228, *1228*, 1229t
extracellular fluid volume in, 1227t, 1227–1228, *1228*
gastrointestinal disorders and, 1227t, 1227–1228, *1228*
kidney role in, 1227t, 1227–1228, *1228*
metabolic, *1222*, 1227t, 1227–1228, *1228*
nomogram for, *1222*
phosphate level in, 1212–1213
potassium level and, 1180, 1180t, 1181, 1227, 1229t
respiratory, *1222*
treatment of, 1228–1229, 1229t
Alkylating agents, 1409t
chemical warfare use of, 48, 52
chemotherapy with, 1409t, 1409–1410
lung affected by, 1409t, 1409–1410
Allen test, 236
Allergy, drug, 1264t, 1264–1265
Alloantibodies, transfusion reaction and, 1381
Almitrine bismesylate, pulmonary hypertension and, 846
Alpha waves, *775*
Alpha-blockers, hypertensive emergency and, 1332
Alpha-receptors, 1703–1704
catecholamines and, *1319*, 1319t, 1320–1322, 1321t, *1322*, 1322t
drug poisoning and, 1703t
Alphavirus, 392t, 397
ALS (amyotrophic lateral sclerosis), 676, 766
Alteplase, 1000
Alternating current, 1645
Altitude, atmospheric pressure and, *44*, 54
body gases and, 54
injuries affected by, 43t, 43–45, *44*
medical equipment affected by, 45, 45t, 54–55
oxygen and, 43, *44*, 54
patient affected by, 43t, 43–45, 54
pulmonary capillary pressure and, 838
Aluminum, dementia caused by, 1270
dialysis water and, 1270
Alveolus(i), airway resistance role of, *730*, 730–731
anatomy of, *720*
barotrauma injury to, 904
capnography and, *208*, 208–209, *209*
dead space and, 208, *208*, 733–734, 742–743, 819

Alveolus(i) *(Continued)*
  defense mechanisms of, *749, 750*, 752–753
  edema of, *788*, 788–789, *789*, 789t
  hypoventilation in, 841–842
  interstitial compartment of, 914, *914, 917*
  oxygen toxicity and, *953*, 953–954
  pressure in, 721, *721*, 737–738, *738*, *789*, 789–790
  pulmonary hypertension and, 841–842
  respiratory failure and, *754*, 754–755, *755*, 761–762
  rupture of, 904
  Starling forces in, 788–789, *789*
  uneven ventilation in, *208*, 208–209, *209*, *730*, 730–731
Amanita phalloides, abdominal pain due to, 1483t, 1484
Amantadine, hyperpyretic-rigidity syndrome and, 703
Amaurosis, pregnancy and, 1608
Ambulances, disadvantages of, 43, 54
Amebiasis, dysentery caused by, 510t, 511
American Association of Critical Care Nurses, 75–76, 76t
American Society of Anesthesia Physical Status Classification, 79, 79t
Amikacin, kidney failure due to, 1261t, 1261–1262
  meningitis therapy and, 461t
  pharmacokinetics of, 1692t, 1693t
Amiloride, diuresis using, 1165, 1165t
Amino acids, excitatory, 633, 667, *667*
  neuron death caused by, 667, *667*
Aminoglycosides, 616t
  dose adjustment for, 1305t
  kidney failure and, 1261t, 1261–1262, 1305t
  pathogen susceptibility to, 614t, 614–615, 616t
  pharmacokinetics of, 1692t, 1693t
Aminophylline, COPD and, 799
Aminoquinolines, *Pneumocystis* pneumonia and, 596
Aminosalicylic acid. See also *Aspirin (acetylsalicylic acid)*; *Salicylates.*
  pharmacokinetics of, 1689t
  side effects of, 427t
  tuberculosis therapy and, 427t
Amiodarone, arrhythmia treated with, 1055, 1056t
  drug interactions of, 1056t
  pulmonary toxicity of, 900
Amitriptyline, pharmacokinetics of, 1689t
Ammeter, oxygen electrode and, 242–243, *243*
Ammonia, acidosis role of, 1225t, 1225–1226
  hepatic encephalopathy role of, 1522–1523, 1523t
Amnesia, alcoholic, 707, 710
  brain hypoxia and, 644
  Wernicke-Korsakoff syndrome and, 710
Amniotic fluid, DIC and, 1601
  embolism of, 1601
Amoxicillin, pathogen susceptibility to, 614t
AMP (adenosine monophosphate), immune response role of, 1655, 1655t
Amphotericin B, candidiasis treated with, 438–442
  fungal infections treated with, 444–447
  kidney failure due to, 1261t, 1261–1262
  lung injury due to, 897t, 898–899
Ampicillin, enterococcal infection and, 411t, 415, 415–416

Ampicillin *(Continued)*
  meningitis therapy and, 460t, 460–462, 461t
  pathogen susceptibility to, 415t, 614t
  pharmacokinetics of, 1689t
  resistance to, 415
Ampicillin-sulbactam, pathogen susceptibility to, 614t
Ampulla of Vater, obstruction of, *1493*, 1500
  stone impaction in, *1493*
Amyl nitrite, cyanide antidote role of, 1712
  cyanide antidote use of, 51, 886
Amylase, conditions affecting, 1501, 1501t
  elevated, 1501, 1501t
  pancreatitis and, 1501, 1501t
  pleural effusion and, 865
Amylopectin, 135
Amyotrophic lateral sclerosis (ALS), 676
  respiratory failure due to, 766
Anaerobes, burn injury and, 524
  granulocytopenia and, 533t
  mixed infections due to, 448–453, 449t
  myositis caused by, 452
  odor due to, 450, 452
  peritonitis and, 514–515
  skin and soft tissue and, 448–453, 449t
  susceptibility testing and, 613
Analgesics, kidney failure dose adjustment for, 1304t
  liver disease and, 1689t
  MI treatment and, 996t, 996–997
  pharmacokinetics of, 1689t
Anaphylaxis, 140–141, 1650–1659
  agents causing, 1651t
  anaphylactoid reaction vs., 1651
  antigens causing, 1652
  clinical features of, 1656
  definition of, 1651
  dextran causing, 134
  dialysis and, 1275
  differential diagnosis for, 1651, 1652t
  drug therapy in, 1655t, 1656–1659, *1657*
  factitious, 1651
  fluid resuscitation in, 140–141
  gelatin infusion causing, 136
  historical aspects of, 1650–1651, *1651*
  immunoglobulins and, 1652–1653, *1653*
  incidence of, 1651–1652
  insect bite and, 1652
  mediators of, *1653*, 1654t, 1654–1655, 1655t
    basophil and, 1654t, 1654–1655
    mast cell and, 1654t, 1654–1655
  parasitism and, 1652
  prevention of, 1659
  sequence of events in, 1652–1656, *1653*
  transfusion and, 1391
  treatment of, 1655t, 1656–1659, *1657*
Anatomic Index, 1575
Anemia, 1370–1386
  chemotherapy-induced, 1405–1406
  hemolytic, 1370–1386
    classification of, 1372t
    diagnosis of, 1370t, 1370–1373
    glucose-6-phosphate dehydrogenase and, 1385t, 1385–1386
    hereditary, 1384–1386, 1385t
    history in, 1371
    immune, 1376–1384
      autoimmune, 1376t, 1376–1378, 1378t
      drug-induced, 1378t–1380t, 1378–1381
      transfusion and, 1381–1384, 1382t
    infection and, 1383

Anemia *(Continued)*
    laboratory tests in, 1370t, 1370–1373
    microangiopathic, 1372t, 1373–1376
      associated conditions and, 1372t, 1373–1376
      carcinoma and, 1372t, 1374–1375
      heart valve prosthesis and, 1376
      hemolytic-uremic syndrome in, 1372t, 1374–1375
      pregnancy and, 1372t, 1374–1375
      thrombotic thrombocytopenic purpura and, 1372t, 1373–1374
    physical examination in, 1371
    spur cell, 1372, 1384
    toxin-induced, 1383
  kidney failure and, 1272, 1298
  myelodysplastic syndrome and, 1364t, 1366, 1367
  pregnancy and, 1372t, 1374–1375, 1612
  preoperative care and, 1563–1564
ANEMIA system, 103t
Anemones, venom of, 1674t, 1674–1675, 1675t
Anesthesia, bronchoscopy procedure and, 194
  physical status classification and, 1568t
Aneurysms, *658*
  aortic, 1479–1480
    abdominal pain of, 1479–1480
    rupture of, 1479–1480
  basilar artery, *658*
  berry, 659
  false, *1150*
    femoral artery and, *1150*
    stab wound and, 1149, *1150*
  intracranial, 659t, 659–660
  mycotic, 571
  Rasmussen's, 423
  saccular, 659t, 659–660
  stroke and, 655–660
    hemorrhagic, 657, *658*, 659t, 659–660
    ischemic, 655–656
  subarachnoid hemorrhage and, 659t, 659–660
Anger camera, 1108
Angina pectoris, 989–1012
  atherosclerosis in, 989–991
  diagnosis of, 991, 993–994
  echocardiography in, 993–994
  management of, 994–1012
    angioplasty in, *1004*, 1004–1005
    anticoagulants in, 1001
    beta-adrenergic blockers in, 997–998, 998t
    calcium channel blockers in, 997, 998t
    initial, 1005, 1005t
    intra-aortic balloon pump in, 1005
    predischarge, 1011–1012
  mechanisms of, 989–991
  pathophysiology of, 989–991
  perioperative risk and, 1557–1558, 1559t
  Prinzmetal's, 997
  unstable, 989
Angiodysplasia. See *Arteriovenous malformations.*
Angiography, aortic aneurysm and, 1137–1138, *1138–1140*
  cerebral, head trauma and, 716
  cineangiography and, 326
  mesenteric ischemia and, 1487, *1488, 1489*
  pulmonary embolism and, *852*, 852–854
  sepsis and, 326
Angioplasty, angina pectoris and, *1004*, 1004–1005

Angiotensin. See also *Renin-angiotensin-aldosterone axis.*
  secretion of, 1310–1311, *1311*
Angiotensin-converting enzyme (ACE) inhibitors, cough and, 900
  heart failure and, 1044–1045
  hypertensive emergency and, 1331
  pregnancy and, 1605
Anhidrosis, coma evaluation and, 636
Animal bites. See also *Envenomation; Snakebite.*
  antimicrobials for, 1571t
  rabies and, 691t
Anion gap, acidosis and, 1223–1224
  widened, 1223–1224
Anion-exchange resins, colitis treated with, 508
Anisocoria, coma evaluation and, 636
Anisoylated plasminogen-streptokinase activator complex, MI and, 999–1001, *1001*
Anistreplase, 1000
Anorectal infections, granulocytopenia with, 542
Anorexia nervosa, phosphate level and, 1213
  potassium level and, 1183, 1185, 1185t
Anoxia. See also *Hypoxia.*
  encephalopathy of, 645t, 645–647
Antacids, gastritis and, 1442
Antecubital vein, central venous catheter in, 181
Anterior horn, disorders related to, 676–677
  hereditary diseases and, 676
  infections in, 676–677
  metabolic syndromes and, 677
  respiratory failure and, 766
  toxins affecting, 677
Anthracyclines, heart affected by, 1411–1412, 1412t
Antiarrhythmic agents, 1054–1055, 1056t–1057t
  class I, 1055, 1056t
  class II, 1055, 1056t–1057t
  class III, 1055, 1056t–1057t
  class IV, 1055, 1057t
  drug interactions of, 1056t–1057t
  heart failure treatment and, 1024
  kidney failure dose adjustment for, 1305t
  liver failure dose adjustment for, 1689t, 1700
  pharmacokinetics of, 1056t–1057t, 1689t, 1700
Antibiotics. See *Antimicrobials.*
Antibodies, digitalis neutralized with, 1707
  endotoxins neutralized with, 369
  Fab, 1707
  hemolytic anemia due to, 1376t, 1376–1377, 1377t
  monoclonal, 828t, 836, 1294
  transfusion reaction and, 1381–1382, 1382t
  warm, 1376t, 1376–1377, 1377t
Anticholinergics, antidotes for, 53
  asthma treated with, 810
  chemical warfare use of, 48–49
  clinical effects of, 52–53
  drug overdose with, 1703t, 1703–1705, 1704t
  hyperpyretic-rigidity syndrome and, 703
Anticoagulants, abdominal wall bleeding due to, 1484
  angina pectoris and, 1001
  blood storage and, 1389
  dialysis and, 1281–1282, 1290, 1290t

Anticoagulants *(Continued)*
  dose adjustment for, 1306t
  endocarditis and, 497
  kidney failure affecting, 1306t
  lung affected by, 900
  pharmacokinetics of, 1689t
  pulmonary embolism and, 570, 855–856
  pulmonary hypertension and, 847
  sepsis treated with, 372, 570
  stroke treated with, 654–655
  thrombosis and, 855–856
Anticonvulsants, kidney failure dose adjustment for, 1306t–1307t
  liver failure dose adjustment for, 1690t, 1692t
  meningitis seizure and, 463
  pharmacokinetics of, 1690t, 1692t, 1695t, 1695–1696
  status epilepticus and, 668t, 668–671, 669t, 671t
Antidepressants, kidney failure dose adjustment for, 1307t
  overdose with, 901
  poisoning due to, 1708–1709
  pulmonary edema and, 901
Antidiarrhetics, hypotonicity and, 1172t, 1173, 1173t
  pseudomembranous colitis and, 508
Antidiuretic hormone, inappropriate secretion of, 1172t, 1173, 1173t
Antidotes, 49–53
  anticholinergics and, 53
  benzilate and, 53
  cyanide and, 886, 1712
  nerve agents and, 49, 51–52
  organophosphates and, 52
Antiemetics, chemotherapy and, 1414
Antiepileptics. See *Anticonvulsants.*
Antifreeze, acidosis caused by, 1223
  metabolites of, 1223, *1716*
  poisoning due to, 712, 1715–1720, *1716*, 1716t, 1718t, 1719–1720
Antifungals, kidney failure dose adjustment for, 1307t
Antigens, anaphylaxis caused by, 1652
  blood groups and, 1387
  Thomsen-Freidenreich, 1374–1375
Antihistamines, kidney failure dose adjustment for, 1307t
Antihypertensives, kidney failure dose adjustment for, 1307t
  pharmacokinetics of, 1307t, 1689t
  pregnancy and, 1605
  treatment principles and, 1330t, 1330–1333, 1331t
Anti-inflammatory drugs, meningitis and, 462–463
  pulmonary edema due to, 899, *899*
  sepsis effects treated with, 372
Antimetabolites, 1409t, 1415t
Antimicrobials. See also *Resistant organisms.*
  antineoplastic chemotherapy with, 1409t, 1410, 1410t
  bactericidal concentration of, 616–620, *618*, *619*
  burn injury and, 525t, 525–526
  catheter-related infections and, 606
  colitis caused by, 500–502
  colitis treated with, 505–509
  cyclosporine interaction with, 587t
  cytochrome system affected by, 587t
  dosage factors and, 415t, 614t, 615–616, 618–620, 1690t, 1692t, 1693–1695
    kidney failure affecting, 1305t–1306t
    liver failure affecting, 1690t
  endocarditis and, 496–497

Antimicrobials *(Continued)*
  enterococcal infection and, 415t, 415–416
  glycopeptide, 616t
  gram-positive organisms and, 410–411, 411t
  hepatic encephalopathy treated with, 1525
  infection-site concentration of, *618*, 618–620, *619*
  inhalation therapy using, 962
  inhibitory concentration of, 415t, 616–620, *618*, *619*
  kidney failure due to, 616
  lung injury due to, 897t, 898–899, *899*
  meningitis treated with, 460t, 460–462, 461t
  minimal concentrations for, 415t, 616–620, *618*, *619*
  monitoring of levels of, 1692t
  ophthalmic, 468, 468t
  peritonitis and, 517, 517t
  pharmacodynamics of, *618*, 618–620, *619*
  pharmacokinetics of, 1305t–1306t, 1690t, 1692t, 1693–1695
  Pneumocystis carinii and, 595–596, 596t
  pneumonia and, 482t, 489, 489t, 595–596, 596t
  pneumonitis induced by, 1409t, 1409–1410, 1410t
  polycationic, 370
  postantibiotic effect of, 615, *617*, 618
  preoperative care and, 1570–1572, 1571t, 1572t
  risks and, 482t
  septic shock treated with, *366*, 366–368, 368t, 370
  staphylococcal infections and, 408–414, 411t
  surgery preparation and, 1570–1572, 1571t, 1572t
  susceptibility to, 614, 614t
    enterococcal, 415t, 415–416
    organisms and, 614, 614t
    testing of, 612–613
  time-kill studies of, 616–618, *617*
  topical, 468, 468t, 525t, 525–526
  transplant patient and, 586–587, 587t
  vegetations and, *619*, 620
Antineoplastics, cardiotoxicity of, 1411–1413, 1412t
  kidney failure dose adjustment for, 1307t–1308t
  lung affected by, 1408–1411, 1409t, 1410t
  mitotic cycle and, 1403–1406, 1404t
  myelosuppression due to, 1403–1406, 1404t
  nephropathy due to, 1406–1408
Antioxidants, agents used as, 955, 955t
  cellular, 951, 952t
  mechanical ventilation and, 955, 955t
  oxygen toxicity and, 951, 952t, 955, 955t
  sepsis effects treated with, 373
Antiparkinsonian drugs, kidney failure dose adjustment for, 1308t
  withdrawal from, 701
Antiperistaltics, colitis and, pseudomembranous, 508
Antipsychotics, kidney failure dose adjustment for, 1308t
Antisepsis, AIDS precautions as, 564
  hand washing as, 386–387, 387t, 409, 411–412
  nosocomial infections and, 386–388, 387t
  staphylococcal infections and, 409, 411–412

Antithrombin, sepsis treated with, 372
Antitrichomonal drugs, kidney failure dose adjustment for, 1308t
Antituberculosis drugs, 425t, 425–426, 427t
kidney failure dose adjustment for, 1308t
Antiulcer drugs, kidney failure dose adjustment for, 1308t
Antivenin, black widow spider and, 1679
pit viper, 1670–1672
Antivirals, kidney failure dose adjustment for, 1308t
Ants, anaphylaxis caused by, 1652
venom of, 1681, 1681t
Aorta, *1138*
abdominal, intestinal ischemia and, 1142–1144
occlusion of, 1142–1144
aneurysm of, 1133–1140, *1138*
abdominal, 1142, *1142*
abdominal pain of, 1479–1480
diagnosis of, 1134–1138, *1135–1140*
imaging of, *1138*
pseudoaneurysm and, 1134, *1139, 1140*
resection of, 1139–1140, 1144
rupture of, 1479–1480
syphilitic, 1134
treatment of, 1138–1140
types of, 1134
balloon catheter in, 188–189, *189*
diastolic pressure in, cardiac arrest and, 21
epinephrine effect on, 21
dissection of, *1134,* 1134–1140, *1138*
abdominal pain of, 1479–1480
classification of, *1134,* 1134
hypertension in, 1328, 1330t
imaging of, *1115,* 1119
radiography in, 1134–1135, *1138*
Doppler studies and, *1115,* 1119
ductus bump of, 1137, *1138, 1139*
knob of, *1135,* 1135, *1136*
rupture of, 892, 1134–1140, *1136, 1137*
radiography in, 1134–1138, *1135–1137*
trauma injury to, 892
APACHE (Acute Physiology and Chronic Health Evaluation), 82–86, 83t, 84t, 1575
Apheresis, 1419–1429
anticoagulation in, 1427
calculations for, 1427–1428
complications of, 1428–1429
cost-benefit and, 1429
historical aspects of, 1420
instrumentation for, 1420–1421, *1421, 1422*
replacement fluids in, 1427
ultrafiltration in, 1421, *1422*
vascular access for, 1425–1427
Apnea, brain death diagnosis and, 646, 646t
Cheyne-Stokes respiration and, 636
rigorous test for, 646, 646t
sleep, 777–781
central, *777,* 777
diagnosis of, 779t, 779–780
obstructive, *778,* 778–781
polysomnography in, *777, 778*
symptoms of, 778–780
treatment of, 780t, 780–781
Apoplexy. See *Cerebrovascular disease; Stroke.*
Appendicitis, abdominal pain of, 1475t, 1476
peritonitis and, 516
pregnancy and, 1610t, 1610–1611
salpingitis vs., 1477

Ara-C (cytosine arabinoside), lung injury due to, 897t, 897–898, *898*
neuropathy due to, 1417
Arachidonic acid, cascade, 304–306, *305*
metabolites of, 304–306, *305*
sepsis role of, 304–306, *305*
Arbovirus, 392t, 397, 398t
encephalitis due to, 692–695
vectors for, 397, 397t, 398t
ARDS. See *Respiratory distress syndrome (adult).*
Arenavirus, 392
Arousal, 631. See also *Coma; Consciousness disorders; Unresponsiveness.*
Arrhythmias, 1049–1077. See also *Tachycardia.*
accessory pathways causing, 1064–1066
atrial, *1051,* 1055–1067, *1061–1063, 1067, 1068, 1076*
atrioventricular node in, 1057–1067, *1064–1066*
block and, 1057–1059, *1059*
first-degree, 1057–1058
second-degree (Wenckebach's), 1058, *1058, 1059*
third-degree (complete), 1058–1059, *1059*
re-entry and, 1063–1064, *1064, 1066*
bradycardic, 635t, 1055, *1058*
bronchoscopy causing, 193, 195
bundle branches in, block and, *1051*
chemotherapy-induced, 1412t, 1412–1413
conduction system and, 1049–1077, *1051, 1064*
electrolytes and, 1051–1054, *1052, 1053*
expert system monitoring of, 100–101, *101, 102,* 104–106, *105*
hypercalcemic, 1053
hyperkalemic, *1052,* 1052–1053, *1053*
hypermagnesemic, 1054
hypocalcemic, 1053–1054
hypokalemic, 1053
MI and, 996–997, 1006–1007
perioperative risk and, 1556, 1556t
radiation therapy causing, 1412t, 1413
sinus node in, 1055–1062
arrest of, 1055
bradycardia and, 1055, *1058*
exit block and, 1055
normal rhythm of, 1055
re-entrant tachycardia and, 1062
supraventricular, 1055–1067, *1061–1063, 1067, 1068, 1076*
ventricular, 1067–1077, *1069, 1070, 1072–1076*
lidocaine treatment of, 996
Wolff-Parkinson-White syndrome and, 1064–1067
Arsenic, abdominal pain due to, 1483, 1483t
ARTEMIS system, 103t
Arteries, atherosclerotic, 989–991, *990, 991*
blood pressure monitoring in, 251–257, *253–256*
brachial, 183
carotid. See *Carotid artery.*
catheterization of, 182–188
complications and, 183–184
contraindications for, 183
indications for, 182
coronary. See *Coronary arteries.*
femoral, 235–236, *1150*
iliac, 1144
innominate, 1146–1147

Arteries *(Continued)*
lung embolism and, *852,* 852–854
popliteal, 1150, *1151*
pressure in, 735–737, *737.* See also *Blood pressure.*
intracranial pressure and, 714–715, *715*
pulmonary. See *Pulmonary artery.*
puncture of, 235–237, *236*
blood gas sample and, 236–237
complications of, 236–237
procedure for, 235–237, *236*
radial, 183, *183,* 235–237, *236,* 1148–1149
renal, 1258
Arteriovenous fistula, hemodialysis and, 1149, *1150*
Arteriovenous malformations, cerebral, *658*
gastrointestinal, 1444, *1460,* 1460–1463, *1463*
coagulation therapy for, 1462–1463, *1463*
hemorrhage of, *1460,* 1460–1463, *1463*
lower tract and, 1460–1463, *1463*
upper tract and, 1444
Arteriovenous shunt, 353
Arthritis, endocarditis causing, 573t, 574
Arthropods, venomous, 1677–1681, 1678t, *1678–1681,* 1681t
Arthus' reactions, 1653
Artificial blood, 151–159
complications and, 153, 158–159
fluorocarbon emulsions as, *151,* 151–153, *152,* 152t, 153t
hemoglobin solution as, 153–159, 154t, *154–157*
Artificial intelligence, 95–98, 103–107
bayesian diagnosis and, 96–98, 97t, 98t
future applications of, 106–107
ICU role of, 95–96, 96t
neural networks and, *103–105,* 103–106, 106t
difficulties with, 104t, 106t
future of, 106–107
learning by, 104–106, *105*
pattern recognition by, 103–106
waveform recognition by, 104t, 104–106
Arytenoid cartilage, anatomy of, 968, *968*
displacement of, 116
endotracheal intubation and, 113, *113,* 116
intubation injury to, 969, *969*
Ascites, differential diagnosis of, 168t
hypervolemia and, 1161
paracentesis and, 167–169
peritonitis and, 515–516
postoperative bleeding and, 1144
Ascorbic acid, 952t, 955t, 1529t
Ash, airway injury due to, 35
volcanic origin of, 28–31, 35
Ashman phenomenon, 1051, *1051,* 1061
Aspergillosis, 446–447
allergic, 446
body sites of, 446
clinical findings in, 446–447
CNS, 447
cutaneous, 447
ocular, 446
pulmonary, 446
sinusitis due to, 446
treatment of, 447
Aspiration, 872–875
bronchoscopy risk of, 194
clinical signs of, 872–875, 873t

Aspiration (*Continued*)
  coffee grounds appearance and, 1440, 1441t
  endotracheal intubation and, 115–116, 872
  enteral nutrition causing, 1543
  gastric contents and, 115–116, 872–875, 873t, 1440, 1441t
  gravity role in, *873*
  mortality rate in, 875
  pneumonia due to, 872–875
  pneumonitis due to, 872–875
  risk factors for, 872, 872t
  treatment of, 875
Aspiration procedure, 482–483, 483t, 610
  pneumonia diagnosis and, 482–483, 483t, 610
  transtracheal, 482–483, 483t
Aspirin (acetylsalicylic acid). See also *Aminosalicylic acid.*
  abdominal pain due to, 1483t, 1483–1484
  lactic acidosis caused by, 1238–1239
  MI and, 1003
  pharmacokinetics of, 1689t
  poisoning due to, *1708*, 1708
  pulmonary edema due to, 899, *899*
Assessment. See *Severity classification.*
Asterixis, 635, 637
  elicitation of, 1524
  encephalopathy and, 1507, 1510, 1524
Asthma, 805–813
  acute severe, 805–813
  cell-derived mediators of, 806–807, 807t
  clinical signs in, 808, 808t
  complications in, 812–813
  differential diagnosis in, 813
  drug therapy in, 809t, 809–810
  epidemiology of, 806
  evaluation of, 808–809
  management of, 809t, 809–812, 811t
  mechanical ventilation in, 811t, 811–812
  pathogenesis of, 806–807, 807t
  pathophysiology of, 807t, 807–808
  pulmonary embolism vs., 813
Astrocytes, hepatic encephalopathy role of, 1520, *1520*
Asystole, cardiac arrest causing, 23–24
  CPR outcome and, 120
  ECG switch mistake and, 23–24
Ataxia, sensory, neuropathy and, 679
Atelectasis, chest physiotherapy and, 958–959
  complete, 277, *277*
  consolidation vs., *282*
  differential diagnosis in, 277–278
  endotracheal tube causing, 271, *274*
  pneumonitis vs., 278
  radiography in, 271–278, *274–277*
  rounded, 278
  ultrasonography in, 271–277
Atenolol, dosage for, 999t
  myocardial ischemia and, 999t
  pharmacokinetics of, 1689t
Atherosclerosis, coronary, 989–991, *990, 991*
  angina and, 989–991
  kidney failure and, 1264
  kidney transplant and, 1296–1297, 1297t
  pathogenesis of, 989–991, *990, 991*
  plaque of, 989–991, *990, 991*
Atlanto-occipital joint, endotracheal intubation and, 109, *112*
Atmospheric pressure. See also *Barotrauma.*
  air transport and, 43–45, 54–55, 909
  altitude and, *44*, 54
  bubble-related disorders and, 902–903

Atmospheric pressure (*Continued*)
  diving and, 902–903
  injuries affected by, 43t, 43–45, *44*
  medical equipment affected by, 45, 45t, 54–55
  oxygen and, 43, *44*
  patients affected by, 43–45, 54
ATP. See *Adenosine triphosphate (ATP).*
Atria (atrium), a wave and, *1017*, 1017–1018, *1079*, 1079–1080, *1080*
  arrhythmias of, 1055–1067
  balloon catheter monitoring and, *1079–1081*, 1079–1087
  bundle branch block and, 1073–1076, *1075, 1076*
  c wave and, *1079*, 1079–1080, *1080*
  central venous pressure waves and, *1079–1081*, 1079–1087
  cv wave and, 1080, *1080*
  digitalis affecting, 1073, *1073*
  dilatation of, heart failure and, 1017, *1017*
  Doppler studies and, 1110–1113, *1112, 1113*
  fibrillation of, 1061–1062, 1067, *1067*
  filling period of, 1110–1113, *1112, 1113*
  flutter of, *1062*, 1062–1077, *1076*
  gallop and, *1017*, 1017–1018
  heart failure and, *1017*, 1017–1018
  natriuretic hormone of, 1156, 1158
  pre-excitation and, 1067, *1067, 1068*
  premature complexes and, *1051*, 1060–1070, *1061*
  s wave and, *1079*, 1079–1080, *1080*
  septal defect of, *1118*, 1118–1119
  tachycardia of, *1051*
  v wave and, *1017*, 1017–1018, *1079*, 1079–1080, *1080*
  waveform analysis and, *1079–1081*, 1079–1087
  wide QRS and, 1073–1077, *1076*
  x descent and, *1079*, 1079–1080, *1080*
  x' descent and, *1079*, 1079–1080, *1080*
  y descent and, *1079*, 1079–1080, *1080*
Atrial septal defect, imaging of, *1118*, 1118–1119
Atrioventricular node, accessory conduction in, 1064–1066
  anatomy and, 1057
  arrhythmias and, 1057–1067, *1064–1066*
  block of, first-degree, 1057–1058
    Mobitz's, 1058, *1059*
    second-degree, 1058, *1058, 1059*
    third-degree (complete), 1058–1059, *1059*
    Wenckebach's, 1058, *1058*
  dissociation in, 1058–1059, *1059, 1079*, 1080
  pathways of, 1063–1066
  re-entry phenomena and, 1063–1064, *1064, 1066*
Atropine, cardiac arrest and, 21, 22t, 125
  COPD and, 798–799
  CPR and, 125
  nerve agent antidote use of, 49, 51–52
Audition, evoked potentials and, 231–232, 624
Auscultation, air embolism and, 907
  blood pressure measurement and, 251–252
  endotracheal intubation and, 113
  gallop and, *1017*, 1017–1018
  heart failure and, *1017*, 1017–1018
  pulmonary hypertension and, 845
Autocannibalism, multiple organ system failure and, 345

Autoimmune disorders, hemolytic anemia and, 1376t, 1376–1378, 1378t
  hypoglycemia and, 1253, 1254t, *1255*
  plasmapheresis in, 1425, 1426t
Automobilie accidents, 32, 32t, 33t
Autonomic nervous system, drug overdose affecting, 1703t, 1703–1704, 1704t
  mechanical ventilation and, 946, 946t
  neuropathy of, 672–673, 681–682
Axons, motor neuron and, 673–674
  myelinated, 673
Azathioprine, kidney transplant and, 1293
  side effects of, 1293
Azoles, candidiasis treated with, 438–442
Azotemia. See also *Uremia.*
  chemotherapy causing, 1406–1408
  definition of, 1269
  prerenal, 1257t, 1257–1260
    diagnosis of, 1258–1259
    etiology of, 1257t, 1257–1260
    treatment of, 1258–1260
Aztreonam, pathogen susceptibility to, 614t

B

B cells, *1340*
  cancer effect on, 546
  granulocytopenia and, 533, 534t
B virus (herpesvirus 1), encephalitis and, 399–400
Bacillus, endophthalmitis due to, 471
Bacitracin, pseudomembranous colitis treated with, 507–508
BACTEC system, tuberculosis diagnosis and, 425
Bacteremia, blood culture in, 608–609
  burn débridement and, 526
  cancer patient and, 548–549
  catheter reservoir for, 609
  clinical data in, 297t
  definition of, 557
  endocarditis and, 492–493
  gram-negative organisms in, 383t
  gram-positive organisms in, 383t
  incidence of, 295
  laboratory diagnosis of, 608–609
  neonatal, 417
  pregnancy and, 1608–1609
  pyomyositis and, 452
  rash due to, 457
  staphylococcal, 408–414, 411t
  streptococcal, 416–420
  trauma patient and, 557–558
Bacteria. See also *Pathogens; Resistant organisms;* specific organisms.
  adherence of, 527, 604–606, 751
  aerobic, 514–515, 524, 533t
  anaerobic. See *Anaerobes.*
  endogenous, 384–385, 388
  lactic acidosis due to, 1236, *1236*
  nosocomial infections and, 384–385, 388
  overgrowth of, 1236, *1236*
  septic shock and, 302, 313t, *366*, 366–368
Bacteriuria, catheter-associated, 527–530
  laboratory diagnosis of, 611
Bacteroides, susceptibility of, 614t
Balloons, altitude effect on, 54–55
  catheter flotation using, 1079–1087, *1083*
  intra-aortic pump and, 188–189, *189*
Bamboo spine, 769, *770*
Barber v Superior Court, 1733, 1734
Barbiturates, intracranial pressure reduction and, 463
  kidney failure dose adjustment for, 1305t
  liver disease and, 1689t, 1690t

Barbiturates (Continued)
pharmacokinetics of, 1689t, 1690t, 1692t, 1696
Barium, hypokalemia caused by, 1183–1184
peritoneum and, 514
poisoning due to, 1183–1184
Barotrauma. See also Atmospheric pressure.
asthma and, 811, 812
ear and, 903
lung overexpansion injury in, 904–905
mechanical ventilation causing, 904, 926–927
nasal sinus and, 903–904, 904
pathophysiology of, 903–904, 926–927
pneumocephalus caused by, 903–904, 904
pneumomediastinum due to, 904, 904
pneumothorax due to, 870, 904–905, 905
Bartling v Superior Court, 1733
Bartter's syndrome, alkalosis and, 1228, 1228
potassium level and, 1186, 1190
Baseline wander, ECG signal and, 100t, 100–101
expert system affected by, 100t, 100–101
Bases. See also Acid-base balance.
alkalosis and, 246, 1226–1227
dietary source of, 1220
excess calculation for, 246
Basilic vein, central venous catheter in, 181
Basophils, 1340
anaphylaxis and, 1654t, 1654–1655
hematopoiesis and, 1336
immune response role of, 1654t, 1654–1655
Bats, rabies and, 691t
Batteries, button/disk, corrosive injury due to, 1433
Battle's sign, 634
Batwing appearance, pulmonary edema and, 279
Bayesian diagnosis, artificial intelligence and, 96–98, 97t, 98t
BCNU (carmustine), bone marrow transplant and, 1348t
gastrointestinal effects of, 1414t, 1414–1415
lung affected by, 1410, 1410t
side effects of, 1348t
Beck, Claude, 19
Beer-Lambert law, oximetry and, 203
Bees, 1681
venom of, 1681, 1681t
Belief network, expert system and, 99, 99
Bell's palsy, blink reflex and, 626
Bell's phenomenon, coma evaluation and, 636
Bends, 902–903
Benzilate (BZ), antidotes for, 53
chemical warfare use of, 49
clinical effects of, 52–53
Benzodiazepines, endotracheal intubation and, 111
hepatic encephalopathy role of, 1524
kidney failure dose adjustment for, 1305t
liver disease and, 1689t
pharmacokinetics of, 1689t
Berger's disease, hypertension in, 1328
Beta-agonists, asthma treated with, 809t, 809–810
Beta-blockers, angina pectoris and, 997–998, 998t
arrhythmia treated with, 1055–1057, 1056t
drug interactions of, 1056t–1057t

Beta-blockers (Continued)
hypertensive emergency and, 1333
kidney failure dose adjustment for, 1308t
pharmacokinetics of, 1689t
Beta-lactam agents, 616t
bactericidal action of, 616t, 616–618, 618t
microbe resistance to, 410, 415
susceptibility testing and, 612–613
Beta-lactamase, pathogens producing, 614
resistance due to, 410, 415, 614
Beta-receptors, agonists for, 809t, 809–810
blocking agents for. See Beta-blockers.
catecholamines and, 1319, 1319t, 1320–1322, 1321t, 1322t
drug poisoning and, 1703t
Bicarbonate, acidosis and, 1042–1044, 1042–1044
carbon dioxide content and, 245–246
cardiac arrest and, 22t, 23, 124
CPR and, 124, 1042–1044, 1042–1044
dialysis solution using, 1280–1282, 1282t
diarrhea and, 1466
Biguanides, lactic acidosis caused by, 1237
Biliary tract, gallstones and, 1491–1493, 1493, 1493t, 1494t
inflammation of, 1494–1497
pancreatitis and, 1491–1493, 1493, 1493t, 1494t
Bilirubin, hemolytic anemia and, 1370t, 1371
hepatic failure grading and, 79t, 1452t, 1561t
jaundice levels and, 401
oximetry affected by, 244
Bioethics. See Ethical issues.
Biofilm, bacterial adherence due to, 527
urinary tract and, 527
Biopsy, bronchoscopic, 199–200, 200t
lung, pneumonia and, 483t, 483–484
Biphosphonates, hypercalcemia treated with, 1401t, 1401–1402
Bite cells, formation of, 1372, 1385
hemolytic anemia and, 1372, 1385
Bites and stings. See Animal bites; Envenomation; Snakebite.
Bitot's spots, 1529
Black widow spider, 1678, 1678–1679
venom of, 1678–1679
abdominal pain due to, 1483t, 1484
antivenin and, 1679
symptoms caused by, 1483t, 1484, 1678, 1678–1679
Blackboard architecture, 99–100, 100
Blackouts, alcoholic, 707, 710
Blades, laryngoscopy and, 112, 112
Blastomycosis, 444
Bleach, chemical exposure decontamination with, 49, 52
esophageal injury caused by, 1432t, 1432–1435, 1434t
ingestion of, 1432t, 1432–1435, 1434t
Bleeding. See Hemorrhage.
Bleeding time, heparin therapy and, 855
kidney failure and, 1271
preoperative care and, 1564–1565
Bleomycin, gastrointestinal effects of, 1414t, 1414–1415
lung affected by, 897t, 897–898, 1410, 1410t
Blindness, methanol poisoning and, 1714
pregnancy and, 1608
Blink reflex, Bell's palsy and, 626
diagnostic studies and, 626
Blood, 1389. See also Hematologic disorders.
artificial, 151–159

Blood (Continued)
banking, 1387–1392
historical aspects of, 4
brain barrier and, fluid resuscitation and, 142
inflammation effects and, 456, 456–457
cellular components of, 1335–1337, 1339, 1440
culture of, 605, 609
formation of, 1335–1337
groups, 1387
growth factors and, 1335–1337, 1336t
hyperviscosity of, 1425, 1426t
microaggregates in, 1391
storage of, 1389, 1391
Blood flow. See also Pulmonary vasculature, blood flow in.
cardiac output and, 1087–1090
cerebral, 224–227
coma and, 632
head trauma and, 1583, 1583–1584
herniation and, 632
hypertension treatment and, 1328, 1328
metabolism and, 639
monitoring of, 224t, 224–227, 225, 225t, 226, 228
pressure and, 714
CPR compressions and, 120–124, 121–123
Doppler principles and, 1104–1105, 1105
intracranial pressure and, 714–715, 715
mechanical ventilation affecting, 946–947
snakebite and, 1670, 1672
systemic vascular resistance and, 1097
Blood gases. See also Carbon dioxide, tension; Oxygen, tension.
base excess calculation and, 246
bronchoscopy effect on, 193, 194
decompression sickness and, 902–909
exchange of, 732–747
bubble-related disorders and, 902–909
clinical assessment in, 743–747
diffusion role in, 739, 739–740
hypoventilation effect on, 217
measurement of. See also Capnography; Oximetry.
accuracy in, 242–243
analyzer for, 240, 242–243
derived parameters of, 244–247
early, 3, 235
electrodes for, 239–243, 240–243
error sources in, 237–239, 238, 239
fluorescent optodes used in, 247–248, 248
intra-arterial device for, 247–248, 248
intravascular, 247–248
ion-selective field effect transistors and, 247
noninvasive monitoring and, 203–220
quality assurance in, 242–243
sample collection for, 235–239, 236, 238, 239
temperature effect on, 217–220, 219, 220, 246–247
mechanical ventilation and, 932–935
respiratory failure and, 759t
Blood pressure. See also Pulmonary vasculature, pressure in.
arterial, 251–257, 253–256
mean calculation for, 1095–1096
burn injury and, 1616, 1617
cardiac resuscitation and, 21, 23
CPR compressions and, 120–124, 121–123
heart failure and, 1021, 1021

Blood pressure *(Continued)*
　intracranial, 227–230, 229t
　measurement of, 251–257
　　cannulation site and, 255
　　damping coefficient in, 253
　　Doppler technology and, 251
　　early technique for, 2–3
　　equipment for, 252–254, *253*
　　finger cuff in, 251–252
　　frequency and, *253*, 253–254, *254*
　　intra-arterial, 252t, 252–257, *253–256*
　　manometry in, 251–252
　　noninvasive vs. invasive, 252
　　plethysmography in, 251
　　waveforms of, 252t, 252–257, *254–256*
　　zero reference point in, 254
　MI and, 995, 995t
　monitoring of, 251–257, *253–256*, 995, 995t
　portal, 1447
　pregnancy-induced hypertension and, 1602t, 1603t
Blood type, 1387
Blood volume, calculation of, 1427
　depletion of, 1159t, 1159–1161, 1163–1164. See also *Hypovolemia.*
　expanded, radiographic indices of, *790*
　fluid physiology and, 129–131, *130*, 1155–1159, *1157*
　hypertonicity and, 1175t, 1175–1178
　hypotonicity and, 1171–1173, 1172t
　increase in, 1161–1164. See also *Hypervolemia.*
　plasmapheresis and, 1427–1428
　regulatory mechanisms for, *1155*, 1155–1159, *1157*
　sodium and, *1155*, 1155–1159, *1157*, 1175–1178
Blue toe syndrome, 1144
Blunt trauma, CPR use in, 16
　prehospital management of, 16–19
　spine immobilization in, 16–19
Body, composition of, malnutrition and, 1532
　surface area of, cardiac output related to, 1096
　　Dubois formula for, 1096
　weight of, nutritional assessment and, 1529t, 1529–1530, 1532t
Bohr equation, 734
Bombs, 32
Bone, calcium distribution and, 1197, *1197*, *1198*
　necrosis of, kidney transplant and, 1300
　phosphate deficit and, 1214
Bone marrow, 1339
　cellular elements of, 1339, *1340*
　failure of, 1339–1344
　　platelet, 1342–1344, 1343t, 1344t
　　red blood cell, 1341
　　white blood cell, 1341–1342
　hematopoiesis and, 1336–1337, *1340*
　proliferative disorders of, 1359–1368
　suppression of, 1348, 1348t, 1357
　transplantation of, 1344–1358
　　allogeneic, 1346, 1346t, 1347t
　　autologous, 1346, 1346t, 1347t
　　chemotherapeutic agents in, 1348, 1348t
　　complications following, 1348–1358, 1349t, 1350t
　　　cytomegalovirus in, 393t, 393–394, 1354
　　　exocrine glands and, 1349t, 1350t, 1355, 1356

Bone marrow *(Continued)*
　　　gastrointestinal tract and, 1349t, 1350t, 1351–1352, 1355, 1356
　　　genitourinary tract and, 1350t, 1352
　　　graft-versus-host disease and, 1349t, 1349–1350, 1350t
　　　heart and, 1350–1351
　　　infection and, 1352–1355
　　　liver and, 1349t, 1350t, 1351, 1355, 1356
　　　lung and, 1349t, 1350t, 1351, 1356–1357
　　　nervous system and, 1352, 1356
　　　skin and, 1349t, 1350t, 1355, 1356
　　immunosuppression and, 1348, 1348t, 1357
　　procedure for, 1346–1347
　　recovery period of, 1347–1348
　　rejection in, 1348–1349
　　syngeneic, 1346, 1346t, 1347t
Boomslang, 1662t, 1672
Botulism, differential diagnosis in, 568
　drug abuse patient and, 568
　neuropathy of, 682
　skin and, 568
　symptoms of, 568, 682
　treatment of, 682
Bouvia v Superior Court, 1733
Bradycardia, comatose patient and, 635t
　sinus nodal, 1055, *1058*
Bradykinin, septic shock and, 334
Brain, abscess of, drug abuse patient and, 567, 567t
　sinusitis and, 475t, 476, *476*
　anoxic injury to, 645–647
　blood flow of, 632, 639, 639t, 714. See also *Blood flow, cerebral.*
　coma evaluation and, 631–638
　death, criteria for, 645t, 645–646, 646t
　　diagnosis of, 645t, 645–646, 646t
　　family and, 646–647
　　laboratory tests in, 646
　　Lazarus sign and, 646–647
　　legal and ethical issues of, 647
　　medical concept of, 645
　　organ donation and, 646–647
　　rigorous apnea test and, 646, 646t
　edema of, diabetic ketoacidosis and, 1251
　　heart failure and, 642
　　hepatic encephalopathy and, 1520, *1520*, 1521, *1521*
　energy needs of, 632
　eye movements and, 636–637
　herniation syndromes affecting, 632, 637, 715
　hypothermia and, 1637
　hypoxia effects in, brain stem reflexes and, 641–642, 642t
　　heart failure causing, 639–647
　　intracranial pressure and, 641t, 642
　　myoclonus and, 642
　　neurologic signs and, 641–642, 642t
　　neuron function and, 639t, 640t, 640–641
　　outcome of, 643–645, 644t, 645t
　　pathophysiology of, 639–641, 640t
　　prevention of, 641t, 641–643
　　prognosis for, 644t, 644–645, 645t
　　sequelae of, 643–644
　infarction in, *222*, 222, *230*
　metabolism of, 632–633, 639t, 639–640
　monitoring of, 221–233
　　blood flow and, 224t, 224–227, *225*, 225t, *226*, *228*
　　EEG in, *231*, 232t, 232–233
　　evoked potentials and, 231t, 231–232

Brain *(Continued)*
　　goals of, 221–222, *222*
　　interventional thresholds and, 221–222, *222*, 223, 224t
　　intracranial pressure and, 227–230, 229t, *230*
　　ischemia and, *222*, 222–223, 223t, *230*, 230–233
　　jugular venous saturation and, *230*, 230t, 230–231
　　near-infrared spectroscopy and, 231, *231*, 231t
　　oxygen and, *230*, 230–233, *231*
　　predictive characteristics and, 223, 223t, 224t
　oxygen consumption in, 632
　physiology of, 639t, 639–640
　TNF effects in, 320t
　trauma, consciousness disorder due to, 634
　　fluid resuscitation and, *142*, 142–143
　ventricles of, hemorrhage in, 657
　weight of, 714
Brain stem, brain herniation affecting, 715
　hemorrhage in, 657
Breath odors, coma evaluation and, 635
　solvent poisoning and, 1718t
Breathing. See *Expiration; Inspiration; Respiration; Ventilation.*
Bretylium, CPR and, 124–125
Bromocriptine, hyperpyretic-rigidity syndrome and, 703
Bronchi (bronchus), anatomy of, *720*
　pneumonia and, 483, 483t
　washings of, 483, 483t
Bronchioles, airway resistance and, 724, *725*
　anatomy of, *720*
　transitional, *720*
Bronchiolitis obliterans, bone marrow transplant and, 1357
Bronchitis, 793–794
　chronic, 793–794
　respiratory failure in, 793–794
Bronchoalveolar lavage, bronchoscopy and, 198–199, 199t
　organisms retrieved in, 199
　pneumonia diagnosis and, 610
Bronchodilators, 1696–1697
　aerosolization of, 961t, 961–962
　COPD and, 798–799
　liver failure dose adjustment for, 1691t, 1692t, 1696
　pharmacokinetics of, 1696–1697
Bronchoscopy, 192–201
　arrhythmia caused by, 193, 195
　bleeding and, 193–194, 196, 200
　blood gases affected by, 193, 194
　bronchoalveolar lavage in, 198–199, 199t
　complications of, 193, 195, 200, 200t
　contraindications for, 192, 193t
　diagnostic applications of, *197*, 197–200
　foreign body removal in, 196–197, *197*
　indications for, 192
　lung biopsy in, 200
　medication for, 194
　monitoring during, 194
　mucus plug removal in, 196
　needle aspiration during, 198, *199*
　open lung biopsy vs., 200, 200t
　patient evaluation for, 193–194
　personnel for, 193, 194
　pneumonia and, 483t, 484–485
　procedure for, 194–195
　protected specimen in, 483t, 484–485
　therapeutic applications of, 196–197, *197*

Bronchoscopy *(Continued)*
  tissue biopsy in, 199–200, 200t
  ventilation during, 194–195
  washings and brushings in, *197*, 197–198
Brophy v New England Sinai Hospital, Inc.,
    1733–1734
Broviac catheter, *602*, 603, *603*
  candidiasis and, 438
Brown recluse spider, *1679*, 1679–1680,
    1680t
Brudzinski's sign, 457
Bubble-related disorders, 902–909. See also
    Decompression sickness; Embolism, air.
Buformin, lactic acidosis caused by, 1237
Building collapse, 28, 28t, 32t, 35
Bullae, clostridial myonecrosis and, 451
  lung and, 292, *292*
Bumetanide, diuresis using, 1165, 1165t
  pharmacokinetics of, 1690t
Bundle branch block, *1051*, 1057
  atrial arrhythmias and, 1073–1076, *1075*,
    1076
  tachycardia and, 1073–1076, *1075–1077*
  wide QRS and, 1073–1076, *1077*
Burn injury, 1616–1625
  air transport affecting, 45
  body surface area and, 1618, *1618*
  chemical, 1616
  circulation and, 1616–1617, *1617*, 1621
  complications of, 1622–1625, *1623*
  electrical, 1616–1617, 1645–1649, 1646t
  energy requirements and, 1624, *1624*
  evaluation of, 1617–1618, *1618*, 1618t
  fluid resuscitation in, 1618–1620, 1619t
  gastrointestinal tract and, 1622
  hemodynamic aberrations in, 1616–1617,
    1617, 1620–1621
  hypermetabolism in, 1624, *1624*
  immune system response to, 522t, 522–
    524
  infection of, 524t, 524–526, 525t, 1623–
    1624
    antimicrobial therapy in, 525t, 525–526
    organisms in, 524–525, 525t
    prophylaxis in, 525t, 525–526
    treatment of, 525t, 525–526
    types of, 524t, 524–525
  inhalation injury with, 883–886, 1622–
    1623, *1623*
  monitoring and, 1620–1622
  pathophysiologic changes of, 1616–1618,
    1617, 1618t
  pneumonia with, 524
  pregnancy and, 1611
  prehospital management of, 18
  respiratory failure in, 1621–1623, *1623*
  rule of nines for, 1617–1618, 1618t
  second-degree, 1618, 1618t
  shock due to, 1618–1620
  skin destruction in, 521–522
  smoke inhalation with, 883–886, 1622–
    1623, *1623*
  third-degree, 1618, 1618t
Burst-forming units, *1340*
Busulfan, bone marrow transplant and,
    1348t
  side effects of, 1348t
Bypass grafts, coronary artery, 1003–1004,
    1004t. See also *Grafts, vascular.*
Bystander, CPR by, *19*, 20, 120
  disaster preparedness and, 38–39

C

C peptide, hypoglycemia and, 1252–1253,
    1255

C wave, atrium and, *1079*, 1079–1080,
    1080
C5a, burn injury and, 522–523
Calcitonin, calcium metabolism and, *1198*,
    1199
  calcium regulation and, *1198*, 1198–1199
  hypercalcemia treated with, 1205, 1401t,
    1402
Calcitriol, calcium metabolism and, 1199
Calcium, 1196–1206
  albumin and, 1197–1198, *1199*
  blood pressure and, 1200, *1200*
  cardiac arrest and, 120, 124
  CPR and, 120, 124
  deficit of. See *Hypocalcemia.*
  distribution of, 1197–1198, *1198*
  excess of. See *Hypercalcemia.*
  extracellular, 1197–1199, *1198*
  gastrointestinal tract and, 1197, *1198*,
    1204
  heart affected by, 120, 124, 1045–1046,
    1046, 1199–1200
  hormone effects and, 1198–1199
  intake of, 1197
  kidney failure and, 1272
  metabolism of, 1197–1199, *1198*
  regulatory mechanisms for, 1196–1199,
    1198
Calcium channel blockers, angina pectoris
    and, 997, 998t
  arrhythmia treated with, 1055, 1057t
  drug interactions of, 1057t
  hyperthyroidism treated with, 1322–1323
  MI treated with, 997, 997t
  stroke treated with, 654
Calculi, biliary tract, 1491–1493, *1493*,
    1493t, 1494t
  renal, abdominal pain due to, 1480
  obstruction and, 1265t, 1265–1266
Calories. See also *Energy requirements.*
  enteral nutrition and, 1533, 1538t
  nonprotein/nitrogen ratio and, 1533t
  parenteral nutrition and, 1547t
Cameras, Anger, 1108
  multicrystal, 1108
Canadian Cardiovascular Society Functional
    Classification, 78t, 78–79
Cancer. See *Neoplasia.*
Candidemia, 434t, 436
  catheter-related, 438–439
Candidiasis, 434–442
  anatomic sites of, 434t, 436–437
  burn injury and, 524, 525t
  clinical manifestations of, 436–437
  diagnosis of, 437–438, 609
  epidemiology of, 434t, 434–435
  esophageal, 439–440
  hepatosplenic, 440
  host defense mechanisms in, 435, 436t
  laboratory testing for, 609
  management of, 437–442
  nosocomial, 382, 383t
  ophthalmic, 470–471
  oral, 439–440
  organisms in, 435
  pathogenesis of, 434t, 436
  peritonitis and, 440–441, 516
  prevention of, 441
  renal, 441–442
  risk factors for, 434t, 434–435
  urinary tract, 441–442
Candiduria, 441
  management of, 441–442
Capillaries, blood gas metabolism in, 217–
    220, *219*, *220*
  cerebral, 142

Capillaries *(Continued)*
  fluid exchange in, 130, *1155*, 1155–1156
  hydrostatic pressure in, 129–131, 1155,
    1155
  leakage from, 136, 1164
  osmotic pressure in, 129–131, *1155*
  pleural, 860–861, *861*
  pulmonary. See *Pulmonary vasculature.*
  renal, *1155*, 1155–1156
  Starling forces and, *1155*, 1155
  volume depletion and, 1164
Capnography, 208–216
  abnormal tracing in, 210–214, *211–216*
  alveoli and, *208*, 208–209, *209*
  definition of, 210
  heartbeat effect in, *215*
  normal tracing in, 210, *210*
  perfusion role in, *208*, 208–209, *209*
  physiologic basis of, 208
  sensor location in, 210
  sidestream analyzer in, *210*, *211*
  ventilation and, *208*, 208–209, *209*
Capreomycin, side effects of, 427t
  tuberculosis treated with, 427t
Captopril, infarction survival and, *1009*
Caput medusae, abdominal, 1446
  portal hypertension and, 1446
Carbamates, anticholinergic intoxication
    and, 53
Carbicarb, acidosis treated with, 1042,
    1042, *1043*
Carbon dioxide, acid-base balance role of,
    1044, 1220–1222, *1221*, *1222*
  bicarbonate and, 245–246
  cutaneous, 220, *220*
  end-tidal, 208–216
    cardiac arrest and, 123–124, *124*, *214*
    CPR assessment and, 123–124, *124*
  measurement of. See also *Capnography.*
    electrode for, *241*, 241–242, *242*
    gas analyzer in, *240*, 241–242
    noninvasive monitoring and, 208–216
  nephron reabsorption of, 1220–1222,
    1221
  tension, *1044*
    base excess calculation and, 246
    cardiac output measurement and, 1094
    depressed, *1044*
    elevated, *1044*
    end-capillary, 741, 741–742
    patient transport and, 56, 56–57
    perfusion and, 739–743, *739–744*
    pulmonary artery stenosis and, *216*
    respiratory failure and, 755–758
    ventilation and, 739–743
  total, 245–246
Carbon monoxide, hemoglobin binding of,
    883, 885–886
  lactic acidosis caused by, 1238
  oximetry and, 244
  poisoning due to, 883, 885–886, 1238
    symptoms of, 883, 885
    treatment of, 885–886
  smoke inhalation role of, 883–884, 885–
    886
Carbonic acid, respiration and, 1220
Carbonic anhydrase inhibitors, diuresis due
    to, 1164–1165, 1165t
Carbonyl chloride (phosgene), 48–51
Carboxyhemoglobin, absorption spectrum
    of, *204*, 244
  burn injury and, 1622
  oximetry and, 203, *204*, 244, *244*
Carcinoma. See *Neoplasia.*
Cardiac index, body surface area and,
    1096

Cardiac index *(Continued)*
  fluid resuscitation and, *140*
  prognostic use of, 77–78, 78t
  pulmonary embolism and, 855
Cardiac output, 1087–1095
  acidosis and, *1040*
  burn injury and, 1616, *1617*
  Fick oxygen method for, 1093, *1094*
  fluid resuscitation effects and, *137*, 137–140
  heart failure and, 1015–1018, *1016*, 1021, *1021*
  indicator dye method for, 1086–1088, *1088*
  measurement of, 1086–1093
  noninvasive methods for, 1094–1095
  septic shock effect on, 323–332
  thermodilution method for, 1088–1093, *1089*, *1092*
Cardiography. See also *Electrocardiography (ECG); Ultrasonography, cardiographic.*
  impedance, 1095
  scintigraphic, 1105–1113, *1108*, *1110*
Cardiomyopathy, 685
  chemotherapy-induced, 1412t, 1412–1413
  perioperative risk and, 1557
  pregnancy and, 1611–1612
  radiation therapy causing, 1412t, 1413
Cardiopulmonary resuscitation, 118–127
  abdominal binding role in, 122–123
  asystole and, 120
  bag volume and, 17
  bicarbonate therapy in, 1042–1044, *1042–1044*
  blood pressure mechanisms in, 120–124, *121–123*
  bystander administering, *19*, 20, 120
  compression rate in, 121–122, 125, *126*
  cough in, *121*, 121
  defibrillation in, *118*, 118–120, *119*
  drugs used in, 21–24, 22t, 124–125
  elderly patient and, 126–127
  electromechanical dissociation and, 120
  EMT administration of, *19*, 19–24, *20*, 22t
  hemorrhage and, 15
  historical aspects of, 1–4
  mortality rate and, *118*, 120t, *123*, 124, 125t, 126, *126*
  myocardial perfusion pressure and, 123–124
  open chest, 125–126
  out-of-hospital, *19*, 19–24, *20*, 22t, 126–127
  pulse absence and, 15
  thoracic pump mechanism in, 121–123, *122*, *123*
  time-to-therapy and, 120, 120t, 125–126
  ventilation role in, 118, 122–123, 125
  vest apparatus in, 122–123, *123*, 125, 125t
Cardioversion, 1072–1073
  EMT administering, 22, 22t
  energy levels used in, 118–119
  implanted device for, *118*, 118
  pacemaker device damaged by, 120
  paddle placement for, *119*, 119–120
Carditis. See *Endocarditis; Pericarditis.*
Carmustine (BCNU), bone marrow transplant and, 1348t
  gastrointestinal effects of, 1414t, 1414–1415
  lung affected by, 1410, 1410t
  side effects of, 1348t

Carotid artery, dissection of, *1147*, 1147–1148, *1148*
  neck fascia and, *477*
  rupture of, 1146
  stroke and, 649, *652*
  trauma to, *1147*, 1147–1148, *1148*
Cartilage, arytenoid, 113, *113*, *968*, 968–969, *969*
  auricular, burn injury to, 524
  corniculate, *113*, *968*, *968*
  cricoid, 111, *115*
  cuneiform, *113*, *968*, *968*
  thyroid, *115*
Catabolism, burn patient and, 1624, *1624*
  kidney failure and, 1273–1274
  multiple organ system failure and, 345
  rate calculation for, 1273
Catalase, antioxidant effect of, 955t
Cataracts, electrical injury causing, 1646, 1646t, 1649
Catatonia. See *Seizures.*
Catecholamines, 1318–1326, *1699*
  adrenal gland secretion of, 1318
  catabolism of, *1318*, 1318–1319
  heart failure and, 1324–1325
  infusion rate for, 1693t, 1697t
  lactic acidosis caused by, 1238
  measurement of, 1319t, 1319–1320, 1320t, 1321t
    factors affecting, 1319–1320, 1320t
    methods for, 1319–1320, 1321t
    normal levels in, 1319t
  MI and, 1007–1008, 1008t
  pathophysiology related to, 1322–1326
  pharmacokinetics of, 1693t, 1696–1698, 1697t, *1699*
  receptors for, *1319*, 1319t, 1320–1322, 1321t, *1322*, 1322t
  shock and, 1325
  synthesis of, *1318*, 1318
  thyroid gland and, 1322–1324
  urinary levels of, 1319t, 1319–1320, 1320t
Catfish, venom of, 1676–1677
Catheter devices, 601–604, *602*, 602t
  bacteria adherence to, 604–606
  balloon flotation, 1079–1087, *1083*
  central venous, 601–604, *602*, 602t, *603*
  cuffed, 602t, *603*, *603*
  dead space of, 238
  double-sheathed, *197*, 197–198
  fragments of, 1141
  Hickman/Broviac, 601–604, *602*, 602t, *603*
  infection due to. See *Infections, catheter-related.*
  materials used in, 601–604, *602*, 606
  multilumen, *602*, *602*
  peritoneal, 1283–1284
  pneumonia diagnosis and, 610–611
  protected brush, *197*, 197–198, 610–611
  totally implanted (port), *602*, 602t, *603*–604
  triple-lumen, *1545*
  tunneled, 602t, *603*, *603*
  urinary tract, 527, 530
Catheterization, aortic balloon pump and, 188–189, *189*, 261
  arterial, 182–184, *183*
    blood gas sample from, 237–238
    blood pressure monitoring and, 252–253, *253*, 255
    femoral, *1149*
    pulmonary. See *Pulmonary artery, catheterization of.*

Catheterization *(Continued)*
  cardiac, fluid resuscitation using, *374*, 374–375, 375t
    historical aspects of, 2–3
    MI monitoring with, 995, 995t
    pericardiocentesis and, 1034–1035, *1035*
    pressure waveforms and, *1079*, 1079–1081, *1080*
    right-sided, *374*, 374–375, 375t, *1079*, 1079–1081, *1080*
    sepsis treatment and, *374*, 374–375, 375t
    tamponade and, 1034–1035, *1035*
  central venous, 177–182, *178–181*, 186
    antecubital entry for, 181
    basilic entry for, 181
    complications and, 182, 186
    contraindications for, 178
    CPR compression and, 121
    femoral, 178–179, *179*
    jugular, 180–181, *181*
    pressure waveforms and, *1079*, 1079–1081, *1080*
    Seldinger technique and, 178, *178*, *179*
    subclavian, 180, *180*
  dialysis access and, 1280–1282, 1281t, 1285, 1290
  infection related to. See *Infections, catheter-related.*
  injury due to, 1140–1152
  intracranial, 558–559
  IV (intravascular), aberrant placement of, 258–261, *259–263*
    blood cultures and, 609
    cancer patient and, 548–549
    cardiac arrest care and, 23
    CT scan in, *261*
    flushing and, 23
    pacemaker and, 184–186, *185*
    plasmapheresis and, 1425–1427
    radiography and, 258–261, *259–263*
    thrombosis and, *1149*
    transtracheal ventilation with, 114–115, *115*
    trauma patient and, 558–559, 562–563
  urinary tract, bacteriuria screening and, 611
    catheter type in, 527, 530
    closed system for, 527
    condom device in, 530
    nosocomial infection and, 527–530
    suprapubic, 530
  vascular emergent disorders due to, 1140–1152
Cats, rabies and, 691t
Causal modeling, expert system and, 99
Caustic agents, esophageal injury due to, 1432t, 1432–1435, 1433t
Cavernous sinus, thrombosis of, orbital cellulitis causing, 473
CD (clusters of differentiation) molecules, HIV infection and, 589–591, 590t, *591*, 591t
Cecum, typhlitis and, 541–542
Cefazolin, pathogen susceptibility to, 614t
Cefipime, endocarditis vegetations and, *619*, 620
Cefoperazone, enterococcal susceptibility to, 415t
  pharmacokinetics of, 1690t
Cefotaxime, enterococcal susceptibility to, 415t
  meningitis therapy and, 460t, 460–462, 461t

Cefoxitin, pathogen susceptibility to, 415t, 614t
Ceftazidime, meningitis therapy and, 461t, 462
  pathogen susceptibility to, 614t
Ceftriaxone, meningitis therapy and, 461t, 462
Cefuroxime, meningitis therapy and, 460t, 460–462, 461t
Cell(s), ATP production in, 354, 355
  glycolysis in, 356, 356–357
  metabolism in, aerobic, 354, 355
    anaerobic, 354, 355
  sepsis effects in, 354–361, 355–359
Cellulitis, 449t, 449–450
  anaerobic, 450
  cervical fascia and, 477, 477–479
  clostridial, 450
  drug abuse patient with, 575–576
  mouth and, 477, 478
  neck and, 477, 477–479
  orbital, 472–473, 475t
  peritonsillar, 477, 478
  preseptal, 472–473
  sinusitis and, 475t, 475–476
  submandibular, 477, 478
  supraglottic, 474–475
Cellulose, dialysis membranes and, 1276t, 1276–1279
Central venous access. See Catheterization, central venous.
Centrifugation, continuous flow, 1421, 1421
Cephalopods, venom of, 1676
Cephalosporins, first-generation, 1694, 1694t
  hemolytic anemia induced by, 1379t
  kidney failure dose adjustment for, 1305t–1306t
  liver failure dose adjustment for, 1690t
  meningitis therapy and, 460t, 460–462, 461t
  pathogen susceptibility to, 614t
  pharmacokinetics of, 1690t, 1694, 1694t
  second-generation, 1694, 1694t
  susceptibility testing and, 612
  third-generation, 614t, 617, 1694, 1694t
Cerebellum, hemorrhage of, 656t, 657
  herniation syndromes and, 632, 637, 714
  tonsillar herniation of, 715
Cerebrospinal fluid (CSF), Landry-Guillain-Barré syndrome and, 622
  lumbar puncture and, 622
  meningitis and, bacterial, 456, 457–459, 458t
    viral, 395
  subarachnoid hemorrhage and, 661t
  xanthochromia of, 458
Cerebrovascular disease, 648–661. See also Stroke.
  causes of, 633
  consciousness and, 633
  examination in, 649t, 649–650
  hemorrhagic, 655–661
    brain stem, 657
    cerebellar, 656t, 657
    clinical manifestations of, 656t, 656–657
    CT scan in, 657, 657–658, 658
    diagnosis of, 657–658
    etiology of, 655t, 655–656
    intraventricular, 657
    lobar, 656t, 657
    management of, 658–659
    MRI scan in, 657–658, 658
    pontine, 656t, 658
    putamenic, 656t, 656–657

Cerebrovascular disease (Continued)
    subarachnoid, 659t, 659–661
    thalamic, 656t, 657
  ischemic, 648–655
    clinical features of, 649t, 649–650, 650t
    CT scan in, 651, 654
    diagnostic procedures in, 651–653, 652t
    Doppler studies in, 651
    hospitalized patient and, 650–651
    mechanisms of, 649, 649t
    MRI scan in, 653, 653
    pathophysiology of, 651–653
    treatment for, 653–655
  monitoring and, 222, 222–223, 223t, 230, 230–233
  preoperative care and, 1552–1553
Cerebrum. See also Cerebrovascular disease.
  anoxic injury to, 645–647
  blood flow in, 224–227, 639t, 639–640
    consciousness and, 632–633
    ischemic stroke and, 651
    meningitis and, 456, 457
    monitoring of, 224t, 224–227, 225, 225t, 226, 228
    normal, 633, 714
    pressure and, 632
  fluid resuscitation and, 142, 142–143
  herniation syndromes and, 632, 637, 715
  hypoxia effects in, 639–645, 640t
  infarction in, 222, 222, 230
  metabolism in, 639t, 639–640
  oxygen and, 222t, 222–223, 223t, 227t, 230, 230–233, 231
Cervical fascia, 477
  infection in, 477, 477–479
Cesarean delivery, NIH Consensus Statement on, 72
  perimortem, 1596
Chain of survival concept, 9
Charcoal, chemical exposure protection and, 49
  hemoperfusion using, 1291–1292, 1705
  plasma endotoxins removed with, 370
  poisoning therapy and, 370, 1291–1292, 1705
Charcot's triad, 1494
Chelation, hypocalcemia caused by, 1202–1203
Chemical agents. See also Drugs; Poisoning; Toxic substance(s); specific agents.
  alkylating, 48, 52
  historical aspects of, 48–49
  incapacitating, 48–49, 52–53
  injury due to, 48–53
    acid/alkali ingestion and, 1432t, 1432–1435, 1434t
    airway support in, 49–50
    clinical effects in, 50–53
    decontamination and, 49
    protective equipment and, 49
    triage for, 49
  nerve-targeted, 48, 51–52
  riot control, 48, 50
  vesicant, 48, 52
  warfare and, 48–49
Chemotaxis, burn injury affecting, 523
Chemotherapy, bone marrow transplant and, 1348, 1348t
  complications of, 1403–1417
  cytotoxic agents in, 897t, 897–898, 898
  dose adjustment for, 1307t–1308t
  electrolytes affected by, 1406–1407
  encephalopathy induced by, 1416t, 1416–1417

Chemotherapy (Continued)
  gastrointestinal effects of, 1413–1416, 1414t
  granulocytopenia due to, 532
  heart affected by, 1411–1413, 1412t
  hemolytic-uremic syndrome due to, 1375
  kidney failure and, 1307t–1308t, 1406–1408
  liver affected by, 1415t, 1415–1416
  lung injury due to, 897t, 897–898, 898
  myelosuppression caused by, 1403–1406
  neuropathy induced by, 1416t, 1416–1417
  noncytotoxic agents in, 897t, 897–898, 898
  nosocomial infections and, 384
  vena cava obstruction and, 1394–1395, 1395t
Chest, 1584t. See also Thorax.
  flail injury to, 1587, 1587
  physiotherapy to, 957–959
    adverse effects of, 959
    atelectasis and, 958–959
    cystic fibrosis and, 959
    goals of, 957, 957t
    hospital utilization of, 958, 958
    incentive spirometry in, 958
    indications for, 958, 958t
    percussion in, 957–958
    postural drainage and, 957–958
  pulmonary hypertension and, 845
  trauma injury to, 1578t, 1579t, 1584t, 1584–1588, 1585–1588
    pain control in, 1586–1587
    pneumothorax due to, 16
    prehospital care in, 16
    radiography findings in, 1584t, 1585–1588
    sucking wound due to, 15–16
  wall of, polysomnography of, 777, 778
    respiration role of, 723, 723, 763–765, 764, 765, 767
Cheyne-Stokes respiration, phases of, 635t, 636
Chickenpox, 394–395
  natural history of, 394
Chilblains, 1643
Children. See also Neonate.
  defibrillation energy level for, 22
  endocarditis in, 492
  mortality risk and, 85
Child's classification, liver disease and, 79, 79t, 1452, 1452t, 1561, 1561t
Chloramphenicol, meningitis therapy and, 460t, 460–462, 461t
  pharmacokinetics of, 1689t
Chloride, acidosis and, 1223t, 1224
  diarrhea and, 1465–1466
  gastrointestinal transport of, 1465–1466
Chloroacetophenone, clinical effects of, 50
  riot control with, 48
Chlorobenzylidenemalononitrile, clinical effects of, 50
  riot control with, 48
Chloroplasts, 352
Chlorothiazide, diuresis using, 1165, 1165t
Chlorthalidone, diuresis using, 1165, 1165t
Choking, chemical warfare agents and, 48
  food causing, 1435t, 1435–1438
Cholangiography, cholangitis and, 1495
  gallstone pancreatitis and, 1491–1493, 1493, 1493t, 1494t
Cholangitis, 1494–1497
  acute suppurative, 1494–1497
  clinical features of, 1494
  diagnostic studies in, 1495

Cholangitis (Continued)
  endoscopic treatment of, 1496, 1496t, 1496–1497, 1497
  etiology of, 1494
  medical approach in, 1495
  organisms in, 1495
  pathogenesis of, 1494–1495
  percutaneous transhepatic drainage for, 1496
  sphincterotomy for, 1496t, 1496–1497, 1497
  surgical approach in, 1495–1496
Cholecystectomy, cholangitis treated with, 1496t, 1496–1497, 1497
  pancreatitis treated with, 1492–1493, 1493t, 1494t
Cholecystitis, abdominal pain of, 1477–1478
  acalculous, 1478
    trauma injury causing, 1590
Cholelithiasis, pancreatitis due to, 1490–1494
Cholera, 510
  diagnosis of, 510
  treatment of, 510
Cholesterol, plaque crystals of, 991
Cholestyramine, pseudomembranous colitis and, 508
Cholinergic receptors, drug poisoning and, 1703t, 1703–1705, 1704t
Chondritis, burn injury causing, 524
Choriomeningitis, lymphocytic, 396–397
Chronic obstructive pulmonary disease (COPD), 793–803. See also Asthma.
  airway infection with, 794–795
  complications and, 800
  cor pulmonale and, 795–796
  costs and, 803
  ethical issues and, 803
  heart function and, 795–796
  mechanical ventilation in, 800–802
  nutrition and, 802
  pulmonary embolism with, 794–795
  respiratory failure in, 793–803
  treatment of, 798–802
Chronotropic agents, 1697t
Chylothorax, pleural effusion of, 867–868
  thoracic trauma and, 890
Ciguatoxin, 1673
Cilia, cytotoxic impairment of, 752
  lung defense mechanism and, 750, 752
Cimetidine, pharmacokinetics of, 1689t
Cineangiography, septic shock and, 326
Ciprofloxacin, enterococcal susceptibility to, 415t
Circadian rhythm, ACTH regulation and, 1310, 1310
Circulation. See also Blood flow.
  burn injury and, 1616–1617, 1621
  functional components and, 978–979, 979
  multiple organ system failure and, 345–348, 347, 347t, 349t, 349–350
  portal, 1445–1446, 1446
  pulmonary. See Pulmonary vasculature.
  systemic perfusion and, 979
  systemic vascular resistance and, 1097
Cirrhosis, ammonia metabolism and, 1522–1523, 1523t
  encephalopathy due to, 1521–1525, 1522t, 1524t
  GABA metabolism and, 1523–1524
  hepatitis B causing, 402
  liver transplant and, 1515–1516
  peritonitis and, 515–516, 1506–1507
  portal-systemic shunting in, 1522

Cirrhosis (Continued)
  sodium balance in, 1162t, 1162–1163
  volume overload of, 1162–1163
Cisplatin, gastrointestinal effects of, 1414t, 1414–1415
  nephropathy caused by, 1407
  side effects of, 1407
Citrate, transfusion toxicity of, 1389
Clark electrode, 215, 219
Clavulanate, pathogen susceptibility to, 614t
Cleaning compounds, corrosive esophageal injury and, 1432t, 1432–1435
Clinitest tablets, ingestion of, 1433
Clonidine suppression test, mechanism of, 1320
  pheochromocytoma and, 1325
Clostridial infections, cellulitis due to, 450
  colitis caused by, 500–503
  culture for, 504–505
  fasciitis due to, 451
  gas gangrene due to, 451–452
  laboratory tests for, 504–505
  myonecrosis due to, 451–452
Clothing, antishock, 15, 16
Clotting factors, 1337
  cryoprecipitate containing, 1390
  preoperative care and, 1565
  sepsis role of, 335, 372
Clupeotoxin, 1673–1674
CO_2. See Carbon dioxide.
Coagulase, staphylococcal, 413–414
Coagulation. See also Anticoagulants.
  dextran impairment of, 134
  disseminated intravascular, 1600–1602
  factors, 1337
    cryoprecipitate containing, 1390
    preoperative care and, 1565
    sepsis role of, 335, 372
  hereditary disorders of, 1337, 1565, 1602
  hetastarch impairment of, 135
  pregnancy and, 1594t, 1594–1595, 1595t, 1600–1602
  retained dead fetus syndrome and, 1601
  shock and, 981
  snakebite and, 1663–1664, 1664, 1671
  thrombosis and, 849–850
  time required for, 855
Cobb angle, kyphoscoliosis and, 768, 769
Cobras, 1662t, 1667–1668
  complement activation and, 307–308
  venom factor of, 307–308
Cocaine, abruptio placentae due to, 1597–1598
  adulterants of, 1710t
  forms of, 1710t
  heart affected by, 989, 989t, 1047
  myocardial ischemia due to, 989, 989t
  poisoning due to, 1709–1710
  smuggler bowel obstruction and, 1482–1483, 1710
  street names for, 1710t
  toxic effects of, 1709–1710
Coccidioidomycosis, 444
Cockcroft-Gault formula, 1269–1270
Coelenterates, venom of, 1674t, 1674–1675
Coffee grounds aspirate, 1440, 1441t
Cohn's fraction V, 1390
Cold exposure, 1633–1643. See also Hypothermia.
Colestipol, pseudomembranous colitis and, 508
Colitis, 500–512
  antimicrobials causing, 500–509
  E. coli in, 511
  hemorrhagic, 511, 1460–1461
  ischemic, 1461

Colitis (Continued)
  pseudomembranous, 500–509
    abdominal pain of, 1479
    anion-exchange resins in, 508
    antimicrobial therapy in, 505–509
    antiperistaltic agents in, 508
    C. difficile in, 500–503
    CT scan in, 503, 503
    diagnosis of, 503–505
    epidemiology of, 501
    flora replacement in, 509
    fulminating, 1479
    historical aspects of, 501
    laboratory tests in, 504–505
    mortality rate in, 503
    nosocomial, 501–502
    pathogenesis of, 501–502
    pathology in, 501
    prophylaxis for, 502, 509
    recurrence of, 508–509
    symptoms of, 502–503
    toxins in, 502
    treatment of, 505–509
  ulcerative, 1470–1473
    fulminant, 1471–1473
    malnutrition in, 1473
Collimator, scintigraphy and, 1108, 1109
Colloids, fluid resuscitation using, 132–134, 137, 137t
  osmotic pressure due to, 129–131, 130, 143–145, 144
  physicochemical properties of, 137t
  pulmonary edema and, 143–145, 144
Colon, abdominal pain related to, 1478–1479
  hemorrhage in, 511, 1457–1463
    arteriovenous malformation and, 1460, 1460, 1462–1463, 1463
    colitis and, 1460–1461
    diverticular, 1459–1460
    management of, 1457–1459, 1458, 1462–1463
  perforation of, 1478–1479
  pseudo-obstruction of, 1479
Colony-forming units, 1340
  antimicrobial activity and, 616, 617
Colony-stimulating factors, sepsis mediation and, 312t
  therapeutic use of, 543
Coma. See also Encephalopathy.
  alcoholic, 706t, 706–707, 707t
  anatomic correlates for, 631–633
  assessment of, 634–637
    brain stem reflexes and, 636–637, 641–642, 642t
    cranial nerve function and, 636–637, 641–642, 642t
    eye movement and, 635, 637, 642t
    initial, 634–635
    laboratory studies in, 634
    motor system function and, 637
    movement and, 635, 637, 642t
    neurologic, 635, 642t
    respiration patterns in, 636
  brain and, 641–642, 642t, 645t, 645–647
  differential diagnosis of, 631–634, 632t
  drug overdose and, 1704–1705, 1705t
  examination in, 634–637
  heart failure and, 642t, 644–647
  hepatic, 634
    pathophysiology of, 1519–1521
    stages of, 1515t, 1519t
  herniation syndromes and, 632, 637
  hypoglycemic, 633
  hypoxic, 633–634, 641–642, 642t
  ischemic, 633–634

Coma *(Continued)*
  metabolic, 632–634
  severity grading for, 79–80, 80t, 1575t
  structural, 631–632, 637
  trauma patient and, 1575t
  uremic, 634
  vegetative state as, 635, 644
  vital sign abnormalities in, 635t
Compartment syndrome, 1149–1151
  etiology of, 1150
  muscle affected by, 1149–1151
  signs in, 1150
COMPAS system, 99–100, *100*
Complement, activation of, *307*, 307–308
  burn injury and, 522t, 522–523
  cobra venom factor and, 307–308
  sepsis role of, *307*, 307–308
  shock and, 981
  terminal complex of, 308
Compromised host. See *Host, compromised.*
Computed tomography (CT), aorta and,
    1135–1137, *1138*
  colitis and, 503, *503*
  head trauma and, 716
  meningitis and, *458*, 459, 460
  pleural effusion and, 281, *282–284*, 864
  pneumothorax and, *287*
  respiratory distress syndrome and, 822,
    824
  septic pulmonary embolism and, *570*
  stroke and, hemorrhagic, *657*, 657–658,
    658
    ischemic, 651, *652–654*
  subarachnoid hemorrhage and, *660*
  transport complications and, 55
Computers, 88–95. See also *Artificial
    intelligence; Expert systems.*
  clinical data storage in, 88–91
  decision assistance from, 91
  equipment management using, 94
  ICU use of, 88–95
  interface requirements and, 89t, 89–90
  inventory control and, 94
  medical data bases accessed with, 91
  quality assurance tasks and, 91–93
  scoring system data in, 82
  software design and, 90
  staff communications using, 93–94
  user interface of, 97t, 97–98, 106–107
Concussion. See also *Head trauma.*
  consciousness disorder due to, 634
Cone shells, venom of, 1676
Confusion, 635. See also *Mental status.*
  coma evaluation and, 635
  hypoglycemic, 633
  unresponsive patient with, 627
Congo-Crimean hemorrhagic fever, 404
Conjunctivitis, 466–468
  anatomy and, *466*, 466–467, *467*
  bacterial, 467–468
  culture in, 467
  follicular, 467
  nosocomial, 467–468
  papillary, 467
  prevention of, 468
  pseudomembranous, 467
  smear sample in, 467–468
  treatment of, 468, 468t
Conn's syndrome, potassium level and,
    1181
Consciousness disorders, 631–638. See also
    Coma; Seizures.
  anatomic correlates for, 631–633
  concussive, 634
  differential diagnosis of, 631–634, 632t
  hypoglycemic, 633

Consciousness disorders *(Continued)*
  hypothermia and, 1637
  hypoxic, 633–634
    heart failure and, 641–642, 642t
    ischemic, 633–634
    metabolic, 632–634
    thiamine deficiency in, 633–634
Consensus process, standards formulation
    and, 71–72
Contrast media, kidney failure due to,
    1261t, 1262
  peritoneum and, 513, 514
Convection, dialysis and, 1275
Convulsions. See *Seizures.*
Coombs' test, direct, 1372–1373
  hemoglobinuria and, paroxysmal noctur-
    nal, 1383
  hemolytic anemia and, 1372–1373, 1382t
  indirect, 1373
  transfusion reaction and, 1382, 1382t
COP (colloid osmotic pressure), 129–131,
    130
  pulmonary edema and, 143–145, *144*
COPD. See *Chronic obstructive pulmonary
    disease (COPD).*
Copper, hemolytic anemia due to, 1384
Cor pulmonale, 838–845
  airway obstruction and, 841
  causes of, 840t, 840–845, 1027t
  COPD and, 795–796
  diagnostic tests in, *1027*, 1027–1028
  hemodynamic profile in, 1098t
  pathogenesis of, 838, 1026–1027, 1027t
  right ventricle in, 1026–1028
  signs and symptoms in, 1027
  treatment in, 1028
Coral snake, bite due to, 1662t, 1668–1669
Corectopia, 636
Cori cycle, 1233
Cornea, cold exposure affecting, 1643
  scleral junction with, *466*, 466–467
  ulcer of, *466*, 468–470
    fungal, 470
    prevention of, 470
    treatment of, 469–470
Corniculate cartilage, *113*, 968, *968*
Coronary arteries, atherosclerosis and, *990*,
    990–991, *991*
  blood flow in, 989–991, *990*, *991*
    stenosis and, 989–991, *990*, *991*
  bypass grafts for, 1003–1004, 1004t
  perioperative risk and, 1558–1559
  thrombosis and, 989–991, *990*, *991*
  vasoconstriction in, 991
  ventricular fibrillation and, 118
Coronary care units, historical aspects of,
    1–2
Corrosives, esophageal injury due to, 1432t,
    1432–1435, 1433t
Corticosteroids, alcoholic hepatitis treated
    with, 1508–1509
  asthma treated with, 809t, 810
  COPD and, 799
  meningitis and, 462–463
  myasthenia treated with, 683–684
  pharmacokinetics of, 1690t
  sepsis treated with, 373
  stroke treated with, 654
Corticotropin. See *Adrenocorticotropic
    hormone (ACTH).*
Cortisol (hydrocortisone), 1310–1317
  binding globulin for, 1310t
  deficiency of, 1313t, 1313–1314, 1314t
  hypothyroidism and, 1324
  metabolism of, 1310
  physiologic actions of, *1311*

Cortisol (hydrocortisone) *(Continued)*
  regulatory factors for, 1310, *1311*
Corynebacterium pseudodiphtheriticum, 419
Costophrenic angle, pleural effusion
    imaging and, 862, *862*
Costs, COPD and, 803
  ethical issues and, 5, 77, 1731
  illness severity scoring and, 77
  intensive care services and, 5, 77, 1731,
    1743
  medical care standards and, 69–71
  nosocomial infection and, 365
Cosyntropin test, 1312
Cough, CPR using, *121*, 121
Counterimmunoelectrophoresis, meningitis
    detection by, 459
Coxsackievirus, 396
CPR. See *Cardiopulmonary resuscitation.*
Cramps, muscle, hyperthermia and, 1628
Cranial nerves, coma evaluation and, 636–
    637
  eye movements and, 636–637
  meningitis affecting, 457
C-reactive protein, burn injury and, 523
Creatine kinase, ATP production and, *355*,
    358, *359*
  MI and, 992–993, 993t
Creatinine, clearance of, 1269–1270, 1304–
    1309
  antimicrobial dosage and, 616
  formula for, 616
  glomerular filtration rate and, 1269–
    1270, 1304–1309, 1309t
  height index and, 1530–1531
  kidney failure assessment and, 1269–
    1270, 1309, 1309t
  malnutrition and, 1530–1531
  urinary excretion of, 1530–1531
Crepitation, cellulitis and, 450
  gangrene and, 451
  necrotizing fasciitis and, 451, 577
CREST syndrome, 842
Cricoid cartilage, anatomy of, *115*
  endotracheal intubation and, 111
Cricothyroid membrane, anatomy of, *115*
  incision of, 115, *115*
  transtracheal ventilation and, 114–115,
    115
Crimean-Congo hemorrhagic fever, 404
Critical care. See *Intensive care services;
    Intensive care unit (ICU).*
Crohn's disease, 1470–1473
  hemorrhage due to, 1460–1461, *1471*
  malnutrition due to, 1473
Crotalid bites, 1662t, 1669–1672,
    1670t
Crush syndrome, 33–35
  clinical manifestations of, 33t, 33–34
  diagnosis of, 34
  management of, 34–35, *35*
Crux phenomenon, 715
Cruzan case, 1734
Cryoprecipitate, 1390
  clotting disorders treated with, 1390
Cryptococcal infections, meningitis and,
    444–445
Cryptococcal infections, meningitis and,
    444–445
Crystalloids, fluid resuscitation using, 131t,
    131–132
CSF. See *Cerebrospinal fluid (CSF).*
CT. See *Computed tomography (CT).*
Cuffing, peribronchial, *788*, 788–789
Cullen's sign, 1159, 1501
Cultures, catheter contamination of, 609
  pneumonia and, 609–611
  septicemia and, 608–609
  surgical wound infection and, 611–612

Cultures *(Continued)*
  urinary tract infection and, 611
Cuneiform cartilage, *113*, 968, *968*
Cuprophane, anaphylatoxins and, 1275
Curariform agents, dose adjustment for, 1309t
  kidney failure and, 1309t
Current, defibrillation levels of, 22, 118–119
  electrical injury and, 1645–1646, 1648
  high-tension, 1646
Cushing's signs, bradycardia and, 635, 1398
  coma evaluation and, 635
Cushing's syndrome, 1315–1316
  clinical manifestations of, 1315–1316
  diagnosis of, 1316
  etiology of, 1315, 1315t
  treatment of, 1316
CV wave, atrium and, 1080, *1080*
Cyanide, antidote for, 886, 1712
  clinical effects of, 49, 51, 883, 884, 1237–1238
  discovery of, 48
  lactic acidosis caused by, 1237–1238
  mechanism of action of, 51
  nitroprusside metabolized to, 1331, *1332*, 1711–1712
  poisoning due to, 883, 884, 1237–1238, 1711–1712
  properties of, 48, 884
  smoke inhalation and, 883, 884
Cyclones, 31, 33t
Cyclooxygenase inhibitors, meningitis and, 461t, 464
Cyclophosphamide, bone marrow transplant and, 1348t
  gastrointestinal effects of, 1414t, 1414–1415
  heart affected by, 1412t, 1413
  lung injury due to, 897t, 897–898, *898*
  pharmacokinetics of, 1689t
  side effects of, 1348t
Cycloserine, side effects of, 427t
  tuberculosis treated with, 427t
Cyclosporine, antimicrobial interaction with, 587t
  drug interactions of, 1294t
  kidney transplant and, 1293–1294, 1294t
  pharmacokinetics of, 1692t, 1700
  side effects of, 1293–1294, 1294t
Cystic fibrosis, chest physiotherapy and, 959
Cytochrome system, antimicrobial effects in, 587t
Cytokines, burn injury and, 523–524
  meningitis effects and, 456
  sepsis mediated by, 311–320, 371
Cytomegalovirus, 392–394, 393t
  clinical effects of, 585, 585t
  drug therapy and, 394
  transfusion and, 1391
  transplant patient and, 392–394, 393t, 584–585, 585t
Cytomegalovirus infection, abdominal pain due to, 1481
Cytosine arabinoside, lung injury due to, 897t, 897–898, *898*
  neuropathy due to, 1417
Cytotoxicity, oxygen level and, 949–954, 951t, 952t, *953*

D

D receptors, catecholamines and, *1319*, 1321t, 1321–1322, 1322t

Damping coefficient, fluid-filled system and, 253
Dantrolene, hyperpyretic-rigidity syndrome and, 703
  hyperthermia treated with, 1632
Daptomycin, enterococcal susceptibility to, 415t
Data bases, clinical information in, 88–91
  expert systems and, 96–97, 97t
  medical, computer interface with, 91
Daunorubicin, gastrointestinal effects of, 1414t, 1414–1415
  heart affected by, 1411–1412, 1412t
Dead space, respiratory, 208, *208*, 733–734, 742–743
Death, legal definition of, 3
  right to, 1742–1743
Débridement, bacteremia and, 526
  burn injury and, 526
  fasciitis treatment and, 577
  peritonitis therapy and, 519
Decerebration, posturing of, 637
Decisions, drug allergy monitoring and, 91
  intensive care patient and, 1732–1744
Decompression sickness, bubble formation in, 902–903
  clinical manifestations of, 905–906
  hyperbaric oxygen in, 906–907, *909*
  nervous system effects of, 906
  pathophysiology of, 902–903
  recompression in, 906–907, *909*
  transportation and, 905, 909
  treatment of, 906–907, *909*
  vestibular effects of, 906
Decontamination, chemical exposure and, 49
Decortication, posturing of, 637
Defense mechanisms, respiratory tract and, 748–753, *749*
  skin and, 522t, 522–524
Deferoxamine, antioxidant effect of, 955t
Defibrillation, *118*, 118–120, *119*, 1072–1073
  EMT administering, 22, 22t
  historical aspects of, 3
  implanted device for, *118*, 118
  pacemaker device damaged by, 120
  paddle placement for, *119*, 119–120
  shock energy levels used for, 22, 118–119
  transthoracic impedance in, 119
Delirium, anticholinergic intoxication and, 52–53
  coma evaluation and, 635
Delirium tremens, 708
  treatment of, 709t, 710
Delivery, cesarean, 72, 1596
Delta waves, *775*
Dementia, uremia causing, 1270
Demyelination, alcoholism causing, 711
  central pontine, 711
  corpus callosum and, 711
  nerve roots and, 677–682
  peripheral nerves and, 677–682
Dengue hemorrhagic fever, 403
Depolarization, heart cells and, *1050*, 1050–1051
  motor neuron and, 673
Dermatitis, cancer patient and, 551–552
DESCL system, 103t
Detergents, diarrhea caused by, 1467
  ingestion of, 1432t
Devices. See also *Catheter devices*; *Pump devices.*
  C. difficile transmission and, 502
  nosocomial infection and, 384, 387–388
  prosthetic heart valves and, 494–495

Dexamethasone, hyperthyroidism treated with, 1322
  meningitis and, 462–463
  suppression test using, 1312
Dextrans, coagulation impaired by, 134
  fluid resuscitation using, 133–134, *137*
  molecular weight of, 133
  monovalent hapten, 134
  production of, 133
  side effects of, 134
Diabetes insipidus, causes of, 1176t
  hypothalamic, 1176, 1176t
  nephrogenic, 1176, 1176t
  polyuria of, 1175–1176
  water balance and, 1176
Diabetes mellitus, endocarditis and, 492
  foot infection and, 450
  ketoacidosis of, 1245–1251. See also *Ketoacidosis.*
  kidney transplant and, 1297
  lactic acidosis in, 1235
  phosphate deficit in, 1214
  preoperative care and, 1562
DIABETEX system, 103t
Diagnosis. See also under specific disorders.
  artificial intelligence and, 96–98, 97t, 98t
  expert systems and, 96–98, 97t, 98t
Dialysis, 1304t–1309t
  continuous arteriovenous, 1287–1288, 1287–1291, *1288*, *1289*
    advantages of, 1287t
    antibiotics in, 1291t
    anticoagulation in, 1290t, 1290–1291
    complications of, 1290t, 1290–1291
    equipment used in, 1287–1288, *1288*, *1289*
    membranes used in, 1287–1288
    physicochemical aspects of, 1288–1290, *1289*
  drug dose adjustment and, 1304t–1309t
  energy requirements and, 1273–1274
  hemodialysis, 1280–1283
    acute, 1280t
    anticoagulation in, 1281–1282
    arteriovenous fistula for, 1149, *1150*
    catheter access in, 1280–1282, 1281t
    complications of, 1282–1283, 1283t
    continuous, *1288*, 1288–1291, *1289*, 1290t, 1291t
    crush syndrome and, 34–35
    equipment for, 1280–1281, *1282*
    historical aspects of, 3–4
    hypotension due to, 1282–1283, 1283t
    indications for, 1280t
    methanol poisoning and, 1717
    patient monitoring in, 1282–1283, 1283t
    procedure in, 1282
    solutions used in, 1280–1282, 1282t
  hemofiltration, 1287–1288, *1288*
  hemoperfusion, 1291–1292, 1292t, 1705
  infection and, 1272–1273
  machines used in, 1275–1276, *1276*, *1282*, 1288, *1288*, *1289*
  membranes used in, 1276t, 1276–1279, *1278*, 1287
  modalities for, 1281t
  peritoneal, 1283–1286
    catheter in, 1283–1284
    complications of, 1285t, 1285–1286
    patient monitoring in, 1284–1285
    solution used in, 1284, *1284*, 1284t, *1285*
  poisoning therapy using, 1291–1292, 1292t

Dialysis *(Continued)*
  principles of, 1275–1279, *1276, 1278, 1279*
  shortcomings of, 1267
  solute clearance rates in, 1276t, 1276–1279, *1278, 1279*
Diaphragm, anatomy of, 763–765, *764*
  paralysis of, 767
  respiration role of, 763–765, *764*
  rupture of, 892, 1600
  trauma injury to, 892
Diarrhea, 1464–1470
  AIDS and, 511–512
  alkalosis and, 1227t, 1227–1228, *1228*
  amebic, 510t, 511
  antibiotic-associated, 500–509
  bacterial enterotoxins and, 1467t, 1467–1469
  bicarbonate transport in, 1466
  bloody, 511
  causes of, 1466t, 1466–1469, 1467t
  C. difficile and, 500–509, 1467t, 1467–1469
  chloride transport in, 1465–1466
  choleric, 510, 510t, 1467t
  detergents causing, 1467
  diagnosis in, 1469
  dysentery and, 510–511, 1467t
  E. coli and, 511, 1467t
  lamina propria cell in, *1468*
  mechanisms of, 1466t, 1466–1468
  neurohumoral agents in, 1466, 1466t, 1467
  osmotic, 1466t
  potassium transport in, 1185, 1466
  pseudomembranous colitis and, 502
  Salmonella and, 511
  Shigella and, 510t, 510–511, 1467t
  sodium transport in, 1160, 1464–1465
Diastole, failing heart and, *1016,* 1016–1018
  left ventricle and, *1017, 1026,* 1026–1027
  pressure-volume relationship and, *1026,* 1026–1028
  right ventricle and, *1026,* 1026–1027
Diazepam, alcoholism treated with, 709t, 709–710
  liver disease and, 1689t
  meningitis seizure and, 463
  pharmacokinetics of, 669t, 1689t
  seizure treated with, 668t, 668–671, 669t
Diazoxide, hypertensive emergency and, 1331t
Dibenzoxazepine, clinical effects of, 50
  riot control with, 48
DIC (disseminated intravascular coagulation), 1600–1602
Dichloroacetate, acidosis treated with, 1042, *1043*
  lactic acidosis treated with, 1241–1242, *1242*
  mechanism of action of, 1241–1242, *1242*
Didanosine, HIV infection and, 594
Diet. See also *Food; Nutrition.*
  enteral nutrition formulations and, *1537,* 1537–1540, 1538t
  hepatic encephalopathy and, 1522–1524
  potassium intake and, 1180, 1182, 1185
  pulmonary hypertension and, 844
Dieulafoy's ulcer, 1461
Diffusion, blood gas, *739,* 739–740
  dialysis and, 1275
Digitalis, antibodies to, 1707
  arrhythmia due to, 1073, *1073, 1074*
  arrhythmia treated with, 1055, 1057t
  drug interactions of, 1057t

Digitalis *(Continued)*
  heart failure treated with, *1023,* 1023t, 1023–1024
  hyperkalemia caused by, 1182
  kidney failure dose adjustment for, 1308t
  monitoring of, 1692t
  overdose of, 1706–1707
  pharmacokinetics of, 1692t, 1698
  toxic effects of, *1023,* 1023, 1706–1707
Digits, arterial insufficiency and, 236
  nodes on, endocarditis and, 493
Diltiazem, arrhythmia treated with, 1055, 1057t
  dosage for, 998t
  MI and, 997, 998t
Dinitrophenol, hypothermia induced by, 217, *218*
Dinoflagellates, poisoning due to, 1672–1674, 1676
Diphenhydramine, pharmacokinetics of, 1689t
Diphosphonates, hypercalcemia therapy with, 1205
Diphtheroids, 419
Direct current, 1645, 1648, 1648t
Disaster preparedness, 36–45
  bystander response and, 38–39
  command system and, 38, 38t
  federal agencies and, 40–42
  hospitals and, 40
  initial field response and, 38–39
  local agencies and, 37t, 37–40
  medical assistance teams in, 41t, 41–42, 42t
  medical response phases and, 38t, 38–40
  military personnel and, 42
  response plan flowchart for, *37*
  scene control and, 38–39
  search and rescue teams and, 42, 42t
  state agencies and, 40
  transportation factors and, 39–40, 42–45
Disasters, 25–45
  first discovery of, 36t
  fluid resuscitation in, 34–35, *35,* 47–48
  human origin, 32, 32t, 33t
  injuries caused by, 29t, 32t, 32–36, 33t
  medical syndromes in, 29t, 32t, 32–36, 33t, 42–45
  nomenclature for, 25–26
  transport of casualties in, 39–40, 42–45
  triage categories and, 39
  types of, 25–32
Disequilibrium, dialysis and, 1270, 1283
Disk diffusion test, antimicrobial susceptibility and, 612–613
Disopyramide, arrhythmia treated with, 1055, 1056t
  drug interactions of, 1056t
Disseminated intravascular coagulation (DIC), 1600–1602
  abruptio placentae and, 1601
  amniotic fluid and, 1601
  hemolysis and, 1601
  pregnancy and, 1600–1602
  trauma and, 1601–1602
Dithionate, oximetry and, 244
Diuretics, 1164–1166, 1165t, 1166t
  dopamine, 1165, 1165t
  heart failure treatment and, 1024
  kidney failure dose adjustment for, 1308t
  loop, 1165, 1165t
  magnesium depletion due to, 1208
  mechanism of action of, 1164–1166, 1165t
  resistance to, 1166, 1166t
  thiazide, 1165, 1165t

Diverticular disease, hemorrhage due to, 1459–1460, *1460*
Diving, breath-hold, 904–905
  bubble-related disorders and, 902–909
  depth and, 902, 904
  scuba, 902–904
Dizziness, hypoglycemic, 633
Dobutamine, heart failure treated with, *1021,* 1021–1022, *1022*
  pharmacokinetics of, 1693t, 1696–1698, 1697t
  septic shock therapy and, 375–377, *376,* 376t
Dogs, rabies and, 691t
Doll's eye maneuver, 636
Done nomogram, *1708*
Donnan equilibrium effect, osmotic pressure and, 130
Donors, organ, heart transplant and, 1126–1127
Do-not-resuscitate orders, 1736–1738
Dopamine, catabolism of, *1318,* 1318–1319
  diuresis using, 1165–1166
  heart failure therapy and, *1021,* 1021–1022
  hyperpyretic-rigidity syndrome and, 698–699
  measurement of, 1319t, 1319–1320, 1320t, 1321t
  pharmacokinetics of, 1693t, 1696–1698, 1697t
  receptors for, *1319,* 1319t, 1320–1322, 1321t, 1322t
  septic shock therapy and, 375–377, *376,* 376t
  sodium balance and, 1158
  synthesis of, *1318,* 1318
Dopexamine, sepsis treated with, 362
Doppler studies. See *Ultrasonography, Doppler.*
Dosage, 1304t–1309t, 1689t, 1692t, 1693t. See also *Pharmacokinetics;* specific drugs.
  commonly used IV drugs and, 1693t
  dialysis affecting, 1304t–1309t
  kidney failure affecting, 1304t–1309t
  liver failure affecting, 1689t–1692t, 1692–1693
  loading, 1687–1688
  range, and, 1692t, 1692–1693
Doxorubicin, gastrointestinal effects of, 1414t, 1414–1415
  heart affected by, 1411–1412, 1412t
Drabick case, 1734
Dressler's syndrome, 1010
Drowning, cyclones and, 31, 33t
  floods and, 31–32, 33t
Drug abuse, brain abscess and, 567, 567t
  cocaine and, 1482–1483, 1709–1710, 1710t
  infection(s) related to, 566–577
    endocarditis as, 494, 572–575, 573t, 574t
    hepatitis C as, 402
    HIV as, 591t, 592t
    nervous system and, 566–568, 567t, 574
    respiratory tract and, 568t, 568–572, *569, 570*
    skin and soft tissue and, 575t, 575–577
  narcotics and, 1711, 1711t
  opiates and, 1711, 1711t
  poisoning due to, 1482–1483, 1709–1711
  smuggler bowel obstruction and, 1482–1483
  stroke due to, 655t, 656, 659t

Drugs. See also *Pharmacokinetics*; *Poisoning*;
  specific drugs.
  absorption of, 1687, 1687t
  anaphylaxis treated with, 1655t, 1656–
    1659, *1657*
  antiarrhythmic, 1054–1055, 1056t–1057t
  antiviral, 405–406
  asthma treatment and, 809t, 809–810
  binding of, 1688–1691, 1689t–1692t
  bioavailability of, 1687, 1687t
  cardiopulmonary resuscitation and, 21–
    24, 22t, 124–125
  clearance of, 1687t, 1688–1691, 1689t–
    1691t
  common intravenous, 1693
  distribution of, 1687t, 1687–1688
  diuretics as, 1164–1166, 1165t, 1166t
  dosage for, 1304t–1309t, 1689t–1692t
    commonly used IV drugs and, 1693t
    dialysis affecting, 1304t–1309t
    kidney failure affecting, 1304t–1309t
    liver failure affecting, 1689t–1692t,
      1692–1693
    loading, 1687–1688
    range and, 1692t, 1692–1693
  first-pass effect of, 1687, 1687t
  genetic polymorphism and, 1700t, 1700–
    1701
  half-life of, 1304t–1309t, 1687t, 1688,
    1689t–1692t
  heart failure therapy and, 21–24, 22t,
    120, 124–125, *1023*, 1023t, 1023–
    1024
  hemolytic anemia due to, 1378t–1380t,
    1378–1381, 1385t
  hypothermia induced by, 1635t
  immunosuppression with, 1293t, 1293–
    1294, 1294t
  infusion rates for, 1693t
  interactions of, cyclosporine and, 1294t
  interstitial nephritis due to, 1264t, 1264–
    1265
  kidney failure due to, 1261t, 1261–1263,
    1264t, 1264–1265
  lung injury due to, 896–901
  monitoring of, 1686–1701
  ophthalmic, 468t
  overdose of, 1702–1712
    approach in, 1702–1705
    hemoperfusion therapy in, 1291–1292,
      1292t, 1705
    laboratory tests and, 1702–1703
    nervous system affected by, 1703t–
      1705t, 1703–1705
    symptoms in, 1702–1705, 1703t
    thermoregulation affected by, 1704,
      1704t
    treatment of, 1291–1292, 1292t, 1702–
      1712
  paralyzing, 811t
  poisoning due to, 1702–1712, 1703t–
    1705t, *1708*
  protein binding of, 1688–1691, 1689t–
    1692t
  smuggling of, 1482
  torsades de pointes due to, 1072, 1072t
  toxic syndromes due to, 1702–1712,
    1703t–1705t, *1708*
  vasoconstriction and, 1693t, 1696–1698,
    1697t
Dubois formula, body surface area and,
  1096
Duchenne's dystrophy, 686
Duodenum, gallstone pancreatitis and,
  1490–1492
  nasogastric tube in, 269

Dust, earthquake generation of, 28, 35
  volcanic ash as, 28–31, 35
Duteplase, 1000
Dye dilution method, cardiac output and,
  1086–1088, *1088*
Dysautonomia, 672–673, 681–682
Dysentery, 510–511
  amebic, 510t, 511
  bacillary, 510t, 510–511
  differential diagnosis in, 510t, 510–511
  E. histolytica and, 510t, 511
  Shigella and, 510t, 511
Dysphagia, candidiasis and, 439
Dysphonia, botulism causing, 568

E

Ear, altitude effects in, 54
  barotrauma effects in, 903
  burn injury to, 524
  coma evaluation and, 637
  ice water irrigation of, 637
  oximetry and, 203, 205, *206*
Early satiety, pulmonary hypertension and,
  845
Earthquakes, 27–28
  injuries caused by, 28, 29t, 33t
  magnitude of, 27t, 28, 28t
  plate tectonics and, 27, *27*
  secondary effects of, 27–28, 28t
  structural damage caused by, 27–28, *28*,
    28t
  ten most lethal, 27t
Eastern equine encephalitis, 693
Echinoderms, venom of, 1675–1676
Echocardiography. See *Ultrasonography,*
  cardiographic.
Eclampsia, 1608
  hypertensive emergency due to, 1329,
    1330t
  pregnancy and, 1608
Edema, capillary leak syndrome with, 1164
  cerebral, diabetic ketoacidosis and, 1251
    heart failure and, 642
    hepatic encephalopathy and, 1520,
      1520, 1521, *1521*
  differential diagnosis in, 1161–1164,
    1162t
  endotracheal intubation prevented by,
    116
  fluid resuscitation and, 143–145, *143–*
    145
  hypothyroidism and, 1161
  hypotonicity and, 1171–1172, 1172t
  kidney failure and, 1257, 1257t
  nonpitting, 1161
  peripheral, 1161, 1162t
  pitting, 1161
  pulmonary, *143*, 143–145, 911–922,
    1162t
    acidemia in, *1044*, 1045, *1045*
    alveolar, *788*, 788–789, *789*, 789t, 917–
      918
    blood pressure and, 143–145, *144*,
      912–915, *913*
    capillary permeability and, 279, *280*,
      912–913, *913*
    cardiogenic, 279, *280*, 920
    causes of, 278–280, 279t, 789t, 1162t
    classification of, 912
    drug abuse patient and, 572
    drug-induced, 896–901
    fluid resuscitation and, 143–145, *143–*
      145, *374*
    formation of, 917–918

Edema *(Continued)*
  heart failure and, *788*, 789t, 789–792,
    1019–1020, 1022
  measurement of, 921t, 921–922, 1092–
    1093
  phosgene exposure causing, 50–51
  pregnancy and, 1605–1606
  protein concentration and, 915–916,
    918, *919*
  radiography in, 278–280, *279*, *280*,
    790, *790*, *791*
  resolution of, 918–920
  respiratory distress syndrome and,
    139–140, 920–921
  septic shock and, 139–140
  Starling forces and, *789*, 789–790,
    911–912
  transplant patient and, 583–584, 584t
  vascular pedicle and, 790, *790*, *791*
  volume overload and, 279, 279t, *280*
  sodium and, 1161–1163, 1162t
  systemic, 145–146
  volume depletion with, 1163–1164
Education programs, expert systems and,
  101–102, *102*
Effusions, pericardial, 173t, *1033–1035*,
  1033–1036
  peritoneal. See *Ascites.*
  pleural. See *Pleura, effusions of.*
Eicosanoids, inhibition of, 371–372
  sepsis role of, 304–306, *305*, 371–372
Ejection fraction, calculation of, 327, 367
  heart failure and, 1016–1018
  imaging studies and, *1111*, 1111–1112,
    1112
  left ventricular, 326–328, *327*, 367
  right ventricular, *1092*
  septic shock and, 326–328, *327*, 367
  thermodilution measurement of, *1092*
Elapids, 1662t, *1666*, 1668–1669
Electric shock cardioversion, 22, *118*, 118–
  120, *119*
Electrical impedance cardiography, 1095
Electrical injury, 1645–1649
  alternating current in, 1645
  clinical manifestations of, 1646t, 1646–
    1649, *1649*
  current intensity and, 1645–1646, 1648
  direct current in, 1645, 1648, 1648t
  lightning causing, 1648t, 1648–1649,
    1649
  treatment of, 1647–1649
Electrocardiography (ECG), arrhythmias
  and, 1051–1077
  artificial neural networks and, 104–105,
    105
  cardiac arrest waveforms in, *20*, 23–24
  expert system interpretation of, 100–101,
    101, *102*, 104–106, *105*
  gating with, 1108, *1109*
  hypercalcemia and, 1045–1046, *1046*
  hyperkalemia and, *1046*, 1046–1047,
    1052, 1052–1053, *1053*
  hypocalcemia and, 1045–1046, *1046*
  hypothermia and, *1635*, 1635–1636
  MI and, 991–992, *993*
  pericarditis and, 1032, *1032*
  potassium level and, *1187*, 1187t, 1187–
    1188
  pulmonary embolism and, 852
Electrocoagulation, peptic ulcer and, 1443
Electrodes, blood gas analyzer and, 239–
  243, *240–243*
  calibration of, 242–243
  calomel, 240
  carbon dioxide, *241*, 241–242, *242*

Electrodes *(Continued)*
  Clark, 215, 219
  defibrillation, *119,* 119–120
  fluorescent optode, 247–248, *248*
  glass characteristics and, 240–242
  ion-selective, 242
  mercury chloride, *240,* 240–241
  output drift of, 247
  oxygen, 242–243, *243*
  paddle, *119,* 119–120
  pH, 239–241, *240, 241*
  polarographic, 242, *243*
  reference, *240,* 240–241, *241*
  silver chloride, *240–243,* 241–242
Electroencephalography (EEG), 622–624
  brain monitoring with, *231,* 232t, 232–233
  clinical value of, 622–624
  electrodes for, 622–623
  frequency spectrum in, *231,* 232t, 232–233
  quantitative aspects of, 623
  sleep apnea and, *777, 778*
  sleep stages and, *775*
  spectral array, 624
Electrogram, atrial flutter and, *1076*
Electrolytes. See also *Hypertonicity;*
    Hypotonicity.
  arrhythmia and, 1051–1054, *1052, 1053*
  cardiac arrest and, 22t, 24
  chemotherapy affecting, 1406–1407
  diarrhea and, 1464–1466
  gastrointestinal transport of, 1464–1466
  heart affected by, 1045–1047, *1046,*
    1051–1054
  hypothermia affecting, 1636
  ion-selective field effect transistors and,
    247
  ketoacidosis and, 1247–1248, 1248t,
    1249t, 1249–1250
  kidney failure and, 1271–1272, 1407
Electromechanical dissociation, CPR
    outcome and, 120
Electromyography (EMG), clinical value of,
    626–627
  expert system recognition of, 104
  sleep apnea and, *777, 778*
  techniques for, 626–627
Electron transport, Krebs' cycle and, 1231,
    1232
Electronic mail systems, computers and,
    93–94
Electro-oculography (EOG), sleep apnea
    and, *777, 778*
Embolism, 849–859
  air, 907–909, 1141
    catheter-related, 1141
    dialysis and, 1283
    etiology of, 907
    hyperbaric oxygen and, 908–909, *909*
    iatrogenic, 908–909, 1141
    oxygen therapy in, 908–909, *909*
    paradoxical arterial, 908
    recompression therapy and, 908–909,
      909
    signs and symptoms of, 907–908
    systemic, 889
    thoracic trauma and, 889
    treatment of, 908–909, *909,* 1141
    volume of, 1141
  amniotic fluid, 1601
  carotid artery and, *652,* 1145–1146
  endocarditis etiology of, 492, 573
  fat, respiration and, 893, *894*
  femoral artery target of, 1151
  kidney failure and, 1264

Embolism *(Continued)*
  mesenteric ischemia and, 1485, *1486,*
    1488, *1489*
  pregnancy and, 1611–1612
  pulmonary, 849–859, 1612
    asthma vs., 813
    COPD with, 794–795
    diagnosis of, 851–854, *852–855*
    drug abuse patient and, 568t, 568–570,
      569, 570, 576
    filter therapy in, 856–857
    hemodynamic profile in, 1098t
    hypertension and, 843
    imaging of, *852,* 852–854, *853*
    incidence of, 850
    mortality rate in, 857, *857*
    pathogenesis of, 849–850
    physiologic effects of, 850–851, *851*
    pleural effusion and, 867
    septic, 568t, 568–570, *569, 570,* 576
    surgical approach in, 857, *857*
    treatment in, 854–859, *857,* 857t, *858*
    ventilation/perfusion ratio and, 850–
      851, *851*
  surgery patient and, 1572, 1572t
Emergency medical services, disasters and,
    37t, 38–40
  historical aspects of, 4
  personnel and training for, 9–11
  system organization in, 9–11
Emergency medical technicians, basic, 10
  cardiac care strategies for, 19–24
  certification of, 10
  deployment strategies for, 11
  on-line physician direction for, 11
  paramedics as, 10
  training level of, 9–10
  trauma care strategies for, 11–19
  triage strategies for, 12–14, *13,* 14t
Emesis, alkalosis and, 1227t, 1227–1228,
    1228
  chemotherapy-induced, 1413–1416,
    1414t
  electrolyte depletion due to, 1160, 1185
  marijuana therapy in, 1414
EMG. See *Electromyography (EMG).*
Emphysema, 793–794
  COPD role of, 793–794
  mediastinal, 889
  respiratory failure in, 793–794
  subcutaneous, 889
Empyema, intrathoracic, trauma patient
    and, 561
  pleural, 281–283, *282–285,* 864, 866
    split appearance and, *285*
  pneumonia causing, 488, 866
  subdural, drug abuse patient and, 567
  sinusitis and, 475t, 476
EMT. See *Emergency medical technicians.*
Encainide, arrhythmia treated with, 1055,
    1056t
  drug interactions of, 1056t
  pharmacokinetics of, 1689t
Encephalitis, 397–401
  arboviral, 692–695
  California, 397–398, 398t
  cercopithecine, 399–400
  differential diagnosis in, 399t
  eastern equine, 397–398, 398t, 693
  enteroviral, 696
  geographic range of, 398t
  herpes simplex, 399, 689t, 689–690, *690*
  herpesvirus 1 (B virus), 399–400
  influenza, 695
  Japanese B, 694
  La Crosse, 397, 398t, 695

Encephalitis *(Continued)*
  measles, 400, 696
  mumps, 696
  parainfectious, 696
  rabies, 400–401, 690–692, 691t, 692t
  reservoir species in, 397t, 397–400, 398t
  St. Louis, 398t, 398–399, 692–693
  varicella, 690
  vectors for, 397t, 397–400, 398t
  Venezuelan equine, 398, 398t, 694–695
  viral, 397–401, 687–697
    approach in, 687
    evaluation protocol for, *688*
    management of, 688–689
    neurologic examination in, 688
  western equine, 398, 398t, 693–694
Encephalopathy. See also *Coma.*
  anoxic ischemic, 632, 633–634
  chemotherapy-induced, 1416t, 1416–
    1417
  hepatic, 634, 1510–1511, 1519–1525
    ammonia in, 1522–1523, 1523t
    brain edema in, 1520, *1520,* 1521,
      1521
    cirrhosis and, 1521–1525, 1522t, 1524t
    clinical signs in, 1519t, 1521, 1522t,
      1524
    dietary protein and, 1522–1524
    differential diagnosis for, 1524, 1524t
    GABA in, 1523–1524
    grading of, 1515t, 1519, 1519t, *1523*
    intracranial hypertension in, *1520,*
      1520–1521, *1521*
    management of, 1521, 1524–1525
    neurotoxins in, 1522–1524, 1523t
    pathophysiology of, 1519t, 1519–1524,
      1522t, *1523,* 1523t
    portal shunting role in, 1522
  hyperpyretic-rigidity syndrome and, 699–
    700
  hypertension and, 1328, *1328,* 1330t
  ifosfamide and, 1416t, 1416–1417
  metabolic, 633–634
    asterixis in, 635, 637
    movement and, 635, 637
  multiple organ system failure and, 342t,
    348
  phosphate deficit causing, 1214–1215
  thiamine deficiency in, 633–634
  uremic, 634
  Wernicke's, 634
End-diastolic pressure, balloon catheter
    and, 1081–1084, *1082*
  left ventricular, 1081–1084, *1082*
  monitoring and, 1081–1084, *1082*
End-diastolic volume, balloon catheter and,
    1081–1084, *1082*
  imaging techniques and, 1111–1112
  left ventricular, 1081–1084, *1082*
  monitoring and, 1081–1084, *1082*
  right ventricular, 1092
  thermodilution measurement of, 1092
Endocarditis, 491–499, 572–575
  age and, 492
  anticoagulants and, 497
  antimicrobials in, 496–497, 575, 1572t
  bone and joint effects of, 573t, 574
  burn injury and, 525
  cancer patient and, 552
  candidal, 437
  clinical syndromes of, 494–497, 573t,
    573–575
  complications of, 494–497, 573t, 573–575
  congestive heart failure due to, 494
  diabetes mellitus and, 492

Endocarditis *(Continued)*
  differential diagnosis in, 493, 572, 574–575
  drug abuse patient with, 494, 572–575
  echocardiography in, 494
  emboli of, 492, 573
  epidemiology of, 492, 572
  gastrointestinal tract and, 573t, 573–574
  kidney affected by, 573t, 574
  laboratory tests in, 493–494, 574t
  management of, 495–499, 575
  meningitis and, 460, 574
  nosocomial, 495
  organisms causing, 491–493, 572–573, 575
  pathogenesis of, 492–493, 572–573
  physical examination in, 493
  pregnancy and, 492
  prevention of, 498–499
  prognosis in, 498
  prosthetic valves in, 494–495
  staphylococcal, 496t, 497, 575
  surgical approach in, 497–498
  symptoms of, 492
  valvular disease due to, 492, 494–495
Endocrine system, adrenal gland and, 1312–1317, 1562–1563
  diabetes mellitus and, 1245–1251, 1562
  parathyroid gland and, *1198*, 1198–1199
  preoperative care and, 1562–1563
  thyroid gland and, 1322–1324, 1563
Endometritis, pregnancy and, 1610
Endophthalmitis, *Bacillus* causing, 471
  bacterial, 471–472
  candidal, 437, 470–471
  treatment of, 472
Endorphins, hemodynamic effects of, 306–307
  sepsis role of, 306–307
  shock and, 981, 985
Endoscopy, cholangitis treatment and, *1496*, 1496t, 1496–1497, *1497*
  esophageal varices and, 1450t, 1450–1451, *1451*, *1452*, 1453
  gallstone pancreatitis and, 1491–1493, 1493t, 1494t
  upper GI hemorrhage and, 1440–1442
Endothelial cells, sepsis and, 335, 363
Endothelins, pulmonary vasculature and, 840
Endothelium-derived relaxing factor, 840
Endotoxins, antibodies to, 369
  cell metabolism affected by, 357–358, *358*
  complement activation due to, *307*, 307–308
  hemodynamic effects of, 303–304, *330*, *333*
  human infused with, *330*, *333*
  neutralization of, septic shock and, *366*, 368t, 368–370
  oxygen metabolism affected by, 353, *354*, *358–362*, 358–363
  sepsis caused by, 303–304, *304*, *330*, 333
  structure of, *304*
  TNF induction by, *313*, 313t, 313–314
Endotracheal intubation, 109–116, 967–976
  airway injury due to, 968–976, *969*, *970*, *972*, *974*
  altitude effect and, 44, 54
  anatomy and, 967–968, *968*, *969*, *971*, *972*, *974*
  anchoring of tube in, 113
  asthma patient and, 809
  auscultation in, 113
  clenched teeth and, 17, 18
  complications of, 115–116, 968–976

Endotracheal intubation *(Continued)*
  confirmation of, 113
  cuff and, 972–974, *972–975*
  difficult, 109–110
  duration of, 970
  EMT use of, 14–15, 17–18
  esophageal breach in, 113, 263
  extubation and, 113, *264*, 942
    patient-induced, 971–972
  glottic injury in, 969–972, *969–972*
  head position in, 111–113, *112*
    movement and, 971–972, *972*
  historical aspects of, 3, 967
  infection associated with, 975–976
  larynx injured by, 968–972, *969*, *972*
  litigation related to, 109
  Mallampati classification in, 109–110, 110t
  malplacement in, 261–264, *263*, *264*
  nasal, 18, 113–114
  oral, 18, 111–113
  prehospital care and, 14–15, 17–18
  radiography and, 261–264, *263*, *264*
  retrograde technique for, 114
  right mainstem bronchus and, *263*, 271, *274*
  sedation for, 110–111, 113
  shock and, 983–984
  sinusitis due to, 974–975
  subglottic injury in, 969–972, *969–972*
  supraglottic injury in, 968–969
  trachea injured by, 972–976, *973*, *974*
  tracheostomy vs., 975–976
  tube changer used in, 111–112, *112*
End-plate potential, motor neuron and, 673
End-systolic volume, *367*
  imaging techniques and, 1111–1112
Energy requirements, ATP and, 354, *355*
  brain, 632–633
  burn injury and, 1624, *1624*
  determination of, 1533, 1533t
  kidney failure and, 1274
  neuronal, 632–633
Entamoeba histolytica, dysentery caused by, 510t, 511
Enteral nutrition. See *Nutrition, enteral.*
Enteritis. See also *Gastroenteritis.*
  radiation causing, 1461
Enterococcal infections, 414–416, 415t
  antimicrobial therapy in, 415t, 415–416, 614t
  clinical presentation of, 414–415
  epidemiology of, 414
  pathogen susceptibility and, 614, 614t
  prevention of, 416
  resistant organisms in, 415t, 415–416, 614t
  species in, 414, 415t
  treatment of, 415t, 415–416, 614t
Enterocolitis, abdominal pain due to, 1481
  C. difficile in, 500–503
  differential diagnosis in, 510t, 510–511
  historical aspects of, 501
  inflammatory, 510t
  neutropenic, 1481
  Salmonella and, 511
Enterovirus, 396
  encephalitis due to, 696
  meningitis due to, 396
Envenomation, 1660–1681
  abdominal pain due to, 1483t, 1484
  ant and, 1681, 1681t
  arthropod and, 1677–1681, 1678t, *1678–1681*, 1681t
  bee and, 1681, 1681t
  coelenterate and, 1674t, 1674–1675

Envenomation *(Continued)*
  echinoderm and, 1675–1676
  fish and, 1676–1677, *1677*
  hemolytic anemia due to, 1383
  insect and, 1652, 1681, 1681t
  jellyfish and, 1674t, 1674–1675
  lizard and, 1672
  mollusk and, 1676, 1676t
  octopus and, 1676
  scorpion and, 1484, 1678t, 1680
  snake and, 1662–1672, 1663t, *1664*, 1668t
  spider and, 1677–1680, *1678*, 1678t, *1679*
  starfish and, 1675–1676
Enzymes, alcoholic hepatitis and, 1507–1508
  lactic acidosis and, 1234, 1235t
  liver, 1507–1508
  MI and, 992–993, 993t
  salivary glands and, 1501, 1501t
Eosinophils, *1340*
  hematopoiesis and, 1336
  pleural effusion and, 864–865
Epidemics, domiciliary, 580
  nosocomial, 383, 388t, 389, 580
Epiglottis, anatomy of, 967–968, *968*
Epiglottitis, 474–475
  granulocytopenia with, 533t, 540–541
  nosocomial, 475
Epinephrine, anaphylaxis treated with, *1657*, 1657–1658
  asthma treated with, 809, 809t
  cardiac arrest and, 21, 22t, 23, 124
  catabolism of, *1318*, 1318–1319
  CPR and, 124
  hemorrhage management and, 15
  hypokalemia caused by, 1183
  lactic acidosis caused by, 1238
  measurement of, 1319t, 1319–1320, 1320t, 1321t
  metabolism of, *1699*
  pharmacokinetics of, 1693t, 1696–1698, 1697t, *1699*
  receptors for, *1319*, 1319t, 1320–1322, 1321t, 1322t
  septic shock therapy and, 375–377, *376*, 376t
  synthesis of, *1318*, 1318
Epithelium, alveolar, 912
Epoxides, sepsis role of, 304–306, *305*
Epstein-Barr virus, transplant patient and, *582*, 584–585
Equation(s), Bohr, 734
  Fick, 733
  Harris-Benedict, 1534
  Henderson-Hasselbalch, 245, *246*, 1220, 1222
  Nernst, 241
  order of, pharmacokinetics and, 1688–1689
  Stewart-Hamilton, 1089–1090
Equipment, airway management and, 111t, 111–113, *112*
  altitude effect on, 45, 45t, 54–55
  chemical exposure protection and, 49
  computer management of, 94
  dialysis and, 1275–1276, *1276*, *1282*, 1288, *1288*, *1289*
Erythrocytapheresis, anticoagulation in, 1427
  complications of, 1428–1429
  instrumentation for, 1420–1421, *1421*, *1422*
  replacement fluids in, 1427
  sickle cell disease and, 1423–1424

Erythrocytapheresis *(Continued)*
  transfusion reaction due to, 1428
  vascular access for, 1425–1427
Erythrocytes. See *Red blood cells.*
Erythrocytosis. See also *Polycythemia.*
  classification of, 1363t
  kidney transplant and, 1298
  polycythemia vera vs., 1362, 1363t
Erythromycin, pharmacokinetics of, 1689t
Erythropoietin, 1336t
Escherichia, 487t, 489t
  hemorrhagic colitis due to, 487t, 488, 489t
  peritonitis due to, 487t, 488, 489t
  pneumonia due to, 487t, 488, 489t
  susceptibility of, 614t
Esmolol, arrhythmia treated with, 1055, 1056t
  drug interactions of, 1056t
  pharmacokinetics of, 1689t
Esophagitis, candidal, 439–440, 535t, 541
  granulocytopenia and, 533t, 541
Esophagus, 1432–1444
  aortic rupture affecting, *1135,* 1135, *1136*
  balloon tamponade of, 170–172, *171, 1449,* 1450, 1451t
  corrosive injury to, 1432t, 1432–1435
    complications of, 1433t
    compounds causing, 1432t
    diagnosis of, 1434
    management of, 1434–1435
    pathophysiology of, 1432t, 1432–1435, 1433t
    signs and symptoms in, 1433t, 1433–1434
  displacement of, *1135,* 1135
  endotracheal tube breach of, 113, 263
  foreign body in, 1435t, 1435–1438
  perforation of, causes of, 1436t
    diagnosis of, 1437–1438
    foreign body causing, 1436t, 1436–1438
    pathophysiology in, 1436t, 1436–1437
    signs in, 1437
  trauma injury to, 892
  varices of, aspirate appearance and, 1441t
    balloon tamponade of, 170–172, *171, 1449,* 1450, 1451t
    endoscopic sclerotherapy for, 1450t, 1450–1451, *1451,* 1453
    explosion of, 1448
    gastrointestinal hemorrhage and, 1439, 1439t, 1442–1443
    hemorrhage of, 170–172, 1448–1452
    ligation of, 1451, *1452*
    mortality rate and, 1441t, 1441–1442
    portal-systemic shunt and, 1452–1455, *1453, 1454*
    treatment of, 1449–1455, *1454*
    vasoconstrictor therapy for, 1448–1450, 1449t
Etappenlavage, peritonitis treated with, 519
Ethacrynic acid, diuresis and, 1165, 1165t
Ethambutol, dosage for, 425t, 426
  side effects of, 425t, 426
  tuberculosis treated with, 425t, 426
Ethanol, *1715.* See also *Alcoholism.*
  absorption of, 706
  ethylene glycol poisoning and, 1717
  intoxication due to, 706t, 706–707
  metabolism of, 707, *1715*
  poisoning due to, 706t, 706–710, 1718t
  therapeutic administration of, 1717

Ethanol *(Continued)*
  withdrawal syndromes and, 708t, 708–710
Ethical issues, 1724–1744
  access to care and, 5
  autonomy and, 1724–1726
  beneficence and, 1724–1726
  brain death and, 647
  COPD and, 803
  costs and, 5, 77, 1731
  do-not-resuscitate order and, 1736–1738
  ICU and, 1731–1744
  informed consent and, 1726–1730, 1735–1736
  legal precedents in, 1732–1735, 1740–1741
  proxy decision makers and, 1726–1729, 1731–1732
  quality of life and, 5, 1731–1732
  rubrics and, 1729–1730, 1735t, 1735–1736
  withdrawing treatment and, 1728, 1732–1744
  withholding treatment and, 1728, 1732–1744
Ethionamide, side effects of, 427t
  tuberculosis treated with, 427t
Ethylene glycol, *1716*
  acidosis caused by, 1223, 1718t
  ethanol administration and, 1717
  lactic acidosis caused by, 1239
  metabolism of, 1223, 1715–1716, *1716*
  poisoning due to, 712, 1223, 1715–1716, *1716,* 1718t
Etidronate, hypercalcemia therapy with, 1205, 1401t
Etoposide, bone marrow transplant and, 1348t
  side effects of, 1348t
Euthanasia, 1742–1743
Evoked potentials, auditory, 231–232, 624
  brain monitoring and, 231t, 231–232
  clinical value of, 624–635
  motor, 625
  sensory, 231–232, 624
  somatosensory, 231–232, 624–625
  visual, 231–232, 624
Evolution, oxygen transport and, 352–353
Excitability, neuronal, 632–633
Excretion, acid, 1221, *1221,* 1225–1226
  creatinine, 1530–1531
  gastrointestinal tract and, 1181, 1185
  kidney and, 1156–1159, 1181, 1185–1186
  magnesium, 1206, 1208
  malnutrition and, 1531
  potassium, 1181, 1185–1186
  sodium, 1156, *1157,* 1158–1159
  urea nitrogen, 1531
  water, 1170
Exercise, function tests using, 1555
  potassium and, 1180
Expert systems, 96–107, 103t
  acceptance of, 106–107
  administrative role of, 102–103
  closed-loop, 98
  components of, 96–97, 97t
  diagnosis using, 96–98, 97t, 98t
  education programs using, 101–102, *102*
  false alarms in, 100–101, 106–107
  knowledge bases of, 96–97, 97t
  neural network approach in, *103–105,* 103–106, 106t
  noise effects in, 100t, 100–101, *102*
  order management by, 101
  reasoning engines of, 96–98, 97t

Expert systems *(Continued)*
  rule-based, *97,* 97t, 97–98, *98,* 98t
  user interface with, 97t, 97–98, 106–107
  ventilator management using, 98–100, *98–100*
  waveform recognition by, 100t, 100–106, *101, 102, 105*
Expiration, 726–731. See also *Respiration.*
  cardiac tamponade and, *1035*
  catheterization tracing affected by, *1080,* 1080–1081, *1085,* 1085–1087
  elastic recoil pressure and, 727, *729*
  equal pressure point theory and, 727, *729*
  flow limitation and, 726–731
  flow-volume loop and, *726,* 726–731, *727*
  function testing and, 1554t, 1555
  isovolume pressure-flow curve and, 727, *728*
  mechanical ventilation and, 928–931, *929, 930*
  muscles of, 764–765
  preoperative function testing and, 1555
  quiet, 727, *727*
  tube law and, 730, *730*
  wave speed theory and, 729–730
Explosive devices, 32
Extracorporeal circulation, CO_2 removal and, 835
  historical aspects of, 4
  membrane oxygenation and, 833–835, *834*
Extravascular lung water. See *Edema, pulmonary.*
Extremities, emergent vascular disorders in, 1145–1148
  trauma injury to, 1580t, 1581t, 1589–1590
  prehospital management of, 18–19
Eye. See also *Vision.*
  air transport affecting, 43
  anatomy of, *467*
  burn injury affecting, 1625
  candidiasis affecting, 437
  cold exposure affecting, 1643
  electrical injury affecting, 1646t, 1647
  infection of, 466–474
  movements of, bobbing, 636
    brain damage and, 636–637
    coma evaluation and, 636–637
    cranial nerves and, 636–637
    dipping, 636
    Wernicke-Korsakoff syndrome and, 710–711
  raccoon, 634
  vesicant effects on, 52
  wrong way, 637
Eyelids, coma evaluation and, 636
  tone of, 636

F

Fab antibodies, digitalis neutralized with, 1707
Face, edema of, 116
  trauma to, air transport affecting, 43
Fallopian tube, abdominal pain and, 1477
  torsion of, 1477
False alarms, expert systems and, 100–101, 106–107
Families, decision making by, 1725–1726, 1732–1744
Famine, disaster nomenclature and, 26
Fanconi's syndrome, phosphate metabolism and, 1213, *1215,* 1216

Fasciitis, 449t
  anatomy and, *477*, 477–478
  cervical region, *477*, 477–478
  clostridial, 451
  infection and, *477*, 477–479
  neck and, *477*, 477–479
  necrotizing, 450–451
    organisms in, 576–577
    pain of, 576–577
    pregnancy and, 1611
    symptoms of, 450–451, 576–577
    trauma wound and, 563
    treatment of, 577
Fasciotomy, compartmental syndrome and, 1150–1151
  crush syndrome and, 34
Fasting, hypoglycemia and, 1252–1253, 1253t, *1255*
Fatigue, respiratory muscle and, 767, 787
Fats. See also *Lipids*.
  embolism and, respiration and, 893, *894*
  emulsion of, overload syndrome and, 901
Feces, black, 1441t
  C. difficile in, 501
  diarrhea and, 1469–1470
  electrolytes in, 1469–1470
  flora replacement using, 509
  pseudomembranous colitis and, 502
  red, 1441t
  sodium loss in, 1160
  upper gastrointestinal bleeding and, 1441t
  volume of, 1160
Feeding tubes. See also *Nasogastric intubation*.
  enteral nutrition access using, *1540*, 1540–1542, *1541*
  fluoroscopy and, 269
  guidable, 269
  lung injury and, 269
  malplacement of, 264–269, *267–269*
  nasoenteric, *1540*, 1540–1542, *1541*
  radiography and, 264–269, *267–269*
  types of, 269
Femoral artery, false aneurysm of, *1150*
  puncture of, 235–236
Femoral vein, central venous catheter in, 178–179, *179*
  dialysis access and, 1281t, *1289*, 1290
Femur, fracture of, compartmental syndrome and, 1149–1151
  ischemia due to, 1149–1151
Fentanyl, pharmacokinetics of, 1689t
Fetus, retained, 1601
Fever. See also *Hyperthermia*; *Temperature*.
  air transport effects and, 43
  bronchoscopy causing, 196
  colitis and, 503
  heat production in, *1627*, 1627–1628
  hemorrhagic, 403–405
  hyperpyretic-rigidity syndrome and, 698–704
  ischemic stroke and, 653
  meningitis causing, 459
  seizure causing, 670
  sepsis and, 297
  transplant patient with, 582–583
Fiberoptics, intra-arterial fluorescent optode and, *248*
Fibrillation, atrial, 1061–1062, 1067, *1067*
  ventricular, 1072–1073
Fibrinogen, cryoprecipitate containing, 1390
  osmotic pressure due to, 130
Fibrinolytic agents, stroke treated with, 653–654

Fibronectin, burn injury and, 522, 522t
  cryoprecipitate and, 1390
Fibrosis, respiratory distress syndrome and, 822–823, *823*, *824*, 835–836
Fibula, fracture of, compartmental syndrome and, 1150
Fick equation, 733
Fick oxygen method, cardiac output and, 1093, 1094
Filovirus, 392t
Filters, electronic noise and, 101–102, *102*
  Greenfield, 856
  pulmonary embolism and, 856
Filtration coefficient, 130
Fingernails, neglect of, CNS compromise and, 635
Fingers, arterial insufficiency and, 236
  nodes on, endocarditis and, 493
Fire ants, *1681*
  anaphylaxis caused by, 1652
  venom of, 1681, 1681t
First-pass effect, 1687, 1687t
First-responders, disaster scene and, 38–39
  training level of, 9–11
Fish, envenomation by, 1676–1677, *1677*, 1677t
  poisoning due to, 1673–1674, 1676
Fistula, aortic-duodenal, 1145, *1145*
  aortic-enteric, 1145, *1145*
    upper GI hemorrhage and, 1444
  arteriovenous, hemodialysis and, 1149, *1150*
    penetrating injury and, 1149, *1150*
  bronchopleural, 870, *870*
  tracheal-innominate arterial, 1146–1147
Flail chest injury, *771*
  pendelluft and, 888
  respiration and, 888–889
  respiratory failure due to, 769, *771*
Flashover, lightning injury and, 1648, 1648t
Flavivirus, 392t, 397
Flecainide, arrhythmia treated with, 1055, 1056t
  drug interactions of, 1056t
Fleisch pneumotachygraph, *210*, *211*
Floods, 31–32, 33t
Flora, gastrointestinal, replacement of, 509
Fluid resuscitation, algorithm for, *35*, 47–48
  blood-brain barrier and, 142
  brain trauma and, *142*, 142–143
  burn injury and, 1618–1620, 1619t
  challenge technique in, 138, 138t
  colloids used in, 132–134, *137*, 137t
  complications of, 143–146
  crush syndrome and, 34–35, *35*
  crystalloids used in, 131t, 131–132
  diabetic ketoacidosis and, 1249t, 1249–1250
  disaster victim and, *35*, 35–36, 47–48
  gelatin used in, 136
  preoperative care and, 1566–1567
  pulmonary edema and, 143–145, *143–145*, *374*
  respiratory distress syndrome and, 141–142
  sepsis and, 139–140, *325*, 325, *326*, 336, *374*, 374–375
  shock and, anaphylactic, 140–141
    cardiogenic, 140
    circulatory, 136–139
    hemorrhagic, *138*, 138–139
    hypovolemic, 984t, 984–985
    septic, 139–140, *140*, *325*, 325, *326*, 336, *374*, 374–375
  starches used in, 134–136

Fluid-filled system, damping in, 253
  ringing in, 253
Fluids, altitude effects and, 54–55
  blunt head injury and, 16, 18
  body compartments and, 129–130, *130*
  distribution of, 129–131, *130*
  extracellular, 129–131, *130*, *1155*, 1155–1159
    alkalosis and, 1227t, 1227–1228, *1228*
    depletion of, 1159t, 1159–1161
    kidney failure and, 1270–1271
    overload of, 1161–1164, 1162t
    sodium and, 1155–1164
  hemorrhage management and, 15
  interstitial, 129–131, *130*, *914*, 914–917, *917*, *1155*, 1155–1159
  intracellular, 129–131, *130*
    sodium and, 1156
  meningitis and, 463
  prehospital use of, 16, 18
  transcapillary exchange and, 130
Fluorescence, intra-arterial optode and, 247–248, *248*
Fluorocarbon emulsions, animal studies with, 152
  artificial blood role of, *151*, 151–153, *152*, 152t, 153t
  clinical trials with, 152t, 152–153, 153t
  oxygen binding by, *151*, 151–153, *152*, 153t
Fluorocrit, 152, 152t
Fluoroscopy, feeding tube and, 269
Fluorouracil, gastrointestinal effects of, 1414t, 1414–1415
  heart affected by, 1412t, 1412–1413
Food. See also *Diet*; *Nutrition*.
  anaphylaxis caused by, 1652
  choking on, 1435, 1435t
  esophageal impaction of, 1435, 1435t
  hepatitis A and, 402
  hypertension induced by, 1329
  marine organisms as, 1672–1674, 1676
  poisoning due to, fish toxicity and, 1672–1674, 1676
    mushroom toxicity and, 1483t, 1484
  tyramine content of, 1329
Foot, infection of, diabetes and, 450
Forced expiratory volume, 1554t, 1555
Forced vital capacity, 1554t, 1555
Forceps, Magill, *112*
  obstetric trauma due to, 1599
Foreign bodies, 1435–1438
  bronchoscopic removal of, 196–197, *197*
  catheter fragment and, 1141
  common, 1435t
  esophageal perforation due to, 1436t, 1436–1438
  food bolus and, 1435, 1435t
  lung containing, *273*
  radiography examination and, 271, *272*, *273*
  swallowed, 1435t, 1435–1438
Formaldehyde, methanol metabolized to, 1714, *1715*
  smoke inhalation and, 884
Formates, methanol ingestion and, 1223, 1714–1715, *1715*
  optic nerve toxicity of, 1223, 1714
Foscarnet, 406
  cytomegalovirus and, 394
Fothergill's sign, 1484
Fournier's gangrene, 451
Foxes, rabies and, 691t
Fractures, compartmental syndrome and, 1149–1151
  extremities and, 1580t, 1581t, 1589–1590

Fractures (Continued)
femoral, 1149–1151
ischemia due to, 1149–1151
pelvic, 1580t, 1589, 1589–1590
rib, 1584t, 1585, 1586
wound infection and, 563
Free radicals, oxygen and, 950–952, 951t, 952t, 953
tissue damage due to, 950–952, 951t, 952t, 953
Frontal lobes, hemorrhage of, 656t, 657
Frostbite, 1641–1643
classification of, 1641t, 1642
pathophysiology of, 1641–1642
predisposing factors for, 1642, 1642t
treatment of, 1643
Fructose, lactic acidosis caused by, 1237, 1238
metabolism of, 1238
Fungal infections, 444–447
aspergillosis and, 446–447
blastomycosis and, 444
bone marrow transplant and, 1352–1353
candidal. See Candidiasis.
coccidioidomycosis and, 444
cryptococcosis and, 444–445
granulocytopenia and, 533t, 534t, 535t, 538t
hepatosplenic abscess due to, 1481
histoplasmosis and, 444
meningitis due to, 459–460
mucormycosis and, 445–446
pancytopenia and, 1352–1353
rhino-orbitocerebral, 445, 473–474
Furosemide, diuresis using, 1165, 1165t
pharmacokinetics of, 1690t
Fuzzy reasoning, 97

G

Gallbladder, abdominal pain related to, 1477–1478
Gallop, atrial contraction and, 1017, 1017–1018
heart failure and, 1017, 1017–1018, 1020
S₃, 1017, 1017–1018, 1020
S₄, 1017, 1017–1018, 1020
Gallstones, 1490–1494
abdominal pain and, 1491
cholangiopancreatography and, 1491–1493, 1493, 1493t, 1494t
clinical features of, 1491
diagnosis of, 1491–1492
incidence of, 1490
natural history of, 1492
pancreatitis due to, 1490–1494
pathogenesis of, 1490–1491
sphincterotomy and, 1492–1493, 1493t, 1494t
treatment of, 1492–1493, 1493t, 1494t
Gamma-aminobutyric acid (GABA), hepatic encephalopathy role of, 1523–1524
Gammopathy, plasmapheresis in, 1425, 1426t
Ganciclovir, 405
cytomegalovirus and, 394
side effects of, 405, 406t
Gangrene, circulatory insufficiency causing, 452
cold exposure causing, 1641t, 1641–1643, 1643
Fournier's, 451
lower extremity, 1152
venous, 1152
Garments, antishock, 15, 16

Gas exchange, bubble-related disorders and, 902–909
clinical assessment of, 743–747
decompression sickness and, 905–906
diffusion role in, 739, 739–740
physiology of, 732–747
Gas gangrene, 451–452
Gases. See also Blood gases; Carbon dioxide; Oxygen.
altitude effects on, 44, 54–55
cellulitis and, 450
clostridial, 450
hypodense, 195
mediastinal, 889, 904
necrotizing fasciitis and, 451, 577
pleural. See Pneumothorax.
toxic, 883–885
Gastric fluid, potassium loss and, 1185
Gastritis, acid-suppressive therapy in, 1442–1443
hemorrhage due to, 1442–1443
stress-related mucosal disease and, 1442–1443
Gastroenteritis, 500–512
AIDS and, 511–512
C. difficile and, 500–509
cancer patient and, 551
E. coli and, 511
E. histolytica and, 511
granulocytopenia and, 533t, 540–542
Salmonella and, 511
Shigella and, 510–511
toxic shock syndrome and, 509–510
V. cholerae and, 510
Gastroesophageal sphincter, ventilation breach of, 110
Gastrointestinal tract, 1432–1525. See also specific structures and disorders.
barrier failure and, 1535, 1535–1536
bone marrow transplant and, 1349t, 1350t, 1351–1352, 1355, 1356
burn injury effect in, 1622
calcium metabolism and, 1197, 1198, 1204
chemotherapy effects in, 1413–1416, 1414t
electrical injury and, 1646t, 1647
endocarditis affecting, 573t, 573–574
fluid balance in, 1464–1465, 1465
hemorrhage in, 1439–1463
hypothermia effect on, 1636, 1636
kidney transplant affecting, 1299
lactic acidosis and, 1235–1236
multiple organ system failure and, 342t, 348
phosphate level and, 1212–1213, 1217
potassium excretion in, 1181, 1185
preoperative care and, 1559–1560
sodium loss from, 1160–1161, 1161t
Gatekeeping, medical director role in, 62t, 62–63
Gating, cardiographic scintigraphy and, 1108, 1109
ECG and, 1108, 1109
Gaze, coma evaluation and, 636–637
dysconjugate vertical, 636, 637
palsies of, 636
ping-pong, 637
Gelatin, anaphylaxis caused by, 136
fluid resuscitation using, 136
pharmacokinetics of, 136
Genes, env, 589
gag, 589
lentiviral, 589–590
nef, 589–590
pol, 589

Genes (Continued)
retroviral, 589
rev, 589–590
tat, 589–590
Genetic factors. See also Race.
drug clearance and, 1700t, 1700–1701
myopathy and, 686
pharmacokinetics and, 1700t, 1700–1701
polymorphism and, 1700t, 1700–1701
Gentamicin, enterococcal infections and, 415
kidney failure due to, 1261t, 1261–1262
meningitis therapy and, 461t, 462
pharmacokinetics of, 1692t, 1693t
resistance to, 415
susceptibility testing and, 612–613
Geographic area, transplantation infection and, 579–580
Ginger jake, 681
Glasgow Coma Scale, 79–80, 80t
trauma assessment and, 1575t, 1575–1576
Glasgow Multifactorial Prognostic Scoring System, 1502, 1502t
Glass, Corning 015 pH, 240
electrode sensitivity and, 240–242
ion-selective, 242
Globulins. See also Immunoglobulin(s).
antilymphocyte, kidney transplant and, 1294
osmotic pressure due to, 130
Glomerular filtration rate, calculation of, 1269–1270
creatinine level and, 1269–1270, 1304–1309, 1309t
drug dose adjustments and, 1304t–1309t, 1304–1309
phosphate reabsorption and, 1212
sodium excretion and, 1156, 1158–1159
Glomerulonephritis, kidney failure and, 1264
rapidly progressive, 1264
Glottis, intubation injury to, 969–972, 969–972
Gloves, nosocomial infections and, 386–387, 387t
Glucocorticoids, 1310–1317
deficiency of, 1313t, 1313–1314, 1314t
excess of, 1315t, 1315–1316
hypercalcemia therapy with, 1206
kidney transplant and, 1293, 1293t
metabolism of, 1310
physiologic actions of, 1311
regulatory factors for, 1310, 1311
side effects of, 1293, 1293t
Glucose, 1232, 1233
cerebrum and, 632
deficit in, 1251–1255. See also Hypoglycemia.
lactic acidosis and, 1231–1233, 1232, 1233
metabolism of, 356, 1231–1233, 1232, 1233
aerobic, 1231, 1232
anaerobic, 1231, 1233
hypothermia and, 1636–1637
pleural effusion and, 865
regulatory mechanisms for, 1251–1252
sepsis effects and, 356
Glucose-6-phosphate dehydrogenase, hemolytic anemia and, 1385t, 1385–1386
hereditary deficiency of, 1385t, 1385–1386
Mediterranean variant of, 1385
Glue sniffing, 1720–1721

Glutathione, oxygen radical scavenging and, 951, 952t

Glycerol phosphate, lactic acidosis and, 1235, *1235*

Glycocalyx, bacterial adherence due to, urinary tract and, 527

Glycols. See *Ethylene glycol*; *Propylene glycol*.

Glycolysis, *356*
  lactic acidosis and, 1231–1233, *1232*, *1233*
  mitochondria and, *356*, 356–357

Glycopeptide antimicrobials, 616t

Glycoproteins, drug binding by, 1691–1692, 1692t
  viral envelope and, 589–590

Goldman's Multifactorial Cardiac Risk Index, 79, 80t, 1556, 1556t

Goodpasture's syndrome, pulmonary hemorrhage in, 879t, 879–881, *881*

Gout, kidney failure dose adjustment and, 1308t
  kidney transplant and, 1300

Gowns, nosocomial infections and, 386–387, 387t

Grafts. See also *Transplantation*.
  vascular, aortic-enteric fistula and, 1145, *1145*
    coronary bypass, 1003–1004, 1004t
    infection of, 1140, 1144
    thrombosis and, 1151–1152, *1152*

Graft-versus-host disease, abdominal pain due to, 1481
  acute, 1349
  bone marrow transplant and, 1349t, 1349–1350, 1350t
  chronic, 1349–1350
  clinical manifestations of, 1349t, 1350t
  hyperacute, 1349
  transfusion causing, 1392

Gram-negative organisms, burn injury and, 525t
  granulocytopenia and, 533t, 534t
  peritonitis and, 516
  pneumonia due to, 383t, 486t, 487, 487t, 489t
  septicemia due to, 383t
  urinary tract infections and, 383t
  wound infection and, 383t

Gram-positive organisms, 408–420
  antimicrobial therapy for, 410–411, 411t
  burn injury and, 525t
  granulocytopenia and, 533t, 534t
  pneumonia due to, 383t
  septicemia and, 383t
  urinary tract infection and, 383t
  wound infection and, 383t

Granulocyte colony-stimulating factor, 1336t

Granulocyte-monocyte colony-stimulating factor, 1336t

Granulocytes, *1340*, 1359
  hematopoiesis and, 1336
  transfusion of, 543

Granulocytopenia, 532–543
  anorectal infections with, 542
  antimicrobial therapy in, 533–536, 538t
    combination, 533–536, 535t
    duration of, 536
    modification of, 534–536, 535t
    prophylactic, 542–543
  bone marrow failure and, 1341–1343
  cancer patient and, 532–543, 546, 546t
  chemotherapy and, 532
  definition of, 532
  epiglottitis with, 533t, 540–541
  esophagitis with, 533t, 541

Granulocytopenia (*Continued*)
  fever in, 536
  gastrointestinal tract and, 533t, 540–542
  infection in, 532–543
    organisms of, 534t, 535t, 538t
    prevention of, 542–543
    sites of, 532, 533t, 536
    treatment of, 533–536, 535t
  meningitis with, 542
  periodontal disease with, 533t, 541
  pulmonary infiltrates in, 536–540
    diagnosis of, 537t
    diffuse, 537t, 538t, 539–540
    early, 537, 537t, 538t
    late, 537t, 538t, 539
    localized, 537, 537t, 538t
    refractory, 537t, 537–539, 538t
  sinusitis and, 533t, 540
  stomatitis with, 533t, 541
  strongyloidiasis with, 542
  typhlitis with, 533t, 541–542

Granulocytosis, 1359

Granulomatosis, pulmonary hemorrhage due to, 879t, 879–881

Gravity, aspiration role of, *873*
  pulmonary perfusion and, 737–738, *738*

Gray matter, 639, 639t
  physiology of, 639, 639t

Greenfield filter, pulmonary embolism and, 856

Grey Turner's sign, 1159, 1501

Growth factors, hematopoiesis and, 1335–1337, 1336t
  sepsis mediation and, 312t
  transforming, 312t

Guanosine monophosphate (GMP), immune response and, 1655, 1655t

Guidelines. See also *Standards*.
  standards vs., 67, 72

Guillain-Barré syndrome, 679–680
  diagnosis of, 679
  management of, 679–680
  Miller Fisher syndrome and, 679
  plasmapheresis in, 1425, 1426t
  respiratory failure due to, 766

Gunshot trauma, intra-abdominal abscess and, 561
  pregnancy and, 1600
  prehospital management of, 15
  spinal injury following, 15

H

H wave, atrium and, *1079*, 1079–1080, *1080*

Haemophilus, epiglottitis and, 474–475
  meningitis and, 454–457, 461t
  pneumonia caused by, 486t, 487t, 488, 489t

Haff disease, 686

Hageman's factor, side effects of, 133

Halberstaedter-Prowazek bodies, 468

Hallucinations, alcoholism and, 708
  anticholinergic intoxication and, 53

Halothane, oxygen measurement and, 239

Hamman's sign, 869, 904

Hampton hump, 852

Hand, arterial insufficiency and, 236
  nosocomial infections and, 386–387, 387t, 409, 411–412
  radial arterial puncture and, 236
  staphylococcal infections and, 409, 411–412
  washing of, 386–387, 387t, 409, 411–412

Hantaan virus, hemorrhagic fever and, 403–404

Haptoglobin, hemolytic anemia and, 1370t, 1371

Harris-Benedict equation, energy requirements and, 1534

Hazardous materials spills, 32, 33t

Head trauma, 714–717
  air transport affecting, 44–45
  assessment scale for, 1576t–1577t
  brain herniation and, 715
  cerebral blood flow and, 224–227, *226*, 227t, 229t, *1583*, 1583–1584
  evaluation in, 715–716
  fluids in, 18
  imaging studies in, 715–716
  intracranial pressure and, 227–230, 229t, 714–715, *715*, *1582*, 1582t, 1582–1584
  management of, 717, 1583
  monitoring and, 716, *1582*, 1582t, 1582–1583
  prehospital care in, 17–19
  respiration and, 893
  serious blunt, 17–19
  ventilation and, 17, 1583

Headache, meningitis causing, 459–460
  mycotic aneurysm causing, 493
  severe and unremitting, 493
  stroke and, 656, 660
  subarachnoid hemorrhage and, 660

Health care workers, AIDS precautions and, 564
  emergency medical services and, 9–11
  hand washing by, 386–387, 387t, 409, 411–412
  HIV infection and, 591t, 596–598, 598t
  nosocomial infections and, 386–387, 387t, 409, 411–412

Hearing, evoked potentials and, 231–232, 624

Heart, action potential of, *1050*, 1050–1051
  anatomy of, 790, *790*, *791*
  arrhythmias of. See *Arrhythmias*.
  assist devices for. See *Intra-aortic balloon pump*; *Pump devices, cardiac-assist*.
  calcium level and, 120, 124, 1045–1046, *1046*, 1199–1200
  catheterization of. See *Catheterization, cardiac*.
  conduction system of, *1051*
    disorders of, 1049–1077, *1051*
    MI and, 1007, 1007t
  congenital disease of, 1028t
    pulmonary hypertension and, 840
    right ventricular dysfunction and, 1028, 1028t
  early resuscitation and, 3
  electrolyte effects in, 1045–1047
  failure of, 841, 1015–1024
    biology of, 19–20, *20*
    brain injury following, 639–647
    brain-protective management of, 641t, 641–643
    catecholamines in, 1324–1325
    causes of, 791t, 1016t
    chemotherapy causing, 1411–1413, 1412t
    chronic, 1022–1024, *1023*, 1023t
    clinical evaluation of, 1020, 1020t
    cocaine causing, 1047
    compensatory mechanisms in, *1016*, 1016–1018, *1017*
    congestive, 841
    cor pulmonale and, 838–839, 846–847, 1026–1028

Heart *(Continued)*
　criteria for, 342t
　decompensated, *1016*, 1016–1018
　definition of, 342t
　dialysis and, 1271
　digitalis in, *1023*, 1023t, 1023–1024
　drugs used in, 21–24, 22t, 120, 124–125, 1023–1024
　ECG in, *20*, 23–24, *121*
　electrical injury causing, 1646t, 1646–1647
　electrolytes in, 22t, 24, 120, 124
　end-tidal CO_2 and, 123–124, *124*, *214*
　endocarditis and, 494
　gallop and, *1017*, 1017–1018
　hemodynamic profiles in, 1098t
　hypothermia causing, 1639, 1639t
　incidence of, 118
　kidney transplant and, 1296–1297, 1297t
　left ventricle in, 1016–1018, *1017*
　metabolic disturbances in, 1044–1045
　MI and, 1007–1008, 1008t
　myocardial response to, 1016–1018, *1017*
　perioperative risk and, 1557
　phonocardiogram in, *1017*
　pleural effusion in, 791–792
　prehospital care in, *19*, 19–24, *20*, 22t
　preoperative care and, 1556t, 1556–1559, 1559t
　pulmonary edema in, 1019–1020, 1022, 1161–1162, 1162t
　renin-angiotensin-aldosterone axis in, 1018
　respiratory failure and, 786–792, 791t
　right-sided, 838–839, 846–847, 1025–1030
　　causes of, 1026–1030, 1027t, 1028t, 1030t
　septic shock and, 323–332
　severity classification in, 77t, 77–80, 78t, 80t
　sodium balance and, 1161–1162, 1162t
　stroke volume and, 1018–1019, *1019*, *1022*, *1023*
　surgical procedure risk of, 79t, 79–80, 80t
　sympathetic nervous system in, 1018
　systemic response to, 1018–1019, *1019*
　tamponade and, 891–892
　time-to-therapy and, 120t
　treatment of, 1020–1024, *1021*, *1023*, 1023t
　　out-of-hospital, 21–24, 22t, 120, 120t, 124–125
　vascular resistance increase in, 1018–1019
　hypertrophy of, *1016*, 1016–1018
　hypothermia effects in, *1635*, 1635–1636, 1639, 1639t
　iatrogenic injury to, 1142
　imaging techniques for, 1103–1120
　inflammatory disease of. See *Endocarditis*; *Pericarditis*.
　ischemic disease of. See *Ischemic heart disease*; *Myocardial infarction (MI)*.
　magnesium level and, 1207, 1208
　mechanical ventilation affecting, 944t, 944–948
　murmurs, air embolism and, 907
　　endocarditis and, 493
　　portal hypertension and, 1446
　penetrating trauma to, 14–15
　potassium level affecting, *1187*, 1187t, 1187–1188

Heart *(Continued)*
　pump failure and, 1007–1008, 1008t
　rupture of, 891
　tamponade of, 891–892
　　diagnosis of, 1395t, 1395–1396
　　echocardiography in, 1034, *1034*, *1035*
　　etiology of, 1032t, 1033, 1395
　　neoplasia causing, 1395t, 1395–1396, 1396t
　　pericardial effusion and, *1033–1035*, 1033–1036, 1395–1396
　　prehospital management of, 14
　　signs and symptoms in, 1033–1034, 1395, 1395t
　　trauma injury and, 891–892
　　treatment of, *1034*, 1034–1036, *1035*, 1396, 1396t
　transplantation of, 1125–1132
　　contraindications for, 1125
　　cytomegalovirus and, 394
　　donor selection and management in, 1126–1127
　　harvesting technique for, 1127–1128, *1128*, *1129*
　　immunosuppression and, 1131–1132
　　implantation technique for, 1128–1131, *1129*, *1130*
　　indications for, 1125–1126
　　postoperative management in, 1131–1132
　　prognosis in, 1132
　　rejection and, 1131–1132
　　trauma injury to, 891–892, *1585*, 1587–1588
　valvular disease of, 1113–1117, 1114t, 1115t, *1115–1117*
　　endocarditis and, 492, 494
　vascular pedicle of, 790, *790*, *791*
Heart-lung machine, historical aspects of, 4
Heat injury. See *Burn injury*; *Heatstroke*; *Hyperthermia*.
Heat regulation, 1626, 1634, *1634*
　hyperthermia and, 1626–1629, *1627*, *1628*
　hypothermia and, 1633–1635, *1634*
　loss mechanisms in, 1626, 1633–1634
　　conduction and, 1633
　　evaporation and, 1626, 1633
　　radiation and, 1626, 1633
Heatstroke, clinical features of, 1629
　cooling methods for, 1630, 1630t
　diagnosis of, 1629–1630, 1630t
　hyperpyretic-rigidity syndrome vs., 700
　hyperthermia and, 1628t, 1629–1631
　management of, 1630t, 1630–1631
　monitoring in, 1630t
　nonexertional, 1629
　pathophysiology of, 1629–1630
Heimlich valve, thoracostomy tube with, *166*
Heinz's bodies, hemolytic anemia and, 1372, 1385
Helicopters, disadvantages of, 43, 54
　patient transport in, 43, 54
Heliox, 962
Helium, hypodense gas mixture and, 195
　oxygen mixed with, 962
HELLP syndrome, pregnancy and, 1607, 1607t
Helminths, granulocytopenia and, 542
　transplant patient and, 580
Hematocrit, burn injury and, 1616, *1617*
　polycythemia and, 1365
Hematologic disorders, 1335–1386. See also specific disorders and cell types.
　bone marrow failure causing, 1339–1345

Hematologic disorders *(Continued)*
　hypothermia causing, 1637
　pregnancy and, 1607, 1607t, 1608t
　preoperative care and, 1563–1566
　proliferative, 1359–1368
Hematoma, brain stem, 657
　central venous catheter causing, 261, *261*, *262*
　intracerebral, 656t, 656–657
　mediastinal, *262*, 1135, *1137*
　pleural, *262*
Hematopoiesis, 1335–1341, *1340*
　cyclicity of, 1359
　disorders of, 1337–1386
　　bone marrow failure and, 1339–1345
　　malignant, 1363–1368, 1364t, 1365t
　　myeloid dysplasia in, 1363–1368, 1364t, 1365t
　　proliferative, 1359–1368
　growth factors in, 1335–1337, 1336t, 1359
　rate of, 1339
　regulatory factors for, 1359
Hemiplegia, differential diagnosis in, 628
Hemodialysis. See *Dialysis, hemodialysis*.
Hemodilution therapy, stroke treated with, 654
Hemofiltration, definition of, 1275
Hemoglobin, absorbance spectra of, *204*, 244
　artificial blood role of, 153–159, *154–157*
　carbon monoxide bound to, 883, 885–886
　dissociation curve for, 745, *1636*
　emulsion preparation of, 154, *154*, 154t
　erythrocytapheresis and, 1423–1424
　fetal, 244
　hypothermia effects and, 1636, *1636*
　immunosuppression caused by, 158–159
　kidney failure due to, 1261t, 1263
　nephrotoxicity of, 158
　oximetry role of, 203–205, *204*, *205*, 244, *244*
　oxygen saturation of, 244–245
　P_{50} value for, 245
　polymerized, *155–157*, 155–159, 157t
　pyridoxylated, 154–159, *155–157*, 157t
　S, 1423–1424
　saturation of, 244–245
　sickle cell disease and, 1423–1424
　species of, 203, *204*, 244
　stored blood and, 1389
　stroma-free, 154, *154*, 154t
Hemoglobinuria, cold exposure and, 1378
　nocturnal, 1383
　paroxysmal, 1378, 1383
Hemolysis, 1370. See also *Anemia, hemolytic*.
　DIC and, 1601
　intravascular vs. extravascular, 1372–1373
　mechanisms of, 1370
　uremia with, 1372t, 1374–1375
　　chemotherapy and, 1375
　　clinical signs in, 1374t, 1374–1375
　　plasmapheresis in, 1425, 1426t
　　thrombocytopenic purpura vs., 1374t, 1374–1375
Hemoperfusion, activated charcoal in, 1291–1292, 1705
　complications of, 1292, 1292t
　poisoning treatment and, 1291–1292, 1292t, 1705
Hemophilia, 1337
　preoperative care and, 1565
Hemoptysis, assessment in, 877–878, 880
　bronchoscopic control of, 196

Hemoptysis *(Continued)*
 causes of, 877t, 879t
 iatrogenic, 877t, 879
 lung carcinoma and, 876–877, 877t
 management of, 878–879, 881
 massive, 876–879, 877t, 1396–1397
 mycotic aneurysm and, 571
 neoplasia causing, 1396–1397
 pulmonary artery rupture and, 1141–
  1142
 pulmonary embolism and, 851
 pulmonary hypertension and, 845
 tuberculosis and, 423, 876, 877t
Hemopump, cardiac assistance using,
  1122–1123, *1123*
Hemorrhage. See also *Coagulation.*
 abdominal vascular surgery and, 1144
 abdominal wall, 1484
 arterial puncture and, 237
 bronchoscopy and, 193–194, 196, 200
 esophageal varices and, 170–172, 1448–
  1452
 fluids contraindicated in, 15
 gastrointestinal tract, 1439–1463
  endocarditis causing, 573
  lower, 1457–1463
   arteriovenous malformation and,
    1460, *1460*, 1462–1463, *1463*
   carcinoma and, 1461
   causes of, 1458t
   colitis and, 1460–1461, 1471
   Crohn's disease and, 1460–1461,
    1471
   diagnosis in, 1458, *1459*, 1461–1462
   diverticular disease and, 1459–1460,
    1460
   hemorrhoids and, 1461
   history in, 1458
   imaging of, 1461–1462
   inflammatory bowel disease and,
    1471
   laboratory tests in, 1458, *1459*,
    1461–1462
   management of, 1458–1459, *1459*,
    1462–1463
   physical examination in, 1458
   rectal ulcer and, 1461, *1461*
  upper, 1439–1444, 1448–1455
   aspirate appearance in, 1441t
   endoscopy in, 1440–1442
   fluid resuscitation in, 1440
   localization of, 1440–1442
   peptic ulcer and, 1439t, 1439–1444
   prognosis in, 1441t
 hemorrhoids and, 1461
 heparin and, 855–856
 hypovolemia and, 1159
 intracranial, 17. See also *Cerebrovascular
  disease, hemorrhagic.*
 kidney failure and, 1271
 platelet level related to, 1343, 1343t
 pregnancy-related, 1593–1612
 prehospital management and, 15, 17
 pulmonary, 876–882
  diffuse alveolar, 879–882
   assessment in, 880, *880*, *881*
   causes of, 879t, 879–880, *880*
   classification of, 879t, 879–880, *880*
   management of, 881
  massive, 876–879, 1396–1397
   assessment in, 877–878
   causes of, 877t
   diagnostic tests in, 877–878
   iatrogenic, 877t, 879
   management of, 878–879

Hemorrhage *(Continued)*
 shock due to, 15, *138*, 138–139, 1098t,
  1159
 snakebite and, 1663–1664, *1664*, *1671*
 stress-related mucosal disease causing,
  1442–1443
 subarachnoid, 659t, 659–661
 thoracic, catheter-related, 1140–1142
  emergent, 1140–1142
 thrombolytic agents and, 856, 857t
 ulcer and, 1439t, 1439–1444, 1461, *1461*
Hemorrhagic fever, Congo-Crimean, 404
 dengue, 403
 Korean, 403
 Lassa, 404–405
 Rift Valley, 404
 sandfly, 404
 viral, 403–405
 yellow fever and, 405
Hemorrhoids, 1461
Hemosiderinuria, 1372
Hemosiderosis, transfusion causing, 1392
Hemostasis. See *Coagulation.*
Hemothorax, atelectasis and, 277, *277*
 pleural effusion of, 867
 thoracic trauma and, 889–890
Henderson-Hasselbalch equation, 245, *246*,
  1220, 1222
Henle loop, diuretics and, 1165, 1165t
 sodium excretion by, 1156
Hepadnavirus, 392t
Heparin, arterial blood sample and, 237,
  238, *239*
 dialysis anticoagulation and, 1281–1282,
  1290, 1290t
 hemorrhage and, 855–856
 MI and, 1001–1002, *1002*
 pharmacokinetics of, 1689t
 pulmonary embolism and, 855–856
 septic pulmonary embolism and, 570
 stroke treated with, 654–655
 thrombocytopenia due to, 855–856
Hepatitis, 401–403
 A, 402
 agents causing, 401t
 alcoholic, 1507–1509
 B, 402, 586
  cirrhosis and, 402
  immunization for, 402
  mortality rate for, 402
  risk factors for, 402
 bacterial, organisms in, 401t
 C (non-A, non-B), 402–403, 586
  risk factors for, 402
 delta, 403
  mortality rate in, 403
  natural history of, 403
 drug therapy causing, 401t
 epidemiology of, 402, 1507
 kidney transplant and, 1298t, 1298–1299
 systemic illness causing, 401t
 toxic chemicals causing, 401t
 transfusion and, 402, 1391
 transplant patient and, *582*, 586
 viral, 401–403, *582*, 586
  mortality rate in, 401–403
  organisms in, 401t, 401–403
  symptoms of, 401
Hepatorenal syndrome, kidney failure and,
  1257–1258
 pathogenesis of, 1258
Hereditary disorders, anterior horn
  affected by, 676
 coagulopathy and, 1337, 1602
 hemolytic anemia and, 1384–1386, 1385t
 myopathy and, 686

Hereditary disorders *(Continued)*
 neuropathy and, 676
Herniation (brain), 632, 637
 cerebellar tonsil and, 715
 cingulate gyrus in, 715
 head trauma and, 715
 mydriasis due to, 715
 stages in, 632, 637
 transtentorial, 715
Heroin, pulmonary edema due to, 899–900
 street names for, 1711t
Herpes simplex, encephalitis due to, 399,
  689t, 689–690, *690*
 keratitis due to, 469–470
 transplant patient and, *582*
Herpes zoster, anterior horn and, 676–677
Herpesvirus 1 (B virus), encephalitis and,
  399–400
Hetastarch, 134–136
 coagulation impaired by, 135
 dosage for, 135
 fluid resuscitation using, 134–136, *137*
 pharmacokinetics of, 135, 137t
 side effects of, 135
Hexobarbital, pharmacokinetics of, 1689t
Hickman catheter, *602*, 603, *603*
 candidiasis and, 438
High-tension current, 1646
Hippus, 636
His bundle, anatomy and, 1057
 block in, 1057–1058
Histamine, immune response and, 1654t,
  1656
Histoplasmosis, 444
HIV infection, 589–598. See also *Acquired
  immunodeficiency syndrome (AIDS).*
 asymptomatic interval of, *590*, *591*, 593
 clinical spectrum of, *590*, *591*, 592–593
 cofactors for, 590
 drug therapy in, 593
 encephalopathy of, 702t
 epidemiology of, 591t, 591–592, *592*,
  592t
 global patterns of, 591t, 592, *592*, 592t
 health care worker and, 596–598, 598t
 immune response to, 589–591, *590*, 590t,
  591, 591t
 intensive care admissions and, 594, 594t
 meningitis due to, 397
 onset syndrome of, 593
 opportunistic infections with, *590*, 590t
 pathophysiology of, 589–591, 590t, 591t
 precautions against, 564
 prevention of, 596–598, 598t
 prognosis in, 596, 597t
 pulmonary disorders with, 594–596,
  595t, 844
 staging of, 597t
 symptomatic disease with, 593
 time course of, 589–591, *591*
 transmission of, 591t, 591–592, 592t,
  596–598
 trauma patient with, 564
 treatment of, 593–594
 virology of, 589–590
Hoarseness, intubation causing, 116
 pulmonary hypertension and, 845
Homosexuality, HIV infection and, 591t,
  592t
Homovanillic acid, 1319t
Honeybee, *1681*
 venom of, 1681, 1681t
Hormones. See also specific hormones,
  glands, and disorders.
 calcium regulation and, *1198*, 1198–1199
 potassium level and, 1179–1180, 1180t

Horner's syndrome, coma evaluation and, 636

Hornets, 1681, 1681t

Hospitals. See also *Intensive care unit (ICU)*.
cybernetic model for, *62*
disaster preparedness and, 40

Host, 383t, 522t
compromised, 546t, 550t, 581t
cancer and, 545–554, 546t, 550t
granulocytopenia and, 532–543
splenectomy and, 533, 546–547
transplant patient as, 579–587, 581t
defense mechanisms of, dermal, 522t, 522–524
respiratory tract, 748–753, *749*
infection risk factors for, 383, 383t

Hot potato voice, 478

Human immunodeficiency virus (HIV). See *HIV infection*.

Humidity, air transport and, 55

Hungry bone syndrome, 1214

Hurricanes, 31

Hydralazine, eclampsia and, 1331t
hypertensive emergency and, 1331t
pregnancy and, 1605

Hydrochloric acid, phosgene production of, 50
respiratory effects of, 50–51

Hydrochlorothiazide, diuresis using, 1165, 1165t
lung affected by, 900

Hydrocortisone. See *Cortisol (hydrocortisone)*.

Hydrogen chloride, effects of, 884
smoke inhalation and, 883, 884

Hydrogen cyanide. See also *Cyanide*.
antidote for, 886
effects of, 884
lactic acidosis caused by, 1237–1238
properties of, 884
smoke inhalation and, 883, 884

Hydrogen ion. See also *pH*.
acid-base balance role of, 1220–1222, *1221, 1222*

Hydrogen peroxide, cell production of, 950, *950*
oxygen reduction producing, 950, *950*

Hydroperoxyeicosatetraenoic acid (HPETE), *305*

Hydrostatic pressure, *1155*
capillary-interstitial exchange and, *1155*, 1155
fluid distribution and, 129–131, *130*
pulmonary edema and, *789*, 789t, 789–790
Starling forces and, *789*, 789–790, 1155, *1155*

Hydroxyeicosatetraenoic acid (HETE), *305*

Hydroxyl radical, oxygen toxicity and, 950

Hydroxynaphthoquinone, *Pneumocystis* pneumonia and, 596

Hygiene, CNS compromise affecting, 635

Hyperbaric oxygen therapy, air embolism and, 908–909, *909*
chamber for, *909*
decompression sickness and, 906–907, *909*

Hypercalcemia, 1203–1206, 1205t
arrhythmia due to, 1053
causes of, 1204t, 1400t
clinical features of, 1203–1205, 1205t, 1401
ECG in, *1046*
gastrointestinal tract and, 1204
heart affected by, *1046*, 1053
malignancy and, 1204–1205
neoplasia causing, 1400t, 1400–1402

Hypercalcemia *(Continued)*
pathophysiology of, 1400–1401
potassium level and, 1186
therapy in, 1205–1206
treatment of, 1401t, 1401–1402

Hypercapnia, *1044*
lactic acidosis and, *1233*, 1233–1234
pulmonary hypertension and, 839
respiratory failure and, *754*, 754–761

Hyperchloremia, acidosis due to, 1223t, 1224

Hypercoagulability, thrombosis and, 849–850

Hyperglycemia, hypertonicity due to, 1177–1178

Hyperinsulinism, hypoglycemia due to, 1252–1253

Hyperkalemia, *1181*
acute, 1188, 1191t, 1191–1193
approach to patient with, 1188–1193, *1189*, 1191t
arrhythmia caused by, *1052*, 1052–1053, *1053*
chronic, 1188–1190, *1189*
clinical manifestations of, *1187*, 1187t, 1187–1188
diabetic ketoacidosis and, 1248, 1248t, 1249t, 1250
digitalis causing, 1182
drug-induced, 1189t
ECG effects of, *1046*, 1046–1047, *1187*, 1187t, 1187–1188
false, 1186–1187
hypertonicity and, 1180, 1182–1183
IV therapy causing, 1182
periodic paralysis and, 1183
spironolactone and, 1185

Hyperlipidemia, kidney transplant and, 1297–1298

Hypermagnesemia, 1208–1209
arrhythmia due to, 1054
causes of, 1208–1209
clinical manifestations of, 1208
treatment in, 1209

Hypermetabolism, burn injury and, 1624, *1624*

Hypernatremia, clinical manifestations of, 1177
euvolemic, 1175t, 1175–1178
hypertonicity and, 1174–1178
hypovolemic, 1176–1177
treatment of, 1177–1178

Hyperosmolar agents, intracranial pressure reduction and, 463

Hyperoxia, 949–956
clinical manifestations of, 951t, 954t, 954–955
extrapulmonary effects of, 949
inflammation due to, 952
lung affected by, 949–956, 951t, *953*, 954t
therapy in, 952t, 955, 955t
tissue damage due to, 949–956, 951t, *953*, 954t

Hyperparathyroidism, hypercalcemia due to, 1203, 1204t
kidney transplant and, 1297

Hyperphosphatemia, 1217–1218
causes of, 1217t, 1217–1218
clinical manifestations of, 1218
diagnostic approach in, *1218*, 1218
treatment of, 1218

Hyperpyretic-rigidity syndrome, 698–704
catatonia vs., 700
clinical features of, 699–700, 702t
CNS infection vs., 701, 702t

Hyperpyretic-rigidity syndrome *(Continued)*
diagnosis of, 699–701, 702t
dopamine role in, 698–699
drug-induced, 698, 701
encephalopathy and, 699–700, 702t
heatstroke vs., 700, 702t
incidence of, 701–702
malignant hyperthermia vs., 700–701, 702t
neuroleptic role in, 698–699, 704
recurrence risk for, 704
treatment of, 702–704

Hypertension, comatose patient and, 635t
drug-induced, 1329
emergencies related to, 1327t, 1327–1333, 1329t, 1330t
associated conditions in, 1328–1330, 1329t, 1330t
cerebral blood flow and, 1328, *1328*
drug therapy in, 1330t, 1330–1333, 1331t
epidemiology of, 1328
nitroprusside in, 1330t, 1330–1331, 1331t, *1332*
treatment principles in, 1330t, 1330–1333, 1331t
encephalopathy due to, 1328, *1328*, 1330t
hemorrhagic stroke and, 655
intracranial, 227–230, 229t
hepatic encephalopathy and, *1520*, 1520–1521, *1521*
kidney transplant and, 1295t, 1295–1296, *1296*
malignant, 1328, *1328*
perioperative risk and, 1557
pheochromocytoma and, 1329
portal, 1445–1455
causes of, 1446t
diagnosis in, 1446–1447
pathophysiology of, 1446–1447
portal-systemic shunt in, 1452–1455, *1453, 1454*
pulmonary hypertension vs., 844
pregnancy-induced, 1602t–1604t, 1602–1607, 1606t
antihypertensive agents and, 1605
complications of, 1603, 1603t, 1605–1607
diagnosis of, 1602t, 1603t
etiology of, 1602t, 1603–1607
fluid resuscitation in, 1604
HELLP syndrome and, 1607, 1607t
hematologic disorders and, 1607, 1607t, 1608t
hemodynamic findings in, 1603t
magnesium sulfate and, 1604, 1608
management of, 1603t, 1603–1607
monitoring in, 1603t
neurologic disorders and, 1607–1608
oliguria in, 1606, 1606t
pulmonary edema and, 1605–1606
respiratory function and, 1604t
work-up for, 1603t
pulmonary, 838–947
causes of, 840t, 840–845
collagen disease and, 842–843
cor pulmonale and, 838–839, 846–847
diagnosis of, 845–846, 846t
diet and, 844
heart failure and, 838–839, 846–847
HIV infection and, 844
pathogenesis of, 839–845, 840t
precapillary, 842–843
primary, 843–845
proximal arterial occlusion and, 843

Hypertension (Continued)
    respiratory distress syndrome and, 819,
       819, 844–845
    signs and symptoms of, 845–846
    thrombosis and, 842–843
    toxic oil syndrome and, 844
    treatment of, 846–847
    veno-occlusive disease and, 842
   rheumatologic disorder causing, 1330
   severe, 1327–1328, *1328*
   spinal cord injury and, 1329
   surgical procedure causing, 1330
   trauma causing, 1329
   tyramine and, 1329
Hyperthermia, 1626–1632. See also *Fever*.
   comatose patient and, 635t
   drug overdose causing, 1704, 1704t
   heat exhaustion and, 1628t, 1628–1629
   heatstroke and, 1628t, 1629–1631
   malignant, 1631–1632
       clinical features of, 1631
       drug-induced, 1631t
       hyperpyretic-rigidity syndrome and,
          700–701, 1632
       management of, 1631–1632
       neuroleptic agents and, 700–701, 1632
       pathogenesis of, 1631
   muscle cramps of, 1628
   pathologic, 1628–1632
   predisposing factors for, 1626–1627,
      1628t
   prognosis in, 1631, 1632
   regulatory mechanisms and, 1626–1627,
      1627
Hyperthyroidism, catecholamines and,
      1322–1323
   preoperative care and, 1563
Hypertonic saline, fluid resuscitation using,
      131–132
   side effects of, 132
Hypertonicity, 1168–1170
   clinical manifestations of, 1177
   conditions associated with, 1175t, 1175–
      1178
   euvolemic, 1175t, 1175–1178
   hyperglycemic, 1177–1178
   hypovolemic, 1176–1177
   potassium level and, 1180, 1182–1183
   treatment of, 1177–1178
Hyperuricemia, chemotherapy causing,
      1406–1408
Hyperventilation, cerebral oxygen and,
      227t
   glucose metabolism affected by, 1236–
      1237, *1237*
   hypoventilation effects and, *742*
   intracranial pressure lowered by, 463
   lactic acidosis and, 1236–1237, *1237*
   meningitis therapy and, 463
   neurogenic, central, 636
   prehospital use of, 17
   therapeutic, 17
Hyperviscosity, plasmapheresis in, 1425,
      1426t
Hypervolemia, ascites due to, 1161
   hypernatremia and, 1177
   hypotonicity and, 1171–1172
   mechanisms of, 1161–1164
Hypoalbuminemia, nephrotic edema and,
      1163
   treatment of, 1163–1164
   volume depletion and, 1163–1164
   volume overload and, 1163–1164
Hypoaldosteronism, 1314–1315
   clinical manifestations of, 1313, 1315
   diagnosis of, 1315

Hypoaldosteronism (Continued)
   etiology of, 1314–1315, 1315t
   treatment of, 1315
Hypocalcemia, 1199–1203
   arrhythmia due to, 1053–1054
   chelation causing, 1202–1203
   clinical manifestations of, 1199–1200
   disorders associated with, 1199–1203,
      1202
   ECG in, 1045–1046, *1046*
   heart affected by, 1045–1046, *1046*,
      1053–1054, 1199–1200
   incidence of, 1200–1201, *1201*
   mortality affected by, 1200–1201, *1202*
   platinum causing, 1407
   vascular disorders and, 1199–1200
Hypocapnia, *1044*
Hypodipsia, etiology of, 1175
Hypoglycemia, 1251–1255
   alcoholic, 711, 1253
   approach to patient with, 1254t, 1254–
      1255, *1255*
   autoimmune, 1253, 1254t, *1255*
   causes of, 1252–1254, 1253t
   clinical presentation of, 1252, 1252t
   coma and, 633
   drug-induced, 1254
   drug therapy in, 1309t
   factitious, 1254, 1254t
   glucose metabolism and, 633, 1251–1252
   hyperinsulinism and, 1252–1253, 1254t
   kidney failure dose adjustment and,
      1309t
   mental status and, 17
   neoplasia causing, 1402
   non–islet cell tumor and, 1253
   reactive, 1254t, 1254–1255
   symptoms of, 633, 1252, 1252t
Hypokalemia, *1181*
   acute, 1190, 1193, 1193t
   approach to patient with, *1190*, 1190–
      1191, 1193, 1193t
   arrhythmia due to, 1053
   causes of, 1185t, 1185–1186
   chronic, *1190*, 1190–1191, 1193
   clinical manifestations of, *1187*, 1187t,
      1187–1188
   diet and, 1185
   drug-induced, 1184–1185, 1186
   ECG effects of, *1187*, 1187t, 1187–1188
   epinephrine causing, 1183
   false, 1187
   heart affected by, *1046*, 1046–1047, 1053
   periodic paralysis and, 1184
   treatment of, *1190*, 1190–1191, 1193,
      1193t
Hypomagnesemia, causes of, 1207t, 1207–
      1208
   clinical manifestations of, 1207
   drug-induced, 1208
   evaluation of, 1208
   heart affected by, 1047, 1207, 1208
   neuromuscular effects of, 1207
   platinum causing, 1407
   potassium level and, 1181, 1186
   treatment of, 1208
Hyponatremia, diabetic ketoacidosis and,
      1247, 1248t, 1250
   diarrhea and, 1160, 1464–1465
   isotonic (pseudo), 1171
   kidney and, 1160
   mechanisms of, 1160
   neoplasia causing, 1402
   vomiting and, 1160
Hypoperfusion, shock and, 978–982, *979*
Hypophosphatemia, 1217–1218

Hypophosphatemia (Continued)
   causes of, 1212–1214, 1213t
   clinical manifestations of, 1214–1215
   diagnostic approach in, *1215*, 1215–1216
   gastrointestinal tract and, 1212–1213
   heart affected by, 1046
   hypothermia and, 1212–1213
   prevention of, 1216
   treatment of, 1216–1217, 1217t
Hypopnea, comatose patient and, 635t
Hypoproteinemia, pulmonary edema and,
      143–145, *144*, *145*
Hypotension, comatose patient and, 635t
   dialysis causing, 1282–1283, 1283t
   kidney failure and, 1257
   orthostatic, 1326
   septic shock and, *366*, *367*, 375–377, *376*,
      376t
   shock and, 978–979
   vasopressor therapy in, 375–377, *376*,
      376t
Hypothalamus, thermoregulation by, 1634,
      1634
Hypothermia, 1633–1643
   associated conditions of, 1638t
   classification of, 1635t, 1638, 1638t
   clinical effects of, 1634t, 1634–1638,
      1635
   comatose patient and, 635t, 1639–1640
   disasters and, 36
   drug-induced, 1635t, 1704, 1704t
   ECG in, *1635*, 1635–1636
   forms of, 1634, 1634t
   frostbite and, 1641t, 1641–1643, *1642*,
      1642t
   laboratory studies in, 1640, 1640t
   localized, 1641t, 1641–1643, *1642*, 1642t,
      1643t
   management of, 1638–1641, 1639t, 1643
   paroxysmal hemoglobinuria due to, 1378
   pathophysiology of, 1634t, 1634–1637,
      1635
   phosphate level in, 1212–1213
   prehospital treatment of, 1638
   rewarming and, 1640–1641, 1641t, 1643
   risk factors in, 1635t, 1638t, 1642t
   sepsis and, 297
   trench foot and, 1641t, 1642–1643, 1643t
Hypothyroidism, catecholamines and,
      1323–1324
   edema of, 1161
Hypotonicity, 1168–1170
   clinical manifestations of, 1173–1174
   conditions associated with, 1171–1174,
      1172t
   diuretic-induced, 1173
   edema with, 1171–1172, 1172t
   euvolemic, 1172–1173
   hypervolemic, 1171–1172
   hypovolemic, 1171
   pathophysiology of, 1168–1169, 1172t
   SIADH and, 1172t, 1173, 1173t
   treatment of, 1174
Hypoventilation, alveolar, 841–842
   blood gases and, *217*, 217–218
   end-tidal CO_2 and, 212, *214*
   obesity and, 769–771, 781
   oxygen tension and, 741–742, *742*
   sleep-associated, 773–783
Hypovolemia, blood pressure measurement
      in, *256*
   crush syndrome causing, 33t, 33–34
   fluid resuscitation and, 136–139, *138*
   hemorrhage and, 1159
   hypernatremia and, 1176–1177
   hypotonicity and, 1171

Hypovolemia (Continued)
  mechanisms of, 1159t, 1159–1164
  shock and, 136–139, 138, 367, 375t, 978–985, 983t
  treatment of, 1160–1161
Hypoxemia, 633
  asthma and, 808
  bronchoscopy causing, 193
  COPD patient with, 797–798
  correction of, 797–798
  head trauma causing, 17
  oxygen therapy in, 963–964
  pulmonary hypertension and, 839
  respiratory failure and, 754, 754–755, 755, 761–762, 797–798
  ventilation-perfusion mismatch and, 17, 743, 743–747, 744
Hypoxia, 633
  acidosis with, 1041–1044, 1041–1044
  anemic, 633
  carbon monoxide poisoning and, 883–886
  consciousness and, 633
  global, 738
  heart failure causing, 639–645, 640t
  hypoxic, 633
  lactic acidosis and, 1233, 1233
  normoxemic, 964
  oxygen therapy in, 963–964
  perfusion affected by, 738
  sepsis and, 354–356, 355
  smoke inhalation and, 883–886

I

Iatrogenic disorders, air embolism and, 908–909
  catheterization causing, 1140–1152
  hemoptysis and, 877t, 879
  vascular emergencies due to, 1140–1152
Ibuprofen, endotoxin effects and, 306, 372
  pharmacokinetics of, 1689t
  prostaglandins inhibited by, 372
  sepsis effects treated with, 372
  thromboxane inhibited by, 306, 372
Ichthyosarcotoxin, 1673–1674, 1676
Ifosfamide, encephalopathy due to, 1416t, 1416–1417
If-then reasoning, 97t, 97–98, 98, 98t
Ileum, hemorrhage of, 1460–1461, 1471
  inflammation of, 1470–1473
Iliac artery, occlusion of, 1144
Illness trajectory management, 62, 62t
Imaging. See also specific techniques.
  cardiographic, 1103–1120
IMEX system, 103t
Imipenem, pathogen susceptibility and, 415t, 614t, 615
  resistant organisms and, 614–615
Immune complexes, pulmonary hemorrhage and, 879t, 879–880, 880
Immune response, 1650–1656, 1653. See also Anaphylaxis.
  burns eliciting, 522t, 522–524
  candidiasis and, 435–436, 436t
  HIV infection and, 589–591, 590, 590t, 591, 591t
  mediators for, 1652–1655, 1653, 1654t, 1655t
  shock and, 981
Immunization, C. difficile, 505
  hepatitis B, 402
  personnel need for, 386
  pneumococcal infections and, 419
  poliovirus, 396

Immunization (Continued)
  rabies, 691, 692t
Immunodeficiency. See also Acquired immunodeficiency syndrome (AIDS).
  cancer patient and, 532–543, 545–554
  granulocytopenic, 532–543
  HIV infection causing. See HIV infection.
  hypothermia causing, 1637
  trauma causing, 556–557
Immunoelectrophoresis, meningitis detection by, 459
Immunoglobulin(s), autoimmune disorders and, 1425, 1426t
  burn injury and, 522t, 522–523
  E, anaphylaxis and, 1652–1653, 1653
    parasitism and, 1652
    structure of, 1653
  plasmapheresis and, 1425, 1426t
  therapeutic use of, 543
Immunosuppression, bone marrow and, 1348, 1348t, 1357
  catheter-related infection and, 536
  chemical exposure and, 50, 52
  drugs used for, 1307t–1308t
  hemoglobin infusion causing, 158–159
  kidney failure affecting, 1307t–1308t
  neurologic disorders and, 1300–1301
  nosocomial infections and, 384
  transplantation and, 579–581
    bone marrow, 1348, 1348t, 1357
    kidney, 1293t, 1293–1294, 1294t
Impedance, blood flow resistance and, 1097
  cardiography using, 1095
  transthoracic, 119
Incapacitating agents, 48–49, 52–53
  antidotes for, 49, 53
  chemical warfare use of, 48–49
  clinical effects of, 52–53
Incentive spirometry, chest physiotherapy using, 958
Indicator dilution, cardiac output and, 1086–1088, 1088
  pulmonary edema and, 921–922
Indocyanine green, cardiac output measurement and, 1086–1088, 1088
Infarction, cerebral, 222, 222, 230
  myocardial. See Myocardial infarction (MI).
Infections, 391–620. See also specific organisms and diseases.
  abdominal, 513–526
  AIDS patient and, 589–598
  anterior horn affected by, 676–677
  antimicrobial selection for, 614–620
  burn patient and, 521–526, 1623–1624
  cancer patient and, 545–554, 546t, 550t, 553t
  candidal, 434–442
  catheter-related, 601–607
    antibiotic lock technique in, 606
    cancer patient and, 548–549
    culture contamination and, 609
    diagnosis of, 605
    granulocytopenia and, 536
    incidence of, 601–604, 602t
    intracranial, 558–559, 562–563
    management of, 605–606
    microbiology of, 604–606
    mortality rate in, 606
    organisms in, 604–605
    parenteral nutrition and, 1550
    pathogenesis of, 604–605
    prevention of, 605–606
    trauma patient and, 558–559, 562–563
    urinary tract, 527–530
  compromised host and, 536, 579–587, 581t

Infections (Continued)
  cutaneous, 551
  definition of, 557
  drug abuse patient and, 566–577
  fungal, 444–453
  gastroenteric, 500–512
  granulocytopenic patient and, 532–543, 545–554
  heart muscle, 491–499
  HIV, 589–598
  laboratory tests and, 608–613
  meningeal, 454–464
  mimickers of, 553t
  mycobacterial, 422–432
  neck, 477, 477–479
  nosocomial, 382t, 383t
    control and prevention of, 381–389, 386t, 387t
    costs of, 365
    domiciliary epidemic and, 580
    endogenous flora causing, 384–385, 388
    endotracheal intubation and, 975–976
    epidemiology of, 381–384, 382t, 383t
    hand washing and, 386–387, 387t
    incidence of, 381, 382t
    isolation and, 386, 387t
    medical devices and, 384, 387–388
    mortality and, 381, 382t
    multiple organ system failure and, 348, 349
    organisms in, 349, 382–385, 383t
    outbreak of, 383, 388t, 389
    pathogenesis of, 382–385, 383t
    personnel and, 386t, 387, 387t
    pneumonia and, 480–490, 486, 486t, 487t
    precautions against, 385–389, 386t, 387t, 388t
    predisposing factors in, 381–384, 383t
    reservoirs for, 385
    resistant strains in, 382–383, 388–389
    sites of, 382, 382t, 383t
    staphylococcal, 411–412
    tracheostomy and, 975–976
    transmission routes for, 384–385
    transplant patient and, 579–580
    urinary tract, 527–530
  ophthalmic, 466–474
  organ transplant patient and, 579–587
  oropharyngeal, 477, 477–479, 541
  pregnancy and, 1593–1594, 1594t, 1600–1601, 1608–1611
  respiratory tract, lower, 480–490
    upper, 474–479
  superinfection, pneumonia and, 489
  transplant patient and, 579–587, 581t, 584t, 587t
  trauma patient and, 556–564
  urinary tract, 382t, 383t, 527–530
  viral, 391–406. See also Viruses.
Inflammation, 346. See also Sepsis.
  asthma role of, 806–807, 807t
  hyperoxia causing, 952
  malignant, 345
  subarachnoid space and, 456, 456
Inflammatory bowel disease, 1470–1473
  hemorrhage due to, 1460–1461, 1471
  malnutrition due to, 1473
  pregnancy and, 1473
Influenza, 391–392
  clinical signs in, 391–392
  encephalitis and, 695
  subtypes of, 391
Informed consent, ethical issues and, 1726–1730, 1734–1736

Infusion rates, commonly used drugs and, 1693t
Inhalation injury, 1622–1623, *1623*
  anatomy and, *1623*
  burn injury with, 1621–1623, *1623*
  smoke and, 883–886
Inhalation therapy, 959t, 959–963. See also *Oxygen, therapy*; *Ventilation*.
  antimicrobial delivery and, 962
  bronchodilators and, 961t, 961–962
  mucolytics in, 962
Inhalers, anaphylaxis treatment and, 1658
  COPD treatment and, 798–799
  metered-dose, 798–799, 961
Inherited disorders. See *Hereditary disorders*.
Injury. See *Trauma*.
Injury Severity Score, 1574–1575, 1575t–1581t
Innominate artery, fistula and, tracheal, 1146–1147
Inotropic agents, acidosis and, 1040–1041
  dosage for, 1693t, 1696–1698, 1697t
  heart failure and, *1022*, 1022–1024, 1023t
  negative, 1024
  pharmacokinetics of, 1693t, 1696–1698, 1697t
  pregnancy and, 1595, 1595t
Insecticides, neuropathy due to, 681, 683
Insects, anaphylaxis caused by, 1652
  venom of, 1652, 1681, 1681t
Insomnia, 631. See also *Sleep*.
Inspiration. See also *Respiration*.
  cardiac tamponade and, *1035*
  catheterization tracing affected by, *1080*, 1080–1081, *1085*, 1085–1087
  chest wall muscle and, 723, *723*
  flow-volume loop and, *726*, 726–731, *727*
  mechanical ventilation and, 928–931, *929*, *930*
  mechanisms of, 763–765, *764*, *765*
Instrumentation, airway management and, 111t, 111–113, *112*
Insulin, antibodies to, 1253–1255, *1255*
  counter-regulatory hormones for, *1246*, 1246t, 1246–1248
  deficiency of, *1246*, 1246t, 1246–1248
  hypersecretion of, 1252–1253
  hypoglycemia due to, 1252–1255
  ketoacidosis role of, *1246*, 1246t, 1246–1250, 1249t
  potassium level and, 1179–1180, 1180t
Insulin tolerance test, adrenal function and, 1312
Insulinoma, hypoglycemia and, 1252–1253, 1254t
Intensive care services, 1–4
  air travel and, 42–45, 43t, *44*, 45t, 54–55
  cost-benefit issues and, 5, 77, 1731, 1743
  goals of, 1731–1732
  growth of, 4
  historical aspects of, 1–4
  patient access to, 5, 62–67
  patient decision making and, 1725–1726, 1732–1744
  rationing of, 1743
  standards development for, 70t–71t, 73–76, 74t–76t
  transport modes and, 42–45, 43t, *44*, 45t, 54–57
  withholding of, 1732–1744
Intensive care unit (ICU), 1–4
  admission and discharge in, 62–65, 74t, 1731–1732, 1743–1744
  closed, 60t, 60–61
  COPD patient and, 796

Intensive care unit (ICU) *(Continued)*
  disaster preparedness and, 40
  ethical issues and, 1731–1744
  historical aspects of, 1–4
  hospital strategy and, 64t, 64–66
  illness severity scoring for, 80–86, 81t, 83t–85t
  management of, 59–66
  medical director role in, 59–66, 60t, 62t
  mortality rate in, 1731–1732
  nosocomial infections in, 381–389, 382t, 383t, 386t, 387t
  nursing director role in, 59, 65
  open, 60, 60t
  organization of, 57–66, 60t
  quality assurance plan for, 70t–71t
  resource allocation in, 62t, 62–65
  sleep deprivation in, 781–782
  types of, 1–3, 60t
Interference, electrical, 100t, 100–101
  expert systems and, 100t, 100–101
Interferons, sepsis mediation and, 312t, 318
Interleukins, burn injury and, 523
  hematopoiesis role of, 1336t
  pulmonary edema due to, 899
  sepsis role of, 312t, *317*, 317–318, 334–335
Internist-1, diagnosis with, 96
Intestine. See also *Gastrointestinal tract*.
  abdominal pain and, 1475t, 1476–1477, 1483
  aortic occlusion and, 1142–1144
  drug smuggler packets in, 1482–1483
  false obstruction of, 1479
  ischemia of, 1142–1144
  obstruction of, 1475t, 1476–1477, 1482–1483
  short bowel syndrome and, 1235–1236
  trauma injury to, 1589, *1589*
Intoxication. See *Poisoning*; *Toxic substance(s)*.
Intra-aortic balloon pump, 188–189, *189*. See also *Pump devices*.
  angina pectoris and, 1005
  complications of, 189, 1122, 1149
  contraindications for, 188, 1121
  heart failure treatment and, 1022, 1121–1122
  indications for, 188, 1121, 1121t
  insertion procedure for, 188–189, *189*, 1122, *1122*
  MI and, 1005, 1121–1122, *1122*
Intracranial hemorrhage. See *Cerebrovascular disease, hemorrhagic*.
Intracranial pressure, arterial pressure and, 714–715, *715*
  autoregulation of, 714–715, *715*
  blood flow and, 714–715, *715*
  brain monitoring for, 227–230, 229t, *1582*
  endotracheal intubation and, 116
  fluid resuscitation and, *142*, 142–143
  head trauma and, 227–230, 229t, 714–715, *715*, 1582t, 1582–1583
  heart failure effect on, 641t, 642
  hepatic encephalopathy and, *1520*, 1520–1521, *1521*
  measurement of, 1582t, 1582–1583
  meningitis affecting, *456*, 457, 463
  monitoring of, 625–626, *1582*, 1582–1583
  neoplasia affecting, 1397t, 1397–1398
  reduction therapy for, 463
Intraocular pressure, endotracheal intubation and, 116
Intrapleural pressure, 861, *861*, 865

Intrapleural pressure *(Continued)*
  distribution and, 734–735, *735*
  expiration and, 727, *727*, 728, 861, *861*
  inspiration and, 727, *727*, 861, *861*
  Starling forces and, 861, *861*
  ventilation and, 734–735, *735*
Intravenous drug abuse. See *Drug abuse*.
Intravenous therapy. See also *Catheterization*; *Drugs*; *Pharmacokinetics*.
  commonly used drugs and, 1693t
Intubation, chest, injury due to, 1142
  endotracheal. See *Endotracheal intubation*.
  Linton-Nachlas tube and, 170
  nasogastric. See *Nasogastric intubation*.
  Sengstaken-Blakemore tube and, 170–172, *171*
Inventory control, computer assistance in, 94
Iodinated compounds, lung affected by, 901
Iodine, hyperthyroidism treated with, 1323
Ions. See also *Electrolytes*.
  action potential and, 1050, *1050*
  electrode glass sensitivity and, 242
  measurement of, 247
  selective field effect transistors and, 247
  transport of, diarrhea and, 1465–1467, 1466t
  intestine and, 1466, 1466t, 1467
Ipratropium bromide, COPD and, 798–799
Iridocyclitis, 470
Iron, abdominal pain due to, 1483t, 1484
  binding capacity for, 1530
  lactic acidosis caused by, 1239
  malnutrition and, 1530
Iron lung machine, 925–926
Ischemia. See also *Cerebrovascular disease, ischemic*.
  brain monitoring and, *222*, 222–223, 223t, *230*, 230–233
  encephalopathy due to, 645t, 645–647
  hand and, 236
  intestinal, 1485t, 1485–1489
    aortic occlusion causing, 1142–1144
    drug-induced, 1484
  kidney and, 1144, 1261
  mesenteric, 1485–1489
    abdominal pain of, 1479–1480, 1486–1487
    management of, *1486*, 1487–1488
    pathophysiology of, 1485–1487
    prognosis in, 1488–1489
  mucosal, intubation causing, 116
  neural, 231t, 231–232
  sensory evoked potentials and, 231t, 231–232
Ischemic heart disease, 989–1012
  atherosclerosis and, 989–991, *990*, *991*
  causes of, 989t, 989–991, *990*, *991*
  chemotherapy-induced, 1412t, 1412–1413
  management of, 994–1012
    angina and, 1005, 1005t, 1011–1012
    angioplasty in, *1004*, 1004–1005
    drug therapy in, 995–1003
    intra-aortic balloon pump in, 1005
    revascularization in, 1003–1004, 1004t
  radiation therapy causing, 1412t, 1413
Islet cells, insulin hypersecretion and, 1252–1253
Isolation, category-specific, 386, 387t
  disease-specific, 386, 387t
  nosocomial infection and, 386, 387t
  precautions for, 386–387, 387t
Isoniazid, dosage for, 425, 425t
  pharmacokinetics of, 1689t

Isoniazid *(Continued)*
  side effects of, 425, 425t
  tuberculosis treated with, 425, 425t, 571
Isopropanol, *1718*
  metabolism of, *1718*
  poisoning due to, 712, *1718*, 1718t,
    1718–1719
  products containing, 1718t
Isoproterenol, asthma treated with, 809,
    809t
  pharmacokinetics of, 1693t, 1696–1698,
    1697t
Isosbestic points, 244
Isovolumic relaxation, left ventricular,
    1113, *1114*
IV. See *Catheterization.*

J

J wave, hypothermia and, *1635*, 1635–1636
Janeway's lesions, endocarditis and, 493
Japanese B encephalitis, 694
Jaundice, bilirubin levels and, 401
  hepatitis and, 401
JCAHO (Joint Commission for the
    Accreditation of Healthcare
    Organizations), quality improvement
    and, 91–92
  standards development by, *68*, 68–69, 69t
Jejunum, enteral nutrition in, *1540*, 1540–
    1542, *1541*
Jellyfish, venom of, 1674t, 1674–1675
Jet nebulizer, aerosols produced by, 960,
    960
Joints, candidiasis affecting, 437
Joule's law, 1645–1646
Jugular vein, brain oxygen monitoring and,
    230, 230t, 230–231
  internal, central venous catheter in, 180–
    181, *181*, 258, *259*
    CPR role of, 122, *122*
    misplaced catheter and, 258, *259*, 260,
      261
    valves of, 122, *122*

K

K complexes, *775*
Kanamycin, side effects of, 427t
  tuberculosis treated with, 427t
Keratitis, 468–470
  bacterial, 469
  culture in, 469
  herpetic, 469
  viral, 469
Keratoconjunctivitis, 469
  herpetic, 470
Kernig's sign, 457
  meningitis and, 457
Kerosene, smoke from, 884
Ketamine, asthma treated with, 812
Ketoacidosis, alcoholic, 710–712
  diabetic, 1245–1251
    biochemistry of, *1246*, 1246t, 1246–
      1248
    cerebral edema due to, 1251
    clinical features of, 1247–1248
    diagnosis of, 1248
    electrolytes in, 1247–1248, 1248t,
      1249t, 1249–1250
    epidemiology of, 1245
    hormonal basis in, 1246, 1246t
    insulin deficiency in, *1246*, 1246t,
      1246–1248

Ketoacidosis *(Continued)*
    insulin therapy in, 1249t, 1249–1250
    magnesium depletion in, 1208, 1248t,
      1250
    mortality rate for, 1251
    phosphate deficit in, 1214, 1248t, 1250
    potassium level and, 1183, 1248, 1248t,
      1250
    precipitating factors for, 1245–1246
    treatment of, 1248–1251, 1249t
Ketoconazole, candidiasis treated with,
    438–442
Kety-Schmidt technique, cerebral blood
    flow and, 224
Kidney, 1155–1333
  failure of, 1256–1266
    abdominal pain and, 1482
    acute, 1256–1266
      intrarenal, 1260–1265, 1261t, 1264t
      postrenal, 1265t, 1265–1266
      prerenal, 1257t, 1257–1260
    anemia and, 1272
    antimicrobial dose factors and, 616
    bleeding time and, 1271
    burn injury causing, 1624
    chemotherapy-induced, 1406–1408
    coma and, 634
    criteria for, 342t
    drug dose adjustment for, 1304t–
      1309t, 1304–1309
    drug-induced, 1261t, 1261–1263,
      1264t, 1264–1265
    edematous disorders and, 1257, 1257t
    electrical injury and, 1646t, 1647
    electrolytes and, 1271–1272
    endocarditis and, 573t, 574
    fluid balance in, 1270–1271
    hemoglobin infusion causing, 158
    hepatorenal syndrome and, 1258
    hypertensive emergency due to, 1328–
      1329, 1330t
    hypocalcemia and, 1202
    hypotension and, 1257
    infection predisposition and, 1272–
      1273
    insufficiency vs., 1269
    interstitial nephritis with, 1264t, 1264–
      1265
    ischemic, 1261
    microemboli in, 1264
    nephrotic syndrome and, 1162t, 1163
    nephrotoxic, 1261t, 1261–1262
    nutrition in, 1273–1274
    obstruction and, 1265t, 1265–1266
    precipitating conditions for, 1267–1268
    pregnancy-induced, 1606, 1606t
    preoperative care and, 1561–1562
    prevention of, 1268–1269
    prostaglandin inhibitors causing, 1258
    pulmonary hemorrhage and, 879t,
      879–881, *880*
    radiation-induced, 1408
    renal artery stenosis and, 1258
    sodium balance and, 1163
    treatment of, 1259–1260, 1263–1264
    tubular necrosis in, 1260–1265
      clinical course of, 1260
      diagnosis of, 1260–1261
      etiology of, 1261t, 1261–1263
      management of, 1263–1264
  hypothermia effect on, 1636, *1636*
  ischemia in, 1144
    causes of, 1267–1268
    occlusive disease and, 1144
  stones in, abdominal pain due to, 1480
    obstruction and, 1265t, 1265–1266

Kidney *(Continued)*
  transplantation of, 1293–1301
    acidosis and, 1298
    anemia and, 1298
    atherosclerosis and, 1296–1297, 1297t
    bone necrosis and, 1300
    complications of, 1293–1301
    cytomegalovirus and, 394
    diabetes mellitus and, 1297
    drug side effects in, 1293t, 1293–1294,
      1294t
    erythrocytosis and, 1298
    gastrointestinal disorders and, 1299
    gout and, 1300
    heart failure and, 1296–1297, 1297t
    hepatitis and, 1298t, 1298–1299
    hyperlipidemia and, 1297–1298
    hyperparathyroidism and, 1297
    hypertension and, 1295t, 1295–1296,
      1296
    immunosuppressive therapy in, 1293t,
      1293–1294, 1294t
    neurologic disorders and, 1300–1301
    pancreatitis and, 1299
    rejection and, 1294–1295
    sexual function affected by, 1298
  trauma injury to, 1589
  tubules of, acid-base regulation and,
    1220–1222, *1221*, 1224t, 1224–1225
    acidosis role of, 1224t, 1224–1225
    acute necrosis of, 1260–1265
    phosphate reabsorption in, 1212, 1217
    potassium excretion by, 1181, 1185–
      1186
    sodium and, 1156–1159
  urine concentration and, 1169
  water and, 1169
Killip's classification, MI and, 77t, 77–78
Kinins, septic shock and, 334
Klebsiella, pneumonia caused by, 487t, 488,
    489t
  susceptibility of, 614t
Knee, candidiasis affecting, 437
  dislocation of, popliteal artery damaged
    by, 1150, *1151*
Knowledge data bases, expert systems and,
    96–97, 97t
Korean hemorrhagic fever, 403
Korotkoff sounds, 251
Korsakoff's disease, features of, 710
Kostmann's syndrome, 1337
Kraits, 1662t, 1667–1668, 1668t
Krebs' cycle, 1231, *1232*
Kupffer's cells, *1340*
Kusivar system, *100*
Kussmaul's sign, waveform tracing in, 1080,
    1080
Kwashiorkor, 1528–1529
Kymograph, historical aspects of, 2
Kyphoscoliosis, 768
  causes of, 768t
  Cobb angle in, 768, *769*
  radiography in, *769*
  respiratory failure due to, 768
Kyphosis, 768

L

La Crosse encephalitis, 695
Labetalol, hypertensive emergency and,
    1331t, 1333
  pharmacokinetics of, 1689t
  pregnancy and, 1605
Lacerations, lung, 891
Lactamase, beta, enterococci and, 415

Lactamase *(Continued)*
 pathogens producing, 614
 resistance due to, 410, 415
Lactate dehydrogenase (LDH), hemolytic
 anemia and, 1370t, 1371
 isoenzymes of, 993, 993t
 MI and, 993, 993t
 pleural fluid and, 861t, 861–862
Lactated Ringer's solution, 131, 131t, *137,*
 138
Lactic acid (lactate), acidosis and, *1041,*
 1041–1044, *1043*
 bacterial production of, 1236
 false-normal and, 1236
 isomeric forms of, 1236
 measurement of, *1240,* 1240–1241
 mitochondria and, *356*
 shock and, 980, *980,* 985
Lactic acidosis, 1231–1242
 bacterial overgrowth and, 1236
 biochemistry of, 1231–1233, *1232, 1233*
 cancer and, 1235, *1235*
 causes of, 1233–1241, 1234t, 1235t,
 1235–1239
 classification of, 1233–1234
 congenital disorders and, 1234, 1235t,
 1240
 diabetes and, 1235
 diagnostic testing in, *1240,* 1240–1241,
 1241
 drug-induced, 1234, 1234t, 1237–1240
 enzyme deficiencies and, 1234, 1235t
 gastrointestinal disorders and, 1235–1236
 hyperventilation causing, 1236–1237,
 1237
 isomeric forms and, 1236
 liver disease and, 1234t, 1234–1235
 oxygen debt in, 1233, *1233*
 shock and, 1233–1234, 1234t
 thiamine deficiency causing, 1236
 treatment of, *1241,* 1241–1242, *1242*
Lactitol, hepatic encephalopathy and,
 1524–1525
Lactobacillus, flora replacement and, 509
 lactic acid produced by, 1236, *1236*
 overgrowth of, 1236, *1236*
Lactrodectus mactans, 1678, 1678–1679
 abdominal pain due to, 1483t, 1484
 antivenin and, 1679
 symptoms and, *1678,* 1678–1679
 venom of, 1678–1679
Lactulose, hepatic encephalopathy and,
 1524–1525
Laetrile, lactic acidosis caused by, 1238
 nitroprusside in, 1238
Lahars, volcanic eruption causing, 29–31
Lambert-Beer formula, 244
Lambert-Eaton syndrome, 682–683
 diagnosis of, 683
 symptoms of, 682–683
Lamina propria cells, diarrhea role of, *1468*
Landry-Guillain-Barré syndrome, CSF in,
 622
Landslides, earthquake and, 27–28
Langerhans' cells, *1340*
Laplace formula, wall stress and, 1016
Laryngoscope, brightness of, 111
 endotracheal intubation and, 111, *113*
Larynx, anatomy of, *115*
 edema of, 116
 endotracheal intubation and, 111–113,
 112, 113, 116
 injury in, 968–972, *969, 972*
 spasm of, rocking-boat motion due to,
 116
Lassa fever, 404–405

Latex agglutination test, *C. difficile* and, 505
Lava flows, *29,* 29–31, *30*
Lavage, bronchoalveolar, 198–199, 199t,
 483t, 484
 peritoneal, 169–170, 519t, 519–520
Lazarus sign, brain death and, 646–647
Lead, abdominal pain due to, 1483t
Legal issues, 1732–1744
 brain death and, 647
 court cases on, 1731–1734
 intensive care services and, 1732–1744
 patient decision process and, 1732–1744
Legionella, bronchoalveolar lavage yield and,
 199
Lentivirus, genes of, 589–590
 immunodeficiency due to, 589–591, *590,*
 590t, *591,* 591t
 replication of, 589–590
Leptomeninges, neoplasia affecting, 1398
Leriche syndrome, 1144
Lethargy, unresponsive patient with, 627
Leukapheresis, 1419–1429
 anticoagulation in, 1427
 calculations for, 1427–1428
 complications of, 1428–1429
 instrumentation for, 1420–1421, *1421,*
 1422
 leukemia and, 1423
 pentastarch used in, 136
 replacement fluids in, 1427
 vascular access for, 1425–1427
Leukemia, 1363–1368
 abdominal pain due to, 1482
 acute myelogenous, 1362t
 leukocytosis of, *1360,* 1360–1362,
 1361, 1362t
 lung affected by, 1361, *1361*
 purpura of, 1360, *1360*
 retina affected by, 1360, *1360*
 B cell, 1368
 erythrocytic, 1364t, 1364–1366, 1365t
 hairy cell, 1368
 hyperleukocytic, *1360,* 1360–1362, *1361,*
 1362t, 1363t
 leukapheresis in, 1423
 lymphocytic, 1367t, 1367–1368
 classification of, 1367t
 myelocytic, 1356t, 1363–1364, 1364t,
 1366–1367
 classification of, 1356t, 1363–1364,
 1364t, 1366–1367
 myelomonocytic, 1364t, 1365t, 1367
 smoldering, 1366, 1367
Leukocytes. See also *Granulocytes;*
 Neutrophils.
 apheresis of, 1419–1429
 transfusion and, 1388
Leukocytosis, 1360–1362
 leukemic, *1360,* 1360–1362, *1361,* 1362t,
 1363t
 leukemoid reaction vs., 1359–1360
 management of, 1361–1362, 1362t, 1363t
 non-neoplastic, 1359–1360
Leukopenia, vesicant exposure causing, 52
Leukotrienes, inhibition of, 371–372
 sepsis role of, 304–306, *305,* 371–372
Levodopa, hyperpyretic-rigidity syndrome
 and, 703
Liddle's syndrome, potassium level and,
 1186, *1190*
Lidocaine, arrhythmia treated with, 1055,
 1056t
 bronchoscopy anesthesia with, 194
 cardiac arrest and, 21, 22t, 23, 124–125
 drug interactions of, 1056t
 MI therapy using, 996, 996t

Lidocaine *(Continued)*
 monitoring of, 1692t
 pharmacokinetics of, 1689t, 1700
Liebermeister's sign, 907
Life-support systems, ethical issues and,
 1736–1744
 historical aspects of, 1–4
 withdrawal of, 1738–1739
 withholding of, 1736–1738
Lightning injury, 1648–1649
 clinical manifestations of, 1648–1649,
 1649
 flashover and, 1648, 1648t
 power line injury vs., 1648–1649
 treatment of, 1649
Limbus, cornea and, 466
Linton-Nachlas tube, *1449,* 1450
Lipase, pancreatitis and, 1501
Lipids, *304, 368, 370*
 A, *370*
 analogues of, 369–370, *370*
 antibodies to, 369
 endotoxic function of, 303–304, 368–
 369
 septic shock and, 368–370
 structure of, *304, 368, 370*
 atherosclerosis and, 990–991, *991*
 embolism and, 893, *894*
 kidney transplant and, 1297–1298
 X, *370*
 septic shock treated with, 369–370
 structure of, *370*
Lipopolysaccharides (LPS), *368*
 endotoxins of, *368,* 368–369
 lipid A moiety of, *368,* 368–370, *370*
 meningitis role of, 456
 R-core of, *368*
 structure of, *368*
Lipoproteins, drug binding by, 1691–1692,
 1692t
Liquefaction, soil, earthquake and, 27–28,
 28
Listeriosis, 419–420
 meningitis due to, 454
 neonatal, 419–420
 risk groups for, 419
 treatment of, 420
Lithium, hyperthyroidism treated with,
 1323
 overdose of, 1710–1711
 toxic effects of, 1710–1711
Litigation, endotracheal intubation and, 109
Liver, candidiasis affecting, 440
 chemotherapy affecting, 1415t, 1415–
 1416
 cirrhosis of. See *Cirrhosis.*
 emergent disorders of, 1506–1512
 failure of, 342t
 causes of, 1509t, 1509–1510, 1514t
 classification of, 79, 79t, 1452, 1452t,
 1561, 1561t
 criteria for, 342t
 drug dose adjustment for, 1689t–
 1692t, 1692–1693
 encephalopathy of, 1510–1511, 1519–
 1525
 fulminant, 1509t, 1509–1512, 1514t,
 1516
 lactic acidosis and, 1234t, 1234–1235
 management of, 1510–1511
 pathology of, 1510
 preoperative care and, 1560–1561,
 1561t
 hypertension and, 844, 1445–1447, 1446t
 hypothermia effect on, 1636, *1636*
 kidney failure and, 1257–1258

Liver *(Continued)*
rupture of, spontaneous, 1599
TNF effects in, 317t
transplantation of. See *Transplantation, liver.*
trauma injury to, 1588–1589
veno-occlusive disease of, 1416
Living wills, 1726–1729, 1732–1735
Lizard, venom of, 1672
Locked-in syndrome, 635
Loop of Henle, diuretics and, 1165, 1165t
sodium excretion by, 1156
Lorazepam, meningitis seizure and, 463
pharmacokinetics of, 669t, 1689t
seizure treated with, 668t, 668–671, 669t
Loxosceles, 1679
envenomation due to, 1679–1680, 1680t
Lucky save syndrome, 12
Ludwig's angina, 478
Lugol's iodine solution, hyperthyroidism treated with, 1323
Lumbar puncture, clinical value of, 622
comatose patient and, 638
complications of, 458
contraindications for, 622
meningitis and, 458, 458–459
Lung. See also *Respiratory tract.*
abscess of, 570–571
aspiration of, needle and, 483
transtracheal, 482–483, 483t
asthma effects in, 807, 807–808
biopsy of, 200, 483t, 483–484
blood from. See *Hemoptysis.*
bronchoalveolar lavage and, pneumonia and, 483t, 484
bullae in, 292, *292*
cancer of, 876–877, 877t
chemotherapy effects in, 897t, 897–898, 1408–1411, 1409t, 1410t
chest physiotherapy and, 957–959
chronic obstructive disease of. See *Asthma; Chronic obstructive pulmonary disease (COPD); Emphysema.*
collapse of, prehospital care in, 16
compliance of, 722, 722–723, 723, 730, 730
time constant and, 735
ventilation and, 735–737, 736, 737
consolidation in, 278, 282
contusions to, 890–891, 891
dead space in, 208, 208, 733–734, 742–743, 819
defense mechanisms of, 748–753, 749
illness effect on, 750–753
impairment of, 750–753
mucociliary transport system and, 750, 752
normal flora and, 749
particle size and, 749–750
secretory, 750
drug-induced injury to, 896–901
edema of. See *Edema, pulmonary.*
elastic properties of, 722, 722–723, 723
embolism of. See *Embolism, pulmonary.*
equation of motion of, 722–726
exercise testing of, 1553–1556, 1554t
fluid dynamics in, 911–917, 912–917, 913, 917
function parameters of, 1553–1556, 1554t
interstitial compartments of, 841, 913–916, 914
laceration of, 891
lymphatic drainage and, 916–917
overexpansion injury in, 904–905

Lung *(Continued)*
oxygen toxicity affecting, 949–956, 953, 954t
preoperative care and, 1553–1556, 1554t
pressure gradients in, 719–722, 721
pressure-volume relationships in, 722, 722–723, 723, 756, 760, 831
radiation therapy effect on, 1411
scan of, 852, 852–853, 1555
secretions from, 482–485, 483t
asthma and, 810
chest physiotherapy and, 957–958
COPD and, 799
postural drainage of, 957–958
spirometry and, 1555
surgery risk factors and, 1553–1556, 1554t
trauma injury to, 890–891, 891
volume, airway obstruction and, 727, 728
equal pressure point theory and, 727, 729
flow-volume loop and, 726, 726–731, 727
isovolume pressure-flow curve and, 727, 728
tube law and, 730, 730
wave speed theory and, 729–730
water balance in, 911–917, 913, 917
Lupus erythematosus, drug-induced, 901
pulmonary hemorrhage due to, 879t, 879–881, 880
pulmonary hypertension and, 842
Lymphatic system, capillary fluid exchange and, 1155, 1155
catheterization injury to, 1142
fluid distribution and, 131, 1155, 1155
interstitial fluid transport and, 1155, 1155
lung and, 916–917
peristalsis of, 1155
peritoneal clearance and, 513
pleural drainage by, 860
pulmonary edema and, 143–145, 145
Lymphocytes, burn injury affecting, 522t, 523
hematopoiesis and, 1336
T. See *T cells.*
Lymphocytosis, benign, 1363
leukemic, 1367t, 1367–1368
malignant, 1367t, 1367–1368
management of, 1368
Lymphohematopoiesis, 1339–1341, 1340
Lymphoma, abdominal pain due to, 1482
Lysolecithin, gallstone pancreatitis and, 1490
Lyssavirus, 392t, 400–401

M

MacIntosh blade, 111, *112*
Macroglobulinemia, plasmapheresis in, 1425, 1426t
Macrophages, *1340*
alveolar, 750, 752–753, 806, 807t
asthma role of, 806, 807t
HIV infection and, 589, 591t
Maddrey's discriminant function, 1508
Mafenide, burn injury and, 525t, 525–526
Magill forceps, *112*
Magnesium, 1206–1209
alcoholism and, 1207–1208
distribution of, 1206
excretion of, 1206, 1208
extracellular, 1206
gastrointestinal loss of, 1208

Magnesium *(Continued)*
heart affected by, 1047, 1054
intake of, 1206
potassium level and, 1181, 1186
regulation of, 1206–1207
Magnesium sulfate, asthma treated with, 810
pregnancy and, 1604, 1608
Magnetic resonance imaging (MRI), head trauma and, 716
pleural effusion and, 283
stroke and, hemorrhagic, 657–658, 658
ischemic, 653, 653
Malabsorption, magnesium depletion in, 1208
Malignancy. See *Neoplasia.*
Mallampati classification, airway and, 109–110, 110t
Mallory-Weiss tear, 1444
Malnutrition, albumin in, 1530
assessment of, 1528–1532, 1529t, 1532t
body composition studies and, 1532
classification of, 1532t
creatinine-height index and, 1530–1531
inflammatory bowel disease and, 1473
laboratory tests for, 1530–1532
methylhistidine excretion and, 1531
physical signs of, 1529t, 1529–1530
protein depletion in, 1528–1532, 1529t, 1532t
retinol-binding protein in, 1531
thyroxine-binding prealbumin in, 1531
transferrin in, 1530
urea nitrogen excretion in, 1531
vitamin deficiencies in, 1529, 1529t, 1531
Mambas, bite of, 1662t, 1667–1668
Management, ICU and, 59–66, 60t
illness trajectory and, 62, 62t
Mannitol, head injury treatment and, 1583–1584
kidney protected by, 1268–1269
Manometer, blood pressure measurement and, 251–252
Mantoux's test, interpretation of, 424
Marasmus, 1528
Marchiafava-Bignami disease, alcoholism and, 711
demyelination of, 711
Marijuana therapy, antiemetic action of, 1414
chemotherapy effects and, 1414
Masks, nosocomial infections and, 386–387, 387t
Mast cells, anaphylaxis and, 1654t, 1654–1655
asthma role of, 806, 807t
immune response role of, 1654t, 1654–1655
Masticator space, *477*
Maxillofacial trauma, air transport affecting, 43
Measles, encephalitis and, 400, 696
incidence of, 400
symptoms of, 400
MEDAS system, 103t
Mediastinum, aberrant air and, 889, 904
aortic rupture affecting, 1135, 1135–1137
barotrauma and, 904, 904
widened, 1135, 1135–1137
Mediators, anaphylaxis and, 1654t, 1654–1655, 1655t
basophil production of, 1654t, 1654–1655
drug modulation and, 1655t, 1656–1659

Mediators (Continued)
immune response and, 1652–1655, 1653, 1654t, 1655t
mast cell production of, 1654t, 1654–1655
Medical devices. See Devices.
Medical ethics. See Ethical issues.
Megakaryocytes, 1340
bone marrow failure and, 1343
neoplasia involving, 1365t, 1366
Membrane potential, motor neuron and, 673
Membranes, artificial, 1275–1276, 1276t, 1287
cellulose-derived, 1276t, 1276–1279
dialysis and, 1275–1279, 1276t, 1278, 1287
continuous arteriovenous, 1287–1288
hydrophobic thermoplastic, 1287
solute clearance rates of, 1276t, 1276–1279, 1278
Meningitis, 395–397
aseptic, 395t, 395–397
coxsackievirus and, 396
differential diagnosis of, 395, 459
HIV and, 396–397
lymphocytic (choriomeningitis), 396–397
mumps and, 396
poliovirus and, 396
symptoms of, 395–397, 459
bacterial, 454–464
antimicrobials in, 460t, 460–462, 461t
clinical presentation of, 457–458
corticosteroids in, 462–463
CSF effects in, 458t, 458–459
CT scan in, 458, 459, 460
diagnosis of, 458, 458t, 458–460
epidemiology of, 454–455
etiology of, 454–455
H. influenzae in, 454–457, 461t
headache in, 459–460
listerial, 454, 461t
meningococcal, 454–455, 461t
mortality rate in, 454–455
pathophysiology of, 455–457, 456
pneumococcal, 454, 461t
prophylaxis for, 463–464
Pseudomonas in, 454–455, 461t
resistant organisms in, 461–462
staphylococcal, 454–455
streptococcal, 454–455
symptoms of, 457–460
treatment of, 460t, 460–464
tuberculous, 428–429, 459
cancer patient and, 552
cryptococcal, 444–445
differential diagnosis in, 395, 459–460
fungal, 459–460
paralysis with, 395t, 396
rickettsial, 460
spirochetal, 459
symptoms of, 395, 457–458, 458t
trauma patient and, 558–559
viral, 395t, 395–397
varicella-zoster, 394–395
Meningococcal infections, bacteremia in, 457
meningitis due to, 454–455, 461t
rash in, 457
Meningoencephalitis, mumps with, 396
Mental status, hyperpyretic-rigidity syndrome and, 699
hypoglycemia and, 17
immunosuppressive drugs affecting, 1300–1301

Mental status (Continued)
legal issues and, 1734
neoplasia affecting, 1397t, 1397–1398
smoke inhalation and, 885
thiamine deficiency affecting, 634
trauma affecting, 14t
uremia affecting, 1270
Mercalli scale, 28, 28t
Mercury, abdominal pain due to, 1483, 1483t
Mercury chloride electrodes, 240, 240–241
Mesa effect, 98t
Mesentery, ischemia of, 1485–1489
abdominal pain of, 1479–1480, 1486–1487
management of, 1486, 1487–1488
pathophysiology of, 1485–1487
prognosis in, 1488–1489
Messengers, second, enterotoxins and, 1467, 1467t
ion transport and, 1466, 1466t, 1467
Metabolism, aerobic, 1231, 1232
anaerobic, 354, 355
burn injury acceleration of, 1624, 1624
glucose, 356, 1231–1233, 1232, 1233
water produced during, 1169
Metals, heavy, 681, 1483, 1483t
kidney failure due to, 1261t, 1262
neuropathy due to, 681
poisoning due to, 1483, 1483t
Metanephrine, 1319t, 1319–1320
pheochromocytoma and, 1325
Metaproterenol, asthma treated with, 809, 809t
Metformin, lactic acidosis caused by, 1237
Methanol, acidosis caused by, 1223, 1239, 1715, 1718t
formic acidosis caused by, 1715
metabolism of, 1715
poisoning due to, 712, 1239, 1714–1717, 1718t
products containing, 1714t
Methemoglobin, absorption spectrum of, 204
cyanide binding by, 51, 1712
oximetry and, 203, 204, 207, 244
Methotrexate, encephalopathy due to, 1416t, 1416–1417
gastrointestinal effects of, 1414t, 1414–1415
intrathecal, 1416t, 1416–1417
kidney failure and, 1265, 1407–1408
lung affected by, 1410–1411
side effects of, 1407–1408
Methoxyhydroxyphenylglycol, 1319t
Methyl tyrosine, pheochromocytoma treated with, 1326
Methyldopa, hemolytic anemia induced by, 1379t, 1380–1381
Methylhistidine, malnutrition affecting, 1531
Methylprednisolone, asthma treated with, 809t, 810
sepsis treated with, 373
Methylxanthines, asthma treated with, 810
Metolazone, diuresis using, 1165, 1165t
Metoprolol, arrhythmia treated with, 1055, 1056t
dosage for, 999t
drug interactions of, 1056t
myocardial ischemia and, 999t
pharmacokinetics of, 1689t
Metronidazole, colitis treated with, 507
meningitis therapy and, 461t
resistant organisms and, 614

Mexiletine, arrhythmia treated with, 1055, 1056t
drug interactions of, 1056t
Mezlocillin, enterococcal susceptibility to, 415t
MI. See Myocardial infarction (MI).
Michaelis-Menten equation order, 1688–1689
Military personnel, disasters and, 42
Miller blade, 111, 112
Miller Fisher syndrome, 679
Mill wheel murmur, 907
Mineral oil, lung affected by, 900
Mineralocorticoids, 1310–1317
deficiency of, 1314–1315, 1315t
metabolism of, 1310, 1311
physiologic actions of, 1311, 1311
potassium level and, 1184t, 1184–1185, 1186
regulatory factors for, 1310–1311, 1311
Minimal antimicrobial concentration, 618
bactericidal level and, 616–620, 618, 619
enterococcal isolates and, 415t
inhibitory level and, 415t, 616–620, 618, 619
Minnesota tube, 1449, 1450
Mitochondria, ATP production by, 354, 355
evolution and, 352
glucose metabolism in, 1232, 1233
glycerol phosphate shuttle in, 1235, 1235
glycolysis in, 356, 356–358, 358
oxygen radical production by, 950
Mitomycin, lung injury due to, 897t, 897–898, 1410
nephrotoxicity of, 1408
Mitotic cycle, chemotherapy and, 1403–1406, 1404t
Mitral valve, regurgitation and, MI and, 1009–1010, 1010t
Mittelschmerz, abdominal pain and, 1477
Mobitz's block, atrioventricular node and, 1058, 1059
Mollusks, envenomation by, 1676, 1676t
poisoning due to, 1672–1673
Monitoring. See also Capnography; Oximetry.
antimicrobial levels and, 1692t
arterial pressure and, 251–257, 253–256
balloon catheter and, 1079–1081, 1079–1082
blood pressure and, 251–257, 253–256
brain and, 222, 222–223, 223t, 230, 230–233
burn injury and, 1620–1622
cerebrovascular disease and, 222, 222–223, 223t, 230, 230–233
dialysis patient and, 1282–1283, 1283t
drug levels and, 1686–1701, 1692t, 1693t
fluid-filled system and, 253
head trauma and, 716, 1582, 1582t, 1582–1583
heatstroke patient and, 1630t
hemodynamic, 1079–1099, 1559t
historical aspects of, 1–4
intracranial pressure and, 227–230, 230, 625–626, 1582, 1582–1583
MI management and, 994, 995, 995t
nutrition and, 1542, 1542, 1549t, 1549–1550
pregnancy and, 1595–1596, 1596t, 1603t
septic shock and, 374, 374–375
venous pressure and, 1079–1081, 1079–1082
Monoclonal antibodies, kidney transplant and, 1294
OKT3, 1294

Monoclonal antibodies (Continued)
respiratory distress syndrome and, 828t, 836
Monocyte colony-stimulating factor, 1336t
Monocytes, 1340
burn injury affecting, 523
hematopoiesis and, 1336
Monocytosis, leukemia and, 1367
Mononeuropathy, monoplex, 678
Monoplegia, diagnosis in, 629
Morbillivirus, 392t
Morphine, street names for, 1711t
Morrhuate sodium, respiratory distress syndrome due to, 900–901
Mortality Probability Model, 85, 85t
Mortality rate, APACHE II score and, 83, 83t
aspiration and, 875
catheter-related infections and, 606
colitis and, pseudomembranous, 503
CPR and, 118, 120t, 123, 124, 125t, 126, 126
diabetic ketoacidosis and, 1251
drug poisoning and, 1702
hypocalcemia effect on, 1200–1201, 1202
ICU and, 1731–1732
illness severity scoring and, 77t, 78t, 82–85, 83t, 85t
maternal, 1593
meningitis and, bacterial, 454–455
MI grading and, 77t, 77–78, 78t
multiple organ system failure and, 343, 343t
pneumonia and, 480, 486
poisoning and, 1702
probability model and, 85, 85t
pulmonary embolism and, 857, 857
respiratory distress syndrome and, 824, 824–827
respiratory failure and, 802
seizures and, status epilepticus, 667, 667
sepsis and, 295, 301, 311, 365
Simplified Acute Physiology Score and, 82–83, 83t
trauma patient and, 1574, 1574, 1575
MOSF. See Multiple organ system failure (MOSF).
Mosquitoes, viruses transmitted by, 397–399, 398t, 403–405
Motor system, coma evaluation and, 637
de-efferentation and, 635
evoked potentials of, 231–232, 624–625
respiratory muscle innervation and, 765
spinal cord levels and, 717
Motor unit, 672–674
failure of, 674–676
Mouth, candidiasis affecting, 439–440
cellulitis and, 477, 478
infections in, 439, 477, 477–479, 541
stomatitis and, 541
Movement, adventitious, 628–629
brain death preceding, 646–647
coma evaluation and, 635, 637
encephalopathy affecting, 635, 637
eye and, 636–637, 710–711
hyperpyretic-rigidity syndrome and, 698–699
jerking, twitching, shaking, 628–629
neuropathy and, 628–629
Mucolytics, inhalation therapy using, 962
Mucormycosis, 445–446
cutaneous, 445
diagnosis of, 445
gastrointestinal, 445
nervous system and, 445
pulmonary, 445

Mucormycosis (Continued)
rhino-orbitocerebral, 445, 473–474
treatment of, 445–446
Mucosa, gastrointestinal tract and, 1442–1443
hemorrhage of, 1442–1443
ischemia of, intubation causing, 116
stress-related disorder of, 1442–1443
Mucositis, bone marrow transplant agents and, 1341–1352
chemotherapy-induced, 1414t, 1414–1415
radiation causing, 1461
Mucus, lung defense mechanism and, 750, 752
pulmonary plug of, 196
Mueller-Hinton broth, cation content of, 613
susceptibility testing and, 613
Multicasualty incidents. See Disasters.
Multifactorial Cardiac Risk Index, 79, 80t
Multiple organ system failure (MOSF), 340–351
circulation and, 345–348, 347, 347t, 349t, 349–350
clinical stages of, 341, 342t
definitions in, 340–341, 342t, 557
failure criteria in, 342t
incidence of, 340–341
individual organs in, 342t, 345–348
management of, 348–351, 349t, 350
mortality rate and, 343, 343t
nervous system in, 342t, 348
nosocomial infection and, 348, 349
nutrition in, 350
pathogenesis of, 343–345, 344
patterns in, 341, 341, 342t
respiratory distress syndrome and, 827t, 828t, 836–837
risk factors for, 341–343, 342t
sepsis and, 340–351, 346
splanchnic organs in, 342t, 348
trauma patient and, 557–558
Mumps, 396
encephalitis and, 696
meningoencephalitis with, 396
natural history of, 396
transmission of, 396
Mupirocin, catheter-related infection and, 606
Murmurs, air embolism and, 907
Cruveilhier-Baumgarten, 1446
endocarditis and, 493
mill wheel, 907
portal hypertension and, 1446
Muscle, abscess in, 452
clostridial myonecrosis and, 451–452
compartment syndrome and, 1149–1151
cramps, 1628
crush syndrome and, 34
electrical injury to, 1646, 1646t, 1649, 1649
heatstroke effects and, 1628
infections of, 449t, 450–452
malnutrition effects in, 1531–1532
necrosis affecting, 451–452, 563
respiratory, 723, 723, 731, 731–732, 763–765, 765, 767
rhabdomyolysis affecting, 1182, 1188, 1214, 1217, 1629
TNF effects in, 317t
trauma and, 34, 1149–1151
Muscle relaxants, endotracheal intubation and, 18, 110–111
kidney failure dose adjustment for, 1309t
Muscular dystrophy, Duchenne's, 686

Muscular dystrophy (Continued)
myotonic, 686
Mushrooms, abdominal pain due to, 1483t, 1484
Mustard agents, chemical warfare use of, 48
clinical effects of, 52
decontamination for, 52
historical aspects of, 48
nitrogen, 48
sulfur, 48
Mutism, akinetic, 635, 644
botulism causing, 568
Myasthenia, 682–684
Lambert-Eaton, 682–683
Myasthenia gravis, 683–684
diagnosis of, 683
management of, 683–684
pathophysiology of, 683
plasmapheresis in, 1425, 1426t
preoperative care and, 1553
respiratory failure due to, 766–767
Mycobacterial disease, avium-intracellulare, 430–431
cancer patient and, 550
chelonei, 431
diagnosis of, 430
epidemiology of, 430
fortuitum, 431
gordonae, 431–432
kansasii, 431
pathogen classification and, 430t
rapid growers in, 431
tuberculosis as. See Tuberculosis.
Mydriasis, coma evaluation and, 636
Myelinolysis, 677–682, 711
Myeloblasts, leukocytosis due to, 1360, 1360–1362, 1361
rigidity of, 1361
Myelocytes, leukemia and, 1356t, 1363–1367, 1364t
maturation of, 1404
Myelodysplastic syndrome, 1364t, 1366, 1367
clinical manifestations of, 1366
management of, 1367
Myelosuppression, chemotherapy-induced, 1403–1406
mitotic cycle and, 1403–1406, 1404t
Myocardial infarction (MI), 989–1012
air embolism causing, 907
cocaine causing, 1047
conduction abnormalities in, 1007, 1007t
diagnosis of, 991–994, 992t
ECG in, 991–992, 993
echocardiography in, 993–994, 994
enzyme levels in, 992–993, 993t
history in, 991, 992t
expansion of, 994, 994, 1009, 1011
heart pump failure in, 1007–1008, 1008t
hemodynamic profile in, 1098t
management of, 995–1012
analgesia in, 996t, 996–997
angioplasty in, 1004, 1004–1005
anticoagulants in, 1001–1003, 1002, 1003
balloon flotation catheter in, 995, 995t
beta-adrenergic blockers in, 997–998, 998t, 999t
calcium channel blockers in, 997, 997t
catecholamines in, 1007–1008, 1008t
complications in, 1006t, 1006–1010
diet in, 995
general measures in, 994–995, 995t
initial, 1005–1006, 1006t
intra-aortic balloon pump in, 1005

Myocardial infarction (MI) (Continued)
  lidocaine therapy in, 996, 996t
  monitoring in, 994, 995, 995t
  nitrate therapy in, 995–996, 996t
  oxygen therapy in, 995
  pacemaker in, 1007, 1007t
  predischarge, 1012
  specific measures in, 995–1006
  surgical approach in, 1003–1004, 1004t
  thrombolytic agents in, 999–1001, 999–1001
  vasodilators in, 1007–1008, 1008t
  non–Q wave, 989–992, 1011, 1011, 1012
  pain due to, 991, 992t, 996–997, 1005, 1006t, 1011
  pathogenesis of, 989–991
  perioperative risk and, 1558
  radionuclide studies in, 994
  recurrent, 1011, 1011, 1011t
  respiratory failure and, 788–789
  right ventricular, 1028–1030
    clinical presentation of, 1029
    diagnosis of, 1029, 1029
    pathophysiology of, 1028–1029
    treatment in, 1030
  rupture following, 1009
  severity classification for, 77t, 77–78
Myocardial ischemia, 989–1012
  atherosclerosis and, 989–991, 990, 991
  causes of, 989t, 989–991, 990, 991
  differential diagnosis in, 992t
  pain due to, 991, 992t, 996–997, 1005, 1006t, 1011
  radiation therapy causing, 1413
Myocardium. See also Cardiomyopathy.
  acidosis affecting, 1039, 1039t, 1039–1041, 1040, 1040t
  action potential of, 1050, 1050–1051
  contractility of, 1039, 1039t, 1039–1041, 1040, 1040t
    fiber-shortening work and, 1016, 1016–1017
    wall stress and, 1016, 1016–1017
  contusion to, 891
  CPR outcome and, 123–124
  depressant substances and, 330–333, 331, 333
  heart failure response in, 1016, 1016–1018
  myocyte of, 331, 331
  perfusion pressure in, 123–124
  rupture of, 1009
  septic shock and, 325–327, 325–332, 331–333
Myoclonus, 628
  brain hypoxia and, 642, 646–647
  encephalopathy and, 637
  multifocal, 637
  status epilepticus and, 664
Myoglobin, kidney failure due to, 1261t, 1263
Myoglobinuria, crush syndrome and, 34
Myonecrosis. See also Rhabdomyolysis.
  clostridial, 451–452
    trauma wound and, 563
  synergistic nonclostridial anaerobic, 452
Myopathy, drug-induced, 686
  EMG in, 626
  genetic factors in, 686
  hereditary, 686
  immune, 685–686
  infectious, 685–686
  inflammatory, 685–686
  metabolic disorders and, 684–685
  nutrition and, 684–685
  pathophysiology of, 684

Myosis, coma evaluation and, 636
Myositis, anaerobic streptococcal, 452
Myotonia, hereditary, 686
Myxedema, 1161
  catecholamines and, 1323–1324
  coma of, 1323–1324

N

Nadolol, dosage for, 999t
  myocardial ischemia and, 999t
Nafcillin, meningitis therapy and, 461t, 462
  pharmacokinetics of, 1689t
Nairovirus, 392t
Naloxone, dosage for, 1711
  endotoxin effects and, 306–307, 373
  sepsis treated with, 306–307, 373
Narcotics. See also Drug abuse.
  illicit, 1711, 1711t
  street names for, 1711t
Nasogastric intubation, duodenum and, 269
  enteral nutrition and, 1540, 1540–1542, 1541
  esophageal varices and, 170–172, 171, 1449, 1450
  malplacement in, 264–269, 267–269
  radiography and, 264–269, 267–269
  Sengstaken-Blakemore tube and, 170–172, 171
Nasopharynx, defense mechanisms of, 749, 749
National Disaster Medical System, 41
Natriuresis, drugs eliciting, 1164–1166, 1165t
Natriuretic hormone, atrial, 1156, 1158
  sodium balance and, 1156, 1158
Natural killer cells, 1340
Near-infrared spectroscopy, brain oxygen and, 231, 231, 231t
Neck, anatomy of, 477
  emergent vascular disorders in, 1145–1148
  infection in, deep, 477, 477–479
  trauma to, 1578t, 1579t, 1584
Necrosis, clostridial infection causing, 451–452
  fasciitis with, 450–451, 563, 576–577, 1611
  muscle affected by, 451–452, 563
  pancreatitis causing, 1504
Needle stick, HIV transmission and, 591, 591t, 597
Negotiated order, ICU management and, 64
Neisseria, meningitis and, 454–455, 461t
Neomycin, burn injury and, 526
Neonate, care units for, 2
  colitis resistance in, 502
  HIV exposure of, 591, 591t
  listeriosis in, 419–420
  oxygen toxicity in, 954
  status epilepticus seizures in, 664t, 665, 671
Neoplasia, 1393–1417
  acute effects of, 1393–1402
    cardiovascular, 1393–1396
    metabolic, 1400–1402
    neurologic, 1397–1400
    pulmonary, 1396–1397
    urologic, 1400
  cardiac tamponade caused by, 1395t, 1395–1396, 1396t
  electrolytes affected by, 1400t, 1400–1402, 1401t
  hemolytic anemia with, 1372t, 1374–1375

Neoplasia (Continued)
  hemoptysis due to, 1396–1397
  hypercalcemia due to, 1204–1205
  hypoglycemia due to, 1402
  impaired immunity in, 546–548
  infections and, 545–554, 546t, 550t, 553t
  intracranial pressure and, 1397t, 1397–1398
  leptomeningeal disease and, 1398
  lymphocytic, 1367t, 1367–1368
  mental status affected by, 1397t, 1397–1398
  myelocytic, 1363–1368, 1364t, 1365t, 1367t
  pericardial, 1395–1396
  polycythemic, 1364–1366, 1365t
  preoperative care and, 1567–1568
  seizures due to, 1398
  spinal cord compression due to, 1398–1399
  therapy-induced complications of, 1403–1417
  thrombocytic, 1366
  vena cava obstruction due to, 1393–1395, 1394t, 1395t
Nephritis, allergic, 1264t, 1264–1265
  drug-induced, 1264t, 1264–1265
  interstitial, 1264t, 1264–1265
Nephron, acid-base regulation and, 1220–1221, 1221
  sodium excretion and, 1156, 1158–1159
Nephropathy, chemotherapy-induced, 1406–1408
  radiation-induced, 1408
  uric acid causing, 1406–1407
Nephrotic syndrome, sodium balance in, 1162t, 1163
Nernst equation, 241
Nerve agents, 48, 51–52
  antidotes for, 49, 52
  clinical effects of, 51–52
  historical aspects of, 48
Nerve endings, motor neuron and, 673
Nerve fibers. See also Neurons.
  conduction studies and, 626
Nerve roots, demyelination in, 677–682
Nervous system. See also Neuropathy.
  activation of, 631–632
  candidiasis affecting, 437
  clinical testing of, 621–630
  decompression sickness and, 906
  dialysis and, 1270
  drug overdose affecting, 1703t–1705t, 1703–1705
  infection in. See also Encephalitis; Meningitis.
    bacterial, 454–464
    drug abuse patient and, 566–568, 567t, 574
    granulocytopenia and, 542
    transplant patient and, 584
    viral, 395t, 395–401
  mechanical ventilation and, 946, 946t
  metabolism in, ATP and, 632–633
    oxygen and, 632
  multiple organ system failure and, 342t, 348
  TNF effects in, 317t
  transmitter substances of, 631, 667, 667
  uremia effects in, 1270
Neuraminidase, influenza virus and, 391
Neurodes, artificial neural networks and, 103, 103, 104
Neuroleptics, alcoholism treated with, 709t, 709–710
  hyperpyretic rigidity due to, 698–704

Neuroleptics *(Continued)*
  malignant syndrome due to, 698–704
Neuromuscular disease, 672–686
  approach to patient with, 674–676
  burn injury and, 1625
  calcium level and, 1200
  magnesium level and, 1207
  respiratory failure due to, 763t, 765–767
  support groups for, 674
Neuromuscular junction, 673–674
  disorders of, 673–676
  dysfunction detection in, 626
  jitter and, 626
  toxins affecting, 683
Neurons, energy requirements of, 632–633
  hypoxia effects in, 639–640
  motor, alpha, 673
    anatomy of, 673
    disorders of, 673–677
    functioning of, 673–674
  seizure cascade in, 667, *667*
Neuropathy, 677–682
  axonal, 680
  botulism causing, 568, 682
  chemotherapy-induced, 1416t, 1416–1417
  demyelinating, 677–682
  diagnostic testing and, 621–630
  dysautonomic, 672–673, 681–682
  electrical injury and, 1646t, 1647, 1649
  evoked potentials and, 231t, 231–232, 624–625
  Guillain-Barré, 679–680
  hypothermia causing, 1637
  immunosuppressive drugs causing, 1300–1301
  inflammatory, 680, 681
  kidney transplant and, 1300–1301
  meningitis and, 457, 459–460
  metabolic, 680–681
  movement disorders and, 628–630
  multiple organ system failure and, 348
  pathophysiology of, 677–678
  pregnancy and, 1607–1608
  preoperative care and, 1552–1553
  toxic substances and, 680, 681, 683, 1522–1524, 1664, 1668t
  unresponsive patient and, 627–628
Neurotoxins, 682–683
  hepatic encephalopathy and, 1522–1524, 1523t
  snake venom and, 1663–1664, 1668, 1668t
Neurotransmitters, consciousness and, 631
  reticular formation and, 631
  seizure cascade and, 667, *667*
Neutropenia, abdominal pain and, 1481
  chemotherapy-induced, 1404–1405
  enterocolitis and, 1481
Neutrophils, *1340.* See also *Granulocytes;*
    Leukocytes.
  burn injury and, 522t, 523
  hematopoiesis and, 1336
  maturation of, 1404
  sepsis role of, 309
New York Heart Association, Functional
    Classification of, 78t, 78–79
Nicardipine, dosage for, 998t
  hypertensive emergency and, 1331t, 1332
  MI and, 998t
Nicoladoni-Branham sign, 1149
Nicotinic acid, pellagra and, 711
Nifedipine, angina and, 997, 998t
  dosage for, 998t
  pharmacokinetics of, 1689t
  pregnancy and, 1605

Nightingale, Florence, 1
NIH Consensus Statement on Cesarean
    Delivery, 72
Nikolsky's sign, 412, 1355
Nitrates, MI and, 995–996, 996t
  side effects of, 995
Nitric oxide, endothelium-derived, 353
  hypotension caused by, 353
Nitrites, cyanide antidote role of, 1712
Nitrofurantoin, lung injury due to, 897t, 898–899, *899*
Nitrogen, atmospheric content of, 902
  solubility of, 902
Nitrogen mustard, 48, 52
Nitroglycerin, dosage for, 996t, 1331t
  forms of, 996t
  heart failure treated with, *1021*, 1021–1022
  hypertensive emergency and, 1331, 1331t
  MI and, 995–996, 996t
  ointment, 996t
  sublingual, 996t
  transdermal, 996t
Nitroprusside, cyanide produced from, 1331, *1332*
  heart failure therapy and, *1021*, 1021–1022
  hypertensive emergency treated with, 1330t, 1330–1331, 1331t, *1332*
  lactic acidosis caused by, 1238
  Laetrile and, 1238
  poisoning due to, 1711–1712
  shock treated with, 985
Nitrosoureas, 1409t, 1415t
Nodes of Ranvier, 673
Noise (electronic), arterial pressure
    monitoring and, 253
  expert systems affected·by, 100t, 100–101, *102*
No-reflow phenomenon, 1583, *1583*
Norepinephrine, catabolism of, *1318*, 1318–1319
  measurement of, 1319t, 1319–1320, 1320t, 1321t
  metabolism of, *1699*
  pharmacokinetics of, 1693t, 1696–1698, 1697t, *1699*
  receptors for, *1319*, 1319t, 1320–1322, 1321t, 1322t
  septic shock therapy and, 375–377, *376*, 376t
  synthesis of, *1318*, 1318
Normal saline, fluid resuscitation using, 131, 131t
  ionic composition of, 131t
Nosocomial disorders, infection and. See
    Infections, nosocomial.
  stroke and, 650t, 650–651
Nuclear studies. See *Scintigraphy.*
Nurses. See also *Personnel.*
  standards developed by, 75–76, 76t
Nutrition, 1528–1550
  assessment of, 1528–1532, 1529t, 1532t
  body weight and, 1529t, 1529–1530, 1532t
  burn patient and, 1624, *1624*
  cardiac failure and, 1547–1548
  COPD patient and, 802
  dialysis patient and, 1273–1274
  energy requirements and, 1533, 1533t
  enteral, 1534–1543
    access and delivery for, *1540*, 1540–1542, *1541*
    aspiration due to, 1543
    complications of, 1542–1543
    contraindications for, 1534

Nutrition *(Continued)*
    dietary formulations for, *1537*, 1537–1540, 1538t
    elemental formulas in, *1537*, 1538t, 1538–1539
    gastrointestinal barrier and, *1535*, 1535–1536
    indications for, 1534t, 1534–1535, *1536*
    monitoring of, 1542, *1542*
    patient assessment for, *1535*, 1536–1537
    polymeric formulas in, *1537*, 1537–1538, 1538t
  glucose regulation and, 1251–1252
  hepatic failure and, 1539, 1547
  immune enhancement and, 1539
  kidney failure and, 1273–1274, 1539, 1546–1547, 1547t
  laboratory tests and, 1530–1532
  neuropathy and, 681
  parenteral, 1543–1550
    amino acids in, 1547t, 1548t
    catheter sepsis and, 1550
    central venous access for, 1543–1545, *1544, 1545*
    electrolytes in, 1546t
    glucose in, 1547t, 1548t
    indications for, 1543, 1543t
    metabolic monitoring in, 1549t, 1549–1550
    peripheral venous, 1548t, 1548–1549
    solution formulation for, 1545t–1548t, 1545–1549
  preoperative care and, 1570
  protein requirements and, 1533, 1533t
  respiratory failure and, 1539, 1548, 1548t
  stress and, 1539
Nutritional Advisor system, 98
Nutritional recovery syndrome, 1183, 1207, 1213
Nystagmus, coma evaluation and, 636–637

O

Obesity, hypoventilation and, 769–771, 781
  respiratory failure due to, 769–771, 781
Obstetric disorders. See under *Pregnancy.*
Obstruction, airway. See *Airway, obstruction
    of.*
  biliary tract, 1490–1493, *1493*
    cholangitis and, 1494–1495
  intestinal, abdominal pain and, 1475t, 1476–1477, 1483
    drug smuggler packets and, 1482–1483
    false, 1479
  pancreatic duct, 1491
  urinary tract, extrarenal, 1265t, 1265–1266
    intrarenal, 1265, 1265t
    kidney failure due to, 1265t, 1265–1266
    kidney transplant and, 1293
    neoplasia causing, 1400
    stones and, 1265t, 1265–1266
Obstructive sleep apnea syndrome, *778*, 778–781
Octopus, venom of, 1676
Odors, 635
  breath, coma evaluation and, 635
    poisoning and, 1718t
    solvents and, 1718t
  cellulitis and, 450
  cyanide and, 48
  gangrene and, 452

Odors *(Continued)*
  mustard gas and, 48
  phosgene gas and, 48
Odynophagia, candidiasis and, 439
Ohm's law, skin resistance and, 1646
Oil, toxicity of, pulmonary hypertension
    due to, 844
OKT3, kidney transplant and, 1294
Oliguria, pregnancy-induced, 1606, 1606t
Oncotic pressure, 130. See also *Osmotic
    pressure.*
  capillary-interstitial exchange and, *1155,*
    1155
  pulmonary edema and, 911, 916
  Starling forces and, 1155, *1155*
Ondansetron, 1414
Opioids, illicit, 1711, 1711t
Optodes, blood gas measurement using,
    247–248, *248*
  quenching and, 248
Oral airway, size estimation for, 110
Orbit, anatomy of, *467*
  apex syndrome of, 473
  infection of, 445, 472–474, 475t, 476
  sinusitis and, 475t, 476
Orders, do-not-resuscitate, 1736–1738
  expert system management of, 101
Organ donation, heart and, 1126–1127
Organ system failure. See *Multiple organ
    system failure (MOSF).*
Organ transplantation. See *Transplantation.*
Organophosphates (OP), antidotes for, 52
  chemical warfare use of, 48
  clinical effects of, 51–52
  neuropathy due to, 681, 683
Oropharyngeal space, *477*
  infection in, *477,* 477–479
Oropharynx, bacterial adherence to, 751
  defense mechanisms of, 749, *749*
Orthopoxvirus, 392t
Ortner's syndrome, 845
Osborn wave, hypothermia and, *1635,*
    1635–1636
Osler's nodes, 493
Osmolality. See also *Hypertonicity;
    Hypotonicity.*
  cerebral edema and, 1251
  colloids and, 137t
  fluid distribution and, 129–131, *130*
  idiogenic agents and, 1251
  intracranial pressure reduction and, 463
  thirst and, 1170
  tonicity and, 1168–1169
  urinary, 1169
Osmotic pressure, alveolus and, *788, 789*
  colloid, 129–131, *130,* 143–145, *144*
  hemoglobin emulsion and, 155, *155, 156*
  protein concentration and, 129–131, *130*
  pulmonary edema and, 143–145, *144*
Osteoclasts, *1340*
Osteomyelitis, cancer patient and, 552
  candidal, 437
  sinusitis and, 475t, 476
Outcome prediction. See *Severity
    classification.*
Ovulation, abdominal pain of, 1477
Owl's eye inclusions, cytomegalovirus and,
    394
Oxacillin, meningitis therapy and, 461t, 462
  susceptibility testing and, 612
Oxidative phosphorylation, 358, *358, 359*
Oximetry, 203–208
  accuracy of, 205–207, *206, 207*
  bilirubin interference in, 244
  ear and, 203, 205, *206*
  error sources in, 205–207, *206, 207*

Oximetry *(Continued)*
  instrumentation for, *244*
  physiologic basis of, 203–205, *204*
  pulse, 203–208, *204–207*
  theory of, 203–205, *204–206,* 243–244
Oxygen. See also *Hypoxemia; Hypoxia;
    Ischemia.*
  airway monitoring of, 215–217, *217*
  altitude and, 43, *44*
  arteriovenous difference in, 222t, *230*
  brain monitoring and, *230,* 230–233, *231*
  cell energy transduction and, 353–354,
    355
  cerebrum and, 222t, 222–223, 223t, 227t,
    230, 230–233, *231*
  consumption of, cardiac output measure-
      ment and, 1093
    hypothermia and, 217, *218*
    measurement of, 359
    shock and, 979–980, *980*
    supply-dependent, 360, 361, *361*
    supply-independent, 360, *360, 361*
  cutaneous, 217–220, *219*
  delivery of, cerebrum and, 222, 222t
    formula for, 222
    hypothermia effects and, 1636, *1636*
  end-tidal, 217, *217*
  evolution of, 352–353
  extraction ratio and, 359–360
  free radicals of, *950,* 950–952, 951t, 952t,
    953
    cell quenching of, 951, 952t
    detoxification of, 951, 952t, 955, 955t
    formation of, 950, *950*
    lung production of, 950, *950*
    scavengers for, 951, 952t
    sepsis role of, 373
    tissue damage due to, 950–952, 951t,
      952t, *953*
  helium mixed with, 962
  measurement of, electrode for, 242–243,
    243
    gas analyzer in, *240,* 242–243, *243*
    halothane interference with, 239
    oximetry and, 203–208, *204–207,* 243–
      244, *244*
  nervous system metabolism and, 632
  sepsis and, *328,* 328, 354–363, *355, 358–
    362,* 373
  singlet, 950
  tension, altitude effect on, 43, *44*
    bronchoscopy effect on, 193, *194*
    cardiac output measurement and, 1093
    end-capillary, *741,* 741–742
    increased. See *Hyperoxia; Oxygen, toxicity
      of.*
    inspired oxygen content and, 786–787,
      787
    oxyhemoglobin and, 745, *745*
    P₅₀ value and, 245
    perfusion and, 739–743, *739–744*
    respiratory distress syndrome and,
      818–819, 828–830, *830*
    respiratory failure and, 755–758
    shunting and, 786–787, *787*
    ventilation and, 739–743
  therapy, air embolism and, 908–909, *909*
    concentration and, 950, 955
    COPD patient and, 797–798
    decompression sickness and, 906–907,
      909
    delivery systems for, *964,* 964–965
    gas supply monitoring in, 215–216
    high-flow, *964,* 965
    hyperbaric, 906–909, *909*
    hypoxemia and, 963–964

Oxygen *(Continued)*
    indications for, 963t, 963–964
    low-flow, *964,* 964–965
    mask in, 964–965
    nasal cannula in, 964
    pulmonary hypertension and, 846
    shock and, 983–984
  toxicity of, 949–956
    antioxidants and, 951, 952t, 955, 955t
    clinical manifestations of, 951t, 954t,
      954–955
    cytotoxic effects and, 949–954, 951t,
      952t, *953*
    diagnosis of, 954t, 954–955
    free radicals and, 373, *950,* 950–952,
      951t, 952t, *953*
    neonate and, 954
    prevention of, 955
    respiratory failure due to, 949, 954t,
      954–956
    secondary changes due to, *953,* 953–
      954
    surfactant affected by, 953–954
    therapy in, 952t, 955, 955t
  transport, 203, 352–353, *359–362,* 359–
      363
    artificial blood and, 151–159
    fluorocarbon emulsion and, 151–153,
      151–154, 153t
    hemoglobin emulsion and, 153–159,
      154t, *154–157*
    physiologic mechanism for, 352–353,
      359, 359–363
    plasma and, 151, *151*
    preoperative maximization of, *362*
    ratio with consumption, *360,* 360–361,
      361
    RBCs and, *151*
    whole blood and, 151, *152, 154,* 154t
Oxyhemoglobin, 203, *204.* See also
    Hemoglobin.
  dissociation curve for, 745, *1636*
  hypothermia effects and, 1636, *1636*
  P₅₀ value and, 245

P

P wave, atrial, 1060–1070, *1061*
Pacemakers, code for, 1059–1060
  defibrillation damage to, 120
  endogenous, 1055
  historical aspects of, 3
  indications for, 1060t
  MI and, 1007, 1007t, 1060t
  perioperative risk and, 1556, 1556t
  permanent, 1059–1060, 1060t
  radiography and, 269–270
  sinus nodal, 1055
  temporary, 1059, 1060t
  transvenous catheter with, 184–186, *185,*
    269–270
Paddles, defibrillator, *119,* 119–120
PAE (postantibiotic effect), 615, *617,* 618
  leukocytes in, 618
Pain, 992t, 1006t, 1475t, 1483t
  abdominal, 1474–1484
    acute, 1474–1484
    AIDS and, 1482
    aortic aneurysm and, 1479–1480
    aortic dissection and, 1479–1480
    appendicitis and, 1475t, 1476
    approach in, 1474–1476
    cause and frequency of, 1475, 1475t
    cholangitis and, 1494
    cholecystitis and, 1477–1478

Pain (Continued)
colitis and, 1479
colon perforation and, 1478–1479
colon pseudo-obstruction and, 1479
cytomegalovirus infection and, 1481
false acute, 1484
gallstones and, 1491
graft-versus-host reaction and, 1481
gynecologic disorders and, 1475t, 1477
immunocompromised patient and, 1480–1482
kidney failure and, 1482
kidney stones and, 1480
kidney transplant and, 1480–1482
leukemia patient and, 1482
lymphoma patient and, 1482
mesenteric ischemia and, 1479–1480, 1486–1487
neutropenic enterocolitis and, 1481
nonspecific, 1475t, 1476
obstruction and, 1475t, 1476–1477
pancreatitis and, 1478, 1491, 1500
testicular torsion and, 1480
toxic agents causing, 1483t, 1483–1484
ulcer and, 1389
urologic disorders and, 1480
wall bleeding and, 1484
back, spinal cord compression causing, 1398–1400, 1399
chest, differential diagnosis in, 992t
myocardial ischemia and, 991, 992t, 996–997, 1005, 1006t, 1011
noncoronary causes of, 992t
pneumothorax and, 992t
pulmonary hypertension and, 845
trauma and, 1586–1587
decompression sickness and, 905–906
fasciitis and, 576–577
pleural, differential diagnosis and, 992t
Palsy, cranial nerve, 457
meningitis causing, 457
Pancreas, trauma injury to, 1589
Pancreatitis, abdominal pain of, 1478, 1491, 1500
associated conditions of, 1500, 1500t
clinical presentation of, 1500–1501
complications of, 1503t, 1503–1504
drug-induced, 1500, 1500t
etiology of, 1499–1500, 1500t
gallstones causing, 1490–1493, 1493, 1493t, 1494t
Glasgow system and, 1502, 1502t
hypocalcemia caused by, 1203
imaging studies in, 1501–1502
kidney transplant and, 1299
laboratory studies in, 1501–1502, 1502t
magnesium depletion in, 1208
medical approach in, 1502–1503
necrotizing, 1504
pathogenesis of, 1499, 1500t
prognosis in, 1502, 1502t
pseudocysts in, 1503–1504
radiography in, 1491–1493, 1493, 1493t, 1494t
severity classification for, 79, 79t, 1502, 1502t
surgical approach in, 1504
Pancuronium, mechanical ventilation and, 811t
pharmacokinetics of, 1691t
Pancytopenia, bone marrow transplant and, 1352–1353
infection and, 1352–1353
Papaverine, mesenteric angiography with, 1487, 1488, 1489
Papillary muscle, MI affecting, 1010, 1010t

Papillary muscle (Continued)
rupture of, 1010, 1010t
Paracentesis, 167–169
complications of, 168, 168t
contraindications for, 168
indications for, 168, 168t
procedure for, 168–169, 169
therapeutic, 169
Paraldehyde, 1719
alcoholism treated with, 709, 709t
lactic acidosis caused by, 1239
metabolism of, 1719, 1719
pharmacokinetics of, 669t
poisoning due to, 1718t, 1719
seizure treated with, 668t, 668–671, 669t
Paralysis, botulism causing, 568
brain herniation causing, 715
calcium and, 1183–1184
cerebral blood flow and, 222
coxsackievirus and, 396
diaphragm affected by, 767
drugs inducing, 811t, 1309t
enterovirus causing, 396
meningitis and, 395t, 396
periodic, 1183–1184
poliomyelitis and, 396
shellfish poisoning and, 1672–1673
slight and generalized, 629–630, 715
vocal cords affected by, 116, 568, 968
Paralyzing agents, 1309t
dose adjustment for, 1309t
mechanical ventilation and, 811t
Paramedics, certification of, 10
deployment strategies for, 11
on-line physician direction for, 11
triage strategies for, 12–14, 13, 14t
Paramyxovirus, 392t
Paraplegia, diagnosis in, 629
Parasitism, IgE and, 1652
strongyloidiasis as, 542, 580
transplant patient and, 580
Parasympathetic nervous system, drug overdose and, 1703–1704, 1704t
Parathyroid hormone, calcium and, 1198, 1198–1199
kidney transplant and, 1297
Parenteral nutrition. See Nutrition, parenteral.
Paresis, brain herniation causing, 715
differential diagnosis of, 629–630
generalized, 629–630
Parkinson's disease, preoperative care and, 1553
Parkland formula, hypotonic resuscitation and, 1619
Parotid gland, 477
mumps and, 396
Partial thromboplastin time (PTT). See also Bleeding time.
heparin therapy and, 855
Pathogens, 614, 614t
antimicrobial selection and, 614t, 614–620
surgery patient and, 1570–1572, 1571t, 1572t
susceptibility of, 614t, 614–620
viral, 392t
Patients, decision making by, 1725–1726, 1732–1744
geriatric. See Age.
ICU access of, 5, 62–67
transportation of, 43–45, 54–57
Pattern generators, respiratory, 765, 777
Pattern recognition, artificial neural networks and, 103–106
Pediatric Risk of Mortality (PRISM), 85

PEEP. See Positive end-expiratory pressure (PEEP).
Pellagra, alcoholism causing, 711
treatment of, 711
Pelvis, open book fracture of, 1589, 1589–1590
trauma injury to, 1580t, 1581t, 1589, 1589–1590
Pendelluft theory, 769, 771
flail chest injury and, 888
Penetrating Abdominal Trauma Index, 1575
Penetrating trauma, arteriovenous fistula and, 1149, 1150
heart affected by, 14–15
intra-abdominal abscess and, 561
pregnancy and, 1600
prehospital care in, 14–15
spinal injury following, 15
sucking chest wound due to, 15–16
Penicillins, hemolytic anemia induced by, 1379t, 1380, 1380t
kidney failure dose adjustment for, 1306t
liver failure dose adjustment for, 1690t
meningitis therapy and, 460t, 460–462, 461t
pathogen susceptibility to, 415t, 614t
pharmacokinetics of, 1690t, 1694
resistant organisms and, enterococcal, 415
staphylococcal, 410–411, 411t
streptococcal, 419
staphylococcal infection and, 410–411, 411t
Pentamidine, Pneumocystis pneumonia and, 595–596, 596t
Pentastarch, fluid resuscitation using, 135–136
leukapheresis using, 136
Pentobarbital, alcoholism treated with, 709t
Pentoxifylline, sepsis effects treated with, 372
Perfluorocarbon emulsions, 151, 151–153, 152, 153t
artificial blood role of, 151, 151–153, 152, 152t, 153t
Perfusion, alveolar, 208
capnography role of, 208, 208–209, 209
circulatory regulation of, 979
distribution of, 737–738, 738
gravity effect on, 737–738, 738
kidney failure and, 1267–1268
lung disease and, 738–739, 739t
pulmonary embolism and, 850–852, 851, 852
shock and, 978–979, 979
ventilation and, 737–738, 738, 740–746
clinical assessment of, 743, 743–747
dead space and, 742–743
mismatch in, 742–746, 743–747
normal matching of, 740, 740–746, 741
ratio of, 740, 740–746, 741
shunt flow and, 741–742, 743, 744
Pericardiocentesis, 172–174
complications of, 172, 173t
contraindications for, 172
indications for, 172
procedure for, 173–174, 174
tamponade treated with, 1034–1035, 1035, 1396, 1396t
Pericardiotomy, inelasticity treated with, 1036–1037, 1396t
syndrome following, 1036
Pericarditis, 1031–1037
acute, 1031–1032, 1032, 1032t

Pericarditis *(Continued)*
  chemotherapy-induced, 1412t, 1412–1413
  constrictive, 1036–1037, *1037*
    diagnosis of, 1036–1037, *1037*
    symptoms in, 1036–1037, *1037*
  effusions and, *1033–1035*, 1033–1036
  etiology of, 1031–1032, 1032t
  MI and, 1032–1033
  purulent, pneumonia causing, 488
  radiation therapy causing, 1412t, 1413
  symptoms and signs in, 1031, 1036–1037
  tuberculous, 429
  viral, *1032*
Pericardium, 1030–1037
  anatomy of, 1030–1031
  effusions of, *1033–1035*, 1033–1036
    differential diagnosis and, 173t
    tamponade and, *1033–1035*, 1033–1036, 1395–1396
  friction rub of, 1032
  function of, 1030–1031, *1031*, 1031t
  inelastic, 1036–1037
  neoplasia of, 1395–1396
  resection of, 1036, 1037, 1396t
Periodontal disease, granulocytopenia with, 533t, 541
Periosteum, abscess under, orbital cellulitis and, 473
  sinusitis and, 476
Peripheral nerves, demyelination in, 677–682
Peripheral vascular resistance index, 1097, 1098t
Peristalsis, lymphatic, 1155, *1155*
Peritoneal lavage, 169–170, 519t, 519–520
  complications of, 169–170
  contraindications for, 169
  indications for, 169
  procedures for, 170
Peritoneum, cavity size and, 513
  clearance in, 513
  contrast media in, 513, 514
  defense mechanisms of, 513
  fluid of, 513
  lymphatic system and, 513
  membrane of, 513
Peritonitis, 513–520
  abscess location and, 516, 516t
  antimicrobial therapy in, 517, 517t
  appendicitis and, 516
  ascites and, 515–516
  barium causing, 514
  candidal, 440–441, 516
  cirrhosis and, 515–516
  classification of, 515t, 515–516
  débridement therapy in, 519
  diagnosis of, 515
  dialysis and, 1285–1286
  diffuse, 515t, 516, 518–520, 519t
  drainage and, 518t, 518–519
  fibrin role in, 514
  hemoglobin role in, 514
  lavage in, 519, 519t
  liver disease and, 1506–1507
  localized, 515t, 516, 516t, 517–518
  open cavity therapy in, 519
  organisms in, 514–516
  pathophysiology of, 513–514
  pneumococcal, 515
  primary, 515t, 515–516
  secondary, 515t, 516
  spontaneous bacterial, 1506–1507
  surgical approach in, 517–518
  symptoms of, 515–516
  treatment of, 516t, 516–520, 518t, 519t

Peroxides, 950, *950*
Personnel, AIDS precautions and, 564
  emergency medical services and, 9–11
  hand washing by, 386–387, 387t, 409, 411–412
  HIV infection and, 591t, 596–598, 598t
  nosocomial infections and, 386–387, 387t, 409, 411–412
pH, acid-base balance and, 1220–1222, *1221*, *1222*
  glucose metabolism affected by, 1236–1237, *1237*
  hypocalcemia and, 1202
  measurement of, electrode for, 239–241, *240*, *241*
  patient transport and, *56*, 56–57
  pulmonary edema and, *1044*, 1045, *1045*
  regulatory mechanisms for, 1219–1221, *1221*
Phagocytic cells, blood cells and, 1336
  burn injury and, 522t, 523
Pharmacokinetics, 1054, 1304t–1309t, 1686–1701, 1689t–1692t. *See also* under specific agents.
  antiarrhythmic agents and, 1056t–1057t, 1689t, 1700
  anticonvulsants and, 669t, 1690t
  dialysis effect on, 1304t–1309t, 1304–1309
  drug level monitoring and, 1686–1701
  first-order, 1688–1689
  genetic polymorphism affecting, 1700t, 1700–1701
  kidney failure effect on, 1304t–1309t, 1304–1309
  liver failure effect on, 1689t–1692t, 1692–1693
  principles of, 1054, 1686–1693
  zero-order, 1688–1689
Pharyngomaxillary space, *477*
  infection in, *477*, 477–479
Pharynx, endotracheal intubation and, 111–112, *112*, 116
  infection of, *477*, 477–479
Phenformin, lactic acidosis caused by, 1237
Phenobarbital, 1696
  pharmacokinetics of, 669t, 1690t, 1692t, 1696
  seizure treated with, 668t, 668–671, 669t, 671t
Phentolamine, hypertensive emergency and, 1331t
Phenylephrine, septic shock therapy and, 375–377, *376*, 376t
Phenytoin, 1695–1696
  liver failure dose adjustment for, 1690t, 1695t, 1695–1696
  meningitis seizure and, 463
  overdose of, 1706
  pharmacokinetics of, 669t, 1690t, 1695t, 1695–1696
  seizure treated with, 668t, 668–671, 669t, 671t
  toxic effects of, 1706
Pheochromocytoma, catecholamines in, 1325
  diagnosis of, 1325
  hypertension caused by, 1329
  imaging of, 1325
  preoperative care and, 1563
  symptoms in, 1325
  treatment of, 1325–1326
Phlebitis. *See Thrombophlebitis.*
Phlebovirus, 392t
Phlegmasia cerulea dolens, 1152
Phonocardiography, heart failure and, *1017*

Phosgene (carbonyl chloride), chemical warfare use of, 48
  clinical effects of, 50–51
  postexposure treatment for, 51
Phosphates, hypercalcemia therapy with, 1205–1206, 1401t, 1401–1402
  oral preparations of, 1216–1217, 1217t
  parenteral preparations of, 1217t
Phosphofructokinase, fructose metabolism and, *1238*
  glucose metabolism and, 1231, *1232*, *1237*
  glycolysis regulation and, *356*, 356–357
  pH effect on, *1237*
Phospholipase, shock and, 981
Phosphorus, 1212–1218
  body content of, 1212
  deficit of, 1212–1217, 1213t, *1215*
  excess of, 1217t, 1217–1218, *1218*
  heart affected by, 1046
  intake of, 1212–1213
  physiology of, 1212
  reabsorption of, 1212
Phosphorylation, oxidative, 358, *358*, *359*
Photopheresis, 1420
Phycomycosis, 445–446
Phylogenetics, viruses and, 392t
Physiotherapy, chest, 957–959
Physostigmine, anticholinergic intoxication and, 53
Picornavirus, 392t
Ping-pong gaze, 637
Piperacillin, enterococcal susceptibility to, 415t
Piriform sinus, anatomy of, 967–968, *968*
Pit vipers, 1662t, *1666*, 1669–1672
Pituitary gland, sphenoid sinus and, *476*
Placenta, abruption of, 1597–1598
Placenta previa, 1597
Plaque, atherosclerotic, 989–991, *990*, *991*
  cholesterol crystals in, *991*
  disruption of, *990*, 990–991, *991*
  fissuring of, *990*, 990–991, *991*
  thrombus formation due to, *990*, 990–991, *991*
Plasma. *See also Transfusion.*
  cryoprecipitate from, 1390
  endotoxins in, 370
  extracorporeal detoxification of, 370
  fresh frozen, 1390
  products from, 1389–1390
  protein fraction of, 133
  side effects of, 133
Plasma volume. *See Blood volume.*
Plasmapheresis, 1419–1429
  anticoagulation in, 1427
  calculations for, 1427–1428
  complications of, 1428–1429
  hyperviscosity treated with, 1425, 1426t
  instrumentation for, 1420–1421, *1421*, *1422*
  pulmonary edema and, 143–145, *144*, *145*
  replacement fluids in, 1427
  septic shock treated with, 370
  ultraviolet light exposure and, 1420
  vascular access for, 1425–1427
Plastics, blood gas sample and, 238–239
  smoke inhalation and, 883–884
  syringes of, 238–239
Plate tectonics, earthquakes and, 27, *27*
Platelets, activating factor for, 309, 372
  apheresis of, 1420–1429
  bleeding related to, 1342–1344, 1343t
  bone marrow failure and, 1342–1344, 1343t, 1344t

Platelets *(Continued)*
  bronchoscopy bleeding and, 193–194, 200
  hematopoiesis and, 1336
  level of, 1343t, 1343–1344
  malignancy and, 1363, 1366
  pentoxifylline effect on, 372
  pregnancy and, 1594–1595, 1595t, 1607, 1608t
  preoperative care and, 1564–1565
  transfusion of, 1389
Platinum, electrodes of, *240*, 242, *243*
  nephropathy caused by, 1407
  side effects of, 1407
Plegia, differential diagnosis in, 628–630
  neuropathy and, 628–630
Plethysmography, blood pressure measurement and, 251
Pleura, 860–871
  barotrauma effect on, 904–905
  blood supply to, 860
  effusions of, 861–871
    abdominal symptoms and, 868
    amylase in, 865
    approach to patient with, 865–868
    atelectasis vs., 277–278
    bloody, 864, 867, *867*, 889–890
    chyle in, 867–868, 890
    clinical signs in, 862
    congestive heart failure and, 791–792
    COPD patient with, 796
    CT scan and, 281, *282–284*
    exudative, 861–862, 866, 866t, 868t
    glucose in, 865
    imaging of, *862*, 862–864, *863*, *867*
    loculated, *862*, 863
    MRI scan and, 283
    pathogenesis of, 861–862
    pneumonia and, 488, 864–865
    pulmonary embolism and, 867
    radiography and, 280–283, *281–285*
    respiratory distress syndrome and, 868
    Starling forces and, 860–861, *861*
    subpulmonic, *862*, 862–863
    transudative, 861t, 861–862, 865t, 865–866
    trauma and, 867–868
    ultrasonography and, *285*
    white blood cells in, 864
  fluid dynamics of, 860–862, *861*
  lymphatic drainage of, 860
  normal fluid of, 860–861, 864–865
  parietal, 860, *861*
  physiology of, 860–861, *861*
  pressure within, hydrostatic, 861, *861*
    oncotic, 861, *861*, 865
    respiration effect on, 727, *727*, 728, 861, *861*
    Starling forces and, 861, *861*
  stoma of, 860
  visceral, 860, *861*
Plicamycin, hypercalcemia therapy with, 1205, 1401, 1401t
Pneumatocele, radiography and, 292, *292*
Pneumocephalus, barotrauma causing, 903–904, *904*
Pneumococcal infections, 411t, 418–419
  clinical features in, 419
  meningitis due to, 454
  pathophysiology in, 418–419
  peritoneal, 515
  pneumonia and, 418, 486–487, 487t
  resistance and, 419
  risk factors for, 418
Pneumocystis, biology of, 594–595
  bronchoalveolar lavage and, 199

Pneumocystis (Continued)
  cancer patient and, 550
  cyst form of, 594–595
  trophozoites of, 594
Pneumomediastinum, barotrauma causing, 904, *904*
  diving (sport) and, 904, *904*
  thoracic trauma and, 889
Pneumonia, 480–490
  antimicrobials in, 489, 489t
    risks due to, 482t
  aspiration causing, 872–875
  cancer patient and, 549t, 549–550, 550t
  community-acquired, *485*, 487t
  complications of, 488–489
  compromised host and, 533t, 535t, 536–540, 537t, 538t
  COPD patient with, 795
  diagnosis of, algorithms for, *485, 486*
    differential, 481t
    patient history in, 481, 482t
    procedures in, 481–485, 483t
    radiography in, 278, 481–482
  epidemiology of, 480
  gram-negative bacillus causing, 486t, 487, 487t, 489t
  granulocytopenia and, 533t, 535t, 536–540, 537t, 538t
  incidence of, 480, 486t, 487t
  laboratory diagnosis of, 609–611
  mortality rate in, 480, 486
  nosocomial, 382, 383t, 480–490, *486*, 486t, 487t
  organisms in, 482t, 485–488, 486t, 487t
  pathogenesis of, 480–481, 485–488
  pleural effusion and, 866–867
  pneumococcal, 418–419, 486–487, 487t
  Pneumocystis carinii etiology of, 199, 571–572, 594–596
    clinical signs in, 595
    differential diagnosis in, 595, 595t
    HIV infection and, 594–596
    intensive care indicated in, 594t
    laboratory findings in, 595
    prognosis in, 596
    treatment of, 595–596, 596t
  staphylococcal, 486t, 487, 487t
  streptococcal, 486t, 487t, 488, 489t
  Toxoplasma gondii and, 572
  transplant patient and, 583–584, 584t
  trauma patient and, 560–561
  treatment of, 489t, 489–490
  viral, varicella-zoster in, 395
Pneumonitis, antimicrobials and, 1409t, 1409–1410, 1410t
  aspiration causing, 872–875
  atelectasis vs., 278
  chemotherapy-induced, 1409t, 1409–1410, 1410t
  nitrofurantoin causing, 897t, 898–899, *899*
Pneumopericardium, chest trauma and, *1585*
Pneumoperitoneum, radiography in, 270–271, *270–272*
Pneumotachygraph, Fleisch, *210*, *211*
Pneumothorax, altitude and, 43
  barotrauma causing, 904–905, *905*
  basilar, *288*
  bronchoscopy causing, 200
  clinical signs in, 869, 992t
  CT scan of, *287*, 287–288
  diving (sport) and, 904–905, *905*
  management of, 870–871
  medial, *289*
  open, 15–16

Pneumothorax *(Continued)*
  pleural fluid with, *286*, *290*, 868–871
  prehospital management of, 16
  radiography in, 283–292, *286–292*, *869*, 869–870, *870*
  tension, 16, *290–292*, 291–292, 869
  thoracentesis causing, 160–161, 864
Poikilocytosis, 1384
Poiseuille's law, 723–724, 839
Poisoning. See also *Envenomation; Toxic substance(s); Toxins.*
  abdominal pain and, 1483t, 1483–1484
  acetaminophen, 1483t, *1708*
  acetone, 1718t, 1719
  aluminum, 1270
  antidepressant, 1708–1709
  antifreeze, 712, 1715–1720, *1716*, 1716t, 1718t
  aspirin (acetylsalicylic acid), 1483t, 1483–1484, *1708*, 1708
  barium, 1183–1184
  carbon monoxide, 883, 885–886, 1238
  carbonyl chloride (phosgene), 48–51
  cholinergic, 1703t, 1703–1705, 1704t
  ciguatera, 1673
  clupeoid, 1673–1674, 1676
  cocaine, 1482–1483, 1709–1710, 1710t
  control centers and, 1661
  cyanide, 883, 884, 1237–1238, 1331, 1711–1712
  digitalis, 1023, 1073, 1706–1707
  dinoflagellate bloom and, 1672–1674, 1676
  drug etiology in, 1703t–1705t, 1703–1712
    approach in, 1703–1704
    laboratory tests and, 1702–1703
    mortality rate and, 1702
    nervous system affected by, 1703t–1705t, 1703–1705
    symptoms and, 1702–1705, 1703t
    therapy in, 1705–1712
    thermoregulation affected by, 1704, 1704t
  envenomation vs., 1661–1662
  esophageal injury and, 1432t, 1432–1435, 1433t
  ethanol, 706t, 706–710
  ethylene glycol, 712, 1715–1717, *1716*, 1716t, 1718t
  fish ingestion and, 1673–1674, 1676
  food toxicity causing, 1483t, 1484, 1672–1674, 1676
  glue inhalation, 1720–1721
  insecticide, 1183–1184
  isopropanol, 712, *718*, 718t, 1718–1719
  marine organisms causing, 1672–1674, 1676
  methanol, 712, 1239, 1714t, 1714–1717, *1715*, 1718t
  mortality rate and, 1702
  mushroom, 1483t, 1484
  narcotic, 1711, 1711t
  nitroprusside, 1711–1712
  paraldehyde, 1718t, 1719
  parasympatholytic, 1703–1704, 1704t
  pharmacologic, 1702–1712
  phenytoin, 1706
  propylene glycol, 1718t, 1719–1720
  rubbing alcohol, 712, *1718*, 1718t, 1718–1719
  salicylate, *1708*, 1708
  scombroid, 1673
  shellfish, 1672–1673
  solvent, 1714–1721

Poisoning *(Continued)*
  sympatholytic, 1703t, 1703–1704, 1704t
  theophylline, 1705
  toluene, *1720*, 1720–1721
  treatment of, 1705–1712
    hemodialysis in, 1291–1292, 1292t,
      1717
    hemoperfusion in, 1291–1292, 1292t,
      1705
Poliovirus, 396
  incidence of, 396
  meningitis due to, 396
  mortality rate and, 396
  myelitis due to, 396
    anterior horn and, 676–677
    early ventilators and, 3
  vaccines and, 396
Polycythemia, 1362–1366
  classification of, 1363t
  diagnosis of, 1362
  secondary and relative, 1362–1363, 1363t
  vera, 1362–1366
    complications of, 1364–1365, 1365t
    criteria for, 1362, 1363t
    diagnosis of, 1362, 1363t, 1364–1365,
      1365t
    management of, 1365t, 1365–1366
    symptoms of, 1364–1365
Polydipsia, 1172
  hypokalemia and, 1188
Polyethylene, catheters made of, *602*, 602–
  604
Polymyxin B, burn injury and, 526
  properties of, 370
  septic shock treated with, 370
Polyneuropathy, 678–679
  acute inflammatory, 679–680, 766
  axonal, 680
  chronic inflammatory, 680
  Guillain-Barré, 679–680
  plasmapheresis in, 1425, 1426t
  respiratory failure due to, 766
Polysomnography, sleep apnea and, *777*,
  778
Polyurethane foam, smoke inhalation and,
  884
Polyuria, diabetes insipidus and, 1175–1176
Polyvinyl chloride, catheters made of, *602*,
  602–604, 606
  smoke inhalation and, 884
Pons, hemorrhage of, 656t
Popliteal artery, knee dislocation and, 1150,
  1151
Portacaval shunt, encephalopathy due to,
  1522
Portal vein, alcoholism and, 1445
  anatomy of, 1445, *1446*
  collaterals of, 1445
Portal-systemic shunt, esophageal varices
  and, 1452–1455, *1453*, *1454*
    portal hypertension and, 1452–1455,
      1453, *1454*
Portuguese man-of-war, venom of, 1674t,
  1674–1675, 1675t
Positive end-expiratory pressure (PEEP),
  927, *927*
  asthma and, 811t, 811–812
  auto-PEEP, 801, 927, *927*
  cardiac effects of, 944t, 944–948
  cardiogenic shock and, 788
  COPD and, 801
  effects of, 944t, 944–948
  emergency ventilation and, 17
  inadvertent, 24
  indications for, 934
  intrapleural pressure and, 861, *861*

Positive end-expiratory pressure (PEEP)
  (Continued)
  intrinsic, 801, 927, *927*
  measurement of, 927, *927*
  mechanical ventilation and, 927, *927*,
    933–935
  optimization of, 934–935
  pulmonary blood pressure affected by,
    1086–1087
  pulmonary edema and, 790–791
  respiratory distress syndrome and, 830–
    833, *831*, *832*
  tissue oxygenation and, 946–948
Postantibiotic effect (PAE), 615, *617*, 618
  leukocytes in, 618
Postprandial state, glucose and, 1251–1252
Postural drainage, lung secretions and,
  957–958
Posturing, decerebrate, 637
  decorticate, 637
Potassium, 1179–1193
  acidosis and, 1180, 1180t, 1181
  aldosterone and, 1181, 1184–1185
  alkalosis and, 1180, 1180t, 1181
  deficit of. See *Hypokalemia.*
  diet and, 1180, 1182, 1185
  excess of. See *Hyperkalemia.*
  excretion of, 1181, 1185–1186
  exercise and, 1180
  heart affected by, *1046*, 1046–1047
  hormone effects and, 1179–1180, 1180t
  intrinsic secretory defect and, 1184t,
    1185
  kidney failure and, 1272
  magnesium and, 1181, 1186
  mineralocorticoid effects and, 1184t,
    1184–1185, 1186
  regulatory mechanisms for, 1179–1181,
    1180t
  transfusion concentration of, 1389
Potentiometer, pH measurement and, 239–
  241
Power of attorney, health care decisions
  and, 1734–1735
Poxvirus, 392t
Prealbumin, thyroxine binding by,
  malnutrition and, 1531
Prednisolone, sepsis treated with, 373
Prednisone, asthma treated with, 810
Pregnancy, abortion sepsis and, 1609
  anemia with, 1612
    hemolytic, 1372t, 1374–1375
  antihypertensive agents and, 1605
  appendicitis and, 1610t, 1610–1611
  burn injury and, 1611
  cardiomyopathy and, 1611–1612
  cesarean section and, 1596
  coagulopathy and, 1594t, 1594–1595,
    1595t, 1601–1602
  ectopic, abdominal pain of, 1477
    management of, 1598
    rupture of, 1477
  endocarditis and, 492
  endometritis and, 1610
  fluid therapy in, 1604
  HELLP syndrome and, 1607, 1607t
  hematologic disorders and, 1372t, 1374–
    1375, 1607, 1607t, 1608t
  hypertension induced by, 1602t–1604t,
    1602–1607, 1606t
    complications of, 1603, 1603t, 1605–
      1607
    diagnosis of, 1602t, 1603t
    management of, 1603t, 1603–1607
    severe, 1602t, 1603t

Pregnancy *(Continued)*
  infection and, 1593–1594, 1594t, 1600–
    1601, 1608–1611
  inflammatory bowel disease and, 1473
  kidney failure and, 1606, 1606t
  magnesium sulfate and, 1604, 1608
  mortality rate and, 1593
  necrotizing fasciitis and, 1611
  neurologic disorders and, 1607–1608
  oliguria in, 1606, 1606t
  platelets and, 1594–1595, 1595t, 1607,
    1608t
  presurgery care and, 1568t, 1568–1569
  pulmonary edema and, 1605–1606
  pulmonary embolism and, 1612
  pyelonephritis and, 1610
  respiratory function and, 1604t
  shock with, 1593–1612
    anaphylactic, 1608
    cardiogenic, 1612
    causes of, 1593t, 1593–1612, 1594t
    inotropic agents and, 1595, 1595t
    monitoring in, 1595–1596, 1596t
    septic, 1608–1609
    supportive therapy in, 1594t–1596t,
      1594–1596
  thrombophlebitis in, 1611
  toxic shock syndrome and, 1611
  transfusion and, 1594–1595, 1595t, 1607,
    1608t
  trauma in, 1598–1600
    forceps causing, 1599
    nonobstetric, 1599–1600
    spontaneous, 1598–1599
    surgical, 1599
  tuberculosis with, 429
  vasopressors and, 1595
Prehospital management, 11–19
  electrical injury and, 1647
  EMT triage decisions and, 12–14, *13*, 14t
  hypothermia and, 1638
  trauma patient and, 11–19, *13*, 14t
Prekallikrein activators, side effects of, 133
Preload, 1081–1082, *1082*
  heart failure and, 1019, *1019*, *1022*
Premature complexes, *1051*
  atrial, *1051*, 1060–1070, *1061*
  ventricular, 1067–1068
Preoperative care, 1552–1572
  cancer patient and, 1567–1568
  cardiac disorders and, 1556t, 1556–1559,
    1559t
  endocrine disorders and, 1562–1563
  fluid resuscitation in, 1566–1567
  gastrointestinal disorders and, 1559–1560
  geriatric patient and, 1568t, 1568–1569
  hematologic disorders and, 1563–1566
  hepatic disorders and, 1560–1561, 1561t
  kidney disorders and, 1561–1562
  neurologic disorders and, 1552–1553
  nutritional support and, 1570
  pregnant patient and, 1568t, 1568–1569
  respiratory disorders and, 1553–1556,
    1554t
  transplant patient and, 1569–1570
Presyncope, pulmonary hypertension and,
  845
Prevertebral space, *477*
Primidone, pharmacokinetics of, 1689t
Prinzmetal's angina, 997
Procainamide, arrhythmia treated with,
  1055, 1056t
  drug interactions of, 1056t
  MI and, 996
  monitoring of, 1692t
  pharmacokinetics of, 1689t, 1692t, 1700
Procarbazine, lung injury due to, 897t,
  897–898

Progenitor cells, hematopoiesis and, 1337, 1339–1341, *1340*
Prognosis indices. See *Severity classification.*
Proinsulin, hypoglycemia and, 1252–1253
Propafenone, arrhythmia treated with, 1055, 1056t
  drug interactions of, 1056t
Propranolol, arrhythmia treated with, 1055, 1056t
  dosage for, 999t
  drug interactions of, 1056t
  hyperthyroidism treated with, 1322
  myocardial ischemia and, 999t
  pharmacokinetics of, 1689t
Propylene glycol, drug vehicle role of, 1239
  lactic acidosis caused by, 1239
  liver metabolism of, 1239, *1239*
  poisoning due to, 1718t, 1719–1720
Propylthiouracil (PTU), alcoholic hepatitis and, 1508
Prostaglandins, inhibition of, 371–372, 1258
  kidney failure and, 1258
  sepsis role of, 304–306, *305*, 371–372
  sodium balance and, 1158
Protamine sulfate, lung affected by, 900
Proteins, C, sepsis treated with, 372
  carrier, 1335, 1688–1691, 1689t–1692t
  dialysis patient and, 1273–1274
  drug binding by, 1688–1691, 1689t–1692t
  fluid distribution and, 129–131, *130*
  hematopoiesis and, 1335
  hepatic encephalopathy and, 1522–1524
  kidney failure and, 1261t, 1263
  malnutrition and, 1528–1532, 1529t, 1532t
  nutrition requirements for, 1533, 1533t
  osmotic pressure due to, 129–131, *130*
Proteus mirabilis, susceptibility of, 614t
Prothrombin time, kidney failure and, 1271
  preoperative care and, 1565
  PTT and, 855
Pruritus, decompression sickness and, 905
Pseudoaneurysm, aorta and, 1134, *1139*, *1140*
Pseudocysts, pancreatitis and, 1503–1504
Pseudohypoparathyroidism, hypocalcemia due to, 1203
Pseudomembranes, colitis and, 500
Pseudomonas, meningitis and, 454–455, 461t
  susceptibility of, 614, 614t
Psychogenic disorders, status epilepticus and, 665, 671
Ptosis, botulism causing, 568
PTT (partial thromboplastin time). See also *Bleeding time.*
  heparin therapy and, 855
PTU (propylthiouracil), alcoholic hepatitis treated with, 1508
Ptyalism, corrosive esophageal injury and, 1433–1434
Pulmonary artery, *913*. See also *Pulmonary vasculature.*
  catheterization of, 186–188, 1079–1087
    apparatus for, *1083*
    balloon inflation in, *1081*, 1081–1083, *1083*
    complications of, 188, 1141–1142
    contraindications for, 186–187
    distances to target in, 187t
    indications for, 186
    procedure for, 187–188, 1079–1087
    respiration effects in, *1080*, 1080–1081, *1085*, 1085–1087

Pulmonary artery *(Continued)*
  waveform analysis in, *1079–1082*, 1079–1087
  wedging technique in, 1081, 1084, 1087
  fluid resuscitation and, 137–140, 138t
  pressure-flow relationship in, 735–737, *737*
  pulmonary edema and, 913, *913*
  rupture of, 1141–1142
Pulmonary hypertension. See *Hypertension, pulmonary.*
Pulmonary vasculature, 735–742. See also *Pulmonary artery.*
  blood flow in, 735–737
    alveolar, 737–738, *738*
    gravity effects and, 737–738, *738*
    resistance to, 736–737, *737*
      calculation of, 839, 1097–1098
      cor pulmonale and, 838–845
      embolism and, 850–851, *851*
      increased, 838–845
      restriction of, 840–845
      shunting and, 741–742, *743*, *744*, 786–787
      ventilation and, 735–737, 828–830, *830*
    fluid resuscitation effects in, 137–140, 138t
  muscle tone and, 839–840
  pressure in, 735–737, *737*
    altitude effects and, 838
    balloon occlusion and, *1081*, 1081–1087, *1083*
    factors affecting, 789, 789t, 789–790, 911–918, *913*, *917*
    fluids and, 137–140, 138t
    heart failure and, 1021, *1021*
    hydrostatic, 789t, 789–790
    PEEP and, 1086–1087
    "pop-off" (nadir) method and, 1086
    prognosis and, 78, 78t
    pulmonary edema and, 143–145, *144*, 912–915, *913*
    respiratory distress syndrome and, 139–140, 835
    wedge technique and, arterial, 1081, 1084
    capillary, 1087, *1087*
  veno-occlusive disease of, 841–842, 843t
Pulse, absence of, 15, 22t, 22–23, 1144
  cardiac arrest and, 22t, 22–23
  CPR contraindicated by, 15
  femoral, 1144
  jugular venous, 845
  oximetry and, 203–208, *204–207*
  pulmonary hypertension and, 845
Pump devices, cardiac-assist, 188–189, *189*, 1120–1125, *1122–1124*
  centrifugal, 1123, *1123*
  electric implantable, 1124, *1124*
  Hemopump, 1122–1123, *1123*
  intra-aortic balloon, 188–189, *189*
    angina pectoris and, 1005
    complications of, 189, 1122, 1149
    indications for, 188, 1121, 1121t
    MI and, 1005, 1121–1122, *1122*
  Novacor, 1124, *1124*
  pneumatic, 1123–1124, *1124*
  pulsatile, 1123–1124, *1124*
  roller, 1123, 1124
  ventricular-assist, *1123*, 1123–1125, *1124*
Pump failure, endogenous, 1007–1008, 1008t
Pupils, brain herniation and, 715
  coma evaluation and, 636

Pupils *(Continued)*
  dilated, 715
  oval, 636
  pear-shaped, 636
  reflexes of, 636–637, 641, 642t
  size oscillations of, 636
Purkinje fibers, anatomy and, 1057
Purpura, leukemia causing, 1360, *1360*
  target appearance in, 1360, *1360*
  thrombotic thrombocytopenic, 1372t, 1373–1374
Putamen, hemorrhage of, 656t, 656–657
Pyelonephritis, pregnancy and, 1610
Pyomyositis, 452
Pyrazinamide, dosage for, 425t
  side effects of, 425t, 426
  tuberculosis treated with, 425t, 426, 571
Pyridostigmine, myasthenia treated with, 683–684
Pyroclastic flows, 29, 29–31, *30*
Pyropoikilocytosis, 1384
Pyruvate, glucose metabolism and, 1231, *1232*
  mitochondria and, *355*, *356*
Pyruvate dehydrogenase, glycolysis regulation and, *356*, 356–357

Q

QMR (Quick Medical Reference), diagnosis with, 96
QRS wave, arrhythmias and, 1073–1077, *1076*
  wide, 1067, 1073–1077, *1076*
QT interval, long, 1071–1072, *1072*
Quadriplegia, respiration and, 893
Quality assurance. See also *Standards.*
  computer assistance in, 91–93
  ICU plan for, 70t–71t
  standards development for, 69t–71t, 73–76
Quality of life, informed choice and, 71
  intensive care services and, 5
  longevity vs., 71
Quenching, fluorescent optode technology and, 248
Quick Medical Reference (QMR), diagnosis with, 96
Quinidine, arrhythmia treated with, 1056t
  drug interactions of, 1056t
  hemolytic anemia induced by, 1378–1379, 1379t
  monitoring of, 1692t
  pharmacokinetics of, 1689t, 1692t, 1700
Quinine, hemolytic anemia induced by, 1378–1379, 1379t
Quinlan case, 1731, 1733, 1740–1741
Quinolones, 616t
  pathogen susceptibility to, 614t, 615
  pharmacokinetics of, 1694–1695
Quinsy throat, 478

R

R wave, ventricular tachycardia and, *1070*
Rabies, animal vectors for, 691t
  anterior horn and, 676–677
  diagnosis of, 691
  encephalitis of, 400–401, 690–692, 691t, 692t
  epidemiology of, 400–401
  incidence of, 400
  no-exposure infection with, 401
  pathology of, 691t

Rabies (Continued)
postexposure prophylaxis in, 691t, 692t
symptoms of, 400, 691
treatment of, 401, 692–693
Raccoon eyes, 634
Raccoons, rabies and, 691t
Race, coccidioidomycosis and, 444
drug clearance and, 1700t, 1700–1701
tuberculosis distribution and, 422, 424
Radial artery, catheter injury to, 1148–1149
puncture of, 235–236, 236
thrombosis of, 1148–1149
Radiation therapy, bone marrow transplant
and, 1348t
heart affected by, 1412t, 1413
nephropathy caused by, 1408
vena cava obstruction and, 1394–1395,
1395t
Radiography, 257–292
abdomen and, 270–272
drug smuggler bowel obstruction and,
1483
pneumoperitoneum and, 270–271,
270–272
aorta and, 1134–1138
aneurysm of, 1134–1135, 1135–1140
dissection of, 1134–1135, 1138
rupture of, 1134–1138, 1135–1137
chest, 257–292
aberrant intubation and, 261–269,
263–269
atelectasis and, 271–278, 274–277
catheter misplacement and, 258–261,
259–263
daily, 258
endotracheal intubation and, 261–264,
263, 264
equipment and technique for, 258
nasogastric intubation and, 264–269,
267–269
normal findings in, 270–271
pacemaker placement and, 269–270
pleural disease and, 280–283, 281, 282
pleural effusion and, 862, 862–863,
863, 867
pneumonia and, 278, 481–482, 595
pneumothorax and, 283–292, 286–
292, 869, 869–870, 870
pulmonary edema and, 278–280, 279,
279t, 280, 790, 790, 791
pulmonary embolism and, 569, 852
respiratory distress syndrome and,
278–280, 279, 822–824, 829, 833,
834
thoracostomy and, 264, 265–267
tracheostomy and, 263, 264, 264
transplant patient and, 584t
trauma and, 1584t, 1585–1588
tuberculosis and, 425–426
contrast media for, kidney failure due to,
1261t, 1262
peritoneum and, 513, 514
spine and, ankylosing spondylitis and,
770
kyphoscoliosis and, 769
Radionuclide studies. See Scintigraphy.
Railroad accidents, 32, 32t, 33t
Ranitidine, pharmacokinetics of, 1689t
Ranson's criteria, pancreatitis and, 1502,
1502t
Ranvier nodes, 673
Rash, meningitis organisms and, 457
rickettsial infection and, 457, 460
Rasmussen's aneurysm, 423
Rats, hemorrhagic fever and, 403–404
rabies and, 691t

Rattlesnakes, 1662t, 1669–1672, 1670t
RBC. See Red blood cells.
Reasoning engines, expert systems and, 96–
98, 97t
Receptors, acetylcholine, 673
alpha, 1703t, 1703–1704
beta, 1703t, 1703–1704
catecholamine, 1319, 1319t, 1320–1322,
1321t, 1322, 1322t
cholinergic, 1703t, 1703–1704
drug overdose affecting, 1703t, 1703–
1704
Recompression therapy, air embolism and,
908–909, 909
decompression sickness and, 906–907,
909
Rectum, hemorrhage in, inflammatory
bowel disease and, 1471
infection of, 542
Red blood cells. See also Erythrocytosis;
Polycythemia.
abnormal shape in, 1372
destruction processes for, 1370, 1372. See
also Hemolysis.
Doppler studies and, 1104–1105, 1105
fragmented, 1372, 1373
frozen, 1388
hematopoiesis and, 1336, 1339, 1440
hemoglobin emulsion from, 154, 154,
154t
kidney transplant and, 1298
oxygen transport and, 151
pentoxifylline effect on, 372
potassium level and, 1183
transfusion of, 1388–1389
velocity of, 1104–1105, 1105
washed, 1388–1389
Red man syndrome, vancomycin and, 410
Refeeding syndrome, magnesium level and,
1207
phosphate level and, 1213
potassium level and, 1183
Reflection coefficient, 130
Reflex(es), auditory, 641, 642t
blink, 626
brain hypoxia affecting, 641, 642t
brain stem, 636–637, 641–642, 642t
absence of, 645t, 645–647
coma evaluation and, 636–637, 641–642,
642t
corneal, 636, 641, 642t
cough, 641, 642t
facial grimace, 641, 642t
gag, 641, 642t
heart failure affecting, 641, 642t
light, 636, 642t
nasal stimulus, 641, 642t
ocular, 636–637, 641, 642t
oculocephalic, 636, 641, 642t
pupillary, 636–637, 641, 642t
respiratory, brain death and, 646, 646t
Refractory period, heart action potential
and, 1051
Rejection, acute, 1295, 1295t
bone marrow transplant and, 1348–1349
chronic, 1295
heart transplant and, 1131–1132
hyperacute, 1294
kidney transplant and, 1294–1295
Renal artery, stenosis of, kidney failure
and, 1258
Renin-angiotensin-aldosterone axis, 1310–
1311, 1312t
alkalosis and, 1227
drug-induced alterations in, 1312t
heart failure and, 1018, 1044

Renin-angiotensin-aldosterone axis (Continued)
laboratory evaluation of, 1312
sodium balance and, 1158
Repolarization, motor neuron and, 673
Rescue workers, disaster response of, 38–
39, 42
Reserpine, catecholamine block and, 1319,
1319
Reservoirs, viral infections and, 397t, 397–
405, 398t
Resistance, airway. See Airway, resistance in.
microbial. See Resistant organisms.
vascular, cor pulmonale and, 838–845
embolism and, 850–851, 851
heart failure and, 1018–1019
pulmonary, 736–737, 737, 1097–1098
systemic, 1097
Resistant organisms, beta-lactamase, 410,
415, 614
enterococcal, 415t, 415–416
laboratory testing for, 612–613
meningitis and, 461–462
staphylococcal, 408–411, 411t
streptococcal, 419
tolerance and, 617
Respiration, 719–732. See also Expiration;
Ventilation.
apneustic, 636
catheterization tracing affected by, 1080,
1080–1081, 1085, 1085–1087
chest anatomy and, 763–765, 764, 765
Cheyne-Stokes, 635t, 636
coma and, 635t, 636
exchange ratio of, 733
hypothermia effects and, 1636, 1636
muscles of, 723, 723, 731, 731–732, 763–
765, 765, 767, 787
pattern generator for, 765, 777
physiotherapy and, 957–959
pneumothorax and. See Pneumothorax.
pulmonary blood pressure affected by,
1080, 1080–1081, 1085, 1085–1087
quotient of, 733
sleep and, 775–777, 776t
work done in, 730, 730–731, 760
Respiratory distress syndrome (adult), 816–
837, 827t, 828t
causal disorders in, 817t, 817–818, 818t,
827t, 828t
clinical course of, 820, 820–824, 827–
828, 828t
complement activation role in, 307–308
CT scan in, 822, 824
definition of, 816–817
exudative phase of, 820–822, 821, 822,
827t, 827–835, 828t
fluid resuscitation in, 141–142
hypoxemia of, 818–819, 828–830, 830
lung compliance and, 819, 819, 831
management of, 826–837, 828t
mortality rate in, 824, 824–827, 828t
multiple organ failure and, 827t, 828t,
836–837
paradigms for, 827t, 827–837, 828t, 829
pathology in, 821–823, 830
pathophysiology of, 818–820, 827–828
pleural effusion and, 868
prognosis in, 824, 824–827, 827t
proliferation and fibrosis phase of, 822–
823, 823, 824, 835–836
pulmonary edema and, 139–140, 920–
921
pulmonary hypertension and, 819, 819,
844–845
radiography in, 278–280, 279, 822–824,
829, 833, 834

Respiratory distress syndrome (adult)
(Continued)
recovery phase of, 823–824, *824*
sepsis and, 828t, 836
trauma risk factor in, 893–894
ventilation therapy for, 830–833
wedge pressure in, 139–140
Respiratory failure, 754–762
acidosis with, 798
acute, 793–803
blood gas changes in, 759t
burn injury and, 1621–1623, *1623*
chemical exposure causing, 48–52
chest abnormalities causing, 763t, 767–771
CNS in, 774–775
COPD and, 793–803
criteria for, 342t
extrapulmonary, 774t
heart failure and, 786–792
hypercapnia of, *754,* 754–761
hypoxemia of, 754, *754,* 761–762, 797–798
management of, 796–802, 797t
mortality rate in, 802
muscle fatigue and, 767, 787
neuromuscular disease causing, 763t, 765–767
patient transport causing, *56,* 56t, 56–57, 57t
precipitating events in, 794, 796
pregnancy and, 1604t
preoperative care and, 1553–1556, 1554t
sleep disorders and, 773–783
surgery risk factors and, 1553–1556, 1554t
Respiratory tract, 719–732
aerosol behavior in, 959–963, 960t
airflow patterns in, 723–725, *724, 725*
airway anatomy and, 719, *720, 721*
chest wall role in, 723, *723*
dead space in, 733–734, 742–743
defense mechanisms of, 748–753, *749*
elastic properties of, *722,* 722–726, *723*
flow-resistive properties of, 723–726
infections of, 474–479
bacterial, 751–752
cancer patient and, 549t, 549–550, 550t
complications of, 474–479
drug abuse patient and, 568t, 568–572, *569, 570*
fungal, 437, 444–447
granulocytopenia and, 533t, 535t, 536–540, 538t
nosocomial, 382, 382t, 383t
trauma patient and, 560–561
viral, 391–395, 393t
pressure relationships in, 719–722, *721, 722*
secretions of, 482–485, 483t
asthma and, 810
chest physiotherapy and, 957–958
COPD and, 799
postural drainage of, 957–958
trauma injury to, 890–892
upper, bacterial adherence to, 751
bacterial colonization of, 751–752
Resuscitation. See *Cardiopulmonary resuscitation; Fluid resuscitation.*
Retained dead fetus syndrome, 1601
Reticular activating system, 631–632
anatomy of, 631
consciousness and, 631–632
dysfunction of, 631–632, 632t
nuclei of, 631

Reticular formation, 631–632
functions of, 631
neurotransmitters of, 631
Reticulocytes, corrected count of, 1371
hemolytic anemia and, 1370t, 1370–1371
Retina, comatose patient and, 635
infection of, 470
leukemia affecting, 1360, *1360*
Retinol, binding protein for, malnutrition and, 1531
Retropharyngeal space, *477*
infection of, *477,* 479
Retrovirus, 589
acute syndrome and, 593
genes of, 589
immunodeficiency due to, 589–590, *590,* 590t, *591,* 591t
symptoms caused by, 593
Revised Trauma Score, 1574, *1575,* 1575t
Reynolds number, 724
Rh system, 1387
Rhabdomyolysis, heatstroke and, 1629
phosphate level and, 1214, 1217
potassium level and, 1182, 1188
Rhabdovirus, 392t
Rhinitis, 475
Rhinovirus, 392t
Rib cage, respiration role of, 763–765, *764*
Ribavirin, 405–406
Congo-Crimean fever and, 404
Hantaan virus and, 404
hemorrhagic fever and, 404–405
Lassa fever and, 405
side effects of, 406
Ribs, fractures of, 888–889
respiration and, 888–889
Richter scale, 27t, 28
Rickettsial infections, meningitis due to, 460
rash in, 460
Rifampin, cross-reactions of, 426t
dosage for, 425, 425t
meningitis and, 461t, 464
pharmacokinetics of, 1689t
resistant organisms and, 615
side effects of, 425t, 425–426
tuberculosis treated with, 425t, 425–426, 426t, 571
Rift Valley hemorrhagic fever, 404
Right-to-die, 1742–1743
Rigors, 628
Ringer's lactate solution, 131, 131t, *137, 138*
ionic composition of, 131t
Riot control agents, 48, 50
clinical effects of, 50
compounds used as, 48
decontamination for, 50
historical aspects of, 48
Risk factors. See also *Severity classification.*
cardiac complications and, 79, 80t, 1556, 1556t
frostbite and, 1642, 1642t
hypothermia and, 1635t, 1638t, 1642t
multiple organ system failure and, 341–343, 342t
preoperative conditions and, 1552–1572
pulmonary complications and, 1554t
sepsis and, 302
tetanus and, 1574t
transplantation and, infection and, 579–580
Rocking-boat motion, laryngospasm causing, 116
Roth's spots, 493, 1360, *1360*
endocarditis and, 493

Rubbing alcohol, poisoning due to, 712, *1718,* 1718t, 1718–1719
Rubivirus, 392t
Rumack-Matthew nomogram, *1708*
Rupture, alveolar, barotrauma causing, 904
aortic, 892
cardiac, 891
diaphragmatic, 892
tracheobronchial, 890, *890*

S

S wave, tachycardia and, *1077*
Sabin vaccine, 396
Saccades, coma evaluation and, 636
Saikewicz v Superintendent of Belcher State School, 1733
St. Louis encephalitis, 692–693
Salicylates. See also *Aminosalicylic acid; Aspirin (acetylsalicylic acid).*
lactic acidosis caused by, 1238–1239
poisoning due to, *1708,* 1708
Saline solutions, fluid resuscitation using, 131t, 131–132
Saliva, corrosives ingestion and, 1433–1434
Salivary glands, amylase and, 1501, 1501t
Salk vaccine, 396
Salmonella, enterocolitis and, 511
gastroenteritis due to, 511
Salpingitis, appendicitis vs., 1477
Sarcolemma, acidosis affecting, *1040,* 1040–1041
Sarin, nerve effects of, 48, 51–52
Satiety, early, 845
pulmonary hypertension and, 845
Sawtooth waves, *775*
Saxitoxin, properties of, 1673
tetrodotoxin vs., 1676
Scalded skin syndrome, staphylococcal infection and, 412
Schistocytes, 1373
Schwann cells, motor neuron and, 673
Scintigraphy, angiographic, 1105–1113, *1108, 1110*
cardiographic, 1105–1113, *1108, 1110*
instrumentation and, 1108–1110, *1109*
MI and, 994
septic shock and, 326
Sclera, cornea junction with, *466,* 466–467
Scleroderma, pulmonary hypertension and, 842
Sclerosis, amyotrophic lateral, 676, 766
progressive, pulmonary hypertension and, 842
Sclerotherapy, esophageal varices and, 1450t, 1450–1451, *1451,* 1453
Scoliosis, 768
Scombrotoxin, 1673
Scorpion fish, venom of, 1676–1677, *1677*
Scorpions, venom of, 1484, 1678t, 1680
Sea snakes, venom of, 1662t, 1664–1665, *1666,* 1668t
Sea urchins, venom of, 1675–1676
Seafood, poisoning due to, 1672–1673, 1676
Search and rescue teams, disaster preparedness and, 42, 42t
Second messengers, enterotoxins and, 1467, 1467t
ion transport and, 1466, 1466t, 1467
Sedation, endotracheal intubation and, 110–111, 113
Seizures, 663–671
alcoholism and, 708–709
consciousness affected by, 634

Seizures (Continued)
cyclosporine and, 1300–1301
definitions and, 664
drug overdose and, 1704–1705, 1705t
eclampsia and, 1329, 1330t, 1608
heart failure and, 642, 646–647
hyperpyretic-rigidity syndrome and, 700
immunosuppressive drugs causing, 1300–1301
kidney transplant and, 1300–1301
lactic acidosis due to, 1234
magnesium sulfate and, 1604, 1608
meningitis and, 459, 463
neoplasia causing, 1398
pregnancy and, 1604, 1608
preoperative care and, 1553
status epilepticus, 663–671
absence and, 664, 664t, 670
classification of, 664t, 664–665
complex partial, 664t, 665, 670
drug therapy in, 667–671, 668t, 671t
epidemiology of, 665–666
etiology of, 665, 666
generalized, 664t, 664–665
management of, 667–671, 668t
mortality rate in, 667, 667
neonatal, 664t, 665, 671
neuronal damage due to, 667, 667
nonconvulsive, 664t, 664–665, 670
psychogenic, 665, 671
simple partial, 664t, 664–665, 670
systemic effects of, 666t, 666–667
tonic-clonic, 664t, 664–665, 668–670
treatment protocol for, 668t
unilateral, 665, 670
unresponsive patient and, 627
Seldinger technique, catheterization and, 178, 178, 179
Selenium, antioxidant effect of, 955, 955t
Sellick's maneuver, 111
Sengstaken-Blakemore tube, 170–172, 171, 1449, 1450
Boyce modification of, 171, 171–172
complications and, 171
contraindications for, 171
indications for, 171
installation of, 171–172
Sensory system, evoked potentials of, 231–232, 624–625
Sepsis, 295–377. See also Infections.
arachidonic acid cascade in, 304–306, 305
catheter-related, 601–607
cell metabolism in, 354–361, 355–359
clinical manifestations of, 297t, 297–300
cardiovascular, 298, 323–337, 365–377, 367
endocrinologic, 299–300
fever and, 297
gastrointestinal, 298–299
hematologic, 299, 335, 372
hepatic, 298–299
metabolic, 299–300
neurologic, 299
renal, 299
respiratory, 297–298, 300
coagulation factors in, 335, 372
complement activation in, 307, 307–308, 371
cytokine mediation of, 311–320, 312t, 370–372
definition of, 295–296, 557
endorphins in, 306–307, 373
endotoxin role in, 303–304, 304, 368, 368–370
epidemiology of, 301–302, 365
hypoxia theory of, 354–356, 355

Sepsis (Continued)
incidence of, 295, 295t, 301–302, 365
mortality rate and, 295, 301–302, 311, 365
multiple organ system failure in, 340–351, 346, 366
neutrophil activation in, 309
organisms in, 302, 313t, 366, 366–368
oxygen metabolism and, 328, 328, 354–363, 355, 358–362, 373
pathogenesis of, 302, 302–309, 303t, 315–319, 365–366, 366, 367
platelet-activating factor in, 309, 372
risk factors for, 302
syndrome of, 295–296, 296t
terminology and, 295–296
trauma patient and, 557–558
Septic shock, 139–140, 140, 323t. See also Toxic shock syndrome.
calcium level in, 1201–1202
cardiovascular dysfunction in, 323–337, 367
canine model for, 328–329
cineangiography of, 326
fluid resuscitation and, 325, 325, 326, 336, 374, 374–375
hemodynamics of, 324–325
management of, 335–337, 336t
myocardium and, 325–327, 325–332, 331–333, 367
oxygen transport and, 328, 328
ventricles and, 326, 326–328, 327, 367
future and, 319–320
historical aspects of, 312t, 313, 323–324
interferons in, 312t, 318
interleukins in, 312t, 317, 317–318, 371
mortality rate and, 301–302, 311
pathogenesis of, 365–366, 366, 367
pregnancy and, 1608–1609
TNF role in, 313, 313–319, 314, 316, 317
treatment of, 365–377, 366, 368t
antibodies used in, 369, 371
anticoagulants in, 372
antimicrobials in, 366, 366–368, 368t, 370
antioxidants in, 373
cardiovascular support in, 368t, 375t, 375–377, 376, 376t
eicosanoid inhibitors used in, 371–372
endotoxin neutralization in, 366, 368t, 368–370
lipid A analogues used in, 369–370, 370
mediator modulation in, 366, 368t, 370–373
monitoring in, 374, 374–375
naloxone in, 373
plasma detoxification in, 370
vasopressor therapy in, 375–377, 376, 376t
Septicemia. See also Bacteremia.
blood culture in, 608–609
incidence of, 295, 365
laboratory diagnosis of, 608–609
neonatal, 417
nosocomial, 382, 382t, 383t
rash due to, 457, 460
Serratia, pneumonia due to, 487t, 488, 489t
susceptibility of, 614, 614t
SESAM-DIABETE system, 103t
Severity classification, 77–86
APACHE system and, 82–86, 83t, 84t, 1575
cardiac disease and, 77t, 77–80, 78t, 80t
coma and, 79–80, 80t
computer data storage and, 82

Severity classification (Continued)
frostbite and, 1641t, 1642
future of, 86
hepatic failure and, 79, 79t
hypothermia and, 1635t, 1638, 1638t
ICU use of, 80–86, 81t, 83t–85t
limitations of, 85–86
outcome determinant factors in, 80–81, 81
outside of ICU, 77–80
pancreatitis and, 79, 79t
pediatric unit and, 85
snakebite and, 1663, 1663t, 1670t
surgical procedure risk and, 79t, 79–80, 80t
surgical unit and, 85
trauma patient and, 1574–1582, 1575t–1581t
Sexual function, HIV infection and, 591t, 592t
kidney transplant affecting, 1298
Shellfish, poisoning due to, 1672–1673
Shigella, dysentery caused by, 510t, 510–511
Shingles, 394–395
varicella and, 394–395
Shipwrecks, 32, 32t, 33t
Shivering, 628
loss of, 1634
thermoregulation and, 1634, 1634
Shock. See also Toxic shock syndrome.
air transport effect on, 43
anaphylactic, 140–141, 1608. See also Anaphylaxis.
burn injury causing, 1618–1620
cardiogenic, 140, 323t, 367, 375t, 983, 983t, 1612
hemodynamic profile in, 1098t
respiratory failure and, 788
care units for, historical aspects of, 1–4
catecholamines in, 1325
circulatory, 136–139, 367, 375t, 978–985, 979
classification of, 323t, 367, 375t, 983, 983t
distributive, 323t, 367, 375t, 983, 983t
fluid resuscitation in, 136–141, 138, 140, 374, 374–375, 375t, 984, 984t
garment therapy for, 15, 16
hemorrhagic, 138, 138–139, 1098t, 1159
prehospital management of, 15
hypocalcemia in, 1202
hypovolemic, 136–139, 138, 367, 375t, 978–985, 983t
cell function affected by, 981–982
fluid resuscitation in, 984t, 984–985
heart affected by, 375t, 978–979, 982
hemodynamic parameters of, 375t, 978–979, 979
mediator systems in, 981, 985
metabolic changes in, 980–982
oxygen metabolism and, 979–980, 980
pathophysiology of, 979
treatment approach in, 983–985
lactic acidosis in, 1233–1234, 1234t
obstructive, 983, 983t
extracardiac, 323t, 367, 375t
pregnancy and, 1593t, 1593–1612, 1594t
prehospital care in, 15–16
septic, 1098t. See also Septic shock.
volume depletion in, 1159–1160
Short bowel syndrome, lactic acidosis in, 1235–1236
Shunts, arteriovenous, 353
intracardiac, 1118t
imaging of, 1118–1119
mesocaval, 1453, 1455

Shunts *(Continued)*
    portacaval, *1453*, 1455
    portal-systemic, cirrhosis causing, 1522
        hepatic encphalopathy and, 1522
        portal hypertension and, 1452–1455,
            1453, 1454
    pulmonary vasculature and, 741–742,
        743, 744
        oxygen tension and, 786–787, *787,*
            828–830, *830*
        respiratory distress syndrome and,
            828–830, *830*
        respiratory failure and, 786–787
        right-to-left, 786–787, *787,* 828–830, *830*
    sepsis and, 353
    splenorenal, *1453*, 1455
    transjugular intrahepatic, 1452, *1454*
Shy-Drager syndrome, 1326
SIADH (syndrome of inappropriate
        antidiuretic hormone), causes of, 1173,
        1173t
    hypotonicity and, 1172t, 1173, 1173t
    neoplasia and, 1402
    treatment of, 1174
Sick euthyroid state, 1563
Sick sinus syndrome, 1055–1057
Sickle cell disease, erythrocytapheresis in,
    1423–1424
Silicone, catheters made of, *602*, 602t, *602–
    604*, 606
Silver chloride, electrodes with, *240–242,*
    241–242
Silver nitrate, burn injury and, 525, 525t
Silver sulfadiazine, burn injury and, 525,
    525t
Simplified Acute Physiology Score (SAPS),
    82–83, 83t
Sinus node, anatomy and, 1055
    arrhythmias and, 1055–1062
        arrest and, 1055
            bradycardic, 1055, *1058*
            exit block, 1055
            re-entrant tachycardic, 1062
        normal rhythm of, 1055
        pacemaker role of, 1055
Sinuses, nasal, barotrauma effects in, 903
    piriform, 968, *968*
    sphenoid, *476*
Sinusitis, brain abscess and, 475t, 476, *476*
    cancer patient and, 549
    complications of, 475t, 476, *476*
    endotracheal intubation causing, 974–
        975
    granulocytopenia with, 533t, 540
    nosocomial, 475–476
    trauma patient and, 559–560
Sjögren's syndrome, bone marrow
        transplant and, 1349t, 1356
Skin, abscess of, 450, 575–576
    aspergillosis and, 447
    blood gas metabolism in, *217*, 217–220,
        219, 220
    botulism in, 568
    burn effects in, 521–522
    candidiasis and, 434t, 435
    carbon dioxide measurement and, 220,
        220
    cold exposure affecting, 1641t, 1642–
        1643
    color of, cherry red, 635
        cyanosis and, 635
        jaundice and, 635
        pallid, 635
        sallow, 635
    coma evaluation and, 635
    defensive barrier role of, 521–522, 522t

Skin *(Continued)*
    electrical injury to, 1646, 1646t, 1649,
        1649
    fungal infections and, 445, 447
    infections of, 448–453, 449t
        clinical syndromes in, 449t, 449–452
        drug abuse patient and, 575t, 575–577
        epidemiology of, 448–449, 449t
        organisms in, 448–449, 449t
        treatment of, 453
    mucormycosis and, 445
    oxygen measurement and, 217–220, *219*
    popping, drug abuse and, 568
    tests, tuberculin, 424
    thermoregulation and, 1634, *1634*
Skull, 714
    fusion of, 714
Skunks, rabies and, 691t
Sleep, 775
    apnea during, 777, 777–781, *778*, 779t,
        780t
        airway obstruction and, 778–781, *779*
        obesity and, 781
        surgical approach in, 780–781
        ventilation therapy in, 781
    deprivation of, 781–782
    disorders of, historical aspects of, 631
        respiratory failure and, 773–783, 777,
            778
        sleep-wake cycle and, 631
    EEG in, *775*
    ICU patient and, 781–782
    non-REM, *775*, 775–777, 776t
    polysomnography and, 777, *778*
    REM, *775*, 775–777, 776t
    spindles on EEG during, *775*
    stages of, 775, *775*
Slime, staphylococcal adhesin and, 604–605
Smears, tuberculosis and, 424–425
Smoke inhalation, 883–886
    carbon monoxide role in, 883–884
    clinical evaluation of, 885
    fire environment and, 883–885
    management of, 885–886
    pathophysiology of, 885
    toxic gases in, 883–884
Snails, venom of, 1676
Snakebite, 1662–1672
    anaphylaxis caused by, 1652
    blood flow affected by, 1670, *1672*
    clinical effects of, 1662–1672, 1663t,
        1664, 1672
    coagulation affected by, 1663–1664,
        1664, 1671
    crotalid, 1662t, 1669–1672
    dry, 1662–1663
    elapid, 1662t, 1668–1669
    fang morphology and, *1666,* 1672
    lethality of, 1663
    management of, *1661,* 1662–1672, 1665t
    neurotoxins of, 1663–1664, 1668, 1668t
    severity of, 1663, 1663t, 1670t
    species and, 1662t, 1663–1672
    toxins of, 1662–1672, 1663t, *1664,* 1668t
    venom in, 1662–1672, 1663t, *1664,* 1668t
    viperid, 1662t, 1665–1668, *1666,* 1670t
Sniffing glue, 1720–1721
Sniffing position, intubation and, 111
Snoring, sleep apnea and, 778, 779t
Society for Critical Care Medicine, historical
        aspects of, 4
    standards development by, 74t, 74–76,
        75t
Sodium, blood volume and, *1155,* 1155–
        1159, *1157*
    deficit of. See *Hyponatremia.*

Sodium *(Continued)*
    edema and, 1161–1163, 1162t
    excess of. See *Hypernatremia.*
    excretion of, 1156, *1157*, 1158–1159
    extracellular, 1155–1159
    gastrointestinal transport of, 1464–1465
    intracellular, 1156
    kidney and, 1156–1159
        failure of, 1272
        wasting mechanisms of, 1160
    natriuretic hormone and, 1156, 1158
    reabsorption of, 1156, 1158–1159
    regulatory mechanisms for, *1155,* 1155–
        1159, *1157*
    urinary, 1156–1159
        concentration of, 1160
        loss of, 1160
    volume depletion and, 1159–1161
Sodium acetylsalicylic acid. See *Aspirin
    (acetylsalicylic acid).*
Sodium channel blockers, arrhythmia
        treated with, 1055, 1056t
    drug interactions of, 1056t
Sodium chloride, fluid resuscitation using,
    131t, 131–132
Sodium nitrite, cyanide antidote use of, 51
Soft palate, airway classification and, 109,
    110t
Soft tissues. See *Subcutaneous tissues.*
Soil liquefaction, 27–28, *28*
Solute flux, dialysis and, 1275–1277
Somatosensory system, evoked potentials of
    231–232, 624–625
Sotalol, arrhythmia treated with, 1055,
    1057t
    drug interactions of, 1055, 1057t
Specific Activity Scale, cardiovascular
        disability and, 78t, 78–79
Spectrophotometry, isosbestic points and,
    244
    oximetry and, *244,* 244
Spectroscopy, brain oxygen and, 231, *231,*
    231t, 625
    near-infrared, 231, *231,* 231t, 625
Speech, akinetic mutism and, 635, 644
    botulism affecting, 568
    de-efferentation and, 635
    hot potato voice and, 478
Spherocytosis, hemolytic anemia and, 1372,
    1384
    hereditary, 1384
Sphincter(s), gastroesophageal, ventilation
        breach of, 110
    of Oddi, pancreatitis and, 1499–1500
Spider bite, abdominal pain due to, 1483t,
    1484
    hemolytic anemia due to, 1383
    management of, 1678–1680, 1680t
    species and, 1677–1680, *1678*, 1678t,
        1679
    symptoms of, 1677–1680, *1678*
    venom in, 1677–1679
Spinal cord, anterior horn disorders and,
    676–677
    compression of, back pain and, 1398–
        1400, *1399*
        evaluation of, *1399*
        neoplasia causing, 1398–1400, *1399*
Spinal nerves, demyelination and, 677–682
    respiratory muscles and, *765*
Spine, 15–17
    abscess of, drug abuse patient and, 567
        epidural, 567
    immobilization of, 16–17
    motor levels of, 717
    trauma injury to, 15–17, 1578t, 1584

Spine *(Continued)*
    air transport affecting, 43–44
    evoked potential and, 232
    management of, 717–718
Spirochetal infections, meningitis due to, 459
Spirometry, chest physiotherapy using, 958
    preoperative function testing and, 1554t, 1555
Spironolactone, diuresis using, 1165, 1165t
    hyperkalemia and, 1185
    pharmacokinetics of, 1691t
Spleen, candidiasis affecting, 440
    enlargement of, 1365
    impaired immunity and, 533, 546–547
    polycythemia vera and, 1365
    resection of, 533, 546–547
    trauma injury to, 588
Spondylitis, ankylosing, 769, *770*
    radiography in, *770*
    respiratory failure due to, 769
    spine affected by, *770*
Spur cells, hemolytic anemia and, 1372, 1384
Sputum, acetylcysteine and, 810, 962
    mucolytic agents and, 810, 962
    pneumonia and, 482
    tuberculosis and, 424–425
    viscosity of, 810, 962
Square root sign, 1081, *1081*
    pericarditis and, 1036, *1037*, 1081, *1081*
Squid, venom of, 1676
Stab wound, intra-abdominal abscess and, 561
    pregnancy and, 1600
Staff. See *Personnel.*
Staining methods, *Pneumocystis carinii* and, 594
Standards, 67–76
    admission and discharge, 74t
    American Association of Critical Care Nurses and, 75–76, 76t
    consensus process for, 71–72
    cost containment and, 69–71
    critical care organizations and, 74t–76t, 74–76
    development process for, *68*, 69–73
    future and, 73
    goal identification and, 69–71
    guidelines vs., 67, 72
    historical aspects of, 67–69
    JCAHO development of, *68*, 68–69, 69t, 91–92
    judicial proceedings and, 67
    nursing care and, 74t–76t, 74–76
    options vs., 67
    physician origination of, 67–68
    policy statements concerning, 72–73
    quality assurance and, 69t–71t
    regulatory agencies and, 69
    social origin of, 67
    Society for Critical Care Medicine and, 74t, 74–76, 75t
Stanford classification system, aortic dissection and, *1134*
Staphylococcal infections, 408–414
    adhesin slime role in, 604–605
    catheter-related, 604–606
    clinical presentation of, 409–410, 413
    coagulase-negative, 413–414
    endocarditis and, 497
    epidemiology of, 409
    historical aspects of, 408–409
    meningitis due to, 454–455
    microbiology of, 408, 413
    nosocomial, 409, 411–412, 413

Staphylococcal infections *(Continued)*
    pathogen susceptibility and, 614, 614t
    pathogenesis in, 409, 413
    pneumonia due to, 486t, 487, 487t
    prevention of, 411–412
    resistant organisms in, 408–411, 411t, 614t
    scalded skin syndrome in, 412
    toxic shock syndrome in, 412t, 412–413
    treatment of, 410–411, 411t, 413–414, 614t
Starches, capillary leak repaired by, 136
    fluid resuscitation using, 134–136
    high-molecular-weight, 136
    hydroxyethyl, 134–136
    low-molecular-weight, 135
Starfish, venom of, 1675–1676
Starling forces, 130, *130*
    capillary-interstitial exchange and, *1155*, 1155
    fluid distribution and, 130, 911–912
    hydrostatic pressure and, *789*, 789–790, 1155, *1155*
    oncotic pressure and, 1155, *1155*
    pleural fluid and, 860–861, *861*
    pulmonary edema and, *789*, 789–790, 911–912
Starvation, magnesium level and, 1207
    phosphate level and, 1213
    potassium level and, 1183, 1185, 1185t
Status asthmaticus. See *Asthma.*
Status epilepticus. See *Seizures, status epilepticus.*
Steakhouse syndrome, 1435, 1435t
Stem cells, hematopoiesis and, 1337, 1339–1341, *1340*
Sternum, fractures of, 888
Steroids, hypercalcemia treated with, 1401t, 1402
Stewart-Hamilton equation, cardiac output and, 1089–1090
Stingrays, venom of, 1676–1677, *1677*
Stings and bites. See *Animal bites; Envenomation; Snakebite.*
Stomach. See also *Nasogastric intubation.*
    bubble in, *862*, 862–863
    endotracheal intubation error and, 110, 113
    insufflation of, 110, 113
    pleural effusion imaging and, *862*, 862–863
    secretions of, potassium loss and, 1185
Stomatitis, granulocytopenia with, 533t, 541
Stones, biliary tract, 1491–1493, *1493*, 1493t, 1494t
    kidney, abdominal pain due to, 1480
    obstruction and, 1265t, 1265–1266
Stools. See *Feces.*
Streptococcal infections, 416–420
    beta-hemolytic, 417–418
    group A, 416–417
    group B, 417
    group C, 417–418
    group D, 418
    group G, 418
    meningitis due to, 454–455
    myositis due to, 452
    neonatal, 417
    pathogen susceptibility and, 614, 614t
    peritonitis and, 516
    pneumonia and, 486t, 487t, 488, 489t
    toxic syndrome and, 417
Streptokinase, 857t
    action of, 856, 857t
    dosage for, 857t
    MI and, 999–1001, *1001*

Streptokinase *(Continued)*
    pulmonary embolism and, 856
Streptomycin, dosage for, 425t
    side effects of, 425t, 426
    tuberculosis treated with, 425t, 426
Stress-related mucosal disease, hemorrhage and, 1442–1443
    prevention of, 1442–1443
String sign, carotid artery and, *1148*
Stroke, 648–661. See also *Cerebrovascular disease.*
    carotid artery and, 649, *652*
    embolic, 649, 649t
    fluctuating, 649
    heat, 1629–1630, 1630t
    in-hospital, 650t, 650–651
    ischemic, 648–655, 649t, 650t, *653*
    lacunar, 649
    vertebrobasilar, 649
    watershed region in, 649t, 649–650
Stroke volume, *367*
    fluid resuscitation and, *140*
    heart failure and, 1018–1019, *1019*, *1022*, *1023*
Stroke work, fluid resuscitation and, *140*
    left ventricular, *140*, 1082, *1082*
    right ventricular, 1096–1097
Strongyloidiasis, granulocytopenia with, 542
    transplant patient and, 580
Stupor, 635
    alcoholic, 706t, 706–707, 707t
    coma evaluation and, 635
Subarachnoid hemorrhage, 659t, 659–661
    cerebrospinal fluid and, 661t
    clinical signs of, 660, 660t
    CT scan in, *660*
    diagnosis of, 660–661
    etiology of, 659t, 659–661
    management of, 661
    staging of, 661t
Subarachnoid space, inflammation of, *456*, *456*, 462–463
    meningitis and, 455–456, *456*, 462–463
Subclavian vein, central venous catheter in, 180, *180*
    misplaced catheter and, 258, *259*, *260*, *263*
    parenteral nutrition in, 1543–1545, *1544*, *1545*
Subcutaneous tissues, 448
    infections of, 448–453, 449t
      clinical syndromes in, 449t, 449–452
      drug abuse patient and, 575t, 575–577
      epidemiology of, 448–449, 449t
      organisms in, 448–449, 449t
      treatment of, 453
Submaxillary space, *477*
Submucosa, dissection in, 116
    edema of, 116
    intubation affecting, 116
Succinylcholine, endotracheal intubation and, 18
Sudden death, cardiac arrest and, 19, 118
Suicide, terminal illness and, 1742–1743
Sulfadiazine, burn injury and, 525, 525t
Sulfhemoglobin, oximetry and, 244
Sulfur mustard, 48, 52
Superinfection, pneumonia and, 489
Superoxide anion, oxygen toxicity and, 950, *950*
Superoxide dismutase, radical scavenging by, 951, 952t, 955, 955t
Support groups, neuromuscular disease and, 674
Supraglottitis, 474–475
Surfactant, inhalation therapy using, 963

Surfactant *(Continued)*
lung, 963
antioxidant effect of, 955t
oxygen toxicity affecting, 953–954
respiratory distress syndrome and, 833
Surgery, antibiotic prophylaxis and, 1570–
1572, 1571t
clean, 1571t
clean-contaminated, 1571t
dirty, 1570–1572, 1571t
noncardiac, cardiac risk in, 79t, 79–80,
80t
Sweating, anticholinergic agent effect on,
52
thermoregulation and, 1634, *1634*
Sympathetic nervous system, drug overdose
affecting, 1703t, 1703–1704
heart failure and, 1018
sodium balance and, 1158
Sympathomimetic agents, action of, 1697t
asthma treated with, 809, 809t
infusion rate for, 1693t
pharmacokinetics of, 1693t, 1696–1697,
1697t
Synaptic cleft, 673
Syncope, pulmonary hypertension and, 845
Syndrome of inappropriate antidiuretic
hormone (SIADH), 1173t
causes of, 1173, 1173t
hypotonicity and, 1172t, 1173, 1173t
neoplasia and, 1402
treatment of, 1174
Syphilis, lumbar puncture reactivation of,
622
Syringes, plastic vs. glass, 238–239
Systemic vascular resistance index, 1097,
1098t
Systole, failing heart and, *1016*, 1016–1018
right ventricle in, *1027*, 1027–1028

T

T cells, *1340*
burn injury affecting, 522t, 523
cancer effect on, 546
CD (clusters of differentiation) molecules
of, 589–591, 590t, *591*, 591t
deficiency of, 589–591, 590t, *591*, 591t
granulocytopenia and, 532–533, 534t
HIV infection and, 589–591, 590t, *591*,
591t
suppressor, 590
TA system, 103t
Tabun, nerve effects of, 48, 51–52
Tachycardia, atrial, 1060–1067, *1061–1067*,
1076, *1077*
AV nodal, 1063–1064, *1064–1066*
bundle branch block and, 1073–1076,
1075–1077
comatose patient and, 635t
mechanisms of, 1054
nonparoxysmal junctional, 1064, *1065*
re-entrant, 1062, 1063–1064, *1064–1066*
sinus nodal, 1060, 1062
supraventricular, 1060–1067, *1061–1067*,
1076, *1077*
treatment of, 1077
ventricular, 1067–1077, *1069*, *1070*,
1072, *1074*, *1075*
Tachypnea, comatose patient and, 635t
Tamponade, balloon, 170–172, *1449*, 1450,
1450t
cardiac, 891–892
echocardiography in, 1034, *1034*, *1035*
etiology of, 1032t, 1033, 1395

Tamponade *(Continued)*
hemodynamic profile in, 1098t
neoplasia causing, 1395t, 1395–1396,
1396t
prehospital management of, 14
signs and symptoms in, 1033–1034,
1395, 1395t
trauma injury and, 891–892
treatment of, *1034*, 1034–1036, *1035*,
1396, *1396t*
esophageal varices and, 170–172, *1449*,
1450, 1450t
Tampons, toxic shock syndrome and, 509
Tea-and-toast syndrome, potassium intake
and, 1185
Tear, Mallory-Weiss, 1444
Technetium-99m, cardiographic
scintigraphy and, 1107
Tectonic plates, earthquakes and, 27, *27*
Teeth, clenched, 17, 18
endotracheal intubation and, 17, 18, 116
reimplantation of, 116
Teflon, catheters made of, *602*, 602–604,
606
Teicoplanin, colitis treated with, 507
enterococcal susceptibility to, 415t
Temperature. See also *Fever; Hyperthermia;
Hypothermia.*
core, 1634, 1638, 1638t
dinitrophenol effect on, 217, *218*
drug overdose affecting, 1704, 1704t
heatstroke and, 1629–1630, 1630t
regulation of, 1626, 1633–1634, *1634*
Terrorism, 32, 33t
Testes, torsion of, 1480
Tetanus, anterior horn and, 676–677
drug abuse patient and, 568
immunization for, 1575t
symptoms of, 568
trauma and, 1574t, 1574–1575, 1575t
withdrawal syndrome vs., 568
Tetracyclines, kidney failure dose
adjustment for, 1306t
Tetradecyl sulfate, respiratory distress
syndrome due to, 900–901
Tetrahydrocannabinol, antiemetic effect of,
1414
Tetrodotoxin, 683, 1676
properties of, 1676
saxitoxin vs., 1676
Thalamus, hemorrhage of, 656t, 657
Theophylline, 1696
asthma treated with, 809t, 810
COPD and, 799
lactic acidosis caused by, 1238
liver failure dose adjustment for, 1691t,
1692t, 1696
overdose of, 1705
pharmacokinetics of, 1691t, 1692t, 1696
toxic effects of, 1705
Therapeutic Intervention Scoring System,
81t, 81–82
Thermodilution, cardiac output and, 1088–
1093, *1089*, *1092*
Thermoregulation, 1634, *1634*
drug overdose affecting, 1704, 1704t
heatstroke and, 1629–1630
hyperthermia and, 1626–1627, *1627*
hypothalamus and, 1634, *1634*
hypothermia and, 1633–1635, *1634*
Theta waves, *775*
Thiamine, alcoholism treated with, 709t,
709–711
deficiency of, alcoholism and, 1236
consciousness disorder due to, 633–634
lactic acidosis due to, 1236

Thiamine *(Continued)*
Wernicke-Korsakoff syndrome and,
710–711
Thiazides, diuresis using, 1165, 1165t
Thiosulfate, cyanide antidote role of, 51,
1712
Thirst, osmotic threshold for, 1170
stimuli for, 1170
Thomsen-Freidenreich antigen, 1374–1375
Thoracentesis, 160–163, 864
complications of, 160–161, 161t, 864
contraindications for, 160
indications for, 160, 864
pleural effusion and, 864
pneumothorax treated with, 163, 864
procedure for, 161–163, *162*, 864
supine position in, 160–161, 163
viscous exudate and, 163
Thoracostomy, 163–167
anchoring of tube for, 166
complications of, 164, 164t
contraindications for, 163–164
drainage systems for, *166*, 166–167, *167*
indications for, 163, 164t
malpositioned tube and, 264, *265–267*
procedure for, 164–167, *165*
radiography in, 264, *265–267*
tube removal and, 167
Thorax, CPR role of, 121–123, *122*, *123*
emergent vascular disorders in, 1133–
1142
trauma to. See *Chest, trauma injury to.*
Thrombocytapheresis, 1419–1429
anticoagulation in, 1427
complications of, 1428–1429
instrumentation for, 1420–1421, *1421*,
1422
replacement fluids in, 1427
vascular access for, 1425–1427
Thrombocytopenia, bone marrow failure
and, 1342–1344, 1344t
causes of, 1344t
chemotherapy-induced, 1405
hemoperfusion causing, 1292, 1292t
heparin causing, 855–856
preoperative care and, 1564
thrombotic purpura of, 1372t, 1373–
1374
clinical signs in, 1373–1374, 1374t
hemolytic-uremic syndrome vs., 1373–
1374, 1374t
plasmapheresis in, 1425, 1426t
treatment of, 1344t, 1373–1374, 1374t,
1425, 1426t
Thrombocytosis, 1363. See also
Thrombocytapheresis.
management of, 1366
neoplastic, 1366
preoperative care and, 1564–1565
Thrombolytic agents, 857t
contraindications for, 1000t
endogenous, 991
hemorrhage and, 856, 857t
MI and, 999–1001, *999–1001*
patient selection and, *999*, 999–1000,
1000
pulmonary embolism and, 856–858, 857t
Thrombophlebitis, burn injury and, 525
drug abuse patient and, 568, 576
pregnancy and, 1611
septic, 568–570, 576
Thrombosis, anticoagulant therapy and,
855–856
atherosclerotic, *990*, 990–991, *991*
cavernous sinus, orbital cellulitis causing,
473

Thrombosis (Continued)
  dissolution and, 855–856
  electrical injury causing, 1646, 1646t
  incidence of, 850
  lytic therapy and, 856–858, 857t
  pathogenesis of, 849–850
  plaque disruption and, 990–991, 991
  pregnancy and, 1611–1612
  pulmonary vasculature affected by, 842–843
  surgery patient and, 1572, 1572t
  vascular grafts and, 1151–1152, 1152
Thromboxanes, inhibition of, 371–372
  sepsis role of, 304–306, 305, 371–372
Thumb sign, epiglottitis and, 474
Thumper, CPR with, 123, 123
Thyroid cartilage, anatomy of, 115
Thyroid gland, catecholamines and, 1322–1324
  hyperfunction of, 1322–1324, 1563
  hypofunction of, 1161, 1323–1324
  preoperative care and, 1562–1563
  sick euthyroid state and, 1563
Thyroxine, prealbumin binding of, malnutrition and, 1531
Tibia, fracture of, compartmental syndrome and, 1150
Ticks, neuropathy and, 680
  viruses transmitted by, 397t, 397–399, 398t, 400, 403–405
Tidal volume, capnography and, 211
  mechanical ventilation and, 931, 931t
Tidal waves, 27, 31
Time-kill studies, antimicrobial action and, 616–618, 617
Timentin, pathogen susceptibility to, 614t
Timolol, dosage for, 999t
  myocardial ischemia and, 999t
Tissue plasminogen activator (TPA), 857t
  action of, 856, 857t
  dosage for, 857t
  MI and, 999–1001, 1001
  pulmonary embolism and, 856
  thrombus and, 849
Tissues, soft. See Subcutaneous tissues.
TNF. See Tumor necrosis factor (TNF).
Tobramycin, kidney failure due to, 1261t, 1261–1262
  meningitis therapy and, 461t, 462
  pharmacokinetics of, 1692t, 1693t
Tocainide, arrhythmia treated with, 1055, 1056t
  drug interactions of, 1056t
  lung affected by, 900
  pharmacokinetics of, 1689t
Tocopherol, 952t, 955, 955t
Togavirus, 392t
Tolbutamide, pharmacokinetics of, 1691t
Toluene, 1720
  metabolism of, 1720, 1720
  poisoning due to, 1720–1721
Tonicity, 1168–1178
  decreased. See Hypotonicity.
  disorders of, 1171–1178, 1172t
  increased. See Hypertonicity.
  osmolality and, 1168–1169
  water balance and, 1168–1170
Tonsils, abscess of, 478
Tornadoes, 31, 33t
Torsades de pointes, 1071–1072, 1072
  drugs associated with, 1072, 1072t
Torsion, fallopian tube and, 1477
  testicular, abdominal pain due to, 1480
Toxic megacolon, 1471–1473
Toxic oil syndrome, pulmonary hypertension in, 844

Toxic shock syndrome, 412t, 412–413, 417, 509
  diagnostic criteria for, 412t, 412–413
  gastroenteritis in, 509–510
  pregnancy and, 1611
  rash with, 509
Toxic substance(s). See also Envenomation; Poisoning; Toxins.
  abdominal pain due to, 1483t, 1483–1484
  acid as, 1432t, 1432–1435, 1433t, 1483, 1483t
  aldehyde as, 883–884
  alkali as, 1432t, 1432–1435, 1433t, 1483, 1483t
  arsenic as, 1483, 1483t
  bleach as, 1432t, 1432–1435, 1433t
  corrosive agent as, 1432t, 1432–1435, 1433t
  digitalis as, 1023, 1023, 1073, 1073, 1074, 1706–1707
  drug as, 1702–1712, 1703t–1705t, 1708
  ethanol as, 706t, 706–707, 707t
  formaldehyde as, 883–884
  formate as, 1223
  gaseous, 883–885
  hydrogen chloride as, 883–884
  hydrogen cyanide as, 883–884. See also Cyanide.
  iron as, 1483t, 1484
  lead as, 1483t
  mercury as, 1483, 1483t
  metal as, 1483, 1483t
  neuropathy due to, 680, 681
  oil as, 844
  oxygen as, 949–956
  smoke inhalation and, 883–885
Toxin(s). See also Envenomation; Poisoning; Toxic substance(s).
  bungarotoxin as, 683, 1668, 1668t
  ciguatera as, 1673
  clostridial, 502
  clupeoid, 1673–1674
  colitis due to, 502
  conotoxin as, 683
  hemolytic anemia due to, 1383–1384
  neuropathy due to, 682–683
    hepatic encephalopathy and, 1522–1524, 1523t
  snakebite and, 1663–1664, 1668, 1668t
  saxitoxin as, 1673, 1676
  scombroid, 1673
  snake venom and, 1662–1672, 1663t, 1664, 1668t
  staphylococcal, 409, 412
  tetrodotoxin as, 683, 1676
Trachea, anatomy of, 968, 968, 971, 974
  aortic rupture affecting, 1135, 1135–1136, 1137
  bacterial adherence to, 751
  cross-sectional shape of, 968, 971, 974
  displacement of, 1135, 1135–1136, 1137
  fistula of, innominate arterial, 1146–1147
  intubation injury to, 972–976, 973, 974
Tracheobronchial tree, 195–196, 196
  rupture in, 890, 890
Tracheomalacia, endotracheal intubation and, 968
  tracheostomy and, 975
Tracheostomy, 975–976
  complications of, 975
  cuff in, 975
  endotracheal intubation vs., 975–976
  infection associated with, 975–976
  radiography and, 263, 264, 264
Train crashes, 32, 32t, 33t

Training, emergency medical services and, 9–11
Tranquilizers, alcoholism treated with, 709t, 709–710
  hyperpyretic-rigidity syndrome due to, 698–704
  neuroleptic malignant syndrome due to, 698–704
Transducers, cardiographic
  ultrasonography and, 1104–1105, 1105t, 1105–1107
  locations for, 1104–1105, 1105t, 1105–1107
Transferrin, malnutrition affecting, 1530
Transforming growth factors, sepsis mediation and, 312t
Transfusion, 1387–1392
  adverse effects of, 1390–1392
  autologous, 1392
  blood products used in, 1388–1390
  bone marrow failure and, 1343–1345
  cancer patient and, 548
  citrate toxicity in, 1389
  granulocyte, 543, 1342–1343
  hemoglobin conformation and, 1389
  hepatitis and, 402, 1391
  HIV transmission and, 591, 591t, 592t, 1391–1392
  hypocalcemia caused by, 1202–1203, 1389
  infection transmitted by, 402, 548, 591, 1391–1392
  microaggregates and, 1391
  plasma products in, 1389–1390
  platelet, 1343–1344, 1389, 1392, 1405
  potassium concentration and, 1389
  pregnancy and, 1594–1595, 1595t, 1607, 1608t
  principles of, 1387–1388
  pulmonary edema and, 900, 1391
  reactions to, 1381–1382, 1390–1392
    anaphylactic, 1391
    Coombs' test in, 1382, 1382t
    delayed, 1382, 1390–1391
    erythrocytapheresis and, 1428
    febrile, 1391
    hemolytic anemia due to, 1381–1382, 1382t, 1390
  red blood cell, 1388–1389
  stored blood and, 1389
Transistors, ion-selective technology and, 247
Transplantation. See also under specific organs.
  bone marrow, cytomegalovirus in, 393t, 393–394
  donors for, brain death and, 646
  fever and, 582–583
  heart, 1125–1132, 1128–1130
  immunosuppression with, 579–581
  infection and, antimicrobial therapy and, 586–587, 587t
    classification of, 581t
    cytomegalovirus and, 392–394, 393t, 582, 584–585, 585t
    Epstein-Barr virus and, 582, 584–585
    fever and, 582–583
    geographic area and, 579–580
    hepatitis virus and, 582, 586
    nervous system and, 584
    nosocomial, 580
    organisms and, 581t, 582
    pneumonia and, 583–584, 584t
    pulmonary edema and, 583–584, 584t
    risk factors and, 579–580
    timetable for, 581–582, 582

Transplantation *(Continued)*
kidney, 1293–1301
abdominal pain and, 1482
liver, 1514–1518
complications of, 1517t, 1517–1518
contraindications for, 1515
fulminant hepatic failure and, 1516
hypertension management and, 1517t, 1517–1518
indications for, 1514t, 1514–1515, 1515t
patient evaluation for, 1514–1515, 1515t
postoperative care in, 1516–1518, 1517t
preoperative care for, 1515–1516
preoperative care and, 1569–1570
Transportation, accidents incurred during, 32, 32t, 33t
airplane mode of, 43t, 43–45, *44*, 45t, 54, 54t
ambulance mode of, 43, 54, 54t
cardiac catheter and, 55
complications of, 55–57, 56t, 57t
CT scanning and, 55
decompression sickness and, 905, 909
disaster casualties and, 39–40, 42–45
helicopter mode of, 43, 54
injuries affected by, 42–45, 54
interhospital, 54–55
intrahospital, 55–57, 56t
patient affected by, 54–57
pregnancy and, 55
ventilation support and, 56, 56–57
Trauma, 1574–1590, 1575t–1581t
abdomen, 892–893, 1578t, 1579t, 1588–1589, *1589*
vascular injury in, 1145
AIDS patient and, 563–564
air transport effects and, 43t, 43–45, *44*, 54
altitude effects and, 42–45, 54
arteriovenous fistula due to, 1149, *1150*
assessment scales for, 1574–1582, 1575t–1581t
carotid artery, *1147*, 1147–1148, *1148*
catheterization and, 558–559, 562–563
deaths due to, 1574, *1574*
earthquake etiology and, 28, 29t, 33t
EMT triage in, 12–14, *13*, 14t
extremities and, 1580t, 1581t, 1589–1590
head. See *Head trauma.*
hepatic, 1588–1589
hypertensive emergency due to, 1329
immunodeficiency due to, 556–557
incidence of, 1574
infection and, 556–564
lung, 890–891, *891*
meningitis and, 558–559
multiple organ system failure and, 557–558
muscle, 34
neck, 1578t, 1579t, 1584
pancreatic, 1589
pelvic, 1580t, 1581t, *1589*, 1589–1590
pleural effusion and, 867–868
pneumonia and, 560–561
pregnancy affected by, 1598–1600
prehospital management of, 11–19, *13*, 14t
pulmonary consequences of, 887–892
renal, 1589
respiratory distress syndrome and, 893–894
sinusitis and, 559–560
spinal, 1578t, 1584

Trauma *(Continued)*
air transport affecting, 43–44
blunt, 16–17
evaluation of, 717
evoked potential studies and, 232
management of, 717–718
penetrating wound causing, 15
prehospital care in, 15
respiratory failure due to, 766
spinal cord length and, 717
splenic, 588
tetanus risk and, 1574t, 1574–1575, 1575t
thoracic, 887–892, 888t, 1578t, 1579t, 1584t, 1584–1588, *1585–1588*
transportation effects and, 42–45, 43t, *44*, 54
wound infection and, 563
Trauma Index, prognostic use of, 85
Trauma Score, 1574, *1575*, 1575t
Trauma unit, historical aspects of, 3
prehospital triage and, 12–14, *13*, 14t
TraumAID system, 103t
Tremor, alcoholism and, 708
hypoglycemic, 633
metabolic encephalopathy and, 637
Trench foot, 1641t, 1642–1643, 1643t
pathophysiology of, 1642–1643, 1643t
Triage, chemical warfare and, 49
disasters and, 39
EMT decisions in, 12–14, *13*, 14t
prehospital trauma care and, 12–14, *13*, 14t
severity scoring systems for, 85
Triage Index, 1575
Triamterene, diuresis using, 1165, 1165t
Tricuspid valve, waveform tracings and, 1080, *1080*
Trimethaphan, hypertensive emergency and, 1331t
Trimethoprim-sulfamethoxazole, meningitis therapy and, 460t, 460–462, 461t
pneumonia and, 595–596, 596t
TRISS survival probability, 1575
Trophozoites, *Pneumocystis carinii* and, 594
Tryptophan, lung affected by, 901
Tsunamis, 27, *31*
T-tube, ventilation weaning and, 939–940
Tuberculosis, 422–430
age and, *424*
AIDS and, 430, 571
clinical features of, 423
diagnosis of, 423–425
drug abuse patient with, 571
drug therapy in, 425t, 425–426, 571, 1308t
preventive, 426
second-line, 426, 427t
epidemiology of, 422, *423*
extrapulmonary, 426–429, 427t
geographic distribution of, *423*
hemoptysis due to, 876, 877t
immunity to, 422
incidence of, 422, *423*, *424*
meningitis and, 428–429, 459
miliary, 427–428
pathophysiology of, 422–423
pericarditis and, 429
pregnancy and, 429
pulmonary, 422–426
race distribution of, 422, *424*
radiography in, 425–426
skin test for, 424
transplant patient and, 580
treatment of, 425t, 425–426, 427t, 571
Tumor lysis syndrome, 1406–1407

Tumor necrosis factor (TNF), biosynthesis of, 312t, *313*, 313t, 313–314
burn injury and, 523
cell sources of, 312t
circulating levels of, 319, 319t, 320t
infusion of, *314*, *317*
metabolic effects of, *314*, 315–317, *316*, 317t, 320t
organisms inducing, 313t
septic shock role of, *313*, 313–319, *314*, *316*, *317*
Twitching. See also *Myoclonus*; *Seizures*; *Tremor.*
coma evaluation and, 635, 637
encephalopathy and, 637
Tympanic membrane, altitude effects and, 54
Typhlitis, granulocytopenia with, 533t, 541–542
Typhoons, 31
Tyramine, foods containing, 1329
hypertension due to, 1329

U

Ulcer(s), cocaine causing, 1482–1483
decubitus, 450
Dieulafoy's, 1461
duodenal, 1439, 1439t, 1443
gastric, 1439, 1439t, 1443
peptic, 1439, 1439t, 1443
abdominal pain of, 1478
hemorrhage from, 1439t, 1439–1444
perforation of, 1478
thermal therapy in, 1443–1444
rectal, hemorrhage due to, 1461, *1461*
skin, drug abuse patient and, 568, 576
Ultrafiltration, apheresis using, 1421, *1422*
Ultrasonography, 1103–1120, *1105*, *1106*
atelectasis and, 271–277
B-mode, 1104
cardiographic, 1103–1120, *1106*
angina pectoris and, 993–994
chamber size and, 1110–1111, 1115t
endocarditis and, 494
MI and, 993–994, *994*
transducer locations in, 1104–1105, 1105t, *1105–1107*
transesophageal, 1105, 1107t, *1108*, 1116, *1117*, 1119, *1119*
valvular function assessment and, 1113–1117, 1114t, 1115t, *1115–1117*
ventricular function assessment and, *1027*, 1027–1028, *1111*, 1111–1113
views in, 1104–1105, 1105t, *1105–1107*
Doppler, blood pressure measurement and, 251
cardiac output measurement and, 1094–1095, *1112*, 1112–1113
cerebral blood flow and, 227t, 227–230, *228*
cerebrovascular disease and, 651
continuous wave, 1104
principles of, 1104–1105, *1105*
pulsed, 1104–1105, *1105*
red blood cell velocity and, 1104–1105, *1105*
transcranial, 625
valvular heart disease and, 1117
instrumentation in, 1104–1105
M-mode, 1104, *1104*
physics of, 1104t, 1104–1105, 1105t, *1106*

Ultrasonography (Continued)
  pleural effusion and, 285, 863, 863–864
Ultraviolet light, apheresis with, 1420
Unresponsiveness. See also Coma;
    Consciousness disorders.
  brain stem reflexes and, 641–642, 642t
  coma evaluation and, 635
  eyes-open, 644
  levels of, 635, 641–642, 642t
  neuropathy and, 627–628
Urea nitrogen, acute kidney failure and,
    1256–1266
  catabolic rate calculation and, 1273
  dialysis and, 1277–1279, 1278, 1289,
    1290t
  kidney failure assessment and, 1269–
    1270
  urinary excretion of, malnutrition and,
    1531
Ureidopenicillins, susceptibility testing and,
    612
Uremia. See also Azotemia.
  assessment of, 1269–1270
  coma and, 634
  creatinine level and, 1269–1270
  definition of, 1269
  dialysis and, 1269–1270
  hemolytic anemia with, 1372t, 1374–1375
  nervous system effects of, 1270
  pulmonary hemorrhage and, 879t, 879–
    881, 880
Ureter, bacteria adhering to, 527
Uric acid, intrarenal crystals of, 1265
Urinary tract infections, cancer patient and,
    552
  candidal, 441–442
  laboratory diagnosis of, 611
  nosocomial, 382, 382t, 383t, 527–530
    catheterization and, 527–530
    diagnosis of, 528
    epidemiology of, 528
    pathophysiology of, 527–528
    prevention of, 528
    symptoms of, 529
    treatment of, 529–530
  trauma patient and, 563–564
Urinary tract obstruction, kidney failure
    and, 1265t, 1265–1266
  kidney transplant and, 1293
  neoplasia causing, 1400
Urine, concentration of, 1169
  water balance and, 1169
Urokinase, 857t
  action of, 856, 857t
  dosage for, 857t
  MI and, 999
  pulmonary embolism and, 856
Urologic disorders, abdominal pain due to,
    1480
Urothorax, pleural effusion and, 865, 865t
Urticaria, transfusion reaction causing,
    1391
Uterus, atony of, 1596–1597, 1597t
  rupture of, 1598–1599
Uveitis, 470
Uvulopalatopharyngoplasty, sleep apnea
    and, 780

V

V wave, atrium and, 1017, 1017–1018,
    1079, 1079–1080, 1080
Vaccines, Sabin, 396
  Salk, 396
Vacor, hypoglycemia caused by, 1254

Valium. See Benzodiazepines.
Vallecula, 111
  anatomy of, 967–968, 968
Valproic acid, 1696
  pharmacokinetics of, 1690t, 1692t, 1696–
    1697
Valve devices, endocarditis due to, 494–495
Valvotomy, endocarditis and, 497–498
Valvular disease, chamber size and, 1115t
  endocarditis causing, 492, 494
  perioperative risk and, 1557
  ultrasonography in, 1113–1117, 1114t,
    1115t, 1115–1117
Vancomycin, colitis treated with, 506–507
  enterococcal infections and, 415t, 415–
    416
  meningitis therapy and, 461, 461t
  pharmacokinetics of, 1690t, 1692t, 1694
  red man syndrome and, 410
  staphylococcal infection and, 410–411,
    411t
Vanillylmandelic acid, 1319t, 1319–1320
Varicella, 394–395
  acyclovir therapy in, 395
  anterior horn and, 676–677
  herpes simplex vs., 395
  natural history of, 394–395
  pneumonia with, 395
  symptoms in, 394
  transmission of, 394
Varicella-zoster (shingles), 394–395
Varices, esophageal. See Esophagus, varices
    of.
  rectal, portal hypertension and, 1447
Vascular disorders, catheterization causing,
    1140–1152
  emergent, 1133–1152
    abdomen and, 1133–1142
    extremities and, lower, 1149–1152
      upper, 1145–1148
    neck and, 1145–1148
    thorax and, 1133–1142
  grafts in, aortic-enteric fistula and, 1145,
    1145
  infection and, 1140, 1144
  thrombosis and, 1151–1152, 1152
  iatrogenic, 1140–1152
  occlusive, abdominal aorta and, 1142–
    1144
    kidney and, 1144
  perioperative risk and, 1557–1558
  stroke and, hemorrhagic, 659t, 659–660
    ischemic, 655t, 655–656
Vasoconstriction, acidosis and, 1041
  pharmacologic agents for, 1693t, 1696–
    1698, 1697t
  portal hypertension therapy and, 1449t,
    1449–1450
  pregnancy and, 1595
  septic shock treated with, 375–377, 376,
    376t
  sodium balance and, 1158
  subarachnoid hemorrhage and, 661
Vasodilation, acidosis and, 1041
  heart failure treatment and, 1024
  MI and, 1007–1008, 1008t
  pulmonary hypertension and, 847
  shock treated with, 985
Vectors. See also specific vectors and
    diseases.
  encephalitis and, 397t, 397–400, 398t
  neuropathy and, 680
  rabies and, 691t
  reservoirs and, 397t, 397–405, 398t
  virus transmission by, 397–405

Vecuronium, mechanical ventilation and,
    811, 811t
Vegetations, antimicrobials and, 619, 620
  endocarditis and, 492–493
  fibrin and platelet, 492–493
Vegetative state, chronic, 635, 644
Veins, acidosis and, 1041
  antecubital, 181
  basilic, 181
  femoral, 178–179, 179, 1281t, 1289, 1290
  imaging of, 852–853, 853
  jugular. See Jugular vein.
  occlusive disease of, 841–842, 843t, 1416
  portal, 1416, 1445, 1446
  pulmonary, 841–842, 843t
  subclavian. See Subclavian vein.
  thrombosis and, 852–853, 853
  vascular access in. See Catheterization.
Vena cava, anatomy of, 1393
  misplaced catheter in, 258, 259
  obstruction of, 1140, 1393–1395
    clinical features of, 1394
    diagnosis of, 1394
    etiology of, 1394, 1394t
    neoplasia causing, 1393–1395, 1394t,
      1395t
    treatment of, 1394–1395, 1395t
  portacaval shunt and, 1522
Venezuelan equine encephalitis, 694
Venom, 1660–1681. See also Envenomation;
    Toxins.
  ant, 1681, 1681t
  arthropod, 1677–1681, 1678t
  bee, 1681, 1681t
  coelenterate, 1674t, 1674–1675
  definition of, 1661
  echinoderm, 1675–1676
  fish, 1676–1677, 1677
  hymenoptera, 1681, 1681t
  jellyfish, 1674t, 1674–1675
  lizard, 1672
  mollusk, 1676, 1676t
  poison vs., 1661–1662
  scorpion, 1484, 1678t, 1680
  snake, 1662–1672, 1663t, 1664, 1668t
  spider, 1677–1680, 1678t
  starfish, 1675–1676
Venous access. See Catheterization.
Venous pressure, balloon catheter and,
    1079–1081, 1079–1082
  monitoring of, 1079–1081, 1079–1082
  ventilation and, 737–738, 738
  waveform analysis and, 1079–1081,
    1079–1081
Ventilation, 719–747
  adjunctive therapies and, 957–963
  alveolar, 208, 208–209, 209
  asthma and, 811t, 811–812
  chest physiotherapy and, 957–959
  COPD and, 800–802
  CPR role of, 118, 122–123, 125
  cricothyrotomy for, 115, 115
  decrease in, 757t
  demand-supply aspects of, 756–758, 757
  distribution of, 734–735, 735
  increase in, 758t
  maximal sustainable, 756–757, 757
  mechanical, 924–942
    adjustments in, 931t, 931–933
    alarms in, 932
    autonomic effects of, 946, 946t
    bag-and-mask, 110
    barotrauma caused by, 904
    blood flow and, 946–947
    blood gases and, 932–935
    bronchoscopy procedure and, 194–195

Ventilation *(Continued)*
capnography and, *208*, 208–209, *209*
cardiac arrest and, 22–23
cardiac effects of, 944t, 944–948
controlled hypercapnia in, 833
controlled hypothermia in, 833
cycling mechanisms of, 928–929
flow, 928, *929*
pressure, 928, *929*
time, 928
volume, 928–929, *929*
devices for. See *Ventilators.*
excess manual pressure in, 110
extracorporeal CO₂ removal and, 835, 937, *937*
extracorporeal membrane oxygenation and, 833–835, *834*
flow rate in, 931, 931t
gastroesophageal sphincter breach in, 110
hemodynamic effects of, *927*, 927–928
high-frequency, 833, *833*
jet, *935*, 935–937, *936*
oscillation, *935*, 935–937
historical aspects of, 1–4
indications for, 924–925, 925t
inspiration-expiration in, 928–931, *929*, *930*
inverse ratio, 832–833
modes of, 929–933
airway pressure release, 937, *937*
assist-control, 930, *930*
continuous positive airway pressure, 941
controlled, 929–930, *930*
full-support, *929*, *930*, 931–933
intermittent mandatory, 930, *930*, 940
mandatory minute volume, *941*, 942
partial-support, 937–942
pressure-support, 940–941
nasal nocturnal, 781, 782t
negative-pressure, 925–926
oxygen fraction in, 931t, 932
PEEP and, *927*, *927*, 933–935. See also *Positive end-expiratory pressure (PEEP).*
physiology of, 926–928
positive-pressure, 928–933, *935*, 935–937
pressure relationships in, *927*, 927–933, *929*, *930*
rate in, 931t, 931–933
respiratory failure and, 800–802
sedation for, 811t
settings for, 931t, 931–933
shock and, 983–984
sleep apnea and, 780, 781
surfactant and, 833, 963
temperature and humidity in, 932
tidal volume in, 931, 931t
tissue oxygenation and, 946–948
trigger sensitivity in, 931t, 932
volutrauma of, 927
weaning from, 937–942
approaches to, 939–942
clinical considerations in, 938–939
failure indicators for, 939t
indications for, 938t, 938–939
respiratory muscles and, 939
T-tube used in, 939–940
mechanisms of, 719–732
metabolic coupling and, 732–733
minute, 732
normal requirements of, 732
obesity affecting, 769–771

Ventilation *(Continued)*
oral airway used in, 110
paresis and, 629–630
patient transport and, *56*, 56–57
perfusion and, 737–738, *738*
alveolar, 737–738, *738*
clinical assessment of, *743*, 743–747
dead space and, 742–743
mismatch of, 208–209, 742–746, *743–747*
normal matching of, *740*, 740–746, *741*
ratio of, 208–209, *740*, 740–746, *741*
shunt flow and, 741–742, *743*, *744*
venous pressure and, 737–738, *738*
poor patient effort in, 629–630
prehospital care and, 17–18
pulmonary embolism and, 850–852, *851*
regulatory mechanisms of, 754–758, *755*, *757*
sleep and, 775–777, 776t, 780, 781
transtracheal, 114, *115*
uneven, *208*, 208–209, *209*
weakness affecting, 629–630
Ventilation Manager (VM) system, *98*, 98–99
Ventilators, cuirass, 926
dependency on, 630
early, 3
iron lung, 3, 925–926
management of, expert systems and, 98–100, *98–100*
negative-pressure, 3, 925–926
tank, 3, 925–926
valves of, 3
VentPlan system, *99*, 99–100
Ventricle(s), 1067–1077
acidosis affecting, *1039*, 1039t, 1039–1041, *1040*, 1040t
arrhythmias and, 1067–1077, *1069*, *1070*, *1072–1076*
compliance in, 1082, *1082*
contractility of, *1039*, 1039t, 1039–1041, *1040*, 1040t
echocardiography of, *1027*, 1027–1028
end-diastolic volume of, *367*, 1011–1012, 1081–1084, *1082*, 1092
end-systolic volume of, *367*, 1011–1012
fibrillation of, 9
biology of, 19–20
cardiac arrest and, 9, 19–24, *20*, 22t
defibrillation and, 118–120, *119*
ECG waveforms of, *20*, 23–24
prehospital management of, 19–24, *20*, 22t
function assessment in, *1027*, 1027–1028, 1110–1113, *1110–1114*
imaging studies in, 1110–1113, *1110–1113*
interdependence of, 945–946, 1025–1026
left, 1015–1024
balloon catheter and, 1081–1084, *1082*
dilatation of, *1016*, 1016–1018
end-diastolic volume of, 1081–1084, *1082*, 1111–1112
filling rate and, 1111–1112, *1112*
function of, 1081–1084, *1082*, *1110–1112*, 1111–1113
heart failure and, 1015–1024
imaging studies in, 1110–1113, *1110–1113*
isovolumic relaxation of, 1113, *1114*
monitoring and, 1081–1084, *1082*
pressure in, *1016*, 1016–1017, *1017*, 1081–1084, *1082*
size determination and, *1110*, 1110–1111

Ventricle(s) *(Continued)*
stroke volume of, 1018–1019, *1019*, *1022*, *1023*
stroke work index of, 1082, *1082*, 1096–1097
mechanical ventilation and, 944t, 944–946
right, 1026–1030
dilatation of, *1026*, 1026–1028
ejection fraction of, 1092, 1112
end-diastolic volume of, 1092
function of, 1026–1027, *1081*, 1081, 1110–1113
heart failure and, 1026–1030
imaging studies in, 1110–1113
pressure monitoring and, 1081, *1081*
pressure waveforms in, 1081, *1081*
pressure-volume relationship in, *1026*, 1026–1027
stroke work index of, 1096–1097
septal rupture and, 1010, 1010t, 1098t
septic shock effects in, *326*, 326–328, *327*, 367
stiffness in, 1082, *1082*
stroke volume of, 367
tachycardia of, 1067–1077
digitalis causing, 1073, *1074*
fibrillation and, 1072–1073
nonsustained, 1068–1070, *1069*
polymorphic, *1069*, 1071–1072, *1072*
premature complexes in, 1067–1068
repetitive monomorphic, 1068–1069, *1069*
sustained, *1070*, 1070–1071
torsades de pointes, 1070–1071, *1072*, 1072t
wide QRS and, 1073–1076, *1075–1077*
Verapamil, arrhythmia treated with, 1055, 1057t
dosage for, 998t
MI and, 997, 998t
pharmacokinetics of, 1689t
pregnancy and, 1605
Vertigo, dialysis and, 1270, 1283
hypoglycemia and, 633
Vesicants, chemical warfare use of, 48, 52
clinical effects of, 48, 52
decontamination for, 52
Vesicles, chickenpox, 394
Vestibular system, coma evaluation and, 636–637
decompression sickness and, 906
Vidarabine, 405
Vincristine, abdominal pain due to, 1484
Violin spider, 1679–1680, 1680t
Viper bites, 1662t, 1665–1668, *1666*, 1670t
Virchow's triad, 849
Viruses. See also specific viruses and diseases.
arbovirus, 692–695
bunyavirus, 392t, 397
coxsackie, 396
cytomegalovirus, 392–394, 393t
enteric, 396, 696
granulocytopenia and, 533t
human immunodeficiency, 589–590
influenza, 391–392
isolation of, 393t
lentivirus, 589–590
lymphocytic choriomeningitis and, 396–397
mumps, 396
nervous system affected by, 395t, 395–401
pathogenic, 392t
phylogenetics of, 392t

Viruses (Continued)
polio, 396
replication of, 589–590
respiratory tract affected by, 391–395, 393t
rhabdovirus, 392t
transplantation and, 393t, 393–394, 582, 584–586
varicella, 394–395
vectors for, 397–405
Viscera. See also Abdomen; Intestine.
portal hypertension and, 1446t
Vision. See also Eye.
anticholinergic intoxication and, 52
evoked potentials and, 231–232, 624
methanol poisoning and, 1714
nerve agent effect on, 51
pregnancy and, 1608
Vital signs, coma and, 635t
trauma and, 13, 14t
Vitamin(s), A, 952t, 955, 955t
C, 952t, 955t
E, 952t, 955, 955t
malnutrition and, 1529, 1529t, 1531
oxygen toxicity treated with, 952t, 955, 955t
Vocal cords, anatomy of, 967–968, 968
false, 967–968, 968
inflammation of, 969
intubation injury to, 111–112, 116, 968, 969
paralysis of, 116, 968
true, 967–968, 968
Voice, akinetic mutism and, 635, 644
botulism affecting, 568
de-efferentation and, 635
hot potato, 478
peritonsillar abscess and, 478
Volcanoes, 28–31
ashfalls of, 28–30, 30
eruptions of, 28–31, 29, 30
fatalities caused by, 28–31
lava flows of, 29, 29–31, 30
mud flows caused by, 29–31
Voltmeter, pH electrode and, 240
Volume depletion, 1159–1161, 1163–1164
capillary leak syndrome with, 1164
causes of, 1159t
edema with, 1163–1164
extracellular fluid overload with, 1163–1164
hypoalbuminemia and, 1163–1164
kidney failure and, 1257
sodium role in, 1159–1161
Volume resuscitation. See Fluid resuscitation.
Vomiting, alkalosis and, 1227t, 1227–1228, 1228
chemotherapy-induced, 1413–1416, 1414t
marijuana therapy in, 1414

Vomiting (Continued)
potassium depletion due to, 1185
sodium loss due to, 1160

W

Wakefulness, 631. See also Consciousness disorders; Sleep.
Waldenström's macroglobulinemia, plasmapheresis in, 1425, 1426t
Wall stress, heart failure and, 1016, 1016–1018
Laplace formula for, 1016
myocardial, 1016, 1016–1018
Warfare, chemical agents used in, 48–53
Warfarin, MI and, 1002–1003, 1003
pharmacokinetics of, 1689t
pulmonary embolism and, 856
Washings, bronchial, pneumonia and, 483, 483t
Wasps, 1681, 1681t
Water, 1168–1178
excretion of, 1170
insensible loss of, 1169
intake of, 1170
metabolic production of, 1169
osmolality and, 1168–1169
reabsorption of, 1169
regulatory mechanisms for, 1169–1171
tonicity and, 1168–1169
Water bottle heart, 1395
Water seal, thoracostomy and, 166, 166–167, 167
Waterhouse-Friderichsen syndrome, 1313
Waveforms, artificial neural networks and, 104t, 104–106
atrial, 1079–1081, 1079–1087
blood pressure measurement and, 252t, 252–257, 254–256
cardiac arrest and, 20, 23–24
cardiac catheterization and, 1079, 1079–1081, 1080
ECG and, 20, 23–24
expert system recognition of, 100t, 100–106, 101, 102, 105
pulmonary artery catheter and, 1079–1082, 1079–1087
venous pressure and, 1079–1081, 1079–1081
ventricular pressure and, 1081, 1081
Weakness. See also Neuromuscular disease.
calcium level and, 1204
differential diagnosis of, 629–630
hypokalemia and, 1188
phosphate deficit causing, 1214–1215
poor ventilatory effort due to, 629–630
Wedging technique, pulmonary arterial catheterization and, 1081, 1084, 1087

Wegener's granulomatosis, pulmonary hemorrhage due to, 879t, 879–881
Wenckebach's block, atrioventricular node and, 1058, 1058
Wernicke-Korsakoff syndrome, 710–711
glucose triggering, 634
treatment of, 710–711
Wernicke's disease, features of, 710–711
Western equine encephalitis, 693–694
Whipple's triad, 1251
White blood cells. See also Granulocytes; Leukocytes; Lymphocytes; Neutrophils.
hematopoiesis and, 1136
pleural effusion and, 864
White matter, 639, 639t
physiology of, 639, 639t
Winters' formula, 1222
Wire basket, foreign body removal by, 196, 197
Withdrawal syndromes, tetanus vs., 568
Wolff-Parkinson-White syndrome, arrhythmias of, 1064–1067
Wood alcohol. See Methanol.
Wound. See also Trauma.
burn injury and, 1620, 1623–1624
infection of, 450
burn patient and, 1623–1624
cultures of, 611–612
laboratory diagnosis in, 611–612
nosocomial, 382, 382t, 383t
trauma patient and, 563
tetanus and, 1574t, 1574–1575, 1575t
Wrong-way eyes, 637

X

X descent, atrium and, 1079, 1079–1080, 1080
Xanthochromia, 458
Xenon-133, cerebral blood flow and, 224t, 224–227, 225
clearance test using, 224t, 224–227, 225

Y

Y descent, atrium and, 1079, 1079–1080, 1080
Yellow fever, 405
Yellow jackets, 1681, 1681t
Yohimbine, catecholamine block and, 1319, 1319

Z

Zidovudine (ZDV), HIV infection and, 594
Zoster, varicella and, 394–395
Zygomycosis, 445–446
Zymosan, complement activation due to, 307, 307